KAPLAN & SADOCK'S

COMPREHENSIVE TEXTBOOK OF PSYCHIATRY

VOLUME I

EIGHTH EDITION

Senior Consulting Editor

Robert Cancro, M.D., Med.D.Sc.

Lucius N. Littauer Professor and Chairman, Department of Psychiatry
New York University School of Medicine
Director of Psychiatry, Tisch Hospital
The University Hospital of the New York University Medical Center
New York, New York
Director, Nathan S. Kline Institute for Psychiatric Research
Orangeburg, New York

Contributing Editors

Hagop S. Akiskal, M.D.

Professor of Psychiatry and Director of the International Mood Center
University of California at San Diego School of Medicine
La Jolla, California
Director of the Mood Disorders Program
San Diego VA Healthcare Systems
San Diego, California

William T. Carpenter, Jr., M.D.

Professor of Psychiatry and Pharmacology
University of Maryland School of Medicine
Baltimore, Maryland
Director of Maryland Psychiatric Research Center
Catonsville, Maryland

Dennis S. Charney, M.D.

Chief, Mood and Anxiety Disorders Program
National Institute of Health
National Institute of Mental Health
Bethesda, Maryland

Kenneth L. Davis, M.D.

Gustave L. Levy Distinguished Professor and Dean
Mount Sinai School of Medicine
President and Chief Executive Officer
Mount Sinai Medical Center
New York, New York

Jack A. Grebb, M.D.

Clinical Professor of Psychiatry
New York University School of Medicine
New York, New York
Vice President
Clinical Design and Evaluations
Neuroscience
Bristol-Myers Squibb
Wallingford, Connecticut

Jerome H. Jaffe, M.D.

Clinical Professor of Psychiatry
University of Maryland School of Medicine
Baltimore, Maryland

W. Walter Menninger, M.D.

Adjunct Professor of Psychiatry
Baylor College of Medicine
Clinical Professor of Psychiatry
University of Kansas School of Medicine
Former Dean, Karl Menninger School of Psychiatry and Mental Health Sciences
Chief of Staff Emeritus, Menninger Clinic and Hospital
Active Staff, Menninger Memorial Hospital
Kansas City, Kansas

Caroly S. Pataki, M.D.

Clinical Professor of Psychiatry and Biobehavioral Science
Associate Director of Training and Education for Child and Adolescent Psychiatry
David Geffen School of Medicine at UCLA
Attending Psychiatrist
UCLA Neuropsychiatric Institute and Hospital
Los Angeles, California

Robert G. Robinson, M.D.

The Paul W. Penningroth Professor and Head of Psychiatry
Roy J. and Lucille A. Carver College of Medicine at University of Iowa
Iowa City, Iowa

Gary W. Small, M.D.

Parlow-Solomon Professor of Aging
Professor of Psychiatry and Biobehavioral Sciences
Director of the UCLA Memory Clinic
David Geffen School of Medicine at UCLA
Los Angeles, California

Norman Sussman, M.D.

Professor of Psychiatry
New York University School of Medicine
Director of Psychopharmacology Research and Consultation Service
Bellevue Hospital Center
New York, New York

Joel Yager, M.D.

Professor and Vice-Chairman for Education and Academic Affairs
Department of Psychiatry
University of New Mexico School of Medicine
Albuquerque, New Mexico
Professor Emeritus of Psychiatry and Biobehavioral Sciences
David Geffen School of Medicine at UCLA
Los Angeles, California

KAPLAN & SADOCK'S
COMPREHENSIVE TEXTBOOK OF PSYCHIATRY

VOLUME I

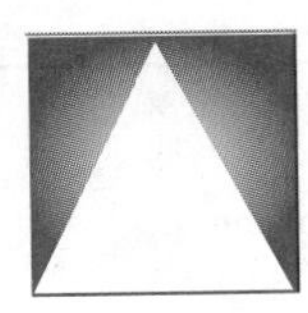

EIGHTH EDITION

EDITORS

Benjamin J. Sadock, M.D.

Menas S. Gregory Professor of Psychiatry and
Vice Chairman, Department of Psychiatry
New York University School of Medicine
Attending Psychiatrist, Tisch Hospital
Attending Psychiatrist, Bellevue Hospital Center
Consulting Physician, Lenox Hill Hospital
New York, New York

Virginia A. Sadock, M.D.

Professor of Psychiatry
New York University School of Medicine
Attending Psychiatrist, Tisch Hospital
Attending Psychiatrist, Bellevue Hospital Center
New York, New York

LIPPINCOTT WILLIAMS & WILKINS
A **Wolters Kluwer** Company
Philadelphia • Baltimore • New York • London
Buenos Aires • Hong Kong • Sydney • Tokyo

Acquisitions Editor: Charles W. Mitchell
Developmental Editors: Joyce Murphy and Lisa Kairis
Supervising Editors: Melanie Bennitt and Nicole Walz
Production Editors: Alyson Langlois and Kate Sallwasser, Silverchair Science + Communications
Senior Manufacturing Manager: Ben Rivera
Marketing Manager: Adam Glazar
Compositor: Silverchair Science + Communications
Printer: Quebecor World Taunton

530 Walnut Street
Philadelphia, PA 19106 USA
LWW.com

Printed in the USA

Library of Congress Cataloging-in-Publication Data

Kaplan & Sadock's comprehensive textbook of psychiatry / editors, Benjamin J. Sadock, Virginia A. Sadock.-- 8th ed.
p. ; cm.
Includes bibliographical references and index.
ISBN 0-7817-3434-7
1. Psychiatry. I. Title: Kaplan and Sadock's comprehensive textbook of psychiatry. II. Title: Comprehensive textbook of psychiatry. III. Sadock, Benjamin J., 1933- IV. Sadock, Virginia A. V. Kaplan, Harold I., 1927-
[DNLM: 1. Mental Disorders. 2. Psychiatry. WM 100 K173 2004]
RC454.C637 2004
616.89--dc22

2004018805

Care has been taken to confirm the accuracy of the information presented and to describe generally accepted practices. However, the authors, editors, and publisher are not responsible for errors or omissions or for any consequences from application of the information in this book and make no warranty, expressed or implied, with respect to the currency, completeness, or accuracy of the contents of the publication. Application of this information in a particular situation remains the professional responsibility of the practitioner.

The authors, editors, and publisher have exerted every effort to ensure that drug selection and dosage set forth in this text are in accordance with current recommendations and practice at the time of publication. However, in view of ongoing research, changes in government regulations, and the constant flow of information relating to drug therapy and drug reactions, the reader is urged to check the package insert for each drug for any change in indications and dosage and for added warnings and precautions. This is particularly important when the recommended agent is a new or infrequently employed drug.

Some drugs and medical devices presented in this publication have Food and Drug Administration (FDA) clearance for limited use in restricted research settings. It is the responsibility of the physician or health care provider to ascertain the FDA status of each drug or device planned for use in their clinical practice.

10 9 8 7 6 5 4 3 2

Dedicated to all those persons who work with and care for the mentally ill

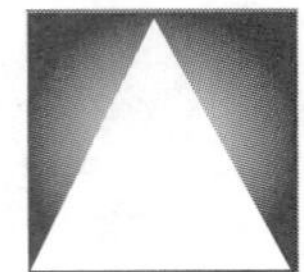

About the Editors

BENJAMIN J. SADOCK, M.D.

Benjamin James Sadock, M.D., is the Menas S. Gregory Professor of Psychiatry and Vice Chairman of the Department of Psychiatry at the New York University (NYU) School of Medicine. He is a graduate of Union College, received his M.D. degree from New York Medical College, and completed his internship at Albany Hospital. He completed his residency at Bellevue Psychiatric Hospital and then entered military service, where he served as Acting Chief of Neuropsychiatry at Sheppard Air Force Base in Texas. He has held faculty and teaching appointments at Southwestern Medical School and Parkland Hospital in Dallas and at New York Medical College, St. Luke's Hospital, the New York State Psychiatric Institute, and Metropolitan Hospital in New York City. Dr. Sadock joined the faculty of the NYU School of Medicine in 1980 and served in various positions: Director of Medical Student Education in Psychiatry, Co-Director of the Residency Training Program in Psychiatry, and Director of Graduate Medical Education. Currently, Dr. Sadock is Director of Student Mental Health Services, Psychiatric Consultant to the Admissions Committee, and Co-Director of Continuing Education in Psychiatry at the NYU School of Medicine. He is on the staff of Bellevue Hospital and Tisch Hospital and is a Consulting Psychiatrist at Lenox Hill Hospital. Dr. Sadock is a Diplomate of the American Board of Psychiatry and Neurology and served as an Associate Examiner for the Board for more than a decade. He is a Distinguished Life Fellow of the American Psychiatric Association, a Fellow of the American College of Physicians, a Fellow of the New York Academy of Medicine, and a member of Alpha Omega Alpha Honor Society. He is active in numerous psychiatric organizations and is president and founder of the NYU-Bellevue Psychiatric Society. Dr. Sadock was a member of the National Committee in Continuing Education in Psychiatry of the American Psychiatric Association, served on the Ad Hoc Committee on Sex Therapy Clinics of the American Medical Association, was a Delegate to the Conference on Recertification of the American Board of Medical Specialists, and was a representative of the American Psychiatric Association Task Force on the National Board of Medical Examiners and the American Board of Psychiatry and Neurology. In 1985, he received the Academic Achievement Award from New York Medical College and was appointed Faculty Scholar at NYU School of Medicine in 2000. He is the author or editor of more than 100 publications, a book reviewer for psychiatric journals, and lectures on a broad range of topics in general psychiatry. Dr. Sadock maintains a private practice for diagnostic consultations and psychiatric treatment. He has been married to Virginia Alcott Sadock, M.D., Professor of Psychiatry at NYU School of Medicine, since completing his residency. Dr. Sadock enjoys opera, golf, skiing, traveling, and is an enthusiastic fly fisherman.

VIRGINIA A. SADOCK, M.D.

Virginia Alcott Sadock, M.D., joined the faculty of the New York University (NYU) School of Medicine in 1980, where she is currently Professor of Psychiatry and Attending Psychiatrist at the Tisch Hospital and Bellevue Hospital. She is Director of the Program in Human Sexuality at the NYU Medical Center, one of the largest treatment and training programs of its kind in the United States. She is the author of more than 50 articles and chapters on sexual behavior and was the developmental editor of *The Sexual Experience*, one of the first major textbooks on human sexuality, published by Williams & Wilkins. She serves as a referee and book reviewer for several medical journals, including the *American Journal of Psychiatry* and the *Journal of the American Medical Association.* She has long been interested in the role of women in medicine and psychiatry and was a founder of the Committee on Women in Psychiatry of the New York County District Branch of the American Psychiatric Association. She is active in academic matters, has served as an Assistant and Associate Examiner for the American Board of Psychiatry and Neurology for more than 15 years, and was also a member of the Test Committee in Psychiatry for both the American Board of Psychiatry and the Psychiatric Knowledge and Self-Assessment Program (PKSAP) of the American Psychiatric Association. She has chaired the Committee on Public Relations of the New York County District Branch of the American Psychiatric Association and has participated in the National Medical Television Network series *Women in Medicine* and the Emmy Award–winning PBS television documentary *Women and Depression.* She has been Vice-President of the Society of Sex Therapy and Research and a regional council member of the American Association of Sex Education Counselors and Therapists, and she is currently President of the Alumni Association of Sex Therapists. She lectures extensively both in this country and abroad on sexual dysfunction, relational problems, and depression and anxiety disorders. She is a Distinguished Fellow of the American Psychiatric Association, a Fellow of the New York Academy of Medicine, and a Diplomate of the American Board of Psychiatry and Neurology. Dr. Sadock is a graduate of Bennington College, received her M.D. degree from New York Medical College, and trained in psychiatry at Metropolitan Hospital. She lives in Manhattan with her husband, Dr. Benjamin Sadock, where she maintains an active practice that includes individual psychotherapy, couples and marital therapy, sex therapy, psychiatric consultation, and pharmacotherapy. She and her husband have two children, James and Victoria, both emergency physicians. In her leisure time, Dr. Sadock enjoys theater, film, golf, reading fiction, and travel.

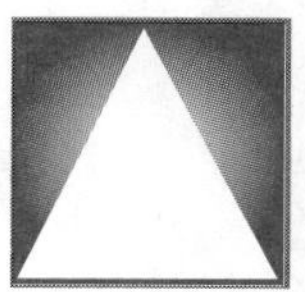

Contents

VOLUME I

VOLUME II

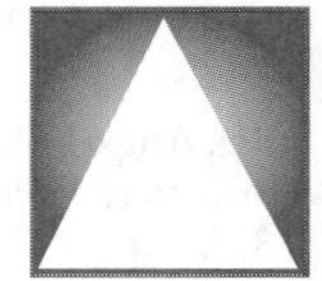

Contributing Authors

Robert C. Abrams, M.D. Associate Professor of Clinical Psychiatry, The Joan and Sanford I. Weill Medical College of Cornell University, New York, New York.
51.3h. Personality Disorders

Russell L. Adams, Ph.D. Professor of Psychiatry and Behavioral Science, University of Oklahoma College of Medicine; Director of the University Hospital Neuropsychology Assessment Laboratory; Director of Psychology Internship and Post Doctoral Neuropsychology Training Program, University of Oklahoma Health Sciences Center, Oklahoma City, Oklahoma.
7.6. Personality Assessment: Adults and Children

W. Stewart Agras, M.D., F.R.C.P.(C) Professor of Psychiatry and Behavioral Sciences, Stanford University School of Medicine; Director of Stanford University Psychiatric Clinics, Stanford, California.
3.3. Learning Theory

Marc E. Agronin, M.D. Assistant Professor of Psychiatry, University of Miami School of Medicine and Director of Mental Health Services, Miami Jewish Home and Hospital for the Aged, Miami, Florida.
51.6g. Sexuality and Aging

Hagop S. Akiskal, M.D. Professor of Psychiatry and Director of the International Mood Center, University of California at San Diego School of Medicine, La Jolla, California; Director of the Mood Disorders Program, San Diego VA Healthcare Systems, San Diego, California.
13.1. Mood Disorders: Historical Introduction and Conceptual Overview; 13.6. Mood Disorders: Clinical Features

Asher Dorell Aladjem, M.D. Clinical Associate Professor of Psychiatry, New York University School of Medicine; Director of Consultation-Liaison Psychiatry and Psychosomatic Medicine; Attending Psychiatrist, Bellevue Hospital Center, New York, New York.
24.11. Consultation-Liaison Psychiatry

Anne Marie Albano, Ph.D. Assistant Professor of Medical Psychology in Psychiatry, Division of Child and Adolescent Psychiatry, Columbia University College of Physicians and Surgeons, New York, New York.
48.3. Cognitive-Behavioral Psychotherapy for Children and Adolescents

Gene E. Alexander, Ph.D. Associate Professor of Psychology and Director of Neuroimage Analysis Laboratory, Arizona State University, Tempe, Arizona; Director of the MRI Morphology Core, Arizona Alzheimer's Research Center, Phoenix, Arizona.
51.2e. Neuroimaging: Overview

George S. Alexopoulos, M.D. Professor of Psychiatry, The Joan and Sanford I. Weill Medical College of Cornell University, New York, New York; Director of the Cornell Institute of Geriatric Psychiatry, New York Hospital-Cornell Medical Center, Westchester Division, White Plains, New York.
51.3d. Mood Disorders

Kenneth Z. Altshuler, M.D. Stanton Sharp Professor of Psychiatry and Former Chairman, Department of Psychiatry, University of Texas Southwestern Medical Center at Dallas; Attending Psychiatrist, Zale Lipshy University Hospital of Southwestern Medical Center, Parkland Health and Hospital System, Presbyterian Hospital of Dallas, St. Paul Medical Center, and Dallas Veterans Affairs Medical Center, Dallas, Texas.
30.10. Other Methods of Psychotherapy

Lori L. Altshuler, M.D. Professor of Psychiatry and Behavioral Sciences and Director of the Mood Disorders Research Program, UCLA Neuropsychiatric Institute and Hospital; Chief, Bipolar Disorder Clinic, Veteran Greater Los Angeles Health Care System, Los Angeles, California.
13.8. Mood Disorders: Treatment of Bipolar Disorders

Stacy S. Amano, Ph.D. Assistant Clinical Professor of Psychiatry and Behavioral Sciences, David Geffen School of Medicine at UCLA, Los Angeles, California.
51.2c. Psychological Changes with Normal Aging

Arnold E. Andersen, M.D. Professor of Psychiatry and Director of Eating Disorder Services, University of Iowa Hospitals and Clinics, Iowa City, Iowa.
19. Eating Disorders

Andrew F. Angelino, M.D. Assistant Professor of Psychiatry and Behavioral Sciences, Johns Hopkins University School of Medicine; Medical Director of Acute Psychiatric Services, Johns Hopkins Bayview Medical Center; Assistant Director of AIDS Psychiatry Services, Johns Hopkins Hospital, Baltimore, Maryland.
2.8. Neuropsychiatric Aspects of HIV Infection and AIDS

Jules Angst, M.D. Emeritus Professor of Psychiatry, Zurich University Psychiatric Hospital, Zurich, Switzerland.
13.2. Mood Disorders: Epidemiology

James C. Anthony, Ph.D., Sc.M. Professor of Psychiatry and Behavioral Sciences, Bloomberg School of Public Health, Johns Hopkins University School of Medicine, Baltimore, Maryland.
11.1. Substance-Related Disorders: Introduction and Overview

Lesley M. Arnold, M.D. Associate Professor of Psychiatry and Director of the Women's Health Research Program, University of Cincinnati College of Medicine, Cincinnati, Ohio.
24.7. Psychocutaneous Disorders

David Axelson, M.D. Assistant Professor of Psychiatry, University of Pittsburgh School of Medicine; Director of Child and Adolescent Bipolar Services, Western Psychiatric Institute and Clinic, University of Pittsburgh Medical Center, Pittsburgh, Pennsylvania.
48.6. Pediatric Psychopharmacology

Alexa Bagnell, M.D. Assistant Professor of Psychiatry, Dalhousie University, Halifax, Nova Scotia, Canada.
49.12. School Consultation

Glen B. Baker, Ph.D., D.Sc. Professor of Psychiatry and Chairman, Department of Psychiatry, Co-Director of the Neurochemical Research Unit; University of Alberta Faculty of Medicine and Dentistry, Edmonton, Alberta, Canada.
31.19. Monoamine Oxidase Inhibitors

Jay M. Baraban, M.D., Ph.D. Professor of Neuroscience and Psychiatry and Behavioral Sciences, Johns Hopkins University School of Medicine, Baltimore, Maryland.
1.8. Intraneuronal Signaling Pathways

David P. Barash, Ph.D. Professor of Psychology, University of Washington, Seattle, Washington.
4.3. Sociobiology

David A. Baron, M.S.Ed., D.O. Professor of Psychiatry and Chairman, Department of Psychiatry, Temple University School of Medicine, Philadelphia, Pennsylvania.
29.2. Other Psychiatric Emergencies

Aaron T. Beck, M.D. Professor Emeritus of Psychiatry and Director of the Psychopathology Research Center, University of Pennsylvania School of Medicine, Philadelphia, Pennsylvania; President, Beck Institute of Cognitive Therapy, Bala Cynwyd, Pennsylvania.
30.6. Cognitive Therapy

Dennis Beedle, M.D. Assistant Professor of Clinical Psychiatry, Chief of General Psychiatry and Attending Psychiatrist, University of Illinois Hospital and Medical Center, Chicago, Illinois.
31.4. Medication-Induced Movement Disorders

Joseph H. Beitchman, M.D. Professor of Psychiatry and Head, Division of Child Psychiatry, University of Toronto Faculty of Medicine; Psychiatrist in Chief, Hospital for Sick Children; and Clinical Director of Child Psychiatry Program, Center for Addiction and Mental Health, Toronto, Ontario, Canada.
37.1. Expressive Language Disorder; 37.2. Mixed Receptive-Expressive Disorder; 37.3. Phonological Disorder; 37.4. Stuttering; 37.5. Communication Disorder Not Otherwise Specified

Carl C. Bell, M.D. Clinical Professor of Psychiatry and Director of Public and Community Psychiatry, University of Illinois College of Medicine; Clinical Professor of Public Health, School of Public Health, University of Illinois of Chicago; Attending Psychiatrist, Jackson Park Hospital and Saint Bernard's Hospital, Chicago, Illinois.
54.3. Correctional Psychiatry

Alan S. Bellack, Ph.D. Professor of Psychiatry and Director of Veteran Capitol Health Care Network Mental Illness Research, Education and Clinical Center, Baltimore, Maryland.
12.13. Psychiatric Rehabilitation

Ruth M. Benca, M.D., Ph.D. Professor of Psychiatry, University of Wisconsin at Madison, Madison, Wisconsin.
1.20. Basic Science of Sleep

David M. Benedek, M.D. Associate Professor of Psychiatry, Uniformed Services University of the Health Sciences, Bethesda, Maryland; Director of the National Capital Consortium Forensic Psychiatry Program, Walter Reed Army Medical Center, Washington, D.C.
28.9. Military and Disaster Psychiatry

Marilyn B. Benoit, M.D. Clinical Associate Professor of Psychiatry, Georgetown University Medical Center, Washington, D.C.
49.2. Adoption and Foster Care

Eugene V. Beresin, M.D. Associate Professor of Psychiatry, Harvard Medical School; Director of Child and Adolescent Psychiatry Residency Training, Massachusetts General Hospital and McLean Hospital, Boston, Massachusetts.
48.10. Psychiatric Treatment of Adolescents

Sarah L. Berga, M.D. Professor and Director of Obstetrics, Gynecology, and Reproductive Sciences, University of Pittsburgh School of Medicine, Magee Women's Hospital, Pittsburgh, Pennsylvania.
28.1. Psychiatry and Reproductive Medicine; 28.2. Premenstrual Dysphoric Disorder

Carlos E. Berganza, M.D. Professor of Psychiatry, Post-Graduate Training Program, San Carlos University School of Medicine, Guatemala City, Guatemala.
9.2. International Psychiatric Diagnosis

R. Lindsey Bergman, Ph.D. Assistant Clinical Professor of Psychiatry and Biobehavioral Science, David Geffen School of Medicine at UCLA; Assistant Clinical Professor of Psychiatry and Associate Director of Childhood Obsessive-Compulsive Disorder, Anxiety and Tourette Disorder Program, UCLA Neuropsychiatric Institute and Hospital, Los Angeles, California.
46.4. Selective Mutism

William Bernet, M.D. Professor of Psychiatry and Director of Forensic Psychiatry, Vanderbilt University School of Medicine, Nashville, Tennessee.
49.3. Child Maltreatment

Gail A. Bernstein, M.D. Professor of Child and Adolescent Psychiatry and Head of Program in Child and Adolescent Anxiety and Mood Disorders, University of Minnesota Medical School; Attending Physician, Fairview-University Medical Center, Minneapolis, Minnesota.
46.3. Separation Anxiety Disorder and Other Anxiety Disorders

Joseph Biederman, M.D. Professor of Psychiatry, Harvard Medical School; Chief, Joint Program in Pediatric Psychopharmacology, Massachusetts General Hospital and McLean Hospital, Boston, Massachusetts.
45.2. Early-Onset Bipolar Disorders

Boris Birmaher, M.D. Professor of Psychiatry, University of Pittsburgh Medical Center; Attending Psychiatrist, University of Pittsburgh Medical Center, Western Psychiatric Institute and Clinic, Pittsburgh, Pennsylvania.
48.6. Pediatric Psychopharmacology

Deborah Blacker, M.D., Sc.D. Associate Professor of Psychiatry, Harvard Medical School; Associate Professor of Epidemiology, Harvard School of Public Health; Director of Gerontology Research Unit, Massachusetts General Hospital; Boston, Massachusetts.
7.9. Psychiatric Rating Scales

Dan G. Blazer II, M.D., Ph.D. J.P. Gibbons Professor of Psychiatry and Behavioral Sciences and Professor of Community and Family Medicine, Duke University School of Medicine, Durham, North Carolina; Adjunct Professor of Epidemiology, University of North Carolina, Chapel Hill, North Carolina.
51.1b. Epidemiology of Psychiatric Disorders

Efrain Bleiberg, M.D. Professor and Vice-Chairman, Department of Psychiatry and Behavioral Sciences, and Director, Division of Child and Adolescent Psychiatry, Department of Psychiatry and Behavioral Sciences, Baylor College of Medicine; Medical Director, Professionals in Crisis, The Menninger Clinic, Topeka, Kansas.
49.8. Identity Problem and Borderline Disorders in Children and Adolescents

Bennett Blum, M.D. Director of Forensic Geropsychiatry Division, Park Dietz and Associates, Inc., Newport Beach, California.
51.6b. Forensic Issues

Omer Bonne, M.D. Senior Lecturer of Psychiatry and Head of Psychiatry Outpatient Services, Hadassah University Hospital, Hebrew University Medical School, Jerusalem, Israel.
14.4. Anxiety Disorders: Neurochemical Aspects

Kyle Brauer Boone, Ph.D. Professor-in-Residence, Department of Psychiatry, David Geffen School of Medicine at UCLA, Los Angeles, California.
51.2d. Neuropsychological Evaluation

Neil W. Boris, M.D. Associate Professor of Community Health Sciences, Tulane University School of Public Health and Tropical Medicine; Assistant Professor of Pediatrics, Psychiatry, and Neurology, Tulane University School of Medicine; Co-Director of Child Psychiatry Consultation-Liaison Service, Tulane University Hospital and Medical Center, New Orleans, Louisiana.
44.1. Reactive Attachment Disorder of Infancy and Early Childhood

Soo Borson, M.D. Professor of Psychiatry and Behavioral Science, University of Washington School of Medicine; Director of Geropsychiatry Services and Director of University of Washington Medical Center Alzheimer's Disease Research Center, Seattle, Washington.
51.3a. Psychiatric Problems in the Medically Ill; 51.3b. Sleep Disorders

Jeff Q. Bostic, M.D., Ed.D. Assistant Clinical Professor of Psychiatry, Harvard Medical School; Director of Psychiatry, Massachusetts General Hospital, Boston, Massachusetts.
49.12. School Consultation

Nashaat N. Boutros, M.D. Associate Professor of Psychiatry, Yale University School of Medicine, New Haven, Connecticut; Director of Dual Diagnostic Program, VA Connecticut Healthcare System; Director of Clinical Electrophysiology and Transcranial Stimulation Laboratory, VA Medical Center, West Haven, Connecticut.
1.14. Applied Electrophysiology

Kathleen T. Brady, M.D., Ph.D. Professor of Psychiatry, Medical University of South Carolina College of Medicine, Charleston, South Carolina.
31.21. Opioid Receptor Agonists: Methadone, Levomethadyl, and Buprenorphine

Elvira Bramon, M.D. Wellcome Research Fellow in Psychiatry, Division of Psychological Medicine, Institute of Psychiatry, De Crespigny Park, London, United Kingdom.
12.5. The Developmental Model of Schizophrenia

Michaeline Bresnahan, Ph.D., M.P.H. Assistant Professor of Epidemiology and Psychiatry, Columbia University College of Physicians and Surgeons, New York, New York.
12.4. Schizophrenia: Environmental Epidemiology

Tim Bressmann, Ph.D. Assistant Professor of Psychiatry, University of Toronto Faculty of Medicine, Toronto, Ontario, Canada.
37.5. Communication Disorder Not Otherwise Specified

Evelyn J. Bromet, Ph.D. Professor of Psychiatry and Preventive Medicine, Stony Brook University Health Science Center School of Medicine, Stony Brook, New York.
12.16b. Schizophreniform Disorder; 12.16c. Delusional Disorder and Shared Psychotic Disorder; 12.16e. Postpartum Psychosis

Kirk J. Brower, M.D. Associate Professor of Psychiatry, University of Michigan Medical School; Executive Director of Chelsea Arbor Addiction Treatment Center, University of Michigan Health System, Ann Arbor, Michigan.
11.13. Anabolic-Androgenic Steroid Abuse

Alan S. Brown, M.D. Associate Professor of Clinical Psychiatry, Columbia University College of Physicians and Surgeons; Deputy Director of Department of Epidemiology of Brain Disorders, New York State Psychiatric Institute, New York, New York.
12.4. Schizophrenia: Environmental Epidemiology

Kelly D. Brownell, Ph.D. Professor and Chairman, Department of Psychology; Professor of Epidemiology and Public Health; and Director of Yale Center for Eating and Weight Disorders, Yale University, New Haven, Connecticut.
24.3. Obesity

Robert W. Buchanan, M.D. Professor of Psychiatry, University of Maryland School of Medicine, Baltimore, Maryland; Chief of Outpatient Research Program, Maryland Psychiatric Research Center, Catonsville, Maryland.
12.1. The Concept of Schizophrenia

Regina Bussing, M.D. Associate Professor of Psychiatry and Director of Division of Child and Adolescent Psychiatry, Departments of Psychiatry, Health Policy and Epidemiology; University of Florida College of Medicine, Gainesville, Florida.
49.15. Child Mental Health Services Research

Juan R. Bustillo, M.D. Associate Professor of Psychiatry and Neurosciences; University of New Mexico School of Medicine, Albuquerque, New Mexico.
12.2. Schizophrenia: Scope of the Problem

William M. Byne, M.D., Ph.D. Associate Professor of Psychiatry, Mount Sinai School of Medicine, New York, New York; Attending Psychiatrist, Bronx Veterans Affairs Medical Center, Bronx, New York.
18.1b. Homosexuality, Gay and Lesbian Identities, and Homosexual Behavior

Shawn P. Cahill, Ph.D. Assistant Professor of Psychology in Psychiatry, University of Pennsylvania School of Medicine, Philadelphia, Pennsylvania.
14.10. Anxiety Disorders: Cognitive-Behavioral Therapy

Gabrielle A. Carlson, M.D. Professor of Psychiatry and Pediatrics and Director of Child and Adolescent Psychiatry, Stony Brook University Health Science Center School of Medicine, Stony Brook, New York.
12.16d. Schizoaffective Disorder

Patrick J. Carnes, Ph.D. Senior Fellow, Compass Point Addiction Foundation, Cave Creek, Arizona; Clinical Director of Sexual Disorders Services, The Meadows, Wickenburg, Arizona.
18.4. Sexual Addiction

William T. Carpenter, Jr., M.D. Professor of Psychiatry and Pharmacology, University of Maryland School of Medicine, Baltimore, Maryland; Director of Maryland Psychiatric Research Center, Catonsville, Maryland.
12.1. The Concept of Schizophrenia

Moses V. Chao, Ph.D. Professor of Cell Biology and Physiology and Neuroscience, Skirball Institute, New York University School of Medicine, New York, New York.
1.7. Neurotrophic Factors

Dennis S. Charney, M.D. Chief, Mood and Anxiety Disorders Program, National Institute of Mental Health, National Institutes of Health, Bethesda, Maryland.
14.1. Anxiety Disorders: Introduction and Overview; 14.4. Anxiety Disorders: Neurochemical Aspects; 14.5. Anxiety Disorders: Neuroimaging

Irene Chatoor, M.D. Professor of Psychiatry and Pediatrics, George Washington University School of Medicine; Director of the Infant and Toddler Mental Health Center, Children's National Medical Center, Washington, D.C.
41. Feeding and Eating Disorders of Infancy and Early Childhood

Domenic A. Ciraulo, M.D. Professor of Psychiatry and Chairman, Boston University School of Medicine; Psychiatrist-in-Chief, Boston Medical Center; Chief of Psychiatry Service, Veterans Affairs Boston Clinic, Boston, Massachusetts.
11.12. Sedative-, Hypnotic-, or Anxiolytic-Related Disorders

Chiara Cirelli, M.D., Ph.D. Assistant Professor of Psychiatry, University of Wisconsin at Madison Medical School, Madison, Wisconsin.
1.20. Basic Science of Sleep

C. Robert Cloninger, M.D. Wallace Renard Professor of Psychiatry, Washington University School of Medicine, Saint Louis, Missouri.
23. Personality Disorders

Judith A. Cohen, M.D. Professor of Psychiatry, University of Pennsylvania School of Medicine, Philadelphia, Pennsylvania; Medical Director of Center for Traumatic Stress in Children and Adolescents, Allegheny General Hospital, Pittsburgh, Pennsylvania.
46.2. Posttraumatic Stress Disorder in Children and Adolescents

Calvin A. Colarusso, M.D. Clinical Professor of Psychiatry and Director of Child Psychiatry Residency Training Program, University of California, San Diego School of Medicine, La Jolla, California; Training and Supervising Analyst, San Diego Psychoanalytic Institute, San Diego, California.
50. Adulthood

Robert F. Cole, Ph.D. Assistant Professor of Psychiatry, University of Connecticut Health Center, Farmington, Connecticut.
52.1. Public and Community Psychiatry

Steven Cole, M.D. Professor of Clinical Psychiatry and Head, Division of Medical and Geriatric Psychiatry, Stony Brook University Health Science Center School of Medicine, Stony Brook, New York.
52.2. Health Care Reform

Ralph Colp, Jr., M.D. Assistant Professor of Clinical Psychiatry, Columbia University College of Physicians and Surgeons; Senior Attending Psychiatrist, St. Luke's-Roosevelt Hospital Center, New York, New York.
55.1. History of Psychiatry

G. Rees Cosgrove, M.D., F.R.C.S.(C) Associate Professor of Surgery, Harvard Medical School, Boston, Massachusetts.
31.31. Neurosurgical Treatments and Deep Brain Stimulation

Paul T. Costa, Jr., Ph.D. Professor of Psychiatry and Behavioral Sciences, Johns Hopkins University School of Medicine; Chief, Laboratory of Personality and Cognition, Gerontology Research Center, National Institute on Aging, National Institutes of Health, Baltimore, Maryland.
6.4. Approaches Derived from Philosophy and Psychology

Jorge Alberto Costa e Silva, M.D. Professor of Psychiatry and Director of International Center of Mental Health Policy and Research, New York University School of Medicine, New York, New York; Former Director of Division of Mental Health and Prevention of Substance Abuse, World Health Organization, Geneva, Switzerland.
55.2. World Aspects of Psychiatry

Louis J. Cozolino, Ph.D. Professor of Psychology, Pepperdine University, Malibu, California; Assistant Clinical Professor of Psychiatry, David Geffen School of Medicine at UCLA, Los Angeles, California.
3.1. Sensation, Perception, and Cognition

Thomas J. Crowley, M.D. Professor of Psychiatry, University of Colorado School of Medicine; Director of Division of Substance Dependence, University of Colorado Health Sciences Center, Denver, Colorado.
11.8. Inhalant-Related Disorders

Jan L. Culbertson, Ph.D. Professor of Pediatrics and Clinical Professor of Psychiatry and Behavioral Sciences, Director of Neuropsychology Services Child Study Center, University of Oklahoma Health Sciences Center, Oklahoma City, Oklahoma.
7.6. Personality Assessment: Adults and Children

John F. Curry, Ph.D. Associate Professor of Psychiatry and Behavioral Sciences, Duke University School of Medicine, Durham, North Carolina.
3.2. Extending Jean Piaget's Approach to Intellectual Functioning

Jill M. Cyranowski, Ph.D. Assistant Professor of Psychiatry, Western Psychiatric Institute and Clinic, University of Pittsburgh Medical Center, Pittsburgh, Pennsylvania.
28.1. Psychiatry and Reproductive Medicine

Catherine J. Datto, M.D. Instructor in Geriatric Psychiatry and Fellow in Clinical Epidemiology, University of Pennsylvania School of Medicine, Philadelphia, Pennsylvania.
51.4f. Electroconvulsive Therapy; 51.6a. Psychiatric Aspects of Long-Term Care

Habib Davanloo, M.D. Professor of Psychiatry, McGill University; Senior Consultant, McGill University Health Center and The Montreal General Hospital, Montreal, Quebec, Canada.
30.9. Intensive Short-Term Dynamic Psychotherapy

David Davis, M.D., F.R.C.Psych. Emeritus Professor of Psychiatry, University of Missouri School of Medicine; Attending Psychiatrist, Psychosomatic Service, University of Missouri Health Sciences Center, Columbia, Missouri.
28.10. Famous Named Cases in Psychiatry

Kenneth L. Davis, M.D. Gustave L. Levy Distinguished Professor and Dean, Mount Sinai School of Medicine; President and Chief Executive Officer, Mount Sinai Medical Center, New York, New York.
10.1. Cognitive Disorders: Introduction and Overview

Mark DeAntonio, M.D. Associate Clinical Professor of Psychiatry and Biobehavioral Sciences, David Geffen School of Medicine at UCLA; Director of Inpatient Adolescent Services, UCLA Neuropsychiatric Institute and Hospital, Los Angeles, California.
48.8. Residential and Inpatient Treatment

Charles DeBattista, M.D., D.M.H. Assistant Professor of Psychiatry and Behavioral Sciences, Director of Depression Clinic and Psychopharmacology Clinic, and Chief of ECT Service, Stanford University School of Medicine, Stanford, California.
31.33. Drug Augmentation

Louisa Degenhardt, Ph.D. Lecturer, National Drug and Alcohol Research Center, University of New South Wales, New South Wales, Australia.
11.5. Cannabis-Related Disorders

Davangere P. Devanand, M.D. Professor of Clinical Psychiatry and Neurology, New York State Psychiatric Institute, Columbia University College of Physicians and Surgeons, New York, New York.
51.2a. Psychiatric Assessment of the Older Patient

Emanuel DiCicco-Bloom, M.D. Associate Professor of Neuroscience and Cell Biology, and Pediatrics, University of Medicine and Dentistry of New Jersey-Robert Wood Johnson Medical School, Piscataway, New Jersey.
1.3. Neural Development and Neurogenesis

Faith B. Dickerson, Ph.D., M.P.H. Director of Psychology and Attending Psychiatrist, Sheppard Pratt Health System, Baltimore, Maryland.
12.11. Schizophrenia: Psychosocial Treatment

Leah J. Dickstein, M.D. Professor of Psychiatry and Associate Chairman for Academic Affairs, Associate Dean for Faculty and Student Advocacy and Director of Division of Attitudinal and Behavioral Medicine, University of Louisville School of Medicine; Staff Psychiatrist, University of Louisville Hospital, Louisville, Kentucky.
25. Relational Problems; 26.4. Other Additional Conditions That May Be a Focus of Clinical Attention

Joel E. Dimsdale, M.D. Professor of Psychiatry, University of California, San Diego; Attending Psychiatrist, University of California, San Diego Medical Center, La Jolla, California.
24.9. Stress and Psychiatry

Lisa Dixon, M.D., M.P.H. Professor of Psychiatry, University of Maryland School of Medicine, Baltimore, Maryland.
12.11. Schizophrenia: Psychosocial Treatment

Christian R. Dolder, Pharm.D. Assistant Clinical Professor of Psychiatry, University of California, San Diego, La Jolla, California; Clinical Pharmacist, Veterans San Diego Health Care System, San Diego, California.
51.3g. Schizophrenia and Delusional Disorders

Robert E. Drake, M.D., Ph.D. Professor of Psychiatry and Community and Family Medicine and Director of New Hampshire-Dartmouth Psychiatric Research Center, Dartmouth Medical School, Hanover, New Hampshire.
12.13. Psychiatric Rehabilitation

Martin J. Drell, M.D. Carl P. Adatto, M.D. Professor of Community Psychiatry and Professor of Head of Infant, Child, and Adolescent Psychiatry, Louisiana State University Medical School; Clinical Director of New Orleans Adolescent Hospital and Community System of Care, New Orleans, Louisiana.
49.4. Children's Reaction to Illness and Hospitalization

Jack Drescher, M.D. Clinical Assistant Professor of Psychiatry, State University of New York Downstate Medical Center College of Medicine, Brooklyn, New York; Training and Supervising Analyst, William Alanson White Institute of Psychiatry, Psychoanalysis and Psychology, New York, New York.
18.1b. Homosexuality, Gay and Lesbian Identities, and Homosexual Behavior

Wayne C. Drevets, M.D. Adjunct Associate Professor of Psychiatry, University of Pittsburgh School of Medicine, Pittsburgh, Pennsylvania; Senior Investigator and Chief, Section of Neuroimaging in Mood and Anxiety Disorder, National Institute of Mental Health, National Institutes of Health, Bethesda, Maryland.
1.15. Nuclear Magnetic Resonance Imaging: Basic Principles and Recent Findings in Neuropsychiatric Disorders; 14.5. Anxiety Disorders: Neuroimaging

Martin Allan Drooker, M.D. Clinical Assistant Professor of Psychiatry, Mount Sinai School of Medicine; Director Division of Behavioral Medicine and Consultation Psychiatry, Mount Sinai Medical Center, New York, New York.
10.5. Other Cognitive Disorders and Mental Disorders Due to a General Medical Condition

William R. Dubin, M.D. Professor of Psychiatry, Temple University School of Medicine; Chief Medical Officer, Temple University Hospital-Episcopal Division, Philadelphia, Pennsylvania.
29.2. Other Psychiatric Emergencies

Steven Dubovsky, M.D. Professor of Psychiatry and Medicine and Vice-Chairman, Department of Psychiatry, University of Colorado School of Medicine, Denver, Colorado.
31.11. Benzodiazepine Receptor Agonists and Antagonists; 31.14. Calcium Channel Inhibitors

Jennifer J. Dunkin, Ph.D. Associate Clinical Professor of Psychiatry and Behavioral Sciences and Director Psychological Services Division of Geriatric Psychiatry and Geriatric Psychology Fellowship Program, David Geffen School of Medicine at UCLA, Los Angeles, California.
51.2c. Psychological Changes with Normal Aging

Elisabeth M. Dykens, Ph.D. Professor of Psychiatry and Behavioral Sciences, David Geffen School of Medicine at UCLA; Attending Psychiatrist, UCLA Neuropsychiatric Institute and Center for Neurobehavioral Genetics, Los Angeles, California.
34. Mental Retardation

James C. Edmondson, M.D., Ph.D. Clinical Assistant Professor of Psychiatry, New York University School of Medicine, New York, New York; Assistant Attending, Department of Neurology, Brooklyn Hospital Center and Long Island College Hospital, Brooklyn, New York.
2.12. Neuropsychiatric Aspects of Neuromuscular Disease; 2.13. Psychiatric Aspects of Child Neurology

Spencer Eth, M.D. Professor of Psychiatry and Vice-Chairman, Department of Psychiatry, New York Medical College; Medical Director of Behavioral Health Services, Saint Vincents Catholic Medical Centers, New York, New York.
54.2. Ethics in Psychiatry

Warachal Eileen Faison, M.D. Assistant Director, Institute for Research Minority Training on Mental Health and Aging, Alzheimer's Research & Clinical Programs, Medical University of South Carolina, Charleston, South Carolina.
51.6d. Minority and Sociocultural Issues

Brian Anthony Fallon, M.D., M.P.H. Associate Professor of Clinical Psychiatry, Columbia University of Physicians and Surgeons; Director Lyme Disease Research Program, New York State Psychiatric Institute, New York, New York.
2.9. Neuropsychiatric Aspects of Other Infectious Diseases (Non-HIV)

Stephen V. Faraone, Ph.D. Professor in the Department of Epidemiology, Harvard School of Public Health; Clinical Professor of Psychiatry, Harvard Medical School; Director of Pediatric Psychopharmacology Research, Massachusetts General Hospital, Boston, Massachusetts.
12.15. Schizophrenia Spectrum: Pathology and Treatment

Armando Favazza, M.D., M.P.H. Professor of Psychiatry and Neurology, University of Missouri Columbia School of Medicine, Columbia, Missouri.
4.1. The Psychiatric Scientist and the Psychoanalyst

Jan Fawcett, M.D. Stanley G. Harris, Sr. Professor of Psychiatry and Chairman, Department of Psychiatry, Rush Medical College; Director of Rush Institute for Mental Well-Being, Chicago, Illinois.
31.26. Sympathomimetics and Dopamine Receptor Agonists

Shmuel Fennig, M.D. Senior Lecturer, Tel Aviv University Sackler School of Medicine, Tel Aviv, Israel; Medical Director of the Adult Outpatient Services, Shalvata Mental Health Center, Hod Hasharon, Israel.
12.16c. Delusional Disorder and Shared Psychotic Disorder; 12.16d. Schizoaffective Disorder; 12.16g. Psychosis Not Otherwise Specified

Wayne S. Fenton, M.D. Associate Director of Clinical Affairs; Deputy Director of the Division of Mental Disorders, Behavioral Research and AIDS, National Institute of Mental Health, National Institutes of Health, Bethesda, Maryland.
12.14. Schizophrenia: Integrative Treatment and Functional Outcomes, 55.3. Future of Psychiatry

Kate Dimond Fitzgerald, M.D. Research Fellow, Department of Psychiatry, University of Michigan Health System, Ann Arbor, Michigan.
49.14. Neuroimaging in Child and Adolescent Psychiatry

Edna B. Foa, Ph.D. Professor of Psychology and Psychiatry and Director of the Center for the Treatment and Study of Anxiety, University of Pennsylvania School of Medicine, Philadelphia, Pennsylvania.
14.10. Anxiety Disorders: Cognitive-Behavioral Therapy

Laura J. Fochtmann, M.D. Professor of Psychiatry and Behavioral Sciences, Pharmacological Sciences and Emergency Medicine, Stony Brook University Health Science Center School of Medicine; Director Electroconvulsive Therapy Service, Stony Brook University Medical Center, Stony Brook, New York.
12.16b. Schizophreniform Disorder; 12.16c. Delusional Disorder and Shared Psychotic Disorder; 12.16d. Schizoaffective Disorder; 12.16e. Postpartum Psychosis; 12.16g. Psychosis Not Otherwise Specified; 12.16h. Treatment of Other Psychotic Disorders

Julian D. Ford, Ph.D. Associate Professor of Psychiatry, University of Connecticut School of Medicine; Medical Staff, University of Connecticut Health Center, Farmington, Connecticut.
52.1. Public and Community Psychiatry

Robert Freedman, M.D. Professor of Psychiatry and Chairman, Department of Psychiatry, University of Colorado School of Medicine; Superintendent, Colorado Psychiatric Hospital; Psychiatrist, Denver Veterans Medical Center, Denver, Colorado.
12.10. Schizophrenia: Sensory Gating Deficits and Translational Research

Nelson B. Freimer, M.D. Professor of Psychiatry and Human Genetics, David Geffen School of Medicine at UCLA; Director of the UCLA Center for Neurobehavioral Genetics, UCLA Neuropsychiatric Institute and Hospital, Los Angeles, California.
1.18. Genetic Linkage Analysis of the Psychiatric Disorders

Mark A. Frye, M.D. Assistant Professor of Psychiatry, David Geffen School of Medicine at UCLA; Director of the UCLA Bipolar Research Program, Los Angeles, California.
31.8a. Carbamazepine; 31.8e. Valproate

Masahiro Fujita, M.D., Ph.D. Staff Scientist, Molecular Imaging Branch, National Institute of Mental Health, National Institutes of Health, Bethesda, Maryland.
1.16. Radiotracer Imaging: Basic Principles and Exemplary Findings in Neuropsychiatric Disorders

Dolores Gallagher-Thompson, Ph.D. Associate Professor of Research, Department of Psychiatry and Behavioral Sciences and Director of the Older Adult and Family Center, Stanford University School of Medicine, Stanford, California.
51.4i. Cognitive-Behavioral Therapy

Thomas R. Garrick, M.D. Professor of Psychiatry and Biobehavioral Sciences, David Geffen School of Medicine at UCLA; Chief of Psychiatry, West Los Angeles Veterans Affairs Ambulatory Care Center, Los Angeles, California.
24.6. Endocrine and Metabolic Disorders

Nori Geary, Ph.D. Research Professor of Psychiatry, The Joan and Sanford I. Weill Medical College of Cornell University, New York, New York; Director of the E. W. Bourne Behavioral Research Laboratory, New York Hospital-Cornell Medical Center, Westchester Division, White Plains, New York.
1.21. Appetite

S. Nassir Ghaemi, M.D. Assistant Professor of Psychiatry, Harvard Medical School, Boston, Massachusetts; Director of the Bipolar Disorder Research Program, Cambridge Hospital, Cambridge, Massachusetts.
31.8f. Other Anticonvulsants: Tiagabine, Zonisamide, Oxcarbazepine, and Levetiracetam

Michael J. Gitlin, M.D. Professor of Clinical Psychiatry and Director of the Division of Adult Psychiatry, Department of Psychiatry and Biobehavioral Sciences, David Geffen School of Medicine at UCLA, Los Angeles, California.
8. Clinical Manifestations of Psychiatric Disorders

Stephen J. Glatt, Ph.D. Assistant Adjunct Professor of Psychiatry, University of California, San Diego, La Jolla, California.
12.15. Schizophrenia Spectrum: Pathology and Treatment

James M. Gold, Ph.D. Associate Professor of Psychiatry, University of Maryland School of Medicine, Baltimore, Maryland; Maryland Psychiatric Research Center, Catonsville, Maryland.
12.9. Schizophrenia: Cognition

Joel Gold, M.D. Clinical Assistant Professor of Psychiatry, New York University Medical Center; Attending Psychiatrist, Bellevue Hospital Center, New York, New York.
28.7. Survivors of Torture

Marion Zucker Goldstein, M.D. Professor of Psychiatry, University of Buffalo State University of New York; Director of the Division of Geriatric Psychiatry, University Psychiatry Practice, Erie County Medical Center, Buffalo, New York.
51.6e. Gender Issues; 51.6f. Elder Abuse, Neglect, and Exploitation

Maureen Fulchiero Gordon, M.D. Assistant Clinical Professor of Psychiatry and Biobehavioral Sciences, David Geffen School of Medicine at UCLA, Los Angeles, California.
32.2. Normal Child Development

Gary L. Gottlieb, M.D., M.B.A. Professor of Psychiatry, Harvard Medical School; Chairman, Department of Psychiatry, Partners Psychiatry and Mental Health System, Partners Health Care System, Inc., Boston, Massachusetts.
51.5a. Financial Issues in the Delivery of Geriatric Psychiatric Care

Jack A. Grebb, M.D. Clinical Professor of Psychiatry, New York University School of Medicine, New York, New York; Vice President, Clinical Design, and Evaluation, Neuroscience, Bristol-Myers Squibb, Wallingford, Connecticut.
1.1. Neural Sciences: Introduction and Overview

Michael F. Green, Ph.D. Professor of Psychiatry, UCLA Neuropsychiatric Institute and Hospital, David Geffen School of Medicine at UCLA; Director of the Treatment Unit, Department of Veterans Affairs VISN 22 Mental Illness, Research Education and Clinical Center, Los Angeles, California.
12.9. Schizophrenia: Cognition

Richard Green, M.D., J.D. Professor of Psychiatry, Imperial College School of Medicine; Head of Gender Identity Clinic and Consultant Psychiatrist, Charing Cross Hospital, London, England; Professor of Psychiatry Emeritus, David Geffen School of Medicine at UCLA, Los Angeles, California.
18.3. Gender Identity Disorders

Benjamin D. Greenberg, M.D., Ph.D. Associate Professor of Psychiatry and Human Behavior, Brown Medical School, Providence, Rhode Island.
31.31. Neurosurgical Treatments and Deep Brain Stimulation

Harvey Roy Greenberg, M.D. Clinical Professor of Psychiatry, Albert Einstein College of Medicine at Yeshiva University, Bronx, New York.
21. Impulse-Control Disorders Not Elsewhere Classified

Robert M. Greenberg, M.D. Clinical Associate Professor of Psychiatry, University of Medicine and Dentistry of New Jersey, Stratford, New Jersey; Director of Geriatric Psychiatry and ECT Services, Bon Secours Health System of New Jersey, Jersey City and Hoboken, New Jersey.
51.4f. Electroconvulsive Therapy

David J. Greenblatt, M.D. Professor and Chairman, Department of Pharmacology and Experimental Therapeutics, Professor of Psychiatry, Medicine and Anesthesia, Tufts University School of Medicine, Boston, Massachusetts.
31.2. Pharmacokinetics and Drug Interactions

Marcia Greenleaf, Ph.D. Assistant Clinical Professor, Department of Psychiatry, Albert Einstein College of Medicine at Yeshiva University, Bronx, New York.
30.3. Hypnosis

Stanley I. Greenspan, M.D. Clinical Professor of Psychiatry and Behavioral Sciences and Pediatrics, George Washington University School of Medicine and Health Sciences; Supervising Child Psychoanalyst, Washington Psychoanalytic Institute, Washington, D.C.
3.2. Extending Jean Piaget's Approach to Intellectual Functioning

John H. Greist, M.D. Clinical Professor of Psychiatry, University of Wisconsin Medical School; Distinguished Senior Scientist, Co-Director of the Lithium Information Center, Madison Institute of Medicine, Madison, Wisconsin.
31.17. Lithium

Roland R. Griffiths, Ph.D. Professor of Psychiatry and Behavioral Sciences, Department of Neurosciences, Johns Hopkins University School of Medicine, Baltimore, Maryland.
11.4. Caffeine-Related Disorders

Christian Grillon, Ph.D. Chief, Unit of Affective Psychophysiology, Mood and Anxiety Disorder Programs, National Institute of Mental Health, Bethesda, Maryland.
14.3. Anxiety Disorders: Psychophysiological Aspects

Hillel Grossman, M.D. Assistant Professor of Psychiatry and Associate Director of Training, Department of Psychiatry, Mount Sinai School of Medicine, New York, New York.
10.4. Amnestic Disorders

Raquel E. Gur, M.D., Ph.D. Professor of Psychiatry and Director of Neuropsychiatry, Department of Psychiatry, University of Pennsylvania School of Medicine, Philadelphia, Pennsylvania.
12.6. Neuroimaging in Schizophrenia: Linking Neuropsychiatric Manifestations to Neurobiology

Ruben C. Gur, Ph.D. Professor of Psychiatry and Director of Neuropsychology and Brain-Behavior Laboratory, Department of Psychiatry, University of Pennsylvania School of Medicine, Philadelphia, Pennsylvania.
12.6. Neuroimaging in Schizophrenia: Linking Neuropsychiatric Manifestations to Neurobiology

Alan S. Gurman, Ph.D. Professor of Psychiatry, Director of Couple-Family Clinic, Chief Psychologist, University of Wisconsin Medical School, Madison, Wisconsin.
30.5. Family Therapy and Couple Therapy

Barry H. Guze, M.D. Professor of Psychiatry, David Geffen School of Medicine at UCLA; Director of the Adult Psychiatry Hospital Service, UCLA Neuropsychiatric Institute and Hospital, Los Angeles, California.
7.8. Medical Assessment and Laboratory Testing in Psychiatry

Kathleen Y. Haaland, Ph.D. Professor of Psychiatry and Neurology, University of New Mexico School of Medicine; Director of Psychology Research, New Mexico Veterans Affairs Healthcare System, Albuquerque, New Mexico.
7.5. Clinical Neuropsychology and Intellectual Assessment of Adults

Donald W. Hadley, M.S. Investigator, Genetic Counseling Research Unit, Medical Genetics Branch, National Human Genome Research Institute; Genetic Counselor, Warren Grant Magnuson Clinical Center, National Institutes of Health, Bethesda, Maryland.
28.3. Genetic Counseling

Wayne Hall, Ph.D. Visiting Professor, National Drug and Alcohol Research Center, University of New South Wales, Sydney, Australia; Professorial Research Fellow: School of Psychology, School of Political Science and International Relations, School of Population Health; and Director of Public Policy and Ethics, Institute for Molecular Bioscience, University of Queensland, St. Lucia, Queensland, Australia.
11.5. Cannabis-Related Disorders

Debra S. Harris, M.D. Assistant Adjunct Professor of Psychiatry, University of California at San Francisco School of Medicine; Attending Psychiatrist, Langley Porter Psychiatric Institute; Courtesy Staff, San Francisco General Hospital, San Francisco, California.
1.11. Psychoneuroendocrinology

Jennifer F. Havens, M.D. Assistant Professor of Clinical Psychiatry, Columbia University College of Physicians and Surgeons; Director of Clinical and Community Services in Child and Adolescent Psychiatry, Children's Hospital of New York Presbyterian, New York, New York.
49.5. Psychiatric Sequelae of HIV and AIDS

Donald P. Hay, M.D. Adjunct Associate Clinical Professor of Psychiatry, Saint Louis University School of Medicine, Saint Louis, Missouri; Clinical Research Physician, Eli Lilly and Company, Indianapolis, Indiana.
51.4f. Electroconvulsive Therapy

Lily Hechtman, M.D., F.R.C.P.(C) Professor of Psychiatry and Pediatrics, Director of Research, Division of Child Psychiatry, McGill University Faculty of Medicine; Director of Adolescent Psychiatry Services, Montreal Children's Hospital, McGill University Hospital Center, Montreal, Quebec, Canada.
39.1. Attention-Deficit/Hyperactivity Disorder

Victoria C. Hendrick, M.D. Associate Professor of Psychiatry and Behavioral Sciences, David Geffen School of Medicine at UCLA; Medical Director of the Center of Women's Well-Being, Los Angeles County Department of Health; and Attending Psychiatrist, UCLA Neuropsychiatric Institute and Hospital, Los Angeles, California.
24.6. Endocrine and Metabolic Disorders

Hugh C. Hendrie, M.B., Ch.B., D.Sc. Professor of Psychiatry, Indiana University School of Medicine; Research Scientist, Indiana University Center for Aging Research, Indianapolis, Indiana.
51.6d. Minority and Sociocultural Issues

Jerry D. Heston, M.D. Professor and Acting Director of Child and Adolescent Psychiatry, Department of Psychiatry, University of Tennessee at Memphis College of Medicine; Medical Director of Child and Adolescent Day Treatment Services, University of Tennessee Medical Center, Memphis, Tennessee.
48.7. Partial Hospital and Ambulatory Behavioral Health Services

John M. Hettema, M.D., Ph.D. Assistant Professor of Psychiatry, Virginia Commonwealth University School of Medicine; Attending Psychiatrist, Virginia Institute for Psychiatric and Behavioral Genetics, Virginia Commonwealth University, Richmond, Virginia.
31.28. Trazodone

Euthymia D. Hibbs, Ph.D. Adjunct Associate Professor of Psychiatry and Behavioral Sciences, George Washington University School of Medicine and Health Sciences, Washington, D.C.
48.2. Short-Term Psychotherapies for the Treatment of Child and Adolescent Disorders

Robert M. Hodapp, Ph.D. Professor of Education and Psychological Studies in Education, David Geffen School of Medicine at UCLA, Los Angeles, California.
34. Mental Retardation

Michael A. Hollifield, M.D. Associate Professor of Psychiatry and Family Medicine and Director of the Special Problems and Behavioral Medicine Clinic, University of New Mexico School of Medicine, Albuquerque, New Mexico.
15. Somatoform Disorders

Harry C. Holloway, M.D. Professor of Psychiatry, Uniformed Services University of the Health Sciences, Bethesda, Maryland.
28.9. Military and Disaster Psychiatry

Andrew Holt, Ph.D. Assistant Clinical Professor of Psychiatry, University of Alberta Faculty of Medicine and Dentistry, Edmonton, Alberta, Canada; Adjunct Professor of Pharmacology, University of Saskatchewan College of Medicine, Head of Drug Discovery, Alviva Biopharmaceuticals Inc., Saskatoon, Saskatchewan, Canada.
31.19. Monoamine Oxidase Inhibitors

Jeffrey Hsu, M.D. Assistant Professor of Psychiatry and Behavioral Sciences, The Johns Hopkins Hospital, Baltimore, Maryland.
2.8. Neuropsychiatric Aspects of HIV Infection and AIDS

James Hudziak, M.D. Assistant Professor of Psychiatry, Director of the Child Psychiatry Division and Behavioral Genetics, University of Vermont College of Medicine; Attending Psychiatrist, Fletcher Allen Healthcare, Burlington, Vermont.
31.12. Bupropion; 31.13. Buspirone

Leighton Y. Huey, M.D. Samuel Birnbaum/Ida, Louis and Richard Blum Professor of Psychiatry and Chairman, Department of Psychiatry, University of Connecticut School of Medicine, Farmington, Connecticut.
52.1. Public and Community Psychiatry; 52.2. Health Care Reform

John R. Hughes, M.D. Professor of Psychiatry, Psychology and Family Practice, University of Vermont; Attending Psychiatrist, Fletcher Allen Healthcare, Burlington, Vermont.
11.9. Nicotine-Related Disorders

Lorie A. Humphrey, Ph.D. Assistant Clinical Professor of Psychiatry and Behavioral Science, David Geffen School of Medicine at UCLA; Attending Psychiatrist, UCLA Neuropsychiatric Institute and Hospital, Los Angeles, California.
7.7. Neuropsychological and Cognitive Assessment of Children

Heidi E. Hutton, Ph.D. Assistant Professor of Psychiatry and Behavioral Sciences, Johns Hopkins University School of Medicine; Staff Clinical Psychologist, AIDS Psychiatry Service, Johns Hopkins Hospital, Baltimore, Maryland.
2.8. Neuropsychiatric Aspects of HIV Infection and AIDS

Celia F. Hybels, Ph.D. Assistant Research Professor of Psychiatry and Behavioral Sciences, Duke University School of Medicine, Durham, North Carolina.
51.1b. Epidemiology of Psychiatric Disorders

Steven E. Hyman, M.D. Provost, Harvard University and Professor of Neurobiology, Harvard Medical School, Boston, Massachusetts.
1.10. Genome, Transcriptome, and Proteome

Robert B. Innis, M.D., Ph.D. Professor of Psychiatry and Pharmacology, Director of Neurochemical Brain Imaging Program, Yale University School of Medicine, New Haven, Connecticut; Chief, Molecular Imaging Branch, National Institute of Mental Health, Bethesda, Maryland.
1.15. Nuclear Magnetic Resonance Imaging: Basic Principles and Recent Findings in Neuropsychiatric Disorders; 1.16. Radiotracer Imaging: Basic Principles and Exemplary Findings in Neuropsychiatric Disorders

Thomas R. Insel, M.D. Director, National Institute of Mental Health, National Institutes of Health, Bethesda, Maryland.
55.3. Future of Psychiatry

Michael Irwin, M.D. Norman Cousins Professor, Cousins Center for Psychoneuroimmunology, UCLA Neuropsychiatric Institute and Hospital, Los Angeles, California.
24.9. Stress and Psychiatry

Keith E. Isenberg, M.D. Professor of Psychiatry, Washington University School of Medicine; Director of Electroconvulsive Therapy (ECT) Service, Barnes-Jewish Hospital, Saint Louis, Missouri.
1.9. Basic Electrophysiology

Rolf G. Jacob, M.D. Professor of Psychiatry and Otolaryngology, University of Pittsburgh School of Medicine, Pittsburgh, Pennsylvania.
30.2. Behavior Therapy

Sandra A. Jacobson, M.D. Associate Professor of Psychiatry, Brown Medical School and Director of Consultation–Liaison Psychiatry, The Miriam Hospital, Providence, Rhode Island.
51.3f. Delirium

Jerome H. Jaffe, M.D. Clinical Professor of Psychiatry, University of Maryland School of Medicine, Baltimore, Maryland.
11.1. Substance-Related Disorders: Introduction and Overview; 11.3. Amphetamine (or Amphetamine-like)–Related Disorders; 11.6. Cocaine-Related Disorders; 11.10. Opioid-Related Disorders

Philip G. Janicak, M.D. Professor of Psychiatry, Medical Director of the Psychiatric Clinical Research Center, Associate Program Director of the General Clinical Research Center, University of Illinois at Chicago College of Medicine, Chicago, Illinois.
31.4. Medication-Induced Movement Disorders

Michael W. Jann, Pharm.D. Professor of Pharmacy Practice and Interim Chairman, Department of Pharmacy Practice, Mercer University Southern School of Pharmacy; Consultant, Peachford Hospital, Atlanta, Georgia.
31.15. Cholinesterase Inhibitors and Similarly Acting Compounds

Lissy F. Jarvik, M.D., Ph.D. Professor Emeritus of Psychiatry and Biobehavioral Sciences, David Geffen School of Medicine at UCLA; Distinguished Physician (Emeritus), UCLA Neuropsychiatric Institute and Hospital, Staff Care Center, Los Angeles, California.
51.1a. Geriatric Psychiatry: Introduction

Daniel Javitt, M.D., Ph.D. Professor of Psychiatry, New York University School of Medicine, New York, New York; Director of the Life Sciences Division, Nathan Kline Institute for Psychiatric Research; Consulting Psychiatrist, Rockland Psychiatric Center, Orangeburg, New York.
11.11. Phencyclidine (or Phencyclidine-like)–Related Disorders

James W. Jefferson, M.D. Clinical Professor of Psychiatry, University of Wisconsin Medical School; Distinguished Senior Scientist, Co-Director of Lithium Information Center, Madison Institute of Medicine, Madison, Wisconsin.
31.17. Lithium

James J. Jenson, M.D. Clinical Associate Professor of Psychiatry, Director of Training Division of Child and Adolescent Psychiatry, University of New Mexico School of Medicine, Albuquerque, New Mexico.
16. Factitious Disorders

Dilip V. Jeste, M.D. Professor of Psychiatry and Neurosciences, Estelle and Edgar Levi Chairman in Aging, Chief, Division of Geriatric Psychiatry, University of California, San Diego School of Medicine, La Jolla, California; Director of Geriatric Psychiatry Clinical Research Center, San Diego VA Healthcare System, San Diego, California.
51.3g. Schizophrenia and Delusional Disorders

Russell T. Joffe, M.D. Professor of Psychiatry and Dean, Department of Psychiatry, University of Medicine and Dentistry of New Jersey–New Jersey Medical School, Newark, New Jersey.
2.7. Neuropsychiatric Aspects of Multiple Sclerosis and Other Demyelinating Disorders; 31.27. Thyroid Hormones

Carla J. Johnson, Ph.D. Associate Professor of Speech-Language Pathology, University of Toronto Faculty of Medicine, Toronto, Ontario, Canada.
37.1. Expressive Language Disorder; 37.2. Mixed Receptive-Expressive Disorder; 37.3. Phonological Disorder

Reese T. Jones, M.D. Professor of Psychiatry, University of California at San Francisco School of Medicine, San Francisco, California.
11.7. Hallucinogen-Related Disorders

Ricardo E. Jorge, M.D. Assistant Professor of Psychiatry, Roy J. and Lucille A. Carver College of Medicine at University of Iowa, Attending Psychiatrist, University of Iowa Hospitals and Clinics, Iowa City, Iowa.
2.2. Neuropsychiatric Aspects of Cerebrovascular Disorders; 2.5. Neuropsychiatric Aspects of Traumatic Brain Injury

Allan M. Josephson, M.D. Professor of Psychiatry and Chief of Psychiatry and Health Behavior, Section of Child, Adolescent and Family Psychiatry, Medical College of Georgia; Chief of Child, Adolescent and Family Psychiatry, Children's Medical Center, and Director of Clinical Services for Psychiatry, Medical College of Georgia Hospital and Clinics, Augusta, Georgia.
48.5. Family Therapy

Nandita Joshi, M.B.B.S. Clinical Fellow, Consultation-Liaison Psychiatry, Department of Psychiatry and Behavioral Sciences, Memorial Sloan-Kettering Cancer Center, New York, New York.
28.4. End-of-Life and Palliative Care

Martha Bates Jura, Ph.D. Associate Clinical Professor of Psychiatry and Biobehavioral Sciences, David Geffen School of Medicine at UCLA; Director of the Psychology Assessment Laboratory, Child Outpatient Department, and Attending Psychologist, Division of Child and Adolescent Psychiatry, UCLA Neuropsychiatric Institute and Hospital, Los Angeles, California.
7.7. Neuropsychological and Cognitive Assessment of Children

John M. Kane, M.D. Professor of Psychiatry, Neurology, and Neuroscience, Albert Einstein College of Medicine at Yeshiva University, Bronx, New York; Chairman, Department of Psychiatry, The Zucker Hillside Hospital, Glen Oaks, New York; Vice President for Behavioral Health Services, North Shore-Long Island Jewish Health System, New Hyde Park, New York.
12.12. Schizophrenia: Somatic Treatment

***Harold I. Kaplan, M.D.** Professor of Psychiatry, New York University School of Medicine, New York, New York.
24.1. History of Psychosomatic Medicine

T. Byram Karasu, M.D. Silverman Professor and Chairman, Department of Psychiatry and Behavioral Sciences, Albert Einstein College of Medicine at Yeshiva University; Psychiatrist-in-Chief, Montefiore Medical Center, Bronx, New York.
30.1. Psychoanalysis and Psychoanalytic Psychotherapy

Niranjan Karnik, M.D., Ph.D. Resident Physician in Psychiatry, Stanford University Hospital and Clinics, Stanford, California.
49.6. Child or Adolescent Antisocial Behavior

Layla Kassem, Psy.D. Senior Research Fellow of the Mood and Anxiety Program, National Institute of Mental Health, National Institutes of Health, U.S. Department of Health and Human Services, Bethesda, Maryland.
14.6. Anxiety Disorders: Genetics

Ira R. Katz, M.D., Ph.D. Professor of Psychiatry, University of Pennsylvania School of Medicine; Director of the Veteran Healthcare Network 4 Mental Illness Research, Education, and Clinical Centers (MIRECC), Philadelphia Veteran Medical Center, Philadelphia, Pennsylvania.
51.6a. Psychiatric Aspects of Long-Term Care

Jeffrey William Katzman, M.D. Assistant Professor of Psychiatry, University of New Mexico School of Medicine; Chief of Psychiatry Service, New Mexico Veteran Healthcare System, Albuquerque, New Mexico.
22. Adjustment Disorders

David L. Kaye, M.D. Associate Professor of Clinical Psychiatry, University of Buffalo State University of New York School of Medicine and Biomedical Sciences; Director of Training in Child and Adolescent Psychiatry, Children's Hospital of Buffalo, Buffalo, New York.
48.1. Individual Psychodynamic Psychotherapy

*Deceased

Francis J. Keefe, Ph.D. Professor of Psychiatry and Behavioral Sciences, Duke University School of Medicine, Durham, North Carolina.
24.9. Stress and Psychiatry

Samuel J. Keith, M.D. Professor of Psychiatry and Psychology and Chairman, Department of Psychiatry, University of New Mexico School of Medicine, Albuquerque, New Mexico.
12.2. Schizophrenia: Scope of the Problem

Allen S. Keller, M.D. Assistant Professor of Clinical Medicine, New York University School of Medicine; Director of the NYU/Bellevue Medical Center Program for Survivors of Torture, Bellevue Medical Center, New York, New York.
28.7. Survivors of Torture

Jeffrey E. Kelsey, M.D., Ph.D. Assistant Professor of Psychiatry and Behavioral Sciences, Director of Mood and Anxiety Disorders Clinical Trials Program, Emory University School of Medicine, Atlanta, Georgia.
31.24. Selective Serotonin Reuptake Inhibitors

John R. Kelsoe, M.D. Professor of Psychiatry, University of California, San Diego School of Medicine; Attending Psychiatrist, San Diego VA Healthcare System, San Diego, California.
13.3. Mood Disorders: Genetics

Kenneth S. Kendler, M.D. Rachel Brown Banks Distinguished Professor of Psychiatry and Human Genetics, Department of Psychiatry; and Director of the Virginia Institute of Psychiatric and Behavioral Genetics, Virginia Commonwealth University Medical Center, Richmond, Virginia.
12.3. Schizophrenia: Genetics

Sidney H. Kennedy, M.D. Professor of Psychiatry, University of Toronto Faculty of Medicine; Psychiatrist-in-Chief, University Health Network, Toronto, Ontario, Canada.
31.19. Monoamine Oxidase Inhibitors

Kimbra Kenney, M.D. Research Medical Officer, Laboratory of Central Nervous System Studies, National Institute of Neurological Disorders and Stroke, National Institutes of Health, Bethesda, Maryland.
2.10. Neuropsychiatric Aspects of Prion Disease

Ronald C. Kessler, Ph.D. Professor of Sociology, Department of Health Care Policy, Harvard Medical School, Boston, Massachusetts.
4.2. Sociology and Psychiatry

Terence A. Ketter, M.D. Associate Professor of Psychiatry and Behavioral Sciences, Chief, Bipolar Disorders Clinic, Stanford University School of Medicine, Stanford, California.
31.8b. Gabapentin; 31.8c. Lamotrigine; 31.8d. Topiramate

Amir Khan, M.D. Assistant Professor of Psychiatry, Brown University Medical School, Providence, Rhode Island.
31.20. Nefazodone

Bryan H. King, M.D. Professor of Psychiatry and Pediatrics, Dartmouth Medical School, Hanover, New Hampshire; Director of Child and Adolescent Psychiatry, Medical Director of the New Hampshire Division of Developmental Sciences, Dartmouth-Hitchcock Medical Center, Lebanon, New Hampshire.
34. Mental Retardation

Deborah A. King, Ph.D. Associate Professor of Psychiatry (Psychology), University of Rochester School of Medicine and Dentistry; Director of Geriatric Psychiatry Services and Clinical Director of Psychology, Strong Memorial Hospital, Rochester, New York.
51.4j. Family Intervention and Therapy with Older Adults

Robert A. King, M.D. Professor of Child Psychiatry, Medical Director of Tourette/Obsessive-Compulsive Disorder Clinic, Yale Child Study Center, Yale University School of Medicine; Associate Director of Child Psychiatry Consultation-Liaison Service in Pediatric, Attending Physician, Yale-New Haven Hospital, New Haven, Connecticut.
33. Psychiatric Examination of the Infant, Child, and Adolescent

Thomas J. Kiresuk, Ph.D. Professor of Clinical Psychology, Department of Psychiatry, University of Minnesota Medical School; Senior Research Scientist, Minneapolis Medical Research Foundation, Minneapolis, Minnesota.
28.8. Alternative and Complementary Health Practices

Brian Kirkpatrick, M.D. Professor of Psychiatry, Maryland Psychiatric Research Center, University of Maryland School of Medicine, Baltimore, Maryland.
12.8. Schizophrenia: Clinical Features and Psychopathology Concepts

Laurel J. Kiser, Ph.D., M.B.A. Associate Professor of Psychiatry, Division of Services Research, University of Maryland Baltimore School of Medicine; Attending Psychologist, University of Maryland Medical System, Baltimore, Maryland.
48.7. Partial Hospital and Ambulatory Behavioral Health Services

Ami Klin, Ph.D. Harris Associate Professor of Child Psychology and Psychiatry, Chief of Psychology, Yale Child Study Center, Yale University School of Medicine, New Haven, Connecticut.
38. Pervasive Developmental Disorders

Alexander Kolevzon, M.D. Fellow in Education, Department of Psychiatry, Mount Sinai School of Medicine, New York, New York.
10.3. Dementia

Alex Kopelowicz, M.D. Assistant Professor of Psychiatry and Biobehavioral Sciences, David Geffen School of Medicine at UCLA, Los Angeles, California; Medical Director of San Fernando Mental Health Center, Mission Hills, California.
52.4. Psychiatric Rehabilitation

Susan G. Kornstein, M.D. Professor of Psychiatry and Obstetrics/Gynecology, Chairman, Division of Ambulatory Care Psychiatry, Executive Director of the Mood Disorders Institute, Executive Director of the Institute for Women's Health, Virginia Commonwealth University School of Medicine, Richmond, Virginia.
31.20. Nefazodone; 31.28. Trazodone

Suchitra Krishnan-Sarin, Ph.D. Assistant Professor of Psychiatry, Yale University School of Medicine, New Haven, Connecticut.
31.22. Opioid Receptor Antagonists: Naltrexone and Nalmefene

Robert Kroll, Ph.D. Assistant Professor of Speech-Language Pathology, Associate Member of Graduate Department of Speech-Language Pathology, University of Toronto; Assistant Professor of Psychiatry, University of Toronto Faculty of Medicine; Director of Stuttering Foundation of Ontario Stuttering Centre; Toronto, Ontario, Canada.
37.4. Stuttering

Akira Kugaya, M.D., Ph.D. Associate Research Scientist, Yale University School of Medicine, West Haven, Connecticut.
1.16. Radiotracer Imaging: Basic Principles and Exemplary Findings in Neuropsychiatric Disorders

Anand Kumar, M.D. Professor of Psychiatry and Behavioral Sciences, David Geffen School of Medicine at UCLA; Director of Geriatric Ambulatory Care Program, UCLA Neuropsychiatric Institute and Hospital, Los Angeles, California.
51.2f. Magnetic Resonance Imaging in Late-Life Mental Disorders

Helen H. Kyomen, M.D. Clinical Instructor, Harvard Medical School, Boston, Massachusetts; Assistant Psychiatrist, McLean Hospital, Belmont, Massachusetts.
51.5a. Financial Issues in the Delivery of Geriatric Psychiatric Care

Brian Ladds, M.D. Associate Professor of Clinical Psychiatry and Associate Chairman, Education and Training, New York Medical College, Valhalla, New York.
54.2. Ethics in Psychiatry

Eugene M. Laska, Ph.D. Professor of Psychiatry, New York University Medical School of Medicine, New York, New York; Director of Statistical Sciences Section, Nathan Kline Institute for Psychiatric Research, Orangeburg, New York.
5.2. Statistics and Experimental Design

John Lauriello, M.D. Associate Professor of Psychiatry and Vice-Chairman, Department of Psychiatry, University of New Mexico School of Medicine, Albuquerque, New Mexico.
12.2. Schizophrenia: Scope of the Problem

Helen Lavretsky, M.D. Associate Professor of Psychiatry, David Geffen School of Medicine at UCLA, Los Angeles, California.
51.4d. Psychopharmacology: Antipsychotic Drugs

Ann E. Layne, Ph.D. Assistant Professor of Child and Adolescent Psychiatry, University of Minnesota Medical School; Associate Psychologist, Fairview-University Medical Center, Minneapolis, Minnesota.
46.3. Separation Anxiety Disorder and Other Anxiety Disorders

Lawrence W. Lazarus, M.D. Staff Psychiatrist, Las Vegas Medical Center, Las Vegas, New Mexico; Past President, American Association for Geriatric Psychiatry, Santa Fe, New Mexico.
51.4h. Individual Psychotherapy

Jay L. Lebow, Ph.D. Clinical Associate Professor of Psychology, Northwestern University; Senior Therapist and Research Consultant, President, Division of Family Psychology APA, the Family Institute at Northwestern University, Chicago, Illinois.
30.5. Family Therapy and Couple Therapy

Barry D. Lebowitz, Ph.D. Chief of Adult and Geriatric Treatment and Preventive Intervention, National Institute of Mental Health, National Institutes of Health, Rockville, Maryland; Adjunct Faculty, Department of Psychiatry, Georgetown University School of Medicine and Health Sciences, Washington, D.C.
51.5d. Community Services for the Elderly Psychiatric Patient

James F. Leckman, M.D. Neison Harris Professor of Child Psychiatry, Pediatrics and Psychology, Program Director of National Institute of Mental Health Research Training Program in Childhood Neuropsychiatric Disorders, Director of Research, Yale Child Study Center, and Associate Program Director of the General Clinical Research Center, Yale University School of Medicine; Attending Physician, Yale-New Haven Hospital; New Haven, Connecticut.
42. Tic Disorders

Marguerite S. Lederberg, M.D. Clinical Professor of Psychiatry, The Joan and Sanford I. Weill Medical College of Cornell University; Attending Psychiatrist, Memorial Sloan-Kettering Cancer Center, New York, New York.
24.10. Psycho-Oncology; 28.4. End-of-Life and Palliative Care

Francis S. Lee, M.D., Ph.D. Assistant Professor of Psychiatry and Pharmacology, Joan and Sanford I. Weill Medical College of Cornell University; Assistant Attending Psychiatrist, New York Presbyterian Hospital, New York, New York.
1.7. Neurotrophic Factors

Anthony F. Lehman, M.D., M.S.P.H. Professor of Psychiatry and Chairman, Department of Psychiatry, University of Maryland School of Medicine; Chief of Psychiatry, University of Maryland Medical Center, Baltimore, Maryland.
12.11. Schizophrenia: Psychosocial Treatment

Ira M. Lesser, M.D. Professor of Psychiatry and Biobehavioral Sciences, David Geffen School of Medicine at UCLA, Los Angeles, California; Vice-Chairman, Department of Psychiatry and Director or Residency and Training, Harbor-UCLA Medical Center, Torrance, California.
51.3c. Anxiety Disorders

Molyn Leszcz, M.D., F.R.C.P.(C) Associate Professor of Psychiatry, Head of Group Psychotherapy Program, University of Toronto Faculty of Medicine, Toronto, Ontario, Canada.
51.4k. Group Therapy

David A. Lewis, M.D. Professor of Psychiatry and Neuroscience, Director of the Center for Neuroscience of Mental Disorders, University of Pittsburgh School of Medicine, Pittsburgh, Pennsylvania.
1.2. Functional Neuroanatomy

Dorothy Otnow Lewis, M.D. Clinical Professor of Psychiatry, Yale University Child Study Center, Yale University School of Medicine; Associate Attending Physician, Yale-New Haven Hospital, New Haven, Connecticut; Attending Physician, NYU/Bellevue Medical Center, New York, New York.
26.2. Adult Antisocial Behavior, Criminality, and Violence

Robert Paul Liberman, M.D. Director of UCLA Psychiatric Rehabilitation Program, UCLA Neuropsychiatric Institute and Hospital, Los Angeles, California.
52.4. Psychiatric Rehabilitation

Walter Ling, M.D. Professor of Psychiatry, Director of Integrated Substance Abuse Programs, Department of Psychiatry and Biobehavioral Sciences, David Geffen School of Medicine at UCLA, Los Angeles, California.
11.3. Amphetamine (or Amphetamine-like)–Related Disorders; 11.6. Cocaine-Related Disorders

Mark S. Lipian, M.D., Ph.D. Assistant Clinical Professor of Psychiatry and Biobehavioral Sciences, David Geffen School of Medicine at UCLA, Los Angeles, California; Assistant Clinical Professor of Psychiatry and Human Behavior, University of California, Irvine College of Medicine, Irvine, California; Medical Director of Conditional Release Program of Orange County, Santa Ana, California.
26.1. Malingering

Judith Eve Lipton, M.D. Clinical Instructor, University of Washington School of Medicine; and Consulting Psychiatrist, Comprehensive Breast Center, Providence Campus, Swedish Medical Center, Seattle, Washington; Faculty, Medical Knowledge Institute, the Netherlands.
4.3. Sociobiology

Benjamin Liptzin, M.D. Professor of Psychiatry and Deputy Chairman, Department of Psychiatry, Tufts University School of Medicine, Boston, Massachusetts; Chairman, Department of Psychiatry, Baystate Medical Center, Springfield, Massachusetts.
51.3f. Delirium

Rodolfo R. Llinás, M.D., Ph.D. Professor of Physiology and Neuroscience and Chairman, Department of Physiology and Neuroscience, Thomas and Suzanne Murphy Professor of Neuroscience, New York University School of Medicine, New York, New York.
3.6. Neuroscientific Bases of Consciousness and Dreaming

Richard J. Loewenstein, M.D. Associate Clinical Professor of Psychiatry and Behavioral Sciences, University of Maryland School of Medicine; Medical Director of the Trauma Disorders Program, Sheppard Pratt Health System, Baltimore, Maryland.
17. Dissociative Disorders

Martha James Love, M.D., J.D. Assistant Clinical Professor of Psychiatry, David Geffen School of Medicine at UCLA; Attending Psychiatrist, UCLA Neuropsychiatric Institute and Hospital, Los Angeles, California.
7.8. Medical Assessment and Laboratory Testing in Psychiatry

Roy H. Lubit, M.D., Ph.D. Assistant Professor of Psychiatry, Mount Sinai School of Medicine, New York, New York.
54.2. Ethics in Psychiatry

Joan L. Luby, M.D. Associate Professor of Psychiatry (Child), Director of Early Emotional Development Program, Washington University School of Medicine, Saint Louis, Missouri.
44.3. Disorders of Infancy and Early Childhood Not Otherwise Specified

Robert J. Lueger, Ph.D. Associate Professor of Psychology and Associate Dean of Academic Affairs, College of Arts and Sciences, Marquette University, Milwaukee, Wisconsin.
30.11. Evaluation of Psychotherapy

Tanya Marie Luhrmann, Ph.D. Max Palersky Chair, Committee on Human Development, The University of Chicago, Chicago, Illinois.
53.3. An Anthropological View of Psychiatry

Constantine G. Lyketsos, M.D., M.H.S. Professor of Psychiatry and Behavioral Sciences, Co-Director of the Division of Geriatric Psychiatry and Neuropsychiatry, Johns Hopkins University School of Medicine, Baltimore, Maryland.
2.8. Neuropsychiatric Aspects of HIV Infection and AIDS

Thomas R. Lynch, Ph.D. Assistant Professor of Psychiatry and Behavioral Sciences and Psychology: Social and Health Sciences, Duke University School of Medicine; Attending Physician, Duke University Medical Center, Durham, North Carolina.
30.8. Dialectical Behavior Therapy

Myrl Manley, M.D. Associate Professor of Psychiatry and Director of Medical Student Education in Psychiatry, New York University School of Medicine, New York, New York.
7.2. Interviewing Techniques with the Difficult Patient

Stephen R. Marder, M.D. Professor of Psychiatry and Biobehavioral Sciences, Department of Psychiatry and Biobehavioral Sciences, David Geffen School of Medicine at UCLA; Director of Section of Psychosis, UCLA Neuropsychiatric Institute and Hospital; Director of Veterans Desert Pacific Mental Health Research, Education and Clinical Center (MIRECC), Los Angeles, California.
12.12. Schizophrenia: Somatic Treatment; 31.16. Dopamine Receptor Antagonists (Typical Antipsychotics); 31.25. Serotonin-Dopamine Antagonists (Atypical or Second-Generation Antipsychotics)

Russell L. Margolis, M.D. Associate Professor of Psychiatry and Neurology, Johns Hopkins University School of Medicine; Attending Physician, Johns Hopkins Hospital, Baltimore, Maryland.
2.6. Neuropsychiatric Aspects of Movement Disorders

Deborah B. Marin, M.D. Blumenthal Professor of Psychiatry, Vice-Chairman for Education, Mount Sinai School of Medicine, New York, New York.
10.3. Dementia

John C. Markowitz, M.D. Associate Professor of Psychiatry, The Joan and Sanford I. Weill Medical College of Cornell University; Research Psychiatrist, New York State Psychiatric Institute; Associate Attending Physician, New York-Presbyterian Hospital, New York, New York.
13.5. Mood Disorders: Intrapsychic and Interpersonal Aspects

Laura Marsh, M.D. Associate Professor of Psychiatry and Neurology, Johns Hopkins University School of Medicine; Director of the Clinical Research Program, Johns Hopkins Morris K. Udall Parkinson's Disease Research Center of Excellence; Attending Physician, Geriatric Psychiatry and Neuropsychiatric Services, Johns Hopkins Hospital, Baltimore, Maryland.
2.6. Neuropsychiatric Aspects of Movement Disorders

Carol A. Mathews, M.D. Assistant Professor of Psychiatry, University of California, San Diego School of Medicine, San Diego, California.
1.18. Genetic Linkage Analysis of the Psychiatric Disorders

Jon M. McClellan, M.D. Assistant Professor of Psychiatry and Behavioral Sciences, University of Washington School of Medicine, Seattle, Washington; Medical Director of the Child Study and Treatment Center, Lakewood, Washington.
47. Early-Onset Schizophrenia

Erin B. McClure, Ph.D. Postdoctoral Fellow, Section on Development and Affective Neuroscience, Mood and Anxiety Disorders Program, National Institute of Mental Health, National Institutes of Health, Bethesda, Maryland.
14.8. Anxiety Disorders: Clinical Features

Cynthia G. McCormick, M.D. Director of the Division of Anesthetic, Critical Care, Addiction Drug Products, Center for Drug Evaluation and Research (CDER), United States Food and Drug Administration, Rockville, Maryland.
31.3. Drug Development and Approval Process in the United States

James T. McCracken, M.D. Joseph Campbell Professor of Child Psychiatry, David Geffen School of Medicine at UCLA, Director of the Division of Child and Adolescent Psychiatry, Department of Psychiatry and Biobehavioral Sciences, UCLA Neuropsychiatric Institute and Hospital, Los Angeles, California.
46.1. Obsessive-Compulsive Disorder in Children

Robert R. McCrae, Ph.D. Research Psychologist, Personality, Stress, and Coping Section, National Institute on Aging, National Institutes of Health, Baltimore, Maryland.
6.4. Approaches Derived from Philosophy and Psychology

Jocelyn Shealy McGee, Ph.D. Postdoctoral Fellow, Clinical Neuropsychiatry, The Institute for Rehabilitation and Research, Baylor College of Medicine, Houston, Texas.
51.4i. Cognitive-Behavioral Therapy

Thomas H. McGlashan, M.D. Professor of Psychiatry, Yale University School of Medicine; Attending Psychiatrist, Yale-New Haven Psychiatric Hospital, New Haven, Connecticut.
12.17. Schizophrenia and Other Psychotic Disorders: Special Issues in Early Detection and Intervention

James J. McGough, M.D. Associate Professor of Clinical Psychiatry, David Geffen School of Medicine at UCLA; Attending Physician, UCLA Neuropsychiatric Institute and Hospital, Los Angeles, California.
39.2. Adult Manifestations of Attention-Deficit/Hyperactivity Disorder

Francis J. McMahon, M.D. Visiting Associate Professor of Psychiatry, The Johns Hopkins University School of Medicine, Baltimore, Maryland; Chief, Genetics Basis of Mood and Anxiety Program, National Institute of Mental Health, National Institutes of Health, U.S. Department of Health and Human Services, Bethesda, Maryland.
14.6. Anxiety Disorders: Genetics

John R. McQuaid, Ph.D. Assistant Professor of Psychiatry, University of California, San Diego; Director of Cognitive and Behavioral Interventions Program, San Diego VA Healthcare System, San Diego, California.
13.9. Mood Disorders: Psychotherapy

Aimee L. McRae, Pharm.D. Assistant Professor of Psychiatry and Behavioral Sciences, Medical University of South Carolina College of Medicine, Charleston, South Carolina.
31.21. Opioid Receptor Agonists: Methadone, Levomethadyl, and Buprenorphine

Morris Meisner, Ph.D. Research Associate Professor of Psychiatry, New York University School of Medicine, New York, New York.
5.2. Statistics and Experimental Design

W. W. Meissner, M.D., S.J. University Professor of Psychoanalysis, Boston College, Chestnut Hill, Massachusetts; Training and Supervising Analyst Emeritus, Boston Psychoanalytic Society and Institute, Boston, Massachusetts.
6.1. Classic Psychoanalysis

Claude Ann Mellins, Ph.D. Associate Professor of Clinical Psychology, Departments of Psychiatry and Sociomedical Sciences, Columbia University; Research Scientist, HIV Center for Clinical and Behavioral Studies, New York State Psychiatric Institute; Co-Director of Special Needs Clinic, Pediatric Psychiatry, Columbia-Presbyterian Medical Center, New York, New York.
49.5. Psychiatric Sequelae of HIV and AIDS

Wallace Mendelson, M.D. Professor of Psychiatry and Clinical Pharmacology, University of Chicago Pritzker School of Medicine, Chicago, Illinois.
20. Sleep Disorders

Mario F. Mendez Ashla, M.D., Ph.D. Professor of Neurobiology, Psychiatry and Biobehavioral Sciences, David Geffen School of Medicine at UCLA; Director of Neurobehavior Unit, Attending Physician, VA Greater Los Angeles Healthcare Center; Attending Physician, UCLA Medical Center, Los Angeles, California.
2.4. Neuropsychiatric Aspects of Epilepsy

Steven J. Mennerick, Ph.D. Assistant Professor of Neurobiology in Psychiatry, Washington University School of Medicine, Saint Louis, Missouri.
1.9. Basic Electrophysiology

W. Walter Menninger, M.D. Adjunct Professor of Psychiatry, Baylor College of Medicine; Clinical Professor of Psychiatry, University of Kansas School of Medicine; Former Dean, Karl Menninger School of Psychiatry and Mental Health Sciences; Chief of Staff Emeritus, Menninger Clinic and Hospital, Active Staff, Menninger Memorial Hospital, Kansas City, Kansas.
52.3. Role of the Psychiatric Hospital in the Treatment of Mental Illness

James R. Merikangas, M.D. Clinical Professor of Psychiatry and Behavioral Science, George Washington University School of Medicine and Health Sciences; Director of Neuropsychiatry Program, Georgetown University Hospital; Attending Physician, George Washington University Hospital, Washington, D.C.
2.11. Neuropsychiatric Aspects of Headache

Kathleen Ries Merikangas, Ph.D. Senior Investigator and Chief, Section on Developmental Genetic Epidemiology, Mood and Anxiety Program, National Institute of Mental Health, National Institutes of Health, Bethesda, Maryland.
2.11. Neuropsychiatric Aspects of Headache; 14.2. Anxiety Disorders: Epidemiology

Jeffrey David Meyerhoff, M.D. Adjunct Assistant Professor, Oregon Health Sciences University School of Medicine; Medical Director, PacifiCare Behavioral Health; Medical Director of Inpatient and Geriatric Psychiatry, Legacy Good Samaritan Hospital, Portland, Oregon.
51.5b. Managed Care

Juan E. Mezzich, M.D., Ph.D. Professor of Psychiatry, Mount Sinai School of Medicine; Director of Division of Psychiatric Epidemiology and International Center for Mental Health, Mount Sinai Medical Center, New York, New York.
5.1. Epidemiology; 9.2. International Psychiatric Diagnosis

Edwin J. Mikkelsen, M.D. Associate Professor of Psychiatry, Harvard Medical School; Medical Director of the Mentor Network, Boston, Massachusetts.
43. Elimination Disorders

Andrew H. Miller, M.D. Professor of Psychiatry and Behavioral Sciences, Emory University School of Medicine; Attending Physician, Emory Healthcare System and Grady Healthcare System, Atlanta, Georgia.
1.12. Immune System and Central Nervous System Interactions

Mark J. Mills, J.D., M.D. Clinical Professor of Psychiatry, Georgetown University School of Medicine, Washington, D.C.
26.1. Malingering

Barbara Milrod, M.D. Associate Professor of Psychiatry, Joan and Sanford I. Weill Medical College of Cornell University; Attending Psychiatrist, New York-Presbyterian Hospital, New York, New York.
13.5. Mood Disorders: Intrapsychic and Interpersonal Aspects

Klaus Minde, M.D., F.R.C.P.(C) Professor of Psychiatry and Pediatrics, McGill University Faculty of Medicine; Director of Department of Psychiatry, Montreal Children's Hospital, Montreal, Quebec, Canada.
49.1. Psychiatric Aspects of Day Care

Jacobo E. Mintzer, M.D. Professor of Psychiatry and Neurology, Director of Geriatric Psychiatry and Fellowship Programs, Director of Geriatric Psychiatry, Medical University of South Carolina College of Medicine, Charleston, South Carolina.
51.6d. Minority and Sociocultural Issues

Mary S. Mittelman, Dr.P.H. Research Associate Professor of Psychiatry, New York University School of Medicine; Director of Caregiving Research, NYU Silberstein Aging and Dementia Research Center, New York, New York.
51.6h. Counseling and Support Needs of Dementia Caregivers

Paul C. Mohl, M.D. Professor and Vice-Chairman of Education, Director of Residency Training, Department of Psychiatry, University of Texas Southwestern Medical Center at Dallas Southwestern Medical School, Dallas, Texas.
6.3. Other Psychodynamic Schools

Ramin Mojtabai, M.D., Ph.D., M.P.H. Assistant Professor of Clinical Psychiatry, Columbia University College of Physicians and Surgeons; Research Scientist, New York State Psychiatric Institute, New York, New York.
12.16a. Acute and Transient Psychotic Disorders and Brief Psychotic Disorder; 12.16f. Culture-Bound Syndromes with Psychotic Features

Steven O. Moldin, Ph.D. Director of the Office of Human Genetics and Genomic Resources and Associate Director of the Division of Neuroscience and Basic Behavioral Science, National Institute of Mental Health, National Institutes of Health, Department of Health and Human Services, Bethesda, Maryland.
1.10. Genome, Transcriptome, and Proteome; 1.17. Population Genetics and Genetic Epidemiology

Michael G. Moran, M.D. Clinical Associate Professor of Psychiatry, University of Colorado School of Medicine; Training and Supervising Analyst, Denver Institute for Psychoanalysis, Denver, Colorado.
24.5. Respiratory Disorders

James Morrison, M.D. Clinical Professor of Psychiatry, Oregon Health & Science University School of Medicine, Portland, Oregon.
53.2. Examining Psychiatrists and Other Professionals

David Mrazek, M.D. Professor of Psychiatry, Psychology and Pediatrics, Mayo Medical School; Chairman, Department of Psychiatry and Psychology, Mayo Clinic, Rochester, Minnesota.
49.13. Prevention of Psychiatric Disorders in Children and Adolescents

Patricia J. Mrazek, M.S.W., Ph.D. Mental Health Policy Consultant, Rochester, Minnesota.
49.13. Prevention of Psychiatric Disorders in Children and Adolescents

Rodrigo A. Muñoz, M.D. Clinical Professor of Psychiatry, University of California, San Diego School of Medicine; Director of Output Services, Scripps Mercy Hospital, San Diego, California.
53.2. Examining Psychiatrists and Other Professionals

Robin M. Murray, M.D., D.Sc., F.R.C.P. Professor of Psychiatry, Institute of Psychiatry, King's College; Consultant Psychiatrist, Maudsley Hospital, De Crespigny Park, London, United Kingdom.
12.5. The Developmental Model of Schizophrenia

Deepa N. Nadiga, M.D. Assistant Professor of Psychiatry, University of New Mexico School of Medicine; Attending Physician, Mental Health Center, Albuquerque, New Mexico.
16. Factitious Disorders

Bushra Naz, M.D. Research Scientist, Suffolk County Mental Health Project, Stony Brook University Health Service Center School of Medicine, Stony Brook, New York.
12.16b. Schizophreniform Disorder; 12.16e. Postpartum Psychosis

J. Craig Nelson, M.D. Professor of Psychiatry, Leon J. Epstein, M.D. Chairman, Department of Geriatric Psychiatry, Director of the Geriatric Psychiatry, University of California at San Francisco School of Medicine, San Francisco, California.
31.29. Tricyclics and Tetracyclics

Charles B. Nemeroff, M.D., Ph.D. Reunette W. Harris Professor of Psychiatry and Behavioral Sciences and Chairman, Department of Psychiatry and Behavioral Sciences, Emory University School of Medicine; Chief, Department of Psychiatry and Behavioral Sciences, Emory University Hospital System, Atlanta, Georgia.
1.6. Neuropeptides: Biology, Regulation, and Role in Neuropsychiatric Disorders; 31.5. α_2-Adrenergic Receptor Agonists: Clonidine and Guanfacine; 31.6. β-Adrenergic Receptor Antagonists; 31.7. Anticholinergics and Amantadine; 31.9. Antihistamines; 31.10. Barbiturates and Similarly Acting Substances

John Case Nemiah, M.D. Professor of Psychiatry, Dartmouth Medical School, Hanover, New Hampshire; Clinical Staff, Mary Hitchcock Memorial Hospital, Lebanon, New Hampshire; Professor of Psychiatry Emeritus, Harvard Medical School, Boston, Massachusetts.
14.7. Anxiety Disorders: Psychodynamic Aspects

Judith A. Neugroschl, M.D. Assistant Professor of Psychiatry, Director of Medical Student Education in Psychiatry, Associate Director Geriatric Psychiatry Fellowship, Mount Sinai School of Medicine; Director of Geriatric Psychiatry Outpatient Clinic, Mount Sinai Hospital, New York, New York.
10.2. Delirium; 10.3. Dementia

Alexander Neumeister, M.D. Professor of Psychiatry, University of Vienna School of Medicine, Vienna, Austria; Attending Physician, Mood and Anxiety Disorders Program, National Institute of Mental Health, Bethesda, Maryland.
14.4. Anxiety Disorders: Neurochemical Aspects

Cory F. Newman, Ph.D. Associate Professor of Psychology, Department of Psychiatry, Director of the Center for Cognitive Therapy, University of Pennsylvania School of Medicine, Philadelphia, Pennsylvania.
30.6. Cognitive Therapy

Dorian S. Newton, Ph.D. Director of the Mills College Counseling and Psychological Services, Oakland, California; Affiliate Member, San Francisco Psychoanalytic Institute, San Francisco, California.
6.2. Erik H. Erikson

Cynthia T. M. H. Nguyen, M.D. Adjunct Clinical Assistant Professor of Psychiatry and Behavioral Sciences, Stanford University School of Medicine, Stanford, California.
51.4c. Psychopharmacology: Antianxiety Drugs

Steven L. Nickman, M.D. Clinical Associate Professor of Psychiatry, Harvard Medical School; Assistant in Psychiatry, Director of Adoption and Custody Unit, Child Psychiatry Clinic, Massachusetts General Hospital, Boston, Massachusetts.
49.2. Adoption and Foster Care

Frank John Ninivaggi, M.D. Assistant Clinical Professor, Yale Child Study Center, Yale University School of Medicine; Associate Attending Physician, Yale-New Haven Hospital, New Haven, Connecticut; Attending Physician in Child Psychiatry, Saint Francis Hospital, Hartford, Connecticut; Director of Psychiatric Services, Devereux Glenholme School, Washington, Connecticut.
26.3. Borderline Intellectual Functioning and Academic Problem

Barry Nurcombe, M.D., F.R.A.C.P. Emeritus Professor of Child and Adolescent Psychiatry, Vanderbilt University, The University of Queensland, Queensland, Australia.
49.7. Dissociative Disorders in Children and Adolescents

M. Kevin O'Connor, M.D. Assistant Professor of Psychiatry, Mayo Medical School, Rochester, Minnesota.
24.8. Musculoskeletal Disorders

Mark Olfson, M.D., M.P.H. Professor of Clinical Psychiatry, Columbia University College of Physicians and Surgeons, New York, New York.
5.3. Mental Health Services

Jason T. Olin, Ph.D. Associate Director, CNS, Clinical Development & Medical Affairs, Forest Research Institute, Jersey City, New Jersey.
51.5d. Community Services for the Elderly Psychiatric Patient

Stephanie S. O'Malley, Ph.D. Professor of Psychiatry and Director of the Division of Substance Abuse Research, Yale University School of Medicine, New Haven, Connecticut.
31.22. Opioid Receptor Antagonists: Naltrexone and Nalmefene

Ekkehard Othmer, M.D., Ph.D. Adjunct Professor of Psychiatry, University of Kansas Medical Center, Kansas City, Kansas; Medical Director of the Othmer Psychiatric Center, Kansas City, Missouri.
7.1. Psychiatric Interview, History, and Mental Status Examination

Johann Philipp Othmer, M.D. Assistant Professor of Psychiatry, University of Pittsburgh Medical Center, Western Psychiatric Institute and Clinic, Pittsburgh, Pennsylvania.
7.1. Psychiatric Interview, History, and Mental Status Examination

Sieglinde C. Othmer, Ph.D. Psychologist, Othmer Psychiatric Center, Kansas City, Missouri.
7.1. Psychiatric Interview, History, and Mental Status Examination

Fred Ovsiew, M.D. Professor of Psychiatry, University of Chicago Division of Biological Sciences Pritzker School of Medicine; Chief, Clinical Neuropsychiatry, and Medical Director of the Adult Inpatient Psychiatry, University of Chicago Hospitals, Chicago, Illinois.
2.1. Neuropsychiatric Approach to the Patient

Michael J. Owens, Ph.D. Associate Professor of Psychiatry and Behavioral Sciences and Associate Director of the Laboratory of Neuropsychopharmacology, Emory University School of Medicine, Atlanta, Georgia.
1.6. Neuropeptides: Biology, Regulation, and Role in Neuropsychiatric Disorders

Ken A. Paller, Ph.D. Professor of Psychology, Director of the Cognitive Neuroscience Program, Weinberg College of Arts and Sciences, Northwestern University, Evanston, Illinois; Fellow of the Cognitive Neurology and Alzheimer's Disease Center, Feinberg Medical School, Northwestern University Medical School, Chicago, Illinois.
3.4. Biology of Memory

Barbara L. Parry, M.D. Professor of Psychiatry, Director of Research, Women's Mood Disorders Clinic, and Associate Director of the Medical Student Clerkship, University of California, San Diego School of Medicine, La Jolla, California.
28.1. Psychiatry and Reproductive Medicine; 28.2. Premenstrual Dysphoric Disorder

Caroly S. Pataki, M.D. Clinical Professor of Psychiatry and Biobehavioral Science, Associate Director of Training and Education for Child and Adolescent Psychiatry, David Geffen School of Medicine at UCLA; Attending Psychiatrist, UCLA Neuropsychiatric Institute and Hospital, Los Angeles, California.
32.1. Introduction and Overview; 32.3. Normal Adolescence; 36. Motor Skills Disorder: Developmental Coordination Disorder

Bradley Dixon Pearce, Ph.D. Assistant Professor of Psychiatry and Behavioral Sciences, Emory University School of Medicine, Atlanta, Georgia.
1.12. Immune System and Central Nervous System Interactions

William E. Pelham, Ph.D. Professor of Psychology and Director of Clinical Training, University of Buffalo State University of New York, Buffalo, New York.
30.2. Behavior Therapy

Ethel Spector Person, M.D. Professor of Clinical Psychiatry, Columbia University College of Physicians and Surgeons; Training and Supervising Analyst, Columbia University Center for Psychoanalytic Training and Research; Attending Psychiatrist, New York Presbyterian Hospital, New York, New York.
18.2. Paraphilias

Eric D. Peselow, M.D. Research Professor of Psychiatry, New York University School of Medicine; Attending Psychiatrist, New York Veterans Affairs Medical Center and Bellevue Hospital Center, New York, New York.
31.32. Other Pharmacological and Biological Therapies

Bradley S. Peterson, M.D. Suzanne Crosby Murphy Associate Professor in Pediatric Neuropsychiatry and Director of Magnetic Resonance Imaging (MRI) Research, Department of Psychiatry, Columbia University College of Physicians and Surgeons; Attending Psychiatrist, New York Presbyterian Hospital, New York, New York.
33. Psychiatric Examination of the Infant, Child, and Adolescent

Betty J. Pfefferbaum, M.D., J.D. Paul and Ruth Jonas Chair, Professor and Chairman, Department of Psychiatry and Behavioral Sciences, University of Oklahoma College of Medicine; Director, Terrorism and Disaster Branch, National Center for Child Traumatic Stress; Attending Physician, OU Medical Center, Oklahoma City, Oklahoma.
49.16. Impact of Terrorism on Children

Suzanne Phelan, Ph.D. Assistant Professor of Psychiatry, Brown Medical School; Staff Psychologist, The Miriam Hospital, Providence, Rhode Island.
24.3. Obesity

Kemuel L. Philbrick, M.D. Assistant Professor of Psychiatry, Mayo Medical School, Rochester, Minnesota.
24.8. Musculoskeletal Disorders

John Piacentini, Ph.D. Associate Professor-in-Residence, Department of Psychiatry and Biobehavioral Science, David Geffen School of Medicine at UCLA; Director of the Child Obsessive Compulsive Disorder (OCD), Anxiety, and Tic Disorders Program, UCLA Neuropsychiatric Institute and Hospital, Los Angeles, California.
46.4. Selective Mutism

Joseph N. Pierri, M.S., M.D. Assistant Professor of Psychiatry, University of Pittsburgh School of Medicine, Pittsburgh, Pennsylvania.
1.2. Functional Neuroanatomy

Daniel S. Pine, M.D. Chief, Section on Development and Affective Neuroscience, Mood and Anxiety Disorders Program, National Institute of Mental Health–Intramural Program, National Institutes of Health, Bethesda, Maryland.
14.8. Anxiety Disorders: Clinical Features

Carlos R. Plata-Salaman, M.D, D.Sc. Executive Director of Scientific Licensing, Pharmaceuticals Group Business Development, Johnson and Johnson Pharmaceutical Research and Development, L.L.C., Spring House, Pennsylvania.
1.5. Amino Acids As Neurotransmitters

Bruce G. Pollock, M.D., Ph.D. Professor of Psychiatry, Pharmacology, and Pharmaceutical Sciences; Chief, Academic Division of Geriatric and Neuropsychiatry and Director of the Clinical Therapeutics Research Program, University of Pittsburgh Medical Center, Pittsburgh, Pennsylvania.
51.4a. Psychopharmacology: General Principles

Harrison G. Pope, Jr., M.D. Professor of Psychiatry, Harvard Medical School, Boston, Massachusetts; Director of the Biological Psychiatry Laboratory, McLean Hospital, Belmont, Massachusetts.
11.13. Anabolic-Androgenic Steroid Abuse

Robert M. Post, M.D. Chief, Biological Psychiatry Branch, Department of Health and Human Services, National Institute of Mental Health, National Institutes of Health, Bethesda, Maryland.
13.8. Mood Disorders: Treatment of Bipolar Disorders; 31.8a. Carbamazepine; 31.8e. Valproate

Karl H. Pribram, M.D., Ph.D. Distinguished Research Professor, Georgetown University School of Medicine, Washington, D.C.; Distinguished Research Professor, George Mason University, Fairfax, Virginia.
3.5. Brain Models of Mind

Trevor R. P. Price, M.D. Professor of Psychiatry and Medicine and Chairman, Department of Psychiatry, University of Pennsylvania School of Medicine; Medical Staff, Hahnemann University Hospital and Medical College of Pennsylvania Hospital, Philadelphia, Pennsylvania.
2.3. Neuropsychiatric Aspects of Brain Tumors

Patricia N. Prinz, Ph.D. Research Professor, Department of Biobehavioral Nursing and Adjunct Professor, Department of Psychiatry and Behavioral Sciences, University of Washington School of Medicine, Seattle, Washington.
51.3b. Sleep Disorders

Ignacio Provencio, Ph.D. Assistant Professor of Anatomy, Physiology and Genetics, Uniformed Services University of the Health Sciences, Bethesda, Maryland.
1.13. Chronobiology

Joan Prudic, M.D. Associate Clinical Professor of Psychiatry, Columbia University College of Physicians and Surgeons, New York, New York.
31.30. Electroconvulsive Therapy

David B. Pruitt, M.D. Professor and Director of the Division of Child and Adolescent Psychiatry, Department of Psychiatry, University of Maryland School of Medicine; Attending Psychiatrist, University of Maryland Medical System, Baltimore, Maryland.
48.7. Partial Hospital and Ambulatory Behavioral Health Services

Andres J. Pumariega, M.D. Professor and Director, Department of Child and Adolescent Psychiatry, James H. Quillen College of Medicine, East Tennessee State University, Johnson City, Tennessee.
48.9. Community-Based Treatment

Frank W. Putnam, M.D. Professor of Pediatrics and Professor of Psychiatry, University of Cincinnati School of Medicine; Director, Center for Safe and Healthy Children, Cincinnati Children's Hospital Medical Center, Cincinnati, Ohio.
17. Dissociative Disorders

Jared S. Putnam, M.D. Attending Psychiatrist, Potomac Ridge Behavioral Health System, Rockville, Maryland.
31.5. α_2*-Adrenergic Receptor Agonists: Clonidine and Guanfacine; 31.6.* β*-Adrenergic Receptor Antagonists; 31.7. Anticholinergics and Amantadine; 31.9. Antihistamines; 31.10. Barbiturates and Similarly Acting Substances*

Robert S. Pynoos, M.D., M.P.H. Professor of Psychiatry and Biobehavioral Science, David Geffen School of Medicine at UCLA; Executive Director of the UCLA Anxiety Disorders Section; Co-Director of the UCLA-Duke University–National Center for Child Traumatic Stress, Los Angeles, California.
49.16. Impact of Terrorism on Children

Charles L. Raison, M.D. Assistant Professor, Mind-Body Program, Department of Psychiatry and Behavioral Sciences, Emory University School of Medicine, Atlanta, Georgia.
1.12. Immune System and Central Nervous System Interactions

Natalie L. Rasgon, M.D., Ph.D. Associate Professor of Psychiatry and Behavioral Sciences; Director of the Behavioral Endocrinology Program; and Associate Director of the Woman's Wellness Center; Stanford University School of Medicine, Stanford, California.
24.6. Endocrine and Metabolic Disorders

Niels C. Rattenborg, Ph.D. Assistant Scientist, Department of Psychiatry, Wisconsin Institute and Psychiatric Clinic, University of Wisconsin Medical School, Madison, Wisconsin.
1.20. Basic Science of Sleep

Scott L. Rauch, M.D. Associate Professor of Psychiatry, Harvard Medical School; Director of Psychiatric Neuroimaging Research and Associate Chief of Psychiatry for Neuroscience Research, Massachusetts General Hospital, Boston, Massachusetts.
31.31. Neurosurgical Treatments and Deep Brain Stimulation

Richard A. Rawson, Ph.D. Associate Director of UCLA Integrated Substance Abuse Programs, David Geffen School of Medicine at UCLA, Los Angeles, California.
11.3. Amphetamine (or Amphetamine-like)–Related Disorders; 11.6. Cocaine-Related Disorders

Stephen L. Read, M.D. Associate Clinical Professor of Psychiatry and Biobehavioral Sciences, David Geffen School of Medicine at UCLA; Attending Psychiatrist, UCLA Neuropsychiatric Hospital and Greater Los Angles Veterans Affairs Health System, Los Angeles, California.
51.6c. Ethical Issues

Richard E. Redding, J.D., Ph.D. Associate Professor of Law and Director of the J.D/Ph.D. Program in Law and Psychology, Villanova University School of Law; Associate Professor of Clinical Health Psychology and Director of the J.D./Ph.D. Program in Law and Psychology, Hahnemann University Medical College of Pennsylvania, Villanova, Pennsylvania.
4.4. Sociopolitical Trends in Mental Health Care: The Consumer/Survivor Movement and Multiculturalism

Eric M. Reiman, M.D. Professor and Associate Head of Psychiatry, University of Arizona College of Medicine, Tucson, Arizona; Scientific Director of the Positron Emission Tomography (PET) Center, Good Samaritan Regional Medical Center and Scientific Director of the Arizona Alzheimer's Research Center, Phoenix, Arizona.
51.2e. Neuroimaging: Overview

David C. Rettew, M.D. Assistant Professor of Psychiatry and Director of the Pediatric Psychopharmacology Clinic, University of Vermont College of Medicine; Attending Physician, Fletcher Allen Health Care, Burlington, Vermont.
31.12. Bupropion

Victor I. Reus, M.D. Professor of Psychiatry, Investigator, Center for Neurobiology and Behavior, Investigator, Program in Pharmacogenomics, University of California at San Francisco School of Medicine; Attending Physician, Langley Porter Hospital, Attending Physician, Moffett-Long Hospital, San Francisco, California.
1.11. Psychoneuroendocrinology

Zoltán Rihmer, M.D., Ph.D. Lecturer in Psychiatry, Department of Psychiatry, Semmelweis University; Director and Head, In- and Outpatient Department of Psychiatry, National Institute for Psychiatry and Neurology, Budapest, Hungary.
13.2. Mood Disorders: Epidemiology

Brien P. Riley, Ph.D. Assistant Professor of Psychiatry and Human Genetics, Director of Molecular Genetics, Virginia Institute of Psychiatric and Behavioral Genetics, Virginia Commonwealth University School of Medicine, Richmond, Virginia.
12.3. Schizophrenia: Genetics

Rosalinda C. Roberts, Ph.D. Professor of Psychiatry, Anatomy and Neurobiology, University of Maryland School of Medicine, Baltimore, Maryland; Director of Maryland Brain Collection, Maryland Psychiatric Research Center, Catonsville, Maryland.
12.7. Schizophrenia: Neuropathology

Robert G. Robinson, M.D. The Paul W. Penningroth Professor and Head of Psychiatry, Roy J. and Lucille A. Carver College of Medicine at University of Iowa, Iowa City, Iowa.
2.2. Neuropsychiatric Aspects of Cerebrovascular Disorders; 2.5. Neuropsychiatric Aspects of Traumatic Brain Injury

David R. Rosenberg, M.D. Professor of Psychiatry and Behavioral Neurosciences, Wayne State University School of Medicine; Miriam L. Hamburger Endowed Chairman, Child and Adolescent Neuropsychiatric Research, Children's Hospital of Michigan and Wayne State University, Detroit, Michigan.
49.14. Neuroimaging in Child and Adolescent Psychiatry

Alvin Rosenfeld, M.D. Formerly Assistant Professor of Psychiatry and Behavioral Sciences, Stanford University School of Medicine, Stanford, California.
49.2. Adoption and Foster Care

M. Zachary Rosenthal, Ph.D. Clinical Associate Professor, Duke University Medical Center, Durham, North Carolina.
30.8. Dialectical Behavior Therapy

Bruce J. Rounsaville, M.D. Professor of Psychiatry, Yale University School of Medicine; Director of the Veterans Affairs, Veteran Integrated Service Network 1 (VISN1) Mental Illness Research, Education and Clinical Center (MIRECC), New Haven, Connecticut.
31.22. Opioid Receptor Antagonists: Naltrexone and Nalmefene

David R. Rubinow, M.D. Chief, Behavioral Endocrinology Branch, National Institute of Mental Health, National Institutes of Health, Bethesda, Maryland.
31.34. Reproductive Hormonal Therapy: Theory and Practice

Teresa A. Rummans, M.D. Professor of Psychiatry, Mayo Clinic and Foundation, Mayo Medical School, Rochester, Minnesota.
24.8. Musculoskeletal Disorders

A. John Rush, M.D. Professor and Vice-Chairman for Research, Betty Jo Hay Distinguished Chairman in Mental Health, and Rosewood Corporation Chairman in Biomedical Science, Department of Psychiatry, University of Texas Southwestern Medical School, Dallas, Texas.
13.7. Mood Disorders: Treatment of Depression; 31.12. Bupropion

Sheila Ryan, C.S.W., M.P.H. Program Director, Special Needs Clinic, New York Presbyterian Hospital, New York, New York.
49.5. Psychiatric Sequelae of HIV and AIDS

Joel Sadavoy, M.D., F.R.C.P.(C) Professor and Sam and Judy Pencer and Family Chairman in Applied General Psychiatry, University of Toronto Faculty of Medicine, Toronto, Ontario, Canada; Psychiatrist-in-Chief, Mount Sinai Hospital, New York, New York.
51.4g. Psychosocial Treatments: General Principles; 51.4h. Individual Psychotherapy

Benjamin J. Sadock, M.D. Menas S. Gregory Professor of Psychiatry and Vice-Chairman, Department of Psychiatry, New York University School of Medicine; Attending Psychiatrist, Tisch Hospital; Attending Psychiatrist, Bellevue Hospital Center; Consulting Physician, Lenox Hill Hospital, New York, New York.
7.3. Psychiatric Report, Medical Record, and Medical Error; 7.4. Signs and Symptoms in Psychiatry; 30.12. Combined Psychotherapy and Pharmacology

Virginia A. Sadock, M.D. Clinical Professor of Psychiatry and Director of Program in Human Sexuality, New York University School of Medicine; Attending Psychiatrist, Tisch Hospital; Attending Psychiatrist, Bellevue Hospital Center, New York, New York.
18.1a. Normal Human Sexuality and Sexual Dysfunctions

Joseph Sakai, M.D. Instructor of Psychiatry, University of Colorado School of Medicine; Associate Director of Adolescent Psychiatric Services, Addiction and Research and Treatment Services, University of Colorado Health Sciences Center, Denver, Colorado.
11.8. Inhalant-Related Disorders

Carl Salzman, M.D. Professor of Psychiatry, Harvard Medical School; Director of Psychopharmacology and Director of Education, Massachusetts Mental Health Center, Boston, Massachusetts.
51.4b. Psychopharmacology: Antidepressants and Mood Stabilizers

Steven C. Samuels, M.D. Assistant Professor of Psychiatry, Program Director of Geriatric Psychiatry Fellowship, Mount Sinai School of Medicine, New York, New York; Staff Psychiatrist, Bronx Veterans Affairs Medical Center, Bronx, New York.
10.2. Delirium; 10.3. Dementia

Ofra Sarid-Segal, M.D. Assistant Professor of Psychiatry, Boston University School of Medicine; Director of Clinical Research, Psychopharmacology Special Programs Section, Boston Medical Center; Staff Psychiatrist, Department of VA Outpatient Clinic, Boston, Massachussetts.
11.12. Sedative-, Hypnotic-, or Anxiolytic-Related Disorders

Sally L. Satel, M.D. Lecturer, Yale University School of Medicine, New Haven, Connecticut; Staff Psychiatrist, Oasis Drug Clinic, W. H. Brady Fellow, American Enterprise Institute, Washington, D.C.
4.4. Sociopolitical Trends in Mental Health Care: The Consumer/Survivor Movement and Multiculturalism

Stephen M. Saunders, Ph.D. Associate Professor and Director of Clinical Training, Clinical Psychology Program, Department of Psychology, Marquette University, Milwaukee, Wisconsin.
30.11. Evaluation of Psychotherapy

S. Alan Savitz, M.D. Consultant, Pacific Care Health Services, Los Angeles, California.
51.5b. Managed Care

Lawrence Scahill, M.S.N., Ph.D. Associate Professor of Nursing and Child Psychiatry, Yale Child Study Center, Yale School of Nursing, New Haven, Connecticut.
42. Tic Disorders

Alan F. Schatzberg, M.D. Kenneth T. Norris, Jr. Professor and Chairman, Department of Psychiatry and Behavioral Sciences, Stanford University School of Medicine; Chief of Service, Stanford University Hospital, Stanford, California.
31.33. Drug Augmentation

Stephen C. Scheiber, M.D. Adjunct Professor of Psychiatry, Northwestern University Medical School, Chicago, Illinois; Adjunct Professor of Psychiatry, Medical College of Wisconsin, Milwaukee, Wisconsin; Senior Attending Physician, Evanston Northwestern Healthcare, Evanston, Illinois.
53.1. Graduate Psychiatric Education

Diane H. Schetky, M.D. Clinical Professor of Psychiatry, University of Vermont College of Medicine, Burlington, Vermont; Psychiatrist, Maine Medical Center, Portland, Maine.
49.10. Forensic Child and Adolescent Psychiatry

Steven C. Schlozman, M.D. Clinical Instructor in Psychiatry, Harvard Medical School; Lecturer in Education, Harvard Graduate School of Education; Staff Child Psychiatrist, Massachusetts General Hospital, Boston, Massachusetts.
48.10. Psychiatric Treatment of Adolescents

Peter J. Schmidt, M.D. Chief, Unit on Reproductive Endocrinology, Behavioral Endocrinology Branch, National Institute of Mental Health, Bethesda, Maryland.
31.34. Reproductive Hormonal Therapy: Theory and Practice

Lon S. Schneider, M.D. Professor of Psychiatry, Neurology, and Gerontology, University of Southern California School of Medicine, Los Angeles, California.
51.4e. Psychopharmacology: Antidementia Drugs

Merritt D. Schreiber, Ph.D. Program Manager, Terrorism and Disaster Branch, National Center for Child Traumatic Stress, David Geffen School of Medicine at UCLA, Los Angeles, California.
49.16. Impact of Terrorism on Children

Marc A. Schuckit, M.D. Professor of Psychiatry, University of California, San Diego School of Medicine; Director of the Alcohol Research Center and Director of the Alcohol and Drug Treatment Program, San Diego VA Healthcare System, San Diego, California.
11.2. Alcohol-Related Disorders

Robert T. Schultz, Ph.D. Associate Professor of Child Study Center and Diagnostic Radiology, Yale University School of Medicine, New Haven, Connecticut.
38. Pervasive Developmental Disorders

Mary E. Schwab-Stone, M.D. Associate Professor of Child Psychiatry and Psychology, Yale University School of Medicine; Attending Physician, Yale-New Haven Hospital, New Haven, Connecticut.
33. Psychiatric Examination of the Infant, Child, and Adolescent

Gary J. Schwartz, Ph.D. Associate Professor of Psychiatry, Joan and Sanford I. Weill Medical College of Cornell University, New York, New York.
1.21. Appetite

William K. Scott, Ph.D. Assistant Research Professor in Medicine and in Biostatistics and Bioinformatics, Duke University School of Medicine, Durham, North Carolina.
51.2g. Genetics of Late-Life Degenerative Disorders

David W. Self, Ph.D. Associate Professor of Psychiatry and Neuroscience, Lydia Bryant Test Professorship, University of Texas Southwestern Medical Center at Dallas Southwestern Medical School, Dallas, Texas.
1.22. Neural Basis of Substance Abuse and Dependence

David Shaffer, M.D., F.R.C.P. Irving Philips Professor of Child Psychiatry; and Professor of Psychiatry and Pediatrics, Columbia University College of Physicians and Surgeons; Director, Division of Child Psychiatry, New York State Psychiatric Institute; and Director, Department of Pediatric Psychiatry, Babies Hospital, New York Presbyterian Hospital, New York, New York.
45.1. Depressive Disorders and Suicide in Children and Adolescents

Bhavik G. Shah, M.D. Associate Clinical Professor, David Geffen School of Medicine at UCLA; Medical Director: Child Inpatient Service, Behavior Genetics Clinic, and Fetal Alcohol Syndrome Clinic, UCLA Neuropsychiatric Institute and Hospital, Los Angeles, California.
44.2. Stereotypic Movement Disorder of Infancy

Richard P. Shank, Ph.D. Consultant, CNS Drug Discovery, Johnson and Johnson Pharmaceutical Research and Development, LLC, Spring House, Pennsylvania.
1.5. Amino Acids As Neurotransmitters

Peter A. Shapiro, M.D. Associate Professor of Clinical Psychiatry, Columbia University College of Physicians and Surgeons; Director of the Transplant Psychiatry Program and Associate Director of the Consultation–Liaison Psychiatry Service, Columbia–Presbyterian Medical Center, New York-Presbyterian Hospital, New York, New York.
24.4. Cardiovascular Disorders

Javaid I. Sheikh, M.D., M.B.A. Associate Professor of Psychiatry, Stanford University School of Medicine, Stanford, California; Chief of Staff, Palo Alto VA Health Care System, Palo Alto, California.
51.4c. Psychopharmacology: Antianxiety Drugs

Mark E. Shelhorse, M.D. Deputy Network Director, Veterans Integrated Service Network 6, Durham, North Carolina.
51.5c. Veterans Affairs Medical Centers and Psychogeriatric Services

Jun Shen, Ph.D. Chief, Unit on Magnetic Resonance Spectroscopy, Molecular Imaging Branch, National Institute of Mental Health, National Institutes of Health, Bethesda, Maryland.
1.15. Nuclear Magnetic Resonance Imaging: Basic Principles and Recent Findings in Neuropsychiatric Disorders

Cleveland G. Shields, Ph.D. Associate Professor of Family Health Medicine and Psychiatry, University of Rochester School of Medicine and Dentistry, Rochester, New York.
51.4j. Family Intervention and Therapy with Older Adults

Stephen R. Shuchter, M.D. Professor of Clinical Psychiatry, University of California, San Diego School of Medicine; Medical Director of the UCSD Outpatient Psychiatry and Associate Director of Residency Training, UCSD Medical Center, San Diego, California.
13.9. Mood Disorders: Psychotherapy

Carole Siegel, Ph.D. Professor of Psychiatry, New York University School of Medicine; Director of the Center for the Study of Issues in Public Mental Health; Director of the Statistical Sciences and Services Research Division, Nathan S. Kline Institute for Psychiatric Research, New York, New York.
5.2. Statistics and Experimental Design

Daniel J. Siegel, M.D. Associate Clinical Professor of Psychiatry and Director of the Center for Human Development, David Geffen School of Medicine at UCLA, Los Angeles, California.
3.1. Sensation, Perception, and Cognition

Steven M. Silverstein, Ph.D. Associate Professor of Psychology in Psychiatry, Weill Medical College of Cornell University; Program Director of the Psychotic Disorders Division, New York Presbyterian Hospital, New York, New York.
52.4. Psychiatric Rehabilitation

Deborah R. Simkin, M.D. Clinical Assistant Professor, Florida State Medical School, Tallahassee, Florida.
49.9. Adolescent Substance Abuse

Robert I. Simon, M.D. Clinical Professor of Psychiatry and Director of the Program in Psychiatry and Law, Georgetown University School of Medicine, Washington, D.C.; Senior Attending and Chairman, Department of Psychiatry, Suburban Hospital, Bethesda, Maryland.
54.1. Clinical-Legal Issues in Psychiatry

Andrew E. Slaby, M.D. Clinical Professor of Psychiatry, New York University School of Medicine; Consulting Physician, Lenox Hill Hospital and Saint Vincent's Hospital and Medical Center, New York, New York; Consulting Physician, Overlook Hospital, Summit, New Jersey.
29.2. Other Psychiatric Emergencies

Gary W. Small, M.D. Parlow-Solomon Professor of Aging, Professor of Psychiatry and Biobehavioral Sciences, Director of the UCLA Memory Clinic, David Geffen School of Medicine at UCLA, Los Angeles, California.
31.15. Cholinesterase Inhibitors and Similarly Acting Compounds; 51.1a. Geriatric Psychiatry: Introduction; 51.3e. Alzheimer's Disease and Other Dementias

Sharon L. Smart, M.D., Ph.D. Clinical Fellow in Biological Psychiatry, University of California at San Francisco School of Medicine, and San Francisco Veterans Medical Center, San Francisco, California.
1.4. Monoamine Neurotransmitters

Virginia L. Smith-Swintosky, Ph.D. Principal Scientist, Johnson and Johnson Pharmaceutical Research and Development, Spring House, Pennsylvania.
1.5. Amino Acids As Neurotransmitters

Solomon H. Snyder, M.D. Distinguished Service Professor, Director of the Department of Neuroscience, Johns Hopkins University School of Medicine, Baltimore, Maryland.
1.23. Future Directions in Neuroscience and Psychiatry

Mariann Sondell, Ph.D. Karolinska Institute, Department of Cell and Molecular Biology, Stockholm, Sweden.
1.3. Neural Development and Neurogenesis

Adrian N. Sondheimer, M.D. Associate Professor of Psychiatry and Training Director of the Division of Child and Adolescent Psychiatry, University of Medicine and Dentistry of New Jersey—New Jersey Medical School, Newark, New Jersey.
49.11. Ethical Issues in Child and Adolescent Psychiatry

Sarah J. Spence, M.D., Ph.D. Assistant Professor, Departments of Psychiatry and Biobehavioral Science and Pediatrics, Divisions of Child Psychiatry and Pediatric Neurology; Medical Director of the UCLA Autism Evaluation Clinic, David Geffen School of Medicine at UCLA, Los Angeles, California.
36. Motor Skills Disorder: Developmental Coordination Disorder

David Spiegel, M.D. Jack, Lulu and Sam Willson Professor in the School of Medicine and Associate Chairman of Psychiatry and Behavioral Sciences, Stanford University School of Medicine; Medical Director of the Center for Integrated Medicine, Stanford University Medical Center, Stanford, California.
30.3. Hypnosis

Herbert Spiegel, M.D. Special Lecturer in Psychiatry, Columbia University College of Physicians and Surgeons, New York, New York.
30.3. Hypnosis

Robert L. Spitzer, M.D. Professor of Psychiatry, Department of Psychiatry, Columbia University College of Physicians and Surgeons; Chief, Biometric Research, New York State Psychiatric Institute, New York, New York.
9.1. Psychiatric Classification

Larry R. Squire, Ph.D. Professor of Psychiatry, Neurosciences and Psychology, University of California, San Diego School of Medicine, La Jolla, California; Research Career Scientist, San Diego VA Healthcare System, San Diego, California.
3.4. Biology of Memory

Murray B. Stein, M.D. Professor of Psychiatry, University of California San Diego; Director of the Anxiety and Traumatic Stress Program, San Diego VA Healthcare System, San Diego, California.
14.9. Anxiety Disorders: Somatic Treatment; 24.9. Stress and Psychiatry

Terry S. Stein, M.D. Professor Emeritus of Psychiatry, Michigan State University, College of Osteopathic Medicine and College of Human Medicine, East Lansing, Michigan.
18.1b. Homosexuality, Gay and Lesbian Identities, and Homosexual Behavior

Alan M. Steinberg, Ph.D. Associate Director, National Center for Child Traumatic Stress, UCLA Neuropsychiatric Institute and Hospital, Los Angeles, California.
49.16. Impact of Terrorism on Children

Hans Steiner, M.D. Professor of Psychiatry, Divisions of Child Psychiatry and Child Development, Stanford University School of Medicine, Stanford, California.
49.6. Child or Adolescent Antisocial Behavior

William S. Stone, Ph.D. Assistant Professor of Psychology, Department of Psychiatry, Harvard Medical School; Director of Neuropsychology Training and Clinical Services, Massachusetts Mental Health Center, Boston, Massachusetts.
12.15. Schizophrenia Spectrum: Pathology and Treatment

Eric C. Strain, M.D. Professor of Psychiatry and Behavioral Sciences, Johns Hopkins University School of Medicine, Baltimore, Maryland.
11.4. Caffeine-Related Disorders; 11.10 Opioid-Related Disorders

Joel E. Streim, M.D. Professor of Psychiatry, University of Pennsylvania and Philadelphia VA Medical Center, Philadelphia, Pennsylvania.
51.6a. Psychiatric Aspects of Long-Term Care

Frederick A. Struve, Ph.D. Senior Research Scientist, Department of Psychiatry, Yale University School of Medicine, New Haven, Connecticut.
1.14. Applied Electrophysiology

Howard S. Sudak, M.D. Clinical Professor of Psychiatry, University of Pennsylvania School of Medicine; Consulting Physician, The Pennsylvania Hospital, Philadelphia, Pennsylvania.
29.1. Suicide

David L. Sultzer, M.D. Associate Professor in Residence, Department of Psychiatry and Biobehavioral Sciences, David Geffen School of Medicine at UCLA; Director of the Gero/Neuropsychiatry Division, West Los Angeles VA Healthcare Center, Los Angeles, California.
51.4d. Psychopharmacology: Antipsychotic Drugs

Stephen J. Suomi, Ph.D. Chief, Laboratory of Comparative Ethology, National Institute of Child Health and Human Development, National Institutes of Health, Bethesda, Maryland.
5.4. Animal Research and Its Relevance to Psychiatry

Ezra S. Susser, M.D., Dr.P.H. Head, Department of Epidemiology, Joseph L. Mailman School of Public Health, Columbia University; Head, Department of Epidemiology of Brain Disorders, New York State Psychiatric Institute, New York, New York.
12.4. Schizophrenia: Environmental Epidemiology

Norman Sussman, M.D. Professor of Psychiatry, New York University School of Medicine; Director of Psychopharmacology Research and Consultation Service, Bellevue Hospital Center, New York, New York.
30.12. Combined Psychotherapy and Pharmacology; 31.1. General Principles of Psychopharmacology

Dragan M. Svrakic, M.D., Ph.D. Associate Professor of Psychiatry, Washington University School of Medicine, St. Louis, Missouri.
23. Personality Disorders

Rex M. Swanda, Ph.D. Adjunct Assistant Professor of Psychiatry, University of New Mexico School of Medicine; Director of Neuropsychology, New Mexico Veterans Healthcare System, Albuquerque, New Mexico.
7.5. Clinical Neuropsychology and Intellectual Assessment of Adults

Zebulon Taintor, M.D. Professor and Vice-Chairman, Department of Psychiatry, New York University School of Medicine; Clinician, Bellevue Hospital Center, Manhattan Psychiatric Center, New York, New York; Clinician, St. Lawrence Psychiatric Center, Ogdensburg, New York.
7.10. Telemedicine, Telepsychiatry, and Online Therapy

Carol A. Tamminga, M.D. Professor of Psychiatry and Communities Foundation of Texas Chairman in Brain Science, University of Texas Southwestern Medical Center, Dallas, Texas.
12.7. Schizophrenia: Neuropathology

Rosemary Tannock, Ph.D. Associate Professor of Psychiatry, University of Toronto; Senior Scientist, Brain and Behavior Research Program, Research Institute of The Hospital for Sick Children, Toronto, Canada.
35.1. Reading Disorder; 35.2. Mathematics Disorder; 35.3. Disorder of Written Expression and Learning Disorder Not Otherwise Specified

Laurence H. Tecott, M.D., Ph.D. Associate Professor of Psychiatry, University of California at San Francisco School of Medicine; Attending Psychiatrist, Langley Porter Psychiatric Institute, San Francisco, California.
1.4. Monoamine Neurotransmitters; 1.19. Transgenic Models of Behavior

Cenk Tek, M.D. Assistant Professor of Psychiatry, University of Maryland School of Medicine, Baltimore, Maryland.
12.8. Schizophrenia: Clinical Features and Psychopathology Concepts

Michael E. Thase, M.D. Professor of Psychiatry, University of Pittsburgh School of Medicine, Pittsburgh, Pennsylvania.
13.4. Mood Disorders: Neurobiology; 31.18. Mirtazapine; 31.23. Selective Serotonin–Norepinephrine Reuptake Inhibitors

Margo L. Thienemann, M.D. Assistant Professor, Division of Child and Adolescent Psychiatry, Department of Psychiatry, Stanford University School of Medicine, Stanford, California.
48.4. Group Psychotherapy

Armin Paul Thies, Ph.D. Associate Clinical Professor, Child Study Center, Yale School of Medicine, New Haven, Connecticut.
33. Psychiatric Examination of the Infant, Child, and Adolescent

Christopher R. Thomas, M.D. Professor of Psychiatry and Behavioral Science, University of Texas Medical Branch at Galveston; Consulting Physician, John Scaly Hospital and Shriners Burns Hospital, Galveston, Texas.
40. Disruptive Behavior Disorders

Larry W. Thompson, Ph.D. Professor of Medicine and Research, Emeritus at Stanford University School of Medicine, Stanford, California; Professor of Psychology, Pacific Graduate School of Psychology, Palo Alto, California.
51.4i. Cognitive-Behavioral Therapy

Joyce A. Tinsley, M.D. Associate Professor of Psychiatry, Director of Psychiatric Residency Training and Director of Addiction Psychiatry Residency Training, University of Connecticut School of Medicine, Farmington, Connecticut.
52.2. Health Care Reform

Oladapo Tomori, M.D. Assistant Professor of Psychiatry, University of New Mexico Health Sciences Center, Albuquerque, New Mexico.
22. Adjustment Disorders

Giulio Tononi, M.D., Ph.D. Professor of Psychiatry, University of Wisconsin-Madison, Madison, Wisconsin.
1.20. Basic Science of Sleep

Alan Trachtenberg, M.D., M.P.H. Adjunct Associate Professor of Community Medicine and Research Director, Indian Health Service, George Washington School of Public Health and Health Services, Washington, D.C.; Adjunct Associate Professor of Preventive Medicine and Biometrics, Uniformed Services University of the Health Sciences, Bethesda, Maryland.
28.8. Alternative and Complementary Health Practices

Glenn J. Treisman, M.D., Ph.D. Associate Professor of Psychiatry and Behavioral Sciences, Associate Professor of Medicine, Johns Hopkins University School of Medicine; Director of AIDS Psychiatry Services, Johns Hopkins Hospital, Baltimore, Maryland.
2.8. Neuropsychiatric Aspects of HIV Infection and AIDS

Robert L. Trestman, M.D., Ph.D. Professor, Clinical Chief and Vice-Chairman of Psychiatry, University of Connecticut School of Medicine, Farmington, Connecticut.
52.2. Health Care Reform

Manuel Trujillo, M.D. Professor of Clinical Psychiatry and Vice-Chairman, Department of Psychiatry, New York University School of Medicine; Director of Psychiatry, Bellevue Hospital Center, New York, New York.
27. Culture-Bound Syndromes

Ming T. Tsuang, M.D., Ph.D. University Professor of Psychiatry and Director of the Institute of Behavioral Genomics, Department of Psychiatry, University of California, San Diego, La Jolla, California; Director of the Harvard Institute of Psychiatric Epidemiology and Genetics, Harvard Departments of Epidemiology and Psychiatry, Harvard University, Boston, Massachusetts.
12.15. Schizophrenia Spectrum: Pathology and Treatment

Jürgen Unützer, M.D., M.P.H. Professor and Vice Chairman, Department of Psychiatry and Behavioral Sciences, Chief of Psychiatry, and Director, Project IMPACT Coordinating Center, University of Washington Medical Center, Seattle, Washington.
51.3a. Psychiatric Problems in the Medically Ill

Robert J. Ursano, M.D. Professor of Psychiatry and Neuroscience and Chairman, Department of Psychiatry, Uniformed Services University of the Health Sciences, Bethesda, Maryland.
28.9. Military and Disaster Psychiatry

Tevfik Bedirhan Üstün, M.D., Ph.D. Head, Office of Classification, Assessment, Surveys and Terminology, World Health Organization, Geneva, Switzerland.
5.1. Epidemiology

Jerome V. Vaccaro, M.D. Associate Clinical Professor of Psychiatry, David Geffen School of Medicine at UCLA, Los Angeles, California; President and CEO, PacifiCare Behavioral Health, Van Nuys, California.
51.5b. Managed Care

Caroline O. Vaillant, M.S.S.W. Research Associate–Emeritus, Study of Adult Development, Harvard University Health Services, Cambridge, Massachusetts.
3.7. Normality and Mental Health

George E. Vaillant, M.D. Professor of Psychiatry, Harvard Medical School, Boston, Massachusetts; Director of the Study of Adult Development, Harvard University Health Services, Cambridge, Massachusetts.
3.7. Normality and Mental Health

Bessel A. van der Kolk, M.D. Professor of Psychiatry, Boston University School of Medicine, Boston, Massachusetts; Medical Director of the Trauma Center, Brookline, Massachusetts.
28.6. Physical and Sexual Abuse of Adults

Daniel P. van Kammen, M.D., Ph.D. Professor Emeritus, University of Pittsburgh School of Medicine, Pittsburgh, Pennsylvania; Adjunct Professor of Psychiatry, University of Pennsylvania Medical School, Philadelphia, Pennsylvania.
31.16. Dopamine Receptor Antagonists (Typical Antipsychotics); 31.25. Serotonin-Dopamine Antagonists (Atypical or Second-Generation Antipsychotics)

William W. Van Stone, M.D. Emeritus Clinical Associate Professor of Psychiatry and Behavioral Sciences, Stanford University School of Medicine, Stanford, California; Associate Chief Consultant, Mental Health Strategic Healthcare Group, Veteran Affairs Central Office, Washington, D.C.
51.5c. Veterans Affairs Medical Centers and Psychogeriatric Services

Jeff Victoroff, M.D. Associate Professor of Clinical Neurology and Psychiatry, Keck School of Medicine of University of Southern California, Los Angeles, California; Director of Neurobehavior, Rancho Los Amigos National Rehabilitation Center, Downey, California.
51.2b. Central Nervous System Changes with Normal Aging

Michael V. Vitiello, Ph.D. Professor of Psychiatry and Behavioral Sciences, Adjunct Professor of Psychology, and Adjunct Professor of Biobehavioral Nursing and Health Systems, University of Washington School of Medicine, Seattle, Washington.
51.3b. Sleep Disorders

Fred R. Volkmar, M.D. Professor of Psychiatry, Pediatrics and Psychology, Yale University School of Medicine; Attending Physician, Yale-New Haven Hospital, New Haven, Connecticut.
38. Pervasive Developmental Disorders

Lisa L. von Moltke, M.D. Research Associate Professor of Pharmacology and Experimental Therapeutics, Tufts University School of Medicine; Associate, Department of Medicine, Tufts-New England Medical Center, Boston, Massachusetts.
31.2. Pharmacokinetics and Drug Interactions

Meena Vythilingam, M.D. Chief, Anxiety Disorders Research Clinic, Staff Physician, Mood and Anxiety Disorders Program, National Institute of Mental Health, National Institutes of Health, Bethesda, Maryland.
1.15. Nuclear Magnetic Resonance Imaging: Basic Principles and Recent Findings in Neuropsychiatric Disorders

Thomas A. Wadden, Ph.D. Professor of Psychology, Department of Psychiatry, University of Pennsylvania School of Medicine, Philadelphia, Pennsylvania.
24.3. Obesity

Dora Wang, M.D. Assistant Professor of Psychiatry, University of New Mexico School of Medicine; Director of the Consultation-Liaison Psychiatry Service, University of New Mexico Health Sciences Center, Albuquerque, New Mexico.
16. Factitious Disorders

G. Scott Waterman, M.D. Associate Professor of Psychiatry, Director of Psychopharmacology, and Director of Medical Student Education in Psychiatry, University of Vermont College of Medicine, Burlington, Vermont.
31.13. Buspirone

Tonya Jo Hanson White, M.D. Assistant Professor of Psychiatry and Pediatrics and Director of Disorders of Cognition, Thought and Social Functioning Clinic, University of Minnesota Medical School, Minneapolis, Minnesota.
49.4. Children's Reaction to Illness and Hospitalization

Denise E. Wilfley, Ph.D. Professor of Pediatrics, Psychiatry, Medicine, and Psychology, San Diego Joint Doctoral Program in Clinical Psychology, and Director of the Center for Eating and Weight Disorders, University of California San Diego School of Medicine, La Jolla, California.
30.7. Interpersonal Psychotherapy

G. Terence Wilson, Ph.D. Oscar K. Buros Professor of Psychology, Rutgers University, Piscataway, New Jersey.
3.3. Learning Theory

Celia Jaffe Winchell, M.D. Instructor, Department of Psychiatry, Johns Hopkins School of Medicine, Baltimore, Maryland.
31.3. Drug Development and Approval Process in the United States

Eve J. Wiseman, M.D. Associate Professor of Psychiatry, University of Arkansas for Medical Sciences; Clinical Chief, Central Arkansas Veterans Healthcare System, North Little Rock, Arkansas.
51.3i. Drug and Alcohol Abuse

Owen M. Wolkowitz, M.D. Professor of Psychiatry, University of California at San Francisco School of Medicine; Director of Psychopharmacology Assessment Clinic, Langley Porter Psychiatric Institute, UCSF Medical Center, San Francisco, California.
1.11. Psychoneuroendocrinology

Normund Wong, M.D. Professor of Psychiatry, Uniformed Services University of the Health Sciences, Bethesda, Maryland; Past Consultant, Officer of the Surgeon General, United States Army, Rockville, Maryland; Consultant, Walter Reed Army Medical Center, Washington, D.C.
30.4. Group Psychotherapy and Combined Individual and Group Psychotherapy

Scott W. Woods, M.D. Associate Professor of Psychiatry, Yale University School of Medicine; Director of the Treatment Research Program, Connecticut Mental Health Center, New Haven, Connecticut.
12.17. Schizophrenia and Other Psychotic Disorders: Special Issues in Early Detection and Intervention

Lyman C. Wynne, M.D., Ph.D. Professor Emeritus, Department of Psychiatry, University of Rochester School of Medicine and Dentistry, Rochester, New York.
51.4j. Family Intervention and Therapy with Older Adults

Joel Yager, M.D. Professor and Vice-Chairman for Education and Academic Affairs, Department of Psychiatry, University of New Mexico School of Medicine, Albuquerque, New Mexico; Professor Emeritus of Psychiatry and Biobehavioral Sciences, David Geffen School of Medicine at UCLA, Los Angeles, California.
8. Clinical Manifestations of Psychiatric Disorders; 19. Eating Disorders

William R. Yates, M.D. Professor of Psychiatry and Family Medicine, Chairman, Department of Psychiatry, University of Oklahoma College of Medicine; Research Consultant, Laureate Psychiatric Clinic and Hospital, Tulsa, Oklahoma.
24.2. Gastrointestinal Disorders

Larry J. Young, Ph.D. Associate Professor of Psychiatry and Behavioral Sciences, Emory University School of Medicine, Atlanta, Georgia.
1.6. Neuropeptides: Biology, Regulation, and Role in Neuropsychiatric Disorders

Charles H. Zeanah, Jr., M.D. Professor and Vice Chairman, Department of Psychiatry and Neurology, and Director of Child and Adolescent Psychiatry, Tulane University School of Medicine, New Orleans, Louisiana.
44.1. Reactive Attachment Disorder of Infancy and Early Childhood

Bonnie T. Zima, M.D., M.P.H. Associate Professor and Director of UCLA Research Program on Advancing Treatment and Health of Children, David Geffen School of Medicine at UCLA, Los Angeles, California.
49.15. Child Mental Health Services Research

Mark Zimmerman, M.D. Associate Professor of Psychiatry and Human Behavior, Brown University School of Medicine; Director of Outpatient Psychiatry, Rhode Island Hospital, Providence, Rhode Island.
9.1. Psychiatric Classification

Sidney Zisook, M.D. Professor of Psychiatry and Director of Residency Training, University of California at San Diego School of Medicine; Attending Physician, UCSD Medical Center and San Diego VA Healthcare System, San Diego, California.
28.5. Death, Dying, and Bereavement

Stephanie A. Zisook, M.D. Fellow in Women's Mental Health, UCLA Neuropsychiatric Institute and Hospital; Associate Physician Diplomat, Student Psychological Services, University of California, Los Angeles, Los Angeles, California.
28.5. Death, Dying, and Bereavement

Charles F. Zorumski, M.D. Samuel B. Guze Professor of Psychiatry and Neurobiology, Washington University School of Medicine; Psychiatrist-in-Chief, Barnes-Jewish Hospital, Saint Louis, Missouri.
1.9. Basic Electrophysiology

Stephen R. Zukin, M.D. Clinical Professor of Psychiatry, Albert Einstein College of Medicine at Yeshiva University, Bronx, New York; Visiting Professor of Psychiatry and Radiology, Johns Hopkins University School of Medicine; Attending Physician, Johns Hopkins Medical Institutions, Baltimore, Maryland.
11.11. Phencyclidine (or Phencyclidine-like)–Related Disorders

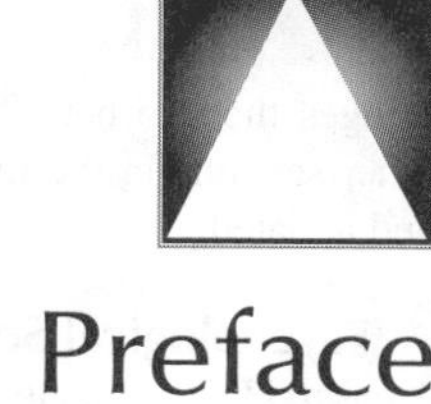

Preface

This is the eighth edition of *Kaplan & Sadock's Comprehensive Textbook of Psychiatry* to appear within a span of 38 years and the second to appear in the 21st century. It has been described as a "university without walls" and has helped educate generations of psychiatrists, other physicians, and mental health professionals from all fields, including psychology, social work, and nursing, among others. Its goal has been and remains to foster professional competence and ensure the highest quality of care to all those persons with mental illness. The textbook has earned a reputation as an encyclopedic compendium of psychiatric knowledge. As editors, we have been extremely gratified by its wide acceptance and use both in this country and around the world.

TEACHING SYSTEM

This textbook forms one part of a comprehensive system developed by the editors to facilitate the teaching of psychiatry and the behavioral sciences. At the head of the system is *Comprehensive Textbook of Psychiatry*, which is global in depth and scope. It is designed for and used by psychiatrists, behavioral scientists, and all workers in the mental health field. *Kaplan & Sadock's Synopsis of Psychiatry* is a relatively brief, highly modified, original, and current version useful for medical students, psychiatric residents, practicing psychiatrists, and mental health professionals. The *Concise Textbook of Clinical Psychiatry*, derived from *Synopsis*, emphasizes clinical psychiatry and includes extensive case studies useful for students and clinical practitioners from all fields. Another component of the system is *Study Guide and Self-Examination Review of Psychiatry*, which consists of more than 1,600 multiple-choice questions and answers, including detailed case histories. It is designed for students of psychiatry and for clinical psychiatrists who require a review of the behavioral sciences and general psychiatry in preparation for a variety of examinations. The questions are modeled after and are consistent with the format used by the American Board of Psychiatry and Neurology and the United States Medical Licensing Examination. Other parts of the system are the pocket handbooks: *Pocket Handbook of Clinical Psychiatry, Pocket Handbook of Psychiatric Drug Treatment, Pocket Handbook of Emergency Psychiatric Medicine*, and *Pocket Handbook of Primary Care Psychiatry.* These books cover the diagnosis and treatment of psychiatric disorders, psychopharmacology, psychiatric emergencies, and primary care psychiatry, respectively, and are concisely written and compactly designed so as to fit in the pockets of clinical clerks and practicing physicians, whatever their specialty, to provide a quick reference. Finally, *Comprehensive Glossary of Psychiatry and Psychology* provides simply written definitions for psychiatrists and other physicians, psychologists, students, mental health professionals, and the general public.

Taken together, these books provide a multiple approach to the teaching, study, and learning of psychiatry.

CHANGES IN THIS EDITION

New Contributors A tradition of inviting a number of new authors to write sections written by prior authors began with the second edition of the textbook. New authors were invited for the same reasons that other great textbooks of medicine do so—to ensure a fresh approach to each topic and to keep the *Comprehensive Textbook of Psychiatry* vital and current. More than 50 percent of the contributors to this edition are new. The editors are deeply grateful to the more than 1,500 psychiatrists and behavioral scientists who contributed to previous editions, all of whom maintained the highest standards of scholarship. Many of their sections remain classics in the field and are accessible to the interested reader. We especially wish to acknowledge John Nemiah, M.D., editor emeritus of the *American Journal of Psychiatry*, who has contributed to every edition of this book.

New Sections More than 50 new sections were written especially for this edition. As a result, this edition is larger than the last by more than 700 pages. This proved necessary because of the enormous increase in the amount of psychiatric knowledge that occurred in the short span of 4 years, especially in the neural sciences and psychopharmacology. Sections were organized to be as succinct as possible through the use of special typeface and new printing techniques; had we attempted to save space by limiting new material and recent advances, we would have done a disservice to the reader and to the field of psychiatry. Almost every chapter has been completely rewritten or revised.

Some of the new additions to the textbook and other highlights are listed below.

Genetics and Neural Science The important role of genetics in the etiology of mental illness is covered in two new sections: *Genome, Transcriptome, and Proteome* and *Transgenic Models of Behavior.* A new section, *Neural Basis of Substance Abuse and Dependence,* describes advances in the neurobiological underpinnings of addictive behavior. Also new to this edition is the section on *Neuropsychiatric Aspects of Prion Disease*. The section *Radiotracer Imaging: Basic Principles and Exemplary Findings in Neuropsychiatric Disorders* appears for the first time. Expanded sections include *Neuropsychiatric Aspects of HIV Infection and AIDS, Neuropsychiatric Aspects of Multiple Sclerosis and Other Demyelinating Disorders,* and *Neuropsychiatric Aspects of Movement Disorders.* A new section, *Neuroscientific Bases of Consciousness and Dreaming,* bridges the gap between the neural and psychological sciences. All other sections in the neural science chapter were completely revised and updated.

Psychological Sciences A new section, *Normality and Mental Health,* deals with the criteria used to define normal and abnormal human behavior across the life cycle. Another new section, *Sociopolitical Trends in Mental Health Care: The Consumer/Survivor Movement and Multiculturalism,* covers highly controversial areas, such as victimology, multiculturalism, and gender issues, among many others. This reflects our view that practitioners have a special obligation to know about the sociopolitical issues that inform the physical and psychological well-being of their patients. The sections *Biology of Memory; Sensation, Perception, and Cognition*; *Learning Theory*; and *Brain Models of Mind* were expanded and updated. *Anthropology and Cultural Psychiatry* and *Sociobiology* have also been expanded. *Mental Health Services* and *Statistics and Experimental Design* were thoroughly revised. The section *Animal Research and Its Relevance to Psychiatry* was rewritten to reflect the latest advances in this important area of study, and the chapter *Classic Psychoanalysis* was completely revised. A new section, *The Psychiatric Scientist and the Psychoanalyst,* examines the role of psychoanalysis and dynamically oriented psychotherapy in modern-day psychiatry.

Clinical Psychiatry A newly written version of *Psychiatric Interview, History, and Mental Status Examination* was prepared for this edition, and a new section, *Interviewing Techniques with the Difficult Patient*, was added. The section *Psychiatric Report and Medical Record* was expanded to cover the important area of medical error. A new section, *Telemedicine, Telepsychiatry, and Online Therapy,* reflects the impact of the electronic revolution on medical and psychiatric practice. The chapter *Delirium, Dementia, and Amnestic and Other Cognitive Disorders* was reorganized completely to provide separate and thorough discussions of each disease entity.

The chapter *Anxiety Disorders* was expanded with new sections added that cover neurochemical aspects, psychophysiological aspects, and neuroimaging. The section *Sexual Addiction* appears for the first time.

The chapter on schizophrenia has been enlarged and reorganized to include two new sections on epidemiology: *Schizophrenia: Genetics* and *Schizophrenia: Environmental Epidemiology.* A new section, *Neurodevelopmental Theory,* has been added in addition to separate new sections on neuroanatomy, neuropathology, and cognition in schizophrenia. Advances in therapy are reflected in the increase from three sections dealing with the treatment of schizophrenia in the last edition to seven sections in this edition.

A new section, *Correctional Psychiatry,* addresses the issues of mental illness in our jails and prisons. Two new sections, *Survivors of Torture* and *Military and Disaster Psychiatry,* reflect the role of psychiatry in caring for victims of war, terrorism, and political upheaval. The editors are also pleased to include the section *Future of Psychiatry,* which reflects the views of the National Institute of Mental Health and its director, Thomas R. Insel, M.D. The section *World Aspects of Psychiatry* has been updated to reflect the increased globalization of mental health issues.

All sections dealing with clinical disorders have been thoroughly updated and follow a similar outline, which includes an introduction and definition of the disorder; a history of the disorder, including comparative nosology, epidemiology, and etiology; diagnosis and clinical features; pathology and laboratory examination; differential diagnosis; and course and prognosis. Treatment strategies for all clinical disorders are presented eclectically to include biological, pharmacological, psychosocial, and psychotherapeutic approaches. The area of psychiatric treatment has been updated and expanded with the addition of a new section, *Dialectical Behavior Therapy.* Another new section, *Famous Named Cases in Psychiatry,* chronicles the important role of individual case reports in the evolution of psychiatry.

Geriatric Psychiatry The chapters on geriatric psychiatry continue to expand in each edition, and the geriatric section can stand alone as a separate textbook in its comprehensive coverage of the psychiatric disorders of old age. Four new sections have been added: *Sexuality and Aging, Delirium, Genetics of Late-Life Degenerative Disorders,* and *Counseling and Support Needs of Dementia Caregivers*. The section *End-of-Life and Palliative Care* appears for the first time to reflect the editors' continued call for psychiatrists to involve themselves in the clinical subspecialty of palliative care and pain control, which is now an interdisciplinary specialty. We especially wish to thank Lissy F. Jarvik, M.D., who first organized this part of the text. Her work has been ably carried on by Gary W. Small, M.D. We thank him for his efforts.

Child Psychiatry As with geriatric psychiatry, the child section stands as a "text within a text." New sections covering child and adolescent psychiatry added to this edition include *Depressive Disorders and Suicide in Children and Adolescents, Early-Onset Bipolar Disorders, Neuroimaging in Child and Adolescent Psychiatry,* and *Child Mental Health Services Research.* A special section on the *Impact of Terrorism on Children* was written to deal with the psychological effects of September 11, 2001, and other acts of terror on this vulnerable population. We especially wish to acknowledge Caroly S. Pataki, M.D., for her extraordinary work organizing the child psychiatry section.

Psychopharmacology The editors continue to use the unique format of discussing drugs used in the treatment of mental disorders on a pharmacological basis rather than under the rubrics of antidepressant, antipsychotic, and the like. Categories such as antidepressants, antipsychotics, anxiolytics, and mood stabilizers are overly broad and do not reflect the clinical use of psychotropic medication. For example, many antidepressant drugs are used to treat anxiety disorders; some anxiolytics are used to treat depression and bipolar disorders; and drugs from all categories are used to treat other clinical disorders, such as eating disorders, panic disorders, and impulse-control disorders. There are also many drugs used to treat a variety of mental disorders that do not fit into any broad classification. Information about all pharmacological agents used in psychiatry, including pharmacodynamics, pharmacokinetics, dosages, adverse effects, and drug–drug interactions, was thoroughly updated and includes all drugs approved since the last edition was published.

Drugs in this text are referred to by their generic name throughout except for their first entry, which is followed by one or more of their proprietary preparations. In some cases, only one proprietary drug exists and, in other cases, more than one exists. In the latter instance, our policy is to list drug names alphabetically. The listing of proprietary names is for educational purposes only and should not be misconstrued as an endorsement of any product. We want to thank Norman Sussman, M.D., for his help in organizing this section of the text.

The section *General Principles of Psychopharmacology* was thoroughly updated for this edition, and several new sections were added. These include *Combined Psychotherapy and Pharmacology, Drug Augmentation, Neurosurgical Treatments and Deep Brain Stimula-*

tion, and *Reproductive Hormonal Therapy: Theory and Practice.* New sections on classes of drugs with unique pharmacological properties were written, including *Opioid Receptor Agonists: Methadone, Levomethadyl, and Buprenorphine* and *Selective Serotonin–Norepinephrine Reuptake Inhibitors,* among others. The most recently developed drugs are covered in detail, and all discussions of other drugs have been thoroughly updated.

A unique aspect of this and other *Kaplan & Sadock* books is the color plates of major drugs used in psychiatry, which show the forms in which they are commercially available and their dose ranges, to help the physician recognize and prescribe the medications. The color plates have also been useful in helping patients identify—to their physicians and therapists—medications that they are taking.

References Following the style of other major medical textbooks, internal literature citations were eliminated, and the number of references at the end of each section was reduced. Contributors were asked to limit references to 30 to 40 major books, monographs, and review articles and to include current references; thus, some citation lists are not as long as some of the authors would have wished. Contributors were also asked to note the five most important references with asterisks. References are as up-to-date as possible. The editors are also mindful that modern-day readers consult internet resources, such as *PsychINFO* and *Medline,* to stay abreast of the most current literature, and they encourage that trend. Cross-references at the end of each section continue to be used to direct the reader to other relevant parts of the text to enhance the learning experience.

DSM and ICD The revised fourth edition of the American Psychiatric Association's (APA) *Diagnostic and Statistical Manual of Mental Disorders* (DSM-IV-TR) was published in 2000. It contains the official nomenclature used by psychiatrists and other mental health professionals; thus, DSM-IV-TR terminology is used throughout the *Comprehensive Textbook.* The DSM classification codes are similar to those in the tenth edition of the *International Statistical Classification of Diseases and Related Health Problems* (ICD-10), published by the World Health Organization (WHO); however, there are differences in some of the diagnostic criteria of mental disorders. Accordingly, we have included tables comparing both DSM-IV-TR and ICD-10 criteria throughout the text. Readers can find tables comparing both nosological systems in Section 9.1.

Although psychiatric disorders discussed in this textbook are consistent with the nosology in DSM-IV-TR, some of our contributors have reservations about the changes introduced into the various editions of DSM. In several sections of the book, these views are clearly stated. DSM-IV-TR is a diagnostic and statistical manual; it is *not* and never claimed to be a textbook. Unfortunately, it is used as a text by some groups, including insurance companies, who believe it to be a comprehensive source of information about mental illness. The reader is referred to Section 9.1, *Psychiatric Classification,* for a thorough discussion of these issues.

As future editions of DSM appear—and the editors believe they are in the offing—the *Comprehensive Textbook of Psychiatry* will continue to allow room for dissent before and especially after every new version appears. It will continue to provide a forum for discussion, evaluation, criticism, and disagreement, while duly acknowledging the official nomenclature.

Case Histories Case histories are used extensively to add clarity to the clinical disorders. They are derived from the DSM and ICD casebooks and the clinical and research experience of the contributors. We wish to thank the APA and WHO for permission to use some of their material. Cases appear in shaded boxes to help the reader find them easily.

CONTINUING CRISIS IN THE FUTURE OF PSYCHIATRY

In the last two editions of the *Comprehensive Textbook of Psychiatry,* the editors included commentary on the crisis in the future of psychiatry. Unfortunately, the situation has not changed since this first appeared in 1995. Excerpts of that commentary appear below.

> The introduction of the American Health Security Bill (the Clinton plan) in 1993 served as a catalyst for dramatic change in the delivery of health care in the United States even though the bill was not enacted into law. In the vanguard of change were the insurance companies and the health maintenance organizations (HMOs), which are, in the main, managed care programs run by large profit-seeking corporations. Managed care has had serious and adverse effects on the practice of psychiatry. For example, most managed mental health care (MMHC) plans restrict the number of outpatient visits for psychotherapy to a small and unpredictable number of sessions, usually 5 to 20 a year. Although some types of psychotherapy can be conducted within that framework, other types (insight oriented) require frequent visits over an extended period.
>
> Prior to consulting the psychiatrist, many HMOs require preauthorization by a panel of so-called behavioral health experts. This panel requires information about the intimate and private details of a person's life to authorize therapy. If the patient or doctor refuses to comply, permission for psychiatric treatment is usually denied. And even if the patient is permitted to enter therapy, the psychiatrist must send frequent written reports to the HMO about the treatment, which breaches the confidentiality and trust of the doctor-patient relationship. Patients usually must be treated by psychiatrists who are enrolled in their particular HMO. They forfeit the right to see a doctor of their own choosing. In the traditional fee-for-service system patients can seek treatment from any psychiatrist they choose and can seek a second or even a third opinion if they so desire. In an HMO the patient does not have these options.
>
> HMOs use from 15 to 30 percent of their revenues to pay for marketing, administration, and the distribution of profits to owners and investors, money that would otherwise be available for clinical care, research, and medical education. Health care in America is being "corporatized," and HMOs reap profits by often eliminating laboratory tests, referrals to specialists, and reducing length of hospital stay to questionable and dangerous proportions. For example, patients with major psychiatric disorders are being forced out of the hospital, often against their will and against the recommendation of their psychiatrists. HMOs also increase their profit margin by paying lower fees to doctors, and since the HMOs control the supply of patients, price control rules the system. [According to the *Wall Street Journal* (February 16, 2000), Aetna/US Health Care corporation reported revenues of $26.5 billion in 2000.]
>
> The issue of financial liability is another area of danger to doctors who work for HMOs. Psychiatrists (and other physi-

cians) who sign contracts with HMOs must agree to accept complete liability if any adverse effects to the patient occur during the course of treatment. Consider this example: A psychiatrist wants to hospitalize a potentially suicidal patient, but the HMO refuses to pay for hospitalization or limits the number of days allowed in the hospital to fewer than the psychiatrist deems necessary. The psychiatrist can be sued for malpractice if the patient ultimately commits suicide because of premature hospital discharge mandated by the HMO. The HMO accepts no liability for any adverse outcome based on their decisions. The only alternative is for the psychiatrist and hospital to treat the patient for no fee or for the patient to pay for treatment out-of-pocket. Neither option is satisfactory.

Currently, the future of psychiatric treatment is of concern. Unfortunately, prejudice toward mental illness still exists in many quarters—political policy makers, insurance companies, the general public, and, sadly, the medical profession itself. Psychiatry and medicine are at a crossroad. It would be tragic to take the path that discards and negates the humanism that psychiatry has brought to medicine. A new concept of *market-driven* medical services now dominates the health care industry and will do so for the foreseeable future. Paradoxically, the role of government must increase to regulate this new industry, whose preoccupation is the *cost* of health care. For example, some states passed legislation allowing patients to sue HMOs. In 2004, however, the U.S. Supreme Court ruled that patients could not sue their health plans in state court for damages incurred when plans refused to pay for doctor-recommended treatment—a ruling criticized by the American Medical Association as allowing "insurance companies to practice medicine without a license." Ultimately, the U.S. Congress will become the arbiter between the consumers of health care (patients), the providers (physicians and other health professionals), and the payers (insurance companies and HMOs). In this sense, society and the body politic will determine the nature and quality of health care in the United States.

The spirit of the Hippocratic oath, written more than 2,000 years ago, continues to inspire the ethics of the medical profession: *To act for the good of my patients according to my ability and my judgment.* As medicine changes, physicians (and other health care professionals) are the last stronghold for humanitarian and compassionate care that stresses the inherent dignity and worth of each person.

CONTRIBUTING EDITORS

In the preparation of this textbook, we have been helped immensely by our distinguished and knowledgeable group of contributing editors. They kept us apprised of new advances in the field and helped obtain contributors with expertise in their respective areas. We thank them for their help and personal involvement. They include Hagop S. Akiskal, M.D., who contributed to *Mood Disorders*; William T. Carpenter, Jr., M.D., who contributed to *Schizophrenia and Other Psychotic Disorders*; Dennis S. Charney, M.D., who contributed to *Anxiety Disorders*; Kenneth L. Davis, M.D., who contributed to *Cognitive Disorders*; Jack A. Grebb, M.D., who contributed to *Biological Psychiatry*; Jerome H. Jaffe, M.D., who contributed to *Substance-Related Disorders*; W. Walter Menninger, M.D., who contributed to *Hospital and Community Psychiatry*; Caroly S. Pataki, M.D., who contributed to *Child Psychiatry*; Robert G. Robinson, M.D., who contributed to *Neuropsychiatry and Behavioral Neurology*; Gary W. Small, M.D., who contributed to *Geriatric Psychiatry*; Norman Sussman, M.D., who contributed to *Psychopharmacology*; and Joel Yager, M.D., who contributed to *Clinical Psychiatry*.

Together, this admirable, talented, and distinguished group helped integrate an immense amount of material into a balanced and consistently styled work. The editors and the field of psychiatry owe them a debt of gratitude for their outstanding help.

ACKNOWLEDGMENTS

In addition to the contributing editors mentioned above, we want to extend our deepest appreciation to Nitza Jones and Yande McMillan, who served as project editors in New York and helped us greatly. Regina Furner was also of great help. Dorice Viera, Associate Curator of the Frederick L. Ehrman Medical Library at the New York University School of Medicine, provided valuable assistance. Others who helped include Victoria Sadock Gregg, M.D., and James Sadock, M.D., experts in pediatric emergency medicine and adult emergency medicine, respectively. They assisted the editors in countless ways.

We want to thank our dear friend Nancy Barrett Kaplan, who gave us her complete support throughout this project. Over the years, she has been an invaluable source of encouragement and understanding.

We also want to take this opportunity to acknowledge those who have translated this and other *Kaplan & Sadock* books into foreign languages, including Croatian, French, German, Greek, Indonesian, Italian, Japanese, Polish, Portuguese, Romanian, Russian, Spanish, and Turkish, in addition to a special Asian and international student edition.

The staff at Lippincott Williams & Wilkins was most efficient. We wish to thank Joyce Murphy and Melanie Bennitt, who were extraordinarily helpful. Alyson Langlois at Silverchair Science + Communications also deserves our thanks. Charley Mitchell, Executive Editor of psychiatry at Lippincott Williams & Wilkins, was of tremendous help, and we thank him for his support and friendship.

Robert Cancro, M.D., Professor and Chairman of the Department of Psychiatry at New York University School of Medicine, participated as Senior Consulting Editor of this edition. Dr. Cancro's commitment to psychiatric education and psychiatric research is recognized throughout the world. He has been a source of great inspiration to the editors and contributed immeasurably to this and previous editions. He is a much valued friend and highly esteemed colleague, and it is a very special privilege to work closely with him. Dr. Cancro has developed a department that represents the very best in American psychiatry. Our collaboration and association with this outstanding American educator have contributed immeasurably to the ideas and directions shaping this textbook.

Finally, we want to express our deepest thanks to our contributors who were extraordinarily cooperative in every aspect of this textbook.

Benjamin James Sadock, M.D.
Virginia Alcott Sadock, M.D.
NYU School of Medicine
New York, New York

KAPLAN & SADOCK'S

Comprehensive Textbook of Psychiatry

Eighth Edition

Drugs Used in Psychiatry

This guide contains color reproductions of some commonly prescribed psychotherapeutic drugs. This guide mainly illustrates tablets and capsules. A † symbol preceding the name of a drug indicates that other doses are available. Check directly with the manufacturer. (*Although the photos are intended as accurate reproductions of the drug, this guide should be used only as a quick identification aid.*)

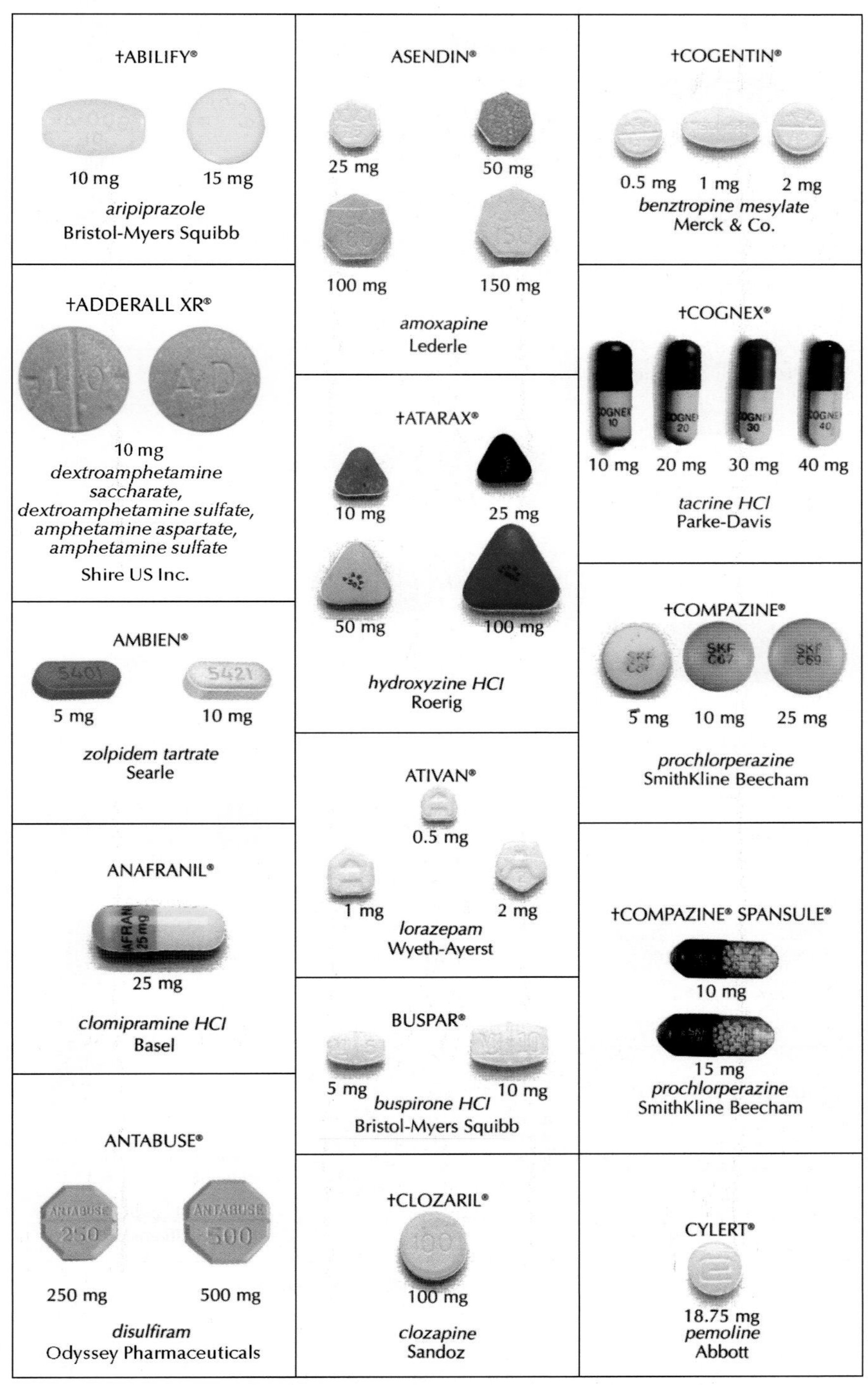

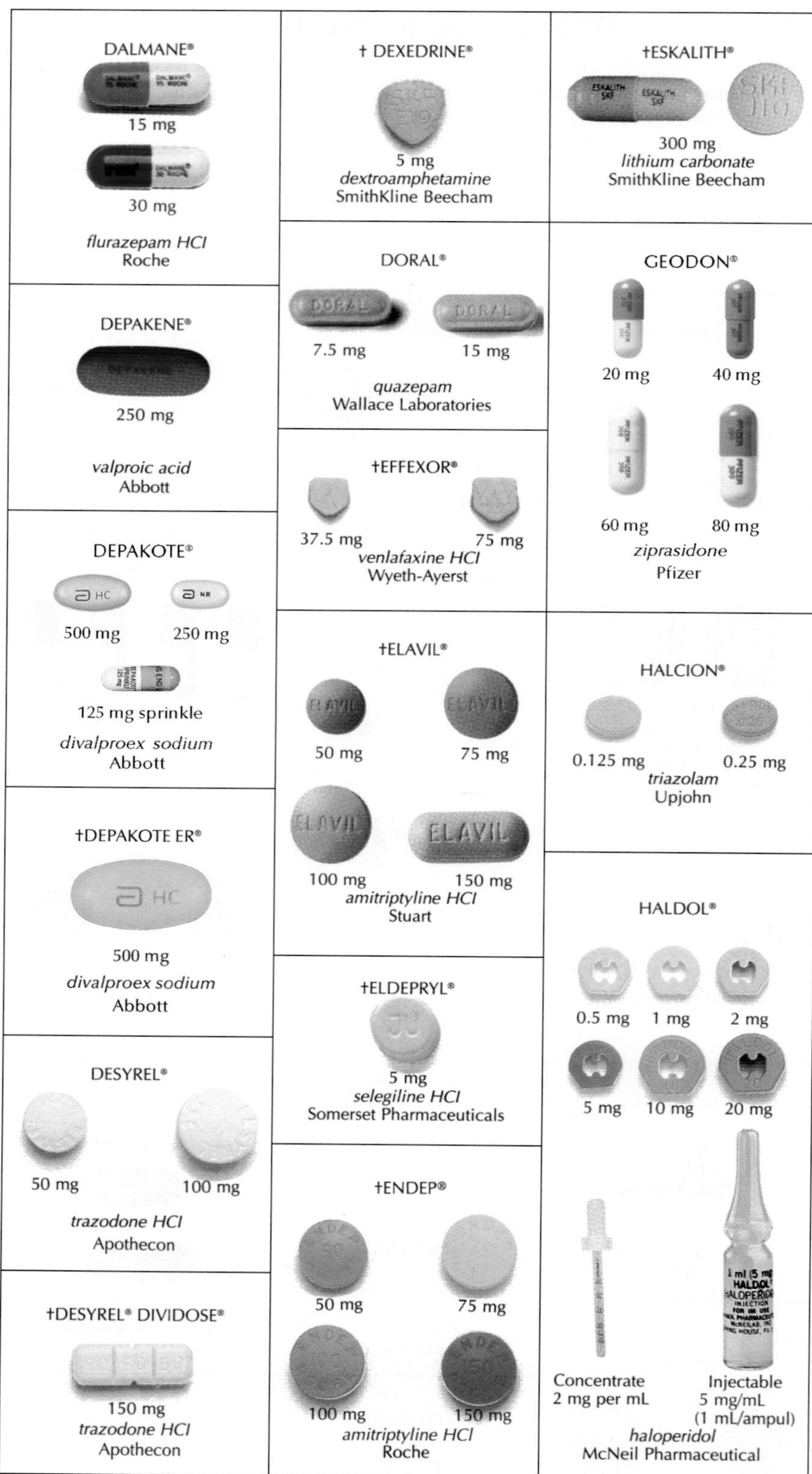

LIPPINCOTT WILLIAMS & WILKINS©

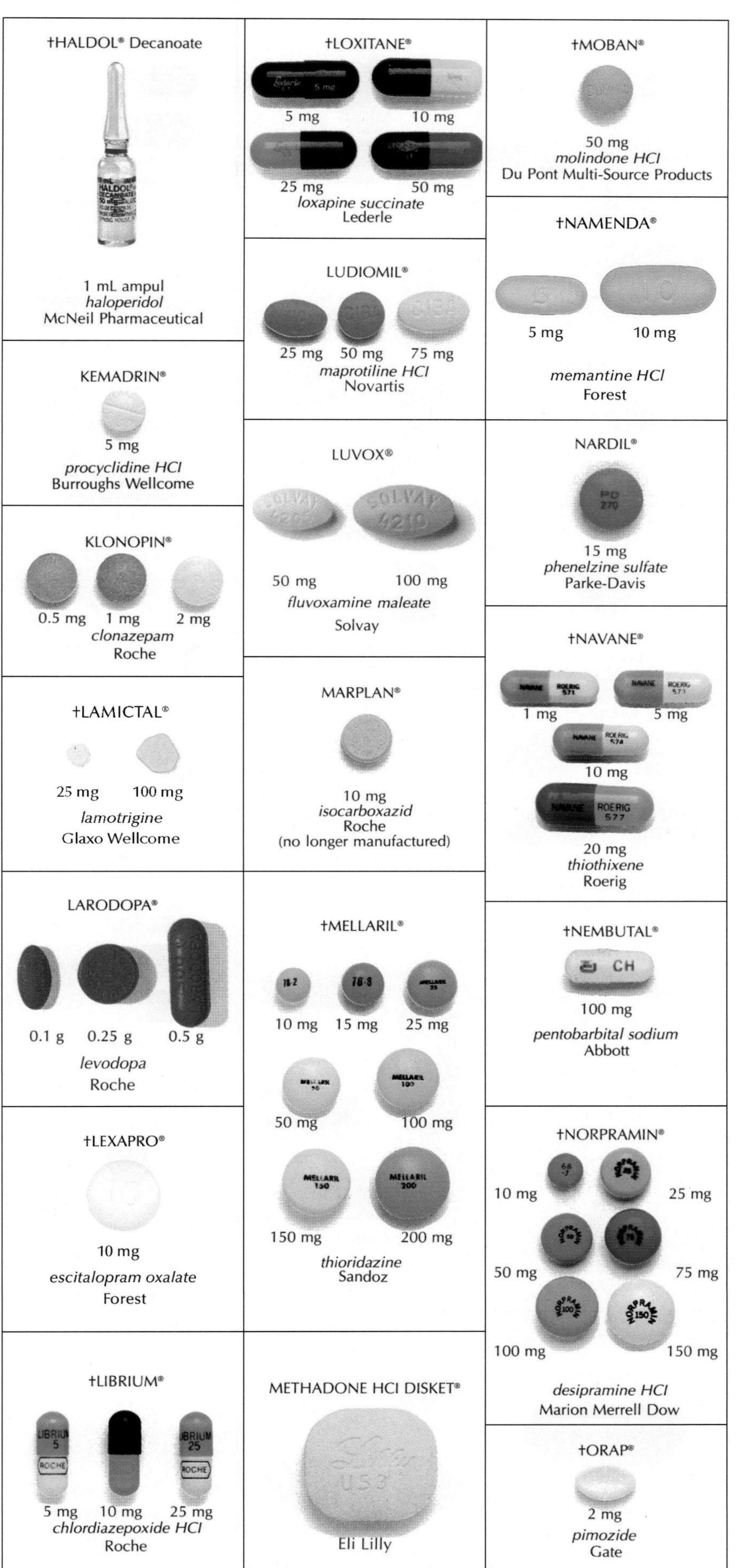
†HALDOL® Decanoate
1 mL ampul
haloperidol
McNeil Pharmaceutical
KEMADRIN®
5 mg
procyclidine HCl
Burroughs Wellcome
KLONOPIN®
0.5 mg 1 mg 2 mg
clonazepam
Roche
†LAMICTAL®
25 mg 100 mg
lamotrigine
Glaxo Wellcome
LARODOPA®
0.1 g 0.25 g 0.5 g
levodopa
Roche
†LEXAPRO®
10 mg
escitalopram oxalate
Forest
†LIBRIUM®
5 mg 10 mg 25 mg
chlordiazepoxide HCl
Roche
†LOXITANE®
5 mg 10 mg
25 mg 50 mg
loxapine succinate
Lederle
LUDIOMIL®
25 mg 50 mg 75 mg
maprotiline HCl
Novartis
LUVOX®
50 mg 100 mg
fluvoxamine maleate
Solvay
MARPLAN®
10 mg
isocarboxazid
Roche
(no longer manufactured)
†MELLARIL®
10 mg 15 mg 25 mg
50 mg 100 mg
150 mg 200 mg
thioridazine
Sandoz
METHADONE HCl DISKET®
Eli Lilly
†MOBAN®
50 mg
molindone HCl
Du Pont Multi-Source Products
†NAMENDA®
5 mg 10 mg
memantine HCl
Forest
NARDIL®
15 mg
phenelzine sulfate
Parke-Davis
†NAVANE®
1 mg 5 mg
10 mg
20 mg
thiothixene
Roerig
†NEMBUTAL®
100 mg
pentobarbital sodium
Abbott
†NORPRAMIN®
10 mg 25 mg
50 mg 75 mg
100 mg 150 mg
desipramine HCl
Marion Merrell Dow
†ORAP®
2 mg
pimozide
Gate

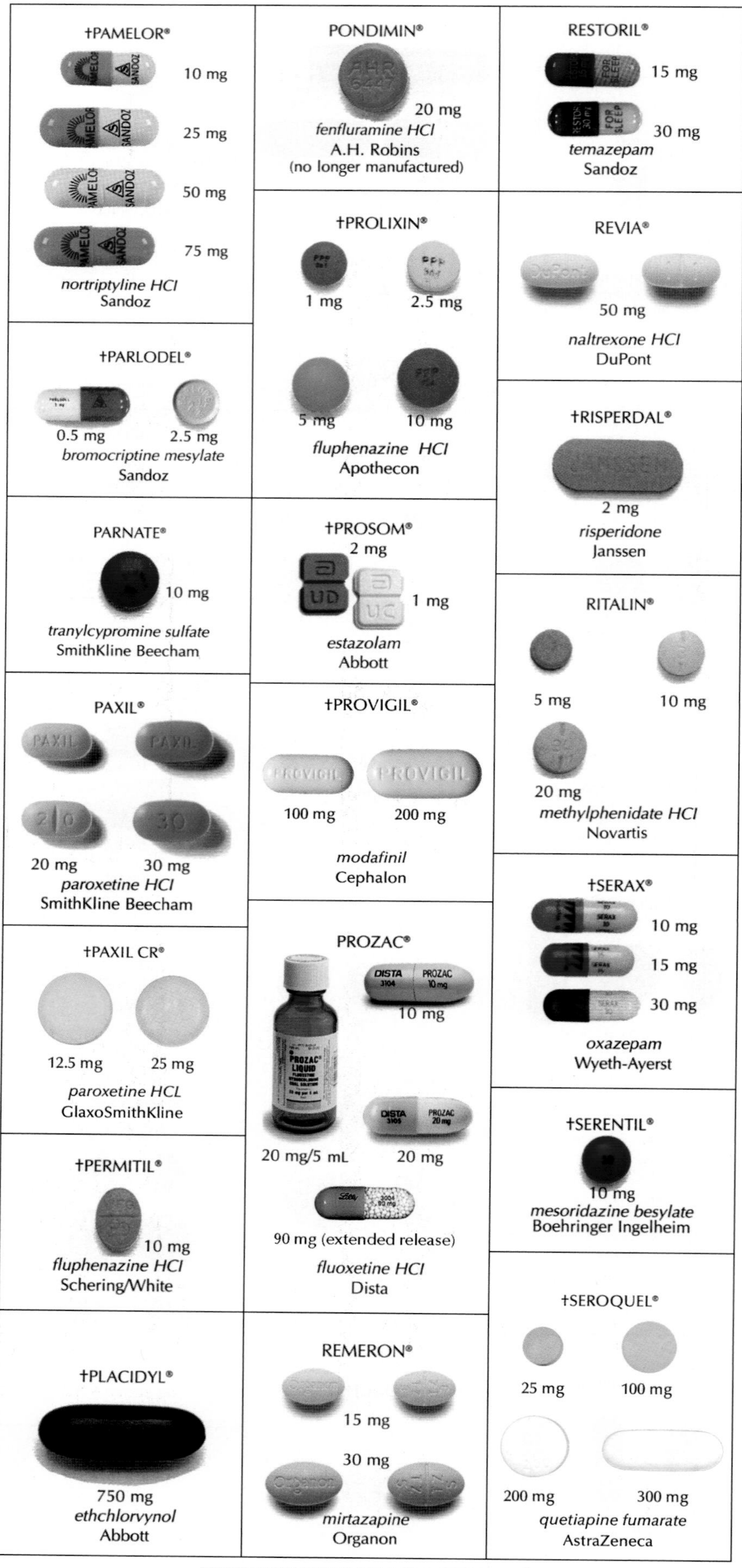

†PAMELOR®
10 mg
25 mg
50 mg
75 mg
nortriptyline HCl
Sandoz
PONDIMIN®
20 mg
fenfluramine HCl
A.H. Robins
(no longer manufactured)
RESTORIL®
15 mg
30 mg
temazepam
Sandoz
†PROLIXIN®
1 mg
2.5 mg
5 mg
10 mg
fluphenazine HCl
Apothecon
REVIA®
50 mg
naltrexone HCl
DuPont
†PARLODEL®
0.5 mg
2.5 mg
bromocriptine mesylate
Sandoz
†RISPERDAL®
2 mg
risperidone
Janssen
PARNATE®
10 mg
tranylcypromine sulfate
SmithKline Beecham
†PROSOM®
2 mg
1 mg
estazolam
Abbott
RITALIN®
5 mg
10 mg
20 mg
methylphenidate HCl
Novartis
PAXIL®
20 mg
30 mg
paroxetine HCl
SmithKline Beecham
†PROVIGIL®
100 mg
200 mg
modafinil
Cephalon
†SERAX®
10 mg
15 mg
30 mg
oxazepam
Wyeth-Ayerst
†PAXIL CR®
12.5 mg
25 mg
paroxetine HCL
GlaxoSmithKline
PROZAC®
10 mg
20 mg/5 mL
20 mg
90 mg (extended release)
fluoxetine HCl
Dista
†SERENTIL®
10 mg
mesoridazine besylate
Boehringer Ingelheim
†PERMITIL®
10 mg
fluphenazine HCl
Schering/White
†SEROQUEL®
25 mg
100 mg
200 mg
300 mg
quetiapine fumarate
AstraZeneca
†PLACIDYL®
750 mg
ethchlorvynol
Abbott
REMERON®
15 mg
30 mg
mirtazapine
Organon

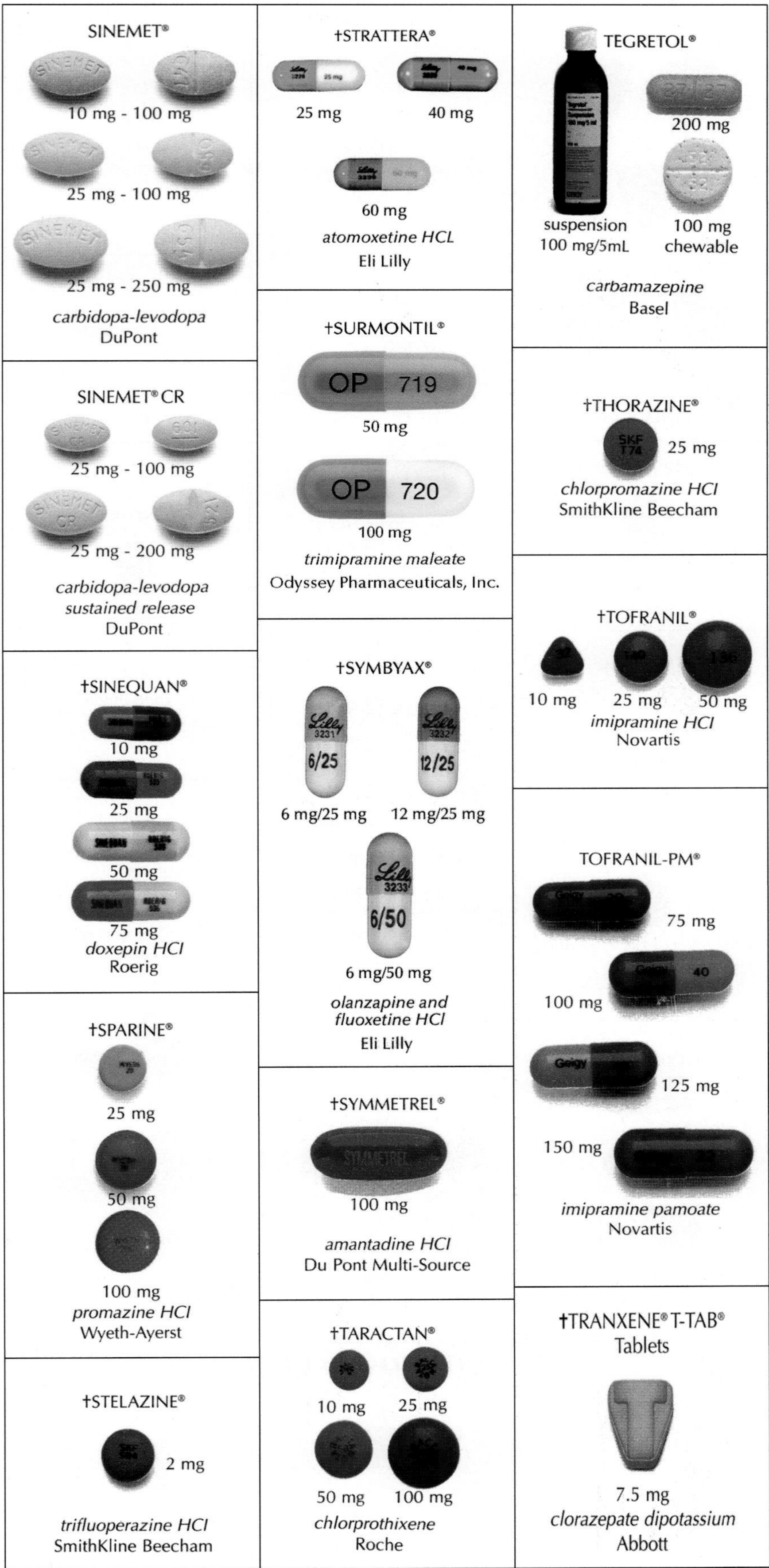

SINEMET®
10 mg - 100 mg
25 mg - 100 mg
25 mg - 250 mg
carbidopa-levodopa
DuPont
SINEMET® CR
25 mg - 100 mg
25 mg - 200 mg
carbidopa-levodopa
sustained release
DuPont
†SINEQUAN®
10 mg
25 mg
50 mg
75 mg
doxepin HCl
Roerig
†SPARINE®
25 mg
50 mg
100 mg
promazine HCl
Wyeth-Ayerst
†STELAZINE®
2 mg
trifluoperazine HCl
SmithKline Beecham
†STRATTERA®
25 mg
40 mg
60 mg
atomoxetine HCL
Eli Lilly
†SURMONTIL®
OP 719
50 mg
OP 720
100 mg
trimipramine maleate
Odyssey Pharmaceuticals, Inc.
†SYMBYAX®
3231
6/25
3232
12/25
6 mg/25 mg
12 mg/25 mg
3233
6/50
6 mg/50 mg
olanzapine and
fluoxetine HCl
Eli Lilly
†SYMMETREL®
SYMMETREL
100 mg
amantadine HCl
Du Pont Multi-Source
†TARACTAN®
10 mg
25 mg
50 mg
100 mg
chlorprothixene
Roche
TEGRETOL®
200 mg
suspension
100 mg/5mL
100 mg
chewable
carbamazepine
Basel
†THORAZINE®
SKF
T74
25 mg
chlorpromazine HCl
SmithKline Beecham
†TOFRANIL®
10 mg
25 mg
50 mg
imipramine HCl
Novartis
TOFRANIL-PM®
75 mg
40
100 mg
Geigy
125 mg
150 mg
imipramine pamoate
Novartis
†TRANXENE® T-TAB®
Tablets
7.5 mg
clorazepate dipotassium
Abbott

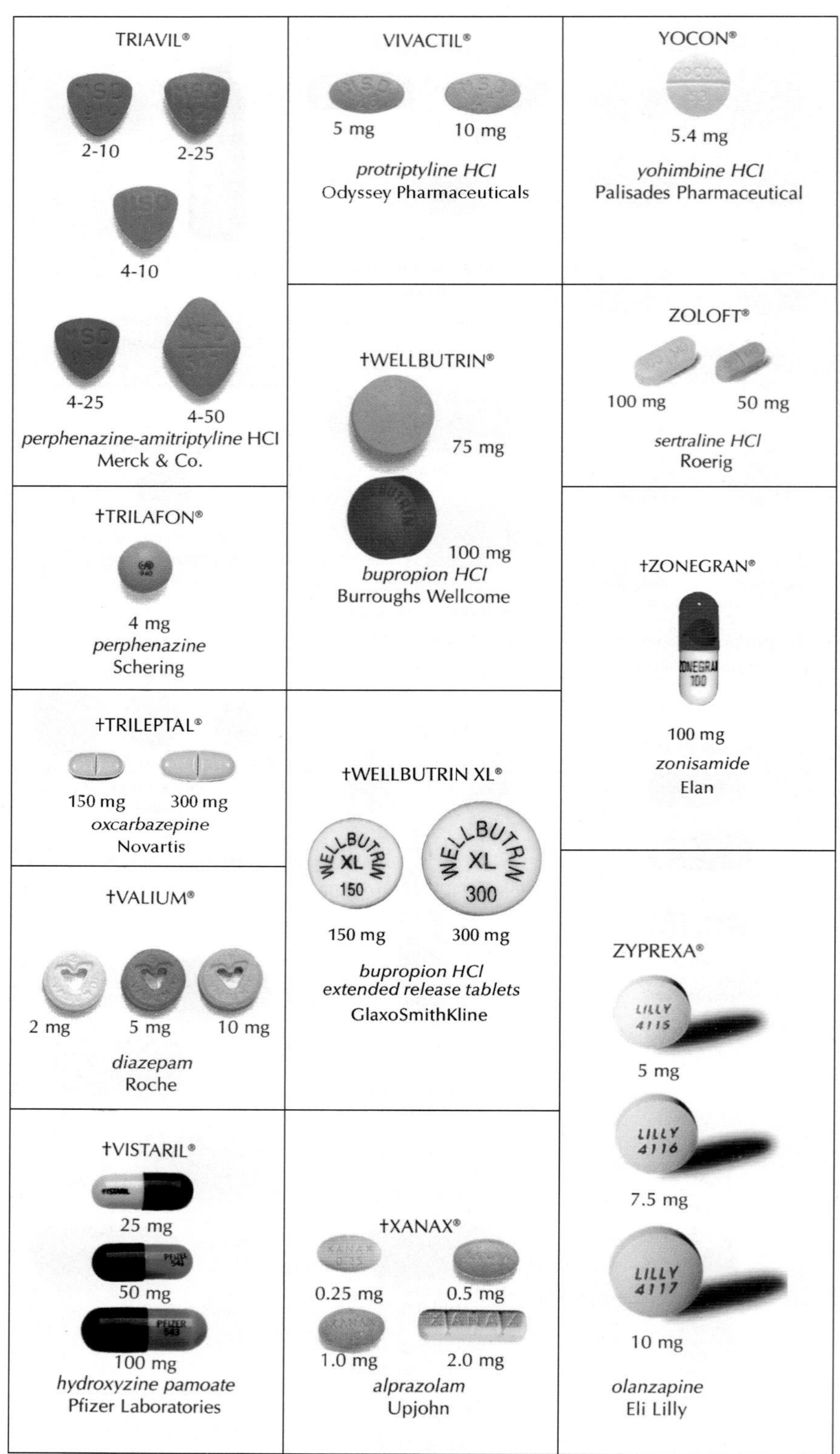

TRIAVIL®
2-10
2-25
4-10
4-25
4-50
perphenazine-amitriptyline HCl
Merck & Co.
†TRILAFON®
4 mg
perphenazine
Schering
†TRILEPTAL®
150 mg
300 mg
oxcarbazepine
Novartis
†VALIUM®
2 mg
5 mg
10 mg
diazepam
Roche
†VISTARIL®
25 mg
50 mg
100 mg
hydroxyzine pamoate
Pfizer Laboratories
VIVACTIL®
5 mg
10 mg
protriptyline HCl
Odyssey Pharmaceuticals
†WELLBUTRIN®
75 mg
100 mg
bupropion HCl
Burroughs Wellcome
†WELLBUTRIN XL®
WELLBUTRIN XL 150
WELLBUTRIN XL 300
150 mg
300 mg
bupropion HCl
extended release tablets
GlaxoSmithKline
†XANAX®
0.25 mg
0.5 mg
1.0 mg
2.0 mg
alprazolam
Upjohn
YOCON®
5.4 mg
yohimbine HCl
Palisades Pharmaceutical
ZOLOFT®
100 mg
50 mg
sertraline HCl
Roerig
†ZONEGRAN®
100 mg
zonisamide
Elan
ZYPREXA®
LILLY 4115
5 mg
LILLY 4116
7.5 mg
LILLY 4117
10 mg
olanzapine
Eli Lilly

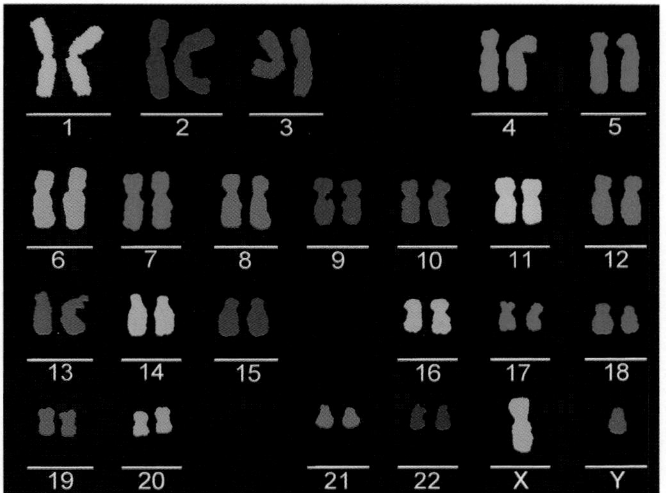

FIGURE 1.10–2 The human karyotype. The normal human genetic material contains two copies of the three billion DNA-base genomic sequence packaged into 22 matched pairs of autosomes and X and Y sex chromosomes. Here the human karyotype has been stained using different-colored chromosome-specific probes. Identical twins share identical copies of genomic DNA. (Adapted from Bentley D. *The Geography of Our Genome*. Supplement to *Nature*, 2001, with permission.)

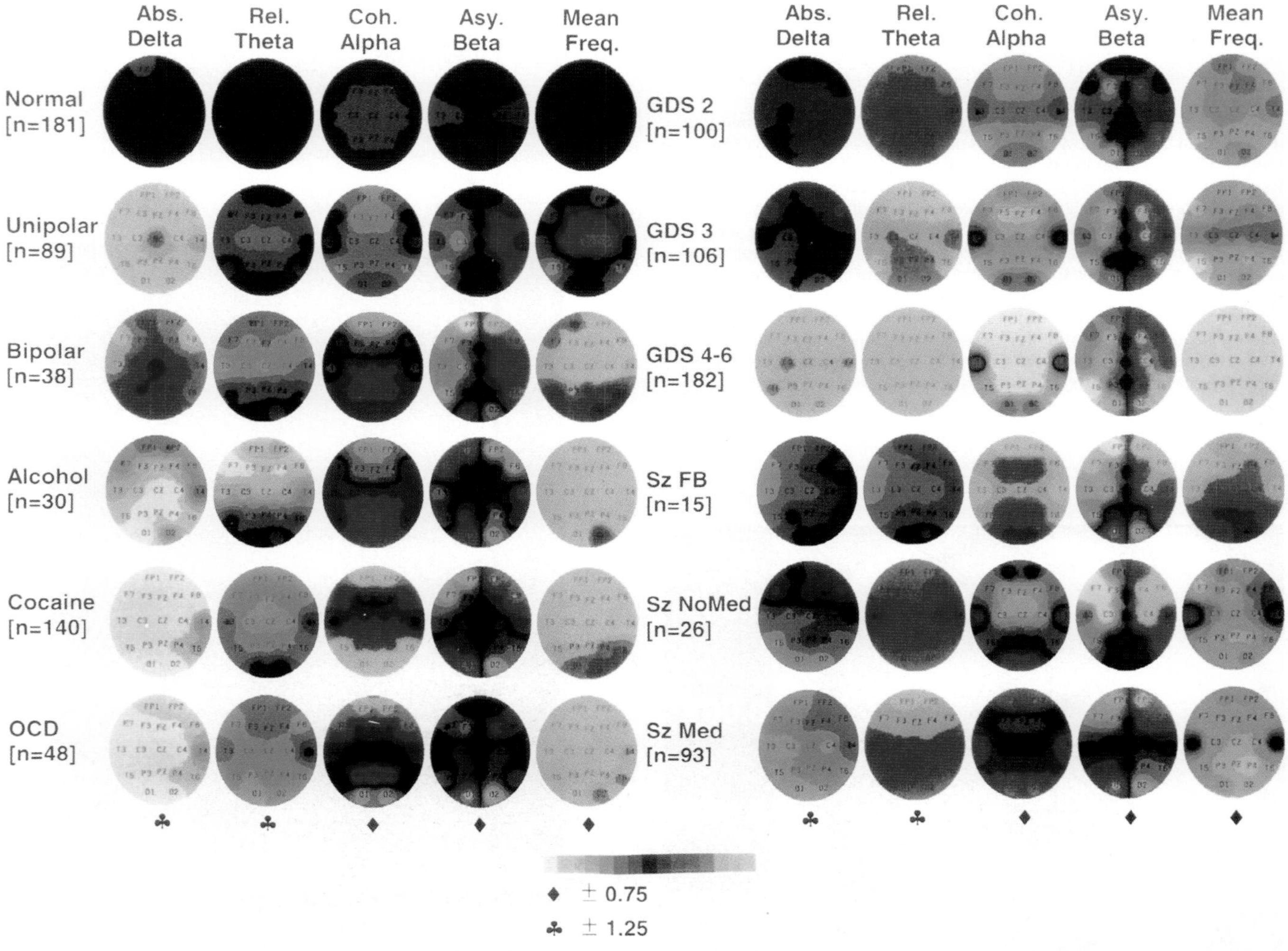

Abs. Delta | Rel. Theta | Coh. Alpha | Asy. Beta | Mean Freq.

Normal [n=181]
Unipolar [n=89]
Bipolar [n=38]
Alcohol [n=30]
Cocaine [n=140]
OCD [n=48]

GDS 2 [n=100]
GDS 3 [n=106]
GDS 4-6 [n=182]
Sz FB [n=15]
Sz NoMed [n=26]
Sz Med [n=93]

♦ ± 0.75
♣ ± 1.25

FIGURE 1.14–20 Baseline group average topographic images of *z* scores for selected quantitative electroencephalography (QEEG) features in different *Diagnostic and Statistical Manual of Mental Disorders*, 4th edition, text revision, psychiatric populations. Successive columns in the left and right panels include absolute (Abs.) power delta, relative (Rel.) power theta, interhemispheric coherence (Coh.) alpha, interhemispheric power asymmetry (Asy.) beta, and total power mean frequency (Freq.). Populations include normal adults; unipolar depressions; bipolar depressions; alcoholics (in withdrawal); cocaine-dependent subjects (5 to 14 days after last drug use); obsessive-compulsive disorder (OCD); global deterioration scale (GDS) 2, which are normal elderly with only subjective cognitive complaints; GDS 3, which meet criteria for mild cognitive impairment; GDS 4 through 6, which meet criteria for dementia; first-break schizophrenics (Sz FB); schizophrenics off medication (Sz NoMed); and schizophrenics on medication (Sz Med). The color scale of each *z* image is in standard deviation units, with a range of +0.75, indicated with a diamond, or +1.25, indicated with a club. To estimate the significance of any regional *z* score for this group average data, the *z* score should be multiplied by the square root of the number of patients in the group. For a group with 100 subjects, the *z* value imaged should be multiplied by 10 to get the estimate of the significance of that *z*. (Courtesy of Dr. E. Roy John, Director, Brain Research Laboratories, Department of Psychiatry, New York University School of Medicine, New York, NY and Nathan S. Kline Institute for Psychiatric Research, Orangeburg, NY.)

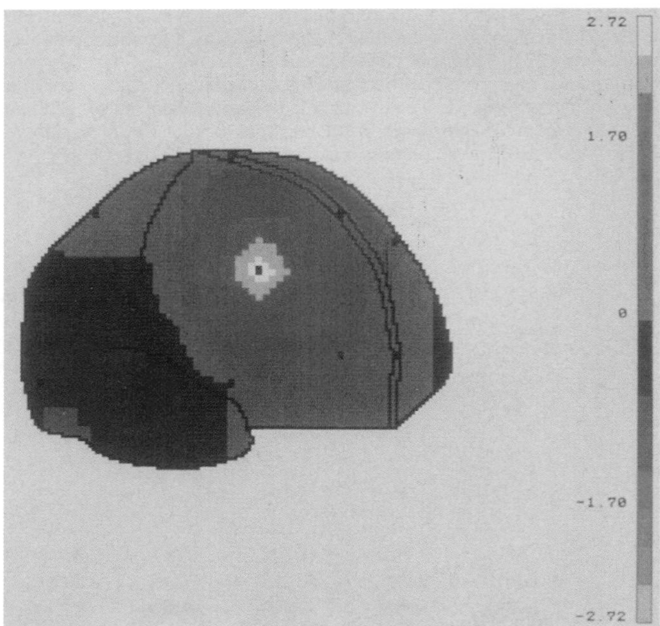

FIGURE 1.14–22 Topographic quantitative electroencephalography map of theta absolute power (*z* score departures from normative database mean). Closed head injury, male patient, 24 years of age. Focus of increased theta voltage is at the locus of an earlier head injury that occurred approximately 2 years before the recording. This was an unexpected finding. After recording and quantification, the color bar scale was adjusted to maximize the bull's-eye localization effect. Theta voltage was also elevated to a lesser extent over a wide, right frontal area and even spread somewhat across the midline. Theta relative power (not shown) was also elevated over the right frontal region, but mapping did not produce a sharp relative power focus at the locus of injury. Important note: A sharply defined bull's-eye can also be produced by artifact from a faulty electrode, and it is imperative to monitor electrical impedance and to check the integrity of the electrode in the event that deviant activity appears confined to only one lead with no spread to adjoining electrodes.

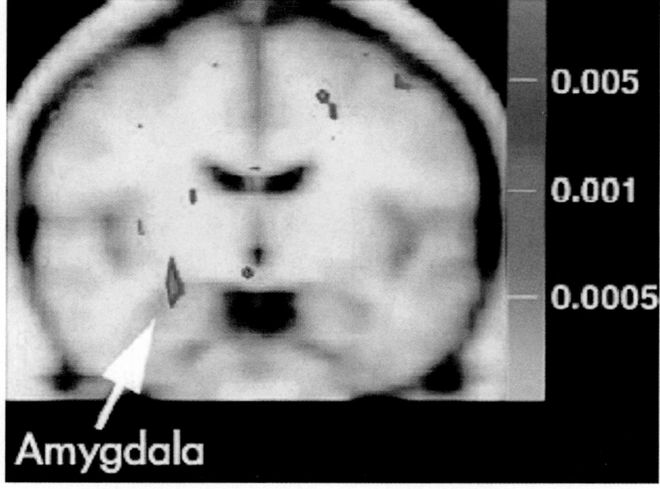

FIGURE 1.15–8 Statistical map of functional magnetic resonance imaging (fMRI) blood oxygenation level–dependent signal intensity differences demonstrating significantly increased activity in the right amygdala in subjects with posttraumatic stress disorder (PTSD) compared to traumatized subjects without PTSD. The response to masked, fearful faces in PTSD and non-PTSD group were compared after normalizing to masked, happy faces. fMRI data are displayed in Talairach template space and are co-registered with structural magnetic resonance imaging data.

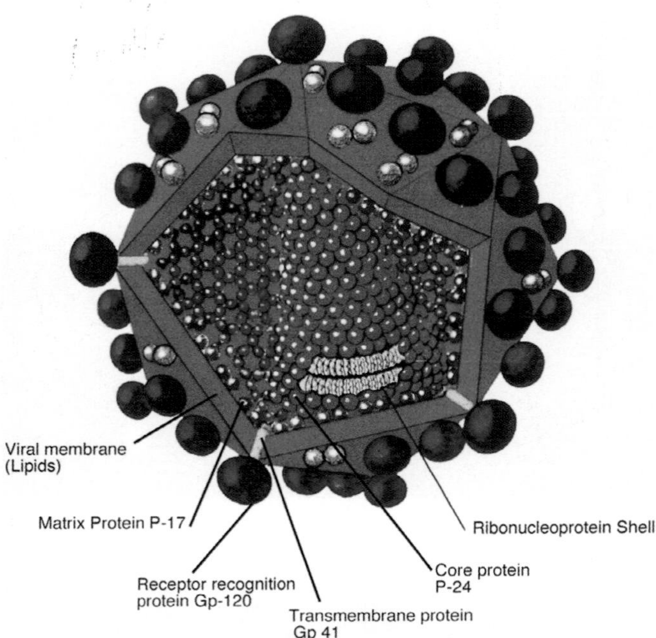

FIGURE 2.8–1 Human immunodeficiency virus viral particle with its lipid envelope. (Courtesy of Milan V. Nermut, M.D., Ph.D., D.Sc.)

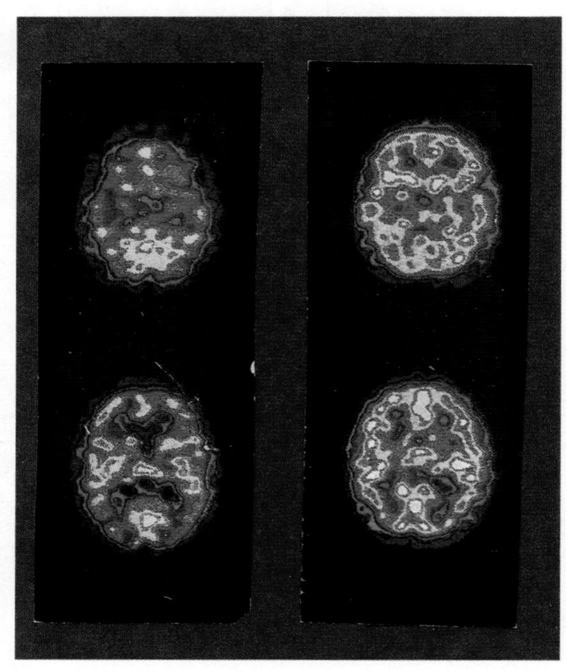

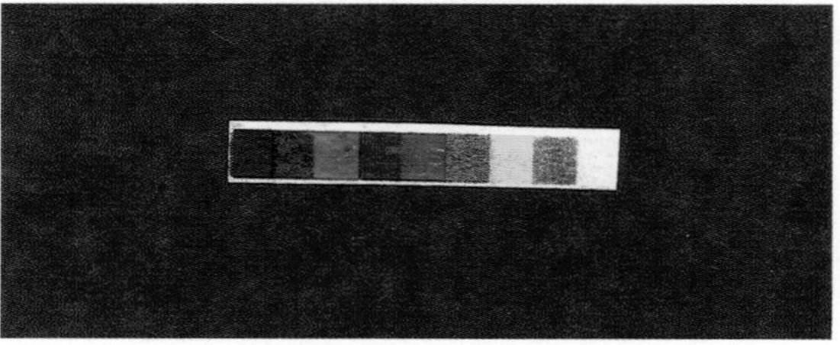

FIGURE 2.9–1 Single photon emission computed tomography scan image demonstrating multiple areas of decreased blood flow in a Lyme disease patient compared to a healthy control.

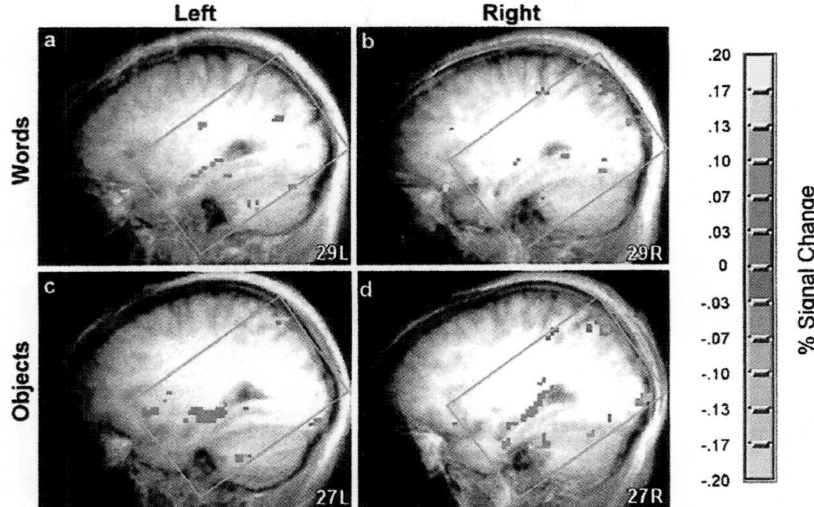

FIGURE 3.4–11 Activity in the left and right hippocampal regions measured with functional magnetic resonance imaging (fMRI) during declarative memory retrieval. Data were collected from 11 participants who saw words at study and test and from 11 different participants who saw pictures of namable objects at study and test. Recognition memory accuracy was 80.2 percent correct for words and 89.9 percent correct for objects. Areas of significant fMRI signal change (targets vs. foils) are shown in sagittal sections as color overlays on averaged structural images. The green box indicates the area in which reliable data were available for all subjects. With words, retrieval-related activity was observed in the hippocampus on the left side **(a)** but not on the right side **(b)**. With namable objects, retrieval-related activity was observed in the hippocampus on the left side **(c)** and the right side **(d)**. [From Stark CE, Squire LR: Functional magnetic resonance imaging (fMRI) activity in the hippocampal region during recognition memory. *J Neurosci.* 2000;20:7776.]

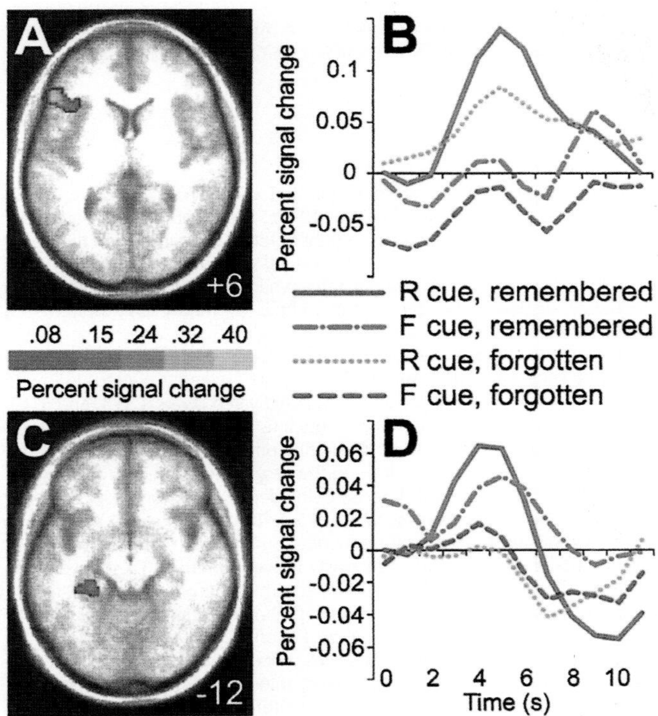

FIGURE 3.4–12 Functional activations of prefrontal and medial temporal regions that were predictive of later memory performance. Single words were presented visually, each followed by an instruction to remember (R cue) or to forget (F cue). Trials were sorted based on the remember or forget instruction and on subsequent recognition performance. Activity in left inferior prefrontal cortex and left hippocampus was predictive of subsequent recognition but for different reasons. Left inferior prefrontal activation **(A)** was associated with the encoding attempt, in that responses were largest for trials with a cue to remember, whether or not the word was actually recognized later. The time course of activity in this region **(B)** was computed based on responses that were time locked to word onset (time 0). Left inferior prefrontal activity increased for words that were later remembered, but there was a stronger association with encoding attempt, as responses were larger for words followed by an R cue that were later forgotten than for words followed by an F cue that were later remembered. In contrast, left parahippocampal and posterior hippocampal activation **(C)** was associated with encoding success. As shown by the time course of activity in this region **(D)**, responses were largest for words that were subsequently remembered, whether the cue was to remember or to forget. (From Reber PJ, Siwiec RM, Gitelman DR, et al.: Neural correlates of successful encoding identified using functional magnetic resonance imaging. *J Neurosci.* 2002;22:9541, with permission. Copyright 2002 by the Society for Neuroscience.)

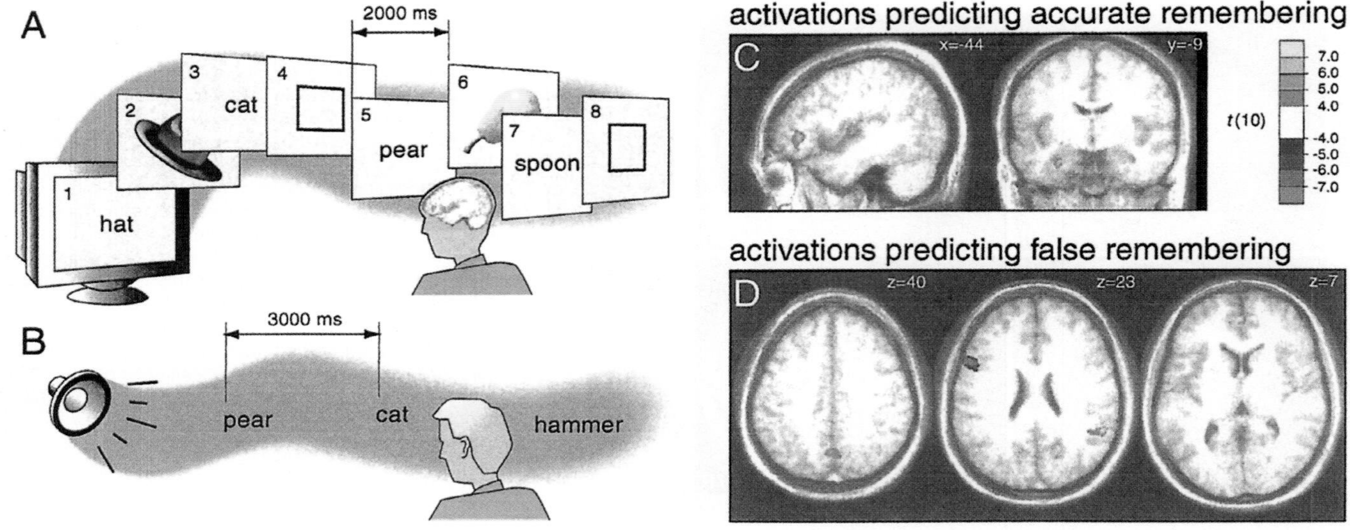

FIGURE 3.4–13 Neural substrates of false memories. **A:** Functional magnetic resonance imaging data were acquired in a learning phase, when subjects read names of objects and visualized the referents. One-half of the names were followed 2 seconds later by a picture of the object. **B:** In a surprise memory test given outside the scanner, subjects listened to object names and decided whether they had seen a picture of the corresponding object. On some trials, subjects claimed to have seen a picture of an object that they had only imagined. **C:** Results showed that left inferior prefrontal cortex and left anterior hippocampus were more active during learning in response to pictures later remembered compared to pictures later forgotten. **D:** Several different brain areas showed a greater response to words in the learning phase that were later falsely remembered as pictures, compared to words not misremembered. Activations that predicted false remembering were found in a brain network important for the generation of visual imagery in response to object names (precuneus, inferior parietal cortex, and anterior cingulate, shown in **left**, **middle**, and **right** images, respectively). (From Gonsalves B, Reber PJ, Gitelman DR, et al.: Event-related fMRI reveals brain activity at encoding that predicts true and false memory for visual objects. *Soc Neurosci Abstr.* 2001, with permission.)

FIGURE 3.6–2 ▶ **A:** Voltage imaging of cortical brain activity in a rodent slice. **Upper left panel:** Averaged snapshots at 5 and 10 milliseconds to stimulation at 10 Hz. **Lower left and right panels:** Averaged snapshots at 5 and 10 milliseconds in response to stimulation at 40 Hz. The color of the image represents membrane potential of the stained neurons, depolarized (*red*) and hyperpolarized (*purple*) (see color bar to the right). Dotted lines indicated the upper and lower cortical borders in the slice. White dots represent the position of the bipolar stimulating electrodes at the subcortical white matter. Note that, at 10 milliseconds after the start of 10-Hz stimulation, the cortical activity covered most of the cortex in the slice **(upper left)**, whereas, at 40 Hz, the activation became columnar, demonstrating that the geometry of cortical activation is frequency dependent. (Adapted from Llinás R, Ribary U, Contreras D, Pedroarena C: The neuronal basis for consciousness. *Philos Trans R Soc Lond.* 1998;353:1841–1849.) **B:** Voltage imaging of thalamocortical activation in the rodent brain slice. Average of a set of single pulse stimulation of thalamic nuclei. Centrolateral (CL) **(left panel)** and ventrobasal (VB) **(right panel)**. The spread of activity after CL and VB stimulation is superimposed on the Nissl's method–stained brain slice. CL and VB stimulation activated reticular nucleus followed by striatum. A different set of patterns of cortical activation was observed for each stimulation site. Although VB stimulation activated layers 4, 2/3, and 5, CL stimulation activated layers 6, 7, and 1. Left and right insets correspond to individual pixel profiles at reticular thalamic nucleus (RTN) (*white lines*), striatum-putamen (Str/Pu) (*blue lines*), layer 5 (*green lines*), and layer 1 (*red lines*) after CL and VB stimulation, respectively, illustrating differences in the latencies. The average delay between the site of stimulation and the point of recording (measured as time between the stimulus and the beginning of the individual pixel responses) is shown in the table under each slice. (Adapted from Llinás R, Leznik E, Urbano IF: Temporal binding via coincidence detection of specific and non-specific thalamocortical inputs: A voltage dependent dye imaging study in mouse brain slices. *Proc Natl Acad Sci U S A.* 2002;99:449–454.) **C:** Voltage imaging of thalamocortical temporal binding in the rodent brain slice. Optically recorded in response to gamma-frequency stimulation in the somatosensory cortex, in response to ten stimuli to CL **(upper panel)**, VB **(middle panel)**, and VB and CL thalamic nuclei simultaneously **(lower panel)**. The response to the fifth stimulus was imaged in each case. Note the marked summation of the response when CL and VB stimuli are presented simultaneously. On the right, the profiles of a single pixel taken from layer 5 are shown for the three different stimulation conditions. Summation was supralinear. (Adapted from Llinás R, Leznik E, Urbano IF: Temporal binding via coincidence detection of specific and non-specific thalamocortical inputs: A voltage dependent dye imaging study in mouse brain slices. *Proc Natl Acad Sci U S A.* 2002;99:449–454.) **D:** Diagram of two thalamocortical systems. Specific sensory or motor nuclei project to cortex layer 4, producing cortical oscillation by direct activation and feedforward inhibition via 40-Hz inhibitory interneurons. Collaterals of these projections produce thalamic feedback inhibition via the reticular nucleus. The return pathway (*circular arrow on the right*) returns this oscillation to specific- and reticularis-thalamic nuclei via pyramidal cells in layer 6 (*blue*). The second loop shows nonspecific intralaminar nuclei projecting to the most superficial layer of the cortex and giving collaterals to the reticular nucleus. Pyramidal cells in layer 5 return the oscillation to the reticular and the nonspecific thalamic nuclei, establishing a second resonant loop. The conjunction of the specific and nonspecific loops is proposed to generate temporal cognitive binding. (Adapted from Llinás R, Leznik E, Urbano IF: Temporal binding via coincidence detection of specific and non-specific thalamocortical inputs: A voltage dependent dye imaging study in mouse brain slices. *Proc Natl Acad Sci U S A.* 2002;99:449–454.) **E:** Magnetoencephalography data from a thalamocortical dysrhythmia (TCD) patient. Power spectra **(upper panels)** and coherence plots **(lower panels)** are displayed. **Top left panel:** Averaged power spectra from control subjects (*blue*) and a TCD patient (*red*). A peak shift into the theta domain and power increase in the theta and beta bands are demonstrated for TCD patients in comparison to controls. **Top right panel:** Power spectrum of a schizoaffective patient presurgery (*red*) and after microsurgery (*blue*). **Bottom panels:** Coherence determined by cross-correlation analysis of the variation along time of the spectral power for frequencies between 0 and 40 Hz. Left panel shows results from a control subject. The middle and right panels illustrate pre- and postsurgical coherence results for the power spectrum shown in the upper right panel. (Adapted from Llinás R, Ribary U, Jeanmonod D, et al.: Thalamocortical dysrhythmia I: Functional and imaging aspects. *Thalamus Related Syst.* 2001;1:237–244.) **F:** Magnetoencephalography source localization for a schizoaffective patient before and after selective miniablation. Projection of 4- to 10-Hz activity onto a magnetic resonance image of the whole brain, before **(top images)** and after **(bottom images)** surgery. The TCD of this patient was localized in the right-sided paralimbic domain comprising the temporopolar, anterior parahippocampal, orbitofrontal, and basal medial prefrontal areas. This low-frequency focus disappears postsurgically. (Adapted from Jeanmonod D, Schulman J, Ramirez R, et al.: Neuropsychiatric thalamocortical dysrythmia: Surgical implications. *Thalamus Related Syst.* 2003;2:103–113.)

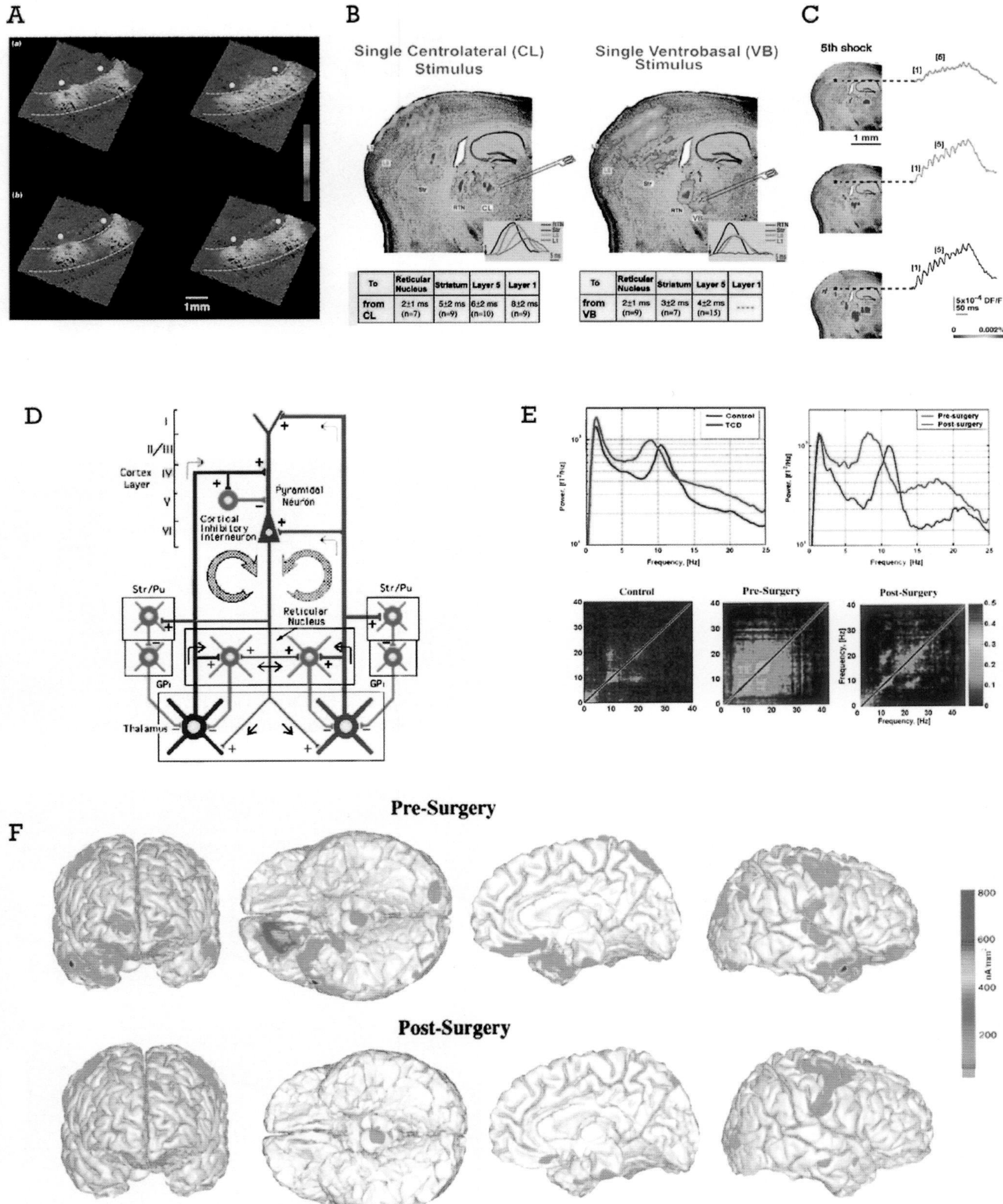

A
(a)
(b)
1mm
B
Single Centrolateral (CL) Stimulus
Single Ventrobasal (VB) Stimulus
RTN
CL
VB
To | Reticular Nucleus | Striatum | Layer 5 | Layer 1
from CL | 2±1 ms (n=7) | 5±2 ms (n=9) | 6±2 ms (n=10) | 8±2 ms (n=9)
To | Reticular Nucleus | Striatum | Layer 5 | Layer 1
from VB | 2±1 ms (n=9) | 3±2 ms (n=7) | 4±2 ms (n=15) | ----
C
5th shock
[1]
[5]
1 mm
50 ms
0
0.002%
D
I
II/III
Cortex Layer
IV
V
VI
Pyramidal Neuron
Cortical Inhibitory Interneuron
Str/Pu
GPi
Reticular Nucleus
Thalamus
E
Control
TCD
Pre-surgery
Post-surgery
Frequency, [Hz]
Control
Pre-Surgery
Post-Surgery
Frequency, [Hz]
F
Pre-Surgery
Post-Surgery
800
600
400
200

FIGURE 5.4–6 Mutual clinging by peer-reared juvenile monkeys. Attachment relationships of these infants are almost always anxious in nature. (Courtesy of Stephen Suomi, Ph.D.)

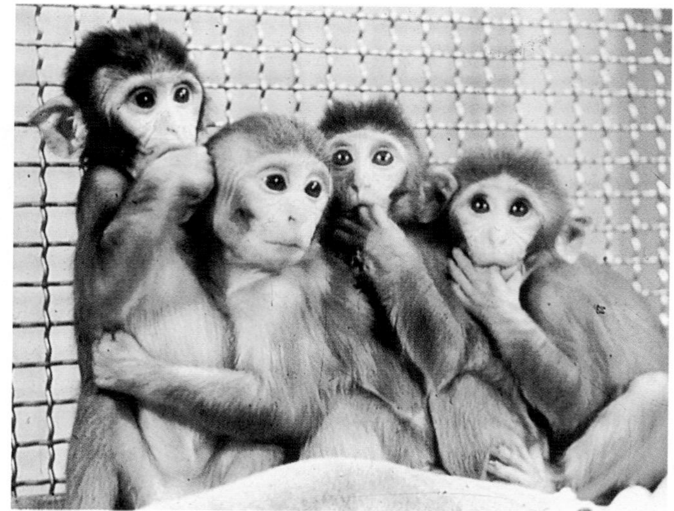

FIGURE 11.3–1 Positron emission tomography scan showing striatal dopamine transporter density in a 33-year-old male methamphetamine (METH) abuser 80 days after detoxification, compared to a 33-year-old male control subject. (From Volkow ND, Chang L, Wang G-J, et al.: Association of dopamine transporter reduction with psychomotor impairment in methamphetamine abusers. *Am J Psychiatry*. 2001;158:377, with permission.)

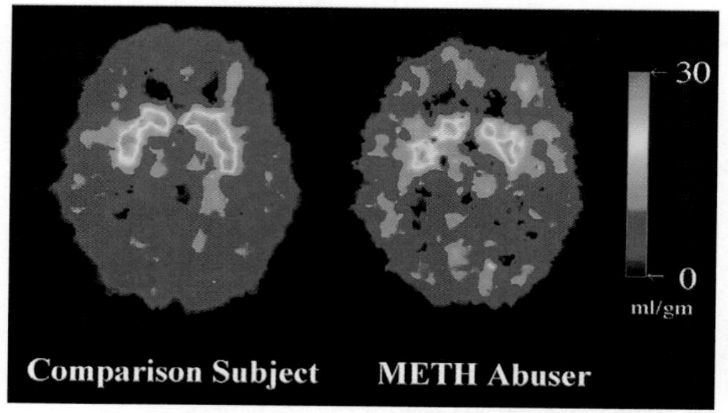

FIGURE 12.1–1 Axial sections demonstrating brain areas with significantly increased activity during auditory verbal hallucinations in the group study. Functional positron emission tomography (PET) results (threshold at Z >3.09, *P* <.001, by reference to the unit normal distribution) are displayed, superimposed on a single structural T1-weighted magnetic resonance imaging scan that has been transformed into the Talairach space for anatomical reference. Section numbers refer to the distance from the anterior commissure–posterior commissure line, with positive numbers being superior to the line. The areas of activation extend into the amygdala bilaterally and into the right orbitofrontal cortex. Although these regions of extension are consistent with the limbic paralimbic component of activity during hallucinations and may contribute to drive and affect in this context, definitive statements cannot be made in the absence of discrete maxima. (From Silbersweig DA, Stern E, Frith C, et al.: A functional neuroanatomy of hallucinations in schizophrenia. *Nature*. 1995;378:1769; with permission.)

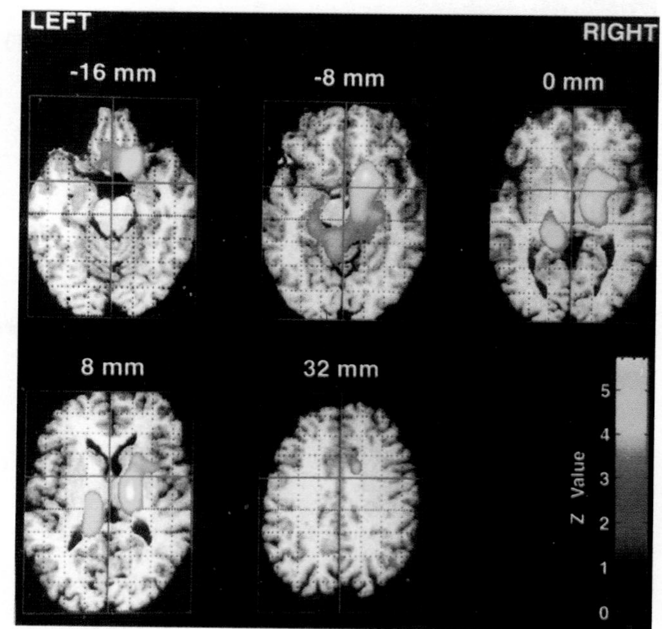

Sensory-Motor Control Task Minus Rest

20 mm

32 mm

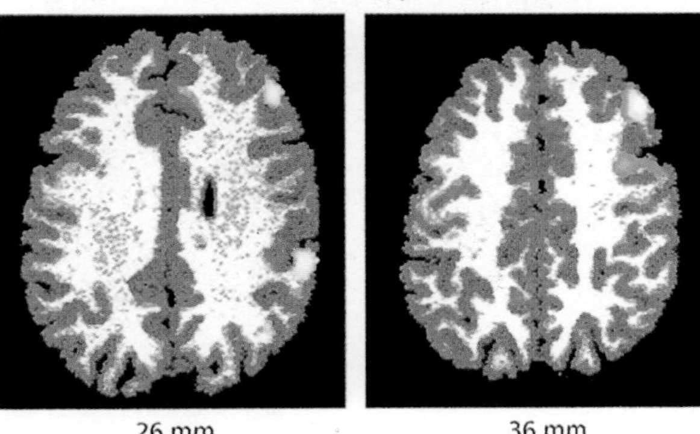

FIGURE 12.1–2 Brain regions activated more in ten schizophrenic patients without primary negative symptoms than in eight patients with primary negative symptoms deficit schizophrenia during a sensory-motor control task and a decision task. As shown in the **left panel**, the regions significantly more activated in nondeficit than deficit patients during the control task were the right and left middle frontal cortex. Right cluster size: 104 voxels with a maximum Z score of 2.61. Left cluster size: 316 voxels with a maximum Z score of 3.98. As shown in the **right panel**, the regions significantly more activated in the nondeficit patients during the decision task were the right middle frontal two clusters and inferior parietal cortices. Right frontal cluster sizes: 299 voxels with a maximum Z score of 4.81 and 138 voxels with a maximum Z score of 3.28. Right inferior parietal cluster size: 185 voxels with a maximum Z score of 3.32. (From Lahti AC, Holcomb HH, Medoff DR: Abnormal patterns of regional cerebral blood flow in schizophrenia with primary negative symptoms during an effortful auditory recognition task. *Am J Psychiatry*. 2001;158:1797–1808, with permission.)

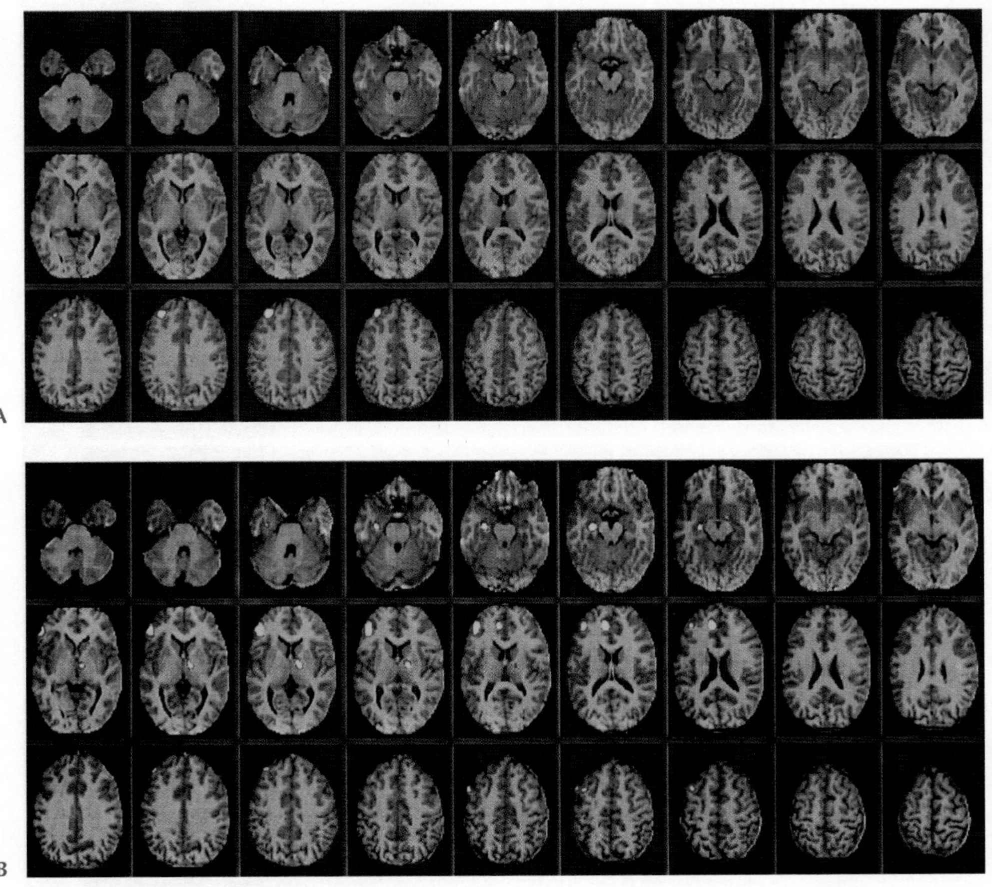

FIGURE 12.6–5 Penn Word Retrieval Test. Positron emission tomography study of memory activation in schizophrenia. **A:** During word encoding, healthy controls (N = 23) show increased activity in the left prefrontal and superior temporal regions relative to patients (N = 23). **B:** During word recognition, controls show greater activation than patients in left prefrontal, left anterior cingulate, left mesial temporal lobe, and right thalamus. (From Ragland JD, Gur RC, Raz J, et al.: Effect of schizophrenia on frontotemporal activity during word encoding and recognition: A PET cerebral blood flow study. *Am J Psychiatry*. 2001;158:1114, with permission.)

FIGURE 12.6–6 Functional magnetic resonance imaging study of emotion processing in schizophrenia, minus age discrimination. Healthy men (control [CNT]) show greater activation in the amygdala relative to men with schizophrenia (SCH). (From Gur RE, McGrath C, Chan RM, et al.: An fMRI study of facial emotion processing in schizophrenia. *Am J Psychiatry.* 2002; 159:1992, with permission.)

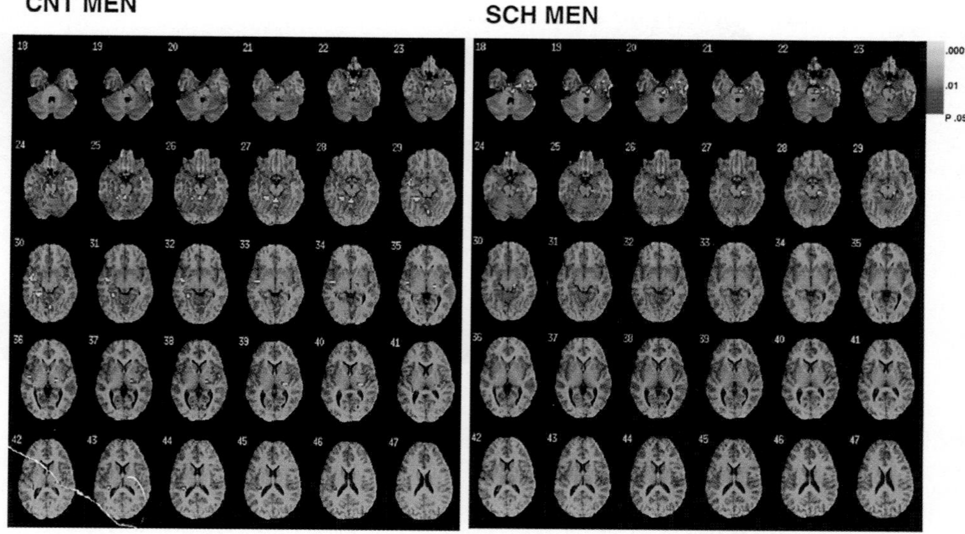

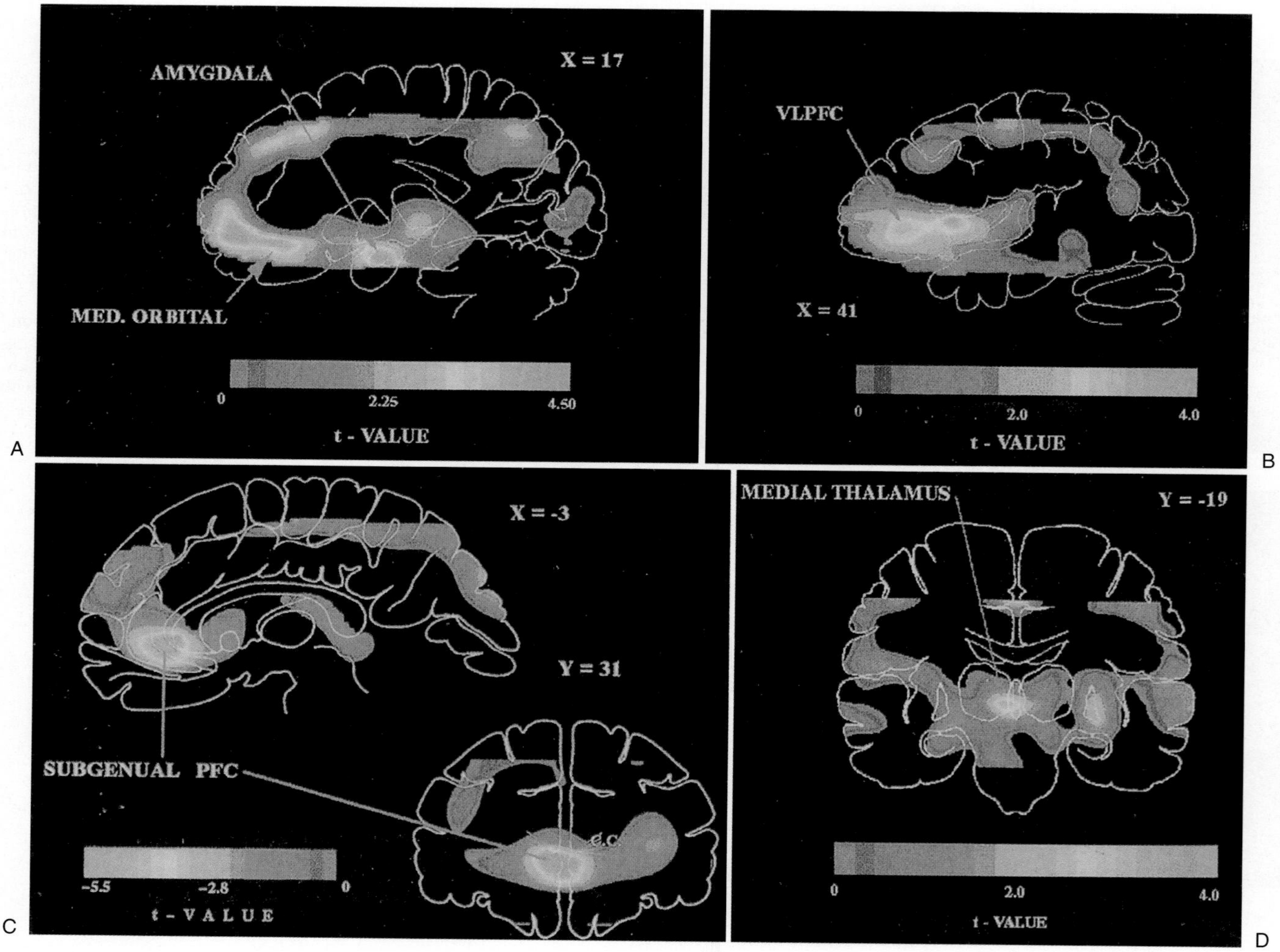

FIGURE 13.4–1 Composite coronal and sagittal sections of positron emission tomography scans show areas in which cerebral glucose metabolism is decreased in depressed patients relative to matched healthy controls. PFC, prefrontal cortex; VLPFC, ventrolateral prefrontal cortex. (From Wayne Drevets, M.D.; and from *Annu Rev Med.* 2002;49 by Annual Reviews, http://www.annualreviews.org, with permission.)

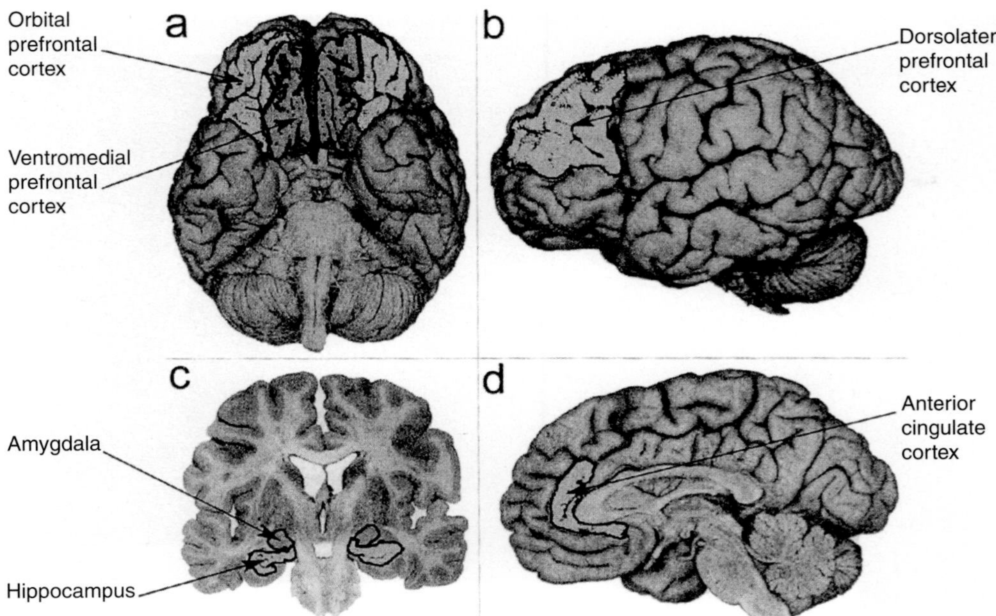

FIGURE 13.4–2 Key brain regions involved in affect and mood disorders. **a:** Orbital prefrontal cortex and the ventromedial prefrontal cortex. **b:** Dorsolateral prefrontal cortex. **c:** Hippocampus and amygdala. **d:** Anterior cingulated cortex.

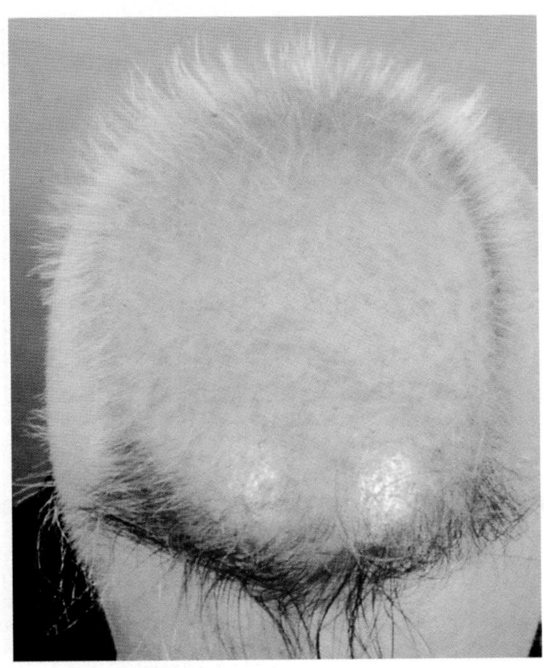

FIGURE 21–4 Example of plucking of the hair of the scalp due to trichotillomania.

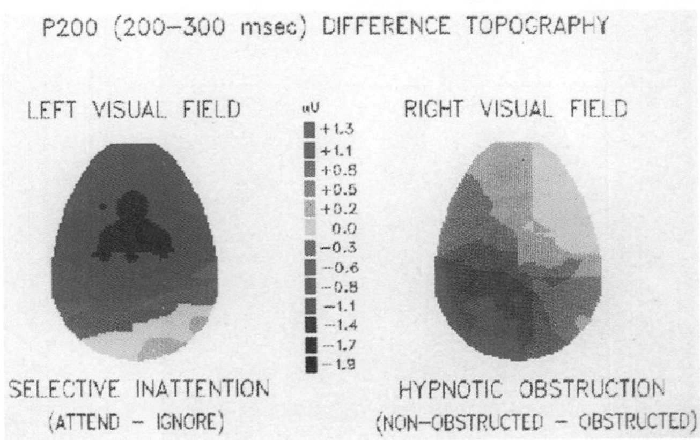

FIGURE 30.3–2 Brain electrical activity mapping of visual event-related potentials comparing the effects of selective inattention to a visual stimulus (attending to the other visual hemifield) and hypnotically hallucinating an obstruction to that stimulus. Selective inattention involves increased amplitude anteriorly, whereas hypnotic hallucination produces decreased amplitude in the occipital cortex.

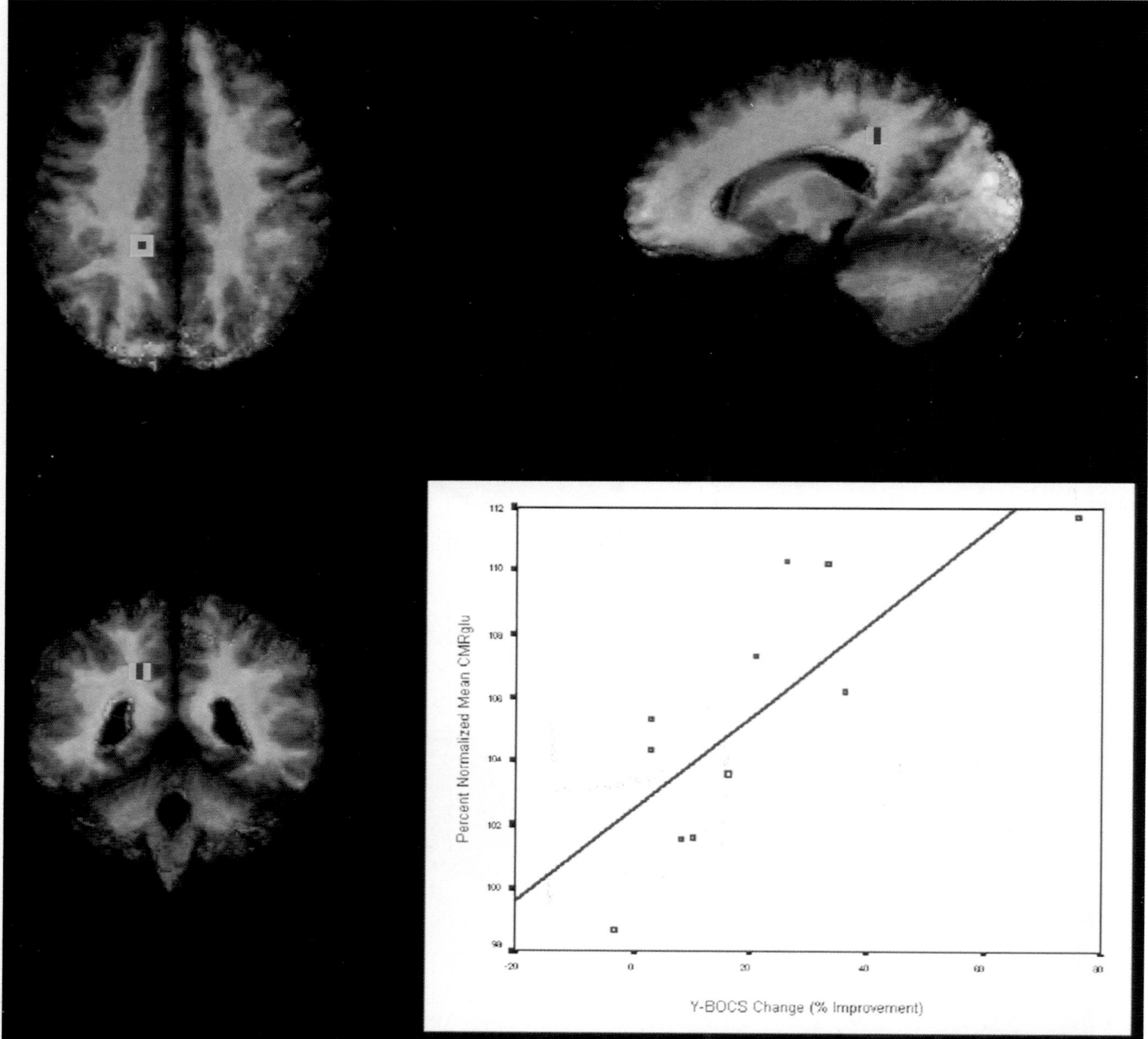

FIGURE 31.31–3 Illustration of the positron emission tomography finding of a statistically significant correlation between preoperative cerebral metabolism within right posterior cingulate cortex and Yale-Brown Obsessive Compulsive Scale (Y-BOCS) improvement after cingulotomy. Left and upper panels show the locus in brain of significant correlation, as viewed from the three conventional orthogonal perspectives. A nominally normal structural magnetic resonance image provides anatomical reference. The red voxel corresponds to the site of peak correlation (*z* score = 3.26). Together with the surrounding eight yellow voxels within the transaxial plane, this defines the region of interest used to generate the data depicted graphically *(lower right panel)*; the Pearson product moment correlation between glucose metabolism and Y-BOCS improvement yielded: $r^2(9) = .79$, $P = .002$. CMRglu, cerebral metabolic rate for glucose. (From Rauch SL, et al.: Cerebral metabolic correlates as potential predictors of response to anterior cingulotomy for obsessive compulsive disorder. *Biol Psychiatry.* 2001;50:659–667, with permission.)

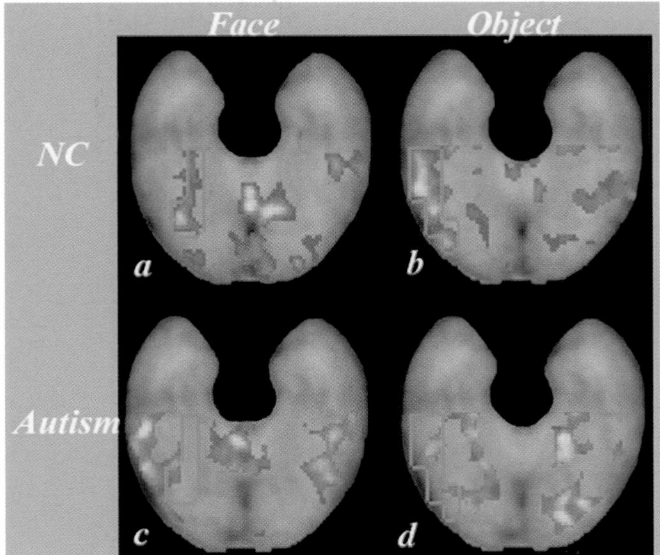

FIGURE 38–1 Composite functional magnetic resonance image comparing a group of 14 normal controls (NC) and 14 individuals with autism or Asperger's syndrome (autism), matched on age and intelligence quotient. Composite images show areas preferentially activated by faces (*a,c*) and nonface objects (*b,d*). Note that the fusiform "face area" has been defined by a green box in *a*. Among individuals with autism or Asperger's syndrome, there is significant underactivation of the fusiform gyrus during face perception and compensatory activation of a region lateral to the fusiform. This more lateral region was most strongly activated by the object task among the NCs. Hypoactivation of the fusiform face area is the best-replicated functional neuroimaging finding in the literature. (Adapted from Schultz RT, Gauthier I, Klin A, et al.: Abnormal ventral temporal cortical activity during face discrimination among individuals with autism and Asperger syndrome. *Arch Gen Psychiatry*. 2000;57:331–340.)

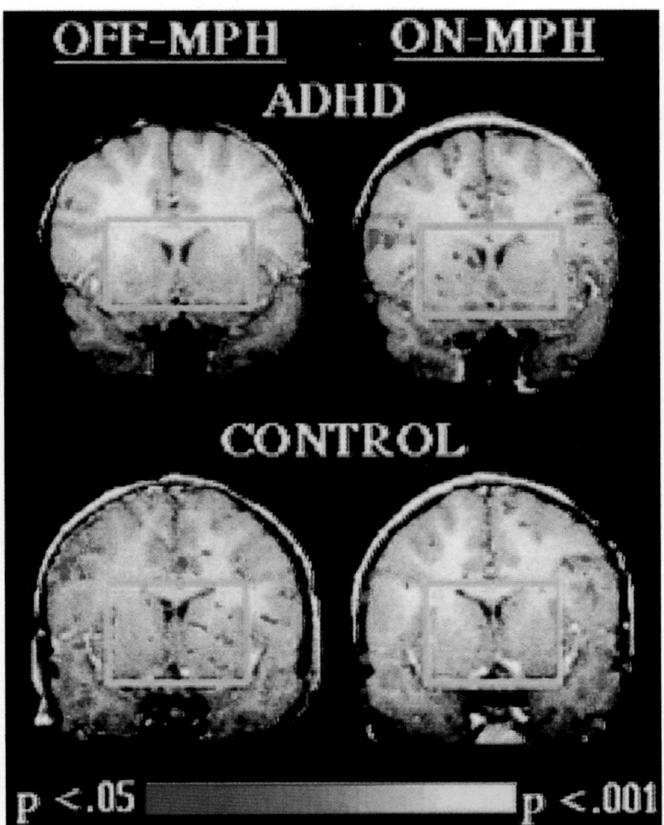

FIGURE 49.14–6 Activation during response inhibition in a coronal slice located 12 mm anterior to the anterior commissure for an attention-deficit/hyperactivity disorder (ADHD) child and a control child. Green squares highlight the opposite effect of methylphenidate (MPH) (Ritalin) in the caudate and putamen in the ADHD and control child. (From Vaidya CH, Austin G, Kirkorian G, et al.: Selective effects of methylphenidate in attention deficit hyperactivity disorder: A functional magnetic resonance study. *Proc Natl Acad Sci U S A*. 1998;95:14494, with permission.)

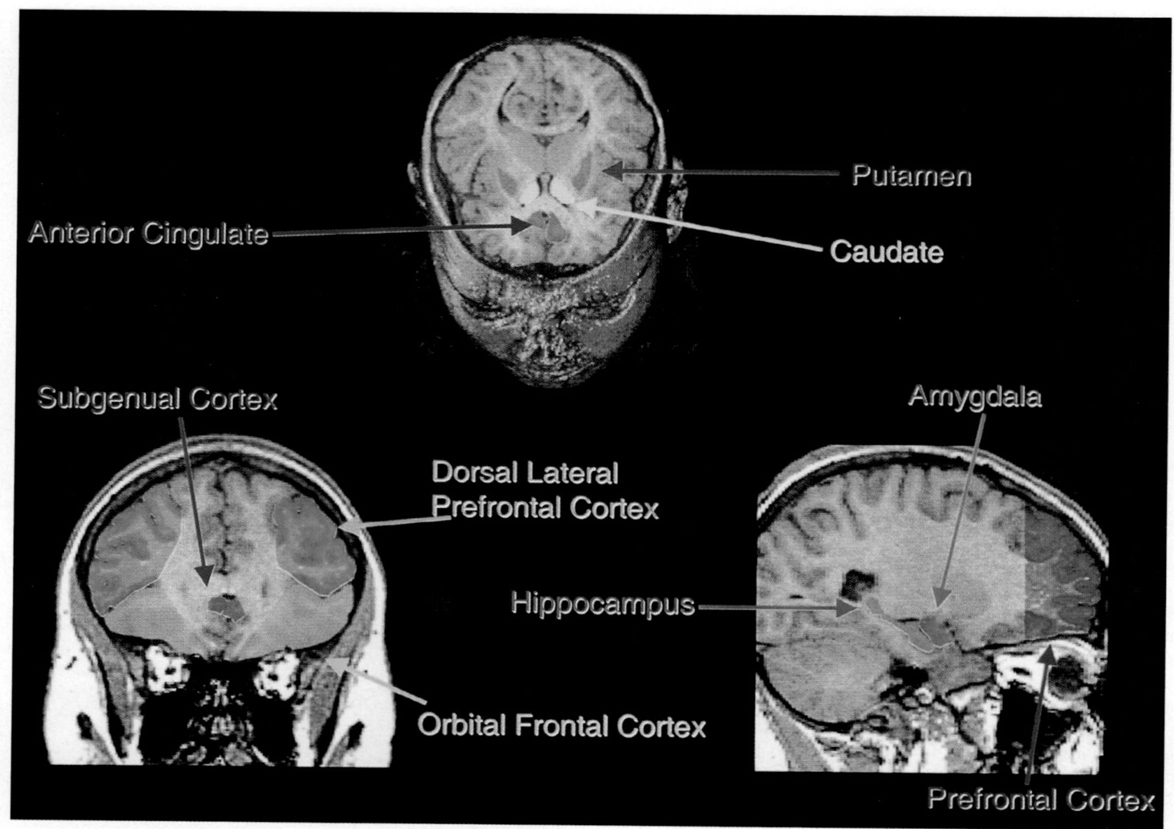

FIGURE 49.14–7 Brain regions implicated in the pathophysiology of major depressive disorder.

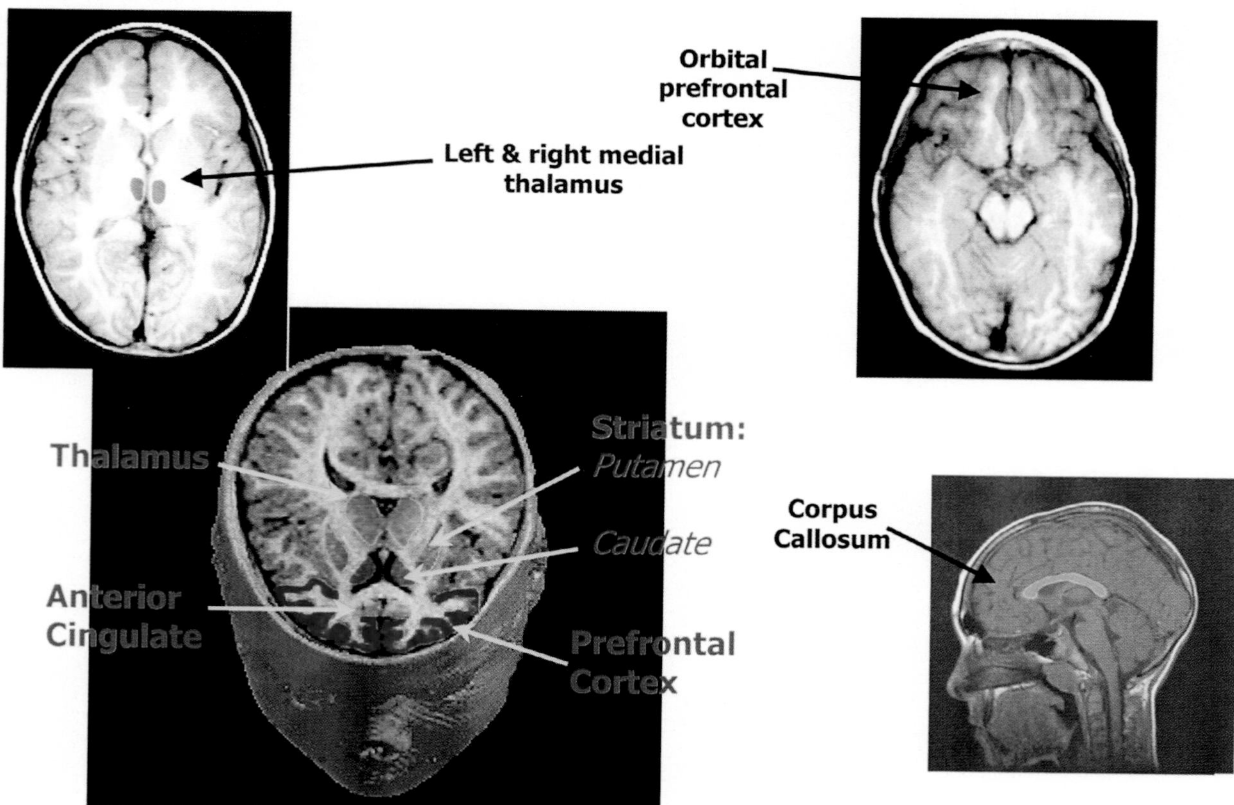

FIGURE 49.14–9 Brain regions implicated in the pathophysiology of obsessive-compulsive disorder. (From Rosenberg DR, MacMillan SN, Moore GJ: Brain anatomy and chemistry may predict treatment response in paediatric obsessive-compulsive disorder. *Int J Neuropsychopharmacol.* 2001;4:179, with permission.)

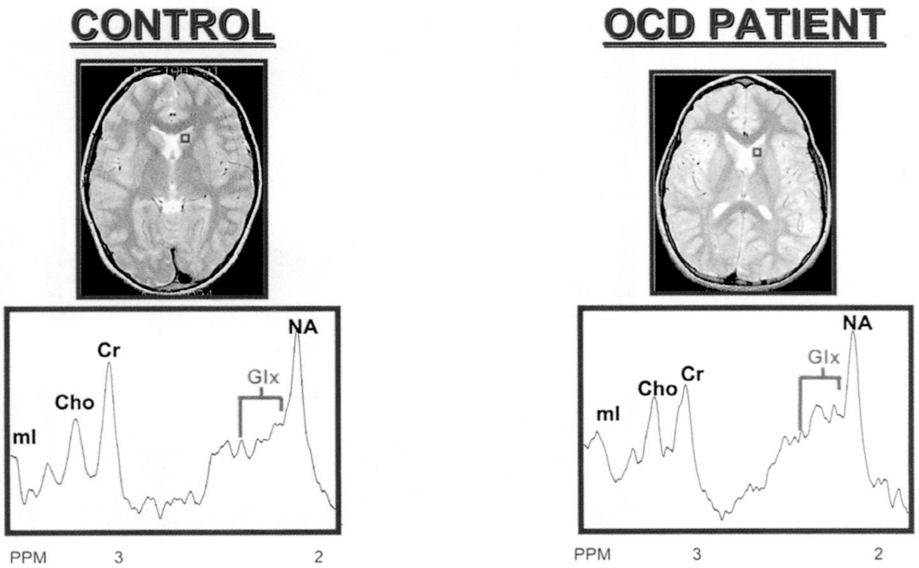

FIGURE 49.14–11 **Top:** Illustration of voxel placement in left caudate nucleus. **Bottom:** H^1-magnetic resonance spectroscopy of a 0.7-mL volume of interest centered in the left caudate in a 10-year-old healthy control and a 9-year-old treatment-naïve patient with obsessive-compulsive disorder (OCD) as shown on the T1-weighted magnetic resonance images. Cho, choline compounds; Cr, creatine/phosphocreatine; Glx, glutamate/glutamine/GABA; ml, myoinositol; NA, N-acetylaspartate. (From Rosenberg DR, MacMillan SN, Moore GJ: Brain anatomy and chemistry may predict treatment response in paediatric obsessive-compulsive disorder. *Int J Neuropsychopharmacol.* 2001;4:179, with permission.)

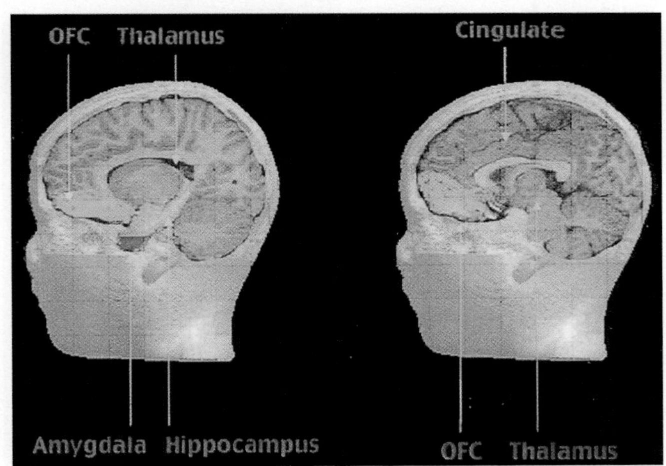

FIGURE 49.14–18 Structures such as the thalamus, cingulate, amygdala, hippocampus, and the orbitofrontal cortex (OFC) are activated in the emotion of fear. (From Rosenberg DR, Paulson LAD, MacMaster FP, et al. Neuroimaging of childhood-onset anxiety disorders. In: Ernst M, Ramsey JM, eds. *Functional Neuroimaging in Child Psychiatry.* New York: Cambridge University Press; 2000, with permission.)

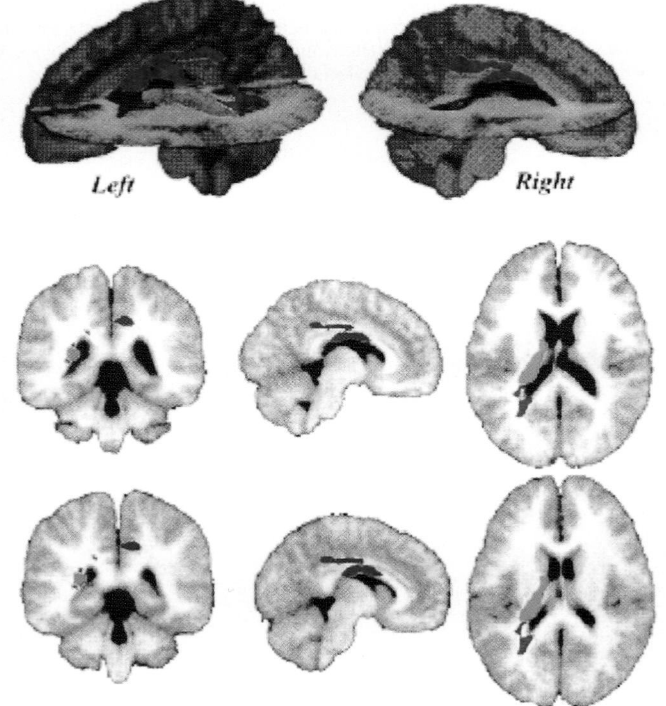

FIGURE 49.14–21 Left and right hemisphere views showing the three-dimensional renderings of the significant clusters from the gray matter (*blue*), white matter (*red*), and cerebrospinal fluid (CSF) (*green*). Statistical parametric maps were mapped into the average brain space for nine childhood-onset schizophrenia patients. **Middle:** Significant voxels form the gray matter (*blue*; voxel threshold $P<.01$, corrected at $P=.05$), white matter (*red*; voxel threshold $P<.01$, corrected at $P=.05$), and CSF (*green*; voxel threshold $P<.01$, corrected at $P=.05$). Statistical parametric maps mapped onto three orthogonal slices from the average schizophrenic brain, and **(bottom)** over the same three slices of the average control brain. (From Sowell ER, Toga AW, Asarnow R: Brain abnormalities observed in childhood-onset schizophrenia: a review of the structural magnetic resonance imaging literature. *Mental Retard Devel Disabil Res Rev.* 2000;6:180, with permission.)

FIGURE 51.2e–1 Whole-brain atrophy in a patient with probable Alzheimer's dementia, computed by the digital subtraction of a baseline magnetic resonance image (MRI) from an MRI acquired 1 year later. Areas in red reflect 1-year reductions in tissue volume and areas in green reflect 1-year gains (e.g., displacement in tissue volume). (Courtesy of N. Fox and colleagues.)

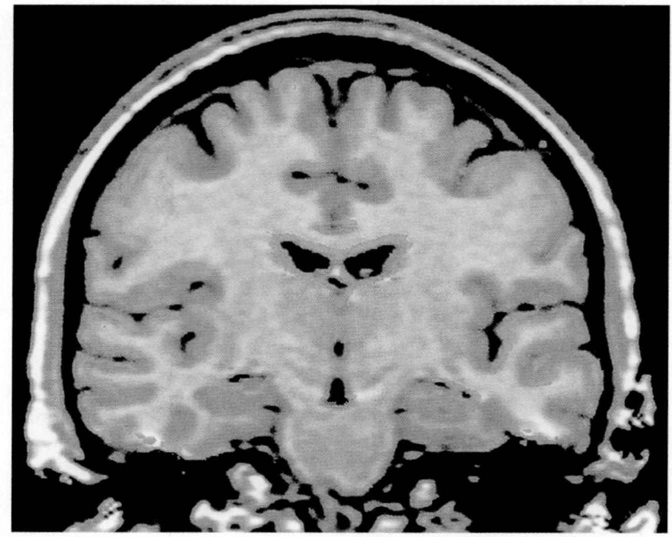

FIGURE 51.2e–2 Fluorodeoxyglucose positron emission tomography (PET) images from a normal elderly volunteer and a patient with probable Alzheimer's dementia. The arrows indicate reductions in the cerebral metabolic rate for glucose (CMRgl) in the patient, which are characteristically observed in patients with Alzheimer's dementia, including in the parietotemporal and frontal association cortices. Orange and yellow reflect higher values of CMRgl, whereas blue and green reflect relatively lower values.

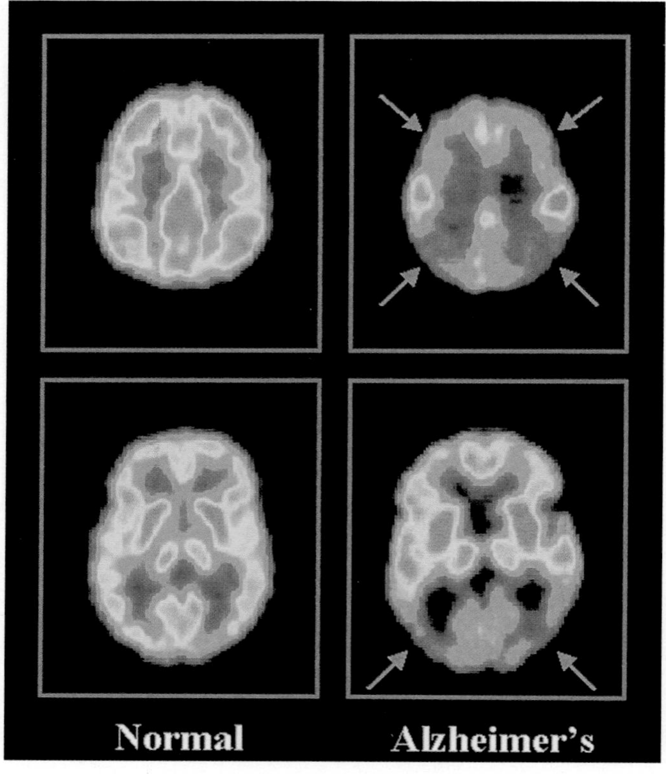

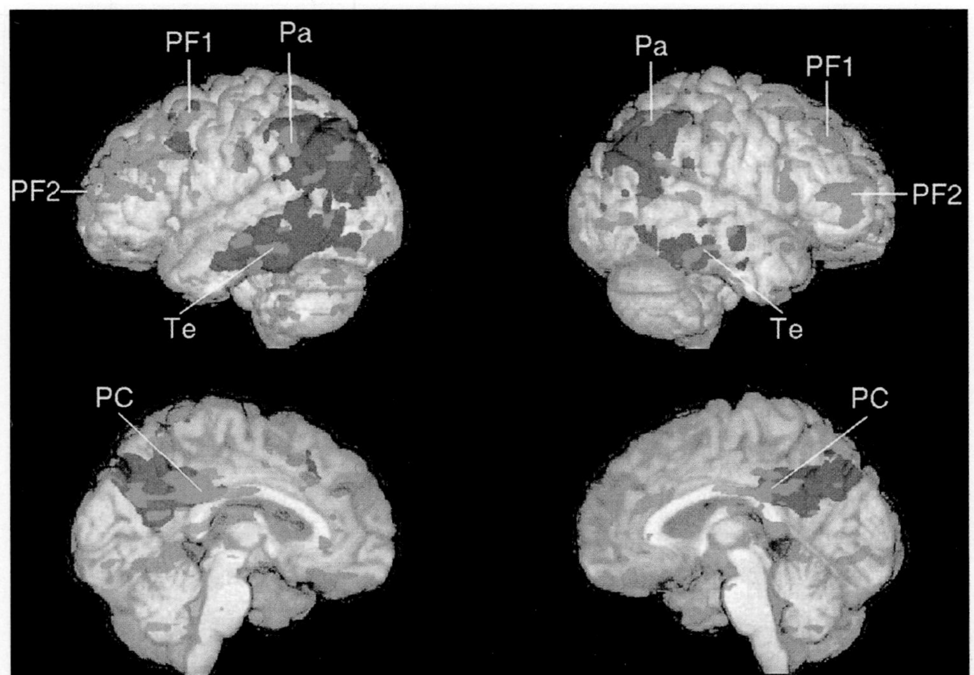

FIGURE 51.2e–3 Regions of the brain with abnormally low positron emission tomography measurements of the cerebral metabolic rate for glucose (CMRgl) in cognitively normal carriers of the apolipoprotein E (APOE) ε4 allele, a common Alzheimer's susceptibility gene. In this composite three-dimensional surface-projection map, purple areas represent abnormally low CMRgl only in the patients with probable Alzheimer's dementia (relative to their own controls); green areas represent abnormally low CMRgl only in the ε4 carriers (relative to their own controls); and blue areas reflect abnormally low CMRgl in both the ε4 carriers and patients. Like patients with probable Alzheimer's dementia, cognitively normal ε4 carriers had abnormally low CMRgl in the same regions of posterior cortex (PC), parietal cortex (Pa), temporal cortex (Te), and prefrontal cortex (PF1) as patients with probable Alzheimer's dementia; they also had abnormally low CMRgl in additional prefrontal regions (PF2), which could reflect accelerated aging. (Adapted from Reiman EM, Caselli RJ, Yun LS, et al.: Preclinical evidence of Alzheimer's disease in persons homozygous for the epsilon 4 allele for apolipoprotein E. *N Engl J Med.* 1996;334:752–758.)

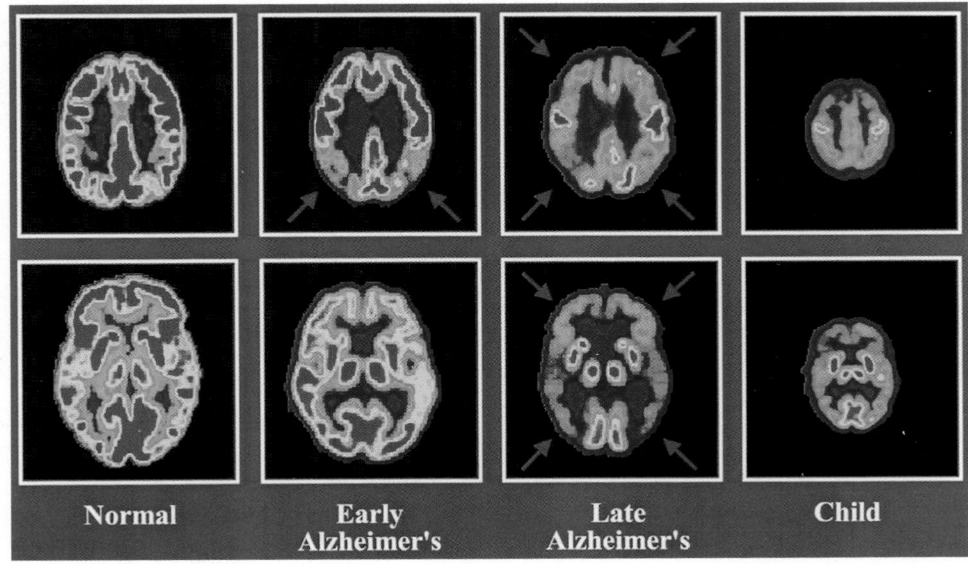

FIGURE 51.3e–1 A positron emission tomography study of glucose metabolism in Alzheimer's disease. The early Alzheimer's study was performed at the stage of questionable Alzheimer's disease and illustrates the characteristic metabolic deficits of Alzheimer's in the parietal and temporal cortices (*arrows*). Over time, the metabolic deficit spreads throughout areas of the cortex, sparing the subcortical structures, as well as the primary sensory areas, such as visual and motor cortices. At the late stage of disease, metabolic function of the brain in Alzheimer's disease is similar to that of the newborn shown to far right, which corresponds to their similar behavior and functional capacity. Magnetic resonance imaging study of the early Alzheimer's patient was normal, and the late Alzheimer's patient had some nonspecific atrophy. (Courtesy of Drs. Daniel Silverman, Gary Small, and Michael Phelps, David Geffen School of Medicine, UCLA, Los Angeles, CA.)

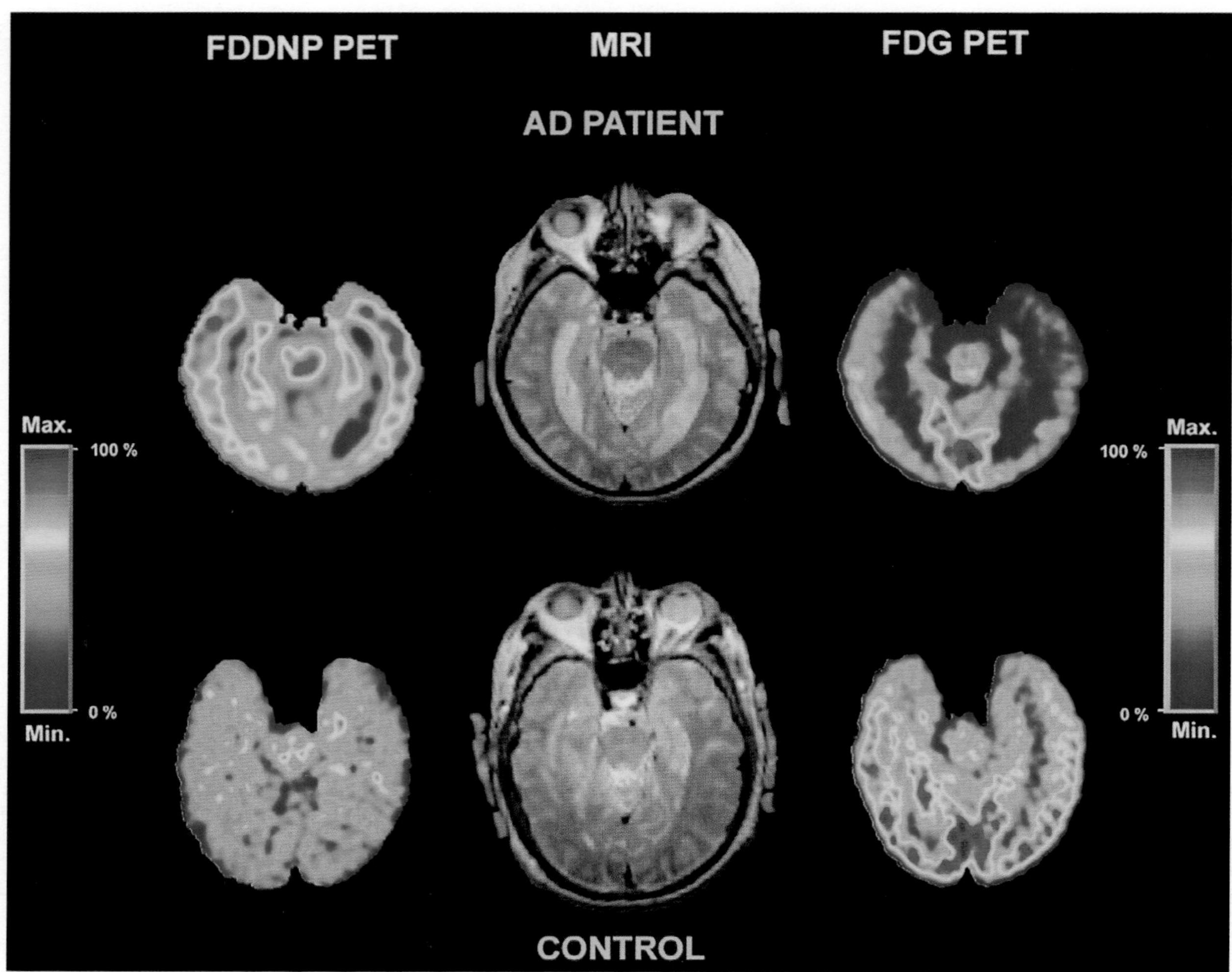

FIGURE 51.3e–2 Fluorine-1,1-dicyano-2-[6-(dimethylamino)-2-naphthalenyl]preopene (FDDNP) positron emission tomography (PET), magnetic resonance imaging (MRI), and fluorodeoxyglucose (FDG) PET images of an Alzheimer's disease (AD) patient and someone without memory loss (control). The FDDNP and FDG images of each stage are co-registered to their respective MRI images. The FDDNP PET of the Alzheimer's patient shows increased signal (*red*) in temporal memory regions compared to the control (*below*). The FDG PET shows glucose metabolism indicating how well the neurons are firing. In the Alzheimer's case (*above*), the FDG PET shows decreased neuronal activity in the brain regions in which FDDNP shows increased activity (i.e., high concentrations of plaques and tangles). (From Shoghi-Jadid K, Small GW, Agdeppa ED, et al.: Localization of neurofibrillary tangles and beta-amyloid plaques in the brains of living patients with Alzheimer disease. *Am J Geriatr Psychiatry.* 2002;10:24–35, with permission.)

1 Neural Sciences

▲ 1.1 Neural Sciences: Introduction and Overview

JACK A. GREBB, M.D.

A paradox in the ongoing effort to understand the human brain is that it is wise to know everything there is to know in the area of neural sciences, but nothing should be believed. Much like Maurits C. Escher's enigmatic illustration of a hand drawing itself, it is up to our own brains to discover and diagram how they are put together. This paradox should not be seen as nihilistic, but rather as reflecting the tremendous excitement regarding neural sciences in the 21st century, which was ushered in by the awarding of the 2000 Nobel Prize in Medicine to three neuroscientists: Arvid Carlsson, Paul Greengard, and Eric Kandel. It is the human brain, after all, that is the biological substrate for emotions, cognitive abilities, and behaviors—that is, everything that humans feel, think, and do. Every week, the scientific journals publish new insights into the neural sciences, many of which conflict with or at least modify previous observations, hypotheses, or theoretical models. Obvious oversimplifications from the past include the absolute demarcation between neurological and psychiatric disorders, the absolute categorization of brain regions as devoted to only motor or emotional activities, and the absolute dogma that axons only release neurotransmitters and dendrites only respond to neurotransmitters. Although the sections in this first chapter on neural sciences do not include everything there is to know, they do provide a framework that outlines much of what is currently known. Moreover, each of the sections provides an insight into the directions in which that particular field is evolving.

NEUROANATOMY AND NEURODEVELOPMENT

Functional neuroanatomy (discussed in Section 1.2) is the study of interacting and interdependent neurons, glia, groups of neurons and glia (e.g., nuclei), and brain regions. The three neural systems of most interest in psychiatry are the thalamocortical system, the basal ganglia, and the limbic system. Although previous generations of neuroanatomists have assigned functions, such as sensation, movement, emotion, cognition, and memory, to specific neuroanatomical structures, a general trend in neuroanatomy is to describe how networks of brain regions interact to produce what is eventually experienced or observed as feelings, thoughts, or behaviors. In addition, as another example of a change to previous dogma, it is increasingly becoming accepted that new neurons can form and function in the adult human brain, especially in regions of the limbic system, such as the hippocampus. This area of neural science is covered in Section 1.3, Neural Development and Neurogenesis, which discusses embryonic neurogenesis, the migration of neurons, and the outgrowth and formation of neuronal axons and dendrites. These developmental processes are of interest to psychiatrists because pathology in neural development might later result in clinical symptoms, or, conversely, clinical pathological states (e.g., excessive stress) could affect these very same neural development and neurogenesis processes in an adverse manner.

INTERNEURONAL MOLECULAR SIGNALS

The two methods for communication among neurons and glia are molecular (or chemical) and electrical. The four most widely recognized classes of molecular signals are the monoamines, amino acids, peptides, and the more recently discovered neurotrophic factors. Although it is reasonable to discuss each of these classes separately, as is done in this textbook, there are a number of common themes relevant to all four classes of molecular signals. First, new molecular signals are being discovered, both within these existing classes (e.g., previously unrecognized amino acid or peptide neurotransmitters), as well as in novel classes of molecular signals (e.g., nitric oxide, carbon monoxide, adenosine, adenosine triphosphate [ATP]). Second, there are hundreds of so-called orphan receptors that have been discovered through examining the sequence of the human genome. These proteins have all the characteristics of receptor proteins, but the endogenous ligands for them have not been discovered, and, in most cases, chemicals that activate or inhibit the receptor function have not yet been synthesized. Third, a general theme among both known and unknown receptors is heterogeneity, such that there are multiple subtypes of receptors for a particular neurotransmitter, such as the α-adrenergic and β-adrenergic receptors for norepinephrine. Similar to heterogeneity in receptors is heterogeneity in the deactivation of neurotransmitter molecules via multiple subtypes of deactivating enzymes (e.g., monoamine oxidase, peptidases) as well as multiple subtypes of transporter proteins (e.g., reuptake pumps). Fourth, any single neuron can release multiple different types of molecular signals (e.g., two different peptides and a monoamine) and also have receptors and receptor subtypes for multiple different molecular signals, thus making each individual neuron capable of exquisite integration and modulation of incoming and outgoing signals.

There are six classic monoamine neurotransmitters: serotonin, the three catecholamines (epinephrine, norepinephrine, and dopamine), acetylcholine, and histamine (Section 1.4). The monoamine neurotransmitters, although present in only a small percentage of neurons localized in small nuclei in the brain, have enormous impact on total brain function because the diffuse projections of axons from these monoaminergic neurons can affect virtually every brain region. In contrast to the monoamine neurotransmitters, the amino acid neurotransmitters are widely distributed in the brain, and it is possible to conceptualize the brain as reflecting the balance between the excitatory amino acid glutamate and the inhibitory amino acid γ-aminobutyric acid (GABA) (Section 1.5). In contrast to the relatively small number of different monoamine neurotransmitters and amino acid neurotransmitters, more than 100 different putative neuropeptide neurotransmitters have been identified (Section 1.6). The neurotrophic factors (Section 1.7) are a class of protein molecular signals that were more recently discovered than the other molecular signals. These proteins are involved in the growth, differentiation, maintenance, and death of neuronal and glial cells and have been demonstrated to be involved in processes such as learning, memory, and complex behaviors.

INTRANEURONAL SIGNALS

The integrative work of an individual neuron is accomplished via intraneuronal molecular signaling pathways, the modulation of the balance between external and internal concentrations of ions, and the conversion of these signals within each individual neuron into the stimulation of axon potentials, the transcription of deoxyribonucleic acid (DNA) into ribonucleic acid (RNA), and the translation of RNA into proteins. When a molecular signal binds to its specific cell surface receptor, a cascade of intraneuronal signals is initiated (Section 1.8). There are multiple interacting signaling pathways within each neuron, and these intraneuronal events should actually be considered the essential sites of action for drugs rather than merely the cell surface receptors. These complex intraneuronal signaling pathways are additional potential sites of interest for understanding the pathophysiology of neuropsychiatric disorders.

The balance between external and internal concentrations of ions is achieved by a wide array of ion channels, some of which are regulated by neurotransmitters and others by voltage gradients directly (Section 1.9). Many of the drugs of interest in psychiatry act directly on ion channels. The benzodiazepines act on GABA type A receptors that are chloride ion channels. Phencyclidine (PCP, or "angel dust") acts on a subtype of glutamate receptors that are calcium ion channels. Nicotine, the active ingredient in tobacco, acts on nicotinic acetylcholine receptors that are sodium and potassium ion channels. A more recently appreciated property of certain neurons and ion channels is the critical role of pacemaker, or oscillatory, activity in normal maintenance of wakefulness, attention, and mood.

Driving the development of the brain as well as the daily maintenance and regulation of brain function is the process of genetic expression (Section 1.10). The basic process of genetics involves the transcription of DNA into RNA and the translation of RNA into a protein. A complex system of regulation exists for transcription and translation, and the newly discovered molecules and pathways for this regulation are sites of investigation and discoveries in the etiology, pathophysiology, and treatment of mental disorders. Alterations in gene expression occur both during development and in adulthood and may be the basis of abnormal and normal development and of abnormal and normal adaptation to stress.

ENDOCRINOLOGY, IMMUNOLOGY, AND CHRONOBIOLOGY

In addition to the central nervous system (CNS), the human body contains two other systems that have a complex, internal communicative network: the endocrine system and the immune system. Mostly because of the discoveries of the involved molecular signals, it is now known that these three systems are integrated with each other, which has given birth to the sciences of psychoneuroendocrinology (Section 1.11) and psychoneuroimmunology (Section 1.12). The interactions between the neuroendocrine system and CNS can most easily be seen in the psychiatric symptoms that can accompany some hormonal disorders (e.g., depression in Cushing's syndrome) and also in the identification of disorders of neuroendocrine regulation as potential markers for state or trait variables in psychiatric conditions. Similarly, the immune system is linked with both the CNS and endocrine system through shared molecular signals. The other property shared by the CNS, endocrine system, and immune system is that they undergo regular changes with time. The study of these changes with time and disorders of time regulation are included in the field of chronobiology (Section 1.13).

BRAIN IMAGING

Current technology allows brain imaging to detect and display electrical brain activity and physical brain structure, as well as functional brain activity. Hans Berger first recorded the human electroencephalogram (EEG) in 1924, and subsequent advances in this area have resulted in the assessment of evoked potentials (visual, auditory, somatosensory, and cognitive), as well as quantitative, computerized assessments of topographic EEG signals (Section 1.14). In addition to the standard X-ray techniques, including computed tomography (CT), a family of brain imaging techniques relies on nuclear magnetic resonance imaging (MRI) to assess both the structure and function of the brain (Section 1.15). These techniques use externally induced manipulations in the magnetic fields of nuclei to image brain structure (sMRI) and brain function (fMRI and magnetic resonance spectroscopy [MRS]). The other major technique for brain imaging uses very small amounts of radioactive compounds introduced into the brain and then visualized by the use of specific imaging cameras (Section 1.16). The two major techniques of this type are positron emission tomography (PET) and single photon emission CT (SPECT). These techniques are particularly well suited for the study of neurotransmitters, receptors, and metabolism. These techniques can measure and visualize brain function during increasingly shorter time periods, allowing researchers to ask specific questions about brain regions and neural networks and their relationships to emotional, cognitive, and behavioral states and activities.

GENETICS

Since the last edition of this textbook, the human, the mouse, and other animal genomes have been sequenced, and, in a sense, the answers are now there, but the right questions must be asked with regard to the genetic basis of mental disorders. By studying the genetics of both populations and individuals, investigators are attempting to "break the code" regarding the etiology of mental disorders (Sections 1.17 and 1.18). Increasingly, investigators conceptualize most complex neuropsychiatric disorders as resulting from the interaction of multiple susceptibility genes rather than a single causal gene or a small number of causal genes. The eventual identification of the key genes, however, would potentially allow an entirely different approach to the diagnosis, prevention, and treatment of mental disorders by using targeted genetic and pharmacological approaches. One of the key experimental approaches on this path of understanding human psychopathology is the use of transgenic animal models of behavior (Section 1.19). The mouse genome is remarkably similar to the human genome, and investigators are now able to make specific manipulations in the mouse genome to produce transgenic mouse models that may evidence behavior and treatment responses that are relevant to understanding and treating human disorders.

COMPLEX HUMAN BEHAVIORS

This textbook contains many chapters describing normal and abnormal complex human behaviors. Three examples of such complex behaviors are sleep (Section 1.20), appetite (Section 1.21), and substance abuse and dependence (Section 1.22). At the beginning of this section, it was mentioned that it is necessary to know everything and believe nothing and also to be wary of oversimplifications from past models of the brain and behavior. Sleep, appetite, and substance abuse are all examples of these lessons, as all three are now conceptualized as involving complex systems within the brain responding to bodily functions outside of the CNS and changing in response to external environmental influences of biological, psychological, and social types.

FUTURE DIRECTIONS

Researchers in neural science will continue to capitalize on the sequencing of the human genome and advances in brain imaging techniques, as well as other advances in experimental neuroscience. Although the ultimate goal of all these efforts is to prevent the development of mental disorders, the immediate goals are to alter disease progression and promote recovery. The pace of discoveries in neural science is, unfortunately, well matched by the complexity of the brain. Nevertheless, neuroscientists are finding ways to challenge their own beliefs in the light of new data, and it may indeed be one of the readers of this textbook that breaks through the current relative ignorance and leads psychiatry into a new paradigm for understanding mental illness in the 21st century.

SUGGESTED CROSS-REFERENCES

Neuropsychiatry and behavioral neurology are discussed in Chapter 2; the neuropsychological and psychiatric aspects of AIDS are discussed in Section 2.8; the neurochemical, viral, and immunological studies of schizophrenia are discussed in Section 12.4; the biochemical aspects of mood disorders are discussed in Section 13.3; biological therapies are discussed in Chapter 31; and Alzheimer's disease is discussed in Section 51.3e. The future of psychiatry is discussed in Section 55.3.

REFERENCES

*Burke W: Genomics as a probe for disease biology. *N Engl J Med*. 2003;349:969.
*Dolan RJ: Emotion, cognition, and behavior. *Science*. 2002;298:1191.
Gingrich JA, ed. Genetically altered mice in the study of neuropsychiatry. *CNS Spectrums*. 2003;8:551.
McKhann GM: Neurology: then, now, and in the future. *Arch Neurol*. 2002;59:1369.
*Rutter M: The interplay of nature, nurture, and developmental influences. *Arch Gen Psychiatry*. 2002;59:996.
*Snyder SH: Forty years of neurotransmitters. A personal account. *Arch Gen Psychiatry*. 2002;59:983.
*Zonta M, Angulo MC, Gobbo S, Rosengarten B, Hossmann K-A, Possan T, Carmignoto G: Neuron-to-astrocyte signaling is central to the dynamic control of brain microcirculation. *Nat Neurosci*. 2003;6:43.

▲ 1.2 Functional Neuroanatomy

JOSEPH N. PIERRI, M.S., M.D., AND DAVID A. LEWIS, M.D.

> The brain, and the brain alone, is the source of our pleasures, joys, laughter, and amusement, as well as our sorrow, pain, grief, and tears. It is especially the organ we use to think and learn, see and hear, to distinguish the ugly from the beautiful, the bad from the good, and the pleasant from the unpleasant. The brain is also the seat of madness and delirium, of the fears and terrors which assail by night or by day, of sleeplessness, awkward mistakes and thoughts that will not come, of pointless anxieties, forgetfulness and eccentricities.
>
> —Hippocrates, ca. 400 BC

The broad range of affective, cognitive, and behavioral characteristics of humans arises as a consequence of specific patterns of activation in networks of neurons that are distributed across the central nervous system (CNS). These patterns of activation are mediated by the connections among specific brain structures. Consequently, understanding the neurobiological bases for the disturbances in affective, cognitive, and behavioral processes present in psychiatric disorders requires an appreciation of the major principles governing the functional organization of these structures and their connections in the human brain. This section reviews some of these anatomical principles and illustrates them in the functional circuitry of several neural systems. These neural systems—the thalamocortical, basal ganglia, and limbic systems—were selected because of their particular relevance for psychiatric disorders.

PRINCIPLES OF BRAIN ORGANIZATION

Cells The human brain contains approximately 10^{11} nerve cells, or *neurons*. In general, neurons are composed of four morphologically identified regions (Fig. 1.2–1): (1) the cell body, or *soma*, which contains the nucleus and can be considered the metabolic center of the neuron; (2) the *dendrites*, processes that arise from the cell body, branch extensively, and serve as the major recipient zones of input from other neurons; (3) the *axon*, a single process that arises from a specialized portion of the cell body (the *axon hillock*) and conveys information to other neurons; and (4) the *axon terminals*, fine branches near the end of the axon that form contacts (*synapses*) generally with the dendrites or the cell bodies of other neurons, release neurotransmitters, and thereby provide a mechanism for interneuronal communication.

The majority of neurons in the human brain are considered to be multipolar in that they give rise to a single axon and several dendritic processes. Although there are a number of classification schemes for neurons in different brain regions, almost all neurons can be considered to be either projection or local circuit neurons. *Projection neurons* have long axons and convey information from the periphery to the brain (sensory neurons), from one brain region to another, or from the brain to effector organs (motor neurons). In contrast, *local circuit* or *interneurons* have short axons and process information within distinct regions of the brain.

Neurons can also be classified according to the neurotransmitters they contain (for example, the dopamine neurons of the substantia nigra). Identification of neurons by their neurotransmitter content in anatomical studies provides a means for correlating the structure of a neuron with certain aspects of its function. However, neurotransmitters have defined effects on the activity of neurons, whereas complex brain functions, such as those disturbed in psychiatric disorders, are mediated by the coordinated activity of ensembles of neurons. Thus, the effects of neurotransmitters (or of pharmacological agents that mimic or antagonize the action of neurotransmitters) on behavioral, emotional, or cognitive states must be viewed within the context of the neural circuits that they influence.

In addition to neurons, the brain also contains several types of *glial* cells, which are at least ten times more numerous than neurons.

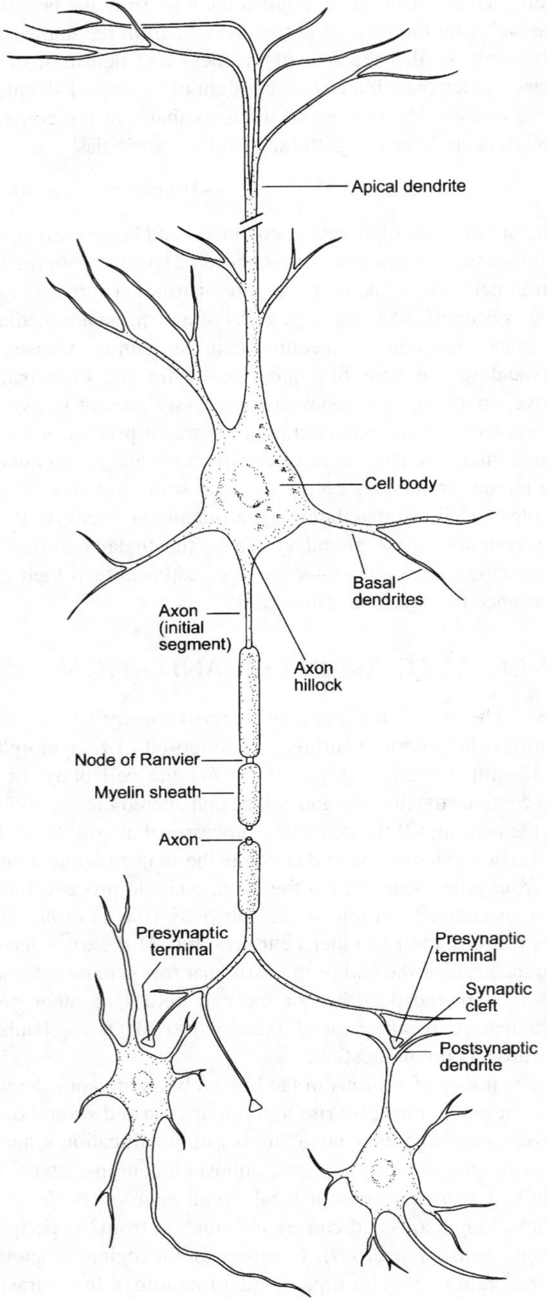

FIGURE 1.2–1 Drawing of the major features of a typical neuron. (Adapted from Kandel ER. Nerve cells and behavior. In: Kandel E, Schwartz J, Jessel T. *Principles of Neural Science.* 3rd ed. New York: Elsevier; 1991:19.)

Oligodendrocytes and *Schwann cells*, found in the CNS and peripheral nervous system, respectively, are relatively small cells that wrap their membranous processes around axons in a tight spiral. The resulting *myelin sheath* facilitates the conduction of action potentials along the axon. *Astrocytes*, the most numerous class of glial cells, appear to serve a number of functions, including participation in the formation of the blood–brain barrier, removal of certain neurotransmitters from the synaptic cleft, buffering of the extracellular potassium (K^+) concentration, and, given their close contact with both neurons and blood vessels, possibly a nutritive function as well. The

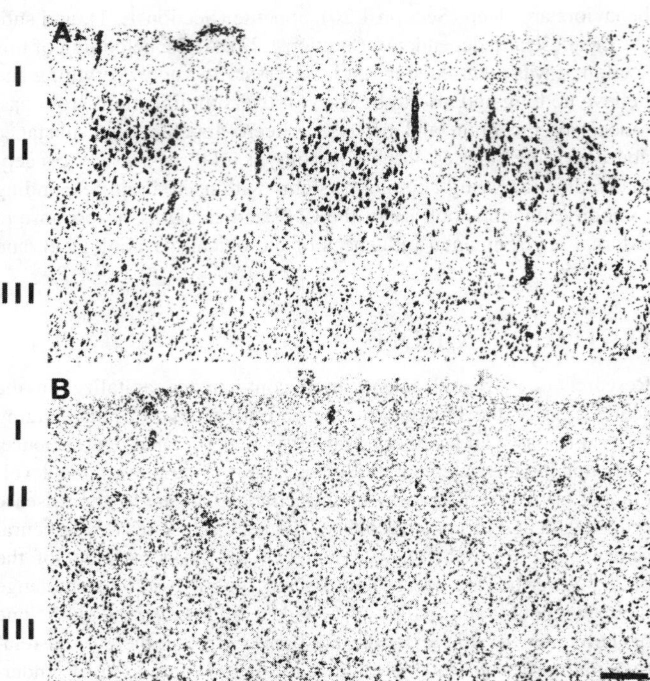

FIGURE 1.2–2 Nissl-stained sections of the superficial layers of the intermediate region of human entorhinal cortex. **A:** In the control brain, layer II contains clusters or islands of large, intensely stained neurons. **B:** In Alzheimer's disease, these layer II neurons are particularly vulnerable to degeneration, and their loss produces a marked change in the cytoarchitecture of the region. Roman numerals indicate the location of the cortical layers. Calibration bar (200 μm) applies to both **A** and **B**.

third class of glial cells, the *microglia*, is actually derived from macrophages and functions as scavengers, eliminating the debris resulting from neuronal death and injury. Recent studies have discovered additional roles for glial cells in brain function and produced data suggesting that alterations in glia may contribute to the pathophysiology of schizophrenia and depression.

Architecture Neurons and their processes form groupings in a number of different ways, and these patterns of organization, or architectures, can be evaluated by several approaches. The pattern of distribution of nerve cell bodies, called *cytoarchitecture*, is revealed by aniline dyes that stain ribonucleotides, Nissl stains, in the nuclei and the cytoplasm of neuronal cell bodies. The Nissl stains demonstrate the relative size and packing density of the neurons and, consequently, reveal, for example, the organization of the neurons into the different layers of the cerebral cortex. In certain pathological states, such as Alzheimer's disease (called dementia of the Alzheimer's type in the fourth revised edition of the *Diagnostic and Statistical Manual of Mental Disorders* [DSM-IV-TR]), neuronal degeneration and loss result in striking changes in the cytoarchitecture of some brain regions (Fig. 1.2–2).

Other types of histological techniques, such as silver stains, selectively label the myelin coating of axons and, consequently, reveal the *myeloarchitecture* of the brain. For example, certain regions of the cerebral cortex—such as area MT, a portion of the temporal cortex involved in processing visual information—can be identified by a characteristic pattern of heavy myelination in the deep cortical layers. The progression of myelination is highly region-specific, may not be

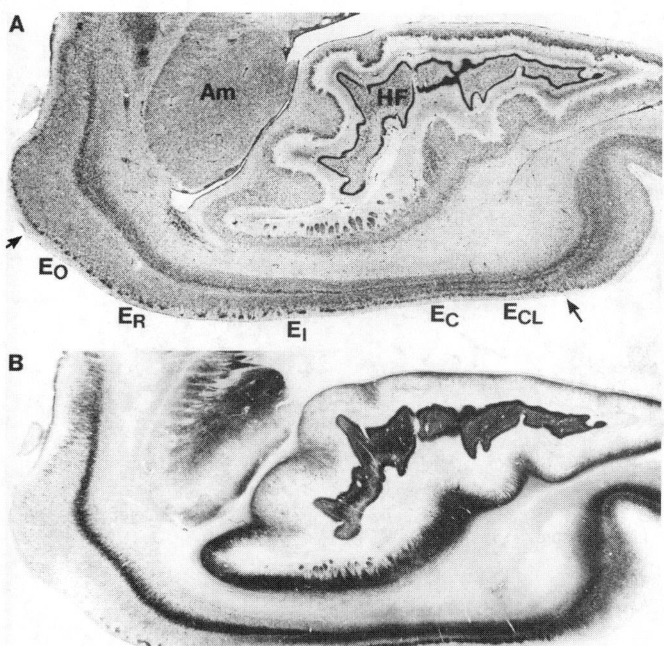

FIGURE 1.2–3 Adjacent sagittal sections through the medial temporal lobe of the human brain labeled to reveal the cytoarchitecture (**A**—Nissl stain) and chemoarchitecture (**B**—nonphosphorylated neurofilament protein immunoreactivity) of the entorhinal (E) cortex. Arrows indicate the rostral (*left*) and caudal (*right*) borders of the entorhinal cortex, and letters indicate some of its subdivisions. Am, amygdala; HF, hippocampal formation. Calibration bar (2 μm) applies to both **A** and **B**. (From Beall MJ, Lewis DA: Heterogeneity of layer II neurons in human entorhinal cortex. *J Comp Neurol.* 1992;321:241, with permission.)

complete for years after birth, and may be a useful anatomical indicator of the functional maturation of brain regions.

Immunohistochemical and other related techniques—which identify the location of neurotransmitters, their synthetic enzymes, or other molecules within neurons—can be used to determine the *chemoarchitecture* of the brain (Fig. 1.2–3B). In some cases, these techniques reveal striking regional differences in the chemoarchitecture of the brain that are difficult to detect in cytoarchitecture.

Connections Every function of the human brain is a consequence of the activity of specific neural circuits. The circuits form as a result of several developmental processes. First, each neuron extends an axon, either after it has migrated to its final location or, in some cases, before. The growth of an axon along distinct pathways is guided by molecular cues from its environment and eventually leads to the formation of synapses with specific target neurons. Although the projection of axons is quite precise, some axons initially produce an excessive number of axon branches, or *collaterals*, and thus contact a broader set of targets than are present in the adult brain. During later development, the connections of particular neurons are focused by the pruning or elimination of axonal projections to inappropriate targets. The developmental timing of synaptic and axonal elimination appears to be highly specific across regions of the brain.

Within the adult brain, the connections among neurons or neural circuits follow several important principles of organization. First, many, but not all, connections between brain regions are *reciprocal*; that is, each region tends to receive input from those regions to which it sends axonal projections. In some cases, the axons arising from one region may directly innervate the reciprocating projection neurons in another region; in other cases, local circuit interneurons are interposed between the incoming axons and the projection neurons that furnish the reciprocal connections. For some projections, the reciprocating connection is indirect, passing through one or more additional brain regions and synapses before innervating the initial brain region.

Second, many neuronal connections are either divergent or convergent in nature. A *divergent* system involves the conduct of information from one neuron or a discrete group of neurons to a much larger number of neurons that may be located in diverse portions of the brain. The *locus ceruleus*, a small group of norepinephrine-containing neurons in the brainstem that sends axonal projections to the entire cerebral cortex and other brain regions, is an example of a highly divergent system. In contrast, the output of multiple brain regions may be directed toward a single area, forming a *convergent* system. Projection from multiple association areas of the cerebral cortex to the entorhinal region of the medial temporal lobe (Fig. 1.2–3A) is an example of a convergent system.

Third, the connections among regions may be organized in a hierarchical or parallel fashion, or both. For example, visual input is conveyed in a serial or hierarchical fashion through several populations of neurons in the retina to the lateral geniculate nucleus, to the primary visual cortex, and then, progressively, to the multiple visual association areas of the cerebral cortex. Within the hierarchical scheme, different types of visual information (for example, motion and form) may be processed in a parallel fashion through different portions of the visual system.

Finally, regions of the brain are specialized for different functions. For example, lesions of the left inferior frontal gyrus (Broca's area, Fig. 1.2–4) produce a characteristic impairment in speech production. However, speech is a complex faculty that depends not only on the integrity of Broca's area, but also on the distributed processing of information across a number of brain regions through divergent and convergent, serial and parallel interconnections. Thus, the role of any particular brain region or group of neurons in the production of specific behaviors or in the pathophysiology of a given neuropsychiatric disorder cannot be viewed in isolation but must be considered within the context of the neural circuits connecting those neurons with other brain regions.

Distinctiveness of the Human Brain Compared with the brains of other primate species, the human brain is substantially greater in size, with certain areas expanded disproportionately. For example, the prefrontal cortex has been estimated to occupy only 3.5 percent of the total cortical volume in cats and 11.5 percent in monkeys but close to 30 percent of the much larger cortical volume of the human brain. Conversely, the relative representation of other regions is decreased in the human brain; for example, the primary visual cortex accounts for only 1.5 percent of the total area of the cerebral cortex in humans, but, in monkeys, a much greater proportion (17 percent) of the cerebral cortex is devoted to this region. Thus, the distinctiveness of the human brain is attributable both to its size and to the differential expansion of certain regions, particularly those areas of the cerebral cortex devoted to higher cognitive functions.

In addition, the expansion and differentiation of the human brain are associated with substantial differences in the organization of certain elements of neural circuitry. For example, when compared with rodents, the dopaminergic innervation of the human cerebral cortex is much more widespread and regionally specific. The primary motor cortex and certain posterior parietal regions receive a dense dopamine innervation in both monkeys and humans, but these areas receive little dopamine input in rats. These types of species differences indicate that there are limits to the accuracy of generalizations made concerning human brain function when using studies in rodents or even nonhu-

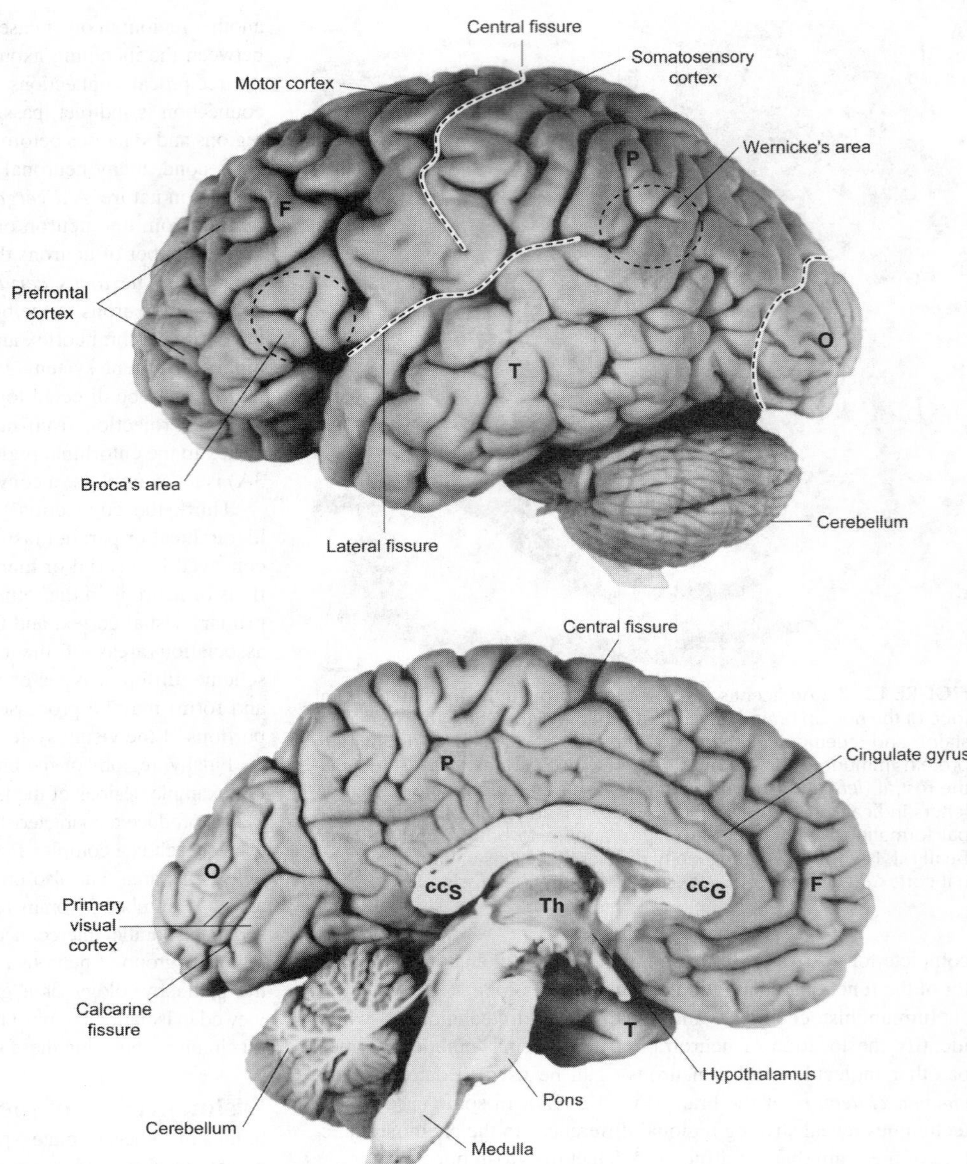

FIGURE 1.2–4 Photographs of the lateral (*top*) and medial (*bottom*) of the left hemisphere of a human brain indicating the location of major surface landmarks. cc_G, genu of the corpus callosum, cc_S, splenium of the corpus callosum; F, frontal lobe; O, occipital lobe; P, parietal lobe; T, temporal lobe; Th, thalamus.

man primates as the basis for the inference. However, direct investigation of the organization of the human brain is obviously restricted and complicated by a number of factors. As indicated above, the expansion of the human brain is associated with the appearance of additional regions of the cerebral cortex. For example, the entorhinal cortex of the medial temporal lobe is sometimes considered to be a single cortical region, yet, in the human brain, the cytoarchitecture and chemoarchitecture of this cortex differ substantially along its rostral–caudal extent (Fig. 1.2–3). It is tempting to identify these regions by their location relative to other structures, but sufficient interindividual variability exists in the human brain to make such a topological definition unreliable. In the case of the entorhinal cortex, the location of its different subdivisions relative to adjacent structures, such as the amygdala and the hippocampus, varies across human brains. Therefore, in all studies, particularly those using the human brain, areas of interest must be defined in a manner (for example, using cyto-, chemo-, or myeloarchitectural features) that allows investigators to accurately identify the same region in all cases.

An additional limitation to the study of the human brain concerns the changes in morphology and biochemistry that can occur during the interval between the time of death and the freezing or fixation of brain specimens. In addition to the influence of the known postmortem interval, such changes may begin to occur during the agonal state preceding death. When comparing aspects of the organization of the human brain with that of other species, the researcher must try to account for changes that may have occurred in the human brain as a result of postmortem delay or agonal state. Furthermore, in the study of disease states, appropriate controls must be used, as differences in neurotransmitter content or other characteristics among cases could be a result of factors other than the disease state, such as methods of tissue preparation (Fig. 1.2–5). Studies of the human brain in vivo—using such imaging techniques as positron emission tomography (PET), magnetic resonance imaging (MRI), and magnetic resonance spectroscopy (MRS)—circumvent many of these problems but are limited by a level of resolution that is insufficient for the study of many aspects of human brain organization.

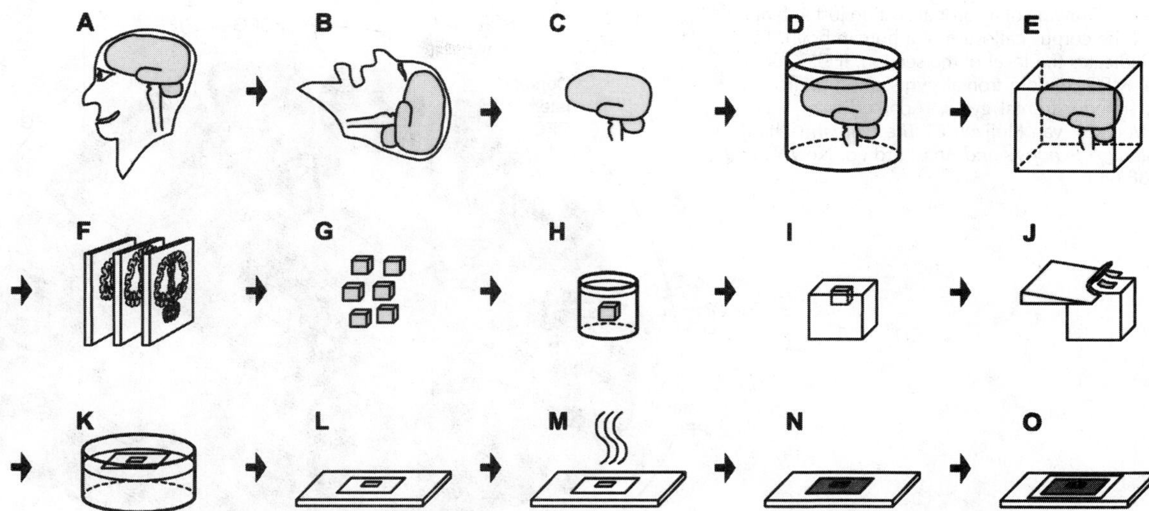

FIGURE 1.2–5 Sequence of drawings depicting selected steps in tissue processing for study of the postmortem human brain. In order to understand how findings from microscopic studies of the human brain reflect in the anatomy of the brain in vivo, an investigator must have knowledge of how each of these steps in tissue preparation affects the anatomical structure of study and how the final product of this process, the microscopic window on the particular brain structure, relates to the intact, functioning, three-dimensional brain. (*A*) brain in living subject; (*B*) brain in deceased subject; (*C*) brain after removal from the body; (*D*) fixation of the brain; (*E*) brain in embedding medium; (*F*) slabbing of embedded tissue; (*G*) blocks of tissue taken from the region of interest; (*H*) dehydration of tissue; (*I*) embedding of tissue in medium for sectioning; (*J*) cutting tissue into sections; (*K*) preparation of sections for staining; (*L*) mounting of sections on a glass slide; (*M*) air drying of section; (*N*) staining of section; (*O*) section covered by coverslip for microscopic study. (Adapted from Dorph-Peteresen K-A, Nyengaard JR, Gundersen HJG: Tissue shrinkage and unbiased estimation of particle number and size. *J Microscopy*. 2001;204:232–246, with permission.)

STRUCTURAL COMPONENTS

Major Brain Structures

In the early stages of human brain development, three primary vesicles can be identified in the neural tube: the *prosencephalon*, the *mesencephalon*, and the *rhombencephalon* (Table 1.2–1). Subsequently, the prosencephalon divides to become the *telencephalon* and the *diencephalon*. The telencephalon gives rise to the cerebral cortex, the hippocampal formation, the amygdala, and some components of the basal ganglia. The diencephalon becomes the thalamus, the hypothalamus, and several other related structures. The mesencephalon gives rise to the midbrain structures of the adult brain. The rhombencephalon divides into the *metencephalon* and the *myelencephalon*. The metencephalon gives rise to the pons and the cerebellum; the medulla is the derivative of the myelencephalon.

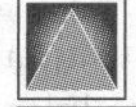

Table 1.2–1
Derivatives of the Neural Tube

Primary Vesicles	Secondary Vesicles	Brain Components
Prosencephalon	Telencephalon	Cerebral cortex
		Hippocampus
		Amygdala
		Striatum
	Diencephalon	Thalamus
		Hypothalamus
		Epithalamus
Mesencephalon	Mesencephalon	Midbrain
Rhombencephalon	Metencephalon	Pons
		Cerebellum
	Myelencephalon	Medulla

Modified from Nolte J. *The Human Brain: An Introduction to Its Functional Anatomy*. 3rd ed. St. Louis: Mosby; 1993:9.

The cerebral cortex of each hemisphere is divided into four major regions: the *frontal, parietal, temporal,* and *occipital* lobes (Fig. 1.2–4). The frontal lobe is located anterior to the central sulcus and consists of the primary motor, premotor, and prefrontal regions (Fig. 1.2–6). The primary somatosensory cortex is located in the anterior parietal lobe; in addition, other cortical regions related to complex visual and somatosensory functions are located in the posterior parietal lobe. The superior portion of the temporal lobe contains the primary auditory cortex and other auditory regions; the inferior portion contains regions devoted to complex visual functions. In addition, some regions within the superior temporal sulcus receive a convergence of input from the visual, somatosensory, and auditory sensory areas. The occipital lobe consists of the primary visual cortex and other visual association areas.

Beneath the outer mantle of the cerebral cortex are a number of other major brain structures, such as the caudate nucleus, the putamen, and the globus pallidus (Fig. 1.2–7). These structures are components of the basal ganglia, a system involved in the control of movement and certain cognitive processes. The hippocampus and the amygdala, components of the limbic system, are located deep in the medial temporal lobe (Figs. 1.2–8, 1.2–9, and 1.2–10). In addition, the derivatives of the diencephalon, such as the thalamus and the hypothalamus, are prominent internal structures; the thalamus is a relatively large structure composed of a number of nuclei that have distinct patterns of connectivity with the cerebral cortex (Figs. 1.2–8, 1.2–9, and 1.2–10). In contrast, the hypothalamus is a much smaller structure involved in autonomic and endocrine functions.

Ventricular System

As the neural tube fuses during development, the cavity of the neural tube becomes the ventricular system of the brain. It is composed of two C-shaped *lateral ventricles* in the cerebral hemispheres that can be further divided into five parts: the anterior horn (which is located in the frontal lobe), the body of the ventricle, the inferior or temporal horn in the temporal lobe, the posterior or

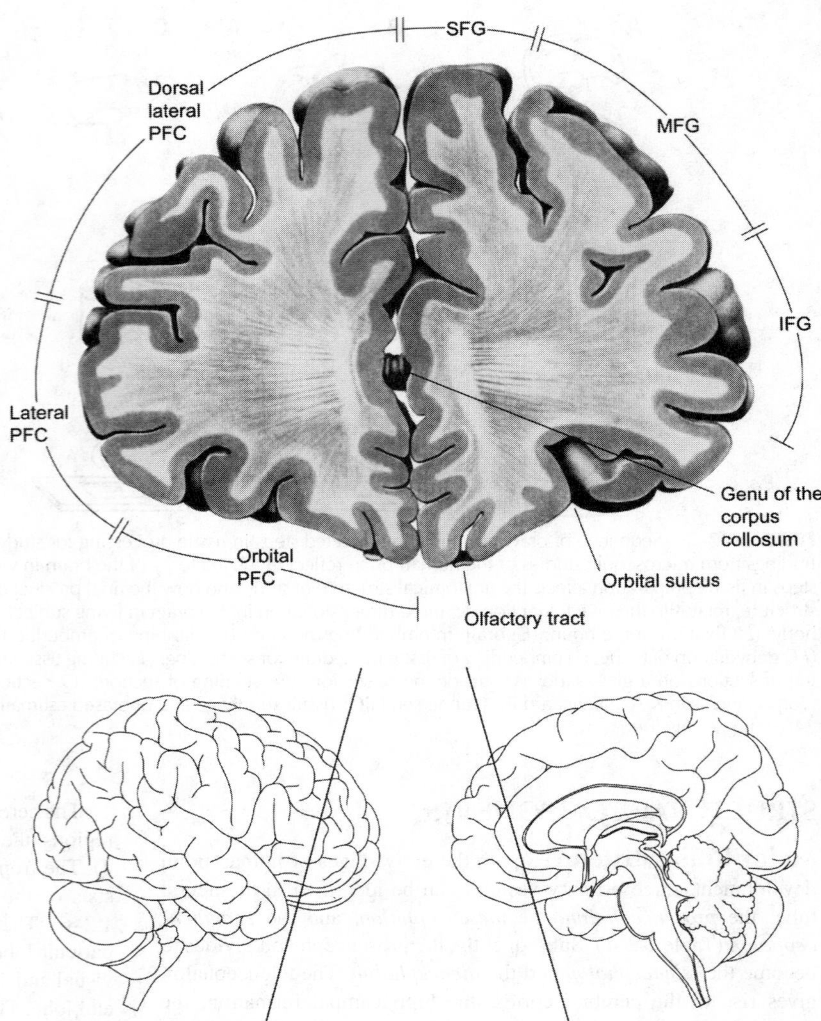

FIGURE 1.2–6 Drawing of a coronal section just anterior to the genu of the corpus callosum of a human brain. The inset below indicates the level of the section. IFG, inferior frontal gyrus; MFG, middle frontal gyrus; PFC, prefrontal cortex; SFG, superior frontal gyrus. (Adapted from Nieuwenhuys R, Voogd J, van Huijzen C. *The Human Central Nervous System: A Synopsis and Atlas.* 3rd ed. New York: Springer; 1988:68.)

occipital horn in the occipital lobe, and the atrium (Fig. 1.2–11). The *foramina of Monro* (interventricular foramina) are the two apertures that connect the two lateral ventricles with the *third ventricle*, which is found on the midline of the diencephalon. The *cerebral aqueduct* connects the third ventricle with the *fourth ventricle* in the pons and the medulla.

The ventricular system is filled with cerebrospinal fluid (CSF), a colorless liquid containing low concentrations of protein, glucose, and potassium and relatively high concentrations of sodium and chloride. The majority (70 percent) of the CSF is produced at the choroid plexus located in the walls of the lateral ventricles and in the roof of both the third and fourth ventricles. The *choroid plexus* is a complex of ependyma, pia, and capillaries that invaginate the ventricle. In contrast to other parts of the brain, the capillaries in the choroid plexus are fenestrated, which allows substances to pass out of the capillaries and through the pia mater. The ependymal or choroid epithelial cells, however, have tight junctions between cells to prevent the leakage of substances into the CSF; this provides what is sometimes referred to as the *blood–CSF barrier*. In other parts of the brain, the endothelial cells of the capillaries exhibit tight junctions that prevent the movement of substances from the blood to the brain; this is referred to as the *blood–brain barrier*.

The CSF is constantly produced and circulates through the lateral ventricles to the third ventricle and then to the fourth ventricle. The CSF then flows through the medial and lateral apertures to the cisterna magna and pontine cistern and, finally, travels over the cerebral hemispheres to be absorbed by the arachnoid villi and released into the superior sagittal sinus. Disruptions in the flow of the CSF usually cause some form of hydrocephalus; for example, if an intraventricular foramen is occluded, the associated lateral ventricle becomes enlarged, but the remaining components of the ventricular system remain normal.

Several functions are attributed to the CSF: it serves to cushion the brain against trauma, to maintain and control the extracellular environment, and to spread endocrine hormones. Because the CSF bathes the brain and is in direct communication with extracellular fluid, it is possible to measure the amount of certain compounds in the CSF as a correlate of the amount of that substance in the brain. For example, levels of homovanillic acid (HVA), a metabolite of the neurotransmitter dopamine, are thought to reflect the functional activity of that neurotransmitter. Thus, the concentration of HVA in samples of the CSF taken in a lumbar puncture may provide a picture of brain dopaminergic function. However, because the CSF bathes the entire brain, the CSF levels of HVA may not be a valid indicator of the activity of dopamine neurons in any particular brain area. Consequently, caution must be exercised in interpreting the findings of investigations that rely on CSF measurements as indicators of neurotransmitter activity.

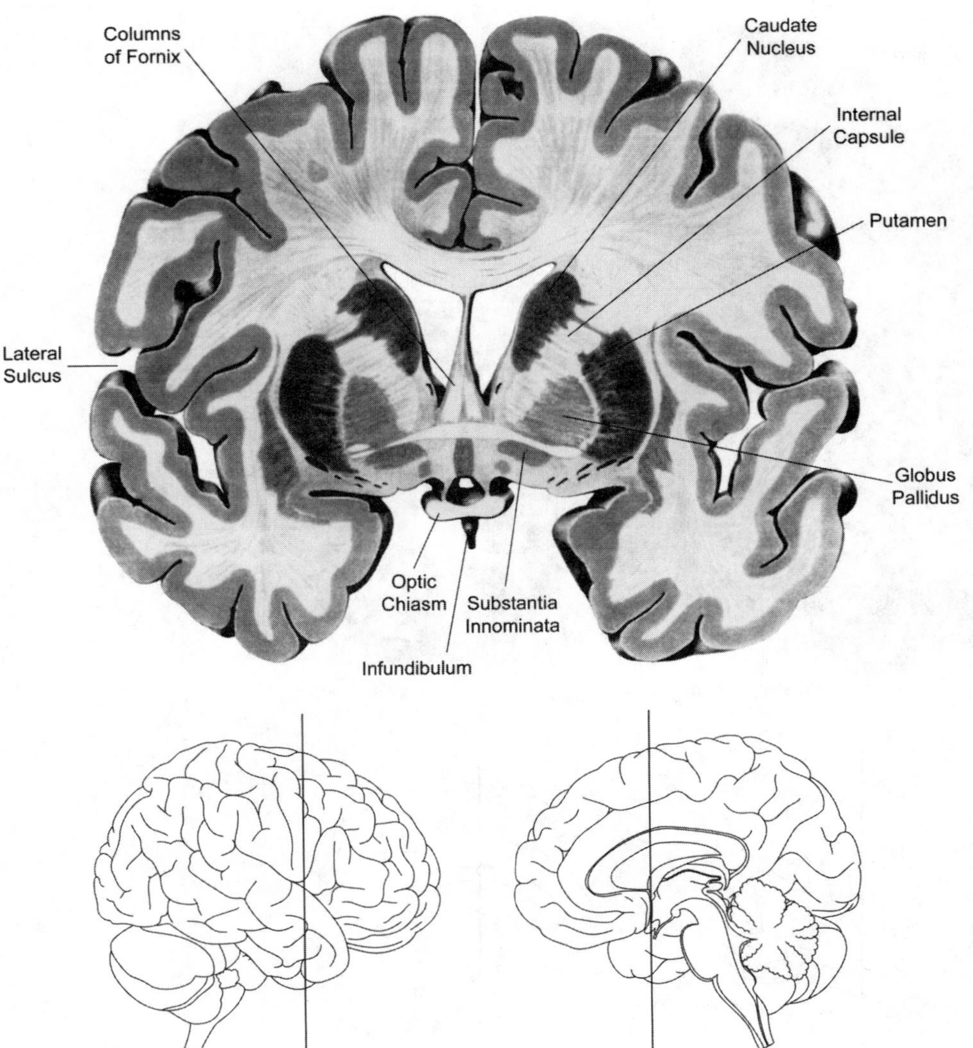

FIGURE 1.2–7 Drawing of a coronal section through the optic chasm of a human brain. The inset below indicates the level of the section. (Adapted from Nieuwenhuys R, Voogd J, van Huijzen C. *The Human Central Nervous System: A Synopsis and Atlas.* 3rd ed. New York: Springer; 1988:70.)

FUNCTIONAL BRAIN SYSTEMS

The relations between the organizational principles and the structural components of the human brain are illustrated in three functional systems: the thalamocortical, basal ganglia, and limbic systems.

Thalamocortical Systems

Thalamus The largest portion of the diencephalon consists of the *thalamus*, a group of nuclei located medial to the basal ganglia that serves as the major synaptic relay station for the information reaching the cerebral cortex (Fig. 1.2–12). On an anatomical basis, the thalamic nuclei can be divided into six groups: anterior, medial, lateral, reticular, intralaminar, and midline nuclei. A thin Y-shaped sheet of myelinated fibers, the *internal medullary lamina*, delimits the anterior, medial, and lateral groups of nuclei (Fig. 1.2–13). In the human thalamus, the anterior and medial groups each contain a single large nucleus, the *anterior* and *medial dorsal nuclei*. The lateral group of nuclei can be further subdivided into dorsal and ventral tiers. The dorsal tier is composed of the *lateral dorsal*, the *lateral posterior*, and the *pulvinar nuclei*; the ventral tier consists of the *ventral anterior*, the *ventral lateral*, the *ventral posterior lateral*, and the *ventral posterior medial nuclei*. The lateral group of nuclei is covered by the *external medullary lamina*, another sheet of myelinated fibers. Interposed between these fibers and the internal capsule is a thin group of neurons forming the *reticular nucleus* of the thalamus. The *intralaminar nuclei*, the largest of which is the *central median nucleus*, are located within the internal medullary lamina. The final group of thalamic nuclei, the *midline nuclei*, covers portions of the medial surface of the thalamus. The midline nuclei of each hemisphere may fuse to form the interthalamic adhesion, which is variably present.

Thalamic nuclei can also be classified into several groups based on the pattern and information content of their connections (Table 1.2–2). For example, *relay nuclei* project to and receive input from specific regions of the cerebral cortex. These reciprocal connections apparently allow the cerebral cortex to modulate the thalamic input it receives. *Specific relay nuclei* process input either from a single sensory modality or from a distinct part of the motor system. For example, the lateral geniculate nucleus receives visual input from the optic tract and projects to the primary visual area of the occipital cortex. As summarized in Figure 1.2–14, neurons of the thalamic relay nuclei furnish topographically organized projections to specific regions of the cerebral cortex, although some cortical regions receive input from more than one nucleus.

In contrast, *association relay nuclei* receive highly processed input from more than one source and project to larger areas of the

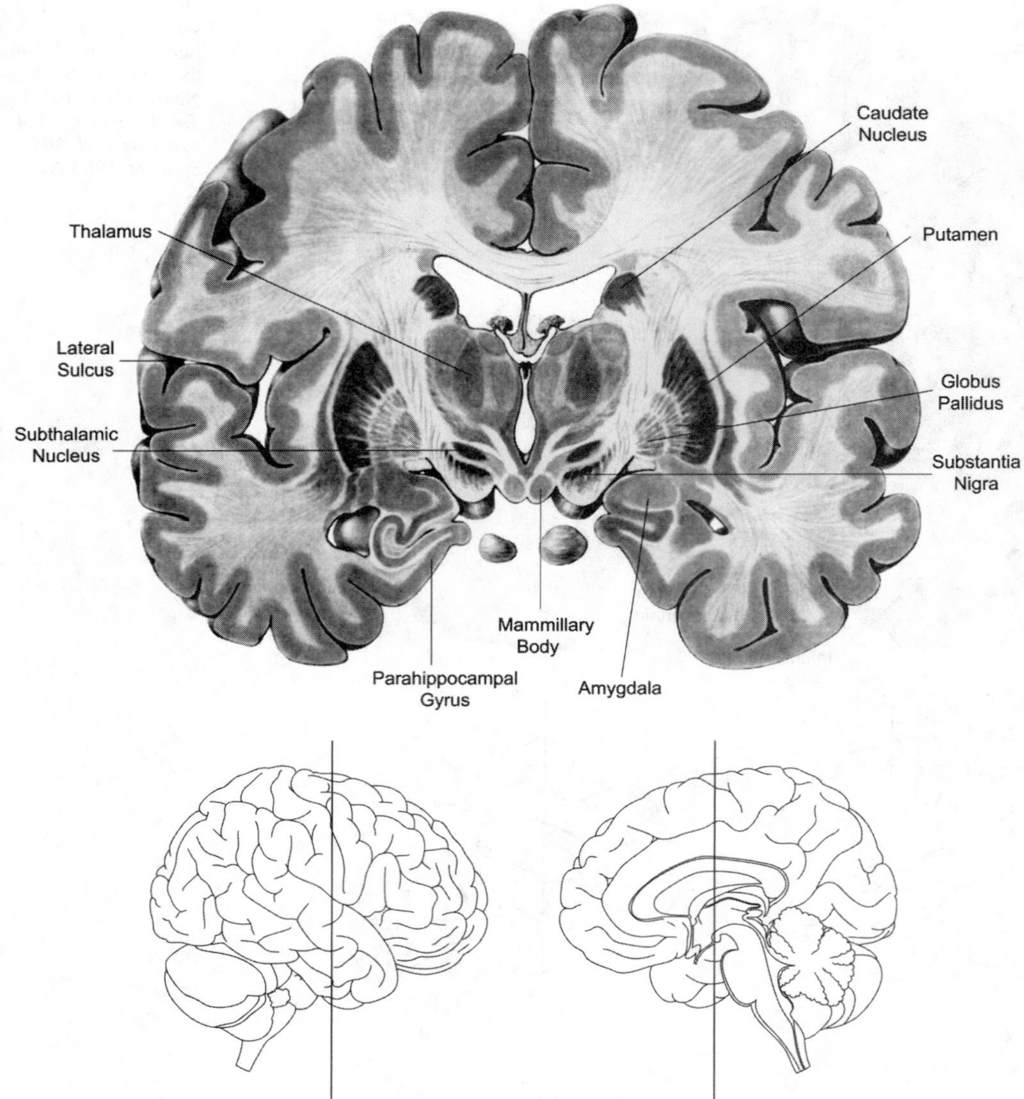

FIGURE 1.2–8 Drawing of a coronal section at the level of the mammillary bodies. The inset below indicates the level of the section. (Adapted from Nieuwenhuys R, Voogd J, van Huijzen C. *The Human Central Nervous System: A Synopsis and Atlas*. 3rd ed. New York: Springer; 1988:72.)

association cortex. For example, the medial dorsal thalamic nucleus receives input from the hypothalamus and the amygdala and is reciprocally interconnected with the prefrontal cortex and certain premotor and temporal cortical regions. In contrast to relay nuclei, *diffuse-projection nuclei* receive input from diverse sources and project to widespread areas of the cerebral cortex and to the thalamus. The divergent nature of the cortical connections of these nuclei indicates that they may be involved in regulating the level of cortical excitability and arousal. Finally, the reticular nucleus is unique in that it contains inhibitory neurons that receive input from collaterals of the axons that reciprocally connect other thalamic nuclei and the cerebral cortex. Each portion of the reticular nucleus then projects to the thalamic nucleus from which it receives input. The pattern of connectivity indicates that the reticular nucleus samples both cortical afferent and efferent activity and then uses that information to regulate thalamic function.

CEREBRAL CORTEX The *cerebral cortex* is a laminated sheet of neurons, several millimeters thick, that covers the cerebral hemispheres. It consists of approximately 22.5 billion neurons communicating via approximately 165 trillion synapses. These neurons have approximately 12 million km of dendrites, and the cerebral cortex and subcortical regions are interconnected by approximately 100,000 km of axons. More than 90 percent of the total cortical area consists of the *neocortex*, which has a six-layered structure (at least at some point during development). The remainder of the cerebral cortex is referred to as the *allocortex* and consists of the *paleocortex* and the *archicortex*, regions that are restricted to the base of the telencephalon and the hippocampal formation, respectively.

Within the neocortex, the two major neuronal cell types are the pyramidal and stellate, or nonpyramidal, neurons (Fig. 1.2–15). *Pyramidal neurons*, which account for approximately 70 percent of all neocortical neurons, usually have a characteristically shaped cell body that gives rise to a single apical dendrite that ascends vertically toward the cortical surface. In addition, the neurons have an array of short dendrites that spread laterally from the base of the cell. The dendrites of pyramidal neurons are coated with short protrusions, called *spines*, that are the sites of most of the excitatory inputs to

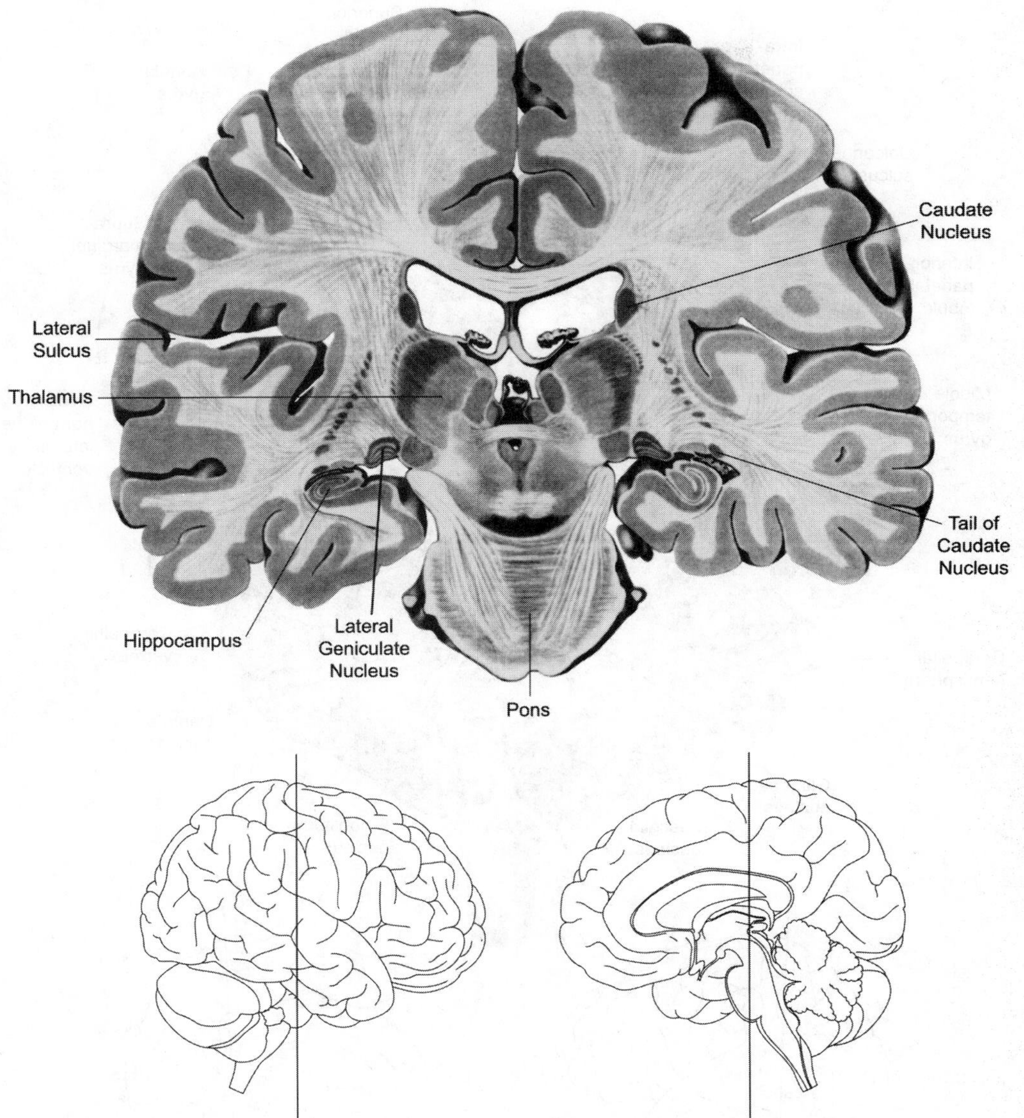

FIGURE 1.2–9 Drawing of a coronal section through the posterior thalamus. The inset below indicates the level of the section. (Adapted from Nieuwenhuys R, Voogd J, van Huijzen C. *The Human Central Nervous System: A Synopsis and Atlas.* 3rd ed. New York: Springer; 1988:74.)

these neurons. Most pyramidal cells are projection neurons that are thought to use excitatory amino acids as neurotransmitters. Interestingly, in postmortem studies, subjects with schizophrenia appear to have fewer spines on the dendrites located at the base of pyramidal neurons in deep layer III of the prefrontal cortex (Fig. 1.2–16).

In contrast, *nonpyramidal cells* are generally small, local circuit neurons, many of which use the inhibitory neurotransmitter γ-aminobutyric acid (GABA). These neurons can be divided into distinct functional subclasses based on their biochemical and morphological features (Fig. 1.2–17). For example, double-bouquet cells contain the calcium-binding protein calbindin and provide inhibitory synapses to the dendritic shafts of pyramidal neurons, as well as other local circuit neurons. In contrast, the chandelier class of GABA neurons contains the calcium binding-protein parvalbumin and exerts powerful inhibitory control over pyramidal neurons through synaptic inputs to the axon initial segment of pyramidal cells (Fig. 1.2–18). Alterations in GABA neurotransmission in the prefrontal cortex in schizophrenia appear to primarily involve disturbances in pre- and postsynaptic markers at chandelier neuron–pyramidal neuron synapses.

Neocortical neurons are distributed across six layers of the neocortex; these layers are distinguished by the relative size and packing density of their neurons (Fig. 1.2–19). Each cortical layer tends to receive particular types of inputs and furnish characteristic projections. For example, afferents from thalamic relay nuclei terminate primarily in deep layer III and layer IV, whereas corticothalamic projections originate mainly from layer VI pyramidal neurons (Fig. 1.2–20). These laminar distinctions provide important clues for dissecting possible pathophysiological mechanisms in psychiatric disorders. For example, reports of decreased somal size and diminished spine density on deep layer III pyramidal neurons in the prefrontal cortex of schizophrenic patients suggest that these changes may be related to abnormalities in afferent projections from the medial dorsal thalamic nucleus. Consistent with this interpretation, the number of neurons in the medial dorsal nucleus has been reported to be decreased in schizophrenia.

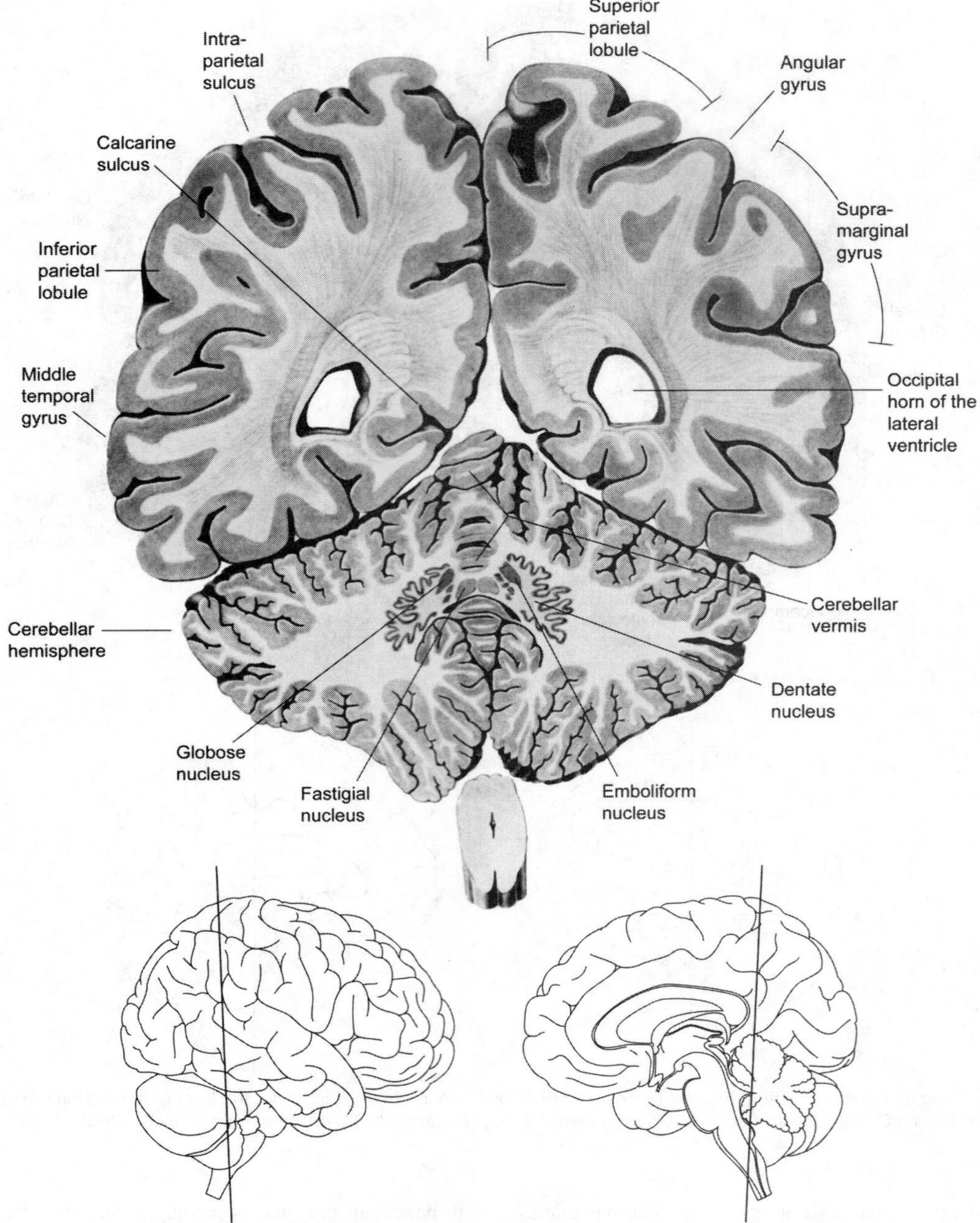

FIGURE 1.2–10 Drawing of a coronal section through the cerebral hemispheres just posterior to the splenium of the corpus callosum and through the deep nuclei of the cerebellum. The inset below indicates the level of the section. (Adapted from Nieuwenhuys R, Voogd J, van Huijzen C. *The Human Central Nervous System: A Synopsis and Atlas.* 3rd ed. New York: Springer; 1988:77.)

In addition to the horizontal laminar structure, many aspects of cortical organization have a vertical or columnar characteristic. For example, the apical dendrites of pyramidal neurons and the axons of some local circuit neurons have a prominent vertical orientation, indicating that these neural elements may sample the input to, or regulate the function of, neurons in multiple layers, respectively. Afferent inputs to the neocortex from other cortical regions also tend to be distributed across cortical layers in a columnar fashion. Finally, physiological studies in the somatosensory and visual cortices have shown that neurons in a given column respond to stimuli with particular characteristics, whereas those in adjacent columns respond to stimuli with different features.

Although best studied in sensory cortices, this pattern of organization is also present in association cortices. For example, recent studies in monkeys using tract-tracing techniques (Fig. 1.2–21) have shown that clusters of prefrontal cortical neurons are organized into reciprocally connected, discrete modular stripes that appear to be the analog of columns identified in the visual cortex. It has been hypothesized that this organization may subserve prefrontal working memory and executive functions.

The neocortex can be divided into two general types of regions. Regions with a readily identifiable six-layer appearance are known as the *homotypical cortex* and are found in association regions of the frontal, temporal, and parietal lobes. In contrast, some regions of the

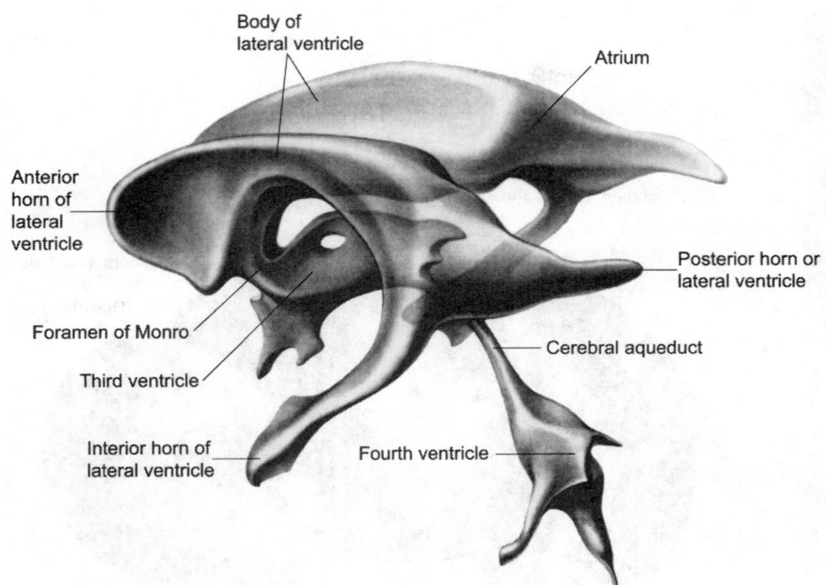

FIGURE 1.2–11 Drawing of a cast of the ventricular system of the human brain. The C shape of the lateral ventricles within the cerebral hemispheres is shown. (Adapted from Nieuwenhuys R, Voogd J, van Huijzen C. *The Human Central Nervous System: A Synopsis and Atlas.* 3rd ed. New York: Springer; 1988:70.)

neocortex do not retain a six-layer appearance. These regions, referred to as the *heterotypical cortex*, include the primary motor cortex, which lacks a defined layer IV, and primary sensory regions, which exhibit an expanded layer IV. The neocortex can be further divided into discrete areas, each area having a distinctive architecture, certain set of connections, and role in particular brain functions. Most subdivisions of the human neocortex have been based on cytoarchitectural features; that is, subdivisions differ in the size, packing density, and arrangement of neurons across layers (Fig. 1.2–19). The most widely used system is that of Korbinian Brodmann (Fig. 1.2–22), who divided the cortex of each hemisphere into 44 numbered areas. Some of these numbered regions correspond closely to functionally distinct areas, such as area 4 (primary motor cortex in the precentral gyrus) and area 17 (primary visual cortex in the occipital lobe). In contrast, other Brodmann's areas appear to encompass several cortical zones that differ in their functional attributes. Although Brodmann's brain map has been extensively used in postmortem studies of psychiatric disorders, many of the distinctions among regions are quite subtle, and the locations of the boundaries between regions vary across individuals.

Although a given cortical area may receive other inputs, it is heavily innervated by projections from particular thalamic nuclei and from certain other cortical regions either in the same hemisphere (*association fibers*) or the opposite hemisphere (*commissural fibers*). The patterns of connectivity make it possible to classify cortical regions into different types. *Primary sensory areas* are dominated by inputs from specific thalamic relay nuclei and are characterized by a topographic representation of visual space, the body surface, or the

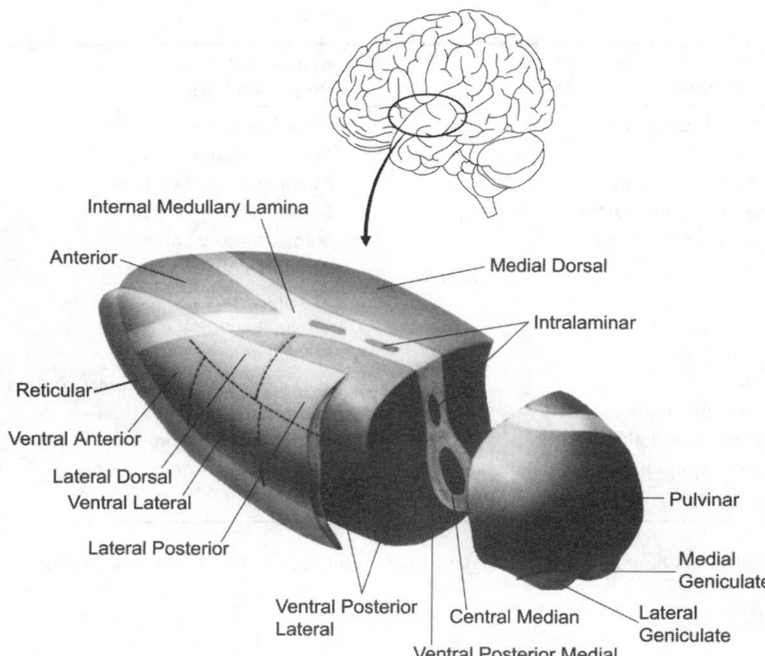

FIGURE 1.2–12 Drawing of the nuclei of the thalamus as seen on the left side of the brain. (Adapted from Kelly JP. The neural basis of perception and movement. In: Kandel ER, Schwartz JH, Jessl TM. *Principles of Neural Science.* 3rd ed. New York: Elsevier; 1991:291, with permission.)

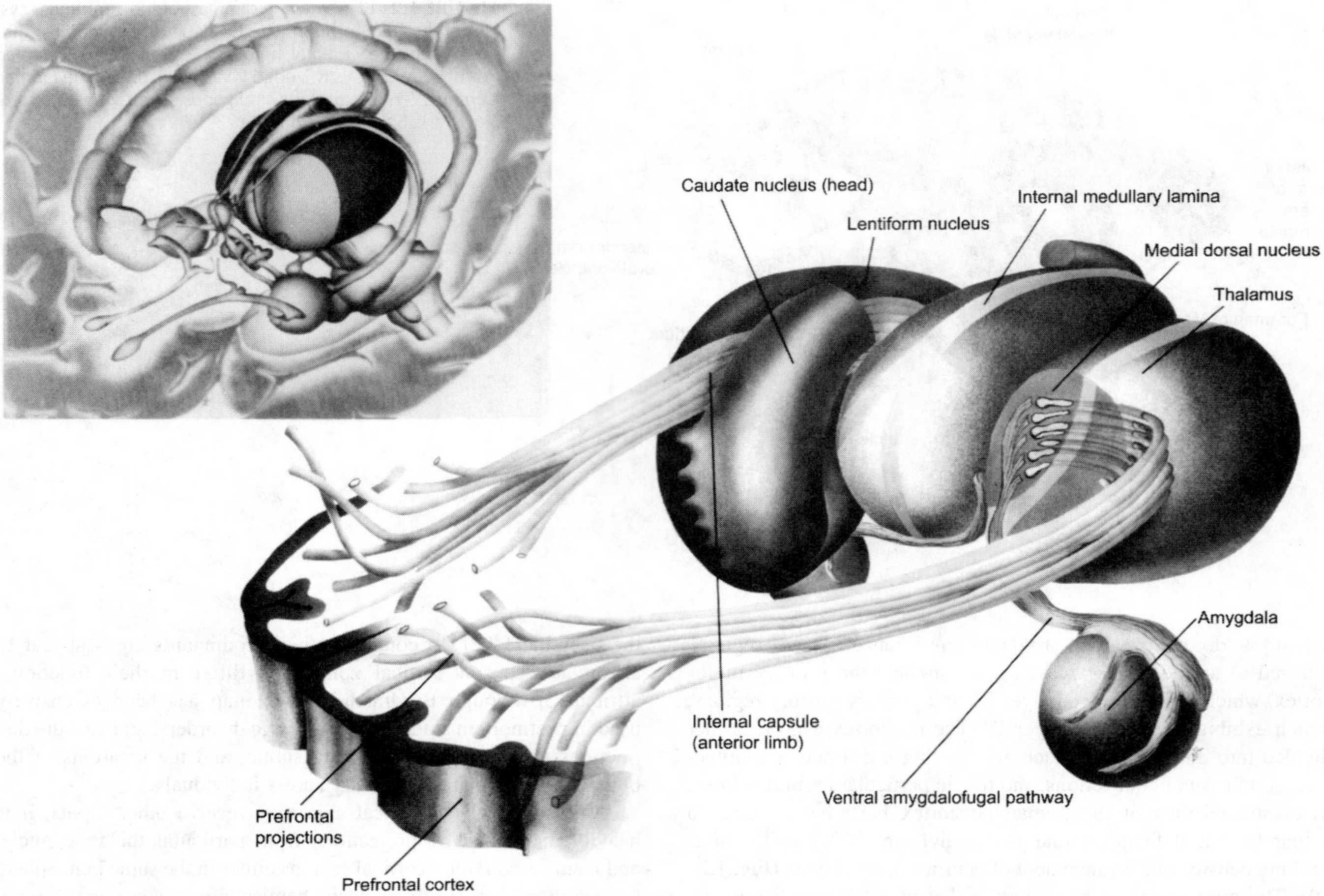

FIGURE 1.2–13 Drawing of the thalamus showing the pathway of projections from the mediodorsal nucleus through lateral thalamic nuclei to the prefrontal cortex. Also shown are afferents from the amygdala to the medial dorsal nucleus. The inset shows the thalamus embedded in the limbic system of which it is a key component. (Adapted from Hendelman WJ. *Student's Atlas of Neuroanatomy*. Philadelphia: W.B. Saunders; 1994:199.)

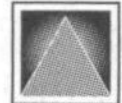

Table 1.2–2
Connections of Thalamic Nuclei[a]

Type	Nuclei	Principal Afferent Inputs	Major Projection Sites
Specific relay	Anterior	Mammillary body of hypothalamus	Cingulate cortex
	Ventral anterior	Globus pallidus	Premotor cortex
	Ventral lateral	Dentate nucleus of cerebellum	Motor, premotor cortices
	Ventral posterior lateral	Medial lemniscal and spinothalamic pathways	Somatosensory cortex
	Ventral posterior medial	Sensory nuclei of trigeminal nerve	Somatosensory cortex
	Medial geniculate	Inferior colliculus	Auditory cortex
	Lateral geniculate	Optic tract	Visual cortex
Association relay	Lateral dorsal	Unknown	Cingulate cortex
	Lateral posterior	Superior colliculus	Parietal cortex
	Pulvinar	Superior colliculus	Temporal, parietal, occipital cortices
	Medial dorsal	Amygdala and hypothalamus	Prefrontal cortex
Diffuse-projection	Midline	Reticular formation, hypothalamus	Basal forebrain, cortex
	Intralaminar	Reticular formation, spinothalamic tract, globus pallidus	Basal ganglia, cortex
	Reticular	Cerebral cortex, thalamus	Thalamus

[a]This table does not include the cortical inputs to each thalamic nucleus.
Adapted from Kelly JP. The neutral basis of perception and movement. In: Kandel ER, Schwartz JH, Jessell TM. *Principles of Neural Science*, 3rd ed. New York: Elsevier, 1991:291.

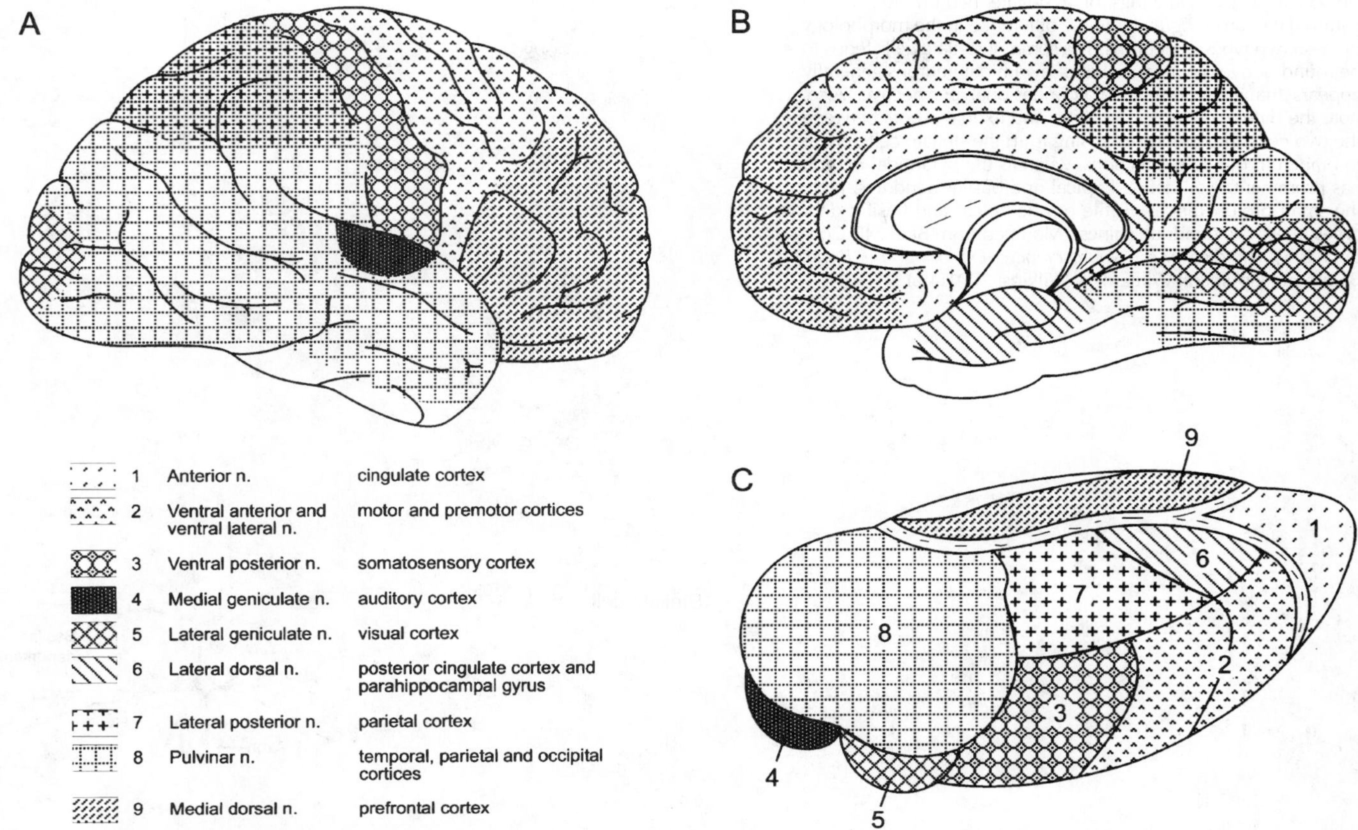

FIGURE 1.2–14 Schematic drawings of the lateral **(A)** and medial **(B)** surfaces of the right cerebral hemisphere and the right thalamus **(C)**. Shading patterns depict the cortical projection zones of some thalamic relay nuclei. n., nucleus. (Modified from Burt AM. *Textbook of Neuroanatomy*. Philadelphia: W.B. Saunders; 1993:443.)

range of audible frequencies on the cortical surface of the primary visual, primary somatosensory, and primary auditory cortices, respectively. These regions project, in turn, to nearby *unimodal association regions*, which are also devoted to processing information from a particular sensory modality. Output from these regions converges in *multimodal association areas*, such as the prefrontal cortex or the temporoparietal cortical regions. Neurons in these regions respond to complex stimuli and are thought to be mediators of higher cognitive functions. Finally, these regions influence the activity of the *motor areas* of the cerebral cortex that control behavioral responses.

Although this classification scheme of cortical regions is accurate in many respects, it fails to account for some of the known complexities of cortical information processing. For example, somatosensory input from the thalamus projects to several distinct topographically organized maps in the cerebral cortex. In addition, information flow within the cortex is not confined to the serial processing route implied in the classification scheme, but also involves parallel processing streams, such as sensory input from the thalamus to both the primary and association areas.

Although this discussion has not distinguished between the cerebral hemispheres, certain brain functions, such as language, are localized to one hemisphere (Fig. 1.2–23). The structural bases for the lateralization of function have not been determined, but some anatomical differences between the cerebral hemispheres have been observed. For example, a portion of the superior temporal cortex, called the *planum temporale*, is generally larger in the left hemisphere than in the right hemisphere. That cortical area, which is located close to the primary auditory cortex and includes the region known as *Wernicke's area* (Fig. 1.2–4), appears to be involved in receptive language functions that are localized to the left hemisphere. In addition, Brodmann's area 44 in the left inferior frontal cortex (Broca's area, Fig. 1.2–4) contains larger pyramidal neurons than the homotopic region of the right hemisphere, a difference that may contribute to the specialization of Broca's area for motor speech function.

Functional Circuitry The connections between the thalamus, the cortex, and certain related brain structures compose three types of thalamocortical systems, each with different patterns of functional circuitry. These three systems—sensory, motor, and association systems—are described separately here but are heavily interconnected.

THALAMOCORTICAL SENSORY SYSTEMS Several general principles govern the organization of the thalamocortical sensory systems. First, sensory receptors transduce certain stimuli in the external environment to neural impulses. The impulses ascend, often through intermediate nuclei in the spinal cord and the medulla, and ultimately synapse in specific relay nuclei of the thalamus.

Second, projections from peripheral sensory receptors to the thalamus and the cortex exhibit topography; that is, a particular portion of the external world is mapped onto a particular region of the brain. For example, in the somatosensory system, axons carrying information regarding a distinct part of the body synapse in a discrete part of

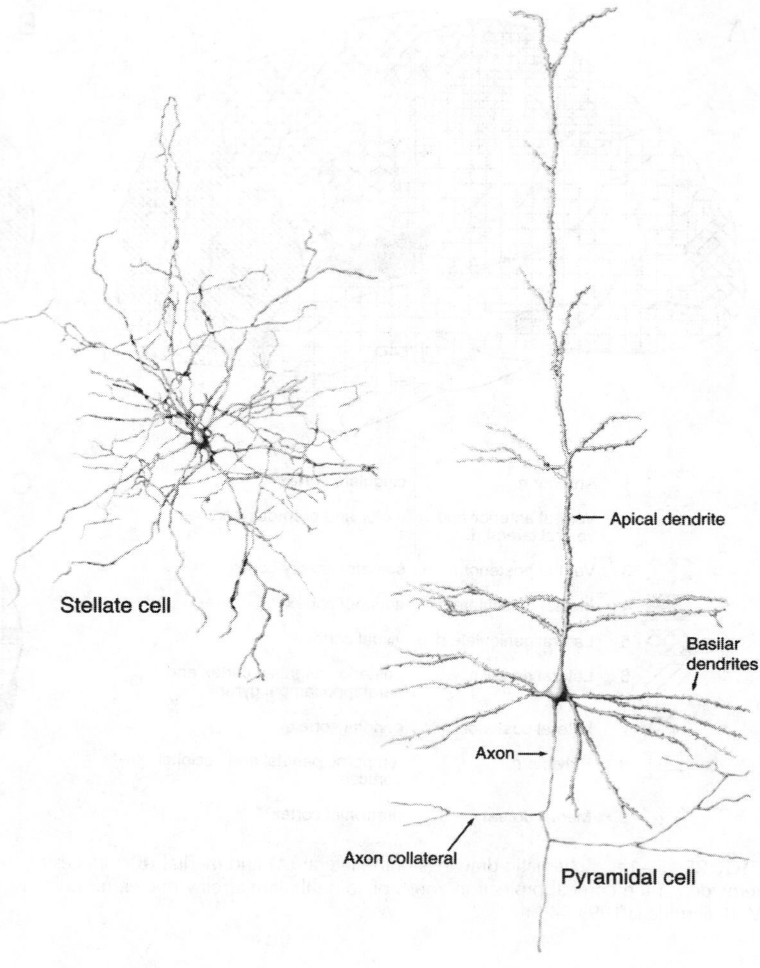

FIGURE 1.2–15 Drawings of a stellate neuron (*left*) and a pyramidal neuron (*right*). Note the difference in the morphology of these two types of neurons. The soma of stellate cells tends to be round or ovoid, whereas that of pyramidal neurons generally appears triangular from a two-dimensional perspective. Also, note the difference in the dendritic and axonal arbors between the two cells. The processes arising from the stellate cell appear to branch in multiple directions, whereas the pyramidal neuron has prominent, well-defined apical and basilar dendrites. Note the small protuberances visible on the apical and basilar dendrites; these are dendritic spines. (Modified from Bear MF, Connors BW, Paradiso MA. *Neuroscience: Exploring the Brain.* Baltimore: Lippincott Williams & Wilkins; 2001:45.)

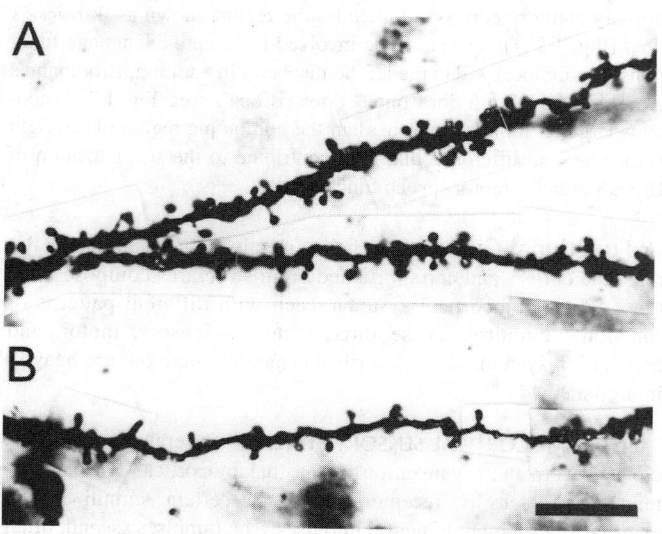

FIGURE 1.2–16 Brightfield photomicrographs of the basilar dendrites of two Golgi-impregnated pyramidal neurons from the human prefrontal cortex. **A:** Basilar dendrites from a normal healthy adult. **B:** Basilar dendrite from a subject with schizophrenia. Note that the number of spines is decreased in the subject with schizophrenia. Calibration bar = 10 μm. (Adapted from Glantz LA, Lewis DA. Decreased dendritic spine density on prefrontal cortical neurons in schizophrenia. *Arch Gen Psychiatry.* 2000;57:65–73.)

the ventral posterior nucleus of the thalamus. Specifically, the ventral posterior medial nucleus receives inputs regarding the head, and the ventral posterior lateral nucleus receives inputs regarding the remainder of the body. The nuclei then project topographically to the primary somatosensory cortex, where several representations of the contralateral half of the body can be found. These representations are distorted; regions heavily innervated by sensory receptors, such as the fingers, are disproportionately represented in the primary somatosensory cortex.

Third, in some cases, sensory inputs travel to the thalamus in a segregated manner according to the submodality of the information conveyed. The inputs are then processed in a parallel fashion; particular pathways may be exclusively devoted to processing a submodality. An example of such segregation is evident in the somatosensory system, where most fibers carrying tactile and proprioceptive information travel in the medial lemniscus, but pain and temperature information is conveyed to the ventral posterior thalamic nuclei through the spinothalamic tract. Although some tactile information is carried in the spinothalamic tract, the submodalities of pain and temperature are largely segregated from tactile and proprioceptive inputs as they ascend to the thalamus.

Finally, sensory pathways exhibit convergence; that is, primary sensory areas process sensory information and then project to unimodal association areas. Subsequently, the unimodal areas project to and converge in multimodal association areas. An illustration of convergence in sensory pathways is found in the somatosensory system.

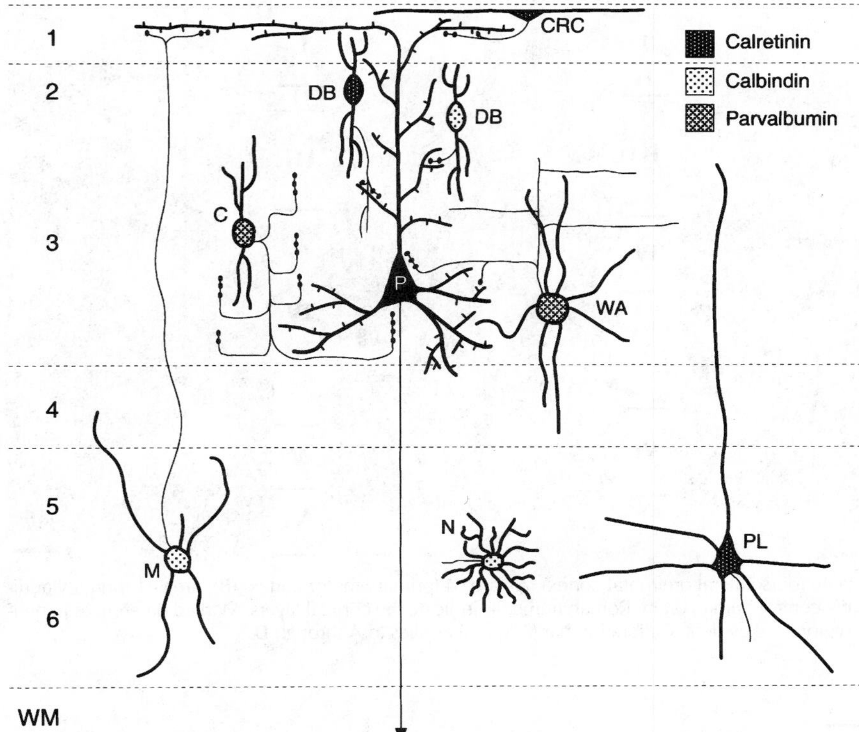

FIGURE 1.2–17 Schematic drawings of different morphological subclasses of γ-aminobutyric acid (GABA)-containing local circuit neurons in the primate prefrontal cortex. As illustrated, the axons of some subclasses of GABA neurons selectively target different portions of pyramidal neurons (P). C, chandelier neuron; CRC, Cajal-Retzius cell; DB, double-bouquet cell; M, Martinotti cell; N, neurogliaform neuron; PL, pyramidal-like; WA, wide arbor. (Adapted from Condé F, Lund JS, Jacobowitz DM, et al.: Local circuit neurons immunoreactive for calretinin, calbindin D-28k or parvalbumin in monkey prefrontal cortex: distribution and morphology. *J Comp Neurol.* 1994;341:95–116.)

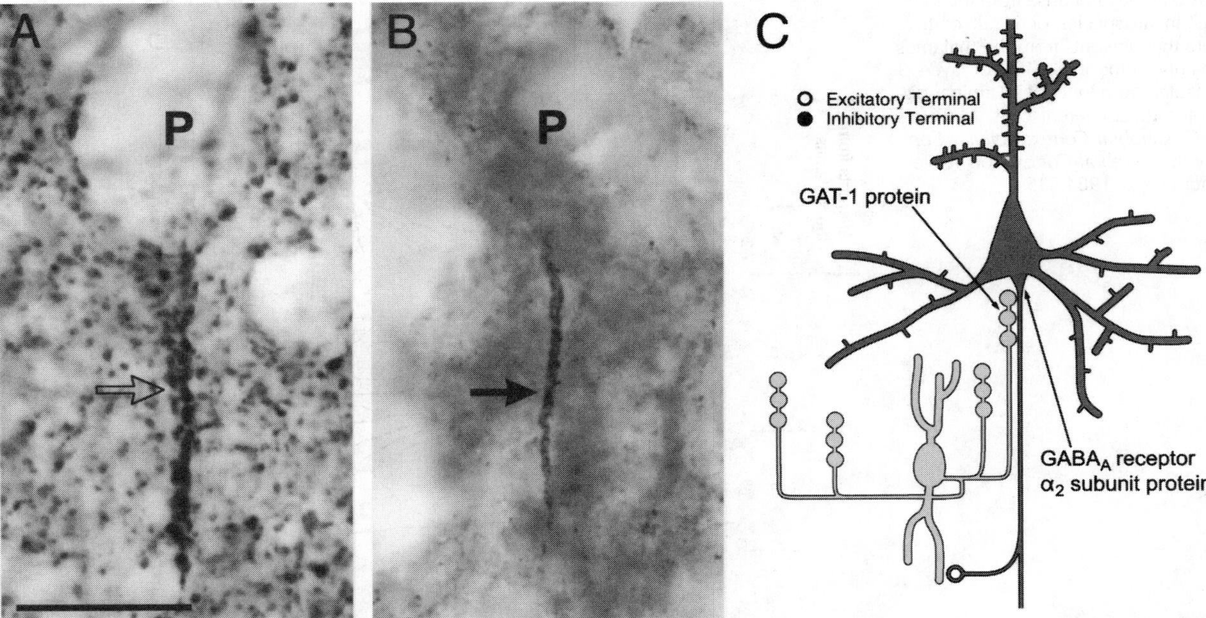

FIGURE 1.2–18 **A:** Brightfield photomicrograph of chandelier neuron axon terminal (*arrow*) immunostained for the γ-aminobutyric acid (GABA) transporter-type 1 (GAT-1). **B:** Brightfield photomicrograph of a pyramidal neuron (P) axon initial segment (the site of action potential generation) immunostained for the α_2 subunit of the GABA$_A$ receptor. **C:** Schematic diagram of the synaptic relationship between a chandelier and a pyramidal neuron. Note the precise relationship between the spatial location of chandelier axon terminals and the receptors located on the axon initial segment. (Adapted from Volk DW, Pierri JN, Fritschy J-N, et al.: Reciprocal alterations in pre- and postsynaptic inhibitory markers at chandelier cell inputs to pyramidal neurons in schizophrenia. *Cereb Cortex.* 2002;12:1063–1070.)

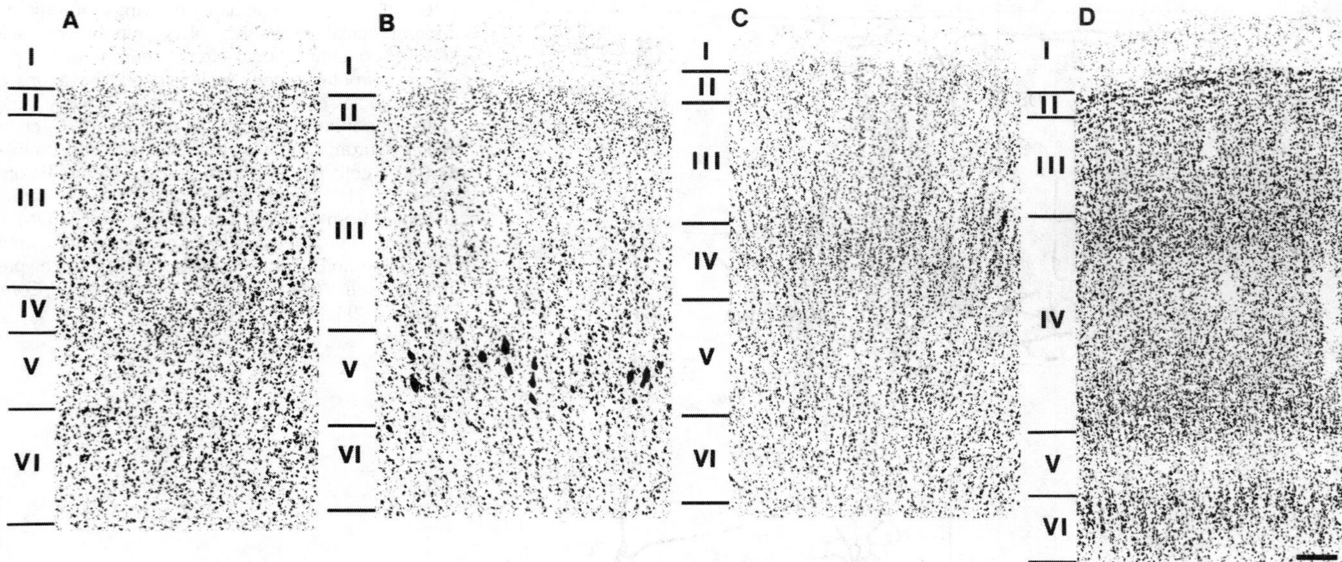

FIGURE 1.2–19 Nissl-stained sections of Brodmann's area 46 (dorsolateral prefrontal cortex) **(A)**, area 4 (primary motor cortex) **(B)**, area 41 (primary auditory cortex) **(C)**, and area 17 (primary visual cortex) **(D)** from a control human brain. Roman numerals indicate the cortical layers. Marked differences in neuronal size and packing density across the layers of the four regions are evident. Calibration bar (200 μm) applies to **A** through **D**.

FIGURE 1.2–20 Schematic diagram of the laminar origins of efferent projections from the cerebral cortex. These data are mainly derived from the study of the monkey via tract-tracing studies. Parentheses indicate projections that may not arise from the identified layer in all species or in all cortical areas. Note that afferents from the thalamus project mainly to the lower half of layers 3 and 4. (Adapted from Jones EG. Laminar distribution of cortical efferent cells. In: Peters A, Jones EG. *Cerebral Cortex: Cellular Components of the Cerebral Cortex*. Vol. 1. New York: Plenum Press; 1984:535.)

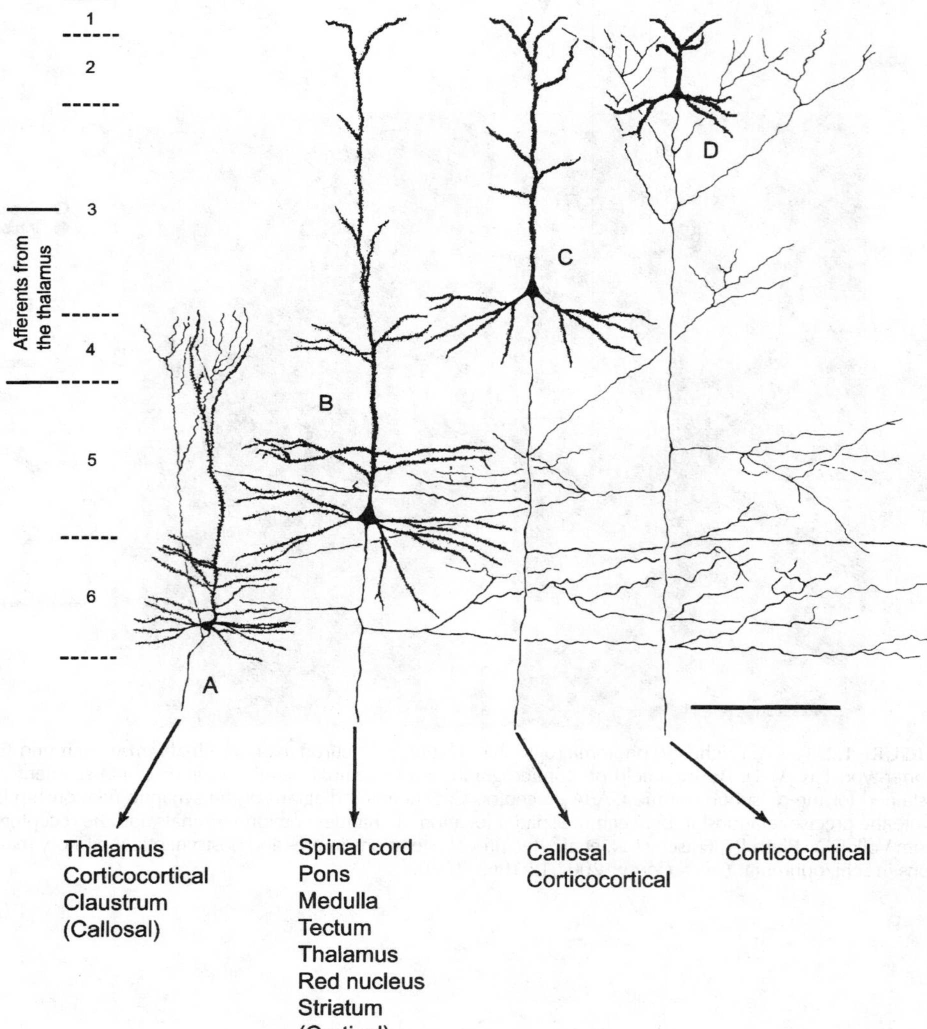

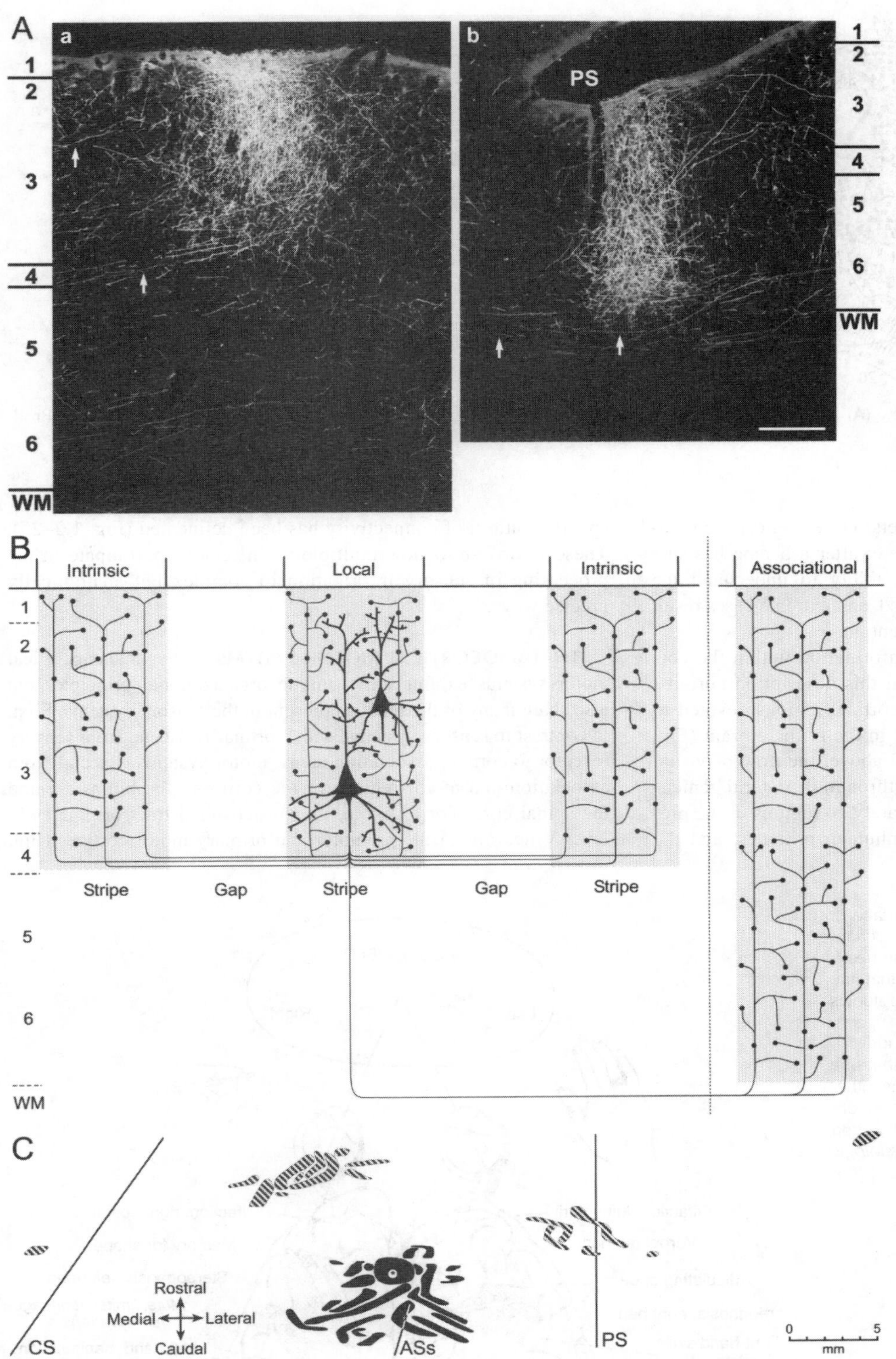

FIGURE 1.2–21 Modular organization of the primate prefrontal cortex (PFC) identified using axon-tracing techniques via localized tracer injection in the monkey. **A:** Darkfield photomicrographs of biotinylated dextran amine (BDA)-labeled axons resulting from an injection site in layer 3 of area 9 of monkey PFC. The horizontally oriented, long-range intrinsic axon collaterals (*a*) travel through the gray matter (*arrows*) and form a stripe-like cluster of labeled axons, and terminals in area 9 are confined to layers 1 through 3. The labeled associational axons from the same injection site (*b*) travel through the white matter (WM) (*arrows*) to the lateral bank of the principal sulcus (PS, area 46) and form a dense cluster that extends across all cortical layers. Calibration bar = 100 μm. (Adapted from Melchitzky DS, Sesack SR, Pucak ML, Lewis DA: Synaptic targets and extrinsic projections of pyramidal neurons providing horizontal connections in monkey prefrontal cortex. *J Comp Neurol.* 1998;390:211–222.) **B:** Schematic diagram illustrating the spatial distribution of the three types of axon terminals furnished by layer 3 pyramidal neurons in monkey PFC. BDA-labeled axons of pyramidal neurons terminate nearby (local) or after traveling horizontally through the gray matter (intrinsic) or through the white matter (associational) to form stripes of labeled terminals. (Adapted from Melchitzky DS, Gonzalez-Burgos G, Lewis DA: Synaptic targets of the intrinsic axon collaterals of supragranular pyramidal neurons in monkey prefrontal cortex. *J Comp Neurol.* 2001;430:209–221.) **C:** Tangential reconstruction of all stripe-like clusters of retrogradely labeled neurons arising from a single injection in area 9. On this unfolded map, the PS is oriented as a vertical line, and all labeled structures and other sulci are shown relative to the PS. The location of the injection site is indicated by the asterisk. Intrinsic stripes are shaded in black, and associational stripes are crosshatched. Note that the associational projections form several distinct groups of stripes, which are located at varying distances from the intrinsic stripes. ASs, superior ramus of arcuate sulcus; CS, cingulate sulcus. (Adapted from Pucak ML, Levitt JB, Lund JS, Lewis DA: Patterns of intrinsic and associational circuitry in monkey prefrontal cortex. *J Comp Neurol.* 1996;376: 614–630.)

The primary somatosensory cortex, located in the anterior parietal lobe, has been divided into four regions on the basis of cytoarchitecture. Each of the cytoarchitectonic regions—numbered 1, 2, 3a, and 3b by Brodmann—contains a topographical representation of the body. The regions are heavily interconnected and all project to the next level of somatosensory processing in area S-II. This type of projection, from one level of processing to a more advanced level, is termed a *feedforward* projection. The reciprocal connection, from the more advanced processing level back to the simpler level, is called a *feedback* projection. Both projections have distinct patterns of laminar termination: feedforward projections originate in the superficial layers of cortex (layer III) and terminate in layer IV; feedback projections originate in layers III, V, and VI and terminate outside layer IV. Further processing of somatosensory information occurs in higher-order somatosensory areas, such as area 7b of the posterior parietal cortex, which receives feedforward projections

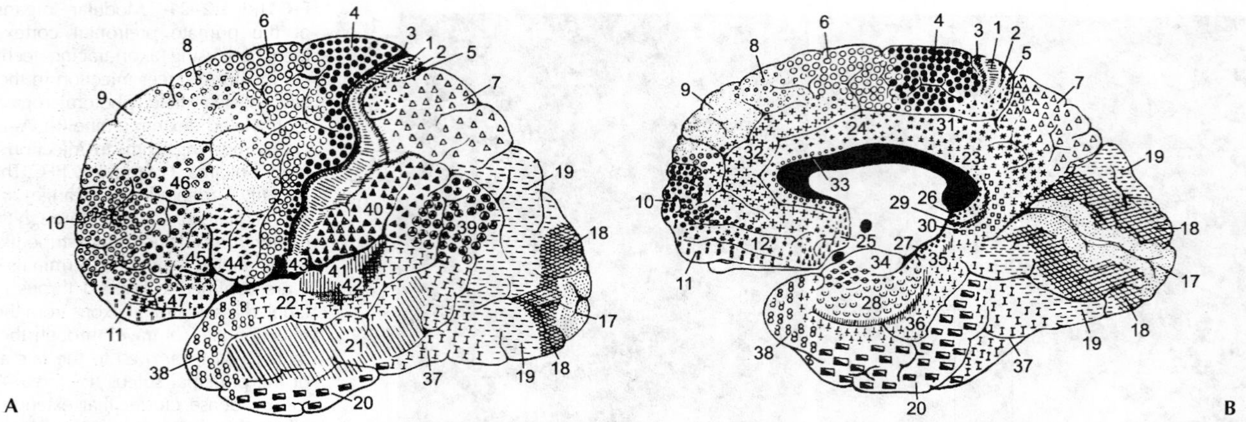

FIGURE 1.2–22 Drawing of the lateral view **(A)** and medial view **(B)** of the cytoarchitectonic subdivisions of the human brain as determined by Brodmann.

from S-II. Lesions of the posterior parietal cortex reflect the complexity of the information processed there; after a person has sustained a posterior parietal lesion, the ability to understand the significance of sensory stimuli is impaired, and extreme cases result in contralateral sensory neglect and inattention.

The processing of somatosensory information within the cortex is clearly much more complex than this description permits. As a case in point, a large number of cortical regions devoted to visual information have been identified in the primate brain (Fig. 1.2–24). Using the principles described above, the flow of visual information from retinal ganglion cells through the lateral geniculate nucleus of the thalamus, and, ultimately, to regions of the prefrontal cortex has been mapped in nonhuman primates, and the specific pattern of connectivity has been delineated (Fig. 1.2–25). These efforts show how multiple brain regions participate in the processing of sensory information in complex but anatomically precise ways.

THALAMOCORTICAL MOTOR SYSTEMS The thalamocortical motor systems exhibit some unique organizational principles but also share many of the features present in the sensory systems. First, in contrast to sensory systems, which primarily ascend from sensory receptor to cortical association areas, motor systems descend from association and motor regions of the cortex to the brainstem and the spinal cord. For example, the corticospinal tract originates in layer V neurons of the premotor and primary motor cortices (Fig.

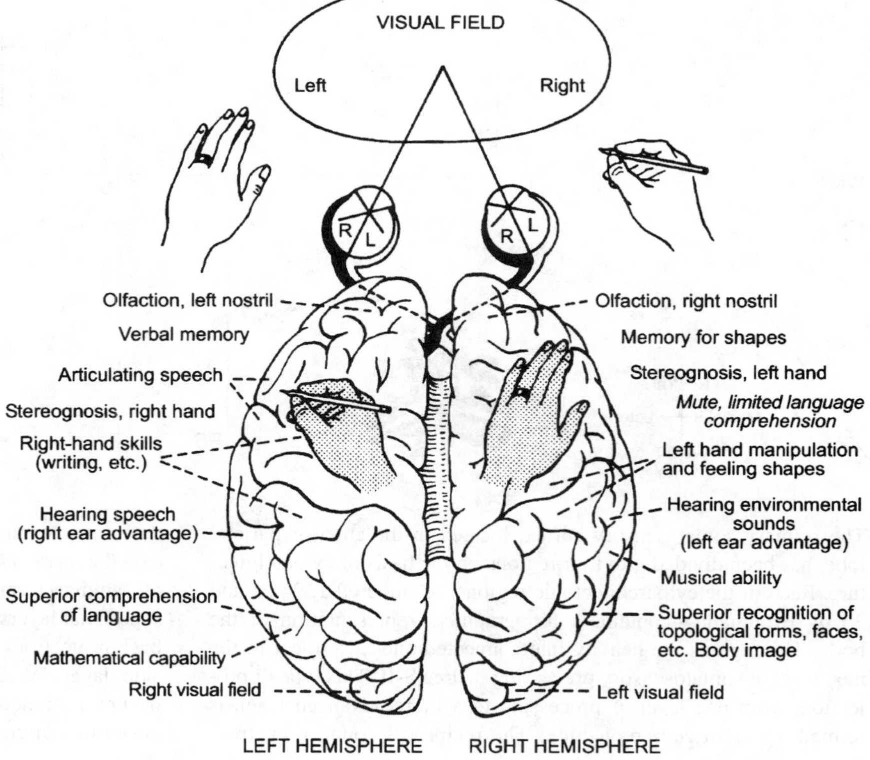

FIGURE 1.2–23 Drawing of the dorsal surface of the human brain showing the tendency for certain functions to be preferentially localized to one hemisphere. However, it is important to note that the intact brain may not be as lateralized as some studies (e.g., of patients with commissurotomies) suggest, that the degree of lateralization differs across individuals, and that, in the intact brain, it is rare that one hemisphere can mediate a function that the other hemisphere is completely unable to perform. (From Fuchs AF, Phillips JO. Association cortex. In: Patton HD, Fuchs AF, Hillie B, et al. *Textbook of Physiology*. Vol. 1, 21st ed. Philadelphia: W.B. Saunders; 1989, with permission.)

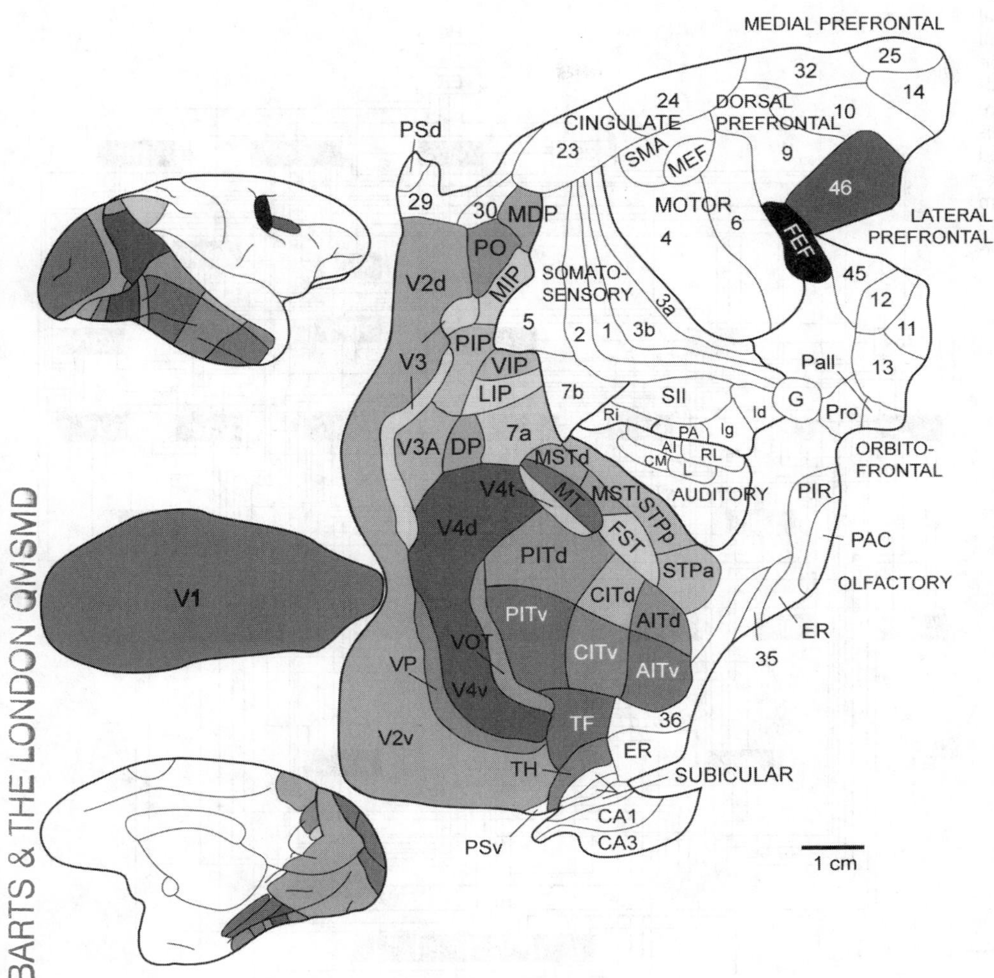

FIGURE 1.2–24 Two-dimensional map of cortical areas in the macaque monkey. The locations of 32 areas likely to be involved in the processing of visual information are identified by shading. Note the number of areas outside the occipital lobe involved in the processing of visual information. The connectivity of this map is illustrated in Figure 1.2–25. The calibration bar applies only to the map. (From Felleman DJ, Van Essen DC: Distributed hierarchical processing in the primate cerebral cortex. *Cereb Cortex.* 1991;1:36, with permission.)

1.2–19B) of the frontal lobe and terminates in the spinal cord to influence motor behavior.

Second, motor systems exhibit strong topography at both the thalamic and cortical levels. For example, the corticospinal tract is organized so that a topographical representation of the contralateral half of the body is evident in the primary motor and premotor cortices. The representation of the body is disproportionate, with large regions of the motor cortex devoted to areas of the body involved in fine movement, such as the face and the hands.

Finally, there is a convergence of projections from several sensory association regions to the motor regions of the frontal cortex. For example, the premotor cortex receives a convergence of afferents from higher-order somatosensory and visual areas of the posterior parietal cortex, whereas afferents from the primary somatosensory cortex converge on the primary motor cortex. In addition to cortical input, the primary motor cortex receives afferents from the ventral lateral nucleus of the thalamus; this nucleus receives afferents predominantly from the cerebellum. The premotor cortex receives input from the ventral anterior thalamic nucleus, which receives much of its input from the globus pallidus.

THALAMOCORTICAL ASSOCIATION SYSTEMS The multimodal association areas of the cortex are organized according to several general principles. First, association regions receive a convergence of input from a variety of sources, including unimodal and multimodal association regions of the cortex, association nuclei of the thalamus, and other structures. For example, the prefrontal cortex receives afferents from higher-order sensory cortices of the parietal and temporal lobes, the contralateral prefrontal cortex, the cingulate cortex of the limbic system, the medial dorsal nucleus of the thalamus (an association relay nucleus), and portions of the amygdala. The medial dorsal nucleus receives highly processed inputs from many sources, including some regions, such as the amygdala, that project directly to the prefrontal cortex. The redundant (direct and indirect) projections may serve to attach additional significance to certain inputs received by the prefrontal cortex. The significance of these inputs may also be influenced by their temporal and spatial coincidence with modulatory inputs from brainstem nuclei that use the monoamine neurotransmitters dopamine, norepinephrine, or serotonin. These monoamine systems project broadly to the cerebral cortex, although with substantial regional differences in density (Fig. 1.2–26). In addition, the innervation density in the cerebral cortex is typically much lower than in some subcortical areas.

Second, the projections that terminate in multimodal association regions exhibit a topographical organization. Because the information conveyed in these projections is highly processed, it does not appear that the topographical organization of the afferents is a representation of the external world. Nonetheless, a distinct pattern is present in the afferents received by association areas. For example, different cytoarchitectonic regions of the medial dorsal nucleus project to discrete regions of the prefrontal cortex. In addition, some of the cortical afferents received by the prefrontal cortex are topo-

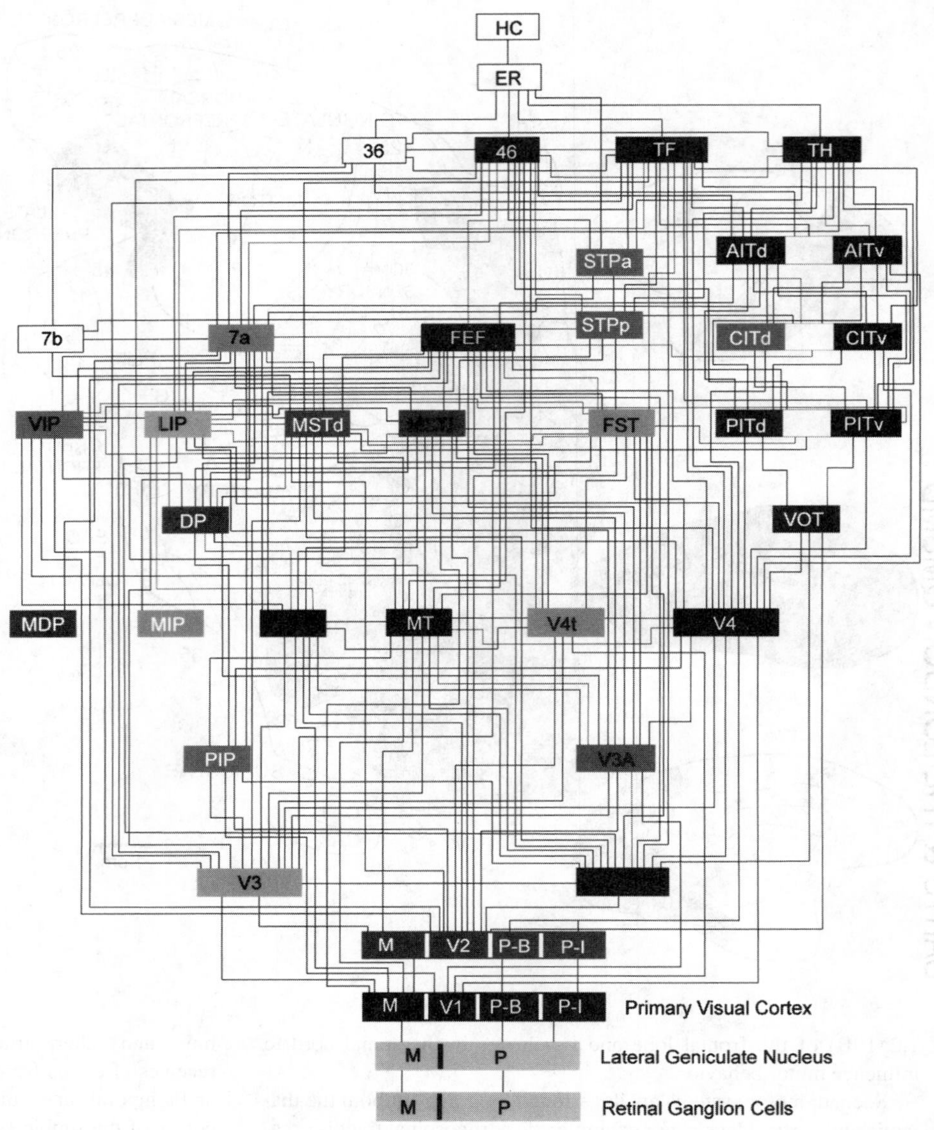

FIGURE 1.2–25 A proposed organizational scheme of the connectivity among cortical areas involved in the processing of visual information, starting with the retinal ganglion cells and extending to area 46 and the frontal eye fields (FEFs). Hierarchical assignments for this scheme were made on the basis of documented feedforward and feedback patterns of connections, as described in the text. (Adapted from Felleman DJ, Van Essen DC: Distributed hierarchical processing in the primate cerebral cortex. *Cereb Cortex.* 1991;1:36.)

graphically organized; certain regions of the prefrontal cortex predominantly receive highly processed information from one modality.

The patterns of connectivity are clearly related to some of the functional characteristics attributed to the prefrontal cortex. For example, in monkeys, lesions of the dorsolateral prefrontal cortex consistently produce impairments in the monkey's ability to perform spatial delayed-response tasks. These tasks require that the monkey maintain a spatial representation of the location of an object during a delay period in which the object is out of sight; it has been suggested that the prefrontal cortex plays a role in maintaining the spatial representation of the object. Such a function would require that the prefrontal cortex receive information regarding the location of objects in space, and, indeed, the dorsolateral prefrontal cortex is innervated by afferents from association regions of the parietal cortex that convey such information. Although the dorsolateral prefrontal cortex is necessary for the performance of delayed-response tasks in the monkey, it is not sufficient for the performance of the task. For example, lesions of the medial dorsal nucleus in the monkey result in similar impairments on the performance of spatial delayed-response tasks. Thus, the functions attributed to the prefrontal cortex are a result of the neural circuitry involving the region.

Knowledge of the integration of afferent inputs into the neural circuitry of certain prefrontal regions may also be important for understanding the nature of prefrontal cortical dysfunction in schizophrenia. Schizophrenic patients perform poorly on tasks that are known to be mediated by the prefrontal cortex. These findings have been correlated with other measures to suggest, albeit indirectly, that the dopamine projections to the prefrontal cortex are impaired in schizophrenia. For example, studies in nonhuman primates have shown that performance of delayed-response tasks, the same type of behaviors that are impaired in schizophrenic subjects, requires an appropriate level of dopamine input to the dorsolateral prefrontal cortex.

CEREBELLO-THALAMOCORTICAL SYSTEMS The cerebellum has traditionally been considered to be involved solely with motor control, regulating posture, gait, and voluntary movements. However, recent studies indicate that the cerebellum may also play an important role in the mediation of certain cognitive abilities through inputs to portions of the thalamus that project to association regions of the cerebral cortex.

The cerebellum is located in the posterior cranial fossa, inferior to the occipital lobes (Figs. 1.2–4 and 1.2–10). The external surface

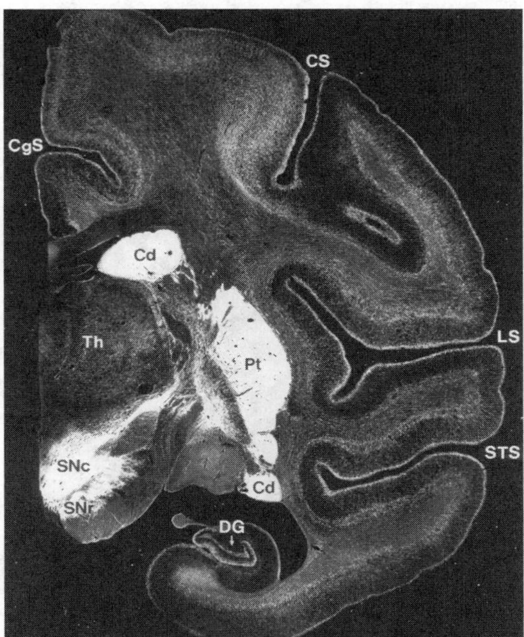

FIGURE 1.2–26 Darkfield photomicrograph of a coronal section through a hemisphere of a macaque monkey immunolabeled for the dopamine transporter. This image illustrates the differential distribution of dopamine-containing axons in different regions of the brain. The brighter the image, the greater the quantity of dopamine-containing axons. Dopamine-rich areas such as the caudate (Cd), putamen (Pt), and substantia nigra (SNc and SNr) appear as white; whereas, dopamine innervation of the cortex and thalamus, although clearly seen, is less dense and varies by the specific cortical and thalamic region. CgS, cingulate sulcus; CS, central sulcus; DG, dentate gyrus; LS, lateral sulcus; STS, superior temporal sulcus; Th, thalamus. Calibration bar = 2 mm. (From Lewis DA, Melchitzky DS, Sesack SR, et al.: Dopamine transporter immunoreactivity in monkey cerebral cortex: regional, laminar and ultrastructural localization. *J Comp Neurol.* 2001;432:119–136, with permission.)

of the cerebellum, the cerebellar cortex, is composed of small folds, termed *folia*, separated by sulci. Viewed from the dorsal surface, the cerebellum contains a raised central portion, called the *vermis*, and lateral portions called the *cerebellar hemispheres* (Fig. 1.2–10). Located within the cerebellum are the deep cerebellar nuclei, which are arranged as follows: the fastigial nucleus is located next to the midline; the globose and emboliform nuclei are located slightly more lateral; and the largest nucleus, the dentate, occupies the most lateral position. In general, the cerebellar cortex can be considered to process the inputs to the cerebellum, and the deep nuclei to process the outputs. Although many portions of the cerebellum are interconnected with brain regions that regulate motor actions, the circuitry of the cerebellum involved in cognitive functions may be of greatest interest from the standpoint of psychiatric illness. For example, the lateral cerebellar cortex and the dentate nucleus are markedly expanded in the primate brain. It has been suggested that these changes are associated with an increase in the size of cortical areas (especially the prefrontal regions) influenced by cerebellar output and an expanded role of the cerebellum in cognitive functions. In fact, recent studies in nonhuman primates have shown that the dorsolateral prefrontal cortex receives inputs from two ipsilateral thalamic nuclei (medial dorsal and ventral lateral), which, in turn, receive inputs from the contralateral cerebellar dentate nucleus. The cells of the dentate nucleus involved in these connections are distinct from those that influence the motor and premotor regions of the cerebral cortex. Interestingly, functional imaging studies in schizophrenic subjects have revealed abnormal patterns of activation in the cerebellum, thalamus, and prefrontal cortex, suggesting that dysfunction of this circuitry might be associated with the disturbances in cognitive processes exhibited by these patients.

Basal Ganglia System

The basal ganglia are a collection of nuclei that have been grouped together on the basis of their interconnections. These nuclei play an important role in regulating movement and in certain disorders of movement (dyskinesias), which include jerky movements (chorea), writhing movements (athetosis), and rhythmic movements (tremors). In addition, recent studies have shown that certain components of the basal ganglia play an important role in many cognitive functions.

Major Structures

The basal ganglia are generally considered to include the *caudate nucleus*, the *putamen*, the *globus pallidus* (referred to as the *paleostriatum* or *pallidum*), the *subthalamic nucleus*, and the *substantia nigra* (Fig. 1.2–27). The term *striatum* refers to the caudate nucleus and the putamen together; the term *corpus striatum* refers to the caudate nucleus, the putamen, and the globus pallidus; and the term *lentiform nucleus* refers to the putamen and the globus pallidus together.

Although these nuclei are generally agreed to belong to the basal ganglia, some controversy exists concerning whether other nuclei should be included in the definition of the basal ganglia. Some investigators believe that additional regions of the brain have anatomical connections that are similar to other components of the basal ganglia and should, therefore, be included in the term. These additional regions are usually termed the *ventral striatum* and the *ventral pallidum*. The ventral striatum includes the nucleus accumbens (Fig. 1.2–27), which is the region where the putamen and the head of the caudate nucleus fuse, and the olfactory tubercle. The ventral pallidum is a region that receives afferents from the ventral striatum and includes, but is not limited to, a group of neurons termed the *substantia innominata* (Fig. 1.2–7). This section focuses on the structures generally accepted as belonging to the basal ganglia but also discusses additional structures when relevant to the functional anatomy of the system.

CAUDATE NUCLEUS

The caudate nucleus is a C-shaped structure that is divided into three general regions. The anterior portion of the structure is referred to as the *head*, the posterior region is the *tail*, and the intervening region is the *body* (Fig. 1.2–27). The caudate nucleus is associated with the contour of the lateral ventricles: the head lies against the frontal horn of the lateral ventricle, and the tail lies against the temporal horn (Figs. 1.2–7, 1.2–8, and 1.2–9). The head of the caudate nucleus is continuous with the putamen; the tail terminates in the amygdala of the temporal lobe.

PUTAMEN

The putamen lies in the brain medial to the insula and is bounded laterally by the fibers of the external capsule and medially by the globus pallidus (Figs. 1.2–7 and 1.2–8). As noted above, the putamen is continuous with the head of the caudate nucleus (Fig. 1.2–27). Although bridges of neurons between the caudate nucleus and the putamen show the continuity of the nuclei, the two structures are separated by fibers of the anterior limb of the internal capsule.

GLOBUS PALLIDUS

In contrast to the caudate nucleus and the putamen, which are telencephalic in origin, the globus pallidus is derived from the diencephalon. The globus pallidus constitutes the inner component of the lentiform nucleus (Fig. 1.2–27, bottom panel);

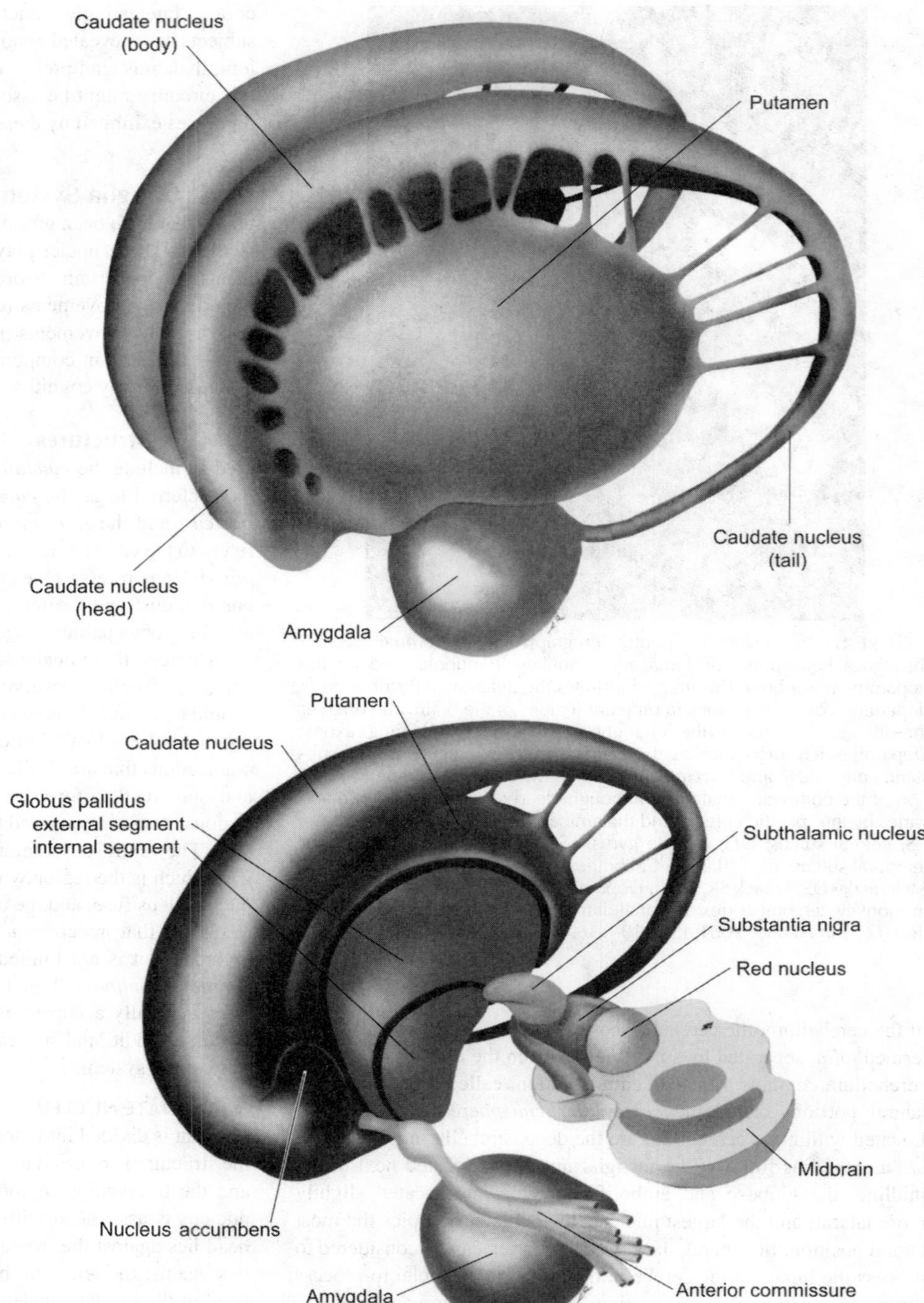

FIGURE 1.2–27 Schematic drawing of the isolated basal ganglia as seen from the dorsolateral perspective, so that the caudate nucleus is apparent bilaterally. In the bottom panel, the left hemisphere of the basal ganglia has been removed, exposing the medial surface of the right putamen and globus pallidus, as well as the subthalamic nucleus and substantia nigra. (Adapted from Hendelman WJ. *Student's Atlas of Neuroanatomy*. Philadelphia: W.B. Saunders; 1994:37.)

with the putamen, it forms a cone-like structure, with its tip directed medially (Figs. 1.2–7 and 1.2–8). The posterior limb of the internal capsule bounds the globus pallidus medially and separates it from the thalamus; the putamen borders the globus pallidus laterally. In the human, the medial medullary lamina divides the globus pallidus into external (lateral) and internal (medial) segments (Fig. 1.2–8).

SUBTHALAMIC NUCLEUS The subthalamic nucleus (of Luys) is also derived from the diencephalon. The large-celled nucleus lies dorsomedial to the posterior limb of the internal capsule and dorsal to the substantia nigra (Figs. 1.2–8 and 1.2–27). Discrete lesions of the subthalamic nucleus in humans lead to hemiballism, a syndrome characterized by violent, forceful choreiform movements that occur on the side contralateral to the lesion.

SUBSTANTIA NIGRA The substantia nigra is present in the midbrain between the tegmentum and the basis pedunculi and is mesencephalic in origin (Fig. 1.2–8). The substantia nigra consists of two components: a dorsal cell–rich portion referred to as the *pars compacta* and a ventral cell–sparse portion denoted the *pars reticulata*. Most of the neurons in the pars compacta of the substantia nigra in humans are pigmented because of the presence of neuromelanin; these cells contain the neurotransmitter dopamine (Fig. 1.2–26). The dendrites of the pars compacta neurons frequently extend into the pars reticulata, where they receive synapses from the neurons of the pars reticulata that use the inhibitory neurotransmitter GABA.

In rodents, the dopamine-containing neurons of the substantia nigra (A9 region) have been distinguished from those located in the ventral tegmental area (A10 region) and the retrorubral field (A8 region), but recent studies in monkeys and humans suggest that dopamine neurons can be more meaningfully organized at a functional level into dorsal and ventral tiers (Fig. 1.2–28). The dorsal tier is formed by a medially–laterally oriented band of neurons that includes the dopamine-containing cells that are (1) located in the medial ventral mesencephalon, (2) scattered dorsal to the dense cell clusters in the substantia nigra, and (3) distributed lateral and caudal to the red nucleus. The ventral tier is composed of the dopamine neurons that are densely packed in the substantia nigra and the cell columns that penetrate into the substantia nigra pars reticulata. Dorsal tier dopamine neurons express relatively low levels of the mRNAs for the dopamine transporter and the dopamine type 2 receptor (D_2), contain the calcium-binding protein calbindin, and send axonal projections to the regions of the striatum that are dominated by input from limbic-related structures and association regions of the cerebral cortex. In contrast, ventral-tier neurons contain high levels of the messenger ribonucleic acids (mRNAs) for the dopamine transporter and the D_2 dopamine receptor, typically lack calbindin, and send axonal projections to the sensorimotor regions of the striatum. Each of these features may contribute to the greater vulnerability of ventral tier neurons to the pathology of Parkinson's disease, whereas dorsal tier neurons may be more likely to be involved in the pathophysiology of schizophrenia.

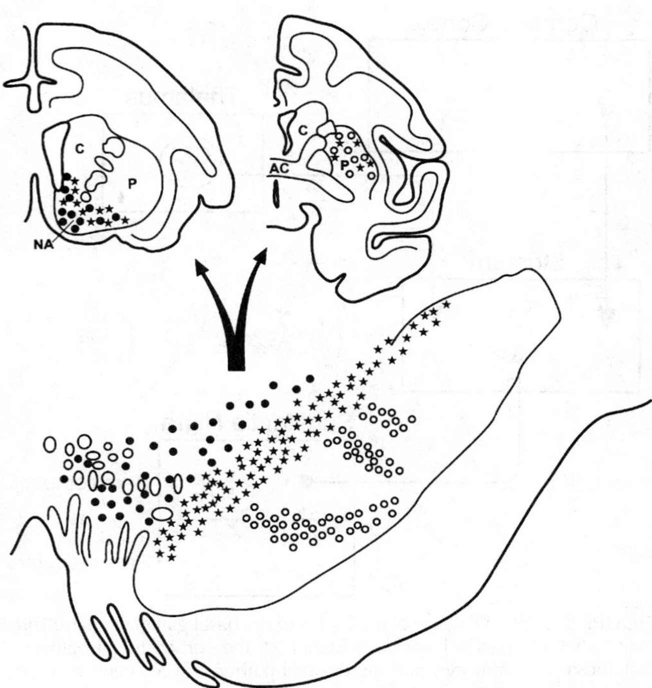

FIGURE 1.2–28 Schematic drawing of the topographic organization of dopamine-containing neurons in the mesencephalon and their projections to the ventral striatum and the sensorimotor-related dorsal striatum. All areas of the ventral striatum receive inputs from the dorsal-tier neurons, with the shell region of the nucleus accumbens innervated almost exclusively by dorsal tier neurons (*filled circles*). In contrast, the ventral columns of cells (*open circles*) in the ventral tier send projections selectively to the sensorimotor-related striatum. The neurons of the densocellular zone (*stars*) of the ventral tier are unique in that they project to both the ventral and sensorimotor-related striatum. AC, anterior commissure; C, caudate nucleus; NA, nucleus accumbens; P, putamen. (Adapted from Lynda-Balta E, Haber SN: The organization of midbrain projections to the ventral striatum in the primate. *Neuroscience.* 1994;59:625–640.)

Internal Organization The caudate nucleus and the putamen are frequently referred to together because of their common characteristics. For example, in the rodent, these nuclei are a continuous structure, and, in all mammals, they are composed of histologically identical cells. The majority of neurons in the striatum are medium-sized cells (10 to 20 μm in diameter) that possess spines on their dendrites; these so-called medium spiny neurons are known to send their axons out of the striatum. In addition to medium spiny neurons, medium-sized cells without spines (medium aspiny neurons) are present, as are large cells with and without spines (large spiny neurons and large aspiny neurons). With the exception of the medium and large spiny cells, most other striatal neurons are local circuit neurons.

Immunohistochemical and receptor-binding studies have shown a discontinuity in the distribution of certain neurotransmitter-related substances that form the functional circuitry of the basal ganglia. For example, in the striatum, zones that contain a low density of acetylcholinesterase (AChE) enzymatic activity are surrounded by regions rich in AChE activity. The AChE-rich regions are referred to as the *matrix*, and the AChE-poor zones are termed either *striosomes* in the primate or *patches* in the rodent. The organization of several neuropeptide systems follows this organization. For example, the distributions of enkephalin, substance P, and somatostatin immunoreactivity show the compartmentalization of the striatum. In addition, in the rodent, certain subtypes of dopamine receptors are present predominantly in one compartment as compared with the other. In addition, the distribution of some afferent systems terminating in the striatum follows the striosome matrix organization. For example, afferents from the thalamus terminate preferentially in the matrix rather than in the striosome.

Functional Circuitry Projections into, within, and out of the basal ganglia are topographically organized and maintain this topography throughout the processing circuits of the basal ganglia. The existence of such patterns of connectivity has resulted in the hypothesis that parallel independent circuits in the basal ganglia process information from different regions of the brain and subserve separate complex functions.

INPUTS TO THE BASAL GANGLIA The striatum is the major recipient of the inputs to the basal ganglia. Three major afferent systems are known to terminate in the striatum: the corticostriatal, nigrostriatal, and thalamostriatal afferents (Fig. 1.2–29). The corticostriatal projection originates from all regions of the neocortex, arising primarily from the pyramidal cells of layers V and VI, which use the excitatory neurotransmitter glutamate. A topography governing corticostriatal projections has been found in the monkey. Afferents from the sensorimotor cortex terminate predominantly in the putamen; association regions of the cortex terminate preferentially in the caudate nucleus. The prefrontal regions, in particular, provide a heavy input to the head of the caudate nucleus. In addition, afferents from the limbic cortical areas, the hippocampus, and the amygdala terminate in the ventral striatum. The second major class of afferents uses the neurotransmitter dopamine. In Fig. 1.2–29, these projections are shown arising from the substantia nigra pars compacta, but, as noted above (Fig. 1.2–28), different portions of the striatum receive input from either the dorsal- or ventral-tier dopamine-containing neurons of the ventral mesencephalon. Electron microscopy studies

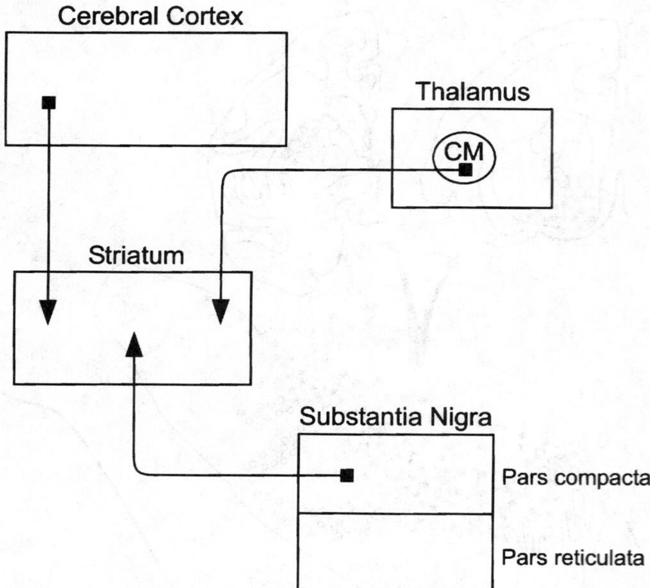

FIGURE 1.2–29 Diagram of the inputs to the basal ganglia system. Three major afferent systems have been identified: the corticostriatal pathways, thalamostriatal pathways, and nigrostriatal pathways. CM, central median nucleus.

have shown that many of the synapses formed by dopamine axon terminals on medium spiny neuron dendrites are immediately adjacent to the synapses provided by corticostriatal axons, suggesting that dopamine may play an important role in modulating the excitatory influence of cortical projections on striatal neurons. The third afferent system originates in the thalamus. The thalamic nuclei providing the projections are the intralaminar nuclei, particularly the central median nucleus.

Disruption of the input pathways of the basal ganglia has been associated with some movement disorders, such as Parkinson's disease, which is characterized by muscular rigidity, fine tremor, shuffling gait, and bradykinesia. The most consistent neuropathological feature of Parkinson's disease is a degeneration of the dopamine neurons in the substantia nigra pars compacta, accompanied by a loss of dopamine terminals in the striatum. The compound levodopa (Larodopa, Dopar), a precursor in the biosynthesis of dopamine, is used as a treatment for Parkinson's disease because of its ability to augment the release of dopamine from the remaining terminals. Conversely, the administration of typical antipsychotic agents in the treatment of schizophrenia is frequently associated with parkinsonian features and other motor system abnormalities; the fact that these agents are D_2 dopamine receptor antagonists is thought to explain their movement-related side effects.

INTERNAL PROCESSING The major processing pathways within the basal ganglia are summarized in Fig. 1.2–30. Within the striatum, the subclass of medium spiny neurons that contain the neuropeptide substance P send inhibitory projections to the internal segment of the globus pallidus in what is termed the *direct pathway*. In contrast, the subpopulation of medium spiny neurons that contain the neuropeptide enkephalin provides inhibitory projections to the external segment of the globus pallidus, which, in turn, sends inhibitory afferents to the internal segment of the globus pallidus in what is termed the *indirect pathway*. The globus pallidus external also projects to the pars reticulata of the substantia nigra. The topography found in the afferent projections to the striatum appears to be main-

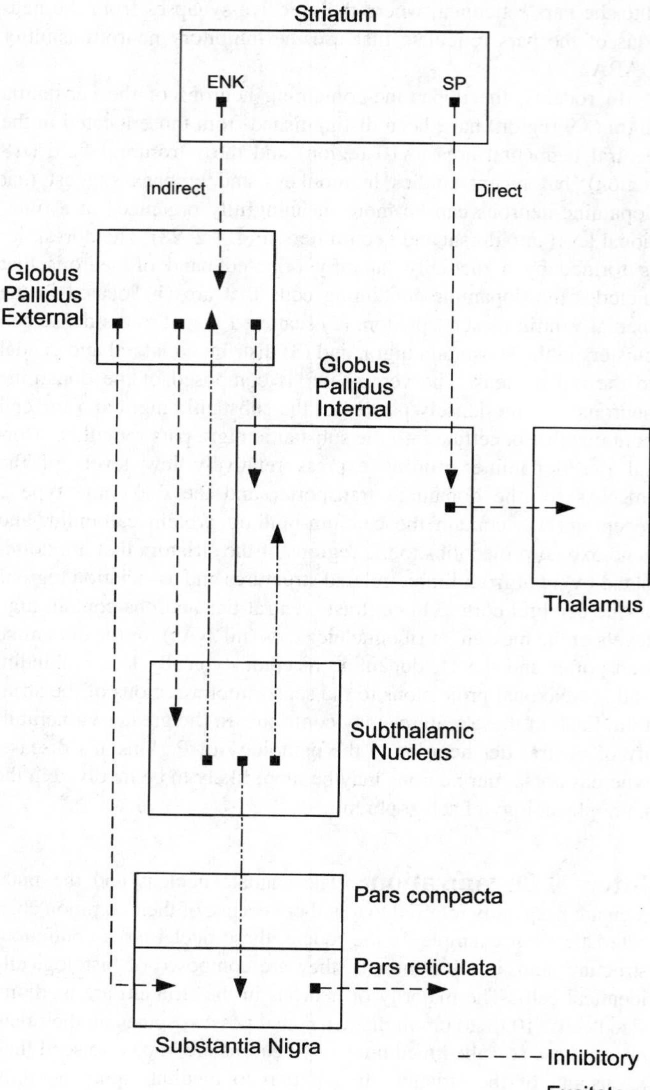

FIGURE 1.2–30 Diagram of the intrinsic circuitry of the basal ganglia. Substance P (SP)–containing striatal neurons send an inhibitory projection directly to the internal segment of the globus pallidus, whereas those containing enkephalin (ENK) provide an inhibitory projection to γ-aminobutyric acid (GABA) neurons in the external segment of the globus pallidus, which, in turn, project to the internal segment of the globus pallidus. The subthalamic nucleus receives a projection from the external segment of the globus pallidus and projects back to both segments. Finally, the subthalamic nucleus and globus pallidus external project to the substantia nigra pars reticulata.

tained in that processing pathway. For example, the sensorimotor territories of the striatum project most heavily to the ventral portion of the globus pallidus, whereas association territories project to the dorsal regions of the globus pallidus.

The external segment of the globus pallidus also gives rise to an inhibitory projection that terminates in the subthalamic nucleus. In contrast, neurons in the subthalamic nucleus provide excitatory projections that terminate in both segments of the globus pallidus and in the pars reticulata. Although most connections within the basal ganglia are unidirectional a reciprocal projection is found between the external segment of the globus pallidus and the subthalamic nucleus.

The intrinsic circuitry of the basal ganglia is disrupted by a severe loss of neurons in the striatum in Huntington's disease. This autoso-

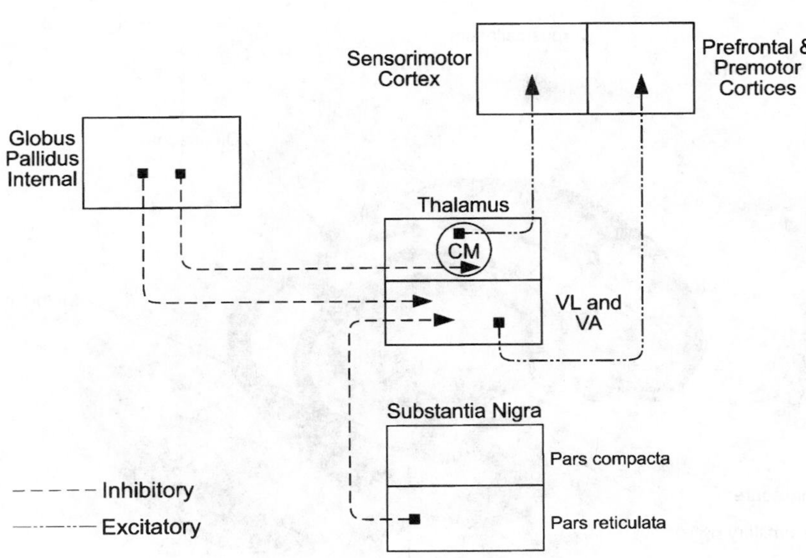

FIGURE 1.2–31 Diagram of the output of the basal ganglia system. The internal segment of the globus pallidus projects to the central median (CM), ventral lateral (VL), and ventral anterior (VA) nuclei of the thalamus. These nuclei then project to sensorimotor, prefrontal, and premotor cortices. The substantia nigra pars reticulata also projects to the VL and VA nuclei.

mal-dominant disorder is characterized by progressive chorea and dementia. Although the Huntington's disease gene has been identified, how the excessive number of trinucleotide repeats in this gene leads to the selective degeneration of striatal cells is currently a matter of intense investigation. Interestingly, recent studies indicate that cortical neurons are also subject to degeneration in Huntington's disease.

OUTPUT OF BASAL GANGLIA The internal segment of the globus pallidus is the source of much of the output of the basal ganglia (Fig. 1.2–31). This segment of the globus pallidus provides a projection to the ventral lateral and ventral anterior nuclei of the thalamus and to the intralaminar thalamic nuclei, particularly the central median nucleus. The pars reticulata of the substantia nigra also provides a projection to the ventral anterior and ventral lateral thalamic nuclei. These portions of the ventral lateral and ventral anterior thalamic nuclei then project to the premotor and prefrontal cortices. As a result of the projections of the premotor and prefrontal cortices to the primary motor cortex, the basal ganglia are able to indirectly influence the output of the primary motor cortex. In addition, the cortical output of the basal ganglia exhibits marked convergence; that is, although the striatum receives afferents from all regions of the neocortex, the eventual output of the globus pallidus and pars reticulata is largely conveyed through the thalamus to a much smaller portion of the neocortex, the premotor and prefrontal regions.

The functional consequences of the neural circuitry of the basal ganglia can also be considered in the context of some of the neurotransmitters used (Figs. 1.2–30 and 1.2–31). Because the afferents from the cortex are thought to use glutamate, which is an excitatory neurotransmitter, cortical afferents presumably excite the structures of the basal ganglia in which they terminate. Many of the processing pathways within the basal ganglia use the inhibitory neurotransmitter GABA. Finally, the output pathways of the basal ganglia—namely, the globus pallidus and the substantia nigra pars reticulata—use GABA as well. Thus, excitation from cortical afferents eventually disinhibits the target structures of the basal ganglia because of the back-to-back inhibitory pathways of the basal ganglia.

Historically, motor systems have been divided into pyramidal (corticospinal) and extrapyramidal (basal ganglia) components; this division is based on clinical findings suggesting that lesions of each system result in distinct motor syndromes. For example, lesions of the extrapyramidal system result in involuntary movements, changes in muscle tone, and slowness of movement; lesions of the pyramidal system lead to spasticity and paralysis. Because of these findings, the pyramidal and extrapyramidal systems were thought to independently control voluntary and involuntary movement, respectively. However, this division is no longer accurate for several reasons. First, other structures of the brain outside the traditional pyramidal and extrapyramidal systems, such as the cerebellum, are involved in the control of movement. Second, the pyramidal and extrapyramidal systems are not independent, but the neural circuits of these systems are interconnected. For example, the basal ganglia influence motor behavior through certain regions of the cerebral cortex, which then directly (through the corticospinal tract) or indirectly (through specific brainstem nuclei) produce motor activity.

Finally, although the basal ganglia are important in the control of movement, this neural system also appears to be involved in other functions of the brain. For example, recent studies of the connections of the basal ganglia in nonhuman primates also support a role for these structures in cognitive functions. The dorsolateral prefrontal cortex has been shown to receive inputs from portions of the thalamus that are the targets of projections from specific locations within the internal segment of the globus pallidus, providing evidence for a distinct pallido-thalamocortical pathway. Thus, in addition to linking association regions of the cerebral cortex, such as the prefrontal and posterior parietal areas, with the control of motor activity in the primary motor cortex, some of the output of the basal ganglia appears to be directed back to regions of the prefrontal cortex. These findings suggest that "closed" loops are present between the prefrontal cortex and basal ganglia, which presumably have a cognitive rather than a motor function.

Limbic System

The concept of the limbic system as a neural substrate for emotional experience and expression has a rich but controversial history. More than 100 years ago, Paul Broca applied the term *limbic* (from the Latin *limbus*, for border) to the curved rim of the cortex, including the cingulate and the parahippocampal gyri, located at the junction of the diencephalon and the cerebral hemispheres (Fig. 1.2–32). In 1937, James Papez postulated, primarily on the basis of anatomical data, that these cortical regions were linked to the hippocampus, mammillary body, and anterior thalamus in a circuit that mediated emotional behavior (Fig. 1.2–33). This concept

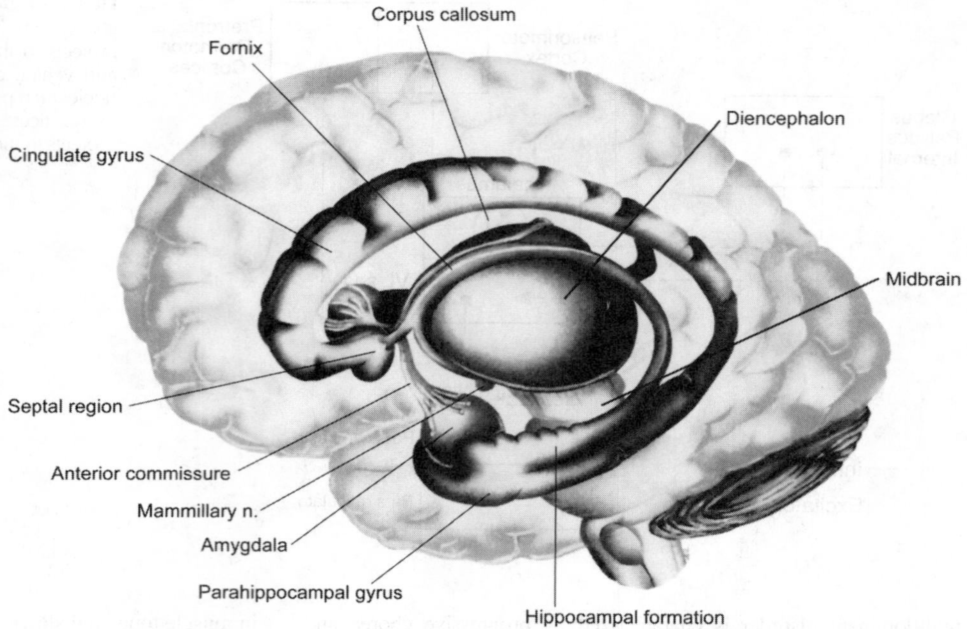

FIGURE 1.2–32 Schematic drawing of the major anatomical structures of the limbic system. Note that the cingulate and parahippocampal gyri form the *limbic lobe,* a rim of tissue located along the junction of the diencephalon and the cerebral hemispheres. n., nucleus. (Adapted from Hendelman WJ. *Student's Atlas of Neuroanatomy*. Philadelphia: W.B. Saunders; 1994:179.)

was supported by the work of Heinrich Klüver and Paul Bucy, who demonstrated that temporal lobe lesions, which disrupt components of the circuit, alter affective responses in nonhuman primates. In 1952, Paul MacLean coined the term *limbic system* to describe Broca's limbic lobe and related subcortical nuclei as the neural substrate for emotion.

However, over the last 40 years, it has become clear that some limbic structures (for example, the hippocampus) are also involved in other complex brain processes, such as memory. In addition, expanding knowledge of the connectivity of traditional limbic structures has made it increasingly difficult to define the boundaries of the limbic system. Despite these limitations, the concept of a limbic system may still be a useful way to describe the circuitry that relates certain telencephalic structures and their cognitive processes with the hypothalamus and its output pathways that control autonomic, somatic, and endocrine functions.

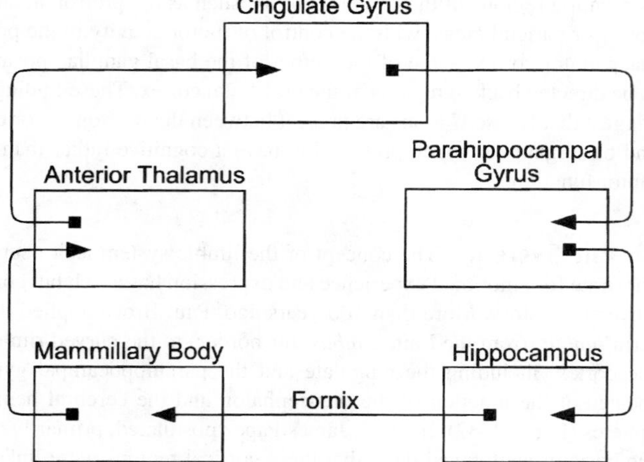

FIGURE 1.2–33 Diagram of the neural circuit for emotion as originally proposed by James Papez.

Major Structures As suggested above, there is no unanimity on the brain structures that constitute the limbic system. This section includes the brain regions that are most commonly listed as components of the limbic system: the cingulate and parahippocampal gyri (limbic cortex), the hippocampal formation, the amygdala, the septal area, the hypothalamus, and related thalamic and cortical areas.

LIMBIC CORTEX The limbic cortex is composed of two general regions, the cingulate gyrus and the parahippocampal gyrus (Fig. 1.2–32). The *cingulate gyrus,* located dorsal to the corpus callosum, includes several cortical regions that are heavily interconnected with the association areas of the cerebral cortex. As the cingulate gyrus travels posteriorly, it becomes continuous (via the cingulum bundle of fibers in the white matter) with the *parahippocampal gyrus,* located in the medial temporal lobe, which contains several distinct cytoarchitectonic regions. One of the most important of these regions is the *entorhinal cortex,* which not only funnels highly processed cortical information to the hippocampal formation, but also is a major output pathway from the hippocampal formation.

HIPPOCAMPAL FORMATION Three distinct zones—the dentate gyrus, the hippocampus, and the subicular complex—constitute the hippocampal formation, which is located in the floor of the temporal horn of the lateral ventricle (Fig. 1.2–9). These zones are composed of adjacent strips of cortical tissue that run in a rostral–caudal direction but fold over each other mediolaterally in a spiral fashion, giving rise to a C-shaped appearance. The *dentate gyrus* is composed of three layers: an outer, acellular molecular layer, which faces the subarachnoid space of the hippocampal fissure; a middle layer composed of granule cells; and an inner polymorphic layer (Fig. 1.2–34). The granule cells extend their dendritic trees into the molecular layer and give rise to axons that form the mossy fiber projection to the hippocampus.

The *hippocampus* is also a trilaminate structure composed of molecular and polymorphic layers and a middle layer that contains pyramidal neurons. On the basis of differences in the cytoarchitecture and connectivity, the hippocampus can be divided into three distinct fields, which have been labeled CA3, CA2, and CA1. (*CA* is

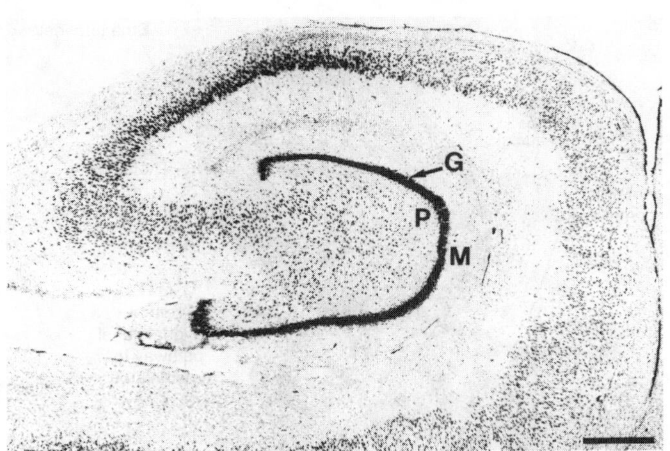

FIGURE 1.2–34 Nissl-stained coronal section through the dentate gyrus of the human hippocampal formation. Medial is to the left. G, granular layer; M, molecular layer; P, polymorphic layer. Calibration bar = 1.0 mm.

derived from the term *cornu ammonis* after the Egyptian deity Ammon, who was depicted with ram's horns, which some early investigators thought described the shape of the hippocampus.) The white matter adjacent to the polymorphic layer of the hippocampus is known as the *alveus*. The axons in this structure contribute to the fimbria, which, at the caudal end of the hippocampus, becomes the crus of the *fornix*. These bilateral structures converge to form the body of the fornix, which travels anteriorly and then turns inferiorly to form the columns of the fornix, which pass through the hypothalamus into the mammillary bodies (Fig. 1.2–35). The *subicular complex* is generally considered to have three components—the presubiculum, the parasubiculum, and the subiculum—that together serve as transition regions between the hippocampus and the parahippocampal gyrus.

The components of the hippocampal formation have a distinct pattern of intrinsic connectivity that is largely unidirectional and provides for a specific flow of information (Fig. 1.2–36). The major input to the hippocampal formation arises from neurons in layers II and III of the entorhinal cortex that project through the *perforant path* (that is, through the subiculum and the hippocampus) to the outer two-thirds of the molecular layer of the dentate gyrus, where they synapse on the dendrites of granule cells. The mossy fiber axons of the granule cells then provide a projection to the pyramidal neurons of the CA3 field of the hippocampus. Axon collaterals from CA3 pyramidal neurons project within CA3 and, through the so-called Schäffer collaterals, to the CA1 field of the hippocampus. This region, in turn, projects to the subicular complex, which provides output to the entorhinal cortex, completing the circuit.

AMYGDALA Located in the medial temporal lobe just anterior to the hippocampal formation are a group of nuclei referred to as the *amygdala* (Fig. 1.2–8). These nuclei form several distinct clusters: the basolateral complex, the centromedial amygdaloid group, and the olfactory group, which includes the cortical amygdaloid nuclei. The *basolateral complex*, the largest of the three groups, differs from the remaining amygdaloid nuclei in a number of respects. Although the basolateral complex is not a laminated structure, its connectivity and some other anatomical characteristics are more similar to cortical regions than to the remaining amygdaloid nuclei. For example,

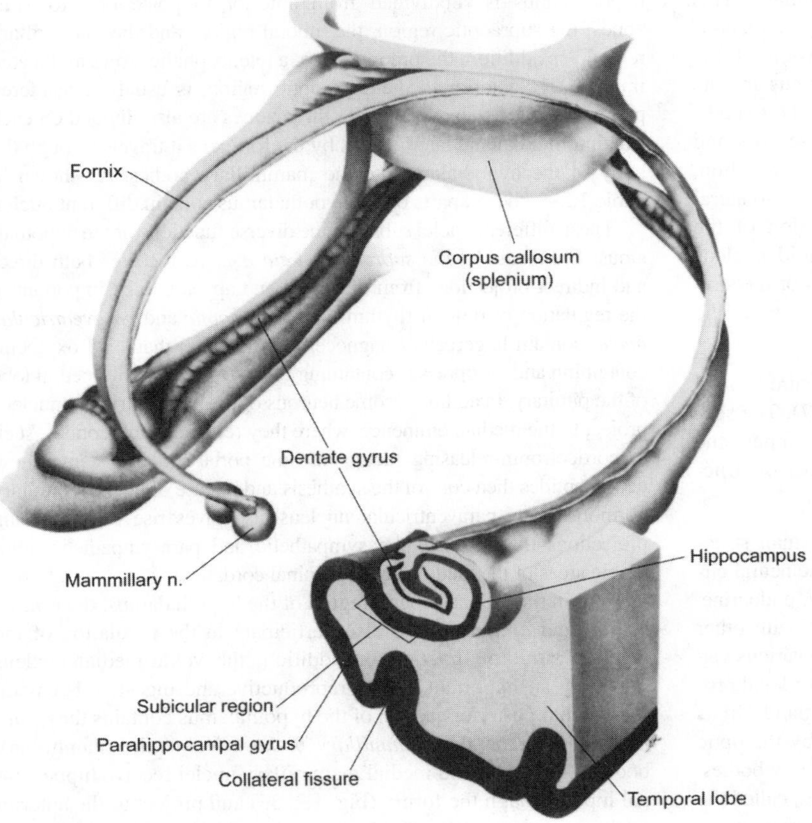

FIGURE 1.2–35 Schematic drawing of a cross-sectional view of the hippocampal formation and the path of the fornix running between this structure and the mammillary bodies. (Adapted from Hendelman WJ. *Student's Atlas of Neuroanatomy*. Philadelphia: W.B. Saunders; 1994:189.)

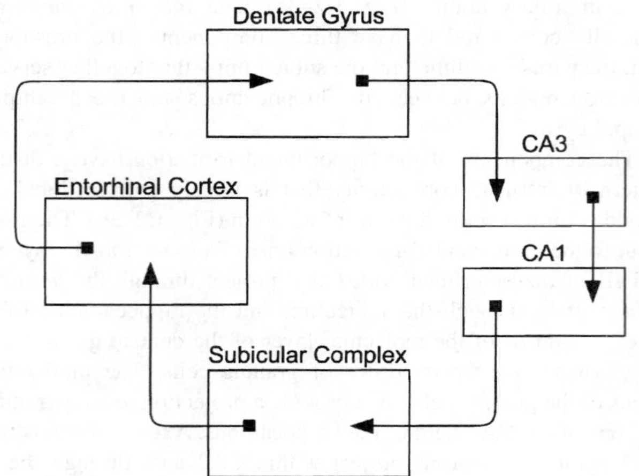

FIGURE 1.2–36 Diagram of the intrinsic neural circuitry of the hippocampal formation.

the basolateral nuclei are directly and reciprocally connected with the temporal, insular, and prefrontal cortices. In addition, like some cortical regions, the basolateral complex shares bidirectional connections with the medial dorsal thalamic nucleus and receives projections from the midline and intralaminar thalamic nuclei. Finally, neurons of the basolateral complex with a pyramidal-like morphology appear to furnish projections to the striatum that use excitatory amino acids as neurotransmitters. Thus, on the basis of these anatomical characteristics, one may hypothesize that the basolateral complex actually functions like a multimodal cortical region.

In contrast, the *centromedial amygdala* appears to be part of a larger structure that is continuous through the sublenticular substantia innominata with the bed nucleus of the stria terminalis. This larger structure, which has been termed the *extended amygdala*, consists of two major subdivisions. The central subdivision of the extended amygdala includes the central amygdaloid nucleus and the lateral portion of the bed nucleus of the stria terminalis. This subdivision is reciprocally connected with brainstem viscerosensory and visceromotor regions and with the lateral hypothalamus. In addition, it receives afferents from cortical limbic regions and the basolateral amygdaloid complex. In contrast, the medial subdivision of the extended amygdala, composed of the medial amygdaloid nucleus and its extension into the medial part of the bed nucleus of the stria terminalis, is distinguished by reciprocal connections with the medial or endocrine portions of the hypothalamus.

SEPTAL AREA The *septal area* is a gray matter structure located immediately above the anterior commissure (Fig. 1.2–37). The septal nuclei are reciprocally connected with the hippocampus, the amygdala, and the hypothalamus and project to a number of structures in the brainstem.

HYPOTHALAMUS The hypothalamus, a relatively small structure within the diencephalon, is a critical component of the neural circuitry regulating not only emotions, but also autonomic, endocrine, and some somatic functions. In addition to its relations with other components of the limbic system, it is interconnected with various visceral and somatic nuclei of the brainstem and the spinal cord and provides an output that regulates the function of the pituitary gland. On its inferior surface, the hypothalamus is bounded rostrally by the optic chiasm and caudally by the posterior edge of the mammillary bodies. The area of the hypothalamus between these two structures, called the *tuber cinereum*, gives rise to the median eminence, which is continu-

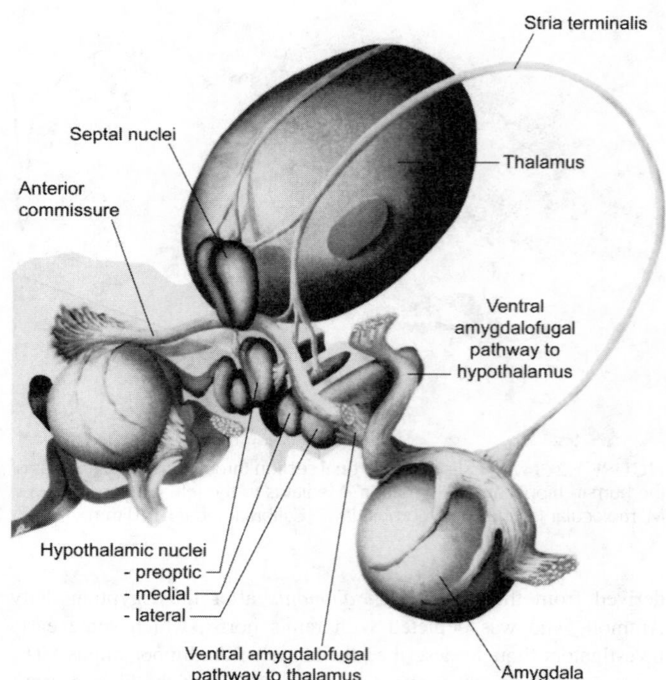

FIGURE 1.2–37 Schematic drawing of some components of the limbic system showing the major output pathways of the amygdala, the stria terminalis, and the ventral amygdalofugal pathway. (Adapted from Hendelman WJ. *Student's Atlas of Neuroanatomy*. Philadelphia: W.B. Saunders; 1994:183.)

ous with the infundibular stalk and then the posterior lobe of the pituitary gland (Fig. 1.2–38). On the basis of these features, the hypothalamus is subdivided from anterior to posterior into three zones: the supraoptic region, the tuberal region, and the mammillary region. (In addition, the preoptic area, a telencephalic structure located immediately anterior to the supraoptic region, is usually considered part of the hypothalamus.) These three zones are also divided on each side into medial and lateral areas by the fornix as it travels through the body of the hypothalamus to the mammillary bodies. As shown in Table 1.2–3, the six parts of the hypothalamus contain different nuclei.

These different nuclei subserve the diverse functions of the hypothalamus. For example, the *suprachiasmatic nucleus* receives both direct and indirect projections from the retina and appears to be important in the regulation of diurnal rhythms. The *supraoptic* and *paraventricular nuclei* contain large cells (magnocellular neurons) that send oxytocin-containing and vasopressin-containing fibers to the posterior neural lobe of the pituitary. In addition, some neurons of the paraventricular nucleus project to the median eminence, where they release neuropeptides, such as corticotropin-releasing factor, into the portal blood system. These neuropeptides then control the synthesis and release of anterior pituitary hormones. The paraventricular nucleus also gives rise to descending projections that regulate the sympathetic and parasympathetic autonomic areas of the medulla and the spinal cord.

Within the medial tuberal region of the hypothalamus, the *ventromedial* and *arcuate nuclei* also participate in the regulation of the anterior pituitary function. In addition, the ventromedial nucleus may play an important role in reproductive and ingestive behavior. The medial posterior section of the hypothalamus contains the *posterior nucleus* and the *mammillary bodies*. Within the mammillary bodies, the lateral and medial mammillary nuclei receive hippocampal input through the fornix (Fig. 1.2–35) and project to the anterior nuclei of the thalamus. The posterior nucleus shares reciprocal con-

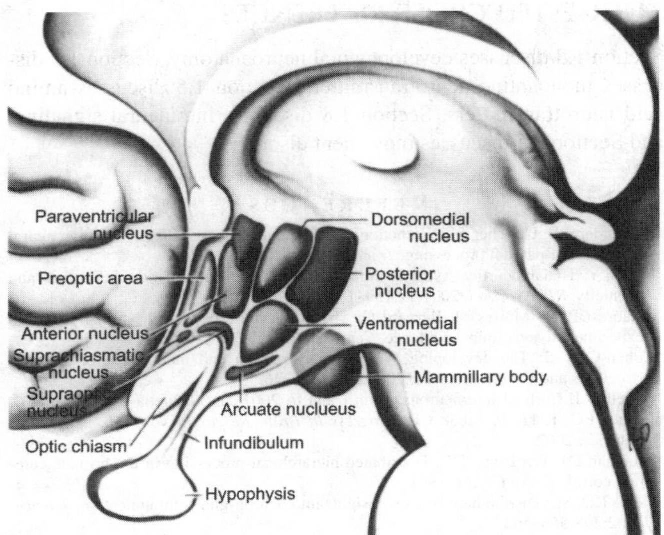

FIGURE 1.2–38 Schematic drawing of the nuclei in the medial hypothalamus. (Modified from Parent A. *Carpenter's Human Neuroanatomy*. 9th ed. Media, PA: Williams & Wilkins; 1996:707.)

nections with the extended amygdala. This nucleus appears to be relatively more developed in primates than in rodents, suggesting that it plays an important but still-to-be-clarified role in the human brain.

The lateral portions of the hypothalamus contain a relatively low density of neurons scattered among longitudinally running fibers of the medial forebrain bundle. This region is interconnected with multiple regions of the forebrain, the brainstem, and the spinal cord.

Functional Circuitry The major structures of the limbic system are interconnected with each other and with other components of the nervous system in a variety of ways. However, several major output pathways of the limbic system are clearly defined. In one pathway (Fig. 1.2–39), highly processed sensory information from the cingulate, the orbital and temporal cortices, and the amygdala is transmitted to the entorhinal cortex of the parahippocampal gyrus and then to the hippocampal formation. After traversing the intrinsic circuitry of the hippocampal formation, information is projected through the fornix either to the anterior thalamus, which, in turn, projects to the limbic cortex, or to the septal area and the hypothalamus. These latter two regions provide feedback to the hippocampal formation through the

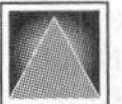

Table 1.2–3
Hypothalamic Nuclei

Region	Medial Area	Lateral Area
Supraoptic	Supraoptic nucleus	Lateral nucleus
	Paraventricular nucleus	Part of supraoptic nucleus
	Anterior nucleus	
	Suprachiasmatic nucleus	
Tuberal	Dorsomedial nucleus	Lateral nucleus
	Ventromedial nucleus	Lateral tuberal nuclei
	Arcuate nucleus	
Mammillary	Mammillary body	Lateral nucleus
	Posterior nucleus	

Adapted from Nolte J. *The Human Brain: An Introduction to Its Functional Anatomy*. 3rd ed. St. Louis: Mosby; 1993:259.

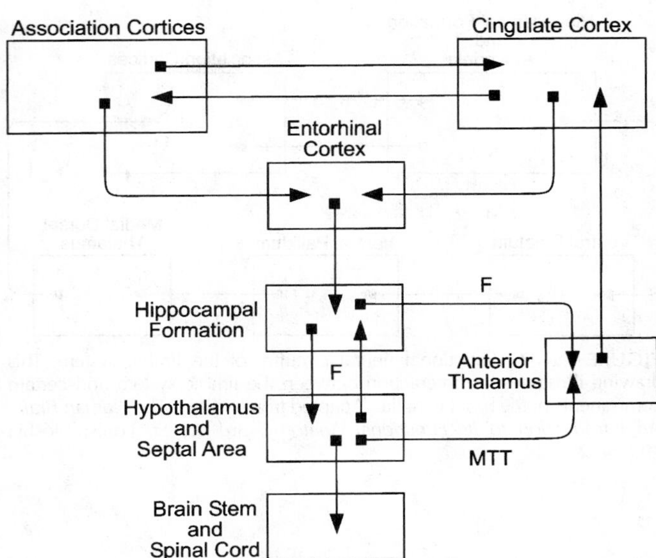

FIGURE 1.2–39 Functional neural circuitry of the limbic system. This diagram illustrates the manner in which the hippocampal formation and the anterior thalamus provide a mechanism for the integration of information between the cerebral cortex and the hypothalamus. F, fornix; MTT, mammillothalamic tract. (Adapted from Nolte J. *The Human Brain: An Introduction to Its Functional Anatomy*. 3rd ed. St. Louis: Mosby; 1993:399.)

fornix. In addition, the mammillary bodies of the hypothalamus project to the anterior thalamus. Finally, the hypothalamus and the septal area project to the brainstem and the spinal cord.

Another major pathway within the limbic system centers on output from the amygdala (Fig. 1.2–40). Highly processed sensory

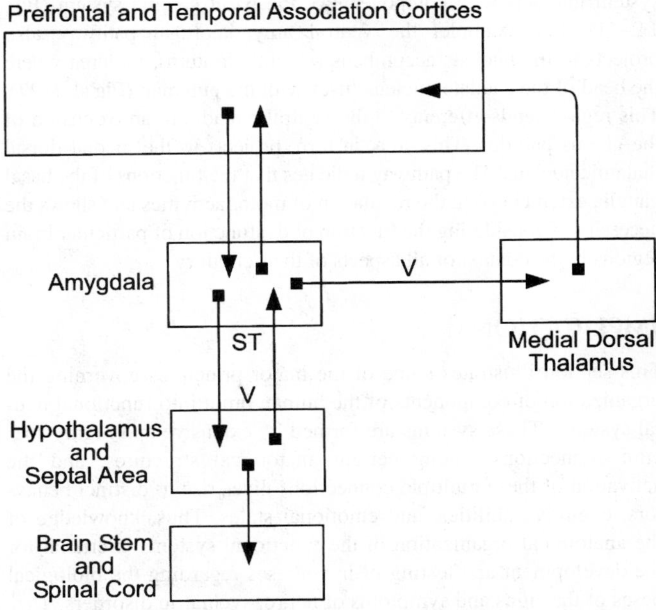

FIGURE 1.2–40 Functional neural circuitry of the limbic system. This diagram illustrates how the amygdala and the medial dorsal thalamus serve to integrate information processing between prefrontal and temporal association cortices and the hypothalamus. ST, stria terminalis; V, ventral amygdalofugal pathway. (Adapted from Nolte J. *The Human Brain: An Introduction to Its Functional Anatomy*. 3rd ed. St. Louis: Mosby; 1993:399.)

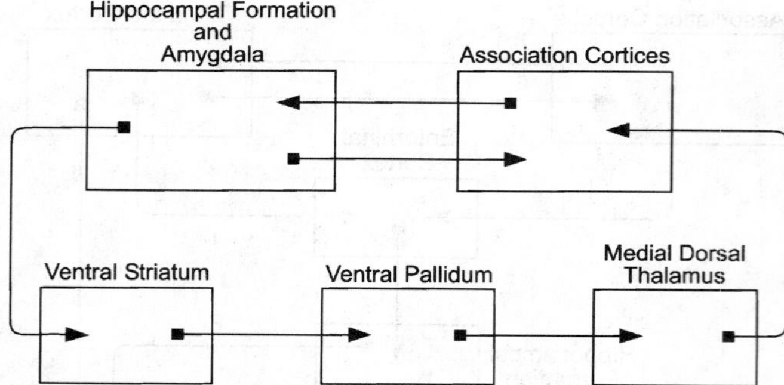

FIGURE 1.2–41 Functional neural circuitry of the limbic system. This drawing illustrates the interaction between the limbic system and certain components of the basal ganglia. (Adapted from Nolte J. *The Human Brain: An Introduction to Its Functional Anatomy.* 3rd ed. St. Louis: Mosby; 1993:412.)

information, primarily from the association regions of the prefrontal and temporal cortices, projects to the amygdala. Output from the amygdala is conducted through two main pathways (Fig. 1.2–37). A dorsal route, the *stria terminalis,* accompanies the caudate nucleus in an arch around the temporal lobe and contains axons that project primarily to the septal area and the hypothalamus. The second major output route, the *ventral amygdalofugal pathway*, passes below the lenticular nucleus and contains fibers that terminate in a number of regions, including the septal area, the hypothalamus, and the medial dorsal thalamic nucleus. The medial dorsal nucleus, in turn, projects heavily to prefrontal and some temporal cortical regions.

Both of these pathways reveal how the limbic system is able to integrate the highly processed sensory and cognitive information content of the cerebral cortical circuitry with the hypothalamic pathways that control autonomic and endocrine systems. In addition, the limbic system interacts with components of the basal ganglia system (Fig. 1.2–41). For example, the ventral amygdalofugal pathway also projects to the nucleus accumbens (ventral striatum), the area where the head of the caudate nucleus fuses with the putamen (Fig. 1.2–27). This region sends efferents to the ventral palladium, an extension of the globus pallidus. This area, in turn, projects to the medial dorsal thalamic nucleus. The pathway indicates that the functions of the basal ganglia extend beyond the regulation of motor activities and shows the necessity of considering the function or dysfunction of particular brain regions in the context of all aspects of their circuitry.

IMPLICATIONS

This section illustrates some of the major principles governing the organization of components of the human brain into functional neural systems. These systems are formed by extensive and highly specific connections among certain anatomical structures, and the activation of these multiple connections gives rise to distinct behaviors, cognitive abilities, and emotional states. Thus, knowledge of the anatomical organization of the functional systems is crucial for the development and testing of hypotheses regarding the biological bases of the signs and symptoms of neuropsychiatric disorders.

SUGGESTED CROSS-REFERENCES

Section 1.3 discusses developmental neuroanatomy, Section 1.4 discusses monoamine neurotransmitters, Section 1.5 discusses amino acid neurotransmitters, Section 1.8 discusses intraneural signaling, and Section 2.5 discusses movement disorders.

REFERENCES

Alexander GE, Crutcher MD: Functional architecture of basal ganglia circuits: neural substrates of parallel processing. *Trends Neurosci.* 1990;13:266.

Amitai Y: Thalamocortical synaptic connections: efficacy, modulation, inhibition, and plasticity. *Rev Neurosci.* 2001;12:159–173.

Calabresi P, De Murtas M, Bernard G: The neostriatum beyond the motor function: experimental and clinical evidence. *Neuroscience.* 1997;78:39.

*Cohen-Cory S: The developing synapse: construction and modulation of synaptic structures and circuits. *Science.* 2002;298:770–776.

DeFelipe J. Cortical interneurons: from Cajal to 2001. In: Azmietia ET, DeFelipe J, Jones EG, Rakic P, Ribak CE. *Progress in Brain Research.* Vol. 136. New York: Elsevier; 2002.

Felleman DJ, Van Essen DC: Distributed hierarchical processing in the primate cerebral cortex. *Cereb Cortex.* 1991;1:36.

Fields RD, Stevens-Graham B: New insights into neuron-glia communication. *Science.* 2002;298:556–562.

Fudge JL, Haber SN: Defining the caudal ventral striatum in primates: cellular and histochemical features. *J Neurosci.* 2002;22:10078–10082.

*Fuster JM: The prefrontal cortex B—an update: Time is of the essence. *Neuron.* 2001;30:319–333.

Gloor P. *The Temporal Lobe and Limbic System.* New York: Oxford; 1997.

*Guillery RW, Sherman SM: Thalamic relay functions and their role in corticocortical communication: generalizations from the visual system. *Neuron.* 2002;33:163–175.

Hashimoto T, Volk DW, Eggan SM, Mirnics K, Pierri JN, Sun Z, Sampson AR, Lewis DA: Gene expression deficits in a subclass of GABA neurons in the prefrontal cortex of subjects with schizophrenia. *J Neurosci.* 2003;23:6315–6350.

Heimer L, Harlan RE, Alheid GF, Garcia MM, De Olmos J: Substantia innominata: a notion which impedes clinical-anatomical correlations in neuropsychiatric disorders. *Neuroscience.* 1997;76:957.

Kandel ER, Schwartz JH, Jessel TM, eds. *Principles of Neural Science.* 4th ed. New York: McGraw-Hill; 2000.

Lewis DA: The human brain revisited: opportunities and challenges in postmortem studies of psychiatric disorders. *Neuropsychopharmacology.* 2002;26:143–154.

Lewis DA, Melchitzky DS, Gonzalez-Burgos G: Specificity in the functional architecture of primate prefrontal cortex. *J Neurocytol.* 2002;31:265–276.

Lewis DA, Sesack SR. Dopamine systems in the primate brain. In: FE Bloom, A Björklund, T Hökfelt. *Handbook of Chemical Neuroanatomy.* Vol. 13. New York: Elsevier; 1997.

Melchitzky DS, Lewis DA: Dopamine transporter-immunoreactive axons in the mediodorsal thalamic nucleus of the macaque monkey. *Neuroscience.* 2001;103:1033–1042.

Middleton FA, Strick PL: Cerebellar projections to the prefrontal cortex of the primate. *J Neurosci.* 2001;21:700–712.

*Nolte J. *The Human Brain: An Introduction to Its Functional Anatomy.* 5th ed. St. Louis: Mosby; 2002.

Ongur D, Price JL: The organization of networks within the orbital and medial prefrontal cortex of rats, monkeys, and humans. *Cereb Cortex.* 2000;10:206–219.

Parent A, Hazrati L-N: Functional anatomy of the basal ganglia. I. The cortico-basal ganglia-thalamo-cortical loop. *Brain Res Rev.* 1995;20:91.

Parent A, Hazrati L-N: Functional anatomy of the basal ganglia. II. The place of subthalamic nucleus and external pallidum in basal ganglia circuitry. *Brain Res Rev.* 1995;20:128.

Risold PY, Thompson RH, Swanson LW: The structural organization of connections between hypothalamus and cerebral cortex. *Brain Res Rev.* 1997;24:197.

Shink E, Bevan MD, Bolam JP, Smith Y: The subthalamic nucleus and the external pallidum: two tightly interconnected structures that control the output of the basal ganglia in the monkey. *Neuroscience.* 1996;73:335.

Simons JS, Spiers HJ: Prefrontal and medial temporal lobe interactions in long-term memory. *Nat Rev Neurosci.* 2003;4:637–649.

Tang Y, Nyengaard JR, De Groot DMG, Gundersen HJG: Total regional and global number of synapses in the human brain neocortex. *Synapse.* 2001;41:258–273.

Tekin S, Cummings JL: Frontal-subcortical neuronal circuits and clinical neuropsychiatry: an update. *J Psychosomatic Res.* 2002;53:647–654.

Toga AW, Thompson PM: Mapping brain asymmetry. *Nat Rev Neurosci.* 2003;4:37–48.

Volk DW, Lewis DA: Deficits in prefrontal inhibition in schizophrenia: relevance for cognitive dysfunction. *Physiol Behav.* 2002;77:501–507.

Volk DW, Pierri JN, Fritschy J-N, Auh S, Sampson AR, Lewis DA: Reciprocal alterations in pre- and postsynaptic inhibitory markers at chandelier cell inputs to pyramidal neurons in schizophrenia. *Cereb Cortex.* 2002;12:1063–1070.

*Young PA, Young PH. *Basic Clinical Neuroanatomy.* Baltimore: William & Wilkins; 1997.

Zigmond MJ, Bloom FE, Landis CS, Roberts JL, Squire LR. *Fundamental Neuroscience.* San Diego: Academic Press; 1999.

▲ 1.3 Neural Development and Neurogenesis

EMANUEL DICICCO-BLOOM, M.D., AND
MARIANN SONDELL, PH.D.

The diverse cognitive, emotional, and sensorimotor functions of the brain depend on multiple networks of interacting neurons, which are positioned within a fabric of glial cells. The neuroanatomical substrates of these functional systems have been described in the previous chapter. The functional networks of the brain emerge from neuron populations that arise during the earliest periods of embryonic development. Indeed, the nervous system begins forming immediately after the primitive gut, or *archenteron*, invaginates the embryonic ball of cells known as the *blastula*. This chapter describes the cellular and molecular processes underlying nervous system formation and introduces the recent discovery that new nerve cell production, or *neurogenesis*, is a life-long process, with important implications for psychiatry.

While many psychiatric diseases become manifest primarily after childhood, such as schizophrenia and depression, others appear within years of birth—for instance, autism and attention-deficit/hyperactivity disorder. Despite the range of presentation, however, increasing evidence suggests that disordered regulation of brain development plays a major role in psychiatric disease by laying down a foundation of altered neuron populations that differ in cell types, numbers, and positions or elaborate abnormal connections. For example, recent models suggest there are important abnormalities in the γ-aminobutyric acid (GABA) interneuron population in schizophrenia, whereas in autism there is dysregulation of early brain growth and cellular organization. With progressive postnatal development, the maturing brain systems call on component neurons to achieve increasing levels of complex information processing. Thus, new neural properties emerge as neuron populations elaborate functional networks based on and modified by ongoing experience. In turn, it is possible that developmental abnormalities in neuron populations, due to genetic or environmental factors, may manifest at diverse times in a person's life. Two genetic disorders, Rett's syndrome and Huntington's disease, illustrate this point: Rett's syndrome, caused by mutations in methyl CpG binding protein—a regulator of DNA methylation that silences genes—presents between the first and second years of life, whereas Huntington's disease, caused by a mutation in the huntingtin protein, manifests in the third to fourth decades.

This chapter's goal is to describe the fundamental events in nervous system development as a basis to consider their possible contributions to psychiatric disease. Although developmental origins have been defined in only a few human brain diseases, an overview of the cellular processes mediating brain formation is provided, and new insights into the molecular and genetic systems underlying the sequence of developmental events are described. In turn, these cellular processes and molecular systems may be considered candidate targets for pathogenetic mechanisms. Disruption or abnormal regulation of these cellular and molecular targets will produce alterations in neuron population formation and function, potentially leading to disease. Finally, an exciting recent discovery regarding brain development is reviewed: Contrary to conventional thought, new neurons are, in fact, generated throughout life in primates—including humans. This discovery is changing current understanding of ongoing brain disease and the locus and action of pharmacological therapies and may provide a previously unrecognized source of new cells to address brain repair.

Nervous system development is traditionally viewed as a sequence of events, including precursor cell proliferation, mitotic cell cycle withdrawal, cell migration, axon and dendrite formation, neurotransmitter system expression, axon outgrowth to targets, synapse elaboration, and selective neuron survival based on appropriate target innervation. Separation of these events into discrete processes is more of a pedagogical convenience than a fact, since many of these processes occur simultaneously, not only within brain regions but even in the same cell. This is important to recognize, since it alters conceptual models about the possible effects of changing one process, and it may, in fact, alter several concurrent processes. For example, the presence of neurotransmitter receptors on very early precursors (those engaged in cell proliferation) allows neurotransmitters themselves—and therapeutic drugs that are administered—to directly affect neuronal cell production during development, an unintended outcome of concern. Of the foregoing events, a subset is discussed, focusing on molecular mechanisms. After a general overview of development comes a description of the critical roles of neural patterning genes, extracellular signals regulating embryonic neurogenesis, molecular mechanisms of cell migration and process growth, neurodevelopmental diseases, and functions and implications of recently discovered adult neurogenesis.

OVERVIEW OF NERVOUS SYSTEM DEVELOPMENT

In considering brain development, several principles guide understanding. First, different brain regions and neuron populations are generated at distinct times of development and exhibit specific temporal schedules. This has implications for the consequences of specific developmental insults, such as production of autism by the drug thalidomide in fetuses exposed only during days 20 to 24 of gestation. Second, the sequence of cellular processes comprising ontogeny predicts that abnormalities in early events necessarily lead to differences in subsequent stages, although not all abnormalities may be accessible to our clinical tools. For example, a deficit in the number of neurons leads to diminished axonal processes and ensheathing white matter in the mature brain. However, at the clinical level, because glial cells outnumber neurons 10 to 1, changes in the majority glial population, oligodendrocytes, and their myelin appear as altered white matter on neuroimaging, with little apparent evidence of neuronal disturbance. Third, it is clear that specific molecular signals, such as extracellular growth factors and cognate receptors, play roles at multiple developmental stages of the cell. For example, both insulin-like growth factor I (IGF-I) and brain-derived neurotrophic factor (BDNF) regulate multiple cellular processes during the generation and function of mature neurons, including cell proliferation, survival promotion, neuron migration, process outgrowth, and the momentary synaptic modifications (plasticity) underlying learning and memory. Thus, changes in expression or regulation of a ligand or its receptor—by environmental insults or genetic mechanisms—will have effects on multiple developmental and mature processes. This chapter addresses these principles and examines cellular and molecular systems regulating development, discussing implications for psychiatric disease.

Neural Plate and Neurulation

The nervous system in the human embryo first appears between $2\frac{1}{2}$ and 4 weeks of gestation.

During development, emergence of new cell types, including neurons, results from interactions between neighboring layers of cells. On gestational day 13, the embryo consists of a sheet of cells. After gastrulation (day 14 to 15), which forms a two-cell–layered embryo consisting of *ectoderm* and *endoderm*, the *neural plate* region of the ectoderm is delineated by the underlying *mesoderm*, which appears on day 16. The mesoderm forms by cells entering a midline cleft in the ectoderm called the *primitive streak*. After migration, the mesodermal layer lies between ectoderm and endoderm and induces overlying ectoderm to become neural plate. Induction usually involves release of soluble growth factors from one group of cells, which in turn bind receptors on neighboring cells, eliciting changes in nuclear transcription factors that control downstream gene expression. In some cases, cell–cell contact-mediated mechanisms are involved. In the gene patterning section below, the important roles of soluble growth factors and transcription factor expression will be described.

The neural plate, whose induction is complete by 18 days, is a sheet of columnar epithelium and is surrounded by ectodermal epithelium. After formation, the edges of the neural plate elevate, forming the neural ridges. Subsequently, changes in intracellular cytoskeleton and cell–extracellular matrix attachment cause the ridges to merge in the midline and fuse—a process termed *neurulation*—forming the *neural tube*, with a central cavity presaging the ventricular system. Fusion begins in the cervical region at the hindbrain level (medulla and pons) and continues rostrally and caudally. Neurulation occurs at 3 to 4 weeks of gestation in humans, and its failure results in anencephaly rostrally and spina bifida caudally. Neurulation defects are well known after exposure to retinoic acid in dermatological preparations and anticonvulsants, especially valproic acid, as well as diets deficient in folic acid.

Another product of neurulation is the *neural crest*, whose cells derive from the edges of the neural plate and dorsal neural tube. From this position, neural crest cells migrate dorsolaterally under the skin to form melanocytes and ventromedially to form dorsal root sensory ganglia and sympathetic chains of the peripheral nervous system and ganglia of the enteric nervous system. Neural crest, however, gives rise to diverse tissues, including cells of neuroendocrine, cardiac, mesenchymal, and skeletal systems, forming the basis of many congenital syndromes involving brain and other organs. The neural crest origin at the border of neural and epidermal ectoderm and its generation of melanocytes forms the basis of the neurocutaneous disorders, including tuberous sclerosis and neurofibromatosis. Finally, another nonneuronal structure of mesodermal origin formed during neurulation is the notochord found on the ventral side of the neural tube. As discussed below, the notochord plays a critical role during neural tube differentiation because it is a signaling source of soluble growth factors, such as sonic hedgehog (Shh), which impact gene patterning and cell determination.

Regional Differentiation of the Embryonic Nervous System

After closure, the neural tube expands differentially to form major morphological subdivisions that precede the major functional divisions of the brain. These subdivisions are important developmentally because different regions are generated according to specific schedules of proliferation and subsequent migration and differentiation. The neural tube can be described in three dimensions, including longitudinal, circumferential, and radial. The longitudinal dimension reflects the rostrocaudal (anterior–posterior) organization, which, most simply, consists of brain and spinal cord. Organization in the circumferential dimension, tangential to the surface, represents two major axes: In the dorso-ventral axis, cell groups are uniquely positioned from top to bottom. On the other hand, in the medial to lateral axis, there is mirror-image symmetry, consistent with right–left symmetry of the body. Finally, the radial dimension represents organization from the inner-most cell layer adjacent to the ventricles to the outer-most surface and exhibits region-specific cell layering. At 4 weeks, the human brain is divided longitudinally into the *prosencephalon* (forebrain), *mesencephalon* (midbrain), and *rhombencephalon* (hindbrain). These three subdivisions, or vesicles, divide further into five divisions by 5 weeks, with the prosencephalon forming the telencephalon (including cortex, hippocampus, and basal ganglia) and the diencephalon (thalamus and hypothalamus), the mesencephalon (which forms the midbrain), and the rhombencephalon forming the metencephalon (pons and cerebellum) and the myelencephalon (medulla). Morphological transformation into five vesicles depends on region-specific proliferation of precursor cells adjacent to the ventricles, the so-called ventricular zones (VZs). As discussed below, proliferation intimately depends on soluble growth factors made by proliferating cells themselves or released from regional signaling centers. In turn, growth factor production and cognate receptor expression also depend on region-specific patterning genes. It is now known that VZ precursors—which appear morphologically homogeneous—express a checkerboard array of molecular genetic determinants that control the generation of specific types of neurons in each domain.

In the circumferential dimension, organization begins very early and extends over many rostrocaudal subdivisions. In the spinal cord, the majority of tissue comprises the lateral plates, which later divide into dorsal or alar plates, composed of sensory interneurons, and motor or basal plates, consisting of ventral motor neurons. Two other diminutive plates—termed the *roof plate* and *floor plate*—are virtually absent in maturity; however, they play critical regulatory roles as growth-factor signaling centers in the embryo. Indeed, the floor plate, in response to Shh from the ventrally located notochord, produces its own Shh, which, in turn, induces neighboring cells in the ventral spinal cord and brainstem to express region-specific transcription factors that specify cell phenotype and function. For example, in combination with other factors, floor plate Shh induces midbrain precursors to differentiate into dopamine-secreting neurons of the substantia nigra. Similarly, the roof plate secretes growth factors, such as bone morphogenetic proteins (BMPs), which induce dorsal neuron cell fate in the spinal cord. In the absence of roof plate, dorsal structures, such as cerebellum, fail to form, and midline hippocampal structures are missing. Finally, in the radial dimension, the organization of layers is subdivision specific, produced by differential proliferation of VZ precursors and cell migration.

Ventricular and Subventricular Proliferative Zones

The distinct patterns of precursor proliferation and migration in different regions generate radial nervous system organization. In each longitudinal subdivision, control of neurogenesis matches production to the final size of a region. Although it is well known that many cells produced during development undergo programmed cell death (up to 10 to 40 percent) regulated by genetic programs, initial cell generation roughly matches regional size requirements. This close relationship indicates that neurogenesis itself is controlled to generate the necessary complement of cells. This contradicts traditional concepts suggesting excess cell production everywhere, with cell number regulation achieved primarily through selective cell death mediated by target-derived survival (trophic) factors. The patterning genes discussed below play major roles in directing regional precursor proliferation that is coordinated with final structural requirements. Consequently, in diseases characterized by brain regions smaller than normal, such as schizophrenia, there may be a failure to generate neurons initially, as opposed to normal generation with subsequent cell loss.

The generation of specific cell types involves proliferation of undifferentiated precursor cells (or *progenitors*), followed by cessation of proliferation (exit from the cell cycle) and expression of specific phenotypic characters, such as neurofilaments and neurotransmitter systems. Precursor proliferation occurs primarily in two densely packed regions during development. The primary site is the VZ lining the walls of the entire ventricular system, which site contributes to all brain regions in the rostrocaudal dimension. For select regions, however—including the cerebral cortex, hippocampus, and cerebellar cortex—precursors from the VZ migrate out to secondary zones where they generate a more restricted range of cell types.

In the early embryo, neural tube VZ progenitors are arranged as a one-cell-layer-thick, pseudostratified neuroepithelium. The bipolar VZ precursors have cytoplasmic processes that span from the ventricular to the pial surface. During the cell cycle, the VZ appears multilayered, or *stratified*, because cell nuclei undergo movements, called *interkinetic nuclear migration*. The cell cycle, by which new cells are produced, comprises four stages, including mitosis (M), when nuclei and cells divide; G_1, when cells grow in size before dividing again; S phase, when cells synthesize DNA and replicate chromosomes; and G_2, a brief period followed by precursor cell division (M phase). M phase occurs at the ventricular margin, producing two new cells. The progeny then re-enter G_1 as they move outward toward the pia. Under the influence of extracellular signals, these cells become committed to another round of division, marked by entry into S phase, which occurs near the upper VZ margin. After DNA replication, during G_2, the nuclei move back down to the ventricular surface, where they undergo mitosis and divide. The role of nuclear migration is not known, although it may allow nuclei access to environmental cues that effect subsequent proliferation and gene expression. Several human genetic mutations interfere with interkinetic nuclear movement and cell migration, producing heterotopic neurons and epilepsy syndromes.

At the earliest stages, VZ cells divide to increase the pool of progenitors before producing postmitotic neurons. Then, during the period of neurogenesis, on average, with each cell cycle, a precursor divides to give rise to both a postmitotic neuron and another dividing precursor. At the end of neurogenesis, precursor division gives rise to two postmitotic neurons only, greatly increasing neuron production and depleting the precursor pool. The newly born neurons do not remain in the VZ, but instead migrate out to their final destinations, such as the cerebral cortical plate, traveling along the processes of radial glial cells (Fig. 1.3–1C). Like the bipolar VZ precursors described above, radial glia have one process associated with the ventricular surface and the other reaching the pial surface—a morphology consistent with the recent discovery that radial glia are, in fact, the dividing VZ precursors. The association between newborn neurons and radial glial process allows cells generated within localized VZ domains, known to express distinct patterning genes, to migrate to specific cortical functional areas, suggesting that VZ precursors already have their phenotypic fate specified at the genetic level prior to ceasing cell division and beginning migration. There is, however, active debate about the relative roles of early expressed VZ genes versus the ingrowing thalamic afferents in determining cortical neuronal fate and function. In rodents, neurons are generated before birth and glia are produced after, whereas in the human brain, neuron production generally occurs for the first 4 months of gestation, and then, from 16 weeks until birth, neurons undergo migration and glial precursors proliferate, migrate, and produce myelin.

In addition to this general plan of neurogenesis, in distinct regions, other cells are produced in secondary proliferative zones. For example, in cerebral cortex and thalamus, the subventricular zone (SVZ) produces astroglial cells, although debate continues whether it also produces oligodendrocytes and neurons. In the hippocampus, the hilus and, later, the subgranular zone produce dentate gyrus granule neurons, a lifelong process of neurogenesis. Finally, in newborn cerebellum, the overlying external germinal layer (EGL) generates granule neurons for several weeks in rodents and for 7 to 20 months in humans, a population likely affected by medical treatments administered in the neonatal intensive care unit. In contrast to the VZ, secondary zone cells do not exhibit nuclear movements, suggesting distinct mechanisms of regulation. After neurogenesis is complete, the VZ differentiates into ciliated epithelial cells of the ependymal lining. Underlying the ependyma, undifferentiated cells of the SVZ—referred to as *subependyma*—have been identified as a neural stem cell population capable of proliferating and generating neurons and glia throughout life.

Radial and Tangential Patterns of Neurogenesis and Migration There are three well-recognized spatiotemporal patterns of neurogenesis that underlie regional brain formation. Although extensive description is not warranted, several examples illustrate common principles concerning relationships of cell cycle exit (cell birthday) to final cell position, the roles of radial glia in migration, and the distinct capacities of secondary proliferative zones. There are two radial patterns of cell migration from the VZ, referred to as *inside-to-outside* and *outside-to-inside*. The third involves nonradial or tangential migration of cells, some of which originate in secondary proliferative zones. Experimentally, these patterns are defined by marking mitotic cells using nuclear incorporation of labeled DNA precursors—either tritiated [^{3}H]thymidine or bromodeoxyuridine (BrdU)—to identify the last day a precursor is in S phase, after which it exits the cell cycle, differentiates, and migrates to its final position.

The two radial patterns of neurogenesis reflect whether a structure is phylogenetically older—such as the spinal cord, tectum, and hippocampal dentate gyrus—or more recently evolved, like the cerebral cortex. In more primitive structures, early-generated cells are positioned on the outside, with later-born cells residing inside, closer to the VZ. This pattern suggests that, as more cells are generated, they passively move previously born cells further away. In the second pattern relevant to the cerebral cortex, early-born cells are located on the inside, with later-born cells migrating past earlier ones to take up position outside. This inside-to-outside gradient requires a more complex mechanism and cannot rely solely on passive cell movement. Although radial glial cell function was initially considered uniquely associated with the inside-to-outside gradient, recent studies indicate that radial glia play roles in both spatiotemporal patterns. Finally, the specific character of a region may be altered by nonradial inward migration of cells generated in other locations, relevant to GABA interneurons in cortex and hippocampus or granule neurons in cerebellum, hippocampal dentate gyrus, and olfactory bulb.

Of interest to psychiatry, the cerebral cortex is the paradigmatic model of inside-to-outside neurogenesis. Derived from the embryonic forebrain telencephalic vesicles, the characteristic six cell layers represent a common cytoarchitectural and physiological basis for neocortical function. Within each layer, neurons exhibit related axodendritic morphologies, use common neurotransmitters, and establish similar afferent and efferent connections. In general, pyramidal

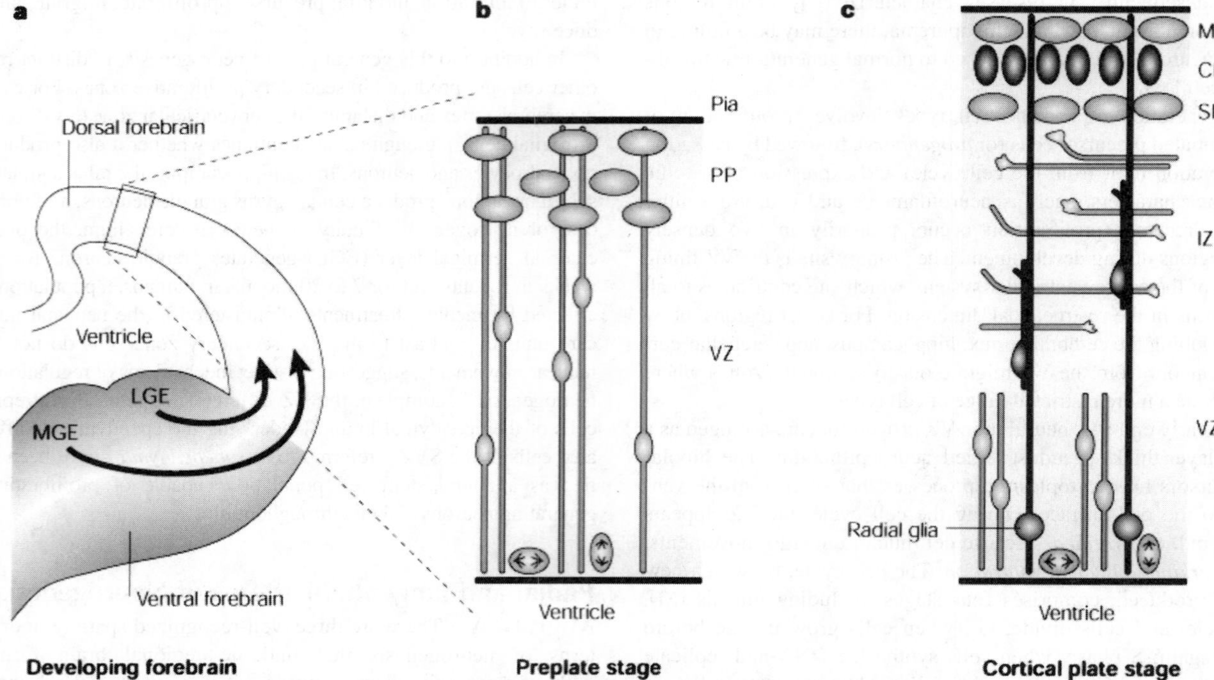

FIGURE 1.3–1 Schematic drawing of radial and tangential migration during cerebral cortex development. **A:** A coronal section of one half of the developing rat forebrain. The dorsal forebrain gives rise to the cerebral cortex. Medial ganglionic eminences (MGEs) and lateral ganglionic eminences (LGEs) of the ventral forebrain generate neurons of the basal ganglia and the cortical interneurons. The arrows indicate the tangential migration route for γ-aminobutyric acid interneurons to the cortex. The boxed area (enlarged in **B** and **C**) shows the developing cortex at early and late stages. **B:** In the dorsal forebrain, the first cohort of postmitotic neurons migrate out from the ventricular zone (VZ) and create a preplate (PP) below the pial surface. **C:** Subsequent postmitotic neurons will migrate along radial glia through the intermediate zone (IZ) and take position in the middle of the preplate, creating a cortical plate (CP) between the outer marginal zone (MZ) and inner subplate (SP). Ultimately, the CP will be composed of six layers that are born sequentially, migrating in an inside-to-outside pattern. Horizontal processes in the IZ represent axon terminals of thalamic afferents. (From Nadarajah B, Parnavelas JG: Modes of neuronal migration in the developing cerebral cortex. *Nat Neurosci.* 2002;3:423, with permission.)

neurons in layer 3 establish synapses within and between cortical hemispheres, whereas deeper layer 5/6 neurons project primarily to subcortical nuclei, including thalamus, brainstem, and spinal cord. The majority of cortical neurons originate from the forebrain VZ. At earliest stages, the first postmitotic cells migrate outward from the VZ to establish a superficial layer termed the *preplate*. Two important cell types compose the preplate: *Cajal-Retzius* cells, which form outermost layer 1, or *marginal zone*, and *subplate* neurons, which lay beneath future layer 6. These distinct regions form when later-born cortical plate neurons migrate within and divide the preplate in two (Fig. 1.3–1B,C).

After preplate formation, the cortical VZ generates, in inside-to-outside fashion, first layer 5/6 neurons and then more superficial layers in temporal sequence. Thus, the day on which a precursor exits the cell cycle in the VZ, its birthday, essentially predicts the kind and localization of the generated neuron. Currently, molecular mechanisms mediating this correlation are being defined, including specific stimulatory and inhibitory proliferative signals. Significantly, the cortical VZ is the primary source of excitatory pyramidal neurons that secrete glutamate.

Recently, the embryonic preplate has taken on clinical significance. Cajal-Retzius cells produce the extracellular glycoprotein reelin, an important signal for neuronal migration. When reelin gene is genetically deleted in mice, cortical neuron migration is inverted. That is, the usual inside-to-outside gradient of cell generation and laminar position becomes inverted, yielding an outside-to-inside pattern. Thus, early born neurons appear furthermost from the VZ, and latest-born cells remain closest to the ventricles. Abnormal levels of reelin protein and mRNA have been found in several diseases, including bipolar depression and schizophrenia, and human reelin mutation is associated with *lissencephaly* (smooth brain), a gyral patterning malformation with loss of gyri and sulci, and abnormalities in cerebellum. On the other hand, the subplate neurons, which persist only until early postnatal development in rodents, play a critical role as temporary targets for thalamic axon terminals on their way to cortex. After pyramidal neurons settle into correct layers in the cortical plate, thalamic processes migrate further to reach layer 4 targets, and subplate neurons undergo programmed cell death.

A recent discovery, postulated for years, has changed our view of the origins of cortical neuron populations involved in human brain disease. Neuron-tracing experiments in culture and in vivo demonstrate that the neocortex, a dorsal forebrain derivative, is also populated by neurons generated in the ventral forebrain (Fig. 1.3–1). Molecular studies of patterning genes, especially *Dlx*, strongly support this model. In contrast to excitatory pyramidal neurons, the overwhelming majority of inhibitory GABA secreting interneurons originate from mitotic precursors of the ganglionic eminences that generate the neurons of the basal ganglia. Subsets of interneurons also secrete neuropeptides—such as neuropeptide Y (NPY) and somatostatin—and express nitric oxide (NO)–generating enzyme, NOS. Not associated with cortical VZ radial glia, these GABA interneurons reach the cortical plate by migrating tangentially, in either the superficial marginal zone or a deep position above VZ, the subplate region where thalamic afferents are also growing. Significantly, in brains from schizophrenic patients, the prefrontal cortex exhibits a reduced density of interneurons in layer 2. In addition, there is upregulation of GABA type A ($GABA_A$) receptor binding, a potential functional compensation, as well as a relative deficiency of NOS-expressing neurons. These observations have led to the hypothesis that schizophrenia is due to reduced GABAergic activity. The origin of GABA interneurons from the ganglionic eminences and their association with specific patterning genes (*Dlx*) raise new genetic models of disease causation and possible strategies for disease intervention. Thus, more broadly, cortical development represents convergence of two principal patterns of neurogenesis, consisting of both radial and nonradial migration of neurons.

In contrast to inside-to-outside neurogenesis observed in the cortex, phylogenetically older regions, such as hypothalamus, spinal cord, and hippocampal dentate gyrus, exhibit the reverse order of cell generation. First-formed postmitotic neurons lie superficially, and last-generated cells localize toward the center. Although this outside-to-inside pattern might reflect passive cell displacement, radial glia and specific migration signaling molecules are clearly involved. Furthermore, cells do not always lie in direct extension from their locus of VZ generation. Rather, some groups of cells migrate to specific locations, as observed for neurons of the inferior olivary nuclei.

Of prime importance in psychiatry, the hippocampus demonstrates both radial and nonradial patterns of neurogenesis. The *pyramidal cell layer*, Ammon's horn CA1–3 neurons, is generated in a typical outside-to-inside fashion in the dorsomedial forebrain from 7 to 15 weeks of gestation, although migration patterns appear complex. However, dentate gyrus granule neurons—the other major population—start appearing at 18 weeks and exhibit prolonged outside-to-inside postnatal neurogenesis, originating from several migrating secondary proliferative zones. In rats, for instance, granule neurogenesis starts at embryonic day 16 (E16) with proliferation in the dentate VZ of the forebrain. At E18, an aggregate of precursors migrates along a subpial route into the dentate gyrus, generating granule cells nearby the dentate. After birth, there is another migration, localizing proliferative precursors to the dentate hilus, which persists until 1 month of life. Thereafter, granule precursors move to a layer just under the dentate gyrus, termed the *subgranular zone* (SGZ), which produces neurons throughout life in adult rats, nonhuman primates, and humans. In rodents, SGZ precursors proliferate in response to cerebral ischemia, tissue injury, and seizures, as well as growth factors. Finally, the diminished hippocampal volume reported in schizophrenia raises the possibility that disordered neurogenesis plays a role in pathogenesis, either as a basis for dysfunction or a consequence of brain injuries, consistent with associations of gestational infections with disease manifestation.

Finally, a different combination of radial and nonradial migration is observed in cerebellum, a brain region recently recognized to play important functions in nonmotor tasks, with particular significance for autism spectrum disorders. Except for granule cells, the other major neurons—including Purkinje and deep nuclei—originate from the primary VZ of the fourth ventricle, coincident with other brainstem neurons. In rats, this occurs at E13 to E15 and in humans, 5 to 7 weeks' gestation. The granule neurons, as well as basket and stellate interneurons, originate in the secondary proliferative zone, the EGL, which covers newborn cerebellum at birth. EGL precursors originate in the fourth ventricle VZ and migrate dorsally through the brainstem to reach this superficial position. The rat EGL proliferates for 3 weeks, generating more neurons than in any other structure, whereas in humans, EGL precursors exist for at least 7 weeks and up to 2 years. When an EGL precursor stops proliferating, the cell body sinks below the surface and grows bilateral processes that extend transversely in the molecular layer, and then the soma migrates further down into the internal granule layer (IGL). Cells reach the IGL along specialized Bergmann glia, which serve guidance functions similar to the radial glia. However, in this case, cells originate from a secondary proliferative zone that generates neurons exclusively of the granule cell lineage, indicating a restricted neural fate. Clinically, this postnatal population in infants makes cerebellar granule neurogenesis vulnerable to infectious insults of early childhood and an undesirable target of several therapeutic drugs—such as steroids—well known to inhibit cell proliferation.

CONCEPT OF NEURAL PATTERNING

The morphological conversion of the nervous system through the embryonic stages, from neural plate through neural tube to brain vesicles, is controlled by interactions between extracellular factors and intrinsic genetic programs. In many cases, extracellular signals are soluble growth factors secreted from regional signaling centers, such as the notochord, floor or roof plates, or surrounding mesenchymal tissues. The precursor's ability to respond (competence) depends on cognate receptor expression, which is determined by patterning genes whose proteins regulate gene transcription. The remarkable new observation is that subdivisions of the embryonic telencephalon—initially based on mature differences in morphology, connectivity, and neurochemical profiles—are also distinguished embryonically by distinct patterns of gene expression. Classic models had suggested that the cerebral cortex was generated as a fairly homogeneous structure, unlike most epithelia, with individual functional areas specified relatively late, after cortical layer formation, by ingrowth of afferent axons from thalamus. In marked contrast, recent studies indicate that proliferative VZ precursors themselves display regional molecular determinants, a "protomap," which the postmitotic neurons carry with them as they migrate along radial glia to the cortical plate. Consequently, innervating thalamic afferents may serve only to modulate intrinsic molecular determinants of the protomap. Indeed, in two different genetic mutants, *Gbx2* and *Mash1*, in which thalamocortical innervation is disrupted, expression of cortical patterning genes proceeds unaltered. On the other hand, thalamic afferent growth may be directed by patterning genes and subsequently plays roles in modulating regional expression patterns. Thus, experience-dependent processes may contribute less to cortical specialization than originally postulated.

The term *patterning genes* connotes families of proteins that primarily serve to control transcription of other genes whose products include other transcription factors or proteins involved in cellular processes, such as proliferation, migration, or differentiation. Characteristically, transcription factor proteins contain two principal domains: one that binds DNA promoter regions of genes and the other that interacts with other proteins, either transcription factors or components of intracellular second messengers. Importantly, transcription factors form multimeric protein complexes to control gene activation. Therefore, a single transcription factor will play diverse roles in multiple cell types and processes, according to what other factors are present. The combinatorial nature of gene promoter regulation leads to a diversity of functional outcomes when a single patterning gene is altered. Furthermore, because protein interactions depend on protein–protein affinities, there may be complex changes as a single factor's expression level is altered. This may be one important mechanism of human variation and disease susceptibility, since polymorphisms in gene promoters, known to be associated with human disease, can alter levels of gene protein products. A transcription factor may associate primarily with one partner at a low concentration but with another at a higher titer. The multimeric nature of regulatory complexes allows a single factor to stimulate one process while simultaneously inhibiting another. During development, a patterning gene may thus promote one event—for example, generation of neurons—by stimulating one gene promoter, while simultaneously sequestering another factor from a different promoter whose activity is required for an alternative phenotype, such as glial cells. Finally, the factors frequently exhibit cross-regulatory functions, where one factor negatively regulates expression of another. This activity leads to establishment of tissue boundaries, allowing the formation of regional subdivisions, such as basal ganglia and cerebral cortex in the forebrain.

In addition to combinatorial interactions, patterning genes exhibit distinct temporal sequences of expression and function, acting in hierarchical fashion. Functional hierarchies were established by using genetic approaches, either deleting a gene (loss of function) or over/ectopically expressing it (gain of function) and defining developmental consequences. At most general levels, genetic analyses indicate that regionally restricted patterning genes participate in specifying the identity and, therefore, function of cells in which they are expressed. Subdivisions of the brain, and of cerebral cortex specifically, are identified by regionalized gene expression in the proliferative VZ of the neural tube, leading to subsequent differentiation of distinct types of neurons in each mature (postmitotic) region. Thus, the protomap of the embryonic VZ apparently predicts the cortical regions it will generate. It appears that different genes underlie multiple stages of brain development, including (1) determining that ectoderm will give rise to nervous system (as opposed to skin); (2) defining the dimensional character of a region, such as positional identity in dorsoventral or rostrocaudal axes; (3) specifying cell class, such as neuron or glia; (4) defining when proliferation ceases and differentiation begins; (5) determining specific cell subtype, such as GABA interneuron; and (6) defining laminar position in the region, such as cerebral cortex. Although investigations are ongoing, studies indicate that these many steps depend on interactions of transcription factors from multiple families. Furthermore, a single transcription factor plays regulatory roles at multiple stages in the developmental life of a cell, yielding complex outcomes—for instance, in genetic loss-of-function studies and human disease.

The numerous transcription factors belong to protein families that have been highly conserved through evolution. Many factors important for brain development were discovered initially in *Drosophila*, where they mediate body and organ segmentation and morphogenesis or regulate neural development. Composed of a DNA binding region and protein–protein interaction domains, many act as heterodimers. In mammals, the *hox* family critically determines the anterior–posterior axis from tail to midbrain, playing major roles in defining segments of the hindbrain (rhombomeres) and its cranial nerves, serving to determine positional identity. The basic helix-loop-helix (bHLH) family—binding DNA and proteins through the basic and helix regions, respectively—regulates multiple stages sequentially from neural plate to neurogenesis. Other gene families bear names reflecting protein interaction domains, including LIM homeodomain (*Lhx*), zinc finger, paired domain (*Pax*), winged helix (*BF1* = *Foxg1*, *Hnf3*β), and *Pou*. Although numerous patterning genes associated with individual regions have been defined and some interactions described, many questions remain about interrelationships among them. However, few factors localize to regions as discrete as Brodmann's areas, which subserve specific cortical functions. Finally, it should be noted that restricting patterning gene discussion to transcription factors only is arbitrary for purposes of simplicity, because downstream target genes and proteins similarly localize to specific regions. Indeed, one of the first described patterning molecules was the *limbic system–associated membrane protein* (LAMP), a classic marker of limbic cortex. LAMP, which appears significantly before extrinsic afferents arrive, is determined in the proliferative VZ precursors, with expression continuing long term. There are numerous patterned downstream proteins that mediate regulatory gene effects, such as cadherins and ephrins, that are important in cell migration and axon pathfinding.

Finally, patterning gene expression in nervous system subdivisions is not insensitive to environmental factors. To the contrary, expression is intimately regulated by growth factors released from regional signaling centers. Indeed, although a century of classic experimental embryology described morphologically induction of new tissues between neighboring cell layers, only recently have molecular identities of soluble protein morphogens and cell response genes underlying development been defined. Signaling molecules from discrete centers establish tissue gradients that provide positional information (dorsal or ventral), impart cell specification, and/or control regional growth. Signals include the BMPs, the Wingless-Int proteins (Wnts), Shh, fibroblast growth factors (FGFs), and epidermal growth factors (EGFs). These signals set up developmental domains characterized by expression of specific transcription factors, which, in turn, control further regional gene transcription and developmental processes. The importance of these mechanisms for cerebral cortical development is only now emerging, altering concepts of the roles of subsequent thalamic innervation and experience-dependent processes. In light of the temporal and combinatorial principals discussed above, brain development can be viewed as a complex and evolving interaction of extrinsic and intrinsic information.

SPECIFIC INDUCTIVE SIGNALS AND PATTERNING GENES IN DEVELOPMENT

Induction of the central nervous system (CNS) begins at the neural plate stage when the notochord, underlying mesenchyme, and surrounding epidermal ectoderm produce signaling molecules that affect the identity of neighboring cells. Specifically, the ectoderm produces BMPs that prevent neural fate, serving to promote and maintain epidermal differentiation. Another way of stating this is that neural differentiation is a default state, which occurs unless it is inhibited. In turn, neural induction proceeds when BMP action is blocked. BMP inhibiting proteins, such as noggin, follistatin, and chordin, are secreted by *Hensen's node* (homologous to amphibian Spemann organizer), a signaling center at the rostral end of the primitive streak, which blocks skin formation and allows ectoderm to adopt a neural fate. Once the neural tube closes, the roof plate and floor plate become new signaling centers, organizing dorsal and ventral neural tube, respectively. As stated earlier, the same ligand/receptor system is used sequentially for multiple functions during development. BMPs are a case in point, since they prevent neural development at neural plate stage, whereas after neurulation, the factors are produced by the dorsal neural tube itself to induce sensory neuron fates.

Spinal Cord

The synthesis, release, and diffusion of inductive signals from signaling sources produce concentration gradients that impose distinct neural fates in the spinal cord. The notochord and floor plate secrete Shh, which induces motoneurons and interneurons ventrally, whereas the epidermal ectoderm and roof plate release several BMPs that impart neural crest and sensory relay interneuron fates dorsally. Growth factor inductive signals act to initiate discrete regions of transcription factor gene expression. For instance, high concentrations of Shh induce winged helix transcription factor *Hnf3β* gene in floor plate cells and *Nkx6.1* and *Nkx2.2* in ventral neural tube, whereas expression of more dorsal genes, *Pax6*, *Dbx1*, *Dbx2*, *Irx3*, and *Pax7*, is repressed. In response to Shh, ventral motoneurons express transcription factor gene *Isl1*, whose protein product is essential for neuron differentiation. Subsequently, ventral interneurons differentiate, expressing *En1* or *Lim1/2* independent of Shh signaling. In contrast, dorsal cord and roof plate release of BMPs induces a distinct cascade of patterning genes to elicit sensory interneuron differentiation. In aggregate, the coordinated actions of Shh and BMPs induce the dorsal–ventral dimension of the spinal cord. In similar fashion, other inductive signals determine rostral–caudal organization of the CNS, such as retinoic acid anteriorly, an upstream regulator of *hox* patterning genes, and the FGFs posteriorly. The overlapping and unique expression of the many *hox* gene family members and *krox20* are important for establishing the segmental pattern in the anterior–posterior axis of the hindbrain and spinal cord, now classic models well described in previous reviews.

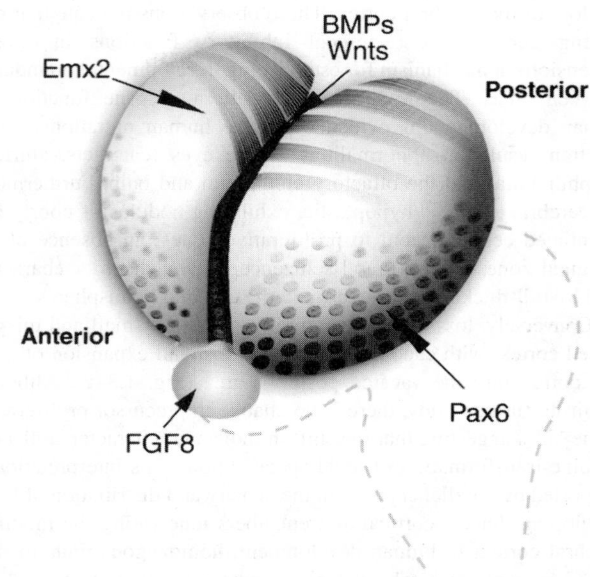

FIGURE 1.3–2 Patterning genes and signaling centers in the developing cerebral cortex. This schematic diagram shows a lateral–superior view of the two cerebral hemispheres of the embryonic mouse, sitting above the midbrain and hindbrain (*broken lines*). The anterior–lateral extent of *Pax6* gene expression is indicated by circles. The posterior–medial domain of *Emx2* expression is indicated by stripes. The genes exhibit continuous gradients of expression that decrease as they extend to the opposite poles. The signaling factor fibroblast growth factor 8 (FGF8) is produced by and released from mesenchymal tissue in the anterior neural ridge, which regulates *Pax6* and *Emx2* expression. In the midline, bone morphogenetic proteins (BMPs) and Wingless-Int proteins (Wnts) are secreted from other signaling centers, including the roof plate and the cortical hems. (Courtesy of E. DiCicco-Bloom and K. Forgash.)

Cerebral Cortex Recent evidence suggests that forebrain development also depends on inductive signals and patterning genes as observed in more caudal structures. In the embryo, the dorsal forebrain structures include the hippocampus medially, the cerebral cortex dorsolaterally, and the entorhinal cortex ventrolaterally, whereas in basal forebrain, the globus pallidus lies medially and the striatum laterally. Based on gene expression and morphological criteria, it has been hypothesized that the forebrain is divided into a checkerboard-like grid pattern of domains generated by the intersection of longitudinal columns and transverse segments, perpendicular to the longitudinal axis. The columns and segments (prosomeres) exhibit restricted expression of patterning genes, allowing for unique combinations of factors within each embryonic subdivision. Many of these genes, including *Hnf3β*, *Emx2*, *Pax6*, and *Dlx2*, are first expressed even before neurulation in the neural plate and are then maintained, providing the protomap determinants of the VZ described above. As in spinal cord, initial forebrain gene expression is influenced by a similar array of signaling center soluble factors, Shh, BMP, and retinoic acid. As the telencephalic vesicles form, signaling centers localize to the edges of the cortex. In the dorsal midline, there is the *anterior neural ridge*, an anterior cranial mesenchyme secreting FGF8, the roof plate, and, at the roof plate–vesicle junction, the cortical hem (Fig. 1.3–2). Other factors originate laterally from the dorsal–ventral forebrain junction, as well as from basal forebrain structures themselves.

Initial forebrain development starts with formation of two telencephalic vesicles from the rostral-most neural tube, the prosencephalon. This process is influenced by secreted signaling molecules, such as FGF8 and Shh, from the anterior neural ridge, followed by the roof plate, the cortical hem, and other cells of the meninges and skin. Disruption of the roof plate is known to cause holoprosencephaly (HPE), characterized by a single forebrain ventricle with a continuous cerebral cortex across the midline. Human HPE is linked to genetic mutations in several components of the inductive cascade, including Shh, its patched (Ptc) receptor, and several transcription factors, including *Six3*, *Zic2*, and *TGIF*, a component of transforming growth factor β (TGFβ) family. Shh and Six3 are coexpressed in the anterior neural ridge and later in the ventral midline, whereas Zic2 is expressed in the dorsal roof plate. Furthermore, HPE is seen in some cases of Smith-Lemli-Opitz syndrome, a defect in biosynthesis of cholesterol, which is necessary for full Shh activity. On the other hand, overexpression of the dorsal signal BMP represses FGF8 and Shh and alters cell proliferation and cell death, eliciting cyclopsia in the embryo. Thus, signaling center growth factors exhibit cross-regulation. In turn, balanced interactions of inductive signals in forebrain development are required for normal growth. Finally, when the anterior neural ridge source of FGF8 is obliterated, there is no induction of *BF1* (*Foxg1*) and an almost complete absence of cerebral cortex results.

Recent genetic studies have begun to provide insight into the mechanisms producing the diversity of cerebral cortical regions. After telencephalic vesicles form, opposing gradients of patterning genes seem to be critical in specifying the rostral–caudal areal characteristics of the cortex. Though likely to become more complex with new discoveries, the current model indicates that rostral–lateral cortex expresses high levels of homeodomain gene *Pax6*, whereas caudal–medial cortex exhibits *Emx2*, *Lhx2*, and *Lhx5* (Fig. 1.3–2). A prediction would be that altering gene expression should cause a change in cortical areas, especially the proportions of motor to sensory cortex. Consistent with this model, expression of motor cortex markers is markedly diminished in mice mutant for *Pax6*, as well as for downstream bHLH transcription factor, *Ngn2*, which it regulates. In addition, the reduction in motor cortex characteristics is accompanied by a proportionate increase in caudal sensory cortex traits. Moreover, there is also change in the dorsal–ventral dimension: Genes usually restricted to the ventral striatum and pallidum, namely *Gsh* and *Dlx*, are now expressed ectopically in dorsal territory. A similar dorsal shift of ventral genes occurs with combined deletion of another set of dorsal transcription factors, *Ngn1/2* and *Gli3*, yielding loss of the cerebral cortex. These observations indicate that patterning genes exert reciprocal inhibitory functions in several dimensions, a mechanism for establishing developmental boundaries between areas. The importance of patterning gene function for human development is evident from the human mutations: *PAX6* deletion results in abnormalities of the eyes (cataracts, aniridia, anophthalmia) and the olfactory epithelium and bulb. Furthermore, the cerebral cortex is hypoplastic, exhibiting nodules of poorly differentiated cells adjacent to proliferative zones, an absence of the marginal zone (layer 1), and schizencephaly, a disorder characterized by full-thickness clefts through the cerebral hemispheres.

Conversely, loss of *Emx2* in mice results in a small and mispatterned cortex, with caudal–medial areas lost and expansion of anterior cortex into the vacated posterior area (Fig. 1.3–2). Although requiring further study, there is no change in precursor proliferation in the VZ, suggesting that the shift in molecular characters reflects a genuine transformation of areal specification. This interpretation is supported by parallel changes in the density and distribution of later-developing thalamocortical afferent fibers innervating the modified cerebral cortex. In human development, homozygous mutations of *EMX2* gene produce schizencephaly, whereas heterozygotes exhibit less severe lesions. The gene dosage effects of human *EMX2* mutations suggest that more moderate changes in *EMX2* expression during development, for example, from promoter polymorphisms, could have more subtle yet widespread effects on cortical cell composition and function. Finally, loss of another medial transcription factor, *Lhx2*, also results in cortical changes in mice, with absent medial and diminished lateral cortex, although manifestations are more complex. Future studies need to characterize the cellular processes underlying the changes, especially distinguishing altered cell specification from changes in proliferation or survival or both.

Finally, the impact of signaling molecules on areal specification has been elegantly demonstrated in experiments genetically altering levels of FGF8. Overexpression of FGF8 in its normal anterior neural ridge location causes a posterior shift of cortical areas, whereas overexpressing a soluble receptor fragment, which sequesters endogenous factor, or reducing FGF8 gene expression shifts borders anteriorly. Furthermore, introducing FGF8 into the posterior cortex where *Emx2* predominates induces a duplication of somatosensory organization. These results suggest that FGF8 alters the ratios of *Pax6* and *Emx2* levels in the cortical neuroepithelium—in other words, changes the gradients—respecifying the rostral–caudal character that emerges. Specifically, FGF8 down-regulates *Emx2*. In contrast, Wnt and BMP signaling positively regulates *Emx2* transcription, indicating combinatorial actions of extracellular signals on patterning gene expression and consequent cortical development. More generally, gradients of patterning genes likely regulate the nature of cortical areas in all three dimensions. Although much remains to be done, critical patterning gene targets will include proteins that mediate cell–cell interactions—such as the adhesive cadherins, membrane-bound ephrins and their Eph receptors, and members of the immunoglobulin superfamily—that play roles in cell differentiation, cell migration, and neuronal process outgrowth.

Do these molecular studies identify how different cortical regions interact with thalamic neurons to establish specific functional modalities, such as vision and sensation? It has been proposed that, initially, there are no functional distinctions in the cortex, but that they are induced by the ingrowth of extrinsic thalamic axons, which convey positional and functional specification, the so-called protocortex model. However, in contrast, the abundant molecular evidence above suggests that intrinsic differences are established early in the neuroepithelium by molecular determinants that regulate areal specification, including the targeting of thalamic axons, termed the protomap model. The foregoing mutants now provide experimental tests of these two alternative models and indicate that neither model is completely correct. Although there is early molecular regionalization of the cortex, the initial targeting of thalamic axons to the cortex is independent of these molecular differences. In the rodent, thalamic afferents first target to their usual cortical regions prenatally, in the late embryo. However, once they reach the cortex, which occurs several days after birth, interactions of thalamic axon branches with local regional cues lead to modifications of initial outgrowth and the establishment of connections that conform to areal molecular identities.

Hippocampus As a region of major importance in schizophrenia and autism, defining mechanisms regulating hippocampal formation may provide clues to developmental bases of these disorders. In mice, the hippocampus is located in the medial wall of the telencephalic vesicle. Where it joins the roof plate—the future roof of the third ventricle—there is a newly defined signaling center, the cortical hem, which secretes BMPs, Wnts, and FGFs (Fig. 1.3–2). Genetic experiments have defined patterning genes localized to the cortical hem and hippocampal primordia, whose deletions result in a variety of morphogenetic defects. In mice lacking Wnt3a, which is expressed in the cortical hem, the hippocampus is either completely missing or greatly reduced, whereas neighboring cerebral cortex is mainly preserved. A similar phenotype is produced by deleting an intracellular factor downstream to Wnt receptor activation, the Lef1 gene, suggesting that the Wnt3a-*Lef1* pathway is required for hippocampal cell specification or proliferation or both—issues remaining to be defined. When another cortical hem gene, *Lhx5*, is deleted, mice lack the hem and neighboring choroid plexus, which are both sources of growth factors. However, in this case, the cortical hem cells may, in fact, proliferate in excess, and the hippocampal primordia may be present but disorganized, exhibiting abnormalities in cell proliferation, migration, and differentiation. A related abnormality is observed with *Lhx2* mutation. Finally, a sequence of bHLH transcription factors plays roles in hippocampal neurogenesis: dentate gyrus differentiation is defective in *NeuroD* and *Mash1* mutants. Significantly, expression of all of these hippocampal patterning genes is regulated by factors secreted by anterior neural ridge, roof plate, and the cortical hem, including FGF8, Shh, BMPs, and Wnts. Moreover, the basal forebrain region secretes an EGF-related protein, TGFα, which can stimulate expression of LAMP. These various signals and genes now serve as candidates for disruption in human diseases of the hippocampus.

Basal Ganglia In addition to motor and cognitive functions, the basal ganglia take on new importance in neocortical function, because they appear to be the embryonic origin of virtually all adult GABA interneurons, reaching the neocortex through tangential migration (Fig. 1.3–1). Gene expression studies have identified several transcription factors that appear in precursors originating in the ventral forebrain ganglionic eminences, allowing interneurons to be followed as they migrate dorsally into the cortical layers. Conversely, genetic deletion mutants exhibit diminished or absent interneurons, yielding results consistent with other tracing techniques. These transcription factors, including *Pax6*, *Gsh2*, and *Nkx2.1*, establish boundaries between different precursor zones in the ventral forebrain VZ through mechanisms involving mutual repression. As a simplified model, medial ganglionic eminence (MGE) expresses primarily *Nkx2.1* and gives rise to most GABA interneurons of the cortex and hippocampus, whereas lateral ganglionic eminence (LGE) expresses *Gsh2* and generates GABA interneurons of the SVZ and olfactory bulb. The boundary between ventral and dorsal forebrain then depends on LGE interaction with the dorsal neocortex, which expresses *Pax6*. When *Nkx2.1* is deleted, LGE transcription factor expression spreads ventrally into the MGE territory, and there is a 50 percent reduction in neocortical and striatal GABA interneurons. In contrast, deletion of *Gsh2* leads to ventral expansion of the dorsal cortical molecular markers and concomitant decreases in olfactory interneurons. Finally, *Pax6* mutation causes both MGE and LGE to spread laterally and into dorsal cortical areas, yielding increased interneuron migration. The final phenotypic changes are complex, as these factors exhibit unique and overlapping expression and interact to control cell fate.

Other transcription factors expressed in the MGE and LGE—including *Mash1*, *Dlx1*, *Dlx2*, *Dlx5*, *Dlx6*, *Lhx6*, and *Lhz7*—appear to regulate both the timing of differentiation as well as the type of interneuron generated. *Mash1* is expressed in early born cells, whereas *Dlx1/Dlx2* appears in later-maturing neurons, having as targets other family members, *Dlx5/Dlx6*. In the *Dlx1/Dlx2* double knock-out, there is a 75 percent reduction in neocortical interneurons and complete absence in the hippocampus, whereas olfactory neurons are preserved. A regulatory cascade has been suggested because *Mash1* can regulate *Dlx* expression, whereas *Dlx2* can induce expression of the GABA synthetic enzyme, glutamic acid decarboxylase (GAD)67. Consistent with this model, the *Mash1* deletion mutant exhibits reduced cortical GABA interneurons and striatal cholinergic interneurons. Similarly, *Nkx2.1* loss also alters neuron subpopulations, leading to complete absence of all cortical interneurons expressing NPY, somatostatin, and NOS. These studies suggest that transcription factors play roles at multiple stages in neuronal production, including generic neuronal fate specification, as well as neuron subtype determination.

Neuronal Specification As indicated for basal ganglia, throughout the nervous system, transcription factors participate in decisions at multiple levels, including determining the generic neural cell, such as neuron or glial cell, as well as neuron subtypes. *Mash1* can promote a neuronal fate over a glial fate, as well as induce the GABA interneuron phenotype. However, another bHLH factor, *Olig1/2*, can promote oligodendrocyte development, whereas it promotes motor neuron differentiation elsewhere, indicating that the variety of factors expressed in a specific cell leads to combinatorial effects and, thus, diverse outcomes for cell differentiation. The bHLH inhibitory factor, *Id*, is expressed at the transition from somatosensory to motor cortex, implying roles of family members in areal characteristics. In the hippocampus, granule neuron fate is dependent on *NeuroD* and *Math1*, with deficient cell numbers when either one is deleted. The role of specific factors in cortical cell layer determination remains an area of active investigation, but likely includes *Tbr1*, *Otx1*, and *Pax6*.

REGULATION OF NEUROGENESIS BY EXTRACELLULAR FACTORS

The interaction of extracellular factors with intrinsic genetic determinants controlling region-specific neurogenesis includes signals that regulate cell proliferation. Patterning genes control the expression of growth factor receptors and the molecular machinery of the cell division cycle. Extracellular factors are known to stimulate or inhibit proliferation of VZ precursors and originate from the cells themselves, termed *autocrine*, from neighboring cells/tissues, or *paracrine*, or from the general circulation (as in endocrine)—all sources known to affect proliferation in prenatal and postnatal developing brain. Although defined initially in cell culture, a number of mitogenic growth factors are now well characterized in vivo, including those stimulating proliferation, such as basic FGF (bFGF), EGF, IGF-I, Shh, and signals inhibiting cell division, such as pituitary adenylate cyclase activating polypeptide (PACAP), GABA, glutamate, and members of the TGFβ superfamily. However, in addition to stimulating re-entry of cells into the cell cycle—termed a *mitogenic effect*—extracellular signals also enhance proliferation by promoting survival of the mitotic population, a trophic action. Stimulation of both pathways is necessary to produce maximal cell numbers. During development, these mitogenic and trophic mechanisms parallel those identified in carcinogenesis, reflecting roles of c-myc and bcl-2, respectively. Several of the neurotrophins, especially BDNF and neurotrophin-3 (NT3), promote survival of mitotic precursors as well as the newly generated progeny.

The developmental significance of extracellular mitogens is demonstrated by factor and receptor expression in regions of neurogenesis and the profound and permanent consequences of altering their activities during development. Changes in proliferation in prenatal cortical VZ and postnatal cerebellar EGL and hippocampal dentate gyrus produce lifelong modifications in brain region population size and cell composition, potentially relevant to structural differences observed in schizophrenia, depression, and autism. In the cerebral cortex VZ of the embryonic rat, proliferation is controlled by promitogenic bFGF and antimitogenic PACAP, which are expressed as autocrine/paracrine signals. Positive and negative effects were shown in living embryos in utero by performing intracerebroventricular (ICV) injections of the factors or antagonists. bFGF produced a larger adult cortex composed of 87 percent more neurons that employed glutamate, thus increasing the ratio of excitatory pyramidal neurons to GABA inhibitory neurons, which were unchanged. Conversely, embryonic PACAP injection inhibited proliferation of cortical VZ precursors by 26 percent, reducing the number of labeled layer 5/6 neurons by 40 percent in the cortical plate 5 days later (Fig. 1.3–3A). A similar reduction was accomplished by genetically deleting promitogenic bFGF, diminishing cortical size. Furthermore, effects of mitogenic signals depended critically on the stage-specific program of regional development, since bFGF injection at later ages, when gliogenesis predominates, affected glial numbers selectively. Thus, developmental dysregulation of mitogenic pathways due to genetic or environmental factors (hypoxia, maternal/fetal infection, drug or toxicant exposure) will likely produce subtle changes in the size and composition of the developing cortex. Other signals likely to play proliferative roles may include Wnts, TGFα, IGF-I, BMPs, and leukocyte inhibitory factor (LIF)/ciliary neurotrophic factor (CNTF).

Similar to cerebral cortex, later-generated populations, such as cerebellar granule neurons and hippocampal dentate gyrus cells, are also sensitive to growth factor manipulation, especially relevant to therapies administered intravenously to premature and newborn infants in the neonatal nursery. As in humans, cerebellar granule neurons are produced postnatally in rats—but for only 3 weeks, whereas in both species, dentate gyrus neurons are produced throughout life. Remarkably, a single peripheral injection of bFGF into newborn rat pups rapidly crossed into the cerebrospinal fluid and stimulated proliferation in the cerebellar EGL by 30 percent, as well as hippocampal dentate gyrus by 100 percent, at 8 hours, consistent with an endocrine mechanism of action (Fig. 1.3–3B). The consequences of mitogenic stimulation in cerebellum were a 33 percent increase in internal granule neuron production and a 22 percent

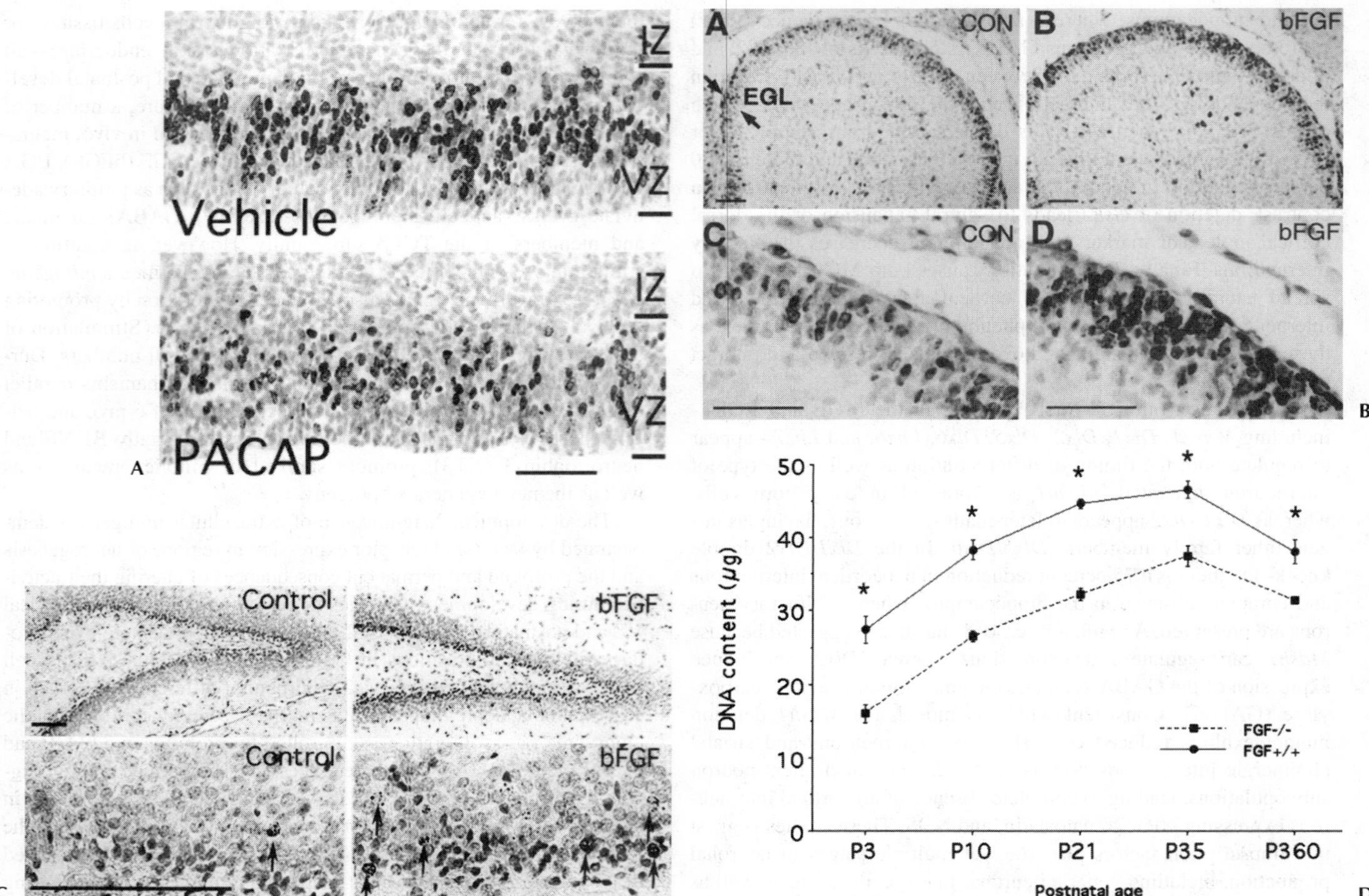

FIGURE 1.3–3 Extracellular growth factors stimulate or inhibit neuronal precursor proliferation during brain development. **A:** Intracerebroventricular injection of antimitogenic peptide, pituitary adenylate cyclase activating polypeptide (PACAP), into the rat embryo in utero inhibits mitosis in ventricular zone (VZ) precursors of the cerebral cortex. Fewer VZ precursors exhibit nuclear labeling with DNA synthesis marker, bromodeoxyuridine (BrdU), in embryos exposed to PACAP, indicating that the cells were prevented from entering S phase of the mitotic cell cycle. Three and 5 days later, there were approximately 40 percent fewer mitotically labeled neurons in the cortical plate. BrdU-positive cells appear brown, and toluidine counterstain appears blue. Scale bar = 50 μm. IZ, intermediate zone. (From Suh J, Lu N, Nicot A, Tatsuno I, DiCicco-Bloom E: PACAP is an anti-mitogenic signal in developing cerebral cortex. *Nat Neurosci.* 2001;4:123, with permission.) **B:** Eight hours after subcutaneous injection of basic fibroblast growth factor (bFGF) in newborn rat pups, 30 percent more cerebellar external germinal layer (EGL) precursors are in mitotic S phase, as indicated by brown nuclear staining compared to saline injected littermates. Thus, peripherally injected factors rapidly alter ongoing neurogenesis in the developing brain. *A* and *B*, low magnification of a single cerebellar folium; *C* and *D*, high magnification; control saline injection (CON) (*A* and *C*); bFGF injected (*B* and *D*). Nuclear BrdU stain appears brown, and basic fuchsin counterstain appears pink. Scale bar = 100 μm. (From Tao Y, Black IB, DiCicco-Bloom E: Neurogenesis in neonatal rat brain is regulated by peripheral injection of basic fibroblast growth factor (bFGF). *J Comp Neurol.* 1996;376:653–663, with permission.) **C:** Three weeks after bFGF injection at birth, there are many more mitotically labeled (*arrows*) dentate gyrus granule neurons in the hippocampal formation. BrdU-positive nuclei indicated by arrows in control and factor-treated animals appear brown, and thionin counterstain appears blue. There were 33 percent more granule neurons quantified by stereological counting, an increase that was maintained throughout life. The postnatal day 21 dentate gyrus is pictured at low (*top*) and high magnification (*bottom*). Scale bar = 100 μm. (From Cheng Y, Black IB, DiCicco-Bloom E: Hippocampal granule neuron production and population size are regulated by levels of bFGF. *Eur J Neurosci.* 2002;15:3, with permission.). **D:** Mice with genetic deletion of bFGF exhibit a lifelong reduction in total cells in the hippocampal formation, reflected by diminished total DNA in μg per hippocampus. Absolute cell counting revealed 30 percent decreases in the number of dentate gyrus granule layer neurons as well as astrocytes at 3 weeks of age. (See Color Plate.) (From Cheng Y, Black IB, DiCicco-Bloom E: Hippocampal granule neuron production and population size are regulated by levels of bFGF. *Eur J Neurosci.* 2002;15:3, with permission.)

larger cerebellum. In hippocampus, mitotic stimulation elicited by a single bFGF injection (Fig. 1.3–3C) increased the absolute number of dentate gyrus granule neurons by 33 percent at 3 weeks, defined stereologically, producing a 25 percent larger hippocampus containing more neurons and astrocytes—a change that persisted lifelong. Conversely, genetic deletion of bFGF resulted in a smaller cerebellum and hippocampus at birth and throughout life, indicating that levels of the growth factor were critical for normal brain region formation (Fig. 1.3–3D). Other proliferative signals regulating cerebellar granule neurogenesis include Shh and PACAP, whose disruption contributes to human medulloblastoma, whereas in hippocampus, the Wnt family may be involved.

There are several clinical implications of these growth factor effects observed in newborns. First, possible neurogenetic effects of therapeutic agents administered in the newborn nursery should be investigated for long-term consequences. Second, bFGF was as effective in stimulating adult neurogenesis as it was at younger ages, since it is specifically transported across the mature blood–brain barrier (BBB), raising the possibility that other protein or peptide growth factors are specifically transported into brain, potentially

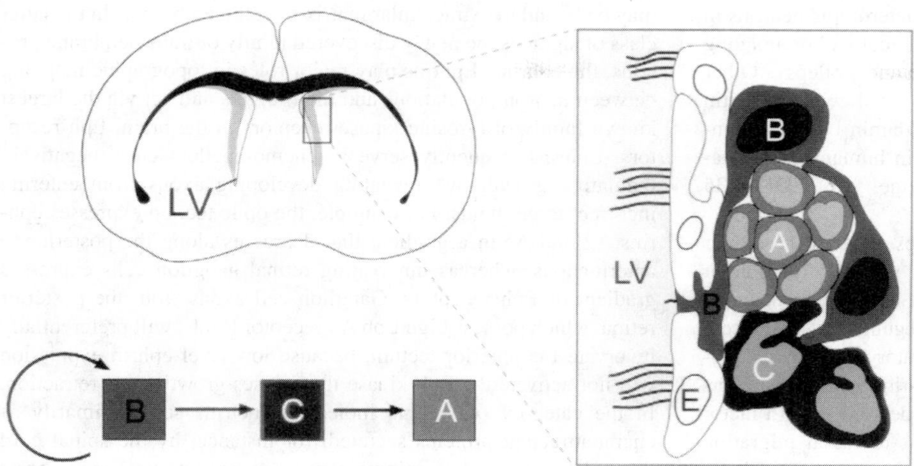

FIGURE 1.3–4 Adult neural stem cells localize to the lateral ventricular wall. This drawing shows a cross section of the adult mouse brain with the boxed area representing an enlargement of the subventricular zone, based on electron microscopic ultrastructural studies. Ciliated ependymal cells (E) line the lateral ventricles (LV) and, behind this lining, astrocytes (B) can be found. These glial cells give rise to dividing precursor cells (C), which, in turn, generate the neuroblasts (A). The neuroblasts migrate to the olfactory bulb by forming chains of cells within glial tunnels composed of astrocytes. The B cell is considered a stem cell that renews itself on each division, indicated by the circular arrow, as well as gives rise to dividing precursors fated to become neurons. (From Alvarez-Buylla A, Seri B, Doetsch F: Identification of neural stem cells in the adult vertebrate brain. *Brain Res Bull.* 2002;57:751, with permission.)

altering ongoing neurogenesis. Indeed, in rats, IGF-I also stimulates mature hippocampal dentate gyrus neurogenesis. Third, other therapeutics, such as steroids, cross the BBB efficiently due to their lipid solubility, which inhibits neurogenesis across the age spectrum. Steroids are frequently used perinatally to promote lung maturation and treat infections and trauma, but effects on human brain formation have not been examined. Finally, it is well known that neurological development may exhibit a delay in children experiencing serious systemic illness, but it is unknown to what degree this reflects interference with neurogenesis and concomitant processes, potentially producing long-term differences in cognitive and motor functional development.

CELL MIGRATION

Throughout the nervous system, newly generated neurons normally migrate away from proliferative zones to achieve final destinations. If disrupted, abnormal cell localization and function result. In humans, more than 25 syndromes with disturbed neuronal migration have been described. In developing cerebral cortex, the most well-characterized mechanism is radial migration from underlying VZ to appropriate cortical layers in inside-to-outside fashion, as described above. In addition, however, the inhibitory GABA interneurons generated in ventrally located MGEs (Fig. 1.3–1) reach the cortex through tangential migration in the intermediate zone along axonal processes or other neurons. The neurons in developing cerebellum also exhibit both radial and tangential migration. Purkinje cells leave the fourth ventricle VZ and exhibit radial migration, whereas other precursors from the rhombic lip migrate tangentially to cover the cerebellar surface, establishing the EGL, a secondary proliferative zone. From EGL, newly generated granule cells migrate radially inward to create the internal granule cell layer. Finally, granule interneurons of olfactory bulb exhibit a different kind of migration, originating in SVZ of the lateral ventricles overlying the striatum. These neuroblasts divide and migrate simultaneously in the rostral migratory stream in transit to the bulb, on a path comprised of chains of cells that support forward movements (Fig. 1.3–4). The most commonly recognized disorders of human neuronal migration are the extensive lissencephalies, although incomplete migration of more restricted neuron aggregates (heterotopias) frequently underlies focal seizure disorders.

Animal models have defined molecular pathways involved in neuronal migration. Cell movement requires signals to start and stop migration, adhesion molecules to guide migration, and functional cytoskeleton to mediate cell translocation. The best characterized mouse model of aberrant neuronal migration is reeler, a spontaneous mutant in which cortical neuron laminar position is inverted, being generated in outside-to-inside fashion. Reelin is a large, secreted extracellular glycoprotein produced embryonically by the earliest neurons in the cortical preplate, Cajal-Retzius cells, and in the hippocampus and cerebellum. Molecular and genetic analysis has established a signaling sequence in reelin activity that includes at least two receptors, the very-low-density lipoprotein receptor (VLDLR) and the apoprotein E receptor 2 (ApoER2), and the intracellular adapter protein, disabled 1 (Dab1), initially identified in the scrambler mutant mouse, a reelin phenocopy. Current thoughts consider the reelin system as one mediator of radial glial-guided neuronal migration, although specific functions in starting or stopping migration remain controversial. The roles of the VLDLR and ApoER2 are intriguing for their possible contributions to Alzheimer's disease risk. Recent studies have found human reelin gene (RELN) mutations associated with autosomal recessive lissencephaly with cerebellar hypoplasia, exhibiting a markedly thickened cortex with pachygyria, abnormal hippocampal formations, and severe cerebellar hypoplasia with absent folia.

With regard to roles of cytoskeletal proteins, studies of the filamentous fungus *Aspergillus nidulans* surprisingly provide insights into molecular machinery underlying the human migration disorder, Miller-Dieker syndrome, a lissencephaly associated with abnormal chromosome 17q13.3. Lissencephaly is a diverse disorder characterized by a smooth cortical surface lacking in gyri and sulci, markedly reducing brain surface area. The absence of convolutions results from a migration defect, the majority of neurons failing to reach final destinations. In classic lissencephaly (type I), cerebral cortex is thick and usually four-layered, whereas in cobblestone lissencephaly (type II), cortex is chaotically organized with a partly smooth and partly pebbled surface and deficient lamination. The most severely affected parts of the brain are the cerebral cortex and hippocampus, with cerebellum less affected. In fungus, the gene *NudF* was found essential for intracellular nuclear distribution, a translocation process also involved in mammalian cell migration. The human homologue of *NudF* is LIS-1 or PAFAH1B1, mutation of which accounts for up to 60 percent of lissencephaly cases of type I pathology. The LIS-1 gene product interacts with microtubules and related motor components dynein and dynactin, as well as doublecortin (DCX), which may regulate microtubule stability. Mutations in DCX gene result in

X-linked lissencephaly in males and bands of heterotopic neurons in white matter in females, appearing as a "double cortex" on imaging studies, producing severe mental retardation and epilepsy. Other migratory defects occur when proteins associated with the actin cytoskeleton are affected, such as mutation in filamin 1 gene responsible for periventricular nodular heterotopias in humans and mutations of a regulatory phosphokinase enzyme, the CDK5/p35 complex.

Cell migration also depends on molecules mediating cellular interactions, which provide cell adhesion or induce attraction or repulsion. *Astrotactin* is a major glial protein involved in neuronal migration on radial glial processes, whereas neuregulins and their receptors, ErbB2–4, play roles in neuronal–glial migratory interactions. Furthermore, some work suggests that early appearing neurotransmitters themselves, GABA and glutamate, and platelet-derived growth factor (PDGF) regulate migration speed. In contrast to radial migration from the cortical VZ, GABA interneurons generated in ganglionic eminences employ different mechanisms to leave the ventral forebrain and migrate dorsally into the cerebral cortex. Several signaling systems have been identified, including the Slit protein and roundabout (Robo) receptor, the semaphorins and their neuropilin receptors, and hepatocyte growth factor and its c-Met receptor—all of which appear to repel GABA interneurons from basal forebrain, promoting tangential migration into cortex (Fig. 1.3–1). Finally, several human forms of congenital muscular dystrophy with severe brain and eye migration defects result from gene mutations in enzymes that transfer mannose sugars to serine/threonine –OH groups in glycoproteins, interrupting interactions with several extracellular matrix molecules and producing type II cobblestone lissencephalies.

DIFFERENTIATION AND NEURONAL PROCESS OUTGROWTH

After newly produced neurons and glial cells reach their final destinations, they differentiate into mature cells. For neurons, this involves outgrowth of dendrites and extension of axonal processes, formation of synapses, and production of neurotransmitter systems, including receptors and selective reuptake sites. Most axons will become insulated by myelin sheaths produced by oligodendroglial cells. Many of these events occur with a peak period from 5 months of gestation onward. During the first several years of life, many neuronal systems exhibit exuberant process growth and branching, which is later decreased by selective "pruning" of axons and synapses dependent on experience, whereas myelination continues for several years after birth and into adulthood.

Although there is tremendous synapse plasticity in adult brain, a fundamental feature of the nervous system is the point-to-point, or topographical, mapping of one neuron population to another. During development, neurons in various brain regions extend axons to innervate diverse distant targets, such as cortex and spinal cord. The structure that recognizes and responds to cues in the environment is the growth cone, located at the axon tip. The growth cone has rodlike extensions called *filopodia* that bear receptors for specific guidance cues, which are present on cell surfaces and in the extracellular matrix. Interactions between filopodial receptors and environmental cues cause growth cones to move forward, turn, or retract. The region-specific expression of extracellular guidance molecules—such as cadherins regulated by patterning genes *Pax6* and *Emx2*—results in highly directed outgrowth of axons, termed *axonal pathfinding*. These molecules affect the direction, speed, and fasciculation of axons, acting through either positive or negative regulation. Guidance molecules may be soluble extracellular factors or, alternatively, may be bound to extracellular matrix or cell membranes. In the latter class of signal is the newly discovered family of transmembrane proteins, the ephrins. Ephrins play major roles in topographic mapping between neuron populations and their targets and act via the largest known family of tyrosine kinase receptors in the brain, Eph receptors. Ephrins frequently serve as chemorepellent cues, negatively regulating growth by preventing developing axons from entering incorrect target fields. For example, the optic tectum expresses ephrins A2 and A5 in a gradient that decreases along the posterior to anterior axis, whereas innervating retinal ganglion cells express a gradient of Eph receptors. Ganglion cell axons from the posterior retina, which possess high Eph A3 receptor levels, will preferentially innervate the anterior tectum, because low-level ephrin expression will not activate the Eph kinase that causes growth cone retraction. In the category of soluble molecules, netrins serve primarily as chemoattractant proteins secreted, for instance, by the spinal cord floor plate to stimulate spinothalamic sensory interneurons to grow into the anterior commissure, whereas Slit is a secreted chemorepulsive factor, which, through its Robo receptor, regulates midline crossing and axonal fasciculation and pathfinding.

In neocortex, layer 5 and 6 axons exit the hemisphere laterally via the internal capsule to reach subcortical destinations, whereas layer 3 axons extend medially through corpus callosum to innervate the opposite hemisphere. The internal capsule carries bidirectional axons—from cortex to thalamus and beyond—as well as thalamocortical processes, exhibiting precise connections between individual thalamic nuclei and distinct cortical domains. During development, thalamic axons must travel a complex route, passing through lateral ventral thalamus, turning to enter the internal capsule, and turning dorsally to reach cortical targets. However, thalamic axons reach the developing neocortex before target neurons have completed their migration to appropriate layers. Instead, the early generated subplate neurons projecting to the internal capsule may function as guidepost cells, serving as temporary targets for thalamic axons. The subplate neurons express two guidance systems, including the chemoattractant netrin 1, and chemorepellant cell surface molecule, ephrin A5, which is complemented by Eph receptor expression by thalamic axon growth cones. After cortical neurons complete laminar migration, thalamic axons leave subplate neurons, which apparently undergo degeneration, and extend into proper cortical layers guided by a number of cues, including chondroitin sulphate proteoglycans, ephrins, and cadherins under patterning gene regulation. In similar fashion, thalamic afferents to limbic cortex, which express Eph A5 receptor, may be repelled from sensorimotor cortex by ephrin A5. Numerous experiments demonstrate misrouted axon terminals in developing brain when ephrin/Eph expression is altered.

NEURODEVELOPMENTAL BASIS OF PSYCHIATRIC DISEASE

Several psychiatric conditions are now considered to originate during brain development, including schizophrenia, autism, and attention-deficit/hyperactivity disorder (ADHD). Defining when a condition begins helps direct attention to underlying pathogenetic mechanisms. The term *neurodevelopmental* suggests that the brain is not formed normally from the very beginning due to abnormal regulation of fundamental processes or their disruption by an insult, in contrast to a normally formed brain injured secondarily. However, the utility of the term *neurodevelopmental* may need reevaluation because of different usage by clinicians and pathologists and recognition that molecular signals function in development and maturity. For example, neurodevelopmental may indicate that (1) the brain is abnormal at disease onset, such as in schizophrenia, where prefrontal cortex and hippocampus are already smaller and ventricles enlarged at presentation in adolescence; or (2) neurons exhibit normal cytoarchitecture but reduced cell diameter that is not associated with glial proliferation or gliosis. According to classic literature, abnormally small neurons unassociated with gliosis signal a nondegenerative mechanism and, therefore, are interpreted as "developmental" in nature. This large range of meanings suggests the term may imply greater understanding than is warranted for several reasons. First, at the basic level, evidence indicates that the same ligand/receptor system or molecular function is employed repeatedly during development and adult function; therefore, a disease considered a neurotransmitter dysfunction in adulthood, such as schizophrenia, will with high likelihood also exhibit developmental abnormalities. As another example, according to the specific genetic polymorphism, hexosaminidase A deficiency presents as a devastating Tay-Sachs disease in infancy or as adult-onset spinal muscular atrophy. Second, classic neurodegenerations exhibit neuronal cell atrophy or loss associated with proliferative gliosis as their hallmark, including alcohol toxicity and Alzheimer's and Parkinson's diseases. However, it is unclear whether adult neurons may progressively atrophy and die without eliciting secondary glial responses. For example, in animal models, interruption of signaling by the survival-promoting neurotrophin BDNF in adult brain results in atrophy of dendrites and neurons in cerebral cortex without eliciting glial proliferation. Thus, the finding of smaller neurons without gliosis in brains of schizophrenic and autistic persons does not necessarily mean the condition is only or primarily developmental in origin. Whereas small neurons may, indeed, reflect an altered developmental program, alternatively, neurons may be produced normally in these conditions, only to undergo atrophy at a later stage due to abnormal regulation of nutrients, synaptic inputs, or survival-promoting neurotrophins. In turn, several etiological assumptions about clinical brain conditions may require reexamination.

Schizophrenia The neurodevelopmental hypothesis of schizophrenia postulates that etiological and pathogenetic factors occurring before the formal onset of the illness—that is, during gestation—disrupt the course of normal development. These subtle alterations in specific neurons and circuits confers vulnerability to other factors, ultimately leading to malfunctions. Schizophrenia is clearly a multifactorial disorder, including both genetic and environmental factors. Clinical studies using risk assessment have identified some relevant factors, including prenatal and birth complications (hypoxia, infection, substance and toxicant exposure), family history, body dysmorphia—especially structures of neural crest origin—and presence of mild premorbid deficits in social, motor, and cognitive functions. These risk factors may impact ongoing developmental processes such as experience-dependent axonal and dendritic proliferation, programmed cell death, myelination, and synaptic pruning.

Neuroimaging and pathology studies identify structural abnormalities at disease presentation, including smaller prefrontal cortex and hippocampus and enlarged ventricles, suggesting abnormal development. More severely affected patients exhibit a greater number of affected regions with larger changes. In some cases, ventricular enlargement and cortical grey matter atrophy increase with time. These ongoing progressive changes should lead us to reconsider the potential role of active degeneration in schizophrenia, whether due to the disease or its consequences, such as stress or drug treatment.

Structural neuroimaging strongly supports the conclusion that the hippocampus in schizophrenia is significantly smaller, perhaps by 5 percent. In turn, brain morphology has been used to assess etiological contributions of genetic and environmental factors. Comparisons of concordance for schizophrenia in monozygotic and dizygotic twins support roles for both factors. Among monozygotic twins, only 40 to 50 percent of both twins have the illness, indicating genetic constitution alone does not assure disease, suggesting that the embryonic environment also contributes. Neuroimaging, pharmacological, and pathological studies suggest that some genetic factors allow for susceptibility and that secondary insults, such as birth trauma or perinatal viral infection, provide the other. This model is consistent with imaging studies showing small hippocampi in both affected and unaffected monozygotic twins. Moreover, healthy, genetically at-risk individuals show hippocampal volumes more similar (smaller) to affected probands than normal controls. Thus, hippocampal volume reduction is not pathognomonic of schizophrenia, but rather may represent a biological marker of genetic susceptibility. It is not difficult to envision roles for developmental regulators in producing a smaller hippocampus, which could result from subtle differences in levels of transcription factors—such as *NeuroD*, *Math1*, or *Lhx*—signaling by Wnt3a and downstream mediator *Lef1* or proliferative control mediated by bFGF. Such genetic limitations may only become manifest after another developmental challenge, such as gestational infection or toxicant exposure.

The locus of schizophrenia pathology remains uncertain but may include hippocampus, entorhinal cortex, multimodal association cortex, limbic system, amygdala, cingulate cortex, thalamus, and medial temporal lobe. Despite size reductions in specific brain regions, attempts to define changes in cell numbers have been unrewarding, because most studies do not quantify the entire cell population but only assess regional cell density. In the absence of regional total volume assessment, cell density measures alone are limited in revealing population size. Most studies have found no changes in cell density in diverse brain regions. A single study successfully examining total cell number in hippocampus found normal neuron density and a 5 percent volume reduction on the left and 2 percent on the right, yielding no significant change in total cell number.

In contrast to total neuron numbers, using neuronal cell type–specific markers, many studies have found a decreased density of nonpyramidal GABA interneurons in cortex and hippocampus. In particular, parvalbumin-expressing interneurons are reduced, whereas calretinin-containing cells are normal, suggesting a deficiency of an interneuron subtype. These morphometric data are supported by molecular evidence for decreased GABA neurons, indicating reduced mRNA and protein for the GABA synthesizing enzyme, GAD67, in cortex and hippocampus. In a recent study, GAD67 mRNA levels were decreased specifically in the parvalbumin interneuron population in layers III and IV. Another product of GABA secreting neurons, reelin, which initially appears in Cajal-Retzius cells in embryonic brain, is reduced 30 to 50 percent in schizophrenia and bipolar disorder with psychotic symptoms. However, this decrease does not appear disease specific and is, in fact, associated with reductions in other general markers of the neuronal compartment, such as synapsin II. However, because cortical GABA neurons produce reelin during adulthood, the data are consistent with an interneuron deficiency. Such a deficiency, leading to diminished GABA signaling, may underlie a potential compensatory increase in $GABA_A$ receptor binding detected in hippocampal CA2–4 fields on both pyramidal and nonpyramidal neurons, apparently selective because benzodiazepine binding is unchanged. More generally, deficiency in a subpopulation of GABA interneurons raises intriguing new possibilities for schizophrenia etiology. As indicated in the gene patterning section above, different subpopulations of forebrain GABA interneurons originate from distinct precursors located in the embryonic basal forebrain. Thus, cortical and hippocampal GABA interneurons may derive primarily from the MGE under control of patterning gene, *Nkx2.1*, whereas SVZ and olfactory neurons derive from *Gsh2*-expressing LGE precursors. Furthermore, the timing and sequence of GABA interneuron generation may depend on a regulatory network including *Mash1*, *Dlx1/2*, and *Dlx5/6*, all gene candidates to examine in schizophrenia. Thus, abnormal regulation of these factors may diminish selectively GABA interneuron formation, which, in turn, may represent a genetically determined vulnerability and may contribute to diminished regional brain size.

Although select cell loss may contribute to disease production, functional deficits in specific neurotransmitters systems certainly play major roles in schizophrenia. Pharmacological evidence of aggravation or relief of the positive and negative symptoms of schizophrenia indicates involvement of dopamine, serotonin, and glutamate systems. The relief of positive symptoms by the dopamine type 2 (D_2) receptor blocker, chlorpromazine (Thorazine), was the first major effective dopamine-related therapy, consistent with symptom exacerbation by dopamine agonism that is induced by amphetamines. Significant therapeutic improvement came with discovery that serotonin drugs relieved both positive as well as negative symptoms, specifically the serotonin type 2 (5-HT_2) receptor blockers, such as clozapine (Clozaril). Finally, glutamate also makes contributions to the disorder, since symptoms can be produced by glutamate antagonism, as caused by the street drug phencyclidine (PCP) or in animal models by partial genetic deletion of the *N*-methyl-D-aspartate (NMDA) glutamate receptor. Therapeutic tools include glutamate receptor modulators glycine, D-serine, and cycloserine. Potentially, a deficiency in GABA signaling may allow these excitatory systems to be relatively overactive, leading, in turn, to the utility of D_2 and 5-HT_2 antagonists. It should be emphasized that abnormalities of these neurotransmitters during development will lead to altered regulation of neurogenesis, cell migration, and survival. Consequently, abnormal development of neural circuitry as well as ongoing adult malfunction may differentially contribute to the positive and negative symptoms of schizophrenia. Furthermore, the characterization of schizophrenia as neurodevelopmental may imply a more limited molecular defect than is warranted.

Deficiencies in these identified transmitter systems may also have genetic bases. Indeed, the known human genetic associations with schizophrenia include neurotransmitters already implicated by pharmacology—specifically, dopamine and serotonin. Dopamine levels are regulated by the catechol-*O*-methyltransferase (COMT) metabolic pathway. Human polymorphisms in the chromosome 22 deletion syndrome (substituting valine for methionine in COMT) alter dopamine levels fourfold in frontal cortex of mice expressing the variant. In families carrying chromosome 22 deletion, the unaffected siblings of schizophrenic patients exhibit poor frontal lobe function for information processing and memory function tasks, suggesting underlying genetic susceptibility. Another human gene associated with schizophrenia is on chromosome 13q, the location of the 5-HT_{2A} receptor, which is the target of the antipsychotic drug clozapine. Future studies should define associations for genes regulating the serotonergic and dopaminergic phenotypic programs, similar to the master regulatory functions defined in mice of *Phox2* in catecholaminergic sympathetic neurons and *Pet1* in serotonergic neurons of the raphe nucleus.

Autism Another condition considered neurodevelopmental in origin is autism, a complex and heterogeneous disorder characterized by abnormalities in social interaction and communication and restricted/repetitive interests and activities. The large diversity of signs and symptoms in autism may reflect the multiplicity of abnormalities observed in pathological and functional studies, which include both forebrain and hindbrain. The functional impairments in autism may be assigned to multiple brain regions. Forebrain neurons in cerebral cortex and limbic system play critical roles in social interaction, communication, and learning and memory. For example, the amygdala, which connects to prefrontal and temporal cortex and fusiform gyrus, plays a prominent role in social and emotional cognition. In autism, the amygdala and fusiform gyrus demonstrate abnormal activation during facial recognition and emotional attribution tasks. On the other hand, neurophysiological tests of evoked cortical potentials and oculomotor responses indicate normal perception of primary sensory information but disturbed higher cognitive processing. The functional impairments in higher-order cognitive processing and neocortical circuitry suggest a developmental disorder involving synaptic organization.

Whereas functional studies indicate broad forebrain dysfunctions in autism, classic pathological studies suggested abnormalities restricted to limbic and cerebellar structures. There were increased densities of small neurons bearing atrophic dendrites in the interconnecting limbic nuclei, including CA fields, septum, mammillary bodies, and amygdala, which potentially reflected failed maturation, although secondary atrophy seems a viable alternative. In cerebellum, there was consistent reduction in Purkinje neurons in the absence of signs typical of acquired postnatal lesions—including gliosis, empty baskets, and retrograde loss of afferent inferior olive neurons—suggesting a prenatal origin at 30 weeks. Finally, discontinuous patches of hypertrophic neurons were observed among normal cell ribbons in olivary and deep cerebellar nuclei present in younger patients (younger than 10 years), whereas atrophy was seen in those older than 25 years. The interpretation was that cell density was increased due to atrophy of neurons, dendrites, and neuropil, without altered cell number, although selective cell deficiencies were observed in adulthood.

In contrast, more recent study identifies widespread and nonuniform abnormalities, suggesting dysregulation of many processes, including neuron proliferation, migration, survival, organization, and programmed cell death. Four of six brains were macrocephalic, consistent with increased size defined by numerous pathology and neuroimaging studies. In the cerebral cortex, there was thickened or diminished gray matter, disorganized laminar patterns, misoriented pyramidal neurons, ectopic neurons in both superficial and deep white matter, and increased or decreased neuron densities. The evidence of abnormal cortical neurogenesis and migration is in accordance with documented cognitive functional deficits. In the brainstem, neuronal disorganization appeared as discontinuous and malpositioned neurons in olivary and dentate nuclei, ectopic neurons in medulla and cerebellar peduncles, and aberrant fiber tracts. There were widespread patchy or diffuse decreases of Purkinje neurons, sometimes associated with increased Bergmann glia without empty baskets or ectopic Purkinje neurons in the molecular layer. Finally, hippocampal neuronal atrophy was not observed, and quantitative stereology found no consistent change in neuron density or number.

Although seemingly incompatible, these various data support a model of developmental abnormalities occurring at different times and altering regions, according to specific schedules of neurogenesis and differentiation. Importantly, a similar range of abnormalities beyond cerebellum and limbic systems were found in classic studies but were excluded because they did not occur in every brain examined. Finally, in 15 children exposed to the teratogen thalidomide during days 20 to 24 of gestation—when cranial and Purkinje neurogenesis occurs in the brainstem—four cases exhibited autism. Based on these data, it can be surmised that autism is associated with insults at 3 weeks for thalidomide, at 12 weeks when inferior olivary neurons are migrating, and before 30 weeks when olivary axons make synapses with Purkinje cells. These diverse abnormalities in cell production, survival, migration, organization, and differentiation in both hindbrain and forebrain indicate disturbed brain development over a range of stages. Although the specific cellular derangements described on pathology may be directly responsible for the core symptoms of autism, there is an alternative hypothesis: Disturbed regulation of developmental processes produces an as-yet-unidentified biochemical cellular lesion(s) to cause autism but also produces the diverse pathology defined to date. This proposal is supported by the currently known genetic causes of autism that account for 10 percent of cases, including tuberous sclerosis, neurofibromatosis, Smith-Lemli-Opitz syndrome, and fragile X mental retardation. These genetic etiologies interfere with cell proliferation control, cholesterol biosynthesis, and Shh function and protein translation involved in dendrite formation—fundamental processes in the sequence of development.

THE REMARKABLE DISCOVERY OF ADULT NEUROGENESIS

In the last decade, there has been a fundamental shift in paradigm regarding the limits of neurogenesis in the brain, with important implications for neural plasticity, mechanisms of disease etiology and therapy, and possibilities of repair. Until recently, it has generally been maintained that new neurons are not produced in the brain after birth (or soon thereafter, considering cerebellar EGL); thus, brain plasticity and repair depend on modifications of a numerically static neural network. Strong evidence to the contrary now suggests that new neurons are generated throughout life in certain regions—well documented across the phylogenetic tree—including birds, rodents, primates, and humans. Because this is an area of intense interest and investigation, rapid progress should occur over the next two decades, likely altering models described herein.

The term *neurogenesis* has been used inconsistently in different contexts, indicating sequential production of neural elements during development—first neurons, then glial cells—but frequently connoting only neuron generation in adult brain, in contrast to gliogenesis. This discussion uses the first, more general meaning, distinguishing cell types as needed. The first evidence of mammalian neurogenesis, or birth of new neurons, in adult hippocampus was reported in the 1960s by Altman and Das, followed by Kaplan and Hinds, in which [^{3}H]thymidine–labeled neurons were documented. As a common marker for cell production, these studies used nuclear incorporation of [^{3}H]thymidine into newly synthesized DNA during chromosome replication, which occurs before cells undergo division. After a delay, cells divide, producing two [^{3}H]thymidine–labeled progeny. *Cell proliferation* is defined as an absolute increase in cell number, which occurs only if cell production is not balanced by cell death. Because there is currently little evidence for a progressive increase in brain size with age—except perhaps for rodent hippocampus—most neurogenesis in adult brain is apparently compensated by cell loss. More recent studies of neurogenesis employ the more convenient thymidine analog BrdU, which can be injected into living animals and then detected by immunohistochemistry.

During embryonic development, neurons are produced from almost all regions of the ventricular neuroepithelium. Neurogenesis in the adult, however, is largely restricted to two regions: SVZ lining the lateral ventricles and a narrow proliferative zone underlying the dentate gyrus granule layer (subgranular zone) in hippocampus. In mice, rodents, and monkeys, newly produced neurons migrate from the SVZ in an anterior direction into the olfactory bulb to become GABA interneurons. The process has been elegantly characterized at both ultrastructural and molecular levels (Fig. 1.3–4). In the SVZ, the neuroblasts (A cells) on their way to olfactory bulb create chains of cells and migrate through a scaffold of glial cells supplied by slowly dividing astrocytes (B cells). Within this network of cell chains, there are groups of rapidly dividing neural precursors (C cells). Evidence suggests that the B cells give rise to the C cells which in turn develop into the A cells, the future olfactory bulb interneurons. The existence of a sequence of precursors with progressively restricted abilities to generate diverse neural cell types makes defining mechanisms regulating adult neurogenesis in vivo a great challenge.

As in developing brain, adult neurogenesis is also subject to regulation by extracellular signals that control precursor proliferation and survival and, in many cases, the very same factors. After initial discovery of adult neural stem cells generated under EGF stimulation, other regulatory factors were defined, including bFGF, IGF-I, BDNF, and LIF/CNTF. Although the hallmark of neural stem cells includes the capacity to generate neurons, astrocytes, and oligodendroglia—termed *multipotentiality*—specific signals appear to produce relatively different profiles of cells that may migrate to distinct sites. Intraventricular infusion of EGF promotes primarily gliogenesis in the SVZ, with cells migrating to olfactory bulb, striatum, and corpus callosum, whereas bFGF favors generation of neurons destined for the olfactory bulb. Both factors appear to stimulate mitosis directly, with differential effects on the cell lineage produced. In contrast, BDNF may increase neuron formation in SVZ as well as striatum and hypothalamus, although effects may be primarily through promoting survival of newly generated neurons that otherwise undergo cell death. Finally, CNTF and related LIF may promote gliogenesis or, alternatively, support self-renewal of adult stem cells rather than enhance a specific cell category.

Remarkably, in addition to direct intraventricular infusions, adult neurogenesis is also affected by peripheral levels of growth factors, hormones, and neuropeptides. Peripheral administration of both bFGF and IGF-I stimulates neurogenesis, increasing selectively mitotic labeling in the SVZ and hippocampal subgranular zone, respectively, suggesting that there are specific mechanisms for factor transport across the BBB. Interestingly, elevated prolactin levels, induced by peripheral injection or natural pregnancy, stimulate proliferation of progenitors in the mouse SVZ (Fig. 1.3–4), leading to increased olfactory bulb interneurons and potentially playing roles in learning new infant scents. This may be relevant to changes in prolactin seen in psychiatric disease. Conversely, in behavioral paradigms of social stress—such as territorial challenge by male intruders—activation of the hypothalamic-pituitary-adrenal axis with increased glucocorticoids leads to reduced neurogenesis in the hippocampus, apparently through local glutamate signaling. Inhibition is also observed after peripheral opiate administration, a model for substance abuse. Thus, neurogenesis may be one target process affected by changes of hormones and neuropeptides associated with several psychiatric conditions.

The discovery of adult neurogenesis naturally leads to questions about whether new neurons can integrate into the complex cytoarchitecture of the mature brain and to speculation about its functional significance, if any. In rodents, primates, and humans, new neurons are generated in the dentate gyrus of the hippocampus, an area important for learning and memory. Some adult-generated neurons in humans have been shown to survive for at least 2 years. Further, newly generated cells in adult mouse hippocampus indeed elaborate extensive dendritic and axonal arborizations appropriate to the neural circuit and display functional synaptic inputs and action potentials. From a functional perspective, the generation and/or survival of new neurons correlates strongly with multiple instances of behavioral learning and experience. For example, survival of newly generated neurons is markedly enhanced by hippocampal-dependent learning tasks and by an enriched, behaviorally complex environment. Of perhaps greater importance, a reduction in dentate gyrus neurogenesis impairs the formation of trace memories—in other words, when an animal must associate stimuli that are separated in time, a hippocampal-dependent task. Finally, in songbirds, neurogenesis is activity dependent and is increased by foraging for food and learning new songs, whether it occurs seasonally or is induced by steroid hormone administration. However, a certain degree of caution is necessary with so many studies focusing on the possible role of neurogenesis in disease and therapeutic response. Specifically, most studies perform only incomplete analysis of new neuron production, relying instead on generally accepted cellular markers. For better confidence, investigators should address the following issues before concluding that neurogenesis has occurred and plays an important role:

1. After incorporating a thymidine analog, such as BrdU or [^{3}H]thymidine, into new DNA, does the cell complete chromosome replication and actually go on to divide, making two new cells? To be definitive, an actual count of neuron numbers will be required to prove actual cell production. It is possible that cells duplicate their chromosomes and then just await in G2, without dividing. Or incorporation may simply reflect DNA repair, although, when examined, this has not been the case in animal models.
2. If mitosis indeed yields two new cells, does the brain region increase in size over time, or, alternatively, do other cells die, keeping a balanced population size? In the rat, the size of the hippocampus in fact enlarges over the animal's lifetime.
3. Are newly generated cells incorporated properly into local circuits, making correct afferent and efferent connections?

In addition to these structural concerns, there are several functional issues under investigation. For example, are new cells required for maintaining ongoing function or information? Or, alternatively, are new cells only required to learn new information? With so many investigators using these approaches, there will be much to consider over the coming decade.

From clinical and therapeutic perspectives, fundamental questions are whether changes in neurogenesis contribute to disease and whether newly formed neurons undergo migration to and integration into regions of injury, replacing dead cells and leading to functional recovery. A neurogenetic response has now been shown for multiple conditions in the adult, including brain trauma, stroke, and epilepsy. For instance, ischemic stroke in the striatum stimulates adjacent SVZ neurogenesis (Fig. 1.3–4), with neurons migrating to the injury site. Furthermore, in a highly selective paradigm not involving local tissue damage, degeneration of layer 3 cortical neurons elicited SVZ neurogenesis and cell replacement. These studies raise the possibility that newly produced neurons normally participate in recovery and may be stimulated as a novel therapeutic strategy. However, in contrast to potential reconstructive functions, neurogenesis may also play roles in pathogenesis: In a kindling model of epilepsy, newly generated neurons were found to migrate to incorrect positions and participate in aberrant neuronal circuits, reinforcing the epileptic state. Conversely, reductions in neurogenesis may contribute to several conditions that implicate dysfunction or degeneration of the hippocampal formation. Dentate gyrus neurogenesis is inhibited by increased glucocorticoids levels observed in aged rats and can be reversed by steroid antagonists and adrenalectomy—observations potentially relevant to the correlation of elevated human cortisol levels with reduced hippocampal volumes and the presence of memory deficits. Similarly, stress-induced increases in human glucocorticoid may contribute to decreased hippocampal volumes seen in schizophrenia, depression, and posttraumatic stress disorder.

A potential role for altered neurogenesis in disease has gained the most support in recent studies of depression. A number of studies in animals and humans suggest a correlation between decreased hippocampal size and depressive symptoms, whereas clinically effective antidepressant therapy elicits increased hippocampal volume and enhanced neurogenesis, with causal relationships still being defined. For example, postmortem and brain imaging studies indicate cell loss in corticolimbic regions in bipolar disorder and major depression. Significantly, mood stabilizers, such as lithium ion and valproic acid, as well as antidepressants and electroconvulsive therapy (ECT) activate intracellular pathways that promote neurogenesis and synaptic plasticity. Furthermore, in a useful primate model, the adult tree shrew, the chronic psychosocial stress model of depression elicited approximately 15 percent reductions in brain metabolites and 33 percent decreases in neurogenesis (BrdU mitotic labeling), which effects were prevented by coadministration of the antidepressant tianeptine (Stablon). More important, whereas stress exposure elicited small reductions in hippocampal volumes, stressed animals treated with antidepressant exhibited increased hippocampal volumes. Similar effects have been found in rodent models of depression.

In addition to the foregoing structural relationships, recent evidence has begun defining the roles of relevant neurotransmitter systems to antidepressant effects on behavior and neurogenesis. One exciting finding is a causal link between antidepressant-induced neurogenesis and a positive behavioral response. In the 5-HT_{1A} receptor–null mouse, fluoxetine (Prozac), a selective serotonin reuptake inhibitor (SSRI), produced neither enhanced neurogenesis nor behavioral improvement. Further, when hippocampal neuronal precursors were selectively reduced (85 percent) by X-irradiation, neither fluoxetine nor imipramine (Tofranil) induced neurogenesis or behavioral recovery. Finally, one study using hippocampal cultures from normal and mutant rodents strongly supports a neurogenetic role for endogenous neuropeptide Y, which is contained in dentate gyrus hilar interneurons. Neuropeptide Y stimulates precursor proliferation selectively via the Y1 (not Y2 or Y5) receptor, a finding consistent with this receptor mediating antidepressive effects of neuropeptide Y in animal models and the impact of neuropeptide Y levels on both hippocampal-dependent learning and responses to stress. In aggregate, these observations suggest that volume changes observed with human depression and therapy may directly relate to alterations in ongoing neurogenesis. More generally, the discovery of adult neurogenesis has led to major changes in our perspectives on the regenerative capacities of the human brain.

References

*Alvarez-Buylla A, Seri B, Doetsch F: Identification of neural stem cells in the adult vertebrate brain. *Brain Res Bull.* 2002;57:751.

Bailey A, Luthert P, Dean A, Harding B, Janota I, Montgomery M, Rutter M, Lantos P: A clinicopathological study of autism. *Brain.* 1998;121:889.

Benes FM, Berretta S: GABAergic interneurons: implications for understanding schizophrenia and bipolar disorder. *Neuropsychopharmacology.* 2001;25:1.

Bishop KM, Goudreau G, O'Leary DD: Regulation of area identity in the mammalian neocortex by Emx2 and *Pax6*. *Science.* 2000;288:344.

Cameron HA, McKay RD: Restoring production of hippocampal neurons in old age. *Nat Neurosci* 1999;2;894.

Cheng Y, Black IB, DiCicco-Bloom E: Hippocampal granule neuron production and population size are regulated by levels of bFGF. *Eur J Neurosci.* 2002;15;3.

Eriksson PS, Perfilieva E, Björk-Eriksson T, Alborn A-M, Nordborg C, Peterson DA, Gage FH: Neurogenesis in adult human hippocampus. *Nat Med.* 1998;4:1313.

Fukuchi-Shimogori T, Grove E: Neocortex patterning by the secreted signaling molecule FGF8. *Science.* 2001;294:1071.

Garel S, Huffman KJ, Rubenstein JLR: Molecular regionalization of the neocortex is disrupted in Fgf8 hypomorphic mutants. *Development*. 2003;130:1903.
Gregg CT, Shingo T, Weiss S: Neural stem cell of the mammalian forebrain. *Symp Soc Exp Biol*. 2001;53:1.
Hashimoto T, Volk DW, Eggan SM, Mirnics K, Pierri JN, Sun Z, Sampson AR, Lewis DA: Gene expression deficits in a subclass of GABA neurons in the prefrontal cortex of subjects with schizophrenia. *J Neurosci*. 2003;23:6315.
Hatten ME, Heintz N: Mechanisms of neural patterning and specification in the developing cerebellum. *Annu Rev Neurosci*. 1995;18:385.
Heckers S, Konradi C: Hippocampal neurons in schizophrenia. *J Neural Transm*. 2002;109:891.
Howell OW, Scharfman HE, Herzog H, Sundstrom LE, Beck-Sickinger A, Gray WP: Neuropeptide Y is neuroproliferative for post-natal hippocampal precursor cells. *J Neurochem*. 2003;86:646.
Jessell TM: Neuronal specification in the spinal cord: inductive signals and transcriptional codes. *Nat Rev Genet*. 2002;1:20.
Kempermann G, Gage FH: Neurogenesis in the adult hippocampus. *Novartis Found Symp* 2000;231:220.
Kintner C: Neurogenesis in embryos and adult neural stem cells. *J Neurosci*. 2002;22:639.
Malberg JE, Duman RS: Cell proliferation in adult hippocampus is decreased by inescapable stress: reversal by fluoxetine treatment. *Neuropsychopharmacology*. 2003;28:1562.
*Marin O, Rubenstein JL: A long remarkable journey: tangential migration in the telencephalon. *Nat Rev Neurosci*. 2001;2:780.
Monuki ES, Walsh CA: Mechanisms of cerebral cortical patterning in mice and humans. *Nat Neurosci*. 2001;4:1199.
Nadarajah B, Parnavelas JG: Modes of neuronal migration in the developing cerebral cortex. *Nat Neurosci*. 2002;3:423.
Noctor SC, Flint AC, Weissman TA, Dammerman RS, Kriegstein AR: Neurons derived from radial glial cells establish radial units in neocortex. *Nature*. 2001;409:714.
Nottebohm F: Why are some neurons replaced in adult brain? *J Neurosci*. 2002;22:624.
Nowakowski R, Hayes NL: CNS development: an overview. *Dev Psychopathol*. 1999;11:395.
O'Leary DDM, Nakagawa Y: Patterning centers, regulatory genes and extrinsic mechanisms controlling arealization of the neocortex. *Curr Opin Neurobiol*. 2002;12:14.
Ragsdale CW, Grove EA: Patterning the mammalian cerebral cortex. *Curr Opin Neurobiol*. 2001;11:50.
Reynolds BA, Weiss S: Generation of neurons and astrocytes from isolated cells of the adult mammalian central nervous system. *Science*. 1992;255:1707.
*Ross ME, Walsh CA: Human brain malformations and their lessons for neuronal migration. *Annu Rev Neurosci*. 2001;24:1041.
Sanes JR, Jessel TM. The guidance of axons to their targets. In: Kandel ER, Schwartz JH, Jessel TM, eds. *Principles of Neural Science*. 4th ed. New York: McGraw-Hill; 2000.
Santarelli L, Saxe M, Gross C, Surget A, Battaglia F, Dulawa S, Weisstaub N, Lee J, Duman R, Arancio O, Belzung C, Hen R: Requirement of hippocampal neurogenesis for the behavioral effects of antidepressants. *Science*. 2003;301:805.
Sawa A, Snyder SH: Schizophrenia: diverse approaches to a complex disease. *Science*. 2002;296:692.
*Schuurmans C, Guillemot F: Molecular mechanisms underlying cell fate specification in the developing telencephalon. *Curr Opin Neurobiol*. 2002;12:26.
Sheline YI, Gado MH, Kraemer HC. Untreated depression and hippocampal volume loss. *Am J Psychiatry*. 2003;160:1516.
*Shors TJ, Miesegaes G, Beylin A, Zhao M, Rydel T, Gould E: Neurogenesis in the adult is involved in the formation of trace memories. *Nature*. 2001;410:372.
Suh J, Lu N, Nicot A, Tatsuno I, DiCicco-Bloom E: PACAP is an anti-mitogenic signal in developing cerebral cortex. *Nat Neurosci*. 2001;4:123.
Vaccarino FM, Schwartz ML, Raballo R, Nilsen J, Rhee J, Zhou M, Doetschman T, Coffin JD,Wyland JJ, Hung YT: Changes in cerebral cortex size are governed by fibroblast growth factor during embryogenesis. *Nat Neurosci*. 1999;2:848.
van Praag H, Schinder AF, Christie BR, Toni N, Palmer TD, Gage FH: Functional neurogenesis in the adult hippocampus. *Nature*. 2002;415:1030.

▲ 1.4 Monoamine Neurotransmitters

Laurence H. Tecott, M.D., Ph.D., and
Sharon L. Smart, M.D., Ph.D.

Historically, the monoamine neurotransmitters and acetylcholine have been strongly implicated in the etiology and treatment of a wide variety of neuropsychiatric disorders. These small molecules—serotonin, norepinephrine, dopamine, histamine, and acetylcholine—are widely distributed throughout the central nervous system (CNS). The activity of each neurotransmitter system modulates multiple neuronal pathways that mediate diverse behavioral and physiological processes. Conversely, each CNS function is regulated by multiple interactive neurotransmitter systems. In light of this complexity, determining the mechanisms through which monoamine systems impact the etiology and treatment of psychiatric disorders poses a major challenge. Advances in molecular neurobiology provide powerful new tools to aid in this endeavor. Molecular cloning studies have led to the identification and functional characterization of gene products that contribute to monoaminergic transmission, such as monoamine receptors, transporters, and synthetic and degradative enzymes. More recently, these genes have provided targets for powerful techniques that enable the precise introduction of mutations into the mouse genome. Thus, the functional consequences of perturbing gene function may be examined in the context of the intact, behaving organism. The molecular cloning of genes involved in monoaminergic transmission has also led to the identification of allelic variants of human genes. This raises the intriguing prospect that the inheritance of particular variants may contribute to disease susceptibility and to the efficacy of therapeutic agents.

ANATOMY OF MONOAMINE SYSTEMS

The anatomical organization of monoaminergic systems shares a number of common features. Monoaminergic systems are strikingly divergent: monoaminergic cell bodies are generally found in aggregates located in a few restricted subcortical brain regions. Individual monoaminergic neurons typically possess long and extensively branched axonal processes, innervating a large number of postsynaptic cells. This organization may permit monoaminergic systems to exert control in a coordinated manner over diverse brain regions. The actions of monoamines in particular brain regions are determined not only by the extent of monoamine innervation, but also by the receptor subtypes expressed in these regions. Monoaminergic receptors are diverse with regard to their regional and synaptic localization within the brain and the intracellular signaling systems to which they couple. This receptor diversity provides a means through which a single signaling molecule may produce effects that vary in different postsynaptic neurons.

Serotonin Although approximately one in a million brain neurons are serotonergic, serotonin systems influence CNS activity at all levels of the neuraxis. Serotonergic neurons are clustered in midline raphe nuclei of the midbrain, pons, and medulla. The tonic firing of these neurons varies across the sleep–wake cycle, with absence of activity during rapid eye movement (REM) sleep. Increase in neuronal firing observed during rhythmic motor behaviors suggests a role for the serotonin system in modulating at least some forms of motor output. Serotonergic projections reach extensively throughout the brain and descend to the spinal cord (Fig. 1.4–1). The majority of the serotonergic innervation of the forebrain arises from the dorsal and median raphe nuclei of the midbrain. Ascending projections from these nuclei course through the medial forebrain bundle before diverging to many target regions. Whereas the median raphe nucleus provides the majority of the serotonergic innervation of the limbic system, including the hippocampus and septum, the dorsal raphe nucleus provides the primary innervation of the striatum and thalamus. In addition to the differences in target areas innervated by the median raphe and dorsal raphe, structural differences in the axonal projections from these nuclei have been observed. Whereas fibers from the dorsal raphe are fine, with small vesicle-containing swell-

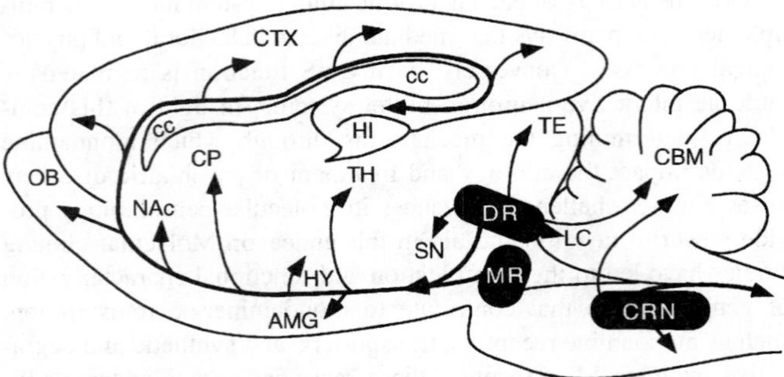

FIGURE 1.4–1 Brain serotonergic pathways (in rats). Serotonergic neurons are located in brainstem midline raphe nuclei and project throughout the neuraxis. (There is an approximate similarity between monoamine pathways in rats and in humans.) AMG, amygdala; CBM, cerebellum; cc, corpus callosum; CP, caudate putamen; CRN, caudal raphe nuclei; CTX, neocortex; DR, dorsal raphe nucleus; HI, hippocampus; HY, hypothalamus; LC, locus ceruleus; MR, median raphe nucleus; NAc, nucleus accumbens; OB, olfactory bulb; SN, substantia nigra; TE, tectum; TH, thalamus; TM, tuberomammillary nucleus of hypothalamus.

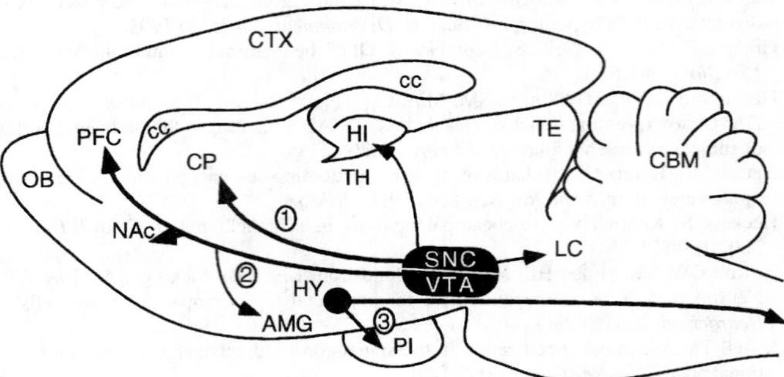

FIGURE 1.4–2 Brain dopaminergic pathways (in rats). The three principal dopaminergic pathways: (*1*) nigrostriatal pathway, (*2*) mesocorticolimbic pathway, and (*3*) tuberohypophyseal pathway. AMG, amygdala; CBM, cerebellum; cc, corpus callosum; CP, caudate putamen; CTX, neocortex; HI, hippocampus; HY, hypothalamus; LC, locus ceruleus; NAc, nucleus accumbens; OB, olfactory bulb; PFC, prefrontal cortex; PI, pituitary; SNC, substantia nigra pars compacta; TE, tectum; TH, thalamus; VTA, ventral tegmental area.

ings called *varicosities*, median raphe axons are beaded, with large spherical varicosities. These axons show differential sensitivity to the neurotoxic effects of the amphetamine analog 3,4-methylenedioxymethamphetamine (MDMA, "ecstasy"). This agent produces a selective loss of fine axons, while sparing the larger beaded projections derived from the median raphe. The significance of the morphological differences in these projection fibers remains to be determined. Both types of fibers are found in the neocortex, which receives a rich serotonergic innervation, derived from both nuclei. The divergent nature of serotonergic projections is illustrated by this innervation; it has been estimated that each serotonergic neuron may influence 500,000 target neurons. Furthermore, each cortical neuron may be associated with more than 200 serotonergic varicosities. This provides a means through which serotonin could effect widespread and coordinated modulation of cortical function. The caudal raphe serotonergic neurons project to the medulla, cerebellum, and spinal cord. Serotonergic efferents to the dorsal horn of the spinal cord have been implicated in the suppression of nociceptive pathways.

Dopamine Dopamine neurons are more widely distributed than those of other monoamines, residing in the midbrain substantia nigra and ventral tegmental area, and in the periaqueductal gray, hypothalamus, olfactory bulb, and retina. In the periphery, dopamine is found in the kidney, where it functions to produce renal vasodilation, diuresis, and natriuresis. Of particular relevance are three CNS dopamine-containing systems: (1) nigrostriatal, (2) mesocorticolimbic, and (3) tuberohypophyseal (Fig. 1.4–2). The nigrostriatal dopamine system has been the most extensively studied of the dopaminergic pathways. Dopamine cell bodies located in the pars compacta division of the substantia nigra send ascending projections to the dorsal striatum, particularly the caudate putamen. This projection modulates motor function, as highlighted by the motor disturbances of Parkinson's disease, a disorder characterized by degeneration of the nigrostriatal system. Prolonged use of dopaminergic agonist agents can result in abnormal movements or dyskinesia. Conversely, the extrapyramidal motor side effects of antipsychotic drugs are believed to result from the blockade of striatal dopamine receptors.

The midbrain ventral tegmental area lies medial to the substantia nigra and contains dopaminergic neurons that give rise to the mesocorticolimbic dopamine system. These neurons send ascending projections that innervate limbic structures, such as the nucleus accumbens and amygdala, as well as associated cortical structures, particularly the prefrontal cortex. The mesoaccumbens projection is believed to regulate the rewarding properties of a wide variety of stimuli, including drugs of abuse. The mesolimbic projection is believed to be a major target for the antipsychotic properties of dopamine receptor antagonist drugs in their control of the positive symptoms of schizophrenia, such as hallucinations and delusions. Conversely, dopamine receptor antagonism in mesocortical circuits believed to be relatively underactive in schizophrenia may, in fact, worsen the negative symptoms of this disorder. In this regard, the decreased predisposition of the atypical antipsychotic clozapine (Clozaril) to produce extrapyramidal motor side effects has been attributed to relatively selective actions on the mesocorticolimbic system versus the nigrostriatal system. The tuberohypophyseal system consists of dopaminergic neurons in the hypothalamic arcuate and periventricular nuclei and their projections to the pituitary gland. These projections provide inhibitory regulation of prolactin release. The administration of dopamine receptor antagonist antipsychotic drugs may lead to a disinhibition of release, resulting in galactorrhea.

Norepinephrine and Epinephrine The postganglionic sympathetic neurons of the autonomic nervous system release norepinephrine, resulting in widespread peripheral effects, including elevated heart rate and blood pressure. Similar responses are seen with adrenal medullary release of epinephrine. Norepinephrine-producing neurons are found within the brain in the pons and medulla, in two major clusterings: the locus ceruleus (LC) and the lateral tegmental noradrenergic nuclei (Fig. 1.4–3). Noradrenergic projections from both of these regions ramify extensively as they project throughout the neuraxis. In humans, the LC is found in the dorsal portion of the caudal pons and contains approximately 12,000 tightly packed neurons on each side of the brain. These cells provide the major noradrenergic projections to the neocortex, hippocampus, thalamus, and midbrain tectum. The activity of LC neurons varies with the sleep–wake cycle, with fastest firing noted when the animal is most awake. The firing rate is responsive to novel and/or stressful stimuli, with largest responses to stimuli that lead to the disruption of ongoing behavior and reorientation of attention. Altogether, physiological studies indicate a role for this structure in the regulation of arousal state, vigilance, and stress response. The projections from

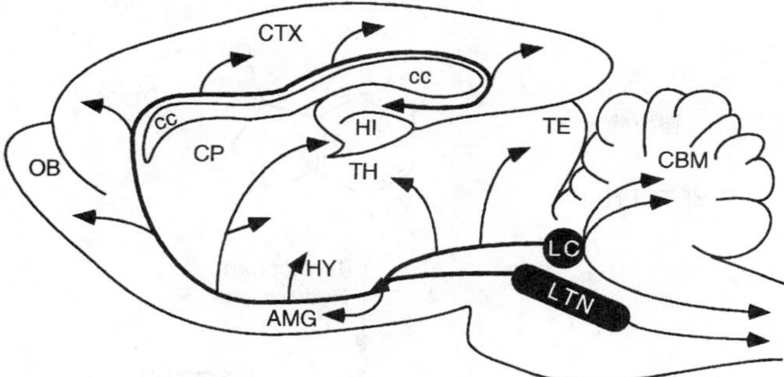

FIGURE 1.4–3 Brain noradrenergic pathways (in rats). Projections of noradrenergic neurons located in the locus ceruleus (LC) and lateral tegmental noradrenergic nuclei (LTN). AMG, amygdala; CBM, cerebellum; cc, corpus callosum; CP, caudate putamen; CTX, neocortex; HI, hippocampus; HY, hypothalamus; OB, olfactory bulb; TE, tectum; TH, thalamus.

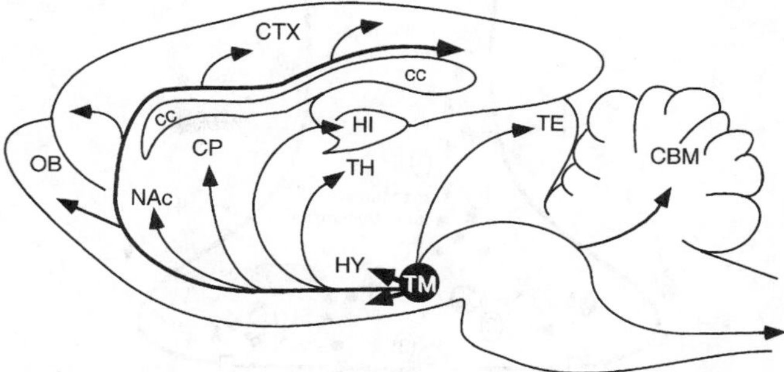

FIGURE 1.4–4 Brain histaminergic pathways (in rats). Histaminergic neurons are located in the tuberomammillary nucleus of the caudal hypothalamus (TM) and project to the hypothalamus (HY) and more distant brain regions. CBM, cerebellum; cc, corpus callosum; CP, caudate putamen; CTX, neocortex; HI, hippocampus; NAc, nucleus accumbens; OB, olfactory bulb; TE, tectum; TH, thalamus.

lateral tegmental nucleus neurons, which are loosely scattered throughout the ventral pons and medulla, partially overlap those of the LC. Fibers from both cell groups innervate the amygdala, septum, and spinal cord. Other regions, such as the hypothalamus and lower brainstem, receive adrenergic inputs predominantly from the lateral tegmental nucleus. The relatively few neurons that use epinephrine as a neurotransmitter are located in the caudal pons and medulla, intermingled with noradrenergic neurons. Projections from these groups ascend to innervate the hypothalamus, LC, and visceral efferent and afferent nuclei of the midbrain.

Histamine Histamine has long been recognized as playing an important role in the allergic response, representing one of the preformed inflammatory mediators stored in mast cells. In contrast, central histaminergic neural pathways have only more recently been characterized, by immunocytochemistry, using antibodies to the synthetic enzyme histidine decarboxylase and to histamine. Histaminergic cell bodies are located within a region of the posterior hypothalamus termed the *tuberomammillary nucleus*. The activity of tuberomammillary neurons is characterized by firing that varies across the sleep–wake cycle, with highest activity during the waking state, slowed firing during slow-wave sleep, and absence of firing during REM sleep. As with other monoaminergic systems, histaminergic fibers project diffusely throughout the brain and spinal cord (Fig. 1.4–4), with considerable variation in regional fiber density among species. Ventral ascending projections course with other monoaminergic fibers in the medial forebrain bundle and provide innervation to the hypothalamus, diagonal band, septum, and olfactory bulb. Dorsal ascending projections innervate the thalamus, hippocampus, amygdala, and rostral forebrain. Descending projections travel through the midbrain central gray to the dorsal hindbrain and spinal cord. The fibers have varicosities that are seldom associated with classic synapses, and histamine has been proposed to act at a distance from its sites of release, like a local hormone. The hypothalamus receives the densest histaminergic innervation, consistent with a role for this transmitter in the regulation of autonomic and neuroendocrine processes. Additionally, strong histaminergic innervation is seen in cholinergic cell and other monoaminergic nuclei.

Acetylcholine Within the brain, the axonal processes of cholinergic neurons may either project to distant brain regions (projection neurons) or contact local cells within the same structure (interneurons). Two large clusters of cholinergic projection neurons are found within the brain: the basal forebrain complex and the mesopontine complex (Fig. 1.4–5). The basal forebrain complex provides the vast majority of the cholinergic innervation to the nonstriatal telencephalon. It consists of cholinergic neurons within the nucleus basalis of Meynert, the horizontal and vertical diagonal bands of Broca, and the medial septal nucleus. These neurons project to widespread areas of the cortex and amygdala, to the anterior cingulate gyrus and olfactory bulb, and to the hippocampus, respectively. In Alzheimer's disease, there is significant degeneration of neurons in the nucleus basalis, leading to substantial reduction in cortical cholinergic innervation. The extent of neuronal loss appears to correlate with the degree of dementia, and the cholinergic deficit is believed to contribute to the cognitive decline characterizing this disease. The mesopontine complex consists of cholinergic neurons within the pedunculopontine and laterodorsal tegmental nuclei of the midbrain and pons and provides cholinergic innervation to the thalamus and midbrain areas (including the dopaminergic neurons of the ventral tegmental area and substantia nigra) and descending innervation to other brainstem regions such as the LC, dorsal raphe, and cranial nerve nuclei. In contrast to central serotonergic, noradrenergic, and histaminergic neurons, cholinergic neurons may continue to fire during REM sleep and have been proposed to play a role in REM sleep induction. Acetylcholine is also found within interneurons of several brain regions, including the striatum. The modulation of stri-

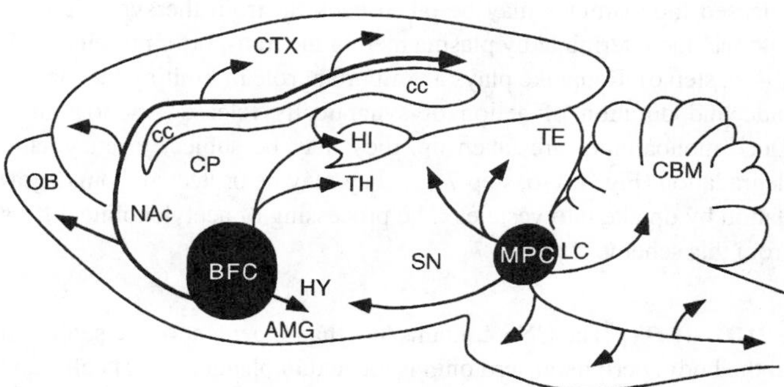

FIGURE 1.4–5 Brain cholinergic projection pathways (in rats). The majority of cholinergic projection neurons are located in the basal forebrain complex (BFC) and the mesopontine complex (MPC). AMG, amygdala; CBM, cerebellum; cc, corpus callosum; CP, caudate putamen; CTX, neocortex; HI, hippocampus; HY, hypothalamus; LC, locus ceruleus; NAc, nucleus accumbens; OB, olfactory bulb; SN, substantia nigra; TE, tectum; TH, thalamus.

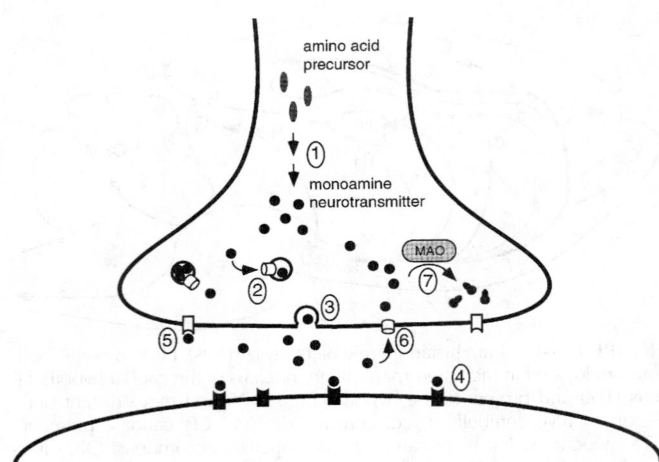

FIGURE 1.4–6 Schematic diagram of monoaminergic synapse. Steps involved in synaptic transmission are described in the text. MAO, monoamine oxidase.

atal cholinergic transmission has been implicated in the antiparkinsonian actions of anticholinergic agents. Within the periphery, acetylcholine is a prominent neurotransmitter, located in motor neurons innervating skeletal muscle, preganglionic autonomic neurons, and postganglionic parasympathetic neurons. Peripheral acetylcholine mediates the characteristic postsynaptic effects of the parasympathetic system, including reduced heart rate and blood pressure and enhanced digestive function.

MONOAMINE SYNTHESIS, STORAGE, AND DEGRADATION

In addition to similarities in neuronal organization, monoaminergic systems are similar with regard to their synthesis, storage, and degradation (Fig. 1.4–6). Monoamines are synthesized within neurons from common amino acid precursors (Fig. 1.4–6, step 1) and taken up into synaptic vesicles via a vesicular monoamine transporter (Fig. 1.4–6, step 2). Upon stimulation, vesicles within nerve terminals release neurotransmitter into the synaptic cleft (Fig. 1.4–6, step 3). Once released, the monoamines interact with postsynaptic receptors to alter the excitability of postsynaptic cells (Fig. 1.4–6, step 4). Monoamines may also interact with presynaptic autoreceptors located on the nerve terminal to suppress further release (Fig. 1.4–6, step 5). In addition, released monoamines may be taken back up from the synaptic cleft into the nerve terminal by plasma membrane transporter proteins (Fig. 1.4–6, step 6). Reuptake plays an important role in limiting the magnitude and duration of action of synaptically released monoamines. Once monoamines are taken up, they may be subject to enzymatic degradation (Fig. 1.4–6, step 7), or they may be protected from degradation by uptake into vesicles. The processing of acetylcholine differs from this scheme.

Serotonin The CNS contains less than 2 percent of the serotonin in the body; peripheral serotonin is located in platelets, mast cells, and enterochromaffin cells of the gastrointestinal system, where serotonin is important for platelet aggregation and modulation of gastrointestinal motility. Despite the abundance of peripheral serotonin, its inability to cross the blood–brain barrier necessitates the synthesis of serotonin within the brain. Serotonin is synthesized from the amino acid tryptophan, which is derived from the diet. The rate-limiting step

TRYPTOPHAN
NH2
CH_2—CH
COOH
N
Tryptophan Hydroxylase
5-HYDROXYTRYPTOPHAN
HO
NH2
CH_2—CH
COOH
N
Amino acid decarboxylase
5-HYDROXYTRYPTAMINE
HO
CH_2—CH_2—NH_2
N
Monoamine Oxidase
Aldehyde Dehydrogenase
5-HYROXYINDOLE-ACETIC ACID
HO
CH_2—COOH
N

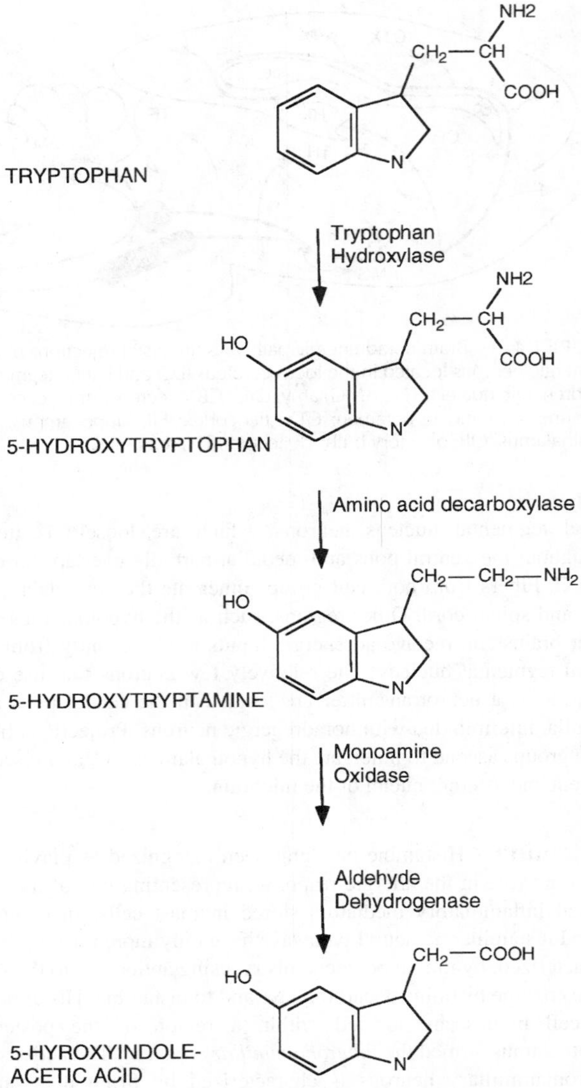

FIGURE 1.4–7 Synthesis and catabolism of serotonin.

in serotonin synthesis is the hydroxylation of tryptophan by the enzyme tryptophan hydroxylase to form 5-hydroxytryptophan (Fig. 1.4–7). A second isoform of the tryptophan hydroxylase enzyme has been identified and shown to be restricted to the CNS; the previously known isoform is found primarily in the periphery. The identification of this second isoform represents an important advance in understanding of the central biosynthesis of serotonin.

Under normal circumstances, tryptophan hydroxylase is not saturated by substrate, so that tryptophan concentration can impact the rate of serotonin synthesis. Therefore, much attention has focused on the factors that determine tryptophan availability. Unlike serotonin, tryptophan is taken up into the brain via a saturable active-carrier mechanism. Because tryptophan competes with other large neutral amino acids for transport, brain uptake of this amino acid is determined both by the amount of circulating tryptophan and by the ratio of tryptophan to other large neutral amino acids. This ratio may be elevated by carbohydrate intake, which induces insulin release and the uptake of many large neutral amino acids into peripheral tissues. Conversely, high-protein foods tend to be relatively low in tryptophan, thus lowering this ratio. Moreover, the administration of specialized low-tryptophan diets has been found to produce significant declines in brain serotonin levels. After tryptophan hydroxylation, 5-hydroxytryptophan is rapidly decarboxylated by aromatic amino acid decarboxylase (an enzyme also involved in dopamine synthesis) to form serotonin.

The first step in the degradation of serotonin is mediated by monoamine oxidase type A (MAO_A), which oxidizes the amino group to form an aldehyde. MAO_A is located in mitochondrial membranes and is nonspecific in its substrate specificity; in addition to serotonin, it oxidizes norepinephrine. The elevation of serotonin levels by MAO inhibitors (MAOIs) is believed to underlie the antidepressant efficacy of these drugs. After oxidation by MAO_A, the resulting aldehyde is further oxidized to 5-hydroxyindoleacetic acid (5-HIAA). Levels of 5-HIAA are often measured as a correlate of serotonergic activity, although the relationship of these levels to serotonergic neuronal activity remains unclear.

Catecholamines

The catecholamines are synthesized from the amino acid tyrosine, which is taken up into the brain via an active transport mechanism (Fig. 1.4–8). Within catecholaminergic neurons, tyrosine hydroxylase catalyzes the addition of a hydroxyl group to the meta position of tyrosine, yielding L-dopa. This rate-limiting step in catecholamine synthesis is subject to inhibition by high levels of catecholamines (end-product inhibition). Because tyrosine hydroxylase is normally saturated with substrate, manipulation of tyrosine levels does not readily impact the rate of catecholamine synthesis. Once formed, L-dopa is rapidly converted to dopamine by dopa decarboxylase, which is located in the cytoplasm. It is now recognized that this enzyme acts not only on L-dopa, but on all naturally occurring aromatic L-amino acids, including tryptophan. Thus, this enzyme is more accurately termed *aromatic amino acid decarboxylase*. In noradrenergic and adrenergic neurons, dopamine is actively transported into storage vesicles, where it is oxidized by dopamine β-hydroxylase to form norepinephrine. This promiscuous enzyme will oxidize most phenylethylamines, producing metabolites that may replace norepinephrine at nerve terminals. These metabolites may act as false neurotransmitters, producing minimal postsynaptic effects themselves, and their accumulation may impair adrenergic synaptic transmission through diminution of norepinephrine content. In adrenergic neurons and the adrenal medulla, norepinephrine is converted to epinephrine by phenylethanolamine *N*-methyltransferase (PNMT), which is located within the cytoplasmic compartment.

Two enzymes that play major roles in the degradation of catecholamines are MAO and catechol-*O*-methyltransferase (COMT). MAO is located on the outer membrane of mitochondria, including those within the terminals of adrenergic fibers, and oxidatively deaminates catecholamines to their corresponding aldehydes. Two MAO isozymes with differing substrate specificities have been identified: MAO_A, which preferentially deaminates serotonin and norepinephrine, and MAO_B, which deaminates dopamine, histamine, and a broad spectrum of phenylethylamines. Neurons contain both isoforms. The blockade of monoamine catabolism by MAOIs produces elevations in brain monoamine levels. Monoamine oxidase is also found in peripheral tissues such as the gastrointestinal tract and liver, where it prevents the accumulation of toxic amines. For example, peripheral MAO degrades dietary tyramine, an amine that can displace norepinephrine from sympathetic postganglionic nerve endings, producing hypertension if tyramine is present in large enough quantities. Thus, patients treated with MAOIs are cautioned to avoid pickled and fermented foods, which typically have high levels of this amine. COMT is located in the cytoplasm and is widely distributed throughout the brain and peripheral tissues, although little to none is found in adrenergic neurons. It has a wide substrate specificity, catalyzing the transfer of methyl groups from *S*-adenosyl methionine to the *m*-hydroxyl group of most catechol compounds. The catecholamine metabolites produced by these and other enzymes are frequently measured as indicators of the activity of catecholaminergic systems. In humans, the predominant metabolites of dopamine and norepinephrine are homovanillic acid (HVA) and 3-methoxy-4-hydroxyphenylglycol (MHPG), respectively.

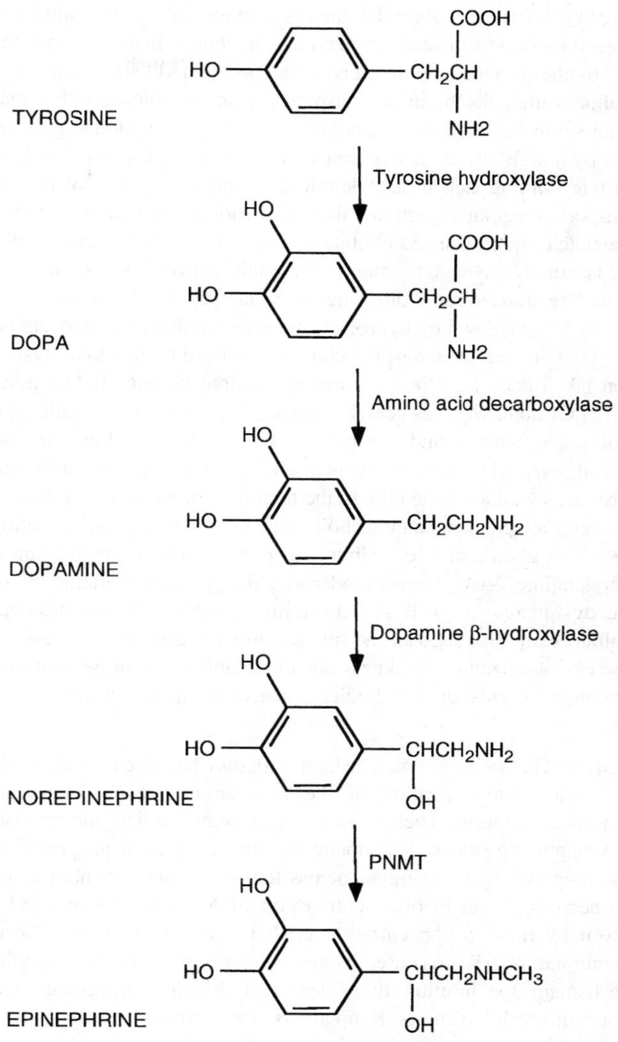

FIGURE 1.4–8 Synthesis of catecholamines.

Histamine

As is the case for serotonin, the brain contains only a small portion of the histamine found in the body. Histamine is distributed throughout most tissues of the body, predominantly in mast cells. Because it does not readily cross the blood–brain barrier, it is believed that histamine is synthesized within the brain. In the brain, histamine is formed by the decarboxylation of the amino acid histidine by a specific L-histidine decarboxylase. As this enzyme is not normally saturated with substrate, histamine synthesis is sensitive to histidine levels. This is consistent with the observation that the peripheral administration of histidine elevates brain histamine levels. Histamine is metabolized in the brain by histamine-*N*-methyltransferase, producing methylhistamine. In turn, methylhistamine undergoes oxidative deamination by MAO_B.

Acetylcholine Acetylcholine is synthesized by the transfer of an acetyl group from acetyl coenzyme A to choline in a reaction mediated by the enzyme choline acetyltransferase (ChAT). The majority of choline within the brain is transported from the blood, rather than being synthesized de novo. Choline is taken up into cholinergic neurons by a high-affinity active transport mechanism, and this uptake is the rate-limiting step in acetylcholine synthesis. The rate of choline transport is regulated such that increased cholinergic neural activity is associated with enhanced choline uptake. After synthesis, acetylcholine is stored in synaptic vesicles through the action of a vesicular acetylcholine transporter. Following vesicular release, acetylcholine is rapidly broken down by hydrolysis, by acetylcholinesterase located in the synaptic cleft. Much of the choline produced by this hydrolysis is then taken back into the presynaptic terminal via the choline transporter. Of note, whereas acetylcholinesterase is primarily localized to cholinergic neurons and synapses, a second class of cholinesterase, termed *butyrylcholinesterase*, is found primarily in the liver and plasma, as well as in the glia. In the treatment of Alzheimer's disease, strategies aimed at enhancing cholinergic function—primarily through the use of cholinesterase inhibitors to prevent normal degradation of acetylcholine—have shown moderate efficacy in ameliorating cognitive dysfunction as well as behavioral disturbances. Cholinesterase inhibitors are also used in the treatment of myasthenia gravis, a disease characterized by weakness due to variable block of neuromuscular transmission by autoantibodies to acetylcholine receptors.

Transporters A great deal of progress has been made in the molecular characterization of the monoamine plasma membrane transporter proteins. These membrane proteins mediate the reuptake of synaptically released monoamines into the presynaptic terminal. The reuptake of monoamines across the presynaptic membrane into the nerve terminal involves cotransport of Na^+ and Cl^- ions and is driven by the ion concentration gradient generated by the plasma membrane Na^+/K^+ ATPase. Monoamine reuptake is an important mechanism for limiting the extent and duration of activation of monoaminergic receptors. Reuptake is also a primary mechanism for replenishing terminal monoamine neurotransmitter stores. Moreover, transporters serve as molecular targets for a number of antidepressant drugs, psychostimulants, and monoaminergic neurotoxins. Whereas transporter molecules for serotonin (SERT), dopamine (DAT), and norepinephrine (NET) have been well characterized, transporters selective for histamine and epinephrine have not been demonstrated.

The molecular cloning of SERT, DAT, and NET has confirmed that all belong to a common gene family of transporter molecules that also includes those for γ-aminobutyric acid (GABA), glycine, and choline. These proteins share strong sequence homologies and are believed to be integral membrane proteins that span the plasma membrane twelve times. In contrast to monoaminergic receptors, there is evidence for only a single type of transporter molecule for serotonin, dopamine, and norepinephrine. The expression of these proteins is localized to the perisynaptic plasma membrane and appears to be restricted to the corresponding class of monoaminergic neurons. For example, the messenger ribonucleic acid (mRNA) encoding the SERT is restricted to serotonergic neurons, the one encoding the DAT is restricted to dopaminergic neurons, and the one encoding the NET is restricted to noradrenergic neurons. However, there is evidence that the norepinephrine transporter may be able to transport dopamine as well as norepinephrine.

Monoaminergic transporters are molecular targets for both psychotherapeutic drugs as well as substances of abuse. The therapeutic effects of tricyclic antidepressants such as amitriptyline and imipramine have been associated with their blockade of the SERT and the NET, although these drugs also interact directly with several monoaminergic receptor subtypes. More selective blockers of the SERT, such as the selective serotonin reuptake inhibitors (SSRIs) (e.g., citalopram [Celexa], fluoxetine [Prozac], fluvoxamine [Luvox], paroxetine [Paxil], and sertraline [Zoloft]), are used in the treatment of depression, anxiety, and a variety of other disorders. Conversely, compounds with relative selectivity for the NET, such as nortriptyline (Pamelor) and desipramine (Norpramin), also have antidepressant efficacy. There is current interest in polymorphic variants of the monoamine transporters as candidate genes involved in various psychiatric illnesses; a recent analysis suggests a positive association between a specific promoter polymorphism of the serotonin transporter gene and suicidal behavior.

Among drugs of abuse, cocaine binds with high affinity to all three known monoamine transporters, although the stimulant properties of the drug have been attributed primarily to its blockade of the DAT. This view has been recently supported by the absence of cocaine-induced locomotor stimulation in a strain of mutant mice engineered to lack the this molecule. In fact, psychostimulants produce a paradoxical locomotor suppression in these animals that has been attributed to the SERT-blocking properties of these compounds. The rewarding properties of cocaine have also been attributed to dopamine-transporter inhibition, although the situation is actually more complex, as demonstrated by persistence of some rewarding effect of this drug in mice lacking the dopamine transporter. It appears that serotonergic as well as dopaminergic mechanisms may be involved. Transporters may also provide routes that allow neurotoxins to enter and damage monoaminergic neurons; examples include the dopaminergic neurotoxin 1-methyl-4-phenyl-1,2,3,6-tetrahydropyridine (MPTP) and the serotonergic neurotoxin MDMA.

Vesicular Monoamine Transporter In addition to the reuptake of monoamines into the presynaptic nerve terminal, a second transport process serves to concentrate and store monoamines within synaptic vesicles. The transport and storage of monoamines in vesicles may serve several purposes: (1) to enable the regulated release of transmitter under appropriate physiological stimulation, (2) to protect monoamines from degradation by MAO, and (3) to protect neurons from the toxic effects of free radicals produced by the oxidation of cytoplasmic monoamines. In contrast with the plasma membrane transporters, a single type of vesicular monoamine transporter is believed to mediate the uptake of monoamines into synaptic vesicles within the brain. Consistent with this, blockade of this vesicular monoamine transporter by the antihypertensive drug reserpine (Serpasil) has been found to deplete brain levels of serotonin, norepinephrine, and dopamine. The molecular cloning of this transporter, termed *VMAT2*, has revealed it to have twelve putative membrane-spanning domains. A second homologous transporter called *VMAT1* is found only in endocrine cells. This class of transporter does not display sequence homology to the plasma membrane transporters. Moreover, it uses a H^+ gradient rather than Na^+/Cl^- gradients. Vesicular transport requires a H^+ pumping ATPase, which establishes a concentration gradient of H^+ across the vesicle membrane. In the presence of this gradient, the vesicular monoamine transporter takes up neurotransmitter in a manner that is coupled to the release of luminal protons. The activity of the transporter is altered by amphetamine-like agents. These compounds are taken up via plasma membrane transporters into monoaminergic terminals, where they act as weak bases to disrupt pH gradients. This produces a reversal of vesicular monoamine transporter activity, leading to monoamine release from vesicles and reversal of plasma membrane transporter activity. The resulting release of monoamines from presynaptic terminals contributes to the stimulant properties of these compounds. The anorectic agent fenfluramine is believed to stimulate serotonin release in an analogous manner. A separate vesicular transporter for acetylcholine (VAchT) has been molecularly cloned; its structure is homologous to that of the vesicular monoamine transmitter, and both are believed to have a common bioenergetic mechanism.

RECEPTORS

Ultimately, the effects of monoamines on CNS function and behavior depend on their interactions with receptor molecules. The binding of monoamines to these plasma membrane proteins initiates a series of intracellular events that modulate neuronal excitability. Unlike the transporters, multiple receptor subtypes exist for each monoamine transmitter (Table 1.4–1). The initial classification of many receptor subtypes was based on radioligand binding studies. Receptor binding sites were identified on the basis of the rank order of binding affinities for a number of agonist and antagonist compounds. More recently, the molecular cloning of monoamine receptors has confirmed that many of the sites initially defined by these binding studies did indeed correspond to distinct receptor proteins encoded by unique genes. In addition, molecular cloning has led to the identification of previously unknown receptors and to the introduction of powerful tools to characterize receptor structure and function.

Neurotransmitter receptors produce intracellular effects by one of two basic mechanisms: (1) via interactions with G proteins that couple receptors to intracellular effector systems and (2) by providing channels through which ions flow when transmitters bind (ligand-gated ion channels). With the exception of the serotonin type 3 (5-HT_3) receptor subtype (a ligand-gated ion channel), all known

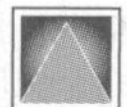

Table 1.4–1
Monoamine Receptors: Overview

Transmitter	Subtype	Primary Effector	Proposed Clinical Relevance
Serotonin	5-HT_{1A}	↓ AC	Antidepressant action; partial agonist; anxiolytic
	5-HT_{1B}	↓ AC	Possible role in locomotor activity, aggression
	5-HT_{1D}	↓ AC	Target of antimigraine drug sumatriptan
	5-HT_{1E}	↓ AC	Unknown
	5-HT_{1F}	↓ AC	Target of antimigraine drug sumatriptan
	5-HT_{2A}	↑ PI turnover	Target of hallucinogens, atypical antipsychotics
	5-HT_{2B}	↑ PI turnover	Regulation of stomach contraction
	5-HT_{2C}	↑ PI turnover	Regulation of appetite, anxiety, seizures; target of hallucinogens, antipsychotics
	5-HT_3	Cation selective Ion channel	Antagonists antiemetic, anxiolytic, cognitive enhancement
	5-HT_4	↑ AC	Modulation of cognition, anxiety
	5-$HT_{5\alpha}$	Unknown	Unknown
	5-$HT_{5\beta}$	Unknown	Unknown
	5-HT_6	↑ AC	Target of hallucinogens, atypical antipsychotics
	5-HT_7	↑ AC	Possible regulation of circadian rhythms
Histamine	H_1	↑ PI turnover	Antagonists produce sedation, weight gain
	H_2	↑ AC	Antagonists for peptic ulcer disease
	H_3	Unknown	Antagonists produce arousal, appetite suppression
	H_4	Unknown	Unknown
Dopamine	D_1	↑ AC	D_1 and D_2 receptor stimulation synergistic; required for stimulant effects of cocaine
	D_2	↓ AC	Target of therapeutic and extrapyramidal effects of dopamine receptor antagonists ("typical antipsychotics")
	D_3	↓ AC	Unknown
	D_4	↓ AC	Target of serotonin-dopamine antagonists ("atypical antipsychotics")
	D_5	↑ AC	Unknown
Adrenergic	$\alpha_{1A,B,D}$	↑ PI turnover	Antagonists antihypertensive
	$\alpha_{2A,B,C}$	↓ AC	Agonists sedative and antihypertensive
	β_1	↑ AC	Regulation of cardiac function
	β_2	↑ AC	Regulation of bronchial muscle contraction
	β_3	↑ AC	Regulation of adipose tissue function
Cholinergic	M1	↑ PI turnover	Regulation of cognition, seizures
	M2	↓ AC	Regulation of cardiac function
	M3	↑ PI turnover	Regulation of smooth muscle contraction
	M4	↓ AC	Target of antiparkinsonian anticholinergic drugs
	M5	↑ PI turnover	Unknown
	NAChR	Cation selective Ion channel	Regulation of tobacco use, seizures; possible cognitive enhancement

↑ AC, increases activity of adenylate cyclase; ↓ AC, decreases activity of adenylate cyclase; ↑ PI turnover, increases turnover of phosphoinositides.

monoaminergic receptors belong to the superfamily of G-protein–coupled receptors. However, within each monoaminergic receptor family, the subtypes are heterogeneous with regard to the G proteins with which they interact and to the second messenger effects that they produce. Monoaminergic receptors are also diverse in their regional patterns of expression within the brain, their neurotransmitter binding affinities, and their synaptic localization. Whereas many receptor subtypes are located exclusively in postsynaptic membranes, others are located presynaptically, in axon terminal membranes. Some receptors on the presynaptic terminal respond to monoamines that are released by that neuron. These presynaptic autoreceptors often act to inhibit neurotransmitter release. A number of monoaminergic receptor subtypes are located presynaptically in some brain regions and postsynaptically in others.

In the wake of the recent proliferation of known receptor subtypes, much work remains to determine the functional roles of individual receptors. In many instances, a paucity of selective agonist and antagonist drugs complicates this effort. Recently, a molecular genetic approach to examining receptor function has been applied to complement pharmacological studies. Gene-targeting procedures have enabled the generation of mouse strains with disruptions in genes that encode individual receptor subtypes. The resulting mutant mice have a complete and specific absence of the targeted receptor. Studies in these animals are providing clues to receptor function and to the contributions of the targeted receptors to the actions of nonspecific drugs. Molecular and pharmacological approaches will guide the generation of subtype-selective compounds and facilitate the development of therapeutic agents that will alter monoaminergic transmission in a more refined manner.

Serotonin Receptors Brain serotonin receptors were initially characterized on the basis of radioligand binding studies into two classes: 5-HT_1 receptors, to which [^{3}H]5-HT bound with high affinity and 5-HT_2 receptors, which were labeled with high affinity by [^{3}H]spiperone. Subsequent binding studies revealed that these classes each consisted of multiple subtypes. The application of molecular cloning techniques has produced a proliferation in the number of known subtypes. The great diversity of serotonin receptors provides a means whereby a single neurotransmitter may produce a wide variety of cellular effects in multiple neuronal systems. At present, at least 14 distinct serotonin receptor subtypes have been identified and molecularly cloned, which has led to rapid advances in determining the structure, pharmacology, brain distribution, and effector mechanisms of these receptors. This information has led to a more precise classification of serotonin receptor subfamilies on the basis of their structural homologies and primary effector mechanisms.

The 5-HT_1 receptors compose the largest serotonin receptor subfamily, with human subtypes designated: 5-HT_{1A}, 5-HT_{1B}, 5-HT_{1D}, 5-HT_{1E}, and 5-HT_{1F}. All five 5-HT_1 receptor subtypes display intronless gene structures, high affinities for serotonin, and adenylate cyclase inhibition. The most intensively studied of these has been the 5-HT_{1A} receptor. This subtype is found on both postsynaptic membranes of forebrain neurons primarily in the hippocampus, cortex, and septum and on serotonergic neurons, where it functions as a somatodendritic autoreceptor. The stimulation of these autoreceptors suppresses the activity of serotonergic neurons. There is significant interest in the 5-HT_{1A} receptor as a modulator of both anxiety and depression. The downregulation of 5-HT_{1A} autoreceptors by the chronic administration of serotonin reuptake blockers has been implicated in their antidepressant effects. In addition, partial 5-HT_{1A} receptor agonists such as buspirone (Buspar) display both anxiolytic and antidepressant properties. The 5-HT_{1B} and 5-HT_{1D} receptors resemble each other in structure and brain localization, although the 5-HT_{1D} receptor is expressed at lower levels. 5-$HT_{1B/D}$ receptors are found on axon terminals of serotonergic and nonserotonergic neurons, where they act to reduce neurotransmitter release. The differentiation of these receptors from each other has been hindered by a lack of selective pharmacological tools. However, the 5-HT_{1B} receptor has been implicated in modulation of locomotor activity levels, consistent with its high level of expression in basal ganglia. It has also been suggested as a modulator of aggression, although 5-HT_{1B} receptor agonist drugs have shown limited clinical efficacy as antiaggressive agents. The functional roles of the 5-HT_{1E} and 5-HT_{1F} receptor subtypes are less well characterized. The highest levels of 5-HT_{1E} receptor expression are found in the striatum and entorhinal cortex, whereas 5-HT_{1F} receptor expression is highest in the dorsal raphe nucleus, hippocampus, cortex, and striatum. In addition, the 5-HT_{1B} and the 5-HT_{1D} and 5-HT_{1F} receptors are found in the cerebral vasculature and the trigeminal ganglion, respectively, and are stimulated by the antimigraine drug sumatriptan (Imitrex). These receptors may therefore be involved in the therapeutic efficacy of this drug, possibly mediating vasoconstriction and inhibition of nociceptive transmission.

At least three receptors mediate the effects previously attributed to a single 5-HT_2 receptor subtype. The classic 5-HT_2 receptor has thus been renamed *5-HT_{2A}* to indicate that it is a member of a serotonin receptor subfamily. A second receptor, initially termed *5-HT_{1C}*, has been renamed *5-HT_{2C}* to indicate its membership within this subfamily. The third known 5HT_2 receptor, termed *5-HT_{2B}*, contributes to the contractile effects of serotonin in the stomach fundus and has limited distribution in the brain. Stimulation of the 5-HT_{2B} receptor appears to underlie the cardiac valve effects of the serotonergic appetite suppressant dexfenfluramine, leading to the discontinuation of its use. All three subtypes exhibit high sequence homology, similar pharmacological binding profiles, and stimulation of phosphoinositide turnover. High levels of 5-HT_{2A} receptors are found in the neocortex and in peripheral locations such as platelets and smooth muscle. Much recent attention has focused on the contributions of 5-$HT_{2A/C}$ receptors to the actions of atypical antipsychotic drugs such as clozapine, risperidone (Risperdal), and olanzapine (Zyprexa). Analysis of the receptor-binding properties of these drugs has led to the hypothesis that 5-HT_{2A} receptor blockade correlates with the therapeutic effectiveness of atypical antipsychotics. Interestingly, the 5-HT_{2A} receptor has also been implicated in the cognitive process of working memory, a function believed to be impaired in schizophrenia. The 5-HT_{2C} receptor is expressed at high levels in many CNS regions, including the hippocampal formation, prefrontal cortex, amygdala, striatum, hypothalamus, and choroid plexus. Stimulation of 5-HT_{2C} receptors has been proposed to produce anxiogenic and anorectic effects. Accordingly, a transgenic mouse strain lacking this receptor subtype exhibits an obesity syndrome associated with overeating. These animals also display an enhanced susceptibility to seizures, implicating this receptor in the regulation of neuronal network excitability. A variety of antidepressant and antipsychotic drugs antagonize 5-HT_{2C} receptors with high affinity. Conversely, hallucinogens such as lysergic acid diethylamide (LSD) display agonist activity at 5-HT_2 (and other) serotonin receptor subtypes. It has recently been reported that the 5-HT_{2C} receptor transcripts undergo RNA editing, producing isoforms of the receptor with altered activity, thereby further expanding the diversity of serotonergic signaling. Postmortem levels of specific 5-HT_{2C} receptor edited transcripts have been found to be elevated in brains of suicide victims with a history of major depression. Work in animals suggests treatment with SSRIs might lower the levels of these same isoforms.

The 5-HT_3 receptor is unique among monoaminergic receptors in its membership within the ligand-gated ion channel superfamily. Rather than activating G proteins, the binding of serotonin to this receptor permits passage of Na^+ and K^+ ions through an ion channel located within the 5-HT_3 receptor complex. This produces rapid excitatory effects in postsynaptic neurons. The 5-HT_3 receptor is expressed within the hippocampus, neocortex, amygdala, hypothalamus, and brainstem, including the area postrema. Peripherally, it is found in the pituitary gland and enteric nervous system. 5-HT_3 receptor antagonists such as ondansetron (Zofran) are used as antiemetic agents and are under evaluation as potential antianxiety and cognitive-enhancing agents. The functional 5-HT_3 receptor appears to comprise at least two distinct subunits, termed *5-HT_{3A}* and *5-HT_{3B}*.

Investigations into the functions of the recently identified 5-HT_4, 5-HT_{5A}, 5-HT_{5B}, 5-HT_6, and 5-HT_7 receptor subtypes are hindered by a lack of selective agonist and antagonists. Studies of the cloned receptors reveal that all but the 5-HT_5 are linked to the stimulation of adenylate cyclase. The primary effector mechanisms of the 5-HT_5 receptors remain to be determined. The 5-HT_4 receptors are expressed in the hippocampus, striatum, substantia nigra, and superior colliculus, and multiple alternatively spliced isoforms have been identified. The 5-HT_4 receptors have been shown to modulate release of neurotransmitters—including acetylcholine, serotonin, and dopamine—and have been implicated in the serotonergic regulation of cognition and anxiety. In the periphery, these receptors are expressed in the cardiac atria and the gut. The 5-HT_4 agonist cisapride (Propulsid) is in clinical use as a gastroprokinetic agent. The two 5-HT_5 receptor subtypes are highly homologous and are expressed in the neocortex, hippocampus, raphe nuclei, and cerebellum. Their neural functions remain unclear, and some reports have indicated they may be predominantly expressed in astrocytes. 5-HT_6 receptors may contribute to the actions of the several antidepressant, antipsychotic, and hallucinogenic drugs that bind with high affinity. These receptors are expressed in the neocortex, hippocampus, striatum, and amygdala. Highest levels of 5-HT_7 receptor expression are found in the hypothalamus and thalamus. These receptors have been proposed to contribute to the serotonergic modulation of circadian rhythms. Although it is premature to assign functional roles to these new receptor subtypes with confidence, it is likely that these receptors will ultimately provide targets for the development of useful therapeutic compounds.

Dopamine Receptors In 1979, it was clearly recognized that the actions of dopamine are mediated by more than one receptor subtype. Two dopamine receptors, termed *D_1* and *D_2*, were distinguished on the basis of differential binding affinities of a series of agonists and antagonists, distinct effector mechanisms, and distinct distribution patterns within the CNS. It was subsequently found that the therapeutic efficacy of antipsychotic drugs correlated strongly with their affinities for the D_2 receptor, implicating this subtype as an important site of antipsychotic drug action. Until recently, these were the only two identified dopamine receptors; however, molecular cloning studies have revealed additional receptor heterogeneity. Three additional dopamine receptor genes have been identified, encoding the D_3, D_4, and D_5 dopamine receptors. Based on their structure, pharmacology, and primary effector mechanisms, the D_3 and D_4 receptors are considered to be "D_2-like," and the D_5 receptor, "D_1-like." The functional roles of the recently discovered subtypes remain to be determined, although several intriguing possibilities are under investigation.

The D_1 receptor was initially distinguished from the D_2 subtype by its high affinity for the antagonist SCH 23390 and relatively low affinity for butyrophenones such as haloperidol (Haldol). Whereas D_1 receptor activation stimulates cyclic adenosine monophosphate (cAMP) formation, D_2 receptor stimulation produces the opposite effect on cAMP formation. In addition to the stimulation of adenylate cyclase, D_1 receptors may also stimulate phosphoinositide turnover and modulate intracellular calcium levels. The D_1 receptor is the most widespread dopamine receptor, and D_1 receptor mRNA is expressed in the terminal fields of the nigrostriatal and mesocorticolimbic pathways, with high levels in the dorsal striatum, nucleus accumbens, and amygdala. In contrast, little D_1 mRNA expression is found in dopamine cell body regions such as the substantia nigra pars compacta and the ventral tegmental area. This finding—and the persistence of D_1 receptor binding after lesions of dopaminergic neurons—suggest that this receptor subtype is not found on dopaminergic neurons and is therefore not an autoreceptor. Dopamine has long been known to have prominent motor effects, well illustrated by the locomotor hyperactivity shown by mice made persistently hyperdopaminergic through lack of the dopamine transporter. Locomotor stimulation appears to involve activation of both D_1 and D_2 receptors. Electrophysiological studies have also indicated that D_1 receptor activation is required for striatal D_2 receptor activation to produce its maximal effect. The proposed synergistic effects of striatal D_1 and D_2 receptor activation have recently received further support from studies in a mouse strain with a targeted elimination of D_1 receptors. The effects of both D_1 and D_2 receptor activation were attenuated in these animals. Moreover, these mice were resistant to the hyperlocomotor effects of cocaine, indicating that D_1 receptors contribute significantly to the CNS effects of cocaine. These animals, however, retain sensitivity to the rewarding properties of cocaine, suggesting involvement of other receptors, perhaps the D_2, in mediating rewarding effects of drugs of abuse. D_1 receptors have also been implicated in cognitive functions of dopamine, such as control of working memory and attention.

The D_5 receptor was molecularly cloned on the basis of its sequence homology with the D_1 receptor. The two receptors have a higher degree of homology with each other than with the $D_{2–4}$ subtypes. This structural similarity is reflected in the similar affinities of a wide variety of dopaminergic drugs for these two receptors. The main distinguishing feature of their binding profiles is that the binding affinity of dopamine is higher for D_5 than for D_1 receptors. Not surprisingly, these two receptors are also similar in that they both stimulate adenylate cyclase activity. However, the D_5 receptor appears to exhibit an increased agonist-independent or constitutive activity when compared with the D_1 receptor, at least in vitro. These receptors also differ with regard to their regional distributions within the CNS. The expression of D_5 receptors appears to be more restricted than that of the D_1 receptor and is found in the hippocampus, hypothalamus, prefrontal cortex, and striatum. A role for the D_5 receptor in inhibition of locomotor activity has recently been suggested.

The dopamine D_2 receptor was initially distinguished from the D_1 on the basis of its high affinity for butyrophenones. Moreover D_2 receptor stimulation was observed to inhibit, rather than stimulate, adenylate cyclase activity. Subsequently, the D_2 receptor subtype was found to display interactions with a variety of G proteins, leading to diverse second messenger effects such as modulation of Ca^{2+} and K^+ channel function and the alteration of phosphoinositide production. The intracellular consequences of D_2 receptor activation appear to depend on the cell type in which the receptor is expressed. In addition to D_2 receptor mRNA expression in brain regions that receive dopaminergic innervation—particularly in the dorsal striatum and nucleus accumbens—D_2 transcripts are found in dopaminergic neurons of the ventral tegmental area and substantia nigra.

Unlike D_1-like receptors, the D_2 receptor may have either a postsynaptic function or an autoreceptor function. D_2 autoreceptors may be found on dopaminergic terminals or on the cell bodies and dendrites of dopaminergic neurons, where they mediate inhibition of evoked dopamine release and inhibition of firing of dopaminergic neurons, respectively. D_2 receptors are also expressed in the anterior pituitary and mediate the dopaminergic inhibition of prolactin and α-MSH release. Molecular cloning has revealed long and short form of the D_2 receptor that differs in length by 29 amino acids, products of alternative splicing of a single gene. Recent work with mice lacking the long form of the D_2 receptor suggests that D_2 autoreceptor functions are mediated by the short form of this receptor. Catalepsy induced by neuroleptics such as haloperidol appears to be largely mediated by the long form of the D_2 receptor.

A great deal of attention has focused on the clinical correlates of D_2 receptor function. Postmortem analyses of schizophrenic brains have revealed elevations in D_2 receptor density. Furthermore, radioligand binding studies have revealed a correlation between the clinical efficacy of antipsychotic drugs and their antagonist affinities for this receptor subtype. This finding has contributed significantly to the "dopamine hypothesis" of schizophrenia. The extrapyramidal side effects of antipsychotic drugs have been attributed to the blockade of striatal D_2 receptors. A significant contribution of D_2 receptors to the dopaminergic regulation of motor function is further highlighted by a parkinsonian movement disorder observed in a mutant mouse strain that lacks this receptor subtype.

The recently identified D_3 and D_4 receptors are considered to be D_2-like on the basis of similarities in their gene structures, sequence homologies, and pharmacology. These receptors are expressed in lower abundance than the D_2 receptor, and their regional distributions are distinct. Whereas D_3 receptor expression is highest in the limbic system nucleus accumbens, highest levels of D_4 receptors are expressed in the frontal cortex, midbrain, amygdala, hippocampus, and medulla. Whereas little D_3 receptor expression has been detected outside the nervous system, D_4 receptors are abundant in the heart and kidney. In recent studies, both the D_3 and D_4 receptors have been shown to inhibit adenylate cyclase activity and therefore cAMP accumulation, as shown previously for D_2 receptors. The extent of action through other intracellular signaling pathways remains to be clarified. The D_3 receptor may play a role in control of locomotion. Recent studies of mice lacking the D_4 receptor have suggested a role in expression of novelty-seeking behavior. Particular attention has also been paid to the D_4 receptor in schizophrenia. As for the D_2 receptor, elevated D_4 receptor levels have been found in postmortem schizophrenic brains. Moreover, the atypical antipsychotic drug clozapine has a high affinity for the D_4 receptor. The D_4 receptor is highly polymorphic in humans, and at least 25 distinct alleles have been identified. Studies were therefore pursued to determine whether particular D_4 alleles are associated with psychotic disorders or with responsiveness to antipsychotic drugs. However, none of the alleles of the D_4 receptor has been found to be associated with an increased risk of schizophrenia, and recent clinical studies have not demonstrated antipsychotic efficacy for a putative D_4-selective antagonist in schizophrenic patients.

Adrenergic Receptors Adrenergic receptor heterogeneity was first appreciated in the 1940s, when α and β subtypes were identified in pharmacological studies of isolated peripheral tissues. Subsequently, radioligand binding and molecular cloning studies have identified three main adrenergic receptor subfamilies: α_1, α_2, and β. Each subfamily consists of at least three distinct receptor subtypes. Receptors within each subfamily share similar sequence homologies, pharmacological binding profiles, and effector mechanisms. A significant amount of information is known about the details of adrenergic receptor function in the peripheral nervous system, whereas their roles are less well understood within the brain. The activation of α_1 receptors (subtypes designated α_{1A}, α_{1B}, and α_{1D}) stimulates phosphoinositide turnover and an increase in intracellular Ca^{2+}. These receptors are believed to play a significant role in regulating smooth muscle contraction and have been implicated in the control of blood pressure, nasal congestion, and prostate function. All three subtypes are expressed in the brain—in areas including the cerebral cortex, hippocampus, septum, amygdala, and thalamus—but their contributions to the central actions of norepinephrine remain to be determined, although some studies point to a role in facilitation of locomotor responses and arousal.

As for the α_1 receptors, the functions of α_2 receptor subtypes (designated α_{2A}, α_{2B}, and α_{2C}) have been difficult to determine due to a lack of selective agonists and antagonists; α_2 receptors display both presynaptic autoreceptor and postsynaptic actions—and all appear to inhibit cAMP formation, as well as activate potassium channels with resultant membrane hyperpolarization. These receptors regulate neurotransmitter release from peripheral sympathetic nerve endings. Within the brain, the stimulation of α_2 autoreceptors (likely the α_{2A} subtype) inhibits firing of the noradrenergic neurons of the LC, which have been implicated in arousal states. This mechanism has been proposed to underlie the sedative effects of the α_2 receptor agonist clonidine (Catapres). In addition, the stimulation of brainstem α_2 receptors has been proposed to reduce sympathetic and to augment parasympathetic nervous system activity. This action may relate to the utility of clonidine in lowering blood pressure and in suppressing the sympathetic hyperactivity associated with opiate withdrawal. Activation of α_2 receptors appears to inhibit the activity of serotonin neurons of the dorsal raphe nucleus, whereas activation of local α_1 receptors appears to stimulate the activity of these neurons. This may represent an important mechanism for crosstalk between the serotonergic and noradrenergic systems.

Like the α-adrenergic receptors described above, the β-adrenergic receptors (subtypes designated β_1, β_2, and β_3) are found both in the brain and in many peripheral tissues. All of the β-adrenergic receptors stimulate adenylate cyclase activity and, thus, cAMP accumulation through G_s. The functional roles of the peripheral β-adrenergic receptors are better understood than are its central functions. Cardiac β_1 receptors play a major role in the regulation of heart function, increasing heart rate and contractility, and β_2 receptors mediate bronchial muscle relaxation. β_3 receptors are found in adipose tissue, where they stimulate fat catabolism. Although β_1 and β_2 receptors are widely distributed in the CNS, their contributions to catecholamine function are not well understood. They have been suggested to play a role in consolidation of memory through actions within the amygdala. Propranolol (Inderal) is a widely used nonspecific antagonist of both β_1 and β_2 receptors. In addition to its utility for the treatment of hypertension and arrhythmias, its effectiveness in blunting autonomic symptoms underlies its utility in the management of social phobia. Moreover, through mechanisms that are currently unknown, it is also effective in the treatment of akathisia.

Histamine Receptors Histaminergic systems have been proposed to modulate arousal, wakefulness, feeding behavior, and neuroendocrine responsiveness. Four histaminergic receptor subtypes have been identified and termed H_1, H_2, H_3, and H_4. The H_4 receptor was identified recently and is detected predominantly in the periphery, in regions such as the spleen, bone marrow, and leukocytes. The other three histamine receptors have prominent expression in the CNS. H_1 receptors are expressed throughout the body, particularly in the smooth muscle of the gastrointestinal tract and bronchial walls, as well as on vascular endothelial cells. H_1 receptors are widely distributed within the CNS, with particularly high levels in the thalamus, cortex, and cerebellum. H_1 receptor activation is associated with G_q activation and stimulation of phosphoinositide turnover and tends to increase excitatory neuronal responses. These receptors are the targets of classic antihistaminergic agents used in the treatment of allergic rhinitis and conjunctivitis. The well-known sedative effects of these compounds have been attributed to their actions in the CNS and implicate histamine in the regulation of arousal and the sleep–wake cycle. Accordingly, a line of mutant mice lacking histamine displays deficits in waking and attention. In addition, the sedation and weight gain produced by a number of antipsychotic and antidepressant drugs have been attributed to H_1 receptor antagonism. Conversely, H_1 receptor agonists stimulate arousal and suppress food intake in animal models.

H_2 receptors are also widely distributed throughout the body and are found in gastric mucosa, smooth muscle, cardiac muscle, and cells of the immune system. Within the CNS, H_2 receptors are abundantly expressed in the neocortex, hippocampus, amygdala, and striatum. Activation of these receptors stimulates adenylate cyclase through G_s and produces excitatory effects in neurons of the hippocampal formation and thalamus. H_2 receptor antagonists are widely used in the treatment of peptic ulcer disease. In contrast, the functional significance of central H_2 receptors is unclear, although several studies indicate that stimulation of these receptors produces antinociceptive effects. H_2 receptors may also be involved in control of fluid balance—possibly along with H_1 receptors—via stimulation of vasopressin release.

Unlike the H_1 and H_2 histamine receptors, H_3 receptors are located presynaptically on axon terminals. Those located on histaminergic terminals act as autoreceptors to inhibit histamine release. In addition, H_3 receptors are located on nonhistaminergic nerve terminals, where they act as heteroreceptors to inhibit the release of a variety of neurotransmitters—including norepinephrine, dopamine, acetylcholine, and serotonin. Particularly high levels of H_3 receptor binding are found in the frontal cortex, striatum, amygdaloid complex, and substantia nigra. Lower levels are found in peripheral tissues such as the gastrointestinal tract, pancreas, and lung. H_3 receptors are coupled to $G_{i/o}$, with inhibition of adenylate cyclase and voltage-activated Ca^{2+} channels. Antagonists of H_3 receptors have been proposed to have appetite suppressant, arousing, and cognitive-enhancing properties.

Cholinergic Receptors Two major classes of cholinergic receptors exist: G-protein–coupled muscarinic receptors and nicotinic ligand-gated ion channels. Muscarinic receptors mediate a response with longer onset latency, which may be either excitatory or inhibitory. In the periphery, muscarinic receptors mediate the effects of postganglionic parasympathetic nerve release of acetylcholine. Central muscarinic receptors have been implicated in learning and memory, sleep regulation, pain perception, motor control, and regulation of seizure susceptibility. Five muscarinic receptor subtypes have been cloned, and these may be divided into two families on the basis of intracellular signaling mechanism: the M_1, M_3, and M_5 receptors activate G_q, leading to phosphatidylinositol turnover and an increase in intracellular calcium; the M_2 and M_4 receptors activate G_i or, possibly, G_o, leading to inhibition of adenylate cyclase. The M_2 and M_4 receptors may act as inhibitory autoreceptors and heteroreceptors to limit presynaptic release of neurotransmitters. The functional roles of the individual subtypes within the CNS are not well understood because highly subtype-selective agonists and antagonists have been unavailable. However, recent development of transgenic mice that lack genes encoding each of the muscarinic receptor subtypes has provided new insights into receptor function.

M_1 receptors are the most abundantly expressed muscarinic receptors in the forebrain, including the cortex, hippocampus, and striatum. Pharmacological evidence has suggested their involvement in memory and synaptic plasticity, and recent evaluation of mice lacking the M_1 receptor gene showed deficits in memory tasks—possibly involving interactions between cortex and hippocampus—but showed normal performance on other memory tasks. These mice were also noted to be resistant to the convulsant effects of muscarinic agonists. In addition to being the predominant muscarinic receptor subtype in the heart—where they function to lower heart rate—M_2 receptors are widely distributed throughout the brain. M_2 receptors appear to mediate tremor, hypothermia, and analgesia induced by muscarinic agonists. M_3 receptors are found extensively in smooth muscle and salivary glands and appear to play a major role in smooth muscle contraction in the gastrointestinal and genitourinary tracts, as well as mediating salivation. Although M_3 receptors are found at modest density in many areas of the CNS, no central role has been elucidated. M_4 receptors are expressed in the hippocampus and cortex and at high levels in the striatum, as well as at lower levels in thalamus and cerebellum. Striatal M_4 receptors may oppose the effects of D_1 dopamine receptors in the striatum and have been implicated as putative targets for anticholinergics used as antiparkinsonian agents—although other muscarinic receptor subtypes may also be involved. M_5 receptors are expressed in various peripheral and cerebral blood vessels and comprise a very small percentage of muscarinic receptors in brain. They may mediate cholinergic cerebral arterial vasodilation.

Nicotinic acetylcholine receptors, like 5-HT_3 receptors, are members of the ligand-gated ion channel superfamily and mediate rapid, excitatory signaling. They are composed of a pentameric complex of membrane protein subunits radially arranged around a central ion pore. The binding of acetylcholine to this receptor induces a conformational change that opens the channel and permits passage of Na^+, K^+, and Ca^{2+} ions through the channel pore, leading to membrane depolarization. Nicotinic acetylcholine receptor subunits are heterogeneous and associate in varied combinations. Thus, the properties of an individual complex—such as cation permeability and rate of desensitization—depend on its particular subunit composition. These various nicotinic acetylcholine receptor subunits can be separated into three general functional classes: (1) skeletal muscle subunits (α_1, β_1, δ, ε), (2) standard neuronal subunits (α_2 through α_6, β_2 through β_4), and (3) subunits capable of forming homomeric receptors (α_7 through α_9).

In the periphery, nicotinic acetylcholine receptors are found in skeletal muscle, autonomic ganglia, and the adrenal medulla. In the brain, they are found in many locations, including the neocortex, hippocampus, thalamus, striatum, hypothalamus, cerebellum, substantia nigra, ventral tegmental area, and dorsal raphe nucleus. Most nicotinic acetylcholine receptors in mammalian brains contain either $\alpha_4\beta_2$ or α_7 subunit combinations. They frequently appear to mediate presynaptic enhancement of neurotransmitter release, influencing the release of acetylcholine, dopamine, norepinephrine, and serotonin, as well as GABA and glutamate. Postsynaptic excitatory transmission is also observed. Nicotinic receptors have been implicated in cognitive function, especially working memory, attention, and processing speed. Cortical and hippocampal nicotinic acetylcholine receptors appear to be significantly decreased in Alzheimer's disease, and nicotine administration improves attention deficits in some patients. The acetylcholinesterase inhibitor, galantamine, used in treatment of Alzheimer's disease, also acts to positively modulate nicotinic receptor function. The α_7 nicotinic acetylcholine receptor subtype has been implicated as one of many possible susceptibility genes for schizophrenia, with lower levels of this receptor being associated with impaired sensory gating observed in some schizophrenic patients and their relatives. Some rare forms of the familial epilepsy syndrome autosomal dominant nocturnal frontal lobe epilepsy (ADNFLE) are associated with mutations in the α_4 or β_2 subunits of the nicotinic acetylcholine receptor. Finally, the reinforcing properties of tobacco use are proposed to involve the stimulation of nicotinic acetylcholine receptors located in mesolimbic dopaminergic reward pathways.

SUGGESTED CROSS-REFERENCES

The intracellular consequences of receptor activation are discussed in Section 1.8. Electrophysiological effects of brain monoamines are described in Section 1.9. Other basic concepts that are relevant to current monoamine research are presented in Sections 1.6, 1.7, and 1.8.

REFERENCES

Anagnostaras SG, Murphy GG, Hamilton SE, Mitchell SL, Rahnama NP, Nathanson NM, Silva AJ: Selective cognitive dysfunction in acetylcholine M1 muscarinic receptor mutant mice. *Nat Neuroscience*. 2003;6:51.

Anguelova M, Benkelfat C, Turecki G: A systematic review of association studies investigating genes coding for serotonin receptors and the serotonin transporter: II. Suicidal behavior. *Mol Psychiatry*. 2003;8:646.

Auld DS, Kornecook TJ, Bastianetto S, Quirion R: Alzheimer's disease and the basal forebrain cholinergic system: relations to β-amyloid peptides, cognition, and treatment strategies. *Prog Neurobiol*. 2002;68:209.

Baik JH, Picetti R, Saiardi A, Thiriet G, Dierich A, Depaulis A, Le Meur M, Borrelli E: Parkinsonian-like locomotor impairment in mice lacking dopamine D_2 receptors. *Nature*. 1995;377:424.

*Barker EL, Blakely RD. Norepinephrine and serotonin transporters: molecular targets of antidepressant drugs. In: Bloom FE, Kupfer DJ, eds. *Psychopharmacology: The Fourth Generation of Progress*. New York: Raven; 1995.

Barnes NM, Sharp T: A review of central 5-HT receptors and their function. *Neuropharmacology*. 1999;38:1083.

Bortolozzi A, Artigas F: Control of 5-hydroxytryptamine release in the dorsal raphe nucleus by the noradrenergic system in rat brain. Role of α-adrenoceptors. *Neuropsychopharmacology*. 2003;28:421.

Brown RE, Stevens DR, Hass H: The physiology of brain histamine. *Prog Neurobiol*. 2001;63:637.

Bymaster FP, McKinzie DL, Felder CC, Wess J: Use of M_1-M_5 muscarinic receptor knockout mice as novel tools to delineate the physiological roles of the muscarinic cholinergic system. *Neurochem Res*. 2003;28:437.

*Cooper JR, Bloom FE, Roth RH. *The Biochemical Basis of Neuropharmacology*. 7th ed. New York: Oxford University Press; 1996.

Dani JA: Overview of nicotinic receptors and their roles in the central nervous system. *Biol Psychiatry*. 2001;49:166.

Durham PL, Russo AF: New insights into the molecular actions of serotonergic antimigraine drugs. *Pharmacol Ther*. 2002;94:77.

*Giros BM, Jaber SR, Jones RM, Wightman, Caron MG: Hyperlocomotion and indifference to cocaine and amphetamine in mice lacking the dopamine transporter. *Nature*. 1996;379:606.

Glickstein SB, Schmauss C: Dopamine receptor functions: lessons from knockout mice. *Pharmacol Ther*. 2001;91:63.

Gould E: Serotonin hippocampal neurogenesis. *Neuropsychopharmacology*. 1999;21:46S.

Gross C, Zhuang X, Stark K, Ramboz S, Oosting R, Kirby L, Santarelli L, Beck S, Hen R: Serotonin 1A receptor acts during development to establish normal anxiety-like behaviour in the adult. *Nature*. 2002;416:396.

Gurevich I, Tamir H, Arango V, Dwork AJ, Mann JJ, Schmauss C: Altered editing of serotonin 2C receptor pre-mRNA in the prefrontal cortex of depressed suicide victims. *Neuron*. 2002;34:349.

Hardman JG, Limbird LE, Molinoff PB, Ruddon RW, Gilman A. *The Pharmacological Basis of Therapeutics*. 9th ed. New York: McGraw Hill; 1996.

*Hartman DS, Civelli O: Molecular attributes of dopamine receptors: new potential for antipsychotic drug development. *Ann Med*. 1996;28:211.

Hoyer D, Hannon JP, Martin GR: Molecular, pharmacological and functional diversity of 5-HT receptors. *Pharmacol Biochem Behav*. 2002;71:533.

Hu XT, Moratalla R, Graybiel AM, White FJ, Tonegawa S: Elimination of cocaine-induced hyperactivity and dopamine-mediated neurophysiological effects in dopamine D1 receptor mutant mice. *Cell*. 1994;79:945.

Lindvall O, Bjorklund A. Dopamine- and norepinephrine-containing neuron systems: their anatomy in rat brain. In: Emson PC, ed. *Chemical Neuroanatomy*. New York: Raven Press; 1983.

Liu Y, Peter D, Merickel A, Krantz D, Finn JP, Edwards RH: A molecular analysis of vesicular amine transport. *Behav Brain Res*. 1996;73:51.

MacKinnon AC, Spedding M, Brown CM: Alpha 2-adrenoceptors: more subtypes but fewer functional differences. *Trends Pharmacol Sci*. 1994;15:119.

Missale C, Nash SR, Robinson SW, Jaber M, Caron MG: Dopamine receptors: from structure to function. *Physiol Rev*. 1998;78:189.

Paterson D, Nordberg A: Neuronal nicotinic receptors in the human brain. *Prog Neurobiol*. 2000;61:75.

*Schwartz JC, Arrang JM, Garbard M, Traiffort E. Histamine. In: Bloom FE, Kupfer DJ, eds. *Psychopharmacology: The Fourth Generation of Progress*. New York: Raven Press; 1995.

Sirvio J, MacDonald E: Central α_1 adrenoceptors: their role in the modulation of attention and memory formation. *Pharmacol Ther*. 1999;83:49.

Tecott LH: Serotonin receptor diversity: implications for psychopharmacology. In: Dickstein LJ, Riba MB, Oldham JM, eds. *Review of Psychiatry*. Vol 15. Washington, DC: American Psychiatric Press; 1996.

Tecott LH, Sun LM, Akana SF, Strack AM, Lowenstein DH, Dallman MF, Julius D: Eating disorder and epilepsy in mice lacking $5HT_{2C}$ serotonin receptors. *Nature*. 1995;374:542.

Tork I: Anatomy of the serotonergic system. *Ann N Y Acad Sci*. 1990;600:9.

Torres GE, Gainetdinov RR, Caron MG: Plasma membrane monoamine transporters: structure, regulation and function. *Nat Rev Neurosci*. 2003;4:13.

Williams GV, Rao SG, Goldman-Rakic PS: The physiological role of 5-HT_{2A} receptors in working memory. *J Neurosci*. 2002;22:2843.

▲ 1.5 Amino Acids As Neurotransmitters

CARLOS R. PLATA-SALAMAN, M.D., D.SC.,
RICHARD P. SHANK, PH.D., AND
VIRGINIA L. SMITH-SWINTOSKY, PH.D.

Interest in amino acids as potential chemical messengers (neurotransmitters or transmitters) at synaptic junctions arose in the 1950s soon after experiments using glass capillary microelectrodes inserted into neuron cell bodies revealed that most synaptic junctions between neurons within the central nervous system (CNS) are not electrically coupled. This realization confirmed that synaptic transmission must be chemically mediated, as was previously demonstrated at neuromuscular junctions. This stimulated research to identify these chemical agents. It was already known that glutamate, when applied to the surface of muscle cells in arthropods, stimulated contraction. This prompted Curtis and Watkins to apply glutamate and several other amino acids to the surface of neurons within the CNS. Their experiments revealed that L-glutamate, L-aspartate, L-cysteate, and L-homocysteate, which are all similar structurally, increased neuronal excitability. In contrast, several other amino acids decreased neuronal excitability, including γ-aminobutyric acid (GABA), glycine, β-alanine, and taurine, which also exhibit structural similarity.

After the effects of these amino acids on the excitability of neurons were reported, a debate arose as to whether these amino acids were really neurotransmitters or served some other undefined function in regulating or modulating the excitability of neurons. Subsequently, criteria were developed and used to establish whether an amino acid or any other chemical functions to transmit signals between neurons at synapses. Criteria used to identify an amino acid as a neurotransmitter include (1) a high concentration within presynaptic terminals (especially within synaptic vesicles), (2) release from

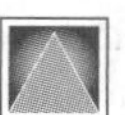

Table 1.5–1
Various Glutamatergic Pathways, Neuron Types, and Behavioral Roles[a]

Anatomical Pathway	Type of Neuron	Behavioral Role
Corticoamygdala	Pyramidal	Emotion
Corticocortical	Pyramidal	Association, perception
Corticonucleus tractus solitarius	Pyramidal	Regulation of breathing, heart rate, taste, olfaction
Corticospinal	Betz	Movement, pain sensation
Corticostriate	Pyramidal	Motor
Corticothalamic	Pyramidal	Relay, integration
Primary sensory afferents	Aδ, C fibers	Sensory input
Intercerebellar	Granule cells	Motor
Entorhinal-hippocampal	Perforant path	Learning, memory, emotion
Intrahippocampal	CA3 pyramidal cells	Learning, memory (Schaffer collaterals)
Dentatohippocampal	Granule cells (mossy fibers)	Learning, memory, association
Hippocampal/subiculoseptal/mammillary	CA1 pyramidal	Learning, memory, emotion
Intraretinal	Photoreceptors, bipolar	Primary visual input
Retinotectal	Ganglion cells	Vision—sensory
Visual geniculocortico	Optic radiation	Vision—integration
Olfactory bulb–olfactory cortex	Mitral cells, tufted cells	Olfaction—integration
Cochlea	Hair cells, spiral cells	Audition—sensory

[a]Pathways and behavioral roles are more complex than indicated.

the presynaptic terminal during membrane depolarization, (3) the presence of specific receptors in the postsynaptic membrane, and (4) an inactivation mechanism (removal of molecules from the synaptic cleft). Three amino acids (glutamate, GABA, and glycine) meet all of these criteria. Glutamate is now regarded as the major excitatory neurotransmitter throughout the CNS, whereas GABA and glycine are regarded as the major inhibitory neurotransmitters in the brain and spinal cord, respectively. Aspartate and taurine likely serve roles in modulating the excitability of neurons that are not yet defined.

NEUROPHYSIOLOGICAL FUNCTIONS OF GLUTAMATE AND ASPARTATE

Glutamate As a Neurotransmitter Glutamate is the principal excitatory neurotransmitter in the mammalian CNS. Most neurons that use glutamate as a neurotransmitter (termed either *glutamatergic* or *glutaminergic*) are projection neurons. These include the pyramidal neurons that arise in the cerebral cortex and project to various subcortical regions or other cortical areas, somatic primary afferent sensory neurons, and retinal ganglion neurons that project to the lateral geniculate (Table 1.5–1). Glutamatergic interneurons include cerebellar granule cells, bipolar cells in the retina, and granule cells in the hippocampus. Glutamatergic neurons are prevalent in the hippocampus, where they appear to have a significant role in memory formation.

Glutamatergic neurons usually synapse on dendritic areas of target neurons. Often, a single postsynaptic neuron may receive synaptic input from many different glutamatergic neurons, with a total number of synaptic contacts in the thousands. The excitatory postsynaptic potentials (EPSPs) generated at each synapse are integrated, and the depolarization is shunted down the dendrite toward the cell body. If the depolarization is sufficient to activate voltage-gated Na^+ channels, an action potential is initiated at the axon hillock. In some neurons, action potentials can be initiated in the dendrites, which facilitates the transfer of membrane depolarization toward the cell body. By virtue of the large number of glutamatergic synaptic contacts, the excitatory influence on the postsynaptic neuron can be precisely controlled. It is estimated that as much as 80 percent of the total number of synapses in the brain are glutamatergic. However, the relative number of neurons that are glutamatergic is much less than 80 percent.

Aspartate As a Neurotransmitter Although aspartate has been shown to potently stimulate neurons in the CNS, its role in the CNS is unclear. No specific receptors for aspartate have been identified, but it may be a physiologically relevant agonist (ligand) at some types of glutamate receptors. Some interneurons within the hippocampus and spinal cord concentrate aspartate within their synaptic terminals and release this amino acid during membrane depolarization. However, it has not been established that aspartate is concentrated in specific types of synaptic vesicles and released from synaptic terminals via controlled exocytosis.

Function of Glutamate in Neurogenesis during Brain Development Glutamatergic neurons develop comparatively late in the development of the CNS, and glutamate may serve a dual role that depends on the stage of development. At an early stage, glutamate can depress the excitability of some neurons, whereas, at later stages, the neuroexcitatory activity is manifest. This excitatory activity promotes neuronal differentiation and migration and is mediated in part by facilitating the influx of Ca^{2+} into neurons. Paradoxically, blockade of the *N*-methyl-D-aspartate (NMDA) subtype of glutamate receptors during the prenatal period can induce apoptosis in vulnerable neurons (the selectivity of the vulnerability depends on the developmental age).

Nontransmitter Functions of Glutamate and Aspartate These amino acids serve several functions in neural tissues unrelated to their role as neurotransmitters. Both are major constituents in proteins and several peptides, including *N*-acetylaspartylglutamate (NAAG), a putative transmitter or cotransmitter. Aspartate is a precursor of *N*-acetylaspartate (NAA), a major organic anion in neurons. Glutamate and aspartate also have a role in energy metabo-

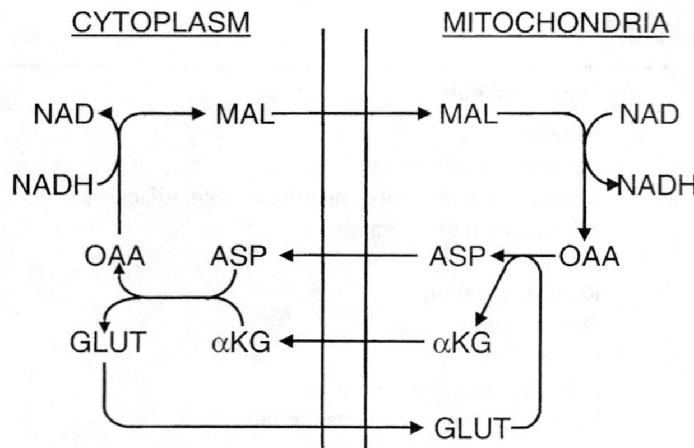

FIGURE 1.5–1 The metabolic components of the malate–aspartate shuttle. Although it is not evident from the diagram, the flux of aspartate (ASP) across the mitochondrial membrane is coupled with the flux of glutamate (GLUT) in the reverse direction. The fluxes of malate (MAL) and α-ketoglutarate (αKG) may be similarly coupled. NAD, nicotinamide adenine dinucleotide; NADH, nicotinamide adenine dinucleotide (reduced); OAA, oxaloacetic acid.

lism; they are intermediates in the malate–aspartate shuttle, a metabolic pathway that reoxidizes cytosolic nicotinamide adenine dinucleotide (NADH) formed as a result of aerobic glycolysis and captures the energy within mitochondria for adenosine triphosphate (ATP) formation (Fig. 1.5–1). Because glucose is rapidly consumed via aerobic metabolism in neural tissues, this pathway is quite active. Another function of glutamate is its role as the immediate metabolic precursor of nearly all the GABA synthesized in neural tissues. Glutamate also can serve as an intermediate in the detoxification of ammonia.

NEUROPHYSIOLOGICAL SIGNIFICANCE OF INHIBITORY AMINO ACIDS

GABA As a Neurotransmitter GABA is prevalent throughout the CNS but is comparatively low in the brainstem and spinal cord. It is generally not present in peripheral neurons but is detected in some endocrine tissues, including β cells in the pancreas and in ovaries. GABA is not an essential amino acid and is not used as a building block for protein, but it is a constituent of some peptides, such as homocarnosine, a dipeptide of GABA and histidine.

Within the CNS, GABA is present at high concentrations in select types of neurons, where it likely functions as a neurotransmitter. Most of these neurons (termed *GABAergic*) are small interneurons with short axons; however, some are projection neurons. These include the Purkinje cells in the cerebellum and the striatonigral and pallidonigral neurons in the basal ganglia (Table 1.5–2). Physiologically, the most common function of GABAergic neurons is to focus and refine the firing pattern (nerve impulse generation) of projection neurons that transfer neural information from one functional unit to another. An example of this is surround inhibition, which occurs when excitatory projection neurons activate inhibitory interneurons via collateral axons, which in turn inhibit surrounding projection neurons via synaptic contacts on the cell soma near the axon hillock. GABAergic neurons can also facilitate the output of excitatory projection neurons through a process of disinhibition, which occurs when two GABAergic neurons are linked synaptically in series. The first inhibits the ability of the second to depress the activity of an excitatory neuron, thereby increasing the excitatory output. GABA also mediates presynaptic inhibition, which occurs when a small presynaptic terminal conjoins with a larger synaptic terminal and inhibits the release of transmitter molecules from the larger one by preventing an action potential in the larger terminal from initiating the process that releases transmitter molecules.

Although GABA functions primarily as an inhibitory neurotransmitter in the mature brain, it can exert an excitatory effect in some instances. An example of this is the pyramidal neurons in the CA1 region of the hippocampus. These neurons are involved in the formation of memory and exhibit long-term potentiation (LTP). When these pyramidal neurons receive a burst of excitatory input from glutamatergic and cholinergic neurons feeding into the CA1 region, GABAergic synaptic activation shifts from hyperpolarizing the membrane to partially depolarizing the membrane, thereby shifting the effect of GABA on the pyramidal neuron from inhibition to excitation. This appears to contribute to the development of LTP. The potential physiological value may be that this can selectively facilitate the excitation of a single neuron.

Function of GABA in Neurogenesis during Brain Development Many GABAergic neurons become functional at an early stage of brain development. During this period, GABA exerts an excitatory effect on developing neurons, which promotes the maturation of these neurons. This neurotrophic effect occurs in part because the GABA-induced depolarization activates voltage-

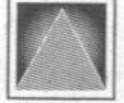

Table 1.5–2
Various GABAergic Neuron Anatomical Locations, Neuron Types, and Neural Pathways Influenced

Anatomical Location	Type of Neuron	Neural Systems Influenced
Cerebral cortex	Inhibitory interneurons	Cortical efferents
Basal ganglia	Neostriatal interneurons	Striatal efferents
	Striatonigral neurons	Extrapyramidal output
	Pallidonigral neurons	Extrapyramidal output
Cerebellum	Purkinje	Cerebellar output
	Basket cells	Cerebellar efferents
	Golgi cells	Cerebellar efferents
	Stellate cells	Cerebellar efferents
Hippocampus	Basket cells	Hippocampal efferents
Retina	Amacrine cells	Retina efferents
Olfactory bulb	Inhibitory interneurons	Olfactory bulb efferents
Brainstem, spinal cord	Inhibitory interneurons	Central integration of sensory afferents; motor neuron output

gated Ca^{2+} channels, which mediate a controlled influx of Ca^{2+} into the postsynaptic neuron. This activates a variety of signal transduction pathways that promote neuronal maturation. This neuroexcitatory effect of GABA is modulated by sex steroids, which may serve a critical role in the sexual differentiation of the brain. It is also at these time periods that the developing brain is especially vulnerable to ethanol, which has a positive modulatory effect on some types of GABA receptors. Such an effect on the neuroexcitatory activity of GABA may participate in the neurodegenerative effects of ethanol that give rise to fetal alcohol syndrome (FAS).

Glycine As a Neurotransmitter Glycine is present throughout the CNS but is more prevalent in the brainstem and spinal cord, which are the principal areas where it serves a transmitter function. As in all tissues, glycine is a major constituent of protein and several peptides, including glutathione. Neurons that utilize glycine as a neurotransmitter (glycinergic neurons) are small inhibitory interneurons. They often are functionally associated with α-motoneurons.

A binding site for glycine exists on the NMDA subtype of glutamate receptors.

Taurine Taurine, a sulfonated amino acid, is prevalent throughout the CNS and many other tissues. It is highly concentrated (10 to 20 mmol/L) in the immature brain and declines gradually during maturation. It is also abundant in white matter and therefore does not have a tissue distribution expected of a neurotransmitter. There is no compelling evidence that taurine activates specific receptors localized to synaptic terminals or that it is concentrated in synaptic vesicles. Therefore, although the inhibitory effects of taurine on neuronal excitability suggest that this amino acid does function to depress neuronal excitability, it is unclear if it serves a function in synaptic signaling.

AMINO ACIDS AS COTRANSMITTERS

Some glutamatergic and GABAergic neurons also utilize another agent, usually a peptide, as a neurotransmitter. An example of this is glutamatergic primary afferent neurons that also release substance P. In addition, enkephalin and cholecystokinin (CCK) have been colocalized with glutamate in the perforant path fibers of the hippocampus. Some glutamatergic neurons may also use aspartate or NAAG as a cotransmitter. CCK, neuropeptide Y (NPY), and galanin are each colocalized with GABA in some cortical, limbic, and spinal neurons, respectively. Enkephalin and thyrotropin-releasing hormone (TRH) are also localized in some spinal GABAergic neurons. Some studies suggest that the peptide neurotransmitters are released from synaptic terminals primarily during periods of high-frequency neuronal firing.

BIOCHEMICAL PROCESSES THAT MEDIATE TRANSMITTER FUNCTION

Synthesis and Regulation of the Neurotransmitter Pool of Glutamate Glutamate is rapidly synthesized from glucose in neural tissues, including synaptic terminals, but this reflects the role of glutamate in energy metabolism. The biochemical process used to replenish the neurotransmitter pool appears to involve a net synthesis of glutamate precursors in astrocytes, which are released and subsequently taken up into glutamatergic synaptic terminals and converted to glutamate. Glutamine is the most firmly established precursor serving this function, but α-ketoglutarate (a tricarboxylic acid [TCA] cycle intermediate) and malate may also be used in this capacity (Fig. 1.5–2).

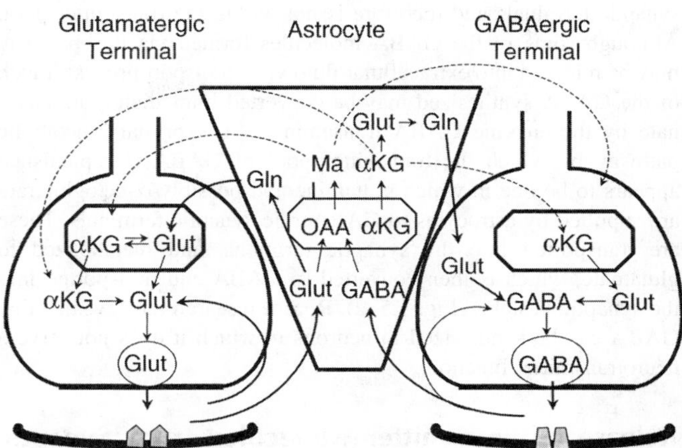

FIGURE 1.5–2 Some biochemical events associated with the neurotransmitter functions of glutamate and γ-aminobutyric acid (GABA). A large portion of the molecules of glutamate (Glut) and GABA released from presynaptic terminals are transported into astrocytes and therein converted to glutamine (Gln) and possibly an intermediate of the tricarboxylic acid cycle and then are released and transported into the nerve terminals for subsequent conversion back into glutamate or GABA. αKG, α-ketoglutarate; Ma, malate; OAA, oxaloacetic acid.

The transmitter pool of glutamate may be defined as the molecules stored within synaptic vesicles. Glutamate is concentrated within vesicles by an ATP-dependent transporter specific for glutamate and present only in the membrane of vesicles in glutamatergic terminals. These transporters are driven by a proton gradient across the vesicle membrane and concentrate glutamate approximately tenfold above the cytosolic level. Because the concentration of glutamate in the cytosol of glutamatergic neurons is approximately 10 mmol/L, the vesicular level is approximately 100 mmol/L. By comparison, the concentration of glutamate in the synaptic cleft when the synaptic terminal is inactive (resting state) is approximately 1 μmol/L. Sodium ion (Na^+)-dependent transporters with high affinity for both glutamate and aspartate also contribute to the regulation of the transmitter function of glutamate. Specific types of transporters are prevalent in the cell membrane of neurons and astrocytes near glutamatergic synaptic terminals. These transporters contribute to neurotransmitter inactivation by maintaining low extracellular concentrations around synapses, whereas neuronal transporters in nonsynaptic regions may contribute to regulating the excitability of neurons by controlling the ratio of the intracellular to extracellular concentration within neurons. In this regard, although the transporters generally function as uptake systems (sometimes termed *reuptake*), they can also serve an export function during membrane depolarization.

Synthesis and Regulation of the Neurotransmitter Pool of GABA Glutamate is the major metabolic precursor of GABA, although a small amount of GABA is derived from polyamines. Glutamate decarboxylase (GAD) catalyzes the reaction, and two distinct forms of this enzyme exist (GAD65 and GAD67). The enzyme requires pyridoxal phosphate (vitamin B_6) as a coenzyme, which also serves a regulatory function. GABA is synthesized from a pool of glutamate that is rapidly formed from α-ketoglutarate. Much of the GABA synthesized via this pathway is probably not in synaptic terminals and therefore is not within the transmitter pool. Although some of the GABA molecules formed via this pathway may be released into extracellular fluid via a transport process, much of the GABA synthesized may be converted immediately to succinate by the enzyme GABA transaminase. The primary metabolic pathway by which the transmitter pool of GABA is replenished appears to be one in which glutamine and possibly α-ketoglutarate are supplied by astrocytes to GABAergic synaptic terminals. These are transported into the synaptic terminals and metabolized to glutamate, which is then converted to GABA and transported into the synaptic vesicles (Fig. 1.5–2). Recent research has revealed that GABA can be synthesized in neurons in which it does not serve a neurotransmitter function.

Release of Transmitter Molecules from Synaptic Terminals

Amino acid neurotransmitters are released from synaptic terminals by a process similar to that for acetylcholine and the monoamine neurotransmitters. Glutamate, GABA, and glycine are each accumulated into their own specific type of synaptic vesicle via a Na^+-independent ATP-dependent transporter (pump). Neurotransmitter molecules are concentrated within synaptic vesicles approximately tenfold over the cytoplasmic concentration, resulting in an intravesicular concentration of nearly 100 mmol/L. Because the diameter of synaptic vesicles is approximately 10^{-7} meter, one vesicle can contain approximately 5,000 molecules.

Transmitter release is triggered by the depolarization of the presynaptic membrane by an action potential. This results in the opening of voltage-dependent Ca^{2+} channels of the N- or P/Q-type, thereby allowing Ca^{2+} to flow into the presynaptic terminal and transiently increase the concentration in close proximity to docking sites where vesicles attach to the inner surface of the presynaptic membrane. The elevation of Ca^{2+} initiates a cascade of events involving at least eight proteins (mostly protein kinases) that enable the vesicles to dock with the membrane and release their contents into the synaptic cleft. Although the presynaptic terminal of neurons within the CNS may contain numerous vesicles, a single action potential typically induces transmitter release from only a few (one to three). This is sufficient to raise the concentration of neurotransmitter molecules within the synaptic cleft to nearly 1 mmol/L for a few milliseconds, which can nearly saturate adjacent postsynaptic receptors.

The release of neurotransmitter molecules is regulated in part by the presence of neurotransmitter or hormone receptors on the surface of presynaptic terminals. These include group II and group III metabotropic glutamate receptors, cholinergic (nicotinic and muscarinic) receptors, adenosine (A1), kappa opioid, $GABA_B$, CCQ, and NPY (Y2) receptors. These receptors may be activated by transmitter molecules released from nearby neurons. Activation of these receptors may affect the activation of Ca^{2+} channels or influence efficiency of vesicle docking. Nitric oxide released from the postsynaptic neuron can also influence neurotransmitter release.

Removal of Transmitter Molecules from the Synaptic Cleft (Neurotransmitter Inactivation)

Transmitter molecules within the cleft can readily diffuse into extracellular fluid (ECF) adjacent to the synapse, where the concentration of transmitter molecules is at least 1,000-fold lower. As long as the 1,000-fold gradient is maintained, diffusion can restore the resting concentration within the cleft to micromolar concentrations within a few milliseconds. Uptake of transmitter molecules back into the presynaptic terminal or into the postsynaptic neuron also contributes to the inactivation process. A key element in the inactivation of the transmitter function of glutamate and GABA is a vigorous uptake by transporters in the cytoplasmic membrane of astrocytes. This is primarily how a low extracellular concentration (≤1 mmol/L) of these amino acids is maintained, thereby allowing diffusion to mediate a rapid removal of molecules from the synaptic cleft.

Five plasma membrane glutamate transporters (EAAT-1 through EAAT-5) have been cloned from the mammalian CNS. They exhibit approximately 50 percent homology, yet possess distinct pharmacology, cellular localization, and regulatory mechanisms. They are all Na^+-dependent, are coupled to G proteins, and are expressed in astrocytes (EAAT-1 [GLAST] and EAAT-2 [GLT-1]) and neurons (EAAT-3 [EAAC-1], EAAT-4, and EAAT-5). In addition, they are known to transport D- and L-aspartate. Recent gene knock-out studies indicate that astrocyte glutamate transporters may have a greater role in regulating extracellular glutamate concentrations than neuronal transporters. In general, EAAT-1 seems to be the most predominant transporter subtype throughout embryogenesis, with a decrease in its expression correlating with an increase in GLT-1 expression postnatally. GLAST expression is maintained at a low level in most of the brain during development, but large increases are seen in the cerebellum after birth. The increases in both GLAST and GLT-1 correlate with the timing of synaptogenesis in specific brain regions. EAAT-4 expression is primarily restricted to the cerebellum, whereas EAAT-5 may be present only in the retina.

AMINO ACID NEUROTRANSMITTER RECEPTORS

Glutamate Receptors

Glutamate receptors are present in synaptic and nonsynaptic regions of neuronal membranes throughout the CNS. Some glutamate receptors are also found in the membrane of astrocytes and oligodendrocytes. There are two general classes of glutamate receptors. The more prevalent are glutamate-gated ion channels selectively permeable to cations and are commonly referred to as *ionotropic glutamate receptors* (iGluR). The second are members of the superfamily of G-protein–coupled receptors (GPCRs) and are commonly referred to as *metabotropic receptors*. The iGluR receptors are currently divided into three types based on pharmacological considerations: NMDA, α-amino-3-hydroxy-5-methylisoxazole-4-propionic acid (AMPA), and kainate (KA). AMPA and KA receptors are sometimes collectively referred to as *non-NMDA receptors*, or *AMPA/KA receptors*. The metabotropic class of receptors (mGluR) are divided pharmacologically into three groups: quisqualate-, (2R,4R)-aminopyrrolidine-2,4-dicarboxylate (APDC)-, and L-2-amino-4-phosphonobutanoic acid (L-AP4)–sensitive receptors. Representative agonists and antagonists for each of these receptor classes are shown in Table 1.5–3.

NMDA Receptors

NMDA receptors are characterized by voltage-dependent block by Mg^{2+}, a high permeability to Ca^{2+}, and slow gating kinetics. The NMDA receptor is a ligand-gated ion channel composed of three different subunits: NMDAR1 (NR1), NMDAR2 (NR2), and NMDAR3A (NR3A). NR1 exists as eight splice variants that are developmentally and regionally expressed in the brain. There are four different genes encoding variants of NR2 (2A, 2B, 2C, and 2D). The NR2 subunits are heterogeneously distributed in the brain, and their distribution correlates with variations in the functional properties that define NMDA receptor heterogeneity. The NR3 subunit is expressed in the developing brain and the adult brain, particularly in the occipital and entorhinal cortices, thalamus, and cerebellum. At present, it is not clear how many NR1, NR2, and NR3 subunits are present in each functional NMDA receptor or if additional subunits exist, although the receptor is thought to

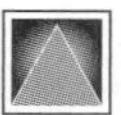

Table 1.5–3
Various Glutamate Receptor Agonists and Antagonists

	NMDA				Metabotropic		
	Glutamate Site	**Glycine Site**	**AMPA**	**KA**	**GrpI**	**GrpII**	**GrpIII**
Receptor-selective agonist	NMDA	Glycine	AMPA	KA	Quis	DCG-IV	L-AP4
		D-Serine	Aniracetam	DA	DHPG	APDC	L-SOP
			BTD	SYM2081	CHPG		
			Ampakines	ATPA			
				5-IW			
				LY339624			
Receptor-selective antagonist	AP-5	KNA	GYKI52466	LY382884	AIDA	MCCG	MeSOP
	CGP39653	7-CKN	NBQX	LY377770	LY367385	LY341495	MAP4
	CGS19755	CNQX	GYKI53655		CPCCOEt	EGLU	CPPG
		MNQX			MPEP		
		HA966					
		GV150526					
		L701324					
		L689560					
Channel blockers	PCP						
	MK801			CP101606			
	Ketamine			Ifenprodil			
	Budipine			Eliprodil			
	Amantadine			Conatokin-			
	Memantine			GConatokin-T			
	TCP						
	Gacyclidine						

AIDA, (R,S)-1 aminoindan-1,5-dicarboxylic acid; AMPA, α-amino-3-hydroxy-5-methylisoxazole-4-proprionic acid; AP-5, 2-amino-5-phosphonopentanoic acid; APDC, (2R,4R)-aminopyrrolidine-2,4-dicarboxylate; ATPA, adenosinetriphosphatase; BTD, benzothiadiazines; CGP39653, (±)-(E)-2-amino-4-propyl-5-phosphonopenoic acid; CGS19755, (±)cis-4-phosphono-methyl-2-piperidine carboxylic acid; CHPG, (R,S)-2-chloro-5-hydroxyphenylglycine; 7-CKN, 7-chlorokynurenic; CNQX, 6-cyano-7-nitroquinoxaline-2,3-dione; CP101606, (1S, 2S)-1-(4-hydroxyphenyl)-2-(4-hydroxy-4-phenylpiperidino)-1-propanol; CPCCOEt, 7-(hydroxylimino)cyclopropa-[b]chromen-1a-carboxylate; CPPG, (R,S)-α-cyclopropyl-4-phosphophenylglycine; DA, domoic acid; DCG-IV, (2S,2'R,3'R)-2-(2',3')-dicarboxycyclopropyl)glycine; DHPG, (S)-3,5-dihydrophenylglycine; EGLU, (2S)-α-ethylglutamic acid; Grp, group; GV150526, 3-[-2(phenylcarbamoyl)ethenyl]-4,6-dichloroindole-2-carboxylic acid; GYKI52466 and GYKI53655, 2,3-benzodiazepines; HA966, 3-amino-1-hydroxypyrrolidin-2; 5-IW, (S)-5-iodowillardiine; KA, kainic acid; KNA, kynurenic acid; L689560, (±)4-(trans)-2-carboxy-5,7-dichloro-4-phenylaminocarbonylamino-1,2,3,4-tetrahydroquinoline; L701324, 7-chloro-4-hydroxy-3-(3-phenoxy)-phenyl-2(H)-quinolone; L-AP4, L-2-amino-4-phosphonobutanoic acid; L-SOP, L-serine-*O*-phosphate; LY339624, (2S,4R,6E)-2-amino-4-carboxy-7-(2-naphthyl)hept-6-enoic acid; LY341495, (2S)-2-amino-2-(1S,2S-2-carboxycyclopropan-1-yl)-3-(xanth-9-yl)propanoic acid; LY367385, (S)-(+)-α-amino-4-carboxy-2-methylbenzeneacetic acid; LY377770 and LY382884, 6-decahydroisoquinolines; MAP4, (S)-2-amino-2-methyl-4-phosphonobutanoate; MCCG, 2S,1'S2S'-2-methyl-2-(2'-carboxycyclopropyl)glycine; MeSOP, (R,S)-α-methylserine-O-phosphate ; MK801, (+)-5-methyl-10,11-dihydro-5H-dibenzo[a,d]cyclohepten-5,10-imine; MNQX, 5,7-dinotroquinoxaline-2,3-dione; MPEP, 2-methyl-6-(phenylethynyl)pyridine; NBQX, 2,3-dihydro-6-nitro-7-sulphamoyl-benzo(f)quinoxaline; NMDA, *N*-methyl-D-aspartate; PCP, phencyclidine; Quis, quisqualate; SYM2081, (2S,4R-4-methylglutamic acid); TCP, 1,-[1-(2-thienyl)cyclohexl]piperidine.

be heteropentameric. However, it is known that NR1 serves as the core subunit of a functional NMDA receptor, with the NR2 and NR3 subunits acting as modulatory components of the receptor. Both NR1 and NR2 proteins are transmembrane proteins with three complete transmembrane regions and an intramembrane loop between the first and second complete transmembrane regions. The amino-terminal region of each protein is extracellular and contains putative ligand-binding regions and multiple glycation sites. The carboxyl-terminal region is intracellular and may control regulation of the receptor by second messenger systems. This intracellular domain anchors NMDA receptors to specific cellular locations via scaffolding proteins such as postsynaptic density protein-95 (PSD-95). NMDA receptor subunits are phosphorylated by either protein kinase C (PKC) or protein kinase A (PKA), which contributes to the heterogeneity of this receptor family. However, the NR2B subunit is phosphorylated by protein tyrosine kinase. In addition, serine/threonine kinases, calcium/calmodulin-dependent protein kinase II (CAMKII), Ras/mitogen-activated protein kinase (MAPK), and the Src family of tyrosine kinases have been implicated in the regulation of NMDA receptor functions. Dephosphorylation by serine/threonine phosphatases, such as calcineurin, or tyrosine protein phosphatases seem to negatively modulate NMDA receptor function.

NMDA receptors have a number of distinct recognition sites for endogenous and exogenous ligands, each with discrete binding domains. At present, there are at least seven pharmacologically distinct sites through which compounds can alter the activity of this receptor (Fig. 1.5–3). Drugs that affect NMDA receptor function are divided into four groups: those acting at (1) the glutamate/NMDA recognition site, which is highly conserved on the NR2 subunits; (2) the strychnine-insensitive glycine binding site (presumably on the NR1 subunit), where glycine is required as a coagonist for channel opening; (3) the intra-ion channel binding site, where Mg^{2+} sits blocking ionic currents through the receptor at resting potentials; and (4) modulatory sites such as the redox modulatory site, the proton-sensitive site, the Zn^{2+} site, and the polyamine site. It is of interest to note that D-serine, an endogenous positive modulator of NMDA receptors secreted by glia, has been found to be threefold more potent than glycine at the coagonist site of NMDA receptors. The extracellular D-serine concentration is similar to or even higher than glycine in the brain and is 100 times more effective than glycine in potentiating NMDA receptor–mediated spontaneous synaptic currents.

The NMDA receptor has three characteristic features: (1) at resting potentials, it remains blocked by Mg^{2+}. Ionic currents through the receptor occur only if the neuronal membrane is partially depo-

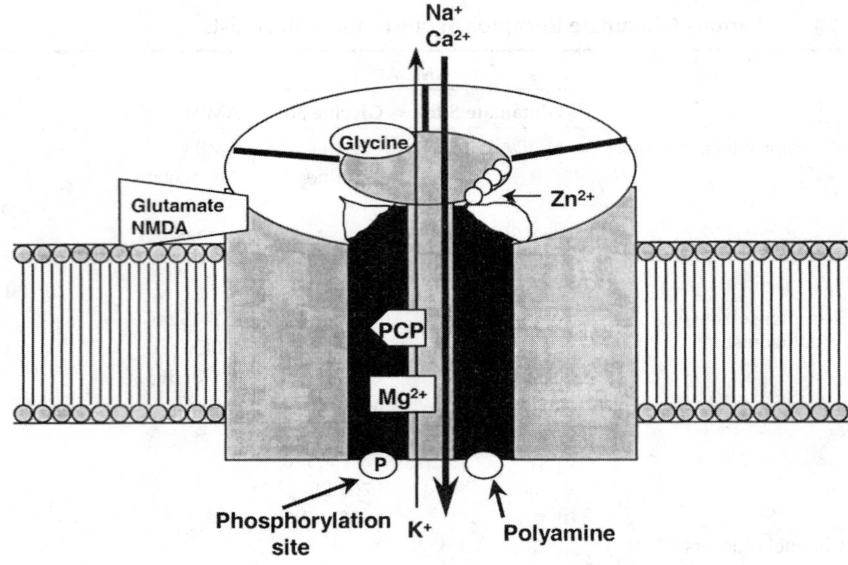

FIGURE 1.5–3 Diagrammatic illustration of the *N*-methyl-D-aspartate (NMDA) receptor/ion channel complex and its modulatory sites. PCP, phencyclidine.

larized; (2) significant amounts of extracellular Ca^{2+} enter the cell interior during activation of the receptor; and (3) the NMDA receptor–mediated neurotransmission occurs slowly and lasts for a prolonged period. Because of these properties, the NMDA receptor serves a critical role in synapse development and plasticity, including the phenomena of LTP and LTD.

AMPA Receptors NMDA receptors mediate excitatory neurotransmission in the CNS in different ways from AMPA and KA receptors, although they are often in close proximity in neuronal membranes and are activated in tandem. Recent cloning efforts have demonstrated that AMPA and KA receptors are distinct receptor complexes, although they can be activated by the same agonists. There are four genes that encode the AMPA receptor (GluR1 through GluR4 or GluRA through GluRD) and five genes that encode the KA receptor (GluR5 through GluR7 and KA1 and KA2). The four AMPA receptor subunits are of similar size, share 70 percent amino acid sequence homology, and are tetra- or pentameric. The receptor subunits have four hydrophobic membrane–associated domains, of which M1, M3, and M4 are membrane spanning, whereas the M2 domain forms a reentrant loop that lines the pore of the ion channel. Both the N-terminal domain and the loop between M3 and M4 domains are extracellular, with consensus glycosylation sequences. These two domains form the agonist binding site of the receptor, and allosteric modulators act on a region in the M3–M4 loop. The C-terminal domain is intracellular and interacts with several cytosolic proteins via PDZ domains. This includes the receptor-clustering proteins glutamate receptor interacting protein (GRIP), protein interacting with C-kinase (PICK1), AMPA receptor–binding protein (ABP), synapse-associated protein-97 (SAP97), and stargazin, which localize and anchor proteins at the synapse. AMPA receptor subunits exist in two different forms, "flip" and "flop," created by alternative splicing. They are expressed predominantly in the "flip" form in embryonic brains and gradually change over to the "flop" form, which dominates in the adult brain. The AMPA receptor channels are permeable to Na^+ and K^+ predominantly but will allow permeability to Ca^{2+} in the absence of the GluR2 (GluRB) subunit. AMPA receptors require higher glutamate concentrations for activation (10 to 100 μmol/L) than the NMDA receptors. The AMPA receptor has at least three binding sites at which agonists or antagonists can interact: glutamate, allosteric, and intra-ion channel binding sites. AMPA receptor function appears to be tightly regulated by various protein kinases. The GluR1 subunit can be phosphorylated by CAMKII, PKC, and PKA, leading to potentiation of AMPA receptor function. Dopamine via D1 receptor activation has been reported to potentiate AMPA currents via phosphorylating the GluR1 subunit (which is linked to LTP) or by inhibiting the activity of protein phosphatase 1 by PKA and the consecutive dopamine- and cyclic adenosine-monophosphate–regulated phosphoprotein 32-kDa (DARPP-32) phosphoprotein activation. Dephosphorylation of the AMPA receptor subunit GluR1 at the PKA phosphorylation site is one possible mechanism for NMDA-induced LTD. Phosphorylation of the GluR2 subunit by PKC has been linked to a disruption in AMPA receptor synaptic clustering and induction of LTD in the cerebellum. Inhibition of GluR2 with antisense oligonucleotides induces cell death in hippocampal neurons. AMPA receptors containing the GluR4 subunit (modulated by phosphorylation) desensitize rapidly.

Kainate Receptors Although KA is an effective agonist of AMPA receptors, it also activates its own distinct class of ionotropic receptors: the KA-preferring receptors. The five subunits are divided into two groups: GluR5 through GluR7 represent the low-affinity kainate binding site (K_d = 50 nmol/L), whereas KA1 and KA2 correspond to the high-affinity kainate binding site (K_d = 5 nmol/L). Each group is of similar size and amino acid sequence identity, with the KA1 and KA2 subunits being slightly larger than the GluR5 through GluR7 subunits. Receptor subunit heterogeneity is increased by alternative splicing and ribonucleic acid (RNA) editing. Kainate receptors desensitize considerably in the presence of glutamate or KA and show various Ca^{2+} permeability states due to alternative splicing and posttranscriptional editing. Concanavalin A has been reported to interact with kainate receptors to decrease their desensitization. KA receptor function seems to be tightly controlled by various protein kinases. The amplitude of the ion current at KA receptors has been reported to be enhanced by PKA-induced phosphorylation of GluR6. KA receptors have been shown to be oppositely modulated by kinases (e.g., CAMKII) and phosphatases (e.g., calcineurin) after Ca^{2+} entry through NMDA receptors or by other routes of Ca^{2+} influx. Despite their wide distribution throughout the CNS, the physiological significance of KA receptors remains largely unknown, although they have been shown to play a role in fast glutamatergic transmission in hippocampal neurons. In addition to postsynaptic functions, KA receptors have been shown to act presynaptically on mossy fiber terminals on CA3 pyramidal neurons within the hippocampus. One unique feature of presynaptic KA receptors is that their activation modulates transmitter release bidirectionally; weak activation enhances glutamate release, whereas strong activation leads to inhibition (GluR6-mediated). Involvement of presynaptic KA receptors in short-term plasticity at the mossy fiber–CA3 synapse suggests that these facilitatory autoreceptors may be important for the induction of LTP and LTD, as these forms of long-term plasticity depend on Ca^{2+} accumulation within mossy fiber terminals. Thus, bidirectional and activity-dependent regulation of transmitter release by KA autoreceptors might have physiological significance in information processing in the hippocampus and other CNS regions, as well as its well-known pathological action contributing to epileptogenesis.

Metabotropic Receptors The metabotropic receptor (mGluR) proteins belong to the superfamily of GPCRs, all of which comprise seven-transmembrane domains. So far, the mGluR gene family has been shown to contain eight members, which are closely related in primary structure and can be divided into three groups according to the extent of amino acid homology of their sequences, agonist sensitivity, and associated signal-transduction mechanisms. Group I receptors (mGlu1, mGlu5) are coupled via G_q to the inositol-1,4,5-triphosphate-Ca^{2+} cascade, whereas group II (mGlu2, mGlu3) and group III (mGlu4, mGlu6 through mGlu8) receptors are coupled to G_i and lead to the inhibition of adenylate cyclase. However, recent evidence suggests that activation of mGluR7 receptors can stimulate phospholipase C (PLC) in addition to reducing cyclic adenosine monophosphate (cAMP) levels. Some members of the mGluR gene families exist in alternatively spliced variants. Several lines of evidence suggest that the N-terminal large extracellular domain of the receptors contains glutamate binding sites, whereas the C-terminal domain plays a role in determining the potency of agonists regulating the transduction mechanisms of the mGluRs.

Group I mGluRs are primarily localized postsynaptically at the periphery of the postsynaptic density, where they can regulate currents through iGluR channels. In contrast, group II and III mGluRs typically function as presynaptic receptors involved in regulating the release of glutamate or other neurotransmitters. The synaptic distribution and functional properties of mGluRs are thought to be regulated by the interaction of various proteins with the C-terminal domain of the mGluR. Group I mGluRs have been shown to interact with several different scaffold proteins, including Homer proteins (1a–c, 2a and 2b, 3), calmodulin (CaM), and Siah-1A. Homers contain an EVH domain that interacts with the proline-rich region at the extreme C-terminus of both group I mGluRs (surface membrane receptors) and IP3 receptors (intracellular receptors) to bring them in close proximity to one another. No proteins have yet been reported to interact directly with the C-termini of group II mGluRs; however, several proteins similar to those interacting with group I mGluRs also interact with group III mGluRs, such as the G protein βγ subunits that interact with PKC, CaM, and PICK1. Generally, mGluR agonists induce a slow membrane depolarization (a rise time of approximately 5 seconds and lasting up to 60 seconds, which is approximately 1,000-fold slower than ionotropic receptors) accompanied by an increase in firing rate in many neurons. These effects are thought to be due to direct inhibitory effects on K^+ channels. In addition to direct excitatory postsynaptic effects, mGluR activation has been shown to suppress both excitatory and inhibitory transmission at synapses by presynaptic mechanisms via an autoreceptor-type mechanism (thought to be mGluR7), thereby modulating presynaptic activity. Similar to other GPCRs, mGluR desensitization is mediated by second messenger–dependent protein kinases and GPCR kinases (GRKs).

Several of the mGluRs have been implicated in synaptic plasticity that occurs in learning and memory. Knock-out of group I mGluRs has resulted in deficits in acquisition and retention of spatial and motor learning. Similar studies in group II and III mGluRs exhibited no learning and memory deficits; rather, deficits were related to visual processing and increased epileptogenesis.

GABA RECEPTORS

There are two major classes of GABA receptors. The more prevalent are ligand-gated channels that are selectively permeable to anions and are termed *$GABA_A$ receptors*. The second class are members of the superfamily of GPCRs, and are termed *$GABA_B$ receptors*. A minor class of GABA receptors that are ligand-gated channels and possess some similarity to $GABA_A$ receptors are termed *$GABA_C$ receptors*.

$GABA_A$ Receptors $GABA_A$ receptors are heteropentameric protein complexes, which, when activated, undergo a series of conformational changes that form an open channel (pore) selectively permeable to anions, specifically chloride anion (Cl^-) and, to a lesser degree, bicarbonate (HCO_3^-). Receptor activation normally results in an influx of Cl^-, which rapidly and transiently hyperpolarizes the membrane, a process generally referred to as the generation of an inhibitory postsynaptic potential (IPSP). The increase in Cl^- flux also decreases the resistance of the membrane, which acts as a shunt to impede the ability of depolarizing excitatory postsynaptic potentials (EPSPs) to elicit action potentials (nerve impulses). For this reason, inhibitory synapses are most effective when located near the point at which action potentials are initiated, usually the axon hillock. Therefore, it is not surprising that GABAergic inhibitory synapses are often concentrated on neuronal cell bodies near the axon hillock.

As noted previously, during early stages of brain development, GABA exerts an excitatory effect on developing neurons, which promotes their maturation. This effect is mediated by the activation of $GABA_A$ receptors, which generates depolarizing synaptic potentials. The synaptic potentials are depolarizing because the concentration of Cl^- in the immature postsynaptic neurons is much higher than in mature neurons, thereby shifting the Cl^- electrochemical equilibrium potential (E_{Cl^-}) to a magnitude more positive than the resting membrane potential (E_m). The high intracellular concentration is maintained by a type of Cl^- transporter in the cell membrane that drives Cl^- into the cell. This transporter, termed *NKCC1*, also carries Na^+ and K^+ into the cell. The energy required to drive the influx of Cl^- is derived from the Na^+ electrochemical potential. When the postsynaptic neuron nears maturity, the NKCC1 transporter declines and is replaced by a transporter that extrudes Cl^-. This transporter, termed *KCC2*, also extrudes K^+, whose electrochemical potential provides part of the energy required to drive the efflux of Cl^-. This results in a gradual decline in the intracellular concentration of Cl^- and shifts the E_{Cl^-} to a magnitude that is negative to the resting E_m.

In mature neurons that express a particular type of $GABA_A$ receptor, depolarizing postsynaptic potentials can be generated by $GABA_A$ receptors during periods in which the postsynaptic neuron is undergoing a high degree of excitatory synaptic input. The mechanistic nature of these depolarizing excitatory potentials has not been clearly established, but it is not due to a change in E_{Cl^-}. In pyramidal

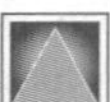

Table 1.5–4
Some γ-Aminobutyric Acid (GABA) Receptor Agonists, Antagonists, and Allosteric Modulators

	GABA$_A$ Receptor Drug Binding Sites				
	GABA sites	**Benzodiazepine**	**Steroid**	**Channel Sites**	**GABA$_B$ Receptor**
Agonists or positive modulators	Muscimol β-Alanine Isoguvacine THIP	Diazepam Lorazepam Clonazepam Alprazolam Zolpidem	Pregnenolone Allopregnenolone Alphaxalone	Pentobarbital Phenobarbital	Baclofen 3-APPA 3-APMPA
Antagonists or channel blockers	Bicuculline Securinine	Flumazenil	PREGS DHEAS	Picrotoxin PTZ TBPS	Phaclofen Saclofen SCH50911
Inverse agonists		Bretazenil β-Carboline			

DHEAS, dehydroepiandrosterone; PREGS, pregnenolone-sulfate; PTZ, pentylenetetrazol; SCH50911, [(+)2S]-5,5-dimethyl-2-morpholineatic acid; TBPS, t-butylbicyclophosphorothionate; THIP, 4,5,6,7-tetrahydroisoxazolo[5,4-c]pyridin-3-ol; 3-APPA, 3-aminopropyl-phosphinic acid; 3-APMPA, 3-aminopropyl, methylphosphinic acid.

neurons within the CA1 region of the hippocampus, these depolarizing potentials may be one of several synaptic events that may contribute to memory formation.

GABA$_A$ receptors are heteromeric in that the receptor can comprise at least four types of subunit proteins, termed α, β, γ, and δ. It is pentameric in that each receptor has a total of five proteins; therefore, all GABA$_A$ receptors have more than one copy of at least one type of subunit protein. There are multiple subtypes of three of the subunit proteins: at least six subtypes of α (α1 through α6), three of β, and three of γ. There are also other subunit subtypes, such as δ, ε, and ρ1 through ρ3. Although, theoretically, there could be many thousands of GABA$_A$ receptor subtypes (based on the possible subunit composition), it seems that a limited number (e.g., ≤20) exist naturally. Most often, the receptors contain two α, two β, and one γ, or one α, two β, and two γ subunits. The different subunits and the different subtypes of each subunit from which a particular type of receptor is formed can influence the physiological properties of the receptor (e.g., channel open time and rate of desensitization) as well as susceptibility to pharmacological agents.

GABA$_A$ receptors are regulated by phosphorylation of some serine hydroxyl residues in the inner loop of most of the subunits. Phosphorylation can be mediated by PKA or protein kinase C (PKC). Depending on the type of subunit, phosphorylation can affect the channel gating properties (e.g., channel open time and rate of receptor desensitization), either positively or negatively.

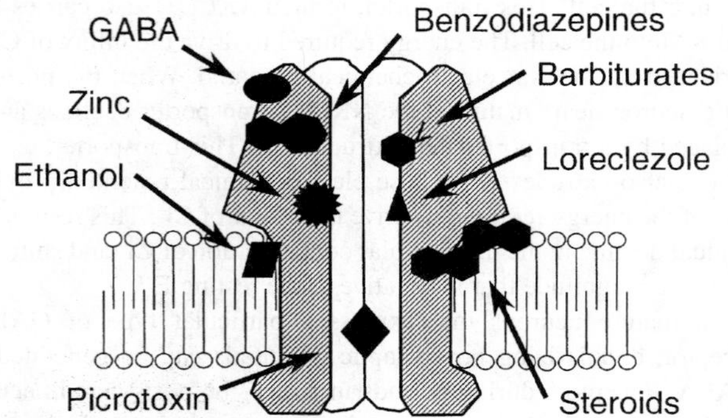

FIGURE 1.5–4 Diagrammatic illustration of the γ-aminobutyric acid type A (GABA$_A$) receptor/ion-channel complex and its modulatory sites.

A variety of pharmacological agents can influence the activity of GABA$_A$ receptors (Table 1.5–4). At least five separate drug binding sites have been identified (Fig. 1.5–4). Among them are the benzodiazepine and barbiturate sites, to which many clinically useful drugs are known to bind. These sites are allosteric to the GABA binding site. Drugs that bind to them influence the ability of GABA to activate the receptor by either altering the affinity between GABA and its binding sites (GABA$_A$ receptors probably possess two GABA binding sites) or by altering the channel open time and rate of receptor desensitization. An unusual characteristic of the benzodiazepine site is that drugs binding to it can exert either a positive modulatory (an agonist) or negative modulatory (an inverse agonist) effect or no effect at all. The steroid binding site probably serves a physiological function in modulating the activity of GABA$_A$ receptors. Several of the pharmacological effects of ethanol are mediated through effects on GABA$_A$ receptors.

GABA$_B$ Receptors The GABA$_B$ receptors generally exert an inhibitory effect on neuronal excitability by generating hyperpolarizing potentials that are much slower (slow IPSPs) in onset and longer in duration than those mediated by GABA$_A$ receptors. GABA$_B$ receptors are GPCRs and activate a type of K^+ channel, thereby hyperpolarizing the membrane. GABA$_B$ receptors are often located on presynaptic terminals, where they serve to inhibit transmitter release by reducing the ability of action potentials to activate Ca^{2+} influx.

CLINICAL CONSIDERATIONS

General Comments Dysregulation and dysfunction of glutamatergic and GABAergic systems are involved in the pathophysiology of multiple neurological and psychiatric disorders. Glutamate involvement in neurotoxicity and neurodegeneration has been extensively studied, and it is known that NMDA receptor–associated excitotoxicity results in apoptosis and necrosis. In neurology, the best studied dysfunctions are those proposed to be associated with epilepsy and status epilepticus, Parkinson's disease, cognitive disorders and dementias, migraine, amyotrophic lateral sclerosis, Huntington's chorea, chronic pain, stroke, traumatic and spinal cord injury, encephalopathies, and other neurodegenerative disorders. In psychiatry, multiple models have been proposed and developed for anxiety disorders and posttraumatic stress disorder, depressive disorders, bipolar disorders, and schizophrenia, including positive and negative symptoms, as well as other psychotic disorders, sleep disorders, and substance abuse such as alcoholism. It is also increasingly recognized that in addition to neurons, glial cells such as oligodendrocytes are highly vulnerable to excitotoxicity mediated by glutamate receptors. Essentially, overactivation of AMPA or KA receptors can induce oligodendrocyte dysfunction and death, resulting in demyelination.

Brain Neuroimaging Approaches Multiple modalities of brain imaging approaches are used in clinical research and for diagnostic purposes. One modality that merits mention in this chapter is the noninvasive proton magnetic resonance spectroscopy that measures the metabolite NAA. NAA is considered an index or marker of neuronal and axonal integrity. A focus of these studies has been the analysis of the relationship between NAA changes with diagnosis and disease progression. Although reported spectroscopic changes need further characterization and the clinical utility is still uncertain, a general pattern has started to emerge. Reduced NAA levels have been consistently reported in specific brain regions of patients with epilepsy, Alzheimer's disease, schizophrenia, and posttraumatic stress disorder (PTSD). NAA is also considered to be an indicator of neuronal development and could have applications in pediatric patients to determine degree of brain dysfunction and damage and as a prognostic tool in early neonatal and infantile periods.

Glutamate

Ischemia- and Injury-Induced Neurodegeneration The events that cause neuronal cell death as a result of stroke, head trauma, or any condition involving a dramatic loss of oxygen or glucose supply to the brain are complex. However, a breakdown in the regulation of glutamate is a major factor. Early metabolic consequences of ischemia or hypoxia include an accumulation of lactic acid and a concomitant decrease in pH and a decrease in energy storage molecules (phosphocreatine and ATP). This has an immediate deleterious effect on the activity of the Na^+/K^+ pump, which accounts for more than 50 percent of ATP-supplied energy use in the CNS. This results in a dissipation of transmembrane gradients for K^+ and Na^+ and a concomitant depolarization of the cell membrane. Dissipation of the Na^+ gradient inhibits the removal of glutamate from extracellular fluid (which depends on vigorous transport systems in the membrane of astrocytes and neurons), and membrane depolarization activates voltage sensitive Ca^{2+} channels in synaptic terminals, thereby promoting excessive glutamate release. Consequently, high levels of glutamate accumulate in the synapse, causing excessive activation of NMDA and AMPA receptors. Because of the prevalence of these receptors, the intracellular accumulation of Ca^{2+} is greatly exacerbated. This pathological accumulation of Ca^{2+} promotes a cascade of events that can result in neuronal cell dysfunction, damage, or death. Neurological disorders in which this pathological cascade may be involved include global and focal ischemia (stroke), hypoglycemia, head trauma, spinal cord injury, status epilepticus, drug abuse, and certain food toxicities (e.g., monosodium glutamate and mussel poisoning).

Chronic Neurodegenerative Disorders Dysregulation of glutamate and aspartate and overactivation of their receptors may contribute to neuronal cell loss in chronic disorders such as acquired immune deficiency syndrome (AIDS) dementia, Parkinson's disease, motor neuron disease (including amyotrophic lateral sclerosis [ALS]), Huntington's disease, and Alzheimer's disease. Tissue-specific defects in glial transporter genes resulting in impaired glutamate uptake (for instance, mutations in the glutamate transporter GLT1 or EAAT-2) have been identified in several cases of the sporadic form of ALS.

Ingestion of β-*N*-oxalylamino-L-alanine (L-BOAA), a naturally occurring excitatory amino acid in the chick pea from the plant *Lathyrus sativus*, induces neurolathyrism, a progressive form of motor neuron disease that is clinically similar to ALS. L-BOAA acts as an agonist at the AMPA receptor. In other motor-impairing disorders, abnormal activation of excitatory pathways within the basal ganglia appears to play a part in the symptom expression of parkinsonism in animal models. In primates, NMDA and non-NMDA antagonists increase the therapeutic efficacy of the dopaminergic drug levodopa (Levodopa).

Epilepsy *Epilepsy* is a group of neurological disorders characterized by spontaneous recurrent seizures. A seizure is an abnormal paroxysmal firing of cerebral neurons in synchronous fashion and is often associated with motor signs and sensory, autonomic, or psychic symptoms. Loss or impairment of consciousness often occurs. Epileptic syndromes are defined based on clusters of signs and symptoms that generally occur together in a patient with recurrent seizures. They are classified based on seizure type: localization related, generalized, undetermined, or a special syndrome. The epileptic syndromes are further divided by a consideration of the etiology: idiopathic, cryptogenic, or symptomatic. Epilepsy occurs in 1 to 2 percent of the population worldwide, and epileptic patients account for a major proportion of the return visits in neurological clinics. Compounds that antagonize the action of glutamate at NMDA receptors or AMPA/KA receptors are generally effective in blocking seizures.

Although many neurobiological factors may contribute to seizure formation, including ictogenesis and epileptogenesis, a prominent feature of most seizures is an abnormal and excessive firing of glutamatergic neural pathways. Therefore, abnormalities in the regulation of glutamate may be a factor in the initiation, spread, and maintenance of seizure activity in some types of epilepsy. The involvement of glutamatergic receptors in seizures and epilepsy is widely accepted based on evidence that injections or focal applications of glutamatergic agonists at NMDA receptors or AMPA/KA receptors seem to produce seizures or epileptic-like activity in numerous in vitro and animal models of epilepsy. Furthermore, selective antagonists to these receptors reduce epileptic activity or are potent anticonvulsants in several models. Some studies using in vitro or ex vivo techniques and studies in animal models indicate that glutamate or aspartate release is increased during seizure activity. In vivo microdialysis performed in epilepsy surgery patients showed marked increases in extracellular glutamate concentrations in epileptic hippocampi immediately before the onset of seizures. Epileptogenic foci in cortical areas, such as temporal or frontal, also release glutamate and aspartate, especially during intense seizures or status epilepticus. Many patients with temporal lobe or complex partial epilepsy are found to have neuronal loss and sclerosis, particularly in mesial hippocampus. Mesial temporal sclerosis is a common finding in surgical specimens removed from patients who experience chronic refractory complex partial seizures. Overall, mesial temporal lobe epilepsy is the most common form of human epilepsy. Neuronal loss is prominent in the CA1, CA3, and dentate regions of the hippocampus. Interestingly, the neuropathology closely resembles the findings seen in model systems of prolonged seizure activity or in those induced by application of excitotoxins.

Kindling, which is a gradual induction of a hyperexcitable neuronal state, can occur by focal repetitive subconvulsive stimulation of the hippocampus, amygdala, or some other brain areas. Kindling results in increased susceptibility to seizures and has been studied extensively in animals, particularly rodents. There is good evidence that glutamatergic receptors, particularly NMDA types, play a role in the development and enhancement of the kindled or seizure-prone state. NMDA receptor antagonists can prevent the kindling phenomenon despite the expression of seizure-like discharges in in vitro models such as hippocampal slices. A variety of NMDA antagonists, including those that act as channel blockers or compete with the glutamate or glycine recognition sites, appear to be highly effective in blocking the development of kindling. They do not appear to be as effective as anticonvulsants in fully expressed seizures unless they are used at dosages that produce significant toxic effects, such as neurological or behavioral impairment. In contrast, AMPA receptor antagonists are highly effective in blocking the expression of seizures but seem to have little effect on the induction of the kindled state. Further research is needed to define the role of excitatory amino acids in kindling and hippocampal injury. Much of the research has focused on ionotropic glutamate receptors.

Schizophrenia Several observations suggest that schizophrenia and other psychotic disorders involve abnormalities (hypofunction) of glutamatergic transmission. This hypothesis has been spurred on by the knowledge that phencyclidine (PCP, "angel dust") and ketamine, both noncompetitive NMDA receptor antagonists, induce schizophrenogenic-like effects. In fact, PCP abuse is associated with positive and negative symptoms and cognitive impairment.

Clinical data supporting a role for glutamate in the etiology of schizophrenia are sparse but interesting. It has been reported that glutamate was reduced in the cerebrospinal fluid (CSF) of schizophrenic patients relative to control patients. These results have not been replicated successfully. Postmortem studies in schizophrenic brains have found reduced concentrations of glutamate in the hippocampus and prefrontal cortex. Various studies have reported an increase in KA receptors in the prefrontal cortex, with a decrease in KA and AMPA receptor binding in the hippocampus and no change in NMDA receptors. Other studies focusing on analysis of receptor mRNA have found a decrease of NMDA, AMPA, and KA receptor mRNAs in specific brain regions. Overall, the results support the hypothesis that schizophrenia involves decreased glutamatergic transmission.

The fact that improvement in symptoms and cognitive function has been observed in schizophrenics receiving antipsychotics together with the use of agents that enhance NMDA receptor function (e.g., glycine and D-serine) as add-on therapy also supports the model of hypoglutamatergic transmission in schizophrenia. These findings also suggest that allosteric-positive modulators of the NMDA receptor may represent an aid in the treatment of schizophrenia. Allosteric modulators of AMPA receptors could also be useful.

Neuropathic Pain Activation of afferent C fibers with nociceptive stimuli produces pain sensations that are enhanced during pathological conditions. Activity-dependent increases in excitability are induced in the spinal dorsal horn neurons by repetitive stimulation of C fibers. This is thought to contribute to the development and maintenance of chronic pain symptoms. The NMDA antagonists, ketamine and D-amino-propyl-valeric acid (D-APV), have consistently reduced this activity in the rat dorsal horn nociceptive neurons, suggesting that the NMDA receptor contributes to this phenomenon. AMPA and KA receptors may also play a role in modulating pain. Overall, NMDA and AMPA receptors are involved in the induction of allodynia, and, in the rostral ventromedial medulla, NMDA and AMPA receptors are proposed to be involved in descending influences after inflammatory hyperalgesia. In situ hybridization studies have revealed that expression of the KA receptor gene GluR5 is particularly prominent in dorsal root ganglion neurons. Animal studies have indicated that KA receptor antagonists significantly reduce nociception, and early human trials with some of these agents show them to be promising for analgesia.

Substance Abuse Evidence indicates that one of the acute effects of ethanol is inhibition of glutamate receptor function, particularly NMDA and KA receptors. Sensitivity of NMDA receptors to ethanol-induced inhibition is influenced by the subunit composition of the receptor. Such inhibition leads to depressed synaptic transmission and may result in ethanol-induced cognitive deficits. Indeed, low concentrations of ethanol are known to inhibit LTP in the hippocampus.

GABA

Epilepsy Like the glutamatergic system, GABA and GABA receptor subtypes play a central role in the expression of seizures. In general, for the mature brain, loss or blockade of GABA inhibition can result in increased hyperexcitability and expression of seizures. Several GABAergic drugs are widely used in the treatment of epilepsy. Clinically effective benzodiazepines and barbiturates likely act at $GABA_A$ receptors to enhance inhibition. Both have been shown to be effective in the control of partial, complex partial, and generalized tonic-clonic seizures. Benzodiazepines also are effective in the acute treatment of generalized absence, but a functional tolerance tends to develop, thereby reducing its efficacy. Benzodiazepines are also effective in the treatment of atypical absence and myoclonic seizures. Anticonvulsant benzodiazepines and barbiturates are highly sedating, which limits their use.

Other evidence that the GABAergic system is important in the expression of seizures is that manipulation of $GABA_A$ receptor function can cause, exacerbate, or reduce seizure activity. The poisons picrotoxin and bicuculline antagonize $GABA_A$ receptors noncompetitively and competitively, respectively, and can elicit seizures. Penicillin given at high doses (especially in renal failure patients or intrathecally) can result in partial or generalized seizures. Penicillin reduces GABA-induced chloride current flow by blocking the ion channel pore. The $GABA_A$ receptor has numerous modulatory sites that can allosterically increase or decrease the chloride ion channel current flow. For example, negative modulators that act at the benzodiazepine site (e.g., β-carbolines) or the steroid site (e.g., pregnenolone-sulfate) can lower seizure thresholds.

In the mature or adult brain, enhancement of $GABA_A$ receptor function generally results in raising of the seizure threshold. Certain naturally occurring and synthetic pregnane-derived steroids are very potent positive modulators, called *neuroactive steroids*, or *neurosteroids*. Not only does positive modulation of these allosteric sites result in anticonvulsant activity, but increases in GABA availability also seem to be of clinical benefit. Reduction of GABA clearance by inhibition of GABA uptake or reduction of GABA degradation by depressing GABA transaminase are both effective mechanisms. Also, some evidence in animal models suggests that modulation of $GABA_B$ receptors may play a role in the treatment of generalized absence seizures.

Progress in the genetics of epilepsy has identified that genetic abnormalities in the $GABA_A$ receptor $\gamma 2$ subunit may be involved in the pathogenesis of generalized epilepsy with febrile seizures plus syndrome, as well as in severe myoclonic epilepsy in infancy. A mutation in the $GABA_A$ receptor $\alpha 1$ subunit has also been implicated in juvenile myoclonic epilepsy. In preclinical models, abnormal (lower) expression of $GABA_A$ receptor subtypes is associated with epileptogenesis; overexpression of the $\alpha 1$ subunit results in seizure resistance, whereas overexpression of the $\alpha2$, $\alpha3$, and $\alpha5$ enhances sensitivity to seizures. Targeted genetic disruption of the δ subunit also results in spontaneous seizures and reduction of neuroactive steroid responsiveness. Thus, evidence indicates that multiple genetic abnormalities of $GABA_A$ receptor subtypes can be involved in epilepsy.

Anesthesia Pentobarbital, an anesthetic barbiturate, has been a popular drug for induction of anesthesia. Like phenobarbital, pentobarbital allosterically enhances $GABA_A$ receptor function, but over a narrow concentration range it also can directly activate $GABA_A$ receptors. Pentobarbital also has activity in blocking glutamate receptors and voltage-gated Ca^{2+} channels. The potent benzodiazepines midazolam (Versed) and lorazepam (Ativan) have replaced diazepam (Valium) as a drug of choice for induction of anesthesia.

In the 1990s, pentobarbital was replaced by propofol, which is more easily titrated and is especially useful in the neurosurgical setting. Propofol, which has a short duration of action, allosterically enhances $GABA_A$ function and directly activates these receptors. Several neurosteroids also can directly activate $GABA_A$ receptors, and it has been proposed that this direct effect is in part responsible for the anesthetic qualities of these agents.

Anxiety- and Sleep-Related Disorders Benzodiazepines and barbiturates have a long history in the treatment of anxiety and insomnia. Diazepam was once the most prescribed medication in the United States. GABA receptor gene-targeting approaches have revealed that $GABA_A$ receptors containing an $\alpha1$ subunit mediate muscle relaxant and sedative effects of benzodiazepines, whereas $GABA_A$ receptors with $\alpha2$ or $\alpha3$ subunits mediate anticonvulsant and anxiolytic effects. Thus, drugs with greater anxiolytic versus sedative–hypnotic properties are related to preferential modulation of particular subtypes of $GABA_A$ receptors. There is an additional level of modulation as it relates to binding and activation of different sites on the same subunit. A prototypical example is zolpidem, a hypnotic agent indicated for the short-term treatment of insomnia, which acts as a selective agonist to the brain $\Omega1$ receptor situated in the $GABA_A$ receptor $\alpha1$ subunit. This is in contrast to benzodiazepines, which nonselectively bind to all Ω receptor subtypes.

Spasticity Loss of spinal and supraspinal inhibition may result in spasticity or hyperreflexic states. One particular disorder, stiff person syndrome, is associated with increased reflexivity, muscle rigidity, episodic muscle spasms, and, occasionally, seizures, diabetes, or both. The disorder is frequently associated with circulating antibodies to glutamate decarboxylase (GAD), the GABA synthesis enzyme. Benzodiazepines, especially diazepam, and baclofen are mainstays in the treatment of spasticity. However, these agents are often only moderately effective, especially in supraspinal forms of spasticity.

Substance Abuse Ethanol enhances GABA receptor function, and chronic ethanol consumption alters $GABA_A$ receptor expression. The $GABA_A$ receptor composition $\alpha4\beta2\delta$ has been proposed to play a pivotal role in ethanol responsiveness, and acute functional tolerance to ethanol seems dependent on the levels of $\gamma2$ subunit. Benzodiazepines and barbiturates that potentiate the activity of $GABA_A$ receptors are known for their development of tolerance and potential addictive activity during chronic administration. Alcohol withdrawal symptoms can be attributed in part to a functional downregulation of some types of $GABA_A$ receptors, which results in a state of hyperexcitability (disinhibition) of some neuronal pathways after ethanol is withdrawn.

Other Conditions It is progressively being recognized that abnormalities of GABA receptor subtypes play a role in other disorders. For instance, the $GABA_A$ $\alpha5$ subunit that is predominantly located in the hippocampus is involved in cognitive processing, and abnormalities of this subunit may be involved in cognitive deficits and bipolar disorders. Abnormalities in the $GABA_A$ receptor $\beta3$ subunit could be involved in anxiety and depressive disorders and insomnia. These few examples bring into context the general concept that specific abnormalities of brain $GABA_A$ receptor subunit subtypes are involved in a pleiotropy of nervous system disorders and neuropsychiatric manifestations.

Fetal Alcohol Syndrome and Fetal Alcohol Effects Ethanol enhances the ability of GABA to activate $GABA_A$ receptors but has an inhibitory effect on the activity of glutamate at NMDA and AMPA receptors. These effects are dose-related and contribute to the pleasurable effects and the mental and motor impairing effects of ethanol. At nontoxic levels, ethanol has little or no permanent deleterious effects on the adult brain; the situation in the developing brain is different. Although the deleterious effects of alcohol on the developing brain have been recognized for many years, major advances in the understanding of the biochemical basis for this have occurred only recently. As discussed previously, GABA has an excitatory effect on immature neurons in the developing brain, which promotes their differentiation and maturation. However, recent studies indicate that pharmacological potentiation of this excitatory effect by ethanol or other $GABA_A$ receptor modulators, such as barbiturates and benzodiazepines, can excessively stimulate the maturing neurons and force them into an apoptotic state. Paradoxically, recent studies also indicate that pharmacological inhibition of the ability of glutamate to activate NMDA receptors can also induce an apoptotic state in immature neurons. The mechanism underlying this effect is unclear. The modulating effects of ethanol on the physiological activity of both GABA and glutamate may account for the exceptionally detrimental effects of ethanol on the development of the CNS.

Glycine

Glycinergic neurotransmission is important in the circuits for local fast inhibitory synaptic control in the spinal cord and areas of the brainstem. Genetic defects in glycine subunit genes have been identified as causes of hypersensitive reflexes and spasticity in both humans and animals. For instance, the major form of hyperekplexia, a hereditary neurological disorder characterized by excessive startle responses, is due to a mutation in the $\alpha1$ subunit of the glycine receptor. Opportunities for pharmacotherapeutic modulation of glycine receptors are expanding based on the molecular knowledge of the receptors. Strychnine, a potent antagonist, has long been used as a poison for rodents and in humans, where it has been used as an instrument of malicious intent. Clinically relevant positive modulators of the glycine receptor include the anesthetic propofol and ethanol.

SUGGESTED CROSS-REFERENCES

The reader is encouraged to refer to the neuroanatomy of specific excitatory and inhibitory projections in Section 1.2 on neuroanatomy. Further information on the receptor transduction mechanisms can be found in Section 1.9 on electrophysiology and on genomes and proteomes in Section 1.10. Information regarding brain neuroimaging approaches can be found in Sections 1.15 and 1.16. Information on sleep mechanisms can be found in Section 1.20, and basic mechanisms of substance abuse in Section 1.22. Other related material includes the contributions of specific cortical regions and pathways in schizophrenia and other psychotic disorders in Sections 12.5 and 12.6 , the role of GABA and receptors in mood disorders in Chapter 13, and their role in anxiety disorders in Chapter 14. The clinical use of benzodiazepines is discussed in Section 31.10. Epilepsy is covered in Section 2.4, substance-related disorders in Chapter 11, and sleep disorders in Chapter 20.

REFERENCES

Barnard EA, Skolnick P, Olsen RW, Mohler H, Sieghart W, Biggio G, Braestrup C, Bateson AN, Langer SN: International Union of Pharmacology. XV. Subtypes of γ-aminobutyric acid A receptors: classification on the basis of subunit structure and receptor function. *Pharmacol Rev*. 1998;50:291.

Barnes GN, Slevin JT: Ionotropic glutamate receptor biology: effect on synaptic connectivity and function in neurological disease. *Curr Med Chem*. 2003;10:2059.

Belsham B: Glutamate and its role in psychiatric illness. *Hum Psychopharmacol*. 2001;16:139.

*Ben-Ari Y: Excitatory actions of GABA during development: the nature of the nurture. *Nat Rev Neurosci*. 2002;3:728.

Betz H, Kuhse J, Fischer M, Schmieden V, Laube B, Kuryatov A, Langosch D, Meyer G, Bormann J, Rundstrum N: Structure, diversity, and synaptic localization of inhibitory glycine receptors. *J Physiol Paris*. 1994;88:243.

Bowery NG, Bettler B, Froestl JP, Gallagher F, Marshall M, Raiteri M, Bonner TI, Enna SJ: International Union of Pharmacology. XXXIII. Mammalian γ-aminobutyric acid B receptors: structure and function. *Pharmacol Rev*. 2002;54:247.

Braithwaite SP, Meyer G, Henley JM: Interactions between AMPA receptors and intracellular proteins. *Neuropharmacology*. 2000;39:919.

Conti P, DeAmici M, De Micheli C: Selective agonists and antagonists for KA receptors. *Mini Rev Med Chem*. 2002;2:177.

*Cull-Candy S, Brickley S, Farrant M: NMDA receptor subunits: diversity, development and disease. *Curr Opin Neurobiol*. 2001;11:327.

Danbolt NC: Glutamate uptake. *Prog Neurobiol*. 2001;65:1.

Davis KM, Wu JY: Role of glutamatergic and GABAergic systems in alcoholism. *J Biomed Sci*. 2001;8:7.

Dickenson AH, Matthews EA, Suzuki R: Neurobiology of neuropathic pain: mode of action of anticonvulsants. *Eur J Pain*. 2002;6(Suppl A):51.

Gottesmann C: GABA mechanisms and sleep. *Neuroscience*. 2002;111:231.

Ikonomidou C, Bittigau P, Koch C, Genz K, Hoerster F, Federoff-Mueser U, Tenkova T, Dikranian K, Olney JW: Neurotransmitters and apoptosis in the developing brain. *Biochem Pharmacol*. 2001;62:401.

Jetty PV, Charney DS, Goddard AW: Neurobiology of generalized anxiety disorder. *Psychiatr Clin North Am*. 2001;24:75.

*Krystal JH, Sanacora G, Blumberg H, Anand A, Charney DS, Marek G, Epperson CN, Goddard A, Mason GF: Glutamate and GABA systems as targets for novel antidepressant and mood-stabilizing treatments. *Mol Psychiatry*. 2002;7(Suppl 1):S71.

Lynch DR, Guttmann RP: Excitotoxicity: perspectives based on *N*-methyl-D-aspartate receptor subtypes. *J Pharm Exp Ther*. 2002;300:717.

McCarthy MM, Auger AP, Perrot-Sinal TS: Getting excited about GABA and sex differences in the brain. *Trends Neurosci*. 2002;25:307.

McKernan RM, Whiting PJ: Which $GABA_A$-receptor subtypes really occur in the brain. *Trends Neurosci*. 1996;19:139.

Michaelis EK: Molecular biology of glutamate receptors in the central nervous system and their role in excitotoxicity, oxidative stress and aging. *Prog Neurobiol*. 1998;54:415.

Moldrich RX, Chapman AG, De Sarro G, Meldrum BS: Glutamate metabotropic receptors as targets for drug therapy in epilepsy. *Eur J Pharmacol*. 2003;476:3.

Najm I, Ying Z, Janigro D: Mechanisms of epileptogenesis. *Neurol Clin*. 2001;19:237.

Ozawa S, Kamiya H, Tsuzuki K: Glutamate receptors in the mammalian central nervous system. *Prog Neurobiol*. 1998;54:581.

Rudolph U, Crestani F, Mohler H: GABA(A) receptor subtypes: dissecting their pharmacological functions. *Trends Pharmacol Sci*. 2001;22:188.

*Sawa A, Snyder SH: Schizophrenia: diverse approaches to a complex disease. *Science* 2002;296:692.

Schoepp DD: Unveiling the functions of presynaptic metabotropic glutamate receptors in the central nervous system. *J Pharm Exp Ther*. 2001;299:12.

Sonnewald U, Qu H, Aschner M: Pharmacology and toxicology of astrocyte-neuron glutamate transport and cycling. *J Pharmacol Exp Ther*. 2002;301:1.

Spooren W, Ballard T, Gasparini F, Amalric M, Mutel V, Schreiber R: Insights into the function of Group I and Group II metabotropic glutamate (mGlu) receptors: behavioural characterization and implications for the treatment of CNS disorders. *Behav Pharmacol*. 2003;14:257.

*Stahl SM: Selective actions on sleep or anxiety by exploiting GABA-A/benzodiazepine receptor subtypes. *J Clin Psychiatry*. 2002;63:179.

Treiman DM: GABAergic mechanisms in epilepsy. *Epilepsia*. 2001;42(Suppl 3):8.

Tzschentke TM, Schmidt WJ: Glutamatergic mechanisms in addiction. *Mol Psychiatry*. 2003;8:373.

Vajda FJ: Neuroprotection and neurodegenerative disease. *J Clin Neurosci*. 2002;9:4.

Wong CG, Gottiglieri T, Snead OC 3rd: GABA, gamma-hydroxybutyric acid, and neurological disease. *Ann Neurol*. 2003;54(Suppl 6):S3.

▲ 1.6 Neuropeptides: Biology, Regulation, and Role in Neuropsychiatric Disorders

LARRY J. YOUNG, PH.D., MICHAEL J. OWENS, PH.D., AND CHARLES B. NEMEROFF, M.D., PH.D.

Over the past 30 years, the complex role of peptides in central nervous system (CNS) function has begun to emerge. Initially, the discovery and characterization of neuropeptides were led by an effort to understand the neuroendocrine regulation of pituitary hormone secretion and subsequent peripheral physiology. However, it soon became clear that many neuropeptides were widely distributed within the CNS, where they are now known to have an extraordinary array of direct or neuromodulatory effects ranging from the modulation of neurotransmitter release to the regulation of emotionality and complex behaviors. More than 100 unique, biologically active neuropeptides have been purified from biological sources (Table 1.6–1). Thus, neuropeptides represent the most diverse class of signaling molecules in the brain. These neuropeptides are often colocalized with other neuropeptide or nonpeptide neurotransmitters, refuting the tenet erroneously attributed to Sir Henry Hallet Dale of "one neuron, one transmitter." In addition to the enormous diversity in neuropeptides distributed in the brain, the actions of many peptides are mediated via multiple receptor subtypes, thereby increasing the complexity of their actions in the brain. In fact, the discovery of new peptides and receptor subtypes has outpaced current understanding of the roles of these peptides in normal or aberrant CNS function, although dysfunction at virtually any level could conceivably lead to neuropsychiatric deficits. The first half of this chapter provides a general overview of neuropeptide biology, including methods for peptide research, biosynthesis, distribution, and signaling. The second half of the chapter provides specific, detailed information for a select group of neuropeptides with special relevance to behavior and psychiatric disorders.

A *neuropeptide*, by definition, is a chain of two or more amino acids linked by peptide bonds and differs from other proteins only in the length of the amino acid chain. Neuropeptides range in length from two (e.g., carnosine and anserine) to more than 40 amino acids (e.g., corticotropin-releasing factor [CRF] and urocortin). Most of the other known active peptides fall within these size limits. By convention, peptides greater than 90 amino acids in length (approximately 10,000 molecular weight) are considered proteins. The neuropeptides highlighted in detail in this chapter include thyrotropin-releasing hormone (TRH), CRF, oxytocin (OT), arginine vasopressin (AVP), and neurotensin (NT). The structures of these neuropeptides are illustrated in Table 1.6–2 and are written, by convention, using the single letter amino acid code from the amino terminus (NH_2-) beginning on the left to the carboxyl terminus (—COOH) on the right. Of course, there are many other examples of neuropeptides of relevance to psychiatric disorders, and a brief discussion of some additional peptides of particular interest is also presented at the end of the chapter. A detailed discussion of all neuropeptide systems of potential relevance to psychiatry is beyond the scope of this chapter. TRH and CRF are hypothalamic hypophysiotropic hormones, which stimulate the release of thyroid-stimulating hormone (TSH) and adrenocorticotropic hormone (ACTH) from the adenohypophysis. OT and AVP are neurohypophysial peptides

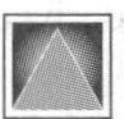

Table 1.6–1
Selected Neuropeptide Transmitters

Adrenocorticotropin hormone (ACTH)
Angiotensin
Atrial natriuretic peptide
Bombesin
Calcitonin
Calcitonin gene-related peptide (CGRP)
Cholecystokinin (CCK)
Cocaine and amphetamine regulated transcript (CART)
Corticotropin-releasing factor (CRF)
Dynorphin
β-Endorphin
Leu-enkephalin
Met-enkephalin
Galanin
Gastrin
Gonadotropin–releasing hormone (GnRH)
Growth hormone
Growth hormone-releasing hormone (GHRH; GRF)
Insulin
Motilin
Neuropeptide Y (NPY)
Neuromedin N
Neurotensin (NT)
Orexin
Orphanin FQ/Nociceptin
Oxytocin (OT)
Pancreatic polypeptide
Prolactin
Secretin
Somatostatin (SS; SRIF)
Substance K
Substance P
Thyrotropin-releasing hormone (TRH)
Urocortin
Vasoactive intestinal polypeptide (VIP)
Vasopressin (AVP; ADH)

that are released directly into the bloodstream under specific physiological conditions. However, all of these peptides, including NT, also function in the CNS as neurotransmitters, neuromodulators, or neurohormones in ways that are often quite distinct and independent from their effects on the peripheral endocrine axes. Neuropeptides have been implicated as chemical mediators in pathways subserving a variety of behavioral and physiological processes, including thermoregulation, food and water consumption, sex, sleep, locomotion, memory, learning, responses to stress and pain, and emotion. Involvement in such behavioral processes has led to the notion that peptidergic neuronal systems may contribute to the symptoms and behaviors exhibited in such major psychiatric illnesses as psychoses, mood disorders, and dementias.

INVESTIGATING NEUROPEPTIDE FUNCTION

The roles of neuropeptides in CNS function and behavior have been examined using a multitude of experimental techniques. The levels of analysis include the following: molecular structure and biosynthesis of the peptide and its receptor(s), the neuroanatomical localization of the peptide and its receptor(s), the regulation of the expression and release of the peptide, and, finally, the behavioral

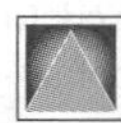

Table 1.6–2
Selected Neuropeptide Structures

Name	Amino Acid Sequence
Thyrotropin-releasing hormone (TRH)	pE-H-P-NH_2
Corticotropin-releasing factor (CRF)	S-E-E-P-P-I-S-L-D-L-T-F-H-L-L-R-E-V-L-E-M-A-R-A-E-Q-L-A-Q-Q-A-H-S-N-R-K-L-M-E-I-I-NH_2
Arginine vasopressin (AVP)	C-Y-I-Q-N-C-P-L-G-NH_2
Oxytocin (OT)	C-Y-F-Q-N-C-P-R-G-NH_2
Neurotensin (NT)	pE-L-Y-E-N-K-P-R-R-P-Y-I-L-OH

Note the cyclized glutamines at the N-terminals of TRH and NT indicated by pE-, the cysteine–cysteine disulfide bonds of AVP and OT, and the amidated carboxy-terminals of TRH, CRF, AVP, and OT.

effects of the peptide. The vast majority of information on neuropeptide biology is derived from laboratory animal studies; however, there is a growing database on the localization, activity, and potential psychiatric relevance of several neuropeptide systems in humans.

Most neuropeptide structures have been identified based on chemical analysis of purified, biologically active peptides, leading ultimately to the cloning and characterization of the genes encoding them. Characterization of the gene structure of peptides and their receptors has provided insight into the molecular regulation of these systems, and their chromosomal localization is useful in genetic studies examining the potential relationships of these genes in psychiatric disorders. Structural characterization permits the production of immunological and molecular probes that are useful in determining peptide distribution and regulation in the brain. Quantitative radioimmunoassay on microdissected brain regions or immunocytochemistry on brain sections is typically used to localize the distribution of peptide within the brain. Both techniques use specific antibodies generated against the neuropeptide to indirectly detect the presence of the peptide. Immunocytochemistry allows researchers to visualize the precise cellular localization of peptide synthesizing cells as well as their projections throughout the brain, although the technique is generally not quantitative. Using molecular probes homologous to the messenger ribonucleic acid (mRNA) encoding the peptides or receptor, in situ hybridization can be used to localize and quantify gene expression in brain sections. This is a powerful technique for examining the molecular regulation of neuropeptide synthesis with precise neuroanatomical resolution, which is impossible for other classes of nonpeptide neurotransmitters that are not derived directly from the translation of mRNAs, such as dopamine, serotonin, and norepinephrine. In addition to immunocytochemistry and in situ hybridization, receptor autoradiography on brain sections or "bind and grind" receptor binding assays on microdissected brain tissue are frequently used to localize and quantify neuropeptide receptors in specific regions of the brain. Receptor autoradiography involves allowing a radiolabeled ligand to bind the receptor on a thin slice of tissue and then detecting the bound by visualizing it on X-ray film or other means. Other molecular techniques, such as Northern blot analysis, ribonuclease protection assay, and polymerase chain reaction, are also commonly used to measure neuropeptide and receptor expression and regulation by quantifying the mRNAs encoding the peptide or receptor. However, quantification of neuropeptide gene expression or immunoreactivity within a cell or tissue homogenate does not provide information on neuropeptide release. In vivo microdialysis, in which peptide concentrated in the extracellular fluid is collected at sequential time intervals using dialysis probes implanted into specific brain regions, may be used to quantify neuropeptide release under defined physiological or behavioral circumstances.

Generally, the behavioral effects of neuropeptides are initially investigated by infusions of the peptide directly into the brain. Unlike many nonpeptide neurotransmitters, neuropeptides do not penetrate the blood–brain barrier in amounts sufficient enough to produce CNS effects. Furthermore, serum and tissue enzymes tend to degrade the peptides before they reach their target sites. The degradation is usually the result of the cleavage of specific amino acid sequences targeted by a specific peptidase designed for that purpose. Thus, intracerebroventricular or site-specific infusions of peptide are generally required to probe for behavioral effects. However, there are some examples of delivery of neuropeptides via intranasal infusions in human subjects, which, in some cases, has been shown to permit access of the peptide to the brain.

In many cases, the interpretation of neuropeptide infusion studies is complicated because of the considerable cross-talk between specific neuropeptides and several heterologous receptors. For example, OT and vasopressin differ at only two of nine amino acids and both peptides cross-react with both receptor types. In some cases, highly selective synthetic agonists or antagonists have been developed that allow researchers to examine the role of specific neuropeptide receptors in the regulation of behavior or physiological processes. In addition, transgenic and knock-out mouse approaches are becoming more and more commonly used as approaches to investigate neuropeptide function. For example, mutant mouse strains with null mutations in either the peptide gene or the corresponding receptor have been developed and have proven quite useful for exploring the role of neuropeptides in behavioral processes.

As noted above, one of the greatest impediments for exploring the role and potential therapeutic value of neuropeptides is the inability of the peptides or their agonists/antagonists to penetrate the blood–brain barrier. Thus, the behavioral effects of most peptides in humans are largely uninvestigated. However, in some instances, small molecule, nonpeptide agonists/antagonists have been developed that can be administered peripherally and permeate the blood–brain barrier in sufficient quantities to affect receptor activation. This will likely lead to a better understanding of the roles of these peptides in both normal human behavior and various psychopathologies.

Humans are less-than-ideal subjects for neuropeptide research for several reasons. First, although blood samples to determine plasma hormone concentrations are relatively easy to obtain, the independent regulation of peripheral and CNS peptide release, the high concentration of plasma peptidases, and the blood–brain barrier make it virtually impossible to infer CNS peptide physiology from plasma hormone concentrations. Also, the use of biopsy to directly assess tissue peptide concentrations is not ideal, as it is not routinely repeatable, is limited to superficial structures, and suffers from potential morbidity. In contrast, however, cerebrospinal fluid (CSF) has been shown to reflect extracellular fluid concentrations of transmitter substances, is in direct contact with the CNS, is screened from peripheral serum sources by the blood–brain barrier, and may be sampled across time. The limitations of human CSF studies include a lack of information about the regional CNS source of any changes in peptide concentration detected; the use of lumbar CSF, which is somewhat removed from higher forebrain CNS sources of peptides and subject to spinal cord peptide contributions; and the potentially confounding effects of previous drug treatments or disease episodes. Postmortem tissue studies of neuropeptide concentration changes in psychiatric disease have been informative in many cases, but interpretation must include consideration of postmortem delay, previous drug treatment, and coexisting illnesses. Most of the data on alterations in CSF or tissue concentrations of neurotransmitters have been derived from comparisons between diagnostically defined psychiatric groups and control groups. However, the controls may be so-called neurological or psychiatric controls, not healthy volunteers, and the accuracy and consistency of the diagnoses may be less than optimal. In addition, the etiology of a syndromal diagnosis may differ among subjects in the same diagnostic group. Even after matching for age, gender, or other demographic variables, heterogeneity among human research populations results in individual variations of absolute peptide values that are often quite wide. Such variances severely reduce the power of group comparisons to detect alterations in peptide concentrations. The use of pretreatment and posttreatment CSF sample or of samples obtained during the active disease state versus when the patient is in remission addresses some of the serious limitations in study design. For such progressive diseases as schizophrenia and Alzheimer's disease, serial CSF samples may be a valuable indicator of disease progression or response to treatment. Even with these constraints, significant progress has been made in describing the effects of various psychiatric disease states on neuropeptide systems in the CNS.

BIOSYNTHESIS

Unlike other neurotransmitters, the biosynthesis of a neuropeptide involves transcription of an mRNA from a specific gene, translation of a polypeptide preprohormone encoded by that mRNA, and then posttranslational processing involving proteolytic cleavage of the preprohormone to yield the active neuropeptide. Over the past 20 years, the gene structures and biosynthetic pathways of many neuropeptides have been elucidated. The gene structure of selected neuropeptides is illustrated in Figure 1.6–1. Neuropeptide genes are generally composed of multiple exons that encode a protein preprohormone. The N-terminus of the preprohormone contains a signal peptide (SP) sequence, which guides the growing polypeptide to the rough endoplasmic reticulum (RER) membrane. The single preprohormone molecule often contains the sequences of multiple peptides that are subsequently separated by proteolytic cleavage by specific enzymes. For example, translation of the gene encoding NT yields a preprohormone, which, on enzymatic cleavage, produces both NT and neuromedin N. Other neuropeptide genes, such as the TRH gene, encode multiple copies of the peptide sequence or, as in the case of OT and vasopressin, also encode other proteins essential in the posttranslational processing and transport of the neuropeptide. The neuroanatomical localization and abundance of neuropeptides are determined primarily by the region-specific expression and regulation of its gene. Each neuropeptide gene is expressed in well-defined populations of neurons within the brain. The precise neuroanatomical pattern of peptide hormone gene expression is determined by regulatory deoxyribonucleic acid (DNA) sequences surrounding the gene. This has been elegantly demonstrated for the OT gene. OT is expressed in a subset of magnocellular neurons in the paraventricular nucleus (PVN) of the hypothalamus. Transgenic mice in which the rat OT gene has been inserted into their genome along with the surrounding regulatory regions express the rat OT transgene specifically in oxytocinergic magnocellular neurons of the hypothalamus. Smaller constructs lacking these regulatory regions did not result in the correct expression patterns in the brain. Transcription factor binding sites located in the promoter of the gene are also involved in the physiological regulation of peptide gene expression. Analysis of promoter sequences of peptide genes has provided insights into the molecular regulation of peptide biosynthesis.

The mRNAs encoding the preprohormone are translated by ribosomes associated with the RER, and the growing polypeptide is

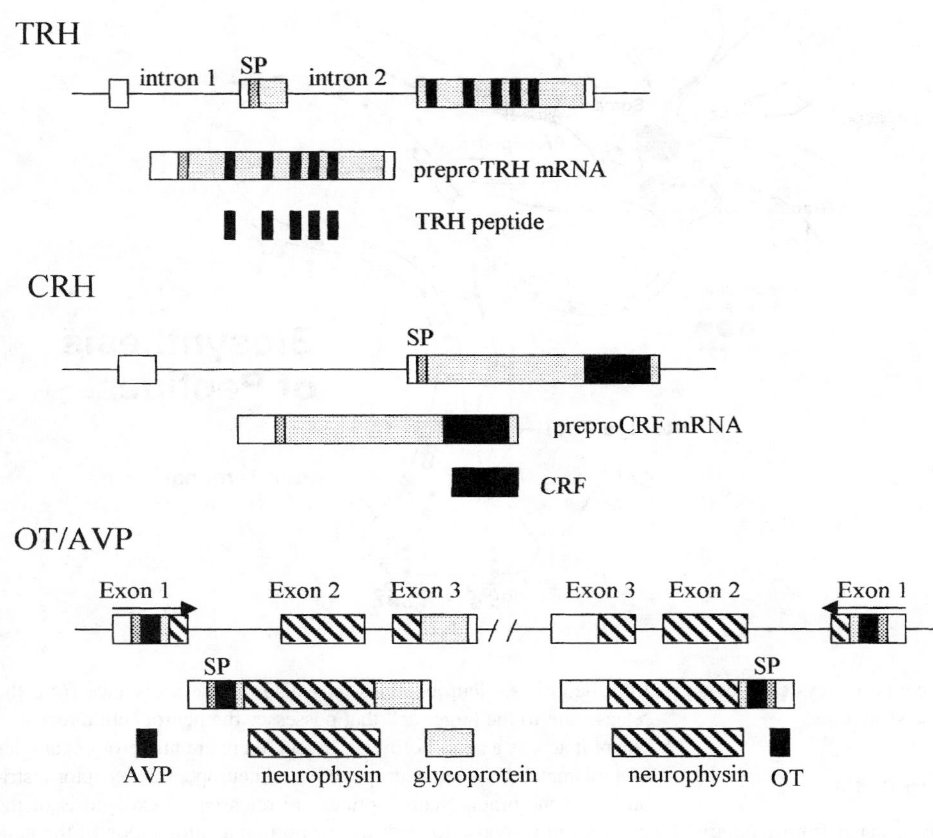

FIGURE 1.6–1 Schematics illustrating the gene structure, preprohormone messenger RNA (mRNA), and processed neuropeptides of thyrotropin-releasing hormone (TRH), corticotropin-releasing factor (CRF), oxytocin (OT), arginine vasopressin (AVP), and neurotensin (NT). Boxed regions indicate the locations of the exons in the respective genes. Shaded regions and hatched regions indicate coding regions. Each preprohormone begins with a signal peptide (SP) sequence. Black boxes indicate the location of the sequences encoding the neuropeptide.

translated into the cisternae of the RER, with SP anchored in the RER membrane. Once translated, the SP of the *pre*prohormone is cleaved by a signal endopeptidase, freeing the *pro*hormone polypeptide. The prohormone is then shuttled to the Golgi apparatus, where packaging into granules or vesicles occurs. Proteolytic cleavage of the prohormone into the biologically active neuropeptide begins in the Golgi and continues in the granules. Production of biologically active neuropeptides from prohormones begins with cleavage at specific sites adjacent to the neuropeptide sequence by specific endopeptidases known as *prohormone convertases*. Prohormone convertases cleave generally at pairs of basic amino acids (e.g., Lys–Arg, Lys–Lys, and Arg–Arg) flanking the neuropeptide sequence. There are at least seven prohormone convertases, each with unique properties, including substrate specificity and neuroendocrine distribution. Prohormone convertases are copackaged with the prohormones in the granules at the Golgi apparatus. The substrate specificity and differential distribution of the prohormone convertases provides a mechanism by which different neuropeptides encoded by a single prohormone can be differentially produced in an active form. After endopeptidase cleavage, the peptide fragments are subjected to exoproteolysis by carboxypeptidases or aminopeptidases or both to remove the residual basic residues on the carboxy or amino terminus of the peptide fragments. The synthesis and processing of neuropeptides is illustrated in Figure 1.6–2.

Although many known peptides are complete and biologically active when cleaved from the prohormone, many others are subjected to additional posttranslational processing. Certain peptides have a metabolically blocked carboxy terminus that is often amidated. A glycine residue in the prohormone sequence often acts as the amide donor and, in the case of TRH, is attacked by a monooxygenase that is contained in secretory granules. TRH is further processed on the N-terminus, where glutamine is cyclized by a glutamylcyclase to yield a pyroglutamyl moiety. These alterations are usually effective in reducing susceptibility to degradation and are often required for biological activity, as is the case for TRH, which is rendered inactive when the C-terminal amide is removed by proline endopeptidase to generate the free-acid structure. Other posttranslational processing events for active peptides include glycosylation, phosphorylation, and the formation of disulfide bonds, which are often required for either biological activity or transport. Several neu-

FIGURE 1.6–2 The peptide neuron. The figure shows the main steps in the chain of events from the information stored in the DNA molecule to the peripherally detected peptide fragments. The DNA sequence in the nucleus is transcribed to the messenger RNA (mRNA) molecule for further transport to the endoplasmic reticulum, where a translation takes place to form a large preproprotein. This protein is prepared for axonal transport by packaging into neurosecretory vesicles or granules within the Golgi complex. During transport, the preproprotein is processed by specific cleavage enzymes into active and inactive peptide fragments. After release, the peptides are further degraded into smaller peptide fragments or constituent amino acids. (Courtesy of Thomas Davis, Ph.D.)

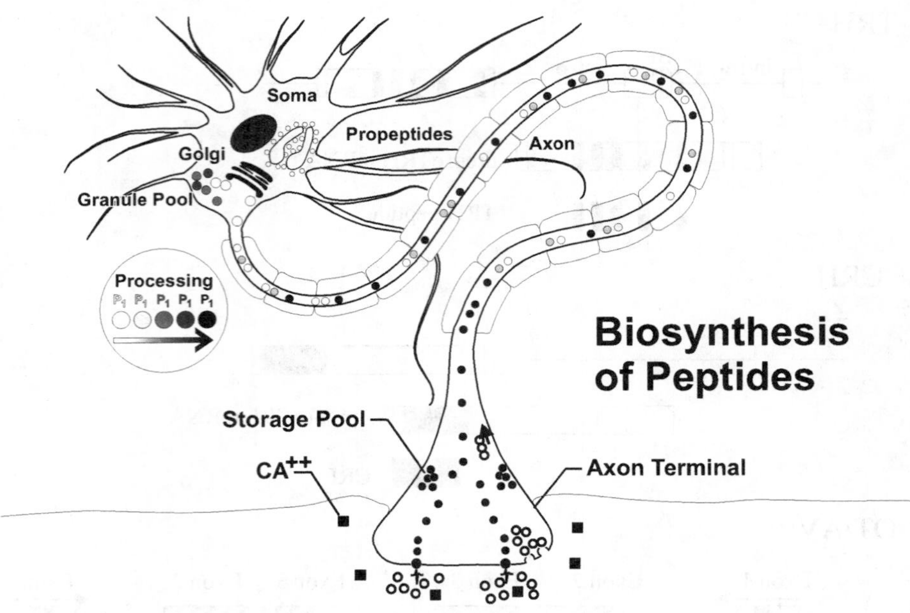

ropeptides, including OT and vasopressin, contain a cysteine–cysteine disulfide bond resulting in cyclic peptide structures.

DISTRIBUTION AND REGULATION

Although many neuropeptides were originally isolated from pituitary and peripheral tissues, the majority of neuropeptides were subsequently found to be widely distributed throughout the brain. These peptides involved in regulating pituitary secretion are concentrated in the hypothalamus. Hypothalamic releasing and inhibiting factors are produced in neurosecretory neurons adjacent to the third ventricle that send projections to the median eminence, where they contact and release peptide into the portal circulatory system. Peptides produced in these neurons are often subject to regulation by the peripheral hormones they regulate. For example, TRH regulates the secretion of thyroid hormones, and thyroid hormones negatively feedback on TRH gene expression. However, neuropeptide-expressing neurons and their projections are found in many other brain regions, including limbic structures, the midbrain, the hindbrain, and the spinal cord. Neuropeptides are often colocalized with other neurotransmitters and other neuropeptides. The colocalization of neuropeptides within classic neurotransmitter circuits suggests an interaction between these systems, and the modulation of monoamine neurotransmitter (e.g., dopamine, norepinephrine) function by neuropeptides is common. These interactions have stimulated speculation concerning the involvement of neuropeptides in the underlying pathophysiology of psychiatric disorders.

NEUROPEPTIDE SIGNALING

Neuropeptides may act as neurotransmitters, neuromodulators, or neurohormones. Neurotransmitters are typically released from axonal terminals into a synapse, where they change the postsynaptic membrane potential, either depolarizing or hyperpolarizing the cell. For classic neurotransmitters, this often involves direct modulation of voltage-gated ion channels. In contrast, neuromodulators and neurohormones do not directly affect the firing of the target cell itself but may alter the response of the cell to other neurotransmitters through modulation of second messenger pathways. Neuropeptide release is not restricted to synapses or axon terminals but may occur throughout the axon or even from dendrites. Neuropeptides may also diffuse a distance from the release site to the target cell that possesses the neuropeptide receptor, where it acts as a neurohormone. In fact, there are numerous examples of a mismatch between neuropeptide and neuropeptide receptor distribution in the brain. Neuropeptides are released by exocytosis of the granules in response to electrical or hormonal stimulation of the neuron containing the neuron. Stimulation results in an increase in intracellular calcium concentrations, which leads to the fusion of the peptidergic granules to the plasma membrane and expulsion of the peptide into the extracellular space.

The cellular signaling of neuropeptides is mediated by specific neuropeptide receptors. Thus, understanding neuropeptide receptor function is essential for understanding neuropeptide biology. Neuropeptide receptors have undergone the same process of discovery and characterization that receptors for other neurotransmitters have enjoyed. The vast majority of neuropeptide receptors are G-protein–coupled, seven-transmembrane domain receptors belonging to the same family of proteins as the monoamine receptors. Each neuropeptide receptor is specifically coupled to one type of G protein (e.g., G_s, G_i, G_q). Depending on the subtype of G protein with which the receptor interacts, receptor activation may result in the stimulation or inhibition of specific second messenger pathways. The most common types of receptor signaling pathways involve the activated G protein modulating the activity of either adenylate cyclase or phospholipase C. Stimulation of adenylate cyclase results in an increase in cyclic adenosine monophosphate (cAMP) concentrations, whereas stimulation of phospholipase C results in an increase in diacylglycerol and inositol triphosphate (IP_3). These responses then lead to increases in intracellular calcium concentrations, activation of protein kinases, and, ultimately, a host of cellular responses, including altered gene expression.

Many neuropeptides exert their effects through multiple different subtypes of receptors, which have different affinities for the peptides and activate different second messenger pathways. These different receptor subtypes are typically differentially distributed throughout the brain. Furthermore, many receptors may be modulated by more than one neuropeptide. For example, there are three subtypes of the vasopressin receptor, the V1a, V1b, and V2 subtypes, with the V1a and V1b predominating in the brain and the V2 localized in the kidney. Each of these receptor subtypes exhibits a unique tissue distribution, interacts with different G proteins, and activates different second messenger systems. In addition, OT may stimulate the vasopressin receptor subtypes, and vasopressin may stimulate the OT receptor. Likewise, the two CRF receptors are differentially localized within the brain, and both receptors can be modulated by both CRF and urocortin, making it difficult to ascertain the relative role of each receptor in CRF functioning.

Molecular technology has made it possible to clone and characterize neuropeptide receptor genes and complementary DNAs (cDNAs). This is most often accomplished in one of three ways. First, the neuropeptide receptor protein is biochemically purified and partially sequenced, which allows the development of oligonucleotide probes that can be used to isolate the cDNA encoding the protein from a cDNA library. A second approach involves producing expression libraries in which cells containing the receptor cDNA can be isolated based on their ability to bind to radiolabeled peptide ligands. Finally, many neuropeptide receptors are isolated based on their sequence homology with other known peptide receptors. Once the cDNA of the receptor has been isolated, it can be used to produce purified receptor protein for structural and functional studies. By mutating specific amino acids in the receptor structure and determining relative binding affinities of peptides with various amino acid substitutions, it is possible to elucidate the nature of the ligand-receptor interaction. This information facilitates the development of drugs that specifically modulate receptor function, leading to the ability to manipulate peptide systems in ways that are currently enjoyed by the more classic neurotransmitters. The availability of cDNAs encoding the receptor also permits the neuroanatomical mapping of the receptor-producing cells in the brain, which is critical for understanding the neural circuits modulated by the peptide. Finally, with the cloned receptor in hand, it is possible to use transgenic techniques, such as targeted gene overexpression, or gene knock-outs to further elucidate the functions of these receptors. However, these techniques cannot provide information on the functions of specific receptor populations within the brain or distinguish the role of developmental versus acute receptor activation.

The three factors that determine the biological role of a neuropeptide hormone are (1) the temporal–anatomical release of the peptide, (2) functional coupling of the neuropeptide receptor to intracellular signaling pathways, and (3) the cell type and circuits in which the receptor is expressed. Genetic studies have demonstrated that regulatory sequences flanking the receptor coding region determine the expression pattern of the receptor and, thus, the physiological and behavioral response to the neuropeptide. For example, mice and voles differ in the localization of AVP receptors in the brain, and they also differ in their behavioral response to AVP. However, when transgenic mice were created carrying the vole AVP receptor gene with the flanking regulatory sequences, the mice expressed the receptor in a pattern similar to that of the vole and then displayed behavioral responses to AVP similar to that of voles. This study suggests that changes in the regulatory region of a neuropeptide receptor gene could result in significant differences in neuropeptide function and, thus, could potentially be relevant to psychiatric disorders. Many receptor genes have now been localized to specific chromosomal loci and are being examined in genetic studies for associations with psychiatric disorders.

Historically, the inability to block specific neuropeptide signals pharmacologically has severely hindered research into the roles of the endogenous peptides in various behaviors and physiological effects. However, for many neuropeptide receptors, selective agonists and antagonists are now available that have been extremely informative in preclinical studies to examine receptor function. As mentioned above, most of these compounds are derivatives of the peptide hormone and therefore do not pass the blood–brain barrier. More recently, a number of pharmaceutical companies have synthesized nonpeptidergic, lipophilic compounds that can pass the blood–brain barrier and may act as neuropeptide agonists or antagonists. The development of these types of compounds is essential for understanding the role of neuropeptide receptor function in human behavior and may also be useful in the development of radioligands for positron emission tomography (PET) to study receptor distribution in living human subjects. These compounds also hold promise as therapeutic agents in the treatment of certain psychiatric disorders.

PEPTIDASES

Unlike monoamine neurotransmitters, peptides are not actively taken up by presynaptic nerve terminals. Rather, released peptides are degraded into smaller fragments and, eventually, into single amino acids by specific enzymes termed *peptidases*. The enzymes may be found bound to post- or presynaptic neural membranes or in solution in the cytoplasm and extracellular fluid and are distributed widely in peripheral organs and serum, as well as in the CNS. As a result, neuropeptides generally have half-lives on the order of minutes, once released. There are several general classes of peptidases, with several distinct enzymes in each class. These classes include the serine endopeptidases, containing such enzymes as trypsin and chymotrypsin; the thiol peptidases, such as pyroglutamate amino peptidase and cathepsin B and C; the acid proteases, such as pepsin and renin; the metalloendopeptidases, such as neural endopeptidase and angiotensin-converting enzymes (ACEs); and the metalloexopeptidases, such as the aminopeptidases and the carboxypeptidases (e.g., enkephalin-convertase and carboxypeptidase A and B). These degradative enzymes are often the same as those used in processing but have different subcellular locations. An example is carboxypeptidase B, which cleaves the dibasic amino acid residues flanking the active peptide sequence in the prohormone during processing or reduces activity at the receptor if the peptide, like NT, contains dibasic amino acids in the active sequence. Peptidases have pH and temperature optimums for activity and can be inhibited by various chemicals or chelators or by amino acid substitution at vulnerable points in the peptide chain. Alterations in peptidase activity or concentration can contribute to alterations in the synaptic availability of a peptide, and the regulation of peptidase levels may be as exquisitely controlled as receptor number and peptide synthesis and release. Cleavage of the actively released form of the peptide usually ends, or significantly reduces, biological activity, but examples abound of partial or complete receptor activation by partially metabolized peptides or their fragments.

Peptidases offer yet another potential opportunity for the integration and regulation of neuropeptide transmitter actions and synaptic availability. Because the present peptidase inhibitors are relatively nonspecific in their ability to inhibit various peptidases, there have been few attempts to influence peptide concentrations by pharmacological blockade of their associated peptidases. The ACE inhibitors, such as captopril, are one exception to this generality. It is expected that second- and third-generation peptidase inhibitors, with discrete peptidase and possibly regional specificity, will be developed that eventually may allow the truly elegant manipulation of endogenous neuropeptide concentrations.

SPECIFIC NEUROPEPTIDES AS PROTOTYPES OF NEUROPEPTIDE BIOLOGY

Thyrotropin-Releasing Hormone In 1969, TRH, a pyroglutamylhistidylprolinamide tripeptide (Table 1.6–2), became the first of the hypothalamic releasing hormones to be isolated and characterized. The discovery of the structure of this hormone led to the conclusive demonstration that peptide hormones secreted from the hypothalamus regulate secretion of hormones from the anterior pituitary. The gene for TRH in humans resides on chromosome 3. In the rat, it consists of three exons (coding regions) separated by two introns (noncoded sequences) (Fig. 1.6–1). The first exon contains the 5' untranslated region of the mRNA encoding the TRH preprohormone; the second exon contains the SP sequence and much of the remaining amino terminal end of the precursor peptide; and the third contains the remainder of the sequence, including five copies of the TRH precursor sequence, the carboxy terminal region, and the 3' untranslated region. The 5' flanking of the gene, or promoter, contains sequences homologous to the glucocorticoid receptor and the thyroid hormone receptor binding sites, providing a mechanism for the regulation of this gene by cortisol and negative feedback by thyroid hormone. Enzymatic processing of TRH begins with excision of the progenitor peptides by carboxy peptidases, amidation of the C-terminal proline and cyclization of the N-terminal glutamine, to yield five TRH molecules per prohormone molecule. TRH is widely distributed in the CNS with TRH immunoreactive neurons located in the olfactory bulbs, entorhinal cortices, hippocampus, extended amygdala, hypothalamus, and midbrain structures. As is the case for most neuropeptides, the TRH receptor is also a member of the seven-transmembrane domain, G-protein–coupled receptor family.

Hypothalamic TRH neurons project nerve terminals to the median eminence, where they release TRH into the hypothalamo-hypophyseal portal system, where it is transported to the adenohypophysis, causing the release of TSH into systemic circulation. TSH subsequently stimulates the release of the thyroid hormones, triiodothyronine (T_3) and thyroxine (T_4), from the thyroid gland. TRH neurons in the PVN contain thyroid hormone receptors and respond to increases in thyroid hormone secretion with a decrease in TRH gene expression and synthesis. This negative feedback of thyroid hormones onto the TRH-synthesizing neurons was first demonstrated by a decrease in TRH content in the median eminence, but not in the PVN of the hypothalamus, after thyroidectomy. This effect can be reversed with exogenous thyroid hormone treatment. The treatment of normal rats with exogenous thyroid hormone decreases TRH concentration in the PVN and posterior nucleus of the hypothalamus. Using a probe against the TRH preprohormone mRNA, in situ hybridization studies have demonstrated that TRH mRNA is increased in the PVN 14 days after thyroidectomy. Unilateral T_3 implants prevent the increase in TRH mRNA observed on the contralateral untreated side in propylthiouracil-induced hypothyroidism. The ability of thyroid hormones to regulate TRH mRNA can be superseded by other stimuli that activate the hypothalamic-pituitary-thyroid (HPT) axis. In this regard, repeated exposure to cold (which releases TRH from the median eminence) induces increases in the levels of TRH mRNA in the PVN despite concomitantly elevated concentrations of thyroid hormones. Further evidence of the different levels of communication of the HPT axis are seen in the ability of TRH to regulate the production of mRNA for the pituitary TRH receptor and for TRH concentrations to regulate the mRNA coding for both the α and β subunits of the TSH molecule. The latter effect has been shown to be dependent on intracellular calcium and protein kinase C. The regulatory interplay also extends to the accessible pools of second messenger phosphoinositides, whose pool size is regulated by TRH receptor number. TRH-containing synaptic boutons have been observed in contact with TRH-containing cell bodies in the medial and periventricular subdivisions of the PVN, thus providing anatomical evidence for ultrashort feedback regulation of TRH concentrations there. Negative feedback by thyroid hormones may be limited to the hypothalamic TRH neurons, as negative feedback on TRH synthesis by thyroid hormones has not been found in extrahypothalamic TRH neurons.

The early availability of adequate tools to assess HPT axis function (i.e., radioimmunoassays, synthetic peptides), coupled with observations that primary hypothyroidism is associated with depressive symptomatology, ensured extensive investigation of the involvement of this axis in affective disorders. Early studies established the hypothalamic and extrahypothalamic distribution of TRH. This extrahypothalamic presence of TRH quickly led to speculation that TRH might function as a neurotransmitter or neuromodulator. Indeed, a large body of evidence supports such a role for TRH. Within the CNS, TRH is known to modulate several different neurotransmitters, including dopamine, serotonin, acetylcholine, and the opioids. TRH has been shown to arouse hibernating animals and counteracts the behavioral response and hypothermia produced by a variety of CNS depressants, including barbiturates and ethanol.

Interest in putative CNS actions of TRH was stimulated by studies of the HPT axis and depression by Arthur Prange and colleagues. Nearly three decades ago, it was hypothesized that thyroid function was integral to the pathogenesis of, and recovery from, affective disorders due to the numerous interactions among thyroid hormones, catecholamines, and adrenergic receptors in the CNS. Overall, these studies suggested a role for thyroid dysfunction in refractory depression and are consonant with clinical studies suggesting the existence of an increased rate of hypothyroidism among patients with refractory depression.

The use of TRH as a provocative agent for assessment of HPT axis function evolved rapidly after its isolation and synthesis. Clinical use of a standardized TRH stimulation test revealed blunting of the TSH response in approximately 25 percent of euthyroid patients with major depression. These data have been widely confirmed. The observed TSH blunting in depressed patients does not appear to be the result of excessive negative feedback due to hyperthyroidism, because thyroid measures, such as basal plasma concentrations, of TSH and thyroid hormones are generally in the normal range in these patients. It is possible that TSH blunting is a reflection of pituitary TRH receptor downregulation as a result of median eminence hypersecretion of endogenous TRH. Indeed, the observation that CSF TRH concentrations are elevated in depressed patients, as compared to controls, supports the hypothesis of TRH hypersecretion but does not elucidate the regional CNS origin of this tripeptide. These elevations of CSF TRH concentration may be relatively specific to depression, as no such alteration has been reported in patients with Alzheimer's disease, anxiety disorders, or alcoholism. However, it is not clear whether elevated TRH activity in the CNS and in the HPT axis represents a causal mechanism underlying the symptoms of depression or simply a secondary effect of alterations in other neural systems affected in depression.

Corticotropin-Releasing Factor In the 1950s, it was observed that pituitary extracts contained a factor, referred to as *CRF*, that could stimulate the release of ACTH from anterior pituitary cells in vivo. After a search spanning nearly three decades, Wylie Vale and colleagues isolated and characterized CRF as a 41–amino acid peptide in 1981. The gene for CRF in humans is located on chromosome 8q13 and is composed of two exons, with the CRF preprohormone being encoded entirely on exon 2 (Fig. 1.6–1). More recently, a related neuropeptide, urocortin, has been identified and shares similar gene structures. CRF is the primary hypothalamic ACTH secretogogue in most species, and it also functions as an extrahypothalamic neurotransmitter in a CNS network that, apparently, coordinates global responses to stressors. There is convincing evidence to support the hypothesis that CRF plays a complex role in integrating the endocrine, autonomic, immunological, and behavioral responses of an organism to stress.

Although it was originally isolated because of its functions in regulating the HPA axis, CRF is widely distributed throughout the brain. The PVN of the hypothalamus is the major site of CRF-containing cells bodies that influence anterior pituitary hormone secretion. These neurons originate in the parvocellular region of the PVN and send axon terminals to the median eminence, where CRF is released into the portal system in response to stressful stimuli. A small group of PVN neurons also project to the brainstem and spinal cord, where they regulate autonomic aspects of the stress response. CRF-containing neurons are also found in other hypothalamic nuclei, the neocortex, the extended amygdala, the brainstem, and the spinal cord. Central CRF infusion into laboratory animals produces physiological changes and behavioral effects similar to those observed after stress, including increased locomotor activity, increased responsiveness to an acoustic startle, and decreased exploratory behavior in an open field.

In a manner similar to that described for TRH, CRF gene expression and content in the PVN are negatively related by glucocorticoids (cortisol) and positively regulated by a wide variety of stressors. Adrenalectomy results in an increase in CRF mRNA content in the PVN, whereas glucocorticoid replacement decreases CRF mRNA content in a dose-dependent manner. Interestingly, glucocorticoids increase, rather than decrease, CRF mRNA content in the amygdala.

CRF is also found in the raphe nuclei and the locus ceruleus (LC), the origin of the major serotonergic and noradrenergic projections to the forebrain, respectively, circuits long postulated to play a role in the pathophysiology of depression and anxiety. Increased anxiety observed after direct CNS administration of CRF has been hypothesized to be associated, in part, with increased noradrenergic activity. Stress has been shown to produce an increase in CRF content in the LC and a decrease in CRF concentrations in the median eminence (consistent with increased release). Other studies have shown that CRF-containing nerve terminals impinge on noradrenergic neurons of the LC and that exogenous CRF applied to those neurons alters their firing rate. Some of the noradrenergic LC neurons, in turn, project to the hypothalamic PVN, where their input increases CRF synthesis and release. Because CRF injection into the LC elicits fearful or anxious behavior, one could postulate that stress activates the CRF neurons terminating on the LC noradrenergic neurons, which may then, acting along with other inputs to the PVN, stimulate the stress-induced increased release of CRF from the median eminence. Interestingly, adult animals exposed to maternal separation early in life, an animal model for early adverse childhood experiences, exhibit elevated CRF concentrations in the LC and exaggerated HPA response to stress.

The actions of CRF and the related urocortin peptide are mediated by at least two receptor subtypes, CRF_1 and CRF_2. The CRF_1 receptor is abundantly expressed in the cerebral cortex, cerebellum, medial septum, and anterior pituitary, whereas the CRF_2 receptor is predominantly found in the lateral septum, ventromedial hypothalamus, and choroid plexus. The CRF_1 receptor appears to be the predominant receptor mediating the effects of CRF in the stress response. The CRF_2 receptor has a 40-fold higher affinity for urocortin relative to CRF. Urocortin has a unique distribution, being concentrated in the Edinger-Westphal nucleus and the lateral superior olive. In the lateral septum, urocortin terminals overlap with the distribution of the CRF_2 receptor. Thus, urocortin has been proposed to be the endogenous ligand for the CRF_2 receptor, but little is known regarding its physiological role. As expected, CRF_1 receptor knock-out mice display decreased anxiety-like behavior, have an impaired stress response, and exhibit elevated CRF mRNA expression in the PVN due to a lack of negative feedback. In contrast, CRF_2 receptor knock-out mice display increased anxiety-like behavior and are hypersensitive to stress.

Hyperactivity of the HPA axis in major depression remains one of the most consistent findings in biological psychiatry. The reported HPA axis alterations in major depression include hypercortisolemia, resistance to dexamethasone suppression of cortisol secretion, blunted ACTH responses to intravenous CRF challenge, and elevated CSF CRF concentrations. The exact pathological mechanism(s) underlying HPA axis dysregulation in major depression and other affective disorders remains to be elucidated.

Once the phenomenon of HPA axis hyperactivity in patients with major depression was established, many research groups utilized various provocative neuroendocrine challenge tests as a "window into the brain" in attempts to elucidate pathophysiological mechanisms. In normal subjects, the CRF stimulation test, using either rat/human or ovine CRF, yields robust ACTH, β-endorphin, β-lipotropin, and cortisol responses after intravenous or subcutaneous administration. However, in patients with major depression, blunting of ACTH or β-endorphin secretion with a normal cortisol response has been repeatedly reported. Patients with posttraumatic stress disorder (PTSD), 50 percent of whom also fulfilled DSM-III (*Diagnostic and Statistical Manual of Mental Disorders*) criteria for major depression, also showed blunted ACTH secretion in response to a CRF challenge. Importantly, researchers have reported normalization of the ACTH response to CRF after clinical recovery from depression, suggesting that the blunted ACTH response, like dexamethasone nonsuppression, may be a state marker for depression. Early-life stress apparently sensitizes the HPA axis and leads to a greater risk of developing depression later in life. Depressed women who were victims of childhood abuse exhibit an exaggerated ACTH and cortisol response to a psychosocial stressor, presumably due to hypersecretion of CRF.

Mechanistically, two hypotheses have been advanced to account for the ACTH blunting after exogenous CRF administration. The first hypothesis suggests that pituitary CRF receptor downregulation occurs as a result of hypothalamic CRF hypersecretion. The second hypothesis postulates altered sensitivity of the pituitary to glucocorticoid negative feedback. Substantial support has accumulated favoring the first hypothesis. However, neuroendocrine studies represent a secondary measure of CNS activity; the pituitary ACTH responses principally reflect the activity of hypothalamic CRF rather than that of the corticolimbic CRF circuits, which are most likely to be involved in the pathophysiology of depression.

A potentially more direct method for the evaluation of extrahypothalamic CRF tone may be obtained from measurements of CSF CRF concentrations. A marked dissociation between CSF and plasma neuropeptide concentrations has been described, thus indicating that neuropeptides are secreted directly into CSF from brain tissue as opposed to being derived from plasma-to-CSF transfer. Evidence that CSF CRF concentrations originate from extrahypothalamic CRF neurons has been obtained from studies in which CSF CRF concentrations were repeatedly measured over the course of the day. Two independent research groups reported that CSF CRF concentrations in rhesus monkeys are not entrained with pituitary-adrenal activity. The proximity of corticolimbic, brainstem, and spinal CRF neurons to the ventricular system of the brain suggests that these areas make substantial contributions to the CSF CRF pool.

A series of studies have demonstrated significant elevations of CSF CRF concentrations in drug-free patients with major depression

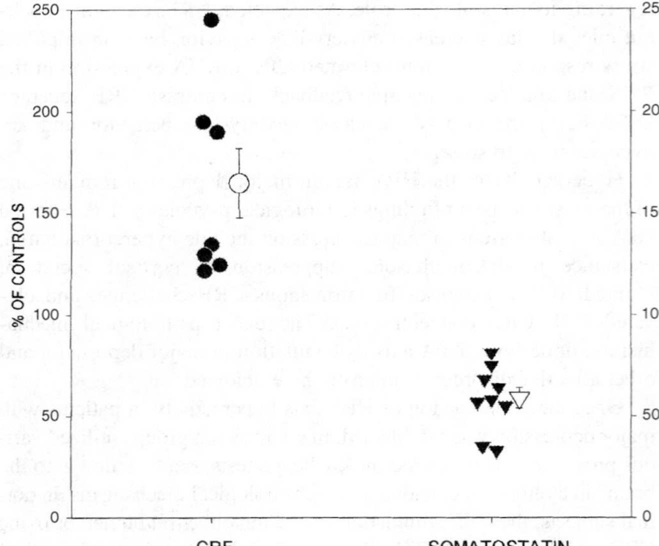

FIGURE 1.6–3 Scatterplot showing the mean cerebrospinal fluid (CSF) corticotropin-releasing factor (CRF) or somatostatin concentrations in patients with major depression. Each individual point represents an individual study. Mean percent control ± standard error of mean for all studies shown by hollow symbols. (Adapted from Owens MJ, Plotsky PM, Nemeroff CB. Peptides and affective disorders. In: Watson SJ, ed. *Biology of Schizophrenia and Affective Disorders.* Washington: American Psychiatric Press Inc., 1996:259.)

or in patients who have committed suicide (Fig. 1.6–3). Additionally, severity of depression appears to correlate significantly with CSF CRF concentrations in patients with anorexia nervosa, multiple sclerosis, and Huntington's disease. The elevation of CSF CRF concentrations in patients with anorexia nervosa reverts to the normal range as these patients approach normal body weight. No alterations of CSF CRF concentrations have been reported in other psychiatric disorders, including mania, panic disorder, and somatization disorders, as compared to controls. A recent study used radioimmunocytochemistry to quantify CRF in specific brain regions of depressed suicide victims. The study reported 30 to 40 percent increases in CRF immunoreactivity in LC and raphe nuclei in depressed suicide victims compared to controls. No differences were found in the dorsal tegmentum or parabrachial nucleus. These findings are consistent with the hypothesis that specific elevations in CRF activity on norepinephrine- and serotonin-containing cells may be associated with the pathophysiology of major depression.

Of particular interest is the demonstration that the elevated CSF CRF concentrations in drug-free depressed patients are significantly decreased after successful treatment with electroconvulsive therapy (ECT), indicating that CSF CRF concentrations, like hypercortisolemia, represent a state, rather than a trait, marker. Other recent studies have confirmed this normalization of CSF CRF concentrations after successful treatment with fluoxetine (Prozac). One group demonstrated significant reduction of elevated CSF CRF concentrations in 15 female patients with major depression who remained depression-free for at least 6 months after antidepressant treatment, as compared to little significant treatment effect on CSF CRF concentrations in nine patients who relapsed in this 6-month period. This suggests that elevated or increasing CSF CRF concentrations during antidepressant treatment may be the harbinger of a poor response in major depression despite early symptomatic improvement. Interestingly, treatment of normal subjects with desipramine (Norpramin) or, as noted above, of depressed patients with fluoxetine, is associated with a reduction in CSF CRF concentrations.

In preclinical studies, CRF hypersecretion is associated with CRF receptor downregulation. Depression is a major determinant of suicide, with more than 50 percent of completed suicides accomplished by patients with major depression. If CRF hypersecretion is a characteristic of depression, evidence of related CRF receptor downregulation should be evident in the CNS of depressed patients who have committed suicide. Indeed, there is a marked decrease in the density of CRF receptors in the frontal cortex of patients who have committed suicide, as compared to matched control samples.

If CRF hypersecretion is a factor in the pathophysiology of depression, then reducing or interfering with CRF neurotransmission might be an effective strategy to alleviate depressive symptoms. Over the past several years, a number of pharmaceutical companies have committed considerable effort to the development of small-molecule CRF_1 receptor antagonists that can effectively penetrate the blood–brain barrier. The recent surge in combinatorial chemistry techniques, coupled with recent technological advances in high-throughput screening, has enabled the field of small-molecule drug discovery. Several compounds have been produced with reportedly promising characteristics. Recently, a small open-label study examining the effectiveness of one such CRF_1 receptor antagonist in major depression was reported. Both standard severity measures of depression and anxiety were reduced after treatment. The drug in that study, R121919, is no longer in clinical development, but it is clear that CRF_1 receptor antagonists represent a potential new class of agents for the treatment of anxiety and depression.

Oxytocin and Vasopressin

The vasopressor effects of posterior pituitary extracts were first described in 1895, and the potent extracts were named *vasopressin*. In 1953, OT became the first peptide hormone to have its structure elucidated and the first to be chemically synthesized. The human OT and AVP genes are situated in tandem in a head-to-tail fashion on chromosome 20p13 separated by a several-kilobase intergenic sequence (Fig. 1.6–1). Both peptides are cyclical nonapeptides containing a cysteine–cysteine disulfide bond and differ at only two amino acid residues (Table 1.6–2). Like the sequence homology of the peptides themselves, the genes for OT and AVP share a common structure, suggesting that the two hormones are derived from a single ancestral hormone as a result of a gene duplication event early in vertebrate evolution. The two genes are transcribed in opposite directions on separate mRNAs. Each gene consists of three exons, with the first exon encoding the 5' untranslated region and the translation initiation codon followed by the SP sequence and the peptide hormone portion of the preprohormone. Exons 2 and 3 encode the neurophysin portion of the prohormone molecule. The AVP prohormone also contains a glycoprotein whose function is unclear. The neurophysin is thought to play a role in the posttranslational processing and transport of the peptides.

OT and vasopressin mRNAs are among the most abundant messengers in the hypothalamus, being heavily concentrated in the magnocellular neurons of the PVN and the supraoptic nucleus of the hypothalamus, which send axonal projections to the neurohypophysis. These neurons produce all of the OT and AVP that is released into the bloodstream, where these peptides act as hormones on peripheral targets. OT and AVP are generally synthesized in separate neurons within the hypothalamus. OT released from the pituitary is most often associated with functions associated with female reproduction, such as regulating uterine contractions during parturition and the milk ejection reflex during lactation. AVP, also known as *antidiuretic hormone*, regulates water retention in the kidney and vasoconstriction through interactions with vasopressin V2 and V1a receptor subtypes, respectively. AVP is released into the bloodstream from the neurohypophysis after a variety of stimuli, including plasma osmolality, hypovolemia, hypertension, and hypoglycemia. The actions of OT are mediated via a single receptor subtype, which is distributed in the periphery and within the limbic CNS. In contrast to OT, there are three AVP receptor subtypes, V1a, V1b, and V2, each of which are G-protein–coupled, seven-transmembrane domain receptors. The V2 receptor is localized in the kidney and is not found in the brain. The V1a receptor is distributed widely in the CNS and is thought to mediate most of the behavioral effects of AVP. The V1b receptor is concentrated in the anterior pituitary, and some reports describe V1b receptor mRNA in the brain, although its function is unknown.

Some parvocellular neurons in the PVN of the hypothalamus also project to the median eminence, where AVP is released into the portal system and delivered to the anterior pituitary. Through interactions with V1b receptors located on corticotrophs in the adenohypophysis, AVP acts to potentiate the effects of CRF on ACTH secretion. AVP is colocalized with CRF in the parvocellular neurons of the PVN. Given the link between HPA axis dysregulation and depression, recent attention has been given to the possible relationship between AVP secretion and psychiatric disorders. Although alterations in CSF AVP concentrations have been reported in patients with major depression, bipolar disorder, schizophrenia, anorexia, and Alzheimer's disease, the findings are not as consistent as for CRF, and many discrepant reports have appeared. In a postmortem study, an increase in the number of paraventricular AVP neurons colocalized with CRF cells has been reported in depressed patients, compared to controls. Recently, a selective, nonpeptide V1b receptor antagonist, SSR149415, has been developed and reported to possess both anxiolytic and antidepressant-like effects in rodent models, raising the possibility of its use as a therapeutic agent to treat stress-related disorders. Microdialysis experiments have demonstrated that AVP is released within the CNS in response to stressful stimuli.

In addition to the hypophyseal OT and AVP systems, parvocellular hypothalamic and extrahypothalamic neurons produce OT and AVP and send projections to the forebrain and brainstem. The release of peptide from these neurons is independent of neurohypophysial release, and it should be noted that OT and AVP released into the bloodstream do not reenter the brain due to the blood–brain barrier. OT and AVP projections from the PVN to the brainstem regulate a host of autonomic functions. However, in the forebrain, these peptides are now known to regulate a number of processes, ranging from anxiety, learning, and memory to complex social behaviors.

Central OT has clear anxiolytic effects in animal models. This is particularly evident during lactation in rats, when OT results in a blunted behavioral and ACTH response to an acoustic stressful stimulus. In contrast, central AVP appears to exert anxiogenic effects. In animal models, OT has been most intensively studied for its role in facilitating specific, complex social behaviors. OT has been reported to facilitate female sexual behavior, increase social interest, and facilitate the onset of maternal behavior. For example, in parturient rats, the onset of maternal behavior is blocked by OT antagonists, whereas maternal behavior can be observed in virgin females after infusion of OT directly into the brain. Likewise, in sheep, mother–infant bonding is facilitated by OT infusions. Studies with OT knock-out mice suggest that this peptide plays a specific role in the processing of socially salient stimuli. For example, OT knock-out mice have normal nonsocial cognitive abilities but have a specific deficit in the ability to recognize previously encountered individuals, even though olfactory processing is intact. Studies in highly social, monogamous rodents suggest that OT is also involved in the formation of selective social attachments between mates. All of these findings have led to the hypothesis that OT is involved in the regulation of the social brain, suggesting that dysregulation of this peptide could potentially explain social deficits in psychiatric disorders such as autism. One study has reported decreased levels of plasma OT in autistic patients and further suggested that this deficit may be due to alterations in the activities of the prohormone convertases responsible for cleaving OT into its active form. However, this observation must be interpreted cautiously, as plasma OT levels are not necessarily an index of CNS concentrations. OT concentrations in the CSF of autistic patients have not yet been measured.

Extrahypothalamic, AVP-producing neurons in the extended amygdala are sexually dimorphic, with males having many more AVP-expressing neurons than females. These neurons project through the ventral forebrain to the lateral septum, where they form a dense plexus of AVP immunoreactive fibers in males but less so in females. Castration diminishes this sex difference, and androgen treatment reestablishes the sexually dimorphic pattern. Thus, extrahypothalamic AVP is predicted to be involved in the regulation of sex-specific behaviors in males. Vasopressin has been reported to modulate a variety of behaviors in males, including anxiety, aggression, affiliation, and social attachment, in several animal models. For example, infusions of AVP into the hamster brain stimulate territorial and aggressive behaviors within minutes of administration. Extending this observation to humans, one study reported that individuals with a history of violent tendencies have elevated levels of AVP in the CSF, compared to nonviolent controls.

One of the most intriguing features of the AVP system is the species specificity in the behavioral effects of AVP. Consistent with this observation, the neuroanatomical localization of V1a AVP receptors is highly species-specific, often with little overlap between even closely related species. In fact, the specific behavioral role of AVP seems to be correlated with the localization of V1a receptors in specific brain regions. For example, AVP facilitates affiliation and social attachment in monogamous mammals. In the prairie vole, a monogamous rodent, AVP has been identified as the neurochemical trigger that stimulates pair bonding between the male and its mate. Comparisons among monogamous rodents and closely related nonmonogamous species have revealed that species differences in social organization are associated with species differences in receptor distribution within the brain. In several monogamous species, including the prairie vole, the vasopressin V1a receptor subtype is abundant in the mesolimbic dopamine reward pathway. In contrast, this region has few V1a receptors in the nonmonogamous, asocial montane vole (Fig. 1.6–4). Infusion of a V1a receptor antagonist directly into the ventral pallidum, a key relay region of the mesolimbic dopamine pathway of the prairie vole, completely blocks pair bonding. Thus, AVP released during mating facilitates social bonding by modulating the mesolimbic dopamine pathway in prairie voles but cannot do so in nonmonogamous species, because of the lack of receptors in that region. Molecular analysis of the V1a receptor genes of these different species have revealed DNA sequences in the promoter of the gene that may be responsible for the differential distribution of the receptor in the brain and, thus, the differences in behavioral patterns. This variability in distribution across species, along with the association between expression patterns and behavior, has led to the hypothesis that individual differences in receptor expression due to individual variation in gene promoter elements could potentially have important behavioral consequences in humans. In fact,

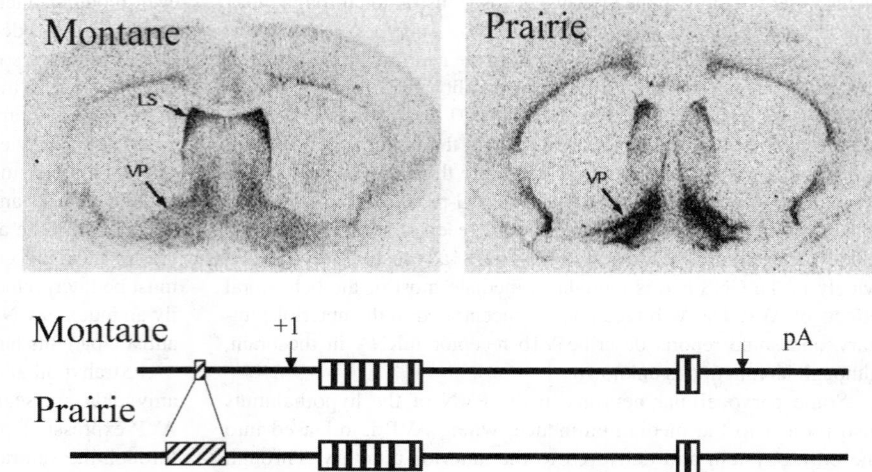

FIGURE 1.6–4 Upper panel depicts receptor autoradiograms illustrating the localization of vasopressin V1a receptor binding in the nonmonogamous montane vole and the monogamous prairie vole. Note the high density of V1a receptor binding in the ventral pallidum (VP) of the prairie vole but not the montane vole. The lower panel illustrates the gene structure of the montane and prairie vole V1a receptor gene, with the large boxed areas indicating exons. The thin hatched box in the 5' flanking region indicates the polymorphic sequence present in the prairie vole thought to be responsible for the species differences in receptor expression patterns and, ultimately, for the different social behaviors exhibited by these species. LS, lateral septum.

one genetic linkage study has found a significant association between a V1a receptor promoter polymorphism and autism.

Neurotensin NT was isolated, based on its hypotensive properties, from bovine hypothalamus in 1973. The NT-neuromedin N gene was originally cloned from canine ileal mucosa, and cDNA probes constructed against this form were used to clone the rat gene. The rat gene contains four exon sequences separated by three introns and spans approximately 10.2 kilobases (Fig. 1.6–1). In the rat, the NT-neuromedin N sequence is contained in the fourth exon, and the single copy of each peptide sequence is bounded and separated by Lys-Arg basic amino pairs. The human NT gene has been localized to chromosome 12 (12q21). In pheochromocytoma (PC-12) neurons in culture, the NT-neuromedin N gene is regulated by lithium, nerve growth factor, cAMP, and dexamethasone through their effects on a 5' flanking promoter region. The distribution of the NT-neuromedin N mRNA is generally the same as described for NT-containing neuronal cell bodies, except in the hippocampus and subiculum, where few neurons stain immunohistochemically for NT and yet an abundance of the NT-neuromedin N mRNA is found. NT-producing cells are found in the midbrain (ventral tegmental area [VTA] and, to a lesser extent, the substantia nigra [SN]), ventral striatum, extended amygdala, lateral septum, and arcuate nucleus. The actions of NT are mediated by three receptors—the NT_1, NT_2, and NT_3 receptor subtypes. The NT_1 and NT_2 receptors are seven-transmembrane, G-protein–coupled receptors, whereas NT_3 is a type 1 amino acid receptor with a single transmembrane domain and is located intracellularly.

Although NT is found in a number of brain regions, it has been most thoroughly investigated in terms of its association with other neurotransmitter systems, particularly the mesolimbic dopamine system, and has gained interest in research on the pathophysiology of schizophrenia. There are several lines of evidence suggesting that NT and its receptors should be considered as potential targets for pharmacological intervention in this disorder. First, the NT system is positioned anatomically to modulate the neural circuits implicated in schizophrenia. Second, peripheral administration of antipsychotic drugs has been shown to consistently modulate NT systems. And third, there is evidence that central NT systems are altered in schizophrenic patients.

Although it is likely that other neurotransmitter systems are involved, one prevalent model of the pathophysiology of schizophrenia is overactivity in the mesolimbic dopamine system. Within the midbrain, NT-producing neurons are found in the VTA and the SN. Within the VTA, NT is found in dense-core vesicles only in tyrosine hydroxylase–positive staining cell bodies, indicating colocalization with dopamine. These NT-dopamine cells project to the prefrontal cortex, striatum, amygdala, and lateral septum. A subset of these NT-dopamine cells projecting from the VTA to the prefrontal cortex also produce cholecystokinin (CCK). In contrast to the VTA, the NT-producing cells in the SN are tyrosine hydroxylase–negative. In addition to the NT-producing cells, dense fibers in the VTA staining positive for NT and originating from projections from the forebrain do not contain tyrosine hydroxylase. The midbrain also expresses NT receptors, with the vast majority of NT receptor–containing neurons in the VTA being dopamine-positive neurons. NT-producing cells, fibers, and NT receptors are also located in the ventral striatum. Thus, NT is colocalized with dopamine in the mesolimbic dopamine system, and this system is, in turn, sensitive to NT modulation, due to the presence of the NT receptors.

NT was first shown to interact with dopamine systems while undergoing characterization of its potent hypothermic and sedative potentiating activity. Subsequent work indicated that NT possessed many properties that were also shared by antipsychotic drugs, including the ability to inhibit avoidance but not escape responding in a conditioned active avoidance task, the ability to block the effects of indirect dopamine agonists or endogenous dopamine in the production of locomotor behavior, and the ability to elicit increases in dopamine release and turnover. Perhaps most importantly, both antipsychotic drugs and NT neurotransmission enhance sensorimotor gating. Sensorimotor gating is the ability to screen or filter relevant sensory input, deficits of which may lead to an involuntary flooding of indifferent sensory data. Increasing evidence suggests that deficits in sensorimotor gating are a cardinal feature of schizophrenia. Both dopamine agonists and NT antagonists disrupt performance on tasks designed to gauge sensorimotor gating. Unlike antipsychotic drugs, NT is not able to displace dopamine from its receptor. As noted above, NT is colocalized in certain subsets of dopamine neurons and is coreleased with dopamine in the mesolimbic and medial prefrontal cortex dopamine-terminal regions that are implicated as the site of dopamine dysregulation in schizophrenia. Antipsychotic drugs that act at dopamine type 2 (D_2) and type 4 (D_4) receptors increase the synthesis, concentration, and release of NT in those dopamine terminal regions but not in others. That effect of antipsychotic drugs in increasing NT concentrations persists after months of treatment and is accompanied by the expected increase in NT mRNA concentrations, as well as expression of the "immediate early gene" c-*fos* and the transcription factor Fos within hours of initial drug treatment. The altered regulation of NT expression by antipsychotic drugs apparently extends to the peptidases that degrade the peptide, as recent reports have revealed decreased NT metabolism in rat brain slices 24 hours after the acute administration of haloperidol. When administered directly into the brain, NT preferentially opposes dopamine transmission in the nucleus accumbens but not the caudate putamen. In the nucleus accumbens, NT receptors are located predominantly on GABAergic neurons, which release GABA on dopamine terminals, thereby inhibiting release.

With regard to schizophrenia, decreased CSF NT concentrations have been reported in several populations of patients, when compared to controls or other psychiatric disorders. Although treatment with antipsychotic drugs has been observed to increase NT concentrations in the CSF, it is not known whether this increase is causal or merely accompanies the decrease in psychotic symptoms seen with successful treatment. Postmortem studies have shown an increase in NT concentrations in the dopamine-rich Brodmann's area 32 of the frontal cortex, but that result may have been confounded by premortem antipsychotic treatment. Other researchers have found no postmortem alterations in NT concentrations of a wide sampling of subcortical regions. Decreases in NT receptor densities in the entorhinal cortex have been reported in the entorhinal cortex of schizophrenic postmortem samples. A comparison of the genomic sequence of the NT-neuromedin N gene in schizophrenic patients compared with age- and sex-matched controls found no differences in the gene sequence in the coding region. A critical test of the hypothesis that NT may act as an endogenous antipsychotic-like substance will be the development of an NT receptor agonist that can penetrate the blood–brain barrier.

OTHER NEUROPEPTIDES

A number of other neuropeptides have been implicated in the pathophysiology of psychiatric disorders. These include, but are not limited to, somatostatin, CCK, substance P, and neuoropeptide Y. A brief overview of the potential involvement of these neuropeptides in psychiatric disorders is provided below.

Somatostatin inhibits growth hormone release from the anterior pituitary but also functions as a neurotransmitter within the CNS. Central somatostatin administration produces changes in sleep patterns, food consumption, locomotor activity, and memory processes. CSF somatostatin concentrations have been reported to be decreased in patients with depression (Fig. 1.6–3), schizophrenia, and Alzheimer's disease.

CCK, originally discovered in the gastrointestinal tract, and its receptor are found in areas of the brain associated with emotion, motivation, and sensory processing (e.g., cortex, striatum, hypothalamus, hippocampus, and amygdala). CCK is often colocalized with dopamine in the VTA neurons that compose the mesolimbic and mesocortical dopamine circuits. Like NT, CCK decreases dopamine release. Infusions of a CCK fragment have been reported to induce panic in healthy individuals, and patients with panic disorder exhibit increased sensitivity to the CCK fragment, compared to normal controls.

The undecapeptide substance P is localized in the amygdala, hypothalamus, periaqueductal gray, LC, and parabrachial nucleus and is colocalized within norepinephrine and serotonin. Substance P serves as a pain neurotransmitter, and administration to animals elicits behavioral and cardiovascular effects resembling the stress response. One study has indicated that a substance P receptor antagonist capable of passing through the blood–brain barrier is more effective than placebo and as effective as paroxetine in patients with major depression with moderate to severe symptom severity. A recent study has also found elevated substance P concentrations in the serum of patients with major depression compared to control patients.

Neuropeptide Y is a 36–amino acid peptide found in the hypothalamus, brainstem, spinal cord, and several limbic structures and is involved in the regulation of appetite, reward, anxiety, and energy balance. Neuropeptide Y neurons innervate CRF-containing neurons in the PVN of the hypothalamus, and neuropeptide Y administration increases hypothalamic CRF levels and promotes CRF release. Neuropeptide Y is colocalized with serotonergic and noradrenergic neurons. Patients diagnosed with major depression who commit suicide are reported to have a pronounced reduction in neuropeptide Y levels in the frontal cortex and caudate nucleus. Furthermore, CSF neuropeptide Y levels are decreased in depressed patients. Chronic administration of antidepressant drugs increases neuropeptide Y concentrations in the neocortex and hippocampus in rats. Recently, a functional polymorphism in the neuropeptide Y gene was found to be associated with alcohol dependence.

It is evident that understanding of the neurobiology of neuropeptides has increased remarkably during the past decade. There is already considerable evidence that these neuroregulators are involved in both the pathophysiology of certain major neuropsychiatric disorders and the mechanism of action of some of the drugs used to treat these disabling illnesses. As further knowledge accrues, it is increasingly likely that neuropeptides will play a greater role in the development of adjunct diagnostic tests and novel treatments for the major psychiatric disorders.

SUGGESTED CROSS-REFERENCES

Section 1.10 discusses basic molecular neurobiology, Section 1.11 discusses psychoneuroendocrinology, and neuropsychiatric aspects of endocrine disorders are discussed in Section 25.6.

References

Austin MC, Janosky JE, Murphy HA: Increased corticotrophin-releasing hormone immunoreactivity in monoamine-containing pontine nuclei of depressed suicide men. *Mol Psychiatry*. 2003;8:324–332.

Binder EB, Kinkead B, Owens MJ, Nemeroff CB: Neurotensin and dopamine interactions. *Pharmacol Rev*. 2001;53:453–486.

Binder EB, Kinkead B, Owens MJ, Nemeroff CB: The role of neurotensin in the pathophysiology of schizophrenia and the mechanism of action of antipsychotic drugs. *Biol Psychiatry*. 2001;50:856–872.

*Bissette G, Nemeroff CB. The neurobiology of neurotensin. In: Bloom FE, Kupfer DJ, eds. *Psychopharmacology: The Fourth Generation of Progress*. New York: Raven Press; 1995:573.

*De Souza EB, Grigoriadis DE. Corticotropin-releasing factor: physiology, pharmacology, and role in central nervous system disorders. In: Davis KL, Charney D, Coyle JT, Nemerof C, eds. *Neuropsychopharmacology: The Fifth Generation of Progress*. Philadelphia: Lippincott, Williams & Wilkins; 2002:91–107.

Gainer H, Wray W. Cellular and molecular biology of vasopressin. In: Knobil E, Neill JD, eds. *The Physiology of Reproduction*. New York: Raven Press; 1994:1099–1129.

Gutman DA, Mussleman DL, Nemeroff CB. Neuropeptide alterations in depression and anxiety disorders. In: denBoer JA, AdSitsen JM, Kasper S, eds. *Handbook of Depression and Anxiety*, 2nd ed. Marcel Dekker, Inc.; 2003:229–265.

Gutman DA, Nemeroff CB. Persistent central nervous system effects of an adverse early environment: clinical and preclinical studies. *Physiol Behav*. 2003;79:471–478.

*Hökfelt TGM, Castel M-N, Morino P, Zhang X, Dagerlind Å. General overview of neuropeptides. In: Bloom FE, Kupfer DJ, eds. *Psychopharmacology: The Fourth Generation of Progress*. New York: Raven Press; 1995:483.

*Insel TR. The neurobiology of affiliation: implications for autism. In: Davidson RJ, Scherer KR, Goldsmith HH, eds. *Handbook of Affective Sciences*. Oxford: Oxford University Press; 2003:1010–1020.

Insel TR, O'Brien DJ, Leckman JF: Oxytocin, vasopressin, and autism: Is there a connection? *Biol Psychiatry*. 1999;443:207–219.

Insel TR, Young LJ: The neurobiology of attachment. *Nat Rev Neurosci*. 2001;2:129–136.

Landgraf R: Neuropeptides and anxiety-related behavior. *Endocr J*. 2001;48:517–533.

Mason GA, Garbutt JC, Prange AJ Jr. Thyrotropin-releasing hormone: focus on basic neurobiology. In: Bloom FE, Kupfer DJ, eds. *Psychopharmacology: The Fourth Generation of Progress*. New York; Raven Press; 1995:493.

Muller MB, Zimmermann S, Sillaber I, Hagemeyer TP, Deussing JM, Timpl P. Kormann MSD, Droste SK, Kuhn R, Reul JMHM, Holsboer F, Wurst W: Limbic corticotrophin-releasing hormone receptor 1 mediates anxiety-related behavior and hormonal adaptation to stress. *Nat Neurosci*. 2003;6:1100–1107.

Scott LV, Dinan TG: Vasopressin as a target for antidepressant development: an assessment of the available evidence. *J Affect Disord.* 2002;72:113–124.

*Strand FL. Neuropeptides: regulators of physiological processes. In: Davis KL, Charney D, Coyle JT, Nemerof C, eds. *Neuropsychopharmacology: The Fifth Generation of Progress.* Philadelphia: Lippincott, Williams & Wilkins; 2002:91–107.

▲ 1.7 Neurotrophic Factors

FRANCIS S. LEE, M.D., PH.D., AND MOSES V. CHAO, PH.D.

Neurotrophins are a unique family of polypeptide growth factors that influence the proliferation, differentiation, survival, and death of neuronal and nonneuronal cells. These proteins do not exist in *Drosophila melanogaster* or *Caenorhabditis elegans*, even though other well-known polypeptide growth factors, such as epidermal growth factor (EGF), fibroblast growth factor, and insulin, are conserved in these species. The evolution of nerve growth factor (NGF), brain-derived neurotrophic factor (BDNF), neurotrophin-3 (NT3), and neurotrophin-4 (NT4) as a family implies that these signaling molecules may act to mediate additional higher-order activities, such as learning, memory, and behavior, in addition to their established functions for cell survival. The effects of neurotrophins depend on their levels of availability, their affinity for binding to transmembrane receptors, and the downstream signaling cascades that are stimulated after receptor activation. Whereas the biological roles for neurotrophins were initially characterized in the development of the nervous system, it is now clear that they have multiple roles in the adult nervous system, such as regulating synaptic connections, synapse structure, neurotransmitter release, long-term potentiation, mechanosensation, pain, and synaptic plasticity. Alterations in neurotrophin levels have been implicated in neurodegenerative disorders, such as Alzheimer's disease and Huntington's disease, as well as psychiatric disorders, such as depression and substance abuse.

NEUROTROPHIN FAMILY

A large number of polypeptide factors affect the survival, growth, and differentiation of the nervous system. The neurotrophins, comprised of NGF, BDNF, NT3, and NT4, are best understood and most widely expressed in the nervous system. The neurotrophins are initially synthesized as precursors or proneurotrophins that are cleaved to release the mature, active proteins. The mature proteins, approximately 12 to 14 kDa in size, form stable, noncovalent dimers and are normally expressed at very low levels during development. Proneurotrophins are cleaved intracellularly by furin or proconvertases using a highly conserved dibasic amino acid cleavage site to release carboxy terminal mature proteins.

The mature proteins mediate neurotrophin actions by selectively binding to members of the tropomyosin-related kinase (Trk) family of receptor tyrosine kinases to regulate neuronal survival, differentiation, and synaptic plasticity. In addition, all mature neurotrophins interact with the p75 neurotrophin receptor ($p75^{NTR}$), which can modulate the affinity of Trk neurotrophin associations. NGF was the first identified neurotrophic factor and has a restricted distribution within the neurotrophin family. In the peripheral nervous system (PNS), it acts on sympathetic neurons, as well as sensory neurons involved in nociception and temperature sensation. In the central nervous system (CNS), NGF promotes the survival and functioning of cholinergic neurons in the basal forebrain. These neurons project to the hippocampus and are believed to be important for memory processes, which are specifically affected in Alzheimer's disease. The other neurotrophins are more widely expressed in the CNS. BDNF and NT3 are highly expressed in cortical and hippocampal structures and have been linked to the survival and functioning of multiple neuronal populations.

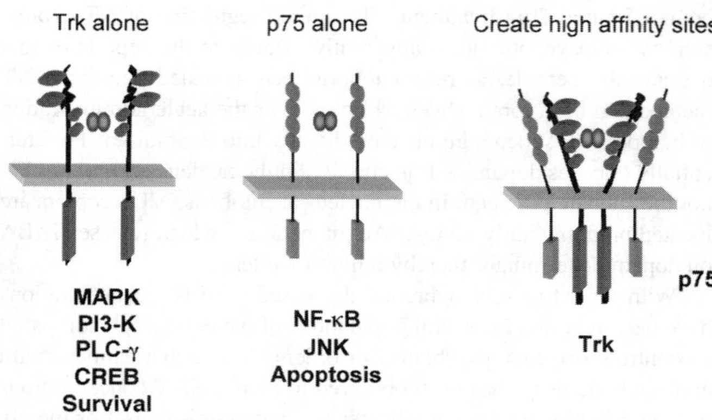

FIGURE 1.7–1 Neurotrophin receptor signaling. Neurotrophins bind to tropomysin-related tyrosine kinase (Trk) receptors (*right*) and p75 neurotrophin receptors ($p75^{NTR}$) (*middle*). Trk receptors mediate differentiation and survival signaling through mitogen-activated protein kinase (MAPK), phosphatidylinositol-3-kinase (PI3-K), and phospholipase C-γ (PLC-γ) pathways, which lead to effects on transcription factors, such as the cyclic adenosine monophosphate response element binding protein (CREB). Trk receptors contain immunoglobulin G domains for ligand binding and a catalytic tyrosine kinase sequence (*left*) in the intracellular domain. $p75^{NTR}$ mediates apoptotic and cell migration responses through nuclear factor κB (NF-κB) and c-Jun N-terminal kinase (JNK) pathways. The extracellular part of $p75^{NTR}$ contains four cysteine-rich repeats; the intracellular domain contains a death domain (*middle*). Interactions between Trk receptors and $p75^{NTR}$ can lead to changes in binding affinity for neurotrophins (*right*).

NEUROTROPHIN RECEPTORS

Neurotrophins are unique in exerting their cellular effects through the actions of two different receptors, the Trk receptor tyrosine kinase and $p75^{NTR}$, a member of the tumor necrosis factor (TNF) receptor superfamily. Trk receptors consist of an extracellular ligand binding region, a single transmembrane domain, and a highly conserved intracellular tyrosine kinase domain. $p75^{NTR}$ consists of an extracellular ligand binding region, a single transmembrane domain, and an intracellular portion containing a protein association region termed the *death domain* (Fig. 1.7–1). All neurotrophins bind to the $p75^{NTR}$. There are three vertebrate *trk* receptor genes, *trkA*, *trkB*, and *trkC*. All Trk receptors exhibit high conservation in their intracellular domains, including the catalytic tyrosine kinase domain, and the juxtamembrane domain. There are no sequence similarities between Trk and $p75^{NTR}$ in either ligand binding or their cytoplasmic domains.

Neurotrophins bind as dimers to Trk family members, leading to the receptor dimerization and activation of the catalytic tyrosine protein kinase domains. The dimerized Trk receptors autophosphorylate several key intracellular tyrosine residues and rapidly initiate intracellular signaling cascades. This is accomplished by the phosphorylated tyrosines on the receptor acting as a recognition site for binding of specific adaptor proteins that contain phosphotyrosine binding motifs, such as src-homology domain 2 (SH2). In particular, the Shc adaptor protein links the activated Trk receptor to two separate intracellular signaling pathways that mediate the majority of biological effects of neurotrophins. The primary survival pathway involves Shc-linking Trk receptor activation to increases in phosphatidylinositol-3-kinase (PI3 kinase) activity, which, in turn, activates another protein kinase, protein kinase B (Akt), which has multiple effects on the cell's apoptotic pathways. Also, Shc phosphorylation by Trk receptor activation leads to increases in Ras and mitogen-activated protein kinase (MAPK) activities. These events, in turn, influence transcriptional events, such as the induction of the cyclic adenosine monophosphate response element binding protein (CREB) transcription factor. CREB produces a multitude of effects on cell cycle, neurite outgrowth, and synaptic plasticity. In addition, phospholipase C-γ (PLC-γ) binds to activated Trk receptors and initiates an intracellular signaling cascade release of inositol phosphates with subsequent activation of protein kinase C (PKC).

NGF binds most specifically to TrkA, BDNF and NT4 to TrkB, and NT3 to TrkC receptors. $p75^{NTR}$ can bind to each neurotrophin but has the additional capability of regulating a Trk's affinity for its cognate ligand. $p75^{NTR}$ and Trk receptors have been referred to as *high-* and *low-affinity receptors*, respectively. However, this is incorrect, as TrkA and TrkB actually bind their ligands with an affinity of 10^{-9} to 10^{-10} M, which is lower than the high-affinity site ($K_d = 10^{-11}$ M). Also, the precursor form of NGF displays high-affinity binding to $p75^{NTR}$. Trk-mediated responsiveness to low concentrations of NGF is dependent on the relative levels of $p75^{NTR}$ and TrkA receptors and their combined ability to form high-affinity sites. This is important, as the ratio of receptors can determine cellular responsiveness and, ultimately, neuronal cell numbers.

Although $p75^{NTR}$ and Trk receptors do not bind to each other directly, there is evidence that complexes form between the two receptors. Perhaps as a result of these interactions, increased ligand selectivity can be conferred onto Trk receptors by the $p75^{NTR}$. One way of generating specificity is by imparting greater discrimination of ligands for the Trk receptors (Fig. 1.7–2). For example, BDNF, NT3, and NT4/5 can each bind to the TrkB receptor, but, in the presence of $p75^{NTR}$ only, BDNF provides a functional response. Likewise, both NGF and NT3 can bind to TrkA, but $p75^{NTR}$ restricts signaling of TrkA to NGF and not NT3 (Fig. 1.7–2). Hence, $p75^{NTR}$ and Trk receptors interact to provide greater discrimination among different neurotrophins.

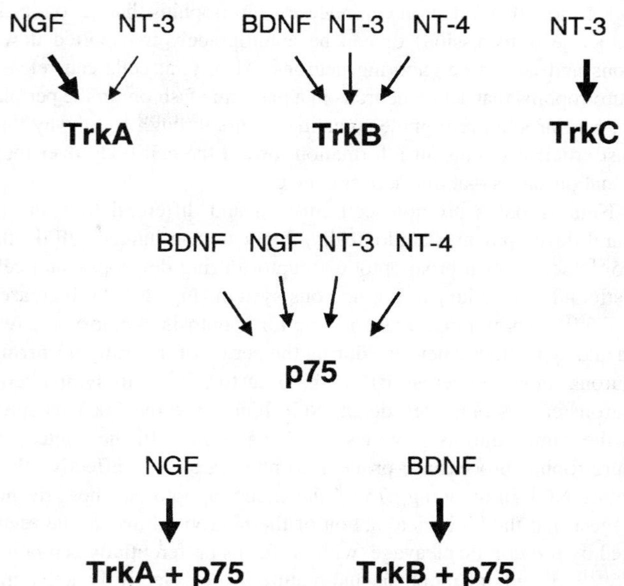

FIGURE 1.7–2 Neurotrophin binding specificities. All neurotrophins bind to p75 neurotrophin receptor ($p75^{NTR}$). Neurotrophins bind selectively to specific tropomyosin-related kinase (Trk) receptors, and this specificity can be altered by $p75^{NTR}$. Several neurotrophins, neurotrophin-3 (NT3) and neurotrophin-4 (NT4), can bind to multiple Trk receptors. BDNF, brain-derived neurotrophic factor; NGF, nerve growth factor.

On one level, neurotrophins fit well with the neurotrophic hypothesis, as many peripheral neuronal subpopulations exhibit a predominant dependence on a specific neurotrophin during the period of naturally occurring cell death. In the CNS, the overlapping expression of multiple neurotrophin receptors and their cognate ligands allows for more diverse connectivity, which extends well into adulthood. In addition, it

NEUROTROPHIC FACTORS AND DEVELOPMENT

The formation of the vertebrate nervous system is characterized by widespread programmed cell death, which determines cell number and appropriate target innervation during development. Neurotrophins are expressed during early development and have been shown to be essential for the survival of selective populations of neurons during different developmental periods. The neurotrophic hypothesis summarizes the role of neurotrophic factors in the development of the nervous system (Fig. 1.7–3) and postulates that during nervous system development, neurons approaching the same final target vie for limited amounts of target-derived trophic factor. In this way, the nervous system molds itself to maintain only the most competitive and appropriate connections. Competition among neurons for limited amounts of neurotrophin molecules produced by target cells accounts for selective cell survival (Fig. 1.7–3). Two predictions emanate from this hypothesis. First, the efficacy of neuronal survival will depend on the amounts of trophic factors produced during development. Second, specific receptor expression in certain cell populations will dictate neuronal responsiveness.

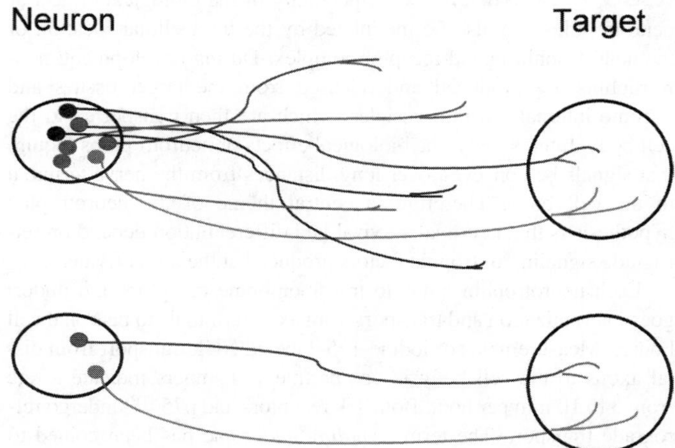

FIGURE 1.7–3 The neurotrophin hypothesis. Neurons compete for limited quantities of neurotrophins in target regions, which leads to selective neuronal survival. Levels of target-derived neurotrophins and neurotrophin receptors will determine efficacy of survival and responsiveness of the neurons. The ability to form high-affinity binding sites allows for greater responsiveness under limited quantities of trophic factors. Lack of trophic support or incorrect targeting of axons to the wrong target results in programmed cell death.

is clear now that a neuron can release neurotrophins that act on itself (autocrine transmission) or can be anterogradely transported down axons and act on neighboring neurons. Also, glial cells can release neurotrophins that act on neurons in a paracrine fashion. In the periphery, neurotrophin retrograde signaling occurs through a pathway that must efficiently transmit information toward the cell body over long axonal distances—at times, over a meter.

Neurotrophins promote cell survival and differentiation during neural development. Paradoxically, they can also induce cell death. $p75^{NTR}$ serves as a proapoptotic receptor during developmental cell death and after injury to the nervous system (Fig. 1.7–1). Increases in $p75^{NTR}$ expression are responsible for apoptosis in embryonic retina and sympathetic neurons during the period of naturally occurring neuronal death. Whereas BDNF binding to $p75^{NTR}$ in sympathetic neurons causes rapid cell death, NGF binding to the TrkA receptor on the same neurons provides a survival signal. In the context of neurotrophin processing, proneurotrophins are more effective than mature NGF in inducing $p75^{NTR}$-dependent apoptosis. These results suggest that the biological action of the neurotrophins can be regulated by proteolytic cleavage, with proforms preferentially activating $p75^{NTR}$ to mediate apoptosis and mature forms selectively activating Trk receptors to promote survival.

What are the reasons for having a Trk receptor that mediates neuronal survival and a $p75^{NTR}$ that mediates apoptosis? Neurotrophins may use a death receptor to prune neurons efficiently during periods of developmental cell death. In addition to competing for trophic support from the target, neurons must establish connections with the proper target. In the event of mistargeting, neurons may undergo apoptosis if the appropriate set of trophic factors is not encountered. In this case, a neurotrophin may not only fail to activate Trk receptors, but also may bind to $p75^{NTR}$ and eliminate cells by an active killing process. For example, BDNF causes sympathetic cell death by binding to $p75^{NTR}$ when TrkB is absent. Likewise, NT4 causes $p75^{NTR}$-mediated cell death in BDNF-dependent trigeminal neurons, presumably due to preferential $p75^{NTR}$ rather than TrkB stimulation. Therefore, Trk receptors and $p75^{NTR}$ can give opposite outcomes in the same cells. Cell death mediated by $p75^{NTR}$ may be important for the refinement of correct target innervation during development.

Retrograde Transport Specificity of the biological effects of neurotrophins can also be modulated by the intracellular location of the neurotrophin ligand-receptor complex. During development, neurotrophins are produced and released from the target tissues and become internalized into vesicles, which are then transported to the cell body. Interestingly, the biological effects of neurotrophins require that signals be conveyed over long distances from the nerve terminal to the cell body. Therefore, a central theme of the neurotrophic hypothesis is that neuronal survival and differentiation depend on retrograde signaling of trophic factors produced at the target tissue.

Each neurotrophin binds to transmembrane receptors and undergoes internalization and transport from axon terminals to neuronal cell bodies. Measurements of iodine-125–labeled NGF transport from distal axons to the cell body in compartment chambers indicate a rate from 3 to 10 mm per hour. Both Trk receptors and $p75^{NTR}$ undergo retrograde transport. The term *signaling endosome* has been coined to describe membrane vesicles that carry Trk, $p75^{NTR}$, and NGF.

A complex of NGF-TrkA has been found in clathrin-coated vesicles and endosomes, giving rise to the model that NGF and Trk are components of the retrograde signal. Several tyrosine-phosphorylated proteins are associated with the TrkA receptor during transport, suggesting that signaling by neurotrophins persists after the internalization of their receptors. Internalization of NGF from axon terminals is necessary for phosphorylation and activation of the CREB transcription factor, which leads to changes in gene expression and increased neuronal cell survival. These events likely require internalization and transport of activated Trk receptors and result in a survival response.

Neurotrophins and Synaptic Plasticity Recent studies have established that neurotrophic factors play significant roles in influencing synaptic plasticity in the adult brain. Many neuronal populations are dependent on these neurotrophins not only for their survival, but also for modulating neuronal activity. Developmental regulation of synaptic plasticity in the visual system is illustrated by the formation of ocular dominance columns in layer IV of the cortex, which can be strongly influenced by exogenous neurotrophins, such as BDNF. Also, the effects on the visual system can be observed using blocking antibodies for the neurotrophins, as well as neurotrophin antagonists (TrkB–immunoglobulin G [IgG] fusion proteins that bind neurotrophins), indicating that an alteration in the levels of endogenous neurotrophins has dramatic consequences.

Modulation of synaptic plasticity in the differentiated adult brain has also been demonstrated in the hippocampus. BDNF promoted the induction of a synaptic strengthening, termed *long-term potentiation* (LTP), in hippocampal slices, whereas blocking reagents, such as the TrkB-IgG fusion protein, interfered with the induction of LTP. In addition, hippocampal preparations containing little or no BDNF gave rise to the same reduction in LTP, suggesting that there was a minimal quantity of BDNF required for the modulation of LTP. Subsequent addition of extra BDNF or adenoviral expression of BDNF to these preparations from mutant mice restored LTP. Neurotrophins have also been shown to evoke other forms of synaptic transmission. Exogenous BDNF or NT3 has been shown to induce enhanced evoked responses in both hippocampal preparations as well as in neuromuscular junction. Thus, neurotrophins can modulate synaptic strengthening and neurotransmission as well as promote cell survival and axonal and dendritic growth.

Neurotrophins and Behavior A series of studies conducted with adult mice with reduced levels of BDNF has indicated that neurotrophins have demonstrable effects on adult brain function and behavior. These studies are important, as earlier homozygous neurotrophin knock-out mice studies were limited due to embryonic lethality or early postnatal death. But heterozygous $BDNF^{+/-}$ mice in which BDNF levels are reduced by approximately half are viable and display a number of behaviors suggestive of impulse control abnormalities. In the absence of normal levels of BDNF, mice exhibit enhanced aggressiveness, hyperactivity, and hyperphagia. Intracerebroventricular infusion of BDNF or NT4 led to a striking reversal of the feeding phenotype. In these heterozygous $BDNF^{+/-}$ mice, serotonergic neuronal function was abnormal in the forebrain, cortex, hippocampus, and hypothalamus. Most strikingly, administration of fluoxetine (Prozac), a selective serotonin reuptake inhibitor (SSRI), ameliorated the aggressive behavior, hyperphagia, and hyperlocomotor activity. In addition, a region-specific conditional deletion of BDNF in the brains of postnatal mice also led to hyperphagia and hyperactivity, as well as higher levels of anxiety as measured by a light/dark exploration test. This study demonstrated that the feeding phenotype, as well as the other behavioral abnormalities, was mediated by the functioning of BDNF in the CNS as compared to any peripheral actions of the neurotrophin.

Lack of BDNF also created defects in memory tasks consistent with defects in LTP found in the hippocampal slice studies. Heterozygous $BDNF^{+/-}$ mice had impairments in spatial memory tasks, such as the Morris water maze. Abnormal behaviors elicited by partial deletion of BDNF indicate a significant role for this neurotrophin in higher-order behaviors, which have clinical correlates to psychiatric disorders, especially those associated with alteration in central serotonergic functioning.

OTHER NEUROTROPHIC FACTORS

Several prominent neurotrophic factor families carry out similar functions as the neurotrophins. Glial-derived neurotrophic factor (GDNF) is an 18-kDa protein, originally isolated from an astrocyte cell line and later shown to be made by many types of neurons, that represents one of the most potent trophic factors for dopaminergic neurons. In both in vitro and in vivo studies, GDNF has been shown to maintain the survival of dopaminergic neurons in the midbrain, as well as of neurons in the myenteric plexus in the gut. Due to its trophic effects on dopaminergic neurons, it has been considered a potential therapeutic agent for Parkinson's disease. GDNF binds to a protein, GFRα1, which is anchored to the plasma membrane by a glycophospholipid. Other ligands in this family have also been discovered—namely, artemin, neurturin, and persephin—that recognize specific GFRα receptors. This ligand-receptor complex then associates with Ret, a receptor tyrosine kinase, which, like the Trk receptors, undergoes dimerization and becomes catalytically active. Phosphotyrosine binding adaptor proteins, such as Shc, then bind to the Ret receptor and mediate downstream signaling cascades, such as the MAPK pathway. Mutations in the Ret receptor and GFRα1 have been associated with Hirschsprung's disease, a disorder caused by the lack of development of myenteric plexus neurons, leading to abnormal gut motility.

Ciliary neurotrophic factor (CNTF) belongs to a family of cytokines, including leukemia inhibitory factor (LIF) and interleukin-6, which maintain the survival of ciliary neurons, as well as motor neurons. Due to its ability to rescue motor neurons after axotomy in animal studies, CNTF has been investigated as a therapeutic agent for motor neuron diseases, such as amyotrophic lateral sclerosis (ALS). These factors use a receptor complex consisting of a plasma membrane–bound CNTF binding protein (CNTFα), a glycoprotein (gp130), and a LIF receptor (LIFR) to transduce signals. Upon formation of this complex, a soluble tyrosine kinase, the Janus kinase (JAK), is activated and leads to the activation of a specific family of transcription factors termed *STATs*.

Therefore, trophic factors exemplified by NGF, CNTF, and GDNF and their family members all utilize intracellular tyrosine phosphorylation to mediate neuronal cell survival. CNTF acts through a complex of a CNTF receptor, gp130, and LIF subunits, which are linked to the JAK/STAT signaling molecules, whereas the GDNF receptor consists of the c-Ret receptor tyrosine kinase and a separate α binding protein.

CLINICAL CORRELATES

Neurotrophic factors regulate numerous neuronal functions in development and adult life and in response to neuronal injury. As a result, neurotrophins have been implicated in the pathophysiology of a wide variety of neurodegenerative and psychiatric disorders and have been considered as a therapeutic strategy for even more neuropsychiatric disorders. The finding that neurotrophic factors modulate neuronal survival and axonal growth was the initial rationale for using these polypeptides to treat neurodegenerative disorders and neuronal injury, such as Alzheimer's disease, Parkinson's disease, Huntington's disease, and ALS, as well as spinal cord injury. The additional effects of neurotrophic factors on synaptic connections, synaptic plasticity, and neurotransmission have formed the basis for their association with psychiatric disorders, such as depression and substance abuse. In these conditions, the response to acute and chronic environmental changes in the setting of a genetic predisposition leads to alterations in neuronal function.

The hypothesis underlying these clinical correlations as well as the development of therapeutic strategies using neurotrophic factors assumes that these disease states result in either (1) decreased availability of neurotrophins for the affected neurons, (2) decreased number of neurotrophin receptors on the affected neurons, or (3) decreased receptor signaling. These deficits can be ameliorated by the addition of neurotrophic factors. In all of these disease states, the assumption has been that exogenous neurotrophic factors would provide symptomatic treatment for the disease state rather than a cure for the core pathophysiology of these nervous system disorders. It should be emphasized, though, that no human disease affecting the nervous system has been shown to be caused by a defect in the neurotrophins or their receptors.

Neurodegenerative Disorders

The initial clinical correlation to Alzheimer's disease was made in the 1980s, based on studies on aged animals that showed that cholinergic neurons in the basal forebrain that are consistently affected in the disease could be rescued with intracerebroventricular NGF with concomitant improvements in memory function. Subsequent animal studies of impaired motor neuron populations demonstrated that other neurotrophins (BDNF, NT3, NT4, and CNTF) could rescue these neurons in axotomized facial and sciatic nerves. In addition, mutant mouse models of motor neuron degeneration (progressive motor neuron disease, wobbler) demonstrated that BDNF and CNTF could increase the number of motor neurons and improve motor performance. These studies led to the therapeutic strategy of using neurotrophins to treat degenerative diseases that affect motor neurons. In the 1990s, great effort was focused on studying whether neurotrophic factors could be used as a treatment strategy for ALS, a progressive neurodegenerative disorder that specifically affects motor neurons and leads to death due to respiratory failure.

With the development of recombinant forms of the neurotrophic factors—namely, BDNF—clinical trials were embarked on in patients with ALS. Subcutaneous or intrathecal BDNF had significant side effects, such as pain and gastrointestinal symptoms, and minimal beneficial effect. It was because of these side effects that decreased doses were used as compared to the doses in the animal studies. Similarly, use of another neurotrophic factor CNTF led to even more significant side effects, such as fever, pain, and anorexia, which also limited the doses used. These multisite clinical trials highlighted the challenges of delivering large quantities of these proteins to CNS and PNS neurons. Clinical studies using NGF for the treatment of patients with Alzheimer's disease and diabetic neuropathy encountered similar hurdles involving problems of delivery and uncertain pharmacokinetics.

Psychiatric Disorders

Many functions of the neurotrophic factors in the adult CNS have been elucidated beyond their effects on survival, such as maintenance of differentiated neuronal phenotypes, regulating synaptic connections, activity-dependent synaptic plasticity, and neurotransmission. These additional functions have made neurotrophins attractive molecular intermediates that may be involved in the pathophysiology of psychiatric disorders in which environmental inputs can presumably lead to alterations in neuronal circuitry and, ultimately, behavior. In particular, it has become clear that neurotrophins can produce long-term changes via regulation of transcriptional programs on the functioning of adult neurons and, thus, may be the molecules that account for the long delay in therapeutic action of many psychiatric treatments. Again, the clinical correlation is based on the assumption that there is a deficit in access or responsiveness to neurotrophic factors contributing to the phenotype of the disease state.

Major Depressive Disorder The strongest evidence for a role for neurotrophins has come from the pathophysiology of depression, especially those associated with stress. In depression, it is believed that there is a fundamental dysregulation of synaptic plasticity and neuronal survival in regions of the brain, such as the hippocampus. There are several lines of evidence suggesting that neurotrophins play a role in depression. First, in animal models, restraint stress leads to decreased expression of BDNF in the hippocampus. In addition, chronic physical or psychosocial stress leads to atrophy and death of hippocampal neurons, especially in the CA3 region in rodents and primates. Also, magnetic resonance imaging (MRI) studies have shown that patients with depressive or posttraumatic stress disorders exhibited a small decrease in hippocampal volume. It is unclear, however, whether the atrophy or death of these neurons is directly related to the decreased availability of BDNF. In addition, not all forms of depression are associated with stress. However, if structural remodeling and synaptic plasticity are involved in the cellular pathophysiology of depression, deficits in BDNF signaling is an attractive candidate molecule to mediate these alterations.

Second, exogenously administered BDNF in the midbrain or hippocampus resulted in antidepressant effects in two animal models of depression (forced swim and learned helplessness paradigms) and was comparable to chronic treatment with pharmacological antidepressants. In addition, BDNF has also been shown to have trophic effects on serotonergic and noradrenergic neurons in vitro and in vivo. Mutant mice with decreased levels of BDNF have been shown to have a selective decrement in serotonergic neuron function and corresponding behavioral dysfunction consistent with serotonergic abnormalities.

Third, SSRIs and norepinephrine reuptake inhibitor antidepressants upregulate and activate CREB, a cAMP-dependent transcription factor, and BDNF in a time course that corresponds to therapeutic action (10 to 20 days). The CREB transcription factor is involved in the induction of BDNF gene expression in neurons. This effect on the cAMP pathway provides a link between monoamine antidepressants and neurotrophin actions. These antidepressant treatments also lead to increases in expression of TrkB receptors in the hippocampus in a time course that also parallels the long time course of therapeutic action of these treatments. Two other antidepressant treatments, monoamine oxidase inhibitors (MAOIs) and electroconvulsive therapy (ECT), also upregulate BDNF transcription. In rodents, long-term ECT has been shown to elicit sprouting of hippocampal neurons, which was attenuated in mutant mice that express lower levels of BDNF. Together, these studies provide a framework to examine further the neurotrophin system as a potential therapeutic target for the treatment of depression. Antidepressants may work by increasing cAMP, activating CREB, and increasing neurotrophin signaling by inducing BDNF and TrkB levels.

NEUROTROPHINS AND GENETICS

Until recently, no genetic associations had been found between neurotrophin genes and any human neurological or psychiatric disorders. A recent series of studies, however, has linked a polymorphism in the BDNF gene with depression, bipolar disorder, and schizophrenia. This polymorphism, identified from a single nucleotide polymorphism (SNP) screen, leads to a single amino acid change from a valine (Val) to a methionine (Met) at position 66 in the pro region of the BDNF protein. This region has been believed to be important in proper folding and intracellular sorting of BDNF. Interestingly, proforms of neurotrophins have recently been shown to act as selective ligands for $p75^{NTR}$. This polymorphism has been associated with increased susceptibility to neurodegenerative and neuropsychiatric disorders, including Alzheimer's disease, Parkinson's disease, bipolar disorder, depression, eating disorder, and obsessive-compulsive disorder (OCD), as well as cognitive impairment. In patients with bipolar disorder or depression, the Val allele appears to confer greater risk for the disease, whereas, in schizophrenic patients, the Met allele appears to be associated with impaired memory functions. Although the molecular mechanism for these alterations is not known, the existence of variants in neurotrophins provides evidence that neurotrophins are implicated in the complex pathophysiology of these diseases. Understanding the molecular mechanism for alterations in BDNF function for these genetic variants will provide invaluable insight into potential pathophysiology for these major psychiatric disorders.

THERAPEUTIC POTENTIAL OF NEUROTROPHINS

The recent clinical trials have highlighted limits in designing therapeutic strategies to use neurotrophic factors for neurodegenerative and psychiatric disorders. First, it has become clear that physical delivery of sufficient polypeptide quantities to target neurons is a major obstacle. Development of small molecules that readily cross the blood–brain barrier to activate neurotrophin receptors or potentiate the actions of neurotrophins is an approach that is in its infancy.

Second, it is also clear that, with neurotrophins having multiple effects on neuronal activity, indiscriminate "flooding" of the CNS with neurotrophic factors likely leads to untoward side effects, such as epileptic activity. In addition, it had been noted in the clinical trials with BDNF that downregulation of the TrkB receptors after unregulated application of BDNF may have also contributed to the minimal therapeutic effects. New strategies include more local and regulated application of neurotrophins through stereotactic injection of regulatable viral vectors or engineered progenitor cells. In particular, this approach is currently being applied to diseases such as Alzheimer's disease, in which there is a defined neuronal population, such as basal forebrain cholinergic neurons, that undergo degeneration and are dependent on one neurotrophin, such as NGF.

Third, activation of the neurotrophin system through other receptor signaling systems offers an alternative strategy. For example, antidepressant agents acting via monoamine G-protein–coupled receptors can lead to increased expression of both neurotrophins and neurotrophin receptors. Importantly, only the neurons that express the monoamine G-protein–coupled receptors will have enhanced production of the neurotrophin or Trk receptor. Recently, it has also been shown that other G-protein–coupled receptors, the purine adenosine 2A receptor and the pituitary adenylate cyclase–activating polypeptide (PACAP) neuropeptide receptor, can activate Trk neurotrophin receptors in the absence of neurotrophins in cultured hippocampal neurons, a process termed *Trk transactivation.* Therefore, small molecules can activate Trk receptors in the absence of neurotrophins. These results raise the possibility that small molecules may be used to elicit neurotrophic effects for the treatment of neurodegenerative diseases by selective targeting of neurons that express specific G-protein–coupled receptors and Trk receptors.

It should be emphasized that all of these strategies using neurotrophic factors are based on an assumption of symptomatic treatment of impaired neurons. This impairment implies not only cell survival, but also proper functioning of these neurons. With greater understanding of the signal transduction pathways that are activated by neurotrophins, alternate strategies can be devised to manipulate these specific pathways through new drug development. In addition, further understanding of the core pathophysiological mechanisms for neurodegenerative and psychiatric disorders will obviously benefit the development of rational therapies that involve engaging the neurotrophin system.

SUGGESTED CROSS-REFERENCES

Related topics include Sections 1.4, 1.5, and 1.6, which cover the role of neurotransmitters in psychiatry.

REFERENCES

Airaksinen MS, Saarma M: The GDNF family: signaling, biological functions and therapeutic value. *Nat Rev Neurosci.* 2002;3:383.

Black IB: Trophic regulation of synaptic plasticity. *J Neurobiol.* 1999;41:108.

Cabelli, RJ, Hohn A, Shatz CJ: Inhibition of ocular dominance column formation by infusion of NT4/5 or BDNF. *Science.* 1995;267:1662.

Chao, MV, Bothwell M: Neurotrophins: to cleave or not to cleave. *Neuron.* 2002;33:9.

Chao MV, Hempstead BL: p75 and Trk: a two-receptor system. *Trends Neurosci.* 1995;18:321.

*Duman RS, Heninger GR, Nestler EJ: A molecular and cellular theory of depression. *Arch Gen Psychiatry.* 1997;54:597.

Egan MF, Kojima M, Callicott JH, Goldberg TE, Kolachana BS, Bertolino A, Zaitsev E, Gold B, Goldman D, Dean M, Lu B, Weinberger DR: The BDNF val66met polymorphism affects activity-dependent secretion of BDNF and human memory and hippocampal formation. *Cell.* 2003;114:521.

Enomoto H, Heuckeroth RO, Golden JP, Johnson EM, Milbrandt J: Development of cranial parasympathetic ganglia requires sequential actions of GDNF and neurturin. *Development.* 2000;127:4877.

*Ginty DD, Segal RA. Retrograde neurotrophin signaling: Trk-ing along the axon. *Curr Opin Neurobiol.* 2002;12:268.

Hariri AR, Goldberg TE, Mattay VS, Kolachana BS, Callicott JH, Egan MF, Weinberger DR: Brain-derived neurotrophic factor val66met polymorphism affects human memory-related hippocampal activity and predicts memory performance. *J Neurosci.* 2003;23:6690–6694.

*Hempstead BL: The many faces of p75NTR. *Curr Opin Neurobiol.* 2002;12:260.

Huang EJ, Reichardt LF: Neurotrophins: roles in neuronal development and function. *Annu Rev Neurosci.* 2001;24:677.

Kaplan DR, Miller FD: Neurotrophin signal transduction in the nervous system. *Curr Opin Neurobiol.* 2000;10:381.

Kernie SG, Liebl DJ, Parada LF: BDNF regulates eating behavior and locomotor activity in mice. *EMBO J.* 2000;19:1290.

Kovalchuk Y, Hanse E, Kafitz KW, Konnerth A. Postsynaptic induction of BDNF mediated long-term potentiation. *Science.* 2002;295:1729.

Lee FS, Chao MV: Activation of Trk neurotrophin receptors in the absence of neurotrophins. *Proc Natl Acad Sci U S A.* 2001;98:3555.

Lee FS, Kim AH, Khursigara G, Chao MV: The uniqueness of being a neurotrophin receptor. *Curr Opin Neurobiol.* 2001;11:281.

Lee R, Kermani P, Teng KK, Hempstead BL: Regulation of cell survival by secreted proneurotrophins. *Science.* 2001;294:1945.

Levi-Montalcini R: The nerve growth factor: thirty-five years later. *Science.* 2001;237:1154.

Lu B: Pro-region of neurotrophins. Role in synaptic modulation. *Neuron.* 2003;39:735–738.

*Lyons WE, Mamounas LA, Ricaurte GA, Coppola V, Reid SW, Bora SH, Wihler C, Koliatsos VE, Tessarollo L: Brain-derived neurotrophic factor-deficient mice develop aggressiveness and hyperphagia in conjunction with brain serotonergic abnormalities. *Proc Natl Acad Sci U S A.* 1999;96:15239.

Minichiello L, Calella AM, Medina DL, Bonhoeffer T, Klein R, Korte M: Mechanism of TrkB-mediated hippocampal long-term potentiation. *Neuron.* 2002;36:121.

*Poo MM: Neurotrophins as synaptic modulators. *Nat Rev Neurosci.* 2001;2:24.

Riccio A, Ahn S, Davenport CM, Blendy JA, Ginty DD: Mediation by a CREB family transcription factor of NGF-dependent survival of sympathetic neurons. *Science.* 1999;286:2358.

Rios M, Fan G, Fekete C, Kelly J, Bates B, Kuehn R, Lechan RM, Jaenisch R: Conditional deletion of brain-derived neurotrophic factor in the postnatal brain leads to obesity and hyperactivity. *Mol Endocrinol.* 2001;15:1748.

Sen S, Nesse R, Stoltenberg SF, Li S, Gleiberman L, Chakravarti A, Weder AB, Burmeister M: A BDNF coding variant is associated with the NEO personality inventory domain neuroticism, a risk factor for depression. *Neuropharmacology.* 2003;28:397–401.

Shirayama Y, Chen ACH, Nakagawa S, Russell DS, Duman RS: Brain-derived neurotrophic factor produces antidepressant effects in behavioral models of depression. *J Neurosci.* 2002;22:3251.

Sklar P, Gabriel SB, McInnis MG, Bennett P, Lim YM, Tsan G, Schaffner S, Kirov G, Jones I, Owen M, Craddock N, DePaulo JR, Lander ES: Family-based association study of 76 candidate genes in bipolar disorder: BDNF is a potential risk locus. *Mol Psychiatry.* 2002;7:579.

Snider WD: Functions of the neurotrophins during nervous system development: What the knockouts are teaching us. *Cell.* 1994;77:627.

Thoenen H, Sendtner M: Neurotrophins: from enthusiastic expectations through sobering experiences to rational therapeutic approaches. *Nat Neurosci.* 2002;5(Suppl):1046.

Xie CW, Sayah D, Chen QS, Wei WZ, Smith D, Liu X: Deficient long-term memory and long-lasting long-term potentiation in mice with a targeted deletion of neurotrophin-4 gene. *Proc Natl Acad Sci U S A.* 2000;97:8116.

Zakharenko SS, Patterson SL, Dragatsis I, Zeitlin SO, Siegelbaum SA, Kandel ER, Morozov A: Presynaptic BDNF required for a presynaptic but not postsynaptic component of LTP at hippocampal CA1-CA3 synapses. *Neuron.* 2003;39:975–990.

▲ 1.8 Intraneuronal Signaling Pathways

JAY M. BARABAN, M.D., PH.D.

Attempting to understand normal and abnormal behavior is futile without an appreciation of the interplay of forces lurking beneath the surface. This notion rings true at the cellular level as well. Thus, deciphering the microscopic world of intraneuronal signaling pathways is critical to understanding how neurons process information. This level of analysis represents a new frontier in dissecting the basis of behavior and psychotropic drug action and is likely to guide development of improved treatment and diagnostic approaches for psychiatric patients in the foreseeable future. Accordingly, this chapter provides an overview of several major intracellular signaling pathways and illustrates their relevance to fundamental issues in psychiatry.

MAJOR SIGNALING PATHWAYS

Before delving into the organization of individual pathways, it is worthwhile to consider why neurons use such a wide variety of intracellular signaling pathways. Perhaps the most straightforward answer is that the multiplicity of intracellular signaling pathways enables cells to maintain separate channels of information processing that can be integrated only when appropriate. Furthermore, each signaling pathway has distinctive spatial and temporal features that have evolved to achieve optimal handling of different types of information. For example, it might be desirable to have extremely high sensitivity to novel stimuli but to ignore repetitive inputs. Alternatively, key information may be coded in the duration of a stimulus, in which case, signaling pathways must integrate the signal over the relevant time scale. Furthermore, use of multiple signaling pathways allows neurons to detect coincident presentation of numerous stimuli and enables them to alter their response accordingly. In brief, intraneuronal signaling pathways make up a microscopic nervous system within each neuron that determines its sensitivity and responsiveness to its environment in light of current circumstances and past experience.

Despite the distinct features found in each signaling pathway, the flow of information from the initial stages of detection to the resultant alterations in neuronal function shares common themes. In general, the organization of these systems can be divided into several layers. Signals are detected by receptors and then funneled into the cell via adapter proteins that link the extracellular signal to one or more intracellular signaling pathways. These, in turn, alter the func-

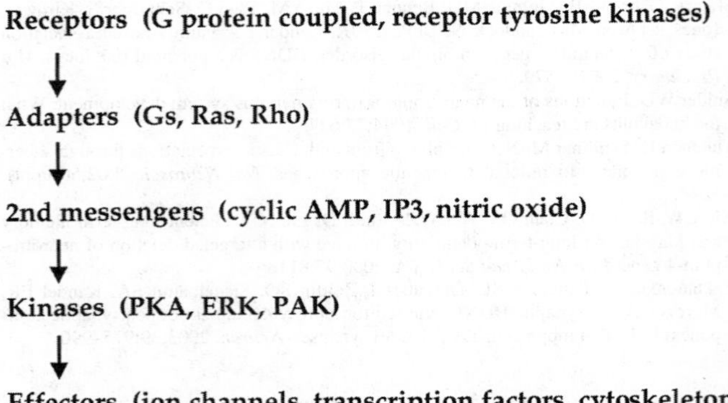

FIGURE 1.8–1 Overview of signaling pathways. Despite marked differences in the organization of distinct signaling pathways, there are common organizational themes linking receptor activation to changes in effector activity. Examples of signaling components that subserve these functions in the major signaling pathways outlined are listed. cyclic AMP, cyclic adenosine monophosphate; ERK, extracellular agonist-regulated kinase; IP_3, inositol trisphosphate; PAK, p21-activated kinase; PKA, protein kinase A.

tion of effector proteins, either directly or via intermediates, such as protein kinases. Like the nervous system, these signaling pathways bridge the spatial and temporal gaps between sensory input and motor output (i.e., receptor activation and changes in effector activity). Examples of how specific signaling pathways fit into this general organizational scheme are presented in Figure 1.8–1.

Cyclic Adenosine Monophosphate (cAMP) System

The classic cross-perfusion experiments conducted by Otto Loewi at the turn of the century led to the first identification of a neurotransmitter substance, acetylcholine, and revolutionized the understanding of synaptic transmission. In a similar manner, the discovery of cyclic adenosine monophosphate (cAMP) by Earl Wilber Sutherland and Theodore Rall nearly half a century later using an analogous approach established the principle that intracellular transmitters or second messengers are instrumental in conveying information from cell surface receptors to their targets within the cell. The accumulation of decades of research on this system has revealed its operating principles in great detail and has served as a blueprint for deciphering other signaling pathways as well.

For this signaling pathway, generation of cAMP is controlled by the balance between the activity of its synthetic enzyme, adenylyl cyclase, which converts adenosine triphosphate (ATP) to cAMP, and phosphodiesterase, which cleaves cAMP to an inactive breakdown product, AMP. Adenylyl cyclase is regulated by cell surface receptors via a family of adapter proteins, referred to as *G proteins* because they bind guanosine triphosphate (GTP) when the receptor is activated. In this activated configuration, the α subunit of the G protein complex dissociates from the βγ subunits, enabling it to regulate cAMP formation. The α subunit possesses an intrinsic GTPase activity that converts GTP to guanosine diphosphate (GDP), allowing the subunits to reassemble into an inactive configuration.

Neurotransmitter receptors couple to adenylyl cyclase via different classes of G proteins, referred to as G_s or G_i, depending on whether they stimulate or inhibit cAMP formation (Fig. 1.8–2). In this way, the net effect of a transmitter on a given neuron or synapse is determined by the specific receptor subtypes expressed on its surface. For example, norepinephrine stimulates adenylyl cyclase via its interaction with β receptors, and it inhibits it via stimulation of α2 receptor subtypes.

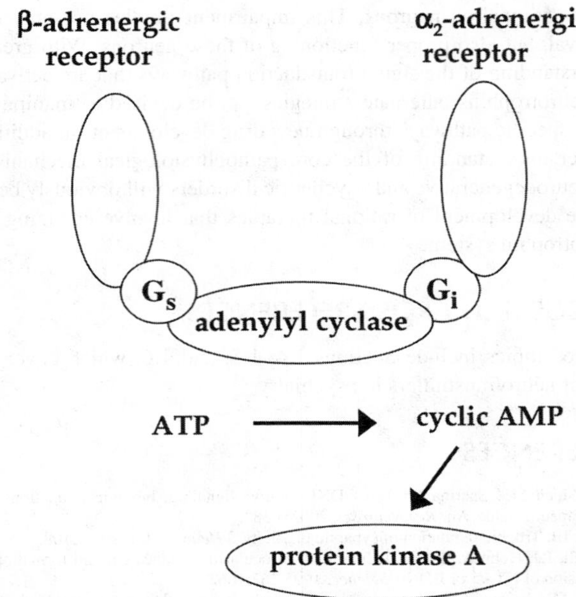

FIGURE 1.8–2 Organization of the cyclic adenosine monophosphate (AMP) system. Generation of cyclic AMP from adenosine triphosphate (ATP) by adenylyl cyclase can be stimulated or inhibited by receptor–G protein linkages. In the example shown, the β-adrenergic receptor couples to G_s to stimulate cyclic AMP formation, whereas the α2 adrenergic receptor inhibits this process via its linkage to G_i. Cyclic AMP exerts many of its cellular actions via its ability to activate protein kinase A.

cAMP exerts a wide variety of actions on neuronal function via its stimulatory effect on cAMP-dependent protein kinase. This enzyme has a broad range of substrate proteins involved in regulating virtually every aspect of neuronal function, from ion channel gating to axonal transport. The divergent actions of the cAMP system inside the cell are reminiscent of the autonomic nervous system, which coordinates the activity of diverse organ systems to achieve a cohesive response. Although cAMP-dependent protein kinase, also referred to as *protein kinase A* (PKA), has a multitude of targets, it is important to emphasize that it is not homogeneously distributed throughout the cell. Instead, a family of scaffolding proteins termed *A-kinase anchoring proteins* (AKAPs) recruits it to the vicinity of substrates. The compartmentalization of key signaling molecules via protein–protein interactions is a recurrent theme in intracellular signaling pathways and has several advantageous features. For example, prepositioning signaling proteins in close proximity to upstream or downstream links in the pathway speeds up the signaling process, eliminating delays due to protein diffusion.

One target of the cAMP system that has been the focus of attention in recent years is a transcription regulatory factor that enables elevations in cAMP to regulate gene expression. This factor, referred to as the *cAMP response element binding* (CREB) *protein*, binds to a short sequence of deoxyribonucleic acid (DNA), called the *CREB response element* (CRE), located in the regulatory regions of its target genes. Phosphorylation of CREB by PKA stimulates its transcriptional activity. Thus, alterations in cAMP levels can affect neuronal function over a broad range of time scales. Rapid effects are achieved by targeting ion channel gating or transmitter release machinery. On a more sluggish time scale, cAMP can influence neurotransmitter synthesis or energy metabolism. Furthermore, cAMP elicits longer-lasting changes in neuronal function as a result of its ability to activate CREB, which controls the expression of specific target genes.

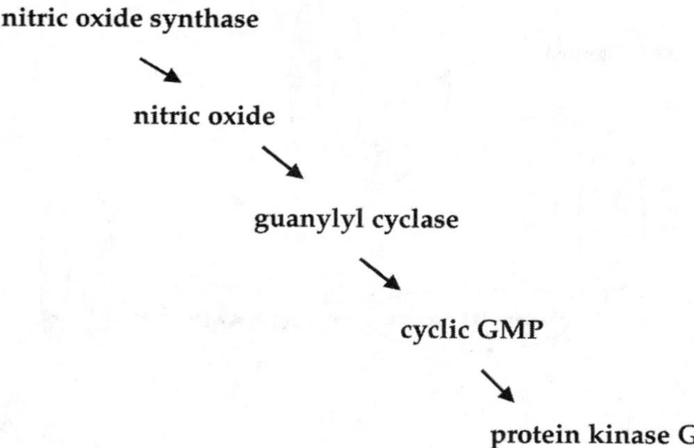

FIGURE 1.8–3 Organization of the cyclic guanosine monophosphate (cyclic GMP) system. In contrast to cyclic adenosine monophosphate (cAMP) formation, which is regulated by G proteins, cyclic GMP synthesis via guanylyl cyclase is stimulated by nitric oxide. Beyond this point in the pathway, cyclic GMP mimics cAMP as it acts by stimulating its cognate kinase, protein kinase G.

Cyclic Guanosine Monophosphate (cGMP) In addition to cAMP, another cyclic nucleotide, cyclic guanosine monophosphate (cGMP), has been identified as a second messenger regulated by neurotransmitter receptor stimulation. The discovery of cGMP-dependent protein kinases suggested that both cyclic nucleotide systems followed similar blueprints. However, subsequent studies have revealed marked contrasts between these systems. The link between neurotransmitter receptor activation and stimulation of guanylyl cyclase is not mediated directly via G-protein coupling. Instead, the available evidence indicates that elevations in intracellular calcium trigger increases in nitric oxide production, which, in turn, activates guanylyl cyclase (Fig. 1.8–3). This demonstration that a gas can act as a second messenger blurs the semantic distinction between extracellular and intracellular messengers, as nitric oxide is capable of diffusing both within cells as well as across cell membranes to act in neighboring cells. Accordingly, nitric oxide has the ability to act in a paracrine fashion to affect cells within its sphere of diffusion.

Studies of the cGMP system have underscored the general principle that regulating degradation of second messengers is a powerful means of modulating the activity of intracellular signaling pathways. One of the best-understood actions of cGMP is its key role in mediating the response of photoreceptor cells to light. In the dark, cGMP levels in these cells are high; activation of rhodopsin by light triggers a rapid decrease in cGMP levels. This effect of light is mediated by activation of a phosphodiesterase that hydrolyzes cGMP to GMP, rather than by suppressing synthesis of cGMP. Thus, linking rhodopsin stimulation to activation of phosphodiesterase allows light to produce rapid drops in cGMP levels and minimizes the delay in visual perception. Conversely, drugs that block cGMP phosphodiesterase provide a convenient way of elevating cGMP levels, as evidenced by the mode of action of antiimpotence drugs, such as sildenafil (Viagra), which exert their vasodilatory effects by blocking cGMP phosphodiesterase in smooth muscle. Thus, this class of drugs illustrates the impressive effects that can be achieved by targeting an intracellular signaling pathway.

Analysis of the role of cGMP in phototransduction also debunked the previously held dogma that all of the actions of cyclic nucleotides are mediated via their corresponding protein kinases. In this system, cGMP acts by directly binding to membrane ion channels. Thus, an important concept to emerge from these studies is that, even though protein kinases play a central role in intraneuronal signaling pathways, second messengers can affect cell function through other means. In a similar vein, it is important to point out that phosphorylation is not the only posttranslational modification that can be used to induce dynamic changes in protein localization or function. Recent studies indicate that nitric oxide may also exert its effects by *S*-nitrosylation of cysteine residues, in addition to its classic effects on cGMP production. Although studies of *S*-nitrosylation are still in their infancy, the available evidence suggests that this posttranslational modification represents an important method of modifying protein function.

Phosphoinositide System Characterization of the neurotransmitter receptors coupled to the cAMP system revealed that there were many receptors that did not act via this second messenger pathway. This discrepancy generated interest in the possible existence of other second messenger systems operating in parallel with the cAMP system. This line of research came to fruition in the early 1980s with the emergence of a coherent view of the phosphoinositide (PI) second messenger system. This system parallels many aspects of the cAMP system but also includes several novel features (Fig. 1.8–4). Neurotransmitter receptor stimulation is coupled, via G proteins, to activation of a second messenger–generating enzyme, phospholipase C. This enzyme cleaves phosphatidylinositol bisphosphate (PIP_2), an inositol-containing phospholipid located in the plasma membrane, into two second messengers, diacylglycerol and inositol triphosphate (IP_3). Thus, activation of neurotransmitter receptors linked to the PI system generates a pair of second messenger signals that can affect cellular processes via distinct pathways.

Because the effects of cAMP are mediated to a large extent via activation of a protein kinase, it was generally assumed that each of these second messengers acted in a similar fashion. This turned out to be true of diacylglycerol, which activates protein kinase C, but not for IP_3. In contrast, IP_3 acts much like an intracellular transmitter. It acts on IP_3 receptors located on the cytoplasmic face of intracellular organelles that store calcium. Binding of IP_3 to its receptor triggers

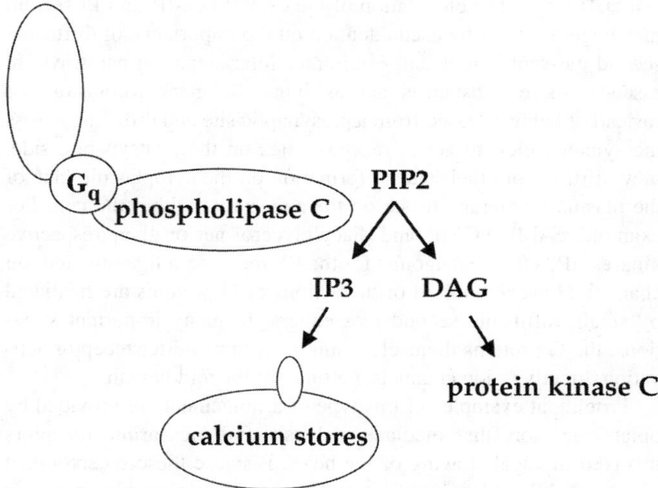

FIGURE 1.8–4 Organization of the phosphoinositide (PI) system. In this system, neurotransmitter receptor stimulation leads, via G-protein coupling, to activation of phospholipase C. This enzyme cleaves the membrane phospholipid, phosphatidylinositol biphosphate (PIP_2), into two second messengers, inositol trisphosphate (IP_3) and diacylglycerol (DAG). IP_3 releases calcium from intracellular stores; DAG stimulates protein kinase C.

release of calcium from these intracellular stores. Calcium, in turn, is a second messenger in its own right. Although it can affect several target proteins directly, such as those involved in triggering neurotransmitter release, its sphere of influence is greatly enlarged by its association with calmodulin, a small, ubiquitous, calcium-binding protein. Calmodulin bound to calcium is able to activate kinases, such as calcium/calmodulin-dependent kinases, as well as phosphatases, including calcineurin. In this way, it is capable of regulating many intracellular processes ranging from ion channel activity to gene expression. Elucidation of the role of IP_3 in liberating calcium from intracellular stores revealed that the regulation of cytoplasmic calcium is more complex than previously appreciated. Thus, in addition to its entry from extracellular fluid via plasma membrane ion channels, calcium can also be released from intracellular stores by cell surface receptors linked to the PI system.

It is noteworthy that lithium (Eskalith) played an important role in the discovery of the PI second messenger system. It had been noted in studies aimed at defining the effects of lithium on the central nervous system (CNS) that lithium caused a modest decrease in concentrations of inositol, a sugar closely related to glucose that is used in the synthesis of membrane PIs. In pursuing the basis for this effect, investigators noted that lithium was an effective inhibitor of a phosphatase that converts inositol phosphate into inositol. Lithium could then be used to enhance accumulation of inositol phosphates, providing a convenient means of measuring activation of the PI system. By using lithium in this way, researchers were able to detect the presence of IP_3.

The discovery that lithium blocks the degradation of inositol phosphates into free inositol needed to replenish inositol phospholipids has prompted the hypothesis that depletion of inositol and subsequent rundown of the PI cycle may underlie lithium's therapeutic action. This view has been challenged by animal studies indicating that inositol levels in the brain are unaffected by lithium concentrations within its therapeutic range. However, recent studies have renewed interest in this hypothesis, as lithium, along with other mood-stabilizing agents, exerts a common effect on axonal outgrowth in vitro that is reversed by treatment with inositol.

Direct Coupling between G Proteins and Ion Channels

The elucidation of the cAMP, cGMP, and PI second messenger systems focused attention on the importance of diffusible second messenger molecules in intracellular signaling pathways. In essence, these substances act as intracellular neurotransmitters. Instead of being released from a presynaptic site and diffusing across the synaptic cleft to act at receptor sites on the postsynaptic side, they diffuse from their site of formation on the cytoplasmic face of the plasma membrane to act on their receptors within the cell. For example, cAMP, cGMP, and diacylglycerol act on their respective kinases; IP_3 acts as an agonist for the IP_3 receptor, a ligand-gated ion channel. However, not all of the actions of G proteins are mediated by small, diffusible second messengers. In many important situations, the G proteins themselves link neurotransmitter receptor activation directly to ion channels, cutting out the middleman.

Prominent examples of this type of arrangement are provided by opiate receptors that mediate analgesia and muscarinic receptors involved in vagal slowing of the heart. Because these receptors act via G_i to inhibit adenylyl cyclase, it was assumed that they regulated ion channels by lowering cAMP levels. However, this theory was shattered by experiments in which restoration of cAMP concentrations was ineffective in reversing this result. Furthermore, patch clamp studies have been used to dissect the role of diffusible second messengers in these responses. Using this approach, one can assess whether channels in the patch are regulated by ligand added to the exterior surface of the patch or to the cell membrane outside of the patch (Fig. 1.8–5). If diffusible second messengers are involved, application of a receptor agonist to the cell membrane outside the patch should be effective, as the signal will be conveyed via intracellular messengers that can diffuse from the receptor to the ion channel. However, in this system, receptor ligands are only effective if applied directly to the exterior surface of the patch, providing compelling evidence that diffusible second messengers are not involved. Subsequent studies confirmed that G_i mediates ion channel regulation via a direct interaction with the channels, a mechanism that is widely used in the nervous system.

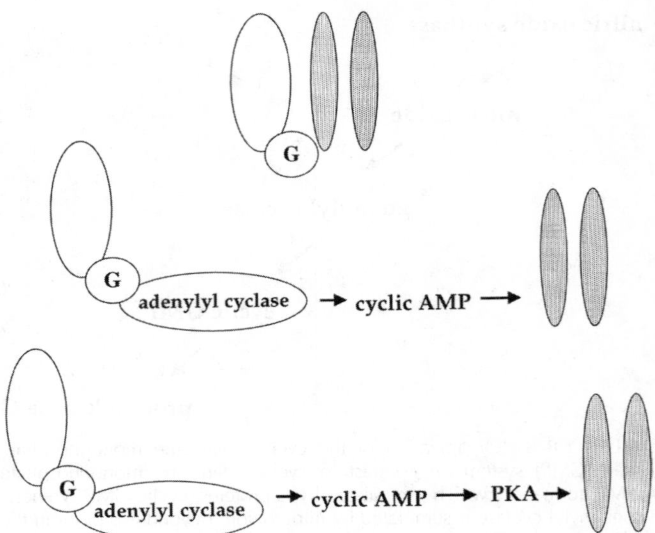

FIGURE 1.8–5 Regulation of ion channels by G-protein–coupled receptors. Not all the effects of cyclic nucleotides are mediated by protein kinases. As shown in the upper panel, G proteins can directly link neurotransmitter receptors to ion channels. This configuration underlies regulation of potassium channels that slow the heart in response to vagal stimulation of muscarinic cholinergic receptors. Alternatively, cyclic nucleotides can directly affect ion channels in a kinase-independent fashion, as illustrated in the middle panel. The conventional kinase-dependent pathway is shown in the bottom panel. This type of arrangement mediates the well-known ability of sympathetic stimulation to speed the heart rate via activation of β-adrenergic receptors. cyclic AMP, cyclic adenosine monophosphate; PKA, protein kinase A.

These findings underscore the concept that intracellular signaling cascades have evolved in ways that heighten their versatility. Although the classic version of the cAMP cascade involves regulation of effector targets via activation of PKA, it is now clear that, as found for cGMP, cAMP can also directly regulate ion channel activity without working via PKA. Furthermore, as described above, cAMP itself is also dispensable, as G proteins can regulate ion channel activity directly without acting via cAMP or other diffusible second messengers. Accordingly, each of these major components of the signaling pathway can act on effector targets themselves or recruit downstream components of the signaling cascade.

Regulation of G-Protein Function

Because G proteins play a central role in linking receptor activation to intracellular signaling pathways, it is not surprising that there is a family of intracellular proteins termed *regulators of G-protein signaling*, or *RGS proteins*, that regulate their activity. They act by accelerating the GTPase activity of G proteins and thereby shorten the duration of the active state. Members of the RGS family are thought to act on different subsets of G proteins. For example, RGS2 interacts with a G protein that couples receptors to phospholipase C. An interesting feature of RGS2 is that its expression can be rapidly increased by neuronal activity and, thus, is thought to provide a feedback mechanism for modulating activation of the PI system. Recent studies have also demonstrated that mice with targeted deletion of the gene encoding RGS2 display alterations in aggression and anxiety. Thus, these findings indicate how RGS proteins can have a major impact on behavior. Another member of this family, RGS9, is highly enriched in the striatum, an area of the brain that receives prominent dopamine innervation. The heterogeneous distribution of RGS family proteins makes them an attractive drug target, as drugs affecting individual isoforms may exert highly selective effects. Certainly, development of selective drugs for individual receptor subtypes (e.g., adrenergic or serotonergic receptor subtypes) has been an effective strategy for developing novel and improved therapeutic agents. In a similar vein, current and future efforts to exploit heterogeneity in intraneuronal signaling pathways will likely be useful as well.

This approach will be applicable not only to RGS proteins, but also to a broad range of intracellular signaling proteins. Many key steps in these pathways are mediated by families of proteins, rather than a single representative. For example, there are nine forms of adenylyl cyclase and more than a dozen genes encoding phosphodiesterases. Each of these has a distinct pattern of expression and regulation. The ability to develop drugs that target individual subtypes selectively is exemplified by sildenafil and related antiimpotence drugs, which selectively inhibit type V phosphodiesterase, an isoform concentrated in vascular smooth muscle. Presumably, these families of proteins have evolved to help tailor the regulation, selectivity, and activity of specific signaling components to the differing needs of distinct cell types. Nature's efforts to expand the versatility of these signaling pathways by generating multiple isoforms of signaling pathway components can be exploited to generate drugs that have a high degree of selectivity.

Tyrosine Phosphorylation

The protein kinases involved in the second messenger pathways discussed above act exclusively on serine or threonine residues. As a result, it was assumed that all protein kinases targeted these residues, as nearly 99 percent of all phosphate groups incorporated into proteins are linked to these amino acids. Thus, it came as quite a surprise that the apparently negligible level of phosphorylation on tyrosine residues reflects the action of a distinct set of signaling pathways (Fig. 1.8–6). Although, from a quantitative point of view, tyrosine phosphorylation is dwarfed by phosphorylation on serine and threonine residues, tyrosine kinase signaling pathways have emerged as playing extremely important roles in intraneuronal signaling. For example, nerve growth factor and other members of the neurotrophin family act via cell surface receptors that are tyrosine kinases. Binding of neurotrophins to the extracellular portion of these receptors leads to activation of a tyrosine kinase domain located in the cytoplasmic portion of these transmembrane proteins. Because neurotrophins have a dimeric structure, their binding to the extracellular portion of their receptor brings together two receptor molecules. This proximity allows their cytoplasmic tyrosine kinase domains to phosphorylate each other on tyrosine residues.

This simple modification of the cytoplasmic tail converts it into a magnet for an array of signaling proteins that are brought together at the inner surface of the membrane. This arrangement triggers activation of multiple, divergent signaling cascades that emanate from this nidus. One of these branches leads to stimulation of the PI system via direct interaction with a phospholipase C isoform without requiring G-protein activation. Thus, both neurotransmitters and growth factors are able to access this intracellular pathway. In addition to the PI system, neurotrophin receptor stimulation also triggers activation of extracellular agonist-regulated kinase (ERK) and phosphatidylinositol 3 (PI3)-kinase pathways.

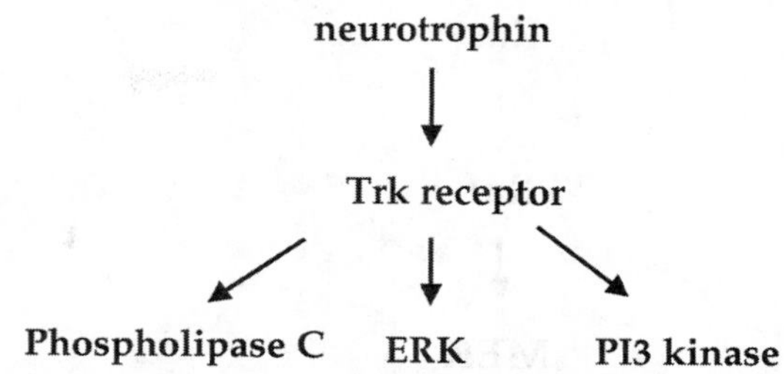

FIGURE 1.8–6 Divergence of signaling pathways from neurotrophin receptors. The cytoplasmic tail of tyrosine receptor kinase (Trk) receptors serves as a staging area for the activation of multiple intracellular signaling pathways. These include the phospholipase C/phosphoinositide (PI) system, the extracellular agonist-regulated kinase (ERK) pathway, which is activated by Ras, and the phosphatidylinositol 3-kinase (PI3) system, which is upstream of Akt.

Another family of tyrosine kinases differs from the transmembrane receptor tyrosine kinases in that its members are cytoplasmic proteins. The absence of an extracellular ligand binding domain has made it difficult to determine how these tyrosine kinases are regulated. Nevertheless, evidence is accumulating that these nonreceptor tyrosine kinases, such as *fyn*, *src*, and *yes*, play a critical role in multiple neuronal responses.

Ras Signaling

Just as classic G proteins play a central role in mediating neurotransmitter receptor activation of intracellular signaling cascades, Ras, the prototype of a distinct family of G proteins characterized by smaller size, plays a similar role in neurotrophin receptor signaling. Like their larger cousins, Ras and other small G proteins are bound to GDP in their inactive state. Stimulation of growth factor receptors initiates a cascade that catalyzes dissociation of GDP and formation of the active GTP-bound form of Ras. In contrast to neurotransmitter receptors, which directly catalyze this activation step when stimulated by receptor agonists, growth factor receptor stimulation triggers activation of a distinct protein referred to as *guanine nucleotide exchange factor* (GEF) that performs this function. While in the active GTP-bound form, Ras is able to activate downstream effector pathways, including the ERK and PI3-kinase pathways. As found for classic G proteins, Ras is inactivated by hydrolysis of GTP. This is achieved with the help of accessory proteins called *GTPase-activating proteins* (GAPs), analogous to the action of RGS proteins on classic G proteins.

Elucidation of the signaling pathways downstream of Ras has revealed two major kinase cascades, the ERK and PI3-kinase pathways that mediate many of the powerful effects of neurotrophins on neuronal differentiation and survival (Fig. 1.8–7). In contrast to the classic second messenger signaling pathways, the ERK pathway does not use a small molecule intermediate. Instead, the signaling pathway is organized as a kinase cascade in which a series of three or more kinases are sequentially regulated by phosphorylation via upstream kinases. One potential advantage of this alternative arrangement is that it has been able to evolve into multiple parallel kinase cascades without being constrained by the availability of distinct small second messengers. Thus, the ERK pathway is one of several parallel kinase cascades, referred to collectively as *mitogen-activated protein* (MAP) *kinase pathways*. Neurotrophins selectively activate the ERK pathway, whereas another MAP kinase pathway, termed the *c-Jun N-terminal kinase* (JNK) *pathway*, is activated by cellular stresses.

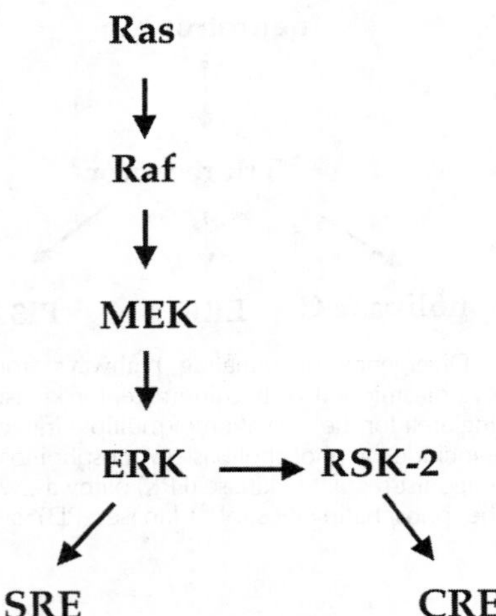

FIGURE 1.8–7 Kinase cascade activated by Ras. Ras, a member of the small G protein family, has been identified as an important mediator of growth factor responses. Activation of Ras stimulates a kinase, Raf, which regulates a series of downstream kinases. In contrast to the "classic" second messenger systems described above, these kinases are directly regulated by upstream kinases, rather than by small second messengers. Extracellular agonist-regulated kinase (ERK) activation plays an important role in regulating rapid changes in gene expression. This effect can be mediated by phosphorylation of factors that act via the serum response element (SRE) or via the CREB response element (CRE). MEK, mitogen-activated protein kinase/ERK kinase; RSK-2, ribosomal S6 kinase-2.

The ERK pathway has received considerable attention because it is involved in regulating a variety of cytoplasmic targets as well as multiple transcription factors. In addition, even though the ERK pathway was initially identified in studies aimed at understanding signaling pathways mediating the effects of receptor tyrosine kinases, subsequent studies have demonstrated that it is also activated by conventional neurotransmitters. Thus, it provides a mechanism for synaptic stimuli to elicit long-term effects on neuronal function. For example, activation of protein kinase C by neurotransmitter receptors linked to the PI system leads to stimulation of the ERK pathway. In turn, this pathway exerts a prominent effect on gene expression by its phosphorylation of two major transcription factor complexes. ERK directly phosphorylates Elk1, a regulator of the transcription factor referred to as *serum response factor*, which mediates rapid increases in gene expression. In addition, ERK can also stimulate the transcriptional activity of CREB via its phosphorylation of an intermediate kinase called *RSK* (ribosomal S6 kinase). Thus, the ERK pathway plays a key role in linking both neurotrophin and neurotransmitter receptor activation to rapid changes in gene expression.

A second pathway that can be activated by Ras is the PI3 kinase pathway. In this pathway, PIP_2, the lipid precursor that is cleaved to DAG and IP_3 in the PI pathway, is phosphorylated by a lipid kinase, PI3 kinase, to yield PIP_3. Because this lipid is restricted to the plasma membrane, it acts by recruiting proteins to the membrane. This translocation yields activation of Akt kinase, which dissociates from the membrane and phosphorylates several substrate proteins important for controlling cell survival. As found for the ERK pathway, recent studies suggest that the PI3 kinase pathway can also be engaged by neurotransmitter receptor activation. In particular, some receptors that act via G_i can trigger activation of PI3 kinase and Akt. Because this pathway plays a central role in mediating cell survival, agonists of these G_i-linked receptors may represent novel strategies for enhancing neuronal survival.

Rho Family of G Proteins The central role that Ras proteins play in neurotrophin signaling has focused attention on elucidating the actions of other small G proteins in the nervous system. In particular, recent studies have implicated the Rho family of small G proteins in mediating the effects of axon guidance signals, proteins that coordinate the incredibly complex task of wiring the nervous system during development. Because developmental abnormalities in neuronal migration or connectivity have been linked to schizophrenia and other psychiatric diseases, this field of research is likely to make important contributions to understanding the pathophysiology of these disorders.

Research in this area has focused on an organelle located at the tip of the growing axon, the growth cone. This highly dynamic structure responds to attractive and repulsive cues in the extracellular milieu via receptors located on its surface. Analysis of two well-studied axon guidance cues, ephrins and semaphorins, indicates that they exert their effects on growth cone behavior via regulation of Rho proteins, which, in turn, act on the actin cytoskeleton to control movement of these organelles. For example, the intracellular segment of one of the ephrin A receptors binds to a RhoGEF protein called *ephexin*, which modulates the exchange of GDP for GTP on Rho proteins. In a similar vein, the intracellular portion of the semaphorin receptor complex is also associated with Rho proteins (Fig. 1.8–8). As found for Ras, the activated forms of Rho act by stimulating protein kinases, which ultimately impact the localization or polymerization state of actin. In this way, external cues steer the growth cone to the vicinity of its target.

The Rho family of small G proteins can be divided into three distinct subgroups—Cdc42, Rac, and RhoA. In general, activation of members of the Cdc42 and Rac subgroups promotes growth cone extension, whereas RhoA arrests growth or triggers retraction. Accordingly, repulsive axon guidance cues have been linked with activation of the RhoA subgroup and inhibition of Rac or Cdc42.

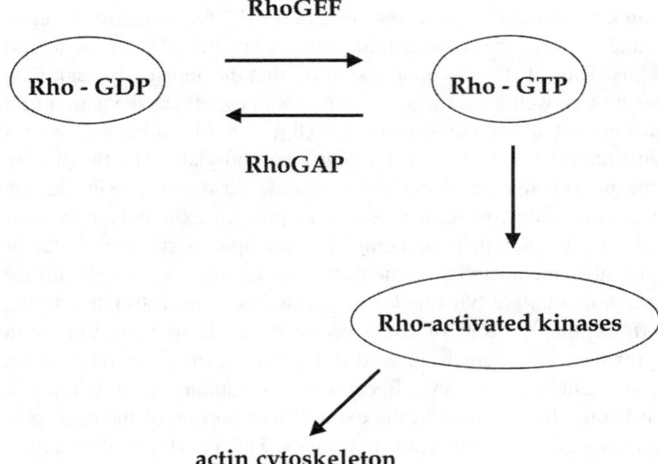

FIGURE 1.8–8 Regulation of the actin cytoskeleton by the Rho family of small G proteins. Like other G proteins, inactive forms of Rho are bound to guanosine diphosphate (GDP). Activation of Rho is catalyzed by RhoGEF proteins, which trigger swapping of GDP for guanosine triphosphate (GTP). Conversely, inactivation of Rho is mediated by RhoGAPs, which enhance the GTPase activity present in Rho proteins. Thus, increases in Rho activity can be achieved by a combination of RhoGEF activation and RhoGAP inhibition. In its GTP-bound form, Rho is able to activate a set of kinases, including PAK and Rho-kinase, which regulate the organization of the actin cytoskeleton. These signaling pathways play a major role in regulating the morphology of growth cones and dendritic spines.

Recent studies indicate that these small G proteins also control extension of regenerating axons. Thus, suppression of axon regeneration induced by components of myelin appears to be mediated by RhoA, as blockade of RhoA has been shown to enable regeneration to occur in vitro. Thus, advances in defining the role of small G proteins in controlling growth cone motility promise to yield exciting new strategies to enhance axonal regeneration.

These findings have focused attention on identifying the downstream signaling pathways that mediate the opposing effects of RhoA and Rac on growth cone behavior. Although these pathways are still being worked out, some of the key initial steps have been clarified. Like their cousin Ras, the active, GTP-bound forms of RhoA and Rac act by binding to and stimulating protein kinases. For example, RhoA activates Rho-kinase; Rac stimulates PAK.

Although the role of Rho proteins in growth cone function has been well established, more recent studies indicate that they play a similar role in regulating dynamic changes in synaptic spines, microscopic outpouchings of dendrites that receive excitatory synaptic inputs. Recent studies indicate that long-lasting changes in synaptic efficacy are associated with changes in spine number or shape. Accordingly, Rho proteins appear to be involved in remodeling synaptic connections in the mature nervous system, as well as in its initial wiring during development. For example, manipulation of Rac expression causes dramatic changes in the shape and density of dendritic spines. In addition, active forms of kalirin, a RacGEF localized to synaptic zones, alters spine morphology.

Because Rho G proteins regulate spine formation and morphology and abnormal spines are observed in many forms of mental retardation, these findings suggest that defects in this signaling pathway may be involved in mental retardation. This inference has been supported by recent genetic studies linking several inherited forms of mental retardation to mutations in genes encoding components of the Rho signaling pathway. These include α PIX, a RacGEF; PAK3, a kinase activated by Rac; and oligophrenin-1, a protein that functions as a GAP for RhoA. In addition, the available evidence indicates that defects in LIM kinase-1, a kinase that is downstream of PAK, plays a central role in the development of Williams syndrome, a form of mental retardation characterized by selective deficiencies in visual–spatial perception with relative preservation of language abilities. Thus, the ability of the Rho signaling pathways to control axon guidance and spine morphology suggests that they play critical roles in normal cognition and in the pathophysiology of cognitive disorders.

Role of Phosphatases Phosphorylation plays a central role in every signaling pathway discussed above. Thus, protein phosphatases, which reverse the effect of protein kinases, can have a major impact on these signaling pathways as well. Accordingly, regulation of phosphatase activity, either by endogenous signaling pathways or by pharmacological agents, provides a powerful mechanism for regulating neuronal responses. Ironically, one key mechanism used to regulate phosphatase activity is phosphorylation itself. A well-studied example of this type of regulation is the control of protein phosphatase 1 (PP1), a major neuronal phosphatase, by PKA. In this scenario, PKA does not phosphorylate PP1 directly but acts via endogenous proteins that inhibit PP1 (Fig. 1.8–9). One of these, dopamine-regulated phosphoprotein-32 (DARPP-32), is of particular interest to psychiatrists, because it is highly enriched in neurons that receive dopaminergic input. Phosphorylation of DARPP-32 by PKA greatly enhances its ability to inhibit PP1. Thus, this indirect mechanism enables PKA to enhance phosphorylation by blocking dephosphorylation. Conceivably, both the direct and indirect mechanisms could impact the same substrate protein. In this case, PKA would both phosphorylate this substrate and

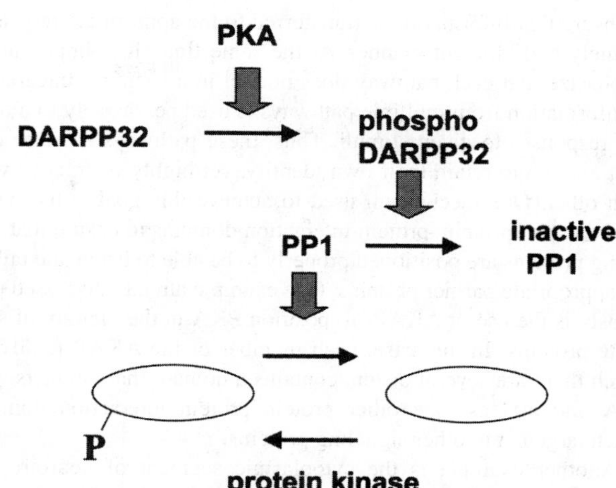

FIGURE 1.8–9 Dynamic regulation of phosphatase activity. Regulation of phosphatase activity can have a major impact on a variety of signaling pathways. As illustrated in this figure, phosphatase activity itself can also be controlled by kinases. In this scenario, protein kinase A (PKA) phosphorylates DARPP-32, which greatly enhances its ability to inhibit the protein phosphatase PP1. Thus, by this indirect mechanism, PKA is able to enhance the phosphorylation of phosphoproteins that are subject to dephosphorylation by PP1.

prevent its dephosphorylation. Alternatively, this indirect mechanism enables PKA to extend its influence by regulating dephosphorylation of substrate proteins acted on by other kinases. Thus, this provides a way for PKA to act synergistically with other kinase pathways.

Phosphatase inhibition by pharmacological agents provides another example of how targeting intracellular signaling pathways can yield important new classes of drugs. FK506, a highly effective immunosuppressant, acts by inhibiting the activity of a phosphatase, calcineurin, which plays a critical role in activation of T lymphocytes. Thus, targeting of phosphatases represents a strategy for manipulating intraneuronal signaling pathways. Support for the relevance of this concept to neuronal systems has been provided by recent studies in which transgenic methods were used to substitute one of the PP1 inhibitor proteins with a constitutively active form. Behavioral testing of these mice indicates that they require fewer task repetitions than wild-type mice do to achieve the same level of learning. In this model, repetition of a task enhances learning by decreasing PP1 activity. Thus, when this inhibition is enhanced genetically, the genetically manipulated mice are able to learn without the need for repetition. In other words, PP1 acts as a suppressor of synaptic modifications underlying learning. Repetition relaxes this suppressor activity and allows learning to occur. Of note, these studies also suggest that memory impairment associated with aging may be mediated, in part, by enhanced PP1 activity, as these genetically altered mice performed better on memory retention as they aged than did control mice. These provocative studies raise the possibility that genetic differences in learning and memory capabilities may be mediated, in part, by polymorphisms or mutations in PP1 and suggest that drugs targeting PP1 may enhance cognitive function in certain settings. These studies also highlight the remarkable potential that transgenic studies have for dissecting the molecular basis of behavior and identifying potential drug targets.

SYNAPTIC SIGNALING COMPLEXES

Given the confusing array of intracellular signaling pathways that are operating simultaneously in a given cell, mechanisms are needed to ensure that information is transferred to the appropriate targets in a timely and efficient manner. At the same time, it is important to emphasize that each pathway does not act in a vacuum. Integration of information from multiple pathways is used pervasively to modulate responses to given stimuli. Thus, these pathways must be distinct enough to retain their own identity, yet highly interactive with each other. One mechanism used to achieve this goal is the widespread use of protein–protein interaction domains to ensure that signaling proteins are positioned properly to be able to listen and talk to the appropriate partner proteins. One example already discussed previously is the use of AKAPs to position PKA in the vicinity of substrate proteins. In this case, each member of the AKAP family, of which there are several dozen, contains a domain that interacts with PKA and at least one other protein–protein interaction domain, which targets it to other signaling proteins.

Another example is the cytoplasmic segment of neurotrophin receptors. Activation of the receptor stimulates phosphorylation of tyrosine residues, which attract adapter proteins containing protein–protein interaction domains that bind to phosphotyrosine residues. In this way, the cytoplasmic portion of the receptor serves as a scaffold for an array of activated signaling molecules.

Scaffolding is also used to organize signaling complexes involving classic neurotransmitter receptors. Analysis of several proteins closely associated with glutamate receptors revealed that they share a distinct protein–protein interaction domain, referred to as the *PDZ domain*, which operates according to a relatively simple recognition rule. This domain binds tightly to the C-terminal segment of proteins in which the last three amino acids match the consensus sequence S/TXV (i.e., serine [S] or threonine [T], followed by any amino acid [X], followed by valine [V] or another hydrophobic residue). Characterization of the growing list of PDZ domain–containing proteins expressed in neurons has revealed that many are targeted to either pre- or postsynaptic elements. Thus, these signature sequences provide a means of forming synaptic signaling complexes.

The recognition that both α-amino-3-hydroxy-5-methyl-4-isoxazole propionic acid (AMPA) and *N*-methyl-D-aspartate (NMDA) glutamate receptors contain the PDZ ligand motif in their C-terminal has fostered an intense search for their partner proteins. The C-terminal of the NR2 NMDA receptor subunits contains a PDZ ligand sequence that interacts with PSD95 and its homologs. These proteins serve as adapters that link the receptor to the cytoskeleton and to other signaling pathways, including Ras and Rho pathways. In a similar vein, the GluR2 and GluR3 AMPA receptor subunits also possess a PDZ ligand motif at their C-terminal and bind to a protein called *glutamate receptor interacting protein* (GRIP), which appears to be composed solely of seven PDZ domains. One of the PDZ domains in GRIP binds to another protein referred to as *GRIP-associated protein* (GRASP), which encodes a Ras GEF. Thus, this adapter protein may enable this receptor-signaling complex to engage the Ras pathway as well. In addition to GRIP, AMPA receptors also bind to another PDZ domain protein termed *protein interacting with C kinase* (PICK1). The mechanisms that regulate AMPA receptor interaction with GRIP or PICK1 appear to play an important role in regulating the functional activity of AMPA receptors. In summary, PDZ domains provide an elegant means of organizing synaptic proteins into efficient signaling modules. In addition to glutamate receptors, many other neurotransmitter receptors are associated with PDZ proteins, indicating that this interaction domain plays a broad role in organizing synaptic signaling pathways.

The physiological importance of synaptic signaling complexes organized by PDZ domains has been underscored by recent studies demonstrating that disruption of the interaction of NMDA receptors with PSD95 produces a marked reduction in neuronal damage caused by ischemia, while having little effect on standard measures of synaptic transmission. Thus, even though attempts to introduce NMDA receptor antagonists into clinical practice have been stymied by the side effects associated with disruption of its essential role in synaptic transmission, uncoupling NMDA receptors from PSD95 represents a potential means of selectively blocking pathways linked to excitotoxicity. Accordingly, drugs designed to interfere with protein–protein interaction domains may yield more selective effects than can be accomplished by directly blocking the function of a signaling protein.

DYNAMIC REGULATION OF PROTEIN EXPRESSION

In the signaling pathways outlined above, the intracellular signal elicited by receptor stimulation is encoded by a change in the level of either a second messenger or the phosphorylation state of a protein, or both. However, there are two major additional mechanisms used by a variety of signaling pathways to influence cellular responses: rapid, stimulus-induced synthesis and degradation of signaling proteins. In the former, signaling pathways can produce robust changes in transcription and translation of messenger ribonucleic acids (mRNAs), within minutes; in the latter, selected proteins can be degraded in the same rapid time frame via the ubiquitination system.

Because neurotrophins produce dramatic long-term effects on neuronal differentiation, it was readily appreciated that these effects are mediated, in part, by changes in gene expression. For example, stimulation of the Ras/MAP kinase signaling pathway by neurotrophins triggers phosphorylation and activation of several transcription factors that mediate long-lasting phenotypic changes induced by these agents. Because the changes in gene expression occur rapidly and are reminiscent of how viruses mobilize transcriptional mechanisms to hijack host cells for their own needs, the initial set of genes induced by cellular stimulation are referred to as *immediate early genes*. Subsequent studies have demonstrated that synaptic activation of neurotransmitter receptors can elicit a comparable transcriptional response and by inference mediate the long-lasting effects of brief synaptic stimuli on neuronal activity or responsivity. A major goal of current research in neuroscience is to identify immediate early genes induced by neuronal stimulation and elucidate how they impact neuronal function. Although this area of investigation is still developing rapidly, several interesting findings have emerged. For example, one immediate early gene, referred to as *Narp*, appears to act by affecting the clustering of AMPA receptors, although the precise effect of Narp on AMPA receptor function remains to be determined. In addition, another immediate early gene product that is rapidly induced by synaptic stimulation is *Homer*. This protein binds to the intracellular domain of metabotropic glutamate receptors. Thus, rapid changes in the expression of Narp and Homer suggest that neurons use transcriptional mechanisms to modify signaling mediated by major classes of glutamate receptors.

In addition to rapid changes in gene transcription, evidence is also emerging for synaptic control of translation of mRNAs that are stored in dendrites. Although it is generally assumed that protein synthesis occurs in the vicinity of the nucleus, numerous studies have provided compelling evidence that the requisite protein translation machinery, including ribosomes and mRNAs, are located in dendrites. Thus, the current working hypothesis is that translation of these dendritic mRNAs is regulated by local synaptic activity, providing an elegant means of tailoring protein synthesis to meet local demands. Although many aspects of this mechanism are still not completely understood, it will likely have important clinical relevance, as the protein affected in the fragile X syndrome of mental retardation, FMRP, appears to be involved in processing dendritic mRNAs.

Conversely, intracellular signaling pathways also use rapid degradation of proteins to exert their effects. Detailed analysis of two signaling pathways in which targeted proteolysis is used has helped reveal how this mechanism operates. In one pathway, a transcription factor, nuclear factor κB (NF-κB), is tethered in the cytoplasm under basal conditions via its association with an inhibitor protein, IκB. Activation of NF-κB is mediated indirectly by phosphorylation of IκB, which triggers its rapid degradation. Degradation of IκB releases NF-κB, enabling it to enter the nucleus to influence transcription.

β-Catenin signaling provides another example of how rapid degradation is used in intracellular signaling pathways. Under normal conditions, β-catenin is a protein with a short half-life, because it is constitutively phosphorylated by a kinase, glycogen synthase kinase (GSK-3), that has a high level of basal activity. This futile cycle of rapid β-catenin degradation is abruptly stopped by activation of upstream signaling pathways that suppress GSK-3 activity. Stabilization of β-catenin allows it to activate transcription. A common feature shared by these and other examples is that phosphorylation can exert dramatic effects on protein turnover. Although, in these two examples, phosphorylation accelerates turnover, it is important to point out that, in other cases, phosphorylation stabilizes the substrate protein.

Although there are numerous transcription factors that regulate gene expression, investigators were surprised to find that there is also a highly sophisticated set of mechanisms controlling protein degradation. Rather than being a passive nonspecific process, it is highly dynamic, energy dependent, and exhibits a high degree of specificity. The pivotal step in the regulated degradation of proteins is the attachment of a small protein called *ubiquitin* to lysine residues of targeted proteins. The specificity of the ubiquitination system is provided by the expression of dozens of ubiquitination enzymes referred to as *ubiquitin ligases*, which have a high degree of specificity, reminiscent of protein kinases. However, unlike protein kinases, whose activity is typically regulated by upstream events, the rate-limiting step in the ubiquitination process appears to be the availability of the appropriate substrate (e.g., phosphorylated β-catenin or IκB). Once proteins are ubiquitinated, they can be rapidly targeted to organelles called *proteosomes*, which contain an efficient array of proteolytic enzymes.

In addition to the important role it plays in a variety of intracellular signaling pathways, the ubiquitination system has also attracted considerable attention because it may play a central role in neurodegenerative diseases. The most direct link between ubiquitination and neurodegeneration has been provided by the identification of two genes linked to familial forms of Parkinson's disease—parkin and synuclein. Although the function of synuclein has not been elucidated, parkin contains domains indicating that it functions as a ubiquitin ligase. Follow-up studies based on this clue have implicated defective ubiquitination in the pathophysiology of this disease. A key pathological finding in Parkinson's disease is the presence of cytoplasmic inclusion bodies, called *Lewy bodies*, in dopaminergic neurons. Both parkin and synuclein are enriched in Lewy bodies, which also stain strongly for ubiquitinated proteins. Furthermore, wild-type parkin ubiquitinates synuclein and its partner protein, synphilin-1, whereas mutant parkins found in patients with familial Parkinson's disease do not. In addition, these patients do not display Lewy bodies, indicating that wild-type parkin is critical for this process. Taken together, these findings indicate that Parkinson's disease may be caused by a defect in protein degradation that is normally mediated by parkin. Mutations in parkin block this process and cause neurodegeneration in the absence of Lewy body formation, whereas other causes of this disease may interfere with protein degradation distal to this point and cause the build up of ubiquitinated proteins in Lewy bodies. These findings in Parkinson's disease have prompted the suggestion that defects in the ubiquitination system may also be involved in other neurodegenerative diseases characterized by the presence of inclusion bodies, such as Huntington's disease.

SYNAPTIC PLASTICITY

Overwhelming evidence indicates that activity-dependent changes in synaptic efficacy play a central role in normal development of the nervous system and in learning and memory. Because defects in these processes play a prominent role in a variety of psychiatric disorders, there has been intense interest in defining the cellular and molecular events mediating these processes. This line of research has highlighted the role of intraneuronal signaling pathways in key aspects of synaptic plasticity. A remarkable convergence of evidence from multiple lines of research indicates that rapid changes in synaptic efficacy, which occur within a few minutes of stimulation, are mediated by insertion or removal of AMPA receptors from postsynaptic sites. The trigger for this rapid change in AMPA receptor localization appears to be mediated by the interplay of signaling pathways located just below the surface of the postsynaptic membrane. Clearly, this process must be tightly regulated, as changes in the functional activity of synapses can have important behavioral implications. One strategy that appears to be used to prevent inadvertent changes in synaptic efficacy is the requirement for concomitant activation of multiple second messenger pathways. Thus, studies of long-term potentiation or enhanced synaptic efficacy have revealed that activation of protein kinase C and calcium–calmodulin kinase II are required for induction of this process. Similarly, dissection of the requirements for triggering long-term depression in cerebellar neurons demonstrated the need for activation of protein kinase C, as well as elevations of intracellular calcium.

Ongoing studies in this field are focusing on defining the molecular events linking activation of specific kinases to AMPA receptor trafficking. Initial results point to the importance of scaffolding proteins tethered to the intracellular tail of AMPA receptors in guiding this process. The C-terminal of AMPA receptors contains a PDZ ligand motif, which mediates its interaction with several PDZ domain proteins, including PICK and GRIP. Current evidence indicates that phosphorylation events trigger a switch in which PDZ proteins bind to the AMPA receptor tail, and this triggers AMPA receptors to be either inserted into or removed from the postsynaptic membrane.

Although these phosphorylation events underlie rapid changes in synaptic efficacy, maintenance of enduring changes in synaptic efficacy appears to depend on targeting of newly synthesized proteins to the synapses being modified. Thus, in addition to local effects on AMPA receptor trafficking, intraneuronal signaling pathways also play a key role in regulating transcriptional events. Transcription factors that bind to the CRE and SRE can be activated by synaptic stimuli that trigger long-lasting changes in synaptic efficacy and, therefore, have been implicated in this process. Several genes that have been induced in synaptic plasticity paradigms have been identified. These include both transcription factors, which presumably trigger another wave of gene expression and "effector" genes, which appear to be involved in producing long-lasting changes in synaptic efficacy. These include Narp, a protein that affects the clustering of

AMPA receptors, and Homer, which binds to the intracellular tail of metabotropic glutamate receptors. Thus, recent studies have begun to delineate a "cell biology" of synaptic plasticity in which changes in the efficacy of specific synapses entail several layers of signaling. Rapid changes are mediated locally in the vicinity of the synapse. Long-lasting changes entail signaling to the nucleus and targeting of newly synthesized proteins back to the affected synapses. Thus, intraneuronal signaling pathways function over a broad range of spatial and temporal domains to control neuronal plasticity.

PSYCHOTROPIC DRUG ACTIONS

In the absence of second messenger systems, drugs would be expected to exert consistent effects with repeated administration. Thus, all of the complex time-dependent changes in psychotropic drug action, such as tolerance to opiates or benzodiazepines or the delayed therapeutic response to antidepressant or antipsychotic drugs, ultimately result from the ability of neurons, through their internal signaling pathways, to mount a compensatory response to this form of stimulation. In some instances, this adaptation may run counter to the desired clinical effect, such as tolerance to the analgesic effects of opioids or substance dependence. Alternatively, this active adaptation can be highly desirable, because it presumably underlies the therapeutic action of antidepressant or antipsychotic agents, which develops after a lag of days to weeks after the onset of treatment.

Development of tolerance to the analgesic effects of opiates is one of the classic adaptation paradigms in psychopharmacology. Tolerance in this system is mediated by phosphorylation of the opiate receptor, which triggers a chain of events that decreases its ability to respond to opiate agonists. In this pathway, occupation of the receptor by ligand leads to its phosphorylation by a class of kinases called *G-protein receptor kinases* (GRKs). The hallmark feature of GRKs is that they only phosphorylate receptors that are occupied by receptor ligands (Fig. 1.8–10). Receptor phosphorylation by GRKs enables arrestin to bind to the receptor and triggers uncoupling of the G protein from the receptor. This provides a use-dependent feedback mechanism for rendering the receptor inactive.

Association of arrestins with G-protein receptors also appears to trigger receptor internalization. In this process, the arrestin/receptor complex interacts with clathrin-coated pits in the membrane that form endocytic vesicles. After internalization, the receptor can be recycled to the cell surface or earmarked for degradation.

Although the role of receptor internalization in the development of opiate tolerance is still being sorted out, there is compelling evidence that arrestins are involved in this process. Mice with a targeted deletion in β2 arrestin do not develop tolerance to the analgesic effects of morphine. Thus, this result indicates that tolerance is mediated via the interaction of GRKs and arrestin with the opiate receptor. Of note, these mice still develop morphine dependence, providing an elegant dissociation between these features of chronic morphine administration.

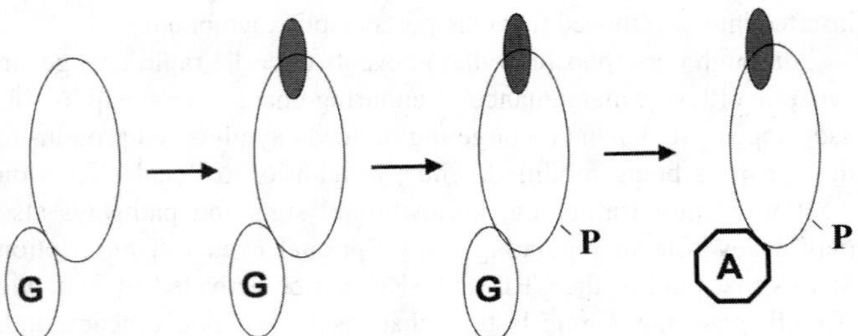

FIGURE 1.8–10 Receptor desensitization mediated by the arrestin pathway. In this pathway, G-protein–coupled receptors that are occupied by their ligand (*darkened oval*) are substrates for phosphorylation by G protein receptor kinases. Allosteric changes triggered by this phosphorylation lead to binding of arrestin (octagonal box labeled A) and uncoupling of the G protein from the receptor. This mechanism of homologous desensitization has been implicated in mediating opiate tolerance.

FUTURE DIRECTIONS

Translating the advances in molecular neurobiology into improved diagnostic and therapeutic capabilities represents the greatest opportunity and challenge facing psychiatry. Although much progress is being made by pursuing traditional classes of drug targets located on the outside of the neuron, intraneuronal signaling pathways represent a new and fertile frontier in this quest. Because dramatic advances have been achieved in other branches of medicine by using knowledge gained from dissecting intracellular signaling pathways used by peripheral cell types, it is reasonable to be optimistic that this strategy will be effective in psychiatry as well. Thus, the increased leverage provided by understanding and being able to manipulate the signaling pathways that neurons use to process information holds out great hope for developing innovative solutions to the daunting problems facing psychiatry.

SUGGESTED CROSS-REFERENCES

The role of intraneuronal signaling pathways in mediating the effects of neurotransmitters on ion channels and gene expression are also discussed in Sections 1.3, 1.4, 1.7, and 1.14. The cellular events underlying memory are discussed in Section 3.5.

REFERENCES

Aarts M, Liu Y, Liu L, Besshoh S, Arundine M, Gurd JW, Wang YT, Salter MW, Tymianski M: Treatment of ischemic brain damage by perturbing NMDA receptor–PSD-95 protein interactions. *Science*. 2002;298:846.

Bohn LM, Gainetdinov RR, Lin FT, Lefkowitz RJ, Caron MG: Mu-opioid receptor desensitization by beta-arrestin-2 determines morphine tolerance but not dependence. *Nature*. 2000;408:720.

Chung KK, Zhang Y, Lim KL, Tanaka Y, Huang H, Gao J, Ross CA, Dawson VL, Dawson TM: Parkin ubiquitinates the alpha-synuclein-interacting protein, synphilin-1: implications for Lewy-body formation in Parkinson disease. *Nat Med*. 2001;7:1144.

Claing A, Laporte SA, Caron MG, Lefkowitz RJ: Endocytosis of G protein-coupled receptors: roles of G protein-coupled receptor kinases and beta-arrestin proteins. *Prog Neurobiol*. 2002;66:61.

Fagni L, Worley PF, Ango F: Homer as both a scaffold and transduction molecule. *Sci STKE*. 2002:RE8.

*Garner CC, Nash J, Huganir RL: PDZ domains in synapse assembly and signaling. *Trends Cell Biol*. 2000;10:274.

Genoux D, Haditsch U, Knobloch M, Michalon A, Storm D, Mansuy IM: Protein phosphatase 1 is a molecular constraint on learning and memory. *Nature*. 2002;418:970.

*Giasson BI, Lee VM: Are ubiquitination pathways central to Parkinson's disease? *Cell*. 2003;112:631.

Hayashi T, Umemori H, Mishina M, Yamamoto T: The AMPA receptor interacts with and signals through the protein tyrosine kinase Lyn. *Nature*. 1999;397:72.

Lee HK, Takamiya K, Han JS, Man H, Kim CH, Rumbaugh G, Yu S, Ding L, He C, Petralia RS, Wenthold RJ, Gallagher M, Huganir RL: Phosphorylation of the AMPA receptor GluR1 subunit is required for synaptic plasticity and retention of spatial memory. *Cell*. 2003;112:631.

*Malinow R, Malenka RC: AMPA receptor trafficking and synaptic plasticity. *Annu Rev Neurosci*. 2002;25:103.

Michel JJ, Scott JD: AKAP mediated signal transduction. *Annu Rev Pharmacol Toxicol*. 2002;42:235.

Miyakawa T, Leiter LM, Gerber DJ, Gainetdinov RR, Sotnikova TD, Zeng H, Caron MG, Tonegawa S: Conditional calcineurin knockout mice exhibit multiple abnormal behaviors related to schizophrenia. *Proc Natl Acad Sci U S A*. 2003;100:8987.

*Nestler EJ, Hyman SE, Malenka RC. *Molecular Neuropharmacology*. New York: McGraw-Hill; 2001.

O'Brien RJ, Xu D, Petralia RS, Steward O, Huganir RL, Worley P: Synaptic clustering of AMPA receptors by the extracellular immediate-early gene product Narp. *Neuron*. 1999;23:309.

*Patapoutian A, Reichardt LF: Trk receptors: mediators of neurotrophin action. *Curr Opin Neurobiol*. 2001;11:272.

Rahman Z, Schwarz J, Gold SJ, Zachariou V, Wein MN, Choi KH, Kovoor A, Chen CK, DiLeone RJ, Schwarz SC, Selley DE, Sim-Selley LJ, Barrot M, Leudtke RR, Self D, Neve RL, Lester HA, Simon MI, Nestler EJ: RGS9 modulates dopamine signaling in the basal ganglia. *Neuron*. 2003;38:941.

Ramakers GJA: Rho proteins, mental retardation and the cellular basis of cognition. *Trends Neurosci*. 2002;25:191.

Shamah SM, Lin MZ, Goldberg JL, Estrach S, Sahin M, Hu L, Bazalakova M, Neve RL, Corfas G, Debant A, Greenberg ME: EphA receptors regulate growth cone dynamics through the novel guanine nucleotide exchange factor ephexin. *Cell*. 2001;105:233.

Sheng M, Kim MJ. Postsynaptic signaling and plasticity mechanisms. *Science*. 2002;298:776.

Shimura H, Schlossmacher MG, Hattori N, Frosch MP, Trockenbacher A, Schneider R, Mizuno Y, Kosik KS, Selkoe DJ: Ubiquitination of a new form of alpha-synuclein by parkin from human brain: implications for Parkinson's disease. *Science*. 2001;293:263.

Thomas MJ, Malenka RC: Synaptic plasticity in the mesolimbic dopamine system. *Philos Trans R Soc Lond B Biol Sci*. 2003;358:815.

Williams RS, Cheng L, Mudge AW, Harwood AJ: A common mechanism of action for three mood-stabilizing drugs. *Nature*. 2002;417:292.

Xia J, Chung HJ, Wihler C, Huganir RL, Linden DJ: Cerebellar long-term depression requires PKC-regulated interactions between GluR2/3 and PDZ domain-containing proteins. *Neuron*. 2000;28:499.

▲ 1.9 Basic Electrophysiology

CHARLES F. ZORUMSKI, M.D., KEITH E. ISENBERG, M.D., AND STEVEN J. MENNERICK, PH.D.

Neurons use electrical signals to send and receive information. These electrical signals determine local and network properties of the central nervous system (CNS) and result from the flow of ions across cell membranes through macromolecular pores called *ion channels*. Neurons possess two classes of ion channels, gated and nongated. Nongated ion channels open spontaneously and contribute to the cellular *resting membrane potential*. The opening of most ion channels is regulated (*gated*) by changes in transmembrane voltage, extracellular neurochemicals, or intracellular second messenger molecules. Certain *voltage-gated sodium channels* allow very rapid movement of ions and provide the basis for communication within and between neurons. These rapid signals (*action potentials*) are generated near the neuronal cell body and are transmitted along the neuron's axon to nerve terminals with little decrement in amplitude. The high-fidelity propagation of the signals results from the regenerative property of action potentials, imparted by the presence of voltage-gated channels along the length of the axon. In myelinated axons, action potential propagation is speeded by *saltatory conduction*, which refers to the ability of electrical signals to "jump" rapidly between axonal nodes of Ranvier.

At nerve terminals, action potential–induced depolarization opens *voltage-gated calcium channels*. The influx of calcium promotes the release of a chemical neurotransmitter into the extracellular space, where the transmitter is able to influence a receiving cell. *Neurotransmitters* bind to specific protein *receptors* and alter neuronal excitability via actions on ion channels. There are two broad classes of neurotransmitter receptors. *Ligand-gated ion channels* are directly opened by the binding of a transmitter, whereas *G-protein–coupled receptors* influence the function of ion channels indirectly via guanine nucleotide binding proteins (G proteins) or chemical second messengers. This chapter presents basic principles of electrophysiology and discusses the relevance of electrical signals to nervous system function and neuropsychiatry.

PRINCIPLES OF CELLULAR ELECTROPHYSIOLOGY

Resting Membrane Potential In cells of most tissues, potassium ion concentration [K^+] is much higher inside the cell than outside. This is achieved by the selective permeability of most plasma membranes, including those of neurons and glial cells, to K^+. The basis for selective permeability is the presence of K^+ ion channels, a class of transmembrane proteins with a hydrophilic pore region that selectively allows K^+ to permeate. Positively charged K^+ is initially attracted into the cell by large, impermeant anions (acids and proteins) within the cell. As K^+ accumulates in the cell, the membrane potential of the cell becomes more depolarized (less negative), and, therefore, K^+ entry is driven less and less by the electrical gradient. Intracellular concentrations of K^+ achieve levels of approximately 100 mmol (extracellular [K^+] is between 2 and 6 mmol in most nervous tissue), setting up a chemical gradient, which, in isolation, would result in net K^+ efflux from the cell. Thus, two gradients act on K^+: the intracellular electronegativity, resulting in K^+ influx, and the chemical gradient on K^+, resulting in efflux. At a specific membrane potential (approximately –96 mV for K^+), the electrical and chemical gradients are exactly equal and opposite. This membrane potential is known as the *equilibrium potential* or *Nernst potential* for K^+. The equilibrium (Nernst) potential is the transmembrane potential at which the electrical and chemical gradients are balanced and there is no net influx or efflux of K^+. Therefore, in a cell whose membrane is only permeable to K^+ and no other ions, the resting potential of the cell would be exactly equal to the Nernst potential for K^+.

The situation in most neurons is not so simple, because other ions, with different electrochemical gradients, are slightly permeant through the ion channels that are open in the resting cell membrane. Each of these ions has its own characteristic Nernst potential, dependent on the concentrations of ion inside and outside the cell. At typical negative resting potentials, calcium (Ca^{2+}) and sodium (Na^+) ions have electrochemical gradients driving them into the cell. These ions are at higher concentrations outside than inside the cell and, therefore, are attracted to flow inwardly down both their electrical gradient and their concentration gradient. Chloride (Cl^-) concentration is usually higher outside the cell, but because of this ion's negative charge, the Nernst potential for Cl^- is near the resting potential (Fig. 1.9–1). The actual resting potential of the membrane is determined by the average of the Nernst potentials of all the permeant ions, weighted by the relative permeability of each species. At rest, K^+ and Cl^- are much more permeant than the other ions and, therefore, typically play the largest role in determining the value of the resting potential, with less-permeant Na^+ and Ca^{2+} contributing less. Typical values for neuronal resting potentials are between –55 and –70 mV.

The concepts of Nernst potential and membrane potential described qualitatively above can be described with more quantitative rigor. The Nernst potential for any ionic species can be calculated based on the ion concentrations on either side of the membrane. For K^+, the Nernst potential (designated E_K) is expressed as: $E_K = (RT/zF) \times \ln([K]_o/[K]_i)$, where R is the ideal gas constant (8.31 joules/degree/mole), T is the temperature in degrees Kelvin, z is the valence of the ion, F is Faraday's constant (96,500 coulombs/mole, the charge on a mole of monovalent ions), and $[K]_o$ and $[K]_i$ are the concentrations of K^+ outside and inside the cell. At 37° C, the Nernst potential for K^+ is –96 mV, E_{Na} is +67 mV, E_{Cl} is –81 mV, and E_{Ca} > +97 mV. These equilibrium potentials are important in determining what happens to the membrane potential when an ion channel that is permeable to a specific ion opens. The opening of a specific ion channel drives the membrane potential toward the equi-

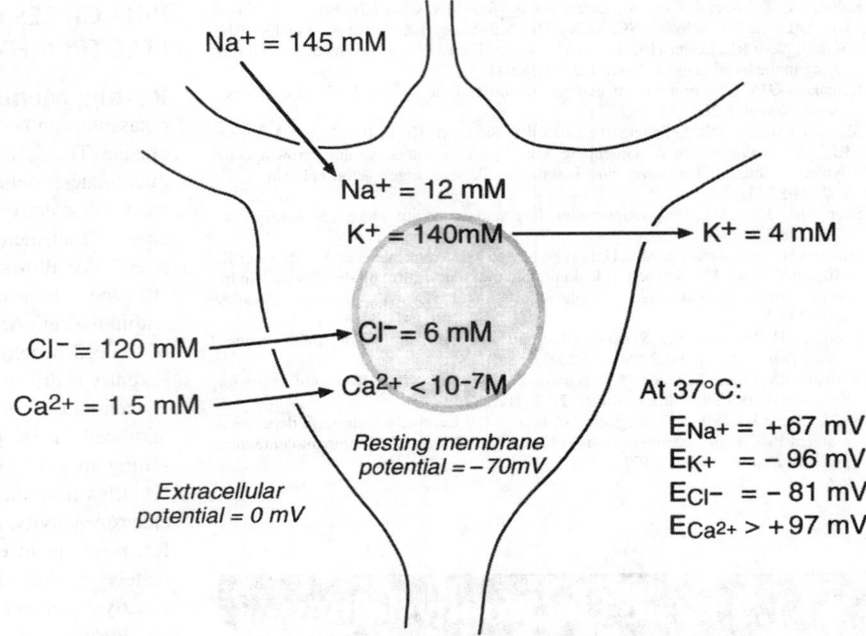

FIGURE 1.9–1 The distribution of Na^+, K^+, Ca^{2+}, and Cl^- across the membrane of a typical neuron; the arrows show the direction of current flow down the chemical gradient. Using the indicated ion concentrations, the equilibrium (Nernst) potentials (E) for these ions at 37°C are shown at the lower right.

librium potential for that ion. For example, when K^+-selective ion channels open, the neuronal membrane potential moves toward –96 mV. This makes the inside of the cell more negative, an effect called *hyperpolarization*. Na^+ and Ca^{2+} channel opening has the opposite effect, making the inside of the cell less negative (*depolarization*).

As mentioned above, because of the membrane's permeability for more than one ion, the true membrane potential is never exactly equal to the Nernst potential for any one ion. The Goldmann/Hodgkin/Katz (GHK) equation quantitatively describes the actual resting potential as the average of permeant ions' Nernst potentials, weighted by the relative permeability of each ionic species. The equation is of the form

$$E_m = \frac{RT}{F}\ln\frac{P_K[K]_O + P_{Na}[Na]_O + P_{Cl}[Cl]_i}{P_K[K]_i + P_{Na}[Na]_i + P_{Cl}[Cl]_O}$$

Most of the variables are familiar from the description of the Nernst equation above. E_m refers to the membrane potential, and P refers to the permeability of the membrane to the ion.

The bulk solutions on either side of the membrane are electrically neutral, with most of the intracellular negative charge being contributed by large intracellular organic anions (acids and proteins). The differential distribution of ions across neuronal membranes is maintained by the action of membrane pumps that use energy from adenosine triphosphate (ATP) hydrolysis to drive ions against a concentration gradient into or out of the cell. The best characterized pump is the Na^+-K^+ ATPase (*sodium pump*) that transports 3 Na^+ out of and 2 K^+ into the cell during each cycle. Because an unequal amount of charge is moved during each cycle, the pump is *electrogenic* and contributes to the intracellular negativity with respect to the extracellular solution. Na^+-K^+ ATPase activity is a major contributor to brain energy utilization, with as much as 40 percent of brain oxygen consumption resulting from pump activity required to reestablish ionic homeostasis after action potential firing and synaptic transmission. The cardiac glycosides, digoxin and ouabain, are effective inhibitors of Na^+-K^+ ATPase in the heart and improve myocardial contractility by depolarizing cardiac myocytes and increasing intracellular Ca^{2+}.

The resting potential is a relatively static entity and represents the potential energy available for neuronal signaling. Transient membrane potential *changes* are the real currency of information exchange in the nervous system. Information processing is typically initiated by a change in current flow across the membrane, usually resulting from the opening or closing of ion channels. The number of ions needed to change the membrane potential is very small relative to concentrations in the bulk solutions. For example, a potential change of 100 mV across a 1 cm^2 area of membrane requires the movement of only approximately 10^{-12} moles of a monovalent ion. By comparison, Na^+ and K^+ are present at approximately 10^{-1} M in the extracellular and intracellular fluids, respectively.

Passive Membrane Properties To understand how ion concentration gradients, electrical gradients, ion channels, and the distribution of charges across the membrane are related, it may be helpful to think of the cell membrane as an electrical circuit consisting of resistors (conductors), batteries, and capacitors. Because ions do not directly penetrate the lipid cell membrane but rather flow through ion channels, ion channels represent variable resistors. Physiologists describe ion channels in terms of their *ion selectivity* (which ions flow through the channel) and their *conductance* (relative ease of passing ions). Conductance (g) is the inverse of *resistance* (R) in an electrical circuit ($g = 1/R$). The presence of a voltage across the membrane provides an electrical driving force for the flow of ions through ion channels, resulting in a transmembrane *current*. The relationship among voltage (V), ionic current (I), and resistance (conductance) is given by the physiologist's version of Ohm's law: $I_{ionic} = g(V_m - E_{rev})$, where V_m is the membrane potential, E_{rev} is the Nernst potential for the ion(s) flowing through the channel, and $(V_m - E_{rev})$ represents the *driving force* for ion flow.

Another important passive electrical property is *capacitance*. A capacitor is an electrical device consisting of two conductors separated by an insulating material that is capable of storing charges of opposite sign on the two conductors. In the case of neurons, the conductors are the extra- and intracellular fluids, and the lipid membrane is the insulator. Whenever current flows through the

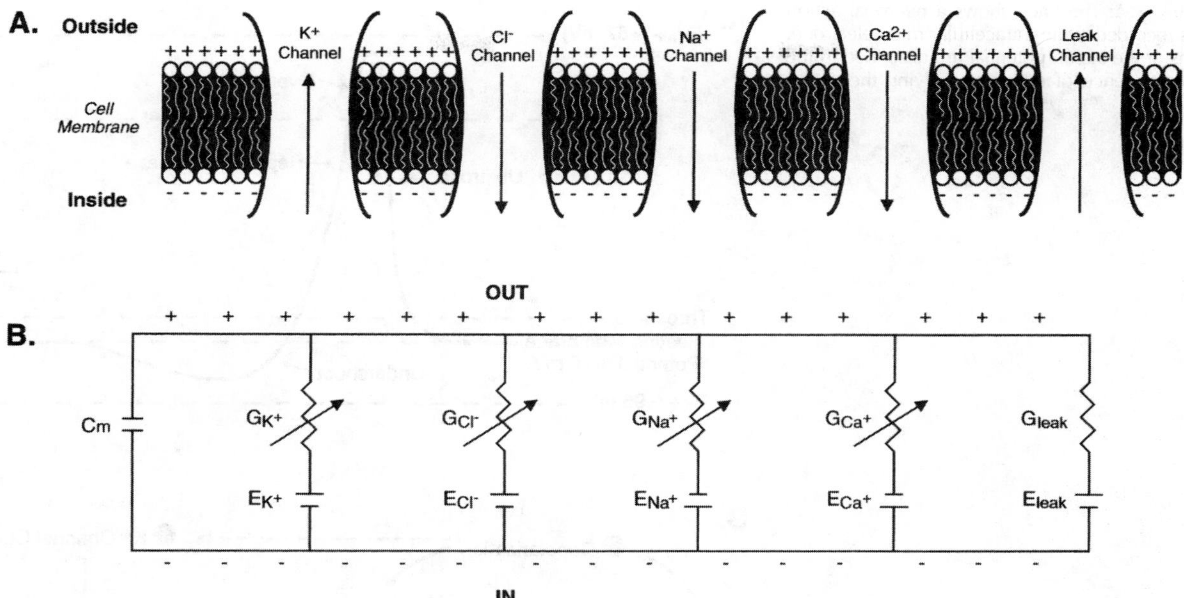

FIGURE 1.9–2 **A:** Ion channels are proteinaceous pores that traverse the lipid bilayer of cell membranes. Because of the action of membrane pumps, the extracellular surface of the membrane has a net positive charge with respect to the intracellular surface. Here is a membrane schematic that includes major ion channels and the predominant direction of ion flux under physiological conditions. **B:** As a result of the transmembrane potential and the presence of ion channels, the neuronal membrane can be depicted as an equivalent electrical circuit in which each ion channel is a variable resistor (conductor, G_x) in series with a battery (E_x). Different ion channels are shown as being in parallel with each other and in parallel with the membrane capacitance (C_m).

membrane, some current must flow to charge the membrane capacitance (C_m). The expression describing this capacitive current is: $I_{cap} = C_m \times (dV/dt)$. Note that capacitive current flows only when the membrane potential is changing (i.e., there is some change in voltage [*dV*] as a function of time [*dt*]). The total current flowing across a membrane at any given time is a sum of I_{cap} and I_{ionic}. One of the major tools used by physiologists to study ionic currents is a *voltage clamp* (or, more recently, a patch clamp). These techniques employ electrical devices to keep the membrane potential constant and eliminate the contribution of capacitive currents during physiological studies, thus making it possible to measure ionic currents directly.

One way to view the operation of an ion channel is as a battery (voltage source) in series with a conductor (resistor). The different types of ion channels are in parallel with each other and with the membrane capacitance. The net result is that the neuronal membrane can be represented by an equivalent electrical circuit (Fig. 1.9–2), which describes how current flows when ions enter and exit the cell in response to various stimuli.

Active Membrane Properties: Action Potentials

Changes in membrane potential have important effects on excitability because certain ion channels are activated (gated) by voltage changes. When neurons depolarize with respect to the resting potential, specific Na^+ channels open rapidly and drive the membrane potential toward the Na^+ equilibrium potential (+66 mV). Because of the leakage channels that are open at rest, there is initially a balance between the leakage currents and the currents flowing through Na^+ channels that are opened by depolarization. However, at a certain depolarized membrane potential, the current flowing through Na^+ channels exceeds the current through the leakage channels. The membrane potential at which Na^+ currents exceed the leakage currents is called the *threshold potential.* This potential is typically between –45 mV and –30 mV in neurons. Importantly, at potentials that are depolarized with respect to threshold, the entry of more Na^+ into the neuron produces further depolarization, which, in turn, opens more Na^+ channels in a positive-feedback cycle. During this process, the neuronal membrane potential depolarizes to potentials > 0 mV but never reaches the Na^+ equilibrium potential for three reasons. First, the leak channels will still play some role in determining the membrane potential during the course of the action potential. Because of the relative K^+ selectivity of these channels, the membrane potential will never achieve the Na^+ Nernst potential. Second, during the depolarization, Na^+ channels not only activate but they also rapidly inactivate. *Inactivation* is a process by which voltage-gated ion channels enter a nonconducting state despite the continued presence of the activating stimulus (depolarization). Third, the depolarization produced by Na^+ entry also opens voltage-gated K^+ channels, which drive the membrane potential toward the K^+ equilibrium potential (–96 mV). The net effect of the activation and inactivation of Na^+ channels and the delayed opening of K^+ channels is that the neuronal membrane potential rapidly changes to values more positive than 0 mV and then returns rapidly to the resting membrane potential. This rapid sequence occurs over several milliseconds and is referred to as an *action potential* (or *spike*) (Fig. 1.9–3). The fact that the membrane potential transiently exceeds 0 mV is called an *overshoot.* Action potentials represent all-or-none increases in electrical excitability and are important contributors to information transfer within and between neurons, allowing the neuronal cell body to communicate rapidly with its terminals and, in the terminals, providing the depolarization that promotes the Ca^{2+}-dependent release of neurotransmitters.

In most neurons, the K^+ equilibrium potential is negative with respect to the resting membrane potential. Thus, the action potential is often followed by a transient *undershoot* (or *afterhyperpolarization*) that decays back to the resting potential as the voltage-sensitive K^+ channels responsible for action potential repolarization close (Fig. 1.9–3). After an action potential, there is a time during which stimulation either cannot elicit an action potential or during which it takes a very strong stimulus to evoke an action potential. These are called the *absolute* and *relative refractory periods.* The absolute refractory

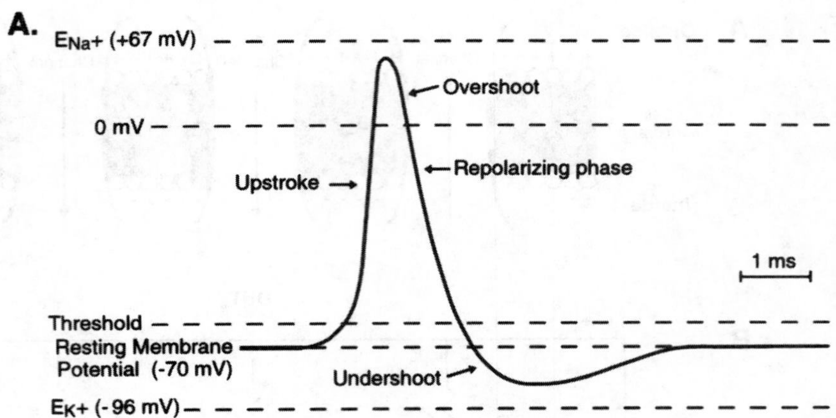

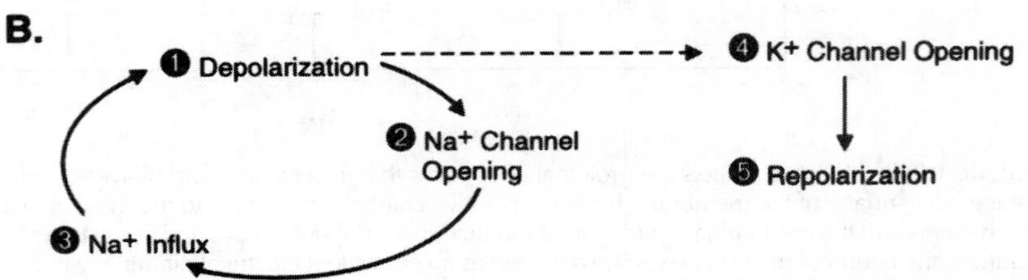

FIGURE 1.9–3 **A:** The trace shows a neuronal action potential as recorded by an intracellular microelectrode. The portions of the action potential are described in the text. **B:** The sequence of events underlying the action potential.

period results from the increased K^+ conductance that repolarizes the action potential and produces the undershoot. The relative refractory period reflects the time it takes for Na^+ channels to recover from inactivation.

Action Potential Conduction in Axons An important characteristic of the action potential is its ability to propagate the length of an axon with little or no decrement in its amplitude. This "regeneration" of the action potential at points down the length of axon is the way in which neurons avoid a decrement in signal (voltage change) over the long distance between cell body and axon terminal. Voltage changes that propagate using purely passive properties of the membrane would die away over short distances because of current loss across the cell membrane. Neurons actually combine passive current flow down the axon with active (depolarization-gated) current flow through membrane ion channels to efficiently propagate action potentials.

Action potentials are typically generated in the neuronal cell body or in the initial segment of the axon (called the *axon hillock*) where there are dense collections of Na^+ channels. Because action potentials are generated at a distance from the nerve terminals where neurotransmitters are released, an important question concerns how action potentials are transmitted to the synaptic terminals. In a strictly passive nerve fiber, leakage of current across the membrane results in *decremental conduction,* with the signal fading over a distance that is determined by the longitudinal (axial) resistance of the fiber, the membrane capacitance, and the transmembrane resistance. Decremental conduction is more typical of the spread of electrical signals along dendrites back to the neuronal cell body, although there is now good evidence that dendrites also have voltage-gated ion channels that can support back-propagating action potentials and that play important roles in modifying electrical/synaptic inputs to the dendrites.

Many axons are encased in myelin sheaths that allow them to send action potentials more efficiently. As a result of myelination, axons are electrically insulated—except at nodes of Ranvier, where there are collections of voltage-gated Na^+ channels involved in action potential generation (Fig. 1.9–4). The myelin sheath greatly increases transmembrane resistance and diminishes leakage of current from the axon, making it easier for current to flow down the length of the axon. Once generated, action potentials propagate rapidly, and the wave of depolarization jumps from node to node in a form that transmits the signal faithfully to the nerve terminals. This process of action potential spread through myelinated axons is referred to as *saltatory conduction* (derived from the Latin word *saltare*, meaning "to jump") and is important because of the speed and fidelity with which electrical information is passed from a nerve cell body to its terminals. Note that although depolarization-gated currents initiate comparatively sluggishly due to the time-dependent changes in channel conformational state required, the passive current flow between nodes occurs essentially instantaneously. Thus, the passive component of action potential propagation is largely responsible for the increase in conduction speed obtained in myelinated axons. A typical value for conduction velocity in large myelinated axons is approximately 100 m per second. The importance of saltatory conduction can be readily appreciated when considering the distances over which impulses must travel from the brain to cause movement in the toes. In several human illnesses, including multiple sclerosis (MS) and Guillain-Barré syndrome, demyelination of axons produces changes in axon conduction and specific neurological defects.

ION CHANNELS

Structure and Function of Voltage-Gated Ion Channels Voltage-gated ion channels allow the flow of ions in response to changes in transmembrane voltage and are key elements in neuronal excitation and inhibition. Although ion channels can usually pass more than a single type of ion, voltage-gated channels are named according to the predominant ion that flows when the

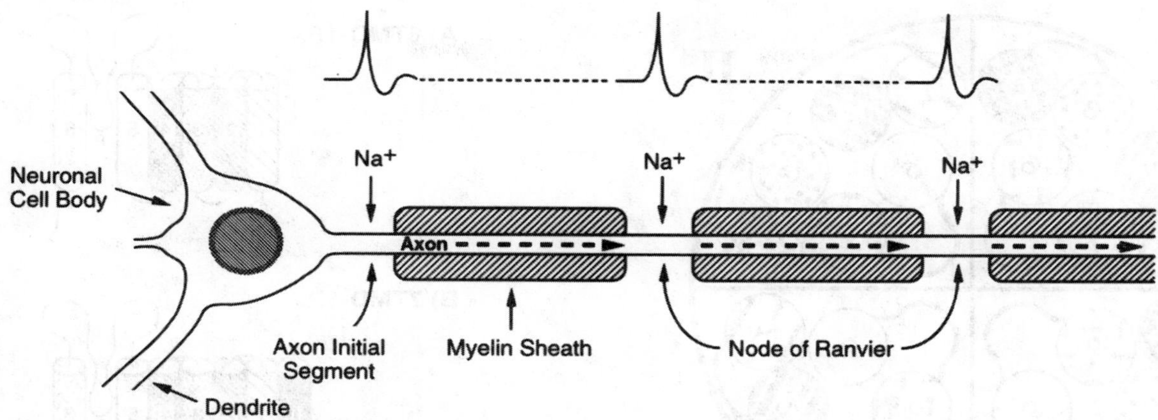

FIGURE 1.9–4 Saltatory conduction of an action potential in a neuron with a myelinated axon. The action potential is generated in the initial segment of the axon. As the signal moves along the axon, current tends to leak from the cell, diminishing the amplitude. However, myelin insulates the axon and markedly diminishes current leakage, thereby enhancing flow to the first node of Ranvier. At the node of Ranvier, Na^+ channels of the type involved in action potential generation open in response to the wave of depolarization and reproduce the all-or-none action potential. The sequence is repeated at subsequent nodes of Ranvier until the action potential reaches the nerve terminal.

channels are open. Ion channels that are selective for Na^+, K^+, Ca^{2+}, or Cl^- have been described in neuronal membranes. Certain ion channels that are gated open by chemical neurotransmitters such as glutamate and acetylcholine are selective for Na^+, K^+, and Ca^{2+} but exclude Cl^- and are called *nonselective cationic channels.*

Sodium (Na^+) Channels Na^+ channels are largely responsible for the fast upstroke of action potentials, although, in some neurons, Na^+ channels also contribute to lower-level depolarization and pacemaker firing. *Pacemaker activity* refers to the ability of certain neurons to depolarize spontaneously and to drive activity in a system of connected cells. Na^+ channels activate (open) rapidly in response to depolarization and also inactivate rapidly and nearly completely in response to prolonged depolarization.

Cloning studies have provided important information about the structure of Na^+ channels. Na^+ channels cloned from rat brain contain three protein subunits—a main (or α) subunit with a molecular weight of 240 to 280 kDa and two minor subunits with molecular weights of 30 to 40 kDa in a 1:1:1 ratio. The α subunit is a glycoprotein consisting of four structurally similar (homologous) domains that each have six proposed membrane-spanning (transmembrane) domains, referred to as S1 through S6 (Figs. 1.9–5 and 1.9–6). The α subunit alone can form a functional channel. Unlike voltage-gated K^+ channels, which are composed of tetramers of subunits each containing six transmembrane domains, functional sodium channels are formed from a single α subunit. There are at least nine genes in mammals that encode sodium channel α subunits. These channels are named *Na_v 1.1* through *1.9*. Some of these are expressed primarily in the CNS, others in the peripheral nervous system (PNS). The properties of voltage dependence, ion permeation, activation, and inactivation are conferred by specific regions of the Na^+ channel protein. However, the exact manner in which the proteins assemble in the lipid membrane remains a matter of active study.

Relationships between primary protein structure and ion channel function in Na^+ channels have been examined using mutations of specific amino acid residues. It appears that both the amino and carboxy terminals of the α subunits are located intracellularly. The fourth membrane-spanning region (S4) plays a key role in sensing

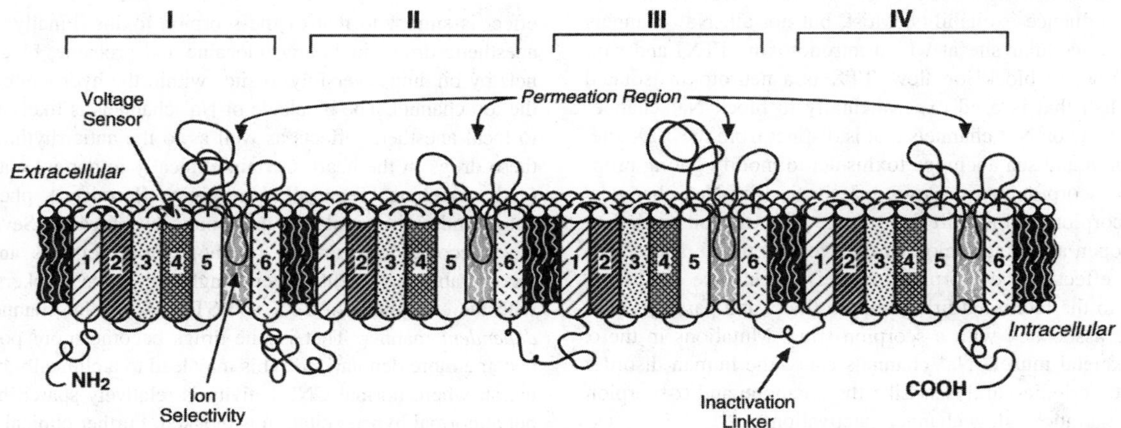

FIGURE 1.9–5 The proposed secondary structure of voltage-gated Na^+ and Ca^{2+} channels, based on analysis of α subunit primary amino acid sequences. Na^+ and Ca^{2+} channels consist of four homologous domains (I–IV), each of which has six membrane-spanning regions (numbered *1* to *6*). Both the amino (NH_2) and carboxy (COOH) terminals are located intracellularly. A stretch of amino acids between S5 and S6, called the *P loop*, forms two antiparallel β sheets that line the ion channel pore. Positive charges in the fourth membrane-spanning (S4) region are believed to comprise the voltage sensor.

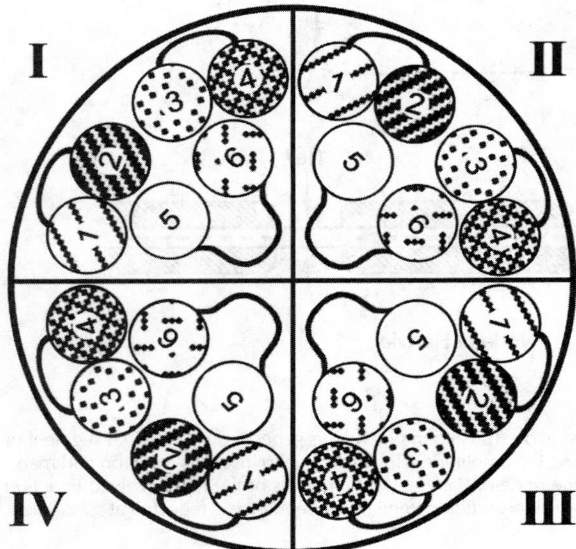

FIGURE 1.9–6 The arrangement of the four homologous repeats (I–IV) in the cell membrane. The view is looking at the channel en face from the outside of the cell. Transmembrane helices are labeled *1* to *6*. Extracellular linker regions are depicted by connecting lines. The P loop is depicted as the linker between the fifth and sixth membrane-spanning regions. Note the P domains from each of the four homologous repeats contribute to lining the ion channel located at the center of the diagram.

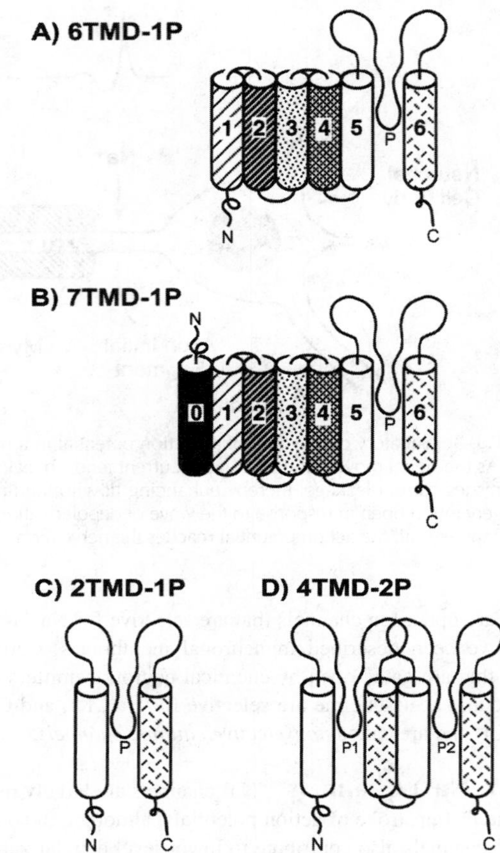

FIGURE 1.9–7 Potassium channels have diverse molecular structures. Depicted are four families of K^+ channels defined by the number of transmembrane domains and number of P domains. **A:** Of the channels described in the text, classic depolarization-gated K^+ channels and KCNQ subunits are members of the six transmembrane domain/1 P-domain family. **B:** Some Ca^{2+}-dependent K^+ channels are also members of this family, but the BK Ca^{2+} and voltage-dependent channels are members of a separate family because of an extra transmembrane domain and an extracellular N-terminus. **C:** Inward rectifiers, including K_{ATP} and astrocyte leak channels, are members of the two transmembrane domain/1 P-domain family. **D:** The tandem pore (TWIK) family of K^+ channels has four membrane-spanning regions and two P domains.

the transmembrane voltage changes that allow channel gating. Between the S5 and S6 membrane-spanning regions, there is a segment of hydrophobic amino acids that does not completely cross the lipid membrane bilayer. This reentrant loop of amino acids (called a *P loop*) appears to form the lining of the ion channel pore (Figs. 1.9–5 and 1.9–6). The P loop is a feature shared by other voltage-gated ion channels and some nonselective cation channels (Fig. 1.9–7).

Na^+ channel β subunits (termed β1 to β3) are glycoproteins with a large amino terminus and a single transmembrane domain. Two β subunits associate with a single α subunit. These auxiliary subunits may serve to increase functional expression of Na^+ channels and regulate the kinetics and gating of the channels. Recently, it has also been proposed that the large extracellular N-terminus is involved in cell adhesion.

Na^+ channels contain several sites at which neurotoxins and drugs act to influence excitability. Most, but not all, Na^+ channels contain an extracellular site at which tetrodotoxin (TTX) and saxitoxin (STX) act to block ion flow. TTX is a neurotoxin isolated from puffer fish that is used experimentally to block Na^+ channel function. At a site on Na^+ channels that is distinct from the TTX site, certain scorpion and sea anemone toxins act to modify gating properties. The α-scorpion toxin slows inactivation of Na^+ channels, whereas β-scorpion toxins shift the voltage of activation and allow channels to open at voltages closer to the resting membrane potential. The net effect of the scorpion toxins is to enhance excitation, contributing to the increased firing in pain fibers and paralysis (tetany) that are associated with a scorpion sting. Mutations in the α subunit of skeletal muscle Na^+ channels cause the human disorder hyperkalemic periodic paralysis. Like the anemone and α-scorpion toxins, these mutations slow channel inactivation.

Other toxins isolated from the buttercup family (*aconitine*), the lily family (*veratridine*), and frogs that are used for arrow poisons in South America (*batrachotoxin*) promote the direct opening of Na^+ channels and prolong the duration that the channels stay open. The net effect is similar to that of the scorpion toxins. Finally, certain local anesthetic drugs, including lidocaine and procaine, block Na^+ channels by binding reversibly to sites within the hydrophobic regions of the ion channel. The blockade of Na^+ channels is likely to contribute to local anesthetic effects as well as to the antiarrhythmic effects of these drugs in the heart. Certain clinically important anticonvulsants (carbamazepine [Tegretol], lamotrigine [Lamictal], phenytoin, riluzole) bind a site similar to that bound by procaine. Several of these have become important in psychopharmacology as antimanic and mood-stabilizing agents. Interestingly, all of the blockers mentioned, with the exceptions of TTX and STX, block Na^+ channels in a *use-dependent* manner. That is, the drugs become more potent as cells become more depolarized. This may lead to a clinically beneficial situation where normal CNS activity is relatively spared by the drugs, but abnormal hyperexcitation is blocked. Further clinical benefit from these drugs may result from their reported ability to dampen excitatory synaptic transmission selectively while sparing inhibitory transmission, a mechanism not fully understood. The rich pharmacology of voltage-gated Na^+ channels provides tools for understanding normal

Na^+-channel function and for manipulating Na^+-channel function therapeutically. It is important to emphasize that not all Na^+ channels in neurons are sensitive to all of the above agents. It is clear that TTX-insensitive Na^+ channels exist in a variety of excitable cells, although their function is not well understood at present.

Potassium (K^+) Channels K^+ channels represent the most diverse family of ion channels in excitable cells and are important participants in determining both the resting and firing properties of neurons. Four or five families with distinct electrophysiological properties and structural motifs are currently known (Fig. 1.9–7). These include the six transmembrane domain/1 P-domain channel subunits (including classic depolarization-gated channels), inwardly rectifying channel subunits with two transmembrane domains, two-pore channel subunits with four transmembrane domains, and two-pore channel subunits with eight transmembrane domains (so far only found in invertebrates). A fifth class of K^+ channels is a class of calcium- and depolarization-gated channels known as *BK channels* (for their big single-channel conductance); these channels are similar in many respects to the six transmembrane domain family but have recently been shown to contain a seventh membrane-spanning domain (S0 region) and an extracellular amino terminus. Based on elegant crystallographic studies, K^+ channels have served as a model for relating the protein structure of membrane ion channels to the functional properties of ion conduction and channel gating (opening and closing) in response to appropriate stimuli. The diversity of neuronal potassium channels can be daunting, and the molecular/structural diversity imparts functional diversity. Perhaps more than any other class of ion channels, K^+ channels shape the pattern of membrane potential changes in response to input signals.

For neurons, six transmembrane domain K^+ channels are a particularly important class, with depolarization-gated channels representing a major subgroup within the family. The voltage-gated K^+ channel subgroup can be divided into molecular subfamilies: K_V1 (sometimes called *Shaker* for the *Drosophila* gene), K_V2 (or *Shab*), K_V3 (or *Shal*), and K_V4 (or *Shaw*), each with constituent subunits (e.g., $K_V1.1$ to 1.4). A functional channel is composed of four subunits (a tetramer) from within the same subfamily. Specific domains within the amino-terminal region of the subunits are responsible for tetramerization. Likewise, domains within the individual subunits modulate gating properties, inactivation properties, and interactions with accessory or interacting proteins.

A common structural motif among subunits in the family of voltage-gated K^+ channels is the presence of six transmembrane domains (S1 through S6) with an intervening reentrant loop (P domain) between S4 and S5. The reentrant loops of the four subunits coordinate to line the pore of the channel. Oxygen atoms from amino acids in the P domain interact with K^+ ions in the pore at various points in the transit of K^+. These interactions mimic the hydration shell for K^+, and the specificity of these interactions within the channel helps to impart the selectivity of the channel for K^+ over other ions. Not surprisingly, the reentrant loop motif is common to K^+ channels of all other families of K^+ channels, including the two P-domain families and the inward rectifying K^+ channels.

Voltage-gated K^+ channels play major roles in defining the electrophysiological "signature" of many neurons. The fast repolarization of neurons produced by certain K^+ channels allows an increased rate of action potential firing that can then be used in frequency-dependent information coding (Fig. 1.9–8). Most neurons express multiple types of K^+ channels that differ in their activation and inactivation kinetics, voltage dependence, and pharmacology. Because the equilibrium potential for K^+ is approximately –90 mV in most neurons, the opening of K^+ channels results in K^+ efflux, membrane hyperpolarization, and a decrease in excitability.

A. Single Action Potentials

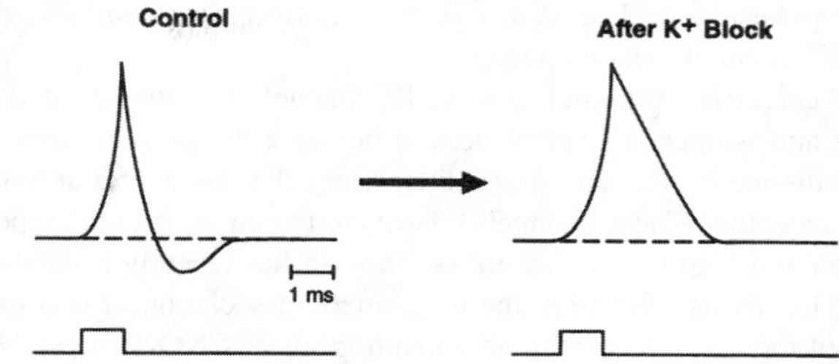

B. Repetitive Firing during Prolonged Depolarization

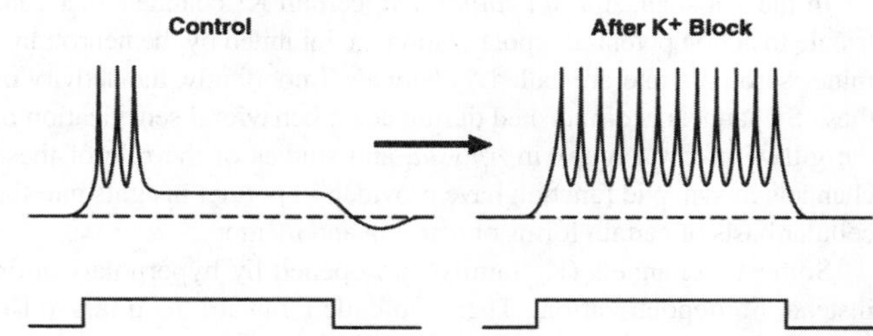

FIGURE 1.9–8 **A:** The traces show the effect of inhibiting K^+ channels involved in action potential repolarization. After K^+ channel block, action potentials are broadened and show a diminished undershoot. **B:** During prolonged depolarizations, Ca^{2+}-activated K^+ conductances diminish repetitive firing by the process of accommodation (or spike adaptation). When these K^+ conductances are inhibited, prolonged depolarization results in repetitive action potential firing for the duration of the depolarizing stimulus.

Historically, the first K^+ channel identified was called a *delayed rectifier*. These channels derive their name from the experiments of Hodgkin and Huxley on squid giant axons and are so named because the currents gated by these channels activate more slowly than the Na^+ channels that produce the upstroke of the action potential (i.e., the K^+ channel opening is "delayed" relative to Na^+ channel opening). A rectifier (or diode) is an electrical device that passes current better in one direction than another. The K^+ current is described as a *rectifier* because, by virtue of its depolarization-gated opening, the channel is more effective in allowing K^+ ions to exit than to enter the cell. Delayed rectifier channels open slowly and show little inactivation during prolonged depolarization. It appears that these channels help to determine the frequency with which neurons fire action potentials. Structurally, delayed rectifiers are members of the six transmembrane K^+ channel subfamily.

In squid giant axons, early experiments indicated that delayed rectifier currents were the primary K^+ currents involved in action potential repolarization. However, in other neurons, the situation is more complex, with several more rapidly activating K^+ channels contributing significantly. These include two classes of calcium-activated K^+ channels that are opened by increases in intracellular Ca^{2+} (some are also gated by depolarization). These channels are important in action potential repolarization and in generating an afterhyperpolarization characteristic of some neuronal types. In cells that possess it, this afterhyperpolarization is responsible for the process of *accommodation* (adaptation) that diminishes repetitive action potential firing during prolonged depolarization (Fig. 1.9–8).

A-type K^+ channels rapidly activate with depolarization to potentials greater than –60 mV and rapidly inactivate at depolarized potentials. *A channels* are involved in setting the interspike frequency with which neurons can fire and contribute to action potential repolarization. The *Shaker* A channel from *Drosophila* was the first K^+ channel to be cloned.

M channels represent a class of K^+ channels that are activated in a time- and voltage-dependent fashion but have the property that they are inhibited by the neurotransmitter acetylcholine, acting at muscarinic receptors. These channels contribute to action potential repolarization and help to slow repetitive firing. It has recently been shown that M currents arise from the heteromeric association of two members of the six transmembrane domain group, KCNQ2 and KCNQ3, and possibly other KCNQ family members. Mutations in the KCNQ subunits are also known to result in benign familial neonatal convulsions, deafness, and a form of cardiac long QT syndrome.

In the sea snail, *Aplysia californica*, certain K^+ channels that contribute to action potential repolarization are inhibited by the neurotransmitter serotonin and are called *S channels*. Importantly, the activity of these S channels is diminished during acute behavioral sensitization of the gill-withdrawal reflex in *Aplysia*, and studies of the role of these channels in synaptic function have provided important insights into the cellular basis of certain forms of learning and memory.

Some K^+ channels (K_{ir} family) are opened by hyperpolarization instead of depolarization. These so-called inward rectifiers (also called *anomalous rectifiers*) allow K^+ to more easily enter rather than exit the cell. Interestingly, many of these channels strongly rectify near the Nernst potential for K^+. Their gating properties are strongly influenced by the extracellular K^+ concentration rather than by the membrane potential alone. Despite the inward rectification of these channels, for neurons, the physiological importance of these channels is likely to lie in the passing of small outward (hyperpolarizing) currents, because neurons are rarely hyperpolarized beyond the K^+ equilibrium potential. These inward rectifiers are now known to be members of the two transmembrane domain group of K^+ channels. This class of K^+ channel contains a single pore region and lacks a voltage sensor (Fig. 1.9–7). Recent studies have shown that the primary mechanism underlying current rectification is channel block by positively charged intracellular magnesium or polyamines.

CNS astrocytes and Müller cells of the retina are known to possess inwardly rectifying K^+ channels of the $K_{ir}4$ subfamily, which may be responsible for helping to buffer extracellular rises in K^+ during neuronal activity. Expression of the inward rectifiers may be localized in these cells to siphon K^+ away from areas (axons and axon terminals) where extracellular accumulation may occur. The unique gating properties of these channels favor influx of K^+ into cells.

An additional feature of K^+ channels is that certain neurotransmitters can alter the function of these channels by activating G-protein–coupled receptors. For example, acetylcholine, acting at muscarinic receptors, blocks several K^+ currents leading to enhanced neuronal excitability. In the hippocampus and other CNS regions, the neurotransmitters γ-aminobutyric acid (GABA), serotonin, and adenosine open the same class of inwardly rectifying K^+ channels. Similarly, acetylcholine activates inwardly rectifying K^+ channels in a variety of tissues, including the heart and brain. These G-protein–regulated, inwardly rectifying channels (called GIRKs) allow divergent synaptic inputs to a single neuron to exert regulatory influences over neuronal firing through a single class of ion channels.

In peripheral tissues and in some neurons, a class of K^+ channels ($K_{ir}6$ subfamily) is regulated by intracellular ATP. These channels are also members of the class of two transmembrane domain inward rectifiers (Fig. 1.9–7). In the pancreas, K_{ATP} channels are important because they are involved in controlling the release of insulin and are a site of action of the hypoglycemic sulfonylurea drugs tolbutamide and glibenclamide, which are used to treat patients with diabetes mellitus. The hypoglycemic drugs promote the release of insulin by blocking ATP-sensitive K^+ channels. This, in turn, leads to membrane depolarization, calcium influx, and release of the hormone. Diazoxide, an antihypertensive drug that, as a side effect, increases blood glucose levels, has the opposite effect on pancreatic ATP-sensitive K^+ channels, opening the channels and diminishing the release of insulin. The sulfonylurea drugs do not interact directly with the K_{ir} subunits that form the K_{ATP} channel but, instead, bind to high-affinity sulfonylurea receptors (SURs) that are expressed with members of the $K_{ir}6$ family in heteromeric combinations of four K_{ir} subunits and four SURs. K_{ATP} channels are expressed in the CNS and appear to be involved in regulating the release of certain neurotransmitters and, perhaps, in determining the response of some neurons to changes in intracellular energy levels. There is also evidence that these channels are expressed intracellularly in mitochondrial membranes and may play a role in regulating apoptotic cell death.

HCN (*h*yperpolarization and *c*yclic-*n*ucleotide-gated) or *H channels* represent a class of nonselective cationic channels that are structurally related to K^+ channels. These channels are strongly expressed in several classes of neurons, including dopaminergic neurons of the substantia nigra and ventral tegmental area. H currents are believed to contribute to the neuronal resting membrane potential and to pacemaker firing in certain neurons. H currents are also found in apical dendrites of some pyramidal neurons and are proposed, along with several other classes of voltage-gated ion channels, to be involved in modulating synaptic signals in dendrites. In terms of gating, HCN channels are similar to K_{ir} channels in that they activate at hyperpolarized voltages and close with depolarization. HCN channels differ in being permeable to both K^+ and Na^+ and in providing a persisting current at membrane potentials near rest. Additionally, these channels have a structure that differs from K_{ir} channels but is similar to typical voltage-activated channels with six membrane-spanning regions, an S4 voltage sensor, and a reentrant P loop. H channels have an intracellular cyclic nucleotide binding domain near the carboxy terminus, and the binding of cyclic adenosine monophosphate (cAMP) shifts the voltage range for channel gating. Four HCN (1 to 4) channels have been cloned to date.

The K^+ channels described above exhibit either two or six transmembrane regions and a single P loop. Another class of K^+ channels has four membrane-spanning regions and two P domains (Fig. 1.9–7). These *tandem pore* (or K_t) channels are widely expressed in the CNS and periphery and appear to serve, at least in part, as leak conductances that help to establish the resting membrane potential. In mammals, more than ten members of this family have been cloned, and it is believed that these proteins form functional dimers. The various tandem pore channels differ in electrical properties and in sensitivity to activating (e.g., neurotransmitters, arachidonic acid, acid, heat, stretch) and modulating stimuli (second messengers). These channels go by a variety of names based on the TWIK channels that were the first cloned. For example, TWIK-related arachidonic acid–sensitive K^+ channels are called *TRAAKs*, and acid-sensitive channels are called *TASKs*. These channels can also be activated by volatile anesthetics and certain anticonvulsants (riluzole), contributing to the CNS-depressant effects of these agents.

Compared to voltage- and transmitter-sensitive channels, members of the TWIK family can be activated by a variety of interesting and novel stimuli, including acid pH, heat, and mechanical activity. Another class of channels, called *ASICs* (acid-sensing ion channels), that is also responsive to these stimuli has been described. These channels have two transmembrane domains with an apparent reentrant loop between. To date, nine mammalian family members falling into five subfamilies have been identified. Unlike the TWIK family, ASICs are voltage-insensitive, nonselective cationic channels that are more permeable to Na^+ than to K^+ and least permeable to Ca^{2+}. Although information about the function of these channels is limited, ASICs appear to participate in peripheral sensory processing, including touch, heat, taste, and pain, and also contribute to certain forms of long-term synaptic plasticity in the hippocampus.

Calcium (Ca^{2+}) Channels Ca^{2+} serves as both an important messenger regulating numerous intracellular events, including excitation-contraction coupling at the neuromuscular junction, metabolism, enzyme activation, gene expression, and neurotransmitter release, and as an electrical signal providing a mechanism for membrane depolarization. In some neurons, Ca^{2+} influx generates a form of action potential ("calcium spike"). Additionally, excessive and prolonged increases in intracellular Ca^{2+} concentrations appear to contribute to neuronal death in acute and chronic human neurodegenerative conditions. These features make the regulation of intracellular Ca^{2+} levels vital to cellular function and survival.

Voltage-activated Ca^{2+} channels provide a major source of the Ca^{2+} signals that are used to activate cellular processes, and, in conjunction with certain Ca^{2+}-permeable ligand-gated ion channels (e.g., *N*-methyl-D-aspartate [NMDA]-type glutamate receptors and neuronal nicotinic acetylcholine receptors), represent major conduits for Ca^{2+} entry from the extracellular environment. Neurons possess multiple classes of voltage-gated Ca^{2+} channels that can be classified based on biophysical and pharmacological properties. Some Ca^{2+} channels are activated by relatively small depolarizations over the range of –80 to –50 mV and are called *low voltage–activated* (LVA) Ca^{2+} channels. These LVA channels inactivate rapidly and are relatively insensitive to dihydropyridine Ca^{2+} channel blockers, such as nifedipine and nimodipine. LVA channels are also called *T-type Ca^{2+} channels* because of their "transient" (inactivating) currents. Because LVA Ca^{2+} channels are activated at membrane potentials near rest, these channels can contribute to burst firing and oscillatory neuronal activity. Oscillatory neuronal firing may be important in driving coordinated movements and in maintaining complex behavioral states such as wakefulness. LVA channels also appear to be present in neuronal dendrites and may contribute to synaptic integration and synaptic plasticity. With a few exceptions, T channels do not generally participate in neurotransmitter release. Recent evidence suggests that LVA channels may be a target for the actions of some antipsychotic drugs. The diphenylbutylpiperidines, pimozide and penfluridol, inhibit LVA channels at concentrations similar to those affecting dopamine type 2 receptors (D_2). Other antipsychotics also inhibit T-type channels but do so at concentrations above those required at dopamine receptors.

A second class of Ca^{2+} channels is activated by stronger membrane depolarizations to potentials that are positive to –50 mV. These are called *high voltage–activated* (HVA) *Ca^{2+} channels*. In many neurons, even when Na^+ channels that are involved in the upstroke of action potentials are blocked, HVA Ca^{2+} channels can produce regenerative spikes. These calcium spikes are typically slower in onset and longer in duration than Na^+ spikes, reflecting the kinetics of HVA channels.

HVA Ca^{2+} channels are heterogeneous, and several channel types contribute to HVA Ca^{2+} currents. *L-type Ca^{2+} channels* (named for their "long-lasting" responses) show slow inactivation during sustained depolarizations and are sensitive to blockade by dihydropyridines. L-type Ca^{2+} channels provide sufficient Ca^{2+} influx during action potentials to activate Ca^{2+}-dependent second messenger systems and gene expression. *N-type Ca^{2+} channels* (named because they are "neither" L nor T type) are also HVA channels that appear to be involved in providing the Ca^{2+} signal necessary for the release of neurotransmitters from some presynaptic terminals. N-type channels are blocked by ω-conotoxin GVIA, a poison derived from the snail, *Conus geographicus*. *P-type Ca^{2+} channels* represent a third class of HVA channels and are so named because of their presence in Purkinje cells of the cerebellum. P-type channels are also found in pyramidal neurons of the hippocampus and cortex and are insensitive to dihydropyridines and ω-conotoxin GVIA but are blocked by a toxin from the funnel web spider, *Agelenopsis aperta*, that is designated *ω-Aga-IVA*. P-type channels, like N-type channels, participate in the release of neurotransmitters in the CNS.

Other classes of HVA Ca^{2+} channels (designated *Q* and *R type*) contribute to CNS function, but their actions are less well understood at present. Q-type channels are blocked by ω-conotoxin-MVIIC isolated from *Conus magus* and participate in transmitter release. It is typically difficult to distinguish P- and Q-type channels and, thus, these channels are often referred to as *P/Q channels*. R-type channels are resistant to the Ca^{2+} channel antagonists described above but are inhibited by SNX-482, a toxin derived from the African tarantula, *Hysterocrates gigas*. R-type channels participate in transmitter release at fast excitatory synaptic synapses in the CNS.

The cloning of specific subunits of Ca^{2+} channels has provided insights into the structural mechanisms of these channels and has highlighted even further complexity than outlined above. Skeletal muscle HVA Ca^{2+} channels were the first cloned and serve as a model for understanding the structure of other voltage-gated Ca^{2+} channels. These channels are involved in excitation-contraction coupling at neuromuscular junctions and consist of five distinct subunits that are termed $\alpha1$ (165 to 195 kDa), $\alpha2$ (approximately 150 kDa), δ (17 to 25 kDa), β (50 to 60 kDa), and γ (25 to 35 kDa) arranged in a 1:1:1:1:1 stoichiometry. The δ subunit arises from cleavage of an $\alpha2/\delta$ peptide, whereas the other subunits are encoded by separate genes. $\alpha1$ Subunits show approximately 30 percent sequence homology to voltage-gated Na^+ channels and form the ion channel pore. A recurring theme in the $\alpha1$ subunits is the existence of four homologous internal repeats that each contain six putative membrane-spanning regions and a pore-forming P loop (Figs. 1.9–5 and 1.9–6). The HVA $\alpha1$ Ca^{2+} channel subunit from skeletal muscle contains the dihydropyridine binding site. Point mutations in the $\alpha1$ subunit of skeletal muscle T-tubule Ca^{2+} channels appear to cause the human disorder, hypokalemic periodic paralysis. The causative mutations occur in the S4 region of the channel involved in voltage sensing. The functions of the β ($\beta1$ to $\beta4$) and γ ($\gamma1$ to $\gamma8$) subunits are less certain but appear to involve membrane expression and trafficking of $\alpha1$ subunits. Interestingly, loss of the $\gamma2$ subunit (*stargazin*) in the stargazer mutant mouse markedly diminishes cell surface expression of certain glutamate receptors.

$\alpha1$ Subunits differ structurally among the different Ca^{2+}-channel subtypes, and ten different $\alpha1$ genes have been cloned. These include four different $\alpha1$ subtypes contributing to L-type channels (termed *α1S* for skeletal muscle channels C, D, and F), three $\alpha1$ genes contributing to P/Q-, N-, and R-type channels (termed *α1A*, *B*, and *E*), and three variants of T-type Ca^{2+} channels (termed *α1G*, *H*, and *I*). Based on the existence of these ten genes that contribute to heterogeneity among voltage-gated Ca^{2+} channels, there has been an effort to develop a simpler standardized nomenclature based on structural similarities. The L-type family (*α1S*, *C*, *D*, and *F*) is referred to as Ca_v *1.1*, *1.2*, *1.3*, and *1.4*. The P/Q, N, and R types (*α1A*, *B*, and *E*) are referred to as Ca_v *2.1*, *2.2*, and *2.3*, and the T-type channel family (*α1G*, *H*, and *I*) is termed Ca_v *3.1*, *3.2*, and *3.3*. Adding further to the complexity, human genes typically go by other, sometimes equally confusing names. For example, the skeletal muscle L-type channel that is referred to an *α1S*, and Ca_v *1.1* is designated *CACNA1S*; other human calcium channel genes are named accordingly. The importance of calcium channels to neuropsychiatric disorders is highlighted by recent evidence demonstrating that mutations in the human CACNA1A gene that encodes the $\alpha 1$ subunit of P/Q-type calcium channels in neurons are associated with familial hemiplegic migraine.

An important question in ion channel biology concerns how channels establish selectivity for one ion over another. At an initial level, ionic charge and charged amino acid residues present on the ion channel proteins help to select for cations over anions. However, it is a more difficult and complex issue to select among different cations. In the case of Ca^{2+} channels, this is particularly vexing because hydrated Ca^{2+} ions are significantly larger than Na^+ or K^+ ions. Thus, the size of the ion channel pore is not helpful for selecting Ca^{2+} over other cations in physiological fluids. Based on a series of elegant biophysical experiments, there is good evidence that selectivity in Ca^{2+} channels results from high-affinity binding sites for the divalent cation within the ion channel pore. When Ca^{2+} is present, its binding within the pore excludes monovalent cations, rendering the channels highly selective for Ca^{2+}. As might be expected, when Ca^{2+} is not present, these channels will readily pass monovalent cations. This principle of ions binding to specific sites within a channel to regulate permeability and gating is an important recurring theme in ion channel biology that can sometimes be exploited for the development of drugs that alter the function of specific channels.

In some regions of the CNS, particularly retinal photoreceptors and olfactory epithelial cells, intracellular cyclic nucleotides (e.g., cAMP and cyclic guanosine monophosphate [cGMP]) gate specific classes of ion channels. These cyclic nucleotide-gated (CNG) channels have structural features that are similar to voltage-gated channels, including the presence of six membrane-spanning regions and a P loop that lines the ion channel. Additionally, CNG channels have an S4-like voltage sensing region, although the channels are not gated by voltage. Three α and three β subunits of CNG channels have been cloned. CNG channels are nonselectively permeable to cations but, like voltage-gated calcium channels, bind divalent cations in the extracellular pore region. The binding of divalent cations restricts the flow of monovalent cations through CNG channels much like voltage-activated Ca^{2+} channels, rendering them somewhat selective for Ca^{2+} over Na^+. In some respects, CNG channels are similar to HCN pacemaker channels but are described here because of their higher calcium permeability. Mutations in retinal photoreceptor CNG channels contribute to colorblindness in humans.

The *TRP superfamily* represents another class of cationic channels with six membrane-spanning regions and high calcium permeability. This family contains at least 20 members in several subfamilies that participate in a variety of cellular processes in the nervous system and in nonexcitable cells ranging from sensory processing to vascular and cell cycle control. TRP channels are named after the first member to be identified, the *trp* (transient receptor potential) gene in *Drosophila*, and have been linked to several human disorders, including polycystic kidney disease and mucolipidosis, a neurodegenerative illness. TRP channels are regulated by intracellular and extracellular signals, including changes in pH, temperature, capsaicin (the active ingredient in hot peppers), and anandamide (an endogenous ligand for cannabinoid receptors). Additionally, a member of the TRP family (TRPV6) appears to contribute to the calcium release–activated calcium (CRAC) channels that mediate extracellular calcium influx after calcium release from intracellular stores. The importance of TRP channels is highlighted by the fact that these proteins may represent the main pathway for calcium entry in nonexcitable cells.

Chloride (Cl^-) Channels In most neurons, Cl^- is present at higher concentrations outside than inside cells, and the equilibrium potential for Cl^- is near the cell resting membrane potential. Thus, the opening of Cl^- channels (ClCs) tends to keep the neuronal membrane potential near rest and, in conjunction with K^+ channels, serves as a mechanism to dampen neuronal excitability. ClCs contribute significantly to the resting membrane potential in certain neurons and muscle cells. These channels are spontaneously open at resting membrane potentials and exhibit weak voltage and time dependence. In certain muscle fibers, the background Cl^- conductance is the largest resting conductance and the distribution of Cl^- is near equilibrium. Multiple (presently nine) human ClCs have been cloned to date, although information about the function and regulation of these channels lags that for cation channels. The ClC family of channels has a structure unlike any cation channel, with eleven membrane-spanning regions. Several of the transmembrane regions participate in ion channel pore formation, but there is no defined S4 voltage-sensing region as there is in the voltage-gated cation channels. Recent crystallographic studies have provided unique insights into the structure and function of bacterial ClC channels. These proteins appear to be double-barreled dimers in which each subunit contains its own pore. In the human illness, myotonia congenita, an abnormality of a muscle ClC (ClC-1) results in abnormally low Cl^- conductance. Symptomatically, these individuals exhibit increased muscular excitability and fatigue with exercise.

There are at least four activating stimuli for ClCs. These include increases in intracellular Ca^{2+}, hyperpolarization, cellular swelling, and phosphorylation by cAMP-dependent protein kinase (PKA). The Ca^{2+}-activated ClCs may help to determine the interspike frequency with which neurons can fire, whereas the swelling-activated channels help to protect cells from damage during osmotic stress. In addition to their roles in neuronal excitability, ClCs serve important functions in secretory cells, providing the major source of Cl^- in tears, sweat, and digestive juices. A defect in secretory ClCs that renders the channels insensitive to normal activating stimuli is important in the pathophysiology of cystic fibrosis. The cystic fibrosis transmembrane conductance regulator (CFTR) has a structure that differs significantly from the ClC family of channels and belongs to a larger family of ATP binding cassette (ABC) proteins that require phosphorylation by protein kinase A and hydrolysis of ATP for activation. Structurally, CFTR has two repeats with six membrane-spanning regions (12 transmembrane regions in total), a nucleotide binding domain, and a regulatory domain.

It is also important to note that intracellular organelles have ion channels. Mitochondrial membranes express voltage-dependent anion channels (VDACs) that pass anions and have unusual gating properties in that they are open at potentials near 0 mV and close with voltage changes in either direction. VDACs (or *porins*) appear to participate in releasing metabolites from mitochondria and are important participants in the mitochondrial permeability transition pore (PTP) that regulates apoptotic cell death. The PTP is a multiprotein complex that includes, at the minimum, adenine nucleotide translocase, hexokinase, cyclophilin D, and a VDAC. Activity of the PTP can be regulated by peripheral benzodiazepine receptors present on mitochondria. There are also suggestions that VDACs are expressed in plasma membranes, particularly in postsynaptic densities, and these channels may complex with some neurotransmitter receptors. The function of VDACs in plasma membranes is uncertain. Three VDACs (VDAC 1 to 3) have been cloned and exhibit interesting structural features. VDACs are β-sheet proteins that clearly differ from the α-helical configuration of most ion channels.

NEUROTRANSMITTERS AND ION CHANNELS

Classes of Neurotransmitters Much of the information transfer between neurons in the CNS occurs via chemical synapses. These synapses use a host of chemical messengers (neurotransmitters) that are released in a Ca^{2+}-dependent fashion from presynaptic terminals and act on specific membrane proteins (receptors) to produce biochemical and excitability changes in the receiving cell. There are two primary groups of neurotransmitters—low-molecular-weight amines and neuroactive peptides. These agents act on two classes of receptors, ligand-gated ion channels, at which the binding of the transmitter directly opens ion channels in the membrane, and G-protein–coupled receptors. The activated G protein then acts on ion channels or alters biochemical *second messenger systems*. Physiologists classify synaptic transmission according to the speed of transmission (fast or slow) and according to the nature of the response (excitatory or inhibitory). Fast synaptic transmission occurs on a time scale of up to several hundred milliseconds and is mediated primarily by amine neurotransmitters acting at ligand-gated ion channels. Slow synaptic communication occurs on the scale of seconds to minutes or longer through the actions of either amines or peptides acting on G-protein–coupled receptors. Different ion channels determine whether transmitter effects are *excitatory* (depolarizing) or *inhibitory* (hyperpolarizing). Moreover, an excitatory synaptic input can exert an inhibitory influence on the firing characteristics of a region. For example, the release of an excitatory neurotransmitter onto an inhibitory neuron can result in the inhibitory neuron diminishing the activity of a population of cells. Conversely, inhibition of inhibitory neurons can enhance regional excitability. This provides a great deal of flexibility in controlling and fine-tuning the inputs and outputs of a region.

There are at least nine low-molecular-weight amines that are likely to serve as neurotransmitters. These include *glutamate*, the major fast excitatory transmitter in the mammalian CNS; *acetylcholine*, the excitatory transmitter at the vertebrate neuromuscular junction; *GABA* and *glycine*, the major fast inhibitory transmitters in the brain and spinal cord, respectively; and the biogenic amines *dopamine*, *norepinephrine*, *epinephrine*, *serotonin*, and *histamine*. It also appears that the purines, *adenosine* and *ATP*, act as transmitters in some regions. A large number of *neuroactive peptides* alter neuronal excitability. However, it is uncertain whether all of these substances function as neurotransmitters. Many of these peptides, including vasopressin and cholecystokinin, were first identified as hormones in the vasculature and gut. ATP and certain neuroactive peptides coexist with amine neurotransmitters in some nerve terminals, and there is evidence for corelease of these agents at particular synapses. These observations suggest that interactions between classes of neurotransmitters may be important in determining the ultimate effects of a presynaptic neuron on its postsynaptic target.

Conductance Mechanisms Underlying Neurotransmitter Actions Physiologists often describe neurotransmitter actions in terms of their effects on membrane conductances. The transmitters that act at ligand-gated ion channels increase the conductance of the cell membrane to specific ions. Excitatory transmitters, such as acetylcholine and glutamate, directly activate nonselective cationic channels, increasing the conductance to Na^+, K^+, and, in some cases, Ca^{2+}, whereas the inhibitory transmitters, GABA and glycine, increase the conductance to Cl^-. A second group of transmitters increases membrane conductance but does so indirectly through a G protein. For example, GABA, serotonin, and adenosine promote G-protein–mediated opening of inwardly rectifying K^+ channels (GIRKs) in a variety of neurons. A third set of transmitter actions results from indirect effects on voltage-gated or leakage ion channels. These transmitters typically decrease membrane conductance by activating chemical second messenger systems via G-protein–coupled receptors. Certain voltage-gated K^+ and Ca^{2+} channels are specific targets of this inhibition, resulting in excitation or inhibition, respectively. Most transmitters that act on G-protein–coupled receptors exert at least some of their effects by these decreased conductance mechanisms. The electrical principles underlying synaptic excitation or inhibition are identical to those described for voltage-gated ion channels and are based on the relative permeabilities of the ion channels and the equilibrium (Nernst) potentials of the ions involved.

Several transmitters (e.g., GABA, glutamate, acetylcholine, serotonin) act at both ligand-gated ion channels and G-protein–coupled receptors. This raises the point that receptors for almost all neurotransmitters and, consequently, the effects of these transmitters are heterogeneous, with the nature of the transmitter effect depending on the specific receptor to which the transmitter binds and the gradients of ions permeant through the channels involved. Molecular cloning studies have demonstrated that receptors for most neurotransmitters are structurally complex, with multiple receptor subtypes being the rule rather than the exception. At the receptor level, there is tremendous flexibility in determining the effects of a given neurotransmitter on a single neuron or on a set of neurons in a CNS region.

Structure of Neurotransmitter Receptors Considerable information now exists about the primary structure of neurotransmitter receptors. Most transmitter-gated ion channels are multimeric proteins consisting of several (usually five) subunits that have multiple (two to five) membrane-spanning regions (Fig. 1.9–9). Functional receptors typically have large amino-terminal regions that extend into the aqueous extracellular environment. In this extracellular region are sites at which neurotransmitters bind and at which sugar molecules are attached to the receptor (glycosylation sites). The function of receptor glycosylation is poorly understood but presumably plays a role in determining optimal conformations for channel gating. The intracellular regions of the receptor often contain sites at which a phosphate group can be attached. Phosphorylation represents an important mechanism by which second messenger systems modulate the function of receptors and ion channels and is likely to be involved in certain forms of short-term learning and memory. Recent studies indicate that many transmitter receptors are multiprotein complexes in which the receptor subunits that compose the ion channel pore are in physical approximation with a variety of intracellular proteins (in some cases, as many as 70 or more intracellular proteins). The intracellular proteins help to regulate receptor trafficking and expression as well as ion channel function and participation in a host of intracellular processes.

The first transmitter-gated channel to be cloned was the muscle-type nicotinic acetylcholine receptor. To date, five neuromuscular nicotinic receptor subunits have been identified. Each of these subunits has four membrane-spanning regions and a pair of cysteine residues located 15 amino acids apart in the extracellular region of the protein (Fig. 1.9–9). These cysteine residues form a disulfide bridged loop that may contribute to transmitter binding. The nicotinic ion channel is a nonselective cation channel that is permeable to Na^+, K^+, and Ca^{2+}. The membrane-spanning regions of the subunits form the ion channel with the second transmembrane region forming the lining of the channel pore. The nicotinic receptor subunits assemble to form a pentamer with the stoichiometry of $\alpha 2$, β, δ, and γ or ε, depending on the age of the animal. Subsequent studies found that muscle-type nicotinic receptors are part of a superfamily that

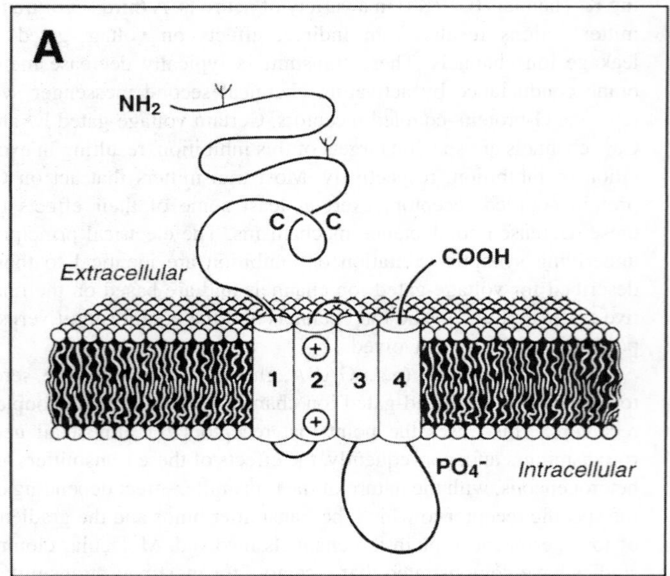

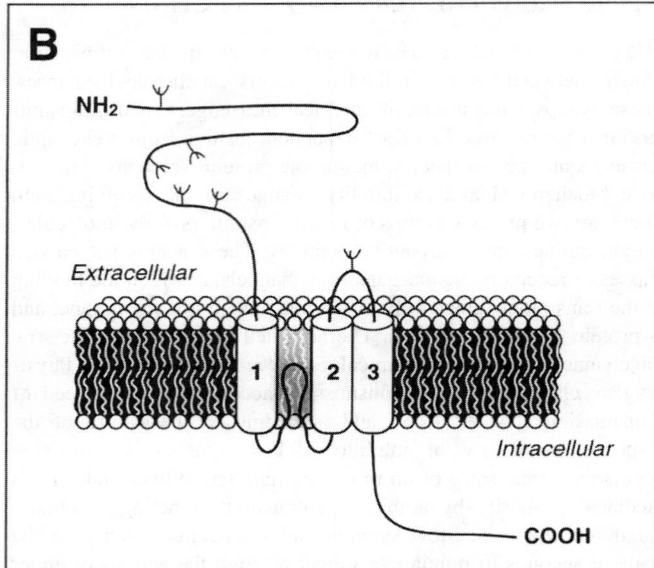

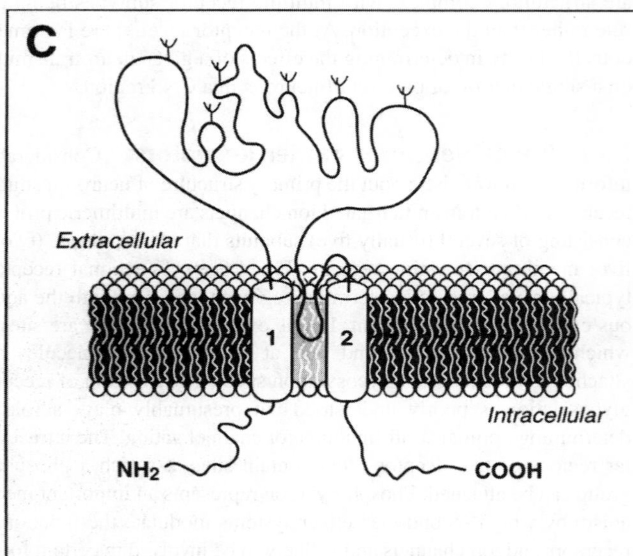

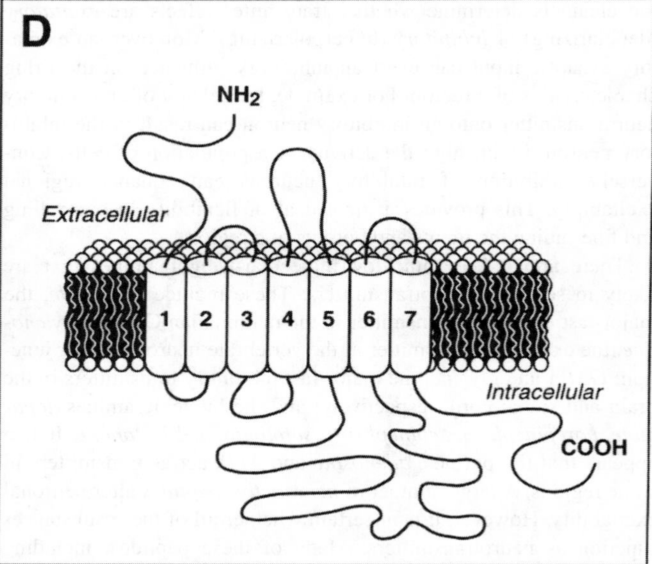

FIGURE 1.9–9 Here is the proposed secondary structure of receptors for several neurotransmitters, including a γ-aminobutyric acid type A receptor **(A)**, an ion channel–linked glutamate receptor **(B)**, a channel gated by extracellular adenosine triphosphate **(C)**, and a G-protein–coupled receptor **(D)**.

includes neuronal nicotinic, GABA type A ($GABA_A$), glycine, and serotonin type 3 ($5\text{-}HT_3$) receptors. Interestingly, $GABA_A$ and glycine receptors are anion selective, passing primarily Cl^- in physiological solutions, whereas nicotinic and $5\text{-}HT_3$ receptors are cation selective. Differences in charges on amino acids at the entrance to the ion channel pore determine whether the channel passes cations or anions. A characteristic of this family of receptors is the presence of the pair of aforementioned cysteine residues in the extracellular domain that are separated by 13 to 15 amino acids. Thus, this receptor family is sometimes referred to as the *CYS loop* receptors.

The ligand-gated ion channels gated by extracellular ATP (called *P2X receptors*) are exceptions to the scheme described above and have structures more typical of the inwardly rectifying K^+ channels (Figs. 1.9–7 and 1.9–9). ATP receptors have two membrane-spanning regions and a pore-forming region (P loop) that are connected by a large loop of extracellularly located amino acids. A major difference between the P2X receptors and the inwardly rectifying K^+ channels is that the bulk of the P2X receptor is extracellular, whereas the majority of the K^+ channel is intracellular. P2X channels are cation selective and have a relatively large permeability to calcium. These receptors appear to play a role in fast excitatory synaptic transmission in certain regions of the CNS, including the thalamus. Native ATP receptors may consist of combinations of P2X subunits.

Ionotropic glutamate receptors are also exceptions to the structural scheme proposed for $GABA_A$ and nicotinic receptors. Glutamate receptor subunits have three membrane-spanning regions and a reentrant P loop between the first and second transmembrane regions that does not completely cross the membrane (Fig. 1.9–9). The P loops in glutamate-gated channels are similar to those found in voltage-gated ion channels and appear to line the ion channel and help to determine channel properties. A difference from voltage-gated channels is that the glutamate receptor P loops enter the membrane from the cytoplasmic side. Recent crystallographic data on the non-NMDA type of glutamate receptor have enhanced understanding of how glutamate binds to its receptors. It appears that functional glutamate channels contain four subunits, each of which binds a glutamate molecule. The glutamate binding region has a bilobed structure resembling a Venus flytrap. When agonists bind, the cleft between the lobes closes to varying degrees, depending on the ligand. This is thought to impart the structural changes necessary for ion channel opening. Interestingly, competitive receptor antagonists that block glutamate binding stabilize the open cleft configuration of the binding pocket, providing a molecular explanation for how an agent can bind to the agonist recognition site but not produce the conformational changes that result in ion channel opening.

G-protein–coupled receptors have structures that differ completely from the ligand-gated ion channels. These receptors are typically single subunit proteins with seven membrane-spanning regions (Fig. 1.9–9). Transmitter binding is believed to occur in a pocket formed by the intramembranous portions of the receptor, except for the glutamate family of G-protein–coupled receptors, where binding occurs in a large amino-terminal region. The coupling of the receptor to a G protein occurs at intracellular loops of the receptor. G-protein–coupled receptors also have sites for glycosylation and phosphorylation.

CLINICAL ASPECTS OF ION CHANNELS

Information processing in the CNS depends critically on the function of ion channels. Most rapid processing involves action potential firing and fast neurotransmission. Although it is beyond the scope of this chapter to detail all of the clinical arenas in which ion channel function is important, the following section highlights some areas where understanding the function of ion channels is important to psychiatry, neurology, and clinical pharmacology.

Electrical Activity and Functional Neuroimaging

The ability to image metabolic activity directly in the brain using positron emission tomography (PET) and functional magnetic resonance imaging (fMRI) has had great impact on current understanding of human cognitive processes and the neurocircuitry of psychiatric disorders. These imaging techniques depend heavily on monitoring changes in regional blood flow and metabolic activity (glucose utilization). Interpretation of results from neuroimaging depends on understanding how changes in blood flow and energy metabolism relate to neuronal activity. It is generally believed that changes observed in functional neuroimaging reflect average neuronal activity in a region of interest. However, it is important to consider how imaging changes relate to neuronal firing and synaptic activity, given differences in temporal resolution for metabolic activity and blood flow on the one hand and ion flux on the other. There have been numerous attempts to estimate principal components contributing to brain energy metabolism at cellular and molecular levels. This task is conceptually and computationally difficult, given the relative contributions of action potential firing, transmitter release, transmitter uptake, and ion pumping required to drive transmission and to reestablish ionic homeostasis in neurons and glia. Importantly, the activity of membrane pumps required to maintain ionic homeostasis is a major contributor to CNS energy consumption. Some evidence suggests that much of the metabolic signaling in the brain results from the activity of fast glutamatergic synapses. Present models suggest that action potential firing and postsynaptic actions of glutamate together account for 80 percent or more of CNS energy consumption. Smaller contributions come from the maintenance of resting ionic conditions and the recycling of glutamate (approximately 15 percent of energy consumption combined). Taken together, these observations suggest that changes detected in functional imaging studies are largely determined by fast excitatory activity in specific brain regions. These observations are of particular importance in attempts to decipher how the neuromodulators involved in the actions of many psychotropic drugs affect CNS processing.

Neuronal Activity and Fetal Alcohol Syndrome

Ion channels play major roles in the development of the mammalian nervous system. During development, more neurons are generated than are needed in the mature nervous system. Depending on the region involved, fifty percent or more of neurons do not survive. This makes it important to understand factors that contribute to neuronal survival and raises important questions about factors that affect neuronal loss in developmental disorders. It is now clear that for neurons to survive and develop mature connections, they must exhibit appropriate levels of activity during critical periods of development. This activity is, in part, the result of intrinsic action potential firing mediated by voltage-activated ion channels. Additionally, appropriate synaptic activity, particularly excitatory synaptic drive, seems to play a significant role in determining neuronal survival during synaptogenesis. When intrinsic neuronal activity is inhibited by blockade of voltage-activated sodium or calcium channels, neurons undergo apoptotic neuronal degeneration. Recent studies in rodents indicate that agents that diminish glutamate-mediated synaptic transmission, particularly the component mediated by NMDA receptors, lead to massive loss of neurons in a variety of brain regions during synaptogenesis. Similarly, treatments that enhance GABA-mediated inhibition also promote massive neuronal apoptosis during the same period of development. A number of clinically used and abused drugs exhibit these same properties. For example, phencyclidine-like drugs that inhibit NMDA ion channels are potently neurotoxic during development in rodents when administered on a single day during synaptogenesis. Similar neurotoxicity is observed with clinically used benzodiazepines and barbiturates that act via $GABA_A$ receptors.

In humans, the period of synaptogenesis extends from the third trimester of pregnancy through the first few years of life. It has been known for some time that exposure of the developing human nervous system to ethanol produces a syndrome referred to as *fetal alcohol syndrome* or, in its milder form, *fetal alcohol effects*. Fetal alcohol syndrome is characterized by microcephaly, short stature, facial abnormalities, and a variety of learning defects. Consistent with the studies outlined above, rodents exposed to intoxicating levels of ethanol for a period of several hours on a single day during synaptogenesis develop widespread apoptotic neurodegeneration, which, in some regions, results in loss of more than half the neurons. Ethanol is a drug with complex effects on the nervous system, including the ability to inhibit NMDA receptors and, in some cases, to enhance $GABA_A$ receptors. In rodents, the developmental damage produced by ethanol appears to reflect a composite of the damage produced by NMDA antagonists and GABA potentiators.

Current models suggest strongly that major psychiatric disorders result from complex interactions of genes with environmental variables. It is interesting to note that some studies indicate that individuals with fetal alcohol effects exhibit significant psychopathology as they mature to adulthood, including increased prevalence of major depression and psychotic disorders. It is reasonable to be concerned that early exposure to drugs that alter neuronal activity during development may have a major impact on the expression of psychiatric syndromes in adulthood. Although this is most clearly the case for abused drugs such as ethanol and phencyclidine, a number of therapeutically used drugs, including anticonvulsants, anesthetics, and sedatives, have similar properties. Recent animal studies indicate that these drugs can also adversely influence the developing nervous system.

Voltage-Gated Sodium Channels and the Actions of Anticonvulsants

Seizures represent a state of hyperexcitability in the CNS and result in complex effects on consciousness and motor activity. Drugs used to treat seizures are generally CNS depressants that act on a variety of ion channels and transmitter systems to enhance inhibition and diminish excitation. $GABA_A$ receptors are favored targets of several anticonvulsants, and effective anticonvulsants enhance GABA-mediated inhibition. Examples of anticonvulsants that act directly on $GABA_A$ receptors include barbiturates and benzodiazepines. Other anticonvulsants affect other aspects of GABAergic neurotransmission. Examples include tiagabine (blocks transporter-mediated uptake of GABA) and γ-vinyl-GABA (inhibits the GABA-degrading enzyme, GABA transaminase).

Voltage-activated Na^+ channels are another target of anticonvulsants. Examples of drugs that alter Na^+ channels include phenytoin, carbamazepine, and lamotrigine. These drugs have complex actions on Na^+ channels but share the property of diminishing ion flow through channels that are responsible for action potential generation. Because action potential–mediated neurotransmitter release is important in transducing neuronal activity into interneuronal signals, it is interesting that anticonvulsant drugs that inhibit Na^+ channels also appear to diminish excitatory (glutamatergic) synaptic transmission preferentially. This has been shown most clearly in hippocampal neurons with the anticonvulsant and neuroprotectant drug, riluzole, which has been used clinically to diminish neuronal loss associated with amyotrophic lateral sclerosis (ALS). Riluzole (and several other anticonvulsants) enhance inactivation of voltage-activated Na^+ channels. Why these agents preferentially diminish glutamatergic transmission remains uncertain but may involve the density of Na^+ channels on glutamatergic versus GABAergic neurons. In effect, excitatory transmission can be diminished by a degree of Na^+-channel inhibition that has little effect on inhibitory transmission.

Given the increasing importance of anticonvulsant drugs as mood stabilizers, these mechanistic observations have relevance for psychiatry. Presently, valproic acid is one of the mainstays in the management of bipolar affective disorder, and other anticonvulsants, including carbamazepine and lamotrigine, are second-line agents. The mechanisms of valproic acid remain uncertain, but effects on GABAergic transmission and sodium channels appear likely to contribute. In contrast, lithium, another mainstay of mood stabilization, permeates sodium channels but is more likely to exert its effects by actions on second messenger systems and perhaps cell survival systems.

GABA Receptors and Benzodiazepines

$GABA_A$ receptors are a type of ligand-gated ion channel that passes chloride ions selectively and is inhibitory in most CNS regions. Additionally, $GABA_A$ receptors are a site of action of many CNS depressants, including barbiturates, neurosteroids, loreclezole, benzodiazepines, and, possibly, ethanol. These agents act at distinct sites within the $GABA_A$ receptor complex. Benzodiazepines, in particular, have complex effects on $GABA_A$ receptors. *Agonists* at benzodiazepine sites (e.g., diazepam [Valium], chlordiazepoxide, alprazolam [Xanax]) increase the apparent affinity of $GABA_A$ receptors for GABA, enhancing responses to low GABA concentrations but not altering the peak responses to maximal GABA concentrations. The net effect of benzodiazepine agonists on $GABA_A$ ion channels is to increase the frequency of channel openings in the absence of changes in intrinsic channel kinetics (e.g., open channel durations). These effects differ from those of the barbiturates and neurosteroids, which prolong channel open times and are capable of directly opening $GABA_A$ channels in the absence of GABA. A second class of benzodiazepines, called *inverse agonists*, bind to benzodiazepine sites but inhibit Cl^- flux. Certain β-carbolines are examples of inverse agonists at benzodiazepine receptors. The inverse agonists have clinical effects that are the opposite of benzodiazepine agonists (e.g., produce anxiety and cause convulsions). Flumazenil (Romazicon) is an *antagonist* at benzodiazepine sites—that is, flumazenil binds to benzodiazepine sites but does not directly alter the flow of Cl^-. Rather, flumazenil blocks the effects of benzodiazepine agonists and inverse agonists. Flumazenil is useful clinically in reversing the effects of sedative benzodiazepines in anesthetic or overdose situations.

The effects of benzodiazepine agonists are heterogeneous and depend on the region of the CNS and the subunit composition of the $GABA_A$ receptors. Certain sites have a high affinity for the hypnotic drug, zolpidem (Ambien), and are referred to as benzodiazepine *type I receptors*. Other sites have a lower affinity for zolpidem and are called *type II receptors*. Type I receptors are the predominant $GABA_A$-benzodiazepine receptors in the CNS, whereas type II sites are found primarily in the hippocampus, neocortex, striatum, and spinal cord.

Studies using recombinant $GABA_A$ receptors have demonstrated that the type I/type II benzodiazepine distinction results from differences in the subunit composition of $GABA_A$ receptors. To date, more than 20 different GABA receptor subunits belonging to eight subclasses have been cloned (termed α1–7, β1–4, γ1–4, δ, ε, π, θ, and ρ1–5), not all of which have been found in mammals. Functional GABA-gated ion channels appear to be pentamers composed of various combinations of these subunits. GABA most likely binds to β subunits, while the presence of a γ subunit is critical for benzodiazepine sensitivity. Benzodiazepine binding likely occurs at the interface between α and γ subunits. The distinction between type I and type II benzodiazepine pharmacology depends on which α subunit is expressed with β and γ subunits. α1-Containing $GABA_A$ receptors exhibit type I pharmacology, whereas α2-, α3-, and α5-containing receptors have type II benzodiazepine responses. Given the number of GABA receptor subunits expressed in the CNS, the number of different pentameric combinations possible is mind-boggling. However, it appears that receptors containing α1β2γ2 and α2β3γ2 account for approximately 80 percent of benzodiazepine-sensitive receptors in the CNS, with α5β3γ2 receptors being the major zolpidem-insensitive GABA receptor expressed in hippocampus. Receptors containing α4 and α6 subunits are insensitive to benzodiazepine agonists. These latter observations have made it possible to engineer GABA receptors with altered benzodiazepine sensitivity.

Recent studies using transgenic mice expressing altered $GABA_A$ receptors have provided some insights into receptor subtypes mediating different behaviors. It appears that mice engineered to express α1 subunits that are insensitive to benzodiazepines by virtue of a single amino acid substitution exhibit diminished sedative, amnestic, and anticonvulsant effects of benzodiazepines but preserved anxiolytic actions. This strongly suggests that it may be possible to create a new generation of benzodiazepine-like drugs that have favorable clinical effects but diminished side effects and abuse potential.

NMDA Receptors and PCP

Direct effects on ion channels are important in understanding the mechanisms of actions of numerous psychoactive drugs. An intriguing observation is that NMDA-type glutamate receptors are an important site of action for the street drug, phencyclidine (PCP, "angel dust"). PCP is abused for its hallucinogenic and dissociative (feelings of unreality) properties. PCP and its structural analogs, dizocilpine (MK-801) and ketamine, bind to a site within the NMDA channel and block ion flow. NMDA channel block by PCP-like drugs has the important property that it is long-lived, with the ion channel closing around the PCP molecule. Relief of PCP block requires that NMDA channels open at depolarized potentials. It is presently uncertain how the NMDA channel blocking effects contribute to the psychotomimetic effects of PCP, although understanding this interaction remains an area of active investigation. The finding that PCP-like drugs produce pathological changes in posterior cingulate cortical neurons suggests the involvement of specific limbic circuits.

An important aspect of NMDA receptors is the role that these ligand-gated channels play in synaptic plasticity. Although the cellular mechanisms underlying learning and memory in the human brain are unknown, it is believed that the changes responsible for certain forms of memory reside in longer-term alterations in synaptic transmission. When glutamate synapses are used at high frequency, they undergo a persistent enhancement of responsivity, referred to as *long-term potentiation* (LTP). In many regions, LTP induction depends on activation of NMDA receptors and requires coincident detection of changes in presynaptic function (glutamate release) and postsynaptic membrane depolarization. NMDA receptors have unique properties that make them potential molecular switches for altering synaptic function. First, NMDA ion channels are highly permeable to calcium ions, and when these channels open, they provide a large calcium signal to neurons. Calcium, in turn, is an important messenger that drives a host of cellular biochemical changes that include activation of specific protein kinases, phospholipases, and other cellular synthetic enzymes. Thus, calcium influx mediated by NMDA channels serves as an important trigger for producing changes in synaptic function. Second, NMDA ion channels are effectively inhibited at membrane potentials near the neuronal resting membrane potential because of a voltage-dependent block by physiological concentrations of extracellular magnesium ions. The magnesium-dependent block of NMDA channels is relieved when the neuronal membrane potential is depolarized. In effect, NMDA receptors serve as "coincidence detectors," requiring for activation both the binding of glutamate and postsynaptic membrane depolarization. When these conditions are met, NMDA receptors participate in synaptic transmission and play key roles in the induction of LTP. Interestingly, NMDA receptors also participate in some forms of long-term synaptic depression (LTD) as well, but in the case of LTD, it appears that the degree of postsynaptic membrane depolarization is less than that which accompanies LTP, resulting possibly in a smaller calcium signal and the preferential activation of protein phosphatases in postsynaptic cells. Presently, LTP and LTD are leading candidates to be cellular mechanisms underlying certain forms of learning in the mammalian nervous system. Given that PCP and ethanol inhibit NMDA receptors, it is tempting to speculate that the amnestic effects of these drugs (called *blackouts* in the case of alcohol) result from blockade of NMDA receptors.

Oscillatory Neuronal Firing and Complex Behavioral States

Certain behavioral states, including wakefulness, attention, mood, and sleep appear to require sustained coherent activity in specific neuronal circuits, particularly corticothalamic networks. Activity in these circuits involves an interplay of the intrinsic electrophysiological properties of specific neurons and sustained effects of more diffusely acting neuromodulator systems, including muscarinic and monoaminergic systems. Certain neurons have specific voltage-gated ionic conductances that allow them to fire rhythmically and spontaneously, thus having properties expected of a *pacemaker* or *oscillator*. For example, neurons in the inferior olivary nucleus fire action potentials spontaneously and sustain this firing for relatively long periods in the absence of outside inputs. These inferior olivary neurons fire conventional fast Na^+ spikes that provide the depolarization needed to open HVA Ca^{2+} channels. In turn, Ca^{2+} influx activates a Ca^{2+}-dependent K^+ conductance that rapidly and effectively hyperpolarizes the membrane. When the membrane hyperpolarizes, LVA Ca^{2+} channels open and bring the membrane potential back to threshold for firing Na^+ spikes, which then activate another cycle. In the case of the inferior olivary neurons, it is the properties of the LVA Ca^{2+} channels that foster oscillatory firing. LVA channels are inactivated at the neuronal resting membrane potential but become activatable when the membrane is hyperpolarized with respect to rest. In effect, hyperpolarization becomes an activating stimulus that allows the LVA channels to open. The oscillatory firing of inferior olivary neurons then drives Purkinje neurons in the cerebellum at the inferior olivary neuron's preferred firing frequency. The Purkinje neurons are thus said to *resonate* in response to the inferior olivary input. This resonating circuit is believed to contribute to the physiological resting tremor, which oscillates at approximately ten cycles per second. In this circuit, the inferior olivary neurons are considered pacemakers.

Pacemaker activity is also found in thalamic neurons where similar, although not necessarily identical, mechanisms are used to drive oscillatory firing. In the thalamocortical system, changes in neuronal activity are associated with the state of behavioral arousal. Network activity in the thalamocortical system is mediated by both intrinsic neuronal conductances and synaptic connections. This activity drives specific changes in the electroencephalogram (EEG) during different stages of sleep and vigilance. Thalamocortical neurons exhibit two distinct activity states. During sleep, the cells show synchronized rhythms that resemble delta, spindle, and other slow waves on the EEG. During awake states and REM sleep, these neurons show tonic activity. LVA calcium channels are important participants in thalamocortical network activity. The transition from sleep to wakefulness is mediated by depolarization of thalamic reticular neurons and inactivation of LVA calcium channels. It also appears that specific abnormalities in thalamocortical neurons may be critical in the generation of the 3-Hz spike-and-wave activity seen during absence seizures.

In some regions of the CNS, the outputs of the pacemaker cells are mediated by fast excitatory or inhibitory transmitters. However, some neurons are capable of firing in bursts of action potentials. *Bursts* are periods of frequent spike firing followed by quiescent periods. This type of firing can be used to drive activity in a local or distributed neural network. Additionally, burst-like firing can provide sufficient intracellular Ca^{2+} signals to stimulate release of peptide transmitters. In turn, the slow synaptic actions of the peptides in combination with or independent of other G-protein–coupled receptor systems can alter the frequency of oscillatory firing and bursting. A clear example of this is the repeated firing that occurs when spike frequency adaptation is inhibited by blocking Ca^{2+}-activated K^+ conductances. In this fashion, both the intrinsic electrical properties of neurons and the effect of modulatory transmitters conspire to determine a background level of activity (or tone) in specific neuronal systems.

Ion Channels and Disease

Over the last several years, there has been increasing evidence that a number of clinical disorders, including neuropsychiatric syndromes, result from heritable or acquired defects in ion channels (called *channelopathies*). These disorders are characterized by altered function of specific ion channels that result from genetic mutations, transcriptional abnormalities, or autoimmune processes. Although most of these illnesses are not considered pure "psychiatric" disorders, the involvement of specific ion channels in illnesses is instructive for understanding the importance of ion channels in physiological function. Furthermore, some channelopathy syndromes suggest ways to think about gene–environment interactions in the production of psychiatric disorders.

The most detailed information about the role of abnormal ion channel function leading to illness exists for cardiac disorders. One example is the long QT syndrome, characterized by defects in cardiac repolarization. Individuals with long QT intervals are predisposed to develop malignant cardiac arrhythmias (e.g., torsades de pointes) either spontaneously or during exposure to certain drugs, including psychotropic medications. Several inherited mutations of cardiac ion channels are implicated in the long QT syndrome. These include mutations in the Na^+ channel gene, SCN5A, or the four genes that contribute to delayed rectifier K^+ currents in the heart. The defect in SCN5A Na^+ channels appears to enhance sodium currents via defects in channel inactivation. Interestingly, a loss-of-function mutation in SCN5A has been associated with Brugada syndrome, a cardiac disorder associated with idiopathic ventricular fibrillation. Given the importance of SCN5A channels in the upstroke of cardiac action potentials, the mechanisms underlying ventricular fibrillation in Brugada syndrome are poorly understood at present. The mutations in delayed rectifier K^+ channels that contribute to long QT syndrome result in loss of channel function and abnormalities of ventricular repolarization. Channel mechanisms contributing to drug-induced long QT syndromes are less well understood but may involve polymorphisms in K^+ channels.

Given the importance of ion channels in determining the firing patterns of neurons, the observation that epilepsy, a group of disorders associated with recurrent episodes of abnormal paroxysmal electrical activity, is associated with mutations in specific ion channels is not surprising. For example, autosomal dominant nocturnal frontal lobe epilepsy is associated with mutations in the neuronal nicotinic acetylcholine receptor $\alpha 4$ gene. The syndrome is characterized by clusters of brief seizures during light sleep and can be confused clinically with nightmares. Mutations reported to date disrupt the second transmembrane domain of the protein that is thought to form the ion channel pore. Benign familial neonatal convulsions are associated with mutations in K^+ channel genes KCNQ2 or KCNQ3. These proteins form M channels that produce slowly activating and slowly inactivating K^+ currents that blunt neuronal firing. The expression of a single mutant allele of either gene—benign familial neonatal convulsions is a dominant disorder with the pathology the product of the mutant allele despite the presence of an allele that is normal on the other chromosome—apparently decreases channel number sufficiently to result in hyperexcitable neurons. Generalized epilepsy with febrile seizures plus is an autosomal dominant syndrome that results from mutations in Na^+ channel subunits. The role that channels play in these rare genetic syndromes suggests that idiopathic epilepsy might be a channelopathy resulting from an interaction between genetic defects in ion channels and adverse environmental effects. Identification of defective channel genes associated with idiopathic epilepsy would offer the opportunity to improve pharmacotherapy by allowing genotyping of individuals to tailor treatment to the specific genes involved.

The calcium channel CACNA1A gene, which encodes the $\alpha 1$ subunit of HVA P/Q-type Ca^{2+} channels, is associated with several rare genetic diseases. Familial hemiplegic migraine is an autosomal dominant form of migraine with childhood onset and an aura that includes a transient hemiparesis or hemiplegia lasting hours to days. Otherwise, the headache is indistinguishable from other migraine syndromes associated with aura, although, in some families, the disorder is associated with progressive ataxia. As is expected in psychiatric disorders, familial hemiplegic migraine is genetically heterogeneous with approximately 50 percent of the cases involving mutations in CACNA1A. The heterogeneity extends to the molecular level with 13 different mutations identified to date. The effect of the mutations was anticipated to be gain of function, given the pathological impact of the single mutant allele on patients. Expression of the various mutant genes in heterologous systems (*Xenopus* oocytes, HEK293 cells) reveals a complex picture with the most frequently identified mutation producing reduced Ca^{2+} currents, presumably a loss of function, and another mutation associated with increased Ca^{2+} flux, or a gain of function. Another dominant disorder associated with mutations in CACNA1A is episodic ataxia type 2. Patients experience episodes of nystagmus and ataxia lasting hours to days; for some, the disorder is progressive with cerebellar atrophy. Approximately 50 percent of the patients experience migraine. Although most of the 15 mutations associated with the disorder grossly disrupt protein expression, several are point mutations that change a single amino acid. Expression of the gene with one of the point mutations in a heterologous system results in complete loss of function without a change in protein expression. Finally, one type of autosomal dominant spinocerebellar ataxia (SCA6) has been linked to the presence of an expansion of CAG repeats (polyglutamine) in the carboxy terminus of the CACNA1A protein. In many ways, it is easier to conceptualize the mutant protein producing a chronic condition such as ataxia rather than an episodic disorder such as migraine, because the P/Q channel is critical for transmitter release in cerebellar circuits responsible for gait. It is conceivable that the P/Q mutations associated with migraine are particularly important to the function of a neural circuit activated by adverse environmental exposure (a precipitant of migraine) or dependent on a transmitter such as serotonin (thought to be involved in pathogenesis of migraine)—or both. Perhaps "knock-out" and conditional expression of the altered CACNA1A genes in mice will further illuminate how molecular pathology translates into symptomatic behavior. The various syndromes associated with altered CACNA1A gene highlight the heterogeneity that is expected from the exploration of genes for psychiatric disorders.

MS produces many types of symptoms, including cerebellar dysfunction, at least partly due to demyelination. Peripheral nerve injury results in changes in Na^+ channel gene expression. Conceptualization of MS as a disorder associated with nerve injury as the result of demyelination suggested that there may be altered Na^+ channel expression in the disorder. Animal models of demyelination revealed the expression of the tetrodotoxin-resistant sensory neuron–specific (SNS) Na^+ channel (Na_v 1.8) in cerebellar Purkinje cells, a type of channel normally not expressed in the brain. Postmortem examination of the brains of patients with MS who exhibited clinical signs of cerebellar dysfunction before death also indicated the expression of the SNS Na^+ channel in Purkinje cells. These findings are apparently specific to MS based on the absence of SNS Na^+ channel expression in the Purkinje cells of cerebellar cortex taken from patients who died as the result of coronary artery disease. This example of an "acquired" channelopathy suggests that gene–environment interaction thought to be so important to the pathophysiology of psychiatric disorders could result in the induction of a channelopathy.

Based on the current status of the field, it appears likely that the diversity of voltage-gated and ligand-gated ion channels will be better understood at structural, biophysical, and genetic levels. Although the electrical events underlying neuronal excitability are relatively stereotyped, the various ion channels contributing to neuronal firing offer a great deal of flexibility in the control of cellular activity. Furthermore, the diversity of ion channels involved in electrical signaling provides a complex and powerful means by which excitability can be modulated by neurotransmitters and therapeutic drugs. Determining how subtle alterations in ion channel function contribute to behavior and clinical syndromes will remain a major goal of work in this field.

SUGGESTED CROSS-REFERENCES

Section 1.4 discusses how monoamine neurotransmitters directly (e.g., 5-HT_3) and indirectly activate (through G proteins) ion channels as an integral part of neurotransmission. Section 1.5 discusses amino acid neurotransmitters—using a similar rationale as for monoamine neurotransmitters (see above). Section 1.6 discusses how neuropeptides alter electrical properties of cells indirectly. Section 1.8 discusses how G proteins, an important intracellular signaling pathways, exert effects on channels as part of signaling. Section 1.14 discusses how applied electrophysiology depends on principles of basic electrophysiology. Section 1.20 discusses the basic science of sleep—how the sleep cycle may be driven by the sustained efforts of neural circuits that, in turn, reflect the electrophysiological properties of specific cells in the network. Section 1.22 discusses neural mechanisms of substance abuse—how several abused drugs affect ion channels.

REFERENCES

Ackerman MJ, Clapham DE: Ion channels—basic science and clinical disease. *New Engl J Med*. 1997;336:1575–1586.

Attwell D, Laughlin SB: An energy budget for signaling in the grey matter of the brain. *J Cereb Blood Flow Metab*. 2001;21:1133–1145.

Bianchi L, Driscoll M: Protons at the gate: DEG/EnaC ion channels help us feel and remember. *Neuron*. 2002;34:337–340.

Cannon SC; Sodium channel defects in myotonia and periodic paralysis. *Annu Rev Neurosci*. 1996;19:141–164.

Catterall WA: From ionic currents to molecular mechanisms: the structure and function of voltage-gated sodium channels. *Neuron*. 2000;26:13–25.

Choe S: Potassium channel structures. *Nat Rev Neurosci*. 2002;3:115–121.

Ducros A, Denier C, Joutel A, Cecillon M, Lescoat C, Vahedi K, Darcel F, Vicaut E, Bousser M-G, Tournier-Lasserve E: The clinical spectrum of familial hemiplegic migraine associated with mutations in a neuronal calcium channel. *N Engl J Med*. 2001;345:17–24.

Dutzler R, Campbell EB, Cadene M, Chait BT, MacKinnon R: X-ray structure of a ClC chloride channel at 3.0A reveals the molecular basis of anion selectivity. *Nature*. 2002;17:287–294.

Fozzard HA, Hanck DA: Structure and function of voltage-dependent sodium channels: comparison of brain II and cardiac isoforms. *Physiol Rev*. 1996;76:887–926.

Heeger DJ, Ress D: What does fMRI tell us about neuronal activity? *Nat Rev Neurosci*. 2002;3:142–151.

Hille B. *Ion Channels of Excitable Membranes*. Sunderland MA: Sinauer Associates Inc.; 2001.

Husi H, Grant SGN: Proteomics of the nervous system. *Trends Neurosci*. 2001;24:259–266.

Jevtovic-Todorovic V, Hartman RE, Izumi Y, Benshoff ND, Dikranian K, Zorumski CF, Olney JW, Wozniak DW: Early exposure to common anesthetic agents causes widespread neurodegeneration in the developing rat brain and persistent learning deficits. *J Neurosci*. 2003;23:876–882.

Jiang Y, Lee A, Chen J, Cadene M, Chait BT, MacKinnon R: Crystal structure and mechanism of a calcium-gated potassium channel. *Nature*. 2002;417:515–522.

Jiang Y, Lee A, Chen J, Cadene M, Chait BT, MacKinnon R: The open pore conformation of potassium channels. *Nature*. 2002;417:523–526.

Jiang Y, Lee A, Chen J, Ruta V, Cadene M, Chait BT, MacKinnon R: X-ray structure of a voltage-dependent K^+ channel. *Nature*. 2003;423:33–41.

Jiang Y, Ruta V, Chen J, Lee A, MacKinnon R: The principle of gating charge movement in a voltage-dependent K^+ channel. *Nature*. 2003;423:42–48.

Jorgensen PL, Hakansson KO, Karlish SJD: Structure and mechanism of Na,K-ATPase: functional sites and their interactions. *Annu Rev Physiol*. 2003;65:817–849.

Karlin A: Emerging structure of the nicotinic acetylcholine receptors. *Nat Rev Neurosci*. 2002;3:102–114.

Koester J. Membrane potential, passive properties of the neuron, and voltage-gated ion channels and the generation of the action potential. In: Kandel ER, Schwartz JH, Jessell TM, eds. *Principles of Neural Science*. 3rd ed. New York: Elsevier; 1991:81–118.

Korpi ER, Grunder G, Luddens H: Drug interactions at $GABA_A$ receptors. *Prog Neurobiol*. 2002;67:113–159.

Madden DR: The structure and function of glutamate receptor ion channels. *Nat Rev Neurosci*. 2002;3:91–101.

Marban E: Cardiac channelopathies. *Nature*. 2002;415:213–218.

McCormick DA, Bal T: Sleep and arousal: thalamocortical mechanisms. *Annu Rev Neurosci*. 1997;20:185–216.

Mennerick S, Zorumski CF: Neural activity and survival in the developing nervous system. *Mol Neurobiol*. 2000;22:41–54.

Montell C, Birnbaumer L, Flockerzi V: The TRP channels, a remarkably functional family. *Cell*. 2002;108:595–598.

Nichols CG, Lopatin AN: Inward rectifier potassium channels. *Annu Rev Physiol*. 1997;59:171–191.

Noebels JL: The biology of epilepsy genes. *Annu Rev Neurosci*. 2003;26:599–625.

Pape H-C: Queer current and pacemaker: the hyperpolarization-activated cation current in neurons. *Annu Rev Physiol*. 1996;58:299–327.

Pietrobon D: Calcium channels and channelopathies of the central nervous system. *Mol Neurobiol*. 2002;25:31–50.

Prakriya M, Mennerick S: Selective depression of low-release probability excitatory synapses by sodium channel blockers. *Neuron*. 2000;26:671–682.

Robbins J: KCNQ potassium channels: physiology, pathophysiology, and pharmacology. *Pharmacol Ther*. 2001;90:1–19.

Sadja R, Alagem N, Reuveny E: Gating of GIRK channels: details of an intricate, membrane-delimited signaling complex. *Neuron*. 2003;39:9–12.

Sather WA, McClesky EW: Permeation and selectivity in calcium channels. *Annu Rev Physiol*. 2003;65:133–159.

Serysheva II, Ludtke SJ, Baker MR, Chiu W, Hamilton SL: Structure of the voltage-gated L-type Ca^{2+} channel by electron cryomicroscopy. *Proc Natl Acad Sci U S A*. 2002;99:10370–10375.

Shulman RG: Functional imaging studies: linking mind and basic neuroscience. *Am J Psychiatry*. 2001;158:11–20.

Steriade M: Corticothalamic resonance, states of vigilance and mentation. *Neuroscience*. 2000;101:243–276.

Szewczyk A, Wojtczak L: Mitochondria as a pharmacological target. *Pharm Reviews*. 2002;54:101–127.

Talley EM, Bayliss DA: Modulation of TASK-1 (Kcnk3) and TASK-3 (Kcnk9) potassium channels. *J Biol Chem*. 2002;277:17733–17742.

Waxman SG: Acquired channelopathies in nerve injury and MS. *Neurology*. 2001;56:1621–1627.

Xia X-M, Zeng X, Lingle CJ: Multiple regulatory sites in large-conductance calcium-activated potassium channels. *Nature*. 2002;418:880–884.

Zagotta WN, Siegelbaum SA: Structure and function of cyclic nucleotide-gated channels. *Annu Rev Neurosci*. 1996;19:235–263.

▲ 1.10 Genome, Transcriptome, and Proteome

STEVEN O. MOLDIN, PH.D., AND STEVEN E. HYMAN, M.D.

This is an era in which the global study of the *deoxyribonucleic acid* (DNA), *ribonucleic acid* (RNA), and protein building blocks of cells has become feasible and increasingly routine, as exemplified by completion of the Human Genome Project (HGP), by large-scale studies of human genetic variation, and by the wide dissemination of DNA microarray technologies and other tools of functional genomics. As a result, it should become increasingly feasible to investigate the genetic underpinnings of mental illness and other genetically complex human diseases. Functional genomics is already becoming routine in brain research and is being applied to the study of postmortem human brains from individuals with mental illness and to animal models of relevance to clinical neuroscience.

What are these "omics" approaches and what do they have in common? All of these approaches are attempts to study a level of biological information from a global perspective. For example, instead of studying the expression of one gene at a time, neuroscientists and other researchers can now study the expression of thousands of genes, which permits the informed selection of a smaller number for detailed investigation.

Genomics is the study of entire *genomes*, and a genome is the sum total of DNA within an organism—with the caveat that higher *eukaryotes* have separate nuclear and mitochondrial genomes. Genomics has been made possible by the technologies of high-throughput DNA sequencing and computation (or *bioinformatics*). The central role of computational methods is not to be underestimated, as many billions of DNA-based pairs are currently in public databases, where they can be readily and rapidly compared and analyzed. *Genetics* and genetic epidemiology (see Section 1.17) is a direct beneficiary of genomics, as genetics is the science that attempts to correlate differences in DNA sequence (*genotype*) with differences in observable traits (*phenotype*). The *transcriptome* is a term that can be applied to the sum total of RNAs expressed (transcribed) in an organism. Studies of gene expression usually focus on *messenger RNA* (mRNA), the intermediate between genes and proteins. Global studies of gene expression compose the field of *functional genomics* and may use such tools as microarrays, in which thousands of gene sequences are etched on a slide or thousands of DNA samples are spotted on a slide and used as a probe to detect and quantify complementary RNA sequences in a sample. The *proteome* denotes the full panoply of proteins expressed in an organism and studied globally by proteomics. Taking this jargon nearer its limit, there is even talk of a *metabolome*, the sum total of enzyme activities. This exuberance and its tortured language can be forgiven, however, if these technologies ultimately live up to their promise. The ability to monitor the expression of thousands of genes, proteins, or enzyme activities at once, along with increasingly powerful computational methods, has given rise to the promise of a new non-reductionist "systems biology" that will increasingly permit us to understand the overall working of cells and even give us glimpses of some aspects of the overall workings of the brain.

The year 2003 is the 50th anniversary of the determination by James Watson and Francis Crick of the structure of DNA and also the year in which the HGP was completed. The HGP yielded a *finished sequence* (highly accurate, contiguous DNA sequence) of the human genome; the sequences of important model organisms such as the mouse are also being produced. The HGP was made possible by the development of technologies to sequence DNA rapidly, accurately, and cheaply. As a result, it has been possible to determine the sequence of large stretches of DNA from many individuals. This has provided an enormous amount of information on human sequence variation, the raw material of genetics. The existence of a human reference sequence, extensive and growing information on human variation, and the genomic sequences of model organisms have given geneticists powerful new tools. Beyond the full sequence of the genome, there are currently intensive efforts to identify all of the actual genes within the genome and to produce and make available *complementary DNA* (cDNA) replicas of all of the mRNAs that are expressed in the human, the mouse, and other species. These collections will facilitate investigation of the biology of the brain and the pathophysiology of mental disorders. Within a reasonably short time, neurobiologists will have access to the cDNAs for every G-protein–coupled receptor encoded in the human genome, all of the ion channels, and all of the protein kinases in cells, to name only a few important classes of proteins.

The study of "normal" species' typical genes and their cDNAs will be complemented by the ability to study variant forms identified by genetics. Thus, it will become clear how slightly different versions of a G-protein–coupled receptor, an ion channel, or a protein kinase alters cellular function and, eventually, the functioning of the brain. More than 1,000 genes in which mutations predispose to human disease have already been identified, and many have been used to produce transgenic mice that can model aspects of the disease. The vast majority of the disease genes that have been identified, however, cause *mendelian* disorders, in which the gene in question exerts a very large effect. Medicine is now turning its attention to the search for the considerably more elusive genes that underlie complex disease phenotypes, including mental disorders.

This chapter begins with an introduction to DNA and the basics of gene expression. It then describes the contribution of the HGP and related large-scale sequencing projects to the toolkit for human genetics and studies of gene expression that are relevant to both mental illness and treatment. What follows is enough detail to permit the reader to begin to evaluate molecular hypotheses that are likely to appear with increasing frequency in the psychiatric literature during the next decade.

DNA AND RNA: BUILDING BLOCKS OF LIFE

Molecular genetics, as it is relevant to psychiatry, is largely concerned with the complex relationships between the information-carrying macromolecules DNA and RNA and their protein products, which are the critical building blocks of all cells, including neurons, in the brain. The genetic blueprint of all living organisms, from bacteria to human beings, is encoded by sequences of DNA. The double helical structure of DNA elucidated by Watson and Crick is well suited to the storage of information, its transfer from generation to generation, and its ability to direct the synthesis of other macromolecules. Each strand of the double helix is a linear polymer constructed of four small building blocks called *nucleotides*. Information is encoded in the linear ordering of these nucleotides.

The four nucleotides that make up DNA are the purines, adenine (A) and guanine (G), and the pyrimidines, cytosine (C) and thymine (T). As shown in Figure 1.10–1, the double helix is constructed of a sugar-phosphate backbone, with the nucleotide bases oriented toward the inside. On the inside of the helix, a *purine* (A or G), the larger type of nucleotide, is always found directly opposite a smaller *pyrimidine* (T or C). The nucleotide A is always paired with T, and G is paired with C—in other words, A is complementary to T, and G complementary to C. A maximum number of stabilizing hydrogen bonds form only between pairs of complementary nucleotides; any other arrangement of bases destabilizes the structure of the DNA.

The principle of complementary base pairing forms the basis of DNA *replication* and of *transcription* of DNA into RNA, which is the first step in gene expression. Because DNA is a linear polymer, it readily serves as a template for the synthesis of other macromolecules. In either DNA replication or RNA synthesis, the double helix unwinds and a new complementary strand of DNA or RNA is synthesized by successively incorporating complementary bases (e.g., an A in the new strand across from a T in the template strand). Since the new strand contains a nucleotide sequence that is the exact complement of the sequence of the template, both strands contain the same information. In DNA replication, each strand of the parent double helix serves as a template for the synthesis of a new complementary strand, resulting in two double helical molecules of DNA identical to the first. In RNA synthesis (*transcription*), only one strand of the DNA serves as a template for the synthesis of a single-stranded RNA, which then dissociates from the template.

Although the structure of DNA is ideally suited for information storage and transfer, its chemical simplicity and its relatively rigid helical structure limit the functions that it can perform within cells. As a result, the information contained within DNA is expressed through RNA and proteins. RNA, like DNA, is a linear polymer of four nucleotides, but unlike DNA, it is a single strand, free to fold into a variety of conformations, making it functionally more versatile. mRNA is RNA that serves as an intermediate between a DNA

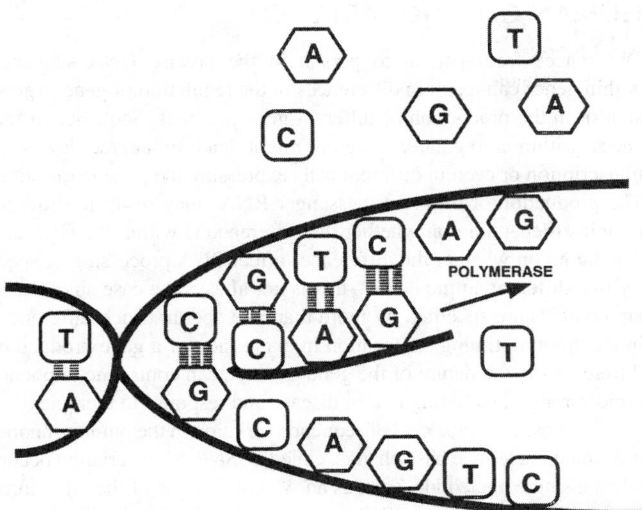

FIGURE 1.10–1 The double helix of DNA. Two complementary strands of DNA hybridize with one another to form a double helix. The backbones of the two strands are formed by alternating sugar and phosphate groups; the nucleotide bases are found on the inside. Formation of a DNA double helix is stabilized when hydrogen bonds form between complementary bases of the two strands. A, adenine; C, cytosine; G, guanine; T, thymine. (Adapted from Hyman SE, Nestler EJ. *Molecular Foundations of Psychiatry*. Washington, DC: American Psychiatric Association; 1993, with permission.)

sequence and the protein it encodes. As in the case of DNA, mRNA carries information encoded in its linear sequence of nucleotides. Other RNA molecules serve structural rather than information-carrying purposes in cells. *Ribosomes*, the organelles on which proteins are synthesized, are constructed out of complexes of ribosomal RNA (rRNA) and proteins. Transfer RNA (tRNA) serves to deliver specific amino acids to ribosomes for incorporation into proteins during the process of *translation* of mRNA into protein.

Proteins are composed of one or more polypeptides, linear macromolecules composed of amino acids that are covalently joined together by peptide bonds. There are 20 amino acids in mammalian cells. These possess chemically diverse side chains that differ in bulk, hydrophobicity, and charge. As a result of this chemical diversity, proteins have much greater functional versatility than either DNA or RNA. The specific properties of proteins (Table 1.10–1) depend not only on the linear sequence of their amino acid building blocks (*primary structure*) but also on their folded, three-dimensional characteristics (*secondary* and *tertiary structure*). In addition, individual proteins (polypeptide chains) may form complexes with other proteins (*quaternary structure*); in such cases, the individual polypeptide chains are called *subunits*. Proteins can interact noncovalently with specific cofactors, for example, ions or small molecules, or can be covalently modified, for example, by the addition of sugar or lipid groups to some of the amino acid side chains. These interactions and modifications influence the conformation of the protein and, therefore, its function. Proteins are involved in essentially all aspects of cellular function.

GENES AND CHROMOSOMES

In *eukaryotes*, the DNA is contained within a membrane-bound organelle, the nucleus. The genome of eukaryotic organisms comprises genes and much intervening DNA. Within the nucleus, DNA is organized into discrete *chromosomes*. The size and number of chromosomes vary greatly between species; human cells have 46—23

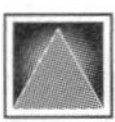

Table 1.10–1
Levels of Protein Structure

Level	Definition
Primary	Linear sequence of amino acids in a polypeptide
Secondary	Path that a polypeptide backbone follows
Tertiary	Overall three-dimensional structure of a polypeptide
Quaternary	Overall structure of a protein, i.e., of a combination of protein subunits

inherited from each parent. Chromosomes are very long DNA molecules that are bound by a variety of structural and regulatory proteins. The most important structural proteins are *histones*, which are small, positively charged proteins that serve to package DNA into structures that fit into the cell nucleus. The DNA helix is wrapped around core histones to form a simple "beads on a string" structure that is then folded into a higher-order structure called *chromatin*. Chromatin contains various additional proteins required for DNA replication, DNA and histone modification, and transcription and processing of RNA.

Each chromosome contains multiple segments of DNA called *genes* (Fig. 1.10–2). The human genome is estimated to have approximately 30,000 genes. Historically, the term "gene" is attributed to Oskar Johannsson and first appeared in the early 1900s as an abstract concept to explain how traits were transmitted across generations. With the advent of molecular biology, it became possible to give physical reality to a gene, as a segment of DNA, and to correlate specific DNA segments with gene products (RNAs and proteins). As a first approximation, one gene was initially said to encode one protein. It was recognized that the sequence of amino acids within a protein was collinear with the sequence of the DNA within the gene that encoded it, except that each amino acid was specific by three consecutive nucleotides (called *codons*). The correlation between codons and amino acids is called the *genetic code*.

Because genes can give rise to multiple RNAs, and RNAs can give rise to multiple proteins, the definition of a gene has grown a bit

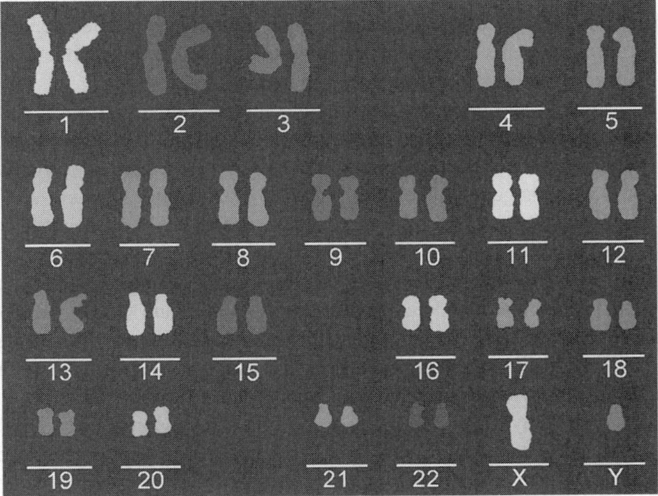

FIGURE 1.10–2 The human karyotype. The normal human genetic material contains two copies of the three billion DNA-base genomic sequence packaged into 22 matched pairs of autosomes and X and Y sex chromosomes. Here the human karyotype has been stained using different-colored chromosome-specific probes. Identical twins share identical copies of genomic DNA. (See Color Plate.) (Adapted from Bentley D. *The Geography of Our Genome*. Supplement to *Nature*, 2001, with permission.)

more complex in recent years. A gene is now understood as a circumscribed chromosomal segment responsible for making specific functional products. Modern definitions of a gene include the following components: the sequence must include both regulatory and coding regions, it must be transcribed (expressed), and the gene product must be functional.

SEQUENCING THE HUMAN GENOME

In 1988, a special committee of the U.S. National Research Council of the U.S. National Academy of Sciences recommended initiation of the HGP to sequence the complete human genome of three billion base pairs. Accomplishments in genomics over the past 15 years as a result of the HGP and other large-scale sequencing projects include the following: construction of a 1-centimorgan (cM)-resolution genetic map with 3,000 markers; construction of a physical map of the human genome containing more than 50,000 sequence-tagged sites; mapping nearly four million human *single nucleotide polymorphisms* (SNPs); identification of more than 15,000 full-length human cDNAs; finished sequences of model organisms, including *Escherichia coli, Saccharomyces cerevisiae, Caenorhabditis elegans,* and *Drosophila melanogaster*; and the development of genomic-scales technologies that include high-throughput oligonucleotide synthesis, DNA microarrays, and normalized, nonredundant cDNA libraries.

Arguably, the most significant milestones in the history of the HGP itself were met in February 2001 with the announcement and publication of the draft version of the human genome sequence and in April 2003 with the announcement that the complete, high-accuracy sequence was available. All of the sequencing, mapping, and SNP data are deposited into National Center for Biotechnology Information (NCBI) public repositories maintained by the five large-scale sequencing centers: the Sanger Institute in the United Kingdom; the Department of Energy's Joint Genome Institute in Walnut Creek, CA; and National Institutes of Health (NIH)-funded centers at Baylor College of Medicine in Houston, TX, Washington University School of Medicine in St. Louis, MO, and the Whitehead Institute in Cambridge, MA. NCBI's GenBank database contains the totality of public DNA and protein sequence information. Human sequencing data generated under HGP are made freely available to the scientific community. Sequencing of the human genome by these publicly funded centers was dramatically accelerated in 1999 and proceeded in competition with efforts of a private company, Celera Genomics.

Now that the HGP has given us a complete human sequence, it is possible, albeit with difficulty, to determine which DNA segments are genes. Michael Synder and Mark Gerstein have described five criteria for identifying genes in the DNA sequence of a genome: (1) *open reading frames* (ORFs), which are strings of codons in the linear sequence of an mRNA molecule encoded by a stretch of DNA (not every codon [group of three nucleotide bases] specifies a tRNA and, therefore, an amino acid; those that do not are called *stop codons* and specify the end of a potential ORF); (2) sequence features, or specific patterns in the DNA sequence (for example, consensus sites for RNA splicing), which can be used to help locate genes; (3) sequence conservation—genes can be identified by comparing multiple sequences among organisms (DNA sequence conservation by evolution is an excellent method to gauge the significance of a DNA region); (4) evidence for transcription—gene identification may be accomplished by searching for RNA or protein expression, the hallmark of a gene product (microarrays, serial analysis of gene expression [SAGE], and sequencing of expressed sequence tags [ESTs] are common approaches); and (5) gene inactivation—a useful method to ascertain if a gene's function is to mutate or inactivate its product, by either direct gene disruption or RNA interference.

HUMAN GENETIC VARIATION

Differences from person to person in the precise DNA sequence within genes can result in differences in the regulation of gene expression or in the production of different gene products. Sequence differences within a regulatory region might lead to altered levels of transcription or even in different cells expressing the gene in question. The production of different messenger RNAs may result in different proteins (depending on whether the difference is within the ORF and depending on whether the differences affect RNA processing or specify two different amino acids—this is not always the case since many amino acids are specified by more than one codon). Such differences in the amount, timing, or location in expression of a gene product, or differences in the nature of the gene product, can contribute to phenotypic variation, including risk of disease and response to therapies.

The most common kind of sequence variation in the human genome is a single nucleotide base change, called an *SNP*. SNP variation occurs when a single nucleotide, such as an A, replaces one of the other three nucleotide bases—C, G, or T. An example of an SNP is the alteration of the DNA segment AAGGTTA to AAGGTTT, where the last A in the first snippet is replaced with a T. On average, SNPs occur in the human population approximately once in every 1,000 bases. Because only approximately 2 percent of a person's DNA sequence represents genes, most SNPs are found in intergenic regions. SNPs found within a coding or regulatory sequence are of particular interest because they are more likely to alter the biological function of a protein.

Because of the potential utility of SNPs for genetic analyses—in other words, to aid in the mapping of genes related to disease—a concerted effort was made to identify and map SNPs in the human genome. In April 1999, ten pharmaceutical companies and the Wellcome Trust formed the *SNP Consortium*, a not-for-profit company whose goal was to contract academic sequencing laboratories funded by the NIH to identify and map SNPs. The SNP Consortium has discovered and mapped nearly four million SNPs to date. Given that it is prohibitively expensive and inefficient to categorize all of these SNPs, analytic strategies have been proposed to reduce the number of SNPs to be analyzed to a more reasonable number. One strategy focuses on sets of nearby SNPs on the same chromosome that are inherited in blocks, or *haplotypes*—representing inherited blocks of ancestral chromosomes that have not been separated by recombination. If, as is now being investigated, human genetic diversity turns out to be represented by a mosaic of haplotypes, it may be possible that different haplotypes at one locus can be efficiently identified by only a small number of SNPs.

SNPs should be useful not only in mapping genetic loci involved in disease risk but also in pharmacogenomics. Because genetic factors affect a person's response to a drug therapy, SNPs will also be useful in helping researchers determine and understand why individuals differ in their risk of adverse effects from a particular drug as well as in their therapeutic responses.

TRANSCRIPTOME: INFORMATION FLOW FROM DNA TO RNA

The expression of genetic information in cells is almost exclusively a one-way system. *Transcription* of DNA into RNA is a basic mechanism by which cells mediate their growth, function, and metabolism. The *transcriptome* can be defined as the complete collection of transcribed elements of the genome. In addition to mRNAs, it also represents noncoding RNAs that are used for structural and regulatory purposes. Alterations in the structure or levels of expression of any one of these RNAs or their proteins can contribute to disease.

Proteins are not synthesized directly from DNA but rather in two sequential processes, transcription of DNA into mRNA, which occurs in the nucleus, and *translation* of the mRNA into protein, which occurs in the cytoplasm. Conceptually, transcription is similar to DNA replication in that one of the two strands of DNA serves as a template to produce an exact complement in terms of nucleotide sequence. However, instead of producing a second strand of nucleic acid that remains annealed to the template strand (as in DNA replication), transcription produces an RNA strand that is released from the template. This allows the DNA of the gene to reanneal into its double helix, and the RNA, which remains single-stranded, to be further processed and then to exit the nucleus for translation. Transcription of genes that encode proteins is carried out by the enzyme RNA polymerase II and associated regulatory proteins. The proteins that are involved in regulating transcription are called *transcription factors*.

The primary control of gene regulation in eukaryotes occurs at the initiation of transcription. Regulation of gene expression depends on regulatory DNA sequences often called *cis-acting elements* that act as binding sites for proteins that mark the start and stop sites of transcription, that recruit RNA polymerase II to the DNA, or that regulate levels of gene expression. Most known *cis*-regulatory elements are relatively short, 8 to 16 nucleotides in length. The role of these elements is to tether the appropriate transcription factors to the correct target genes but not to other genes. In analogy with neuropharmacology, the specific DNA sequences of *cis*-regulatory elements act as receptors for transcription factors. The specificity of the binding site for a given protein is determined by the particular order of bases in that short stretch of DNA. The *cis*-regulatory sequences that are most critically involved in transcription initiation are called the core *promoter* of the gene. The particular *cis*-regulatory elements within a gene and the particular transcription factors found in a given cell determine whether that gene can be expressed in that cell type and, if so, under what circumstances. Cells contain a large number of transcription factors with diverse properties. Some interact with many genes, others with only a small number. Transcription factors can increase or decrease the rate of expression of genes with which they interact—in other words, they can act as transcriptional activators or repressors. The ability of some transcription factors to activate or repress the expression of genes is regulated by physiological signals.

To adapt appropriately to environmental signals, cells must be able to activate or repress the expression of genes. In the nervous system, regulation of gene expression by extracellular signals (i.e., neurotransmitters) is a critical mechanism underlying long-term neural plasticity to permit long-term memory.

RNA Processing After transcription of DNA into RNA, several mechanisms are employed at the level of RNA processing to generate a variety of different gene products. Eukaryotic cells have far more DNA than is needed for genes. In the human genome, it appears that the approximately 30,000 genes that encode proteins take up no more than 2 percent of the DNA. This "extra" DNA is found not only between genes but also within them. While in bacteria, proteins are almost invariably encoded by a single uninterrupted stretch of DNA; in higher organisms, most genes have their protein coding sequences, called *exons* (because these sequences are *ex*ported from the nucleus in the form of mRNA), interrupted by noncoding sequences called *introns*. When a gene is transcribed, a long RNA is produced that is colinear with the DNA and, therefore, contains both exons and introns. This is called the *primary transcript*. Before this RNA leaves the nucleus, RNA processing enzymes remove the introns, and the exons are joined to form a mature mRNA. This process is called *RNA splicing* (Fig. 1.10–3). In some cases, primary transcripts may be spliced in alternative ways, depending on the cell type or the stage of development, to produce different mRNAs and, hence, different proteins. This mechanism enables more than one protein to be synthesized from a single gene and primary transcript, depending on which exons are retained or spliced out.

One of the best studied examples of alternative splicing concerns calcitonin and calcitonin gene related peptide (CGRP): certain cells within the nervous system form CGRP, which serves as a neurotransmitter, whereas medullary cells in the thyroid gland form calcitonin, which serves as a hormone, from the same gene. Once splicing is completed, the mRNA leaves the nucleus and binds to a ribosome in the cytoplasm, where it can direct the synthesis of a protein.

Genetic and Epigenetic Regulation of Gene Expression Cells of multicellular organisms have the same DNA in their nuclei but have different structure and functions because of differential gene expression. Epigenetic mechanisms are essential for development and differentiation, but they may also arise in mature humans either by random changes (*stochastic* processes) or under environmental influences. Stable epigenetic alterations are heritable in the short term but do not involve mutations of the DNA itself. Two interdependent molecular mechanisms are involved in chromatin silencing and mediate epigenetic phenomena: *DNA methylation* and *histone modification*. The modification of core histones at their amino-terminal tails by acetylation, phosphorylation, methylation, and ubiquitylation has a fundamental role in gene regulation, with the combined acetylation, phosphorylation, and methylation status of the histone tails determining gene activity. DNA methylation in humans is a general mechanism for repressing transcription. DNA methylation is one component of a wider epigenetic program that includes other postsynthesis modifications of chromatin. Chromosomes are organized into functional domains of gene expression (*chromatin domains*), which differ in regard to transcriptional activity. Chromatin structure exerts long-range control over gene expression. Because all cells of an organism contain the same DNA (i.e., a complete copy of the organism's genome), individual genes must contain regulatory elements that permit selective expression of the genes during development and adult life. Differential expression of a common genome is required for the formation of distinct cell types during development (e.g., neuron versus kidney versus liver cells), including the differentiation of thousands of distinct types of neurons found in the brain. Differential gene expression also underlies the unique functional properties of these various cell types.

The long-term control of gene expression within cells is also controlled by covalent modification of DNA (e.g., by the addition of methyl groups to cytosine residues) and by chromatin structure. Some of these long-term mechanisms can be transmitted to progeny cells after cell division. Such mechanisms that are not directly attributable to the DNA sequence are described as *epigenetic* mechanisms. Table 1.10–2 presents an overview of mechanisms regulating gene expression in human cells.

Regulation of Gene Expression by Neurotransmitters and Second Messengers Gene expression in the brain can be activated by normal physiological processes, by experience, and by pharmacologic agents. The general mechanism by which synaptic signals are transduced to the genome involves the activation of intracellular second messenger systems and their cognate protein kinases. The protein kinases then phosphorylate specific transcription factors (or associated proteins) that alter their transcriptional activity. Phosphorylation of a transcription factor can alter its binding to the appropriate

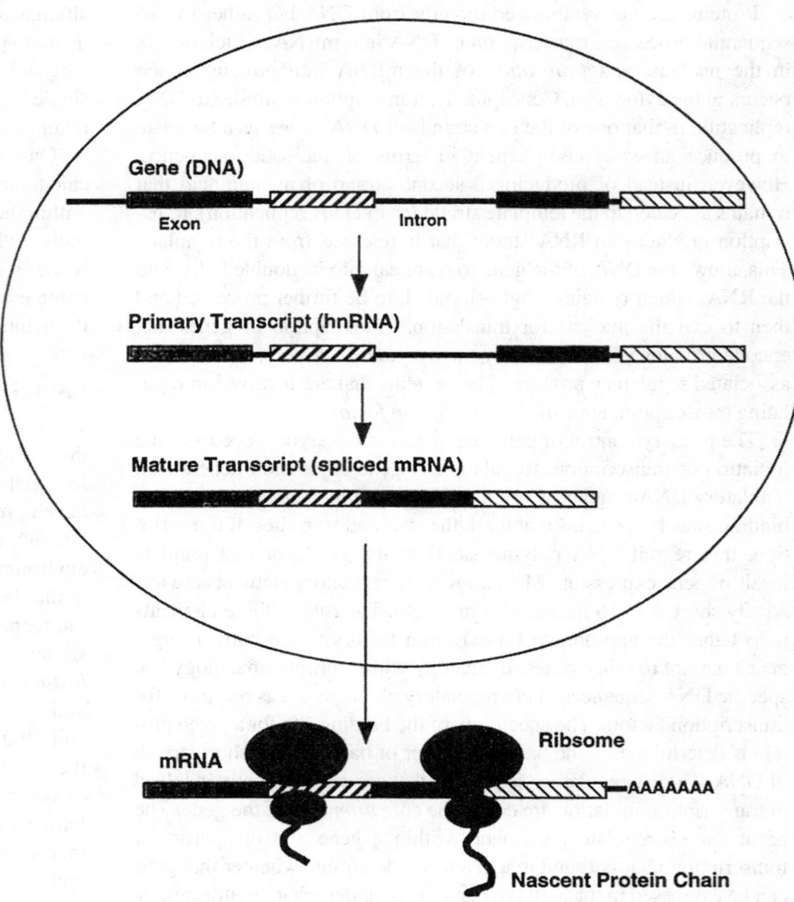

FIGURE 1.10–3. Schematic illustration of RNA splicing. DNA contains both exons, which encode polypeptides, and introns, which do not. The primary RNA transcript produced by RNA polymerase II contains both exons and introns. Before the transcript leaves the nucleus, a series of enzymes (themselves partly composed of RNA) recognize particular sequences as exon–intron boundaries and splice out the intron sequences. The mature messenger RNA (mRNA), containing only exons, is then exported from the nucleus into the cytoplasm, where it can bind to ribosomes and be translated into protein. hnRNA, heterogeneous nuclear RNA. (Adapted from Hyman SE, Nestler EJ. *Molecular Foundations of Psychiatry.* Washington, DC: American Psychiatric Association; 1993, with permission.)

cis-regulatory element or, if already bound to DNA, its ability to regulate the activity of the polymerase II complex (Fig. 1.10–4). Within this schema, there are two major variants. One involves direct activation of a transcription factor that preexists within the neuron even under basal conditions, for example, by phosphorylation. The other mechanism is indirect; phosphorylation activates a preexisting transcription factor that, in turn, activates the expression of genes that encode additional transcription factors. These newly synthesized factors can then activate or repress an additional set of "target" genes. The first mechanism occurs more rapidly than the second and partly explains the widely different time courses observed for transsynaptic regulation of gene expression. Thus, some neurotransmitter receptor–stimulated changes in gene expression occur within minutes, whereas others may require many hours and depend on new protein synthesis.

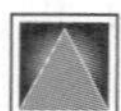

Table 1.10–2
Regulation of Gene Expression in Human Cells

Mechanism	Examples
Transcriptional	
Binding of tissue-specific transcription factors to *cis*-acting elements of a single gene	Erythroid-specific transcription factor NF-E2
Direct binding of hormones or growth factors to response elements in inducible transcription elements	Steroid hormone response elements
Use of alternative promoters in a single gene	Eight distinct promoters generate cell-type–specific expression of the dystrophin gene
Posttranscriptional	
Alternative splicing	Differential splicing in the *WT1* Wilms' tumor gene
Tissue-specific RNA editing	Expression of apolipoprotein B gene in the intestine
Translational control mechanisms	IRE binding protein regulates production of ferritin heavy chain and transferrin receptor
Epigenetic and long-term control of gene expression by chromatin structure	
Allelic exclusion	Imprinting exclusively in brain of *UBE3A* gene
X chromosome inactivation	Inactivation of many X chromosome genes by XIST gene product
Long-range control by chromatin structure	Suppression of expression of the *SOX9* gene in campomelic dysplasia
Short-range cell–cell signaling	Mammalian embryo cells

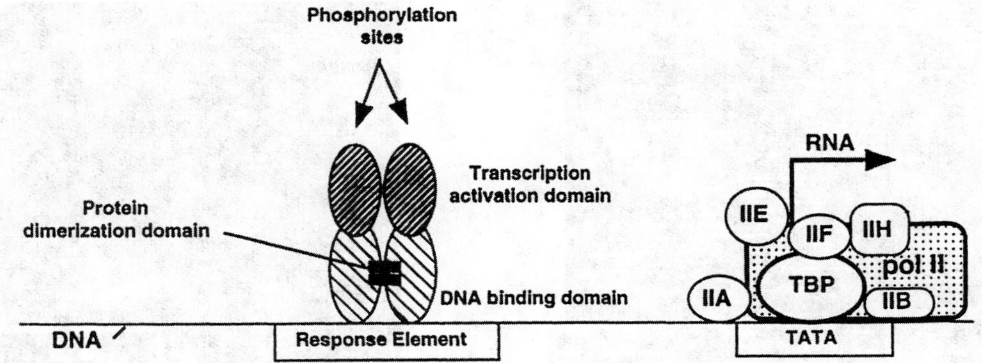

FIGURE 1.10–4 Schematic illustration of the translation of messenger RNA (mRNA) into protein. Ribosomal subunits bind together on mature mRNAs to form actively translating ribosomes. The ribosome begins adding amino acids when it reaches a start codon on the mRNA and moves down the mRNA, one codon at a time, adding the appropriate amino acid as it is delivered by a transfer RNA. When a stop codon is reached, the ribosome releases the polypeptide chain and dissociates from the mRNA. Each mRNA that is being actively translated has multiple ribosomes moving sequentially down its length, forming a polyribosome complex. (Adapted from Hyman SE, Nestler EJ. *Molecular Foundations of Psychiatry*. Washington, DC: American Psychiatric Association; 1993.)

Both direct and indirect mechanisms are widely used by neurons to regulate their long-term responses to environmental signals.

Direct Activation of Gene Expression by Cyclic Adenosine Monophosphate

The first type of second messenger response element to be characterized was one that conferred activation by cyclic adenosine monophosphate (cAMP) on the genes in which it was found. Similar cAMP response elements (CREs) have now been found within many neural genes, including those for proenkephalin, somatostatin, vasoactive intestinal polypeptide, tyrosine hydroxylase, and c-fos. By comparing response element sequences within many genes, an idealized "consensus" sequence can be derived. For CREs, the consensus nucleotide sequence is TGACGTCA, and the nucleotides CGTCA are absolutely required.

The major transcription factor that binds to CREs is called CREB (for CRE binding protein). When bound to a CRE, CREB activates transcription when it is phosphorylated by cAMP-dependent protein kinase and also by calcium/calmodulin-dependent protein kinases. The potential complexity of this regulation is likely to result in a great deal of flexibility and specificity in the way in which different types of cells respond to the environment.

Gene Expression Patterns

cDNA or oligonucleotide microarrays have proved invaluable for analyzing RNA transcript levels in a growing number of biological systems. DNA microarrays, or DNA (gene) chips, are fabricated by high-speed robotics on glass or nylon substrates, for which probes are used to determine complementary binding (Fig. 1.10–5). Hundreds of thousands of gene sequences may be represented on a single array. When a gene is activated, cellular machinery begins to copy certain segments of that gene. The mRNA produced by the cell is complementary and, therefore, will bind to the original portion of the DNA strand from which it was copied. To determine which genes are turned on and which are expressed in a given cell, a researcher must first collect the mRNA molecules present in that cell. The researcher then labels each mRNA molecule by attaching a fluorescent dye. Next, the researcher places the labeled mRNA onto a DNA microarray slide. The mRNA that was present in the cell will then hybridize—or bind—to its cDNA on the microarray, leaving its fluorescent tag. A researcher must then use a special scanner to measure the fluorescent areas on the microarray. If a particular gene is very active, it produces many molecules of mRNA, which hybridize to the DNA on the microarray and generate a very bright fluorescent area. Genes that are somewhat active produce fewer mRNAs, which results in dimmer fluorescent spots. If there is no fluorescence, none of the messenger molecules have hybridized to the DNA, indicating that the gene is inactive. Researchers frequently use arrays to examine gene expression patterns at different developmental periods or in response to different environmental stimuli.

Constructing a Transcript Map in the Nervous System

As described, many and, possibly, most genes contain *cis*-regulatory elements that confer responsiveness to physiological signals. Such *cis*-elements are often called *response elements.* Response elements work by binding transcription factors that are activated (or inhibited) by specific physiological signals, such as by second messenger–dependent phosphorylation or hormone binding. This type of regulatory mechanism, which transduces physiological signals mediated by neurotransmitters, hormones, growth factors, or drugs into changes in gene expression, may prove relevant to the etiology and course of mental disorders and the therapeutic actions of psychotropic medications. Microarrays are likely to be a powerful first step in constructing transcript maps in the brain. Altered gene expression in response to stress, drugs, lesions, learning patterns, or even the activation of a transgene can be investigated in animal models through the use of arrays. Confirmation of potentially significant examples of gene regulation, whether in animal models or human postmortem brain, can then be confirmed and mapped in detail using such techniques as in situ hybridization.

PROTEOME: INFORMATION FLOW FROM RNA TO PROTEIN

Although many RNAs have biological functions other than carrying information for the synthesis of proteins, proteins carry out the major biological work of cells. *Proteomics* is a still nascent field focused on the systematic study of a large number of proteins in a parallel manner with the aims of providing detailed descriptions of the structure, function, and control of biological systems. Technological and methodological advances are increasingly making it possible to move from studies of individual proteins to proteome-wide

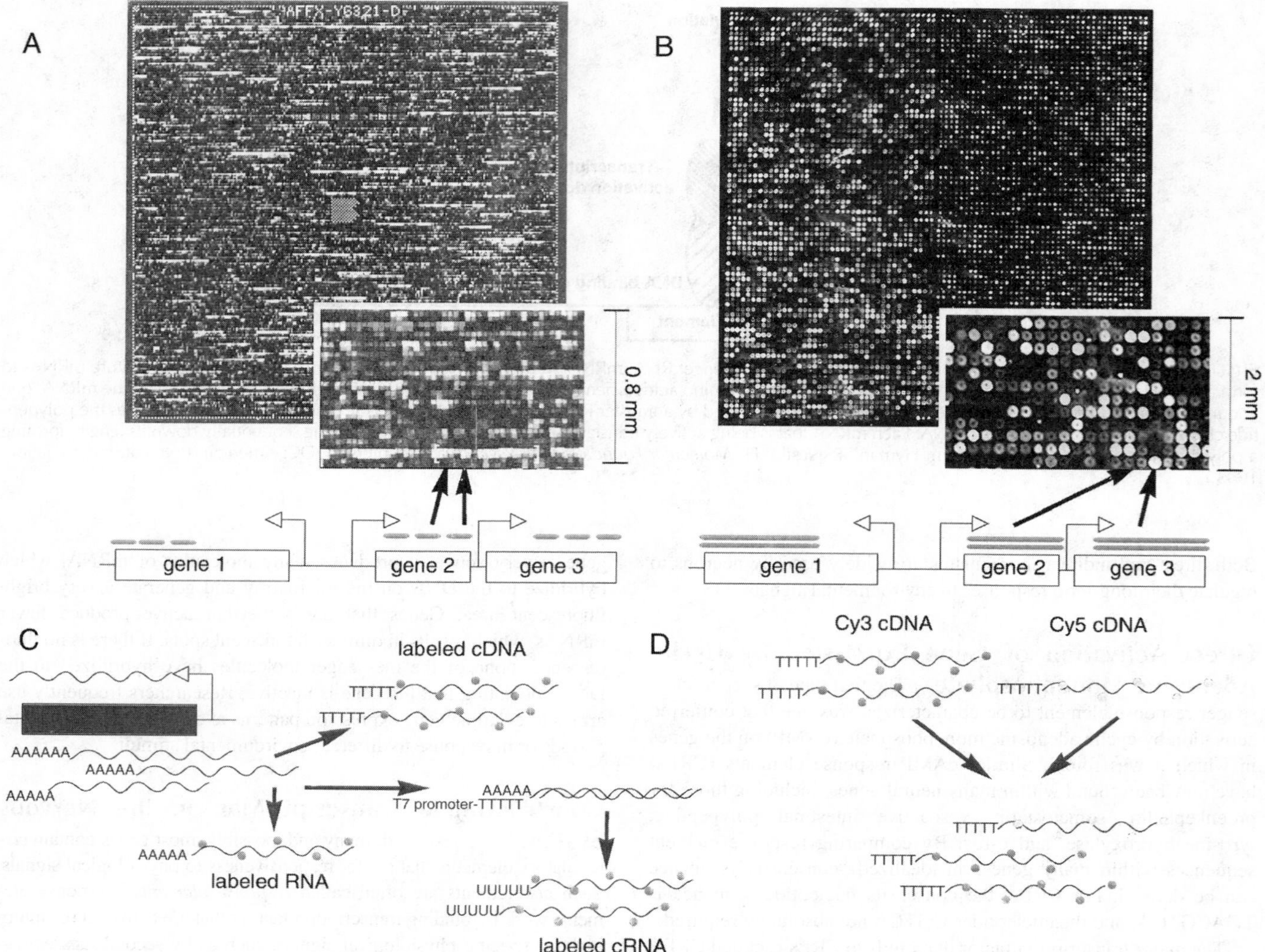

FIGURE 1.10–5 Principal types of DNA arrays used in gene expression monitoring. **A:** An oligonucleotide array from the company Affymetrix. **B:** A complementary DNA (cDNA) array. Images are shown after hybridization of labeled samples and fluorescence detection. In the case of photolithographically synthesized arrays, approximately10^7 copies of each selected oligonucleotide (usually 25 nucleotides in length) are synthesized base by base in a highly parallel, combinatorial synthesis strategy in hundreds of thousands of different areas on a 1.28 cm × 1.28 cm glass surface (some current arrays are even higher density, using more than 400,000 different probes). **C:** Different methods for preparing labeled material for measurements of gene expression (messenger RNA [mRNA] abundance) levels. RNA can be labeled directly using chemical or enzymatic methods. In the protocol used most frequently for oligonucleotide arrays, cDNA is generated from cellular mRNA. The double-stranded cDNA intermediate serves as template for a reverse transcription reaction in which labeled nucleotides are incorporated into complementary RNA (cRNA). **D:** Two-color hybridization strategy often used with cDNA microarrays. cDNA from two different conditions is labeled with two different fluorescent dyes, and the two samples are cohybridized to an array. (From Lockhart DJ, Winzeler EA: Genomics, gene expression and DNA arrays. *Nature.* 2000;405:827, with permission. cDNA array image courtesy of J. DeRisi and P. O. Brown.)

measurements. Proteomics is an essential component of an emerging "systems biology" approach in science that seeks to comprehensively describe biological systems.

Translation of RNA Transcripts into Proteins

As described above, the rules governing the translation of mRNA into protein are called the *genetic code*. The sequence of nucleotides in the mRNA is read on ribosomes in serial order in groups of three. Each triplet of nucleotides specifies one amino acid and is called a *codon*. The codons within an mRNA do not interact directly with the amino acids they specify; the translation of mRNA into protein depends on the presence of adaptor RNA molecules, called tRNAs, which recognize the three bases within a codon and carry a corresponding amino acid. tRNAs do this by providing a covalent attachment for a specific amino acid and a loop of RNA with a sequence complementary to a particular codon (Fig. 1.10–6). This loop is called an *anticodon* and allows the tRNA to interact with the mRNA and to deliver its amino acid to the growing peptide chain. There is a specific tRNA species for each codon triplet that specifies an amino acid.

Ribosomes, which are, themselves, composed of both proteins and specific ribosomal RNAs, provide the structure on which tRNAs can interact (via their anticodons) with the codons of an mRNA in sequential order. The ribosome finds a specific start site on the mRNA and then moves along the mRNA molecule translating the nucleotide sequence one codon at a time, using tRNAs to add amino acids to the growing end of the polypeptide chain (Fig. 1.10–3). When the ribosome reaches the end of the message, both the mRNA and the newly synthesized protein are released from the ribosome, which then dissociates into individual subunits. After (and often coincident with) translation, proteins are further processed: by specific cleavages to produce

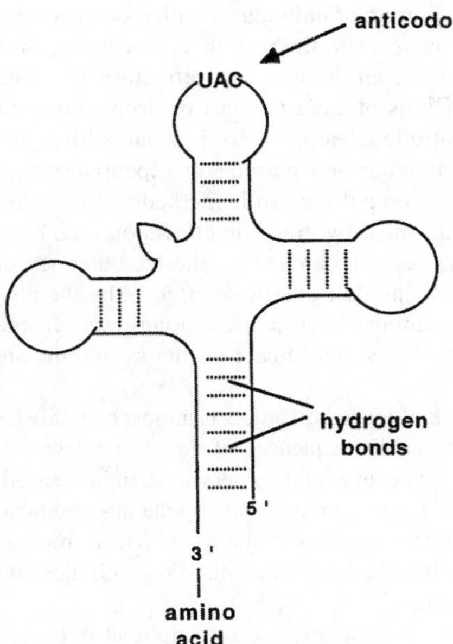

FIGURE 1.10–6 Chemical structure of transfer RNA (tRNA). tRNA is a single strand of RNA that folds on itself through the apposition of complementary base pairs and the subsequent formation of hydrogen bonds, indicated by the dashed lines in the figure. One of the loops formed contains the anticodon, the sequence of three nucleotides on the tRNA that binds to the complementary codon on a messenger RNA (mRNA) molecule. For the anticodon UAC shown in the figure, the corresponding codon on the mRNA would be AUG. The free 3-foot end of the tRNA binds to a specific amino acid. Each tRNA, with a given anticodon, binds only one type of amino acid determined by the genetic code. (Adapted from Hyman SE, Nestler EJ. *Molecular Foundations of Psychiatry.* Washington, DC: American Psychiatric Association; 1993.)

smaller peptides and proteins, by covalent modification (e.g., glycosylation) of particular amino acid residues within the protein, and by specific folding mechanisms. At this point, proteins are targeted to their proper location within the cell, for example, within the cell membrane or membranes of particular organelles, within the cytoplasm, to other cellular locations, or to secretory pathways.

In summary, information within the genome is read out by a series of processes, each of which is highly regulated by the cell. These processes include transcription of DNA into mRNA, mRNA splicing, translation of mRNA into protein, and posttranslational modification of proteins.

Structural and Functional Analysis of Proteins The three-dimensional structural analysis of proteins is called *structural genomics*. The field of structural genomics arose out of a desire of scientists to obtain structural data and, eventually, functional information about all known proteins based on the identification of protein families. The explosion of genetic sequences from the HGP and a number of technical advances in structure determination have made such an effort possible. A protein's genetic sequence can provide clues about its function, but a protein's structure can better illuminate its biological action and its role in human disease. Determining high-resolution protein structures is often difficult and time consuming, however. The essential tools of structural biology—X-ray crystallography and nuclear magnetic resonance spectroscopy (MRS)—each have their drawbacks. The former requires crystallization of the proteins, a laborious task, and the latter, although it uses proteins in solution, is usually slower and is limited to solving the structures of small and medium-sized molecules. Examples of useful new technologies include an improved method for growing crystals, a new system to select target molecules, and the use of robotics for faster and less costly data collection.

Currently, there is funding for structural genomics projects in the United States, the European Union, Japan, China, Canada, and Israel. Pharmaceutical companies and biotechnology startups are also committing to structural genomics, primarily to aid drug discovery. The publicly funded U.S. effort is spearheaded by the National Institute of General Medical Sciences (NIGMS), which, in 2000, launched a Protein Structure initiative. The goals of this very large effort are to develop new techniques to streamline and accelerate every step in structural genomics, from choosing which protein structures to solve to cloning and purifying the proteins, determining the structures, and depositing the data into the Protein Data Bank, an online public database of macromolecular structures maintained by the Research Collaboratory for Structural Bioinformatics. Another long-term goal of the NIGMS project is to develop a public library of nature's protein shapes that integrates sequence, structural, and functional information. This library should enable researchers to use genetic sequences to predict the approximate structures—and, possibly, the function—of any protein. To build this public resource, researchers funded under this initiative will determine the structures of one or two representative proteins from each of thousands of different structural families. Ten thousand unique protein structures are expected to be solved over the next decade.

In comparison to its nucleic acid–based counterpart, the experimental complexity of proteomics is far greater. Owing to the lack of amplification techniques analogous to the polymerase chain reaction (PCR), only proteins isolated from a natural source can be analyzed. Complexities arise because most proteins seem to be modified in complex ways and can be the products of differential splicing. Consequently, the relatively low number of human genes (approximately 30,000) has a very high potential to generate an enormous proteome of great complexity.

Two-dimensional gel electrophoresis is a highly robust technique for the quantitative analysis of protein expression patterns that is unmatched for separating intricate patterns of differentially modified and processed proteins. However, it is highly technical, low throughput, and quite expensive; consequently, vigorous investigation of alternative methods for large-scale protein expression analysis has been undertaken. A combination of sequence database searching and capillary, high-pressure liquid chromatography is an approach widely adopted for gel-independent quantitative profiling of the proteome. Often referred to as "shotgun" proteomics, it has the ability to catalog thousands of components in samples isolated from different sources. Mass spectrometry–based proteomics is becoming the method of choice for analyzing functional protein complexes. Given that this approach permits identification of multiple members of complexes, it complements the view of Leland Hartwell and colleagues and Scott Patterson and Ruedi Aebersold that a cell is a collection of groups of proteins with many interconnections, acting synergistically to execute cellular activities. Two large-scale protein complex studies in yeast used mass spectrometry to identify thousands of previously unknown protein interactions in isolated complexes. Although these experimental approaches require further optimization, it is clear that quantitative proteomic technologies will mature to become a clear choice for the systematic characterization of proteins.

GENES, BRAIN, AND BEHAVIOR

Based on family, twin, and adoption studies, it is apparent that both genetic and environmental factors play important roles in the normal development of temperament, personality, and attitudes as well as in the pathogenesis of major mental disorders (see Section 1.17).

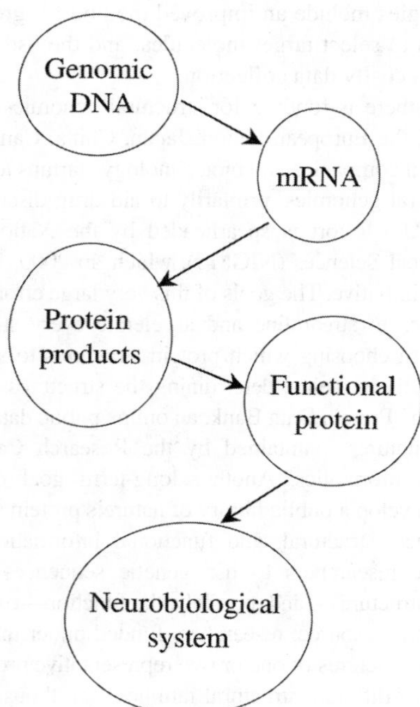

FIGURE 1.10–7 Complex pathway from genomic sequence to neurobiological systems. mRNA, messenger RNA.

Before the advent of molecular genetics, human behavioral genetics, including investigations of mental illness, were limited to quantitative analyses of twin studies, adoption studies, and multigenerational family designs that attempted to discriminate genetic from nongenetic influences on behavioral phenotypes and to determine the modes of inheritance. Historically, the most common designs were the comparison of monozygotic twins versus dizygotic twins raised together. On the assumption of a shared environment, one could then examine the role of genes based on the fact that monozygotic twins share 100 percent of their DNA, whereas dizygotic twins share, on average, 50 percent of their DNA. Multiple studies confirm that genes exert a potent influence on the risk of many mental disorders, but at the same time, there is no common mental disorder for which monozygotic twins are 100 percent concordant. Thus, there is an important role not only for genes but also for environmental factors and for stochastic and chaotic factors that act in brain development (even with identical genes, it is not possible to wire up 100 trillion synapses identically). Studies of individuals who had been adopted away from their biological families early in life better separate heredity and environment than studies of twins raised together. Such studies confirm a role for genes in such disorders as schizophrenia and alcoholism.

The fundamental challenges facing psychiatric genetics are the difficulty of defining phenotypes and the apparently large number of genetic and nongenetic risk factors involved in producing mental illness phenotypes. Without the technologies and information that have resulted from the HGP, the SNP Consortium, and related large-scale projects, it is difficult to imagine how risk genes would have been identified for mental disorders. As it is, there are still enormous difficulties based on the likely multiplicity of many genetic risk factors of small individual effect.

Gene–environment interactions may play a role not only in the initial expression of mental disorders but also in their course. For example, a subgroup of individuals with mood disorders exhibits a worsening course over time, with episodes becoming progressively more frequent, severe, and refractory to treatment. Other disorders, such as bulimia nervosa or drug abuse, may begin as relatively controlled, learned behaviors but, with repetitive experience (either binging and purging or repetitive drug administration), become compulsive, with markedly diminished voluntary control accompanied by dramatic effects on mood and cognition. In all of these cases, it can be hypothesized that neurotransmitters or hormones released or otherwise affected by the disease, behavior, or drug administration produce long-term changes in neural functioning that have an impact on the symptoms and course of the disorder.

In sum, risk of mental disorders is almost certainly based, in part, on differences in the sequences of genes at relevant loci (genetic effects). Risk and course of disorders are also influenced by environmental effects that may be mediated by the up- or downregulation of expression of certain genes in the brain. Thus, the brain integrates effects due to inherited sequence variation with those due to quantitative regulation.

Alterations in gene expression might also be central to the mechanism of action of many psychotherapeutic drugs. Most of the drugs used in psychiatric treatment, such as antidepressants, antipsychotics, and lithium, exert their therapeutic effects over a period weeks, rather than minutes to hours. Thus, it would appear that the direct, rapidly occurring effects of these drugs on neurotransmitter reuptake transporters, neurotransmitter receptors, and intracellular signaling cascades do not represent their ultimate therapeutic mechanism but rather serve as initial stimuli for slower-onset therapeutic actions. A current hypothesis is that drug-induced alterations in neural gene expression ultimately lead to alterations in synaptic strength within relevant neural circuits, resulting in a reduction in symptoms. Although the activation or suppression of genes begins within minutes of drug stimulation, the time delay is thought to reflect the need to go from gene transcription to remodeling of synapses.

FUTURE DIRECTIONS

As described in the introduction, there is an increasing realization that long-term changes in brain function brought about by both endogenous and environmental stimuli are likely to be mediated in large part by alterations in neural gene expression. This chapter describes the complex pathways that extend from the basic level of genetic structure (the genome) through the transcription of DNA into RNA (transcriptome), to the transcription of mRNA into proteins (proteome). As shown in Figure 1.10–7, ultimate characterization of protein function will have a fundamental effect on the understanding of neural pathways, circuits, and systems—and, ultimately, on the understanding of pathophysiological mechanisms in mental disorders. Although the precise mechanisms by which those stimuli directly relevant to mental disorders and psychotherapeutic drug administration act on the genome—transcriptome and proteome remain speculative at the present time—the mechanisms described in this chapter are likely to prove critical. Extending what is known about these mechanisms at a basic level to the problems of psychiatry is becoming an intense focus of research and is a necessary complement to the search for disease genes. Given the rapid technological advances that are occurring in human molecular genetics, all basic and clinical neuroscientists should make liberal use of resources on the World Wide Web (Table 1.10–3).

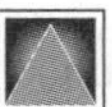

Table 1.10–3
Scientific Resources on the World Wide Web

Electronic Address	Description
http://www.ncbi.nlm.nih.gov	National Center for Biotechnology Information
http://www.hgmp.mrc.ac.uk/	U.K. Human Genome Mapping Project
http://www.ornl.gov/hgmis/	U.S. Human Genome Mapping Project
http://www.gdb.org/	The Genome Database
http://www.wellcome.ac.uk/en/genome/index.html	Wellcome Trust genome research primer
http://snp.cshl.org/	The SNP Consortium
http://www.genome.gov/	National Human Genome Research Institute
http://www.rcsb.org/pdb/	Protein Data Bank
http://www.nigms.nih.gov/funding/psi.html	National Institute of General Medical Sciences (NIGMS) Protein Structure Initiative
http://pir.georgetown.edu/	Protein Information Resource
http://www.ncbi.nlm.nih.gov/disease/Brain.html	Genes and diseases of the nervous system
http://www.nature.com/neurosci/	Nature Publishing Group neuroscience resources
http://www.sciencemag.org/feature/plus/sfg/	*Science* magazine: functional genomics

SUGGESTED CROSS-REFERENCES

Classic epidemiological genetic principles and methods are discussed in Section 1.17. Findings related to the epidemiology of schizophrenia, mood disorders, and anxiety disorders are presented in Section 12.4, Section 13.2, and Section 14.2, respectively. Findings from the study of the genetics of schizophrenia, mood disorders, and anxiety disorders are presented in Section 12.3, Section 13.3, and Section 14.6, respectively. Transgenic animals and related approaches are discussed in Section 1.19.

References

Berke JD, Paletzki RF, Aronson GJ, Hyman SE, Gerfen CR: A complex program of striatal gene expression induced by dopaminergic stimulation. *J Neurosci.* 1998;18:5301.

Boguski MS, McIntosh MW: Biomedical informatics for proteomics. *Nature.* 2003;422:233.

Botstein D, Risch N: Discovering genotypes underlying human phenotypes: past successes for mendelian disease, future approaches for complex disease. *Nat Genet.* 2003;33[Suppl]:228.

Bouchard TJ Jr, Lykken DT, McGue M, Segal NL, Tellegen A: Sources of human psychological differences: the Minnesota study of twins reared apart. *Science* 1990;250:223.

Bunney WE, Bunney BG, Vawter MP, Tomita H, Li J, Evans SJ, Choudary PV, Myers RM, Jones EG, Watson SJ, Akil H: Microarray technology: a review of new strategies to discover candidate vulnerability genes in psychiatric disorders. *Am J Psychiatry.* 2003;160:657.

*Chin HR, Moldin SO. *Methods in Genomic Neuroscience.* Boca Raton, FL: CRC Press; 2001.

Collins FS, McKusick VA: Implications of the Human Genome Project for medical science. *JAMA.* 2001;285:540.

Collins FS, Morgan M, Patrinos A: The Human Genome Project: lessons from large-scale biology. *Science.* 2003;300:286.

Couzin J: Human genome. HapMap launched with pledges of $100 million. *Science.* 2002;298:941.

*Cowan WM, Kopnisky KL, Hyman SE: The human genome project and its impact on psychiatry. *Annu Rev Neurosci.* 2002;25:1.

Gauss C, Kalkum M, Lowe M, Lehrach H, Klose J: Analysis of the mouse proteome. (I) Brain proteins: separation by two-dimensional electrophoresis and identification by mass spectrometry and genetic variation. *Electrophoresis.* 1999;20:575.

Gavin AC, Bosche M, Krause R, Grandi P, Marzioch M, Bauer A, Schultz J, Rick JM, Michon AM, Cruciat CM, Remor M, Hofert C, Schelder M, Brajenovic M, Ruffner H, Merino A, Klein K, Hudak M, Dickson D, Rudi T, Gnau V, Bauch A, Bastuck S, Huhse B, Leutwein C, Heurtier MA, Copley RR, Edelmann A, Querfurth E, Rybin V, Drewes G, Raida M, Bouwmeester T, Bork P, Seraphin B, Kuster B, Neubauer G, Superti-Furga G: Functional organization of the yeast proteome by systematic analysis of protein complexes. *Nature.* 2002;415:141.

Green ED: Strategies for the systematic sequencing of complex genomes. *Nat Rev Genet.* 2001;2:573.

Hartwell LH, Hopfield JJ, Leibler S, Murray AW: From molecular to modular cell biology. *Nature.* 1999;402:C47–C52.

Ho Y, Gruhler A, Heilbut A, Bader GD, Moore L, Adams SL, Millar A, Taylor P, Bennett K, Boutilier K, Yang L, Wolting C, Donaldson I, Schandorff S, Shewnarane J, Vo M, Taggart J, Goudreault M, Muskat B, Alfarano C, Dewar D, Lin Z, Michalickova K, Willems AR, Sassi H, Nielsen PA, Rasmussen KJ, Andersen JR, Johansen LE, Hansen LH, Jespersen H, Podtelejnikov A, Nielsen E, Crawford J, Poulsen V, Sorensen BD, Matthiesen J, Hendrickson RC, Gleeson F, Pawson T, Moran MF, Durocher D, Mann M, Hogue CW, Figeys D, Tyers M: Systematic identification of protein complexes in *Saccharomyces cerevisiae* by mass spectrometry. *Nature.* 2002;415:180.

*Hyman SE, Nestler EJ. *The Molecular Foundations of Psychiatry.* Washington, DC: American Psychiatric Press; 1993.

Jaenisch R, Bird A: Epigenetic regulation of gene expression: how the genome integrates intrinsic and environmental signals. *Nat Genet.* 2003;33[Suppl]:245.

Li E: Chromatin modification and epigenetic reprogramming in mammalian development. *Nat Rev Genet.* 2002;3:662.

Lonze BE, Ginty DD: Function and regulation of CREB family transcription factors in the nervous system. *Neuron.* 2002;35:605.

Mirnics K, Middleton FA, Marquez A, Lewis DA, Levitt P: Molecular characterization of schizophrenia viewed by microarray analysis of gene expression in prefrontal cortex. *Neuron.* 2000;28:53.

Pandey A, Mann M: Proteomics to study genes and genomes. *Nature.* 2000;405:837.

Patterson SD, Aebersold RH: Proteomics: the first decade and beyond. *Nat Genet.* 2003;33[Suppl]:311.

*Reich DE, Schaffner SF, Daly MJ, McVean G, Mullikin JC, Higgins JM, Richter DJ, Lander ES, Altshuler D: Human genome sequence variation and the influence of gene history, mutation and recombination. *Nat Genet.* 2002;32:135.

Snyder M, Gerstein M: Genomics. Defining genes in the genomics era. *Science.* 2003;300:258.

*Strachan T, Read AP. *Human Molecular Genetics.* 2nd ed. New York, NY: Wiley-Liss; 1999.

Venter JC, Levy S, Stockwell T, Remington K, Halpern A: Massive parallelism, randomness and genomic advances. *Nat Genet.* 2003;33[Suppl]:219.

Wolfsberg TG, Wetterstrand KA, Guyer MS, Collins FS, Baxevanis AD: A user's guide to the human genome. *Nat Genet.* 2002;32[Suppl]:1.

Wolters DA, Washburn MP, Yates JR, III: An automated multidimensional protein identification technology for shotgun proteomics. *Anal Chem.* 2001;73:5683.

▲ 1.11 Psychoneuroendocrinology

DEBRA S. HARRIS, M.D., OWEN M. WOLKOWITZ, M.D., AND VICTOR I. REUS, M.D.

The term *psychoneuroendocrinology* expresses an appreciation of inextricable structural and functional relationships between hormonal systems and the central nervous system (CNS) and the behaviors that modulate and are derived from both. Endocrine disorders are frequently associated with secondary psychiatric symptoms, such as depressed mood and disturbances in thought, although a significant percentage of patients who have defined psychiatric syndromes display distinct patterns of endocrine dysfunction. In the classic conception, *hormones* were defined as products of endocrine glands that were transported by blood to exert their action at sites distant from their release. Advances in neuroscience have shown, however, that in the CNS, the brain not only serves as a target site for regulatory control of hormonal release but also has secretory functions of its own, making classic distinctions between the origin, structure, and function of neurons and those of endocrine cells dependent on physiological context.

HORMONE EVOLUTION

Over the course of evolution, as organisms have increased in complexity, hormones that first appeared in unicellular organisms have been recruited to serve a multiplicity of functions, a quality that is referred to as *pleiotropy*. A single hormone may act at multiple sites, including binding to receptors on the membrane, cytoplasm, or nucleus, each with different effects, and subtle differences in molecular structure or metabolic processing can have profound physiological consequences. Hormones are thus ideally suited to regulate complex behavioral activities and to play a role in the *plasticity* of the organism, allowing it to adapt to the changing demands of the environment, as, for example, in the alteration of sexual phenotype in certain amphibians and reptiles in response to changing environmental conditions. This chapter emphasizes neuroendocrine systems that have been most directly linked to specific behavioral functions, particularly those involved in the organism's response to stress, and the principles underlying their regulation and interaction.

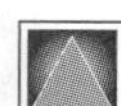

Table 1.11–2
Classification of Hormones by Location of Function

Hormone Classification	Function
Autocrine	Self-regulatory effects
Paracrine	Local or adjacent cellular action
Endocrine	Distant target site

HORMONE CLASSIFICATION

Hormones are divided into two general classes by structure—(1) proteins, polypeptides, and glycoproteins; and (2) steroids and steroid-like compounds—and into three classes by location of function (Tables 1.11–1 and 1.11–2). In addition to classical action on a target tissue, hormones may also act as *neuromodulators,* regulating the effects of neurotransmitters and, in rare cases, meeting criteria for neurotransmitter function independently.

HORMONE SECRETION

Hormone secretion is stimulated by the action of a neuronal secretory product of neuroendocrine transducer cells of the hypothalamus. Examples of hormone regulators (Table 1.11–3) include corticotropin-releasing hormone (CRH), which stimulates adrenocorticotropin (adrenocorticotropic hormone [ACTH]); thyrotropin-releasing hormone (TRH), which stimulates release of thyroid-stimulating hormone (TSH); gonadotropin-releasing hormone (GnRH), which stimulates release of leuteinizing hormone (LH) and follicle-stimulating hormone (FSH); and somatostatin (somatotropin release-inhibiting factor [SRIF]) and growth hormone-releasing hormone (GHRH), which influence growth hormone (GH) release. Chemical signals cause the release of these neurohormones from the median eminence of the hypothalamus into the portal hypophyseal bloodstream and subsequent transport to the pituitary to regulate the release of target hormones. Pituitary hormones in turn act directly on target cells (e.g., ACTH on the adrenal gland) or stimulate release of other hormones from peripheral endocrine organs. In addition, these hormones have feedback actions that regulate secretion and exert neuromodulatory effects in the CNS.

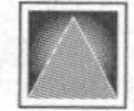

Table 1.11–1
Classification of Hormones by Structure

Structure	Examples	Storage	Lipid Soluble
Proteins, polypeptides, and glycoproteins	Adrenocorticotropic hormone, beta-endorphin, thyrotropin-releasing hormone, leuteinizing hormone, follicle-stimulating hormone	Vesicles	No
Steroids and steroid-like compounds	Cortisol, estrogens, testosterone, progesterone, dehydroepiandrosterone	Diffusion after synthesis	Yes

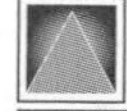

Table 1.11–3
Examples of Regulating Hormones

Regulating Hormone	Hormone Stimulated (or Inhibited)
Corticotropin-releasing hormone	Adrenocorticotropic hormone
Thyrotropin-releasing hormone	Thyroid-stimulated hormone
Luteinizing hormone-releasing hormone	Luteinizing hormone
Gonadotropin-releasing hormone	Follicle-stimulating hormone
Somatostatin	Growth hormone (inhibited)
Growth hormone-releasing hormone	Growth hormone
Progesterone, oxytocin	Prolactin
Arginine vasopressin	Adrenocorticotropic hormone

HORMONE SYNTHESIS AND STRUCTURE

Peptide hormones represent subsections of larger amino acid chains or polypeptides called *prohormones*. Production of a peptide hormone occurs by the cleavage of its prohormone chain at a given site on the chain by the appropriate enzyme. Proopiomelanocortin (POMC) is an example of a prohormone that contains the sequences for ACTH, beta-endorphin, β-lipotropin, and melanocyte-stimulating hormone (MSH). Some hormones, called *dimers*, contain two or more peptide chains (e.g., FSH, LH, TSH). Further cleavage of these hormone peptide chains in the course of metabolism may create additional biologically active peptides that have different effects from those of the parent peptide, and even minor modifications of structure can drastically change binding properties and metabolic processing.

Tropic hormones, such as ACTH and gonadotropins, in turn, induce steroidogenesis in two distinct ways. Acute regulation occurs through activation and rapid synthesis (over minutes) of steroidogenic acute regulatory (StAR) protein, which regulates the rate-limiting step of steroid hormone synthesis, the transport of cholesterol from the outer to the inner mitochondrial membrane. In contrast, chronic stimulation induces transcription, increased P450scc protein, and steroidogenesis over hours to days.

CELLULAR MODE OF ACTION

Genomic The first known mode of action of steroid hormones (glucocorticoids, estrogen, testosterone) and thyroid hormones (triiodothyronine [T_3] and thyroxine [T_4]) is by binding to intracellular receptors in the cytoplasm. The hormone-receptor complex in turn binds to common response elements on chromosomal deoxyribonucleic acid (DNA) and alters transcription through a conformational change that unmasks the binding site. The hormone complex can also interact with transcription factors such as those produced by c-*fos*, c-*jun*, or activator protein-1 (AP-1) to amplify or to inhibit gene expression and, by these mechanisms, to regulate the induction of such gene products as enzymes and other cell proteins that effect metabolic change.

Nongenomic Alternatively, as in the case of estrogen-stimulated prolactin release, certain hormones may exert a physiological effect within seconds to minutes, a time course precluding a genomic mechanism. Nongenomic action is hypothesized to involve membrane hormone receptors, but none as yet has been cloned. Some nongenomic effects appear to be mediated through distinct, nonclassical membrane receptors in that they are not blocked by classical receptor inhibitors and do not require gene transcription, protein synthesis, or a coagonist. Hormones may also act through ion-gated neurotransmitter receptors as coagonists or antagonists, as in the modulation of γ-aminobutyric acid (GABA) type A ($GABA_A$) receptors by neurosteroids, or by altering the fluidity and microenvironment of membrane receptors through intercalation of the steroid in the phospholipid bilayers. Genomic and nongenomic mechanisms may be active simultaneously, with cross-talk a likely occurrence.

CHARACTERISTICS OF ENDOCRINE ACTIVITY

In general, most hormonal compounds exert their effect in a tonic, rather than phasic, fashion, being diffused in a less precise manner than a neurotransmitter and over a longer time period. Theoretically, such a characterization would allow hormones to be more closely linked to integrated behavioral responses. Release of many hormones is pulsatile, and the pattern of these pulses (i.e., duration, interpulse interval, slope of increase or decrease in rate, and amplitude) is crucial to their effects. Other factors that can influence the regulation and effect of a hormone in a given individual include a history of exposure to the hormone during critical developmental encoding periods, the frequency and chronicity of past exposure, the time since last exposure, and the status of other influences on the target system. A decrease in the amplitude of response after repeated exposure is referred to as *habituation*, and an enhancement is termed *sensitization*. Facilitation of a habituated response after exposure to a novel stimulus or more severe stressor is called *dishabituation*. In the case of the hypothalamic-pituitary-adrenal (HPA) system, the release of cortisol by the adrenal gland is dependent on an integration of three separate control systems. These include an underlying circadian rhythm regulated by the suprachiasmatic nucleus; a stress-responsive circuit involving inputs to the hypothalamus from the brainstem, limbic system, and cerebral cortex; and a feedback control system exerted through two classes of corticosteroid receptor.

DEVELOPMENTAL PSYCHONEUROENDOCRINOLOGY

Although a review of the effect of hormones on brain development is beyond the scope of this chapter, it is important to note that hormones can have organizational as well as activation effects. Exposure to gonadal hormones during critical stages of neural development directs changes in brain morphology and function (e.g., sex-specific behavior in adulthood) and differentiation of dopaminergic neurons. Similarly, thyroid hormones are essential for the normal development of the CNS, and thyroid deficiency during critical stages of postnatal life severely impairs growth and development of the brain, resulting in behavioral disturbances that may be permanent if replacement therapy is not instituted. Prenatal exposure in animals to endogenous or exogenous glucocorticoids or to stressful circumstances reduces offspring birth weight and may result in long-lasting changes in immune response, hypertension, hyperglycemia, hyperinsulinemia, cardiovascular function, and altered neuroendocrine responses and behavior, including attentional deficits, increased anxiety, and disturbed social behavior. Maternal deprivation in strains of rats with increased glucocorticoid response to stress has similarly been shown to lead to increased startle responses, anxiety-like behavior, increased alcohol preference, and difficulties with spatial learning in adulthood.

PSYCHONEUROENDOCRINOLOGY METHODOLOGY

Human studies are often limited to examining the relationship between hormone concentrations or changes in concentration and psychiatric disease states, symptoms, neurotransmitter function, or response to treatment. Concentrations may be measured in plasma, urine, saliva, cerebrospinal fluid (CSF), or postmortem tissue and are sometimes used as indicators of regulatory neurotransmitter function in response to a given stimulus. For example, cortisol response to d-fenfluramine has been used to assess serotonin activity and GH response to clonidine (Catapres) to assess dopaminergic function.

One example of a provocative psychoendocrine test used to assess the HPA system is the combined dexamethasone–corticotropin-releasing hormone (CRH) test, which assesses response to two hormonal stimuli, one inhibiting (dexamethasone [Decadron]) and the other stimulating (CRH), for cortisol secretion. Typically, 1.5 mg of dexamethasone is given in the evening, and plasma cortisol concentration is measured 16 hours later on the following day. An infusion of 100 μg of CRH is then given, and cortisol level and ACTH are measured again. Abnormalities in this test are found in a variety of psychiatric illnesses, including bipolar disorder, major depression, schizophrenia, and posttraumatic stress disorder (PTSD). Sustained alteration in inhibitory response is predictive of poor prognostic outcome.

HYPOTHALAMIC-PITUITARY-ADRENAL AXIS

Since the earliest conceptions of the stress response by Hans Selye and others, investigation of HPA function has occupied a central position in psychoendocrine research. CRH, ACTH, and cortisol are all elevated in response to a variety of physical and psychological stresses and serve as prime factors in the maintenance of homeostasis and the development of adaptive responses to novel or challenging stimuli. The hormonal response is dependent not only on the characteristics of the stressor itself, but also on how the individual assesses and is able to cope with it. Aside from generalized effects on arousal, distinct effects on sensory processing, stimulus habituation and sensitization, pain, sleep, and memory storage and retrieval have been documented. In primates, social status can influence adrenocortical profiles and, in turn, can be affected by exogenously induced changes in hormone concentration.

Exposure to chronic stress produces increased concentrations of CRH and arginine vasopressin (AVP) in the paraventricular nucleus of the hypothalamus and, over time, leads to a reduction in CRH receptor number in the anterior pituitary. Release of CRH results in a simultaneous activation of the locus ceruleus noradrenergic circuit, which functionally increases arousal and selective attention and decreases vegetative functions, such as appetite and sex drive. In contrast, ACTH concentrations are increased in acute stress but diminish over time in chronic stress.

Glucocorticoid receptors (GRs) are ubiquitously distributed throughout the body. At least two intracellular receptor subtypes bind corticosteroids: the mineralocorticoid receptor (MR) (or type I receptor) and the GR (or type II receptor). The human GR has an α and a β form, the α form showing high affinity for dexamethasone, modest affinity for cortisol, and low affinity for aldosterone, deoxycortisol, and the sex steroids, and the β form acting as a negative regulator. Owing to the difference in affinity, low corticosteroid levels generally result in a predominant MR occupation, with higher steroid levels shifting the balance in favor of the GR. "Permissive actions" of MR activation before the onset of stress are tonically involved in the mediation of the initial stress response. When more GRs become occupied, local excitability may decrease or, in some cases, may increase on a short-term basis to inhibit or to enhance the initial effects of stress responsive hormones. Over time, continued stress produces increasing "allostatic load," the sustained effects of hypercortisolemia giving rise to hyperglycemia, increased visceral fat, elevated blood pressure, decreased bone density, hyperlipidemia, and changes in electrolytes and immune response. Interactions between MR and GR in the hippocampus may be relevant to understanding the regulation of stress response in depression and the efficacy of antidepressants.

Glucocorticoid release is amplified by serotonergic and cholinergic input and is inhibited by GABA and opioids. Three types of inhibitory feedback of glucocorticoids on CRH and ACTH have been characterized. Fast, rate-sensitive feedback occurs while plasma concentrations of the glucocorticoid are rising and regulates release, rather than synthesis, of CRH and ACTH. Intermediate, delayed feedback occurs from 1 to 2 hours after steroid administration, is dose sensitive and duration sensitive rather than rate sensitive, and inhibits release of CRH and ACTH, as well as synthesis of CRH. Slow feedback is similar to intermediate feedback but occurs over a longer period of time (hours) and is distinguished by decreased synthesis of CRH and ACTH (and other POMC derivatives).

Similarities in the changes in neuroendocrine systems after chronic stress and in depressive disorders suggest that some psychiatric syndromes may not be distinct disease states per se but rather exist on a continuum with normal functioning. In support of such a conception are a variety of studies showing that, although immediate release of glucocorticoids serves homeostatic needs, more prolonged activation can result in structural neuropathology, glutamate toxicity, damage to CA1 and CA4 hippocampal neurons, and, speculatively, lasting behavioral change. Some of the neuropathological sequelae of normal human aging parallel such stress-induced adaptations in the HPA system and may produce or may be secondary to changes in neuroendocrine function and stress responsivity.

Pathological alterations in HPA function have been associated primarily with mood disorders, PTSD, and dementia of the Alzheimer's type, although recent animal evidence also points toward a role of this system in substance use disorders as well. Disturbances of mood are found in more than 50 percent of patients with Cushing's syndrome (characterized by elevated cortisol concentrations), with psychosis or suicidal thought apparent in more than 10 percent of cases studied. Cognitive impairments similar to those seen in major depressive disorder are common and relate to the degree of hypercortisolemia present and the possible reduction in hippocampal size. In general, reductions in cortisol level result in a normalization of mood and mental status. Conversely, in Addison's disease (characterized by adrenal insufficiency and diminished glucocorticoid output), apathy, social withdrawal, impaired sleep, and decreased concentration frequently accompany prominent fatigue. Replacement of glucocorticoid results in resolution of behavioral symptomatology, although correction of the associated electrolyte disturbances by itself does not. Exogenous administration of synthetic corticosteroids is commonly associated with mild activation, but a higher dose and more sustained treatment may produce depression, mood lability, memory and attentional impairment, and, rarely, psychosis. Alterations in HPA function associated with depression include elevated cortisol concentrations, failure to suppress cortisol in response to dexamethasone, increased adrenal size and sensitivity to ACTH, a blunted ACTH response to CRH, and elevated CRH concentrations in brain. In addition to altered slow feedback, several groups have demonstrated decreased sensitivity to glucocorticoid fast feedback as well. The pattern of these abnormalities has not, thus far, led to a definitive theory of mechanism, and other elements, such as AVP, may be important to understanding the change in homeostasis. For instance, it has recently been noted that individuals with depression have impaired secretion of pro–γ-MSH and beta-endorphin, but not ACTH, after metyrapone inhibition of cortisol synthesis. The finding that corticosteroids have multiple regulatory effects on serotonergic function, particularly on the serotonin (5-hydroxytryptamine type 1A [5-HT_{1A}]) receptor, may also be relevant, as may be the state-dependent stimulant-like effects that glucocorticoids can exert on mesencephalic dopamine transmission.

Studies of GR function have pointed to a relevant decrement in response to agonist in depressed patients, but MR function is generally preserved. The change in MR to GR ratio may be relevant to understanding the potential antidepressant benefit of GR antagonists, such as mifepristone (RU-486). Patients with PTSD may exhibit low cortisol levels despite high CRH activity.

Alcohol usage and withdrawal produce profound changes in HPA regulation; pseudocushingoid features are a phenotypic feature of chronic alcohol intake, and HPA adaptation to alcohol withdrawal varies by family history of alcoholism. There is also suggestive evidence that alteration in HPA response to acute alcohol challenge may represent an endophenotype of genetic risk of dependence.

ENDOGENOUS OPIOIDS

Since the discovery of endogenous opioid receptors and their endogenous ligands in the early 1970s, research into the possible behavioral roles of such compounds has grown at a rapid pace. Beta-endorphin is the principal opioid peptide prototype and, like ACTH, MSH, and β-lipotropin, is derived from POMC. Methionine enkephalin (met-enkephalin) and leucine enkephalin (leu-enkephalin) are two small pentapeptides that also possess direct opioid activity, met-enkephalin being contained in POMC and another precursor, proenkephalin, and leu-enkephalin being contained in the prohormones proenkephalin and prodynorphin. At least three different receptor systems for these ligands have been identified (μ, δ, and κ), and it is likely that each of these has subtypes. The best-documented function of the endogenous opiates is analgesia and alteration of pain perception, but effects on stress, appetite regulation, learning and memory, motor activity, and immune function also appear to be of physiological importance.

In animal models, a number of stressors, including those that are purely psychological, induce opiate-mediated effects such as analgesia and hypomotility that are reversed by the opiate antagonist naloxone (Narcan). Several studies have found that concentrations of plasma beta-endorphin in humans are correlated with measures of stress elicited by surgery, exercise, parachuting, or pain. Short-term administration of opioid agonists also increases eating, whereas antagonists reduce food intake by as much as 30 percent, diminish intake of fats and highly palatable foods, and increase caloric expenditure. Thus far, however, their long-term use in obesity and eating disorders has not proven clinically useful. Some studies of opioid antagonist treatment have found certain binge parameters (e.g., duration) to be reduced in bulimia, but no studies have demonstrated weight loss in obese subjects. Naltrexone (ReVia) has recently been demonstrated in double-blind trials to be an effective adjunct in the treatment of alcohol dependence, reducing drinking, craving, the high derived from drinking alcohol, and the likelihood that sampling alcohol would precipitate a relapse.

It is well known that exogenous opioids (e.g., heroin and morphine) can induce a euphoric mood state and that exercise increases release of endogenous opioids and is associated with mood enhancement; these observations, together with findings that exercise-induced mood enhancement is blocked by naloxone, suggest that endogenous opioids are also involved in the mediation of mood. Such conclusions must be moderated, however, by the recognition that additional specific and nonspecific effects on other neurochemical systems are possible contributors to exercise-related mood effects.

Early enthusiasm for the idea that a dysfunctional opiate system was etiologically related to mental illness, particularly schizophrenia, has waned in the face of contradictory findings. Increases in various endorphin compounds have been reported in plasma, as well as in postmortem brain tissue of patients with schizophrenia, but studies of short-term and long-term treatment with opioid antagonists show no consistent or reproducible effects on psychopathology. In rhesus monkeys, however, naloxone has been shown to reduce maternal affect and social grooming.

NEUROPEPTIDE Y, GALANIN, AND INSULIN

Neuropeptide Y is widely distributed throughout the CNS and is one of the most conserved peptides in evolution, suggesting an important role in the regulation of basic physiological function, including learning and memory. Neuropeptide Y and neuropeptide Y–related peptide bind at three receptors, neuropeptide Y type 1 (Y_1) (postsynaptic), type 2 (Y_2) (presynaptic and postsynaptic), and type 3 (Y_3), which are widely distributed but relatively concentrated in the hippocampus. Neuropeptide Y is synthesized in the arcuate nucleus of the hypothalamus, has a mutually inhibitory relation with insulin, and is stimulated by stress and corticosteroids. It has been studied for its potential anxiolytic, antinociceptive, antihypertensive, and memory-enhancing effects and for a possible role in seizure disorder, schizophrenia, and depression. Immunoreactive neuropeptide Y is found in the serotonin-containing raphe nucleus, and treatments for depression (antidepressants, lithium [Eskalith], and electroconvulsive therapy [ECT]) increase neuropeptide Y concentrations in many brain areas in rats. Reduced concentrations of neuropeptide Y have been found in the brains of suicide victims and of depressed individuals who died of other causes, and significantly low levels have been found in the temporal cortex of patients with schizophrenia. Neuropeptide Y has been found to increase feeding, particularly carbohydrate ingestion, and to counteract leptin effects in a variety of animal models. Neuropeptide Y also suppresses the thermogenic activity of brown fat and increases the storage of white fat.

Galanin is an inhibitory peptide that is stimulated in a coordinated fashion with gonadal steroid release. Its documented actions include increased release of GH and inhibition of insulin release, locus ceruleus noradrenergic firing, and acetylcholine release, as well as impairment of memory. Galanin can dramatically increase food consumption, partly because of an increased preference for fats over carbohydrates. Work on identifying receptor subtypes and developing specific antagonist ligands for them is in the early phase but holds promise for the treatment of obesity and eating disorders.

Insulin is a protein hormone secreted by the beta cells of the pancreas in response to elevations of glucose and amino acids; insulin receptors occur in high density in the hippocampus and are believed to help neurons metabolize glucose by controlling the transport across cell membranes. Increasing evidence indicates that insulin may be integrally involved in learning and memory. Depression is frequent in patients with diabetes, as are indices of impaired hormonal response to stress, but it is not known whether these findings represent direct effects of the disease or are secondary, nonspecific effects. Some atypical antipsychotics impair response to insulin and raise blood glucose, increasing the risk of developing type II diabetes. Antidepressants, which predominantly increase catecholamine activity, such as many of the tricyclics, also reduce sensitivity to insulin. Those that increase serotonergic function, such as the serotonin reuptake inhibitors, increase sensitivity to insulin and are preferred in the treatment of depression comorbid with diabetes.

LEPTIN

Leptin is a protein hormone synthesized and secreted in a pulsatile fashion by adipose tissue and involved in the regulation of food intake. Obesity is associated with leptin resistance, principally its metabolic actions, because sympathetic effects are preserved. Leptin also affects the hypothalamic-pituitary-gonadal (HPG) axis, inhibits insulin-induced steroidogenesis and human chorionic gonadotropin–induced testosterone secretion, and may play a role in menstruation, pregnancy, lactation, puberty, and amenorrhea due to weight loss in anorexia nervosa. Leptin stimulates hematopoiesis, T-cell activation, phagocytosis, and cytokine production and decreases susceptibility to infection. Mediators of leptin action include orexigenic neuropeptides, such as neuropeptide Y, galanin and galanin-like peptide, and melanin-concentrating hormone, and anorexigenic neuropeptides, such as CRH and alpha-MSH hormone. A melanin-concentrating hormone-1 receptor antagonist has been shown not only to inhibit food intake and to reduce body weight in rats, but also to produce effects similar to antidepressants in animal models of depression. Weight gain produced by some atypical antipsychotics may be mediated, at least in part, through increases in leptin.

HYPOTHALAMIC-PITUITARY-GONADAL AXIS

GnRH is a decapeptide that was sequenced and synthesized by Schally et al. in 1971. GnRH administration results in the rapid release of LH and FSH from the pituitary in healthy subjects and, in some pathological states, such as acromegaly, an abnormal release of GH or prolactin. The cell bodies of GnRH are located principally over the optic chiasm in the arcuate area, with projections to the median eminence, and in the lamina terminalis. GnRH release is stimulated by norepinephrine and is inhibited through negative feedback of gonadal steroids. Administration of GnRH can result in a depressive-like state, characterized by hot flashes, anxiety, insomnia, decreased libido, and fatigue in euthymic subjects, but it is not known whether this is a direct effect of the agent or is caused by the hypoestrogenic state that is produced when GnRH is given continuously. By decreasing testosterone, a GnRH analog has been found to have some efficacy in the treatment of paraphilia. In contrast to other neuroendocrine systems, there is relatively little evidence for a disturbance in the HPG axis in depression, with normal LH and FSH responses being observed after administration of even supramaximal doses of GnRH.

The gonadal hormones (progesterone, androstenedione, testosterone, E_2, and others) are steroids that are secreted principally by the ovary and testis, but significant amounts of androgens arise from the adrenal cortex as well. The prostate gland and adipose tissue are also involved in the synthesis and storage of dihydrotestosterone and contribute to individual variance in sexual function and behavior.

The timing and presence of gonadal hormones play a critical role in the development of sexual dimorphisms in the brain. Developmentally, these hormones direct the organization of many sexually dimorphic CNS structures and functions, such as the size of hypothalamic nuclei (INAH3) and corpus callosum, the neuronal density in the temporal cortex, the organization of language ability, and the responsiveness in Broca's area. Women with congenital adrenal hyperplasia, a deficiency of the enzyme 21-hydroxylase leading to high exposure to adrenal androgens in prenatal and postnatal life, have been found to be more aggressive and less interested in traditional female roles than control female subjects. Sexual dimorphisms may also reflect acute and reversible actions of relative steroid concentrations (e.g., higher estrogen levels transiently increase CNS sensitivity to serotonin).

Testosterone

Testosterone is the primary androgenic steroid, having androgenic (i.e., facilitating male gonadal development) and anabolic (i.e., facilitating linear body growth and somatic growth) functions. It also has modulating effects on AVP synthesis and ACTH release. Testosterone administration has been shown to result in increased violence and aggression in animals, and testosterone level tends to be correlated with aggression in humans, but anecdotal reports of increased aggression with testosterone treatment have not been uniformly substantiated in human scientific investigations. Reports may be confounded by factors such as past history and social factors, which are particularly important determinants of the effects of hormones in primates and in humans. For instance, in the cynomolgus monkey, administration of testosterone increases dominant behavior in dominant monkeys and submissive behavior in submissive monkeys; in hypogonadal men, it improves mood and decreases irritability. Varying effects of anabolic-androgenic steroids on mood have been noted anecdotally. In one prospective placebo-controlled study of anabolic-androgenic steroid administration in normal subjects, positive mood symptoms, including euphoria, increased energy, and sexual arousal, were reported, in addition to increases in negative mood symptoms of irritability, mood swings, violent feelings, anger, and hostility. Studies of testosterone treatment in depression have generally been inconclusive, although two randomized, placebo-controlled trials found intramuscular (IM) therapy effective in eugonadal men with late-life depression and testosterone gel supplementation efficacious in refractory depression.

Testosterone is important for sexual desire in men and women. In males, muscle mass and strength, sexual activity, desire, thoughts, and intensity of sexual feelings are dependent on normal testosterone levels, but these functions are not clearly augmented by supplementing testosterone in those with normal androgen levels. The addition of small amounts of testosterone to normal hormonal replacement in postmenopausal women has, however, proven to be as beneficial as its use in hypogonadal men.

Anabolic steroids are synthetic derivatives of testosterone modified to enhance their anabolic actions, such as muscle growth, rather than their androgenic actions. In addition to a variety of physical adverse effects, anabolic steroids can cause a variety of psychiatric effects, including aggressive behavior, mood and psychotic disturbances, and psychological dependence, particularly when taken in high doses.

Dehydroepiandrosterone (DHEA)

DHEA and DHEA sulphate (DHEA-S) are adrenal androgens secreted in response to ACTH and represent the most abundant circulating steroids. DHEA is also a neurosteroid that is synthesized in situ in the brain. DHEA has many physiological effects, but behavioral interest has centered on its steady decrement over the life span in humans and its possible involvement in memory and mood. It has been shown to act as an excitatory neurosteroid and to enhance memory retention in mice, but studies of DHEA administration to humans have not consistently shown any improvement in cognition. Several controlled trials of DHEA administration point to an improvement in well-being, mood, and functional status, however, in depressed as well as healthy individuals. Administration of DHEA to women with adrenal insufficiency (e.g., Addison's disease) has repeatedly been demonstrated to enhance mood, energy, and sexual function; effects in men remain to be assessed. Mood, fatigue, and libido improved in human immunovirus–positive patients treated with DHEA in one study, and DHEA and DHEA-S have been found to be inversely correlated with severity in attention-deficit/hyperactivity disorder (ADHD). Several cases of possible DHEA-induced mania have been reported.

Double-blind treatment studies have shown antidepressant effects of DHEA in patients with major depression, midlife-onset dysthymia, and schizophrenia, although beneficial effects on memory have not been reliably demonstrated. A small double-blind trial of DHEA treatment of Alzheimer's disease failed to reveal significant benefit, although a near-significant improvement in cognitive function was seen after 3 months of treatment. Beneficial effects on mood, energy, libido, and well-being in healthy controls, even in elderly ones with low serum DHEA levels, are occasionally but not uniformly reported.

Animal studies suggest that DHEA may be involved in eating behavior, aggressiveness, and anxiety as well, with its effects resulting from its transformation into estrogen or testosterone, from its antiglucocorticoid activity, or from direct effects on $GABA_A$, *N*-methyl-D-aspartate (NMDA), and sigma receptors. Because of the antiglucocorticoid effects, the ratio of cortisol to DHEA levels may be particularly important in understanding adaptive responses to stress.

Estrogen and Progesterone The primary estrogens are estradiol (E_2), estrone (E_1), and estriol (E_3), with E_2 being the major secretory product of the ovaries. Two different estrogen receptors have been identified (α and β), each with different anatomical distribution and physiological effects. Estrogens can influence neural activity in the hypothalamus and limbic system directly through modulation of neuronal excitability and have complex multiphasic effects on nigrostriatal dopamine receptor sensitivity. Estrogens also enhance dopamine synthesis and release, modify basal firing rates, and can lead to stereotypic behavior in rodents. Accordingly, there is evidence that the antipsychotic effect of psychiatric drugs may change over the menstrual cycle and that the risk of tardive dyskinesia is partly dependent on estrogen concentrations. However, studies of symptom changes in schizophrenic women show significant differences for anxiety-depression and withdrawal-retardation subscales but not for psychotic subscales across the menstrual cycle. Several studies have suggested that gonadal steroids modulate spatial cognition and verbal memory and are involved in impeding age-related neuronal degeneration. There is also increasing evidence that estrogen administration may decrease the risk and delay onset of dementia of the Alzheimer's type in postmenopausal women, but acute treatment in dementia has been ineffective in reducing symptoms. Estrogen has mood-enhancing properties and can also increase sensitivity to serotonin, possibly by inhibiting monoamine oxidase; in animal studies, long-term estrogen treatment results in a decrease in $5\text{-}HT_1$ and an increase in $5\text{-}HT_2$ receptors. In oophorectomized women, significant reductions in tritiated imipramine binding sites (which modulate presynaptic serotonin uptake) were restored with estrogen treatment. Estrogen deficiency in severe postpartum depression has been successfully treated with sublingual 17-β-estradiol, as have depressive disorders in perimenopausal women in a large, randomized, double-blind trial.

Progesterone, the primary progestin, is produced by the corpus luteum of the ovary. Although progesterone itself may be anxiogenic, metabolites of progesterone (allopregnanolone and pregnenolone) appear to have anxiolytic and hypnotic properties via $GABA_A$ agonistic activity. Progesterone is colocalized with serotonin in cells of the median raphe and causes increased serotonin uptake and turnover in the brain in several species. The ratio of estrogen to progestin in oral contraceptives may be associated with negative mood change, although this effect varies with depression history.

The association of these hormones with serotonin is hypothetically relevant to mood change in premenstrual and postpartum mood disturbances. Women with a history of depression have higher FSH and LH and lower E_2 levels and are at risk to begin perimenopause at a younger age. Similarly, the 2:1 female to male ratio in depression prevalence may speculatively be related to the rapid changes in hormone levels in menarche. Premenstrual dysphoric disorder is a disorder in which a constellation of symptoms resembling major depressive disorder occurs in most menstrual cycles, appearing in the luteal phase and disappearing within a few days of the onset of menses. No definitive abnormalities in estrogen or progesterone levels have been demonstrated in women with premenstrual dysphoric disorder, but decreased serotonin uptake with premenstrual decreases in steroid levels have been correlated with severity of symptoms in some studies. Progesterone downregulates the estrogen receptor, and it has been suggested that, despite high circulating concentrations of estrogen, the luteal phase is a period of functional estrogen withdrawal, with concomitant effects on the serotonergic system. Recent evidence indicates that the abrupt decline of progesterone and allopregnanolone in the luteal phase results in increased production of the $\alpha 4$ subunit of the $GABA_A$ and changes in receptor sensitivity that could account for the typical behavioral symptoms noted. This effect is correlated with insensitivity of the GABA receptor to modulation by the benzodiazepine class of tranquilizers (and hence is anxiogenic). Selective serotonin reuptake inhibitors (SSRIs), particularly fluoxetine (Prozac), have demonstrated efficacy, and as many as 50 percent of women may respond to fluoxetine administered only in the second half of each cycle. Alprazolam (Xanax), a $GABA_A$ agonist, has been found to be more effective than placebo in several studies for the treatment of premenstrual dysphoric disorder and may be an alternative for women who do not respond to treatment with SSRIs. In women with severe symptoms that are not responsive to these treatments, the long-term use of a GnRH agonist to abolish menstrual cycling, with added estrogen-progestin, may be therapeutic.

Menstrual phase has been associated with aspects of substance abuse. Although reports vary, craving for cigarettes and tobacco withdrawal appear to vary with menstrual phase (worse in luteal). Women show greater heart rate and pleasurable drug effects after cocaine administration during the follicular phase but report that cocaine improves dysphoric mood during the luteal phase.

The bulk of psychological symptoms associated with the menopause are actually reported during perimenopause rather than after complete cessation of menses. Although studies suggest no increased incidence of major depressive disorder, reported symptoms include worry, fatigue, crying spells, mood swings, diminished ability to cope, and diminished libido or intensity of orgasm. Estrogen replacement alone maybe beneficial, but combination androgen-estrogen replacement may be superior for reinstating energy, a sense of well-being, and libido. In women with an intact uterus, the addition of progestin is necessary to protect against endometrial hyperplasia but can attenuate the beneficial effects of estrogen on mood.

Women with bipolar disorder appear to be particularly sensitive to alterations in gonadal steroid level. A high risk for relapse during the postpartum period has been observed and appears to be maintained over subsequent pregnancies; evidence for familial preponderance of the puerperal trigger also exists, suggesting a genetic contribution.

PREGNENOLONE AND ALLOPREGNANOLONE

Neuroactive steroids, such as pregnenolone and allopregnanolone, modulate activity at $GABA_A$, NMDA, sigma-1, $5\text{-}HT_3$, nicotinic, kainate, oxytocin, and glycine receptors, among others. Pregnenolone is a neurosteroid synthesized from cholesterol in the brain and is partially metabolized to all subsequent steroids. It appears to have memory-enhancing properties in animal studies and increases the rate and extent of formation of microtubules, important in neuronal plasticity and function. Progesterone counteracts this effect. Pregnenolone-sulphate is an excitatory neurosteroid and has GABA inhibitory effects.

Allopregnanolone is a neurosteroid derived from progesterone with high concentrations in the CNS. It acts as a $GABA_A$ agonist, decreases CRH concentrations in the hypothalamus, and reduces the anxiety evoked by CRH in rats. Fluoxetine and paroxetine (Paxil) increase brain allopregnanolone levels in rats, and CSF levels of allopregnanolone in humans have been correlated with clinical improvement over the first 8 to 10 weeks of SSRI treatment, an effect that appears to be independent of the serotonin reuptake inhibition. Allopregnanolone increases in response to ethanol administration and may play a role in ethanol withdrawal through modulation of $GABA_A$. Administration of allopregnanolone has also been shown to reduce anxiety and hyperlocomotion associated with benzodiazepine withdrawal in animals.

PROLACTIN

Since its identification in 1970, the anterior pituitary hormone prolactin has been examined as a potential index of dopamine activity, dopamine receptor sensitivity, and antipsychotic drug concentration in studies of CNS function in psychiatric patients and as a correlate of stress responsivity. The secretion of prolactin is under direct inhibitory regulation by dopamine neurons located in the tuberoinfundibular section of the hypothalamus. Prolactin also inhibits its own secretion by means of a short-loop feedback circuit to the hypothalamus. In addition, a great number of prolactin-releasing or -modifying factors have been identified, including estrogen, serotonin (particularly through the 5-HT_2 and 5-HT_3 receptors), norepinephrine, opioids, TRH, T_4, histamine, glutamate, cortisol, CRH, and oxytocin, with interaction effects possible. For example, estrogen may promote the serotonin-stimulated release of prolactin.

Prolactin is primarily involved in reproductive functions. During maturation, prolactin secretion participates in gonadal development, whereas, in adults, prolactin contributes to the regulation of the behavioral aspects of reproduction and infant care, including estrogen-dependent sexual receptivity and breast-feeding. In female rats, prolactin secretion is strongly stimulated with exposure to pups. In women, basal prolactin levels are elevated in the postpartum period before weaning, and prolactin release is stimulated by suckling. Hyperprolactinemia is associated with low testosterone in men and reduced libido in men and women. In rodents, prolactin is increased along with corticosterone in response to such stressful stimuli as immobilization, hypoglycemia, surgery, and cold exposure and may be specifically associated with the use of passive coping in the face of a stressor. Prolactin promotes various stress-related behaviors in rats, depending on the condition, such as increasing object-directed exploration while decreasing other exploration. Although prolactin has been described as being relatively less responsive to psychological stress, some human studies do show psychological stress–induced increases.

Prolactin metabolism is not clearly altered in psychiatric disorders, but hyperprolactinemic patients often complain of depression, decreased libido, stress intolerance, anxiety, and increased irritability. These behavioral symptoms usually resolve in parallel with decrements in serum prolactin when surgical or pharmacological treatments are used. Serum prolactin concentrations have also been positively correlated with severity of tardive dyskinesia, particularly in women who have been exposed to antipsychotic medication. Studies in psychiatric populations have attempted to use prolactin response to infusions of dopaminergic agonists as an index of central neurotransmitter activity. Thus far, the conclusions to be drawn from this strategy are not clear because widely discrepant and contradictory results have been reported.

HYPOTHALAMIC-PITUITARY-THYROID AXIS

Thyroid hormones are involved in the regulation of nearly every organ system, particularly those integral to the metabolism of food and the regulation of temperature, and are responsible for optimal development and function of all body tissues. Moreover, rates of secretion and metabolism of all other major hormones and catecholamines (cortisol, gonadal hormones, insulin) depend on thyroid status. The thyroid gland secretes two thyroid hormones: T_3 and T_4. T_3 is the more potent of the two, and most of the T_3 circulating in the blood is created by the peripheral metabolism of T_4. The brain relies on its own conversion of T_4 to T_3, rather than on circulating T_3. The hypothalamus secretes TRH into the capillaries of the pituitary portal venous system, and the pituitary responds with synthesis and secretion of TSH, which stimulates thyroid cells. Negative feedback regulation occurs when T_3 and T_4 act in the pituitary and hypothalamus to inhibit TSH and TRH, respectively. Finally, a corticotropin release-inhibiting factor (CRIF) has recently been identified in the rat that inhibits synthesis and secretion of ACTH. This peptide, prepro-TRH 178-199, is derived from the prohormone TRH and may play a role in integrating the regulation of the HPA and hypothalamic-pituitary-thyroid axes. Receptors for thyroid hormones are encoded by two genes, TR_α and TR_β, the expression of which plays a major role in the regulation of neuronal differentiation and the action of immediate early genes. As in the case of steroids, thyroid hormones regulate the transcription of a variety of genes through binding to thyroid response elements (TREs) in regulatory sequence elements.

There is general agreement that central noradrenergic systems are primarily stimulatory to TSH secretion and that central dopamine neurons inhibit TSH release. Thyroid hormones, in turn, are important regulators of central adrenoreceptor function, generally decreasing presynaptic noradrenaline release and increasing postsynaptic β-adrenergic receptor number. Hypothyroidism is conversely associated with decreased beta receptor number. Changes in serotonin function are also apparent, with T_3 increasing 5-HT in frontal cortex and inducing downregulation of 5-HT_{1A} autoreceptors. These changes in neurotransmitter release and receptors in response to thyroid hormones parallel the alteration in α- and β-receptor sensitivity associated with pharmacological and electroconvulsive antidepressant treatments and may explain the therapeutic efficacy of supplemental thyroid hormone in treatment-resistant depression. Alternatively, therapeutic benefit may be secondary to alteration of gene expression and a remodeling of synaptic connectivity. In addition to its prime endocrine function, TRH has direct effects on neuronal excitability, behavior, and neurotransmitter regulation, particularly on central cholinergic systems located in the septohippocampal band and on mesolimbic and nigrostriatal dopamine systems. In lower animals, TRH possesses mild stimulant properties. Initial reports of its mood-elevating effects in healthy human subjects led to a number of projects investigating its short-term and long-term antidepressant effects in clinical populations. Despite some initial enthusiasm, the degree of mood alteration does not seem to be great nor is its occurrence reliable.

Given these observations, it is not surprising that alterations in behavioral function have been observed in patients with primary thyroid gland dysfunction, beginning with the earliest reports in the medical literature. It has been noted that thyroid disorders may induce virtually any psychiatric symptom or syndrome, although regular associations of specific syndromes and thyroid conditions are not consistently found. Hyperthyroidism is commonly associated with fatigue, irritability, insomnia, anxiety, restlessness, weight loss, and emotional lability; marked impairment in concentration and memory may also be evident. Such states can progress into delirium or mania, or they can be episodic in nature. On occasion, a true psychosis develops, with paranoia being a particularly common presenting feature. In some cases, psychomotor retardation, apathy, and withdrawal, rather than agitation and anxiety, are the presenting features. Symptoms of mania have also been reported after rapid normalization of thyroid status in hypothyroid individuals and may covary with thyroid level in individuals with episodic endocrine dysfunction. In general, behavioral abnormalities resolve with a normalization of thyroid function and are responsive symptomatically to traditional psychopharmacological regimens. Long-term residual complaints of fatigue, cognitive impairment, and emotional distress have been reported in some individuals even after remission of the precipitating thyroid dysfunction. Caution should be exerted, however, regarding use of antidepressant medications in hyperthyroid states because of possible synergistic cardiotoxicity. In several case reports, haloperidol (Haldol) has been linked to increasing thyrotoxicity, and hyperthyroidism has been associated with an enhancement of the neurotoxic effects of antipsychotic medications.

The psychiatric symptoms of chronic hypothyroidism are generally well recognized. Most classically, fatigue, decreased libido, memory impairment, and irritability are noted, but a true secondary psychotic disorder or dementia-like state can also develop. In milder, subclinical states of hypothyroidism, the absence of gross signs accompanying endocrine dysfunction may result in its being overlooked as a possible cause of a mental disorder. Accordingly, the evaluation of basal TSH concentration or the TSH response to TRH infusion is necessary to arrive at the proper diagnosis. Figure 1.11–1 illustrates a characteristic physical sign of advanced hypothyroidism.

A blunted response of TSH to TRH infusion has been found in a significant percentage of patients with a variety of disorders, including eating disorders, panic disorder, alcoholism, schizophrenia, and, most commonly, major depressive disorder, and probably reflects a transient hyperthyroxinemia. No evidence of TRH hypersecretion has been shown. Large-scale studies suggest that such subjects are in fact euthyroid, and predictive sensitivity of the test is low. Antithyroid antibodies are found more frequently in women with depression than control subjects and may contribute to relative treatment resistance as well as to postpartum behavioral disturbance. Patients with major depression have also been found to have low levels of CSF transthyretin, a protein involved in thyroid transport. Basal T_3 level has been inversely related to time to episode recurrence, and basal TSH positively correlated with overall severity of depressed mood in an unselected inpatient population. Depressed patients who show an improvement in mood after one night of sleep deprivation also appear to have lower T_3 uptake at baseline and greater nocturnal TSH release. In recent years, several investigators have presented evidence that ADHD may be associated with a generalized resistance to thyroid hormone due to a genetic mutation of the β-thyroid receptor.

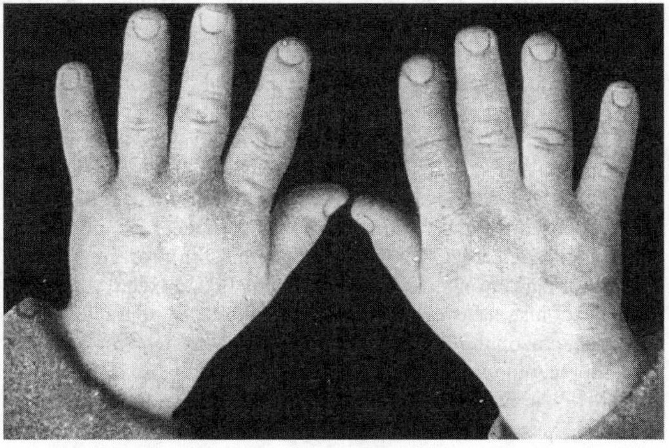

FIGURE 1.11–1 Hands of a patient who has hypothyroidism (myxedema), illustrating the swelling of the soft parts, the broadening of the fingers, and their consequent stumpy or pudgy appearance. (From Waterfield RL. Anæmia. In: Douthwaite AH, ed. *French's Index of Differential Diagnosis.* 7th ed. Baltimore: Williams & Wilkins; 1954, with permission.)

Most antidepressant therapies have some influence on thyroid concentrations at baseline; T_4 and T_3 concentrations have been correlated with antidepressant response, as have antidepressant-induced changes in thyroid hormones, as well as changes induced by ECT. Lithium increases antithyroid antibodies and inhibits iodine uptake into the thyroid, iodination of tyrosine, release of T_3 and T_4 from the thyroid, and peripheral breakdown of thyroid hormones. It also regulates *TR* gene expression, blocks the thyroid-stimulating effects of TSH through interference with adenylate cyclase, and may, in certain circumstances, precipitate a rebound thyrotoxicosis. Approximately 30 percent of patients receiving lithium have an elevated TSH level during treatment, and approximately one-sixth of these patients go on to develop frank hypothyroidism. Attention to subtle alteration in thyroid status induced by lithium treatment is important in the clinical evaluation of symptomatic complaints, such as fatigue, memory impairment, and anhedonia; a specific association between lower serum T_4 and mood instability during lithium maintenance suggests even subclinical changes may be clinically relevant. Carbamazepine (Tegretol), an anticonvulsant shown to have antimanic properties akin to lithium, also decreases peripheral thyroid hormone concentrations while increasing TSH. Administration of T_3 accelerates clinical response to tricyclic antidepressants and is sometimes helpful in patients with treatment-resistant depression, whereas adjunctive T_4 contributes to decreasing cycling in patients with rapid-cycling bipolar I disorder. Supraphysiologic dosing is sometimes required, with 200 to 500 μg per day being given as an adjunct in treatment-resistant depression and intractable bipolar disorder. One study has also documented a rapid improvement in mood and suicide tendency with intrathecal TRH.

PARATHYROID HORMONE

Parathyroid hormone (PTH) was originally isolated as an endocrine factor having effects on bone, gut, and kidney and contributing to calcium and phosphorus homeostasis. However, the frequent, and often profound, neuropsychiatric changes that can result from altered parathyroid gland function are consistent with other central actions of PTH that have been described in recent years. Hyperparathyroidism can cause lethargy, stupor, coma, depression, delirium, psychosis, or anxiety and hypoparathyroidism, cognitive impairment, psychosis, depression, or anxiety by alterations in calcium and magnesium levels. PTH administration can impair the active uptake and release of norepinephrine and dopamine and result in adrenergic-like effects (not blocked by β-adrenergic antagonist), learning and memory problems, and a state of hyperalgesia.

Lithium treatment can raise the concentrations of serum calcium and may increase PTH over a period of months to years by a direct stimulation of PTH secretion and through a shift in the set-point for inhibition of PTH secretion by calcium. When such effects are associated with somatic or behavioral change, discontinuation of lithium should result in rapid symptomatic improvement. When this does not happen, a parathyroid adenoma is sometimes discovered fortuitously. Primary hyperparathyroidism most commonly occurs secondary to a single parathyroid adenoma, the removal of which almost invariably results in a lysis of behavioral symptoms, regardless of severity or chronicity. Animal studies suggest that long-term lithium administration can stimulate the development of extant parathyroid tumors but does not induce tumors in normal parathyroid tissue. Thus, reinstitution of lithium treatment after surgical removal of the tumor should be possible.

GROWTH HORMONE

Somatotropin or GH, a hormone required for normal growth, is synthesized and released by the anterior pituitary gland. Dopamine, serotonin acting at the 5-HT_{1D} receptor, and norepinephrine, acting at the α_2-adrenergic receptor, appear to play a role in its release. GH acutely stimulates lipolysis and ketogenesis, important in the adaptation to stress, and prevents hypoglycemia. Most psychiatric studies of the regulation of GH have used strategies similar to those described for prolactin. Accordingly, studies of GH response to various provocative stimuli, such as to GHRH or psychotherapeutic drugs, have been seen as a means to evaluate central neurotransmitter function. Augmentation of GH secretion in response to GHRH, LH-releasing hormone (LHRH), or TRH in patients with schizophrenia or dementia of the Alzheimer's type has been interpreted as reflecting an alteration in catecholamine and, possibly, prostaglandin regulation, which facilitate the secretion of human GH. In general, however, there is a large variation in GH response to GHRH; a blunted response has been variably linked to length of illness, presence of negative symptoms, and platelet monoamine oxidase activity, but the validity of the conclusions drawn from this test is controversial.

The stress responsiveness of somatotrophs is well established but species dependent, with increases in circulating GH noted in humans and inhibition of secretion noted in rodents. In humans, the direction of the GH stress response may depend on the persistence of the stressor. GH appears to be relatively more responsive to exercise and hypoglycemic stress than to psychological stress. On the other hand, GH has been reported to increase in response to psychological stress in anxious subjects, perhaps due to hyperactivity of the noradrenergic system. Case reports have documented reversible GH deficiencies and marked growth retardation and delay of puberty secondary to stressful experience. Administration of GH to individuals with GH deficiency has a beneficial effect on cognitive function in addition to its more obvious somatic effects. Some prepubertal, as well as adult, patients with diagnoses of major depressive disorder show hyposecretion of GHRH during an insulin tolerance test, a deficit that has been interpreted as reflecting alterations in cholinergic and serotonergic mechanisms. Blunted response to 5-HT_{1D} agonists has also been found. Panic disorder patients may have a blunted GH response to clonidine, an α_2-adrenergic agonist, which does not normalize with antidepressant treatment. A number of GH abnormalities have also been noted in patients with anorexia nervosa, but secondary factors, such as weight loss, may be responsible for such alterations in endocrine release in depression and eating disorders. At least one study has reported that GHRH stimulates food consumption in patients with anorexia nervosa and attenuates elevated food consumption in patients with bulimia. Administration of GH to elderly men results in an increase in lean body mass, but controlled trials have been unable to replicate anecdotal reports of improved mental clarity, muscle strength, or vigor. Recent evidence indicates that a novel growth hormone secretagogue, ghrelin, may represent an important alternative regulatory influence over food intake and sleep pattern.

SOMATOSTATIN

Somatostatin (SRIF) is a hypothalamic tetradecapeptide that is located principally in the nerve endings of the median eminence and in neurosecretory neurons located in the paraventricular nucleus. SRIF inhibits anterior pituitary secretion of ACTH, thyrotropin, GH, and prolactin and alters release of catecholamine neurotransmitters. Five receptor subtypes have been cloned, and receptor-specific ligands have been developed. *SRIF* was so named because of its action in inhibiting the release of immunoreactive GH, a function that is subserved by SRIF-2 receptors.

In rats, SRIF delays the extinction of active avoidance behavior and antagonizes amnesia induced by electric shock. Alterations in the concentration of SRIF have been associated with an number of conditions in which cognitive dysfunction is present, including Huntington's disease, Parkinson's disease, multiple sclerosis, and Alzheimer's disease. Decreases in SRIF are highly correlated with decreases in acetylcholinesterase, suggesting a close relationship between the cholinergic and somatostatinergic systems. Decreased concentrations of SRIF in CSF are inconsistently found in patients with depression, and central injection of SRIF in rats causes decreased slow wave and rapid eye movement (REM) sleep, altered appetite and locomotor activity, impaired cognition, and decreased sensitivity to pain. Early stressful experiences have also been related to sustained elevations of CRH and somatostatin in the CSF of adult primates.

CHOLECYSTOKININ

Cholecystokinin (CCK) is a peptide neurotransmitter originally isolated from the gut but abundantly distributed in the CNS. In addition to its presence in pancreas and the gastrointestinal (GI) tract, CCK has been identified in mammalian brain, with high concentrations found in the cerebral cortex, limbic system, and hypothalamus. In animal studies, CCK is involved in the regulation of such behavioral functions as inhibition of intake of solid and liquid food, production of satiety, and pain relief. Of the two identified receptor subtypes, CCK type A (CCK-A) is found primarily in the periphery and in some discrete brain areas, whereas CCK type B (CCK-B) is plentiful in the brain. The primary form of CCK, CCK-8S (a sulphated octapeptide), coexists with dopamine in the ventral tegmental area and substantia nigra, and its interactions with dopamine are context and location specific. CCK-A and CCK-B receptors have a high affinity for CCK-8S. CCK-B receptors also have high affinity for CCK-8SUS (unsulphated), CCK-4, and pentagastrin, whereas CCK-A receptors do not. In addition, CCK stimulates synthesis of nerve growth factor and plays a neuroprotective role.

Of particular interest to psychiatry is the coexistence of CCK with dopamine in mesolimbic and mesocortical, but not in nigrostriatal, systems. This suggests that CCK-8 activity might be dysregulated in psychiatric syndromes thought to involve altered dopamine transmission or that CCK analogs could be used therapeutically in the treatment of these syndromes. CCK-A receptor antagonists have been proposed for the treatment of schizophrenia, and initial evidence suggests that CCK agonists may be useful for decreasing the severity of parkinsonian symptoms. Caerulein, a mixed CCK-A and CCK-B agonist, has weak, neuroleptic-like effects on prepulse inhibition in schizophrenic patients. Evidence is stronger for a role of CCK-B receptor antagonists in the treatment of anxiety. Several small-scale human studies have demonstrated that administration of CCK-4 or pentagastrin can induce panic attacks and can increase neurosteroid release in a significant percentage of healthy volunteers, as well as anxiety disorder patients, even in the absence of arousal or environmental stress. Panic attacks in subjects with preexisting panic disorder can be elicited at doses of CCK-4 that do not reliably induce panic in healthy subjects, indicating enhanced sensitivity. Not only can selective CCK-B antagonists completely abolish the anxiogenic effects of CCK-4, but, in an animal model of anxiety used to evaluate the efficacy of benzodiazepines, CCK-B antagonists also demonstrated independent anxiolytic properties. Pretreatment with atrial natriuretic peptide has similarly been shown to decrease panic attacks in patients and controls given CCK-4.

MELATONIN

Melatonin is a pineal hormone that is derived from the serotonin molecule and controls photoperiodically medicated endocrine events (particularly those of the HPG axis). It also modulates immune function, mood, and reproductive performance; is a potent antioxidant and free-radical scavenger; and may have oncostatic effects. Melatonin has a depressive effect on CNS excitability and exerts neuroprotective effects against excitotoxicity. Melatonin has analgesic effects through its actions on opiate receptors and has regulatory effects on serotonin metabolism. Altered secretory patterns and levels of melatonin have been found in various psychiatric disorders, such as unipolar and bipolar depression, seasonal affective disorder, bulimia, anorexia, schizophrenia, panic disorder, and obsessive compulsive disorder. Although suppression of melatonin is not necessary for the efficacy of light therapy in seasonal affective disorder, melatonin can be a useful therapeutic agent in the treatment of circadian phase disorders, such as jet lag, and intake of melatonin increases the speed of falling asleep, as well as its duration and quality.

ARGININE VASOPRESSIN

AVP (or antidiuretic hormone [ADH]) is a posterior pituitary hormone that maintains plasma osmolarity through regulation of renal water excretion. AVP release is triggered by pain, emotional stress, dehydration, increased plasma osmolarity, or decreases in blood volume and acts synergistically with CRH to control ACTH release. Alprazolam, an inhibitor of CRH secretion, inhibits vasopressin (Pitressin)-stimulated release of ACTH and cortisol.

Profound alterations in fluid ingestion and excretion have been observed in psychiatric patients throughout most of the 20th century. Polydipsia occurs in 10 to 15 percent of hospitalized psychiatric patients and is unrelated to diagnosis; in many cases, the syndrome is secondary to inappropriate secretion of AVP, which occurs as a feature of the altered behavioral state itself and resolves with treatment or, conversely, is precipitated by a variety of antidepressant or antipsychotic agents.

Animal and normal human studies of AVP administration (or longer-acting synthetic analog compounds) have indicated that the hormone may enhance the consolidation and retrieval of memory, particularly that associated with aversive learning. Assessments of attention, concentration, and memory in the elderly, those with depression, or those with dementia have had more mixed results. Although positive results exist, the effect is small and has yet to be consistently reproduced; it may be that such reported effects are secondary to a general arousal effect. However, AVP has also been shown to prevent the loss of tolerance to the incoordinating, sedative-hypnotic, and hypothermic effects of alcohol after cessation of ingestion and to delay the loss of sexual behavior after castration, both of which suggest involvement of a learning mechanism.

Altered AVP function has been reported in depression and in eating disorders. Anorexic and bulimic patients show hypersecretion of centrally directed AVP, and patients with bulimia nervosa or depression may have an attenuated AVP response to hypertonic saline. Vasopressin delays the extinction of behaviors acquired during aversive conditioning and may be related to obsessional preoccupation with the aversive consequences of eating and weight gain. An inverse relation between AVP concentration and motor activity in depression and an increased number of vasopressin and oxytocin neurons have also been reported in the hypothalamus of depressed patients. Although dexamethasone suppression of ACTH and cortisol release is attenuated in depressed patients, suppression of ACTH and cortisol release in response to vasopressin is not; fluoxetine treatment of depression, however, decreases CSF vasopressin levels.

OXYTOCIN

Oxytocin is a posterior pituitary hormone that is involved in osmoregulation, the milk ejection reflex, food intake, and female maternal and sexual behaviors and has many effects reciprocal to those of vasopressin. Convergent evidence, using a range of methodologies, indicates that oxytocin inhibits food and sodium intake. Oxytocin binding in the hypothalamus is increased by estrogen and glucocorticoids and in estrogen-primed women. Oxytocin has anxiolytic activity and promotes a variety of reproductive (grooming, arousal, lordosis, orgasm, nesting, and birthing) and maternal behaviors (breast-feeding and mother–infant bonding), although the former may be restricted to nonmonogamous species. Infusion of oxytocin in female subjects of monogamous species facilitates pair bonding in the absence of mating, and administration of an oxytocin antagonist prevents pair bonding. AVP serves a similar pair-bonding function in male subjects and promotes monogamy and paternal behavior in male prairie voles. Oxytocin can also act as a neuromodulator of limbic dopamine concentrations and thus may be involved in adaptation to substances of abuse, and it can act as a mediator of the effect of CRH on ACTH. It has been called the *amnestic neuropeptide* owing to its ability to attenuate memory consolidation and retrieval. Patients with autism and anorexia have been reported to have reduced levels of oxytocin, whereas those with obsessive-compulsive disorder (OCD) have been reported to have a vasopressin-oxytocin ratio that was negatively correlated with symptom severity.

SUBSTANCE P

The neurokinin substance P, an 11–amino acid peptide discovered originally in 1930, has neurotrophic effects and acts as an excitatory transmitter in primary afferent nerve terminals in mammalian spinal cord, helping regulate sympathetic noradrenergic function. Depending on the pain paradigm used, administration of substance P can produce hyperalgesia or analgesia. Substance P also has been found to have memory-promoting effects, possibly through increases in acetylcholine in the frontal cortex produced by the N-terminal fragment, and to have reinforcing effects, possibly through increases in dopamine in the nucleus accumbens, produced by the C-terminal fragment. The unexpected finding that an antagonist (MK869) of the substance P receptor (neurokinin$_1$, or NK$_1$) was shown to have significant antidepressant effect in a well-controlled clinical trial has stimulated scientific investigation of the antidepressant and antianxiety effects of a number of NK$_1$ antagonist compounds, as well as preclinical development of NK$_2$ and NK$_3$ receptor antagonists.

Substance P receptors are localized to neuroanatomic regions involved in the regulation of affective behavior and stress (amygdala, hippocampus, raphe nuclei, locus ceruleus, and hypothalamus) and are involved in the modulation of serotonin and norepinephrine release. A small-scale study has shown that NK$_1$ receptors are decreased in major depressive disorder, although most behavioral evidence linking substance P to mood and anxiety disorders derives from rodent models.

NEUROTENSIN

Neurotensin is a tridecapeptide that appears to play a role in neuroendocrine regulation and coordination as a signaling molecule. Gonadal and adrenal steroids and thyroid hormones alter neurotensin levels in the hypothalamus, preoptic area, and arcuate nucleus. Neurotensin has a close neuroanatomical relation with serotonin and dopaminergic pathways and is involved in the control of anterior pituitary activity, stimulating release of prolactin and TSH, as well as in the regulation of a subpopulation of serotonergic neurons in the dorsal raphe and frontal cortex and GABAergic and glutamatergic neurons. Stimulation of serotonin neurons may be responsible for its analgesic effects and reduction of stress response, whereas the dopaminergic effects suggest a possible antipsychotic role. Subgroups of drug-free schizophrenic patients have low neurotensin CSF concentrations and altered neurotensin receptor binding in entorhinal cortex, and psychotogenic drugs (e.g., methamphetamine) inhibit the release of striatal neurotensin via an inhibitory effect of the dopamine type 1 (D_1) receptor. Most antipsychotic drugs increase neurotensin concentrations in the nucleus accumbens and caudate nucleus; schizophrenic patients with decreased CSF neurotensin show an increase compared to control values after antipsychotic drug treatment and clinical improvement. Because of neurotensin's association with the nigrostriatal dopamine and the serotonin systems, it is suspected of playing a role in movement disorders caused by antipsychotic drugs. Central administration of neurotensin in rats produces motor effects seen in animal models of parkinsonian and dystonic reactions (catalepsy) and tardive dyskinesia. Neurotensin may exert an antipsychotic action through intramembrane receptor interactions that reduce affinity of the dopamine type 2 (D_2)-agonist binding site.

An involvement in the development of drug dependence has also been hypothesized. Blocking the effects of neurotensin with antiserum or a receptor antagonist enhances dopamine release in the nucleus accumbens, and neurotensin itself blocks stimulant-induced motor activity. However, doses that block hyperlocomotion do not attenuate self-administration of cocaine and even enhance conditioned place preference, an animal model of rewarding effects. Neurotensin's modulating effects on dopamine activity may depend on stimulus intensity, enhancing the rewarding properties of a subthreshold stimulus from intracranial self-stimulation (ICSS), as do psychostimulants, but decreasing maximal stimulation rate, as do antipsychotic drugs. Acute administration of stimulants increases neurotensin in the nucleus accumbens, but, with chronic administration, levels return to normal. Ibogaine, a hallucinogen used in indigenous religious ceremonies, has been shown to interrupt cocaine and methamphetamine abuse in patients and may act similarly to ICSS, increasing neurotensin concentrations in the nucleus accumbens when given alone but attenuating cocaine-induced increases in neurotensin.

MELANOCYTE-STIMULATING HORMONE

MSH, an anterior pituitary peptide, controls secretion of melatonin (and melanin) and, in some paradigms, exerts opposite effects on behavior. Intraperitoneal administration of α-MSH delays extinction in a passive-avoidance paradigm and increases emotional response. In a double-blind, crossover trial in humans, an infusion of α-MSH resulted in a significant improvement in verbal memory but little change in mood. Because phenothiazines increase pituitary MSH secretion and pigmentation in patients in proportion to their therapeutic potency, it has been suggested that MSH peptides may possess some therapeutic properties. A dose-related biphasic effect on mood has also been reported for MSH release-inhibiting factor. Recent data indicate that MSH interacts with leptin to counteract neuropeptide Y, decrease food intake, and increase energy expenditure. Levels of MSH have also been associated with dyskinesia in animals.

SUGGESTED CROSS-REFERENCES

Section 1.12 on the immune system contains information on the interaction between endocrine, immune, and neural systems, and Section 1.13 contains information on chronobiology, a more detailed analysis of circadian regulation. Section 1.21 discusses endocrine involvement in eating behavior more extensively, whereas Section 1.6 provides a more comprehensive discussion of neuropeptide effects on behavior. Section 11.13 discusses anabolic-androgenic steroid abuse. Chapter 13 discusses further aspects of mood disorders, and Section 31.27 presents the therapeutic use of thyroid hormones.

REFERENCES

Altshuler LL, Bauer M, Frye MA, Gitlin MJ, Mintz J, Szuba MP, Leight KL, Whybrow PC: Does thyroid supplementation accelerate tricyclic antidepressant response? A review and meta-analysis of the literature. *Am J Psychiatry.* 2001;158:1617.

Bailer UF, Kaye WH: A review of neuropeptide and neuroendocrine dysregulation in anorexia and bulimia nervosa. *Curr Drug Target CNS Neurol Disord.* 2003;2:53.

Bauer M, Whybrow PC: Thyroid hormone, neural tissue and mood modulation. *World J Biol Pyschiatry.* 2001;2:59.

Blackburn-Munro G, Blackburn-Munro RE: Chronic pain, chronic stress and depression: Coincidence or consequence? *J Neuroendocrinol.* 2001;13:1009.

*Blanchard RJ, McKittrick CR, Blanchard DC: Animal models of social stress: effects on behavior and brain neurochemical systems. *Physiol Behav.* 2001;73:261.

Brambilla F: Psychoneurendocrinology: A science of the past or a new pathway for the future? *Eur J Pharmacol.* 2000;405:341.

*Christiansen K: Behavioral effects of androgen in men and women. *J Endocrinol.* 2001;170:39.

Drolet G, Dumont EC, Gosselin I, Kinkead R, Laforest S, Trottier JF: Role of endogenous opioid system in the regulation of the stress response. *Prog Neuropsychopharmacol Biol Psychiatry.* 2001;25:729.

Ferguson JN, Young LJ, Insel TR: The neuroendocrine basis of social recognition. *Front Neuroendocrinol.* 2002;23:200.

Gass P, Reichardt HM, Strekalova T, Henn F, Tronche F: Mice with targeted mutations of glucocorticoid and mineralocorticoid receptors: models for depression and anxiety? *Physiol Behav.* 2001;73:811.

Genazzani AR, Monteleone P, Gambacciani M: Hormonal influence on the central nervous system. *Maturitas.* 2002;43[Suppl 1]:S11.

Gerra G, Zaimovic A, Timpano M, Zambelli U, Delsignore R, Brambilla F: Neuroendocrine correlates of temperamental traits in humans. *Psychoneuroendocrinology.* 2000;25:479.

*Gispen-de Wied CC, Jansen LM: The stress-vulnerability hypothesis in psychotic disorders: focus on the stress response systems. *Curr Psychiatry Rep.* 2002;4:166.

Gold PW, Gabry KE, Yasuda MR, Chrousos GP: Divergent endocrine abnormalities in melancholic and atypical depression: Clinical and pathophysiologic implications. *Endocrinol Metab Clin North Am.* 2002;31:37.

*Habib KE, Gold PW, Chrousos GP: Neuroendocrinology of stress. *Endocrinol Metab Clin North Am.* 2001;30:695.

Halbreich U, Kahn LS: Hormonal aspects of schizophrenias: An overview. *Psychoneuroendocrinology.* 2003;28[Suppl 2]:1.

Hogervorst E, Yaffe K, Richards M, Huppert F: Hormone replacement therapy to maintain cognitive function in women with dementia. *Cochran Database Syst Rev.* 2002:CD003799.

Holsboer F: The role of peptides in treatment of psychiatric disorders. *J Neural Transm Suppl.* 2003;64:17.

Kask A, Harro J, von Horsten S, Redrobe JP, Dumont Y, Quirion R: The neurocircuitry and receptor subtypes mediating anxiolytic-like effects of neuropeptide Y. *Neurosci Biobehav Rev.* 2002;26:259.

Losel RM, Falkenstein E, Feuring M, Schultz A, Tillmann HC, Rossol-Haseroth K, Wehling M: Nongenomic steroid action: Controversies, questions, and answers. *Physiol Rev.* 2003;83:965.

McEwan BS: Mood disorders and allostatic load. *Biol Psychiatry.* 2003;54:200.

Mormede P, Courvoisier H, Ramos A, Marissal-Arvy N, Ousova O, Desautes C, Duclos M, Chaouloff F, Moisan MP: Molecular genetic approaches to investigate individual variations in behavioral and neuroendocrine stress responses. *Psychoneuroendocrinology.* 2002;27:563.

*Reus VI, Wolkowitz OM: Antiglucocorticoid drugs in the treatment of depression. *Expert Opin Invest Drugs.* 2001;10:1789.

Reus VI, Wolkowitz OM. DHEA effects on human behavior and psychiatric illness. In: Morfin R, ed. *DHEA and the Brain.* Vol 1. New York: Taylor and Francis; 2002.

Rupprecht R: Neuroactive steroids: Mechanisms of action and neuropsychopharmacological properties. *Psychoneuroendocrinology.* 2003;28:139.

Santarelli L, Gobbi G, Blier P, Hen R: Behavioral and physiologic effects of genetic or pharmacologic inactivation of the substance P receptor. *J Clin Psychiatry.* 2002;63[Suppl 11]:11.

Seidman SN: Testosterone deficiency and mood in aging men: Pathogenic and therapeutic interactions. *World J Biol Psychiatry.* 2003;4:14.

Steiner M, Dunn E, Born L: Hormones and mood: From menarche to menopause and beyond. *J Affect Disord.* 2003;74:67.

Stevens JR: Schizophrenia: Reproductive hormones and the brain. *Am J Psychiatry.* 2002;159:713.

Wolkowitz OM, Rothschild AJ, eds. *Psychoneuroendocrinology: The Scientific Basis of Clinical Practice.* Washington, DC: American Psychiatric Press, Inc.; 2003.

Young EA, Korszun A: The hypothalamic-pituitary-gonadal axis in mood disorders. *Endocrinol Metab Clin North Am.* 2002;31:63.

▲ 1.12 Immune System and Central Nervous System Interactions

CHARLES L. RAISON, M.D., BRADLEY DIXON PEARCE, PH.D., AND ANDREW H. MILLER, M.D.

An ever-growing database demonstrates that interactions between the immune system and the central nervous system (CNS) play a critical role in the maintenance of bodily homeostasis and the development of diseases, including psychiatric disease. Alterations in CNS function brought about by a variety of stressors have been clearly shown to influence the immune system as well as diseases that involve the immune system. Moreover, many of the relevant hormonal and neurotransmitter pathways that mediate these effects have been elucidated. Of considerable interest are recent data outlining the impact of soluble factors (cytokines) derived from immune cells and glia, which, in turn, have profound effects on the CNS. The relative roles of these factors in the various psychiatric diseases are an area of active investigation, as is the role of infectious and autoimmune diseases in the pathophysiology of psychiatric disorders. Taken together, these findings highlight the importance of interdisciplinary efforts involving the neurosciences and immunology for gaining new insights into the etiology of psychiatric syndromes.

OVERVIEW OF IMMUNE SYSTEM

The immune system has the capacity to protect the body from the invasion of foreign pathogens, such as viruses, bacteria, fungi, and parasites. In addition, the immune system can detect and eliminate cells that have become neoplastically transformed. These functions are accomplished through highly specific receptors on immune cells for molecules derived from invading organisms and a rich intercellular communication network that involves direct cell-to-cell interactions and signaling between cells of the immune system by soluble factors called *cytokines.* The body's absolute dependence on the efficient functioning of the immune system is illustrated by the less than 1-year survival rate of untreated infants born with severe combined immunodeficiency disease and the devastating opportunistic infections and cancers that arise during acquired immune deficiency syndrome (AIDS).

CELLS AND TISSUES

The immune system must be able to survey all tissues of the body for the presence of infectious agents or neoplastic cells and to mobilize its effector components to specific sites in the body at which infectious agents may invade. Therefore, an important requirement of the immune system is that it be systemic and mobile. Cells of hematopoietic origin largely accomplish this function. Like all other blood cells, immune cells are derived from hematopoietic precursor stem cells, which, in the adult, originate in the bone marrow. The stem cells are pluripotent and are capable of differentiating into any one of the various mature hematopoietic cells. There are two major paths of differentiation that are regulated in part by cytokines and other factors (Fig. 1.12–1). The lymphoid path leads to the formation of the mature lymphocytes—B cells, T cells, and natural killer (NK) cells; the myeloid path of differentiation leads to the other cells of the blood (some of which participate in the immune response), including monocytes and granulocytes, which include neutrophils, eosinophils, and basophils. Monocytes and basophils may further differentiate into macrophages and mast cells, respectively, which take up residence in tissues throughout the body.

Lymphocyte maturation occurs in *primary immune tissues.* In humans, the bone marrow serves as the primary site for B-cell maturation, and the thymus is the primary site for T-cell maturation. An important part of the maturation process is the screening out of cells that are reactive to the body's own constituents (*self-reactive*). On maturation, lymphocytes exit the primary immune tissues and circulate through the bloodstream and the lymphatic system into and out of the secondary immune tissues, including the spleen and widely distributed lymph nodes. *Secondary immune tissues* provide a structure for interactions between different immune cells and circulating pathogens.

NATURAL AND ACQUIRED IMMUNITY

The immune system is often divided on a functional basis into two separate categories: natural or innate immunity and specific or acquired immunity (Table 1.12–1). The components of natural immunity act in a relatively nonspecific manner against pathogens or infected cells and may be evolutionarily more primitive than the specialized T and B lymphocytes that mediate specific immunity; operationally, however, the two modes of immunity interact and cooperate.

Natural Immunity The cells mediating natural immunity do not require prior activation or specific recognition of invading pathogens, or both, to be functional; they therefore provide an important first line of defense against infectious agents during the early stages of an immune response. Mononuclear phagocytic cells and NK cells are examples of immune cells that mediate nonspecific immunity. Mononuclear phagocytic cells, such as macrophages, microglia, certain endothelial cells, and reticular cells of lymphoid organs, are collectively referred to as the *reticuloendothelial system.* These cells recognize extracellular pathogens (e.g., bacteria and parasites) through relatively crude pattern recognition molecules and destroy these pathogens by engulfing and degrading them. Mononuclear phagocytes also release type I interferons (IFNs), which have direct antiviral properties, and proinflammatory cytokines, including tumor necrosis factor (TNF), interleukin (IL)-1, and IL-6. TNF is the principal mediator of the response to gram-negative bacteria and is one of the earliest cytokines released in the proinflammatory cascade that includes IL-1 followed by IL-6. TNF is an endogenous pyrogen

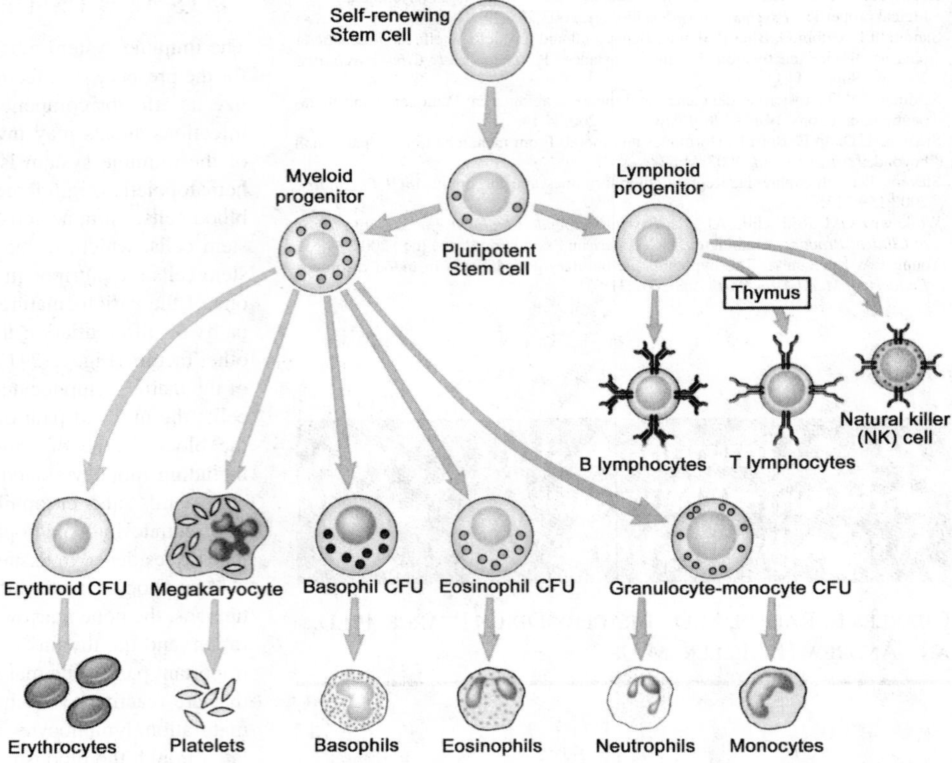

FIGURE 1.12–1 Hematopoietic tree. The development of different lineages of blood cells is depicted in this hematopoietic tree. CFU, colony-forming unit. (From Abbas AK, Lichtman AH, Pober JS. *Cellular and Molecular Immunology.* Philadelphia: WB Saunders; 2000, with permission.)

that, along with IL-1, is capable of inducing fever by increasing the synthesis of prostaglandins by cytokine-stimulated hypothalamic cells. TNF also leads to cachexia, characterized by wasting of muscle and fat cells, in part, secondary to appetite suppression.

The combination of liver-derived plasma proteins induced by TNF and IL-1 with those induced by IL-6 constitutes the acute-phase response (Fig. 1.12–2). The acute-phase response is designed to limit tissue damage, to isolate and destroy invading organisms, and to set repair functions in motion. These objectives are achieved by rapid changes in plasma protein composition characterized by increases in the so-called acute-phase reactants: C-reactive protein (which coats bacteria to facilitate phagocytosis-opsonization), macroglobulin and other antiproteases (which neutralize tissue destructive proteases), and the clotting protein fibrinogen. Albumin and transferrin, the iron transport protein, decline during the acute-phase response and are therefore called *negative acute-phase reactants.* During the acute-phase response, inflammatory cytokines also coordinate the systemic response to infection, having potent effects on the neuroendocrine system (especially the hypothalamic-pituitary-adrenal [HPA] axis) and the CNS, where they mediate many symptoms of illness, including fever, loss of appetite, social withdrawal, and sleep changes.

Complement factor proteins, which are produced by the liver, provide another important humoral component of nonspecific immunity. These functionally linked proteins interact with one another in a highly regulated manner and subserve many of the effector functions of the immune system, including cell lysis, opsonization, activation of inflammation by attracting inflammatory cells (chemotaxis), stimulation of immune cells to release chemical mediators of inflammation, and neutralization of antigen-antibody complexes that can damage tissues.

NK cells are also an important component of natural immunity. These cells can destroy virally infected cells by binding to them and releasing cytolytic factors, including perforin. NK cells also have the ability to recognize and destroy neoplastically transformed host cells, especially those of hematopoietic origin, thus providing protection against some cancers.

Acquired Immunity

T and B lymphocytes are the crowning achievement of immune cell specialization and evolution. These cells account for the diversity and the specificity of the immune response and for the adaptive aspect of the immune system. Furthermore, T and B cells are responsible for directing the immune response against foreign targets, rather than self components. An effective specific

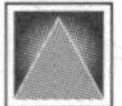

Table 1.12–1
Divisions of the Immune System: Innate versus Acquired

	Innate	Acquired
Physicochemical barriers	Skin, mucous membranes	Cutaneous and mucosal immune systems
Cells	Phagocytes (macrophages, neutrophils, and natural killer cells)	Lymphocytes (B and T cells)
Soluble mediators that affect other cells	Macrophage-derived cytokines (i.e., IL-1, IL-6, tumor necrosis factor-α, and interferons)	Lymphocyte-derived cytokines (i.e., IL-2, IL-4, IL-5, IL-6, IL-10, and interferon-γ)
Circulating molecules	Complement	Antibodies

IL, interleukin.

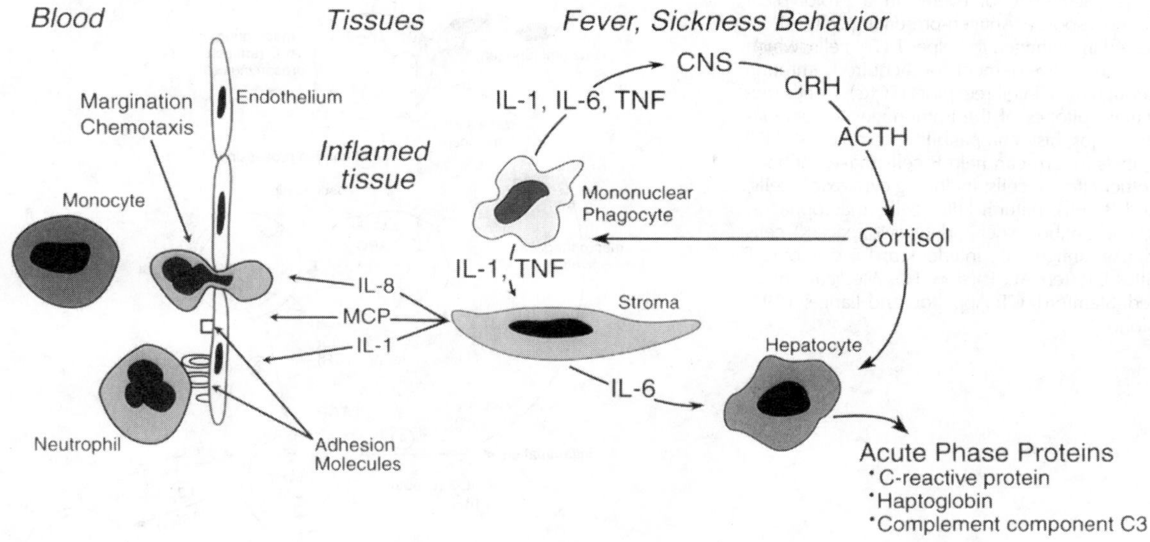

FIGURE 1.12–2 Schema for cell and cytokine interaction in the acute-phase response. Mononuclear phagocytes release early cytokines, such as interleukin (IL)-1 and tumor necrosis factor (TNF), at the site of tissue damage. These cytokines stimulate the accumulation of inflammatory cells in several ways; they activate adjacent stroma to elicit other chemotactic cytokines (such as monocyte chemotactic protein [MCP], IL-1, and IL-8), and they induce endothelial cells to express adhesion molecules that bind inflammatory cells. The hepatic response is activated by other cytokine mediators, as is the activation of the hypothalamic-pituitary-adrenal axis to release corticotropin-releasing hormone (CRH), adrenocorticotropic hormone (ACTH), and, subsequently, cortisol. CNS, central nervous system. (From Raison CL, Gumnick, JF, Miller AH. Neuroendocrine–immune interactions: implications for health and behavior. In: Pfaff DW, Arnold AP, Etgen AM, et al., eds. *Hormones, Brain and Behavior.* Vol 5. San Diego, CA: Academic Press; 2002, with permission.)

immune response includes three conceptually separate phases: an induction phase, in which the presence of an infectious agent or antigen is detected; an activation phase, which includes the proliferation and the mobilization of the immune cells relevant to the eradication of the infectious agent; and an action or effector phase, in which the infectious agent is neutralized and eliminated.

Induction Phase Recognition of pathogens or neoplastically transformed cells is achieved through specialized receptors for antigens on the surface of B and T lymphocytes. Antigens are foreign substances that induce specific immunity and typically include molecules derived from pathogens, such as viral subunits, enzymes, and bacterial cell wall glycoproteins. The B-cell antigen receptor is a membrane-

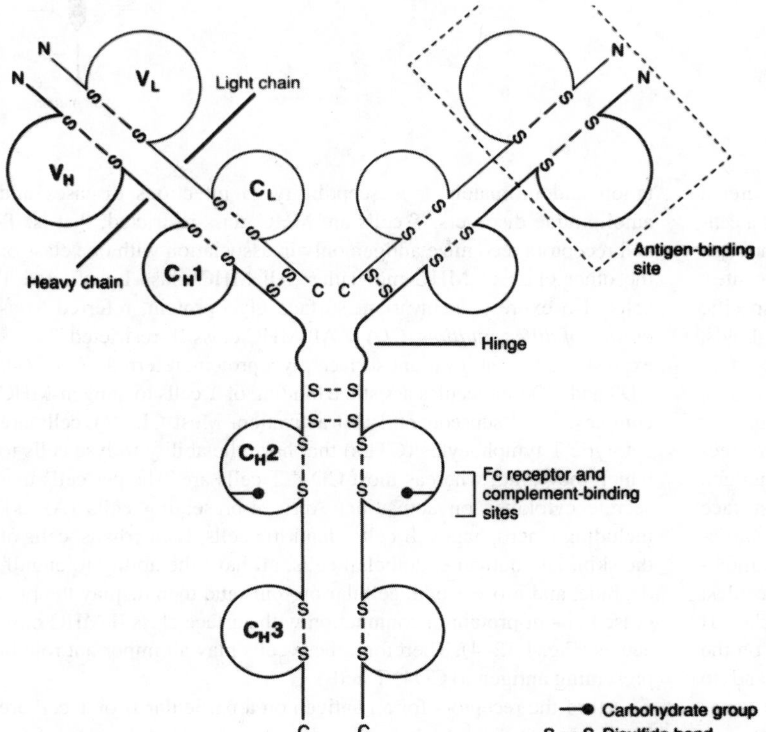

FIGURE 1.12–3 Schematic diagram of an immunoglobulin (Ig) molecule. In this drawing of an IgG molecule, the antigen-binding sites are formed by the juxtaposition of variable region of the light chain (V_L) and variable region of the heavy chain (V_H) domains. The locations of complement and Fc receptor-binding sites within the heavy chain constant regions are approximations. S--S refers to intrachain and interchain disulfide bonds; N and C refer to amino and carboxy termini of the polypeptide chains, respectively. C_H, constant region of the heavy chain; C_L, constant region of the light chain. (From Abbas AK, Lichtman AH, Pober JS. *Cellular and Molecular Immunology.* Philadelphia: WB Saunders; 1991, with permission.)

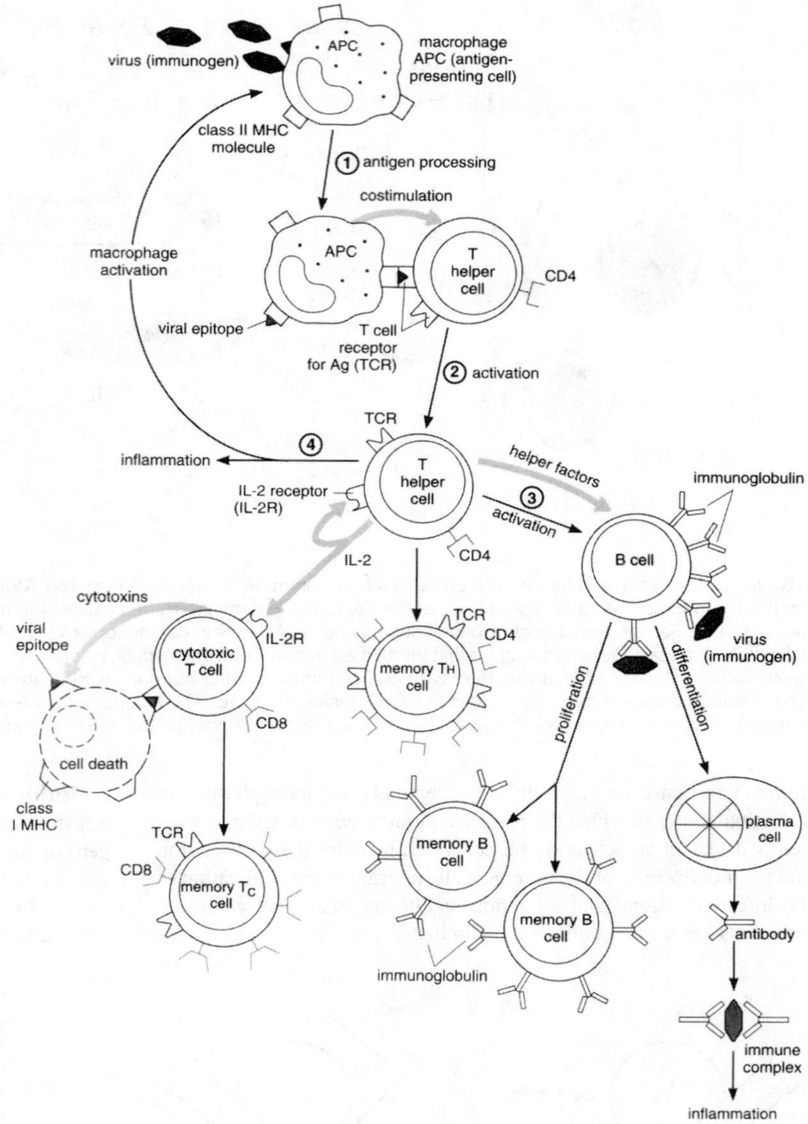

FIGURE 1.12–4 Sequence of events in a prototypical acquired immune response. Antigen-presenting cells (APCs) present processed immunogen to helper T (T_H) cells, which are central to the development of acquired immune responses. Through their T-cell receptors (TCRs), T cells recognize particular epitopes of the immunogen in association with the major histocompatibility complex (MHC) molecule. T_H cells in turn can help B cells make antibody and activate other effector cells, including cytotoxic T cells, memory T and B cells, natural killer cells, macrophages, granulocytes, and antibody dependent cytotoxic (K) cells (not pictured). Ag, antigen; IL, interleukin; T_C, cytotoxic T cell. (From Sites DP, Terr AL, Parslow TG. *Medical Immunology*. 9th ed. Stamford, CT: Appelton and Lange; 1997, with permission.)

bound form of immunoglobulin (Ig). A related form of Ig is secreted as antibody by mature B cells (plasma B cells). Antibodies play a central role in humoral immunity and help kill a variety of pathogens. Each Ig or antibody molecule has two identical antigen-binding sites, and those binding sites can recognize the tertiary structure of specific proteins and other molecules, such as polysaccharides and lipids, which are important components of infectious agents (Fig. 1.12–3).

The T-cell antigen receptor has a single antigen binding site. Antigen recognition by T cells takes on an added level of complexity that is not inherent to B cells (Fig. 1.12–4). The T-cell receptor recognizes only fragments of protein antigens. In addition, the antigen fragments must be present in association with a class of cell surface molecules called *major histocompatibility complex* (*MHC*) *molecules*. Virtually all nucleated cells of the body express MHC molecules on their surface. Most cells express class I MHC molecules; some cells, usually of immune system origin, also express class II MHC molecules. The induction of a T-cell response depends on the ability and the effectiveness of MHC molecules to bind and to present antigen. Therefore, the repertoire of MHC molecule genes that a person inherits can contribute significantly to antigen presentation and ultimately to susceptibility to infectious diseases and autoimmune disorders. T cells are MHC class-restricted; that is, T-cell receptors recognize antigen only in association with one class or the other class of MHC molecules. All MHC class I–restricted T cells also express an invariant surface glycoprotein, referred to as *cluster of differentiation* (*CD*) *8*. All MHC class II–restricted T cells express a different invariant surface glycoprotein, referred to as *CD4*. CD8 and CD4 molecules assist the binding of T cells to antigen-MHC complexes and subsequent T-cell activation. Most $CD8^+$ T cells are cytolytic T lymphocytes (CTLs) that have the ability to lyse cells to which they bind, whereas most $CD4^+$ T cells are T-helper cells that secrete cytokines on activation. Antigen-presenting cells (APCs), including macrophages, B cells, dendritic cells, Langerhans' cells of the skin, and human endothelial cells, all have the ability to engulf, degrade, and process extracellular proteins and then display the processed bits of protein in conjunction with surface class II MHC molecules (Fig. 1.12–4). Therefore, these cells play an important role in presenting antigen to $CD4^+$ T cells.

All of the receptors for an antigen on a particular B or T cell are identical and unique to that cell and its descendants (*clones*). A fam-

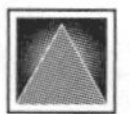

Table 1.12–2
Cytokine Mediators of Natural Immunity and Inflammation

Cytokines	Source	Target	Primary Effect
Type I interferon (IFN-α, IFN-β)	Monocyte, macrophage, and others	All	Antiviral, increased class I MHC expression
		NK cell	Activation
Tumor necrosis factor (TNF)	Monocyte, macrophage, T cell	Neutrophil	Activation (inflammation)
		T cell and B cell	—
		Liver	Acute-phase reactants
		Hypothalamus	Fever
		Adipose, muscle	Catabolism
Interferon γ (IFN-γ)	T cell and NK cell	Macrophage and others	Activation, upregulation of class I and II MHC molecules
Interleukin-1 (IL-1)	Monocyte, macrophage, and others	T cell and B cell	Costimulator
		Hypothalamus	Fever
Interleukin-6 (IL-6)	Monocyte, macrophage, and T cell	T cell and B cell	Costimulator
		Mature B cell	Growth
Interleukin-10 (IL-10)	Macrophage and T cell	Macrophage	Inhibition of IL-12, upregulation of class II MHC molecules
		B cells	Activation
Interleukin-12 (IL-12)	Macrophage	NK cell	Activation
		T cell	Growth and activation
Macrophage migration inhibitory factor (MIF)	Macrophage, pituitary, and liver	Multiple	Overrides activity of glucocorticoids, promotes inflammatory responses

MHC, major histocompatibility complex; NK, natural killer.
Adapted from Abbas AK, Lichtman AH, Pober JS. *Cellular and Molecular Immunology.* Philadelphia: WB Saunders; 2000.

ily of lymphocytes with identical antigen receptor specificity is called a *clonal line.* Diversity in antigen recognition is derived from the vast number of different B-cell and T-cell clonal lines present in each person. Such diversity is achieved by semirandom mixing and matching of sequences of DNA that code for the antigen-binding portion of the T-cell and B-cell receptors. That process of genetic diversity has been estimated to have the capacity to generate in each person more than 10^8 different receptors with functionally distinct antigenic specificity. Such high diversity makes it likely that each person possesses some clonal line of lymphocytes with an antigen receptor specificity capable of binding to a portion of any pathogen that may be encountered. Thus, the specific recognition of pathogens by the immune system entails the clonal selection of lymphocytes that are specifically responsive to the infectious agent.

Activation Phase The binding of foreign antigens by B cells and T cells is usually not sufficient to produce cell activation; an accessory signal must also be provided. Important accessory signals are generated by a group of cytokines called *ILs* that are secreted by T-helper cells and APCs, such as macrophages. T-helper cells and APCs cooperate (Fig. 1.12–4); APCs secrete IL-1 and other cytokines that stimulate T-helper cells to secrete a host of cytokines, including IFN-γ, which then increases the phagocytic ability of APCs and increases their class II MHC expression, thus improving their antigen-presenting capacity. IFN-γ also has direct antiviral properties. In addition, IL-1 stimulates T cells to produce IL-2 and to express IL-2 receptors on their surface. IL-2 is an important cytokine that activates multiple lymphocyte functions.

Recent evidence indicates that two subclasses of T-helper cells secrete different cytokine profiles after stimulation. These T-helper cell subsets have been best characterized in the mouse. Type 1 T-helper (Th-1) cells primarily secrete IL-2 and IFN-γ and are involved in cell-mediated inflammatory reactions and result in activation of CTLs. Type 2 T-helper (Th-2) cells primarily secrete IL-4, IL-5, IL-6, and IL-10, and encourage antibody formation, particularly IgE responses. Thus, Th-2 cytokines are found in association with strong antibody responses and allergic responses. Cytokines can be broadly divided into categories based on their role in the initiation, regulation, and maintenance of the immune response. Hence, there are sets of cytokine mediators involved in natural immunity and inflammation (Table 1.12–2), other sets involved in adaptive immunity (Table 1.12–3), and sets of cytokines that control proliferation and differen-

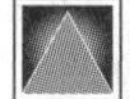

Table 1.12–3
Cytokine Mediators of Adaptive Immunity

Cytokines	Source	Target	Primary Effect
Interleukin-2 (IL-2)	T cell	T cell	Growth and cytokine production
		Natural killer cell	Growth and activation
		B cell	Growth and antibody production
Interleukin-4 (IL-4)	CD4⁺ T cell	T cell	Growth and differentiation
		B cell	Isotype switching to IgE
Interleukin-5 (IL-5)	T cell	Eosinophil	Activation
		B cell	Growth and IgA production
Transforming growth factor β (TGFβ)	T cell and others	T cell	Inhibition of growth and activation
		B cell	Inhibition of growth
		Macrophage	Inhibition of activation

Ig, immunoglobulin.
Adapted from Abbas AK, Lichtman AH, Pober JS. *Cellular and Molecular Immunology.* Philadelphia: WB Saunders; 2000.

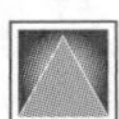

Table 1.12–4
Cytokine Mediators of Immune Cell Growth and Differentiation

Cytokines	Source	Target	Primary Effect
Interleukin-3 (IL-3)	T cell	Immature progenitor	Growth and differentiation to many cell lines
Granulocyte-monocyte CSF (GM-CSF)	T cell, monocyte, macrophage, and others	Immature and committed progenitor and macrophage	Growth and differentiation to all cell lines
Macrophage CSF	Macrophage and others	Committed progenitor	Differentiation to monocyte and macrophage
Granulocyte CSF	Monocyte, macrophage, and others	Committed progenitor	Differentiation to neutrophil, eosinophil, and basophil
Interleukin-7 (IL-7)	Fibroblast and bone marrow stromal cell	Immature progenitor	Growth of T and B cell lines
Leukemia inhibitory factor (LIF)	Fibroblast and bone marrow stromal cell	Immature progenitor and others	Governs growth and differentiation of hematopoietic and monocyte cell lines

CSF, colony-stimulating factor.
Adapted from Abbas AK, Lichtman AH, Pober JS. *Cellular and Molecular Immunology.* Philadelphia: WB Saunders; 2000.

tiation of immature immune cells (Table 1.12–4). Nevertheless, these sets overlap in function and act together to govern the dynamic events of immunity.

After binding antigen in the presence of stimulatory cytokines, T and B lymphocytes with the appropriate binding sites are activated, leading to cell growth, division, and proliferation. Activation also results in the clonal expansion of immune cells with the identical high-affinity specificity for the foreign antigen. Some of the progeny during clonal expansion undergo further differentiation into mature effector cells, such as antibody-secreting plasma B cells, and CTLs. By contrast, some descendants of activated B cells or T cells become memory cells that are primed for activation on further stimulation by the same antigen. Reexposure to that antigen results in a secondary immune response (*acquired immunity*), which is usually more rapid and more robust than the first or primary immune response to that antigen. Memory cells may live for many years, thus providing long-lasting acquired immunity, as is evident in individuals who received a vaccine or had their first contact with a specific infectious agent during infancy.

Effector Phase The ultimate aim of an immune response is the neutralization and elimination of pathogens. The principal effector mechanisms of acquired immunity are mediated by antibodies (*humoral immunity*) secreted from B cells and by cytolytic T cells (*cellular immunity*). Humoral immunity is especially effective in combating extracellular pathogens, such as bacteria and parasites; cellular immunity is effective in protecting against viral infection and, as with NK cells, may provide some protection against tumor cells.

The effector components of natural immunity are also recruited, enhanced, and directed toward specific pathogens as a result of the actions of B and T cells. For example, circulating antibodies can neutralize pathogens by binding to and coating the pathogens (*opsonization*). Pathogens that are opsonized are made susceptible to lysis by complement factors and phagocytosis. NK cells and *phagocytic cells*, such as neutrophils and macrophages, have receptors for the Fc fragment of antibodies. Furthermore, complement proteins bind to and are activated by the Fc fragments of some types of antibodies. Thus, antibodies can link effector cells and cytolytic proteins of natural immunity with pathogens, lending a level of specificity that is not inherent in the effector processes themselves. Although a large diversity of antigen-binding domains is present in different antibodies, the remainder of the molecule is highly conserved, and there are a limited number of different types of Fc fragments (*isotypes*) of the molecule. Because the Fc fragment of the antibody is the effector portion of the molecule, antibodies with different isotypes have different effector features (Table 1.12–5).

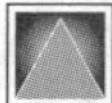

Table 1.12–5
Antibody Isotypes and Their Features

Properties	IgM	IgD	IgG	IgA	IgE
Human adult serum level (Ig makes 20% of all serum protein)	0.5–2.0 mg/mL	0–0.4 mg/mL	8–16 mg/mL	1–4 mg/mL	10–400 ng/mL
Activates complement	++++	–	++	–	–
Crosses placenta	–	–	+	–	–
Binds to macrophages, neutrophils, and natural killer cells	–	–	+	–	–
Binds to mast cells and basophils	–	–	–	–	+
Primary role	Primary immune response	?	Secondary immune response	Mucosal immunity	Immediate hypersensitivity (allergic response); protects against parasites

Ig, immunoglobulin.
Adapted from Abbas AK, Lichtman AH, Pober JS. *Cellular and Molecular Immunology.* Philadelphia: WB Saunders; 1991.

IMMUNE SYSTEM AND DISEASE

The general effectiveness of the immune system in protecting the body against pathogens has been made dramatically clear by the extensive pathology that characterizes AIDS in persons infected by the human immunodeficiency virus (HIV). HIV selectively binds to the CD4 molecule on T-helper cells via the gp120 protein on its membrane envelope and thereby gains entry and inhibits T-helper cell function. Because T-helper cells play a critical role in facilitating all aspects of specific immunity, the incapacitation of T-helper cells by HIV has catastrophic effects on the immune system. AIDS patients become susceptible to a wide spectrum of pathogens, such as protozoa (*Pneumocystis*), bacteria (*Mycobacterium tuberculosis*), fungi (*Candida*), and viruses (herpes simplex). Furthermore, AIDS patients have a high incidence of malignant tumors, especially those known to result from virally induced cellular proliferation and transformation. The nervous system is also affected in many AIDS patients, as evidenced by memory loss and other nonspecific neuropsychiatric disorders. No evidence indicates that HIV directly infects neurons; however, the infection of macrophages in neural tissues may lead to the impairment of neuronal function through the release of cytokines.

At the other end of the spectrum from immunodeficiency is autoimmunity. A number of relatively common diseases, such as type I diabetes, rheumatoid arthritis, and systemic lupus erythematosus have been shown to result from a specific autoimmune response directed against self-antigenic components. Clear genetic links to the expression of autoimmune disorders are often associated with specific types of MHC molecules. In most cases, however, a genetic background is not sufficient for the expression of disease. For example, the much greater prevalence of rheumatoid arthritis and systemic lupus erythematosus in women than in men suggests that, at least in some cases, there may be a hormonal component to the expression of these diseases.

The extent to which the immune system provides protection against cancer is still undetermined. Several effector mechanisms of the immune system are capable of destroying tumor cells in vitro (NK cells, CTLs, and TNF). The relatively rare occurrence of nonvirally induced tumors in immunodeficient patients suggests that the immune system plays a role primarily in protecting against tumor-inducing viruses rather than providing widespread tumor surveillance and elimination. Nevertheless, the extensive use of a variety of cytokines and other immune modulators in the treatment of neoplastic diseases underlines the importance of these factors in cancer therapy.

METHODS USED IN STUDYING THE IMMUNE SYSTEM

In Vitro Assays Much of the understanding of the immune system has been derived from in vitro studies. In vitro assays may be especially useful in dissecting the direct and indirect mechanisms by which neurally controlled factors can influence immune cell function. Two of the most widely used assays in the study of neural–immune interactions assess the proliferative capacity of lymphocytes and determine the cytolytic capability of CTLs and NK cells.

For proliferative assays, mononuclear cells, including lymphocytes, are removed from the experimental subject and are challenged in vitro with a mitogenic stimulus. Commonly used mitogenic stimuli (including concanavalin A, phytohemagglutinin, pokeweed mitogen, and lipopolysaccharide) are glycoproteins derived from plant lectins or bacterial cell walls that have been found to polyclonally stimulate lymphocyte proliferation. Proliferation is monitored by the incorporation of $[^3H]$thymidine into the DNA of the dividing cells. The limitations of proliferative assays are their notorious interassay variability and a limited understanding of the relationship between the polyclonal proliferative response to a mitogen and the clonally selective proliferative response to a specific antigen or pathogen.

NK cell assays have been widely applied to studies of neural–immune interactions. Typically, immune cells isolated from a subject are incubated in vitro with chromium 51–labeled target cells. Lysis of target cells results in the release of chromium 51 into the incubation medium, which is then collected and measured.

Flow Cytometry The development of monoclonal antibodies against specific immune cell surface markers, such as the various CD determinants, has been useful in monitoring and sorting subclasses of immune cells (Table 1.12–6). Fluorescently tagged monoclonal antibodies and the cells to which they bind can be detected by a laser-controlled flow cytometer. Clinically, flow cytometry has important applications in monitoring the proportion of subsets of immune cells in patients' peripheral blood. For example, a diagnostic feature of the onset of AIDS is the precipitous decline in the proportion of circulating $CD4^+$ cells. Experimentally, flow cytometry may be useful in studying the effects of various treatments and environmental factors on the proportion or number of immune cell subpopulations present in the various immune compartments. However, changes in the number and the percentage of a given subset are independent phenomena and may involve different mechanisms: for example, the increased percentage of one subset may actually be related to a decrease in the percentage of other subsets of lymphocytes.

In Vivo Assays Results from in vitro assays can be difficult to interpret, because the relation between changes in these assays and the capability of the immune system to exert effective responses in vivo is still unclear. To address this issue, studies exploring the immune system in humans (e.g., evaluating the consequences of stressors) have used several different approaches for the examination of the immune system in vivo, including examination of (1) the antibody response to antigen challenge, such as a vaccination; (2) antibody titers to latent viruses; (3) cutaneous delayed-type hypersensitivity (DTH); and (4) wound healing. All of these approaches allow evaluation of multiple phases of the immune response, including antigen presentation, B- and T-cell cooperation, and humoral immunity. Wound healing also represents an excellent assessment of inflammatory responses, as well as tissue growth and remodeling. Finally, plasma measures of circulating cytokines and their soluble receptors, as well as acute-phase proteins, provide information on the status of the immune system in situ.

REGULATION OF THE IMMUNE RESPONSE

An effective immune response requires the cooperation of many components of the immune system, often resulting in the augmentation of each component's contribution to the overall immune response. However, the simultaneous indiscriminate amplification of all aspects of the immune system would not be efficient and could even be disastrous. An overactive immune system may contribute to autoimmunity; furthermore, the inflammatory component of immune responses can be damaging if not controlled, as is seen in immune complex diseases and septic shock. Therefore, regulation of the immune response is necessary to make sure that the response is energy efficient, focused on the infectious agent, counterbalanced in

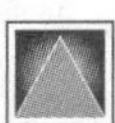

Table 1.12–6
Examples of Some Defined CD Molecules and Their Known Functions

CD Designation	Main Cellular Expression	Known Function
CD2	T cells and NK cells	Adhesion molecule, binds CD58 and sheep red blood cells
CD3	T cells and thymocytes	Signal transduction from T-cell receptor to cytoplasm
CD4	T-helper cells	Involved in MHC class II restricted antigen recognition
CD5	T cells, thymocytes, and B-cell subset	Cell signaling molecule
CD7	Some T cells	Cell signaling molecule
CD8	Cytotoxic and suppressor T cells	Involved in MHC class I restricted antigen recognition
CD16, CD32, and CD64	NK cells, neutrophils, macrophages, and B cells	Low-, intermediate-, and high-affinity receptors for IgG; CD64 is an Fc receptor
CD21	Mature B cells	Complement factor (C3d) receptor; Epstein-Barr virus receptor
CD23	Activated B cells and macrophages	Low-affinity receptor for IgE
CD25	Activated T and B cells and macrophages	Low-affinity IL-2 receptor
CD54	Broad	Adhesion molecule (intercellular adhesion molecule-1)
CD58	Broad	Adhesion molecule (lymphocyte function–associated antigen-3) for CD2
CD71	Activated T and B cells and macrophages	Transferrin receptor

Ig, immunoglobulin; IL, interleukin; MHC, major histocompatibility complex; NK, natural killer.
Adapted from Abbas AK, Lichtman AH, Pober JS. *Cellular and Molecular Immunology.* Philadelphia: WB Saunders; 1991.

a fashion that does not cause self-damage, and reversible once the pathogen has been eliminated.

Probably the most important form of *intrinsic regulation* of the immune system is mediated by the various cytokines. Several examples of the facilitatory effects of cytokines have been cited; however, some cytokines, such as transforming growth factor β (TGFβ), also produce potent inhibitory effects on lymphocyte activation and proliferation (Table 1.12–3). In addition, there is clear evidence for the existence of a subclass of $CD4^+$ and $CD8^+$ T cells (suppressor T cells) that act primarily to suppress the function of other T cells, by secreting inhibitory cytokines or by cytolysis. However, the isolation of a unique subset of T cells that have a predominant suppressor action has been elusive. Another important mode of intrinsic regulation results from the production of antibodies or T cells that bind to determinants (idiotypes) in the antigen-binding domain of other antibodies or T-cell antigen receptors and serve to influence (inhibit) further antigen–antibody interactions.

The relative significance of *extrinsic regulation* of the immune response remains to be fully established. However, the increasing evidence of neural–immune interactions indicates that extrinsic factors of CNS origin play an important role in the modulation of the immune system. These data provide the foundation for nervous, endocrine, and immune system interactions (Table 1.12–7).

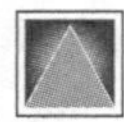

Table 1.12–7
Foundations of Nervous, Endocrine, and Immune System Interactions

Expression of receptors for neurotransmitters, hormones, and neuropeptides on immune cells
Autonomic nervous system innervation of lymphoid tissues
Conditioning of the immune response
Stress effects on immune function
Expression of cytokines and their receptors in the central nervous system
Influence of the immune system on neurotransmitter turnover, neuroendocrine function, and behavior

EVIDENCE OF NERVOUS SYSTEM AND IMMUNE SYSTEM INTERACTIONS

Immune Cell Receptors As outlined in Table 1.12–8, cells from the immune system express receptors for a wide variety of molecules that are, in part, regulated by or derived from the nervous system. One of the first receptors to be characterized in lymphocytes was the β-adrenergic receptor, which is the predominate adrenergic receptor subtype expressed on T and B cells. Subsequently, receptors for the other classic neurotransmitters have been described. As in the nervous system, receptors for the neurotransmitters in immune cells are located in the cell membrane and, in most cases, are coupled to G proteins and associated second-messenger pathways. Nevertheless, the biochemical mechanisms for the receptor-mediated activity of the majority of the molecules listed in Table 1.12–8 have yet to be fully elucidated.

Several important concepts from research on receptors in immune cells and tissues are central to understanding the effects of neurally derived molecules on immune function. First, the expression of receptors is heterogeneous. For example, of the two types of receptors for adrenal steroids, mineralocorticoid receptors and glucocorticoid receptors (GRs), only GRs are expressed in the thymus, whereas glucocorticoid and mineralocorticoid receptors are expressed in the spleen. Related to heterogeneity in receptor expression in immune cells and tissues is heterogeneity in receptor density.

Heterogeneity of receptor expression and density is relevant for determining the net effect of circulating transmitters on immune function. For example, the β_2-adrenergic receptor is expressed on resting and activated B cells, naive $CD4^+$ T cells, newly generated Th-1 cells, and Th-1 cell clones. However, it is not expressed on newly generated Th-2 cells or Th-2 cell clones. Consistent with these findings, norepinephrine (NE) has been found to enhance IL-12–induced differentiation of naive $CD4^+$ T cells into Th-1 cells and to promote production of IFN-γ by these cells. No effect was found on IL-4–induced Th-2 cell differentiation. The effect of NE on Th-1 type responses is also manifested by the ability of NE to help Th-1 cells support B-cell antibody production.

Another important concept is that a change in circulating concentrations of a hormone or transmitter is not necessarily reflected

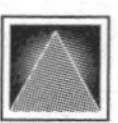

Table 1.12–8
Receptors for Neurotransmitters, Hormones, and Peptides on Immune Cells

Neurotransmitters	Hormones	Peptides
Acetylcholine Dopamine Histamine Norepinephrine Serotonin	Corticosteroids—glucocorticoids and mineralocorticoids Gonadal steroids—estrogen, progesterone, and testosterone Growth hormone Prolactin Opioids (endorphins and enkephalins) Thyroid hormone	Adrenocorticotropin hormone α-Melanocyte-stimulating hormone Arginine vasopressin Calcitonin Calcitonin gene-related peptide Corticotropin-releasing hormone Growth hormone-releasing hormone Gonadotropin-releasing hormone Insulin-like growth factor-1 Melatonin Neuropeptide Y Parathyroid hormone Somatostatin Substance P Thyrotropin-releasing hormone Thyroid-stimulating hormone Vasoactive intestinal peptide

equally in all immune compartments. For example, stress-related increases in glucocorticoids are more effective in activating GRs in the peripheral blood and the thymus than in the spleen. Thus, the microenvironment of any given tissue is critical in determining hormonal or neurotransmitter influences on immune function. Taken together with the heterogeneity in receptor expression and density, the data demonstrate that the influence of any given molecule on the immune system is a function of (1) the type of cell that exhibits the relevant receptor, (2) the density of the receptors on that cell, and (3) whether that cell is located in an immune compartment that allows access of the relevant molecule to the receptor under the conditions being studied.

Cross-talk between receptor-associated second-messenger pathways is another important mechanism by which neurally derived or regulated molecules can influence the immune response, and vice versa. For example, activation of p38 mitogen-activated protein kinase by IL-2 and IL-4 (as well as IL-1) has been shown to lead to disruption of GR function and may account for the glucocorticoid resistance seen in some inflammatory disorders and, possibly, major depression.

IN VITRO AND IN VIVO EFFECTS

Numerous chemical messengers derived from or regulated by the nervous system are capable of altering immune cell function and distribution. Table 1.12–9 provides a necessarily simplified, representative listing of selected hormones and their immune effects, and Table 1.12–10 lists some of the immune activities of neurotransmitters and neuropeptides. The immunological effects of these agents depend on

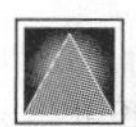

Table 1.12–9
Representative Listing of Hormone Messengers and Their Immunological Effects

Chemical Messengers (Hormones)	Immunological Activity	
	In Vitro	**In Vivo**
Adrenal steroids	Inhibition of IL-1, IL-2, interferon; augmentation of IL-4 production; inhibition of NK-cell activity, mitogen proliferation, and antigen presentation; promotion of T-cell differentiation toward Th-2 profile and away from Th-1 profile	Thymic involution; lymphopenia; monocytopenia; neutrophilia; suppression of inflammation and cell-mediated immunity during chronic exposure; enhancement of immune responsiveness during acute exposure, modulation of apoptosis, and immune cell trafficking
Estrogen	Inhibition of suppressor T-cell and NK-cell activity; increased macrophage phagocytosis and lysosomal activity; promotion of T-cell differentiation toward Th-1 profile; increased IL-6 and IL-10; inhibition of B-cell apoptosis	Lymphopenia; decreased mitogen responsiveness, NK-cell activity, and macrophage phagocytosis; increased plasma cells in spleen; promotion of autoantibodies
Progesterone	Decreased mitogen responsiveness at high concentrations; inhibition of T-cell activation and cytotoxicity; inhibition of NK-cell activity; inhibition of prostaglandin synthesis; promotion of T-cell differentiation toward Th-2 profile	Increased skin graft survival; increased survival of xenographic tumor cells; increased risk of viral infection; decreased $CD4^+$ cell numbers
Growth hormone	Enhancement of mitogen responsiveness and cytotoxic T-cell activity; priming of macrophages and neutrophils for superoxide anion release; augmentation of neutrophil differentiation; enhancement of neutrophil and macrophage phagocytosis; increased synthesis of interferon γ	Increase of thymus and spleen size and cellularity; augmentation of antibody synthesis, T- and B-cell proliferation, IL-2 production, mitogen responsiveness, NK-cell activity; promotion of survival during bacterial infection
Insulin-like growth factor	Prevention of promyeloid cell apoptosis; promotion of priming of macrophages and neutrophils for superoxide anion release; enhancement of neutrophil and macrophage phagocytosis	Promotion of hematopoiesis and lymphopoiesis; increase of thymus and spleen size and cellularity; enhancement of overall immune responsiveness in aged animals
PRL	Removal of PRL from culture media inhibits DNA synthesis and cell proliferation; comitogenic with IL-2; inhibition of T-cell apoptosis; promotion of Th-2 cytokine production from T cells	Increase of thymus and spleen size and cellularity; counteraction of glucocorticoid-mediated immunosuppression; PRL removal reduces NK-cell activity and T-cell proliferation and increases lethality of *Listeria* challenge; stimulation of autoimmunity

IL, interleukin; NK, natural killer; PRL, prolactin; Th-1, type 1 T-helper cell; Th-2, type 2 T-helper cell.

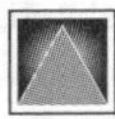

Table 1.12–10
Immunological Effects of Representative Neurotransmitters and Neuropeptides

Chemical Messengers	Immunological Activity	
	In Vitro	**In Vivo**
Neurotransmitters		
Norepinephrine	Stimulation of T-cell proliferation at low concentrations; inhibition of T-cell proliferation at high concentrations; enhancement of IL-12–induced differentiation of naive CD4 cells into Th-1 cells; stimulation of IFN-γ production by Th-1 cells	Influence on immune cell trafficking; redistribution of NK cells from spleen to blood; inhibition of NK-cell activity and cytolytic T-cell activity; inhibition of generation of antigen-specific T cells in draining lymph nodes, but increase in inflammation in joints during autoimmune arthritis
Serotonin	At suprapharmacologic concentrations: suppression of lymphocyte reactivity to mitogens and antigens At physiological concentrations: inhibition of monocyte-induced suppression of NK-cell activity; promotion of capacity of macrophages to enhance T-cell activation; enhancement of macrophage superoxide production and IFN-γ–induced phagocytosis; stimulation of chemotactic factors; contribution to DTH	Suppression of humoral and cellular immune responses; enhancement of immune activity when serotonin availability is decreased
Neuropeptides		
Opioids	Enhancement of T-cell proliferation, NK-cell activity, cytokine production, and generation of cytotoxic T cells	Mediation of immunosuppressive effects of stress on NK-cell activity; inhibition of mitogen-induced lymphocyte proliferation and phagocytic cell function; inhibition of antibody production; diminished DTH; promotion of splenic immune cell apoptosis
Substance P	Enhancement of lymphocyte proliferation, lymphocyte and monocyte chemotaxis, and monocyte production of IL-1, IL-6, and tumor necrosis factor; augmentation of IgA synthesis; enhancement of IL-2 production; induction of mast cell degranulation; promotion of superoxide anion release from neutrophils and eosinophils	Increased severity of adjuvant-induced arthritis; association with hypersensitivity reactions and chronic inflammatory disorders
Adrenocorticotropic hormone	Suppression of antibody production and disruption of macrophage-mediated tumoricidal activity	Activation of immunoregulatory glucocorticoids
Corticotropin-releasing hormone	Stimulation of T- and B-cell proliferation; enhancement of IL-1 and IL-6 secretion but inhibition of IFN-γ secretion	Exertion of mixed proinflammatory (e.g., in the periphery) and immunosuppressive (central) actions; promotion of IL-1 production in central nervous system and increase in IL-2; activation of the hypothalamic-pituitary-adrenal axis; suppression of NK-cell activity in the spleen; inhibition of antibody production and decrease in T-cell numbers; inhibition of mitogen-induced T-cell proliferation
Vasoactive intestinal peptide	Enhancement of monocyte chemotaxis; inhibition of Ig and IL-2 production; inhibition of NK-cell activity and one-way mixed lymphocyte reaction	Inhibition of egress of lymphocytes from sheep lymph nodes
α-Melanocyte-stimulating hormone	Inhibition of proinflammatory cytokine release from peripheral blood mononuclear cells	Antipyretic and antiinflammatory

DTH, delayed-type hypersensitivity; IFN, interferon; Ig, immunoglobulin; IL, interleukin; NK, natural killer; Th-1, type 1 T-helper cell.

a number of factors, aside from those involving the relevant expression, density, and activation of receptors on target immune cells. For example, the effect of any given molecule on the immune system depends on the phase of the immune response that is involved. As previously noted, the major phases of an immune response include the induction phase, the activation and proliferation phase, and the effector phase. NE, for example, has been found to promote immune function during the induction phase, to potentiate and inhibit immune function during the activation and proliferation phase, and to inhibit the effector phase. The potentiation of the proliferative phase occurs at low concentrations of NE, but inhibition occurs at high NE concentrations. These findings indicate that the timing of exposure as well as the dose are important.

Issues of timing are also relevant in terms of development and aging. In aged rats, for example, a progressive loss of noradrenergic innervation of the spleen is accompanied by a progressive increase in the density of β receptors on splenic lymphocytes. However, there is also an age-related dysfunction that involves impaired coupling between the β receptor and adenylate cyclase, indicating that noradrenergic agents may have variable, unpredictable effects on immune function in aged animals.

Related to the phase of the immune response and the developmental stage of the animal is the type of immune response as it relates to pathophysiology. Substances that are primarily inhibitory to immune function may promote tumor development in animals with cancer but may attenuate the development of autoimmune disease. For example, the administration of glucocorticoids accelerates the growth of tumors in mice. But glucocorticoids inhibit the development of several types of autoimmune disorders, including experimental allergic encephalitis (a model of multiple sclerosis) and streptococcal cell wall–induced polyarthritis (a model of rheumatoid arthritis). Relevant to the effects of gonadal steroids on immune function, estrogens tend to promote Th-1–type responses, whereas progesterone tends to promote Th-2–type responses. Accordingly, during pregnancy, Th-2–type immune responses prevail (possibly secondary to the increased influence of progesterone), and autoimmune disorders related to excessive Th-1–like activity (multiple sclerosis and rheumatoid arthritis) improve. In contrast, diseases related to Th-2–like activity (systemic lupus erythematosus) are exacerbated during pregnancy.

Another important factor in determining the immunological effect of a particular molecule is its indirect effects, as well as its direct effects, on the immune system. In vitro studies provide important information on the direct effects of the various chemical messengers, but the influence of those agents in vivo may be completely different. For example, a number of in vitro studies have shown that opioid peptides are capable of enhancing NK-cell activity (NKCA). However, in vivo, opioid peptides play an important role in mediating the inhibitory effects of shock stress on NKCA, most likely through effects in the brain. In vivo, neurally derived molecules act against a complicated background of multiple hormones that may have synergistic or antagonist effects, or both. For example, prolactin antagonizes the effects of glucocorticoids on spleen mitogen responses in mice. Furthermore, many of the hormones and transmitters influence other bodily systems, including the cardiovascular system, which may influence the traffic of immune cells to various organs, immunological and otherwise. Changes in immunocyte distribution may ultimately have effects on cellular function.

NEURAL INNERVATION OF LYMPHOID TISSUES

Historically, the identification of nerve fibers derived from the sympathetic nervous system (SNS) in immune tissues was one of the first indications that communication between the CNS and the immune system was possible. Sympathetic nerve fibers have been identified in organs that are responsible for the development, education, and function of lymphocytes. Specifically, nerve fibers are found in the bone marrow, thymus, spleen, and lymph nodes. The nerves that innervate the thymus gland are derived from the vagus, phrenic, and recurrent laryngeal nerves and from the stellate and other small ganglia of the thoracic sympathetic chain. The nonmyelinated nerves that innervate the bone marrow arise from the level of the spinal cord associated with the location of the bone. The spleen obtains its sympathetic nerves from the celiac ganglion. Autonomic nervous system (ANS) innervation of the lymph nodes is not as dense or as uniquely distributed as noted for the spleen and the thymus.

In general, sympathetic nerve fibers enter the lymphoid tissues in association with the vascular supply. Because those nerves play an important role in vascular tone, their presence in association with the smooth muscle cells of the blood vessels is not unexpected. However, the nerve fibers travel with small blood vessels devoid of smooth muscle cells and are present in the parenchyma of the lymphoid tissue, associated not only with blood vessels but with lymphocytes and other immune cells (Fig. 1.12–5). Electron microscopy has shown that sympathetic nerve terminal endings exist in close approximation with lymphocytes and macrophages. This suggests that the SNS can influence the immune system by changing the vascular tone and blood flow into lymphoid organs or by directly influencing immune cell function via locally released neurotransmitters that, in turn, interact with specific receptors on nearby immune cells and ultimately influence their function. Although not as well characterized, recent data support an immune modulatory role for the parasympathetic branch of the ANS. Stimulation of the vagus nerve (a primary parasympathetic outflow pathway) has been shown to attenuate the systemic response to endotoxin administration, an effect believed to be secondary to local release of acetylcholine, given that acetylcholine inhibits endotoxin-stimulated TNF-α production from macrophages in vitro.

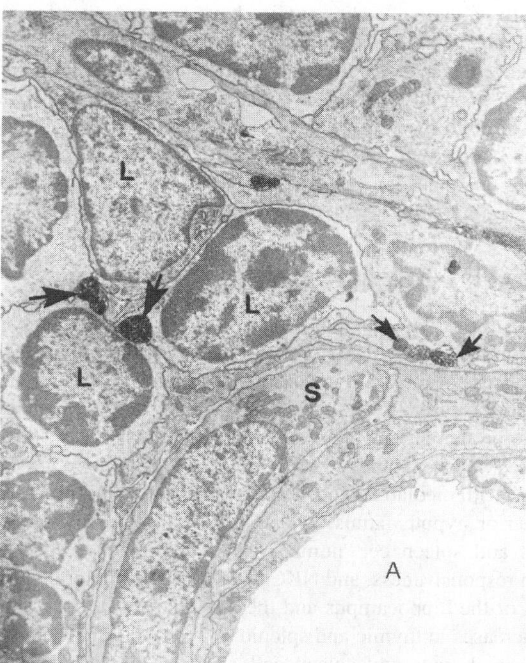

FIGURE 1.12–5 Sympathetic nervous system innervation of lymphoid tissue. Tyrosine hydroxylase–immunoreactive nerve processes (*small arrows*) in contact with the smooth muscle (S) of the central arteriole (A), and nerve processes (*large arrows*) in direct contact with lymphocytes (L) in the periarteriolar lymphatic sheath of the rat spleen. Transmission electron micrograph, × 6,732. (Courtesy of Denise L. Bellinger, Center for Neuroimmunology, Loma Linda University, Loma Linda, CA, and Suzanne Y. Felten, Department of Neurobiology and Anatomy, University of Rochester School of Medicine and Dentistry, Rochester, NY.)

Since catecholamines (including NE) have stimulatory effects on immune function at low concentrations and inhibitory effects at high concentrations, differential SNS effects on the immune response are possible, depending on local concentrations of catecholamines and the location of the immune cell relative to the point of neurotransmitter release. Chemical sympathectomy has variable effects on immune function, depending in part on the phase of the immune response studied. The reported effects of sympathectomy include suppressed antibody responses to sheep red blood cells, suppressed cytolytic T-cell activity, and enhanced NKCA. Splenic sympathectomy also leads to an upregulation of β-adrenergic receptors on lymphocytes and a decrease in suppressor lymphocyte function. Aside from the phase of the immune response, other factors that may influence the effects of nervous innervation on immune function include the animal's age, sex, and strain.

A variety of neuropeptides, including neuropeptide Y, substance P, vasoactive intestinal peptide, calcitonin gene-related peptide, and corticotropin releasing hormone, are colocalized with neurotransmitters in nerves innervating immune tissues. The distribution of these peptides has not been extensively studied, and their relative significance has yet to be determined.

Data suggest that local immune responses within the microenvironment of the immune tissues also may be able to interact directly with nerve fibers through the effects of cytokines on neurotransmitter release. Neurotransmitters may, in turn, regulate immune function or the sensitivity of cells to local immunomodulatory factors.

Finally, although earlier studies have focused on efferent nerve fibers, more attention is now being paid to sensory afferent fibers and their relevance to immune system communication with the brain. For example, sensory afferent fibers appear to relay immune signals through the vagus nerve, to the nucleus of the solitary tract. From the nucleus of the solitary tract, there are pathways to other brain regions that may be relevant to the CNS response to immune system activation.

CNS LESIONS AND CELLULAR IMMUNITY

Some of the earliest studies demonstrating CNS involvement in the regulation of immune phenomena were those involving lesions in specific areas of the brain in laboratory animals. In a series of experiments in the early 1960s, lesions of the anterior hypothalamus were found to protect guinea pigs from death by anaphylactic shock when compared to sham and control lesions. Such protection was not apparent with median and posterior hypothalamic lesions. Lesions of the anterior hypothalamus were also accompanied by decreases in thymus and spleen cell number, splenic mitogen responsiveness, antigen responsiveness, and NKCA. In contrast, bilateral electrolytic lesions of the hippocampus and the amygdala have been associated with increases in thymic and splenic mitogen responsiveness and no change in thymus and spleen cell number. Left-sided neocortical lesions have been associated with decreases in spleen T-cell numbers, T-cell mitogen proliferation, T-cell cytotoxicity (measured in mixed lymphocyte cultures), and NKCA; these immune parameters were unchanged or enhanced by right-sided lesions. B-cell and macrophage responses were not affected by right-sided or left-sided neocortical ablations.

Some investigators have reported an increased prevalence of immune disorders in humans, especially those disorders involving the thyroid and the gastrointestinal (GI) tract, in association with atypical cerebral dominance (left-handedness). The relation between cerebral dominance and immune dysfunction in humans lends support to the notion that lateralized alterations in CNS function may have differential effects on the immune response. However, some patients with brain tumors and head injuries have gross disturbances of in vitro lymphocyte function, and there is no evidence that the immune changes are related to the laterality of the lesion.

BEHAVIORAL CONDITIONING

Demonstration that learning processes are capable of influencing immunological function is another example of interactions between the immune system and the nervous system. Several classical conditioning paradigms have been associated with the suppression or enhancement of the immune response in various experimental designs. The conditioning of immunological reactivity provides further evidence that the CNS can have significant immunomodulatory effects.

Some of the first experiments on immunological conditioning were derived from the serendipitous observation that animals undergoing extinction in a taste-aversion paradigm with cyclophosphamide (Cytoxan), an immunosuppressive agent, had unexpected mortality. In that taste-aversion paradigm, the animals were simultaneously exposed to an oral saccharin solution (the conditioned stimulus) and an intraperitoneal injection of cyclophosphamide (unconditioned stimulus). Because the animals experienced considerable physical discomfort from the cyclophosphamide injection, through the process of conditioning, they began to associate the ill effects of cyclophosphamide with the taste of the oral saccharin solution. If given a choice, the animals avoided the saccharin solution (taste aversion). Conditioned avoidance can be eliminated or extinguished if the saccharin is repeatedly presented in the absence of cyclophosphamide. However, it was observed that animals undergoing extinction of cyclophosphamide-induced taste aversion unexpectedly died, leading to the speculation that the oral saccharin solution had a specific conditioned association with the immunosuppressive effects of cyclophosphamide. Repeated exposure to the saccharin-associated conditioned immunosuppression during extinction might explain the unexpected death of animals. To test that hypothesis, researchers conditioned the animals with saccharin (conditioned stimulus) and intraperitoneal cyclophosphamide (unconditioned conditioned stimulus) and then immunized them with sheep red blood cells. At different times after immunization, the conditioned animals were reexposed to saccharin (conditioned stimulus) and examined. The conditioned animals exhibited a significant decrease in mean antibody titers to sheep red blood cells as compared to the control animals. Thus, the evidence demonstrated that immunosuppression of humoral immunity was occurring in response to the conditioned stimulus of saccharin alone.

Because the immunological effects of conditioned immunosuppression were not large, the influence of immunological conditioning on the development of a spontaneously occurring autoimmune disease in New Zealand mice was investigated. These animals provide a standard model for the study of systemic lupus erythematosus, a fatal autoimmune disorder that is similar to that found in humans. Death in the New Zealand mice can be delayed by weekly injections of cyclophosphamide. In the initial studies, the animals were first conditioned with saccharin and cyclophosphamide and then divided into three groups: (1) saccharin only (conditioned stimulus group), (2) saccharin and cyclophosphamide (conditioned stimulus plus unconditioned stimulus group), and (3) no treatment. As shown in Figure 1.12–6, animals given saccharin alone had a mortality rate as low as the animals receiving saccharin plus weekly injections of cyclophosphamide; these findings supported the notion that conditioned immunosuppression was occurring in response to saccharin alone, and the effects were of sufficient magnitude to powerfully influence disease expression.

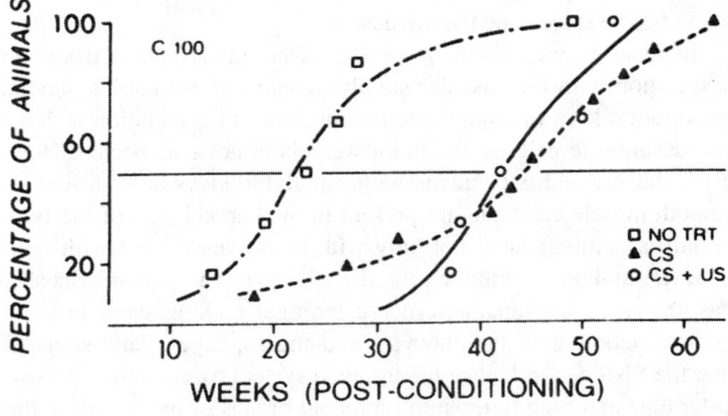

FIGURE 1.12–6 Conditioned immunosuppression. Mortality rate in first filial generation female mice (New Zealand black × New Zealand white) treated with saccharin and cyclophosphamide (CY) weekly and then continued on a regimen of saccharin and CY (group conditioned stimulus [CS] + unconditioned stimulus [US], N = 6), continued on saccharin alone (group CS, N = 11), or deprived of saccharin and CY (no treatment [TRT], N = 6). (From Ader R. Behaviorally conditioned modulation of immunity. In: Guillemin R, Cohen M, Melnechuk T, eds. *Neural Modulation of Immunity.* New York: Raven Press; 1985, with permission.)

The ability to condition immunosuppression using T-cell–independent antigens and a graph-versus-host response (T cells present in transplanted bone marrow attack the host) has indicated that conditioned immunosuppression generalizes to humoral and cell-mediated immunity. Furthermore, conditioned enhancement of NKCA in response to the conditioned stimulus, camphor, has been found after repeated pairing of the immunostimulant poly I:C with camphor odor. Finally, studies of conditioning of immune responses have been expanded to include environmental stimuli, such as those inherent in passive avoidance paradigms. In these studies, certain aversive environments can be associated with conditioned immunosuppression.

STRESS AND THE IMMUNE RESPONSE

Stress and Illness Interest in the effects of stress on the immune system grew out of a series of animal and human studies suggesting that stressful stimuli can influence the development of immune-related disorders, including infections, cancer, and autoimmune diseases. Experiments conducted on laboratory animals in the late 1950s and the early 1960s, for example, indicated that a wide variety of stressors—including isolation, rotation, crowding, exposure to a predator, and electric shock—increased morbidity and mortality in response to several types of tumors and infectious disease caused by viruses and parasites. However, as research progressed it became increasingly clear that *stress* is too variegated a concept to have singular effects on immunity and that, in fact, the effects of stress on immunity can be opposite depending on a number of factors. Chief among these factors is whether a stressor is acute or chronic. Other critical variables include stressor severity and type, as well as the timing of stressor application and the type of tumor or infectious agent investigated. For example, mice subjected to electric grid shock 1 to 3 days before the injection of Maloney murine sarcoma virus–induced tumor cells exhibited a decreased tumor size and incidence. In contrast, mice exposed to grid shock 2 days after tumor cell injection exhibited an increase in tumor size and number.

Fewer studies have been carried out on the relation between stress and immune-related illnesses in humans, and, not infrequently, these studies are difficult to interpret because of the many factors that can influence illness and illness behavior. Nevertheless, mounting data support a relationship between chronic stress and increased immune-related disorders. For example, a series of prospective studies on experimentally induced upper respiratory virus infection have demonstrated that stressful life events can increase the susceptibility to infectious disease in humans. Investigators found that infection rates by five separate rhinoviruses administered intranasally were significantly greater in persons experiencing a high degree of psychological stress than in those experiencing low stress. Chronic stress also has been found to correlate with decreased antibody responses to vaccines and delayed wound healing. Similarly, naturalistic studies indicate that psychological stress hastens progression to AIDS in HIV-infected individuals. Indeed, after 5 years of follow-up, individuals above the median in terms of life stress were two to three times more likely to have developed AIDS than were patients below the median. In terms of autoimmune disorders, a number of studies have noted that increased life stress correlates with worsening of symptom expression (although effects may be dependent on stressor severity). Prospective studies in humans on the effect of stress on cancer development are mixed. Some studies have indicated a relationship between life stress or depression, or both, (presumably, secondary to increased stress and inability to cope) and cancer development; others have been unable to replicate these findings. Pointing to the complexity of the issue, a recent study found that, although not affecting cancer development per se, stress synergistically increased breast cancer development in women with physical risk factors, such as smoking, family cancer history, and early menstruation. Once cancer has developed, however, it appears more certain that stress and related factors, such as personality and coping styles, influence the development of disease-related morbidity and survival. In keeping with this, several studies suggest that psychotherapeutic interventions can lengthen survival time in cancer patients. However, other studies have been unable to confirm these findings. This discrepancy might result from several factors, including the type of therapy used, the length of therapeutic intervention, and differences in patient groups, especially given that most of these studies did not select subjects based on psychosocial stress or depressive symptoms, or both.

Immune Parameters during Stress In an attempt to understand the effects of stress on illness, a number of studies have examined the effect of stress on a variety of disease-relevant immune parameters. Nevertheless, even a moment's reflection suggests that stress is a protean entity that defies easy classification. Although generally considered to be any external or internal event that challenges organismal homeostasis, stress has been used to label a wide array of phenomena, from mild environmental perturbations to life-threatening cataclysms. In addition, stress is sometimes confined to actual internal or external stressors and is sometimes broadened to include an organism's perception of a stressor. Given all this, it is not surprising that, when stress is taken in its broadest sense, no consistent pattern of stress-induced immune alterations is readily apparent. However, when stress is divided into acute or mild, or both, versus severe or chronic, or both, forms, a clearer relationship between stress and immune functioning becomes manifest (Table 1.12–11). In general, acute or mild stressors tend to enhance aspects of cellular and humoral immunity, whereas severe or chronic stressors tend to suppress these same parameters.

Acute or Mild Stress Increasingly, it is recognized that in addition to contributing to medical morbidity, the body's stress response system plays a central role in maintaining an organism's functional integrity in the face of shifting environmental conditions. Thus, although chronic stress system activation has been found to correlate with medical morbidity, appropriate and time-limited stress system activation does not appear to carry a similar risk and, in fact, may be associated with positive psychological functioning. In keeping with this, data from laboratory animals suggest that brief or mild stressors may actually enhance acquired immunity. For example, in a series of elegant experiments in rats, it has been shown that a brief stressor (i.e., 2 hours of physical restraint or shaking) applied before antigen challenge significantly enhances DTH, an antigen-specific reaction mediated by CD4 T lymphocytes. Similarly, rodents exposed to an acute or mild stressor, or both, before antigen presentation have been reported to demonstrate enhanced humoral immunity by producing more antibodies than animals exposed to the same antigen in the control condition. Interestingly, the enhanced DTH and humoral immunity observed with mild or acute stressors is opposite to the effects seen if the stress intensity or duration is increased, even if the stressor type remains the same. In the case of DTH, the enhancing effect of acute stress depends on a stress-related release of corticosterone. Similarly, acute administration of epinephrine also increases DTH. However, chronic administration of corticosterone suppresses DTH in much the same manner as does chronic stress, strongly suggesting that stress hormones, even ones classically considered to be immunosuppressive, may have different, even

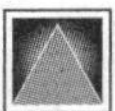

Table 1.12–11
Effects of Acute Stress, Chronic Stress, and Depression on Immune Parameters in Humans

Immune Variable	Acute Stress	Chronic Stress	Major Depression
White blood cells	↑/↑	↑/↑	↑/↑
Lymphocytes	→	→	↓/↓
Monocytes	→	→	→
T lymphocytes	→	↓/↓	→
B lymphocytes	↓/↓	↓/↓	→
CD4$^+$ cells	→	↓/↓	→
CD8$^+$ cells	↑/↑	↓/↓	→
NK cells	↑/↑	↓/↓	→
CD4$^+$/CD8$^+$	↑	↓/↓	→
Percentage of B cells	→	→	→
Percentage of T cells	→	↓/↓	→
Percentage of CD4$^+$	↓	→	→
Percentage of CD8$^+$	↑	↓/↓	→
Percentage of CD4$^+$/CD8$^+$	→	→	→
Percentage of NK cells	?	→	→
NKCA (total)	↑/↑	↓/↓	↓/↓
NKCA (per cell)	→	↓	↓
Mitogen-induced proliferation	↓	↓/↓	↓/↓
Response to vaccine	?	↓	?
Antibody titers to Epstein-Barr virus	?	↓/↓	?
Cytolytic T-cell response to antigen	?	↓	?
Wound healing	?	↓	?
Ratio of type 1 T-helper cell cytokines to type 2 T-helper cell cytokines	↑	↓	?
Delayed-type hypersensitivity	?	→	↓

↑/↑, positive effect confirmed by metaanalysis; ↑, majority of studies suggest positive effect; ↓/↓, negative effect confirmed by metaanalysis; ↓, majority of studies suggest negative effect; →, conflicting findings; ?, not enough data to suggest positive or negative relationship; CD4/CD8, ratio of CD4$^+$ T lymphocytes to CD8$^+$ T lymphocytes; NK, natural killer; NKCA, natural killer–cell activity.

Reprinted with permission from Raison CL, Gumnick JF, Miller, AH. Neuroendocrine–immune interactions: implications for health and behavior. In: Pfaff DW, Arnold AP, Etgen AM, Fahrbach SE, Rubin RT, eds. *Hormones, Brain and Behavior.* Vol 5. San Diego, CA: Academic Press; 2002, with permission.

opposite, effects on immune functioning, depending on the severity and duration of the stress that leads to their production.

Although many studies have examined the immune effects of brief, mild stressors in humans, little of this data bears directly on potential enhancements in naturalistic measures of actual immune functioning, such as the DTH or antibody production. Rather, studies of acute stress in humans have focused on changes in enumerative and in vitro immune system functional assessments. Based on many studies and two metaanalyses, a clear pattern of immune changes emerges from a host of acute stressors, ranging from mental arithmetic and public speaking to first-time parachute jumping (Table 1.12–11). Enumerative changes include increased numbers of white blood cells, CD8 T lymphocytes, and NK cells and decreased numbers of total T and B lymphocytes. Functional changes associated with acute stressors in humans include a decrease in lymphocyte responses to several nonantigenic mitogens and an increase in NKCA, although it should be noted that this increased activity may only reflect an increase in NK-cell number and not an increase in activity per NK cell. It is important to note that this pattern of immune changes is seen most consistently in response to brief, *laboratory*-type stressors, such as brief public speaking or role playing tasks. Relatively short duration naturalistic stressors, such as taking examinations, produce immune changes similar to those seen with more chronic forms of stress, indicating that, in humans at least, stress rapidly becomes *chronic* in terms of immune system effect.

Chronic or Severe Stress In keeping with the well-documented health risks associated with chronic or severe stress, many studies confirm that, in animals and humans, these more pernicious types of stressors are associated with immune alterations that may predispose toward disease development and that are, in some cases, opposite to the changes seen in the context of acute or mild stress, or both (i.e., laboratory stressors in humans) (Table 1.12–11). Many individual studies and two large metaanalyses find that, in humans, naturalistic stressors lasting from days to years evince a consistent pattern of in vitro enumerative and functional immune changes. Enumerative changes include an increase in circulating white blood cells and a decrease in CD4 and CD8 cells, with a decrease in the ratio of CD4 (helper) to CD8 (cytotoxic) T cells. Functional changes associated with chronic stress include a decrease in NKCA and in the proliferation of lymphocytes after mitogen stimulation. One, but not both, of the metaanalyses also found chronic stress to be associated with a decreased number of B cells, T cells, and NK cells.

In animals and humans, chronic or severe stress has been found to affect humoral (i.e., antibody) and cellular immunity in ways directly relevant to real world immune functioning. Stressors such as exam taking or caring for a demented spouse have been repeatedly shown to impair the body's ability to suppress the activity of latent viruses (especially Epstein-Barr virus), as measured by an increase in latent viral antibodies, and have been shown to interfere with antibody development after vaccination. Consistent with these findings, examination and caregiving stress are associated with decrements in memory T cell responses to latent virus antigens and to vaccines, in terms of antigen-induced T-cell proliferation and T-cell–mediated killing of virally transformed B lymphocytes. DTH is the standard test of in vivo cell-mediated immunity, and, as discussed previously, animal studies suggest that chronic or severe stress impairs DTH, as would be predicted by latent virus and vaccine-related findings in humans. However, little is known about the effect of chronic or severe stress on DTH in humans, and the available results are equivocal. Thus, although relatively brief naturalistic stressors, such as exam taking, marathon running, or surgery, appear to suppress DTH, longer stressors, such as bereavement or caregiving, have been reported not to affect DTH, even while being associated with suppression of nonspecific T-cell proliferation and other typically stress-related abnormalities in T-cell function and enumerative measures.

In addition to effects on enumerative, functional, and naturalistic measures of immune functioning, it has become increasingly recognized that acute and chronic stress alter the mix of cytokines produced by T lymphocytes and that this alteration may contribute to the effects of stress on immunity. It appears that acute or mild stress in animals and humans favors the in vitro production of the Th-1 cytokine IFN-γ without increasing the Th-2 cytokine IL-4. Interestingly, the increase in DTH observed in rodents under conditions of brief, mild stress also depends on a stress-associated increase in IFN-γ, suggesting that in vitro measures of Th-1–Th-2 balance are relevant to naturalistic immune functioning. On the other hand, chronic or severe stressors in animals and humans tend to suppress lymphocyte production of the Th-1 cytokines IFN-γ and IL-2, while not affecting or actually increasing the Th-2 cytokines IL-4 and IL-10. In addition to in vitro lymphocyte cytokine production, other findings consistent with chronic or severe stress-enhancing activity of Th-2 cytokines include a decrease of IL-2 receptor–positive lymphocytes after mitogen stimulation and a reduced response of NK cells to IFN-γ and IL-2.

Stress Activates Innate Immunity Although stress has been most often seen as suppressing immune function, recent data indicate that a wide variety of stressors may activate innate immunity (especially the production of proinflammatory cytokines), even while suppressing in vitro and in vivo measures of acquired immunity. For example, in rodents, brief electric foot and tail shock increases alveolar macrophage production of proinflammatory cytokines and augments nitric oxide (NO) release from macrophages stimulated in vitro with lipopolysaccharide. Enhanced macrophage NO release has been observed in infant squirrel monkeys separated for 24 hours from their mothers, suggesting that stress-induced augmentation of innate immunity cannot be accounted for by any physical damage that might ensue from electric shock. In humans, peripheral production of IL-1β or IL-1 soluble receptor antagonist (sIL-1ra) has been reported to be increased in the context of several acutely stressful situations, including medical school examinations and brief laboratory stressors.

Recent data indicate that acute laboratory stressors also activate intracellular transcription factors that play a central role in mediating the physiological effects of proinflammatory cytokines. In response to a public speaking and mental arithmetic task, 17 out of 19 subjects demonstrated activation of nuclear factor κB (NF-κB) in parallel with stress-induced increases in cortisol and catecholamines. Corollary animal data demonstrated that stress-related NF-κB activation could be reduced by blockade of α_1-adrenergic receptors, suggesting that, although sympathetic nervous system activity may inhibit certain immune functions, it may also be a primary player in stress-related enhancement of innate immunity.

Chronic stress may also be associated with enhanced proinflammatory activity. For example, increased chronic stress before experimental inoculation with influenza A virus was found to correlate with higher IL-6 concentrations in nasal lavage and with increased symptom scores, suggesting that stress-related inflammatory activation may impair the body's ability to fight viral infection. In a longitudinal study, elderly persons undergoing the stress of caring for a spouse with dementia demonstrated significantly increased serum levels of IL-6 over a 6-year period when compared to matched, noncaregiving controls. This fourfold difference in IL-6 increase over the study period could not be accounted for by factors such as differences between groups in chronic health problems, medication status, or health-relevant behaviors (e.g., smoking and so forth). Interestingly, caregiving for a spouse with dementia has been associated with increased medical morbidity, suggesting that stress-induced increases in proinflammatory activity may have demonstrable effects on real-world health outcomes.

Immunological Mechanisms Only recently have investigators begun to examine the immunological mechanisms through which stress may affect the immune system. In general, a stressor can alter immune function in two major ways. First, the stressor can lead to changes in the distribution of immune cells in any given part of the body. Second, stress can alter the function of the immune cells themselves. Because the immune response depends on the interplay of various immune cell subtypes, a redistribution of relevant cell types into or out of a particular immune compartment can directly influence the local immune response. For example, significant and selective changes in immune cell distribution have been described in rats undergoing a mild acute stress (2 hours of restraint), including decreased numbers and percentages of cells in the peripheral blood and a concomitant increase in immune cells in the skin. It appears that cells leaving the blood during acute stress may migrate to the skin, where they might be more likely to encounter pathogens.

In addition to redistribution effects, stressors have also been shown to alter a variety of cell-specific activities, including IL-2 production and expression of the IL-2 receptor gene. In a study examining the biochemical mechanisms of stress-induced impairment of T-cell mitogenesis, spleen cells isolated from rats exposed to two brief stressors (5 minutes of restraint or 2 minutes of foot shock) exhibited a diminished response to T-cell mitogens and a combination of the phorbol ester tetradecanoylphorbol acetate and the calcium ionophore ionomycin. Because stimulation with the latter two agents mimics early signals generated by mitogen surface receptor binding, including increased intracellular calcium and protein kinase C activation, the data indicate that stress-related defects in T-cell proliferation occur at sites beyond or in addition to the early events in cellular activation. Intriguing data suggest that stress-induced activation of proinflammatory elements may contribute to many classical immunosuppressive findings associated with stress. For example, production of NO by macrophages (an early step in inflammatory activation) has been shown to be involved in the biochemical mechanisms underlying the ability of stress to reduce lymphocyte proliferation. Depletion of macrophages and inhibition of NO synthesis have been shown to attenuate stress-induced changes in acquired immunity. Consistent with this finding, it is known that chronic proinflammatory cytokine production inhibits several indices of T-cell–mediated immunity.

POTENTIAL NEUROENDOCRINE MECHANISMS AND MEDIATORS

A number of studies have focused on the neuroendocrine mechanisms by which stress and stress-related alterations in CNS function may influence the immune response. The two systems that have received the most attention are the endocrine system, especially the HPA axis and the ANS. These two systems are intimately associated with the organism's response to stress, and immune cells and tissues not only express receptors for the transmitters and hormones emanating from these systems, but also receive direct innervation from ANS fibers.

The interplay of the HPA axis and ANS with the immune system has been the focus of numerous experiments. The data indicate that the HPA axis and the ANS have specific and selective effects on the immune system that are determined in part by which immune compartment and which type of immune response are examined. For example, after mild foot shock, investigators have found suppression of splenic and peripheral blood lymphocyte responses to nonspecific T-cell mitogens. Removing endogenous corticosteroids by adrenalectomy prevents shock-induced suppression of the proliferative response of T cells in the peripheral blood. However, adrenalectomy has no effect on the stress-induced suppression of T-cell proliferation in the spleen. On the other hand, β-adrenergic receptor blockade attenuates shock-induced suppression of T-cell proliferation in the spleen but has no effect on stress-induced T-cell proliferation in the peripheral blood. In addition to body compartment specificity, stress system effects on immunity are time dependent. Early immune responses to a stressor, in animals and humans, have been repeatedly shown to depend on ANS activity (activation of the SNS), whereas later responses to a stressor are more profoundly influenced by HPA axis activity.

A central factor in the regulation of the response to stress is *corticotropin-releasing hormone* (*CRH*). In addition to modifying a number of animal behaviors, CRH is a pivotal molecule in mediating the HPA axis and SNS outflow of the stress response to peripheral tissues. The effects of CRH on an array of immune functions have been well characterized. CRH administered intracerebroventricularly (ICV) was first shown to have a powerful immunosuppressive effect on NKCA in the rat spleen that was dependent on CRH activation of the SNS. Follow-up studies have shown that CRH is also capable of inhibiting in vivo antibody formation, specifically, the generation of an IgG response to immunization with keyhole limpet hemocyanin. The influence of CRH on antibody responses is also apparent in CRH-overproducing mice whose immune deficits are characterized by a profound decrease in B-cell number and severely diminished primary and memory antibody responses. Chronic ICV administration of CRH and acute infusion of CRH into the locus ceruleus have been shown to suppress lymphocyte proliferative responses to nonspecific mitogens and antibody to the T-cell receptor (anti-CD3).

Interestingly, CRH also stimulates the release of proinflammatory cytokines in laboratory animals and humans. Long-term ICV administration of CRH to rats led to induction of IL-1β messenger ribonucleic acid RNA (mRNA) in splenocytes, and intravenous (IV) infusion of CRH in humans led to an almost fourfold induction of IL-1α. Both treatments also led to significant increases in the immunoregulatory cytokine IL-2. Finally, the proinflammatory effects of CRH are manifested in the direct autocrine or paracrine inflammatory actions of this peptide at peripheral sites of inflammation, such as in an inflamed arthritic joint. Taken together, these results demonstrate that CRH has well-documented immunosuppressive effects on in vivo cellular and humoral responses, while having a stimulatory effect on cytokine production and local inflammation.

The mechanisms by which centrally acting CRH influences the immune response have been increasingly elucidated. Two major outflow pathways stimulated by hypothalamic CRH are the HPA axis, which ultimately releases glucocorticoids, and the SNS, which releases catecholamines. Both factors (i.e., glucocorticoids and catecholamines) are known to influence multiple aspects of cellular and humoral immune responses, as well as the production and release of cytokines. Activation of the SNS by ICV CRH has been shown to be a major regulator of the suppressive effects of CRH on splenic NKCA. The HPA axis also contributes to CRH effects on immunity, as demonstrated by the finding that CRH-mediated attenuation of splenic proliferative responses was eliminated by adrenalectomy. In addition, B-cell decreases observed in CRH-overproducing mice are consistent with the marked reduction of rodent B cells found after chronic exposure to glucocorticoids. Pathways by which CRH stimulates proinflammatory cytokines are not well delineated, but it is interesting to note that catecholamines have been shown, in some studies, to promote cytokine production.

In addition to potentially mediating depressive symptoms in the context of cytokine activation, hyperactivity of CRH pathways at baseline, before cytokine exposure, may represent a risk factor for the development of depression during immune activation, based on recent data demonstrating that patients who respond to an initial dose of IFN-α-2β with increased production of adrenocorticotropic hormone (ACTH) and cortisol (both resulting from CRH release from the hypothalamus) are at markedly increased risk of developing major depression after 8 weeks of IFN-α-2β treatment. In this study, patients who subsequently developed depression did not evince elevated IL-6 responses to the first dose of IFN-α-2β, suggesting that depression during immune activation may more directly result from neuroendocrine responses to inflammatory mediators than from the degree of inflammatory activity per se.

Endorphins also appear to play a role in stress effects on NKCA in the spleen. Rats subjected to a foot-shock paradigm known to be associated with opioid analgesia exhibited decreased NKCA that was prevented by injections of the long-acting opioid antagonist naltrexone (ReVia).

Much of the focus of CNS–immune system interactions has been on the inhibitory immunological effects of neurally derived or regulated molecules, but several pituitary hormones, including prolactin and growth hormone, appear to have immune-enhancing or immunoprotective properties. For example, removal of the pituitary before stress results in an augmented inhibitor effect of stress on a variety of immune parameters, suggesting that pituitary hormones may restrain stress-induced effects.

Finally, the effects of cytokines on the nervous system and the endocrine system close the loop between the brain and the immune system and indicate that neural–immune interactions are bidirectional (Fig. 1.12–7).

IMMUNE SYSTEM EFFECTS ON CNS AND ENDOCRINE FUNCTION

Cytokine Effects on the Neuroendocrine System

Tremendous interest has been generated in the neurosciences by the discovery that cytokines are capable of exerting profound effects on the CNS and neuroendocrine system. Acting at the level of the CNS, the pituitary, and the adrenal glands, cytokines are involved in the regulation of sleep, temperature, feeding behavior, and other homeostatic mechanisms not only in the context of infection, but also in response to circadian changes in these vital functions. In addition, cytokines play a role in the regulation of neurotransmission and the secretion of multiple peptides and hormones, including CRH, ACTH, prolactin, leuteinizing hormone, follicle-stimulating hormone (FSH), growth hormone, thyroid-stimulating hormone, and glucocorticoids. For example, IL-1 has been shown to potently stimulate the secretion of hypothalamic CRH and therefore is capable of activating the neuroendocrine cascade, resulting in increased glucocorticoid release and SNS activation. In addition, IL-1β and its mRNA (as well as other cytokines, including TNF-α, IL-6, and IL-2) have been found in nerve cell bodies and nerve fibers within the hypothalamus, the hippocampus, and other regions in human and rodent brains, suggesting that IL-1 and other cytokines may play a role in neurotransmission.

Further evidence that the immune system exerts a powerful regulatory influence on neuroendocrine function is provided by data showing the effects of cytokines on the pituitary gland. For example, in vitro studies have shown that IL-1 is capable of enhancing the release of corticotropin (ACTH), luteinizing hormone, growth hormone, and thyroid-stimulating hormone, while inhibiting the release of prolactin from rat pituitary cells. Evidence of direct interactions between the immune system and the adrenal gland also exists. In particular, it has been shown that immune cells can produce ACTH-like and beta-endorphin–like hormones. The simultaneous release of ACTH-like and beta-endorphin–like products in response to a variety of stimuli, including CRH, indicates that immunocytes (probably macrophages), like pituitary cells, are capable of transcribing the proopiomelanocortin gene, which is responsible for coding the precursor protein from which ACTH and beta-endorphin are derived. Lymphocyte production of an ACTH-like hormone suggests that immunocytes may be capable of tapping directly into the HPA axis at the level of the adrenal gland, giving rise to a so-called lymphoid-adrenal axis. Nevertheless, the physiological relevance of the lymphoid-adrenal axis has not been established. Other hormones found to be secreted by immunocytes include somatostatin, vasoactive intestinal polypeptide, thyrotropin, prolactin, and growth hormone.

Finally, based on recent data from mice infected with a virus, it appears that, depending on the type of immune stimulus (i.e., bacterial versus viral), different cytokine pathways may be involved in neuroendocrine activation. Early glucocorticoid responses to viral infections and virus-type stimuli, for example, seem to involve preferentially IL-6, whereas TNF-α and IL-1β may play a greater role in glucocorticoid release during bacterial infections.

Cytokine to Brain Signaling and the Cytokine Network within the Brain Significant evidence indicates that the CNS is a primary site for the mediation of cytokine effects on

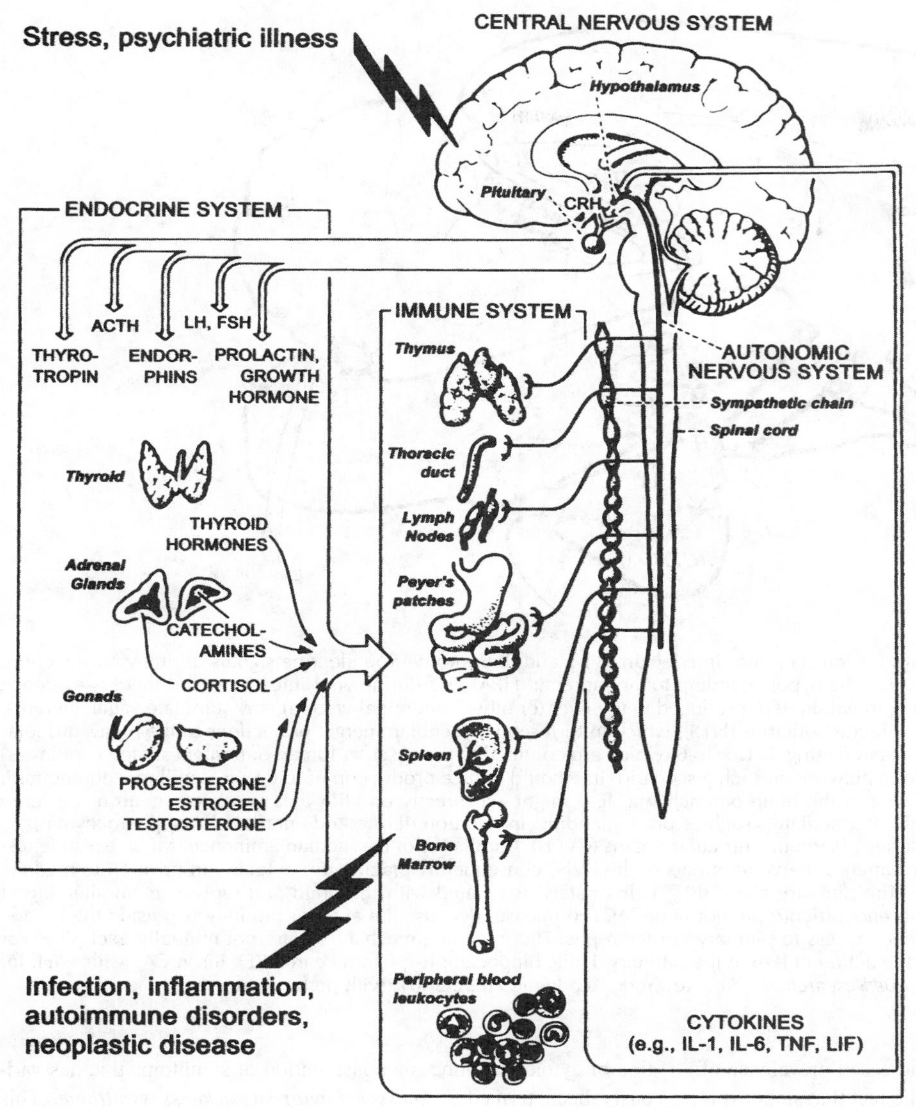

FIGURE 1.12–7 Diagram of bidirectional communication between the central nervous system (CNS) and the immune system. The endocrine system and the autocrine nervous system are depicted as important mediators of CNS effects on the immune system. Inflammatory cytokines, including interleukin (IL)-1, IL-6, tumor necrosis factor (TNF), and leukemia inhibitory factor (LIF), are shown closing the loop and interacting with the brain. ACTH, adrenocorticotropic hormone; CRH, corticotropin-releasing hormone; FSH, follicle-stimulating hormone; LH, leuteinizing hormone. (Drawn by Ellen Felten, Medical Arts Department, Mount Sinai Medical Center, New York and labeled by David Purselle, Department of Psychiatry and Behavioral Sciences, Emory University School of Medicine, Atlanta.)

behavior. Consistent with this, proinflammatory cytokines released in the periphery rapidly affect CNS functioning. However, because cytokines are large molecules that do not readily cross the blood–brain barrier, considerable attention has been paid to the mechanisms by which peripherally released cytokines might communicate with the brain, especially during infections (Fig. 1.12–8). Four major pathways have been identified, including (1) active transport of cytokines across the blood–brain barrier; (2) access of cytokines to brain areas in which the blood–brain barrier is relatively porous, such as the organum vasculosum of the lamina terminalis; (3) conversion of cytokine signals into secondary signals, such as prostaglandin or NO signals, by endothelial cells that line the blood vessels of the brain; and (4) transmission of cytokine signals (through cytokine receptor binding) along sensory afferents of the vagal nerve to the nucleus of the solitary tract and then via ascending catecholaminergic pathways on to relevant brain regions, including the paraventricular nucleus of the hypothalamus. There are data to support each of these mechanisms, and it appears that the various effects of cytokines on the CNS may each be mediated by one or more of these pathways, depending on the site of initial peripheral cytokine production and the strength of the peripheral proinflammatory signal. Once these peripheral signals reach the brain, it appears that, in many instances, these signals are translated back into cytokine signals (i.e., peripheral cytokines induce new central cytokines). For example, peripheral administration of IL-1 itself or substances such as endotoxin that induce IL-1 is associated with a rapid increase in IL-1 immunoreactivity and bioactivity in several brain regions, including the hippocampus and hypothalamus. Cytokines mediate their effects through specific receptors that are members of several classes of receptor gene families, including the Ig family (for IL-1 and IL-6), the hemopoietin family (for IL-2 through IL-7), and the nerve growth factor family (for TNF and nerve growth factor). There is a widespread and anatomically unique distribution of cytokine receptors in the brain. For instance, especially high concentrations of IL-1 and its receptors are found in rat hippocampus. Of note, soluble receptors exist for many cytokines, as do decoy (inactive) receptors (such as the IL-1 receptor type II), both of which serve to limit cytokine action. A specific endogenous soluble IL-1 receptor antagonist has also been described.

INFLAMMATION AND DEPRESSION IN MEDICAL ILLNESS

Depression is far more common in the context of medical illness than in healthy people, with rates of major depression in some medical conditions being as much as ten times greater than the rate

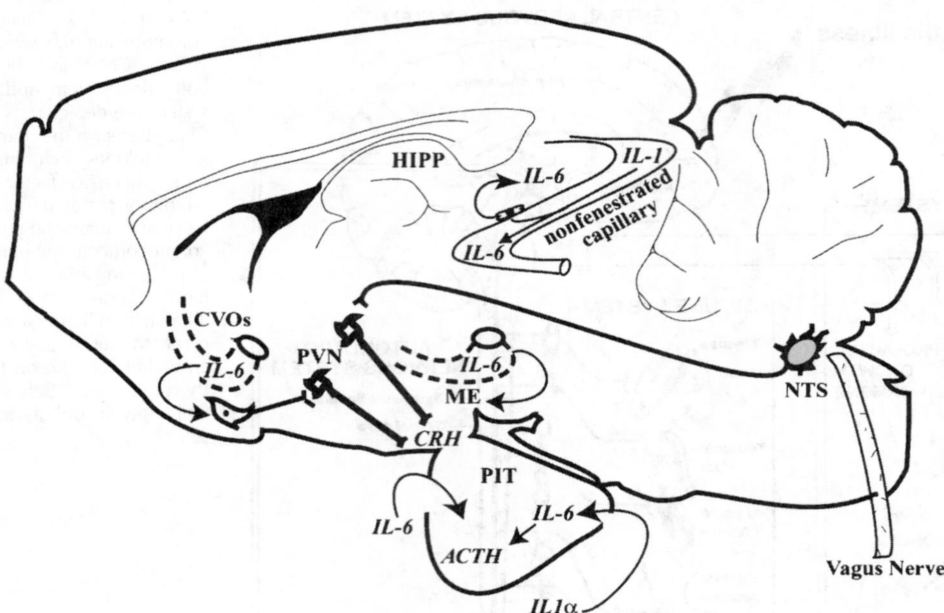

FIGURE 1.12–8 Schematic of possible pathways for translation of interleukin (IL)-1 and IL-6 into neuroendocrine signals during viral infection. IL-1 and IL-6 are thought to play a role in activating the hypothalamic-pituitary-adrenal (HPA) axis during viral infections, and there is evidence for various pathways by which this occurs. During infection, IL-6 produced in the liver (or other abdominal viscera) may stimulate vagal afferents, thereby activating central neurons in the nucleus tractus solitarius (NTS), which in turn send catecholaminergic projections to the paraventricular nucleus (PVN) of the hypothalamus. Alternatively, circulating IL-1 or IL-6 (which are confined to the vascular lumen of nonfenestrated capillaries) may act indirectly by recruiting the brain's cytokine network. In such a scenario, IL-1 could induce production of IL-6 from capillary endothelium, microvascular pericytes, or perivascular glia. Once in the brain parenchyma, IL-6 might act directly on HPA axis regulatory neurons or, more likely, might modulate HPA axis activity through intermediates, such as prostaglandins. In addition, IL-6 could enter the brain parenchyma passively by diffusing through the fenestrated capillaries of circumventricular organs (CVOs). Capillaries of the median eminence (ME) are also fenestrated, allowing IL-6 to travel from the vascular lumen to nerve terminals of the PVN, consequently placing this cytokine in position to mediate corticotropin-releasing hormone (CRH) release. The pituitary gland (PIT) is intimately associated with the brain and represents another site at which virus-induced cytokines could mediate adrenocorticotropic hormone (ACTH) release. Because the anterior pituitary is outside the blood–brain barrier, IL-1 and IL-6 presumably have direct access to pituitary corticotrophs. The foregoing mechanisms are not mutually exclusive. For example, CRH could play a permissive role for the action of IL-6 at the pituitary. HIPP, hippocampus. (From Pearce BD, Biron CA, Miller AH. In: Buchmeier MJ, Campbell IL, eds. *Advances in Virus Research.* Vol 56. NewYork: Academic Press; 2001, with permission.)

observed in healthy subjects. Although this increased prevalence of depression has been traditionally ascribed to the fact that sickness is a profound psychosocial stressor, growing data indicate that pathophysiologic processes inherent to sickness, especially inflammation, may alter CNS and hormonal functioning in ways that biologically predispose a person to develop depressive symptoms. These notions are derived from data indicating relevant immune-to-brain signaling that can powerfully influence neuroendocrine function and neurotransmission. Further evidence for the role of an activated immune response in mood dysregulation in the medically ill comes from findings that rates of depression are especially high in conditions such as multiple sclerosis, lupus erythematosus, and cardiovascular disease, in which inflammatory activity is critically involved in disease pathology. Moreover, in conditions characterized by episodic immune dysregulation, such as multiple sclerosis or herpes infection, depression typically precedes, rather than follows, episodes of disease exacerbation, suggesting that depressive symptoms associated with these conditions result from underlying immune system activity, rather than arising as a psychological reaction to being sick.

Sickness Behavior Direct evidence that proinflammatory cytokine exposure predisposes toward depression comes from studies that examine the effect of cytokine administration in animals and cytokine therapy in humans. In animals and humans, the administration of cytokines induces a constellation of symptoms that has variously been termed *sickness behavior* or *sickness syndrome*. This syndrome is characterized by weakness, malaise, listlessness, anhedonia, hypersomnia, anorexia, social isolation, hyperalgesia, and poor concentration. These symptoms are also typically seen during infections but may occur in a wide variety of clinical settings, including any medical condition or treatment that leads to significant inflammation or the release of proinflammatory cytokines (e.g., TNF, IL-1, and IL-6). The role of cytokines in promoting sickness behavior has probably been best characterized in patients receiving IFN-α-2β (IFN-α) for the treatment of hepatitis C or various cancers. INF-α is expressed by the body early in viral infections and has antiviral and antiproliferative properties. IFN-α also potently induces proinflammatory cytokines, especially IL-6, but also IL-1 and TNF-α, and hence represents a unique model system for understanding the effect of cytokine exposure in humans. IFN-α induces symptoms of sickness behavior in a majority of patients. Indeed, as many as 80 percent of patients receiving chronic IFN-α therapy develop fatigue sufficient to interfere with daily functioning. On the other hand, major depression occurs in fewer patients—30 to 50 percent, depending on dosage. This raises the possibility that, rather than directly causing major depression, chronic cytokine production may predispose toward the development of depression in patients with preexisting vulnerabilities exposed during the course of ongoing immune activation. Consistent with this, a recent study demon-

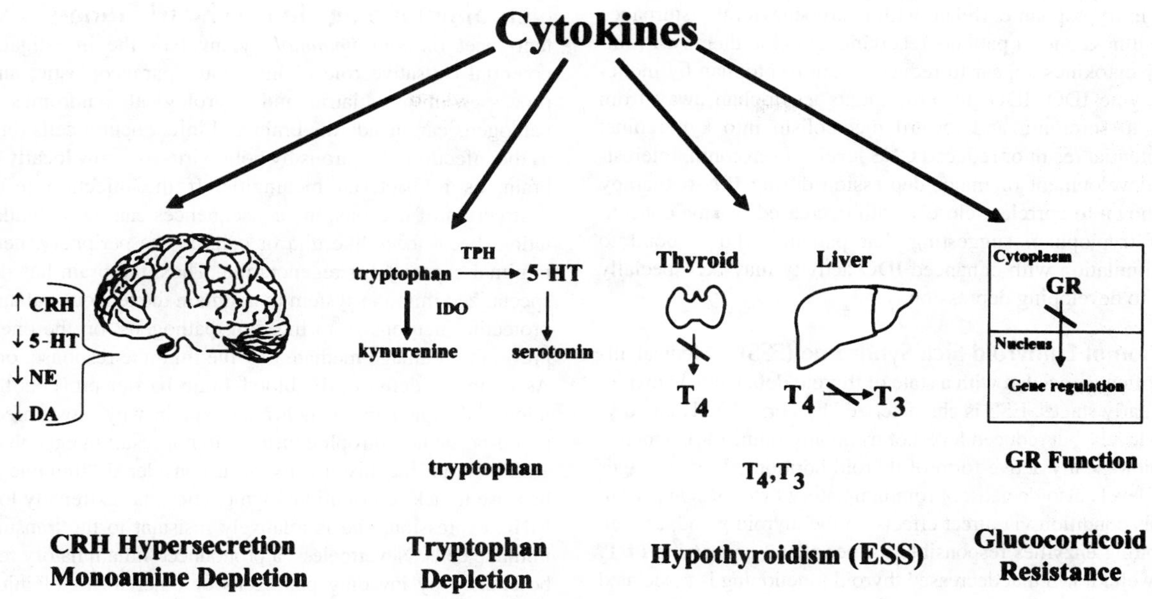

FIGURE 1.12–9 Pathways by which cytokines can cause sickness behavior and depression. There are several pathways by which cytokines can lead to behavioral changes that overlap with those found in major depression. From left to right, cytokines are potent inducers of corticotropin-releasing hormone (CRH), and chronic cytokine exposure may reduce availability of monoamines that are important in mood regulation. Cytokine induction of the enzyme, indolamine 2,3-dioxygenase (IDO), which metabolizes tryptophan to kynurenine, may lead to tryptophan depletion, which has been shown to induce depression in vulnerable individuals. Cytokines can also disrupt thyroid function directly or indirectly by impairing peripheral conversion of thyroxine (T_4) to triiodothyronine (T_3), leading to the euthyroid sick syndrome (ESS). Finally, cytokines can directly inhibit glucocorticoid receptor function, thereby disrupting negative feedback pathways that regulate CRH and further cytokine production. DA, dopamine; GR, glucocorticoid receptor; 5-HT, 5-hydroxytryptamine; NE, norepinephrine; TPH, tryptophan hydroxylase. (From Raison CL, Gumnick, JF, Miller AH. Neuroendocrine–immune interactions: Implications for health and behavior. In: Pfaff DW, Arnold AP, Etgen AM, Fahrbach SE, Rubin RT, eds. *Hormones, Brain and Behavior.* Vol 5. San Diego, CA: Academic Press; 2002, with permission.)

strates that antidepressant pretreatment effectively blocks the development of IFN-α–induced major depression, but it does so by preventing symptoms, such as depressed mood and anxiety, rather than blocking the development of symptoms more directly shared by illness and depression, such as fatigue and anorexia. These findings suggest that proinflammatory cytokine activation may directly induce sickness symptoms (including symptoms shared by illness and depression) but may induce depression-specific symptoms in humans by affecting CNS and neuroendocrine systems known to be affected by immune system activation.

Putative Mediators of Cytokine-Induced Behavioral Alterations

At least five mechanisms have been identified by which proinflammatory cytokines may induce depression in the context of therapeutic cytokine treatment and medical illness (Fig. 1.12–9). These mechanisms include (1) stimulation of CRH with resultant HPA axis activation, (2) alteration of CNS monoamine neurotransmission, (3) reduction of serum concentrations of L-tryptophan via activation of the enzyme indolamine 2,3-dioxygenase (IDO), (4) induction of euthyroid sick syndrome (ESS), and (5) development of tissue resistance to glucocorticoids.

Activation of CRH Pathways Proinflammatory cytokines potently stimulate the production and release of CRH within the CNS and especially within the paraventricular nucleus of the hypothalamus from which CRH serves as the primary secretagogue for the HPA axis. CRH has been shown, in animals, to play a key role in mediating symptoms associated with cytokine-induced sickness behavior, such as fever and sleep disturbance. Moreover, CRH administered ICV produces behavioral effects in animals that resemble those seen in patients with major depression. Of particular interest, CRH antagonists have been shown to block the behavioral effects of IFN-α in rodents.

Alteration of CNS Monoamine Neurotransmission Currently available antidepressants work via effects on monoamine (i.e. NE, serotonin, and dopamine) neurotransmitters in the CNS, providing strong evidence that these systems are involved in the pathophysiology of major depression. Moreover, patients with depression frequently demonstrate increased NE in cerebrospinal fluid (CSF) and plasma, and decreased production of serotonin's primary metabolite, 5-hydroxyindoleacetic acid (5-HIAA). Consistent with the high rate of behavioral disturbance during immune activation, proinflammatory cytokine administration to laboratory animals has been shown, in many studies, to acutely alter monoamine metabolism in the CNS. When administered ICV to rodents, IL-1 produces regionally specific increases in NE and serotonin turnover. Less is known about the effects of chronic cytokine exposure on NE and serotonin metabolism, although evidence suggests that chronic cytokine administration may decrease, rather than increase, serotonin turnover. Consistent with this evidence, chronic administration of IFN-α has been shown to diminish dopaminergic signaling capacity in the CNS of rats.

IDO-Induced Depletion of L-Tryptophan During medical illness and therapeutic cytokine therapy, the ability of proinflammatory cytokines to reduce serum levels of L-tryptophan has been well documented. Moreover, as one might predict from the known mood-lowering effects of tryptophan depletion, cytokine-induced reductions in tryptophan correlate with neurobehavioral disturbance in medical illness and in patients receiving cytokine therapy. Proinflammatory cytokines appear to reduce serum tryptophan by inducing the enzyme IDO. IDO, in turn, shunts tryptophan away from conversion to serotonin and toward metabolism into kynurenine, with the potential result of reduced CNS levels of serotonin. Interestingly, the development of major depression during IFN-α therapy has been shown to correlate closely with decreased plasma concentrations of tryptophan, suggesting that patients who respond to immune stimulation with enhanced IDO activity may be especially vulnerable to developing depression.

Induction of Euthyroid Sick Syndrome (ESS) Medical illnesses are often associated with a state of thyroid deficiency known as *ESS*. In its early stages, ESS is characterized by normal TSH and thyroxine (T_4) levels, but reduced levels of triiodothyronine (T_3), which is the more biologically active form of thyroid hormone. In later stages of ESS, T_4 levels also decrease. Proinflammatory cytokines appear to promote this condition via direct effects on the thyroid gland, as well as by inhibiting enzymes responsible for peripheral conversion of T_4 to T_3. It is well known that decreased thyroid functioning is associated with the development of depressive symptoms.

Development of Glucocorticoid Resistance In addition to promoting CRH hyperactivity in the CNS, in vivo and in vitro studies suggest that proinflammatory cytokines may induce resistance to the negative feedback effects of circulating glucocorticoids in nervous, endocrine, and immune tissues. These observations are especially salient given the high rates of relative glucocorticoid resistance seen in patients with major depression and in animals and humans exposed to chronic or severe stressors. Mechanisms by which proinflammatory cytokines may decrease tissue sensitivity to glucocorticoids include reducing the functional capacity of GRs. In animal models, proinflammatory cytokines downregulate GR expression in the CNS. Two isoforms for the GR exist: an active alpha isoform and an inert beta isoform. TNF-α and IL-1β have been found to promote production of the inert beta isoform, with a resultant decrease in GR function. Overproduction of the beta GR isoform may have clinically relevant effects on glucocorticoid sensitivity, given findings that patients with a variety of inflammatory and immune system disorders, including asthma, ulcerative colitis, and chronic lymphocytic leukemia, who are resistant to steroid treatment demonstrate a significantly increased GR-β to GR-α ratio. Finally, proinflammatory cytokines may induce glucocorticoid resistance by affecting the intracellular functioning of GR without altering GR receptor number. IL-1α has been shown in in vitro studies to block the ability of dexamethasone to induce translocation of the GR from cytoplasm to its site of action in the nucleus. This cytokine-induced embargo on nuclear translocation, in turn, inhibits GR activity, as indicated by a decrease in the ability of dexamethasone to activate a glucocorticoid-sensitive reporter gene construct.

RELEVANCE OF IMMUNE–CNS INTERACTIONS TO PSYCHIATRY

Given that CNS processes appear to be involved in immune regulation and that the immune system can influence CNS function, it is logical to consider that disorders of the CNS may contribute to the development, course, or outcome of immunological disorders and that the pathophysiology of some neuropsychiatric disorders may involve significant contributions from the immune system.

Neuroimmunology in Psychiatric Illness An important facet of *neuroimmunology* involves the investigation of the potential causative role of infectious, paraneoplastic, and immune processes in psychiatric and neurological syndromes. Microbial pathogens can invade the brain and infect neural cells directly, such as the infection of neurons by polio virus, or grow locally outside the brain, as in bacterial meningitis. If the infection results in the destruction of neurons, the consequences can be particularly devastating, because, unlike glia or cells in the periphery, neurons have minimal capacity for regeneration. Thus, the brain has developed a specialized immune system to maintain the tenuous balance between protecting neurons from invading pathogens, on the one hand, and preventing damage mediated by the immune response, on the other. As an initial defense, the blood–brain barrier prevents the entry of microbial organisms, which may explain why most infections with blood-borne neurotrophic viruses do not result in encephalitis.

The brain has historically been considered "immune privileged" because it lacks conventional lymphatics, has extremely low levels of MHC expression, and is relatively resistant to the transmigration of immune cells. Nevertheless, a pronounced inflammatory response can be elicited by invading pathogens or other forms of injury. During CNS infection, extracellular antigens are thought to drain to cervical lymphatics, glia are induced to express MHC class I and II molecules, and activated T cells enter the CNS. Local induction of cytokines helps orchestrate the immune response, and adhesion molecules are upregulated on endothelium and perivascular glia to facilitate the entry of macrophages and other leukocytes. Besides being major sources of proinflammatory cytokines, astrocytes and microglia become activated during inflammation and can produce other diffusible mediators such as NO, prostaglandins, and excitatory amino acids. Such inflammatory reactions can occur even in the absence of an infectious agent, as exemplified in postischemic brain injury in which there is a rapid induction of cytokines, extravasation of leukocytes, and gliosis. Which aspects of this immune reaction are deleterious and which aspects are the immunological accouterments of the remains of tissue repair have not been entirely deciphered.

The idea that infectious agents can lead to psychiatric disorders has been well established. Obvious examples include the mental retardation that may develop after congenital infection with rubella or cytomegalovirus, the delirium that accompanies acute meningoencephalitis after CNS infection by herpes simplex virus type 1, dementias due to slow viruses, such as kuru and Creutzfeldt-Jakob disease, and the neuropsychiatric manifestations that occur during neurosyphilis. Other conditions that have received significant interest relevant to neuroimmunology and the bidirectional communication between the brain and immune system are reviewed in the following discussion.

Major Depression

The neuropsychiatric disorder that has been best characterized in terms of the bidirectional influence of the brain on the immune system and vice versa is major depression. For many years, major depression was seen as a quintessential example of how stress-related disorders may decrease immunocompetence. More recently, researchers have also become aware that stress may activate inflammatory pathways, even while suppressing measures of acquired immunity. Not surprisingly, studies now indicate that, in addition to immunosuppression, major depression may also be associated with inflammatory activation. Recent research showing that proinflammatory cytokines are capable of suppressing many of the immune measures examined in major depression may supply a mechanism to account for how chronic stress system–induced inflammatory activity may give rise to depression-related suppression of in vitro functional assays, such as lymphocyte proliferation and NKCA.

Immunosuppression Despite heterogeneity across individual studies, significant evidence indicates that major depression is associated with a number of immunosuppressive changes that are also seen in individuals without depression but who are undergoing chronic or severe stress, or both (Table 1.12–11). Enumerative immune changes shared by major depression and severe or chronic stress include a decrease in serum concentrations of lymphocytes, B cells, and T cells. Functional changes include a decrease in NKCA and lymphocyte proliferation in response to nonspecific mitogens. Less is known about the effects of major depression in vivo (i.e., naturalistic immune functioning); however, available evidence suggests that depression may impair T-cell function in ways relevant to disease vulnerability. For example, one study reports that patients with major depression have a marked decrement in their ability to generate lymphocytes that respond to the herpes zoster virus. Also consistent with impaired T-cell function is the observation that depressed patients, especially those with melancholia, demonstrate impaired DTH.

Because major depression is a heterogenous condition, immune changes are not uniform across all patients. In general, these changes tend to be most robust in patients who are older, who are hospitalized, or who have more severe or melancholic, or both, types of depression. There is also some indication that certain depressive symptoms might disproportionately account for immune alterations. For example, it should be noted that patients with primary sleep disorders who are not depressed exhibit immune alterations similar to those seen in major depression. Nevertheless, data from a metaanalysis of relevant literature indicate that age, hospitalization status, depression severity, or specific symptoms of depression cannot completely account for the association between major depression and alterations in enumerative and functional immune measures.

Inflammatory Activation Growing evidence suggests that major depression may be associated with inflammatory activation, even in the absence of medical illness. This is in keeping with recent studies showing that psychological stressors are capable of activating inflammatory pathways. Although the mechanism is unknown, it has been observed that CRH and catecholamines—both of which appear elevated in major depression—are capable of inducing proinflammatory cytokine production. Inflammatory changes reported in medically healthy patients with major depression include increases in plasma and CSF concentrations of proinflammatory cytokines (especially IL-1β in CSF and IL-6 in plasma), increased in vitro production of proinflammatory cytokines from stimulated peripheral blood mononuclear cells, increased plasma acute-phase proteins and decreased negative acute-phase proteins, increased production of prostaglandins, decreased tryptophan and increased kynurenine, and decreased zinc. In addition, depression has been associated with an increase in activated T cells and autoantibodies. Also consistent with immune activation in major depression is the observation that proinflammatory cytokines are capable of inducing pathophysiological changes common in patients with depression, including insulin resistance, cachexia, bone loss, increased body temperature, and cell loss in the CNS.

As with studies of immunosuppression, not all studies find evidence of immune activation in depression. Indeed, a recent large and well-controlled study failed to detect proinflammatory cytokine alterations in major depression when controlling for known potential confounders, such as gender, age, smoking status, body mass index, ongoing or recent infections, and medication usage. Nonetheless, using a random effects paradigm, a metaanalysis of published studies found evidence that ongoing studies will confirm the presence of inflammatory activation in major depression, based on the strength of the association already observed between depression and increased plasma concentrations of IL-6, prostaglandin E_2, and the acute-phase protein, haptoglobin.

Given the known antiinflammatory properties of glucocorticoids, it might be predicted that depressed patients who are resistant to cortisol, as assessed in vivo by the dexamethasone-suppression test (DST), might be especially likely to exhibit inflammatory activation. Some evidence suggests this is the case. Compared to depressed patients with normal glucocorticoid sensitivity, depressed patients who were DST nonsuppressors demonstrated increased plasma concentrations of the acute-phase reactant α_1-glycoprotein, as well as increased mitogen-stimulated IL-6 production. It should be noted, however, that a recent study failed to replicate this relationship in depressed patients with cancer. Nevertheless, given evidence that glucocorticoid resistance is associated with treatment nonresponse, it is intriguing that depressed patients with treatment resistance have been reported to be more likely than treatment responders to demonstrate increased proinflammatory cytokine activity, including increased plasma concentrations of acute-phase proteins, IL-6 and the soluble receptor for IL-6, which synergistically enhances IL-6 bioactivity.

Although most research has focused on immune activation in medically healthy subjects with depression, recent work suggests that proinflammatory cytokine production may also contribute to major depression in patients who are medically ill. For example, plasma concentrations of IL-6 were found to be significantly elevated in patients with pancreatic, esophageal, or breast cancer compared to cancer patients without depression.

As for infectious diseases contributing to the pathophysiology of major depressive disorders, the potential contribution of a virus to the etiology of depression has long been considered. There has been renewed interest in this area based on the isolation of Borna disease virus from immune cells of patients with depression. Borna disease virus was primarily of interest as a pathogen of horses and sheep until recent serological and virological data demonstrated that it can infect humans and may be associated with psychiatric diseases. The neurotrophic and immunopathogenic capabilities of Borna disease virus have been well studied in the rat model. During the initial phase of Borna disease in rats, the infection of neurons and glia is accompanied by a robust inflammatory response with participation of T cells, B cells, and macrophages. Rats that recover from the initial phase may develop chronic symptoms, including behavioral abnormalities and obesity; further studies are needed to clarify the importance of Borna disease virus in human neuropsychiatric disorders, such as major depression.

Schizophrenia Since the 1980s, there has been growing interest in the idea that infectious agents, particularly viruses, may underlie at least some cases of schizophrenia. Although it is well established that viral encephalitis can present clinically as psychosis, the primary focus of the *viral hypothesis* for schizophrenia has been on infections during neurodevelopment, because this is congruent with the emerging consensus that schizophrenia originates in prenatal or early postnatal development. Several lines of indirect evidence suggest that viral infection during CNS development may be involved in the pathogenesis of schizophrenia. The data include (1) an excess number of patient births in the late winter and early spring, suggesting possible exposure to viral infection in utero during the fall and winter peak of viral illnesses; (2) an association between exposure to viral epidemics in utero and the later development of schizophrenia; (3) a higher prevalence of schizophrenia in crowded urban areas, which have conditions that are particularly conducive to the transmission of viral pathogens; and (4) seroepidemiological studies indicting a higher infection rate for certain viruses in schizophrenia patients or their mothers.

In addition, schizophrenia is associated with indices of immune activation, including elevations in proinflammatory cytokines and the soluble IL-2 receptor. A shift in the Th-1–Th-2 cytokine profile has also been reported in some patients. Although these immune findings in schizophrenia patients may indicate evidence of immune system activation secondary to infection, it should be noted that they might also indicate that an autoimmune process is involved in the disorder. Thus, despite the plethora of studies pointing to abnormalities in cellular and humoral immunity in schizophrenia, the data have not been uniform or conclusive, and there is a need for more studies that account for confounding variables, such as medication status and tobacco smoking. Moreover, attempts to isolate infectious agents from schizophrenic brain tissue or to detect viral nucleic acids in the CNS or peripheral blood of schizophrenic patients have generally yielded negative results.

Because the initial neuronal abnormalities in schizophrenia have been proposed to arise during neurodevelopment, a perinatal viral infection could insidiously disrupt development and then be cleared by the immune system before clinical diagnosis. In such a scenario, host factors, such as cytokines, could be responsible for causing the developmental abnormality by interacting with growth factors or adhesion molecules. Various animal models using influenza virus, Borna disease virus, or lymphocytic choriomeningitis virus in rodents have demonstrated that prenatal or postnatal viral infections can lead to neuroanatomical or behavioral alterations that are somewhat reminiscent of schizophrenia in humans. As mentioned previously, epidemiological studies also support the link between infection with a teratogenic virus and the development of psychotic disorders later in life. Associations have been observed between maternal infection with rubella or influenza during gestation and the development of a schizophrenia spectrum disorder in the offspring. Similarly, maternal antibodies to herpes simplex virus that develops during pregnancy are correlated with increased rates of psychosis during adulthood in the offspring.

Non-HIV retroviruses might also play a role in the pathogenesis of schizophrenia. Retroviruses integrate into host DNA and can disrupt the function of adjacent genes. Moreover, the genomes of all humans contain sequences of *endogenous retroviruses* that hold the capacity to alter the transcriptional regulation of host genes. If genes controlling the development or function of the brain undergo transcriptional disruption by retroviral effects, this might lead to a cascade of biochemical abnormalities eventually giving rise to schizophrenia.

As previously noted, an autoimmune cause has been suspected in some patients with schizophrenia. Nevertheless, attempts to isolate autoantibodies to CNS tissue constituents in schizophrenia patients have not consistently identified an antigen that bears a crucial relationship to the brain alterations found in the disease. Furthermore, because schizophrenia may involve various forms of CNS tissue damage, with the resultant release of brain antigens, autoantibodies to CNS tissues in those instances may be the result of CNS pathology rather than the cause.

Autism Autism is associated with a number of immune abnormalities, including unbalanced cytokine production, reduced NK- and T-cell activation, and the production of autoreactive antibodies. An immunogenetic basis for autism is supported by the high rate of autoimmune diseases in first degree relatives of autism patients. Still, although a convincing case can be made for a significant immune component to autism, the relationship of immune abnormalities to the neurobehavioral symptoms of the disease remains controversial. The claim that autism is triggered by childhood vaccines has not been substantiated by recent epidemiological studies, and immune-based therapies for autism have not been reliably effective. Thus, although it is tempting to speculate that the immune system holds the clue to a cure for autism, there are currently not even enough data to determine whether immune anomalies cause autism, or are *caused by* autism, or are just adventitiously associated with the disease.

Multiple Sclerosis Multiple sclerosis is a demyelinating disease characterized by disseminated inflammatory lesions of white matter. Since the mid-1970s, considerable progress has been made in elucidating the immunopathology of myelin destruction that occurs in multiple sclerosis and, in the animal model for the disease, *experimental allergic encephalomyelitis*. Although the initial step in lesion formation has not been determined, disruption of the blood–brain barrier and the infiltration of T cells, B cells, plasma cells, and macrophages all appear to be associated with lesion formation. Proinflammatory cytokines, notably TNF-α, IFN-γ, and IL-1, are believed to participate in the immunopathology by activating glia, inducing MHC class II molecules, or mediating cytotoxicity by stimulation of free radical formation. Conversely, treatment with IFN-β decreases lesions and has been used clinically in multiple sclerosis. Current therapeutic strategies are focusing on preventing the transmigration of leukocytes into the brain by targeting chemokines (a type of cytokine that mediates chemoattraction) or by blocking adhesion molecules on endothelium or glia. Several viruses have been suggested to trigger multiple sclerosis, most recently, human herpesvirus 6. One mechanism by which a virus could trigger multiple sclerosis is by molecular mimicry in which a shared epitope between a virus and the host allows for self-tolerance to myelin to be broken. The selective depletion of autoreactive T cells or induction of immune tolerance by oral administration of myelin proteins is also under investigation.

Alzheimer's Disease Although Alzheimer's disease is not considered primarily an inflammatory disease, emerging evidence indicates that the immune system may contribute to its pathogenesis. The discovery that amyloid plaques are associated with acute-phase proteins, such as complement proteins, α_1-antichymotrypsin, and C-reactive protein, suggests the possibility of an ongoing immune response. Furthermore, gliosis and increased levels of proinflammatory cytokines are found in and around plaques. Interestingly, the induction of IL-6 has been proposed to precede neuritic degeneration in nascent (diffuse) plaques, and IL-1β can increase mRNA for amyloid precursor protein. Thus, immune mediators have been theorized to have an early role in plaque formation. The idea that inflammatory processes are involved in Alzheimer's disease has been bolstered by recent studies showing that the long-term use of nonsteroidal antiinflammatory drugs is negatively correlated with the development of Alzheimer's disease. Studies are underway to determine whether immune suppression can improve disease outcome.

HIV Infection HIV infection is an immunological disease associated with a variety of neurological manifestations, including dementia. Although some neurological symptoms may be a consequence of opportunistic infections, accumulating evidence indicates that HIV itself can produce encephalitis. Infected microglia can be readily identified in the brain, whereas infection of neurons does not appear to occur in vivo. Nevertheless, HIV encephalitis results in synaptic abnormalities and loss of neurons in the limbic system, basal ganglia, and neocortex. Current research examining the mechanism of this neurodegeneration has focused on a network of interactions between viral products (e.g., gp120 and tat), glia, macrophages, and neurons. In this regard, soluble factors, such as cytokines (IL-1, IL-6, TNF, and TGFβ), free radicals, and excitatory amino acids, have all been proposed as intermediaries in HIV-induced neuropathology. Studies in rodents have demonstrated that viral gp120 can induce IL-1β expression, activate glia, and cause neuronal damage. Antagonists of the *N*-methyl-D-aspartate (NMDA) excitatory amino acid receptor can ameliorate this damage, although many aspects of this neuropathogenic pathway are unclear. Neuroendocrine abnormalities have also been described after HIV infection, perhaps as a result of cytokine activation. Thus, although the complex interactions between viral and host factors in HIV encephalitis may be perplexing, current research is revealing a variety of potential targets for therapeutic intervention in the disease.

Recent studies have demonstrated that life stress and major depression hasten development of AIDS in patients who are HIV positive. Although the mechanism by which stress worsens disease outcome is unknown, one interesting possibility is suggested by a recent study showing that patients with heightened autonomic arousal, such as occurs during stress, had a significantly impaired response to antiretroviral medications.

Other Disorders Several autoimmune disorders, including autoimmune disorders of the thyroid and collagen vascular diseases, such as systemic lupus erythematosus and Behçet's syndrome, are capable of indirectly or nonspecifically altering CNS function, but only a few autoimmune conditions directly involve brain antigens. Neural cells are the target for autoantibodies in the paraneoplastic syndromes. For example, autoantibodies to cytoplasmic proteins of Purkinje cells are associated with subacute cortical cerebellar degeneration, which is a rare complication of breast or ovarian cancers. Autoantibodies to γ-aminobutyric acid (GABA)–ergic neurons in the serum and the CSF appear to be the mechanism behind the stiff person syndrome, a rare disorder characterized by progressive rigidity, accompanied by recurrent painful muscle spasms. Antineuronal antibodies can also arise after infection with group A β-hemolytic streptococcal infections, as exemplified by Sydenham's chorea. Considering that children with Sydenham's chorea frequently exhibit obsessive-compulsive symptoms, emotional lability, and hyperactivity, there appears to be a spectrum of pediatric autoimmune neuropsychiatric disorders associated with streptococcal infections (PANDAS). In particular, sudden onset of obsessive-compulsive disorder (OCD), tics, attention-deficit/hyperactivity disorder (ADHD), and other psychiatric syndromes has been characterized in children following infection with group A β-hemolytic streptococcus. These findings, in conjunction with the indication of a genetic vulnerability to this condition (high frequency of binding of a monoclonal antibody designated D8/17), represent an exciting new development in the etiology and possible treatment of these disorders.

Finally, there are several disorders in which neural–immune interactions are suspected but not well documented. Chronic fatigue syndrome is an illness with controversial etiology and pathogenesis. Besides persistent fatigue, symptoms frequently include depression and sleep disturbances. Tests of immune function have found indications of immune activation and immunosuppression. Neuroendocrine assessments indicate that patients with chronic fatigue syndrome may be hypocortisolemic because of impaired activation of the HPA axis. Although an acute viral infection frequently precedes the onset of CFS, no infectious agent has been definitively identified as causing the disease. In contrast, Lyme disease, in which sleep disturbances and depression are also common, is clearly caused by infection with the tick-borne spirochete, *Borrelia burgdorferi.* The organism can invade the CNS and cause encephalitis and neurological symptoms. Lyme disease is remarkable, because it has been claimed to produce a spectrum of neuropsychiatric disorders including anxiety, irritability, obsessions, compulsions, hallucinations, and cognitive deficits. Immunopathology of the CNS may be involved, because symptoms can persist or reappear even after a lengthy course of antibiotic treatment, and the spirochete is frequently difficult to isolate from the brain. Gulf War syndrome is a controversial condition with inflammatory and neuropsychiatric features. The condition has been attributed variously to combat stress, chemical weapons, infections, and vaccines. Given the impact of stress on neurochemistry and immune responses, these pathogenic mechanisms are not mutually exclusive.

THERAPEUTIC IMPLICATIONS

The bidirectional nature of CNS–immune system interactions implies the therapeutic possibility that agents known to positively alter stress system activity might benefit immune functioning and, conversely, that agents that modulate immune functioning may be of potential benefit in the treatment of neuropsychiatric disturbance, especially in the context of medical illness. Increasing evidence supports both of these hypotheses.

Antidepressants and the Immune System Emerging data indicate that, in animals and humans, antidepressants are able to attenuate or abolish behavioral symptoms induced by proinflammatory cytokine exposure. For example, pretreatment of rats with imipramine (Norfranil) or fluoxetine (Prozac) (a tricyclic and serotonin reuptake inhibitor, respectively) for 5 weeks before endotoxin administration significantly attenuated endotoxin-induced decrements in saccharine preference (commonly accepted as a measure for anhedonia), as well as weight loss, anorexia, and reduced exploratory, locomotor, and social behavior. Similarly, several studies in humans suggest that antidepressants are able to ameliorate mood disturbances in the context of chronic cytokine therapies, especially if given prophylactically before inflammatory exposure. In the largest such study to date, the serotonin reuptake inhibitor paroxetine (Paxil) significantly decreased the development of major depression in patients receiving high doses of IFN-α for malignant melanoma. After 3 months of IFN-α, 45 percent of patients receiving placebo developed major depression, compared to only 11 percent of patients receiving paroxetine. Moreover, patients on placebo had significantly higher rates of IFN-α treatment discontinuation secondary to depression when compared to patients receiving paroxetine, suggesting that, by blocking cytokine-induced mood disturbance, antidepressants may contribute to treatment success. Interestingly, in a dimensional analysis, it became apparent that paroxetine prevented major depression by blocking mood, anxiety, and cognitive symptoms. In contrast, the antidepressant was no more effective than placebo in preventing neurovegetative symptoms, such as fatigue and anorexia. These findings raise the possibility that major depression in the medically ill represents a phenomenon comprised of at least two separate syndromes mediated by two distinct pathways: an affective syndrome that is antidepressant responsive and a neurovegetative syndrome that is antidepressant resistant. Importantly, recent evidence suggests that affective, but not somatic, symptoms account for depression-associated increases in mortality in hospitalized, medically ill patients, raising the possibility that, by specifically targeting these symptoms, antidepressants may improve survival in the context of medical illness.

Many studies indicate that, in general, antidepressants decrease immune system responsivity in ways that are likely to be of benefit in the context of immune activation. A number of antidepressants have been shown to diminish proinflammatory cytokine production, not just from peripheral immune cells, but also within the CNS, where desipramine has been reported to attenuate TNF-α release within the locus ceruleus. Rolipram, a phosphodiesterase type IV inhibitor, has antidepressant properties and has been shown to suppress NF-κB activity, which is a primary pathway for the induction of genes that encode proinflammatory cytokine production. Concomitant with attenuating proinflammatory cytokine production, antidepressants enhance production of the antiinflammatory cytokine IL-10. Antidepressants are also known to enhance activity in intracellular second messenger pathways (such as the cyclic adenosine monophosphate [cAMP] cascade) known to suppress production of proinflammatory cytokines.

Finally, antidepressants also reverse the relative glucocorticoid resistance found in many patients with major depression, suggesting that antidepressants may diminish activity in CRH and immune pathways by restoring normal glucocorticoid-mediated feedback inhibition.

Immune Modulators and Psychiatric Illness A logical correlate to the idea that antidepressants modulate inflammation is that agents with the capacity to directly diminish cytokine production may be of value in stress-related conditions, such as depression. Evidence supportive of this idea comes from animal studies showing that, in addition to attenuating cytokine-induced sickness behavior, endogenous inhibitors of proinflammatory cytokines, such as the sIL-1ra, block many of the sequelae of psychological stress in rodents. For example, administration of IL-1 receptor antagonist diminishes HPA axis responses to psychological stressors, such as restraint, and prevents stress from causing learned helplessness, which is an animal model for depression. Consistent with this, etanercept (Enbrel), a soluble receptor that decreases TNF-α activity has been reported to improve emotional well-being in patients with rheumatoid arthritis, a condition characterized by chronic proinflammatory cytokine overproduction. Finally, a study demonstrating increased antipsychotic efficacy in schizophrenic patients treated with the combination of the cyclooxygenase-2 inhibitor celecoxib (Celebrex), an antiinflammatory drug, and risperidone (Risperdal) (versus risperidone plus placebo) suggests that antagonizing inflammatory pathways may have a broad spectrum of activity in neuropsychiatric disorders.

Behavioral Interventions and Immunity It has been known for years that psychosocial factors can mitigate or worsen the effects of stress, not only on immune functioning, but also on the long-term outcomes of medical conditions in which the immune system is known to play a role. Therefore, behavioral interventions aimed at maximizing protective psychosocial factors might be predicted to have a beneficial effect, not only in terms of mitigating the effect of stress on immune functioning, but perhaps also on diminishing emotional disturbances that arise in the context of immune system dysregulation.

Two factors that have been repeatedly identified as protecting against stress-induced immune alterations are social support and the ability to see stressors as being, to some degree, under the individual's control. Interestingly, the two types of psychotherapy most often examined in illnesses associated with immune dysregulation are group therapy, which provides social support, and cognitive behavioral therapy, which provides cognitive reframing techniques aimed at enhancing one's sense of agency (and hence control).

Consistent with the known benefits of social support and sense of control on disease progression, studies suggest that psychotherapeutic interventions in the context of illness are capable of improving not just depressive symptomatology, but also immune functioning and physical symptoms as well. For example, group psychotherapy has been reported to decrease stress-related immune alterations after an acute laboratory stressor in patients with breast cancer. In addition to treating depression, cognitive behavioral and group therapy have also been shown to diminish IFN-γ production in patients with multiple sclerosis over a 12-week treatment course. Finally, two well-designed studies suggest that group therapy may prolong survival in cancer patients, an effect that was correlated in one study with enhancement of NKCA in patients with malignant melanoma.

SUGGESTED CROSS-REFERENCES

Functional neuroanatomy is discussed in Section 1.2. Psychoneuroimmunology is discussed in Section 1.11, and neuropeptides are covered in Section 1.6. Schizophrenia is covered in Chapter 12, mood disorders are covered in Chapter 13, and anxiety disorders are covered in Chapter 14. Alzheimer's disease is presented in Chapter 10 and Section 51.3e.

REFERENCES

*Abbas AK, Lichtman AH, Pober JS. *Cellular and Molecular Immunology.* 4th ed. Philadelphia: WB Saunders; 2000.

Ader R, Felten DL, Cohen N. *Psychoneuroimmunology.* 3rd ed. New York: Academic Press; 2001.

Avitsur R, Stark JL, Sheridan JF: Social stress induces glucocorticoid resistance in subordinate animals. *Horm Behav.* 2001;39:247.

Ben-Eliyahu S, Page GG, Yirmiya R, Shakhar G: Evidence that stress and surgical interventions promote tumor development by suppressing natural killer cell activity. *Int J Cancer.* 1999;80:880.

Berkenbosch F, Oers JV, Del Rey A, Tilders F, Besedovsky H: Corticotropin-releasing factor-producing neurons in the rat activated by interleukin-1. *Science.* 1987;238:524.

Bierhaus A, Wolf J, Andrassy M, Rohleder N, Humpert PM, Petrov D, Ferstl R, von Eynatten M, Wendt T, Rudofsky G, Joswig M, Morcos M, Schwaninger M, McEwen B, Kirschbaum C, Nawroth PP: A mechanism converting psychosocial stress into mononuclear cell activation. *Proc Natl Acad Sci U S A.* 2003;100:1920.

Capuron L, Gumnick JF, Musselman DL, Lawson DH, Reemsnyder A, Nemeroff CB, Miller AH: Neurobehavioral effects of interferon-alpha in cancer patients: Phenomenology and paroxetine responsiveness of symptom dimensions. *Neuropsychopharmacology.* 2002;26:643.

Capuron L, Neurauter G, Musselman DL, Lawson DH, Nemeroff CB, Fuchs D, Miller AH: Interferon-alpha-induced changes in tryptophan metabolism: Relationship to depression and paroxetine treatment. *Biol Psychiatry.* 2003;54:906.

Capuron L, Raison CL, Musselman DL, Lawson DH, Nemeroff CB, Miller AH: Association of exaggerated HPA axis response to the intial injection of interferon-alpha with development of depression during interferon-alpha therapy. *Am J Psychiatry.* 2003;160:1342.

Cohen S, Tyrell D AJ, Smith AP: Psychological stress and susceptibility to the common cold. *N Engl J Med.* 1991;325:606.

Cole SW, Naliboff BD, Kemeny ME, Griswold MP, Fahey JL, Zack JA: Impaired response to HAART in HIV-infected individuals with high autonomic nervous system activity. *Proc Natl Acad Sci U S A.* 2001;98:12695.

Dantzer R: Cytokine-induced sickness behavior: Where do we stand? *Brain Behav Immun.* 2001;15:7–24.

Dhabhar FS, McEwen BS: Enhancing versus suppressive effects of stress hormones on skin immune function. *Proc Natl Acad Sci U S A.* 1999;96:1059.

Fatemi SH, Earle J, Kanodia R, Kist D, Emamian ES, Patterson PH, Shi L, Sidwell R: Prenatal viral infection leads to pyramidal cell atrophy and macrocephaly in adulthood: Implications for genesis of autism and schizophrenia. *Cell Mol Neurobiol.* 2002;22:25.

Glaser R, Kiecolt-Glaser JK, Marucha PT, MacCallum RC, Laskowski BF, Malarkey WB: Stress-related changes in proinflammatory cytokine production in wounds. *Arch Gen Psychiatry.* 1999;56:450.

Goebel MU, Mills PJ, Irwin MR, Ziegler MG: Interleukin-6 and tumor necrosis factor-alpha production after acute psychological stress, exercise, and infused isoproterenol: Differential effects and pathways. *Psychosom Med.* 2000;62:591.

Karalis K, Muglia LJ, Bae D, Hilderbrand H, Majzoub JA: CRH and the immune system. *J Neuroimmun.* 1997;72:131.

Keller S, Schleifer SJ, Liotta AS, Bond RN, Farhoody N, Stein M: Stress-induced alterations of immunity in hypophysectomized rats. *Proc Natl Acad Sci U S A.* 1988;85:9297.

Kiecolt-Glaser JK, Preacher KJ, MacCallum RC, Atkinson C, Malarkey WB, Glaser R: Chronic stress and age-related increases in the proinflammatory cytokine IL-6. *Proc Natl Acad Sci U S A.* 2003;100:9090.

Krueger JM, Obal FJ, Fang J, Kubota T, Taishi P: The role of cytokines in physiological sleep regulation. *Ann N Y Acad Sci.* 2001;933:211.

Leo NA, Bonneau RH: Chemical sympathectomy alters cytotoxic T lymphocyte response to herpes simplex virus infection. *Ann N Y Acad Sci.* 2000;917:923.

Leonard HL, Swedo SE: Paediatric autoimmune neuropsychiatric disorders associated with streptococcal infection (PANDAS). *Int J Neuropsychopharmacol.* 2001;4:191.

*Maier SF, Watkins LR: Cytokines for psychologists: Implications of bidirectional immune-to-brain communication for understanding behavior, mood, and cognition. *Psychol Rev.* 1998;105:83.

Muller N, Riedel M, Gruber R, Ackenheil M, Schwarz MJ: The immune system and schizophrenia: An integrative view. *Ann N Y Acad Sci.* 2000;917:456.

*Musselman DL, Lawson DH, Gumnick JF, Manatunga AK, Penna S, Goodkin RS, Greiner K, Nemeroff CB, Miller AH: Paroxetine for the prevention of depression induced by high-dose interferon alfa. *N Engl J Med.* 2001;344:961.

Pearce DB: Schizophrenia and viral infection during neurodevelopment: A focus on mechanisms. *Mol Psychiatry.* 2001;6:634.

*Raison CL, Gumnick JF, Miller, AH. Neuroendocrine–immune interactions: implications for health and behavior. In: Pfaff DW, Arnold AP, Etgen AM, Fahrbach SE, Rubin RT, eds. *Hormones, Brain and Behavior.* Vol 5. San Diego, CA: Academic Press; 2002.

Raison CL, Miller AH: When not enough is too much: The role of insufficient glucocorticoid signaling in the pathophysiology of stress-related disorders. *Am J Psychiatry.* 2003;160:1554.

Rivest S, Lacroix S, Vallieres L, Nadeau S, Zhang J, Laflamme N: How the blood talks to the brain parenchyma and the paraventricular nucleus of the hypothalamus during systemic inflammatory and infectious stimuli. *Proc Soc Exp Biol Med.* 2000;223:22.

*Sheridan JF, Stark JL, Avitsur R, Padgett DA: Social disruption, immunity, and susceptibility to viral infection: Role of glucocorticoid insensitivity and NGF. *Ann N Y Acad Sci.* 2000;917:894.

Spiegel D: Effects of psychotherapy on cancer survival. *Nat Rev Cancer.* 2002;2:383.

Spiegel D, Kraemer HC, Bloom JR, Gotheil E: Effects of psychosocial treatment on survival of patients with metastatic breast cancer. *Lancet.* 1989;2:888.

Wong ML, Bongiorno PB, Rettori V, McCann SM, Licinio J: Interleukin (IL) 1beta, Il-1 receptor antagonist, Il-10, and Il-13 gene expression in the central nervous system and anterior pituitary during systemic inflammation: Pathophysiological implications. *Proc Natl Acad Sci U S A.* 1997;94:227.

Yolken RH, Karlsson, H, Yee F, Johnston-Wilson NL, Torrey, EF: Endogenous retroviruses and schizophrenia. *Brain Res Rev.* 2000;31:99.

*Zorilla E, Luborsky L, McKay J, Roesnthal R: The relationship of depression and stressors to immunological assays: A meta-analytic review. *Brain Behav Immun.* 2001;15:199.

▲ 1.13 Chronobiology

IGNACIO PROVENCIO, PH.D.

Chronobiology is the study of biological time. A manifestation of biological timing is biological rhythmicity. Periods of biological rhythmicity vary widely, ranging from seconds to days and even months. For example, the period of respiratory rhythms is in the realm of seconds, whereas bouts of depression associated with *seasonal affective disorder* (SAD) recur with a period of approximately 1 year. Among biological rhythms, *circadian* (Latin: *circa*, about; *dies*, day) *rhythms* are the most extensively studied. As the term implies, these rhythms have periods of approximately 24 hours. The activity–rest cycle is the most apparent of all circadian rhythms. Daytime and nighttime temporal niches are different, each offering distinct challenges and opportunities. Hence, animals have evolved to restrict the active portion of the activity–rest cycle to a particular phase with respect to the transition between day and night. Accordingly, nocturnal animals become active as night falls, whereas diurnal animals become active around daybreak. In reality, more complex phase relationships between activity cycles and the astronomical day exist in nature. In fact, many mammals are crepuscular, only becoming active at twilight.

A defining feature of circadian rhythms is that they persist in the absence of time cues and are not simply driven by the 24-hour environmental cycle. Experimental animals housed for several months under constant darkness, temperature, and humidity continue to exhibit robust circadian rhythms. Maintenance of rhythmicity in a "timeless" environment points to the existence of an internal biological timing system that is responsible for generating these endogenous rhythms.

The site of the primary circadian oscillator in mammals, including humans, is the suprachiasmatic nucleus (SCN), located in the anterior hypothalamus (Fig. 1.13–1). The mean circadian period generated by the human SCN is approximately 24.18 hours. Like a watch that ticks 10 minutes and 48 seconds too slowly per day, an individual with such a period gradually comes out of synchrony with the astronomical day. In slightly more than 3 months, a normally diurnal human would be in antiphase to the day–night cycle and thus would become transiently nocturnal. Therefore, a circadian clock must be reset on a regular basis to be effective at maintaining the proper phase relationships of behavioral and physiological processes within the context of the 24-hour day.

Although factors such as temperature and humidity exhibit daily fluctuations, the environmental parameter that most reliably corresponds to the period of Earth's rotation around its axis is the change in illuminance associated with the day–night cycle. Accordingly, organisms have evolved to use this daily change in light levels as a time cue or *zeitgeber* (German: *zeit*, time; *geber*, giver) to reset the endogenous circadian clock. Regulation of the circadian pacemaker through the detection of changes in illuminance requires a photoreceptive apparatus that communicates with the central oscillator. This apparatus is known to reside in the eyes, because surgical removal of the eyes renders an animal incapable of resetting its clock in response to light.

The circadian clock drives many rhythms, including rhythms in behavior, core body temperature, sleep, feeding, drinking, and hormonal levels. One such circadian regulated hormone is the indoleamine, melatonin. Melatonin synthesis is controlled through a multisynaptic pathway from the SCN to the pineal gland. Serum levels of melatonin become elevated at night and return to baseline during the day. The nocturnal rise in melatonin is a convenient marker of circadian phase. Exposure to light elicits two distinct effects on the daily melatonin profile. First, light acutely suppresses elevated melatonin levels, immediately decreasing them to baseline levels. Second, light shifts the phase of the circadian rhythm of melatonin synthesis. Because melatonin can be assayed easily, it provides a convenient window into the state of the circadian pacemaker. Any perturbation of the clock is reflected in the melatonin profile; thus, melatonin offers an output that can be used to study the regulation of the central circadian pacemaker.

Taken together, the circadian axis of mammals can be divided into three distinct functional components: (1) a master pacemaker situated in the SCN, (2) a photoreceptive input to the SCN that originates in the eye, and (3) the myriad of rhythmic outputs that provide insight into the clockwork of the circadian pacemaker.

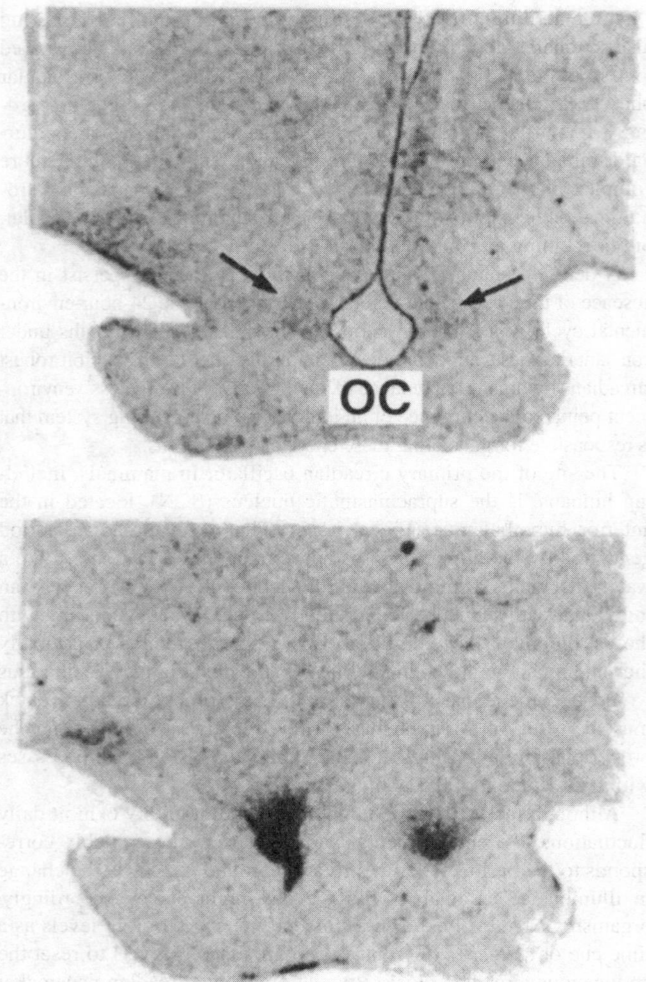

FIGURE 1.13–1 The human suprachiasmatic nucleus. **Top:** Nissl's stain of section through the human hypothalamus. The suprachiasmatic nuclei are indicated by arrows and are located dorsal to the optic chiasm (OC). **Bottom:** Autoradiograph of same section. Specific binding of a radioiodinated analog of melatonin is indicated by the darkening of the suprachiasmatic nuclei. (From Reppert SM, Weaver DR, Rivkees SA, Stopa EG: Putative melatonin receptors in a human biological clock. *Science.* 1988;242:78, with permission.)

CIRCADIAN PACEMAKERS

Anatomy The mammalian circadian system is organized as a hierarchy of pacemakers. The SCN is the master oscillator that orchestrates a multitude of slave oscillators. These slave oscillators are found in a wide range of peripheral tissues including kidney, liver, lung, and other sites in the brain. Because most of the current understanding of the SCN and its slave oscillators is derived from rodent studies, the information presented here is largely based on these findings.

The SCN are small, paired, hypothalamic structures situated immediately dorsal to the optic chiasm. They were recognized as the site of the primary circadian pacemaker, because lesions in the ventral hypothalamus that encompassed the SCN rendered rodents behaviorally arrhythmic. Transplantation of SCN tissue from mutant hamsters that expressed abnormally short circadian periods into the brains of SCN-lesioned host hamsters with normal prelesion circadian periods resulted in a transfer of the abnormally short period.

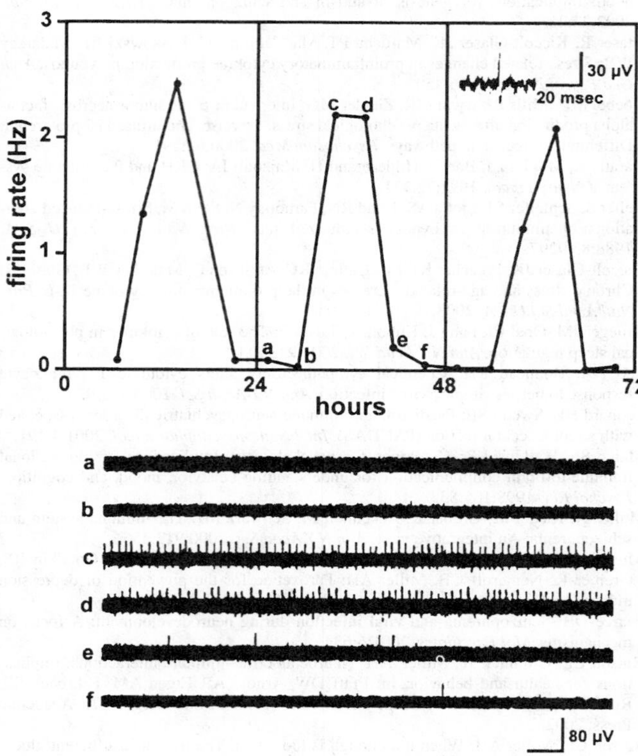

FIGURE 1.13–2 Circadian rhythm in the firing rate of an individual suprachiasmatic nucleus (SCN) neuron. **Top:** Firing rate of an individual SCN neuron over 3 successive days. Inset shows waveform of a single action potential. **Bottom:** Extracellular recording traces corresponding to the labeled times indicated during day 2 in the top panel. (From Welsh DK, Logothetis DE, Meister M, Reppert SM: Individual neurons dissociated from rat suprachiasmatic nucleus express independently phased circadian firing rhythms. *Neuron.* 1995;14:697, with permission.)

This transfer of a distinguishing parameter of the circadian clock indicated that the SCN is a true biological pacemaker and not simply a neural relay for a rhythm generator located elsewhere in the brain. Although long suspected of being the primary circadian pacemaker, these studies firmly established the central role of the SCN in driving circadian rhythmicity in mammals.

Metabolically, the SCN show peak activity during the subjective day. This increased level of metabolism is paralleled by increased electrophysiological activity evident from brain slice recordings. SCN neurons that are isolated and maintained in culture for several days also continue to show approximately 24-hour rhythms in action potential frequency (Fig. 1.13–2).

This observation indicates that the rhythmicity of the SCN is not an emergent property of the system but rather an inherent feature of individual SCN neurons. Molecular studies have confirmed that the oscillatory machinery of the SCN is indeed contained within the individual neurons. It is likely, however, that the general output of the SCN is a result of coupling between individual cellular oscillators, resulting in a coordinated rhythmic signal. The prevailing view of SCN oscillator organization is that the individually oscillating neurons are largely synchronized and the composite output of the SCN reflects the mean phase of these oscillators. Recent studies, however, have shown that discrete phase groupings of oscillators exist. The relative contributions of these "phase ensembles" to the overall rhythmic output of the SCN are likely to be modulated by entraining agents such as light. In addition to the variable contributions of the ensembles to the global output of the SCN, the amplitude and relative phase of the ensembles may also be modified by entraining agents. The potential to manipulate so many parameters of these sets of oscillatory neurons affords a tremendous degree of flexibility with respect to clock-resetting mechanisms. Furthermore, the relative phasing of heterogeneous oscillator groups provides a strategy by which seasonality can be transduced into a biological signal.

The neurons of the SCN are among the smallest neurons in the entire brain. They possess short dendrites that are not extensively branched. A consequence of these cellular dimensions is the high packing density of the nucleus. Virtually every neuron in the SCN is immunopositive for the inhibitory neurotransmitter γ-aminobutyric acid (GABA). The subdivisions of the SCN have also been defined according to immunohistochemical and neural tract tracing criteria. Perhaps the most obvious anatomical subdivision is the *core* of the SCN, defined by the presence of calbindin-positive neurons. The remainder of the SCN that surrounds the core is considered the *shell*. Discrete functions have not been firmly assigned to subdivisions of the SCN, but the afferent and efferent projections to and from these subdivisions are beginning to provide insights into their putative functions.

Afferent Projections The retinohypothalamic tract is the primary afferent input to the SCN. It originates in the retina from a small subset of retinal ganglion cells and innervates the entire volume of the SCN, although the specific subregions of the SCN that are most heavily innervated vary among different species of mammals. Each retina sends a similar number of projections to each SCN, resulting in an approximately bilaterally balanced input. This is in contrast to the projections of the visual system, which tend to be heavily weighted toward the contralateral side. The degree of contralateralism of the visual system is inversely related to the number of retinal ganglion cell axons crossing over at the chiasmatic midline, which, in turn, is directly related to the degree of visual field binocularity. For example, humans have forward-set eyes and, therefore, well-developed binocular vision, allowing excellent perception of depth of field at the expense of a wide visual field. Rodents, on the other hand, have laterally set eyes, resulting in little overlap of each eye's respective visual field. This is manifested as a low degree of binocularity, which is reflected anatomically in the optic chiasm as a large number of axons crossing over the chiasmatic midline. Hence, in rodents, a preponderance of visual system projections targets central structures in the contralateral side of the brain. No such relationships exist in the projections of the retinohypothalamic tract. The lack of contralateralism is consistent with a system optimized for simple irradiance detection rather than visual tracking.

The excitatory neurotransmitter, glutamate, is the primary neurotransmitter of the retinohypothalamic tract, with pituitary adenylyl cyclase activating peptide (PACAP) modulating glutamate's effect in the SCN. Glutamate receptor antagonists can block the effects of light on the circadian axis, illustrating the importance of this neurotransmitter in conveying photic information from the retina to the SCN.

The SCN also receives afferents from the ipsilateral intergeniculate leaflet (IGL), a subnucleus of the lateral geniculate complex. The IGL, in turn, receives input directly from the retina, thus providing a secondary indirect pathway from the retina to the SCN. Neuropeptide Y is the predominant transmitter of the IGL-to-SCN projection. Although the function of the IGL is not well established, it is purported to be involved in encoding environmental luminance. Other, less understood projections to the SCN are known to exist.

Most prominent among these is a distinct serotonergic projection from the midbrain raphe. Serotonin (5-hydroxytryptamine [5-HT]) is known to modulate light's effect on SCN function. Systemic administration of a 5-HT_{1B} receptor agonist before the application of a light pulse attenuates light-induced phase shifts of circadian locomotor activity in hamsters and mice. Light-induced expression of *Fos* (an immediate early gene) within the SCN is also attenuated with this agonist. 5-HT_7, a novel serotonin receptor subclass, has also been implicated in mediating serotonin's modulation of the glutamatergic input to the SCN. Electron microscopy has been used to localize 5-HT_{1B} and 5-HT_7 receptors in pre- and postsynaptic membranes within the SCN. The behavioral data, in conjunction with the pharmacological and anatomical findings, highlight the importance of serotonin in regulating the photic information reaching the SCN via the retinohypothalamic tract. It has been hypothesized that serotonin may adjust the gain of the circadian system's response to light.

Efferent Projections Most SCN efferent projections remain within the limits of the hypothalamus. The best-studied projection originating in the SCN is the multisynaptic projection to the pineal gland. Axons of inhibitory GABAergic SCN neurons traverse the hypothalamus dorsally to the autonomic division of paraventricular nucleus (PVN). The tonic activity of the PVN is suppressed during the day, when the SCN firing rate is high, and is uninhibited during the night, when the SCN is quiescent. The PVN sends a descending glutamatergic projection through the medial forebrain bundle to the intermediolateral cell column of the spinal cord at the upper thoracic levels (T-1 and T-2). Cholinergic preganglionic sympathetic neurons propagate this signal by synapsing on adrenergic postganglionic sympathetics within the superior cervical ganglion. These postganglionic fibers finally innervate pinealocytes to stimulate melatonin synthesis. Norepinephrine release from the terminals of these fibers increases intracellular cyclic adenosine monophosphate (cAMP) levels and, consequently, the activity of melatonin synthetic pathway. Melatonin is not stored or released via a secretory pathway. Its lipophilic nature permits it to passively diffuse through membranes. Thus, the release of melatonin is directly related to its rate of synthesis.

The action of norepinephrine is mediated through β- and α_1-adrenergic receptors. β-Adrenergic receptors stimulate the production of cAMP, whereas the α_1-adrenergic receptors potentiate the action of β-adrenergic receptors. The ultimate outcome of this efferent pathway is that increased melatonin synthesis occurs when SCN activity is low. This antiphasic relationship is established by the GABAergic sign-changing synapse at the PVN. Melatonin receptors localized to the SCN are likely to provide a feedback mechanism by which the antiphasic relationship between the SCN and pineal gland is maintained and possibly reinforced.

A second, less understood efferent pathway from the SCN plays an important role in the control of cortisol. Systemic cortisol levels increase in response to stress. However, these levels also have a strong circadian component, being highest in the early morning in humans. Peak cortisol levels occur at approximately 6 AM to 8 AM, just as melatonin levels approach baseline. This stress-independent component was identified through SCN-lesion studies in rodents that abolished circadian rhythms of cortisol but left the acute response to stress intact. An inhibitory GABAergic projection from the SCN to the hypothalamic PVN is the first element in the neural pathway regulating rhythmic cortisol levels. Axons of this projection synapse on the parvicellular neurons of the PVN that contain corticotropin-releasing hormone (CRH). The terminals of these CRH-containing neurons reside in the median eminence, where they release CRH into the pituitary portal system and stimulate the release of adrenocorticotrophic hormone (ACTH) from the adenohypophysis. ACTH, in turn, acts on the zona fasciculata of the adrenal gland to release cortisol.

A secondary inhibitory pathway to the PVN via a vasopressinergic projection through the dorsomedial hypothalamus has been implicated in cortisol regulation. Analogous to the circuit controlling pineal melatonin, the circuit regulating cortisol contains a single inhibitory synapse. Accordingly, one would expect a circadian cortisol secretion profile similar in phase and shape to that of pineal melatonin. This is not the case, suggesting the presence of other factors that may be involved in shaping the circadian profile of cortisol. First among these is the mechanism of information transfer. Although the SCN-pineal circuit is exclusively neural, the SCN-adrenal circuit involves the stimulated release of hormones that are subject to the vagaries of diffusion and transport through the circulation. Second, the sensitivity of the adrenal cortex to ACTH also exhibits a circadian variation. Finally, it has been proposed that cortisol itself may feed back on the brain to inhibit CRH and ACTH production.

Molecular Clockwork As mentioned previously, isolated SCN neurons can generate circadian rhythms. For decades, however, the lack of knowledge regarding the inner clockwork of the circadian pacemaker forced investigators to treat the SCN as a "black box." Since the mid-1980s, progress in understanding rhythmic biochemical processes has led to advances in the identification and characterization of the molecular gears of circadian pacemakers. A cohort of principal clock genes has been identified in mammals since 1997. Many of these molecular components were initially discovered in the fruit fly, *Drosophila melanogaster*, leading to the discovery of mammalian orthologs. The basic architecture of the circadian clockwork is generally conserved among species of the animal kingdom; however, some of the clock genes have been duplicated in the mammalian genome. These duplications have added another level of complexity and the possibility of partially redundant functions.

The molecular clockwork of the master clock in the SCN is virtually identical to that of the peripheral slave oscillators. The SCN are so small that their size precludes most biochemical analyses. However, investigators have been able to characterize clock proteins from abundant clock-containing peripheral tissues, such as liver, to understand the workings of the central clock in the SCN. From these and other studies, the following concepts are now established.

The mammalian circadian clockwork consists of interacting positive and negative transcriptional and translational feedback loops. The expression of three homologs of the *Drosophila* period gene (*Per1*, *Per2*, and *Per3*) and two homologs of the *Drosophila* cryptochrome gene (*Cry1* and *Cry2*) are positively regulated by the binding of CLOCK-MOP3 (*MOP3* is also known as *BMAL1*) heterodimers to E-box enhancers in the promoters of these genes. The products of the *Per* and *Cry* genes translocate back into the nucleus and repress their own transcription. This series of events constitutes the negative feedback limb of the core oscillation.

In addition to activating the transcription of the *Per* and *Cry* genes, the CLOCK-MOP3 complex also activates expression of the orphan nuclear receptor gene, *Rev-Erbα*. The gene product of *Rev-Erbα* in turn, translocates into the nucleus and represses transcription of the *MOP3* gene through *Rev-Erb/ROR* response elements in the *MOP3* gene promoter. MOP3 subsequently heterodimerizes with CLOCK and again activates expression of the *Per*, *Cry*, and *Rev-Erbα* genes. This derepression (or activation) of the *MOP3* gene, subsequent heterodimerization with CLOCK, and activation of the *Per*, *Cry*, and *Rev-Erbα* genes constitutes the positive feedback limb of the core oscillator.

The interactions of clock proteins and the translocations of these proteins between cellular compartments are tightly regulated by posttranslational modifications. For example, phosphorylation of some of the PER proteins by casein kinase Iε is important for their translocation into the nucleus. Other kinases, and presumably phosphatases, are emerging as critical regulators of the circadian molecular clockwork. More global regulatory mechanisms, such as histone acetylation or phosphorylation, are also likely to control the rhythmic expression and function of clock genes.

RESETTING THE CIRCADIAN CLOCK

Sensory Parameters In humans and other mammals, light perceived through the eyes is the most effective agent for entraining (synchronizing) the circadian system to the 24-hour day. Bilateral removal of the eyes renders an individual incapable of resetting the circadian clock, indicating that the photosensitive apparatus necessary for resetting must be ocular. However, several lines of evidence suggest that this apparatus is distinct from the rod and cone photoreceptors that are required for vision.

First, the photic sensitivities of the visual and circadian systems are quite different (Fig. 1.13–3). The visual system can be activated by intensities of light ranging from dim starlight to bright daylight. This dynamic range represents approximately 14 log units of light intensity measured in photons per second per cm^2. The dynamic range of the circadian system is only 3 log units, and the activation threshold is much higher than the visual system. Additionally, the circadian system requires light stimuli of much longer duration to activate clock resetting than that required by the visual system to construct images.

These differences in activation parameters are consistent with the differences in the photoreceptive tasks performed by these functionally distinct systems. The principal task of the visual system is to construct a spatiotemporal representation of the environment. In this sense, the eye functions like a movie camera, acquiring a series of still shots that the

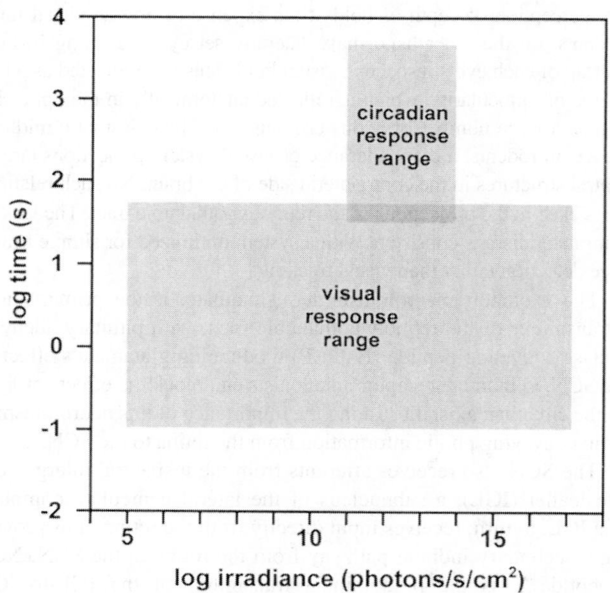

FIGURE 1.13–3 Graphical representation of the response ranges of the visual and circadian systems. The response ranges of sensitivity (x-axis) and integration time (y-axis) of the circadian and visual systems are contained within the boundaries of their respective rectangles. Note that the circadian system is insensitive to light and requires stimuli of longer durations relative to the visual system.

brain can interpret as a dynamic visual scene. Thus, information about the relative positions of different stimuli within the visual field must be maintained throughout processing. The ability to detect motion within the visual field also requires a relatively fast integration time analogous to a fast International Standards Organization (ISO) rating for a roll of 35-mm film. These spatial and temporal requirements can be satisfied by a fine two-dimensional array of narrow-capture, highly sensitive, photoreceptive elements, such as the photoreceptor layer of the retina that contains the rod and cone photoreceptors.

By contrast, the task of the photoreceptive input to the circadian system is the measurement of ambient illumination. In essence, the circadian photoreceptive system must function as a light meter rather than a camera. The requirements of a light meter are different than those of a camera. Spatial information is not important and may, in fact, confound the system. Luminous point sources of light, such as the moon, could prove confusing for narrow-capture photoreceptive elements. If, however, the system used relatively insensitive, broad-capture photoreceptive elements capable of integrating large sectors of visual space, the relative contribution of the moon's irradiance to the total ambient irradiance would be minimized and thus would not be mistaken for a daytime light level. Theoretically, a fine, two-dimensional array of narrow-capture photoreceptive elements could serve in this capacity if the output of the array were averaged. Alternatively, an anatomically distinct, coarse array of relatively few broad-capture photoreceptive elements would be optimal for wide spatial integration at a reduced absolute sensitivity. Lightning could also potentially baffle the circadian system. Ambient levels of illumination achieved by lightning can equal those levels of daylight. However, the circadian system's insensitivity to stimuli of short duration essentially filters out this source of photic noise. Taken together, the spatial and temporal stimulus parameters required to activate the circadian photic input system ensure that only relevant stimuli are conferred to the central circadian pacemaker.

The different sensory demands of the circadian and visual systems raise the possibility that a novel photoreceptive apparatus subserves light-mediated entrainment of the circadian system to the day–night cycle. Visually blind rodents that have a genetically induced loss of rods and cones remain capable of light-mediated circadian clock resetting. Paradoxically, the loss of rods and cones has no effect on the sensitivity of the circadian system to light, despite the fact that these animals are incapable of forming images. A similar situation has been observed in blind humans. A subset of blind individuals retain the ability to photically regulate the rhythmic synthesis of melatonin.

Some blind individuals report no cognitive visual perception, show no electrophysiological evidence for ocular light detection as determined by electroretinogram analysis, and exhibit no pupillary light response. However, some of these individuals continue to show an acute suppression of nocturnal melatonin and a phase shift in the circadian rhythm of melatonin production. All too frequently, blind individuals are bilaterally enucleated and fitted with prosthetic eyes for purposes ranging from susceptibility to ocular infections to reasons of aesthetics. Perhaps some of these decisions should be reconsidered in light of the fact that the eyes may retain a function in clock resetting despite being useless for vision.

Extraocular Photoreception In recent years, it has been suggested that photic stimulation of extraocular tissues is sufficient to shift the human circadian clock. Specifically, blue light illumination of highly vascularized tissue, such as the popliteal region behind the knee, was shown to phase shift the nightly increase of melatonin. This remarkable result was challenged by multiple studies in humans and rodents that failed to replicate the original finding of extraocular circadian photoreception. One such study involved exposing bilaterally enucleated hamsters to irradiances equivalent to sunlight levels at noon. These animals were also completely shaved to maximize transcutaneous transmission of light. Even these extraordinary measures were not sufficient to demonstrate any evidence of extraocular circadian photoreception in these eyeless rodents. Subsequently, a human study designed to replicate the protocol of the original study failed to reproduce the results of the initial work. Currently, the concept of extraocular circadian photoreception in humans and other mammals is not widely accepted among those investigating entrainment mechanisms.

NOVEL CLASS OF RETINAL PHOTORECEPTOR

Intrinsically Photosensitive Retinal Ganglion Cells

The findings from retinally degenerate animal models and blind humans indicate that photoreceptors other than rods and cones are likely to be involved in the photoregulation of the circadian axis. Blue wavelengths of light most efficiently suppress melatonin in humans. However, the spectral profile of melatonin suppression does not match that of any of the photopigments found in human rods or cones. A small subset of rodent retinal ganglion cells recently has been shown to be intrinsically photosensitive. The spectral sensitivity of these cells matches the spectral sensitivity of the circadian system. Most compelling, however, is that the intrinsically photosensitive retinal ganglion cells project directly to the SCN. They also project to the IGL and the olivary pretectal nuclei, other brain structures involved in the interpretation of illuminance information. The intrinsically photosensitive cells contain melanopsin, a photopigment initially discovered in the pigmented skin cells (melanophores) of tadpoles and subsequently identified in human and mouse retinas. The anatomy and physiology of melanopsin-containing retinal ganglion cells are consistent with the previously described characteristics expected of cells involved in illuminance detection. Namely, these cells are few in number. They represent 1 to 2 percent of all of the retinal ganglion cells in the rodent retina. These cells are also distributed over the entire retinal expanse. The dendritic arbors of melanopsin-containing retinal ganglion cells are vast, with arbors in the mouse retina ranging from 400 to 500 μm in diameter. Melanopsin itself is localized to the plasma membrane of the cell body, axons, and dendrites. The size of the receptive fields of these cells matches the size of the dendritic arbors, indicating that the entire arbor has the ability to initiate phototransduction and therefore is capable of spatially integrating large sectors of the visual field. The average mouse eye is approximately 3 mm in diameter. Therefore, a photoreceptor with a receptive field diameter of 400 to 500 μm is able to spatially integrate 15 to 20 degrees of visual space. By comparison, the diameter of the full moon at its highest point in the sky is approximately equivalent to 1 degree of the human visual field. Melanopsin-containing retinal ganglion cells are clearly broad-capture photoreceptors. Furthermore, because the dendritic arbors overlap, these cells form a photoreceptive net in the inner mammalian retina. This complex of cells represents the coarse array of photoreceptive elements expected of an irradiance detector. In addition, the activation parameters of these cells parallel the parameters observed for the circadian system as a whole. The melanopsin-containing ganglion cells are significantly less sensitive to light compared to the rod and cone photoreceptors of the visual system, and they require light stimuli of relatively long duration to be activated. Finally, these cells are maximally sensitive to wavelengths of light similar to those required to acutely suppress nocturnal melatonin levels in humans.

Function Although the anatomy and physiology of melanopsin retinal ganglion cells are highly suggestive that these cells function as circadian photoreceptors, recent studies provide the most compelling evidence. Mice with a targeted disruption of both copies of the

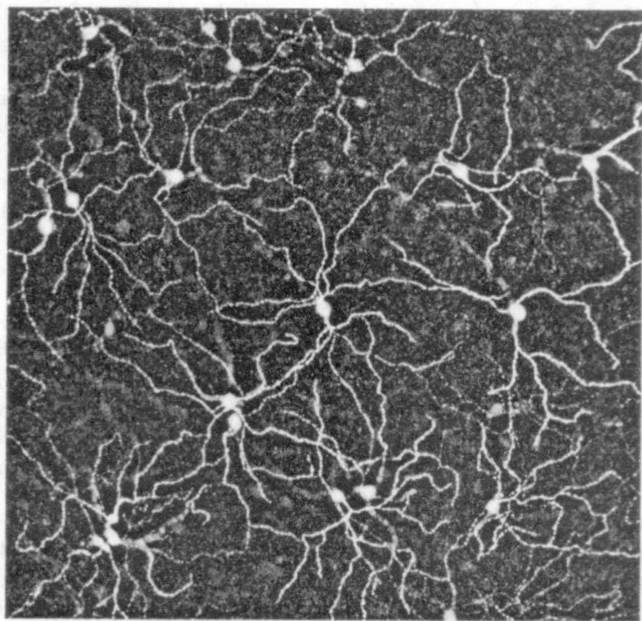

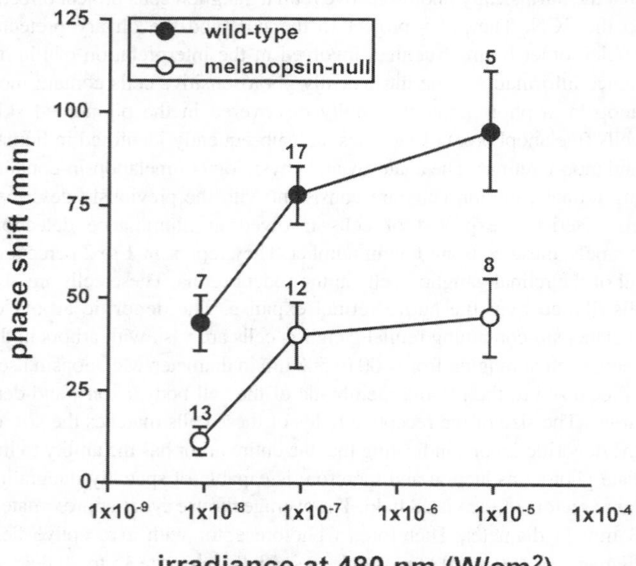

FIGURE 1.13–4 Melanopsin in the mouse. **Top:** Retinal ganglion cells in a flat-mounted mouse retina labeled by indirect immunofluorescence with an antibody against melanopsin. Note the *photoreceptive net* formed by the overlapping dendritic arbors. (Courtesy of Dr. Ana Castrucci.) **Bottom:** Fluence-response relationship in wild-type and melanopsin-null mice in response to a 15-minute pulse of blue (480-nm wavelength) light at circadian time 15 hours. Melanopsin-null mice exhibited attenuated phase shifting of circadian locomotor rhythms relative to wild-type siblings at all irradiances tested. (Adapted from Panda S, Sato TK, Castrucci AM, et al.: Melanopsin [*Opn4*] requirement for normal light-induced circadian phase shifting. *Science.* 2002;298:2213.)

melanopsin gene show profound deficits in their ability to phase shift circadian locomotor rhythms in response to pulses of light. These deficits were observed at all irradiances tested (Fig. 1.13–4). Thus, the photopigment melanopsin and, presumably, the retinal ganglion cells containing melanopsin are required for normal photic regulation of circadian rhythms. Perhaps the most surprising aspect of these "knock out" studies is that disrupting both copies of the

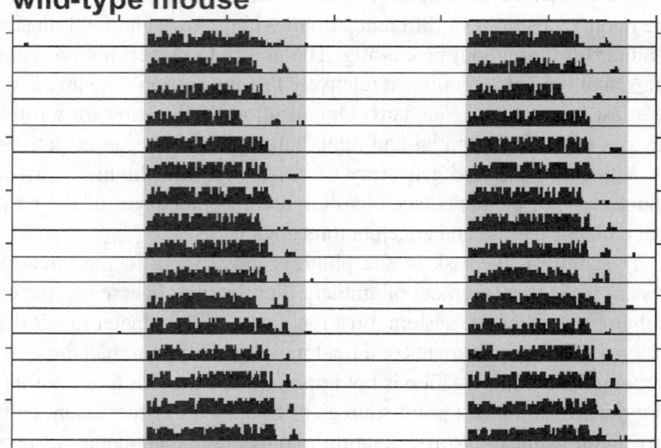

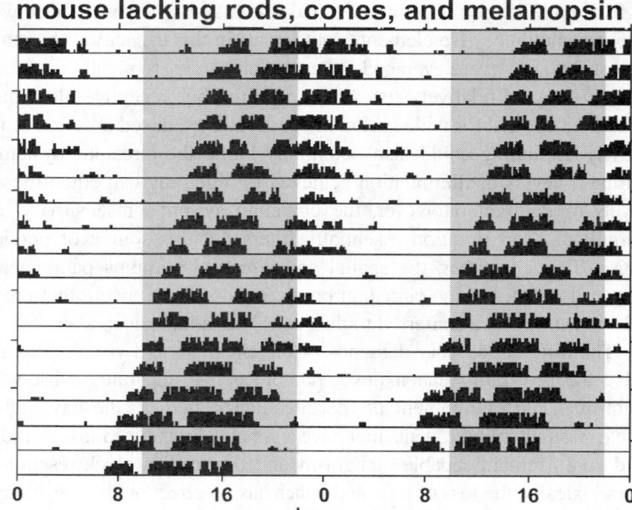

FIGURE 1.13–5 Wheel running activity records of a wild-type mouse and a mouse lacking rods, cones, and melanopsin. **Top:** Representative double-plotted activity record of a wild-type mouse under entraining conditions of 12 hours of white light (800 lux) and 12 hours of darkness (*grey box*). **Bottom:** Representative double-plotted activity records of a mouse lacking rods, cones, and melanopsin under identical entraining conditions. Whereas wild-type mice consolidate their activity to the dark phase, and the time of activity onset is coincident with the light to dark transition, the mice lacking rods, cones, and melanopsin continue to free run with an intrinsic period length of less than 24 hours. (Adapted from supplementary data from Panda S, Provencio I, Tu DC, et al.: Melanopsin is required for non-image-forming photic responses in blind mice. *Science.* 2003; 301:525.)

melanopsin gene does not completely abolish light-induced circadian phase shifting; some capacity for phase shifting remains. The photoreceptors mediating this residual sensitivity are likely to be the rods or the cones; however, one cannot exclude the possibility that an unrecognized class of ocular photoreceptor fulfills this role.

To test the contribution of rod and cone photoreceptors to photoentrainment, melanopsin-null mice were crossed with mice lacking rods and cones. The progeny of this cross that were rodless, coneless, and melanopsin-null were incapable of photoentrainment, even at high irradiances of ambient light (Fig. 1.13–5). Other nonvisual photophysiology was also abolished in these mice, such as the photoregulation of the melatonin biosynthetic pathway, the pupillary light response, and the acute light-induced inhibition of activity. From these studies, it can be concluded that at least partial functional redundancy exists for nonvisual photoreception between rods, cones, or both and the melanopsin-containing retinal ganglion cells. It should be noted that the relative contribution of the visual photoreceptors versus that of the melanopsin retinal ganglion cells appears to be different among the various nonvisual responses. For example, melanopsin plays a rather significant role in the phase shifting of circadian locomotor activity, however, the pupillary light response is relatively insensitive to the loss of melanopsin. Importantly, the complete loss of photic responses in melanopsin-null mice lacking rods and cones demonstrates that no additional photopigments, such as cryptochromes, are required for nonvisual photic signaling. Thus, it appears that multiple photoreceptor systems subserve nonvisual photoreception, a phenomenon observed across phylogeny.

The dawn of air travel has introduced society to the phenomenon of jet lag, a dramatic example of circadian desynchrony. Simply stated, jet lag is the condition of one's circadian clock being desynchronized from the local time. Shift work can also cause circadian desynchrony. The invention of artificial lighting has permitted the manufacturing and service industries to work around the clock. As a result, shift workers are constantly experiencing the effects of circadian desynchrony as they try to entrain to an ever-changing light–dark cycle. Some deleterious effects of shift work include elevated stress, deficits in alertness, decreased cognitive function, and gastric distress. Although no therapy currently exists for jet lag or shift work, an efficacious treatment ultimately must involve the appropriate resetting of the clock. Such a treatment may include timed administration of light stimuli of spectrally optimal wavelengths. A more complete understanding of how melanopsin-containing retinal ganglion cells convert such stimuli into neural signals may present investigators with pharmacological entry points against which chronobiotic drugs can be designed.

SLEEP AND CIRCADIAN RHYTHMS

Sleep Regulation Restful consolidated sleep is most appreciated when sleep disturbances are experienced. Sleep is the integrated product of two oscillatory processes. The first process, frequently referred to as the *sleep homeostat*, is an oscillation that stems from the accumulation and dissipation of sleep debt. The biological substrates encoding sleep debt are not known, although adenosine is emerging as a primary candidate neuromodulator of the sleep homeostat. The second oscillatory process is governed by the circadian clock and controls a daily rhythm in sleep propensity or, conversely, arousal. These interacting oscillations can be dissociated by housing subjects in a timeless environment for several weeks.

The circadian cycle in arousal (wakefulness) steadily increases throughout the day, reaching a maximum immediately before the circadian increase in plasma melatonin (Fig. 1.13–6). Arousal subsequently decreases to coincide with the circadian trough in core body temperature. Experiments imposing forced sleep schedules throughout the circadian day have shown that an uninterrupted 8-hour bout of sleep can only be obtained if sleep is initiated approximately 6 hours before the temperature nadir. This nadir typically occurs at approximately 5:00 AM to 6:00 AM. In healthy individuals, initiating sleep between 11:00 PM and 12:00 AM affords the highest probability of getting 8 solid hours of sleep.

It should be stressed that diurnal preference varies among individuals as a function of age, endogenous circadian periods, and other factors. This variability is paralleled by physiology. Clinically, diurnal preference can be quantified using the Horne-Östberg (HO) questionnaire. In qualitative terms, *morning people* or *morning larks* tend to awaken earlier and experience the core body temperature minimum at an earlier clock time relative to *night people* or *night owls*. Sleep deprivation studies have shown that the homeostatic component of sleep is remarkably similar among individuals of similar age. (It should be noted that there is a well-established age-dependent decline in sleep need.) Therefore, diurnal preference is dictated almost exclusively by the circadian component of sleep regulation.

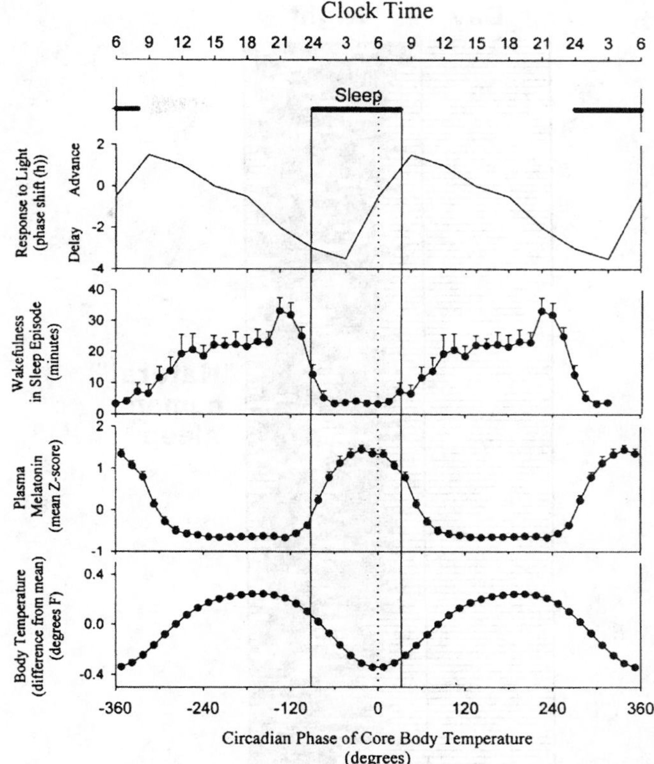

FIGURE 1.13–6 Relative phase relationship of sleep in young adults to other circadian phase markers. (From Dijk D-J, Lockley SW: Invited review: Integration of human sleep-wake regulation and circadian rhythmicity. *J Appl Physiol.* 2002;92:852, with permission.)

Circadian Sleep Disorders Advanced sleep phase syndrome (ASPS) is a pathological extreme of the morning lark phenotype. An autosomal-dominant familial form of ASPS (FASPS) recently has been genetically characterized. Afflicted family members exhibit a striking 4-hour advance of the daily sleep–wake rhythm. They typically fall asleep at approximately 7:30 PM and spontaneously awaken at approximately 4:30 AM. Affected individuals have a single nucleotide polymorphism in the gene encoding hPER2, the human homolog of the mouse *Per2* clock gene. This adenine-to-guanine nucleotide polymorphism results in serine-to-glycine amino acid substitution that causes the mutant protein to be inefficiently phosphorylated by casein kinase Iε, an established component of the circadian molecular clockwork. Similarly, delayed sleep phase syndrome (DSPS) has been shown to be influenced by genetics. A length polymorphism in a repeat region of the *hPER3* gene appears to be associated with diurnal preference in DSPS patients, the shorter allele being associated with evening preference.

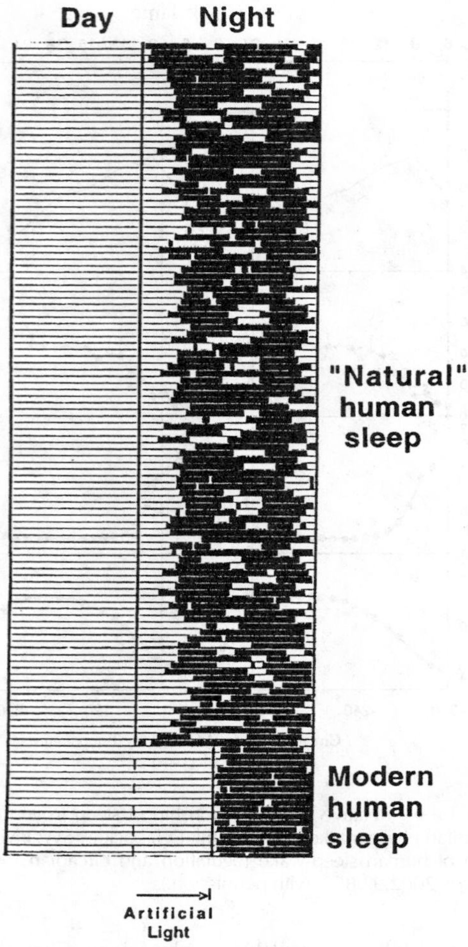

FIGURE 1.13–7 Change of sleep structure in response to artificial lighting. Total sleep time is reduced, and periods of quiet wakefulness are abolished by extending daytime into nighttime through artificial lighting. (From Wehr TA, Moul DE, Barbato G, et al.: Conservation of photoperiod-responsive mechanisms in humans. *Am J Physiol.* 1993;265:R846, with permission.)

The advent of the light bulb has extended the human day into the natural night. This encroachment on the night, although increasing productivity, has affected human sleep patterns (Fig. 1.13–7). Typical use of artificial lights results in a single, consolidated bout of sleep lasting approximately 8 hours. This pattern of sleep is uncommon among most other mammals, which typically experience more fractured sleep. Human sleep under more natural photoperiods, where the duration of the night is longer, becomes decompressed. Specifically, a bimodal distribution of sleep is observed; bouts of sleep occur in early and late night. Periods of *quiet wakefulness* are interspersed between the two primary bouts of sleep. This natural sleep pattern is more similar to the sleep patterns of other mammals.

SEASONALITY

The 24-hour period of the Earth's rotation around its axis is unchanging. However, the Earth's axis is tilted 23.45 degrees from the plane of its own orbit around the sun (the ecliptic). As a result, the relative proportion of daytime to nighttime within the 24-hour astronomical day varies as the Earth proceeds through its orbit of the sun. Many organisms are capable of synchronizing physiology to the seasonal cycle to maximize survival. For example, precise seasonal cycles in reproduction are seen throughout the plant and animal kingdoms. Large mammals that typically have long gestation periods, such as sheep, conceive in the fall when the nights are long and the days are short, so birth occurs during the relatively mild season of spring. These animals are referred to as *short-day breeders*. Conversely, mammals with gestation periods of only a few weeks, such as hamsters, conceive and give birth during spring and summer, when the days are long and the nights are short. Hence, these animals are referred to as *long-day breeders*. Like circadian rhythms, many of these yearly (circannual) rhythms tend to persist in the absence of seasonal cues with endogenous periods of approximately 1 year.

Melatonin and Seasonality

The most reliable environmental parameter providing a faithful representation of the solar day is the day–night cycle. Similarly, the most reliable environmental parameter reflecting the progression through the seasons is the change in day length, the fraction of the 24-hour day between sunrise and sunset. In seasonally breeding animals, day length is physiologically encoded through the melatonin profile. As described previously, melatonin levels are elevated during the night. A long night, such as that experienced during the short day lengths of winter, results in an elevated melatonin profile of relatively long duration. A short summer night, by contrast, results in a short duration of elevated melatonin. This seasonal signal is interpreted by the reproductive axis, resulting in an appropriate reproductive response. Melatonin's role in transducing day length was elucidated by pinealectomizing seasonally breeding animals, thereby removing the primary endogenous source of melatonin. Melatonin was then infused in profiles mimicking long days or short days. The duration of elevated melatonin was the primary determinant of seasonal reproductive status, even when the infused profile was administered under a conflicting day length. Variations in other parameters, such as the amplitude of the melatonin profile, the amount of total melatonin synthesized, or the phase relationship of the profile to the light–dark cycle, are of limited importance in producing a humoral signal that transduces day length.

Reproductive responses to changing day length can be dramatic. A male Siberian hamster (*Phodopus sungorus*) maintained in long days is reproductively competent and typically has a testicular weight of approximately 250 mg per testis. Under short days, however, the testes regress to approximately 15 mg per testis, representing a 94 percent decrease in testicular mass. The same degree of regression is observed in response to melatonin infusions that mimic short days. Communication of the hormonally transduced day length to the reproductive axis is likely to be mediated, at least partially, through melatonin receptors in the *pars tuberalis* of the pituitary gland. The exact mechanism remains unknown, but activation of these receptors is hypothesized to indirectly regulate an unidentified factor putatively named *tuberalin*. Tuberalin, in turn, controls gene expression and prolactin release from lactotrophs in the adenohypophysis of the pituitary.

Seasonality in Humans

Whether humans are truly seasonal is still a point of considerable debate. Several lines of evidence exist that suggest the presence of a residual tendency toward seasonality. A peak in the rate of suicide occurs in the summer; this peak is cross-cultural. Birth rates also tend to show a seasonal variation; a small but distinguishable peak in the rate of births occurs in spring and summer. This pattern, however, is itself variable and is heavily influenced by unknown cultural and geographic factors. Interestingly, the amplitude of the spring-summer birth rate peak has diminished as societies have become industrialized.

The decompressed bimodal structure of human sleep during long nights indicates that the length of natural sleep is related to the length of the night. Potentially, a two-oscillator system could function to maintain proper sleep patterns during changing photoperiods. Such a proposed system would consist of an evening oscillator that tracks the transition from day to night (dusk) and a morning oscillator that tracks the transition from night to day (dawn). The relative phase differences between these oscillators may encode the changing day lengths associated with the passing of the seasons. Biological evidence for a two-oscillator system exists in rodents and humans.

The melatonin profile of many vertebrates, including some humans, is bimodal, with evening and morning peaks. In rodents, metabolic and electrophysiological studies of the SCN typically have been done in brain slices cut in the coronal plane. Results of electrophysiological studies conducted in brain slices cut in the horizontal plane have provided new insights. The action potential frequency in SCN neurons from horizontally cut preparations is bimodal, with peaks in the early and late subjective day. Furthermore, the interpeak interval varies as a function of the photoperiod in which the animal was housed. These studies lend credence to long-standing suspicions that the SCN of seasonally breeding mammals and, perhaps, nonseasonal mammals harbor a morning and evening oscillator that interact to convey day length information.

In seasonally reproductive mammals, the duration of the nightly increase in melatonin effectively encodes day length (or, more accurately, night length). By contrast, in the vast majority of humans, the duration of elevated melatonin is invariant throughout the year. Recent studies have shown that healthy men living in their usual home environment had winter and summer melatonin profiles that were indistinguishable. However, healthy men enrolled in a carefully controlled photoperiod experiment gave surprisingly different results. In this cohort, long nights elicited an extended period of melatonin elevation. Conversely, short nights produced a compressed period of elevated melatonin. In essence, humans retain the capacity to encode day length, although this capacity is masked by the self-imposed artificial lighting regimens of modern society. It should be noted that a small percentage of individuals residing in their usual environment exhibits melatonin profiles that track day length, much like seasonally breeding mammals. Of particular interest are male patients experiencing SAD, some of whom exhibit this apparent seasonality.

SEASONAL AFFECTIVE DISORDER AND CIRCADIAN RHYTHMS

SAD is the most overt manifestation of seasonality in humans. It is characterized by recurrent major depressive episodes followed by periods of remission that occur on a seasonal basis. SAD is not categorized as a distinct mood disorder in the fourth revised edition of the *Diagnostic and Statistical Manual of Mental Disorders* (DSM-IV-TR). Rather, once the diagnostic criteria for a *major depressive episode* have been met, then it can be determined whether the *seasonal pattern specifier* criteria are present, thus indicating a diagnosis of SAD. The SAD specifier criteria are

A. Regular temporal relationship between the onset of major depressive episodes and a particular time of the year (unrelated to obvious season-related psychosocial stressors).
B. Full remissions (or a change from depression to mania or hypomania) also occur at a characteristic time of the year.
C. Two major depressive episodes meeting criteria A and B have occurred in the last 2 years, and no nonseasonal episodes have occurred in the same period.
D. Seasonal major depressive episodes substantially outnumber the nonseasonal episodes over the individual's lifetime.

Winter SAD

The most prevalent form of SAD has an onset in the late fall and early winter and remits in the late spring and early summer. This condition is frequently referred to as *winter SAD*, *winter depression*, or the *winter blues*. Symptoms atypical of major depression can present with winter SAD. These include, but are not restricted to, a significant increase in weight, hyperphagia, an increase rather than decrease in sleep, a heightened sensitivity to interpersonal rejection, and a leaden feeling in the extremities. Most distinct, however, is a craving for carbohydrates.

Surveys indicate the prevalence of winter SAD among the general population to be between 4 and 9 percent. Women are four times as likely as men to be affected, and as much as 20 percent of the population may have subsyndromal features. Rates of SAD are slightly higher among relatives of those with a confirmed diagnosis of SAD. This could be attributed to a genetic influence or environmental influences, given shared environmental exposure among families.

The gold standard treatment for winter SAD is light therapy. A typical prescription for light therapy involves 45 to 90 minutes daily exposure to a broad spectrum, ultraviolet-filtered, white light source of relatively high irradiance (5,000 to 10,000 lux). Recent studies have suggested that a combination treatment of light therapy in conjunction with cognitive-behavioral therapy may be more efficacious than light therapy alone. Monoamine oxidase inhibitors (MAOIs) have also been used successfully to treat winter SAD. The antidepressant effect of phototherapy in winter SAD patients has given rise to several hypotheses regarding the etiology of the disorder. One hypothesis proposes that SAD patients experience the consequences of a chronically phase delayed circadian clock, suggesting that the aberrant phase angle between the clock and the environment is causative of winter SAD. Consistent with this hypothesis is that the offset of the nightly release of melatonin is delayed among some winter SAD patients relative to healthy controls (Fig. 1.13–8). However, the onset of melatonin increase is not phase shifted relative to controls. In essence, these patients have a longer duration of elevated melatonin that increases at the same clock time as that of controls but stays elevated longer, thus impinging on the morning hours. Although these data are not consistent with the phase delay hypothesis, they may explain the effectiveness of morning bright light therapy that would acutely suppress the extended melatonin profile of winter SAD patients. It should be noted that the sculpting of the melatonin profile by morning light exposure cannot entirely explain the proven success of phototherapy. In some winter SAD patients, bright light administered during the evening is also antidepressant. In fact, some phototherapy treatment paradigms prescribe morning and evening light exposures.

The success of light therapy administered at various clock times suggests that winter SAD may not have a circadian-based etiology. An alternate hypothesis proposes that patients experiencing winter SAD are generally less sensitive to light than healthy counterparts. Such photic insensitivity would become apparent during the decreased light levels of late fall and early winter, depriving these individuals of the threshold of light required to stave off depression. Accordingly, daily supplementation of light through bright photo-

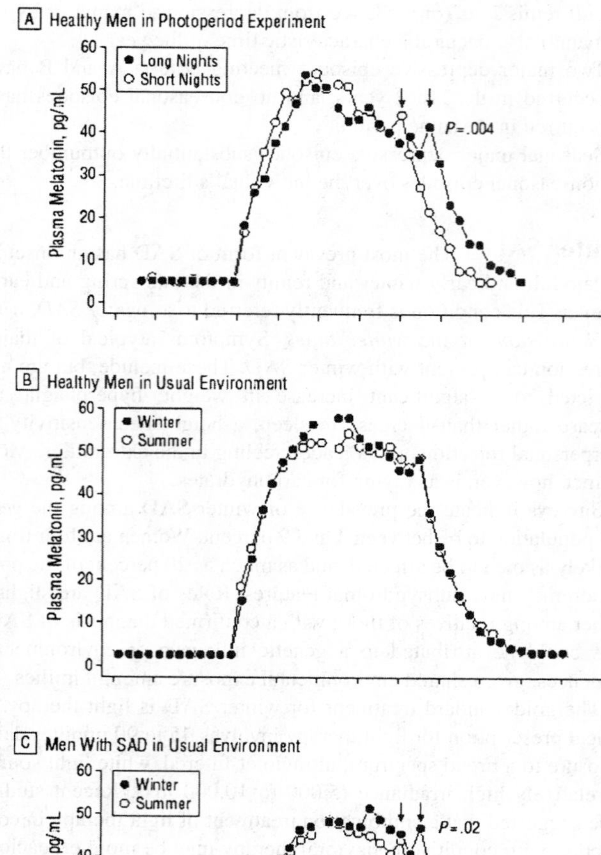

FIGURE 1.13–8 Seasonal variation in melatonin profiles of healthy men and men with seasonal affective disorder (SAD). **A:** The melatonin profiles of healthy men vary as a function of the experimentally controlled photoperiod. Winter-like long nights produce a longer profile of elevated melatonin relative to summer-like short nights. **B:** Healthy men did not show a seasonal variation of the melatonin profile when they had been living under the lighting cycle of their usual environment. **C:** By contrast, men with SAD exhibited a seasonal variation of the melatonin profile when they had been living under the lighting cycle of their usual environment. (From Wehr TA, Duncan WC Jr, Sher L, et al.: A circadian signal of change of season in patients with seasonal affective disorder. *Arch Gen Psych.* 2001;58:1108, with permission.)

therapy would be expected to exceed this theoretical threshold. This hypothesis predicts that the incidence of winter SAD among blind individuals would be much higher than that experienced among the sighted population. This correlation has not been observed. However, it should be remembered that a portion of the blind population still retains a residual ability to detect light for purposes of melatonin suppression and circadian phase shifting, despite an inability to construct visual images. It must be emphasized that a lack of cognitive vision should not be equated with a diminished or abolished capacity to detect gross environmental illuminance changes.

A basic tenet in the development of pharmacological treatments is that a dose dependence must exist to implicate the effectiveness of the drug in question. Similarly, a dose or fluence dependence should be observed with respect to treatment of winter SAD with bright phototherapy. Several studies attempting to document a fluence-response relationship in the treatment of winter SAD have provided the field with conflicting data. Moreover, light therapy, like other photobiological responses, should show a wavelength dependence that reflects the spectral sensitivity of the photopigments mediating that response. Several investigators have attempted to establish the relative efficacy of colored-light treatments. Taken together, these studies have provided equivocal results with no clear range of wavelengths proving to be most effective.

It has been proposed that winter SAD patients do not experience an inherent insensitivity to light but rather fail to respond appropriately to light. Several physiological responses to light have been tested among SAD patients, and no striking deficits in photoresponsiveness were observed relative to healthy controls. Light exposure, however, elicits a myriad of biological responses, some of which are subtle. Studies comparing the photoresponsiveness of SAD and control subjects are far from comprehensive.

In general, it cannot be denied that phototherapy has proven to be an effective treatment for winter SAD. The mechanisms by which bright light ameliorates the symptoms of this disease remain unknown. Experimentally, it has proven difficult to select an appropriate control treatment to assess the contribution of the placebo effect of light therapy. SAD patients tend to be educated about their malady and the available treatment paradigms, making experimental design difficult and subsequent interpretation of results necessarily cautious.

NONSEASONAL DEPRESSION AND CIRCADIAN RHYTHMS

Aberrations in the timing and amount of sleep are frequently part of the symptomology of depression, including nonseasonal depression. For example, the circadian phase angle of sleep onset can vary in bipolar I disorder, depending on the state; depression causes a phase delay, whereas mania results in a phase advance. In addition, sleep disturbances can contribute to the pathogenesis of the disease. A curious phenomenon related to depression and sleep is that total sleep deprivation can provide a transient antidepressant effect in a majority (approximately 60 percent) of depressed patients. No difference was observed between medicated and nonmedicated patients in the efficacy of sleep deprivation treatment.

Relapse occurs after the following night of sleep. Even short, daytime naps can cause relapse. This tendency of nap-induced relapse varies as a function of time of day during which the nap is taken. Early morning appears to be a critical time during which naps have a high tendency of causing relapse. Using this information, a treatment paradigm was developed combining total sleep deprivation, a phase advance of the sleep schedule, and slow resetting to the original sleep schedule.

Patients who have just initiated a regimen of antidepression medication are sleep deprived for one night and are allowed to sleep on the following day from 5:00 PM to midnight. This constitutes a 6-hour phase advance relative to the sleep schedule observed before the night of sleep deprivation. Sleep onset and offset are subsequently delayed 1 hour each day for 1 week until a conventional bedtime of 11:00 PM to 6:00 AM is achieved. This paradigm ensures that sleep is avoided during the critical morning period when relapse tendency is high. It also provides an acute antidepressant effect during the lag time typically observed between initiation of pharmacotherapy and the onset of symptom improvement.

FUTURE CONSIDERATIONS

Just as air travel presented the novel phenomenon of jet lag, commercial space travel will introduce new challenges. Space shuttle astronauts experience 90-minute "days" as the shuttle orbits the Earth. The confounding temporal environment of space will require space travelers to be vigilant about resetting their internal clocks. The health consequences of not doing so in such a hazardous environment are potentially life threatening. A better understanding of photic and nonphotic entrainment of circadian rhythms will provide the tools for resetting. Many of these issues are currently being addressed in the atemporal environs of the nuclear submarine. It is hoped that these lessons will prove valuable as an age of interplanetary travel begins.

SUGGESTED CROSS-REFERENCES

Sleep is discussed in Section 1.20, sleep disorders are discussed in Chapter 20, and mood disorders are discussed in Chapter 13.

REFERENCES

Berger M, Vollmann J, Hohagen F, Konig A, Lohner H, Voderholzer U, Riemann D: Sleep deprivation combined with consecutive sleep phase advance as a fast-acting therapy in depression: An open pilot trial in medicated and unmedicated patients. *Am J Psychiatry.* 1997;154:870.

Berson DM: Strange vision: Ganglion cells as circadian photoreceptors. *Trends Neurosci.* 2003;26:314.

Berson DM, Dunn FA, Takao M: Phototransduction by retinal ganglion cells that set the circadian clock. *Science.* 2002;295:1070.

Brainard GC, Hanifin JP, Greeson JM, Byrne B, Glickman G, Gerner E, Rollag MD: Action spectrum for melatonin regulation in humans: Evidence for a novel circadian photoreceptor. *J Neurosci.* 2001;21:6405.

Campbell SS, Murphy PJ: Extraocular circadian phototransduction in humans. *Science.* 1998;279:396.

Carter DS, Goldman BD: Antigonadal effects of timed melatonin infusion in pinealectomized male Djungarian hamsters (*Phodopus sungorus sungorus*): Duration is the critical parameter. *Endocrinology.* 1983;113:1261.

Czeisler CA, Duffy JF, Shanahan TL, Brown EN, Mitchell JF, Rimmer DW, Ronda JM, Silva EJ, Allan JS, Emens JS, Dijk DJ, Kronauer RE: Stability, precision, and near-24-hour period of the human circadian pacemaker. *Science.* 1999;284:2177.

*Dijk DJ, Lockley SW: Integration of human sleep-wake regulation and circadian rhythmicity. *J Appl Physiol.* 2002;92:852.

Hattar S, Liao HW, Takao M, Berson DM, Yau KW: Melanopsin-containing retinal ganglion cells: Architecture, projections, and intrinsic photosensitivity. *Science.* 2002;295:1065.

Hattar S, Lucas RJ, Mrosovsky N, Thompson S, Douglas RH, Hankins MW, Lem J, Biel M, Hofmann F, Foster RG, Yau KW: Melanopsin and rod-cone photoreceptive systems account for all major accessory visual functions in mice. *Nature.* 2003;424:75.

*Herzog ED, Schwartz WJ: A neural clockwork for encoding circadian time. *J Appl Physiol.* 2002;92:401.

*Klein DC, Moore RY, Reppert SM, eds. *Suprachiasmatic Nucleus: The Mind's Clock.* New York: Oxford University Press; 1991.

Klerman EB, Shanahan TL, Brotman DJ, Rimmer DW, Emens JS, Rizzo JF III, Czeisler CA: Photic resetting of the human circadian pacemaker in the absence of conscious vision. *J Biol Rhythms.* 2002;17:548.

Menaker M: Circadian rhythms. Circadian photoreception. *Science.* 2003;299:213.

Miller JD, Morin LP, Schwartz WJ, Moore RY: New insights into the mammalian circadian clock. *Sleep.* 1996;19:641.

Moore RY: Circadian rhythms: Basic neurobiology and clinical applications. *Annu Rev Med.* 1997;48:253.

Morin LP: The circadian visual system. *Brain Res Rev.* 1994;19:102.

Muscat L, Huberman AD, Jordan CL, Morin LP: Crossed and uncrossed retinal projections to the hamster circadian system. *J Comp Neurol.* 2003;466:513.

Nelson DE, Takahashi JS: Sensitivity and integration in a visual pathway for circadian entrainment in the hamster (*Mesocricetus auratus*). *J Physiol.* 1991;439:115.

Panda S, Provencio I, Tu DC, Pires SS, Rollag MD, Castrucci AM, Pletcher MT, Sato TK, Wiltshire T, Andahazy M, Kay SA, Van Gelder RN, Hogenesch JB: Melanopsin is required for non-image-forming photic responses in blind mice. *Science.* 2003;301:525.

*Panda S, Sato TK, Castrucci AM, Rollag MD, DeGrip WJ, Hogenesch JB, Provencio I, Kay SA: Melanopsin (*Opn4*) requirement for normal light-induced circadian phase shifting. *Science.* 2002;298:2213.

Provencio I, Rodriguez IR, Jiang G, Hayes WP, Moreira EF, Rollag MD: A novel human opsin in the inner retina. *J Neurosci.* 2000;20:600.

Provencio I, Rollag MD, Castrucci AM: Photoreceptive net in the mammalian retina. This mesh of cells may explain how some blind mice can still tell day from night. *Nature.* 2002;415:493.

Quintero JE, Kuhlman SJ, McMahon DG: The biological clock nucleus: A multiphasic oscillator network regulated by light. *J Neurosci.* 2003;23:8070.

Ralph MR, Foster RG, Davis FC, Menaker M: Transplanted suprachiasmatic nucleus determines circadian period. *Science.* 1990;247:975.

Reppert SM, Weaver DR: Coordination of circadian timing in mammals. *Nature.* 2002;418:935.

Rohan KJ, Tierney LK, Roecklein KA, Lacy TA: Cognitive-behavioral therapy, light therapy, and their combination in treating seasonal affective disorder: A pilot study. *J Affect Disord.* 2004 (*in press*).

Ruby NF, Brennan TJ, Xie X, Cao V, Franken P, Heller HC, O'Hara BF: Role of melanopsin in circadian responses to light. *Science.* 2002;298:2211.

Smith BN, Sollars PJ, Dudek FE, Pickard GE: Serotonergic modulation of retinal input to the mouse suprachiasmatic nucleus mediated by 5-HT1B and 5-HT7 receptors. *J Biol Rhythms.* 2001;16:25.

*Takahashi JS, Turek FW, Moore RY, Takahashi JS, Turek FW, Moore RY, eds. *Handbook of Behavioral Neurobiology: Circadian Clocks.* New York: Kluwer Academic Publishers; 2001.

Thapan K, Arendt J, Skene DJ: An action spectrum for melatonin suppression: Evidence for a novel non-rod, non-cone photoreceptor system in humans. *J Physiol.* 2001;535:261.

Toh KL, Jones CR, He Y, Eide EJ, Hinz WA, Virshup DM, Ptacek LJ, Fu YH: An hPer2 phosphorylation site mutation in familial advanced sleep phase syndrome. *Science.* 2001;291:1040.

Turek FW, Dugovic C, Zee PC: Current understanding of the circadian clock and the clinical implications for neurological disorders. *Arch Neurol.* 2001;58:1781.

Wehr TA: Melatonin and seasonal rhythms. *J Biol Rhythms.* 1997;12:518.

Wehr TA: Effect of seasonal changes in day length on human neuroendocrine function. *Horm Res.* 1998;49:118.

Wehr TA: Photoperiodism in humans and other primates: evidence and implications. *J Biol Rhythms.* 2001;16:348.

Wright KP Jr, Czeisler CA: Absence of circadian phase resetting in response to bright light behind the knees. *Science.* 2002;297:571.

Yamazaki S, Goto M, Menaker M: No evidence for extraocular photoreceptors in the circadian system of the Syrian hamster. *J Biol Rhythms.* 1999;14:197.

▲ 1.14 Applied Electrophysiology

NASHAAT N. BOUTROS, M.D., AND
FREDERICK A. STRUVE, PH.D.

HISTORY AND OVERVIEW

Over a span of more than 70 years, the field of human scalp electroencephalography (EEG) has expanded from its beginnings as a highly controversial phenomenon to its maturity as an investigative and clinical method with wide applications in medicine and neuroscience. Originally tied to neurology and psychiatry, EEG methods have enjoyed expanded use in the study of central nervous system (CNS) effects of a variety of metabolic, endocrinological, toxic, pharmacological, and traumatic events. Recent decades have witnessed the development and refinement of topographic quantitative EEG (QEEG) methods applied to clinical and research problems, and the present era promises the technology to simultaneously record multichannel EEG and functional imaging during magnetic resonance imaging (MRI) scanning. Furthermore, the basic field of EEG has given birth to the emergence of significant sister fields of polysomnography and magnetoencephalography.

Origins The lengthy transition from laboratory experiment to eventual acceptance of EEG was plagued by intense controversy.

Despite the continuing accumulation of experimental evidence of brain-derived electrical potentials, beginning with Richard Caton's discovery in 1874 of spontaneous electrical activity recorded from the exposed cortex of cats, rabbits, and monkeys, the notion that electrical potentials emanated from the brain was rejected for nearly 50 years by leading authorities. Caton's work was replicated by Vasili Danilevsky's 1877 report that electrical oscillations recorded from the animal brain could be altered by strong sensory stimuli, and, later, in 1883, Fleischl von Marxow demonstrated that changes in brain electrical activity produced by sensory stimulation could be abolished by chloroform. Three further historical highlights of note include (1) the 1891 demonstration by Adolph Beck that the dog visual cortex produced large electrical potentials when the eyes were rhythmically illuminated (thus laying the experimental foundation for EEG photic driving), (2) Beck and Napoleon Cybulski's 1892 report that local injury to the cortex could alter the characteristics of recorded spontaneous electrical activity, and (3) Cybulski's 1914 report that brain-wave seizure discharges could be induced in the cortex by applying electrical stimulation to the cortex (thus presaging the use of EEG in epilepsy). Despite this stream of successful experimental work, the EEG phenomenon remained largely insecure.

The focused perseverance of Hans Berger, a biologically oriented Professor of Psychiatry and Director of the Psychiatric Clinic in Jena, Germany, finally brought EEG to a position of acceptance and clinical usefulness. After years of unsuccessful attempts to record brain waves from humans (he was able to obtain recordings from animals), he finally succeeded in recording the human EEG in 1924, and, in 1929, he published the first in his classic series of 23 papers describing many aspects of the human EEG. Among his vast achievements, he demonstrated that brain electrical activity came from neurons and not blood vessels or connective tissue, that recordings from patients with brain tumors contained high-voltage slow waves (his recording technique did not permit localization), that waking *alpha* waves were blocked by eye opening, and that the characteristics of EEG activity change with age, sensory stimulation, state of consciousness, and physiochemical state of the body. He coined the word *electroencephalogram.* However, acceptance was still temporarily delayed when Lord Adrian, a Nobel laureate neurophysiologist, claimed that Berger's findings "were impossible." Later, in 1934, Adrian publicly confirmed Berger's work, and the field of EEG was born.

Epilepsy and Classical Neurology

Despite the fact that EEG originated in psychiatry, the strongest initial impetus for its use came from neurology, particularly the study of epilepsy. The years from 1934 to 1940 saw a marked proliferation of EEG studies focused on structural brain lesions and a variety of seizure disorders. In 1934, the team led by Fred Gibbs discovered the classic three-per-second spike-and-wave complex, which proved to be specific to petit mal absence attacks. Before the decade ended, they had described EEG patterns associated with grand mal and myoclonic seizures and a diffuse spike-and-wave pattern that was slower in frequency than petit mal (and given the confusing name of petit mal variant) and that was associated with grand mal seizures and a high incidence of mental retardation. They also introduced the term *psychomotor seizures* (now *complex partial seizures* [CPSs]) and described the EEG manifestations characterizing an ictal psychomotor attack. Later, in 1947 and 1948, they described the anterior temporal spike focus that became the interictal EEG correlate of this disorder. The other side of the neurological coin, structural brain lesions, was also advanced through landmark, new EEG discoveries during this early decade. In 1935, O. Foerster and H. Altenberger reported from Germany that focal slow waves in the EEG recording often appeared near brain tumors, and, later, Grey Walter made a major advance by demonstrating a technique for EEG localization of brain tumors. Under the leadership of Herbert Jasper in Montreal, direct cortical EEG recording began to be introduced during neurosurgery, and, by the close of the decade, in 1941, Denis Williams at Oxford began using EEG recordings to study and localize traumatic intracranial injuries received during World War II.

Psychiatry

Starting in approximately 1938, a flurry of continuing EEG investigations began to reveal an increase in the overall prevalence of minor abnormalities in almost all psychiatric populations as compared to healthy or nonpsychiatric controls, a finding that remains undisputed today. On the other hand, two major factors led to the rapid disillusionment of the field of psychiatry with EEG. The first was the lack of specificity of EEG abnormalities to known psychiatric syndromes. The second factor, alluded to previously, was the continuing discovery of EEG abnormalities correlating with epilepsy, tumors, encephalopathies, stroke syndromes, and coma. The fact that discoveries of significant EEG changes accompanying neurological problems were occurring while those EEG abnormalities associated with psychiatric symptomatology continued to be minimal (compared to those related to neurological disorders) and noncontributory to the diagnostic process led the field of *clinical EEG* (and later *clinical neurophysiology*) to become squarely a subspecialty of the field of neurology, with nearly a complete lack of interest in EEG among psychiatrists.

The recent significant surge of interest in the neurobiology of psychiatric disorders, the emergence of the clinical field of *neuropsychiatry*, and the unprecedented advances in computerized analyses of EEG and other neurophysiological signals have resulted in a strong rekindling of interest in electrophysiology among psychiatrists. Less than a decade ago, John Hughes undertook the mammoth task of compiling a comprehensive outline of the broad area of EEG and psychiatry with 181 significant references selected for citation from before 1950 until 1994. When such compilations are inspected, the findings reveal that more than one-half of the EEG-psychiatry references appear after 1980, and one-third were written within the 5 years preceding Hughes' 1995 report. Continued inspection of the literature indicates that this trend has not abated.

ELECTROENCEPHALOGRAPHY

A given brain wave is no more than the transient difference in electrical potential (greatly amplified) between any two points on the scalp or between some electrode placed on the scalp and a reference electrode located elsewhere on the head (i.e., ear lobe or nose). In a simplistic sense, the EEG is nothing more than an extremely sensitive voltmeter, with the unit of measurement being the microvolt, or millionth of a volt. Typical EEG signals range from approximately 30 to 80 μV, but they can be as low as 10 μV in some tracings or as high as 150 or 200 μV in some high-voltage "spike" discharges. The difference in electrical potential measured between any two EEG electrodes fluctuates or oscillates rapidly, usually many times per second. It is this oscillation that produces the characteristic "squiggly line" that even many lay persons now recognize as the appearance of "brain waves."

The earliest EEG recordings involved only one pair of electrodes, or one *channel* of recording, and although this could detect certain normal and abnormal features, effective clinical application remained for the future. Soon, the breakthrough ability to record two channels of brain waves emerged, and it became possible to record activity simultaneously from homologous locations in each hemisphere. Before long, the rapid advances in recording technology allowed four- and eight-channel recordings to be made, and EEG became a viable clinical tool. Eventually, 10-, 12-, and 16-channel recording machines became the standard work horses of clinical and research EEG laboratories around the world. EEG equipment capable of simultaneous recording from 64 (or even many more) channels is available but is largely confined to special research applications. The ability to simultaneously record brain waves from many scalp locations is important, because it allows direct comparisons between homologous cortical regions, permits recording arrays to locate focal or regional abnormal features more clearly, and increases the ability to detect various artifacts (i.e., waveforms of non-brain origin) that can contaminate the recording.

Scalp EEG cannot detect the electrical activity generated by a single neuron or even by several neurons close to the scalp. Rather, the recorded EEG signals that are seen are the result of summated field potentials generated by excitatory postsynaptic potentials (EPSPs) and inhibitory postsynaptic potentials (IPSPs) in vertically oriented pyramidal cells of the cortex. An EPSP in a dendrite produces electrical negativity in the immediately surrounding area, but the electrical field becomes positive with increasing distance from the source. The reverse occurs with an IPSP, generating an electrical positivity nearby and a negative field at a distance. The summation of EPSPs and IPSPs is enhanced, because the neurons are tightly packed together and oriented vertically in parallel. In addition, large aggregates of these neurons may receive similar input, thus making it likely that they may respond in unison over time. Because of the manner in which the dominant intrinsic brain waves are generated, EEG is maximally sensitive to cortical neuronal activity and relatively insensitive to electrical potentials generated from subcortical regions. However, there are some minor exceptions, because subcortical neuronal events can sometimes influence cortical neuronal firing via afferent transmissions along subcortical-cortical tracts.

Probably the first observation about brain waves, going back to the time of Caton, was that the recorded potentials oscillate and repeat in a rhythmic fashion. Indeed, the term *intrinsic rhythms* is often used for normal activity, and the term *dysrhythmic* is used for activity that might be abnormal. Within reasonable limits, the repetitive rhythmic nature of the EEG is stable across individuals and within individuals over time, barring the introduction of pathophysiologic events.

Limitations of Scalp Electroencephalography

EEG continues to be one of the few objective measures of brain function. However, appreciation of its strengths in clinical and research settings must also be tempered with recognition of its limitations.

Because of the limitations of scalp EEG, a normal EEG can never constitute positive proof of absence of brain dysfunction. With several diseases with established brain pathophysiology, such as multiple sclerosis, deep subcortical neoplasm, some seizure disorders, and Parkinson's disease and other movement disorders, to name only a few, a substantial incidence of patients with normal EEGs may be encountered. Nonetheless, as is discussed later in the chapter, a normal EEG can often provide convincing evidence for excluding certain types of brain pathology that may present with behavioral or psychiatric symptoms.

Brain Coverage and Impedance

Because the human brain is encased and protected in a bony skull, large areas of cortex are inaccessible to scalp EEG recording. Although approximately one-third of the outer convexity of the cortex may be within reach, much cortical area consists of mesial, inferior, and deep buried cortical tissue that is removed from the proximity of electrodes that are confined to external scalp placement. Electrical events generated in these areas may not be detected by scalp electrodes. Furthermore, substantial impedance to electrical conduction from skin, skull, dura, and brain tissue exists between the source of generated electrical potentials and the detecting electrode on the scalp. Weak electrical signals, even those close to the surface, may escape detection. It has been demonstrated that electrical potentials recorded from the cortical surface are much higher in voltage than potentials recorded simultaneously at the surface of the scalp and that depth electrode recordings often show activity that is attenuated and distorted or not visible at the scalp.

Paroxysmal Discharges and Recording Length

Many types of EEG abnormality, particularly abnormalities of brain wave frequency, such as generalized or focal slowing, tend to be present from the beginning of the recording, and the recording length generally is not a limiting factor in their detection. For example, in several clinical situations, such as suspected delirium or suspected nonconvulsive status, a 10-minute wake EEG often provides the needed diagnostic information. However, other significant abnormalities, including focal and diffuse spike or spike-wave complexes and several controversial paroxysmal dysrhythmias, occur episodically against a background of more or less normal activity. In cases in which sporadic paroxysmal discharges occur frequently during a tracing, a limited recording length may not be problematic. However, paroxysmal abnormal discharges are often widely spaced, may occur only a few times in a long tracing, or may be confined to certain recording states, such as stage I or II sleep. In these cases, a short recording may fail to detect infrequent sporadic discharges and thus are falsely negative.

Nonspecificity of Results

There are only a limited number of ways in which brain electrical activity can respond to normal or pathological influences. Brain waves can only reflect change by becoming faster or slower in frequency or lower or higher in voltage, or perhaps some combination of these two responses. Thus, the same or similar abnormal EEG patterns can emerge from different etiological causes. For example, a neoplasm, subdural hematoma, brain abscess, cerebral vascular accident (CVA), closed head injury, or aneurysm may result in similar, although not always identical, focal EEG slowing. Generalized slowing is a common abnormal finding for which the etiological causes are legion and include cortical atrophy, drug-induced encephalopathy, electroconvulsive therapy (ECT), encephalitis, certain endocrine disorders (hypothyroidism and hypopituitarism), porphyria, head trauma, lead exposure, hypocalcemia, and Wernicke's encephalopathy, to name but a few. The nonspecificity of results or the failure to specifically denote etiology is a genuine limitation but one that is not as bleak as this paragraph suggests. More often than not, information from the patient's symptoms, clinical course and history, and other laboratory results identifies a probable cause for the EEG findings. Furthermore, EEGs are often ordered for specific reasons in cases in which a pathophysiological process is already suspected.

RECORDING

Much has been written about the complexities of EEG recording and interpretation and the corresponding high level of skill needed to obtain an adequate EEG. What may be insufficiently recognized is the fact that there are also clinical situations in which a greatly simplified EEG secured by a properly trained registered nurse or resident can have substantial diagnostic usefulness. There are some important EEG findings of particular relevance to emergency room settings and, possibly, even to some acute psychiatric admission or triage units that can be assessed in only 10 minutes by using only a 10- or 12-channel recording instrument by those with a minimum level of technical skill. Cases presenting with moderate to marked confusion and agitation, delirium, or possible nonconvulsive status may have diffuse EEG abnormalities that are more or less continuous in the tracing, once the recording is turned on. Such findings (if present) do not require sophisticated localization studies, and their presence, as well as their absence, is diagnostically relevant. Prompt access to an EEG laboratory may not always be possible, especially on weekends or evenings, and on-site screening may thus be helpful.

Other than the circumscribed (yet potentially highly useful) screening EEGs described previously, recording the EEG does, in fact, require a considerable amount of skill and experience. It is not merely a technical act performed by a technician. The unfolding clinical EEG tracing is a constantly moving and shifting parade of complex waveforms recorded simultaneously from numerous scalp locations, and the EEG patterns differ dramatically during wakefulness, drowsiness, and various sleep levels. The appearance of the EEG also changes from one recording montage to another while a host of normal and abnormal EEG waveforms and contaminating artifacts must be identified in their obvious and subtle forms. In addition to the necessary skills of accurate electrode application and machine operation, the better technologists are also capable of sophisticated EEG interpretation. It may not be obvious how important this is. EEG abnormalities do not always emerge in clear-cut, textbook form but instead may be distorted and, hence, ambiguous. Interpretative ability is necessary to recognize probable abnormalities and then to arrange recording montages and states of patient alertness (wake or sleep) in ways that might enhance or bring out the patterns and allow a more definite interpretation by the electroencephalographer. A minimum of 1 year of full-time training, including didactic instruction and supervised, hands-on recording and interpretation experience, is necessary for an EEG technologist to achieve competence. Formal training schools for EEG technologists exist in many places, and the graduates can become registered EEG technologists by taking and passing a two-part written and practical examination.

Electrode Placement As EEG emerged into the clinical arena, electrodes were simply placed on the scalp symmetrically by eye, using salient landmarks on the head as reference points, and not all laboratories used the same placement system. Eventually, in 1947, it was decided at an International EEG Congress held in London that some effort should be made to standardize the system of electrode placement, so that clinical and research findings would be more directly comparable across different laboratories. The challenge was taken up by Jasper, who developed the 10/20 International System of Electrode Placement, which has become standard worldwide since 1958. Without going into lengthy technical detail, the 10/20 system simply measures the distance between readily identifiable landmarks on the head and then locates electrode positions at 10 percent or 20 percent of that distance in an anterior-posterior or transverse direction (Fig. 1.14–1). Electrodes are then designated by an uppercase letter denoting the brain region beneath that electrode and a number, with odd numbers used for the left hemisphere and with even numbers signifying the right hemisphere (the subscript Z denotes midline electrodes). Thus, the O2 electrode is placed over the right occipital region, and the P3 lead is found over the left parietal area.

Although most laboratories use 21 scalp electrodes for standard recordings, the 10/20 system provides for additional electrodes to provide greater coverage, if needed, and the American EEG Society has even developed a nomenclature for the designation of as many as 75 defined electrode locations (Fig. 1.14–2). However, it must be stressed that extremely large numbers of scalp electrodes, although no doubt impressive, are unnecessary for currently established clinical EEG applications. For currently accepted clinical indications,

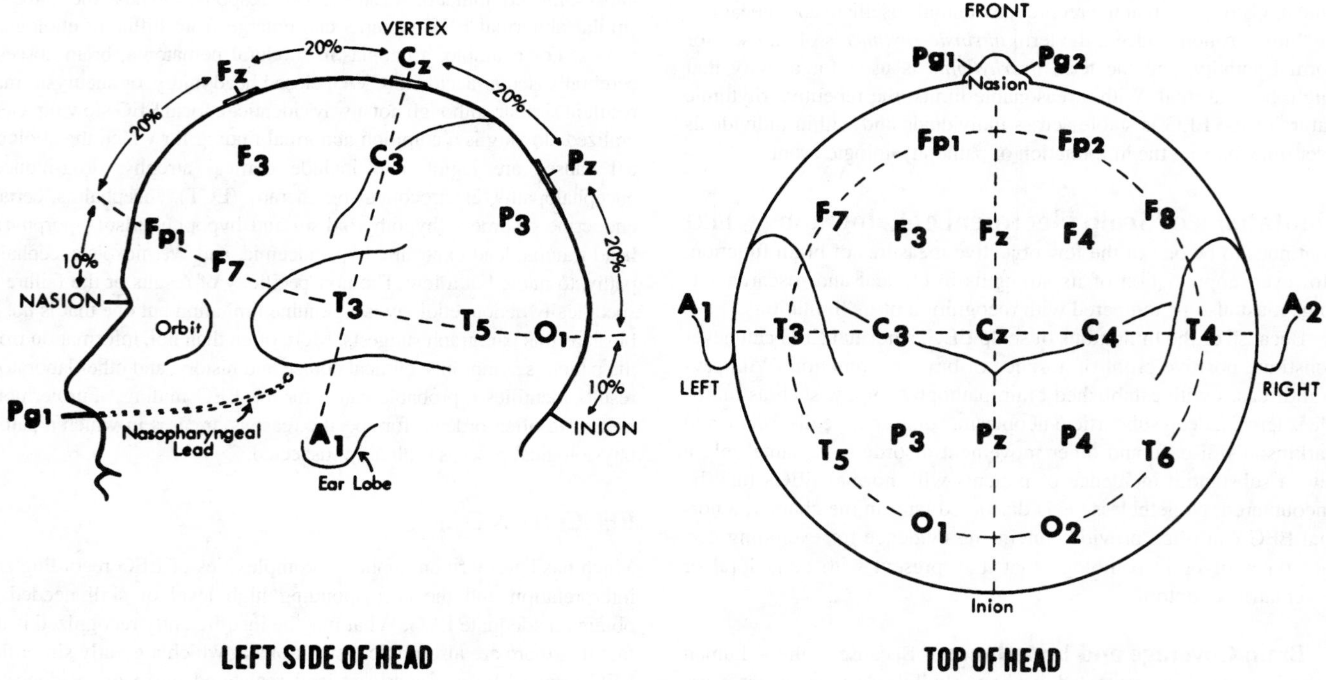

FIGURE 1.14–1 International 10/20 Electrode Placement System. (Courtesy of Grass, Astro-Med, Inc. Product Group.)

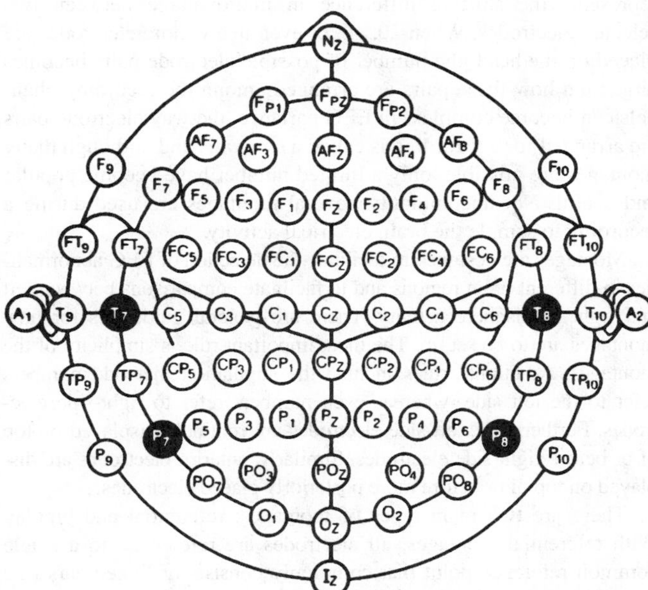

FIGURE 1.14–2 An expanded 75-electrode array developed by the Electrode Nomenclature Committee of the American Electroencephalography Society. The four electrode positions in black are given new names. Previous designations of T3 and T4 have been renamed (*black electrodes*) as T7 and T8. The T5 and T6 locations in the original placement system are now renamed (*black electrodes*) as P7 and P8. Such extensive placement systems are primarily used for special research studies and are only rarely used for clinical recordings.

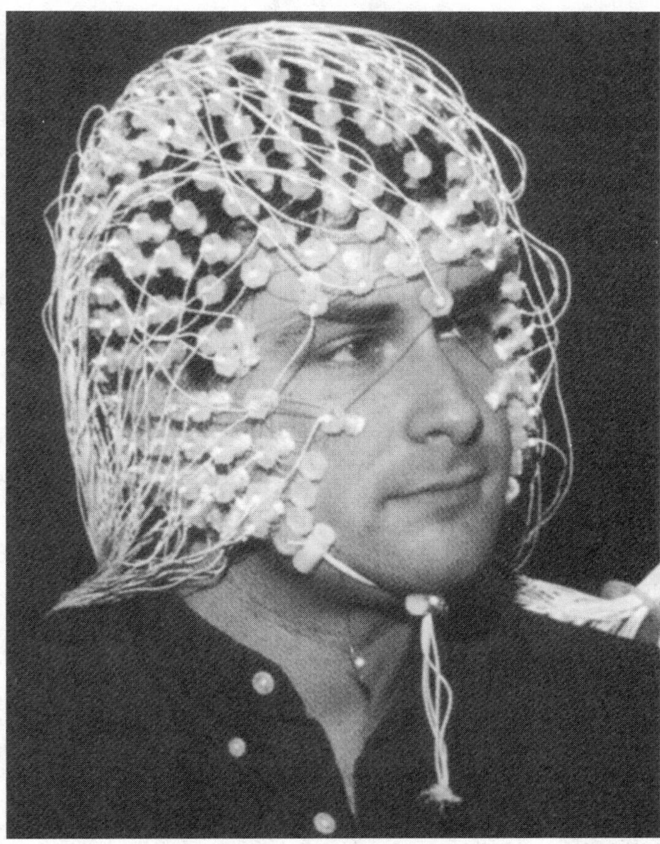

FIGURE 1.14–3 A 256–electrode-dense sensor array. Such large arrays are often used in research requiring optimal resolution for source analyses and three-dimensional dipole localization. (Courtesy of Electrical Geodesies, Inc.)

optimally useful EEG recordings can be achieved with only 21 or, at the most, 32 scalp electrodes. However, large electrode sensor arrays, including 125 or even 256 scalp leads (Fig. 1.14–3), may be needed for specialized research applications involving source analyses and three-dimensional dipole characterization in which it has been estimated that the limit at which additional unique information may be obtained is between 200 and 300 electrodes.

Although tedious, the 10/20 placement system has several advantages. Because the placement system is based on rigorous measurements, electrode placement error, particularly asymmetrical placement of electrodes for homologous electrode pairs, is greatly minimized. The system also renders recordings entirely comparable between laboratories, as well as across serial tracings obtained from a single subject. Because percentages of distances between landmarks on the head are used for placement locations, scalp electrodes overlie the same cortical regions despite differences in head size. Furthermore, the relationships between electrodes placed on the scalp and underlying brain structures have been well established (Fig. 1.14–4) by using placements on cadavers (with holes drilled at the electrode sites to later identify the cortical area under the electrode), as well as recent studies using computed tomography (CT) scanning.

It has been suggested that, in cases of suspected temporal lobe abnormality unconfirmed by traditional electrodes, a closer examination of the temporal area should be attempted, because the anterior temporal lobe is not well covered by the standard 10/20 placement system. The F7 and F8 electrodes are over the posterior-inferior-frontal lobe and, hence, forward of the temporal pole, whereas the T3 and T4 electrodes are behind the anterior temporal region. Some laboratories now add new electrodes (T1 and T2) or simply relocate the F7 and F8 electrodes to this new position. The placement of the T1 and T2 anterior temporal electrodes is based on the distance from the lateral canthus of the eye to the external auditory canal, with electrodes placed at one-third of this total distance anterior to the auditory canal and 1 cm up from a line connecting these two landmarks (Fig. 1.14–4). However, the F7 and F8 electrodes may detect potentials spreading from the anterior temporal cortex, particularly if the voltages of the discharges are high.

Scalp electrodes must be applied carefully. The skin under the electrode must be clean and completely free of oil or grease. A common practice is to rub the area with a slightly abrasive cleansing electrolyte material that also removes some of the superficial epidermis. When this is done, a metal disc electrode can be applied to the scalp by using a conducting electrode paste. Electrode impedance should be maintained at equal to or less than 3,000 Ω. The whole electrode application procedure should not be uncomfortable for the subject. In some laboratories, subdermal needle electrodes are used. Although they can reduce the electrode application time, they have the significant disadvantage of coming loose spontaneously or when the head is moved. They also involve a concern about transmission of disease, especially human immunodeficiency virus (HIV).

Special Electrodes

Nasopharyngeal (NP) electrodes can be inserted into the NP space through the nostrils and can be closer to the temporal lobe than scalp electrodes (Fig. 1.14–1; these leads are designated Pg1 and Pg2 in the 10/20 placement system). No actual penetration of tissue occurs. The NP lead is a long (as long as 15 cm for adults), curved S- or Z-shaped insulated wire with a silver ball (the electrode) on the tip, which is inserted in the nostril and then rotated laterally, so that

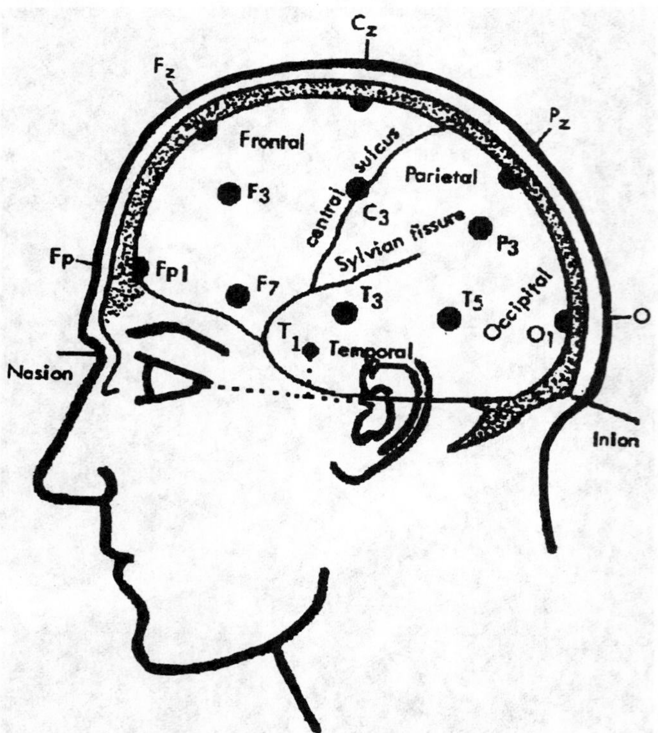

FIGURE 1.14–4 A left-lateral diagram of the head showing the locations of the routine 10-20 electrodes (left-side electrode locations F7 and T3 and the new electrode placement [T1]) in relation to the temporal pole. (Modification of figure printed courtesy of Grass, Astro-Med, Inc. Product Group.)

the ball is in contact with the roof of the nasopharynx. With a cooperative patient and a skilled technologist, the procedure can be well tolerated. Although this lead is presumed to be better positioned to detect activity from the orbitofrontal cortex, temporal pole, and hippocampus, it has numerous disadvantages. Chief among these are a high propensity to produce pulse and respiration artifact and the fact that NP leads cannot be used when a deviated septum or nasal inflammatory process is present. They are also contraindicated with many psychiatric patients displaying behaviors, such as confusion, agitation, or belligerence, that could pull the leads out, possibly lacerating the nasal passage. Their use may also interfere with obtaining a sleep-activated EEG, and, not infrequently, otherwise cooperative patients simply refuse the procedure.

Sphenoidal electrodes use a hollow needle through which a fine electrode that is insulated, except at the tip, is inserted between the zygoma and the sigmoid notch in the mandible, until it is in contact with the base of the skull lateral to the foramen ovale. This is an invasive procedure that must be done by a physician and requires a signed consent form. The yield of positive results from these specialized electrodes, over and above findings present in conventional scalp recordings, is still controversial. In general, the yield from NP leads has not been high, although, with sphenoidal leads, positive results as great as 40 percent have been reported from seizure patients who had no other specific changes in the waking or sleep EEG.

Montage Selection

A common misconception is that the EEG records the voltage detected at each electrode site. Instead, each "squiggly line" on the EEG chart represents the shifting or oscillating difference in electrical potential *between* two electrodes. Thus, in a multichannel recording, the activity from each channel represents the shifting difference in microvoltage between two selected electrodes. When 10, 16, or even many more electrodes are placed on the head, the number of possible electrode pairs becomes large, and how these pairs are arranged among the recording channels can become complex. In EEG parlance, the way electrode pairs are arranged for a recording is called a *montage*, and, although many montages are possible, only a limited number have become popular and useful. Not uncommonly, several montages are used during a recording to sample the brain electrical activity.

Montages are designed to facilitate the detection of EEG abnormalities in different brain regions and to facilitate comparisons between left and right hemisphere activity. There are general guidelines for how montages are to be set up. The most important rule is simplicity of the montages. Additional rules include the stipulation that odd numbers refer to the left side, whereas even numbers refer to right-side electrodes. Furthermore, left-side electrodes are routinely displayed on top of or before right-side electrodes. Similarly, anterior electrodes are displayed on top of or before more posteriorly placed electrodes.

There are two main types of montages: referential and bipolar. With referential montages, all electrodes are referenced to a single common reference point that commonly consists of linked ears (the mastoid prominence can be used in place of the ear lobe), with variations being left or right ear reference alone, ipsilateral ear reference in which all electrodes in one hemisphere are referenced to the ear on that side, or a contralateral ear reference in which all electrodes in one hemisphere are referenced to the opposite-side ear. Referential montages are useful for judging the magnitude of the abnormality (in terms of how large a sharp wave or slow wave is in microvolts). Bipolar montages, on the other hand, are useful (and, indeed, are much more widely used than referential montages) for pinpointing the area of maximal abnormality or the exact source of an abnormal activity. In bipolar montages, electrodes are referenced from one scalp location to a nearby scalp location in chains of electrodes going across the head from front to back (Fig. 1.14–5) or from left to right (Fig. 1.14–6).

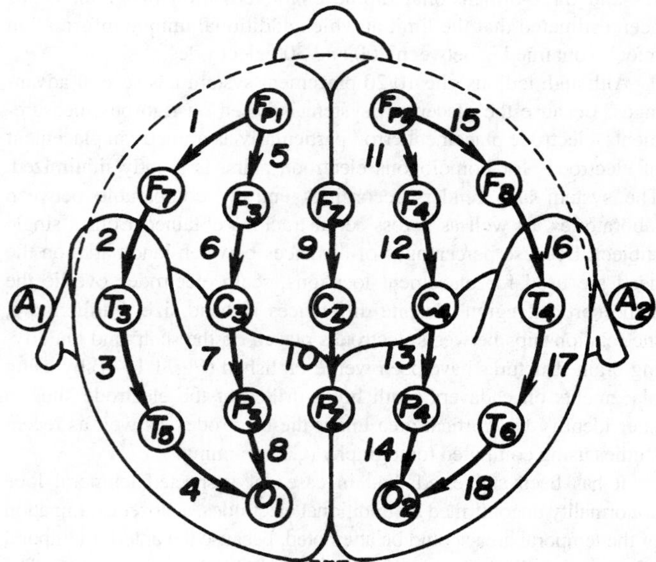

FIGURE 1.14–5 Example of an 18-channel bipolar montage with anterior to posterior linkages. The numbers between electrode locations designate recording channels. Thus, the number 6 means channel 6, which measures the difference in electrical potential between the F3 and C3 electrodes. (From Tyner FS. *Fundamentals of EEG Technology: Basic Concepts and Methods.* Vol 1. New York: Raven Press; 1985, with permission.)

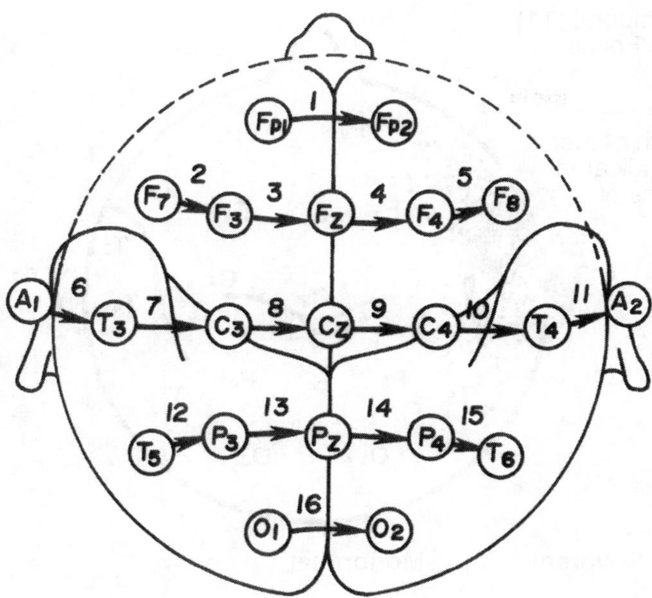

FIGURE 1.14–6 Example of a 16-channel transverse bipolar montage. (From Tyner FS. *Fundamentals of EEG Technology: Basic Concepts and Methods.* Vol 1. New York: Raven Press; 1985, with permission.)

The majority of abnormal cerebral activities tend to appear at the surface as negative potentials. One can think of a given channel of EEG activity as being derived from two inputs. By convention, the first electrode of a pair constitutes input 1, whereas the second electrode provides input 2. Thus, in the electrode pair C3-P3, the first electrode C3 constitutes input 1. The direction of the pen deflection is based on whether input 1 (the first electrode in a pair) is, *relatively speaking*, "more negative" or "less negative" (i.e., relatively more "positive") than the second electrode (input 2). If the first electrode in a recording pair (input 1) is *closer* to the source of a negative field and, hence, more "negative" than the second electrode (input 2), even though both electrodes may be within the field, there is an upward pen deflection. Conversely, if the first electrode of a pair is more distant from the source of the field than the second electrode and, hence, less negative than the second electrode (which is the same as saying that it is, *relatively speaking*, more "positive"), the pen deflection is downward. There is no denying that it takes some time to become accustomed to these polarity principles. However, they lead to important techniques for localizing certain abnormal features. As bipolar pairs of electrodes move in a longitudinal or transverse direction from one side of a strong and highly localized negative field to the other side, the pen deflection changes direction as the first electrode in a given pair (input 1) shifts from being relatively more negative to relatively more positive than the second electrode (input 2). This change of pen deflection is called a *phase reversal* and is a powerful method for localization of sharply focal abnormalities. By contrast, monopolar montages localize by identifying the electrode with the highest amplitude of the abnormality (Fig. 1.14–7).

With rapidly advancing computer technology, it is possible today to record the EEG with one montage and to reconnect digitally the electrodes in any sequence desired. This has the advantage of being able to examine the entire EEG record in all possible configurations. One particular montage configuration deserves special mention, for it may be particularly useful in psychiatric EEG. This is a montage that combines referential and bipolar electrode arrangements. Following four bipolar connections from the frontal regions through the temporal areas and ending in the occipital region, a referential placement connects each posterior temporal region (T5 and T6) to the opposite ear. This arrangement allows activity of low amplitude to be highlighted by the referential electrodes for further examination via the bipolar electrode pairs. This montage is commonly referred to as the *Queen Square montage* (Fig. 1.14–8).

The appearance of EEG activity varies greatly from one recording montage to another. Large interelectrode distances often (but not always) yield higher voltages, whereas a close spacing between electrodes in a pair tends to reduce voltage, because when both electrodes overlie nearly the same portion of an electrical field the potential difference between them is small. Furthermore, specific EEG patterns visible in one montage may be distorted or even completely canceled out in another montage. Although some montages may permit a differentiation of activity between two or more brain regions, other montage choices may not do so. For example, EEG sleep patterns are well visualized and well differentiated in central and occipital regions when a common (monopolar) reference recording is made. However, differentiation between central and occipital sleep activity is no longer possible when bipolar anterior-posterior linkages are used (C3-O1 and C4-O2), and, with transverse bipolar links between homologous electrodes, the sleep patterns may not be visible at all (Fig. 1.14–9). The issue is not merely academic. Discharges of interest to the electroencephalographer, whether they be clinically abnormal or controversial, that are detectable in some recording montages may be completely or nearly undetectable, even though they are currently "firing" when a different montage is being used (Fig. 1.14–10).

Sensitivity

The amplification used in EEG recording is adjustable and can be increased to visualize low-voltage signals or decreased to prevent recording pens from reaching their deflection limits and "squaring off," thus distorting the shape of the top of the waveform. Although the accepted standard sensitivity across laboratories for most recording situations is 7 μV for each mm of pen deflection, the sensitivity may be altered, if necessary, to increase the clarity of the EEG information being obtained. For example, it may be necessary to sharply decrease the amplification to 10, 15, or even 20 μV per mm to visualize the complete waveform shape in certain high-voltage seizure discharges. Conversely, there are situations, such as recordings to document electrocerebral silence, in which it is important to maximize the ability to detect brain wave activity. In such situations, a high amplification of 1.0 or 0.5 μV per mm might be selected, along with the use of referential montages or bipolar runs with large interelectrode distances, to further enhance low-voltage registration. The EEG recording indicates the sensitivity setting at the beginning of the record and at any point in the recording at which the sensitivity was changed.

Frequency Filter Settings

Nearly all of the EEG activity that is analyzed for clinical or research purposes falls within the frequency range of 0.5 to 40.0 or 50.0 Hz. Conventional EEG recordings usually use a high-frequency filter setting of 70 Hz, which means that brain waves become progressively attenuated in amplitude the more that they increase above this filter setting. At the other end of the spectrum, most laboratories set the low-frequency filter at 1.0 Hz to reduce the registration of frequencies below this level. Unfortunately, scalp electrodes pick up a variety of electrical potentials of nonbrain origin, and many of these have frequencies within or close to the EEG frequency spectrum. Frequency filters may, to

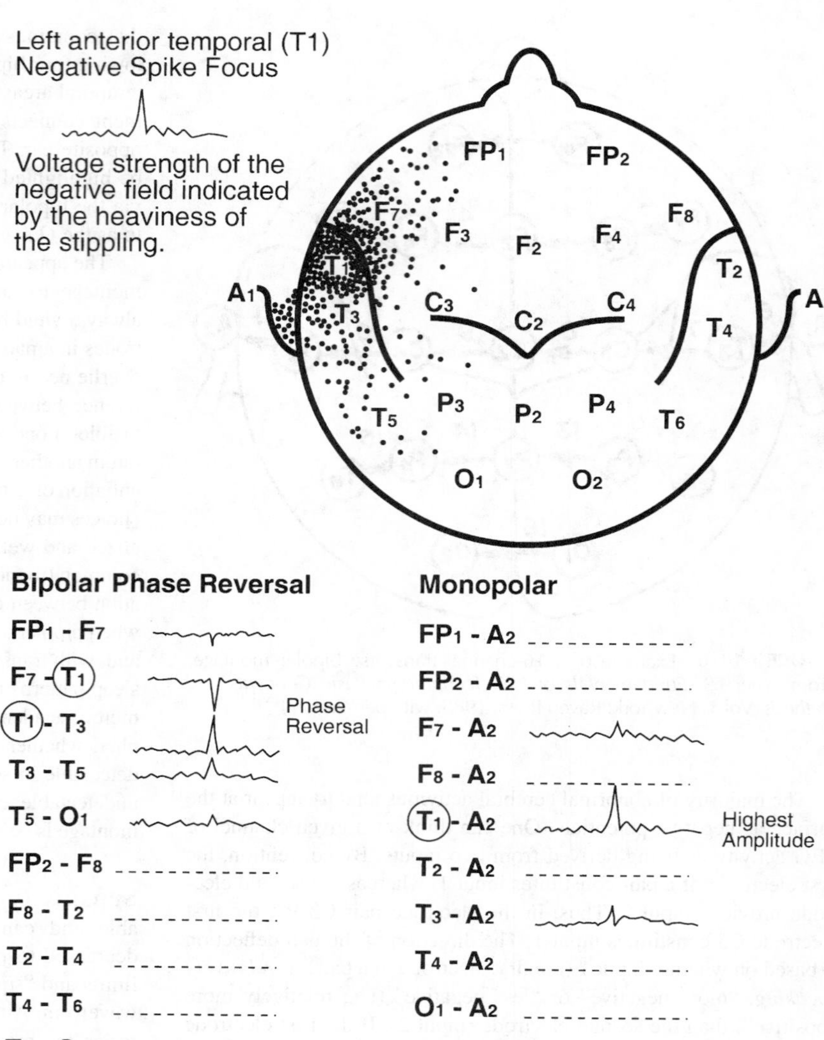

FIGURE 1.14–7 Illustration of bipolar (phase-reversal) and monopolar (highest amplitude) localization of a focal negative spike discharge at the left anterior temporal (T1) electrode. See the text for an explanation.

some degree, mitigate against the distorting effects of frequencies generated by nonbrain sources. However, filters must be used judiciously and with caution, because they can also filter out real brain waves that one wishes to see.

Although the low-frequency filter can be adjusted downward to 0.3 Hz or even 0.1 Hz to capture slow waves, this is seldom done in routine recordings. More commonly, the low-frequency filter is moved upward to 5 Hz to eliminate unwanted slow potentials known to be artifact. Chief among these unwanted slow waves are those generated by electrical activity of the skin during sweating (galvanic skin response), and they can be of sufficiently high amplitude that they completely obliterate genuine EEG activity in the affected recording channels (usually bilateral frontal-anterior temporal areas). Increasing the low-frequency filter setting to 5 Hz totally eliminates this source of contamination in the recording (Fig. 1.14–11) but does so at the expense of attenuating any real generalized or focal slow activity that may also be present. It is much more common to adjust the high-frequency filter downward from 70 Hz to 35 Hz or even 15 Hz to eliminate or reduce unwanted muscle potential from the recording (Fig. 1.14–12). Again, the choice to do this involves a compromise, because such lowering of the high-frequency filter setting may make the accurate detection of certain fast spike discharges problematic.

Special Activations Over the years, electroencephalographers have recognized that certain activating procedures tend to increase the probability that abnormal discharges, particularly spike or spike-wave seizure discharges, will occur. Some activating techniques remain standard in many laboratories, others are used only rarely for specific purposes, and still others introduced in the past have largely been abandoned, because they were not easy to use or involved risk.

Medication Activation Although the use of drugs to induce EEG changes enjoyed a certain vogue in the past, this type of activation is essentially no longer used in clinical work today. During the 1940s and 1950s, the convulsant drug, pentylenetetrazol (Metrazol), was sometimes used to activate seizure discharges in the EEG, but, if not used with caution, it could precipitate actual overt grand mal seizures during the EEG recording. The use of bemegride, another drug with convulsant properties, was also used, and, although it was presumed to be safer, it also was not without risk. Of particular relevance to psychiatry, Russell Monroe began using α-chloralose in the 1960s as a specific activator of EEG abnormalities in psychiatric patients. Although it was reported to be effective with psychiatric patients, it was said to be particularly effective in activating paroxysmal EEG discharges in a high proportion of patients with aggressive episodic dyscontrol syndromes.

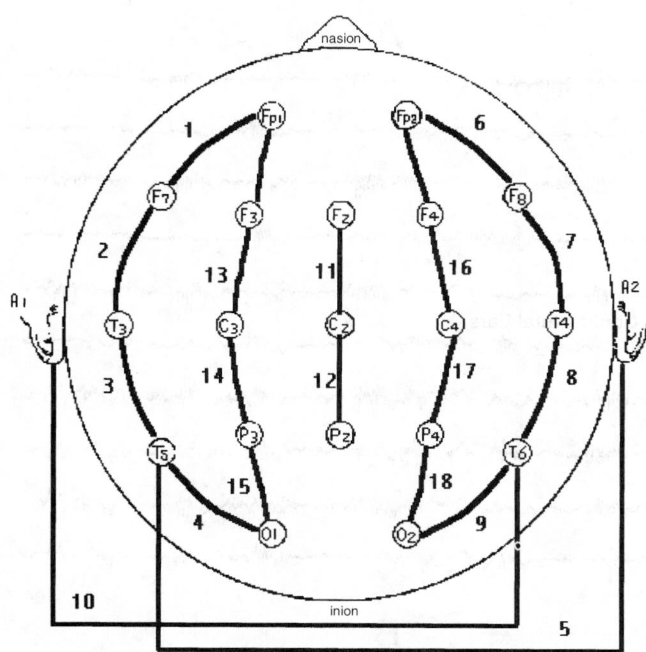

FIGURE 1.14–8 Diagram of the Queen Square montage. This is an 18-channel montage modified to include two referential leads to highlight temporal lobe activity.

Hyperventilation Strenuous hyperventilation is one of the oldest, and still one of the most frequently used, activation procedures in clinical laboratories. While remaining reclined with the eyes closed, the patient is asked to overbreathe through their open mouth with deep breaths for 1 to 4 minutes, depending on the laboratory (3 minutes is common). The normal EEG response to hyperventilation (referred to in EEG parlance as a *build-up*) consists of an increase in generalized medium- to high-voltage synchronous slow waves in the delta range, which then quickly subside when overbreathing stops. Not everyone has a build-up response to hyperventilation, and children are far more likely to respond with diffuse EEG slowing than are adults. In terms of activating EEG abnormality, hyperventilation is especially effective in eliciting the classic diffuse three-per-second spike-and-wave complex of petit mal seizures when the pattern does not first appear in the standard wake tracing, and, to a lesser degree, it may activate other synchronous diffuse spike-wave patterns. Activation of focal seizure activity has been reported much less frequently. An interesting observation is that significantly low blood glucose levels have been associated with large, synchronous delta wave hyperventilation build-ups, and, because of this, a large delta wave build-up in an adult may signal the existence of covert, unsuspected pathological hypoglycemia. If this suspicion should present itself during a recording, a good idea would be to give a sugar drink to the patient and then to repeat hyperventilation later. If the glucose ingestion reduces or abolishes the large hyperventilation build-up, the suspicion of hypoglycemia is reinforced. In general, hyperventilation is one of the safest EEG activating procedures, and, for the majority of the population, it presents no physical risk. However, it may pose a risk for patients with cardiopulmonary disease or risk factors for cerebral vascular pathophysiology.

Photic Stimulation In the earliest days of EEG, it was known that the frequency of normal EEG activity recorded from posterior scalp regions could be made (within narrow limits) to follow the frequency of a flickering light that was flashed slightly faster or slower than the intrinsic brain wave frequencies, a phenomenon that came to be referred to as *photic-driving*. When it also became known that photic-driving would sometimes cause paroxysmal discharges to occur in the EEG, photic stimulation (PS) emerged as a technique for eliciting EEG abnormalities. Although there is some variation between laboratories, PS generally involves placing an intense strobe light approximately 12 inches in front of the subject's closed eyes and flashing at frequencies that can range from 1 to 50 Hz, depending on how the procedure is carried out. Retinal damage does not occur, because each strobe flash, although intense, is extremely brief in duration. Some laboratories sample independent flash frequencies separately and randomly, although almost no one samples all frequencies between 1 and 50 Hz. Other laboratories use a *zoom technique* in which the flashes start at a low frequency, such as 1 Hz, and are then gradually and continuously increased to much higher flash frequencies. In some individuals, PS produces facial and eye muscle jerks, called a *photomyoclonic response* (PMR). More than 40 years ago,

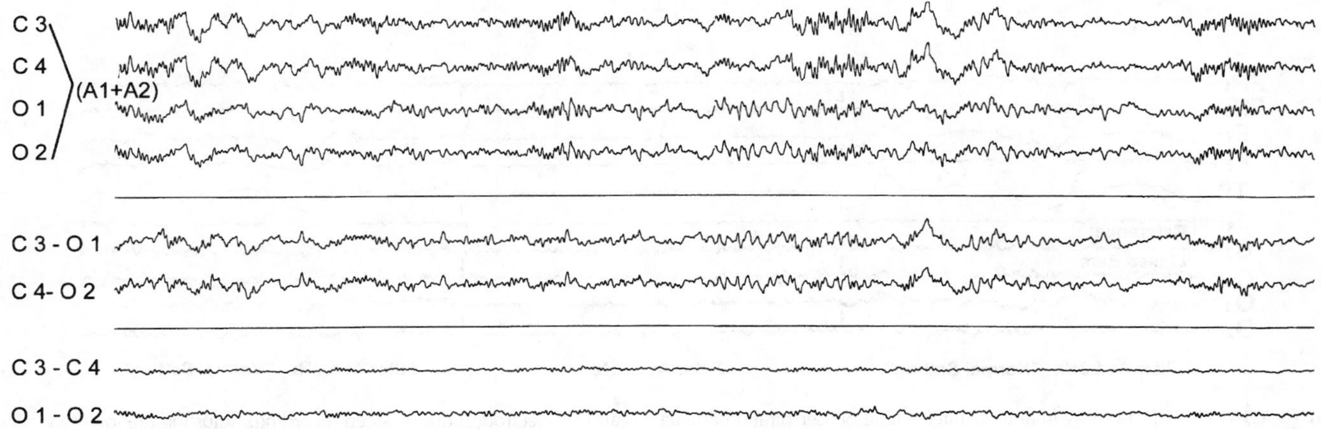

FIGURE 1.14–9 Alteration of appearance of brain waves (sleep patterns) with change in recording montage. Note that the monopolar montage (*top four channels*) yields higher amplitudes and greater differentiation between central and occipital activity. Similar input to members of an electrode pair (C3-O1 and C4-O2) can reduce voltage in the bipolar derivation. Note the absence of differentiation between central and occipital activity in the bipolar derivation. Note the extreme cancellation of activity in the last two bipolar derivations.

FIGURE 1.14–10 **A:** Fourteen-per-second and six-per-second positive spike discharges (a controversial pattern), independent left and right temporal-parietal-occipital area (monopolar montage). **B:** The top two channels show these discharges with the same monopolar montage as channels 3 and 4 in **A**, whereas lower channels show bipolar cancellation of the discharges, even though all electrodes in montage **A** are present. The female patient was 32 years of age with a closed head injury.

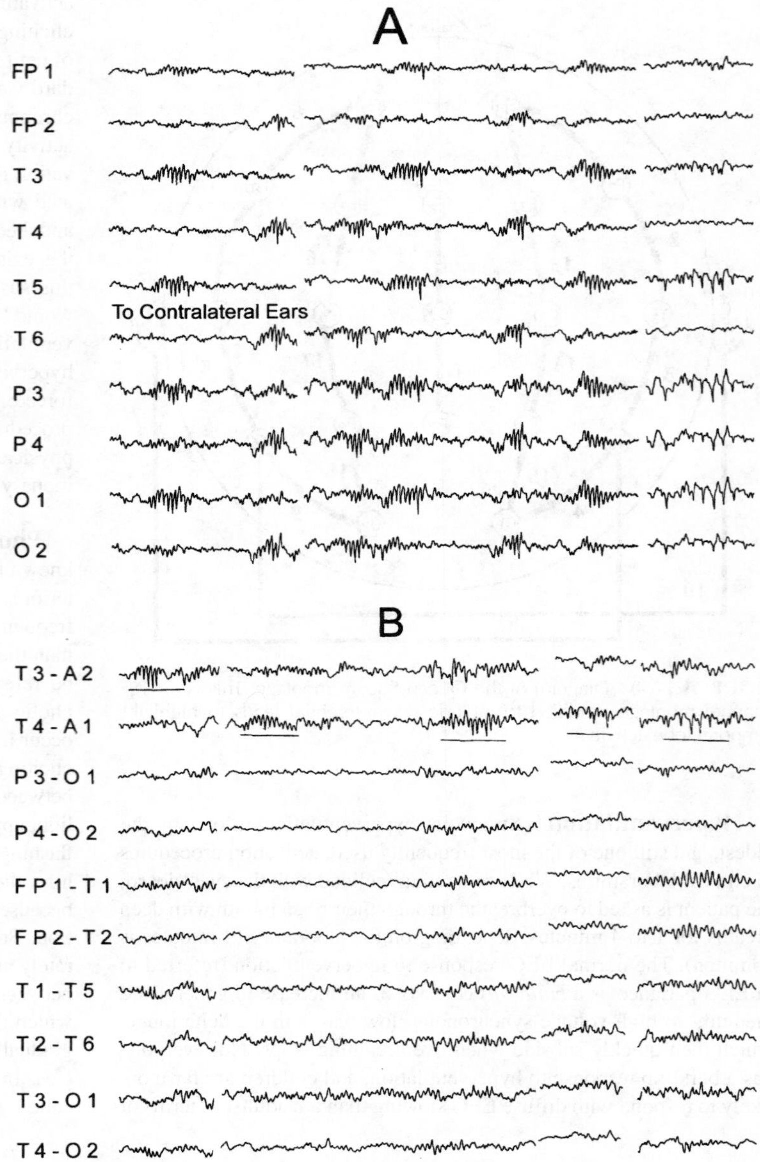

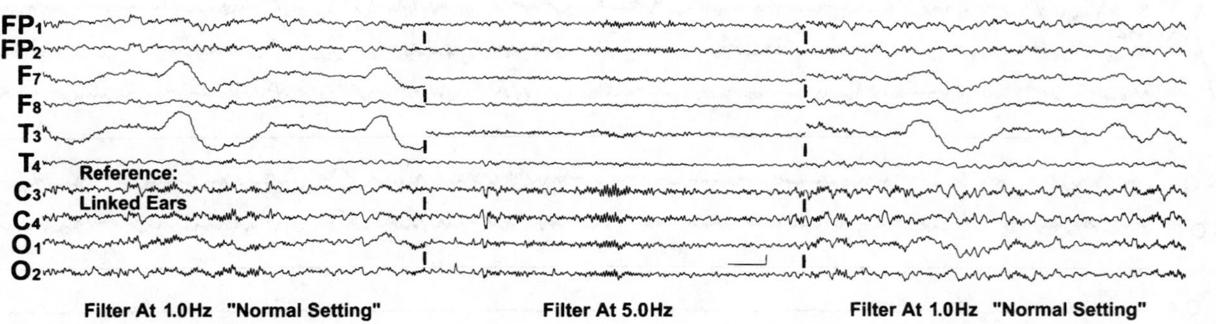

FIGURE 1.14–11 Effect of low-frequency filter setting on perspiration artifact (F7 and T3 electrodes) during sleep recording. Adjusting the low-frequency filter upward to 5 Hz completely eliminates the artifact and also eliminates the normal slow wave components of sleep but does not alter the 14-Hz sleep spindles.

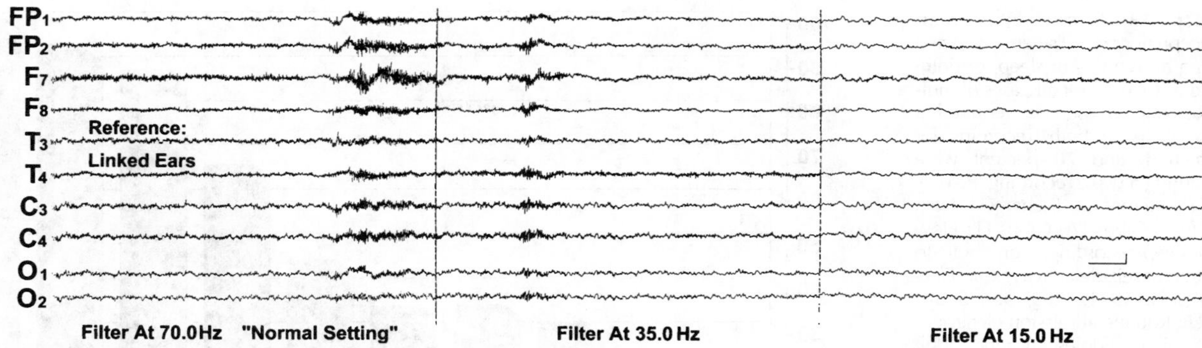

FIGURE 1.14–12 Effect of adjusting the high-frequency filter setting on muscle potential artifact (generated by having the patient grind his teeth repeatedly). Muscle potential seen at the "normal" filter setting of 70 Hz is attenuated when the filter setting is lowered to 35 Hz and is completely removed when it is set at 15 Hz. Lowering the high-frequency filter introduces the risk of attenuating or removing (i.e., filtering out) abnormal spike discharges from the tracing.

Henri Gastaut observed that PMR occurs in 0.3 percent of normal subjects, 3 percent of epileptic patients, and 17 percent of patients with psychiatric disorders. The PMR is also enhanced in early stages of alcohol withdrawal in chronic alcoholics and after a sudden withdrawal from barbiturates and other sedatives. The clinical relevance of PMR is yet to be fully explored in systematic research.

In terms of activating EEG abnormalities, one looks for a photoconvulsive response that consists of bilaterally synchronous, usually diffuse, spike-and-wave discharges of various frequencies or diffuse, multiple spike-wave complexes. When the resting EEG is normal, and a seizure disorder or behavior that is suspected to be a manifestation of a paroxysmal EEG dysrhythmia is suspected, PS can be a valuable activation to use. Its primary limitation, especially as a routine procedure, is the not insignificant "false positive" incidence of photoconvulsive EEG responses in individuals with no history of seizure disorder and no current symptoms suggestive of such. The persistence of the spike-wave discharges after the cessation of the PS may also be indicative of a photoconvulsive response. Moreover, the spread of the spike-wave activity to other leads besides the occipital leads may also be indicative of a pathological process.

Sleep Largely because of the pioneering studies and perseverance of Fred and Erna Gibbs, EEG recording during sleep, natural or sedated, is now widely accepted as an essential technique for eliciting a variety of paroxysmal discharges, when the wake tracing is normal, or for increasing the number of abnormal discharges to permit a more definitive interpretation to be made. A variety of focal and diffuse spike and spike-wave discharges, as well as several minor or controversial paroxysmal patterns, occurs much more often during drowsiness and light sleep than during the wake recording, and some of them are seen almost exclusively during the sleep recording. Paroxysmal patterns differ substantially among themselves in the degree to which their appearance in the tracing is sleep activation dependent (Fig. 1.14–13). Although most clinical EEGs should contain a drowsy- and light-sleep tracing to be complete, deep stages III and IV sleep with generalized high-voltage delta slowing has almost no activating property and is not clinically useful.

Sleep Deprivation It has been shown that the CNS stress produced by 24 hours of sleep deprivation alone can lead to the activation of paroxysmal EEG discharges in some cases. This effect is presumably independent of the known activating properties of natural or sedated sleep itself. Sleep deprivation is without risk for the healthy patient but may be contraindicated for patients medically or physically compromised. The primary disadvantage is the tendency for sleep deprived individuals to enter into deep sleep (stages III and IV) immediately at the start of the recording, thus reducing the chances of detecting spike activity. The optimal method is to ensure that the subject stays awake until the recording begins and remains so for the initial recording period, after which a gradual transition into drowsy sleep can be observed.

Miscellaneous Special Activations It has long been recognized that seizure manifestations or aberrant behaviors that might rest on a seizure basis can be triggered by specific stimuli. In this regard, cases of audiogenic, musicogenic, photogenic, and reading epilepsy readily come to mind, even though such cases are rare, and most practitioners have never encountered them. Seizure phenomena related to other sensory system input (e.g., somatosensory and gustatory) are even more rare. Sometimes, it may be possible for laboratory personnel to duplicate or approximate sensory triggers in various modalities to determine if they activate EEG seizure discharges combined with overt symptoms. Psychiatrists evaluating a patient with an atypical behavioral reaction to a drug (for example, an unusually explosive reaction after a small amount of alcohol or other abused drug or some other highly idiosyncratic response) may want to consider a drug-activated EEG to determine if ingestion of the drug activates any type of seizure or other paroxysmal abnormality in the tracing that might have explanatory clinical value.

NORMAL ANALOG EEG TRACING

Although the appearance of the EEG tracing may vary somewhat between individuals, the range of frequencies, voltages, and waveforms that characterize the normal EEG during wake and sleep has been well established. Nonetheless, there are certain waveforms that continue to engender disagreements regarding their place on the normal-abnormal continuum, and several of these controversial waveforms may have significant importance to psychiatry. Stated somewhat differently, the normal boundaries of the EEG, although well established for evaluating neurological or medical disorders, are not nearly as well established for psychiatric disorders. Furthermore, the dynamic nature of many psychiatric disorders, combined with the fact that many EEG findings and their associated symptoms are known to cut across specific psychiatric diagnostic categories, makes the electroclinical relationships between psychiatric syndromes and EEG more complex. Nonetheless, normative patterns that are not controversial are discussed in this section.

Normal Intrinsic Frequencies The normal EEG tracing is composed of a complex mixture of many different frequencies.

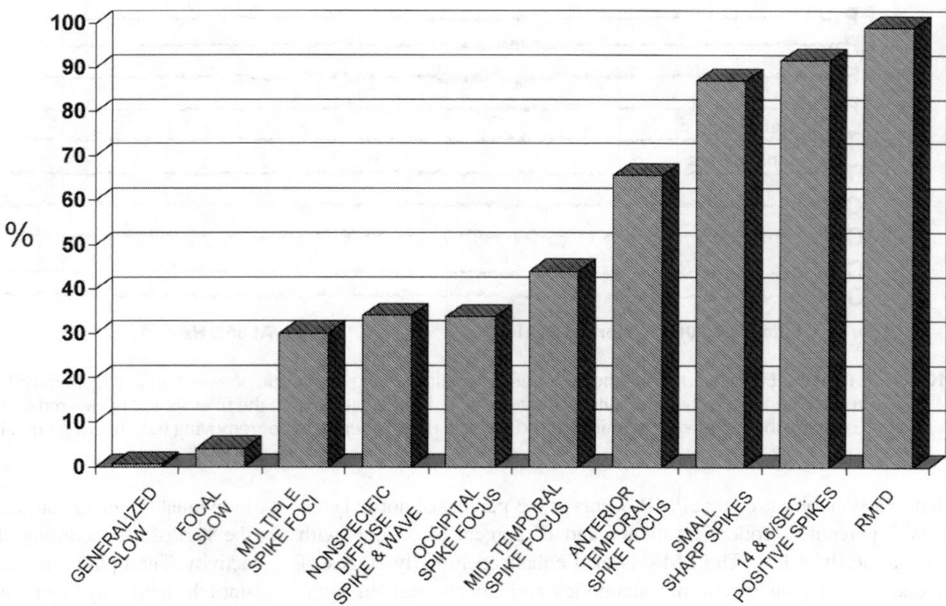

FIGURE 1.14–13 Percent of various electroencephalography patterns detected only during drowsiness or sleep, or both. To be read as follows: Of all cases of multiple spike foci, 30 percent required a drowsy or sleep, or both, recording for their detection, and 70 percent were detected during a wake recording. RMTD, rhythmic mid-temporal discharges. (Data abridged from Gibbs FA, Gibbs EL: How much do sleep recordings contribute to the detection of seizure activity? *Clin Electroencephalogr.* 1971;2:169; and Struve FA, Pike LE: Routine admission electroencephalograms of adolescent and adult psychiatric patients awake and asleep. *Clin Electroencephalogr.* 1974;5:67. A greatly expanded graph with 27 electroencephalography patterns can be found in Struve FA. Clinical electroencephalography as an assessment method in psychiatric practice. In: Hall RCW, Beresford TP, eds. *Handbook of Psychiatric Diagnostic Procedures.* Vol 2. New York: Spectrum Publications, 1985.)

Furthermore, some frequency bands are expressed more strongly over some cortical regions than others, and, in addition, the frequency profile varies considerably as the recording moves from alert wakefulness into sleep. Following the lead of Berger, discrete frequency bands within the broad EEG frequency spectrum are designated with Greek letters.

Alpha Highly rhythmic alpha waves with a frequency range of 8 to 13 Hz constitute the dominant brain wave frequency of the normal eyes-closed wake EEG. Through middle age, the vast majority of normal adults have an alpha frequency at, or close to, 10 Hz, whereas, with normal geriatric populations, a slower alpha frequency of 8 to 9 Hz is not uncommon. Alpha activity is also most prominent over the posterior cortex, particularly the parietal, posterior temporal, and occipital cortex, with the occipital region being best suited to show this activity. The registration of alpha activity diminishes as one records from more anterior locations, and this frequency is rare at prefrontal electrode sites. Alpha activity is abolished, or at least severely attenuated, by eye opening, and alpha activity also disappears with drowsiness and sleep. It is often not appreciated that alpha activity can be highly responsive to cognitive activity, such as focused attention or concentration. For example, under eyes-closed recording conditions, alpha can be blocked or attenuated by engaging in visual imagery, numeric calculation, or almost anything requiring significant concentration (Fig. 1.14–14). Alpha frequency can be increased or decreased by a wide variety of pharmacological, metabolic, or endocrine variables.

Theta Waves with a frequency of 4.0 to 7.5 Hz are collectively referred to as *theta activity*. A small amount of sporadic, arrhythmic, and isolated theta activity can be seen in many normal waking EEGs, particularly in frontal-temporal regions. Although theta activity is limited in the waking EEG, it is a prominent feature of the drowsy and sleep tracing. Excessive theta in wake, generalized or focal in nature, suggests the operation of a pathological process.

Delta Delta activity (equal to or less than 3.5 Hz) is not present in the normal waking EEG but is a prominent feature of deeper stages of sleep. The presence of significant generalized or focal delta in the wake EEG is strongly indicative of a pathophysiological process.

Beta Frequencies that are faster than the upper 13 Hz limit of the alpha rhythm are termed *beta waves*, and they are not uncommon in normal adult waking EEGs, particularly over frontal-central regions. It is also not uncommon for beta to appear as runs of rhythmic activity as opposed to sporadic isolated waves. Although there is no real upper limit designation for beta activity, the practical constraints of recording apparatus and filtering requirements tend to restrict beta activity to less than 40 or 50 Hz. The voltage of beta activity is also almost always lower than that of activity in the other frequency bands described previously. Researchers sometimes divide beta activity into *low* and *high* beta frequencies, and some have even specified the higher frequencies by using designations, such as gamma 1 (25 to 35 Hz), gamma 2 (35 to 50 Hz), and gamma 3 (50 to 100 Hz).

Changes with Age The appearance of the EEG tracing changes dramatically from birth to advanced age. From a preponderance of irregular medium- to high-voltage delta activity in the tracing of the infant, EEG activity gradually increases in frequency and becomes more rhythmic with increasing age. Rhythmic activity in the upper theta–lower alpha range (7 to 8 Hz) can be seen in posterior areas by early childhood, and, by the time mid-adolescence is reached, the EEG essentially has the appearance of an adult tracing. The interpretation of EEGs secured from children demands a solid grounding in the age-related changes during this period and is best performed by one specializing in pediatric EEG.

Sleep Patterns The EEG patterns that characterize drowsy and sleep states are different from the patterns seen during wake state. A detailed accounting of the nuances of sleep patterns would exceed the scope of this chapter. In simplistic terms, the rhythmic posterior alpha activity of the waking state subsides during drowsiness and is replaced by irregular low-voltage theta activity. As drowsiness deepens, slower frequencies emerge, and sporadic vertex

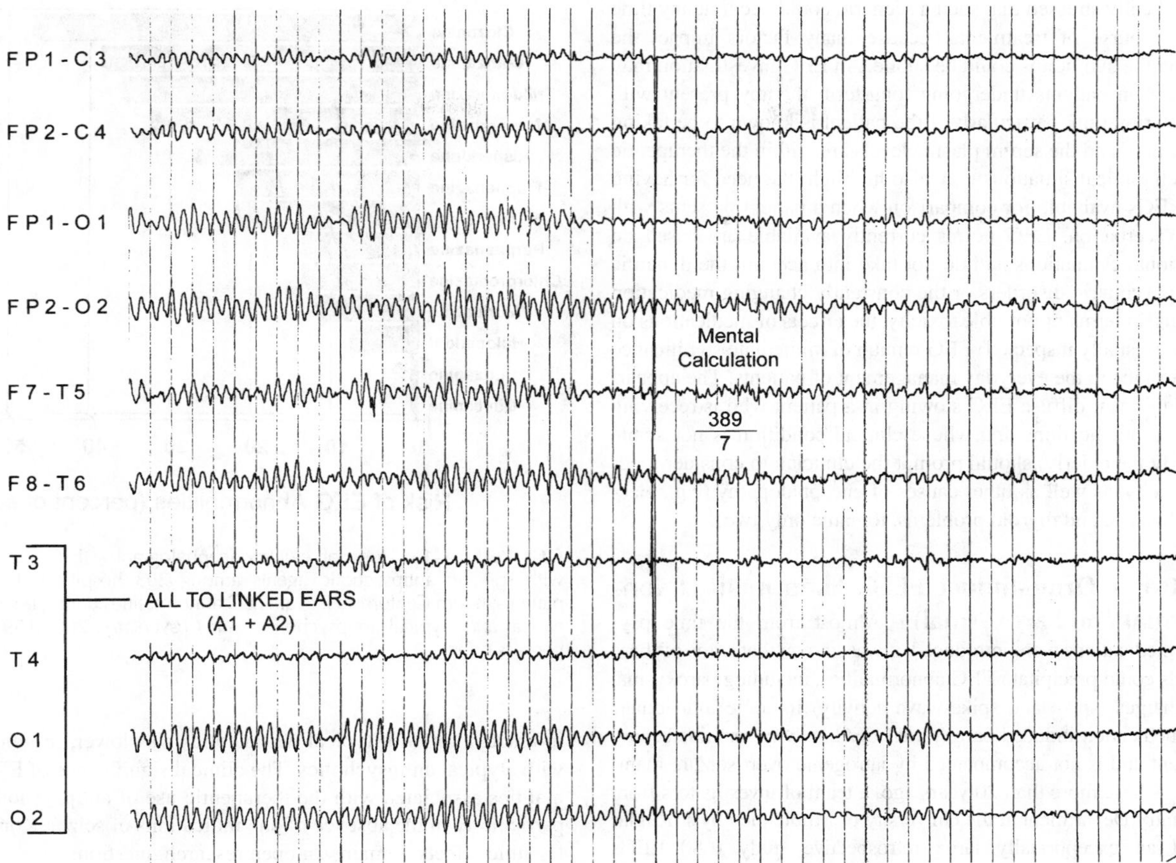

FIGURE 1.14–14 Resting, eyes-closed, awake electroencephalography recording. Effect of mental concentration on alpha activity. While instructed to keep the eyes closed, at the heavy vertical line, the patient is asked to divide 389 by 7. Note the immediate blocking of alpha activity.

sharp waves may appear at central electrode sites, particularly among younger persons. Finally, the progression into sleep is marked by the appearance of 14-Hz sleep spindles (also called *sigma waves*), which, in turn, gradually become replaced by high-voltage delta waves as deep sleep stages are reached.

Artifacts Artifacts are electric potentials of nonbrain origin that are in the frequency and voltage range of EEG signals and that are detected by scalp electrodes. Most EEGs contain some artifacts, and the electroencephalographer must identify them, particularly those that can closely mimic "real" brain waves, before making an interpretation. Common artifacts include eye blinks, vertical or lateral eye movements, frontalis EMG, muscle potentials from jaw clenching, perspiration artifact (galvanic skin response), and head movement. Less frequently seen are artifacts from electrocardiogram (ECG) (especially in heavy "barrel-chested" subjects recorded with a monopolar EEG montage), lateral rectus eye muscle "spikes," lingual movements, and a variety of electrode and amplifier problems. The competent technologist is capable of modifying recording conditions and patient instructions to distinguish artifact from brain waves when necessary, and, when this competence is not available, the quality of the EEG may become compromised. Automatic artifact rejection programs exist for some computerized research applications, but they have not strongly entered the clinical arena.

EEG ALTERATIONS FROM MEDICATIONS AND DRUGS

A great many medications, as well as substances consumed for recreational or abuse purposes, can produce some degree of alteration in the EEG. This section attempts to highlight those compounds most relevant to clinical and research psychiatry.

Psychotrophic Medications (General Considerations) It is well known that psychotropic agents can affect the EEG. For the routine EEG, with the exception of the benzodiazepines and some compounds with a propensity to induce paroxysmal EEG discharges, there is little, if any, clinically relevant effect when the medication is not causing any toxicity. Benzodiazepines, even in small doses, always generate a significant amount of beta activity that is seen diffusely. This response is so universal that it has been suggested that, if a particular brain region fails to exhibit the expected benzodiazepine-induced beta activity, that area may be dysfunctional.

Psychotropic Medications (Toxic Effects) For a long time, it has been accepted that the EEG is sensitive to the neurotoxic effects of psychotropic medications, and clinical vignettes illustrating the value of EEG in detecting a neurotoxic reaction to medications when a clinical deterioration was evident have been reported. It is often specifically stressed that such a scenario could occur at any time during the course of treatment, because many factors impact the patient, and the symptoms could be subtle. An EEG investigation may be useful when patients undergoing long-term therapy present with clinical deterioration, particularly if the patient is known to be taking the medication, and the serum plasma levels are within the therapeutic range. Such clinical situations may also highlight the need for having baseline EEGs available for comparison when a patient presents with clinical exacerbation. EEG norms currently available are based on cross sectional evaluations and do not take into account the dynamic nature of psychiatric disorders or the constantly changing medication status. Thus, in terms of possible toxicity, the effects of medications on the routine (visually inspected) EEG remain of immediate significance and of relevance to the everyday management of patients. The appearance of significant diffuse EEG slowing in a patient who is receiving psychotropic medications and whose clinical condition is not stable (particularly the elderly) should prompt the clinician to consider medication toxicity, as well as other causes of encephalopathy (e.g., electrolyte imbalance and thyroid problems, to name only two).

Psychotropic Drug–Induced EEG Abnormality (Nonparoxysmal and Paroxysmal) Almost from the time psychotropic medications were introduced, it was known that some of these compounds could precipitate EEG abnormalities, including paroxysmal EEG discharges (spike and spike-wave activity) in some individuals. Usually, medication-induced paroxysmal EEG activity remains behaviorally silent and is not accompanied by iatrogenic overt seizure manifestations. A little more than 20 years ago, a team of investigators from the Psychiatry Department at the University of Munich led by J. Kuglar conducted an exceptionally large retrospective study (680 EEGs obtained from 593 patients) of the effects of psychotropic agents on the EEG and reported that the highest proportion of abnormal EEGs occurred in clozapine (Clozaril)–treated patients (59 percent), followed by lithium (Eskalith, Lithobid) (50 percent). The overall proportion of paroxysmal EEG discharges was 13 percent, and actual seizures were witnessed with treatment with clozapine, lithium, and maprotiline (Ludiomil). Lithium continues to be widely used in the treatment of bipolar disorder, as well as other episodic behavioral syndromes, including aggressive tendencies. This compound is capable of causing abnormal generalized slowing or paroxysmal activity, or both, including a 10 percent incidence of toxic delirium, in normal research volunteers and patients undergoing lithium treatment.

Recent times have seen the emergence of several new atypical antipsychotic compounds. Although clozapine has received extensive EEG study and is now recognized as a compound highly associated with risk of induced EEG abnormality, information regarding the other new compounds remains sparse. A research team led by Franca Centorrino recently made a substantial effort to fill this knowledge gap. In their study, the effects of typical and atypical antipsychotic medications were compared using EEG recordings from 323 hospitalized psychiatric patients (293 on antipsychotic medications and 30 not receiving antipsychotic drugs) who were graded blind to diagnosis and treatment for type and severity of EEG abnormalities. Abnormal EEGs occurred in 19 percent of treated patients and 4 percent of untreated patients; however, the risk for EEG abnormality varied widely among the different types of medication (Fig. 1.14–15). The highest incidence of EEG abnormalities was associated with clozapine (47 percent) and was somewhat lower with olanzapine (Zyprexa) (38.5 percent) and risperidone (Risperdal) (28 percent). There were no EEG abnormalities seen in association with quetiapine (Seroquel). The incidence of EEG abnormalities in association with typical neuroleptics was lower, in general, than with atypical antipsychotics. The clinical significance of EEG abnormalities associated with the therapeutic use of antipsychotic agents, particularly in the absence of any indications of seizures or encephalopathic effects, remains an open research question.

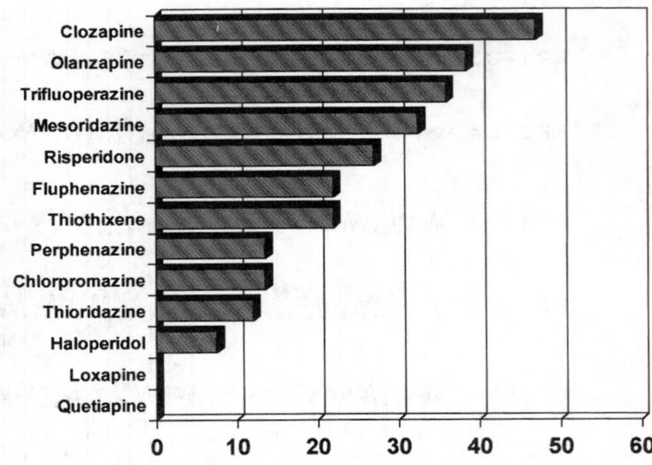

FIGURE 1.14–15 Risk of electroencephalography (EEG) abnormalities with specific antipsychotic agents among 293 hospitalized psychiatric patients. (From Centorrino F et al.: EEG abnormalities during treatment with typical and atypical antipsychotics. *Am J Psychiatry.* 2002;159:109, with permission.)

Pharmaco-EEG The effects of psychotropic drugs on the frequency and power distribution of the different EEG spectra, using topographic QEEG methods, is the subject of a vast and growing field entitled *pharmacoelectroencephalography* (*pharmaco-EEG*). The focus of this field is to be able to predict the likely psychotropic effect of newly developed agents (i.e., antipsychotic vs. antidepressant vs. anxiolytic). Researchers in this field are also developing methods to predict the responsiveness of a particular patient to a particular compound by using test doses with the hopes of avoiding having to subject patients to 3 to 6 weeks of a medication trial before realizing that this agent is not helpful.

Drugs of Abuse Recreational and addictive involvement with abuse drugs is a significant phenomenon in society today, and it is becoming of increasing concern for those involved in the assessment and treatment of psychiatric disorders. Nearly all abuse drugs are capable of altering the frequency spectrum of the EEG, and the degree of alteration varies with recreational versus heavy use and whether the EEG was secured during or close to acute exposure (intoxication), during intervening nonintoxication states, or during clinical withdrawal in the addicted individual.

With only infrequent exceptions, the use of an abuse drug does not introduce frank clinical abnormalities into the visually analyzed EEG tracing. This is especially true for recreational drug use and is even largely true for dependent and addictive use, as well, and, for this reason, drug abuse alone is not a sufficient reason for EEG referral. Although the alterations of EEG frequency and voltage in the visually analyzed EEG produced by many abuse drugs are often unimpressive, topographic QEEG analyses often reveal marked alterations of the EEG spectrum that constitute significant deviations from population norms, even though the clinical implications may not be clear. Because of this, they constitute significant problems for researchers using topographic QEEG measures in their work. For example, if one wants to establish a QEEG profile for a particular diagnostic group or a particular psychotropic medication (i.e., as in pharmaco-EEG research), the QEEG effects of certain abuse drugs may constitute serious methodological confounds, rendering any results scientifically uninterpretable.

Alcohol There is considerable consensus that an increase in the amount of alpha activity and a slight slowing of alpha frequency typically accompany alcohol consumption and that higher blood alcohol levels increase the amount of theta in the tracing. Some reports have indicated that chronic alcohol consumption may be associated with a lower voltage and slightly faster resting EEG, although the clinical relevance of this remains obscure. Higher-frequency beta activity may be substantially increased in the addicted alcoholic undergoing withdrawal, and, if delirium tremens complicates the clinical picture, excessive fast activity may dominate the EEG tracing (whereas delirium from other causes is associated with generalized slowing).

Opiates Opiate effects on the EEG are similar to those of alcohol and involve slight reductions in alpha frequency. They may also increase the voltage of the EEG, particularly the power of theta and delta activity. However, when an opiate overdose produces a comatose clinical presentation, the EEG usually consists of clinically abnormal diffuse slowing.

Barbiturates When barbiturates are taken for medical purposes or for recreational or habitual abuse, beta activity is introduced into the EEG, particularly over frontal regions. The barbiturate effect on the EEG is thus opposite to that of alcohol. However, sudden, abrupt withdrawal from barbiturates after long-term dependence can produce EEGs containing generalized paroxysmal activity and spike discharges, which are often not associated with overt motor seizure manifestations, and these effects may be seen for days or even a few weeks after last drug exposure.

Marijuana Use of marijuana (tetrahydrocannabinol [THC]) is widespread in society and not infrequently constitutes a comorbid feature of psychiatric conditions. Exposure to THC produces highly characteristic alterations of the waking EEG that can be appreciated visually but are best documented through use of topographic QEEG study. The EEG response to smoking THC is rapid. The voltage, amount, and interhemispheric coherence of alpha activity increases dramatically over the bilateral frontal cortex (areas in which alpha activity normally is only rarely seen) within 2 minutes of the first THC inhalation. The frequency of the alpha activity also slows by as much as 0.5 Hz. Some studies have shown that increases in frontal alpha are accompanied by subjective feelings of euphoria. With the chronic user, the EEG always shows increased frontal alpha and slowed alpha frequency, even when THC urine levels are absent, to the degree that a suspicion of THC use from mere inspection of the tracing would not be unreasonable.

Cocaine Chronic cocaine exposure produces topographic QEEG changes similar (but not identical) to those seen with marijuana abuse, and the EEG effects can last throughout 6 or more months of abstinence. Primary effects are reported to consist of increased relative power (i.e., amount, abundance) of alpha activity seen maximally over the frontal cortex combined with a deficit of the amount and voltage of theta and delta frequencies.

Inhalants Inhalation abuse of volatile substances (e.g., airplane glue, cleaning fluid, paint thinner, and gasoline) can produce a nearly instantaneous sensation of euphoria, and, in the early period of use, there may be no obvious residuals after the acute response subsides. However, with continued inhalant abuse, neurological and neurocognitive deficits, which are often quite serious, can emerge, and they are not always completely reversible with abstinence. The immediate effects of inhalation of volatiles on the human EEG appear not to have been well studied. Where persistent neurological or neurocognitive sequelae follow chronic inhalant abuse, clinically abnormal diffuse EEG slowing in the lower theta to upper delta range may be seen.

Hallucinogens Drugs, such as lysergic acid diethylamide (LSD) and mescaline, appear to have only minor effects on the visualized EEG and do not produce clinically relevant changes.

Tobacco Like many of the drugs reviewed previously, tobacco does not appear to produce dramatic alterations in the analog EEG. However, topographic QEEG analyses reveal striking EEG changes with acute exposure to, as well as withdrawal from, tobacco. The immediate effects of smoking include a decrease in slower frequencies (especially theta), increased power of frequencies in the upper one-half of the alpha frequency band, and beta activity. Twenty-four hours of tobacco deprivation produce a marked decrease in alpha frequency, with a corresponding marked increase in the relative power (amount) of theta activity. The effects of acute smoking and abstinence are essentially opposite to one another.

Caffeine Coffee and products containing caffeine are also ubiquitous in this culture. The use of caffeine is of little concern to the electroencephalographer interpreting the visually analyzed EEG. Withdrawal from caffeine in the caffeine-dependent individual, however, produces a markedly significant increase in the amplitude, or voltage, of theta activity—an effect that is reversible within 15 minutes of consuming one cup of coffee.

CLINICAL INTERPRETATION OF THE EEG

The interpretation of the standard or analog EEG tracing is essentially a problem of learning to recognize all of the myriad intrinsic waveforms, their expected distributions over the various cortical regions, and their range of variation in amplitude and degree of symmetry. Although there is little doubt that 16, 32, or even 64 channels of oscillating waves appear quite confusing to the beginner, there is an inherent regularity to the brain's electrical output that the experienced electroencephalographer comes to recognize. Because of this inherent regularity, the intrinsic EEG rhythms and their range of variation that characterizes the wake, drowsy, and various sleep states become easily recognized through practice and experience. Furthermore, various artifacts (electrical potentials of nonbrain origin) produce localized or regional waveforms of distinctive shapes, allowing for their identification. The primary job of the interpreter is to identify those EEG waveforms that appear to fall outside of what one might call the *normal range of variation* of the intrinsic background activity and that are therefore (1) frankly abnormal with known pathophysiological correlates or (2) controversial abnormal waveforms of potential clinical relevance, pending the results of further continuing clinical investigation. The number of accepted and still controversial EEG abnormalities is quite large and well beyond the scope of this chapter. For the purpose of illustration only, four classic abnormal EEG patterns are shown (Figs. 1.14–16, 1.14–17, 1.14–18, and 1.14–19).

FIGURE 1.14–16 Diffuse three-per-second spike-and-wave discharge of the petit mal type with a multiple spike component. Female patient, 16 years of age. Previous history of petit mal seizures and rare grand mal attacks. At a previous psychiatric facility, the diagnosis was changed to "hysterical seizures" after a psychological evaluation.

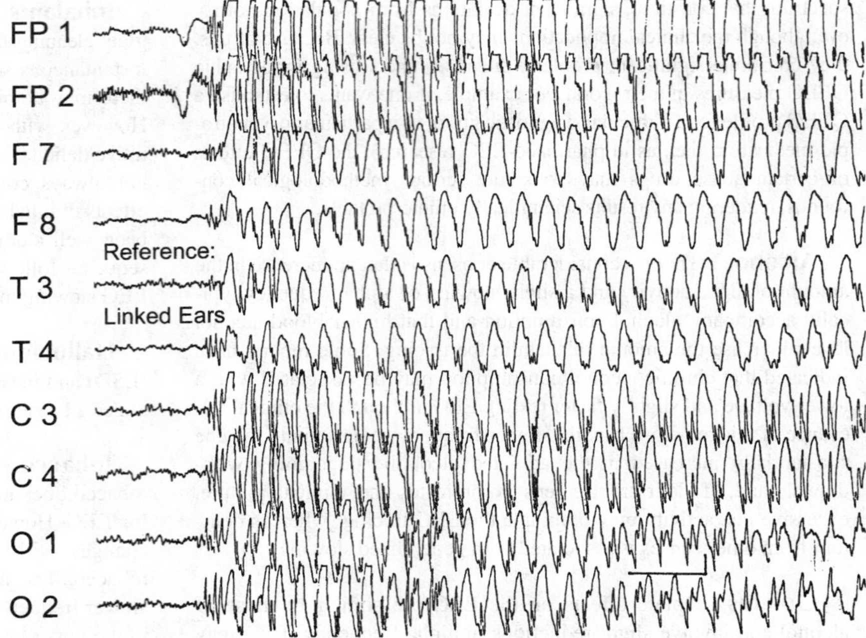

Interpreter Reliability

Because the EEG record is obtained by precisely measuring the microvolt fluctuations of electrical potentials over the scalp, a misconception often emerges that EEG interpretation is purely objective in the sense that measurements of temperature, weight, length, and volume are objective. In truth, there is a large, subjective element of judgment in EEG interpretation, and the achievement of skill in this area only follows a period of thorough training and the guiding hand of clinical experience. Accepted EEG abnormalities do not always appear in the EEG tracing in clear-cut textbook form, and there is always a gray area in which EEG activity that is clearly normal becomes blurred and shades off into waveforms that are unequivocally abnormal.

FIGURE 1.14–17 Focal slow (delta), right prefrontal spreading with reduced voltage to right anterior and mid-temporal and right central. During the sleep recording (not shown), sleep spindles were absent in the right hemisphere. Female patient, 49 years of age. No prior psychiatric history. Recent emergence (over 6 months) of depression, mild episodic confusion, symptoms of hyperthyroidism, and pathological crying. Glioblastoma found at surgery.

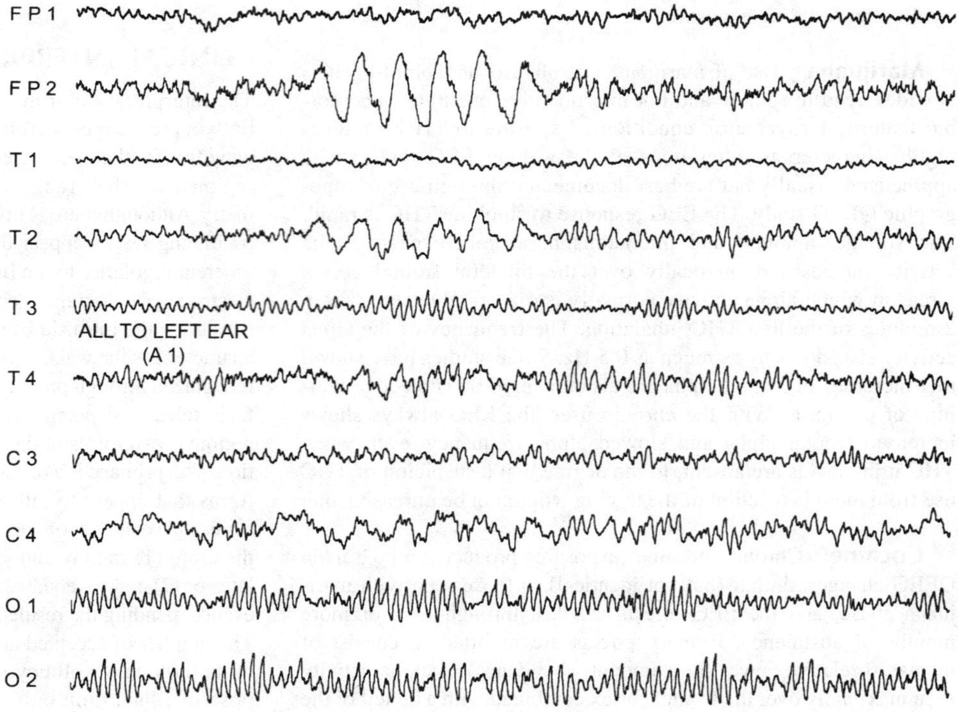

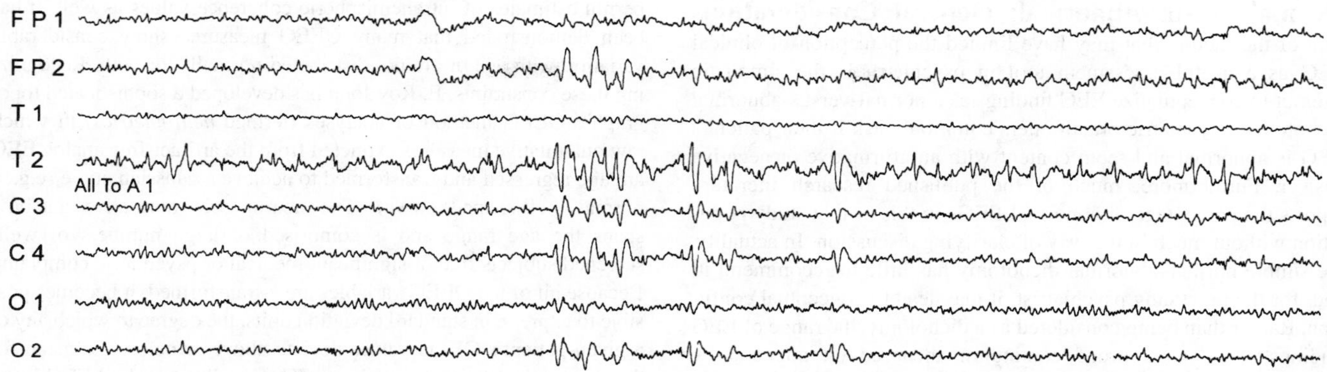

FIGURE 1.14–18 Focal negative spike and spike-wave discharges in the right anterior temporal cortex and often spreading with reduced voltage throughout the right hemisphere. Adult male patient. Complex partial seizures (psychomotor). Psychiatric outpatient with infrequent periods of sudden unresponsiveness during which time he would make grunting and guttural sounds and speak with incoherent words and syllables with amnesia for these events. (His girlfriend, who was involved in New Age phenomena, was convinced that he was communicating with spirits during these unresponsive spells and did not want him to be medicated.)

Although the important area of reliability of clinical EEG interpretation has not enjoyed extensive study over the years, the balance of available evidence suggests that high levels of statistically (and clinically) significant interpretation reliability can be obtained. The two methods for assessing reliability involve comparing the independent readings of two or more EEG interpreters (interjudge reliability) and asking one electroencephalographer to blindly reinterpret a sample of EEGs after an elapsed time (intrajudge reliability). A review of interjudge and intrajudge interpretative comparisons involving 1,567 clinical standard EEGs revealed a weighted average of 91 percent interpretive agreement over 11 separate studies (see the 1985 article by Frederick Struve). It should be noted that interpretive differences usually involve disagreements over gray areas in which alterations in the frequency, symmetry, or amplitude of the intrinsic EEG activity begin to shade off into what, by consensus, would be considered outside of normal limits. In such transition areas in which the dividing line is not sharply precise, statements such as *borderline slowing* are sometimes used to denote the understandable uncertainty that is involved. When disagreements in this borderline region are removed from consideration, interpretive agreements ranging from 95 to 98 percent are not uncommon.

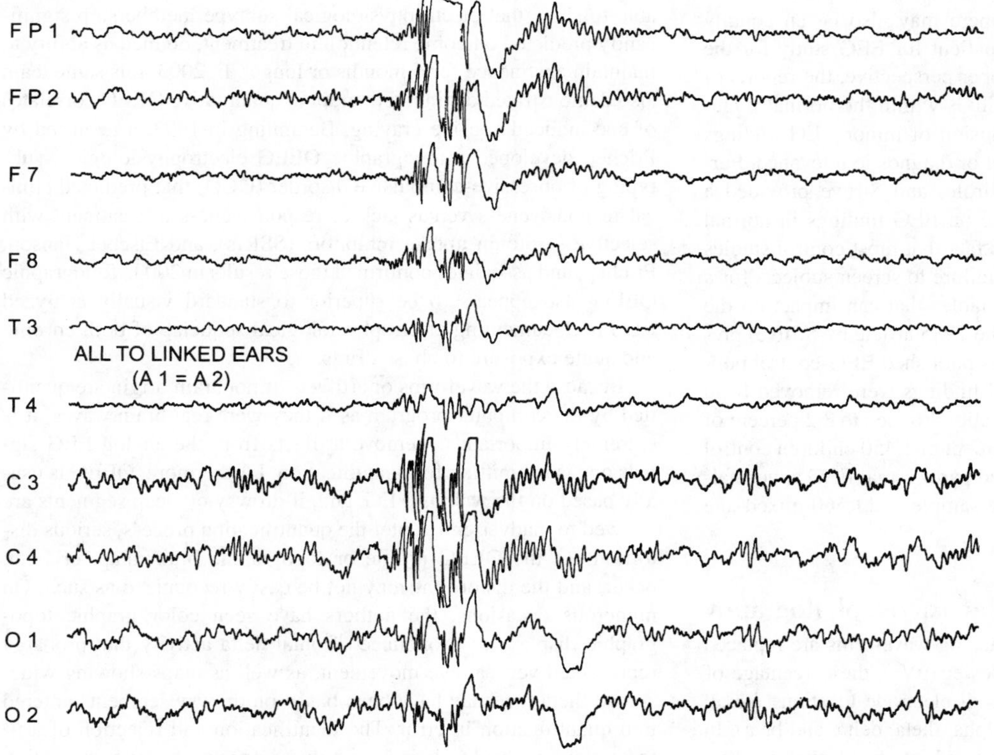

FIGURE 1.14–19 Diffuse spike-and-wave discharges during the sleep recording. The waking electroencephalography (EEG) was within normal limits. Female patient, 15 years of age. Admitted to inpatient adolescent psychiatric unit with the complaint of serious temper dyscontrol and episodic dizzy spells.

Normal versus Abnormal: General Considerations

One of the factors that may have limited the perception of clinical EEG as a useful assessment tool in psychiatry is the simplistic attempt to conceptualize EEG findings as a normal-versus-abnormal dichotomy. Psychiatric practitioners commonly ask if their patient's EEG is abnormal and seem content with an affirmative or negative answer. Furthermore, much of the published research literature reports the percentage of abnormal EEGs in this or that study population without much in the way of clarifying discussion. In actuality, the simple normal–abnormal dichotomy has little to recommend it, and, for the practicing psychiatrist, it may lead to conceptual confusion. Rather than being considered as a dichotomy, the range of EEG findings exists on a broad continuum anchored on one end by unequivocally normal EEGs and extending in the other direction through a long parade of findings from those with unclear yet potential clinical relevance all the way to findings that correlate with life-threatening pathology. Some EEG patterns that are correctly classified as abnormal are on the low end of the continuum of clinical expressivity and may not always contribute strongly to diagnostic decisions. The psychiatrist receiving a report (without clarification) of a minor finding of limited clinical relevance may understandably begin to question the value of EEG when no current or past history organic signs are detected. The bottom line is that one should not ask simply if an EEG is abnormal, as if it were one side of a dichotomy, but instead should ask what specific kind of finding was present and what is the range of possible clinical correlates associated with it.

An additional confusion caused by unwise reliance on the normal-abnormal dichotomy involves reports in review articles and book chapters stating that 10 percent, 15 percent, or even 20 percent of the normal population have abnormal EEGs. Because such statements are almost never properly clarified, they tend to be terribly misleading. Clearly, there can be an understandable reluctance to follow up an abnormal EEG report if one has read in a presumably authoritative source that 20 percent of the normal population have abnormal EEGs. More importantly, there may also be an equally understandable reluctance to refer a patient for EEG study for the same reason. To place the issue in proper perspective, the reports of substantial percentages of abnormal EEGs within the normal population are heavily skewed by the inclusion of minor EEG findings which often have low levels of clinical or diagnostic relevance. Furthermore, Nashaat Boutros, Hugh Mirolo, and Struve provided a comprehensive review of the literature on EEG findings in normal control populations that highlights the fact that most control studies have been seriously compromised by failure to screen subjects for a variety of medical and psychiatric variables that can impact on the EEG results. One of the authors (see the 1985 article by Struve) previously reanalyzed data from numerous published EEG-control population studies. When borderline EEG findings were removed from the data, the incidence of EEG abnormality dropped to 3.2 percent of 6,182 adult control subjects and 3.5 percent of 1,450 children control subjects, and the prevalence of accepted paroxysmal EEG abnormalities dropped to only 1.14 percent of a sample of 11,560 mixed-age control subjects.

Topographic Quantitative Electroencephalography (QEEG)

In QEEG analyses, raw analog waveforms are replaced by quantitative estimates of absolute power (μV^2), the percentage of relative power and mean frequency at all electrode locations for all four standard EEG frequency bands (alpha, theta, delta, and beta). In addition, estimates of power asymmetry and interhemispheric coherence between homologous regions can be obtained, and some systems permit estimates of intrahemispheric coherence values as well. It has been demonstrated that many QEEG measures show considerable variation with age or are not distributed normally, or both. Recognizing these constraints, E. Roy John has developed a sophisticated topographic QEEG method of analyses (termed *neurometrics*) in which raw quantitative measures extracted from the artifact-free analog EEG are age regressed and transformed to achieve a gaussian curve (e.g., a normal, bell-shaped curve). The neurometric normative database spans the age range and is comprised of large numbers of well-screened subjects free of significant medical or psychiatric complaint. Because all of the QEEG variables are z-transformed, it becomes possible to express, in standard deviation units, the degree to which any of a given patient's QEEG values deviate above or below the mean for the normal population for their age. Thus, unlike standard EEG interpretation, which relies on waveform recognition, interpretation of the QEEG involves an assessment of the statistical degree of congruence or lack of congruence between a patient and the normal population or the degree of similarity between a given patient and a QEEG profile that may be characteristic of some defined clinical group. Typically, the interpretive results can be displayed numerically or with topographic color-graphic brain maps. Among many other things, the quantitative approach can display variations in QEEG profiles (which presumably reflect variations in neurophysiological function) across primary diagnostic groups (Fig. 1.14–20). It can also display progressive change in neurophysiological function over time.

Recent years have seen a substantial growth in research and attempted clinical applications involving topographic QEEG. Such methods hold considerable promise for psychiatry, particularly in terms of possibly establishing neurophysiological subtypes of certain psychiatric disorders and in seeking electrophysiological indicators of clinical outcome. For example, in papers published in 1999 and 2002, Leslie Prichep, Kenneth Alper, and their colleagues successfully used topographic QEEG methods to derive three distinct electrophysiological subtypes of cocaine dependence. They were able to show that electrophysiological subtype membership significantly predicted outcome retention in treatment, defined as ability to maintain abstinence for 6 months or longer. In 2003, this same team also demonstrated distinct topographic quantitative QEEG correlates of cue-induced cocaine craving. Beginning in 1993, a team led by Prichep developed a topographic QEEG electrophysiological subtyping of obsessive-compulsive disorder (OCD) that predicted clinical responsiveness versus lack of responsiveness to treatment with selective serotonin uptake inhibitors (SSRIs), and Elsebet Hanson, Prichep, and associates confirmed those results in 2003. Topographic QEEG also appears to be superior to standard visually analyzed EEG in documenting electrophysiological sequelae of both chronic and acute exposure to abuse drugs.

Because the waveforms of artifacts of nonbrain origin are quantified by the computer program as if they were real brain waves, it is extremely important to remove artifacts from the analog EEG signals one is submitting for quantification. Furthermore, QEEG is usually based on the waking EEG, and, if drowsy or sleep segments are allowed to inadvertently enter the quantification process, serious distortions of the QEEG profile or topographic brain map, or both, occur, and the distortions may not be easily recognized as such. On numerous occasions, the authors have seen color graphic topographic displays of pronounced frontal delta activity that probably represented vertical eye movement, as well as maps showing widespread theta that may have been based on drowsy segments entered into quantification in error. The identification and rejection of artifacts is an involved task and can only be done with visual inspection of the analog tracing by experienced electroencephalographers or

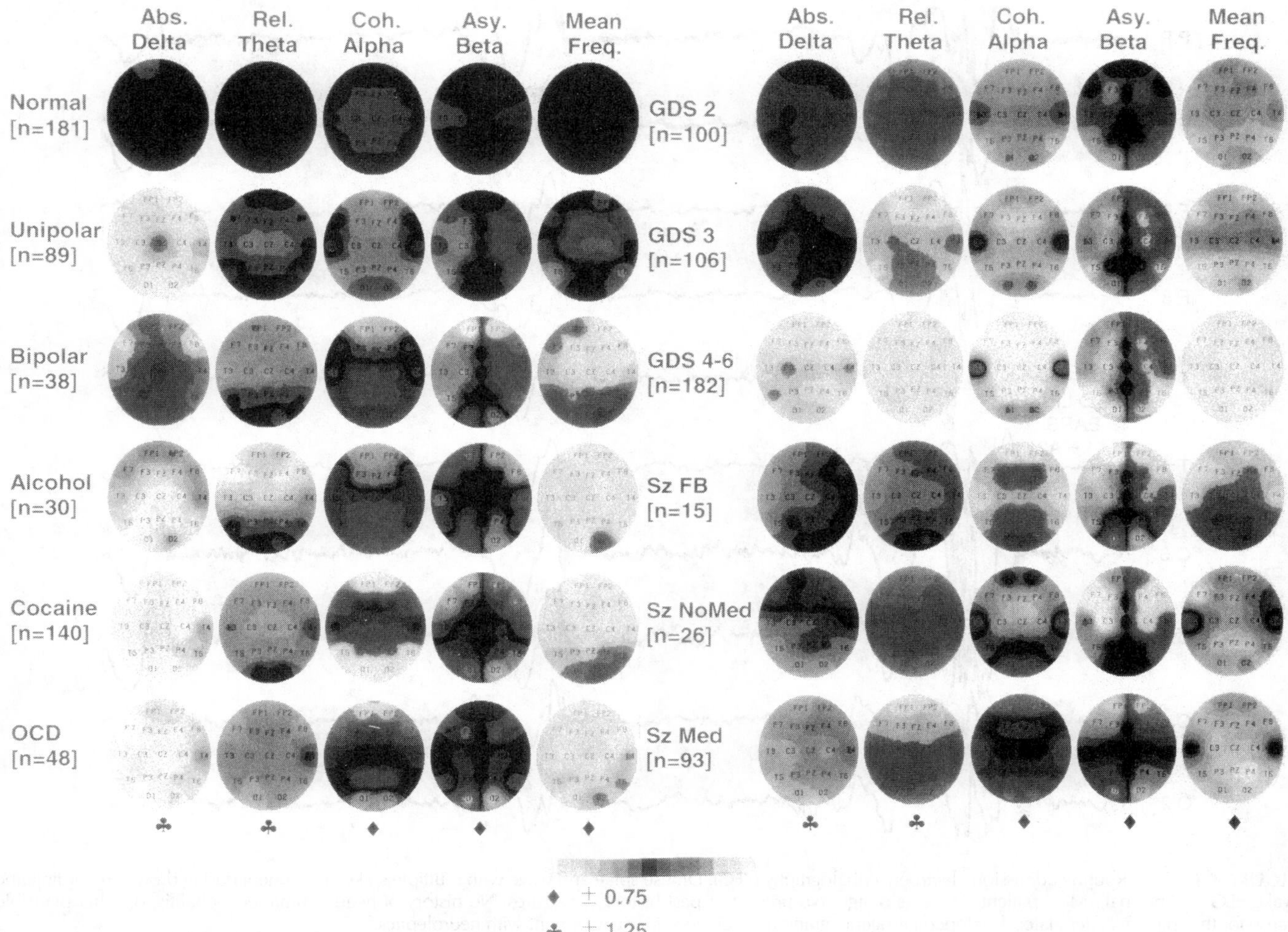

FIGURE 1.14–20 Baseline group average topographic images of *z* scores for selected quantitative electroencephalography (QEEG) features in different *Diagnostic and Statistical Manual of Mental Disorders*, 4th edition, text revision, psychiatric populations. Successive columns in the left and right panels include absolute (Abs.) power delta, relative (Rel.) power theta, interhemispheric coherence (Coh.) alpha, interhemispheric power asymmetry (Asy.) beta, and total power mean frequency (Freq.). Populations include normal adults; unipolar depressions; bipolar depressions; alcoholics (in withdrawal); cocaine-dependent subjects (5 to 14 days after last drug use); obsessive-compulsive disorder (OCD); global deterioration scale (GDS) 2, which are normal elderly with only subjective cognitive complaints; GDS 3, which meet criteria for mild cognitive impairment; GDS 4 through 6, which meet criteria for dementia; first-break schizophrenics (Sz FB); schizophrenics off medication (Sz NoMed); and schizophrenics on medication (Sz Med). The color scale of each *z* image is in standard deviation units, with a range of +0.75, indicated with a diamond, or +1.25, indicated with a club. To estimate the significance of any regional *z* score for this group average data, the *z* score should be multiplied by the square root of the number of patients in the group. For a group with 100 subjects, the *z* value imaged should be multiplied by 10 to get the estimate of the significance of that *z*. (See Color Plate.) (Courtesy of Dr. E. Roy John, Director, Brain Research Laboratories, Department of Psychiatry, New York University School of Medicine, New York, NY and Nathan S. Kline Institute for Psychiatric Research, Orangeburg, NY.)

technologists skilled in EEG interpretation. When the issue of artifact contamination of the QEEG is not properly addressed, one has a situation described a generation ago by computer programmers, namely, *garbage in–garbage out*. Several commercial QEEG instruments also have programs for automatic artifact rejection. Although some of these may be useful to some degree for major high-voltage artifacts, such as vertical eye blinks, seldom are they completely effective with all sources of contamination.

CLINICAL FINDINGS (GENERAL OVERVIEW)

The routine EEG is a completely noninvasive test that is even available in out-of-the-way rural areas. It is a relatively inexpensive test, with charges of $200 for the test and $100 for the interpretation being common (in some instances a range of $500 to $600). Furthermore, any psychiatrist can be fully trained to interpret EEGs, and, with skill, useful EEG data can often be obtained from agitated and psychotic patients.

Brief Synopsis of EEG Findings in Organic Pathophysiology The standard clinical EEG has a high degree of sensitivity to a wide variety of medical conditions and events that impinge on CNS function. For this reason, EEGs have sometimes contributed to the detection of unsuspected organic pathophysiologies influencing the psychiatric presentation. However, the range of EEG findings in medical disease is enormous and far beyond the scope of this chapter. The reader is referred to the large edited volume by Ernst Niedermeyer and Fernando Lopes da Silva for more in-depth coverage.

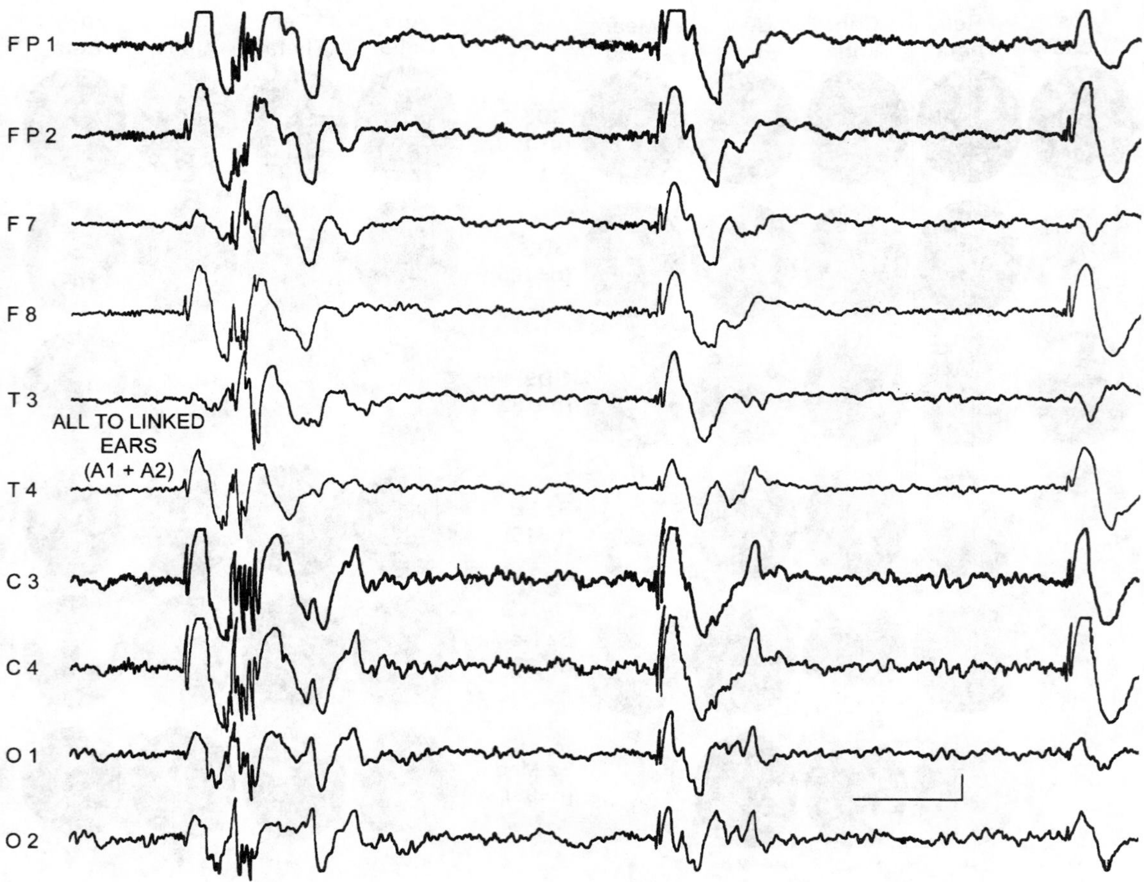

FIGURE 1.14–21 Routine admission electroencephalography (EEG). Diffuse spike and wave with multiple spike component during drowsy recording (the wake EEG was normal). Male patient, 16 years of age. No present or past history of seizures. No history of head trauma, encephalitis, or other plausible cause for the spiking. Patient later developed iatrogenic grand mal seizures during treatment with neuroleptics.

Findings with Seizures The hallmark EEG finding for a seizure disorder is the generalized, hemispheric, or focal spike or spike-wave discharge, or both (Figs. 1.14–16, 1.14–18, and 1.14–19). However, this statement constitutes a large oversimplification, because many types of EEG abnormalities have been associated with seizures at one time or another, and some patients with a bona fide seizure disorder have been known to have normal interictal EEG tracings. Furthermore, seizure disorders can be associated with an extremely wide range of etiologies (idiopathic or genetic, closed or open head trauma, cerebrovascular pathophysiology, metabolic disorders, structural brain lesions, infectious or toxic encephalopathies, certain drug-abuse withdrawal states, iatrogenic causes, to name only a few), and these considerations may modify the nature of the EEG-seizure disorder association.

The classification of seizure types is also wide, and the majority of specific seizure manifestations may be of little concern to the practicing psychiatrist. One of the exceptions may be petit mal status, which can last from less than 1 hour to longer than 1 day, during which time the patient presents with grossly impaired consciousness marked by pronounced confusion, greatly slowed mental processes, or stuporous or somnolent behavior, or both. The psychiatrist is most likely to encounter this clinical presentation in the emergency room, where it is often confused with other functional or organic syndromes or intoxicant states. If suspected, the status can be confirmed quickly by an EEG demonstration of continuous, diffuse spike-wave activity. Typical petit mal seizures (i.e., nonstatus) may also be of relevance to the child psychiatrist, because this type of epilepsy has a peak age distribution during childhood and early adolescence, and, in some cases, the absence attack may be mistaken for inattention or other functional behavioral reactions. Spike foci, usually anterior temporal, associated with CPSs (psychomotor) should also interest the psychiatrist, because the wide range of possible seizure manifestations is truly amazing, and almost any combination of "automatic" motor movements, sensory disturbances, seemingly psychiatric symptoms, or autonomic signs may be seen. The symptom cluster almost always remains the same from one attack to another, and the "automatic" behavior during the ictal event may, at times, be bizarre, with the patient undressing, picking at clothing and lip smacking, walking in circles and yelling, trying to climb on a table while making guttural noises, experiencing hallucinatory symptoms, or almost any other action. When continuous or closely spaced CPS attacks (complex partial status) lasting hours or longer than a day occur, they may mimic hysterical dissociative states.

Spike activity of various kinds and locations is sometimes found in the EEGs of psychiatric patients with no obvious seizure manifestations. In such cases, one might consider possible relationships to episodic aberrant behavior (particularly explosive aggressiveness), if present, followed by an empirical trial with an anticonvulsant. Sometimes, such spike discharges in the nonseizure psychiatric patient may indicate an elevated risk for iatrogenic seizures after treatment with neuroleptic medication (Fig. 1.14–21).

Findings with Structural Lesions Structural and space-occupying lesions are typically associated with focal slowing in the EEG (Fig. 1.14–17). The magnitude of the slowing may correspond to the extent of the pathology. When the lesion is also irritating to surrounding tissue, the focal slowing may be accompanied by focal spike activity as well. In this respect, a cerebral abscess is space occupying and highly irritating and can produce the most dramatic EEG abnormality in terms of profound focal slowing and spiking. If the structural lesion is small or is located in deeper subcortical regions, it may remain invisible to scalp EEG. Sometimes, minor focal slowing, often in temporal regions, without any clinical expressivity is found in the routine EEG. However, it should be recognized that a large neoplasm generating marked focal slowing must have started out earlier as a small lesion producing only minor focal EEG effects. For this reason, it would be a wise precaution in cases of minor focal slowing to repeat the EEG after a reasonable period of time. An increase in the magnitude of focal slowing on the repeat exam might suggest a growing or expanding lesion. Newer scanning techniques have largely supplanted the EEG as a first line assessment tool for space-occupying lesions. Nonetheless, it should be noted that 90 percent of cortical brain tumors can be detected and localized on the scalp with routine EEG.

Findings with Closed Head Injuries Focal slowing is the expected EEG sequela of sharply focal head trauma, and it may appear over the site of the trauma or over a contracoup location. The EEG change may be relatively transient with resolution over days or weeks, or it may persist for extended periods of time. If a gradual appearance of focal spiking occurs, it may herald the subsequent onset of a posttraumatic seizure disorder. Subdural hematomas after head injury may present with focal delta slowing or more widespread slowing, and, on occasion, a primary finding may consist of amplitude asymmetry of waking intrinsic EEG frequencies with the voltage decreased over the site of the subdural. In psychiatry, alcoholics, in particular, may be susceptible to closed head injury during bouts of intoxication.

Topographic QEEG may be especially useful in the assessment of the closed head injury patient. Numerous studies by Robert Thatcher and his colleagues, as well as others, have shown that there are characteristic QEEG findings that are frequently associated with the postconcussion syndromes after mild to moderate closed head trauma. Often, these QEEG changes involve a combination of increased theta power, decreased alpha power, and decreases in coherence, and serial changes in these measures over time may reflect the clinical course and recovery process. Topographic QEEG is also useful in cases of closed head trauma, because the quantification process can sometimes identify and document sharply focal or regional alterations in intrinsic analog EEG activity that are just below the threshold of resolution with visual inspection of the EEG tracing yet represent statistically significant deviations from normative database means (Fig. 1.14–22). When sharply focal QEEG findings correlate precisely with the locus of the trauma on the scalp, the presumption that neuronal injury has occurred can be compelling.

Findings with Infectious Disorders Most infectious disorders involving the brain produce EEG abnormalities. The existence of diffuse, often hypersynchronous, high-voltage slowing is, for all practical purposes, a universal finding during the acute phase of encephalitis, and similar diffuse slowing is usually present in early meningitis as well. This type of finding gradually

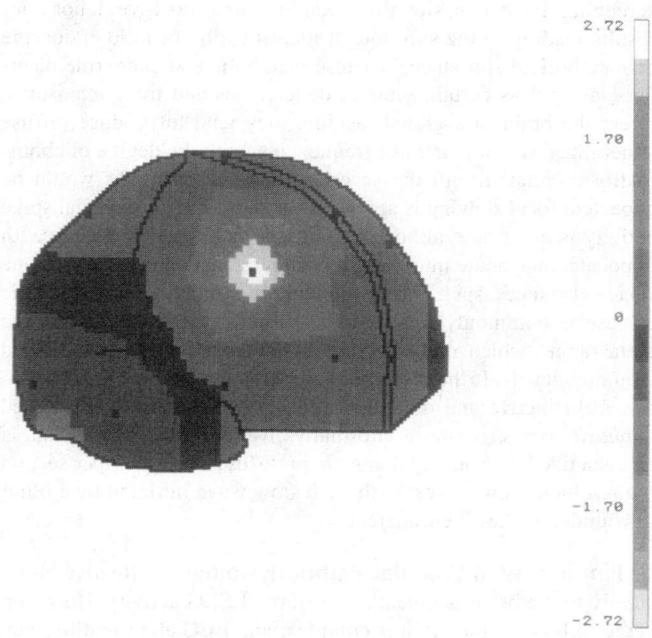

FIGURE 1.14–22 Topographic quantitative electroencephalography map of theta absolute power (*z* score departures from normative database mean). Closed head injury, male patient, 24 years of age. Focus of increased theta voltage is at the locus of an earlier head injury that occurred approximately 2 years before the recording. This was an unexpected finding. After recording and quantification, the color bar scale was adjusted to maximize the bull's-eye localization effect. Theta voltage was also elevated to a lesser extent over a wide, right frontal area and even spread somewhat across the midline. Theta relative power (not shown) was also elevated over the right frontal region, but mapping did not produce a sharp relative power focus at the locus of injury. Important note: A sharply defined bull's-eye can also be produced by artifact from a faulty electrode, and it is imperative to monitor electrical impedance and to check the integrity of the electrode in the event that deviant activity appears confined to only one lead with no spread to adjoining electrodes. (See Color Plate.)

resolves over time with recovery, and the EEG may return to normal. Focal slow wave findings may be superimposed on this picture if focal neurological symptoms are present. Not uncommonly, the magnitude of EEG abnormality is greater with children than with adults. Postencephalitic EEG or symptomatic sequelae, or both, are always possible, of course, and, if focal or diffuse EEG spiking should emerge during or after resolution of generalized slowing, a subsequent postencephalitic seizure disorder may develop. Regrettably, a brief synopsis cannot do justice to the complexities of EEG manifestations of all CNS infectious processes. A wide variety of electroencephalographic features, some highly unique with differential diagnostic implications, are found with Creutzfeldt-Jakob disease, subacute sclerosing panencephalitis, neurosyphilis, herpes simplex encephalitis, Sydenham's chorea, Reye's syndrome, and neuro-Behçet's syndrome, to name a few. These are discussed in depth in specialty reference sources (see the 1993 article by Niedermeyer and Lopes da Silva).

Findings with Metabolic and Endocrine Disorders

EEG is not a tool that one would use in assessing endocrine or metabolic disorders. Yet the majority of these conditions alter the EEG, and unexpected abnormal findings during routine EEG screening have occasionally been the first positive laboratory results leading to the subsequent identification of mild endocrine or metabolic disturbance. Because metabolic and endocrine disorders, as well as certain vitamin deficiencies and toxic exposures, affect the brain in a global fashion, they tend to produce diffuse generalized slowing of wake frequencies, with the degree of abnormality correlated with the severity of the disorder. As would be expected, focal slowing is almost never seen, and paroxysmal spike activity is quite rare, although spike activity may be possible with hypocalcemia, acute intermittent porphyria, and exposures to some toxic substances, such as lead and carbon monoxide. Early hepatic disease is commonly associated with generalized slowing in the theta range, which may increase in severity with elevated blood ammonia levels. If the disorder progresses to hepatic encephalopathy, a distinctive and diagnostically relevant EEG pattern, called *triphasic waves* (or, more informally, *liver waves*), emerges that is characterized by frontally dominant or diffuse 1.5- to 3.0-per-second high-voltage slow waves, with each slow wave initiated by a blunt or rounded spike-like transient.

Findings with Vascular Pathophysiology Effective blood supply to the brain is essential for normal EEG activity. However, cerebral blood circulation is complex, and EEG abnormalities can be focal, regional, or generalized, depending on the particular vascular pathology present, and the degree of EEG abnormality can range from minor to extreme. The EEG of the older person with diffuse cerebral arteriosclerosis usually shows a slowed alpha frequency and an increase in generalized theta slowing, particularly if mild cognitive changes have been detected. A frontally dominant EEG slowing in the theta-delta range, termed *anterior bradyrhythmia*, may appear with worsening diffuse cerebrovascular disorder. To the disappointment of many, EEG findings in transient ischemic attacks are highly variable, with normal EEGs being not unusual, thus limiting the diagnostic usefulness of this test for these events. In contrast, CVAs can produce profound EEG abnormality consisting of marked focal or regional delta activity, with the degree of EEG abnormality bearing a rough correspondence to the severity of the clinical event.

CLINICAL FINDINGS (EEG IN PSYCHIATRIC DISORDERS)

Given that the fourth revised edition of the *Diagnostic and Statistical Manual of Mental Disorders* (DSM-IV-TR) requires the exclusion of general medical conditions as being responsible for the presenting behavioral changes, attention to possible medical problems is essential. However, beyond the exclusion of certain general medical conditions, the routine EEG has a limited role in the diagnosis of most axis I or axis II disorders, and it provides little in the way of differentiating major depression from bipolar disorder or any of the schizophrenia spectrum disorders. However, it should also be noted that a rather voluminous literature exists in which the EEGs of variably well-characterized groups of psychiatric patients were examined, and, in almost all of the studies, the rates of EEG abnormalities tended to be higher in patient than in nonpatient populations. This is particularly true for a group of controversial waveforms, which are discussed in a special section that follows. For a more detailed account of the various specific types of EEG abnormalities reported in different psychiatric disorders, the reader is referred to the excellent 1993 review by Joyce Small. Despite the many incidence studies performed, it should be noted that research focused on identifying the clinical meaning of these various EEG abnormalities and their diagnostic and prognostic value in a psychiatric context has been largely lacking. Furthermore, the small amount of research that does address this area was performed in the 1950s and 1960s, well before the advent of more sophisticated and restrictive diagnostic criteria and standardized diagnostic scales. Also, the research that was done suffered from the lack of ability for factor analysis of symptom clusters, lack of other diagnostic technology, such as MRI, and the ability to quantify EEG data collected from large numbers of electrodes.

The previously stated comments are not applicable to the rapidly advancing field of topographic quantified EEG. In subjects with psychiatric disorders, high sensitivity and specificity of quantifiable EEG profiles, as well as evoked response deviations, are being reported across numerous studies, and an excellent in-depth review of this literature has been recently provided by John R. Hughes and Erwin R. John. Although, by and large, QEEG remains a research tool, its promise for aiding the differential diagnostic process and predicting treatment response to pharmacological agents is evident.

The standard routine EEG can be most useful when the presenting symptoms, age of first symptom onset, or response to treatment is atypical, suggesting that a more structural cerebral pathology may be contributing to the syndrome being evaluated. In such cases, the presence of paroxysmal EEG activity or focal or diffuse slowing should be ruled out (see the example in Figure 1.14–23). If paroxysmal activity is identified, it is important to be clear that such an EEG finding is not sufficient grounds to diagnose epilepsy, unless, retrospectively, the symptoms can be seen as being of an epileptic nature. The presence of a paroxysmal EEG abnormality in a patient who has presented with an atypical presentation, particularly in the absence of a family history of the diagnosis that is being considered, should lead the clinician to be wary of and less confident in the diagnosis. It may be a good practice at this state of knowledge of the significance of such findings to take advantage of the *not otherwise specified* category. Whether anticonvulsants are indicated in these situations remains an open research question, and only a limited number of studies addressing this important question have been conducted. Monroe was an early pioneer in this area, and he demonstrated that anticonvulsants can sometimes block electroencephalographic epileptiform discharges and can also lead to dramatic clinical improvement in individuals exhibiting repeated and frequent aggressive behavior. Other reports tend to confirm the possibility that carbamazepine (Tegretol) may be clinically useful in schizophrenics with temporal lobe EEG findings, but no history of seizure disorder, who show aggressive tendencies. On the other hand, other studies suggest that anticonvulsant therapy may have a beneficial effect on aggressive tendencies irrespective of the presence or absence of EEG abnormalities. Until definitive studies are performed, patients should be given the benefit of the doubt, and a trial of anticonvulsant should be offered when an EEG proves to be abnormal, particularly if it is focally and paroxysmally abnormal.

Similar comments can be made regarding the presence of a focal slow wave abnormality in the EEG. A minimal focal slow wave abnormality is unlikely to reflect a serious space-occupying lesion in a patient with a normal neurological examination. However, if no logical explanation for the minor focal slowing is apparent (e.g., old head injury), and the finding did not appear on earlier EEGs, a repeat EEG at some future date may be valuable to document that the finding is static and is not increasing in magnitude. Clinicians should use their clinical judgment regarding when imaging (and what imaging) should be performed. If a space-occupying

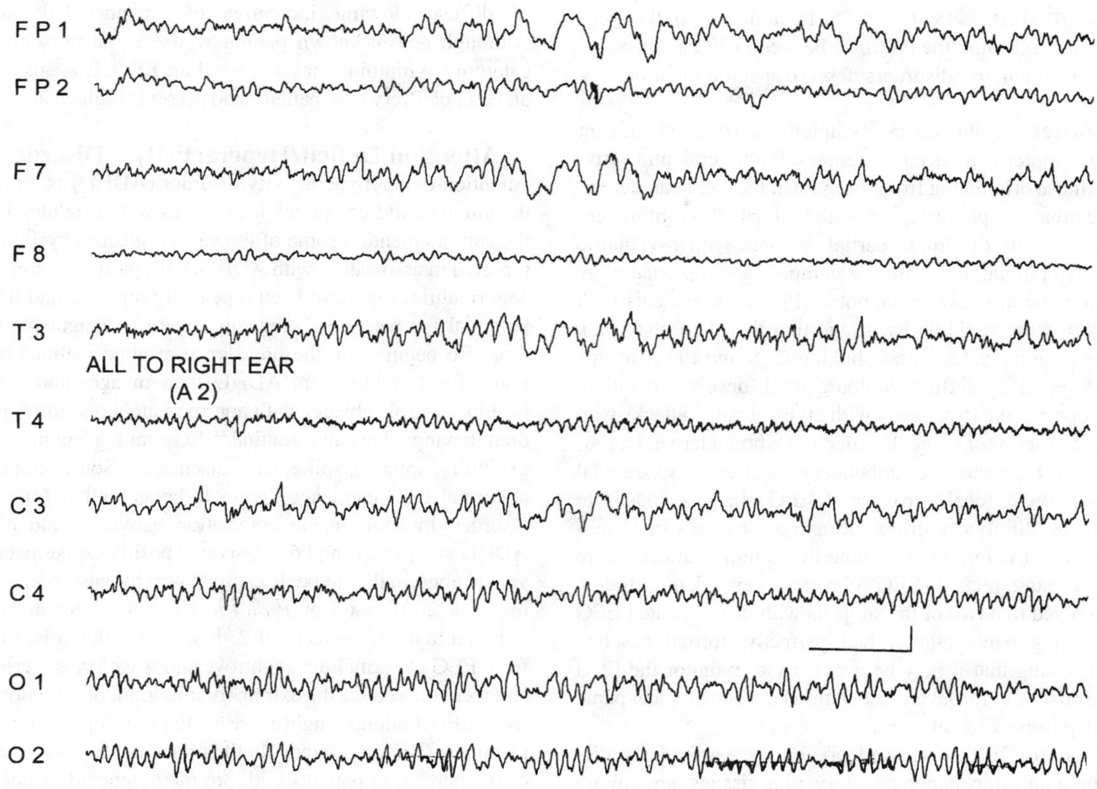

FIGURE 1.14–23 Single female patient, 40 years of age. Admitted to psychiatry for "functional" anorexia nervosa. First episode with no prior psychiatric history. Patient would frequently vomit after meals and insisted that it was not self-induced. Medical examination before admission was negative. Routine admission electroencephalography: focal slowing (delta), left frontal-temporal with reduced voltage spread through left hemisphere. Left frontal-temporal deep neoplasm found. Neurosurgical intervention was unsuccessful.

lesion is suspected, a CT scan is usually sufficient. An MRI is more likely to yield abnormalities if the nature of the lesion is likely to be less dramatic (e.g., old head injury). The presence of a focal slow abnormality, similar to the presence of paroxysmal activity, should cause the clinician to be wary of the diagnosis. Consideration should also be given to obtaining a neuropsychological evaluation to assess whether the focal cerebral abnormality identified by the EEG has any clinically correlating deficits.

The situation is different when an EEG is obtained in the course of managing an unstable or nonresponsive patient. The most important data to be gained from an EEG performed on an acutely agitated patient are the presence of diffuse slowing (indicating a delirious encephalopathic state) or ongoing epileptic activity (nonconvulsive status epilepticus). In both conditions, the EEG abnormality is fairly obvious, and patients can be restrained temporarily, and electrode caps can be used, thus minimizing the time during which a patient's mobility is restricted. The EEG can be extremely useful in ruling out delirium secondary to medication toxicity, and, in this respect, it should be noted that diffuse EEG slowing (suggestive of a diffuse encephalopathic process) may be seen despite serum plasma levels within the therapeutic range. When dealing with geriatric populations, sensitivity to organic pathology should be particularly heightened. In addition to the evaluation for dementia and delirium, EEG could be invaluable when there is a suspicion of seizures, and, in this respect, it is noted that elderly patients may account for as many as one-fourth of the cases of new onset epilepsy. One must also keep in mind that a normal EEG in a patient diagnosed with dementia that is advanced passed a mild stage should raise the suspicion that a depressive disorder may be contributing to the clinical picture.

A summary of the "red flags" that may alert the psychiatrist to the possibility of the presence of covert medical or organic factors causing or contributing to the psychiatric presentation is given in Table 1.14–1.

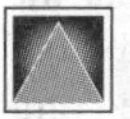

Table 1.14–1
Warning Signs of the Presence of Covert Medical or Organic Factors Causing or Contributing to Psychiatric Presentation

Atypical age of onset (i.e., anorexia nervosa beginning at mid-adulthood [Figure 1.14–23])
Complete lack of positive family history of the disorder when a positive family history is expected
Any focal or localized symptoms (i.e., unilateral hallucinations)
Focal neurological abnormalities
Catatonia
Presence of any difficulty with orientation or memory (in general, Mini-Mental State Examination should be normal)
Atypical response to treatment
Atypical clinical course

Note: Clinicians should have a high index of suspicion for suspecting underlying medical conditions and a low threshold for initiating appropriate workups.

Specific Psychiatric Disorders

In addition to the general considerations regarding the interface between EEG and psychiatry, a number of psychiatric disorders deserve specific mention.

Panic Disorder

Panic attack symptoms carry a significant resemblance to symptoms induced by temporolimbic epileptic activity, particularly those originating from the sylvian fissure. Fear, derealization, tachycardia, diaphoresis, and abdominal discomfort are characteristic symptoms of simple partial seizures with psychiatric and autonomic symptomatology. Studies comparing symptomatology of patients with panic disorder agoraphobia (PDA) and patients with CPSs have reported much similarity, suggesting that there may be a common neurophysiological substrate linking CPS and PDA. In this respect, a 1995 report by Jeffrey Weilburg et al. deserves mention. These authors reported on 15 subjects with atypical panic attacks who met DSM-III-TR criteria for panic disorder and who underwent a routine EEG followed by prolonged ambulatory EEG using sphenoidal electrodes. They found focal paroxysmal EEG changes consistent with partial seizure activity occurring during a panic attack in 33 percent of the patients. It is important to note that multiple attacks were recorded before panic-related EEG changes were demonstrated. Moreover, they noted that two of the subjects with demonstrated EEG abnormalities during panic attacks had perfectly normal baseline EEGs, thus suggesting that it may be necessary to monitor the EEG during multiple attacks to reveal an association between atypical panic attacks and epileptiform EEG changes.

The limitations of EEG discussed previously, particularly distance from source and impedance of intervening tissues, are among the reasons why it has been difficult to establish a relationship between some forms of panic attack and seizure activity.

In a different vein, a number of reports provide evidence that EEG abnormalities are not infrequent in panic disorder patients. However, the specific EEG findings differ from study to study and range from paroxysmal epileptiform discharges to asymmetrical increases in slow wave activity. Focal slow wave abnormalities are also detected in as much as 25 percent of this population. The fact that reports of EEG abnormalities in panic disorder patients continue to appear in the literature indicates the need for a detailed workup of every panic disorder patient. This is reinforced by reports that some of these patients may respond well to valproic acid (Depakene) therapy.

Panic attacks have also been demonstrated to occur more frequently in epileptic patients. In some cases, these attacks could lead to overmedication for seizures if their nature is not precisely defined. Again, EEG monitoring during multiple attacks is indispensable in rendering such an evaluation. Other reports have concluded that the most common psychiatric disorder that must be differentiated from temporal lobe epilepsy is panic disorder. Epileptic seizures are commonly briefer and more stereotyped than panic attacks. Additionally, aphasia and dysmnesia often accompany seizure activity.

Finally, topographic QEEG promises a further refinement of the usefulness of EEG in detecting abnormalities in panic disorder, as well as improvements in defining the diagnostic accuracy overall. In 1991, Henry Abraham and Frank Duffy were able to use QEEG methods to differentiate between panic patients and control subjects with 92.5 percent accuracy.

Catatonia

Although the routine EEGs of catatonic patients with known functional etiology tend to be normal, catatonia could be a symptom of a number of serious medical conditions, including epilepsy and encephalopathy secondary to a variety of general medical conditions. Neuroleptic malignant syndrome has presented, at times, as catatonia, and, in such cases, the EEG is likely to show a picture of diffuse slowing indicative of an encephalopathic process. Although a well-known patient whose usual presentation includes catatonic symptoms may not need an EEG, it is advisable to obtain an EEG on every new patient who presents with catatonic symptoms.

Attention-Deficit/Hyperactivity Disorder (ADHD)

Attention-deficit/hyperactivity disorder (ADHD) is a prevalent disorder among children and adolescents, as well as adults. In this section, the authors mention some of the various electrophysiological findings reported in association with ADHD, with particular emphasis on those abnormalities that have been repeatedly reported and thus have some potential for becoming clinically useful as diagnostic or prognostic tools. To begin with, the prevalence of abnormalities in the conventional EEG is higher in ADHD than in age- and gender-matched healthy control subjects, with approximately one-third of ADHD children having abnormal routine EEGs and a significant proportion exhibiting spike or spike-wave discharges. Some studies even report abnormal EEG incidence figures to be as high as 60 percent for this disorder. In addition, an association between child and adolescent ADHD and the 14- and 6-per-second positive spike pattern (a controversial abnormality to be discussed later) has also been reported. Writing in a 2001 issue of *Pediatric Neurology*, Sarah Hemmer et al. reported that 15.4 percent of 234 ADHD children had frank epileptiform EEG abnormalities (controversial waveforms were not included) and went on to offer the extremely important observation that epileptiform EEG findings might increase the risk for seizures with methylphenidate (Ritalin) therapy. In their data, there was a seizure incidence of 0.6 percent in patients with pre-methylphenidate normal EEGs, as contrasted with a 10 percent seizure incidence in patients with pre-methylphenidate epileptiform EEGs (an example of premedication seizure discharges in a patient developing iatrogenic grand mal seizures after neuroleptic treatment was given earlier in Figure 1.14–21).

Quantitative spectral analysis has demonstrated that increased theta activity, particularly in the frontal lobe regions, is a rather promising QEEG finding in ADHD. Even when learning disability is removed as a confounding variable, increased theta remains as one of the most consistent EEG findings in this disorder, and this EEG association with ADHD has been replicated by a number of groups from different parts of the world. In addition to being a consistent finding, the theta increase seen in ADHD is resistant to age effects, whereas abnormalities of beta EEG frequency tend to decrease with age. It should also be noted that early work suggests that increased theta abnormality frontally may be a strong predictor of response to methylphenidate and other psychostimulants and that favorable clinical responses may be associated with a normalization of the EEG abnormality. Because decreased beta activity has sometimes been reported in ADHD, some investigators have tried to examine the theta to beta ratio as a stronger measure of ADHD-related EEG abnormality with a higher detection power. There are additional QEEG reports of an increase (instead of decrease) in beta activity in similar patients. However, whether or not a distinct subgroup of ADHD patients with increased beta activity exists must await further replication of this finding and the identification of clinical correlates, if any, for this EEG subcluster. As stated previously, QEEG methods hold a highly significant promise for developing increased specificity of EEG associations to psychiatric dysfunction. In regard to the present disorder, discriminant function analyses of QEEG data have been shown to be capable of significantly discriminating between normals, attention deficit disorder and ADHD, and learning disability subpopulations.

Antisocial Personality Disorder

Patients diagnosed with antisocial personality disorder also frequently harbor organic brain pathology that can be assessed with the help of EEG, along with other neuroevaluative tools. Within the antisocial personality diagnostic category, aggressive or even violent behavior is often of clinical concern, and several reports suggest an increased incidence of EEG abnormality associated with significant aggressive behavior. Some of these studies report an increased hemispheric asymmetry (usually delta activity) for frontotemporal regions, and others report correlations between conventional EEG slow wave abnormality, as well as CT scan abnormality, and the degree of symptomatic violence in incarcerated patients. Although the significance of these findings is yet to be fully explored, the presence of diffuse or focal slowing should lead to a complete neuropsychological evaluation. Additionally, the presence of paroxysmal EEG activity may indicate that an anticonvulsant regime may help decrease the frequency or severity of violent episodes.

Borderline Personality Disorder Standard EEG studies have been carried out based on the hypothesis that abnormal brain electrical activity or focal brain dysfunction, or both, particularly in the temporal lobes, plays a significant role in the pathogenesis of borderline personality disorder characterized by impulsiveness and affective instability. A number of case reports have described patients who were diagnosed with borderline personality disorder who were subsequently found to have CPSs documented by epileptic discharges over one or both temporal regions. As early as the mid-1980s, the presence of significant EEG abnormalities, definitive and less definitive, in borderline personality disorder patients was well documented. Furthermore, minor EEG abnormalities that are not suggestive of epilepsy but may be contributing to episodic behavior disorder (e.g., 14- and 6-per-second positive spikes) are seen in more than one-fourth of borderline personality disorder patients, as well as in some other personality disorders. In this latter respect, the presence of these controversial waveforms may be associated with elevations of specific behaviors (e.g., impulsivity) found within the overall borderline personality disorder symptom cluster profile.

Studies have also reported between a 40 and 80 percent incidence of generalized slowing of the intrinsic background activity in borderline personality disorder patients, with the lower incidence figures being derived from studies that exclude subjects with comorbid axis I disorders, current drug abuse, or known neurological problems.

In summary, two types of standard EEG abnormalities seem to be observable in some borderline personality disorder patients. The first is the presence of epileptiform discharges. This type of abnormality is likely to indicate a decreased threshold for seizure activity or cortical excitability and may be predictive of responsiveness to anticonvulsant therapy. The second type of standard EEG abnormality is the presence of diffuse EEG slowing. If significant diffuse slowing (not just minor alteration of background alpha activity) is present in the unmedicated subject, it may indicate the presence of a metabolic or a degenerative brain disorder or mental retardation. The presence of this EEG abnormality should prompt further workup of the patient in an effort to identify causes of possible encephalopathy. The presence of static-(nonprogressive), nonmetabolic-, and nonencephalopathic-based diffuse EEG slowing could be indicative of a more difficult group of borderline personality disorder patients who are less likely to respond to pharmacotherapy.

Chronic Alcoholism Niedermeyer and his colleagues described a state of subacute encephalopathy with seizures in chronic alcoholic patients that is not related to withdrawal from alcohol. Lethargy, confusion, and neurological deficits, including seizures, usually accompany this condition. The EEG shows prominent slowing and periodic lateralized paroxysmal discharges. The occurrence of partial seizures should lead to full neurological workup including brain imaging.

Alcohol Withdrawal Alcohol withdrawal seizures need to be differentiated from seizures in epileptics who happen to be alcoholics. Routine EEG can be extremely helpful in this regard. A normal EEG during periods of sobriety, particularly if associated with an abnormal EEG during early withdrawal, strongly suggests that the seizures are withdrawal induced. It should be noted that the EEG tends to normalize faster (with the exception of generalized decrease in amplitude) during withdrawal from alcohol as compared to barbiturates.

The differential diagnosis of acutely disturbed and disorganized patients often includes delirium. In acutely agitated delirious patients, the EEG is often helpful in indicating whether the alteration in consciousness is due to (1) a diffuse encephalopathic process, (2) a focal brain lesion, or (3) continued epileptic activity without motor manifestations. Most often, patients with delirium have a toxic-metabolic encephalopathy. In general, with the progression of the encephalopathy, there is diffuse slowing of the background rhythms from alpha (8 to 13 Hz) to theta (4.0 to 7.5 Hz) activity. Delta activity (<3.5 Hz) usually does not become prominent until the patient approaches nonresponsiveness. The major exception to this rule is seen during withdrawal from alcohol and during delirium tremens. Instead of diffuse slowing, as described previously, excessive fast activity dominates the EEG in patients with alcohol withdrawal delirium. Patients in alcohol withdrawal who are not delirious could have a normal EEG. Low-voltage fast activity can also be induced by benzodiazepines, and this should be borne in mind when interpreting the EEG. The EEG thus can be helpful in differentiating between alcohol withdrawal delirium tremens and encephalopathies from other causes, including iatrogenic encephalopathy.

Dementia Because patients with advanced dementia rarely have a normal EEG, a normal electroencephalogram can play an important role in diagnosing cases of pseudodementia (symptoms of dementia secondary to depression or psychosis). When dementia and depression coexist, it becomes important to have some idea about the relative contribution of each disorder to the overall clinical presentation. In a comparison of the EEGs of patients with depression, dementia, pseudodementia, and dementia plus depression with the EEGs of normal age-matched controls, the degree of EEG abnormality shows a significant inverse association with clinical response to antidepressants.

The routine EEG is also useful in following the progression of Alzheimer's disease. On the other hand, patients with frontopolar dementia may have normal routine EEGs, despite the progressive behavioral deterioration that they exhibit.

CONTROVERSIAL SHARP WAVES OR SPIKE PATTERNS

Early in the emergence of clinical EEG, a considerable amount of heated controversy developed around the clinical significance of certain sharp wave or spike patterns that were easily identified in the EEG tracing. These so-called controversial patterns deserve a specific mention here, because they have been consistently observed in numerous studies to be more prevalent in psychiatric populations than healthy or nonpsychiatric patient control populations. Despite the increased prevalence in psychiatric patients, defining the clinical and neurobiological correlates of these patterns has proved to be an elusive goal. The task is made difficult because none of these patterns are specific for a diagnostic category, and none predictably correlate with seizure disorders. Because the physiological or pathological correlates of these patterns have not been well studied using currently available improved methodologies and assessment

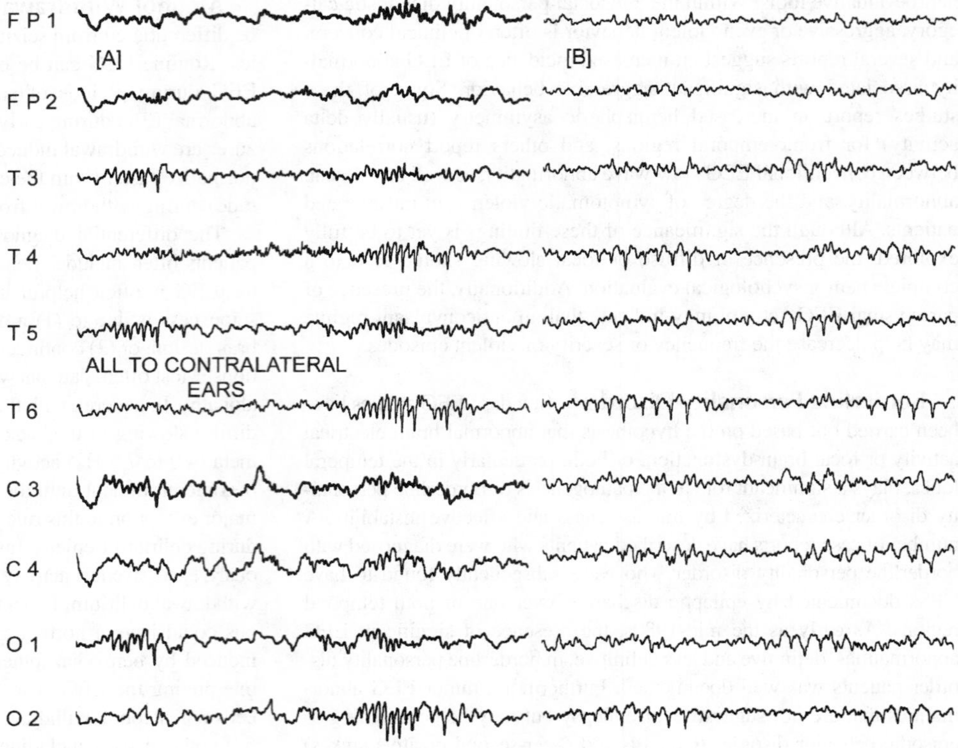

FIGURE 1.14–24 Fourteen- and six-per-second positive spikes, independent left and right mid-temporal-posterior temporal-occipital. **A:** Fourteen-per-second variety; female patient, 13 years of age. **B:** Six-per-second variety; male patient, 24 years of age. An electroencephalograph may contain either variety alone or both combined.

techniques, the assertion that they are irrelevant to neuropsychiatric conditions is not fully supportable. At a minimum, the appearance of such patterns may give support to the possible organic nature of presenting symptoms. This assertion may strengthen the alliance between the patient and the psychiatrist, as compared to the assumption that the patient is in control of his or her symptoms, which tends to put the patient and the psychiatrist at opposite sides of the therapeutic effort. Whether these patterns predict a favorable response to anticonvulsant treatment is not known and awaits well-designed controlled studies. Until such time, patients harboring one of these patterns should be given the benefit of the doubt and allowed a trial of anticonvulsant treatment. The reader should note that each of these four patterns has two different labels. One label is usually used by those who ascribe clinical significance to the pattern (i.e., *small sharp spikes* [SSSs]) and the other is used by those who consider these patterns to be normal variants (i.e., *benign epileptiform transients of sleep* [BETS]). Labels given in parentheses in the following section are the ones used by those who reject the potential clinical significance of the patterns.

Fourteen- and Six-per-Second Positive Spikes (Ctenoids) Since its description by Fred and Erna Gibbs 50 years ago, the 14 and 6 positive spike pattern (hereafter called *PS*) has become the most frequently encountered of the controversial waveforms and the one with the most extensive literature (Fig. 1.14–24). For reasons that are unclear, the controversy over this pattern has continued despite excellent reviews by Charles Henry in 1963 and Hughes in 1983, as well as several later studies, pointing to areas of potential clinical relevance for this EEG finding. Unfortunately, major EEG reference works describe the PS pattern as irrelevant or normal.

The accumulated PS literature is too voluminous for a comprehensive review in this space. To avoid listing numerous specific citations, the highlights regarding this pattern (and the three that follow) are derived from and discussed more fully in the recent 2002 paper by Boutros and Struve. Nearly everyone agrees that this pattern is highly age related. It is rarely encountered in the very young. During childhood, it gradually increases in incidence to a peak prevalence in adolescence, after which the pattern then becomes increasingly rare throughout adulthood, with a 1.3 percent prevalence at 25 years of age and a 0 percent prevalence at 40 years of age. Because of the rarity of PS in normal adults, it may be easier to demonstrate associations between this pattern and clinical phenomenon by studying older people—a research strategy that has seldom been used. Investigators using this strategy compared the incidence of PS in the routine wake and sleep EEGs of 2,888 consecutively admitted psychiatric patients 20 years of age and older and found the elevated incidence of PS among adult psychiatric admissions compared to the adult normal control population to be overwhelmingly significant at all age categories. Others have found that 85 percent of a sample of 460 adults with PS complained of neurovegetative or psychiatric symptoms.

PS discharges are presumed to originate in subcortical regions, with thalamic or hypothalamic regions frequently being implicated, and this observation may be of potential relevance to some of the symptoms attributed to this dysrhythmia. The presumed subcortical locus has been supported by results from a small number of brain tumor location and depth electrode recordings from patients who display this pattern. In a 1972 paper, O. Andy and M. Jurko used neurosurgical depth electrode recording methods to provide clear evidence of a phase reversal (a localizing method used in EEG; Fig. 1.14–7) of PS activity occurring within the thalamus. The patient complained of severe visceral and pain symp-

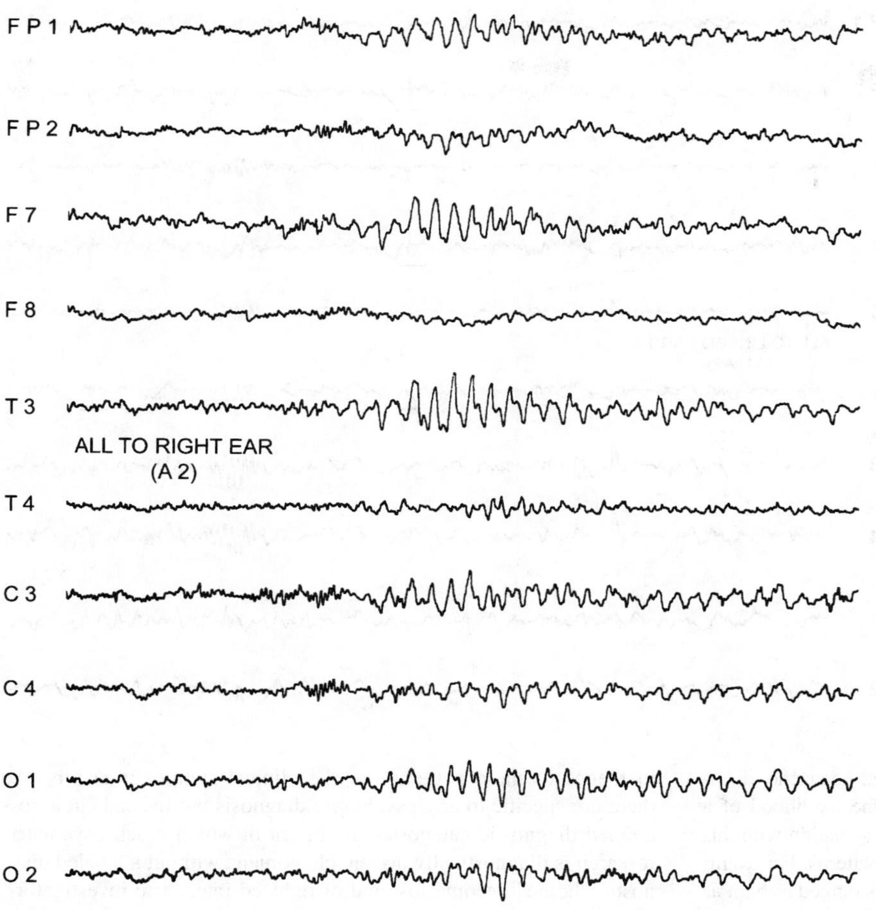

FIGURE 1.14–25 Rhythmic mid-temporal discharges (psychomotor variant) during drowsy recording. Left mid-temporal focus. Male patient, 20 years of age. Episodic temper dyscontrol, frequent intense homicidal urges, paresthesias, headaches, abdominal pain, suicide plans (as a way of avoiding acting on strong homicidal impulses). Patient responded well to phenytoin (Dilantin) therapy.

toms, and the PS discharges and the symptoms were no longer present.

The presumed causes of the PS pattern range from sequelae of encephalitis to closed head trauma, but, often, no plausible etiological cause can be found. A small literature argues for genetic factors playing a role. Support for head trauma constituting at least one etiological cause emerged when a large sample of 2,000 head injury cases collected by Fred Gibbs was subjected to rigorous statistical analyses by other investigators. It was shown that PS incidence increased significantly (while normal EEG incidence decreased) as the severity of skull fractures increased from linear to depressed to basal. The incidence of PS also significantly increased (while normal EEGs decreased) as the severity of immediate posttraumatic states increased from conscious to dazed to unconscious. Furthermore, postinjury symptom presence (e.g., headache, temper dyscontrol, nausea, and many others) was always significantly associated with the PS pattern, as contrasted with normal postinjury EEGs.

Previous reviews and a large number of anecdotal clinical reports suggest that PS may be associated with discrete symptoms that cut across psychiatric diagnostic boundaries and can be found in people with almost any condition, or for that matter, no psychiatric diagnosis at all. When all of the available literature is reviewed, PS symptoms appear to cluster into two categories. The first symptom cluster includes a variety of physiological or autonomic symptoms, or both, such as headache, stomachache, nausea, flushing, spells of dizziness, and paresthesias, with headache being the most common, followed by abdominal symptoms. The second grouping includes temper dyscontrol and related phenomena, such as irritability and emotional lability. It is important to recognize that symptoms of PS may range in severity from being mildly expressed, in which case they may cause the individual little difficulty, to being so strongly expressed that they form the basis for clinical complaint.

Rhythmic Mid-Temporal Discharges (RMTDs [Psychomotor Variant]) One-third to one-half of subjects exhibiting rhythmic mid-temporal discharges (RMTDs) were found to have psychiatric problems, particularly symptoms of anxiety. RMTDs (Fig. 1.14–25) have also been associated with increased somatization. Earlier studies reported an increased incidence of seizures in patients with RMTD, but the association of this pattern with ictal phenomena remains controversial. Although there have been several efforts to link this EEG dysrhythmia with behavioral symptoms, such as temper dyscontrol, personality disorder, or autonomic phenomena, other studies have not been able to demonstrate such associations. There have been rare documented cases of RMTD status epilepticus associated with prolonged periods of confusion.

Small Sharp Spikes (SSS) (Benign Epileptiform Transients of Sleep [BETS]) The SSS pattern consists of rather low-voltage sharp negative or biphasic spikes that are best seen over the frontal-temporal cortex, sometimes alternating between the left and right hemisphere (Fig. 1.14–26). They have also been associated

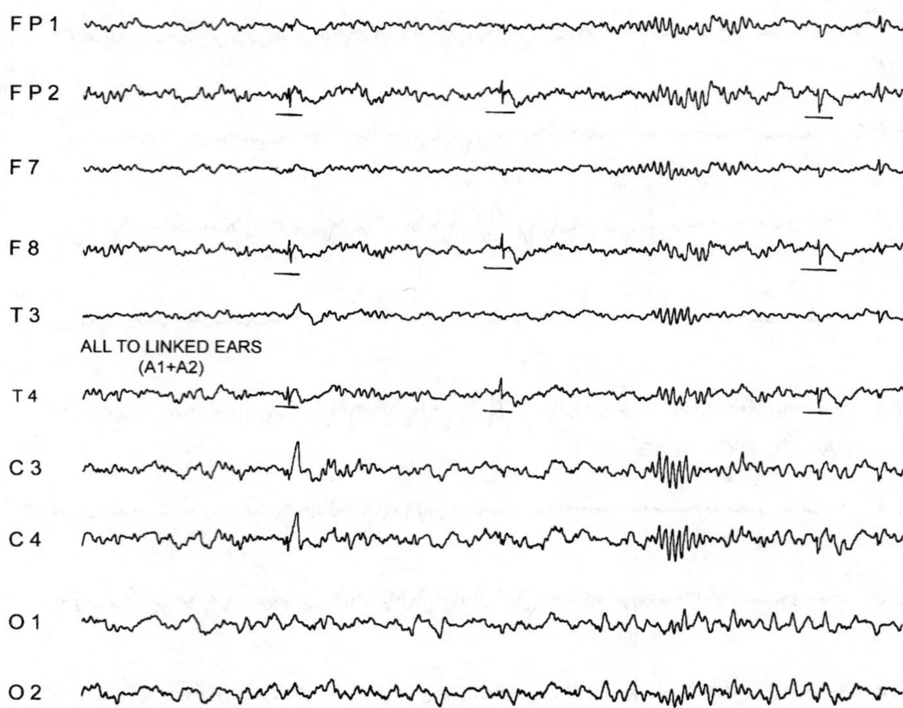

FIGURE 1.14–26 Small sharp spikes (underlined), right frontotemporal during spindle sleep. Female patient, 24 years of age. History was negative for head trauma, encephalitis, or seizures. Psychiatric diagnosis: major depression. Patient also complained of headaches and infrequent paresthesias.

with the presence of neurovegetative symptoms (i.e., headache, dizziness, and episodic abdominal pain). Furthermore, the likelihood of a patient experiencing epileptic seizures is higher in association with this pattern as compared to the other three controversial patterns. For example, the incidence of seizures in patients with SSS has ranged as high as 53 percent and even 67.4 percent, thus stressing the moderate degree of epileptogenicity of this pattern. Small and her colleagues have studied the SSS pattern within psychiatric patient populations and reported an association between this pattern and depressive symptoms. However, the view that this controversial pattern has potential clinical relevance has not always been universally shared.

Six-per-Second Spike and Wave (Phantom Waves)

Finally, the six-per-second spike and wave pattern (also called *spike-wave phantom*) is often difficult to recognize, because the discharges tend to be low in amplitude (Fig. 1.14–27). Like other controversial waveforms, they have been correlated with increased impulsivity and neurovegetative symptoms, as well as elevated scores on the Minnesota Multiphasic Personality Inventory (MMPI) hysteria scale. The prevalence of this pattern among psychiatric patients varies widely, with a range extending from a low of 1.5 percent to a high of approximately 20 percent.

The recent advances in the ability to localize neural source generators of activity recorded on the scalp can be illuminating, once the clinical correlates of these controversial patterns are elucidated more clearly. Further probing into the clinical correlates of these EEG patterns can also be facilitated by recent developments in standardized psychiatric rating scales and methods of investigating symptom clusters in psychiatric populations. For reasons that are unclear, basic clinical and empirical research focused on the relevance of the four controversial EEG patterns described previously has declined since the mid 1970s and now seems to be nearly abandoned. It should be noted that many early negative studies contained recognizable methodological flaws that could be corrected with further study. One possible contributing factor for the declining interest is that neither the incidence of these patterns nor the clinical symptoms ascribed to them are specific to any psychiatric diagnosis but instead cut across defined diagnostic categories. In an era in which much psychiatric research is diagnostically driven, phenomena without a labeled diagnostic "home" become lost and of reduced interest to investigators. This neglect is unfortunate, because much of the past work appears to point strongly to several clinically relevant symptomatic correlates that stand a good chance of being substantiated if subjected to additional methodologically sound, well-controlled investigations.

EEG: CLINICAL PSYCHIATRY FLOW CHART

There is little doubt that the field of EEG, including what may seem to be complex and esoteric technical aspects, myriad clinical and research applications from historical times to the present (and future!), and controversies still unresolved, may appear formidable to those outside of the field. Because of this, EEG assessment may fall far short of being optimally used in psychiatric diagnoses and treatment. Apart from some of the obvious indications for an EEG study (i.e., suspected seizures), EEG is likely to be a valuable assessment tool in many clinical situations in which the initial presentation or the clinical course appear to be unusual or atypical—"red flags" suggesting the possible operation of organic pathophysiological variables (Table 1.14–1). The EEG flow chart presented in Figure 1.14–28 is prepared to illustrate some of the assessment strategies that may prove useful in evaluating the unusual or difficult patient presenting with atypical clinical features.

CEREBRAL EVOKED POTENTIALS

Cerebral evoked potentials (EPs) are a series of surface (scalp) recordable waves that result from brain stimulation (visual, auditory, somatosensory, and cognitive). These EPs are usually of small magnitude as compared to the ongoing EEG activity. When the stimuli are repeated, and the resulting EEG activities after each stimulus are

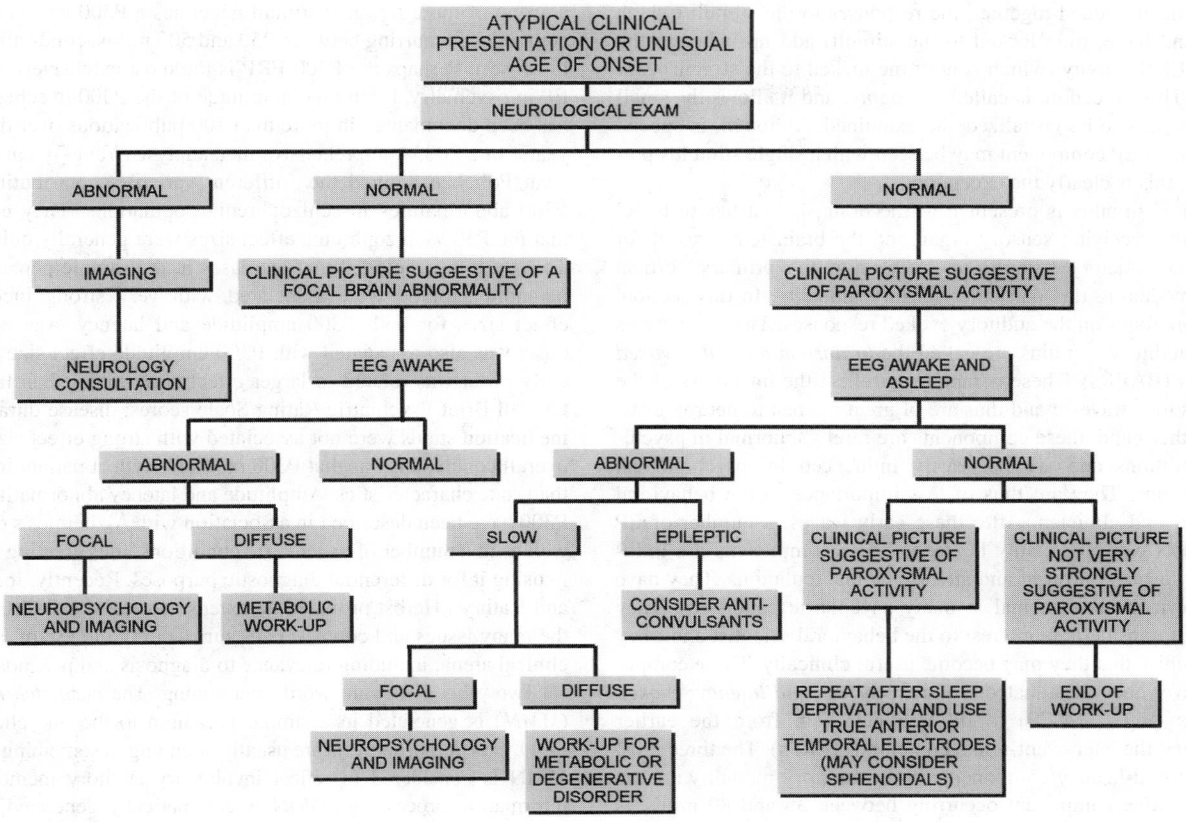

FIGURE 1.14–28 A flow chart for electroencephalography (EEG) evaluations in neuropsychiatric patients.

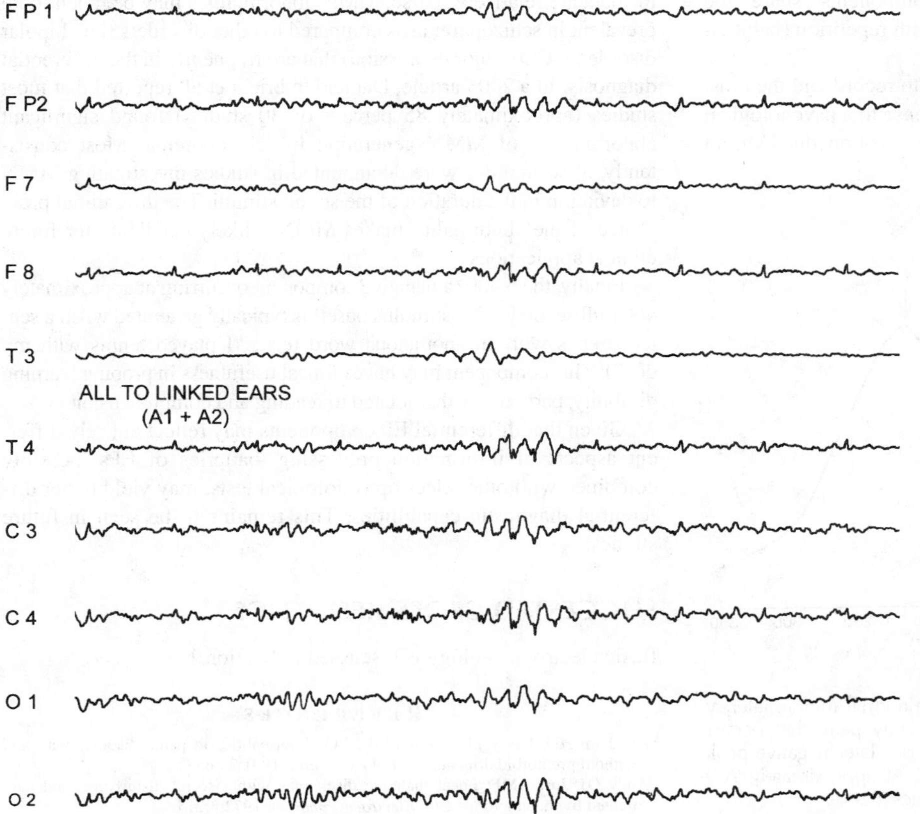

FIGURE 1.14–27 Six-per-second spike and wave (spike-wave phantom) during drowsy recording. Small electrocardiogram artifact present. Male patient, 24 years of age. Diagnosis: schizophrenia.

mathematically added together, the responses to the stimuli (which are, by and large, time locked to the stimuli) add up, whereas the ongoing EEG activity (which is not time locked to the stimuli) cancels out. This procedure is called *averaging*, and it allows the small magnitude EPs to be visualized and examined. Although, in special situations, an EP component may be seen with a single stimulus presentation, this is clearly the exception.

When a stimulus is presented to the brain, it first has to travel through the receiving sensory organ and the brainstem (except for visual and olfactory stimuli) on its way to the primary cortical regions mediating this particular sensory modality. In this section, the authors focus on the auditory evoked responses. The early waves after an auditory stimulus are called the *brainstem auditory evoked responses* (BAERs). These components reflect the intactness of the pathways they traverse and thus are of great interest to neurologists. On the other hand, these components are rarely abnormal in psychiatric conditions and are not easily influenced by psychological manipulations. They are thus of less importance to the behavioral researcher and clinician. After these early waves, a number of EP components can predictably be seen. These components are influenced by levels of arousal and attentional manipulations. They have been shown to be abnormal in many psychiatric conditions. They thus are of considerable interest to the behavioral scientist and carry some promise that they may become useful clinically. These components have been designated collectively as *mid-latency evoked responses* (Fig. 1.14–29) to differentiate them from the earlier BAERs and the later event-related potentials (ERPs). The three most examined mid-latency components in the auditory modality are the P50 (a positive component occurring between 35 and 80 milliseconds after stimulus onset), the N100 (a negative component occurring between 80 and 150 milliseconds after stimulus onset), and P200 (a positive component occurring between 150 and 250 milliseconds after stimulus onset). Figure 1.14–29 shows a typical example of these mid-latency EPs. These components share the characteristic that their amplitude decreases with repetition (habituation or sensory gating).

The ERPs are by far the most challenging to record and the most promising clinically. ERPs occur only in response to a psychological event. For example, the detection of a rare stimulus imbedded within a group of more frequent stimuli generates a P300 wave (a positive component occurring between 250 and 500 milliseconds after stimulus onset). Perhaps the P300 ERP is the most extensively examined EP in psychiatry. Decreased amplitude of the P300 in schizophrenia has been documented in more than 100 publications over the last 30 years. In a 2003 comprehensive metaanalysis, Yang-Whan Jeon and John Polich examined the different variables contributing to the P300 abnormalities in schizophrenia populations. They concluded that the P300/schizophrenia effect sizes were generally quite robust. They further concluded that increases in the sample percentages of paranoid subtype were associated with very strong increases in effect sizes for both P300 amplitude and latency. Age of disease onset was also associated with P300 amplitude effect size such that early onset was related to larger effect sizes rather than late onset. Overall Brief Psychiatric Rating Scale scores, disease duration, and medication status were not associated with strong effect sizes. Their overall conclusion was that P300 measures reflect patient trait rather than state characteristics. Amplitude and latency abnormalities of the P300 have been described in association with Alzheimer's disease as well as in a number of psychiatric conditions, thus creating difficulty in using it for differential diagnostic purposes. Recently, John Polich and Kathryn Herbst provided an extensive review and discussion of the many issues and controversies surrounding the use of EPs in the clinical arena, including relevance to diagnosis and prognosis.

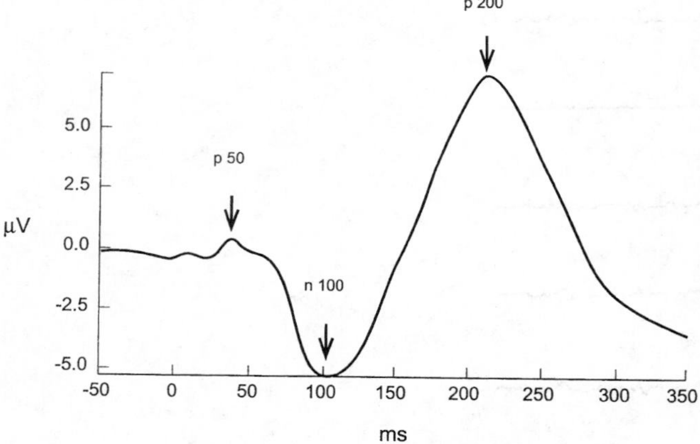

FIGURE 1.14–29 Waveform morphology of the normal middle latency auditory evoked potential. P50 is a positive polarity peak that occurs approximately 50 msec after the stimulus. N100 is a later negative peak seen approximately 100 msec after the stimulus. At approximately 200 msec after the stimulus, a large positive peak emerges (P200).

Two other ERPs are worth mentioning. The *mismatch negativity* (*MMN*) is generated in a similar paradigm to the one eliciting the P300, except that subjects are usually attending to something else. The MMN is considered to reflect involuntary auditory memory–based information processing. MMN is automatically generated when an incoming auditory stimulus deviates in some physical feature, such as frequency, duration, or intensity, from previous repeatedly presented standard stimuli. A comprehensive detailed presentation of the methodology can be found in the 1992 book by Risto Naatanen. Although the data are relatively sparse, MMN abnormalities may be much more prevalent in schizophrenia as compared to other disorders (i.e., bipolar disorder, OCD, major depression) that are frequently in the differential diagnosis. In a 2003 article, Daniel Umbricht et al. reported that most studies (approximately 85 percent of 30 studies) found significant abnormalities of MMN generation in schizophrenia. Most consistently, abnormalities were documented in studies investigating MMN to deviation in the duration of the sound stimuli. The differential prevalence of the abnormality makes MMN a likely candidate for future clinical applications.

Finally, the N400 (a negative component occurring at approximately 400 milliseconds after stimulus onset) is typically generated when a sentence ends with an anomalous word (e.g., "I played tennis with my dog"). This component may have clinical usefulness in probing learning disability, particularly that related to reading and comprehension.

Given that differential EP components may reflect entirely different aspects of information processing, batteries of EPs, possibly combined with other electrophysiological tests, may yield better differential diagnostic capabilities. This remains to be seen in future studies.

SUGGESTED CROSS-REFERENCE

Basic electrophysiology is discussed in Section 1.9.

REFERENCES

Abraham HD, Duffy FH: Computed EEG abnormalities in panic disorder with and without premorbid drug abuse. *Biol Psychiatry.* 1991;29:687.

Andy OJ, Jurko MF: Focal thalamic discharges with visceral disturbance and pain treated by thalamotomy. *Clin Electroencephalogr.* 1972;3:215.

Bauer LO. Electroencephalographic studies of substance use and abuse. In: Kaufman MJ, ed. *Brain Imaging in Substance Abuse.* Totowa, NJ: Humana Press; 2001.

Boutros NN: Diffuse electroencephalogram slowing in psychiatric patients: A preliminary report. *J Psychiatry Neurosci.* 1997;21:259.

Boutros NN, Mirolo HA, Struve FA: Normal analog EEG in neuropsychiatry. *J Neuropsychiatry Clin Neurosci.* Fall 2004 *(in press).*

*Boutros NN, Struve F: Electrophysiological assessment of neuropsychiatric disorders. *Sem Clin Neuropsychiatry.* 2002;7:30.

Centorrino F, Price BH, Tuttle M, Bahk W, Hennen J, Albert MJ, Baldessarini RJ: EEG abnormalities during treatment with typical and atypical antipsychotics. *Am J Psychiatry.* 2002;159:109.

Duffy FH, Iyer VG, Surwillo WW, eds. *Clinical Electroencephalography and Topographic Brain Mapping.* New York: Springer-Verlag; 1989.

Gibbs FA, Gibbs EL. *Atlas of Electroencephalography. Neurological and Psychiatric Disorders.* Vol 3. Reading, MA: Addison Wesley; 1964.

Gibbs FA, Gibbs EL: How much do sleep recordings contribute to the detection of seizure activity? *Clin Electroencephalogr.* 1971;2:169.

Gloor P, ed. *Hans Berger on the Electroencephalogram of Man.* Amsterdam: Elsevier Science; 1969.

Hanson ES, Prichep LS, Bolwig TG, John ER: Quantitative electroencephalography in OCD patients treated with Paroxetine. *Clin Electroencephalogr.* 2003;34:70.

Hemmer SA, Pasternak JF, Zecker SG, Trommer BL: Stimulant therapy and seizure risk in children with ADHD. *Pediatr Neurol.* 2001;24:99.

Henry CE: Positive spike discharges in the EEG and behavior abnormality. In: Glaser GH, ed. *EEG and Behavior.* New York: Basic Books; 1963.

Hughes JR: A review of the positive spike phenomenon: recent studies. In: Hughs JR, Wilson WP, eds. *EEG and Evoked Potentials in Psychiatry and Behavioral Neurology.* Boston: Butterworth-Heinemann; 1983.

Hughes JR: The EEG in psychiatry: An outline with summarized points and references. *Clin Electroencephalogr.* 1995;26:92.

*Hughes JR, John ER: Conventional and quantitative electroencephalography in psychiatry. *J Neuropsychiatry Clin Neurosci.* 1999;11:190.

*Hughes JR, Wilson WP. *EEG and Evoked Potentials in Psychiatry and Behavioral Neurology.* Boston: Butterworth-Heinemann; 1983.

Jacobsen T, Schroger E: Is there pre-attentive memory-based comparison of pitch? *Psychophysiology.* 2001;38:723.

John ER, Prichep LS. Principles of neurometrics and neurometric analysis of EEG and evoked potentials. In: Niedermeyer E, Lopes da Silva F, eds. *Electroencephalography: Basic Principles, Clinical Applications and Related Fields.* Baltimore: Williams & Wilkins; 1993.

*John ER, Prichep LS, Fridman J, Easton P: Neurometrics: Computer-assisted differential diagnosis of brain dysfunctions. *Science.* 1988;239:162.

Korzyukov O, Alho K, Kujala A, Gumenyuk V, Ilmoniemi J, Virtanen J, Kropotov J, Naatanen R: Electromagnetic responses of the human auditory cortex generated by sensory-memory based processing of tone-frequency changes. *Neurosci Lett.* 1999;276:169.

Kuglar J, Lorenzi E, Spatz R, Zimmerman H: Drug-induced paroxysmal EEG activities. *Pharmakopsychiatry.* 1979;12:165.

Naatanen R. *Attention and brain function.* Hillsdale, NJ: Erlbaum; 1992.

Niedermeyer E. The EEG signal: polarity and field determination. In: Niedermeyer E, Lopes da Silva F, eds. *Electroencephalography: Basic Principles, Clinical Applications and Related Fields.* 2nd ed. Baltimore: Urban & Schwarzenberg; 1987.

*Niedermeyer E, Lopes da Silva F, eds. *Electroencephalography: Basic Principles, Clinical Applications and Related Fields.* Baltimore: Williams & Wilkins; 1993.

Polich J: P300 clinical utility and control of variability. *J Clin Neurophysiology.* 1998;15:14.

Polich J, Herbst KL: P300 as a clinical assay: Rationale, evaluation, and findings. *Int J Psychophysiol.* 2000;38:3.

Prichep LS, Alper KR, Kowalik SC: Prediction of treatment outcome in cocaine dependent males using quantitative EEG. *Drug Alcohol Depend.* 1999;54:35.

Princhep LS, Alper KR, Sverdlov L, Kowalik SC, John ER, Merkin H, Tom M, Howard B, Rosenthal MS: Outcome related electrophysiological subtypes of cocaine dependence. *Neurosci Lett.* 1999;276:169.

Prichep LS, John ER: QEEG profiles of psychiatric disorders. *Clin Electroencephalogr.* 2002;33:8.

Prichep LS, Mas F, Holander E: Quantitative electroencephalographic subtyping of obsessive-compulsive disorder. *Psychiatr Research: Neuroimaging.* 1993;50:25.

Reid MS, Prichep LS, Ciplet D, O'Leary S, Tom ML, Howard B, Rotrosen J, John ER: Quantitative electroencephalographic studies of cue-induced cocaine craving. *Clin Electroencephalogr.* 2003;34:110.

Small J. Psychiatric disorders and EEG. In: Niedermeyer E, Lopes da Silva F, eds. *Electroencephalography: Basic Principles, Clinical Applications and Related Fields.* Baltimore: Williams & Wilkins; 1993.

Struve FA. Clinical electroencephalography as an assessment method in psychiatric practice. In: Hall RCW, Beresford TP, eds. *Handbook of Psychiatric Diagnostic Procedures.* Vol 2. New York: Spectrum Publications; 1985.

Struve FA, Manno BR, Kemp P, Patrick G, Manno JE: Acute marijuana (THC) exposure produces a "transient" topographic quantitative EEG profile identical to the "persistent" profile seen in chronic heavy users. *Clin Electroencephalogr.* 2003;34:75.

Struve FA, Pike LE: Routine admission electroencephalograms of adolescent and adult psychiatric patients awake and asleep. *Clin Electroencephalogr.* 1974;5:67.

Struve FA, Straumanis JJ, Patrick G, Leavitt J, Manno JE, Manno BR: Topographic quantitative EEG sequelae of chronic marijuana use: A replication using medically and psychiatrically screened normal subjects. *Drug Alcohol Depend.* 1999; 56:167.

Takahashi T. Activation methods. In: Niedermeyer E, Lopes da Silva F, eds. *Electroencephalography: Basic Principles, Clinical Applications and Related Fields.* 2nd ed. Baltimore: Urban & Schwarzenberg; 1987.

Thatcher RW, North D, Curtin R, Walker RA, Biver CJ, Gomez JF, Salazar AM: An EEG severity index of traumatic brain injury. *J Neuropsychiatry Clin Neurosci.* 2001;13:77.

Umbricht D, Koller R, Schmid L, Skrabo A, Grubel C, Huber T, Stassen H: How specific are deficits in Mismatch Negativity generation to schizophrenia? *Biol Psychiatry.* 2003;53:1120.

Weilburg JB, Schachter S, Worth J, Pollack MH, Sachs GS, Ives JR, Schomer DL: EEG abnormalities in patients with atypical panic attacks. *J Clin Psychiatry.* 1995;56:358.

Yang-Whan J, Polich J: Meta-analysis of P300 and schizophrenia: Patients, paradigms, and practical implications. *Psychophysiology.* 2003;40:684.

▲ 1.15 Nuclear Magnetic Resonance Imaging: Basic Principles and Recent Findings in Neuropsychiatric Disorders

MEENA VYTHILINGAM, M.D., JUN SHEN, PH.D., WAYNE C. DREVETS, M.D., AND ROBERT B. INNIS, M.D., PH.D.

This chapter reviews the underlying physical principles and applications (clinical and research) of imaging methods whose signals derive from *nuclear magnetic resonance* (NMR). For each of these methods, the source of the signal is the magnetic field in nuclei of certain atoms and its interaction with the local environment and with externally induced manipulations of the magnetic field. The three in vivo methods that are reviewed are (1) *structural magnetic resonance imaging* (sMRI), (2) *functional magnetic resonance imaging* (fMRI), and (3) *magnetic resonance spectroscopy* (MRS). The companion chapter on positron emission tomography (PET) and single photon emission computed tomography (SPECT), neuroimaging techniques that use radiotracers, is intended to complement the current chapter and to provide a thorough overview of the most common neuroimaging methods used in psychiatric research and, to a lesser extent, in psychiatric care.

sMRI was the first of the three NMR methods to be developed. Today, it is widely used for brain imaging, and, in fact, sMRI has all but replaced the once common computed tomography (CT) imaging. CT's advantage is that it clearly differentiates and separates the skull from the brain, but it is unable to yield discreet delineation of substructures within the brain, such as gray and white matter. sMRI, on the other hand, provides clearer images of specific tissues than CT and therefore is commonly used for detection and localization of neurological anomalies, such as tumors, cerebral infarcts, and plaques characteristic of multiple sclerosis (MS). Initially, sMRI was used as a noninvasive "rule out" diagnostic tool in psychiatry. For example, using sMRI, one could exclude the presence of a temporal lobe tumor in a patient presenting with psychotic symptoms. Formerly, the belief was that psychiatric disorders were a result of abnormal brain *function*, rather than structural abnormalities. Data provided by the magnetic resonance (MR) studies have exposed many underlying structural abnormalities in various psychiatric disorders.

For example, alcoholism and Alzheimer's disease are clearly associated with brain atrophy. Furthermore, "pure" psychiatric disorders, such as schizophrenia, depression, and *posttraumatic stress disorder* (PTSD) have all been associated with sMRI abnormalities. For instance, global loss of gray matter has been reported in schizophrenia and depression; schizophrenia also exhibits relatively selective deficits surrounding the lateral ventricles, and the hippocampus and the subgenual prefrontal cortex are smaller in depression. Finally, recent studies in animals and humans have clearly shown that new neurons can grow in the hippocampal formation and that physical activity in animals can stimulate this neurogenesis. Thus, structural imaging studies are clearly within the purview of psychiatry, not only as a correlate of disease, but also possibly even for restorative and preventive interventions.

fMRI is one of several techniques used to measure local neuronal activity. The electroencephalogram (EEG) is perhaps the oldest method used to provide data on brain functioning. Today, it remains a common clinical tool, primarily used to obtain measures of electrical fields at the scalp surface originating from the firing of millions of neurons in the brain. Although EEG techniques allow rapid measurements (because they have excellent temporal resolution), the precise source of electrical fields is typically difficult, if not impossible, to identify.

Later, other methods were developed to measure neuronal activity, including PET and SPECT. These techniques were based on theories of autoregulation of cerebral blood flow (CBF), by which increased neuronal activity has a direct, linear relationship to blood flow in any given region of the brain. Radioactive *tracers* (such as radiolabeled water or xenon gas) were administered to subjects, and measures of radioactivity in the brain were obtained over the course of several hours by using PET or SPECT cameras. Similar techniques were developed for radiolabeled glucose analogs and were based on the premise that glucose metabolism and neuronal activity were also directly correlated.

fMRI is a recent NMR technique that was developed to measure neuronal activity in the brain. fMRI signal reflects the level of oxygenated hemoglobin in the blood, and, thus, this technique also rests on the principle of autoregulation. That is, areas of increased activity have increased blood flow and increased concentration of oxygenated hemoglobin. The major advantages of fMRI over older radiotracer methods are that (1) the subjects are not exposed to radioactivity, (2) the measurements can be repeated many times, and (3) the temporal resolution (time required to obtain data) is much smaller (approximately 1 to 2 seconds for fMRI vs. 45 minutes for PET glucose measurements). However, despite its advantages, the time resolution of fMRI is much smaller than that of EEG (millisecond range), and it currently lacks the level of absolute quantifiability of radiotracer methods. Nevertheless, fMRI research has markedly expanded over the past decade and is used at the neural systems level not only to pinpoint areas in the brain associated with movement, cognition, and emotion, but also to discover the relationships between multiple regions that cooperate in execution of simple and complex tasks.

In vivo MRS is kindred to various in vitro analytical chemistry techniques that have been used to identify specific chemical compounds. In short, this method is an in vivo neurochemical technique that can measure neurochemicals, such as levels of γ-aminobutyric acid (GABA), creatine (Cr), choline (Cho), glutamate (Glu), and other compounds present at relatively high concentrations in the brain (greater than approximately 10^{-3} M).

To summarize, as a broad generalization, sMRI is used to evaluate the structure of the brain, fMRI measures functional activity of discrete brain regions associated with increased blood flow, and MRS provides chemical measurements of specific molecules in the brain. In comparison to radiotracer methods described in the next chapter, all three of the aforementioned NMR methods are capable of excellent anatomic resolution and can be repeated multiple times within a short time span, in part, because they do not involve exposure to radioactivity. However, the major physical limitation of these NMR methods is their relatively low sensitivity. That is, NMR techniques can be used only when the component to be measured (water that provides the signal in sMRI, oxyhemoglobin for fMRI, and the specific chemical targets for MRS) is present in relatively high concentrations. Although radiotracer methods have lower anatomic resolution, they have much higher sensitivity (approximately 10^{-12} to 10^{-14} M) than these NMR techniques.

HISTORY OF MRI

Felix Block from Stanford University and Edward Purcell from Harvard University independently demonstrated the NMR phenomena by extending Isidor Isaac Rabi's discovery of *molecular beam* MR. They found that, when certain nuclei were placed in a magnetic field, they absorbed and later emitted this energy when the nuclei transferred back to their original state. The *nuclear* in *NMR* refers to the observation that only the nuclei in certain atoms have this response. *Magnetic* refers to the fact that a magnetic field is required. *Resonance* refers to the frequency dependence of the magnetic and radio frequency fields. The findings led to the discovery of NMR spectroscopy and analytical methods to study the composition of chemicals. In recognition of this landmark discovery, Block and Purcell were awarded the Nobel Prize for physics in 1952.

Over the next two decades, NMR spectroscopy was developed and used for the noninvasive chemical, physical, and molecular analysis of compounds. The application of NMR to distinguish between tumor tissue and healthy tissue came from an in vitro demonstration by Raymond Damadian, a physician of the State University of New York in Brooklyn, who demonstrated that cancerous rat tissue had a longer relaxation time than normal tissue. In 1972, Paul Lauterbur of the State University of New York at Stonybrook bridged the gap between NMR and imaging by combining three-dimensional magnetic field gradient and computed axial tomography (CAT) scan back projection techniques. This revolutionary extension of physics to imaging led to the first MR image of two test tubes of water. The combination of a weak gradient magnetic field with a stronger magnetic field to help localize the two test tubes of water led to the term *zeugmatography*, in which the Greek word *zeugma* refers to the joining of strong and weak fields. The applications of MR principles to imaging quickly became obvious. In 1977, Damadian performed the first magnetic resonance imaging (MRI) of the chest cavity of a live man. Subsequently, others focused on reducing imaging time without compromising image quality. Richard Ernst proposed using phase and frequency encoding and Fourier transformation. This technology forms the basis of current MRI techniques and was the reason that he won the Nobel Prize in chemistry in 1991. The word *nuclear* was eventually dropped from NMR, presumably because of its potential confusion with radioactivity (such as that associated with the nuclear bomb), and the acronym *MRI* was adopted instead. The development of echo-planar imaging by Peter Mansfield reduced the time required to obtain images and extended the use of MRI beyond the detection of structural changes to the evaluation of brain function. Peter Mansfield and Paul Lauterbur shared the 2003 Nobel Prize in physiology of medicine for their important contributions to the development and application of MRI techniques to clinical imaging. George Radda and colleagues from University of Oxford found that MRI could detect changes in the level of oxygen in the blood, which in turn reflects physiological activity. In

1990, Seiji Ogawa from the AT&T Bell laboratory demonstrated that an area containing deoxygenated hemoglobin distorts the magnetic field and reported variations in local tissue oxygenation using blood oxygen level dependent (BOLD) contrast. This series of discoveries set the stage for the burgeoning field of fMRI over the last two decades.

GENERAL PHYSICAL PRINCIPLES OF NUCLEAR MAGNETIC RESONANCE

NMR imaging and MRS are based on the predictable and measurable effects of high frequency radio waves on the alignment of the protons in an atom exposed to a strong magnetic force. Fortunately, most elements have at least one naturally occurring isotope that has a nonzero nuclear spin; thus, many elements can interact with an external magnetic field generated by a magnet that produces NMR signals. In principle, most elements in nature can be studied using MRI or MRS. Like many similar methods, NMR is an excite-and-detect technique.

Magnetic Nuclei

In general, each nucleus is composed of two types of fundamental particles: protons, which possess a positive charge, and neutrons, which have no charge. The nucleus can be regarded as constantly rotating around an axis; that is, it behaves as though it were a spinning particle. One physical characteristic of a spinning body is its *angular momentum*, referring to the characteristics of a body revolving around a fixed point. (This is important because, owing to this innate characteristic, certain elements cannot be studied using NMR.) For example, in nature, there are a limited number of values for *angular momentum* of the nucleus (designated as I). Values of angular momentum are based on the composition of the nucleus and are quantized or subdivided into discreet values. There are three groups of values for the nucleus spin I: zero, half-integers, and nonzero integers. A nucleus has no spin ($I = 0$) if it has an even number of protons and an even number of neutrons, because the fundamental particles tend to pair up. Such nuclei cannot interact with an external magnetic field and therefore cannot be studied using MRI or MRS. A nucleus has an integral value of I (for example, $I = 1, 2, 3$, etc.) if it has an odd number of protons and an odd number of neutrons. A nucleus has a half-integral value for I (for example, $I = 0.5, 1.5, 2.5$, etc.) if it has either an odd number of protons and an even number of neutrons or an even number of protons and an odd number of neutrons. The nuclear spins I for elements commonly found in biological systems are tabulated in Table 1.15–1.

A spinning positively charged nucleus is accompanied by a local magnetic field (*magnetic moment*) that functions like a loop of current. The *magnetic moment* associated with a spinning nucleus is fundamental to the NMR phenomenon. A nuclear spin behaves in many ways like a tiny bar magnet. Just as a bar magnet can be described as having a north and south pole and a certain value of magnetic moment or, more precisely, a vector with a direction and magnitude, so can the nuclear spin be described through a vector with a spinning axis having a definite orientation and magnitude of angular momentum. The associated magnetic field generated by the spinning nucleus halos the proton and lies parallel to the axis of self-rotation for the nucleus. All NMR signals are based on the orientation of the magnetic nuclear spins with respect to an external magnetic field and the induced changes the nucleus undergoes in interactions with external or local radiofrequency (RF) energies.

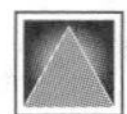

Table 1.15–1
Nuclear Magnetic Resonance Properties of Some Biologically Common Nuclei

Nucleus	Spin	Gyromagnetic Ratio (MHz/T)	Natural Abundance (%)	Relative Sensitivity (%)
Hydrogen-1	0.5	42.58	100	100
Lithium-7	1.5	16.55	92.58	29
Carbon-12	0	[a]	[a]	0
Carbon-13	0.5	10.71	1.11	1.6
Nitrogen-14	1	3.08	99.63	0.1
Nitrogen-15	0.5	4.31	0.37	0.1
Oxygen-16	0	[a]	[a]	0
Fluorine-19	0.5	40.05	100	83.4
Sodium-23	1.5	11.26	100	9.2
Phosphorus-31	0.5	17.24	100	6.6

[a]Nonmagnetic nucleus; nuclear magnetic resonance invisible.

Generation of Net Magnetization

Rather than focusing on a single type of nucleus, MR experiments group data from similar type nuclei. Considering an arbitrary volume of tissue, the three basic characteristics of every nucleus that play a part in NMR signal computation are (1) the specific *spin vector*, (2) its *orientation*, and (3) its *magnitude*. The magnitude of all spin vectors is the same for all nuclear spins. However, in nature, when there is no internal or external force acting on them, protons are oriented in random fashion, so the directions of the spins are also random. It follows that if a vector addition of all spin vectors in nature is performed, a zero sum is obtained, and there is no net (or bulk) magnetization.

A strong, stable, and homogeneous magnet is necessary to align or to orient protons in a way that they can send signals detectable by NMR. Most MR scanners use superconducting magnets because of their strong fields and optimal stability. Current-day commercial MR scanners generate a magnetic field (represented as B_0) approximately 10,000 to 100,000 times greater than Earth's magnetic field. These magnets consist of circular coils surrounding the bed (gantry) of the machine. To maintain their superconductivity, these coils are immersed in liquid helium reservoirs at 4°K. Because there is no factor of physical resistance in this amazing coil system, it can perpetuate an electrical current indefinitely without an external power supply. As electricity moves through the coils, a magnetic field is produced that parallels the axis of the gantry. This parameter, by convention, is identified as the z-coordinate in the cartesian system.

When an object (e.g., a patient) is placed into the hollow core of an MR magnet, the strong magnetic field causes the spinning nuclei to move in a fashion called *precession*, which is likened to the movement of a wobbly, spinning top (Fig. 1.15–1). The axes of self-rotation of the nuclei tilt slightly away from the axis of the magnetic field B_0, but the axis of precession (or wobbling) is parallel to B_0 (the z-axis). Just like the wobbling that is caused by the interaction of gravity with the mass of the spinning top, the cause of the precession is the interaction of the external magnetic field with the spinning, positively charged nuclei. The perpendicular, or transverse components of the precession (x- and y-components perpendicular to B_0) of an individual nucleus are nonzero and change over time as the nucleus precesses. The parallel or longitudinal component of the precession (z-component parallel to B_0) is constant across time. The frequency of precession is proportional to the strength of B_0 and is called the *Larmor frequency*, represented as ω_0, where $\omega_0 = \gamma B_0$, with γ being the constant for each nucleus and termed the *gyromagnetic ratio*. Mathematically speaking,

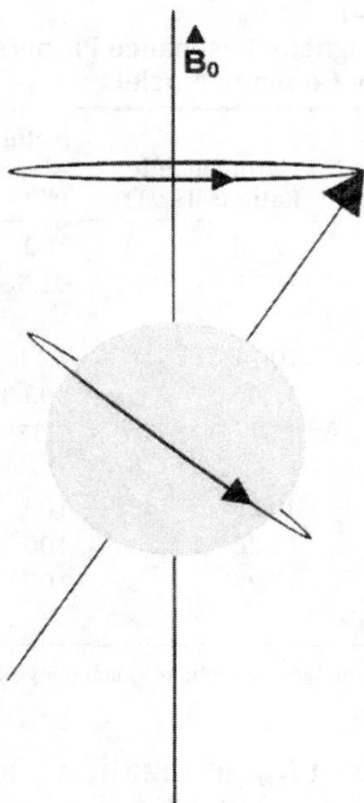

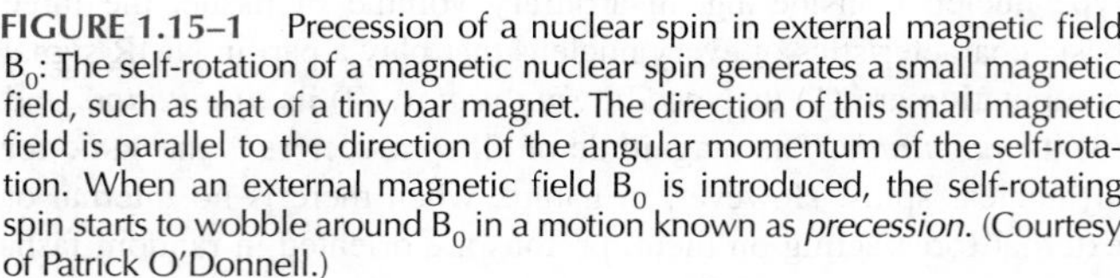

FIGURE 1.15–1 Precession of a nuclear spin in external magnetic field B_0: The self-rotation of a magnetic nuclear spin generates a small magnetic field, such as that of a tiny bar magnet. The direction of this small magnetic field is parallel to the direction of the angular momentum of the self-rotation. When an external magnetic field B_0 is introduced, the self-rotating spin starts to wobble around B_0 in a motion known as *precession*. (Courtesy of Patrick O'Donnell.)

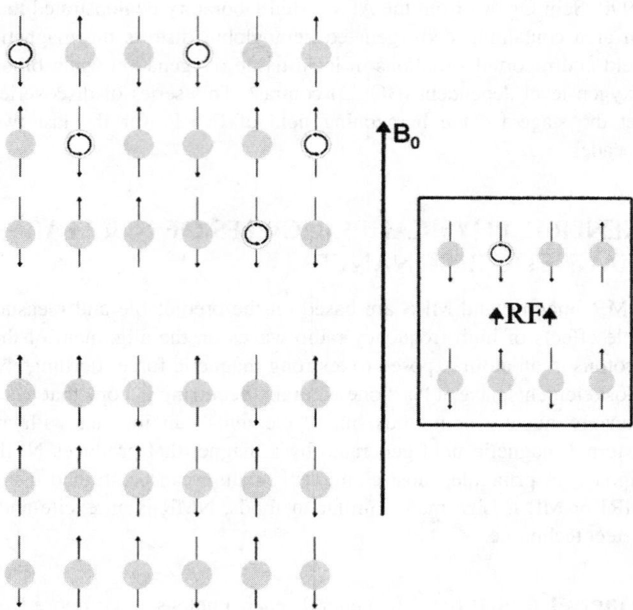

FIGURE 1.15–2 The Zeeman effect: Magnetic nuclei, such as hydrogen-1, make magnetic resonance imaging and spectroscopy possible, because they are similar to a bar magnet. Under the influence of an external magnetic field, B_0, the magnetic nuclei are aligned parallel or antiparallel to B_0. When the nuclei are irradiated with a radiofrequency (RF) pulse at their resonant frequency, they become activated and flip from parallel alignment to antiparallel alignment with respect to B_0. (Courtesy of Patrick O'Donnell.)

the *gyromagnetic ratio* signifies the ratio of the angular momentum of the nucleus to its magnetic moment. Its unit is MHz per T, with ω_0 in MHz but B_0 in T. The larger the γ, the more NMR-sensitive the nucleus is in a certain external B_0. Table 1.15–1 lists values for γ for those nuclei common to biological systems.

As mentioned previously, not all magnetic nuclei are useful for applications of NMR imaging or spectroscopy techniques (Table 1.15–1). The level of NMR sensitivity to a particular isotope depends on its gyromagnetic ratio, γ; spin quantum number, *I*; abundance; and the strength of the external magnetic field, B_0, or *Larmor frequency*, ω_0. For a given nucleus, the only way to increase NMR sensitivity is to increase B_0 or the quantity of the isotope, or both. Because of the high sensitivity of hydrogen-1 (^1H) and the prevalence of water in tissues, protons in water have served as the primary signal source for most medical applications of NMR. ^1H protons have a spin of 0.5 and are the most abundant isotope for hydrogen. ^1H is also sensitive to the external magnetic field due to its large gyromagnetic ratio, γ. General NMR principles apply to all magnetic nuclei, but, for the remainder of this chapter, the ^1H proton serves as an example.

If an addition for proton spin vectors is performed again after the tissue is placed inside the magnetic field, the results are somewhat different from the sum obtained outside the magnetic field. Perpendicular to B_0, the spin orientations are still randomly distributed just as they were outside the magnetic field. There is still no net magnetization perpendicular to B_0 inside the magnetic field. However, along the direction parallel to the magnetic field B_0, the result of vector addition is quite different from outside the magnetic field. The time-independent orientation of the proton to the axis of procession, which is parallel to B_0, generates a quantum interaction between the spin and B_0. This interaction is known as the *Zeeman effect*, as depicted in Figure 1.15–2. The *Zeeman effect* creates the difference in potential energy between protons aligned parallel to the magnetic field B_0 and those aligned antiparallel to it. This energy difference between parallel and antiparallel spins, depicted as ΔE, is proportional to the strength of the external magnetic field B_0.

As shown in Figure 1.15–2, because of the Zeeman effect, the protons with orientation parallel to B_0 reside in a lower-energy state than protons in antiparallel orientation. It follows that, because less energy is required to hold protons in parallel orientation, more protons are oriented parallel to the magnetic field B_0 than antiparallel to it. The change in proton orientation in the tissue is effected by the magnetic field. The exact number of protons in the two energy levels is determined by ΔE (therefore, also by B_0) and temperature. For protons at room temperature, there is approximately one proton in every one million protons at the lower energy level. This tiny lower-energy proton group means that the vector addition of spins inside the magnetic field B_0 is nonzero and parallel to B_0. That is, in the presence of the strong external magnetic field B_0, the tissue becomes slightly magnetized with a net magnetization of M_0. The orientation M_0 is parallel to B_0. This M_0–parallel to–B_0 configuration, with no transverse components, is the most probable state for the protons at thermal equilibrium and in the presence of the external B_0. It has the lowest energy and is the configuration to which the protons naturally return (through relaxation) after termination of any disturbances, such as an RF pulse. The net magnetization, M_0, is the source of signal for all three NMR methods. The greater the external magnetic field, B_0, the greater the net degree of alignment and the greater the magnetization of the bulk sample (i.e., the greater M_0 or NMR signal becomes). This aside, because the sum of the difference between the two Zeeman energy levels for the total proton population is so small, NMR's overall sensitivity is lacking.

Radiofrequency (RF) Excitation NMR experiments can be understood in terms of energy transfer or excite and detect. During the procedure, the object, or patient, absorbs energy of a specific frequency when exposed to irradiation. Subsequently, this energy is emitted, detected, and processed. To the advantage of NMR imaging and spectroscopy, the absorbed energy is nonionizing. This energy is a short burst oscillating in the range of *RF*. RF pulses are generated by the RF transmitter system, which contains a frequency synthesizer, a waveform generator, a high-power amplifier, and a coil (also called an *antenna*). The frequency synthesizer produces the carrier frequency for the RF pulse, and the waveform generator mixes the RF pulse before amplification to produce an amplitude-modulated pulse at the desired frequency. Then, the RF power amplifier must sufficiently magnify the signal emitted from the frequency synthesizer to excite the nuclei. Typical RF amplifiers for MR scanners are rated at 1 to 4 kW of output power. The final component of the RF system is the RF transmitter coil, which irradiates the RF energy to the object. Although the low-energy RF electromagnetic pulse is not ionizing, and it poses no known hazards to biological tissues, the absorbed RF power does generate heat in the patient. Generally, MR systems are designed to limit this effect to less than approximately 1°C.

During the RF pulse, a proton absorbs the energy at the Larmor frequency. This boosts the proton from the lower-energy orientation (parallel to B_0) to the higher-energy orientation (antiparallel to B_0). At the same time, a proton in the higher energy level is compelled to release energy and falls to the lower energy level. Owing to the quantized nature of the nuclear spin angular momentum, only the energy at the frequency defined by ΔE (i.e., ω_0) is absorbed; this energy level is known as the *resonant frequency*. Different magnetic nuclei respond to different *resonant frequencies*, or Larmor frequencies, while being exposed to the same external magnetic field.

Macroscopically, significant energy absorption and emission occur when the RF pulse is emitted. Because an excess of protons are present at the lower energy level, there is a net energy absorption in the tissue being irradiated. Energy is applied as an RF pulse with a carrier frequency ω_0 and an orientation perpendicular to B_0, as indicated by an effective field B_1 that rotates around B_0 at, or close to, the Larmor frequency. Absorption of the RF energy frequency ω_0 can throw the magnetization M_0 out of alignment with B_0 to such an extent that it can even temporarily reverse the alignment. The amount of energy transmitted can be changed by varying the duration of the RF pulse, which determines the degree to which the protons are tipped. For example, a 90-degree pulse refers to the energy required to cause M_0 to rotate entirely to the transverse plane, perpendicular to B_0 and B_1 (Fig. 1.15–3). If the same RF pulse is left on twice as long, M_0 is rotated to align antiparallel to B_0, resulting in an

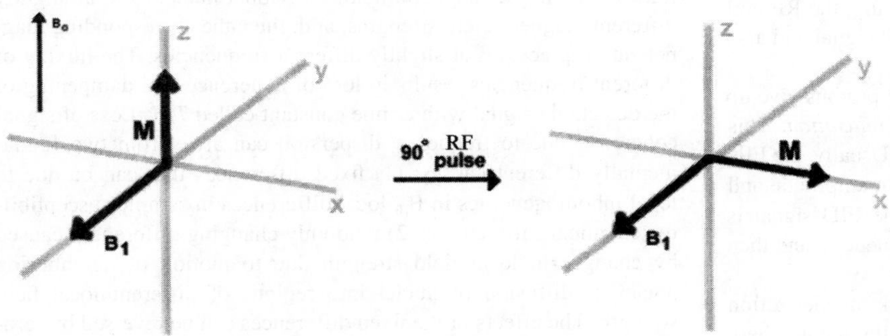

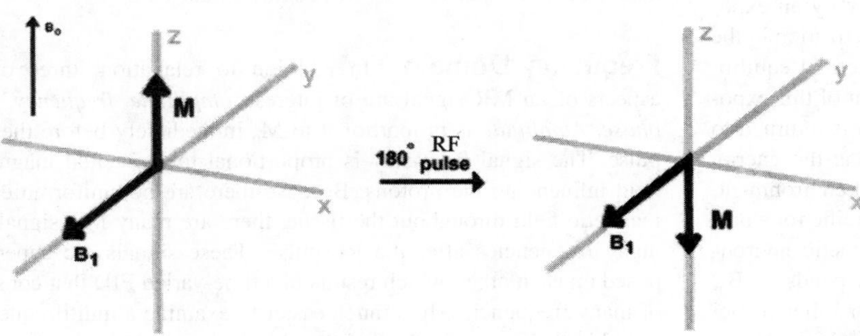

FIGURE 1.15–3 At thermal equilibrium, magnetic nuclei, such as hydrogen-1, are aligned parallel to the magnetic field, B_0. The bulk magnetization is depicted as *M*. When the sample is irradiated with a radiofrequency (RF) pulse (B_1) at the resonant frequency, the bulk magnetization is rotated away from its equilibrium alignment. If the action of the RF pulse is to rotate the magnetization exactly to the transverse plane, the RF pulse is referred to as a *90-degree pulse*; if the magnetization is rotated to the antiparallel alignment position, the RF pulse is referred to as a *180-degree pulse*. (Courtesy of Patrick O'Donnell.)

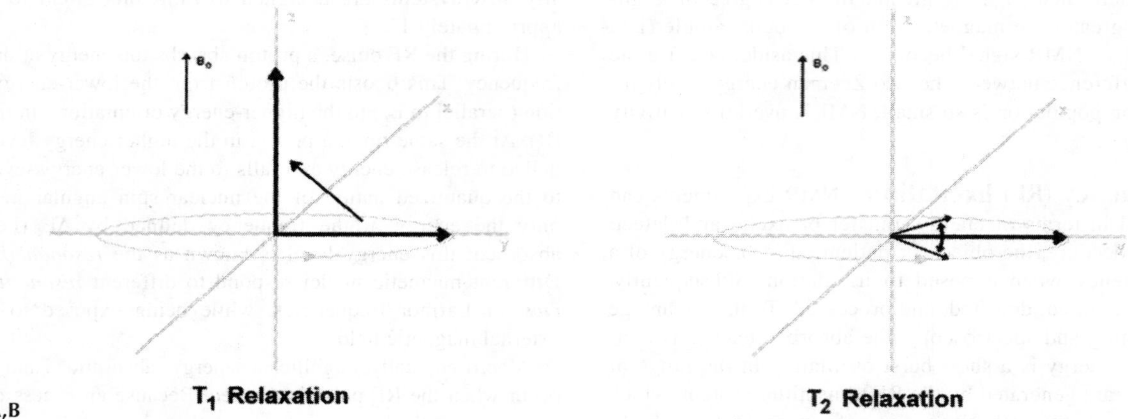

FIGURE 1.15–4 When rotated away from its thermal equilibrium position, magnetization gradually relaxes back toward its equilibrium. There are two simultaneous magnetization relaxation processes: The longitudinal magnetization along the z-axis relaxes toward its full strength when magnetization is at its thermal equilibrium in a process referred to as *T_1 relaxation* **(A)**; the transverse magnetization at the xy-plane relaxes toward zero in a process referred to as *T_2 relaxation* **(B)**. B_0, magnetic field. (Courtesy of Patrick O'Donnell.)

inverted population of the spins at both energy levels. In this instance, the RF pulse is a 180-degree pulse (Fig. 1.15–3).

Free Induction Decay and Relaxation After the RF excitation field is switched off, the protons immediately start to realign themselves with B_0, and they return to their original equilibrium orientation. At the same time, they give off energy at frequency ω_0. Macroscopically, the precession motion of the bulk magnetization M_0 creates a weak, but detectable, electromagnetic RF signal, which is detected by an RF coil in the magnet. Usually, the RF coil has the dual purpose of detecting the electromagnetic signal and also transmitting the RF pulse into the tissue.

The NMR signal decays over time as more of the protons give up their absorbed energy through a process known as *relaxation.* This NMR signal is called the *free induction decay* (*FID*). Usually, the FID produced by protons is between 10^{-9} and 10^{-6} volts in amplitude and 20 to 300 MHz in frequency (radio frequency). The FID signal is amplified, demodulated to kHz frequency (audio frequency), and then processed by the analog-to-digital converters (ADCs).

As discussed previously, once perturbed, the bulk magnetization gradually relaxes back to its thermal equilibrium alignment. There are two different types of *relaxation* processes. Both are important in producing contrast in MRI images. The first type is called *T1 relaxation* (or *longitudinal relaxation* or *spin-lattice relaxation*). *T1 relaxation* only concerns the longitudinal (parallel to the direction of B_0) component of the magnetization relaxing back to its magnitude M_0 at thermal equilibrium. It is described mathematically by an exponential curve that increases with time as the net magnetization in the longitudinal axis returns to its original strength at thermal equilibrium (Fig. 1.15–4A). T1 is defined as the time constant of this exponential process when 63 percent of the magnetization is returned to the thermal equilibrium. The T1 relaxation process is the energy exchange between higher-energy spins and their local environment. To clarify, this means that T1 relaxation time is not specific for a particular type of nucleus but rather is affected by the magnetic environment of neighboring atoms and molecules. Thus, it depends on B_0, molecular size, temperature, presence of electrons or other nuclei with magnetic moments, and other factors at the molecular level.

The second type of relaxation process is called *T2 relaxation* (or *transverse relaxation* or *spin-spin relaxation*). In contrast to T1 relaxation, *T2 relaxation* only concerns the transverse (perpendicular to the direction of B_0) component of magnetization relaxing back to zero after excitation by an RF field at the Larmor frequency. It is described mathematically as an exponential curve that decreases with time until the transverse magnetization approaches zero (Fig. 1.15–4B). T2 is defined as the time constant of this exponential process when 63 percent of the transverse magnetization is lost. Initially, when the RF field is turned off, all of the magnetization is coherent, and a detectable signal is produced. However, nonuniformities exist in the magnetic field. Individual nuclei exist at slightly different magnetic field strengths, and, thus, the corresponding magnetization precesses at slightly different frequencies. The mixing of different frequencies results in loss of coherence and dampening of the detectable signal with a time constant called *T2**. Loss of signal coherence due to frequency dispersion can arise from two fundamentally different causes: (1) fixed differences that can be due to local inhomogeneities in B_0, local differences in sample susceptibility, chemical shift, etc. or (2) randomly changing differences caused by changes in local field strength due to motion of neighboring nuclei or diffusion of nuclei into regions of different local field strength. The effects of the fixed differences can be reversed by refocusing techniques, such as the spin-echo method, which is discussed later in this chapter. Signal decay resulting from randomly changing differences is an entropic, irreversible loss of signal coherence. The time constant describing the irreversible signal loss, which depends on the local molecular environment and molecular motions, is the actual T2. Note that T2* is always shorter than T2.

Frequency Domain In addition to relaxation, three other aspects of an MR signal are of interest: *amplitude*, *frequency*, and *phase*. *Amplitude* is proportional to M_0 immediately before the RF pulse. The signal *frequency* is proportional to the actual magnetic field influencing the protons. Because there are nonuniformities of magnetic field throughout the tissue, there are many MR signals at many frequencies after the RF pulse. These signals are superimposed on each other, which results in a time-varied FID that consists of many frequencies. It is much easier to examine a multifrequency signal in the frequency domain than in the time domain.

The conversion of the digitized time domain FID to a frequency domain presentation is accomplished by using a mathematical oper-

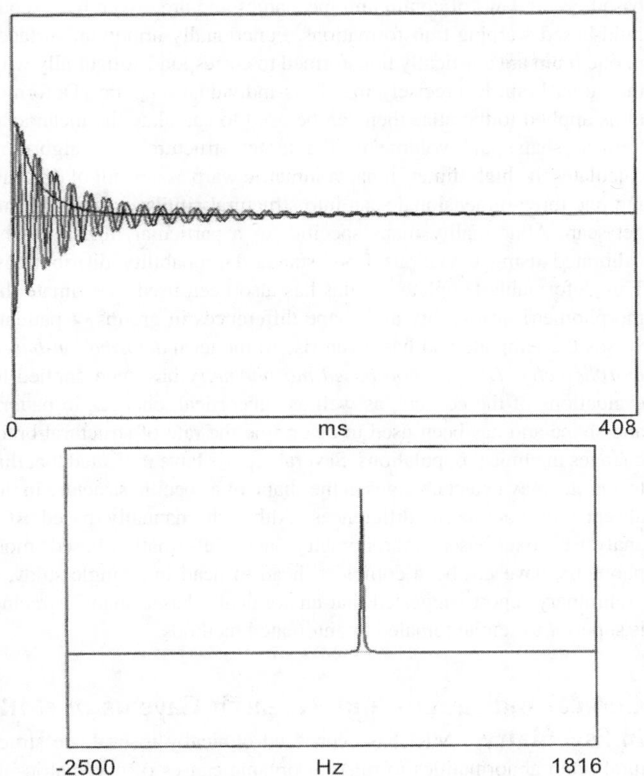

FIGURE 1.15–5 Time domain free induction decay (FID) versus frequency domain presentation: The Fourier transformation converts a time domain signal (FID) into the corresponding frequency domain signal (spectrum). (Courtesy of Patrick O'Donnell.)

ation called the discrete *Fourier transformation.* Figure 1.15–5 shows the relationship between a time domain FID and the corresponding frequency domain data obtained using the *Fourier transformation.* In the frequency domain, the NMR signal is mapped according to its frequency relative to the carrier frequency.

The specific frequency that a proton emits depends on magnetic fields that affect it. The bulk of the magnetic field is the external magnetic field B_0 generated by the magnet. This field can be changed slightly by the sample as well as by the use of external field gradients, a concept that is examined more fully later in this chapter. For each type of magnetic nucleus, the static magnetic field it experiences is slightly modified by the circulating currents of electrons in close proximity to it. As electrons move, they create their own small, regional, magnetic fields that, to a slight degree, alter the final magnetic field experienced by the nucleus. This can shift the magnetic field value B_0 by a few or tens of parts per million (ppm). Thus, the Larmor frequency of the nucleus is changed. This change is termed *chemical shift* and is a phenomenon of molecular origin associated with the chemical environment of the nucleus. Because the spatial configuration of electrons is unique for a given molecule, precessing nuclei take on altered frequencies that correlate with their chemical environment. Because different chemical environments shield the external magnetic field, B_0 acts on an element in a molecule, or on different molecules, in different ways. Thus, in MRS, *chemical shifts* enable the different locations of elements within the same molecule to be probed and different molecules to be distinguished.

In most other types of diagnostic imaging, signal localization is achieved by geometric means. In NMR, the precession frequency of the magnetic nuclei depends on the strength of the external magnetic field. This field dependence can also be used to assign frequencies to different regions of space and therefore to create an image. Unlike the chemical shift in which variations in the magnetic field are intrinsically caused by electrons circulating around the nuclei, in the case of imaging (and localized spectroscopy and spectroscopic imaging [SI] as well, the magnetic field is made spatially dependent by superimposing the so-called *magnetic field gradients* on the static magnetic field B_0. *Magnetic field gradients* can be regarded as small disturbances or perturbations in the static magnetic field B_0. These perturbations are linearly dependent on their position inside the magnet. A typical field gradient produces a maximum field distortion of less than 1 percent, which is many orders of magnitude greater than the chemical shift difference between protons. They are active for short periods of time and are referred to as *gradient pulses* (as opposed to the RF pulses). Ordinarily, three gradients are used to produce the orthogonal field distribution required for imaging; these gradients correspond to the x-axis, the y-axis, and the z-axis, respectively. They are each generated by the flow of electrical current through separate loops of wire mounted into a single hardware component known as the *gradient coil.* Variations in gradient amplitude are produced by changes in the amount or direction of the electrical current flowing through the gradient coil. In the presence of a magnetic field, protons at the same point along the gradient, corresponding to a plane perpendicular to the direction of the gradient, share the same resonant frequency, whereas those in the neighboring planes precess at different frequencies. Gradients are easily produced in multiple directions. Quite simply, the MR image is a map of nuclear frequencies emitted through unique magnetic fields that correspond to each pixel (i.e., point element) throughout the image. The pixel intensity is proportional to the number of nuclei contained within each voxel (i.e., volume element) weighted by the T1 and T2 or T2* relaxation times for the tissue within the voxel. The field gradients are also used in localized spectroscopy and SI to differentiate spectroscopic signals from various locations in the tissue.

STRUCTURAL MRI

MRI Analysis Earlier imaging studies in psychiatric disorders used qualitative and subjective methods (such as visual inspection) to detect differences in the size of particular brain structures between patients and controls. The qualitative methods gave rise to more objective quantitative methods in which investigators determined the size of structures by outlining the gray matter, white matter, or cerebrospinal fluid (CSF) borders. Recently, voxel-based and deformation-based morphometric techniques provide automated measures of shape and volume and are less labor-intensive compared to manual methods. Many of the automated or semiautomated methods of analysis include steps to standardize the spatial orientation of the brain, which reduces variability due to differences in head positioning during scan acquisition. MRI scans are usually aligned vertically to the interhemispheric plane and horizontally to the line connecting the anterior and posterior commissures, or, in the case of a longitudinal structure, such as the hippocampus, scans are resliced in the coronal plane perpendicular to the longest axis of the structure. The anatomical boundaries of the region are defined using specific criteria and are manually traced in each slice (Fig. 1.15–6). The areas of the manually segmented region are then calculated by a computer algorithm and multiplied by the thickness of each slice to give the volume. The volumes of the individual slices are then summed to give a total volume of the *region of interest* (*ROI*). Although results based on manually based ROI performed by trained raters are accurate, this method is time consuming, labor intensive, and amenable to rater bias and depends on varying a priori anatomical criteria amongst groups.

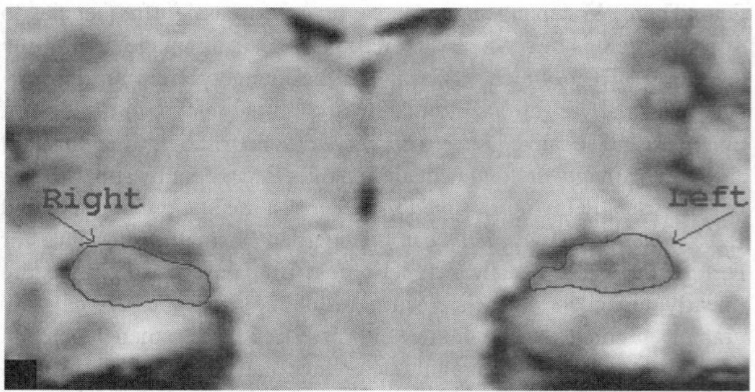

FIGURE 1.15–6 Region of interest (right and left) hippocampal morphometry based on manual techniques. Boundaries of the target structure are manually outlined by a trained rater blind to the diagnosis of the subject by using a priori anatomical criteria. The volume of each slice is calculated by a computer algorithm and is summed across the structure to result in the final volume.

Although the majority of published MRI studies continue to rely on manually traced ROI methods, semiautomated and automated morphometric techniques and analysis have become increasingly popular. These newer techniques make it possible to quantify the volume and to identify the shape of structures, such as hippocampi, and to provide information on sulcal patterns and the thickness of the cortex. These semiautomated techniques also help eliminate rater bias, and they allow for the identification of structural abnormalities that cannot be picked up with visual inspection.

One of the earliest semiautomated methods is *voxel-based morphometry*. This technique is often used for analysis of functional imaging data and is based on statistical parametric mapping (SPM) methods. It provides voxel-by-voxel comparisons of gray matter concentration between groups. MRI scans are preprocessed to reduce interindividual variations in brain size and shape. Structural data are spatially transformed into a standard stereotactic space. The standard spatial normalization process involves superimposing an index MRI on an atlas, such that the MRI data are transformed to the space occupied by the atlas. The atlas used for this purpose is called the *Talairach template* and is based on postmortem sections of the brain of a 60-year-old female subject. This transformation to a *Talairach template* vertically aligns the interhemispheric plane and horizontally aligns the line connecting the anterior and posterior commissures, creating a customized template. To overcome the limitations of the Talairach template, the International Consortium for Brain Mapping (ICBM) constructed a composite MRI data set from young normal subjects whose scans were individually mapped into the Talairach system. The normalized sMRI scan therefore conforms to a standard anatomical space but also represents local MRI scanner features. After this intermediate step of spatial normalization, scans are then segmented into gray matter, white matter, and CSF partitions by using SPM. Differences among image intensities in the MRI are normalized by using nonuniformity correction. The normalized and segmented images are then smoothed to conform to the gaussian model used for statistical analysis to detect regional differences. Statistical maps created in the standardized brain space confirm the exact anatomical location of the voxel clusters having significantly different gray matter volume.

A fixed brain atlas cannot accurately reflect the complex and subtle structural differences among subjects. Variations in cortical patterns between normal subjects and subjects with disorders cannot easily be identified using a standard anatomical template. To overcome this limitation, *deformable atlases* have been developed. These atlases are based on the laws of continuum mechanics and are driven by viscous fluid-based warping transformations. Functionally important surfaces in one brain are elastically transformed to correspond structurally with the target brain to precisely match its individual anatomy. Deformations applied to the atlas then can be used to calculate the mean anatomical shape and volume of the target structure. The algorithm calculates the high-dimensional volumetric warp as a result of deforming one three-dimensional scan into structural similarity with the target scan. Abnormality maps specific for a particular illness can be calibrated using deviations from standard probability distributions. This deformable template or atlas has also been used to estimate the morphometric variability and shape differences in groups of patients versus the template and has given rise to the term *deformation-based morphometry*. *Deformation-based morphometry* has been applied to evaluations of the cortical, as well as subcortical, changes in pattern and shape and has been used to determine the rate of structural brain changes in clinical populations. Several reports have indicated that this technique may detect changes in the shape of a specific structure in the absence of volumetric differences. Although manually based ROI analysis, voxel-based morphometry, and deformation-based morphometry have not been compared head to head in a single study, a preliminary report suggested that anatomically based manual tracing is superior to semiautomated or automated methods.

Clinical Indications and Research Caveats of sMRI in Psychiatry

MRI has been used clinically to evaluate structural brain abnormalities to rule out organic causes of psychiatric illness. Other clinical indications include the evaluation of an abrupt change in mental status, new-onset dementia or psychosis, and new-onset memory loss. Research studies that have used sMRI to evaluate brain abnormalities have reported group differences between patients and controls. However, sMRI abnormalities are not diagnostic of any particular psychiatric illness. With the exception of dementia and, perhaps, schizophrenia, structural abnormalities in other psychiatric disorders are mixed. Factors contributing to inconsistencies in sMRI findings include differences in image acquisition and image analysis, as well as differing anatomical criteria used for defining the regions of interest. Results are further confounded by clinical characteristics, such as duration and severity of illness, comorbid disorders, and medication status. This heterogeneity and variance in sMRI findings could be reduced by collaboration and communication among researchers studying well-defined groups of subjects. Finally, even when an abnormality has been reported consistently, it is not clear whether the structural change is a consequence, a correlate, or a risk factor for developing the illness. Longitudinal studies in high-risk populations, family studies, and studies combining neuroimaging with genetics could help tease out "the chicken and the egg" dilemma facing sMRI studies in psychiatric illness.

sMRI Findings in Psychiatric Disorders

Dementias Together with a clinical history and a neurological examination, sMRI could serve as a diagnostic tool for Alzheimer's disease and other dementias. The majority of sMRI studies of Alzheimer's disease found atrophy of the whole brain along with enlargement of the ventricular and sulcal CSF spaces. Alzheimer's disease is characterized by amyloid plaques and neurofibrillary tangles that could result in the loss of neurons in the cortex as well as the subcortical limbic system. In addition to global atrophy and reduction in gray matter, focal atrophy has been found in the frontal, temporal, and parietal lobes. Although most studies in Alzheimer's disease did not confirm changes in white matter, it is possible that subjects with early-onset Alzheimer's disease have a decrease in white matter in addition to reductions in gray matter. Patients with Alzheimer's disease have been distinguished from healthy subjects with 92 percent accuracy based on large temporal and parietal ventricular CSF space along with small temporal gray matter. Increasing demential severity was shown to be related to decreased gray matter volume.

Of the various medial temporal lobe structures evaluated in Alzheimer's disease, the hippocampus has been the main focus, given its crucial role in mediating declarative memory. Several groups have consistently found a reduction in hippocampal volume in subjects with Alzheimer's disease. This volumetric reduction was most prominent in the head of the hippocampus. The range of volume reduction of the hippocampus in Alzheimer's disease was approximately 19 to 40 percent. Hippocampal volume has been correlated with neuronal counts in patients with Alzheimer's disease and directly correlated with poor performance on delayed-recall memory tasks. Although several longitudinal studies have shown that the rate of volume loss for the hippocampus is greatest in Alzheimer's disease when compared to healthy subjects and subjects with mild cognitive impairment, a single report suggested that accelerated temporal lobe atrophy may be more prominent in Alzheimer's disease than atrophy of the hippocampus. Longitudinal volumetric changes in the hippocampus have also been used to evaluate patients with mild cognitive impairment who are at risk for developing dementia. According to various published studies, subjects with mild cognitive impairment who have significant hippocampal atrophy are at a higher risk for developing Alzheimer's disease. Smaller hippocampal volume in Alzheimer's disease was also associated with apo E ε4 allele. Patients who carried two copies of the apo E ε4 allele had greater hippocampal volume loss than subjects who carried one or no apo E ε4 allele. However, not all studies have been able to replicate this genetic association in Alzheimer's disease.

Other medial temporal lobe structures have also been evaluated in Alzheimer's disease. A 15 to 20 percent reduction in the volume of the parahippocampal gyrus, a 30 to 40 percent smaller amygdala volume, a decreased entorhinal cortical volume (38 to 61 percent), and a smaller subiculum have also been reported in patients with Alzheimer's disease. Although entorhinal cortical measurements could differentiate mild Alzheimer's disease from normal elderly and could potentially be a tool for early detection of Alzheimer's disease, the anatomical definitions make manual tracing of this structure difficult. Reduction in the volume of the corpus callosum as a result of white matter degeneration is a consistent finding in Alzheimer's disease; however, the exact focal location of volumetric reduction in the corpus callosum has been debated. Longitudinal studies in patients with Alzheimer's disease have demonstrated a progressive loss of whole brain volume at 1.0 to 2.8 percent per year for whole brain volume and an approximately 4 percent annual loss in volume for the hippocampus, with an increase in temporal horn volume at approximately 14 percent. Deformation-based morphometry has also been used to longitudinally evaluate changes in cortical and subcortical maps in Alzheimer's disease and minimal cognitive deficits.

sMRI has also been used in the diagnosis of other kinds of dementias, such as frontotemporal dementia and Huntington's disease. Selective atrophy of the frontal and temporal lobes is characteristic of frontotemporal dementia, whereas atrophy of the putamen and caudate nucleus is more characteristic of dementia related to Huntington's disease.

Psychotic Disorders: Schizophrenia Johnstone and coworkers' initial report of enlarged ventricles, as seen with CT in the mid 1970s, has subsequently been replicated numerous times using CT and sMRI. The expanding fluid-filled spaces in the schizophrenic brain are now considered characteristic of the disease observed; they are observed not only in the ventricles, but also in the sulci (gaps between adjacent gyri in the neocortex). However, increases in ventricular size are often relatively modest (10 to 20 percent), and most patient values overlap those of healthy subjects. Thus, increased ventricular size is not diagnostic of the disorder. Furthermore, increased ventricular volume is not specific to schizophrenia, because it is found in many other disorders of diverse developmental or degenerative etiologies (e.g., Alzheimer's disease, hydrocephalus, and bipolar disorder).

The increased fluid spaces in the presence of a normal-sized cranial vault means that there must be less brain tissue in this disorder. Is there less brain tissue because of atrophy or were there fewer brain cells at birth or during the brain's development? Researchers continue to debate this question along lines that can be described as the *neurodegenerative* versus the *neurodevelopmental hypothesis*. The *neurodevelopmental hypothesis* is supported by the higher incidence of gross structural abnormalities in the disorder, including cavum septum pellucidum (a fluid-filled cyst forming in the septum located in the midline between the hemispheres) and callosal agenesis (an underdevelopment of the corpus callosum, the wide tract of axons that connect the two hemispheres). Evidence for a *neurodegenerative process* is controversial and difficult to confirm, because it involves the repeated scanning of subjects over time. Nevertheless, some studies have been able to confirm the progression of ventricular enlargement, and loss of frontal lobe volume is greater in patients with schizophrenia than in healthy subjects. However, these results are not consistent across patient populations, occurring most often in chronic schizophrenia and in patients with prominent negative symptoms.

Serial MRI studies of childhood-onset schizophrenia performed at the National Institute of Mental Health (NIMH) provide some insight into the neurodevelopmental and neurodegenerative hypotheses. Childhood-onset schizophrenia is a severe illness with onset of psychosis occurring before 12 years of age. Even at the time of the initial psychotic break, patients with childhood-onset schizophrenia have smaller brain volume than age-matched controls, exhibiting an overall 10 percent decrease in total gray matter volume. Furthermore, childhood-onset schizophrenia patients show a progressive loss in frontal and temporal gray matter volumes during late adolescence that is appreciably greater than the gray (and white) matter loss typical of normal brain development in late adolescence. Thus, childhood-onset schizophrenia patients exhibit initial development abnormality at the onset of early symptoms, as well as a progressive component. Should this latter progression, however, be termed *neurodegeneration* or *abnormal development*? In fact, selection between these two terms may be rather arbitrary and off the point. Instead, research efforts should be and are being focused on the mechanisms for these losses in the hope that therapeutics can reverse them. Finally, the structural neurological changes seen in childhood-onset schizophrenia may not reflect changes seen in the adult-onset disorder. It is quite possible that childhood-onset schizophrenia is a severe and etiologically distinct disorder.

Because the studies of enlarged ventricles have been well replicated, and because these studies imply lower brain tissue volumes, can one assume that this deficit is localized to one region, or is it a generalized loss in all regions? A small, global (approximately 5 percent) volume loss has been reported in some, but not all, sMRI studies. Disproportionately large volume losses (10 to 15 percent) are commonly seen in medial temporal lobe structures (including amygdala, hippocampus, and parahippocampal gyrus) and the superior temporal gyrus. However, a smaller percentage of studies also report tissue deficits in frontal and parietal cortices, as well as the corpus callosum. Most of these localized volume deficits are found not only in chronic schizophrenics, but also in patients exhibiting first-break psychosis, suggesting that peripheral changes could predispose subjects to psychosis. Furthermore, because ventricular enlargement and regional brain volume losses are commonly found in studies of first-break patients who were previously pharmacologically naive, these abnormalities are most likely not caused by neuroleptic medications. However, typical (but not atypical) antipsychotic medications have been frequently reported to increase the size of human basal ganglia (caudate, putamen, and globus pallidus).

A so-called two-hit model is sometimes used to explain the typical age of onset of schizophrenia in late adolescence or early adulthood. Genetic or early neurodevelopmental abnormalities are the so-called first hit that predisposes subjects to the disorder. Later, a variety of potential stressors in adolescence, including hormonal influences on the brain and the social stress of this age group, may act as the second hit to precipitate a psychotic episode.

Do regional brain volume losses correlate with specific symptoms of schizophrenia? Although not consistently replicated, negative or deficit symptoms may be associated with enlarged lateral ventricles and decreased volume of medial temporal lobe structures. In a similar, but not uniform, manner, positive symptoms may correlate with decreased volume of the superior temporal gyrus.

Mood Disorders Affective disorders are a heterogeneous group of illnesses with no apparent single etiology. Various functional abnormalities in the limbic-thalamic-cortical and the limbic-cortical-striatal-pallidal-thalamic circuits or their components have been reported in major depressive disorder and bipolar disorder. sMRI studies of mood disorders have investigated individual components of these circuits. Unlike schizophrenia, several controlled MRI studies have confirmed normal total brain volumes in bipolar and unipolar disorders. The findings of earlier CAT scan findings, as well as more recent MRI studies evaluating third and lateral ventricular volumes in major depressive disorder and bipolar patients, are mixed. In contrast, the majority of MRI studies in late-onset depressed elderly subjects have consistently confirmed larger third and lateral ventricles and cortical atrophy. It is possible that contradictory sMRI findings in mood disorders could be due to varying sociodemographic and illness characteristics of the study samples. In fact, lateral ventricles were significantly larger in patients with bipolar disorder with recurrent episodes as compared to first-episode patients or healthy subjects (see the 2002 article by Strakowski et al.), suggesting that brain morphology can change over time.

Because the prefrontal cortex plays a critical role in emotion and cognition, several groups have investigated volumetric changes in affective disorders using sMRI. Studies confirmed a volumetric reduction in the frontal lobes in unipolar depression. Subsequent sMRI studies localized atrophy in the frontal lobe to the prefrontal cortical region. When subregions of the prefrontal cortex were examined, focal reductions in volume were observed in the left subgenual prefrontal cortex (an area of the anterior cingulate cortex [ACC] ventral to the genu of the corpus callosum) in familial unipolar and bipolar disorder. Postmortem studies confirmed a reduction in glia in the subgenual prefrontal cortex. This defect may alter synaptic transmission and may disrupt reciprocal connections with other regions of the brain, including the limbic system, thereby resulting in affective, neuroendocrine, and autonomic dysfunction characteristic of depression. However, more recent studies evaluating the volume of the subgenual prefrontal cortex have been unable to replicate the volume reduction seen in earlier studies. Postmortem studies also confirmed a reduction of neuropil in the posterior orbital cortex in unipolar and bipolar disorders. The volume of the orbital frontal cortex, specifically the gyrus rectus, was reduced in elderly and nonelderly unipolar depressed subjects compared to controls. Because the orbital cortex is reciprocally connected to the amygdala and modulates behavioral and cognitive responses related to fear and reward, structural abnormalities in this region could underlie behavioral and autonomic symptoms related to depression.

Based on the preclinical literature supporting hippocampal neuronal damage secondary to elevated levels of steroids, several groups evaluated hippocampal volume in unipolar depression. Reductions in the left, right, and bilateral hippocampi in the range of 6 to 20 percent were confirmed in several, but not all, studies on unipolar depression (Fig. 1.15–7A). Using deformation-based morphometric techniques, an abnormality of the shape of the subiculum was identified in the absence of smaller hippocampal volumes in depressed patients compared to controls. Hippocampal volume reduction correlated with length of the affective illness and total duration of depression in elderly women, suggesting that cumulative hippocampal damage occurred with repeated episodes. Depressed subjects with treatment-resistant chronic depression had reduced the gray matter density in the left temporal cortex using voxel-based morphometry. However, the inconsistencies in the hippocampal volume data require more explanation. Close examination of MRI studies of patients with major depressive disorders suggests that smaller hippocampal volume is restricted to subjects with treatment-resistant depression, older women with major depression, women with treatment-resistant depression, depressed women with a history of childhood sexual abuse, and elderly depressed patients. This conclusion has been challenged by the recent finding that male patients with a first episode of major depression have significantly smaller left hippocampal volumes as compared to healthy male patients. In contrast to the mixed findings of hippocampal volume in unipolar disorders, hippocampal volumes in bipolar patients are similar to normals; moreover, two groups reported an increase in hippocampal volume.

Future longitudinal studies in medication-naive subjects may shed light on the question of hippocampal volume and its role as a predisposing factor or as a consequence of repeated episodes of major depression. Earlier studies evaluating hippocampal and amygdalar measures grouped these structures together, because it was not possible to define the exact anatomical separation. A recent study of unipolar major depression demonstrated a volume reduction in core nuclei in the amygdala in the absence of a reduction in the total volume of the amygdala. In bipolar disorder, two studies demonstrated amygdalar enlargement, whereas others studies confirmed a decrease or no change. The anterior portion of the superior temporal gyrus was enlarged in one study of bipolar disorder; however, volumetric differences were not seen in other subregions, including the planum temporale or the Heschl's gyrus. Of note, hippocampal and amygdalar abnormalities in depressed patients occurred in the absence of volumetric changes in the temporal lobes, suggesting that anatomical abnormalities may be restricted to the mesial temporal lobe.

Decreased putaminal and caudate volumes have been reported in unipolar depression. In contrast, increased caudate and putaminal volumes have been reported by some, but not all, studies of bipolar disorder. With regard to affective disorders, thalamic volume data are also mixed, with some studies reporting an increase, whereas others reported a decrease or no change. Volumetric reductions have been reported in the cerebellum and the vermis in affective disorders, particularly in familial bipolar disorder. One study showed unipolar depressed subjects had larger pituitary volumes, although this finding was not reflected in subsequent studies. On the other hand, bipolar disorder was associated with decreased pituitary volume. The finding of subcortical white matter hyperintensities on T2-weighted sMRI in late-life depression has received increasing attention. The term *vascular depression* has been coined to distinguish subjects with late-onset depression from early-onset mood changes.

Despite the various structural changes observed in mood disorders, it is not clear whether a focal brain abnormality is central to the

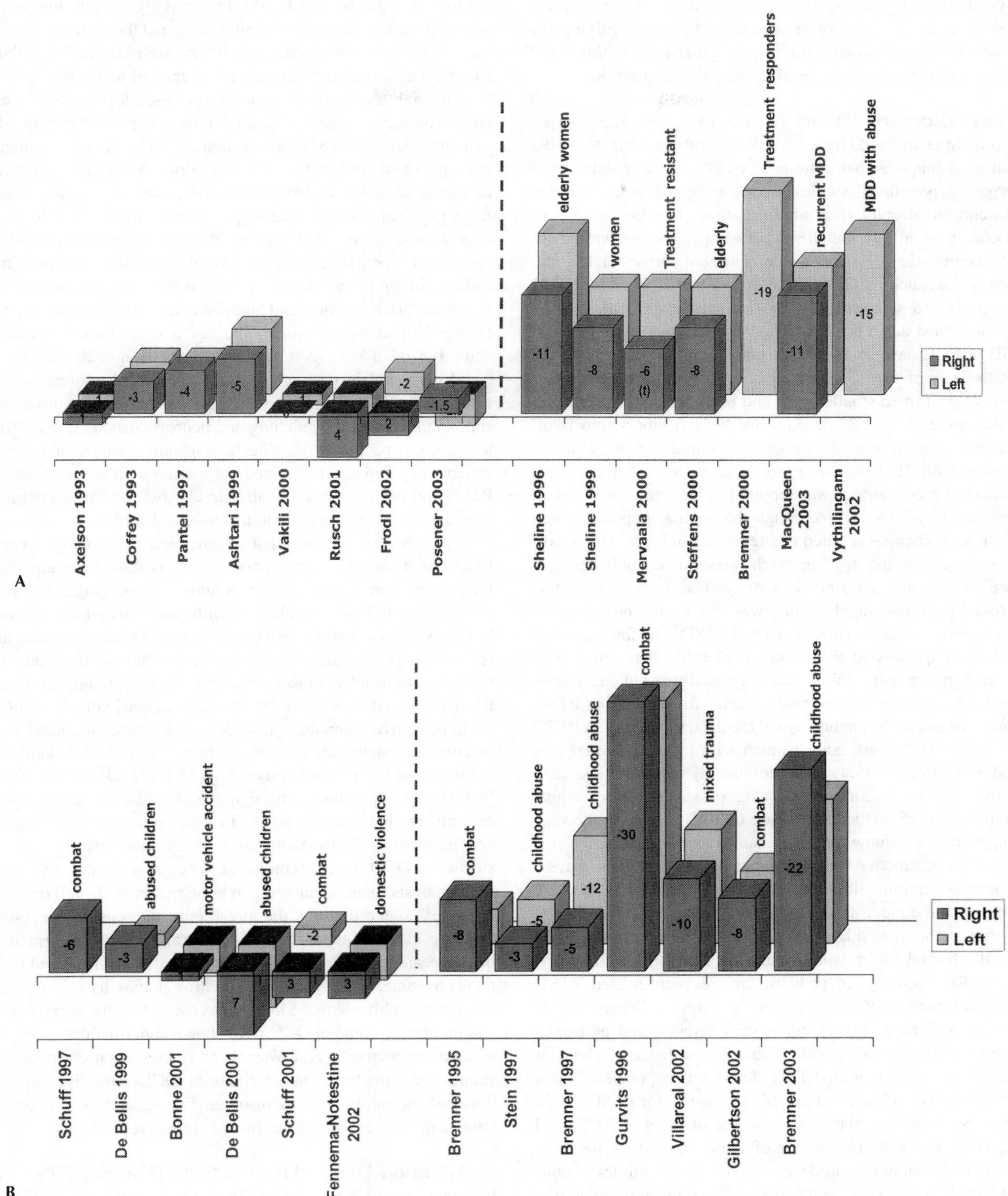

FIGURE 1.15–7 Depicts the percentage difference in hippocampal volume between patients and controls. Hippocampal volume findings using structural magnetic resonance imaging studies in unipolar major depressive disorder (MDD) **(A)** and posttraumatic stress disorder (PTSD) **(B)** are mixed. Studies on the left of the dotted line demonstrate no significant differences between groups, whereas the studies on the right confirm a significant reduction in left and/or right hippocampal volume in MDD and PTSD, respectively. Clinical characteristics, including frequency and duration of depression, treatment response, early childhood trauma, age, and gender, contribute to variable findings in MDD, whereas type and frequency of trauma, subtype of trauma, and comorbid disorders contribute to the variability in PTSD.

pathophysiology of depression. It is also unclear whether these morphometric changes are primary or secondary to the underlying illness. Prospective morphometric studies of high-risk populations and twin studies will help clarify some of the remaining questions.

Anxiety Disorders Of the various anxiety disorders, structural abnormalities in PTSD have been extensively investigated. MRI investigation of hippocampal volume in PTSD was stimulated by a large corpus of preclinical studies reporting hippocampal neuronal loss and dendritic atrophy after administration of hydrocortisone or psychosocial stress in rats. Smaller hippocampal volume was attributed to the neurotoxic effects of elevated levels of cortisol and excitatory amino acids, such as Glu release during stress. Because PTSD follows exposure to an overwhelming traumatic event that involves actual or threatened death or serious injury, researchers hypothesized that PTSD patients have smaller hippocampal volume because of the neurotoxic effects of stress. As anticipated, early studies of combat-related PTSD confirmed smaller right and bilateral hippocampal volumes in the range of 5 to 26 percent. Smaller left hippocampal volume was also reported in adult women with childhood sexual abuse and in women with PTSD secondary to childhood sexual abuse, and a smaller bilateral hippocampus was reported in men and women with mixed trauma (Fig. 1.15–7B). Although the popular hypothesis was that stress-related changes resulted in a reduction in hippocampal volume, "the chicken or the egg" research question has only recently been clarified in a monozygotic twin study. The findings from this study reveal that hippocampal volume was smaller in untraumatized monozygotic twins if their twin siblings had PTSD. The findings from this novel study questioned the causal relationship between trauma and smaller hippocampal volume and suggested that smaller hippocampal volume could be a predisposing factor for developing PTSD after trauma. To add to the conundrum of the data, subjects with PTSD secondary to the Holocaust, adult women with intimate partner violence, and a longitudinal study in predominantly motor vehicle accident victims did not confirm the finding of smaller hippocampal volume reported in prior studies. Because only 40 percent of the variance in hippocampal volume was attributable to genetic influence, it is possible that the interaction between genes and environment plays a crucial role in determining the sinus of the hippocampus.

In contrast to the majority of studies in adults with PTSD, sMRI abnormalities in children with PTSD are mainly restricted to the cerebrum and the frontal lobes, whereas the hippocampus is normal. A series of studies focusing on pediatric maltreatment-related PTSD repeatedly confirmed smaller volume of the corpus callosum and its subregions as well as a smaller intracranial cerebral and prefrontal cortex despite normal hippocampal volume. The absence of a smaller hippocampus in children with PTSD defies the hypothesis that a smaller hippocampal volume is a reliable risk factor for PTSD. Brain volume was positively correlated with the age of onset of PTSD and negatively correlated with the duration of abuse, suggesting that there are brain maturational and neurodevelopmental abnormalities in children with PTSD secondary to maltreatment. The only adult report that supports frontal cortical and cerebral abnormalities came from a recent study of adult women with PTSD secondary to intimate partner violence in which, despite normal hippocampal volume, PTSD subjects had a smaller supratentorial cranial vault and smaller frontal and occipital gray matter volume as compared with abused women without PTSD. Cranial vault volume was negatively correlated with severity of childhood physical abuse, but no correlation was seen with PTSD after adulthood trauma, thus supporting a neurodevelopmental etiology for this observation. Recent sMRI studies revealed a focal reduction in the volume of the anterior cingulate cortex, particularly the left, in patients with PTSD. Interestingly, despite the prominent role of the amygdala in fear conditioning and the increased activity of the amygdala in functional neuroimaging PTSD studies, volumetric structural abnormalities have not been reported in this region.

Although nonstandard methodologies used for the aforementioned brain volumetric analysis could, in part, explain the contradictory structural data on PTSD, various trauma, clinical, and treatment variables may also contribute to the conundrum. For example, differences in trauma variables, including mode of trauma (e.g., sexual abuse and rape, physical abuse, witnessing violence, motor vehicle accident, combat, and victim of mugging), duration of trauma (repeated episodes over a period of years vs. a single episode), severity of trauma, and the timing of trauma with regard to development (prepubertal vs. postpubertal), may confound analysis and decrease the ability to generalize hippocampal volume findings across studies. Additionally, comorbid disorders, such as major depression with alcohol abuse, could also explain the variance in hippocampal volume. Moreover, antidepressants may contribute to hippocampal volume differences by stimulating dendritic branching and neurogenesis. Future sMRI studies that prospectively evaluate homogenous groups of traumatized patients exposed to similar kinds of trauma with and without current PTSD and healthy subjects will help clarify the relative contributions of genetics and environment to this unique disorder.

It appears that hippocampal volume reduction could be specific to PTSD, as it was not seen in another anxiety disorder: panic disorder. Despite smaller temporal lobe volumes, hippocampal volume was within normal limits in subjects with panic disorders compared to healthy subjects. A single MRI study in social phobia revealed an age-related smaller putamenal volume in patients with social phobias compared to healthy subjects. However, there were no significant differences in total cerebral and subcortical regional volume. sMRI studies in obsessive-compulsive disorder (OCD) have attempted to detect whether volumetric changes in the front subcortical thalamic circuit are implicated in the pathophysiology of OCD. Decreased total cerebral white matter volume and significantly greater total cerebral cortical volumes have been reported in subjects with OCD compared to healthy subjects. Furthermore, left orbital frontal cortical regions were smaller in OCD patients compared to controls. A recent voxel-based MRI analysis found an increase in brain matter in the left orbital frontal cortex, suggesting that the global reduction could be a result of a decrease in white matter density. Abnormalities in the striatum have been repeatedly confirmed with reduction in the caudate and the putamenal volume, although several control studies have not replicated this finding. Other single MRI studies evaluating the corpus callosum and pituitary volume in OCD have shown abnormalities in length and volume, respectively. However, these studies require replication. To summarize, structural abnormalities in OCD partially mirror functional abnormalities in this disorder. Future studies evaluating thalamic and other regions of the frontal cortex are warranted.

Attention-Deficit/Hyperactivity Disorder The NIMH has conducted sMRI studies evaluating brain maturational changes in a large cohort of healthy children and children with attention-deficit/hyperactivity disorder (ADHD). The normal trajectory of brain development shows increased cortical gray and white matter volumes from 5 years of age, with a peak at approximately 12 to 15 years of age. These volumes decrease in later adolescence, presumably reflecting pruning of synaptic connections, programmed neuronal loss, and decreased white matter connections. From early onset, ADHD is associated with slightly smaller (4 percent) total brain volume, affecting gray and white matter regions. The only exception to this small, but widespread, loss is a striking (15 percent) decrease in the volume of the posterior inferior cerebellar vermis. Prospective studies in ADHD over several years with serial sMRI acquisitions demonstrated that the overall trajectory of brain development was essentially parallel to that of healthy subjects but slightly lower. This parallel trajectory of brain development was seen in drug-treated and untreated patients, suggesting that the ADHD-related abnormalities are fixed, nonprogressive, and unrelated to stimulant treatment.

FUNCTIONAL MRI

fMRI refers to a class of measures in which MRI technology is applied to noninvasively assess neurophysiology in terms of regional hemodynamic parameters. By imaging local changes in hemodynamic activity, fMRI enables delineation of the neuroanatomical correlates of various mental processes. Because fMRI permits measures at higher spatial and temporal resolution than can be achieved using PET and obviates the need for radiation exposure, the majority of tomographic, human brain mapping studies are now performed using fMRI rather than PET.

Susceptibility Contrast Based fMRI Of the various fMRI techniques developed for investigating neurophysiology, imaging changes in the bulk magnetic susceptibility parameter of blood during neuronal activation is currently the method most commonly applied in human brain mapping studies. The volume magnetic susceptibility of a substance is the measure (dimensionless) of the extent to which that substance modifies the strength of a magnetic field strength passing through it. The magnetic susceptibility of blood results from the distortion of the magnetic field (B_0) by the small fraction of paramagnetic iron atoms present in deoxyhemoglobin in resting state blood, which alters T2* over blood vessels. Oxygenated hemoglobin, in contrast, is isomagnetic, so the susceptibility parameter of blood decreases as the oxyhemoglobin to deoxyhemoglobin ratio increases. Increases in oxygen saturation are consequently evidenced by elevations in the MR signal intensity (T2*) in the vicinity of the affected blood vessel. This sensitivity of T2*-weighted images (commonly acquired using echo-planar or spiral imaging pulse sequences) to variations in the oxygen saturation of blood affords the opportunity to map changes in neuronal activation via the blood oxygenation level–dependent (BOLD) signal.

When neuronal activity increases during physiological activation, the local CBF, cerebral blood volume (CBV), and cerebral oxygen use also increase. The relationships between these parameters are complex, however. The proportionate magnitude of increase is much greater for CBF than for CBV, although these changes are directly related. In contrast, during the initial minutes after activation, glucose use and oxygen use become uncoupled, and CBF—which remains coupled to glucose metabolism—increases at a greater rate than oxygen metabolism. This rapid, initial elevation of CBF increases the amount of oxyhemoglobin supplied to the tissue at a rate exceeding that of the concomitant elevation in oxygen extraction. Consequently, the local oxyhemoglobin to deoxyhemoglobin ratio increases, resulting in an elevation of the BOLD signal.

Temporal Resolution of fMRI The hemodynamic response to increasing neuronal activity lags the onset of the associated electrophysiological activity by approximately 500 milliseconds and persists for a few seconds beyond the cessation of neuronal electrical activity. Although this temporal resolution is inadequate to delineate network dynamics in real time (which requires the millisecond resolution afforded by electroencephalography or magnetoencephalography), it is high enough to permit imaging of neural responses to single events. The temporal course of the BOLD signal also permits repeated imaging of the same event during a single scan session. Repeated measurement of changes in the BOLD (ΔBOLD) parameter between experimental and control tasks is critical to the design of fMRI studies to achieve an adequate signal to noise ratio, because the magnitude of the ΔBOLD response is relatively small (ranging from a fraction of a percent to a few percent) and variable (within and across subjects).

The types of tasks that lend themselves particularly well to this type of design involve sensorimotor and cognitive operations that can be repeatedly performed without the occurrence of significant habituation or alteration of the underlying neural activity over the testing period. In contrast, mental events that cannot be initiated and discontinued in a rapid and controlled manner are less well suited for BOLD signal imaging. Examples of the latter include emotional provocation using contemplation of sad or traumatic memories, which elicit emotional states that cannot be rapidly terminated in a controlled manner.

Nevertheless, even in the case of neural responses that are known to habituate during repeated stimulation, the time course of habituation may be slow enough to permit repeated, reliable measurement of the ΔBOLD response. Serial imaging can be exploited to investigate the biphasic neural response during habituation, in terms of the rate at which the initial, positive ΔBOLD response attenuates and then becomes increasingly negative during repeated stimulation. For example, such a design has been used to demonstrate differential rates of extinction of the neural responses to aversively conditioned stimuli (measured during repeated exposure to a conditioned stimulus without reinforcement by the unconditioned, aversive stimulus) in the amygdala, prefrontal cortex, and temporal lobe visual association cortices. Investigating rates of habituation to emotionally salient stimuli may prove fruitful in assessing the capability for modulating emotional responses in anxiety and mood disorders.

The duration of the BOLD response to single events can be studied to elucidate the temporal characteristics of neural activity during cognitive processing. For example, tasks requiring working memory have been shown to result in prolonged BOLD signal increases in dorsolateral prefrontal cortex (PFC) areas of humans that appear homologous to areas at which sustained neuronal firing activity has been demonstrated in depth electrode studies of comparable working memory tasks in monkeys.

Measuring the duration of the BOLD response may prove fruitful in studies of psychopathology as well. For example, the duration of the amygdala's hemodynamic response to sadly valenced words was shown to persist for several seconds longer in major depressives relative to healthy controls. This finding was associated with differential activity between depressives and controls in PFC regions thought to modulate emotional thought and experience.

Other Limitations of Susceptibility Contrast Imaging Partly because the BOLD signal constitutes a complex hemodynamic parameter reflecting a combination of local CBF, CBV, and oxygen extraction, the BOLD signal fluctuates across relatively short time periods in association with a variety of nonspecific physiological and technical factors. The measurement of the basal or resting BOLD effect is thus unstable and has not proven useful for reliable quantitation of resting physiology. The sensitivity for detecting ΔBOLD instead depends on comparing images in experimental versus control conditions that are acquired within the same, few-minute epoch. Moreover, the reproducibility of the ΔBOLD response within individuals across separate days has not been well established, so the usefulness of treating ΔBOLD responses as trait-like biomarkers of neural responsiveness that can be meaningfully associated with temperament or genotype remains unclear.

The elevation of CBF and metabolism during neuronal activity predominantly occurs in the terminal projection fields of activated neurons, because it is largely influenced by energy use during synaptic transmission and only slightly by energy use within cell bodies. The CBF increase accompanying terminal field synaptic activity primarily occurs in the local capillaries and arterioles supplying the involved tissue, rather than at the levels of the larger arteries and veins. The true localizing capability for imaging neuronal activity in terms of changes in local hemodynamic activity depends, therefore, on detection of changes in CBF and oxygen extraction within local arteriolar and capillary beds supplying the activated tissue. However, because the BOLD signal reflects oxygen saturation of blood rather than CBF or oxygen use per se, the ΔBOLD signal is also evident (and generally most prominent) in the larger veins draining a region. This effect shifts the spatial location of the centroid of the area of BOLD signal change toward the larger draining vein and away from the relevant capillary bed. The spatial location of the hemodynamic correlate of neural activity obtained using CBF imaging has thus been shown to differ by as much as 1 cm from that obtained using BOLD imaging. The impact of this draining vein effect on the spatial information obtained from BOLD contrast imaging can be reduced by altering some MR image acquisition parameters.

Another limitation of susceptibility and contrast-based fMRI has been that the MR signal obtained using T2*-weighted images is also sensitive to other sources of magnetic susceptibility. One of the most problematic artifacts in these images has been the susceptibility artifact associated with air in the bony sinuses of the skull (e.g., sphenoid sinus), which markedly attenuates the MR signal in the orbitofrontal cortex, ventromedial PFC, and basotemporal cortex. The extent of MR signal dropout from such susceptibility artifacts worsens as the magnetic field strength of the MRI scanner increases.

MRI-Based Perfusion Imaging Because imaging CBF alone could potentially provide measures of neural activation characterized by having a greater magnitude of change and a higher spatial accuracy (i.e., freedom from draining vein and signal susceptibility artifacts) than BOLD contrast imaging, a variety of MR methods have been developed to image perfusion. Unfortunately, these methods have thus far proven less useful than BOLD contrast imaging for brain mapping studies, because their signal to noise ratio and temporal resolution have been inferior to that of BOLD imaging. Nevertheless, some of these techniques have proven useful in clinical and research applications that require information about vascular perfusion. One type of perfusion imaging that is in widespread clinical use to provide MRI-based visualization of the cerebral vasculature involves intravenous (IV) infusion of paramagnetic contrast agents, such as gadolinium.

For research applications aimed at quantitating regional CBF at higher spatial resolution, some promising techniques involve arterial spin labeling or tagging. This method uses a surface coil to continuously label arterial spins, while a standard head coil is used to transmit and receive RF signals. The quantitative accuracy of arterial spin tagging measures of CBF have been validated against PET-$H_2{}^{15}O$ measures of CBF. Although the temporal resolution of this technique (which requires approximately 10 minutes for multislice image acquisition) is inadequate for most brain mapping studies, arterial spin labeling appears particularly useful for measurement of baseline physiology.

This type of imaging may prove particularly useful for measuring basal differences in resting CBF in psychiatric disorders. For example, PET measures of resting CBF and glucose metabolism were abnormal in the amygdala, the anterior and posterior cingulate cortex, the ventral striatum, the medial thalamus, and multiple areas of the prefrontal cortex during the depressed phase of some subtypes of primary mood disorders (for example, the major depressive disorder melancholic subtype, the depressed phase of bipolar disorder, and familial pure depressive disease). In the amygdala, the magnitude of the abnormal elevation of flow and metabolism in these groups, measured using PET, ranged from 5 to 7 percent. When corrected for the relatively low spatial resolution (i.e., partial volume effects) of PET, this difference would reflect an increase in the actual CBF and metabolism of 50 to 70 percent. These magnitudes are in the physiological range, as CBF increases approximately 50 percent in the rat amygdala during exposure to fear-conditioned stimuli, as measured by tissue autoradiography. Because MRI-based perfusion imaging using arterial spin labeling can be performed at high spatial resolution (e.g., as voxels 3 to 4 mm in all orthogonal planes), it may be possible to identify differences between depressives and controls at magnitudes closer to this putative, physiological difference.

Technical Issues Related to Image Analysis Strategies The precision of anatomical localization in fMRI images has been enhanced by progressive improvements in spatial resolution (to <1 mm for high-resolution fMRI), techniques for co-registering functional images to higher-resolution anatomical images, and statistical mapping methods that delimit inherent physiological differences between patients and controls. However, in most studies, the fMRI images are blurred (by filtering) to a lower spatial resolution before analysis to enhance signal to noise ratio or to reduce the effects of anatomical variability across subjects, or both. This practice reduces the capability for resolving hemodynamic changes in small structures of interest.

The method for detecting differences in regional physiology between groups or conditions also influences type II error (i.e., the sensitivity for detecting true differences). The more anatomically precise techniques involve ROI analysis in which ROI are predefined on each subject's own anatomical MRI image and then transferred to co-registered, lower-resolution fMRI images. This approach can, nevertheless, miss an intergroup difference that is not located within the ROI and can excessively dilute an intergroup difference if the ROI defined is excessively large. Voxel-by-voxel approaches (e.g., SPM) were thus developed to survey entire data sets and to localize peak, inherent differences between conditions. These approaches, nevertheless, reduce sensitivity for detecting abnormalities in structures that are small (e.g., amygdala) or characterized by a high degree of anatomical variability (e.g., orbital cortex), because they depend on spatial transformation of the primary images into a standardized stereotaxic space using algorithms that do not precisely align small structures or variable gyral patterns across subjects. To reduce the effects of this misalignment error, images are blurred (filtered) before analysis to a lower spatial resolution, sacrificing the spatial resolution advantage of fMRI over PET. Some state-of-the-art image analysis approaches apply principles from ROI and voxel-by-voxel analyses by constraining the voxel-by-voxel search to voxels located within an ROI that has been anatomically predefined in the native image (i.e., avoiding the alignment imprecision and blurring involved in stereotaxic transformation).

Because of the extremely large number of independent measurements obtained within each fMRI image, the assignment of statistical significance to apparent differences between conditions poses a major challenge to data analysis. For example, voxel-by-voxel approaches typically compute thousands (or even hundreds of thousands) of independent statistical comparisons per image set, yielding a high probability that an apparent difference between groups or conditions reflects multiple comparison artifacts. The significance of findings must therefore be established by applying appropriate corrections of *P* values for multiple comparisons or by replication in independent samples.

Interpreting Changes in Local Hemodynamic Activity in fMRI Studies Local CBF and glucose metabolism predominantly reflect a summation of the metabolic activity associated with terminal field synaptic transmission within each image volume element or voxel. Elevated regional CBF, metabolism, or BOLD contrast may thus signify increased neurotransmission from afferent projections arising from within the same structure or from a distal structure. Conversely, reductions in these physiological parameters may reflect a decrease in afferent transmission (e.g., due to inhibitory transmission at upstream synapses). Dynamic brain images may thus provide maps of regional neural function associated with ongoing mental activity. Metabolic and CBF images are also affected by the integrity of the cerebrovascular system, the amount of viable gray matter within an image voxel, and other factors that may be abnormal in some psychiatric disorders. Differences in CBF or metabolic images between psychiatrically ill subjects and controls may therefore reflect the neurophysiological correlates of emotional, behavioral, or cognitive symptoms associated with an illness episode; the pathophysiological changes that predispose to or result from recurrent disease; or the compensatory mechanisms invoked to modulate or inhibit psychopathological processes.

The physiological correlates of ongoing psychiatric symptoms and behaviors putatively appear as abnormalities of local CBF or metabolism that normalize after effective treatment and that may, to some extent, be reproduced in healthy subjects imaged while performing tasks that mimic the corresponding clinical manifestation. Neuroimaging abnormalities in psychopathology may alternatively reflect pathophysiological changes in synaptic transmission associated with altered neurotransmitter synthesis, receptor sensitivity and binding, or neuronal arborization. Such defects may, in some cases, be evident as trait-like abnormalities that persist whether subjects are symptomatic or asymptomatic. Irreversible abnormalities in CBF and metabolism have been associated with gray matter volume reductions in familial mood disorders or cerebrovascular disease in elderly depressives with a late age of depression onset.

Effect of Behavioral State and Basal Metabolism on Hemodynamic Response Because of the sensitivity of CBF, metabolism, and BOLD contrast to changes in neural activity, the behavioral state in which subjects are imaged profoundly influences functional imaging data. The ability to detect differences between depressives and controls is thus dependent on the behavioral state under which image data are acquired. For example, some limbic and paralimbic regions, including the amygdala, ventromedial prefrontal cortex, lateral orbital cortex, and posterior cingulate cortex normally deactivate (seen as a dynamic, reduction in CBF and BOLD) during performance of tasks demanding attention. Interpreting differential changes in CBF or metabolism between patients and controls in association with performing experimental tasks is thus specific to the experimental and control tasks under which subjects were imaged. Moreover, the neural response to both conditions is influenced by the basal or resting neurophysiological state.

When basal neuronal activity is already increased in a region because of the pathophysiology associated with a psychiatric illness or symptom, mental operations that would further activate the same neuronal fields are expected to result in an attenuated metabolic, CBF, and BOLD response. Knowledge about differences in basal CBF or glucose metabolism between psychiatric and control samples thus becomes critical to interpreting differences in the BOLD response obtained during performance of a neuropsychological task. For example, in the left amygdala, the hemodynamic response to viewing fearful faces (relative to viewing smiling or neutral faces) was blunted in depressed children and depressed adults relative to age-matched controls. This finding was consistent with the elevation of basal CBF and glucose metabolism seen in the *left* amygdala in such cases (as was demonstrated using PET in the adult depressives). As a noteworthy contrast, fMRI studies of PTSD—in which the basal amygdalar CBF or metabolism has not been found to differ between depressives and controls—found exaggerated hemodynamic responses in the amygdala in PTSD subjects relative to trauma-matched, non-PTSD controls during exposure to pictures of fearful faces presented using a backward masking technique.

Effects of Structural Abnormalities in Functional Brain Images The neuromorphological abnormalities seen in the sMRI images of some psychiatric disorders can also influence functional imaging measures. The tissue reductions reflected by ventricular and sulcal enlargement and the reductions in some lobar or gyral volumes in depressives who are elderly with a late age-of-depression onset, bipolar, or psychotic decrease the magnitude of tomographic measures from the corresponding regions via *partial volume averaging* effects. This problem diminishes as spatial resolution of the image data increases. Nevertheless, because the cortex is normally only 3 to 4 mm thick, reductions in the proportion of gray matter relative to CSF or white matter, or both, within corresponding image voxels reduce the measured physiological signal via partial volume averaging effects in standard-resolution fMRI images (which are generally filtered to spatial resolutions of ≥7 mm). By adding greater contributions from CSF, which is metabolically inactive, or white matter, which is one-fourth as metabolically active as gray matter and which shows a negligible change in CBF and metabolism during neuronal activation, relative to a diminished contribution of gray matter, cortical thinning can reduce BOLD responses measured over the affected area. Evidence that focal areas of reduced gray matter volume exist in some psychiatric disorders emphasizes the importance of considering such abnormalities as a source of difference in the ΔBOLD signal observed between ill and control samples.

For example, basal glucose metabolism and CBF were shown to be abnormally decreased in the dorsomedial or dorsal anterolateral prefrontal cortex and the ACC ventral to the corpus callosum (i.e., subgenual ACC) in PET studies of depressed subjects with major depressive disorder. In most studies, these abnormalities did not normalize during effective antidepressant drug treatment. These persistent deficits in metabolism were associated with a reduction in gray matter volume in morphometric MRI and postmortem neuropathological studies of clinically similar individuals. Neuropsychological tasks that involve processing of emotional stimuli or memories activate these regions in dynamic PET and fMRI studies of healthy subjects. In contrast, remitted major depressive disorder subjects showed an abnormal blunting of the ΔBOLD signals obtained in these regions during the same emotional tasks, which could conceivably be accounted for by the histopathological abnormalities reported in this cortex or by partial volume effects of the reduction in gray matter.

Applications of fMRI in Psychiatric Research fMRI research holds great promise for elucidating the pathophysiology of psychiatric disorders that have been associated with disruptions of brain function, based on neurochemical, neuroendocrine, or neurophysiological data, or a combination of these, but that have also

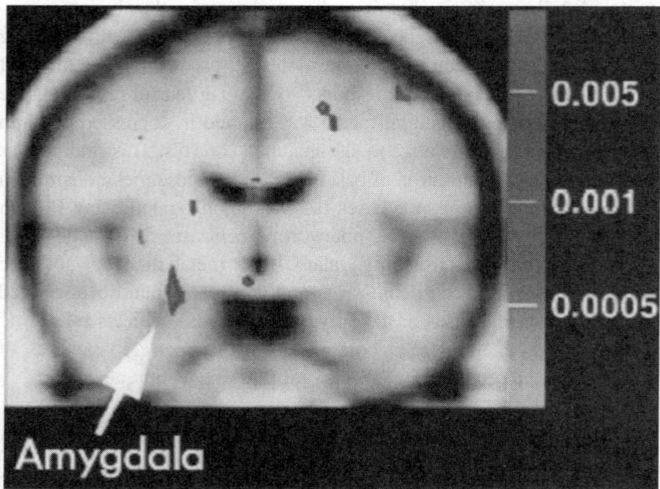

FIGURE 1.15–8 Statistical map of functional magnetic resonance imaging (fMRI) blood oxygenation level–dependent signal intensity differences demonstrating significantly increased activity in the right amygdala in subjects with posttraumatic stress disorder (PTSD) compared to traumatized subjects without PTSD. The response to masked, fearful faces in PTSD and non-PTSD group were compared after normalizing to masked, happy faces. fMRI data are displayed in Talairach template space and are co-registered with structural magnetic resonance imaging data. (See Color Plate.)

shown a relatively well-preserved, gross brain morphology, based on structural imaging and postmortem studies. The insights gained from fMRI studies of such conditions are already being used to elucidate the pathophysiology of mood, anxiety, psychotic, and addictive disorders and the mechanisms of psychopharmacological treatments for these conditions (Fig. 1.15–8). They may ultimately guide pathophysiology-based classification of psychiatric phenotypes for genetic and treatment outcome studies.

Psychiatric disorders that manifest a recurrent, episodic nature and responsiveness to treatment (e.g., mood and anxiety disorders arising in early to midlife) appear particularly tractable to fMRI studies, because they permit imaging in symptomatic and asymptomatic states. The physiological correlates of symptoms or state-related cognitive biases and emotional responses can be distinguished from the pathophysiological changes that may underlie the tendency to develop illness episodes. Moreover, because many symptoms of these disorders (e.g., depressed and anxious mood) reflect distortions of emotional states that can be expressed by healthy subjects, the nature of neurophysiological changes related to the pathological emotional state can be explored by imaging healthy subjects during experimentally induced sadness or anxiety.

In contrast, some other psychiatric conditions are less well suited for application of some fMRI techniques. For example, depression arising secondary to cerebrovascular disease presents serious problems for studies assessing BOLD contrast, because varying degrees of cerebrovascular involvement of tissue alter the relationships between CBF, CBV, and oxygen extraction in complex ways, potentially confounding interpretation of abnormalities in the ΔBOLD signal. This problem appears to extend to depressives whose age-at-illness onset is older than 55 years of age, who are highly likely to exhibit more numerous and extensive MR signal hyperintensities in the deep and periventricular white matter in T2-weighted structural images compared to age-matched, healthy controls or age-matched, early-onset depressives. Tissue acquired postmortem from subjects manifesting patch- and cap-shaped areas of MR signal hyperintensity consistently show arteriosclerosis, gliosis, white matter necrosis, and axon loss within the affected areas but not in surrounding tissue in which the MRI signal appears normal. Regional CBF is decreased in the areas at which patches or large caps of white matter hyperintensity (WMH) are evident in MR images. The personal and family risk factors for developing such WMH patches and late-onset depression are risk factors for cerebrovascular disease, and the left frontal cortical areas at which infarction has been associated with an increased risk of major depression are the areas most commonly affected by WMH in late-onset major depressive disorder. Such cases must be studied separately from early-onset cases in a variety of neuroimaging studies, because cerebrovascular disease profoundly alters the relationships between CBF, metabolism, oxygen extraction, and hemodynamic regulation.

Psychotropic Drug Effects on fMRI A variety of psychotropic drugs are also expected to influence hemodynamic parameters, potentially confounding the results of fMRI studies. For example, CBF and metabolism can be reduced by acute and chronic administration of benzodiazepine receptor agonists and antipsychotic drugs. In addition, agents that affect vascular tone may alter CBV, especially in the venous blood pool. Furthermore, chronic treatment with antidepressant, antipsychotic, and antianxiety drugs exerts regionally specific effects on CBF, metabolism, or neuronal activity, or a combination of these, in prefrontal cortical or limbic areas of interest that cannot be factored out simply by applying global scaling. Consequently, studying subjects in a condition in which they are medication free (for a period long enough to avoid treatment withdrawal effects) becomes critical to the design of experiments involving psychiatric subjects.

fMRI studies can conversely be designed to investigate neurophysiological effects of psychotropic treatments. By imaging before and during treatment, the effects of psychotropic drugs on basal perfusion or hemodynamic responses to sensory and cognitive events can be characterized. For example, chronic treatment with a variety of antidepressant drugs reduces the abnormal elevation of amygdala CBF and metabolism in major depressive disorder toward normal, an effect that is expected to be robust in images acquired using arterial spin labeling. Moreover, the amygdala's hemodynamic response to emotionally valenced stimuli (e.g., fearful faces) has been shown to be markedly attenuated in major depressive disorder subjects after chronic antidepressant drug treatment.

Application of fMRI in Clinical Psychiatry In contrast to the use of fMRI in research applications, the clinical capabilities of these tools for guiding diagnostic or treatment decisions have not been established. The abnormalities identified by imaging studies of depression have thus far lacked effect sizes sufficient to provide sensitive and specific discrimination of individual patients from healthy subjects or from subjects with other illnesses. It remains unclear whether MRI techniques for high-resolution perfusion imaging may ultimately identify abnormalities that can sensitively and specifically classify individual patients.

MRS

The phenomenon known as *chemical shift* allows detection of different nuclei, as well as differentiation of the same nuclei in different chemical environments. Unlike MRI, in which the resonance frequency of dominant water protons is detected, MRS detects signals as much as 10,000 to 100,000 times less concentrated, allowing noninvasive assay of specific, biologically relevant molecules in vivo.

Hence, MRS is widely appreciated as a method of noninvasive biopsy. However, because metabolite concentrations are typically low, the voxel size in MRS is usually approximately 1 mL or larger for ^{1}H MRS. Much larger volume elements are necessary for other nuclei (often referred to as *X nuclei*). Therefore, MRS studies are limited to the examination of relatively large regions of tissue.

The most interesting nuclei for psychiatric research using MRS are ^{1}H, phosphorus-31 (^{31}P), fluorine-19 (^{19}F), and lithium-7 (^{7}Li). Recent improvement in carbon-13 (^{13}C) MRS methods also makes it possible to study ^{13}C-enriched metabolites in psychiatric disorders. Although the number of relevant nuclei is limited, a wealth of information is available, because, often, a large number of molecules can be detected simultaneously for each type of nucleus. ^{1}H MRS allows detection of a number of important metabolites and amino acid neurotransmitters. ^{31}P MRS provides information about energetically important phosphorus-containing metabolites and intracellular pH. ^{19}F and ^{7}Li MRS can be used in vivo to monitor the pharmacokinetics of certain drugs. ^{13}C MRS offers the possibility to study instability in important metabolic pathways, such as the tricarboxylic acid (TCA) cycle, as well as the Glu-Gln cycle between neurons and astrocytes.

The basic principles of MRS are similar to those of MRI. Bulk magnetization detected in an ensemble of spins in a magnetic field represents the change between RF energy absorption and T1 and T2 relaxations, this concept being identical for MRS and MRI. However, there are two marked differences between MRS and MRI. First, unlike MRI, which uses relaxation to generate intensity contrasts, relaxation effects (T1, T2, or T2* weighting) are avoided as much as possible in MRS, because relaxation effects distort the true concentration of metabolites and therefore should be minimized whenever possible. Second, MRS signals are detected in the absence of a gradient pulse. All molecules are detected in the presence of the same base magnetic field B_0 from the magnet. Ideally, the chemical shift should be the only source of magnetic field variations present during signal acquisition.

For multiple reasons, MRS faces more stringent technical requirements than does MRI. Because the differences in resonant frequencies caused by chemical shifts are small, MRS requires a much greater temporal and spatial uniformity in the applied magnetic field. Furthermore, the external magnetic field used in MRS tends to be of greater strength (e.g., 1.5 to 4.0 T). The greater field strength increases the frequency separation between spectral peaks. Although not universally true, MRS measures are generally enhanced at higher field strength. This enhancement is often essential for detection of dilute metabolites or for improvement of spatial resolution or sensitivity, or both. Furthermore, manufacturers of MR scanners usually provide only a few basic MRS sequences. As a result, time-consuming technical developments are often necessary for more advanced MRS studies.

Techniques used for basic spatial localization of the MRS signals are also derived from similar techniques used in MRI. In the same manner as in MRI, slice-selective excitation pulses, in conjunction with gradient pulses, are used to focus the RF pulses in the desired tissue slice.

There are two categories of localization methods that are based on the number of voxels from which MRS spectra are obtained in each measurement. The first category is the single voxel, or single volume method, that acquires spectra from a single small volume of tissue. The most common approaches collect signals from discrete tissue volumes at the intersection of three selected slices. Each RF pulse is applied using a different gradient for slice selection. Only magnetic nuclei located at the intersection of all three slices contribute to the observed signal. The second category is the multiple voxel technique from which multiple MRS spectra are acquired during each measurement. The most common of these methods is known as *chemical shift imaging* (CSI) or *SI*. *CSI* methods are similar to standard imaging techniques in that slice-selective and phase-encoding gradients are used for spatial localization. Unlike MRI, no readout gradient is used in CSI. Instead, two orthogonal phase-encoding gradients are used to label a particular in-slice frequency. Figure 1.15–9 shows an example of ^{1}H CSI.

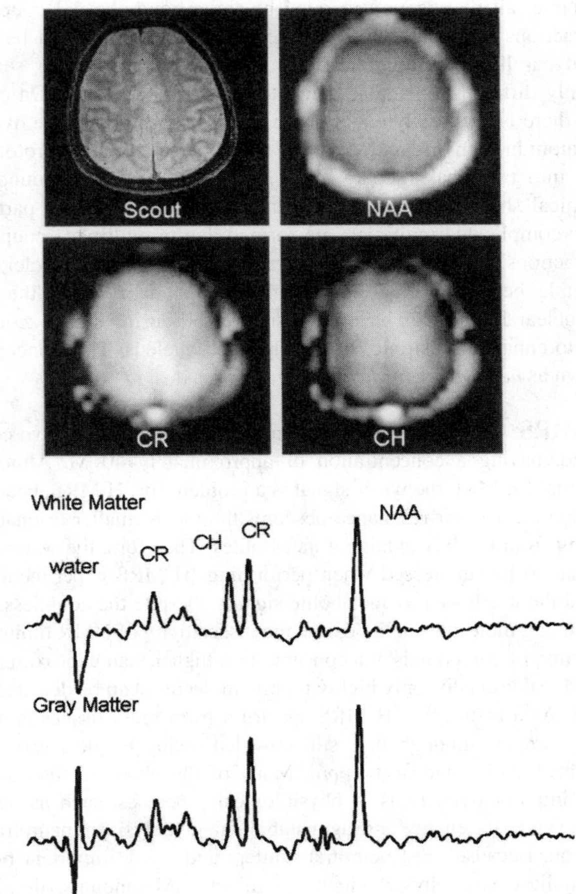

FIGURE 1.15–9 Hydrogen-1 (^{1}H) chemical shift imaging (CSI) and corresponding anatomical image and ^{1}H spectra from two pixels located in the white matter and gray matter, respectively. The CSI data were acquired with a spatial resolution of 0.5 mL. For each peak in the spectra, a chemical shift image can be generated. CH, choline-containing compounds; CR, creatine; NAA, *N*-acetylaspartate. (From Shen J, Rothman DL, Hetherington HP, et al.: Linear projection method for automatic slice shimming. *Magn Reson Med.* 1999;42:1082, with permission.)

In addition to the chemical shift, there is another molecular interaction that modifies the environment of a nucleus. The local magnetic field of any nucleus is affected by the local magnetic field of any other nucleus located on the same molecule. In biological systems, the most common instance of this is facilitated electron bonding in the molecule and is known as *scalar coupling* or *J coupling*. *J coupling* differs from the chemical shift in two significant ways: J coupling is independent of magnetic field strength, whereas spectral separation caused by chemical shifts increases linearly with B_0. Conversely, in the case of chemical shift, there is always another spin involved in the coupling. J coupling causes the MR signal of the coupled spins to be divided. The number of resultant signals and their relative amplitudes depends on the number of spins of each type. In principle, all hydrogens separated by three bonds have J coupling interactions between them. For one hydrogen atom, it can be oriented parallel or antiparallel to B_0. Its J coupling partner senses slightly different molecular magnetic fields in each case. On average, there is a virtually equal number of possibilities for the hydrogen atom in each orientation, so the signal detected for the protons is split into two peaks separated by a few Hz, centered around its chemical shift. If the proton has more than one coupling partner, more complicated multiplets are formed due to multiple J coupling interactions. There are also J couplings between heteronuclei; for example, between ^{1}H and ^{13}C or between ^{1}H and ^{31}P. Often, the heteronuclear J couplings have to be suppressed during signal acquisition to enhance sensitivity of the observed nucleus. This concept is known as *heteronuclear decoupling*.

^{1}H MRS Water is the most abundant ^{1}H-containing in vivo compound, having a concentration of approximately 40 M. Although essential for MRI, the water signal is a problem for ^{1}H MRS, because the dominant water resonance obscures the much smaller resonances arising from the ^{1}H-containing metabolites. Therefore, the water signal has to be suppressed when performing ^{1}H MRS experiments to reveal the much weaker metabolite signals. Despite the countless ^{1}H-containing molecules in the tissue, the insensitivity of NMR limits the detection of compounds at a concentration higher than approximately 1 mM. Additionally, only highly mobile molecules can be detected by MRS. As a result, the ^{1}H MRS spectrum from brain tissues is relatively simple, although it is still crowded owing to the narrow ^{1}H chemical shift range of 10 ppm. Many of the observed resonances have important functions in physiological processes, such as membrane synthesis, energy or drug metabolism, glycolysis, or neurotransmission. Because most neurotransmitters and many important brain metabolites exist physiologically in minute nM amounts, they are undetectable by MRS.

As shown in Figure 1.15–9, in ^{1}H NMR spectra of normal brain tissue, the most pronounced resonance originates from the methyl group of *N*-acetylaspartate (NAA) at 2 ppm (to a small degree, *N*-acetylaspartylglutamate and, possibly, *N*-acetylneuraminic acid). NAA is a relatively inactive amino acid derivative. Even though there is a substantial amount of literature on the synthesis, distribution, and possible function of NAA, the *exact* function of NAA remains a mystery. For in vivo ^{1}H MRS, because there is evidence that NAA is found almost exclusively in neurons and their processes with the highest concentrations in pyramidal Glu neurons, NAA resonance has been used as a neuronal marker. Furthermore, its concentration correlates well with neuronal density. It is absent when neurons die but persists in the brain for 24 hours postmortem. As a result, NAA is a nonspecific, but highly sensitive, marker of neuronal pathology. Virtually all conditions involving neuronal pathology that have been studied show changes in NAA signals in regions of brain pathology. Recent data have established that NAA reductions can reverse after various forms of brain damage and can change with clinical improvement and treatment.

In ^{1}H NMR spectra of normal brain tissue, the single Cr resonance at 3 ppm and 3.9 ppm arises from the methyl and methylene protons of Cr and phosphocreatine (PCr). The chemical difference between corresponding protons in Cr and PCr is indiscernible at field strengths available in the current clinical realm. Therefore, measures reflect total Cr (tCr). tCr concentration is relatively constant over time. It is often used as an internal standard for quantitation of other metabolites.

Most of the Cho in the brain is in the form of the membrane phospholipid phosphatidylcholine, but major contributors to the Cho peak in a ^{1}H MRS spectrum come from the mobile phosphorylcholine (PC) and glycerophosphorylcholine (GPC). Cho itself is below MRS visibility in normal brain tissue. Only a small portion of the Cho signal arises from acetylcholine. Because there are a number of resonances contributing to the observed signal, Cho is often referred to as *Cho-containing compounds*. In vivo ^{1}H MRS spectra do not distinguish the different Cho compounds because of the small chemical shift differences relative to line width. Together, they form a single sharp line at 3.2 ppm. Cho-containing compounds are involved in pathways of phospholipid synthesis and degradation, therefore reflecting membrane turnover. In pathological conditions associated with membrane turnover, or gliosis, the Cho peak tends to be elevated.

Glu is the major excitatory neurotransmitter in the central nervous system (CNS) that can be found in all brain cell types, although the concentration is the highest in neurons. Glutamine (Gln) is mostly found in astrocytes. Glu and Gln are involved in glutamatergic neurotransmission through the Glu-Gln cycle between neurons and surrounding astrocytes. The ^{1}H MRS spectrum of Glu and Gln is entirely composed of J-coupled resonances. Collectively, they are often referred to as *Glx*, because, at magnetic field strengths available in clinical studies, Glu and Gln overlap with each other at all resonant positions. Moreover, their ^{1}H spectra appear different in different echo times and different field strengths. These factors make their observation and quantification difficult with ^{1}H MRS. The minute concentrations, as well as the metabolic fluxes involving Glu and Gln, are best studied using ^{13}C MRS.

Inositol metabolites are of considerable interest because of the role of inositol phosphates in intracellular message transduction via the phosphatidylinositol cycle. In this context, myoinositol (MI) may be regarded as a reservoir for inositol diphosphate. MI also maintains cell osmolarity. It serves as a glial cell marker and, possibly, as an indicator of neurotoxicity. MI resonates at four distinct chemical shift positions. At short echo time (TE), the most pronounced resonance of MI is from protons at 3.5 ppm. Although other complex inositol phosphates also contribute to the observed signal, MI itself accounts for the majority of the peaks at 3.5 ppm.

Lactate (Lac) is a product of anaerobic glycolysis. It serves as a metabolically significant marker of tissue ischemia and hypoxia, because its concentration increases markedly in aerobic tissues, such as brain and muscle, when deprived of oxygen for a short period of time. Under normal aerobic conditions, Lac concentration is close to the NMR detection limit of 1 mM. Except when using a small surface coil, it is normally not detected in healthy brain tissues in ^{1}H MRS spectra. It has a doublet at 1.3 ppm that is readily observable when cerebral Lac is elevated in ischemia, hypoxia, or in tumors. Elevated brain Lac measured by ^{1}H MRS during functional stimulation has also been reported.

GABA is the major inhibitory neurotransmitter in brain. GABA resonates at three chemical shift positions: a triplet at 2.3 ppm, a quintet at 1.9 ppm, and another triplet at 3 ppm. The resonances at 1.9 ppm and 2.3 ppm overlap with resonances of Glu, Gln, and NAA. The resonances at 3 ppm, which overlap with the tCr peak, have been detected through the aid of spectral editing. Editing suppresses the dominant noncoupled Cr methyl signal at 3 ppm and reveals the J-coupled GABA signal buried underneath.

The potential of in vivo ^{1}H MRS has not been fully exploited, because, owing to the mere 10-ppm chemical shift range, many of the numerous metabolite resonances overlap and therefore obscure their presence. A typical case is the GABA triplet at 3 ppm that underlies the dominant noncoupled Cr methyl signal, which also resides at 3 ppm.

Many important features of J coupling have been used to differentiate coupled spins from noncoupled spins, a technique that is generally known as *spectral editing*. For example, evolution of J coupling is not reversed by the application of a nonselective 180-degree refocusing pulse, but the evolution of chemical shift and frequency differences caused by local susceptibility and B_0 nonhomogeneity are refocused. J-coupled spins can also form unique spin states known as *multiple quantum coherences*, whereas noncoupled spins can only exist as single quantum coherences on the transverse plane. For a given gradient filter, only the selected quantum coherence can be detected, therefore achieving *spectral editing*.

^{31}P Spectroscopy ^{31}P has been a popular nucleus for in vivo MRS studies of tissue metabolism. It is naturally abundant and has a sensitivity that is roughly one-fifteenth that of ^{1}H. The ^{31}P chemical shift range of tissue metabolites is approximately 30 ppm. In just a few minutes, it is possible to obtain ^{31}P spectra containing relatively few, but, nonetheless, important, intermediates of energy metabolism. Several resonance peaks are discernible in a typical ^{31}P spectrum. Three resonances arise from the α, β, and γ phosphates of adenosine triphosphate (ATP) and any other nucleoside triphosphates at –7.8 ppm, –16.3 ppm, and –2.7 ppm, respectively. The α and γ phosphate resonances also contain contributions from any nucleoside diphosphates at the α and β phosphate resonances, respectively. The α phosphate peak of ATP is further overlapped by signals from nicotine adenine dinucleotide and reduced nicotine adenine dinucleotide. The β phosphate resonance of ATP, which is relatively free from contaminating resonances, is used to quantify changes in ATP concentration. A distinctively sharp PCr peak, which is used as the 0 ppm chemical shift reference, represents PCr only. The inorganic phosphate (P_i) peak at 4.9 ppm accounts for free intracellular P_i.

ATP, PCr, and P_i provide information about high-energy phosphate metabolism. Concentrations of ATP are closely regulated and are mainly related to the demands for ATP hydrolysis and the rate of ATP production via the Krebs cycle. Energy is released from conversion of ATP into adenosine diphosphate (ADP) accompanied by the release of P_i. PCr shuttles energy from subcellular sources to sites of use. The Cr kinase reaction essentially acts as a buffer to prevent short-term ATP deficits. The P_i resonance position is determined by the acid–base equilibrium between PO_4^{2-} and PO_4^- ions and is used to calculate intracellular pH. Metabolite ratios, such as those of PCr to P_i, ATP to P_i, and PCr to ATP, can be calculated to provide information about the energy state in brain tissues.

The phosphomonoester (PME) peak is poorly resolved. It contains phosphorylethanolamine (PEt) and PC, both of which are essentially precursors of myelin and membrane phospholipids, such as phosphatidylcholine, phosphatidylethanolamine, and phosphatidylserine. The phosphodiester (PDE) peak is also poorly resolved. The majority of brain PDE is believed to originate from the more mobile phospholipids. The rest is from membrane degradation products, such as the freely soluble GPC and glycerophosphorylethanolamine. The relative concentrations of PME and PDE are closely related to the metabolic activity of membrane phospholipids. The ratio of PDE to PME may reflect turnover of neuronal cell membranes in the brain. The clinical use of the PME and PDE peaks lies in the fact that they represent markers for disturbances in membrane metabolism in disease states.

^{19}F MRS A number of fluorinated psychopharmacological drugs are currently in clinical use. ^{19}F MRS offers a safe and powerful technique to monitor their pharmacokinetics directly in the brain. ^{19}F is naturally abundant and has an NMR sensitivity of 83 percent relative to proton. Its chemical shift range is more than four times that of phosphorus, whereas line widths are comparable. Because there are no endogenous fluorine-containing compounds in biological tissues, ^{19}F MRS cannot be used for studying endogenous metabolites. The advantageous side of this is that interference of background signals, such as tissue water and extracranial fat in ^{1}H MRS, is never a problem in ^{19}F MRS measurement of pharmacokinetics. ^{19}F MRS studies have been conducted in patients being treated with many ^{19}F-containing drugs, such as the selective serotonin reuptake inhibitor (SSRI) fluoxetine (Prozac) and fluvoxamine (Luvox). This technique is particularly valuable because of the unreliable relationship between the serum concentrations of neuroleptic agents and their clinical effects. Therefore, the pharmacokinetic monitoring of tissue concentrations of fluorinated pharmaceuticals with ^{19}F MRS represents a potentially promising technique in clinical psychopharmacology.

^{7}Li MRS ^{7}Li MRS has been used for in vivo studies of the pharmacokinetics of lithium. Because ^{7}Li is not normally present in the human brain, ^{7}Li MRS, like the ^{19}F MRS, is free from interference from endogenous MRS signals. When exogenously administered to patients, ^{7}Li can reach the necessary concentration in the brain to be detected by MRS. Because of difficulties in accurate quantitation, determination of the exact lithium concentrations in the human brain is not yet possible with MRS. Nevertheless, brain ^{7}Li concentrations have been estimated to be approximately one-half of those in serum. ^{7}Li MRS has also been used to demonstrate that brain lithium concentrations vary at different affective states and may correlate with clinical improvement.

^{13}C MRS Carbon is one of the elements that occurs in virtually all molecules in biological systems. The isotope carbon-12 (^{12}C), which exists with the highest natural abundance, has a spin quantum number $I = 0$, and, thus, it has no interaction with an external magnetic field. The isotope ^{13}C has a natural abundance of 1.1 percent. Its gyromagnetic ratio, γ, is only one-fourth that of a proton. This makes ^{13}C a relatively insensitive nucleus for NMR measurement. However, as in the case of ^{19}F and ^{7}Li MRS, the low natural abundance of ^{13}C can be used to an advantage in that ^{13}C-enriched precursors can be used to study metabolic pathways with little background interference from endogenous signals; this is despite that fact that subcutaneous fat signals still have to be eliminated by using proper spatial localization or by subtraction of the background spectrum. The sensitivity of ^{13}C MRS is also significantly increased by isotope enrichment. Even still, a large volume of ^{13}C and high magnetic field strength is necessary for achieving good sensitivity in ^{13}C MRS.

In biological systems molecules, one or several hydrogen atoms are directly bound to most carbon atoms and interact with them through the ^{1}H-^{13}C J-coupling effect. The splitting of ^{13}C resonance lines provides only trivial information—that is, the reduction of in vivo intensity or sensitivity. ^{13}C MRS must suppress the line splitting by proton decoupling during signal acquisition. If one irradiates for a sufficient time in the frequency range of proton resonance before data acquisition, the sensitivity of ^{13}C can be enhanced through a process known as the *nuclear Overhauser effect* (NOE). With small molecules, a NOE enhancement factor of 3 can be obtained. The actual enhancement of sensitivity obtained, however, depends on many factors that determine the magnitude of the NOE. A more robust sensitivity enhancement can be achieved by sophisticated RF pulse schemes, known as *^{1}H-^{13}C heteronuclear polarization transfer*, with which an enhancement factor of 4 can be achieved.

An advantage of ^{13}C MRS is certainly the large range of chemical shifts of more than 200 ppm. The large chemical shift dispersion allows

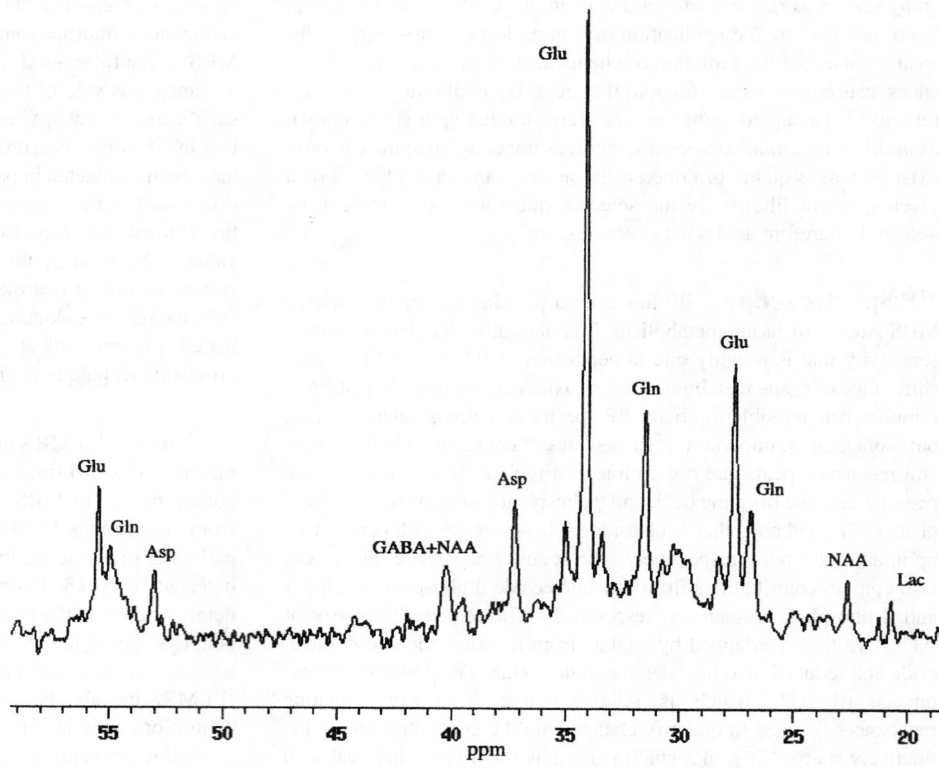

FIGURE 1.15–10 In vivo carbon-13 (^{13}C) spectrum from the occipital and parietal lobes of human brain using hydrogen-1(^{1}H)-^{13}C polarization transfer and ^{1}H decoupling for sensitivity enhancement after intravenous 1-^{13}C-glucose infusion. The following are some of the labeled peaks: Glutamate (Glu): 4-^{13}C-glutamate at 34.2 ppm, 3-^{13}C-glutamate at 28.7 ppm, and 2-^{13}C-glutamate at 55.6 ppm. Glutamine (Gln): 4-^{13}C-glutamine at 31.6 ppm, 3-^{13}C-glutamine at 27.9 ppm, and 2-^{13}C-glutamine at 55.1 ppm. 2–^{13}C-γ-aminobutyric acid (GABA) at 35.3 ppm is overlapped by the down-field sideband of the isotopomer 3, 4-$^{13}C_2$-glutamate; 4-^{13}C-GABA at 40.4 ppm is overlapped by 3-^{13}C–*N*-acetylaspartate (NAA). Asp, aspartic acid; Lac, lactate. (From Shen J, Petersen KF, Behar KL, et al.: Determination of the rate of the glutamate-glutamine cycle in the human brain by in vivo ^{13}C NMR. *Proc Natl Acad Sci U S A.* 1999; 96:8235, with permission.)

the discrimination of carbon atoms that are chemically similar. Many overlapping metabolite signals in the ^{1}H MRS spectrum are well resolved in the corresponding ^{13}C spectrum. Figure 1.15–10 shows a typical ^{13}C MRS spectrum obtained from the occipital and parietal lobes of the healthy human brain during an IV infusion of 1-^{13}C-glucose. The α and β anomeric carbons of glucose are located in 92.7 ppm and 96.6 ppm, respectively. Markedly, the 4-^{13}C-Glu, at 34.2 ppm, and the 4-^{13}C-Gln, at 31.6 ppm, are clearly resolved from each other.

The administration of appropriate ^{13}C-enriched precursors can provide specific and quantitative information about metabolic pathways, such as glycolysis, TCA cycle, and Glu-Gln cycle between neurons and surrounding astrocytes. In the case of the 1-^{13}C-glucose infusion, because Glu is a large pool residing mostly in neurons and in rapid exchange with TCA cycle intermediate α-ketoglutarate, Glu acts as an effective trapping pool for ^{13}C labels in the TCA cycle. The rate of label incorporation into Glu largely reflects the rate of neuronal TCA cycle. The rate of label incorporation into Gln, which is located mostly in astrocytes, is tightly associated with the rate of Glu-Gln cycle between neurons and astrocytes. Using sophisticated mathematical models, the TCA cycle and the Glu-Gln cycle allow simultaneous extraction of the rates of TCA cycle and the Glu-Gln cycle from the kinetics of ^{13}C label incorporation into Glu and Gln. Because glutamatergic abnormalities are involved in many psychiatric diseases, the recently developed ^{13}C MRS technique has potential as a useful tool for studying brain Glu neurotransmission.

MRS Applications in Psychiatric Research

Dementia Dementia, especially Alzheimer's disease, has been studied extensively using MRS. In Alzheimer's disease, NAA loss has been consistently identified by using proton MRS, indicating reduced neuroviability. NAA loss has also been found in other dementia syndromes, such as Parkinson's disease and Huntington's disease. Significantly elevated MI has been found in gray matter of patients with Alzheimer's disease. Reduction in NAA and elevation in MI can be used to detect neural tissue that is at risk, preceding observable structural changes. The results from phosphorus MRS studies, however, have been less consistent.

Schizophrenia Many ^{31}P MRS studies of dorsolateral prefrontal cortex in schizophrenia patients have found decreased PME and increased PDE. These findings have been interpreted to reflect decreased synthesis and increased breakdown of neuronal membrane phospholipids. This is consistent with the hypothesis about exaggeration in schizophrenics of normal synaptic pruning; however, some other studies have failed to replicate these findings. In terms of changes in P_i and ATP peaks, in schizophrenics, the reported data in literature are inconsistent. In some cases, a decrease in P_i and an increase in ATP were reported in first-episode patients. This has been interpreted as evidence for decreased frontal lobe metabolism.

Most of the ^{1}H MRS studies that have examined cortical regions in frontal and temporal lobes of schizophrenia patients, regardless of their treatment status, have reported reduced NAA signals in these regions. Results of other peaks in the proton spectra of schizophrenics, such as Cho, Cr, and MI, have been controversial. Several studies have also reported the measurement of the Glx peak. Due to the severe spectral overlap and strong J-coupling effects at and around the Glx resonance position, data fitting methods based on a priori knowledge of the relative contributions of the different spectral components must be used. The reliability of Glx measurements is limited at the low magnetic field strength currently available for clinical studies. At the current time, all interpretations of MRS results in schizophrenia are tentative. Nevertheless, there has been a significant push toward understanding and interpretation of MRS data, especially with regard to the fairly consistent NAA decrease in schizophrenics. It is possible that the reduced NAA signal reflects temporal and frontal cortical volume loss because of a reduced number of synaptic neuropil. However, postmortem studies have not provided any convincing evidence of neuronal loss or of neuronal degeneration in the areas of NAA signal reduction. The NAA decrease in schizophrenia patients may actually reflect more subtle aspects of neuronal biology rather than neuronal degeneration or neuronal loss.

Affective Disorders Primarily due to the considerable heterogeneity of mood disorders, application of MRS to research on affective disorders is still in its infancy. Nevertheless, the somewhat limited number of studies of affective disorders that have been done using MRS have suggested several possible abnormalities. Specifically, in the case of bipolar disorder in the euthymic state, decreased PME and increased PDE levels in the frontal lobes and decreased PME levels in the temporal lobes seem to be standard MRS observations. Increased peak for Cho-containing compounds in the basal ganglia and anterior cingulate has also been relatively consistently observed in depressed adults, in bipolar disorder and major depression; these data support the pathophysiological role of Cho-containing compounds in depression. In some reports, decreased intracellular pH and decreased PCr peak are observed in the frontal lobes in bipolar disorder in the euthymic state. Decreased NAA and Cr concentrations have also been observed in dorsal lateral prefrontal cortex of bipolar disorder patients. In contrast, increased NAA and Cr concentrations have been reported in the thalamus of familial bipolar patients. Studies using ^{7}Li MRS and ^{19}F MRS in the treatment of affective disorders have elucidated the pharmacokinetics of lithium and fluoxetine. It has been suggested that lithium, which inhibits Cho transport, increases the PME peak during the treatment of mania, but it does not increase the Cho peak in basal ganglia or cerebral cortex. More recent studies of patients with affective disorders have shown significant reduction in the concentration of occipital cortical GABA. This is consistent with lowered plasma and CSF GABA concentrations in depressed patients, as well as the mood-stabilizing and antidepressant effects of some GABA-mimetic and anticonvulsant drugs.

Anxiety Disorders Because of the anxiogenic environment of MR scanners, thus far there have been far fewer MRS studies of anxiety disorders. Nevertheless, an elegant ^{1}H MRS study has examined metabolic abnormalities in panic disorder using Lac-induced panic attacks. In unmedicated panic disorder patients, it was reported that the Lac level was elevated as compared to healthy controls. In comparison, medicated patients with panic disorder showed no increase in Lac levels. This study demonstrated that IV infusion of Lac is associated with an excessive increase in brain Lac concentrations in patients who experience a panic attack during the Lac infusion. In a subsequent controlled hyperventilation experiment, patients with panic disorder had a similar disproportionate increase in Lac. These studies provide evidence of a generalized metabolic or vascular dysfunction in response to panicogenic stimuli. They also highlight the capability of MRS as a useful tool in studying the potential neurochemical mechanisms in panic disorder.

A reduction of occipital cortical GABA has also been observed in panic disorder that is consistent with previous evidence implicating GABAergic dysfunction in the pathophysiology of panic disorder. Preliminary ^{1}H MRS studies of patients with OCD showed essentially no change in lenticular concentrations of NAA, Cr, or Cho. In contrast, in childhood PTSD, decreased NAA in the anterior cingulate has been measured.

Limitations and Future Directions MRS has proven to be a useful tool for the study of psychiatric illness. It has provided a better understanding of the associated neurochemical changes and has helped track those changes during the progression of disease. MRS is also becoming a valuable tool in assessing pharmacokinetic and pharmacodynamic properties of psychiatric drugs and the metabolic effects of psychiatric treatment. Moreover, its psychiatric applications are gradually evolving beyond research. As new treatments for psychiatric disorders become available, MRS is certain to have more clinical use in the future. Still, two limitations that must be conquered are its low sensitivity and poor spatial resolution. Many of the controversial results in MRS, especially in ^{31}P MRS, can largely be attributed to insufficient sensitivity and localization problems. However, MRS technology is developing rapidly, and some exciting new techniques are ready to be used in psychiatric research. For example, in a high-strength magnetic field, a nominal spatial resolution of 0.5 mL has been achieved for ^{1}H CSI. Dramatic reduction of partial volume effect can be achieved by combining CSI localization with T1- or T2-based anatomical image segmentation. Recent improvements in ^{13}C MRS techniques have made it possible to use this noninvasive technology to study Glu metabolism and Glu neurotransmission in normal brain function and in neurological brain disorders. Sophisticated MRS techniques are also being developed to measure GABA metabolism and GABA neurotransmission at high magnetic field strength. In the near future, direct application of these techniques will probe glutamatergic and GABAergic pathophysiology and psychopharmacology of many psychiatric disorders, including schizophrenia, depression, and anxiety. It is possible that future endeavors in MRS neurochemical profiling will lead to classification of psychiatric disease based on neurochemistry. Noninvasive MRS technology also holds great potential for short-term and long-term neurochemical characterization and optimization of pharmacological treatment of psychiatric illness.

SUGGESTED CROSS-REFERENCES

Genetic mechanisms of schizophrenia are discussed in Section 12.3, bipolar I disorder is discussed in Chapter 13, and OCD is presented in Chapter 15. Chapters 35 through 49 discuss childhood psychiatric disorders, substance abuse is discussed in Chapter 11, and Alzheimer's disease is discussed in Section 51.3e.

References

Bertolino A, Weinberger DR: Proton magnetic resonance spectroscopy in schizophrenia. *Eur J Radiol.* 1999;30:132.

Beyer JL, Krishnan KR: Volumetric brain imaging findings in mood disorders. *Bipolar Disord.* 2002;4:89.

Canli T, Zhao Z, Brewer J, Gabrieli JD, Cahill L: Event-related activation in the human amygdala associates with later memory for individual emotional experience. *J Neurosci.* 2000;20:99.

Drevets WC: Neuroimaging studies of mood disorders. *Biol Psychiatry.* 2000;48:813.

Drevets WC: Neuroimaging abnormalities in the amygdala in mood disorders. *Ann N Y Acad Sci.* 2003;985:420.

Frangou S, Williams SC: Magnetic resonance spectroscopy in psychiatry: Basic principles and applications. *Br Med Bull.* 1996;52:474.

Good CD, Ashburner J, Frackowiak RS: Computational neuroanatomy: New perspectives for neuroradiology. *Rev Neurol (Paris).* 2001;157:797.

Hariri AR, Weinberger DR: Imaging genomics. *Br Med Bull.* 2003;65:259.

Hsu YY, Du AT, Schuff N, Weiner MW: Magnetic resonance imaging and magnetic resonance spectroscopy in dementias. *J Geriatr Psychiatry Neurol.* 2001;14:145.

*Hull AM: Neuroimaging findings in post-traumatic stress disorder. Systematic review. *Br J Psychiatry.* 2002;181:102.

Krystal JH, D'Souza DC, Sanacora G, Goddard AW, Charney DS: Current perspectives on the pathophysiology of schizophrenia, depression, and anxiety disorders. *Med Clin North Am.* 2001;85:559.

*Lyoo IK, Renshaw PF: Magnetic resonance spectroscopy: Current and future applications in psychiatric research. *Biol Psychiatry.* 2002;51:195.

*McEwen BS: The neurobiology and neuroendocrinology of stress implications for posttraumatic stress disorder from a basic science perspective. *Psychiatr Clin North Am.* 2002;25:469.

*Moonen CT, Bandettini PA. *Functional MRI.* New York: Springer-Verlag; 1999.

Moore GJ, Bebchuk JM, Hasanat K, Chen G, Seraji-Bozorgzad N, Wilds IB, Faulk MW, Koch S, Glitz DA, Jolkovsky L, Manji HK: Lithium increases *N*-acetyl-aspartate in the human brain: In vivo evidence in support of bcl-2's neurotropic effects? *Biol Psychiatry.* 2000;48:1.

*Morris JS, Buchel C, Dolan RJ: Parallel neuronal responses in amygdala subregions and sensory cortex during implicit fear conditioning. *Neuroimage.* 2001;13:1044.

Nasrallah HA, Pettegrew JW. *NMR Spectroscopy in Psychiatric Brain Disorders.* Washington, DC: American Psychiatric Press; 1995.

Rauch SL, Whalen PJ, Shin LM, McInerney SC, Macklin ML, Lasko NB, Orr SP, Pitman RK: Exaggerated amygdala response to masked facial stimuli in posttraumatic stress disorder: A functional MRI study. *Biol Psychiatry.* 2000;47:769.

Sapolsky RM: Glucocorticoids and hippocampal atrophy in neuropsychiatric disorders. *Arch Gen Psychiatry.* 2000;57:925.

Sapolsky RM: Chickens, eggs and hippocampal atrophy. *Nat Neurosci.* 2002;5:1111.

Saxena S, Rauch SL: Functional neuroimaging and the neuroanatomy of obsessive-compulsive disorder. *Psychiatr Clin North Am.* 2000;23:563.

Schneider F, Weiss U, Kessler C, Muller-Gartner HW, Posse S, Salloum JB, Grodd W, Himmelmann F, Gaebel W, Birbaumer N: Subcortical correlates of differential classical conditioning of aversive emotional reactions in social phobia. *Biol Psychiatry.* 1999;45:863.

Sheline YI, Barch DM, Donnelly JM, Ollinger JM, Snyder AZ, Mintun MA: Increased amygdala response to masked emotional faces in depressed subjects resolves with antidepressant treatment: An fMRI study. *Biol Psychiatry.* 2001;50:651.

Shen J: Slice-selective J-coupled coherence transfer using symmetric linear phase pulses: Applications to localized GABA spectroscopy. *J Magn Reson.* 2003;163:73.

Shen J, Rothman DL, Brown P: In vivo GABA editing using a novel doubly selective multiple quantum filter. *Magn Reson Med.* 2002;47:447.

Shenton ME, Dickey CC, Frumin M, McCarley RM: A review of findings in schizophrenia. *Schizophr Res.* 2001;49:1.

Siegle GJ, Steinhauer SR, Thase ME, Stenger VA, Carter CC: Can't shake that feeling: Event-related fMRI assessment of sustained amygdala activity in response to emotional information in depressed individuals. *Biol Psychiatry.* 2002;51:693.

Strakowski SM, Adler CM, DelBello MP: Volumetric MRI studies of mood disorders: Do they distinguish unipolar and bipolar disorder? *Bipolar Disord.* 2002;4:80.

Thomas KM, Drevets WC, Dahl RE, Ryan ND, Birmaher B, Eccard CH, Axelson D, Whalen PJ, Casey BJ: Abnormal amygdala response to faces in anxious and depressed children. *Arch Gen Psychiatry.* 2001;58:1057.

Toga AW, Thompson PM: New approaches in brain morphometry. *Am J Geriatr Psychiatry.* 2002;10:13.

Vythilingam M, Charles HC, Tupler LA, Blitchington T, Kelly L, Krishnan KR: Focal and lateralized subcortical abnormalities in unipolar major depressive disorder: An automated multivoxel proton magnetic resonance spectroscopy study. *Biol Psychiatry.* 2003;54:744.

Vythilingam M, Heim C, Newport J, Miller AH, Anderson E, Bronen R, Brummer M, Staib L, Vermetten E, Charney DS, Nemeroff CB, Bremner JD: Childhood trauma associated with smaller hippocampal volume in women with major depression. *Am J Psychiatry.* 2002;159:2072.

Yamasue H, Kasai K, Iwanami A, Ohtani T, Yamada H, Abe O, Kuroki N, Fukuda R, Tochigi M, Furukawa S, Sadamatsu M, Sasaki T, Aoki S, Ohtomo K, Asukai N, Kato N: Voxel-based analysis of MRI reveals anterior cingulate gray-matter volume reduction in posttraumatic stress disorder due to terrorism. *Proc Natl Acad Sci U S A.* 2003;100:9039.

▲ 1.16 Radiotracer Imaging: Basic Principles and Exemplary Findings in Neuropsychiatric Disorders

MASAHIRO FUJITA, M.D., PH.D., AKIRA KUGAYA, M.D., PH.D., AND ROBERT B. INNIS, M.D., PH.D.

Radiotracer imaging can be understood from the two components of its name. *Radio* refers to the use of unstable atoms that decay and release radiation, which is detected after it leaves the body. *Tracer* refers to the fact that the radioactive compound is almost always administered in *trace* amounts that are too low to cause any pharmacological effects. Many of the principles of radiotracer methods derive from George de Hevesy, who received the Nobel Prize in chemistry in 1943 for the use of radioactive compounds to mirror the disposition of naturally occurring cognate nonradioactive compounds. For example, tritium-labeled glucose given in trace amounts can be used to monitor the disposition and metabolism of nonradioactive glucose present in much higher concentrations. The radioactive compound is typically administered in tracer doses, so that it does not significantly increase the total amount or concentration of the cognate compound. That is, the radiotracer accurately reflects the disposition of the cognate compound without significantly altering the endogenous situation. Because the radiotracer is merely a proxy for the cognate nonradioactive compound, why not directly measure the nonradioactive compound itself? There are two major reasons: (1) the feasibility of external measurements and (2) the high sensitivity of radiotracer methods. The direct measurement of nonradioactive glucose, for example, would presumably entail a sampling of the tissue and the use of an in vitro analytical method. Although blood can easily be used to obtain these measures, sampling directly in the brain would be problematic, because it is safely ensconced in the skull, and because such sampling might cause damage to brain tissues. In comparison, the γ-rays emitted by radiotracers travel through the skull, and nuclear medicine cameras are used to obtain external γ-ray measures. Second, radioactivity can be measured in low concentrations compared to many other analytical chemistry techniques. That is, radiotracer methods have high sensitivity. For example, the sensitivity of in vivo radiotracer imaging with positron emission tomography (PET) is approximately 10^{-12} to 10^{-14} mol. In comparison, the in vivo nuclear magnetic resonance (NMR) techniques described in the previous chapter have a sensitivity of approximately 10^{-4} mol. For example, in vivo NMR can measure brain levels of γ-aminobutyric acid (GABA) (present in mmol concentration) but lacks the sensitivity to measure most proteins in the brain that are often present at concentrations of less than 10^{-9} mol.

The two typical radiotracer methods used for neuroimaging are PET and single photon emission computed tomography (SPECT). Both are *tomographic* techniques, meaning that they can be used to reconstruct multiple image *slices* from successive depths in the brain. These tomographic methods differ from *planar* methods, such as X-ray imaging, in which, for example, the chest X-ray melds visual images of anterior bones into the same plane as images of posterior bones, resulting in a single, flat image. This chapter reviews the different types of radioactivity used in PET versus SPECT. PET uses a positron (i.e., nuclear particle) emitter, and, when positrons collide with electrons, two photons (i.e., two γ-rays) are released. In contrast, SPECT uses a nuclide that decays with the release of a single high-energy photon.

ADVANTAGES AND DISADVANTAGES

PET and SPECT have advantages and disadvantages relative to other neuroimaging modalities. Because both are radiotracer techniques, they have high sensitivity, with PET being approximately 100 times more sensitive than SPECT. Another advantage is pharmacological specificity. For example, a radioactive PET tracer can be made that binds to a small percentage of dopamine type 2 (D_2) receptors. Such a tracer, when used in conjunction with proper tracer methodology, can measure the total population or density of such receptors in a target region. PET probes can be made with such great specificity that they only bind to D_2 receptors and not to other subtypes of dopamine receptors, but, certainly, they also do not bind to other unrelated receptors, such as those for serotonin (5-HT). However, despite the positive aspects of sensitivity and pharmacological specificity of PET and

SPECT imaging, their two major disadvantages are limited resolution and radiation exposure. In the 1980s, early PET and SPECT cameras provided spatial resolutions in the range of 1 to 2 cm. Improvement has been made, as current commercial cameras now provide a resolution of approximately 3 to 5 mm for PET and 7 to 10 mm for SPECT. Nevertheless, these resolutions are still inferior in contrast to magnetic resonance imaging (MRI) (<1 mm). Another disadvantage of radiotracer techniques is that subjects are exposed to radioactivity. Exposures to radioactivity for clinical nuclear medicine procedures are not specifically regulated. In contrast, the vast majority of PET and SPECT imaging of psychiatric patients is for research purposes. Agencies of the federal government, such as the U.S. Food and Drug Administration (FDA) and Nuclear Regulatory Commission (NRC), as well as international agencies, have established guidelines (although not consistent) on the levels of radioactivity that provide a small, yet acceptable, risk of exposure for research subjects. However, this topic remains controversial among scientists and is also inflammatory among the lay public. Although all aspects of this dispute cannot be adequately reviewed here, certain generalizations can be made. First, most people in the general population do not understand that radiation exposure occurs to all of us—at the rate of approximately 1 mrem (millirem, a measure of radiation dose) per day from cosmic sources. Furthermore, the risk of radiation exposure during PET and SPECT scans can only be estimated, not immediately assessed. The levels of exposure during these procedures are far too low to cause immediate effects, such as radiation burn or radiation sickness. Instead, the most serious biological side effect is a potential increase in the likelihood of cancer (especially leukemia and lymphoma) that may develop as much as 10 to 30 years later because of radiation-induced mutations in deoxyribonucleic acid (DNA). There is a great deal of debate among scientists as to whether typical exposures of PET or SPECT actually increase the rate of developing cancer. However, there is consensus that, if the rate of cancer is increased, it is quite small and could only be measured in prospective studies by using extraordinarily large sample populations. For example, current statistics indicate that approximately one in four Americans dies of cancer. If radiotracer imaging increases this death risk, it is probably on the order of approximately 0.1 percent. This suggests an increase from 25 to 25.1 percent. Statistically significant measurement of such a small increase would require a study with a large sample size, and the existing prospective studies have been too small to detect any effect. Thus, current risk estimates have largely relied on follow-up studies of World War II survivors of Hiroshima and Nagasaki and have been calculated by using a linear back-extrapolation of data from persons with much higher levels of exposure with significantly increased rates of cancer. However, this back-extrapolation has been the crux of much controversy, and some scientists feel that a linear extrapolation is not appropriate. In contrast to estimates yielded by back-extrapolation, one school of thought (called *hormesis*) cites a substantial body of data from plants and animals that indicate low-level radiation exposure actually decreases genetic malformations by inducing the synthesis of DNA repair enzymes. In the end, psychiatrists must understand and then appropriately communicate to their research subjects that the increased risk of developing cancer, if it exists, is quite small and has not yet been adequately measured in prospective studies.

PSYCHIATRY FOLLOWS NEUROLOGY AND RADIOTRACER IMAGING FOLLOWS MRI

As a broad generalization, psychiatry's use of neuroimaging has largely followed and mirrored that in neurology. In a similar manner, PET and SPECT imaging modalities have followed and mirrored MRI applications. The first generalization can be seen in the clinical use of MRI in neurology. MRI has well-established usefulness for the diagnosis of disorders, such as stroke and multiple sclerosis (MS). The clinical usefulness of MRI for psychological disorders is still quite limited but is, nonetheless, following the example set by neurology. As described in the previous chapter, structural MRI research has demonstrated that many psychiatric illnesses, including schizophrenia, depression, and posttraumatic stress disorder (PTSD), are associated with structural abnormalities of the brain. Such findings have been shown to be statistically significant when comparing groups of subjects (e.g., patients vs. controls) but have not yet achieved usefulness for individual patients. In a similar manner, radiotracer imaging was initially applied largely to neurological patients (such as central nervous system [CNS] tumors, stroke, Alzheimer's disease, and Parkinson's disease), and psychiatry has followed suit with comparable studies in their patient population. Thus, psychiatry's use of MRI and radiotracer imaging has followed models initially applied in neurology.

Similarly, radiotracer imaging appears to follow the path of MRI. Structural MRI was initially used only for research purposes but then demonstrated clear superiority to computed tomography (CT) imaging of the brain. FDA approval of clinical use of MRI markedly stimulated technological advancement in the 1980s. The resolution and speed of image acquisition was improved, and, today, at least one MRI scanner can be found in almost every medium-sized to large hospital in America. The prevalence of these devices in university hospital centers allowed faculty to quickly implement functional MRI (fMRI) research studies when that technique was developed in the 1990s. Insurance reimbursement of the structural MRI scans served to inspire commercial interest and brought further improvements in the technology, which ultimately spurred the widespread acquisition of these devices worldwide. Comparatively, PET imaging has undergone a slower, more localized evolution of acceptance into clinical and commercial realms, and, until recently, it served only as a research tool. However, in the late 1990s, the FDA approved PET imaging of increased glucose metabolism for the localization of several primary tumors and their metastases. Subsequently, approval of reimbursement by insurance companies and the federal government's Center for Medicare and Medicaid Services (CMS), formerly the Health Care Financing Administration, led to improvements in PET technology, and it is now widespread in the United States. If a medium-sized hospital does not currently have a PET camera, it is likely considering its acquisition or has made plans for routine visits by a mobile PET device in a large truck. This recent expansion in PET technology was driven by clinical usefulness for oncology and has made this modality widely available for research. Analogous to fMRI development in existing MRI centers, one can now expect a marked expansion of research neuroimaging with PET.

CHALLENGES

A recent wave of medical specialties and general research fields have glibly, and even sometimes paradoxically, attached the word *molecular* to their professional designation to enhance prestige. It seems that *molecular neurobiology* is more fashionable, and perhaps more futuristic, than mere *neurobiology*. Some in psychiatry have even adopted the oxymoron *molecular psychiatrist* as their preferred title. With due acknowledgment of its fashionably excessive usage, the authors believe that radiotracer imaging could be legitimately characterized as *molecular imaging*. Despite the fact that there is no universally accepted definition of the phrase, this two-word title has recently been adopted by at least two new scientific societies, a few new journals, and many university departments. A reasonable stab at the definition would posit that the targets to be imaged are specific molecules—for example, specific proteins, fatty acids, carbohydrates, or nucleic acids. In the case of neuroimaging, the targets have been almost exclusively protein molecules (such as a specific enzyme, receptor, or transporter). Conversely, relatively little work has been done to measure fatty acids and carbohydrates in the brain, and radiolabeled probes for nucleic acids are not currently useful for brain imaging, because the probes themselves are charged and cannot cross the blood–brain barrier or cell membranes. Thus, radiotracer imaging in the brain could be defined as a subset of molecular imaging that focuses on specific proteinaceous molecular targets. Despite the lack of consensus on the definition of *molecular imaging*, it should surely be contrasted with *functional imaging*, which is commonly understood to measure localized neuronal brain activity. Because of the collinear relationship between neuronal activity and localized blood flow, oxygen extraction, and glucose use, increased neuronal activity can be implied using PET and fMRI. Because blood and glucose are present in high concentrations in brain, high sensitivity is not required for such measurements. Thus, most functional neuroimaging studies have switched from PET to fMRI, which has no radiation exposure and much better spatial and temporal sampling resolution. In summary, *molecular imaging* is used to reflect specific molecular targets and is contrasted with *functional imaging* of local neuronal activity.

With this definition of radiotracer imaging as *molecular imaging*, the major challenges to the field become more obvious. Which specific protein targets in brain should be measured and can this be done? PET imaging in schizophrenia exemplifies these dilemmas. Many initial PET studies in schizophrenia in the 1980s and 1990s focused on the dopamine D_2 receptor, because clinically useful antipsychotic agents act as antagonists at this site, and because PET tracers could be relatively easily developed as radiolabeled analogs of neuroleptic medications. Numerous controversial studies were performed, but the current consensus is that patients with schizophrenia have minimal, if any, increase in dopamine D_2 receptors and that such alterations are certainly not required to develop the disorder. So, which proteins should now be measured in schizophrenia? In addition, the development for PET probes for these new protein targets is expensive and time consuming.

The usefulness of radiotracer imaging in psychiatry is based on the assumptions that protein abnormalities are associated with psychiatric illnesses and that medications need to be developed for these protein targets. Both of these assumptions are adequately justified to devote personal careers and major resources to this area. The challenges that are now faced are numerous. Broadly trained and clever scientists are needed to determine relevant research findings from basic neurobiology that justify the effort to translate such measurements to living subjects with PET. Substantial medicinal chemistry and radiochemistry efforts are needed to develop new PET probes for selected protein targets. Clinical nuclear medicine expertise and sophisticated methods of digital image quantitation are required to evaluate the safety and efficacy of new PET probes. Finally, almost a new breed of psychiatrists must be trained in neuroimaging techniques to be able to design and to apply radiotracer imaging methods. In fact, if clinical usefulness is demonstrated for radiotracer imaging in psychiatry, subspecialty training in neuroimaging may be required for some psychiatrists, just as neuroradiology is a subspecialty in that field of medicine.

This overview has now come almost full circle, and the purpose of the chapter has become clear. That is, this text is designed as an introduction to the field of molecular neuroimaging, which offers great promise to understand the protein abnormalities that underlie psychiatric illness, in the hope that this knowledge will enhance diagnosis, guide treatment, and assist in the development of improved treatments.

BASIC PRINCIPLES

In PET and SPECT, a biological process of interest is studied by synthetically incorporating a radionuclide into a molecule of known physiological relevance. The so-called radiopharmaceutical is then administered to a patient by inhalation, ingestion, or, most commonly, intravenous (IV) injection. As radioactivity distributes within the subject, the radiotracer's uptake into the brain is measured over time and is used to obtain information about the physiological process of interest. Because of the high-energy γ-ray emissions of the specific isotopes used and the sensitivity and sophistication of the instruments used to detect them, the two-dimensional distribution of radioactivity within a brain slice may be inferred from information obtained outside the head. For this reason, PET and SPECT are referred to as *emission tomographic* (from the Greek *tomos* for cut) techniques. (The data of PET and SPECT are actually collected as three-dimensional volumes, and two-dimensional images can be created on any plane.) In contrast to more conventional radiographic methods, such as a chest X-ray, in which an external source of radiation merely casts a shadow of the body's organs and cavities onto a planar film, PET and SPECT rely on more sophisticated principles to produce three-dimensional information. To understand this process, a basic understanding of the physics of photon emission is required.

Physics of Photon Emission

Radioactive decay is a process in which an unstable nucleus transforms into a more stable one by emitting particles or photons, or both, and releasing nuclear energy. For the radionuclides used in PET, a proton is converted to a neutron, and a particle called a positron (denoted e^+ or β^+) is emitted. A positron may be thought of as the antimatter equivalent of an electron, possessing identical mass but opposite charge. When ejected from the nucleus, a positron travels until it collides with an electron. This collision results in the annihilation of both particles and the conversion of mass into energy (Fig. 1.16–1). The energy produced has a characteristic profile consisting of two γ-photons (rays) of equivalent energy (511 keV) and opposite trajectory (180 degrees apart, although this is actually not exactly 180 degrees; see the following discussion). These dual photons distinguish PET from SPECT and have implications for camera design. The most commonly used positron-emitting nuclides in PET include carbon-11 (^{11}C), nitrogen-13 (^{13}N), oxygen-15 (^{15}O), and fluorine-18 (^{18}F).

PET scanners take advantage of the unique spatial signature of "back-to-back" photons by using a method known as *coincidence detection* to locate the source of an annihilation event, (Fig. 1.16–2). Coincidence detection is an efficient technique and contributes to PET's superior sampling rates, sensitivity, and spatial resolution compared to those of SPECT. In a typical configuration, a PET scanner consists of a circular array of highly sensitive scintillation detectors that surround the head. These detectors are made of dense crystalline materials (e.g., bismuth germanium oxide [BGO], sodium iodide, or cesium fluoride) that trap the invisible, high-energy γ-rays and convert them to visible light. This brief flash of light is then converted into an electrical pulse by an immediately adjacent photomultiplier tube (PMT), and the electrical pulse is then registered by the scanner's computer. When the scanner detects two electronic signals from two radiation detectors that coincide (to within 3 to 10 nanoseconds, for practical purposes), an

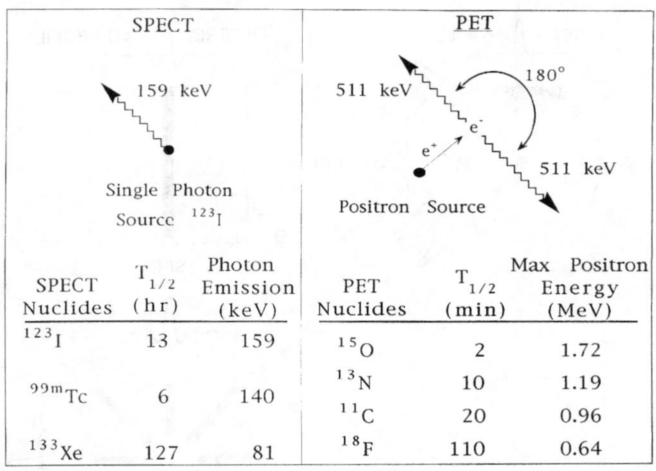

SPECT Nuclides	$T_{1/2}$ (hr)	Photon Emission (keV)
^{123}I	13	159
^{99m}Tc	6	140
^{133}Xe	127	81

PET Nuclides	$T_{1/2}$ (min)	Max Positron Energy (MeV)
^{15}O	2	1.72
^{13}N	10	1.19
^{11}C	20	0.96
^{18}F	110	0.64

FIGURE 1.16–1 The decay of a single photon emission computed tomography (SPECT) radiopharmaceutical results in the emission of a high-energy photon directly from the radionuclide. In contrast, the decay of a positron emission tomography (PET) radiopharmaceutical results in the emission of a positron (e^+), which travels a variable distance before annihilating with an electron (e^-), which then yields two 511-keV photons at 180-degree angles to each other. The distance traveled by the positron decreases the resolution of PET images, when using the typical nuclides listed, by 0.2 to 1.3 mm, with resolution measured as full width at half maximum. The longer-lived SPECT radionuclides emit single photons of different energies, whereas the PET radionuclides consistently yield two photons of 511 keV. ^{11}C, carbon-11; ^{18}F, fluorine-18; ^{123}I, iodine-123; ^{13}N, nitrogen-13; ^{15}O, oxygen-15; $T_{1/2}$, terminal half-life; ^{99m}Tc, technetium-99m; ^{133}Xe, xenon-133.

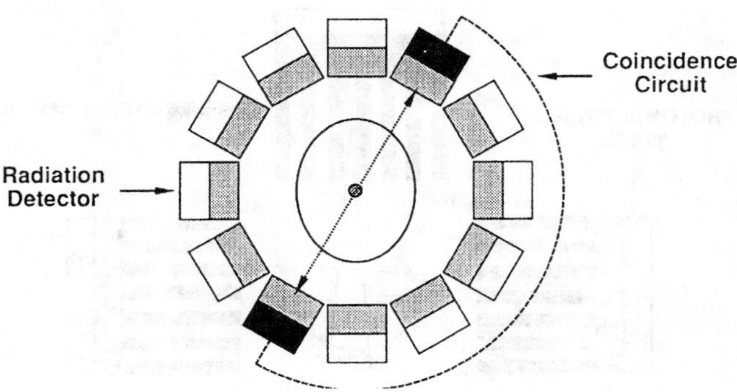

FIGURE 1.16–2 A positron emission tomography scanner consists of a ring of radiation sensors that are designed to detect the simultaneously emitted, characteristically "back-to-back" (180 degrees apart) dual photons that are created by the annihilation of a positron and an electron. Opposing detectors are electronically coupled to form a coincidence circuit. Thus, when separate scintillation events in paired detectors coincide, an annihilation event is presumed to have occurred at some point along a line connecting the two. This information is registered by a computer and later is used to reconstruct images using the principles of computed tomography. (From Malison RT, Laruelle M, Innis RB. Positron and single photon emission tomography: Principles and applications in psychopharmacology. In: Bloom F, Kupfer D, eds. *Psychopharmacology: The Fourth Generation of Progress.* New York: Raven Press; 1995, with permission.)

annihilation event is presumed to have occurred at some point along an imaginary line connecting the detectors. In contrast, single events are ignored. Although any two crystal detectors may be activated by coincident photons, the most straightforward conceptual configuration for a PET camera is one in which only opposing detectors are electronically connected. Although it is the case that two unrelated photons from spatially separate annihilation events can reach opposing detectors concurrently, such accidental coincidences are much less frequent than true ones. Nevertheless, random coincidences constitute one source of the background noise in PET images.

Because PET detects the site at which a positron annihilates and not the site of its emission, there exists an intrinsic theoretical limit on the spatial resolution of PET. Specifically, a positron generally travels a finite distance before coming to rest in a tissue and colliding with an electron (positron range). Thus, an annihilation typically occurs some distance away from the site of radioactive decay. This distance is proportional to the positron's average kinetic energy as it is emitted from the nucleus and is characteristic of the specific isotope used (Fig. 1.16–1). For example, the average range for ^{11}C decay is 1.1 mm. An additional limitation placed on PET is that photons are emitted at an angle slightly different than 180 degrees (noncollinear annihilation). The residual momentum of the electron pair at annihilation results in γ-rays being emitted with a small deviation from the assumed 180 degrees. Thus, positron range and noncollinear annihilation are factors that theoretically limit PET's achievable spatial resolution.

For the radionuclides used in SPECT, a somewhat opposite type of radioactive decay occurs. Instead of a proton-rich radionuclide ejecting a positron (i.e., e^+), it "captures" an orbiting electron (denoted e^-). Once again, the net result is transformation of a proton into a neutron. For some radionuclides, the radioactive progeny of this process remains in a residually excited, so-called metastable state. With the dissipation of this metastable arrangement, the daughter nucleus achieves a ground state, and a single γ-photon is produced. Thus, SPECT uses isotopes that decay by electron capture or γ-photon emission, or both, including iodine-123 (^{123}I) and the long-lived metastable nuclide technetium-99m (^{99m}Tc). A theoretical limit on spatial resolution, which is comparable to the positron range, exists for SPECT, because the site of γ-photon emission and the site of radioactive decay are synonymous.

The emission of only a single photon fundamentally distinguishes SPECT from PET and necessitates an intrinsically different approach to ascertaining the origin of a decay event and, therefore, camera design. Specifically, SPECT uses a method know as *collimation* (Fig. 1.16–3). In a manner analogous to the effects of a polarizing filter for visible light, a collimator is a physical filter that permits only γ-rays of a specific spatial trajectory to reach the SPECT scanner's detector. Most commonly, a collimator is a lead structure that is interposed between the subject and the radiation detector. The collimator contains many holes of sufficiently long and narrow dimension, so that only photons of a parallel trajectory are allowed through. In contrast to parallel photons, γ-rays that deviate slightly are absorbed by the lead and go undetected (Fig. 1.16–3). Different collimators (e.g., parallel, fan-beam, and cone-beam) have holes of differing orientations (e.g., perpendicular to the detector, focused in two dimensions, and focused in three dimensions, respectively). Given a known geometric configuration for the specific collimator's holes, the original path of a detected photon is linearly extrapolated. As might be imagined, collimation is much less efficient than coincidence detection, because many potentially informative photons are lost. Although the sensitivity of SPECT has been largely overcome by advances in collimator design and increases in the number of detectors surrounding the body, the sensitivity is still much lower than that of PET, as described in the introduction. As one can imagine from the difference between coincidence detection (PET) and collimation (SPECT), PET has higher spatial resolution.

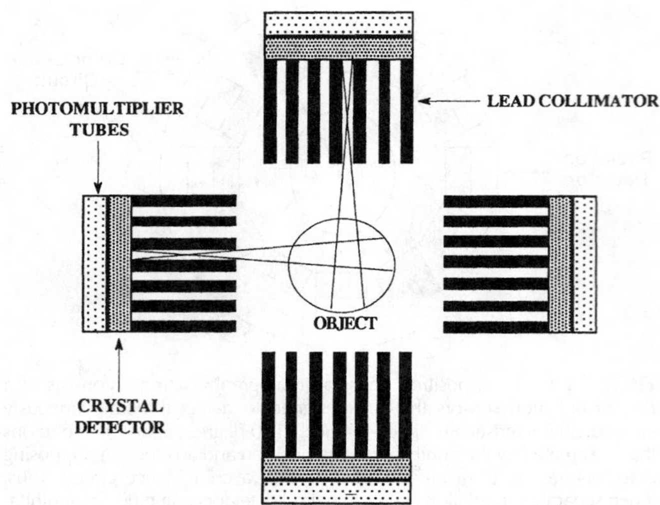

FIGURE 1.16–3 The method of image reconstruction from back projection in single photon emission computed tomography uses a collimator placed between the object and the crystal detector. The area of the object that is viewed by the underlying detector is decreased by having longer and narrower holes in the collimator. By moving the detector-collimator complex around the object, multiple views are obtained and provide the primary data for image reconstruction.

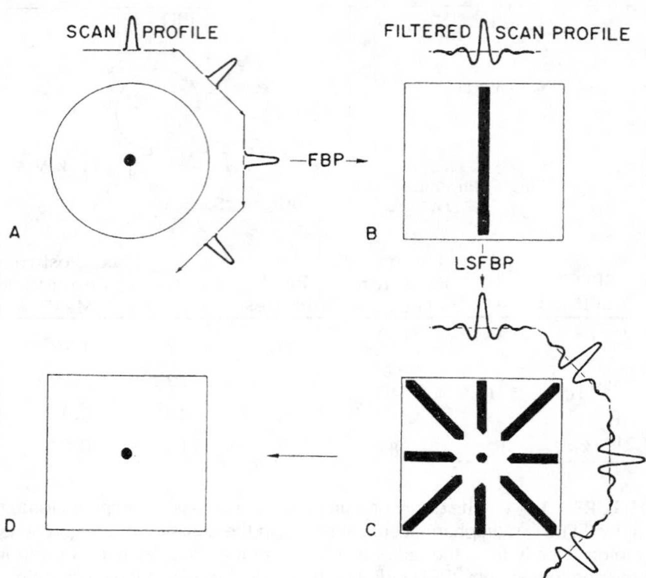

FIGURE 1.16–4 Example of Fourier-based reconstruction technique, linear superposition of filtered back-projection (LSFBP). Detector readings are zero, except when a small object at center is encountered. **A:** Object and scan profiles. **B:** Single filtered scan profile projected back across the cross-sectional plane. **C:** Four filtered scan profiles projected back across the plane and added together (superposition). **D:** Image produced when sufficient angles are used to remove defocusing. (From Phelps ME, Hoffman EJ, Gado M, Ter-Pogossian MM. Computerized transaxial transmission reconstruction tomography. In: DeBlanc HJ Jr, Sorenson JA, eds. *Noninvasive Brain Imaging, Computed Tomography and Radionuclides.* Reston, VA: Society of Nuclear Medicine; 1975, with permission.)

Image Reconstruction Although the nature of photon emission and detection are different in PET and SPECT, both techniques rely on the same principles of CT when translating information about photon paths into brain images (Fig. 1.16–4). Briefly, CT is based on the premise that an appreciation of an object's two- or three-dimensional distribution in space may only be inferred by viewing it from multiple vantage points (Fig. 1.16–4A). More specifically, because information about a photon's direction, not depth, is known, views of photon trajectories from multiple angles around the entire head are required. In PET and SPECT, such a set of measurements from a given angle or viewpoint is referred to as a *projection* or *scan profile* (Fig. 1.16–4B). A ring of essentially contiguous radiation detectors in a PET scanner provides multiple scan profiles in this modality. In contrast, SPECT cameras usually rely on several (typically two to four) detector "heads" that rotate around the subject in synchrony, collecting data over an entire 360 degrees. A picture of the distribution of radioactivity within a given brain slice is then inferred by retracing or *back-projecting* the trajectories (typically thousands) of γ-rays across the field of view for every imaging angle (Fig. 1.16–4C). Conceptually analogous to the simple childhood puzzle in which numbers in a square grid (e.g., 3 × 3) are inferred from their sums along each row, PET and SPECT images require fast computer coprocessors and efficient mathematical algorithms (fast Fourier transformations) to handle the considerably larger matrices (e.g., 128 × 128 or 256 × 256 elements) of radiation density values and the correspondingly more intensive calculations. In this manner, individual radiation values (i.e., counts of detected events) are determined for each cell of the matrix (also known as a picture element or *pixel*), corresponding shades of color are assigned, and an image of the distribution of radioactivity within the brain is produced.

Despite its complexity and computational intensity, back-projection is an imperfect process and, in fact, introduces known artifacts into the images themselves. As the back-projection algorithm retraces a photon's path, it cannot be sure of the actual point of decay. Therefore, the algorithm is forced to assume an equal probability of radioactive decay and, hence, radiation value for every point along the line of trajectory. Areas of the brain in which radioactivity is highly concentrated stand out as many trajectories from multiple projections are superimposed and their probability values are summed (Fig. 1.16–4C,D). In the process, however, those areas containing no radioactivity now bear the statistical imprint of the algorithm's guess. Thus, small, but finite, values are ascribed to areas at which none should exist. By increasing the density of spatial sampling through greater numbers of projections, the impact of these spurious values on image quantitation can be minimized but not eliminated. Therefore, a filter is still required to restore quantitative accuracy to images by erasing counts in those areas that should have none. Several filters have been developed (e.g., Ramp, Butterworth, and Hanning) in an effort to overcome these limitations, and these techniques remain the mainstay of the field of image reconstruction. Although the considerations involved in the choice of a filter are beyond the scope of this chapter, suffice it to say that trade-offs exist with respect to their relative impact on spatial resolution and noise amplification, and filter selection depends on the imaging context. Alternative reconstruction methods (e.g., restorative and iterative techniques) are the current focus of much research, and simple filtered back-projection is likely to be superseded by more quantitatively accurate methods in the near future.

Factors Affecting Image Quantitation Several physical factors affect the quantitative accuracy of PET and SPECT images. Among these are the statistics of radioactive decay, attenuation, scatter, limited spatial resolution, and partial volume effects.

Statistics of Radioactive Decay Mathematically, radioactive decay is described by an exponential curve. The rate at which a specific radionuclide decays is expressed in terms of its radioactive half-life ($T_{1/2}$) value, a parameter defined as the time required for one-half of the radioactive atoms to decay. Values of $T_{1/2}$ vary between species and are characteristic of a given nuclide. The characteristic $T_{1/2}$ values of several commonly used PET and SPECT isotopes are listed in Figure 1.16–1. Although a given isotope's $T_{1/2}$ is constant, the nature of radioactive decay is intrinsically statistical. This phenomenon is most readily conceptualized by imagining an isotope of infinite $T_{1/2}$ (i.e., unchanging levels of radioactivity). In struggling to measure the precise amount of radioactivity during a fixed period of time, one's efforts invariably lead to variations in the individually recorded values. Only by taking the statistical average of multiple measurements is the true amount of radioactivity (and $T_{1/2}$ value) inferred. The variation in sampling derives from the intrinsic probabilistic nature (mathematically described by a Poisson distribution) of radioactive decay and the random fluctuation in individual decay events from moment to moment, and it occurs irrespective of detection method.

The manifestations of this effect are most readily appreciated by imaging an object that contains a uniform concentration of radioactivity. The Swiss cheese appearance of the resulting images is the spatial equivalent of this temporal variation in PET and SPECT images. The probabilistic inaccuracies or *statistical noise* introduced is, by virtue of its random nature, easily surmountable through the collection of more counts. Longer sampling times and greater instrument sensitivity are the principal ways in which counting statistics are improved. In the former, longer acquisition times improve statistical noise at the expense of temporal resolution. Conversely, increased sensitivity (e.g., larger collimator holes in SPECT) is traded for poorer spatial resolution (i.e., because slightly-less-than-parallel photons are detected).

Photon Attenuation Although the high energies of photons emitted by PET and SPECT nuclides enable their penetration of brain structures, a significant number of γ-rays escape detection by both types of scanners based on their interactions with surrounding tissues. These interactions fall into one of two general categories—Compton scattering and photoelectric absorption. In Compton scattering, a collision occurs between the photon and an atomic electron. The photon is deflected from its original trajectory and, in the process, loses a fraction of its original energy. Alternatively, in photoelectron absorption, the photon's energy is completely absorbed by the atom, and an electron may be ejected from its orbit. For the latter reason, γ-radiation is said to be *ionizing*.

Because the chances of scatter or absorption decrease with increasing photon energy and increase with distance, photon attenuation is energy and depth dependent. On both counts, PET has distinct advantages. Because photons in PET have higher energies (i.e., 511 keV) than those in SPECT (typically 80 to 160 keV), they are less prone to attenuation (Fig. 1.16–1). Nevertheless, activity at the brain's center is disproportionately underestimated (by roughly four to five times) in comparison to its surface for PET and SPECT. Compensating for undetected photons is therefore crucial for comparing radioactive densities in different brain regions. The most commonly used method with SPECT is *uniform* attenuation correction. In uniform attenuation correction, an ellipse is fitted to the brain's contour, and the same attenuation value (typically equal to that of water) is assigned to all points within the ellipse. A commonly used method for attenuation correction in PET (and with some recent SPECT devices) is *nonuniform* (*measured*) attenuation correction, which relies on a preceding transmission study similar to a CT scan. An external source of radiation is transmitted through the subject's head, creating a precise attenuation map for that individual. Because the sizes and shapes of patients' heads vary, and because the attenuation properties of bone, tissue, fluid, and air differ, such an approach has clear theoretical advantages.

Photon Scatter In PET and SPECT, instrumentation and image reconstruction are based on the underlying assumptions that detected photons retain their linear paths. As noted previously, however, Compton effects cause photons to deviate from their original trajectories. Although these photons lose energy to atoms in the tissue, many scattered photons retain sufficient energy to enable their escape from the brain. The detection of scattered events therefore leads to errors in image reconstruction as a result of false assumptions about the photon's original path. Much like accidental coincidences, scattered photons increase the background noise and compromise image contrast.

Because radionuclides emit photons of a known energy, scattered photons may be distinguished from true ones by the loss of energy they sustained from collisions with electrons. In an attempt to exploit this principle, PET and SPECT cameras measure the energy spectrum of their detected photons. In practice, however, accurately discriminating between true and scattered photons is often difficult. First, the energy resolution of current PET and SPECT scanners is limited. Second, the photopeak energies of true photons are not identical but rather normally distributed around a mean value. Thus, scattered and photopeak photons inevitably overlap in their energy distributions. Current algorithms subtract a *scatter fraction* from the photopeak counts in an attempt to compensate for this problem. However, these methods have obvious limitations. As for attenuation correction, advances in scatter correction offer the promise of incorporating a priori information about the head's structure and density in achieving more faithful image reconstruction.

Spatial Resolution In contrast to the fine visual detail seen in MRI, pictures created using SPECT and PET appear blurred. The visual sense of imprecision is the qualitative consequence of limited spatial resolution. Equally important, however, is the quantitative impact of finite resolution on the measured radioactivity in individual brain regions. The latter, so-called *partial volume effects* have important consequences for image quantitation and require a clearer understanding of spatial resolution and its definition.

In PET and SPECT, *spatial definition* is defined in practical terms—the distance by which two objects must be separated to perceive them as discrete (Fig. 1.16–5). In a SPECT or PET camera with perfect resolution, a point source of radioactivity would be depicted as a vertical line of infinitely narrow width. In such an ideal device, two point sources could be distinguished from each other as long as they were not superimposed. In the real world, however, PET and SPECT scanners perceive the radioactivity from such a point source as a gaussian curve. The radioactivity from the point is spread out. This so-called point spread function characterizes a camera's resolving capacity. This spatial diffusion of imaged radioactivity is expressed in terms of the *full width at half maximum* (FWHM), or the width of the gaussian curve at one-half of the curve's peak activity. The FWHM is the parameter most commonly used to define resolution in emission tomography, because this is the distance at which the peaks of both sources become distinguishable from one another (Fig. 1.16–5).

Excluding issues of positron range, image resolution is primarily influenced by issues of instrumentation. For example, the precision of collimation, the number and size of detectors, and the accuracy with which scintillation events are localized within the crystalline elements all contribute to limited spatial resolution. In the case of

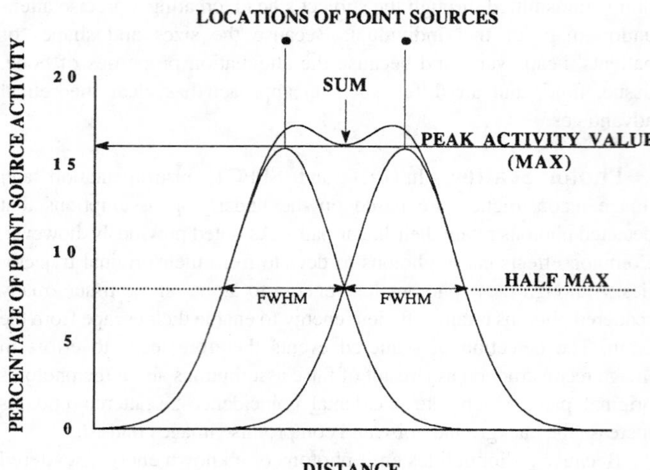

FIGURE 1.16–5 The limited resolution of positron emission tomography and single photon emission computed tomography cameras blurs the activity of single point sources into adjacent regions with no activity. Viewed in just one dimension, a point source is visualized by the camera as a gaussian curve. Resolution is defined as the width of the curve at half maximum measured peak levels (full width at half maximum [FWHM]). For two point sources of equal intensity separated by a distance equal to the FWHM of the camera, the sum of the activities begins to show a modest decrease at the midpoint. Thus, two point sources separated by a minimum distance equal to the FWHM begin to appear as two separate points rather than just one.

PET, state-of-the-art devices have yielded resolutions close to the theoretical limits of accuracy (2 mm). However, the average PET and SPECT cameras are currently capable of 5 to 6 mm and 7 to 9 mm FWHM, respectively.

Partial Volume Effects In its simplest terms, partial volume effects create one of two problems for image quantitation: the appearance of radioactivity where there was none and the impression of less radioactivity than truly exists. For example, just as the brightness in a part of a room depends on the intensity and distance separating two lamps, so too does the measured radioactivity in a given brain region reflect the relative activity and proximity of nearby structures. Thus, brain regions having relatively lower concentrations of radioactivity appear "hotter" in PET and SPECT images as imaged activity "spills over" from adjacent (more active) areas. Conversely, as the size of a radioactive region becomes smaller than two to three times the FWHM, true activity is effectively diluted by nonradioactive areas within the field of resolution. In the latter case, regions containing equal concentration of radioactivity appear to have declining levels with decreasing size. Together, these two effects result in, by visual analogy, sharp peaks and steep canyons of brain activity being rendered as short hills and shallow valleys in PET and SPECT images.

Several approaches are currently taken to compensate for errors resulting from limited spatial resolution and partial volume effects. One method attempts to simulate errors created by partial voluming by creating a plastic model or phantom. Models can be designed to approximate the structures or activity distributions, or both, of interest in the brain. For example, finely machined, polycarbonate brain phantoms are commercially available that recreate the geometry of gray and white matter. Once imaged, regionally specific correction factors, or recovery coefficients, are derived that relate units of measured activity to known activity. Such methods, however, are unable to account for intersubject variations in brain anatomy, whether pathological or nonpathological. A more modern way to correct partial volume effect is to use structural information (e.g., CT or MRI scans) of individual subjects for quantifying functional information. More specifically, partial volume errors may be mathematically compensated for by registering a subject's MRI scan with his or her own PET or SPECT scan and incorporating a priori functional (e.g., relative blood flow ratios in gray and white matter) and physical information (e.g., a PET or SPECT camera's three-dimensional point spread function). Although more complicated than the former technique, the latter approach has obvious advantages for conditions, such as Alzheimer's disease, in which cortical atrophy is present.

Radiopharmaceuticals The versatility and sensitivity of PET and SPECT arise largely from the ability of talented radiochemists to synthesize a radiopharmaceutical of high chemical purity, high radioactive yield, and small mass dose. Expressed differently, to ensure that a specific biological system of interest is adequately measured, yet unperturbed, by the tracer, a high purity and high specific activity (expressed in units of radioactivity per chemical quantity; e.g., Ci/mmol) are paramount. However, the physical nature of radioactive decay and the short $T_{1/2}$ of most suitable radionuclidic species (Fig. 1.16–1) constantly challenge the radiochemist's efforts. Specifically, chemical yield generally improves with increasing reaction times; however, radioactivity (and specific activity) diminishes with increasing decay times. Thus, an optimal synthetic scheme is a balanced one in which chemical yield is maximized, radioactive byproducts are minimized, and the final product is capable of prompt purification. Given the high affinity of many radiopharmaceuticals (e.g., neurotransmitter receptor ligands) for their physiological targets, specific activities of greater than 1,000 to 2,000 Ci/mmol are generally required. Although most radiopharmaceuticals are still manually prepared by radiochemists racing against the clock of a nuclide's decay, a limited number of radiochemical syntheses are now automated and performed in robotically controlled hot cells (e.g., [^{18}F]-2-fluoro-2-deoxyglucose [(^{18}F)FDG]; [^{11}C]raclopride).

In the case of positron-emitting radionuclides (e.g., ^{15}O, ^{13}N, ^{11}C, and ^{18}F), the particularly short $T_{1/2}$ (2, 10, 20, and 109 minutes, respectively) has special implications for the design of PET imaging facilities. Most PET centers have an on-site cyclotron that generates radionuclides for real-time use. An exception to this is ^{18}F, whose nearly 2-hour $T_{1/2}$ permits a local regional facility to produce quantities for a large or nearby metropolitan center. The significant expense of a cyclotron (typically $1 million to $2.5 million) and its highly skilled support staff are relative disadvantages for PET. In contrast, SPECT isotopes, such as ^{99m}Tc ($T_{1/2}$, 6 hours), may be obtained from inexpensive molybdenum generators located in many hospital radiopharmacies. Alternatively, ^{123}I has a sufficiently long $T_{1/2}$ (13 hours) to permit centralized production at distant (>3,000 miles) commercial reactors. The radionuclide may then be delivered via overnight express mail and may still meet the radiochemical needs of high activity.

The choice of a candidate molecule for radiopharmaceutical development depends primarily on the physiological process that one is interested in studying. In the case of regional cerebral blood flow, relatively nonspecific, and often nonorganic, diffusible tracers may be used (e.g., the gaseous tracer xenon-133 [^{133}Xe]). In contrast, the measurement of aspects of brain neurochemistry requires much greater biochemical selectivity. Thus, PET and SPECT radiopharmaceuticals are most often naturally occurring substances, structural analogs, or ligands that selectively label a particular brain target. In this regard, PET has significant advantages over SPECT, because ^{11}C can be directly substituted for carbon-12 (^{12}C) in existing organic molecules without altering their intrinsic biochemical properties. Alternatively, fluorine is frequently substituted for native hydrogen atoms without significant isotopic effects (e.g., [^{18}F]FDG). In contrast, SPECT nuclides (i.e., ^{123}I and ^{99m}Tc) are uncommon elements of organic substrates. The metallic nature and multiple valence states of ^{99m}Tc necessitate bulky complexing groups for its molecular stabilization. These barriers have largely limited the initial uses of ^{99m}Tc to nonselective processes (e.g., the blood flow agent [^{99m}Tc]-hexamethyl propyleneamine oxime [(^{99m}Tc)HMPAO]). However, ^{99m}Tc-labeled probes of the dopamine transporter (DAT) have recently been developed, and SPECT imaging has demonstrated appropriate labeling in human and monkey brains. Extension of these efforts is certain to result in the development of many other ^{99m}Tc-labeled probes in the future.

Many ^{123}I-containing radiopharmaceuticals have been developed as a result of rapid advances in iododemetallation procedures and increasing knowledge of the structure–activity relationships of pharmacologically active compounds. In fact, the lipophilic nature of ^{123}I may actually facilitate transfer across the blood–brain barrier and, in some instances, may improve affinity of the parent compound at its site of action. In particular, SPECT imaging of brain receptors and uptake sites with ^{123}I-containing radiopharmaceuticals is routine at many university medical centers.

Successful in vivo radiopharmaceuticals must fulfill several stringent pharmacokinetic criteria. Because a radiopharmaceutical must easily enter the brain, tracer binding to plasma proteins must be readily reversible, and its transport across the blood–brain barrier must be favorable. Although some tracers (e.g., [^{18}F]FDG) may have facilitated carriers, most ligands must be sufficiently lipid-soluble to permit passive diffusion across the blood–brain barrier. However, as tracer's lipophilicity increases, its *signal-to-noise* properties may be degraded as nonspecific binding increases. If lipophilicity is too high, passive diffusion across the blood–brain barrier is also impaired owing to increased binding to plasma proteins and blood cells. Therefore, a certain level of lipophilicity (typically a log D [log of ratio of radioligand in oil and water measured at pH 7.4] of 1 to 3 is required). Higher affinity is required to obtain higher levels of specific binding. Thus, lipophilicity (brain uptake and nonspecific binding) and affinity (specific binding) are important factors influencing an imaging agent's signal levels and signal to noise ratio. Lastly, tracer metabolism may also limit a ligand's in vivo usefulness. For example, rapid degradation, lipophilic radioactive metabolites, and pharmacologically active metabolites may all confound central measurements.

Small Animal PET and SPECT Imaging

PET devices designed to image small animals, such as rodents, were brought into operation in the early 1990s. During the last few years, significant improvements in imaging devices and data processing algorithms, as well as the development of various strains of genetically modified mice, spurred a quickly growing interest in small animal imaging techniques in various fields besides nuclear medicine, including basic science, clinical medicine, and the pharmaceutical industry. These techniques provide valuable information from living animals that is hard to obtain using conventional in vitro procedures, such as homogenate receptor binding assay and autoradiography. However, one should be aware of current limitations of small animal imaging that are occasionally overlooked, such as high receptor occupancy by imaging ligands.

Although small animal imaging devices have reached a spatial resolution of FWHM 2 mm, autoradiography provides, and probably will continue to provide, information with greater spatial resolution. However, to perform autoradiography, animals must be sacrificed to prepare brain slices. Therefore, small animal imaging is particularly useful when performing repeated measurements within a single experiment or across multiple experiments on the same animals over time. Imaging studies are particularly valuable when availability of animals, such as genetically engineered mice, is limited.

In addition to repeated measurements, small animal imaging may also be useful to detect in vivo biochemical processes that are difficult to study using other techniques. For example, small animal imaging can be used to evaluate the usefulness of imaging agents that label amyloid plaques in mice that have been genetically engineered to overexpress amyloid plaques. Although radioligand binding to amyloid plaques can be confirmed by in vitro binding assay and autoradiography, it is difficult to study kinetic properties of the radioligand by sacrificing animals at multiple time points after radioligand injection. Desired properties of imaging agents are (1) rapid passage of blood–brain barrier, (2) quick washout of nonspecifically bound tracer, (3) low nonspecific uptake, and (4) dissociation of specifically bound tracer within the time frame for PET or SPECT scans. Fifty to 100 times more animals are required to obtain the desired information when sacrificing animals at multiple time points after tracer injection than with small animal imaging; thus, small animal imaging offers great advantage, as it is often difficult to obtain a large number of genetically engineered animals. However, it is important to note that small animal imaging does not completely replace the need for classic techniques. In the case of amyloid imaging, binding characteristics first need to be studied by in vitro binding assay and autoradiography. In vivo radioligand binding must be confirmed by sacrificing animals after ligand injection and examining the coincidence of radioactivity and amyloid plaque location on brain slices. Therefore, small animal imaging and classic procedures together provide the essential information. Another thing that should not be overlooked is that imaging data do not provide information on chemical properties of the radioactivity. For example, it is necessary to know if the radioligand produces labeled metabolites that enter the brain and increases nonspecific radioactive signals. To obtain such information, radioactive compounds in plasma and the brain must be analyzed with high-performance liquid chromatography.

Whole-body distribution studies are required to estimate radiation-absorbed doses. By imaging the whole body by using small animal imaging devices, such studies can be performed much quicker than the classic methods that entail dissecting individual animals. Additionally, use of high-resolution human imaging devices (e.g., CTI's HRRT) for small animal whole-body imaging is more efficient than using small animal PET devices, because several animals can be scanned at the same time.

Another use is the detection of in vivo biochemical processes. Reporter gene imaging is a common application for small animal imaging devices. The basic design of this technique is to deliver a fusion of a reporter and a therapeutic gene. Thus, one can indirectly monitor the transcription of the therapeutic gene by using a radiolabeled tracer that is specifically metabolized by or that specifically binds to the product of the reporter gene. The final goal of these techniques is to monitor gene therapy in humans. These techniques were recently modified to noninvasively detect endogenous biological processes. Endogenous gene expression is monitored by administering transgenes containing endogenous promoters fused to a reporter gene. The transcription of the fused gene is then expected to mimic that of endogenous genes connected to the same promoter. Modifications of reporter gene imaging techniques have also been used to detect protein–protein interaction, which induces transcription of a reporter gene.

To image small animals, such as mice and rats, high resolution, preferably at a submillimeter level, is required. Resolution of small animal PET is limited by three factors: (1) positron range (see the previous discussion), (2) noncollinear annihilation (see the previous discussion); and (3) intrinsic spatial resolution of the imaging device. By applying new techniques and materials, as described in the following discussion, FWHM of current small animal PET cameras has been refined to 2 mm, and further improvement of spatial resolution and sensitivity is expected. The new scintillator material lutetium oxyorthosilicate (LSO) possesses significantly higher scintillation efficiency and shorter light decay time than BGO, which is typically used in human scanners. These beneficial characteristics resulted in an increased counting rate and a reduction in random coincident rate. Conventional methods using a filtered back-projection algorithm are being replaced by iterative reconstruction methods to improve spatial resolution. To reduce errors caused by noncollinear annihilation and also to reduce cost, small animal PET devices have a small diameter, which makes the depth-of-interaction (DOI) effect significant. The DOI effect results in an increased uncertainty in the location of endpoints of the line of response connecting detector pairs. Several methods have been proposed to reduce DOI error, such as multiplayer scintillation crystal arrays in which the layer of interaction is determined by differences in light decay time between the scintillator in each layer.

As compared to in vitro and ex vivo autoradiography, which have higher spatial resolution, one advantage of small animal imaging is that it can provide pharmacokinetic information by repeated measurement in a single animal. On the other hand, one pitfall is that theories of pharmacology assume the use of negligible amounts of imaging ligand. If a large amount of imaging ligand is required to obtain adequate counts, this would violate assumptions of these theories. Assuming a consistent relationship between injected dose of radioligand and its concentration at the site of action, and using a method analogous to Michaelis-Menten equation kinetics, the following formula was derived to estimate receptor occupancy:

$$\text{Occupancy} = (\text{injected radioactivity})/(\text{body weight} \times \text{median effective dose } [ED_{50}] \times \text{specific activity} + \text{injected radioactivity})$$

To achieve low receptor occupancy in small animal imaging studies, high specific activity is required. A low level of receptor occupancy, which would fulfill tracer conditions, must be confirmed beforehand by estimating occupancy from specific activity and ED_{50}.

Although PET is clearly more advantageous than SPECT for achieving higher spatial resolution and high sensitivity, there have been some attempts to develop SPECT devices for small animal imaging.

Quantification of Receptor Densities

In vitro receptor binding assays characterize receptors and ligands by measuring receptor density (B_{max}) and affinity (K_D). To obtain these measurements, various concentrations of radiolabeled and nonlabeled ligand must be used in the reactions. Although possible, it is usually difficult to measure each of B_{max} and K_D in human molecular imaging studies by administering various levels of ligands, because substantial levels of receptor occupancy can cause serious pharmacological effects. Limiting dose of ligand administration makes it impossible to measure each of B_{max} and K_D, and only a ratio of B_{max}/K_D (which equals specific binding distribution volume, V_S) can be measured. Therefore, in most human studies, V_S is the measure used to reflect changes in receptors and transporters. This ratio indicates that, when there is an increase in V_S, it is caused by an increase in B_{max} or a decrease in K_D.

Theoretical foundations for the calculation of V_S are beyond the scope of this chapter. Nevertheless, in brief, V_S is calculated as a ratio of specific binding in the brain to the parent ligand level in arterial plasma under equilibrium conditions (i.e., C_s^e/C_a^e, where C_s^e and C_a^e are the specific binding in the brain and the parent ligand level in arterial plasma under equilibrium conditions, respectively). An intuitive way of understanding V_S is that, under equilibrium conditions, specific binding in the brain is normalized to the radioligand level in arterial plasma. The level of specific binding in the brain is determined by the injected amount and the clearance of the radioligand, as well as the receptor parameter, B_{max}/K_D. For example, under tracer conditions, if the dose of injected radioligand is higher, specific binding in the brain becomes higher. Therefore, to measure the receptor parameter V_S, the level of specific binding in the brain needs to be normalized to the radioligand level in plasma.

The measurement of V_S requires accurate measurement of parent radioligand levels in plasma by metabolite analysis. A less labor intensive way to measure a receptor parameter is to calculate the ratio of specific to nonspecific binding under equilibrium conditions (i.e., C_s^e/C_{NS}^e, where C_{NS}^e is the nonspecific binding in the brain under equilibrium conditions). This parameter is often called the *binding potential* (*BP*). In analogy to V_S, an intuitive way to understand BP is that, under equilibrium conditions, the level of specific binding is normalized to that of nonspecific binding in the brain. If a greater amount of radioligand enters the brain, specific and nonspecific binding increase, and the level of specific binding is influenced by the amount of radioligand entering the brain. Therefore, to obtain measures that reflect binding of the targeted receptor or transporter, the level of specific binding needs to be normalized to the amount of the radioligand entering the brain. Hence, one must compare measures of nonspecific binding in a brain region that does contain a negligible level of the targeted receptor or transporter. For example, to study dopamine receptors, the cerebellum is often used as a region that contains few receptors. An assumption to use BP to compare groups of subjects is that, under equilibrium conditions, there is no difference in nonspecific binding per plasma radioligand level among groups. On the other hand, such an assumption is not required to use V_S.

This equilibrium ratio V_S is calculated through mathematical modeling or by experimentally achieving equilibrium conditions. In many studies, the radioligand is administered as an IV bolus. In such studies, brain and plasma parent ligand activity change dynamically over time, and a true equilibrium condition is never achieved (Fig. 1.16–6). In bolus injection studies, the ratio under equilibrium conditions, V_S, is calculated mathematically. There is another method to calculate V_S. Instead of calculating the equilibrium ratio V_S mathematically, the true equilibrium condition is achieved experimentally

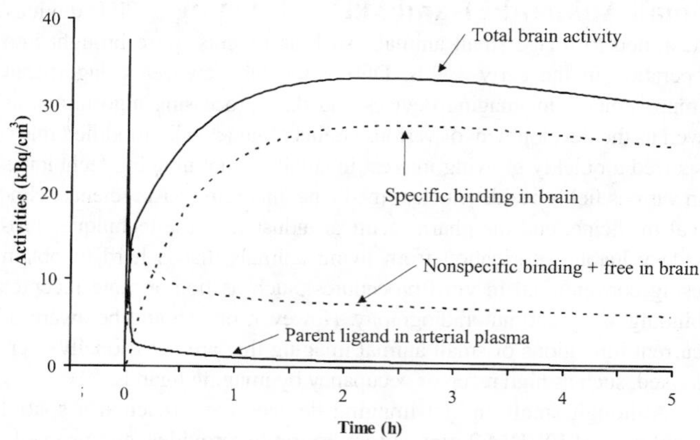

FIGURE 1.16–6 An example of brain and plasma parent ligand levels after a bolus injection. Levels of each component change dynamically over time. Note that all activities are decay corrected to time zero.

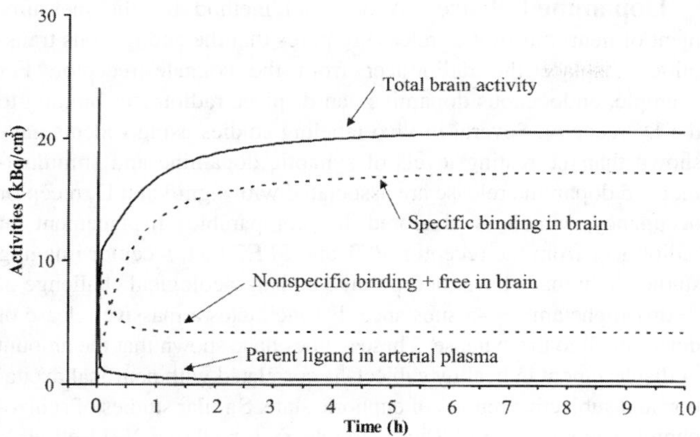

FIGURE 1.16–7 An example of brain and plasma parent ligand levels after a bolus injection and constant infusion. The same set of kinetic parameters is used to create curves of Figures 1.16–6 and 1.16–7. After prolonged infusion, an equilibrium condition is experimentally achieved—that is, all components reached stable levels. Note that all activities are decay corrected to time zero.

by performing an initial bolus injection of the radioligand, followed by a prolonged constant infusion (i.e., bolus plus constant infusion; Fig. 1.16–7). BP can also be calculated in these two ways—mathematically or experimentally.

SAFETY

With regard to studies in humans, PET and SPECT share similar safety concerns for radiation exposure and pharmacological toxicity of the injected radiopharmaceutical. The radiation exposures from typical PET and SPECT scans are thought to be reasonably safe within the context of present knowledge of radiation biology. The FDA has established limits of radiation exposure to various organs of the body and the body as a whole that are applied to research studies and that are often lower than exposures in routine clinical nuclear medicine procedures. Although the FDA limits are presently thought to provide adequate safety, the long-term biological effects of ionizing radiation remain an area of active investigation and even controversy. Although the estimation of the dose received by the body has multiple factors (including the amount of activity, the type of emission, and the residence time in the body), the shorter $T_{1/2}$ of PET radionuclides and the higher sensitivity of the method generally yield lower radiation burdens than a comparable SPECT study. A useful guideline is to use doses of radiotracer that are "as low as reasonably allowable" to provide useful results.

Fortunately, the pharmacological toxicity of radiopharmaceuticals is usually not a significant issue. The sensitivity of molecular imaging is so high that minuscule mass doses of compound may be injected, although that small mass is associated with significant levels of radioactivity. For example, some radiopharmaceuticals are injected at doses (in μg/kg and ng/kg) that are a millionfold lower than the minimal effective dose to cause any pharmacological effect. In such situations, no pharmacological toxicity would be expected, and only an unusual immunological adverse side effect could be anticipated. Nevertheless, the potential pharmacological effects and toxicity of radiopharmaceuticals need to be evaluated relative to previously established criteria for nonradioactive pharmaceuticals. Of course, the final formulation of any radiotracer must meet established guidelines for purity, sterility, and lack of pyrogenicity.

CLINICAL APPLICATION OF NEURORECEPTOR IMAGING

The use of PET and SPECT brain imaging can be roughly divided into measurements of local neuronal activity, neurochemistry, and in vivo pharmacology.

Local Neuronal Activity

Local neuronal activity is directly correlated with energy consumption and can be calculated using (1) direct measures targeting glucose metabolism or (2) indirect measures of cerebral blood flow (CBF). Tandem fluctuations of CBF and glucose metabolism are regulated via an autoregulatory mechanism that has not yet been identified. Tracers used in PET imaging for measurement of local neuronal activity include [^{18}F]FDG (fluorodeoxyglucose) for glucose metabolism, and [^{15}O]H_2O for measures of blood flow. With regard to SPECT imaging, ^{99m}Tc- and ^{123}I-labeled agents, as well as ^{133}Xe gas, are used to calculate CBF, but no comparable tracer has yet been developed for glucose metabolism in SPECT imaging.

Neuronal metabolic demands are believed to reflect primarily terminal, rather than cell body, activity. This conclusion is based on a limited number of studies of nerve cells whose cell bodies are anatomically distant from their terminals. Given this hypothesis, in any specified volume of brain tissue, the majority of [^{18}F]FDG uptake in PET glucose metabolism studies is in the terminal, rather than in the cell body. Another important factor in understanding the big picture reflected by these measures is that metabolic analyses cannot distinguish activity of excitatory neurons from that of inhibitory neurons. Thus, although increased [^{18}F]FDG uptake is usually interpreted as a regional increase in functional activity, it may ultimately reflect overall systemic inhibition as a result of increased firing of inhibitory interneurons.

In the clinical setting, PET and SPECT are primarily used to target and to assess local neuronal abnormalities, including those associated with cerebral ischemia and epilepsy, and, furthermore, can also be used to distinguish radiation necrosis from tumor growth. These imaging results can significantly impact decisions on clinical care. For example, the neurosurgical treatment of patients with medically refractory epilepsy requires precise localization of seizure foci. Because foci are often distant from the surface of the brain, PET and SPECT modalities are uniquely suited for this task, and, in comparison, localization using scalp electrode electroencephalography (EEG) is crude. During the interictal period, the seizure focus is hypometabolic, exhibiting decreased blood flow. Conversely, blood flow increases in the focus during the ictal period, and the region becomes hypermetabolic. Thus, because of their dual use in assessment of glucose metabolism and blood flow, imaging with PET and SPECT not only has served as primary means of localization of seizure foci, but also confirm other diagnostic tests required to pinpoint the portion of the brain that is subsequently resected.

PET imaging using [^{15}O]H_2O has been elegantly used in neuropsychological activation studies to identify areas of the brain that perform cognitive and sensory functions, including reading, speaking, word association, visual identification, and spatial localization. The short $T_{1/2}$ of ^{15}O ($T_{1/2}$ of 2 minutes) is optimal for these studies, as it allows for multiple (often eight to ten) bolus injections of the tracer in one experimental session. Thus, baseline scans and those following neuropsychological tasks can be repeated and averaged.

PET imaging has also been used to determine the physiology and anatomy of depression. In patients diagnosed with major depression, neuronal activity assessments using measures of CBF glucose metabolism revealed decreased activity in several areas of the brain, including regions of the frontal and temporal cortices and caudate nucleus. In familial major depressive disorders (unipolar or bipolar depression), metabolism in the prefrontal cortex, ventral to the genu of the corpus callosum (i.e., subgenual prefrontal cortex), was significantly lower as compared to controls. It was discovered, however, that gray matter volume in that region was less than normal and that, after corrections for volumetric differences were made, neuronal activity was actually higher in the patients than in healthy subjects. Thus, metabolism in the right subgenual prefrontal cortex correlates positively with depression severity, and this area, along with the other aforementioned brain regions, is now known to play a significant role in emotional processing. Further investigation of the anomalies in neural circuitry exposed by these imaging studies will hopefully lead to discovery of more precise mechanisms of the pathophysiology of depression and improved treatment of these disorders.

Neurochemistry Two important aspects in PET and SPECT imaging are high sensitivity and chemical selectivity, both of which are fundamental to reliable in vivo neurochemical measures. The sensitivity of PET and SPECT to detect radiotracers is less than 10^{-12} mol, which is several orders of magnitude greater than that of NMR methods. The term *sensitivity* refers to the minimal concentration of the tracer compound that can be reliably measured. For example, the minimal concentration of [^{11}C]chlorpromazine that can be measured with PET in the human brain within acceptable imaging time (e.g., 15 to 30 minutes) is less than 10^{-12} mol. In contrast, the minimal concentration of GABA that can be measured with magnetic resonance spectroscopy (MRS) is approximately 10^{-4} mol.

Radiotracers used to label specific target sites in the brain can be developed in a manner analogous to the development of therapeutic drugs selective for specific receptor sites. Radiotracers can then illuminate neurochemical pathways and mechanisms in the brain, including sites of neurotransmitter synthesis, reuptake and release, receptors, and metabolic enzymes. Additionally, researchers also hope to develop imaging techniques that could be used to investigate second messenger systems.

Of the various neurochemical systems in the brain, the greatest effort has been devoted to those that involve dopaminergic and serotonergic transmission. Current radiotracer development for these two systems focuses primarily on the pathophysiology of psychological disorders. The three principal research goals for these imaging studies are (1) to discover correlations between imaging results and clinical symptoms, (2) to measure effects of psychotropic or therapeutic drugs, and (3) to predict the clinical course of the disorder. However, except for imaging of the DAT in Parkinson's disease, existing neuroreceptor imaging agents have not demonstrated clinical usefulness for the diagnosis or management of neuropsychiatric disorders.

Dopamine Research for Parkinson's Disease 6-[^{18}F]Fluoro-L-3,4-dihydroxyphenylalanine ([^{18}F]FDOPA) has been used successfully in human studies to provide measures of dopaminergic terminals in the striatum. Results indicated significantly decreased striatal uptake in patients with Parkinson's disease compared to healthy subjects. Data from these studies have challenged the previously accepted notion that parkinsonian symptoms develop only after depletion of 85 to 90 percent of endogenous dopamine levels, as they illustrate that early signs of the disorder may appear after a decrease of only 50 to 60 percent in striatal dopamine terminal innervation. Conversely, studies of patients with schizophrenia revealed that neuroleptic-naive patients had an approximately 15 percent higher [^{18}F]FDOPA uptake in the putamen.

Dopamine Release A potential method for the measurement of neurotransmitter release requires that the endogenous transmitter displace the radiotracer from the cognate receptor. For example, endogenous dopamine can displace radiotracer binding to the D_2 receptor. Several in vivo labeling studies using rodents have shown that the resting levels of synaptic dopamine and stimulant-induced dopamine release are associated with significant D_2 receptor occupancy, which is mirrored by comparable displacement of radiotracer from the receptor. PET and SPECT D_2 receptor imaging studies in humans have incorporated a pharmacological challenge of dextroamphetamine—a substance that facilitates a massive release of dopamine into the synapse. These studies have shown that the amount of displacement in healthy subjects is correlated with neuronal excitation and subjective reports of euphoric state. Similar studies of schizophrenia patients using [^{123}I]iodo-2-hydroxy-6-methoxy-*N*-([1-ethyl-2-pyrrolidinyl]methyl)benzamide ([^{123}I]IBZM) as a D_2 receptor ligand have revealed that the amount of dopamine released is two and one-half times higher than that in healthy subjects (Fig. 1.16–8) and that the amount of the release is correlated with a transient increase in positive symptoms (Fig. 1.16–9). The same method was applied to a study of unipolar depressed patients that found unaltered release of dopamine. Another study looked at resting levels of dopamine in the synapse. Comparisons of D_2 receptor availability measures before, and during, α-methyl-*para*-tyrosine–induced dopamine depletion were performed on data from schizophrenia patients and healthy controls. Elevated synaptic dopamine was observed in patients and correlated with good response of positive symptoms to antipsychotic drugs. These imaging studies have provided further evidence of dopamine's role in psychotic symptoms.

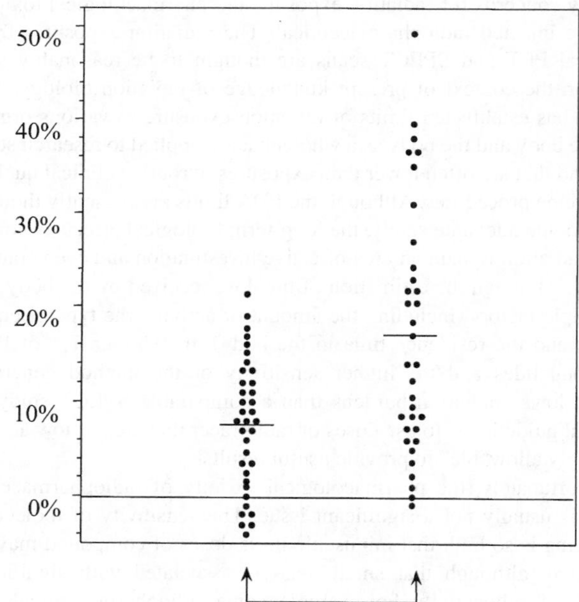

FIGURE 1.16–8 Effect of amphetamine (0.3 mg/kg) on [^{123}I]iodo-2-hydroxy-6-methoxy-*N*-([1-ethyl-2-pyrrolidinyl]methyl)benzamide([^{123}I]IBZM) binding in healthy control subjects and untreated patients with schizophrenia. The y-axis shows the percentage decrease in [^{123}I]IBZM binding potential induced by amphetamine, which is a measure of the increase occupancy of dopamine type 2 receptors by dopamine after the challenge. (From Laruelle M, Abi-Dargham A, Gil R, et al.: Increased dopamine transmission in schizophrenia: Relationship to illness phases. *Biol Psychiatry.* 1999;46:56, with permission.)

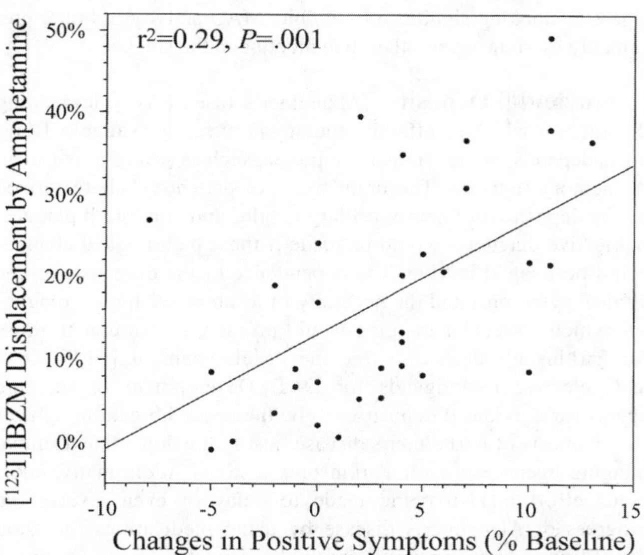

FIGURE 1.16–9 Relationship between striatal amphetamine-induced dopamine release and amphetamine-induced changes in positive symptoms. [^{123}I]IBZM, [^{123}I]iodo-2-hydroxy-6-methoxy-*N*-([1-ethyl-2-pyrrolidinyl]methyl)benzamide. (From Laruelle M, Abi-Dargham A, Gil R, et al.: Increased dopamine transmission in schizophrenia: Relationship to illness phases. *Biol Psychiatry.* 1999;46:56, with permission.)

Receptors Among all of the potential targets of neurochemical imaging, receptors have probably received the most attention. If a receptor is selectively altered in a specific disease, then imaging of this site may provide diagnostic information about the disorder.

Dopamine Type 1 (D_1) Receptor Because of its role in cognitive function in the prefrontal cortex and occupancy by some antipsychotic drugs, the dopamine type 1 (D_1) receptor has received considerable attention. Among the receptor ligands developed for D_1-like receptors (D_1 and D_5 subtypes), [^{11}C]SCH23390 came first. In the initial human study using this radiotracer, schizophrenic patients showed lower D_1 receptor binding in the prefrontal cortex as compared to controls, and these lower measures correlated with negative symptoms of the disease.

Later, a more selective D_1 radiotracer, [^{11}C]NNC-112, was developed and used in schizophrenia studies. This tracer yields a higher ratio of specific to nonspecific uptake than [^{11}C]SCH23390 and is able to provide measures of D_1 receptors in low-density regions. As opposed to [^{11}C]SCH23390, [^{11}C]NNC-112 showed a moderate *increase* in receptor binding in the dorsolateral prefrontal cortex of patients with schizophrenia. This increase was negatively correlated with patients' performance on a working memory task. Researchers hypothesized that increased prefrontal D_1 receptor binding was a compensatory upregulation resulting from long-term decreases in dopamine innervation of the cortex, but future studies are needed to solidify and confirm this important conjecture.

Dopamine Type 2 (D_2) Receptor The D_2 receptor, a known target of antipsychotic drugs, was the first receptor to be extensively studied with preponderance on schizophrenia beginning in the 1980s. Initial studies investigated baseline levels of D_2 receptor binding, looking for differences between normal patients and patients with schizophrenia. Contradictory findings were reported by investigators in the United States (elevated striatal D_2 receptors) and in Sweden (no elevation). Although this controversy is still not completely resolved, the general consensus is that schizophrenia is associated with no or, at most, small elevations of striatal D_2 receptor binding.

Subsequent studies have focused on endogenous measures of dopamine itself (see the previous discussion) or on development of new PET tracers for quantification of low-density D_2 receptors found in extrastriatal regions, such as the temporal cortex. Among the newly discovered PET ligands are agents, such as [^{18}F]fallypride and [^{11}C]FLB-457, both of which have demonstrated low enough nonspecific uptake so as not to obscure low levels of receptor binding in cortical regions. More recently, in drug-naive schizophrenia patients, [^{11}C]FLB-457 binding in the anterior cingulate was found to be lower compared to measures in healthy controls. Current trends in research convey increasing interest in extrastriatal D_2 receptors, and the results of these studies are anticipated in the near future.

Serotonin Type 1A (5-HT_{1A}) Receptor The serotonin type 1A (5-HT_{1A}) receptor is found at postsynaptic sites in areas such as the hippocampus and at presynaptic sites on 5-HT neurons in the dorsal raphe nucleus of the midbrain. In presynaptic (i.e., somatodendritic) locations, the 5-HT_{1A} receptor functions as an inhibitory autoreceptor to decrease 5-HT neural firing, thereby reducing the release of 5-HT at distal terminal regions. Animal and human studies suggest that the 5-HT_{1A} receptor may play a critical role in the mechanisms of action of selective serotonin reuptake inhibitors (SSRIs). During the first few weeks of SSRI treatment, the postsynaptic 5-HT_{1A} receptor is thought to increase in sensitivity as the 5-HT_{1A} presynaptic autoreceptor decreases in functional activity. The net result is a marked enhancement in 5-HT neurotransmission: enhanced postsynaptic activity and decreased autoinhibition. This fundamental outcome has made the 5-HT_{1A} receptor subtype a popular target of PET imaging, especially with regard to mood disorder research. This receptor is a major player in the regulation of serotonergic neuronal activity. Abnormalities in this receptor have been inferred by clinical observations of treatment of major depression. ^{11}C-labeled WAY-100635 (*N*-[2-(4-[2-methoxyphenyl]-1-piperazinyl)ethyl]-*N*-[2-pyridyl] cyclohexane carboxamide) was developed expressly for 5-HT_{1A} receptor imaging. Results from two PET studies using this radiotracer indicated reduction in receptor binding in patients with unipolar major depression. One of these studies indicated more pronounced reduction in the presynaptic region (dorsal raphe), whereas both studies demonstrated moderate reduction in the postsynaptic regions (neocortex and hippocampus). Furthermore, one study showed minimal change in the receptor after chronic SSRI treatment, suggesting that binding decreases are a trait-dependent, rather than a state-dependent, abnormality.

Transporters In addition to receptors, transporters (reuptake sites) have also been imaged.

Dopamine Transporter When dopamine is released from neuron terminals into the synaptic cleft, this chemical signal is deactivated by reuptake into presynaptic terminals by the DAT. This transporter plays a fundamental role in affecting the physiological and subsequent psychological outcomes of therapeutic agents and drugs of abuse. For example, amphetamine causes DAT to operate in reverse, thereby ejecting large quantities of dopamine into the synapse. Cocaine and methylphenidate act to halt the function of DAT, leading to a buildup of dopamine in the synaptic cleft.

Several radiotracers have been developed for DAT, including: [^{11}C]cocaine, [^{11}C]methylphenidate, 2β-carbomethoxy-3β-(4-fluorophenyl) tropane ([^{11}C]CFT) (also designated *WIN 35,428*), and (1*R*)-2β-carbomethoxy-3β-(4-iodophenyl) tropane ([^{123}I]β-CIT), which is also designated *RTI-55*. Research involving these new tracers has shown that striatal uptake of [^{11}C]CFT and [^{123}I]β-CIT is markedly decreased in patients with Parkinson's disease in comparison to healthy subjects of similar age. Although much is still to be learned, DAT imaging with these tracers offers new hope for early diagnosis and tracking disease progress. Additionally, a new SPECT tracer for DAT was recently approved for use in the European Union to aid in the diagnosis of Parkinson's disease.

In another realm of current research, [^{123}I]β-CIT and other tropane analogs are being used to investigate DAT function in psychiatric disorders, such as schizophrenia, acute cocaine abstinence, and Tourette's syndrome. In patients with schizophrenia, no apparent change was observed in levels of DAT protein, which have been imaged and quantified with SPECT or PET. Imaging in abstinent cocaine addicts has shown contradictory results of increased, versus decreased, DAT binding. However, this discrepancy could be caused by inconsistencies in subject selection concerning the period after cocaine discontinuation. Immediately after discontinuation, DAT levels may be elevated, and these elevations reflect changes stemming from a short-term physiological adaptation responding to the abruptly unmet demands of a firmly established chronic DAT blockade. Finally, in at least two studies of Tourette's syndrome, reports have shown significant (35 percent) elevations of DAT levels in the striatum. Elevated levels in this context may reflect enhanced dopamine neurotransmission in this disorder and may be the key to the partial success of dopamine blocking therapies, as with neuroleptic medications.

Serotonin Transporter Similar to mechanisms involved in termination of dopamine synaptic signaling, the activity of 5-HT is terminated by its reuptake into 5-HT terminals via the serotonin transporter (SERT). The antidepressant actions of SSRIs are mediated by a SERT blockade, thereby leading to a buildup of 5-HT in the synapse. SERT imaging may be important to elucidate the pathophysiology of the disorder and to monitor treatment. Before the recent development of PET radiotracers selective for SERT, [^{123}I]β-CIT and other tropane analogs that bind SERT *and* DAT have been studied in patients with depression. Despite their lack of selectivity, the inherent difference in regional distributions of DAT and SERT has made it possible to arrive, at least, at ballpark measures of each transporter type. The binding of [^{123}I]β-CIT predominantly reflects SERT in midbrain and diencephalon and DAT in striatum. In reference to clinical symptoms, these data have inferred irregularities of SERT in several disorders, including alcoholism, major depression, and cocaine abuse. In an early study in patients with major depression, midbrain SERT binding was found to be lower in patients as compared to healthy controls. In patients with behavioral problems, such as binge eating and impulsivity, lower SERT binding was found by using the radiotracer. Still, one must remember that these are no more than rudimentary applications and that cross-reactivity of these tropane analogs with SERT and DAT precludes a precise measurement of SERT levels. Fortunately, more selective SERT ligands have recently been developed and will provide valuable information on this target for mood and other psychiatric disorders. An initial report of one of these new selective agents, *N,N*-dimethyl-2-(2-amino-4-cyanophenylthio) benzylamine ([^{11}C]DASB), found no change in SERT levels in frontal cortex, caudate, or thalamus.

Metabolism The fate of a neurotransmitter can be studied by injection of selective inhibitors of its catabolic enzymes. For example, ^{11}C-labeled suicide enzyme inactivators, clorgyline and L-deprenyl, are used to image monoamine oxidase (MAO) types A and B, respectively. In this regard, PET imaging unexpectedly revealed that cigarette smoking significantly inhibits MAO activity in brain, presumably by some agent other than nicotine in the smoke.

Amyloid-β Deposits Alzheimer's disease is a devastating disorder for which no effective therapy is currently available. Diagnosis depends on the clinical symptoms, such as severe impairment of memory function. The brain tissue of patients is characterized by the deposition of neurofibrillary tangles and amyloid-β plaques. Subjective diagnosis would be made if these pathological changes could be imaged in vivo. The dependence of the diagnosis on the clinical symptoms and the necessity of a subjective tool of diagnosis, which molecular imaging would provide, are similar to those for Parkinson's disease before the development of [^{18}F]FDOPA and selective radioligands for DAT. Development of imaging agents for amyloid-β deposits will be the needed breakthrough for the diagnosis of Alzheimer's disease, just as the dopamine terminal imaging agents were for Parkinson's disease. Additionally, enormous effort is also being made to delay or even reverse the progress of Alzheimer's disease by using medications that stop deposition of or even remove amyloid-β deposits. Therefore, imaging agents for amyloid-β deposits will also provide tools to track progress of such therapies, as well as to diagnose the disease. From this perspective, such imaging agents may also follow the same path of clinical use as dopamine terminal imaging agents, which now provide a means to monitor implanted cells in Parkinson's diseased patients and to monitor possible delays of the progress of disease by new therapeutics. After years of trials based on the structures of dyes used in postmortem studies, some progress is now being seen with radioligands, developed during the first years of this century, that show hope for successful imaging of amyloid-β deposits in vivo.

Intracellular Signal Transduction Systems Although only a limited number of studies have been performed in human subjects, attempts to image intracellular signal transduction systems should be noted. Cyclic adenosine monophosphate (cAMP) and phosphoinositides are two major second messengers in neurotransmission systems, and arachidonate also plays a role in intracellular signal transduction systems. [^{11}C]Rolipram is the most widely used ligand for signal transduction system imaging. This ligand is an inhibitor of phosphodiesterase IV, which specifically metabolizes cAMP in the brain. Therefore, the binding of [^{11}C]rolipram reflects levels of the feedback system of the cAMP pathway. Other, less widely used tracers are [^{11}C]diacylglycerol and [^{11}C]arachidonate. Injected [^{11}C]diacylglycerol is incorporated into phosphoinositides and is expected to reflect their turnover.

In Vivo Pharmacology

Because receptors are frequently the targets of therapeutic medications, several investigators have argued that receptor imaging may be used to monitor drug treatment more accurately than is possible with measurement of plasma levels of the medications. However, the rationale for this argument is flawed from the theoretical perspective. Under steady-state conditions achieved with long-term treatment, the level of free (i.e., not protein bound) drug in plasma should achieve equilibrium with the free level of drug in the extracellular space of the brain. Thus, under steady-state conditions, there is little apparent value in performing expensive neuroreceptor imaging studies instead of simple measurements of the free level of drug in plasma. However, for non–steady-state conditions (e.g., beginning or discontinuing treatment), receptor imaging can provide valuable kinetic information.

The brain uptake and washout of many psychoactive agents can be markedly delayed compared to the rapid peak and fast clearance of the drug from plasma. For example, the maximal brain uptake of the potent cocaine analog, cocaine-iodo-tropane, occurs approximately 12 hours after IV administration as compared to plasma levels, which peak at 2 minutes. In addition, significant D_2 receptor occupancy has been reported to last for several weeks after discontinuation of antipsychotic agents, even when plasma levels are almost undetectable.

Several pharmaceutical companies and academic researchers have begun to explore the role of receptor imaging in new drug development. Two fundamental methods used in this investigation are (1) the radiolabeling of a target compound (e.g., labeled with ^{11}C) and (2) the in vivo screening of the effects of IV administered nonradioactive compounds with previously developed radiotracers. An example of the first method would be the use of ^{11}C-labeled fluoxetine (Prozac); an example of the second method would be the use of nonradioactive fluoxetine that would interact with another radiolabeled probe (e.g., [^{11}C]DASB for SERT).

Antipsychotic occupancy of the D_2 receptor has been extensively investigated using [^{11}C]raclopride. Studies have demonstrated occupancy of the D_2 receptor by typical and atypical antipsychotic medications, such as haloperidol (Haldol), clozapine (Clozaril), quetiapine (Seroquel), risperidone (Risperdal), olanzapine (Zyprexa), and loxapine (Loxitane). Data have shown that D_2 receptor occupancy of therapeutic doses of atypical antipsychotic agents is lower (approximately 40 to 60 percent) than with comparable doses of typical neuroleptic medications (70 to 90 percent). The lower incidence of extrapyramidal symptoms with atypical agents may be due, in part, to their lower D_2 receptor occupancy.

In a similar manner, SERT occupancy by SSRIs has been measured by using PET. Recent studies have shown that even low doses of SSRIs cause nearly complete (80 to 90 percent) occupancy of brain SERT. This conclusion, in turn, now raises the question of the functional usefulness of higher SSRI doses. However, as in most avenues of research, many new questions arise in the search for empirical confirmation of current hypotheses, and, thus, knowledge is refined, and improved clinical treatment of disease is pushed ever closer.

SUGGESTED CROSS-REFERENCES

Brain-imaging techniques are discussed in Section 1.15. Electrophysiology in clinical practice is discussed in Section 1.14, and neuroimaging in geriatric assessment is discussed in Sections 51.2e and 51.2f. The other sections of Chapter 1 discuss related neural sciences, particularly Section 1.2 on functional neuroanatomy and Section 1.14 on applied electrophysiology.

REFERENCES

Abi-Dargham A, Mawlawi O, Lombardo I, Gil R, Martinez D, Huang Y, Hwang DR, Keilp J, Kochan L, Van Heertum R, Gorman JM, Laruelle M: Prefrontal dopamine D1 receptors and working memory in schizophrenia. *J Neurosci.* 2002;22:3708.

Bacskai BJ, Klunk WE, Mathis CA, Hyman BT: Imaging amyloid-beta deposits in vivo. *J Cereb Blood Flow Metab.* 2002;22:1035.

Blasberg R: Imaging gene expression and endogenous molecular processes: Molecular imaging. *J Cereb Blood Flow Metab.* 2002;22:1157.

*Carson RE. Parameter estimation in positron emission tomography. In: Phelps ME, Mazziotta JC, Schelbert HR, eds. *Positron Emission Tomography and Autoradiography: Principles and Applications for the Brain and Heart.* New York: Raven Press; 1986.

Carson RE, Channing MA, Blasberg RG, Dunn BB, Cohen RM, Rice KC, Herscovitch P: Comparison of bolus and infusion methods for receptor quantitation: Applications to [^{18}F]cyclofoxy and positron emission tomography. *J Cereb Blood Flow Metab.* 1993;13:24.

Drevets WC, Frank E, Price JC, Kupfer DJ, Holt D, Greer PJ, Huang Y, Gautier C, Mathis C: PET imaging of serotonin 1A receptor binding in depression. *Biol Psychiatry.* 1999;46:1375.

Farde L, Nordstrom AL, Wiesel FA, Pauli S, Halldin C, Sedvall G: Positron emission tomographic analysis of central D1 and D2 dopamine receptor occupancy in patients treated with classical neuroleptics and clozapine. Relation to extrapyramidal side effects. *Arch Gen Psychiatry.* 1992;49:538.

Farde L, Wiesel FA, Stone-Elander S, Halldin C, Nordstrom AL, Hall H, Sedvall G: D2 dopamine receptors in neuroleptic-naive schizophrenic patients. A positron emission tomography study with [^{11}C]raclopride. *Arch Gen Psychiatry.* 1990;47:213.

*Huang S-C, Phelps ME. Principles of tracer kinetic modeling in positron emission tomography and autoradiography. In: Phelps M, Mazziotta J, Schelbert H, eds. *Positron Emission Tomography and Autoradiography: Principles and Applications for the Brain and Heart.* New York: Raven Press; 1986.

*Hume SP, Gunn RN, Jones T: Pharmacological constraints associated with positron emission tomographic scanning of small laboratory animals. *Eur J Nucl Med.* 1998;25:173.

Kung HF, Kim HJ, Kung MP, Meegalla SK, Plossl K, Lee HK: Imaging of dopamine transporters in humans with technetium-99m TRODAT-1. *Eur J Nucl Med.* 1996;23:1527.

Laruelle M: Imaging synaptic neurotransmission with in vivo binding competition techniques: A critical review. *J Cereb Blood Flow Metab.* 2000;20:423.

*Laruelle M, Abi-Dargham A, Gil R, Kegeles L, Innis R: Increased dopamine transmission in schizophrenia: relationship to illness phases. *Biol Psychiatry.* 1999;46:56.

Mathis CA, Wang Y, Holt DP, Huang GF, Debnath ML, Klunk WE: Synthesis and evaluation of ^{11}C-labeled 6-substituted 2-arylbenzothiazoles as amyloid imaging agents. *J Med Chem.* 2003;46:2740.

Meltzer CC, Zubieta JK, Links JM, Brakeman P, Stumpf MJ, Frost JJ: MR-based correction of brain PET measurements for heterogeneous gray matter radioactivity distribution. *J Cereb Blood Flow Metab.* 1996;16:650.

Okubo Y, Suhara T, Suzuki K, Kobayashi K, Inoue O, Terasaki O, Someya Y, Sassa T, Sudo Y, Matsushima E, Iyo M, Tateno Y, Toru M: Decreased prefrontal dopamine D1 receptors in schizophrenia revealed by PET. *Nature.* 1997;385:634.

Parkinson Study Group PS: Dopamine transporter brain imaging to assess the effects of pramipexole vs. levodopa on Parkinson's disease progression. *JAMA.* 2002;287:1653.

Sargent PA, Kjaer KH, Bench CJ, Rabiner EA, Messa C, Meyer J, Gunn RN, Grasby PM, Cowen PJ: Brain serotonin 1A receptor binding measured by positron emission tomography with [^{11}C]WAY-100635: Effects of depression and antidepressant treatment. *Arch Gen Psychiatry.* 2000;57:174.

Seibyl JP, Marek KL, Quinlan D, Sheff K, Zoghbi SS, Zea-Ponce Y, Baldwin RM, Fussell B, Smith EO, Charney DS, Hoffer PB, Innis RB: Decreased single-photon emission computed tomographic [^{123}I]β-CIT striatal uptake correlates with symptom severity in idiopathic Parkinson's disease. *Ann Neurol.* 1995;38:589.

*Sorensen JA, Phelps ME. *Physics in Nuclear Medicine.* 2nd ed. Philadelphia: WB Saunders; 1987.

Ungerleider LG: Functional brain imaging studies of cortical mechanisms for memory. *Science.* 1995;270:769.

Whone AL, Watts RL, Stoessl AJ, Davis M, Reske S, Nahmias C, Lang AE, Rascol O, Ribeiro MJ, Remy P, Poewe WH, Hauser RA, Brooks DJ: Slower progression of Parkinson's disease with ropinirole versus levodopa: The REAL-PET study. *Ann Neurol.* 2003;54:93.

Wong DF, Wagner HN Jr, Tune LE, Dannals RF, Pearlson GD, Links JM, Tamminga CA, Borussolle EP, Ravert HT, Wilson AA, Toung T, Malat J, Williams MA, O'Tuama LA, Snyder SH, Kuhar MJ, Gjedde A: Positron emission tomography reveals elevated D2 dopamine receptors in drug naive schizophrenics. *Science.* 1986;234:1558.

Zubieta JK, Heitzig MM, Smith YR, Bueller JA, Xu K, Xu Y, Koeppe RA, Stohler CS, Goldman D: COMT val158met genotype affects mu-opioid neurotransmitter responses to a pain stressor. *Science.* 2003;299:1240.

▲ 1.17 Population Genetics and Genetic Epidemiology

STEVEN O. MOLDIN, PH.D.

The human genome's 35,000 genes are located on 22 pairs of autosomal chromosomes and two sex chromosomes, comprising approximately three billion base pairs of *deoxyribonucleic acid* (DNA). The coding regions of these genes take up less than 5 percent of the genome. The pace of the molecular dissection of human disease, through the application of powerful quantitative analytic methods, new technologies such as microarrays, and the nearly completed sequence of the human genome, has permitted identification of mutations for more than one-fourth of the roughly 4,000 genetically inherited diseases currently recorded in databases, such as Victor McKusick's Online Mendelian Inheritance in Man (OMIM).

There are major public health implications of identifying the genes and, specifically, the genetic variants that influence risk for the more common familial mental disorders, such as autism, bipolar and other mood disorders, panic and other anxiety disorders, schizophrenia, eating disorders, and alcoholism. Such findings ultimately will be of relevance to many affected individuals and their relatives, because they will allow the development of genetic tests to identify individuals at risk and, most important, will provide the pharmaceutical industry with new drug therapeutic targets. The application of population genetic and genetic epidemiologic methods to the emerging data is expected to usher in an era of genomic medicine in which knowledge of our genetic uniqueness will alter most aspects of the diagnosis, treatment, and prevention of clinical disorders. This section is meant for psychiatric clinicians and researchers who want to understand the basic mathematical principles and quantitative methods of population genetics and genetic epidemiology, so that they are able to judge and appreciate the relevance of new data derived from the genetic analysis of mental disorders.

SUBFIELDS OF GENETICS

The scientific study of heredity, which arguably began with Gregor Mendel's work on peas in 1865, gradually developed into five major disciplines. *Biochemical genetics* is concerned with the biochemical reactions by which genetic determinants are replicated and produce their effects. *Developmental genetics* is the study of how the expression of normal genes controls growth and other developmental processes, often by the study of mutations that produce developmental abnormalities. *Molecular genetics* studies the structure and the functioning of genes at the molecular level. *Cytogenetics* deals with the chromosomes that carry those determinants. *Population genetics*, which deals with the mathematical properties of genetic transmission in families and populations, can be subdivided into the partially overlapping fields of evolutionary genetics, genetic demography, quantitative genetics, and genetic epidemiology. The primary goal of *evolutionary genetics* is to understand changes in gene frequency across generations. *Genetic demography* is primarily concerned with differential mortality and fertility (fitness) in human populations.

Quantitative genetics and genetic epidemiology are the fields of genetics that are highly relevant to the study of mental disorders. Both provide the mathematical methods to aid in the identification of genetic factors that influence risk to mental disorders. The goal of *quantitative genetics* is to partition the observed variation of phenotypes into its genetic and environmental components. Quantitative genetics was developed largely to improve animals and plants through artificial selection and usually deals with continuous traits (for example, milk yield or egg size), rather than discrete traits. *Genetic epidemiology* is explicitly directed toward understanding the causes, distribution, and control of disease in groups of relatives and the multifactorial causes of disease in populations. The mathematical principles of genetic epidemiology and quantitative genetics are central to risk analysis, which is the essential element in genetic counseling for familial disease, and to *linkage analysis*, which is an important statistical procedure used to implicate a particular chromosome as containing a putative disease gene.

Figure 1.17–1 shows the focus of genetic epidemiology to be on genetic and environmental factors that interact in determining observed behavioral outcomes (disease). Differences between common and individual-specific environmental effects and between genes of major versus minor effect are discussed in the section Multilocus Models. *Psychiatric genetics* involves the specific application of genetic principles and methods to the study of mental disorders. *Genetic medicine* is the application of genetic principles and knowledge about genetic differences among individuals to the practice of clinical medicine. It includes *pharmacogenetics*, the study of how genetic differences influence the variability in a patient's response to therapeutic compounds and how genetic information may be used to construct personalized therapeutic regimens.

BASIC ELEMENTS

A fundamental distinction in population genetics, dating to Wilhelm Johannsen's work in 1909, is between *genotype* (a pair of realizations of possible forms of a gene) and *phenotype* (an observed effect of those genes); the distribution of the frequencies of the various phenotypes constitutes the essential description of a population. When there is a simple mapping between genotypes and phenotypes, gene frequencies can be used to predict frequencies of genotypes and phenotypes, and vice versa, under a set of assumptions that include the following:

1. From the pattern of familial inheritance, the genotypes can be distinguished unequivocally, such that the frequencies of phenotypes are the same as those of the underlying genotypes. This relationship between phenotypic and genotypic frequencies requires the related assumptions of negligible mutation rates and the occurrence of segregation of genes according to Mendel's laws.

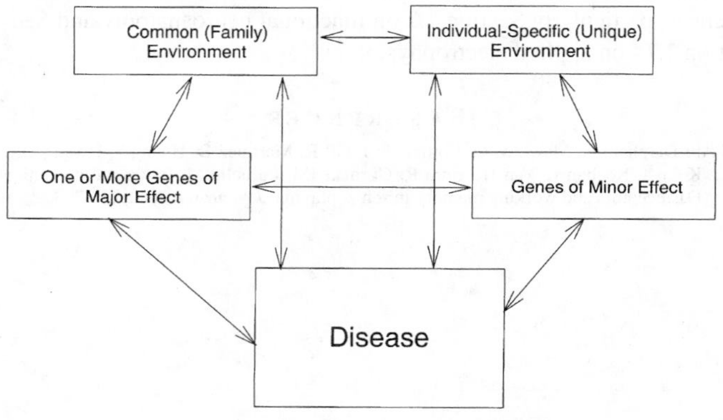

FIGURE 1.17–1 The network of genetic epidemiology.

2. There is no selection—that is, the expected number of fertile progeny from a mating that reaches maturity does not depend on the genotypes of the mates.
3. The population structure is such that all matings take place at random with respect to the genetic differences being considered in a population of infinite size. Consequently, the probability of mating between persons is in no way influenced by their genotype at a given *locus* or position on a chromosome.

A general theorem formulated independently in 1908 by Godfrey Harold Hardy and Wilhelm Weinberg is derived from those assumptions and fits the facts well in many cases. In its simplest form, the *Hardy-Weinberg law* states that, if respective gene frequencies of two alternative forms of a gene (*alleles*) *A* and *a* are *p* and *q*, the respective genotypic frequencies among progeny with genotypes *AA*, *Aa*, and *aa* are p^2, $2pq$, and q^2. This relationship between gene frequencies and genotype frequencies is of the greatest importance, because many of the deductions in quantitative and population genetics rest on it.

Linkage disequilibrium (LD) is the nonrandom association of alleles at adjacent loci. When a given allele at locus *M* is found together on the same chromosome with a specific allele at a second locus *N* at a frequency greater than that expected by chance, then alleles at loci *M* and *N* are in disequilibrium. At the heart of all measures of LD is the difference, *D*, between the observed frequency of a two-locus *haplotype*—closely linked loci at which alleles tend to be inherited together and not separated by recombinations now or in the recent evolutionary history of human populations—and the frequency it would be expected to show if the alleles were independent. Assuming two adjacent loci *M* and *N* with alleles (1,2 and 3,4) at each respective locus, the observed frequency of the *1,3* haplotype is represented by $P_{1,3}$. Given that P_1 is the frequency of allele *1*, and P_3 is the frequency of allele *3*, $D = P_{1,3} - (P_1 \times P_3)$.

A proposed strategy to detect some of the genetic variants affecting liability to mental disorders and other common diseases is to test many common genetic variants evenly spaced throughout the genome for their association with disease. If enough variants are tested, the thinking goes, even if the causal variants were not tested, disease association would still be detected, because variants in LD with the causal variants would be tested. Most human sequence variation is in the form of *single nucleotide polymorphisms* (SNPs), of which ten million are estimated to exist in the human genome. These are places in the genome at which the DNA sequence varies by a single base. Recent evidence from SNP data suggests that there is substantial heterogeneity of LD across the genome, with numerous regions of substantial LD, such that sets of mapped and ordered SNP variants can be grouped into blocks as distinct haplotypes. Recently, the National Human Genome Research Institute (NHGRI) has proposed an international effort (the *HapMap project*) to characterize the patterns of LD across the human genome and thus develop a map of common haplotype patterns in at least three ethnic populations. In principle, this HapMap project will accelerate the discovery of genetic variants affecting susceptibility to disease by providing a roadmap, loosely speaking, of what SNPs should be genotyped to characterize any particular region of the genome. A basic distinction in population genetics of direct relevance for the analysis of mental disorders is that between *quantitative* and *qualitative* phenotypes. That is to say, can persons be classified to one of a small number of discrete classes of disease status, or can they be assigned a continuous score on an observed continuum of disease susceptibility, a quantitative phenotype? Disease phenotypes are qualitative—persons are classified, according to diagnostic criteria, as affected or unaffected. However, contemporary genetic analysis usually posits that underlying disease status is a liability to affection that is continuous and, possibly, unobservable, with affected individuals at one extreme end of the continuum. In some instances, the liability score can be inferred by other attributes of individuals in addition to their affection status. When the liability is completely unobservable, it is analogous to having height as the phenotype but only being able to measure it as tall versus nontall, rather than measuring height in centimeters. Many quantitative phenotypes are directly observable and measured on some relevant continuous scale; lipoprotein levels, body mass index, scores determined from an intelligence test, and blood pressure are typical examples.

When a continuous variable is dichotomized, substantial information can be lost relative to what would be encoded by the variable in its original scale. For this reason, it is reasonable to predict that quantitative traits that are highly correlated with liability to an illness can make important contributions to genetic analysis. Highly specific and sensitive biological measures of quantitative processes have not yet been found for many mental disorders; rather, qualitative determinations (affected versus unaffected status) established through a structured diagnostic interview are the typical source of phenotypic data for genetic analysis. Evaluation of the usefulness of quantitative traits for inclusion in genetic studies of several mental disorders is the focus of several ongoing research efforts. Such traits include measures of neurophysiology (prepulse inhibition and eye tracking) and neurocognition (sustained attention and verbal and working memory) in schizophrenia and measures of language dysfunction in autism.

GENETIC MODELS OF FAMILIAL TRANSMISSION

Mathematical models are required in population genetics to represent the ways in which genes and the environment interact to form complex phenotypes transmitted within families (Table 1.17–1). These models quantify changes transmitted in families that depend on DNA sequence.

Single Major Locus Model The single major locus model assumes that all relevant genetic variations are due to the presence of alleles at a single locus and that environmental variations are unique to an individual. With two alleles, *A* and *a*, with respective frequencies *p* and *q*, three genotypes are possible: *AA*, *Aa*, and *aa*. When both alleles are the same, it is a *homozygous* genotype; when two alleles are different, it is a *heterozygous* genotype. The sum of the allele frequencies totals unity, or $p + q = 1$. If the environment is constant, such that each genotype corresponds to only one phenotype, the gene at a given locus is *completely penetrant*.

Diseases transmitted through a single major locus are referred to as *Mendelian diseases*, as the pattern of inheritance in families follows the rules of Mendelian segregation and can usually be recognized through visual inspection of pedigrees. Characteristic single locus diseases include retinitis pigmentosa, Duchenne's muscular dystrophy, polycystic kidney disease, Huntington's disease, phenylketonuria, and cystic fibrosis. The important discovery in 1991 of intraallelic expansion of highly unstable trinucleotide (triplet) repeat sequences helps explain the variations in age of onset and severity, without invoking an additional modifying locus. Huntington's disease, fragile X syndrome, myotonic dystrophy, spinobulbar muscular atrophy, spinocerebellar ataxia type I, and Machado-Joseph disease are examples of clinical disorders caused by the expansion of unstable repeat sequences.

Familial patterns of simple mendelizing inheritance can be characterized by whether the disease gene is on an autosome or on a sex chromosome and by whether both alleles are required for expression

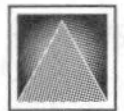

Table 1.17–1
Genetic Models of Disease Transmission

	Source of Familial Resemblance			
Model	**Genes of Major Effect (No.)**	**Genes of Minor Effect**	**Common Environment**	**Individual-Specific Genetic Environment**
Single major locus	Yes (1)	No	No	Yes
Allelic heterogeneity	Yes (1)	No	No	Yes
Locus heterogeneity	Yes (>1)	No	No	Yes
Multilocus models				
Multifactorial	No	Yes	Yes	Yes
Mixed	Yes (1)	Yes	Yes	Yes
General multilocus	Yes (>1)	Yes	Yes	Yes

(*recessive* inheritance) or only one allele is sufficient (*dominant* inheritance). The liability distributions in the general population resulting from a diallelic major locus in Hardy-Weinberg equilibrium are shown in Figure 1.17–2.

The following criteria for different single locus models of disease transmission are required: (1) In *autosomal dominant* transmission, (a) transmission continues from generation to generation without skipping; (b) except for freshly mutated cases (or nonpaternity), every affected child has an affected parent; (c) the two sexes are affected in equal numbers; and (d) in marriages of an affected heterozygote to a normal homozygote, the probability that a child born into that family is affected (the *segregation ratio*) is 0.5. (2) In *autosomal recessive* transmission, (a) if the disease is rare, parents and relatives (except siblings) are usually normal; (b) all children of two affected parents are affected; (c) in marriages of two healthy parents, the probability an offspring is affected is 0.25; and (d) the two sexes are affected in equal numbers. (3) In *sex-linked recessive* transmission, (a) if the disease is rare, parents and relatives (except maternal uncles and other male relatives in the female line) are usually healthy; (b) hemizygous affected men do not transmit the disease to children of either gender, but all their daughters are carriers; (c) heterozygous carrier women are normal but transmit the disease to their

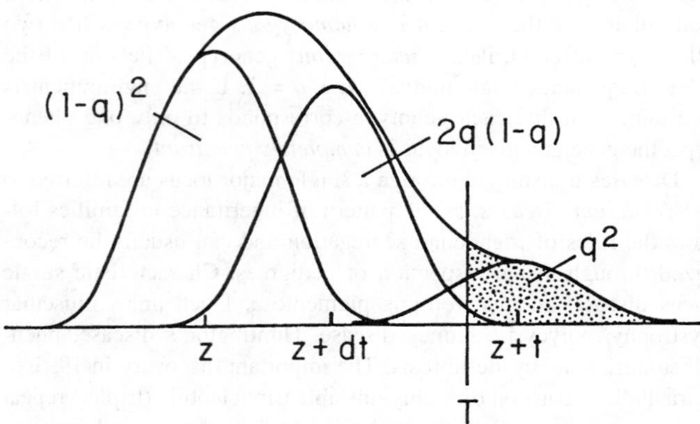

FIGURE 1.17–2 Liability distributions resulting from a single major locus in Hardy-Weinberg equilibrium. The locus has two alleles, *A* and *a*, with frequency *p* and *q*. The three genotypes (*AA*, *Aa*, and *aa*) have respective means of z, z + dt, and z + t; $d = 0$ results in a recessive locus, whereas $d = 1$ results in a dominant locus. Given that $p + q = 1$, and assuming the Hardy-Weinberg law holds, the respective genotypic frequencies are $(1 - q)^2$, $2q(1 - q)$, and q^2. The shaded area gives the lifetime morbid risk of the disease (K_p). The proportion of persons with a given genotype who are above the threshold (*T*) gives the penetrance of that genotype.

sons with a probability of 0.5 (and with a probability of 0.5 the daughters are normal carriers); and (d) except for mutants, every affected male child comes from a carrier mother.

The concept of *incomplete penetrance* has been introduced to cover the case in which persons with identical genotypes can have different phenotypes due to variability in nontransmissible environmental factors or transmissible modifiers of gene expression that contribute to the phenotype. The *penetrance*, often denoted by f, is the probability that a person with a given genotype manifests the illness. The lifetime cumulative incidence or morbid risk of a disease is frequently denoted by K_p. In the case of a disorder caused by a diallelic autosomal single major locus in which the respective gene frequencies of the *A* and *a* alleles are p and q, the respective penetrances associated with the *AA*, *Aa*, and *aa* genotypes are f_1, f_2, and f_3. Assuming the Hardy-Weinberg law holds, $K_p = f_1p^2 + f_22pq + f_3q^2$. Current generalized single major locus models allow for incomplete penetrance (i.e., one or more fs are not equal to 0 or 1), with transmission of a fully penetrant major locus contained as a submodel.

Elucidation of abnormal protein products and subsequent resolution of pathophysiology is theoretically more straightforward in the case of disease transmission through a single major gene than in the case of disease transmission through polygenes. However, the genetics of single major locus diseases can still be complicated, as exemplified by Huntington's disease. Clinical characterization first occurred in the 1800s, a dominant disease locus was linked to genetic markers on chromosome 4 in 1983, and the precise gene was identified 10 years later.

Multilocus Models

Multilocus models specify the effects of multiple loci, with or without contributions from environment factors, on susceptibility to disease. It is useful to distinguish *familial (common) environmental effects* from *individual-specific (idiosyncratic) environmental effects*. The latter refer to environmental experiences that are unique to the individual and are not shared among family members; this is also called the *within-family environment*. The former refer to environmental influences that are common to or shared by family members; this is also called the *between-family environment*.

Genetic influences in multilocus models may arise from the effects of *genes of major effect* versus *genes of minor effect*. The former refer to genes that make a large relative contribution to the total variance in the disease attributable to genetic influences; the latter refer to genes that each make a small relative contribution to the total variance attributable to genetic factors. The individual unit for each—a gene—is, of course, the same; the distinction between genes of major versus minor effect refers exclusively to the relative degree of influence that they have on the final behavioral outcome. Most common human diseases are inherited under a multilocus model; examples include hypertension, insulin-dependent diabetes mellitus, pyloric stenosis, rheumatoid arthritis, peptic ulcer, most cases of breast cancer, coronary artery disease, spina bifida, late-onset Alzheimer's disease, multiple sclerosis (MS), and most mental disorders. Multilocus model variants may be distinguished in regard to the number (if any) of loci that exert a larger influence on the phenotype relative to the influence of other genes.

Knowledge of the number of causative loci is necessary to design and estimate the power of mapping studies of complex diseases produced under multilocus models. Different methods have been developed to make these estimates, and recent work suggests that the best-fit estimates of causative loci for cleft lip and cleft palate and schizophrenia in a genetic isolate of Finland were three and four loci, respectively.

Multifactorial Model The multifactorial model assumes that all genetic variance is attributable to genes that each exert a small relative effect (*polygenes*). All relevant genetic and environmental contributions to variation can be combined into a normally distributed variable termed *liability*. There are one or more threshold values on the liability scale, such that affected individuals are those with liability values that exceed the threshold. Familial inheritance is modeled through correlations in liability between family members, with the following assumptions: (1) Relevant genes act additively and are each of small effect in relation to the total variation, (2) environmental contributions are due to many events whose effects are additive, and (3) there may be multiple thresholds, such that individuals with scores between threshold values represent milder phenotypic or *spectrum* cases. When all transmissible effects are genetic (i.e., the common environment exerts no influence), this is called the *polygenic model*. One or more threshold values are on the liability scale; affected persons are those with liability values that exceed the threshold. Familial inheritance is modeled through correlations in liability between family members. There may be multiple thresholds, such that persons with scores between threshold values represent mild phenotypic or spectrum cases. Normal traits inherited in this way include intelligence, stature, skin color, and total dermal ridge count. When the phenotype is qualitative (presence or absence of disease), a continuous liability distribution is unobservable but assumed to underlie the discrete phenotypic events that are observed. Liability distributions in the general population for single-threshold and two-threshold multifactorial models are shown in Figure 1.17–3.

Mixed Model The mixed model is a marriage of the single major locus model and the multifactorial model. A distribution of liability is determined by the effects of a major locus, a multifactorial transmissible background (polygenes or environmental factors), and residual individual-specific environmental factors. The mixed model differs from the multifactorial model regarding the presence of a single genetic locus of major effect. Because the single major locus model and the multifactorial model are submodels, the mixed model provides a statistical advance in permitting the rigorous testing of whether a single major locus or a multifactorial component (or both) contributes to familial resemblance.

General Multilocus Model The general multilocus model differs from the mixed model by the inclusion of more than one locus of relative major effect. The major assumption is that the marginal effects of these genes are detectable and separable from the background effects of other genetic loci of minor effect or environmental

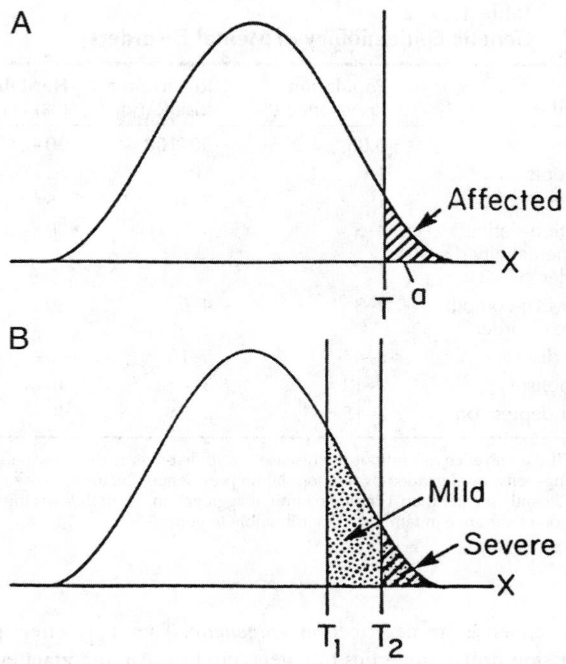

FIGURE 1.17–3 The unobserved liability (*x*) underlying a multifactorial disease with **(A)** a single threshold (*T*) and a mean liability of affected persons, denoted by *a*, and **(B)** two thresholds, T_1 and T_2, used to model severity, such that persons with a liability score above T_2 have a core (severe) phenotype, and persons whose liability is between T_1 and T_2 have a milder form of the illness (spectrum condition). The shaded areas give the lifetime cumulative incidences (K_p).

contributors. Complex interactions among loci of major or minor effect (*epistasis*) may occur. Alternatively, each locus of relative major effect may be an independent and sufficient cause of disease; such multilocus models are referred to as *genetic heterogeneity models*—an individual can be affected if he or she possesses a predisposing genotype at any one of the loci of relative major effect. *Locus heterogeneity* applies when a clinical disorder is caused by mutations at different loci (e.g., different forms of mental retardation); *allelic heterogeneity* applies when a disease is caused by different mutations at the same locus (e.g., breast cancer and cystic fibrosis).

The general multilocus model is the most comprehensive and realistic transmission model, because common illnesses are likely to be influenced by major and minor genetic effects and by the common environment. One way to quantify the relative effect of one locus versus others in multilocus models is to consider the proportion of disease risk that is attributable to that locus. This may be accomplished through consideration of the risks to different classes of relatives (i.e., siblings, monozygotic twins, and cousins) of affected individuals conferred by that specific locus as compared to the population prevalence. Locus-specific risk ratios for siblings of an affected individual (frequently denoted as λ) on the order of 1.5 to 2.0 may be expected for many mental disorders and other complex diseases. Table 1.17–2 shows recurrence risk ratios for first-degree relatives and other genetic epidemiological data for several mental disorders.

EPIGENESIS

In addition to genetic effects transmitted in families under the preceding models, additional factors that can be transmitted to progeny cells after cell division but that are not directly attributable to the

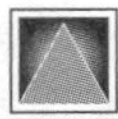

Table 1.17–2
Genetic Epidemiology of Mental Disorders

Disorder	Population Prevalence (%)	Recurrence Risk Ratio	Heritability (%)
Autism	0.05	50–100	90+
Schizophrenia	1	10	75+
Bipolar disorder	1	7–10	75+
Attention-deficit/hyperactivity disorder	3–5	4–6	60+
Obsessive-compulsive disorder	1–3	4–6	60+
Panic disorder	2–4	5–10	40+
Alcoholism	7–12	3	40+
Major depression	5–15	3	40+

Note: The recurrence risk ratio is the disease risk to first-degree relatives (parents, siblings, offspring) divided by the population prevalence. Recurrence risk ratios significantly greater than 1 indicate familial aggregation. *Heritability* is the proportion of variance in familial risk attributable to genes.

DNA sequence are described as *epigenetic*. They may effect gene expression or the properties of a gene product. An important epigenetic mechanism of potential relevance to mental disorders is *DNA methylation*. Silencing of an intact gene by methylation of adjacent control sequences is a normal component of development, differentiation, and X-chromosome inactivation. Methylation can cause pathological loss of function. For example, in fragile X syndrome, the *FMR1* gene is silenced by methylation triggered by a local DNA sequence change (a trinucleotide expansion).

Imprinting is another important epigenetic mechanism that affects several human genes. The expression of imprinted genes is controlled by methylation patterns that differ according to the parental origin of the genes. Malfunctioning of the imprinting mechanism or unexpected parental origin results in a pathological loss of function or inappropriate gene expression. Prader-Willi, Angelman's, and Beckwith-Wiedemann syndromes are classic examples of clinical disorders in which imprinted genes are involved.

RESEARCH DESIGNS

Population, epidemiological, family, twin, adoption, linkage, and association studies can each contribute evidence to evaluate the involvement of genetic factors in the cause of an illness (Table 1.17–3). In many cases, substantial increases in power are afforded when research designs are combined, for example when linkage studies are conducted in pedigrees identified in epidemiological samples.

Population and Epidemiological Studies

Prevalence and incidence rates of mental and other disorders derived from community-based surveys have important scientific and health policy implications. Variations in such rates can provide clues to causes and can be used as base rates for comparative purposes in family genetic studies. Epidemiological studies of all affected individuals in populations isolated by geography, culture, or other factors have the potential to be particularly useful. Use of such *population isolates* increases the chance that a greater fraction of affected individuals have a disease for the same reason—that is, etiologic heterogeneity is decreased. In some population isolates, the entire population is essentially one large pedigree. Typically, increases in genetic homogeneity in isolates are accompanied by increases in homogeneity of cultural and other environmental risk factors as well, and complexities engendered by gene–environment interactions could be diminished. Some population isolates are characterized by large regions of LD around disease alleles, such as the populations on the Micronesian islands of Palau and Yap. The enriched LD is presumably due to a small population at the founding of these relatively young (approximately 100 generations) populations. Genetic studies of mental disorders are being conducted in population isolates in Costa Rica, Micronesia, Sweden, Iceland, and other localities.

Family Studies

If genetic factors are involved in illness transmission, the illness should occur in the families of affected members at a higher rate than in appropriate control populations. However, relatives who share a number of genes also tend to share common environments, so familial aggregation by itself does not necessarily implicate a genetic mechanism; culture, family environment, or infectious agents may be responsible. Family studies for mental and other disorders begin with affected persons (*probands*) selected from patient pools such as consecutive hospital inpatient admission and a psychiatric case registry. Available relatives are located and assessed for psychopathology with structured or semistructured diagnostic instruments. Countries with national health insurance and psychiatric registers can provide morbidity information across generations. Recurrence risks are expected to increase as the degree of relatedness between relatives decreases. The closest degree of relatedness is that of monozygotic twins (zero degree), who are 100 percent identical at the level of their genes (barring early mutation). Dizygotic twins, full siblings, parents, and children are first-degree relatives who, on average, have one-half of their genetic material in common. Second-degree relatives of affected individuals—grandparents,

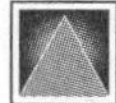

Table 1.17–3
Study Designs for Genetic Research on Mental Disorders

Study	Unit of Analysis	Goal
Population	Subjects in the general population	Establish lifetime incidence
Family	Pedigrees	Establish familiarity Estimate mode of transmission and risks to relative classes
Twin	Monozygotic and dizygotic twins	Distinguish genetic from environmental effects
Adoption	Adoptees; adoptive and biological relatives of adoptees	Distinguish genetic from environmental effects
Linkage	Nuclear or extended pedigrees, or both	Establish chromosomal location of a disease locus
Association	Unrelated affected individuals and controls	Identify a specific disease locus
Transgenic	Gene expression in animals	Implicate genes, molecules, pathways, and circuits

grandchildren, uncles, aunts, nieces, nephews, and half-siblings—have one-fourth of their genetic materials in common.

A variety of factors tend to make comparisons of familial risk to mental disorders across studies difficult. Those factors include differences in sample characteristics, methods of age correction, ascertainment schemes, and diagnostic procedures. For example, such methodological heterogeneity provides a partial explanation for why the risk for depression in first-degree relatives of depressive probands varies between 10 and 20 percent in different studies, whereas the risk to relatives of healthy controls varies between 1 and 10 percent. Comparison of healthy controls and high-risk relatives by similar case-finding and diagnostic methods are essential when interpreting mean risk estimates. Likewise, the ideal family study uses double-blind, case-controlled methods in which diagnoses of relatives are made independently of the proband's diagnosis.

Family studies permit determination of morbid risk estimates in different relative classes. A simple tally of the frequency of a disorder in relatives underestimates the true morbid risks, because not all unaffected individuals have passed through the period of risk for mental disorders at the time of examination. Quantitative methods have been developed that permit estimation of morbid risks with suitable *age correction*—that is, morbid risk estimation that takes into account the fact that some of the unaffected individuals now observed as unaffected will develop illness at a later point in time. Weinberg's short method of age correction was the first devised; this simple procedure assigns weights to the number of unaffected persons in different age groups. Weinberg's method was followed by one developed by Eric Strömgren, which uses the ages at onset in the proband samples to obtain an age-at-onset distribution. Each unaffected relative is weighted by the proportion of the risk period through which he or she has passed, and the lifetime morbid risk is then computed as the number of affected individuals divided by the number at risk (the number affected plus the weighted sum of unaffected relatives).

Survival curve estimation methods are now applied to determine age-corrected lifetime morbid risks in relatives. *Survival analysis* is a mathematical technique that models time to an event (e.g., illness onset) while paying special attention to incomplete (censored) data in which the event is not observed for all individuals. Covariates that influence the time to the event may be modeled in the Cox proportional hazards model. The nonparametric Kaplan-Meier curve estimate of time to onset of illness is typically used to estimate lifetime morbid risk; only onsets in relatives (and not in the probands) are considered.

Twin Studies

The twin method has been a popular research design to implicate or exclude genetic factors in the cause of a disease. Because monozygotic twins have identical genotypes, any dissimilarity between pair members must be due to the action of the environment during prenatal or postnatal development. Such developmental instability is due to pure *stochastic* (random) effects or stochastic effects involving gene–environment interaction. Customarily, it is assumed that anything less than 100 percent concordance among monozygotic pairs living through the period of risk excludes genetic factors as sufficient determinants of that disease. Thus, if genetic differences are not important for the familial clustering of a disorder, no differences should be seen in the monozygotic and dizygotic concordance rates. This is what occurs in twin studies of diseases caused by infectious agents (e.g., measles). Conversely, if genes are important in causing a disease, the monozygotic concordance rate is significantly higher than the dizygotic rate. A genetic basis is the most likely explanation for the higher monozygotic concordance rate if (1) monozygotic twins are not more predisposed to having the disease and (2) monozygotic twin environments are not more alike in features that cause the disease.

The twin method in psychiatry has also been useful in identifying spectrum conditions that are alternative manifestations of the disease genotype that occur in monozygotic twins discordant for the core illness. A variant of the twin design is to include the offspring of concordant versus discordant twins to identify environmental factors of importance in increasing susceptibility to illness or modifying clinical course or outcome.

Critics of the twin method have argued that monozygotic pairs share more similar environments than do dizygotic pairs and that is responsible for the higher monozygotic concordance rate for mental disorders. Three ways in which environmental factors may increase the rate have been advanced: (1) monozygosity per se, (2) the effects of identification by one twin with another, and (3) the sharing of a similar ecology, with enhanced exposure to triggering events. No conclusive evidence exists that those limitations have substantially or consistently biased the results of twin studies of mental disorders. Likewise, the role of the twinning process itself as a substantial risk factor for mental disorders (e.g., autism) is not supported.

Adoption Studies

Whereas monozygotic and dizygotic twin studies endeavor to hold the family environment constant to compare the resemblances between persons with the same and different genotypes, adoption studies permit the comparison of the effects of different types of rearing on groups who are assumed to be similar in their genetic predispositions. Such studies attempt to separate the effects of genes and the familial environment by capitalizing on the adoption process, in which children receive their environment from a source that is different from their gene source. Consequently, adoption study designs permit the disentangling of genetic and environmental factors that contribute to the familial aggregation of a disease. The ability to draw inferences from an adoption study is strongest when the adopted children are separated from their biological parents at birth. Potential problems of the research design are that (1) any parent–child interaction from the time of birth to the separation confounds a clear demarcation of genetic and environmental aspects; and (2) the environmental circumstances of biological parents may be associated with prenatal and perinatal events relevant to the cause of the disease.

Three major designs of adoption studies have been used to study mental disorders: (1) The parent-as-proband design compares the rate of illness in the adopted-away offspring of ill and well persons. Support for a genetic component is indicated if the risk of illness among adopted-away children of ill parents is greater than the risk of illness among adopted-away children of well parents. (2) The adoptee-as-proband design uses ill and well adoptees as probands. Genetic factors are implicated if (a) the risk of illness in the biological relatives of ill probands is greater than that in the adoptive relatives of well probands and (b) the risk of illness is greater in the biological relatives of ill probands than that in the biological parents of well adoptees. (3) The seldom-used cross-fostering approach compares rates of illness in two groups of adoptees. One group of adoptees has ill biological parents and is raised by well adoptive parents; the other group has well biological parents and is raised by ill adoptive parents.

A famous adoption study in psychiatry was started in the 1960s by David Rosenthal, Seymour Kety, Paul Wender, and their colleagues to study schizophrenia in Denmark. Major accomplishments of the project were to rule out some alleged environmental factors (being reared by a schizophrenic parent) as necessary or sufficient for the development of schizophrenia in the offspring of schizophrenic parents and to confirm the validity of family and twin results in implicating genes. The data have held up remarkably well, even after probands and relatives were classified with criteria used in the third edition of the *Diagnostic and Statistical Manual of Mental Disorders* (DSM-III). The data also provided an opportunity to develop operational criteria for schizotypal personality disorder as a spectrum condition genetically related to the core schizophrenic phenotype, because it occurred at a higher rate in the biological relatives of adopted-away schizophrenic persons than in the adoptive relatives of schizophrenic persons and the relatives of control adoptees.

Association Studies

The standard method for mapping Mendelian disease loci applies classic parametric or nonparametric methods to family data in a search for linkage between the disease and a *marker locus* (a gene or DNA sequence of known location). An alternative approach, especially for diseases with a more complex genetic basis, is to look for statistical associations in the general population between the disease and a marker. These studies typically involve the analysis of unrelated affected individuals and a control sample (the control sample can be parents or other relatives of affected individuals). Linkage analysis of family data implicates a chromosomal region by assuming a relationship between a disease locus and marker loci in that region; association analysis implicates a specific gene by assuming a relationship between a disease and alleles at a specific genetic locus (or, at most, a small set of genes with the association induced by local LD).

Population associations can generally arise for three reasons: (1) The implicated locus is itself a disease susceptibility locus—possession of the particular allele associated with the disease is neither necessary nor sufficient, but the likelihood of becoming ill is increased. (2) A disease locus and the associated marker locus are tightly linked—that is, physically close to each other—and are in LD. LD can persist for many generations as a function of the physical distance between the disease locus and the marker locus. (3) Individuals with the disease and those without may be genetically different subsets of the population that coincidentally differ in allele frequencies (*population stratification*)—in this case, the implicated locus is likely unrelated to the disease.

Classic disease-marker studies have been conducted by studying a sample of unrelated affected persons and by comparing the frequency of a particular marker allele in the affected group versus its frequency in a control sample. This is a *population-based case control study* of disease-marker association. Associations have been found between the human leukocyte antigen (HLA) system on chromosome 6 and a few diseases (e.g., ankylosing spondylitis); weaker associations have more typically been found for complex diseases, such as insulin-dependent diabetes mellitus and MS. However, causal inferences based on genetic differences between cases and controls drawn from a heterogeneous population have been difficult to replicate or to interpret in the study of mental disorders. This may result for several reasons: (1) Problems with selections of controls lead to difficulties in distinguishing linkage disequilibrium from population stratification, (2) inadequate statistical correction for the testing of association at many loci leads to an increased type I error rate and chance findings (i.e., falsely concluding that a disease-marker association exists when there truly is none), (3) there is limited statistical power in small samples, (4) laboratory and data analytic errors exist, and (5) the challenge of identifying excellent candidate genes exists.

Selecting suitable controls for population-based association studies is crucial to minimize the chances that the study and control groups are drawn from genetically distinct subpopulations. Methods have been recently applied to largely circumvent this problem, and the focus is on the use of association tests as a means of locating disease genes through detection of linkage disequilibrium. *Family-based association studies* use disease and marker data within families. Comparisons are made by comparing genetic material from a sample of patients with genetic material obtained from their two parents. A single affected individual and his or her two parents identified for family-based association studies are frequently referred to as a *trio*. Given that data from parents may be difficult or impossible to obtain (e.g., in studies of Alzheimer's disease), methods for family-based association analysis have been extended to permit the use of data from unaffected siblings.

An important spin-off effort of the Human Genome Project is a massive government and industry-sponsored effort to develop a dense set of biallelic SNP markers across the human genome. These efforts have been accelerated owing to the realization that a dense set of SNPs across the genome may yield critical information for mapping genetically complex diseases, in large part through population-level association. One possibility for using SNP technologies and discoveries efficiently is to incorporate it into case-control samples. New methods for incorporating SNPs within a case-control association design, which have the advantages of case-control and family-based association designs, recently have been developed. A new approach developed by Bernie Devlin and colleagues for case-control association studies, termed *genomic control*, takes into account the impact of population substructure by using the distribution of multiple polymorphisms throughout the genome (only some of which are pertinent to the disease of interest).

QUANTITATIVE METHODS

Data from many of the research designs described previously can be analyzed by taking advantage of recent advances in statistical methods and computer science. The methods most typically used in the study of genetic factors are presented in Table 1.17–4.

Path Analysis

Path analysis was introduced as a technique (1) to explain the interrelations among variables by analyzing their correlational structure and (2) to evaluate the relative importance of varying causes influencing a certain variable. The primary goal of path analysis in genetic epidemiology is to distinguish genetic effects from common environmental effects that contribute to the familial aggregation of a disease. Twin and adoptive data are necessary to separate nature from nurture in path analysis. When genetic transmission is present, additive genetic effects cannot be distinguished from other

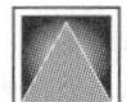

Table 1.17–4
Quantitative Methods of Genetic Analysis

Method	Data Source	Goal
Path analysis	Twin, adoption	Distinguish transmissible environment from polygenes
Segregation analysis	Pedigree	Distinguish a major locus from polygenes or transmissible environment
Linkage analysis	Pedigree	Establish chromosomal localization of a putative disease susceptibility locus
Association analysis	Unrelated affecteds, controls	Implicate a specific gene as a disease susceptibility locus, given linkage disequilibrium

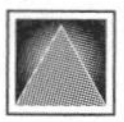

Table 1.17–5
Genetic and Environmental Contributions to the Variance in Liability of Several Traits, Assuming Etiological Homogeneity

Trait	Genes	Common Environment	Individual-Specific Environment
Intelligence	0.52	0.34	0.14
Personality (extroversion)	0.60	0.00	0.40
Religious devotion	0.29	0.24	0.47
Bipolar disorder	0.86	0.07	0.07
Major depression	0.45	0.00	0.55
Neurotic depression	0.08	0.54	0.38
Schizophrenia	0.63	0.29	0.08
Alcoholism (women)	0.50	0.00	0.50
Late-onset Alzheimer's disease	0.58	0.39	0.03
Tuberculosis	0.06	0.62	0.32

genetic effects (i.e., single major locus models and multilocus models cannot be distinguished).

Familial correlations are estimated through *maximum likelihood techniques*, statistical procedures for estimating parameters, such that the best-fitting estimates are those that maximize the probability of the observations. Comparisons of competing models are made by fitting a general model and alternative submodels. Because log likelihoods are calculated for the general model (L_1) and the submodel (L_2), then $-2(L_1 - L_2)$ is approximately distributed as a chi-square with the degrees of freedom equal to the difference in the number of estimated parameters. This is the *likelihood ratio test*, the test statistic for comparing alternate models. Qualitative (affected or unaffected status) and quantitative phenotypes may be analyzed, and examples of the results of applying path models of multifactorial transmission to analyze several traits are given in Table 1.17–5.

A useful application of complex path models was exemplified by the analysis of twin and family data from a variety of published sources for tuberculosis and schizophrenia. The results showed that the major contribution to phenotypic variance for tuberculosis came from the shared family environment rather than from genes; that result is expected for an illness caused by an infectious agent. Results from twin data alone would have been misleading in implicating a significant genetic effect. By contrast, the largest contribution to the variance in schizophrenia and bipolar disorder comes from genes, with suggestion of a modest role for the common environment.

Segregation Analysis

Segregation analysis is a method for resolving a single major locus effect, but it leaves cultural inheritance confounded with additive polygenes. The unit of analysis is an entire pedigree, and the goal is to statistically assess evidence for the segregation of a major gene in the presence of other sources of familial resemblance. The application of segregation analysis to psychiatric family data has led to disappointing results, in the sense that no single gene effect has been consistently identified for any mental disorder. Given the conceptual sophistication of multilocus genetic models and the introduction of cheap, fast, and highly automated approaches to genotyping, the added value of segregation analysis for implicating major gene effects in the analysis of complex disorders is further diminished.

Linkage Analysis

Segregation analysis is an analytical tool for identifying the effect of a major locus in terms of the covariance of ill and well individuals within and between families, but phenotypic segregation patterns alone do not provide opportunities for its localization and ultimate identification of genetic variants affecting disease susceptibility. Linkage analysis is a statistical procedure by which pedigree data are examined to determine whether a disease phenotype is cosegregating with a genetic marker of known chromosomal location. Linkage analysis allows an investigator to infer that two loci (a genetic marker locus and a putative disease susceptibility locus) are located close enough together on the same chromosome that their alleles tend to be transmitted together from parent to child more frequently than would occur by random assortment. The demonstration of linkage between a putative disease susceptibility locus and one or more genetic markers thus determines in which chromosomal region the disease locus lies. Chromosomal localization through linkage analysis is the first essential step in the process of identifying, isolating, and cloning a disease susceptibility locus.

Genetic markers are entities known to follow a simple Mendelian mode of inheritance with an identified chromosomal location. At least one parent must be doubly heterozygous for mating to be informative for linkage. Therefore, a genetic marker locus' usefulness for linkage depends on the number of alleles and the gene frequencies (its degree of *polymorphism*). A common measure of the degree of polymorphism is the marker's *heterozygosity*, which is defined as the probability of randomly drawing two different alleles from the population. This is easily calculated as 1 minus the probability of drawing identical alleles, or $1 - \Sigma P_i^2$. Within limits, the probability of informative matings, with respect to linkage, increases with increasing heterozygosity.

Thirty years ago, the number of available polymorphic genetic markers was severely limited to blood cell antigen loci (ABO, Rh, and HLA) now known to lie on chromosomes 1, 6, or 9. Some of those markers were highly polymorphic, but their limited number and restricted coverage of the genome meant that even linkage studies with excellent family data had little prospect for success. However, in the late 1970s and early 1980s, geneticists proposed to treat differences in the DNA sequence as allelic variants and to use them as genetic markers. Through molecular genetic techniques, *restriction fragment length polymorphisms* (RFLPs) were obtained and were well suited as genetic markers in linkage analysis. RFLP markers are highly polymorphic and are available in great numbers that saturate the genome.

A variety of other types of genetic markers have since been developed. These include minisatellite *variable number tandem repeat* (VNTR) markers, which have many alleles and high heterozygosity. Technical problems have limited their use. The advent of polymerase chain reaction (PCR) methods finally made mapping relatively quick and easy and led to the identification of *microsatellite* markers. Shorter than minisatellites, they amplify well and are mostly cytosine-adenine $(CA)_n$ repeats. Much effort has been devoted to producing sets of microsatellite markers that can be amplified together in a multiplex PCR reaction. Automated, high-throughput genotyping technologies now permit conduction of whole genome scans in a matter of weeks, as opposed to the months that were required 2 years ago. Genotyping costs are further reduced through *DNA pooling*, in which DNA from multiple subjects is pooled by using approximately equal amounts of DNA from each individual, and the fraction of genotypes in each pool is estimated. DNA pooling has been proposed for linkage, association, and physical mapping studies.

Three analytical strategies (Table 1.17–6) are used to search for linkage to mental disorders and to locate disease susceptibility genes: (1) application of parametric maximum likelihood methods to analyze data in small or extended pedigrees, (2) application of non-

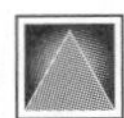

Table 1.17–6
Quantitative Methods to Locate Disease Susceptibility Genes

Method	Unit of Analysis	Mode of Inheritance	Multipoint Analysis	Computational Load	Typical Statistic	Target
Parametric	Pedigree	Required	Yes (<4)	Intensive	LOD score	Chromosomal region
Allele-sharing	Affected sibling pairs and pedigrees	Not required	Yes	Not intensive	Identical-by-descent–sharing probability; nonparametric linkage statistic	Chromosomal region
Linkage disequilibrium	Unrelated affecteds, controls	Not required	No	Not intensive	Chi-square	Individual gene

Note: *Multipoint analysis* refers to the simultaneous use of information provided by more than one genetic marker.
LOD, logarithm of odds.

parametric methods to study allele sharing among affected siblling pairs, or (3) application of family-based or case-control association tests to detect linkage, given LD.

Parametric Methods In principle, a doubly heterozygous person—for example, *Aa*, *Bb*—received the *A* allele with the *B* or *b* allele from one parent. If two loci (with alleles *A* or *a* at one locus and *B* or *b* at the other) are inherited independently of each other, a father passes the four haplotypes *AB*, *ab*, *Ab*, and *aB* to his offspring in the ratio of 1:1:1:1. If the *AB* and *ab* haplotypes look the same as the ones he received from his parents, the children receiving them are called *parental types*. The other two haplotypes (*Ab* and *aB*) in this case are unlike any haplotypes received by the father from the grandparents of the child and contain one allele from each grandparent (a recombination of grandparental alleles must have occurred in the father). The nonparental types (*Ab* and *aB*) are called *recombinants,* and the other two haplotypes are called *nonrecombinants*. A *recombination* between two genes denotes the event that two different grandparents contributed one allele at each of the two loci to a haplotype in a person, whereas a *nonrecombination* is said to have occurred when a haplotype in a person contains two alleles that originated from the same grandparent of that person. A mating is potentially informative for linkage between two specific genes when at least one of the parents is a double heterozygote.

When two genes are inherited independently of each other, recombinants and nonrecombinants are expected in equal proportions among the offspring. Some pairs of genes consistently deviate from the 1:1 ratio of recombinant to nonrecombinant offspring; in other words, alleles of different genes appear to be genetically coupled. That is called *genetic linkage*. The extent of genetic linkage is measured by the *recombination fraction*, which is the probability that a gamete produced by a parent is a recombinant. The recombination fraction is frequently denoted by the Greek letter *theta* (θ). Genes segregating independently are unlinked with θ equaling 0.5, whereas linked genes are characterized by a θ of less than $1/2$. Some pairs of genes are tightly linked, so that θ approaches 0—that is, only rarely does a recombination occur between them. The estimation of θ and the test of the hypothesis of free recombination ($\theta = 1/2$) versus linkage ($\theta < 1/2$) are the goals of linkage analysis.

Recombination fractions reflect *genetic* distance on a chromosome, which is not exactly the same as *physical* distance. *Genetic distance* refers to a mathematical estimate of distance between markers and reflects the number of recombinant events (values of θ greater than $1/2$ are not meaningful); *physical distance* reflects the actual number of base pairs on the chromosome. Two loci that show 1 percent recombination are defined as being 1 centimorgan (cM) apart on a genetic map (100 cM define a Morgan, which was named in honor of Thomas Hunt Morgan—these are the units that measure genetic distance along a chromosome). However, for distances greater than approximately 5 cM, genetic distance is not a simple reflection of the number of recombinant events. A mathematical equation called the *mapping function* defines the relationship between the recombination fraction and genetic distance.

A nonconstant relationship exists between genetic distance, as measured in cM, and physical distance, which is measured in DNA base pairs or megabases (Mb; 1 Mb = one million base pairs). The entire human genome is 3,000 Mb, or three billion base pairs. A sex-averaged figure that relates physical and genetic distance is 1 cM equals 0.9 Mb, but the actual correspondence varies widely for different chromosomal regions.

Figure 1.17–4 shows in a simplified manner the chromosomal interpretation of recombination. In *meiosis* (cell division leading to the formation of gametes), homologous chromosomes pair up. At that point, each homologous chromosome consists of two strands (*chromatids*), so that a chromosome pair consists of four. In the course of meiosis, the two homologous chromosomes separate from each other at most places but maintain, at most, a few zones of contact (*chiasmata*). Chiasmata reflect the occurrence of *crossing over* between chromatids. Figure 1.17–4 shows one (1) or two (2) chiasmata; a single crossover generates two recombinant and two nonrecombinant chromatids (1), whereas a two-strand double crossover leaves four nonrecombinant chromatids (2). The overall effect averaged over all double crossovers is to generate 50 percent recombinants.

Because recombination events can be recognized only on the basis of haplotypes passed from parents to children, linkage analysis requires phenotypic observations on pedigree members. Estimation of θ can be accomplished by using the method of maximum likelihood. A relevant quantity is the likelihood ratio that is obtained by dividing the likelihood of a given family $L(\theta)$ by its value under free recombination $L(1/2)$. A common practice is to work not with the likelihood ratio but with its logarithm to the base 10. This is the *logarithm of odds* (LOD) *score* $Z(\theta)$, such that $Z(\theta) = \log_{10} [L(\theta)/L(0.5)]$.

The LOD score serves as a measure of the weight of the data in favor of the hypothesis of linkage. The critical value generally adhered to as the criterion for significant evidence for linkage to simple, monogenic diseases with unambiguous phenotypes and established modes of transmission is 3 for autosomal loci. The one-sided type I error rate associated with that value when θ is the only estimated parameter (i.e., the mode of disease transmission is known) and when the linkage test is conducted at a single marker is 0.0001 in large samples. Appropriate LOD score criteria for the analysis of complex diseases, such as mental disorders, in which linkage results are evaluated using markers across the entire genome are described in the following discussion.

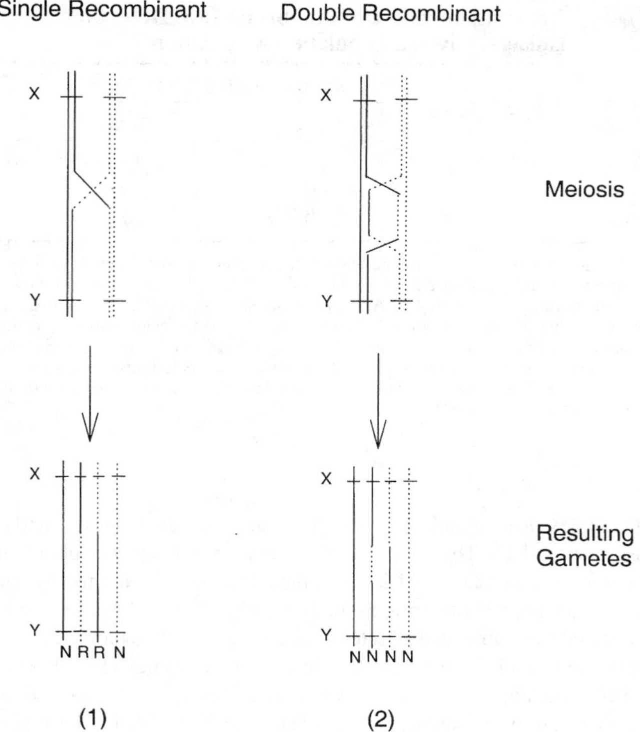

FIGURE 1.17–4 Schematic representation of a pair of homologous chromosomes, each consisting of two strands. Single-strand (1) and two-strand double (2) crossovers involve two of the four chromatids; the solid line chromosome carries alleles X_1 and Y_1 at two loci, whereas the dotted line chromosome carries alleles X_2 and Y_2. Gametes (sperm and ovum) in which the chromatid is the same line type at the two loci are nonrecombinant (N) for these loci; those in which the chromatids are different line types are recombinant (R).

The traditional advantages of LOD score methods for linkage analysis include the following: (1) Because it is a parametric approach, LOD score methods have high power to detect a true linkage, given knowledge of the true mode of disease inheritance; (2) if affected sibling pairs are rare and etiologic heterogeneity is likely, multigenerational pedigrees with multiple affected relatives of various classes (uncles, grandparents, cousins, and so forth) can be analyzed; (3) linkage to a particular chromosomal region can be excluded; and (4) a measure of the distance between two loci—the recombination fraction θ—can be estimated.

A consideration when applying LOD score methods for linkage analysis is that the mode of inheritance is assumed to be known. When single major locus inheritance parameters (gene frequencies and penetrances) are estimated jointly with θ in linkage analysis, the LOD score value does not have the same statistical meaning. One conservative correction for maximizing a LOD score over *t* different transmission models is to subtract $\log_{10}(t)$ from the result—for example, a LOD score of 3 maximized over five transmission models is reduced to approximately 2.3.

Allele-Sharing Methods Allele-sharing methods assume that a disease susceptibility locus can be identified given that a pair of affected relatives—typically a sibling pair, but other relative pairs may also be considered—tends to inherit the same allele more often than expected under random Mendelian assortment. Each pair shares 0, 1, or 2 alleles *identical by descent* at a given locus, and the *allele-sharing proportion* is defined as the proportion of affected relative pairs that share a single allele identical by descent at that locus. Genotyping parents and other individuals in a pedigree allow determination of whether given alleles are actually inherited from a common ancestor, that is, identical-by-descent status can be deduced. In practice, the situation is more complicated, because one cannot unambiguously determine the number of alleles shared identical by descent at all of the loci in the genome. In such cases, inferences are drawn based only on identical-by-state information—that is, it is determined whether individuals show the same allele at a given locus, regardless of whether the allele came from a common ancestor. Identical-by-descent methods have greater power to detect linkage and are less sensitive to misspecification of marker allele frequencies (which can lead to false-positive results) as compared to identical-by-state methods.

Tracing the inheritance pattern in the affected sibling pair method uses perturbations in the distribution of identical-by-descent scores at a marker locus to detect the presence of a linked disease locus. In the absence of linkage, the probability that two siblings share neither, one, or both marker alleles identical by descent is independent of their disease phenotypes. Consequently, if pairs of siblings are studied because they are both affected, they have 2, 1, or 0 alleles identical by descent with probabilities 0.25, 0.5, and 0.25, respectively. Various statistics for linkage can be defined on the basis of affected sibling pair identical-by-descent sharing, and they have different power depending on the true, underlying genetic model affecting liability at the tested locus. For example, the means test is simple to understand. For a single affected sibling pair and complete identical-by-descent information, the mean identical-by-descent sharing (in the absence of linkage) is calculated as $0(1/4) + 1(1/2) + 2(1/4) = 1$, and the variance of the mean is $1/2$. For *N* sibling pairs with observed total identical-by-descent sharing *O*, then, the test statistic is $t = (O - N)/(N/2)^{**}(1/2)$, which is distributed as a standard normal deviate for large *N* under the null hypothesis of no linkage. Of the numerous test statistics available, a few have good properties over a wide range of genetic models, as evaluated by Haydar Sengul and colleagues.

The specific advantages of affected sibling pair methods in the study of mental disorders are the following: (1) Specification of complex nonMendelian modes of transmission is not required. Concomitantly, several confounding factors that make it difficult to accurately estimate the mode of transmission in segregation analysis (e.g., complex ascertainment strategies, cohort effects, environmental effects, sex effects, variable age of onset) do not have to be modeled. (2) The practice of testing for linkage under several transmission models, which necessitates some downward correction to the linkage statistic to prevent inflation in the type I error rate for testing across multiple disease transmission models, is now unnecessary. (3) Large multigenerational families with many affected persons, which are typically difficult to locate in family studies of mental disorders, are not required. (4) Complete extraction of multipoint inheritance information and estimation of disease gene location is possible using new nonparametric methods.

Linkage Disequilibrium Analysis Parametric and nonparametric linkage methods, as described previously, are useful in the search for disease susceptibility genes. However, these methods may require large sample sizes to detect the modest gene effects that are most likely operative in most mental disorders (recurrence risk ratios on the order of 1.5 or less; Fig. 1.17–5). In addition, isolation of a specific disease gene knowing only its subchromosomal location (*positional cloning*) depends on high-resolution mapping of the chromosomal regions detected through linkage analysis. With current technologies, in the absence of fortuitous events, such as the presence

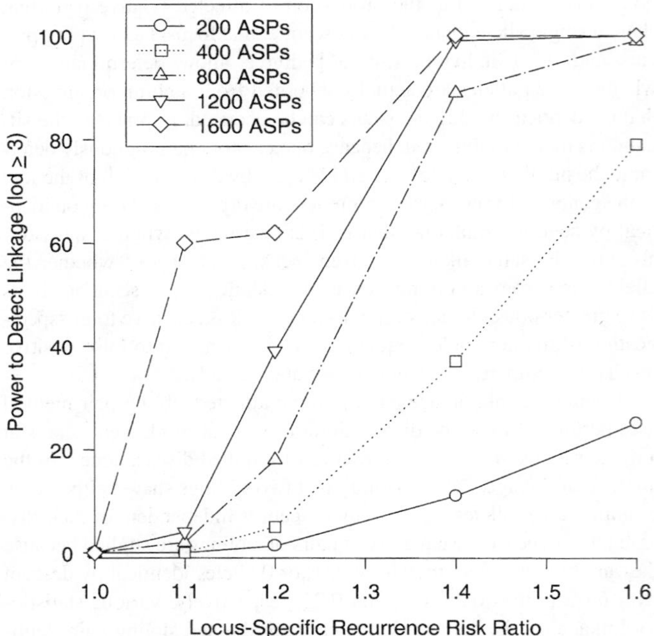

FIGURE 1.17–5 Morbid risk conferred by a specific susceptibility locus to first-degree relatives of an affected individual, divided by the lifetime cumulative incidence of the disease. Figures displayed are percentages. Linkage detection is defined as a logarithm of odds (LOD) score greater than or equal to 3. ASP, affected sibling pair. (From Hauser ER, Boehnke M, Guo S-W, Risch N: Affected-sib-pair interval mapping and exclusion for complex genetic traits: Sampling considerations. *Genet Epidemiol.* 1996;13:117, with permission.)

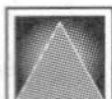

Table 1.17–7
Transmission and Disequilibrium Test: Detecting Linkage, Given a Population Association

Transmitted Allele	Nontransmitted Allele A_1	A_2	Total
A_1	a	b	$a + b$
A_2	c	d	$c + d$
Total	$a + c$	$b + d$	$2n$

Note: Combinations of transmitted and nontransmitted marker alleles A_1 and A_2 among $2n$ biological parents of n affected individuals. The notation is as follows: *a*, the number of times that an A_1A_1 parent transmits A_1 to affected offspring; *b*, the number of times that an A_1A_2 parent transmits A_1 to affected offspring; *c*, the number of times that an A_1A_2 parent transmits A_2 to affected offspring; and *d*, the number of times that an A_2A_2 parent transmits A_2 to affected offspring. For the hypothesis of no linkage (and no allelic association), χ^2 (one degree of freedom) $= (b - c)^2/(b + c)$.

of a trinucleotide repeat expansion or gross deletion, a gene most likely must be localized to a region of approximately one million base pairs before it is practical to identify it. Given the magnitude of the genetic effects found in mental disorders, localization to regions of this size may require well more than 1,000 affected sibling pairs.

An alternative approach to parametric and nonparametric linkage methods for gene mapping is LD analysis (however, linkage and LD may be analyzed on any given data set). When a new mutation arises on a chromosome, it is in complete LD with other alleles at adjacent loci. When this new allele is transmitted to the next generation, the haplotype of alleles of linked polymorphisms is also transmitted. In LD analysis, the standard study design is to collect a number of unrelated affected and unaffected individuals from the same population. Then, the genotypes at a marker locus are tested to determine whether they are more similar within the sample of affected individuals than within the entire sample of affected and unaffected individuals. An alternative strategy as described previously in the section Association Studies is to collect trios, consisting of two parents and one affected offspring. Catherine Falk and Pablo Rubenstein proposed the haplotype relative risk (HRR) method as a family-based test of association. The control sample is the alleles at different loci that are received from one parent (the parental haplotype; see the following discussion) and are not present in the affected person, which represents a random sample of haplotype pairs from the same genetic population. They did not focus on the use of the HRR as a test for linkage. The key advantage of this method is that it ensures that case and control samples come from the same genetic population.

Richard Spielman and colleagues developed a related method—the transmission/disequilibrium test (TDT)—as a test for linkage between a complex disease and a marker, given an established disease-marker association (LD). The TDT is a test of linkage that is powerful only in the presence of LD. The TDT uses the alleles not transmitted by parents to an affected offspring as the "controls." Thus, DNA needs to be collected from unrelated affected subjects and their two biological parents. Table 1.17–7 shows the simple 2 × 2 contingency table that can be constructed, given a marker with two alleles A_1 and A_2; the significance test uses the simple chi-square statistic. The TDT has been generalized to the case of an arbitrary number of marker alleles.

Use of the TDT does not solve the issue of inadequate statistical correction, given conduction of a large number of association tests at many loci. A conservative approach is to divide the desired type I error probability by the number of tests conducted. For example, maintenance of a 5 percent false-positive rate (significance level = 0.05) when 50 independent tests have been conducted would require a significance level of 0.001 for each test.

Neil Risch has advocated LD studies as viable alternatives to linkage approaches for the genetic analysis of complex diseases and, perhaps, the study design of choice in this setting. He has discussed the intriguing possibility of eventually testing for disease associations in all of the human genes that will eventually be identified. LD analysis can be powerful when the affected individuals in a sample share the same allele identical by descent at the same disease locus from some common ancestor. This approach has been successful in mapping genes for rare Mendelian disorders, especially in homogeneous, isolated populations, such as those in Finland (e.g., diastrophic dysplasia). An efficient design for psychiatric genetic studies may be to use a multistage strategy for genotyping and analysis of extended pedigrees that incorporates linkage and family-based association methods.

Rapid advances in engineering and genomic technologies stimulated an effort by a consortium of researchers (SNP Consortium) funded by the NHGRI and private industry to identify and characterize high-density maps of SNPs with high heterozygosities, based on the belief that common variants play an important role in the etiology of common human diseases and, in this case, that genome-wide associations could have greater power for gene mapping. More than four million of the estimated ten million SNPs have been identified by and placed in a public repository.

Given that it is prohibitively expensive and inefficient to categorize all of these, the question has been raised regarding the minimum number of SNPs required for whole-genome association studies—recent estimates have focused on 300,000 to 500,000. One strategy to reduce the number of SNPs to this more reasonable number is to

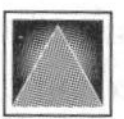

Table 1.17–8
Criteria for Evaluating Reports of Linkage to Mental Disorders

Linkage Method	Nominal *P* Value	Genome-Wide *P* Value	Number of Random Occurrences per Genome Scan	Equivalent LOD Score	Decision Classification
LOD score analysis	1.70×10^{-3}	.632	1.000	1.86	Suggestive
	4.88×10^{-5}	.049	0.050	3.30	Significant
	6.37×10^{-7}	.001	0.001	5.10	Highly significant
Allele-sharing methods	7.36×10^{-4}	.632	1.000	2.20	Suggestive
	2.25×10^{-5}	.049	0.050	3.61	Significant
	3.02×10^{-7}	.001	0.001	5.41	Highly significant

Note: *LOD score analysis* refers to methods in which LOD scores are determined in whole pedigrees; *allele-sharing methods* refer to the analysis of pairs of affected relatives (thresholds shown are for affected sibling pairs)—an equivalent LOD score that yields the comparable nominal *P* value is also shown. Displayed LOD scores are those calculated assuming the absence of genetic heterogeneity (i.e., all families are assumed to be linked).
LOD, logarithm of odds.
Adapted from Lander E, Kruglyak L: Genetic dissection of complex traits: Guidelines for interpreting and reporting linkage results. *Nat Genet.* 1995;11:241.

focus on sets of nearby SNPs on the same chromosome that are inherited in blocks. This pattern of SNPs on a block forms a distinct haplotype. Blocks may contain a large number of SNPs, but a few SNPs are enough to uniquely identify the haplotypes in a block.

Recently, NHGRI has proposed the development of a map, termed *HapMap*, of common haplotypes comprised of blocks of LD among tightly linked SNPs. HapMap is expected to make much more efficient and comprehensive genome scan approaches to finding regions with genes that affect diseases, because effort will not be wasted typing more SNPs than necessary, and all regions of the genome can be included. Costs would be greatly reduced, given that markers could be chosen much more wisely to capture the haplotype structure of the human genome. Haplotype information may also be well recovered from certain DNA pooling designs, thereby resulting in further savings in genotype costs. In addition to its use in studying genetic associations with disease, HapMap should be a powerful resource for studying the forces shaping the distribution of variation in the human genome. If it proves successful at identifying genetic factors for disease, it likely will also contribute to the understanding of variation in response to environmental factors. Finally, it should contribute to the knowledge of the effectiveness of and adverse responses to therapeutic compounds.

Whether association analysis will prove successful at finding genetic variants affecting liability to mental disorders is highly dependent on the existence of detectable LD, the number of loci involved, the number of disease-producing alleles per locus (allelic heterogeneity), the role of environment, and the degree of gene–environment interactions. Despite the technological and other advances offered by HapMap, underlying biological complexities that result in weak correlations between genetic variation and complex disease phenotypes will remain and will pose challenges for researchers, as they will for any approach for the genetic analysis of mental disorders and other complex diseases.

Criteria for Declaring Linkage to Mental Disorders

It is crucial in the genetic investigation of mental disorders that a sufficiently stringent standard is adopted for the declaration of linkage to maintain a high likelihood that the assertion will be true and will stand the test of time. As discussed previously, the LOD score criterion for declaring a linkage is 3 in the study of classic Mendelian diseases with known modes of familial transmission.

Ever-evolving genetic methods and technologies now permit systematic screening of the entire human genome. The increased number of markers being tested inflates the type I error rate. Using theoretical results from stochastic processes and assuming complete identical-by-descent information throughout the genome, Eric Lander and Leonid Kruglyak have proposed a set of guidelines for interpreting linkage results of complex diseases. They differentiate the *nominal* significance level, which is the probability of encountering a linkage statistic of a given magnitude at one specific locus, from the *genome-wide* significance level, which is the probability that one would encounter such a deviation somewhere in a whole genome scan. A given linkage statistic, such as a LOD score, has a corresponding nominal *P* value and a genome-wide *P* value.

Lander and Kruglyak further proposed that genome-wide *P* values be interpreted to evaluate the magnitude of linkage evidence and classify it as *suggestive*, *significant*, or *highly significant*. Suggestive linkage reports, with lower LOD scores (larger *P* values), often reflect chance findings and often are wrong but are worth reporting as tentative findings. Table 1.17–8 shows equivalent LOD score values and associated nominal and genome-wide *P* values for these different categories. A more stringent LOD score criterion (3.3 for LOD score methods; 3.6 for allele-sharing methods) than the traditional value of 3 is required to claim significant linkage evidence in the analysis of mental disorders and other complex diseases. Confirmation of linkage requires a two-step process: (1) Significant linkage is found in at least one study, and (2) evidence of linkage to the same region is obtained by an independent group of investigators in an independent sample.

EPISTASIS

Epistasis—defined as the interaction between different loci—is important, because its existence can alter or mask the effect of one locus by another, thereby reducing the power to detect the first and confounding elucidation of the joint effects at the two loci. Such gene–gene interactions have been detected for the *IDDM1* and *IDDM2* loci in diabetes mellitus and the *NAT1* and *NAT2* enzyme polymorphisms in colorectal cancer. Genetic interactions between mutations in the *RET* and *EDNRB* genes are a recently identified mechanism in Hirschprung's disease, a genetically complex and common congenital malformation.

A variety of statistical methods exist to detect or to control for the presence of epistasis. By allowing for epistatic interactions among loci that produce disease susceptibility, it may be possible for researchers to identify genetic variants that otherwise may have been undetected. On the other hand, allowing for interaction magnifies the problem of multiple testing already inherent in the search for single-gene effects. Exciting benefits that may result from the identification of robust statistical models of the joint effects of several loci are the prediction of phenotype and targeting of therapeutic interventions.

Ultimately, however, there are limits to the knowledge of biological mechanisms that is produced from statistical modeling alone. A combination of molecular and statistical studies offers the best approach to resolving true biological interactions that occur in complex diseases.

GENE–ENVIRONMENT INTERACTION

Gene–environment interactions pose major challenges for the identification of genetic variants producing liability to mental disorders and other complex diseases. In genetic studies of model organisms, researchers measure phenotypes under carefully controlled environmental conditions or design experiments in such a way as to measure the effect of the environment. It is easy to imagine scenarios in which there is little power to detect modest genetic effects, because they are obscured by environmentally mediated variation. A useful approach for the study of mental disorders is to measure as many potential environmental events and risk factors that may contribute to disease vulnerability. Controlling for environmental variation will decrease residual variance in the phenotype, resulting in increased power to identify and characterize underlying genetic factors. Because the environmental factors operative in the etiology of mental disorders are likely of modest effect and, in many cases, may be idiosyncratic (nonfamilial), controlling for environment could be a daunting task. On the other hand, if the effect of the environment is small, controlling for such effects may not be so critical for gene discovery.

MULTIVARIATE ANALYSIS INCORPORATING QUANTITATIVE TRAITS

Traditional approaches in genetic epidemiology focus on the qualitative determination of disease status as the exclusive source of data for genetic analysis. That approach is problematic in the case of mental disorders, in which phenotypic assessment through structured and semistructured interviews is potentially complicated by diagnostic error and misclassification. Quantitative traits that cosegregate with the disease phenotype (so-called endophenotypes, as discussed in the following section) provide greater information content than do groupings of persons into affected or unaffected classes. The informativeness of pedigrees is increased, as a greater range of information is available on unaffected persons who are not yet through the risk period. Thus, the power to initially map a susceptibility locus of small relative effect may be enhanced through consideration of the effects of such loci on quantitative traits correlated with disease. The application of such multivariate methods in the genetic analysis of mental disorders has yet to reach its full potential. Examples of such traits include psychophysiological abnormalities in alcoholism and attentional impairments in schizophrenia.

PSYCHIATRIC GENETIC EPIDEMIOLOGY: A STUDY DESIGN FOR THE 21ST CENTURY

Although multiple linkages have been reported for several mental disorders, it is still unclear which are real, and the goal of positionally cloning susceptibility genes remains elusive. Joseph Terwilliger and colleagues argue that many of the failures in gene mapping of complex diseases in the late 20th century have resulted from an overemphasis on the ultimate clinical phenotype—and its importance on the public health burden—and insufficient attention to what is practical and powerful, given the inability to perform controlled breeding experiments in humans. One alternative study design focuses on the collection of genetically informative families (i.e., those with large sibships and multiple generations) drawn from the general population and not identified on the basis of a clinical phenotype. Family members would then be characterized on a rich array of phenotypic and environmental measures that can be reliably made, such as those measured on a quantitative scale (in an analogous fashion to blood pressure, body mass, etc.) The ideal phenotypes to be measured would be those that are more closely related to underlying biological mechanisms and that lie closer to the level of genes and their products in the gene–phenotypic pathway. A potentially useful and powerful strategy is to find such traits—defined by many as *endophenotypes*—that are correlated with underlying disease susceptibility and that may be reliably measured. As discussed previously, promising active areas of inquiry are focused on measures of neurophysiology (prepulse inhibition and eye tracking) and neurocognition (sustained attention and verbal and working memory) in schizophrenia and measures of language dysfunction in autism. As the genetic bases of these and other complex traits (e.g., hippocampal volume) are elucidated, it is expected that this knowledge will provide insights into multiple neurobiological circuits and pathways that are implicated in the pathophysiology of mental disorders. These insights, in turn, will provide molecular targets for the development of new therapeutic compounds, thereby improving disease diagnosis, treatment, and, ultimately, prevention.

EXPERIMENTAL SYSTEMS: THE MOUSE AND OTHER ORGANISMS

A variety of experimental systems (e.g., mouse, rat, zebra fish, frog, songbird, flatworm, and fruit fly) have played and will continue to play a pivotal role in elucidating basic neurobiological mechanisms and pathways, thereby providing important insights into the etiology and pathophysiology of mental disorders. Studies of the mouse undoubtedly will make critical contributions to our understanding of the function of mammalian genes. Major technological advances in the last decade have been developed that enable researchers to manipulate the mouse genome in a highly targeted and predictable way. Such advances include transgenics, capitalization on the pluripotency and germline potential of embryonic stem cells, gene targeting, and the discovery of the highly potent chemical mutagen *N*-ethyl-*N*-nitrosourea (ENU). Such technologies, in combination with the mouse genome sequence, will provide researchers with unprecedented opportunities for global analyses of mammalian gene and protein function.

Given the conservation of cellular and developmental processes from mouse to humans, an important approach to studying the genetic basis of human disease is to map and to characterize genes influencing related biological processes in the mouse. Isolating, in population genetic and genetic epidemiologic studies, human variants of newly identified genes in a mouse pathway can, in turn, elucidate the corresponding human pathway.

MICROARRAYS AND GENOMIC MEDICINE

A new technology is revolutionizing how researchers study genes. DNA microarrays, or DNA (gene) chips, are fabricated by high-speed robotics on glass or nylon substrates, for which probes are used to determine complementary binding. This technology provides a systematic way to survey DNA and ribonucleic acid (RNA) variation across the entire genome. An experiment with a single DNA array can dramatically increase throughput and can provide researchers information on thousands of genes simultaneously. These arrays are likely to become a standard tool for molecular biological research and clinical diagnostics. DNA microarrays are currently being used for genome-wide genotyping and gene expression profiling; protein microarrays are being actively explored. This high-throughput approach is being used for a multiplicity of applications, ranging from specific hypothesis-testing and hypothesis-generating efforts to identify and to characterize functions of newly identified genes to the identification of therapeutic drug targets and the characterization of complex patterns of gene expression as a molecular profile of disease pathophysiology.

One of the most exciting applications of great interest to psychiatry is the key role that gene expression analysis using microarrays now plays in many stages of the drug development pipeline—that is, as a tool for the identification of genes with altered expression as targets, as an evaluative tool to determine whether a gene product is causative, and as a comparative methodology to determine which drug, among several drug candidates, is the most specific for a given protein implicated in disease pathophysiology.

The resulting information from microarrays studies will generate literally thousands of individual measurements and will provide a detailed quantitative assessment of biological properties of central nervous system (CNS) and other tissue. As discussed by Geoffrey Duyk, such an avalanche of data in the next decade will be overwhelming, emphasizing a need to shift the focus beyond studying individual molecules and toward pathways, networks, and, eventually, the cell itself.

PHARMACOGENOMICS AND THE PRACTICE OF PSYCHIATRY

The sequencing of the human genome and the increasingly widespread availability of high-throughput technologies, such as microarrays, now have made possible the global analysis of DNA and the simultaneous analysis of multiple genes. *Pharmacogenetics*, a term used to describe the prediction of medication response using inherited differences in genetic information, has now given way to *pharmacogenomics*, as the logical extension of this work to large-scale and genome-wide analysis. Current research is focused on allelic variation in specific genes associated with interindividual variability in drug uptake, transport, and metabolism. This includes well-studied examples, such as cytochrome P450 polymorphisms, and more recent work on the importance of genetic variation in drug transporters, ion channel molecules, and nuclear receptors. The identification of genes and gene products involved in the absorption, distribution, metabolism, and excretion (ADME) of psychoactive drugs that predict therapeutic response will be an important advance.

One of the most exciting anticipated uses of genetic information in clinical therapeutics is the use of SNPs or haplotypes to develop a personalized genetic profile—in practice, this could extend to the full genome, that is, specification of genetic variation in all 35,000 human genes for a single individual. It would then be possible, in principle, to tailor therapeutic regimens, such that individuals would be prescribed particular medications—and not prescribed others—based on the prediction from gene expression profiles of efficacy (or adverse events). For example, in recent studies, combinations of multiple SNPs were predictive of bronchodilator response to a β agonist (albuterol [Proventil]) in asthmatics, and association studies in multiple candidate genes have been used to identify the combination of polymorphisms that give the best predictive value of response to clozapine (Clozaril) in schizophrenic patients.

POPULATION GENETICS AND GENETIC EPIDEMIOLOGY IN HEALTH CARE

The clinical application of population genetic and genetic epidemiological principles in genomic medicine offers great potential for ameliorating the public health burden caused by mental disorders and other common diseases. One area in which the anticipated impact is great is diagnosis. It has been proposed by Dennis Charney and colleagues that future multiaxial systems of classification in psychiatry include one axis devoted to a patient's genotype, based on the presence or absence of specific disease susceptibility genes, resiliency genes, and genes related to therapeutic responses and side effects to specific psychoactive drugs.

Another area in which the anticipated impact will be immense is the area of preventive medicine. Increased genetic information resulting from SNP or haplotype profiling may play a great role in genetic counseling in which a goal is to quantify the risk of unborn individuals or other individuals for developing disease. Current practice in genetic counseling scenarios involves the estimation of disease risk based on empirical risks for different relative classes. Increased refinement in recurrence risk estimation is afforded through analysis of phenotypic information on relatives through a computer program written 30 years ago by the animal-breeding geneticist Charles Smith for use with polygenic traits. This program takes into account the number of affected and unaffected pedigree members, as well as their gender and age (or age of onset).

Figure 1.17–6 shows a hypothetical pedigree in which the goal is to determine the risk to an unborn child. The knowledge that the unborn child has one affected sibling results in a risk figure close to that predicted by consideration of empirical risk figures alone (siblings of an individual affected with schizophrenia have a risk of approximately 10 percent of developing the disorder). If the unborn child in this pedigree had an affected mother, the risk increases to 23 percent; the existence of an affected sister of the affected mother increases risk to 27 percent. Predictions of risk based on the genotype of the child may not be highly accurate, given the small gene effects and complex interactions between genes and environment found in schizophrenia. More accurate risk estimation could result if relatives' genetic and endophenotypic information (e.g., verbal memory performance and attention) was taken into account. Obtaining genetic and phenotypic information (diagnosis and related endophenotypic traits) from relatives may add considerable power for recurrence risk estimation.

If an individual were to be identified as being at increased genetic risk, there is the theoretical opportunity to provide preventive interventions. However, the potential of generating all of this genetic information about individuals raises serious questions of potential discrimination and other misuse; this strongly demonstrates that all patients and psychiatric caregivers must be informed about the meaning of genetic risk and genetic testing. To prepare for the issues associated with genetic testing for psychiatric diseases in the future, psychiatrists and other mental health professionals will need more training in genetics and genetic counseling.

FUTURE DIRECTIONS

With the full anatomy of the human genome at hand, researchers for the first time will be able to move beyond traditional gene-by-gene approaches and to take a global view of gene expression patterns crucial for neurobiological processes. This chapter has provided an overview of state-of-the-art methods in population genetics and genetic epidemiology that are being applied to the genetic analysis of mental disorders. Table 1.17–9 shows a variety of relevant resources on the World Wide Web. As information on an ever-increasing number of SNPs and haplotypes (HapMap) are identified and placed in public repositories, and as the completed human genome sequence is available, gene mapping in mental disorders will be accelerated.

Gene discovery in mental disorders has been complicated by etiologic heterogeneity, the need for large samples, the influence of

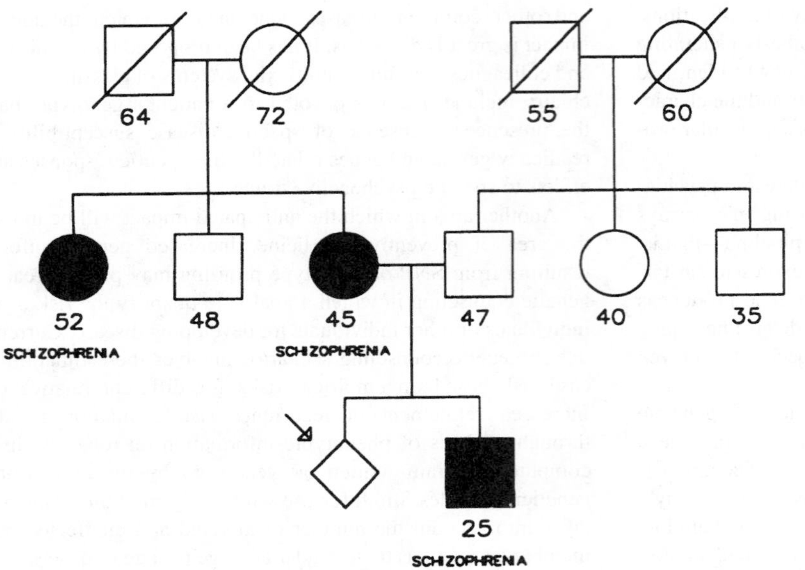

FIGURE 1.17–6 Risk to an unborn child of unknown sex (denoted by arrow) in a hypothetical pedigree. Men are denoted by squares, and women are denoted by circles. Shaded symbols denote affected individuals. Current ages are shown beneath symbols. Slashed symbols denote deceased individuals.

multiple genes of small relative effect, incomplete penetrance, and environmental effects. The mapping of susceptibility loci may be made more difficult by diagnostic error and misclassification, the involvement of rare genetic variants in producing disease, genetic (allelic and locus) heterogeneity, epistasis, gene–environment interactions, and epigenesis. As a result, positional cloning of genes producing susceptibility to mental disorders has proved much more difficult than originally envisioned, with linkage detection and positional cloning remaining elusive goals. Present challenges may be overcome with the following:

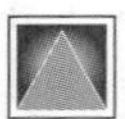

Table 1.17–9
Scientific Resources on Genetics and Genomics

Electronic Address	Description
http://www.nature.com/ng/	*Nature Genetics*
http://www.genome.org/	*Genome Research*
http://www.journals.uchicago.edu/AJHG/home.html	*The American Journal of Human Genetics*
http://www.blackwellmunksgaard.com/g2b	*Genes, Brain and Behavior*
http://www.faseb.org/genetics/ashg/ashgmenu.htm	The American Society of Human Genetics
http://www.biostat.wustl.edu/~genetics/iges/	International Genetic Epidemiology Society
http://linkage.rockefeller.edu/	Web resources of genetic linkage analysis
http://linkage.rockefeller.edu/soft/list.html	Genetic analysis software
http://snp.cshl.org/	Single Nucleotide Polymorphism (SNP) Consortium
http://watson.hgen.pitt.edu/T32/	University of Pittsburgh NIMH postdoctoral training program in statistical genetics
http://psychiatric-genetics-training.bsd.uchicago.edu/information.html	University of Chicago NIMH training program in psychiatric genetics
http://www.genomicglossaries.com/	Genomics glossary
http://www.ornl.gov/TechResources/Human_Genome/publicat/primer/index.html	Genome programs of the U.S. Department of Energy Office of Science
http://www.ncbi.nlm.nih.gov/genome/guide/human/	NCBI Human Genome Resources
http://genecards.weizmann.ac.il/udb/	Database for human genome mapping
http://genome.ucsc.edu/cgi-bin/hgGateway?db=hg12	Human genome browser
http://www.ornl.gov/hgmis/research/centers.html	Human Genome Project information
http://www.genome.gov/	The National Human Genome Research Institute
http://zork.wustl.edu/nimh/NIMH_initiative/NIMH_initiative_link.html	NIMH Human Genetics Initiative
http://www.nih.gov/science/models/	Model organisms for biomedical research
http://www.ncbi.nlm.nih.gov/disease/Brain.html	Genes and diseases of the nervous system
http://www.ncbi.nlm.nih.gov/omim/	Online *Mendelian Inheritance in Man*
http://www.rcsb.org/pdb/	Protein Data Bank
http://www.cidr.jhmi.edu/	Center for Inherited Disease Research

NCBI, National Center for Biotechnology Information; NIMH, National Institute of Mental Health.

1. Collections of sufficiently large samples of genetically informative pedigrees ascertained through affected individuals are required to obtain sufficient power to detect linkage and to map loci to small chromosomal regions. Selection of such pedigrees from genetically homogenous populations may offer distinct advantages. Such samples provide the opportunity for a search for linkage and for LD, with added value offered for large-scale family-based association tests across the whole genome.

2. Collection of an epidemiologically based large sample of genetically informative pedigrees drawn from the general population (not ascertained through affected individuals) and characterized on a large number of phenotypic measurements of relevance to mental disorders (e.g., attention, fMRI measures of brain structure and function) may prove extremely valuable. Insights into the pathways, molecules, and circuits involved in one or more mental disorders—even including those that are less common (e.g., schizophrenia and bipolar disorder)—will be generated.

3. Independent confirmation by at least one independent group of investigators must remain the standard to establish the validity of an initial linkage report. The linkage evidence in at least one report needs to be significant and must remain so after sample augmentation (more families, or more subjects per family, are analyzed).

4. Given the avalanche of data expected from studies of thousands of gene expression patterns, SNPs, and haplotypes, appropriate statistical corrections need to be developed to maintain the type I error rate at appropriate levels.

5. Resolution of genetic and etiologic heterogeneity is essential and will require further work on phenotypic classification to identify clinical characteristics that can delineate genetically distinct subgroups.

6. Genotypic and phenotypic (diagnostic and endophenotypic traits) data should be deposited in the public scientific domain. This will facilitate efforts to understand discrepancies between studies, accelerate efforts to replicate initial results, and enable metaanalytic studies of combined data sets.

7. State-of-the-art techniques for molecular and quantitative genetic analysis must continue to be rapidly applied to the genetic analysis of mental disorders. These include new methods for haplotype analysis, DNA pooling techniques, advances in high-throughput SNP genotyping, and the development and application of DNA and protein microarrays. Data mining and other analytic methods are required to detect true biological signals of relevance for understanding the neurobiology of mental disorders.

8. Cross-talk between basic neuroscientists, geneticists, and clinicians offers a great opportunity to anchor genetic studies of mental disorders to fundamental brain neurocircuitry and clinical phenomena. Animal models of constituent behavioral and other defects found in mental disorders will be key. The availability of full genomic sequence for the mouse and other key organisms (e.g., zebra fish) will be a critical factor in realizing the potential of these model organisms. Basic neuroscience research can direct attention to biochemical pathways and molecules that could provide multiple targets for developing new therapies for these disabling conditions.

SUGGESTED CROSS-REFERENCES

Findings related to the epidemiology of schizophrenia, mood disorders, and anxiety disorders are presented in Sections 12.4, 13.2, and 14.2, respectively. Findings from the study of the genetics of schizophrenia, mood disorders, and anxiety disorders are presented in Sections 12.3, 13.3, and 14.6, respectively. Transgenic animals and related approaches are discussed in Section 1.19.

References

Altmüller J, Palmer LJ, Fischer G, Scherb H, Wjst M: Genome-wide scans of complex human diseases: True linkage is hard to find. *Am J Hum Genet.* 2001;69:936.

Ardlie KG, Kruglyak L, Seielstad M: Patterns of linkage disequilibrium in the human genome. *Nat Rev Genet.* 2002;3:299.

Carlson CS, Eberle MA, Rieder MJ, Smith JD, Kruglyak L, Nickerson DA: Additional SNPs and linkage-disequilibrium analyses are necessary for whole-genome association studies in humans. *Nat Genet.* 2003;33:518.

Carrasquillo MM, McCallion AS, Puffenberger EG, Kashuk CS, Nouri N, Chakravarti A: Genome-wide association study and mouse model identify interaction between RET and EDNRB pathways in Hirschsprung disease. *Nat Genet.* 2002;32:237.

Chakravarti A: To a future of genetic medicine. *Nature.* 2001;409:822.

Chakravarti A, Little P: Nature, nurture, and human disease. *Nature.* 2003;421:412.

Charney DS, Barlow DH, Botteron K, Cohen JD, Goldman D, Gur RE, Lin K-M, López JF, Meador-Woodruff JH, Moldin SO, Nestler EJ, Watson SJ, Zalcman SJ. Neuroscience research agenda to guide development of a pathophysiologically based classification system. In: Kupfer DJ, First MB, Regier DA, eds. *A Research Agenda for DSM-V.* Washington, DC: American Psychiatric Press; 2002.

Collins FS, McKusick VA: Implications of the Human Genome Project for medical science. *JAMA.* 2001;285:540.

Cordell HJ: Epistasis: What it means, what it doesn't mean, and statistical methods to detect it in humans. *Hum Mol Genet.* 2002;11:2463.

Couzin J: Human genome. HapMap launched with pledges of $100 million. *Science.* 2002;298:941.

Devlin B, Roeder K, Wasserman L: Genomic control, a new approach to genetic-based association studies. *Theor Popul Biol.* 2001;60:155.

Duyk GM: Sharper tools and simpler methods. *Nat Genet.* 2002;32[Suppl]:465.

Falk CT, Rubinstein P: Haplotype relative risks: An easy reliable way to construct a proper control sample for risk calculations. *Ann Hum Genet.* 1987;51:227.

Gabriel SB, Schaffner SF, Nguyen H, Moore JM, Roy J, Blumenstiel B, Higgins J, DeFelice M, Lochner A, Faggart M, Liu-Cordero SN, Rotimi C, Adeyemo A, Cooper R, Ward R, Lander ES, Daly MJ, Altshuler D: The structure of haplotype blocks in the human genome. *Science.* 2002;296:2225.

Geschwind DH, Gregg JP. *Microarrays for the Neurosciences: An Essential Guide.* Boston: MIT Press; 2002.

Haines JL, Pericak-Vance MA. *Approaches to Gene Mapping in Complex Diseases.* New York: Wiley-Liss; 1998.

Hauser ER, Boehnke M, Guo S-W, Risch NJ: Affected-sib-pair interval mapping and exclusion for complex genetic traits: sampling considerations. *Genet Epidemiol.* 1996;13:117.

Hyman SE, Moldin SO. Genetic science and depression: Implications for research and treatment. In: Weissman MM, ed. *The Treatment of Major Depression: Bridging the 21st Century.* Washington, DC: American Psychiatric Press; 2001.

International SNP Map Working Group: A map of human genome sequence variation containing 1.42 million single nucleotide polymorphisms. *Nature.* 2001;409:928.

Kalow W, Meyer UA, Tyndale RF. *Pharmacogenomics.* New York: Marcel Dekker Inc; 2001.

Lander ES, Kruglyak L: Genetic dissection of complex traits: Guidelines for interpreting and reporting linkage results. *Nat Genet.* 1995;11:241.

Lynch M, Walsh B. *Genetics and Analysis of Quantitative Traits.* Sunderland, MA: Sinauer Associates; 1998.

Matise TC, Sachidanandam R, Clark AG, Kruglyak L, Wijsman E, Kakol J, Buyske S, Chui B, Cohen P, de Toma C, Ehm M, Glanowski S, He C, Heil J, Markianos K, McMullen I, Pericak-Vance MA, Silbergleit A, Stein L, Wagner M, Wilson AF, Winick JD, Winn-Deen ES, Yamashiro CT, Cann HM, Lai E, Holden AL: A 3.9-centimorgan-resolution human single-nucleotide polymorphism linkage map and screening set. *Am J Hum Genet.* 2003;73:271.

McGuffin P, Owen MJ, Gottesman II. *Psychiatric Genetics and Genomics.* New York: Oxford University Press; 2002.

McGuffin P, Riley B, Plomin R: Genomics and behavior. Toward behavioral genomics. *Science.* 2001;291:1232.

Mitchell AA, Cutler DJ, Chakravarti A: Undetected genotyping errors cause apparent overtransmission of common alleles in the transmission/disequilibrium test. *Am J Hum Genet.* 2003;72:598.

Moldin SO: National Institutes of Health Statistical Genetics Initiative Symposium. *Genet Epidemiol.* 2000;19[Suppl 1]:S1–S105.

Moldin SO: Neurobiology of anxiety and fear: Challenges for genomic science of the new millennium. *Biol Psychiatry.* 2000;48:1144.

Moldin SO, Farmer ME, Chin HR, Battey JF Jr: Trans-NIH neuroscience initiatives on mouse phenotyping and mutagenesis. *Mamm Genome.* 2001;12:575.

Ott J. *Analysis of Human Genetic Linkage.* 3rd ed. Baltimore: Johns Hopkins University Press; 1999.

Peltonen L, McKusick VA: Genomics and medicine. Dissecting human disease in the postgenomic era. *Science.* 2001;291:1224.

Plomin R, McGuffin P: Psychopathology in the postgenomic era. *Annu Rev Psychol.* 2003;54:205.

Rao DC, Province MA. *Genetic Dissection of Complex Traits.* San Diego, CA: Academic Press; 2002.

Reich DE, Cargill M, Bolk S, Ireland J, Sabeti PC, Richter DJ, Lavery T, Kouyoumjian R, Farhadian SF, Ward R, Lander ES: Linkage disequilibrium in the human genome. *Nature.* 2001;411:199.

Reik W, Walter J: Genomic imprinting: Parental influence on the genome. *Nat Rev Genet.* 2001;2:21.

Risch NJ: Searching for genetic determinants in the new millennium. *Nature.* 2000;405:847.

Roses AD: Pharmacogenetics and the practice of medicine. *Nature.* 2000;405:857.

Sengul H, Weeks DE, Feingold E: A survey of affected-sibship statistics for nonparametric linkage analysis. *Am J Hum Genet.* 2001;69:179.

Spielman RS, McGinnis RE, Ewens WJ: Transmission test for linkage disequilibrium: The insulin gene region and insulin-dependent diabetes mellitus (IDDM). *Am J Hum Genet.* 1993;52:506.

Terwilliger JD, Göring HH: Gene mapping in the 20th and 21st centuries: statistical methods, data analysis, and experimental design. *Hum Biol.* 2000;72:63.

Terwilliger JD, Ott J. *Handbook of Human Genetic Linkage.* Baltimore: Johns Hopkins University Press; 1994.

Wang S, Kidd KK, Zhao H: On the use of DNA pooling to estimate haplotype frequencies. *Genet Epidemiol.* 2003;24:74.

Waterston RH, Lindblad-Toh K, Birney E, Rogers J, Abril JF, Agarwal P, Agarwala R, Ainscough R, Alexandersson M, An P, Antonarakis SE, Attwood J, Baertsch R, Bailey J, Barlow K, Beck S, Berry E, Birren B, Bloom T, Bork P, Botcherby M, Bray N, Brent MR, Brown DG, Brown SD, Bult C, Burton J, Butler J, Campbell RD, Carninci P, Cawley S, Chiaromonte F, Chinwalla AT, Church DM, Clamp M, Clee C, Collins FS, Cook LL, Copley RR, Coulson A, Couronne O, Cuff J, Curwen V, Cutts T, Daly M, David R, Davies J, Delehaunty KD, Deri J, Dermitzakis ET, Dewey C, Dickens NJ, Diekhans M, Dodge S, Dubchak I, Dunn DM, Eddy SR, Elnitski L, Emes RD, Eswara P, Eyras E, Felsenfeld A, Fewell GA, Flicek P, Foley K, Frankel WN, Fulton LA, Fulton RS, Furey TS, Gage D, Gibbs RA, Glusman G, Gnerre S, Goldman N, Goodstadt L, Grafham D, Graves TA, Green ED , Gregory S, Guigo R, Guyer M, Hardison RC, Haussler D, Hayashizaki Y, Hillier LW, Hinrichs A, Hlavina W, Holzer T, Hsu F, Hua A, Hubbard T, Hunt A, Jackson I, Jaffe DB, Johnson LS, Jones M, Jones TA, Joy A, Kamal M, Karlsson EK, Karolchik D, Kasprzyk A, Kawai J, Keibler E, Kells C, Kent WJ, Kirby A, Kolbe DL, Korf I, Kucherlapati RS, Kulbokas EJ, Kulp D, Landers T, Leger JP, Leonard S, Letunic I, LeVine R, Li J, Li M, Lloyd C, Lucas S, Ma B, Maglott DR, Mardis ER, Matthews L, Mauceli E, Mayer JH, McCarthy M, McCombie WR, McLaren S, McLay K, McPherson JD, Meldrim J, Meredith B, Mesirov JP, Miller W, Miner TL, Mongin E, Montgomery KT, Morgan M, Mott R, Mullikin JC, Muzny DM, Nash WE, Nelson JO, Nhan MN, Nicol R, Ning Z, Nusbaum C, O'Connor MJ, Okazaki Y, Oliver K, Overton-Larty E, Pachter L, Parra G, Pepin KH, Peterson J, Pevzner P, Plumb R, Pohl CS, Poliakov A, Ponce TC, Ponting CP, Potter S, Quail M, Reymond A, Roe BA, Roskin KM, Rubin EM, Rust AG, Santos R, Sapojnikov V, Schultz B, Schultz J, Schwartz MS, Schwartz S, Scott C, Seaman S, Searle S, Sharpe T, Sheridan A, Shownkeen R, Sims S, Singer JB, Slater G, Smit A, Smith DR, Spencer B, Stabenau A, Stange-Thomann N, Sugnet C, Suyama M, Tesler G, Thompson J, Torrents D, Trevaskis E, Tromp J, Ucla C, Ureta-Vidal A, Vinson JP, Von Niederhausern AC, Wade CM, Wall M, Weber RJ, Weiss RB, Wendl MC, West AP, Wetterstrand K, Wheeler R, Whelan S, Wierzbowski J, Willey D, Williams S, Wilson RK, Winter E, Worley KC, Wyman D, Yang S, Yang SP, Zdobnov EM, Zody MC, Lander ES: Initial sequencing and comparative analysis of the mouse genome. *Nature.* 2002;420:520.

Wolfsberg TG, Wetterstrand KA, Guyer MS, Collins FS, Baxevanis AD: A user's guide to the human genome. *Nat Genet.* 2002;3[Suppl]:1.

▲ 1.18 Genetic Linkage Analysis of the Psychiatric Disorders

CAROL A. MATHEWS, M.D., AND NELSON B. FREIMER, M.D.

Although the etiology of neuropsychiatric disorders remains poorly understood, genetic epidemiologic investigations have suggested that there is a prominent genetic component in the causation of most, if not all, of these disorders. Efforts to identify specific genetic variants that cause susceptibility have been successful in only a few cases, such as Alzheimer's disease. However, advances in technology and analytical approaches to genetic mapping encourage optimism that there will soon be breakthroughs in the field of psychiatric genetics.

Genetic mapping studies are based on the idea that specific inherited mutations in the genetic material (the *genome*) of an individual are ultimately responsible for disease causation. These studies aim to isolate the responsible genes by identifying their chromosomal location through investigation of affected individuals and their families. All cells contain two copies of each chromosome (called *homologs*), one inherited from the mother and one inherited from the father. During meiosis, the parental homologs cross over, or recombine, creating unique new chromosomes that are then passed on to the progeny. Genes that are physically close to one another on a chromosome are genetically linked, and those that are farther apart or are on different chromosomes are genetically unlinked. Genes that are unlinked recombine at random (i.e., there is a 50 percent chance of recombination). Genes that are linked recombine less frequently than expected by random segregation; how much less often is proportional to the physical distance between them. Genetic mapping studies identify regions of the genome at which recombination between two genetic loci is less than would be expected by chance, that is, areas of linkage. The chromosomal location of disease genes is identified by comparing the inheritance pattern of the disease within a family to the inheritance pattern of genetic markers in that family.

Genetic markers are segments of deoxyribonucleic acid (DNA) of known chromosomal location that contain variations or polymorphisms. Historically, a number of different types of markers have been used in genetic mapping studies, including the blood group antigens and other antigenic markers, as well as restriction fragment length polymorphisms (RFLPs) (naturally occurring genomic sequence differences resulting in variations in restriction enzyme cutting sites in the genome). However, the low variability, small number, and uneven distribution of these markers have limited their power in linkage studies. More recently, microsatellite markers (also called *simple sequence length polymorphisms* [SSLPs]) and single nucleotide polymorphisms (SNPs) have been widely used. SSLPs are stretches of variable numbers of repeat nucleotides that are two to four base pairs in length. These markers are highly polymorphic, that is, the number of repeat units varies a great deal between individuals. *SNPs*, as the name implies, are single base pair changes at a specific nucleotide and are the most common form of sequence variation in the genome. SSLPs and SNPs are widely used for genetic mapping studies because they are numerous and distributed widely throughout the genome, and because they can be amplified with a technique called *polymerase chain reaction*, which provides opportunities for high throughput and automation.

It is now straightforward to identify linkage for Mendelian traits (traits for which a specific genotype at one particular locus is necessary and sufficient to cause the trait). However, psychiatric diseases do not follow simple Mendelian inheritance patterns but rather are examples of complex traits. Etiological complexity may be due to many factors, including incomplete penetrance (expression of the phenotype in only some of the individuals carrying the disease genotype), the presence of phenocopies (forms of the disease that are not caused by genetic factors), locus heterogeneity (different genes causing the same disease in different families or populations), or polygenic inheritance (the presence of multiple genes acting together to cause disease). Mapping a complex disorder involves several components, including definition of the phenotype to be studied, epidemiological studies to determine the evidence for genetic transmission of the phenotype, choice of an appropriate study population, and determination of correct technical and statistical approaches. Because it allows for close examination of virtually all chromosomal regions of interest by using multiple markers, the construction of a genetic map that densely covers the genome with a large number of highly polymorphic markers has been a pivotal development in the study of complex traits.

EPIDEMIOLOGICAL APPROACHES

Epidemiological studies, including twin studies, relative risk determinations, and segregation analyses, are primarily used to suggest whether a given disease or phenotype is likely to have a genetic etiology. They may also be useful for estimating the likely degree of the genetic contribution to the disorder, as well as possible modes of inheritance. Twin studies examine the concordance rates of a particular disorder (the percentage of twin pairs in which both twins have the disorder) in monozygotic and dizygotic twins. For a disorder that is strictly determined by genetic factors, the concordance rate should be 100 percent in monozygotic twin pairs (who share 100 percent of their genetic material) and 25 percent or 50 percent in dizygotic twin pairs (who are no more closely related than any siblings), depending on whether the disease is recessive or dominant, respectively. For a disorder in which genetic factors play important, but not exclusive, roles in disease causation, the concordance rates should be greater for monozygotic than for dizygotic twins. When genetic factors do not play a role, the concordance rates should not differ between the twin pairs, assuming that the environment for monozygotic twin pairs is no more similar than that for dizygotic twin pairs (which may not be true).

Relative risk (λ) is defined as the rate of occurrence of a disease for the relatives of an affected individual divided by the rate of occurrence of the disease for the general population. A relative risk of greater than 1 suggests a genetic etiology, and the magnitude of the measure gives an estimate of the genetic contribution to the disease. Relative risks can be calculated for sibling pairs, parent–offspring pairs, and various other types of family relationships. The likely mode of transmission can be assessed by comparing the degree of relative risk for each type of relationship.

Segregation analysis compares the observed number of affected individuals within a given family to the expected number of affected individuals within that family, assuming a particular mode of inheritance, and then compares the likelihood of observing these data under the given genetic model to the likelihood of observing the data under other genetic models. These studies not only establish whether there is a genetic component to the disorder in question but can also be used to estimate the likely genetic model or mode of inheritance. Because segregation analysis can be used to calculate the likelihood of a particular genetic model for individual families under specified parameters, it is useful for choosing families for a genetic study when previous studies have indicated that the disease is Mendelian in only a proportion of affected families and for choosing appropriate statistical models when studying a particular set of families.

Defining a Phenotype for Genetic Studies Because complex diseases, by definition, are not inherited in a simple Mendelian manner, they are often difficult to map genetically. One approach to simplifying the genetic mapping process is to carefully define the disease phenotype. This is a particularly important step in the study of psychiatric disorders, because they are defined empirically rather than on the basis of anatomic or physiological indices.

There are several elements to phenotype definition. The first involves deciding on the appropriate diagnostic criteria for the study in question and deciding how these criteria are applied to individuals in the study. One way of standardizing the procedures used to identify and to assess potential study subjects is to use only experienced clinicians in the diagnostic process and to train them in the administration of the instruments and the diagnostic criteria to be used. Additionally, a "best-estimate" procedure or a consensus diagnosis is helpful. The best-estimate process involves making use of every piece of available information, including medical records, interviews, and videotapes, when appropriate, to arrive at a diagnosis. For a consensus diagnosis, two or more diagnosticians independently review the material and make a diagnosis for each individual. The diagnoses are then compared, and individuals for whom an agreement in diagnosis cannot be reached are not entered into the study.

The second element in phenotype definition involves making use of all available information about the genetic epidemiology of the disorder to choose a sample of affected individuals to study. It is often the case that a subset of families carries the disorder in what appears to be a simple Mendelian pattern, whereas the inheritance pattern is less clear for other families or groups. In a disorder for which there are likely to be multiple genes contributing to the phenotype, it makes sense to begin with a study sample in which there may be major loci. Redefining the disease phenotype can often simplify the mapping process by identifying such groups or families. For example, in the search for a genetic defect for Alzheimer's disease, the process was advanced enormously by limiting the study population to those individuals who had early age of onset (before 65 years of age); the early-onset trait segregated in an autosomal-dominant fashion. Other ways of redefining the phenotype include focusing on specific ethnic groups; subgrouping by genetic epidemiology (family history and maternal or paternal inheritance), age of onset, treatment response, symptom severity, or the presence of comorbid disorders; or by using endophenotypes. *Endophenotypes* are defined as alternative phenotypes that are related to a disease phenotype but are hypothesized to demonstrate a more straightforward inheritance pattern. Another advantage is that endophenotypes can usually be assessed quantitatively (as opposed to disease phenotypes, which are typically qualitative). Endophenotypes include biochemical measures, such as serum or cerebrospinal fluid (CSF) levels of metabolites or hormones, and biophysical markers, such as responses to evoked potentials. Analysis of endophenotypes has been a useful strategy in identifying susceptibility genes for some complex disorders, including non–insulin-dependent diabetes mellitus, which was mapped to chromosome 12 in a sample of affected individuals only after the phenotype was modified to account for mean insulin levels. Although the overall genome screen provided no significant evidence of linkage, significant evidence of linkage was found on chromosome 12 when the study was limited to those individuals with the lowest mean insulin levels.

Narrowing the phenotype by using the approaches discussed previously may increase the chances of finding a genetic defect in complex diseases, but it can also greatly reduce the power of the study by limiting the number of available affected individuals. For this reason, it has been argued that, for some disorders, broadening the phenotype is an appropriate strategy. The suggestion is that, for some complex diseases, the phenotype of interest may represent the extreme end of a spectrum and that, to have enough power to identify a gene, other disorders within the spectrum must also be included. This argument has been particularly favored in the study of schizophrenia. Family studies have indicated that there is an increased incidence of schizoaffective disorder, schizotypal personality disorder, and paranoid personality disorder in the biological families of schizophrenic patients, and individuals with these disorders are often included as affected subjects in genetic studies of schizophrenia. The primary disadvantage of using a broadly defined phenotype is that it may lead to an increase of etiologic heterogeneity and, consequently, an increased rate of phenocopies, making detection of linkage more difficult.

Although the two approaches of narrowing the disease phenotype and broadening the disease phenotype may seem to be mutually exclusive, many groups studying complex disorders are attempting to incorporate both approaches into their study designs. One way to do this is to create stratified diagnostic categories, ranging from a narrow diagnostic category to a broad diagnostic category, and to test for genetic linkage under each of these schemas. There is currently a great deal of debate about whether this strategy is useful or not. Some investigators argue that, for complex diseases that may actually be part of a spectrum, this strategy decreases the rate of false negatives, that is, of missing an existing linkage because of misspecification. Others argue that using several models and picking the one that gives the highest scores statistically greatly increases the rates of false positives, that is, of identifying an area of linkage where none exists. One problem that clearly exists with the use of multiple diagnostic categories is that, as more models are used, increasingly stringent levels of significance are also required.

The issues involved in phenotype definition are complicated and difficult, and, within the field of genetics, there is a disagreement about the best way to approach studies of complex traits. Because of the number of unknowns in other aspects of these studies, however, it is clear that the problem of how to define the disease to be studied is perhaps the single most difficult issue.

Genome Screen Versus Candidate Gene Approach

Once genetic epidemiology has provided as much information as possible about the genetic basis of a trait, and the phenotype to be studied has been defined, the next step is to search for regions of the genome that may be linked to the disorder, by examining candidate regions or by performing a screen of the entire genome. For disorders for which the pathophysiology is known or partially understood, one or several candidate genes for the disorder may already have been identified. A *candidate gene* is one whose location has already been determined and whose protein product is known and that is hypothesized to play a role in the pathophysiology of the disorder in question. Genes with unknown functions that are located in a particular chromosomal region of interest are often also considered via this approach. Candidate genes for the neuropsychiatric disorders have traditionally been derived from pharmacological information or from cytogenetic data (including translocations and deletions) indicating a candidate region.

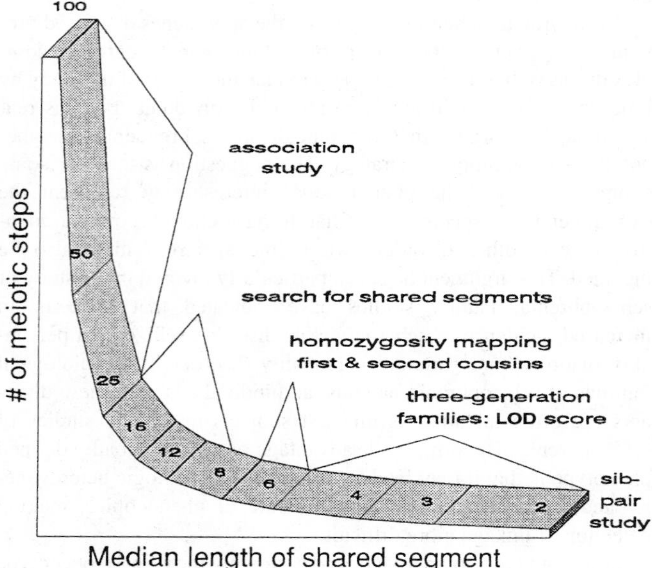

FIGURE 1.18–1 Depiction of the median lengths of the chromosomal segments inherited identical by descent around a disease gene by two individuals separated from a common ancestor by differing numbers of meiotic steps. LOD, logarithm of odds; sib, sibling. (From Houwen RHJ, Baharloo S, Blankenship K, et al.: Genome screening by searching for shared segments: Mapping a gene for benign recurrent intrahepatic cholestasis. *Nat Genet.* 1994;8:380, with permission.)

The other approach to searching for linkage is to conduct a whole genome screen. This approach assumes that there are no known specific areas of interest within the genome and therefore involves screening the entire genome with evenly spaced markers in an attempt to find an area or areas of potential linkage. Strategies to map disease genes are based on identifying genetic marker alleles that are shared by affected individuals identical by descent, that is, that are inherited from a common ancestor along with a linked disease gene. The optimal method used for genetic mapping is determined by the composition of the study sample. Methods that are useful for samples of individuals who are closely related to one another may be inappropriate for samples whose members are only distantly related. For example, methods for analyzing samples of affected sibling pairs (ASPs) are based on the idea that they are only one generation removed from their common ancestor and therefore share large regions of the genome identical by descent. At the other extreme, methods for analyzing samples drawn from a population are based on the idea that the affected individuals are separated from their common ancestor by perhaps hundreds of generations and therefore are identical by descent for only small segments of the genome (Fig. 1.18–1). Methods for analyzing population samples are best suited to identifying identical-by-descent regions for fine-scale mapping, whereas ASP approaches are well suited to initial localization of broad areas of linkage.

PEDIGREE ANALYSIS

Searching for areas of linkage to the disorder of interest, in a whole genome screen or in a candidate area, has traditionally been done using pedigree analysis. This type of study is done in families comprising three or four generations, in which affected individuals are separated by two to six meiotic steps. The primary goal of pedigree analysis is to determine if two or more genetic loci (i.e., a genetic marker and the disease of interest) are cosegregating within a pedigree. For each marker locus, the number of recombinants within the pedigree is compared to the number of nonrecombinants within the pedigree, and a recombination fraction (θ) is estimated. The recombination fraction represents the percent recombination between two loci—in this case, the hypothetical disease locus and the marker locus—and is equal to the genetic distance between the two loci (1 percent of recombination equals 1 centimorgan [cM] in genetic distance and, on average, covers a physical distance of approximately 1 megabase [Mb] of DNA). A recombination fraction of 0.5 percent or 50 percent indicates that the two loci are not linked but rather that they are segregating independently. A logarithm of odds (LOD) score is then calculated to determine the likelihood that the two loci are linked at the distance suggested. The LOD score is calculated by dividing the likelihood of acquiring the data if the loci are linked at a given recombination fraction by the likelihood of acquiring the data if the loci are unlinked ($\theta = 0.5$). This step gives an odds ratio, and the $\log_{10}$ of this odds ratio is the LOD score.

A LOD score can be obtained for various values of the recombination fraction, from 0 (completely linked) to 0.5 (unlinked). In addition, data from multiple family pedigrees can be combined to derive a cumulative LOD score (designated by Z). The value of θ that gives the largest LOD score is considered to be the best estimate of the recombination fraction between the disease locus and the marker locus. This recombination fraction can then be converted into a genetic map distance. In general, the likelihood that any two given loci are linked (the prior probability of linkage) is expected to be approximately 1:50, based on the genetic length of the genome. To compensate for the prior probability of linkage and to bring the posterior (or overall) probability of linkage to approximately 1:20, which corresponds to the commonly accepted significance level of P equals .05, a conditional probability of 1,000:1 odds in favor of linkage (corresponding to a LOD score of 3 and a P value of .0001) is required. Therefore, under ideal conditions, for simple Mendelian disorders, a LOD score of 3 is considered to be significant evidence for linkage.

A pedigree analysis consists of scanning the genome or a portion of the genome with a series of markers in one or more affected pedigrees, calculating a LOD score at each marker position, and identifying the chromosomal regions that show a significant deviation from what would be expected under the conditions of independent assortment. Because many hundreds of markers and multiple genetic models are frequently used in genome screens, and because of uncertainties in estimates of penetrance level and allele frequencies for many disorders, the question arises as to what represents acceptable evidence for linkage. In the instances in which multiple genetic markers are tested, a LOD score of 3.4 has been suggested as providing sufficient evidence for linkage. The problem of using multiple genetic models is somewhat more difficult. One suggestion has been to use the formula $3 + \log(t)$, where t is the number of tests performed. Under these parameters, a LOD score of 3.4 or higher would be required to provide significant evidence of linkage if more than one model is used, and a LOD score of 4 would be required if ten models are used. Many investigators argue that these criteria are, in fact, too stringent, as they assume that each model is independent of the others, which is not the case in mapping studies.

It is important, however, to account for the increased likelihood of obtaining a false positive in the context of multiple tests. In a standard genome screen of several hundred markers, one can expect to find false positives (regions that are significant at $P < .05$, corresponding to a LOD score of >1) by chance alone approximately 24 times (once per chromosome) (Fig. 1.18–2). This is important because some investigators have argued that a LOD score of greater than 1 is a significant LOD score in genetic studies of a complex disease. For this reason, a classification system for reporting linkage based on dense genome scans has been proposed (Table 1.18–1). These criteria, although used by some investigators, are not universally accepted. Because the techniques and statistical methods used in the study of complex diseases are being developed at a rapid pace, as of 2003, there is no universally accepted standard for evaluating the significance of findings in such studies.

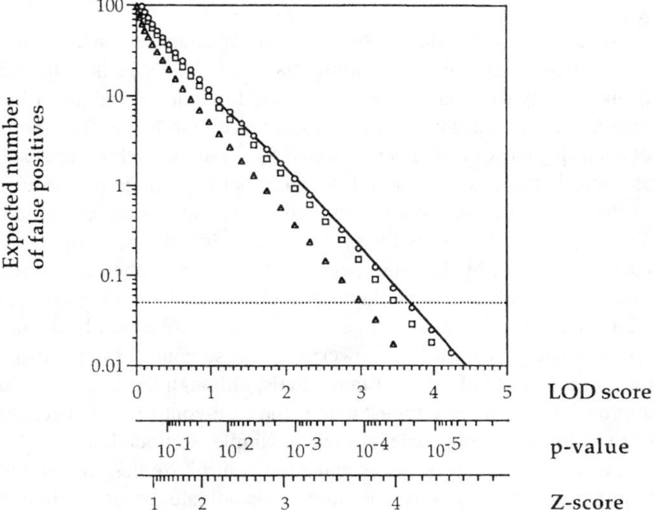

FIGURE 1.18–2 Number of false positives expected in a whole genome scan for a given threshold of logarithm of odds (LOD) score. Solid line represents the expectation for a perfect genetic map. Symbols represent the results for 100 sibling pairs using genetic maps with markers spaced every 0.1 centimorgan (cM) (*circles*), every 1 cM (*squares*), and every 10 cM (*triangles*). The dotted line indicates the 5 percent genome-wide significance level. (Courtesy of Dr. Eric Lander.)

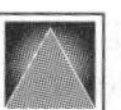

Table 1.18–1
Suggested Criteria for Statistical Evidence of Linkage in Genetic Studies of Complex Traits

Suggestive linkage	Statistical evidence that would be expected to occur one time at random in a genome screen	$P \leq .001$
Significant linkage	Statistical evidence that would be expected to occur approximately 0.05 times in a genome screen	$P \leq .0001$
Highly significant linkage	Statistical evidence that would be likely to occur 0.001 times in a genome screen	$P < .00002$
Confirmed linkage	Significant linkage from one or a combination of initial studies that has subsequently been confirmed in a further sample	—

Courtesy of Dr. Eric S. Lander.

Although replication of a finding in a separate sample has been suggested as one way of confirming linkage, it is important to note that failure to replicate a linkage finding in another population does not necessarily mean that there is not linkage at that locus. Failure to replicate the finding may be due to genetic heterogeneity, diagnostic differences between the study populations, or stochastic (statistical) fluctuation. In such cases, extension studies in the original population or a metaanalysis of all studies may help confirm or refute the initial finding.

NONPARAMETRIC APPROACHES

Multiple nonparametric approaches have also been developed to address the problem of searching for linkage in the presence of genetic heterogeneity, incomplete penetrance, and unknown modes of transmission. These are called *model-free tests for linkage* because they do not require the specification of a model or the attendant parameters (such as mode of inheritance, type of penetrance, allele frequencies, and mutation and recombination rates). Nonparametric methods are less powerful in their ability to detect linkage than LOD score analysis using a correctly specified linkage model, but they are more robust than the LOD score approach in the face of unknown parameters. For this reason, they are best used when the genetic etiology of the disorder is complex, that is, when simple Mendelian inheritance patterns are not observed. Another advantage of nonparametric methods is that LOD score analysis of a small number of large families can be sensitive to small changes in a few data points (for example, a change from unaffected status to affected status), whereas nonparametric analyses, because they are usually done on a large number of small families, tend to normal distributions and are thus less affected by such changes. The most commonly used nonparametric method in the study of psychiatric disorders is sibling-pair analysis.

Sibling-Pair Analysis

ASP analysis, first proposed in 1935, is a nonparametric method that is widely used in genetic studies of complex traits. Sibling-pair analysis examines the frequency with which sibling pairs concordant for a trait share a particular region of the genome compared to the frequency that is expected under random segregation. Although it is possible to do this test by using affected and unaffected siblings, usually only affected-affected sibling pairs are evaluated, because little information is gained by including unaffected sibling pairs, and because excluding these individuals alleviates the need to consider possible incomplete penetrance for the trait in question.

Sibling-pair analysis is based on the concept that siblings share approximately 50 percent of their genomes identical by descent. Therefore, if a group of unrelated sibling pairs with a certain trait shares a particular area of the genome significantly more than 50 percent of the time (the proportion of sharing expected under conditions of random segregation), that area of the genome is likely to be linked to the trait in question. In this method, siblings are genotyped, and population frequencies and parental genotypes are used to estimate the proportion of genes shared identical by descent at each site for each sibling pair. Those pairs concordant and discordant for each genetic locus are then compared via analytical methods.

Association Studies Whereas linkage studies attempt to find cosegregation of a genetic marker and a disease gene within a family or families, association studies examine whether a particular allele occurs more frequently than expected in affected individuals within a population. One type of association study is based on the idea that certain alleles at markers closely surrounding a disease gene are in linkage disequilibrium (LD) with the disease gene—that is, that these alleles are carried more often than expected by random segregation in affected individuals because they are inherited identical by descent. Association studies of candidate genes make a different assumption—that a particular variant allele is actually causative of the disease.

LD studies have traditionally been used to complement traditional pedigree analyses, to narrow a region of interest that has already been identified or to confirm a previous finding. However, these methods are now being used for whole genome screens, particularly for diseases for which traditional linkage studies have been unsuccessful. These studies have one great advantage over a traditional pedigree analysis—because affected individuals are chosen from an entire population rather than from one or a few pedigrees, the number of potential subjects is limited only by the size of the population and the frequency of the disease. For disorders in which genetic heterogeneity or incomplete penetrance are likely to be factors, maximizing the potential number of affected individuals that can be included in the analysis is extremely important.

Genome-wide LD studies are perhaps most readily implemented in relatively recently founded isolated populations, because the relative homogeneity of such populations and the high degree of relatedness of affected individuals in these populations may enable LD studies to be conducted with fewer markers than in outbred populations. On the other hand, it is possible that variant alleles that are important in such isolates may be relatively unimportant in large outbred populations. For this reason, there is increasing interest in carrying out association studies in both isolated and outbred populations.

Isolated Populations Genetically isolated populations are those that are descended from a small number of original founders with little or no subsequent immigration or admixture. As a population gets older, recombination across the generations gradually diminishes the length of the chromosomal regions that are shared identical by descent, and individuals several generations away from the founding of the population should therefore share few regions of the genome by chance. Individuals who share a common trait or disease in such a population are thus likely to have inherited the same genetic defect as well as specific alleles for markers in the region surrounding the putative disease gene. In general, such LD approaches require that the population under investigation has undergone rapid expansion from a small original founding population and that there has been minimal immigration subsequent to the founding. For a genome screen attempting to find shared segments of the genome using currently practical numbers of markers, the ideal population should be less than 100 generations distant from its founders. A population that is older than this is likely to have conserved areas that are extremely small and that may be missed using even dense marker maps. For studies that are attempting to further delineate an area already identified by a traditional linkage study by examining associations between the disease gene and particular alleles at one or a few markers, an older population may be more appropriate, as the smaller regions of sharing between affected individuals help narrow the region of interest.

Outbred Populations As the available genetic marker maps become denser with the continuing discovery of SNPs, association studies in outbred populations are now becoming feasible. There are two common approaches to association studies in outbred populations—case-control studies and family-based or trio studies. In a case-control study, allele frequencies between a group of affected individuals and a matched control sample are compared. Case-control studies have the potential for being powerful, as large samples can often be collected with relative ease. Case-control samples are particularly useful for traits with a late age of onset, as they do not require the participation of parents or additional family members. The biggest disadvantage to using a case-control approach is the problem of stratification. If the control sample is not carefully chosen to match the case sample, the chance of false-positive associations is increased because of underlying differences in allele frequencies between the cases and controls. One way that has been proposed to control for this genetically is to genotype some number of extra markers distributed randomly throughout the genome to determine if stratification is present and then to statistically control for any background differences in allele frequencies that are identified between the groups.

Another way to address the problem of stratification is to use small nuclear families. In a family-based study, DNA is collected from a family trio, that is, from an affected individual and his or her parents. In this design, the nontransmitted chromosomes (the copy of each chromosome that is not passed from parent to child) are used as control chromosomes, and differences between allele frequencies in the transmitted and nontransmitted chromosomes are examined. This approach eliminates the problem of stratification, as the comparison group is, by definition, genetically similar to the case group. The main disadvantage of this approach is that it is less powerful than a case-control study. In general, a family-based study is only approximately two-thirds as powerful as a case-control sample using the same number of affected individuals, although the family-based approach is much more robust than is the case-control study because of the elimination of problems such as sample stratification.

As of 2003, family-based and case-control studies in outbred populations are primarily focusing on candidate genes. Although there is potential to use such samples for complete genome screens, the problems of stratification and marker map density have, in practice, not been fully addressed. For a genome screen using a case-control approach, it has been estimated that at least 50,000 markers are required, at an average distance of 50 kilobases (kb). Although sufficient markers exist to complete such a genome screen, the effort and expense required to genotype and analyze such a large number are substantial. However, as technology advances, and as high-throughput automated genotyping becomes more easily available, such studies will become more feasible.

Although, in linkage studies, each marker or genetic model, or both, that is tested is not completely independent of the other markers and models that are tested, for association studies in candidate genes, each test performed carries an independent risk of a false-positive result. It has been suggested that the threshold for significance for such studies should be set at $P = .05/n$, where n is the number of independent tests, or, in the case of testing for multiple alleles at multiple markers, $P = .05/n(m - 1)$, where n is the number of markers, and m is the number of alleles per marker. This approach assumes that only one polymorphism is being tested in each candidate gene, however, and that the candidate genes of interest are not physically close to each other. The issue becomes more complex when association studies are used for genome screens. In this situation, as with genome screens using linkage analysis, the markers are closely spaced and thus are not completely independent of one another.

Conclusion

Genetic mapping has undergone a number of important advances in the last several years, making it possible to find the genetic basis for many complex traits, including familial breast cancer, diabetes mellitus, and, more recently, neuropsychiatric disorders, such as Alzheimer's disease. For the neuropsychiatric disorders, as for other complex traits, however, geneticists are no longer searching for one definitive genetic defect, as was the case with simple Mendelian diseases. Rather, the search has shifted to identifying susceptibility genes, with the understanding that there are likely to be several such genes for each clinical entity, acting in concert with one another within a population or independently in different populations, and that these gene effects are likely to be modified by environmental phenomena. Several neuropsychiatric diseases that have been extensively studied genetically, with varying degrees of success, include Alzheimer's disease, bipolar disorder, schizophrenia, Tourette's syndrome, and autism. Each of these disorders has provided a somewhat different insight into the difficulties inherent in the genetic mapping of complex disorders.

ALZHEIMER'S DISEASE

Alzheimer's disease provides an excellent example of how advances in available technologies and methods have aided genetic mapping studies of complex diseases. The search for the genetic basis of Alzheimer's disease began with a traditional linkage study using a candidate area on chromosome 21. This effort evolved over time into a study of a number of other areas of the genome using several different approaches, culminating in the identification of defects in three unique genes that are responsible for Alzheimer's disease.

Alzheimer's disease is a form of dementia characterized by progressive impairment of memory and intellectual functioning. The clinical signs and symptoms, although characteristic, are not limited to Alzheimer's disease but are also found in several other types of dementia. For this reason, the diagnosis of Alzheimer's disease can only be confirmed histopathologically at autopsy. The presence of senile plaques (made up of a core of β-amyloid fibrils surrounded by dystrophic neurites), tau-rich neurofibrillary tangles, and congophilic angiopathy in the brain parenchyma and associated blood vessels are pathognomonic for Alzheimer's disease.

Alzheimer's disease occurs in familial and sporadic forms. Approximately 60 percent of cases appear to be sporadic (do not have a family history). A variable age of onset has been noted, ranging from onset as early as 35 years of age to onset as late as 95 years of age. The concordance rate for Alzheimer's disease in monozygotic twin pairs is approximately 50 percent, indicating a moderately strong genetic component. Other factors that may play a role in the development of Alzheimer's disease include age, gender, previous head injury, years of education, and cardiovascular disease.

Although, phenotypically, Alzheimer's disease appears to be a fairly homogenous disorder, epidemiological studies have indicated that it is genetically heterogeneous. To more clearly define a phenotype that would be amenable to genetic studies, investigators initially divided Alzheimer's disease into early and late onset categories. Early-onset Alzheimer's disease consists of individuals affected before 65 years of age, whereas late-onset Alzheimer's disease consists of individuals affected after 65 years of age. No consistent phenotypic differences between early and late onset have been noted. However, in a substantial number of families, the early-onset form of the disorder appears to be inherited in an autosomal-dominant fashion with age-dependent penetrance. In late-onset Alzheimer's disease, the etiology is less clear—although some cases are probably inherited in a Mendelian manner, it is likely that most cases are not caused by a major susceptibility locus. As knowledge about the genetic etiology of Alzheimer's disease has progressed, the terminology for this classification has changed somewhat. As of 2003, Alzheimer's disease is now usually divided into familial Alzheimer's disease and sporadic Alzheimer's disease.

Chromosome 21

It has long been recognized that many individuals with Down syndrome (trisomy 21) develop an early-onset dementia that is clinically and histopathologically indistinguishable from Alzheimer's disease. For this reason, chromosome 21 was considered to be an excellent candidate region for initial genetic studies of Alzheimer's disease. Amyloid β-peptide (a proteolytic product of amyloid precursor protein [APP]) is present in the senile plaques characteristic of Alzheimer's disease and was known to map to chromosome 21q11-q21.2. It was hypothesized that a defect in this gene, leading to overexpression of normal β-amyloid or to expression of an abnormal form of β-amyloid, was responsible for Alzheimer's disease. Mutations were subsequently found in coding regions within the APP gene, resulting in amino acid substitutions, and in areas that lie outside the β-amyloid sequence, resulting in overproduction of β-amyloid or production of longer fragments in individuals with Alzheimer's disease. Transgenic mice with different APP mutations have been shown to produce β-amyloid deposits and senile plaques, as well as showing synapse loss, astrocytosis, and microgliosis, all part of the pathology of Alzheimer's disease. Mutations in the genes that encode β-APP all lead to an increase in the extracellular concentration of longer fragments of β-amyloid ($A\beta_{42}$). Most of the strains of transgenic mice with mutations in APP exhibit increased rates of behavioral changes and impairment in several memory tasks, indicating dysfunction in object-recognition memory and working memory, among others. Although no neurofibrillary tangles are observed in most of the different transgenic mice, these findings nevertheless represent striking evidence that mutations in the β-amyloid gene are indeed responsible for at least some of the histopathological elements of Alzheimer's disease. To date, there have been a number of missense mutations identified near or within the β-amyloid sequence of the APP on chromosome 21 that are present in early-onset Alzheimer's disease families.

Chromosome 14

Because linkage to chromosome 21 was excluded in a number of early-onset Alzheimer's disease families, genome screening was done to search for evidence of linkage elsewhere. As a result of these studies, linkage on chromosome 14 was independently identified in early-onset Alzheimer's disease by four teams studying a large number of families from several populations and was found to be the strongest at 14q24.3. Using linkage analysis, investigators were able to narrow the region of interest on chromosome 14 to 8.9 cM. Haplotype inspection further delineated the region, and a physical map of this area was constructed using yeast artificial chromosomes (YACs). Exon trapping and direct selection of coding DNA from the YACs then identified several new genes. Five missense mutations were found in early-onset Alzheimer's disease families in one of these transcripts, containing a previously uncharacterized gene that was subsequently named *presenilin-1* (*PS-1*). The *PS-1* gene on chromosome 14 has since been recognized as a major locus for Alzheimer's disease in early-onset familial Alzheimer's disease, contributing to as much as 70 percent of cases. More than 70 mutations of *PS-1* have been identified. This area of chromosome 14 has also been examined in late-onset Alzheimer's disease families; however, as of 2003, there is no evidence for linkage in these families.

Chromosome 1 Although the *PS-1* gene accounts for a significant proportion of families with early-onset Alzheimer's disease, it does not account for all familial early-onset Alzheimer's disease. In particular, *PS-1* does not account for Alzheimer's disease in a group of large families of Volga-German descent. These families, which have a high incidence of early-onset Alzheimer's disease, are known to be descended from one German family that emigrated to Russia from Germany and then emigrated to the United States. In this group, Alzheimer's disease segregates in an autosomal-dominant fashion, and this was hypothesized to be due to a single gene defect inherited from a common ancestor. Initial linkage results from a genome search in several Alzheimer's disease families of Volga-German descent did not show linkage to the chromosome 14 site or to the chromosome 21 site but did identify yet another region, this time on chromosome 1 in the area of 1q31-q42. After this linkage study and the identification of *PS-1*, a search of a publicly available database identified a coding DNA sequence showing high homology to the *PS-1* gene on chromosome 14, which was found to map to within the chromosome 1 region of interest for Alzheimer's disease. This gene was subsequently named *presenilin-2* (*PS-2*). Two missense mutations have been found in *PS-2* in the Volga-German families and in several Italian families with early-onset Alzheimer's disease.

Presenilin-1 and -2 Mutations *PS-1* and *PS-2* are integral transmembrane proteins with at least seven transmembrane domains. Although their exact functions are unknown, the presenilin (PS) proteins associate with the plasma membrane of cells, suggesting that their expression at the cell surface might mediate cell–cell contacts that are responsible for adhesion or transcellular binding. Studies of transfected cell lines and transgenic mice suggest that mutations in the PS genes may lead to an increase in $A\beta_{42}$, although how this occurs is not yet known.

PS-1 mutations account for Alzheimer's disease in between 18 and 70 percent of early-onset Alzheimer's disease families. As of 2003, more than 70 missense mutations and at least one in-frame splice site mutation in *PS-1* have been found; all of the missense mutations involve amino acids that are conserved between *PS-1* and *PS-2*. *PS-1* mutations are, for the most part, fully penetrant with a narrow age-of-onset range (35 to 55 years of age). It appears that, for Alzheimer's disease owing to this gene, age of onset is determined by the nature of the mutation and by the position of the mutation within the gene. In addition, although most mutations result in early-onset Alzheimer's disease, some *PS-1* mutations may also result in late-onset Alzheimer's disease. Although less is currently known about *PS-2* mutations, they do appear to result in a later and more variable age of onset (as late as the seventh and eighth decades of life) than do *PS-1* mutations.

Chromosome 19 For early-onset Alzheimer's disease, traditional linkage studies were successful in identifying linkage to the three genes noted previously, in part because careful phenotype definition allowed investigators to identify large families in which the disease appeared to segregate in a Mendelian fashion. However, these approaches were unsuccessful in studies of late-onset or sporadic Alzheimer's disease, in part because the mode of inheritance was less clear in individuals with this disorder. For this reason, investigators used a nonparametric linkage approach to search for evidence of linkage in a large number of small families with late-onset Alzheimer's disease. In 1991, the results of a linkage study using 36 markers in late-onset Alzheimer's disease families provided evidence ($P < .001$) for a susceptibility gene on the long arm of chromosome 19. Subsequent multipoint LOD score analysis gave a LOD score of 4.6 on chromosome 19 between two markers in the area of 19q13.2. There were several candidate genes known to map to this area, including growth factors, proteases, and apolipoprotein E (apoE). The major known function of apoE is in lipid transport, but other functions have also been suggested. Although apoE has no known specific causal relationship to Alzheimer's disease, it is found in senile plaques, neurofibrillary tangles, and vascular amyloid deposits in Alzheimer's disease brains. In addition, apoE in the CSF binds to β-amyloid with high affinity. For this reason, studies were undertaken to determine if an association between Alzheimer's disease and any of the expressed alleles of apoE was present.

Apolipoprotein E In 1993, several epidemiological studies identified the *ε4* allele of the apoE gene as a genetic risk factor for late-onset Alzheimer's disease. There are three known alleles of this gene—*ε2*, *ε3*, and *ε4*. In most populations, the *ε3* allele is the most common. However, in familial late-onset Alzheimer's disease, the incidence of *ε4* is approximately 50 percent, and, in sporadic late-onset Alzheimer's disease, it is 40 percent, compared to 16 percent in normal controls. Epidemiological studies suggest that between 30 and 60 percent of late-onset Alzheimer's disease cases have at least one *apoE-ε4* allele. The *ε4* genotype appears to be a more important risk factor for Alzheimer's disease in populations of European and Asian origin when compared to populations of African origin. There does appear to be a gene dose effect for the *ε4* allele in late-onset Alzheimer's disease families, with the risk for Alzheimer's disease increasing and the mean age of onset decreasing with increasing number of *ε4* alleles. In the late-onset Alzheimer's disease families, those who are homozygous for *e4* are affected 91 percent of the time with a mean age of onset at 68.4 years of age. Those who are heterozygous for *ε4* are affected 47 percent of the time with a mean age of onset at 75.5 years of age, and those with no *ε4* are affected 20 percent of the time with a mean age of onset at 84.3 years of age. *Apo-ε4* binds more readily to β-amyloid than does *apoE-ε3*, and patients homozygous for *apoE-ε4* have more β-amyloid deposited in senile plaques and cerebral blood vessel walls than do those homozygous for *apoE-ε3*, providing support for the hypothesis that apoE plays a role in the etiology of Alzheimer's disease.

Genome Screens Complete genome screens for Alzheimer's disease, particularly for late-onset Alzheimer's disease, have been technically difficult to accomplish, for a variety of reasons. Because of the late age of onset, it has been difficult to sample complete families, making traditional linkage analyses relatively uninformative. However, recent advances in statistical methodologies for linkage analysis now permit investigation of such families, and genome screening studies of late-onset Alzheimer's disease are now being undertaken.

At least four genome screens for late-onset Alzheimer's disease have now been completed. These studies have generally examined late-onset Alzheimer's disease by using a modified ASP or a case-control design. Sample sizes have ranged from 50 to more than 700 cases or sibling pairs. Regions of interest with varying levels of statistical significance have been identified on 14 chromosomes, including the apoE region on chromosome 19. The strongest findings have been on chromosome 9 (two-point maximum LOD score [MLS] of 4.31), chromosome 10 (multipoint maximum LOD score [MMLS] of 3.9), and chromosome 12 (MMLS of 3.5). Of these regions, only the chromosome 10 locus has shown evidence for association in follow-up studies. Three of four replication studies have shown some continued evidence for association with Alzheimer's disease. In a linkage study that used plasma $A\beta_{42}$ levels as a surrogate trait for Alzheimer's disease and examined the chromosomal areas of interest identified by the genome screens, a MLS of 3.93 was found on chromosome 10. This study is significant not only because it provides support for a previous linkage finding for Alzheimer's disease, but also because it successfully uses a biological marker as a quantitative trait. This approach sidesteps the problem created by the fact that Alzheimer's disease can only be definitively diagnosed posthumously. It has been suggested that the chromosome 10 locus may act synergistically with *apoE-ε4*. In a prospective, longitudinal follow-up of 325 asymptomatic first-degree relatives of Alzheimer's disease patients older than 11 years of age, the age-specific risk of developing Alzheimer's disease was the greatest for those relatives with the *apoE-ε4* allele and the chromosome 10 allele (risk ratio of 16.2).

In summary, Alzheimer's disease is a neuropsychiatric disorder with multiple etiologies, presumably genetic and environmental. Although the genetics of this complex disorder are not fully elucidated, the history of the search for disease genes for Alzheimer's disease illustrates how important each phase of the approach can be, from carefully defining the phenotype to making use of available epidemiologic studies, as well as the importance of using all available data, including the public databases. As of 2003, genes have been identified on chromosomes 21, 14 and 1, coding for the β-amyloid peptide of APP, *PS-1*, and *PS-2*. Together, mutations in these genes account for approximately 5 percent of affected individuals, primarily those with familial early-onset disease. An additional 15 percent of affected individuals have sporadic early-onset disease, whereas 30 percent have familial late onset, and 45 percent have sporadic late onset. In addition, chromosome 19q has been identified as being linked to Alzheimer's disease in the late-onset familial form of the disease. This area is the location of the gene coding for apoE, which was previously shown to be related to Alzheimer's disease. Presence of the *ε4* allele of this gene in these families correlates with increased risk of getting the disease and decreased age of onset of the symptoms in a dose-effect manner. Figure 1.18–3 shows the locations of the susceptibility genes that have been identified for Alzheimer's disease.

Although the pathophysiology of Alzheimer's disease remains a mystery, β-amyloid, in particular, the overexpression of the $A\beta_{42}$

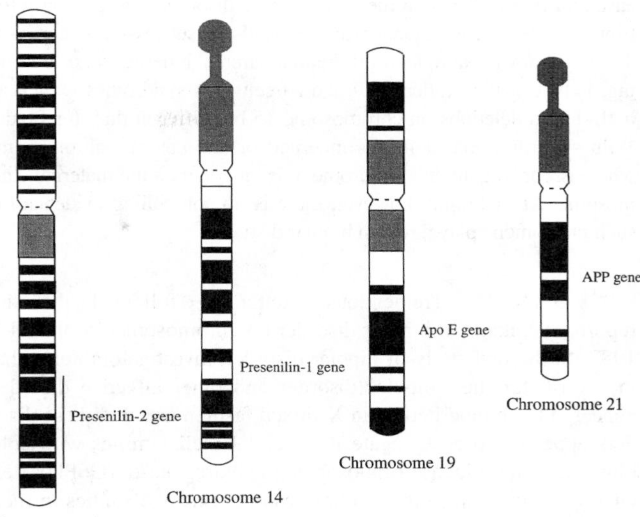

FIGURE 1.18–3 Chromosomal location of the genes implicated in Alzheimer's disease. ApoE, apolipoprotein E; APP, amyloid precursor protein.

form of the protein, appears to play a significant role in the course of the disease. The role of the PS proteins and *apoE-ε4* is less clear. The PSs are thought to play a role in controlling the maturation of β-APP: Mutations in either of these genes lead to an increased production of $A\beta_{42}$ in vitro. The *ε4* allele of apoE may act in a similar manner, promoting the precipitation of Aβ into the insoluble plaques.

BIPOLAR DISORDER

The search for the genetic basis of bipolar disorder has been less successful than that for Alzheimer's disease. Fraught with missteps and partial answers, the history of genetic mapping attempts for bipolar disorder illustrates not only the extreme complexity of the psychiatric disorders, but also the evolution of genetic approaches to such diseases. Bipolar disorder is an episodic illness characterized by recurrent periods of mania and depression. Psychotic symptoms are often a part of the clinical picture, particularly in more severely affected individuals. Although there is still disagreement, bipolar disorder is considered by many to be part of a spectrum of affective illnesses ranging from unipolar depression through bipolar disorder types I and II to schizoaffective disorder, manic type.

Genetic epidemiology studies strongly support a genetic contribution to bipolar disorder, although the mode of transmission has not been determined. Concordance rates for bipolar disorder range between 65 and 100 percent in monozygotic twins and between 10 and 30 percent for dizygotic twins, indicating that the disorder is highly heritable. Some, but not all, segregation analyses have provided support for a locus of major effect for bipolar disorder and have suggested a variety of inheritance patterns, including autosomal dominant, X-linked, and recessive inheritance. Other studies have suggested that a more realistic model involves several genes acting in a multiplicative way. It is currently believed that bipolar disorder is genetically heterogeneous, with a number of genes playing at least some role in its etiology. In addition, phenomena such as anticipation (where successive generations of affected individuals experience an earlier onset or a more severe form of the disorder because of instability in the genetic mutation) and differential maternal and paternal inheritance have also been hypothesized. Anticipation is seen in several neuropsychiatric disorders, such as Huntington's disease and fragile X syndrome and, in these disorders, is secondary to a trinucleotide repeat sequence that expands in successive generations. The best known example of differential parental inheritance, or imprinting, is that of the Prader-Willi and Angelman's syndromes, which are both due to deletions on chromosome 15 but differ in that, for Prader-Willi syndrome, the defect is inherited on the paternal chromosome, whereas, for Angelman's syndrome, it is inherited on the maternal chromosome. At this point, however, there is no compelling evidence that such phenomena play a role in bipolar disorder.

Early Studies Tremendous excitement followed the first reports of linkage to bipolar disorder on chromosomes X and 11 in 1987. In the first study of bipolar disorder, investigators noted that, in several families, bipolar disorder and other affective disorders appeared to be inherited in an X-linked fashion and that these disorders appeared to cosegregate in several Israeli families with color blindness and glucose-6-phosphate dehydrogenase (G6PD) deficiency, which map to the X chromosome. Linkage studies in these pedigrees, using color blindness or G6PD deficiency as marker loci, gave LOD scores between 4 and 9, the first reported significant evidence of linkage for bipolar disorder. Early studies of chromosome 11 were similar to those for the X chromosome in that they used a few markers in a particular genomic area of interest. These studies, which were done in large Old Order Amish pedigrees heavily loaded for bipolar disorder and were based on previous suggestions of linkage to this region, reported initial LOD scores between 4 and 5.

Not surprisingly, these findings generated a great deal of interest. Both studies showed high LOD scores and seemed to provide clear evidence for linkage, the first reported for bipolar disorder. However, replication studies in other populations failed to produce positive results for the X chromosome or for chromosome 11, and extension and reanalysis of the original data also failed to support the findings. With reevaluation of chromosome X in the original Israeli pedigrees using DNA markers, evidence for linkage disappeared in all but one family, and, in this family, the LOD score dropped to 2. The most likely explanation for this is that the initial linkage studies used variations in phenotype (color blindness and G6PD deficiency) as markers rather than DNA polymorphisms. Such markers are less informative, and recombinations are frequently missed. Also, errors in G6PD status of some individuals were identified, and some previously unaffected individuals later developed bipolar disorder. These changes in phenotype also affected the linkage results. Unfortunately, in the one family that continued to have a suggestive LOD score in the reanalysis, the pedigree could not be extended for further study, making confirmation impossible.

For chromosome 11, the most significant change between the original study and the follow-up was a change in affection status. When the original Amish pedigrees were reevaluated, the phenotype of two members changed from unaffected to affected. These two individuals did not share the alleles of interest in the original two markers, and this single change lowered the LOD scores from close to 5 to less than 2. Attempts to extend the study by adding a new branch of the pedigree with affected and unaffected members also provided no significant evidence for linkage. As there was evidence that bipolar illness might segregate separately in this new branch, it was analyzed alone and as a part of the larger kindred. In both instances, linkage of bipolar disorder to the original area on chromosome 11 was excluded.

Candidate Gene Studies To date, a number of candidate genes for bipolar disorder have been examined, primarily involving receptor, transporter, or enzymatic and metabolic genes in the serotonergic, dopaminergic, and adrenergic systems. Candidate gene studies have principally been based on association analyses in case-control or family-based samples. Of the 20 or more genes that have been examined, none have so far provided strong evidence for a role in bipolar disorder susceptibility. The most widely studied has been the serotonin transporter gene (*5HTT*) on chromosome 17q. The promoter region of the *5HTT* gene has an insertion-deletion polymorphism that causes differential gene expression, leading to speculation that it may be a functional (causative) polymorphism for bipolar disorder. Although positive associations have been reported for *5HTT*, numerous negative studies also exist. These mixed results may mean that the *5HTT* gene is a risk factor for some individuals with bipolar disorder and that the variation between studies is due to genetic heterogeneity among affected individuals, but it is more likely that the findings are false positives. Most of the positive associations have occurred in case-control studies, which are subject to high false-positive rates owing to underlying differences in allele frequency between cases and controls for reasons unrelated to disease status. Family-based studies, which control for the problems of differential allele frequencies by using parental chromosomes as controls, have been negative or equivocal for linkage to *5HTT*. The *5HTT* gene has been examined in nearly every neuropsychiatric phenotype known, with similar results.

Brain-derived neurotrophic growth factor (BDNF) is another gene that has excited some interest as a potential candidate gene for bipolar disorder. Initially thought to be a strong candidate gene for schizophrenia, most association studies for that disorder were negative or equivocal. However, two studies examining the relationship between BDNF and bipolar disorder suggest that there may be an association. In the first study, which examined probands with bipolar disorder I, bipolar disorder II, and schizoaffective disorder, manic type, weak evidence for an association between one SNP in BDNF and bipolar disorder was found ($P < .05$) in a study that examined 76 candidate genes for bipolar disorder. Follow-up studies in additional samples did not strengthen this association. In the second study, the evidence for association was stronger, with P values between .04 and .0004 for the two single markers examined and for a particular haplotype of the markers. BDNF is considered to be a good candidate gene for bipolar disorder because of its postulated role in the action of antidepressants. Intracerebral administration of BDNF to animals causes a phenomenon that has been likened to depression, and administration of antidepressants to BDNF knockout mice can reverse some of the behavioral changes observed in these strains. At this point, however, the genetic evidence that BDNF is a susceptibility gene for bipolar disorder is not conclusive.

For other proposed candidate genes for bipolar disorder, positive and negative studies have been reported. Because of the problems in interpreting such contrasting results, several investigators have used metaanalysis as a way to assess the association data for a particular candidate gene. This approach has the advantage of increased power by combining data from a number of small (and presumably underpowered) studies, although problems leading to false-positive results in the original studies may be compounded in a metaanalysis. To date, metaanalyses have been done for several candidate genes for bipolar disorder, and all have been negative or inconclusive.

The lack of success in the early linkage studies and in the candidate gene studies illustrates the importance of considering the entire genome in linkage studies of complex traits. Genome-wide screens have now become the approach of choice for bipolar disorder, given the relative lack of information about pathophysiology and the lack of success with candidate gene approaches. These studies have an important advantage in that they do not require a priori knowledge of the biological underpinnings of bipolar disorder. Complete genome screens provide an opportunity to compare LOD scores (or *P* values) in potential areas of interest to LOD scores in other areas of the genome, thus giving an estimate of the level of background noise and the chances that the results of interest represent a false-positive rather than a true area of linkage or association. For example, a LOD score of 1.5 would be of more interest in a genome screen in which only a few LOD scores are greater than 0.5 than it would in a genome screen in which a large number of LOD scores are greater than 1.

Most of the genome screens done to date support the idea that bipolar disorder is genetically heterogeneous and suggest that many, if not all, of the genes for bipolar disorder confer a modest susceptibility risk rather than being genes of major effect. So far, there are at least three chromosomal areas that show some evidence for linkage in more than one study—chromosome 18, chromosome 4p, and chromosome 21q.

Chromosome 18 Pericentromeric There are several studies suggesting that there is at least one susceptibility gene for bipolar disorder on chromosome 18, although the precise location remains unclear, and there may, in fact, be more than one important region on this chromosome. The first report of linkage came from a partial genome screen that examined 11 markers on chromosome 18 and identified a region of interest near the centromere. This study was a linkage analysis using pedigree data, meaning that model specification was required. Because the inheritance patterns for bipolar disorder are unknown, the results were analyzed using recessive and dominant models. Of the positive LOD scores reported (the highest was 2.38), no clear pattern of inheritance was observed. Some of the markers were positive under a recessive model in some families, some under a dominant model in other families, and some markers gave positive LOD scores in some families under both models. Nonparametric tests, which do not require a mode of inheritance to be specified, provided somewhat stronger evidence for linkage.

These data may represent evidence for a susceptibility locus for bipolar disorder in the pericentromeric region of chromosome 18, indicating a small gene effect present in many families or a major locus responsible for the phenotype in a few particular families. However, as with many studies of complex disorders, the data do not clearly point to a specific mode of inheritance or to linkage to specific markers in the area. Because multiple markers and multiple genetic models were used, a statistical correction is necessary, reducing the statistical significance of the findings. In addition, the LOD scores were highest under a broad diagnostic category, which included bipolar disorder I, bipolar disorder II, schizoaffective disorder, and recurrent unipolar major depression. The LOD scores were lower under a narrow diagnostic category, calling into question the hypothesis that these LOD scores reflect a susceptibility gene specific to bipolar disorder. Additional genotyping in the original sample in the area of interest has continued to support the linkage finding, however.

Attempts to replicate this finding in other populations have been mixed. So far, at least two groups have found no evidence for linkage to the pericentromeric region of chromosome 18 in their samples, although one other group has found evidence to support linkage to this region. Hypothesizing that a parent-of-origin effect might play a role in the genetics of bipolar disorder, they divided their sample into those families in which the disorder appeared to be inherited from the paternal side and those in which it appeared to be inherited from the maternal side, and they analyzed these groups together and separately. Using nonparametric methods, they found evidence for excess allele sharing in the paternal pedigrees for several markers in the pericentromeric area of chromosome 18 (18p11) using a broad diagnostic category, which included bipolar disorder I, bipolar disorder II, and recurrent major depression. Since this finding, two other groups have also reported evidence of a parent-of-origin effect in this area of chromosome 18.

Chromosome 18q and 18p The same group that initially reported support for a parent-of-origin effect near the centromere also analyzed markers all along chromosome 18 in their families, and found excess allele sharing in the area of 18q as well. Although the supporting evidence for linkage on 18p11 described previously was obtained under a broad diagnostic category, the evidence for linkage on 18q was found under a relatively narrow diagnostic category, which included only bipolar disorder I and bipolar disorder II. The results for 18q were also somewhat strengthened when the pedigrees were divided into paternal and maternal samples. Although the original MLS was 1.45 in the overall sample, two-point LOD scores in the area of 18q were between 2.6 and 3.5 in the paternal-inheritance pedigrees, the MMLS in this area was 3.11, and there was evidence of excess allele sharing for several markers in the area. When this group attempted to replicate their findings in a new sample of bipolar disorder pedigrees using the same diagnostic criteria as the original study, they found evidence for excess allele sharing among ASPs in two markers in the region of interest on 18q (18q21) but little evidence for linkage on 18p. Support for the parent-of-origin effect was also reduced in this new sample. Analysis of these bipolar disorder families combined with the original study set strengthened the evidence for linkage on 18q, although most of the linkage was shown to come from allele sharing between sibling pairs with bipolar disorder II and not from those with bipolar disorder I.

A complete genome screen in two large Costa Rican pedigrees (Fig. 1.18–4) also gave evidence for linkage on chromosome 18q22-q23, as well as in an area on 18p. Under a narrow diagnostic model that included only bipolar disorder I and schizoaffective disorder, manic type, three consecutive markers on chromosome 18 in the area of 18q22-q23 had LOD scores exceeding 1.6. When this area was further examined, a shared haplotype (composed of several alleles that are relatively rare in the general population of Costa Rica) was found in the majority of affected individuals.

Because of the continued suggestion of one or more susceptibility loci located on chromosome 18, other groups have also examined this area for evidence of linkage. Several of these groups have found some evidence for linkage, although weak, at or near 18q23, as well as near 18q12. Support for linkage at 18p has been more uncertain. In an attempt to consolidate the various results, a metaanalysis of some of the chromosome 18 linkage data was conducted. This study did not include data from all of the chromosome 18 studies but did include approximately 700 families, and attempted to standardize the data for pooling and comparison. This study found evidence of excess allele sharing at the tip of 18p, as well as in the pericentromeric region of 18 when a broad phenotype was used. There was less evidence for excess allele sharing on chromosome18q from this study, although there were some isolated markers that showed evidence of excess sharing under one model or another. Results of the metaanalysis under a narrow phenotypic model were not reported.

The combined evidence of these studies, although somewhat contradictory and confusing, points to at least two different susceptibility loci on chromosome 18, one on 18p and one on 18q. These loci, if they do indeed represent true areas of linkage, are different in intriguing ways. The 18p finding is perhaps the most difficult to explain, as, for most studies, a single marker generates the majority of the positive findings, and each study points to a different marker. In addition, the evidence for a locus in this area appears to be stron-

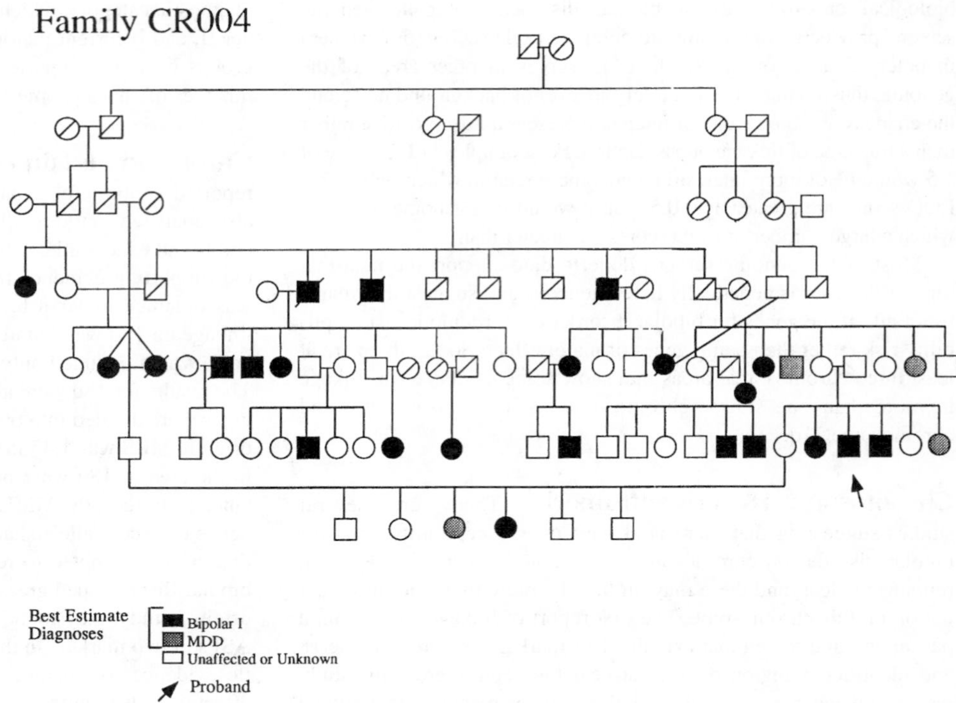

FIGURE 1.18–4 Pedigree of a large Costa Rican family containing multiple members affected with bipolar disorder and major depressive disorder (MDD). (From Freimer NB, Reus VI, Escamilla M, et al: An approach to investigating linkage for bipolar disorder using large Costa Rican pedigrees. *Am J Med Genet.* 1996;67:254, with permission.)

gest in individual families—the evidence actually diminishes when families are combined, and it is strongest under a broad phenotype definition that includes not only bipolar disorder, but also major depression, suggesting that this area may harbor a susceptibility locus for affective disorders in general rather than for bipolar disorder specifically.

In contrast, the 18q finding extends over several markers and is robust to the addition of new families. Although different markers were tested in the different studies, they all lie within the area of the larger haplotype originally noted in the Costa Rican families. Finally, this finding is dependent on a narrow phenotypic definition—the evidence weakens or disappears when the phenotype is expanded to include major depression, suggesting that this putative locus may be more specific for bipolar disorder.

Chromosome 4p Another possible susceptibility locus for bipolar disorder is located on chromosome 4p16. This locus was originally identified in a genome screen of 12 Scottish families with bipolar disorder I, bipolar disorder II, and recurrent major depression. One of the 12 families had an MLS of 4.1 in one marker, as well as positive LOD scores in the flanking markers under an autosomal-dominant model. The peak multipoint LOD score in this region was 4.8. In all cases, the LOD score was highest under the narrow phenotypic model, which included bipolar disorder I and bipolar disorder II only. Haplotype analysis identified seven markers that were shared by all of the individuals with bipolar disorder and by the majority of those with recurrent major depression. Extended relative pair analysis also provided evidence for linkage, although this result was not statistically significant. When the other 11 families were added, the MLS dropped to between 2.9 and 3.3. However, there was evidence for locus heterogeneity in these families, with only approximately 30 to 35 percent of the families likely to be linked to this locus. Under the assumption of genetic heterogeneity, the MLS for the combined families increased to 4.1.

At least two other studies have also provided supporting evidence of a potential susceptibility locus at 4p. A LOD score of 2 was found at the original marker of interest in a subsequent study of Danish families, and study of German families showed evidence of allele sharing at the same marker. The group that performed the original study has now reportedly narrowed the area of interest on chromosome 4p to approximately 9 cM using haplotype analysis.

Chromosome 21 The initial report of linkage on chromosome 21 came from a partial genome screen of 47 multigenerational bipolar disorder families. This study initially gave high LOD scores for ten markers on 21q22.3 in one family (MLS of 3.41) under an autosomal-dominant model, as well as significant results in this region using an affected pedigree member (APM) approach. However, as with many of the initial genetic findings in bipolar disorder, attempts to replicate this finding have been inconsistent. Although the LOD score analysis and the APM method in the original study gave evidence for linkage that was significant or at least suggestive, they were found in only one pedigree. Early attempts to strengthen the finding by adding other families to the sample significantly diminished evidence for this finding rather than enhancing it. A recent replication study by the same group in an additional 40 families reported a peak heterogeneity LOD score of 3.35, with 50 percent of the families studied contributing to the linkage results. Other studies examining this region have been equivocal. Although there have been two reports of excess allele sharing among individuals with bipolar disorder, there have also been studies that have found no evidence for linkage to bipolar disorder in this region.

Other Regions of Interest Interest in the X chromosome as a potential region of linkage for bipolar disorder continues, despite the revision of the findings of the early studies. At least two groups have reported linkage to Xq24-27, with one group reporting a LOD score of 3.9 in one bipolar disorder family. However, these reports have not been replicated, and X-linked inheritance does not appear to be a major mode of transmission in the majority of bipolar families.

Linkage to chromosome 22q11-3 (LOD scores of between 2 and 3.5) has also been reported by at least one group. This region may be of particular interest, because it has also been linked to schizophrenia and has been reported to harbor genes that are induced in studies of methamphetamine-treated rats, which have been used as a model of psychosis. Although the linkage findings to bipolar disorder have not been replicated, it is possible that 22q11 may harbor a gene that confers risk for psychosis, rather than being specific for bipolar disorder.

In addition to traditional linkage studies using large pedigrees, LD-based genome screening approaches are also being used to study the genetics of bipolar disorder. A complete genome screen using family trios from the recently founded isolate of the Central Valley of Costa Rica and a particularly narrow diagnostic classification (bipolar disorder I with at least two psychiatric hospitalizations) has recently been reported. Although this study reports several areas of interest, the most interesting localization to emerge so far from these studies is on 8p12-21. As with the region on 22q11, this region has also been identified as a potential area of linkage in schizophrenia and may represent a more general susceptibility locus for psychotic disorders.

The early genetic studies of bipolar disorder in the Amish illustrate many of the inherent difficulties of doing genetic analysis in complex disorders. The Amish appear to be a perfect population for such investigations; they are an isolated population with known genealogies, clean phenotypes with little comorbidity, and large extended families. However, the findings for bipolar disorder in this group have so far been inconsistent or contradictory, or both, and, even in this seemingly ideal population, there has been no strong evidence for linkage that has withstood attempts at confirmation or replication.

The failure to identify unequivocal susceptibility loci for bipolar disorder may reflect uncertainty about the "true" affected phenotype. For example, there is significant symptom overlap between bipolar disorder and other affective and psychotic disorders, and, currently, as the different inclusion criteria in the previous studies imply, there is also disagreement about the degree of relationship between these disorders. One recent study using monozygotic and dizygotic twins with bipolar disorder, schizophrenia, or schizoaffective disorder suggests that there is genetic overlap between these syndromes. This study found that bipolar disorder and schizophrenia had evidence of syndrome-specific and shared genetic components and that all of the genetic contribution for schizoaffective disorder appeared to be shared with the other two syndromes. The difficulty in interpreting the genetic studies points to the importance of carefully following up isolated positive results by examining flanking markers, by adding new families or affected individuals, and by attempting replication of significant or near significant results in an independent sample. Despite the uncertainties and contradictions, however, these studies indicate several promising areas of the genome that warrant further examination. In addition, new approaches to the study of bipolar disorder, such as population-based studies and large-scale sibling-pair analyses, may allow for the implementation of strategies, such as stricter phenotype definition without a concomitant loss of power. These strategies, in turn, may increase the likelihood of finding loci that have a small gene effect or are present in only a small proportion of affected individuals.

SCHIZOPHRENIA

Although no genes predisposing to schizophrenia susceptibility have yet been definitely identified, the genetic study of this neuropsychiatric disorder has been relatively successful, particularly given its phenotypic and etiologic complexity, and there are several strong candidates. The phenotype for schizophrenia is broad, and can be difficult to define. The cardinal symptoms, delusions and hallucinations, are also found in other psychiatric disorders, and a number of secondary symptoms that are normally found primarily in nonpsychotic disorders, such as mood abnormalities and anxiety, are also frequently seen in schizophrenia, complicating the diagnosis. More specific characteristics of schizophrenia, such as negative symptoms (for example, flat or inappropriate affect, social isolation, and poverty of thought) and a progressive downhill course, can be difficult to recognize or to quantify, or both. Although the genetic boundaries of schizophrenia are still debated, it is thought by most investigators to represent the extreme end of a spectrum of psychotic disorders that also includes schizoid, schizotypal, and paranoid personality disorders and schizoaffective disorder.

The genetic contribution to schizophrenia may be weaker than that for bipolar disorder, but epidemiological studies have nevertheless strongly supported a genetic component to its etiology. Relative risk studies indicate that the lifetime expectancy of developing schizophrenia among first-degree relatives of affected individuals is between 5 percent (for the parent of an affected child) and 46 percent (for the child of two affected parents) as compared to the population risk of 1 percent. Concordance rates for schizophrenia are approximately 40 to 50 percent in monozygotic twins and 9 to 10 percent for dizygotic twins. Furthermore, the risk of developing schizophrenia in the children of unaffected individuals with a schizophrenic monozygotic twin is the same as for the children of the affected twin (17 percent). Environment also appears to play a role in the development of schizophrenia, however. This is best demonstrated by the findings that high-risk offspring (children of a biological parent with schizophrenia) are more likely to develop a thought disorder if they are raised by adoptive parents with high levels of communication abnormalities than if they are raised by adoptive parents with low levels of communication abnormalities.

Recent linkage and association studies indicate that it is unlikely that schizophrenia is caused by a single gene of major effect. A more likely model encompasses multiple susceptibility genes, each with a number of different, relatively common, variants. Unfortunately, most current genetic approaches are not powerful enough to identify genes of small effect without enormous sample sizes. Investigators have continued to pursue the identification of susceptibility genes for schizophrenia by using these techniques, however, with some positive results.

Although early linkage studies of schizophrenia pointed to some potentially interesting areas, most notably chromosomes 5 and 22, the most promising evidence of linkage for schizophrenia susceptibility genes has come from complete genome screens. Over ten independent genome screens have been completed so far for schizophrenia. These studies have identified a number of chromosomal regions of interest, and as many as ten regions have been implicated in multiple studies. Of these, 6p, 1q, and 8p have been the most consistently positive, and there is some evidence for linkage on chromosomes 5, 13, and 22 from the genome screen data as well.

Chromosome 6p The short arm of chromosome 6 was the first region to be implicated by a complete genome screen for schizophrenia, and the initial findings have been supported by follow-up replication and extension studies. Positive LOD scores were initially obtained on 6p25-p24, and follow-up studies gave an MLS of 3.51 under the assumption of 50 percent heterogeneity (i.e., only 50 percent of the study families were considered linked to the locus). Sibling-pair analysis provided additional support for linkage in the study families, although the overall results were weaker. As has been the case in many schizophrenia studies, all of the results were strongest for broad diagnostic categories. Although suggestive for linkage in the region of 6p24-22, these studies provided little information about the likely mode of inheritance—for a given diagnostic category, the LOD scores for the codominant, dominant, and recessive models were often similar.

A follow-up study that attempted to replicate the finding of linkage in the 6p area used sibling-pair analysis and a narrow diagnostic phenotype (schizophrenia and schizoaffective disorder only). This study found excess allele sharing in ASPs at one of the original markers and several additional markers in the region, with an MLS of 2.2. Further support for a susceptibility locus on 6p came from a second complete genome screen. Investigators in this study found preliminary evidence of linkage on 6p in five Icelandic pedigrees using a nonparametric method called *weighted-rank pair-wise correlation* (WRPC). Follow-up of this finding in an additional 65 families also pointed to the 6p25-p24 region, and, when the two samples were combined, a slight increase in the probability of linkage in this area was obtained but did not meet stringent criteria for significant linkage. Because of the previous work on chromosome 6 and these positive findings, 6p25-p24 was examined in a third sample using association methods. In this sample, evidence of LD on 6p was obtained. These data were combined with the data from the original Icelandic study and gave significant evidence of association (P = .00004) at one marker. Attempts at replication in a fourth sample were unsuccessful, however, and a separate replication study in a sample of 57 pedigrees gave only mildly positive evidence of linkage (MLS of 1.17). Yet another study that focused on 6p took a slightly different approach. After traditional pedigree and sibling-pair analysis produced no significant evidence for linkage in ten large Canadian families with schizophrenia, this group used a quantitative trait approach to examine the positive symptoms of schizophrenia, including disorganized thinking, hallucinations, and delusions. Using this phenotype they found significant evidence for linkage (nominal P values were .000012 and .0000054, and empirical P values were .034 and .0085 after corrections, respectively) for two markers in the 6p11 to 6p21 region, slightly more centromeric than the area implicated in the other studies, but adjoining it.

Using families that showed evidence of linkage to 6p24-21 from the original genome screen, further studies attempting to narrow the region of interest or to identify candidate genes, or both, have been conducted. Multipoint LOD scores were positive (MMLS was 2.22) in four consecutive markers in two regions, 6p22.3 and 6p24.3. SNPs were then identified in the region with the highest LOD scores, which was found to contain two genes, *jumonji* and *dysbindin*. Positive association was found for a number of SNPs in the *dysbindin* gene, under all phenotypic categories (P values were between .05 and .00004). Several three-marker haplotypes within this region were found to be transmitted to affected individuals more often than expected by chance alone (P values were .09 and .0001). As of 2003, the association between schizophrenia and dysbindin has been replicated in multiple independent samples. However, this association is not between schizophrenia and any specific SNP or haplotype but rather varies with the study. In addition, none of the SNPs appears to cause functional mutations within the *dysbindin* gene, nor do they affect transcription, making the significance of this finding unclear.

Chromosome 1q

The first evidence of a schizophrenia susceptibility locus on chromosome 1 came from significant linkage findings (MLS of 6) between schizophrenia and a variety of other neuropsychiatric disorders (including affective disorders and conduct disorder) and a balanced translocation between 1q42 and chromosome 11q14 in a large Scottish pedigree in the early 1990s. Although the high LOD score and the strong pattern of cosegregation between the translocation and mental illness suggest that genes in this region of chromosome 1 are in some way related to the development of neuropsychiatric symptoms, follow-ups of these findings in other samples have been negative, suggesting that this finding may not represent a general locus for schizophrenia but rather may be specific to the original Scottish family. Recent cloning efforts have identified two novel genes on chromosome 1 that are interrupted by the breakpoints of the translocation; these have been named disrupted in schizophrenia 1 (DISC1) and DISC2 and are currently under investigation as potential candidate genes for schizophrenia and other neuropsychiatric disorders.

The next indication of linkage to schizophrenia on chromosome 1q came from a complete genome screen in 22 Canadian families. This study was unique in two important ways: The families were all of primarily Celtic origin, minimizing the likely genetic heterogeneity, and only four genetic models were tested (autosomal-dominant and -recessive inheritance using a narrow and a broad phenotype) to minimize the problems of multiple testing. The two-point MLS for this study (5.79) was seen on chromosome 1q21-q22 under a narrow phenotype and recessive inheritance model. LOD scores were greater than or equal to 2 for five adjacent markers covering a 39 cM region. Multipoint analysis of these markers yielded an MLS of 6.5, with 75 percent of families estimated to be linked to this locus.

This study was the first complete genome screen to show evidence of linkage for schizophrenia that met the criteria for highly significant linkage (P <.00002). Two subsequent replication studies using the same genetic models and phenotype definitions failed to find evidence of linkage in 21 large French Canadian families and in 779 smaller schizophrenia families with 984 ASPs. In a separate complete genome screen in 13 densely affected British and Icelandic families with schizophrenia, however, a peak heterogeneity LOD score of 2.9 was obtained at 1q22-q23 using a narrow phenotype. Follow-up studies using a multipoint analysis with the same genetic markers gave a peak heterogeneity LOD score of 3.2 and a peak homogeneity LOD score of 2.8 at 1q32.

A second region on chromosome 1q, 1q32-q42, has also been identified as a possible linkage region of schizophrenia, this time in a number of schizophrenia families collected from Finland. This region was initially identified in a three-stage genome screen that used linkage and association studies to take advantage of the unique features of the genetically isolated Finnish population. Stage I consisted of a complete genome screen using schizophrenia cases and controls from a population subisolate in northern Finland, as well as a linkage analysis using nine individuals from two large pedigrees from this region. In stages II and III, positive markers from stage I were further examined with additional families and additional markers and analyzed using ASP and linkage approaches. The most significant linkage results were found at 1q32-q41. Three markers in this region gave LOD scores greater than 3 (MLS = 3.82), and a common haplotype spanning 6.6 cM was seen in most affected members (and some unaffected members) of 3 of the 20 families, including the largest pedigree.

At least three follow-up studies or independent genome screens have provided additional support for a schizophrenia susceptibility locus at 1q32-42. A second genome screen, this time in ASP families from the general Finnish population rather than the subisolate, identified a positive region approximately 15 cM distal to the original linkage area (LOD score 2.62 under a broad phenotype). Fine mapping of 1q32-42 was subsequently conducted in families from the subisolate and from the general Finnish population, including the families from the original genome screen. Two linkage peaks within the broader region of interest on 1q were identified. The first was found in the combined sample (MLS = 2.71) and spanned approximately 8 cM. The second linkage peak was 21 cM centromeric and appeared to be specific to the subisolate families and, in particular, to the large schizophrenia pedigree that provided most of the evidence for linkage in the original genome screen (MLS = 2.30).

As several investigators have suggested, the disparate findings on chromosome 1q are somewhat confusing. The linkage peaks that span 1q from 1q21 to 1q42 could represent multiple lines of evidence for one schizophrenia susceptibility locus on 1q, muddied by genetic heterogeneity and stochastic variation in linkage findings, or two (or more) separate linkage findings, each specific to a different study sample. The LOD score from the Canadian study was high and, because it was seen in a complete genome screen, was fairly convincing. It is complicated, however, by the fact that all of the individuals in the original pedigrees who were not phenotyped as having schizophrenia were considered to be unaffected rather than unknown. As was seen with the early studies of the genetics of bipolar disorder, diagnostic misspecifications or changes (i.e., from unaffected to affected) in just a few individuals can have an important effect on linkage results, leading to false positives with high LOD scores at times. Replication studies of chromosome 1q have been inconsistent, and a specific location has been hard to identify, although, in general, the data have provided support for one or more schizophrenia susceptibility loci somewhere in this region.

Chromosome 8p Interest in 8p22-21 began after a complete genome screen for schizophrenia gave a LOD score of 2.35, and a follow-up of this region using the same families but different genetic markers resulted in a LOD score of 3.64. Three additional studies, including two complete genome screens, also found LOD scores between 2.0 and 3.5. In one of the most carefully controlled studies, a LOD score of 3.49 was found in 22 Canadian families of Celtic origin, using a narrow phenotype. Follow-up studies on the region of interest on 8p were done in more than 500 schizophrenia pedigrees from different research groups (including those used in the original study) to confirm the finding and to narrow the region. Heterogeneity LOD scores of 2.22 and 3.06 were obtained in the new sample (without the original families) and in the combined sample, respectively. Because of the multiple lines of evidence supporting a susceptibility locus on 8p, additional follow-up studies using 13 British and Icelandic pedigrees were conducted. These studies gave MLSs of 3.5 and 3.6 for two markers on 8p using a narrow phenotype and a recessive mode of inheritance. Multipoint linkage analyses, which incorporate genetic information available from surrounding markers, gave peak LOD scores of 2.8 and 3.2.

Although there was no evidence of linkage to 8p in any of the Finnish schizophrenia genome screens, this region was positive in a genome screen in another genetically isolated population, that of Iceland. In this study, 950 markers were genotyped in 476 individuals with schizophrenia from a number of extended pedigrees. Linkage and association studies were done, with an initial MMLS of 3.06 in a region approximately 10 to 15 cM centromeric to the previously reported region of 8p21-p22. The addition of several markers in this new region caused the two-point MLS to decrease to 2.53, with a multipoint LOD score of 3.48. Further increasing the density of the markers on 8p led to the identification of two shared haplotypes, however, each of which appeared in multiple families. Examination of the region of overlap between the haplotypes narrowed the region of interest to approximately 600 kb. An exon from a gene called *neuregulin 1* (*NRG1*) and an expressed tag sequence, or presumed gene of unknown function, were found to be located within the haplotype region. *NRG1* is expressed at synapses in the central nervous system (CNS), and plays a role in the expression and activation of neurotransmitter receptors, including glutamate receptors. Defects in glutamatergic neurotransmission have been postulated to play a role in the development of schizophrenia because of the effects of known glutamate antagonists, such as phencyclidine (PCP), which induces psychosis in normal individuals and can exacerbate symptoms of schizophrenia through actions at the *N*-methyl-D-aspartate (NMDA) receptor. Mutant mice that are heterozygous for *NRG1* have a behavioral phenotype that has been postulated to overlap with mouse models for schizophrenia, including hyperactivity (which is traditionally used in animal models to evaluate the impact of antipsychotics on dopaminergic tone) and impaired prepulse inhibition (PPI) to an acoustic startle paradigm. PPI is a measure of sensory gating that is defined as an inhibition of the startle response when a low-intensity stimulus (a prepulse) precedes an acoustic startle stimulus. Abnormalities in PPI have been consistently found to be increased in individuals with schizophrenia when compared to controls.

To determine whether *NRG1* was indeed associated with schizophrenia in the Icelandic sample, 58 SNPs located in the exons and the promoter region of this gene were genotyped in all affected individuals, and an additional 123 SNPs were genotyped in a subset of patients and controls. Association studies and haplotype analyses were performed. No single marker within *NRG1* showed significant evidence of association to schizophrenia (the lowest *P* value was .003). However, a core haplotype that consisted of five SNPs and SSLPs was identified that did show evidence of association to schizophrenia (*P* values were between .0000067 and .000087). The association between this core haplotype and schizophrenia was subsequently replicated in two additional independent samples, with odds ratios of approximately 1.5. The high-risk haplotype, which has no mutations thought to be causative for schizophrenia, has an estimated frequency of 7.5 percent in the general population and an estimated frequency of 15.4 percent in individuals with schizophrenia. If it is in fact associated with an increased risk for schizophrenia, it would account for only a 9 percent increase in risk for siblings of an affected individual, however, and therefore, although potentially important, does not fully explain the linkage results on 8p.

Because of the difficulty in proving causation of a particular candidate gene in complex disorders using standard genetic techniques, the Icelandic investigators used animal models to support their hypothesis that *NRG1* was associated with schizophrenia. They tested the effects of clozapine (Clozaril), an atypical antipsychotic drug that facilitates glutamatergic transmission, on heterozygous *NRG1* mutant mice and in wild-type mice (homozygous *NRG1* mutations are lethal). They found that clozapine had no effect on the spontaneous activity level of the wild-type mice, but that it reversed the hyperactivity seen in the *NRG1* mice. The PPI abnormalities were not reversed by administration of clozapine, however. Binding studies of the forebrains of *NRG1* mutant mice and wild-type mice revealed that the *NRG1* mutants had 16 percent fewer functional NMDA receptors than did the wild-type mice, suggesting that *NRG1* may be involved in expression of NMDA receptors.

The Icelandic study did not definitively show that defects in *NRG1* cause schizophrenia. Despite this, it is an important study, because it provides several compelling lines of evidence for an association and, ultimately, for a causative role between *NRG1* and schizophrenia. The use of a combination of approaches, including linkage and association studies in humans and knock-out studies in mice, is likely to become more standard in studies of complex disorders, as it becomes clearer that disease variants in many neuropsychiatric disorders are unlikely to be traditional mutations causing coding changes in exons and are more likely to be difficult-to-identify mutations in intronic sequences or promoter regions leading to variations in splicing or gene expression.

Chromosome 5 Early studies of chromosome 5 were based on a report of a chromosomal translocation in an uncle–nephew pair with schizophrenia-like symptoms, which prompted several linkage studies in the area of 5q11-q13. Although the first linkage studies reported high LOD scores (4.33 to 6.49) using an extremely broad definition of affected status that included essentially all psychiatric disorders, subsequent linkage and association studies of 5q11-q13 have been negative. To date, there has been no follow-up to this finding in the form of extension or fine mapping studies in the original population, making interpretation of the original finding difficult.

In addition to the early studies of schizophrenia that reported linkage to 5q11-q13, linkage to chromosome 5 has also been reported for 5q22-31. Linkage to 5q22-31 was initially identified in a study of Irish families with two-point heterogeneity LOD scores of 3.04 and 3.35 for two markers. Follow-up studies found that four of eight additional independent schizophrenia samples gave LOD scores of greater than 1 in this region, although none were statistically significant. Although this region has not been as well studied as others, further support for 5q22-q31 has been seen in a large schizophrenia kindred from Palau (another genetic isolate) with a LOD score of 3.4, in the Finnish genome screens discussed previously (LOD scores >3), and in a set of German families (LOD score of 1.8).

Chromosome 22q11 Interest in chromosome 22 initially came from the results of a partial genome screen in a subset of families with multiple cases of schizophrenia or schizoaffective disorder. Although the LOD scores were fairly low (three contiguous markers gave LOD scores between 0.94 and 1.54), they were located on 22q13, near the velocardiofacial syndrome (VCFS) region. VCFS is a disorder caused by microdeletions in 22q11 in which as many as 30 percent of affected individuals meet diagnostic criteria for schizophrenia or have schizophrenia-like symptoms beginning in adolescence or early adulthood. Microdeletions in 22q11 are 80 times more common in individuals with schizophrenia than in the general population and 240 times more common in those with childhood-onset schizophrenia.

Because of the increased incidence of microdeletions in individuals with schizophrenia, interest in 22q11 has continued. Several candidate genes have been identified in the VCFS region of 22q11. Two of these have shown some evidence of association to schizophrenia, *COMT* and *PRODH2*. *COMT* has been considered to be a good candidate for many neuropsychiatric disorders because of its role in dopaminergic and noradrenergic neurotransmission and has been extensively studied in schizophrenia. Initial association studies using a polymorphism that causes a valine-to-threonine substitution and a decrease in available enzyme were negative. However, a recent association study using additional SNPs in the gene is more promising. This study used 12 SNPs within and around *COMT* and found significant evidence for association with three. Sex-specific differences in allele frequency were noticed in the control population, so all studies were done in men and women separately. Associations were significant for each polymorphism separately and for a haplotype consisting of all three SNPs (*P* values were between .001 and .0000091), and the odds ratio or effect size for this haplotype was calculated at approximately 1.6. Follow-up studies examining the association between *COMT* and schizophrenia have been inconsistent, and the positive studies have shown relatively weak associations.

PRODH2 encodes proline dehydrogenase, a mitochondrial enzyme that is involved in transfer of redox potential across the mitochondrial membrane. It was identified as a candidate gene for schizophrenia through screening of the 22q11 region. Initial analysis of 18 SNPs in 107 schizophrenia family trios gave nominally significant evidence for linkage in one marker in *PRODH2*. Eight SNPs in and around *PRODH2* were then tested in an independent sample of schizophrenia patients. Evidence for LD ($P < .01$) was found for the majority of SNPs in this gene, and one haplotype (of a total of 17 detected in the sample) showed statistical evidence of preferential transmission to schizophrenia subjects in the sample ($P = .003$). Because of the overrepresentation of the 22q11 microdeletion in childhood-onset schizophrenia patients, the association study using the *PRODH2* SNPs was repeated in a sample of nuclear trios with childhood-onset schizophrenia. In these families, the same pattern of preferential transmission was seen (*P* values were between .06 and .001). In individuals in the sample who had early-onset of deviant behaviors predisposing to schizophrenia, the presence of the risk haplotype was associated with an approximate relative risk of 4.6, 2.4 times larger than the relative risk calculated for the entire sample.

PRODH2 has a nearby duplicate gene, *PRODH2-P*, which has accumulated a number of point mutations, as well as some deletions and insertions (one large deletion removes exons 2 through 5 and part of exon 6). This duplicated gene is not transcribed and thus is considered a pseudogene. Several of the affected individuals in the study sample were noted to have one copy of a single pseudogene-like single base-pair substitution or of a cluster of such substitutions in *PRODH2*. Seven distinct haplotypes were identified that carried these substitutions, and several of the heterozygous carriers of these haplotypes had plasma proline levels at the high end of the normal range, suggesting that the mutations may affect the function of the PRODH2 enzyme, although this has not been conclusively demonstrated.

Confirmation of the association findings was then sought in a third sample of schizophrenia cases and controls from the genetically isolated Afrikaner population. This sample showed a trend for overtransmission of the risk haplotype found in the other samples, although the association was not statistically significant. When a subset of the affected individuals with early-onset symptoms was examined, the frequency of the risk haplotype increased from 15 percent in the complete sample of schizophrenia cases to 20 percent, compared to a frequency of 9 percent in the controls. Of the three pseudogene-like variants that appeared to be enriched in the original samples, two were also enriched among the Afrikaner cases, especially among those with an early onset of symptoms.

As with *NRG1*, there is some evidence for association between *PRODH2* and schizophrenia, although it is not conclusive. The association studies are consistent across several independent study samples, and the convergence of mutations in the pseudogene and in *PRODH2* itself strengthens the finding. As with *NRG1*, additional, although indirect, support for a role of *PRODH2* in schizophrenia comes from animal studies, as mice that are homozygous for *PRODH2* deficiency exhibit the type of PPI abnormalities seen in individuals with schizophrenia.

Chromosome 13q Two complete genome screens have suggested that yet another susceptibility locus for schizophrenia may reside on chromosome 13q32-34. The first study, in 1998, provided significant evidence for linkage in this region in 56 multiplex pedigrees with at least two affected members. The second genome screen, conducted on the cohort of Canadian families of Celtic origin discussed earlier, gave an MLS of 3.81 in this region. Subsequent studies identified haplotypes within a 5-mb region on 13q that were strongly associated with schizophrenia ($P = 3 \times 10^{-6}$). Two overlapping genes, designated *G30* and *G72*, were identified, one of which, *G72*, was found to interact with D-amino acid oxidase, which itself is associated with schizophrenia. However, these findings, although interesting, are very preliminary and have yet to be replicated in follow-up samples.

The genetic studies of schizophrenia have progressed enormously in the past several years. Multiple genome screens have given consistent evidence for several chromosomal regions that are likely to harbor schizophrenia susceptibility loci. Although no definitive schizophrenia susceptibility genes have yet been identified, there are several reasonable candidates. The studies of *NRG1* and *PRODH2* are particularly interesting, not only because they are good candidates for schizophrenia, but also because they represent the beginnings of a paradigm shift toward the application of adjunctive strategies for strengthening the evidence for association, such as evaluation of animal models, cytogenetic abnormalities, and the complete genomic sequence surrounding particular candidate genes. For schizophrenia, as with Alzheimer's disease and many other neuropsychiatric disorders, any individual loci that are identified are likely to account for only a small proportion of cases. In addition, the variability of the genetic findings in schizophrenia using different phenotype definitions and the association of these findings with associated abnormalities in physiological traits, such as PPI, suggest that, when the genetic underpinnings are finally elucidated, they will change the current understanding of schizophrenia. The categorical definitions that are currently in use may be supplanted or supplemented by definitions of disease based on other, more continuous phenotypes, such as are seen in measures of blood pressure or intelligence.

TOURETTE'S SYNDROME

Tourette's syndrome is a neuropsychiatric disorder characterized by chronic intermittent motor and vocal tics with onset in childhood. The genetic epidemiology of Tourette's syndrome was thought for many years to be fairly straightforward, with clear Mendelian inheritance patterns. Early segregation analyses supported the idea that Tourette's syndrome was inherited in a Mendelian pattern and indicated that the most likely mode of inheritance was autosomal dominant with incomplete penetrance (with a lower penetrance for women than for men) and variable phenotypic expression (including chronic motor tic syndrome and obsessive-compulsive disorder [OCD]). However, linkage analyses using this model have consistently failed to uncover any areas suggestive of linkage, prompting the data from these studies to be reanalyzed and the underlying assumptions to be more closely examined.

In the first such study, a single large pedigree that appeared to follow the autosomal-dominant model was reanalyzed under an assumption of assortative mating when it was noticed that a higher-than-expected number of married-in spouses were also affected (36 percent). Reanalysis indicated that the correlation due to assortative mating was significant and suggested an additive model of inheritance in which heterozygotes (who carry one copy of the disease allele) had a lower risk of developing Tourette's syndrome than homozygotes (who carry two copies of the disease allele). Bilineal transmission of Tourette's syndrome has since been noted in approximately 25 percent of families. Other groups have since provided support for an additive rather than dominant or recessive model of inheritance, as well as evidence for the presence of a strong multifactorial background. Extrapolating from the results of one study, investigators hypothesized that, under an additive model, all individuals homozygous for a Tourette's syndrome allele would be affected, but only 2.2 percent of men and 0.3 percent of women heterozygous for a Tourette's syndrome allele would be likely to be affected. Other segregation analyses of Tourette's syndrome have been less clear, and the only current consensus is that Tourette's syndrome susceptibility is probably genetic in etiology but that it is unlikely to follow Mendelian patterns of inheritance.

At the same time as some investigators were reevaluating the assumptions underlying the presumed genetic models of Tourette's syndrome, others were reevaluating the assumptions underlying the presumed phenotype. Because of the strong phenotypic similarities between Tourette's syndrome and other tic disorders, such as chronic motor tic syndrome, and because chronic motor tic syndrome and OCD cosegregate in Tourette's syndrome families, many investigators have suggested that these disorders represent alternate phenotypes of a common Tourette's syndrome susceptibility gene. Twin studies of Tourette's syndrome have supported this hypothesis: The monozygotic concordance rate for Tourette's syndrome and chronic motor tic syndrome together is 77 percent, and the dizygotic concordance rate is 23 percent, whereas the concordance rates for Tourette's syndrome alone are 53 and 8 percent, respectively.

Early Studies

As with bipolar disorder and schizophrenia, early studies of Tourette's syndrome were based on observed cytogenetic abnormalities in a few individuals with tic symptoms. Linkage studies based on these findings initially focused on chromosomes 3, 8, 9, and 18 and have been persistently negative. In addition, despite evidence of sufficient power based on segregation analyses, complete genome screening efforts using large pedigrees also initially failed to find evidence of linkage. Candidate gene studies examining the dopamine receptors (D_1 through D_5), the dopamine transporter protein, prodynorphin, proopiomelanocortin, gastrin-releasing peptide, tyrosine hydroxylase, dopamine β-hydroxylase, and *COMT* have also been negative. Because of the lack of success with linkage and candidate gene studies, despite evidence of a strong genetic contribution to Tourette's syndrome and, ostensibly, sufficient power in several large Tourette's syndrome pedigrees, investigators have had to reexamine their assumptions about the presumed genetic homogeneity of this disorder. More recent studies have turned to approaches, such as sibling-pair analysis and association studies, in genetically isolated populations.

Affected Sibling-Pair Analysis

ASP analysis has become one of the most popular approaches for investigating the genetics of complex traits, in part because this approach is robust to genetic heterogeneity and because it does not require specification of a genetic model. A complete genome screen in 110 sibling pairs (91 independent sibling pairs) with narrowly defined Tourette's syndrome was completed in 1999 by an international consortium of scientists and clinicians. Two areas, one on chromosome 4q and one on chromosome 8p, gave evidence that was suggestive for linkage. The peak MLS score on chromosome 4 was 2.3, with scores greater than or equal to 2 for a region spanning 12 cM. Peak MLS scores of 2 were also found in two adjacent regions on chromosome 8. These regions also showed increased evidence of identical by descent sharing by affected siblings. Follow-up of these regions and confirmation by a second genome screen in a new sample of ASP are under way.

Isolated Populations

In the first study of Tourette's syndrome to use a genetically isolated population, a group from South Africa reported positive associations for Tourette's syndrome on three chromosomal regions—chromosomes 2p, 8q, and 11q. The first stage of this study used two independent sets of cases and a single group of controls from the genetically isolated Afrikaner population to look for evidence of association (as measured by differences in allele frequencies between cases and controls) in a genome screen of more than 1,100 markers. Four markers showed evidence of association in both sets of cases. In a follow-up study, linkage analyses were done for the five strongest regions of interest from either of the two case-control studies or from the combined sample. Two methods of analysis were used, the transmission/disequilibrium test (TDT) and the haplotype relative risk (HRR) analysis. Both of these analyses compare the number of times a particular allele is transmitted from a parent to an affected offspring to the number of times it is not transmitted. Three markers on chromosomes 2, 8, and 11 showed nominal evidence for association ($P = .05$) with one method of analysis but not with the other. The strongest finding was on chromosome 2, with P values of .007 and .025, using versions of the TDT and HRR that incorporate data from adjacent markers.

Interpretation of these results is complicated for a number of reasons. Nonstandardized ascertainment and diagnostic procedures were used, calling the phenotype into question, and the sampling design did not guard against population stratification, an important problem in case-control studies. In addition, the authors used DNA pooling to combine DNA from the cases and from the controls. This approach saves time and expense, as it requires genotyping two samples rather than hundreds, but it can cause artifactual results due to differential amplification of alleles in the different groups.

An independent follow-up of the original association results was also conducted in a large family of French-Canadian origin. In this family, which had 20 individuals affected with Tourette's syndrome and another 20 with tic-related disorders, such as chronic motor tic syndrome and OCD, the 24 markers that were suggestive in the original Afrikaner sample were genotyped, plus an additional two markers on chromosome 13. The family in this study was well suited for linkage analysis of Tourette's syndrome for two reasons: It was a large (and thus potentially powerful) family with multiple affected and unaffected members, and it came from the genetically isolated population of Quebec, decreasing the likely genetic heterogeneity. Because of the multiple phenotypes seen among family members, the authors used a graded approach to phenotype definition and examined a narrow phenotype (Tourette's syndrome only), an intermediate phenotype (Tourette's syndrome, chronic motor tic syndrome, chronic single tic disorder, and OCD), and a broad phenotype (including nonspecific tic disorder). Two-point and multipoint linkage analyses were conducted using three inheritance models (autosomal dominant with different degrees of penetrance). The highest multipoint LOD score obtained under these conditions was 3.24 on chromosome 11q23 (two-point MLSs of 2.4 and 1.27) using the narrow phenotype. Chromosome 13 also showed suggestive results, with a two-point LOD score of 3.2. A sensitivity analysis aimed at assessing the impact that individual family branches had on the linkage findings indicated that when two branches of the family were eliminated, the MMLS on chromosome 11 reached 5.94. The significance of this finding is unclear, however, as each of the branches that were eliminated contained a subject who met narrow-definition Tourette's syndrome, as well as unaffected individuals and those with other tic phenotypes. In addition, the most common haplotype seen on chromosome 11 was found in some affected individuals but not in others, suggesting that, if the linkage is a true finding, there is genetic heterogeneity even in this large family from an isolated population.

There are currently no significant linkage or association findings for Tourette's syndrome, but there are several regions that warrant follow-up. The current approach among investigators is to continue to do complete genome screens, in additional sibling-pair samples and in samples from genetically isolated populations, with the idea that the data will begin to converge, helping identify susceptibility loci that have a relatively large effect. Follow-up studies of regions of interest are also being pursued, with traditional linkage studies in large pedigrees and with LD studies in nuclear families from isolated populations, such as the Afrikaners and the Central Valley of Costa Rica. The genetic study of Tourette's syndrome is unique among the neuropsychiatric disorders in that essentially all of the investigators who are involved in the genetic study of Tourette's syndrome internationally have agreed to collaborate, sharing data and samples in an attempt to clearly elucidate the susceptibility loci for this disorder.

AUTISM

Autism is a severe neurodevelopmental disorder that is characterized by three primary features: impaired language and communication, abnormal or impaired social interaction, and restricted, repetitive, and stereotyped patterns of behavior. Understanding of the etiology of autism has proceeded slowly, but there is now strong evidence that autism is at least partly genetic in etiology. The sibling recurrence risk for autism, autism spectrum disorders, or both is between 2 and 6 percent. Given the population prevalence of 1 in 2,000 (0.04 percent), this means that the siblings of autistic individuals are approximately 50 to 100 times more likely to develop autism than a person in the general population. Twin studies also support a genetic component to the etiology of autism and show a consistently higher concordance rate in monozygotic twins (36 to 91 percent) than in dizygotic twins (0 to 23 percent).

Epidemiologic studies strongly suggest that the genetics of autism are likely to be complex, however. For example, although the risk of autism in first-degree relatives is high, there is a substantial fall-off for second- and third-degree relatives of autistic probands, suggesting that multiple interacting genes may be required to produce the syndrome. Segregation analysis of the autism phenotype also indicates that it is a heterogeneous disorder and likely the result of multiple genes of small effect. A latent class analysis performed to study possible modes of transmission suggested that the most likely scenario was an epistatic model with between two and ten interacting loci, and a recent genome screen for autism has estimated that as many as 15 genes may be involved.

Between 10 and 25 percent of autism cases are associated with medical disorders with known genetic causes, most commonly fragile X syndrome or tuberous sclerosis. The genetic underpinnings of each of these disorders are relatively well understood. Fragile X syndrome, which is involved in 3 to 4 percent of autism cases, is caused by an unstable trinucleotide repeat in the *FMR1* gene at Xq27.3. This repeat expands as it is passed to succeeding generations and causes methylation and inhibition of expression of *FMR1*. *FMR1* produces an ribonucleic acid (RNA) binding protein that acts as a chaperone for the transport of RNA from the nucleus to the cytoplasm. Tuberous sclerosis accounts for 2 to 10 percent of autism cases (the rate of tuberous sclerosis is higher among autistic individuals with seizure disorders). Tuberous sclerosis is caused by mutations in one of two genes, *TSC1* on 9q34 and *TSC2* on 16p13. *TSC1* codes for hamartin, whose function is currently unknown. *TSC2* codes for tuberin, which has a role in tumor suppression and vesicular trafficking in cells.

Cytogenetic abnormalities associated with autism have also been reported on almost every chromosome. Between 1 and 6 percent of autistic individuals have been found to have chromosomal abnormalities (excluding fragile X syndrome and tuberous sclerosis). Approximately 2 percent of individuals with autistic features have abnormalities of the sex chromosomes, including Turner's syndrome (Xp22.3) and Rett's syndrome (Xq28). The most common cytogenetic abnormalities in autism are duplications of chromosome 15q11-q13 (as much as 6 percent of autism cases).

Chromosome 15q11-q13 Chromosome 15q11-q13 is one of the most complex regions of the genome. It has a high rate of genomic instability, including frequent duplication and deletion events, and imprinting plays an important role in the expression of genes in this region. The 15q11-q13 region is the critical region for the Angelman's and Prader-Willi syndromes, neurologic disorders that are due to deletions or mutations in this region that occur on maternally and paternally inherited chromosomes, respectively.

Despite the high rate of duplications of 15q11-13 among autistic individuals, genome screens have not shown strong support for linkage or association to this region. Candidate gene studies continue, however, in part because a rate of 6 percent of autistic individuals with duplications in this region is hard to ignore. Association studies with the Angelman's syndrome gene (*UBE3A*), the most obvious candidate in the region, have been consistently negative. The candidate genes that have excited the most interest are the γ-aminobutyric acid (GABA) type A receptor ($GABA_A$) genes, including the α5, β3, and γ3 receptor subunits. GABA is an important inhibitory neurotransmitter in the CNS, and is responsible for controlling excitability in mature brains. Of the three receptor genes located on 15q, the gene coding for the β3 subunit is the most interesting in autism, as it is expressed early in development, and because mice with mutations leading to loss of this gene have seizures and a phenotype that resembles some autistic features. Association studies for markers in this gene have been equivocal, however.

Genome Screens At least nine complete genome screens have been published in the last several years as a part of the search for autism susceptibility genes. Many of the larger studies have been conducted collaboratively, and the majority of studies have used similar approaches, usually a two-stage genome screen in ASP families, facilitating comparisons between them. In a two-stage genome screen, the entire genome is examined at approximately a 10 cM interval in a small number of families (usually approximately 50). The power of a genome screen to detect linkage depends primarily on the number of families studied and on the genetic heterogeneity of the disorder, although, to a lesser extent, the density of the markers also plays a role. Areas of the genome that meet a predetermined significance threshold (e.g., an MLS score of ≥0.5) are then examined more closely, using additional families and additional markers. Areas of potential linkage that have been previously identified by other groups may also be examined. Results of the currently completed genome screens for autism are summarized in Table 1.18–2. These studies point to potential areas of linkage on twenty chromosomes. Although several chromosomal regions have been the focus of further study on the basis of these results, the strongest evidence from the cumulative data points to the presence of at least one susceptibility locus for autism on chromosome 7q.

Chromosome 7q Because several complete genome screens implicated chromosome 7q as a potential area of linkage for autism, a number of groups have further explored this area in an attempt to identify susceptibility genes. Part of the problem with interpreting the previous studies has been that, although 7q has repeatedly been identified in genome screens for autism, the area of linkage is broad, spanning from 7p through 7qter. Additional exploration has taken four paths—further linkage studies using ASP or other multiplex families, association studies using nuclear families or case-control samples, investigation of regions of interest from known chromosomal abnormalities, and investigation of candidate genes.

Although follow-up studies have consistently provided at least moderate evidence for a susceptibility gene (or possibly several) on chromosome 7q, attempts to narrow the region of interest have been relatively unsuccessful. The region of interest (7p to 7q36) on chromosome 7 can be perhaps narrowed somewhat using the cumulative data (e.g., 7p was identified in only one study, making it a less likely region than 7q), but it still spans approximately 70 cM. For complex, multilocus disorders, such as autism, precise localization for relatively weak loci may be difficult, and linkage peaks may be tens of cM away from the true disease locus. In fact, even in the presence of a single disease locus, localization can be imprecise for studies using less than 200 ASP families, as is the case for all of the current genome screens and follow-up studies for autism. In a disorder as genetically complex as autism, approaches such as linkage analyses and association studies may thus be limited to a fairly general localization. Other approaches, such as the examination of chromosomal abnormalities to narrow the region, or the identification of likely candidate genes from animal or other biological models, may provide the necessary next step.

In general, individuals with the cooccurrence of a particular phenotype and a specific chromosomal abnormality can be useful in the understanding of that phenotype. A number of cases of chromosomal inversions, translocations, or other rearrangements associated with autism or speech and language abnormalities, or both, have been reported over the years, and at least six have focused in particular on the area of 7q. Of the cases reported involving 7q, one had a complex rearrangement between chromosomes 1, 7, and 21 (two areas of chromosome 7 were involved, 7pter to 7q11.23 and 7q36.1 to 7qter), three carried an inversion of 7q22-q31.2, one had a balanced pericentric inversion of 7p12.2 -q31.1, one had a balanced translocation between chromosomes 2p23 and 7q31.3, and the last had a translocation between 7q31.3 and 13q21. These cases, when combined with the results of the linkage studies described previously, have provided increased evidence that at least one susceptibility gene for autism lies somewhere along chromosome 7q. Although some of the chromosomal rearrangements point to the area of 7q31, taken in sum, these cases do not narrow the area of interest significantly and, in fact, implicate the entire area of 7q.

Candidate Genes on 7q The linkage area on chromosome 7q is rich in potential candidate genes for autism. At least 12 genes have been examined to date, ranging in location from 7q22 to 7q36; of these, there is some evidence of association to autism for two, *WNT2* and *RELN*.

WNT2 (wingless-type murine mammary tumor virus [MMTV] integration site family member 2) is located on 7q31 and is part of a family consisting of structurally related genes encoding secreted signaling proteins that have been implicated in several developmental processes, including regulation of cell fate and patterning during embryogenesis. Two families have been identified in which nonconservative (potentially functional or causative) coding sequence variants in *WNT2* segregate with autism. LD between an SNP in the 3' untranslated region of *WNT2* and autism is also present in a subgroup of families with severe language abnormalities that accounted for almost all of the evidence for linkage on chromosome 7q in one of the original genome screens. Of note, this gene is 20 cM distal to the

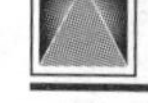

Table 1.18–2
Areas of Potential Linkage for Autism

Chromosome	1	2	3	4	5	6	7	8	9	10	11	13	15	16	17	18	19	20	22	X
IMGSAC				1.55 (B)			2.53 (B)			1.36 (B)				1.51 (B)			1.11[d] (B)		1.39 (B)	
Philippe et al.						2.23[a] (N)							1.10 (N)				1.37[a] (N)			
Barrett et al.		1[b] (N)		1.5[b] (N)			2.2 (N)	1[b] (N)			1.5[b] (N)	3[a] (N)		1[b](N)						
Risch et al.	2.15[a] (N)						1.01 (N)						1.75 (N)		1.21 (N)	1 (N)				
Buxbaum et al.	1.24[c] (B)	2.25[a] (N)			1.46[c] (B)				1.89[a,c] (B)											
Alarcon et al.	2.2[b,e]		2.2[b]				2.98			2.10[e]	2.19[e]					2.3[b]		2.29[e]		
Auranen et al.	2.63 (N)		4.81 (B)				3.04 (B)													2.75 (B)
Liu et al.					2.55 (B)		2.13 (B)	1.66 (B)						1.93 (N)			2.46 (N)			2.67 (N)
Shao et al.			2.02[c] (N)				1.66 (N)										1.21 (N)			2.49 (N)
IMGSAC II		4.8 (N)					3.2 (B)							2.93[a] (B)	2.34[a] (B)					

Note: The first eight studies are complete genome screens, and the last is a follow-up study. The Liu et al. study is a complete genome screen plus a follow-up of chromosome 7. All values are the maximum multipoint logarithm of odds scores reported, with the exceptions noted. All other values in this study are quantitative trait locus analyses using age at first word.
B, broad phenotype; N, narrow phenotype.
[a]More than one area on this chromosome met minimum significance criteria.
[b]Values are approximate.
[c]Single point analysis.
[d]Significant only when a subset of families from the United Kingdom was analyzed separately.
[e]Quantitative trait locus analysis using age at first phrase.

strongest area of linkage, perhaps supporting the idea that linkage studies may not allow for precise localization in complex disorders.

RELN (Reelin) is a signaling protein secreted by Cajal-Retzius cells located in the marginal zone of the developing brain. It plays an important role in neuronal migration, as well as in the development of neural connections. *Reeler* mice, which have spontaneous deletions of *RELN*, have cytoarchitectonic alterations in their brains during development that are similar to those that have been described in autistic brains. The *RELN* gene maps to chromosome 7q22. Only one of two groups that have examined polymorphisms within or near *RELN* has found evidence of an association with autism. Association studies used three polymorphisms in and around *RELN*. These studies suggested that autistic individuals were more likely to have a long allele for the CGG repeat (greater than ten repeats) in one of the polymorphisms than were controls in a family-based design and a case-control design, although there were no differences for the other two polymorphisms tested. In addition, transmission disequilibrium patterns significantly differed between affected and unaffected siblings. The studies suggested that the odds of having autism with the transmission of a long allele were between 2.2 (case-control study) and 3.2 (family study). Preferential transmission was found in all samples examined (odds ratio, 1.6 to 19.2). Haplotype frequencies based on all three polymorphisms also differed significantly in cases and controls. However, the long triplet repeat was found in only 20 percent of patients, suggesting that if *RELN* does contribute to the development of autism, it plays only a small role.

Of the ten other candidate genes on chromosome 7q that have been examined so far, none has shown evidence for association with autism. Two of these genes, *MEST* (mesoderm specific transcript) and *COPG2* (coatomer protein complex, subunit gamma 2), were initially of interest, in part because they are paternally imprinted. Imprinting has been of great interest in the field of autism genetics, because it has been suggested that the linkage to autism on 7q is primarily paternal in origin and because of the strong role of imprinting in the 15q11-q13 region, which has also been implicated in autism.

Although no definitive susceptibility genes have yet been identified for autism, the evidence for such loci on chromosome 7 is compelling. Autism genetics is proceeding at a rapid pace, and multiple approaches, in animals and in humans, are being aggressively pursued. Given the pace at which research in this field is progressing, it would not be surprising if one or more susceptibility loci for autism were identified within the next few years.

FUTURE DIRECTIONS

The field of genetics has developed a great deal in the last several years, and continues to grow at a rapid pace. For many diseases and traits of interest, it is not possible to rely exclusively on traditional linkage studies assuming Mendelian inheritance. New approaches and methodologies that address or circumvent the problems inherent in the study of complex disorders, such as genetic heterogeneity, unknown genetic parameters, uncertain inheritance patterns, and variable phenotypes, have previously led to the identification of genetic defects for complex disorders, such as breast cancer and diabetes. These methods are also successfully being applied to the genetic study of neuropsychiatric disorders, such as Alzheimer's disease, bipolar disorder, schizophrenia, Tourette's syndrome, and autism. Neuropsychiatric disorders have not only provided the impetus but have also served as models for the development and use of new genetic approaches, such as complete genome screens using LD and sibling-pair analyses; in addition, they have emphasized the importance of epidemiological studies, phenotype definition, and careful selection of the study sample. Additional approaches, such as studies in animal models and careful examination of surrounding regions of the genome, are being used to support or refute initial linkage findings. In particular, the genetic studies of Alzheimer's disease have clearly illustrated the value of careful phenotype definition and the use of a variety of methodological approaches, as well as the importance of incorporating all available information into the study. In the next several years, the use of these tools will help elucidate the genetic bases for a number of other neuropsychiatric diseases, including, but not limited to, those discussed here.

SUGGESTED CROSS-REFERENCES

Section 1.10 on genome, transcriptome, and proteome; Section 1.17 on population genetics; and Section 1.19 on transgenic models of behavior provide basic information on the mechanisms of cell division and genetic recombination, as well as the required elements of genetic study in humans and animals.

REFERENCES

Alarcon M, Cantor RM, Liu J, Gilliam TC, Geschwind DH: Evidence for a language quantitative trait locus on chromosome 7q in multiplex autism families. *Am J Hum Genet.* 2002;70:60.

Cardno AG, Rijsdijk FV, Sham PC, Murray RM, McGuffin P: A twin study of genetic relationships between psychotic symptoms. *Am J Psychiatry.* 2002;159:539.

Dracopoli NC, Haines JL, Korf BR, Moir DT, Morton CC, Seidman CE, Seidman JG, Smith DR. *Current Protocols in Human Genetics.* Bethesda, MD: John Wiley and Sons; 1996.

Ertekin-Taner N, Graff-Radford N, Younkin LH, Eckman C, Baker M, Adamson J, Ronald J, Blangero J, Hutton M, Younkin SG: Linkage of plasma A[beta]42 to a quantitative locus on chromosome 10 in late-onset Alzheimer's disease pedigrees. *Science.* 2000;290:2303.

*Folstein SE, Rosen-Sheidley B: Genetics of autism: complex aetiology for a heterogeneous disorder. *Nat Rev Genet.* 2001;2:943.

Freimer NB, Reus VI, Escamilla M, Spesny M, Smith L, Service S, Gallegos A, Meza L, Batki S, Vinogradov S, Leon P, and Sandkuijl L: An approach to investigating linkage for bipolar disorder using large Costa Rican pedigrees. *Am J Med Genet.* 1996;67:254.

Hallmayer J: The epidemiology of the genetic liability for schizophrenia. *Aust N Z J Psychiatry.* 2000;34[Suppl]:S47.

Harnson PJ, Owen MJ: Genes for schizophrenia? Recent findings and their pathophysiological implications. *Lancet.* 2003;361:417.

Holmes C: Genotype and phenotype in Alzheimer's disease. *Br J Psychiatry.* 2002;180:131.

Houlden H, Crook R, Backhovens H, Prihar G, Baker M, Hutton M, Rossor M, Martin JJ, Van Broeckhoven C, Hardy J: ApoE genotype is a risk factor in nonpresenilin early-onset Alzheimer's disease families. *Am J Med Genet.* 1998;81:117.

Houwen RHJ, Baharloo S, Blankenship K, Raeymaekers P, Juyn J, Sandkuijl LA, Freimer NB: Genome screening by searching for shared segments: Mapping a gene for benign recurrent intrahepatic cholestasis. *Nat Genet.* 1994;8:380.

Lamb JA, Moore J, Bailey A, Monaco AP: Autism: Recent molecular genetic advances. *Hum Mol Genet.* 2000;9:861.

Lander E, Kruglyak L: Genetic dissection of complex traits: Guidelines for interpreting and reporting linkage results. *Nat Genet.* 1995;11:241.

Lander E, Shork NJ: Genetic dissection of complex traits. *Science.* 1994;265:2037.

Leckman JF, Sholomskas D, Thompson WD, Belanger A, Weissman MM: Best estimate of lifetime psychiatric diagnosis. *Arch Gen Psychiatry.* 1982;39:879.

Liu H, Heath SC, Sobin C, Roos JL, Galke BL, Blundell ML, Lenane M, Robertson B, Wijsman EM, Rapoport JL, Gogos JA, Karayiorgou M: Genetic variation at the 22q11 PRODH2/DGCR6 locus presents an unusual pattern and increases susceptibility to schizophrenia. *Proc Natl Acad Sci U S A.* 2002;99:3717.

Neves-Pereira M, Mundo E, Muglia P, King N, Macciardi F, Kennedy JL: The brain-derived neurotrophic factor gene confers susceptibility to bipolar disorder: Evidence from a family-based association study. *Am J Hum Genet.* 2002;71:651.

*O'Donovan MC, Williams NM, Owen MJ: Recent advances in the genetics of schizophrenia. *Hum Mol Genet.* 2003;12:125.

Ott J. *Analysis of Human Genetic Linkage.* Revised Edition. Baltimore: The Johns Hopkins University Press; 1992.

*Pauls DL: An update on the genetics of Gilles de la Tourette syndrome. *J Psychosom Res.* 2003;55:7.

Pericak-Vance MA, Grubber J, Bailey LR, Hedges D, West S, Santoro L, Kemmerer B, Hall JL, Saunders AM, Roses AD, Small GW, Scott WK, Conneally PM, Vance JM, Haines JL: Identification of novel genes in late-onset Alzheimer's disease. *Exp Gerontol.* 2000;35:1343.

Potash JB, DePaulo JR Jr: Searching high and low: A review of the genetics of bipolar disorder. *Bipolar Disord.* 2000;2:8.

Risch N: Genetic linkage: Interpreting lod scores. *Science.* 1992;255:803.

Shifman S, Bronstein M, Sternfeld M, Pisante-Shalom A, Lev-Lehman E, Weizman A, Reznik I, Spivak B, Grisaru N, Karp L, Schiffer R, Kotler M, Strous RD, Swartz-

Vanetik M, Knobler HY, Shinar E, Beckmann JS, Yakir B, Risch N, Zak NB, Darvasi A: A highly significant association between a COMT haplotype and schizophrenia. *Am J Hum Genet.* 2002;71:1296.
Simonic I, Nyholt DR, Gericke GS, Gordon D, Matsumoto N, Ledbetter DH, Ott J, Weber JL: Further evidence for linkage of Gilles de la Tourette syndrome (GTS) susceptibility loci on chromosomes 2p11, 8q22 and 11q23-24 in South African Afrikaners. *Am J Med Genet.* 2001;105:163.
*Sklar P: Linkage analysis in psychiatric disorders: the emerging picture. *Annu Rev Genomics Hum Genet.* 2002;3:371.
Stefansson H, Sigurdsson E, Steinthorsdottir V, Bjornsdottir S, Sigmundsson T, Ghosh S, Brynjolfsson J, Gunnarsdottir S, Ivarsson O, Chou TT, Hjaltason O, Birgisdottir B, Jonsson H, Gudnadottir VG, Gudmundsdottir E, Bjornsson A, Ingvarsson B, Ingason A, Sigfusson S, Hardardottir H, Harvey RP, Lai D, Zhou M, Brunner D, Mutel V, Gonzalo A, Lemke G, Sainz J, Johannesson G, Andresson T, Gudbjartsson D, Manolescu A, Frigge ML, Gurney ME, Kong A, Gulcher JR, Petursson H, Stefansson K: Neuregulin 1 and susceptibility to schizophrenia. *Am J Hum Genet.* 2002;71:877.
*Strachan T, Read AP. *Human Molecular Genetics.* 2nd ed. New York: Wiley-Liss; 1999.
Straub RE, Jiang Y, MacLean CJ, Ma Y, Webb BT, Myakishev MV, Harris-Kerr C, Wormley B, Sadek H, Kadambi B, Cesare AJ, Gibberman A, Wang X, O'Neill FA, Walsh D, Kendler KS: Genetic variation in the 6p22.3 gene DTNBP1, the human ortholog of the mouse dysbindin gene, is associated with schizophrenia. *Am J Hum Genet.* 2002;71:337.
Suh YH, Checler F: Amyloid precursor protein, presenilins, and alpha-synuclein: Molecular pathogenesis and pharmacological applications in Alzheimer's disease. *Pharmacol Rev.* 2002;54:469.
Van Broeckhoven CL: Molecular genetics of Alzheimer's disease: Identification of genes and gene mutations. *Eur Neurol.* 1995;35:8.
Wassink TH, Piven J: The molecular genetics of autism. *Curr Psychiatry Rep.* 2000;2:170.

▲ 1.19 Transgenic Models of Behavior

LAURENCE H. TECOTT, M.D., PH.D.

Recent developments in the characterization of mammalian genomes reveal a remarkable degree of similarity in the genetic endowments of humans and mice. Although the human genome project is exerting a profound impact in accelerating the search for genes associated with susceptibility to disease (see Sections 1.17 and 1.18), the recent publication of the mouse genome has been heralded by some as a development of comparable importance for the future of biomedical research. It is likely that the use of mice will contribute substantially to the application of advances in genomics to benefit all fields of medicine. This chapter provides an overview of recent advances in mouse molecular genetics and their promise for elucidating biological processes relevant to mammalian central nervous system (CNS) function and to the pathophysiology and treatment of psychiatric disease.

GENOMES OF HUMANS AND MICE

A major surprise provided by the sequencing of the 3.2 billion nucleotide-long human genome was a downward revision in the estimate of the number of human genes. Whereas, previously, estimates typically ranged between 50,000 and 150,000, the sequence revealed a much more likely estimate of approximately 30,000. This was disconcertingly similar to the number of genes seen in some so-called simpler organisms. For example, the number of genes estimated for the fruit fly *Drosophila* and the nematode *Caenorhabditis elegans* is 13,000 and 20,000, respectively. This has lent support to the view that increases in organismal complexity are not primarily achieved by the addition of genes but by increasing sophistication in the manner in which they are regulated, that is, turned on and off.

As the human genome project progressed, parallel efforts were under way to determine the genomic sequence of the mouse. Priority was given to the mouse over other mammals owing to the development of technologies that made its genome most accessible to experimental manipulation. As expected, the number of genes possessed by the mouse, a fellow mammal, was estimated at approximately 30,000, similar to the human gene number. However, further comparisons between the species revealed that many additional features of their genomes shared a remarkable degree of similarity. For example, approximately 99 percent of mouse genes have readily identifiable human counterparts. Conversely, a mouse version can be identified for 99 percent of human genes. Furthermore, long stretches of mouse and human deoxyribonucleic acid (DNA) are syntenic, that is, they possess chromosomal regions with the same sequence of genes. Approximately 96 percent of mouse genes are found in such syntenic regions. In accord with these similarities, comparative genomic analyses indicate that mammalian lineages giving rise to mice and humans diverged from a common ancestor 75 to 125 million years ago, relatively recently by evolutionary standards.

BRAIN STRUCTURE AND FUNCTION IN HUMANS AND MICE

The high level of similarity between the genomes of humans and mice reflects the extensive similarities that exist across mammalian species in the structures and functions of organ systems, and this includes the CNS. The brains of all vertebrates have a common structural organization, consisting of six primary divisions: the medulla, pons, cerebellum, midbrain, diencephalons, and cerebral hemispheres. Among mammals, the neural structures within these divisions and the circuits that interconnect them are similar to a high level of detail. Moreover, mammalian brains share similar neurochemical features, such as neuromodulatory signaling molecules. For example, the substantia nigra appears in reptilian evolution, and this nucleus has a similar organization among marsupial and placental mammals, including a pars compacta subdivision containing dopaminergic neurons displaying similar patterns of projection to other brain regions.

Of course, substantial differences exist in the structure of human and mouse brains—the most apparent differences relate to the high degree of elaboration of the cerebral hemispheres in humans, a feature proposed to contribute to the enhanced cognitive abilities of this species. In light of these differences and the obvious differences in the behavioral repertoires of humans and mice, what evidence exists that an understanding of mouse brain function may be pertinent to human behavior? Functionally, the brains of mice and humans share a large number of tasks. The primary senses and the brain structures relaying sensory information in humans are also found in mice, albeit the relative levels of development of particular senses vary in accord with the ecological niches inhabited by the two species. The CNS regulation of sympathetic and parasympathetic autonomic function in the two species regulates neuroendocrine responses to stress and the function of peripheral organ systems in a similar manner. Moreover, the CNS coordinates complex behaviors observed in both species, such as feeding, drinking, sleep, circadian rhythms, and sexual function. Such functional similarities frequently generalize to behavioral responses to drugs. For example, sedative, activating, anorectic, addicting, and other behavioral effects of drugs observed in humans are frequently observed in mice. Such species similarities in behavioral pharmacology are recognized by the pharmaceutical

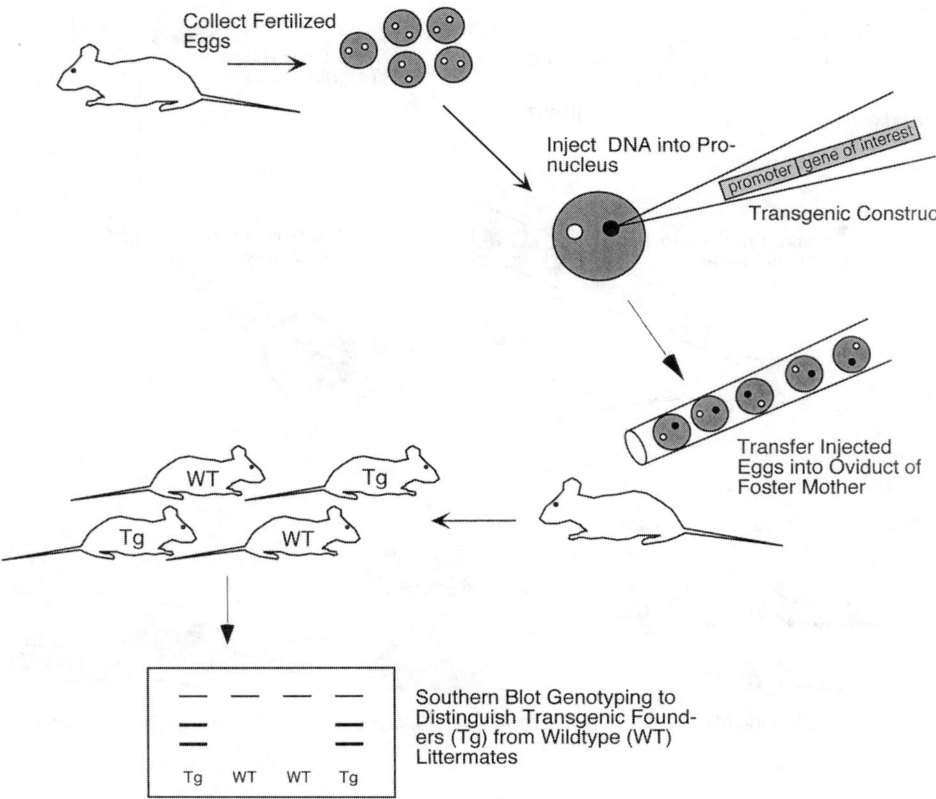

FIGURE 1.19–1 Procedures required for the generation of transgenic mouse lines. DNA, deoxyribonucleic acid.

industry, in which rodent behavioral assays are an important part of the drug development process.

MOUSE MOLECULAR GENETIC APPROACHES

A major factor accounting for the rapid growth in the use of mice is the *genetic tractability* of the species, that is, that it is possible to use gene targeting and transgenic methods to generate mice with planned alterations of any gene or sets of mice in which large numbers of genes are randomly mutated. This enables gene function to be examined in the context of an intact organism in which mammalian behaviors can be modeled, providing unprecedented opportunities to characterize the influence of genes on neural systems implicated in psychiatric illnesses. In addition to *transgenic* and *gene targeting* approaches, *phenotype-based* strategies are also increasingly used. In these approaches, attempts are made to determine the genes responsible for differences in the expression of a particular behavioral trait (behavioral phenotype) of interest. The most commonly used phenotype-based approaches use quantitative trait locus analysis (QTL) and random mutagenesis.

Transgenic Procedures Procedures for introducing exogenous DNA into the mouse genome for the production of *transgenic* animals are in widespread use. Transgenes are typically introduced by microinjection of DNA constructs into the male pronuclei of fertilized mouse eggs (Fig. 1.19–1). DNA constructs commonly consist of a gene of interest linked to promoter sequences that regulate the anatomical distribution and timing of transgene expression. The injected eggs are then surgically placed into the oviducts of foster mothers. To determine whether the transgene has been incorporated into the germ cells of offspring, DNA is isolated from tail tissue and analyzed using Southern blot or polymerase chain reaction (PCR) techniques, or both. Often, the transgene integrates at a single random chromosomal location in multiple copies, permitting high levels of transgene expression. The resulting transgenic mice are heterozygous for transgene insertion and may be used as founders, that is, they are bred to propagate the transgene to the next generation.

Transgenic techniques may be used in a wide variety of experimental strategies. Because transgenic mice often possess multiple copies of the transgene, they have been used to examine the consequences of enhancing the function of a particular gene of interest through its overexpression. It is also possible to engineer *dominant negative* mutations: mutations that induce loss of gene function when expressed in the heterozygous state. In addition, hypotheses regarding mechanisms of gene action can be tested by expressing modified forms of gene products. For example, a line of mice was generated bearing a transgene composed of the Ca^{2+}-calmodulin–dependent protein kinase α subunit (CaMKIIα) promoter driving expression of a mutant form of CaMKIIα. These mice exhibited altered hippocampal physiology, as well as deficits in spatial memory. These studies led to an enhanced understanding of the role of CaMKIIα in synaptic plasticity and cognition.

It is also possible to study the functional roles of particular cell types in the brain by selectively manipulating their gene expression using transgenic methods. This may be achieved by using DNA constructs in which promoter regions directing gene expression to a selected cell type are fused with coding sequences of genes that impact cell function. For example, a transgenic line was developed in which the promoter for the dopamine type 1 (D_1) receptor was used to drive expression of a cholera toxin subunit to stimulate cells that express D_1 dopamine receptors. Chronic overstimulation of forebrain neurons expressing D_1 receptors was found to produce an

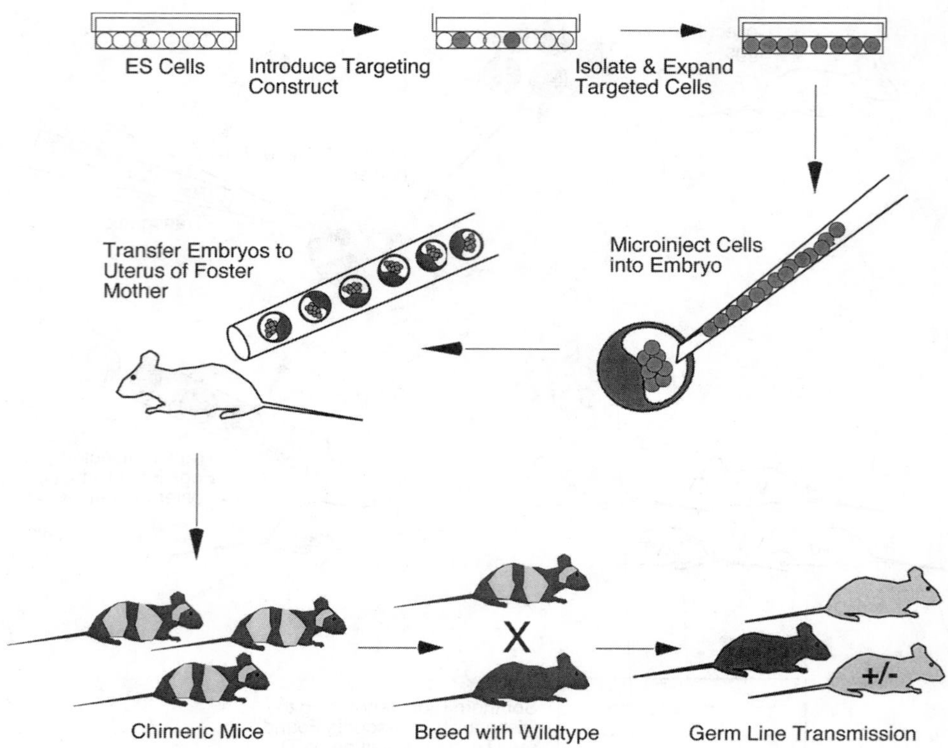

FIGURE 1.19–2 Procedures required for the generation of mouse lines with targeted mutations. ES, embryonic stem.

abnormal behavioral phenotype that was likened to human compulsive behaviors. Conversely, it is also possible to make cell type–selective lesions by using DNA constructs in which promoter sequences are fused with genes encoding toxic proteins, such as diphtheria toxin.

Because transgenes are commonly expressed throughout development, transgenic mouse phenotypes could reflect the adult function of the gene or an indirect consequence of perturbed brain development, or both. To minimize developmental effects, strategies have been developed permitting inducible expression of transgenes in the adult animal. For example, a line of transgenic mice has been developed with inducible expression of ΔFosB, a transcription factor implicated in the stimulant and reward effects of cocaine. The expression system was designed so that chronic treatment with a tetracycline analog (doxycycline [Doryx]) during early development suppressed expression of ΔFosB. Cessation of doxycycline treatment induced ΔFosB expression and increased the behavioral responsiveness of the animals to cocaine, supporting a role for this gene in the reinforcing properties of cocaine.

Gene Targeting Procedures Gene targeting procedures enable the introduction of planned mutations into predetermined sites in the genome. Commonly, mutations are designed to eliminate gene function, resulting in the generation of *knock-out* mice. It is also possible to introduce mutations that alter, but do not eliminate, gene function. The initial step in the generation of gene-targeted mice is the introduction of mutation-bearing DNA sequences (targeting construct) into embryonic stem (ES) cells (Fig. 1.19–2). ES cells are derived from 3- to 4-day-old mouse embryos and are totipotent, that is, they retain the ability to contribute to all tissues of the developing fetus. ES cells are rendered permeable to exogenous DNA by exposing them to an electrical current. The targeting construct typically consists of target gene sequences into which loss-of-function mutations have been engineered. Targeting constructs are designed to achieve homologous recombination, a process through which construct DNA precisely replaces its homologous gene sequence within the mouse genome. Most frequently, the exogenous DNA incorporates in a nontargeted manner at random locations throughout the genome at frequencies greatly exceeding homologous recombination. Therefore, drug selection strategies are used to select those rare cells in which homologous recombination has occurred. After selection, genomic DNA is extracted from ES cell clones and is screened for homologous recombination by PCR or Southern blot analysis.

The homologous recombinant cells are then used to generate mice through microinjection into 3- to 4-day-old mouse embryos. The injected embryos are surgically transferred into the uteri of surrogate mothers, which give birth to *chimeric* mice that are partly derived from the injected ES cells and partly derived from the host embryo. If the coat color of the mouse strain from which the ES cells were derived differs from that of the strain of the injected embryo, then the resulting chimeric mice have a patchy coat color, reflecting contributions from both lineages. Chimeras are mated with wild-type mice, and genomic DNA obtained from the progeny is screened for the presence of the mutation. The resulting heterozygous mice are bred to produce homozygous mutant mice bearing two copies of the mutant gene. Animals bearing mutations that completely eliminate gene function are termed *null mutant* or *knock-out* mice.

Although gene targeting methods are most commonly used to produce animals with null mutations, subtle mutations may also be introduced to alter, but not eliminate, gene function. For example, a single amino acid change was engineered in a gene encoding the α1 subunit of the γ-aminobutyric acid (GABA) type A ($GABA_A$) receptor, rendering $GABA_A$ receptors containing this subunit insensitive to benzodiazepines. Whereas the resulting animals displayed reduced sensitivity to the sedative and amnestic effects of diazepam (Valium), no change in sensitivity to the anxiolytic-like effects of this drug was observed. By

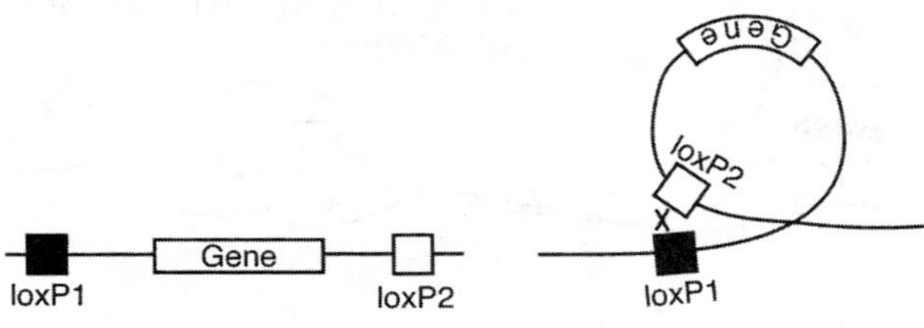

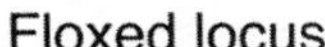

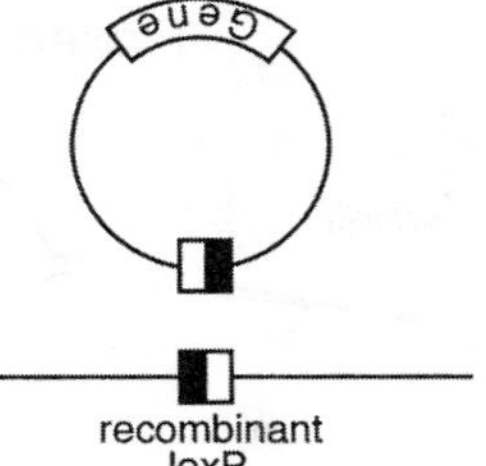

FIGURE 1.19–3 Cyclization of recombination (Cre)–mediated recombination. A gene of interest is flanked by locus of crossing over of P1 (loxP) sites ("floxed"). In the presence of the Cre enzyme, a recombination event results in the excision of the flanked sequences, leaving behind a single loxP site.

contrast, mice bearing a corresponding mutation in the α2 subunit were insensitive to the anxiolytic-like effects of diazepam. These results indicate that the development of benzodiazepine site ligands active at α2 subunit–containing $GABA_A$ receptors, while devoid of activity at receptors containing the α1 subunit, warrants consideration for the production of anxiolytic agents without side effects typically associated with benzodiazepines.

Conditional Gene Targeting

Caveats in the interpretation of phenotypic abnormalities in gene-targeted mouse lines can arise, not only through developmental considerations as described previously, but also because the gene is mutated in every cell in which it is normally expressed in the mouse. Therefore, abnormal phenotypes may arise from the absence of the functioning gene product in a peripheral organ system or in any of its sites of CNS expression. It is possible that the absence of a gene product in the periphery may lead to embryonic lethality, precluding use of the mutant for studies of behavior. For genes that are widely expressed within the CNS, it may be difficult to pinpoint neural circuits through which mutations produce particular aspects of behavioral phenotypes. To address these issues, "conditional" gene targeting approaches have been devised, in which targeted mutations are produced in a restricted subpopulation of cells or induced at predetermined developmental stages.

Recent efforts have focused on mutational strategies developed to exert spatial control over the pattern of expression of mutations introduced into mice. These approaches use somatic cell recombination rather than germ cell (or ES cell) recombination to inactivate a gene in restricted populations of cells or tissues. Commonly, tissue-specific promoter sequences are used to direct expression of a site-specific recombinase to limit gene inactivation to only those cells expressing the recombinase. Most frequently, the cyclization of recombination (Cre)–locus of crossing over of P1 (loxP) system is used for this purpose. Cre recombinase is a protein from bacteriophage P1 that recognizes and excises DNA regions that are flanked by two loxP sites, the recognition sequences for Cre (Fig. 1.19–3).

Typical approaches involve the generation of two independent lines of mice—a line bearing a genetic region of interest flanked by loxP sites ("floxed") and a transgenic line in which Cre expression is driven by a tissue-specific promoter (Fig. 1.19–4). Floxed mice bearing a genetic region of interest flanked by loxP sites are generated by gene targeting. Because the loxP sites are relatively small and are placed in intronic regions, they do not typically interfere with normal gene transcription. A second line of *Cre* mice is most commonly generated by creating a transgenic line in which Cre expression is driven by a tissue-specific promoter. Once a line exhibiting the desired pattern of Cre expression is identified, it is crossed with an appropriate floxed line to commence a breeding strategy resulting in the generation of animals with a restricted pattern of gene inactivation.

Several lines of Cre mice have been reported in which expression is restricted to subpopulations of cells within the CNS. For example, a line of mice was generated in which inactivation of the glutamate receptor subunit *N*-methyl-D-aspartate (NMDA) receptor type 1 (NMDAR1) was restricted to CA1 pyramidal neurons of the hippocampus. NMDAR1 is the predominant NMDAR subunit and is widely expressed in most CNS neurons. It had been previously demonstrated that widespread gene inactivation in NMDAR1 null mutants resulted in perinatal lethality. By contrast, when the mutation was restricted to hippocampal CA1 neurons, animals were viable and exhibited impaired spatial learning and impaired plasticity of CA1 synapses. This was the initial demonstration that spatial restriction of neural mutations can be used to uncover particular brain regions through which gene inactivation alters behavior.

The usefulness of this approach for producing cell type–specific inactivation of genes is enhanced by the fact that lines of floxed and Cre mice produced in one laboratory can be mixed and matched with those from another laboratory. In this way, Cre lines generated for use with a particular floxed gene may also be used with other floxed genes when a similar pattern of gene inactivation is desired. Collaborative efforts to generate databases of Cre and floxed lines will speed the generation of animals with restricted patterns of gene inactivation. Moreover, lines of mice in which Cre recombinase is under the control of an inducible promoter (such as the tetracycline-responsive system described previously) will allow investigators temporal, as well as spatial, control of gene inactivation.

Quantitative Trait Locus Analysis

In human populations, it has been estimated that 40 to 90 percent of phenotypic variations in traits of temperament and susceptibility to psychiatric disease are under the control of genetic factors. Quantitative measures of complex behavioral traits, such as those reflecting affective and cognitive responses, reveal continuous distributions across a population. Graded distributions of phenotypes are consistent with polygenic, rather than single-gene, regulation of traits. Each of the many genes influencing a complex trait may influence a small portion of its distribution across a population, complicating attempts to determine the genetic determinants of complex behavioral traits. To address this challenge, QTL analysis procedures have been developed for the identification of genetic factors accounting for variability in behavioral trait. A *QTL* is a chromosomal region containing genes that contribute a portion of the genetic variation for a particular phenotype.

Typically, mouse QTL experiments are designed to identify genes that underlie variation in a phenotype of interest that differs between two inbred strains of mice. This depends on the availability of mouse strains that are extensively inbred, so that animals within a strain have two identical copies of each gene (i.e., homozygous at all

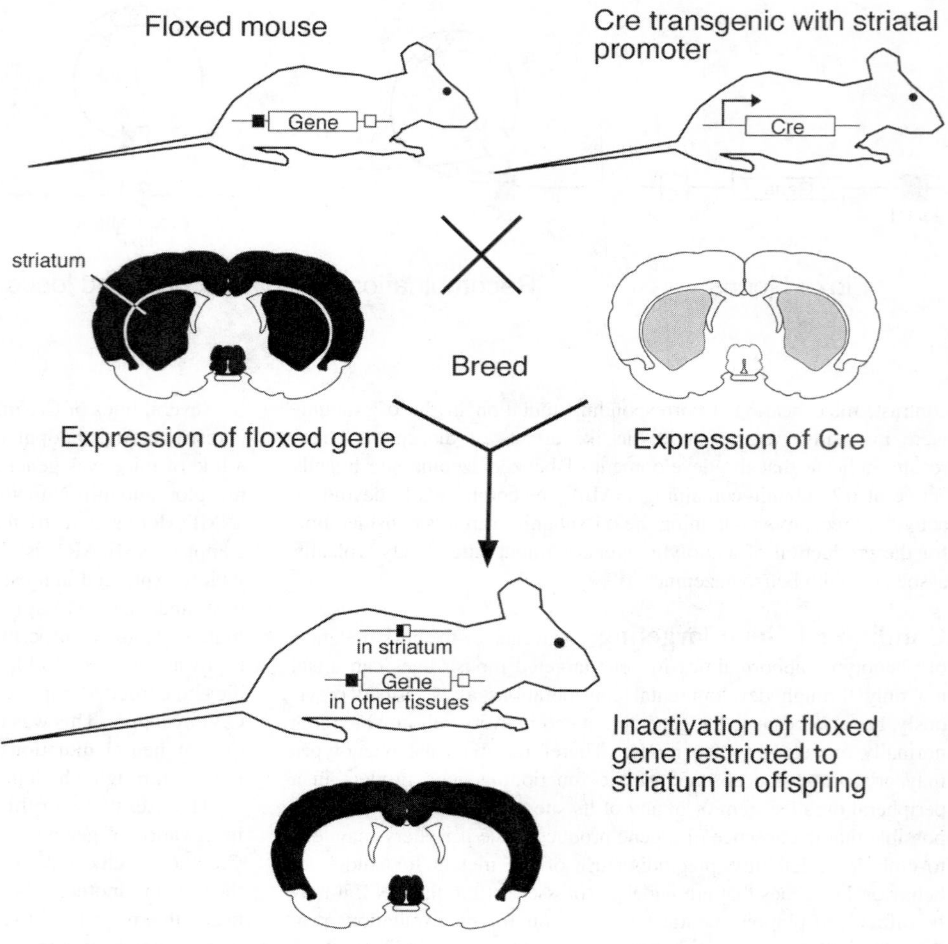

FIGURE 1.19–4 An example of region-specific gene inactivation. A mouse with a floxed gene of interest is bred with an animal bearing a transgene driven by a promoter directing expression to the striatum. In the offspring, cyclization of recombination (Cre)–mediated recombination leads to the selective loss of striatal expression of the gene of interest.

autosomal loci). A mating strategy is pursued in which mice of the two strains are interbred, creating a generation of hybrid mice that is designated F_1 for *first filial generation*. In F_1 mice, all genes that differ between the parental strains occur in a heterozygous state, because the animals received one intact chromosome from each of the two inbred parents. F_1 animals are then crossed, and genetic recombination occurs during gamete formation, resulting in an second filial generation (F_2) with animals possessing varying contributions of genes from the two parental strains.

F_2 mice are then tested in a behavioral assay of phenotype of interest, in which the two parental strains perform differently. A continuous distribution of behavioral scores is usually found, and animals at the extremes of the distribution are selected for further genetic analysis. Correlations are sought between behavioral scores and the inheritance patterns of particular genetic loci that differ between strains. This requires an extensive set of DNA marker sequences throughout the genome that are *polymorphic*, that is, that differ between the parental strains. Commonly, DNA polymorphisms that occur in repeats of DNA known as *microsatellites* are used as markers. These polymorphisms, termed *simple sequence length polymorphisms* (SSLPs), are widely distributed throughout the entire genome and may be readily assayed. QTL analyses are performed using a variety of statistical techniques to test the probability that a variation in the phenotype is associated with a particular mapped polymorphism. The strength of an association of a QTL with a phenotype is reported using logarithm of odds (LOD) scores or standard alpha levels (*P* values). After identification of QTLs that contribute significantly to phenotypic variation, a variety of strategies are used to precisely identify the gene bearing the functional polymorphism. Approaches include analysis of previously unknown genes in the QTL region, sequencing of known candidate genes, and determination of differential gene expression.

QTL analyses allow for the identification genes influencing phenotypic variation without a priori knowledge of the genes themselves. This is particularly advantageous for the study of complex behaviors, because the precise mechanisms through which they are regulated remain unclear. QTL analyses are under way to identify genes contributing to emotionality, learning, seizure sensitivity, sensorimotor gating, and responses to drugs of abuse. Several limitations to the QTL approach exist. For traits that are regulated by a large number of genes with miniscule effect sizes, large, impractical sample sizes may be required. In addition, QTL analysis does not detect all genes that are essential to neurobiological pathways regulating behavior but rather only those that determine variation between the particular parental strains.

Random Mutagenesis Random mutagenesis strategies have been gaining popularity as an alternative approach for identifying novel genetic regulators of complex behavior. Typically, large numbers of animals bearing randomly induced mutations are generated using chemical mutagens. These animals may be screened for mutations that alter complex behaviors of interest. An advantage of the chemical mutagenesis approach is that the entire genome may be screened for genes influencing a particular behavioral process, as opposed to QTL strategies, which are limited to the more restricted set of genes that are polymorphic between two parental strains.

To chemically produce mutations, male mice are treated with *N*-ethyl-*N*-nitrosourea (ENU) to induce single base-pair mutations in the spermatogonia. These mice are then mated with wild-type females, and offspring (first generation, or G1 generation) are screened for phenotypes of interest. Because all mutations in G1 offspring will be in the heterozygous state, phenotypic screening of these mice would detect only dominant mutations. To detect recessive mutations (mutations that only produce phenotypic abnormalities in the homozygous state), additional crosses of G1 mice would be required to generate and behaviorally screen offspring that are homozygous for induced mutations.

In typical screens for dominant mutations, G1 mice are tested in a battery of developmental, physiological, and behavioral assays. Because mutations are random and not restricted to genes regulating the behavior of interest, interpretation of the resulting behavioral data must be performed with care. For example, genetic perturbations producing illness, motor impairment, blindness, poor olfaction, or dysregulated anxiety could alter behavior in an assay intended to assess memory. In such cases, test performance would be altered by primary mutations affecting genes other than those controlling biochemical pathways important for anxiety. Therefore, tests of peripheral organ system function and a global neurological assessment are usually incorporated in the primary mutagenesis screen.

After screening, mice with behavioral scores near the extremes of the population distribution are selected for further breeding. Progeny of mice bearing true positive mutations will be found to transmit the altered behavioral trait between generations. Once identified, these mutations are localized to chromosomal regions using gene mapping methods as in QTL analyses. Ultimately, sequencing of the gene in the normal and mutant states is required to identify the actual mutation.

Alternative methods, such as "gene trapping," have recently been developed to facilitate identification and characterization of randomly induced mutations. ES cells are transfected with DNA vectors that integrate randomly throughout the genome. The gene trap vectors are designed so that, on integration into an intron, a fusion protein is generated between the endogenous ("trapped") gene and a reporter gene, allowing detection of cells in which the endogenous gene is expressed. The insertion of the gene-trapped DNA may disrupt function of the endogenous gene (and thus behavior) in mice generated from these ES cells and may serve as a tag for rapid identification of the trapped gene.

The potential usefulness of the random mutagenesis approach has been demonstrated by the *CLOCK* mutant mouse. This mutation, produced by ENU mutagenesis, resulted in a line of mice with profound abnormalities of circadian rhythms. The responsible mutation was subsequently mapped, and the *CLOCK* gene was molecularly cloned, setting the stage for subsequent studies that are providing novel insight into neural mechanisms that underlie circadian rhythms. Enthusiasm for chemical mutagenesis approaches has led to the establishment of several international centers devoted to mutagenesis screens. It is anticipated that current large-scale efforts will result in thousands of single gene mutants, many of which will provide novel insights into neural processes that regulate behavior.

NEUROBEHAVIORAL ASSESSMENT OF GENETICALLY MODIFIED MICE

Evaluating Behavioral Models The careful design and implementation of mouse behavioral analysis procedures are essential for translating the rapid advances in mouse molecular genetics for insights into psychiatric disease susceptibility and treatment. It is useful to distinguish the variety of purposes for which behavioral assays are used. Three classes of uses have been proposed: screening tests, behavioral bioassays, and models of clinical features of psychiatric disorders. Behavioral screening tests are commonly used in the pharmaceutical industry and have one main requirement—that they accurately predict the efficacy of compounds for the treatment of clinical disorders. An example of such a test is the forced-swim *behavioral despair* model of depression discussed in the section Depression. Behavioral bioassays use a behavioral readout to measure the impact of experimental manipulations on particular brain systems. For example, the influence of novel compounds on brain dopaminergic neurotransmission may be studied by examining their effects on circling behavior in animals with unilateral lesions of the nigrostriatal pathway. A third class of behavioral assays attempts to model the clinical phenomenology of psychiatric disorders. Considerations in the use of mouse genetic models for simulating human psychiatric disease are discussed below.

The potential for mouse models to mimic multiple aspects of complex neuropsychiatric disorders is illustrated by studies of mutant mice lacking the hypothalamic neuropeptide orexin. Observations of these animals revealed a dramatic behavioral syndrome, characterized by frequent episodes of inactivity, manifested by the sudden collapse of the head and buckling of extremities. Electroencephalogram (EEG) analysis revealed instances in which attacks were accompanied by sudden transitions into rapid eye movement (REM) sleep in a pattern similar to narcoleptic attacks observed in humans and in a strain of narcoleptic dogs. Moreover, a mutation of an orexin receptor gene was found to underlie the canine syndrome, and clinical studies subsequently revealed orexin deficiencies in narcoleptic humans. Thus, studies of orexin null mutant mice revealed a novel role for orexin in the regulation of arousal and an important animal model for examining the pathophysiology and treatment of narcolepsy.

There are significant obvious limitations in the extent to which mice may be used to develop similarly compelling models that mimic signs and symptoms of common psychiatric disorders. Owing to difficulties in obtaining self-reported data from mice, many phenomenological aspects of psychiatric disorders, such as feelings of guilt, self-esteem obsessions, hallucinations, and delusions, may not be assessed. In mice, perturbations of psychological processes must be inferred from behavior. Available behavioral assays relating to clinical conditions, such as anxiety and depression, appear to have some validity as screening tests; that is, they predict the anxiolytic and antidepressant efficacy of compounds. However, their face validity, the degree to which the measured behaviors resemble these human disorders, and their construct validity, the degree to which the assays reproduce the etiology and pathophysiology of human psychiatric disorders, are questionable. With few exceptions, current mouse models may be most productively used to examine the neural bases of particular behavioral elements relevant to psychiatric disorders rather than as comprehensive models of complex psychiatric syndromes. Examples of mouse models currently used to model clinical features of psychiatric illnesses are described in the following sections.

Anxiety Behavioral assays of anxiety have typically focused on attempts to model anxiety states rather than the complex symptom clusters associated with particular anxiety disorders. Because it is not possible to gain detailed insight into the subjective experiences of mice, internal state must be inferred from patterns of behavior. Rather than concluding that experimental treatments have altered anxiety, this important caveat is acknowledged through references to their influences on *anxiety-like* or *anxiety-related* behaviors. The most frequently used class of tests assesses exploratory behavior, relying on the innate predisposition of rodents to avoid open or brightly lit spaces, or both. For example, when placed in a novel open field chamber, mice exhibit thigmotaxis, an affinity for the periphery of the behavioral arena rather than the center. The proportion of time spent in the periphery is proposed to correlate with anxiety state.

Perhaps the most commonly used screening test for examining the effects of pharmacological and genetic manipulations on anxiety-like behavior is the elevated plus maze. This consists of an elevated plus-shaped platform with four arms, two of which are walled and two of which are open. The predisposition of mice to prefer the closed to the open arms is proposed to correlate with anxiety state. The responses of rodents to pharmacological agents in this assay are predictive of the effects of these compounds on human anxiety states. Thus, the administration of anxiolytic drugs, such as diazepam, increases the proportion of time that the animals spend exploring the open arms. A variant of this assay, the elevated zero maze, consisting of an annular platform divided into two opposing walled quadrants and two open quadrants, is used for a similar purpose.

The light–dark exploration test is another assay of anxiety-related behavior in common use. The test enclosure consists of two chambers with an opening enabling mice to travel between them. One of the chambers is covered and dark, and the other is open and brightly lit. Mice typically display a strong preference for the dark compartment, and the time spent there is interpreted to correlate with anxiety state. The number of transitions mice make between the chambers has been interpreted to correlate inversely with anxiety state.

The previously mentioned assays assess locomotor behavior, leading to a potential confound if a drug or mutations produce nonspecific changes in activity levels. In contrast to anxiety tests that assess exploratory behavior, an alternative strategy focuses on the ability of anxiety or fear states to augment the startle response to stimuli, such as sound. After pairings of a conditioned stimulus, such as light, with foot shock, acoustic startle responses are elevated in the presence of the light. Much has been learned about the neural circuitry associated with the fear-potentiated startle response. These studies have been extended to reveal that acoustic startle responses are enhanced under bright light conditions. The potentiation of the startle response by light has been proposed as a model of anxiety that does not depend on locomotor responses.

In another class of assays, animals are exposed to conflict situations in which the animals must expose themselves to an aversive stimulus to obtain a reward. For example, water-restricted animals are provided access to an electrified drinking spout, or food-restricted animals are provided access to food placed in the center of an open, brightly lit arena. Treatments with anxiolytic compounds suppress punishment- or novelty-induced behavioral inhibition, resulting in increased drinking or feeding behavior.

To date, behavioral assessments have revealed phenotypes consistent with anxiety dysregulation in at least 30 lines of mice. For example, marked enhancements of anxiety-related behaviors were observed in three different laboratories that had independently generated mice bearing a targeted null mutation of the serotonin type 1A (5-HT_{1A}) receptor gene. These animals may be used to examine mechanisms through which serotonin systems regulate anxiety. Insights into the role of the neuropeptide corticotropin-releasing factor (CRF) in the regulation of anxiety have also been provided by genetic studies—whereas enhanced anxiety-like behaviors were observed in mice bearing mutations that enhance CRF function, reduced anxiety-like behaviors were exhibited by mice with genetic perturbations that reduce brain CRF signaling. Mutations impacting the signaling of acetylcholine, dopamine, GABA, neuropeptide Y, cholecystokinin, nitric oxide, and other neuromodulators have been found to impact anxiety-related behaviors.

Depression

There is a great deal of variability in the extent to which various features of depressive syndromes may be modeled in animals. Whereas simulations of subjective feelings, such as depressed mood, diminished self-esteem, guilt, and suicidal ideations, are inaccessible in the mouse, prospects are better for gaining insights into a number of neurovegetative symptoms. These include perturbations of psychomotor behavior, feeding, diurnal rhythmicity, sleep, and the pursuit of natural rewards, such as food and sexual activity. Among the first attempts to simulate depression in animals was the learned helplessness model. This was originally developed in dogs and subsequently was applied to a variety of species, including rodents. It was observed that, after inescapable shocks, animals display a number of behavioral perturbations, including apparently reduced motivation to escape aversive stimuli, such as shock. In addition, animals display reduced appetite and weight loss, as well as reductions in appetite-motivated tasks that have been proposed to simulate anhedonia. Moreover, many of these effects are reversed by treatment with a variety of antidepressant drugs. Despite the apparent face validity and predictive validity of this model, several factors have limited its use as a depression model. In contrast with the chronicity of human depressive states, learned helplessness effects are typically short lived. In addition, many investigators prefer assays that do not require subjecting animals to inescapable shock.

Some investigators have attempted to model the proposed contribution of chronic stress to depressive disorders by exposing animals to a series of varied and unpredictable environmental stressors. Such chronic exposure produces a putative anhedonic state characterized by reduced consumption of a highly palatable sucrose solution. This behavioral deficit persists after cessation of the stress regimen and is reversible by chronic, but not acute, treatment with tricyclic antidepressants and selective serotonin reuptake inhibitors (SSRIs), mimicking the time course of antidepressant action in humans. Although the chronic mild stress procedure may be considered to simulate more plausibly factors conferring susceptibility to depression, its use has been limited by problems of reliability and reproducibility of results. Despite the apparent construct validity of this model, further efforts will be needed to overcome such limitations.

The two most frequently used depression-related mouse behavioral assays are the forced-swim and the tail suspension *behavioral despair* paradigms. For the forced-swim test, mice are placed for several minutes in a water-containing cylinder from which they cannot escape. Initially, animals display high levels of activity in apparent attempts to escape, followed by increasing episodes of immobility during which they appear to float at the surface. This immobile state was initially proposed to reflect behavioral despair—the loss of hope of escaping. Because immobility in this assay is reduced by a wide variety of antidepressant drugs, the assay is used in the pharmaceutical industry to predict potential antidepressant efficacy of novel compounds. However, limitations do exist in the predictive validity of the test. False-negative responses to a variety of serotonergic antidepressants have been observed, as well as false-positive responses to a number of convulsants, antihistamines, and opiates. A variant of this assay, the tail suspension test, is more sensitive to serotonergic antidepressants. In this test, animals are suspended by the tail for several minutes, and the time spent immobile (absence of apparent escape attempts) is measured.

The utility of these behavioral assays as models of depression has been a matter of debate, because their face and construct validity are limited. It is unlikely that a single forced-swim or tail suspension experience closely models the process through which clinical depression develops. It is also unclear whether immobility in these assays reflects a state of despair, because immobility may be alternatively viewed as an adaptive strategy for coping with these experimental situations. Moreover, whereas the therapeutic effects of antidepressants typically require several weeks of treatment, acute drug responses are typically assessed in these assays. Despite these limitations, the significant predictive validity of these tests indicates that insights into the neural mechanisms underlying these behaviors may shed light on neural pathways pertinent to the pathophysiology or treatment, or both, of depression. To date, mutations of at least 20 genes have been associated with abnormal responses to these tests, including those encoding the 5-HT_{1A} and serotonin type 1B (5-HT_{1B}) receptors, α-adrenergic receptors, the norepinephrine plasma membrane transporter, monoamine oxidases A and B, and others.

Schizophrenia Given the nature of the clinical manifestations of schizophrenic disorders and the uncertainty regarding their pathophysiological bases, the challenge of modeling schizophrenia in mice may seem daunting. Many features of these disorders, such as delusions, hallucinations, bizarre ideations, loosening of associations, and abnormalities of speech, cannot be examined in mice and may involve brain regions that are relatively underdeveloped in rodents. Moreover, limited understanding of the etiology of schizophrenia presents a major challenge in the development of models with credible construct validity. Nevertheless, investigators have noted many features of schizophrenic disorders that are more amenable to modeling in mice, and molecular genetic approaches are yielding insights into their underlying neural substrates.

Following observations that psychostimulants can produce a behavioral syndrome mimicking schizophrenia and that dopamine receptor blockade is a feature shared by many antipsychotic compounds, brain dopamine systems have been strongly implicated in the pathophysiology and treatment of schizophrenia. Behavioral manifestations of hyperdopaminergic states in mice include elevated locomotor activity levels and increased rates of stereotypic motor patterns. Although hyperactivity and increased motor stereotypes are not considered to be cardinal manifestations of schizophrenia, these behaviors have predictive value in assessing the antipsychotic potential of compounds. However, their benefit may be limited to only those compounds that alter dopaminergic function.

Another behavioral assay is used to model the proposed deficits in sensorimotor gating that occur in schizophrenia. It has been proposed that an impaired ability to filter or gate sensory information leads to sensory overload and to the cognitive disorganization observed in these disorders. To probe this function, assays focused on the prepulse inhibition (PPI) of startle have been developed for humans and mice. PPI procedures are commonly based on the observation that a weak sensory stimulus presented before a strong stimulus reduces the magnitude of the startle response to the strong stimulus. PPI deficits have been observed in schizophrenic patients and as a result of psychostimulant administration. In mice, the assay typically involves the presentation of a mild auditory prestimulus before a strong auditory startle stimulus to a mouse on a force detector that can measure the amplitude of startle responses. The ability of the prestimulus to reduce the force of the subsequent startle response is used to quantitate PPI magnitude. It is important to note that abnormalities of PPI in clinical populations are not limited to schizophrenia but can also be seen in amphetamine psychosis, mania, and obsessive-compulsive disorder (OCD). In addition, PPI magnitude can be influenced by a wide variety of neurotransmitter systems.

Phenotypes proposed to relate to schizophrenia have been observed in several lines of mutant mice. Phenotypic characterization of mice with targeted mutations of genes involved in dopaminergic neurotransmission has revealed a variety of neurobehavioral perturbations. For example, animals bearing a targeted null mutation of the dopamine transporter gene display a *hyperdopaminergic* phenotype with markedly elevated extracellular dopamine levels. These mice display locomotor hyperactivity, motor stereotypes, and a PPI deficit that are reversed by selective D_2 receptor antagonists and by antipsychotic drugs. However, additional aspects of the phenotype, such as its amelioration by psychostimulants and the absence of social interaction deficits, do not mimic features of schizophrenia and have led some to consider these animals a model of attention-deficit/hyperactivity disorder (ADHD).

In addition to the hyperdopaminergic hypothesis of schizophrenia, a more recent proposal focuses on a potential contribution of diminished glutamatergic neurotransmission. This idea arose from observations of the psychotomimetic properties of glutamate NMDA receptor antagonists, such as phencyclidine (PCP). Accordingly, a relevant set of phenotypic abnormalities was observed in a line of mice bearing a mutation that markedly reduced NMDA receptor numbers. These animals exhibited normal extracellular dopamine levels yet displayed locomotor hyperactivity, motor stereotypes, and diminished social interactions, all of which were reversed by clozapine treatment. Further studies of these mice may be useful for illuminating functional relationships between glutamatergic and dopaminergic signaling.

Future Directions The application of mouse molecular genetic technologies promises to provide useful insights into the biology of neural processes relevant to the pathophysiology and treatment of psychiatric disorders. Continuing technological advances in this field will accelerate the use of these approaches. Advances in procedures for the precise restriction of mutations to particular neuronal cell types and brain regions will facilitate studies of the roles of gene products in defined neuronal circuits. The further development of inducible systems will facilitate studies of the developmental contributions of gene function to behavior. In addition, the growing accessibility of gene chip technologies will allow simultaneous examination of the influence of targeted mutations on the expression of thousands of genes.

Technological advances will also facilitate the performance of phenotype-based genetic screens. The characterization of single nucleotide polymorphisms (SNPs) will enable genomic mapping with high precision. Gene chip technology will enable simultaneous analysis of thousands of SNPs, accelerating gene mapping and QTL analyses. Sequence information provided by the Mouse Genome Project will further facilitate the process of mapping QTLs and ENU-induced mutations.

To maximize the benefits of mouse molecular genetics to neuropsychiatric research, more rapid progress must be made in establishing mouse behavioral assays with demonstrated relevance to psychiatric phenomena that are not effectively addressed by current models. These include tests of attention, psychosis, impulsivity, compulsions, panic, social withdrawal, and feeding regulation. Prospects of generating mouse models that more fully mimic the complex constellations of features characterizing human psychiatric disorders will improve with advances in the development and application of mouse molecular genetic technologies, combined with advances in understanding the neurobiology and genetics of psychiatric disorders. Altogether, the rapid progress in this field bodes well for its potential to contribute key insights into neural and genetic mechanisms underlying psychiatric disease etiology and treatment.

SUGGESTED CROSS-REFERENCES

Neurotrophic factors are covered in Section 1.7. Further information about the genome is found in Section 1.10. Genetic linkage of psychiatric disorders is discussed in Section 1.18.

REFERENCES

Belknap JK, Hitzemann R, Crabbe JC, Phillips TJ, Buck KJ, Williams RW: QTL analysis and genome-wide mutagenesis in mice: complementary genetic approaches to the dissection of complex traits. *Behav Genet.* 2001;31:5–15.
Bradley A: Mining the mouse genome. *Nature.* 2002;420:512–514.
Campbell KM, de Lecea L, Severynse DM, Caron MG, McGrath MJ, Sparber SB, Sun LY, Burton FH: OCD-like behaviors caused by a neuropotentiating transgene targeted to cortical and limbic D1+ neurons. *J Neurosci.* 1999;19:5044–5053.
Chemelli RM, Willie JT, Sinton CM, Elmquist JK, Scammell T, Lee C, Richardson JA, Williams SC, Xiong Y, Kisanuki Y: Narcolepsy in orexin knockout mice: molecular genetics of sleep regulation [See comments]. *Cell.* 1999;98:437–451.
Crabbe JC: Genetic contributions to addiction. *Annu Rev Psychol.* 2002;53:435–462.
Cryan JF, Markou A, Lucki I: Assessing antidepressant activity in rodents: Recent developments and future needs. *Trends Pharmacol Sci.* 2002;23:238–245.
Finn DA, Rutledge-Gorman MT, Crabbe JC: Genetic animal models of anxiety. *Neurogenetics.* 2003;4:109–135.
Francis DD, Szegda K, Campbell G, Martin WD, Insel TR: Epigenetic sources of behavioral differences in mice. *Nat Neurosci.* 2003;6:440–442.
Gainetdinov RR, Mohn AR, Caron MG: Genetic animal models: focus on schizophrenia. *Trends Neurosci.* 2001;24:527–533.
Geyer MA, Krebs-Thomson K, Braff DL, Swerdlow NR: Pharmacological studies of prepulse inhibition models of sensorimotor gating deficits in schizophrenia: a decade in review. *Psychopharmacology (Berl).* 2001;156:117–154.
Holmes A: Targeted gene mutation approaches to the study of anxiety-like behavior in mice. *Neurosci Biobehav Rev.* 2001;25:261–273.
Hrabe de Angelis MH, Flaswinkel H, Fuchs H, Rathkolb B, Soewarto D, Marschall S, Heffner S, Pargent W, Wuensch K, Jung M: Genome-wide, large-scale production of mutant mice by ENU mutagenesis. *Nat Genet.* 2000;25:444–447.
Keltz MB, Chen J, Carlezon WA, Whisler K, Gilden L, Beckmann AM, Steffen C, Zhang YJ, Marotti L, Self DW: Expression of the transcription factor ΔFosB in the brain controls sensitivity to cocaine. *Nature.* 1999;401:272–275.
King DP, Zhao Y, Sangoram AM, Wilsbacher LD, Tanaka M, Antoch MP, Steeves TD, Vitaterna MH, Kornhauser JM, Lowrey PL: Positional cloning of the mouse circadian clock gene. *Cell.* 1997;89:641–653.
Kwan KM: Conditional alleles in mice: practical considerations for tissue-specific knockouts. *Genesis.* 2002;32:49–62.
Lewandoski M: Conditional control of gene expression in the mouse. *Nat Rev Genet.* 2001;2:743–755.
McGuffin P, Riley B, Plomin R: Toward behavioral genomics. *Science.* 2001;291:1232–1249.
Mohn AR, Gainetdinov RR, Caron MG, Koller BH: Mice with reduced NMDA receptor expression display behaviors related to schizophrenia. *Cell.* 1999;98:427–436.
Muller U: Ten years of gene targeting: targeted mouse mutants, from vector design to phenotype analysis. *Mech Dev.* 1999;82:3–21.
Munroe RJ, Bergstrom RA, Zheng QY, Libby B, Smith R, John SW, Schimenti KJ, Browning VL, Schimenti JC: Mouse mutants from chemically mutagenized embryonic stem cells. *Nat Genet.* 2000;24:318–321.
Nolan PM, Peters J, Strivens M, Rogers D, Hagan J, Spurr N, Gray IC, Vizor L, Brooker D, Whitehill E: A systematic, genome-wide, phenotype-driven mutagenesis programme for gene function studies in the mouse. *Nat Genet.* 2000;25:440–443.
Peyron C, Faraco J, Rogers W, Ripley B, Overeem S, Charnay Y, Nevsimalova S, Aldrich M, Reynolds D, Albin R: A mutation in a case of early onset narcolepsy and a generalized absence of hypocretin peptides in human narcoleptic brains. *Nat Med.* 2000;6:991–997.
Rudolph U, Crestani F, Mohler H: GABA(A) receptor subtypes: dissecting their pharmacological functions. *Trends Pharmacol Sci.* 2001;22:188–194.
Shekhar A, McCann UD, Meaney MJ, Blanchard DC, Davis M, Frey KA, Liberzon I, Overall KL, Shear MK, Tecott LH, Winsky L: Summary of a National Institute of Mental Health workshop: Developing animal models of anxiety disorders. *Psychopharmacology (Berl).* 2001;157:327–339.
Tarantino LM, Bucan M: Dissection of behavior and psychiatric disorders using the mouse as a model. *Hum Mol Genet.* 2000;9:953–965.
Tecott LH: The genes and brains of mice and men. *Am J Psychiatry.* 2003;160:646–656.
Tecott LH, Wehner JM: Mouse molecular genetic technologies: promise for psychiatric research. *Arch Gen Psychiatry.* 2001;58:995–1004.
Tsien JZ, Huerta PT, Tonegawa S: The essential role of hippocampal CA1 NMDA receptor-dependent synaptic plasticity in spatial memory. *Cell.* 1996;87:1327–1338.
van der Weyden L, Adams DJ, Bradley A: Tools for targeted manipulation of the mouse genome. *Physiol Genomics.* 2002;11:133–164.
Venter JC, Adams MD, Myers EW, Li PW, Mural RJ: The sequence of the human genome. *Science.* 2001;291:1304–1351.
Waterston RH, Lindblad-Toh K, Birney E, Rogers J, Abril JF, Agarwal P, Agarwala R, Ainscough R, Alexandersson M, An P: Initial sequencing and comparative analysis of the mouse genome. *Nature.* 2002;420:520–562.
Willner P: Animal models of depression: an overview. *Pharmacol Ther.* 1990;45:425–455.
Willner P. Behavioral models in psychopharmacology. In: Willner P, ed. *Behavioral models in Psychopharmacology: Theoretical, Industrial and Clinical Perspectives.* Cambridge, UK: Cambridge University Press; 1991:3–18.

▲ 1.20 Basic Science of Sleep

RUTH M. BENCA, M.D., PH.D., CHIARA CIRELLI, M.D., PH.D., NIELS C. RATTENBORG, PH.D., AND GIULIO TONONI, M.D., PH.D.

Sleep is a universal behavior that has been demonstrated in every animal species studied, from insects to mammals. It is one of the most significant of human behaviors, occupying roughly one-third of human life. Although the exact functions of sleep are still unknown, it is clearly necessary for survival, because prolonged sleep deprivation leads to severe physical and cognitive impairment and, finally, death. Sleep is particularly relevant to psychiatry, because sleep disturbances occur in virtually all psychiatric illnesses and are frequently part of the diagnostic criteria for specific disorders. Sleep disturbance has predictive value in identifying individuals at risk for the development of psychiatric illness. Specific changes in sleep architecture, identified particularly in relation to mood disorders, serve as biological markers that may provide insights into pathophysiology of these disorders. Furthermore, manipulations of sleep have profound impacts on mood, memory, and behavior that can influence the course of an illness; sleep deprivation, for example, produces immediate antidepressant effects in depressed patients or even mania in bipolar patients. Virtually all psychiatric medications have effects on sleep, further underscoring the strong relationships between the neurobiology of sleep and the pathophysiology of psychiatric disorders.

NORMAL HUMAN SLEEP

Definition of Sleep From a behavioral standpoint, sleep is a state of decreased awareness of environmental stimuli that is distinguished from states such as coma or hibernation by its relatively rapid reversibility. Sleeping individuals move little and tend to adopt stereotypic postures. Although sleep is characterized by a relative unconsciousness of the external world and a general lack of memory of the state, unlike people who have been comatose, a person generally recognizes when he or she feels sleepy and is aware that he or she has been asleep at the termination of an episode.

For clinical and research purposes, sleep is generally defined by combining behavioral observation with electrophysiological recording. Humans, like most other mammals, express two types of sleep: rapid eye movement (REM) and nonrapid eye movement (NREM) sleep. These states have distinctive neurophysiological and psychophysiological characteristics. *REM sleep* derives its name from the frequent bursts of eye movement activity that occur. It is also referred to as *paradoxical sleep*, because the electroencephalogram (EEG) during REM sleep is similar to that of waking. In infants, the equivalent of REM sleep is called *active sleep* because of prominent phasic muscle twitches. NREM sleep, or *orthodox sleep*, is characterized by decreased activation of the EEG; in infants, it is called *quiet sleep* because of the relative lack of motor activity.

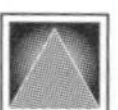

Table 1.20–1
Stages of Sleep—Electrophysiological Criteria

	Electroencephalogram	Electrooculogram	Electromyogram
Wakefulness	Low-voltage, mixed frequency activity Alpha (8–13 cps) activity with eyes closed	Eye movements and eye blinks	High tonic activity and voluntary movements
Nonrapid eye movement sleep			
Stage I	Low-voltage, mixed frequency activity Theta (3–7 cps) activity, vertex sharp waves	Slow eye movements	Tonic activity slightly decreased from wakefulness
Stage II	Low-voltage, mixed frequency background with sleep spindles (12–14 cps bursts) and K complexes (negative sharp wave followed by positive slow wave)	None	Low tonic activity
Stage III	High-amplitude (≥75 μV) slow waves (≤2 cps) occupying 20 to 50 percent of epoch	None	Low tonic activity
Stage IV	High-amplitude slow waves occupy >50% of epoch	None	Low tonic activity
REM sleep	Low-voltage, mixed frequency activity Saw-tooth waves, theta activity, and slow alpha activity	REMs	Tonic atonia with phasic twitches

REM, rapid eye movement.
Criteria from Rechtchaffen A, Kales A. *A Manual of Standardized Terminology, Techniques, and Scoring System for Sleep Stages of Human Subjects.* UCLA, Los Angeles: Brain Information Service/Brain Research Institute; 1968.

Stages of Sleep Within REM and NREM sleep, there are further classifications called *stages* (Table 1.20–1, Fig. 1.20–1). For clinical and research applications, sleep is typically scored in epochs of 30 seconds, with stages of sleep defined by the visual scoring of three parameters: EEG, electrooculogram (EOG), and electromyogram (EMG) recorded beneath the chin. The criteria defined by Allan Rechtschaffen and Anthony Kales in 1968 are accepted in clinical practice and for research around the world (Table 1.20–1).

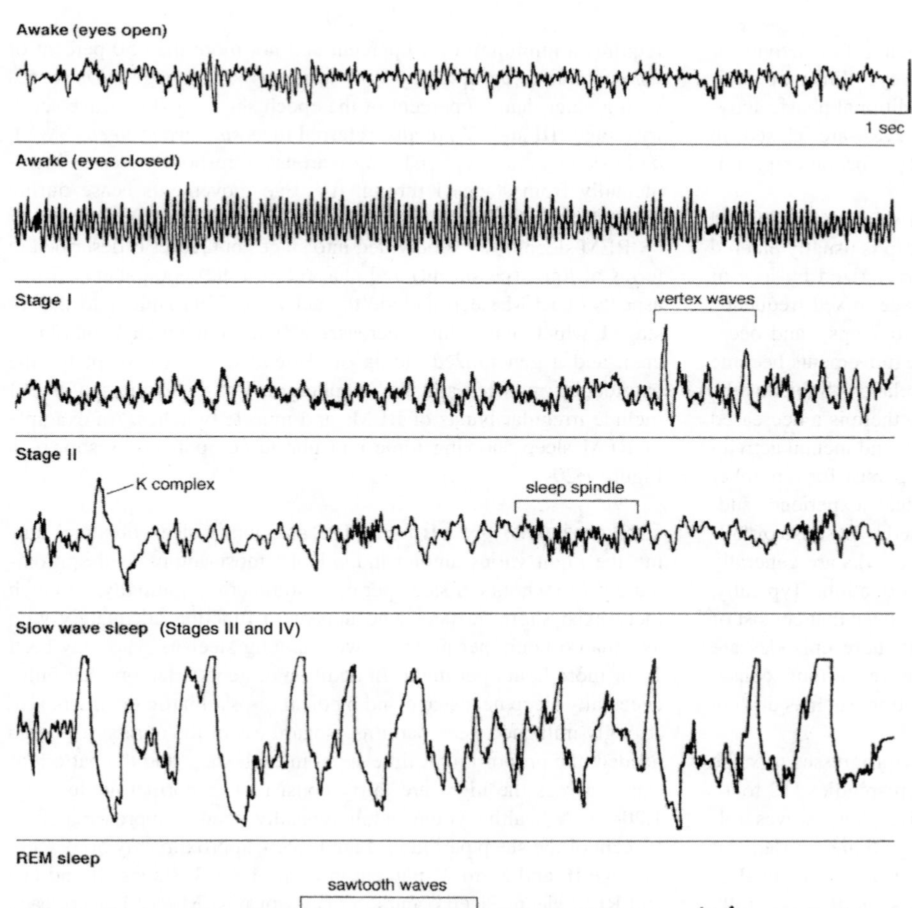

FIGURE 1.20–1 Electroencephalogram patterns for stages of human sleep and wakefulness. REM, rapid eye movement. (From Butkov N. *Atlas of Clinical Polysomnography*. Medford, Oregon: Synapse Media; 1996, with permission.)

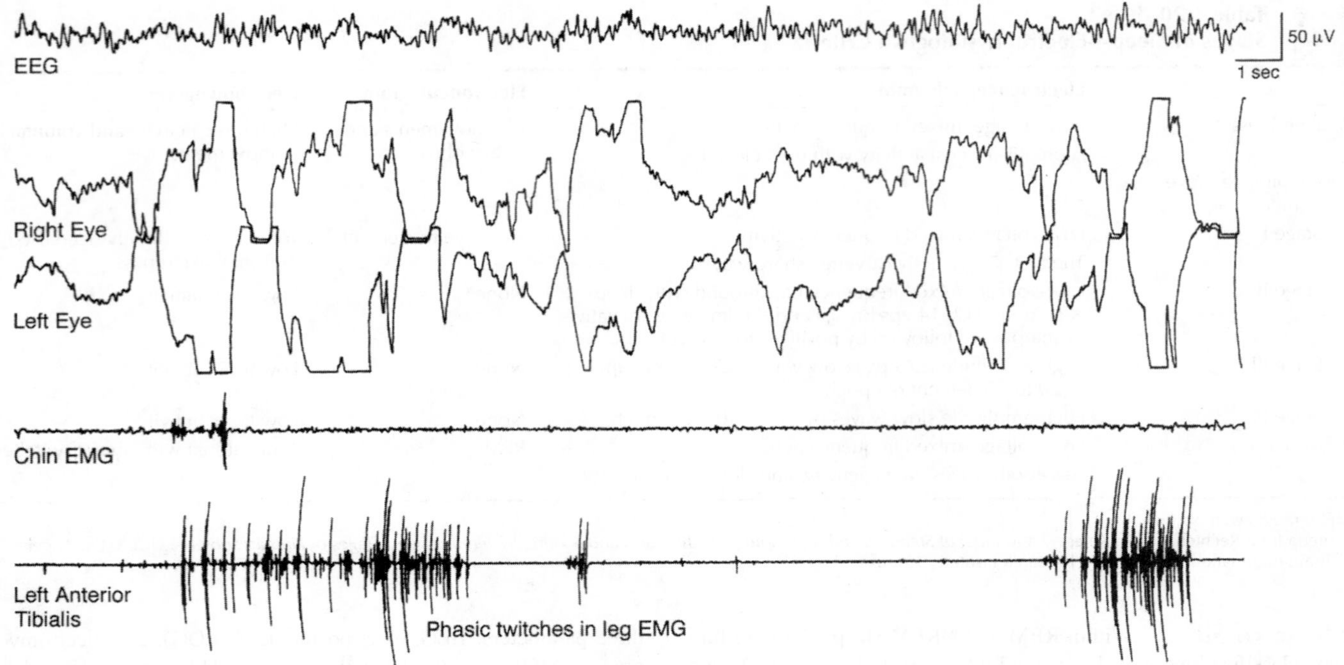

FIGURE 1.20–2 Example of human rapid eye movement (REM) sleep. EEG, electroencephalogram; EMG, electromyogram. (From Butkov N. *Atlas of Clinical Polysomnography*. Medford, Oregon: Synapse Media; 1996, with permission.)

During wakefulness, the EEG shows a low-voltage fast activity or activated pattern. Voluntary eye movements and eye blinks are obvious. The EMG has a high tonic activity, with additional phasic activity related to voluntary movements. When eyes are closed in preparation for sleep, alpha activity (8 to 13 cps) becomes prominent, particularly in occipital regions.

NREM sleep, which usually precedes REM sleep, is subdivided into four stages (Table 1.20–1, Fig. 1.20–1). Sleep is usually entered through a transitional state, stage I sleep, characterized by loss of alpha activity and the appearance of a low-voltage mixed frequency EEG pattern with prominent theta activity (3 to 7 cps), and occasional vertex sharp waves may also appear. Eye movements become slow and rolling, and skeletal muscle tone relaxes. Subjectively, stage I may not be perceived as sleep, although there is a decreased awareness of sensory stimuli, particularly visual, and mental activity becomes more dream-like. Motor activity may persist for a number of seconds during stage I. Occasionally, individuals experience sudden muscle contractions, sometimes accompanied by a sense of falling or dream-like imagery, or both; these hypnic jerks are generally benign and may be exacerbated by sleep deprivation. Typically, sleep-deprived individuals enter periods of *microsleep* that consist of brief (5 to 10 seconds) bouts of stage I sleep; these episodes are unavoidable in sleepy individuals and can have serious consequences in situations that demand constant attention, such as driving a motor vehicle.

After a few minutes of stage I, sleep usually progresses to stage II, which is heralded by the appearance of sleep spindles (12 to 14 cps) and K complexes (high-amplitude negative sharp waves followed by positive slow waves) in the EEG. Stage II and subsequent stages of NREM and REM sleep are all subjectively perceived as sleep. Particularly at the beginning of the night, stage II is generally followed by a period comprised of stages III and IV. Slow waves (≤2 cps in humans) appear during these stages, which are subdivided according to the proportion of delta waves in the epoch; stage III requires a minimum of 20 percent and not more than 50 percent of the epoch time occupied by slow waves, whereas stage IV is scored with greater than 50 percent of the epoch showing slow wave activity. Stages III and IV are also referred to as *slow wave sleep* (SWS), *delta sleep*, or *deep sleep*, because arousal threshold increases incrementally from stages I through IV. Eye movements cease during stages II through IV, and EMG activity decreases further.

REM sleep is not subdivided into stages but rather is described in terms of tonic (persistent) and phasic (episodic) components. Tonic aspects of REM sleep include the activated EEG similar to that of stage I, which may exhibit increased activity in the theta band (3 to 7 cps), and a generalized atonia of skeletal muscles, except for the extraocular muscles and the diaphragm. Phasic features of REM include irregular bursts of REMs and muscle twitches. An example of REM sleep showing tonic and phasic components is shown in Figure 1.20–2.

Organization of Sleep

The amount of sleep obtained during the night varies among individuals; most adults need approximately 7 to 9 hours of sleep per night to function optimally, although there exist short sleepers who appear to function adequately with less than 6 hours per night, as well as long sleepers who may need 12 or more hours per night. In addition to genetic factors that influence daily sleep needs, age and medical or psychiatric disorders also strongly influence sleep patterns. Regardless of the number of hours needed, the proportion of time spent in each stage and the pattern of stages across the night are fairly consistent in normal adults (Fig. 1.20–3). A healthy young adult typically spends approximately 5 percent of the sleep period in stage I sleep, approximately 50 percent in stage II, and 20 to 25 percent in each of SWS (stages III and IV) and REM sleep. Sleep occurs in cycles of NREM-REM sleep, each lasting approximately 90 to 110 minutes. SWS (stages III and IV) is most prominent early in the night, especially during the first NREM period, and diminishes as the night progresses. As SWS wanes, peri-

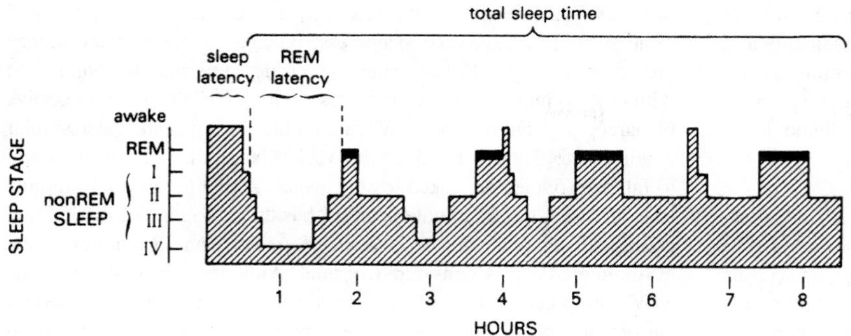

FIGURE 1.20–3 Sleep pattern in a young, healthy subject. REM, rapid eye movement. (From Gillian JC, Seifritz E, Zoltoltoski RK, Salin-Pascual RJ. Basic science of sleep. In: Sadock BJ, Sadock VA, eds. *Kaplan & Sadock's Comprehensive Textbook of Psychiatry*. 7th ed. Vol 1. Baltimore: Lippincott Williams & Wilkins; 2000:199, with permission.)

ods of REM sleep lengthen, showing greater phasic activity and generally more intense dreaming later in the night.

EFFECTS OF AGE ON SLEEP

Sleep patterns change markedly across the lifespan, with the most rapid changes occurring during the first years of life. Development of EEG patterns of sleep and wakefulness begins at approximately 24 weeks of gestational age, and differentiation into active (REM) and quiet (NREM) sleep occurs during the last trimester. Newborn infants spend 16 to 18 hours per day sleeping, and premature infants may sleep even more. Infants do not show evidence of strong diurnal sleep patterns for the first several months of life; they exhibit short sleep–wake cycles of approximately 3 to 4 hours, as well as reduced length of active–quiet sleep cycles (approximately 50 minutes). Active sleep occupies approximately one-half of their sleep time, and they tend to enter sleep through active rather than quiet sleep. At approximately 3 to 4 months of age, several important developmental changes occur: babies shift to the adult-like pattern of initiating sleep with NREM, sleep starts to become consolidated during the night, and the sleep EEG shows more mature waveforms characteristic of NREM and REM sleep.

During early childhood, total sleep time decreases, and REM sleep proportion drops to adult levels (20 to 25 percent). Napping normally continues during the preschool years but is often abandoned once children begin school full-time. Young children show the highest percentages of SWS, with particularly high arousal thresholds; this accounts for the difficulty in arousing them at the beginning of the sleep period, as well as the high incidence of bedwetting and SWS-related parasomnias, such as sleepwalking and night terrors.

SWS amounts diminish significantly during adolescence, possibly related to cortical synaptic pruning. Irwin Feinberg has suggested that abnormalities in synaptic elimination may account for the seemingly coincidental timing of maturation of sleep patterns and the increasing incidence of schizophrenia in late adolescence and early adulthood. Adolescents often decrease their total sleep time significantly, although this is probably due to behavioral changes rather than representing a true decrease in sleep need. They also show a tendency to become "night owls," preferring to stay up late rather than wake up early. This shift to "eveningness" may be related to an increase in the intrinsic period of the circadian clock.

Older adults show an increased incidence of primary sleep disorders (e.g., sleep apnea and periodic limb movements), medical illnesses, and psychiatric disorders that all may interfere with sleep; it is therefore difficult to determine which sleep changes represent normal aging. SWS continues to decline across adulthood and may disappear entirely by 60 years of age. Sleep also becomes more fragmented, with prolonged latency to sleep onset, increased numbers of arousals, more time spent awake during the sleep period, and increased daytime napping. Older individuals thus may spend more time in bed but obtain less sleep. They also show a trend to wake up earlier and feel more alert in the morning in comparison to the evening. Although the amount of REM sleep is preserved in normal elderly individuals, patients with Alzheimer's disease and other degenerative disorders of the central nervous system (CNS) show loss of REM sleep and a deterioration in diurnal patterns of sleep-wakefulness; this deterioration may become so severe that nursing home patients may not spend a single hour of the day in which they are consistently asleep or awake.

MONITORING HUMAN SLEEP

Sleep-wakefulness related alterations in the human EEG were first reported by Hans Berger in 1928. Since this discovery, the EEG and other electrophysiological parameters have been used to investigate normal human sleep. Starting in the 1970s, researchers and clinicians began to use similar monitoring techniques to characterize and to diagnose sleep disorders. In addition to the EEG, the EOG and EMG are recorded to measure eye movements and muscle activity, respectively, both requisites to distinguish wakefulness and the stages of sleep. The EEG is recorded from electrodes affixed to the scalp overlying specific regions of the brain according to the International 10/20 system of electrode placement. Because the EEG features that define wakefulness and the stages of sleep are most readily recorded from different regions of the brain, a minimum of two strategically chosen regions are studied. Sleep spindles and K complexes, transient EEG activity that characterize stage II sleep (Fig. 1.20–1), are recorded from electrodes placed over the central region. The central electrode also registers the relatively high-voltage, low-frequency activity originating from the frontal lobes during sleep stages III and IV. The second electrode is placed over the occipital lobe to optimize detection of alpha activity, a correlate of a relaxed waking state with closed eyes. Under certain research or clinical circumstances (e.g., diagnosis of sleep-related seizure disorders) additional electrodes are applied to obtain higher spatial resolution of EEG activity. The EOG recording is used to detect REMs associated with wakefulness and REM sleep, as well as the slow rolling eye movements that occur during stage I sleep. Because the retina is electrically negative when compared to the cornea, eye movements generate small electrical fields that can be detected from electrodes attached to the skin near the eyes. The EMG recording is used to detect tonic and phasic changes in muscle activity that correlate with changes in behavioral state. In particular, during REM sleep, skeletal muscle tone reaches the lowest tonic levels, reflecting the general paralysis associated with this stage of sleep. Typically, the EMG is recorded from electrodes attached to the chin.

In clinical settings, additional EMG electrodes are placed over the anterior tibialis and intercostal muscles to detect leg movements and respiratory effort, respectively. Depending on the presenting symptoms, clinical monitoring may also include additional respiratory effort and airflow sensors, electrocardiogram (ECG), oxyhemoglobin saturation, esophageal pH, and penile erections.

Standard Sleep Stage Scoring Standardized visual scoring rules instituted by Rechtschaffen and Kales in 1968 are used to quantify time spent in wakefulness and each sleep stage, as well as the temporal distribution, or architecture, of sleep across the recording period. Although computer-assisted algorithms for automated sleep stage scoring are currently being developed, none has gained widespread use among sleep researchers or clinicians. Nevertheless, mathematical techniques, such as power spectral analysis based on the fast Fourier transformation, are frequently used to quantify the relative contribution of various brain wave frequencies to the overall EEG recording. For example, power spectral analysis has shown that slow wave activity is greatest early in the sleep period and progressively declines across successive periods of stages III and IV sleep.

Sleep stage scoring yields several measures of sleep quantity and quality, including clinically relevant markers of sleep and psychiatric disorders. For each sleep measure, specific clinical or research circumstances may call for slightly different definitions. *Sleep latency* is the time elapsed from the start of the recording to the onset of sleep. *Sleep onset* is usually defined as the first three consecutive epochs of stage I sleep or any single epoch of a deeper sleep stage. *REM latency* is defined as the time elapsed from sleep onset to the first epoch of REM sleep. *Total sleep time* is the cumulative time spent in all sleep stages, and *sleep efficiency* is the proportion of the recording period spent asleep. Other measures of interest include the proportion of sleep spent in each sleep stage.

Measuring Daytime Sleepiness In addition to characterizing sleep patterns across the major sleep period, researchers and clinicians are sometimes interested in quantifying daytime sleepiness. Daytime sleepiness manifests as an increased propensity to fall asleep or a decreased ability to maintain wakefulness, or both. Sleepiness can be measured by using subjective questionnaires or objective electrophysiological monitoring. Sleep questionnaires, such as the Stanford Sleepiness Scale (SSS) or Epworth Sleepiness Scale (ESS), are easy to use in the laboratory or physician's office. The SSS asks the individual to rate his or her current level of sleepiness, whereas the ESS asks the individual to rate his or her probability of falling asleep under various circumstances. Both questionnaires may be influenced by the individual's ability to assess his or her own level of alertness or propensity to fall asleep, as well as his or her motivation to obtain treatment.

Objective measures of sleepiness generally require time-consuming laboratory-based testing but yield a more reliable estimate of sleepiness. Two standardized objective tests are typically used to measure daytime sleepiness: The Multiple Sleep Latency Test (MSLT) measures the propensity to fall asleep, whereas the Maintenance of Wakefulness Test (MWT) measures the ability to maintain wakefulness. Both tests use the electrophysiological sleep monitoring techniques described previously. The MSLT consists of four or five sleep latency tests spaced 2 hours apart. At the start of each test, individuals are asked to lie quietly in a darkened room and to allow themselves to fall asleep. The latency to sleep onset is recorded, and, if sleep does not occur within 20 minutes, the test is terminated. In the clinical setting, patients that fall asleep are usually allowed to sleep for 15 minutes to determine whether they exhibit a tendency to enter REM sleep in an abnormally short period of time. The mean sleep latency is calculated, as well as the number of tests in which REM sleep was detected. A mean sleep latency of less than 5 minutes reflects excessive sleepiness, whereas a mean sleep latency greater than or equal to 15 minutes is considered normal. In conjunction with other symptoms, two or more tests with REM sleep are suggestive of narcolepsy. During the MWT, individuals are placed under similar conditions to that described for the MSLT, but, rather than being asked to fall asleep, they are asked to stay awake. Although 20- to 40-minute tests are used, the 40-minute protocol has the advantage of minimizing ceiling effects. A mean sleep latency of greater than 35 minutes on the 40-minute MWT is considered normal. Although the MSLT and the MWT are objective tests of sleepiness, the results can be influenced by various factors, such as an individual's prior sleep history. In the clinical setting, in particular, the goal is to assess whether a patient exhibits a pathological degree of sleepiness despite obtaining normal amounts of sleep; short sleep latencies on the MSLT are of limited clinical use if the patient is clearly sleep deprived. Consequently, it is critical that the patient's prior sleep history be evaluated by monitoring in the sleep laboratory during the preceding night, as well as by questionnaires logging sleep habits for the previous week. Under certain circumstances, patients may wear small devices on their wrists that detect and log motion, a correlate of wakefulness, for several days or weeks before undergoing laboratory testing. Such activity monitoring (or actigraphy) is also used to obtain objective measures of sleep at home in patients complaining of insomnia. Other objective measures of sleepiness based on power spectral analysis of the EEG, pupillary activity, and performance on cognitive tests are currently under development.

PHYSIOLOGY IN SLEEP

An appreciation of the physiological changes that occur during sleep is helpful for understanding the effects of normal and disturbed sleep on medical disorders. Various parameters of neuroendocrine and autonomic nervous system physiology show changes related to circadian rhythms or sleep itself (Table 1.20–1).

Autonomic Nervous System During NREM sleep and tonic REM sleep, there is a relative increase in parasympathetic activity relative to sympathetic activity. The autonomic nervous system reaches its most stable state during SWS in comparison to wakefulness. During phasic REM sleep, however, there are brief surges in sympathetic and parasympathetic activity, resulting in a high degree of autonomic instability.

Cardiovascular System Blood pressure, heart rate, and cardiac output decrease during NREM sleep, reaching their lowest average values and least variability in SWS. Although these parameters remain reduced on average during REM sleep in comparison to waking, they attain their peak values during REM. Arrhythmias are also more prevalent in REM sleep, which may contribute to the increased rate of cardiovascular mortality in the early morning, the time of greatest REM sleep propensity. It is also possible that increased rates of mortality related to cardiovascular causes seen in major depression might be related to the tendency of depressed patients to have increased amounts of REM sleep with greater phasic activity.

Pulmonary System Temporary breathing instability or periodic breathing, or both, may occur at the onset of sleep related to the loss of waking-related respiratory drive, as well as a decreased sensitivity of central chemoreceptors to partial pressure of carbon dioxide (P_{CO_2}); sensitivity to P_{CO_2} declines further during REM sleep, along with a decrease in the ventilatory response to reduced partial pressure of oxygen (P_{O_2}). Respiratory rate and minute ventilation decrease during sleep, and upper airway resistance increases as a result of muscle relaxation, most significantly during REM sleep. These changes contribute to exacerbations of underlying pulmonary disease, as well as sleep-related breathing disorders, such as sleep apnea.

Thermoregulation In addition to the circadian-related nocturnal decrease in body temperature, sleep has direct effects on thermoregulation. Brain and body temperature are downregulated during NREM sleep, particularly SWS, as a result of a decreased hypothalamic temperature set point, as well as active heat loss. People commonly experience this phenomenon when they go to sleep feeling somewhat cold and wake up several hours later to throw off their extra covers because they feel too warm. During REM sleep, there is a decreased ability to regulate body temperature through sweating and shivering.

Neuroendocrine Changes Most hormones that are regulated by the circadian system also show significant interactions with sleep-wakefulness patterns. *Growth hormone* (GH) is released primarily during the early part of the night, and its secretion is enhanced by SWS. Sleep also stimulates *prolactin* secretion, although prolactin peaks after GH, usually during the middle portion of the night. Pulses of GH and prolactin can occur after the onset of sleep, regardless of its timing, however. GH and prolactin may have feedback effects on sleep as well; GH seems to enhance SWS, whereas prolactin may increase REM sleep. In contrast, *thyroid-stimulating hormone* (TSH) reaches its peak level in the evening just before sleep onset; its secretion is inhibited by sleep and is stimulated by sleep deprivation. The *hypothalamic-pituitary-adrenal* (HPA) *axis* is usually at its most inactive state at nocturnal sleep onset. Sleep onset inhibits cortisol release, whereas *adrenocorticotropic hormone* (ACTH) and *cortisol* levels rise at the end of the sleep period, shortly before awakening, and likely contribute to morning arousal. Severe sleep disruption or sleep deprivation may have significant clinical effects on the endocrine system; for example, patients with obstructive sleep apnea show decreased levels of GH and prolactin, and sleep deprivation produces evidence of HPA axis activation in the evening of the day after deprivation.

Melatonin secretion is mediated by a combination of circadian control and effects of the light–dark cycle. It can only be released at night if it is dark; darkness during the day does not stimulate melatonin secretion. Thus, melatonin can transduce the duration of the photoperiod; it has a significant role in timing reproductive function in some mammals, although its function in humans is less clear. Melatonin can feed back on the circadian clock and may serve to maintain entrainment, which is why is it sometimes recommended for treatment of jet lag or sleep schedule disorders. It may also have a modest hypnotic effect in humans but can produce arousal in nocturnal animals, suggesting that it acts as a modulator of nocturnal behaviors.

Sexual Function One of the characteristics of REM sleep in men is the occurrence of penile erections, beginning in infancy and persisting into old age. Nocturnal penile tumescence studies are therefore helpful in determining whether cases of impotence are related to organic or psychogenic etiologies. In women, REM sleep produces increased vaginal blood flow and clitoral erection. These changes are not necessarily linked to sexual content in associated dreams.

NEUROBIOLOGY OF SLEEP AND WAKEFULNESS

Sleep and wakefulness are governed by separate, yet interacting, systems. Although the specific mechanisms are not fully understood, it is clear that multiple structures and systems in the brainstem, hypothalamus, and basal forebrain are involved in the orchestration of wakefulness, NREM sleep, and REM sleep. No single brain lesion has been able to produce persistent insomnia or sleep. Given the importance of these behaviors to survival, it is not surprising that there is a certain amount of apparent redundancy in their mechanisms.

Wakefulness As mentioned previously, the waking EEG is characterized by an activated pattern with low-voltage fast activity. Correspondingly, positron emission tomography (PET) studies show that, during resting wakefulness, blood flow and metabolic activity are higher than in NREM sleep. The most active brain areas include the prefrontal cortex, the anterior cingulate parietal cortex, and the precuneus, as indicated by increased regional cerebral blood flow (rCBF); these areas are known to be involved in attention, cognition, and memory.

Maintenance of wakefulness is dependent on the *ascending reticular activating system* (ARAS), which is comprised of inputs from the oral pontine and the midbrain tegmentum, as well as the posterior hypothalamus (Fig. 1.20–4). In animals, electrical stimulation of these regions produces an activated EEG pattern and behavioral arousal. Lesions may produce a coma-like state, although recovery of cortical activity can sometimes occur given sufficient time, suggesting that structures outside the brainstem reticular formation are also involved in maintaining wakefulness. Clinically, lesions in the midbrain or posterior hypothalamus can produce somnolence, stupor, or coma.

It is now known that several distinct structures and neurochemical systems with diffuse projections are involved in wakefulness, including noradrenergic cells in the *locus ceruleus* (LC), cholinergic cells in the *pedunculopontine tegmental* (PPT) and *lateral dorsal tegmental* (LDT) nuclei, histaminergic cells in the *tubero-*

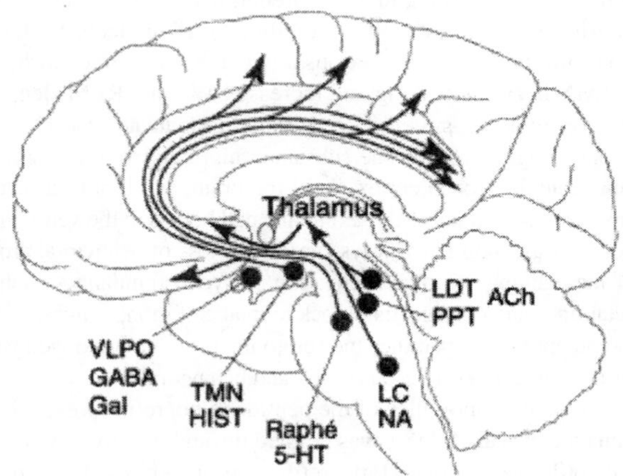

FIGURE 1.20–4 The ascending arousal system sends projections from the brainstem and posterior hypothalamus throughout the forebrain. Neurons of the laterodorsal tegmental (LDT) nuclei and pedunculopontine tegmental (PPT) nuclei send cholinergic fibers (Ach) to many forebrain targets, including the thalamus, which then regulate cortical activity. Aminergic nuclei diffusely project throughout much of the forebrain, regulating the activity of cortical and hypothalamic targets directly. Aminergic neurons of the tuberomammillary nucleus (TMN) contain histamine (HIST), neurons of the raphe nuclei contain serotonin (5-HT), and neurons of the locus ceruleus (LC) contain noradrenaline (NA). Sleep-promoting neurons of the ventrolateral preoptic (VLPO) nucleus contain γ-aminobutyric acid (GABA) and galanin (Gal). (From Saper CB, Chou TC, Scammell TE: The sleep switch: Hypothalamic control of sleep and wakefulness. *Trends Neurosci.* 2001;24:726, with permission.)

mammillary nucleus (TMN) of the posterior hypothalamus, and glutamatergic neurons in various structures in the CNS. The ARAS produces cortical activation via input to the thalamus, as well as through an extrathalamic pathway with projections to the hypothalamus and basal forebrain.

Noradrenergic cells from the LC project directly throughout the brain and show their highest discharge rates during wakefulness, decrease their firing during NREM sleep, and cease firing altogether during REM sleep. Recent evidence suggests that wakefulness and sleep differ not only in terms of behavior, metabolism, and neuronal activity, but also in terms of gene expression. LC cells are responsible for at least some of the changes in gene expression that occur in the brain between wakefulness and sleep.

Cholinergic cells from the oral pontine region (LDT, PPT) fire at high rates when the EEG is activated, that is, in wakefulness and REM sleep, but reduce firing in NREM sleep. They promote cortical activation through inputs to the thalamus, hypothalamus, and basal forebrain. In addition, cholinergic cell bodies in the basal forebrain, including the nucleus basalis, substantia innominata, diagonal band of Broca, and septum receive input from the ARAS and, in turn, provide excitatory input to the entire cortex. Loss of cholinergic cells in Alzheimer's patients is associated with slowing of the cortical EEG. Drugs with anticholinergic activity, including tricyclic antidepressants, can cause sedation and can increase slow wave activity. On the other hand, cholinergic agonists (e.g., nicotine) or anticholinesterase inhibitors (e.g., neostigmine [Prostigmin]) enhance arousal.

Histaminergic neurons in the TMN of the posterior hypothalamus also appear to have an important wakefulness-promoting function, in part inferred from the fact that antihistaminergic drugs typically produce sedation. The significance of this region for waking was first identified by Constantin von Economo in the early part of the 20th century after an outbreak of viral encephalitis; *encephalitis lethargica*, as it was called, produced lesions of the posterior hypothalamus and profound somnolence. Histaminergic TMN neurons project throughout the cortex and, like noradrenergic cells, fire at the highest rates during wakefulness and are inhibited during sleep. Histamine infusion into the CNS causes arousal, whereas experimental lesions of the TMN decrease waking and increase SWS and REM sleep.

The dopaminergic system also appears to modulate arousal. Dopamine-containing neurons in the substantia nigra and ventral tegmental area innervate the frontal cortex, basal forebrain, and limbic structures. Lesions of areas containing dopaminergic cell bodies in the ventral midbrain or their ascending pathways can lead to loss of behavioral arousal while maintaining cortical activation. Psychostimulants, such as amphetamines and cocaine, that block reuptake of monoamines, including norepinephrine, dopamine, and serotonin, promote prolonged wakefulness and increase cortical activation and behavioral arousal.

Recently, the importance of the peptide hypocretin (orexin) in the maintenance of wakefulness was defined through discovering its role in the disorder narcolepsy. Hypocretin is produced by cells in the lateral hypothalamus that provide excitatory input to all components of the ARAS, including the LC, PPT, and LDT, ventral tegmental area, basal forebrain, and TMN. These neurons also appear to be most activated during waking, especially with motor activity. Animal models of narcolepsy are related to deficits in the hypocretin system; canine narcolepsy is caused by a mutation in the hypocretin type II receptor gene, whereas narcoleptic symptoms (sleep attacks and sleep-onset REM periods) occur in hypocretin knock-out mice. Human narcoleptics show loss of hypocretin cells in the brain, loss of hypocretin protein in the cerebrospinal fluid (CSF), or both.

Serotonergic cells from the *dorsal raphe* nucleus also project widely throughout the cortex. Serotonergic neurons, like noradrenergic neurons, fire at higher levels in waking and lower levels in NREM sleep and fall silent during REM sleep. However, in sharp contrast to noradrenergic neurons, serotoninergic neurons are inactivated during orientation to salient stimuli and are activated instead during repetitive motor activity, such as locomotion, grooming, or feeding. Selective serotonin reuptake inhibitors (SSRIs) tend to decrease sleep time and increase arousal during sleep. The role of serotonin in sleep is not straightforward, however, because there is also evidence that serotonin may be involved in sleep induction.

A number of other neurotransmitters and neuromodulators appear to have wakefulness-promoting effects. These include substance P, neurotensin, epinephrine, and hypothalamic peptides, such as corticotropin-releasing factor, vasoactive intestinal peptide, and thyrotropin-releasing factor, all of which can increase arousal levels. Cortisol also promotes wakefulness. It is thus possible that sleep disturbance in depression, including early morning awakening, could be related, in part, to the associated hyperactivity of the HPA axis.

NREM Sleep

The EEG of NREM sleep is dramatically different from waking and is characterized by oscillatory waveforms, such as sleep spindles, K complexes, delta waves (1 to 4 cps), and slow oscillations (mainly, 0.7 to 1.0 cps). Brain activation generally decreases in NREM sleep, particularly SWS, which is characterized by an overall decrease in cerebral blood flow. PET imaging studies show deactivation of many structures, including the brainstem, thalamus, anterior hypothalamus, basal forebrain, basal ganglia, cerebellum, and frontal, parietal, and mesiotemporal cortical areas.

The control of NREM sleep, like wakefulness, involves multiple structures ranging from the lower brainstem to the thalamus, hypothalamus, and forebrain. Electrophysiological studies in animals have clarified the generation of various thalamocortical oscillations that result in the characteristic waveforms in NREM sleep. The generation of sleep oscillations requires the interplay between intrinsic cellular properties and synaptic activity mediated by corticocortical, corticothalamocortical, and thalamoreticular loops. Work in animals has shown that, shortly before the transition from waking to sleep, changes in the activity of cholinergic, noradrenergic, histaminergic, and glutamatergic neuromodulatory systems with diffuse projections belonging to the ARAS bring about a change in firing mode of thalamic and cortical neurons. Thalamocortical cells are hyperpolarized, whereas reticulothalamic cells are facilitated and further inhibit thalamocortical cells, with the consequence that sensory stimuli are gated at the thalamic level and often fail to reach the cortex. Rebound firing due to the activation of intrinsic currents in thalamocortical cells leads to the emergence of oscillations in the spindle frequency range within local thalamoreticular circuits. Local thalamic spindle sequences are globally synchronized and grouped with other rhythmic activities by the slow oscillations that originate in the cortex. Intracellular recordings have shown that the slow oscillation is the result of a prolonged hyperpolarization of cortical neurons (approximately 0.5 seconds), which is seen in the surface EEG as a high-amplitude negative wave. The hyperpolarization phase is followed by a slightly longer depolarization phase, during which the firing of cortical neurons entrains and synchronizes spindle sequences in thalamic neurons, resulting in EEG-detectable spindles. K complexes are made up of the cortical depolarization phase followed by its triggered spindle. The slow oscillation also organizes delta waves, which can be generated within the thalamus and the cortex. The hyperpolarization phase of the slow oscillation is associated with the virtual absence of synaptic activity within cortical networks. By contrast, during the depolarized phase, cortical cells fire at rates that can be higher than those seen in waking. Moreover, during the depolarized phase, thalamocortical neurons often fire rhythmically in the gamma range (approximately 40 cps), which was previously thought to be exclusively associated with activated states, such as wakefulness and REM sleep. The slow oscillation is found in virtually every cortical neuron and is synchronized across the cortical mantle by corticocortical connections. Intrinsic currents are also involved in initiating and terminating the oscillation.

The importance of hypothalamic structures for sleep induction was recognized in early studies in which electrical stimulation of the anterior hypothalamus resulted in increased slow wave activity in the cortex. Conversely, some cases of encephalitis lethargica, in which lesions occurred in the anterior, rather than posterior, hypothalamus, were characterized by severe insomnia. Recently, attention has focused on the *ventrolateral preoptic* (VLPO) *area* as a possible sleep switch. The expression of the gene *c-fos*, whose induction is often associated with neural activation, is increased during sleep in VLPO neurons. The VLPO area has important inhibitory inputs (through release of γ-aminobutyric acid [GABA] and galanin) to wakefulness-promoting centers in the TMN, LC, dorsal raphe, and cholinergic regions in the pons and basal forebrain (Fig. 1.20–5); all of these regions provide reciprocal inputs to the VLPO area, also probably of an inhibitory nature. It has been suggested that this strong bidirectional inhibitory relationship between sleep and wakefulness provides state stability, in that each state reinforces itself as well as inhibits the opponent state. Experimental ablation of the VLPO area in animals leads to reductions in NREM and REM sleep, and VLPO neurons show increased activity in REM as well as NREM, suggesting that this area may modulate both types of sleep.

In terms of NREM sleep neurochemistry, many substances modulate sleep, but no unique sleep factor has been identified. GABA, the major inhibitory neurotransmitter in the CNS, appears to be involved in thalamocortical oscillations and VLPO-mediated inhibition of waking centers. Most hypnotics, including barbiturates, benzodiazepines, and several of the newer nonbenzodiazapine hypnotics act by enhancing GABA transmission.

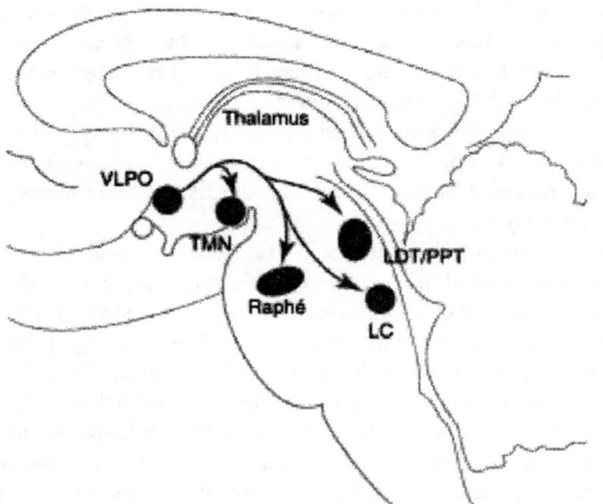

FIGURE 1.20–5 The projections from the ventrolateral preoptic (VLPO) nucleus to the main components of the ascending arousal system. LC, locus ceruleus; LDT, lateral dorsal tegmental nuclei; PPT, pedunculopontine tegmental nuclei; TMN, tuberomammillary nucleus. (From Saper CB, Chou TC, Scammell TE: The sleep switch: Hypothalamic control of sleep and wakefulness. *Trends Neurosci.* 2001;24:726, with permission.)

Adenosine has been increasingly recognized as having a role in sleep. Caffeine probably exerts its stimulant effects by blocking adenosine receptors. Adenosine, a degradation product of adenosine triphosphate (ATP), accumulates in the basal forebrain during prolonged wakefulness and decreases during sleep, suggesting that it may serve to transmit the homeostatic signal for sleep. Adenosine infusion promotes SWS sleep, and adenosine inhibits cholinergic neurons in the pons and basal forebrain.

Early studies raised the possibility that serotonin might also be involved in SWS, because lesions of serotoninergic nerve cells in the dorsal raphe led to insomnia. Serotoninergic neurons decrease firing rates in NREM sleep and are completely inhibited during REM. However, they inhibit cholinergic neurons and produce behavioral inhibition, raising the possibility that they help facilitate sleep onset, although they may not be involved in directly inducing or maintaining sleep. It remains controversial as to how much serotonin contributes to sleep versus arousal.

A large number of other substances, including peptides and neuromodulators, have been attributed with sleep-promoting properties. These include a variety of hormones, such as melatonin, α-melanocyte-stimulating hormone, GH-releasing factor, insulin, cholecystokinin, and bombesin; cytokines, such as interleukin-1, interleukin-6, and tumor necrosis factor; muramyl peptides produced from gut bacteria; and dozens of other substances. Most of these factors have mild hypnotic or circadian effects, or both, consistent with the usual timing of their release (e.g., melatonin or GH-releasing factor, which is normally released at night) or the physiological state of the organism (e.g., cytokines produced during infectious illness promote sleep).

REM Sleep REM sleep is characterized by an activated EEG and increased neuronal activity and cerebral blood flow. Recent studies using functional imaging techniques have shown that, during REM sleep, there are some brain regions showing increased activation as well as others with decreased activation in comparison to wakefulness. Areas involved in REM sleep generation in the mesopontine tegmentum, thalamus, posterior cortical areas, and limbic areas, particularly the amygdala, are highly activated during REM sleep. In contrast, frontal and parietal cortices are relatively deactivated.

REM sleep is somewhat unique because specific brain regions—the *pons* and *caudal midbrain*—are necessary and sufficient to generate the features of REM sleep and represent the final common pathway for the induction of REM sleep. A series of transection studies has demonstrated that REM sleep is preserved only in the portion of the CNS containing these structures. Bilateral lesions within the pons and caudal midbrain can completely eliminate REM sleep. Although these findings have created a tendency to focus on brainstem mechanisms of REM sleep, more rostral brain regions are also important in organizing REM episodes across the night.

As in wakefulness, cholinergic neurons produce EEG activation and hippocampal theta rhythm during REM sleep. LDT and PPT neurons provide input to the thalamus and cholinergic basal forebrain neurons that, in turn, activate the limbic system and cortex. J. Allan Hobson and Robert McCarley proposed the reciprocal interaction hypothesis to explain NREM-REM cycles based on interactions between cholinergic and aminergic neurons in the mesopontine junction. Cholinoceptive or cholinergic, or both, REM-on cells in the PPT and LDT regions become activated during REM sleep, whereas noradrenergic or serotoninergic REM-off cells are inhibitory of the REM-on cells. The aminergic cell groups are most active during waking; they decrease activity somewhat during NREM sleep. Meanwhile, cholinergic activity increases to turn on REM sleep.

REM sleep episodes are terminated because REM-on cells are self-inhibitory and provide excitatory input to the REM-off cells.

The role of cholinergic–monoaminergic interactions in regulating REM sleep is supported by a variety of experimental data. Local infusion of cholinergic agonists, such as carbachol (Carbastat), in the region of the LDT and PPT of cats or systemic administration of physostigmine (Eserine Salicylate), arecoline, pilocarpine (Salagen), or other cholinergic agonists in humans produces prolonged REM sleep episodes and reduced latency to REM sleep. Cholinergic induction of REM sleep appears to be related primarily to activation of muscarinic type 2 (M2) receptors in pontine reticular formation. Facilitation of REM sleep also results from depletion of brainstem monoaminergic activity, for example, in human subjects with an acute depletion of serotonin after being fed a tryptophan-deficient diet. Most antidepressants cause significant reductions in REM sleep, particularly those that increase synaptic availability of norepinephrine or serotonin, or both; anticholinergic effects seen in tricyclics and monoamine oxidase inhibitors (MAOIs) may also contribute to REM sleep suppression.

Muscle atonia in REM sleep can be eliminated by small lesions in the pontine reticular formation lateral to the LC or by lesions in the medial medulla that eliminate inhibitory input from this area to the spinal motoneurons. Tonic hyperpolarization of spinal motoneurons during REM sleep appears to be mediated by glycine, whereas the phasic muscle twitches may be mediated by glutamate acting at *N*-methyl-D-aspartate (NMDA) receptors. Disfacilitation of spinal motoneurons resulting from decreased monoaminergic activity also contributes to suppression of muscle tone during REM sleep. Several clinical conditions illustrate how atonia may be separated from the state of REM sleep. In narcolepsy, muscle atonia can occur during wakefulness as cataplexy, a sudden loss of muscle tone usually brought on by emotional stimuli, or sleep paralysis, in which atonia persists briefly after waking out of REM sleep. In contrast, patients with REM sleep behavior disorder do not develop atonia during REM sleep and act out their dreams, sometimes with such violence that they may injure themselves or their bed partners. REM sleep-suppressing antidepressants, such as tricyclics, MAOIs, and SSRIs, may induce REM sleep behavior disorder in some individuals.

In animals, pontogeniculooccipital (PGO) waves that occur sequentially in the pons, lateral geniculate nucleus of the thalamus, and occipital cortex appear just before the initiation of REM periods and in conjunction with phasic activity in REM sleep, including eye movements and muscle twitches. They originate from cholinergic cells in the peribrachial region and are suppressed by serotonergic cells in the raphe nuclei. Eye movements during REM sleep are tightly linked to PGO waves and are mediated by inputs to vestibular neurons that, in turn, activate oculomotor cells. PGO waves are thought to be the internal representation of orienting responses, because they can also be observed during a startle response during waking.

In addition to recent imaging data showing dramatically increased activity in forebrain structures during REM sleep, previous work has also suggested forebrain involvement in REM sleep regulation. Transection studies that separate forebrain from pons disrupt NREM-REM cycling caudal to the transection. The amygdala has reciprocal connections with REM-generating brainstem regions, and electrical stimulation or infusion of carbachol into the amygdala can increase REM sleep. Abnormal activation of limbic structures occurs in depression and may contribute to associated changes in REM sleep.

CIRCADIAN AND HOMEOSTATIC REGULATION OF SLEEP

The regulation of sleep—NREM and REM—involves at least two key components: a circadian one and a homeostatic one. The circadian component is responsible for the change in sleep propensity that is tied to the time of day, with obvious adaptive advantages. The homeostatic component refers to the fact that the longer one stays awake, the greater the propensity to sleep, and it represents the essential aspect of sleep whose function remains mysterious.

Two-Process Model Several models of sleep regulation positing a circadian and a homeostatic process have been proposed and validated on the basis of a large amount of data. One of the most influential is the *two-process model* developed by Alexander A. Borbély and colleagues, which predicts sleep propensity based on the interaction between the homeostatic *process S* and the circadian *process C*. Process S builds up across the day in response to the increase in sleep pressure caused by wakefulness and decreases during sleep. The circadian process C, on the other hand, reaches its peak during the latter half of the night. Thus, nocturnal sleep onset is primarily driven by process S, whereas process C maintains sleep through the latter part of the night. It is common for humans to have a brief period of arousal in the middle of the night, possibly related to a reduction in overall sleep drive from the fall in process S before process C has reached its maximal values. Similarly, the tendency for afternoon napping may be caused by the increase in process S across the day before process C has reached its lowest values in the late afternoon or early evening. Although napping during the day has become relatively uncommon in industrialized societies, most people experience a period of increased sleepiness in the afternoon. This afternoon dip can produce significant daytime sleepiness in individuals who are already somewhat sleep deprived, are taking sedating medications, or have sleep disorders causing excessive daytime sleepiness, such as sleep apnea, or a combination of these.

Circadian Rhythms In humans and other mammals, the primary pacemaker for generating circadian rhythms lies in the *suprachiasmatic nucleus* (SCN) of the hypothalamus. As described in Section 1.13, the SCN regulates a number of neuroendocrine and behavioral parameters, including sleep propensity as measured by process C, to coordinate the state of the organism with the 24-hour light–dark cycle. Circadian sleep regulation is strongly linked to the endogenous temperature rhythm; subjective sleepiness, sleep propensity, and REM sleep propensity are all maximal at the minimum (nadir) of core body temperature, usually in the very early morning, several hours before waking up. Sleep tendency is greater on the falling phase of the temperature curve, during the night. When core body temperature begins its rising phase in the morning hours, people tend to wake up; arousal levels, performance, and cognitive function are maximal in association with the rise of body temperature across the day.

In animals in which the SCN has been lesioned, sleep is no longer concentrated in one main episode but is dispersed across the entire 24-hour cycle. Still, in these animals, sleep propensity increases as a function of previous waking. Thus, although process C and process S normally work together and interact significantly, they can, to a large extent, be separated. Several approaches have been used to investigate specifically the circadian regulation of sleep in humans. The *constant routine* protocol was designed to minimize the influences of factors other than the circadian clock on behavioral state. In this protocol, subjects are kept awake, usually for more than 24 hours, while sitting in bed in a dimly lit room. This technique has been used successfully to demonstrate the persistence of various circadian outputs in the absence of external cues, but the need to enforce sleep deprivation limits the duration of the experiment. With *temporal isolation*, subjects are placed in an environment without time cues for periods of weeks to months. Although circadian rhythms of sleep persist, the *day length*, as defined by the period between successive bedtimes, is close to 25 hours. These results led to the conclusion that the endogenous period of the human circadian clock is approximately 25 hours, and that the light–dark cycle serves to entrain it to the 24-hour day.

To accurately determine the endogenous period of the circadian pacemaker, it is necessary to disentangle the circadian output from the effects of sleep or prolonged sleeplessness; however, neither of the two protocols discussed previously can satisfactorily achieve this. The *forced desynchrony* protocol, originally developed by Nathaniel Kleitman in 1938, consists of having subjects live on a 28-hour day in temporal isolation. Because it is not possible to entrain the human circadian clock to a period of 28 hours, after a sufficient period of time, sleep periods occur at all phases of the circadian cycle. Thus, circadian and homeostatic influences on human sleep organization can be teased apart. Data from forced desynchrony studies suggest that the endogenous human circadian period is, in fact, close to 24 hours (24.1 to 24.2 hours). Moreover, they show that SWS is primarily regulated by the homeostatic sleep drive, whereas REM sleep is primarily regulated by the circadian clock. However, REM sleep is also homeostatically regulated, as indicated by the rising number of attempts to initiate REM sleep if that stage of sleep is prevented.

HOMEOSTATIC REGULATION OF SLEEP AND THE EFFECTS OF SLEEP DEPRIVATION

In humans, as well as in virtually all animal species in which sleep has been carefully studied, sleep deprivation produces sleepiness and increased sleep pressure that soon become overwhelming. Sleep deprivation is followed by a *sleep rebound*—that is, a compensatory increase in the duration or the intensity of sleep, or both. After sleep deprivation, sleep latency is decreased, and sleep efficiency is increased, that is, sleep is less fragmented. The amount of NREM sleep (especially stages III and IV in humans) increases, together with markers of NREM sleep intensity, such as slow wave activity in the cortical EEG. REM sleep amount also increases, but it is unclear whether this is also true for REM sleep intensity. Such exquisite homeostatic regulation is one of the most important indications that there must be a distinct physiological, biochemical, or molecular process that builds up beyond its usual level in the brain if sleep initiation is postponed. As discussed at the end of this chapter, it is this process that is still not understood.

The most prominent effect of total sleep deprivation in humans is cognitive impairment, with striking practical consequences. Each year, errors due to sleep deprivation and sleepiness cause 25,000 deaths and 2.5 million disabling injuries and cost more than $56 billion in the United States alone. Moreover, the National Highway Traffic Safety Administration estimates conservatively that, each year, drowsy driving is responsible for at least 100,000 automobile crashes, 71,000 injuries, and 1,550 fatalities. A sleep-deprived person tends to take longer to respond to stimuli, particularly when tasks are monotonous and low in cognitive demands. However, sleep deprivation produces more than just decreased alertness. Tasks emphasizing higher cognitive functions, such as logical reasoning; encoding, decoding, and parsing complex sentences; complex subtraction tasks; and tasks requiring divergent thinking, such as those involving a flexible thinking style and the ability to focus on a large number of goals simultaneously, are all significantly affected even after one single night of sleep deprivation. Tasks requiring sustained attention, such as those including goal-directed activities, can also be impaired by even a few hours of sleep loss. Thus, sleep loss causes attention deficits, decreases in short-term memory, speech impairments, perseveration, and inflexible thinking. These deficits can explain why sleep-deprived subjects underestimate the severity of their cognitive impairment, often with tragic consequences. Another reason is the fact that the lack of sleep does not completely eliminate the capacity to perform but rather makes the performance inconsistent and unreliable. Thus, a sleepy driver responds normally to an emergency or not at all, owing to rapid changes in vigilance state and the sudden intrusion of microsleeps during waking. Similarly, subjects may still be able to transiently perform at baseline levels in short tests even after 3 to 4 days of sleep deprivation. However, the same subjects perform very poorly when engaged in tasks requiring sustained attention. New evidence suggests that not just a few hours of sleep, but several days of normal sleep–wake patterns are required to normalize cognitive performance after sleep deprivation.

Cognitive impairment is unfortunately not only a consequence of total sleep deprivation. Cognitive performance is also affected by sleep restriction (5 hours per night) if it continues for several days and by chronic sleep discontinuity, such as that occurring in patients with chronic pain or sleep apnea. According to the 2002 "Sleep in America" poll conducted by the National Sleep Foundation, United States residents of at least 18 years of age slept on average 6.9 hours during weekdays and 7.5 hours on weekends. Twenty-four percent of the respondents in this poll reported that, during weekdays, they slept less than they needed to not feel sleepy the next day. Whether this chronic sleep restriction is sufficient to affect objective measures of cognitive performance is not known but is certainly concerning given the data from sleep restriction studies.

Brain and peripheral tissues respond differently to sleep loss. As in sleep-deprived animals, the peripheral metabolic rate is increased in sleep-deprived human subjects, as well as in insomniacs, relative to normal sleepers and in normal sleepers on nights of poor sleep relative to baseline nights. In animals and humans, glucose metabolism is higher in many brain regions in waking than in NREM sleep. After one day of sleep deprivation, selective brain areas can still be activated metabolically when the subject is engaged in specific tasks. However, global cerebral metabolic rate does not increase and actually decreases relative to normal waking values in brain areas such as the thalamus and the midbrain. Thus, although peripheral metabolic rate is persistently increased during sleep deprivation, brain metabolic rate is not. This may be an indication that the brain cannot sustain high-energy metabolism for too long.

In addition to cognitive impairment, sleep deprivation in humans may also affect various physiological systems with impacts on overall health. It has been suggested that sleep loss can affect host defense systems; for example, sleep-deprived rats show increased rates of bacteremia. Sleep deprivation has also been shown to lead to decreased glucose tolerance, increased sympathetic nervous system activation, and elevated cortisol levels, suggesting that it may contribute to disorders such as diabetes, hypertension, and obesity. Patients with insomnia have increased rates of health problems, including cardiac disease, further suggesting a possible causal relationship between reduced sleep amounts and health outcomes. Some studies have linked long-term disturbances in sleep with reduced longevity. Others have suggested that, in fact, short sleep and insomnia are associated with little risk distinct from comorbidities. This issue remains controversial; additional longitudinal studies to determine the specific contributions of sleep loss on health are needed.

The most extreme case of prolonged sleep loss in humans is observed in patients affected by fatal familial insomnia (FFI), a prion disorder characterized by near-complete loss of sleep associated with various neurological symptoms and spongiform degeneration in select brain regions. The disease is invariably fatal after a course of a few months to 2 to 3 years. In FFI with a short clinical course (death in <1 year), insomnia is almost complete from the onset, and spongiform degeneration is mainly restricted to the thalamus and inferior olive but does not extend to the cerebral cortex. In FFI cases with longer clinical course (death in 2 to 3 years), insomnia develops more gradually, and spongiform degeneration is found in most cortical regions. Although several clinical aspects of FFI can be attributed to diffuse spongiform degeneration, it is likely that sleep loss per se plays an important role in determining the evolution of the disease, especially in short course FFI. Indeed, the severity of the clinical course correlates with the severity of the insomnia rather than with the accumulation of prion protein.

In humans, sleep deprivation is never enforced for more than 3 to 4 days (the record is 11 days, but in only one subject), making it impossible to determine whether there are other more severe effects of prolonged sleep loss. Prolonged sleep deprivation is possible in animals, in which several techniques have been used, from forced locomotion to pharmacological stimulation with amphetamines. Irrespective of the method used, an important and consistent finding is that even drastic manipulations, such as brain electrical stimulation, are unable to enforce complete and uninterrupted wakefulness after the first 24 hours. Evidently, sleep pressure overcomes whatever method is used to maintain wakefulness in animals as well as in humans.

The most comprehensive series of sleep deprivation studies in animals has been performed using the *disk-over-water* (DOW) *apparatus*, which can prevent sleep for days and even weeks. This method uses minimal stimulation to enforce chronic sleep deprivation in the sleep-deprived rat, while it simultaneously applies the same stimulation to the control rat, but without severely limiting its sleep. Sleep deprivation with the DOW apparatus produces a series of dramatic physiological changes that culminate invariably in death after 2 to 3 weeks of sleep loss. Within the first 1 to 2 days, rats develop a syndrome characterized by an increase in food intake, energy expenditure, and heart rate, followed by a decrease in body weight and a decline in body and brain temperature. The sleep deprivation syndrome and its lethal consequences have also been observed after selective REM sleep deprivation; although the pathology associated with the loss of sleep takes longer to appear, the survival time is longer (4 to 5 weeks instead of 2 to 3 weeks), and body and brain temperature are not significantly decreased. Despite a long series of studies, the DOW sleep deprivation syndrome has not been fully explained nor it is clear why the animals die of sleep deprivation. It is evident, however, that the syndrome produced by the DOW is not unique, and other methods of chronic sleep deprivation used in different animal species have produced similar effects. In dogs, rabbits, and, to a lesser extent, cats, sleep deprivation for several days also causes an increase in food intake and heart rate, weight loss, and eventually death. Even fruit flies, if prevented from sleeping for several days, die of sleep deprivation. Again, these findings suggest that there must be at least one potentially vital function for sleep and that this function is conserved across different animal species.

DREAMING

For a long time, sleep has been regarded as the annihilation of consciousness, save for the occasional dream that is remembered on awakening. Just as the old notion that the brain is silent during sleep has been disproved, so has the myth of cognitive death during sleep. Most subjects, if awakened and asked to report whatever may be going through their minds, report some kind of mental activity most of the time. Often, such mental activity constitutes a dream, which can be defined as a complex, temporally unfolding, hallucinatory episode that occurs during sleep.

Differences between Dreaming and Normal Waking Consciousness

Dream hallucinations are typically more vivid than waking images. Images are predominantly visual, although all modalities can be represented, and impossible motor activities, such as flying, may occur. Hearing speech or conversation is extremely frequent. Dreaming is generally delusional—events and characters in the dream are taken for real—and confabulatory—a dream involves making up a story. There is often disorientation, that is, uncertainty about space (where one is in the dream), about time (when the dream is taking place in personal history), and confusion about the gender, age, and identity of dream characters. However, dreams appear to run in real time, as there are good correlations between the subjective duration of a dream, the length of the dream report, and the time it would take to reenact a dream. Emotions are prominent in many dreams, especially fear and anxiety. Although the self is almost always at the center of the dream, there is some reduction of reflective consciousness. Dreams have been described as single-minded, that is, missing the alternation of primary and reflective consciousness that characterize wakefulness. Self-monitoring, directed thinking, and volition are reduced, leading to an inability to analyze situations, to question assumptions, and to make appropriate decisions. The ability to form new memories is drastically impaired (dream amnesia). Not surprisingly, psychiatrists have pointed out similarities between some aspects of dreaming cognition and certain psychotic symptoms, as well as delirium.

Similarities between Dreaming and Waking Consciousness

Despite these psychopathological traits, perhaps the most important fact about dreaming consciousness is how remarkably similar it can be to waking consciousness. That is, the sleeping brain, disconnected from the "real" world, is capable of generating an imagined world, a virtual reality that is fairly similar to the "real" one and is indeed experienced as equally real. When they consider them in the waking state, people are often intrigued by the bizarre quality of some dreams, especially morning dreams, but it should be kept in mind that, if collected systematically throughout the night, dreams are much more mundane—they are a faithful replica of waking life. The ingredients of sleep are much the same as the ingredients of waking consciousness or waking imagery. As a rule, one can dream what one can imagine, although dreams are much more vivid, probably because of the reduced competition from external signals. If blind people can still construct visual images, they have visual dreams, otherwise not. If a stroke abolishes the ability to perceive color during waking, visual images, as well as dreams, become achromatopsic. Like the ability to form mental images, dreaming seems to depend most strongly on the integrity of cortical areas higher than the primary visual cortex. Similarly, somatosensory motor and audioverbal motor imagery are normal in the dreams of hemiplegic and aphasic patients. Another example of the close connection between waking and dreaming cognitive competence comes from the study of children's dreams. Dream reports are rare and extremely short until 4 to 5 years of age—in agreement with the limited ability of children of that age to imagine and to narrate complex stories with high emotional content. Finally, there is a good correlation between waking and dreaming mood, imaginativeness, and personality. Studies of dream content in psychiatric populations, especially in depression and posttraumatic stress disorder (PTSD), have generally been unremarkable. However, some intriguing findings have been reported, for example, that changes in dream content may anticipate changes in the course of the disorder.

Dreaming and Sleep Stages

It was initially suggested that full-fledged dreams could be elicited almost exclusively during REM sleep. Later studies have shown conclusively, however, that dream-like mental activity can be elicited also from NREM sleep, especially at sleep onset and during the last part of the night—the times when NREM sleep is less deep. As much as 15 percent of subjects, however, never recall any mental content when awakened from NREM sleep. Moreover, typical REM dream reports can easily be distinguished from NREM ones by being, on average, much longer (as much as seven times longer). When dream reports are longer, this suggests longer duration of the actual dream, but they may also be due to an increased density or bizarreness of the experienced scenes. Whether REM dreams are not just longer, but also qualitatively different—more bizarre, hallucinatory, delusional, narrative, and emotional than NREM—dreaming remains controversial. So is the suggestion that NREM dreams may be covert REM dreams, due to an intrusion of REM characteristics in NREM sleep. There is no doubt, however, that typical dreams, as well as nightmares, can be experienced in certain phases of NREM sleep. Dream-like mental activity having a hallucinatory-delusional character can also occur during quiet wakefulness, especially under conditions of reduced sensory input (daydreaming). Conversely, some waking-like mental activity—nonhallucinatory and nondelusional—is occasionally reported at sleep onset. A good example of a mixed state is lucid dreaming, where dreamers are aware that they are dreaming and, to some extent, can control the course of their dreams.

The initial equating of the cognitive state of dreaming with the physiological state of REM sleep was encouraged by the remarkable similarity between the EEG of REM sleep with that of conscious waking and by their equivalent differences from the NREM sleep EEG. It seemed natural to infer that the activated (low-voltage, high-frequency) EEG of waking and REM sleep would support vivid conscious experience, whereas the deactivated (high-voltage, low-frequency) EEG of NREM sleep would not. Although frequent dream reports at sleep onset could still be reconciled with the mixed EEG of stage I sleep, the presence of dream-like experiences, although shorter, during NREM stages characterized by EEG slow waves seemed paradoxical. This paradox may be resolved by considering the time course of neural excitability during the slow oscillation of NREM sleep. It is now known that, during the depolarized phase of the slow oscillation, neural activity is as intense as in waking or REM sleep, and neurons are highly excitable. However, the depolarized phase is interrupted, roughly once a second, by a hyperpolarized phase during which neural activity ceases throughout the cerebral cortex, and neurons are much less excitable. If dream-like experiences occur during the depolarized phase, they cannot be long or rich because of the interruption of experience associated with the hyperpolarized phase. Altogether, it would seem that the likelihood of conscious experience during sleep is related to moment-to-moment cortical activation, indicated by the readiness of cortical neurons to respond to incoming signals.

Neural Correlates of Dreaming Consciousness

Recently, lesion and imaging studies have provided new insights into brain correlates of the characteristic differences between dreaming and waking consciousness. The most obvious difference is that dreaming consciousness is only marginally influenced by external stimuli, few of which are incorporated into the dream narrative. During NREM sleep, partial functional disconnection is mediated by thalamic inhibition. During REM sleep, external stimuli more easily pass the thalamic gate and reach primary cortical areas, but they do not seem to influence higher cortical areas, as if the brain were not paying attention to them. The hallucinatory character of dreams is obviously facilitated by such sensory disconnection. Visual hallucinosis of dreams is indeed associated with increased activity in higher visual areas, whereas the primary visual cortex is less active, as indicated by PET studies. Whether the intense visual experience and scene changes characteristic of dreams are triggered primarily by phasic signals from the brainstem or by areas involved in visual imagery, or both, is an unresolved issue.

Another relevant difference between dreaming and waking consciousness concerns the ability to reflect on oneself and one's experience, especially the ability to judge the verisimilitude of dreaming experience. Imaging studies indicate that the dorsolateral prefrontal cortex, a brain region implicated in volitional control and self-monitoring, is less active in sleep compared to waking. Reduced activation of the dorsolateral prefrontal cortex may also contribute to the disorientation and reduction of directed thinking and working memory observed in dreams and may contribute to dreaming amnesia. Recent episodic memories are conspicuously absent in dreams, and memory for dreams is strikingly labile, unless one wakes up and rehearses the dream.

Dreams are also characterized by a high degree of emotional involvement, especially fear and anxiety. Correspondingly, imaging studies have revealed a marked activation of limbic and paralimbic structures, such as the amygdala, the anterior cingulate, and the insular and medial orbitofrontal cortex, during REM sleep. Altogether, cognitive activity during sleep provides a powerful indication of the extent to which fluctuating levels of several neuromodulators, whose dysfunction is implicated in several psychiatric disorders, can affect mental function in healthy subjects. Indeed, Hobson has suggested that most aspects of dreaming cognition can be explained by considering the level of three processes—brain activation, input source (external or internal), and neuromodulation—across the sleep–waking continuum.

Theories of Dreaming

In what he considered his most important work—*The Interpretation of Dreams*—Sigmund Freud suggested that dreams provide disguised wish fulfillment and, if properly interpreted, would provide essential clues to the most profound determinants of psychic life, "the royal road to the unconscious." The systematic investigation of dreams has not provided much support for this notion.

A radically different suggestion was made by Hobson and McCarley based on their neurophysiological studies of REM sleep–generating mechanisms in the brainstem. According to their activation-synthesis hypothesis, dreams were the forebrain's attempt to make sense of the random activation of thalamocortical networks by the upper brainstem, like the music produced by unmusical fingers wandering over the keys of a piano. Another suggestion, based on a comprehensive evaluation of dream reports, was made by David Foulkes and others. According to this view, dreams reveal not so much the psychodynamic unconscious, but instead, the cognitive development, competence, and style of the dreamer, just as in waking cognition. This view carefully eschews the one-to-one conflation of dreams with REM sleep.

Along these lines, Mark Solms has recently reviewed neuropsychological evidence and shown that the ability to dream depends not on the upper brainstem but on forebrain regions. In more than 100 cases of cessation of dreaming, the responsible lesion was the parietotemporooccipital junction (unilaterally or bilaterally) or the white matter near the orbitomesial prefrontal cortex (bilaterally). Despite the cessation of dreaming, REM sleep was almost always preserved. The parietotemporooccipital junction is important for mental imagery, for spatial cognition (on the right side), and for symbolic cognition (on the left side), all central features of dreaming. The white matter underlying the ventromesial prefrontal cortex that is necessary for dreaming is the same brain area that is targeted by modified prefrontal leucotomy. Its lesion reduces the positive symptoms of schizophrenia but produces adynamia. Chemical activation of these circuits by stimulants, such as amphetamines, as well as by levodopa (L-dopa), can produce hallucinations and delusions, suggesting that dreams may be facilitated by the activation of the mesolimbic and mesocortical dopaminergic systems.

SLEEP IN ANIMALS

The study of sleep in animals has influenced the understanding of human sleep at many levels. The ubiquitous nature of sleep in the animal kingdom, even under circumstances in which sleep is dangerous, underscores the fundamental biological importance of sleep. Comparisons of sleep across animals from diverse taxonomic groups have revealed ecological and physiological correlates of sleep that may yield insight into the purpose of sleep. Finally, the discovery of remarkable adaptations, such as unihemispheric sleep, has been of significant heuristic value for conceptualizing the functional basis of sleep.

Sleep in Mammals Sleep behavior and electrophysiology have been studied most extensively in mammals. NREM and REM sleep have been found in every placental and marsupial mammal investigated. (In the animal literature, *SWS* usually refers to all sleep that is not REM sleep.) Even fossorial mammals, such as moles, with a regressed visual system display periods of REM-like EEG activation with elevated arousal thresholds, indicating that REMs are not a necessary feature of REM sleep. The diversity of reported sleep behaviors parallels the diversity of ecological niches occupied by mammals; rodents sleep curled up in burrows, bats sleep hanging from cave ceilings, and great apes sleep in freshly made beds of leaves. Giraffes, elephants, and horses can engage in SWS while standing but must lie down for REM sleep owing to the loss of skeletal muscle tone occurring during this state. Interestingly, when the brainstem regions actively involved in inhibiting muscle tone during REM sleep are lesioned, cats in REM sleep stand up and stalk imaginary prey, as if acting out a dream. Humans with similar lesions experience REM sleep behavior disorder, a parasomnia characterized by the behavioral enactment of dreams.

The amount of time spent in SWS and REM sleep varies across mammals. For a given size, when compared to mammals with lower metabolic rates, mammals with higher metabolic rates spend less total time sleeping and less time in SWS in particular. The amount of REM sleep in mammals is strongly correlated with maturational patterns; when compared to precocial mammals (those which undergo relatively small amounts of postnatal brain development), altricial mammals (those which undergo relatively large amounts of postnatal brain development) spend more time in REM sleep as neonates and adults. Along with experimental data, this relationship between REM sleep and maturational pattern suggests that REM sleep plays a critical role in early brain development in altricial mammals, such as humans.

Unihemispheric Slow Wave Sleep in Aquatic Mammals Aquatic mammals have developed several adaptations that mitigate the conflict between the simultaneous need to sleep and to breathe in the water. Cetaceans (dolphins, porpoises, and whales) are able to swim to the surface to breathe while sleeping with only one-half of their brain at a time, a unique state that is referred to as *unihemispheric SWS* (Fig. 1.20–6). During unihemispheric SWS, the eye contralateral to the awake hemisphere is usually open and presumably is scanning the environment. Dolphins alternate sleeping with each hemisphere on an hourly basis, and, if sleep is experimentally prevented in only one hemisphere, only that hemisphere shows a compensatory rebound in SWS. Manatees and certain seals also engage in unihemispheric SWS, and, unlike cetaceans, bihemispheric SWS and REM sleep. Interestingly, most investigators have not detected electrophysiological signs of REM sleep in cetaceans. Nevertheless, REM sleep may occur in small amounts or in a modified form, because cetaceans display rare twitches similar to those observed in terrestrial mammals during REM sleep. The small amount of REM sleep in cetaceans, animals thought to be highly intelligent, challenges current theories that suggest REM sleep is involved in memory consolidation. The preservation of SWS and REM sleep, often in a modified form, in aquatic mammals underscores the biological importance of both states. Moreover, the presence of unihemispherically regulated SWS indicates that SWS may serve a local function for the brain.

Monotremes The few extant species of monotremes, an evolutionary ancient group of egg-laying mammals, provide a unique opportunity to explore the evolution of sleep states in mammals. An

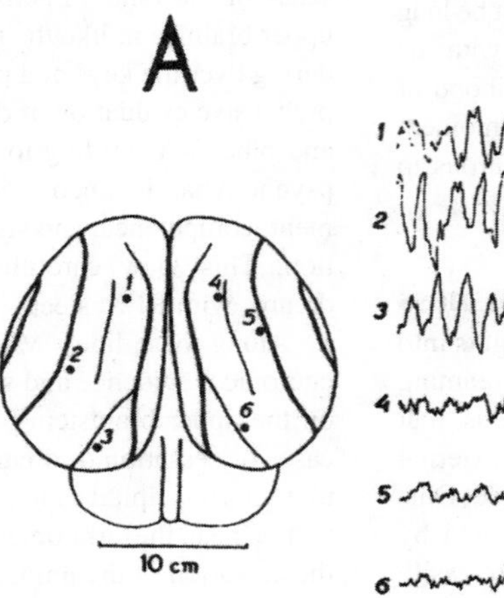

FIGURE 1.20–6 Electroencephalogram (EEG) recorded from the parietooccipital cortex **(A)** of a bottlenose dolphin (*Tursiops truncatus*) during unihemispheric slow wave sleep with the left **(B)** or right **(C)** hemisphere asleep. Note the high-voltage, low-frequency EEG activity in the sleeping hemisphere and the low-voltage, high-frequency EEG activity in the awake hemisphere. (From Mukhametov LM, Supin AY, Polyakova IG: Interhemispheric asymmetry of the electroencephalographic sleep patterns in dolphins. *Brain Res.* 1977;134:581, with permission.)

early report of SWS, but not REM sleep, in the echidna suggested that REM sleep evolved after the evolutionary line leading to marsupial and placental mammals diverged from that leading to the extant monotremes. Recent studies of the echidna and the duck-billed platypus, however, suggest that monotremes exhibit a heterogeneous sleep state with concurrent slow cortical activity indicative of SWS and brainstem neuronal discharge patterns and associated twitching indicative of REM sleep. According to this scenario, this heterogeneous state diverged into temporally distinct states of SWS and REM sleep with cortical activation in marsupial and placental mammals.

Sleep in Birds Despite having diverged from a common reptilian ancestor more than 310 million years ago, the sleep patterns of mammals and birds resemble each other more than reptiles. Birds are the only taxonomic group other than mammals to exhibit unequivocal SWS and REM sleep. When compared to mammals, birds spend similar amounts of time sleeping, but have approximately one-fourth the amount of REM sleep. As in mammals, muscle tone is reduced, and thermoregulation is impaired during REM sleep. Although circumstantial evidence suggests that some birds sleep in flight, this remains unconfirmed. As in aquatic mammals, birds frequently keep one eye open during SWS, a behavior associated with greater EEG activation in the contralateral hemisphere. The proportion of sleep spent with one eye open increases when birds sleep under riskier situations, such as on the edge of a group of birds. Moreover, birds sleeping at the group edge direct the open eye away from the other birds, as if watching for approaching predators. This ability to switch from sleeping with both eyes closed to sleeping with one eye open when sleeping under dangerous circumstances underscores the fact that sleep serves a vital function for the brain that can only be performed while in a potentially dangerous state of reduced environmental awareness.

The presence of SWS and REM sleep in mammals and birds suggests that both states were inherited through common descent from a reptilian ancestor with similar states. Alternatively, either or both states may have arisen independently in mammals and birds. Distinguishing between these alternatives is important, because common descent suggests that SWS and REM sleep may serve a fundamental function for vertebrates, whereas convergent evolution suggests that the function of SWS and REM sleep are linked to specific shared aspects of mammals and birds (e.g., homeothermy). Studies of sleep in reptiles, amphibians, and fish have revealed clear signs of behavioral sleep, but the electrophysiological correlates of sleep and the presence or absence of SWS, REM sleep, or a monotreme-like heterogeneous sleep state remain controversial and in need of further investigation. Consequently, it is unclear whether SWS and REM sleep evolved in mammals and birds through common descent or through convergent evolution.

Sleep in Invertebrates Until recently, relatively little research had focused on sleep in invertebrates, such as insects. Given the difficulty of recording brain activity in small insects, most studies have focused on determining whether insects display behavioral signs of sleep. Periods of sleep-like behavioral quiescence with elevated arousal thresholds have been described in several species of insect. In bees and fruit flies, the only insects in which sleep-related brain activity has been recorded, brain activity shows distinct changes between wakefulness and sleep. In bees, neurons in the visual system show reduced responsiveness to visual stimuli during sleep when compared to wakefulness. Fruit flies also show reduced brain activity during sleep. Thus, although the insect brain is not capable of generating the state-related EEG patterns observed in mammals or birds, it nevertheless shows similar changes in spontaneous activity and responsiveness to the environment. Insects experimentally deprived of sleep also show a compensatory rebound in sleep duration and intensity, indicating that, as in vertebrates, sleep is homeostatically regulated in insects. Other parallels between sleep in insects, such as the fruit fly, and mammals include a reduction in sleep time and continuity with increasing age; alerting responses to pharmacological agents, such as caffeine; and similar behavioral state-related changes in gene expression within the brain. The presence of sleep in the fruit fly provides an unparalleled opportunity to explore the function of sleep through identifying and manipulating the genetic and molecular correlates of sleep.

FUNCTIONS OF SLEEP

Why humans and animals sleep is still a mystery. Sleep may have evolved from the circadian rest–activity cycle and may thus represent a default state. However, it is likely that sleep serves some more fundamental function. Otherwise, why should animals engage in prolonged periods of quiescence with increased arousal thresholds, during which they cannot monitor potential dangers in the environment? Sleep seems to be universal. All animal species studied so far sleep, from invertebrates, such as fruit flies and bees, to birds and mammals. Mammals and birds generally display more elaborate sleep cycles that include an alternation of NREM and REM sleep. Getting rid of sleep does not seem to be easy. Some marine mammals that may need continuous vigilance while swimming, such as certain dolphins and porpoises, have developed alternating unihemispheric sleep rather than eliminating sleep altogether. Sleep deprivation leads to an increase in sleep pressure, manifested as sleepiness, which rapidly becomes irresistible. Sleep pressure may lead to microsleeps or piecemeal sleep that result in cognitive impairment. Sleep deprivation is followed by longer and more intense sleep, suggesting a regulated need for sleep. If sleep is prevented for several weeks, the consequences are fatal. Rats deprived of sleep for more than 2 weeks invariably die. Humans affected by a rare prion disorder called *FFI* also die, although it is not certain whether death is due to sleep deprivation per se.

Many hypotheses have been formulated about the functions of sleep. A good hypothesis should account for the following facts: (1) Sleep involves partial disconnection from the environment, which is potentially dangerous; sleep must therefore provide something not provided by quiet waking. (2) Sleep is accompanied by intense neural activity in most brain regions; one needs to explain why the brain should be active in the absence of overt behavior. (3) Sleep seems to constitute a universal requirement, but its amount varies a great deal across different species; one must explain why this is so. (4) In most species, sleep is prevalent early in life; sleep should perform important functions during development and in the adult. (5) Sleep is often made up of NREM and REM stages; it must be explained whether the sequence of the two stages is important or whether both stages serve a similar function—for example, in both stages, the animal is disconnected from the environment, neural activity is intense, and monoaminergic discharge is reduced. No single hypothesis has been proposed that can account for all of these facts.

Sleep and Brain Restitution Most hypotheses currently under investigation are concerned with a role of sleep in restoring some metabolic function or in serving neural plasticity. It is likely that sleep may preserve energy by enforcing body rest in animals with high metabolic rates. Indeed, animals and humans eat more during sleep deprivation. However, in humans, the metabolic efficiency of sleep is only marginally better than that of quiet waking. Most bodily organs can obtain rest through quiet wakefulness, except for the brain; thus, sleep may be especially important for the brain. Some molecular pathway or chemical in the brain may be wasted during waking and restored during sleep. For example, it has been suggested that sleep may favor the replenishment of glycogen in glial stores, although recent evidence shows that this may only be true in a few brain regions. Alternatively, sleep could prevent synaptic overload or counteract synaptic fatigue by favoring the replenishment of calcium in presynaptic stores, the replenishment of glutamate vesicles, the resting of mitochondria, the recycling of membranes, or the transfer of proteins along axons and dendrites. Although recent studies have revealed that molecular changes do occur between sleep and waking and after sleep deprivation, the significance of such changes is still unknown. If sleep restores something, it is still not known what this is.

Sleep and Memory A connection between sleep and memory was noted a long time ago. After struggling to learn a new piece of music for much of the day, an individual often plays it better after a night of sleep. Recently, the importance of sleep, and even naps, occurring after certain types of declarative and nondeclarative learning has been documented in well-controlled experiments. Sleep could indeed offer a favorable context for certain aspects of learning and memory. The sensory disconnection associated with sleep reduces interference between ongoing activities and the consolidation of previously acquired memories. Moreover, sleep permits the repeated reactivation, in an off-line mode, of the neural circuits originally activated during the memorable experience. Studies using multielectrode recordings in animals and PET in humans have shown that brain areas or cells activated during waking are preferentially reactivated during subsequent sleep. A further advantage of sleep is that the relevant neural circuits can be reactivated in a spaced and interleaved fashion. This would favor the integration of new memories with old memories and would avoid catastrophic interference. The intense, high-frequency bursts of spontaneous neural activity that occur during sleep may be particularly important for triggering molecular mechanisms of synaptic consolidation and to enlarge the network of associations.

Many unknowns remain, however. Whether sleep may favor the consolidation of newly established memories or the maintenance of older ones is not clear. The molecular correlates of such processes are still not known. Molecular markers of memory acquisition are turned off during sleep, which may be advantageous, given that the intense neural activity of sleep occurs while the animal is disconnected from the environment. Much of the early literature connecting sleep and memory was concerned with REM sleep. However, prolonged inhibition of REM sleep in humans through MAOIs does not seem to disrupt memory, nor does the complete disappearance of REM sleep after certain brainstem lesions. Perhaps the most convincing evidence concerns the role of sleep in developmental plasticity. Recent experiments have shown that REM sleep deprivation in newborn rats and NREM sleep deprivation in kittens influence the activity-dependent development of visual system circuits. If sleep affects synaptic maturation and plasticity, one can expect that sleep disturbances in early life may affect psychopathological development.

SLEEP AND PSYCHIATRY

Historically, psychiatrists have been interested in sleep and dreaming and their relationship with mental illness. Beginning with Freud and Carl Jung in the latter part of the 19th century, the interpretation of dreams became an important tool in psychoanalytic psychotherapy. After the discovery of REM sleep in 1953, psychiatrists began to explore whether specific sleep abnormalities could be correlated with psychiatric disorders. One of the first questions addressed was whether schizophrenia might represent a disorder of REM sleep, given the similarities between dreaming and psychosis. Although psychosis could not be explained as an REM sleep disorder, REM sleep and schizophrenia were later found to be associated with decreased activity in dorsolateral prefrontal cortex. Narcolepsy, on the other hand, turned out to be caused by abnormal intrusion of REM sleep phenomena into wakefulness.

By far, the greatest amount of investigation has been done on sleep in depression. Even before the discovery of REM sleep, depressives were known to have disrupted sleep. Sleep EEG recordings in the 1950s and 1960s also showed that they had a relative loss of SWS, in comparison to age-matched control subjects, and specific changes in REM sleep, including reduced latency to REM sleep, greater proportion of REM sleep during the first third of the night, increased frequency of REMs during REM sleep (i.e., increased REM density), and increased percentage of sleep time spent in REM sleep. Although not every patient with depression shows changes in REM sleep, and not every patient with short REM latency has depression, REM sleep abnormalities are one of the more robust biological markers for depression. Reduced REM sleep latency and loss of SWS appear to be trait markers for depression in that they persist even during clinical remission and are found at higher rates in first-degree family members of depressives with these features. Although the mechanisms for sleep changes in depression are not fully understood, there is a convergence of data suggesting that sleep and mood are regulated by common systems. For example, the cholinergic-monoaminergic imbalance hypothesis of depression is consistent with the observed increase in REM sleep and reduction in SWS that would be caused by increased cholinergic activity. Depressives show a heightened sensitivity to REM sleep induction by cholinergic drugs in comparison to nondepressed control subjects as well.

Sleep deprivation studies are even more suggestive of a functional relationship between sleep and mood. Total deprivation of a single night of sleep, or even partial deprivation of sleep in the latter half of the night, can have an immediate antidepressant response in many moderately to severely depressed individuals. Sleep loss can induce or perpetuate mania in bipolar patients, who may go for periods of several days with little or no sleep. In contrast, even a short bout of sleep can reverse the antidepressant effect of sleep deprivation, and prolonged sleep can induce depression in some individuals. Functional imaging studies have shown that sleep deprivation, like antidepressant drug therapy, normalizes the increased metabolic activity seen in the anterior cingulate gyrus in depressives. Selective REM sleep deprivation has also been shown to have antidepressant effects, and it has been suggested that REM sleep-suppressing antidepressants may act, in part, through their effects on sleep. REM sleep suppression, however, is not a requirement for antidepressant efficacy, because some newer agents, such as bupropion (Wellbutrin) and nefazodone (Serzone), appear to cause no significant reduction of REM sleep.

Although therapeutic sleep deprivation may be beneficial for some cases of depression, the preponderance of evidence suggests that disturbed sleep is a risk factor for the development of psychiatric illness. People with insomnia have higher rates of psychiatric disorders, particularly mood and anxiety disorders; in primary care settings, insomnia is more strongly associated with depression than with any other medical disorder. Individuals who have insomnia or even difficulty sleeping during times of stress are significantly more likely to develop depression in the future. A causal link between sleep and depression has not yet been established, but the fact that sleep deprivation and depression are becoming more prevalent in society suggests that the relationship between the two must be clarified.

From an epidemiological perspective, although sleep disturbance is most strongly associated with psychiatric disorders, there are a number of other significant health-related correlates. People with insomnia have higher rates of other medical illnesses; use more health care services; have higher rates of absenteeism, accidents, and disability; and have poorer outcomes with some medical disorders, including cardiac disease. Whether treatment of sleep problems can prevent the development of any of these comorbidities remains to be seen.

Sleep abnormalities are also seen in virtually all other psychiatric disorders, particularly disturbances in sleep continuity, including prolonged latency to sleep onset, diminished efficiency of sleep, and decreased amounts of total sleep. REM sleep abnormalities similar to depression have been described in some studies of patients with schizophrenia, alcoholism, eating disorders, and borderline personality disorder. Patients with panic disorder may have panic attacks arising from sleep, usually at the transition into SWS, which further emphasizes the biological etiology of this disorder.

An appreciation of sleep neurobiology is essential for clinicians, because psychiatric patients often have sleep problems associated with their illnesses, and most psychiatric drugs have significant effects on sleep; these range from sedation caused by many antipsychotics, benzodiazepines, tricyclic antidepressants, and antiparkinsonian agents to sleep disturbance caused by MAOIs, SSRIs, and psychostimulants. Antidepressants may precipitate some sleep disorders, such as periodic movements in sleep and REM sleep behavior disorder, and abrupt withdrawal of REM-suppressing antidepressants, including tricyclics, MAOIs, and SSRIs, can lead to REM sleep rebound, characterized by increased duration and intensity of REM sleep and sleep disruption. Sleep apnea may be exacerbated by drugs that produce muscle relaxation (e.g., benzodiazepines or barbiturates) or weight gain (e.g., antipsychotics, antidepressants, and mood stabilizers).

Sleep is a revealing, although not yet transparent, window into the functional state of the human brain. The study of sleep has shed light on many aspects of consciousness and the workings of the human brain. Clarifying the functions and mechanisms of sleep will undoubtedly provide a greater understanding of psychiatric disorders and their treatments.

SUGGESTED CROSS-REFERENCES

The reader is encouraged to refer to Section 1.13 for more extensive information on chronobiology. Section 1.14 discusses electrophysiology and its applications to sleep deprivation. Chapter 20 discusses sleep disorders. Section 51.3b focuses on sleep disorders in the elderly.

REFERENCES

Aserinsky E, Kleitman N: Regularly occurring periods of ocular motility and concomitant phenomena during sleep. *Science.* 1953;361.

BBS Special Issue: Sleep and dreaming. *Behav Brain Sci.* 2000;23.

Benca RM, Obermeyer WH, Thisted RA, Gillin JC: Sleep and psychiatric disorders: A meta-analysis. *Arch Gen Psychiatry.* 1992;49:651.

Borbely AA, Achermann P: Sleep homeostasis and models of sleep regulation. *J Biol Rhythms.* 1999;14:557.

Carskadon M. *Adolescent Sleep Patterns: Biological, Social, and Psychological Influences.* Cambridge, UK: Cambridge University Press; 2002.

Dijk DJ, Lockley SW: Integration of human sleep-wake regulation and circadian rhythmicity. *J Appl Physiol.* 2002;92:852.

Ferber R, Kryger MH. *Principals and Practice of Sleep Medicine in the Child.* Philadelphia: WB Saunders; 1995.

Foulkes D. *Dreaming: A Cognitive-Psychological Analysis.* Hillsdale, NJ: L. Erlbaum Associates; 1985.

Graves L, Pack A, Abel T: Sleep and memory: A molecular perspective. *Trends Neurosci.* 2001;24:237.

*Harrison Y, Horne JA: The impact of sleep deprivation on decision making: A review. *J Exp Psychol Appl.* 2000;6:236.

Hobson JA. *Dreaming as Delirium: How the Brain Goes Out of Its Mind.* Cambridge, MA: The MIT Press; 1999.

Hobson JA, McCarley RW, Wyzinski PW: Sleep cycle oscillation: Reciprocal discharge by two brainstem neuronal groups. *Science.* 1975;189:55.

*Hobson JA, Pace-Schott EF: The cognitive neuroscience of sleep: Neuronal systems, consciousness and learning. *Nat Rev Neurosci.* 2002;3:679.

Horne J. *Why We Sleep: The Functions of Sleep in Humans and Other Mammals.* Oxford: Oxford University Press; 1988.

Jouvet M: Paradoxical sleep mechanisms. *Sleep.* 1994;17:S77.

Kilduff TS, Peyron C: The hypocretin/orexin ligand-receptor system: Implications for sleep and sleep disorders. *Trends Neurosci.* 2000;23:359.

*Kryger MH, Roth T, Dement WC. *Principles and Practices of Sleep Medicine.* Philadelphia: WB Saunders; 2000.

Lydic R, Baghdoyan HA. *Handbook of Behavioral State Control: Molecular and Cellular Mechanisms.* Boca Raton, FL: CRC Press; 1999.

Maquet P: Functional neuroimaging of normal human sleep by positron emission tomography. *J Sleep Res.* 2000;9:207.

Mignot E, Taheri S, Nishino S: Sleeping with the hypothalamus: Emerging therapeutic targets for sleep disorders. *Nat Neurosci.* 2002;5[Suppl]:1071.

Pace-Schott EF, Hobson JA: The neurobiology of sleep: Genetics, cellular physiology and subcortical networks. *Nat Rev Neurosci.* 2002;3:591.

Rattenborg N, Amlaner C. Phylogeny of sleep. In: Lee-Chiong T, Sateia M, Carskadon M, eds. *Sleep Medicine.* Philadelphia: Hanley & Belfus, Inc; 2002.

*Rechtschaffen A: Current perspectives on the function of sleep. *Perspect Biol Med.* 1998;41:359.

Rechtschaffen A, Bergmann BM: Sleep deprivation in the rat: An update of the 1989 paper. *Sleep.* 2002;25:18.

Rechtschaffen A, Kales A. *A Manual of Standardized Terminology, Techniques, and Scoring System for Sleep Stages of Human Subjects.* UCLA, Los Angeles: Brain Information Service/Brain Research Institute; 1968.

Rye DB, Jankovic J: Emerging views of dopamine in modulating sleep/wake state from an unlikely source: PD. *Neurology.* 2002;58:341.

Saper CB, Chou TC, Scammell TE: The sleep switch: Hypothalamic control of sleep and wakefulness. *Trends Neurosci.* 2001;24:726.

Steriade M. *The Intact and Sliced Brain.* Cambridge, MA: The MIT Press; 2001.

*Steriade M: Coherent oscillations and short-term plasticity in corticothalamic networks. *Trends Neurosci.* 1999;22:337.

Sutcliffe JG, de Lecea L: The hypocretins: Setting the arousal threshold. *Nat Rev Neurosci.* 2002;3:339.

Tononi G, Cirelli C: Modulation of brain gene expression during sleep and wakefulness: A review of recent findings. *Neuropsychopharmacology.* 2001;25:S28.

Tononi G, Cirelli C: Sleep and synaptic homeostasis: A hypothesis. *Brain Res Bull.* 2004 (*in press*).

Van Dongen HP, Maislin G, Mullington JM, Dinges DF: The cumulative cost of additional wakefulness: Dose-response effects on neurobehavioral functions and sleep physiology from chronic sleep restriction and total sleep deprivation. *Sleep.* 2003;26:117.

▲ 1.21 Appetite

NORI GEARY, PH.D., AND GARY J. SCHWARTZ, PH.D.

New methodologies and new conceptual schema have led to rapid advances in the behavioral neuroscience of eating. The traditional view that food intake is tightly controlled by hypothalamic neural centers reacting to the state of energy balance has been replaced by a more complex perspective of a widely distributed neural network in the brain that integrates oropharyngeal food stimuli (including those giving rise to hedonic perceptions), gastrointestinal (GI) signals, metabolic signals (including signals related to body adiposity), and environmental and experiential contingencies. This new perspective emphasizes peripheral signals, their specific effects on eating, and their peripheral and central mediating mechanisms rather than the idea that one or a few circumscribed integratory sites in the brain produce a unitary motive state that can be labeled *appetite*.

MEALS

Meal as the Unit of Analysis The behavioral neuroscience of eating focuses increasingly on the individual meal as the unit of analysis rather than on measures of food intake over extended periods, for example, kilocalories per day. This change is based on the realization that understanding the physiology of individual meals is necessary for understanding disordered and normal eating and the contribution of eating to body weight. The meal is the biological unit of eating, because, in humans as well as the vast majority of animal species, ingestive behavior is organized as discrete bouts, or meals, that are separated by intervals of noneating. The meal is the functional unit of eating, because the timing, size, and content of meals provides a complete description of the organism's response to the basic challenge of nutrition, namely what to eat and how much to eat. In addition, abnormally large meals are the defining behavioral change in bulimia nervosa and in the binge-eating disorder displayed by many obese people; abnormally small meals are the defining behavioral change in restricted eating and anorexia nervosa. Therefore, this chapter approaches the basic science of eating from the perspective of the individual meal.

A distinction is often drawn between *short-term* and *long-term* influences on eating. *Long-term* influences are supposed to have biological prepotency because of their relation to energy balance, that is, to the matching of energy intake in the form of food to energy output in the forms of physical or metabolic work and heat. Furthermore, long-term influences are supposed to be fundamentally independent from those influences affecting individual meals. Implicit in this perspective is the idea that the science of eating can advance without direct measures of behavior; rather, indirect measures, such as amounts eaten per day or week, are sufficient. This strategy can provide a net accounting of long-term changes of eating and their implications for energy balance (Fig. 1.21–1D), but it fails to provide an explanation of eating in terms of the actual behavioral output of the brain. In contrast, meal analysis measures behaviors whose biological bases can be sought at the level of the central nervous system (CNS). Furthermore, the amount eaten over any period of time is completely determined by the number and size of meals. Therefore, all influences on eating, including long-term influences, must affect the timing or size of meals.

Short-term controls, conversely, are supposed to act on individual meals and to be independent of energy balance. This again suggests that the behavioral science of the meal is biologically unimportant. However, this is not the case. Individual meals are indeed affected by signals related to long-term controls, such as body adiposity. Thus, the analysis of eating is best approached from the perspective of the meal.

Analysis of the Meal

The behavioral phases of the meal that require analysis are the initiation of eating, the maintenance of eating during the meal, and the termination of eating (Fig. 1.21–1A). Ingestion of food during the meal stimulates positive feedback signals from the mouth that contribute to the maintenance of eating and negative feedback signals from the mouth, stomach, small intestine, and, perhaps, postabsorptive sites that ultimately terminate eating (Fig. 1.21–1B). The temporal organization of eating movements during the meal is the microstructure of eating (Fig. 1.21–1C). Food is licked, sucked, bitten, or masticated before being moved by lingual and palatal movements to the oropharynx and swallowed. The chief advantage of the analysis of these movements is the potential to track their neural control through the lower motor neurons of the fifth, seventh, ninth, tenth, and twelfth cranial nerves into (1) the local circuits in the motor nuclei of these nerves, (2) the central pattern generators in the hindbrain that project onto these nuclei, (3) the interneuronal networks upstream of this motor outflow, and (4) ultimately, sensory inputs. One of the basic goals of the behavioral neuroscience of eating is to use this strategy to link the signals controlling the timing or size of meals to the motor controls of the movements of eating.

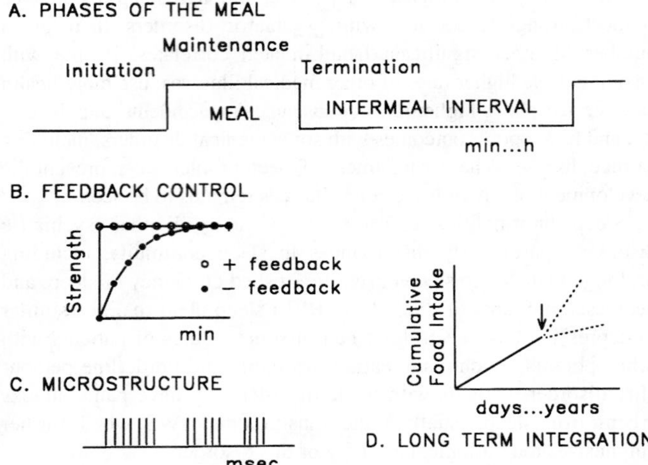

FIGURE 1.21–1 **A:** The meal is the functional unit of eating. The physiological mechanisms of eating control the initiation, maintenance, and termination of eating and, consequently, the size of meals and the duration of intermeal intervals. **B:** Meal size is a function of positive and negative feedbacks elicited by preabsorptive food stimuli arising during meals. Positive feedback, shown in hypothetical units, begins as soon as eating begins and is thought not to decrease significantly during the meal. Negative feedback increases in strength gradually as eating continues. When the strength of negative feedback equals that of positive feedback, eating stops and the meal ends. **C:** Microstructural analyses are based on the patterns of the individual movements of eating, for example, the temporal organization of individual licks of liquid foods on an event recorder. **D:** Amount eaten in the long term is simply the sum of the sizes of many individual meals. This schematic demonstrates the typically constant increase in cumulative intake evident on a macroscopic scale (e.g., kilocalories per day). This rate is increased or decreased if energetic demands are increased or decreased, for example, by changing physical activity, as shown to the right of the arrow.

Subjective Experience of Eating

The subjective experiences associated with meals are scientifically accessible in humans and provide important insights into the expression of normal and disordered eating (for example, Fig. 1.21–2). Their analysis is most productive when it has been based on operationally defined categories of subjective experience rather than theoretical categorizations.

PERIPHERAL SIGNALS FOR MEAL INITIATION

Because the frequency of meals is a determinant of intake, it is important to identify the adequate stimuli and mechanisms for the initiation of eating. The adequate stimuli for meal initiation include olfactory, visual, auditory, temporal, circadian, metabolic, cognitive, and social stimuli. Most of these are conditioned stimuli (CS) whose potency to stimulate eating depends on prior eating experience. The following paragraphs describe the few candidate unconditioned stimuli (UCS) for meal initiation. Note that these do not include gastric contractions. Despite the referral of some visceral sensation to the stomach area and persistent citations of flawed early work in many texts, there is no evidence that gastric contractions are adequate stimuli for meal initiation.

Metabolism

Signals resulting from decreased glucose or fatty acid use may be UCS for meal initiation. Whether these signals operate under normal physiological conditions remains to be determined. They may operate only under rarely occurring extremes of nutrient depletion, such as biochemical hypoglycemia.

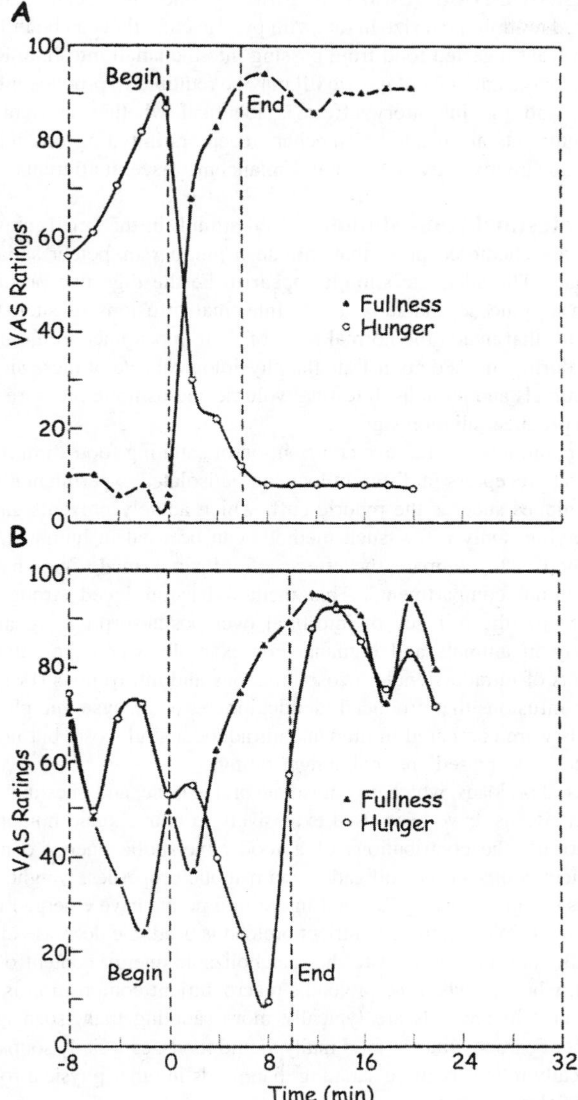

FIGURE 1.21–2 Example of the use of the visual analog scale (VAS) (essentially a 100-mm line that the subject marks with a pencil to indicate the momentary intensity of a percept; the line is anchored with descriptors, such as "most possible" or "not at all") to measure meal-related changes in hunger and fullness in a healthy woman **(A)** and a woman with anorexia nervosa **(B)**. In the healthy woman **(A)**, hunger is high before the meal, fullness is low before the meal, and the two percepts change in a reciprocal fashion before, during, and after eating; this is typical of most healthy subjects. In contrast, in this patient with anorexia nervosa **(B)**, hunger and fullness change irregularly before, during, and after the meal and are often not reciprocally related; other patients with anorexia nervosa showed a variety of responses, some more and some less normal than these. Note that the figure does not show some crucial experiences associated with eating, such as pleasure and tranquilization. The challenge for this research is to disentangle the various psychological and physiological influences producing these percepts. (From Owen WP, Halmi KA, Gibbs J, Smith GP: Satiety responses in eating disorders. *J Psychiatr Res.* 1985;19:279, with permission.)

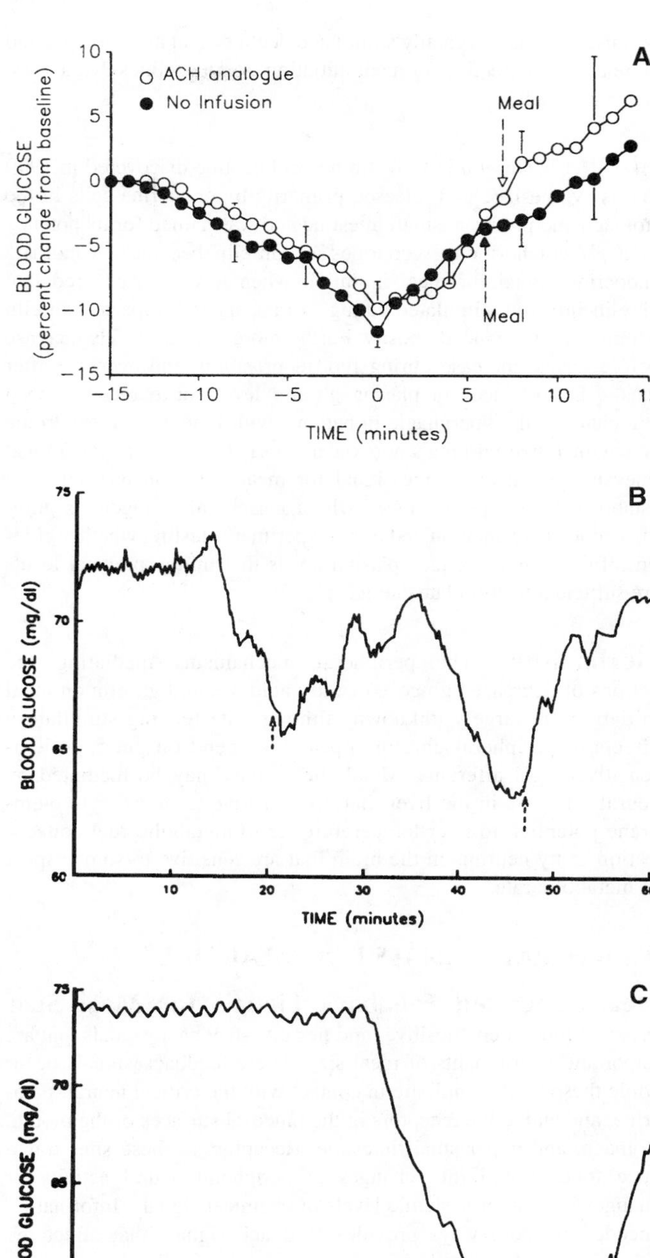

FIGURE 1.21–3 The premeal transient decline in blood glucose in rats and humans. **A:** Filled circles represent the percent deviations from baseline blood glucose during undisturbed spontaneous feeding in rats. Note that meals begin several minutes after the nadir. Open circles represent intravenous infusions of an insulin secretogogue that produced similar declines and also elicited meal initiation. ACH, acetylcholine. (From Campfield LA, Smith FJ: Meal initiation occurs after experimental induction of transient declines in blood glucose. *Am J Physiol.* 1993;265:R1423, with permission.) **B,C:** Blood glucose changes preceding requests for morning meals (*arrows*) in two normal weight volunteers spending the night in a metabolism laboratory. (From Campfield LA, Smith FJ, Rosenbaum M, Hirsch J: Human eating: Evidence for a physiological basis using a modified paradigm. *Neurosci Biobehav Rev.* 1996;20:133, with permission.)

A physiological stimulus for the initiation of eating related to glucose is the transient decline in plasma glucose that has been recorded before spontaneous meals in rats and humans (Fig. 1.21–3). The decline is too small to influence cellular glucose availability. Instead, the temporal dynamics of the decline appear crucial. This is because pharmacologically stimulated declines that are too rapid and large are as ineffective for meal initiation as are declines that are too slow and small.

Ghrelin *Ghrelin* is a 28–amino acid peptide discovered in 1999 that is synthesized and released primarily by endocrine cells in the stomach and proximal small intestine and was named for its potency as a growth hormone secretogogue. Ghrelin became a candidate endocrine signal for meal initiation when it was discovered that ghrelin infusion stimulated eating in rats; indeed, repeated ghrelin administration induced obesity. Furthermore, ghrelin levels increase before meals, increase during food deprivation, and decrease after meals. Disturbances in plasma ghrelin levels have recently been associated with hyperphagia in patients with Prader-Willi syndrome and with binge-purging anorexia nervosa. Ghrelin's physiological relevance as an endocrine signal for meal initiation has not been established by experiments in which peripheral endogenous ghrelin's actions are antagonized or by experiments testing whether ghrelin infusions that produce plasma levels that mimic premeal levels are sufficient to stimulate eating.

Mechanisms The peripheral mechanisms mediating the actions of decreased glucose or fatty acid use and ghrelin on meal initiation are largely unknown, although the feeding-stimulatory effects of peripheral ghrelin appear to depend on gut capsaicin-sensitive vagal afferents. Metabolic signals may be mediated by neural afferents in the liver that are sensitive to hepatocyte membrane potential, to liver temperature, or to metabolic fuel concentration or by neurons in the brain that are sensitive to some aspect of metabolic rate.

PERIPHERAL SIGNALS FOR MEAL SIZE

Meal-Generated Feedback Signals for Meal Size

Ingested food elicits positive- and negative-feedback signals that are important determinants of meal size. These feedback signals occur while these food stimuli are in contact with the critical neural, paracrine, and endocrine receptors in the mucosal surfaces of the mouth, stomach, and upper small intestine. Receptors at these sites transduce food stimuli into changes in peripheral neural activity or changes in local or systemic levels of chemical signals. Information encoded in these ways provides feedback signals that affect the maintenance of eating during the meal and the termination of eating at the end of the meal. The process mediating the termination of eating is technically known as *satiation*.

Oropharyngeal Food Stimuli Flavors provide the only known positive-feedback signals facilitating eating once it has begun. These signals arise from olfactory, gustatory, tactile, and thermal oropharyngeal food stimuli and reach the brain via the olfactory, trigeminal, facial, glossopharyngeal, and vagus nerves. This afferent information (except for olfactory stimuli) is initially processed in the hindbrain. The potency of oropharyngeal food stimuli to maintain eating is dramatically demonstrated by the sham feeding technique, in which ingested food is diverted via esophageal or gastric cannulas. As originally observed by Ivan Petrovich Pavlov, after overnight food deprivation, animals sham feed nearly continuously for hours. After short periods of food deprivation in rats, however, sham feeding terminates in satiation, suggesting that oropharyngeal food stimuli can also produce satiation signals.

Gastric Food Stimuli Gastric volume has been demonstrated to limit meal size in rats with pyloric cuffs that can be inflated to prevent ingested food from passing into the small intestine. Relatively large amounts of gastric fill may be required to produce inhibition, and the inhibitory effect is identical whether nutrients or nonnutrients are used. The mechanoreceptors initiating this inhibition apparently activate vagal and splanchnic visceral afferents.

Intestinal Food Stimuli Food stimuli in the small intestine activate chemoreceptors that initiate a number of potent satiation signals. The adequate stimuli appear to be the digestive products, such as glucose and fatty acids. Intestinal infusions of such food stimuli that match the normal rates of their appearance in the intestine during meals demonstrate the physiological role of these signals in animals and humans. Intestinal volume and osmotic pressure may also produce satiation signals.

In animals, the relative contribution of satiating food stimuli that activate receptors in different loci can be isolated experimentally by techniques such as the pyloric cuff, which acutely prevents gastric emptying. Only a few such methods can be used in humans. One method is to compare the effects of infusions made into distinct functional compartments. This method has produced strong evidence for the primacy of intestinal over postabsorptive signals in satiety in animals and humans. For example, when the satiating effects of intraduodenal glucose infusions and intravenous (IV) glucose infusions that produced identical increases in systemic glucose levels were compared in humans, intraduodenal glucose, but not IV glucose, decreased premeal hunger ratings.

Oral preloads, which do not isolate oral, gastric, and intestinal satiation signals, have been used extensively in animals and humans to determine the contributions of a food's metabolic energy content, nutrient composition, colligative and osmotic properties, weight, etc., to its satiating potency. Several interesting points have emerged from this work. When a mixed nutrient preload is used, the decrease in eating is often proportional to the metabolizable energy content of the load, whereas, when the preload's macronutrient composition is varied, protein preloads are typically more satiating than isoenergetic loads of carbohydrate or fat. Finally, liquid foods, especially soups, are typically relatively more satiating than foods in other physical forms, especially in women.

Mechanisms

Vagal and Splanchnic Nerves Negative-feedback signals elicited by gastric and intestinal food stimuli are carried by afferent vagal and splanchnic afferents to hindbrain sites, including the nucleus tractus solitarius (NTS), the primary sensory nucleus of the vagus. The NTS is an important integratory site that receives sensory input from the oral cavity as well as descending inputs from hypothalamic nuclei and other sites important in determining food intake. The relative role of vagal and nonvagal gut sensory neurons may vary for different food-elicited stimuli. The sensory gut vagus is necessary for the satiating actions of the gut peptides cholecystokinin (CCK) and pancreatic glucagon in the rat (see the next section). However, vagal and nonvagal gut sensory fibers appear to be necessary for the full satiating effect of intestinal food stimuli, because surgical transection of gut vagal afferents or upper gut splanchnic nerves completely reverses the feeding-inhibitory effects of intraduodenal nutrient infusions in rats (Fig. 1.21–4). Finally, selective surgical section of sensory abdominal vagal fibers is sufficient to increase meal size.

Gut afferent nerve endings appear to be stimulated directly by food stimuli in the intestinal lumen and indirectly by signaling molecules that

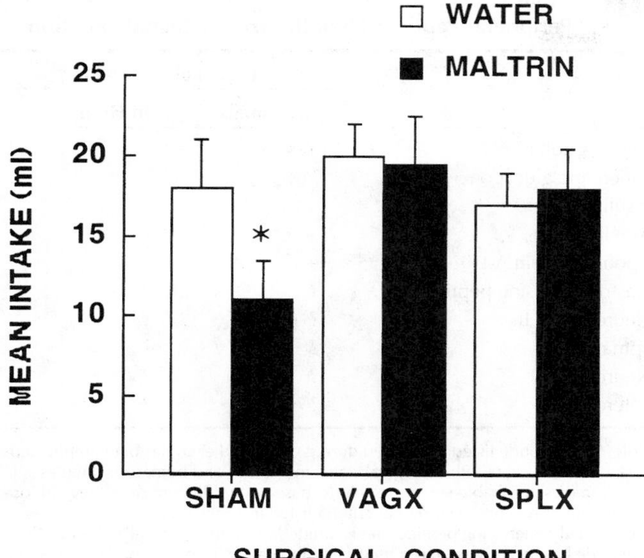

FIGURE 1.21–4 Vagal and splanchnic gut sensory nerves are necessary for intraduodenal carbohydrate infusions to reduce food intake. Vertical axis indicates intake of a saccharin-flavored maltose-dextrin solution (maltrin) after intraduodenal infusions of water (*open bars*) or maltrin (*filled bars*) in intact rats (SHAM), rats with gut vagal afferent transactions (VAGX), or rats with splanchnic nerve transection (SPLX). Note that transection of either gut vagal afferents or gut nonvagal splanchnic afferents completely reverses the ability of duodenal infusions to reduce subsequent food intake. (From Sclafani A, Ackroff K, Schwartz GJ: Selective effects of vagal deafferentation and celiac-superior mesenteric ganglionectomy on the reinforcing and satiating action of intestinal nutrients. *Physiol Behav.* 2003;78:285, with permission.)

are released by luminal food stimuli, such as CCK and serotonin (5-HT). Evidence for the indirect mechanism includes demonstrations that (1) duodenal vagal afferents are responsive to CCK and 5-HT, and (2) administration of peripherally acting CCK or 5-HT receptor antagonists reduces the effects of CCK or 5-HT on meal size and on gut vagal afferent neurophysiological responses.

Gut Peptides Gut peptides are important signal mechanisms for the transmission of negative-feedback information from meal-related food stimuli from the periphery to the brain. One gut peptide, CCK, has been proven to be a physiological control of meal size in animals and humans, based on fulfillment of the empirical criteria listed in Table 1.21–1. (Note that analogous criteria could be applied to the analyses of meal initiation and postprandial satiety, although this has not been done.)

CCK is synthesized by endocrine cells dispersed along the small intestine and is released by preabsorptive, intestinal food stimuli. In animals, CCK injections elicit dose-related decreases in meal size. This inhibitory effect of CCK is highly specific. Two examples are that CCK inhibits intake of liquid food but does not inhibit water intake in water-deprived rats and that CCK elicits the behavioral signs of satiation, including grooming and sleep, in rats that are sham feeding with open gastric cannulas that otherwise sham feed essentially indefinitely. IV CCK infusion in normal weight and obese humans in doses that mimic meal-stimulated levels are sufficient to inhibit eating without side effects. Most important, in animals and humans, premeal treatment with antagonists of the CCK-1 receptor (formerly called the CCK-A receptor) blocks the satiating

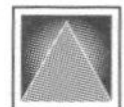

Table 1.21–1
Empirical Criteria for a Peripheral Molecular Satiation Signal

The molecule is released during meals.
Cognate receptors for the molecule are expressed at its site of action.
Administration of the molecule to its site of action in amounts that reproduce prandial levels at that site are sufficient to reduce meal size.
Administration (or ingestion) of secretogogues for the molecule produces effects similar to its administration.
The inhibitory effects on eating occur in the absence of abnormal behavioral, physiological, or subjective side effects.
Premeal administration of selective agonists and antagonists to the receptors for the molecule produces effects on eating consistent with their receptor pharmacologies; in particular, administration of a specific and potent receptor antagonist must increase meal size.

Note: Molecular satiation signals may have endocrine, paracrine, or neurocrine modes of action. These criteria have shaped the analysis of the gut peptides listed in Table 1.21–2 that are hypothesized to signal satiation.

action of exogenous CCK in animals and, when injected alone, increases meal size (Fig. 1.21–5).

Local infusion experiments reveal that the receptors sufficient to initiate CCK's satiating action are located in the proximal small intestine, not in the brain. Activation of these abdominal receptors increases neural activity in the vagal afferents innervating this site, and transection of these vagal afferent fibers abolishes the satiating action of CCK.

Spontaneous mutations have been identified in the CCK-1 receptor. Rats without CCK-1 receptors overeat at every meal and develop obesity and diabetes. Humans without CCK-1 receptors are also obese. These data indicate that CCK is an important part of the natural process of satiation. They also indicate that the physiological system controlling food intake, however complicated, is not completely redundant. Rather, the lack of a single basic control of meal size can produce uncompensated hyperphagia and obesity.

The study of CCK's satiating action has been paradigmatic for the study of a number of other candidate satiation signals. The present status of these peptides as physiological satiation signals lags behind that of CCK by varying degrees (Table 1.21–2). The probable existence of numerous peptide signal mechanisms for satiation raises the question of their interactions and their relative contributions in various normal and pathophysiological contexts. As yet, however, little is known about these questions. Finally, the peripheral origin and, in most cases, peripheral actions of these peptides make them attractive targets for the development of pharmacological therapies.

Other Signals for Meal Size

Meal size is also influenced by a panoply of signals that are not of alimentary origin and do not change during individual meals. These include (1) delayed negative feedbacks from physiological stimuli that are indirectly related to eating, but are not related to the ongoing meal, such as signals originating in the adipose tissue; (2) physiological signals not related to eating, such as circadian signals and signals from reproductive hormones; (3) signals related to increased immune system function during stress, infection, etc., including cytokines and other immune system mediators, which can acutely and chronically inhibit eating; and (4) conditioned signals, including signals conditioned to nonphysiological stimuli, such as social and cultural stimuli, as well as those conditioned to more physiological stimuli. The most important of these are described in the subsequent sections.

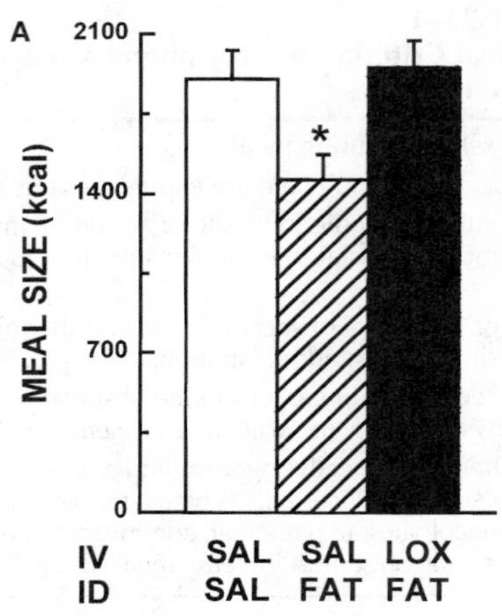

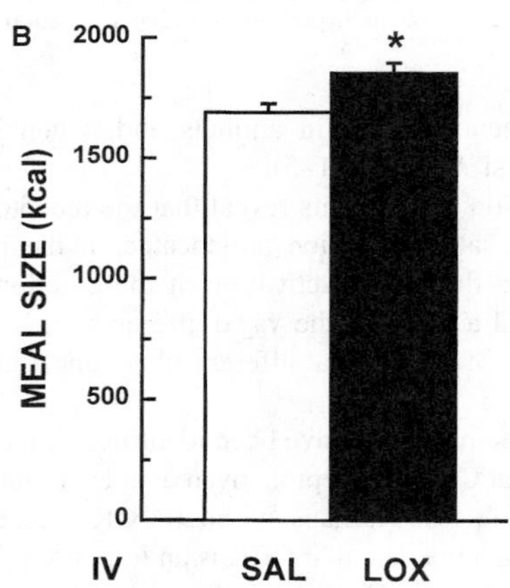

FIGURE 1.21–5 Demonstration of the physiological role of cholecystokinin (CCK) in human satiation. **A:** Normal-weight adult men began a noontime lunch buffet 4 hours after a standard breakfast, 90 minutes after beginning an intravenous (IV) infusion of the CCK-1 receptor antagonist loxiglumide (LOX) (10 μmol/kg-h) or saline (SAL), 60 minutes after an intraduodenal (ID) infusion of corn oil (FAT) or SAL (0.4 mL per minute), and 20 minutes after an oral preload of 400 mL of a low-fat banana milkshake. The infusions were continued throughout the meal. *Intraduodenal fat infusion significantly reduced the size of the lunch meal (expressed as total energy content of the various foods) without producing physical or subjective side effects, and this inhibition of eating was reversed by LOX infusion. (From Matzinger D, Gutzwiller J-P, Drewe J, et al.: Inhibition of food intake in response to intestinal lipid is mediated by cholecystokinin in humans. *Am J Physiol.* 1999;277:R1718, with permission.) **B:** Normal-weight adult men began a noontime lunch buffet 4 hours after a standard breakfast and 60 minutes after beginning an IV infusion of LOX (22 μmol/kg-h) or SAL. Infusions were continued throughout the meal. *LOX significantly increased meal size without affecting the subjects' enjoyment of their meals or their subjective sense of normal satiation. (From Beglinger C, Degen L, Matzinger D, et al.: Loxiglumide, a CCK-A receptor antagonist, stimulates calorie intake and hunger feedings in humans. *Am J Physiol.* 2001;280:R1149, with permission.)

ADIPOSITY SIGNALS

Adiposity signals are related to the mass of the adipose tissue. Adiposity is the only large bodily reserve of stored energy and is related to eating by the basic energy equation:

Stored Energy = Energy Intake – Energy Expenditure

Food is the only source of metabolically useful energy; energy expenditure includes physical work and heat production. Thus, signals that are related to adipose tissue mass may be considered delayed, indirect feedbacks from past eating that influence current eating.

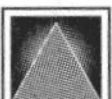

Table 1.21–2
Peripheral Peptides Hypothesized to Signal Satiation

	Physiological Status	
	In Animals	**In Humans**
Cholecystokinin	Yes	Yes
Pancreatic glucagon	Yes	+
Insulin	+	?
Amylin	+	?
Apolipoprotein A-IV	+	?
Gastrin-releasing peptide	?	?
Neuromedin B	?	?
Somatostatin	?	?
Neurotensin	?	?
Enterostatin	?	?

Note: Each peptide listed is released during meals and each has been implicated as a satiation signal. Physiological status in animals and humans is rated as proven (Yes), probable (+), or unclear (?) based on fulfillment of all, several, or only one or two of the empirical criteria listed in Table 1.21–1.

A potentially interesting peptide that is omitted from this table is PYY(3-36). This peptide has recently been reported to inhibit eating in rodents and humans, but PYY(3-36) is released mainly from the distal small intestine and colon, and PYY(3-36) levels usually increase only slowly after eating, making it unlikely that this peptide contributes to satiation.

Is Adiposity Regulated? *Energy balance* refers to the relation between energy intake and energy expenditure. When intake equals expenditure, the organism is in energy balance, and adipose tissue mass and body weight are stable. The nature of the influence of energy balance on eating is controversial. The relative constancy of body weight through adulthood has encouraged the view that a negative-feedback control system actively determines eating so as to maintain stored energy (which translates essentially to adipose tissue mass) within a narrow envelope. It is clear that body weight often maintains an impressive constancy. It is also clear that negative-feedback signals produced by body adiposity affect eating. What is not clear is whether these signals contribute to an active regulation produced by a negative-feedback control system that, like the thermostatic control of a centrally heated building, includes set points, comparators, and error signals. A simpler alternative hypothesis is that the relative constancy of body weight results from a passive steady state. This hypothesis seems to fit better the common observation that a laboratory animal's body weight is easily increased by offering it palatable, energy-dense foods. The dramatic increase in obesity in the United States in the past decades and the increased access to highly palatable, energy-dense foods suggests that the same is true of humans. Consequently, the role of adiposity-related negative-feedback signals in eating is best understood without the hypothesis of an active regulation of body weight.

Leptin Leptin is a secretory product of the adipose tissue, especially visceral or abdominal adipose tissue, that was discovered in 1994. Leptin appears to act as a negative-feedback signal for meal size (recall that this feedback does not arise from stimuli generated during the meal but is indirectly related to eating through its effect on adiposity). Single gene mutations that disrupt the leptin signaling pathway produce dramatic syndromes of increased meal size, hyperphagia, obesity, and diabetes of obese (*ob/ob*) and diabetic (*db/db*) mice. The wild-type *ob* gene, *Lep*, encodes the peptide leptin, and

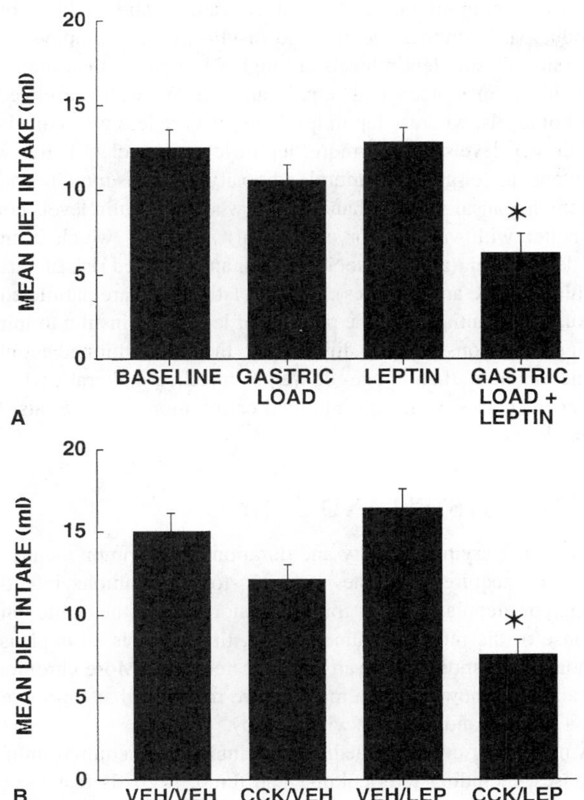

FIGURE 1.21–6 Leptin administration increases the satiating effects of intragastric nutrient preloads and of cholecystokinin (CCK) injections. **A:** Intracerebroventricular administration of leptin increases the satiating potency of nutrient preloads in rats. Intragastric infusion of a complete liquid nutrient (Ensure; Ross Products, Abbott Laboratories, Abbott Park, IL) alone had only a small inhibitory effect on the size of subsequent test meals, and intracerebroventricular infusions of leptin had no significant effect, whereas the gastric loads plus brain leptin administration significantly reduced meal size (*). (From Emond M, Schwartz GJ, Ladenheim EE, Moran TH: Central leptin modulates behavioral and neural responsivity to CCK. *Am J Physiol.* 1999;276:R1545–R1549, with permission.) **B:** Leptin increases the satiating potency of CCK in rats. Compared to control tests in which only drug vehicles were administered (VEH/VEH), intraperitoneal injection of 4 μg/kg CCK alone (CCK/VEH) significantly reduced subsequent liquid nutrient intake, intracerebroventricular injection of leptin alone (VEH/LEP) was without effect, and the combination of CCK and leptin (CCK/LEP) produced a significantly larger reduction in test meal size than did CCK treatment alone (*). (From Emond M, Ladenheim EE, Schwartz GJ, Moran TH: Leptin amplifies the feeding inhibition and neural activation arising from a gastric nutrient preload. *Physiol Behav.* 2001;72:123–128, with permission.)

the wild-type *db* gene, *Lepr*, encodes the leptin receptor. Plasma leptin levels are closely correlated with body fat mass. Leptin acts in the brain to inhibit eating. It is transported across the blood–brain barrier by a specific transport mechanism to reach leptin receptors in several brain loci, and eating is reduced by administration of leptin directly into the cerebral ventricles, the hypothalamus, or the NTS area of the caudal brainstem. Furthermore, at least in the short term, central administration of leptin antibodies stimulates eating. Leptin also appears to have other functions related to nutritional status, including reduction of the neuroendocrine responses to food deprivation and regulation of the onset of puberty.

Central and peripheral administration of leptin reduces eating by selectively decreasing meal size. How does increased leptin, a presumably tonic signal produced by increased adipose mass, decrease meal size? Presumably, leptin increases the activity of brain interneuronal networks that mediate satiation. Recent evidence suggests that this may occur in the caudal brainstem areas that receive negative-feedback signals from the gut. First, leptin increases the satiating potency of gastric loads and CCK (Fig. 1.21–6). Second, leptin increases the neuronal activation produced by gastric loads and CCK in the caudal brainstem region that receives these gut negative-feedback signals.

Leptin receptors in the arcuate nucleus of the hypothalamus have been localized to neurons that express various interneuronal signaling molecules that have been linked to the control of eating, including neuropeptide Y (NPY), α-melanocyte-stimulating hormone, and agouti-related peptide. The neuroanatomical, neuropharmacological, and neurophysiological analyses of the brain networks in which these neurons function are areas of intense investigation and have not yet revealed how leptin reduces eating.

Numerous questions remain for the hypothesis that leptin plays a physiological role in the determination of meal size. One question regards leptin resistance. In humans and animals, the inhibitory effect of exogenous leptin on eating usually decreases as overweight and hyperleptinemia increase. Decreased leptin transport into the brain may be part of the mechanism for this resistance. This phenomenon may also explain leptin's apparent inability to decrease eating sufficiently to prevent weight gain. Animals and humans with apparently normal leptin systems can easily be induced to overeat and to become obese, for example, by easy access to palatable, energy-rich foods. It has been suggested that these data may reflect a fundamental asymmetry in leptin physiology, such that leptin levels below a critical threshold stimulate eating and reduce energy expenditure in defense of body fat stores, whereas leptin levels above this threshold provoke little or no reciprocal response, allowing adiposity to increase.

Disturbed leptin signaling may also be a factor in human obesity. A few humans with homozygous mutations of the leptin or leptin receptor gene have been identified; not surprisingly, these rare individuals display dramatic syndromes like *ob/ob* and *db/db* mice. Perhaps more relevant to obesity are the reports that heterozygosity for mutations in *Lep* or *Lepr* is associated with increased body weight.

Insulin and Amylin There is substantial evidence that two other peripheral peptides act as negative-feedback signals relating eating to adiposity. These peptides, insulin and amylin, are synthesized and cosecreted by the pancreatic beta cells. Their apparent function as adiposity signals appears to be independent of their possible role in satiation (Table 1.21–2). That is, their adiposity signaling is related to tonic plasma levels (which are positively correlated with adiposity for both), and their direct satiating signaling is related to phasic, meal-related levels. For both peptides, chronic peripheral or central administration decreases eating and body weight, and central administration of antagonists to them increases eating. Like leptin, insulin and amylin selectively decrease meal size. It is important that centrally administered insulin inhibits feeding without eliciting the hormone's peripheral metabolic effects. Furthermore, because adipocytes require insulin to deposit fat, weight gain cannot occur during peripheral insulin insufficiency, even if food intake increases, as occurs in uncontrolled diabetes mellitus.

SEXUAL DIFFERENTIATION OF EATING

Ovarian cycling and other reproductive states affect eating. Adult female mammals of many species decrease eating during the periovulatory phase of the cycle. In rats, this is the day of estrus (i.e., of sexual receptivity) in their 4-day cycle, but the change in eating is independent of the change in sexual receptivity. The decreased eating is caused by the increase in estradiol levels in the diestrus and proestrus phases preceding estrus. There is also a periovulatory decrease in eating in monkeys and in women, which is presumably also caused by the increased estradiol levels during the follicular phase. In women, the effect is at most a few hundred kcal per day and is not consciously appreciated. In cycling animals, oophorectomy causes increased eating and weight gain, both of which are normalized by estradiol treatment (but not by treatment with other reproductive hormones). The periovulatory decrease and the postoophorectomy increase are caused by selective changes in meal size; meal frequency does not contribute. Indeed, when the hyperphagia of oophorectomized rats abates after they have increased body weight by approximately 25 percent, it is because meal frequency decreases; the oophorectomy-induced increase in meal size is permanent. This is a good example of the importance of meal pattern analysis in understanding the controls of eating. Estradiol decreases meal size during the periovulatory phase in rats at least in part by selectively increasing the potency of the satiation signals of CCK and pancreatic glucagon (Fig. 1.21–7).

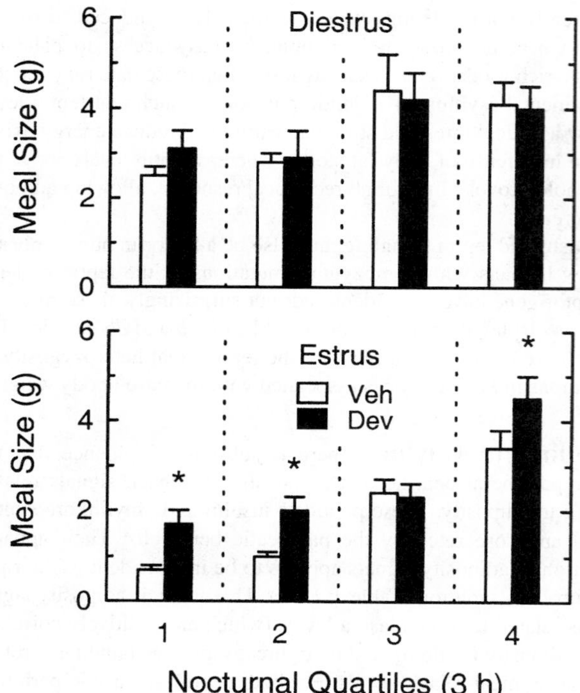

FIGURE 1.21–7 Endogenous cholecystokinin (CCK) contributes to the control of meal size more during the periovulatory phase than the early preovulatory phase (diestrus 2) in rats. Intraperitoneal injection of the CCK-1 receptor antagonist devazepide (Dev) (1 mg/kg) at the onset of the night of estrus significantly increased nocturnal spontaneous meal size (*), but Dev injection at the onset of the second night had no effect. Data are the mean sizes of spontaneous meals initiated during each 3-hour quartile of the dark phase. Meal frequency was not affected by Dev, so that total food nocturnal food intake increased significantly in rats treated with Dev during estrus. Note that, during estrus, Dev significantly increased meal size early in the dark, when control meals were small, and later in the dark, when control meals were as large as those during early dark in diestrus. Thus, Dev's effect was not an artifact of the smaller average meal size during estrus. Veh, vehicle. (From Eckel LA, Geary N: Endogenous cholecystokinin's satiating action increases during estrus in female rats. *Peptides.* 1999;20:451, with permission.)

An emerging literature connects estradiol (and perhaps other reproductive hormones), leptin, and insulin in the pathophysiology of obesity. Plasma leptin levels are higher in women than men, and leptin levels in women and female animals are well correlated to estradiol levels, whereas leptin levels in men are less well correlated to androgen levels. Furthermore, leptin levels correlate better with subcutaneous (or gluteal-femoral) adiposity, which is more prevalent in premenopausal women than in men, whereas insulin levels correlate better with visceral (or abdominal) adiposity, which is more prevalent in men (and is associated with an increased risk of cardiovascular disease and diabetes). These relationships are paralleled by a sexual differentiation in the potency of leptin and insulin to inhibit feeding: Injections of leptin directly into the brain inhibited eating in female rats more than in age- or weight-matched male rats, whereas similar injections of insulin inhibited eating more in male rats than in female rats.

IMMUNE SYSTEM AND EATING

Anorexia of varying intensity and duration is a common element of innate and acquired immune responses to, for example, infection, trauma, or neoplasm. The transient anorexia of the acute phase response of the innate immune system, like fever, is an unpleasant but adaptive response that can facilitate recovery. More chronic illness anorexia, however, is a maladaptive response that can increase illness severity and interfere with therapy.

A number of cytokine mediators of innate and acquired immune responses, including interleukin-1 and tumor necrosis factor-α, are involved in illness anorexia in animals. Peripherally released cytokines apparently affect the brain directly and indirectly via endocrine and peripheral neural responses. Peripheral immune responses can also lead to de novo production of cytokines within the CNS. In animals, these various cytokine responses can lead to reduced meal size or reduced meal number, or both. Illness anorexia in humans remains poorly understood but is presumably equally complex.

CENTRAL MECHANISMS THAT INFLUENCE MEAL SIZE

Brainstem The afferent signals arising from peripheral influences of meal size are initially processed in the hindbrain by a local interneuronal network that consists of sensory neurons that receive afferent stimuli from the gut, interneurons that integrate these stimuli, and premotor and motor neurons of the cranial nerves that produce the rhythmic oral movements of eating. Although this hindbrain network is the lowest level of the neural hierarchy mediating meal size, it alone is sufficient to produce many of the integrated aspects of the control of meal size. This has been elegantly demonstrated in decerebrate rats, in which supracollicular transections of the brainstem disconnect the hindbrain from the diencephalon and telencephalon. Decerebrate rats do not search for food and do not initiate eating, except, when liquid food is delivered into the mouth, they eat and swallow discrete meals that are terminated by passive rejection of delivered food. Most importantly, the size of these meals is normally responsive to some of the same oropharyngeal and GI feedback signals of meal size that operate in the intact rat, including the stimulatory effect of sucrose and the inhibitory effect of CCK on eating (Fig. 1.21–8).

Forebrain Experimental manipulations of the hypothalamus can dramatically affect eating. Lateral hypothalamic damage produces

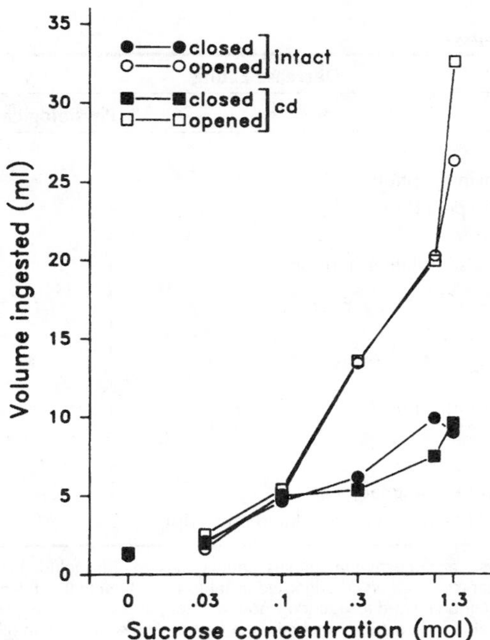

FIGURE 1.21–8 Eating behavior in intact and chronic decerebrate (cd) rats. Various concentrations of sucrose were delivered by intraoral catheters so that rats could ingest it or passively reject it by allowing it to drip from the mouth. Intake is an increasing function of sucrose concentration in cd rats that feed normally (closed condition). The gain of this function is dramatically increased in sham feeding rats in which postingestive controls of meal size are minimized by opening a gastric cannula (opened condition). Note the close correspondence, in intact and cd rats, of the stimulatory effect on eating of increasing sucrose concentration and the interaction of this stimulatory effect with the inhibitory effect of normal postingestive food stimuli. (From Grill HJ, Kaplan JM: Sham feeding in intact and chronic decerebrate rats. *Am J Physiol.* 1992;262:R1070, with permission.)

hypophagia, whereas electrical stimulation in this area elicits eating. Lesion and stimulation of the ventromedial hypothalamus have the opposite results. Originally presented as explanations of how eating was organized neurologically into a lateral hunger center reciprocally connected with a medial satiety center, these hypothalamic effects are now seen as problems to be solved in terms of hypothalamic functions in the distributed neural network that mediates eating. As mentioned previously, most contemporary analyses seek to identify the sites of actions and functional roles of particular signaling molecules in the brain. This work has led to increased understanding of the roles in eating of other hypothalamic areas, including the arcuate, paraventricular, and dorsomedial nuclei, as well as an increasing roster of telencephalic sites, including the nucleus accumbens, ventral pallidum, amygdala, olfactory cortex, visceral sensory cortex, and orbitofrontal cortex. The increasing sophistication of this work implicates increasingly widespread neuronal networks in the mediation of eating. This blurs apparent functional boundaries between the neurobiological substrates of eating, arousal, reward, learning, etc., because a local neuronal network in a specific site can be part of several larger networks that mediate these functions.

Brain Signaling Molecules Central administration of numerous neurochemicals has been shown to stimulate eating, to inhibit eating, or, depending on the situation or the site of administration, to do both. The extent to which the endogenous neurochemical plays a physiological role in eating can be assessed by using criteria derived from the classical criteria for neurotransmitter or neuromodulatory function (Table 1.21–3). Although much has been accomplished, these stringent criteria make clear that much remains to be done (Table 1.21–4). The following paragraphs give examples of recent progress made by examining one neurochemical that stimulates eating, one that inhibits eating, and one that can do both.

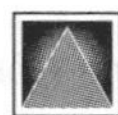

Table 1.21–3
Empirical Criteria for the Physiological Status of Interneuronal Signaling Molecules in the Mediation of Eating

1. The molecule's synaptic activity changes at the appropriate brain site at the appropriate time. For example, for molecules mediating satiation, this could be increased release or decreased inactivation during meals, and, for molecules mediating meal initiation, this could be such changes during the intermeal interval.
2. Cognate receptors for the molecule are expressed at its site(s) of action.
3. Administration of the molecule at its brain site(s) of action in amounts that reproduce the changes in (1) is sufficient for the appropriate behavioral effect.
4. Administration of the molecule as in (2) is sufficient to produce postsynaptic ionotropic or metabotropic effects in the neurons expressing the cognate receptors.
5. The molecule's behavioral effect occurs in the absence of pathophysiological behavioral, physiological, or subjective side effects.
6. Administration of selective agonists and antagonists to these receptors produces effects on eating consistent with their receptor pharmacologies.

Note: These criteria closely parallel the criteria for proof of a neurotransmitter or neuromodulator. No interneuronal signaling molecules have yet met all of these criteria for proof of physiological status as part of the mechanism of eating.

Neuropeptide Y (NPY) NPY is a potent stimulant of eating. Acute central NPY administration increases feeding in numerous animal species, although it had no effect in the single test in nonhuman primates. Chronic central NPY administration leads to sustained hyperphagia and increased body weight in rats. Although NPY is frequently described as a hunger signal, its major effect is to increase meal size rather than to increase the frequency of meal initiation.

The paraventricular nucleus and the adjacent perifornical hypothalamus, which receive projections from NPY cells in the hindbrain and in the arcuate nucleus of the hypothalamus, are considered the most likely sites for a physiological action of NPY. NPY concentrations in this area change during meals, and administration of NPY antibodies or antisense NPY deoxynucleotides here decreases feeding.

The analysis of NPY in eating has also, however, produced some surprises. For example, transgenic knock-out of NPY does not noticeably affect eating or body weight in mice. In addition, when liquid food is infused intraorally, rats do not increase ingestion after NPY administration (in this situation, rats ingest the intraoral infusate or let it drain from their mouths). This result suggests that NPY may selectively stimulate the consummatory phase of eating without affecting the *appetitive* processes mediating the search and acquisition for food.

Serotonin (5-Hydroxytryptamine [5-HT]) The prototypical 5-HT agonist D-fenfluramine, which releases synaptic 5-HT and blocks 5-HT reuptake, inhibits eating in animals and humans. The inhibitory effect in rodents can be blocked by antagonism of two 5-HT receptor subtypes, 2C (5-HT_{2C}) and 1B (5-HT_{1B}) (which is the

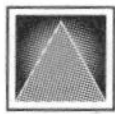

Table 1.21–4
Interneuronal Signaling Molecules Implicated in the Control of Eating

Increase Eating		Decrease Eating	
Molecule	**Physiological Status**	**Molecule**	**Physiological Status**
Dopamine	++	Serotonin	++
Neuropeptide Y	++	Gastrin-releasing peptide	++
Norepinephrine	++	Glucagon-like peptide 1	++
Endogenous opioids	++	Acetylcholine	++
Agouti-related peptide	+	α-Melanocyte-stimulating hormone	+
Growth hormone-releasing hormone	+	γ-Aminobutyric acid	+
Galanin	+	Dopamine	+
Melanin-concentrating hormone	?	Oxytocin	+
		Neuromedin B	+
		Gastrin-releasing peptide	+
		Glutamate	+
		Urocortin	+
		Corticotropin-releasing factor	+
		Cocaine- and amphetamine-regulated transcript	?

Note: Each signaling molecule listed occurs in the brain and has been implicated in the central physiology of eating in animals. Endogenous opioids include beta-endorphin and dynorphin. Physiological status in animals is rated as very likely (++), likely (+), or unclear (?), based on criteria listed in Table 1.21–3. Note that the molecules' hypothetical functional roles are not specified and range from controls of meal initiation (e.g., NE), food reward (e.g., endogenous opiates), and satiation (e.g., serotonin) to aversion anorexia (e.g., glucagon-like peptide-1). Furthermore, some molecules, such as dopamine, may act in some brain loci to stimulate eating and in other brain loci to inhibit eating. Finally, the table does not include signaling molecules that act on the brain but originate in the periphery, such as leptin, or in nonneural cells, such as immune system signaling molecules.

It is important to note that what is known derives mainly from animal studies, in which it is now possible to manipulate and to measure brain neurochemicals at the sites of their biological action during meals. In contrast, only indirect methods are possible in humans, such as measurements of the concentrations of neurotransmitters or their metabolites in the cerebrospinal fluid, and these cannot usually be done in the context of eating.

homolog of the 1D subtype in other mammals). Complementary work with 5-HT agonists indicates that 5-HT_{1B} receptors primarily affect meal size, and 5-HT_{2C} receptors affect eating rate. Endogenous 5-HT appears to have a physiological role in satiation, because meal size is increased by intraventricular injection of 5-HT_{2C} receptor antagonists and by direct injection of 5-HT type 1A receptor antagonists in the brainstem raphe, where they stimulate autoreceptors on 5-HT perikarya and decrease 5-HT release in the forebrain. Additionally, mutant mice without 5-HT_{2C} receptors are hyperphagic, overweight, and unresponsive to 5-HT agonists. There is also evidence that part of CCK's satiating action is mediated by central 5-HT_{2C} receptors. 5-HT may be also be involved in the stimulatory effect of sweet taste on eating. The paraventricular nucleus appears to be an important, but not the sole, site of 5-HT effects on eating in animals.

Dopamine Dopamine appears to play an important role in mediating the rewarding effects of food that maintain eating, produce pleasure, and reinforce learning about food. In animals, dopamine antagonists markedly decrease the appetitive and consummatory responses maintained by food. For example, in rats sham feeding with open gastric cannulas, dopamine antagonists selectively reduce sham intake of concentrated sucrose solutions by selectively decreasing the size of bursts of licks. This is the same microstructural change that characterizes rats' intake of less concentrated sucrose solutions and is different from the microstructural change associated with increased satiation, thus suggesting that dopamine decreases the orosensory positive-feedback effect of sucrose solutions. Furthermore, dopamine antagonists inhibit eating without altering the postingestive satiating potency of food, without impairing oromotor movements, and without creating aversions. Dopamine is released in several brain areas thought to mediate reward functions, including the medial hypothalamus, amygdala, and nucleus accumbens, where its release increases as a monotonic function of sucrose concentration.

Dopamine may also be involved in the inhibition of eating. Dopamine inhibits intake when injected into perifornical sites in the hypothalamus. This is a good example of how the effect of a transmitter on eating depends on site of action and on the neurobiological context provided by the activities of other aspects of the network it acts in. The role of hypothalamic dopamine in the inhibition of eating may explain the clinical finding that neuroleptics that antagonize dopamine increase body weight, apparently by increasing food intake.

LEARNING

Meal initiation, food selection, and meal size are all readily conditionable in animals and humans. Classical (or pavlovian) and instrumental (or operant) procedures are effective. Environmental context and flavor usually provide the CS for these learned controls. For example, when a sound or light CS was presented to rats before each of six scheduled meals for several days and then was tested during *extinction*, that is, when the rats had free access to the same diet, the CS elicited initiation of a large meal on each daily presentation for 3 weeks. Thus, cues that predict food availability during food deprivation can provoke the initiation of a large meal in the absence of deprivation. The UCS for this learning has not been identified.

Satiation is also conditionable. The UCSs for conditioned satiation are the postingestive consequences of eating. For example, rats that drink flavored water while proteins, carbohydrates, or fats are intragastrically infused subsequently eat less food with that flavor. This is satiation, not aversion. When preference is tested, the rats choose the flavor associated with the nutrient infusion. Interestingly, different neural mechanisms appear to mediate conditioned satiation and conditioned preference (Fig. 1.21–9). The importance of conditioned controls can be demonstrated in the absence of explicit learning contingencies, for example, by using the sham feeding procedure to extinguish conditioned controls of meal size (Fig. 1.21–10).

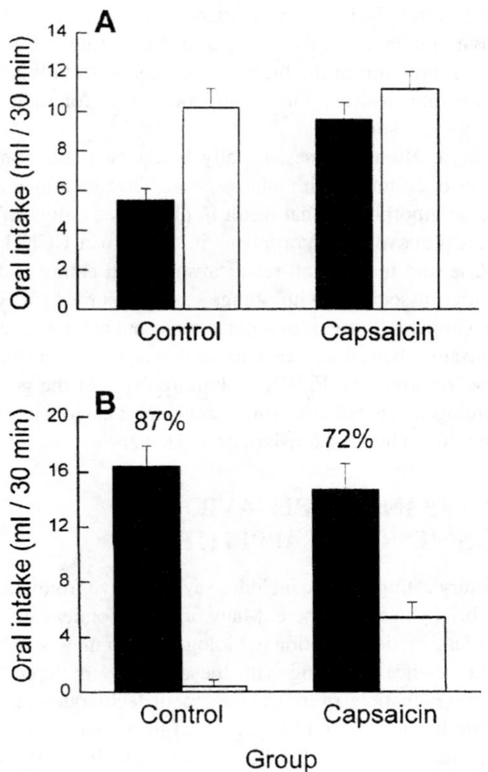

FIGURE 1.21–9 Intraduodenal carbohydrate conditions satiation and preference in rats by at least partially distinct gut afferent mechanisms. Rats were trained to drink a flavored saccharin solution during intraduodenal infusions of carbohydrate and, on other days, a differently flavored solution during control water infusions. One group of rats was first treated with capsaicin, a neurotoxin that produced partial visceral deafferentation by destroying unmyelinated sensory fibers. **A:** During training tests, intraduodenal carbohydrate infusions (*filled bars*) reduced saccharin intake in intact rats but not in capsaicin-treated rats. **B:** During subsequent choice tests during which both flavors were presented, and no infusions were done, intact and capsaicin-treated rats strongly preferred the flavor previously paired with intraduodenal carbohydrate (percentages are the intake of carbohydrate-paired flavor divided by the total intake). (From Lucas F, Sclafani A: Capsaicin attenuates feeding suppression but not reinforcement by intestinal nutrients. *Am J Physiol.* 1996;270:R1059, with permission.)

Higher-order conditioning is likely to play important roles in human eating. For example, cultural socialization may result in a preference for the flavor of capsaicin (chili), which all infants avoid. Indeed, with the exception of a few unconditioned gustatory preferences and aversions (such as for sweet and bitter tastes), *all* food selection appears to be learned. Some forms of learned controls of eating are special forms of conditioning. Flavor aversions conditioned by upper GI food poisoning, for example, can be learned after only one CS-UCS pairing, despite extraordinarily long CS-UCS delays (hours), and are extremely resistant to extinction.

The analysis of the influence of learning on human eating should be a high priority. The number of unconditioned brain mechanisms, through which all learned influences of meal size presumably operate, is small enough to imagine achieving control of them in humans. Furthermore, behavior therapy programs, because they are relatively highly structured and can present specific food stimuli, should provide excellent opportunities for the clinical use of conditioned physiological controls of eating.

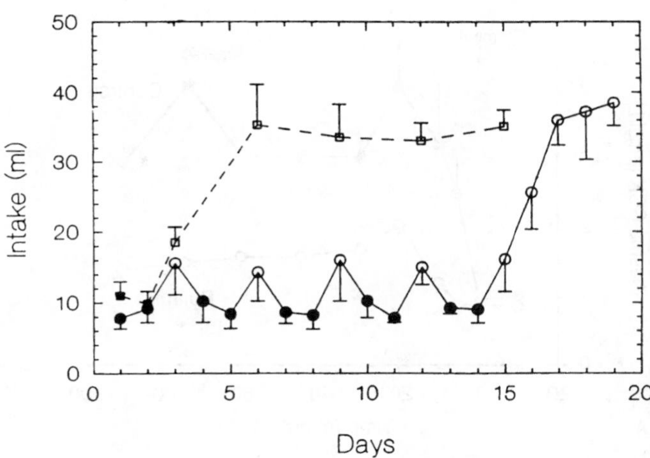

FIGURE 1.21–10 The role of conditioned satiation in eating in the rat. Data are 30-minute intakes of 0.8 mol sucrose in two groups of rats in successive tests. Rats were prepared with steel gastric cannulas that were closed (*closed symbols*) during real feeding tests or open (*open symbols*) for sham feeding tests, during which sucrose did not accumulate in the stomach or enter the intestines. One group (*squares*) real fed sucrose once and then sham fed. The other group (*circles*) alternated real and sham feeding tests. The progressive increase in sucrose intake in the first two tests in which rats sham fed was prevented by interspersing two normal feeding tests between each sham feeding test. When this is done, sham intake is significantly larger than real intake but is significantly smaller than the asymptotic sham intake. These data reveal that normal feeding of sucrose produces a learned association between the taste of the sucrose and its postingestive effects, that this association limits intake, and that it extinguishes during consecutive sham feeding tests. (From Davis JD, Smith GP: Learning to sham feed: Behavioral adjustments to loss of physiological postingestional stimuli. *Am J Physiol.* 1990;259:R1228, with permission.)

BEHAVIORAL NEUROSCIENCE OF DISORDERED EATING

The translation of the behavioral neuroscience of eating into clinical research has opened new perspectives on eating disorders. This is exemplified by recent progress in the analysis of eating in patients with disordered eating. Two demonstrations that patients with bulimia nervosa binge in the laboratory were especially important. First, it was discovered that, under laboratory conditions, patients with bulimia nervosa eat significantly larger meals than do normal volunteers. This difference can be obtained in individual test meals of a single test diet or in residential laboratory settings in which subjects have free access to a variety of foods for one or more days. A study of the latter design by Walter H. Kaye and colleagues showed that patients with bulimia and control subjects took similar numbers of meals and that most of the meals taken by patients with bulimia were within the range of meal sizes displayed by the controls, but that approximately one-fourth of the meals taken by the patients were larger than any meal taken by control subjects, on average by a factor of ten. The second discovery was that cognitive stimuli are sufficient to induce binges in the laboratory. That is, when subjects are instructed to eat large meals, patients with bulimia nervosa eat much larger meals than do controls and report that these meals have the same subjective character as binges.

There is considerable evidence that the postingestive negative-feedback satiation signals are less potent in patients with bulimia: (1) Equivalent preloads of food decrease intake less in bulimic patients than in controls, particularly when the patients are eating large meals. (2) Patients with bulimia must eat larger amounts of

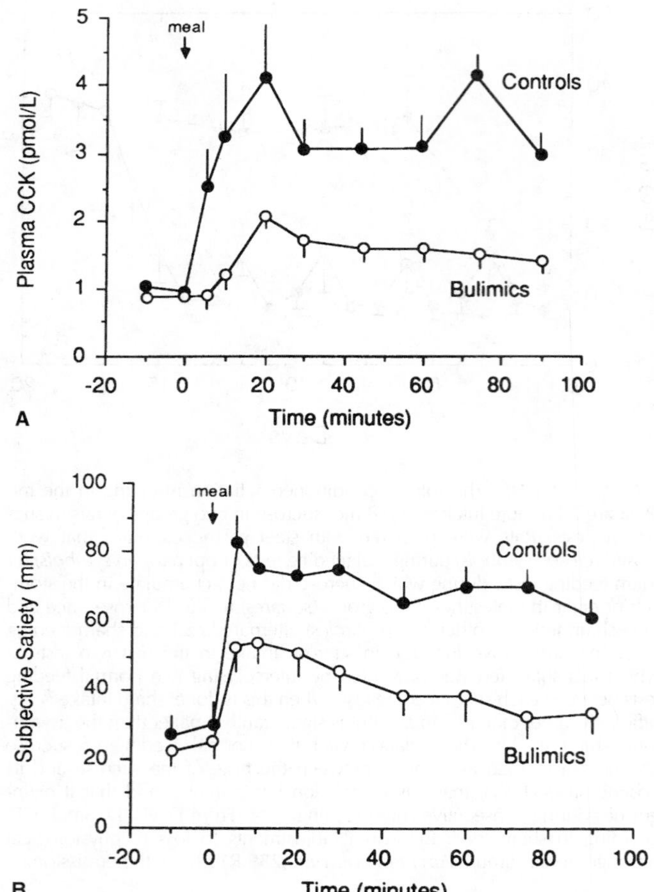

FIGURE 1.21–11 Prandial concentrations of cholecystokinin (CCK) **(A)** and the subjective experience of satiety **(B)** are reduced in patients with bulimia nervosa. Fourteen patients and ten control women matched for age and weight were offered a 400-mL liquid meal after an overnight fast (*arrows*) and ate it in 1 to 2 minutes. Plasma CCK was measured with a selective bioassay. Satiety was measured by a 100-mm visual analog scale (0 = empty and 100 = full). The peak CCK concentration and the integrated CCK response (*area under the curve*) were significantly reduced in bulimic patients, and this correlated with reports of significantly less satiety beginning 5 minutes after meal onset. (From Geracioti TD Jr, Liddle RA: Impaired cholecystokinin secretion in bulimia nervosa. *N Engl J Med.* 1988;319:683, with permission.)

food to produce equivalent self-reports of fullness during a meal. (3) Volume distention of the stomach produces a decreased perceptual and mechanical response in patients with bulimia, presumably because the stomachs are larger than normal as the result of accommodation to the frequent ingestion of large meals. (4) Food-stimulated CCK release is less in bulimic patients than in controls (Fig. 1.21–11). These abnormalities appear to resolve as bingeing decreases, suggesting that they are not the initial cause of bulimia. Nevertheless, it is possible that they facilitate the development of the disorder once it has begun and impede recovery from it.

Several results indicate that the abnormal central processing of meal-generated negative-feedback information in patients with bulimia nervosa may be due to decreased brain serotoninergic function. If central 5-HT function is decreased in bulimic patients, then they should be more vulnerable than controls to a further decrease in 5-HT function produced by acute 5-HT depletion. This prediction has been confirmed: Acute tryptophan depletion that probably decreased central 5-HT activity increased meal size in bulimic patients but not in controls. Studies documenting reduced 5-HT transporter expression in the brains of women with bulimia nervosa and binge-eating disorder further support a role for reduced 5-HT activity in these disorders.

Gene segregation analyses, usually based on predictions arising from studies of animals with mutated genes, have identified a number of genetic polymorphisms that result in disordered eating in humans. As mentioned above, polymorphisms in the human CCK-1 receptor gene, in *Lep*, and in *Lepr*, all result in increased eating and obesity. Obesity, often associated with binge-eating disorder (in which the binges are similar to those of bulimia nervosa but are not accompanied by compensatory behaviors), also accompanies melanocortin 4 receptor gene polymorphisms. Finally, polymorphisms of the gene encoding the endogenous melanocortin 4 receptor antagonist AGRP are associated with an increased risk of anorexia nervosa.

FRONTIERS IN THE BEHAVIORAL NEUROSCIENCE OF APPETITE

Contemporary eating science includes several active frontiers, a few of which are briefly described here. Many of these frontiers are related to the molecular genetic revolution in biology, which may be said to have reached the science of eating with the discovery of leptin in 1994. Innovative combinations of molecular genetic techniques and sophisticated classic behavioral and physiological techniques have produced particularly interesting results. Functional brain imaging is another frontier that has just begun to focus on evaluating brain networks that influence eating. Finally, improved measurements of eating behaviors and the feelings associated with them are also contributing to more rapid progress.

Molecular Genetics

Gene Therapy The first generation of molecular genetic techniques permitted targeted deletion, or knock out, of specific genes, thus providing a molecule-specific lesion. Current refinements of this method include procedures to make tissue-specific and environmentally inducible knock outs. In addition, it is now possible to reinsert or to rescue a missing gene. The first report of this in behavioral neuroscience of eating was tissue-specific reinsertion of *Lepr* in *db/db* mice, which lack it. The tissue specificity was provided by linking *Lepr* to an enolase gene that is expressed mainly in neurons. This procedure resulted in a nearly complete normalization of eating and body weight. A second strategy involved insertion of *Lep* linked to a retrovirus into the brains of *ob/ob* mice, which lack functional *Lep*. Again, a dramatic reversal of the *ob/ob* hyperphagia and obesity phenotype resulted. Such methods provide powerful tools for the behavioral neuroscience of eating and important potentials for future translation of basic research results into therapies for genetically based eating disorders.

Hybrid Techniques Molecular technology has begun to be combined with neurophysiological and neuroanatomical techniques. For example, targeted knock outs of mouse genes have been used in conjunction with tract-tracing viruses and fluorescent markers to reveal new aspects of the neural networks mediating eating. One such study demonstrated that hypothalamic neurons containing the feeding-stimulatory peptide NPY received neural inputs from limbic and cortical areas previously not known to influence hypothalamic NPY neurons. Furthermore, in a refinement of classical lesion strategies, novel biochemical conjugates are being applied to destroy selectively neurons with particular neurochemical phenotypes in living animals. To test the role of endogenous NPY in eating, neurotoxins conjugated to NPY that bind to and destroy only NPY-receptive neurons were injected into the brain, resulting in reduced food intake and body weight.

Nature and Nurture The interaction of genotype and environment is, of course, the gordian knot of biology. Two recent results highlight the unexpected ways in which gene–environment interactions determine normal eating. The first deals with melanocortins (MCs), a family of peptides derived from the proopiomelanocortin gene that is expressed in neurons and many other cell types. Brain MCs reduce food intake, and mice lacking a subpopulation of central MC receptors (MC3/4 knock-out mice) are typically obese and hyperphagic, suggesting that central MC signaling is involved in eating. However, merely providing access to a running wheel normalizes eating and body weight. These data reveal how the influence of genes on ingestion is modified by environmental variables.

A similar point emerges from a study of Otsuka Long-Evans Tokushima Fatty (OLETF) rats, which spontaneously fail to produce the CCK-1 receptor subtype that mediates the satiating action of peripheral CCK. Adult OLETF rats are hyperphagic owing to increased meal size and develop obesity and diabetes in adulthood. Providing young OLETF rats with access to running wheels before obesity develops normalizes their meal size and daily food intake and prevents the development of obesity and diabetes. Furthermore, eating and body weight remain normal after the wheels are removed. This suggests that temporary gene–environment interactions can have persisting behavioral influences. In addition, the potency of these interactions between physical activity and signaling molecules related to eating provides a compelling rationale for investigating the role of exercise in the development of anorexia nervosa.

Functional Brain Imaging Advances in positron emission tomography (PET), single photon emission computed tomography (SPECT), and functional magnetic resonance imaging (fMRI) technologies produce images of correlates of human brain activity, such as regional cerebral blood flow, with increasingly greater spatial and temporal resolutions. Such images have begun to provide detailed characterizations of the brain networks producing the subjective and behavioral phenomena of eating. Eating increases neuronal activity in prefrontal cortex in normal weight and obese humans and decreases activity in several limbic system structures, including insular cortex, parahippocampal gyrus, and hypothalamus. Conversely, fasting increases the neuronal activity produced by the sight of food in several limbic forebrain areas that are involved in processing alimentary tract information, including the amygdala and parahippocampal gyrus. These are encouraging beginnings in the search for differences in activation of eating-related brain networks as a function of meals, metabolic state, gender, disordered eating, etc. Progress in this field demands studies that probe satiation directly by sampling brain activation after eating different types and quantities of foods.

Behavioral and Subjective Measures The advent of high-technology molecular and genetic and imaging methodologies does not diminish the importance of developing improved methods to measure the behavioral and subjective phenotyping of eating. To the contrary, the need for new methods in these domains is only increased by such new developments. Two examples are the complexities of behavioral phenotypes exhibited by genetically modified animals and the temporal sampling constraints imposed by functional brain imaging techniques. Results from studies that apply reductionist molecular technologies are limited in their interpretational strength to the extent that they fail to assess eating behavior as an integral set of dependent measures. Eating is an integrative function of the CNS, and a systems-level synthesis is required to provide a full account of it. Such an account will require continued efforts to develop experimental techniques for laboratory measurements of behavioral and subjective responses in animals and in humans that capture the richness of the phenomenology of eating and that permit translation from the biology of the brain to the eating problems that bring patients to clinics.

SUGGESTED CROSS-REFERENCES

Sections 1.4, 1.5, and 1.6 contain further information on the physiology of neurotransmitters. Section 1.19 describes transgenic models of behavior. Basic learning theory is covered in Section 3.3. Eating disorders are reviewed in Chapter 19, and Section 24.3 includes background information on obesity.

References

Asakawa A, Inui A, Kaga T, Katsuura G, Fujimiya M, Fujino MA, Kasuga M: Antagonism of ghrelin receptor reduces food intake and body weight gain in mice. *Gut.* 2003;52:947.

Banks WA: Is obesity a disease of the blood brain barrier? Physiological, pathological and evolutionary considerations. *Curr Pharm Des.* 2003;9:801.

Batterham RL, Cohen MA, Ellis SM, Le Roux CW, Withers DJ, Frost G, Ghatei MA, Bloom SR: Inhibition of food intake in obese subjects by peptide YY3-36. *N Engl J Med.* 2003;349:941.

*Berthoud H-R: Multiple systems controlling food intake and body weight. *Neurosci Biobehav Rev.* 2002;26;393–428.

Booth DA, ed. *Neurophysiology of Ingestion.* New York: Pergamon Press; 1993.

Branson R, Potoczna N, Kral JG, Lentes KU, Hoehe MR, Horber FF: Binge eating as a major phenotype of melanocortin 4 receptor gene mutations. *N Engl J Med.* 2003;348:1096.

Clegg DJ, Reidy CA, Blake Smith KA, Benoit SC, Woods SC: Differential sensitivity to central leptin and insulin in male and female rats. *Diabetes.* 2003;52:682–687.

Cowley MA, Smart JL, Rubinstein M, Cerdan MG, Diano S, Horvath TL, Cone RD, Low MJ: Leptin activates anorexigenic POMC neurons through a neural network in the arcuate nucleus. *Nature.* 2001;411:480.

DeFalco J, Tomishima M, Liu H, Zhao C, Cai X, Marth JD, Enquist L, Friedman JM: Virus-assisted mapping of neural inputs to a feeding center in the hypothalamus. *Science.* 2001;291:2608.

Devlin MJ, Walsh BJ, Guss JL, Kissileff HR, Liddle RA, Petkova E: Postprandial cholecystokinin release and gastric emptying in patients with bulimia nervosa. *Am J Clin Nutr.* 1997;65:114.

Dhillon H, Kalra SP, Prima V, Zolotukhin S, Scarpace PJ, Moldawer LL, Muzyczka N, Kalra PS: Central leptin gene therapy suppresses body weight gain, adiposity and serum insulin without affecting food consumption in normal rats: A long term study. *Regul Pept.* 2001;99:69.

Fairburn CG, Brownell KD, eds. *Eating Disorders and Obesity: A Comprehensive Handbook.* 2nd ed. New York: The Guilford Press; 2002.

Farooqi IS, Keogh JM, Yeo GS, Lank EJ, Cheetham T, O'Rahilly S: Clinical spectrum of obesity and mutations in the melanocortin 4 receptor gene. *N Engl J Med.* 2003;348:1085.

Friedman JM: Leptin and the regulation of body weight. *The Harvey Lecture Series.* 2001;95:107.

*Geary N: Effects of glucagon, insulin, amylin and CGRP on feeding. *Neuropeptides.* 1999;33;400.

Geary N: Estradiol, CCK and satiation. *Peptides.* 2001;22:1251.

*Grill HJ, Kaplan JM: The neuroanatomical axis for control of energy balance. *Front Neuroendocrinol.* 2002;23:2–40.

Heymsfeld SB, Greenberg AS, Fujioka K, Dixon RM, Kushner R, Hunt T, Lubina JA, Patane J, Self B, Hunt P, McCamish M: Recombinant leptin for weight loss in obese and lean adults: A randomized, controlled, dose-escalation trial. *JAMA.* 1999;282:1568.

Kaye WH, Weltzin TE, McKee M, McConaha C, Hansen D, Hsu LKG: Laboratory assessment of feeding behavior in bulimia nervosa and healthy women: Methods for developing a human-feeding laboratory. *Am J Clin Nutr.* 1992;55:372.

Kissilef HR, Wentzlaff TH, Guss JL, Walsh BT, Devlin JJ, Thornton JC: A direct measure of satiety disturbance in patients with bulimia nervosa. *Physiol Behav.* 1996;60:1077.

*Kowalski TJ, Liu SM, Leibel RL, Chua SC Jr: Transgenic complementation of leptin-receptor deficiency. I. Rescue of the obesity/diabetes phenotype of LEPR-null mice expressing a LEPR-B transgene. *Diabetes.* 2001;50:425.

*Langhans W, Hrupka B: Cytokines and appetite. 2004 *(in press).*

Lavin JH, Wittert G, Sun W-M, Horowitz M, Morley JE, Read NW: Appetite regulation by carbohydrate: role of blood glucose and gastrointestinal hormones. *Am J Physiol.* 1996;271:E209.
Leibel RL: The role of leptin in the control of body weight. *Nutr Rev.* 2002;60:S15.
List JF, Habener JF: Defective melanocortin 4 receptors in hyperphagia and morbid obesity. *N Engl J Med.* 2003;348:1160.
Masuzaki H, Paterson J, Shinyama H, Morton NM, Mullins JJ, Seckl JR, Flier JS: A transgenic model of visceral obesity and the metabolic syndrome. *Science.* 2001;294:2166.
*Moran TH: Cholecystokinin and satiety: Current perspectives. *Nutrition.* 2000;16:858.
Rinaman L, Rothe EE: GLP-1 receptor signaling contributes to anorexigenic effect of centrally-administered oxytocin in rats. *Am J Physiol.* 2002;283:R99.
Robinson SW, Dinulescu DM, Cone RD: Genetic models of obesity and energy balance in the mouse. *Annu Rev Genet.* 2000;34:687.
Rushing PA: Central amylin signaling and the regulation of energy homeostasis. *Curr Pharm Des.* 2003;9:819.
*Scharrer E: Control of food intake by fatty acid oxidation and ketogenesis. *Nutrition.* 1999;15:704.
Sclafani A: Psychobiology of food preferences. *Int J Obes.* 2001;25:S13.
Smith GP. Dopamine and food reward. In: Fluharty SJ, Morrison AR, Sprague J, eds. *Progress in Physiological Psychology and Psychobiology.* Vol 16. San Diego, CA: Academic Press; 1995:83.
*Smith GP, ed. *Satiation from the Gut to the Brain.* New York: Oxford University Press; 1998.
Tanaka M, Naruo T, Yasuhara D, Tatebe Y, Nagai N, Shiiya T, Nakazoto M, Matsukura S, Nozoe S: Fasting ghrelin levels in subtypes of anorexia nervosa. *Psychoneuroendocrinology.* 2003;28:829.
Vink T, Hinney A, van Elburg AA, van Goozen SH, Sandkuijl LA, Sinke RJ, Herpertz-Dahlmann BM, Hebebrand J, Remschmidt H, van Engeland H, Adan RA: Association between an agouti-related protein gene polymorphism and anorexia nervosa. *Mol Psychiatry.* 2001;6:325.
Weingarten HP: Conditioned cues elicit feeding in sated rats: a role for learning in meal initiation. *Science.* 1983;220:431–433.
Weltzin TE, Fernstrom MH, Fernstrom JD, Neuberger SK, Kaye WH: Acute tryptophan depletion and increased food intake and irritability in bulimia nervosa. *Am J Psychiatry.* 1995;152:1668.
Woods SC, Stricker EM. Food intake and metabolism. In: Zigmond MJ, Bloom FE, McConnell SK, Roberts JL, Spitzer NC, Zigmond MJ, eds. *Fundamental Neuroscience.* 2nd ed. San Diego, CA: Academic Press; 2002:991–1009.

▲ 1.22 Neural Basis of Substance Abuse and Dependence

DAVID W. SELF, PH.D.

Over the past few decades, tremendous advances have been made in understanding the neurobiological basis of substance abuse and dependence. These advancements stem from early psychopharmacological studies on the neural substrates of drug and alcohol reinforcement to recently discovered molecular alterations that accompany chronic substance abuse. In addition, recent studies have begun to differentiate the role that specific neurobiological changes play in discrete behavioral changes that accompany substance dependence in animals, and the combination of this animal work with advancements in human neuroimaging has led to an integrative systems level view of the addicted brain.

This chapter begins by defining some of the fundamental behavioral changes underlying substance abuse and dependence, followed by an overview of the neurobiological substrates of drugs and alcohol reinforcement, and craving and relapse. Adaptations in these substrates are discussed in terms of alterations at the systems, synaptic, and molecular levels, using exemplary changes commonly found across multiple abused substances. Finally, the perplexing, but important, question of why patients experience relapse after abstaining for prolonged periods is discussed in light of learning- and memory-based theories recently modeled in animals. In many instances, human studies have corroborated certain findings and added complementary information to form a more comprehensive view of functional abnormalities and brain changes in dependent patients.

REINFORCEMENT, INCENTIVE MOTIVATION, AND ADDICTION

The fact that animals learn to self-administer virtually every substance abused by humans has been an enormous advantage for basic research on substance abuse and dependence. Thus, drug and alcohol self-administration in animals precisely emulates many features of human substance abuse. Abused substances are defined as reinforcing if they increase and maintain the occurrence of specific behaviors in animals, such as a lever press response that delivers drug injections. Such rapid and powerful associations between a reinforcing drug stimulus and the drug-seeking response reflect an ability to directly modulate preexisting brain reinforcement mechanisms. Under normal circumstances, these mechanisms reinforce the pursuit of food, water, and sexual and social interaction. Although this definition of reinforcement is purely operational, most abused substances are thought to function as positive reinforcers, because they produce a positive affective state (e.g., reward or euphoria), most notably during the initial stages of drug use. However, some substances are thought to possess negative reinforcing properties, thereby alleviating pain, anxiety, or distress attributed to an underlying depression or to withdrawal from chronic substance use.

Appetitive and Consummatory Phases

Self-administration is a complex behavior, but critical features are represented by two behaviorally distinct phases. The first phase is referred to as an *appetitive phase* and is reflected when animals engage in behavior aimed at obtaining drugs, such as approaching and responding at a lever previously associated with delivery of intravenous (IV) drug injections. The pursuit of further reinforcement is thought to represent incentive motivation or drive elicited by environmental cues previously associated with drugs through pavlovian conditioning. In humans, the appetitive phase often is described by subjective qualities, such as wanting or craving, and objectively is indicated by *drug-seeking behavior.* Basic research on craving and relapse is aimed at understanding the neurobiological events that trigger and maintain drug-seeking behavior during the appetitive phase. Drug-seeking behavior can be measured in a variety of animal self-administration paradigms, many of which focus on the triggers of relapse after prolonged periods of withdrawal from chronic drug or alcohol self-administration.

The appetitive phase culminates with delivery of the drug injection and is immediately followed by a *consummatory phase* (referring to consummation of the act or receiving the goal). In humans, subjective descriptions of the consummatory phase include "rush," "high," euphoria, and temporary satiation of craving. In animals, the consummatory phase is characterized by a notable absence, or pause, in further drug-seeking behavior. The postinjection pause is tightly regulated by the amount of drug received in the injection, such that increasing the injection dose also increases the length of the pause between successive self-injections. Thus, higher injection doses actually decrease the number of injections self-administered over a given period of time, despite their increasing reinforcement value. This inverse relationship produces an inverted U-shaped self-administration dose–response curve (Fig. 1.22–1A), spanning thresh-

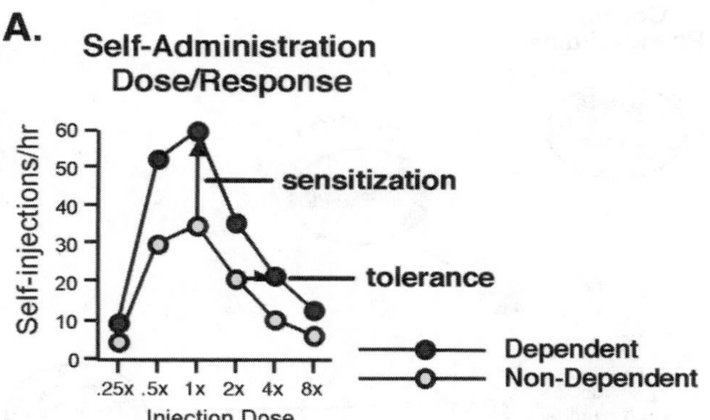

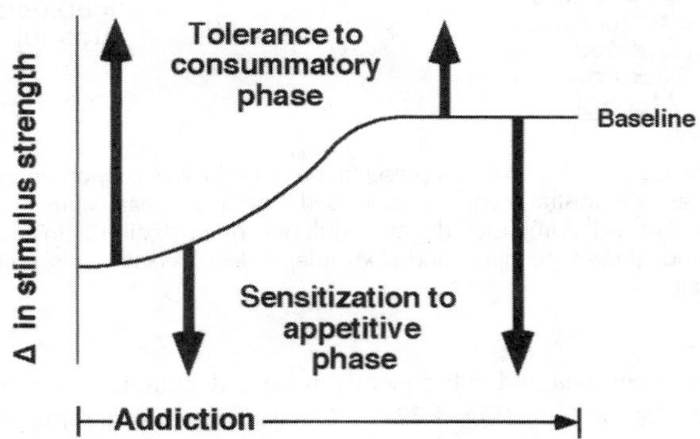

FIGURE 1.22–1 Comparison of the self-administration dose–response relationship in dependent versus nondependent animals **(A)**. The addicted phenotype is indicated by a vertical and rightward shift in the inverted U-shaped dose–response curve typical of drug and alcohol self-administration. These alterations result from opposing changes in appetitive and consummatory phases of drug self-administration as the addiction process develops **(B)**. Tolerance reduces the signal strength of drug during the consummatory phase of self-administration, resulting in a rightward shift in the descending limb of the curve. Sensitization increases the signal strength of stimuli that elicit drug seeking during the appetitive phase. This latter change is reflected by a vertical shift in the peak rate of drug self-administration, an index of increased motivation to maintain brain levels of drug as the injection dose is lowered.

old doses for maintaining self-administration, and a descending limb at higher doses, reflecting drug-induced inhibitory regulation (pause) of further drug intake.

Transition from Substance Abuse to Dependence

Chronic substance use leads to behavioral and neurobiological alterations referred to as *dependence* and is indicated by multiple psychiatric criteria listed in the text revision of the fourth edition of the *Diagnostic and Statistical Manual of Mental Disorders* (DSM-IV-TR), including an escalation in drug intake during self-administration, impulsive and compulsive drug use, markedly increased craving, or withdrawal symptoms, including dysphoria and anxiety, or a combination of these. In contrast, pharmacologists describe these phenomena as *addiction* in *Goodman and Gilman's the Pharmacological Basis of Therapeutics* to distinguish the psychological component of dependence from a broader spectrum of substances that produce physical, but not psychological, dependence. Certain psychiatric criteria for substance dependence have been modeled in animal self-

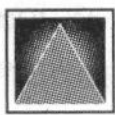

Table 1.22–1
Pharmacological and Psychiatric Changes of Addiction and Substance Dependence

Drug Addiction (Pharmacological)	Drug Dependence (Psychiatric)
Tolerance	Escalating intake (amount and frequency)
Reduced substance effectiveness	
Sensitization	Compulsive drug use (loss of control)
Increased substance effectiveness	Impulsivity
	Increased craving (positive affect)
Dependence	Dysphoria
Manifestation of opponent withdrawal symptoms	Anxiety
	Increased craving (negative affect)

administration experiments in attempts to dissociate *addicted* from *nonaddicted* states. In these studies, the addicted state is induced by increasing daily access to drug self-administration or is selected from outbred animal populations based on higher preferred levels of drug intake. Importantly, high levels of drug intake have been specifically related to increased drug-seeking behavior during withdrawal (compulsive drug use and craving), thereby encompassing major criteria for psychiatric dependence in animal models (Table 1.22–1).

From a strictly pharmacological viewpoint, escalating drug intake in dependent animals reflects the development of tolerance to the consummatory phase of self-administration, resulting in a rightward shift in the descending limb of the self-administration dose–response curve (Fig. 1.22–1). This view is supported by the fact that drug intake also increases with antagonist treatment, and the length of the postinjection pause in dependent animals becomes shorter in a manner that resembles reducing the injection dose. Tolerance to these rate-limiting drug effects may reflect tolerance to the euphorigenic or satiating effects of some drugs or tolerance to the sedative or aversive effects of other drugs.

While tolerance develops to certain consummatory properties of abused substances, sensitization (or reverse tolerance) simultaneously develops to the appetitive phase (Fig. 1.22–1B) as the incentive properties of abused substances and substance-related stimuli gain motivational salience. Thus, the ability of stimuli to trigger and maintain drug-seeking behavior is enhanced and is thought to contribute to compulsive substance use and progressive intensification of craving in humans. In animal studies, sensitization to the appetitive phase is reflected by progressive increases in the amount of effort (e.g., lever pressing) animals exert to obtain drugs or alcohol when reinforcement is withheld. This enhancement in the motivation to obtain reinforcement is also reflected by a vertical shift in the peak response rate a drug maintains in self-administration dose–response studies, because animals exert even greater effort to maintain blood levels as the injection dose is reduced (Fig. 1.22–1A). However, neither the dose thresholds nor the peak dose are shifted leftward, as should occur with an overall *pharmacological* sensitization to the drug. Therefore, maximal reinforcing efficacy is sensitized in the dependent state but without an increase in drug sensitivity. The concurrent development of tolerance to consummatory effects of drugs and sensitization to appetitive stimuli produces a vertical and rightward shift in self-administration dose–response curves in drug-dependent animals (Fig. 1.22–1A).

These changes in animal self-administration behavior are reflected in dependent patients by self-reports of dramatically increased wanting or craving but reduced euphoria during substance use when compared to earlier stages of their drug use history. Importantly, the psychological construct shown in Figure 1.22–1B suggests that escalating drug intake (tolerance) and increased craving (sensitization) results from mechanistically and, possibly, neurobiologically distinct phenomena that are studied independently to gain better access to their underlying neural substrates. Another notable aspect of substance dependence is the appearance of withdrawal symptoms (the pharmacological definition of *drug dependence*). These withdrawal symptoms typically oppose the acute physiological and behavioral effects of drugs and alcohol. For example, withdrawal from chronic benzodiazepine use is associated with anxiety, opiate withdrawal is associated with hyperalgesia, and most abused substances produce at least some degree of dysphoria or depression with abrupt discontinuation from chronic or repeated use. Although these withdrawal symptoms are often encountered in the clinic, their role in maintaining ongoing substance use and their contribution to craving and relapse in abstinent patients are subjects of much study and debate among behavioral neuroscientists. Although many argue that the negative reinforcing properties of drugs, for example, their ability to alleviate withdrawal symptoms, represent the primary motivation for continued use in dependent patients, others contend that sensitization to the positive reinforcing aspects, as discussed previously, plays a major role in relapse to substance use.

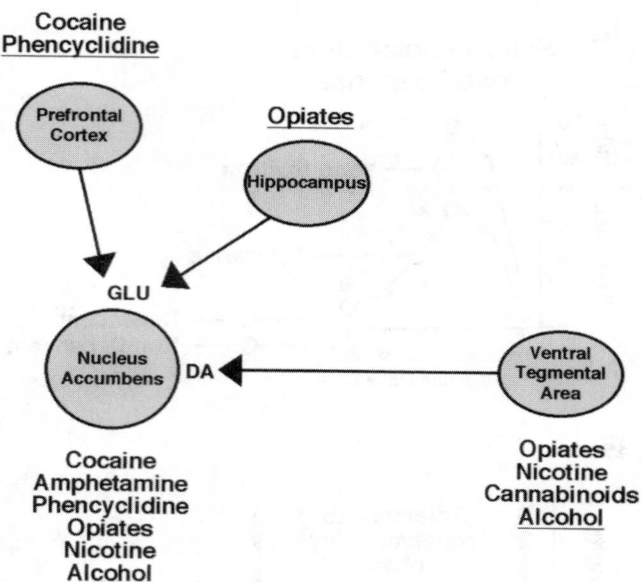

FIGURE 1.22–2 Schematic representation of brain sites supporting intracranial self-administration of several abused substances. Many abused substances are self-administered into multiple brain regions, involving dopamine (DA)-dependent and DA-independent mechanisms. GLU, glutamate.

NEURAL SUBSTRATES OF SUBSTANCE ABUSE

Mesolimbic Dopamine System

Studies in laboratory animals have produced a wealth of information on the neural substrates of drug and alcohol reinforcement. The most common finding is that many abused substances activate the mesolimbic dopamine system, and this system plays a critical role in the reinforcing effects of natural and drug reinforcers. Thus, the mesolimbic dopamine system and its associated limbic circuitry represent a point of convergence onto a common neural substrate for behavioral reinforcement. This system consists of dopaminergic neurons in the A9 and A10 regions of the ventral tegmental area (VTA) and their axon projections to forebrain regions, such as the nucleus accumbens (NAc) and the prefrontal cortex (PfC). Numerous intracranial self-administration studies have indicated the brain regions that support self-administration and have revealed the cellular mechanism used by opiates, psychostimulants, alcohol, nicotine, and cannabinoids drugs to activate the mesolimbic dopamine system. For example, rats self-administer dopamine, amphetamine that releases dopamine, and cocaine that elevates dopamine levels by blocking reuptake all directly into the NAc (Figs. 1.22–2 and 1.22–3B), indicating that dopamine receptors in the NAc are fully capable of mediating the primary reinforcing properties of drugs. Although substances, such as amphetamine and cocaine, also elevate the monoamines norepinephrine and serotonin, these neurotransmitters have little, if any, ability to produce primary reinforcing effects in the NAc or other brain regions. However, norepinephrine and serotonin can act indirectly to increase dopamine release in the NAc or to modulate the reinforcing effects of dopamine in the NAc. For example, animals self-administer cocaine directly into the PfC, where elevated norepinephrine levels activate excitatory glutamatergic projections to dopamine neurons in the VTA, thereby indirectly leading to dopamine release in the NAc. In contrast, global depletion of forebrain serotonin actually enhances cocaine reinforcement, indicating a negative modulatory role for serotonin on dopamine reinforcement mechanisms.

Several other abused substances are self-administered directly into the dopamine cell body region in the VTA, where they activate dopamine neurons and subsequently release dopamine in terminal regions like the NAc (Fig. 1.22–2). Opiates, such as morphine and heroin, activate VTA dopamine neurons indirectly by removing the dopamine neurons from tonic inhibition provided by local γ-aminobutyric acid (GABA)ergic interneurons in the VTA (Fig. 1.22–3A). The μ opiate receptors are coupled to inhibitory G proteins that reduce cyclic adenosine monophosphate (cAMP) formation and activate hyperpolarizing potassium channels that inhibit the GABAergic interneurons. The reinforcing substances in cannabis act on cannabinoid CB1 receptors (cannabinoid receptor type 1) coupled to similar inhibitory G proteins on GABAergic interneurons and also disinhibit the VTA dopamine neurons. Low to moderate doses of alcohol can have a similar disinhibitory effect by selectively facilitating GABA-mediated inhibition of the GABAergic interneurons, without directly inhibiting VTA dopamine neurons. Nicotine, on the other hand, depolarizes VTA dopamine neurons directly via agonist action at nicotinic cholinergic receptors located on the dopamine neurons, but nicotine also facilitates dopamine release in the NAc via nicotinic receptors on dopamine nerve terminals (Fig. 1.22–3B). These and other findings have led investigators to suggest that dopamine release in the NAc is a final common event in the reinforcing effects of opiates, psychostimulants, and other abused drugs.

Dopamine-Independent Reinforcement

There also is substantial evidence for reinforcement mechanisms that are independent of dopamine through direct actions on NAc neurons or by actions in other brain regions (Figs. 1.22–2 and 1.22–3B). For example, opiates such as morphine, in addition to their ability to disinhibit VTA dopamine neurons, are self-administered directly into the NAc, where μ and δ opiate receptors inhibit NAc neurons similar to dopamine itself (dopamine can also excite NAc neurons depending on the receptor subtype and activation state of NAc neurons). Animals self-administer noncompetitive *N*-methyl-D-aspartate (NMDA) glutamate receptor antagonists, such as phencyclidine (PCP) and ketamine, directly into the NAc, where

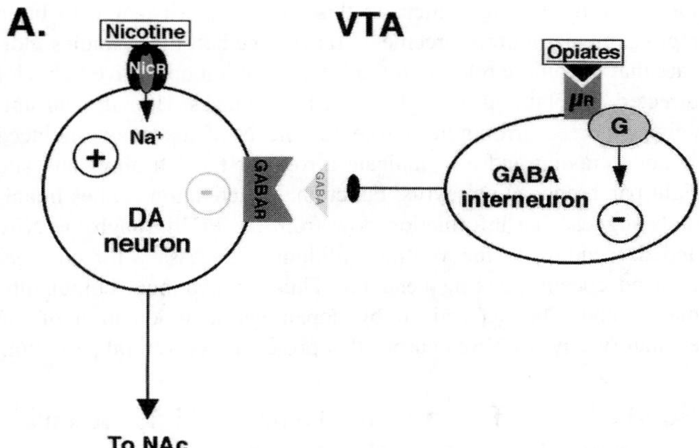

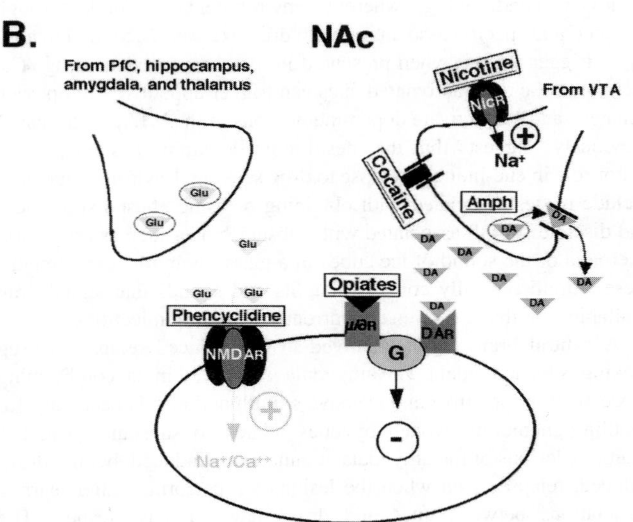

FIGURE 1.22–3 Mechanism of action underlying drug and alcohol reinforcement in the ventral tegmental area (VTA) and nucleus accumbens (NAc). In the VTA **(A)**, opiate drugs activate VTA dopamine cells by removing the tonic inhibitory influence of γ-aminobutyric acid (GABA)ergic interneurons (disinhibition). μ Opiate receptors (μRs) are coupled to inhibitory G proteins that reduce cyclic adenosine monophosphate formation and activate hyperpolarizing K^+ channels to inhibit the GABA interneurons. Low to moderate doses of alcohol also disinhibit VTA dopamine neurons. Nicotine acts on nicotinic cholinergic receptors (NicRs) that directly depolarize VTA dopamine neurons. In the NAc **(B)**, psychostimulants, like cocaine, block dopamine (DA) reuptake into DA nerve terminals, whereas amphetamine (Amph) releases vesicular DA that is reverse transported to the synaptic cleft. Nicotinic receptors also facilitate DA release from nerve terminals. DA receptors (DARs) and opiate μ and δ receptors (μ/δRs) located on NAc neurons are coupled to G proteins that generally act to inhibit NAc neurons. Phencyclidine and other drugs with *N*-methyl-D-aspartate glutamate receptor (NMDAR) antagonist-like properties (alcohol) attenuate excitatory glutamatergic (Glu) input to NAc neurons. GABAR, γ-aminobutyric acid receptor; PfC, prefrontal cortex.

reinforcement is thought to involve blockade of afferent excitation emanating from PfC, hippocampus, amygdala, and thalamus. In effect, attenuation of this excitatory input can potentiate the inhibitory influence of dopamine or other neurotransmitters, leading some investigators to suggest that drug reinforcement ultimately involves inhibition of NAc neurons. Similarly, alcohol reinforcement could involve NMDA antagonist-like properties in the NAc in addition to its ability to stimulate dopamine release. NMDA antagonists also are self-administered in the PfC, and opiates are self-administered in the hippocampus; whether these effects ultimately involve dopamine or other neurotransmitters in the NAc is unknown.

Dual Role for Dopamine Natural rewards, such as food and copulation, also stimulate dopamine release in the NAc to reinforce behavior in animals. In experienced animals, even the sight of food or a receptive female is sufficient to elevate dopamine levels in the NAc. This indicates that environmental cues that are predictive of reward availability also can stimulate dopamine release.

In contrast, natural rewards eventually lose their ability to activate dopamine neurons with repeated reinforcement training (habituation). Instead, the dopamine signal is transferred to environmental cues that predict reward availability (e.g., a cue light that indicates when responding will be reinforced) through the process of pavlovian conditioning. When animals are presented with the cues, dopamine signals in the NAc increase, and animals exhibit appetitive behavior and approach the rewards. Thus, for natural rewards, dopamine plays a dual role by acting first as a neurochemical signal for novel rewards when new learning is important and then as a neurochemical signal to trigger appetitive behavior when the response is learned. In a series of elegant experiments, Wolfram Schultz and colleagues have shown that dopamine neurons respond to natural rewards according to the following equation:

$$\text{Dopamine Response} = \text{Reward Received} - \text{Reward Expected}$$

Thus, when animals are presented with unanticipated or novel rewards, dopamine is released in the NAc. When environmental cues predict reward availability, the cues trigger a dopamine response, but there is no dopamine response to the expected reward. In contrast, when a reward is expected but is not received, the dopamine neurons actually decrease their firing rates. Dopamine neurons, in effect, convey information on error to the brain.

In contrast to natural rewards, abused substances continue to produce dopamine signals even after reinforcement is learned, and, thus, the brain continues to perceive drug and alcohol reward as novel or unexpected. This artificial extension of incentive learning during substance use could facilitate drug craving in prolonged abstinence. The transfer of the dopamine response to environmental cues associated with, or predictive of, substance availability represents a neurobiological trigger for relapse to drug seeking, although the amount of dopamine release in the NAc is substantially less than that produced by the abused substances themselves. Indeed, the amount of dopamine release after several drug injections is actually high enough to suppress appetitive behavior until much of the drug effect has waned, leading to the postinjection pause described previously. Thus, appetitive and consummatory phases of self-administration are regulated by NAc dopamine levels, with moderate increases inducing drug-seeking and saturating dopamine levels suppressing it. Lowered basal levels of dopamine in early stages of drug or alcohol withdrawal also suppress appetitive behavior, an effect thought to represent anhedonia, dysphoria, and depression.

NEURAL SUBSTRATES OF CRAVING AND RELAPSE

Desire, want, or craving for abused substances are cognitive states described by subjective self-reports in humans and cannot be directly measured in laboratory animals. However, drug- or alcohol-seeking behaviors are operant events that provide objective measurements when laboratory animals engage in appetitive responses in pursuit of drugs or alcohol. To measure relapse to drug or alcohol seeking in an experimental setting, investigators first introduce extinction conditions leading to a decline in behavior to low, virtually nonexistent, levels.

Then, specific environmental, neural, or pharmacological stimuli are tested for their ability to reinstate or to induce relapse to drug or alcohol seeking, and the magnitude and persistence of this behavior is measured while reinforcement is withheld. In essence, this approach separates the appetitive from consummatory phases of drug self-administration for study as a discrete event.

Generally, there are only a few stimuli known to induce relapse to drug seeking in animals. These stimuli consist of environmental cues predictive of drug availability as described previously, stressful situations, and low, "priming" doses of abused substances themselves. Because these stimuli also trigger self-reports of wanting and craving in human substance abusers, these paradigms have gained validity as animal models of craving. Moreover, given that relapse to substance use in humans is not always associated with self-reports of substance craving, these animal models offer a more objective measure of the propensity for relapse in laboratory settings.

Drug-Induced Relapse to Drug-Seeking Behavior

A powerful trigger of drug and alcohol seeking in animal models is the administration of low-dose priming with the drug that was self-administered on previous occasions. Interestingly, priming injections of opiates and cannabinoids can trigger relapse to cocaine-seeking behavior, and vice versa, probably reflecting their common ability to activate the mesolimbic dopamine system (Fig. 1.22–4). Indeed, microinfusion of amphetamine directly into the NAc, where it causes local dopamine release from nerve terminals within the NAc, effectively induces relapse to heroin-seeking behavior, and microinfusion of morphine directly into the VTA, where it disinhibits dopamine neurons, induces relapse to heroin- and cocaine-seeking behavior. In contrast, morphine microinfusions into other brain regions, such as the NAc, do not release dopamine from nerve terminals and are ineffective at inducing relapse to drug-seeking behavior, despite their ability to reinforce self-administration behavior in these brain regions.

Several directly acting dopaminergic agonists are powerful inducers of relapse to cocaine- and heroin-seeking behavior. Direct activation of dopamine receptors in the NAc and PfC is sufficient to

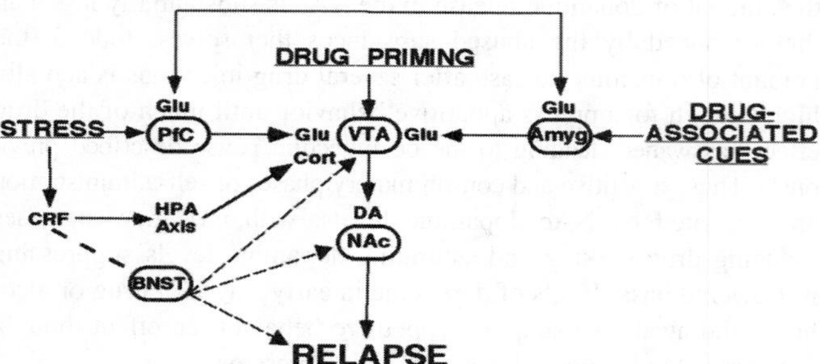

FIGURE 1.22–4 Schematic representation of the primary pathways used by stress, drug priming, and drug-associated cues to trigger relapse to drug and alcohol seeking. Stress- and drug-associated (learned) cues activate descending excitatory glutamate (Glu) projections from the prefrontal cortex (PfC) and amygdala (Amyg), respectively, to the ventral tegmental area (VTA), whereas drugs of abuse activate VTA dopamine (DA) neurons or stimulate DA release from nerve terminals in the nucleus accumbens (NAc). Reciprocal connections between the Amyg and PfC form secondary pathways for activation of VTA DA neurons. Stress-induced activation of the hypothalamic-pituitary-adrenal (HPA) axis and subsequent corticosterone (Cort) secretion in the periphery also facilitate excitatory drive of VTA dopamine neurons. In addition, stress-induced release of corticotropin-releasing factor (CRF) in the bed nucleus of the stria terminalis (BNST) could produce DA-dependent and DA-independent effects that contribute to relapse.

initiate drug seeking, which, in this case, is consistent with brain regions mediating reinforcement. Taken together, these studies indicate that dopamine release in the NAc can elicit appetitive behavior directed at obtaining multiple abused substances. Human neuroimaging studies corroborate a role for the NAc in cocaine-induced cocaine craving and also indicate a role for the left amygdala and right parahippocampal gyrus. Functional inactivation studies in animals suggest that information flow from the PfC through the NAc and descending to the ventral pallidum is necessary for cocaine-induced cocaine-seeking behavior. Thus, motivational output ultimately could be determined by dopaminergic modulation of the excitatory drive of NAc neurons that project to the ventral pallidum.

Cue-Induced Relapse to Drug-Seeking Behavior

Cue-induced relapse to drug-seeking behavior involves the process of pavlovian conditioning, whereby environmental stimuli, through repeated and specific association with drug exposure, acquire the ability to trigger relapse when presented in the absence of the drug. The fact that these drug-associated cues can trigger appetitive or approach behavior and can activate dopamine neurons in the VTA, as discussed previously, suggests that the mesolimbic dopamine system plays a major role in cue-induced relapse to drug seeking. Environmental cues include places associated with obtaining or using abused substances and discrete stimuli associated with substance use, such as drug paraphernalia or the sound of ice cubes in a glass. In animal experiments, these stimuli typically consist of lights and sounds that signal drug availability or that are given concurrently with drug injections.

A central brain region involved in cue-induced relapse to drug seeking is the amygdala. The amygdala is involved in the conditioning processes for appetitive and aversive stimuli and also is necessary for recalling memories evoked by cues related to substance use. For example, lesions of the amygdala attenuate cue-induced, but not drug-induced, relapse, even when the lesions are performed after learned associations between cues and drugs have already formed. The amygdala is thought to process the motivational relevance of environmental cues and subsequently accesses the motivational systems involved in approach and avoidance behavior. Descending neuronal projections from the amygdala activate VTA dopamine neurons through monosynaptic and polysynaptic pathways, leading to increased dopamine levels in the NAc (Fig. 1.22–4). These pathways involve excitatory (glutamatergic) inputs from the central nucleus of the amygdala and the PfC to VTA dopamine neurons. Cue elicitation of drug-seeking behavior is generally, but not always, associated with cue-induced dopamine release in the NAc, suggesting that other non-dopaminergic pathways could also be involved. Indeed, several other brain regions, including the anterior cingulate cortex, hippocampal regions, and central gray area, are activated during cocaine-seeking behavior elicited by contextual (environmental) cues.

Human neuroimaging studies also show that cue-elicited cocaine craving is associated with activation of the amygdala (right greater than left) and NAc, paralleling brain regions activated during drug-induced cocaine craving, and are consistent with animal studies suggesting that drug- and cue-induced relapses ultimately converge onto similar pathways. The anterior cingulate cortex is activated during cue-elicited craving in humans and when animals are placed in an environmental context associated with drug use. The coactivation of anterior cingulate or other medial prefrontal cortical areas, along with the amygdala, may reflect reciprocal connectivity between these structures and their roles in associative processes controlling craving and relapse. However, lesions of the anterior cingulate and medial PfC lead to persevering drug-seeking behavior, and, thus, these structures also exert some inhibitory control over the motivation to seek drugs.

Stress-Induced Relapse to Drug-Seeking Behavior

A major precipitant of relapse to substance use in humans is stress. In animals, stress-induced relapse is triggered after a brief period of mild intermittent and unpredictable footshocks. Presentation of this stressor effectively induces relapse to cocaine-, heroin-, nicotine-, and alcohol-seeking behavior. Interestingly, stress is equally effective at inducing relapse to heroin seeking, whether animals are opiate-dependent or non–opiate-dependent, suggesting that opiate withdrawal symptoms do not contribute to this effect. The neural pathways of stress-induced relapse overlap substantially with pathways activated by cues and drugs but also use different pathways. Thus, stress is similar to drugs and cues, because it activates the mesolimbic dopamine system. Stress-induced dopamine release in the NAc correlates temporally with relapse to heroin seeking, and stress-induced relapse is partially attenuated by pretreatment with dopamine antagonists. The excitatory projection from the PfC to the VTA is a major pathway whereby stress stimulates dopamine release in the NAc (Fig. 1.22–4).

Another major mechanism for stress-induced relapse involves the neuropeptide corticotropin-releasing factor (CRF). Stress-induced CRF release produces multiple effects that contribute to relapse in animal studies. First, hypothalamic CRF activates the hypothalamic-pituitary-adrenal (HPA) axis, and peripheral glucocorticoid release induces relapse to drug seeking by facilitating excitatory input to VTA dopamine neurons (Fig. 1.22–4). However, adrenalectomy fails to block relapse to heroin seeking induced by central CRF injections, suggesting that central stress and CRF mechanisms are sufficient for inducing relapse. In contrast, adrenalectomy attenuates stress-induced relapse to cocaine seeking, but the fact that replacement of basal glucocorticoid levels restores this effect suggests that normal glucocorticoid levels may be necessary, but stress-induced elevations in glucocorticoids are not needed for stress to induce cocaine seeking.

Central mechanisms for CRF-induced relapse involve CRF release in the bed nucleus of the stria terminalis (BNST), probably due to stress-induced activation of the noradrenergic system that innervates CRF neurons in the amygdala and BNST. The BNST neurons project to the VTA, the NAc, and several other brain regions, where central pathways of CRF-induced relapse could involve dopamine-dependent and -independent mechanisms (Fig. 1.22–4).

Negative Reinforcement and Relapse to Drug Seeking

In humans, craving often is associated with negative affect, anxiety, and dysphoria during early stages of withdrawal from drugs and alcohol, and these negative symptoms are thought to spur motivation for maintaining daily substance use. However, precipitation of opiate withdrawal with antagonists, such as naltrexone (ReVia), fails to precipitate relapse in opiate-dependent animals, despite their ability to produce adverse withdrawal signs. Similarly, drugs that block dopamine receptors fail to induce drug-seeking behavior, despite their ability to produce aversive effects. Therefore, the motivation to alleviate dysphoria or anxiety (negative reinforcement) is not a substantial impetus for relapse in animal studies. In addition, early stages of drug and alcohol withdrawal are associated with an increase in the electrical stimulus required to maintain self-stimulation of the brain, an effect thought to reflect anhedonia that is contrary to facilitation of appetitive behavior. Finally, drug- and alcohol-seeking behavior progressively increase after substantially longer abstinent periods and at times when early withdrawal symptoms have completely subsided, suggesting that these withdrawal symptoms and their neurobiological correlates are not primary mediators of relapse. These findings, although contrasting with self-reports of craving in humans, agree with the high prevalence of protracted abstinence at later times and are difficult to reconcile with negative reinforcement theories of addiction. However, negative reinforcement mechanisms may contribute to relapse indirectly through their effects on incentive learning.

From a neurobiological standpoint, early phases of drug withdrawal are associated with marked depletions in extracellular dopamine and serotonin levels in the NAc that are thought to contribute to anhedonia and depression, whereas stimuli that induce relapse all increase dopamine levels in the NAc. Thus, drug-like or *proponent* neurobiological processes appear to underlie appetitive behavior in animals, whereas drug-opposite or *opponent* neurobiological processes actually attenuate this behavior. Stressful stimuli and subsequent CRF release are characteristic of drug-like and withdrawal-like effects. Thus, cocaine acutely elevates CRF levels in the brain, and cocaine and CRF activate central dopamine release, but withdrawal from drugs and alcohol is also associated with elevated CRF levels in the amygdala, and this effect may underlie the anxiogenic effects of withdrawal. The ability of stress to stimulate dopamine release could override anxiogenic or other negative effects in precipitating relapse.

Dopamine and Glutamate Receptor Regulation of Relapse

Studies described in preceding sections suggest that dopamine release in the NAc is sufficient and, in some cases, necessary for environmental stimuli or drugs to induce relapse to drug-seeking behavior. Dopamine acts on two major classes of dopamine receptors that are distinguishable by their opposite or differential effects on cellular excitability and intracellular second messenger systems, including cAMP formation. Striatal dopamine type 1 (D_1) receptors (D_1 and type 5 [D_5]) stimulate adenylyl cyclase and cAMP formation and can facilitate excitatory input, whereas striatal dopamine type 2 (D_2) receptors (D_2, type 3 [D_3], and type 4 [D_4]) inhibit cAMP formation and generally inhibit neurons. Neurons intrinsic to the NAc express D_1 and D_2 classes of dopamine receptors but on somewhat different populations of NAc neurons with distinct peptide content and efferent projections.

Animal studies suggest that D_1 and D_2 receptors are involved in regulating drug-seeking behavior, although the exact brain sites at which these effects are mediated are not fully known. Stimulation of D_2 receptors in the NAc triggers relapse to cocaine seeking, whereas generalized (systemic) D_1 receptor stimulation prevents relapse induced by priming injections of cocaine and conditioned cues. Hence, NAc D_2 receptors could mediate appetitive behavior elicited by cues, stress, and drug or alcohol priming that elevate dopamine levels, whereas D_1 receptors in NAc and other brain regions could mediate certain consummatory aspects of drugs and alcohol, such as reward, reduction in craving, or satiety, or a combination of these. However, blockade of either D_1 or D_2 receptors attenuates relapse to cocaine seeking, suggesting that D_1 receptors may have a permissive action on cocaine seeking elicited by D_2 receptors.

This D_1-D_2 dichotomy is paralleled to some extent in human studies. For example, pretreatment with a D_1 agonist suppresses craving for nicotine and, to a lesser degree, cocaine, whereas nonselective or D_2-preferring agonists induce cravings for cocaine, nicotine, and ethanol. Conversely, D_1 receptor antagonists are reported to attenuate the euphorigenic effects of cocaine and to increase cocaine self-administration, whereas several D_2 selective antagonists (neuroleptics) generally fail to attenuate the euphorigenic effects of cocaine and amphetamine.

Given that glutamate receptors are intimately involved in regulating mesolimbic dopamine neurons, it is perhaps not surprising that they also play a role in regulating relapse to substance use. The ionotropic glutamate receptors (α-amino-3-hydroxy-5-methyl-4-isoxazolepropionic [AMPA] and NMDA) are located on dopamine neurons in the VTA, where they mediate excitatory input from cortical and other areas. Blockade of NMDA receptors in the VTA attenuates relapse induced by electrical stimulation of the PfC or hippocampus, suggesting that these effects involve glutamatergic modulation of mesolimbic dopamine neurons. Conversely, systemic administration of an NMDA antagonist actually induces relapse to cocaine seeking, suggesting actions in other brain regions, such as the NAc, at which NMDA antagonists facilitate reinforcement. The role of excitatory neurotransmission in the NAc in regulating relapse is unclear, because generalized activation of AMPA glutamate receptors triggers cocaine seeking, but facilitation of endogenous glutamate activity at AMPA receptors reduces cocaine seeking. These discrepancies suggest a complex role for glutamatergic input to the NAc in regulating the motivation to seek abused substances, with glutamatergic involvement in triggering relapse but also in exerting control over such urges. The sources of glutamatergic input emanate from cortical, hippocampal, amygdala, and thalamus, and temporal and spatial integration of these inputs with dopamine signals may determine whether drug seeking is induced or attenuated.

The circuitry regulating drug and alcohol reinforcement, craving, and relapse could explain the potential therapeutic efficacy of drugs, such as naltrexone and acamprosate (Campral), in treating craving and relapse. For example, naltrexone blocks endogenous opiate activity in the VTA, where opiates disinhibit VTA dopamine neurons. The subsequent blunting of dopaminergic responses to alcohol and conditioned cues could blunt alcohol reinforcement and cravings for alcohol in protracted abstinence, respectively. Drugs such as acamprosate, which have antagonist properties at glutamate receptors, also could interfere with excitatory drive of VTA neurons. The use of dopamine receptor antagonists has been limited by undesirable side effects, but full or partial dopamine agonists could have potential for replacement pharmacotherapy, producing low-level tonic stimulation and blunting phasic dopamine responses to drugs, stress, and conditioned stimuli. As studies continue to unravel the complex neural circuitry involved in drug and alcohol reinforcement and pathways of craving and relapse, other possible pharmacological treatments could be based on targeted sites that interrupt reinforcement and craving or restore deficits in these circuits.

NEUROADAPTATIONS IN SUBSTANCE DEPENDENCE

Chronic drug and alcohol use produces numerous neurobiological changes in several brain regions, including brain regions involved in regulating addictive behavior. These changes occur at virtually every level of information processing, ranging from neurotransmitters and receptors to intracellular signaling pathways and regulation of gene expression to long-term structural changes that alter synaptic plasticity. These changes ultimately could alter entire neural networks with impact on motivation, emotion, decision making, and other cognitive processes. Such changes are usually referred to as *neuroadaptations*, because they often reflect a compensatory biological response to the direct pharmacological influence of drugs and alcohol in an attempt to regain homeostasis (as found in mechanisms of tolerance). However, in many instances, neuroadaptations to chronic substance use sensitize the system to drugs and alcohol, reflecting an overall change in responsiveness rather than a correction to regain a normal state. There are far too many known changes to describe here, but certain neuroadaptations in the mesolimbic dopamine system, especially the NAc, are commonly found with chronic exposure to several abused substances. This may reflect their ability to activate a common reinforcement substrate and to produce similar symptoms characteristic of dependence. The following sections highlight some of these changes, with special emphasis given to neuroadaptations that have been causally related to dependence-like alterations in self-administration or the propensity for relapse to drug and alcohol seeking.

Adaptations in NAc Neurotransmitter and Receptor Systems

One of the most common and persistent behavioral changes that occurs after chronic exposure to abused substances is psychomotor sensitization. Thus, repeated exposure to cocaine, amphetamine, opiates, nicotine, and alcohol produces progressively larger psychomotor responses to a fixed challenge dose. Sensitization involves the development of hypersensitivity in the mesolimbic dopamine system to drugs, stress, and drug-associated stimuli (Fig. 1.22–5). Hypersensitivity in the dopamine system is related to greater dopamine release from dopamine nerve terminals in the NAc, although repeated exposure to drugs, such as morphine, amphetamine, and cocaine, also facilitates the psychomotor response to D_2 receptor agonists, reflecting hypersensitivity in the postsynaptic response of NAc neurons. Studies on dopamine receptor densities have produced mixed results, depending on drug, exposure, and withdrawal time. In fact, neuroimaging studies generally find decreases in D_2 receptor densities in the NAc and cortical regions in human substance abusers. The development of D_2 recep-

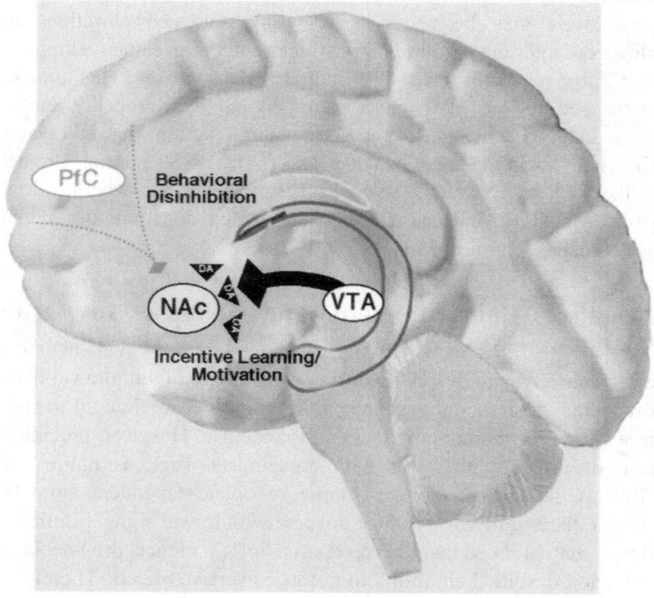

FIGURE 1.22–5 Addiction-related changes in cortical and subcortical systems involved in regulating addictive behavior in the nucleus accumbens (NAc). Chronic drug and alcohol abuse is associated with hypofrontality in several regions, including the prefrontal cortex (PfC) in human studies, and long-term depression (LTD) in corticoaccumbal synapses in animals. Conversely, ventral tegmental area (VTA) dopamine (DA) neurons exhibit sensitized responses to drugs and drug-related environmental stimuli in animal studies. The weakening of cortical glutamatergic input is thought to contribute to behavioral disinhibition (impulsivity), whereas enhancement of DA input is thought to facilitate incentive learning and motivational responses to relapse-inducing stimuli. These changes may persist for at least 1 month into abstinence in dependent patients.

tor supersensitivity despite decreases in receptor density could involve neuroadaptations in dopamine receptor signaling pathways, or an imbalance between dopamine and glutamate inputs to NAc.

Chronic drug and alcohol treatment also produces alterations in glutamatergic input to the mesolimbic dopamine system. VTA dopamine neurons are supersensitive to excitation by glutamate after chronic psychostimulant treatment, but this effect does not persist for long after cessation of drug exposure. In the NAc, however, a longer lasting reduction in glutamatergic neurotransmission persists for at least 1 month of withdrawal. This reduction involves lower basal levels of glutamate released from cortical and other inputs (Fig. 1.22–5). There are also reductions in glutamate receptors on NAc neurons, and NAc neurons are subsensitive to the excitatory influence of glutamate after chronic cocaine and amphetamine. At the synaptic level, excitatory synapses emanating from the PfC enter a state of long-term depression (LTD) after chronic cocaine and, possibly, other drugs. Thus, the balance of input to the NAc shifts in favor of dopamine over glutamate in dependent animals, especially at later withdrawal times.

In addition, several human neuroimaging studies have found reduced metabolic activity in the PfC and other frontal cortical areas, and these changes persist for at least 1 month into drug and alcohol abstinence. This "hypofrontality" syndrome is hypothesized to contribute to compulsive and impulsive behavior, an inability to make appropriate choices, and a loss of inhibitory control over craving. In contrast, hyperactivity in mesolimbic dopamine systems is thought to enhance mechanisms of incentive learning during drug and alcohol self-administration and incentive motivational responses to stimuli that activate the dopamine system in withdrawal. The combination of hypoactive glutamate and hyperactive dopamine input to NAc could account for many of the most persistent and difficult behavioral changes associated with substance dependence (Fig. 1.22–5).

Adaptations in Dopamine Receptor Signaling The prominent role for dopamine in substance dependence could involve receptor regulation of intracellular second messenger responses, such as cAMP formation. D_1 and D_2 receptors are coupled to the cAMP second messenger system but in opposite ways. D_1 receptors are coupled to stimulatory G proteins (G_s and G_{olf}) that stimulate cAMP formation by activating adenylate cyclase. In contrast, D_2 receptors are coupled to inhibitory G proteins (G_i and G_o) that inhibit adenylate cyclase activity and cAMP formation. Elevations in intracellular cAMP levels activate cAMP-dependent protein kinase (PKA). PKA, in turn, regulates cellular activity through phosphorylation of numerous intracellular proteins, including ion channels, glutamate receptors, and transcription factors, such as cAMP response element binding protein (CREB). Acute PKA activation in the NAc can facilitate the rewarding effects of conditioned cues (secondary reinforcement) and drug rewards. In contrast, sustained or tonic PKA activation reduces the rewarding effects of drugs, such as cocaine and morphine.

Previous work has shown that repeated exposure to opiates, cocaine, and ethanol produces relatively long-term (approximately 1 month) neuroadaptations in the cAMP signaling pathway in NAc neurons. These neuroadaptations are characterized by reduced levels of G proteins that inhibit cAMP formation and increased levels of adenylyl cyclase and PKA. Decreased levels of G proteins that inhibit cAMP formation coupled with an increase in the biochemical machinery to synthesize (adenylate cyclase) and to respond to cAMP (PKA) all contribute to a generalized upregulation of the NAc-cAMP pathway. These neurobiological changes have been specifically related to addiction-related changes in drug and alcohol self-administration. For example, experimental inactivation of inhibitory G proteins in the NAc increases cocaine and heroin intake, producing a rightward shift in the descending limb of self-administration dose–response curve. A similar increase in cocaine, heroin, and alcohol self-administration is produced when PKA is continuously activated by experimental manipulation. Thus, artificially mimicking drug- and alcohol-induced upregulation of cAMP signaling in the NAc increases self-administration in a manner reminiscent of substance dependence. This effect is thought to reflect a reduction in reward, and animals compensate by taking drugs or alcohol at a faster rate. Taken together, these studies suggest that neuroadaptations in the NAc-cAMP pathway caused by repeated drug and alcohol use represent an intracellular mechanism of tolerance, leading to escalating drug and alcohol consumption as dependence develops (Fig. 1.22–6).

Possible mechanisms for PKA-mediated tolerance could involve reciprocal negative feedback on dopamine receptor responses themselves. For example, sustained PKA activity desensitizes D_1 dopamine receptors through phosphorylation mechanisms and reduces the ability of D_1 receptors to modulate cellular responses through cAMP-dependent and cAMP-independent mechanisms. Indeed, chronic exposure to cocaine reduces the ability of D_1 receptors to phosphorylate AMPA and NMDA glutamate receptors, an effect that reduces excitatory glutamatergic responses in NAc neurons.

In NAc neurons containing D_2 receptors, similar upregulation in cAMP signaling could oppose D_2 responses that inhibit cAMP formation, but, given that supersensitivity develops to the psychomotor effects of D_2 agonists, sensitization rather than tolerance to D_2 responses apparently occurs, possibly as a compensatory response to the cAMP upregulation. Furthermore, supersensitivity in D_2 receptor responses, which are capable of triggering relapse, would facilitate the ability of stimuli that release dopamine in the NAc to trigger drug- and alcohol-seeking responses. Thus, opposite neuroadaptations in D_1 and D_2 responsiveness could produce tolerance to the rewarding effects of drugs and alcohol while simultaneously enhancing the incentive to seek them.

Adaptations in Gene Expression Another consequence of upregulation in cAMP signaling in the NAc involves sustained activation of the transcription factor CREB (Fig. 1.22–7). CREB is phosphorylated by PKA and Ca^{2+}-calmodulin–dependent protein kinase IV (CaM-KIV). PKA and CaM-KIV are activated by D_1 (cAMP) and NMDA (Ca^{2+}) glutamate receptors, respectively, during drug exposure, and chronic upregulation in cAMP signaling could lead to prolonged CREB phosphorylation. When CREB is phosphorylated, its transcriptional regulation is activated, and CREB subsequently alters expression of numerous genes containing cAMP response elements (CREs) in their regulatory regions. The contribution of increased CREB activity to drug and alcohol dependence is not fully understood, but studies suggest that NAc CREB activity is involved in regulating sensitivity to drug reward. Increasing NAc CREB activity reduces sensitivity to cocaine and morphine reward, whereas reducing CREB activity facilitates sensitivity to these drugs. Thus, sustained or repeated activation of CREB with chronic drug and alcohol use also could contribute to the development of tolerance.

The mechanism for CREB regulation of drug sensitivity is thought to involve a transsynaptic effect that reduces dopamine release from presynaptic nerve terminals in the NAc. CREB increases expression of the opiate peptide transmitter dynorphin in

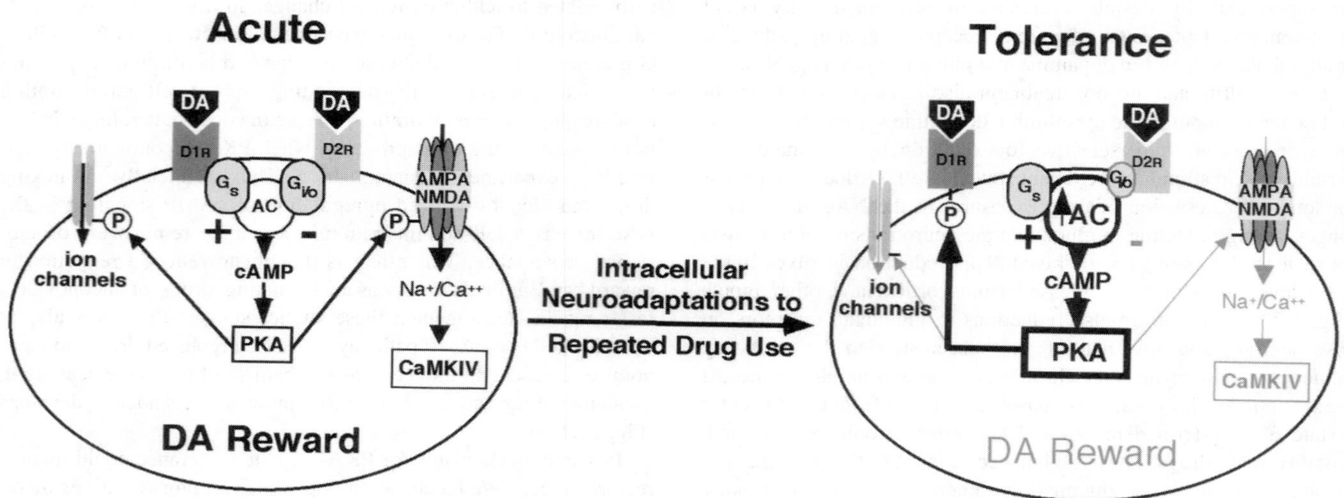

FIGURE 1.22–6 Intracellular mechanism of tolerance to drug and alcohol reward. In the acute state **(left)**, abused substances release dopamine (DA) in the nucleus accumbens (NAc) that activates DA type 1 (D_1) and type 2 (D_2) receptors on distinct subpopulations of NAc neurons. D_1 receptors are coupled to the cyclic adenosine monophosphate (cAMP) pathway via stimulatory G proteins (G_s or G_{olf}) that activate adenylyl cyclase (AC) and cAMP formation. cAMP, in turn, activates cAMP-dependent protein kinase (PKA), which modulates neuronal activity through phosphorylation (P) of various ion channels and glutamate receptors (α-amino-3-hydroxy-5-methyl-4-isoxazole propionate [AMPA] and *N*-methyl-D-aspartate [NMDA]). D_2 receptors (located on different NAc cells) are coupled to inhibitory G proteins ($G_{i/o}$) that inhibit AC and cAMP formation. Repeated drug use leads to chronic upregulation in cAMP signaling characterized by increased levels of AC or PKA, or both, and decreased levels of inhibitory G proteins **(right)**. Sustained upregulation of this pathway produces tolerance to drugs and alcohol, possibly by desensitizing D_1 receptors through PKA-mediated phosphorylation. Reduced coupling of D_1 receptors to G proteins blunts DA reward signals; these signals use other D_1 cellular responses that do not involve cAMP and PKA (not shown). In NAc neurons expressing D_2 receptors, upregulation of cAMP signaling could oppose D_2 receptors that inhibit the pathway. Animals and people compensate for a decrease in DA input during self-administration by increasing their drug and alcohol intake. CaMKIV, Ca^{2+}-calmodulin–dependent protein kinase IV.

NAc neurons. When dynorphin is released from NAc neurons, it activates inhibitory kappa (κ) opiate receptors located on dopamine nerve terminals, thereby reducing dopamine release in the NAc. Increased CREB activity has been shown to potentiate the dysphoria and aversive effects of early withdrawal from cocaine and morphine via the dynorphin pathway and subsequent dopamine depletion.

Another downstream target of CREB is the neurotrophin brain-derived neurotrophic factor (BDNF) that is involved in dendritic structural changes and synaptic plasticity (Fig. 1.22–7). BDNF promotes neurite outgrowth, suggesting that a CREB-BDNF signaling cascade contributes to dendritic sprouting and branching in NAc neurons after chronic psychostimulant self-administration. Behaviorally, infusions of BDNF into the NAc facilitate drug sensitization and appetitive responses to conditioned cues. Thus, although CREB regulation of dynorphin expression may contribute to tolerance- and dependence-like processes, CREB regulation of BDNF expression could contribute to incentive sensitization and incentive learning and could promote cocaine seeking in withdrawal. Taken together, these effects illustrate how neuroadaptations in transcription factors, such as CREB, can differentially alter discrete behavioral aspects of addiction through changes in multiple downstream target genes.

The transcription factor ΔFosB also is upregulated as a consequence of chronic, but not acute, drug and alcohol exposure. ΔFosB is induced by a cascade of events involving repeated activation of D_1 receptor–cAMP–CREB–mediated signaling pathways. ΔFosB is a highly stable protein and is degraded slowly. Thus, repeated substance use leads to a substantial accumulation of this transcription factor in NAc neurons that lasts for several weeks into withdrawal. ΔFosB forms dimers with other members of the activating protein-1 (AP1) family of transcription factors that bind to specific AP1 binding sites on DNA to regulate gene expression. ΔFosB overexpression has been shown to increase the pursuit of cocaine in animals but does not alter the amount of drug consumed, and, thus, would represent a neuroadaptation underlying sensitization of appetitive processes rather than tolerance and escalating drug consumption. These changes, as discussed previously, are thought to facilitate the propensity for craving and relapse in withdrawal.

When ΔFosB accumulates in NAc neurons, its AP1 binding activity induces or alters expression of numerous genes that fall under AP1 regulation (Fig. 1.22–7). One downstream target gene induced by ΔFosB in the NAc is cyclin-dependent kinase 5 (CDK-5). ΔFosB-induced expression of CDK-5 represents yet another pathway for negative feedback signaling, because CDK-5 phosphorylation converts an important dopamine signaling protein (dopamine-regulated phosphoprotein 32 [DARPP-32]) into an endogenous PKA inhibitor. Thus, CDK-5 expression may counteract the acute effects of D_1 receptor–mediated cAMP formation and upregulation of cAMP signaling proteins produced by chronic drug and alcohol exposure. However, CDK-5 may also be involved in growth-related changes in dendritic spines in NAc neurons that accompany behavioral sensitization, as described previously.

LEARNING AND MEMORY IN SUBSTANCE DEPENDENCE

When considering the persistent nature of substance dependence and the high prevalence of relapse from months to years of abstinence, it is important to note that most neurobiological changes inevitably revert to normal within a month or two after cessation of chronic drug and alcohol use. However, even transient changes in receptor signaling and gene expression can lead to long-term consequences, such as dendritic arborization and synaptic plasticity, that produce relatively permanent changes in synaptic organization. These changes outlast neuroadaptations in signal transduction and gene expression themselves. Subtle changes in synaptic effi-

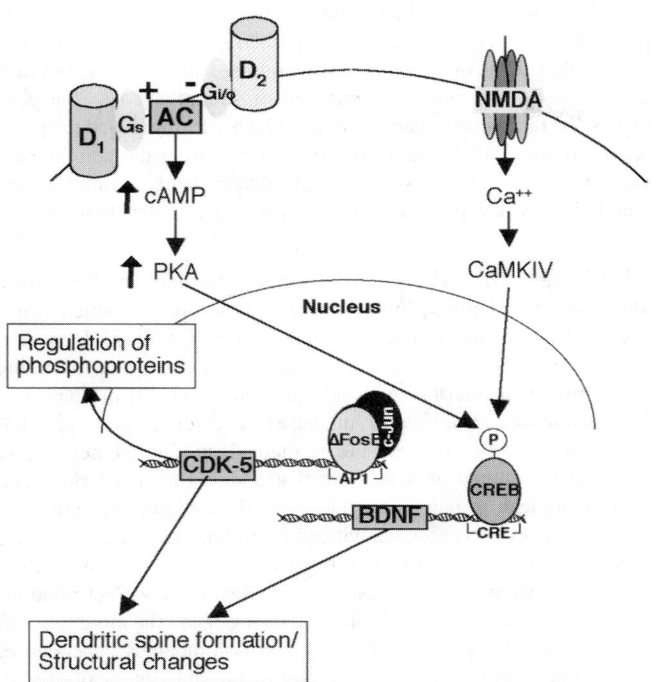

FIGURE 1.22–7 Chronic drug and alcohol exposure upregulates the transcription factors ΔFosB and cyclic adenosine monophosphate (cAMP) response element binding (CREB) protein in the nucleus accumbens (NAc) and other brain regions. Upregulation in the cAMP signaling pathway increases CREB phosphorylation (activation) and transcriptional regulation of genes containing cAMP response elements (CREs) in upstream regulatory regions. Similarly, chronic, but not acute, drug and alcohol exposure leads to accumulation of the transcription factor ΔFosB. ΔFosB forms dimers with other activator protein-1 (AP1) family members, such as c-*Jun*, and regulates transcription of genes containing AP1 binding domains. Two downstream targets of ΔFosB and CREB are cyclin-dependent kinase 5 (CDK-5) and brain-derived neurotrophic factor (BDNF), respectively. Both target proteins may be involved in dendritic spine formation in medium spiny NAc neurons and synaptic plasticity. In addition, CDK-5 phosphorylation of dopamine-regulated phosphoprotein 32 (DARPP-32) (not shown) provides negative feedback regulation of cAMP-dependent protein kinase (PKA) activity. AC, adenylyl cyclase; CaMKIV, Ca^{2+}-calmodulin–dependent protein kinase IV; D_1, dopamine type 1 receptor; D_2, dopamine type 2 receptor; G_s, stimulatory G protein; $G_{i/o}$, inhibitory G protein; NMDA, *N*-methyl-D-aspartate receptor.

cacy multiplied across numerous synaptic connections and brain regions would profoundly influence neural networks and global brain activity. Many of these changes could have direct consequences on addictive behavior, whereas others could influence incentive learning and could strengthen drug- and alcohol-related memories. Several current studies are aimed at (1) understanding the interaction between such short-term neuroadaptations and incentive learning during active substance use that may indirectly facilitate relapse in the long term and (2) identifying other long-lasting or late-forming neuroadaptations in withdrawal that directly facilitate motivational responses to stimuli that trigger relapse. Such efforts are based on two recently developed animal models that illustrate the distinction between learning- and memory-based interactions in substance dependence.

Contribution of Incentive Learning In the initial phases of drug and alcohol use, self-administration is maintained primarily by the positive reinforcing effects of the abused substance. As dependence develops, the negative aspects of withdrawal could play an increasingly important role in increasing the motivation for substance use. However, as discussed previously, animal studies have been unable to show that relapse is facilitated by the negative aspects of drug or alcohol withdrawal, despite clear signs of anxiety and dysphoria. One possibility is that negative and positive reinforcement processes act in concert to facilitate incentive learning during ongoing substance use. In this scenario, the negative aspects of withdrawal do not function as direct triggers of drug- or alcohol-seeking behavior but rather act indirectly to enhance the reinforcing efficacy of abused substances.

This concept is illustrated in a recent study by Anthony Dickinson and colleagues in which some opiate-dependent animals were allowed to alleviate negative withdrawal symptoms on a few occasions by self-administering heroin, whereas other opiate-dependent animals were not allowed to alleviate withdrawal symptoms through self-administration. Several weeks later, when withdrawal symptoms were no longer evident, animals that experienced this negative reinforcement exhibited markedly greater heroin-seeking behavior than those prevented from alleviating withdrawal symptoms. These findings are remarkable because both groups had equivalent levels of heroin self-administration and were equally opiate dependent, as indicated by the manifestation of early physical withdrawal signs. The findings suggest that the positive and negative reinforcing effects of heroin summate during self-administration or that the negative reinforcing effects of heroin are stronger than the positive reinforcing effects in opiate-dependent animals. It is important to reiterate that testing was conducted weeks later when animals were no longer in an opiate-dependent state, so withdrawal symptoms, per se, could not directly explain the differences.

Studies like this suggest that incentive learning during the active self-administration phase is a major determinant of the propensity for relapse in prolonged abstinence. Thus, the ability of relatively transient neuroadaptations to influence the strength of reinforcement learning could underlie persistent craving and relapse in abstinent patients and not the neuroadaptations themselves. This interaction is illustrated in Figure 1.22–8A, whereby neuroadaptations to chronic substance use that facilitate the negative aspects of drug withdrawal (e.g., CREB) could greatly increase the magnitude of the reinforcing stimulus and, thus, incentive learning, leading to stronger drug-related memories and craving in prolonged abstinence. Conversely, other neuroadaptations could potentiate the positive reinforcing stimulus of drugs (e.g., ΔFosB) and would also facilitate incentive learning even in the absence of prominent negative symptoms. Although the former scenario could play a greater role in opiate and alcohol dependence, the latter may be more likely in psychostimulant dependence. In either case, incentive learning is directly related to the overall strength of the reinforcing stimulus, and enhancement of this stimulus leads to stronger craving responses (memories) long after the neuroadaptations normalize in prolonged abstinence.

Sensitization of Memory in Withdrawal Recent animal studies have discovered another important phenomenon that could underlie the difficulty in treating substance dependence even after long periods of abstinence. The phenomenon is indicated when animals develop progressively greater levels of drug- and alcohol-seeking behavior with progressively longer periods of forced abstinence. In essence, the memory of prior drug use seems to be strengthened, rather than weakened, as the time since substance use becomes longer. In some cases, increases in drug and alcohol seek-

A.

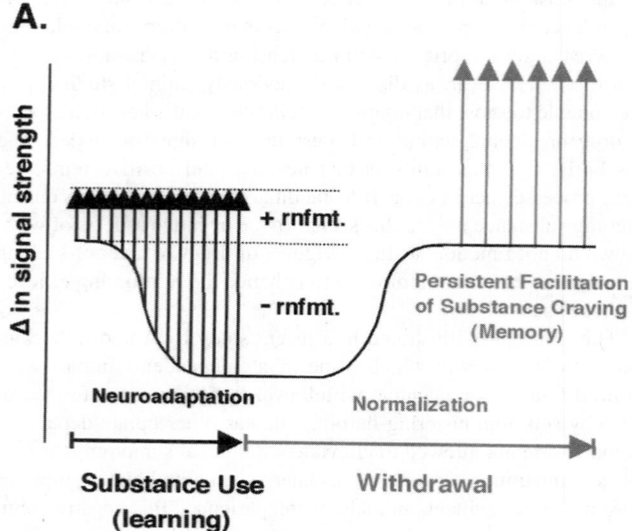

B.

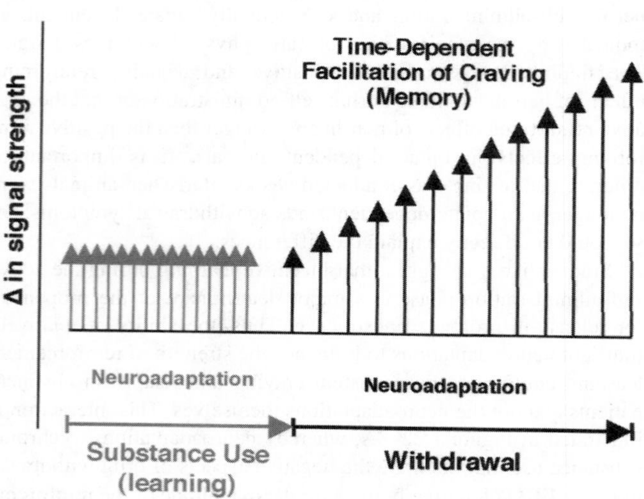

FIGURE 1.22–8 Possible interactions between neuroadaptations to chronic substance use and mechanism of learning and memory. **A:** Neuroadaptations during chronic substance use contribute to dysphoria, anxiety, and depression in early withdrawal, thereby facilitating negative reinforcement mechanisms during self-administration. Summation of positive and negative reinforcement facilitates incentive learning, leading to persistent increases in the motivational strength of memories related to substance use, even after neuroadaptations normalize in long-term withdrawal. **B:** Time-dependent changes in neuroadaptations during long-term withdrawal directly facilitate the motivational strength of memories related to substance use, leading to a greater propensity for relapse in prolonged abstinence.

ing continue to develop over several weeks to months after chronic self-administration, and current efforts are aimed at identifying the specific neuroadaptations during abstinence that coincide with time-dependent enhancement of drug- and alcohol-seeking behavior (Fig. 1.22–8). Time-dependent increases in cocaine seeking are paralleled by increases in amygdala dopamine release when animals are placed back into the environmental context in which cocaine was self-administered. Given the role of the amygdala in conditioned responses to abused substances, progressive increases in the dopamine response could augment the ability of the cocaine-related environmental stimuli to elicit drug-seeking behavior as abstinence proceeds. Another possibility is that certain genes regulated by drugs and alcohol act as memory repressors during substance use, but then drug-related memories are unmasked or strengthened as the gene expression fades in abstinence. These and other learning- and memory-based animal models are useful for understanding the neurobehavioral basis for the persistence of the disease and, in some cases, could identify new potential targets for medication development.

Challenge for Future Treatment Earlier studies have identified the pharmacological mechanisms through which drugs and alcohol activate brain reinforcement pathways. This information has led to pharmacological approaches for intervention, stemming from drugs that interfere with primary reinforcement mechanisms, (e.g., naltrexone, disulfiram [Antabuse]), and replacement pharmacotherapies during withdrawal (e.g., methadone [Dolophine]). Other potential treatments in development are aimed at interfering with neurobiological triggers of relapse (CRF antagonists), although attempts to reverse neuroadaptations to chronic substance use with pharmacotherapy have not yet proved successful. A remaining challenge for basic neuroscientists is to establish cause–effect relationships between critical neurobiological changes and the more relevant and persistent behavioral pathology that accompanies dependence. These studies will benefit by investigating possible interactions with incentive learning and long-term memory that have an indirect but prolonged influence in addition to more straightforward cause–effect relationships. Similarly, development of new pharmacological treatments should be considered in view of possible enabling interactions as adjuncts to behavior-based approaches, in addition to their efficacy alone. Pharmacological and behavioral therapies, in turn, can now be studied in the context of their enduring neurobiological consequences, as advances in neuroimaging permit detection of subtle brain changes that accompany symptom improvement. The combination of these approaches could provide an invaluable bidirectional flow of information between the neurobiological changes associated with dependence and treatment outcome. In this sense, efforts to treat substance abuse and dependence ultimately can follow the biomedical model used to treat other organic diseases.

SUGGESTED CROSS-REFERENCES

The basic neuroscience of monoamine, amino acid, and neurotrophic factors is discussed in Sections 1.4, 1.5, and 1.7, respectively. The basic neuroscience of intraneuronal signaling pathways and molecular biology of gene regulation is discussed in Sections 1.8 and 1.10. Further information of substance-related disorders is given in Chapter 11.

REFERENCES

Ahmed SH, Koob GF: Transition from moderate to excessive drug intake: Change in hedonic set point. *Science.* 1998;282:298.

Baker DA, McFarland K, Lake RW, Shen H, Tang XC, Toda S, Kalivas PW: Neuroadaptations in cystine-glutamate exchange underlie cocaine relapse. *Nat Neurosci.* 2003;6:743.

*Bardo MT: Neuropharmacological mechanisms of drug reward: Beyond dopamine in the nucleus accumbens. *Crit Rev Neurobiol.* 1998;12:37.

Beninger RJ, Miller R: Dopamine D_1-like receptors and reward-related incentive learning. *Neurosci Biobehav Rev.* 1998;22:335.

Bindra D: A motivational view if learning, performance, and behavior modification. *Psychol Rev.* 1974;81:199.

Brauer LH, Goudie AJ, De Wit H: Dopamine ligands and the stimulus effects of amphetamine: Animal models versus human laboratory data. *Psychopharmacology.* 1997;130:2.

Breiter HC, Gollub RL, Weisskoff RM, Kennedy DN, Makris N, Berke JD, Kantor HL, Gastfriend DR, Riorden JP, Mathew RT, Rosen BR, Hyman SE: Acute effects of cocaine on human brain activity and emotion. *Neuron.* 1997;19:591.

Colby CA, Whisler K, Steffan C, Nestler EJ, Self DW: Striatal cell type-specific overexpression of ΔFosB enhances incentive for cocaine. *J Neurosci.* 2003;23:2488.
Di Chiara G: Nucleus accumbens shell and core dopamine: Differential role in behavior and addiction. *Behav Brain Res.* 2002;137:75.
Everitt BJ, Wolf ME: Psychomotor stimulant addiction: A neural systems perspective. *J Neurosci.* 2002;22:3312.
*Goldstein RZ, Volkow ND: Drug addiction and its underlying neurobiological basis: Neuroimaging evidence for the involvement of the frontal cortex. *Am J Psychiatry.* 2002;159:1642.
Haney M, Collins ED, Ward AS, Foltin RW, Fischman MW: Effect of a selective D_1 agonist (ABT-431) on smoked cocaine self-administration in humans. *Psychopharmacology.* 1999;143:102.
Hutcheson DM, Everitt BJ, Robbins TW, Dickinson A: The role of withdrawal in heroin addiction: Enhances reward or promotes avoidance? *Nat Neurosci.* 2001;4:943.
Kilts CD, Schweitzer JB, Quinn CK, Gross RE, Faber TL, Muhammad F, Ely TD, Hoffman JM, Drexler KP: Neural activity related to drug craving in cocaine addiction. *Arch Gen Psychiatry.* 2001;58:334.
Koob GF, Le Moal M: Drug abuse: Hedonic homeostatic dysregulation. *Science.* 1997;278:52.
Kosten TR, George TP, Kosten TA: The potential of dopamine agonists in drug addiction. *Expert Opin Invest Drugs.* 2002;11:491.
Kreek MJ, Koob GF: Drug dependence: Stress and dysregulation of brain reward pathways. *Drug Alcohol Depend.* 1998;51:23.
Krystal JH, Petrakis IL, Webb E, Cooney NL, Karper LP, Namanworth S, Stetson P, Trevisan LA, Charney DS: Dose-related ethanol-like effects of the NMDA antagonist, ketamine, in recently detoxified alcoholics. *Arch Gen Psychiatry.* 1998;55:354.
London ED, Ernst M, Grant S, Bonson K, Weinstein A: Orbitofrontal cortex and human drug abuse: Functional imaging. *Cereb Cortex.* 2000;10:334.
McBride WJ, Le AD, Noronha A: Central nervous system mechanisms in alcohol relapse. Alcoholism. *Clin Exp Res.* 2002;26:280.
McFarland K, Kalivas PW: The circuitry mediating cocaine-induced reinstatement of drug-seeking behavior. *J Neurosci.* 2001;21:8655.
Neisewander JL, Baker DA, Fuchs RA, Tran-Nguyen LT, Palmer A, Marshall JF: Fos protein expression and cocaine-seeking behavior in rats after exposure to a cocaine self-administration environment. *J Neurosci.* 2000;20:798.
*Nestler EJ: Molecular basis of long-term plasticity underlying addiction. *Nat Rev Neurosci.* 2001;2:119.
Nestler EJ, Barrot M, Self DW: ΔFosB: A molecular switch controlling compulsive and impulsive behaviors. *Proc Natl Acad Sci U S A.* 2001;98:11042.
Nicola SM, Surmeier J, Malenka RC: Dopaminergic modulation of neuronal excitability in the striatum and nucleus accumbens. *Annu Rev Neurosci.* 2000;23:185.
O'Brien CP. Drug addiction and drug abuse. In: Hardman JG, Limbird LE, Gilman AG, eds. *Goodman and Gilman's the Pharmacological Basis of Therapeutics.* 10th ed. New York: McGraw-Hill; 2001.
Piazza PV, Le Moal M: The role of stress in drug self-administration. *Trends Pharmacol Sci.* 1998;19:67.
Robbins TW, Everitt BJ: Neurobehavioural mechanisms of reward and motivation. *Curr Opin Neurobiol.* 1996;6:228.
Robinson TE, Berridge KC: Incentive-sensitization and addiction. *Addiction.* 2001;96:103.
Romach MK, Glue P, Kampman K, Kaplan HL, Somer GR, Poole S, Clarke L, Coffin V, Cornish J, O'Brien CP, Sellers EM: Attenuation of the euphoric effects of cocaine by the dopamine D1/D5 antagonist ecopipam (SCH 39166). *Arch Gen Psychiatry.* 1999;56:1101.
Saal D, Dong Y, Bonci A, Malenka RC: Drugs of abuse and stress trigger a common synaptic adaptation in dopamine neurons. *Neuron.* 2003;37:577.
Schultz W: Predictive reward signal of dopamine neurons. *J Neurophysiol.* 1998;80:1.
See RE: Neural substrates of conditioned-cued relapse to drug-seeking behavior. *Pharmacol Biochem Behav.* 2002;71:517.
*Self DW, Nestler EJ: Relapse to drug seeking: Neural and molecular mechanisms. *Drug Alcohol Depend.* 1998;51:49.
Shaham Y, Erb S, Stewart J: Stress-induced relapse to heroin and cocaine seeking in rats: A review. *Brain Res Rev.* 2000;33:13.
Sinclair J: The alcohol-deprivation effect. Influence of various factors. *Q J Stud Alcohol.* 1972;33:769.
Sutton MA, Schmidt EF, Choi KH, Schad CA, Whisler K, Simmons D, Karanian DA, Monteggia LM, Neve RL, Self DW: Extinction-induced upregulation in AMPA receptors reduces cocaine-seeking behavior. *Nature.* 2003;421:70–75.
Tran-Nguyen LT, Fuchs RA, Coffey GP, Baker DA, O'Dell LE, Neisewander JL: Time-dependent changes in cocaine-seeking behavior and extracellular dopamine levels in the amygdala during cocaine withdrawal. *Neuropsychopharmacology.* 1998;19:48.
*Vanderschuren LJ, Kalivas PW: Alterations in dopaminergic and glutamatergic transmission in the induction and expression of behavioral sensitization: A critical review of preclinical studies. *Psychopharmacology.* 2000;151:99.
Volkow ND, Chang L, Wang GJ, Fowler JS, Ding YS, Sedler M, Logan J, Franceschi D, Gatley J, Hitzemann R, Gifford A, Wong C, Pappas N: Low level of brain dopamine D2 receptors in methamphetamine abusers: Association with metabolism in the orbitofrontal cortex. *Am J Psychiatry.* 2001;158:2015.
Wand G, Levine M, Zweifel L, Schwindinger W, Abel T: The cAMP-protein kinase A signal transduction pathway modulates ethanol consumption and sedative effects of ethanol. *J Neurosci.* 2001;21:5297.
White FJ, Kalivas PW: Neuroadaptations involved in amphetamine and cocaine addiction. *Drug Alcohol Depend.* 1998;51:141.
Wise RA: Drug-activation of brain reward pathways. *Drug Alcohol Depend.* 1998;51:13.

▲ 1.23 Future Directions in Neuroscience and Psychiatry

SOLOMON H. SNYDER, M.D.

The goal of basic biological research in psychiatry is to elucidate fundamentals of brain structure and function with a goal of identifying molecular substrates that are disordered in mental illness. Another thrust takes advantage of molecular neuroscience to develop novel therapies, which may be effective even without the underlying cause of diseases being known. An underlying assumption of much of this research is that the predisposition to these conditions lies in aberrations in one or more genes. In recent years, numerous candidate genes have emerged. In some instances, the protein products of these genes are beginning to make sense in terms of the signaling systems that they regulate and which may be disordered in mental illness.

LINKING ABNORMAL GENES TO ABNORMAL SIGNALING

Unlike Huntington's disease, a genetically dominant disorder caused by mutation of a single gene, most investigators suspect that the principal disorders in psychiatry are multigenic, with aberrant genes contributing to a predisposition to respond to environmental stress with mental breakdown. The technique of reverse genetics has led to associations of a number of genetic loci to psychiatric disturbances. The number is sufficiently large, so this brief essay does not attempt to enumerate them. Instead, the author focuses on disease-associated genetic loci related to signaling systems of which impairments might plausibly explain patient symptoms. In other, less frequent, instances, investigators have identified single gene mutations associated with neuropsychiatric disturbances, which occur only in a very small percentage of patients. Nonetheless, insight into these rare disorders may shed light on the much larger population of patients whose specific molecular abnormalities remain to be determined.

The classic paradigm of a rare form of a disease shedding light on more common forms involves Alzheimer's disease. Amyloid plaques are characteristic of all patients. A small number of patients with familial Alzheimer's disease display mutations of enzymes that process the amyloid precursor protein, leading to accumulation of the neurotoxic amyloid-β peptide and plaque deposition. Until these rare forms of the disease were identified, many researchers were skeptical as to whether amyloid plaques caused the disease or were merely "scars" secondary to some other fundamental disturbance.

More recently, a similar situation has arisen in the case of Parkinson's disease. Rare familial forms of the disease are associated with mutations in the proteins α-synuclein or parkin. Parkin is a ubiquitin-3-ligase associated with protein degradation but with no obvious link to Parkinson's disease. By contrast, the α-synuclein protein is concentrated in the Lewy bodies that are characteristic of almost all patients with the disease. Recent protein–protein interaction studies reveal that both α-synuclein and parkin bind to a recently discovered protein, synphilin, providing clues to how parkin may contribute to the etiology of the disease.

An analogous situation may occur in schizophrenia. Disrupted-in-schizophrenia-1 (DISC-1) was identified as the product of a gene whose translocation in a Scottish family is very strongly associated with major psychiatric illness with a preponderance of schizophrenic symptoms. The translocation in patients interrupts the coding sequence of DISC-1, leading to the loss of the C-terminal 257 amino acids. Protein–protein interaction studies, analogous to the studies linking synphilin with parkin and α-synuclein, have revealed binding of DISC-1 to several cytoskeletal proteins, especially NUDEL. NUDEL interacts selectively with the portion of DISC-1 that is deleted in patients, so that NUDEL fails to bind to DISC-1 with the diseased mutation. Transfection of the mutant DISC-1 into neuronal-like cultures leads to abnormalities in neuronal outgrowth. This fits with the association of DISC-1 with cytoskeletal elements in cells that are well known to regulate neuronal migration and axonal outgrowth during development. It also accords with the notion that schizophrenia is a developmental disorder with aberrations in cytoskeletal proteins that regulate neuronal outgrowth. Association of NUDEL with other proteins fits with this concept. Thus, NUDEL binds to LIS-1, which is mutated in a form of lissencephaly, a disease with altered cerebral cortical development. Additionally, NUDEL occurs downstream of a signaling cascade derived from Reelin, whose mutations are associated with lissencephaly. Interestingly, Reelin expression is diminished in the schizophrenic brain.

In reverse genetic approaches, chromosome 22Q11 appears associated with schizophrenia. Moreover, individuals with deletion of this chromosome display a very high incidence of schizophrenia, approximately 25 to 30 percent, whereas in 2 percent of diagnosed schizophrenics, 22Q11 deletion has been detected. Although the exact gene on 22Q11 responsible for disease predisposition is not yet established, there are some interesting candidates. Particularly tantalizing is catechol-*O*-methyltransferase (COMT), whose gene is located on 22Q11. COMT is one of the major catecholamine metabolizing enzymes and is polymorphic. One of the two alleles of the COMT gene is associated with augmented enzyme activity and related to poor performance and inefficient brain activation during memory tests. This allele occurs more often in schizophrenics than in matched controls. Interestingly, COMT does not influence catecholamine disposition in most areas of the brain but is a major determinant of dopamine inactivation in the prefrontal cerebral cortex, which mediates the cognitive functions that are impaired in schizophrenia. Augmented COMT, with reduced cortical dopamine, seems to be associated with impaired brain function, suggesting therapeutic efficacy for COMT inhibitors that penetrate into the brain.

Proline dehydrogenase oxidizes the amino acid, leading to ring cleavage, formation of glutamate γ-semialdehyde, and transformation to glutamate. Like COMT, the gene for proline dehydrogenase is localized to 22Q11. A family with a high incidence of schizophrenia displays a deletion of 350 kilobases in the 22Q11 region, which involves the locus for the proline dehydrogenase gene, whereas missense mutations associated with high plasma protein levels occur in other schizophrenics. Moreover, genetic variations at this locus have been associated with schizophrenia in large population studies. Interestingly, proline dehydrogenase knock-out mice display deficits in sensorimotor gating, which are characteristic of schizophrenic patients.

Deoxyribonucleic acid (DNA) microarray analysis facilitates screening thousands of genes in disease states. In some instances, abnormalities discovered in such studies intersect with other genetic influences. A tantalizing example is the regulator of G-protein–signaling-4 (RGS-4). Microarray analysis reveals a decrease of RGS-4 expression in schizophrenic prefrontal cerebral cortex, whereas ten other members of the RGS family display normal levels. RGS-4 maps to locus 1Q21-22, a chromosome region that is strongly linked to schizophrenia. Interestingly, the RGS family of 20 proteins is a class of guanosine triphosphatase activating proteins (GAPs), which enhance the breakdown of guanosine triphosphate (GTP) when it is bound to G proteins, thus shortening the duration of G-protein–related synaptic signaling. All of the major biogenic amine and amino acid neurotransmitters signal to some extent via G-protein–coupled receptors. If diminished RGS-4 activity is indeed related to schizophrenic disturbances, agents that enhance its activity should be therapeutic. Schizophrenic brains also display diminished expression of genes associated with neurotransmitter release such as *N*-ethylmaleimide sensitive factor (NSF) and synapsin II. Drugs that augment actions of these two proteins may be clinically relevant.

NEUROTRANSMITTERS AND DRUGS

Virtually every drug that influences mental function does so by interacting with one or another neurotransmitter system. Almost all of the drugs in psychiatry influence a handful of neurotransmitters, especially the biogenic amines serotonin, dopamine, and norepinephrine as well as the amino acid neurotransmitter γ-aminobutyric acid (GABA). Few, if any, drugs have been developed to target the roughly 50 other known neurotransmitters. Hence, developing therapeutic agents by influences on neurotransmitters is hardly a "mature" field. Recent findings point to a number of novel promising targets.

The classic neuroleptics block dopamine type 2 (D_2) receptors with potencies that correlate with their therapeutic efficacy. This conclusion has held fast for almost 30 years, although many nuances have been advanced to explain phenomena such as the lag in therapeutic response and the variable incidence of extrapyramidal side effects. The atypical neuroleptics, exemplified by clozapine and more recent agents, such as risperidone, olanzapine, quetiapine, and ziprasidone, also block dopamine receptors but display behavioral effects differing somewhat from classic drugs, such as exerting favorable influences on certain negative symptoms. Clozapine often benefits patients who do not respond to classic neuroleptics. It is not known for certain what accounts for the unique properties of the atypical drugs, although some investigators feel that blockade of serotonin type 2, as well as dopamine receptors, is important. Clarifying the mechanism of action of clozapine may lead to newer, more effective, and safer agents.

In the case of tricyclic antidepressants, there is agreement that inhibiting the reuptake inactivation of norepinephrine or serotonin, or both, is of importance. Various mechanisms have been proposed to explain the therapeutic lag with antidepressant therapy. Insights into this process could have major therapeutic benefit. Recent studies suggest that blockade of substance P receptors may provide antidepressant effects.

A role for glutamate in schizophrenia stems predominantly from evidence that phencyclidine (PCP) produces a psychotic state that mimics schizophrenia better than other drug psychoses. The discovery that PCP blocks the *N*-methyl-D-aspartate (NMDA) subtype of glutamate receptor has provoked major interest in glutamate in schizophrenia. The NMDA receptor functions via its ion channel that admits sodium and calcium. By contrast, metabotropic glutamate receptors are G-protein–coupled and influence adenosine 3',5'-cyclic monophosphate (cAMP) or inositol 1,4,5,-triphosphate (IP-3) formation. Group II metabotropic glutamate receptors (mGluR2/3) are localized presynaptically on nerve endings of glutamate neurons, so that their activation inhibits glutamate release. PCP blocks NMDA receptors on GABA inhibitory neurons that synapse on glutamate neurons and thus enhances glutamate release in the prefrontal cerebral cortex. mGluR2/3 agonist drugs inhibit the increased glutamate release provoked by PCP as well as PCP-elicited behavioral abnormalities. Accordingly, these drugs offer promise as novel antischizophrenic agents.

The NMDA receptor provides yet another avenue to novel therapy in schizophrenia. This receptor is unique in possessing distinct recognition sites for two neurotransmitters, glutamate and glycine. Because of the extremely high brain levels of glutamate, one might reason that the requirement for two agents to activate the receptor is a "fail safe" mechanism to protect against excess glutamate. However, like glutamate, glycine is an abundant dietary amino acid. Recent evidence indicates that D-serine, the "abnormal" isomer of the amino acid, is the physiological ligand for the "glycine site" in most brain regions. D-Serine is synthesized in a unique population of glial cells, protoplasmic astrocytes that ensheath the synapse. D-Serine is formed by a novel enzyme, serine racemase, which converts L- to D-serine. If functional blockade of NMDA receptors is associated with schizophrenic symptomatology, agents that stimulate NMDA receptors might be therapeutic. Glutamate cannot be readily used. Several clinical trials have reported therapeutic responses to administration of glycine or D-serine together with classic neuroleptics. Negative, as well as positive, symptoms responded. Moreover, D-cycloserine, an antituberculosis drug that is a partial agonist at the glycine site of the receptor, is also therapeutically effective in patients.

Acetylcholine has recently emerged as a potentially important neurotransmitter in schizophrenia, both from the perspective of drug development and as a possible molecular abnormality that predisposes to disease development. Schizophrenics smoke more than other psychiatric patients, and this behavior is not easily explained as an effort to relieve the sedating effects of neuroleptics. Nicotine administration does transiently relieve some schizophrenic symptoms. Behavioral studies in animals and humans indicate that nicotinic cholinergic receptors mediate a type of sensory processing that is altered in schizophrenics. Schizophrenics have difficulty in screening out extraneous sensory information. The P50 electroencephalogram (EEG) response to repeated auditory stimuli, which reflects inhibition of excess auditory stimulation, is diminished in schizophrenics. Abnormalities in this form of auditory gating occur frequently in first-degree relatives of schizophrenics. Nicotine gum treatment normalizes the deficient auditory gating in patients and their relatives. Auditory gating can be readily monitored in mice and is abnormal in strains of mice possessing the fewest number of the $\alpha 7$ subtype of nicotinic cholinergic receptor. Moreover, agonists at the $\alpha 7$ receptors normalize the deficient auditory gating. Conventional nicotinic agonists are not acceptable therapeutic drugs because of their nicotine-like side effects. Strikingly, $\alpha 7$ selective nicotinic agonists do not manifest the cardiovascular and addictive properties of nicotine and, accordingly, are undergoing clinical trials in schizophrenia. A possible role of $\alpha 7$ receptors in schizophrenic pathophysiology stems from observations of a higher prevalence of functional promoter mutations in $\alpha 7$ nicotinic receptors in schizophrenics than in control subjects. Moreover, one of these mutations influences the P50 auditory evoked response.

In summary, recent developments may portend a convergence of basic molecular neuroscience research and explorations of genetic loci associated with mental disturbance. In the interest of brevity, the chapter focuses more on research in schizophrenia than other conditions. However, similar patterns are evident in studies of affective and anxiety disorders. At an earlier stage of genetic investigation, one could worry that finding the "abnormal gene" in a major mental disorder would fail to provide an insight into specific molecular mechanisms that account for symptoms and afford no suggestions for novel therapy. Such a situation has to some extent been the case in Huntington's disease, in which the specific genetic abnormality and its encoded protein huntingtin were identified in 1993. Yet, for a decade thereafter, researchers failed to elucidate a specific function of this protein that could fully explain patient symptoms and lead to novel drug therapy. The numerous "coincidences" of genetic loci in mental illness being associated with proteins that could be relevant to pathophysiology afford promise for major beneficial advances in psychiatry in the finite future.

SUGGESTED CROSS-REFERENCES

Sections 1.4, 1.5, and 1.6 discuss neurotransmitters. Section 1.7 covers neurotrophic factors, and Chapter 2 covers the entire field of behavioral neurology. Schizophrenia is discussed in Chapter 12, and cognitive disorders, including delirium and dementia, are covered in Chapter 10.

References

Baldessarini RJ, Tondo L: Suicide risk and treatments for patients with bipolar disorder. *JAMA.* 2003;290:1517–1519.

Baranano DE, Ferris CD, Snyder SH: Atypical neural messengers. *Trends Neurosci.* 2001;24:99–106.

Berrettini WH: Are schizophrenic and bipolar disorders related? A review of family and molecular studies. *Biol Psychiatry.* 2000;48:531–538.

*Blackwood DH, Fordyce A, Walker MT, St. Clair DM, Porteous DJ, Muir WJ: Schizophrenia and affective disorders—cosegregation with a translocation at chromosome 1q42 that directly disrupts brain-expressed genes: Clinical and P300 findings in a family. *Am J Hum Genet.* 2001;69:428–433.

Brzustowicz LM, Hodgkinson KA, Chow EW, Honer WG, Bassett AS: Location of a major susceptibility locus for familial schizophrenia on chromosome 1q21-q22. *Science.* 2000;288:678–682.

Chang KK, Zhang Y, Lim KL, Tanaka Y, Huang H, Gao J, Ross CA, Dawson VL, Dawson TM: Parkin ubiquitinates the alpha-interacting protein, synphilin-1: Implications for Lewy-body formation in Parkinson disease. *Nature Med.* 2001;1:1144–1150.

Chowdari KV, Mirnics K, Semwal P, Wood J, Lawrence E, Bhatia T, Deshpande SN, B K Thelma, Ferrell RE, Middleton FA, Devlin B, Levitt P, Lewis DA, Nimgaonkar VL: Association and linkage analyses of RGS4 polymorphisms in schizophrenia. *Hum Mol Genet.* 2002;11:1373–1380.

Coyle JT, Duman RS: Finding the intracellular signaling pathways affected by mood disorder treatments. *Neuron.* 2003;38:157–160.

Egan MF, Goldberg TE, Kolachana BS, Callicott JH, Mazzanti CM, Straub RE, Goldman D, Weinberger DR: Effect of COMT Val108/158 Met genotype on frontal lobe function and risk for schizophrenia. *Proc Natl Acad Sci U S A.* 2001;98:6917–6922.

*Goff DC, Coyle JT: The emerging role of glutamate in the pathophysiology and treatment of schizophrenia. *Am J Psychiatry.* 2001;158:1367–1377.

Gogos JA, Santha M, Takacs Z, Beck KD, Luine V, Lucas LR, Nadler JV, Karayiorgou M: The gene encoding proline dehydrogenase modulates sensorimotor gating in mice. *Nat Genet.* 1999;21:434–439.

Guidotti A, Auta J, Davis JM, DiGiorgi-Gerevini V, Dwivedi Y, Grayson DR, Impagnatiello F, Pandey G, Pesold C, Sharma R, Uzunov D, Costa E, DiGiorgi-Gerevini V: Decrease in reelin and glutamic acid decarboxylase67 (GAD67) expression in schizophrenia and bipolar disorder: A postmortem brain study. *Arch Gen Psychiatry.* 2000;57:1061–1069.

Hariri AR, Weinberger DR: Imaging genomics. *Br Med Bull.* 2003;65:259–270.

Jacquet H, Raux G, Thibaut F, Hecketsweiler B, Houy E, Demilly C, Haouzir S, Allio G, Fouldrin G, Drouin V, Bou J, Petit M, Campion D, Frebourg T: PRODH mutations and hyperprolinemia in a subset of schizophrenic patients. *Hum Mol Genet.* 2002;11:2243–2249.

Javitt DC, Zukin SR: Recent advances in the phencyclidine model of schizophrenia. *Am J Psychiatry.* 1991;148:1301–1308.

Kapur S, Remington G: Atypical antipsychotics: New directions and new challenges in the treatment of schizophrenia. *Annu Rev Med.* 2001;52:503–517.

Leonard S, Gault J, Logel J, Short M, Berger R, Drebing C, Oliney A, Ross RG, Adler LE, Freedman R: Promoter mutations in the alpha7 nicotinic acetylcholine receptor subunit gene are associated with a schizophrenia. *Am J Med Genet.* 2002;114:749.

*Liu H, Heath SC, Sobin C, Roos JL, Galke BL, Blundell ML, Lenane M, Robertson B, Wijsman EM, Rapoport JL, Gogos JA, Karayiorgou M: Genetic variation at the 22q11 PRODH2/DGCR6 locus presents an unusual pattern and increases susceptibility to schizophrenia. *Proc Natl Acad Sci U S A.* 2002;99:3717–3722.

Meltzer HY. Atypical antipsychotic drugs. In: Davis KL, Charney D, Coyle JT, Nemeroff C, eds. *Psychopharmacology: The Fourth Generation of Progress.* New York: Raven Press; 2002:1277–1286.

Millar JK, Wilson-Annan JC, Anderson S, Christie S, Taylor MS, Semple CA, Devon RS, Clair DM, Muir WJ, Blackwood DH, Porteous DJ: Disruption of two novel genes by a translocation co-segregating with schizophrenia. *Hum Mol Genet.* 2000;9:1415–1423.

Mirnics K, Middleton FA, Marquez A, Lewis DA, Levitt P: Molecular characterization of schizophrenia viewed by microarray analysis of gene expression in prefrontal cortex. *Neuron.* 2000;28:53–67.

Mirnics K, Middleton FA, Stanwood GD, Lewis DA, Levitt P: Disease-specific changes in regulator of G-protein signaling 4 (RGS4) expression in schizophrenia. *Mol Psychiatry.* 2001;6:293–301.

Moghaddam B, Adams BW: Reversal of phencyclidine effects by a group II metabotropic glutamate receptor agonist in rats. *Science.* 1998;281:1349–1352.

*Murphy KC: Schizophrenia and velo-cardio-facial syndrome. *Lancet.* 2002;359:426–430.

Murphy KC, Jones LA, Owen MJ: High rates of schizophrenia in adults with velo-cardio-facial syndrome. *Arch Gen Psychiatry.* 1999;56:940–945.

Ozeki Y, Tomoda T, Kleiderlein J, Kamiya A, Bord L, Fujii K, Okawa M, Yamada N, Hatten ME, Snyder SH, Ross CA, Sawa A: Disrupted-In-Schizophrenia-1 (DISC-1): Mutant truncation prevents binding to NUDEL and inhabits neurite outgrowth. *Proc Natl Acad Sci U S A.* 2003;100:289–294.

*Sawa A, Snyder SH: Schizophrenia: Diverse approaches to a complex disease. *Science.* 2002;296:692–695.

Schoepp DD, Marek, JG: Preclinical pharmacology of mGlu2/3 receptor agonists: Novel agents for schizophrenia? *Curr Drug Target CNS Neurol Disord.* 2002;1:215–225.

Simosky JK, Stevens KE, Freedman R: Nicotinic agonists and psychosis. *Curr Drug Target CNS Neurol Disord.* 2002;1:149–162.

Thaker GK, Carpenter WT Jr: Advances in schizophrenia. *Nature Med.* 2001;7:667–671.

2 Neuropsychiatry and Behavioral Neurology

▲ 2.1 Neuropsychiatric Approach to the Patient

FRED OVSIEW, M.D.

INTRODUCTION

Neuropsychiatry is the psychiatric subspecialty that deals with the psychological and behavioral manifestations of brain disease. Neuropsychiatry is closely allied with the neurological subspecialty that interests itself in psychological phenomena in patients with brain disease, namely cognitive and behavioral neurology. The care of patients with identifiable, acquired brain disease—such as those with epilepsy, movement disorders, and traumatic brain injury—requires the physician to have a knowledge base and a familiarity with assessment and treatment methods not usually required for patients with primary psychiatric disorders. Patients with organic mental syndromes are common in clinical practice and often are difficult to manage for the generalist or for the general psychiatrist in consultation with specialists in other fields. In addition to expert management of patients with organic mental disorders, from its clinical vantage point, neuropsychiatry can offer a distinctive perspective on idiopathic psychiatric disorders. Moreover, neuropsychiatry draws on a knowledge base in the cognitive neurosciences that has the potential to broaden, sharpen, and modernize assessment and nosology in general psychiatry.

This chapter provides information about assessment by history, examination, and paraclinical investigations in neuropsychiatry and describes neuropsychiatric psychopathology from three perspectives: anatomy, symptom or syndrome, and disease. Coverage from each vantage point is panoramic in the hope that the three perspectives, by triangulation, produce an image of how a neuropsychiatrist thinks when assessing a patient—the cerebral substrate of behavior, the plausible consequences of disease processes, the clinical phenomena, and their elucidation at the bedside. Some of the points made in the description of clinical techniques are illustrated in vignettes in the final section of the chapter that focus on assessment issues.

The seemingly obvious view that neuropsychiatry is the offspring of psychiatry and neurology is historically mistaken. Psychiatry differentiated itself as a medical specialty in the early part of the 19th century and neurology somewhat later. Ample evidence shows that early asylum physicians, the precursors of psychiatrists, considered their patients to have brain diseases and, moreover, that a large proportion of their patients evinced organic disease, even as it could be identified with the tools of that time. General paresis of the insane (neurosyphilis, as it was later discovered to be), epilepsy, mental retardation, and the complications of alcohol abuse were all common in the 19th-century asylum. On this evidence, one might say that general psychiatry, as it was understood for the larger part of the 20th century, derived from an earlier neuropsychiatry.

Early neurology, on the other hand, took little part in the care of patients with major psychiatric disorders, at least those requiring hospitalization; but what would later become outpatient psychiatry—the care of patients with milder mood and anxiety disorders not requiring asylum management, for example—fell into the province of the early neurologists. The theories by virtue of which they understood their patients have, fortunately, been consigned to the dustbin of history. The mainstream of Anglo-American neurology was ill equipped to give rise to a scientific neuropsychiatry, and it was not until (as a convenient and meaningful landmark) Norman Geschwind in 1965 awakened interest in the continental tradition of a behavioral neurology *avant la lettre* that the contributions of John Hughlings Jackson, Ludwig Lichtheim, Hugo Carl Liepmann, Karl Wernicke, and others could provide impetus for the development of a clinical specialty devoted to scientific understanding of the cerebral basis of mental and behavioral disorder.

To say that neuropsychiatry is devoted to the care of patients with brain disease is not to depreciate the role of psychological and social factors in the understanding of the genesis of symptoms or in the formulation of interventions to assist patients. To the contrary, patients with brain disease are often inordinately reactive to or dependent on influences from the outside world, notably the social world. Neuropsychiatric case formulation takes into account both the vulnerability and the setting. To the extent that patients suffer from brain-based impairments in processing information from their environment, their need for assistance in dealing with instrumental and interpersonal tasks increases. Much of the brain, after all, is devoted to processing social information and devising ways of meeting internal needs in a social context. The neuropsychiatrist requires a detailed assessment of the patient's functional deficits and the contexts in which they arise.

To say that the neuropsychiatrist regards deficits, or for that matter intact behavior, as the manifestation of brain-based processes is not to imply that idiopathic psychiatric disorders occur in people with normal brains nor that general psychiatrists are unaware of the cerebral origin of these disorders. To the contrary, the evidence for abnormal brain structure and function in the major psychiatric disorders is unmistakable, and general psychiatrists often assert the neurobiological nature of these illnesses. However, evidence for such assertions is often not demonstrable in the individual case, all available laboratory investigations characteristically falling within the broad range of normal. Moreover, the neurobiological abnormalities in question are believed to be, at least in large part and at least in most illnesses, genetic in nature and developmental in pathogenesis. The recognition and understanding of the mental consequences of *acquired* diseases of the brain—which form the bulk of the neuropsychiatrist's concern—are likely to require different tools from those required by the general psychiatrist treating idiopathic disorders. Although a bright line between the two situations is not possible, and although many neuropsychiatrists maintain a lively interest in such disorders as schizophrenia and autism, the distinction supports the continued use of the term *organic* to refer to these acquired disorders with pathology identifiable at the bedside and by the clinical laboratory, as much as some want to see the term interred.

To define neuropsychiatry by how the clinician thinks, however, may be less telling than to define it by what the clinician does. Neuropsychiatrists perform physical examinations, not just a focused screen for extrapyramidal signs, such as is within the ambit of most general psychiatrists, but a broad assessment of cerebral function using the tools available. Neuropsychiatrists not only order neuroimaging and electroencephalographic studies but also review them personally, not just to "rule out organic disease" but to see which organic disease is present and where.

NEUROANATOMICAL BASIS OF THE NEUROPSYCHIATRIC EXAMINATION

The neuropsychiatric brain is more complex than the general psychiatric brain. The latter is a soup of neurotransmitters, perhaps in "chemical imbalance" (as patients are wont to say), with considerable pharmacological, but little anatomical, specificity. Although the benefits of psychopharmacological intervention are indisputable, the locus of these effects is rarely of concern to clinicians. A neuropsychiatric approach relies on greater differentiation among brain circuits and systems. The chapter considers several major brain systems of key importance to neuropsychiatric case formulation.

Lateralization The two hemispheres differentially subserve many cerebral functions, although in many instances, both hemispheres participate in naturally occurring behavior, albeit contributing differently to the complex outcome. Brain asymmetries arise early in vertebrate evolution, and the two hemispheres display regional lateral asymmetries in size and differentially innervate viscera and peripheral endocrine tissues. For example, the pars opercularis of the third frontal gyrus (Broca's area) and the planum temporale (infolded cortex in the posterior portion of the sylvian fissure) are typically larger on the left, with greater dendritic branching of the neurons therein (for simplicity's sake, "left" and "right" here refer to the situation in the average dextral patient). These cortical regions are parts of the substrate of language processing. Insular cortex of the right hemisphere regulates cardiac sympathetic drive and of the left hemisphere, parasympathetic drive. In consequence, left hemisphere stroke involving insula produces more cardiac destabilization and morbidity than right, and lateralization of seizure discharges may have implications for autonomic function and unexplained sudden death in patients with epilepsy. Lateral differences in limbic (hypothalamic and amygdalar) regulation of sexual function also have clinical implications; for example, polycystic ovary syndrome in females may be more commonly associated with left-sided limbic epilepsy. Hemispheric side of lesion also affects the immunological consequences of brain injury.

Whether a single tag can accurately contrast the processing "styles" of the hemispheres—"local versus global" or "linear versus context dependent," for example—across multiple functions is doubtful. Although left lateralization of language and right lateralization of visuospatial function are widely recognized, lateral specialization in the prefrontal regions is less obvious but of clinical significance. Frontal lobe degeneration involving the right, more than the left, frontal lobe is particularly associated with disinhibition. Traumatic injury to the right hemisphere is more associated with depression and anxiety, to the left with anger and hostility. Women and sinistrals tend to show less lateralization of language (and perhaps of other functions), so that left hemisphere lesions are less likely to produce severe impairment.

Of considerable importance for neuropsychiatric practice is the question of lateralization of emotional processing. An array of evidence supports the notion of differential emotional valences in the two hemispheres. On this account, the left hemisphere is specialized for positive emotions, the right for negative emotions. Thus left hemisphere destructive lesions are associated with pathological crying and right hemisphere ones with pathological laughing; contrariwise, left hemisphere discharging lesions produce gelastic (laughing) epilepsy and right hemisphere ones, dacrystic (crying) epilepsy. In this context, the reported association of left anterior stroke with depression makes sense.

However, much evidence favors assigning a prepotent role in emotional processing in general to the right hemisphere. Patients with right hemisphere damage appear to be more impaired at perceiving emotion regardless of the valence or input medium. Lesions of the right hemisphere are associated with impairments in processing emotion in speech, a defect known as *aprosodia*. Patients may lack the capacity to modulate prosody, so as to encode emotional information into speech, or the capacity to recognize emotional intonations produced by others. Subtler clinically may be deficits in recognizing emotion in faces or visual scenes. Such deficits may be part of the basis for a finding that may seem counterintuitive, namely that patients with right hemisphere injury have a poorer rehabilitation outcome than their left hemisphere counterparts.

Frontosubcortical Circuits The projection of prefrontal cortex to subcortical structures in multiple closed loops is a crucial feature of behavioral neuroanatomy. The key concept is that, in each loop, a distinct region of prefrontal cortex projects to a distinct portion of the striatum, then to an output nucleus of the basal ganglia, then, in turn, to a specific nucleus of the thalamus, which itself projects to the given area of cortex. Thus, a set of parallel closed loops of frontosubcortical connections processes information in separate domains. In the motor system, premotor cortex and supplementary motor area project primarily to putamen, the output of which projects via ventrolateral globus pallidus and caudolateral substantia nigra pars reticulata (SNr) to ventrolateral-ventroanterior and centromedian nuclei of thalamus and then back to the originating cortical structures. Of particular interest to neuropsychiatrists are the loops involving dorsolateral prefrontal, medial and lateral orbitofrontal, and anterior cingulate cortex:

Dorsolateral prefrontal cortex projects to dorsolateral caudate; projections from caudate go to dorsolateral globus pallidus and SNr. The output from basal ganglia flows primarily to ventrolateral and ventroanterior nuclei of thalamus (but also to dorsomedial nucleus of thalamus), whence it projects to areas 9 and 46 of dorsolateral prefrontal cortex.

Lateral orbitofrontal cortex projects to ventromedial caudate, thence to the caudomedial aspect of SNr. The thalamic level of this loop is represented in ventral anterior and dorsomedial nuclei, whence projections arise back to the lateral aspect of area 12 in orbitofrontal cortex.

The medial orbitofrontal cortex loop features projections from gyrus rectus and medial orbital gyrus to ventromedial caudate; output from the basal ganglia arises in SNr and flows to dorsomedial nucleus of thalamus, as well as ventrolateral and ventroanterior nuclei, thence back to medial orbitofrontal cortex. Anterior cingulate cortex, in the dorsomedial aspect of the hemisphere, projects to ventral striatum, including nucleus accumbens and olfactory tubercle (termini of the mesolimbic dopamine system), with output from SNr flowing through ventroanterior thalamus on its way back to anterior cingulate cortex.

Disruption of each of these loops produces a distinctive clinical syndrome. As is implied by the concept of a circuit, deficits similar to those produced by cortical damage can also occur with damage to the subcortical connections of the cortical region. Before a sketch of each of these syndromes, note must be made that most naturally occurring lesions do not respect the anatomic boundaries, so that clinical presentations are commonly mixed. Nonetheless, for analytical purposes, the anatomical specificity is of interest and importance.

Interference with the loop involving dorsolateral prefrontal cortex prominently produces executive cognitive impairment, with decrements in working memory, problem solving, and related capacities. Damage to this loop commonly arises from traumatic brain injury, stroke, and basal ganglion degenerative diseases such as Parkinson's disease. Involvement of the white matter of the frontal lobes by small-vessel disease commonly leads to interruption of corticosubcortical connections in this circuit and the picture of subcortical dementia.

Damage to orbitofrontal cortex and its connections produces impulsivity, disinhibition, dampening of the experience of emotion, irritability and lability of affect, poor judgment and decision making (especially in regard to social behavior), and insightlessness about these impairments. These impairments are generally seen with bilateral damage, although unilateral right-sided injury may also produce them. As a neighborhood sign, damage often involves the olfactory nerve (which runs along the orbital surface of the brain) with consequent anosmia—at times the only neurological sign. Cognitive function, as tested by the usual bedside or neuropsychological probes, may be unaffected even in the presence of devastating personality change. Trauma is a common etiology.

Damage to dorsomedial prefrontal structures may arise from tumor or stroke. Abulia and apathy, disorders of the initiation of action and the experience of motivation, are the result. Abnormalities of initiation of movement, with akinetic mutism as the most extreme state, may occur. Cingulate cortex is a structure of particular interest. Evidence from animal and imaging studies demonstrates its importance in orienting attention under conflicting stimulus demands, modulating focused problem solving, and monitoring performance to optimize reward. A cell type seen only in cingulate cortex, the spindle cell, appears in evolution only with the great apes and in ontogeny only at 4 months of age, concomitant with the infant's increasing capacity to focus attention. Interference with the output of cingulate gyrus, namely by interrupting the cingulum—the procedure of cingulotomy—appears to be beneficial in a disorder of excessive attention, namely obsessive-compulsive disorder (OCD).

Limbic System *Le grand lobe limbique* was delineated in the mid-19th century (by Paul Broca of aphasia fame) as a ring of cortical and subcortical structures on the medial aspect of the hemispheres. James Papez drew attention to the circuit formed by projections from hippocampus via fornix to mamillary bodies of hypothalamus, thence to anterior nucleus of thalamus, thence via the anterior limb of internal capsule to cingulate gyrus, thence back to hippocampus via presubiculum, entorhinal cortex, and the perforant pathway. In addition to this "Papez circuit," amygdala and its reciprocally connected orbitofrontal cortex are taken to form part of a *limbic system*, a term first used by Paul MacLean one-half century ago. Although some anatomists bristle at its inclusiveness, the concept is nearly universally used, probably because it focuses attention on the "emotional brain."

The core limbic structures are characterized by rich reciprocal monosynaptic connections with hypothalamus; these are

Hippocampus
Amygdala
Piriform cortex anterior to amygdala on the medial surface of the temporal lobe
Septal nuclei in the medial wall of the hemispheres, immediately rostral to lamina terminalis
Substantia innominata in the basal forebrain

Paralimbic cortices reside in temporopolar, insular, and orbitofrontal regions, which have primary affiliations with amygdala, and in parahippocampal, retrosplenial/posterior cingulate, and subcallosal regions, with primary affiliations with hippocampus.

In the limbic system, broad and direct input from sensory cortices into amygdala and hippocampus is extensively processed on its way to effector neurons in hypothalamus regulating autonomic and endocrine activity. In addition to this mediation of the regulation of the internal milieu, the limbic system gates the activity of the motor systems in the basal ganglia, regulating action in the external milieu. This occurs by prefrontal cortical integration of information in the limbic frontosubcortical circuit, which reaches the cortex via projections from ventral pallidum to mediodorsal nucleus of thalamus.

One reason for the central importance of the limbic system in neuropsychiatry is that the threshold for production of epileptic discharges is lowest in amygdala and hippocampus. Thus, most epilepsy in adults is limbic epilepsy. One consequence is the "voluminous mental state," first identified by Hughlings Jackson. This refers to the range of experiential phenomena encountered as auras in limbic epilepsy: *déjà vu*, depersonalization/derealization, micropsia, and macropsia, and so forth. Such symptoms are seen not only in epilepsy, but also in mood disorders and as putative pointers to limbic involvement in paroxysmal disorders not of clear epileptic nature, including those associated with borderline personality disorder and with childhood abuse. Their presence, therefore, does not unequivocally mark an organic diagnosis.

Another reason for the centrality of the limbic system is that hippocampus, in particular, has a crucial role in explicit memory, further discussed below. Persisting substantial amnestic deficits in multiple modalities require limbic system damage.

Cerebellum Against the prevailing notion that the cerebellum is a motor structure, anatomical evidence shows that cerebellar inputs access areas of prefrontal cortex, with a relay in thalamus. These areas of cortex project reciprocally to cerebellum, creating, as with the prefrontal-basal ganglia circuits previously discussed, a set of parallel (relatively) closed loops, or channels. These crossed connections from the cerebellar hemispheres and the further crossing of descending cerebrofugal long tracts mean that motor deficits are manifest ipsilateral to lateralized cerebellar injuries. Additional reciprocal connections link cerebellum with hypothalamus monosynaptically and with other areas of the limbic system via a relay in the basis pontis. The phylogenetically older vermis and fastigial nucleus can be differentiated from the neocerebellum of the cerebellar hemispheres and considered a "limbic cerebellum."

Growing evidence of cerebellar contributions to cognition and affect comes from clinical data and neuropsychological studies. The data are fraught with uncertainty, however, because many cerebellar patients have disorders that may not be limited to cerebellum; for example, cerebellar degenerations may include cortical degeneration, and tumors (and their treatment with radiation and chemotherapy) may have remote effects. Moreover, the phenomenon of crossed cerebellar diaschisis—the reduction in blood flow to connected neocortical areas after cerebellar damage—means that interpretation of deficits as due to abnormal *cerebellar* processing, as compared to shutdown of cerebral cortical processing, is treacherous. Nonetheless, patients with stroke lesions clinically and by neuroimaging limited to cerebellum may have deficits in executive cognitive function, memory, language, and visuospatial function. The data suggest that lateralized cerebellar damage is associated with the predicted lateralized cognitive phenomena (right cerebellar damage with language impairment, left with visuospatial impairment). Reports of an affective syndrome after cerebellar injury are less systematic. Defects in affect regulation, with irritability and lability, are proposed to be associated with damage to the limbic cerebellum, notably the vermis.

White Matter and Cerebral Connectivity

Whereas the volume of neocortex has increased over the course of phylogenetic history, the volume of white matter has increased disproportionately. In humans, the white matter tracts occupy some 42 percent of the volume of the hemispheres. The great majority of these fibers serve corticocortical connectivity rather than projections between cortical regions and subcortical sites; for example, thalamic input is estimated to represent only 5 percent of the total input into primary sensory cortex, the remainder being from other cortical areas.

The fibers in white matter are of several types. First are the longer intrahemispheric fiber tracts:

Arcuate fasciculus, which connects superior and middle frontal gyri to the temporal lobe and (via a superior portion of the fasciculus called *superior longitudinal fasciculus*) the parietal and occipital lobes

Uncinate fasciculus, which connects orbitofrontal cortex to temporal cortex and (via an inferior portion of the fasciculus called *inferior occipitofrontal fasciculus*) the occipital lobe

Cingulum, which lies medially beneath cingulate cortex in cingulate gyrus and connects frontal and parietal lobes with parahippocampal gyrus and adjacent structures

Second are the long projection systems linking cortex, subcortical nuclei, and lower portions of the neuraxis. Medial forebrain bundle is the primary connection between limbic structures and the brainstem and carries projections from the monoaminergic cells in the midbrain and pons. Others are the thalamic peduncle with reciprocal fibers between thalamus and parietal lobe and the corticopontine and corticospinal tracts descending through corona radiata and internal capsule. Fibers from prefrontal cortex descend in the anterior limb of internal capsule, so that lesions there may have predominant behavioral and a paucity of elementary sensorimotor effects.

Lacunes and degeneration of the white matter due to hypertensive small-vessel disease (Binswanger's disease) interrupt these corticocortical fibers and corticosubcortical projections. The result of progressive loss of communication among cortical regions and between cortex and subcortical gray matter is the clinical state of subcortical dementia, which is prominently characterized by slowing of mental processing and failure of executive control processes. The latter may be explained in part by the preferential occurrence of lacunes in frontal locations but also by the impairment of connectivity.

Third, *U fibers* are the short, juxtacortical fibers connecting adjacent cortical regions. These fibers are characteristically spared in Binswanger's disease, cerebral autosomal dominant arteriopathy with subcortical infarction and lacunes (CADASIL), and certain other disease processes.

Fourth are the many specific projection systems linking delimited regions such as mammillothalamic tract, which connects mammillary bodies with anterior nucleus of thalamus, and fornix, which connects mammillary bodies with hippocampus. Interesting neurobehavioral syndromes have been described related to rare cases of focal interruption of such pathways. For example, interruption of mammillothalamic tract or of fornix is implicated in amnesia.

Fifth, several pathways connect the two hemispheres, notably corpus callosum but also anterior and posterior commissures and massa intermedia of thalamus. Syndromes due to interruption of the smaller commissures have not so far been described, although absence of massa intermedia is reported to be associated with schizophrenia in women, and anterior commissure and massa intermedia are larger in women than in men. Corpus callosum is congenitally absent in numerous neurodevelopmental syndromes, and its absence has been associated with schizophrenia. Congenital absence is not, however, associated with the interesting disconnection symptoms seen in lesional interruption of the callosum such as by anterior or posterior cerebral artery stroke or by surgical callosotomy for control of epilepsy.

Two callosal disconnection syndromes are worthy of specific mention. After anterior cerebral artery occlusion with anterior callosal infarction, the right hemisphere is deprived of verbal information; a left-hand apraxia is seen, and the patient cannot name unseen objects placed in the left hand. Reciprocally, the right hand shows constructional apraxia. This is the *anterior disconnection syndrome*. After occlusion of the left posterior cerebral artery with infarction of the left occipital lobe and the splenium (posterior portion) of corpus callosum, the language cortices of the left hemisphere lose access to visual information: The left visual cortex is damaged, as are the projections from the right visual cortex, which cross in the splenium. Thus, reading becomes impossible, although other language functions are unaffected—the syndrome of *alexia without agraphia*.

Cerebral Cortex

The cerebral cortex develops through complex but increasingly well-understood processes of cell proliferation and migration, axonal projection, and dendritic proliferation and pruning. Abnormalities in these processes lead to cortical dysplasia with clinical consequences, including mental retardation and epilepsy. Some 10 percent of intractable epilepsy may be due to such disorders, and increasingly, migration abnormalities are recognizable by imaging before neuropathological examination. Failure of normal pruning of synapses by elimination of dendrites is now known to be crucial in the pathogenesis of the fragile X syndrome and has been speculatively linked to schizophrenia. Rarely, cortical dysplasia may be present without epilepsy or mental retardation; the neurobehavioral consequences of this abnormality are just coming under investigation.

The organization of sensory cortices follows a regular plan. Each primary sensory cortical area projects to unimodal association cortices specialized for the extraction of features in that particular modality; the unimodal association cortices are densely and reciprocally interconnected. For example, visual association cortex has specialized regions for color, motion, and shape. This creates an intricate web of sensory processing; the visual cortex in the cat, for example, is believed to have 19 processing regions. Unimodal association cortices project, in turn, to heteromodal cortices, which receive inputs from more than a single sensory modality. Heteromodal cortices are located in prefrontal, posterior parietal, lateral temporal, and parahippocampal regions. Unimodal cortices do not project to unimodal cortices in other modalities, only to the higher-level heteromodal cortices. Further, widespread hippocampal projections to cortex arrive only at association cortices, not primary sensory cortices. These structural features amount to the isolation of sensory processing from top-down influences over the first several synaptic stages and presumably increase its fidelity to external phenomena.

Lesions of cortical association areas produce an array of behavioral and cognitive disorders of intriguing specificity. The specificity can be demonstrated by the occurrence of double dissociations: A lesion in area A produces a deficit in function x but not y; a lesion in area B produces a deficit in function y but not x. This pattern of findings provides crucial confirmation that the deficits arise not from task difficulty (if y were simply more difficult than x, then y would always be disturbed when x was disturbed), but from separable processing components. For example, some patients show a greater impairment for naming living things than for naming artifacts after a brain injury. However, occasionally, patients show the opposite pattern, greater impairment in naming living things: a double dissociation. The explanation of the discrepancy thus cannot depend on insufficient processing resources but must reveal a property of the organization of the semantic system.

Cognitive disorders of the visual system can serve as a paradigm of the syndromes seen with damage to the association cortex. Lesions of primary visual cortex (V1, or Brodmann's area [BA] 17) produce cortical blindness in a quadrant, hemifield, or the entire visual field. Despite the genuine blindness, accuracy above chance in localizing visual stimuli can be achieved without awareness of vision, the phenomenon of *blindsight*, which testifies to subcortical visual processing inaccessible to consciousness. V1 projects to adjacent cortical regions (BA18 and BA19), which contain neurons that respond to specific features of visual stimuli such as color, movement, or shape. Lesions in these cortices produce deficits in identification of these features. Thus arise syndromes such as central achromatopsia, demonstrated by inability to sort (as well as to name) colors. The stream of information transfer divides into dorsal and ventral streams, the former specialized for localization of visual stimuli ("where") and the latter for identification of the stimuli ("what"). Dorsal lesions involving superior parietal lobule can produce impaired reaching under visual guidance (optic ataxia), a part of Balint's syndrome; the deficit testifies to the integration of visual information with motor output in association cortex. Ventral lesions, involving inferotemporal cortex, produce defects in recognition (agnosia). Agnosic patients are not only unable to name elements within the domain of agnosia but also are unable to demonstrate their use or show recognition of the items in other nonverbal ways.

Central auditory disorders include cortical (or central) deafness; pure word deafness, the inability to recognize words presented in the auditory modality despite preserved visual–verbal function; and auditory agnosia, the inability to recognize words or complex sounds (e.g., the meaning of the ringing of a telephone). Central deafness requires bilateral lesions involving primary auditory cortex in superior temporal gyrus or auditory radiations in white matter. Patients with pure word deafness generally have bilateral lesions of association cortex more anteriorly in superior temporal gyrus, although unilateral left lesions, presumably disconnecting left from right cortices by subcortical damage, also are reported. Primary auditory cortex is partially spared in these cases. In agnosia for nonverbal environmental sounds, right hemisphere damage is sufficient to produce the deficit. Amusia, the incapacity to recognize musical sounds, is associated with cortical damage, but the issue of laterality is complex, dependent in part on the preinjury level of musical skills.

Full evaluation of these disorders requires techniques that go well beyond bedside examination or routine paraclinical tools. At issue in the agnosic disorders is the extent to which a deficit is apperceptive—that is, due to impairment in analysis of subtle perceptual elements presumably dependent on more upstream cortical regions—and associative—that is, occurring in the absence of definable perceptual abnormalities and presumably due to dysfunction of more downstream cortical analyzers. This distinction requires detailed neuropsychological and often psychophysical assessment.

Modulators of Brain States

This account of cognitive processing in cortex seems to many psychiatrists to leave out of consideration the matters with which they are most concerned: pervasive states of altered mood, drive, and behavior. That such states are behaviorally pervasive does not argue that they are anatomically global. Limbic structures discussed above provide in part the anatomical substrate for emotional states. Further, several systems with diffuse cortical projections have the capacity to modulate processing in widespread brain regions. These originate in

- Intralaminar thalamic nuclei, which project to cortex (especially prefrontal and cingulate cortex) and to striatum
- Histaminergic cells in posterior hypothalamus
- Serotonergic cells in pontine raphe nuclei
- Noradrenergic cells in locus ceruleus
- Dopaminergic cells in the midbrain ventral tegmental area giving rise to the mesocortical and mesolimbic systems
- Cholinergic cells in basal forebrain nuclei such as nucleus basalis of Meynert

The last of these is of relevance to cholinesterase inhibitor treatment of dementia, the preceding three of relevance to treatment of mood, anxiety, and psychotic disorders. The hypothalamic histaminergic projections are involved in arousal. "Nonspecific" thalamic projections may have an important role in executive dysfunction seen after thalamic lesions. So as not to become complacent about current understanding of such pathways, recall that only within the past few years were a previously unknown neurotransmitter and its pathways recognized, and the discovery of orexin/hypocretin and its hypothalamic anatomy exposed the secrets of narcolepsy. Neuropsychiatric anatomy is not a closed book.

MODULARITY AND NEUROPSYCHIATRY

These focal behavioral syndromes, and many others, compel attention to local processing in the brain and almost irresistibly suggest a particular model of brain organization. One imagines a box-and-arrow diagram, in which each box—representing an elementary cognitive function—maps on to a specialized region of cortex. Each area of cortex has its job to do, and a lesion of any area produces a distinctive, delimited, and predictable deficit.

This model raises the issue of modular organization of the brain. The general topic of modularity in cognitive processing deserves further consideration because it is crucial to the theoretical perspective of neuropsychiatry and, in particular, because it bears on the value of neuropsychiatric data for the understanding of idiopathic psychiatric disorders. *Modularity* in cognitive neuroscience refers to a brain organization characterized by multiple computational devices, each of which operates on characteristically encapsulated input with prewired (perhaps innate) rules, thus being rapid, efficient, and reliable. For example, elementary visual processing can be considered modular, inasmuch as it uses restricted input with hard-wired feature extraction (e.g., motion, color, shape). In another domain, consider that it is easier to teach an animal to associate a taste than a visual stimulus with the aversive effects of an ingested toxin. This finding implies domain-specific, innate learning constraints. The classic cognitive example of domain-specific prewiring is language—for example, Chomsky's observation that children generate language errors that they have never heard: "He bringed me here," the small child might say, although he or she has never heard an adult say "bringed." The implication is that a language-processing module possesses innate grammatical rules that have generated a grammatical form without experiential foundation.

Evolutionary psychologists have forcefully argued the case for modular processing, as opposed to domain-general problem-solving devices. The core of the evolutionary argument is that cerebral organization is the result of natural selection operating on the adaptational fitness of humans' Pleistocene hunter-gatherer ancestors. Domain-specific processing has advantages of speed and efficiency that necessarily lead to an advantage in fitness. The availability of preexperiential information about the content of domain-specific processing carries a large advantage over the "combinatorial explosion" of informational possibilities requiring evaluation by a domain-general processor. For example, detection of cheating in social exchanges is an essential element of adaptation in a population group featuring cooperative behavior. Is it a function of a domain-general logical problem-solving device, or is there a "cheater-detection" module? Cross-cultural evidence shows that people are far better at detecting violation of social exchange rules than at solving problems of equivalent logical complexity when posed in other terms, and focal lesions can differentially affect cheater detection. The implication is that prewired mechanisms, presumably located in a particular brain area, are "tuned" to recognize and reason about this adaptationally crucial behavior, just as innate mechanisms subserve language learning and toxin recognition. One of the strengths of the evolutionary approach is to direct attention to processing domains the modularity of which is plausible on adaptational grounds.

However, many of the "modules" that have attracted clinical interest are *not* plausibly directly the objects of natural selection. Reading and writing are clear examples. These have arisen too recently in evolutionary time to have been the product of natural selection and, thus, must depend on the workings of processors that are, at least to this extent, domain general.

Moreover, much of the literature on modularity is written from a cognitive-psychological or philosophical perspective, with less attention to the "wetware" (i.e., actual brain substance) implementation of the processing devices. A foundation in cognitive neuroscience and evolutionary biology can enrich clinical theories, but it creates the potential for misunderstanding by clinicians interested in the functioning of patients with brain lesions. The modules of the evolutionary biologists and philosophically inclined cognitivists do not map directly onto brain areas. One of the striking results of functional neuroimaging experiments is that, however the function under study is delimited, multiple areas of brain activation are found. A metaanalysis of reports of positron emission tomography (PET) studies of cognition found that the mean number of activation peaks per experiment was 10.24! Each task engaged a mean of 3.3 Brodmann's areas; contrariwise, each Brodmann's area was engaged by a mean of 3.42 perceptual or cognitive tasks. Even functions that seem psychologically fundamental are not implemented in a simple way, and local processing components may be recruited into networks subserving a variety of tasks. This seems to be the case in respect to the limited number of frontal sites involved in a wide range of executive tasks. The specialization of regions is dependent on input from other regions; specialization is not entirely dependent on intrinsic properties but partially on top-down influences.

The issue is not whether different cerebral regions carry out different modes of information processing. This is unquestionably so, and neither unreconstructed holists who believe in the equipotentiality of cortex nor strict localizationists who believe only in fully autonomous processing devices figure on the current neuroscientific scene. The question is how regions are linked in carrying out tasks. Functions are implemented by networks, most or all of the nodes of which participate in multiple functional networks. This pattern of cerebral organization has been termed *selectively distributed processing* or *sparsely distributed networks.* Although cortical regions have specialized capacities for information processing, functions cannot be localized to regions (as Hughlings Jackson explicitly warned a century and a half ago). It is erroneous, for example, to believe that an area crucial for face recognition contains all of the neurons, and only neurons, that respond to faces.

Moreover, normal individuals may differ in how they recruit regions into networks. The methods used in studying groups of subjects in functional imaging experiments may obscure such individual differences. For example, robust individual differences in patterns of activation emerged in a memory task, differences putatively reflecting different strategies in performing the task. The differences were stable within individuals over time, yet analysis of group data revealed activations in regions activated in only some of the subjects and failed to disclose activations in regions consistently activated in others. Individual differences in organization of language cortex are evident clinically in the unusual, but not negligible, occurrence of crossed aphasia (aphasia due to right hemisphere injury in a dextral), crossed nonaphasia (lack of aphasia with a left hemisphere injury that "ought" to cause aphasia in a dextral), and aphasic deficits anomalous in respect to the predicted effects of lesions in both dextrals and sinistrals.

Another crucial critique for neuropsychiatry of the modularity hypothesis derives from developmental psychology. Trenchant arguments contradict the assumption that a mapping of deficits to specific brain structures could be static over developmental time. To the contrary, how the brain performs cognitive tasks changes with development. Development entails changing patterns of interaction among brain components, and localization may alter as neurons and regions become "tuned" in responsiveness based on their initial characteristic processing biases and their patterns of inputs and connectivity. This reorganization of cortical function could mean that the same behavior has different substrates at different developmental epochs. For example, in adult subjects with Williams syndrome, poor number processing and good language skills are characteristic; however, in infancy, the opposite pattern is seen. Whatever the fundamental processing disorder of genetic origin may be, it cannot be seen as having "knocked out" a module. A large expanse of nonlinear brain development lies between the gene and the clinical phenomena, an expanse that can be understood only with a better theory than neophrenology (Fig. 2.1–1). The very development of modularity can be anomalous. Indeed, in the Williams syndrome cases, magnetic resonance imaging (MRI) data disclose an anomalous, diffuse pattern of activation for music perception, an area of preserved or enhanced ability in these patients. Focal syndromes in adults provide an appropriate place to start in formulating hypotheses, but a deficit seen in an idiopathic disorder cannot be assumed to have its basis in dysfunction in the same simple locus as a phenomenologically similar deficit seen after a focal brain lesion occurring in an adult.

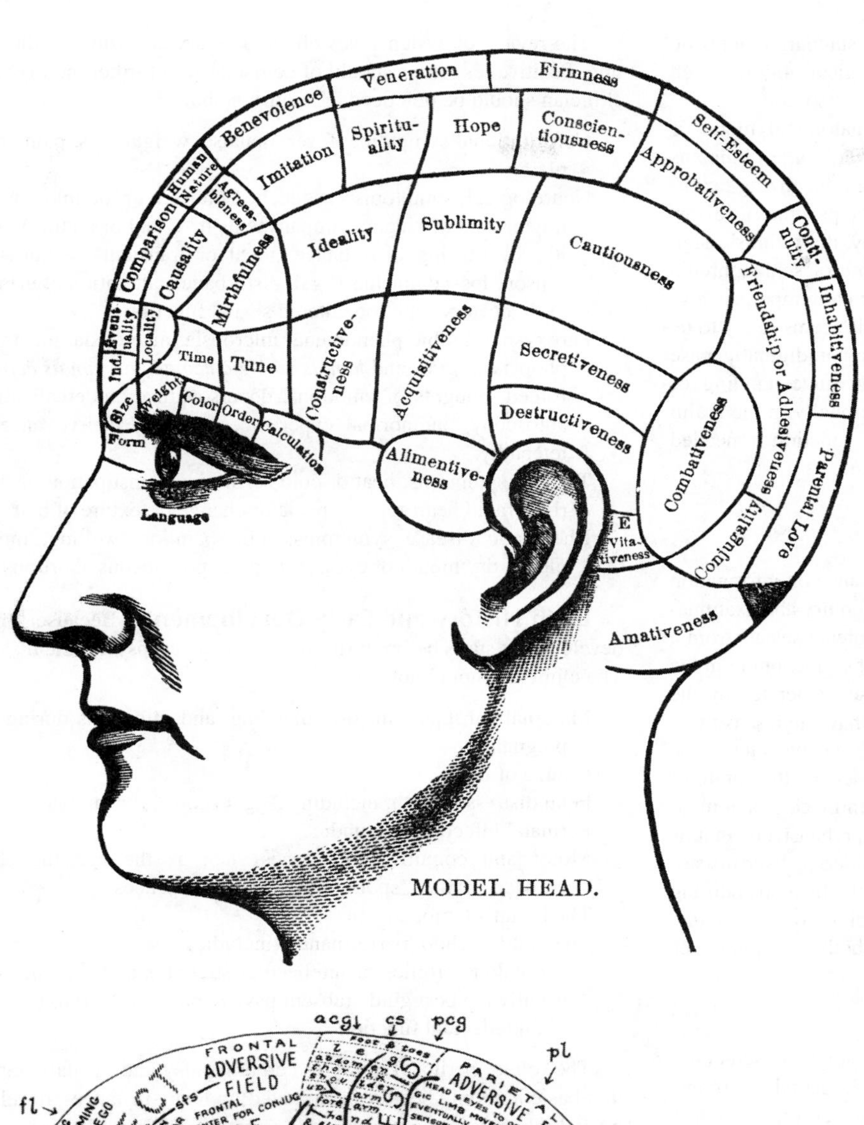

A

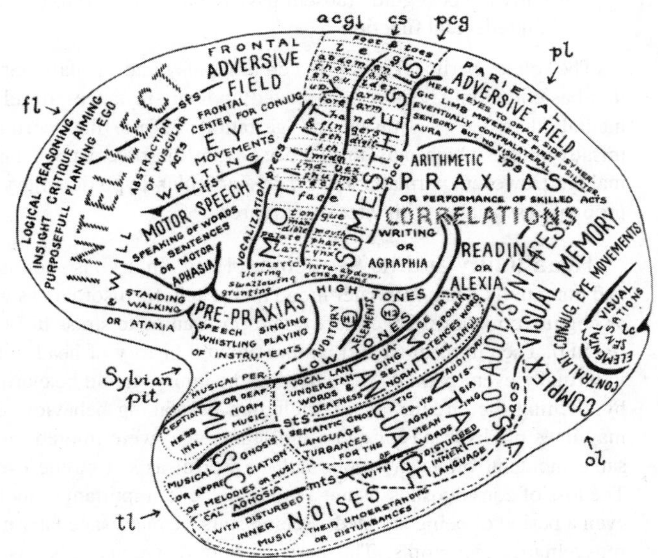

B

FIGURE 2.1–1 A phrenological head as pictured in 1890 **(A)** and 1957 **(B)**. Despite the interval of 67 years, they are suspiciously alike. (From Fowler OS, Fowler LN. *The Self-Instructor in Phrenology and Physiology*. New York: Fowler & Wells; 1890:iii; and Polyak S. *The Vertebrate Visual System*. Chicago: The University of Chicago Press; 1957:456, with permission.)

Nothing in this line of argument diminishes the interest of focal neurobehavioral syndromes, which are clinical facts and have a substantial heuristic value for the cognitive neurosciences. Neuropsychiatry, along with other brain specialties, has the task of importing into clinical theory the understanding of the mind and brain that is developing in cognitive neuroscience. The search for psychopathological understanding based on identification of deficits in cognitive modules that are relatively well understood in normal subjects has been termed *cognitive neuropsychiatry*. This pursuit inevitably results in deconstruction of the psychiatric diagnoses of the revised fourth edition of *Diagnostic and Statistical Manual of Mental Disorders* (DSM-IV-TR) or the International Classification of Diseases

(ICD) into symptoms or syndromes because the standard diagnostic categories are generally based on folk-psychological notions (such as the division between "thought" and "affective" disorders).

Much of this chapter is devoted to the anatomical mode of thought practiced by neuropsychiatrists. However, some clinicians appear to hope that neuropsychiatry will provide a localizing taxonomy of behavioral syndromes, so that particular psychiatric disorders will carry the same localizing power as, say, the Babinski sign for the corticospinal tract—the nuclear syndrome of schizophrenia to the left temporal lobe, for example. From the contemporary cognitive neuroscience perspective just reviewed, this seems likely to be false hope. The Babinski sign is a limiting, not a paradigmatic, case of brain–behavior relationships. For the fullest understanding of complex mental syndromes, notably those traditionally in the realm of psychiatry, a more adequate theory of brain function is needed than can be offered by the localizationist tradition.

CLINICAL EVALUATION

The neuropsychiatric perspective places great reliance on information that can be gathered at the bedside. No practical inquiry and examination can include all possible items; rather, the clinician selects from a toolbox of probes of the history and of the patient's functioning in the examination room to confirm or refute hypotheses generated by the emerging clinical picture. Screening items should have high sensitivity but not necessarily high specificity. Beyond screening, elements of the history and examination that might potentially elucidate the nature of the disease process under consideration form the entire corpus of medical assessment and cannot be dealt with comprehensively in this chapter. For example, the neuropsychiatrist considering liver disease as the explanation for delirium wants to estimate the liver span during the physical examination, but techniques for doing so are not discussed below. The discussion here is focused on both common issues and techniques distinctive to neuropsychiatry.

Neuropsychiatric History The initial steps in screening for the presence of organic disease in patients with mental symptoms are easily taken. The physician should obtain a general medical history, including a history of diseases possibly relevant to the neuropsychiatric symptoms under consideration, and a review of systems in potentially relevant areas. With a cognitively impaired or psychotic patient, such history taking may be unreliable. Collateral history from a family member or other informant and review of medical records are almost always essential.

With virtually every patient, the clinician should inquire as to a history of

- Heart, lung, liver, kidney, skin, joint, and eye disease
- Hypertension
- Diabetes
- Traumatic brain injury
- Seizures, including febrile convulsions in childhood
- Unexplained medical symptoms
- Substance misuse
- Current medication
- Family history of neuropsychiatric disorder

The inquiry about these disorders in some settings can be quite general. For example, the question "have you ever had heart problems?" along with a few questions in the review of systems may suffice to screen for heart disease in a young, apparently healthy patient. In other settings, more detailed information must be gathered.

The review of systems as well should vary according to the setting. Positive responses should of course lead to further inquiry. The clinician should be practiced in inquiring about

- Constitutional symptoms: fever, malaise, weight loss, pain complaints
- Neurological symptoms: headache, blurred or double vision, impairment of balance, impairments of visual or auditory acuity, swallowing disturbance, focal or transient weakness or sensory loss, clumsiness, gait disturbance, alteration of urinary or defecatory function, altered sexual function
- Paroxysmal limbic phenomena: micropsia, macropsia, metamorphopsia, *déjà vu* and *jamais vu*, *déjà écouté* and *jamais écouté*, forced thoughts or emotions, depersonalization/derealization, autoscopy, paranormal experiences such as clairvoyance or telepathy
- Thyroid symptoms: heat or cold sensitivity, constipation or diarrhea, rapid heart rate, alopecia or change in texture of hair
- Rheumatic disease symptoms: joint pain or swelling, mouth ulcers, dry mouth or eyes, rash, past spontaneous abortions

Birth History and Early Development Because brain development starts before birth, so does the neuropsychiatric history. The clinician should note

- Maternal substance misuse, bleeding, and infections during the pregnancy
- Course of labor
- Fetal distress at birth, including Apgar scores, if available
- Perinatal infection or jaundice
- Motor and cognitive milestones such as the age the child crawled, walked, spoke words, spoke sentences
- The infant's temperament
- The child's school performance (including special education and anomalous profiles of intellectual strengths and weaknesses), usually the best guide (absent psychometrical data) to premorbid intellectual function

The role of perinatal injury in cerebral palsy and mental retardation has commonly been overestimated; in many instances, developmental disorder is present in gestation before the perinatal misadventure, which may in fact arise from the preexisting abnormality. However, perinatal injury, in particular hypoxic injury, is probably associated with later schizophrenia.

Head Injury and Its Sequelae Head injury is common and potentially a factor in later mood and psychotic disorders as well as cognitive impairment, epilepsy, and posttraumatic stress disorder (PTSD). The clinician should inquire about a history of head injury in virtually every patient. The nature of the injury should be clarified by eliciting the circumstances, including risk-taking behaviors that may have predisposed to injury and others who were injured in the same incident, often an emotionally powerful aspect of the event. The loss of consciousness is not a prerequisite to important sequelae; even a period of being stunned, "seeing stars," can presage later neuropsychiatric symptoms. The period of loss of consciousness, or coma, should be established, ideally with the assistance of contemporaneous medical records. The period of retrograde amnesia—from last memory before the injury to the injury itself—and of anterograde amnesia—from injury to recovery of the capacity for consecutive memory—should be noted.

Attack Disorders Paroxysmal disorders of neuropsychiatric interest include epilepsy, migraine, panic attacks, and episodic dyscontrol of aggression. Taking a history of an attack has common features irrespective of the nature of the disorder. The clinician should track through the chronology of the attack. This starts with the possible presence of a prodrome, a warning of an impending attack in the hours or days before one. The attack itself may be presaged by an aura, lasting seconds to minutes. In the case of an epileptic seizure, this represents the core of the seizure itself and may carry important localizing information about the side and site of the focus. The pace of buildup, from onset to peak of the ictus, is of differential diagnostic importance. For example, epileptic seizures begin abruptly; panic attacks may have a more gradual development to peak intensity. The mental and behavioral features of the ictus itself should be elicited in detail from collateral informants as well as from the patient, if possible. The duration of the spell and the mode of its termination should be elicited. Inquiring whether the patient has just one sort of spell or more than one is an essential prelude to establishing the frequency of episodes, both at present and at maximum and minimum in the past.

By interviewing the patient and collateral informants, information necessary to make a differential diagnosis can usually be elicited. The differential diagnosis between epilepsy and pseudoseizures can be difficult, but at times, if asked properly, the patient makes the diagnosis for the clinician by reporting "two kinds of seizures," one of which is clearly epileptic and the other of which is clearly dependent on emotional states.

Cognitive Symptoms Recognizing cognitive symptoms in patients without established dementia is a crucial element of neuropsychiatric history taking. Such symptoms may be outweighed by more dramatic behavior or mood change, but identification of cognitive impairment can reorient the diagnostic evaluation of a late-life depression, for example. No doubt the most common complaint along cognitive lines is of memory problems. In the setting of depression, the more intense the complaint of memory impairment, the less likely it is to have an organic basis and the more likely to testify to depressive ideation and attentional failure. The clinician should establish whether forgotten material (for example, an acquaintance's name or a task meant to be performed) comes to the patient later, as a matter of absentmindedness rather than amnestic failure. Certain other complaints are highly characteristic of organic disease. These include a loss of the capacity for divided attention or for the automatic performance of familiar tasks. A patient might report, for example, no longer being able to read and listen to the radio at the same time. Getting lost or beginning to use aids for recall, such as a notebook, are suggestive of organic cognitive failure.

Appetitive Symptoms and Personality Change Alterations of sleep, appetite, and energy are common in idiopathic psychiatric disorders, as well as transiently in the healthy population, and cannot be interpreted as implying brain disease. Certain patterns of altered sleeping and eating behavior and personality, however, are pointers to organic disease. Excessive daytime sleepiness or sleep attacks raise the question of sleep apnea or narcolepsy or, in a different temporal pattern, Kleine-Levin syndrome. Abnormal behavior during sleep raises the question of a parasomnia. Of particular interest is rapid eye movement (REM) behavior disorder, which may be due to a pontine lesion but, when a focal lesion is absent, strongly points to ingravescent Lewy body disease. Much more rarely, nocturnal oneiric behavior represents a prion disease, notably fatal familial insomnia. Loss of dreaming occurs with parietal or bifrontal damage; loss of visual imagery in dreams occurs with ventral occipitotemporal damage, part of the Charcot-Wilbrandt syndrome (loss of visual imagery with brain damage). In medial hypothalamic disease, eating behavior is marked by lack of satiety and resultant obesity. In the Klüver-Bucy syndrome of bilateral anterior temporal damage (involving amygdala), patients mouth nonfood items. With frontal damage, patients may stuff food into the mouth, a form of utilization behavior, sometimes with alarming or even fatal consequences. A "gourmand" syndrome of excessive concern with fine eating has been associated with right anterior injury.

Changes in sexual behavior are common consequences of brain disease. Hyposexuality is common in epilepsy, possibly as a consequence of limbic discharges. A change in habitual sexual interests, quantitative or qualitative, developing in midlife suggests organic disease. It is possible, although understudied, that relevant organic disease, such as the sequelae of traumatic brain injury, is common in sexual offenders. Other changes in personality, such as the development of shallowness of affect, irritability, loss of sense of humor, or a coarsening of sensibilities, may indicate ingravescent organic disease, for example, frontotemporal dementia.

Handedness Approximately 90 percent of people designate themselves as dextral, almost all the rest as sinistral, and a very few as ambidextrous. The true state of affairs is somewhat more complicated, in that handedness may be considered more dimensionally—that is, as a matter of degrees rather than categories. A patient may call himself or herself right-handed but use the left hand preferentially for certain tasks. Inquiring about a few specific tasks—writing, throwing, drawing, using scissors or a toothbrush—yields helpful information. A family history of sinistrality may also be relevant.

Neuropsychiatric Physical Examination

To the neuropsychiatrist, the physical examination is a central feature of clinical evaluation. In principle, any aspect of the general physical or neurological examination may be relevant to neuropsychiatric diagnosis, if only in revealing an incidental clinical problem in a neuropsychiatric patient. Here, the focus is on elements of the physical examination with specific relevance to detection and identification of organic disease in patients with mental presentations. The mental examination, including the cognitive examination, is discussed below in association with syndromes of behavioral disorder and insofar as it can elicit or elucidate these syndromes in the consultation room.

General Physical Examination

GENERAL APPEARANCE *Dysmorphic features* include so-called minor physical anomalies, some of which are captured in the widely used Waldrop scale. These are associated with developmental disorders, including schizophrenia. Some of these features are listed in Table 2.1–1. These features center on the head, hands, and feet. No single minor anomaly is diagnostic of pathological development, but the coincidence of multiple anomalies argues that development has gone awry. Many specific developmental disability syndromes can be diagnosed by the constellation of dysmorphic features presented. *Cleft lip or palate* is associated with brain malformations and frontal cognitive impairment. *Asymmetry* of the extremities, often best seen in the thumbnails, or of the cranial vault points to a developmental abnormality. Occasionally, a patient even reports wearing shoes of different sizes on the two feet. The larger extremity and the smaller side of the head are ipsilateral to the abnormal cerebral hemisphere. *Short stature* is an important feature of many developmental syndromes, both common, such as fetal alcohol syndrome and Down syndrome, and uncommon, such as mitochondrial cytopathies. *Abnormal habitus*, such as the marfanoid habitus of homocystinuria, may be a clue to diagnosis. *Weight loss* is an impor-

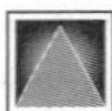

Table 2.1–1
Selected Minor Physical Anomalies

Head and face	Mouth
Head circumference[a]	High arch of palate[a]
Hair whorls[a]	Furrowed tongue[a]
Fine electric hair that will not comb down[a]	Geographical tongue[a]
Frontal bossing	Abnormal philtrum
	Cleft uvula
Eyes	Extremities
Wide-spaced eyes[a]	Clinodactyly[a]
Epicanthus[a]	Abnormal palm crease[a]
Short palpebral fissures	Toe 3 longer than toe 2[a]
Iris discoloration or defect	Partial syndactyly[a]
Ears	Gap between toes 1 and 2[a]
Adherent lobes[a]	Small nails
Malformation[a]	Single crease finger 5
Asymmetry[a]	
Soft and pliable[a]	
Low seated[a]	
Preauricular skin tag	

[a]Anomaly is part of Waldrop scale.

tant clue to systemic disease, such as neoplasia; it should not be dismissed, even in a patient with depression, which may—but may not—account for the weight loss. *Weight gain* equally may point to limbic or systemic disease, especially an endocrinopathy, or may reflect toxicity of psychotropic drugs.

VITAL SIGNS *Elevated temperature* or *heart or respiratory rate* should never be ignored, even in a patient whose agitation or anxiety might seem to explain the abnormality. Doing so risks missing infection, neuroleptic malignant syndrome, connective tissue disease, or other important causes of morbidity. *Abnormal respiratory patterns* occur in hyperkinetic movement disorders (including tardive dyskinesia). *Yawning* is a feature of opiate withdrawal and serotonergic toxicity.

SKIN *Alopecia* or *rash* may point to systemic connective tissue disease. Alopecia is also a feature of drug toxicity and hypothyroidism (where thinning of the lateral part of the eyebrow is characteristic). The malar rash of systemic lupus erythematosus is typically slightly raised and tender and extends to both cheeks in a "butterfly" pattern while sparing the nasolabial folds. Discoid rashes in lupus are characterized by hyperkeratosis, atrophy, and loss of pigment; the strong tendency to scarring means that the presence of a discoid rash does not necessarily indicate active disease. A pink periungual rash is also characteristic of lupus. A vasculitic rash is classically palpable purpura and may be seen in lupus or other connective tissue diseases. Livedo reticularis, a net-like violaceous pattern on the trunk and lower extremities, is not specific but raises the question of Sneddon's syndrome, in which stroke or dementia is a clinical accompaniment. The neurocutaneous syndromes have typical skin manifestations: adenoma sebaceum (facial angiofibromas), ash-leaf macules, depigmented nevi, and shagreen patches (thickened, yellowish skin over the lumbosacral area) in tuberous sclerosis; a port-wine stain (typically involving both upper and lower eyelids) in Sturge-Weber syndrome; neurofibromas, café au lait spots, and axillary freckling in neurofibromatosis.

HEAD *Head circumference* should be measured in patients with a question of developmental disorder. Most reference works give normal ranges for head circumference in developing children but not for adults, and extrapolation is inaccurate. Fortunately, adequate data to establish normal ranges do exist. Although height and weight need to be taken into account along with gender, the normal range for adult men is approximately 54 to 60 cm (21.25 to 23.50 in.), for women, 52 to 58 cm (20.50 to 22.75 in.). *Old skull fracture or intracranial surgery* usually leaves palpable evidence.

EYES *Exophthalmos* usually indicates Graves' disease, although it may reveal a space-occupying lesion, especially if unilateral. *Dry eyes*, along with dry mouth, raise the question of Sjögren's syndrome, although drug toxicity or the aging process is a common confound. Inflammation in the anterior portion of the eye, *uveitis*, can be appreciated at the bedside by the presence of pain, redness, and a constricted pupil; this is commonly associated with connective tissue disease. The *Kayser-Fleischer ring* is a brownish-green discoloration at the limbus of the cornea; it sensitively and specifically indicates Wilson's disease. The pupils, optic disks, visual fields, and eye movements are discussed below.

MOUTH *Oral ulcers* can be seen in lupus, Behçet's syndrome, and other connective tissue disease. *Dry mouth* is a part of the sicca syndrome along with dry eyes, discussed above. Vitamin B_{12} deficiency produces *atrophic glossitis*, a smooth, painful, red tongue.

HEART AND VESSELS A *carotid bruit* indicates turbulent flow in the vessel but is a poor predictor of the degree or potential risk of the vascular lesion. A thickened, tender *temporal artery* points to giant cell arteritis; here, the physical examination is an excellent guide to clinical significance. Cardiac valvular disease, marked by cardiac *murmurs*, is important in assessing the cause of stroke, and congestive failure may be relevant in delirium. In a schizophrenic patient, a murmur may imply the velocardiofacial syndrome. Patients with developmental disabilities may have multiple anomalies, including structural heart disease.

EXTREMITIES *Joint inflammation* as an indication of systemic rheumatic disease is distinguished from noninflammatory degenerative joint disease (osteoarthritis) by the presence of swelling, warmth, and erythema and is characteristically seen in wrists, ankles, and metacarpophalangeal joints, as compared with the involvement of the base of the thumb, distal interphalangeal joints, and spine in degenerative joint disease. *Raynaud's phenomenon* and *sclerodactyly* are signs of connective tissue disease.

Neurological Examination

OLFACTION *Hyposmia* is common in neurological disease but even more common in local disease of the nasal mucosa, which must be excluded before a defect is taken to be of neuropsychiatric significance. Assessment of olfaction is often ignored (cranial nerves II through XII normal), but it is easily performed and gives clues to the integrity of regions otherwise hard to assess, notably orbitofrontal cortex. The olfactory nerve lies underneath orbitofrontal cortex; projections go to olfactory tubercle, entorhinal and piriform cortex in the temporal lobes, amygdala, and orbitofrontal cortex. Testing of olfaction is best performed using a floral odorant such as scented lip balms, which are inexpensive and simple to carry. Although a distinction can be made between the threshold for odor detection and that for identification of the stimulus with differing anatomies, at the bedside without special equipment, the best one can achieve is recognition of a decrement in sensitivity—that is, whether the patient smells anything, even without being able to identify it.

EYES *Pupillary* dilation may indicate anticholinergic toxicity; pupillary constriction is a characteristic feature of opiate toxicity. Argyll Robertson pupils are bilateral, small, irregular, and reactive to accommodation but not to light; the finding is characteristic of pare-

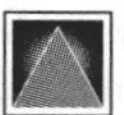

Table 2.1–2
Speech Syndromes

Syndrome	Output	Characteristic Lesion Location or Associations
Aphemia	Initial mutism, recovery without agrammatism	Broca's area (BA44), foot of left third frontal gyrus
Apraxia of speech	Inconsistent and slowed articulation, flattened volume, abnormal prosody	Left insula
Ataxic dysarthria	Slowed, equalization of or erratic stress (scanning), imprecise articulation	Cerebellum, especially superior anterior vermis, left hemisphere > right
Pyramidal dysarthria	Slowed, strained, slurred	Anterior hemispheres, usually bilateral; may be accompanied by pseudobulbar palsy (dysphagia, drooling, pathological laughing and crying)
Extrapyramidal dysarthria	Hypophonia, monotony of intonation, trailing off with longer phrases	Basal ganglia
Bulbar dysarthria	Nasality, breathiness, slurred articulation	Brainstem
Foreign accent syndrome	Phonetic and prosodic alterations like those of dysarthria after cortical damage but giving listener feeling of foreign accent	Motor or premotor cortex or subjacent white matter of left hemisphere
Developmental stuttering	Repetition, prolongation, arrest of sounds; if overcome in childhood, may reemerge after stroke, onset of Parkinson's disease	?
Acquired stuttering	No dystonic facial movements as are seen in developmental stuttering	Various hemisphere sites
Cessation of stuttering	Not an abnormality but the reversal of an abnormality	Various hemisphere sites
Echolalia	Automatic repetition of interlocutor's speech or words heard in environment, sometimes with reversal of pronouns, correction of grammar, completion of well-known phrases	Various anatomies, but seen in frontotemporal dementia, transcortical aphasias, other settings
Palilalia	Automatic repetition of own final word or phrase, with increasing rapidity and decreasing volume	Usually extrapyramidal system
"Blurting," "echoing approval"	Automatic utterance of stereotyped or simple responses (e.g., "yes, yes")	Frontal system

tic neurosyphilis but also is present in other conditions. *Papilledema* indicates elevated intracranial pressure; the earliest and most sensitive feature is loss of venous pulsations at the optic disk. A homonymous upper quadrantic *field defect* is present when temporal lobe disease affects Meyer's loop, the portion of the optic radiation that dips into the temporal lobe. A field defect in a delirious patient may point to an etiology in focal vascular disease (as discussed below). The normal spontaneous *blink rate* is 16 ± 8 per minute. Hypodopaminergia is associated with a reduction in blink rate. Impairment of voluntary eye opening is seen in association with extrapyramidal signs, making the common denomination of "apraxia" of eye opening a misnomer. Impairment of voluntary eye closure is seen after frontal or basal ganglia damage.

Both saccadic and pursuit *eye movements* should be examined. The former are assessed by asking the patient to look to the left and the right, up and down, and at the examiner's finger on the left, right, up, and down. Pursuit eye movements are examined by asking the patient to follow a moving stimulus in both the horizontal and vertical planes. These maneuvers test supranuclear control of eye movements; the oculocephalic maneuver (doll's-head eyes)—that is, moving the patient's head—tests the brainstem pathways and may be added to the assessment if saccades or pursuit is abnormal. Limitation of voluntary upgaze is common in the normal elderly. A limitation of voluntary downgaze, however, in a patient with extrapyramidal signs or frontal cognitive impairment may suggest progressive supranuclear palsy. Slowed saccades are characteristic of Huntington's disease. Impairment of initiation of voluntary saccades, requiring a head thrust or head turning, amounts to apraxia of gaze and is seen in developmental disorders as well as Huntington's disease and parietal damage. Contrariwise, impairment of inhibition of saccades represents a visual grasp, with forced gaze at environmental stimuli. This can be usefully tested by placing stimuli (a finger and a fist) in the left and right visual fields of the patient and asking the patient to look at the fist when the finger moves and vice versa. The patient's inability to perform horizontal pursuit or saccadic movements without turning the head may represent the same impairment of inhibition.

FACIAL MOVEMENT Both spontaneous movements of emotional expression and movement to command should be tested. In pyramidal disorders, spontaneous movements may be relatively spared when the face is hemiparetic for voluntary movements. Contrariwise, in nonpyramidal motor disorders, voluntary movement may be possible despite a hemiparesis of spontaneous movement. The latter situation is seen *inter alia* in temporal lobe disease, including temporal lobe epilepsy, for which it has lateralizing value. Vertical furrowing between the eyebrows is known as *Veraguth folds* and is associated with depression.

SPEECH A variety of speech abnormalities is tabulated in Table 2.1–2. A systematic examination of speech may include asking the patient to produce a sustained vowel ("ahhh . . ."), the performance being assessed for voice quality, steadiness, and loudness; then strings of consonants ("puh-puh-puh") and alternating consonants ("puh-tuh-kuh-puh-tuh-kuh"), the performance being assessed for rate, rhythm, and clarity.

The *mute patient* poses a special problem in neuropsychiatric assessment. Mutism may occur at the onset of aphemia or transcortical aphasia due to vascular lesions, and it commonly develops late in the course of patients with frontotemporal dementia or primary progressive aphasia. The examiner should assess nonspeech movements of the relevant musculature, for example, tongue movements, swallowing, and coughing. Other means of communication should be attempted such as gesture, writing, or pointing on a letter board or word board.

ABNORMALITIES OF MOVEMENT The neuropsychiatric examiner should pay attention to weakness, abnormality of muscle tone, abnormal gait, and involuntary movements. *Weakness* due to muscle, peripheral nerve, or lower motor neuron disease is associated with atrophy, fasciculations, characteristic distributions, loss of reflexes, and tenderness in the case of muscle disease. Of greater relevance to cerebral mechanisms, pyramidal weakness, greatest in the distal musculature, is accompanied by increased muscle tone in a spastic pattern (flexors in the upper extremity, extensors in the lower extremity, with the sudden loss of increased tone during passive movement, the "clasp-knife" phenomenon), loss of control of fine movements, brisk tendon jerks, and the presence of abnormal reflexes such as the Babinski sign (discussed below). Less well recognized is the nonpyramidal motor syndrome such as is seen in caudate or premotor cortical lesions: clumsiness, decreased spontaneous use of effected limbs, apparent weakness but production of full strength with coaxing. Mild degrees of impairment can be elicited with the pronator test by seeking pronation of the outstretched supinated arms; the forearm rolling test, by asking the patient to roll the forearms around each other first in one direction then in the other, looking for one side that moves less, thus, appearing to be an axis with the other circling around; or fine finger movements, with the hands resting facing up on the thighs, the patient touching each finger to the thumb in turn and repeatedly.

Muscle tone can be increased not only in the pyramidal fashion just described but also as a manifestation of extrapyramidal or diffuse brain disease. In the latter case, paratonic rigidity, or Gegenhalten, is manifested by an erratic, "pseudoactive" increase in resistance to passive movement. The fluctuating quality of the resistance reflects the presence of both oppositional and facilitory aspects of the patient's response to passive movement. The facilitory aspect can be evoked by repeatedly flexing and extending the patient's arm at the elbow, then abruptly ceasing and letting go when the arm is extended; the abnormal response, facilitory paratonia, is for the patient to continue the sequence by flexion. In the case of extrapyramidal disease, tone is increased in both extensors and flexors and throughout the range of movement, so-called lead-pipe rigidity. The "cogwheel" or ratchety feel to the rigidity is imparted by a coexisting tremor and is not intrinsic to the hypertonus; when paratonic rigidity co-occurs with a metabolic tremor, a delirious patient may mistakenly be believed to have Parkinson's disease.

Gait should always be tested, if only by focused attention to the patient's entering or leaving the room. Attention should be paid to the patient's station, postural reflexes, stride length and base, and turning. *Postural reflexes* can be assessed by asking the patient to stand in a comfortable fashion, then pushing gently on the chest or back, with care taken to avoid a fall. Gait should be stressed by asking the patient to walk in tandem fashion and on the outer aspects of the feet. This may reveal not only mild ataxia (representing cerebellar vermis dysfunction), but also asymmetric posturing of the upper extremity (in nonpyramidal motor dysfunction).

Akinesia is manifested by delay in initiation, slowness of execution, and difficulty with complex or simultaneous movements. Mild akinesia may be observed in the patient's lack of spontaneous movements of the body while sitting or of the face or elicited by asking the patient to make repeated large amplitude taps of the forefinger on the thumb (looking for decay of the amplitude). Akinesia is characteristically accompanied by rigidity. These signs, plus rest tremor and postural instability, represent the core features of the parkinsonian syndrome, seen not only in idiopathic Parkinson's disease (IPD), but in several other degenerative, "Parkinson-plus" disorders, such as progressive supranuclear palsy and multiple system atrophy, as well as in vascular white matter disease. Rest tremor is less common in these other disorders than in IPD.

Dystonia is sustained muscle contraction with consequent twisting movements or abnormal postures. Typically, dystonia in the upper extremity is manifested as hyperpronation, in the lower extremity as inversion of the foot with plantar flexion. Dystonia may occur only with certain actions, such as writer's cramp; focally, such as blepharospasm or oculogyric crisis; or in a generalized pattern, such as torsion dystonia associated with mutations in the *DYT1* gene. The symptoms and signs often do not comport with a naïve idea of how things ought to be in organic disease; only expert knowledge suffices for recognition. For example, a patient with early torsion dystonia may be able to run but not walk because the latter action elicits leg dystonia. Or a patient with intense neck muscle contraction may be able to bring the head to the midline by a light touch on the chin, a "*geste antagoniste*" diagnostic for dystonia.

Tremor is a regular oscillating movement around a joint. In *rest tremor*, the movement occurs in a relaxed, supported extremity and is reduced by action. Often an upper extremity rest tremor is exaggerated by ambulation. The frequency is usually 4 to 8 Hz. This is the distinctive tremor of Parkinson's disease. In *postural tremor*, sustained posture elicits tremor. It may be amplified if obscured by placing a sheet of paper over the outstretched hand. Hereditary essential tremor presents as postural tremor, predominantly in upper extremities but also at times involving head, jaw, and voice. A coarse, irregular, rapid postural tremor is often seen in metabolic encephalopathy. In *intention tremor*, the active limb oscillates more prominently when approaching its target, such as touching the examiner's finger with the index finger. Maximizing the range of movement increases the sensitivity of the test. Intention tremor is one form of *kinetic tremor*—that is, tremor elicited by movement; another sort of kinetic tremor is that elicited by a specific action, such as writing tremor or orthostatic tremor on standing upright. The examiner can characterize tremor by observing the patient with arms supported and fully at rest, then with arms outstretched and pronated, then with arms abducted to 90 degrees at the shoulders and bent at the elbows while the hands are held palms down with the fingers pointing at each other in front of the chest. The patient should also be observed during ambulation. Anxiety exaggerates tremor; this normal phenomenon, for example, when the patient is conscious of being observed, should not be mistaken for psychogenesis. A good test for psychogenic tremor relies on the fact that, although organic tremor may vary in amplitude, it varies little in frequency. A patient can be asked to tap a hand at a frequency different from the tremor frequency; if another tremulous body part entrains to the tapped frequency, psychogenic tremor is likely.

Choreic movements are random and arrhythmic movements of small amplitude that dance over the patient's body. They may be more evident when the patient is engaged in an activity such as ambulation. When the movements are of large amplitude and forceful, the disorder is called *ballism*. Ballistic movements are usually unilateral.

Myoclonus is a sudden, jerky, shock-like movement. It is more discontinuous than chorea or tremor. The negative of myoclonus is asterixis, a sudden lapse of muscle contraction in the context of attempted maintenance of posture. Both phenomena, but more sensitively asterixis, are common in toxic-metabolic encephalopathy (not just hepatic encephalopathy). Asterixis should be carefully sought by observation of the patient's attempt to maintain extension of the hands with the arms outstretched because it is pathognomonic for organic disease and is never seen in acute idiopathic psychosis or other nonorganic disorders. Myoclonus is additionally an important feature of nonconvulsive generalized status epilepticus, Hashimoto's encephalopathy, and Creutzfeldt-Jakob disease. Unilateral asterixis rarely may be seen in parietal, frontal, or (most often) thalamic structural disease.

Tics are sudden, jerky movements as well, but they may be more complex than myoclonic jerks and are subjectively characterized by an impulse to perform the act and a sense of relief for having done so (or mounting tension if restrained from doing so). Compulsions are not easy to differentiate from complex tics; the tiqueur may, like the patient with compulsions, report deliberately performing the act. Repetitive behavior superficially similar to compulsions may occur in organic disease but represents environment-driven behavior and does not have the same subjective structure as compulsive behavior. For example, a patient with frontal disease may repeatedly touch an alluring object without an elicitable subjective impulse and without anxiety if separated from the object. Organic obsessions and compulsions occur as well and have been associated with globus pallidus lesions, among others.

Akathisia is defined by both its subjective and its objective features. The patient exhibits motor restlessness, for example, by shifting weight from foot to foot while standing, and expresses an urge to move. At times, psychotic or cognitively impaired patients cannot convey the subjective experience clearly, and the examiner must be alert for the objective signs to differentiate akathisia from agitation due to anxiety or psychosis. The complaints and the signs in akathisia are referable to the lower, not the upper, extremities; the anxious patient may wring his or her hands, the akathisic patient shuffles his or her feet. Myoclonic jerks of the legs may be evident in the recumbent patient. The phenomenon occurs in IPD and with drug-induced dopamine blockade but also rarely with extensive frontal or temporal structural lesions.

Ataxia is a disorder of coordinating the rate, range, and force of movement and is characteristic of disease of cerebellum and its connections. In the limbs, dysmetria represents disordered determination of the distance to be moved, so that the patient overshoots or undershoots the target; if the reaching limb oscillates in the process, the clinician observes intention tremor. Asking the patient to touch the examiner's finger and then his or her own nose tests this system. Accurately touching one's own nose with eyes closed requires both cerebellar and proprioceptive function. Eye movements also may be hypermetric or hypometric. The patient's difficulty in performing rapid alternating movements, such as supination/pronation of the hand or tapping of the foot, is called *dysdiadochokinesia*. The failure of coordination of movement is also demonstrated by loss of check, which should not be elicited by arranging for the patient to hit himself or herself when the examiner's hand is removed. In the normal situation, if the outstretched arms are tapped, only a slight waver is produced; the ataxic patient does not damp the movement. Gait may be affected by midline cerebellar (vermis) disease in the absence of limb ataxia, which is related to cerebellar hemisphere disease. Gait is unsteady, with irregular stride length and a widened base. (In the normal subject, the feet nearly touch at their nearest point; even a few inches of separation represents widening of the base.) Gait and limb ataxia may be complemented by cerebellar dysarthria (described in Table 2.1–2) and by eye movement disorders, including nystagmus (usually gaze paretic), slowed saccades, saccadic pursuit, and gaze apraxia.

The *catatonic syndrome* has been variously defined. The core of the syndrome is a mute motionless state; variably added are abnormal movements, including grimacing, stereotypy, echopraxia, and catalepsy. The latter, known also as *flexibilitas cerea* (waxy flexibility), refers to posturing of a limb in the position in which it is placed by the examiner or in some other unnatural position. It is not seen in all or even most cases of catatonia, and it can be seen apart from the catatonic syndrome in patients with contralateral parietal lesions (as described below as the avoidance sign of parietal disease). *Catatonic excitement* refers to the sudden eruption into overactivity of a catatonic patient; this probably usually represents psychotic mania. The catatonic syndrome occurs in the course of schizophrenia or mood disorder, or without other psychopathology as idiopathic catatonia, or in the setting of acute cerebral metabolic or structural derangements. In the latter case, it is best thought of as a nonspecific reaction pattern, such as is delirium, requiring a comprehensive clinical and laboratory evaluation to seek the cause of the behavioral disturbance. An important instance is catatonia as part of the neuroleptic malignant syndrome, the diagnosis of which requires exclusion of other metabolic encephalopathy, notably systemic infection. Catatonia is thus a medical emergency, requiring prompt attention to diagnostic evaluation as well as supportive care (fluids, nutrition, measures to avoid complications of immobility, including venous thrombosis).

Motor sequencing tests assay function of premotor cortical areas and striatum and are related to deficits in executive cognitive function seen with dysfunction of the dorsolateral prefrontal loop. The ring/fist test involves asking the patient to alternate between making a ring with his thumb and first finger and making a fist with the same hand: "ring, fist, ring, fist . . ." The abnormal response is perseveration of one or the other posture or disorganization of the sequence. At times, patients are unable to perform the correct series even when repeating the verbal cues aloud. A more complex alternation is between striking the table gently with the fist, then the edge of the hand, then the palm: "fist, edge, palm, fist, edge, palm . . ." A different approach is to ask the patient to extend the arms, make a fist with one hand while keeping the other hand flat, then switch hands. The abnormal response has the patient ending up with two fists or two palms outstretched.

Much can be accomplished in the neurological examination by asking the patient to stretch out his or her arms. With a few additional maneuvers (tapping the outstretched pronated hands, supinating them and asking the patient to close his or her eyes, then asking the patient to touch his or her nose with the eyes still closed, then asking the patient to perform the alternating fists test), all of the following can be assessed in a matter of a minute or so: postural and intention tremor, loss of check, asterixis and myoclonus, a pronator sign, dysmetria, and motor sequencing. Doing this, plus testing muscle tone, plus observing the patient's natural and stressed gait, plus checking tendon jerks and abnormal reflexes, takes just a few minutes and does not elucidate disorders of muscle, nerve, and spinal cord but represents a rather extensive assessment of the central organization of the motor system.

ABNORMALITIES OF SENSATION Disorders of sensation are sometimes difficult to assess reliably in patients with cognitive and behavior disorders. Nonetheless, several points should be familiar to the neuropsychiatrist. Distal loss of sensation, often accompanied by loss of ankle jerks, is characteristic of peripheral neuropathy. Often, all modalities of sensation are disturbed. If proprioception is sufficiently severely reduced, Romberg's sign is present. *Romberg's sign* means that closing the eyes produces substantial impairment of balance; it is elicited by asking the patient to stand, allowing the patient to seek a comfortably balanced position, then asking the patient to close the eyes (ensuring against a fall).

Loss of sensation from sensory cortex injury is classically limited to complex discriminations such as graphesthesia (recognizing numbers written on the palm), stereognosis (identifying unseen objects in the hand), and two-point discrimination (telling whether the examiner is touching with one or two points, as these come closer together in space). However, patients with parietal stroke may have a pseudothalamic sensory syndrome (with impairments in elementary sensory modalities and subsequent dysesthesia) or other anomalous patterns of sensory loss. At times, these patients present with pseudomotor deficits: ataxia, fluctuating muscle tone and strength (dependent in part on visual cueing), and "levitation" and awkward positioning of the arm contralateral (or at times ipsilateral) to the lesion. In the acute phase, the combination of deficits can amount to "motor helplessness." These deficits result from the loss of sensory input to regions in which motor programs arise. The lessons are that "cortical" sensory deficits should be sought if there is a question of cortical involvement and that more dramatic or unusual sensory abnormalities may also occur with cortical lesions.

SOFT SIGNS An extensive literature about "soft signs" of neurological dysfunction is difficult to comprehend because of the varied definitions and batteries used in the various studies. Most of the signs sought in these batteries are discussed in this chapter under their more specific headings, such as graphesthesia under Abnormalities of Sensation and the alternating fist (Oseretsky) test in the paragraph on motor sequencing. From the corpus of test batteries, a few simple maneuvers can be extracted that may make a contribution to the neurological examination of the patient with a mental presentation.

While the patient is touching each finger to the thumb, the examiner can watch the opposite hand for mirror movements. Obligatory bimanual synkinesias are seen specifically in disorders of the pyramidal pathways, such as the Klippel-Feil syndrome, and in agenesis of the corpus callosum but also in putative neurodevelopmental disorders such as schizophrenia. Asking the patient, with eyes closed, to report whether the examiner is touching one or the other hand (with the patient's hands on the lap), or one or the other sides of the face, or a combination, is called the face–hand test. The examiner touches the left hand and right face simultaneously. If the patient reports only the touch on the face—that is, extinguishes the peripheral stimulus—then the examiner can prompt (once): "Anywhere else?" Then the examiner touches the right hand and left cheek, left hand and left cheek, right hand and right cheek, both hands, and both cheeks. Extinction of the peripheral stimulus is the pathological response and has been associated with schizophrenia and dementia.

ABNORMAL REFLEXES The Babinski sign is the shibboleth of the neurological examination. It should be elicited by stroking the lateral aspect of the foot from back to front, with the leg extended at the knee, using a pointed object such as an orange stick or a key. The response of extension of the great toe with or without fanning of the other toes indicates corticospinal tract disease. Two confounding factors in assessment of the Babinski sign are the striatal toe and the plantar grasp. The striatal toe is extension of the hallux without fanning of the other toes or a flexion synergy in the other muscles of flexion of the leg. It may occur spontaneously or on elicitation in patients with Parkinson's disease in the absence of evidence of pyramidal dysfunction. The plantar grasp, the equivalent of the familiar palmar grasp, may mask an extensor response to lateral foot stimulation when stimulation in the midfoot brings about flexion of the toes.

Other important reflexes for the neuropsychiatrist are

Myerson's sign, a failure to habituate to regular, one-per-second taps on the glabella (with the tapping hand outside of the patient's visual field), present in parkinsonism and diffuse brain disease

Hoffmann's sign, flexion of the thumb with snapping of the distal phalanx of the patient's middle finger, an upper extremity sign of pyramidal dysfunction, although sometimes present bilaterally in normal subjects

Grasp, flexion of the fingers with stroking of the patient's palm toward the fingers during distraction and despite instructions to relax, associated with disease of the contralateral supplementary motor area

Avoidance, extension of the wrist and fingers to the same stimulus as the grasp, a less well-known sign that points to contralateral parietal cortex abnormality

Several other "primitive reflexes" are less specific in that they are commonly present in the normal subject and, thus, are less useful for diagnostic purposes. These include the suck, snout, and palmomental reflexes.

FOCAL NEUROBEHAVIORAL SYNDROMES

The idea that the brain is regionally specialized had a difficult gestation in the 19th century, and the key to its acceptance lay in recognition of the effects of focal brain lesions. At the end of the 18th century and early in the 19th century, phrenology drew adherents to the claim that personality traits could be inferred by inspection of the cranium. This claim was faulty, but phrenology had an underlying theory that was an important step forward for the brain sciences; in particular, the beliefs that the brain was the organ of the mind and that the mind could be fractionated into functions gave impetus to the development of neuroscience in a modern form. In the middle of the 19th century, the gradual realization that aphasia occurred with damage to specific areas of the left hemisphere was another crucial step. The subsequent identification of numerous syndromes of localized damage—such as apraxia, agnosia, visuospatial impairment in its various forms, and so forth—is a fascinating story of astute and painstaking clinicopathological, and later clinicoradiological, correlation.

Patients' introspective access to their deficits may be limited. Much of cognitive processing is unconscious, not in the sense of being excluded from awareness by motivated defense, but in the sense that it is not even in principle open to introspection. Jonathan Miller, in his television show *The Body in Question*, displayed this point by asking passersby in a person-in-the-street interview, "Sir, where is your spleen?" No one can say from introspection where the spleen is. The same is true of much of cognitive processing. Explanations provided by patients may be confabulations that fill in such introspective gaps in a situation in which the brain is functioning abnormally in a way not foreseen in its design. In neuropsychiatry, subjective experience and behavior are separate *explicanda*. For instance, in the realm of emotion, the networks subserving conscious experience—"feelings"—and those underlying the emotional forces influencing behavior are distinct, although overlapping, with the amygdala notably absent from the former. The patient's appraisal of his or her own situation is always relevant to collaboration with treatment and its outcome and should be explored in every clinical encounter.

Dementia

Although dementia is characteristically considered a syndrome of "global" cognitive impairment, implying global or diffuse brain dysfunction, each dementing disorder produces a distinct pattern of brain pathology and corresponding pattern of cognitive dysfunction. For this reason, and against tradition, dementia is discussed under the rubric of focal neurobehavioral syndromes.

In Alzheimer's disease, the earliest neuropathological abnormality is characteristically medial temporal accumulation of plaques and tangles, initially in entorhinal cortex and subiculum (the input and output zones of hippocampus). The disease progressively involves association cortices in temporoparietal and prefrontal regions. This burden of pathology determines the characteristic early memory impairment with ensuing anomia, failure of grasp, and coarsening of personality. On occasion, Alzheimer's disease pathology is predominantly posterior, with concomitant predominance of visuospatial impairment in the clinical course. By contrast, in frontotemporal dementia, the earliest disease manifestations are pathologically in frontal or temporal cortex, clinically presenting as primary progressive aphasia, semantic dementia, or a frontal apathy or disinhibition syndrome. In none of these situations is a view of dementia as a "global" impairment of brain function justified by the clinical or pathological facts; rather, selective disruption of anatomical networks corresponds to symptomatic features.

Extensive subcortical white and gray matter damage due to small-vessel disease is a common cause of dementia, and, in this situation, the clinical picture is dominated by slowed mental processing, forgetfulness with relative preservation of recognition memory (as opposed to free recall), and executive cognitive dysfunction. "Strategically" located single infarctions can also produce dementia. These strokes can involve left angular gyrus, genu of internal capsule, and (perhaps most commonly) medial thalamus. The thalamic and internal capsule strokes may produce cognitive impairment by interfering with frontal networks.

Delirium Classically a syndrome of "global" brain dysfunction due to toxic-metabolic infectious encephalopathy, delirium may also point to focal brain disease. Delirium may be due to infarction in the right posterior superior temporal gyrus caused by occlusion of the inferior division of the right middle cerebral artery or to infarction in the inferior temporo-occipital cortex on the left or bilaterally due to posterior cerebral artery occlusion. In both instances, focal neurological signs may be limited to a visual field cut or absent entirely. Finding bilateral asterixis or multifocal myoclonus strongly indicates a toxic-metabolic brain derangement, and the history and physical examination should provide pointers for the essential laboratory confirmation of the abnormality. Features of the mental state are of little use in determining the cause of the syndrome except that agitation is far more common in certain disorders such as substance withdrawal, hypoxia, and the syndromes of left posterior cerebral artery stroke or of right middle cerebral artery territory stroke with involvement of the temporal lobe.

Aphasia Acquired impairment of lexical or syntactical performance is termed *aphasia*. Lexicon and syntax do not exhaust the domain of language, and attention is devoted below to prosody and discourse pragmatics. At the bedside, the clinician should be able to distinguish language impairment from other sources of abnormal discourse (such as psychosis), delineate the features of abnormality in the patient's linguistic function, and tentatively identify the locus of brain injury.

A simple distinction between "expressive" and "receptive" defects has some power to distinguish between anterior and posterior lesion sites, but it is not in current use in aphasiology because most aphasiogenic lesions produce some impairment in both production and comprehension of language, and these impairments are of multiple sorts.

A widely accepted approach to examination and classification in aphasia identifies six domains for elucidation: *spontaneous speech, naming, comprehension, repetition, reading,* and *writing.* Attention to spontaneous speech reveals dysfluency and word-finding difficulties. The dysfluent speaker produces shorter phrases and utterances without a natural "flow." Substantives (nouns and verbs) may be preserved at the expense of function words (such as prepositions) and grammatical morphemes (such as tense endings), leading to agrammatical utterances that are nonetheless relatively information rich. Lesions disrupting fluency are characteristically anterior in the left hemisphere or involve putamen. Naming performance requires the adequate functioning of a network, including posterior temporal, temporoparietal, and inferior frontal sites. This is ordinarily tested by confrontation ("What do you call this?"), which can be conveniently done using body parts or common items at the bedside. Naming from description ("What do you call the vehicle that travels under water?") is an alternative mode of testing, particularly useful for visually impaired or agnosic patients. Comprehension is tested best using probes with minimal demand on output, so "yes/no" questions ("Does a stone sink in water?") are better than motor commands, which may be impaired by concurrent apraxia. Impairment of comprehension results from posterior temporal lesions. Disordered repetition is disclosed by asking the patient to produce progressively longer utterances, reiterating the examiner: "airplane, he and she are here . . ." Repetition may be surprisingly spared (the so-called transcortical aphasias) or disproportionately affected (conduction aphasia). The latter depends on lesions of insula or external capsule. Reading comprehension (not reading aloud, a different skill) tests comprehension with a different input modality from aural comprehension, and some patients show significant dissociations. Similarly, writing tests output in a different modality from speech. Writing is a particularly sensitive probe for the anomia seen in early Alzheimer's disease and the disorganization seen in delirium.

A classification of the aphasias using the data from an examination as just outlined is shown in Table 2.1–3. Clinicians recognize, however, that many patients do not fit well into the categories created by this scheme.

Ideomotor apraxia commonly occurs together with aphasia. This is a disorder of performance of skilled movements to command in the absence of explanatory elementary sensory and motor disturbances. Oral apraxia is revealed by the patient's incapacity to show, for example, how to blow out a match or lick a postage stamp. Limb apraxia is shown by the patient's incapacity to show, for example, how to wave good-bye or use a hammer or screwdriver. Patients with these deficits may, nonetheless, be able to follow whole body commands: "Show me how a boxer stands," for example. Patients rarely complain of apraxic deficits, in part because they are artifacts of the examination in the sense that they may not be present in the use of real-world items.

Attention Several related phenomena cluster under the clinical description of attentional disorders. At the most fundamental level, alertness represents a continuum ranging from coma to normal wakefulness. The clinician faced with a patient who is less than fully alert should quantify the disorder by assessing the patient's response to a graded series of probes: Does the patient orient to the examiner's presence in the room; what does the patient do when his or her name is called or when touched or when shaken or when a (harmless) painful stimulus is applied; and so forth. These responses should be recorded in detail, rather than summarized by ambiguous terms such as "lethargic."

Alert patients may show deficits in sustained attention to external stimuli (vigilance) or internal stimuli (concentration). Attentional deficits of these sorts are characteristic of delirium. Vigilance can be assessed with a bedside adaptation of a continuous performance task, for example, by asking the patient to lift a hand each time the examiner says the letter "A" or, to increase the difficulty, each time

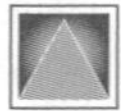

Table 2.1–3
Aphasia Syndromes

Aphasic Syndrome	Spontaneous Speech	Repetition	Naming	Aural Comprehension	Reading for Comprehension	Writing	Additional Features	Characteristic Lesion Location
Global	Impaired	Impaired	Impaired	Impaired	Impaired	Impaired	Right hemiplegia, hemisensory loss, hemianopia	Extensive anterior and posterior perisylvian cortex
Broca's	Dysfluent, effortful, agrammatic	Impaired	Impaired	Spared	Spared	Impaired	Frustration, right hemiparesis, buccofacial and limb apraxia	Anterior perisylvian cortex and insula
Wernicke's	Fluent, paraphasic, absence of substantive words	Impaired	Impaired	Impaired	Impaired (but not always to the same degree as aural comprehension)	Impaired	Unawareness of illness, paranoia, visual field defect	Wernicke's area (posterior superior temporal gyrus)
Conduction	Fluent, paraphasic with phonemic errors	Impaired	Impaired	Spared	Spared	Impaired	—	Supramarginal gyrus or primary auditory cortex
Transcortical motor	Dysfluent	Spared	Impaired	Spared	Spared	Impaired	—	Anterior/superior to Broca's area or medial surface of hemisphere involving supplementary motor area
Transcortical sensory	Fluent, paraphasic	Spared	Impaired	Impaired	Impaired	Impaired	—	Temporoparietal or occipitotemporal cortex posterior and inferior to Wernicke's area
Mixed transcortical	Dysfluent	Relatively spared	Impaired	Impaired	Impaired	Impaired	Echolalia	Isolation of perisylvian cortex by extensive watershed infarction
Anomical	Fluent, paraphasic	Spared	Impaired	Spared	Spared	Spared	—	Nonspecific within language areas

the examiner says the letter "A" after the letter "D." The examiner then produces a series of random letters at a deliberate and steady rate over an extended period. Any error of omission or commission represents a failure. By asking the patient to count from 20 to 1 or give the days of the week or the months of the year in reverse, the examiner can appraise concentration. Digit span—asking the patient to repeat a list of numbers spoken at a slow, steady rate without separation into chunks—is a classic test of attention; the lower limit of normal for digit span is five.

A "higher" level of attentional function is the capacity to manipulate information kept in consciousness over a short period—a test of working memory. An excellent example is alphanumeric sequencing. The patient is asked to alternate between numbers and letters; the examiner provides "1-A-2-B-3-C" as a model, then allows 30 seconds for the patient to start at 1 and give as many alternations as possible. If only the number of correct alternations is counted (ignoring errors), the lower limit of normal is 15. A comparable, simple task is alphabetizing the letters of the word "world" (or any similar word). Working memory is known to require intact processing in dorsolateral prefrontal cortex.

Hemineglect is a focal disorder of attention almost always of left hemispace in a patient with acute right hemisphere disease. Most characteristically, the lesion is parietal, but distinguishable patterns of hemineglect occur with frontal and cingulate lesions. Gross neglect can be recognized in the patient's ignoring, or even denying the ownership of, the left limbs or not attending to objects and people in left hemispace. Subtler degrees of neglect can be elicited by presenting an array in which the patient must search into both hemifields to point to items, for example, all the yellow dots in a stimulus card with dots of varied colors to both left and right.

In the phenomenon of hypermetamorphosis, part of the Klüver-Bucy syndrome of bilateral anterior temporal damage, animals or patients exhibit an increased level of attention to individual items in the environment.

Amnesia The term *memory* is used in several ways by clinicians and psychologists. The amnestic syndrome features impairment of learning of new material (anterograde amnesia) and a variable period of impaired recall before the onset of the syndrome (retrograde amnesia). It is due to damage to hippocampus or to anterior thalamus (including mammillothalamic tract). Memory proper is distinguished from retention in consciousness of material over the course of a few seconds, which may be called "working" or "iconic" or "short-term" memory. This function is spared in the amnestic syndrome because it depends on frontoparietal mechanisms distinct from the hippocampal and thalamic pathways damaged in amnesia. Deficits due to hippocampal and thalamic lesions are dependent on the lateralization of the damage, left-sided damage producing verbal and right-sided damage producing figural memory impairments.

A distinction between free recall and recognition memory is of neuropsychological significance and generally can be made adequately, if imperfectly, at the bedside. Hippocampal and thalamic patients show accelerated forgetting, so that cues (such as providing the semantic category) are relatively ineffective in aiding recall. Recognition memory is always better than free recall on an absolute scale; exaggeration of the disparity—that is, sparing of recognition memory—is characteristic of memory impairment due to dysfunction of frontal mechanisms of effortful search.

In addition, frontal patients show impairments of memory for the temporal context or source of information. This deficit is probably relevant to the occurrence of confabulation. Spontaneous confabulation occurs in only a minority of amnestic patients and depends on ventromedial frontal damage.

Memory is so commonly impaired in brain disorders that it should be tested in all patients undergoing neuropsychiatric evaluation. Recall of a test phrase (for example, a name and address) over a several-minute distraction is a valid and simple screening test. However, more detailed analysis of memory is necessary in patients with disorders likely to affect memory mechanisms, including (among many others) head injury, epilepsy, and dementing disorders. Testing should include both verbal and nonverbal material. For example, testing recall of three words and three shapes or three words and three pointed directions over several minutes' delay is easily performed. Further, the examiner should be prepared with cues, including appropriate (incorrect) foils, to assess sparing of the capacity to make use of cues in frontal memory impairment. For example, if one of the words provided is "piano," the examiner could cue, "One was a musical instrument," and further provide "guitar, piano, violin" as multiple-choice options. Only rough inferences can be drawn from this bedside assessment, as compared with formal neuropsychological evaluation.

Apart from patients with persisting amnestic syndromes, the neuropsychiatrist may be presented with patients who experienced an amnestic state transiently or rarely may see one during a transient amnestic state. The syndromes of transient global amnesia and transient epileptic amnesia and their differentiation have been fully described and require thorough history taking, neuropsychological evaluation, and electroencephalography (EEG) recordings. The neuropsychiatrist should also know that amnesia for criminal offenses is common; certainly it is not confined to those who committed a crime while in a delirious, ictal, or postictal state, as is sometimes claimed for legal reasons.

Visuospatial Dysfunction The requirement to test visual, as well as verbal, memory has just been mentioned. Drawing and copying tasks can further the assessment. Copying intersecting pentagons (as in the Mini-Mental State Examination [MMSE]) or (as an incidental performance) the shapes used in the memory task begins the assessment. With more complex figures, failures with a slavish element-by-element strategy are characteristic of patients with right hemisphere damage, as is neglect of the left side of the stimulus.

The variety of disorders of higher visual function has already been mentioned in describing the complex structure of visual association cortices. *Prosopagnosia* is a defect in recognition of faces. Such a defect may be obvious from the history or may be a more subtle abnormality; it can be spotted at the bedside, albeit insensitively, with the use of a few pictures of famous people. *Defects of topographical skill*, although rarely presenting in an isolated form, also occur with right hemisphere dysfunction. The patient can be asked to describe a route between familiar places or a geographical question believed to be within premorbid capacities ("If you're going from New York to Los Angeles, is the Atlantic Ocean in front of you, behind you, to your left, to your right?").

The incapacity to grasp in attention multiple visual objects at once is known as *simultanagnosia*. The patient may fail in describing a complex visual scene by virtue of reporting only a single, perhaps peripheral, element. Together with psychic paralysis of gaze (inability to direct gaze voluntarily, or ocular apraxia) and optic ataxia (a disorder of misreaching under visual guidance), it makes up Balint's syndrome, the archetypal disorder of the dorsal visual pathway. The patient with impairment of reaching under visual guidance should be examined without visual guidance (e.g., pointing to parts of his or her own body with eyes closed) to confirm the defect.

Executive Cognitive Dysfunction *Executive cognitive dysfunction* refers to initiation of cognition and action, their maintenance in the face of distraction, organized but flexible pursuit of goals, and self-monitoring with error correction. Executive processes are crucial in adaptive function, and performance in this realm is better correlated with real-world outcomes of brain-injured patients than are many other domains traditionally analyzed in neuropsychology or many psychosocial variables. Bedside exploration of executive function is of central importance in the neuropsychiatric examination. Analysis of behavioral disturbance and neuropsychological deficits in patients with cerebral injury suggests that multiple dissociable processes compose executive cognitive function, and certainly these processes are instantiated by anatomically distributed systems. Curiously, however, many different tasks recruit a similar or identical set of regions in the middorsolateral prefrontal cortex, midventrolateral prefrontal cortex, and anterior cingulate. Nonetheless, the clinical examiner must know that no single probe can screen for all dysfunctions.

Many aspects of executive function are illuminated by attention to the patient's performance of elements of the history taking and examination. *Disinhibition* may be noted in abnormalities of comportment during social interaction. *Motor impersistence*, the failure to sustain actions that can be undertaken properly, may be noted in the patient's "peeking" when asked to keep the eyes closed, repeatedly looking back at the examiner's face when lateral gaze (especially to the left) is attempted, or not keeping the arms extended or the tongue protruded when instructed to do so. *Perseveration* is the continuation of elements of past actions into present activity. Perseverative responses may be noted when testing naming or attention. *Echopraxia*, for example, the patient crossing his or her arms when the examiner (spontaneously) does so, even when some other behavior has been requested, can be observed during the interview and examination. *Utilization behavior* is an automatic tendency to make use of objects in the environment, for example, picking up a pen and starting to write despite this behavior's being inappropriate to the setting.

More focused efforts to assess executive function are almost always indicated in the neuropsychiatric examination. Perseveration may be specifically sought in the motor sequencing tasks described above or with a sample of spontaneous writing. A tapping task with conflicting instructions may illuminate the inflexibility of goal-directed behavior that gives rise to perseverative responding. The patient is instructed to tap once if the examiner taps twice, and twice if the examiner taps once. The examiner then taps on the table in a random series of one or two taps. This can be directly followed by a go/no-go tapping task, in which the patient is instructed to tap once if the examiner taps once, not at all if the examiner taps twice. Intrusions from the previous task's instructions represent perseverative responding; echopraxic responses (tapping just like the examiner) represent failures of inhibition. Inhibition of reflexive gaze can be tested during the examination of eye movements. Looking at the moving stimulus rather than in the opposite direction as instructed amounts to a visual grasp response and represents failure of inhibition. Spontaneous word-list generation ("Tell me all the animals you can think of" or "Tell me all the words that start with 's'") depends on the capacity for effortful search of semantic stores. A greater decrement in fluency to semantic cues ("animals") than to phonemic cues ("words with 's'") is seen in Alzheimer's disease because of the degradation of semantic stores due to temporoparietal damage. Working memory can be assessed with the alphanumeric sequencing task described above.

Anatomical inferences from dissociations in performance on these tasks are limited. Go/no-go tasks depend on the integrity of orbitofrontal cortex, other tasks on the dorsolateral prefrontal cortex and its circuit. Impersistence is associated with right hemisphere dysfunction. A further dissociation is between executive cognitive impairments and personality change in frontal injury. Especially with orbitofrontal lesions, executive function can be spared even in the face of grave alterations in emotion and comportment; the two domains cannot simply be considered two sides of the same coin. Nonetheless, it bears repeating that neuropsychiatric examiners always should consider executive cognitive function in their formulation of cases.

Disordered Mood and Emotion Several syndromes of disordered emotion in organic disease can be delineated. *Disturbances of recognition and expression of emotion* with right hemisphere lesions have already been mentioned. Patients and their familiars are rarely aware of these deficits and do not complain of them; rather, the examiner must recognize the deficit and figure it into a formulation of the patient's social and functional decline. Impairment of prosodic expression should not be mistaken for depressed affect. Testing of affective prosody can be undertaken at the bedside without special equipment. The examiner should ask the patient to say emotionally loaded sentences in a emotional manner, expressing surprise, fear, pleasure, and anger. People vary considerably in their native acting talents, and the range of normal performance is wide. The examiner also can utter neutral sentences in various emotional tones: "I am going to the store," stated with surprise, and so forth, with the examiner's face turned away from the patient to avoid providing a second input channel. Patients should be able to recognize the affect. Separately, if testing materials are available, the examiner can assess the patient's capacity to identify emotions in visual scenes and facial expressions. Lesions that involve both limbic and heteromodal cortices in the right hemisphere especially impair performance in recognizing emotional facial expressions.

Pathological laughing and crying also are mentioned as lateralized behavioral disturbances. The phenomena are displays of affect incongruent with inner experience and elicited by inappropriate, nonemotional, or inadequate stimuli. The examiner may, in the extreme, be able to elicit full displays of affect by waving a hand in front of the patient's face. The patient is often embarrassed by the pathological expression of affect. The traditional explanation is that a lesion of descending frontopontine pathways releases from inhibition a "laughing center" or "crying center" in the brainstem. Indeed, features of pseudobulbar palsy are often present in these patients. However, the relevant centers have never been identified, and the possibility that the phenomena result from cerebellar disconnection has been raised. A broader form of *affective dysregulation*, which may be called "emotionalism," is commonly seen, usually in the direction of tearfulness. Patients report that they are more emotional than previously and that the tears are sudden, unexpected, and uncontrollable. However, they are generally congruent with the patient's subjective state. Such patients are often cognitively impaired; lesions favor the left frontotemporal region. The rare phenomenon of *fou rire prodromique* (mad prodromal laughter) presages acute vascular lesions of the brainstem or thalamus.

Apathy is an emotional disturbance marked by reduction of affect and motivation. Goal-directed behavior is reduced, and emotional responses are lacking. The distinction from depression is crucial: Patients do not report negative emotional states or ideational content. Although they may meet criteria for depression because of the loss of interest in activities, they are mentally empty rather than full of distress. Recognizing apathy rather than mistaking it for depression may imply treatment with different pharmacological agents, for example, use of dopamine agonists. *Euphoria* refers to a persistent and unrealistic sense of well-being without the increased mental or motor rate of mania. Although often mentioned in connection with multiple sclerosis, it is unusual and almost always associated with extensive disease and substantial cognitive impairment.

The *Klüver-Bucy syndrome*, as described in the captive monkey, includes reduction in aggression (tameness), excessive and indiscriminate sexual behavior, hypermetamorphosis (forced attention to environmental stimuli), and hyperorality (mouthing nonfood items). This mixture of emotional, perceptual, and motivational changes is dependent on bilateral damage to amygdala. In human patients, pathologies including trauma, herpes simplex encephalitis, and frontotemporal dementia can produce the syndrome, usually in partial form.

Depression is common in patients with brain diseases, including stroke, multiple sclerosis, traumatic brain injury, and Parkinson's disease. Certainly, this is in part a reaction to altered circumstances and distressing disability. Nonetheless, the syndromal nature of the depressed state and its imperfect correlation with measures of disability have prompted extensive efforts to seek anatomical correlations. Converging evidence leads to a model of alterations in a distributed network involving neocortical and limbic elements. In particular, a dorsal compartment involving dorsolateral prefrontal cortex, inferior parietal cortex, and the dorsal and posterior portions of cingulate gyrus shows underactivity in the depressed state; these regions are believed to mediate the cognitive alterations and impairments of depression. Inversely, a ventral compartment containing anterior insula, subgenual cingulate, hippocampus, and hypothalamus is overactive; these elements are believed to mediate somatic ("vegetative") features of the depressed state. Interactions between the two compartments are mediated through thalamus, basal ganglia, and, especially, rostral cingulate.

Mania is substantially less common than depression after brain injury. Mania is associated with right-sided lesions involving paralimbic cortices in orbitofrontal or basotemporal regions or subcortical sites in caudate or thalamus. Some evidence suggests that subcortical lesions are more likely to produce a bipolar picture, cortical lesions unipolar mania. As with depression, the abnormal mood state does not necessarily appear in close temporal association with the injury, so determining whether the mood disorder is organic or idiopathic is not always straightforward. The absence of a personal history of mood disorder is an obvious criterion, but the presence of a family history of mood disorder may mark a vulnerability factor not operative in the absence of the brain lesion. Age of onset is relevant, especially for mania: The onset of idiopathic mania after 40 years of age is rare.

A particularly common issue in neuropsychiatric assessment is the patient with late-onset depression in whom evaluation reveals executive cognitive dysfunction and subcortical white matter disease. This state of "vascular depression" is marked by the presence of vascular risk factors, notably hypertension, a tendency to psychomotor retardation and anhedonia and not psychosis or guilty ideation, and poor outcome with usual treatments. Some, but not all, of these patients have apathy rather than depression.

Abnormalities in Agency

Ordinarily, the person performing an action has the sense of being the one performing it. The prototype abnormality of this normal subjective sense is the "alien hand" phenomenon. Patients with parietal lesions may report a sense of strangeness of the hand, and the limb may exhibit levitation or avoidance reactions. More dramatically, with medial frontal or callosal lesions, the hand may engage in unwilled behavior (representing unilateral utilization behavior), or intermanual conflict may occur.

Abnormal Social Behavior

The multitude of behaviors exhibited in social interaction has, of course, multiple underpinnings. Several behavioral complexes, the neurobiology of which has come under scrutiny, can be observed in their abnormal form in patients and, at times, understood from an anatomical and physiological point of view.

The intensity of social interaction manifested by patients with temporal lobe epilepsy may be due to deficits in social cognition or to a limbic lesion reinforcing social cohesiveness. Failures of empathic understanding are common in patients with frontal injury. These impairments result both from cognitive inflexibility in assessing complex social situations, especially in patients with dorsolateral prefrontal lesions, and from emotional impoverishment, especially in patients with orbitofrontal lesions.

The capacity of humans to understand the mental states of others—and thus to recognize not just another's goals or intentions but also the other's deceptions or pretense—has been termed *mentalization* or *theory of mind.* Imaging and lesion data suggest that this capacity depends critically on prefrontal cortex (particularly right medial prefrontal cortex adjacent to anterior cingulate gyrus), right temporoparietal cortices, and amygdala. Patients with isolated lesions of amygdala are rare, but deficits in theory of mind are seen in patients with frontal disease and may contribute to their social failure. Patients with right hemisphere lesions have a range of deficits in social interaction that may be characterized as a disorder of pragmatics. Although they may grasp the propositional content of language correctly, they mistake aspects of communication that require appraisal of the interlocutor's intent, for example, whether an utterance was intended as a joke. Pragmatic disorders due to frontal and right hemisphere damage may impair narrative coherence through verbosity, vagueness, and disregard for the listener's informational needs. Thus, for example, pronoun use may be syntactically correct but the referents of pronouns obscure to the listener. Although language itself is normal, the way language is embedded in social interaction is not.

Abnormal Beliefs and Experiences

Hallucinations are a common feature of diseases of the brain. *Visual hallucinations* in the absence of auditory hallucinations are suggestive of organic disease. Visual hallucinations may occur in a hemifield blind from cerebral disease, so-called release hallucinations. Visual hallucinations in the setting of visual impairment due to ocular disease, usually in the elderly, are known as the *Charles Bonnet syndrome*. The hallucinations are characteristically vivid images of living figures, and the patient is aware of their unreality. Other psychopathology is absent, but treatment aimed at the hallucinations is usually ineffective. Elaborate-formed visual hallucinations may occur with lesions of thalamus or upper brainstem, so-called peduncular hallucinosis. The symptoms are worse in the evening (crepuscular), and again, the patient is aware of the unreality of the visual experiences. Prominent, early visual hallucinations in the context of progressive dementia may suggest dementia with Lewy bodies.

Auditory hallucinations occur rarely with pontine lesions. More common are musical hallucinations in the setting of hearing impairment, akin to the Charles Bonnet syndrome. Unilateral hallucinations are characteristically ipsilateral to the deaf ear. Olfactory hallucinations occur as a limbic aura in partial epilepsy, but they also occur in idiopathic psychiatric illness.

Palinopsia and *palinacousis* refer to persisting or recurrent perceptual experiences after the object is gone in the visual and auditory domains, respectively. Lesions in association cortex—parieto-occipital and temporal, respectively—are responsible, although (for the visual sphere more than the auditory) drug toxicity is often the explanation.

The content of *delusions* may yield clues to causative organic disease and its nature. Most notably, misidentification delusions have been associated with dysfunction of face processing and clearly linked—in many but not all cases—to right hemisphere dysfunction. Misidentification of place is regularly associated with visuospatial and executive cognitive dysfunction. Misidentification delusions have been of special interest in cognitive neuropsychiatry, with a focus on face recognition impairment in such patients. Perceptual recognition without a sense of familiarity (as in Capgras' syndrome and perhaps the nihilistic delusions of Cotard's syndrome) may reflect a disruption of visual–limbic connections. In a sense, it is the reverse of *déjà vu*, which amounts to familiarity without perceptual recognition. However, many patients with misidentification delusions have no evidence of organic disease. Although such patients may have dysfunction of similar underlying mechanisms to patients with ascertainable organic disease, the similarity of clinical phenomena cannot be taken to prove an identity of mechanism.

Particular delusional themes may mark delirious thinking, such as a focus on danger or harm to others, as opposed to the more self-centered constructions in idiopathic psychotic disorders. However, most delusions in patients with brain disease are of more banal nature, often with persecutory elements that bespeak cognitive failure (the theft of one's purse, for example, representing a failure of memory as to its location). Complexity or elaborateness of delusional ideation is associated with preservation of intellect, and delusions tend to become less complex with progression of dementia.

LABORATORY INVESTIGATIONS

Specialized laboratory investigation forms a major part of the neuropsychiatrist's arsenal. Sometimes patients are referred for neuropsychiatric consultation when a routine investigation—such as a screening MRI or EEG—gives an unexpected abnormal result; the neuropsychiatrist is called on to assess the meaning of the finding in the psychiatric context.

Neuroimaging

Structural neuroimaging with computed tomography (CT) and later with MRI revolutionized practice in the clinical neurosciences. No longer was the organ of interest invisible within the carapace of the skull. CT relies on the differential absorption of X-rays by brain tissues and on the power of computerized methods to integrate data from multiple perspectives. The strengths of CT are its speed and its sensitivity to blood and bone. Thus, for neuropsychiatric purposes, situations in which a patient cannot tolerate a prolonged imaging procedure may mandate CT. This problem often arises with an agitated demented or psychotic patient. Bony abnormalities, parenchymal deposition of calcium, and intracranial hemorrhage are particularly well assessed by CT. Such questions arise in the acute aftermath of trauma in particular.

The advent of MRI was an advance over CT in several respects. The anatomical resolution is substantially better, and the discrimination of white matter abnormalities exceptionally so. The capacity to display data from a single acquisition in multiple views—sagittal, axial, and coronal—allows improved anatomical understanding. T1 (or short relaxation time [TR]) images give maximal anatomical resolution. T2 (or long TR) images and intermediate-weighted (proton density) images give maximum salience to areas of abnormality, characteristically bright against a darker parenchyma. Fluid attenuation inversion recovery (FLAIR) images mark out the lesions even better, with dark cerebrospinal fluid (CSF) providing better contrast with regions of abnormality than the bright CSF of T2 images. Gradient echo images sensitively reveal the sequelae of hemorrhage and may be useful in assessing the damage from trauma. Infusion of gadolinium for contrast enhancement is not necessary for delineation of nonvascular anatomical structures, such as is the goal in the case of atrophy or old stroke or trauma, but can identify areas of breakdown of the blood–brain barrier such as in the meninges in meningitis or in parenchymal lesions of active multiple sclerosis, tumor, or acute stroke. Special imaging sequences should be used for the identification of cortical dysplasia or mesial temporal sclerosis. Volumetric MRI allows diagnosis by quantitative assessment of delineated brain structures such as hippocampus in the case of temporal epilepsy and potentially Alzheimer's disease. One imagines the day in the near future when the scans come (as electrocardiograms now do) with quantitative information routinely accompanying the analog image. Magnetic resonance angiography (MRA) allows the delineation of medium and large vessels without the administration of contrast material, as is required for conventional angiography. Stenosis of these vessels, such as the vessels of the neck, or the presence of vascular malformations or aneurysms is reliably ascertained. However, resolution is not sufficient to allow assessment of small vessels; thus, some forms of vasculitis cannot be excluded with MRA and require contrast angiography.

Additional MRI sequences include diffusion-weighted imaging, which captures acute vascular injury; diffusion tensor imaging, which discloses patterns of connectivity in white matter; and magnetization transfer imaging, which promises even greater sensitivity to brain lesions than FLAIR imaging. Except for diffusion-weighted imaging in acute stroke, none has an established clinical use. Magnetic resonance spectroscopy is a method for analyzing the regional chemical composition of the brain. The benefits of its ability to identify neuronal loss and glial proliferation are still under investigation, although in certain circumstances, such as distinguishing radiation necrosis from recurrent brain tumor, it is of proven usefulness.

Functional Neuroimaging Four methods of functional neuroimaging are available: single photon emission computed tomography (SPECT), PET, functional MRI, and brain mapping by quantitative EEG. All are exciting research avenues, but the established clinical role for functional imaging is limited. All the techniques have a place in the presurgical evaluation of epileptic patients. SPECT or PET in the patient with frontotemporal dementia typically discloses the lobar nature of the dysfunction, although their value diagnostically over and above neuropsychological demonstration of the same phenomenon is questionable. Similarly, in exactly which circumstances demonstrating bilateral temporoparietal hypoperfusion advances the diagnosis of Alzheimer's disease is not yet clear. The demonstration of occipital hypoperfusion strongly supports a diagnosis of dementia with Lewy bodies. The evidence for other clinical uses of functional imaging is at present limited or anecdotal.

Electroencephalography The expectation of the originators of EEG was that it would allow tracking of mental processes. This hope has not been realized. EEG does have the advantage over other clinically available brain imaging tools that it reflects function at high temporal resolution, resolution corresponding to the time course of mental processing. Thus, at least from a research perspective, measurement of brain potentials in relation to stimuli—the technique of evoked potentials—has the capacity to identify anomalous modes of cerebral processing. Recordings from electrode placements in subdural or cortical sites provide irreplaceable information about the origin and spread of epileptic discharges, but this invasive technique is justified only under exceptional circumstances. From today's practical point of view, scalp EEG has several uses:

- Investigation of epilepsy to confirm the diagnosis and clarify the type of epilepsy
- Differentiation of delirium from acute nonorganic psychosis
- Recognition of Creutzfeldt-Jakob disease
- Distinction of frontotemporal dementia

Only 30 to 50 percent of patients with epilepsy show an epileptic abnormality on a single interictal waking EEG. With sleep deprivation, sleep during the recording, and repeated recordings, sensitivity improves to 70 to 80 percent. Anterior temporal electrodes add to the sensitivity and localizing power of the EEG, but nasopharyngeal electrodes, which are quite uncomfortable for the patient, do not provide additional sensitivity, and are not recommended. A reasonable protocol starts with a routine EEG, including anterior temporal leads; if this is negative but suspicion remains high, a second EEG with sleep deprivation can be undertaken. A third and fourth EEG may be useful, but the rate of discovery of abnormalities decreases after that. Even then, some epileptic patients will not have been shown to have interictal abnormalities. At times, ambulatory EEG is of use to ascertain the epileptic nature of undiagnosed events, but the restricted montage of the ambulatory equipment limits its usefulness. Hospitalization for video-EEG recording may be essential for clarifying the nature of puzzling spells.

Delirium is characterized by slowing of the EEG, a finding never seen in acute idiopathic psychosis. This differential point can be decisive in a confusing clinical setting. However, EEG is not indicated as a routine in the screening of psychotic patients. Among the dementing disorders, frontotemporal dementia is distinctive in having a normal EEG even as the clinical state becomes moderately severe. In Creutzfeldt-Jakob disease, the EEG is always slow and may ultimately (not necessarily immediately) show the diagnostic feature of pseudoperiodic complexes. Repeated EEGs at weekly intervals may clinch this diagnosis in a puzzling case.

Evoked potentials can identify abnormalities in neural transmission along myelinated pathways such as the visual pathway or the sensory pathways of the spinal cord and brainstem. This can help in the diagnosis of disorders such as multiple sclerosis or vitamin B_{12} deficiency.

Laboratory Investigations

In general, empirical evidence for the usefulness of laboratory studies supports only a limited role for "routine" or screening investigations; for the most part, laboratory tests should be performed as guided by the history and examination. A full discussion of laboratory strategies for all neuropsychiatric situations is beyond the scope of this chapter. In regard to dementia, a complete blood cell count (CBC), chemistry panel, vitamin B_{12} assay, and thyrotropin (TSH) assay are indicated as screening tests in addition to a test for syphilis (the fluorescent treponemal antibody test [FTA]) in those areas of the United States in which the prevalence of syphilis justifies the testing. (The region of high incidence is a broad belt across the South, in addition to some urban areas in the North; 30 U.S. counties contribute more than one-half of the national total of cases.) The reason the FTA is the test of choice is that reagin tests (the Venereal Disease Research Laboratory [VDRL] or Rapid Plasma Reagin [RPR]) revert to normal after intercurrent antibiotic treatment or with the passage of time and, thus, are insufficiently sensitive to serve as screening tests for neurosyphilis.

Appropriate screening tests for mental presentations other than dementia, for example, first episode psychosis, are less well established. Unfortunately, no cohort studies applying a consistent laboratory diagnostic approach are available to provide guidance as to the sensitivity and specificity of testing or even as to the prevalence of organic disease in this situation. The first step should be a neuropsychiatric history and examination. A reasonable laboratory screen might include CBC, chemistry panel, TSH, urinalysis, and urine toxicology. If it is considered justified to screen for rheumatic disease, an antinuclear antibody test (ANA) is adequate for this purpose, being abnormal in almost all cases of lupus, although not sufficient to confirm that diagnosis. (False positives from psychotropic drug–induced ANA tests are an important confound.)

Excessive laboratory testing is to be deplored; on the other hand, limiting laboratory testing to generally familiar diseases is inexpert. Consideration of rare metabolic diseases should be within the neuropsychiatrist's routine. Ruling out aminoacidurias or organic acidurias in patients with adolescent or young-adult onset of psychosis should be considered, especially if unexplained fluctuations possibly due to dietary factors, unexplained physical signs, or unexplained cognitive impairment is present. A reasonable broad screen includes ammonia, plasma for amino acids, and urine for organic acids, although this fails to detect such conditions (known to be associated with psychiatric presentations) as GM_2 gangliosidosis (hexosaminidase A deficiency) and adrenoleukodystrophy. Further testing with specific metabolic or genetic assays should be performed as circumstances indicate.

Examination of the Cerebrospinal Fluid

Examination of CSF obtained through lumbar puncture is sometimes a crucial element of the diagnostic process, in particular to diagnose infection or inflammation, more rarely in neuropsychiatric practice to seek evidence of neoplasia (such as meningeal carcinomatosis). Specific assays are available for the diagnosis of neuropsychiatrically relevant infectious agents such as polymerase chain reaction (PCR) for the herpes simplex virus (HSV) genome to diagnose herpes encephalitis or cryptococcal antigen assay to diagnose this fungal meningitis. In rheumatic diseases involving the brain, the white cell count may not be elevated, but elevated protein and evidence of intrathecal elaboration of antibodies may give evidence of inflammatory activity. The latter is sought by the ratio of immunoglobulin G (IgG) to albumin or, better, by the IgG index, which requires measurement of serum IgG by immunoelectrophoresis. CSF antineuronal antibodies are uncommon but specific for cerebral lupus. In the future, assay of CSF cytokines may provide assistance in the difficult diagnosis of these inflammatory diseases.

Measurement of the neuron-derived 14-3-3 protein has adequate specificity and sensitivity to assist in the diagnosis of Creutzfeldt-Jakob disease as long as the pretest probability of this rare disease is sufficiently high. In practice, this means that use of the test should be confined to patients with a progressive dementia of less than 2 years' duration. Measurement of tau and amyloid peptides is not yet of satisfactory validity for general use in the diagnosis of Alzheimer's disease.

Removal of CSF by lumbar puncture or external drainage also plays an important role in the evaluation of patients suspected of shunt-reversible normal pressure hydrocephalus.

Neuropsychological Assessment

Neuropsychological evaluation has an important role to play in neuropsychiatric care, both for diagnosis and for management. Sound use of the clinical neuropsychologist as a consultant requires, as a first step, formulation of a cogent consultative question. The more specific the consultant's question, the more able the neuropsychologist is to integrate the psychometric data with the rest of the clinical picture. Much of the early literature on neuropsychological assessment focused on identifying and localizing organic brain disease. With the advent of neuroimaging, neuropsychological testing is seldom the most powerful means of addressing this issue, although it certainly continues to play such a role, for example, in lateralizing cognitive deficits as a preoperative tool in epileptic patients. Nor is the role of the neuropsychologist to make a disease diagnosis, although at times the psychometric picture is strongly suggestive of a particular diagnosis.

In several areas of assessment, the neuropsychiatrist has particular reason to turn to the neuropsychologist. If substantial confounds make bedside diagnosis difficult, neuropsychological data may be of considerable assistance. For example, identifying supervening cognitive impairment in a mentally retarded or poorly educated patient or subtle impairment in a highly intelligent patient may be impossible for the clinician to do with confidence, whereas quantitative assessment may allow these diagnoses. Another example of using neuropsychological assessment as a probe of brain function is disclosing a pattern of cognitive strengths and weaknesses amounting to right hemisphere learning disabilities in a patient with a clinical picture suggestive of pervasive developmental disorder or a cluster A personality disorder. Obtaining neuropsychological data about a dementing patient often allows more precise targeting of behavioral interventions, more specific education of families, and more confident assessment of decline or of benefit from pharmacological treatments.

One common use of neuropsychological assessment requires a word of caution: identifying cognitive impairment in an older patient presenting with mood disorder or psychosis. No neuropsychological findings should deter the clinician from aggressive treatment of the psychiatric symptoms, and nonspecific, state-dependent attentional and motivational factors may confound the neuropsychological results. Rather than devoting resources of time and energy to pinpointing a moving target in the acute phase, deferring the assessment until symptoms are reduced is often the wiser course.

Another caution about neuropsychological assessment falls under the rubric of *ecological validity*. This term refers to the extrapolation of results obtained in the neuropsychological laboratory by artificial "paper-and-pencil" methods to real-world performance. The concern arises in particular with orbitofrontal lesions, which may produce a paucity of cognitive findings but devastating personality change. Deriving clinical measures from the developing realm of affective neuroscience suitable to characterize such patients is a current challenge to neuropsychology.

Brain Biopsy Biopsy of the brain has a limited role in neuropsychiatric evaluation. The morbidity and mortality of the procedure, as performed by an experienced neurosurgeon, are low, but the sensitivity of the procedure is lower than one might expect. For example, the sensitivity of biopsy for primary angiitis of the central nervous system (CNS) may be only 75 percent. In some circumstances, biopsy of a peripheral tissue can substitute for brain biopsy in a patient with primarily cerebral symptoms at lower risk. For example, lung or muscle biopsy may make a diagnosis of sarcoid, skin biopsy a diagnosis of vasculitis if a rash is present or of CADASIL, temporal artery biopsy of giant cell arteritis. In neuropsychiatric situations, the major indication for biopsy of the brain is consideration of inflammatory disease when the nature and aggressiveness of treatment depend on a tissue-proven diagnosis.

Although of course it cannot be considered a clinical diagnostic test, autopsy should not be overlooked by the neuropsychiatrist as a learning tool.

COMMON NEUROPSYCHIATRIC CONDITIONS

This section provides a survey of some issues commonly brought to the attention of neuropsychiatrists. The emphasis is on the priorities for clinical and laboratory assessment for a variety of presentations. The organization is by disease and syndrome, as a complement to the anatomical and symptom-oriented discussion provided so far. This perspective is distinctive for neuropsychiatry within psychiatry; the disease processes underlying symptoms in the idiopathic disorders are unknown. For neuropsychiatric patients, one can hope and work to uncover the disease causing the symptoms and, on fortunate occasions, to provide disease-specific treatment.

Dementia An extensive list of diseases produces the clinical state of dementia. A shotgun laboratory approach to "ruling out treatable disease" is unwise, if only because finding reversibility is so unusual. Moreover, clinical clues to reversible disease are available in the history and examination: use of psychotoxic medicines, rapid course, mildness of cognitive impairment (even short of fully meeting criteria for dementia), subcortical features of the cognitive disorder, and presence of motor signs. Table 2.1–4 provides specific guidance to be gained from clinical clues. The differential diagnosis of dementia needs to include differential diagnosis among the degenerative disorders, an exercise that depends very largely on clinical findings rather than imaging or laboratory data. In particular, apolipoprotein E testing is by consensus not recommended for routine diagnostic purposes at the present time.

The clinician needs to gather data relevant to management issues other than purported reversibility, such as safety of living arrangements, driving ability, and preparation of a will and advance directives. Dementing patients often develop psychiatric symptoms, which respond to pharmacological and behavioral treatment. All these considerations should prompt the clinician to cast a wide net in data gathering regarding the demented patient.

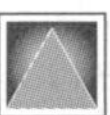

Table 2.1–4
Clues to the Differential Diagnosis of Dementia in the Neurological Examination

Abnormal eye findings
- Celiac disease
- Gaucher's disease type 3
- Mitochondrial cytopathy
- Multiple sclerosis
- Niemann-Pick disease type C
- Progressive supranuclear palsy
- Syphilis
- Vascular dementia
- Wernicke-Korsakoff syndrome
- Whipple's disease
- Wilson's disease

Ataxia
- Celiac disease
- Cerebellar degenerations
- GM_2 gangliosidosis
- Hypothyroidism
- Multiple sclerosis
- Niemann-Pick disease type C
- Prion disease
- Progressive multifocal leukoencephalopathy
- Toxic-metabolic encephalopathy
- Wernicke-Korsakoff syndrome
- Wilson's disease

Dysarthria
- Cerebellar degenerations
- Dementia pugilistica
- Dialysis dementia
- Motor neuron disease
- Multiple sclerosis
- Niemann-Pick disease type C
- Neuroacanthocytosis
- Pantothenate kinase–associated neurodegeneration
- Progressive multifocal leukoencephalopathy
- Progressive supranuclear palsy
- Wilson's disease

Extrapyramidal signs
- Alzheimer's disease
- Cerebellar degenerations
- Dementia pugilistica
- Dementia with Lewy bodies
- Fahr's syndrome
- GM_1 gangliosidosis, type III
- Huntington's disease
- Multiple system atrophy
- Neuroacanthocytosis
- Niemann-Pick disease type C
- Normal pressure hydrocephalus
- Pantothenate kinase–associated neurodegeneration
- Parkinson's disease
- Progressive supranuclear palsy
- Postencephalitic parkinsonism
- Subacute sclerosing panencephalitis
- Toxic-metabolic encephalopathy
- Vascular dementia
- Wilson's disease

Gait disorder
- Adrenomyeloneuropathy
- Cerebellar degenerations
- Dementia pugilistica
- HIV encephalopathy
- Multiple sclerosis
- Normal pressure hydrocephalus
- Parkinson's disease
- Progressive supranuclear palsy
- Syphilis
- Vascular dementia
- Wernicke-Korsakoff syndrome

Myoclonus
- Alzheimer's disease
- Celiac disease
- Dialysis dementia
- Kufs' disease
- Lafora's body disease
- Mitochondrial cytopathy
- Prion disease
- Subacute sclerosing panencephalitis

Peripheral neuropathy
- Adrenomyeloneuropathy
- B_{12} deficiency
- HIV encephalopathy
- Metachromatic leukodystrophy
- Porphyria
- Toxic-metabolic encephalopathy

Pyramidal signs
- Adrenomyeloneuropathy
- B_{12} deficiency
- Cerebellar degenerations
- GM_2 gangliosidosis
- HIV encephalopathy
- Kufs' disease
- Metachromatic leukodystrophy
- Motor neuron disease
- Multiple sclerosis
- Pantothenate kinase–associated neurodegeneration
- Polyglucosan body disease
- Progressive multifocal leukoencephalopathy
- Syphilis
- Vascular dementia

HIV, human immunodeficiency virus.
Modified from Sandson TA, Price BH: Diagnostic testing and dementia. *Neurol Clin.* 1996;14:45–59.

Epilepsy Major concerns in patients with epilepsy include differential diagnosis, psychosis, personality change, depression, violence and other episodic behaviors, and pseudoseizures. The last will be dealt with below along with other conversion disorders.

A 67-year-old woman presented with at least 1 year of progressive memory impairment, confusion, then irritability and suspiciousness. The mental state was typical of Alzheimer's disease, and the physical examination disclosed only brisk tendon jerks. An EEG, done earlier because of a spell of uncertain nature, had shown left temporal spikes. Neuropsychological assessment had shown a pattern typical for Alzheimer's disease, with memory impairment characterized by rapid forgetting, semantic–phonemic verbal fluency deficits, and anomia. MRI, however, demonstrated extensive white matter disease, with bilateral confluent hyperintensities, which extended into the gyri and involved U fibers. CSF examination was entirely normal. Skin biopsy for CADASIL and screening genetic assay for CADASIL were negative. Repeat EEG showed bilateral temporal spikes, and carbamazepine (Tegretol) was begun. The clinical diagnosis was leukoencephalopathy due to cerebral amyloid angiopathy, possibly with Alzheimer's disease. The patient's mother had died at 86 years of age, having suffered from "the same thing" as the patient. Four of the mother's five siblings demented in the 8th or 9th decade of life, none earlier, in most cases with a diagnosis of Alzheimer's disease. The patient was an only child. The patient's two daughters, both young adults, were very concerned that they might inherit the same disease as their mother, and they insisted the patient undergo the brain biopsy that a geriatrician had recommended. This disclosed pronounced congophilic angiopathy. Immunostaining for A-beta confirmed the vessel abnormality and showed neuropil plaques; immunostaining for tau did not reveal neuritic plaques. Nonetheless, Alzheimer's disease could not be excluded. No inflammation was seen. However, several days after the biopsy, she developed status epilepticus.

Patients with attack disorders can be misdiagnosed as having epilepsy when they do not or as having a different disorder when epilepsy is the correct diagnosis. Paroxysmal symptoms from panics, cardiac disease with syncope or near syncope, endocrine disorders (pheochromocytoma, carcinoid, systemic mastocytosis), or conversion disorder can be mistakenly labeled epileptic; contrariwise, epilepsy can be missed when a diagnosis of panic disorder, in particular, is accepted.

A 59-year-old man was evaluated for 7 years of memory problems and spells refractory to treatment on a diagnosis of panic disorder. These spells characteristically lasted 5 to 10 seconds and recurred as often as hourly; he was sometimes amnestic for the spells afterward. During an attack, he had gooseflesh, and his speech became garbled; once at church, he was believed to be speaking in tongues. Extensive treatment trials with benzodiazepines and serotonergic drugs had given no consistent benefit. Apart from hyperlipidemia, he had no significant medical history. EEG had been negative on three occasions, MRI on two, Holter monitoring and SPECT on one each. The neurological and mental state examinations were normal. An attack was witnessed during the examination: He showed 10 seconds of facial flushing and stereotyped hand movements. The attacks were subsequently abolished by a trial of an antiepileptic drug. The case illustrates that epilepsy is primarily a clinical, not an EEG, diagnosis.

A 52-year-old woman was referred for the evaluation of spells. In her 30s she had been hospitalized for depression and was subsequently treated intermittently as an outpatient. The family history included several members with depression or bipolar disorder. Two years before evaluation, she presented with headache and proved to have an unruptured aneurysm, which was clipped through a craniotomy. Several months later, she had a generalized convulsion. She went on to have spells at a rate of up to six a day. They were stereotyped and abrupt in onset and termination; she could not identify provocative factors or social contexts. During a spell, she felt cold and had gooseflesh for approximately 3 minutes. Then she become rigid and unable to speak or interact, although she could hear others' speech. This lasted several minutes. Then she began to cry. The whole sequence lasted 6 to 10 minutes. She was on phenytoin with a therapeutic serum level. Previous trials of divalproex (Depakote) and topiramate (Topamax) were not tolerated. EEGs had shown only right frontal slowing with no epileptic features on several tracings. The neurological and cognitive examinations were normal, and she was not depressed at the time of evaluation. The clinical picture was inconclusive: In favor of epilepsy were the abrupt onset and termination, stereotyped nature of the spells, and background of craniotomy; against epilepsy were the weeping, length of the ictus (if all the phenomena were taken to be ictal), lack of response to treatment, relatively inactive EEG, and background of depression. Video EEG done after medication withdrawal recorded three complex partial seizures with right anterior inferior temporal onset with her typical semiology and no pseudoseizures.

In exploring the psychiatric concomitants of epilepsy, the clinician needs to be aware of the nature of the epilepsy. Most adult epilepsy is focal ("localization-related epilepsy"), with the ictal onset in the temporal lobe. However, other forms of epilepsy, including frontal epilepsy and primary generalized epilepsy, are common. These distinctions, and the laterality of the focus, can often be inferred from the semiology of the seizures as reported or as observed clinically. A history of febrile convulsions in childhood and age of onset of epilepsy are relevant to the likelihood of mesial temporal sclerosis as the underlying pathology. Body asymmetry and dissociated facial paresis should be sought as indicators of laterality. The MRI and EEG provide crucial information on pathology and seizure type. Almost all the findings relating psychiatric disorder to epilepsy are concerned with partial epilepsy of temporal onset; linking psychiatric symptoms to epileptic syndromes other than temporal lobe, or limbic, epilepsy generally goes beyond the evidence. Further, to what extent psychopathology is associated with the epilepsy per se and to what extent with the underlying brain disease remain controversial. Without question, cognitive impairments are related to the lateralization of the temporal focus.

Psychotic states in epileptic patients are usually divided into those occurring during the epileptic ictus, often called *epileptic twilight states*; those occurring for a delimited period in the aftermath of a seizure or, more commonly, a flurry of seizures, so-called *postictal psychosis*; and those that are chronic, called *interictal psychosis*. Usually, this chronology can be ascertained by inquiry, but at times, EEG monitoring is necessary to identify the occurrence of seizures in relation to psychopathological phenomena, especially because patients can be amnestic for complex partial seizures. A further issue to be elucidated from the history is of a relationship between seizure treatment and control and the level of psychopathology, especially psychosis. An inverse relationship is sometimes noted, better seizure control being associated with occurrence of psychosis, a phenomenon known as *forced normalization*. On the other hand, frequent seizures certainly can cause an increase in confusion and related failure in functional capacity.

A 35-year-old woman with lupus and intractable epilepsy was admitted several times with persecutory and nihilistic delusions ("I'm dead") and depressive symptoms. Investigations to identify active cerebral lupus were unrevealing, even when she had evidence of peripheral activity of the disease. In fact, MRI disclosed the findings of hippocampal sclerosis, suggesting that the epilepsy was idiopathic and not due to old cerebral lupus. Without specific treatment, the psychotic symptoms diminished over the course of several days; this also was believed to make a diagnosis of cerebral lupus unlikely. Between episodes, she showed no psychotic phenomena.

The interictal personality syndrome of temporal lobe epilepsy (the Gastaut-Geschwind syndrome) is characterized by hypergraphia; religiosity or deepened metaphysical interest; intensified emotionality with a tendency to holding grudges and aggression; hyposexuality; and an alteration of social behavior with intensity of interaction, an inability to end interactions, and circumstantiality of discourse (phenomena confusingly denominated as "viscosity"). The syndrome remains controversial; what is of importance for neuropsychiatric assessment is that inquiry be directed to phenomena, such as hypergraphia, that are not included in the review of symptoms of idiopathic psychiatric disorder.

Episodic aggression is often suspected of being ictal but very rarely is. Aggression occurring during seizures is almost always disorganized, not carefully directed. A high threshold is justified in attributing a violent act to epilepsy in the absence of typical epileptic features. Amnesia for serious violence is common and not a strong pointer to an epileptic origin.

A special issue in neuropsychiatric assessment of the epileptic patient is the presurgical evaluation. Surgical treatment, especially of temporal lobe epilepsy due to mesial temporal sclerosis, is underused; ideally, more and more patients with medically refractory epilepsy will be evaluated for their suitability for surgery. Along with intensive electroencephalographic evaluation, volumetric MRI, and neuropsychological assessment, the patient's psychiatric state should be systematically evaluated. The patient's ability to consent and issues such as the patient's capacity to cope with the stress of monitoring and surgery as well as the expectations held for surgery should be addressed. Neither depression nor psychosis is an absolute contraindication to surgery, although a chronic psychosis probably will not be alleviated by surgery. Indeed, few, if any, psychiatric findings contraindicate surgery, but psychiatric evaluation may well reveal deficits that need to be taken into account in developing a treatment plan.

Traumatic Brain Injury Traumatic brain injury is epidemic in society, with advances in emergency medical care leading to growth in the prevalence of survivors of severe injury. Issues commonly facing the neuropsychiatrist include aggression, depression and anxiety, and the delineation of deficits (sometimes for legal purposes) in patients with mild traumatic injury. The features of the head injury should be ascertained, ideally with confirmation from medical records.

The altered behavior and personality common after traumatic brain injury are more burdensome for families than are the physical disabilities. Disinhibition and aggression are particularly uncomfortable and often hard to treat. A complicating factor is that preinjury impulsivity and substance abuse are common, as they predispose to head injury.

A 24-year-old woman was seen 19 months after an automobile collision in which she was an unrestrained passenger. She was comatose for 3 months and underwent surgical evacuation of a left-sided intracranial hematoma. She had a few weeks of rehabilitation after regaining consciousness and returned home after spending most of a year in a nursing home. The family was at wits' end over episodes of aggression, which appeared to be directed angry behavior elicited by frustration. She did not have depressive symptoms. On examination, she showed severe bilateral spasticity, including spastic dysarthria, drooling, and a brisk jaw jerk. She was able to recall dates and other details of her illness accurately, but she disclaimed behavioral or emotional alterations. Her language comprehension was adequate, but output was telegraphic. Affect was labile. Behavior during the consultation was initially appropriate, with an obvious effort to cooperate with the evaluation, although she had greeted the examiner with, "I love you." At the end of the examination, however, she urgently requested the examiner's business card and rammed him with her wheelchair while cutting off his access to the door. Chronic-phase CT showed atrophy and left temporal encephalomalacia.

A 59-year-old man was referred by a court for assessment of his ability to take part in proceedings related to his divorce. Three months before evaluation, he was struck several times by an unknown assailant during an altercation regarding who was to get the use of a taxi. He suffered contusions of the left periorbital area but no other overt injury. He was able to recount the events in some detail, but he explained that this was because, over time, by comparing notes with others, he had "put it all back together"; of his own recollection, he could remember the first punch that struck him but not the second or subsequent events of the altercation. Although he could not be certain of the duration of the gap in his recollection, it was clearly a matter of some seconds, conceivably a minute or two, and at no time was he unconscious. In the aftermath, he was "confused" and had a headache. He found that he could not come up with names, dates, or numbers, although this information generally came back to him later or with considerable unaccustomed effort. He also noticed that he "couldn't visualize" geographical scenes, so that in planning to go to a familiar place, he was unable to picture it in his mind. Although he did not get lost, he found that he turned the wrong way or missed a turn because of inattention and had to correct himself. He noted that his memory, previously highly trustworthy, could not be counted on: "I had to write everything down." He found that he had to "take time to think," "strain my brain to focus." He distanced himself from business decisions and relied on trusted subordinates to counsel him. He acknowledged sensitivity to light, noting that he had begun to wear sunglasses even when the weather was cloudy and to turn off the room lights when he was watching television. To a lesser extent, he was bothered by noise. He noted that he was more readily irritated than was characteristic of him. He did not have depressive symptoms, intrusive recall of the altercation, or nightmares. The symptoms had gotten gradually less severe. The history included several head injuries in adolescence, two of which resulted in loss of consciousness of a few hours without recognized sequelae. The noncognitive mental state and neurological examinations were normal. He scored 21 on the Mental Alternation Test, a clearly normal performance on a task of mental speed and working memory. He scored 16 out of 18 on the Frontal Assessment Battery, a collection of tasks assessing executive cognitive function. The two lost points were on the go/no-go task, on which he made perseverative errors. He was mildly disorganized on performing the ring/fist test of motor sequencing. MRI and EEG had been normal. The picture was believed to be consistent with organic sequelae of traumatic brain injury. The case underlines the importance of prior traumatic brain injury in determining the effects of seemingly mild trauma and that loss of consciousness is not a prerequisite for significant sequelae.

Movement Disorders Cognitive impairment due to involvement of subcortical structures is a common neuropsychiatric feature of the movement disorders. This applies to cerebellar, as well basal ganglia, diseases for the anatomical reasons described above. The anatomy of the close relation between emotion and movement was also described above. Clinically, mood disorders are common in IPD and other movement disorders. Anxiety disorders, although less emphasized in the literature than depression, are also common. The evaluator should take into account that mood and anxiety can fluctuate according to the timing of doses of dopaminergic drugs. A mood disorder can occasionally present in advance of overt movement abnormalities, so IPD must be considered in the differential diagnosis of late-onset mood disorders.

A 43-year-old woman with no personal or family history of psychiatric illness developed a psychotic depression. She had a severe extrapyramidal reaction to risperidone (Risperdal). Two years later, when euthymic and unmedicated, she developed progressive shuffling gait, upper-extremity tremor, and micrographia. She then suffered another episode of depression. Three years later, she had severe anxiety, no cognitive impairment, and the motor features of IPD.

Psychotic reactions to dopaminergic drugs are an important feature of movement disorders. Sometimes this is the result of overuse of prescribed dopaminergic agents in an effort to increase time in the "on" state.

A 63-year-old man with long-standing IPD developed delusions while being treated with high-dose carbidopa-levodopa (Sinemet) on a five-times-a-day schedule, pramipexole (Mirapex), tolcapone, and amantadine (Symmetrel). Under inpatient observation for several days on the prescribed doses, he remained psychotic. He responded well to quetiapine (Seroquel).

Developmental Disabilities Adult patients with developmental disabilities are enormously underserved by the medical and social service communities and are frequently referred for neuropsychiatric attention. Few of these patients have had adequate diagnostic evaluation for the cause of the disability. Beyond clinical assessment, with particular attention to dysmorphology because features of the mental state and neurological examination are generally nonspecific, the most useful diagnostic tests are MRI and karyotyping. Specific genetic probes can confirm tentative clinical recognition of syndromes of mental retardation. Patients with developmental disabilities are vulnerable—indeed, especially vulnerable—to the mood, anxiety, and psychotic disorders that can afflict anyone and can be treated effectively for these; diagnostic overshadowing (attributing all psychological and behavioral disturbance to "retardation" *tout court*) is to be avoided. These syndromes may present atypically in the developmentally disabled population, and the clinician must be alert to indirect indicators of mood disturbance or psychotic experience. For example, although the patient may not report depressed mood verbally, the caregivers may report the loss of interest in favorite activities and the other features of a depressive syndrome.

Of particular neuropsychiatric interest is the question of behavioral phenotypes, specific psychological correlates of developmental syndromes. Syndromes recognized to have behavioral phenotypes (and their correlates) include

Lesch-Nyhan syndrome (self-injury)
Prader-Willi syndrome (excessive eating)
Williams syndrome (anomalous cognitive profile, elevated sociability)
Velocardiofacial syndrome (schizophrenia)

Infectious and Inflammatory Diseases Infectious and inflammatory diseases of the brain need always to be considered in acutely or subacutely evolving mental disorders. Among the infectious diseases, HSV encephalitis has a particular claim on attention because delay in diagnosis, even by hours, can lead to substantially increased morbidity and mortality. Definitive diagnosis is possible without biopsy by assaying for HSV in the CSF with the PCR, but treatment may be indicated if suspicion is high in advance of firm diagnosis. Chronic meningitis, for example, from infection with fungi, is a rare consideration in subacutely evolving dementia; the definitive diagnostic tests are CSF assays or serological tests (e.g., for toxoplasmosis). In the acquired immunodeficiency syndrome (AIDS) era, infection with opportunistic agents and with the human immunodeficiency virus itself needs to be kept in mind, even in circumstances not immediately suggestive of AIDS.

Noninfectious inflammatory diseases include the rheumatic diseases, of which the prototype is systemic lupus. A rheumatic disease review of systems is always of importance in exploring the differential diagnosis of a puzzling case, especially in a young woman. Although psychosis is often considered the psychiatric hallmark of lupus, in fact, psychotic states (other than delirium) are unusual, and a variety of other psychiatric pictures need to be included in the clinician's consideration. Few clinical features of lupus are risk factors for cerebral disease, not even disease activity, which may be misleading in either a positive or a negative direction. One feature that is a risk factor for neuropsychiatric symptoms, including cognitive impairment, is the presence of antiphospholipid antibodies; the primary antiphospholipid syndrome similarly carries mental risk.

A 40-year-old woman presented with the typical features of a psychotic depression. There was a family history of depression, and she had suffered two episodes of depression earlier in her adult life, both of which were brief, nonpsychotic, and responsive to treatment. For the previous year, however, her depression had been poorly responsive to pharmacological and electroconvulsive therapy (ECT) treatment

Examination disclosed no definite cognitive abnormality and brisker reflexes on the left. Review of MRI obtained at her previous treatment venue, presumably performed as a routine before the administration of ECT, evinced striking areas of white matter abnormality in the right hemisphere. Extensive laboratory investigation, short of angiography and biopsy, revealed only high-titer IgA anti-β2-glycoprotein-1 antibodies. Neuropsychological assessment performed after partial remission of the depression showed deficits in attention and mental processing speed. The working diagnostic formulation was that an otherwise ordinary idiopathic depressive disorder had been rendered treatment resistant and gravely severe by a wave of cerebral injury due to the antiphospholipid syndrome. One lesson of the case is to always look at the imaging.

Other rheumatic diseases, such as Sjögren's syndrome and the vasculitides, are also of neuropsychiatric importance. Hashimoto's encephalopathy—subacutely developing cognitive impairment and myoclonus or seizures with high-titer antithyroid antibodies—is important in the differential diagnosis of Creutzfeldt-Jakob disease and of subacute confusional states. Prominent among nonrheumatic inflammatory diseases is paraneoplastic limbic encephalitis, an autoimmune complication of several tumors, notably small cell carcinoma of the lung.

A 60-year-old woman was admitted for confusion. She had been drinking more heavily than usual after a forced retirement several months earlier. The family noted that she had been forgetful and behaviorally erratic for 1 to 2 months. She smoked cigarettes and had hypertension. On examination, she had mild gait instability but no other physical signs. Thought was disorganized, but no psychotic ideas were present. Psychomotor rate and affect were normal. She showed verbal memory impairment and disinhibition, with many errors of commission on a go/no-go task and inability to inhibit reflexive gaze. CSF examination revealed a mild lymphocytic pleocytosis with no other abnormalities. EEG showed intermittent frontal slowing. The following were negative or normal: serological studies, thyroid function and antibody tests, anti-Hu, MRI, MRA, chest and abdominal CT (except a benign adrenal tumor), and cerebral angiogram. The patient's family refused brain biopsy. On a differential diagnosis of primary angiitis and paraneoplastic encephalitis, the patient received a pulse of intravenous (IV) methylprednisolone, without benefit, then a course of oral cyclosphosphamide and prednisone, again without benefit. Some months after discharge, she died suddenly. Autopsy revealed pulmonary embolus to be the cause of death. Perivascular T-cell infiltrates and activated microglia were seen in the medial temporal lobes and to a lesser degree widespread in the cortex. No tumor was found in the lungs or elsewhere. Nonetheless, the pathology supported the clinical consideration of "paraneoplastic" encephalitis, which has been reported to occur in otherwise typical form but without a discoverable tumor. Often, extensive evaluation is necessary for patients suspected of inflammatory brain disease; at times, even extensive evaluation does not suffice.

Conversion Disorder Neuropsychiatrists often see patients whose symptoms appear to arise from brain disease but do not. These patients' conditions have been described under various names: hysteria, functional disorder, psychogenic disorder, conversion disorder, and medically unexplained symptoms. None of the designations is entirely satisfactory. For example, the DSM-IV-TR denomination of *conversion disorder* is based on an outmoded notion of the conversion of emotions into physical form. Whatever the designation, such patients are not uncommon. Complicating matters is the common coexistence of organic disease and conversion symptoms. For example, a sizable minority of patients with pseudoseizures have epilepsy as well. Brain disease may, in some of these patients, have produced organic personality change with a reduction in the maturity of defenses and the too-easy resort to somatization.

Various techniques have been advocated for identification of nonorganic disease by the physical examination. These have several shortcomings. First, they easily lend themselves to a countertherapeutic alliance in which the examiner is trying to trick the patient—not a good start for the treatment, whatever the findings. Second, they fail to distinguish deliberate falsification on the patient's part—that is, malingering—from conversion disorder. Third, most such findings are commonly present in patients with organic disease who are trying to help the examiner make the diagnosis. That is, they may mark a patient as histrionic or suggestible but fail to rule out organic disease. Thus, for example, reporting a difference in vibratory sensation between the two sides of the sternum is by no means confined to patients with conversion disorder. Exceptions to this caution occur in cases in which the nonphysiological finding is precisely the phenomenon of the complaint. Even then, however, the phenomena of brain disease are sufficiently odd that the examiner should maintain an attitude of humility about achieving diagnostic certainty by recognizing the nonphysiological at a glance. Of the described "signs of hysteria," perhaps the best is Hoover's sign. The examiner places a hand underneath the heel of the affected leg of a supine patient who complains of leg weakness. Asked to press down with the heel, the patient does not generate power with the leg. Asked to raise the opposing leg, however, the patient produces an automatic synergistic downward movement of the affected leg.

Recent systematic findings of progressively greater methodological sophistication confirm the belief that experiences of abuse in childhood are common in the background of patients with conversion disorder. This may indirectly account for another progressively more solidly substantiated finding, namely, that the prognosis of conversion disorder is poor. Although a given symptom may wax and wane or disappear, patients commonly have a chronic course of disability, interpersonal difficulties, psychiatric symptoms, and fruitless seeking after medical help. Although hysterical symptoms have often been taken to represent symbolically a psychological conflict, the fundamental difficulty is that patients who make prominent use of somatization have a disorder of the symbolic function itself. The goal of the examiner should not be to catch the patient out but to establish an alliance that allows exploration of areas of the patient's life outside the presenting symptoms and construction of a plan to reduce distress (including focused treatment of commonly coexisting depressive disorder) and to develop alternative ways of seeking attention and assistance for distress.

NEUROPSYCHIATRIC PERSPECTIVE

The neuropsychiatrist thinks anatomically about mental state disorders, even as cognitive neuroscientists attempt to construct a sufficiently sophisticated model of large-scale brain function to do justice to the complex mental states of neuropsychiatric interest. The neuropsychiatrist relies on rich data gathered at the bedside and on laboratory methods of investigating brain structure and function and of diagnosing disease. The effort is to identify not just behavioral syndromes as found in DSM-IV-TR or ICD, but the pathological processes underlying them in two senses. First, neuropsychiatry seeks medical diagnoses of systemic or brain diseases to account for the patient's illness. Second, neuropsychiatry seeks to understand clinical phenomena in terms of the disruption of elementary mental processes, the nature of which is beginning to be elucidated by the cognitive neurosciences. The result is a highly differentiated diagnostic enterprise. With continual refreshment from a multidisciplinary base—ranging from cognitive neuroscience to general medicine—the neuropsychiatric approach to the patient is certain to remain exciting.

SUGGESTED CROSS-REFERENCES

Section 1.2 provides a review of neuroanatomy. Section 1.15 discusses nuclear MRI and Section 1.16 covers radiotracer imaging. The other sections in this chapter deal in detail with neuropsychiatric aspects of various disease processes. The sections in Chapter 7 deal with the diagnostic process in general psychiatry, including the examination of the mental state (see Sections 7.1 and 7.3), neuropsychological evaluation (see Section 7.5), and laboratory testing (see Section 7.8).

REFERENCES

*Bogousslavsky J, Cummings JL, eds. *Behavior and Mood Disorders in Focal Brain Lesions*. Cambridge: Cambridge University Press; 2000.

D'Esposito M, ed. *Neurological Foundations of Cognitive Neuroscience*. Cambridge, MA: MIT Press; 2003.

Dolan RJ: Emotion, cognition, and behavior. *Science*. 2002;298:1191.

Duchaine B, Cosmides L, Tooby J: Evolutionary psychology and the brain. *Curr Opin Neurobiol*. 2001;11:225.

Duncan J, Owen AM: Common regions of the human frontal lobe recruited by diverse cognitive demands. *Trends Neurosci*. 2000;23:475.

Duus P. *Topical Diagnosis in Neurology*. 3rd ed. New York: Thieme; 1998.

Friston KJ, Price CJ: Dynamic representations and generative models of brain function. *Brain Res Bull*. 2001;54:275.

Geschwind N: Disconnexion syndromes in animals and man. I. *Brain*. 1965;88:237.

Geschwind N: Disconnexion syndromes in animals and man. II. *Brain*. 1965;88:585.

Golomb M: Psychiatric symptoms in metabolic and other genetic disorders: Is our "organic" workup complete? *Harv Rev Psychiatry*. 2002;10:242.

Halligan PW, David AS: Cognitive neuropsychiatry: Towards a scientific psychopathology. *Nat Rev Neurosci*. 2001;2:209.

Johnson MH, Halit H, Grice SJ, Karmiloff-Smith A: Neuroimaging of typical and atypical development: A perspective from multiple levels of analysis. *Dev Psychopathol*. 2002;14:521.

Kopelman MD: Disorders of memory. *Brain*. 2002;125:2152.

Levitin DJ, Menon V, Schmitt JE, Eliez S, White CD, Glover GH, Kadis J, Korenberg JR, Bellugi U, Reiss AL: Neural correlates of auditory perception in Williams syndrome: An FMRI study. *Neuroimage*. 2003;18:74.

Liddle PF. *Disordered Brain and Mind: The Neural Basis of Mental Symptoms*. London: Gaskell; 2001.

*Lishman WA. *Organic Psychiatry: The Psychological Consequences of Cerebral Disorders*. Oxford: Blackwood Science; 1998.

Lloyd D: Terra cognita: From functional neuroimaging to the map of the mind. *Brain Mind*. 2000;1:93.

*Mesulam MM. Behavioral neuroanatomy: Large-scale networks, association cortex, frontal syndromes, the limbic system, and hemispheric specializations. In: Mesulam MM, ed. *Principles of Behavioral and Cognitive Neurology*. London: Oxford University Press; 2000.

Mesulam MM: From sensation to cognition. *Brain*. 1998;121:1013.

Middleton FA, Strick PL: Basal ganglia and cerebellar loops: motor and cognitive circuits. *Brain Res Brain Res Rev*. 2000;31:236.

Miller MB, Van Horn JD, Wolford GL, Handy TC, Valsangkar-Smyth M, Inati S, Grafton S, Gazzaniga MS: Extensive individual differences in brain activations associated with episodic retrieval are reliable over time. *J Cogn Neurosci*. 2002;14:1200.

*Ovsiew F. Bedside neuropsychiatry: Eliciting the clinical phenomena of neuropsychiatric illness. In: Yudofsky SC, Hales RE, eds. *American Psychiatric Publishing Textbook of Neuropsychiatry and Clinical Neurosciences*. Washington, DC: American Psychiatric Publishing; 2002.

Ovsiew F: Seeking reversibility and treatability in dementia. *Semin Clin Neuropsychiatry*. 2003;8:3.

Ovsiew F, Bylsma FW: The three cognitive examinations. *Semin Clin Neuropsychiatry*. 2002;7:54.

Ovsiew F, Jobe T. Neuropsychiatry in the history of mental health services. In: Ovsiew F, ed. *Neuropsychiatry and Mental Health Services*. Washington, DC: American Psychiatric Press; 1999.

Paterson SJ, Brown JH, Gsodl MK, Johnson MH, Karmiloff-Smith A: Cognitive modularity and genetic disorders. *Science*. 1999;286:2355.

Schmahmann JD, Sherman JC: The cerebellar cognitive affective syndrome. *Brain*. 1998;121:561.

*Shallice T. *From Neuropsychology to Mental Structure*. Cambridge: Cambridge University Press; 1988.

Silver JM, McAllister TW: Forensic issues in the neuropsychiatric evaluation of the patient with mild traumatic brain injury. *J Neuropsychiatry Clin Neurosci*. 1997;9:102.

Stone VE, Cosmides L, Tooby J, Kroll N, Knight RT: Selective impairment of reasoning about social exchange in a patient with bilateral limbic system damage. *Proc Natl Acad Sci U S A*. 2002;99:11531.

Sugiyama LS, Tooby J, Cosmides L: Cross-cultural evidence of cognitive adaptations for social exchange among the Shiwiar of Ecuadorian Amazonia. *Proc Natl Acad Sci U S A*. 2002;99:11537.

▲ 2.2 Neuropsychiatric Aspects of Cerebrovascular Disorders

ROBERT G. ROBINSON, M.D., AND
RICARDO E. JORGE, M.D.

Cerebrovascular disease encompasses a wide range of disorders, including atherosclerotic changes of cerebral blood vessels leading to thrombus formation and cerebral infarction or embolic events resulting from the breakup of thrombi within the heart or large cervical arterial vessels that travel to the brain. These ischemic phenomena constitute approximately 85 percent of cerebrovascular disorders and may produce large infarcts or small lacunar lesions. Cerebral vascular disease also includes hemorrhagic disorders caused by weakness of the vascular wall resulting in bleeding under the brain's covering—that is, subarachnoid bleeding or bleeding into the brain itself (i.e., intraparenchymal hemorrhage). They constitute approximately 15 percent of all cerebrovascular disease. Cerebral vascular disease is the third leading cause of mortality in the United States and, therefore, represents a major public health problem.

Stroke is defined as a sudden loss of blood supply to the brain leading to permanent tissue damage caused by thrombotic, embolic, or hemorrhagic events. Stroke is the most common serious neurological disorder in the world and accounts for one-half of all the acute hospitalizations for neurological disease. The age-specific incidence of stroke varies dramatically over the life course. The annual incidence in developed countries for those 55 to 64 years of age ranges from 10 to 20 per 10,000, whereas for those older than 85 years of age, the incidence is almost 200 per 10,000 population.

The association of neuropsychiatric disorders with cerebrovascular disease has been recognized by clinicians for more than 100 years, but it is only within the past 30 years that systematic studies have been conducted. The vast majority of studies, however, have focused on neuropsychiatric disorders associated with stroke.

HISTORY

Early reports of depression after brain damage (usually caused by cerebrovascular disease) were made by neurologists and psychiatrists in case descriptions. Adolf Meyer warned that new discoveries of cerebral localization in the early 1900s, such as language function, led to an over-hasty identification of centers and functions of the brain. He identified several disorders, such as delirium, dementia, and aphasia, which were the direct result of brain injury. In keeping with his view of biopsychosocial causes of most mental "reactions," however, he saw manic-depressive illness and paranoiac conditions as arising from a combination of brain injury (specifically citing left frontal lobe and cortical convexities) as well as family history of psychiatric disorder and premorbid personal psychiatric disorders to produce the specific mental reaction. Eugen Bleuler noted that, after stroke, "melancholic moods lasting for months and sometimes longer appear frequently." Emil Kraepelin recognized an association between manic-depressive insanity and cerebrovascular disease. He stated that "the diagnosis of states of depression may offer difficulties, especially when arteriosclerosis is involved." Kraepelin concluded that cerebrovascular disorder may be an accompanying phenomenon of manic-depressive disease or may itself produce depressive disorder.

Another emotional disorder that has been historically associated with brain injury, such as cerebral infarction, and represents one of the differential diagnoses for depression is pathological crying. Redvers Ironside described the clinical manifestations of this disorder. Patients' emotional displays were characteristically unrelated to their inner emotional state. Crying may have occurred spontaneously or after some seemingly minor provocation. This phenomenon has been given various names, including emotional incontinence, emotional lability, pseudobulbar affect, and pathological emotionalism. Some investigators have differentiated pseudobulbar disorder, which is characterized by bilateral brain lesions and subjective feelings of being forced to laugh or cry, from emotional lability, in which there is an easy and sometimes rapid vacillation between euthymic appearance and laughing or crying.

Another emotional abnormality also believed to be characteristic of brain injury is the indifference reaction described by Derek Denny-Brown. Associated with right hemisphere lesions, this reaction consists of symptoms of indifference toward failures, lack of interest in family and friends, enjoyment of foolish jokes, and minimization of physical difficulties. In the late 19th century, Leonore Welt first described euphoria and loquaciousness associated with orbital frontal injury. Hermann Oppenheim used the term *Witzelsnicht* to refer to the inappropriate humor in these patients, and Karl Kleist stated that the orbital frontal cortex was the center of emotional life and the dorsal lateral frontal cortex was the source of psychomotor and intellectual activity.

Another neuropsychiatric disorder historically associated with disorders such as stroke was first described by Kurt Goldstein. He characterized the catastrophic reaction as an emotional outburst involving various degrees of anger, frustration, depression, tearfulness, refusal, shouting, swearing, and sometimes aggressive behavior. Goldstein ascribed this reaction to the inability of the organism to cope when faced with a serious defect in its physical or cognitive functions.

COMPARATIVE NOSOLOGY

The revised fourth edition of the *Diagnostic and Statistical Manual of Mental Disorders* (DSM-IV-TR) defines *poststroke psychotic disorder*, *mood disorders*, and *anxiety disorders* as disorders due to cerebral vascular disease or stroke with delusions or hallucinations for psychotic disorders with depressive features, major depressive-like episode, manic features, or mixed features for mood disorder; and with generalized anxiety, panic attacks, or obsessive-compulsive symptoms for anxiety disorders. The only disorder that is specific for cerebrovascular disease is vascular dementia, which may be uncomplicated or occur with delirium, delusions, or depressed mood. The other DSM-IV-TR–defined disorder that is commonly used in patients with cerebrovascular disease is minor depression. This diagnosis is classified as a "research diagnosis" but is a subsyndromal form of major depression. Patients with more than two but fewer than five of the required symptoms for major depression meet the criteria for this diagnosis. The neuropsychiatric disorders that are specific to brain injury do not have defined diagnostic criteria such as pathological laughing or crying or catastrophic reactions.

Investigators of depression associated with physical illness have debated the most appropriate method for the diagnosis of these disorders when some symptoms (e.g., sleep or appetite disturbance) could result from the physical illness. Four approaches have been used to assess depression in the physically ill. These approaches are the "inclusive approach," in which depressive diagnostic symptoms are counted regardless of whether they may be related to physical illness; the "etiological approach," in which a symptom is counted only if the diagnostician feels that it is not caused by the physical illness; the "substitutive approach," in which other psychological symptoms of depression replace the vegetative symptoms; and the "exclusive approach," in which symptoms are removed from the diagnostic criteria if they are not found to be more frequent in depressed than nondepressed patients.

Paradiso and colleagues have examined the usefulness of these methods in the diagnosis of depression during the first 2 years after stroke. Among 205 patients with acute stroke, 142 patients were followed up for examination at 3, 6, 12, or 24 months after stroke. The patients who were not included in the follow-up had died, could not be located, or refused to attend follow-up evaluations. Of 142 patients with follow-up, 60 (42 percent) reported the presence of a depressed mood (depressed group) while they were in the hospital, and the remaining 82 patients were nondepressed. There were no significant differences in the background characteristics between the depressed and nondepressed groups except that the depressed group was significantly younger (P = .006) and had a significantly higher frequency of personal history of psychiatric disorder (P = .04).

Throughout the 2-year follow-up, depressed patients showed a higher frequency of both vegetative and psychological symptoms compared with the nondepressed patients (Table 2.2–1). The only symptoms that were not more frequent in the depressed, compared with nondepressed, patients were weight loss and early awakening at the initial evaluation; weight loss and early-morning awakening at 6 months; weight loss, early-morning awakening, anxious foreboding, and loss of libido at 1 year; and weight loss and loss of libido at 2 years. Among the psychological symptoms, the depressed patients had a higher frequency of most psychological symptoms throughout the 2-year follow-up. The only psychological symptoms that were not significantly more frequent in the depressed than in the nondepressed group were suicidal plans, simple ideas of reference, and pathological guilt at 3 months; pathological guilt at 6 months; pathological guilt, suicidal plans, guilty ideas of reference, and irritability at 1 year; and pathological guilt and self-depreciation at 2 years.

The effect of using each of the proposed alternative diagnostic methods for poststroke depression using DSM-IV-TR criteria was examined. Compared with diagnoses based solely on the existence of five or more specific symptoms for the diagnosis of DSM-IV-TR

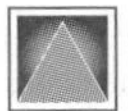

Table 2.2–1
Number of Patients with Vegetative Depressive Symptoms at Each Poststroke Evaluation

	Initial Evaluation		3-Month Follow-Up		6-Month Follow-Up		1-Year Follow-Up		2-Year Follow-Up	
Symptom	Dep Mood	Non-Dep Mood	Dep Mood	Non-Dep Mood	Dep Mood	Non-Dep Mood	Dep Mood	Non-Dep Mood	Dep Mood	Non-Dep Mood
Autonomic anxiety	23 (39)	4 (5)[a]	15 (52)	5 (11)[a]	18 (58)	7 (15)[a]	9 (45)	6 (12)[a]	16 (64)	8 (20)[a]
Anxious foreboding	21 (36)	8 (10)[a]	13 (46)	3 (6)[a]	9 (29)	7 (15)	4 (20)	4 (8)	11 (44)	2 (5)[a]
Morning depression	38 (63)	4 (5)[a]	17 (67)	2 (4)[a]	20 (65)	2 (4)[a]	11 (55)	2 (4)[a]	17 (68)	0 (0)[a]
Weight loss	20 (34)	16 (20)	6 (22)	3 (6)	10 (32)	11 (24)	4 (20)	2 (4)	7 (28)	6 (15)
Delayed sleep	24 (40)	12 (15)[a]	10 (36)	9 (19)	15 (48)	7 (15)[a]	8 (40)	5 (10)[a]	11 (44)	2 (5)[a]
Subjective anergia	35 (58)	16 (20)[a]	17 (61)	12 (28)[a]	19 (61)	10 (22)[a]	10 (50)	8 (16)[a]	15 (60)	10 (24)[a]
Early awakening	16 (27)	13 (16)	9 (32)	8 (17)	4 (13)	7 (15)	3 (15)	3 (6)	11 (44)	5 (12)[a]
Loss of libido	16 (27)	7 (9)[a]	12 (46)	12 (11)[a]	12 (39)	6 (14)[a]	5 (25)	7 (14)	11 (44)	10 (24)

Note: Number and percentage (in parentheses) of patients with or without depressed mood presenting definite symptoms.
Dep, depressed.
[a]Significant at the .05 level.
Courtesy of T. E. Oxman.

major depression, diagnoses based on unmodified symptoms (i.e., early awakening and weight loss included) had a specificity of 98 percent and a sensitivity of 100 percent.

Similar results were found at 3, 6, 12, and 24 months' follow-up. The sensitivity of unmodified DSM-IV-TR criteria consistently showed a sensitivity of 100 percent and a specificity that ranged from 95 percent to 98 percent, compared with criteria only using specific symptoms. Thus, one could reasonably conclude that modifying DSM-IV-TR criteria because of the existence of cerebrovascular disease is probably unnecessary.

EPIDEMIOLOGY

Vascular Dementia In a review of population-based studies, the European Community Concerted Action on Epidemiology and Prevention of Dementia found a consistent increase in the lifetime prevalence of vascular dementia with advancing age. Prevalence rates ranged from 1.5 per 100 for women 75 to 79 years of age in the United States to 16.3 per 100 for men older than 80 years of age in Italy (Table 2.2–2). In most age groups, men had a higher prevalence of vascular dementia than women. Vascular dementia is the most common type of dementia in Japan, representing up to 50 percent of all clinical cases and from 54 to 65 percent of all autopsy-confirmed dementia cases.

In two autopsy series, stroke accounted for approximately 20 to 25 percent of all dementia cases, and 10 to 15 percent of cases were believed to be the result of a combination of vascular disease and dementia of the Alzheimer's type. In a clinical series using in vivo imaging, the proportion of dementia that was directly attributable to stroke was 10 to 15 percent.

Depression Depressive disorders are probably the most common emotional disorder associated with cerebrovascular disease. The prevalence depends on whether community-based samples or hospitalized patients are examined or whether patients with acute stroke or those with chronic stroke are evaluated. Based on the world's literature, the pooled data mean prevalence for major depression in community samples is 14.1 percent and for minor depression 9.1 percent (Table 2.2–2). For hospitalized patients, the pooled data mean for major depression is 19.3 percent and for minor depression 18.5 percent. The similar data for outpatient studies are 23.3 percent for major depression and 15.0 percent for minor depression.

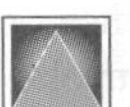

Table 2.2–2
Prevalence Studies of Psychiatric Disorders after Stroke

Disorder	Prevalence Rate	Studies
Vascular dementia	1.5/100.0; women 75–79 yrs of age in United States	Rocca et al. 1991
	16.3/100.0 men >80 yrs of age in Italy	Rocca et al. 1991
	10/100 dementia cases in United States	Katzmen et al. 1988
Major depression	15/100 strokes in community	Burville et al. 1995
	20/100 strokes in acute hospital	Robinson 1998
Mania	<1/100 strokes in acute hospital	Robinson, Starkstein 1997
Anxiety	6/100 strokes in acute hospital	Castillo et al. 1993
	27/100 anxiety ± depression acute	Castillo et al. 1993
	28/100 anxiety ± depression acute	Astrom et al. 1996
	3.5/100.0 anxiety neurosis in community	House et al. 1991
Psychosis	<1/100 strokes in acute hospital	Robinson, Starkstein 1997
Apathy	11/100 apathy only in acute hospital	Starkstein et al. 1993a
	11/100 apathy ± depression in acute hospital	Starkstein et al. 1993a
Catastrophic reaction	19/100 strokes in acute hospital	Starkstein et al. 1993b
Pathological emotions	15/100 acute stroke in community	House et al. 1991
	21/100 6-mo poststroke	House et al. 1991
	14/100 first stroke in community	Andersen 1995
	18/100 rehabilitation hospital	Morris et al. 1993
Anosognosia	24/100 strokes in acute hospital	Starkstein et al. 1992

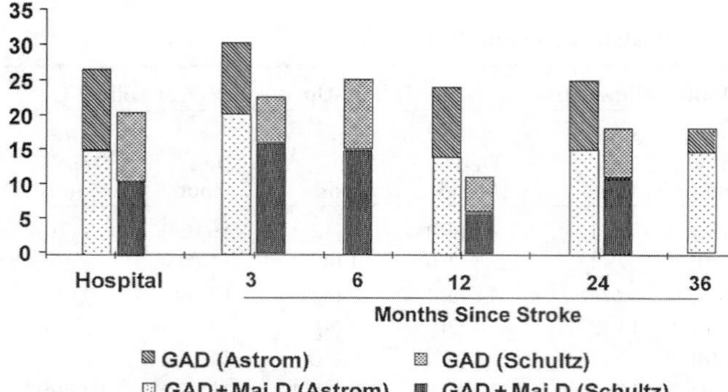

FIGURE 2.2–1 The frequency of generalized anxiety disorder (GAD) with and without major depression (Maj D) over the 3 years after acute stroke. Results obtained from Schultz et al. (1997) using the revised fourth edition of the *Diagnostic and Statistical Manual of Mental Disorders* (DSM-IV-TR) criteria were compared to the results of Astrom (1996) using DSM-IV-TR criteria. Results indicate a slightly lower frequency of GAD using DSM-IV-TR criteria and emphasize the prominence of major depression in this population of patients with poststroke anxiety disorder. (From Robinson RG. *The Clinical Neuropsychiatry of Stroke*. Cambridge University Press; 1998, with permission.)

Mania Mania occurs much less frequently than depression after stroke (only three cases were identified among a consecutive series of more than 300 acute stroke patients, including 143 patients with longitudinal assessment). Although numerous case reports and empirical studies document that stroke is associated with mania, there are no epidemiological studies that document the incidence or prevalence of this condition. Approximately one-half of the reported cases involve single or repeated manic episodes without major depression.

Anxiety In a consecutive series of 301 patients with first episode acute stroke lesions, Castillo reported that 10 percent met the DSM-IV-TR criteria for generalized anxiety disorder in the absence of any mood disorder. On the other hand, 12 percent met DSM-IV-TR criteria for generalized anxiety disorder (excluding the 6-month duration criteria) comorbid with major depression. Thus, the majority of patients with generalized anxiety disorder also had major depression. A Swedish study found also that 28 percent of 80 patients with acute stroke had generalized anxiety disorder, and 55 percent of the patients with generalized anxiety disorder also had major depression (Fig. 2.2–1). A community-based study reported that 3.5 percent of 89 patients with stroke met International Classification of Diseases (ICD)–9 criteria for anxiety neurosis at 1 month poststroke (Table 2.2–2). Thus, anxiety disorder after stroke is frequently comorbid with depressive disorder, although a significant number of patients have anxiety alone.

Psychosis Although rare, case reports and empirical studies have documented that psychosis may occur after stroke. No epidemiological study has documented the incidence or prevalence of psychosis after stroke.

Apathy *Apathy* is the absence or lack of feeling, emotion, interest, concern, or motivation and has been reported frequently among patients with brain injury. Using an apathy scale, in 80 consecutive patients with single stroke lesions, nine (11 percent) showed apathy as their only psychiatric disorder, whereas another 11 percent had both apathy and depression (Table 2.2–2).

Catastrophic Reaction *Catastrophic reaction* is a term first used by Goldstein to describe anxiety, tears, aggressive behavior, swearing, displacement, refusal, renouncement, and, sometimes, compensatory boasting, which he attributed to an "inability of the organism to cope when faced with physical or cognitive deficits." Using a Catastrophic Reaction Scale (CRS), which was developed to assess the existence and severity of catastrophic reactions, 12 of 62 consecutive patients (19 percent) with acute stroke lesions had catastrophic reactions (Table 2.2–2).

Pathological Emotions Pathological emotions are characterized by episodes of laughing or crying, or both, that are not appropriate to the context. They may appear spontaneously or may be elicited by nonemotional events and do not correspond to underlying emotional feelings. It was found in 13 of 89 patients (15 percent) seen at 1 month poststroke, 21 percent at 6 months, and 12 percent at 1 year (Table 2.2–2). Other studies have reported frequencies of 18 percent in a rehabilitation hospital and 14 percent of patients in a community-based study.

Anosognosia *Anosognosia* is a term first used by Joseph Babinski (1914) to indicate the lack of awareness of hemiplegia. It has been used, however, to refer to unawareness of other poststroke deficits such as cortical blindness, hemianopia, and amnesia. Among 80 acute stroke patients, 24 percent had moderate or severe anosognosia (Table 2.2–2).

ETIOLOGY

Poststroke Depression Although the etiology of poststroke depression is unknown, a number of studies have suggested that location of brain injury may play an important role. One of the first studies to report a significant role for lesion location in poststroke depression examined 36 patients with single stroke lesions of the left (N = 22) or right (N = 14) hemisphere documented by computed tomography (CT) scan but without prior history of psychiatric disorder. There was a significant inverse correlation between the severity of depression and the distance of the anterior border of the lesion from the frontal pole in the left hemisphere and positive correlation in the right hemisphere (Fig. 2.2–2). This surprising finding led to a number of subsequent examinations of this phenomenon in other populations. A recent metaanalysis of 13 studies examining 163 patients found that the correlation between severity of depression and distance of the lesion from the left frontal pole, using both fixed and random models, was −0.53 fixed and −0.59 random ($P < .001$) (Fig. 2.2–3). The correlations in the right hemisphere, however, were not significant.

Other studies of patients with acute stroke have also found an important role of hemispheric lesion location and poststroke depression. For example, a study of 45 patients with single lesions restricted to either cortical or subcortical structures in the left or right hemisphere found that significantly more (44 percent) patients with left cortical lesions or left subcortical lesions (39 percent) were depressed, compared with patients with right cortical lesions (11 percent) or patients with right subcortical lesions (14 percent) (Table 2.2–3).

Although significantly more patients with left anterior lesions developed poststroke depression during the acute stroke period, compared with other lesion locations, not every patient with a left anterior lesion developed a depressive disorder. That raised the question of why some, but not all, patients with lesions in these locations develop depression. Therefore, 13 patients with major poststroke

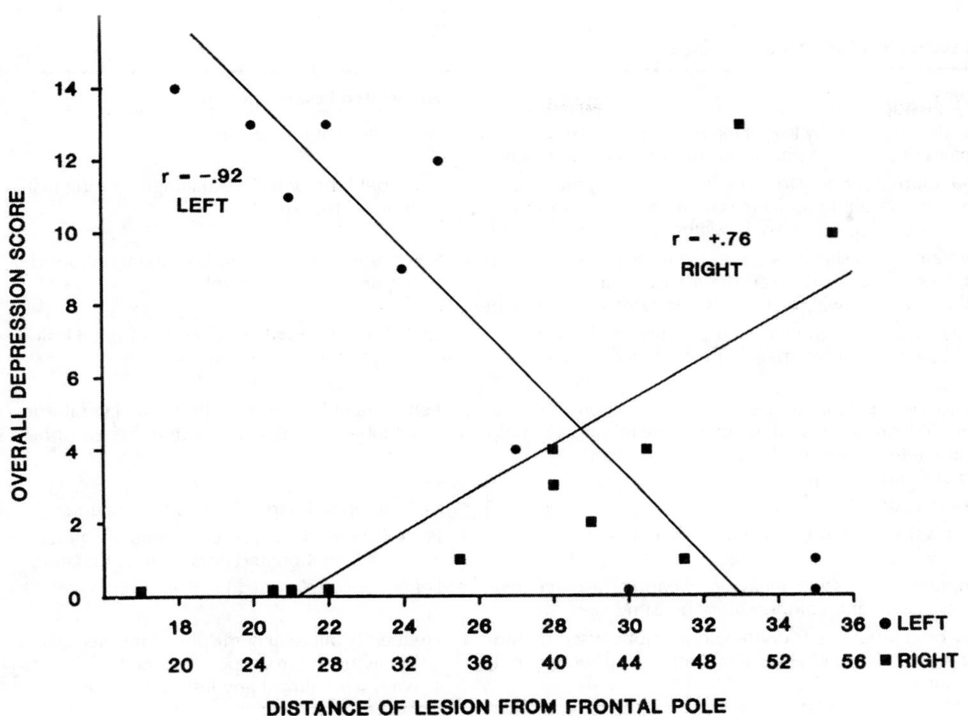

FIGURE 2.2–2 Scattergram showing the correlation between severity of depression (overall score based on a combination of Hamilton depression and present state examination scores) and proximity of the anterior border of the lesion to the frontal pole. Patients had single lesions of the right or left hemisphere and no risk factors (e.g., family or personal history of psychiatric disorder) for depression and were right-handed. Left hemisphere lesions were all anterior to 40 percent of the overall anterior-posterior brain measurement. The severity of depression increased with proximity of the lesion to the frontal pole in patients with left hemisphere lesions; however, for those with right hemisphere lesions, depression increased with the proximity to the occipital pole. (From Robinson RG, Kubos KL, Starr LB, Rao K, Price TR: *Brain.* 1984;107:81–93, with permission.)

depression were compared with 13 stroke patients without depression who were matched for lesion size and location. Patients with major depression had significantly more subcortical atrophy as measured both by the ratio of third ventricle to brain (i.e., the area of the third ventricle divided by the area of the brain at the same level) and the ratio of lateral ventricle to brain (i.e., the area of the lateral ventricle contralateral to the brain lesion divided by the brain area at the same level). It is likely that the subcortical atrophy preceded the stroke because it was visible within a few days after the stroke and was found on the side of the brain opposite the lesion.

Several studies have reported that depressed patients were more likely than nondepressed patients to have either a personal history or a family history of psychiatric disorders. For example, an Australian study of 99 patients in a poststroke rehabilitation hospital found that 11 of 16 patients (69 percent) with major depression after right or left hemisphere stroke had a family history of mood or anxiety disorder, compared with 5 of 18 with minor depression (28 percent) and 20 of 54 (37 percent) who were not depressed (Fig. 2.2–4). There were similar findings for major depression and personal history of psychiatric disorder (i.e., 8 of 16 with major depression vs. 14 of 54 nondepressed; $P = .04$).

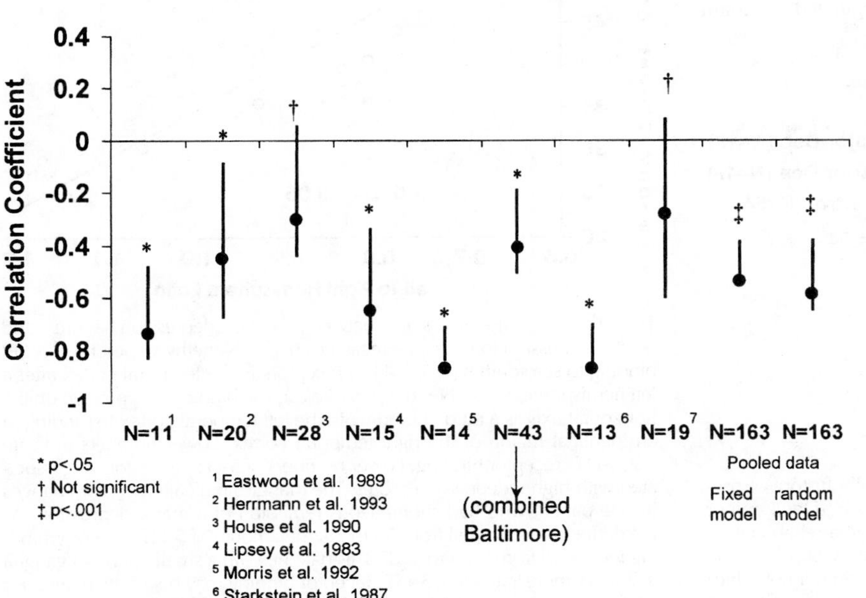

FIGURE 2.2–3 Correlation coefficients between severity of depression and the distance of the anterior border of stroke lesion from the frontal pole in the left hemisphere. The correlation coefficient for each published study and the upper and lower estimates are shown on the figure. Metaanalysis of these studies found a significant inverse correlation using either the random or fixed-model analyses. (From Narushima K, Robinson J: *Neuropsychiatry Clin Neurosci.* 2003, with permission.)

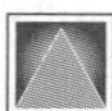

Table 2.2–3
Clinical Syndromes Associated with Cerebrovascular Disease

Syndrome	Clinical Symptoms	Associated Lesion Location
Vascular dementia	Cognitive decline demonstrated by loss of memory and at least one other deficit in domains of aphasia, apraxia, agnosia, or executive function	Multiple ischemic lesions
Major depression	Depressed mood, diurnal mood variation, loss of energy, anxiety, restlessness, worry, weight loss, decreased appetite, early-morning awakening, delayed sleep onset, social withdrawal, and irritability	Left front lobe or left basal ganglia during first 2 mos poststroke
Minor depression	Depressed mood, anxiety, restlessness, worry, diurnal mood variation, hopelessness, loss of energy, delayed sleep onset, early-morning awakening, social withdrawal, weight loss, and decreased appetite	Left posterior parietal and occipital regions during first 2 mos poststroke
Mania	Elevated mood, increased energy, increased appetite, decreased sleep, feeling of well-being, pressured speech, flight of ideas, grandiose thoughts	Right basotemporal or right orbitofrontal lesions or right subcortical lesions
Anxiety disorder	Symptoms of major depression, intense worry, and anxious foreboding in addition to depression, associated light-headedness or palpitations and muscle tension or restlessness, and difficulty concentrating or falling asleep	Left cortical lesions, usually dorsal lateral frontal lobe; anxiety alone with right hemisphere lesions
Psychotic disorder	Hallucinations or delusional	Right temporal parietal occipital junction
Apathy (without depression, with depression)	Loss of drive, motivation, interest, low energy, unconcern	Posterior internal capsule or cingulate gyrus ventral striation and dorsomedial thalamus
Catastrophic reaction	Anxiety reaction, tears, aggressive behavior, swearing, displacement, refusal, renouncement, and compensatory boasting	Left anterior subcortical
Pathological laughing and crying	Frequent, usually brief laughing or crying; crying not caused by sadness or out of proportion to it; and social withdrawal secondary to emotional outbursts	Frequently bilateral hemispheric lesions; lesions involving the frontopontine cerebellar pathways with almost any lesion location

It has been suggested that some cases of poststroke depression may be the consequence of severe depletions of norepinephrine or serotonin, or both, produced by frontal or basal ganglia lesions. In support of this hypothesis, a positron emission tomography (PET) study found that patients with left hemisphere stroke showed a significant inverse correlation between the amount of *N*-methylspiperone binding (predominantly serotonin type 2 [5-HT_2] receptor binding) in the left temporal cortex and severity of depression as measured by the Zung depression scale (i.e., higher depression scores were associated with lower serotonin receptor binding) (Fig. 2.2–5). Patients with right hemisphere lesions, on the other hand, had an increase in 5-HT_2 receptor binding in the temporal and parietal cortex. Thus, an upregulation of serotonin receptors might protect against depression. Patients with left hemisphere lesions, however, may not have upregulated serotonin receptors, therefore producing a dysfunction of biogenic amine systems in the left hemisphere.

This dysfunction in the serotonergic pathways must also be related to the growing consensus about the anatomical circuits that seem to play a dynamic role in the mechanism of both primary (i.e.,

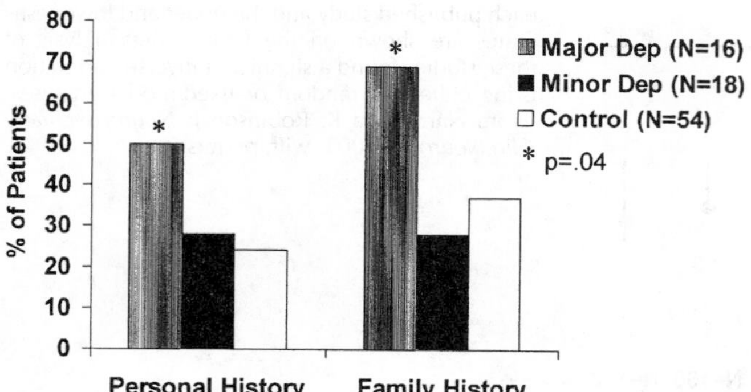

FIGURE 2.2–4 Frequency of a personal history or family history of psychiatric disorder among patients with major depression (Dep), minor depression, or no mood disorder who were hospitalized in a rehabilitation hospital after stroke. Both personal history and family history of psychiatric disorder were significantly associated with major depression but not minor depression. (From Robinson RG. *The Clinical Neuropsychiatry of Stroke.* Cambridge University Press; 1998, with permission.)

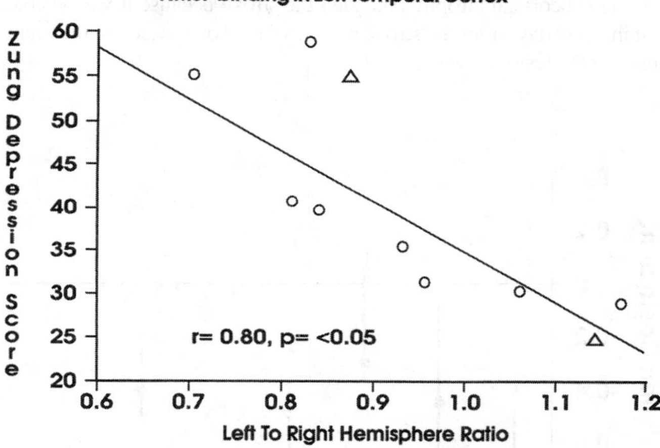

FIGURE 2.2–5 Relationship between Zung depression score and positron emission tomography measures of [11]C-*N*-methylspiperone (NMSP) binding to serotonin type 2 (5-HT_2) receptors in the temporal cortex after a left hemisphere stroke (N = 8; *open circles*). The binding is expressed on the horizontal axis as a ratio of binding in the left temporal cortex to binding in an identical region of the right temporal cortex. Lower numbers indicate less 5-HT_2 receptor binding. Lower numbers of 5-HT_2 receptors are associated with higher depression scores. The triangles indicate receptor changes in one patient who had spontaneous remission of a major depression. As the depression score fell from 55 to 25, the amount of 5-HT_2 receptor binding increased from 0.86 to 1.15. This patient, with a small left basal ganglia infarct, demonstrated that 5-HT_2 receptor binding may be a state marker for poststroke depression. (From Robinson RG. *The Clinical Neuropsychiatry of Stroke.* Cambridge University Press; 1998, with permission.)

no brain lesion) and secondary (i.e., known structural abnormality) depression. There are five cortical basal ganglia circuits that have been shown to play an important role in types of neuropsychiatric disorders. The lateral orbital frontal circuit receives input from the dorsolateral temporal pole (BA38), as well as the inferior and superior temporal cortex (BA20 and BA22), terminating in the magnocellular mediodorsal thalamus with projections back to the orbital frontal cortex. Based on the lesion data and receptor binding data already presented, disruption of the temporal input to this dynamic circuitry may play an important role in the etiology of some poststroke depressions.

Mania A study of 17 patients with secondary mania (mood disorder due to stroke with manic features) found that 12 had unilateral right hemisphere lesions. The frequency of right hemisphere lesions was significantly higher, compared with 28 patients with major depression who tended to have left frontal or basal ganglia lesions or patients with no mood disorder after stroke (Table 2.2–3). Lesions associated with mania were either cortical (basotemporal cortex or orbitofrontal cortex) or subcortical (frontal white matter, basal ganglia, or thalamus). A PET study using [^{18}F]fluorodeoxyglucose (FDG) showed a focal hypometabolic deficiency in the right basotemporal cortex in three patients with right subcortical lesions not seen in seven age-comparable, normal controls.

Thus, mania appears to be provoked by injury to specific right hemisphere structures that have connections to the limbic system. The right basotemporal cortex may be particularly important because direct lesions, as well as distant hypometabolic effects (diaschisis), of this cortical region were associated with secondary mania.

Not every patient with a lesion in limbic areas of the right hemisphere develops secondary mania. Therefore, there must be risk factors for this disorder. One study found that patients with secondary mania had a significantly higher frequency of positive family history of affective disorders than did depressed patients or patients with no mood disturbance (Fig. 2.2–6). Another study compared patients with secondary mania to patients with no mood disturbance who were matched for size, location, and etiology of brain lesion. Patients with secondary mania had significantly greater degree of subcortical atrophy, as measured by bifrontal and third ventricular to brain ratio. Moreover, of the patients who developed secondary mania, those who had a positive family history of psychiatric disorders had significantly less atrophy than those without such a family history, suggesting that genetic predisposition to affective disorders and brain atrophy may be independent risk factors for poststroke mania.

Although the mechanism of secondary mania remains unknown, both lesion studies and metabolic studies have suggested that the right basotemporal cortex may play an important role. The basotemporal cortex has strong efferent connections to the orbital frontal cortex, suggesting that the lateral orbital frontal circuit in the right hemisphere may play a role in the etiology of mania. A combination of biogenic amine system dysfunction and release of tonic inhibitory input to the orbital frontal thalamic circuit may lead to the production of mania.

Poststroke Psychosis Information about the mechanism of poststroke psychosis is derived from anecdotal or small case series. One study of five patients with psychosis after stroke found that all patients had right hemisphere lesions, primarily involving frontoparietal regions (Table 2.2–3). When compared with five patients matched for age, education, and lesion size and location, but no psychosis, patients with secondary psychosis had significantly greater subcortical

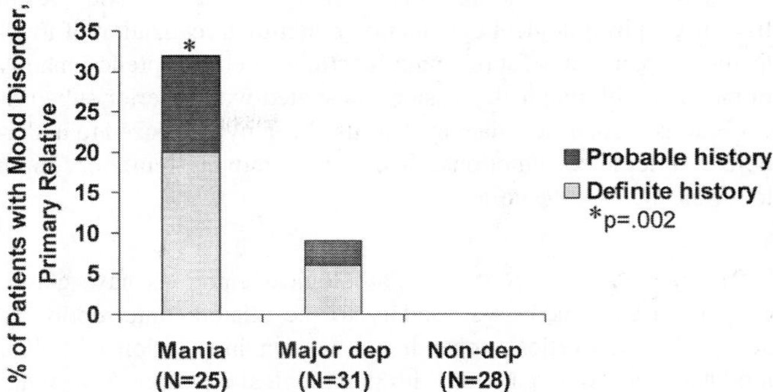

FIGURE 2.2–6 The frequency of family history (definite or probable) of mood disorder in the primary relatives of patients with mania after stroke (N = 15), tumors (N = 6), or trauma (N = 4), compared with poststroke major depression (dep) or no mood disorder (non-dep) after stroke. Patients with mania were significantly more likely to have a family history of mood disorders than the other two groups. (From Robinson RG. *The Clinical Neuropsychiatry of Stroke*. Cambridge University Press; 1998, with permission.)

atrophy, as manifested by larger areas of both the frontal horn of the lateral ventricle and the body of the lateral ventricle (measured on the side contralateral to the brain lesion). Several investigators have also reported a high frequency of seizures among patients with secondary psychosis. These seizures usually started after the brain lesion but before the onset of psychosis. A study of patients with poststroke psychoses compared with lesion-matched controls found seizure disorder among three of five patients with poststroke psychosis, as compared with zero of five stroke patients without psychosis.

It has been hypothesized that three factors may be important in the mechanism of organic hallucinations, namely, a right hemisphere lesion involving the temporoparietal cortex, seizures, or subcortical brain atrophy.

Apathy A previously mentioned study of 80 patients with single stroke lesions found that apathetic patients showed a significantly higher frequency of lesions involving the posterior limb of the internal capsule, as compared with patients with no apathy. Lesions in the internal globus pallidus and the posterior limb of the internal capsule have been reported to produce behavioral changes such as motor neglect, psychic akinesia, and akinetic mutism (Table 2.2–3). The ansa lenticularis is one of the main internal pallidal outputs, and it ends in the pedunculopontine nucleus after going through the posterior limb of the internal capsule. Overall, lesions along the anterior cingulate subcortical circuit (including cingulate gyrus, ventral striatum, ventral pallidum, and magnocellular dorsomedial thalamus) have been repeatedly associated with the occurrence of apathetic syndromes.

Catastrophic Reaction In a study of 62 patients with acute stroke, those demonstrating catastrophic reactions had a significantly higher frequency of lesions involving the basal ganglia, compared with acute stroke controls. When ten depressed patients with a catastrophic reaction were compared with ten depressed patients without a catastrophic reaction, the catastrophic reaction group had significantly more anterior lesions, which were mostly located primarily in subcortical regions (i.e., eight of nine depressed patients with catastrophic reaction had subcortical lesions; three of nine depressed patients without catastrophic reaction had subcortical lesions) (Table 2.2–3).

Based on these findings, the catastrophic reaction may result from neurophysiological dysfunction rather than realization of intellectual impairment. Catastrophic reactions occurred predominantly in patients with major depression associated with anterior subcortical lesions. Subcortical damage has also been hypothesized to underlie the "release" of emotional display by removing inhibitory input to limbic areas of the cortex.

Pathological Emotions Pathological emotions have classically been explained as secondary to the bilateral interruption of descending neocortical upper motor neuron innervation of bulbar motor nuclei. Some patients with pathological emotions have bilateral lesions and pseudobulbar palsy, but others do not. One study found that patients with frontal or temporal lesions in either hemisphere had a significantly increased frequency of pathological emotions (Table 2.2–3). Examination of lesion size and location in 12 patients with pathological crying found that patients with the most frequent crying episodes had relatively large bilateral pontine lesions. The intermediate group had large bilateral lesions. The least affected patients had relatively large unilateral subcortical lesions. It was hypothesized that pathological emotions may arise from partial destruction of raphe serotonergic neurons or their projections. More recently, investigators at the University of Iowa suggested that the critical lesions eliciting pathological laughing and crying are located along frontopontocerebellar pathways.

DIAGNOSIS AND CLINICAL FEATURES

Vascular Dementia *Dementia* is a syndrome that includes both deterioration of intellectual ability and alterations in the patient's emotional and personality functions. Multiinfarct dementia is characterized by an abrupt onset, stepwise deterioration of intellectual function, and gradual accumulation of neuropsychological deficits in which some cognitive functions are more impaired than others. It results from ischemic injury in multiple brain regions. To make the diagnosis, these deficits must not be limited to a period of depression or delirium and must be of sufficient degree to impair work, usual social activities, or interpersonal relations.

Based on DSM-IV-TR criteria, cognitive decline should be demonstrated by loss of memory and at least one other deficit, including aphasia, apraxia, agnosia, or deterioration in executive function. Multifocal deficits are expected, and single defects in cognition, such as amnestic states, aphasia, and apraxias, do not fulfill the criteria. Single lesions may produce vascular dementia if they lead to loss of both memory and some other cognitive function of sufficient severity to produce impairment in daily living.

Poststroke Depression The frequency of depressive symptoms in a group of 43 patients with major poststroke depression were compared with those in a group of 43 age-matched patients with "functional" (i.e., no known brain pathology) depression. The main finding was that both groups showed almost identical profiles of symptoms, including those that were not part of the diagnostic criteria. More than 50 percent of the patients who met the diagnostic criteria for major poststroke depression reported sadness, anxiety, tension, loss of interest and concentration, sleep disturbances with early-morning awakening, loss of appetite with weight loss, difficulty concentrating and thinking, and thoughts of death.

Another study examining the phenomenology of poststroke depression used a Poststroke Depression Rating Scale (PSDRS). The scale included ten items: depressed mood, guilt feelings, thoughts of death or suicide, vegetative symptoms, apathy and loss of interest, anxiety, catastrophic reactions, hyperemotionalism, anhedonia, and diurnal mood variations. The last section on diurnal mood variations is scored between +2 and –2, with +2 indicating a motivated depression associated with situational stresses, handicaps, or disabilities and –2 indicating a lack of associated motivation, with depression being more prominent in the early morning. Patients with poststroke major depression less than 2 months (N = 58), 2 to 4 months (N = 52), and more than 4 months (N = 43) after stroke were compared with 30 patients admitted to a psychiatric hospital with a diagnosis of endogenous major depression. Although the two groups looked identical on most scales, patients with poststroke depression had higher scores on catastrophic reaction, hyperemotionalism, and association with stress or handicap, suggesting an association with disability. Both catastrophic reactions and hyperemotionalism, however, occurred in patients without depression, indicating the comorbid nature of these conditions. The symptoms that are integral to the DSM-IV-TR diagnosis of depression do not include catastrophic reactions or hyperemotionalism. Validation of this new form of depressive disorder remains to be demonstrated.

Mania The symptoms of mania were examined in a series of 25 consecutive patients who met DSM-IV-TR criteria for a mood disorder due to brain injury with manic features. These patients, who developed mania after a stroke, traumatic brain injury, or tumors, were compared to 25 patients with primary mania (i.e., no known neuropathology). Both groups of patients showed similar frequencies of elation, pressured speech, flight of ideas, grandiose thoughts, insomnia, hallucinations, and paranoid delusions (Fig. 2.2–7). Thus, the symptoms of mania that occurred after brain damage (secondary mania) appeared to be the same as those found in mania without brain damage (primary mania).

Anxiety The diagnosis of generalized anxiety disorder based on DSM-IV-TR criteria is termed "anxiety disorder due to stroke with generalized anxiety." It requires the presence of anxiety and worry

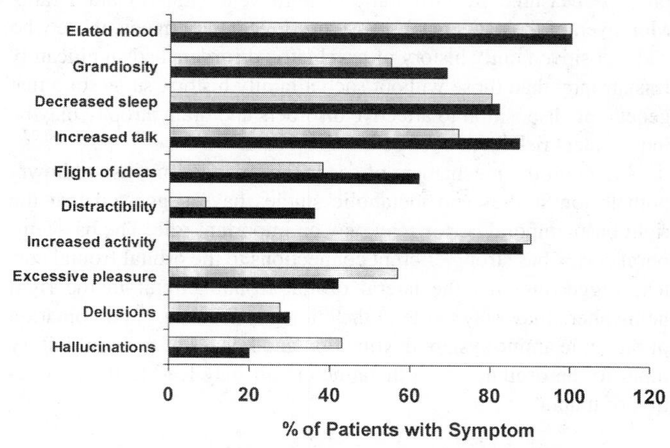

FIGURE 2.2–7 The frequency of manic symptoms found in patients with mania after brain injury (secondary), compared with patients with mania not associated with brain injury (primary). There were no significant differences in the frequency of any of the symptoms, which suggests that the clinical presentation of secondary mania is very similar to that of primary mania. (From Robinson RG. *The Clinical Neuropsychiatry of Stroke.* Cambridge University Press; 1998, with permission.)

for the majority of the time over 6 or more months and the presence of three or more of these symptoms: restlessness or being keyed up, early fatigue, difficulty concentrating, irritability, muscle tension, or sleep disturbance. A study of patients with acute stroke lesions for the presence of anxiety and depressive symptoms found that generalized anxiety disorder (excluding the 6-month duration criteria) was associated with a history of alcohol abuse significantly more frequently than among depressed or control patients. A subsequent in-hospital study found that patients with both generalized anxiety disorder and major depression were significantly more impaired in their activities of daily living (ADL) and social functioning at 1 to 2 years' follow-up than patients with depression alone. Patients with in-hospital generalized anxiety disorder, however, were not more impaired in their ADL or social function than non–generalized anxiety disorder patients. These findings suggest that impairment does not cause generalized anxiety disorder, but generalized anxiety disorder, particularly with comorbid depression, impacts physical and social recovery from stroke.

The patient was a 71-year-old farmer who suffered a basilar artery thrombosis. He developed visual blurring, gait disturbance, and paresthesias of his face. Within 2 months after the stroke, the patient developed panic attacks and generalized anxiety disorder. Generalized anxiety disorder was characterized by almost constant anxiety, worry about minor issues, insomnia, agitation, and restlessness and poor concentration. The panic attacks were characterized by rapid onset of anxiety, with tachycardia, shortness of breath, sweating, and fears that he would pass out or die from another stroke or heart attack. The panic attacks occurred first when he was away from home and later while he was at home. The panic attacks were controlled by alprazolam (Xanax), but, in spite of taking this medication four times per day, he continued to have significant anxiety symptoms of worry, restlessness, nervous tension, poor concentration, and insomnia. Approximately 2 months later, the patient also developed depression, with symptoms of low mood, loss of interest, poor concentration, self-blame, hopelessness, and psychomotor slowing. He responded to electroconvulsive therapy (ECT) but relapsed quickly. He was then treated with nortriptyline (Pamelor), which led to remission of both his depression and anxiety disorder.

Apathy

In a study of 80 acute stroke patients, 18 had apathy, compared with 62 stroke patients without apathy. Apathetic patients (with or without depression) were significantly older than nonapathetic patients. Also, apathetic patients showed significantly more severe deficits in ADL, and there was a significant interaction between depression and apathy. Of the 18 patients with apathy, nine were found to meet criteria for both apathy and depression, and the patients with comorbid apathy and depression were significantly more impaired in their ADL than patients with apathy or depression alone.

Catastrophic Reactions

Catastrophic reactions occurred in 12 of 62 patients (19 percent) admitted to the hospital with acute stroke. Patients with catastrophic reactions were found to have a significantly higher frequency of familial and personal history of psychiatric disorders (mostly depression) than patients without catastrophic reactions. Catastrophic reactions, however, were not significantly more frequent among aphasic, compared with nonaphasic, patients. This finding did not support the contention that catastrophic reactions represent an understandable psychological response of "frustrated" aphasic patients. Furthermore, 9 of 12 patients with catastrophic reactions also had poststroke major depression, two had minor depression, and only one was not depressed. Thus, catastrophic reaction was significantly associated with poststroke depression.

Pathological Emotions

A study of the clinical correlates and treatment of emotional lability (including pathological laughter and crying) was conducted in 28 patients with either acute or chronic stroke. A Pathological Laughter and Crying Scale (PLACS) was developed to assess the existence and severity of pathological emotions. Although there are no generally accepted criteria for the diagnosis of pathological emotions, patients with this condition acknowledged an inability to control their crying or laughter, an increased frequency of emotional display, and a recognition that the emotional display was inconsistent or excessive to their underlying emotional feelings.

PATHOLOGY AND LABORATORY EXAMINATION

Vascular Dementia

The clinical identification of vascular dementia requires a medical history, neurological examination, psychiatric interview, and neuropsychological assessment. Structural imaging studies using CT or magnetic resonance scan should document the existence of one or several cerebrovascular lesions. Laboratory data that can be helpful are blood chemistries (including B_{12}, folate, thyroid function), cerebrospinal fluid (CSF) analysis, an electroencephalogram (EEG) and an EEG with evoked responses, CT, magnetic resonance imaging (MRI), and, in certain cases, cerebral angiography. These laboratory data usually identify potentially treatable forms of dementias caused by tumor; vascular malformation; cerebral hematoma; normal pressure hydrocephalus; infections; and metabolic, toxic, and drug-induced encephalopathy as well as dementia due to vitamin or endocrine deficiencies.

Poststroke Depression

The dexamethasone-suppression test (DST) has been investigated as a possible biological marker for functional melancholic depression. Several studies have demonstrated a statistical association between major poststroke depression and failure to suppress serum cortisol in response to administration of dexamethasone. The specificity of the test, however, has generally been insufficient to allow it to be diagnostically useful. In a study of 65 patients whose acute strokes had occurred within the preceding year, 67 percent of the patients with major depression did not suppress serum cortisol, compared with 25 percent of patients with minor depression and 32 percent of nondepressed patients. The sensitivity of the DST for major depression was 67 percent, but the specificity was only 70 percent. False-positive tests, found in 30 percent of patients, seemed to be related to large lesion volumes.

A study of growth-hormone response to desipramine (Norpramin) found that growth-hormone responses were significantly blunted in patients with poststroke depression, suggesting that diminished α_2-adrenergic receptor function may be an important marker for poststroke depression. The sensitivity of the test was 100 percent, and the specificity was 75 percent. Future studies may further examine the validity of endocrine responses as markers of poststroke depression.

Other Disorders

The usefulness of laboratory examinations in the diagnosis or prognosis of mania, anxiety disorder, psychosis, apathy, catastrophic reactions, or anosognosia has not been established except as discussed in the section Etiology.

COURSE AND PROGNOSIS

Vascular Dementia The course of vascular dementia is characterized by current stroke with associated deterioration of cognitive function. The probability of recurrent stroke is approximately 7 percent per year. The course and prognosis, however, can be influenced by prevention. A longitudinal study of 173 patients examined the frequency of risk factors for stroke and cerebral atherosclerosis among patients with vascular dementia. Although hypertension was the single most potent risk factor for cerebral atherosclerosis and stroke, hypotension, present in 66 percent of cases, was, by far, the most common risk factor for vascular dementia in this sample. Heart disease of the atherosclerotic type, with or without cardiac arrhythmia, was also present in the majority of cases of vascular dementia. Cardiac disease may provide a source of cerebral emboli leading to vascular dementia. Cigarette smoking of one or more packs per day was a risk factor in 21 percent of the patients. Hyperlipidemia of the type 4 form (hypertriglyceridemia) was present in 29 percent of cases. Diabetes mellitus of sufficient clinical severity to require medical treatment was found in 20 percent of the cases, and symptomatic peripheral vascular disease with ischemic symptoms referable to the lower extremities was present in 6 percent of the cases. The association with limited education suggested that prevention efforts that are related to education may be effective in slowing or preventing the disease. Alternatively, the association with limited education may suggest some social or neurobiological benefits of learning that may inhibit the development of this disease.

Depression In a 2-year longitudinal study, a consecutive series of 103 acute stroke patients was examined for depression at 3, 6, 12, and 24 months' follow-up. At the time of the initial in-hospital evaluation, 26 percent of the patients had the symptom cluster of major depression, whereas 20 percent had the symptom cluster of minor depression. Although both major and minor depressive disorders were still present in 86 percent of patients at 6 months' follow-up, only one of five patients with in-hospital major depression continued to have major depression at 1 year of follow-up (two cases had minor depression) (Fig. 2.2–8).

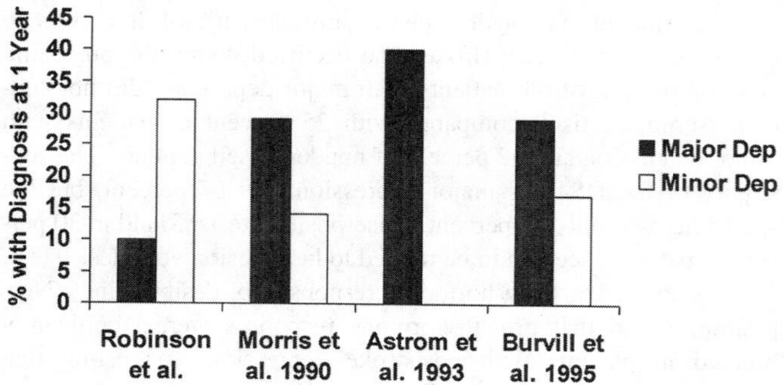

FIGURE 2.2–8 The percentage of patients with an initial assessment diagnosis of major poststroke depression (Dep) who continued to have a diagnosis of major depression or had improved to a diagnosis of minor depression at 1 year's follow-up. Note that the number of chronic cases varies among studies, probably reflecting a mixture of etiologies among the group with an in-hospital diagnosis of major poststroke depression. The mean frequency of persistent major depression at 1 year's follow-up across all studies was 26 percent. (From Robinson RG. *The Clinical Neuropsychiatry of Stroke.* Cambridge University Press; 1998, with permission.)

Another group of 99 patients was studied in a stroke rehabilitation hospital in Australia. Those with major depression had a mean duration of major depression of 40 weeks, whereas those with adjustment disorders (minor depression) had a mean duration of depression of only 12 weeks. These findings confirm that major depression has a duration of approximately 9 months to 1 year but suggest that less severe depressive disorders may be more variable in their duration. Another group of 80 Swedish patients with acute stroke contained 27 (34 percent) with major depression in hospital or at 3 months' follow-up. Of these patients with major depression, 15 (60 percent) had recovered by 1 year of follow-up, but by 3 years' follow-up, only one more patient had recovered. This finding indicates that there may be a minority of patients with either major or minor depression who develop prolonged depression after stroke (Fig. 2.2–8).

Mortality is certainly the most important outcome after stroke. One study of 976 patients with stroke found that patients with depression, assessed at 3 weeks' poststroke using the Wakefield Self-Assessment Depression Inventory, had a 50 percent higher mortality at 1 year, compared with nondepressed patients. Another study of 103 acute stroke patients followed up at 10 years' poststroke found that patients with major or minor depression during in-hospital evaluation had a significantly increased mortality rate over the 10 years (odds ratio, 3.4; confidence interval [CI], 1.4 to 8.4; $P = .007$). A 9-year follow-up of patients who had been treated for poststroke depression found that active treatment with nortriptyline or fluoxetine (N = 69) versus placebo (N = 35) over 12 weeks resulted in increased probability of survival at 6 years' follow-up (Kaplan-Meier log rank, $\chi^2 = 7.3$; degrees of freedom [df] = 1; $P = .006$). The survival rate among patients given antidepressants was 61 percent, whereas the survival rate among patients given placebo was 34 percent. A logistic regression that examined the effects of age, diabetes, relapsing depression, and antidepressant use found that antidepressant use was independently associated with increased survival.

The course of poststroke mood disorders is exemplified by the following case history.

> A 52-year-old married man suffered a heart attack while playing basketball. Two nights later, he had a cardioembolism, producing a large right middle cerebral artery infarct with left hemiparesis and sensory deficit. He developed a depression within 2 months that lasted for several months. After a course of antidepressant medication, he became manic with grandiose ideas, pressured speech, decreased sleep, and increased energy. This was effectively treated with lithium, but another depression ensued with prominent suicidal thoughts and delusional beliefs. This was treated effectively with ECT, and the patient remained euthymic on lithium and nortriptyline.

Mania The course of mania after stroke has not been systematically examined. Anecdotal cases have been reported indicating that recurrent episodes of mania or depression may occur in these patients. The course of this disorder for individual patients with single or recurrent episodes of mania suggests that most patients respond to lithium, although some do not respond to either lithium or carbamazepine.

Anxiety A 2-year follow-up of 142 patients with acute stroke found that 39 patients (27 percent) had the symptoms of generalized anxiety disorder during their acute in-hospital evaluation, whereas

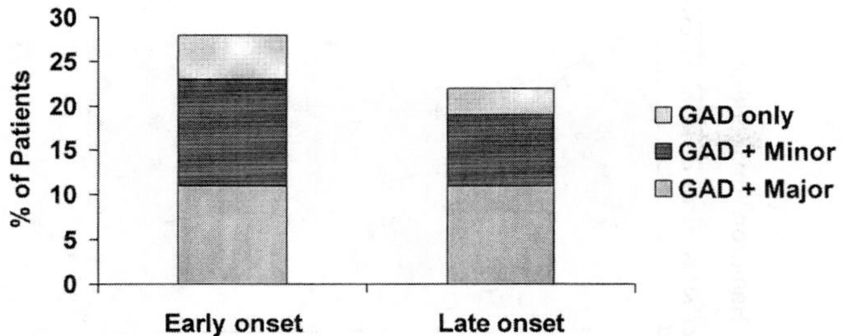

FIGURE 2.2–9 The frequency of generalized anxiety disorder (GAD) with or without depression during the acute hospital period (early onset) and 3 to 24 months (late onset) after stroke. Of 142 patients seen acutely and at follow-up, the number of early- and late-onset cases associated with depression was quite similar. The great majority of GAD cases had associated depression. (From Robinson RG. *The Clinical Neuropsychiatry of Stroke*. Cambridge University Press; 1998, with permission.)

another 31 patients (23 percent) developed generalized anxiety disorder after the initial in-hospital evaluation (i.e., between 3 and 24 months poststroke) (Fig. 2.2–9). Early onset, but not late onset, was associated with history of psychiatric disorder, including alcohol abuse. Early-onset anxiety disorder without depression had a mean duration of 1.5 months, whereas delayed onset generalized anxiety disorder without depression had a mean duration of 3 months. In addition, the existence of anxiety disorder also influenced the duration of depression. Patients with generalized anxiety disorder and major depression had a mean duration of depression that was significantly longer than the duration of depression without anxiety disorder.

Other Disorders

The course and prognosis of patients with psychosis, apathy, catastrophic reaction, pathological emotion, and anosognosia have not been systematically studied.

TREATMENT

Vascular Dementia

Some of the risk factors for stroke can be effectively treated, thus giving hope that the natural progression or even pathogenesis of vascular dementia might be effectively treated. Stroke of cardioembolic origin is responsible for approximately 15 percent of all ischemic strokes, and this percentage is even higher among younger patients. After cardioembolic stroke, anticoagulation is an effective treatment to reduce the risk of recurrence.

In the past decade, treatment with antiplatelet aggregate drugs has reduced the number of repeated ischemic vascular episodes in patients with transient ischemic attacks (TIAs). Acetylsalicylic acid (ASA) and other antiplatelet drugs have been shown to be effective in secondary prevention of stroke. The United Kingdom TIA Aspirin Trial, with 2,435 patients using two different dosages of ASA, found that there was a 21.7 percent and 25.1 percent (depending on dosage) reduction in the risk of nonfatal strokes, myocardial infarction, or death, compared with placebo treatment.

Other therapeutic measures that may be helpful in vascular dementia include antihypertensives (e.g., angiotensin-converting enzyme inhibitors and calcium channel blockers), lipid-lowering agents (e.g., statins), smoking cessation, and prevention or careful management of diabetes mellitus. For patients who are in a "predementia" stage (i.e., history of TIAs, stroke, previous cognitive impairment, or silent cerebral infarctions, but without global cognitive impairment), prevention may include carotid endarterectomy (when carotid stenosis is from 70 to 99 percent). Finally, for patients who are in the dementia stage (i.e., patients who have already shown evidence of cognitive decline in several areas of intellectual functioning), treatment measures may include antidepressant drugs, antihypertensives, cholinergic agonists, antiplatelet aggregation agents, statins, and neurotrophic factors.

Depression

At the present time, there are five placebo-controlled, randomized, double-blind treatment studies on the efficacy of antidepressant treatment of poststroke depression. The first study, reported in 1984, examined 14 patients treated with nortriptyline and 20 patients given placebo. The 11 patients treated with nortriptyline who completed the 6-week study showed significantly greater improvement in their Hamilton Rating Scale for Depression (HAM-D) scores than did 15 placebo-treated patients ($P <.01$). Successfully treated patients had serum nortriptyline levels of 50 to 150 ng/mL. Three patients experienced side effects (including delirium, confusion, drowsiness, and agitation) that were severe enough to require the discontinuation of nortriptyline.

Another study examined 27 patients who were approximately 6 weeks poststroke and were enrolled in a stroke rehabilitation program. They were randomly assigned to trazodone (50 to 20 mg) or placebo. When the analysis was restricted to 16 patients with abnormal DST, seven patients receiving trazodone had greater improvement in Barthel ADL scores than did nine placebo-treated control subjects during 4 to 5 weeks of treatment ($P <.05$).

Another double-blind, controlled trial compared 33 poststroke patients with Hamilton depression scores greater than 13 given citalopram (Celexa) (20 mg for patients younger than 66 years of age and 10 mg for patients older than 66 years of age) with 33 similar patients given placebo. The patients were between 2 and 4 months after acute stroke. Among the study completers, Hamilton depression scores were significantly more improved over 6 weeks in patients receiving active treatment (N = 27) than placebo (N = 32). The response rate to citalopram was 59 percent and to placebo, 28 percent ($P <.05$). This study established for the first time the efficacy of selective serotonin reuptake inhibitors (SSRIs) in the treatment of poststroke depression. Side effects included nausea, vomiting, and fatigue.

Lauritzen and colleagues compared combined treatment with imipramine (Tofranil, 75 mg) plus mianserin (Bolvidon, 10 mg; N = 10) with treatment with desipramine (Norpramin, 66 mg) plus mianserin (27 mg; N = 10). The melancholia scale (MES) showed a greater change in the imipramine than the desipramine group. There were no differences using the Hamilton depression scale.

The most recent treatment study, however, compared depressed patients treated with fluoxetine (Prozac) (N = 23), nortriptyline (N = 16), or placebo (N = 17) in a double-blind, randomized treatment design. Patients were enrolled if they had a diagnosis of either major or minor poststroke depression and had no contraindication to the use of fluoxetine or nortriptyline, such as intracerebral hemorrhage (fluoxetine) or cardiac induction abnormalities (nortriptyline). Patients were treated with 10-mg doses of fluoxetine for the first 3 weeks, 20 mg for weeks 4 through 6, 30 mg for weeks 7 through 9, and 40 mg for the last 3 weeks, 10 through 12. The nortriptyline-treated patients were given 25 mg for the first week, 50 mg for weeks 2 and 3, 75 mg for weeks 4 through 6, and 100 mg for weeks 7 through 12. Patients treated with placebo were given identical capsules of the same number used for the active-treated patients. Intention-to-treat analysis demonstrated significant time-by-treatment interaction with patients treated with nortriptyline, showing a significantly greater decrease in Hamilton depression scores than either the pla-

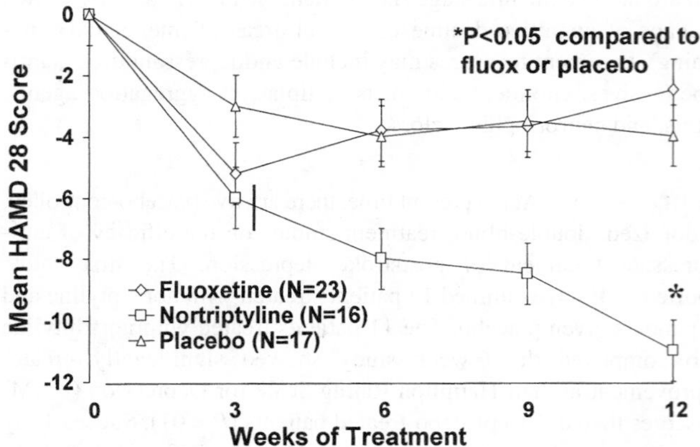

FIGURE 2.2–10 Intention-to-treat analysis. Change in (28-item) Hamilton Rating Scale for Depression (HAMD) score over 12 weeks of treatment for all patients who were entered in the study. Fluox, fluoxetine. (From Robinson RG, Schultz SK, Castillo C, Kopel T, Kosier JT, Newman RM, Curdue K, Petracca G, Starkstein SE: *Am J Psychiatry*. 2000;157:351–359, with permission.)

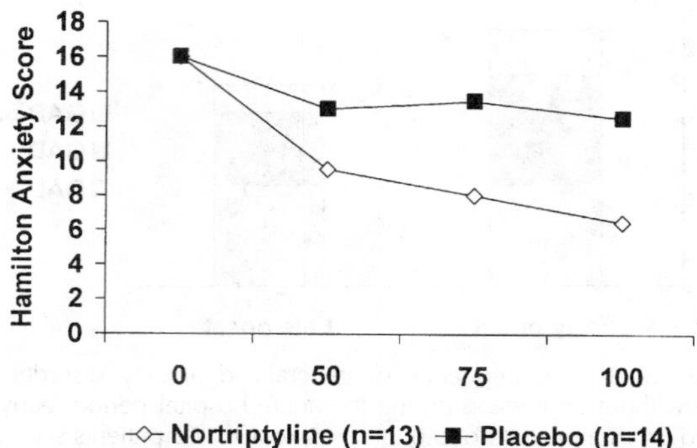

FIGURE 2.2–11 Mean Hamilton Anxiety Scale scores in patients with generalized anxiety disorder and comorbid depression after stroke after double-blind treatment with nortriptyline or placebo. The data are based on a merged analysis of three prior double-blind treatment trials. (From Robinson RG, Starkstein SE. In: Yudofsky SC, Hales RE, eds. *Textbook of Neuropsychiatry and Clinical Neurosciences.* 4th ed. American Psychiatric Press; 2002, with permission.)

cebo- or fluoxetine-treated patients at 12 weeks of treatment (Fig. 2.2–10). There were no significant differences between the fluoxetine and the placebo groups.

Anxiety Disorders

Benzodiazepines are the most commonly used medications in generalized anxiety disorder. Effects include sedation, ataxia, disinhibition, and confusion. As with tricyclics, very conservative dosage and careful monitoring must be used.

Recently, data from three randomized, double-blind treatment studies were merged to evaluate nortriptyline (N = 13) versus placebo (N = 14) in the treatment of patients with comorbid generalized anxiety disorder and depression after stroke. Severity of anxiety was measured using the Hamilton Rating Scale for Anxiety (HAM-A), and severity of depression was measured using HAM-D. Although there were no significant differences between the nortriptyline and placebo groups in demographic characteristics, stroke type, and neurological findings, patients receiving nortriptyline treatment showed significantly greater improvement on the HAM-A and HAM-D scales than patients receiving placebo (Fig. 2.2–11). Furthermore, the anxiety symptoms showed earlier improvement than depressive symptoms, suggesting that anxiety disorders and depressive disorders may be separate but frequently are comorbid illnesses. Finally, buspirone may be useful in reducing anxiety without many of the adverse side effects, such as sedation, and without the risk of development of tolerance. This medication, however, has not been empirically evaluated in poststroke anxiety disorders.

Psychosis

There are no controlled treatment trials among patients with delusions or hallucinations after stroke. Anecdotal reports have suggested two basic approaches to treatment, one using anticonvulsant therapy and the other neuroleptic therapy. The use of anticonvulsants has its rationale in the frequent coexistence of seizures with psychotic disorders after stroke.

Apathy

There have been no controlled trials for treatment of apathy after stroke. Patients have been treated with nortriptyline, apomorphine, and amphetamine with some success. Because this is a relatively common consequence of stroke, treatment trials are urgently needed to address a problem that can be devastating to the recovery of physical and social activities after stroke.

Pathological Emotions

The treatment of pathological laughter and crying in patients with stroke has been assessed in two double-blind, placebo-controlled trials. Using a standardized PLACS, a double-blind drug trial of nortriptyline versus placebo was conducted. The dose of nortriptyline was titrated from 20 mg in week 1 to 50 mg in weeks 2 and 3 to 70 mg in week 4 to 100 mg in weeks 5 and 6. Twenty-eight patients completed the 6-week protocol (four dropped out). Patients on nortriptyline showed significantly greater improvement in PLACS scores, compared with placebo-treated controls. These group differences were statistically significant at weeks 4 and 6. Although a significant improvement in depression scores was also observed, improvements in PLACS scores were significant for both depressed and nondepressed patients with pathological emotions. This indicates that treatment response was not simply related to treatment of depression.

Citalopram, an SSRI, has also been evaluated in the treatment of pathological emotion after stroke. In a double-blind, placebo-controlled crossover study, 16 patients were evaluated. Treatment was given for 3 weeks after a week of washout. All of the citalopram-treated patients reported a greater than 50 percent reduction in the number of crying episodes. There were eight patients who responded within 24 hours of taking citalopram (20 mg), three patients who responded within 3 days, and only four patients who took more than 1 week to respond. None of the patients had major depression, but Hamilton scores dropped significantly during citalopram treatment.

The clinical manifestations of this disorder can be appreciated in a case history.

> A 64-year-old, right-handed, married woman with no history of stroke suffered a thrombotic right hemisphere stroke with a hemiparesis but no sensory deficit. Beginning within a few days after the stroke, the patient had uncontrollable crying episodes that occurred five to ten times per day and lasted approximately 1 to 2 minutes. She and her husband were retired and had an active social life. In addition to the crying episodes, the patient had major depression, with a Hamilton score of 19. She stated that she felt sad, but the crying was greatly in excess

of her sadness at the time, and she had no sense of being able to control the crying. Her PLACS score was 24, which was severe. She showed no improvement over 6 weeks while treated with placebo but improved greatly after a course of nortriptyline. The pathological emotions were more troublesome to her than the depression. She stopped seeing any friends or even leaving the house for fear of being embarrassed socially by these crying episodes.

Thus, citalopram, as well as nortriptyline, appears to be an effective method of treatment for pathological crying after stroke. In addition, poststroke depression and pathological laughing and crying appear to be independent phenomena, although they may coexist. Both depression and pathological laughing and crying, however, are amenable to treatment.

Other Disorders Effective treatments have not been established for catastrophic reactions or anosognosia.

SUGGESTED CROSS-REFERENCES

Basic neurological issues are discussed in Section 1.2. Neuroimaging is covered in Sections 1.15 and 1.16. Neuropsychological tests used to evaluate neurological and psychiatric patients are described in Sections 7.5, 7.6, and 7.7. Delirium, dementia, and amnestic disorders are covered in Chapter 10. Neuropsychiatric complications of epilepsy and traumatic brain injury are discussed in Sections 2.4 and 2.5, respectively.

REFERENCES

Andersen G, Vestergaard K, Ingemann-Nielsen M, Lauritzen L: Risk factors for poststroke depression. *Acta Psychiatrica Scandinavica.* 1995;92:193–198.

*Andersen G, Vestergaard K, Lauritzen L: Effective treatment of poststroke depression with the selective serotonin reuptake inhibitor citalopram. *Stroke.* 1994;25:1099–1104.

Astrom M: Generalized anxiety disorder in stroke patients: A 3-year longitudinal study. *Stroke.* 1996;27:270–275.

Bleuler EP. *Textbook of Psychiatry.* New York: Macmillan; 1951.

Burvill PW, Johnson GA, Jamrozik KD, Anderson CS, Stewart-Wynne EG, Chakera TMH: Prevalence of depression after stroke: The Perth Community Stroke Study. *Br J Psychiatry.* 1995;166:320–327.

Castillo CS, Starkstein SE, Fedoroff JP, Price TR, Robinson RG: Generalized anxiety disorder following stroke. *J Nerv Ment Dis.* 1993;181:100–106.

Denny-Brown D, Meyer JS, Horenstein S: The significance of perceptual rivalry resulting from parietal lesions. *Brain.* 1952;75:434–471.

Eastwood MR, Rifat SL, Nobbs H, Ruderman J: Mood disorder following cerebrovascular accident. *Br J Psychiatry.* 1989;154:195–200.

Goldstein K. *The Organism: A Holistic Approach to Biology Derived from Pathological Data in Man.* New York: American Books; 1939.

Herrmann M, Bartles C, Wallesch C-W: Depression in acute and chronic aphasia: symptoms, pathoanatomical-clinical correlations and functional implications. *J Neurol Neurosurg Psychiatry.* 1993;56:672–678.

House A, Dennis M, Warlow C, Hawton K, Molyneux K: Mood disorders after stroke and their relation to lesion location. A CT scan study. *Brain.* 1990;113:1113–1130.

House A, Dennis M, Mogridge L, Warlow C, Hawton K, Jones L: Mood disorders in the year after stroke. *Br J Psychiatry.* 1991;158:83–92.

Jorge RE, Robinson RG, Arndt S, Starkstein S: Mortality and poststroke depression: A placebo-controlled trial of antidepressants. *Am J Psychiatry.* 2003;160:1823–1829.

Katzman R, Lasker B, Bernstein N. Advances in the diagnosis of dementia: Accuracy of diagnosis and consequences of misdiagnosis of disorders causing dementia. In: Terry RD, ed. *Aging and the Brain.* New York: Raven Press; 1988:17–62.

Kraepelin E. *Manic Depressive Insanity and Paranoia.* Edinburgh: E & S Livingstone; 1921.

Lipsey JR, Robinson RG, Pearlson GD, Rao K, Price TR: Mood change following bilateral hemisphere brain injury. *Br J Psychiatry.* 1983;143:266–273.

Meyer A: The anatomical facts and clinical varieties of traumatic insanity. *Am J Insanity.* 1904;60:373.

Morris PLP, Robinson RG, Raphael B: Lesion location and depression in hospitalized stroke patients: Evidence supporting a specific relationship in the left hemisphere. *Neuropsychiatry Neuropsychol Behav Neurol.* 1992;3:75–82.

Morris PLP, Robinson RG, Andrezejewski P, Samuels J, Price TR: Association of depression with 10-year post-stroke mortality. *Am J Psychiatry.* 1993;150:124–129.

Narushim K, Chan KL, Kosier JT, Robinson RG: Does cognitive recovery after treatment of poststroke depression last? A 2-year follow-up of cognitive function associated with poststroke depression. Am J Psychiatry. 2003;160:1157–1162.

*Narushima K, Kosier JT, Robinson RG: A reappraisal of post-stroke depression, intra and inter-hemispheric lesion location using meta-analysis. *J Neuropsychiatry Clin Neurosci.* 2003.

O'Brien JT, Erkinjuntti T, Reisberg B, Roman G, Sawada T, Pantoni L, Bowler JV, Ballard C, DeCarli C, Gorelick PB, Rockwood K, Burns A, Gauthier S, DeKosky ST: Vascular cognitive impairment. *Lancet Neurol.* 2003;2:89–98.

Paradiso S, Ohkubo T, Robinson RG: Vegetative and psychological symptoms associated with depressed mood over the first two years after stroke. *Int J Psychiatry Med.* 1997;27:137–157.

Ramasubbu R, Patten SB: Effect of depression on stroke morbidity and mortality. *Can J Psychiatry.* 2003;48:250–257.

*Robinson RG. *The Clinical Neuropsychiatry of Stroke.* Cambridge University Press; 1998:491.

Robinson RG: Poststroke depression: prevalence, diagnosis, treatment, and disease progression. *Biol Psychiatry.* 2003;54:376–387.

Robinson RG, Kubos KL, Starr LB, Rao K, Price TR: Mood disorders in stroke patients: Importance of location of lesion. *Brain.* 1984;107:81–93.

*Robinson RG, Schultz SK, Castillo C, Kopel T, Kosier T: Nortriptyline versus fluoxetine in the treatment of depression and in short term recovery after stroke: a placebo controlled, double-blind study. *Am J Psychiatry.* 2000;157:351–359.

Robinson RG, Starkstein SE. Neuropsychiatric aspects of cerebrovascular disorders. In: Yudofsky SC, Hales RE, eds. *Textbook of Neuropsychiatry.* 3rd ed. Washington, DC: American Psychiatric Press; 1997:607–633.

Robinson RG, Starkstein SE. Neuropsychiatric aspects of cerebrovascular disorders. In: Yudofsky SC, Hales RE, eds. *The American Psychiatric Publishing Textbook of Neuropsychiatry and Clinical Neurosciences,* 4th ed. Washington, DC: American Psychiatric Press; 2002:723–752.

Robinson RG, Parikh RM, Lipsey JR, Starkstein SE, Price TR: Pathological laughing and crying following stroke: Validation of measurement scale and double-blind treatment study. *Am J Psychiatry.* 1993;150:286–293.

Rocca WA, Hofman A, Brayne C, Breteler MM, Clarke M, Copeland JR, Dartigues JF, Engedal K, Hagnell O, Heeren TJ: The prevalence of vascular dementia in Europe: Facts and fragments from 1980–1990 studies. *Ann Neurol.* 1991;30:817–824.

Sinyor D, Jacques P, Kaloupek DG, Becker R, Goldenberg M, Coopersmith H: Poststroke depression and lesion location: An attempted replication. *Brain.* 1986;109:539–546.

Starkstein SE, Robinson RG, Price TR: Comparison of cortical and subcortical lesions in the production of post-stroke mood disorders. *Brain.* 1987;110:1045–1059.

Starkstein SE, Fedoroff JP, Price TR, Leiguarda R, Robinson RG: Anosognosia in patients with cerebrovascular lesions: A study of causative factors. *Stroke.* 1992;23:1446–1453.

*Starkstein SE, Fedoroff JP, Price TR, Leiguarda R, Robinson RG: Apathy following cerebrovascular lesions. *Stroke.* 1993;24:1625–1630.

Starkstein SE, Fedoroff JP, Price TR, Leiguarda R, Robinson RG: Catastrophic reaction after cerebrovascular lesions: Frequency, correlates, and validation of a scale. *J Neurol Neurosurg Psychiatry.* 1993;5:189–194.

Welt L: Ueber charakterveranderungen des Menschen infolge von lasionen des stirnhirns. *Dtsch Arch Klin Med.* 1888;42:339–390.

UKTIA Study Group: United Kingdom transient ischaemic attack (UK-TIA) aspirin trial: Interim results. *Br Med J.* 1988;296:316–320.

▲ 2.3 Neuropsychiatric Aspects of Brain Tumors

TREVOR R. P. PRICE, M.D.

DEFINITIONS AND COMPARATIVE NOSOLOGY

Tumors of the brain are of two types: those that originate within the brain and the meninges, that is, primary brain tumors, and those that result from metastases to the brain from malignant tumors outside the neuraxis.

Primary and metastatic brain tumors are frequently associated with secondary psychiatric and behavioral symptoms. These symptoms may include neurocognitive changes, changes in personality, perceptual abnormalities and disturbances of thought content and processes, anxiety and agitation, and mood and affective changes.

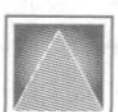

Table 2.3–1
Primary Brain Tumor Frequency

Tumor Type	Frequency (Percent)
Meningiomas	24
Glioblastomas	23
Astrocytomas	12
Pituitary tumors	10
Nerve sheath tumors and primary acoustic neuromas	7
Medulloblastomas and pinealomas	5
Anaplastic astrocytomas and lymphomas	4
Oligodendrogliomas	3
All others	12

Adapted from Yudofsky SC, Hales RE, eds. *Textbook of Neuropsychiatry.* 4th ed. Washington, DC: American Psychiatric Association Press; 2002 and American Brain Tumor Association. *Primer of Brain Tumors.* 7th ed. Des Plaines, IL: American Brain Tumor Association; 2002.

These symptoms often mimic the clinical features of primary psychiatric disorders.

EPIDEMIOLOGY, NATURAL HISTORY, AND PROGNOSIS

Statistical data indicated that, in 2002, more than 186,000 new brain tumors would be identified in the United States, with more than 36,000 being primary cerebral tumors, half of which were benign and half malignant. The remaining 150,000 were metastatic tumors, with breast and lung cancers being the most common primaries. Incidence rates are estimated to be 12.8 and 52.4 per 100,000 person years, respectively, for primary and metastatic brain tumors, with an overall rate of 65.2 per 100,000 person years. Childhood brain tumors, the majority of which are primary, occur at a rate of 3.7 per 100,000 person years.

Brain tumors occur slightly more often in men than in women, and their incidence has been stable in recent years across most age groups, except for those older than 85 years of age, in whom they have been reported to be increasing. This may reflect the increased use of less invasive, more sensitive brain imaging in this age group, resulting in increased tumor detection, rather than a real change in tumor incidence.

The most common types of brain tumors and predominant tumor types by age group are listed in Tables 2.3–1 and 2.3–2, respectively.

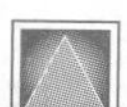

Table 2.3–2
Most Common Brain Tumor Types by Age Groups

Age Range (Yr)	Tumor Types
0–9	Primitive neuroectodermal tumors and medulloblastomas
10–19	Astrocytomas
20–34	Pituitary tumors
35–44	Meningiomas
45–75	Glioblastomas
76 and older	Meningiomas

Adapted from Yudofsky SC, Hales RE, eds. *Textbook of Neuropsychiatry.* 4th ed. Washington, DC: American Psychiatric Association Press; 2002 and American Brain Tumor Association. *Primer of Brain Tumors.* 7th ed. Des Plaines, IL: American Brain Tumor Association; 2002.

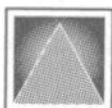

Table 2.3–3
Anatomic Location of Brain Tumors and Frequency of Neuropsychiatric Symptoms

Anatomic Location	Percentage of All Brain Tumors	Percentage with Psychiatric and Behavioral Symptoms (Estimated)
Frontal lobes	22	As much as 90
Temporal lobes	22	50–55
Parietal lobes	12	As much as 16
Pituitary	10	As much as 60
Occipital lobes	4	As much as 25
Diencephalic region	2	50 or more
Posterior fossa, cerebellum, and brainstem	28	Uncertain; numerous neuropsychiatric symptoms reported

Adapted from Lohn JB, Cadet JK. Neuropsychiatric aspects of brain tumors. In: Yudofsky SC, Hales RE, eds. *Textbook of Neuropsychiatry.* 4th ed. Washington, DC: American Psychiatric Association Press; 2002:754.

Brain tumors vary in frequency across different brain regions. As Table 2.3–3 indicates, they are most common in the frontal and temporal lobes and least common in the occipital lobes and diencephalic regions, with pituitary, parietal, and infratentorial tumors being intermediate in frequency.

The prevalence rate for primary brain tumors in the year 2000 was 130.8 per 100,000 persons, which translates into 375,000 people in the United States with medical and neuropsychiatric complications of brain tumors, of which 25 percent are malignant and 75 percent are benign. Notably, the 5-year survival rate for individuals diagnosed with malignant brain tumors has improved from 22 to 32 percent since the 1980s. This increased survival rate translates into a growing number of brain tumor patients who have secondary psychiatric and behavioral symptomatology and require sophisticated neuropsychiatric diagnosis and treatment to enjoy an optimal quality of life.

NEUROPSYCHIATRIC SYMPTOMATOLOGY AND BRAIN TUMORS

A wide variety of psychiatric and behavioral symptoms, often indistinguishable from those associated with primary psychiatric disorders, are associated with cerebral tumors in 47 to 94 percent of cases. The frequency of this association depends importantly on the location of the tumor, with frontal, temporal, and diencephalic neoplasms being most commonly associated with neuropsychiatric symptoms. Based on older studies, it has been suggested that, in as many as 18 percent of brain tumor patients, psychiatric and behavioral symptoms may have been the first indication of a tumor. Making the appropriate diagnosis in such cases is difficult on clinical grounds alone but can be greatly facilitated by the use of the highly accurate, noninvasive brain imaging capabilities now available to the clinician.

Brain Tumor–Associated Neuropsychiatric and Behavioral Symptoms: Anatomical Considerations

Supratentorial Tumors

TUMORS OF THE FRONTAL LOBE Frontal lobe tumors have been reported to be associated with psychiatric and behavioral symptoms in as much as 90 percent of cases, although they may be clinically silent for many years before an accurate diagnosis is made; this often occurs only when focal signs or symptoms emerge or the patient has a seizure. Frequently, frontal lobe tumors are associated with symptoms suggestive of mood disturbances and psychoses, including mania and hypomania, depression, catatonia, delusions, and hallucinations. Tumors of the frontal lobes tend to produce characteristic symptom complexes that reflect their anatomical locations.

Patients with orbitofrontal tumors often exhibit personality changes, irritability and mood lability, behavioral disinhibition and impulsivity, lack of insight, and poor judgment, with consequent social inappropriateness characterized by unaccustomed profanity, tactless jocularity, and inappropriate sexuality.

Tumors involving the dorsolateral prefrontal convexities are typically associated with apathy, abulia, lack of spontaneity, psychomotor retardation, reduced ability to plan ahead, motor impersistence, and impaired attention and concentration. This constellation of symptoms may often be mistakenly diagnosed as a major depressive disorder.

Frontal lobe tumors involving the anterior cingulate may be associated with akinetic mutism, whereas tumors of the falx frequently cause deficits in complex attentional functions. Tumors of the ventral right frontal lobe are often associated with euphoria and secondary hypomania or mania, especially in patients with family histories of mood disorders. Tumors of the left frontal lobe often cause decreased speech fluency and diminished verbal output, word-finding problems, and circumlocutory speech, whereas tumors affecting both frontal lobes are often associated with confabulation, Capgras' syndrome, or reduplicative paramnesias, or a combination of these.

Although frontal lobe tumors do not generally cause a decline in IQ or focal neurological signs or symptoms, they may significantly impair concentration and attentional processes and may interfere with frontally mediated executive functions, which disrupt patients' abilities to think abstractly, plan complex activities, integrate and synthesize information, organize time sequences and complicated behavioral strategies, solve complicated problems, and conceptualize, initiate, organize, and carry through to completion various work and non–work-related tasks.

Such deficits may cooccur with expressive aphasia and dysprosodic speech. Taken together, this constellation of neurocognitive dysfunctions, by themselves or in conjunction with the various other psychiatric and behavioral manifestations associated with frontal lobe tumors, can have catastrophic efforts on the ability of patients experiencing them to function normally in day-to-day life.

A woman who was 51 years of age developed florid schizophrenic symptomatology in association with a possible local recurrence of a temporal lobe tumor that had been removed 2 years previously. There was no family history of schizophrenia, and her premorbid personality had shown no schizoid traits.

She had presented originally with a 15-year history of attacks of visual disturbance in the right field of vision and a 1-year history of grand mal epilepsy. A slow-growing astrocytoma of the left temporal lobe was discovered and was partially removed. She made an excellent recovery, apart from transient dysphasia in the early postoperative period, but, 2 years later, she became depressed for several weeks after her husband had a stroke. As the depression receded, she gradually developed a number of strange ideas—she believed that strangers could read her thoughts and could communicate with her, became distressed when she saw the color red, and felt that words had special significance for her if they contained A as the second letter. With this, she developed occasional hallucinations in the right half-field of vision—of an eye, of a man standing in a room or by a car, or of a sepia-colored scene.

These disturbances increased over several months until she was admitted to hospital. She then showed many of the first rank symptoms of schizophrenia. She believed that her thoughts were read by some radio mechanism and that others betrayed this by gestures; she believed that her husband could alter the train of her thoughts and cause them to block and that he had taken over control of the limbs on the left of her body; she felt that other patients were talking about her and looking at her in a special way and that, when she put on her spectacles, a neighboring patient and her doctor could see more clearly. She also felt strongly attracted to a certain doctor in the ward, but she saw an orange light which meant "no" to her wish to see him alone. She felt that she was caught up in some ill-defined plan involving many people.

Her speech was somewhat circumstantial with loosening of associations, tangential thinking, and occasional thought block. However, her affect remained warm, her personality was intact, and she preserved a certain measure of insight into the abnormal nature of her beliefs and experiences.

Examination revealed a new upper quadrantic visual field defect, a return of her dysphasia, some defect of recent memory, and a slight dropping away of the outstretched right arm. The EEG also showed an increase in slow activity in the left frontotemporal region. A local extension of the tumor was suspected, but angiography failed to give definite evidence of this.

She was started on chlorpromazine (Thorazine), increased to 100 mg three times a day, and, over the next 2 weeks, the schizophrenia-like symptoms began to recede. Coincidentally, her dysphasia and right arm weakness also began to resolve, and the EEG improved to its base-line state. Within 2 months, all psychotic symptoms had disappeared, and she had regained full insight. She remained well when followed up at 6 months after starting chlorpromazine, apart from occasional grand mal and other minor epileptic attacks and a persistent mild defect of recent memory. Residual dysphasic symptoms were again evident, especially when she was tired.

One year later she was readmitted with increasing dysphasia and frequent attacks of falling. She developed increasing drowsiness and a right hemiparesis and died after 3 weeks in hospital. At autopsy, recurrence of the tumor was found in the left frontotemporal region.

(From Lishman WA. *Organic Psychiatry: The Psychological Consequences of Cerebral Disorder.* 2nd ed. Oxford, England: Blackwell Science; 1987, with permission.)

A man who was 58 years of age presented with a 12-month history of extravagance, boastfulness, excessive drinking, marital discord, unrealistic planning, and several changes of job. He had previously held a responsible job in a senior position. He showed a happy, confident manner and believed he was rich but was self-neglectful and grossly lacking in insight. The plantar reflexes were up-going, and there was left papilledema with reduced visual acuity. A left olfactory groove meningioma was discovered.

(From Lishman WA. *Organic Psychiatry: The Psychological Consequences of Cerebral Disorder.* 2nd ed. Oxford, England: Blackwell Science; 1987, with permission.)

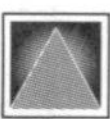

Table 2.3–4
Features of the Interictal Personality of Temporal Lobe Epilepsy

Interpersonal stickiness and viscosity
Increased emotionality with depression, elation, or irritability, or a combination of these
Hostility and aggressiveness
Humorlessness
Hyperreligiosity
Excessive philosophical concerns
Hyposexuality
Hypergraphia

Adapted from Yudofsky SC, Hales RE, eds. *Textbook of Neuropsychiatry.* 4th ed. Washington, DC: American Psychiatric Association Press; 2002 and Strub RL, Black FW. *Neurobehavioral Disorders: A Clinical Approach.* Philadelphia: Davis; 1998;410.

TEMPORAL LOBE TUMORS As many as 50 to 55 percent of patients with temporal lobe tumors experience psychiatric, behavioral, or personality changes. Psychopathology related to temporal lobe tumors can be *ictal*, that is, seizure associated, or *interictal*, completely unrelated to seizure activity.

Patients with tumors of the temporal lobe who have temporal lobe seizures often have seizure-associated schizophrenia-like psychotic symptoms, including auditory hallucinations and atypical dream-like episodes, depersonalization, blanking-out spells, and dazed feelings. The interictal mood reactivity and variability, normal affect, and retained ability to relate to others in a relatively normal fashion that are frequently encountered in such patients help distinguish them from patients with primary psychoses. Olfactory, gustatory, visual, and tactile hallucinations may occur in such patients, with olfactory hallucinations often being part of the preictal aura.

Other patients with temporal lobe seizures may present with depression and frontal lobe–like apathy and irritability, on the one hand, or with features suggesting hypomania or mania, on the other hand. There have been reports over the years that schizophrenia-like symptoms are more frequently seen with left-sided temporal lobe tumors, whereas affectiform symptoms are more common with tumors on the right side. Anxiety symptoms and panic attacks may also be seen with temporal lobe tumors, with the latter being more often associated with right-sided than left-sided tumors.

Personality changes commonly occur and may be one of the earliest indications of an undiagnosed temporal lobe tumor. Personality changes that are seen range from the characteristic symptomatology of the so-called interictal personality, first described by Norman Geschwind (Table 2.3–4), to that more typically seen in conjunction with frontal lobe tumors, such as mood lability, irritability, anger, impulsiveness, disinhibition and behavioral dyscontrol, and socially inappropriate behavior.

Neurocognitive changes due to temporal lobe tumors also occur frequently. These include memory deficits, which may be primarily verbal or nonverbal, depending on whether the tumor involves the dominant or nondominant temporal lobe. Receptive aphasias may also be seen with tumors on the dominant side, whereas impaired ability to discriminate among nonspeech sounds may be seen with nondominant lesions.

A 53-year-old woman was admitted to the hospital after attacking her husband with a knife. She had recently been behaving bizarrely, accusing her family of trying to poison her, and refusing to eat in self-defense. She believed they were spraying the house with poison gas in an attempt to harm her and that her son was turning her into a dog. She also complained of severe headache and pains in the chest and stomach. Immediately before admission, she spent two nights in an alley improperly dressed. Her previous personality had been that of a sociable, quick-tempered, and outspoken woman.

On examination, there were no abnormal neurological signs. Speech was incoherent, but she was mostly unresponsive to questioning. She showed bizarre facial mannerisms and sudden unexpected actions from time to time, for example, sudden rolling of the eyes or abrupt attempts at undressing. After 3 weeks in the hospital, she became stuporose and died. A glioblastoma was found in the right temporal lobe.

(From Lishman WA. *Organic Psychiatry: The Psychological Consequences of Cerebral Disorder*. 2nd ed. Oxford, England: Blackwell Science; 1987, with permission.)

DIENCEPHALIC, THIRD VENTRICULAR, AND HYPOTHALAMIC TUMORS Tumors involving the diencephalon, which includes the thalamus, hypothalamus, and other structures surrounding the third ventricle, are less common than those involving other regions of the brain. They account for only 1 to 2 percent of brain tumors, affecting mainly children, adolescents, and young adults; nonetheless, because they occur in such close proximity to the limbic system and its efferent and afferent tracts, they are frequently associated with psychiatric and behavioral symptoms. In some case series, 50 percent or more of patients have been reported to have had such symptoms. Psychotic and schizophreniform symptoms, depression, mood lability, euphoria, hyperactivity, personality changes, and akinetic mutism have all been described, as have hyperphagia and anorexia nervosa–like restrictive eating patterns. Sleep disturbances characterized by hypersomnia also may occur with such lesions.

Neurocognitive changes due to tumors in this region typically involve memory dysfunction. Other characteristic clinical features of subcortical dementias may also be seen. These include bradyphrenia, bradykinesia, depression, apathy, and amotivational states. Tumors involving the periventricular structures and ventricular system may interfere with normal flow of cerebrospinal fluid (CSF), which may, in turn, cause secondary psychiatric and neurocognitive changes.

A woman who was 24 years of age complained of increasing depression, sleepiness, loss of interest and energy, and recurrent memory lapses. Her depression had been coming on gradually over several months. On examination, she was disoriented for the day of the week and showed poor recall of objects but had no neurological abnormalities. She was apathetic, spoke slowly, and stared impassively. A diagnosis was made of severe depression.

Further examination confirmed marked impairment of judgment and recent memory, and she was considered to be affectively flat rather than depressed. The possibility was raised of hysteria or an organic brain syndrome. Skull X-ray surprisingly showed evidence of raised intracranial pressure, and a computed tomography (CT) scan showed dilated lateral ventricles and a spherical mass in the third ventricle. A colloid cyst was removed, and she ultimately made a full recovery.

(From Lishman WA. *Organic Psychiatry: The Psychological Consequences of Cerebral Disorder*. 2nd ed. Oxford, England: Blackwell Science; 1987, with permission.)

PITUITARY TUMORS Although they only constitute approximately 10 percent of brain tumors, pituitary tumors are associated with prominent behavioral symptomatology in as much as 60 percent of cases. The spectrum of neuropsychiatric symptoms associated with pituitary tumors may mimic a broad range of psychiatric disorders. These include anxiety, depression, and psychotic symptoms due to the direct effects of the pituitary tumor itself, including the neuroendocrine abnormalities it may cause, as well as the frequent secondary involvement of contiguous diencephalic structures as the tumor grows and expands.

Neurocognitive abnormalities accompanying the secondary neuropsychiatric syndromes and neuroendocrine disturbances caused by pituitary tumors, including attentional problems and delirium, are also quite common.

PARIETAL LOBE TUMORS Psychiatric and behavioral symptomatology occurring in conjunction with parietal lobe tumors is less common than it is with frontal, temporal, diencephalic, and pituitary tumors. Patients with parietal lobe tumors have been reported to have secondary psychopathology in as few as 16 percent of cases. The observed symptoms have been primarily affective in nature, with depressive features being more common than hypomania or mania. Psychotic symptoms may also occur but are less common than affective symptoms. Reported psychotic manifestations have included paranoid delusions and Cotard's syndrome, a condition in which patients experience nihilistic delusions that they have lost everything, are dead, and no longer exist.

Although relatively silent with respect to psychiatric symptoms, parietal lobe tumors are associated with multiple neurocognitive abnormalities, many of which have important lateralizing characteristics. They may cause contralateral disturbances in two-point discrimination, joint position sense and stereognosis, and graphesthesia. Tumors of the dominant parietal lobe may cause difficulties with reading and spelling, receptive aphasias, and Gerstmann's syndrome (Table 2.3–5). Nondominant parietal lobe tumors typically cause problems with visuospatial discrimination and anosognosia characterized by a lack of awareness, denial, or complete neglect of obvious contralateral neurological deficits. Various types of apraxias may also be seen in patients with parietal lobe tumors.

OCCIPITAL LOBE TUMORS Patients with occipital lobe tumors also have relatively few psychiatric and behavioral symptoms with the exception of mood variability and visual hallucinations, which may be seen in as much as 25 percent of cases. Typically, the visual hallucinations are simple light flashes, not the complex visual hallucinations of figures and forms that tend to occur in conjunction with primary psychiatric disorders or delirium. Seizure-like visual phenomena, such as simple geometric and color patterns, may also occur as a result of occipital lobe tumors.

Neurocognitive abnormalities are common with occipital lobe tumors. These include homonymous hemianopsia (loss of sight in the same half of the visual field in both eyes) and visual agnosia, in which patients are unable to recognize the objects that they are looking at. A particularly striking instance of this type of dysfunction is the phenomenon of prosopagnosia in which patients are unable to recognize the faces of people who are well-known to them.

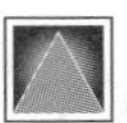

Table 2.3–5
Features of the Gerstmann Syndrome

Finger agnosia
Dysgraphia
Right–left confusion
Acalculia

CORPUS CALLOSUM TUMORS Tumors of the corpus callosum, especially those involving the anterior portion, frequently cause psychiatric and behavioral symptoms. These include depression and psychotic symptoms, as well as personality changes. Neuropsychological abnormalities also often occur with callosal tumors. Depending on the extent and specific location of the tumor, various elements of the callosal disconnection syndrome may be demonstrated on formal neuropsychological testing.

Infratentorial and Posterior Fossa Tumors

Tumors involving structures located in the posterior fossa can be associated with a variety of psychiatric and behavioral symptoms, although it is generally believed that such symptoms are less common with infratentorial tumors as compared to supratentorial tumors. In several case series of patients with tumors involving structures in this area, affective symptoms in the form of depression, mania, and mixed manic and depressive states; phobic anxiety; somatization; personality changes; sleep disturbances; and auditory and visual hallucinations, as well as other psychotic manifestations including paranoid delusions, have been reported. Despite the broad range of reported neuropsychiatric symptoms in patients with infratentorial tumors, no clear association between specific psychiatric symptoms and particular tumor types or locations has been established.

A woman who was 59 years of age with no previous or family history of mental disorder became increasingly depressed and unable to manage her housework after the unexpected death of her mother. Her family noted marked memory impairment. She would put household utensils and money carefully away and then forget where they were, which upset her greatly. When first examined, there were no abnormal physical signs, and her symptoms were considered to be a psychological reaction to the death of her mother 2 months before.

Over the next 6 months, she developed occasional incontinence of urine and some ill-defined difficulty with walking. She was now euphoric and showed much emotional lability. There was a marked memory defect for recent events, some nominal dysphasia, and a suggestion of constructional apraxia. Neurological examination showed a fine tremor of the outstretched hands, brisk tendon jerks, and a shuffling gait, but no papilledema or other abnormal signs. The CSF protein was 90 mg/100 mL but under normal pressure.

She was considered to have an early organic dementia, but, in view of the high CSF protein, ventriculograms were carried out when lumbar air encephalograms proved unsatisfactory. A posterior fossa tumor was found, and, at operation, a hemangioblastoma of the right cerebellar lobe was successfully removed. Over the next 3 months, she improved rapidly and steadily, and, on discharge, she was sensible and fully orientated and had normal memory with formal testing. She returned to full household duties and social life and maintained the improvement when followed up 3 years later.

(From Lishman WA. *Organic Psychiatry: The Psychological Consequences of Cerebral Disorder*. 2nd ed. Oxford, England: Blackwell Science; 1987, with permission.)

PSYCHIATRIC AND BEHAVIORAL COMPLICATIONS OF MEDICAL AND SURGICAL TREATMENTS FOR BRAIN TUMORS

From the foregoing information, it is clear that brain tumors can be associated with a broad range of psychiatric and behavioral symptoms and syndromes. Making the relationship between brain tumors and secondary behavioral changes even more complex is the fact that complications of various therapeutic interventions may also result in behavioral and neurocognitive abnormalities.

These may be similar or dissimilar to the symptoms associated with the tumor that is being treated. Incidental, intraoperative injury to normal brain tissue in the course of surgical resection or debulking of a tumor or tissue injury resulting from peri- or postoperative bleeding or infarction may, on occasion, result in the appearance of behavioral symptoms that are entirely new or represent a worsening of preexisting symptoms. Hopefully, highly accurate preoperative mapping and more precise surgical resection that will be made possible by the use of new technologies such as magnetoencephalography (MEG) will minimize such complications in the future.

In addition, ionizing radiation can damage normal neurons as well as tumor cells. Although every attempt is made to limit exposure to radiation to abnormal tumor cells, normal neurons may be inadvertently damaged, resulting in behavioral symptoms or neurocognitive abnormalities, or both. These may become apparent immediately after the radiation treatment or may be delayed in appearance. Radiation-induced tissue damage and secondary behavioral changes due to it may be transient and reversible, presumably occurring as result of localized edema, which usually rapidly resolves, or it may be permanent and irreversible as a result of radiation-induced brain cell necrosis, in which case secondary psychiatric and neurocognitive changes may be persistent. In rare cases in which severe tissue damage from radiation therapy has been reported, progressive dementia, coma, and eventual death have occurred.

It is important to keep in mind that treatment of malignant brain tumors with various chemotherapeutic agents may be associated with reversible delirium and that treatment of increased intracranial pressure or cerebral edema, or both, with corticosteroids can result in a variety of psychotic and affective symptoms, including mania or depression, or a mixture of both. Typically, such behavioral complications of steroid therapy occur relatively early in the course of treatment when relatively high doses of steroids, that is, 40 mg per day or more of prednisone (Deltasone, Orasone) or its equivalent, are being given. Treatment includes discontinuation of steroid medication, if possible, or, if not possible, reduction in dose to as low a level as possible. If, with the lowered dose of steroids, symptoms persist, antipsychotic medication or mood stabilizers, or both, may be necessary, alone or in combination.

CONTRIBUTING FACTORS IN THE DEVELOPMENT OF NEUROPSYCHIATRIC MANIFESTATIONS OF BRAIN TUMORS

General Considerations

Brain tumors are found more frequently in patients who have psychiatric and behavioral symptomatology than in those who do not. In fact, psychiatric patients are ten times more likely to have brain tumors than are individuals from nonpsychiatric control populations. Autopsy data from chronic psychiatric patients dying in mental hospitals from other causes have shown that unsuspected and undiagnosed brain tumors were present in as much as 3 percent of the patients examined. In contrast, brain tumor prevalence rates indicate that cerebral tumors occur in only 0.13 percent of the general population. Furthermore, neuropsychiatric or neurocognitive symptoms are not infrequently the earliest indication of the presence of a previously unsuspected brain tumor. As previously noted, older studies have indicated that this may be the case in as many as 18 percent of patients with brain tumors.

In reports regarding patients who had experienced early neuropsychiatric symptoms that later turned out to have been the earliest manifestation of underlying, but as-yet undiagnosed, brain tumors, the patients frequently had attributed their psychiatric symptoms to various environmental or situational stresses, such as economic difficulties, losses of loved ones, or other major life stresses.

Much of the discussion thus far regarding the relationships between brain tumors and psychiatric symptomatology has been based on older studies, because there is a paucity of recent reports of large samples of brain tumor patients describing the onset and clinical course of behavioral and neuropsychiatric symptoms occurring in them.

Recent studies of psychiatric patients who had been screened with CT or magnetic resonance imaging (MRI) scanning, or both, suggest that occult cerebral neoplasms may be found in as few as 0.1 to 0.4 percent of unselected psychiatric patients. Clearly, the availability of modern brain imaging techniques has enhanced the likelihood of earlier diagnosis of previously unsuspected brain tumors in psychiatric patients and has led to the much earlier initiation of potentially curative treatments as well.

Anatomical Localization

The notion that certain behavioral aberrations might be specific to brain tumors occurring in particular anatomical locations has for many years been a kind of Holy Grail for neuropsychiatrists studying the association between brain tumors and abnormal behaviors. Most of the available literature, new and old, suggests that, although anatomical localization may be an important factor, it is only one of many factors that must be taken into account in understanding the nature and severity of neuropsychiatric and neurocognitive symptoms that cooccur with brain tumors.

Thus, for example, limbic and infratentorial tumors may cause a broad array of psychiatric symptoms, which are highly inconsistent in their relation to the involvement of particular anatomical structures or regions.

Similarly, although the literature has suggested a tendency for left-sided tumors to cause dysphoria and depression and for right-sided tumors to cause euphoria and symptom denial and neglect, the association between laterality and behavioral symptomatology is by no means consistent. An important issue in understanding the relationship between anatomical localization of tumors and associated psychopathology is that much of the available literature that addresses this issue is old and antedates the application of more recent psychiatric and neuropsychiatric diagnostic classification schema, making many of the clinical inferences from this literature difficult to interpret in current terms.

Neuropsychiatric and behavioral symptoms may arise from structures far removed from the location of a tumor, presumably as a result of the neural phenomenon known as *diaschisis* and the various disconnection syndromes that result from damage to or disruption of interconnecting neural pathways caused by tumors, especially those involving the corpus callosum. Thus, future attempts to more fully understand the etiological relationship of various neuropsychiatric and neurocognitive symptoms to the localization of the brain tumors causing them will need to take into account more sophisticated connectivity models.

Tumor Growth The aggressiveness of the tumor itself and the rapidity and extent of its spread are also believed to be important factors in the type, acuity, and severity of psychiatric and behavioral symptoms that may be associated with it. Thus, rapidly growing tumors are frequently associated with more acute psychiatric symptomatology, as well as significant neurocognitive impairment. Patients with more slowly advancing tumors tend to present with more vague and subtle behavioral changes that are less likely to be accompanied by acute neurocognitive disturbances. Metastatic lesions involving multiple anatomical locations in the brain, in contrast to those occurring in single locations, are more often associated with psychiatric and behavioral symptoms.

Tumor Type In general, the specific histological characteristics of brain tumors have not been shown to be correlated with specific psychiatric and behavioral symptoms. However, as noted previously, more aggressive tumors, such as high-grade gliomas, are more likely to be associated with acute psychiatric and behavioral symptoms than are slower growing malignant and benign tumors. The older literature has suggested that meningiomas are more likely than other types of brain tumors to be associated with psychiatric and behavioral symptomatology. This observation may be less related to histological tumor type than to the tendency of meningiomas to occur disproportionately in frontal regions and to grow slowly and to be relatively silent with respect to focal neurological signs and symptoms; thus, they present more often with vague and subtle psychiatric and behavioral symptomatology.

Other Medical Factors Data from various sources have suggested that changes in intracranial pressure may play an important role in determining the nature and severity of neuropsychiatric and neurocognitive symptoms in brain tumor patients. Increased intracranial pressure due to brain tumors can cause acute central nervous system (CNS) changes that can result in focal and nonfocal neurological signs and symptoms, including diffuse cognitive impairment with changes in attention and concentration and alterations in the level of consciousness, as well as nonspecific behavioral changes ranging from anxiety, agitation, and irritability, on the one hand, to a depression-like state of apathy, on the other hand.

Premorbid Patient Characteristics and Psychosocial Factors The patient's premorbid psychiatric status and history of prior psychiatric illness can have a major impact on the psychiatric and behavioral symptoms that may occur when a brain tumor develops. Acute exacerbations of preexisting psychiatric conditions may occur as a result of the stress of having a life-threatening illness, such as a brain tumor. The patient's premorbid cognitive capacity, coping skills, and adaptive or maladaptive behavioral styles, in conjunction with the adequacy and availability of psychosocial support systems, play important roles in determining the impact and degree of dysfunction caused by brain tumor–associated psychiatric and behavioral complications.

Acute psychiatric symptomatology in patients with brain tumors may be a direct or indirect result of the neuropathological effects of the tumor or may be related to the acute stress of coping with a new brain tumor diagnosis or the ongoing stresses of coping with the various challenges of living with a brain tumor. The latter include the tumor's clinical progression and the mounting neurocognitive and physical disabilities that result, as well as the morbidity that may occur with surgery, radiotherapy, or chemotherapy, or a combination of these.

Although the anatomical location of brain tumors is undoubtedly an important contributing factor in determining the type and severity of psychiatric and behavioral symptoms that may be associated with any given brain tumor, its role is probably less important than that of many of the other factors just discussed.

To summarize, the contributing factors that determine the type and severity of psychiatric and behavioral symptoms that cooccur with brain tumors are multiple and complex. They include, to varying degrees, the tumor type, the rate and extent of tumor growth, the anatomical location, the presence or absence of increased intracranial pressure, and the types of treatment used and the type and severity of complication associated with them, as well as premorbid patient characteristics, psychiatric history, the adequacy of coping skills, and the availability and intactness of psychosocial and family support systems.

A few generalizations with respect to tumor-associated behavioral symptoms appear to be supported by the available literature. These include a higher frequency of psychiatric and behavioral symptoms and neurocognitive dysfunctions with supratentorial tumors, as compared to infratentorial tumors; with frontotemporolimbic and deep midline tumors, as compared to parietooccipital and posterior fossa tumors; with increased intracranial pressure, as opposed to normal intracranial pressure; with multifocal tumors, as compared to unifocal tumors; with rapidly and aggressively growing malignant tumors, as compared to slower-growing malignant and benign tumors; with more aggressive surgical and nonsurgical interventions; and in patients with preexisting psychiatric illnesses and less robust premorbid intellectual capabilities, less adaptive coping skills, and less adequate family and psychosocial supports.

DIAGNOSTIC CONSIDERATIONS

Brain tumors can cause specific focal and localizing neurological and neuropsychological signs and symptoms (Table 2.3–6), as well as nonspecific, nonfocal psychiatric, behavioral, and neurocognitive symptoms and disturbances of functional capacity.

Although newer, more sophisticated, and less invasive brain imaging capabilities have led to earlier diagnosis of many brain tumors, psychiatrists must still be cognizant of the fact that brain tumors may initially present with vague, subtle, and nonspecific psychiatric and behavioral changes. Thus, the psychiatrist must have a high index of suspicion and a low threshold for considering the possibility of a brain tumor in the differential diagnosis of patients with new-onset psychiatric symptoms, especially if they have a negative past personal and family history for psychiatric illnesses, and especially if the symptoms have atypical features and are associated with otherwise unexplained personality changes or newly appearing neurological or neurocognitive abnormalities and dysfunction, or a combination of these.

In such instances, the psychiatrist should inquire carefully of the patient and family members who know the patient well about any of the symptoms that are commonly associated with brain tumors, including motor, sensory, gait, and equilibrium changes; seizures (or seizure-like activity); new-onset headaches; visual or auditory changes; unexplained nausea and vomiting; or subtle cognitive, memory, behavioral, personality, or functional changes; or a combination of these.

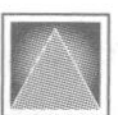

Table 2.3–6
Neurological and Neuropsychologic Findings with Localizing Value

Brain Region	Neurological and Neuropsychological Findings
Frontal lobes	
Prefrontal	Contralateral grasp reflex, executive functioning deficits (inability to formulate goals, to plan, and to effectively carry out these plans), decreased oral fluency (dominant hemisphere), decreased design fluency (nondominant hemisphere), motor perseveration or impersistence, and inability to hold set
Posterior	Contralateral hemiparesis; decreased motor strength, speed, and coordination; and Broca's aphasia
Temporal lobes	Partial complex seizures, contralateral homonymous inferior quadrantanopsia, Wernicke's aphasia, decreased learning and retention of verbal material (dominant hemisphere), decreased learning and retention of nonverbal material (nondominant hemisphere), amusia (nondominant hemisphere), and auditory agnosia
Parietal lobes	Partial sensory seizures, agraphesthesia, astereognosis, anosognosia, Gerstmann's syndrome (acalculia, agraphia, finger agnosia, and right–left confusion), ideomotor and ideational apraxia, constructional apraxia, agraphia with alexia, dressing apraxia, prosopagnosia, and visuospatial problems
Occipital lobes	Partial sensory seizures with visual phenomena, homonymous hemianopsia, alexia, agraphia, prosopagnosia, color agnosia, and construction apraxia
Corpus callosum	Callosal apraxia
Thalamus	Contralateral hemisensory loss and pain
Basal ganglia	Contralateral choreoathetosis, dystonia, rigidity, motor perseveration, and parkinsonian tremor
Pituitary	Bitemporal hemianopia, optic atrophy, hypopituitarism, and hypothalamus and diabetes insipidus
Pineal	Loss of upward gaze (Parinaud's syndrome)
Cerebellum	Ipsilateral hypotonia, ataxia, dysmetria, intention tremor, and nystagmus toward side of tumor
Brainstem	
Midbrain	Pupillary and extraocular muscle abnormalities and contralateral hemiparesis
Pons	Sixth and seventh nerve involvement (diplopia and ipsilateral facial paralysis)

From Lohn JB, Cadet JK. Neuropsychiatric aspects of brain tumors. In: Yudofsky SC, Hales RE, eds. *Textbook of Neuropsychiatry.* 4th ed. Washington, DC: American Psychiatric Association Press; 1987:354, with permission.

Indications for Brain Imaging and Further Neurological Evaluation to Rule Out Brain Tumors in Psychiatric Patients Established, as well as newly identified, psychiatric patients presenting with specific neurological complaints suggesting the possibility of an intracranial process in conjunction with focal neurological findings on examination usually rapidly receive definitive diagnostic evaluation in the form of computerized axial tomography (CAT) or MRI scanning, or both. Patients with more subtle, nonspecific, and atypical features, including behavioral symptoms on clinical evaluation, present a more difficult problem. These patients raise the important question as to when patients with psychiatric and behavioral symptoms should be referred for brain imaging or more specific neurological evaluations, or both.

Certain clinical characteristics should be carefully sought in such patients and, if present, should strongly indicate the need to rule out an underlying brain tumor with appropriate brain imaging studies. These features include the symptoms listed in Table 2.3–7.

The presence of these symptoms, alone and especially if multiple, should lead to prompt neurological evaluation, including a careful assessment of the nature and time course of neurological symptoms, physical and neurological examinations, neurocognitive screening with the Mini-Mental State Examination (MMSE), and specifically targeted formal neuropsychological testing, as indicated. Based on the initial clinical information elicited by these assessments, structural and functional brain imaging, electrophysiological studies, or lumbar puncture and laboratory examination of the CSF, or a combination of these, may be indicated.

It is important for the clinician to bear in mind that even a careful neurological assessment may not initially or even for a considerable period of time elicit focal neurological signs with localizing values like those listed in Table 2.3–6 in patients with brain tumors. Such signs may only be elicited after the tumor has been present for a considerable period of time, especially with slow-growing tumors involving a relatively silent brain region, including the posterior fossa, corpus callosum, prefrontal regions, and nondominant temporal and parietal lobes. It is patients with these types of tumors who may frequently have psychiatric and behavioral symptoms as the first indication of an underlying brain tumor. Definitive brain imaging studies are indicated in psychiatric patients with new or preexisting psychiatric and behavioral symptoms accompanied by focal neurological findings and also in those in whom focal signs are not present but in whom one or more of the symptoms listed in Table 2.3–7 are present.

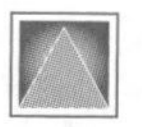

Table 2.3–7
Symptoms Suggestive of Brain Tumors in Psychiatric Patients

A history of newly appearing focal, partial, or generalized seizures or seizure-like phenomena in adult patients, because the first occurrence of a seizure in an adult may indicate the presence of a brain tumor
A history of recent onset, increased frequency, or progression in severity of headaches, or combination of these, particularly if the headaches are persistent and nonmigrainous in character, and especially if they are nocturnal, present on awakening, or worsened by positional changes or Valsalva's maneuver, or a combination of these
Nausea and vomiting, especially if associated with nonmigrainous headaches
Decrease in visual acuity, field cuts, and double vision
Unilateral high-frequency hearing loss, intermittent tinnitus, vertigo
Focal weakness
Focal sensory loss, paresthesias, and dysesthesias
Gait disturbances, incoordination, ataxia, and dysarthria

DIAGNOSTIC STUDIES

Structured Imaging

General Considerations The introduction of CAT scanning in the 1970s and the later development of MRI scanning in the 1980s have vastly improved the diagnosis of brain tumors, have led to earlier initiation of definitive treatments, have enhanced clinical outcomes, and have improved overall rates of survival. The enormous advances in recent decades in image resolution, ease of administration, enhanced patient safety and acceptance with CAT and MRI scanning in comparison to older, less accurate, more dangerous, and less well-tolerated diagnostic approaches, such as plain skull films, radioisotope brain scans, pneumoencephalography (PEG), and cerebral arteriography, have made a remarkable difference in reducing morbidity and mortality in patients with brain tumors.

Plain Skull X-Ray Skull X-rays are now only infrequently used in the diagnosis of brain tumors. They may play an important role in the tomographic evaluation of tumors, such as pituitary adenomas and craniopharyngiomas involving the sella turcica, and in the evaluation of intracranial calcifications or bony metastases involving the skull, although bone scanning is the preferred means of evaluation of the latter.

Computerized Axial Tomography: CAT Scanning Widespread use of the CAT scan, beginning in the 1970s, significantly improved the clinician's ability to diagnose small, soft tissue lesions in the brain. Although CAT scans are effective in diagnosing 90 percent of cerebral tumors, their diagnostic efficacy has been further enhanced by the use of intravenous (IV) contrast material that enhances the visibility of tumors that might otherwise not be identified.

Certain types of tumors are difficult to identify with CAT scans. These include lesions less than 0.5 cm in diameter; tumors occurring in close proximity to bony structures, such as acoustic neuromas, pituitary tumors, and skull base tumors, such as clival chordomas and some meningiomas; low-grade astrocytomas; tumors involving brainstem structures; tumors that are isodense in relation to CSF or brain parenchyma, or both; and carcinomatosis of the meninges, in which tumor involvement is diffuse and nonlocalized. Such tumors are often not identified by CAT scanning and require MRI scanning for optimal diagnosis. Although CAT scan image acquisition requires less time in the scanner than does MRI, which is an advantage, CAT scanning does involve radiation exposure, although of a relatively low degree, whereas MRI scanning does not.

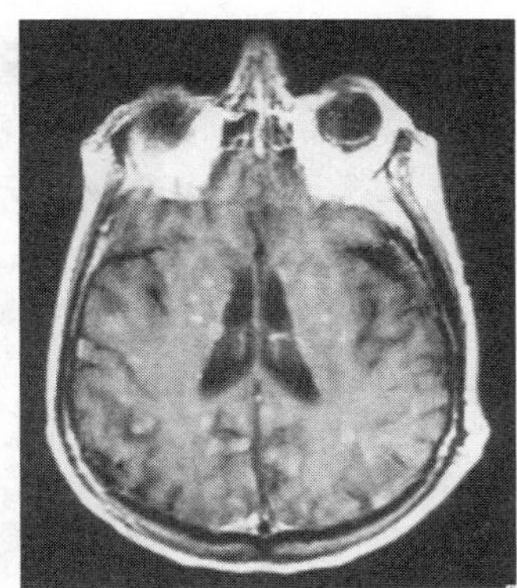

FIGURE 2.3–1 Diffuse metastatic disease (small cell carcinoma of the lung) in a 66-year-old man, as seen with magnetic resonance imaging. A computed tomography scan had not shown any metastatic lesions. (Courtesy of Dr. A. Goldberg, Department of Radiology, Allegheny General Hospital, Pittsburgh, PA.)

CAT scans may be useful in the evaluation of tumors having calcifications, erosion of bony intracranial structures by tumors, the presence of focal or diffuse cerebral edema, shifts in middle cerebral structures due to the presence of a tumor, and abnormalities involving the ventricular system, such as tumor-associated obstructive hydrocephalus.

Magnetic Resonance Imaging (MRI) MRI scans are superior to CAT scans in the diagnosis of small neoplasms, that is, those less than 0.5 cm in diameter; skull base tumors and infratentorial and posterior fossa tumors involving cerebellar, midbrain, and brainstem structures (Figs. 2.3–1 and 2.3–2). As with CAT scanning, the ability of MRI to identify small intracranial tumors is enhanced by the use of IV contrast material (Fig. 2.3–3). As a result of its greater image resolution capability, MRI is superior to CAT scanning in identifying the specific nature of brain tumors,

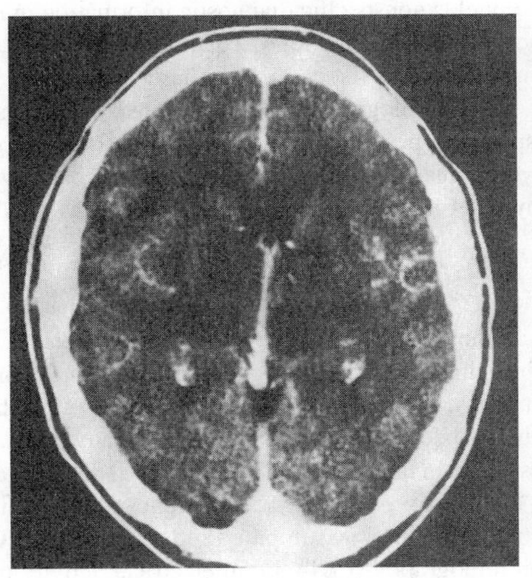

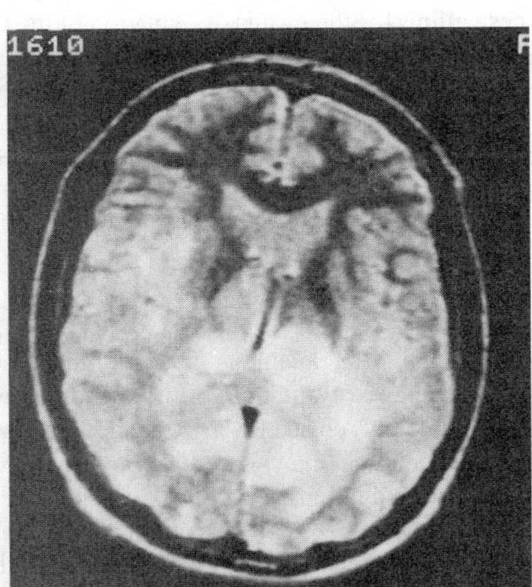

A,B

FIGURE 2.3–2 Brain images of a 50-year-old man with a multicentric glioma. A computed tomography scan shows no evidence of tumor **(A)**. In a magnetic resonance imaging scan, the tumor is clearly evident **(B)**. (Courtesy of Dr. A. Goldberg, Department of Radiology, Allegheny General Hospital, Pittsburgh, PA.)

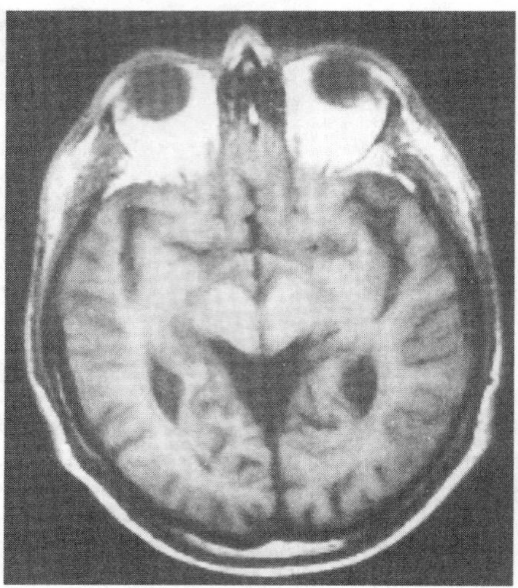
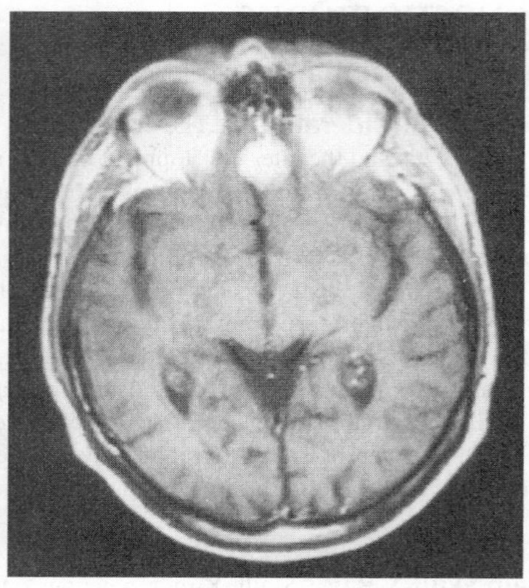

A,B

FIGURE 2.3–3 Brain images of a 70-year-old man with a meningioma. This tumor was not evidenced on an unenhanced magnetic resonance imaging (MRI) scan **(A)** but was seen clearly with a gadolinium-enhanced MRI scan **(B)**. (Courtesy of Dr. A. Goldberg, Department of Radiology, Allegheny General Hospital, Pittsburgh, PA.)

that is, whether they are solid or cystic, or both, and in more precisely defining the relationship of a given tumor to nearby vascular structures.

Potential clinical applications of newer MRI-based diagnostic techniques, including MRI spectroscopy, as well as fast and echoplanar MRI scanning, are currently being studied. In the future, these newer techniques will enhance the ability to evaluate in vivo tumor properties, such as blood supply, perfusion, and tissue metabolism, and may assist in the differentiation of radiological changes indicative of extension, recurrence, and regrowth of a tumor previously treated with radiation therapy from benign scarring consequent to that treatment. Intraoperative MRI scans with open MRI scanning have shown considerable promise in enhancing image-guided surgery, in terms of improved surgical outcomes as well as reduced postsurgical morbidity.

Although, in terms of diagnostic sensitivity and lack of exposure to radiation, MRI is superior to CAT scanning, it is more expensive, involves considerably longer image acquisition time, and is often less well-tolerated by patients because of the confined space and loud noises in the scanner and the resultant anxiety and claustrophobia that some patients experience during the scanning procedure.

CT and MRI Cisternography CT and MRI cisternography techniques are used in special circumstances calling for the evaluation of the circulation of CSF, the morphology of the ventricular system, the subarachnoid spaces, and the basilar cisterns. They may be helpful in diagnosing tumor-associated hydrocephalus and CSF leaks, as well as the presence of intraventricular tumors. MRI cisternography is noninvasive, does not involve radiation exposure, and provides better resolution than does CT cisternography. These newer techniques have completely replaced pneumencephalography in the diagnostic evaluation of brain tumors.

Cerebral Angiography Although functional MRI imaging techniques are being increasingly used in the preoperative evaluation of tumor vascular supply and may eventually completely replace traditional cerebral angiography in the diagnosis and surgical management of brain tumors, the latter is still used in certain situations.

Electroencephalography (EEG) Electroencephalography (EEG) is a noninvasive diagnostic procedure that may be helpful in the initial assessment of whether significant brain pathology is present. The EEG most often yields information that is nonspecific and of relatively little value in defining the specific nature and precise location of intracranial pathology. In 10 to 25 percent of patients with undiagnosed brain tumors, the EEG may reveal no abnormal findings at all or only abnormalities that are nonspecific and nondiagnostic, unless the tumor is causing seizure activity. In such cases, paroxysmal or continuous discharges, such as spikes, sharp waves, and slow wave activity, focal or diffuse, may be seen.

EEG abnormalities are more common with rapidly growing, aggressive tumors and less common with slow-growing tumors, such as low-grade astrocytomas, meningiomas, pituitary tumors, and posterior fossa tumors. To summarize, although helpful in determining the presence of significant brain pathology, the EEG is of relatively little value in the differential diagnosis of its specific nature and etiology.

Lumbar Puncture and CFS Examination Clinicians currently have a wide variety of safe, well-tolerated, noninvasive diagnostic studies that often yield highly specific information in the evaluation of brain tumors. Lumbar punctures are invasive and involve a certain degree of risk in brain tumor patients, especially those with increased intracranial pressure. Because laboratory examination of the CSF yields nonspecific diagnostic information in most cases, it is a procedure that is used less frequently in the evaluation of brain tumors now than was the case in the past. However, it may be quite helpful when cytology studies are required in the assessment of certain specific types of neoplasms involving the CNS, such as leukemias, lymphomas, and meningeal carcinomatosis, which may be missed by other neurodiagnostic approaches.

Other Diagnostic Procedures Given the fact that 80 percent of metastatic tumors in the brain originate from lung, breast, kidney, and gastrointestinal (GI) cancers and malignant melanomas, obtaining a chest X-ray, urinalysis, and stool guaiac, ensuring that a recent breast exam has been done, and inquiring about any suspicious skin lesions are essential in the evaluation of possible CNS metastases.

Other newer, quantitative, computerized, diagnostic capabilities, including single photon emission computed tomography (SPECT), positron emission tomography (PET), brain electrical activity mapping (BEAM), and MEG, hold considerable promise for improving the diagnosis and treatment of brain tumors in the future.

Although not currently in routine clinical use, these techniques may have a unique use in special situations in the future. Thus, for example, SPECT and PET may enhance the ability to differentiate tumor recurrence from radiation necrosis and scarring in patients who have received prior radiation therapy and have new radiological changes on structural imaging studies (Figs. 2.3–2 and 2.3–3). They may also allow differentiation between the occurrence of CNS lymphoma and opportunistic infections, such as toxoplasmic encephalitis, in acquired immune deficiency syndrome (AIDS) patients. Also, MEG may be helpful in more precisely characterizing the phenomenon of diaschisis and the various disconnection syndromes, which frequently occur in brain tumor patients. It also promises to allow for noninvasive in vivo localization of specialized cortical function, such as motor, speech, vision, etc., preoperatively in brain tumor patients to plan for surgical resections that remove as much pathological tissue as possible with minimal risk of inadvertently damaging these and other critical cortical functions as a result.

TREATMENT OF BRAIN TUMOR–ASSOCIATED PSYCHIATRIC AND BEHAVIORAL SYMPTOMS

When a psychiatric disturbance is directly caused by a cerebral tumor, surgical removal of the neoplasm may lead to complete remission of the patient's behavioral and neurocognitive symptoms. In cases in which complete removal of the tumor is not possible, various treatment interventions, whether operative, chemotherapeutic, or with radiation therapy alone, in combination, or sequentially, aimed at decreasing the size (debulking) of the tumor or inhibiting its growth or potential for further spread may favorably impact the patient's psychiatric and behavioral status. In addition, in brain tumor patients, drug treatments that reduce increased intracranial pressure and cerebral edema, as well as shunting procedures that relieve hydrocephalus, may be quite effective in rapidly reducing psychiatric and neurocognitive symptomatology, even though the brain tumor itself is unchanged.

The psychiatrist is most often consulted when the patient's behavior or neurocognitive symptoms persist or become more severe after treatment of the brain tumor itself has been initiated. Appropriate diagnosis and treatment of such patients may reduce symptomatic distress, improve functional ability, and enhance overall well-being and quality of life. Optimal treatment interventions typically involve pharmacotherapy and supportive psychotherapy of the patient, psychoeducation and support of the family, and clear communication regarding treatment recommendations with the patient's neurosurgeon. Ameliorating nonspecific agitation, irritability, dysphoria, and anxiety, as well as any specific psychiatric symptomatology that may be present, with appropriate medication therapy in conjunction with psychological support for the patient and education of family members is often enormously helpful.

The proportion of brain tumor patients with psychiatric disturbances exclusively due to the direct effects of the tumor is relatively small. Given the high lifetime prevalence of mood and anxiety disorders, as well as other psychiatric disorders, in the general population at large and, hence, in patients who eventually develop brain tumors, symptoms indicative of such disorders in brain tumor patients are likely to have resulted from exacerbations of psychiatric illnesses present before the development of the tumor.

In many instances, acute exacerbations of these disorders have emerged in response to the fear and stress of being diagnosed with a brain tumor, having to undergo a variety of painful and unpleasant surgical or medical treatments, or both, having an uncertain prognosis, or the possibility of facing an untimely and likely painful death. In many brain tumor patients, psychiatric and behavioral symptoms result from increasing dysfunction and disability due to the tumor itself or from side effects or complications related to the various therapeutic interventions that have been part of its treatment.

In developing a treatment approach, the psychiatrist should make every effort to characterize the patient's psychiatric and behavioral symptoms as being primarily tumor-associated, with no prior psychiatric history; due to an exacerbation of a preexisting psychiatric condition; or largely due to a psychological reaction to illness-related stressors. Although frequently unclear, such diagnostic differentiation can be helpful in planning optimal pharmacological and psychotherapeutic treatment interventions with patients and their families.

DRUG AND OTHER SOMATIC TREATMENTS OF ACUTE EXACERBATIONS OF PREEXISTING PSYCHIATRIC ILLNESSES IN BRAIN TUMOR PATIENTS

In general, drug treatments of acute exacerbations of preexisting psychiatric disorders in patients with cerebral neoplasms should, with a few notable exceptions, follow the same general principles as treatment of clinically similar patients who are tumor free. These exceptions relate to the fact that patients with brain tumors, as is the case in many patients with other coarse brain diseases, are more susceptible to the CNS side effects of psychotropic medications. These include acute metabolic encephalopathy and delirium, which occur very frequently in brain tumor patients during the early postoperative period after craniotomy for tumor resection or in those who have received radiation therapy or chemotherapeutic agents as nonsurgical treatments of their brain tumors.

Many of the older psychopharmacological agents, including the tertiary amine tricyclic antidepressants (TCAs), the low-potency typical antipsychotics, the anticholinergic antiparkinsonian drugs, the benzodiazepines as a group, and lithium carbonate, are all potentially deliriant and should probably be used only in brain tumor patients in whom they have had documented prior efficacy and have been well tolerated. If any of these medications are to be used in patients who have received them before and have subsequently developed a brain tumor, they should be introduced in low doses and should be gradually titrated to effective dose levels to avoid precipitation of a drug-induced delirium.

In patients who fail to respond adequately to or are intolerant of the side effects of previously effective drug treatments, and in those who have not responded well to them in the past, newer alternatives, such as second and third generation antidepressants, atypical antipsychotics, nonbenzodiazepine anxiolytics, nonanticholinergic antidepressants, and anticonvulsant mood stabilizers, are the drug treatments of choice. Although less deliriant and generally possessing lower side effect profiles, these agents should be used with the same start-low, slowly titrate approach, especially in elderly patients and those with multiple medical conditions who are frequently already on numerous other medications. Atypical antipsychotics should be used in preference to the older typical antipsychotics in brain tumor patients with chronic schizophrenia, acute psychotic episodes, and other psychotic disorders, although high-potency agents, such as haloperidol (Haldol) and fluphenazine (Prolixin), orally or in depot form, may still be necessary and, with appropriate dosage adjustments, may be reasonably well tolerated.

In general, the second generation and heterocyclic antidepressants are preferable to the tricyclics in the treatment of depression in brain tumor patients, although TCAs, monoamine oxidase inhibitors (MAOIs), and various combinations of antidepressants, alone and with various other adjunctive drug treatments, as well as nonpharmacological treatments, such as electroconvulsive therapy (ECT), transcranial magnetic stimulation (TMS), or vagal nerve stimulation (VNS), or a combination of these, may be necessary in cases of refractory depression. ECT was once thought to be absolutely contraindicated in the treatment of depression in brain tumor patients. However, several studies appearing in the literature in recent years have reported that unilateral brief pulse ECT is safe, effective, and well tolerated in selected patients with brain tumors in whom appropriate precautions have been taken.

In patients with preexisting anxiety disorders, such as generalized anxiety disorder, obsessive-compulsive disorder (OCD), posttraumatic stress disorder (PTSD), and panic disorder, one or more of the selective serotonin reuptake inhibitors (SSRIs), buspirone (BuSpar) or clonazepam (Klonopin), alone or in combination, may be highly effective and well tolerated in treating acute symptomatic exacerbations. This is especially true in comparing them with benzodiazepines and tertiary amine tricyclics, such as imipramine (Norfranil) and clomipramine (Anafranil), which were widely used in the past with various of the anxiety disorders.

In bipolar brain tumor patients with acute mania, if lithium (Eskalith) is ineffective or poorly tolerated, mood-stabilizing agents, such as valproic acid (Depakene), carbamazepine (Tegretol) or oxcarbazepine (Trileptal), gabapentin (Neurontin), clonazepam, or topiramate (Topamax), or a combination of these, may be efficacious and well tolerated. Lithium and atypical antipsychotics, including quetiapine (Seroquel), risperidone (Risperdal), olanzapine (Zyprexa), and ziprasidone (Geodon), may also be effective in conjunction with the antimanic anticonvulsants in controlling acute mania. In medication-refractory acute mania, ECT, in selected patients with proper precautions, may be rapidly effective, although ECT-treated brain tumor patients need to be monitored carefully for post-ECT delirium, especially if bilateral ECT is being used.

Treatment of acute depression in bipolar brain tumor patients may be difficult. In such patients, there is a risk of precipitating secondary mania or rapid-cycling, or both, when the TCAs or SSRIs are used, although there is a substantially greater risk of this with the former class of drugs as compared to the latter. Recent data suggest that the anticonvulsant lamotrigine (Lamictal) may be more effective in the treatment of bipolar depression than standard antidepressants, new or old, and it appears to have the distinct advantage of not precipitating secondary mania or causing rapid cycling, although it also has the potential for causing serious and, in some cases, potentially fatal dermatological side effects.

Treatment with anticonvulsants to achieve mood stabilization in bipolar brain tumor patients may be necessary when lithium is ineffective or poorly tolerated, as is frequently the case in such patients. In addition, the use of anticonvulsants may have obvious additional advantages in patients with tumor-associated seizures.

The frequent occurrence of seizures in brain tumor patients is another concern when choosing specific drug treatments for psychiatric disturbances. Many psychotropic drugs have the potential to variably lower seizure threshold and should be used with care in such patients. Although the available literature is not clear on the relative risks of inducing seizures with various psychotropic medications, in general, the newer atypical antipsychotics and antidepressants are believed to have less potential for doing so than do the older, low-potency, typical antipsychotic and tertiary amine tricyclics. High-potency antipsychotics, including molindone (Moban), fluphenazine, and haloperidol, are believed to have less seizure-producing potential than do others of the older typical antipsychotics, whereas bupropion (Wellbutrin) and maprotiline (Ludiomil) are believed to have a greater risk of inducing seizures than do other antidepressants and should therefore be avoided in brain tumor patients with a history of seizures. Lithium carbonate, which is known to be seizure producing, should also be avoided in brain tumor patients with seizures. One or more of the anticonvulsant mood-stabilizing agents previously listed should be used in preference to lithium in such cases.

In brain tumor patients being treated with anticonvulsants for associated seizure disorders, care should be taken in adding psychotropic agents as treatment for psychiatric symptoms. In such clinical situations, drug–drug interactions may occur through mechanisms, including differential protein binding of various drugs and inhibition or enhancement of the cytochrome P450 system metabolism of one of the coadministered drugs by the other.

Although using psychotropic medications with little or no potential for drug–drug interactions with anticonvulsants is preferable, when this is not possible, anticonvulsant drug levels should be carefully monitored. In such situations, anticonvulsant levels may be increased or decreased, with resulting signs of drug toxicity or loss of seizure control that call for reduction or increase in the dosage of the anticonvulsant in question or, in some cases, substitution of another anticonvulsant.

DRUG AND SOMATIC TREATMENT OF SECONDARY MENTAL DISORDERS DUE TO BRAIN TUMOR

In brain tumor patients with psychiatric and behavioral disorders that are not preexisting, definitive treatment of the tumor in the form of complete removal may result in complete elimination of the secondary psychiatric symptomatology, whether it is directly due to the tumor itself and its direct effects on the brain or a result of the psychological stress of and reaction to having been diagnosed with a brain tumor.

In cases in which treatments, whether surgery, chemotherapy, or radiotherapy, or a combination of these, have been only partially effective in eliminating the tumor, psychiatric syndromes with variable behavioral symptomatology may persist and also may benefit significantly from psychopharmacological treatment. As noted previously, the symptomatology of these secondary syndromes may be predominantly psychotic, affective, or neurocognitive or may be characterized by generalized anxiety and agitation. In prescribing drug treatment for patients with one or more of these conditions, the psychiatrist must, as with brain tumor patients with recurrent episodes of preexisting primary psychiatric syndrome, be cognizant of the fact that they may require, tolerate, and benefit from lower than usually expected doses of psychotropic medication, especially if they are elderly.

In addition to judicious dosing, the choice of specific medications in the treatment of such patients should take into consideration the side effect profiles of potential agents, especially in relation to their likelihood of causing deliriant, epileptogenic, extrapyramidal, or sedating side effects, or a combination of these. Careful attention to these factors can minimize morbidity while optimizing therapeutic benefit from pharmacological interventions.

DRUG TREATMENT OF DELIRIUM IN BRAIN TUMOR PATIENTS

As in all delirious patients, the identification and elimination of its causes are key to successful treatment of delirium in brain tumor patients and usually lead to the clearing of associated psychiatric and behavioral symptoms within a few days to 2 to 3 weeks. Agitation, anxiety, hallucinations, paranoid delusions, confusion, and dissociative symptoms are commonly part of the clinical picture with delirium. In addition to the usual environmental reorienting measures—a clock, a calendar, a radio or television, and low lights on in the room; safety measures, such as side rails, Posey belts, etc.; and brief, frequent, reorienting, supportive contacts—psychotropic medications may also be quite helpful.

High-potency, standard neuroleptics, such as haloperidol, and several of the newer atypical antipsychotics, such as olanzapine and risperidone, in low doses may be helpful in the treatment of agitation and psychotic symptoms. In some cases, the use of a short-acting benzodiazepine, such as lorazepam (Ativan), alone or in combination with an antipsychotic may be necessary to achieve satisfactory relief of anxiety and agitation. In some delirious patients who are inadequately responsive to standard oral doses of these medications, IV administration of haloperidol and lorazepam in high doses every 1 to 2 hours until the patient is calmed and behaviorally stabilized may be necessary.

DRUG TREATMENT OF PSYCHOTIC DISORDERS IN BRAIN TUMOR PATIENTS

Tumor-associated secondary psychotic symptoms often respond to antipsychotic medications in lower doses than are required in patients with primary psychotic disorders. These lower effective doses are generally in the range of one-tenth to one-fourth of the standard dose. Although low-dose, high-potency, standard neuroleptics are clearly preferable to the low-potency typical agents and are often helpful in the treatment of psychotic symptoms in many patients, they frequently cause significant extrapyramidal side effects in brain tumor patients. These symptoms may be quite distressing, because they frequently are more severe and persistent and may require aggressive treatment with antiparkinsonian agents. Because of the increased risk of drug-induced delirium in brain tumor patients, treatment of extrapyramidal side effects should preferably be with nonanticholinergic agents, such as diphenhydramine (Benadryl) or amantadine (Symmetrel), for dystonic and pseudoparkinsonian symptoms and benzodiazepines or β-blockers for akathisia.

Although there has been more experience over the years in the use of high-potency, typical neuroleptics in brain tumor patients with psychotic symptoms, in view of their lower overall side effect profile, the substantially lower likelihood of extrapyramidal symptoms, the greater patient tolerability and acceptance, and the reported effectiveness in treating psychotic symptoms associated with many other medical and neurological disorders, many clinicians feel that the atypical antipsychotic medications are the treatments of first choice at this point. Even with these agents, lower starting doses and gradual titration are recommended, especially in elderly patients, unless there is an urgent need for rapid symptom control.

DRUG TREATMENT OF ANXIETY DUE TO BRAIN TUMOR

Nonpsychotic agitation and anxiety may be directly related to the presence of a brain tumor but more commonly are indirect results of the fear, agitation, uncertainty, and stress that occur in many people when they are first diagnosed with a brain tumor, especially if it is malignant, or, later, when they must undergo and cope with painful or invasive diagnostic studies or treatments as a part of the management of their disease.

With respect to tumor-associated anxiety symptoms, most clinicians feel that antipsychotics should be avoided, unless specific psychotic symptoms are associated with the patient's anxiety and agitation. This is clearly the case with typical antipsychotics, which are usually ineffective with nonpsychotic anxiety symptoms and are often poorly tolerated by nonpsychotic patients, because they often cause dysphoric reactions in them. Such a proscription is less clear with respect to the atypical antipsychotics, which have been reported to have substantial beneficial effects as adjunctive treatments in some primary mood and anxiety disorders.

With regard to anxiety occurring in reaction to the psychological stress of being diagnosed with and being treated for a malignant brain tumor, full and detailed explanations of all diagnostic procedures and proposed treatments, with opportunities for the patient and family to have their questions fully answered, are essential first steps. In patients who are experiencing reactive agitation and anxiety, supportive psychotherapy for them and psychoeducation for their families may be quite beneficial in reducing their stress and anxiety and in helping their families to be optimally supportive of them.

The mainstays of anxiolytic drug treatment in brain tumor patients are the SSRIs, buspirone, and low-dose, long-acting benzodiazepines, such as clonazepam, in conjunction with supportive psychotherapy. In certain instances, alternative medications, such as hydroxyzine (Vistaril), or low-dose tertiary amine TCAs may be helpful, as may be gabapentin.

Patients with acute fear, anxiety, or panic disorder symptoms occurring as a part of a temporal lobe tumor-induced complex partial seizure disorder, may respond to antiepileptic drug treatment with carbamazepine or oxcarbazepine, which has fewer side effects and a lower risk of agranulocytosis; valproic acid; or primidone (Myidone). If such symptoms occur during the interictal period, the anxiolytic agents discussed previously may be helpful. If psychotic symptoms occur interictally, the use of antipsychotics, preferably with minimal potential for inducing seizures, is indicated. Brain tumor patients with temporal lobe seizures and psychotic or nonpsychotic anxiety symptoms frequently require combined antiepileptic, antianxiety, and antipsychotic drug treatments. As noted previously, in such cases, the clinician should be vigilant with regard to possible drug–drug interactions.

DRUG TREATMENT OF MOOD DISORDERS DUE TO BRAIN TUMORS

Antidepressant medications are helpful in treating depressive symptoms occurring as part of brain tumor–induced mood disturbances, and, given that depression plays a major role in decreasing the overall quality of life that many brain tumor patients experience, early recognition and rapid institution of effective treatment for depression, when it is present, is critical. Because of their substantial side effect profile, which includes sedation, anticholinergic effects, orthostatic hypotension, and weight gain, which often lead to poor patient acceptance, the TCAs have been largely abandoned in the treatment of depression in brain tumor patients in favor of the newer, atypical antidepressant agents. The main exception to this generalization is the secondary amine TCA, nortriptyline (Aventyl), which has relatively few side effects, is generally well tolerated, even in medically ill elderly patients, and has a well-defined relationship between blood levels and therapeutic response, which is helpful in optimizing therapeutic response while minimizing side effects.

The SSRIs have largely supplanted the TCAs as first-line treatments for depressive syndromes in brain tumor patients, because they are safe, effective, relatively free of significant side effects and are therefore generally well-tolerated and less likely to cause delirium in such patients. The main drawbacks with these agents are their high cost, the frequent occurrence of sexual side effects, and potential weight gain, which many patients find unacceptable.

Methylphenidate (Ritalin) has been shown to be an effective antidepressant in brain tumor patients and is being used increasingly in treating depression in them. It has the advantages of having a rapid onset of therapeutic effect, no effect on seizure threshold, and no sedating or deliriant properties. Moreover, it is generally well tolerated by patients of all ages, including those who are quite elderly and frail. Although most of the clinical experience to date has been with regular methylphenidate, long-acting forms, such as Concerta, which can be given once daily, may have a future role in such patients. If it is as effective with depressive symptoms as regular methylphenidate is, Concerta may provide depressed brain tumor patients with some unique advantages vis-à-vis regular methylphenidate in the form of single daily dosing, improved treatment compliance, and fewer arousal and activation side effects.

When the atypical antidepressants and secondary amine TCAs are ineffective in alleviating depression in brain tumor patients, MAOIs may be effective and do not pose any undue risks as long as coadministration of potentially dangerous medications is avoided and a tyramine-free diet is maintained. Before using these agents, it is important to assess the patient's cognitive capacity with respect to successfully observing these restrictions.

When single agents are ineffective, combinations of antidepressant drugs, preferably from different pharmacological classes, or combinations of antidepressants and other adjunctive medications, such as lithium carbonate, thyroid hormone, or atypical antipsychotics, may be helpful.

When depressed patients are refractory to pharmacological treatment, ECT may play an important role in selected patients with appropriate precautions. The potential roles of VNS or TMS, or both, in the treatment of brain tumor patients with refractory depression are unclear at present, because both are still largely experimental treatments. Nevertheless, both have been shown to be safe, well tolerated, and effective in many depressed patients who have been previously unresponsive to or intolerant of other antidepressant treatment interventions. Their place in the treatment of depression in brain tumor patients remains to be defined by future research.

As noted previously, mania or hypomania in brain tumor patients is relatively uncommon in comparison to depression. However, in manic brain tumor patients who do not have seizures, lithium carbonate alone or in combination with other adjunctive antimanic agents, including typical or atypical antipsychotics, lorazepam, or clonazepam may be beneficial. In manic patients who fail to respond to lithium carbonate or who have a history of seizures, mood stabilizers in the anticonvulsant category, such as carbamazepine, oxcarbazepine, valproic acid, topiramate, or gabapentin, alone or in combination, may be effective alternatives. When these alternatives are ineffective in such patients, ECT administered with appropriate precautions may have rapid antimanic effects without worsening any underlying seizure disorder that may be present, because it has anticonvulsant properties of its own.

DRUG TREATMENT OF PERSONALITY CHANGES DUE TO BRAIN TUMORS

As previously described, a variety of subtle or not-so-subtle personality changes may be associated with brain tumors, especially those involving the frontal and temporolimbic regions of the brain. Personality changes with impulsivity and lability of mood may respond to treatment with lithium, carbamazepine, oxcarbazine, or valproic acid; whereas those with psychomotor retardation, abulia, and apathy may respond to dopamine agonists, such as bromocriptine (Parlodel), or stimulants, such as methylphenidate or modafinil (Provigil).

In patients in whom the observed personality changes include features suggestive of an intermittent explosive disorder with sudden, angry, impulsive, aggressive, and violent behavioral dyscontrol with rage and explosive outbursts, a variety of agents that have been previously used successfully in patients with similar behaviors occurring in conjunction with other neurological conditions may be helpful. These include various anticonvulsants that were discussed previously, phenytoin (Dilantin), lithium carbonate, atypical antipsychotics, β-blockers, or short-acting benzodiazepines.

As with much of current psychopharmacology, there are no clear guidelines as to which specific drug or combination of drugs to use first in the treatment of intermittent explosive disorder. The clinician needs to identify and carefully quantify the occurrence, frequency, and severity of episodic target behaviors and then carry out systematic treatment trials with gradual upward titration of selected agents until optimal therapeutic doses have been established by minimizing the severity or frequency, or both, of target symptoms or causing the emergence of intolerable side effects that prevent further dose increases. Such empirical therapeutic trials should be systematically carried out until the optimal types and doses of single medications or combinations of medications have been established for the individual in question.

DRUG TREATMENT OF COGNITIVE AND NONSPECIFIC NEUROBEHAVIORAL SYMPTOMS DUE TO BRAIN TUMORS

A variety of nonspecific neurobehavioral changes may be seen in patients with brain tumors, as a result of the tumor itself as well as the result of various surgical and nonsurgical treatment interventions. These include postoperative anxiety and depression in patients who have undergone surgical resection involving heteromodal association cortex in frontal, parietal, and paralimbic regions; impairment of attention, concentration, and various other cognitive functions, which can be assessed and monitored with serial neuropsychological testing; abulia and amotivational states; excessive fatigue that negatively impacts almost all aspects of patients' lives; and decreased energy and physical stamina, which can significantly interfere with day-to-day functioning and overall quality of life.

Recently, there have been reports of malignant glioma patients with many of these symptoms who have shown significant improvement with low-dose methylphenidate treatment. Despite MRI-proven progression of these tumors over time, many of the patients who were receiving methylphenidate experienced continued improvement in attention, concentration, and cognitive function, as well as decreased fatigue, enhanced motivation, increased energy, and greater physical stamina.

Few side effects, no seizures, and the ability to reduce ongoing doses of steroids were also observed in many of these methylphenidate-treated patients. Whether other stimulants, such as dextroamphetamine (Dexedrine), combined amphetamine and dextroamphetamine, or modafinil, might have similar or additional benefits is unclear at present but is an important question for further research.

Additionally, whether modafinil might have the same kind of beneficial effect on nonspecific, brain tumor treatment-associated fatigue as it does with the profound, although nonspecific, fatigue that is often seen in multiple sclerosis patients is also unclear but is another important area for future study.

PSYCHOTHERAPEUTIC TREATMENT OF PATIENTS WITH BEHAVIORAL DISTURBANCES ASSOCIATED WITH BRAIN TUMORS

Supportive psychotherapy is a critical part of the overall management of most, if not all, malignant brain tumor patients, especially those in whom the tumor is inoperable or incurable. Psychotherapeutic interventions should take into account the types of treatment, surgical and otherwise, the patient has undergone; the types of complications that may have occurred as a result of the tumor and its treatment; the patient's anticipated short- and long-term prognosis; the patient's psychiatric history and the type and severity of current psychopathology that he or she may be manifesting; the concomitant pharmacological treatments that are being administered; and the patient's cognitive and intellectual capabilities and emotional needs. It is also important for the psychiatrist to be fully aware of the adequacy of social supports with respect to the intactness of interpersonal relationships and the availability of family members, as well as the patient's current day-to-day functioning, with a particular emphasis on any physical or behavioral disability. All of these factors must be carefully considered in developing and integrating an optimally helpful psychotherapeutic approach into the overall management of the brain tumor patient.

Being diagnosed with a malignant and, therefore, potentially fatal brain tumor causes enormous psychological stress, as does subsequently having to undergo surgical, radiotherapeutic, or chemotherapeutic courses of treatment, or a combination of these. These stressors may trigger reoccurrences of preexisting psychiatric disorders in patients with a history of psychiatric disorder or may cause acute reactive psychiatric and behavioral disturbances in previously psychiatrically healthy individuals. These stressors can also have a profound and devastating effect on patients' families. Thus, providing supportive psychotherapy to patients, as well as their families, is important and is likely to be beneficial and appreciated by both.

Supportive psychotherapy, whether for the patient or for those close to him or her, should generally focus on concrete, reality-based issues, as well as the feelings that patients and their families are experiencing in relation to various treatment decisions and choices they are facing and the expected benefits or potential complications of various diagnostic procedures or treatment interventions that are being proposed. It is important that psychotherapeutic interventions take into account the level of understanding that patients and their families are capable of, as indicated by the premorbid intellectual and cognitive capacities of both, as well as any cognitive changes that may have occurred in the patient as a result of surgery, radiotherapy, or chemotherapy or progression of the tumor itself.

Although, at first, psychotherapy often focuses on the shock, fear, and denial that often accompany the initial diagnosis of a malignant brain tumor, as the patient begins to undergo various procedures and treatments for it, the focus is likely to shift to the concrete day-to-day impact of the tumor and its management on the patient's functional status, emotional and physical, which, in large part, determines the overall quality of his or her life. Over time, the impact of these factors on the patient's spouse, significant other, or family takes on increasing importance, as do anticipatory discussions of the challenges inherent in coping with and adapting to existing or anticipated physical or neurocognitive dysfunctions and disabilities and their implications for the patient's future.

Brain tumor patients whose tumors are incurable struggle with anticipatory grief in relation to potential losses of function, independence, and autonomy and their eventual death and tend to experience a great deal of worry, fear, sadness, and anger in relation to these issues. The skilled therapist can empathically help the patient address these frightening realities and be able to recognize, acknowledge, and express his or her feelings about them. These kinds of therapeutic interactions may help the patient deal more appropriately with painful feelings and affects and, by so doing, may decrease the common tendency for emotional responses to them to be inappropriately displaced onto caregivers and loved ones.

Patients with malignant brain tumors differ greatly in their capacity to cope with and adapt to major life stressors. For them, however, dealing with the daily reality of coping with a potentially or actually incurable disease is unavoidable and continuing. Their ability to cope with this reality, in large measure, depends on their premorbid capacity to deal adaptively with other major life stresses. The adaptiveness of the individual's coping mechanisms reflects his or her native intelligence, creativity, flexibility, problem-solving capacity, temperament, characterological and personality styles, interpersonal relatedness, sense of individual autonomy, level of self-esteem, and capacity for patience and perseverance. It is important for the therapist to assess each of these areas and to help the patient develop and strengthen effective coping strategies by building on existing strengths while minimizing the impact of ineffective coping mechanisms.

In interactions with the clinician, some patients give the impression of being relatively unaffected by the diagnosis of a malignant brain tumor. Such patients often are in denial with respect to the potentially grave implications of their disease. Denial may initially be desirable and helpful to some patients in coping with the emotional impact of the frightening diagnostic and prognostic information they have been given and the associated fears and anxieties it arouses in them. However, continuing denial in patients or their families becomes maladaptive when it results in compromised treatment compliance or failure to deal with any of a host of important, reality-based, legal, family, or interpersonal issues, or a combination of these, that are affected by the patient's increasing disability or eventual death and that need to be addressed in a timely fashion while he or she is still cognitively intact. In such circumstances, the clinician may need to directly, although gently, confront the patient and his or her family, regarding the potential consequences of not dealing with such issues, in a sensitive and supportive fashion and then may proceed to explore with them optimal ways of dealing with these issues.

Others may be emotionally devastated and overwhelmed when they learn they have a malignant brain tumor and may develop severe psychiatric symptomatology as a result. These psychiatric symptoms may require intensive psychological support and aggressive treatment with psychotropic medication to minimize their impact on the patient's ability to function at home and at work and to make necessary decisions with regard to his or her illness and its treatment.

The issue of discussing the anticipated prognosis of a malignant brain tumor with patients and families is a difficult one. To begin with, the prognosis is not always clear nor, for that matter, is the likely outcome of various therapeutic interventions that may be proposed, because patient variables make a substantial difference in the outcome of individual cases. Most clinicians, as well as patients and their family members, feel that the presentation of information regarding prognosis and potential outcomes of various treatment options should be direct and open, presented in a caring and sensitive fashion, at a level that patients and families can fully comprehend, and should be as accurate as possible in addressing those things that are known, as well as those about which uncertainties exist. These discussions should provide the patient and family with realistic hope, if not for a cure, then at least for active care and support, continued preservation of the patient's dignity, and effective pain relief as the disease progresses, if it is incurable.

Such discussions and opportunities for the questions that patients and families may have should be provided by the treating neurosurgeon, so that they are fully answered. After such discussions, the psychiatrist can be helpful to the patient and family in further clarifying and reinforcing diagnostic, prognostic, and treatment-related information conveyed by the neurosurgeon, as well as in addressing the emotional reactions and concerns it may have aroused. Such information processing may go on over a considerable period of time and working through the information and their emotional reactions to it may help patients and families in making critical treatment decisions and in cooperating with diagnostic procedures or treatments for which compliance might otherwise have been an issue.

Occasionally, patients with benign tumors or malignant neoplasms that have been completely removed, thereby effecting a complete cure, may also experience psychiatric and behavioral symptoms. These may take the form of nonspecific depressive symptoms or persistent generalized anxiety and fear, or both, which may benefit from supportive psychotherapy or short-term cognitive behavioral therapy. Although these interventions are generally the preferred treatments for such symptoms and often lead to rapid symptom reduction and resolution, in those cases in which symptoms are severe and persistent, are having an impact on the patient's capacity to function at home or at work, or have evolved into a more clearly defined, autonomous psychiatric disorder with characteristic clinical features, appropriately targeted pharmacotherapy as an adjunct to ongoing supportive or cognitive behavioral therapy, or both, may be helpful in enhancing the patients' recovery.

Because brain tumor patients who are being treated for psychiatric and behavioral symptoms may have a variety of neurocognitive abnormalities affecting attention, concentration, and higher-level abstracting capabilities, supportive or cognitive behavioral psychotherapeutic approaches, or both, are preferred over psychodynamically oriented psychotherapeutic approaches. Having said that, it is still incumbent on the treating psychiatrist to be fully aware of important dynamic factors in the patient's history to formulate a treatment approach that is optimally effective and efficient in light of them.

Brain tumor patients with neurocognitive dysfunctions are often unable to take full advantage of psychodynamic psychotherapy as a result of tumor-associated memory and attentional dysfunctions, frontal and prefrontal lobe executive dysfunctions, or other neurocognitive dysfunctions, or a combination of these, which may have resulted from surgery, radiation therapy, or the brain tumor itself. If such patients are confronted with the psychological demands inherent in the traditional, dynamically oriented psychotherapy that typically requires intact neurocognitive capabilities, including attention and concentration, long- and short-term memory, executive capacities, and a substantial degree of psychological mindedness, they may experience considerable frustration, a sense of failure, and acute distress as a result of their inability to meet the demands and expectations of this type of therapy.

In addition to emphasizing active supportive psychotherapy and reality-based, cognitive behavioral therapy as the cornerstones of the psychotherapeutic management of brain tumor patients, the psychiatrist should adopt an active, supportive "here and now," psychoeducationally oriented therapeutic stance vis-à-vis patients and their families. In general, the psychiatrist should eschew more traditional, dynamically oriented psychotherapy in which the psychiatrist is typically a relatively passive observer of reported psychiatric symptoms, free associations, and dream material and an interpreter of psychological conflicts, defenses, and transference issues, which provide the patient with insights that can lead to changes in his or her behavior.

Brain tumor patients with psychiatric and behavioral symptoms generally benefit greatly from active "here and now" therapeutic and psychoeducational approaches focusing on concrete day-to-day issues related to their illness or its treatment, alone or in conjunction with appropriately targeted pharmacotherapy. Although there are no data that speak to the relative efficacy of combined psychotherapy and pharmacotherapy in brain tumor patients in comparison to these individual treatment approaches used separately, there appear to be no contraindications to combining them. If, as seems likely, psychiatric and behavioral symptoms in brain tumor patients are similar in their response to treatments to those that occur in non–tumor-associated psychiatric and behavioral syndromes, then combining them is likely to be more effective than using either of them separately.

FUTURE DIRECTIONS

Brain tumors, whether benign or malignant, can directly or indirectly cause a host of psychiatric, behavioral, and neurocognitive symptoms. The presence of a brain tumor should be a differential diagnostic consideration in any patient presenting with new-onset behavioral or neurocognitive symptomatology, especially if the symptoms are atypical or associated with any of the varied neurological signs and symptoms that may be suggestive of an underlying brain tumor. Appropriate diagnostic evaluation of such patients should include full physical, neurological, and mental status examinations; structural and functional brain imaging; and other specialized neurological studies and formal neuropsychological assessments, as indicated by the clinical history and physical examination.

The aggressiveness, tumor cell type, size, rate of growth, and anatomical location of brain tumors are all factors that influence the type and severity of psychiatric symptoms that may be associated with them. Although, in general, the relationship between anatomical location of tumors and specific behavioral manifestations related to them is not robust, tumors involving the frontal and temporal lobes and the thalamus and hypothalamus are most frequently associated with psychiatric and behavioral manifestations. Small, slow-growing tumors and tumors with associated behavioral symptomatology involving the posterior fossa, anterior frontal lobes, nondominant temporal and parietal lobes, and the corpus callosum, the so-called silent brain regions, because tumors occurring in them rarely cause focal signs and symptoms, are most often missed or misdiagnosed as psychiatric disorders.

Treatment of brain tumor–associated psychiatric, behavioral, and neurocognitive symptoms, if it is to be optimal, should be multimodal and should include appropriate psychopharmacological treatment and supportive and cognitive behavioral psychotherapeutic interventions.

Selection of drugs for the treatment of various tumor-associated psychiatric syndromes should be based on standard drug treatments of analogous primary psychiatric disorders. However, the clinician must bear in mind that the dose and type of medication used often need to be modified, given brain tumor patients' increased sensitivity to many psychotropic agents and their increased risk of developing acute metabolic encephalopathies and seizures.

Psychotherapeutic intervention should be based on supportive and cognitive behavioral therapy principles, not on more traditional psychodynamic approaches, and the psychiatrist should adopt an active role in providing support and cognitive behavioral interventions to patients and psychoeducation and psychological support to their families in relation to concrete, "here and now" problems and issues related to the brain tumor, its treatment, complications, and anticipated prognosis.

When a thoughtful and carefully planned multimodal psychopharmacological and psychotherapeutic treatment approach is coordinated with ongoing cognitive, physical, and vocational rehabilitative efforts, and when these are tightly integrated with the patient's ongoing neurosurgical and medical care, the expected outcome should be substantial improvement in the quality of patients' lives, their sense of well-being, and the ability of their loved ones to be available as sources of support.

SUGGESTED CROSS-REFERENCES

Functional neuroanatomy is discussed in Section 1.2, neuroimaging is discussed in Sections 1.15 and 1.16, schizophrenia is discussed in Chapter 12, and mood disorders are discussed in Chapter 13.

REFERENCES

American Brain Tumor Association. Facts and statistics. In: *Primer of Brain Tumors.* 7th ed. Des Plaines, IL: American Brain Tumor Association; 2002:1–7.

*Armstrong CL, Goldstein B, Shera D, Ledakis GE, Tallent EM: The predictive value of longitudinal neuropsychologic assessment in the early detection of brain tumor recurrence. *Cancer.* 2003;97:649–656.

Bear DM, Fedio P: Quantitative analysis of interictal behavior in temporal lobe epilepsy. *Arch Neurol.* 1977;34:454–467.

Burkle FM, Lipowski ZJ: Colloid cyst of the third ventricle presenting as psychiatric disorder. *Am J Psychiatry.* 1978;135:373–374.

Chipkevitch E: Brain tumors and anorexia nervosa syndrome. *Brain Dev.* 1994;16:175–179.

Cummings JL: Frontal-subcortical circuits and human behavior. *Arch Neurol.* 1993;50:873–880.

Cummings JL, Mendez MF: Secondary mania with focal cerebrovascular lesions. *Am J Psychiatry.* 1984;141:1084–1087.

Davies E, Hall S, Clarke C: Two year survival after malignant cerebral glioma: Patient and relative reports of handicap, psychiatric symptoms, and rehabilitation. *Disabil Rehabil.* 2003;25:259–266.

Dubovsky SL. Psychopharmacological treatment in neuropsychiatry. In: Yudofsky SC, Hales RE, eds. *The American Psychiatric Press Textbook of Neuropsychiatry.* Washington, DC: American Psychiatric Association Press; 1992:663–701.

Fox S, Lantz C: The brain tumor experience and quality of life: A qualitative study. *J Neuroscience Nurs.* 1998;30:245–252.

Frazier CH: Tumor involving the frontal lobe alone: A symptomatic survey of 105 verified cases. *Arch Neurol Psychiatry.* 1935;35:525–571.

Hahn CA, Dunn RH, Logue PE, Edwards CL, Halperin EC: Prospective study of neuropsychologic testing and quality-of-life assessment of adults with primary malignant brain tumors. *Int J Radiat Oncol Biol Phys.* 2003;55:992–999.

Hobbs GE: Brain tumors simulating psychiatric disorder. *Can Med Assoc J.* 1963;88:186–188.

Hollister LE, Boutros N: Clinical use of CT and MR scans in psychiatric patients. *J Psychiatry Neurosci.* 1991;16:194–198.

Hustinx R, Alavi A: SPECT and PET imaging of brain tumors. *Neuroimaging Clin North Am.* 1999;9:751–766.

Kaplan CP, Miner ME: Anxiety and depression in elderly patients receiving treatment for cerebral tumours. *Brain Inj.* 1997;11:129–135.

*Keschner M, Bender MB: Mental symptoms associated with brain tumor: A study of 530 verified cases. *JAMA.* 1938;110:714–718.

Keschner M, Bender MB, Strauss I: Mental symptoms in cases of tumor of the temporal lobe. *Arch Neurol Psychiatry.* 1936;35:572–596.

Klotz M: Incidence of brain tumors in patients hospitalized for chronic mental disorders. *Psychiatr Q.* 1957;31:669–680.

*Lishman WA. Cerebral tumours. In: *Organic Psychiatry: The Psychological Consequences of Cerebral Disorder.* 2nd ed. Oxford, England: Blackwell Science; 1987:187–206.

*Meyers CA, Hess KR: Multifaceted end points in brain tumor clinical trials: Cognitive deterioration precedes MRI progression. *Neuro-oncol.* 2003;5:89–95.

Meyers CA, Wietzner MA, Valentine AD, Levin VA: Methylphenidate therapy improves cognition, mood, and function of brain tumor patients. *J Clin Oncol.* 1998;16:2522–2527.

Nakawatase TY. Frontal lobe tumors. In: Miller BL, Cummings JL, eds. *Human Frontal Lobes Functions and Disorders.* New York: The Guilford Press; 1999:436–445.

Nasrallah HA, McChesney CM: Psychopathology of corpus callosum tumors. *Biol Psychiatry.* 1981;16:663–669.

Patton RB, Sheppard JA: Intracranial tumors found at autopsy in mental patients. *Am J Psychiatry.* 1956;113:319–324.

Pollak L, Klein C, Rabey JM, Schiffer J: Posterior fossa lesions associated with neuropsychiatric symptomatology. *Int J Neurosci.* 1996;87:119–126.

*Price TRP, Goetz KL, Lovell MR. Neuropsychiatric aspects of brain tumors. In: Yudofsky SC, Hales RB, eds. *The American Psychiatric Publishing Textbook of Neuropsychiatry and Clinical Neurosciences.* 4th ed. Washington, DC: American Psychiatric Publishing; 2002:753–781.

Pringle AM, Taylor R, Whittle IR: Anxiety and depression in patients with an intracranial neoplasm before and after tumor surgery. *Br J Neurosurg.* 1999;13:46–51.

Ricci PE: Imaging of adult brain tumors. *Neuroimaging Clin North Am.* 1999;9:651–669.

Ruiz A, Ganz WI, Post J: Use of thallium-201 brain SPECT to differentiate cerebral lymphoma from toxoplasma encephalitis in AIDS patients. *Am J Neuroradiol.* 15:1885–1994.

Selecki BR: Intracranial space occupying lesions among patients admitted to mental hospitals. *Med J Aust.* 1965;1:383–390.

Strauss I, Keschner M: Mental symptoms in cases of tumor of the frontal lobe. *Arch Neurol Psychiatry.* 1935;33:986–1005.

Weitzner MA: Psychosocial and neuropsychiatric aspects of patients with primary brain tumors. *Cancer Invest.* 1999;4:285–291.

Yudofsky SC, Hales RE. Neuropsychiatric aspects of brain tumors. In: Yudofsky SC, Hales RE, eds. *Textbook of Neuropsychiatry.* 4th ed. Washington, DC: American Psychiatric Association Press; 2002:753–782.

Zwil AS, Bowring MA, Price TRP: ECT in the presence of a brain tumor: Case report and a review of the literature. *Convuls Ther.* 1990;6:299–307.

▲ 2.4 Neuropsychiatric Aspects of Epilepsy

MARIO F. MENDEZ ASHLA, M.D., PH.D.

Epilepsy is associated with a range of psychiatric disorders. Studies from communities, epilepsy clinics, and psychiatric hospitals demonstrate an increased prevalence of psychiatric problems among epileptic patients as compared to nonepileptic patients. Among epileptic patients, much of the psychopathology results from electrophysiological, structural, or chemical changes in the temporal limbic system, and, possibly, the frontal lobes.

Although most patients with epilepsy are healthy, one-fourth or more have schizophreniform psychoses, depression, personality changes, or hyposexuality. These behavioral changes may be chronic and present between seizure episodes. Other behaviors are episodic and directly related to the seizure discharges. Epileptic patients may have auras with psychic content, nonconvulsive status epilepticus, prodromal symptoms, postictal confusion, and a periictal psychosis that usually occurs in the postictal period and is distinct from the schizophreniform psychosis of epilepsy.

There are important implications for the management of epileptics with psychopathology. These include maximizing the mood stabilizing and other psychotropic effects of anticonvulsant drugs, such as carbamazepine (Tegretol), valproate (Depakene), lamotrigine (Lamictal), and clonazepam (Klonopin). Psychotropic medications can also lower the seizure threshold, an important consideration in choosing a psychotropic drug for a brittle epileptic patient. Finally, the clinician must consider the potential interaction of anticonvulsant and psychotropic medications and must monitor their respective drug levels.

DEFINITION

Epileptic *seizures* are sudden, involuntary behavioral events associated with excessive or hypersynchronous electrical discharges in the

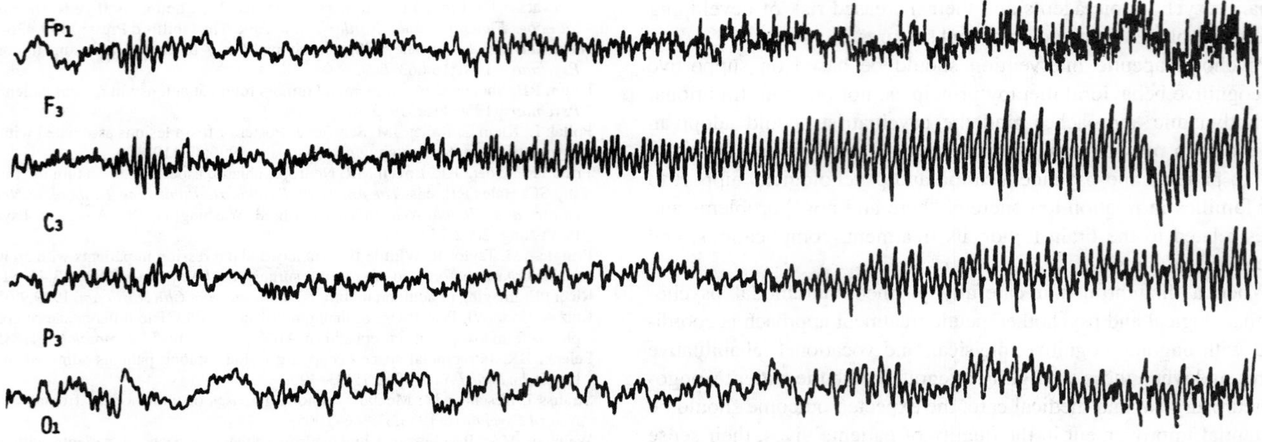

FIGURE 2.4–1 Electroencephalogram demonstrating the focal onset of seizure discharges from the left frontotemporal region that are consistent with the onset of complex partial seizures.

brain. The seizure itself is known as the *ictus*. The *interictal period* refers to the period between the postictal abnormalities and the next ictus, and the *periictal period* refers to the period just before or after the ictus and is applied when there is insufficient information to know when the ictus ends or begins. Epileptic seizures can be primary, secondary to a neurological condition, or reactive to a situational factor, such as sleep deprivation or drug withdrawal. *Epilepsy* is the recurrent tendency to seize, and *status epilepticus* is prolonged or repetitive seizures without intervening recovery.

In epilepsy, abnormal electrical discharges are due to hyperexcitable neurons with sustained postsynaptic depolarization. Proposed mechanisms for this sustained depolarization include changes in ionic conductance, decreased γ-aminobutyric acid (GABA) inhibition of cortical excitability, and increased glutamate-mediated cortical excitation. In animals, alumina-induced membrane changes alter the ratio of intracellular to extracellular ionic concentrations and result in abnormal neuronal firing. Anticonvulsants, such as phenytoin (Dilantin), carbamazepine, and valproate, reduce this repetitive firing through effects on sodium channels. Ethosuximide (Zarontin) works through blockage of calcium currents. Penicillin-induced cortical injury causes seizures through decreased GABA inhibition. Barbiturates and benzodiazepines may reduce seizures by enhancing GABA receptor current and valproate through blockage of GABA catabolism. Kainic acid, a glutamate agonist, induces seizures through increased synaptic action at its *N*-methyl-D-aspartate (NMDA) receptors. Much work is underway on potential anticonvulsants that may work through inhibition of this excitatory receptor mechanism.

The electroencephalogram (EEG) is a surface recording of brain wave activity used in the evaluation of seizures. Basic waves include normal waking alpha waves (8 to 13 Hz), which are most prominent over the occipital region, high frequency beta waves (greater than 13 Hz), and theta waves (4.0 to 7.5 Hz) and delta slowing (3.5 Hz or less). Seizures are manifest as multiple spikes of spike and wave discharges on the EEG (Fig. 2.4–1). A spike is a sharp transient with a duration of 20 to 70 milliseconds. Interictally, single spikes and other markers of abnormal electrical activity may be seen, often emanating from a temporal lobe.

HISTORY

In his book on epilepsy, *On The Sacred Disease*, Hippocrates (460 to 377 BC) attacked the prevailing belief that those afflicted with epilepsy were possessed by gods or goddesses. He proposed that epilepsy was a brain disease caused by the blockage by phlegm of air-carrying vessels to the brain. Despite this initial view, throughout most of human history, epilepsy constituted demonic possession or the accumulation of bad humors, and attempts at exorcism involved trephination, cautery of the back of the skull, diuretics, emetics, bloodletting, purging, sweating, and even intercourse to release sperm. In the 18th century, the first so-called scientific treatise on epilepsy since ancient times attributed seizures to masturbation. By happenstance, bromides, which were introduced to diminish libido and masturbation, proved to be the first successful anticonvulsant medication. With the development of effective anticonvulsants and the introduction of EEG, physicians have come full circle to Hippocrates' belief that epilepsy is rooted in organic brain disease.

The purported association of epilepsy with behavioral disorders also dates to antiquity. The brain was the seat of the falling sickness and madness, and both were related to phlegm. With demonic possession as a form of punishment, unusual or abnormal behaviors became associated with seizure patients, even during their seizure-free periods. At the turn of the 19th century, the psychiatric writings of Emil Kraepelin emphasized that epileptic patients possessed personality changes and a predisposition to psychosis. With the greater understanding of the physical basis of epilepsy, many clinicians sought to protect epileptic patients from the demonic stigma of their disease; in their view, psychiatric problems resulted from the psychosocial difficulties associated with having seizures rather than any unique relationship of epilepsy with psychiatric illness. The current age was initiated by the definition of temporal lobe epilepsy and the concept of a physiological disturbance in the limbic or emotional brain.

NOSOLOGY

The International Classification of Epileptic Seizures divides seizures into *generalized* and *partial* (Table 2.4–1). Generalized seizures are those with an initial widespread bihemispheric involvement, and partial seizures are those that emanate from a focus limited to part of one hemisphere. In adults, most generalized seizures are *tonic-clonic* seizures (grand mal seizures or convulsions) and are characterized by an abrupt loss of consciousness with tonic rigidity followed by a synchronous, clonic release. Partial seizures are *complex partial seizures* (psychomotor or temporal lobe epilepsy) or *simple partial seizures*, depending on whether there is complex symptoma-

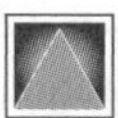

Table 2.4–1
International Classification of Epileptic Seizures

Partial (focal, local) seizures
- Simple partial seizures
  - Motor, somatosensory, autonomic, or psychic symptoms
- Complex partial seizures
  - Begin with symptoms of simple partial seizure but progress to impairment of consciousness
  - Begin with impairment of consciousness
- Partial seizures with secondary generalization
  - Begin with simple partial seizure
  - Begin with complex partial seizure (including those with symptoms of simple partial seizures at onset)

Generalized seizures (convulsive or nonconvulsive)
- Absence (typical and atypical)
- Myoclonus
- Clonic
- Tonic
- Tonic-clonic
- Atonic/akinetic

Unclassified

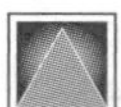

Table 2.4–2
Psychic Auras

Type	Symptoms	Probable Source
Dysphasic[a]	Nonfluent Impaired comprehension	Left perisylvian language areas
Dysmnesic	*Déjà vu, déjà vécu, déjà pensé, déjà entendu, jamais vu,* etc., prescience, illusion of memory	Mesobasal temporal,[b] especially on right
Cognitive	Dreamy state, altered time sense, derealization, depersonalization	Mesobasal temporal and temporal neocortex
	Forced thinking, forced actions, and altered or obscure thoughts	Frontal association cortex
Affective	Fear, anxiety, apprehension, depression, pleasure, displeasure	Mesobasal temporal and temporal neocortex
Illusions[c]	Macropsia, micropsia, teleopsia, movement, metamorphopsia, increased color intensity, increased stereopsis intensity	Lateral superior temporal neocortex, especially on right for visual illusions
Hallucinations[c]	Structured, hallucinatory remembrances, autoscopy	Mesobasal temporal and temporal neocortex

[a]Does not include speech arrest or simple vocalizations.
[b]Includes hippocampus, amygdala, and the parahippocampal gyrus.
[c]Includes interpretive (size, motion, shape, and stereopsis) or experiential (elements of past experience or involvement).

tology, such as an alteration of consciousness or psychic symptoms (Table 2.4–2). Simple partial seizures produce isolated motor, sensory, autonomic, psychic, or mixed symptoms in a clear sensorium. Simple partial seizures that evolve to complex partial seizures are considered *auras.* Complex partial seizures are usually characterized by motionless staring combined with simple automatisms, or automatic motor activity, and last approximately 1 minute. Complex partial seizures that evolve to generalized tonic-clonic seizures are *secondarily generalized.* Finally, there is a second form of generalized seizures, *absence* (petit mal) seizures, which occur less commonly in adults and are characterized by brief lapses of consciousness. Absence seizures differ from complex partial seizures in being short (10 seconds long) and repetitive; in lacking auras, postictal confusion, or complex automatisms; and in having characteristic 2 to 4 cps spike and wave discharges on EEG.

EPIDEMIOLOGY

Seizure disorders are common and usually have an early onset. Epilepsy affects 20 to 40 million people worldwide and has a prevalence of at least 0.63 percent and an annual incidence of approximately 0.05 percent. The overall incidence is high in the first year, drops to a minimum in the third and fourth decades of life, then increases again in later life. More than 75 percent of patients have their first seizure before 18 years of age, and 12 to 20 percent have a familial incidence of seizures. Among adults, the most common seizures are complex partial and generalized tonic-clonic seizures.

Psychopathology Epidemiological studies from communities, psychiatric hospitals, and epilepsy clinics report a 20 to 60 percent prevalence of psychiatric problems among epilepsy patients. Epilepsy patients are prone to psychosis, depression, personality disorders, hyposexuality, and other behavioral disorders. These problems are approximately equally divided between those that occur ictally or periictally and those that occur interictally or are variably related to the ictus. The percentage of epilepsy patients in psychiatric hospitals was also higher than the general prevalence of epilepsy and ranged from 4.7 percent of all inpatients in a British psychiatric hospital to 9.7 percent in a U.S. Veterans Affairs psychiatric facility. Among patients attending epilepsy clinics, approximately 30 percent had a prior psychiatric hospitalization, and 18 percent were on at least one psychotropic drug. Furthermore, epidemiological studies indicate an increased interictal psychopathology among head-injured patients with epilepsy compared to head-injured patients without epilepsy. Despite criticisms of selection bias, these studies constitute a broad spectrum of sources that indicate greater overall psychopathology in epilepsy patients.

Do epilepsy patients have greater psychopathology than other similarly impaired patients? If this were so, it would suggest that the psychopathology is of biological origin rather than a less specific reaction to chronic disease. Although disputed by some investigators, several studies report more psychopathology among epileptic patients than among patients with chronic diseases that do not directly affect the brain. Furthermore, the pattern of behavioral changes in seizure patients appear specific to epilepsy. For example, on the Minnesota Multiphasic Personality Inventory (MMPI) 2, despite a lack of difference in overall psychopathology, patients with epilepsy have higher schizophrenia scale and paranoia scale scores than patients with other neurological disabilities.

Many studies found a special relationship to psychopathology in patients whose seizures emanated from mediobasal temporal lesions. Psychiatric disturbances, primarily psychosis and personality disorders, are two to three times more common in patients with complex partial seizures, most of whom have a temporal focus, compared to those with generalized tonic-clonic seizures; other studies have failed to find a difference. Nevertheless, 60 to 76 percent of adults with epilepsy, regardless of seizure type, have a temporal lobe focus, and many generalized tonic-clonic seizures are secondarily generalized from a temporal lobe focus without a preceding complex partial seizure. Moreover, psychic auras from the temporal lobe, particularly if associated with negative feelings (e.g., *jamais vu* and fear), predispose to psychosis or personality disorders.

Psychosis Psychosis is the specific psychiatric disorder most clearly associated with epilepsy. The lifelong prevalence of all psychotic disorders among epileptic patients ranges from 7 to 12 percent. In a follow-up of 100 children with complex partial seizures for as long as 30 years, of the 87 patients who survived to adulthood and who did not have mental retardation, 9 (10 percent) experienced a psychotic illness. Moreover, in temporal lobectomy studies, in which there is surgical removal of an epileptic focus, psychosis occurred in 7 to 8 percent of patients, even long after the seizures were arrested. That percentage represents approximately a twofold or greater risk of psychosis for epileptic patients than for the general population; patients whose epilepsy has a mediobasal temporal focus are especially at risk.

Studies on the laterality of the seizure focus suggest an association of a left-sided focus with psychosis. Although conclusions derived from surface EEG recording are open to criticism, depth recordings of presurgical patients show that twice as many patients with left temporal lesions have psychosis. Positron emission tomography (PET) scans and single photon emission computed tomography (SPECT) scans may show predominant left temporal hypometabolism in epilepsy patients with psychosis.

Depression The prevalence of depression in various studies varies and may range from 7.5 to 34 percent of patients with epilepsy. Those with complex partial seizures and poor seizure control are more likely to have mood disorders. Psychological studies also suggest a greater incidence of ideational orientation, self-criticism, and depression among epilepsy patients with a left hemisphere focus. Patients with complex partial seizures of temporal limbic origin have a higher incidence of depression than do patients with other types of seizure disorders.

Other Behaviors The prevalence of other specific behavioral disorders among patients with epilepsy is less well established. There is convincing evidence, however, that personality disorders, suicidal behavior, and hyposexuality are more prevalent among epilepsy patients than among those without seizure disorders.

ETIOLOGY

Most new-onset epilepsy is idiopathic, but other frequent causes include trauma in the third and fourth decades of life, neoplasms in the fifth and sixth decades of life, and cerebrovascular disease in the elderly. Although some complex partial seizures originate from frontal or temporal neocortex and other areas, at least two-thirds of complex partial seizures and generalized tonic-clonic seizures originate from the mediobasal temporal limbic structures (hippocampus, amygdala, and parahippocampal gyrus).

Psychopathology The relationship of seizures, psychiatric syndromes, and the mediobasal temporal lobes implies that many behavioral changes are more than psychological reactions to the psychosocial stressors of epilepsy. Stimulation and ablation studies in humans and animals link temporal limbic structures to emotional behavior.

For example, temporal limbic stimulation in a person evokes psychic auras and automatisms, and amygdalar stimulation and ablation in animals results in aggression or placidity. Moreover, psychotic behavior in cats occurs when their limbic structures undergo kindling (that is, the repeated application of epileptic agents to induce lasting behavioral changes).

There are several potential organic causes of psychiatric disturbances in epilepsy (Table 2.4–3). First, the pathology itself could be the source of seizures and behavioral changes. Left hemisphere and temporal lobe lesions may be associated with a schizophreniform psychosis, and psychosis in epilepsy may be particularly frequent if there is specific underlying pathology or ventricular enlargement. Psychotic disorders may be more common with temporal dysplasia or neurodevelopmental abnormalities and depression with mesial temporal sclerosis. Second, ictal or subictal epileptiform activity may promote behavioral changes by facilitating distributed neuronal connections, increasing limbic-sensory associations, or changing the overall balance between excitation and inhibition. This may occur not only with temporal lobe seizures, but also with those that originate in the frontal lobes. Third, the absence of function, such as the interictal hypometabolism observed on PET scans (Fig. 2.4–2), may lead to depression or other interictal behavioral changes. Among epileptic patients with a schizophreniform psychosis, SPECT scans have shown reductions in cerebral blood flow in the left medial temporal region. Fourth, seizures may result in neuroendocrine or neurotransmitter changes, such as increased dopaminergic or inhibitory transmitters, decreased prolactin, increased testosterone, or increased endogenous opioids, all of which can affect behavior. Furthermore, neurobiological factors may be potentiated by psychodynamic factors, such as feelings of helplessness, learned helplessness, dependency, low self-esteem, and the disruption of reality testing. In sum, the psychiatric manifestations of epilepsy are heterogeneous disorders with a multiplicity of causes.

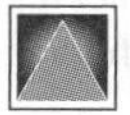

Table 2.4–3
Proposed Relationships of Psychiatric Disturbances to Epilepsy

Common neuropathology, genetics, or developmental disturbance
Ictal or subictal discharges potentiate abnormal behavior
Kindling or facilitation of a distributed neuronal matrix
Changes in spike frequency or inhibitory–excitatory balance
Altered receptor sensitivity, for example, dopamine receptors
Secondary epileptogenesis
Absence of function at the seizure focus
Inhibition and hypometabolism surrounding the focus
Release or abnormal activity of remaining neurons
Dysfunction or downregulation of associated areas
Neurochemical
Dopamine and other neurotransmitters
Endorphins
Gonadotrophins and other endocrine hormones
Psychodynamic and psychosocial effects of living with epilepsy
Dependence, learned helplessness, low self-esteem, weak defense mechanisms
Disruption of reality testing
Neurobiological and psychodynamic factors potentiate each other
Sleep disturbance
Anticonvulsant drug related

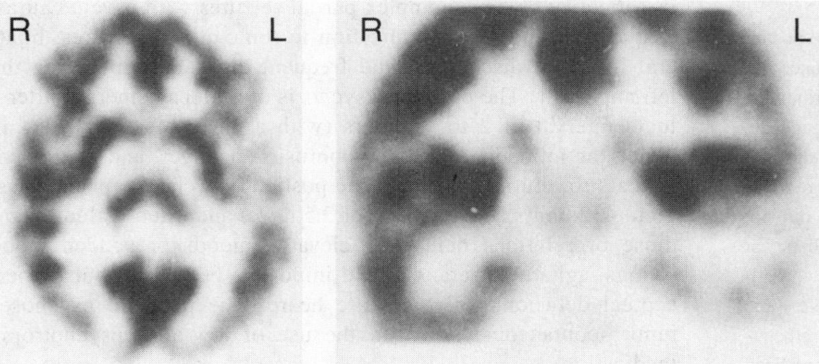

FIGURE 2.4–2 [18]Fluorodeoxyglucose positron emission tomography scans demonstrating interictal hypometabolism in the left temporolimbic region. This is evident as an area of decreased signal uptake (*lighter*) in the left temporal lobe. (From Engel J Jr, ed. *Seizures and Epilepsy*. Philadelphia: FA Davis Co; 1989, with permission.)

DIAGNOSIS

In epilepsy, psychiatric behaviors can be conceptualized in relation to the ictus or seizure discharges. These behaviors occur as part of the ictus, periictally, or during the interictal period (Table 2.4–4). Moreover, a range of other behaviors appear to have some relation to the ictus but do not clearly fall into one of the former three categories.

Ictal Features Seizure discharges can produce semipurposeful automatisms and psychic auras, such as mood changes, derealization and depersonalization, and forced thinking. Ictal fear, which ranges from a vague apprehension to abject fright, has occurred without any other seizure manifestation, and ictal depression has extended days or longer after the seizure has passed. Some patients have pleasurable auras. Fyodor Dostoyevsky had "ecstatic auras" in which he felt in perfect harmony with the entire universe and "would give 10 years of this life, perhaps all of it, for a few seconds of such bliss." The experience of epileptic derealization or depersonalization could impair reality testing. Another psychic aura is "forced thinking," characterized by recurrent intrusive thoughts, ideas, or crowding of thoughts. Forced thinking must be distinguished from obsessional thoughts and compulsive urges. Epileptic patients with forced thinking experience their thoughts as stereotypical, out-of-context, brief, and irrational, but not necessarily as ego dystonic.

A 36-year-old right-handed man presented with frontal headaches and 5 years of complex partial seizures. His seizures began with 15 seconds of a sense of "impending doom," speech arrest, and orobucchal movements followed by 30 seconds of altered consciousness. At seizure onset, the patient felt forced to think the phrase "tell me yes." The phrase repeated several times without his being able to control it. Concomitantly, his mouth would open, and he would attempt to say the phrase but could utter only unintelligible sounds. The patient interpreted this phrase as a call for help. On examination, he had a mild memory deficit, normal language testing, a right facial droop, and brisk right-sided reflexes with a right Babinski sign. Neuroimaging revealed a left frontal mass lesion. EEGs showed amplitude attenuation and polymorphic delta in the left frontal area, and intraoperative electrocorticography disclosed polyspike and spike-wave discharges and impaired language from just below the lesion. The patient underwent subtotal resection of a $4.3 \times 3 \times 3$ cm oligodendroglioma. Postoperatively, his forced thinking and seizures resolved, but he had a nonfluent aphasia.

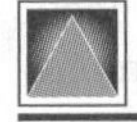

Table 2.4–4
Behavioral Disorders in Epilepsy

Ictal
- Ictal psychic symptoms
- Nonconvulsive status: simple partial seizures, complex partial seizures, and periodic lateralizing epileptiform discharges

Periictal (includes prodromal, postictal, and mixed ictal)
- Prodromal symptoms: irritability, depression, headache, etc.
- Postictal confusion
- Periictal psychoses
  - Concomitant with increased seizure frequency
  - Concomitant with decreased seizure frequency
  - Postictal psychoses

Interictal psychosis and personality disturbances
- Schizophreniform psychosis
- Personality disorders
- Gastaut-Geschwind syndrome

Behavioral disturbances variably related to ictus
- Mood disorders (depression and mania)
- Dissociative states
- Aggression and violence
- Hyposexuality
- Suicide
- Other behaviors

Cognitive disorders follow status epilepticus with simple partial seizures, complex partial seizures, or absence seizures. Recurrent or prolonged simple partial seizures do not result in alteration of consciousness or invariable abnormalities on EEG, and, if manifested by psychic auras, simple partial seizures may be difficult to distinguish from primary psychiatric disturbances. Status epilepticus from complex partial seizures and absence seizures results in prolonged alterations of responsiveness. With the addition of various ictal auras, complex partial status epilepticus can appear psychotic. Occasionally, EEGs and a therapeutic trial of anticonvulsant medications may be the only way to distinguish behavioral disturbances due to nonconvulsive status epilepticus. Finally, recurrent EEG complexes, known as *periodic lateralizing epileptiform discharges*, may also be associated with prolonged confusional behavior and focal cognitive changes.

A 68-year-old man had a left temporal-parietal hemorrhagic stroke. An initial fluent aphasia and right hemiparesis completely resolved, but he developed poststroke epilepsy. His seizures began with speech arrest and were followed by secondary generalization to tonic-clonic seizures. The postictal periods lasted days due to continued left-hemisphere periodic lateralizing epileptiform discharges. During these prolonged postictal periods, he was confused and placid and had a return of his aphasia. One year later, after achieving seizure control, the patient developed mania for the first time in his life. His mania was in a clear sensorium without a change in his neurological examination or epileptiform activity on EEG. He did not sleep, had flight of ideas, and had grandiose ideation, including beliefs that he was a three-star general, had killed Adolph Hitler, and was now a millionaire. He exposed himself to everyone, including his daughter, and inserted pencils up his penis, because he believed that he needed catheterization. His psychosis lasted for 3 months until he had two generalized tonic-clonic seizures. Postictally, for 10 days he remained placid, confused, and aphasic, with a right beating nystagmus and periodic lateralizing epileptiform discharges maximal in the left temporal region (Fig. 2.4–3). With a new anticonvulsant medication, he returned to normal with total resolution of his mania.

Periictal Features Psychiatric disturbances can occur before seizures (prodromal), after seizures (postictal), or during intermittent seizure activity. Some patients experience prodromal symptoms that begin at least 30 minutes before seizure onset, last 10 minutes to 3 days, and are continuous with irritability, depression, headache, confusion, and other symptoms. The postictal period is characterized by a confusional state lasting minutes to hours or, occasionally, days. Prolonged, postictal confusion may particularly follow right temporal complex partial seizures. Some "twilight states" result from a protracted period of intermixed ictal and postictal changes.

Periictal psychotic symptoms often worsen with increasing seizure activity. Rarely, psychotic symptoms alternate with seizure activity. In this *alternating psychosis*, when patients are having seizures, they are free of psychotic symptoms, but when they are seizure free and their EEG has *forced* or *paradoxical normalization*, they manifest psychotic symptoms. This alternating pattern is much less common than the increased emergence of psychotic behavior with increasing seizure activity.

An important periictal psychiatric disorder consists of brief psychotic episodes that follow clusters of generalized tonic-clonic seizures (i.e., postictal psychosis). These psychotic episodes occur in patients who have complex partial seizures with psychic auras, frequent secondary generalization to tonic-clonic seizures, bilateral interictal discharges, and frequent discharges involving the left amygdala. The postictal psychosis of epilepsy emerges after a lucid interval of 2 to 72 hours (with a mean of 1 day), during which the immediate postictal confusion resolves, and the patient appears to return to normal. The postictal psychotic episodes last 16 to 432 hours (with a mean of 3.5 days) and often include grandiose or religious delusions, elevated moods or sudden mood swings, agitation, paranoia, and impulsive behaviors, but no perceptual delusions or voices are heard. The postictal psychoses remit spontaneously or with the use of low-dose psychotropic medication.

A 33-year-old man with a 15-year history of generalized tonic-clonic seizures and a 4-year history of periictal psychotic episodes had several hospitalizations for recurrent postictal psychosis. The initial flurry of generalized tonic-clonic seizures was followed by a 24- to 48-hour latency period, and, subsequently, 2 to 7 days of delusions, hallucinations, and disordered thought processes. He believed that people could transmit messages and could read his thoughts, and voices commanded him to love his neighbor. The patient claimed to read the future and to communicate with a dead grandfather who voiced dissatisfaction with things on earth. During these episodes, the patient had loose associations, euphoria, agitation, and occasional spike and waves on EEGs. Between psychotic episodes, he was psychiatrically and neurologically normal, and his EEGs showed left temporal interictal spikes. After the postictal psychosis, the patient returned to baseline without residual changes in behavior.

Interictal Features

Schizophreniform Psychosis Most epilepsy patients with a schizophreniform psychosis have a chronic interictal illness without a known direct relationship to seizure events or ictal discharges. Many of these patients, however, develop worsening psychotic symptoms that are concomitant with an increase in seizure frequency or with anticonvulsant withdrawal, and a few others have worsening psychotic symptoms on control of the seizures (alternat-

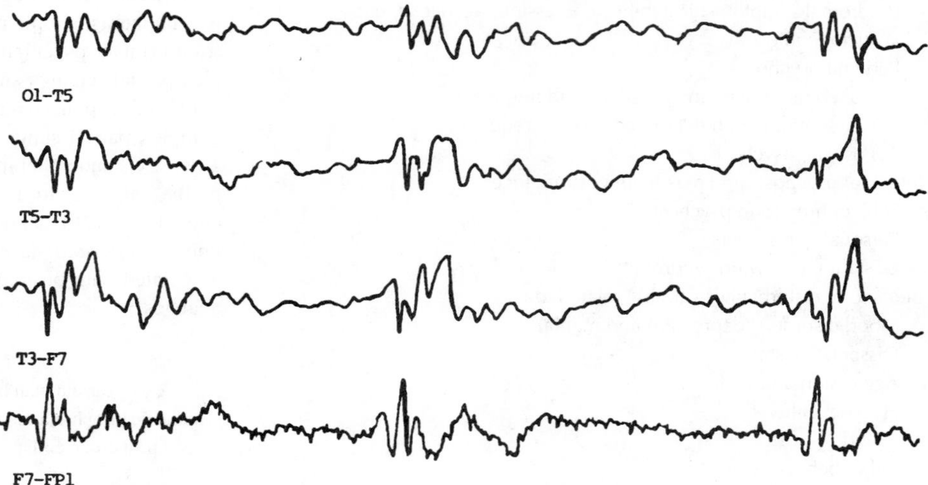

FIGURE 2.4–3 Periodic lateralizing epileptiform discharges. Left-sided electrodes per the International 10/20 System.

ing psychosis). The terms *alternating psychosis* and *forced* or *paradoxical normalization* refer to this demonstrable antagonism between the psychosis and the seizures or EEG discharges. Epilepsy patients with this chronic interictal psychosis often have an early age of onset of seizures and a decade or more of poorly controlled partial complex seizures, usually with secondary generalized tonic-clonic seizures. This interictal psychosis may evolve from prior recurrent postictal psychotic episodes. Seizure control with anticonvulsants or removal of the seizure focus does not prevent the development of the interictal psychosis, which occasionally emerges for the first time after successful seizure treatment. This disorder sometimes resembles a schizoaffective psychosis with intermixed affective symptoms. In addition, there are prominent paranoid delusions, relative preserved affect, normal premorbid personality, and no family history of schizophrenia. Other reported differences with idiopathic schizophrenia are outlined in Table 2.4–5.

A 23-year-old man developed paranoid delusions after his daily complex partial seizures were controlled for the first time. His seizures dated from 8 years of age and consisted of a rising epigastric sensation and facial flushing followed by a motionless stare and automatisms, often culminating in secondary generalized tonic-clonic seizures. Before initiating anticonvulsant therapy, there was no history of paranoid or psychotic behavior. Afterward, he believed that people were sending energy to him through small concealed batteries. He believed that he was able to work this energy off with his fluorescent watch dial and a one-armed plastic crucifix in his boot. The patient also felt that people were observing him, trying to manipulate him, and were threatening him through telephone lines and telephone poles. His examination was remarkable for the degree of emotion when relating his bizarre ideas. He had a lesion in the left anterior temporal area, probably consistent with an old calcified cyst, and left temporal spikes on EEG. His paranoid delusions subsequently abated with antipsychotic therapy.

Personality Disorders Among epileptic patients, there is a high prevalence of personality disorders, including borderline, atypical or mixed, histrionic, and dependent disorders. Patients with personality disorders tend to show dependent and avoidant personality traits. The most common personality disorder in epilepsy is a borderline personality. Not surprisingly, epileptic patients frequently lack a stable character structure and can be immature and impulsive. This personality constellation partially explains the increased incidence of irritability, suicide attempts, and intermittent explosive disorder. Those with epilepsy are stigmatized, feared, and subject to difficulties in obtaining a job, driving an automobile, and maintaining a marriage. These psychosocial difficulties, along with any associated mental retardation, contribute to the dependency, low self-esteem, and overall borderline personality traits present in many such patients. In addition, the experience of epileptic auras may contribute to the development of personality disorders.

Gastaut-Geschwind Syndrome Although there is no general epileptic personality, a group of traits termed the *Gastaut-Geschwind syndrome* occurs in a subset of patients with complex partial seizures. Some epilepsy patients with a temporal limbic focus develop a sense of the heightened significance of things. These patients are serious, humorless, overinclusive, and have an intense interest in philosophic, moral, or religious issues. Occasionally, epilepsy patients experience multiple religious conversions or experiences. In interpersonal encounters, they demonstrate *viscosity*, the tendency to talk repetitively and circumstantially about a restricted range of topics. They can spend a long time getting to the point, give detailed background information with multiple quotations, or write copiously about their thoughts and feelings (hypergraphia). Viscosity may particularly occur in patients with left-sided or bilateral temporal foci.

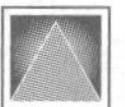

Table 2.4–5
Proposed Predisposing Factors for the Interictal Schizophreniform Psychosis of Epilepsy

Epilepsy characteristics
- Complex partial seizures with secondary generalized tonic-clonic seizures
- More auras and automatisms than nonpsychotic epilepsy patients
- Epilepsy present for 11 to 15 years before psychosis
- Long interval of poorly controlled seizures
- Recently diminished seizure frequency, especially generalized tonic-clonic seizures
- Left temporal focus
- Mediobasal temporal lesions, especially tumors

Psychosis characteristics
- Atypical paranoid psychosis-paranoia with sudden onset
- Psychosis alternating with seizures
- Preserved affective warmth
- Failure of personality deterioration
- Less social withdrawal than schizophrenia
- Less systematized delusions than schizophrenia
- More hallucinations and affective symptoms than schizophrenia
- More religiosity than schizophrenia
- More positive, as opposed to negative, symptoms
- Few schneiderian first-rank symptoms

A 39-year-old man developed seizures after a contusion of the left temporal region. His seizures began with stereotypical voices and generalized to tonic-clonic seizures. He was extremely circumstantial and tangential, stressed every detail, and had difficulty getting to the point. Ironic and minor philosophical insights were fascinating to him. He wrote 30-page rambling letters to his physician, and his writings were full of metaphors and quotes. An example of his writing was as follows: "I became overwhelmed by the sentiment of a letter composed in my head before reaching paper. The sentiment of this letter continued to expand in all dimensions until it seemed no longer connected to any specific ideal, but more to an all pervasive color, yellow, and a smell, like burning leaves. I felt deliriously happy, but I felt in danger as well. Afterwards I got an acute attack of aphasia and could do nothing but shrug. My prior prophet voices which went away with the Dilantin were saying something profound that I needed to get down on paper. It seems as though I am a prophet and I will never have another problem for the rest of my life."

Conclusive proof that epileptic patients with a temporal lobe foci are disproportionately prone to the Gastaut-Geschwind syndrome has remained illusive. Most of the early studies used the MMPI, a test that proved insensitive to most of the specific traits attributed to epilepsy. Studies with the Bear-Fedio Inventory, an MMPI-like instrument developed to assess these "epileptic traits," found that epileptic patients with temporal lobe foci were sober and humorless, dependent, and circumstantial and had strong philosophical interests. In addition, those with a left-sided focus had a more reflective ideational style and maximized their problems, whereas those with a right-sided focus had emotional tendencies and minimized their problems. Further investigations with the Bear-Fedio Inventory described these seizure patients as having viscosity in interactions, prominent religious interests, a pronounced sense of personal destiny, and deepened affect. However, other applications of this inventory found the same characteristics in nonepileptic patients with psychiatric disorders or with comparable physical disabilities. Although these personality characteristics do occur in some epileptic patients, they may not be specific for patients with seizure disorders.

Behavioral Disturbances Variably Related to Ictus

Mood Disorders Depressive disorder is the most prevalent neuropsychiatric disorder in epilepsy, occurring in 7.5 to 25 percent of epileptic patients. Depression is also the main diagnosis among epileptic patients in mental hospitals. Depression is twice as common in epilepsy patients as in comparably disabled populations, suggesting that much of the depression in epilepsy patients is more than just a psychological reaction to a disability.

Most patients with epilepsy have a chronic interictal depression or dysthymia. Some investigators refer to this condition as the *interictal dysphoric disorder of epilepsy* and emphasize associated paroxysmal irritability or agitation along with a good therapeutic response to antidepressant medications. These patients may have accompanying paranoia and hallucinations, emphasizing the continuum with psychotic disorders. Patients with interictal dysphoria tend to have frequent complex partial seizures, possibly with greater left-sided temporal foci, although this lateralization is not established. The experience of certain psychic auras, especially those with cognitive content, may predispose to interictal depression. Several investigators also report increased seizure control or a decrease in seizures before the onset of interictal depressive symptoms. Patients with this "alternating depression" experience relief with a seizure or electroconvulsive therapy (ECT).

There are other associations of depression with epilepsy. The rare occurrence of ictal depression may not only outlast the actual ictus but also may lead to suicide. Depression also occurs periictally. Episodic mood disturbances, often with agitation, suicidal behavior, and psychotic symptoms, may occur with increasing seizure activity. Finally, postictal depression is common, and a prolonged depressive state occasionally follows complex partial seizures, even when ictal experiences do not include depression.

Mood disorder due to epilepsy with manic features or with mixed features is much rarer than mood disorder due to epilepsy with depressive features or with major depressive-like features. Rarely, manic symptoms may emerge with an increase in seizure frequency or after seizure control. Although a right temporal focus is a possible source of mania in epilepsy, this laterality is not established.

Dissociative States A specific association of epilepsy with dissociative identity disorder, depersonalization disorders, possession states, fugue states, and psychogenic amnesia is intriguing but unresolved. Studies of patients with multiple personality disorder reveal frequent EEG changes but few actual seizures. It is conceivable that temporary personality disintegration occurs in some patients as part of postictal confusion or periictal psychosis, particularly in those with a right temporal focus. In one intracarotid amobarbital (Amytal) study of multiple personality in two seizure patients, the different personalities were precipitated without seizure activity. Persistent alterations in the experience of self and feelings of being taken over by others may occur in patients with auras of derealization and depersonalization. In epilepsy, prolonged periods of compulsive wandering with amnesia have resulted from an admixture of ictal and postictal changes and have been termed *poriomania*. Finally, some patients may have periods of amnesia or lost time, possibly due to complex partial seizures without surface EEG abnormalities.

Aggression Lay people have accredited to epilepsy aggressive and violent acts and have even used this epilepsy defense in criminal proceedings. This belief peaked in the 19th century when the criminologist Cesare Lombroso promoted the association of epilepsy with aggressive, sociopathic tendencies. Investigators have bolstered this association with studies showing aggressive verbalizations with stimulation of the amygdala and interictal defensive rage in cats with epileptic hippocampal lesions. A minority of violent epilepsy patients have left-sided amygdalar atrophy probably from a prior encephalitis. Among patients in a maximum-security mental hospital, the violent patients had focal temporal slowing or sharp waves on EEG and dilated temporal horns or small temporal lobes on computed tomography (CT) scans. These results suggest that high violence rating scores are associated with abnormal temporal electrical discharges on EEG and temporal lobe abnormalities on CT. Moreover, patients with left temporal lobe seizure foci have higher scores on hostile feelings than other patients with epilepsy.

> A 37-year-old left-handed man with epilepsy presented with aggressive episodes. The seizures consisted of an olfactory aura followed by "spacing out" or alteration of consciousness for approximately 1 minute. In addition to these complex partial seizures, the patient had occasional secondary generalized tonic-clonic seizures with urinary incontinence and tongue biting. During the postictal period, as he began to recover consciousness, he experienced an overwhelming sense of threat or of having been harmed. These feelings became focused on any individual who was in his immediate environment. That person was believed to have beaten or otherwise hurt him and was going to harm him further. The patient felt compelled to attack these individuals, often inflicting significant physical injury. Although his postictal confusion would clear in approximately 1 hour, his sense of being harmed or threatened slowly diminished over approximately 24 hours after a seizure. After the resolution of these feelings, he felt great remorse over the harm that he had done. Nevertheless, on several occasions, he was charged with aggravated assault. Sleep-deprived EEGs confirmed the presence of left anterior temporal epileptiform activity. The patient's aggressive postictal episodes abated with control of his complex partial seizures with carbamazepine.

Although aggression can occur in relation to an ictus, as exemplified by this patient's subacute postictal aggression, most aggression among epilepsy patients is not related to epileptiform activity. Aggression in epilepsy is usually associated with psychosis or intermittent explosive disorder and correlates with subnormal intelligence, lower socioeconomic status (SES), childhood behavior problems, prior head injuries, and possible orbital frontal damage. Moreover, although the prevalence of epilepsy among prison inmates has been two to four times that among the general population, studies from

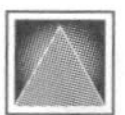

Table 2.4–6
Criteria for the Assessment of Ictal Violence in Epilepsy

The diagnosis of epilepsy is established by at least one specialist in epilepsy.

The presence of epileptic automatisms are documented by history and by closed circuit television EEG telemetry.

The presence of violence during epileptic automatisms is verified in a videotape-recorded seizure in which ictal epileptiform patterns are also recorded on the EEG.

The aggressive act is characteristic of the patient's habitual seizures, as elicited by history.

A clinical judgment is made by the epilepsy specialist attesting to the possibility that the aggressive act was part of a seizure.

EEG, electroencephalogram.

the United Kingdom and the United States have not found more violent crimes among prisoners with epilepsy than among prisoners without epilepsy.

Can violence itself be a seizure? After the 1976 case of a New York City policeman who had never had seizures and successfully claimed the epilepsy defense, criteria for ictal violence were proposed that included video-EEG telemetry (Table 2.4–6). Since then, epilepsy has rarely, if ever, been proved to directly result in premeditated violence. Such acts require a series of coordinated steps that rarely occur as manifestations of seizures. Simple violent automatisms, such as spitting or flailing the arms, can occur at the onset of complex partial seizures, and secondary violent automatisms can occur as a response to an unpleasant or emotional aura or periictal sensation (Table 2.4–7). More commonly, nondirected violent movements, aimless destructive behavior, or angry verbal outbursts occur during postictal delirium when patients misinterpret attempts to protect or restrain them or as a manifestation of postictal psychosis and subacute postictal aggression.

Sexuality Patients with epilepsy tend to be hyposexual. Men and women experience disturbances of sexual arousal and a lower sexual drive. Some patients have a disinterest in "all the usual libidinous aspects of life," including loss of erotic fantasies or dreams, and may experience impotence or frigidity. Men have an increased risk of erectile dysfunction, suggesting a neurophysiological component, and studies of sex hormones suggest the possibility of a subclinical hypogonadotropic hypogonadism. Substantial improvement to the point of public hypersexuality can occur after seizures are brought under control. Moreover, before temporal lobectomy, most epileptic patients are hyposexual, but nearly one-third of them have an increase in libido after the operation, providing that their seizures are controlled.

Other sexuality changes are rare. Individual cases of homosexuality, transvestism, fetishism, and gender dysphoria are not frequent enough to exclude a coincident association. True ictal sexual manifestations are also unusual; however, libidinous feelings, erotic sensations, sexual remembrances, and even orgasm rarely occur, primarily in women and probably from seizure discharges in the amygdala. In addition, ictal masturbation has occurred with absence status. A woman with nymphomania proved to have incidental sexuality from sensory simple partial seizures caused by a tumor in the sensory cortex representing her genital region.

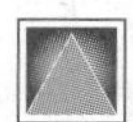

Table 2.4–7
Mechanisms of Aggression Among Epilepsy Patients

Period	Cause
Interictal	Impulse-control disorder
	Mental retardation or cognitive impairments
	Personality disorders
	Schizophrenia-like psychosis of epilepsy
	Medication related
Prodrome	Mounting tension, irritability
Ictal	Direct manifestation of the seizure
	Violent automatism
	Reaction to a negative aura
	Subtle seizure equivalents
Postictal	Resistive
	Postictal psychosis
	Subacute postictal aggression
	Poriomania and somnambulism

Suicide The risk of completed suicide in epilepsy patients is four to five times greater than among the nonepileptic population, and those with complex partial seizures of temporal lobe origin have a particularly high risk, as much as 25 times greater. Death by suicide occurs in 3 to 7 percent of epilepsy patients. A comparison of suicide attempts among patients with epilepsy and comparably handicapped nonepileptic controls has reported that 30 percent of those with epilepsy had attempted suicide as compared to 7 percent of the controls. This increased risk of suicide continues even long after temporal lobectomy and successful control of seizures. Most suicidal behavior among epileptic patients is not directly due to reactions to the psychosocial stressors of having a seizure disorder. Rather, these patients are likely to attempt suicide in conjunction with borderline personality behaviors and are likely to complete suicide during postictal psychosis. Contributors to successful suicides include paranoid hallucinations, agitated compunction to kill themselves, and occasional ictal command hallucinations to commit suicide.

A 26-year-old woman had her initial seizure during her first pregnancy at 18 years of age. Her seizures included echoing sounds "like walking in a cave," a motionless stare with stereotypical automatisms, postictal confusion, and occasional secondary generalized tonic-clonic seizures. Because of a variable anticonvulsant response, she underwent EEG and closed-circuit television video-EEG (CCTV-EEG) telemetry that documented complex partial seizures from a right temporal focus and nonepileptic seizures. The patient, who had six children by six different individuals, had prominent feelings of inadequacy and isolation and was considering cutting her wrists "just to see if anyone cared." Her multiple suicide attempts and threats resulted in five psychiatric hospitalizations. During one period of time, she complained of decreased menses, weight gain, stretch marks, increased appetite and sleep, and exhaustion. She insisted that she was pregnant despite six negative pregnancy tests and multiple evaluations.

Other Behavioral Changes Other psychiatric disorders may be associated with epilepsy or epileptiform EEG activity. Anxiety and panic disorders occur among epileptic patients and must be distinguished from simple partial seizures manifesting as anxiety or panic. Among the impulse control disorders, intermittent explosive disorder is characterized by a prodromal mounting tension and irritability, postictal remorse, and increased temporal spikes on EEG. Among the somatoform disorders, some epileptic patients have a conversion disorder, often manifested as nonepileptic seizure events. Finally, patients with epilepsy are subject to other behavioral difficulties stemming from their epilepsy, such as adjustment disorders, subtle cognitive effects of seizures, and the potential behavioral effects of anticonvulsant medications.

PATHOLOGY AND LABORATORY EXAMINATION

Neurodiagnostic Tests In addition to the routine laboratory data and toxicology screens used to exclude reactive seizures, several neurodiagnostic tests are useful in the assessment of epilepsy. EEG is the most widely used confirmatory test for seizures; however, single EEGs are frequently normal and must be repeated, particularly with provocative maneuvers, such as sleep. Occasionally, CCTV-EEG telemetry for an extended period of time is necessary to capture seizure activity. Neuroimaging procedures, such as CT scans and magnetic resonance imaging (MRI), can more precisely visualize a seizure focus or even mesial temporal sclerosis (Fig. 2.4–4). Other tests that occasionally aid in localizing the seizure focus include quantitative EEG, SPECT scans, and PET scans. PET scans may show interictal hypometabolism around the temporal seizure focus and are also useful in the presurgical assessment of medically intractable seizure patients. Neuropsychological examinations, particularly during a Wada's test, further help in localizing and lateralizing memory and language before surgery.

Neuropathology The common pathological findings in epilepsy are mediobasal temporal lobe lesions. Approximately two-thirds of epileptic adults have a temporal lobe focus, and two-thirds of these have mesial temporal sclerosis with pyramidal cell loss in the hippocampus. Theories about the cause of mesial temporal sclerosis include perinatal insults, dysgenesis, and kindling from reactive seizures. Another 20 to 25 percent of those with temporal lobe lesions have tumors, such as hamartomas and gangliogliomas. The rest have scars from trauma and other causes or lack a distinct histological lesion.

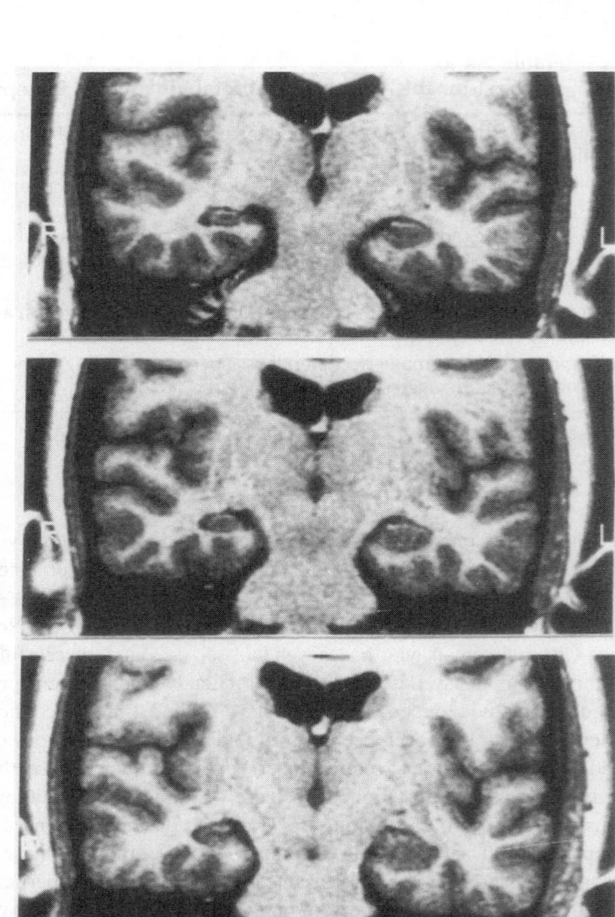

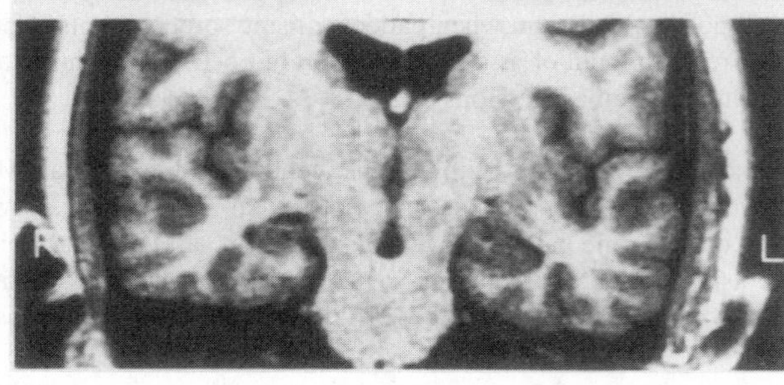

FIGURE 2.4–4 A series of magnetic resonance imaging scans demonstrating mesial temporal sclerotic changes in the left hippocampal region. (From Engel J Jr. In vivo imaging the temporal lobe limbic system. In: Trimble MR, Bolwig TG, eds. *The Temporal Lobes and the Limbic System.* Petersfield, England: Wrightson Biomedical Publishing; 1992, with permission.)

DIFFERENTIAL DIAGNOSIS

Clinicians must distinguish epileptic seizures from two other transient behavioral events, syncope and nonepileptic seizures (pseudoseizures). *Syncope* is a loss of consciousness, usually with premonitory lightheadedness, autonomic reactivity, a brief atonic ictus, and little or no postictal confusion. Syncope lacks the many characteristic features of seizures and a clear epileptiform EEG. *Nonepileptic seizures*, on the other hand, are involuntary, psychogenically induced spells that, by definition, mimic many epileptic behaviors.

Differentiating epileptic seizures from nonepileptic seizures can be extremely difficult, and even epileptologists are incorrect 20 to 30 percent of the time. Patients with nonepileptic seizures are most commonly women between the ages of 26 and 32 years of age with psychological stressors and poor coping skills. Approximately 10 to 15 percent of these patients have a true seizure disorder as well, and nonepileptic seizures may result from the elaborating or "highlighting" of their epileptic seizures. Nonepileptic seizures are most commonly characterized by unresponsiveness with motor activity that does not fit a typical complex partial or generalized tonic-clonic seizure (Table 2.4–8). In children, pseudoseizures are usually characterized by unresponsiveness, with violent and uncoordinated movements of the whole body. However, every epileptic behavior can occasionally occur, including tongue biting and incontinence, and nonepileptic events are especially difficult to differentiate from the atypical motor behavior of frontal lobe epilepsy. The most helpful differentiation feature may be an ictal duration of 2 minutes or more. In addition, nonepileptic seizures usually occur in the presence of a witness; can often be induced with injections, hypnosis, or sug-

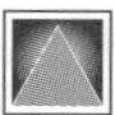

Table 2.4–8
Nonepileptic Seizures versus Epileptic Seizures

Nonepileptic Seizures	Epileptic Seizures
Preceding ictus	
Absence of explanatory disease or signs	Frequent evidence of neurological disease
Anxiety auras: palpitations, choking, etc.	Wide range of epileptic auras
Seizures may be induced or provoked	Rarely induced except for reactive seizures
During ictus	
Inconsistencies in clinical presentation	Fit specific seizure types
Seizures may differ from attack to attack	Stereotypical seizure pattern
Only occur when others are present	Often occur without witnesses or at night
Gradual onset, prolonged duration (>2 min)	Abrupt onset, short duration (<2 min)
Asymmetrical, out-of-phase movements, pelvic thrusts, and hyperarching	Decrescendo, symmetrical clonic activity in GTC seizure
Rare whole body rigidity	Tonic rigidity at onset of GTC seizure
Rare incontinence, tongue biting, self-injury	Incontinence, tongue biting if generalized
Normal autonomic reactivity, corneal reflex, and pupillary responses	Disturbed autonomic reactivity, corneal reflexes, and pupillary responses
Avoids noxious stimuli or eye opening	Cannot avoid noxious stimuli
Vocalizations may occur throughout ictus	Single vocalization, if present, at onset
Normal ictal EEG	Abnormal ictal EEG
After ictus	
No postictal delirium	Typical postictal delirium
No increase in prolactin	Prolactin >1,000 IU/L, 10 to 20 min postictally
Normal postictal EEG	Postictal slowing on EEG
Subsequent recall of events during ictus	No or fragmentary recall of ictal events
No relationship of ictal frequency to anticonvulsant medications	Diminished seizure frequency with anticonvulsant medications

EEG, electroencephalogram; GTC, generalized tonic-clonic.

gestions; and are poorly responsive to anticonvulsant medications. Ultimately, the differentiation may require CCTV-EEG telemetry along with the assessment of the absence of a seizure-induced rise in serum prolactin levels.

Nonepileptic seizures result from a variety of psychiatric conditions. The most common psychiatric disturbance among these patients is conversion disorder. Patients with nonepileptic seizures who have conversion disorder have a high incidence of prior trauma or sexual or physical abuse. The remaining patients with nonepileptic seizures have depression, dissociative disorders, anxiety disorders, posttraumatic stress disorder (PTSD), or borderline or other personality disorders. Additional diagnoses associated with nonepileptic seizures are psychosis, impulse control problems, and mental retardation.

Nonepileptic seizures must be differentiated from those specifically due to the malingering or feigning of epilepsy for secondary gain (Table 2.4–9). Epileptic seizures lend themselves to malingering because of their behavioral and episodic nature and the lack of consistent physical or diagnostic findings.

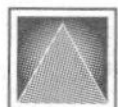

Table 2.4–9
Malingered Seizures versus Nonmalingered Nonepileptic Seizures

Malingered Seizures	Nonmalingered Nonepileptic Seizures
Preceding ictus	
More common in men	Marked female predominance
Less likely to obtain prior abuse history	Prior history of physical or sexual abuse
Less likely to obtain prior psychiatry history	Prior psychiatric history
Evident secondary gain	No clear secondary gain
No clear emotional precipitants	Frequent emotional precipitants
Seizures are not suggestible	Seizures may be easily suggested
During ictus	
Seizures under volitional control	Seizures not under volitional control
Conscious awareness of seizures	Subconscious awareness of seizures only
Cannot maintain deficits over time	Able to maintain deficits over time
Errors in seizure behavior are likely to be major distortions	Errors in seizure behavior are likely to be omissions, perseverations, near misses
After ictus	
Angry, anxious on confrontation, with a lack of evidence for epileptic seizures	Indifferent, detached
Uncooperative, including circumstantial and evasive answers; may leave against medical advice	Cooperative with the workup, but answers may be devoid of content

A 33-year-old veteran of the Persian Gulf War presented with a complaint of epileptic spells, beginning 3 years after returning home. The patient claimed that the stress of the war induced his seizure disorder, and he requested disability compensation. He described his seizures as the abrupt loss of consciousness associated with jerking movements of his extremities. His episodes occurred irregularly with a frequency of two to four per week. On admission to the hospital, medical staff observed several seizure-like spells in which the patient assumed a flexed posture of his upper and lower extremities and then shook them uncontrollably and in an asynchronous fashion. During this ictal period, the patient had normal pupillary and corneal reflexes. His seizures lasted nearly 5 minutes and then immediately resolved without postictal confusion. Postictally, he recalled comments and other environmental events that occurred during his seizure-like episodes. EEGs obtained immediately after an event did not reveal postictal slowing, and prolactin levels obtained 15 minutes after a seizure episode were not significantly elevated over baseline levels. His seizures did not respond to anticonvulsant medications, but they abated after he changed his strategy and began to explore compensation for other reasons.

COURSE AND PROGNOSIS

Most epileptic patients have a good prognosis. The majority of seizures can be controlled sufficiently with anticonvulsant medications so that the patient can live a productive life. Some seizures, such as absence seizures, tend to disappear by adulthood. For epileptic patients who are medically intractable, epilepsy surgery offers a good alternative (that is, temporal lobectomy or corpus callosot-

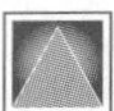

Table 2.4–10
Seizure Threshold Lowering Effect of Psychotropic Medications

Potential	Antipsychotic	Antidepressant	Other Psychotropic
High	Chlorpromazine (Thorazine) Clozapine (Clozaril)	Bupropion (Wellbutrin) Imipramine (Norfranil) Maprotiline (Ludiomil) Amitriptyline (Elavil) Amoxapine (Asendin) Nortriptyline (Aventyl)	
Moderate	Most piperazines Thiothixene (Navane)	Protriptyline (Vivactil) Clomipramine (Anafranil)	Lithium (Eskalith)
Low	Fluphenazine (Prolixin) Haloperidol (Haldol) Loxapine (Loxitane) Molindone (Moban) Pimozide (Orap) Thioridazine (Mellaril) Risperidone (Risperdal) Olanzapine (Zyprexa) Ziprasidone (Geodon)	Doxepin (Sinequan) Desipramine (Norpramin) Trazodone (Desyrel) Trimipramine (Surmontil) Selective serotonin reuptake inhibitors	Ethchlorvynol (Placidol) Glutethimide (Doriden) Hydroxyzine (Vistaril) Meprobamate (Equanil) Methaqualone (Quaalude)

omy), provided that the focus can be localized or lateralized. In addition, most epileptic patients do not have psychiatric disorders, and others have psychiatric difficulties only if they endure many years of poorly controlled seizures. For those with behavioral problems, anticonvulsant drugs or epilepsy surgery may relieve some symptoms, such as hyposexuality and aggression, but may not affect the emergence of others, such as psychosis and suicidal behavior.

TREATMENT

Anticonvulsant Medications

In the treatment of psychiatrically disturbed epileptic patients, a first consideration is the behavioral effects of anticonvulsant medications. Carbamazepine, valproate, lamotrigine, and gabapentin (Neurontin) have significant antimanic and modest antidepressant properties, probably through mood stabilization effects. They have some efficacy in the long-term prophylaxis of manic and depressive episodes. Carbamazepine and valproate may also ameliorate some dyscontrolled, aggressive behavior in brain-injured patients. Clonazepam, in addition to its anxiolytic properties, can serve as a supplement to other antimanic therapies. Gabapentin also decreases anxiety and improves general well-being in some epilepsy patients. Carbamazepine and ethosuximide may have value for borderline personality disorder.

Encephalopathic changes occur at toxic levels of all anticonvulsant drugs. Even at therapeutic levels, barbiturates may need discontinuation because of drug-induced depression, suicidal ideation, sedation, psychomotor slowing, and paradoxical hyperactivity in the very young and the very old. Gabapentin may induce aggressive behavior or hypomania, and vigabatrin (Sabril) may precipitate depression. In addition, clinicians need to be aware of the potential emergence of psychopathology on withdrawal of anticonvulsant medications. Anxiety and depression are the most common emergent symptoms, but psychosis and other behaviors may also occur.

Psychotropic Medications

A second consideration is the seizure threshold lowering effect of psychotropic medications (Table 2.4–10). This is usually not a problem but can occasionally reach clinical significance in poorly controlled epilepsy. Psychotropic drugs are most convulsive with rapid introduction of the drug and in high doses. Clozapine (Clozaril), for example, has induced seizures in 1.0 to 4.4 percent of patients, particularly when the dose was rapidly increased. When initiating psychotropic therapy, it is best to start low and go slow while monitoring anticonvulsant levels and EEGs.

Drug Interactions

A third treatment consideration is the potential for interaction of anticonvulsant and psychotropic medications (Table 2.4–11). Most commonly, an anticonvulsant drug increases the metabolism of a psychotropic drug with a consequent decrease in its therapeutic efficiency. Conversely, withdrawal of anticonvulsant drugs can precipitate rebound elevations in psychotropic levels. Moreover, the initiation of a psychotropic drug may result in competitive inhibition of anticonvulsant metabolism with elevations of anticonvulsant levels to toxicity.

Compared to older drugs, the new anticonvulsant medications have fewer potential interactions with psychotropic medications. Gabapentin, lamotrigine, vigabatrin, and tiagabine (Gabitril) are relatively free of enzyme-inducing or -inhibiting properties. Felbamate (Felbatol), however, has been withdrawn in the United States, because some patients developed fatal aplastic anemia and liver disease.

Surgery

Epilepsy surgery is a fourth treatment consideration and is limited to patients with medically intractable seizures. The main operation involves resection of epileptogenic tissue by removal of 4 to 6 cm of the anterior temporal lobe. More than 80 percent of temporal lobectomy patients experience some reduction in their seizure frequency, and more than 50 percent of patients are entirely seizure free. Removal of the amygdala and most of the hippocampus may have postoperative behavioral effects. Some patients have an anomia or a verbal memory deficit after resection of the dominant hemisphere, and patients occasionally develop a transient postoperative affective disorder. Others experience a reduction in postictal psychosis, depression, and hyposexuality, but epileptic patients may continue to develop interictal psychosis, personality changes, and suicidal behavior even long after the temporal lobectomy. Moreover,

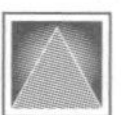

Table 2.4–11
Anticonvulsant-Psychotropic Drug Effects on Blood Levels

Anticonvulsant	Indication	Effects of Psychotropic Drug on Anticonvulsant Drug[a]	Effects of Anticonvulsant Drug on Psychotropic Drug[a]
Carbamazepine (Tegretol)	SPS, CPS, GTCS	Potentially decreased	Decreased
Phenytoin (Dilantin)	SPS, CPS, GTCS	Potentially decreased or increased, rarely toxic levels	Decreased
Phenobarbital (Barbita) and primidone (Myidone)	SPS, CPS, GTCS	Potentially decreased	Significantly decreased
Valproic acid (Depakene)	CPS, GTCS, absence	Potentially increased, rarely toxic levels	Potentially decreased
Ethosuximide (Zarontin)	Absence	None known	None known
Clonazepam (Klonopin)	Myoclonic	Potentially decreased	Potentially decreased
Gabapentin (Neurontin)	Add on: CPS, SPS, ±2nd GTCS	No significant interactions known	No significant interactions known
Lamotrigine (Lamictal)	Add on: CPS, SPS, ±2nd GTCS	No significant interactions known	No significant interactions known
Vigabatrin (Sabril)	Add on: CPS, SPS, ±2nd GTCS	No significant interactions known	No significant interactions known
Tiagabine (Gabitril)	Add on: CPS, SPS, ±2nd GTCS	No significant interactions known	No significant interactions known

CPS, complex partial seizure; GTCS, generalized tonic-clonic seizure; SPS, simple partial seizure.
[a]Antipsychotic and antidepressant drugs; lithium and the minor tranquilizers have few drug interactions with anticonvulsant drugs.

patients with preoperative psychotic symptoms are at higher risk for a poor surgical outcome and postoperative psychosis.

Less common epilepsy surgeries include resection of extratemporal lesions, removal of the epileptogenic hemisphere, and ligation of the corpus callosum. Corpus callosotomy, which aims to prevent the interhemispheric spread of seizures, results in a unique, transient disconnection syndrome of mutism, apathy, agnosia, apraxia of the nondominant limbs, difficulty naming, and writing with the nondominant hand.

Seizure Management

In treating the neuropsychiatric disorders of epilepsy, a final consideration is altering the seizure management itself. In addition to the occasional behavior alleviated by strict seizure control, allowing seizures under carefully controlled conditions, much like ECT, relieves some cases of periictal psychosis, depression, or other behaviors.

SUGGESTED CROSS-REFERENCES

Most of the specific psychiatric syndromes associated with epilepsy are discussed in more detail in the appropriate sections devoted to them. Personality disorders are discussed in Chapter 23, mood disorders are discussed in Chapter 13, and sexual disorders are discussed in Chapter 18. The rest of the neuropsychiatric sections of Chapter 2 are also pertinent to epilepsy.

REFERENCES

Adachi N, Matsuura M, Okubo Y, Oana Y, Takei N, Kato M, Hara T, Onuma T: Predictive variables of interictal psychosis in epilepsy. *Neurology.* 2000;55:1310.

Adachi N, Onuma T, Nishiwaki S, Murauchi S, Akanuma N, Ishida S, Takei N: Interictal and post-ictal psychoses in frontal lobe epilepsy: A retrospective comparison with psychoses in temporal lobe epilepsy. *Seizure.* 2000;9:328.

Alper K, Devinsky O, Perrine K, Vazquez B, Luciano D: Psychiatric classification of nonconversion nonepileptic seizures. *Arch Neurol.* 1995;52:199.

*Bear D, Fedio P: Quantitative analysis of interictal behavior in temporal lobe epilepsy. *Arch Neurol.* 1977;34:454.

Benbadis SR, Agrawal V, Tatum WO IV: How many patients with psychogenic nonepileptic seizures also have epilepsy? *Neurology.* 2001;57:915.

*Blumer D: Dysphoric disorders and paroxysmal affects: Recognition and treatment of epilepsy-related psychiatric disorders. *Harv Rev Psychiatry.* 2000;8:8.

Cockerell OC, Moriarty J, Trimble M, Sander JW, Shorvon SD: Acute psychological disorders in patients with epilepsy: A nation-wide study. *Epilepsy Res.* 1996;25:119.

Dongier S: Statistical study of clinical and electroencephalographic manifestations of 536 psychotic episodes occurring in 516 epileptics between clinical seizures. *Epilepsia.* 1959;1:117.

Gerard ME, Spitz MC, Towbin JA, Shantz D: Subacute postictal aggression. *Neurology.* 1998;50:384.

Jones JE, Hermann BP, Gilliam FG, Kanner AM, Meader KJ: Rates and risk factors for suicide, suicidal ideation, and suicide attempts in chronic epilepsy. *Epilepsy Behav.* 2003;4[Suppl 3]:31.

Kanemoto K, Kawasaki J, Kawai I: Postictal psychosis: A comparison with acute interictal and chronic psychoses. *Epilepsia.* 1996;37:551.

Kanner AM, Stagno S, Kotagal P, Morris HH: Postictal psychiatric events during prolonged video-electroencephalographic monitoring studies. *Arch Neurol.* 1996;53:258.

Lancman ME, Asconape JJ, Graves S, Gibson PA: Psychogenic seizures in children: Long-term analysis of 43 cases. *J Child Neurol.* 1994;9:404.

Lesser RP: Psychogenic seizures. *Neurology.* 1996;46:1499.

*Lindsay J, Ounsted C, Richards P: Long-term outcome in children with temporal lobe seizures: III. Psychiatric aspects in childhood and adult life. *Develop Med Child Neurol.* 1979;21:630.

Lopez-Rodriguez F, Altshuler L, Kay J, Delarhim S, Mendez MF, Engel J Jr: Personality changes among medically-refractory epileptic patients. *J Neuropsychiatry Clin Neurosci.* 1999;11:464.

Manchanda R, Freeland A, Schaefer B, McLachlan RS, Blume WT: Auras, seizure focus, and psychiatric disorders. *Neuropsychiatry Neuropsychol Behav Neurol.* 2000;13:13.

Mandelbaum DE, Burack GD: Pre-existing or epilepsy related problems have attributed to AEDs. Antiepileptic drugs. *Epilepsia.* 1999;40:389.

*Marsh L, Rao V: Psychiatric complications in patients with epilepsy: A review. *Epilepsy Res.* 2002;49:11.

*Mendez MF, Cummings JL, Benson DF: Depression in epilepsy, significance and phenomenology. *Arch Neurol.* 1986;43:766.

Mendez MF, Doss RC, Taylor JL: Interictal violence in epilepsy. Relationship to behavior and seizure variables. *J Nerv Ment Dis.* 1993;181:566.

Mendez MF, Engebrit B, Doss R, Grau R: The relationship of epileptic auras and psychological attributes. *J Neuropsychiatry Clin Neurosci.* 1996;8:287.

Morrell MJ, Guldner GT: Self-reported sexual function and sexual arousability in women with epilepsy. *Epilepsia.* 1996;37:1204.

Murialdo G, Galimberti CA, Fonzi S, Manni R, Costelli P, Parodi C, Solinas GP, Amoretti G, Tartara A: Sex hormones and pituitary function in male epileptic patients with altered or normal sexuality. *Epilepsia.* 1995;36:360.

Ott D, Siddarth P, Gurbani S, Koh S, Tournay A, Shields WD, Caplan R: Behavioral disorders in pediatric epilepsy. *Epilepsia.* 2003;44:591.

Paradiso S, Hermann BP, Blumer D, Davies K, Robinson RG: Impact of depressed mood on neuropsychological status in temporal lobe epilepsy. *J Neurol Neurosurg Psychiatry.* 2001;70:180.

Perez MM, Trimble MR: Epileptic psychosis—diagnostic comparison with process schizophrenia. *Br J Psychiatry.* 1980;37:245.

Perini GL, Tosin C, Carraro C, Bernasconi GFG, Canevini MP, Canger R, Pellegrini A, Testa G: Interictal personality disorders in temporal lobe epilepsy and juvenile myoclonic epilepsy. *J Neurol Neurosurg Psychiatry.* 1996;61:601.

Pollack MH, Scott EL: Gabapentin and lamotrigine: Novel treatments for mood and anxiety disorders. *CNS Spectrums.* 1997;2:56.

Rao SM, Devinsky O, Grafman J, Stein M, Usman M, Uhde TW, Theodore WH: Viscosity and social cohesion in temporal lobe epilepsy. *J Neurol Neurosurg Psychiatry.* 1992;55:149.

Reuber M, Pukrop R, Bauer J, Helmstaedter C, Tessendorf N, Elger CE: Outcome in psychogenic nonepileptic seizures: 1 to 10-year follow-up in 164 patients. *Ann Neurol.* 2003;53:305.

Sachdev P. Schizophrenia-like psychosis and epilepsy: The status of the association. *Am J Psychiatry.* 1998;155:325.
Scheepers M, Kerr M: Epilepsy and behaviour. *Curr Opin Neurol.* 2003;16:183.
Slater E, Beard A: The schizophrenia-like psychosis of epilepsy: Psychiatric aspects. *Br J Psychiatry.* 1963;109:95.
Smith DB, Treiman DM, Trimble MR, eds. *Neurobehavioral Problems in Epilepsy.* New York: Raven Press; 1991.
Swanson SJ, Rao SM, Grafman J, Salazar AM, Kraft J: The relationship between seizure subtype and interictal personality. Results from the Vietnam Head Injury Study. *Brain.* 1995;118:91.
Tarulli A, Devinsky O, Alper K: Progression of postictal to interictal psychosis. *Epilepsia.* 2001;42:1468.
Trimble MR, ed. *The Psychosis of Epilepsy.* New York: Raven Press; 1991.
Tucker GJ: Seizure disorders presenting with psychiatric symptomatology. *Psychiatr Clin North Am.* 1998;21:625.
Williams D: The structure of emotions reflected in epileptic experiences. *Brain.* 1956;79:29.
Wong MT, Lumsden J, Fenton GW, Fenwick PB: Electroencephalography, computed tomography and violence ratings of male patients in a maximum-security mental hospital. *Acta Psychiatr Scand.* 1994;90:97.

▲ 2.5 Neuropsychiatric Aspects of Traumatic Brain Injury

RICARDO E. JORGE, M.D., AND ROBERT G. ROBINSON, M.D.

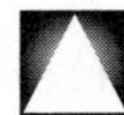

Table 2.5–1
DSM-IV-TR Classification of Some Behavioral Syndromes Occurring after Traumatic Brain Injury

Delirium due to traumatic brain injury
Amnestic disorder due to traumatic brain injury
Transient and chronic types
Dementia due to traumatic brain injury
Personality change due to traumatic brain injury
Labile, disinhibited, aggressive, apathetic, paranoid, combined, other, and unspecified types
Mood disorder due to traumatic brain injury
With depressive features
With major depressive-like episode
With manic features
With mixed features
Anxiety disorder due to traumatic brain injury
With generalized anxiety
With panic attacks
With obsessive-compulsive symptoms
Posttraumatic stress disorder
Psychotic disorder due to traumatic brain injury
With delusions
With hallucinations

The neuropsychiatric consequences of traumatic brain injury (also referred to as TBI) may be divided into disorders that are also seen in patients without brain injury and those that are unique to patients with brain damage. The disorders that are also seen in patients without brain injury cover the whole spectrum of psychiatric disorders, including substance abuse, mood, anxiety, psychotic, and personality disorders. Many of these disorders are included in the revised fourth edition of the *Diagnostic and Statistical Manual of Mental Disorders* (DSM-IV-TR) as disorders due to a medical condition, in this case, traumatic brain injury (Table 2.5–1). Most of these disorders have not been extensively studied in the traumatic brain injury population, and much research is still needed in this area. The disorders that are unique to brain injury also cover a wide range of disorders, including pathological laughing or crying, apathy, anosognosia, aprosody, and neglect. Most of these disorders have not been extensively examined in patients with traumatic brain injury. This chapter focuses on the neuropsychiatric consequences of traumatic brain injury as defined by DSM-IV-TR but also addresses some of the disorders that are unique to brain injury.

HISTORY

The earliest physical evidence of traumatic brain injury due to assault occurred one million years ago. A damaged skull from an early hominid found in South Africa showed two posterior fractures that matched with the condylar surfaces of an antelope humerus discovered nearby. The earliest written evidence of brain injuries was found on the Edwin Smith Papyrus, dated 5,000 years ago, which contained the first 27 head injury records. The Hippocratic Corpus included a treatise on head injury with thoughtful comments on skull fractures, delirium, seizures, and coma.

Associations between traumatic brain injury and a variety of neuropsychiatric disorders have been reported in the medical literature for many years. Adolf Meyer, for example, identified a number of disorders that he referred to as the "traumatic insanities." Although he believed that these disorders were determined by a combination of psychological, social, historical, and biological factors, he suggested that there may be some unique associations between these disorders and specific lesion locations. Studies of war-related head injuries identified the high prevalence of psychiatric complications after traumatic brain injury. Several of these studies emphasized the importance of frontal lesions in the pathogenesis of behavioral disturbances. The most famous case of frontal lobe injury, however, was Phineas Gage, who suffered a penetrating frontal brain injury after an explosion that shot an iron bar through his skull. After the injury, he was described as childish, capricious, inconsiderate, and profane and as having poor judgment.

Analysis of large series of cases, such as the Oxford Collection of Head Injury Records, suggests that biological variables, such as the extent of brain damage, lesion location, and the presence of posttraumatic epilepsy, were important etiological factors in determining the type and duration of psychiatric syndromes.

COMPARATIVE NOSOLOGY

The neurological and neurosurgical literature abounds with clinical descriptions of early and delayed behavioral abnormalities that follow traumatic brain injury. Acute syndromes include confusional states, agitation, restlessness, irritability, and posttraumatic amnesia. Delayed, often irreversible, consequences of traumatic brain injury include cognitive disorders (e.g., amnesia and executive dysfunction), traumatic dementia, and organic personality change.

The spectrum of psychiatric disorders that are attributable to traumatic brain injury spans almost the entire spectrum of psychiatric disorders. According to the DSM-IV-TR, these disorders are categorized as due to traumatic brain injury if there is evidence from the history, physical examination, or ancillary studies that the disturbance is the direct physiological effect of brain trauma (Table 2.5–1).

EPIDEMIOLOGY

In the United States, the annual incidence of closed head injuries admitted to a hospital can be conservatively estimated as 200 per

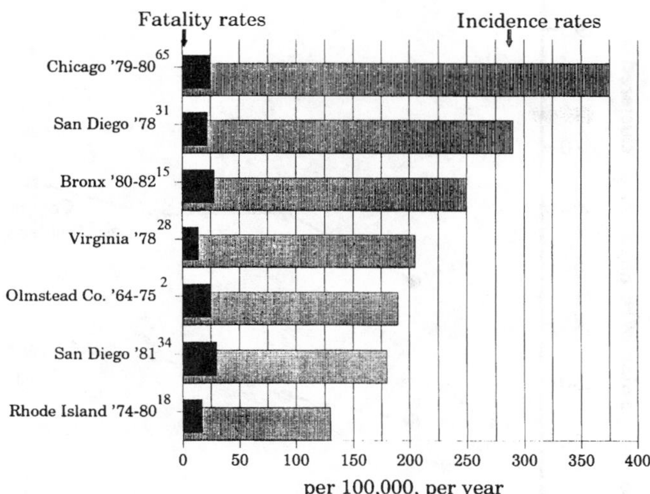

FIGURE 2.5–1 Brain injury incidence and fatality rates from selected U.S. studies. (From Kraus JF, McArthur DL. Epidemiology of brain injury. In: Evans RW, ed. *Neurology and Trauma.* Philadelphia: WB Saunders; 1996:7, with permission.)

100,000 population. The incidence of penetrating head injury has been estimated to be 12 per 100,000. According to these rates, there are approximately 500,000 new cases each year, a significant proportion of which results in long-term disabilities. Figure 2.5–1 shows the annual incidence of new cases of traumatic brain injury leading to death or to admission to hospital. Approximately 80 percent of traumatic brain injury patients had mild head injury, 10 percent experienced moderate head injury, and the remaining 10 percent were categorized as severe. Most of these injuries occurred among adolescents and young adults, with a second peak occurring among elderly subjects. There was also a significant gender difference. Men were two to three times more likely to experience brain injury than women. Blacks also had higher rates of traumatic brain injury than other groups, a finding that may be explained by increased firearm exposure and higher homicide rates among this group.

Low socioeconomic status (SES) constitutes another independent risk factor for traumatic brain injury. The single greatest risk factor for traumatic brain injury, however, is alcohol and drug abuse. Close to one-third of brain injury patients had an identifiable alcohol problem before trauma, and more than 50 percent were intoxicated at the time of injury. Transportation-related cases (i.e., motor vehicle accidents and pedestrians hit by vehicles) are the most important cause of injury, particularly in younger adults. Falls associated with older age are the second most prevalent cause of injury. Assaults (especially penetrating injuries involving firearm use), as well as sports- and recreation-related injuries, are the next most common causes of traumatic brain injury.

CLINICAL FEATURES

Acute Behavioral Consequences

Head injury encompasses a wide range of severity, from patients who die at the moment of trauma to those who do not require medical evaluation or assistance. Most of the patients admitted to hospital with a head injury diagnosis have a mild injury. A minority of these mildly affected patients develop acute complications (e.g., brain swelling, delayed hematoma, and intracranial infection) or prolonged postconcussional symptoms. Neuroimaging studies (computed tomography [CT], magnetic resonance imaging [MRI]) have demonstrated the presence of structural brain lesions in some mild head injury patients who have not experienced clinical complications.

The most common consequence of head injury is impairment of consciousness, ranging from transient confusion to protracted coma. The Glasgow Coma Score (GCS) is commonly used to grade the severity of traumatic brain injury. The scale gives a quantitative estimate of level of consciousness and neurological status based on patterns of eye opening, as well as best verbal and motor responses. GCS scores between 13 and 15 define *mild brain injury*, whereas scores between 9 and 12 define *moderate brain injury*, and scores between 3 and 8 define *severe brain injury*.

The early phase of recovery from traumatic brain injury is characterized by disorientation, confusion, and impaired memory function. Apathetic withdrawal, agitation, or severe delirium may also be observed in these patients.

Posttraumatic amnesia occurs during the period when the patient (who is usually emerging from coma) is disoriented and confused and has disrupted memory functioning. Deficits are observed in declarative memory (i.e., memory of recent events and times), affecting anterograde and retrograde processes. Procedural memory, in contrast, appears to be relatively spared. Duration of posttraumatic amnesia has been widely used as a measure of traumatic brain injury severity. It may be assessed using the Galveston Orientation and Amnesia Test (GOAT), which evaluates orientation to person, place, and time, as well as awareness of the accident and its consequences. Alternatively, retrospective structured questionnaires have shown an excellent correlation with this prospective determination. Duration of posttraumatic amnesia has proved to be a good predictor of the degree of disability, vocational outcome, and severity of personality change after traumatic brain injury.

Clinical features of the early phase of recovery from traumatic brain injury are not exclusively characterized by memory impairment. Patients frequently have a decreased level of consciousness and meet DSM-IV-TR criteria for delirium. In addition, patients may present with perceptual disturbances (i.e., illusions or hallucinations), delusional thoughts, psychomotor agitation or retardation, affective lability, and neurovegetative symptoms (e.g., tachycardia, hypertension, diaphoresis, and sleep-wake cycle disruption). Symptoms usually have an acute onset and a fluctuating course. Delirium is most frequently observed in severe traumatic brain injury cases.

A 19-year-old man was admitted to a trauma center after a motorcycle accident. He presented with a right epidural hematoma and bilateral contusions in the anterior temporal lobes. He had also a scalp laceration and right maxillary and zygomatic fractures. The postresuscitation GCS score was 8. The hematoma was surgically evacuated, and the patient was transferred to the intensive care unit. Two days later, the patient became restless and agitated. He removed his intravenous (IV) lines and monitoring devices and tried to get out of bed. He was disoriented, incoherent, and aggressive. His behavior suggested that he was experiencing frightening visual hallucinations. A coarse, rapid tremor was noted in both hands, and he was diaphoretic and mildly hypertensive. He responded well to a short course of high-potency antipsychotic agents.

There are multiple conditions that may contribute to the development of delirium in traumatic brain injury patients. These include structural brain damage, cerebral edema, brain hypoxia, seizures, electrolyte imbalance, infections, medications (e.g., barbiturates, opiates, and steroids), and drug or alcohol withdrawal. Old age, coexistent severe medical disease, polypharmacy, basal ganglia, and right hemisphere lesions have also been shown to be significant risk factors.

Chronic Behavioral Consequences

Cognitive Disorders Cognitive disturbances are some of the most important long-term sequels of severe traumatic brain injury. A seminal study reported on the cognitive outcome of 127 severely brain injured patients who were capable of completing serial neuropsychological assessments during a 1-year follow-up period (i.e., excluding those patients with a persistent vegetative state or with severe intellectual impairment). At 1-year follow-up, the brain injured patients showed slower information processing and greater impairment in memory function compared to a neurologically intact control group. In contrast, linguistic and visuospatial abilities were found to be within the normal range. Patients with mild or moderate head injuries may also show cognitive impairment after brain trauma. These patients complain of lack of concentration and memory deficits during the first weeks after traumatic brain injury. However, spontaneous recovery is the rule for the majority of these patients. Repetitive, mild head injury, such as that observed among certain athletes (e.g., soccer and football players), requires special attention. A recent study among college football players showed that a history of multiple concussions was associated with reduced cognitive performance. In addition, there is evidence indicating that repeated concussions among amateur soccer players is associated with deficits in memory and executive functions.

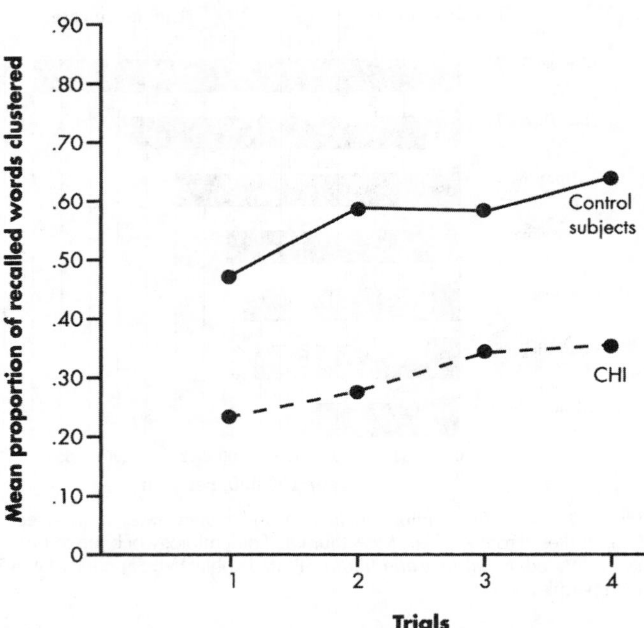

FIGURE 2.5–2 Proportion of clustered recall by patients with closed head injury (CHI) as compared with uninjured control subjects, plotted across trials. The proportion of words clustered has been corrected for the absolute number of words recalled. (From Kraus MF, Levin HS. The frontal lobes and traumatic brain injury. In: Salloway SP, Malloy PF, Duffy JD, eds. *The Frontal Lobes and Neuropsychiatric Illness.* Washington, DC: American Psychiatric Publishing Inc; 2001:204, with permission [http://www.appi.org].)

Attentional deficits are among the most frequent neuropsychological symptoms observed in traumatic brain injury patients after resolution of posttraumatic amnesia. Attention consists of multiple processes subserved by interrelated neural networks. Traumatic brain injury patients may present with restricted verbal or visuospatial attention span, altered vigilance patterns (i.e., sustained attention deficits), or slowed information processing. The most consistent findings, however, are associated with performance in the most demanding tasks (e.g., in divided attention paradigms, such as the Paced Auditory Serial Addition Task).

Memory functions are also distinctively impaired in traumatic brain injury patients. Memory deficits are the most frequent cognitive disturbances reported by patients and relatives in the chronic phase of traumatic brain injury. Memory dysfunction is characterized by anterograde and retrograde deficits, faulty sequencing of events, and inefficient encoding and storage strategies. For instance, Harold Levin and Felicia Goldstein demonstrated that, when compared to control subjects, traumatic brain injury patients were unable to organize recall of words by clustering them in appropriate semantic categories (Fig. 2.5–2). A DSM-IV-TR diagnosis of amnesic disorder due to traumatic brain injury and chronic subtype may be made for those nondemented patients in whom the memory disturbance causes significant impairment in social or vocational functioning and represents a significant decline with respect to previous levels of performance. However, patients manifesting an isolated memory deficit are rare.

Linguistic competence is also frequently affected by traumatic brain injury. Approximately one-third of severely brain injured patients admitted to a rehabilitation facility showed fluent (51 percent), nonfluent (35 percent), or global (14 percent) aphasic syndromes. Aphasia tends to resolve in the majority of cases during the first year after trauma. Anomia, however, constitutes the most prevalent long-term linguistic deficit after trauma. Traumatic brain injury patients may also have high-order language alterations and present with a defective narrative discourse, a lack of semantic coherence, aprosody, and impaired pragmatics of communication. All of these result in impoverished and disorganized language and in a reduced proficiency in communication.

A prominent defect in control or executive functions has been consistently described in patients surviving severe head injury. Executive functions include goal formation, planning, selection of adequate response patterns, and monitoring of ongoing behavior. Several neuropsychological tasks were specifically designed to quantify these deficits. These include the Wisconsin Card Sorting Test, the Goldberg Executive Control Battery, the Tower of London Test, and the Trail-Making Test. Simple cognitive tests, such as the verbal and figural fluency tasks, can document the lack of spontaneity and perseverative tendencies frequently observed in patients with traumatic brain damage (Fig. 2.5–3). The executive dysfunction observed in traumatic brain injury patients is strongly associated with dysfunction of frontosubcortical pathways. When confronted with a demanding environment, the adaptive functioning of traumatic brain injury patients is also often impaired.

In contrast to what happens with memory and control functions, visuospatial and praxis abilities are usually preserved during the chronic phase of traumatic brain injury. This finding is probably due to the relative sparing of posterior association cortices in traumatic brain injury.

Finally, unawareness (anosognosia) or denial of deficits is a cognitive disorder frequently observed in traumatic brain injury patients, particularly in those who have experienced extensive frontal lobe damage. This constitutes a severe behavioral sequel that impedes realistic goal setting and interferes with the rehabilitation process.

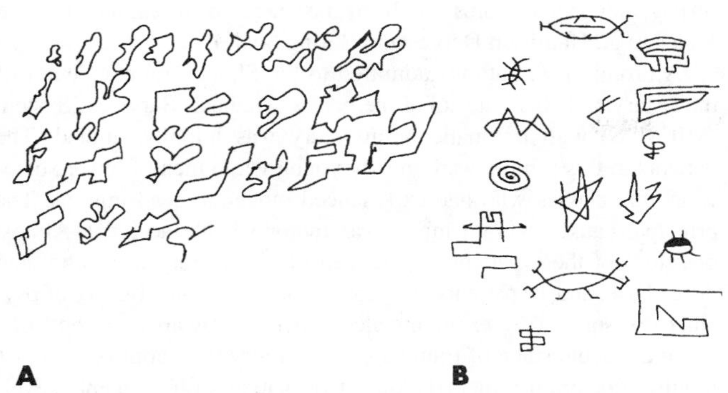

FIGURE 2.5–3 **A:** Lack of spontaneity and perseverative performance in a design fluency task by a patient with bilateral traumatic frontal lesions. **B:** Figures created by a control subject matched for age and education. (From Kraus MF, Levin HS. The frontal lobes and traumatic brain injury. In: Salloway SP, Malloy PF, Duffy JD, eds. *The Frontal Lobes and Neuropsychiatric Illness.* Washington, DC: American Psychiatric Publishing Inc; 2001:202, with permission [http://www.appi.org].)

Cognitive impairment after traumatic brain injury is determined by the type and extent of brain damage. However, genetic factors may also play a significant role in cognitive outcome, perhaps because of their effect on repair processes. For instance, recent studies demonstrated a strong association between the apolipoprotein E–epsilon 4 allele and a poor clinical outcome, implying genetic susceptibility to the effect of brain injury.

Dementia *Dementia* is a syndrome defined in DSM-IV-TR by impairment of memory and at least one other cognitive domain in the absence of an alteration of consciousness. The cognitive defect must have a significant impact on the social and occupational functioning of the involved subject. Dementia due to head trauma is characterized by prominent memory and executive dysfunction with relatively preserved visuospatial, praxis, and primary linguistic functions. In addition, these patients may be severely apathetic and withdrawn and may demonstrate markedly slow information processing. Physical examination may reveal the presence of extrapyramidal signs. Of note, a chronic subdural hematoma in the elderly may present as a progressive dementia.

A 40-year-old white man was severely injured in a motor vehicle accident and experienced protracted coma of 1-month duration. An MRI performed at 2 weeks from injury revealed the presence of widespread diffuse axonal injury. At 6-month follow-up, the patient presented with a mild left hemiparesis, right hemidystonic symptoms, and a left peripheral facial palsy. Neuropsychological testing disclosed substantial memory deficits, frontal lobe dysfunction, and significantly impaired problem-solving ability. Visuospatial and linguistic skills ranked within the lower average range. His hygiene and self-care were poor, and he hoarded garbage in his pockets and under his bed. He had frequent bursts of severely aggressive behavior, but, overall, he remained abulic and withdrawn. Lithium (Eskalith) was effective in controlling his aggressive behavior.

There is consistent evidence that previous traumatic episodes constitute a risk factor for the development of Alzheimer's disease. Traumatic brain injury is associated with expression of amyloid precursor protein, oxidative stress, and an increased deposition of amyloid-β peptides that might ultimately lead to the onset of dementia. Dementia pugilistica is another related condition. Multiple traumatic brain injuries associated with boxing occur in approximately 20 percent of professional boxers. The diagnosis of this severe complication is dependent on documenting progressive dementia that is associated with chronic and repeated brain trauma and that is unexplainable by an alternative pathophysiological process. Pathologically, dementia pugilistica shares many characteristics with Alzheimer's disease (i.e., neurofibrillary tangles, diffuse amyloid plaques, or tau immunoreactivity, or a combination of these).

Personality Changes Traumatic brain injury patients may experience significant personality changes. These patients have been described as irritable, childish, inconsiderate, capricious, anxious, or aggressive. They lack foresight and misjudge the consequences of their actions. Disinhibition is a frequent and striking clinical feature that may lead to antisocial behavior. On the other hand, they may become apathetic, abulic, and withdrawn.

Some investigators group these changes into two distinct syndromes: a pseudodepressed personality syndrome, which is characterized by apathy and blunted affect, and a pseudopsychopathic personality syndrome, which has disinhibition, egocentricity, and sexual inappropriateness as its outstanding features.

DSM-IV-TR defines *personality change due to traumatic brain injury* as a persistent personality disturbance that represents a change from the individual's previous personality profile (or a deviation of normal development in children) and that is attributable to the pathophysiological changes triggered by brain trauma (Table 2.5–1). The disturbance must not occur exclusively during the course of delirium and cannot be diagnosed if dementia is present. In addition, the disturbance must not be better accounted for by another mental disorder (e.g., mood disorder or substance abuse).

A 42-year-old construction worker fell from the second floor of a new building. He was in coma for 3 days and remained amnestic and disoriented for approximately 3 weeks. A CT scan showed bilateral orbitofrontal and anterior temporal hemorrhagic contusions.

Six months after the injury, he had undergone a significant personality change. He spent most of his day watching television and refused to reinitiate his usual activities. He ate and gained excessive weight. His wife complained of his frequent and often inappropriate sexual demands and stressed his lack of intimacy. He was also easily upset, shouting and making threats when he felt provoked. He was less sensitive to other people's feelings. A trial of carbamazepine (Tegretol) with therapeutic blood concentrations and the maintenance of a numerical record of outbursts resulted in significantly reduced irritability and outbursts.

DSM-IV-TR further categorizes this condition into the following subtypes: labile (if the predominant symptom is affective lability), disinhibited, aggressive, apathetic, paranoid, combined, and unspecified (other) types (e.g., personality changes associated with a seizure disorder). Disinhibition, poorly modulated emotional reactions, disturbances in decision making and goal-directed behavior, social inappropriateness, hypersexuality, and lack of empathy and insight have all been linked to the occurrence of ventromedial frontal lesions (Fig. 2.5–4). In addition, aggression and poor impulse control have been associated with lesions in the anterior temporal lobe.

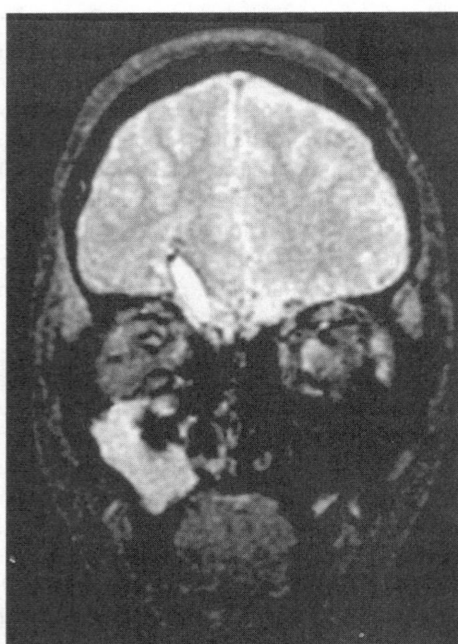

FIGURE 2.5–4 Coronal magnetic resonance image showing right orbitofrontal contusions in a patient with prominent personality change after traumatic brain injury.

Mood Disorders

DEPRESSIVE DISORDERS Depressive disorders appear to be frequent psychiatric complications among patients with traumatic brain injury. Using DSM-IV-TR diagnostic criteria, depressive disorders associated with traumatic brain injury are categorized as *mood disorder due to traumatic brain injury* with the following subtypes: (1) with major depressive-like episode (if the full criteria for a major depressive episode are met) or (2) with depressive features (prominent depressed mood, but the full criteria for a major depressive episode are not met).

The reported frequency of depressive disorders after traumatic brain injury has varied from 6 to 77 percent. This variability in the reported frequency of depressive disorders, particularly major depression, may be due to the lack of uniformity in the psychiatric diagnosis. Most of the early studies relied on rating scales or relative's reports rather than on structured interviews and established diagnostic criteria (e.g., DSM-IV-TR).

A recent study used a structured interview and DSM-IV-TR criteria to identify Axis I psychopathology in 100 adults with traumatic brain injury who were evaluated, on average, 8 years after trauma. The prevalence of major depression in this series was 61 percent. Other investigators studied the prevalence of major depressive disorder among a sample of 722 outpatients with traumatic brain injury, who were evaluated at an average of 2.5 years after brain injury. *Major depression*, defined using DSM-IV-TR criteria, was diagnosed in 303 patients (42 percent).

For the past few years, the prevalence, duration, and clinical correlates of mood disorders after traumatic brain injury have been studied. Rather than using a dimensional approach to characterize the behavioral disturbance occurring after traumatic brain injury, a disease perspective has been adopted, assuming that mood disorders, although diagnosed through a recognized constellation of symptoms, have an identifiable biological substrate, a distinct clinical prognosis, and a predictable treatment response. In studies by Ricardo Jorge and Robert Robinson, psychiatric diagnosis has been made using semistructured interviews and DSM-IV-TR criteria, and the severity of psychiatric symptoms has been measured using validated rating scales (e.g., Hamilton Depression Rating Scale).

A group of 66 patients admitted to the Shock Trauma Center of the Maryland Institute of Emergency Medical Services System (MIEMSS) with traumatic brain injury was initially studied. The patients in this sample were mostly young white men of lower socioeconomic classes who had experienced moderate head injuries. The principal cause of brain injury was motor vehicle accident. Almost one-third of these patients (30 percent) had a history of alcohol and drug abuse, and 11 patients (17 percent) had a personal history of psychiatric disorder (i.e., excluding alcoholism or drug abuse, or both).

In the acute stage of traumatic brain injury (i.e., approximately 1 month after brain injury) 17 out of 66 patients (26 percent) developed major depression. Another two patients (3 percent) developed minor (dysthymic) depression.

The prevalence of major depression during the year after traumatic brain injury remained stable at 25 percent, with some patients recovering from major depression and other patients developing delayed-onset depressions. There were 11 patients who developed delayed-onset major depression at some point during the follow-up period. Thus, 28 of the 58 patients (47 percent) for whom follow-up data were available met revised third edition of the *Diagnostic and Statistical Manual of Mental Disorders* (DSM-III-TR) criteria for major depression during the first year after the traumatic episode. Patients who developed major depression during the acute period had an estimated mean duration of depression of 4.7 months, with a minimum of 1.5 months and a maximum of 12 months.

Under current analysis are the findings from a new group of 91 consecutive patients with closed head injuries who were admitted to the University of Iowa Hospitals and Clinics and the Iowa Methodist Medical Center, in Des Moines, Iowa, and who were examined in a 2-year prospective observational study. In addition, 27 patients with multiple traumas but without clinical or radiological evidence of central nervous system (CNS) involvement (i.e., without primary or secondary brain damage or spinal cord injury), who were consecutively admitted to the University of Iowa Hospitals and Clinics, constituted the control group. Severity of traumatic brain injury was classified as moderate in 37 patients (40.6 percent), whereas 32 patients (35.2 percent) had mild brain injuries, and 22 patients (24.2 percent) were categorized as severe head injuries. Out of the 91 traumatic brain injury patients enrolled in the study, 47 (51.6 percent) developed mood disorders during the first year after traumatic brain injury, compared to 6 out of 27 patients (22.2 percent) in the control group. Thus, the frequency of mood disorders was significantly higher in brain injured patients compared to patients having a similar severity of physical impairment but without brain damage. Of the 47 patients with post–traumatic brain injury mood disorders, major depressive disorder occurred in 30 patients (33 percent), nine patients (9.9 percent) developed minor depression, and the remaining eight patients (8.8 percent) presented with manic or mixed episodes. Among this group of patients, duration of major depression was estimated to be approximately 6 months. Thus, these new data replicate many of the results from a first study, including the findings that approximately one-half of traumatic brain injury patients developed a depressive disorder during the first year after traumatic brain injury (Fig. 2.5–5).

A 42-year-old engineer had a motor vehicle accident when returning from a convention. He had multiple injuries, including a diaphragmatic rupture and a left frontotemporoparietal subdural hematoma. When admitted to the hospital, the patient was hypotensive and hypoxic. His diaphragm was repaired, and the subdural hematoma was evacuated with the urgent intervention of two surgical teams. The patient remained in coma during the following 72 hours. Posttraumatic amnesia lasted for almost 3 weeks. At this point, the neurological examination disclosed a right hemiparesis and a left lateral rectus palsy. The patient was mildly hypophonic and dysarthric. Forty days after the accident, he was transferred to a specialized rehabilitation unit. A neuropsychiatric evaluation was completed once his posttraumatic amnesia had cleared. Neuropsychological tests were within normal limits. The patient conveyed a profoundly depressed mood and feelings of hopelessness. He stated that he would never be able to recover, that his career was ruined, and that it would have been better if he had died in the accident. He had no appetite and refused to participate in physical rehabilitation. He also had significant sleep problems. Treatment of depression was initiated with paroxetine (Paxil) at a dosage of 20 mg per day. After 3 weeks, the patient's mood was significantly improved, and he became involved in the rehabilitation program. At 6-month follow-up, he was no longer depressed and had returned to work.

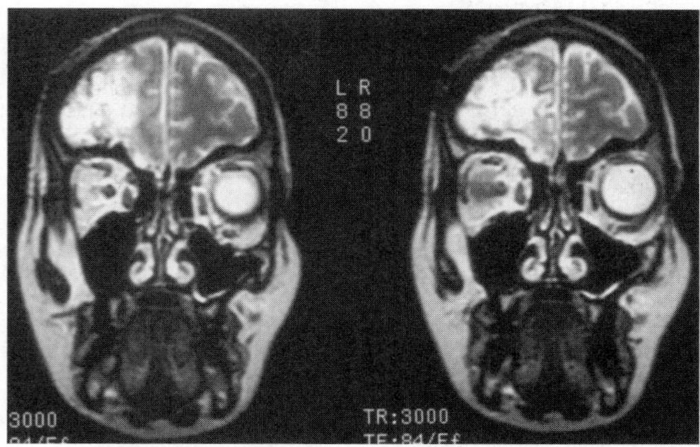

FIGURE 2.5–6 Coronal magnetic resonance images from a patient who developed pathological laughter and crying 3 months after a closed head injury secondary to a motor vehicle accident. Abnormal emotional control was associated with prefrontal damage.

The differential diagnosis of post–traumatic brain injury major depression includes adjustment disorder with depressed mood, apathetic syndromes, and emotional lability. Patients with adjustment disorders develop short-lived and relatively mild emotional disturbances within 3 months of a stressful life event. Although they may present with depressive symptoms, they do not meet DSM-IV-TR criteria for major depression. Pathological laughter and crying is characterized by the presence of sudden and uncontrollable affective outbursts (e.g., crying or laughing), which may be congruent or incongruent with the patient's mood. These emotional displays are recognized by the patient as being excessive to the underlying mood and can occur spontaneously or may be triggered by minor stimuli. A recent study examined the prevalence and clinical correlates of pathological laughter and crying assessed using the Pathological Laughter and Crying Scale in a group of 92 consecutive patients with traumatic brain injury. Pathological laughter and crying were diagnosed in 10 of the 92 patients (10.9 percent) during the first year after traumatic brain injury. Pathological laughter and crying were associated with the presence of anxiety disorders and frontal lobe lesions involving the lateral and ventral aspects of the prefrontal region (Fig. 2.5–6). In addition, patients with pathological laughter and crying had significantly more frequent aggressive outbursts and poorer social functioning. On the other hand, pathological laughter and crying lack the pervasive alteration of mood, as well as the specific vegetative symptoms associated with a major depressive episode. This condition has been shown to respond to treatment with antidepressants in other neurological disorders, such as stroke and multiple sclerosis.

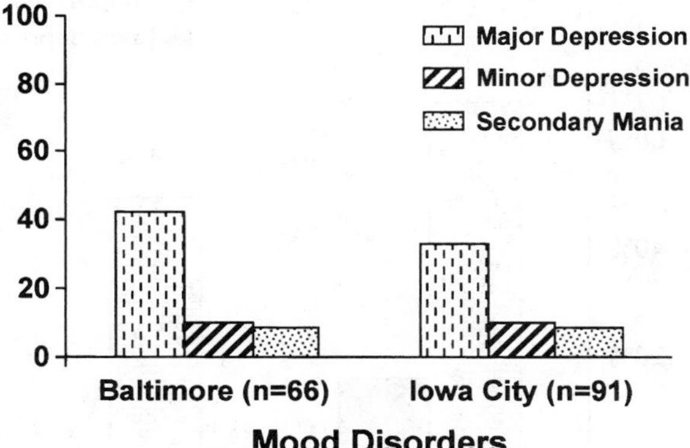

FIGURE 2.5–5 Frequency of mood disorders in two independent series of patients with traumatic brain injury during the first year after brain trauma. Mood disorders were diagnosed using criteria from the revised fourth edition of the *Diagnostic and Statistical Manual of Mental Disorders.*

Finally, traumatic brain injury patients may present with apathetic syndromes that interfere with the rehabilitation process. Apathy is frequently associated with psychomotor retardation and emotional blunting. In addition, a significant proportion of these patients also have a depressed mood. Among patients with stroke, one-half of the patients with apathy were also reported to have met diagnostic criteria for major or minor depression. A recent study of 83 consecutive traumatic brain injury patients seen in a neuropsychiatric clinic showed that 59 patients (71.1 percent) were apathetic. However, 50 of these 59 patients were also depressed. Thus, although apathy is often comorbid with depression, it can be distinguished from depression by adhering to appropriate diagnostic criteria. Apathy is frequently associated with medial prefrontal lobe damage; the relationship between apathy and the type, extent, and location of traumatic brain injury, however, has not been systematically studied.

Is there a particular group of patients who are more prone to develop depressive disorders after traumatic brain injury? When compared with traumatic brain injury patients who did not develop mood disorders, depressed traumatic brain injury patients were not significantly different with regard to demographic variables (i.e., age, sex, educational level, and marital status), severity of brain injury, or the degree of functional disability. Depressed patients were more likely to have a personal history of mood or anxiety disorders than the nondepressed group. The frequency of personal history of substance abuse, however, was not significantly different between the depressed and the nondepressed groups (Table 2.5–2).

Analysis of the Oxford Collection of Head Injury Records suggested that depressive symptoms were more common among patients with right hemisphere lesions. Depressive symptoms were also more frequent among patients with frontal and parietal lesions than among patients with other lesion locations. Furthermore, a

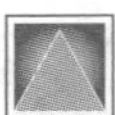

Table 2.5–2
History of Psychiatric Illness

Variable	Major Depression (%) (N = 30)	Nondepressed (%) (N = 44)
History of mood disorders[a]	36.7	11.4
History of anxiety disorders[a]	20.0	4.4
History of alcohol abuse	20.0	15.9
History of drug abuse	20.0	6.8
Concurrent alcohol abuse	6.7	2.3
Concurrent drug abuse	6.7	2.3

[a]$P = .03$.

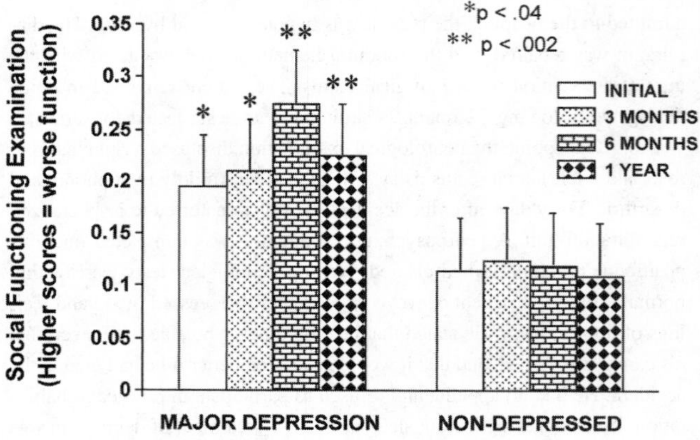

FIGURE 2.5–7 Social functioning examination scores over the first year after traumatic brain injury in patients with major depression or no mood disturbance. Social functioning during the initial evaluation reflected impairment before traumatic brain injury, whereas the follow-up evaluations reflected social functioning in the month before evaluation. Depressed patients consistently had more impairment in social functioning than nondepressed traumatic brain injury patients.

study of Vietnam War veterans conducted several years after head injury reported that depressive and anxiety symptoms were more frequently associated with penetrating injuries involving the right orbitofrontal cortex than with any other lesion location.

On the other hand, in the first series by Jorge and Robinson of 66 traumatic brain injury patients, a logistical regression model taking all of the sites of brain injury into account showed that major depression after acute traumatic brain injury was associated with the presence of left dorsolateral frontal or left basal ganglia lesions, or both, and, to a lesser extent, with right hemisphere and parietooccipital lesions. Left dorsolateral frontal and left basal ganglia lesions were strongly associated with major depression during the initial in-hospital evaluation. By 3-month follow-up, however, the major correlates of depression were previous history of psychiatric disorder and impaired social functioning. In a more recent study, major depressive disorder occurring during the first year after traumatic brain injury was significantly associated with decreased gray matter volumes in the left prefrontal cortex as measured by a research MRI scan obtained 3 months after traumatic brain injury (Table 2.5–3).

Overall, the most consistent clinical correlate of depressive disorder is poor psychosocial adjustment. It appears that traumatic brain injury patients who develop depression after trauma tend to have poor premorbid social functioning, and their social functioning worsens after the onset of depression (Fig. 2.5–7). Several studies have demonstrated that major depression has a deleterious effect on psychosocial outcome and activities-of-daily-living outcome. Depressive disorders might negatively influence patient's participation in rehabilitation efforts and social interaction early during their course of recovery. Furthermore, patients might be unable to recover these early losses even when the depression is over (Fig. 2.5–8).

Secondary Mania Secondary mania and hypomanic states have been reported in a number of organic disorders, such as thyroid disease, uremia, and vitamin B_{12} deficiency, or after open heart surgery. Mania has also been associated with traumatic brain injury.

A 1987 study reported on 20 patients who developed manic syndromes after closed head trauma. There was a significant association between mania and the presence of posttraumatic seizures, predominantly of the partial complex type (temporal lobe epilepsy). There was no association, however, with family history of bipolar disorder among first-degree relatives.

A more recent study, using DSM-III-TR criteria for manic episode, reported that 6 out of 66 traumatic brain injury patients (9 percent) developed secondary mania at some point during the first year after traumatic brain injury. Although manic episodes were short

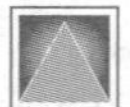

Table 2.5–3
Volumetric Analysis

Variable	Nondepressed	Major Depressed
Whole brain (cc)	1,398.2 (133.4)	1,407.4 (132.1)
Total gray matter (cc)	788.9 (90.2)	774.9 (69.8)
Total white matter (cc)	506.3 (56.2)	500.0 (65.6)
Left frontal gray matter (percentage of total gray matter)[a]	16.6 (0.63)	15.9 (0.74)
Right frontal gray matter (percentage of total gray matter)	17.2 (0.82)	16.9 (1.1)
Left frontal white matter (percentage of total white matter)	16.7 (0.84)	16.9 (0.90)
Right frontal white matter (percentage of total white matter)	17.2 (1.15)	17.1(1.25)

[a]$P \leq .008$.

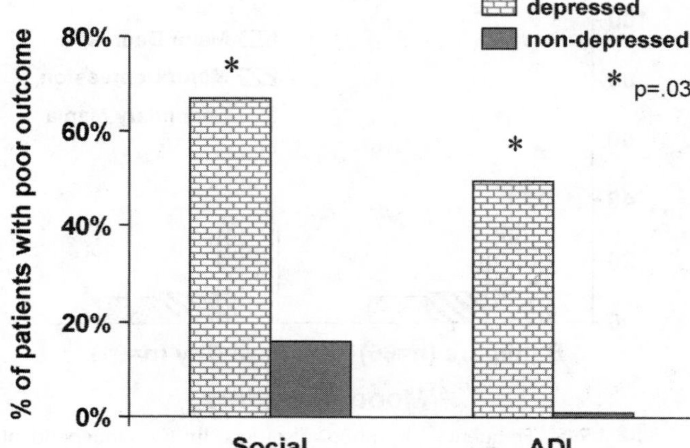

FIGURE 2.5–8 Impact of depressive disorders on psychosocial outcome and activities of daily living (ADL) outcome. The percentage of patients with a poor outcome was significantly higher in the depressed group.

lasting (approximately 2 months), the presence of an expansive mood or irritable mood had a mean duration of 5.7 months. Secondary mania was not related to the type or severity of brain injury, the presence of posttraumatic epilepsy, the degree of physical or intellectual impairment, the level of social functioning, or the presence of family or personal history of psychiatric disorder. Secondary mania was, however, associated with the presence of lesions in the ventral and anterior aspects of the temporal lobe. This is consistent with the findings in patients with mania secondary to stroke. The development of abnormal electrical activation patterns in limbic networks, functional changes in aminergic inhibitory systems, and the presence of aberrant regeneration patterns may all play a role in the genesis of these syndromes.

The diagnosis of mania after traumatic brain injury is based on DSM-IV-TR criteria for mood disorder due to traumatic brain injury with manic or mixed features (Table 2.5–1). As in the case of depressive disorders, the mania must be thought to be a direct physiological consequence of the brain injury. The diagnosis only requires that the predominant mood be elevated, euphoric, or irritable. This obviously does not require the same specificity of syndrome as a manic episode or a major depressive episode.

A 31-year-old married man with two children was struck in the head when a welding tank exploded, sending large and small pieces of metal in all directions. He experienced an intracerebral bleed in the right basal ganglia and white matter surrounding the anterior horn of the right lateral ventricle. Within a few days, he became manic, staying up all night, selling things he owned for ridiculously low prices, and buying a new car he could not afford. He believed that he would become a famous songwriter and was hypersexual. He was admitted to a hospital, where he was treated successfully with lithium and low-dose haloperidol (Haldol). He remained euthymic for approximately 6 months, and he discontinued his medications. Although he continued to experience significant behavioral changes, manic symptoms did not recur during a 2-year follow-up period.

The differential diagnosis of mania after traumatic brain injury should include substance-induced mood disorder, psychotic syndrome associated with epilepsy, and personality change due to traumatic brain injury. Substance-induced mood disorder occurs after intoxication or withdrawal from drugs and is another important differential diagnosis among patients with traumatic brain injury who frequently have a prior history of substance abuse.

Anxiety Disorders There is a paucity of studies on the prevalence and clinical correlates of anxiety disorders in the traumatic brain injury population. The available data, however, suggest that post–traumatic brain injury anxiety disorders are a frequent psychiatric complication of traumatic brain injury. DSM-IV-TR classifies anxiety disorders due to a medical condition (i.e., traumatic brain injury) according to the predominance of generalized anxiety, panic attacks or obsessive-compulsive symptoms (Table 2.5–1).

Anxiety disorders after traumatic brain injury may manifest themselves in a variety of ways. Pathological worrying, anxious foreboding, and autonomic symptoms are commonly associated with anxious depressions. A prospective study of 66 patients with traumatic brain injury found that 7 out of 17 patients (41.2 percent) with acute major depressive disorder met DSM-III-TR criteria for generalized anxiety disorder. In this study, anxious depressions had a more prolonged course. The mean duration of depression associated with generalized anxiety disorder was 7.5 months, whereas depression alone had a mean duration of 1.5 months. In a more recent prospective study of 92 traumatic brain injury patients, major depressive disorder was associated with prominent anxiety symptoms. Of the 30 patients who developed major depression during the course of a year of follow-up, 23 (76.7 percent) met DSM-IV-TR criteria for anxiety disorder compared to 9 out of 44 patients (20.4 percent) who did not develop a mood disorder but met criteria for anxiety disorder. Of the 23 patients with a coexistent anxiety disorder, 14 patients presented with generalized anxiety features, two patients had generalized anxiety and panic attacks, and the remaining seven patients met diagnostic criteria for posttraumatic stress disorder (PTSD). Other authors reported a relatively high prevalence of panic disorder after traumatic brain injury. For instance, in a recent study, panic disorder was observed in 18 of 196 patients (9 percent) hospitalized with traumatic brain injury.

Rigidity of thinking, obsessions, and ritualistic compulsions may also be observed after brain trauma. The onset of obsessive-compulsive symptoms, however, is usually preceded by generalized anxiety.

The prevalence of obsessive-compulsive disorder (OCD) occurring after traumatic brain injury has been estimated to be 2 to 4 percent. A recent article described the clinical characteristics of 10 patients who developed OCD after traumatic brain injury. Severity of traumatic brain injury was considered mild in six of the ten patients, two patients had moderate traumatic brain injury, and two patients had severe injuries. MRI scans were abnormal in patients with moderate and severe traumatic brain injury, demonstrating lesions involving the frontotemporal cortex or the caudate nucleus, or both. The global severity of OCD assessed using the Yale-Brown Obsessive Compulsive Scale ranged from moderate to severe.

PTSD is characterized by recurrent intrusive recollections, distressing dreams, and flashbacks of the traumatic event. Patients with PTSD show features of increased arousal, such as difficulty falling or staying asleep, exaggerated startle response, and irritability. Patients lose interest in social activities and avoid thoughts, feelings, or circumstances associated with the event.

There is controversy regarding whether PTSD can develop after traumatic brain injury. It has been proposed that loss of consciousness and posttraumatic amnesia after traumatic brain injury prevent the development of PTSD in moderate and severe traumatic brain injury. In addition, the significant symptomatic overlap between PTSD and postconcussive symptoms makes diagnosis of the former more difficult and unreliable among patients with mild head injury. For those who endorse this view, the prevalence of PTSD after traumatic brain injury might be less than 1 percent of cases. On the other hand, other investigators reported that PTSD is a relatively frequent complication of traumatic brain injury. They argue that traumatic brain injury patients can encode and retrieve trauma memories at an implicit level and that these memories can influence ongoing emotions and behaviors. Fear conditioning to a traumatic experience is mediated in limbic structures that are independent of higher cortical processes, and this mechanism might elicit PTSD symptoms among traumatic brain injury patients with loss of consciousness or severe posttraumatic amnesia. In addition, traumatic brain injury patients might have partial recollection of the circumstances of trauma (e.g., being on an ambulance or arriving at an emergency room), or, during the recovery process, they can reconstruct distressing memories of the traumatic event. According to these studies, the prevalence of PTSD after traumatic brain injury varies between 27 to 38 percent.

In a recent series by Jorge and Robinson, PTSD occurred in 13 out of 92 patients (14.1 percent) during the first year after traumatic brain injury. This frequency was not significantly different than the one observed in a control group of trauma patients without brain injury (i.e., 11.5 percent).

A 33-year-old certified nurse was assaulted while walking to her job in a small hospital. She received several blows to her head and was admitted unconscious to the emergency room. A CT scan showed a depressed skull fracture and right temporal and parietal contusions. She regained consciousness during the first 12 hours of admission and was confused and disoriented for the following 3 days. After this, she had an uneventful course and a good recovery. One month after trauma, she received a complete neuropsychiatric evaluation. She complained of intrusive recollections of the moments previous to the assault, which were associated with great psychological distress, sweating, and palpitations. She was also disturbed by nightmares in which she suddenly found herself in an intensive care unit connected to a ventilator, incapable of talking or asking for help. She avoided the hospital's surroundings and was unable to walk alone. She also complained of decreased concentration and memory impairments. The results of her neuropsychological tests, however, were within the normal range.

Is there a particular group of patients who are more vulnerable to develop anxiety disorders after traumatic brain injury? Overall, the presence of anxiety disorder has not been associated with any background characteristic, including severity of head injury or severity of social, physical, or cognitive impairment resulting from traumatic brain injury. The aforementioned study of Vietnam War veterans with penetrating brain injuries found that anxiety symptoms were associated with the presence of right orbitofrontal cortex lesions.

In addition, other studies found that patients with anxious depressions were more likely to have focal right hemisphere lesions. Taken together, these findings suggest that anxiety disorders may be mediated by pathophysiological changes provoked by right hemisphere lesions.

Psychotic Disorders The reported frequency of psychotic disorders after traumatic brain injury has varied from approximately 7 percent in retrospective reviews of World War II records to as much as 20 percent in medical populations of closed head injury patients. A recent study reviewed the clinical characteristics of 69 cases reported in the literature from 1971 to 1997. The majority of these patients were men who developed psychotic symptoms within the first 2 years after moderate or severe head injury. Positive symptoms (e.g., paranoid delusions and auditory hallucinations) were more prominent, whereas negative symptoms (e.g., alogia, avolition, and affective flattening) were relatively infrequent. A majority of these patients showed frontal or temporal lesions, or both. Posttraumatic psychosis has been associated with seizure disorder in 33 to 58 percent of cases. In addition, the epileptic foci are often located in limbic or paralimbic cortical regions. Psychotic episodes may be temporally linked to seizures or may have a more prolonged interictal course. In the latter case, the clinical picture is characterized by the presence of partial or complex-partial seizures, or both, and by a schizoaffective syndrome. Electroencephalographic and functional neuroradiological studies (e.g., single photon emission computed tomography [SPECT] and positron emission tomography [PET]) usually define ictal and interictal disturbances.

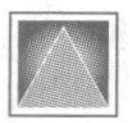

Table 2.5–4
Neuropathological Classification of Traumatic Brain Injury Lesions

Focal lesions
Intracranial-extracerebral hemorrhage (epidural and subdural hematomas and subarachnoid hemorrhage)
Intracerebral hemorrhage
Focal ischemic lesions
Diffuse lesions
Diffuse axonal injury
Diffuse ischemic damage

PATHOLOGY

Types of Primary and Secondary Brain Injury The first level of categorization of head injuries divides them into *closed* or *penetrating injuries* depending on the integrity of meningeal coverings. Missile wounds are the most frequent cause of penetrating brain injuries. They tend to produce discrete lesions that may be complicated by infection or hemorrhage. On the other hand, motor vehicle accidents are the most frequent cause of closed trauma, which represents the majority of traumatic brain injuries. Diffuse brain damage is a prominent feature of closed head injury (Table 2.5–4).

Primary brain damage is produced by contact and inertial forces that occur at the time of injury. Contact forces may result in laceration to the scalp, skull fractures, intracranial hemorrhages, contusions, and intracerebral hemorrhages. Inertial loading consists of acceleration, deceleration, and rotational forces that result in diffuse axonal injury and, eventually, acute subdural hematoma from the tearing of subdural bridging veins. Secondary brain damage is produced by pathological processes that are initiated at the moment of injury but span a variable period after the traumatic episode. These include brain damage secondary to ischemia (e.g., that resulting from associated hypotension or hypoxia, or both), brain swelling, raised intracranial pressure (with consequent reduction of cerebral perfusion pressure), and infection.

Focal lesions consist of contusions and lacerations that usually occur at the surface of the brain. They are more prominent at the crest of cerebral gyri and have a predilection for the frontal and temporal poles. Lacerations are usually accompanied by extracerebral hemorrhages (burst lobe). Intracranial-extracerebral hemorrhages occur in the epidural space (i.e., between the skull and the dura), the subdural space (i.e., between the dura and the arachnoid), or the subarachnoid space. Intracerebral hemorrhages are often multiple, involving the frontal and temporal lobes and basal ganglia, and may have a delayed onset (i.e., hours or days after trauma). Finally, ischemic damage may result from traumatic vascular lesions (e.g., arterial dissection, vascular distortion and compression, and venous thrombosis) or from arterial vasospasm.

Diffuse lesions include diffuse axonal injury, which occurs preferentially within the corpus callosum, thalamus, and dorsolateral quadrants of the upper brainstem. Pathologic processes include fragmentation of the axolemma, axonal transport disruption, axonal bulb formation, astrogliosis, and microglial activation. Although usually associated with immediate and persistent coma, lesser degrees of axonal disruption may also be seen in patients with a lucid interval or even in patients who experienced mild brain injuries (Fig. 2.5–9). Diffuse injury also includes ischemic damage. Ischemic damage is highly prevalent among patients with severe head injuries. David E.

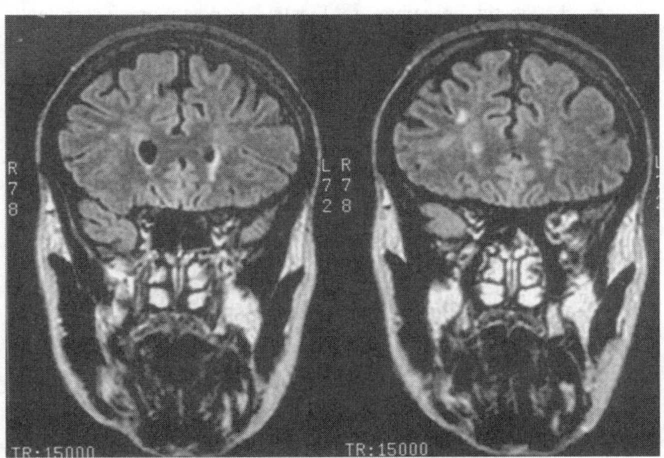

FIGURE 2.5–9 Coronal magnetic resonance images of the frontal lobes showing bilateral white matter lesions consistent with the presence of diffuse axonal injury.

Graham and colleagues reported that severe ischemic damage was present in 27 percent of their 151 pathologically examined cases, moderately severe ischemic damage was present in 43 percent, and mild damage was present in another 30 percent of cases.

The influence of these different patterns of injury on the psychiatric disorders after traumatic brain injury has not been extensively studied. Previous studies have stressed the importance of diffuse brain injury as a predictor of long-term disability of traumatic brain injury patients. A recent study, however, did not find significant differences in neuropsychological outcome between two groups of patients with focal or diffuse patterns of injury. Furthermore, focal and diffuse lesions usually coexist in traumatic brain injured patients.

Neurobiological Changes During the last decade, numerous studies have identified the complex pathological processes occurring after brain trauma with the hope of designing effective specific interventions to prevent neuronal death and to foster restorative change. These processes include an array of neurochemical and structural changes, including the release of neurotransmitters and neuropeptides, the expression of several transcription factors, and the activation of the molecular cascades associated with necrotic cell death and neuronal apoptosis. Other complex delayed processes include microglial activation and release of inflammatory cytokines, as well as mechanisms of repair and regeneration that include reactive synaptogenesis and axonal sprouting. The role that these changes play in mediating the behavioral outcome of traumatic brain injury patients, particularly in relation to the onset and course of psychiatric disorders, has not been elucidated and represents a fertile area of research.

During the past few years, there have also been numerous examinations of posttraumatic changes in the major neurotransmitter systems in the brain. Glutamate has been extensively studied because of its role in excitotoxic injury. Excitotoxic injury has a sequential mechanism that includes, first, sodium and chloride influx with resultant cytotoxic edema and, second, calcium influx leading to increased expression of early transcription factors, acute phase proteins, caspases, and proteolytic enzymes that mediate neuronal apoptosis. Clinical studies have reported that glutamate concentrations are significantly elevated for several days in the cerebrospinal fluid (CSF) of traumatic brain injury patients. Thus, it is conceivable that excitotoxic injury could be prevented through pharmacological intervention. Glutamate antagonists have shown a beneficial effect in experimental models of traumatic brain injury. In addition, inhibitors of glutamate release, such as riluzole (Rilutek), may be an alternative to postsynaptic glutamatergic blockade, which is known to be associated with severe psychiatric side effects. There is also evidence that magnesium chloride administered early after traumatic brain injury attenuates cortical histological damage and improves behavioral outcome.

Cholinergic neuronal activity appears to be increased immediately after traumatic brain injury. Blockade of massive acetylcholine release resulting from pathologic excitation of basal forebrain nuclei at the time of injury may prevent neuronal cell loss and associated behavioral deficits. There is also evidence of a hypofunctional cholinergic state occurring later in the course after traumatic brain injury. A reduction of cholinergic transmission in hippocampal and neocortical areas has been observed after cortical contusion brain injury. In addition, experimental models in rats have demonstrated dysfunction of the septohippocampal cholinergic pathway, which might play a significant role in the development of posttraumatic cognitive and behavioral deficits. Although cholinergic systems have not been systematically studied in clinical populations of traumatic brain injury patients, cholinergic deficits observed in patients with Alzheimer's disease have been associated with behavioral changes, including lack of motivation and anhedonia, as well as agitation and disinhibited behavior.

Ascending biogenic amine pathways have also been implicated in the pathophysiological processes underlying the clinical presentation and even the long-term outcome of traumatic brain injury patients. Circulating levels of catecholamines have been shown to significantly correlate with traumatic brain injury severity as measured by the GCS score. A recent study found that traumatic brain injury patients showed an increase in serotonergic and noradrenergic metabolites in the CSF. The investigators hypothesized that prolonged increase of the synaptic concentration of these neurotransmitters would result in subacute or chronic downregulation of aminergic transmission and, eventually, depressive symptoms.

Dysregulation of mesolimbic and mesocortical dopaminergic pathways, perhaps as a result of prefrontal damage, might also be involved in the mechanisms underlying manic and hypomanic syndromes. In addition, aminergic neurotransmitters may be implicated in the restorative processes occurring in the chronic phase of traumatic brain injury, an effect that may be mediated by neurotrophic factors.

LABORATORY TESTS

During the past few years, there has been extensive research on the diagnostic and predictive value of serum markers for traumatic brain injury. These include neuronal (e.g., neuron specific enolase, creatine kinase-BB isoenzyme) and glial (e.g., myelin basic protein, S-100B) proteins. For instance, serum S-100B is reported to have 90-percent sensitivity and 99-percent sensitivity for detecting intracranial pathology on head CT scans. In addition, serum S-100B levels greater than 2.0 μg/L predicted unfavorable outcome among patients with moderate to severe brain injury even more accurately than traditional clinical measures, such as the GCS. In mild head injury, early detection of serum S-100B levels greater than 0.2 μg/L predicted long-term neuropsychological dysfunction, even in cases in which MRI was negative. Thus, serum markers may objectively diagnose traumatic brain injury in symptomatic patients with normal neuroimaging findings. In addition, sustained or secondary release of serum markers may prove useful in detecting disease progression or monitoring treatment response. Early identification of patients at high risk for long-term neurobehavioral dysfunction could greatly assist with the development of effective therapeutic interventions for traumatic brain injury.

Head trauma has been also associated with neuroendocrine dysfunction, particularly with pituitary hormone deficiencies. Diabetes insipidus is easily recognized in the acute stage, but other pituitary hormone deficits may present insidiously, escaping detection for months or years. The potential importance of such deficiencies is increased by the emergence of the syndrome of growth hormone deficiency (GHD) in adults, which is characterized by decreases in strength, energy, and sense of well-being. A recent study assessed neuroendocrine disturbances in a group of 70 traumatic brain injury patients evaluated at approximately 30 months after their injuries. The frequency of GHD was estimated at 15 percent in this series.

In addition, thyroid-stimulating hormone (TSH) or free thyroxine (FT_4) values, or both, were below the normal range in 22 percent of subjects, suggesting partial central hypothyroidism. The authors hypothesized that a loss of cholinergic neurons secondary to traumatic brain injury might disinhibit hypothalamic somatostatin secretion, resulting in suppression of growth hormone (GH) and TSH levels. Other investigators have reported low cortisol levels and decreased gonadotropin secretion, resulting in hypogonadism.

Neuroimaging There have been recent advances in neuroimaging techniques that will certainly increase the understanding of the relationship between structural abnormalities and behavioral disturbances after traumatic brain injury. CT and MRI are routinely used for the evaluation of traumatic brain injury patients. CT is still the most efficient means of detecting surgically treatable hematomas and is the study of choice for evaluating patients with rapid changes in their neurological status. MRI, however, is more sensitive in detecting the more prevalent posttraumatic nonhemorrhagic lesions (e.g., cortical contusions and deep white matter lesions) and in identifying small subdural collections. A delayed MRI scan (i.e., 2 weeks after injury) would be indicated in those patients whose initial instability favored an emergency CT scan but were later treated medically or were left with persistent neurological deficits after a neurosurgical procedure. There is also some evidence that functionally significant lesions may be better evaluated by late MRI scanning.

Functional neuroimaging studies, for example, PET and SPECT, provide additional information with regard to the metabolic rates of cortical and subcortical structures and of the status of specific neurotransmitter systems. PET and SPECT have greater sensitivity than CT and MRI in detecting local abnormalities in chronic traumatic brain injury patients. The correlation between these radiological abnormalities and specific neurobehavioral deficits, however, has generally been weak and requires further study.

Recently, proton magnetic resonance spectroscopy (MRS) has demonstrated abnormalities in regions of gray and white matter that appeared normal in other conventional imaging studies. Early MRS alterations correlated with outcome in patients after traumatic brain injury. *Diffusion tensor MRI* is another imaging technique that might prove to be useful to quantify the degree of diffuse axonal injury and white matter pathology that would otherwise be underestimated with routine MRI scans. These new imaging developments may be relevant to understanding the behavioral consequences of traumatic brain injury.

Electrophysiological Studies Conventional electroencephalogram (EEG) recordings are currently used in trauma intensive care units for monitoring procedures and for brain death diagnosis. The EEG is also invaluable in the diagnosis of status epilepticus and is the primary diagnostic procedure to localize a posttraumatic epileptic focus. The chance of finding an abnormality on routine EEG can be increased by using nasopharyngeal, anterior temporal, or sphenoidal leads. Video-EEG monitoring and 24-hour ambulatory recordings may be useful in the differential diagnosis of patients presenting with unclear paroxysmal behavioral disturbances. Quantitative EEG (QEEG) is currently used as an adjunctive diagnostic technique in the evaluation of slow wave abnormalities associated with brain injuries and in the diagnosis of posttraumatic temporal lobe epilepsy. Polysomnography permits the diagnosis of atypical sleep disturbances that may occur in traumatic brain injury patients. These include atypical night terrors, sleep apnea, nocturnal myoclonus, and restless leg syndrome. Visual, auditory, and somatosensory evoked potentials are useful to localize the level of injury to the CNS. Auditory evoked potentials are particularly effective in detecting brainstem pathology. There has also been increasing interest in more complex electrophysiological responses. A recent study evaluated P50 physiology and sensory gating mechanisms in traumatic brain injury patients. The P50 ratio might serve as a marker of hippocampal dysfunction in this population.

COURSE AND PROGNOSIS

Course and prognosis of traumatic brain injury patients involve the longitudinal analysis of neurological, neuropsychological, psychiatric, and psychosocial variables. Some of these variables are readily operationally defined, whereas others are more elusive and difficult to quantify. The Glasgow Outcome Scale (GOS) has been widely used as a measure of the long-term outcome of traumatic brain injury patients. It consists of five levels of outcome: (1) death, (2) persistent vegetative state, (3) severe disability (conscious but dependent in activities of daily living), (4) moderate disability (disabled but living independently), and (5) good recovery (mild neuropsychiatric sequels but able to resume an otherwise normal life). Although crude, the scale is appreciated for its validity and high reproducibility.

The long-term outcome of traumatic brain injury patients is primarily related to severity of brain injury, type and location of intracranial lesion, patient age, and efficacy of acute medical and surgical treatment (Fig. 2.5–10). Outcome is also influenced by concurrent factors that include socioeconomic status, educational level, previous psychiatric disorders (e.g., history of alcohol and drug abuse and personality disorders), and premorbid social functioning levels. Finally, the quality and extent of rehabilitation services and the availability of social and vocational support also play significant roles in traumatic brain injury outcome.

The National Institutes of Health Traumatic Coma Data Bank was initiated by the National Institute of Neurological Disorders and Stroke to characterize the natural history of traumatic head injury and to evaluate the determinants of recovery. Of 746 severe head injured patients studied in this cohort, 243 patients (32.5 percent) died, 325 patients (42 percent) were severely disabled or in a vegetative state, 138 (18 percent) had moderate disability, and the remaining 50 (7 percent) had a good recovery, as measured by the GOS at the time of hospital discharge. Another study analyzed the outcome of 170 patients with moderate head injuries at 3 months after traumatic brain injury. According to the GOS, 38 percent of moderate head injury patients made a good recovery, 49 percent were left with moderate disability, and 10 percent of patients had severe disability. The mortality rate was 3 percent. The same authors found that the majority of mild head injury patients (78 percent) made a good recovery, 22 percent of patients were left with moderate disability, and there were no patients experiencing severe disability.

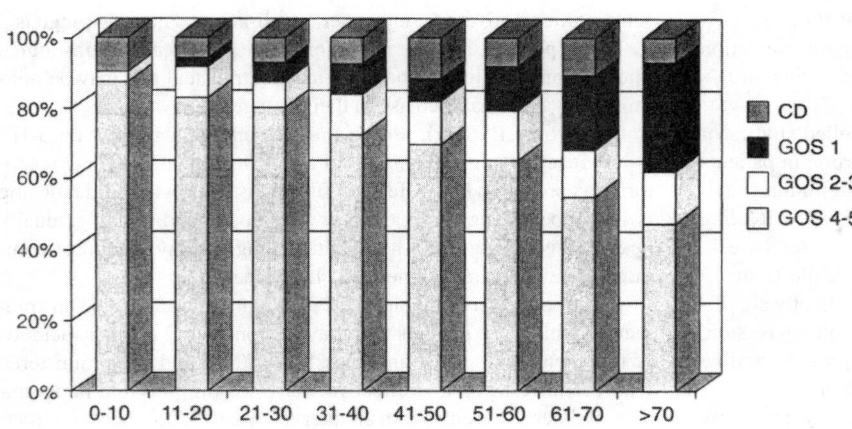

FIGURE 2.5–10 Final outcome assessed using the Glasgow Outcome Scale (GOS) (percentage of distribution) in eight age groups in 1,508 patients. CD, cerebral death. (From Rudehill A, Bellander BM, Weitzberg E, Bredbacka S, Backheden M, Gordon E: Outcome of traumatic brain injuries in 1,508 patients: Impact of pre-hospital care. *J Neurotrauma.* 2002;19:855–868, with permission.)

Cognitive disturbances are among the most important factors in long-term disability after severe traumatic brain injury. A previous study reported on a group of 50 mild and moderate head injury patients and correlated different neuropsychological measures obtained in-hospital and at 1- and 3-month follow-ups with serial MRI findings. The traumatic brain injury group had significantly greater neuropsychological impairment than a control group. These cognitive deficits showed an impressive recovery during follow-up and were not consistently related to specific lesion locations. MRI abnormalities were present at baseline in 40 (80 percent) of these patients and gradually resolved by 3 months. Other studies have reported that 18 percent of severe head injury patients had returned to gainful employment, and 62 percent of former students had returned to school by 6-month follow-up. For those not back to work or school at 6 months, 31 percent of the former workers and 66 percent of the former students had returned by 12 months. The three most significant predictors for returning to work or school were age, intact verbal abilities, and speed of information processing. A series of moderate head injury cases revealed that 69 percent of patients who had been gainfully employed before the injury were unemployed at 3-month follow-up.

Furthermore, behavioral changes associated with traumatic brain injury may disrupt interpersonal relationships and may pose a great burden to family members. During the first year after the injury, more than two-thirds of relatives experienced moderate to severe degrees of burden as a consequence of the behavioral changes in their family member. Thus, it is not surprising that psychosocial adjustment and community reentry have become the targets of rehabilitation efforts after traumatic brain injury. Patient motivation and a history of alcohol and drug abuse, as well as awareness of cognitive and physical impairments, have been shown to exert a significant effect on rehabilitation outcome.

TREATMENT OF NEUROPSYCHIATRIC COMPLICATIONS

Organic Therapies Treatment of psychiatric disorders occurring after traumatic brain injury involves different pharmacological and nonpharmacological strategies. One would assume that treatment of the neurobehavioral consequences of traumatic brain injury should begin early in the acute phase after injury. If it is possible to modify the processes associated with neuronal damage, the intervention should be started as early as possible. This would presumably lead to the greatest amount of recovery in cognition, motivation, activity levels, and emotional disorder.

Despite the progress observed in elucidating neuronal pathologic mechanisms at a biomolecular level, however, therapeutic interventions based on experimental models have been disappointing. Although calcium kinetics and the production of reactive oxygen species (ROS) have been consistently implicated in cellular injury, controlled trials have shown no clinical benefit from calcium channel blockers or ROS scavenger agents. Further interventions at different points in the pathological cascades (e.g., inhibition of caspases) might be more successful.

Another critical area for potential therapeutic intervention involves the plastic and restorative changes occurring in the brain after brain damage. Investigators are also starting to depict the behavioral consequences of these changes. One of the most active fields of research involves the biology of neurotrophic factors. These factors support neuronal survival and facilitate neuronal plasticity. Expression of different growth factors is enhanced in the acute period of experimental trauma, and there is some evidence that post-traumatic administration of neurotrophic factors is protective to the injured brain. For example, central *nerve growth factor* (NFG) administration can reduce the extent of programmed apoptotic cell death in septal cholinergic neurons after experimental brain trauma. Preliminary studies using hippocampal precursor cells transfected with NFG and transplanted to cortical areas of injury have been found to improve neurobehavioral outcome. In addition, continuous subcutaneous administration of *insulin-like growth factor-1* (IGF-1) for 7 days dramatically accelerated neurological motor recovery and attenuated cognitive deficits after lateral fluid percussion brain injury in rats. It is worthy to note that antidepressants, through their action on noradrenergic and serotonergic receptors, enhance the expression of neurotrophic factors and that this effect may be a substantial contributor to their clinical efficacy.

Although progress in basic research allows a promising future for therapeutic intervention after traumatic brain injury to be envisioned, there is a lack of adequately controlled clinical studies that are needed to provide a solid scientific basis for neuropsychiatric treatment. Currently, anecdotal cases and clinical experience are the only things that support many daily treatment decisions.

Patients with brain injury are more sensitive to the side effects of medications, especially psychotropics. Jonathan Silver and Stuart Yudofsky proposed several general guidelines for their use in this population. Doses of psychotropics must be prudently increased, minimizing side effects (i.e., start low, go slow). The patient must receive, however, an adequate therapeutic trial with regard to dosage and duration of treatment. Brain injured patients must be frequently reassessed to determine changes in treatment schedules. Special care must be taken in monitoring drug interactions. Finally, if there is evidence of a partial response to a specific medication, augmentation therapy may be warranted, depending on the augmenting drug's mechanism of action and potential side effects.

There have been no double-blind, placebo-controlled studies of the efficacy of pharmacological treatments of depression in patients with acute traumatic brain injury. There is some preliminary evidence that desipramine (Norpramin) may be effective for treating depression in patients with severe traumatic brain injury. An 8-week, nonrandomized, placebo, run-in trial of sertraline (Zoloft) in 15 patients with mild traumatic brain injury showed statistically significant improvement in psychological distress, anger, and aggression, as well as in the severity of postconcussive symptoms. Sertraline may also lead to a beneficial effect on cognitive functioning.

Selection among competing antidepressants is usually guided by their side effect profiles. Mild anticholinergic activity, minimal lowering of seizure threshold, and low sedative effects are the most important factors to be considered in the choice of an antidepressant drug in this population. Tricyclic antidepressants (TCAs) have important anticholinergic effects that may interfere with cognitive and memory functions. In addition, they may lower the seizure threshold. If, however, a decision is made to administer TCAs, nortriptyline (Aventyl) (starting at 10 mg per day) constitutes a reasonable alternative, provided that blood levels and toxic effects are carefully monitored. Selective serotonin reuptake inhibitors (SSRIs) are antidepressants that appear to have a less adverse side effect profile. The most common side effects include headache, gastrointestinal (GI) complaints, insomnia, diminished libido, and sexual dysfunction. Escitalopram (Lexapro) (10 mg per day), sertraline (25 to 200 mg per day), or paroxetine (starting at 5 to 40 mg per day) are among the most useful drugs in this group. Trazodone (Desyrel) and nefazodone (Serzone) are alternative antidepressants that block serotonin (5-HT) type 2 receptors and also inhibit serotonin reuptake. These can be useful for the treatment of patients with prominent anxiety symptoms and sleep disturbance. Nefazodone dose should be gradually increased from 100 mg per day to 500 mg per day. Trazodone is also started at low doses (50 to 100 mg) at bedtime after a snack. The dose may be gradually increased every 3 to 4 days to 400 mg. The most troublesome side effects are sedation and orthostatic hypotension.

There are case reports of successful treatments of post–traumatic brain injury depression with psychostimulants. These include dextroamphetamine (Dexedrine) (8 to 60 mg per day) and methylphenidate (Ritalin) (10 to 60 mg per day). They are given twice a day with the last dose at least 6 hours before sleep to prevent initial insomnia. Dextroamphetamine and methylphenidate might also be useful to treat deficits in attention and apathetic symptoms that are frequently seen in patients with traumatic brain injury. However, the magnitude and temporal course of their therapeutic effect is still a matter of controversy. Treatment is begun at lower doses, which are then gradually increased. Patients taking stimulants need close medical observation to prevent abuse or toxic effects. The most common side effects are anxiety, dysphoria, headaches, irritability, anorexia, insomnia, cardiovascular symptoms, dyskinesias, or even psychotic symptoms.

Amantadine (Symmetrel), a drug with a complex pharmacological effects on dopaminergic, cholinergic, and *N*-methyl-D-aspartate (NMDA) receptors, might be of some use for the treatment of motivational and executive deficits. It is usually started at low doses (50 mg twice a day) and gradually increased to 200 mg twice a day.

There is also some empirical evidence of the beneficial effects of cholinesterase inhibitors, such as donepezil (Aricept), on cognitive functioning, motivation, and general well-being. The dose range is 5 to 10 mg per day, and the more common side effects are insomnia, diarrhea, and dizziness. These are usually transient and may be minimized by a gradual increase in their dosage.

Buspirone (BuSpar), a drug that has an agonist effect on 5-HT type 1 receptors and an antagonist effect on dopamine type 2 receptors, has proved to be a safe and efficacious anxiolytic. Initial dosing is 15 mg per day, given in three divided doses, and it may gradually be increased (5 mg every 4 days) to 60 mg per day. The most common side effects are dizziness and headaches.

Electroconvulsive therapy (ECT) is not contraindicated in traumatic brain injury patients and may be considered if other methods of treatment prove to be unsuccessful. ECT should be administered with the lowest possible effective energy, using pulsatile nondominant unilateral currents, with an interval of 2 to 5 days between treatments and 4 to 6 treatments for a complete course. Finally, the role that social intervention and adequate psychotherapeutic support may play in the treatment of depression after traumatic brain injury has already been mentioned.

There have been no systematic studies of the treatment of secondary mania. Lithium, carbamazepine, and valproic acid (Depakene) therapies have also been reported to be efficacious in individual cases. Lithium has been reported to impair cognitive performance in traumatic brain injured patients. In addition, it may lower the seizure threshold. Some authors limit its use to patients in whom bipolar disorder preceded the onset of traumatic brain injury. The mood stabilizer and anticonvulsant carbamazepine should be gradually increased to obtain therapeutic blood levels (i.e., 8 to 12 μg/mL). Complete blood counts should be obtained every 2 weeks for the first 2 months of therapy and every 3 months thereafter. Liver function tests should be obtained every 3 months. Frequent side effects include sedation, dry mouth, GI upset, drowsiness, impaired concentration, ataxia, nystagmus, and rash. Severe complications include pancytopenia, aplastic anemia, and cholestatic jaundice. Valproic acid (Depakene) may be progressively increased from 500 mg per day to the dose necessary to obtain plasma levels between 50 and 100 μg/mL. The maximum recommended dose is 60 mg/kg per day divided into two to four doses. Valproic acid may have potentially serious side effects, including hepatotoxicity, which ranges from a discrete elevation of transaminases and serum ammonia levels to irreversible liver failure. Hemorrhagic pancreatitis has also been reported. The most common side effects are drowsiness, tremor, gastritis, and increased weight. Liver function tests and serum amylase levels should be monitored. The role of other anticonvulsants, such as lamotrigine (Lamictal) or topiramate (Topamax), as mood stabilizers has not been tested in traumatic brain injury populations.

Finally, pathological emotions may respond to treatment with antidepressants, particularly SSRIs. There is, however, a great variability in treatment response among brain injured patients, with some showing a rapid response at relatively low doses, whereas others require more time and higher doses.

Based on this discussion of therapeutic interventions, it is obvious that treatment options are based on logic and current standards of practice rather than empirically based controlled treatment trials. There is a great need for randomized, double-blind, placebo-controlled trials to establish the most effective treatments for the variety of psychiatric disorders that occur in traumatic brain injury patients.

Behavioral and Psychotherapeutic Treatment Behavioral deficits in self-care habits (e.g., feeding or personal hygiene), interpersonal skills (e.g., disinhibited behavior), problem solving, or response to environmental stress may be amenable to behavioral intervention. Behavioral rehabilitation programs shape behavior based on the principles of operant conditioning (e.g., contingency contracts and token economies). Their goal is to increase the patient's repertoire of social and independent living skills, generalizing their use from the rehabilitation environment to the more demanding conditions of community life.

Controlled treatment trials of psychotherapy in any of the neuropsychiatric disorders resulting from brain injury have not been conducted. There are, however, reports of the use of cognitive behavioral therapy, group therapy, and family therapy in the treatment of depression or other neuropsychiatric disorders. The use of specific psychological interventions for each neuropsychiatric disorder needs to be developed.

SUGGESTED CROSS-REFERENCES

Basic neurological issues are discussed in Section 1.2. Neuroimaging is covered in Section 1.15 and Section 1.16. Neuropsychological tests used to evaluate neurological and psychiatric patients are described in Chapter 7.

Delirium, dementia, and amnestic disorders are covered in Chapter 10 and Chapter 51. Neuropsychiatric complications of stroke and epilepsy are discussed in Section 2.2 and Section 2.4, respectively.

References

Arciniegas DB, Topkoff JL, Rojas DC, Sheeder J, Teale P, Young DA, Sandberg E, Reite ML, Adler LE: Reduced hippocampal volume in association with p50 nonsuppression following traumatic brain injury. *J Neuropsychiatry Clin Neurosci.* 2001;13:213.

Bombardier CH, Temkin NR, Machamer J, Dikmen SS: The natural history of drinking and alcohol-related problems after traumatic brain injury. *Arch Phys Med Rehabil.* 2003;84:185.

Brooks WM, Friedman SD, Gasparovic C: Magnetic resonance spectroscopy in traumatic brain injury. *J Head Trauma Rehabil.* 2001;16:149.

Dixon CE, Bao J, Long DA, Hayes RL: Reduced evoked release of acetylcholine in the rodent hippocampus following traumatic brain injury. *Pharmacol Biochem Behav.* 1996;53:679.

Feinstein A, Hershkop S, Ouchterlony D, Jardine A, McCullagh S: Posttraumatic amnesia and recall of a traumatic event following traumatic brain injury. *J Neuropsychiatry Clin Neurosci.* 2002;14:25.

*Graham DI, Gentleman SM, Nicoll JA, Royston MC, McKenzie JE, Roberts GW, Griffin WS: Altered beta-APP metabolism after head injury and its relationship to the aetiology of Alzheimer's disease. *Acta Neurochir Suppl (Wien).* 1996;66:96.

Hattori N, Huang SC, Wu HM, Yeh E, Glenn TC, Vespa PM, McArthur D, Phelps ME, Hovda DA, Bergsneider M: Correlation of regional metabolic rates of glucose with Glasgow Coma Scale after traumatic brain injury. *J Nucl Med.* 2003;44:1709.

Hillary FG, Steffener J, Biswal BB, Lange G, DeLuca J, Ashburner J: Functional magnetic resonance imaging technology and traumatic brain injury rehabilitation: Guidelines for methodological and conceptual pitfalls. *J Head Trauma Rehabil.* 2002;17:411.

*Jorge RE, Robinson RG, Moser D, Tateno A, Crespo-Facorro B, Arndt SE: Major depression following traumatic brain injury. *Arch Gen Psychiatry.* 2004;61:42.

Jorge RE, Robinson RG, Starkstein SE, Arndt SV: Influence of major depression on 1-year outcome in patients with traumatic brain injury. *J Neurosurg.* 1994;81:726.

Jorge RE, Robinson RG, Starkstein SE, Arndt SV, Forrester AW, Geisler FH: Secondary mania following traumatic brain injury. *Am J Psychiatry.* 1993;150:916.

Kreutzer JS, Seel RT, Gourley E: The prevalence and symptom rates of depression after traumatic brain injury: A comprehensive examination. *Brain Inj.* 2001;15:563.

Levin HS: Neurobehavioral recovery. *J Neurotrauma.* 1992;9[Suppl 1]:S359.

Levin HS, Hanten G, Chang CC, Zhang L, Schachar R, Ewing-Cobbs L, Max JE: Working memory after traumatic brain injury in children. *Ann Neurol.* 2002;52:82.

*Lishman WA: Psychiatric disability after head injury: The significance of brain damage. *Proc R Soc Med.* 1966;59:261.

Lishman WA: Psychiatric sequelae of head injuries: Problems in diagnosis. *Ir Med J.* 1978;71:306.

Maxwell WL, Dhillon K, Harper L, Espin J, MacIntosh TK, Smith DH, Graham DI: There is differential loss of pyramidal cells from the human hippocampus with survival after blunt head injury. *J Neuropathol Exp Neurol.* 2003;62:272.

McAllister TW: Neuropsychiatric sequelae of head injuries. *Psychiatr Clin North Am.* 1992;15:395.

*McIntosh TK, Saatman KE, et al.: The Dorothy Russell Memorial Lecture. The molecular and cellular sequelae of experimental traumatic brain injury. 1998.

Pelinka LE, Toegel E, Mauritz W, Redl H: Serum S 100 B: A marker of brain damage in traumatic brain injury with and without multiple trauma. *Shock.* 2003;19:195.

Povlishock JT, Hayes RL, Michel ME, McIntosh TK: Workshop on animal models of traumatic brain injury. *J Neurotrauma.* 1994;11:723.

Raghupathi R, Graham DI, McIntosh TK: Apoptosis after traumatic brain injury. *J Neurotrauma.* 2000;17:927.

Rapoport MJ, McCullagh S, Streiner D, Feinstein A: The clinical significance of major depression following mild traumatic brain injury. *Psychosomatics.* 2003;44:31.

Rosenthal M, Christensen BK, Ross TP: Depression following traumatic brain injury. *Arch Phys Med Rehabil.* 1998;79:90.

Royo NC, Shimizu S, Schouten JW, Stover JF, McIntosh TK: Pharmacology of traumatic brain injury. *Curr Opin Pharmacol.* 2003;3:27.

Seel RT, Kreutzer JS, Rosenthal M, Hammond FM, Corrigan JD, Black K: Depression after traumatic brain injury: A National Institute on Disability and Rehabilitation Research Model Systems multicenter investigation. *Arch Phys Med Rehabil.* 2003;84:177.

Silver JM, Yudofsky SC: The Overt Aggression Scale: Overview and guiding principles. *J Neuropsychiatry Clin Neurosci.* 1991;3:S22.

*Silver JM, Yudofsky SC, Hales RE, eds. Neuropsychiatry of traumatic brain injury. Washington, DC: American Psychiatric Press, 1994.

Wilson JT, Pettigrew LE, Teasdale GM: Emotional and cognitive consequences of head injury in relation to the Glasgow Outcome Scale. *J Neurol Neurosurg Psychiatry.* 2000;69:204.

Yan HQ, Kline AE, Ma X, Li Y, Dixon CE: Traumatic brain injury reduces dopamine transporter protein expression in the rat frontal cortex. *Neuroreport.* 2002;13:1899.

▲ 2.6 Neuropsychiatric Aspects of Movement Disorders

Laura Marsh, M.D., and Russell L. Margolis, M.D.

Emotion, cognition, and movement are controlled by a series of interrelated and interdependent circuits that link the fields of psychiatry and neurology. Thus, patients presenting with disorders of emotion or cognition frequently have motor abnormalities, and patients presenting with motor abnormalities often have emotional or cognitive disorders. The motor status of patients presenting to psychiatrists is, therefore, of utmost relevance, and the motor examination is an essential component of the psychiatric examination.

The complex relationship between psychiatric phenomena and movement abnormalities can be simplified into at least five overlapping categories. First, medications used to treat psychiatric conditions often cause abnormal movements as side effects, some of which may be long lasting or even permanent. Second, abnormal movements may be evident in patients with psychiatric disorders before drug exposure, a point that underscores the need for baseline motor screening in all patients. Abnormal movements in such patients may indicate the presence of gross congenital disorders (such as cerebral malformations), developmental disorders without gross brain malformation (such as the often subtle "soft signs" seen in patients with schizophrenia or autism), neurodegenerative disorders (such as Huntington's disease or Parkinson's disease), other cerebral insults (including strokes and tumors), or even normal aging. Third, movement abnormalities may reflect the presence of powerful emotional influences in normal individuals (e.g., tremulousness with anxiety). Fourth, movement abnormalities may be the physical manifestations of a primary psychiatric disorder, as illustrated by the motor slowing seen with depression or the motor hyperactivity seen with mania. Finally, psychiatric disturbances are commonly associated with neurological diseases initially presenting with abnormal movements and may aggravate the primary motor deficits. Thus, although often relegated to the specialty of neuropsychiatry, the careful appraisal and appreciation of movement abnormalities and movement disorders in psychiatric patients should be considered an important aspect of general psychiatric practice.

This chapter addresses the neuropsychiatric aspects of *movement disorders*, a term that typically refers to a diverse group of diseases of the central nervous system (CNS), primarily involving neurodegeneration of the basal ganglia or cerebellum or both. In addition to the motor abnormalities, psychiatric and cognitive abnormalities are very common in these conditions and contribute significantly to morbidity and caregiver burden. However, diagnosis of psychiatric conditions in patients with primary movement disorders is challenged by the interplay of motor, cognitive, and psychiatric features over the course of the disease and their overlap at the time of examination such as the masked face of parkinsonism and the flat affect in depressive disorders. Management of psychiatric disorders is often complex because treatments for the motor symptoms, when available, may aggravate or cause cognitive or psychiatric symptoms. In turn, psychiatric treatments may result in adverse motor and cognitive side effects. Appreciation of the distinctive motor, cognitive, mood, and behavioral aspects of the various movement disorders and their underlying pathophysiology helps to target therapies that are effective and limited in their risks.

COMPARATIVE NOSOLOGY

Classification of Movement Disorders Movement disorders can be classified using several different approaches (Table 2.6–1), each with advantages and limitations. From the phenomenological standpoint, movement disorders can be grouped into three main categories. Parkinsonian disorders are characterized by reduced amplitude of movements (hypokinesia), slowness of movements (bradykinesia), and difficulty initiating movements (akinesia). Dyskinetic disorders are characterized by increased motor activity and excessive (hyperkinetic) involuntary movements, including tremor, chorea, ballism, tics, dystonia, or myoclonus. Ataxias are characterized by problems with gait, dysmetria, and dysdiadokinesis. Nosologically, this scheme is problematic because the clinical features overlap across diseases. In addition, many syndromes involve several types of movement abnormalities, such as akinesia, dystonia, and tremor in Wilson's disease, whereas others, such as focal dystonia, consist of a single movement abnormality. Classification schemes based on neuropathological findings generally distinguish extrapyramidal diseases, in which the primary pathology is in the basal ganglia system, from diseases that primarily affect the cerebellum, cerebral cortex, or motor neurons. Again, common clinical features and neuronal system involvement across the different neuropathological groups limit this approach. An etiological classification has the advantage of linking a syndrome directly to its cause and directing attention at specific modes of pathogenesis, treatment, and prevention. On the other hand, the cause of many diseases is unknown (e.g., idiopathic Parkinson's disease), and an etiological nosology can lead to confusion, as entities with clinical similarities are separated into multiple different categories.

Classification of Psychiatric Disturbances Associated with Movement Disorders In accordance with the revised fourth edition of the *Diagnostic and Statistical Manual of Mental Disorders* (DSM-IV-TR), movement disorders are considered neurological disorders and are classified in DSM-IV-TR on Axis III as general medical conditions. Axis I psychiatric disturbances associated with movement disorders should generally be classified as "secondary to a general medical condition" such as depression secondary to Huntington's disease, psychosis secondary to dementia with Lewy bodies, or anxiety disorder secondary to Parkinson's disease. Additional qualifiers can be used to designate specific features of the presentation such as with hallucinations, with major depressive-like features, or with panic attacks. For research purposes, it is common to use the phenomenological criteria for DSM-IV-TR idiopathic psychiatric conditions to establish diagnoses while ignoring the general medical exclusion criterion. The prominence of psychiatric and cognitive manifestations in movement disorders, however, points out the arbitrariness of this scheme; it is equally valid for many of the movement disorders to be considered on Axis I as dementias, with associated movement and psychiatric phenomena. Another shortcoming of the DSM-IV-TR nosological system is that the nuances of many psychiatric disturbances are not captured by its terminology. Examples include the disruptive perseverative behaviors seen with Huntington's disease or pathological laughter or crying syndromes that may occur with progressive supranuclear palsy.

BEDSIDE ASSESSMENT OF MOVEMENT DISORDERS

Screening for motor deficits in psychiatric practice is straightforward, involves little extra time, and should be a standard component of patient assessment because the results affect treatment decisions. When the motor examination is accompanied by an adequate history and suspicion, overlapping motor and psychiatric signs can be recognized and distinguished according to the relative influences of the primary motor disorder, a psychiatric disturbance, a drug effect, or some interaction among them. For example, an elderly patient with melancholic depression may also show evidence for early Parkinson's disease, which requires additional treatment beyond antidepressant agents.

In patients with known movement disorders, the initial history and physical examination should first seek to confirm the presence of the diagnosed movement disorder. It is important to remember that movement disorders often share similar features, but their causes are diverse, and the course and treatment response vary over time and across the different disorders. Given this, there is frequent misdiagnosis of movement disorders; only 75 to 80 percent of patients with Parkinson's disease are correctly diagnosed with idiopathic Parkinson's disease during life by movement disorder specialists, and the rate of misdiagnosis is probably higher among nonspecialists. Examples of disorders that mimic Parkinson's disease, especially early in their course, are progressive supranuclear palsy, dementia with Lewy bodies, and neuroleptic drug effects. A second goal of the motor examination is to evaluate the extent of motor deficits relative to the patient's reported impairment. Complaints of motor dysfunction can be exaggerated in patients with depression, whereas dementia or lack of insight, as is often the case with Huntington's disease, can contribute to denial of illness or impulsive behaviors that increase the risk of falls. Last, as mentioned above, serial motor examinations provide a barometer of motor side effects due to agents used to treat psychiatric conditions.

The main elements of a motor function screen (Table 2.6–2) include assessment of gait, involuntary movements, coordination, muscle tone, and strength. Gait provides clues to the presence of upper versus lower motor neuron disease, sensory loss, and cerebellar versus extrapyramidal pathology and should first be observed when a patient walks to the examining room. Ability to rise indepen-

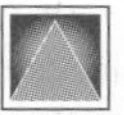

Table 2.6–1
Classification Schemes for Movement Disorders with Examples

- Major clinical feature
  - Hypokinetic movements
    - Idiopathic Parkinson's disease
    - Parkinsonian syndromes
    - Progressive supranuclear palsy
    - Corticobasal degeneration
    - Frontotemporal dementia
    - Dementia with Lewy bodies
    - Multiple-system atrophy—parkinsonian type
  - Hyperkinetic movements (see also Table 2.6–4)
    - Huntington's disease
    - Wilson's disease
    - Essential tremor
    - Dystonias
  - Ataxia
    - Spinocerebellar ataxia
    - Multiple-system atrophy—cerebellar type
- Location of primary neuropathology
  - Basal ganglia
    - Idiopathic Parkinson's disease
    - Parkinsonian syndromes
    - Progressive supranuclear palsy
    - Huntington's disease
    - Wilson's disease
    - Dystonias
  - Cerebellum (see also Table 2.6–5)
    - Friedreich's ataxia
    - Some spinocerebellar ataxias
  - Cerebral cortex
    - Frontotemporal dementia
  - Motor neuron
    - Amyotrophic lateral sclerosis
  - Multiple affected regions
    - Multiple-system atrophy—both types
    - Corticobasal degeneration
    - Dementia with Lewy bodies
    - Some spinocerebellar ataxias
- Etiological
  - Genetic
    - Huntington's disease
    - Parkinson's disease secondary to α-synuclein or Parkin mutations
    - Friedreich's ataxia
    - Some spinocerebellar ataxias
    - Frontotemporal dementia with parkinsonism linked to chromosome 17
    - Familial amyotrophic lateral sclerosis
    - Wilson's disease
    - Familial essential tremor
    - Some dystonias
  - Medication induced
    - Neuroleptic-induced parkinsonism or dystonia
  - Toxin induced
    - 1-Methyl-4-phenyl-1,2,3,6-tetrahydropyridine, manganese, or carbon monoxide–induced parkinsonism
  - Infectious
    - Postencephalitic parkinsonism
  - Traumatic
    - Posttraumatic parkinsonism, tremor, dystonia, or frontotemporal dementia
  - Vascular
    - Vascular parkinsonism or ataxia
  - Idiopathic
    - Most Parkinson's disease
    - Progressive supranuclear palsy
    - Corticobasal degeneration
    - Some cases of frontotemporal dementia
    - Dementia with Lewy bodies
    - Multiple-system atrophy
    - Essential tremor
    - Sporadic spinocerebellar ataxia

dently from a chair and without pushing off the armrests is a common, but nonspecific, screen for gait difficulties and increased fall risk in the geriatric population. Balance should be examined separately. Hyperkinetic and hypokinetic movement abnormalities can be observed during the interview while the patient rests comfortably in a chair. The five main types of abnormal hyperkinetic involuntary movements are tremor, chorea, myoclonus, tics, and dystonia. Asking the patient to hold his or her arms outstretched reveals forms of nonrest tremor and other adventitious movements as well as motor weakness. Finger-to-nose testing permits examination of large proximal arm movements, kinetic tremor, and dysmetria. Hypokinesia, characteristic of parkinsonian syndromes, is manifest by bradykinesia and akinesia. There is a relative absence of spontaneous movements or gestures, slowed movements, decreased arm swing, and diminished facial expressiveness (masked face) and spontaneous blinking. Gait disturbances are related to difficulties initiating and sustaining movements and turning. Coordination can be assessed with finger–thumb tapping. Motor tone is tested by passive movement of an extremity or the neck while the patient is at rest. When assessing tone, the examiner should note whether there is increased resistance to the passive movements and whether that resistance is active, spastic, or "lead pipe" in character. Cogwheeling, a feature of a tremor, is often mistaken for a measure of tone.

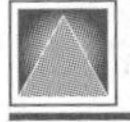

Table 2.6–2
Screening Examination for Motor System Dysfunction

- Gait—observe walking, including on tiptoes and heels
- Station—observe balance and ability to arise from chair, pull test
- Abnormal movements
  - At rest—observe for excessive movements, hypokinesia, or dystonic features
  - Hold arms outstretched
- Coordination—rapid finger tapping, finger-to-nose test
- Tone—passive movement of limbs and neck
- Strength

PARKINSON'S DISEASE

Parkinson's disease is a progressive neurodegenerative disorder that is associated with loss of dopaminergic neurons in the substantia nigra pars compacta (SNpc). The hallmarks of the disease are its triad of motor features—resting tremor, rigidity, and akinesia/bradykinesia (inability to initiate movement and slowness of movement, respectively). Gait and postural disturbances also characterize the disease. *Parkinsonism*, or *parkinsonian syndromes*, refers to the clinical appearance of Parkinson's disease without implying causation. Some patients, for instance, have parkinsonism secondary to antidopaminergic drugs without pathology of the substantia nigra.

History Descriptions of parkinsonian syndromes are found in the earliest medical writings. Idiopathic Parkinson's disease is named after James Parkinson, a general practitioner in London who wrote about paralysis agitans as a distinct disease separate from other causes of tremor in his classic 1817 article "Essay on the Shaking Palsy." Parkinson's description of the disease, based on six cases, made a point of distinguishing the resting tremor and festinating gait as major symptoms of the disease and highlighted the cardinal motor signs that remain characteristic of the disease today. Anticholinergic belladonna alkaloids were used to treat Parkinson's disease in the 19th century. The discovery that dopaminergic precursors reversed reserpine (Serpalan)-induced parkinsonism led to treatment of Parkinson's disease with levodopa (Larodopa), which is still the gold standard of antiparkinsonian medications. Although Parkinson reported the "senses and intellect being uninjured," subsequent descriptions recognized memory loss and other neuropsychiatric features. Until effective treatment with levodopa became available in the 1960s, profound akinesia and speech difficulties limited evaluation of the mental state in Parkinson's disease patients, and psychiatric disorders were often unrecognized.

Epidemiology Parkinsonian syndromes are frequently present in the elderly, and their prevalence increases with advancing age, affecting up to 15 percent of individuals up to 74 years of age and more than one-half of those older than 85 years. The most common parkinsonian syndrome is Parkinson's disease. It is the second most common neurodegenerative disease after Alzheimer's disease, and it affects more than 1 percent of the population older than 55 years and nearly 3 percent of the population older than 70 years. The mean age of onset for Parkinson's disease is 60 years, and 80 percent of individuals develop the disorder between the ages of 40 and 70 years. Approximately 5 percent of patients have symptom onset before 40 years of age, and, in such cases, the disease is classified as young-onset Parkinson's disease. Juvenile onset occurs in less than 1 percent of cases. The wide range in the age of onset of Parkinson's disease also contributes to its misdiagnosis, especially in younger patients.

Sex and ethnic differences in the frequency of Parkinson's disease are important sources of variation because of the association of Parkinson's disease with genetic and environmental factors. The prevalence is highest in Europe and North America, with lower rates in Asia and Africa. Men are affected slightly more often than women. In most studies, the incidence is lower among blacks than whites. These discrepant rates may be due to socioeconomic factors such as access to health care and perception of the disease.

Etiology The primary pathology in Parkinson's disease is loss of dopaminergic neurons in the ventral tier of the SNpc (Fig. 2.6–1A), but what leads to this selective and progressive cell death is unknown. Most cases of Parkinson's disease are sporadic and believed to be caused by exogenous environmental factors or their interactions with genetic vulnerability factors. A number of risk factors have been proposed, but the only unequivocal risk factor for Parkinson's disease is increasing age. Dopaminergic cell loss also occurs with normal aging, although the loss is less severe and involves different subpopulations of SNpc neurons than Parkinson's disease. Proposed pathogenic mechanisms in Parkinson's disease include free radical–mediated oxidative injury, mitochondrial abnormalities, perturbations of the neuronal cytoskeleton/axonal transport, excitotoxicity, calcium-induced injury, and programmed cell death. Toxins associated with parkinsonism include viral infection of the CNS and industrial exposures, including manganese, carbon monoxide, organophosphates, and 1-methyl-4-phenyl-1,2,3,6-tetrahydropyridine (MPTP). Higher prevalence rates in industrialized regions and associations with well water consumption, farming, and rural living may reflect exposure to neurotoxins contained in pesticides and other agricultural agents that contain homologs of MPTP. By contrast, other environmental factors or behaviors, such as caffeine use and cigarette smoking, are associated with a reduced risk to develop Parkinson's disease.

Familial forms of Parkinson's disease are less common, but several causative genes have been identified in affected families with early-onset Parkinson's disease. Mutations in the α-synuclein gene, located on chromosome 4q21-q23, are associated with autosomal dominant Parkinson's disease. Mutations in a gene on chromosome 6 that codes for parkin, a protein involved in the ubiquitination pathway, are the most common inherited defects and are particularly associated with a juvenile autosomal recessive form of early-onset Parkinson's disease. Gene loci on chromosome 4 that affect ubiquitin processing are also linked to Parkinson's disease. Because patients with sporadic Parkinson's disease who have normal α-synuclein genes have Lewy bodies that stain positive for α-synuclein and ubiquitin, it is possible that neuronal cell death in Parkinson's disease is related to abnormal accumulations of these proteins. Family and twin studies suggest presence of genetic risk factors for idiopathic Parkinson's disease, with greater heritability for younger onset cases.

Contemporary models of basal ganglia/cortical physiology suggest the presence of five adjacent but anatomically distinct frontocortico-striato-thalamic loops with motor, oculomotor, limbic, anterior cingulate, and prefrontal targets and that dysfunction of these neural loops is linked to the motor and nonmotor features in Parkinson's disease and other basal ganglia disorders. A common feature of these cortical-subcortical loops is their projection from higher-level cortical areas to the basal ganglia via striatal areas with outflow through the internal globus pallidum (Gpi) or its histological analog, the substantia nigra pars reticulata (SNpr) (Fig. 2.6–2). Gpi/SNpr outputs then project to specific areas of the thalamus that complete the loops through projections to the original cortical area. Within each loop, the striatonigral component includes a "direct" pathway that projects directly from striatum to Gpi/SNpr and an "indirect" pathway that flows from the striatum through the subthalamic nucleus (STN) to reach Gpi/SNpr.

Motor Manifestations Human and animal models of Parkinson's disease demonstrate that loss of SNpc dopaminergic neurons affects frontocortico-striato-thalamic circuits sufficiently to result in the motor manifestations of Parkinson's disease. The best studied of these neuronal circuits is the "motor circuit," as illustrated in Figure 2.6–2. In Parkinson's disease, dopaminergic degeneration appears to have differential effects on the nigrostriatal pathway. Projections from SNpc to striatal targets are inhibitory in the dopamine

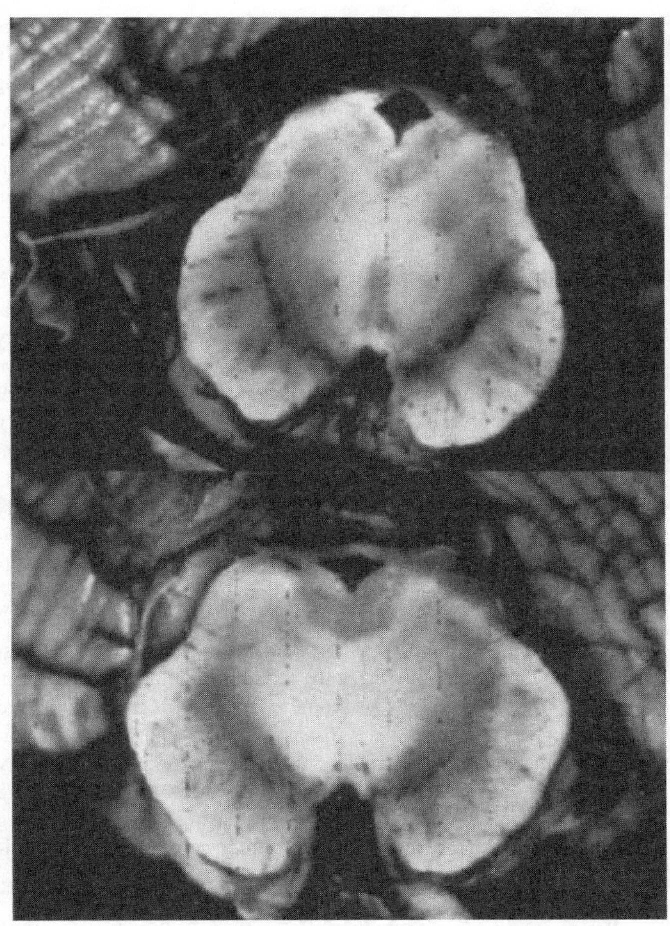

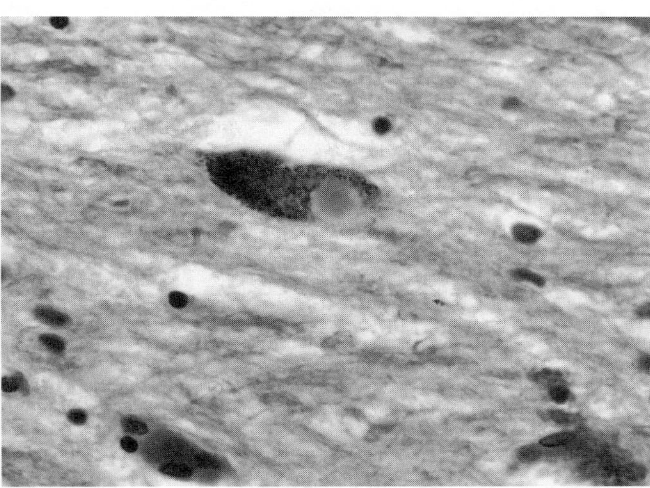

FIGURE 2.6–1 Parkinson's disease neuropathology. **A:** Gross pathology in cross section of the midbrain. Note pallor and depigmentation of the substantia nigra in Parkinson's disease (*bottom*), compared with control (*top*) brain. **B:** Lewy body in a pigmented neuron of the substantia nigra. Lewy bodies are cytoplasmic inclusions with a dense eosinophilic core surrounded by a clear halo. (See Color Plate.) (Photographs courtesy of The Morris K. Udall Parkinson's Disease Research Center and the Alzheimer's Disease Research Center at Johns Hopkins and Drs. Olga Pletnikova and Juan Troncoso.)

type 1 (D_1) receptor–mediated direct path and excitatory in the dopamine type 2 (D_2) receptor–mediated indirect path. Normal movement results from coordinated regulation of thalamocortical excitation by the direct and indirect pathways, with the presence of nigrostriatal dopaminergic projections tending toward increased movement by facilitation of the direct pathway and inhibition of the indirect pathway. Loss of dopamine results in hypokinetic symptoms secondary to overactivity of the STN and Gpi via the indirect path, which increases inhibitory input to the thalamus and then reduces the excitatory thalamocortical activity that ordinarily facilitates motor movements. Hyperkinetic movements, such as levodopa-induced dyskinesias, occur with overactivation of the direct pathway.

Cognitive Manifestations Dementia in Parkinson's disease is associated with increasing age, a family history of dementia, depression, and more severe motor dysfunction. Neuropathological and imaging studies in Parkinson's disease patients with dementia are associated with neuronal loss in cholinergic cells of the basal forebrain, suggesting a role for cholinergic deficits in Parkinson's disease–related cognitive impairment. Cortical Lewy bodies may also be associated with dementia. The histopathological changes of Alzheimer's disease—neurofibrillary tangles and senile plaques—are seen in some patients with Parkinson's disease and dementia. Other cognitive impairments, in which higher-order associative functions are preserved, may involve dysfunction of nonmotor neural circuits, including mesocortical and mesolimbic dopaminergic projections. Bradyphrenia may be associated with noradrenergic cell loss.

Psychiatric Manifestations Other than Parkinson's disease itself, there are no known specific risk factors for psychiatric disturbances in Parkinson's disease. Although psychological reactions influence occurrence of depression, most evidence suggests that depressive disorders are intrinsic to the disease processes of Parkinson's disease. In particular, development of depressive and anxiety disorders before motor symptoms suggests that these mood symptoms are either neurological signs of the disease or a risk or causative factor for development of Parkinson's disease. Cross-sectional studies do not show consistent relationships between the age onset or severity of depression to the age onset, severity, duration, or subtype (tremor dominant versus akinetic rigid) of Parkinson's disease. Several studies link depression with excessive serotonergic loss from the midbrain raphe. Depression in Parkinson's disease is also associated with decreased blood flow in frontal regions, a finding also seen in idiopathic depression. In apathetic syndromes, a role for noradrenergic dysfunction is suggested by a relationship between bradyphrenia and neuronal loss in the locus ceruleus. Several studies implicate noradrenergic dysfunction in anxiety disorders, including an imbalance in noradrenergic/dopaminergic tone. Psychosis in Parkinson's disease is most often associated with dopaminergic therapy, which may lead to hypersensitivity of mesocortical and mesolimbic dopaminergic receptors. Other factors related to the incidence of psychosis are cognitive impairment, disease severity, mood disorders, impaired visual acuity, other psychoactive medications, and delirium. The association of psychosis with cognitive impairment and mood disorders implicates more widespread brain pathology involving other neurotransmitter systems, including cholinergic deficits or a serotonergic/dopaminergic imbalance.

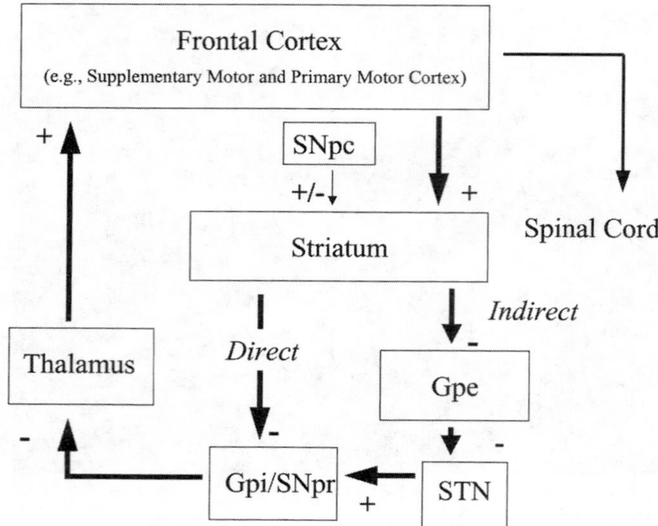

FIGURE 2.6–2 Cortico-striatal-thalamic circuits. In the motor circuit, the supplementary motor area and primary motor cortices in frontal regions project mainly to putamen and then "directly" to the internal globus pallidum (Gpi) or "indirectly" via the external globus pallidus (Gpe) and then the subthalamic nucleus (STN) to reach Gpi. Excitatory (glutamatergic) cortical projections generally decrease Gpi activity through the direct pathway and increase Gpi activity through the indirect pathway. Inhibitory (γ-aminobutyric acid–ergic) Gpi projections to thalamus and excitatory thalamocortical projections result in net excitation (increased motor activity) or net inhibition (decreased movement) through the direct and indirect pathways, respectively. Dopamine has differential inhibitory and excitatory effects on the nigrostriatal pathway. SNpc, substantia nigra pars compacta; SNpr, substantia nigra pars reticulata.

Diagnosis and Clinical Features

Motor Manifestations Motor symptoms initially affect one-half of the body and gradually progress to the contralateral side but remain asymmetric. The slow (3- to 6-Hz) classic resting tremor is often the presenting feature of Parkinson's disease, but other types of tremor may be present, and 20 to 30 percent of cases have no tremor at all. Bradykinesia and akinesia are the most disabling aspects of Parkinson's disease and contribute to problems with dexterity and gait. Patients typically walk in a flexed forward posture without swinging their arms. The gait is slow and shuffling, with small steps and a tendency to fall forward and hasten the rate of walking (festination). Difficulty initiating movements leads to start hesitation and "freezing." For example, a patient may suddenly be unable to move his or her legs while walking or move his or her hands when reaching into a pocket. Deteriorated handwriting, weakness, and clumsiness in one limb are also common initial symptoms of bradykinesia. Rigidity is appreciated as increased muscle tone on examination. Patients often note muscle cramps, weakness, or stiffness as the first indication of rigidity.

The diagnosis of Parkinson's disease is clinically based because there is no biological marker for the disease. Most experts require the presence of two of the three cardinal motor signs to diagnose the disease along with a robust response to an initial trial of levodopa. Early in its course, Parkinson's disease can be difficult to diagnose because the signs of the disease may be subtle and not even perceived by the patient. Parkinsonian signs can also be a feature of normal aging. The initial symptoms in up to 20 percent of patients are nonmotor, including fatigue, musculoskeletal complaints, and depression. Other nonmotor somatic symptoms include sialorrhea, dysarthria, visual and genitourinary dysfunction, sleep disturbances, sweating, seborrhea, edema, constipation, paresthesias, and a decreased sense of smell. In many patients, there is clear evidence for a prodromal phase, lasting approximately 4 to 8 years before the onset of obvious motor signs and often characterized by depression, anxiety, and musculoskeletal discomfort. Heightened vigilance for signs of Parkinson's disease during this phase might result in earlier disease detection, especially in older adult patients who present with depression.

Cognitive Manifestations Some degree of cognitive impairment, ranging from mild executive dysfunction to dementia, affects nearly all patients with Parkinson's disease; approximately 25 to 40 percent of patients develop dementia. Commonly, cognitive decline is not obvious clinically, and scores on tests that screen for dementia, such as the Mini-Mental State Examination (MMSE), remain in the "normal" or nondemented range for some patients who nonetheless have dementia. The concept of "subcortical dementia" has been used to describe the cognitive impairment that is frequently associated with the various movement disorders characterized primarily by subcortical neuropathology. Executive dysfunction is especially common, resulting from deficits that affect the ability to process new information and anticipate, plan, initiate, maintain, and change behaviors. Memory, visuospatial skills, information processing speed, attention, explicit recall, spatial planning, perseveration, verbal fluency, and poverty of thought are also affected. Compared with patients with Alzheimer's disease, recognition memory, aphasia, agnosia, apraxia, and higher language functions are relatively spared. There are patients with Parkinson's disease, however, who demonstrate wider involvement of cortical functions, including aphasia, apraxia, and memory deficits, and, in some cases, the cognitive presentation is indistinguishable from Alzheimer's disease.

Psychiatric Manifestations Psychiatric disturbances affect up to 90 percent of patients at some point during the course of Parkinson's disease, and more than one psychiatric disturbance is often present. Early in the disease process, adult-onset anxiety and depressive disorders precede the obvious onset of motor symptoms in up to 30 percent of patients.

DEPRESSION Normal psychological reactions to the illness can result in low mood, grief, demoralization, frustration, and embarrassment. Depressive disorders in Parkinson's disease involve more pervasive mood changes and generally resemble idiopathic forms of depression. Reported prevalence rates range from 20 to 90 percent, with an average reported frequency of 40 to 50 percent. Up to one-half of those with depression, in most studies, have major depression. The majority of Parkinson's disease patients with depression have nonmajor depressive syndromes that are variably referred to as *minor depression, dysthymia*, or *subsyndromal depression*. Nonmajor forms of depression often progress to major depression if untreated. Anxiety symptoms and comorbid anxiety syndromes, such as panic disorder, are especially prominent, but self-blame, guilt, delusions, a negative self-attitude, self-destructive thoughts, a sense of failure, and anhedonia may be less evident. Suicide can occur but at a similar rate as for the general population. Other psychological, vegetative, and autonomic features of depression are also common, but early-morning awakening, anergia, and retardation occur at comparable rates in nondepressed Parkinson's disease patients. Depression is generally not associated with a family history of mood disorders.

APATHY Apathy occurs in at least 25 percent of patients and often coexists with depression. It is manifest as indifference and a lack of motivation, initiative, perseverance, interest in new things, or concern for one's health. In most cases, apathy is not distressing to the patient, but the absence of spontaneous effort and interest can be frustrating for caregivers who may perceive the patient as depressed. Inactivity, deconditioning, and fatigue contribute to further loss of function and increased disability and suffering. Other neurological signs and symptoms, such as akinesia, hypomimia, hypophonia, cognitive dysfunction, and bradyphrenia, can confound recognition of apathy. Selective serotonin reuptake inhibitors (SSRIs), the most frequently prescribed antidepressants for Parkinson's disease patients, can also cause apathy, although this has not been demonstrated in Parkinson's disease specifically.

ANXIETY Difficulties initiating movements can frequently lead to anxiety-provoking circumstances in the course of living with Parkinson's disease, but pathological anxiety is still more common compared with other parkinsonian syndromes. Particularly common are generalized anxiety disorder, social phobia, and panic disorder, which has a prevalence rate of 25 percent in some series. In general, the anxiety syndromes in Parkinson's disease resemble those in idiopathic conditions and frequently cooccur with depression. Anxiety can also be associated with fluctuations in levodopa levels and motor function, although there is not always a strict temporal relationship between anxiety and motor "off" states. Some patients describe episodic panic attack–like states that develop at the same time every day and can be associated with motor deficits. Sleep difficulties are very common and seem to aggravate daytime anxiety.

PSYCHOSIS Psychosis affects approximately 25 percent of patients. "Benign" visual hallucinations are the most common psychotic symptom in Parkinson's disease and are related to dopaminergic medications. They typically include well-delineated animals or people who occur in a clear sensorium and with retained insight. They are rarely distressing. Auditory and tactile hallucinations also occur. Next, occurring later in the disease in some patients, are persistent hallucinations or delusions in a clear sensorium but with diminished insight. Aggression, delusional jealousy, and other paranoid accusations (delusional fears about eating or medications, inappropriate sexual behaviors, and confusion) are frequent manifestations that can be difficult to manage and may require hospitalization. Some patients develop chronic paranoid syndromes that resemble schizophrenia. Hallucinations and delusions also occur with major depression, mania, or anxiety disorders and may be overlooked when patients are especially agitated. Fragmented sleep, vivid dreams, and nightmares may herald the onset of chronic psychosis. Hallucinations and delusions associated with advanced Parkinson's disease are a major reason for nursing home placement. A third category includes hallucinations or delusions in the context of delirium related to antiparkinsonian medications or other causes.

PREMORBID PERSONALITY There is controversy over whether certain premorbid personality characteristics prevail in patients with Parkinson's disease. Many observers have noted premorbid personality features that include industriousness, cautiousness, perfectionism, and punctuality in individuals who ultimately develop Parkinson's disease and persistence of these traits over the course of the illness. One argument is that these traits represent a consequence of premorbid reductions in dopaminergic tone.

OTHER DISTURBANCES Disinhibited behaviors are relatively uncommon but often lead to psychiatric referral. Hypersexuality is seen in 2 to 6 percent of Parkinson's disease patients and is usually related to antiparkinsonian therapy. Usually, this presents as an increase from baseline sexual activity, but elevated mood, compulsive behaviors, and paraphilias can occur. Mania or euphoric syndromes are generally related to dopaminergic medications and are often associated with mood swings and on–off phenomena but can reflect a premorbid disorder. Pathological gambling and other disinhibited behaviors are also reported. *Emotionalism* refers to heightened and excessive sentimentality, often with pathological tearfulness (emotional incontinence) that can be precipitated by a variety of emotions; it can be a feature of a depressive disorder.

Pathology and Laboratory Examination

Unlike other common neurodegenerative disorders, there are no accepted neuropathological criteria for Parkinson's disease. Most neuropathologists agree that dopaminergic neuronal loss in the SNpc is a requisite finding. However, the pathological process precedes the clinical presentation because classic motor signs of Parkinson's disease are not evident until there is a 70 to 80 percent loss of nigral neurons. In addition to dopaminergic cell loss, Lewy bodies, which are intraneuronal aggregates of the protein α-synuclein, are present in most forms of Parkinson's disease (Fig. 2.6–1B) and are seen in the substantia nigra, locus ceruleus, dorsal vagal nucleus, and nucleus basalis of Meynert. Lewy bodies are not specific to Parkinson's disease and are seen in a variety of conditions, including Alzheimer's disease. Parkinson's disease is also accompanied by degeneration of noradrenergic neurons in the locus ceruleus, serotonergic neurons in the dorsal raphe, and cholinergic neurons in the nucleus basalis and their attendant projection systems. Alzheimer-type neuropathological changes (e.g., senile plaques and neurofibrillary tangles) are present in some patients with Parkinson's disease and dementia. Differential degrees of pathology among affected neuronal systems are believed to underlie the heterogeneous motor, cognitive, and psychiatric features of Parkinson's disease.

It is important to rule out other causes of parkinsonism. Laboratory tests should be conducted to rule out Wilson's disease and hypothyroidism. Neuropsychological testing can help to clarify the extent of cognitive deficits, evaluate cognitive status in potential candidates for neurosurgical treatments, or establish alternative diagnoses. Dementia, in particular, is an exclusionary criterion for surgical therapies because it is associated with a poor motor outcome but also limits compliance. An atypical cognitive profile for Parkinson's disease also predicts a poor outcome. Structural neuroimaging studies may help exclude other diagnoses, such as vascular disease, normal pressure hydrocephalus, and other parkinsonian conditions, but are generally indicated for classic Parkinson's disease. With functional imaging, decreased dopaminergic uptake in the putamen is characteristic of Parkinson's disease, and subclinical dopaminergic changes are evident in some at-risk relatives in kindreds with familial Parkinson's disease. Single photon emission tomography (SPECT) and positron emission tomography (PET) can be helpful for diagnosing Parkinson's disease in unclear cases with atypical signs and a poor response to levodopa and for assessing presynaptic dopaminergic integrity as a marker of disease progression.

Differential Diagnosis

Several clinical features help distinguish Parkinson's disease from other parkinsonian disorders. Parkinson's disease progresses more slowly, postural instability is a later finding, and there is an excellent and sustained response to levodopa. Alternative diagnoses, such as progressive supranuclear palsy or multiple system atrophy, are suggested by rapid progression with development of postural instability and early falls (within 3 years), a poor or transient response to levodopa, orthostatic hypotension, and other signs of autonomic dysfunction, early dysphagia, and supranuclear gaze palsy. Early hallucinations unrelated to treatment and early dementia suggest dementia with Lewy bodies or Alzheimer's disease with associated Parkinson's disease. Myoclonic jerks, pyramidal signs (e.g., Babinski sign), and cerebellar signs (e.g., wide-based gait) are not features of Parkinson's disease but are seen in other parkinsonian disorders. Other non–Parkinson's disease–associated findings include alien limb syndrome or ideomotor apraxia.

It is always important to consider alternative diagnoses to depression. Apathetic syndromes, dementia, or delirium can all cause changes in mood that are usually more apparent to families than the patient. The differential diagnosis of depression in Parkinson's disease also includes bipolar disorder, adjustment disorders, anxiety syndromes, psychosis, pathological tearfulness (emotional incontinence), substance abuse or dependence, mood lability associated with parkinsonian motor fluctuations, and increased medical debility. Independent of a depressive disorder, sleep disturbances and daytime fatigue in Parkinson's disease can impair function and lead patients to feel discouraged. Parkinson's disease–related depression is also frequently associated with anxiety disorders (e.g., panic disorder) and dementia. The somatic and autonomic symptoms of anxiety can overlap with features of other medical conditions. Psychosis in the early stages of Parkinson's disease suggests alternative diagnoses such as dementia with Lewy bodies or Alzheimer's disease with extrapyramidal features. In some cases, preexisting psychopathology emerges with dopaminergic treatment.

Course and Prognosis

Parkinson's disease is clinically heterogeneous. In each case, there is a different clinical presentation, age onset, natural history, and response to levodopa. Many cases of Parkinson's disease can be subdivided into either a tremor-predominant form or one characterized by prominent gait disorder and postural instability, the former having a more benign prognosis. Heterogeneity in clinical onset, progression, and levodopa response also influences the natural history of Parkinson's disease. This includes the onset of motor fluctuations and other treatment-related complications, longevity, and functional impairment. The rate and course of cognitive deterioration is also highly variable, ranging from mild to severe. Successful treatment of depression improves motor status, but medical treatment of motor symptoms does not usually improve depressive syndromes. Even in the absence of depression, antidepressant medications and ECT have been shown to improve motor function. As in the general population, anxiety disorders often coexist with depressive episodes, but anxiety disorders tend to be chronic. The need for nursing home placement, often triggered by psychosis, is associated with a higher mortality rate.

Treatment

Motor Symptoms

PHARMACOLOGICAL TREATMENTS Current treatment options for Parkinson's disease provide only symptomatic relief of the motor deficits, as there are no known preventative or regenerative strategies. The gold standard of treatment is levodopa, which increases the life expectancy among patients and significantly improves function and quality of life. During early stages, anticholinergic medications, such as trihexyphenidyl (Artane) or benztropine (Cogentin), amantadine (Symmetrel), and selegiline (Eldepryl), provide mild to moderate reductions in motor symptoms. Dopamine agonists, such as pramipexole (Mirapex), ropinirole (Requip), and pergolide (Permax), or levodopa may then be added to address progressive disability. Dopamine agonists are especially effective early treatments that can delay initiation of levodopa therapy. Postural instability does not usually respond to antiparkinsonian medications.

There is debate over when to begin levodopa therapy because it is associated with dose-limiting motor side effects (in addition to psychosis). Initially, there is tremendous improvement in motor function, but higher doses of levodopa are gradually required to achieve similar benefit, and the duration of the motor response wanes. Fluctuating motor effects then replace sustained motor benefits, with improved motor function in response to medications (the "on" state) and reduced mobility when medication effects subside (the "off" state). Patients also develop abnormal involuntary hyperkinetic choreiform or dystonic movements during the "on" state, referred to as *drug-induced dyskinesias*. Relatively newer agents that inhibit dopamine metabolism via catechol-*O*-methyltransferase inhibition, such as tolcapone (Tasmar) and entacapone (Comtan), can reduce motor fluctuations.

PSYCHIATRIC DISTURBANCES RELATED TO FLUCTUATING EFFECTS OF DOPAMINERGIC THERAPY Emotional influences can trigger or intensify motor fluctuations, and drug-induced dyskinesias themselves can be distressing or embarrassing. In the extreme, "on-off" fluctuations range from states of complete immobility or "freezing" to severe writhing. Fluctuating motor states may be accompanied by nonmotor phenomena, including akathisia, anxiety, dysphoria, autonomic symptoms, irritability, apathy, hallucinosis, psychosis, screaming, and cognitive slowing during "off" periods; hypersexuality, hypomania, and thought racing may occur during "on" periods.

Surgical Treatments

Before the availability of levodopa in the 1960s, neurosurgical procedures were standard treatments for tremor and rigidity in Parkinson's disease. More refined stereotactic neurosurgical therapies currently used for Parkinson's disease involve high-frequency deep brain stimulation (DBS) of the STN and Gpi or ablative procedures that target the Gpi (pallidotomy) or thalamus (thalamotomy). Both improve motor function because they reduce the hyperactivity of the STN and its efferent targets, thus partially restoring thalamic outflow. Thalamotomy and thalamic DBS are indicated for disabling tremor. STN, DBS, and pallidal interventions also improve tremor but are mainly indicated for severe dyskinesias, bradykinesia/akinesia, and rigidity. The procedures are aimed at alleviation of contralateral symptoms, but bilateral benefits are seen for dyskinesias and bradykinesia. Embryonic cell transplantation of dopamine neurons, first performed in the 1980s, remains an experimental procedure.

NEUROPSYCHIATRIC EFFECTS OF NEUROSURGICAL THERAPY FOR PARKINSON'S DISEASE Initial studies showed limited, if any, adverse cognitive effects after ablative or DBS procedures when surgical candidates underwent careful screening for dementia. Some pallidotomy studies found changes in executive function, memory, verbal fluency, and attentional set shifting, but lesion size may have been influential. Stimulation parameters, laterality and site-specific effects, electrode placement, and stimulation sites may also affect cognitive outcomes.

Although many patients report improved quality of life after surgery, acute stimulation with DBS can be associated with profound depressive or manic symptoms, including in patients with no prior psychiatric history. In some patients, preexisting disorders, such as depression, anxiety, or drug dependence, and interpersonal conflicts can worsen and overshadow any motoric benefits. DBS treatment-emergent sexually deviant behaviors, gambling, mood lability, apathy, and aggression are also described. Reductions in anxiety and depression, unrelated to improved motor status, are reported after unilateral pallidotomy, but bilateral pallidotomy can result in depression and apathy. Studies of pallidotomy show no consistent effects on depression or anxiety, but a history of a prior or active affective disturbance at the time of surgery may be associated with development of a mood disorder.

Cognitive Manifestations There are no standard treatments for cognitive deficits in Parkinson's disease. Evidence for cholinergic deficits in Parkinson's disease and their relationship to dementia suggests a role for cholinesterase inhibitors. A few small clinical trials showed cognitive benefits with donepezil and tacrine, although cholinesterase inhibitors cause confusion and aggravate motor symptoms in some patients. Patients and families benefit from education about cognitive deficits in Parkinson's disease, especially their consequences on executive functioning and strategies for minimizing distress related to selective cognitive impairments, and, later in the course, dementia.

Psychiatric Manifestations A first step in the treatment of psychiatric disorders is to evaluate the contribution of the antiparkinsonian medications, fluctuating medication effects, other medical conditions, cognitive deficits, and caregiver and other psychosocial variables to the presenting problem. The common occurrence of more than one psychiatric disturbance also influences treatment. Sleep is commonly disrupted in Parkinson's disease, independent of psychiatric problems, and addressing it alone can reduce daytime mood lability, psychosis, and motor impairments. Initial treatment involves consideration of the antiparkinsonian regimen, sleep hygiene practices, and use of a low-dose sedating antidepressant or hypnotic such as trazodone (Desyrel) (e.g., 25 to 100 mg). Benzodiazepines can be used judiciously but are not considered first-line therapy for anxiety, agitation, or sleep disturbances because of effects on cognition, falls, and interdose withdrawal symptoms. Patient and caregiver education, especially about the psychiatric condition and its overlap with parkinsonian features, and supportive therapy are cornerstones of effective treatment. Parkinson's support groups can be invaluable sources of education and community support. Ancillary treatment by speech, physical, and occupational therapists can help patients to maximize function, even early in the disease and periodically as the disease progresses and new impairments emerge. Regular exercise helps motor symptoms and overall well-being.

DEPRESSION Despite the prevalence and seriousness of affective disorders in Parkinson's disease, research on their treatment is limited, and controlled trials are still needed to provide guidelines. Published controlled trials on antidepressant treatment in Parkinson's disease are of poor quality but show efficacy with imipramine (Tofranil), nortriptyline (Aventyl, Pamelor), desipramine (Norpramin), and bupropion (Wellbutrin). No trials have been conducted using the newer antidepressants available since 1990. Several open-label studies and case reports suggest that SSRIs improve depressive symptoms in both major and nonmajor depressive syndromes. As with primary depression, antidepressant selection is usually based on consideration of side effect profiles. SSRIs can aggravate motor symptoms, but this is not especially common. Use of selegiline with antidepressants carries the risk of inducing a serotonin syndrome or hypertensive reactions, but most patients tolerate this combination. ECT is safe and effective for depression in Parkinson's disease.

ANXIETY Treatment of Parkinson's disease–related anxiety has not been studied in clinical trials. As with idiopathic anxiety, antidepressants are often effective. Buspirone (BuSpar), a nonbenzodiazepine anxiolytic, has been used in Parkinson's disease, but its specific effects on anxiety are not obvious. There is recent use of gabapentin for anxiety disorders, but its use in Parkinson's disease has not been examined. The usefulness of antipsychotic medications as adjunctive therapy is also not known.

APATHY There have been no studies on the treatment of apathy in Parkinson's disease. Treatment of comorbid depression is an obvious initial approach, but there may be residual or SSRI-induced apathy. Antidepressants that inhibit dopamine or norepinephrine reuptake are suggested by neurochemical theories of apathy. If depression is not an issue, dopaminergic agents, including levodopa, dopamine receptor agonists, selegiline, amphetamines, and amantadine, have been most consistently effective; the absence of cognitive dysfunction predicts a better response. In Alzheimer's disease, cholinesterase inhibitors reduce apathy and may similarly benefit Parkinson's disease patients.

PSYCHOSIS Treatment of psychosis in Parkinson's disease is challenged by the delicate balancing act between the use of medications that relieve psychosis without aggravating motor or cognitive dysfunction and the treatment of motor symptoms without exacerbating the mental status. Caregiver safety is also an issue because of immobility, directed aggression, and combativeness during care. Reducing or simplifying the antiparkinsonian regimen usually involves elimination of anticholinergics, amantadine, and selegiline because levodopa is generally preferred to dopamine agonists and controlled-release levodopa when there is psychosis. When higher doses of levodopa are required or disruptive symptoms persist, treatment usually requires addition of an atypical antipsychotic. In contrast to the other psychiatric disturbances in Parkinson's disease, there are evidence-based data on treatment of psychosis in Parkinson's disease. The gold standard is clozapine (Clozaril); it is effective even at low doses (less than 25 mg), does not block D_2 receptors, and has been evaluated in several controlled trials. Because of the requisite blood monitoring with clozapine, quetiapine (Seroquel) is usually the initial drug of choice, but some patients eventually experience worsened motor function, and patients with dementia may be especially vulnerable. Anecdotally, aripiprazole (Abilify), available more recently, has had favorable antipsychotic effects in some patients without increasing motor deficits. In other patients, it has not been tolerated or had no effect. Orthostatic hypotension, headache, and nausea also contribute to intolerance. Other "atypical" neuroleptic agents (olanzapine [Zyprexa] and risperidone [Risperdal]) reduce or eliminate psychosis at low doses, but their effects on striatal D_2 receptors are frequently associated with significant motor deterioration. ECT can be used to treat psychotic depression as well as dopamine-induced psychosis. Cholinergic agents can also have antipsychotic effects.

Other Parkinsonian Conditions

Progressive Supranuclear Palsy

EPIDEMIOLOGY AND ETIOLOGY Progressive supranuclear palsy, an important cause of parkinsonism, was first described in 1964. The prevalence is 5 to 6 cases per 100,000, and progressive supranuclear palsy accounts for 4 percent of all cases with parkinsonism. Onset of symptoms is usually after 60 years of age in all races and both genders, but men tend to be affected more often than women. There are rare familial cases of progressive supranuclear palsy, but its development is usually sporadic. Progressive supranuclear palsy is classified as a *tauopathy*, a term referring to neurodegenerative disorders characterized by intracellular aggregations of abnormally phosphorylated tau protein. Tau normally stabilizes microtubules, and its aggregation leads to formation of abnormal cytoskeletal fibrils. The cause of the tauopathy in progressive supranuclear palsy, and its role in neurodegeneration, remains uncertain.

CLINICAL FEATURES The defining motor features of progressive supranuclear palsy are progressive parkinsonism with symmetric bradykinesia, axial rigidity, and paralysis of downward vertical gaze. The problems with ocular motility may not be evident for several years but cause problems with walking down stairs. Dysphagia develops over the course of the illness. Unlike Parkinson's disease, postural instability leading to falls and dysarthria are early and often presenting features. Also, there is a poor response to levodopa, tremor is uncommon, and stride length is erratic. Posture tends to be upright or sometimes opisthotonic because of axial rigidity. Instead of a lack of facial expression (hypomimia), patients appear "worried" or "astonished," resulting from dystonic contractions of facial muscles between the eyebrows, reduced blinking, lid retraction, and gaze palsy.

Cognitively, patients show features of a subcortical dementia with bradyphrenia, memory deficits, and predominant frontal lobe dysfunction with executive and attentional deficits. Aphasia, apraxia, and agnosia, the classic features of "cortical dementias," are not evident. Apathy and disinhibition, compatible with damage to orbitofrontal and medial frontal circuits, are the most common psychiatric features. There are also sleep disturbances; depression; emotional lability, including pathological laughter and crying (emotional incontinence); irritability; and, occasionally, schizophreniform psychotic symptoms.

PATHOLOGY AND LABORATORY EXAMINATION Neuropathologically, there is broader involvement of the basal ganglia in progressive supranuclear palsy than in Parkinson's disease. Progressive supranuclear palsy affects the substantia nigra as well as the striatum, thalamus, subthalamus, other brainstem nuclei, and periaqueductal gray matter. The main pathological findings are high-density, tau-positive neurofibrillary tangles; neuronal loss; and gliosis. There is pronounced dopamine depletion in the striatum, decreased density of striatal D_2 receptors, widespread cholinergic neuronal damage, and effects on serotonergic and γ-aminobutyric acid (GABA)–ergic systems. Structural imaging studies initially reveal midbrain atrophy followed by third ventricular enlargement and pontine and frontotemporal atrophy. PET studies show decreased striatal dopamine binding and fluorodopa uptake and frontal and temporal hypometabolism.

DIFFERENTIAL DIAGNOSIS After Parkinson's disease, which is at least ten times more prevalent, progressive supranuclear palsy is the second most common parkinsonian syndrome. Frontotemporal dementia and corticobasal ganglionic degeneration manifest similar clinical and pathological features, including parkinsonism, frontal executive impairments, apathy, and tau-positive inclusions. Although apathy is the predominant psychiatric feature, it is often mistaken for depression, which occurs with apathy in a minority of cases.

COURSE AND PROGNOSIS Progressive supranuclear palsy is a rapidly progressive and devastating degenerative disease. Life expectancy is generally 5 to 7 years after onset, with death often related to dysphagia.

TREATMENT There are no specific treatments for the motor or cognitive aspects of Parkinson's disease. Levodopa is ineffective, probably because of the reduced number of postsynaptic striatal D_2 receptors. Despite extensive cholinergic damage, cholinergic-enhancing agents provide little or no benefit for cognition and can be poorly tolerated. The psychiatric symptoms can be difficult to treat but include standard targeted pharmacological and psychosocial approaches aimed at reducing apathy, irritability, agitation, mood lability, and so forth in neuropsychiatric populations.

Corticobasal Ganglionic Degeneration Originally termed *corticodentatonigral degeneration*, corticobasal ganglionic degeneration was first described in 1968 as a syndrome of involuntary movements and slowed voluntary movements. Corticobasal ganglionic degeneration is classified as a sporadic tauopathy and shares common clinical and pathological features with other tauopathies, including progressive supranuclear palsy and certain forms of frontotemporal dementia. Corticobasal ganglionic degeneration affects adults, with gradual onset usually after 40 years of age and steady progression until death within 2 to 12 years. Median survival is approximately 8 years. The pathological findings include ballooned achromatic neurons, frontoparietal atrophy, pronounced cortical neuronal loss, cortical astrocytic plaques, and tau inclusions in the substantia nigra, basal ganglia, and along dentatorubrothalamic tracts. Neuroimaging studies show asymmetric frontoparietal atrophy and subcortical hypometabolism contralateral to the more affected side along with bifrontal-parietal hypometabolism.

The clinical manifestations reflect both basal ganglia and cortical dysfunction. Motor signs almost invariably include asymmetric motor signs of parkinsonism (rigidity, bradykinesia/akinesia, and postural or action tremor). There is also postural instability, focal reflex myoclonus, and limb dystonia. Oculomotor motility may be impaired, similar to progressive supranuclear palsy. The most prominent neuropsychiatric features are lateralized ideomotor and ideational apraxia and the "alien hand syndrome." As with other subcortical motor disorders, there are multiple cognitive deficits, including predominant executive, memory, and attentional dysfunction, that may be severe enough to amount to dementia. Aphasia may also be present. Depression is much more common in corticobasal ganglionic degeneration relative to progressive supranuclear palsy, which is characterized by apathy. In corticobasal ganglionic degeneration, apathy, disinhibition, and delusions are also common and may co-occur but appear distinct from depression, suggesting different underlying mechanisms. There are no definitive treatments for the motor or cognitive symptoms in corticobasal ganglionic degeneration, but the parkinsonism may have a limited response to levodopa. Antidepressants are used for depression and anxiety but are not always effective. Caregiver education and assessment for depression are important aspects of patient care.

PRIMARY DEMENTIA SYNDROMES WITH PARKINSONIAN SIGNS

Frontotemporal Dementia Frontotemporal dementia is a clinical syndrome characterized by prominent behavioral or personality changes, language dysfunction, and neuronal loss, spongiosis, and gliosis in the frontal and temporal cortices. However, frontotemporal dementia is both pathologically and genetically heterogeneous, divided by the presence or absence of tau pathology and by the presence or absence of linkage, in familial cases, to chromosomes 17, 9, and 3. Most, but not all, cases linked to chromosome 17 have mutations in the gene encoding the cytoskeletal protein tau, and this form of frontotemporal dementia is now generally referred to as frontotemporal dementia *and parkinsonism linked to chromosome 17* (FTDP-17) because parkinsonian manifestations are common. Mutations in other familial forms of frontotemporal dementia have yet to be identified. Onset of frontotemporal dementia is usually after 50 years of age but ranges from 35 to 75 years of age. Life expectancy after diagnosis is 3 to 15 years.

Symptom onset is insidious, with behavioral and personality changes such as apathy, impulsive disinhibition (e.g., shoplifting or grabbing food off another person's plate), loss of personal awareness (e.g., neglect of personal grooming), stereotyped and perseverative behaviors, delusions, depression, affective lability, overeating and other signs of hyperorality, social inappropriateness, and lack of tact or empathy. A second variant presents with a progressive nonfluent aphasia and a third variant with a semantic dementia with receptive language impairments. Cognitive testing reveals profound impairment on tests of executive function but relative preservation of other cognitive domains, including memory. Motor deficits vary by frontotemporal dementia subtype and may include symptoms of motor neuron disease or parkinsonism, especially rigidity or akinesia. Structural imaging studies may show frontal and anterior temporal atrophy; functional imaging typically reveals hypoperfusion in the same regions, although there may be pronounced asymmetry. More widespread involvement of parietal regions is suggestive of Alzheimer's disease. The electroencephalogram (EEG) may be normal in early stages. The differential diagnosis in younger people includes schizophrenia, mood disorders, addictions, and personality disorders. When onset is later, the diagnosis is often confused with Alzheimer's disease, late-life depression, and, when there are prominent motor features, corticobasal ganglionic degeneration and progressive supranuclear palsy. These conditions resemble one another in their advanced stages but are distinguished by the course of the disease before the advanced stage. There are no treatments for the underlying disease process and no definitive evidence supporting the use of cholinergic treatments. The behavioral symptoms may improve with SSRIs. Aggressive behaviors can be managed with low doses of atypical antipsychotics or trazodone, and antiseizure medicines can reduce agitation and aggression. Family counseling is a critical part of treatment so that the safety of the patient and others is maintained in the setting of their poor judgment and to provide caregiver support and assist with psychosocial issues.

Dementia with Lewy Bodies

Dementia with Lewy bodies is a dementia syndrome with Lewy bodies in the cerebral cortex, brainstem, thalamus, and striatum. It is now regarded as the second most common form of dementia after Alzheimer's disease. Symptom onset is usually after 50 years of age, and the disease is more common in men. Average survival is less than 10 years. Both genetic and sporadic forms of dementia with Lewy bodies exist, and there is overlap in the clinical and pathological findings of dementia with Lewy bodies, Alzheimer's disease, Parkinson's disease, and other α-synucleinopathies. Approximately one-half of the patients with dementia with Lewy bodies also have Alzheimer's pathology. Up to one-third of cases show microvascular ischemic pathology. Neurochemically, there is evidence of a cholinergic deficit.

Although the defining feature of dementia with Lewy bodies is progressive cognitive impairment, its association with extrapyramidal signs and hallucinations leads to its inclusion in the differential diagnosis of parkinsonian movement disorders with psychiatric presentations. In the earlier stages, cognitive deficits often involve attentional, visuospatial, or frontal-subcortical skills, and memory impairment may only become apparent with progression. Cognition is often described as fluctuating with variations in attention and alertness, but a reliable definition of fluctuating cognition has been difficult to establish. With progression, there are the usual cortical features of dementia (aphasia, apraxia, and agnosia). The psychiatric symptoms present early in the course and often include dramatic visual hallucinations, depression, or paranoid delusions. Motor features include myoclonus and parkinsonian signs of bradykinesia, rigidity, and gait difficulties, with early falls in approximately two-thirds of patients. Resting tremor is uncommon. There may be an early but limited response to levodopa. As a general rule, the occurrence of psychosis unrelated to medications and early dementia with spontaneous parkinsonism, especially within the first year, should lead to consideration of dementia with Lewy bodies. The diagnosis of dementia with Lewy bodies remains clinically based and neuroimaging studies are not especially helpful in distinguishing dementia with Lewy bodies from Alzheimer's disease. Treatment of dementia with Lewy bodies requires a target approach. Motor symptoms can be treated with antiparkinsonian therapies, although this may aggravate the psychiatric symptoms, especially psychosis. Atypical neuroleptics can reduce psychosis but are often not tolerated, and cases of neuroleptic malignant syndrome are reported. The most promising treatments include cholinergic therapies, which can benefit cognitive and psychiatric symptoms. Antidepressants and stimulants can also be helpful.

Multiple System Atrophy

The term multiple system atrophy was introduced in 1969 and operationally defined in 1999 to describe a clinically heterogeneous neurodegenerative disorder with variably present parkinsonian, autonomic, cerebellar, and pyramidal manifestations. Multiple system atrophy is now used in place of three older diagnoses: olivopontocerebellar atrophy (OPCA), Shy-Drager syndrome, and striatonigral degeneration, which could not be reliably distinguished from one another. Two types of multiple system atrophy have been defined: autonomic dysfunction with predominant cerebellar findings (multiple system atrophy–cerebellar [multiple system atrophy–C]) and autonomic dysfunction with predominant parkinsonian findings (multiple system atrophy–P). The disease is rare and affects both sexes equally. It typically begins in late middle-age, with a median survival of approximately 9 to 10 years after symptom onset. The cause is unknown, but almost all cases are sporadic. The neuropathology consists of glial cytoplasmic inclusions (that contain tau, synuclein, and ubiquitin, among other proteins) in the presence of neurodegeneration in a variable combination of CNS structures, potentially including the putamen, caudate, globus pallidus, substantia nigra, inferior olives, brainstem nuclei, cerebellum, and spinal cord. Although magnetic resonance imaging (MRI) may reveal typical signs (hyperintense portions of the putamen, "hot-cross-bun" sign in the basis pontis), the diagnosis is essentially made clinically or neuropathologically.

Psychiatric and cognitive manifestations of multiple system atrophy have received little systematic attention. Sleep disorders and subcortical cognitive impairment appear to be common, personality change is probably frequent, and affective syndromes may be elevated beyond baseline. Treatment is symptomatic. Levodopa may improve parkinsonian features in some patients. Orthostatic hypotension and urinary symptoms may respond to both pharmacological agents and environmental manipulations, and such treatment may substantially improve patient and caregiver quality of life. There are no clear guidelines for treating psychiatric disorders; it is likely that strategies useful for Parkinson's disease, Huntington's disease, or cerebellar disease will also prove to be of value in multiple system atrophy. A small case series has demonstrated the usefulness and safety of ECT in patients with multiple system atrophy.

Encephalitis Lethargica Encephalitis lethargica, described by Constantin von Economo, presented as a worldwide epidemic between 1917 and 1929, but isolated cases have been reported in the last decade. It is important historically as an early example of the relationship between brain disease and psychopathology. The acute phase was characterized by profound lethargy, hence its name, along with other mental status changes, such as psychosis or catatonia, and various movement abnormalities, including parkinsonism, choreoathetosis, and myoclonus. The mortality rate was approximately 30 percent during the acute phase. Survivors returned to normal for several months to years, then many developed a chronic postencephalitic syndrome characterized most commonly by parkinsonism (usually without tremor) and less commonly by hyperkinetic movements resembling tardive dyskinesia and episodic oculogyric and respiratory crises. Psychiatric manifestations included disinhibition, mania, attentional deficits, apathy, narcolepsy, verbal tic-like behaviors, executive dysfunction, and bradyphrenia. Hyperactivity and oppositional behaviors developed in children. Postmortem studies of acute patients showed inflammatory changes in the substantia nigra, globus pallidus, and subthalamic, red, and brainstem nuclei. Postencephalitic cases showed degenerative changes and depigmentation of the same subcortical areas, with neurofibrillary tangles but without Lewy bodies. The etiology has never been determined.

HUNTINGTON'S DISEASE

Huntington's disease (formerly Huntington's chorea) is an autosomal dominant neurodegenerative disorder characterized by midlife onset, a relentlessly progressive course, and a combination of motor, psychiatric, and cognitive symptoms. The disease is caused by a CAG repeat expansion mutation in the huntingtin gene on chromosome 4. For 130 years, Huntington's disease has been recognized as one of the most terrible yet enlightening of all medical disorders, and now, as in the past, the approach to Huntington's disease provides a model for the development of clinical, scientific, and ethical strategies in other genetic diseases of the brain. Huntington's disease remains an important example of subcortical dementia and the prominence of the psychiatric consequences of neurodegenerative disorders.

History George Huntington first described the disease that now bears his name in 1872. His original paper, which noted the salient features that still define Huntington's disease, remains a model of clarity and clinical observation. After serving as the textbook case of dominant inheritance for 100 years, Huntington's disease again made news in 1983 as the first disorder mapped to a specific chromosomal locus using anonymous deoxyribonucleic acid (DNA) markers and then again in 1993 when the genetic etiology was discovered to be a member of a new class of mutations referred to as *repeat expansion* or *dynamic mutations*. Current research focuses on understanding Huntington's disease pathogenesis, and the use of this knowledge to develop rationale therapeutics for the underlying disease process.

Epidemiology The prevalence of Huntington's disease in the United States is approximately 5 cases per 100,000 individuals, with similar rates found in most European countries. The prevalence in Japan is approximately tenfold less, and prevalence also appears to be low in China, Finland, and Africa. As with many rare autosomal disorders, pockets of high prevalence exist. The most famous concentration is in the villages surrounding Lake Maracaibo in Venezuela; analysis of this population led to the discovery of the Huntington's disease mutation and has contributed greatly to the clinical understanding of Huntington's disease.

Etiology Huntington's disease is one of a group of eight neurodegenerative diseases caused by a mutation in which consecutive codons consisting of the nucleotides cytosine, adenine, and guanine (a so-called CAG repeat) increase in number. This is referred to as a *CAG trinucleotide repeat expansion mutation.* Because the codon CAG encodes for the amino acid glutamine, the result of the expansion is a protein with an excessively long stretch of glutamine residues. The CAG repeat expansion occurs in different and unrelated genes in each of the CAG repeat diseases. The only similarity among the genes is the repeat itself. This and other lines of evidence has led most investigators to conclude that proteins with stretches of more than approximately 35 to 40 consecutive glutamine residues become neurotoxins. The differences among the CAG repeat expansion diseases, particularly concerning which brain regions are most prominently affected and the precise threshold for toxicity, are believed to derive from other aspects of protein expression and structure.

The CAG repeat expansion in Huntington's disease is located in exon 1 of the huntingtin gene (formerly referred to as *IT15*) on the short arm of chromosome 4. Like the genes associated with other polyglutamine disorders, huntingtin is widely expressed and is not limited to the CNS. The normal function of huntingtin remains unknown, although it has been associated with vesicular transport and regulation of growth factors. Like many of the other repeat expansion diseases, the phenomenon of anticipation (younger age of onset in subsequent generations of a family) occurs in Huntington's disease. The explanation derives from a strong correlation between repeat length and younger age of onset and a tendency for repeat length to increase during paternal transmission of the gene (Fig. 2.6–3A,B).

The investigation into the pathway that leads from the CAG repeat expansion to clinical phenotype in Huntington's disease and related diseases is among the most exciting and fast-moving research endeavors in medicine. Proteins with expanded stretches of polyglutamine appear to take on an abnormal configuration, which results in the formation of polyglutamine aggregates that can be visualized with immunohistochemical stains in postmortem brain from Huntington's disease patients (Fig. 2.6–4A). Whether the toxicity is a direct result of the aggregates or results from intermediary structures formed during the process of aggregation remains to be determined. One proposal is that the long glutamine stretches sequester other proteins, including transcription factors. These proteins become unavailable to perform their normal cellular duties, with potentially lethal consequences. Alternatively, proteins with long polyglutamine expansions or aggregates of these proteins may interfere with function of the ubiquitin-dependent proteasome pathway, which normally functions to degrade aberrantly folded proteins. Failure of this system might lead to an accumulation of a variety of toxic proteins. It has also been proposed that polyglutamine expansions interfere with mitochondrial energy metabolism.

Diagnosis and Clinical Features Typically, the diagnosis of Huntington's disease is made by a genetic test in the setting of motor signs and symptoms in an individual with a family history of Huntington's disease. The advent of genetic testing now makes diagnosis possible in presymptomatic patients or those with unusual presentations or no known family history of a movement disorder.

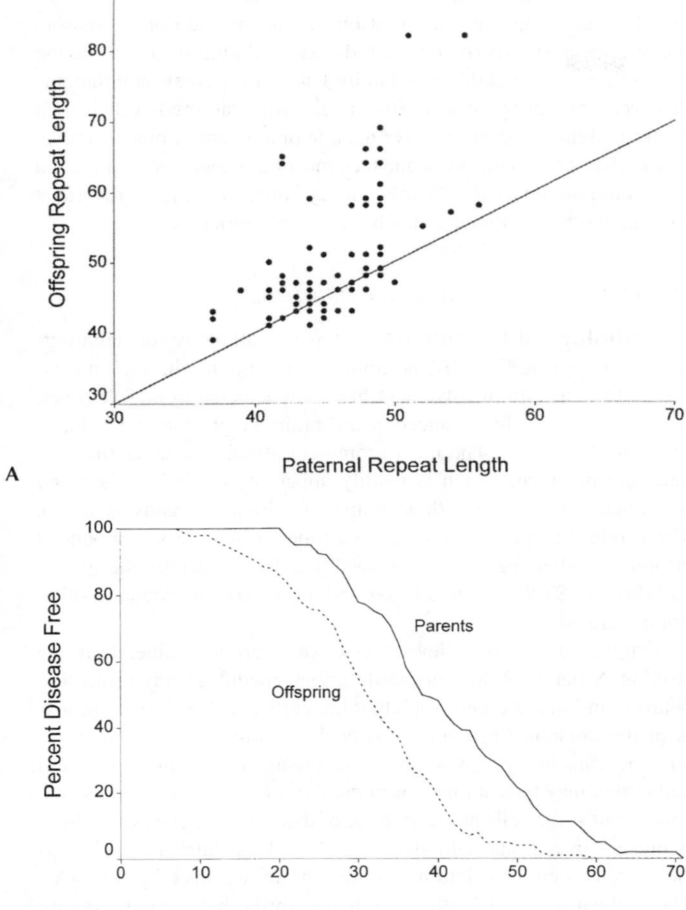

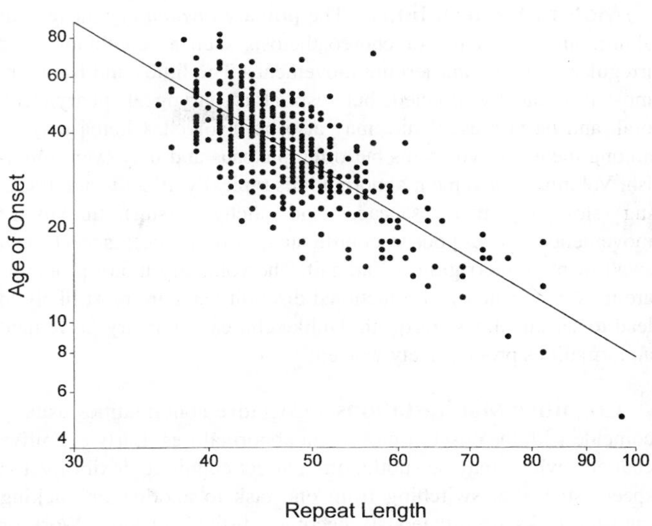

FIGURE 2.6–3 Repeat length as an important variable in Huntington's disease. **A:** Repeat length increases in paternal transmission of the expanded allele. Points above the diagonal line represent cases in which the repeat length increases during paternal transmission. Expansion occurs in most cases, and in some instances the expansion is substantial. N = 84 pairs; mean ± standard deviation increase of repeat length = 4.2 ± 0.8 triplets. **B:** Correlation of repeat length with a younger age of onset. As repeat length increases, age at disease onset decreases. N = 480; r^2 = 0.57. **C:** Anticipation in Huntington's disease. The age at which affected parents and their affected offspring first develop disease symptoms is depicted as a survival curve. The younger generation develops the disease at a substantially younger age, a result of increasing repeat length during paternal transmission and the correlation of repeat length with younger age of onset. N = 61 parents, 82 offspring. (From the Baltimore Huntington's Disease Center, courtesy of Drs. Adam Rosenblatt and Christopher A. Ross, with permission.)

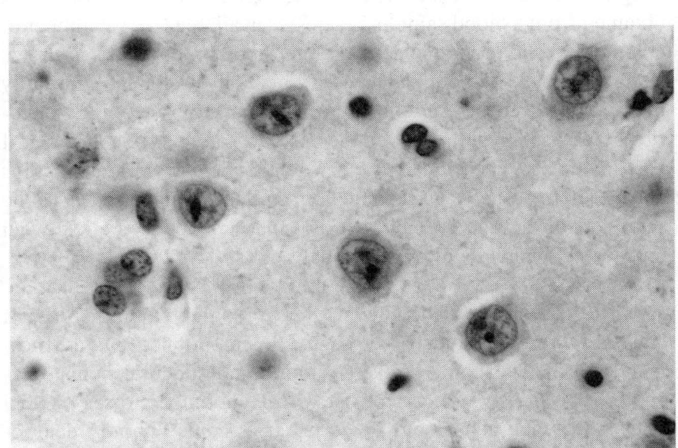

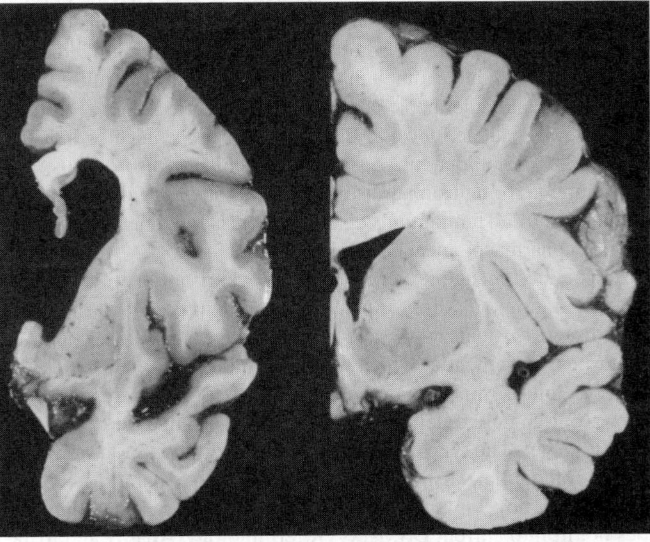

FIGURE 2.6–4 Huntington's disease neuropathology. **A:** Intranuclear inclusions in Huntington's disease. Immunohistochemical staining of cerebral cortex from a Huntington's disease patient with an antibody that labels the huntingtin protein demonstrates prominent intranuclear inclusions in neurons. **B:** Gross pathology. Huntington's disease case on the left, control brain on the right. Note the enlarged lateral ventricle, nearly absent caudate and putamen, and atrophy of the cerebral cortex. (See Color Plate.) (Photographs courtesy of Dr. Christopher A. Ross.)

Motor Manifestations The primary *involuntary* movement abnormality is chorea or choreoathetosis such as continuous and irregular writhing and jerking movements. The limbs and trunk are most prominently affected, but respiratory, laryngeal, pharyngeal, oral, and nasal musculature may also be involved. Chorea may be among the early symptoms but often plateaus and may even diminish. Voluntary movement abnormalities typically affect visual tracking (slow hypometric saccades and catchy pursuit), fine motor movements (slow, poorly coordinated, arrhythmic), speech and swallowing, tone (rigidity), and gait. The voluntary motor problems are most associated with functional disability and are most likely to lead to serious illness or death. Unlike chorea, voluntary movement abnormalities progressively worsen.

Cognitive Manifestations Cognitive abnormalities usually coincide with the onset of movement abnormalities. Early cognitive changes, which may be subtle, often affect cognitive flexibility and speed, such that switching from one task to another or tracking multiple tasks simultaneously becomes difficult or slow. Work or school performance may suffer to the point that colleagues notice. A four-domain model of cognitive deficits suggests that in early- to middle-stage Huntington's disease, visuospatial deficits are the most pronounced deficits, followed by executive dysfunction, and then less prominent memory and verbal deficits. The dementia becomes more global as the disease progresses, but aphasia and agnosia are less evident than in Alzheimer's disease, as in other subcortical dementias. MMSE scores typically decline by 1 to 2 points per year.

Psychiatric Manifestations As many as 80 percent of Huntington's disease patients develop some form of noncognitive psychiatric disorder within 10 to 15 years of disease onset. The consequences of these disorders may be devastating to the patient and family, perhaps more so than either the cognitive or motor dysfunction. The suicide rate is higher than in the general population, with an average across studies of 4.6 percent of all deaths. Because, at present, it is the psychiatric aspects of Huntington's disease that are most amenable to treatment, at present, psychopathology should be sought for diligently. Thirty to 40 percent of Huntington's disease patients develop major depression, and another 10 to 20 percent have a nonmajor form of depressive syndromes. Up to 10 percent of Huntington's disease patients develop mania, although this diagnosis may be confused with disinhibition and other personality changes. Less frequently, Huntington's disease patients develop disorders that are clinically indistinguishable from idiopathic obsessive-compulsive disorder (OCD), schizophrenia, or delusional disorder. As in patients with other types of brain damage, Huntington's disease patients are vulnerable to delirium from pharmacological or medical illness.

Personality change is very common, occurring in up to 50 percent of Huntington's disease patients by midcourse. Most Huntington's disease patients with personality change also have cognitive impairment or dementia (which would technically exclude the DSM-IV-TR diagnosis of personality change due to a general medical condition), but cognitive deficits and personality change do not always occur together. The types of change would fall into DSM-IV-TR categories of labile, disinhibited, apathetic, and paranoid. Other patients may develop a naïve, superficial, child-like personality that does not fit into current DSM-IV-TR terminology. Apathy and irritability are particularly common and troublesome states and may exist as either separate syndromes (currently ill-defined under DSM-IV-TR) or symptoms of other disorders.

The many psychosocial issues that accompany Huntington's disease increase the chance for adjustment disorders, relationship disorders, and other behavioral disorders. Caring for a cognitively impaired, irritable, or apathetic family member may result in emotional turmoil and financial hardship. Frequent additional stressors include social stigma (real or feared), parental guilt over passing the disease gene on to children, a family legacy of secrecy, and the burden faced by young gene-positive adults who can predict their own future in light of the progressive decline of a parent or other relative. These issues and their consequences must be recognized and treated but should not be used to "explain away" other psychiatric disorders for which other treatments may be more appropriate.

Pathology and Laboratory Examination

Pathological Examination Gross pathology of Huntington's disease (Fig. 2.6–4B) is limited to the brain, although microscopic or metabolic involvement has been detected in muscle, liver, and lymphocytes. In advanced cases, brain weight may be reduced by 25 to 30 percent. The most prominent atrophy involves the caudate and putamen, which is readily apparent on MRI scans or on gross pathology, along with accompanying hydrocephalus ex vacuo. The cerebral cortex becomes quite atrophied, with less pronounced atrophy in other regions of the basal ganglia (especially the globus pallidus and STN) and, to a lesser and more variable extent, in other brain regions.

On the microscopic level, selective neuronal vulnerability is striking. Striatal cell loss primarily affects medium spiny projection neurons and in a gradient such that the earliest and most severe loss is in the dorsomedial region. Cortical cell loss consists mostly of large neurons in layers 3, 4, and 5. Surviving neurons in the striatum and cortex may have an increased number of dendrites and dendritic spines, but some cells have evidence of dystrophic processes. Gliosis is present in regions with significant cell loss. Intranuclear inclusions are evident in striatum and other brain regions (Fig. 2.6–4A). The inclusions consist of amyloid-like fibrils that contain, among other proteins, mutant huntingtin, ubiquitin, and synuclein but not tau. Inclusions may also be detected in neuronal cytoplasm and processes.

Laboratory Evaluation Since 1993, it has been possible to directly test for the Huntington's disease repeat expansion, using a simple polymerase chain reaction (PCR)–based assay on DNA obtained from a blood sample. The test is available from a number of commercial and academic centers. Interpretation of results is shown in Table 2.6–3. Although the test is generally reliable, ambiguity may arise if a repeat length is on the borderline of one of the categories because the results of even the best laboratories have an error of ±1 triplet. Also, occasionally, only a single allele of normal length is detected. This usually means that both alleles contain a repeat of the same length, but the possibility exists that an expanded allele went undetected, which requires additional assays.

Ancillary Tests MRI, computed tomography (CT), SPECT, and PET were previously of diagnostic importance but are now mainly used to exclude strokes, tumors, and subdural hematomas and other lesions that may coexist with Huntington's disease. MRI scans should be considered if the patient's course rapidly deteriorates or in the presence of signs and symptoms not typical for Huntington's disease.

Presymptomatic Testing The availability of a diagnostic test for Huntington's disease has made presymptomatic testing readily available. Only a minority of individuals at risk for Hun-

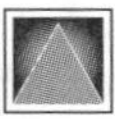

Table 2.6–3
Interpretation of Repeat Length (Longest of the Two Alleles)

Repeat Length (CAG Triplets)	Interpretation	Comments
<29	Unaffected	Repeat length stable
29–35	Unaffected	Rare expansions in paternal transmission
36–40	May develop HD	Increasing risk with longer repeats
≥41	Will develop HD	Earlier age of onset with longer expansions

HD, Huntington's disease.

tington's disease desire presymptomatic testing, often for psychological and practical reasons related to childbearing, long-term planning about caring for a relative with Huntington's disease, and finances. Perhaps because of the self-selected nature of those seeking presymptomatic testing and the exclusion from testing of those who are suffering from major depression, most patients feel relieved to learn of their status, whether testing positive or negative. Careful protocols for pre- and posttest counseling have been developed to ensure that patients understand the potential psychological risks and risks of discrimination (employment and insurance) that may arise from the test results. Expert counseling is mandatory before presymptomatic testing is obtained. For known gene carriers, it is possible to obtain prenatal diagnosis early in pregnancy. A few centers offer preimplantation testing of embryos generated by in vitro fertilization.

Differential Diagnosis

The availability of a definitive diagnostic test leaves two issues in Huntington's disease differential diagnosis: when to consider a diagnosis of Huntington's disease and what diagnoses to consider if a patient with Huntington's disease–like symptoms tests negative for Huntington's disease. Huntington's disease may occasionally present with rigidity, dystonia, athetosis, or tic-like movements rather than chorea, sometimes in every member of a pedigree. At other times, patients present with typical clinical manifestations, but they have no known family history of Huntington's disease. This may arise when disease onset occurs earlier in a child than his or her parent, a parent carrying the mutation has died from other causes before the onset of clinical Huntington's disease, there is false paternity or adoption, or, in very rare cases, a new mutation arises that is not present in previous generations. Genetic testing should be considered in any of these situations. Table 2.6–4 lists some of the disorders that present with Huntington's disease–like symptoms. Notably, any disease or insult that affects the basal ganglia might lead to chorea or dystonia.

Course and Prognosis

Huntington's disease is relentlessly progressive and fatal (Fig. 2.6–3C). Onset is typically insidious, with early complaints of clumsiness, jerks, and tremor. Whereas the chorea tends to plateau and may even decline by later in the course, the voluntary motor abnormalities progress, paralleled by cognitive decline. Patients with late-stage Huntington's disease require complete care for all activities of daily living. They are mostly nonverbal, rigid, and akinetic but may make whole-body movements resembling myoclonic jerks when disturbed. Dementia is global and severe but may be less severe than the patient's appearance suggests.

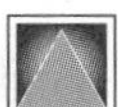

Table 2.6–4
Differential Diagnosis of Choreiform Disorder

Disorder	Comment
Family history of movement disorder	
Dentatorubral pallidoluysian atrophy	Autosomal dominant, rare in the United States, more common in Japan, variable presentation
HD-like 2	Rare autosomal dominant disorder clinically indistinguishable from HD
Spinocerebellar ataxia types 2 and 3	Autosomal dominant, each may present with prominent chorea or dystonia
Hereditary Creutzfeldt-Jakob disease	Autosomal dominant, 85% of cases are sporadic
Wilson's disease	Autosomal recessive, distinguished by eye and liver abnormalities, abnormal copper metabolism
Ceroid neuronal lipofuscinoses	Usually childhood-onset autosomal recessive, rarely adult-onset autosomal dominant
Neuroacanthocytosis	Recessive and dominant forms, distinguished by abnormal red blood cells (acanthocytes)
Benign hereditary chorea	Usually childhood onset
Pantothenate kinase–associated neurodegeneration	Childhood onset, recessive
Fahr's disease	Basal ganglia calcification, usually autosomal dominant, adult onset
Mitochondrial diseases	Maternal inheritance, heterogeneous phenotypes
No family history	
Tardive dyskinesia	Common
Sydenham's chorea	Poststreptococcal complication
Systemic lupus erythematosus	May occur in 1–7% of cases
Neurosyphilis	Also human immunodeficiency virus infection in most cases
Thyroid disease	Typically hyperthyroidism
Drug induced	Anticonvulsants, lithium, stimulants

HD, Huntington's disease.

Death usually occurs 15 to 20 years after disease onset, often from the consequences of swallowing difficulties (suffocation or aspiration pneumonia) or general debilitation. Juvenile-onset Huntington's disease often presents with bradykinesia, rigidity, dystonia, and sometimes seizures or myoclonus. Chorea may be minimal or absent. The course seems to be more rapid and severe than typical Huntington's disease.

Treatment

There is currently no treatment for the underlying neurodegeneration of Huntington's disease. However, the quality of life for the patient and his or her family can be substantially improved by medical intervention. Some patients are concerned about the social implications of chorea, and others may find chorea functionally impairing. Chorea may respond to low doses (0.5 to 2.0 mg per day) of typical high-potency antipsychotics, such as haloperidol or fluphenazine; other neuroleptics; benzodiazepines; dopamine-depleting agents, such as tetrabenazine or reserpine; or amantadine. Care must be taken because these medicines may worsen voluntary movement abnormalities or apathy or cause akathisia or excess sedation. Clonazepam has been reported to help in later stages of the illness when dopamine antagonists may lose effectiveness. The simple mechanical strategy of weights strapped to the wrists can often prove of considerable value without causing side effects. Environmental interventions, such as removal of throw rugs, adding grab bars in bathrooms, and avoidance of stairs, are always essential to reduce falls. Other common symptoms can also be at least partially ameliorated. Swallowing abnormalities can be assessed by pharyngeal esophagram and treated with thickened liquid and softened solid diet. Botulinum injections may be useful for dystonia. Myoclonus has been successfully treated with valproate (Depakote) and clonazepam, and valproate may also be effective for seizures.

There are no established pharmacological treatments for cognition. In particular, the effect of anticholinesterase inhibitors is unknown. Simple education interventions may prove helpful, as in other forms of dementia. Early in the disease, patients can be taught to write notes and to limit the number of tasks undertaken at once. Patients, and especially family members and care providers, need to be told about the progressive cognitive decline so that they can learn to phrase questions more simply, provide cues for recall, and keep cognitive demands on the patient at a level commensurate with cognitive capacity. The topic of guardianship or power of attorney for legal, financial, and medical decisions should be raised before the patient is too incapacitated to participate in the discussion.

Depression may be treated with any of the standard antidepressants, with the caveat that, as in any patient with brain damage, starting doses should be low, and doses should be increased slowly, with careful monitoring for delirium. SSRIs are often useful and, given the higher suicide risk in Huntington's disease patients, are notably less toxic in overdose than tricyclic antidepressants or monoamine oxidase inhibitors (MAOIs). SSRIs may occasionally cause akathisia, insomnia, or dyskinesias. Other antidepressants, including venlafaxine (Effexor), bupropion, and nefazodone (Serzone), have been used successfully. ECT has been used successfully to treat life-threatening or intractable depression and, other than an increased risk of delirium, is generally well tolerated. Mild mood elevations may not warrant treatment, but mania, like depression, can be treated with standard pharmacological agents; limited data and anecdotal accounts suggest that divalproex sodium or carbamazepine are better tolerated and more effective than lithium. Benzodiazepines or antipsychotics (the atypical agents may have fewer negative effects on movement than the typical agents) may be helpful adjuncts.

Aggression and irritability stem from multiple causes, including psychiatric syndromes, cognitive and personality changes, and environmental precipitants such as hunger, thirst, pain, frustration over an inability to communicate, boredom, or unexpected change in routine. Treatment of any underlying psychiatric disorder and careful attention to possible precipitants are the first approach. When necessary, anecdotal evidence supports the effectiveness, in some patients, of SSRIs, antipsychotics, anticonvulsants, β-blockers, and benzodiazepines. Apathy probably responds best to family education combined with a structured and stimulating environment. SSRIs, stimulants, and dopaminergic agents, such as amantadine and bromocriptine (Parlodel), may be of value, although the latter agents may increase chorea.

WILSON'S DISEASE

Wilson's disease (hepatolenticular degeneration) is an autosomal recessive disorder in which mutations in the gene ATP7B result in abnormal copper accumulation in the liver, brain, and other tissues, with consequent hepatic cirrhosis and neuronal degeneration. Psychiatric and movement abnormalities are common, and patients may present to a psychiatrist first. Wilson's disease is treatable yet fatal without treatment. Recognition of the characteristic signs, symptoms, and laboratory abnormalities is therefore essential.

History The disease was named after Samuel Alexander Kinnier Wilson, who first recognized the syndrome, including a high rate of psychiatric abnormalities, in 1912. In 1948, the role of copper in disease pathogenesis was established; in 1952, I. Herbert Scheinberg and David Gitlin discovered the deficiency of ceruloplasmin in Wilson's disease patients (establishing a test that is still in use); and in 1960, Alexander Bearn definitively established the recessive nature of the disorder. The molecular basis of the disease emerged first with linkage to the esterase D locus on chromosome 13 in 1985, and then, in 1993, with the discovery of causative mutations in ATP7B.

Epidemiology Wilson's disease is found worldwide, with a frequency estimated at approximately 1 per 30,000 in most populations. Approximately 1 in 90 individuals are heterozygous carriers.

Etiology More than two hundred mutations associated with Wilson's disease have been described in ATP7B. A few mutations are common (H1069Q accounts for more than 40 percent of mutations in northern European populations), whereas most are rare. The result is that most individuals with Wilson's disease are compound heterozygotes, carrying a different mutation on each allele. The Wilson's protein, an adenosine triphosphatase (ATPase) involved in copper transport, functions to maintain copper homeostasis by facilitating excretion of copper from hepatocytes into bile. In patients with Wilson's disease, this function fails, resulting in accumulation of copper in the liver, brain, and other tissues, eventually leading to hepatic failure and neurological and psychiatric signs and symptoms. In the brain, the basal ganglia appear to be particularly affected.

Clinical Features Approximately 40 percent of patients first present with liver abnormalities, 40 percent with neurological abnormalities, and 20 percent with psychiatric abnormalities. Liver dysfunction, the most common childhood presentation of Wilson's disease, may be manifest as mild elevations of serum transaminases, chronic active hepatitis, cirrhosis, or acute and fulminant liver failure. Copper toxicity may also lead to cardiac arrhythmias, renal disease, rhabdomyolysis, joint disease, anemia, and thyroid and parathyroid dysfunction. Neurological signs and symptoms, which strongly correlate with brain and cerebrospinal fluid (CSF) copper levels, generally reflect the multiple brain regions involved and include dysdiadochokinesia, dysarthria, tremor, dystonia, rigidity, choreoathetosis, bradykinesia, masked facies, and micrographia. Seizures occur in 6 percent of patients.

Cognition in Wilson's disease has not been well studied. Relatively mild cognitive impairment is believed to be present in approximately 25 percent of patients, worsening with time and in conjunction with accumulating neurological symptoms.

Two-thirds of patients may have psychiatric symptoms by first presentation, and 10 to 20 percent of patients seek psychiatric treatment before the diagnosis of Wilson's disease is established (a stage at which the diagnosis is often missed). Eventually, psychiatric manifestations affect nearly all patients with Wilson's disease, and the psychiatric profile generally resembles Huntington's disease. The most common symptoms are personality changes (often described as irritability, aggressiveness, and emotional lability) and depression (ranging from subsyndromal mood changes to major depression, at times with suicidality). It is likely that anxiety disorders, psychotic disorders (and individual psychotic symptoms), and catatonia are more common than in the general population. The severity of psychiatric symptoms correlates more strongly with the extent of neurological findings than with the liver disease, providing evidence that the psychiatric symptoms reflect the brain damage rather than a psychological reaction to the severity of illness.

Diagnosis Because the hepatic, neurological, and psychiatric manifestations of copper toxicity are only partially reversible, prompt diagnosis of Wilson's disease is essential. The key step is considering the diagnosis. Elevated liver transaminases are nonspecific but may be the first diagnostic clue. Kayser-Fleischer rings, copper deposits in the limbus of the cornea, may be detected by inspection or with a slit-lamp examination but are often absent early in the disease. Serum ceruloplasmin is below normal in 95 percent of Wilson's disease patients but is also low in newborns and 20 percent of heterozygous Wilson's disease carriers and may be misleadingly normal in the setting of infection or inflammation. The absence of serum ceruloplasmin oxidase activity is a useful test in the latter cases. Urinary copper concentration is generally elevated. A liver biopsy reveals increased hepatic copper concentration in addition to evidence of hepatitis or cirrhosis. Genetic testing for Wilson's disease mutations has been limited due to the many possible mutations in ATPB7, although increasingly efficient methods for detecting mutations should make this a critical laboratory test in the near future.

In patients with neurological or psychiatric disorders and sometimes in patients without clinical evidence of brain disease, a head MRI reveals generalized atrophy and increased T2-weighted signal in the basal ganglia (most typically the putamen) secondary to copper deposition. Atrophy may also be detected in the cerebral cortex (especially the frontal lobe), brainstem, and cerebellum. PET, SPECT, and magnetic resonance spectroscopy (MRS) have been used to reveal functional abnormalities in these regions. The most prominent pathological changes involve cavitary degeneration of the basal ganglia, with neuronal loss, gliosis, and high levels of copper.

Differential Diagnosis Elevated hepatic copper may also result from cholestatic liver disease (normal or elevated ceruloplasmin) or idiopathic childhood cirrhosis (elevated ceruloplasmin). Aceruloplasminemia may result in neurological symptoms but results in elevated liver iron rather than copper. Urine copper excretion may be elevated secondary to metal chelation therapy or in the presence of acute liver failure or cirrhosis with cholestasis or nephrotic syndrome.

Course, Prognosis, and Treatment Onset of Wilson's disease is usually in the second or third decade, with a mean onset age of 17 years. Without treatment, death may occur within 5 years or sooner for patients with CNS disease. However, Wilson's disease is one of the few neurodegenerative diseases in which the fundamental pathogenic process, copper accumulation, is amenable to treatment. If caught early enough, many of the manifestations of the disease, including the neurological and psychiatric consequences, can be at least partially reversed. Treatment strategies involve either removing copper (chelation) by agents such as D-penicillamine, trientine, and tetrathiomolybdate or blocking copper absorption by zinc salts. Except for patients in areas with high levels of copper in the drinking water, it appears that dietary control of copper is not helpful. D-Penicillamine, which is poorly tolerated by some patients and prone to induce hypersensitivity reactions, and trientine have been noted to occasionally increase neurological and psychiatric symptoms acutely, as hepatic copper is mobilized and deposited in the brain. For patients with end-stage liver disease, orthotopic liver transplantation has proved successful. All treatment modalities appear to improve neurological and psychiatric symptoms, but the response may only be partial if disease was at an advanced stage by the time therapy was instituted.

There are no controlled trials regarding the symptomatic treatment of the psychiatric manifestations of Wilson's disease. Anecdotal evidence suggests that Wilson's disease patients may be particularly vulnerable to extrapyramidal side effects of neuroleptics. It seems prudent to treat psychiatric syndromes with standard psychiatric treatment modalities, both pharmacological and psychotherapeutic, but to choose lower doses of medicines, increase doses slowly, and avoid high-potency neuroleptics.

CEREBELLAR DISORDERS

The cerebellum has long been considered a modulator of motor function. Over the past 10 years, it has become increasingly clear that the cerebellum also modulates cognition and affect and that damage to the cerebellum from many different causes can result in cognitive deficits and psychiatric syndromes.

History A role for the cerebellum in regulating motor function was established early in the 19th century, beginning with the studies of Luigi Rolando. By the early 20th century, the effect of cerebellar degenerative disease on coordination of the limbs, gait, posture, and speech was appreciated. By 1939, the work of Sir Gordon Holmes established much of the terminology and methods of examination of the cerebellum still in use. Simultaneously, diseases that affect the cerebellum were delineated, including hereditary disorders described by Nikolaus Friedreich in 1863 and Pierre Marie in 1893. Anecdotal reports of cognitive and psychiatric disorders arising from cerebellar damage have been noted since the early days of cerebellar research. However, systematic investigation of this link only began in the 1980s, stimulated by a series of neuroanatomical studies, still ongoing, that demonstrated connections between the cerebellum and multiple other brain regions.

Epidemiology The overall prevalence of cerebellar disorders is difficult to determine because many different diseases may affect the cerebellum. As many as 50 percent of patients who have alcohol dependence syndromes develop clinical or histological evidence of cerebellar pathology; this may be the single most common cause of cerebellar damage worldwide. The cerebellum is affected in 1.5 to 8.0 percent of all strokes, so this is probably the second most common cause of cerebellar damage. In children, the annual incidence of tumors affecting the cerebellum is between 0.25 and 1.00 per 100,000 per year. In adults, primary tumors of the cerebellum are more rare, but metastases are more common. The prevalence of recessive (primarily Friedreich's ataxia), dominant, and sporadic neurodegenerative diseases that primarily affect the cerebellum is, in each case, approximately 2 per 100,000. Other causes of cerebellar lesions are rare.

Etiology Table 2.6–5 lists many of the diseases that cause permanent injury to the cerebellum. With the exception of some strokes, tumors, and degenerative conditions, most of these disorders are

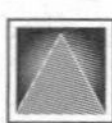

Table 2.6–5
Diseases That Cause Cerebellar Damage

Hereditary degenerative autosomal dominant	Nutritional/dietary
Spinocerebellar ataxia types 1–23	Vitamin E
Dentatorubral pallidoluysian atrophy	Thiamine (often in association with alcoholism)
Huntington's disease (uncommonly)	Celiac disease
Hereditary prion diseases	Toxic
Episodic ataxias types 1 and 2	Ethanol
Hereditary autosomal recessive (metabolic)	Phenytoin
Abetalipoproteinemia	Lithium
Friedreich's ataxia	Organic solvents
Niemann-Pick type C	Oncological
Hexosaminidase A deficiency (Tay-Sachs)	Primary tumors
Glutamic aciduria	Metastases
Hydroxyglutamic aciduria	Paraneoplastic (small cell carcinoma of lung, breast, female genital tract, lymphomas)
Cholestanolosis (cerebrotendinous xanthomatosis)	
Metachromatic leukodystrophy	Infectious/postinfectious
Galactocerebrosidase deficiency (Krabbe's disease)	Abscesses
α-Tocopherol deficiency (vitamin E deficiency)	Whipple's disease
Hartnup disease	Subacute sclerosing panencephalitis
Refsum's disease (phytanic acid oxidase deficiency)	Progressive rubella panencephalitis
Biotinidase deficiency	Infectious prion disease
Hereditary autosomal recessive, deoxyribonucleic acid repair	Other
Ataxia-telangiectasia	Multiple sclerosis
Xeroderma pigmentosum	Sporadic late-onset cerebellar degeneration
Cockayne's syndrome	Multiple system atrophy
Hereditary X linked	Trauma
Pelizaeus-Merzbacher disease	Radiation
Adrenoleukodystrophy	Vascular
Rett's syndrome	Embolic, hemorrhagic, or occlusive
Mitochondrial	Congenital (some autosomal recessive or X-linked hereditary)
Kearns-Sayre syndrome	Marinesco-Sjögren's syndrome
Myoclonic epilepsy associated with ragged-red fibers	Joubert's syndrome
Neuropathy, ataxia, and retinitis pigmentosa	Disequilibrium syndrome
Leber's hereditary optic neuropathy	Early-onset ataxia with hypogonadism, retinopathy, or deafness

unlikely to affect the cerebellum in isolation. Therefore, cognitive and psychiatric manifestations of these diseases may derive from damage to multiple brain regions. However, based on recently established neuroanatomical links between the cerebellum and other regions of the brain and analysis of focal cerebellar lesions, it is now clear that damage to the cerebellum itself is sufficient to cause cognitive and emotional disturbance.

The pathway from the cerebral cortex to the cerebellum originates with projections from neurons in cortical layer Vb in motor, somatosensory, association, and paralimbic regions, including posterior parietal association cortex; portions of the superior temporal sulcus and gyrus; parastriate and parahippocampal regions; and dorsolateral, medial, and, to a lesser extent, ventral lateral prefrontal regions. After synapse in the pons, where topographical distinctions among the different sources of input are maintained, the pathway continues as projections into the cerebellar cortex. Feedback to the cortex begins with axons projecting from cerebellar Purkinje cells to the deep cerebellar nuclei, where the pathway again remains topographically defined. These nuclei then project to both "motor" and "nonspecific" nuclei of the thalamus. Axons in neurons from both types of thalamic nuclei project to posterior parietal, superior temporal, and prefrontal association regions of the cerebral cortex, and the intralaminar nuclei also project to limbic regions. This cerebro-cerebellar pathway appears to consist of a series of discrete and relatively closed loops, similar to the loops connecting the basal ganglia and the cerebral cortex. Other pathways of potential relevance include reciprocal connections between the cerebellum and brainstem catecholaminergic (locus ceruleus) and serotoninergic nuclei (dorsal raphe), the hypothalamus, and the brainstem reticular formation.

In addition to its connections to multiple other brain regions, the other aspect of cerebellar anatomy important to affect and cognition are the "cerebellar cortical modules." These modules exist as radially oriented, structurally identical units that comprise the cerebellar cortex. Each module consists of a Purkinje cell (numbering approximately 15 to 30 million in the human cerebellum), granule cells that receive input from outside of the cerebellum and innervate the Purkinje cell, and inhibitory interneurons (basket, stellate, and Golgi cells). The Purkinje cell thus serves to integrate excitatory and inhibitory input.

It is generally believed that these units perform the same type of transform for all information coming into the cerebellum, with the specificity of information processing provided by the unique connections of each region of the cerebellum to other brain structures. Jeremy Schmahmann has therefore proposed that just as the "cerebellum regulates the rate, force, rhythm, and accuracy of movements, so may it regulate the speed, capacity, consistency, and appropriateness of mental or cognitive processes." He has termed this the *dysmetria of thought hypothesis* and suggests that damage to the cerebellum leads to an "unpredictability and illogic to social and societal interaction," just as it leads to poorly coordinated and misjudged movements. Although intriguing, it remains uncertain to what extent this hypothesis can explain the multitude of cognitive and psychiatric phenomena that accompany cerebellar disease.

Diagnosis and Clinical Features

The diagnosis of cerebellar disorders involves narrowing the complicated differential: Is onset age at birth (congenital), childhood (metabolic, oncological, Friedreich's ataxia), middle age (spinocerebellar ataxias), or elderly age (oncological, vascular)? What other organ systems or regions of the nervous system are affected? Is the process acute (vascular, toxic, infectious), subacute (infectious, oncological), chronic (hereditary, toxic, nutritional), or episodic? Is there progression or have symptoms remained static? Is there a family history of a similar disorder? Have there been exposures to drugs, alcohol, or toxins? The history and examination, followed by an MRI scan (and potentially other imaging modalities such as PET, SPECT, or angiography) and then specific genetic or metabolic tests, often, but by no means always, provide a final diagnosis.

Motor Features

Problems with balance and speech are often the presenting complaints in disorders with primarily cerebellar involvement. The "cerebellar gait" is wide based and staggering. Patients may complain of walking as if they were drunk, and stairs are particularly difficult. On examination, patients are unable to perform a tandem walk and may sway or display titubation, a low-frequency tremor of the body. The dysarthria is characterized by slurred speech of irregular rhythm and with incorrect emphasis of syllables. Speech may be slowed and monotonic (scanning speech) in compensation.

Cerebellar damage is also manifest in other ways. Eye movement abnormalities vary and may include nystagmus, square wave jerks (inability to maintain fixation when gazing at a specified point), dysmetria (over- or undershoot when making rapid eye movements [REMs] from one target to another), and uneven smooth pursuit. Limb incoordination may be manifest as trouble with fine motor tasks. Tremor may be either postural or kinetic, the latter often observable as an intention tremor during finger-to-nose testing. The presence of other signs or symptoms signals the possibility that other regions of the CNS are also involved, more the rule than the exception with diseases affecting the cerebellum.

Cognitive Features

The cerebellum is involved in a variety of cognitive tasks, including procedural learning, executive function, language processing, visuospatial orientation, sensory processing, timing, and attention. Within 10 to 15 years of disease onset, approximately 20 percent of patients with cerebellar degeneration meet DSM-IV-TR criteria for cognitive decline or dementia, and the rate presumably increases significantly later in the disease course. The pattern of deficits is consistent with a subcortical dementia, with deficits in verbal and nonverbal intelligence and, especially, executive function in the absence of aphasia, apraxia, or agnosia. Cognitive deficits in these patients, particularly when subtle, may not be detected on simple clinical mental state examinations that focus on language and memory. Executive functions impaired in cerebellar degeneration include attention, sequencing, and timing. Executive, visuospatial, verbal, and visual memory and language deficits also frequently follow focal lesions of the cerebellum. It has been suggested that cognitive deficits are more likely to follow lesions of the cerebellar hemisphere, whereas vermal lesions result in psychiatric disturbances.

Psychiatric Features

Many anecdotal reports, but only a few small systematic studies, have examined the frequency and nature of psychiatric syndromes in patients with cerebellar disease. After strokes restricted to the posterior circulation (cerebellum and brainstem), approximately 35 percent of patients develop either a major or minor depression acutely, with the frequency declining to approximately 20 percent 6 months after the stroke and 10 percent 12 to 24 months later. Personality changes, particularly blunted affect and disinhibition, may be prominent in patients with large posterior circulation infarcts, whereas anterior lobe or very small cerebellar infarcts elsewhere are less likely to produce personality change.

In degenerative disorders predominately limited to the cerebellum, approximately 75 percent of patients develop one or more psychiatric syndromes within 10 to 15 years of disease onset. As many as one in three experience at least one episode of major depression, and another one-third experience other forms of depression (including brief recurrent depression, minor depressive disorder, and dysthymia). Approximately 25 percent develop persistent personality changes, similar in type to those found in Huntington's disease and, as in Huntington's disease, not limited to patients with cognitive decline. The frequency of mania, anxiety syndromes, and psychotic syndromes may all be somewhat elevated.

Pathology and Laboratory Examination

The pathology of cerebellar disorders depends on the underlying disease. Even with signs and symptoms relatively specific to the cerebellum, pathological examination is likely to reveal noncerebellar findings. Laboratory evaluation, including genetic testing for hereditary disorders and metabolic screens for metabolic disorders, is based on clinical and MRI findings. Neuropsychological testing, with a focus on executive function, may help detect subtle cognitive difficulties of considerable clinical relevance. In addition to the diagnostic workup, imaging studies are important if the nature or severity of signs and symptoms change unexpectedly to exclude the presence of new subdural hematomas, infarcts, or tumors.

Differential Diagnosis

The differential diagnosis of the underlying disease for a patient presenting with cerebellar signs and symptoms is depicted in Table 2.6–5. Similar to other movement disorders, the differential diagnosis of affective symptoms is perhaps the most important issue facing the psychiatrist. Delirium must always be considered, regardless of whether the criteria for DSM-IV-TR major depression are met. Isolated affective symptoms in the absence of delirium and major depression may reflect a subsyndromal depressive disorder but could also be manifestations of a personality change or cognitive deficits either resulting in affective change (particularly apathy or irritability) or fueling demoralization.

Course and Prognosis

The course of cerebellar diseases varies widely by etiology, ranging from steadily progressive to intermittent to completely static. Personality and cognitive change are likely to follow the underlying disease course, whereas major depression may be more intermittent, suggesting differences in pathophysiology among these disorders.

Treatment

Determining the cause of the underlying disorder is essential because cerebellar degeneration secondary to nutritional, dietary, and some metabolic disorders may be treatable and at least partially reversible. Cognitive treatments are supportive and educational, as described for Huntington's disease. Little is known about the treatment of psychiatric disorders. Anecdotal accounts indicate that patients respond to standard treatments, including various classes of antidepressants and ECT. Caution is necessary with agents that may increase ataxia.

Essential Tremor Essential tremor (ET) has been well characterized since 1887, but controversy remains over its definition, whether it represents a symptom, syndrome, or disease entity, and the basis for associated neuropsychiatric abnormalities. ET affects approximately 5 percent of individuals older than 65 years of age and is the most common type of movement disorder. Its etiology and pathophysiology are unclear, but, traditionally, ET has been regarded as a benign condition presenting as a monosymptomatic disorder without other neurological involvement or nonmotor effects. It is commonly familial, and linkage to two different loci (3q13 and 2p25-p22) indicates that is it genetically heterogeneous. The main clinical sign is a predominantly postural and kinetic tremor affecting the hands, head, or both that is either sporadic or genetic in origin and is not associated with other known causes of tremor. There is now increasing evidence that ET is associated with the development of other motor abnormalities, including comorbid diseases, such as Parkinson's disease or dystonia, as well as cognitive and psychiatric features. The kinetic component of ET, as well as subtle signs of ataxia, suggests cerebellar involvement, and neuroimaging studies suggest nigrostriatal damage. Several recent studies have identified selective and sometimes subtle cognitive deficits that suggest frontocerebellar dysfunction in association with ET, including executive dysfunction and impairment in attention, verbal fluency, verbal learning, and verbal memory. High levels of depressive symptoms are also reported in ET, but the epidemiology and features of discrete psychopathological syndromes have not been examined in ET. No studies have addressed treatment of neuropsychiatric features in ET.

Dystonias Dystonia is characterized by involuntary, sustained muscle contractions that result in twisting, torsional, repetitive movements of one or more body parts and frequently appear as abnormal and sometimes painful or awkward positions and postures. It is the third most common movement disorder after Parkinson's disease and ET. Like ET, it can present as a monosymptomatic condition or as a feature of a broader syndrome. Any part of the body can be affected, including the limbs, trunk, neck, eyelids, face, or vocal cords. There are three categories used to classify each patient with dystonia: age of onset, body distribution of symptoms, and etiology. Age of onset is defined as childhood, adolescence, or adulthood (older than 28 years of age) and is an important predictor of whether symptoms will spread to other body parts. Distribution of dystonia is categorized as generalized, focal, segmental, multifocal, or hemidystonic and is one indicator of disease severity. The etiologic classification scheme is evolving due to ongoing discovery of different genetic forms of dystonia. Primary dystonias are defined by the existence of dystonia as the major symptom and include both hereditary and sporadic forms. In dystonia-plus syndromes, dystonia is accompanied by another prominent neurological feature such as parkinsonism or myoclonus. At least ten genes or chromosomal locations are associated with primary dystonias and dystonia-plus conditions, including early-onset generalized dystonia, dopa-responsive dystonia, paroxysmal dystonia, X-linked dystonia-parkinsonism (Lubag), myoclonic dystonia, and rapid-onset dystonia-parkinsonism. Secondary dystonias can be attributed to numerous cerebral insults, including perinatal injury, trauma, toxins, or infarction, or as a dopaminergic medication–related effect in Parkinson's disease or schizophrenia. Dystonia also may occur in association with neurodegenerative conditions such as Wilson's disease and Parkinson's disease. Neurophysiological dysfunction in dopaminergic neurotransmission and basal ganglia output activity are believed to underlie primary dystonia and dystonia-plus disorders, in which there is no evidence of nerve cell loss.

Dystonic movements begin with a particular motor action but eventually generalize to multiple actions and are then present at rest. The contractions may be extreme, usually resulting in muscle hypertrophy and often pain or an oppositional tremor. Certain postures or sensory tricks can reduce dystonic contractions. Anticholinergic medications used to treat dystonia can affect memory, but cognitive impairment is not a general feature of dystonias. There is limited information about the relationship between dystonia in general and psychopathology, and even less is known about the psychiatric phenomena in the clinically or genetically distinct subtypes of dystonia. Demoralization appears to be common, and major depression may be elevated beyond population norms. Anxiety and depression have pronounced effects on quality of life. Alcohol may be misused to self-treat motor symptoms. Obsessive-compulsive disorder may be overrepresented in families with myoclonic dystonia.

The prognosis of dystonia and rate of progression vary with the underlying condition and age of onset. Often, it stabilizes within 5 years of onset, but stressful circumstances provoke symptoms. Most therapy is symptomatic. Strategies include medications to reduce spasms and pain (e.g., anticholinergics, benzodiazepines, and muscle relaxants). Dopamine and dopamine-blocking agents have either negative or beneficial effects on dystonias. Botulinum toxin injections into selected muscles are used extensively to treat the various forms of dystonia. Exercise programs are an important component of therapy. When medical approaches are inadequate, surgery includes thalamotomy, pallidotomy, and DBS procedures. There have been no studies of the treatment of psychiatric disorders associated with dystonia, but care must focus on identifying and treating psychiatric disorders or psychological distress. For example, botulism injections may reduce torticollis and depressive symptoms, but self-perceptions remain impaired. SSRIs can precipitate, aggravate, or improve dystonia. ECT may benefit motor and mood symptoms.

SUGGESTED CROSS-REFERENCES

Age-related changes in motor function are discussed in Section 51.2b. Motor abnormalities associated with Alzheimer's disease and other dementias are included in Section 51.3e. Tardive dyskinesia and tic disorders are discussed in Chapter 42. Conversion disorders are included in Chapter 15.

References

Aarsland D, Andersen K, Larsen JP, Lolk A, Kragh-Sorenson P: Prevalence and characteristics of dementia in Parkinson's disease. *Arch Neurol.* 2003;60:387–392.

Aarsland D, Litvan I, Larsen JP: Neuropsychiatric symptoms of patients with progressive supranuclear palsy and Parkinson's disease. *J Neuropsychiatry Clin Neurosci.* 2001;13:4–49.

Albers DS, Augood SJ: New insights into progressive supranuclear palsy. *Trends Neurosci.* 2001;24:3471.

*Bates G, Harper P, Jones L, eds. *Huntington's Disease.* 3rd ed. Oxford, UK: Oxford University Press; 2002.

*Bedard, M-A, ed. *Mental and Behavioral Dysfunction in Movement Disorders.* New Jersey: Human Press; 2003.

Cummings JL, Chow T, Masterman D: Encephalitis lethargica: Lessons for neuropsychiatry. *Psychiatric Ann.* 2001;31:165.

Dekker MCJ, Bonifati V, van Duijn CM: Parkinson's disease: Piecing together a genetic jigsaw. *Brain.* 2003;126:1722–1733.

GeneTests. Available at: http://www.genetests.org.

Gwinn-Hardy, K: Genetics of parkinsonism. *Mov Disord.* 2002;17:645.

Joseph AB, Young RR. *Movement Disorders in Neurology and Neuropsychiatry.* 2nd ed. Malden, MA: Blackwell Science; 1999.

Kashmere J, Camicoli R, Martin W: Parkinsonian syndromes and differential diagnosis. *Curr Opin Neurol.* 2002;15:461.

Lauterbach EC, Cummings JL, Duffy J, Coffey CE, Kaufer D, Lovell M, Malloy P, Reeve A, Royall DR, Rummans TA, Salloway SP: Neuropsychiatric correlates and treatment of lenticulostriatal diseases: A review of the literature and overview of research opportunities in Huntington's, Wilson's, and Fahr's diseases. *J Neuropsychiatry Clin Neurosci.* 1998;10:249, 266.

*Leroi I, O'Hearn E, Marsh L, Lyketsos CG, Rosenblatt A, Ross CA, Brandt J, Margolis

RL: Psychopathology in degenerative cerebellar diseases: A comparison to Huntington's disease and normal controls. *Am J Psychiatry*. 2002;159:1306.

Margolis RL, Ross CA: The diagnosis of Huntington's disease. *Clin Chem*. 2003;49:1726–1732.

Marsh L, Berk A: Neuropsychiatric aspects of Parkinson's disease: Recent advances. *Curr Psychiatry Rep*. 2003;5:68–76.

McKeith IG, Perry EK, Perry RH: Report of the second dementia with Lewy body international workshop. Diagnosis and treatment. *Neurology*. 1999;53:90.

McKhann GM, Albert MS, Grossman M, Miller B, Dickson D, Trojanowski JQ: Clinical and pathological diagnosis of frontotemporal dementia. *Arch Neurol*. 2001;58:1803.

*Parent A, Cicchetti F: The current model of basal ganglia organization under scrutiny. *Mov Disord*. 1998;13:199–202.

Perry RJ, Miller BL: Behavior and treatment in frontotemporal dementia. *Neurology*. 2001;56[Suppl 4]:S46–S51.

Peyser CE, Naimark D, Zuniga R, Jeste DV: Psychoses in Parkinson's disease. *Semin Clin Neuropsychiatry*. 1998;3:41–50.

Rosenblatt A, Ranen NG, Nance MA, Paulsen JS. *A Physician's Guide to the Management of Huntington's Disease*. 2nd ed. Huntington's Disease Society of America; 1999.

Ross CA: Polyglutamine pathogenesis: Emergence of unifying mechanisms for Huntington's disease and related disorders. *Neuron*. 2002;35:819.

Saint-Cyr JA, Trépanier LL: Neuropsychologic assessment of patients for movement disorder surgery. *Mov Disord*. 2000;15:771–783.

Sawamoto N, Honda M, Hanakawa T, Fukuyama H, Shibasaki H: Cognitive slowing in Parkinson's disease: A behavioral evaluation independent of motor slowing. *J Neurosci*. 2002;22:5198–5203.

Schilsky ML: Diagnosis and treatment of Wilson's disease. *Pediatr Transpl*. 2002;6:15.

Schmahmann JD, ed. *The Cerebellum and Cognition*. *Int Rev Neurobiol*. Vol 41. San Diego: Academic Press; 1997.

Schmahmann JD: The cerebrocerebellar system. *Int Rev Psychiatry*. 2001;13:247.

Schmahmann JD, Sherman JC: The cerebellar cognitive affective syndrome. *Brain*. 1998;121:561.

Schulz JB, Klockgether T, Petersen D, Jauch M, Müller-Schauenburg W, Spieker S, Voigt K, Dichgans J: Multiple system atrophy: Natural history, MRI morphology, and dopamine receptor imaging with 123-IBZM-SPECT. *J Neurol Neurosurg Psychiatry*. 1994;57:1047–1056.

Schuurman AG, van den Akker M, Ensinck KTJL, Metsemakers JFM, Knottnerus JA, Leentjens AFG, Buntinx F: Increased risk of Parkinson's disease after depression. A retrospective cohort study. *Neurology*. 2002;58:1501.

Simard M, van Reekum R, Cohen T: A review of the cognitive and behavioral symptoms in dementia with Lewy bodies. *J Neuropsychiatry Clin Neurosci*. 2000;12:425.

Tison F, Yekhlef F, Chrystostome V, Balestre E, Quinn NP, Poewe W, Wenning GK: Parkinsonism in multiple system atrophy: Natural history, severity (UPDRS-III), and disability assessment compared with Parkinson's disease. *Mov Disord*. 2002;17:701.

Weiner WJ, Lang AE, eds. *Behavioral Neurology of Movement Disorders* in *Advances in Neurology Series*. Vol 65. New York: Raven Press; 1995.

*Wichmann T, Vitek JL, DeLong MR: Parkinson's disease and the basal ganglia: Lessons from the laboratory and from neurosurgery. *Neuroscientist*. 1995;1:236.

Wolters ECH, Scheltens PH, Berendse HW, eds. *Mental Dysfunction in Parkinson's Disease II*. Utrecht: Academic Pharmaceuticals Productions; 1999.

▲ 2.7 Neuropsychiatric Aspects of Multiple Sclerosis and Other Demyelinating Disorders

RUSSELL T. JOFFE, M.D.

The demyelinating disorders, including *multiple sclerosis* (MS), are a heterogeneous group of disorders of the central nervous system (CNS), which share a common pathology, namely, the partial or complete loss of the myelin sheath surrounding axons in the white matter of brain and spinal cord. As these axons are widely disseminated throughout the brain and spinal cord, lesions may occur diffusely, resulting in complex and widespread neurological symptoms.

The etiology of the demyelinating disorders is diverse and largely conforms to the traditional, binary classification of etiology of disorders, that is, congenital and acquired. Under the congenital disorders are included presumed genetic and chromosomal abnormalities. The chromosomal abnormalities include the gangliosidoses, such as Tay-Sachs disease, which usually presents in infancy or early childhood. Another group of disorders includes the leukodystrophies, of which there are numerous subtypes, such as metachromatic, globoid cell, and adrenoleukodystrophy, as well as Hurler's syndrome. Among the acquired conditions, there are a variety of demyelinating disorders. These include infectious disease, particularly acquired immune deficiency syndrome (AIDS); trauma, including open and, especially, closed brain trauma; vascular disorders, including the vascular dementias; toxins, including alcohol and other solvents; and autoimmune disorders, the most prominent of which is MS. This list is certainly not inclusive, and many disease types may cause a demyelinating encephalopathy. By far, the most common of these disorders is MS. This disease is described in greater detail.

MULTIPLE SCLEROSIS

MS is a demyelinating disorder of the brain and spinal cord that has been described in the literature for more than 150 years. The French neurologist Jean-Martin Charcot first established diagnostic criteria for MS in the middle of the 19th century. His original diagnostic triad is now known not to be specific, and, in fact, over the years, numerous other diagnostic criteria were developed, all of which had a lack of specificity for the illness, thus including many false positives.

The epidemiology of MS has been studied in most countries, but a clear geographic distribution remains difficult to clarify. The highest prevalence rates appear to occur in whites of northern European descent and in the United States, where a clear north–south gradient has been demonstrated. The disease is particularly rare in certain Asian populations, such as Uzbekistans, native Siberians, North and South American Indians, Chinese, and Japanese, as well as African Americans and New Zealand Maoris. The data suggest more than just a geographical vulnerability, but also strong genetic influences. The disease is far more common in women and, most commonly, is diagnosed in the age group of 20 to 50 years of age.

The diagnosis of MS is a largely clinical one, although the advent of magnetic resonance imaging (MRI) has greatly supported, but not superseded, the clinical diagnosis. MRI is not always specific for the diagnosis of MS and may lead to false-positive diagnosis if it is relied on exclusively.

Currently, the diagnosis of MS is clinically defined as the presence of two attacks, involving different parts of the CNS, separated by a period of at least 1 month, and lasting a minimum of 24 hours. The laboratory support for the diagnosis of MS, apart from MRI lesions, consists of demonstration in cerebrospinal fluid (CSF) of at least two oligoclonal bands or increased CNS synthesis of immunoglobulin G (IgG). In addition to this evidence, evoked potentials, particularly visual or somatosensory evoked potentials, are slowed or absent and may contribute or support the clinical diagnosis. The clinical diagnostic criteria specified allow one to distinguish MS from disseminated encephalomyelitis, which is most commonly a single episode of illness, with all lesions occurring within a few weeks, although multiple separate lesions do sometimes occur. The initial symptoms of MS are nonspecific and heterogeneous and may include a broad range of somatosensory, ocular, and motor symptoms. The motor symptoms could include transient hemiparesis and various forms of seizure, among others. Symptoms of cerebellar dysfunction may occur, including scanning speech, gait ataxia, and various tremors. Although these are common in the initial presentation, almost any neurological symptom can be the first presentation of MS.

MS has a variable course over time. The most common course is the relapsing-remitting form. In this type, the patient has relapses of illness that can present with a broad range of neurological symptoms leading to remission and almost complete recovery. The secondary progressive form may evolve from the relapsing-remitting form, leading to incomplete recovery after acute exacerbations of illness. Occasionally, the secondary progressive form can occur at the outset of the illness, and the disorder then takes on a chronic progressive nature. The last type is quite uncommon, occurring in no more than 10 percent of cases, and is known as the *primary progressive type* in which there is a steady worsening of course from the outset of the disease. This form may be rapidly progressive and is rarely seen in patients younger than 40 years of age.

The relationship between these different forms is not clearly understood, and it is uncertain to what extent they represent different types of illness with regard to etiology. The etiology of MS is now more fully understood. It is known to be an autoimmune disorder, whereby T cells and, to a lesser extent, B lymphocytes invade the CNS, attaching to and destroying axons. Damage to the myelin leads to an inflammatory reaction, and resolution of this leads to the formation of plaque in various parts of the brain.

Neuropsychiatric Aspects of Multiple Sclerosis

There are three broad groups of mental symptoms that affect patients with MS. These include (1) fatigue, (2) psychiatric symptoms, and (3) cognitive impairment.

Fatigue Fatigue is one of the most common presenting symptoms of patients with MS. It also substantially contributes to the disability and poor quality of life that these patients experience. Fatigue of MS has been extensively described. It is referred to as a physical fatigue, in which the patient feels unable to perform physical activity because of his or her profound fatigue, as well as mental fatigue, which makes the patient unable to participate in his or her usual activities, including work. The extent of fatigue is not directly related to neurological lesions as seen by the MRI nor to the degree of disability or neurological dysfunction. It is estimated that more than 80 percent of patients with MS complain of fatigue as one of their most predominant symptoms.

Fatigue in MS appears to have a reverse diurnal rhythm in that it is worse as the day progresses. Furthermore, heat, exhaustion, and stress may also aggravate the fatigue associated with MS. Patients often learn to alter their lifestyle and to do much of their activities early in the day before the fatigue of the later day and evening becomes disabling.

The reason for the etiology of fatigue in MS remains an area of active research. There are no clear etiological factors identified. In particular, the fatigue does not appear to be related to depression, in which fatigue is also a common symptom. Treatment of depression does not necessarily alleviate the symptom of fatigue, which is often the most prominent symptom for the MS patient. A broad range of psychiatric symptoms may occur in patients with MS. The most prominent among them are mood symptoms, particularly depression. A large number of patients with MS report symptoms of depression. When the diagnosis of major depressive disorders is considered, MS patients experience a high rate of this psychiatric illness. Various studies have reported that between 20 and 50 percent of patients with MS have a major depression at some point during the course of their illness.

Psychiatric Symptoms The occurrence of depressive symptoms or a major depressive syndrome in MS patients is not directly related to severity of illness, location of lesions, neurological symptomology, or degree of disability. However, depressive symptomology may substantially add to the disability and the burden of illness associated with MS. Besides the classic features of a major depressive disorder, affective lability, sadness or depression, and debility may be prominent features of the disorder.

Patients with depressive symptoms and, particularly, with major depressive disorders respond to treatment with antidepressants. There are limited data on the use of tricyclic antidepressants. However, these drugs should be used with caution in patients with MS because of their side effects. These particularly include the anticholinergic effects, which can inhibit bladder and bowel function, both of which may already be compromised by the neurological illness. The selective serotonin reuptake inhibitors (SSRIs) offer an alternative and are generally better tolerated by patients with MS. They can substantially improve depressive symptoms or the depressive syndrome and improve quality of life and functioning.

In addition to depression, the syndrome and the symptoms, it has been observed that bipolar affective disorder may occur to a greater degree in patients with MS. This may be a phenomenon secondary to the MS with periods of depression, alternating with periods of emotional dyscontrol or irritability. In addition, in bipolar patients with a rapid-cycling course, the possibility of MS as a course-modifying factor for the bipolar disorder should be seriously considered.

In addition to mood symptoms, any CNS illness, including the demyelinating disorders, as well as MS, can lead to a broad range of heterogenous psychiatric symptoms, such as psychosis, anxiety, and cognitive difficulties, among others.

Cognitive Impairment Cognitive impairment is common in patients with MS. It has been estimated that as many as 70 percent of patients with MS show evidence of cognitive impairment on an appropriate battery of neuropsychological tests. As with other psychiatric symptoms, there are inconclusive data to support a clear correlation between these cognitive difficulties and other clinical variables, such as neurological dysfunction, CNS lesions, and degree of disability. Nonetheless, cognitive symptoms contribute substantially to the dysfunction and to poor quality of life that occurs in patients with MS.

Cognitive dysfunction in MS may be broad based and may include many different features. For example, all aspects of memory function may be impaired. Moreover, higher-order functions, such as information processing or executive function, may also be impaired, and there is evidence in some cases of MS of subcortical dementia. In addition, abnormalities of attention and concentration may be evident, and these may contribute substantially to work impairment. Abnormalities of language are less common, although some dysfunction may be determined on broad-based neuropsychological tests. Tests of intelligence quotient (IQ) yield substantial deficits, although scores on tests of verbal IQ are generally higher than on performance IQ.

Most of the studies of cognitive impairment in MS are cross-sectional in nature. There are limited data on longitudinal course of cognitive difficulty. In general, however, these studies show a gradual decline in all aspects of cognitive function in the patient with MS.

MS presents a substantial challenge as far as differential diagnosis is concerned. In those with the common relapsing-remitting course of illness, together with typical clinical, paraclinical, and laboratory, as well as MRI, findings, the diagnosis is easily made. However, in atypical cases, differential diagnosis can be difficult. This applies particularly at the onset of the disease, during the first episode, when the conventional clinical criteria are hard to apply. With the first attack of MS, it is difficult to differentiate this illness from the other demyelinating disorders.

Differential Diagnosis

There are a variety of other conditions to consider in the differential diagnosis. These include

A single episode of acute disseminated encephalomyelitis: factors that may point to this diagnosis include systemic symptoms, signs of cortical dysfunction, and, perhaps, bilateral optic neuritis. MRI may be quite characteristic of this disorder and helps distinguish it from MS.

Cerebral vasculitis: This has numerous courses. They include primary *cerebral vasculitis*, which is extremely rare, associated with *systemic lupus erythematosus*, AIDS, *lymphoproliferative disorders*, and *Wegener's granulomatosis*. Various ancillary laboratory findings may help distinguish these various forms of disease. Rarer forms of vasculitis may include Behçet's disease and also *CNS sarcoidosis*.

The leukodystrophies: These disorders are characterized by the accumulation of unchanged saturated fatty acids, which are detectable in plasma or fibroblasts and include adrenoleukodystrophy, which may have an adult-onset form. These conditions are rare and can usually be identified by the presence of the family history.

Chronic fatigue syndrome: It has been previously emphasized that fatigue is one of the most predominant symptoms of MS. Chronic fatigue syndrome, also known as *fibromyalgia*, requires differentiation, especially if no focal neurological symptoms are found. Failure to elicit specific neurological symptoms, as well as the presence of other associated features of fibromyalgia, including sleep disturbance, myalgias, and arthralgias, among other relatively nonspecific symptoms, is supportive of this diagnosis.

In summary, the diagnosis of MS, particularly a first episode, remains a substantial clinical challenge.

Treatment of Multiple Sclerosis In the last 10 to 15 years, the treatment of MS has evolved from nonspecific symptomatic treatment to specific treatments, which may actually impact the course and prognosis of the disorder.

There are nonspecific symptomatic treatments. As previously mentioned, antidepressants, particularly SSRIs, may be used to treat mood symptoms. Amantadine (Symmetrel) has been used to treat the fatigue with mixed results. Glucocorticoids have been used to treat the acute inflammatory responses associated with the damage to the myelin sheath; although causing some symptomatic relief, they do not impact the long-term course or outcome of the disorder.

The interferon compounds have substantially changed the approach to the treatment of patients with MS. These include interferon-β-1b (Betaseron), interferon-β-1a (Avonex), glatiramer acetate (also known as *copolymer-1* [Copaxone]), and mitoxantrone hydrochloride (Novantrone). These drugs can be classified as *immunosuppressive* or *immunomodulatory agents*. They have substantial impact on the course of illness by reducing the number of relapses, preventing disability, and stabilizing changes observed with MRI. They are, however, only affective to a partial degree in patients with the disorder.

The most common form of MS, the relapsing-remitting form, may be treated with one of several agents. First, interferon-β-1b, a recombinant form derived from bacterial cells, has been shown to reduce annual relapse rates when compared to placebo. In addition to changing the course of the disorder, there are preliminary data that this compound may also ameliorate the cognitive symptoms associated with this form of illness.

The second compound, interferon-β-1a, is also a recombinant form of interferon. It, too, has been shown to reduce disability and relapse in patients with the relapsing-remitting form of illness. Like the previous compound, interferon-β-1a may also have beneficial effects on cognitive function. Another recombinant form of interferon, which is produced in mammalian cells, is identical in structure to the other interferon-β-1a, which is produced in Chinese hamster ovary cells. This compound is also identical in structure to the human interferon-β. This compound has been approved in Canada and Europe but not in the United States, but it has shown similar effects compared to the other two interferon compounds. The fourth compound is glatiramer acetate. This is a four–amino acid polymer. This, too, has effects on reducing relapse and improving disability, and, like the others, it also has stabilizing affects on MRI changes. These interferons have also been applied to other forms of the illness with variable effects but, generally, with some evidence of partial improvement.

CONCLUSION

The demyelinating disorders present a diagnostic challenge. The most common of them, MS, requires differentiation from other disorders because of its distinct clinical presentation and course of illness. Moreover, there are now specific treatments that may reduce relapse rates and degree of dysfunction, and, therefore, a definitive diagnosis is necessary. MS can present with a variety of psychiatric symptoms, particularly depressive symptoms, which may require specific intervention or psychotropic agents.

SUGGESTED CROSS-REFERENCES

Neuroimaging is described in Sections 1.15 and 1.16, neuroanatomy is described in Sections 1.2 and 1.3, schizophrenia is described in Chapter 12, mood disorders are described in Chapter 13, AIDS is described in Section 2.8, exposure to alcohol is described in Section 11.2, and exposure to volatile inhalants is described in Section 11.8.

REFERENCES

Amato MP, Ponziani G, Siracusa G, Sorbi S: Cognitive dysfunction in early-onset multiple sclerosis: A reappraisal after ten years. *Arch Neurol.* 2001;58:1602.

Bashir K, Whitaker JN: Current immunotherapy for demyelinating diseases. *Arch Neurol.* 2001;58:1611.

*Brinar VV: The differential diagnosis of multiple sclerosis. *Clin Neurol Neurosurg.* 2002;104:211.

Feinstein A, Feinstein K: Depression associated with multiple sclerosis: Looking beyond diagnosis to symptom expression. *J Affect Disord.* 2001;66:193.

Gold SM, Schulz H, Monch A, Schulz KH, Heesen C: Cognitive impairment in multiple sclerosis does not affect reliability and validity of self-report health measures. *Mult Scler.* 2003;9:404.

*Holmes G, Kaplan J, Gantz N: Chronic fatigue syndrome: A working case definition. *Ann Int Med.* 1988;108:387.

Janculjak D, Mubrin Z, Brzovicz Z, Birnar V: Change in short-term memory processes in patients with multiple sclerosis. *Eur J Neurol.* 1999;6:1.

Janssens AC, van Doorn PA, de Boer JB, Kalkrs NF, van der Meche FG, Passchier J, Hintzen RQ: Anxiety and depression influence the relation between disability status and quality of life in multiple sclerosis. *Mult Scler.* 2003;9:397.

*Joffe RT, Ippert GP, Gray T, Sawa G, Horvath Z: Mood disorder multiple sclerosis. *Arch Neurol.* 1987;44:376.

Kesseloring J, Miller D, Robb S: Acute disseminated encephalomyelitis, MRI findings and the distinction for multiple sclerosis. *Brain.* 1990;113:291.

Lamberg L: Psychiatric symptoms common in neurological disorders. *JAMA.* 2001;286:711.

McDonald W, Holliday A: Diagnosis and classification of multiple sclerosis. *Br Med Bull.* 1977;33:4.

Miller A, Galboyz Y: Multiple sclerosis: From basic immunopathology to immune intervention. *Clin Neurol Neurosurg.* 2002;104:117.

Minden SL, Roav J, Reich P: Depression in multiple sclerosis. *Gen Hosp Psychiatry.* 1987;9:426.

Minden SL, Schiffer RB: Affective disorders in multiple sclerosis. Review and recommendations for clinical research. *Arch Neurol.* 1990;47:98.

*Mohr DC, Hart SL, Goldberg A: Effects of treatment for depression on fatigue in multiple sclerosis. *Psychosom Med.* 2003;65:542.

Poser CM: Onset symptoms in multiple sclerosis. *J Neurol Neurosurg Psychiatry.* 1995;58:253.

Poser CM, Brinar VV: Multiple sclerosis 2001. *Clin Neurol Neurosurg.* 2002;104:165.

Pugliatti M, Sotgiu S, Rosati G: The worldwide prevalence of multiple sclerosis. *Clin Neurol Neurosurg.* 2002;104:182.

Pullicino PM, Ostrow PT, Kwen PL: Cerebral white matter disease: Imaging, clinical and pathological aspects. *Neurologist.* 1996;2:288.

Rabins PV, Brooks BR, O'Donnell P, Parlson GD, Mobr GP, Jublet B, Coyle P, Dalos N, Folstein MF: Structural brain correlates of emotional disorder in multiple sclerosis. *Brain.* 1986;109:585.

Rao SM, Leo GJ, Burnardin L, Unvrzagt F: Cognitive dysfunction in multiple sclerosis. 1. Frequency, patterns and prediction. *Neurol.* 1991;41:685.

Shafey H: The effect of fluoxetine in depression associated with multiple sclerosis. *Can J Psychiatry.* 1992;37:147.

Triulzi F, Scotti G: Differential diagnosis of multiple sclerosis: Contribution of magnetic resonance techniques. *J Neurol Neurosurg Psychiatry.* 1998;64[Suppl]:6.

Zarei M, Chandran S, Compston A, Hodges J: Cognitive presentation in multiple sclerosis: evidence for a cortico variant. *J Neurol Neurosurg Psych.* 2003;74:872.

*Zephir H, De Seze J, Stojkovic T, Dellise R, Ferriby D, Cabaret M, Vernersch P: Multiple sclerosis in depression. Influence of interferon beta therapy. *Mult Scler.* 2003;9:284.

▲ 2.8 Neuropsychiatric Aspects of HIV Infection and AIDS

Glenn J. Treisman, M.D., Ph.D., Andrew F. Angelino, M.D., Heidi E. Hutton, Ph.D., Jeffrey Hsu, M.D., and Constantine G. Lyketsos, M.D., M.H.S.

The human immunodeficiency virus (HIV) epidemic was identified in the 1980s and neurologists described several HIV-related central nervous system (CNS) syndromes within the first several years of the epidemic. Mental health professionals from nursing, social work, psychology, and psychiatry followed the plight of patients of the epidemic and helped to mobilize interest and galvanize a response. Initially, much of the work focused on grief and loss issues, as well as supportive psychotherapy, but quickly broadened to recognize a number of specific psychiatric conditions, including acquired immune deficiency syndrome (AIDS) dementia, the associated AIDS mania, increased rates of major depression, and psychiatric consequences of CNS injuries.

It is apparent now that psychiatric issues play a central role in this epidemic in developed countries. HIV is transmitted almost entirely by specific risk behaviors, and populations with high rates of these behaviors have been targeted for education and prevention since the mid-1980s. Because of this, HIV, at least in the United States, has become a condition predominantly of vulnerable people who demonstrate difficulty changing behaviors and acting in a safer manner. Whereas transfusion recipients and homosexual men who were unaware of the risk of HIV were the early patients, many current patients are aware of the risks but unable to decrease their risk behaviors because of addictions, personality vulnerabilities, affective disorders, psychological maladaptations, cognitive impairment, social isolation and disenfranchisement, or other barriers to behavioral change. In addition, HIV-infected patients with psychiatric vulnerabilities may have great difficulty in modifying behaviors so as not to infect others. Although there are also cases of infection contracted by single impulsive acts, the impact of psychiatric disorders demands attention and intervention. Moreover, psychiatric disorders lead to vulnerabilities that affect the treatment of HIV infection. Taking medications as prescribed (now referred to as *medication adherence*) is critical to successful treatment of HIV. Psychiatric disorders have been identified as a central barrier to adherence in all the studies that have examined the problem. Thus, the same psychiatric disorders that prevent patients from reducing their risk prevent them from obtaining benefit from their treatment. Untreated patients with high viral loads are more infectious than those on effective treatments with undetectable viral loads, leading to an increased potential for the spread of the HIV epidemic.

This chapter is organized around those conditions commonly seen in the HIV clinic and those that are clearly involved in risk for HIV or that are barriers to HIV treatment. The introductory part of the chapter is a medical overview of HIV. The second part considers psychiatric conditions associated with HIV, and the third part considers related neurological issues that have an impact on psychiatric function and are part of the differential diagnosis of any patient presenting with HIV and psychiatric complaints. For greater detail on psychiatric treatment of HIV patients, please refer to the practice guidelines of the American Psychiatric Association (APA).

OVERVIEW OF HIV INFECTION AND AIDS

Epidemiology HIV was originally recognized through a series of case descriptions involving young homosexual men with *Pneumocystis carinii* pneumonia in the early 1980s in Los Angeles. Subsequently, it became clear that these patients had severe immune system compromise and were vulnerable to infections that had been seen in other immunocompromised individuals. Recent estimates indicate that up to 40 million people are infected worldwide, and another 20 million have died from HIV disease. Currently, 750,000 babies are born each year with HIV infection. Some estimate that 16,000 new infections occur each day, and that one individual is infected with HIV approximately every 10 seconds.

In the United States, there were 711,344 identified cases of HIV by 1999. Most estimates suggest that approximately one million people in the United States are infected with HIV. Some populations within the United States are at increased risk for infection. The originally identified high-risk populations were the so-called 4-H club: *h*omosexual men, *h*eroin (or any intravenous [IV] drug) users, *h*emophiliacs (anyone requiring frequent transfusions), *H*aitians, and *h*ealth care workers (there were five subgroups in the 4-H club). However, the high-risk population has changed. Homosexual men have reduced their high-risk behaviors substantially but, as a group, continue to have high seroprevalence. IV drug users and their sexual partners are currently the population with the greatest risk for infection, particularly among certain racial and ethnic minority populations. Blood product screening has made transfusion risk negligible. Vertical transmission risk from mother to fetus, which occurs in approximately 25 to 30 percent of live births, is influenced by delivery type, severity of HIV, and the availability of antiviral treatment. The frequency of vertical transmission in the United States has decreased dramatically in the last decade but remains a significant problem in many other parts of the world and in some U.S. communities. Efforts at promoting safer sex practices, clean needle and drug paraphernalia use, and prenatal assessment had an impact on behaviors in a great many individuals. However, psychiatric disorders continue to play a significant role in thwarting prevention efforts by making vulnerable patients unable to access or benefit from prevention efforts.

Virology HIV is a single-stranded ribonucleic acid (RNA) virus that selectively infects immune cells, particularly T lymphocytes and macrophages. RNA viruses use several strategies to infect cells and reproduce themselves. HIV is one member of a class of RNA viruses called *retroviruses*, all of which carry the enzyme reverse transcriptase (RNA-dependent deoxyribonucleic acid [DNA] polymerase) in the viral particle and depend on this enzyme for successful infection. Reverse transcriptase synthesizes viral DNA from the viral RNA strand. This DNA is then transported into the nucleus of the cell and directs the production of more viral RNA using the cell's synthetic machinery. This DNA also may become inserted into the cellular DNA (where it is referred to as a *provirus*) and lie dormant, only to be activated at a much later time. The mechanism by which some cells become "latently infected" whereas others become active producers of virus is poorly understood. It is believed that this latent infection is one of the key factors that make it so difficult for HIV infection to be eradicated even when it is adequately treated.

An icosahedral envelope derived from the host cell membrane coats the HIV virus. It is studded with viral gp120 and transmembrane gp41 proteins, which perform specific roles in receptor binding, internalization, and subsequent viral budding. The core contains

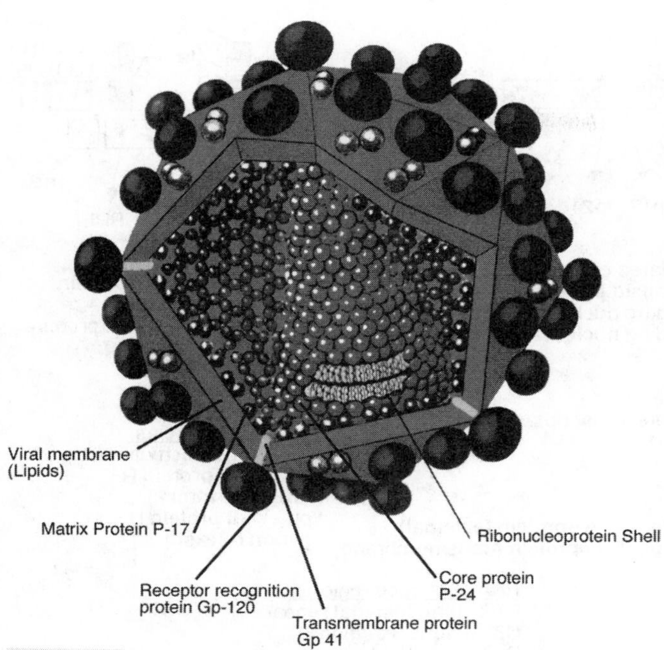

FIGURE 2.8–1 Human immunodeficiency virus viral particle with its lipid envelope. (See Color Plate.) (Courtesy of Milan V. Nermut, M.D., Ph.D., D.Sc.)

two copies of single-stranded viral RNA, several nucleic capsid proteins (p24, p17, p9, and p7), and reverse transcriptase. The virus is most specifically bound by the CD4 receptor on T lymphocytes expressing the CD4 protein (these are usually called *T-helper cells*) and by the CCR5 receptors on macrophages. Patients with certain genetic variants of these receptors may be less susceptible to infection; at least one mutation of the CCR5 receptor has been associated with reduced susceptibility to infection (Fig. 2.8–1).

The steps by which human cells are infected are summarized in Figure 2.8–2. As previously described, virus binds to specific recognition proteins found on the surface of certain cells of the immune system. Once bound, the virus is taken into the cell. At the same time, the outer coating of the viral particle is removed. The enzyme reverse transcriptase carried within the viral particle then begins the process of transcribing the viral RNA into DNA. This DNA moves to the nucleus of the cell where it directs the cell machinery to produce large quantities of viral messenger RNA (mRNA). The viral RNA then uses the cell's own machinery to produce the proteins required to make viral particles and other viral proteins. The viral particles are assembled around viral RNA, and the mature virions bud outward from the cell's surface. Finally, viral particles are cleaved from the cell surface and released into the host to infect other immune cells.

The viral genome of HIV has been extensively investigated. Figure 2.8–3 shows its approximate structure. As can be seen, several critical sites may be targets for medication development. These include the *gag* region that codes for nucleocapsid proteins, the *pol* region that codes for reverse transcriptase and related enzymes, and the *env* region that codes for the surface proteins that allow cell recognition and binding. The *tat* and *rev* proteins regulate the rate of transcription and posttranscriptional activity, respectively. *Nef* seems to enhance the infectivity of HIV and leads to downregulation of expression of CD4 antigen on the cell surface. *Vif* enhances infectivity, *Vpr* promotes nuclear entry of viral transcribed DNA, and *Vpu* enhances viral budding. The exact mechanisms by which the protein products of each of these genes functions are not fully elaborated, and each may have several different actions.

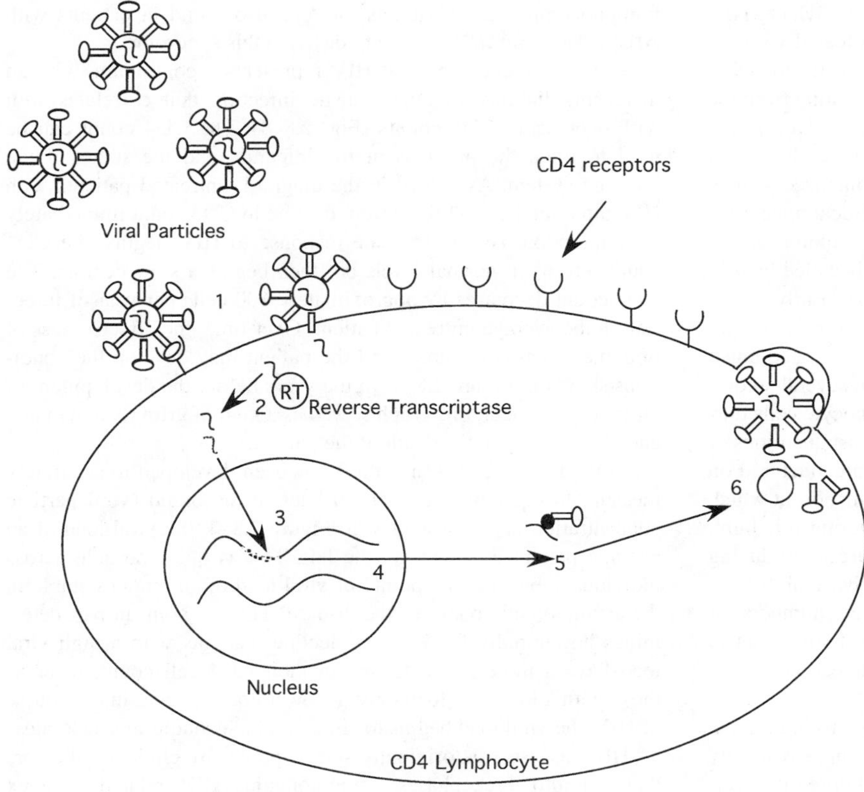

FIGURE 2.8–2 The human immunodeficiency virus life cycle. 1: Viral binding to cell surface receptors and internalization of viral content (site of action of fusion inhibitors). 2: Reverse transcriptase makes viral DNA (site of action of nonnucleoside reverse transcriptase inhibitors and nucleoside reverse transcriptase inhibitors). 3: Viral integration into host genome. 4: Transcription of DNA to RNA. 5: Translation of viral RNA to protein components. 6: Protein processing, cleavage, viral assembly, and budding (site of action of protease inhibitors). (Courtesy of Glenn Treisman, M.D., Ph.D., and Andrew F. Angelino, M.D.)

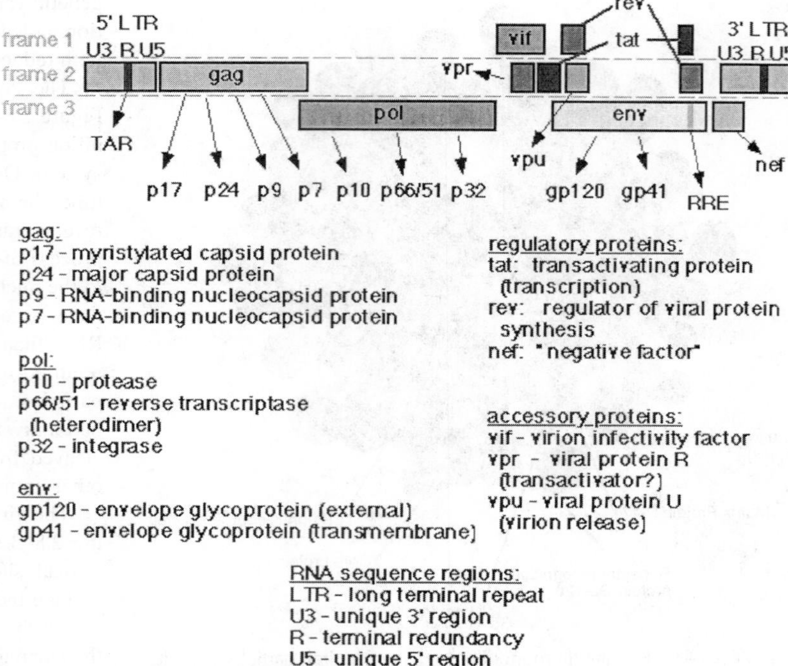

FIGURE 2.8–3 Human immunodeficiency virus 1 (HIV-1) genome organization.

The HIV virus itself is believed to have originated in Africa. It is genetically related to a family of retroviruses that all infect immune cells that have been extensively researched and mapped. The generic term *HIV* usually refers to HIV-1, whereas a second genetically distinct type of human-specific immune virus called *HIV-2* also targets humans. HIV-2 is prevalent in a region in western Africa. Several "species-specific" immune viruses target other animals, and primates are believed to be the original source from which HIV evolved. It has been postulated that humans were infected with the genetically similar simian viruses, and based on genetic mapping and the identification of cases of confirmed infection dating from the late 1950s, the suggestion has been made that HIV evolved in the early 20th century. The hypothesis that HIV was a result of oral polio vaccine trials contaminated by infected chimpanzee kidney cells in the Belgian Congo still has tremendous political appeal for some but seems unlikely to most virologists and epidemiologists.

The retrovirus subfamily to which HIV belongs is called *lentivirus* (from the Latin word *lentus*, which means *slow*). Early in the HIV epidemic, it was believed that HIV was a "slow virus" that integrated into the cell genome and then was latent until activated much later. In the early 1990s, this idea was changed when several studies demonstrated very large rates of turnover of T-lymphocyte cells during the course of HIV infection, with production of vast quantities of virus. Approximately ten billion viral particles are manufactured on an average day. HIV infection is a vicious war of attrition in which the virus gradually depletes the immune system. During this fight, the body mobilizes enormous immune system resources, producing up to two billion CD4 cells a day. HIV has a relatively high transcriptional error rate and therefore produces large numbers of mutants, thus giving rise to strains of virus that can be resistant to drugs, target different cell receptors, and generally defeat the body's strategies for defense.

HIV causes the lysis of CD4 lymphocytes. These cells are critical in cell-mediated immunity. The average person has approximately 1,000 CD4 lymphocytes per mm^3 (or μL) of blood. Before the development of effective treatment for HIV, the average patient's CD4 cell count dropped approximately 100 CD4 cells per mm^3 (or μL) per year, and, thus, over a 10-year course was completely decimated. The immune system becomes quite compromised as the CD4 cell count drops below 200 per μL, and "cellular" immunity diminishes and is finally lost. At this point, the patient becomes vulnerable to opportunistic infections. There are also several tumors that occur in immunocompromised patients that are also found in patients with AIDS. The term *AIDS* is used to describe this syndrome.

It is now recognized that HIV represents a continuum, with an increasing liability to opportunistic infection that correlates well with decreasing CD4 counts (Fig. 2.8–4). The CD4 count can be used to track the progress of the infection and the status of the immune system. As shown in the diagram, untreated patients with HIV infection have a brief severe decline in CD4 count immediately after infection. As the immune response to HIV begins, the CD4 count returns to normal levels but then begins a slow decline. The CD4 count decreases by approximately 100 cells per year of infection in the average untreated patient. Over time, the effectiveness of immune function declines, and the patient may develop the conditions shown in Figure 2.8–4. In the years before the development of effective treatment, this graph served as a kind of grim road map that ended inevitably in the death of the patient.

In the last several years, a test has been developed to accurately measure the quantity of viral particles in the blood (viral particle concentration or "viral load"). In Figure 2.8–4, the viral load of an average patient is shown on the left. This is quite variable across individuals, but the "set point" of viral load often remains stable in the asymptomatic phase of the disease. This set point in part determines how rapidly CD4 counts decline. Patients with a high viral load have a more rapid decline in their CD4 cell count, whereas those with a low viral load have a slower course. Later in the course of HIV, the viral load begins to climb, and the condition accelerates.

HIV disease was originally staged purely by clinical indicators that fell into three phases: asymptomatic, AIDS-related complex

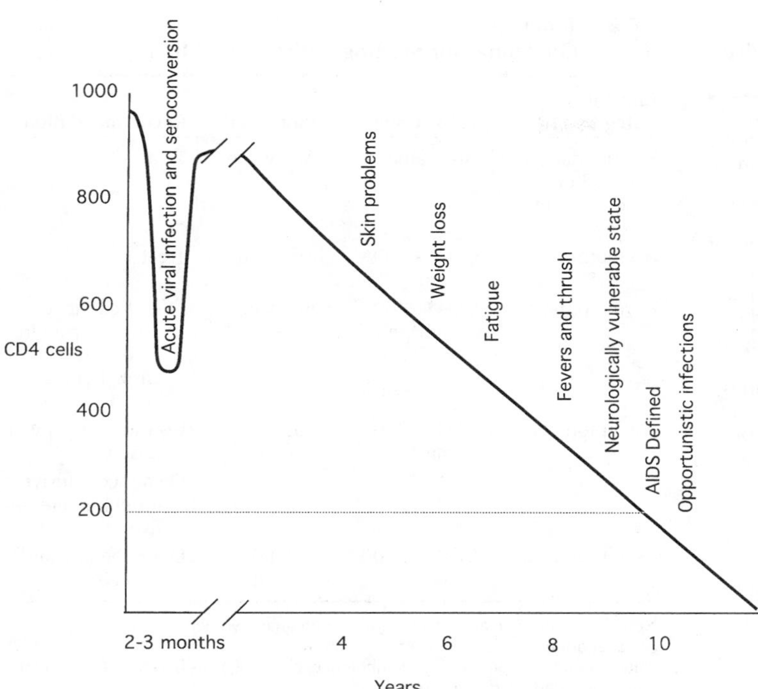

FIGURE 2.8–4 Schematic CD4 count decrease and the points below which opportunistic diseases may be expected to occur. AIDS, acquired immune deficiency syndrome. (Courtesy of John G. Bartlett, M.D.)

(ARC), and, finally, AIDS. More recently, the U.S. Centers for Disease Control and Prevention (CDC) has defined three categories along the lines of the historically relevant clinical stages (Table 2.8–1). Category A includes those with early disease who are either asymptomatic or have only lymphadenopathy or only an acute retroviral syndrome. Category B includes those who were originally referred to as having ARC because they developed conditions shown in Table 2.8–1. Category C includes those often described as having AIDS. These categories are often used as research tools but have been made less relevant by the development of viral particle concentration measurements and CD4 counts. The definition of *AIDS* now is any individual whose CD4 cells have fallen below 200 per μL or individuals with higher CD4 cell counts who develop opportunistic infections. The development of any "AIDS-defining illness" leads to a formal diagnosis even in patients with CD4 counts greater than 200 per μL.

TREATMENT OF HIV DISEASE AND AIDS

Each of the steps in the process of HIV infection provides a potential target for antiviral agents. Reverse transcriptase, an enzyme not normally found in eukaryotic cells, was the target for the first effective HIV drugs. In theory, drugs that inhibit this enzyme should have no impact on normal cellular function because, in normal cells, RNA is not transcribed into DNA. The first agents widely used (such as azidothymidine [AZT]), the nucleoside reverse transcriptase inhibitors (NRTIs; often called *nucs* and pronounced *nukes*), worked to inhibit reverse transcriptase. Two newer types of agents, the nonnucleoside reverse transcriptase inhibitors (NNRTIs, or non-nucs) and, finally, nucleotide reverse transcriptase inhibitors, have all been developed. A later target was the protease enzyme necessary for the virus to be cleaved from the cell membrane and become infective. Another class of antiviral drugs called the *protease inhibitors* (PIs) has been developed, which inhibits the virus at this site. The latest addition to the anti-HIV armamentarium is a fusion inhibitor, enfurvitide (Fuzeon), which inhibits HIV particle fusion to CD4 cells, which is only available as a twice-daily injection and currently is adjunctive to standard therapies.

The treatment of HIV has undergone rapid evolution over the few years since the recognition of the epidemic. Guidelines for initiating therapy and current treatments are shown in Tables 2.8–2, 2.8–3, and 2.8–4. The initial clinical use of these agents began in the late 1980s with AZT (originally called *azidothymidine* and now called *zidovudine*), which delayed the onset of AIDS and prolonged the lives of most patients by approximately 1 to 2 years or led to significant improvement in immune function in some patients. As new agents emerged, they were also deployed sequentially as monotherapy.

In the mid-1990s, several investigations studied combination therapies of two reverse transcriptase inhibitors and a PI. This "triple therapy" was later referred to as *highly active antiretroviral therapy* (HAART). HAART dramatically reduced viral load (often to levels that were undetectable by the standard polymerase chain reaction [PCR] assay of the time) and often resulted in an increase in CD4 cell count. Subsequent studies have shown that extended treatment does not result in a cure but that effective continued treatment results in years or even decades of time with little clinical disease manifestation. This is now understood to be the result of successful suppression of viral production to minimal levels, leading to the production of very few viral mutations. It takes several mutations in the viral genome to produce drug resistance, so in the presence of effective treatment, these mutations occur very slowly.

Currently recommended treatments shown in Table 2.8–3 include those combinations that have been shown to be effective by producing a sustained response in viral load and clinical disease. Most consist of two NRTIs and a third agent that can be an NNRTI, a PI, or another agent. An ideal response to treatment is suppression of viral replication to a level at which virus particles are undetectable by ultrasensitive assay of a patient's serum. If this occurs, patients who continue to take their medications are most likely to continue to have undetectable viral loads without the emergence of resistant mutations. However, even a few missed doses were shown to be associated with viral production and, thus, emergence of mutations. HAART combinations were initially

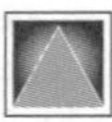

Table 2.8–1
Clinical Categories of Human Immunodeficiency Virus (HIV) Infection

Category A consists of one or more of the conditions listed below in an adolescent or adult (13 years of age or older) with documented HIV infection. Conditions listed in Categories B and C must not have occurred.
- Asymptomatic HIV infection
- Persistent generalized lymphadenopathy
- Acute (primary) HIV infection with accompanying illness or history of acute HIV infection

Category B consists of symptomatic conditions in an HIV-infected adolescent or adult that are not included among conditions listed in clinical Category C and that meet at least one of the following criteria: (1) The conditions are attributed to HIV infection or are indicative of a defect in cell-mediated immunity; or (2) the conditions are considered by physicians to have a clinical course or to require management that is complicated by HIV infection. Examples of conditions in clinical Category B include, but are not limited to
- Bacillary angiomatosis
- Candidiasis, oropharyngeal (thrush)
- Candidiasis, vulvovaginal; persistent, frequent, or poorly responsive to therapy
- Cervical dysplasia (moderate or severe)/cervical carcinoma in situ
- Constitutional symptoms, such as fever (38.5°C) or diarrhea, lasting longer than 1 mo
- Hairy leukoplakia, oral
- Herpes zoster (shingles) involving at least two distinct episodes or more than one dermatome
- Idiopathic thrombocytopenic purpura
- Listeriosis
- Pelvic inflammatory disease, particularly if complicated by tubo-ovarian abscess
- Peripheral neuropathy

You are in Category C (i.e., you have acquired immune deficiency syndrome) if
- Your T cells have dropped below 200, *OR*
- You have had at least one of the following defining illnesses:
  - Candidiasis of bronchi, trachea, or lungs
  - Candidiasis, esophageal
  - Cervical cancer, invasive[a]
  - Coccidioidomycosis, disseminated or extrapulmonary
  - Cryptococcosis, extrapulmonary
  - Cryptosporidiosis, chronic intestinal (more than 1 mo's duration)
  - Cytomegalovirus disease (other than liver, spleen, or nodes)
  - Cytomegalovirus retinitis (with loss of vision)
  - Encephalopathy, HIV related
  - Herpes simplex: chronic ulcer(s) (more than 1 mo's duration); or bronchitis, pneumonitis, or esophagitis
  - Histoplasmosis, disseminated or extrapulmonary
  - Isosporiasis, chronic intestinal (more than 1 mo's duration)
  - Kaposi's sarcoma
  - Lymphoma, Burkitt's (or equivalent term)
  - Lymphoma, immunoblastic (or equivalent term)
  - Lymphoma, primary, of brain
  - *Mycobacterium avium-intracellulare* complex or *Mycobacterium kansasii*, disseminated or extrapulmonary
  - *Mycobacterium tuberculosis*, any site (pulmonary[a] or extrapulmonary)
  - *Mycobacterium*, other species or unidentified species, disseminated or extrapulmonary
  - *Pneumocystis carinii* pneumonia
  - Pneumonia, recurrent[a]
  - Progressive multifocal leukoencephalopathy
  - *Salmonella* septicemia, recurrent
  - Toxoplasmosis of brain
  - Wasting syndrome due to HIV

[a]Added in the 1993 expansion of the acquired immune deficiency syndrome surveillance case definition.

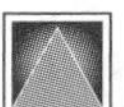

Table 2.8–2
Guidelines for Starting Antiretroviral Therapy

Clinical Category	CD4+ Count	Viral Load	Recommendation
Symptomatic (AIDS or severe symptoms)	Any value	Any value	Treat
Asymptomatic, AIDS	CD4+ <200/mm³	Any value	Treat
Asymptomatic	CD4+ >200/mm³ but <350/mm³	Any value	Offer treatment especially if viral load is >20,000 c/mL, but controversial[a]
Asymptomatic	CD4+ >350/mm³	>55,000 c/mL	Consider therapy or observe[a] Data inconclusive for either alternative
Asymptomatic	CD4+ >350/mm³	<55,000 c/mL	Defer therapy and observe

Note: There are special considerations for pregnant women.
AIDS, acquired immune deficiency syndrome.
[a]Patient readiness, probability of adherence, and prognosis based on CD4 count and HIV load need to be considered.
From Bartlett JG. *Pocket Guide to Adult HIV/AIDS Treatment.* (*in press*), with permission.

quite burdensome for patients, as some drugs required special diets, refrigeration, very specific timing, and large numbers of pills. All of these interfered with the ability of patients to take treatment as prescribed. Newer treatments take advantage of drug combinations, drug–drug interactions that increase blood levels of some medications, and sustained-release preparations.

Several controversial issues face clinicians as they begin to treat a patient for HIV. The first is when to treat patients with HAART in the course of HIV. The second is which antiviral agents to use, and the third is when to change treatment. When HAART therapy was first described, some clinicians hoped that aggressive early treatment would result in a cure. Because there has been little evidence that early treatment has improved the course for patients and because all treatments have significant toxicity, current recommendations for treatment suggest beginning late in the course of HIV. Treatment recommendations are usually based on CD4 cell counts tempered by viral load. Several sets of treatment recommendations from different organizations have had minor differences, but most suggest waiting until CD4 counts fall below 350, a number that has fluctuated over the years. The decision is also tempered by other factors for many clinicians, including patient readiness for treatment evidenced by the ability to adhere to a regimen. In addition, the presence of comorbid diagnoses, such as hepatitis C infection, substance use, psychiatric disorders, and other medical conditions, influence the decision.

The choice of regimen balances the complexity of the regimen, the side effects of the agents, and the type of mutations that arise if a patient develops resistance. It is important to know if the patient has had prior antiretroviral treatment and therefore may have developed resistance already. Specific drugs select for certain mutations, and some of the mutations confer resistance to whole classes of agents, whereas others may actually select for mutations that can increase sensitivity to other drugs. With currently available drugs, clinicians balance convenience and ease of a regimen, ability to preserve treatment options, toxicity and tolerability, and, sometimes, cost in trying to select a regimen.

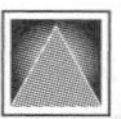

Table 2.8–3
Starting Regimens for Antiretroviral-Naïve Patients

Regimen	Drugs	No. of Pills Per Day
NNRTI-based regimens		
Preferred regimens	Efavirenz + lamivudine + (zidovudine or tenofovir DF or stavudine), except for pregnant women or women with pregnancy potential	3–5
Alternative regimens	Efavirenz + (lamivudine or emtricitabine) + didanosine, except for pregnant women or women with pregnancy potential	3–4
	Efavirenz + emtricitabine + (zidovudine or tenofovir or stavudine[a])	3
	Nevirapine + (lamivudine or emtricitabine) + (zidovudine or stavudine[a] or didanosine)	5
PI-based regimens		
Preferred regimens	Lopinavir/ritonavir + lamivudine + (zidovudine or stavudine)	8–10
Alternative regimens	Amprenavir + ritonavir[b] + (lamivudine or emtricitabine) + (zidovudine or stavudine[a])	4–10
	Atazanavir + (lamivudine or emtricitabine) + (zidovudine or stavudine[a])	4–5
	Indinavir + (lamivudine or emtricitabine) + (zidovudine or stavudine[a])	8–10
	Indinavir + ritonavir[b] + (lamivudine or emtricitabine) + (zidovudine or stavudine[a])	8–11
	Nelfinavir + (lamivudine or emtricitabine) + (zidovudine or stavudine[a])	6–14
	Saquinavir (soft gel capsule or hard gel capsule) + ritonavir + (lamivudine or emtricitabine) + (zidovudine or stavudine[a])	14–16
	Lopinavir/ritonavir + emtricitabine + (zidovudine or stavudine[a])	8–9
Triple NRTI regimen as alternative to PI- or NNRTI-based regimens		
Alternative regimens	Abacavir + lamivudine + (zidovudine or stavudine[a])	2–6

NNRTI, nonnucleoside reverse transcriptase inhibitor; NRTI, nucleoside reverse transcriptase inhibitor; PI, protease inhibitor.
[a]Stavudine is associated with higher rates of lipoatrophy and mitochondrial toxicity than other NRTIs.
[b]Low-dose (100–400 mg) ritonavir.
From Bartlett JG. *Pocket Guide to Adult HIV/AIDS Treatment.* (*in press*), with permission.

Special Considerations

Once-daily regimens
- Preferred: efavirenz + lamivudine + (didanosine or tenofovir DF)
- Alternative:
  - Nevirapine + 2 NRTIs (lamivudine, didanosine, tenofovir DF)
  - Ritonavir boosted saquinavir + 2 NRTIs (lamivudine, didanosine, tenofovir DF)
  - Ritonavir boosted amprenavir + 2 NRTIs (lamivudine, didanosine, tenofovir DF)

Drug interactions
- Rifampin, use:
  - Efavirenz (consider efavirenz dose of 800 mg qd)
  - Nevirapine
  - Saquinavir (as Fortovase or Invirase) 400 mg bid + ritonavir 400 mg bid
  - Substitute rifabutin plus PI in modified doses
- Ribavirin increases levels of didanosine—do not coadminister. Ribavirin increases bone marrow suppression with zidovudine—use combination with caution.
- Methadone levels are decreased by efavirenz and nevirapine—monitor for withdrawal. Nelfinavir, lopinavir/ritonavir, and ritonavir need to be monitored. Methadone decreases buffered didanosine levels—consider using didanosine EC (no interaction).

Acute human immunodeficiency virus infection
- Similar to regimens recommended for chronic human immunodeficiency virus infection.

Women with child-bearing potential
- Avoid efavirenz-based highly active antiretroviral therapy, especially in first trimester.

Several key studies have shown that the single most important factor in successful treatment is the ability to accurately and completely take the prescribed medications. The term *treatment adherence* has replaced the older term *compliance* in the HIV literature and refers to measurements of how accurately patients follow their prescription. Several studies show that adherence correlates highly with treatment success in terms of viral load reduction. Research in this area is complicated by difficulties in accurately assessing adherence. Clinician and patient assessments of adherence are often inaccurate. This problem was circumvented in a study of prison inmates treated with directly observed therapy and mouth checks in which 100 percent of patients were able to achieve undetectable viral loads, presenting some of the strongest evidence that adherence is the key to successful treatment.

Patients who are likely to have poor adherence and therefore do not respond to treatment may be excluded from treatment. These include IV drug users, mentally ill patients, or patients with high risk for poor outcomes, of whom there have been relatively few studies of treatment success. Resources are often scarce in HIV clinics, and patients who are "high-cost users" and "resource intensive," such as the above groups, are the least likely to receive effective treatment. Therefore, the ability to provide adequate psychiatric care to HIV-infected patients is critical for effective treatment of HIV. Psychiatric disorders compromise the ability to take medications, adhere to treatment, practice safer sexual behaviors, and stop using IV drugs. Although they are not the only factors driving the HIV epidemic, they have been largely overlooked as a critical factor in the continued spread of HIV.

Outside of the United States, financial issues have a greater impact on treatment decisions, and the ability to dramatically reduce perinatal transmission with even one drug has complicated public health approaches to HIV care. Also, the pharmaceutical companies have patents and attempt to recover research and development costs and profit on HIV medications, leading some governments to nationalize the manufacture of HIV drugs to reduce costs. In these settings, mental health issues may have an even greater impact on treatment selection decisions.

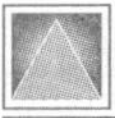

Table 2.8–4
Antiretroviral Regimens or Components That Are Not Generally Recommended

	Rationale	Exception
Antiretroviral regimens not recommended		
Monotherapy	Rapid development of resistance. Inferior antiretroviral activity when compared to combination with 3 or more antiretrovirals.	Pregnant women with HIV-RNA <1,000 copies/mL using AZT monotherapy for prevention of perinatal HIV transmission.
Two-agent drug combinations	Rapid development of resistance. Inferior antiretroviral activity when compared to combination with three or more antiretrovirals.	For patients currently on this treatment, it is reasonable to continue if virologic goals are achieved.
ABC + TDF + 3TC as a triple-NRTI regimen	High rate of virologic failure and resistance.	—
ATV + IDV	Potential for additive hyperbilirubinemia.	No exception.
FTC + 3TC	No potential benefit.	No exception.
Antiretroviral components not recommended as part of antiretroviral regimen		
SQV hard gel capsule (Invirase) as single PI	Poor oral bioavailability (4%). Inferior antiretroviral activity when compared to other PIs.	No exception.
d4T + ddI in pregnancy	Reports of serious, even fatal, cases of lactic acidosis with hepatic steatosis with or without pancreatitis in pregnant women.	When no other antiretroviral options are available and potential benefits outweigh the risks (reasonable to use in unusual circumstances).
Efavirenz in pregnancy	Teratogenic in nonhuman primate.	When no other antiretroviral options are available and potential benefits outweigh the risks (reasonable to use in unusual circumstances).
APV oral solution in (1) pregnant women, (2) children <4 yrs old, (3) patients with renal or hepatic failure, and (4) patients treated with metronidazole or disulfiram	Oral liquid contains large amount of the excipient propylene glycol, which may be toxic in the patients at risk.	No exception.
d4T + AZT	Antagonistic.	No exception.
ddC + d4T or ddC + ddI	Additive peripheral neuropathy.	No exception.
Hydroxyurea	Decreases CD4 count. Augments d4T- and ddI-associated side effects, such as pancreatitis and peripheral neuropathy. Inconsistent evidence of improved viral suppression. Contraindicated in pregnancy (pregnancy category D).	No exception.
Not recommended as part of initial antiretroviral regimen		
APV as single PI	Pill burden of 16 caps/day.	Reasonable to use in unusual circumstances.
DLV	Modest antiretroviral effect.	Reasonable to use in unusual circumstances.
RTV as single PI	Gastrointestinal intolerance.	Reasonable to use in unusual circumstances.
d4T + ddI	Increased peripheral neuropathy, lactic acidosis, and pancreatitis.	Reasonable to use in unusual circumstances.
NFV + SQV	High pill burden of 16–22 caps/day.	Reasonable to use in unusual circumstances.
AZT + ddC	Modest antiretroviral effect.	Reasonable to use in unusual circumstances.

ABC, abacavir; APV, amprenavir; ATV, atazanavir; AZT, zidovudine; ddC, zalcitabine; ddI, didanosine; DLV, delavirdine; d4T, stavudine; FTC, emtricitabine; HIV, human immunodeficiency virus; IDV, indinavir; NRTI, nucleoside reverse transcriptase inhibitor; PI, protease inhibitor; RTV, ritonavir; SQV, saquinavir; 3TC, lamivudine; TDF, tenofovir DF.
From Bartlett JG. *Pocket Guide to Adult HIV/AIDS Treatment.* (*in press*), with permission.

PSYCHIATRIC CONDITIONS IN PATIENTS WITH HIV

Delirium

Delirium is a state of global derangement of cerebral function. It occurs more frequently in medically ill, brain-injured, or metabolically unstable patients. Prevalence of delirium in HIV-infected populations has been reported between 43 and 65 percent. The clinical presentation and significance of delirium in HIV patients are the same as in non-HIV–infected individuals and are characterized by inattention, disorganized thinking or confusion, and fluctuations in level of consciousness. Emotional changes are common and often unpredictable, and hallucinations and delusions are frequently seen. The syndrome has an acute or subacute onset and remits fairly rapidly once the underlying etiology is treated. If untreated, patients have a marked increased risk of mortality, with estimates of approximately 20 percent in hospitalized inpatients.

Aside from general risk factors, such as older age, multiple medical problems, multiple medications, impaired visual acuity, and previous episodes of delirium, patients with HIV-associated dementia are at increased risk to develop delirium. The differential diagnosis of delirium includes HIV-associated dementia, especially with AIDS mania, minor cognitive-motor disorder, major depression, bipolar disorder, panic disorder, and schizophrenia. Delirium can usually be differentiated from the above conditions based on its rapid onset, fluctuating level of consciousness, and link to a medical etiology.

The cause of delirium should be aggressively sought by intensive medical examination. Vital signs and oxygen saturation, careful history and physical examination, laboratory tests, electrocardiogram (ECG), radiological examinations, and critical review of all medications are essential to the workup. Possible etiologies include toxic (poisonings; drugs; and new, recently changed, or interacting medications, especially medications with potent anticholinergic activity), metabolic (electrolyte disturbances), infectious (CNS infections or sepsis), endocrine (especially thyroid and adrenal axes), neoplastic (especially CNS), cardiovascular (myocardial infarction, arrhythmia), neurological (seizure, stroke), pulmonary (hypoxia, hypercapnia), and traumatic (head injury, burns) causes. In toxic/metabolic causes especially, the electroencephalogram (EEG) may show diffuse slowing of the background alpha rhythm, which resolves as confusion clears.

Treatment consists of three parts. The first is the identification and removal of the underlying cause. The second is the reorientation of the patient by maintaining a normal diurnal variation of light cycles; providing orienting stimuli, such as calendars, clocks, and a view of the outside world; and active engagement and reorientation by staff members, family, and friends. The third, if necessary, is the management of behavior or psychosis. Low doses of high-potency antipsychotic agents work well. Newer, atypical antipsychotics are currently being used with some success, but those with more anticholinergic activity may worsen the condition. Benzodiazepines should be used with caution, as they may contribute to delirium in some patients but are of particular use in alcohol or benzodiazepine withdrawal deliria. Physical restraint may be necessary if the patient becomes violent, but all attempts should be made to use this at a minimum, not only because of the legal issues it poses but because restriction of movement or access to orienting stimuli worsens delirium.

HIV-Associated Dementia

Introduction and Neuropathology Early in the AIDS epidemic, some patients presented with rapidly progressing neurocognitive disturbances, leading to an intensive search for etiology. Several CNS opportunistic conditions were identified, including cytomegalovirus (CMV) encephalitis, progressive multifocal leukoencephalopathy (PML), cerebral toxoplasmosis, cryptococcal meningitis, and CNS lymphoma. However, a subset of patients remained for which no identifiable pathogen could be found, and it was deduced that HIV itself was the causative factor behind the dementia. Autopsy studies of demented AIDS patients revealed characteristic white matter changes and demyelinization, microglial nodules, multinucleated giant cells, and perivascular infiltrates but a marked absence of HIV within neurons. This has led to the current theories of neuronal loss through action of macrophages and microglial cells, through activation of cytokines and chemokines that trigger abnormal neuronal pruning, or through both. It appears that basal ganglia and nigrostriatal structures are affected early in the dementia process, with diffuse neuronal losses following. Typical late findings show an approximate 40 percent reduction in frontal and temporal neurons.

Epidemiology, Risk Factors, and Clinical Course The cumulative prevalence of HIV dementia in the lifetime of an infected adult has been reported to be near 15 percent, although the incidence has decreased by approximately 50 percent since the introduction of HAART. HIV-associated dementia is generally seen in late stages of HIV illness, usually in patients who have had a CD4 cell count nadir less than 200 cells per μL. Furthermore, certain risk factors have been associated with eventual development of HIV dementia, namely higher HIV RNA viral load, lower educational level, older age, anemia, illicit drug use, and female sex. High cerebrospinal fluid (CSF) HIV RNA levels may be present in patients with relatively low serum HIV RNA levels and may correlate more directly with severity of neurological deficits.

Clinically, the dementia presents with the typical triad of symptoms seen in other subcortical dementias—memory and psychomotor speed impairments, depressive symptoms, and movement disorders. Initially, patients may notice slight problems with reading, comprehension, memory, and mathematical skills, but because these symptoms are subtle, they may be overlooked or discounted as fatigue and illness. Usually, early cases show impairments in timed trials such as a timed oral trail-making task or grooved pegboard. The Modified HIV Dementia Scale is a very useful bedside screen and can be administered serially to document disease progression. Later, patients develop more global dementia, with marked impairments in naming, language, and praxis.

Motor symptoms are also often subtle in early stages, including occasional stumbling while walking or running; slowing of fine repetitive movements, such as playing the piano or typing; and slight tremor. On examination, patients demonstrate impaired saccadic eye movements, dysdiadochokinesia, hyperreflexia, and, especially in later cases, frontal release signs (grasp, root, snout, and glabellar reflexes). In late stages, motor symptoms may be quite severe, with marked difficulty in smooth limb movements, especially in the lower extremities. Impairments on tests of psychomotor speed in patients at the time of AIDS diagnosis with no memory complaints have been shown to predict development of HIV-associated dementia up to 2 years before memory is affected.

Apathy is a common early symptom of HIV-associated dementia, often causing a noticeable withdrawal by the patient from social activity. A frank depressive syndrome also commonly develops, typically with irritable mood and anhedonia instead of sadness and crying spells. Sleep disturbances are common, as is weight loss. Restlessness and anxiety may be complicating factors. Psychosis develops in a significant number of patients, typically with paranoid ideas, although hallucinations are seen. In approximately 5 to 8 percent of patients, a syndrome known as *AIDS mania* develops. Overall, HIV-associated dementia is rapidly progressive, usually ending in death within 2 years.

Treatment of HIV-Associated Dementia Initial open-label studies using AZT (zidovudine, Retrovir) showed promising results, with patients improving on neuropsychological tests. At first, it was believed that only antiretroviral agents with good penetration into the CNS would be useful in treating HIV-associated dementia, but later efforts revealed that HAART in many different combinations, including in those with poor CNS levels, could provide some relief. Patients started on HAART may improve clinically, and magnetic resonance imaging (MRI) confluent signal abnormalities in the deep white matter may reverse. Further, studies have shown a normalization of cerebral metabolites associated with progression of dementia after 9 months of treatment with HAART.

Standard of care for patients with HIV-associated dementia is to ensure an optimal HAART regimen and treat associated symptoms aggressively. Depression can be treated with standard antidepressants, and in some cases, methylphenidate (Ritalin) or other stimulants may be useful in treatment of apathy. Safety assessments should be done when indicated, and patients requiring intensive monitoring should be referred to appropriate facilities.

Minor Cognitive-Motor Disorder Whereas HIV-associated dementia is a late-stage disorder, there is a less severe neurocognitive disorder emergent in earlier HIV infection known as *minor cognitive-motor disorder* or *mild neurocognitive disorder.* The symptoms of minor cognitive-motor disorder are often overlooked, as they may be very subtle, but they are essentially mild manifestations of the same symptoms seen in HIV-associated dementia: cognitive and motor slowing. Often, the disorder is discovered as a result of a singular minor complaint by a patient, such as taking longer to read a novel; dysfunction when performing fine motor tasks, such as playing the piano; an increased tendency to stumble or trip; or more mistakes when balancing the checkbook. The disorder is confirmed when mild impairments are present in at least two of the following domains: verbal/language, attention, memory (recall or new learning), abstraction, and motor skills.

Prevalence data for minor cognitive-motor disorder are variable, often suggesting up to 60 percent prevalence by late-stage AIDS. Prevalence in earlier stages is not well defined, but the disorder has been anecdotally reported preceding a diagnosis of AIDS by 11 years. Whether minor cognitive-motor disorder predisposes to HIV-associated dementia is also of some debate. It appears that some patients may continue to have minor problems, whereas another group progresses to frank dementia.

With regard to treatment, there are no controlled data available. HAART may be of some benefit in slowing progression, but this conclusion is confounded by a lack of understanding of factors that lead some patients to progress, whereas others remain static.

Major Depression

Epidemiological Considerations Depressive symptoms are the most common complication of chronic medical illness. Depression has a negative impact on adherence with medical treatments, quality of life, and treatment outcome. Despite all of this important evidence, depression remains underrecognized, underdiagnosed, and undertreated in medical clinics. Depression is a significant problem in HIV/AIDS. The question of whether there is increased incidence and prevalence of major depression in HIV-infected patients has been a controversial topic. Several factors complicate this issue. First, identification of major depression as a specific condition, as opposed to the assessment of depressive symptoms, is a methodological barrier to cross-sample comparison. Additionally, populations at risk for HIV infection have elevated rates of major depression. High rates of major depression have been found in homosexual men and patients with substance use disorders. A recent metaanalysis of ten studies comparing HIV-positive and at-risk HIV-negative patients demonstrated a twofold increase in the prevalence of major depression in patients infected with HIV.

Major depression is a risk factor for HIV infection by virtue of its impact on behavior, intensification of substance abuse, exacerbation of self-destructive behaviors, and promotion of poor partner choice in relationships. In this way, depression can be seen as a vector of HIV transmission. Depression has been clearly shown to hinder effective treatment of infected individuals. Patients with major depression have been shown to be at increased risk for disease progression and mortality. HIV increases the risk of developing major depression through a variety of mechanisms, including direct injury to subcortical areas of brain, chronic stress, worsening social isolation, and intense demoralization. Although direct evidence for a relationship between worsening HIV disease and the development of major depression is limited, there are several studies that support this link, particularly the study based in the Multicenter AIDS Cohort Study (MACS) showing that there is a two and one-half–fold increase in rates of depression as patients' CD4 cell counts fall below 200 per μL just before they develop AIDS.

Taken together, these lines of evidence suggest that HIV is a causal factor in depression and that depression is a causal factor in the transmission of HIV and in HIV morbidity, making the patients with these disorders a treatable vector for the HIV epidemic and suggesting an important role for mental health care in HIV treatment and prevention.

Differential Diagnosis of Major Depression The differential diagnosis of depression includes nonpathological states of grief and mourning (sometimes made quite severe by the vulnerabilities of the person) and a variety of disorders related to both psychological and physiological disturbances. Patients with complaints of depressive syndromes can have dysthymia, dementia, delirium, demoralization, intoxication, withdrawal, CNS injury or infection, acute medical illness, and a variety of other conditions. AIDS dementia and other HIV-related CNS conditions can produce a flat, apathetic state that is often misdiagnosed as depression. Cocaine withdrawal produces a depressive syndrome, and delirium can mimic many psychiatric conditions. CNS syphilis, a condition that had become quite rare, has been reappearing in medical centers with HIV specialty services and remains "the great imitator" as it was called when it was originally described.

The diagnosis of major depression in the HIV clinic is complicated by the high frequency of depressive symptoms that are associated with chronic illness, significant losses and isolation, and complex medical treatments. The diagnosis may be further complicated by the presence of comorbid neurological illness, comorbid substance use, and the use of many medications that can alter mental function. Despite this, studies of patients with major depression have shown that the response to treatment is similar to that expected in other populations.

Mood is the feature of affective life that describes the prevailing emotional tone a patient experiences. Patients express depression as feeling blue, low, sad, or, sometimes, flat, devoid of emotion, or empty. A patient may say that he or she is miserable, in agony, anxious, worried, or angry, upset, and irritable. Although some are apathetic, most find the state extremely uncomfortable. Moods may vary with the time of day but are usually worse in the morning and better in the afternoon; sometimes, other patterns may occur. Pleasure (or a sense of reward) is associated with many behaviors of life, including those driven by appetite, such as sleeping, eating, and sex, and those associated with function, such as work, hobbies, dress, social activity, and artistic expression. This is suppressed or absent in depression and is a cardinal feature.

Vital sense is the subjective sense of well-being. Depressed patients say they are sick, have a heavy pressure in their chest, have low energy, and even feel themselves dying. *Self-attitude* is the feelings directed at the self. Depressed patients feel guilty, that they are bad or evil, that they are undeserving of things they have, or that they have failed those they love.

Neurovegetative symptoms are commonly associated with this cardinal syndrome. These include difficulties with sleep, appetite, concentration, and memory. Sleep disturbances can include insomnia or hypersomnia, but most characteristically, patients describe waking early in the morning with difficulty falling back to sleep. Appetite may be decreased or increased significantly, and patients often complain that food has lost its flavor. Appetite changes result in corresponding weight changes if untreated for long periods. Patients report slowed thought processes, with impairments in concentration and short-term memory and, occasionally, generalized confusion.

HIV patients with major depression frequently present to internists and family practitioners with multiple somatic symptoms. These include, but are not limited to, headache, gastrointestinal (GI) disturbances, inexplicable musculoskeletal or visceral pain, cardiac symptoms, dizziness, tinnitus, weakness, and anesthesia. Given the burdens of HIV, the medical problems associated with it, and the side effects of medications, depression may be very low on the list of considered causes of the patient's complaint. Even patients complaining of depressive symptoms may have depression overlooked or discounted due to the presence of a plethora of other diagnoses. Nonspecific somatic symptoms are often the result of depression rather than HIV infection in patients who do not have concurrent medical illness.

As an example, fatigue has been found to be associated with depression and not HIV progression. Worsening of fatigue and insomnia at 6-month follow-up was highly correlated with worsening depression but not CD4 count, change in CD4 count, or disease progression by CDC category. These findings support the notion that somatic symptoms generally suggestive of depression should trigger a full psychiatric evaluation. In later-stage HIV infection, a variety of illnesses are common, often moving depression down on the differential diagnosis list. Somatic symptoms should always be evaluated carefully and considered in context—that is, either with other indicators of progression of HIV or with other indicators of depression.

Certain HIV-related medical conditions and medications can cause depressive symptoms. These include CNS disorders such as toxoplasmosis, cryptococcal meningitis, lymphoma, syphilis, and others. Some investigators have found significant rates of depressive symptoms among male HIV patients with low testosterone levels. A number of treatments used for HIV disease or comorbid conditions—efavirenz (Sustiva), interferon, metoclopramide (Reglan), clonidine (Catapres), propranolol (Inderal), sulfonamides, anabolic steroids, corticosteroids, muscle relaxants, and many others—have all been reported to produce major depression or similar syndromes. Although these depressive syndromes often respond to withdrawal of the offending drug, when they do not, they should be treated as major depression with appropriate antidepressant medication. The experience with the depressive syndromes caused by efavirenz and interferon indicates that treatment with antidepressant medications is well tolerated and often necessary for success.

Routine screening for psychiatric disease in HIV clinical patients can effectively preempt urgent referrals for rapidly progressing disorders. Several screening tools for depression in medical settings have been studied, and in one study specifically looking at HIV-infected patients, the combination of two brief self-administered questionnaires, the Beck Depression Inventory (BDI) and the General Health Questionnaire (GHQ), prospectively predicted a psychiatric disorder (other than substance abuse) with a sensitivity of 81 percent, specificity of 61 percent, and positive predictive value of 71 percent.

Treatment of Major Depression

PHARMACOTHERAPEUTIC TREATMENT Pharmacotherapy is the mainstay of treatment for major depression. Several studies have demonstrated efficacy of various antidepressant agents in HIV patients, but no single antidepressant has been found superior in treating HIV-infected patients as a group.

Aside from how well the pharmacology of the antidepressant matches a patient's disease, the engine that drives effectiveness is patient adherence. Patients who reliably take adequate doses of antidepressants have the best chance of improvement. A general rule is to start at low doses of any medication, titrating up to a "full" dose or therapeutic serum level (when meaningful) slowly, so as to minimize early side effects that may act as obstacles to adherence.

Table 2.8–5 lists antidepressants often used in HIV disease, their dosages, and common side effects. In many patients, side-effect profiles of certain agents may be used to an advantage, and these "good-match" agents should be tried first. Second choices are medications that do not have side effects that might worsen the patient's symptoms (e.g., a medication that is not associated with insomnia for a patient having difficulty falling asleep). Later choices include medications that have side-effect profiles that would likely exacerbate a patient's symptoms (e.g., a medication associated with increased GI motility for a patient with chronic diarrhea).

The first week of treatment with a medication usually determines whether a patient is able to tolerate the medication at all. After this brief period, the dosage of any antidepressant should be increased slowly to either a typical full dose or a therapeutic serum level. Once at this level, patients should be encouraged to wait as long as possible for the therapeutic effect, which may take longer than 6 weeks to achieve in some patients. Side effects should be assessed at every visit, and attempts should be made to treat any side effects the patient finds bothersome. For example, insomnia caused by selective serotonin reuptake inhibitors (SSRIs) may respond well to low doses of trazodone (25 to 150 mg at bedtime). Constipation from a tricyclic antidepressant (TCA) often is relieved by increased water and fiber intake. Sexual side effects from SSRIs are common; impotence may be treated with sildenafil (Viagra) in select patients, whereas decreased libido and delayed orgasm may be alleviated with a drug holiday or by the addition of bupropion (Wellbutrin), buspirone (BuSpar), cyproheptadine (Periactin), or ginkgo biloba.

Patients who show only partial response to antidepressant medication should be offered an augmentation strategy or an alternative treatment. There are several agents that have been used for antidepressant augmentation. The best studied is lithium, but its side-effect profile often prevents its use in the HIV setting. Thyroid preparations, especially L-triiodothyronine, have also been shown to be of benefit and may be of particular advantage in patients complaining of fatigue. Olanzapine (Zyprexa), risperidone (Risperdal), and pindolol (Visken) have also been reported to be effective augmenting agents, although many others have also been used without support from the literature, including a second antidepressant, other mood stabilizers, trazodone, other antipsychotic medications, methylphenidate, benzodiazepines, sleep deprivation, and bright light therapy.

If no benefit is gained from the primary antidepressant, even after augmentation, or if it must be abandoned due to intolerable side effects, a new primary agent should be chosen, titrated slowly, and augmented as necessary. Although medications in the same class may produce similar side effects and, therefore, may not be tolerated, there is evidence to suggest that a response may be seen from one drug when none was seen from another in the same class.

Finally, clinicians often wonder about the interaction of antidepressant medications and HAART medications. Some potential interactions are listed in Table 2.8–4, but two points deserve emphasis. First, because depression is associated with reductions in adherence to HAART, untreated depression may be equally or more detrimental to disease progression than any medication interaction. Second, experience in working with comorbid HIV and depression has not yet shown clinical significance to the drug–drug interaction—that is, need for dose adjustments for either antidepressants or HAART for successful outcomes.

PSYCHOTHERAPEUTIC TREATMENT Psychotherapy is an important and integral part of the treatment of major depression. Treatment

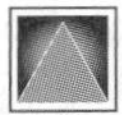

Table 2.8–5
Antidepressant Use in HIV-Infected Patients

Drug	Starting Dosage	Usual Therapeutic Dosage	Serum Level	Advantages	Interactions with HIV Medicines
Nortriptyline (Pamelor)	10–25 mg qhs	50–150 mg qhs	70–125 ng/dL	Promotes sleep, weight gain, decreases diarrhea	Increases nortriptyline levels: fluconazole, lopinavir/ritonavir, ritonavir
Desipramine (Norpramin)	10–25 mg qhs	50–200 mg qhs	>125 ng/dL	Promotes sleep, weight gain, decreases diarrhea	Increases desipramine levels: lopinavir/ritonavir, ritonavir
Imipramine (Tofranil)	10–25 mg qhs	100–300 mg qhs	>225 ng/dL	Promotes sleep, weight gain, decreases diarrhea	Increases imipramine levels: lopinavir/ritonavir, ritonavir
Amitriptyline (Elavil)	10–25 mg qhs	100–300 mg qhs	200–250 ng/dL	Promotes sleep, weight gain, decreases diarrhea	Increases amitriptyline levels: lopinavir/ritonavir, ritonavir
Clomipramine (Anafranil)	25 mg qhs	100–200 mg qhs	150–400 ng/dL	Promotes sleep, weight gain, decreases diarrhea	Increases clomipramine levels: lopinavir/ritonavir, ritonavir
Doxepin (Sinequan)	10–25 mg qhs	150–250 mg qhs	100–250 ng/dL	Promotes sleep, weight gain, decreases diarrhea	Increases doxepin levels: lopinavir/ritonavir, ritonavir
Fluoxetine (Prozac)	10 mg qam	20 mg qam	Unclear	Activating	Increases HIV medication levels: amprenavir, delavirdine, efavirenz, indinavir, lopinavir/ritonavir, nelfinavir, ritonavir, saquinavir; decreases fluoxetine levels: nevirapine
Sertraline (Zoloft)	25–50 mg qam	50–150 mg qam	Unclear	—	Increases sertraline levels: lopinavir/ritonavir, ritonavir
Citalopram (Celexa)	20 mg qam	20–60 mg qam	Unclear	—	Increases citalopram levels: lopinavir/ritonavir, ritonavir
Escitalopram (Lexapro)	10 mg qam	20 mg qam	Unclear	—	Unknown
Paroxetine (Paxil)	10 mg qhs	20–40 mg qhs	Unclear	Somewhat sedating	Increases paroxetine levels: lopinavir/ritonavir, ritonavir
Fluvoxamine (Luvox)	50 mg qhs	150–250 mg qhs	Unclear	Somewhat sedating	Increases HIV medication levels: amprenavir, delavirdine, efavirenz, indinavir, lopinavir/ritonavir, nelfinavir, ritonavir, saquinavir; decreases fluvoxamine levels: nevirapine
Venlafaxine XR (Effexor)	37.5 mg qam	75–300 mg qam	Unclear	—	Increases venlafaxine levels: lopinavir/ritonavir, ritonavir
Mirtazapine (Remeron)	7.5–15.0 mg qhs	15–45 mg qhs	Unclear	Promotes sleep, weight gain	—
Nefazodone (Serzone)	50 mg b.i.d.	300–400 mg/day in divided doses	Unclear	Somewhat sedating	Increases HIV medication levels: efavirenz, indinavir
Trazodone (Desyrel)	50–100 mg qhs	50–150 mg qhs for sleep; 200–600 mg qhs for depression	Unclear	Promotes sleep	Increases trazodone levels: lopinavir/ritonavir, ritonavir
Bupropion SR (Wellbutrin)	100 mg qam	150–400 mg/day in divided doses	Unclear	Activating, no sexual side effects	—

HIV, human immunodeficiency virus.

with medication plus psychotherapy has been shown to be more effective for patients than either modality alone. A major open question continues to be which type of psychotherapy is most appropriate to provide. Among the individual psychotherapies, interpersonal psychotherapy and cognitive-behavioral psychotherapy are quite popular for treatment of depression and have the best evidence to support their efficacy.

The literature on the use of psychotherapy for treatment of depression in HIV patients is extensive, but clinical trial data are sparse. One study showed that imipramine (Tofranil) with either interpersonal or supportive psychotherapy had better efficacy than those therapies used alone. Group cognitive-behavioral therapy has also demonstrated efficacy for HIV patients used alone or in combination with medication. Improvements have been demonstrated as well for HIV patients treated with group cognitive-behavioral therapy either as a single treatment modality or combined with medication.

Supportive psychotherapy helps patients with major depression who interpret their suffering to be a reaction to the diagnosis or morbidity of HIV infection. These patients often believe they can pull themselves out of depression and get frustrated when they continue to expend effort with little result. They need education about the disease nature of their depression, encouragement to keep going, and therapeutic optimism that the treatments will work.

In addition, psychotherapy applied judiciously and in combination with effective antidepressant medication provides patients with a framework for the provider–patient relationship that is so crucial to success. The medical providers who keep the concept of psychotherapy in mind structure their interactions with patients to slowly empower and enable the patients to take control of their lives, thus enabling them to rely on the providers less and less.

Bipolar (Manic-Depressive) Illness

Bipolar disorder is a condition in which patients experience episodic alterations in mood that cause disorder. Manic episodes are associated with increased rates of substance abuse and impulsive behavior, and there has been speculation that bipolar disorder may be a risk factor for HIV infection. To date, there has been no unequivocal evidence to show that bipolar illness directly increases the risk for HIV infection, but the technical difficulties in demonstrating this link are considerable.

In the classic presentation, patients alternate between extended episodes of depression, similar to major depression, and briefer episodes of increased mood, increased energy, and increased confidence and well-being, often with grandiose ideas about themselves and their circumstances. The synonymous appellation "manic-depressive insanity" is a reminder that many patients have auditory hallucinations and frank delusions when they are ill. Most often, patients cycle from one type of mood state to the other, at times interspersed with periods of normal mood, but occasionally show features of both depressive and elevated mood states simultaneously (mixed states) or in very rapid succession (rapid cycling). Milder forms of mania are seen in a condition termed *bipolar illness type II*. The spectrum of bipolar illness is broad, ranging from a severely crippling and chronic mental illness to a mildly disordering alternating experience of prevailing mood. This has made it difficult to accurately measure prevalence and incidence and to explore the relationship of bipolar illness with HIV. Additionally, it is difficult to distinguish severe bipolar illness from schizophrenia even in studies that use rigorous research approaches. Thus, investigators looking at the relationships between HIV and mental illness often use the term *chronically mentally ill* for patients with severe disability from either schizophrenia or bipolar disease.

The elevated mood states form a continuum from increased energy, euphoria, irritability, and decreased sleep called *hypomania* to a more extreme condition complicated by hallucinations, delusions, disordered thinking, and disorganized and sometimes violently agitated behavior called *mania*. Hypomania is characterized by euphoria, an improved self-attitude, and an elevated vital sense. Patients feel elated, energized, and as if they are functioning better than usual. Thoughts speed up and horizons expand, such that the patient feels many brilliant things are coming to him or her in rapid succession. Often, there is a noticeable increase in the amount and speed of speech; interrupting these patients may be necessary and hard to accomplish. Because energy is so high, patients feel a decreased need for sleep and occasionally do not sleep at all. When these symptoms impair judgment and function is lost, the patient is seen to be further down the spectrum in the syndrome of mania. Manic patients not only have pressured speech, they often demonstrate a thought disorder in which ideas come so quickly that it is impossible to see the connections between them, the so-called flight of ideas. The expansive self-attitude may take on proportions outside the realm of reality, known as *grandiose delusions*. Paranoid delusional thoughts may be seen, and hallucinatory experiences occur in some patients.

In contrast to this type of bipolar disorder, there is a type of mania that appears to be specifically associated with late-stage HIV infection and is associated with cognitive impairment and a lack of previous episodes or family history. This syndrome is called *AIDS mania* and may represent a related but different condition. Studies of this form of mania are less common, as HAART has had a significant impact on both the frequency of AIDS dementia and mania.

Mania can occur anytime in the course of HIV infection, but AIDS mania has been described in late HIV infection, allowing stratification of patients with mania into two groups: preexisting bipolar disorder and secondary mania (or AIDS mania), which appears to be a consequence of HIV brain involvement. In general, manic syndromes in HIV patients occur with higher frequencies after the onset of AIDS. Furthermore, AIDS patients develop mania at rates substantially greater than the general population: in one series, 8 percent of all AIDS patients seen at the HIV clinic over 17 months (more than ten times the 6-month general population prevalence). The study grouped mania patients into those whose first manic episode came late in their HIV course with a CD4 count less than 200 cells per μL and those whose episode came early with a CD4 count greater than 200 cells per μL. The late-onset patients were less likely to have a personal or a family history of mania or any mood disorder, which presumably means they were less likely to have bipolar disorder or a genetic predisposition to mania. They were also more likely to have dementia or other cognitive impairment, indicating brain damage.

AIDS mania seems to have a somewhat different clinical profile than bipolar mania. Patients tend to have cognitive slowing or dementia. Without a previous dementia diagnosis, however, this may be difficult to ascertain in the midst of an acute manic episode, and the history usually reveals progressive cognitive decline before the onset of mania. Irritable mood is more characteristic than euphoria. Sometimes, prominent psychomotor slowing accompanying the cognitive slowing of AIDS dementia replaces the expected hyperactivity of mania, which complicates the differential diagnosis. Clinical experience has suggested that AIDS mania is usually quite severe in its presentation and malignant in its course. In one series, late-onset patients had a greater total number of manic symptoms than early-onset patients. They were also more commonly irritable and less commonly hypertalkative. AIDS mania seems to be more characteristically chronic than episodic, has infrequent spontaneous remissions, and usually relapses with cessation of treatment. Because of their cognitive deficits, patients have little functional reserve with which to begin. Also, they are less able to pursue treatment independently or consistently.

One clinically described presentation of mania, either early or late, is the delusional belief that one has discovered a cure for HIV or has been cured. Although this may serve to cheer otherwise demoralized and depressed patients, it may also result in the resumption of high-risk behavior and lead to the spread of HIV and exposure to other infectious entities. When euphoria is a prominent symptom in otherwise debilitated late-stage patients, caregivers may wistfully question the humaneness of robbing patients of the illusion of happiness. It is the clearly impairing, often devastating, effects of the other symptoms of mania that tip the balance of the risk/benefit equation toward treatment.

The treatment of mania in early-stage HIV infection is not substantially different than the standard treatment of bipolar disorder. It relies on the use of mood-stabilizing medications, particularly lithium salts and the anticonvulsants valproic acid (Depakene), carbamazepine (Tegretol), and lamotrigine (Lamictal) and antipsychotic agents, now more commonly atypical agents. These medications decrease manic symptoms and may prevent recurrence.

As HIV infection advances with lower CD4 counts, more medical illnesses, more CNS involvement, and greater overall physiological vulnerability, treatment strategies may be somewhat different. Although treatment with traditional antimanic agents may be preferred, it can be very difficult in patients with advanced disease. AIDS mania patients may respond to treatment with antipsychotic agents alone. In general, late-stage patients are far more sensitive to the therapeutic effects, but even more so to the toxic side effects, of antipsychotic agents. In late-stage disease, the dose of antipsychotic needed may be much lower than customarily used for mania in other settings. The more advanced the patient's HIV or dementia, the more sensitive he or she is to dosage changes that might otherwise seem trivial. These patients can develop extrapyramidal symptoms but also prove very sensitive to the side effects, especially delirium, of anticholinergic agents.

In recent years, the atypical antipsychotics, such as risperidone, olanzapine, quetiapine (Seroquel), and now ziprasidone (Geodon), have taken the place of the older agents. These agents have fewer side effects than traditional antipsychotics but have fewer data and less experience to support their use. The side-effect issue has been important enough that these agents are now first line and may be primary treatment in most advanced cases. Starting doses should be low and titrated to effectiveness.

There has been considerable experience with traditional mood-stabilizing agents in selected AIDS mania patients but with relatively sparse documentation. Lithium use has been problematic for several reasons, including high rates of associated delirium and cognitive difficulty, GI symptoms (including nausea and diarrhea), and polyuria resulting in dehydration. Lithium is also associated with the development of diabetes insipidus in rare patients. The major problem with lithium in AIDS patients has been rapid fluctuations in blood level, occurring even in the hospital on previously stable doses, causing lithium intoxication. Valproic acid has been used with success, titrating to the usual therapeutic serum levels of 50 to 100 ng/dL. Enteric-coated Depakote is better tolerated in most patients. This is sometimes limited by side effects, especially hepatotoxicity in the setting of chronic viral hepatitis. Monitoring of liver function tests is essential, but hepatic toxicity is not often a problem. In cases of severe hepatic *Mycobacterium avium-intracellulare* complex (MAC) infiltration, such as with portal hypertension, valproic acid should likely be avoided, but this and related considerations have not been formally studied. Depakote can also affect hematopoietic function, so white blood cell and platelet counts must be monitored. Carbamazepine may also be effective but more poorly tolerated because of sedation and the presumed potential for synergistic bone marrow suppression in combination with antiviral medications and HIV itself. There are little data for the newer anticonvulsants, such as gabapentin (Neurontin) and lamotrigine (Lamictal), but these agents look promising to some clinicians.

Schizophrenia

The literature on patients with severe and chronic mental illnesses, accounted for primarily by schizophrenia and bipolar I disorder, reports prevalence rates of between 4 percent and 19 percent in both inpatient and outpatient samples. There is no evidence that HIV infection causes schizophrenia, but there are data to show that schizophrenia contributes to behaviors that may lead to HIV infection. Although injection drug use accounts for the majority of infections in many studies, there has also been a wealth of information published regarding the sexual risk factors for patients with schizophrenia. In particular, data reveal high rates of unprotected sex, multiple sex partners, trading sex for money or other goods, and sex while intoxicated. Further, there is evidence that patients with more positive symptoms and impulse control problems are at increased risk for high-risk sexual behavior despite demonstration of adequate knowledge of HIV risk factors.

Practitioners who see patients with schizophrenia should be sensitive to the risk for acquiring HIV and should screen patients carefully for risk behaviors in addition to inquiring about patients' knowledge of HIV transmission routes. A screening tool called the Risk Behaviors Questionnaire (RBQ) consists of 13 questions and has been validated for use in psychiatric patients.

The principles of treatment for HIV-infected patients with schizophrenia follow the same basic principles as any other patient with schizophrenia, namely, control of symptoms with medications and psychosocial support and rehabilitation. In these cases, however, close ties with HIV providers are strongly suggested, so that HIV treatment can be coordinated and monitored.

ISSUES OF PERSONALITY IN PATIENTS INFECTED WITH HIV

A disturbing trend in the HIV epidemic has been the persistence of high-risk behaviors among individuals who are HIV infected. Such individuals, who report high rates of sex or drug risk behaviors, include HIV-infected drug users, patients presenting at HIV primary care clinics for medical treatment, and HIV-infected men who have sex with other men. Apparently, knowledge of HIV and its transmission is insufficient to deter these individuals from engaging in HIV risk behaviors, suggesting that certain personality characteristics may enhance their vulnerability to practice such behaviors.

Traditional approaches in risk reduction counseling emphasize the avoidance of negative consequences in the future, such as using a condom during sexual intercourse to prevent sexually transmitted diseases (STDs). Such educational approaches have proved ineffective for individuals with certain personality characteristics. Effective prevention and treatment programs for HIV-infected individuals must consider specific personality factors that render them vulnerable to practicing risky behaviors that further endanger their health as well as the health of others. This purpose of this section is to review the dimensional nature of personality: extroversion–introversion and stability–instability; outline the role of personality characteristics and personality disorder in HIV risk behavior; and highlight specific interventions to reduce HIV risk behaviors that are formulated for individuals whose personality characteristics place them at increased risk.

Dimensional Nature of Personality

Personality is defined by the emotional and behavioral characteristics or traits that constitute stable and predictable ways that an individual relates to, perceives, and thinks about the environment and the self. Personality is a blend of inherited temperament and learned characteristics. Traits are not positive or negative; they are adaptive in one setting and maladaptive in another. Individuals vary in the degree to which they possess a given trait and in the way it influences their behavior. When traits found in certain individuals exceed the levels found in most of society and are sufficiently rigid and maladaptive to cause subjective distress or functional impairment, a *personality disorder* is usually diagnosed.

Most personality models depict individuals along temperamental dimensions of extroversion–introversion and stability–instability. The dimension of *extroversion–introversion* refers to the individual's basic tendency to respond to stimuli with either excitation or inhibition. Individuals who are *extroverted* are (1) present oriented, (2) feeling directed, and (3) reward seeking. His or her chief focus is the immediate and emotional experience. Feelings dominate thoughts, and the primary motivation is immediate gratification or relief from discomfort. Extroverts are sociable, crave excitement, take risks, and act impulsively. They tend to be carefree, inconsistent, and optimistic. By contrast, *introverted* individuals are (1) future and past oriented, (2) cognition directed, and (3) consequence avoidant. Logic and

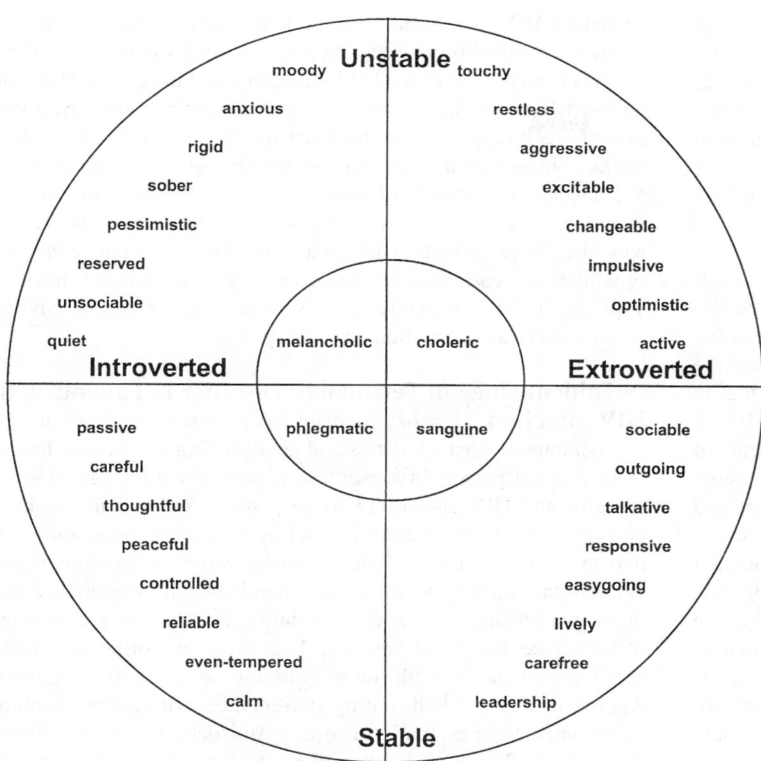

FIGURE 2.8–5 Hans Eysenck's circle. (From Eysenck HJ. Principles and methods of personality description, classification and diagnosis. In: Eysenck HJ, ed. *Readings in Extroversion-Introversion, I. Theoretical and Methodological Issues*. New York: Wiley-Intersciences; 1970:36, with permission.)

function predominate over feelings. Introverts are motivated by appraisal of past experience and avoidance of future adverse consequences. They do not engage in a pleasurable activity if it might pose a threat in the future. Introverted individuals are quiet, dislike excitement, and distrust the impulse of the moment. They tend to be orderly, reliable, and rather pessimistic. The second personality dimension, *stability–instability*, defines the degree of emotionality or lability. The emotions of *stable* individuals are aroused slowly and minimally and return quickly to baseline. By contrast, *unstable* individuals have intense, mercurial emotions that are easily aroused and return slowly to baseline. If these two personality dimensions are juxtaposed, four personality types emerge (Fig. 2.8–5).

Personality Models, Their Instruments, and Findings Related to HIV Risk Behaviors After the higher-order traits of extroversion and neuroticism, personality models have elaborated other trait domains and developed personality inventories to empirically assess these traits. The major models and their inventories are

The three-factor model (Eysenck & Eysenck): extroversion, neuroticism, and psychoticism; measured by the Eysenck Personality Questionnaire (EPQ)

The five-factor model (Costa & McCrae): neuroticism, extroversion, openness, agreeableness, conscientiousness; measured by the Neuroticism, Extroversion, Openness Scale (NEO-AC)

The alternative five-factor model (Zuckerman): neuroticism-anxiety, sociability, impulsive sensation seeking, aggression-hostility, activity; measured by the Zuckerman Kuhlman Personality Questionnaire (ZKPQ)

The seven-dimension model (Cloninger): novelty seeking, harm avoidance, reward dependence, persistence, self-directedness, cooperativeness, self-transcendence; measured by the Tridimensional Personality Questionnaire (TPQ)

A relevant addition to each of these models for understanding HIV risk behavior is the sensation or novelty-seeking trait. Although defined somewhat differently in each model (psychoticism, openness to experience, [low] conscientiousness, impulsive sensation seeking, or novelty seeking), it describes the individual's motivation to seek varied, intense experiences and the corresponding lack of regard for the potential negative consequences. In the authors' view, a combination of extreme extroversion and instability (neuroticism) can account for the observation that certain individuals are more prone to seek novel and intense experiences. Whether it is an extreme form of two combined traits or an independent trait, personality inventories show that sensation seeking in particular and, to a lesser extent, extroversion and neuroticism are correlated with HIV risk behaviors.

Personality traits appear to influence a variety of sexual risk behaviors, yet there is relatively little research on sexual risk taking from the major personality models. On the EPQ, extroversion is associated with sexual promiscuity, desire for sexual novelty, and multiple sex partners and, in a quantitative review of overall sexual risk taking, shows a modest effect size. Neuroticism is related to unprotected anal sex. Psychoticism is associated with number of sexual partners and unprotected sex in several studies. On the NEO-AC, neuroticism is associated with unprotected sex and, to a lesser extent, sex with multiple partners. Low conscientiousness is also associated with unprotected sex. Low openness to experience is associated with the denial of risk of HIV infection. The TPQ has minimal research on sexual risk taking, but one study shows that novelty seeking is associated with unprotected sex. The impulsive sensation seeking scale of the ZKPQ has received the most research attention and predicts number of sex partners, unprotected sex, and high-risk sexual encounters, such as sex with a stranger, across a variety of populations.

Research on personality traits links extroversion and neuroticism to drug and alcohol addiction. On the EPQ, psychoticism and, to a lesser extent, neuroticism have been linked prospectively to alcohol dependence in a 6-year study. On the ZKPQ, impulsive sensation seeking is consistently associated with addiction severity as well as amount and variety of illegal drug use. Although there is no specific "alcoholic" or "drug-using" personality, there appears to be a modest link between substance abuse and either impulsivity/high novelty seeking or neuroticism/negative emotionality. Individuals with *both* of these traits may be at the greatest risk for addiction.

Implications for HIV Risk Behavior There has been relatively little empirical investigation of the influence of personality characteristics on HIV risk behavior; however, clinical observation suggests that of the four temperaments, unstable extroverts are the most prone to engage in HIV risk behavior. It is estimated that in the Psychiatry Service of the Johns Hopkins AIDS Service (JHAS), approximately 60 percent of patients present with this blend of extroversion and emotional instability. These individuals are preoccupied by, and act on, their feelings, which are evanescent and changeable. Thus, their actions tend to be unpredictable and inconsistent. Most striking is the inconsistency found between thought and action. Regardless of intellectual ability or knowledge of HIV, unstable extroverts can engage in behavior associated with extreme risk of HIV infection. Past experience and future consequences have little salience in decision making for the individual who is ruled by feeling; the present is paramount. The patient's overarching goal is to achieve immediate pleasure or removal of pain, regardless of circumstances. Furthermore, as part of their emotional instability, they experience intense fluctuations in mood. It is difficult for them to tolerate painful affect, such as boredom, sadness, or unresolved drive; they want to escape or avoid such feelings as quickly and easily as possible. Thus, he or she is motivated to pursue pleasurable experiences, however risky, and eliminate low moods.

Unstable extroverts are more likely to engage in behavior that places them at risk for HIV infection. They are less likely to plan ahead and carry condoms and more likely to have unprotected vaginal or anal sex. They are more fixed on the reward of sex and remarkably inattentive to the STD they may acquire if they do not use a condom. Unstable extroverts are also less likely to accept the diminution of pleasure associated with the use of condoms or, once aroused, to interrupt the "heat of the moment" to use condoms. Similarly, unstable extroverts are more vulnerable to alcohol and drug abuse. They are drawn to alcohol and drugs as a quick route to pleasure. They are more likely to experiment with different kinds of drugs and to use greater quantities. Unstable extroverts are also more likely to become injection drug users because the experience is more intense. They are also less likely to defer this intensity in the interest of safety.

The second most common personality type observed in this group, which may represent approximately 25 percent of JHAS patients referred to psychiatry, is that of the *stable* extrovert. Stable extroverts are also present oriented and pleasure seeking; however, their emotions are not as intense, as easily provoked, or mercurial. Hence, they are not as strongly driven to achieve pleasure. Their emotional "flatness" may generate a kind of indifference to HIV risk more than a drive to seek pleasure at any cost. Stable extroverts may be at risk because they are too optimistic or sanguine to believe that they will become HIV infected.

Introverted personalities appear to be less common among this study of psychiatric patients. Their focus on the future, avoidance of negative consequences, and preference for cognition over feeling render them more likely to engage in protective and preventive behaviors. HIV risk for introverts is determined by the dimension of emotional instability–stability. Approximately 14 percent of JHAS patients present with a blend of introversion and instability. Unstable introverts are anxious, moody, and pessimistic. Typically, these patients seek drugs, sex, or both not for *pleasure,* but for relief or distraction from pain. These patients are concerned about the future and adverse outcomes but believe that they have little control over their fates. Stable introverts comprise the remaining 1 percent of patients. These patients, with their controlled, even-tempered personalities, are least likely to engage in risky or hedonistic behaviors. Typically, these individuals are HIV positive as a result of a blood transfusion or an occupational needle stick.

Epidemiology of Personality Disorder in Patients with HIV Infection Personality disorders represent extremes of normal personality characteristics and are disabling conditions. Prevalence rates of personality disorders among HIV-infected (19 to 36 percent) and HIV at-risk (15 to 20 percent) individuals are high and significantly exceed rates found in the general population (10 percent). Antisocial personality disorder is the most common and is a risk factor for HIV infection. Individuals with personality disorder, particularly antisocial personality disorder, have high rates of substance abuse and are more likely to inject drugs and share needles, compared with those without an Axis II diagnosis. Approximately one-half of drug abusers meet criteria for a diagnosis of antisocial personality disorder. Antisocial personality disorder individuals are also more likely to have higher numbers of lifetime sexual partners, engage in unprotected anal sex, and contract STDs compared with individuals without antisocial personality disorder.

Implications for Medication Adherence Average medication adherence across a variety of diseases and patient populations has been consistently estimated at 50 percent. Adherence is especially challenging in HIV, which is associated with all of the components of low adherence: long duration of treatment, preventative rather than curative treatment, asymptomatic periods, and frequent and complex medication dosing. Average rates of nonadherence to antiretroviral therapy range from 50 to 70 percent, with adherence rates of less than 80 percent associated with detectable viremia in a majority of patients.

Personality factors have received little investigation in relation to adherence and antiretroviral therapy; however, the authors' clinical experience suggests that nonadherence is more common among extroverted or unstable patients. The same personality characteristics that place patients at risk for HIV also reduce their ability to adhere to demanding drug regimens. Specifically, their present-time orientation, combined with reward seeking, makes it more difficult for these patients to tolerate uncomfortable side effects from antiretroviral drugs whose treatment effects may not be immediately apparent. It is also difficult for feeling-driven individuals to maintain consistent, well-ordered routines. Hence, following frequent, rigid dosing schedules can also be problematic. These unstable, extroverted patients are usually intent on following the schedule, but their chaotic and mercurial emotions are more likely to interfere and disrupt daily routines. For example, a patient may report that he or she felt very upset and nihilistic after a fight with a family member and missed several doses of his or her antiretroviral medicines. Missed doses of HAART can increase the chance of HIV resistance developing. Identifying factors that influence adherence in HIV disease is important in improving overall health outcomes.

Treatment Implications Psychiatric and medical treatment of patients with extroverted or emotionally unstable personalities, or both, is challenging. Such patients are often baffling or frustrating for physicians and other medical providers because they engage in high-risk sex and drug behaviors in spite of knowing the risks or do not adhere to treatment regimens for HIV infection in spite of knowing the consequences. A patient may stop his or her antidepressant medicine because of a headache, but be perfectly willing to inject heroin into multiple sites on the body. After 6 months of missed medical appointments, a patient may impulsively leave the clinic if the primary care provider is 15 minutes late for the appointment. Such personality traits reflect relatively stable, lifelong modes of responding; thus, direct efforts to change these traits are unlikely to be successful. It is possible, however, to modify the behavior that is an expression of the trait. By recognizing individual differences in risk-related personality characteristics, interventions can be better targeted, and their impact maximized.

The authors have found that a cognitive-behavioral approach is most effective in treating patients who present with extroverted or emotionally unstable personalities, or both. Six principles guide standard care:

1. Focus on thoughts, not feelings. Individuals with unstable, extroverted personalities benefit from learning how they are predisposed to act in certain ways. Often, they do not recognize the extent to which their actions are driven by the impulse or feeling of the moment. These patients may not understand why they intend to stay clean but later find themselves "shooting dope." Treatment helps to identify the role that strong feelings play, so that these patients can begin the process of understanding their own chaotic, often irrational behavior.

   Simultaneously, treatment encourages the patient's cognitive, logical side. This process begins by identifying what the patient thinks *in* a given situation, as opposed to what he or she thinks *about* the situation: "I deserve some cocaine because I have had a difficult day." The influence of the patient's assumption on feelings, behavior, and, ultimately, the consequences of behavior is examined. Through the treatment dialogue, patients understand that the notion of a "cocaine reward" creates a feeling of urgency and entitlement to getting high. As a consequence of using cocaine, the development of other more constructive reward systems or coping methods is preempted, a relapse into cocaine dependence can occur, or family or employers may be alienated. Through treatment, patients learn to identify maladaptive assumptions that drive feeling and behaviors, so that they can either lessen the force of these assumptions or substitute more constructive assumptions to guide their life experience.
2. Use a behavioral contract. A behavioral contract is developed with all patients. The contract outlines goals for treatment, often only a day or a week at a time. Although patients and mental health professionals may develop the contract, the focus of treatment is *not* on what patients *want* or *are willing to do* to get off of drugs but rather on established methods such as drug treatment and Narcotics Anonymous (NA) or Alcoholics Anonymous (AA). The importance of the behavioral contract lies in the creation of a *stable* plan that supersedes the emotional meanderings of these patients. Unstable extroverts present an ever-changing array of concerns and priorities. The task of the treatment is to order the priorities with patients and help them follow through on these regardless of changing emotions. In short, behavioral contracts provide consistent, cognitive focus to patients' bewildering emotional experience of life.
3. Emphasize constructive rewards. In developing the behavioral contract and in treatment, the purpose is cast in terms of the rewards that will follow from their behavioral change. Positive outcomes, not adverse consequences, are salient to extroverts. Most of the patients have already experienced negative consequences from their behavior, HIV, drug addiction, homelessness, and such. Exhortations to use condoms to avoid STDs are unpersuasive. More success has been achieved with extroverts by eroticizing the use of condoms or by the addition of novel sexual techniques (erotic massage, use of sex toys) into sexual repertoires. Similarly, the rewards of abstaining from drugs or alcohol are emphasized, such as having money to buy clothing, having a stable home, or maintaining positive relationships with children.
4. In building adherence to antiretroviral therapies, the focus is on the rewards of an increased CD4 count and reduced viral load rather than avoiding illness. Using the viral load as a strategy to build adherence can increase acceptance in all patients but is especially effective in reward-driven extroverts.
5. Use relapse prevention techniques. The relapse prevention model, originally developed for treatment of substance abuse behavior, is an effective method for changing any habitual way of behaving. This intervention trains individuals to recognize and interrupt the sequence of behaviors that link to the final high-risk behavior. Behavioral therapy methods are also used to teach individuals how to recognize and avoid situations that trigger high-risk behaviors.
6. Coordinate with medical care providers. Medical care providers are often frustrated or discouraged when treating unstable, extroverted patients. It is useful to provide education about a patient's personality and how it influences behavior. Particularly effective is the development of a coordinated treatment plan in which the medical care provider and mental health professional work in tandem to develop behavioral contracts to reduce HIV risk behaviors and build medication adherence.

Personality characteristics and personality disorders reflect relatively stable, lifelong propensities that are difficult to change. This does not mean, however, that HIV risk-reduction efforts are necessarily futile. Rather, by understanding personality characteristics and their role in HIV risk behavior and medication adherence, the mental health professional can develop more effective, specific treatment strategies. Similarly, the HIV-infected patient who can identify aspects of his or her personality that might interfere with intentions to practice safer behavior and who knows strategies for dealing with these situations is less likely to practice high-risk behaviors. Finally, the mental health professional can provide valuable assistance to medical care providers to improve health outcomes for these patients.

ISSUES OF SUBSTANCE ABUSE AND ADDICTION IN PATIENTS WITH HIV INFECTION

Substance abuse is a primary vector for the spread of HIV. This impact is directed at those who use IV drugs and their sexual partners and those who are disinhibited by intoxication or driven by addiction to unsafe sexual practices. It has a further impact, as those who are infected by HIV are often demoralized and may become hopeless and engage in risk behaviors. Patients with substance use disorders may not seek health care or may be excluded from health care. In addition, intoxication and the behaviors necessary to obtain drugs interfere with health care.

Injection drug use is obviously a primary risk factor for contracting HIV. In the United States, the proportion of injection drug users with HIV infection markedly increased from 17 percent during 1981 to 1987 to 33 percent during 1993 to 1995. Even among non–injection drug users, substance abuse plays a major, albeit more subtle, role in HIV transmission. Addiction and high-risk sexual behavior have been linked across a wide range of settings. For example, crack cocaine abusers are more likely to engage in prostitution to obtain money for drugs. Men who use crack cocaine are more likely to engage in unprotected anal sex with casual male contacts. Alcohol intoxication can also lead to risky sexual behaviors by way of cognitive impairment and disinhibition.

A multifactorial matrix of influences initiate, drive, and exacerbate substance abuse and addiction. Many of these are intrinsic to the substances and behaviors themselves, but many are characteristic of the host or the environment. Behavioral approaches to understanding addictions have been particularly fruitful, as seen in the work of Joseph Brady and his colleagues. This approach allows the development of animal models of self-administration and the measurement of reinforcing properties of drugs, many of which are profoundly predictive of human behavior. On the other hand, the understanding of the individual and cultural and social forces that impact substance use is essential to translation of those models into human settings.

Psychiatric and psychological comorbidity render people more vulnerable to substance use disorders. Personality factors may lead to more risk taking, and therefore more likelihood to experiment with behaviors, and more sensitivity to rewards, and therefore more sensitivity to the reinforcing properties of drugs and less sensitivity to the consequences of drug use. Other personality types are consequence and risk avoidant and are relatively protected from addiction. Depression makes the ordinary rewards of life less rewarding and makes people more sensitive to the rewarding effects of drugs. Life experiences that expose people to drugs and social acceptance of drug use also increase risk of addiction. Individual biology is involved in several ways. In the case of alcohol, genetic factors may affect the degree to which alcohol is rewarding, so that some patients report that their first drink was so rewarding that they began a lifetime of heavy drinking immediately. Others say they never really liked drinking all that much and, therefore, are surprised as they become more and more dependent on alcohol to control the emotional discomforts of their lives. Cocaine is less affected by genetics, and patients with exposure to cocaine are extremely rewarded, such that the use to abuse ratio is quite high. Finally, other medical conditions, such as chronic pain, a variety of disease states, and surgical procedures, may result in exposure to addictive drugs. Such patients may be developing iatrogenic addiction and then persistent drug use problems. All of these factors enhance or diminish the risk of the addictive cycle getting out of control.

Finally, choice involves the free will of the individual to initiate and continue using the drug. That choice becomes narrower as addiction progresses by way of stronger drive and conditioned learning, but it is only through the individual's choice that he or she decides to enter treatment and change his or her lifestyle.

Research on substance use and HIV is complicated by the same problems of definition, detection, and methodology that impede research on the other areas discussed here. All drug use disorders are on a spectrum of increasing use, dependence, and increasing impairment of function that blend gradually into one another. Indeed, it is often difficult to define precisely when the transition from heavy drinker to alcoholic occurs. Some patients use heavily but never actually become disordered by their use. Others are disordered by a surprisingly modest use of a substance. The *Diagnostic and Statistical Manual of Mental Disorders* (DSM-IV-TR) divides disorders related to the use of psychoactive substances into two main categories: primary substance use disorders and secondary substance-induced disorders. Substance use disorders include substance abuse and substance dependence. Substance-induced disorders include substance intoxication, substance withdrawal, substance-induced psychotic disorder, substance-induced mood disorder, substance-induced anxiety disorder, substance-induced sleep disorder, substance-induced persisting dementia disorder, substance-induced amnestic disorder, and substance-induced sexual dysfunction.

To satisfy the criteria for substance dependence, an individual must have tolerance or dependence. *Tolerance* refers to the need for using increasing amounts of the substance to achieve the same effect. Dependence is usually divided into two components: physiological and psychological. Physiological dependence occurs when the individual has physically adapted to the substance to the point that he or she must continue to use the substance to feel "normal." If the individual stops using the substance abruptly, he or she experiences uncomfortable physical withdrawal symptoms, and the substance itself is used to prevent the individual from going into withdrawal. Psychological dependence occurs when the individual believes that he or she needs to continue using the substance to feel emotionally stable.

Substance abuse, on the other hand, is a maladaptive pattern of using the substance that becomes socially, legally, or occupationally problematic for the individual. For example, a college student who becomes intoxicated at a fraternity party and behaves badly constitutes alcohol abuse, whereas the retired businessperson who drinks martinis on a daily basis and experiences tremors and anxiety when he or she stops drinking constitutes alcohol dependence.

Substance Use Disorders and Their Interaction with HIV Treatment Ongoing substance abuse has grave medical implications for HIV-infected individuals. Many physical symptoms of HIV infection overlap with those of substance abuse or dependence, including malaise, fatigue, weight loss, fevers, and night sweats. The accumulation of medical sequelae from chronic substance abuse accelerates the process of immunocompromise and amplifies the progressive burdens of the HIV infection itself. Injection drug users, for example, are at higher risk for developing bacterial infections such as pneumonia, sepsis, soft tissue infections, and endocarditis. Tuberculosis, STDs, viral hepatitis infection, and coinfection with human CD4 cell lymphotrophic virus also occur more commonly in injection drug users who are infected with HIV. Certain malignancies, lymphomas in particular, occur more frequently in HIV-infected drug users.

Neurological symptoms can overlap between HIV infection and substance abuse. For instance, both AIDS dementia and drug intoxication can present with apathy, disorientation, aggression, and an altered level of consciousness. Drug withdrawal can present with seizures and neurovegetative symptoms, as can opportunistic infections of the CNS. In addition, HIV-infected injection drug users tend to be at higher risk for developing fungal or bacterial infections of the brain and spinal cord.

Because the HIV-infected patient is likely to be on a variety of antiretroviral agents and prophylactic agents for opportunistic infections, the clinician must be especially mindful of interactions between these medications and the abused substances. Opioid users are at particular risk for medication interactions. Rifampin (Rifadin), for example, increases the elimination of methadone (Dolophine,

Methadose) from the body and may result in the rapid onset of withdrawal symptoms in opiate addicts on maintenance therapy. Decreased plasma levels of methadone also occur with concurrent administration of ritonavir (Norvir), nelfinavir (Viracept), efavirenz, and nevirapine (Viramune), necessitating adjustments in methadone dosage should withdrawal symptoms occur. This has important implications for treatment compliance in that the patient in a methadone program is less likely to take a medication because of the fear of withdrawal. HIV medications, such as dideoxyinosine, may also cause peripheral neuropathies, which may be worsened by the neurotoxic effects of alcohol and malnutrition related to chronic substance abuse.

The term *dual diagnosis* refers to a patient who has both a drug use disorder and another psychiatric disorder; *triple diagnosis* refers to a dual diagnosis patient who also has HIV. Such patients are overrepresented in treatment settings because of their symptom severity and chronicity. For instance, in inner-city Baltimore, as many as 44 percent of new entrants to the HIV medical clinic at Johns Hopkins Hospital had an active substance use disorder. Twenty-four percent of these patients had both a current substance use disorder and another non–substance-related Axis I diagnosis.

Difficulties in the realm of personality are among the most common psychiatric problems seen in this population. Although personality disorder diagnoses are currently described in a categorical fashion in the DSM-IV-TR, it is probably more useful to view personality as being dimensional in nature. Using this model, personality traits exist along a continuum, which predicts habitual maladaptive approaches to life's difficulties.

Unstable extroversion has important implications for the HIV-positive addict. These traits are generally found in the so-called cluster B personality disorders in the DSM-IV-TR (antisocial, borderline, narcissistic, and histrionic), which can be found in as many as 49 percent of all substance abusers. Not only do these traits result in a vulnerability to addiction and other risky behaviors that predispose one to become infected with HIV, but they also pose significant barriers to treatment. These patients tend to act on strong, impulsive feelings rather than on carefully considered treatment instructions. Their behavior tends to be driven by the transient, immediate rewards of drugs rather than by their lasting future consequences. Such patients tend to get bored easily, and treatment is often unexciting. They tend to "want what they want when they want it" rather than when it may be good for them. It is critical to identify these personality vulnerabilities in this patient population because they can have a profound effect on treatment engagement and prognosis.

Affective disorders, especially major depressive disorder, are also found in these patients, with studies estimating a prevalence of 15 to 30 percent. Diagnosing affective disorders (and other psychiatric disorders) in drug users can be difficult and even controversial. This controversy stems from the problem in determining the causal, or even chronological, relationship between drug disorders and affective disorders. Although some theorists want to emphasize the primacy of one or the other in guiding treatment, this "chicken or egg" approach is not especially productive. Given the very high prevalence of overlapping addictive and affective disorders in clinical settings, as well as the very poor prognosis associated with untreated affective disorders, a treatment approach should necessarily emphasize simultaneous and equal treatment of both entities. This is not to suggest that it is easy to distinguish transient depressive symptoms, such as those presenting in drug withdrawal, demoralization, or grief reactions, from persistent depressive symptoms indicating a major affective disorder. It often becomes necessary to observe the patient over a period of abstinence in a confined treatment setting, if necessary, before this can be elucidated. Features of the clinical history may also be supportive of an affective disorder.

The importance of identifying affective disorders lies not only in their own well-known sequelae, including suicide, but also in their complex interactions with addiction. Depression is associated with worsening of addiction and resistance to treatment. The anhedonia of depression makes it difficult for addicts to respond to and enjoy life's other rewards. These pale in comparison to the intense, although ephemeral, charge of intoxicating drugs, which stimulate the mesolimbic reward system of the brain. Depressed patients are more difficult to engage and are less likely to invest in and sustain treatment, given their anergy and negativism. It is essential, therefore, for the clinician to recognize and treat depression early to maximize successful treatment outcome.

Treatment of Substance Use Disorders in Patients Infected with HIV

Although oversimplified, the steps for treatment of substance use can be outlined in this simple way. These steps often occur at the same time as treatment begins but are described as a sequence:

1. Induction of patient role
2. Detoxification
3. Treatment of comorbid conditions
4. Rehabilitation
5. Relapse prevention

Role Induction and Motivation to Change

The initial, and often most daunting, task of treating the addict is engagement and induction of the patient role. The general rule is that addicts and treatment providers begin with differing agendas—addicts tend to come to treatment settings seeking comfort and crisis relief, whereas physicians and other health providers look at long-term goals of improvement in the patient's health and overall functioning. One of the critical initial tasks of the health provider is to engender the gradual evolution of the patient's attitudes to coincide with those of the treatment plan.

Many authors, most notably James Prochaska and Carlo DiClemente, have described a "transtheoretical stages of change" model to elucidate the addiction and recovery process. The patient progresses through several different stages of change in the recovery process: (1) precontemplation—the patient has no intention to change his or her addictive behavior; (2) contemplation—the patient considers change because of the negative consequences of his or her drug use but is ambivalent about it; (3) preparation—the patient shows intention to change and takes initial steps to seek treatment; (4) action—the patient decides to modify behavior, environment, and circumstances to relinquish the addictive lifestyle; and (5) maintenance—the patient works to prevent relapse and consolidate his or her changed behavior and lifestyle. The most difficult task faced by most clinicians is in preparing and moving the patient from a contemplative stage to an action stage. A technique known as *motivational interviewing,* developed by William Miller and Stephen Rollnick, facilitates the patient's readiness to change by using empathy and gentle confrontation to amplify the discrepancy between the substance abuser's current lifestyle and long-term life-enhancing goals.

Detoxification

For intoxicated patients to understand and process the cognitive steps needed for recovery, detoxification is the first step. Many HIV-positive substance abusers benefit from a brief hospital stay to stabilize their psychiatric and medical comorbidities. Slowly tapering either the drug of dependence or using a cross-dependent drug that has a similar pharmacological mechanism of action best accomplishes detoxification.

Detoxification is often unpleasant, and there has been no evidence to support the idea that noxious withdrawal during detoxification improves outcome. In fact, some behavioral studies suggest that patients with severe withdrawal may actually develop conditioned withdrawal, such that exposure to environments similar to the one experienced during "cold-turkey withdrawal" can bring withdrawal symptoms back months later. Benzodiazepine, barbiturate, and alcohol withdrawal can be life-threatening. Active tapers using slow downward titration of the dose of a drug from the class to which the patient is addicted are recommended for opiates and sedative-hypnotics. Drugs such as dicyclomine (Bentyl), prochlorperazine (Compazine), promazine (Sparine), and clonidine (Catapres) can ameliorate the unpleasant symptoms of withdrawal. Some clinicians have used antidepressants to help patients detoxify from psychomotor stimulant classes of drugs (amphetamines and cocaine), but data to support this practice are controversial. This approach may work best for patients with clear evidence of major depression.

Sedative-hypnotics or alcohol is best detoxified through the use of a long-acting benzodiazepine such as diazepam (Valium), chlordiazepoxide (Librium), or oxazepam (Serax). Detoxification of opiates is accomplished through a taper of long-acting opioid agonists such as methadone. Alternative agents that can be used include buprenorphine (Buprenex), a partial opioid agonist; clonidine; and α_2-agonists that can bring symptomatic relief of heroin withdrawal.

Treatment of Comorbid Psychiatric Conditions As stated earlier, many patients with HIV and addictions often have comorbid psychiatric conditions that need to be treated to maximize compliance and abstinence. Conditions such as major depression, bipolar disorder, and schizophrenia are best managed with pharmacological treatment and psychotherapies tailored to the individual patient. Because these patients tend to have multiple medical complications, it is important to remember to start medications at low dosages and to titrate slowly to minimize the risk of developing adverse side effects and delirium.

Disorders of personality, in particular unstable extroversion, are managed with psychotherapy. The ways that unstable extroverts may sabotage treatment include staff splitting, doctor shopping, general noncompliance, and manipulative behavior. Therapy addressing these personality issues should include firm limit setting and a devotion to consistency on the part of all health care providers involved. To this end, a documented treatment plan with clear goals agreed on by all the treatment staff is essential. The treatment plan should be reviewed with the patient at the initiation treatment, so that the patient understands clearly what is expected of him or her and what can be expected from the treatment providers if the patient adheres to these goals.

Maintenance Treatment and Relapse Prevention After role induction, detoxification, and treatment of comorbid conditions, long-term treatment is necessary for patients to begin the process of lifestyle change and recovery. Because this patient population is complicated and especially vulnerable to recidivism, one must take an integrated approach to treatment. To this end, a "one-stop shopping" model is especially useful to maintain treatment engagement. Thus, a treatment center catering to HIV-positive addicts should ideally include medical providers, psychiatrists, social workers, housing counselors, and day care workers in addition to substance abuse counselors. This integrated approach helps bring order out of these patients' chaotic lifestyles.

It is important to remember that addiction treatment is active rather than passive and entails transforming previously held beliefs, attitudes, and personal identity into a new way of life. To this end, group therapy is a necessary part of all substance use disorder treatment, whether it is one of the 12-step models, network therapy, rational recovery, therapeutic community, or SMART recovery (*s*elf-*m*anagement *a*nd *r*ecovery *t*raining). In group therapy, the more experienced members of the group provide both confrontation and support for the newly initiated member. Group support also provides the newly recovering addict with a hopeful view of the benefits to be achieved with recovery. A commitment to a community of recovery protects the patient from the influences of the drug community and provides the patient with new bonds that help maintain a sense of purposefulness and hopefulness. Specific HIV-positive recovery groups are now widely available, and although they may be of particular benefit in addressing HIV-related issues, they are not necessary to successful recovery.

Therapy should focus on identifying triggers to substance use, on minimizing or decreasing exposure to substances, and on defining a clear plan of action if relapse occurs. It is important to realize that relapse is often the rule and not the exception, and plans should be in place for early intervention. Monitoring measures such as urine and serum toxicology and breathalyzer tests can help to enforce compliance. Contingency management using a variety of positive and negative reinforcers tied to urine toxicology results has also been shown to be highly effective in maintaining sobriety.

Individual and family therapies can enhance the effectiveness of treatment but should not take the place of group therapy. In individual treatment, it is important that the treatment provider remain flexible in the treatment approach. Thus, although a cognitive-behavioral approach may work for some types of patients, others may do better with a modified psychodynamic approach. Treatment failures often result when the therapist adheres too rigidly to one model of therapy. Pharmacological treatments should be seen as enhancements to the overall treatment plan and not as a replacement. Pharmacological treatment can be divided into the following categories:

- Aversive conditioning: disulfiram (Antabuse) (alcohol)
- Blockade of reinforcement: naltrexone (ReVia) (opioids)
- Drive suppression: bupropion (tobacco), buprenorphine (cocaine), naltrexone (tobacco)
- Substituted addiction: methadone, levomethadyl acetate (Orlaam), buprenorphine (opioids)

Relapse can occur impulsively, and some patients are eager for a type of insurance so that they will not relapse in a single weak moment. They have often had experience with this in the past and know their weak moments. Drugs such as disulfiram (an inhibitor of acetaldehyde dehydrogenase) can be very effective. Disulfiram is taken once daily at doses from 250 to 500 mg and causes a very unpleasant reaction when alcohol is ingested due to the buildup of acetaldehyde in the body. Symptoms include nausea, flushing, headaches, and hypotension. Liver enzymes should be monitored because of the risk of hepatotoxicity. Naltrexone is an opioid antagonist that has high affinity for blocking μ receptors. It is taken once daily, orally, at doses ranging from 50 to 100 mg. The medication blocks the euphoric effects of opioids when taken; however, it also can precipitate withdrawal symptoms in dependent individuals because it also displaces opioids from the μ receptors. As with disulfiram, liver function tests are monitored in patients on naltrexone because of the risk of hepatotoxicity. Naltrexone has been shown to reduce alcohol cravings across a number of studies. In opiate-dependent individuals, pharmacotherapy includes both opioid agonist and antagonist medications. Methadone is the opioid agonist most often used for maintenance treatment. This medication is given to the patient at varying dosages from 40 to 140 mg daily. The medication is administered daily under supervision until the patient has established a pattern of abstinence. At this point, take-home doses are often allowed. A newer partial agonist, buprenorphine, is undergoing clinical trial for oral administration and may be a useful alternative to methadone. Several agents used to treat HIV and related infections induce methadone metabolism. Providers should investigate drug–drug interactions before prescribing and monitor patients closely for signs of withdrawal once therapy has been initiated.

PSYCHOLOGICAL PROBLEMS IN PATIENTS INFECTED WITH HIV

In the context of the psychological realm of living with HIV, it is difficult to distinguish which came first: the variety of psychiatric disorders the patient has, the HIV risk behaviors, the losses and psychological traumas, or the impact of having HIV itself. A common sentiment from patients, to echo one of the patients at the authors' clinic, is: "HIV is not even one of my biggest problems." Each of these factors seems to be both a consequence and an antecedent to all the others. The DSM-IV-TR provides the opportunity to choose between "adjustment disorder" and posttraumatic stress disorder (PTSD) for patients living with violence, despair, and loss of unthinkable proportion. However, the psychological difficulties of living with HIV are infinitely more complex than this.

Patients with HIV have been shown to have more severe trauma, high rates of PTSD and anxiety, economic and social disenfranchisement, and high rates of interpersonal instability. Cognizance of the psychological issues in the care of patients with HIV is essential. On the other hand, the treatment of these problems is well within the scope of most clinicians in the field. The psychotherapy for patients infected with HIV can be broadly divided three categories:

1. Psychotherapy for the problems of life encountered by patients infected with HIV
2. Psychiatric treatment for specific psychiatric conditions associated with HIV infections
3. Specific psychoeducational and psychotherapeutic interventions associated with specific types of interactions with HIV-infected patients

For the first two categories listed, the psychotherapeutic issues are largely similar to those seen in patients who are not infected with HIV. Although specific papers have been written regarding coping skills, social isolation, grief, PTSD, intimate relationships, family problems, and many others, these recommendations are largely similar to those found in patients coping with other chronic medical conditions or chronic impoverishment elsewhere in this text. The psychotherapy issues of conditions commonly seen in HIV clinics have been reiterated when appropriate but are also similar to those issues for patients with the same conditions but without HIV infection. The section Posttraumatic Stress Disorder (PTSD) is included because of the high prevalence and special issues for HIV patients.

Posttraumatic Stress Disorder (PTSD)

Traumatic events that are life-threatening provoke terror, anxiety, and stress in most people. In some individuals, the chronicity, intensity, frequency, and comorbidity of these symptoms can become psychiatrically disabling. Specifically, patients have intrusive intense recollections of the traumatic event, sometimes to the point at which they feel as if they are experiencing the event again, and there is persistent avoidance of stimuli associated with the trauma and persistent symptoms of increased arousal not present before the trauma. When these symptoms persist for more than 1 month and interfere with social, familial, or occupational functioning, PTSD may be diagnosed (DSM-IV-TR). PTSD has a current prevalence of less than 1 percent and a lifetime prevalence of 1 to 9 percent, with a female to male lifetime prevalence ratio of 2:1. In civilian populations, rape is the event most likely to produce PTSD, particularly if it occurs before or during adolescence.

PTSD increases the likelihood of engaging in destructive behaviors such as alcohol and other drug abuse, sexual promiscuity, or prostitution. PTSD is of particular concern in HIV treatment and research because it may engender or exacerbate HIV risk behaviors and worsen health outcomes.

Cross-sectional research has shown that both symptoms of PTSD and a diagnosis of PTSD have been associated with HIV risk behaviors and markers of HIV progression. Symptoms of PTSD in adolescence have been associated with prostitution, injection drug use, and choice of a high-risk sex partner in young adults. HIV-infected adults who have a history of childhood sexual or physical abuse have reported engaging in more HIV risk behaviors, such as drug abuse and sexual compulsivity, than people with no history of trauma. A high prevalence (42 percent) of HIV-infected women attending county medical clinics had PTSD symptoms severe enough to meet a diagnosis of PTSD. In HIV treatment, traumatic stressors and PTSD symptoms have also been associated with lower CD4 T-cell to CD8 T-cell ratio at 1 year's follow-up. The relationship between a psychiatric diagnosis of PTSD and HIV risk behavior or infection has received less attention. Veterans with a diagnosis of PTSD are at greatly increased risk of HIV infection, particularly if they are also diagnosed with a substance abuse disorder. Female prisoners with a lifetime history of PTSD are more likely to have engaged in prostitution and receptive anal intercourse before incarceration, compared with women prisoners without PTSD. These studies of PTSD and PTSD symptoms and HIV risk behaviors have been cross-sectional; thus, a causal relationship cannot be inferred. It may be that HIV risk behaviors, such as prostitution or drug abuse, increase exposure to trauma and, thus, the likelihood of developing PTSD. Alternatively, PTSD that stems from early trauma may predispose an individual to engage in sex or drug behaviors that can increase the risk of HIV infection.

The presence of PTSD in an at-risk or HIV-positive individual is of particular concern because of high rates of comorbidity (up to 80 percent) with other psychiatric disorders. Specifically, PTSD is most often comorbid with depression and cocaine/opioid abuse, both risk factors for HIV. Prior depression may be either a risk factor for the development of PTSD after a traumatic event or a co-occurring response with PTSD to a trauma. Substance abuse may be either an attempt to "self-medicate" suffering after a traumatic experience or a lifestyle that increases exposure to traumatic events such as robbery or assault.

PTSD and substance abuse disorders that occur together can also adversely affect treatment. Comorbid conditions have been associated with poorer treatment adherence and motivation, quicker relapse, more inpatient hospitalizations and medical problems, and lower global functioning than either disorder alone. Thus, treatment of PTSD that does not address coexisting depression or substance abuse may be insufficient or even worsen psychiatric status. PTSD treatment that typically involves behavioral exposure and flooding has been reported to exacerbate emotional arousal and precipitate relapse, although this has not yet been shown in experimentally controlled investigations. Likewise, the AA philosophy of surrender and sharing one's story may be counterproductive to substance-abusing HIV-infected individuals with PTSD.

HIV at-risk or HIV-infected individuals should be routinely screened for PTSD. Instruments such as the Trauma History Questionnaire and the PTSD Checklist have improved detection rates of the disorder. Similarly, any individuals presenting with symptoms of PTSD should routinely be screened for depression and substance abuse. For HIV-infected individuals with PTSD and another concurrent psychiatric disorder, treatment that simultaneously addresses both disorders is likely to be more effective and practical.

Pretest, Test, and Posttest Counseling and Education Patients at risk for HIV infection are often reticent to get testing. Surveys suggest that they fear the results of the test or are too overwhelmed by the issues of their current life and behavior to present for testing. Before 1993, patients who received a positive HIV test result saw their diagnosis as essentially fatal. Additionally, many patients believed it would be burdensome to know that they were placing others at risk for infection. In more recent years, with the advent of HAART, HIV has become a chronic treatable illness. In this setting, it seems more reasonable for patients to get tested and engage in treatment. Nonetheless, survey data show that a large number of patients who are at significant risk are not getting tested. Psychoeducational psychotherapy directed at encouraging patients to get tested has been offered to a variety of at-risk populations of patients. The outcomes of these intervention studies show that such psychotherapy does result in patients getting tested and diagnosed earlier.

Pretest counseling has been described in a number of papers. Before testing, patients need informed consent regarding the meaning of a positive and a negative test. It should be stressed that a negative test does not mean that a patient is immune and cannot become infected later and that a positive does not mean that a person has AIDS, is going to die, or will contract opportunistic infections. It should also be stressed that the test remains negative for a time after infection (the time it takes for antibody to develop); therefore, after a recent exposure, a patient may have a negative test but, in fact, be infected. Pretest counseling should also include safe sex, safe needle, and other risk-reduction interventions. This is because a significant percentage of patients who obtain testing do not return for their results for extended periods and sometimes not at all.

A number of articles have described posttest counseling psychotherapy issues and interventions. These include both psychoeducational interventions regarding the meaning of test results, recommendations for treatment, and, importantly, risk reduction interventions to stem the spread of HIV infection. These posttest interventions should occur in both HIV-negative and HIV-positive patients.

The current protocol for testing HIV-infected patients involves initial enzyme-linked immunoabsorbent assay (ELISA) that detects antibodies made by the patient to the HIV virus. Because this test has false-positives, before notifying a patient of a positive test result, confirmation is made using a second technique to detect HIV antibodies called a *Western blot*. Both of these tests look for antibodies; therefore, the results of these tests are negative immediately after infection when patients have not yet developed antibodies to HIV, despite the fact that the patient is infected.

At the time that test results are given to patients, it is not uncommon for patients to have a variety of intense psychological reactions, including suicidal feelings, anger, homicidal thoughts directed at potentially infecting partners, overwhelming grief, and complete psychological breakdown. Patients with poor coping skills, poor impulse control, history of suicidal feelings and behaviors, substance abuse disorders, and lack of social supports are at increased risk for impulsive and self-destructive behaviors. Because of these circumstances, availability of psychological interventions at the time of HIV testing and result provision are critical.

Although a separate matter, bad news regarding progression of HIV disease can provoke a similar response in patients and probably should be considered in a similar way. Transition from the asymptomatic phase to the development of an opportunistic infection or to a formal diagnosis of AIDS because of a decrease in CD4 cells may provoke similar reactions to those described above. Again, the presence of psychological intervention is extremely critical in this setting. Patients may be overwhelmed by the news that they need to start antiretroviral drugs and therefore need emergent attention at this time.

Psychotherapy to Prevent HIV Transmission in Selected Populations of Patients Men who have sexual contacts with other men may be either exclusively homosexual, bisexual, or heterosexual men. Men with sexual contacts with other men continued to be the largest subgroup for new AIDS diagnoses in the United States in 2000. In states in which HIV is reported, this group continues to be the largest subgroup of newly reported HIV infections. In intervention studies of men who have sex with other men, many interventions have shown a decrease in either risk behaviors or infection. Studied interventions include stress management and relaxation techniques, cognitive self-management training, negotiation skills training, psychotherapy directed at emotional distress reduction, relapse prevention models of high-risk behavior reduction, education directed at eroticizing safer sex, assertiveness training, and peer education in bars. Outcomes of these interventions showed that all have a modest impact on either risk behavior or HIV infection. Although there are fewer data, similar studies have been done targeting heterosexually transmitted HIV, substance-related risk behaviors, women, and IV drug users. It is unclear from the data what the best intervention is and how to stratify the interventions. More important, the results of these studies are quite modest, with a 25 percent reduction in risk being quite a good outcome.

Studies of rates of psychiatric disorders in at-risk populations show impressively high rates of affective disorder substance abuse, personality disorders, and psychological distress. As yet, no systematic study with treatment and targeted intervention methods based on psychiatric diagnosis has been reported. It is clear from the data on risk and epidemiology that this is the direction that needs to be taken to try to improve prevention.

Partner Notification The landmark legal decision in the *Tarasoff v. Regents of the University of California* case has resulted in the increased scope of responsibility for care providers. A variety of legislation differing from state to state has afforded practitioners an increased number of options with regard to confidential situations. In some states, *Tarasoff* statutes (those statutes providing duty to warn vulnerable individuals of imminent danger from a patient overriding issues of confidentiality) have completely changed the way in which mental health professionals handle confidential issues.

Numerous articles have been written about the issues of ethics, confidentiality, duty to warn, and medical/legal aspects of this element of practice. Although no clear consensus has been reached, recommendations are that patients who are sexually active and infected with HIV should be counseled about potential risk to their sexual partners. Additionally, known partners should be notified of exposure risk and potential infection as well. Partner notification has been an extremely hotly debated topic; however, many states have developed legislation requiring or allowing either physicians or health department officials to notify partners of HIV-infected patients of their risk. The current standard, despite the controversy, appears to be an obligation on the part of health care professionals to notify anyone who could be construed as clearly at risk and clearly identifiable and who may be unaware of their risk.

A particularly difficult situation is that of sex-industry workers known to be HIV infected and known to be working actively as prostitutes. There are public health issues that pose a risk both for these patients and, depending on the politics of the circumstances, for their potential partners, clients, customers, victims, or victimizers. The response to this problem has ranged from a sense that sex-industry workers and their clients can make their own decisions and should be responsible for their own behavior all the way to the sentiment that such people should be arrested and jailed for attempted murder. It has additionally been noted that some sex-industry workers are impaired by a variety of psychiatric conditions, including cognitive impairment, major mental illness, personality disorder, and substance abuse disorders. These may further contribute to the sense that some sex-industry workers may be less than fully responsible for their behavior. Recommendations have been made for voluntary and involuntary interventions regarding these patients. Specific psychiatric interventions regarding competency, ability to consent, capacity, and, most important, treatment for the conditions that impair such people are critical to the mental health needs of patients with HIV.

Capacity to Consent/Competence Patients with psychiatric disorders in HIV clinics often have a variety of difficulties with medical care provision. In some of these settings, the patient's capacity or competence to make medical decisions regarding his or her health care can be in doubt. Provision of mental health care evaluations to determine this is an often unmet need in HIV clinics. The issues of competence and capacity in these patients are often no different than those described elsewhere in this textbook; however, the consequences of inadequate assessment of patients' competency and capacity can have grave consequences in this clinical setting. HIV dementia and delirium can be overlooked in this population, as can intoxication with substances. This is a problem in obtaining meaningful consent.

The question of capacity and consent involves several issues and, to some extent, varies with state law. The most important question is the specific question of what the patient is being asked. In many cases, medical providers want a judgment about competence as a general rule—a judgment impossible to make. It is usually straightforward to ask if a patient can understand the issues of consenting to a specific procedure and the risks and benefits involved and can arrive at a decision that is reasoned and clearly communicated.

In many cases, dangerousness, patterns of prior behavior, severity of illness, poor judgment, and psychiatric vulnerabilities complicate these decisions and play an important role in tempering the way in which patients are managed. The ethics of a particular case may get very complex when a patient understands the issues in a cognitive way, but their judgment is colored by their affective state, temperament, drug cravings, social situation, or, simply, difficulty with tolerating discomfort. These cases often divide medical teams and require consultation and a group conference to resolve. It is critical to get all providers to discuss the most difficult cases, clarify the issues, and come to a decision based on the patient's best interest, not the most expedient management.

Adherence Counseling The single most important factor regarding outcome of HIV treatment is the patient's ability to adhere to a prescribed regimen. Although this has been debated in the literature, a recent study by Margaret Fischel showed that looking at HIV-infected prisoners revealed that 100 percent of patients who received directly observed therapy in a prison setting developed undetectable viral loads. This strongly supports adherence as the major feature of treatment. There are compelling studies suggesting that major depression, substance abuse, personality disorder, and psychosocial disruption all affect adherence. We have discussed intervention in these conditions above. More subtle factors affecting adherence include psychosocial support networks, individual coping skills, life structure, access to resources, and behavioral control. Interventions such as cognitive behavioral psychotherapy, structured psychoeducational psychotherapy, supportive psychotherapy, and group intervention have all been used to improve patient adherence to medication regimens.

The current literature on HIV medication adherence focuses on technical interventions such as pill box and timer reminders, less complex pharmacological interventions, decreased pill burdens, and increased access to care. A growing literature examines psychosocial interventions, relationship with care providers, case management, and psychiatric disorders as barriers to adherence. It is in this arena that mental health care can have an enormous impact on outcome. Psychotherapy has been shown to improve clinic visit adherence, the best indirect predictor of medication adherence.

NEUROLOGICAL COMPLICATIONS OF HIV AND AIDS

Opportunistic Infections

Toxoplasmosis *Toxoplasma gondii is* a protozoan acquired most commonly from cat feces or uncooked meat. Infection generally occurs in patients with fewer than 200 CD4 cells per μL. In AIDS patients, toxoplasmosis is the most common reason for intracranial masses, affecting between 2 and 4 percent of the AIDS population. Other manifestations are possible, including hepatosplenomegaly, myositis, pneumonitis, myocarditis, and maculopapular rash. Lymphadenopathy may be present in cutaneous cases. Symptoms of CNS infection are fever, change in level of alertness, headache, focal neurological signs (approximately 80 percent of cases), and partial or generalized seizures (approximately 30 percent of cases). Computed tomography (CT) and MRI scans usually show multiple, ring-enhancing lesions in the basal ganglia or at the gray/white matter junction. CSF studies are normal in 20 to 30 percent of cases but more often show a mild monocytosis. Serum *T. gondii* immunoglobulin G (IgG) is generally helpful in the diagnosis but has a false-negative rate of 5 to 10 percent. Brain biopsy provides the definitive diagnosis, but because this invasive procedure carries some risks, empirical treatment is often offered if the clinical and radiographical pictures suggest infection.

Treatment consists of pyrimethamine plus sulfadiazine or clindamycin. Clinical and radiological improvement is seen in more than 85 percent of patients by day 7. Because these medications are effective only against the tachyzoite form of the protozoan, they must be continued for a full 6 weeks, and then prophylaxis, usually with the treating agents, must be prescribed to prevent recrudescence. The use of trimethoprim-sulfamethoxazole as prophylaxis has reduced the incidence of *T. gondii* infection. Patients with hypersensitivity to sulfa drugs may use pyrimethamine plus dapsone.

Cytomegalovirus (CMV) CMV infection is found at autopsy in approximately 30 percent of brains from HIV-infected patients. However, the development of clinically evident CMV encephalitis is fairly rare and most often occurs in patients with CD4 counts less than 50 cells per μL. Of particular note, CMV infection of other tissue, such as retina, blood, adrenal glands, or GI tract, is often found at the time of encephalitis.

There are two distinct syndromes of CMV CNS infection. The first and more common is encephalitis with dementia, which presents with subacute onset accompanied by periods of delirium, confusion, apathy, and focal neurological deficits. The second is a ventriculoencephalitis in which CMV infects the ependymal cells lining the ventricles, causing a rapid progression from delirium to death, with cranial nerve deficits and ventriculomegaly developing quickly.

Investigation of CMV encephalitis begins with examination for signs of CMV infection of the retinae, electrolyte studies to look for adrenal insufficiency, and viral blood cultures. CT scan may show ventriculomegaly or decreased attenuation diffusely throughout the parenchyma. MRI may show increased signal intensity around the ventricles. CSF studies may be normal or show high protein, low glucose, and pleocytosis. CSF CMV cultures are usually negative, but PCR may reveal the presence of the virus. Brain biopsy provides a definitive diagnosis.

Treatment is mostly supportive. Ganciclovir and foscarnet may be prescribed but are of questionable benefit. Trials of a promising new medication, cidofovir, are under way.

Cryptococcal Meningitis Although meningitis caused by *Cryptococcus neoformans* is rare in immunocompetent people, it occurs in approximately 8 to 10 percent of AIDS patients and may be devastating. Patients generally present with fever and delirium. In contrast, meningeal signs (headache, stiff neck, photophobia, and nausea) are not universally seen. Seizures and focal neurological deficits occur in approximately 10 percent of patients. CT scans are normal, but gadolinium-enhanced MRI may show meningeal inflammation. Intracranial pressure is elevated in 50 percent of patients. CSF studies are normal in approximately 20 percent but otherwise show mild to moderate monocytosis, elevated protein, decreased glucose, and positive fungal cultures. The fungus can be seen on india ink stain of CSF approximately 60 to 80 percent of the time. There is also a test for *C. neoformans* antigen, which is usually positive in both serum and CSF.

Treatment for cryptococcal meningitis requires amphotericin B (Fungizone) and flucytosine (Ancobon). Patients who survive must receive prophylaxis against recurrence because this is very common. Some authors suggest that patients who receive HAART for 6 months with an increase in CD4 count to more than 100 cells per μL may terminate secondary prophylaxis. Prophylaxis can be prescribed as oral fluconazole or intermittent IV amphotericin B. Primary prophylaxis for *C. neoformans* is not recommended.

Progressive Multifocal Leukoencephalopathy PML is a demyelinating disease of white matter in immunocompromised patients. First described in cancer patients, the causative agent is a polyoma virus named *JC virus* after a patient (not to be confused with Creutzfeldt-Jakob disease, caused by a prion). Its transmission route is unclear but may be respiratory, and there is no known clinical syndrome of acute infection. The prevalence of PML in AIDS is between 1 and 10 percent of patients, although AIDS patients account for almost three-fourths of PML cases seen in the United States. Typically, PML affects AIDS patients with fewer than 100 CD4 cells per μL.

The pathology of PML consists of demyelination and death of astrocytes and oligodendroglia, with a multifocal presentation. The clinical syndrome consists of multiple focal neurological deficits, such as mono- or hemiparetic limb weakness, dysarthria, gait disturbances or sensory deficits, and progressive dementia, with eventual coma and death. Occasionally, there may be seizures or visual losses. There is usually no fever or headache.

MRI is more useful than CT in diagnosis, displaying multiple areas of attenuated signal on T2 images primarily in the white matter of brain, although gray matter, brainstem, cerebellar, and spinal cord lesions are possible. CSF studies are generally unhelpful except for PCR evaluation for the presence of JC virus, which is sensitive and specific. Brain biopsy provides the definitive diagnosis but is rarely used. Trials of antiviral agents for the treatment of PML are under way but have been largely unsuccessful.

CNS Neoplasms Lymphoma is the most common neoplasm seen in AIDS patients, affecting between 0.6 and 3.0 percent. AIDS is the most common condition associated with primary CNS lymphoma. The patient is generally afebrile and may develop a single lesion with focal neurological signs or small, multifocal lesions most commonly presenting with a mental status change. Seizures present in approximately 15 percent of patients. CNS lymphoma is at times misdiagnosed as toxoplasmosis, HIV dementia, or other encephalopathy. CT scan of the brain may be normal or show multiple hypodense or patchy, nodular enhancing lesions. MRI generally shows enhanced lesions that may be difficult to differentiate from CNS toxoplasmosis, but thallium single photon emission computed tomography (SPECT) scanning may help differentiate the two disorders and is 90 percent sensitive and specific for lymphoma. CSF studies may be normal or show a moderate monocytosis; cytology studies reveal lymphoma cells in less than 5 percent of patients. Brain biopsy is required for confirmation of the diagnosis of CNS lymphoma. As this procedure carries some morbidity, clinicians should weigh the clinical presentation carefully, suspecting lymphoma in afebrile patients with a negative toxoplasma IgG screening test, patients with a single lesion, and patients who do not respond to empirical therapy for toxoplasmosis as demonstrated by clinical examination and repeat MRI at 2 weeks. The differential diagnosis of CNS neoplasm also includes metastatic Kaposi's sarcoma and primary glial tumors. Lymphoma may respond in part to radiation therapy, thus alleviating high intracranial pressure and its associated symptoms. Chemotherapy is generally adjunctive for lymphoma. Although CNS lymphoma had a grim prognosis with an average survival of 3 to 5 months before the advent of HAART, the prognosis is now dependent on the HAART response, with considerable improvement possible in patients who respond to HAART.

Direct CNS Manifestations of HIV

Guillain-Barré Syndrome A small percentage of patients, usually young men, present with Guillain-Barré syndrome associated with early HIV infection. Guillain-Barré syndrome is an inflammatory demyelinating polyneuropathy causing symmetrical paralysis and few, if any, sensory symptoms, usually beginning in the lower extremities and progressing upward. The condition becomes especially serious if abdominal musculature is involved, as it may impair respiration. The disorder is believed to be autoimmune in etiology and generally self-limited. IV Ig and plasmapheresis have been used to shorten the course, but neither treatment has been studied well in HIV-infected individuals.

Vacuolar Myelopathy Vacuolar myelopathy is highly prevalent among patients with AIDS, being found in up to approximately 50 percent of patients at autopsy. Clinical manifestation of this disease is much less common, affecting 20 to 30 percent of end-stage AIDS patients. The presence of vacuolar myelopathy has been associated with a history of *P. carinii* and *M. avium-intracellulare* infections, suggesting that the development of vacuolar myelopathy is related to more severe immunosuppression. The mechanism of the disease is unclear but appears similar to the myelopathy of combined systems disease associated with vitamin B_{12} deficiency. Multinucleated giant cells are seen on histological examination, and theories about mechanism focus on immunological activation damage, direct toxicity of HIV products, and metabolic dysfunction of transmethylation processes.

The clinical manifestations of vacuolar myelopathy appear when the disease progresses to affect the lateral and posterior columns and, thus, includes spastic paraparesis, loss of proprioception and vibration sense, bowel and bladder urgency or incontinence, and impotence. To date, no data exist to suggest that HAART has any effect on incidence or course, but one open pilot study showed promising results using L-methionine.

Special Issues in HIV

Fatigue Fatigue is a common symptom in HIV-infected patients that is often overlooked, improperly assessed, or inadequately investigated. Several authors have commented on the high prevalence of fatigue as a symptom of HIV infection, especially in later stages. Fatigue may be mild and annoying, or it may be severe enough to impair function. Several scales have been published to assess fatigue symptoms and severity. Fatigue is a nonspecific symptom and may have a single or multifactorial etiology. Medical causes include pneumonia, bronchitis, hypothyroidism, hepatitis, heart failure, renal failure, many cancers, and myopathy. In a sample of ambulatory AIDS patients, fatigue significantly correlated with anemia and pain. In addition to disease causes, patients may present with fatigue as a side effect of medications such as antihypertensives, anticonvulsants, benzodiazepines, antidepressants, narcotic analgesics, antipsychotics, antiemetics, antihistamines, and, most important for HIV patients, HAART. In fact, fatigue has been found to be one of the most common side effects of PIs and may be a reason for nonadherence.

Fatigue may also be the result of a psychiatric disorder. Alcohol and substance use disorders may lead to fatigue, either related to the use or withdrawal of the substance or as a symptom of demoralization in addicts. Most important, fatigue is caused by major depression. HIV patients with major depression are much more likely to complain of fatigue than patients without depression. Many depression screening tools, such as the BDI and Hamilton Depression Rating Scale, have not been very useful in distinguishing fatigue from major depression, usually because fatigue symptoms are present on the screening tools.

In general, the evaluation of a patient complaining of fatigue should include a careful history of its temporal characteristics, severity, and associated symptoms. It should also include careful review of current and recent medications, physical examination, and a mental status examination. The latter should carefully examine for anhedonia; diminished sense of self-worth; guilty feelings; sleep disturbance, especially early-morning awakening with inability to return to sleep; appetite changes, especially a recent, more than 5 percent change in body weight; thoughts of death or suicide; and impairments in concentration or memory. Certain laboratory studies should also be obtained, including complete blood cell count, electrolytes, liver tests, oxygen saturation, and thyroid function tests.

If fatigue is believed to be related to a medical or medication cause, all attempts should be made to treat the illness or modify the medication so as to alleviate the fatigue. In this context, testosterone is a successful treatment for fatigue in HIV-infected men, even when depressive symptoms are present. Of course, a clinical major depression should be treated with standard therapies. More activating antidepressants, such as fluoxetine (Prozac), citalopram (Celexa), escitalopram (Lexapro) or bupropion SR, may be better tolerated by fatigued depressed patients. Some authors have reported that dextroamphetamine (Dexedrine) may be useful in treating fatigue and depression in HIV. Care must be exercised in using stimulants, as long-term use may lead to dependence or worsening depression on some occasions.

HIV/HCV Coinfection Hepatitis C virus (HCV) is a blood-borne pathogen that is currently most commonly transmitted by injection drug use but may be transmitted sexually, although far less commonly than HIV. Some clinics have reported that 50 percent of HIV-infected patients are also infected with HCV. The natural history of HCV infection in HIV-negative individuals is that 15 percent of patients clear the infection after the acute phase, whereas 85 percent progress to a chronic infection. Hepatic fibrosis develops, often requiring approximately 10 years to reach significant levels, with cirrhosis following approximately 20 years from time of infection. Hepatocellular carcinoma (HCC) has been linked to chronic HCV infection and usually develops approximately 30 years after infection. However, HIV infection is likely to make individuals more susceptible to contract HCV if exposed, likely due to immunosuppression, and also to cause more rapid progression of liver disease, cutting the above approximate timetable in half (i.e., fibrosis in 5 years, cirrhosis in 10, HCC in 15). Liver failure is a growing cause of death in HIV patients.

Very little has been written about the specific psychiatric disturbances seen in HIV/HCV coinfected patients. However, a fair amount has been described regarding the development of neuropsychiatric complications of treatment with interferon alpha, a mainstay of therapy for HCV. In particular, interferon alpha has been associated with depressive syndromes, suicide, and, on rare occasions, mania. Patients with preexisting depression or bipolar disorder are more likely to develop affective symptoms while receiving the drug but may not be more likely to stop treatment than patients developing these symptoms de novo. Further, depressive symptoms associated with interferon alpha have been successfully treated with both SSRIs and TCAs.

Coinfected HIV/HCV patients should be screened for the presence of psychiatric disturbance like any other patient with HIV, but special monitoring should be performed during the period of treatment with interferon alpha for the purpose of early recognition and treatment of affective symptoms. Alcohol hastens the progression of HCV disease and should be strongly discouraged in any amount. Drug use other than alcohol may exacerbate neuropsychiatric side effects of interferon alpha, and patients should be stabilized before this antiviral treatment. Although no data exist yet, methadone maintenance may be a good option for patients who cannot achieve abstinence from opiates but need to start interferon therapy due to precipitous declines in liver function.

FUTURE DIRECTIONS

HIV and AIDS are conditions intimately linked to psychiatry. In a sense, psychiatric disorders can be seen as vectors of HIV transmission and additionally complicate the treatment of HIV. Also, HIV produces a number of psychiatric conditions and exacerbates many others. This chapter has attempted to show the intense comorbidity and links among various types of psychiatric conditions, the way depression exacerbates addictions, the way personality disorder exacerbates addictions, and the way in which addictions exacerbate both personality vulnerabilities and depression. HIV is driven by behaviors that are intimately connected with all of these conditions.

The authors see HIV as a model for the way in which psychiatry needs to speak to the rest of medicine about the role of psychiatry in general medicine and health care. It is a sad symptom of the problems in U.S. health care that there are abundant data showing the need for psychiatric presence in every phase of HIV care, and yet there is a poverty of funding and availability of psychiatric care in HIV clinics.

The authors' experience in caring for HIV patients is that by developing a comprehensive diagnostic formulation on which to base treatment, there is significant success with even difficult patients. The formulation includes disease syndromes such as major depression and schizophrenia, personality vulnerabilities such as unstable extroversion, behavioral disorders such as addictions, and problems of life experience such as trauma and trust issues. Each problem has the potential to sabotage treatment for all the remaining conditions. The treatment plan must be comprehensive in scope to address the whole person.

The authors have had the privilege of watching patients face their own certain death as their CD4 cell counts drop and the ominous specter of opportunistic conditions arise. The authors have then watched the nearly miraculous medical advances save these patients, only to find them facing life again and completely unprepared to meet the challenges this imposes on them. These same patients must now press on in the face of daily burdens of ongoing treatment, side effects, stigma, and ongoing injury. To help them with this is a monumental task, but the lessons from the field of psychiatry are there that have helped patients shoulder the same burdens from mental illness. At the heart of the work, the authors try to give hope for the future, therapeutic optimism, advocacy, sanctuary, and rehabilitation—the approaches psychiatry has discovered as the field has evolved.

SUGGESTED CROSS-REFERENCES

Some of the specific syndromes associated with HIV infection are discussed in Chapter 10 on delirium, dementia, and other cognitive disorders; in Chapter 11 on substance-related disorders; in Chapter 12 on schizophrenia; in Section 12.5 on other psychotic disorders; in Chapter 13 on mood disorders; in Chapter 14 on anxiety disorders; and in Chapter 18 on human sexuality. Treatment of specific disorders is reviewed in Chapter 30 on psychotherapies and in Chapter 31 on biological therapies. Detailed information on neuropsychological assessment is provided in Chapter 7 on diagnosis and psychiatry. Psychoneuroendocrinology is covered in Section 1.11 and the immune system is discussed in detail in Section 1.12. Additional topics in neuropsychiatry are treated in Chapter 2 on neuropsychiatry and behavioral neurology. Discussion of neuroimaging is provided in Sections 1.15 and 1.16 on neuroimaging in clinical practice. Detailed discussion of life adversity and immunity is provided in Section 24.9 on behavior and immunity.

REFERENCES

American Psychiatric Association. *The Diagnostic and Statistical Manual of Mental Disorders.* 4th ed. Washington, DC: American Psychiatric Press; 1994.

*Angelino AF, Treisman GJ: Management of psychiatric disorders in patients infected with human immunodeficiency virus. *Clin Infect Dis.* 2001;33:847–856.

Astemborski J, Vlahov D, Warren D, Solomon L, Nelson KE: The trading of sex for drugs or money and HIV seropositivity among female intravenous drug users. *Am J Public Health.* 1994;84:382–387.

Avants SK, Warburton LA, Hawkins KA, Margolin A: Continuation of high-risk behavior by HIV-positive drug users. *J Substance Abuse Treat.* 2000;19:15–22.

Breitbart W, McDonald MV, Rosenfeld B, Monkman ND, Passik S: Fatigue in ambulatory AIDS patients. *J Pain Symptom Manage.* 1998;15:159–167.

Brooner RK, Greenfield L, Schmidt, CW, Bigelow GE: Antisocial personality disorder and HIV infection among intravenous drug users. *Am J Psychiatry.* 1993;150:53–58.

Ciesla JA, Roberts JE: Meta-analysis of the relationship between HIV infection and risk for depressive disorders. *Am J Psychiatry.* 2001;158:725–730.

Costa PT Jr, Widiger TA, eds. *Personality Disorders and the Five-Factor Model of Personality.* Washington, DC: American Psychological Association; 1994.

Cournos F, Guido JR, Coomaraswamy S, Meyer-Bahlburg H, Sugden R, Horwath E: Sexual activity and risk of HIV infection among patients with schizophrenia. *Am J Psychiatry.* 1994;151:228–232.

*Davis HF, Skolasky RL Jr, Selnes OA, Burgess DM, McArthur JC: Assessing HIV-associated dementia: Modified HIV dementia scale versus the grooved pegboard. *AIDS Reader* 2002;12:29–31, 38.

Dinwiddie SH, Cottler L, Compton W, Ben Aabdallah A: Psychopathology and HIV risk behaviors among injection drug users in and out of treatment. *Drug Alcohol Depend.* 1996;43:1–11.

Edlin BR, Irwin KL, Faruque S, McCoy CB, Word C, Serrano Y, Inciardi JA, Bowser BP, Schilling RF, Holmberg SD, Multicenter Crack Cocaine and HIV Infection Study Team: Intersecting epidemics—crack cocaine use and HIV infection among inner-city young adults. *N Engl J Med.* 1994;331:1422–1427.

Eysenck HJ: Genetic and environmental contributions to individual differences: The three major dimensions of personality. *J Pers.* 1990;58:245–261.

Ferrando S, Evans S, Goggin K, Sewell M, Fishman B, Rabkin J: Fatigue in HIV illness: Relationship to depression, physical limitations, and disability. *Psychosom Med.* 1998;60:759–764.

Golding M, Perkins DO: Personality disorder in HIV infection. *Int Rev Psychiatry.* 1996;8:253–258.

Gourevitch MN, Friedland GH: Interactions between methadone and medications used to treat HIV infection: A review. *Mt Sinai J Med.* 2000;67:429–436.

Hutton, HE, Treisman GJ, Hunt WR, Fishman M, Kendig N, Swetz A, Lyketsos CG: HIV risk behaviors and their relationship to posttraumatic stress disorder among women prisoners. *Psychiatr Serv.* 2001;52:508–513.

*Ickovics JR, Hamburger ME, Vlahov D, Schoenbaum EE, Schuman P, Boland RJ, Moore J: HIV Epidemiology Research Study Group: Mortality, CD4 cell count decline, and depressive symptoms among HIV-seropositive women: Longitudinal analysis from the HIV epidemiology research study. *JAMA* 2001;285:1466–1474.

Johnson JG, Williams JB, Rabkin JG, Goetz RR, Remien RH: Axis I psychiatric symptomatology associated with HIV infection and personality disorder. *Am J Psychiatry.* 1995;152:551–554.

Kalichman SC Heckkman T, Kelly JA: Sensation-seeking as an explanation for the association between substance use and HIV-related risky sexual behavior. *Arch Sexual Behavior.* 1996;25:141–154.

Lyketsos CG, Hanson A, Fishman M, McHugh PR, Treisman GJ: Screening for psychiatric morbidity in a medical outpatient clinic for HIV infection: The need for a psychiatric presence. *Int J Psychiatry Med.* 1994;24:103–113.

Lyketsos CG, Hoover DR, Guccion, M, Dew MA, Wesch J, Bing EG, Treisman GJ: Changes in depressive symptoms as AIDS develops. *Am J Psychiatry.* 1996;153:1430–1437.

Lyketsos CG, Schwartz J, Fishman M, Treisman G: AIDS mania. *J Neuropsychiatry Clin Neurosci.* 1997;9:277–279.

McArthur JC, McClernon DR, Cronin MF, Nance-Sproson TE, Saah AJ, St. Clair M, Lanier ER: Relationship between human immunodeficiency virus-associated dementia and viral load in cerebrospinal fluid and brain. *Ann Neurol.* 1997;42:689–698.

*McCown W: Contributions of the EPN paradigm to HIV prevention: A preliminary study. *Pers Individ Dif.* 1991;12:1301–1303.

McCown W: Personality factors predicting failure to practice safer sex by HIV-positive males. *Pers Individ Dif.* 1993;14:613–615.

McDaniel JS, Chung JY, Brown L, Cournos F, Forstein M, Goodkin K, Lyketsos C, Work Group on HIV/AIDS: Practice guidelines for the treatment of patients with HIV/AIDS. *Am J Psychiatry.* 2000;157:1–62.

McKinnon K, Cournos F, Sugden R, Guido JR, Herman R: The relative contributions of psychiatric symptoms and AIDS knowledge to HIV risk behaviors among people with severe mental illness. *J Clin Psychiatry.* 1996;57:506–513.

Novotna L, Wilson TE, Minkoff HL, McNutt LA, DeHovitz JA, Ehrlich I, Des Jarlais DC: Predictors and risk-taking consequences of drug use among HIV-infected women. *J Acquir Immune Defic Syndr Hum Retrovirol.* 1999;20:502–507.

Perkins DO, Davidson EJ, Leserman J, Liao D, Evans DL: Personality disorder in patients infected with HIV: A controlled study with implications for clinical care. *Am J Psychiatry.* 1993;150:309–315.

Perkins DO, Leserman J, Stem RA, Baum SF, Liao D, Golden RN, Evans DL: Somatic symptoms and HIV infection: Relationship to depressive symptoms and indicators of HIV disease. *Am J Psychiatry.* 1995;152:1776–1781.

Prochaska JO, DiClemente CC, Norcross JC: In search of how people change. Applications to addictive behaviors. *Am Psychol.* 1992;47:1102–1114.

*Rees V, Saitz R, Horton NJ, Samet J: Association of alcohol consumption with HIV sex- and drug-risk behaviors among drug users. *J Subst Abuse Treat.* 2001;21:129–134.

Rutter M: Temperament, personality and personality disorder. *Br J Psychiatry.* 1987;150:443–458.

Stein MD, Hanna L, Natarajan R, Clarke J, Marisi M, Sobota M, Rich J: Alcohol use patterns predict high-risk HIV behaviors among active injection drug users. *J Subst Abuse Treat.* 2000;18:359–363.

Tourian K, Alterman A, Metzger D, Rutherford M, Cacciola JS, McKay JR: Validity of three measures of antisociality in predicting HIV risk behaviors in methadone-maintenance patients. *Drug Alcohol Depend.* 1997;47:99–107.

*Treisman G, Fishman M, Schwartz J, Hutton H, Lyketsos C: Mood disorders in HIV infection. *Depress Anxiety*. 1998;7:178–187.

Trobst KK, Wiggins JS, Costa PT Jr, Herbst JH, McCrae RR, Masters HL II: Personality psychology and problem behaviors: HIV risk and the five-factor model. *J Personality*. 2000;68:1232–1252.

Volavka J, Convit A, O'Donnell J, Douyon R, Evangelista C, Czobor P: Assessment of risk factors for HIV infection among psychiatric inpatients. *Hosp Comm Psychiatry*. 1992;43:482–485.

Wagner GJ, Rabkin JG, Rabkin R: Testosterone as a treatment for fatigue in HIV+ men. *Gen Hosp Psychiatry*. 1998;20:209–213.

Weissman MM: The epidemiology of personality disorders: A 1990 update. *J Pers Disord*. 1993;7[Suppl]:44–62.

Zuckerman M: Good and bad humors: Biochemical bases of personality and its disorders. *Psychol Sci*. 1995;6:325–332.

Zuckerman M: Sensation seeking: A comparative approach to a human trait. *Behav Brain Sci*. 1984;7:413–471.

▲ 2.9 Neuropsychiatric Aspects of Other Infectious Diseases (Non-HIV)

Brian Anthony Fallon, M.D., M.P.H.

Since 1990, microbes have been connected with a variety of medical disorders previously considered outside the domain of infectious disease, such as *Chlamydia* contributing to atherosclerotic heart disease and *Helicobacter pylori* contributing to gastric and duodenal ulcers. On the neuropsychiatric front, compelling evidence links streptococcal infection with the onset of obsessive-compulsive disorder (OCD) and tic disorders in susceptible children and *Borrelia* infection with the onset of irritability, mood swings, and cognitive problems. The search for infectious causes of neuropsychiatric disorders is a logical enterprise, given the increasing recognition of the importance of environmental factors in the development of psychiatric disorders. For example, prenatal exposure to infection is considered one of the strongest candidate risk factors for the development of schizophrenia, based on observations linking schizophrenia with birth during the winter and in urban areas and ecological studies demonstrating associations between influenza and rubella epidemics and births of preschizophrenic patients.

The link between severe neuropsychiatric disorders and infectious disease was established in the early 1900s by the identification of a spirochete as the cause of syphilis and was reinforced in the 1920s after severe neurobehavioral syndromes were observed among people affected by the viral influenza epidemic. At times, the link between an infectious agent and a neuropsychiatric disorder is obvious, as in the case of the current human immunodeficiency virus (HIV) and the Lyme disease epidemics. At other times, the link is less clear but strongly suspected, as has been true for chronic fatigue syndrome.

Infectious agents may affect the central nervous system (CNS) directly or indirectly. Direct involvement by a neurotropic agent may result from attachment of the microbe to neuronal tissue, eliciting a local inflammatory response and immediate dysfunction, or by integration of the microbial genome into the cellular deoxyribonucleic acid (DNA), resulting in long-term alternations in brain function. Alternatively, the microbe may have indirect effects through its impact on the host-determined cellular, humoral, or cytokine immune responses. The quality and intensity of the immune response, modulated by genetic factors, may be perpetuated by the continued presence of a viable organism, a piece of a nonviable organism, or a misdirected cross-reactive autoimmune process that was initiated by prior infection. The immune response in its effort to protect may thereby provoke neuropsychiatric disorders.

This section focuses on selected infectious diseases other than HIV that invade the CNS and that have been directly associated with neuropsychiatric syndromes. Particular attention is paid to the neuropsychiatric aspects of Lyme disease, because it is a disease that has spread rapidly during the past two decades in various parts of the world and has been associated with a plethora of neuropsychological and neurobehavioral problems in children and adults. The concluding portion of this section briefly addresses a few areas of emerging interest into the overlap of infectious disease and neuropsychiatry.

SPIROCHETAL DISEASES

Under the umbrella of the order of spirochetes are three agents that are known to invade the CNS. These include *Borrelia*, *Treponema*, and *Leptospira*. *Borrelia*, which require an arthropod vector and a mammalian or bird reservoir, are commonly known to cause relapsing fever and Lyme disease. *Treponema*, which are spread person to person and do not use an arthropod vector, are the spirochetes responsible for syphilis. *Leptospira*, which are spread by contaminated water, are the agents of Weil's syndrome, which can have CNS manifestations.

Lyme Disease (Lyme Borreliosis)

Lyme disease, transmitted by the bite of an infected *Ixodes* tick, can cause a vast array of neuropsychiatric disorders, ranging from mild mood changes to psychosis and severe memory loss. Lyme disease has been reported throughout the United States and in numerous countries throughout the world. The causative agent of Lyme disease, *Borrelia burgdorferi*, is initially inoculated into the skin by an infected tick, typically inducing a local bull's-eye–like rash, known as *erythema migrans*, which is recalled by approximately two-thirds of infected patients. Rapidly disseminated by the blood stream through the body, *B. burgdorferi* has been found in the CNS as soon as 3 weeks after initial skin infection. Known to be neurotropic, *B. burgdorferi* may reside in the CSF or may adhere to glial cells or other brain tissue. Like its spirochetal counterpart, *Treponema pallidum*, *B. burgdorferi* may remain latent, causing illness months to years later. Partly because of this latency in disease expression, patients may be unable to recall the initial tick bite or rash. Antigenic variability, that is, the ability to express different surface antigens and thus to evade the immune response, is a feature of *Borrelia* organisms that *B. burgdorferi* shares.

Diagnosis

The epidemiological surveillance criteria for the diagnosis of Lyme disease in the United States require a history of exposure to a Lyme endemic area and a physician-diagnosed erythema migrans rash or serological evidence of exposure to *B. burgdorferi* and at least one of the following three clinical features: (1) arthritis, (2) neurologic symptoms (cranial or peripheral neuropathy, meningitis, encephalomyelitis, or encephalitis with evidence of intrathecal antibody production), or (3) cardiac conduction defects. Although useful for epidemiologic monitoring, these criteria are unduly restrictive for clinical purposes, excluding patients who might not recall the rash as well as seropositive patients who have diffuse arthralgias but not frank arthritis or patients who have encephalopathy without objective CSF abnormalities. Further complicating the diagnosis is the unreliability of the serological tests. False-positive results might result because of cross-reactivity with other spirochetal organisms. False-negative results may occur because the patient is tested too soon after infection before an appropriate antibody response is mounted or because the patient's immune response has been abrogated. It is not uncommon for a patient with Lyme disease to test negative or equivocally in one laboratory but positive in another or for a patient to test negative initially but positive several months later after antibiotic treatment has been initiated. For these reasons, a rational approach to the diagnosis of Lyme disease must be based on the clinical presentation primarily, followed by the supportive evidence supplied by laboratory tests. Laboratory tests that can be helpful include indirect tests, such as enzyme-linked immunosorbent assay (ELISA) and Western blot test, and direct tests, such as polymerase chain reaction (PCR) for *Borrelia* DNA or antigen detection assays. A newer ELISA, based on an invariant C6 region, is a highly specific, adjunctive test for Lyme disease. Bands of particular significance on the Western blot test include the ones identified by the Centers for Disease Control (CDC) as being most frequent and specific, as well as the 31-kDa (OspA) and 34-kDa (OspB) bands. The PCR assay, although highly specific for *B. burgdorferi* DNA, has low sensitivity.

Clinical Manifestations The erythema migrans rash is the hallmark feature of early Lyme disease. Antibiotic treatment at this stage often results in cure. Because patients may not recall or see the rash, the flu-like symptoms that often occur shortly after the rash may be ignored, only to be followed several months to years later by the emergence of a multisystem disease affecting the joints, the heart, the eyes, or the peripheral nervous system or the CNS, or a combination of these. Fifteen to 40 percent of patients may have neurological signs as their presenting feature. Headaches may be followed by meningitis, cranial neuritis, motor or sensory radiculitis, or an encephalitis characterized by mood lability and disturbances of memory or sleep, or a combination of these. Although suggestive of Lyme disease, seventh cranial nerve palsy may occur in only 5 to 10 percent of a sample of patients with neurological Lyme disease. Symptoms of radiculoneuropathy and peripheral nerve involvement include sharp stabbing or deep boring pains that may radiate from the spine into an extremity or the trunk; areas of numbness, burning, or tingling; weakness; and fasciculations. In later stages of Lyme disease, a minority of patients may develop a chronic meningoencephalomyelitis characterized by somnolence, confusion, poor concentration, impaired memory, myoclonus, apraxia, ataxia, paraparesis, dysarthria, dysphasia, seizures, or bladder abnormalities, or a combination of these. Some of these patients may be misdiagnosed as having multiple sclerosis (MS) because of the overlapping features of a relapsing and remitting course and the concurrence of spinal motor signs, ataxia, bladder dysfunction, and, less often, optic neuritis.

The profile of neuropsychiatric Lyme disease typically includes disturbances of cognition and mood. On formal neuropsychological testing, more than 50 percent of patients with chronic neurological Lyme disease show impairment in short-term memory, processing speed, or attention, or a combination of these. This cognitive impairment, although worsened by marked pain, severe fatigue, sensory hyperacusis, or mood disorders, exists independently of the number of physical symptoms or the severity of concurrent depression. Typical cognitive symptoms include word-finding problems, word substitutions, new-onset dyslexia, transient episodes of geographical disorientation, marked inattention and distractibility, difficulty with organization, and the sensation that one's brain is in a fog. Less commonly, the severity of the cognitive disturbance causes a global impairment, suggestive of a new-onset dementia.

Although the full spectrum of psychiatric disorders has been associated with *B. burgdorferi* infection, by far the most frequent are disturbances of mood, characterized by irritability, mood swings, and sleep loss. The majority of controlled studies in which patients with Lyme disease are compared to healthy controls or to patients with other illnesses reveals that depression occurs more frequently in the group with Lyme disease. Children with neurological Lyme disease typically present with complaints of headaches as the most common symptom, followed by behavioral, attentional, or mood disturbance as the next most prevalent symptom. Common behavioral problems include agitation, falling asleep in class, and poor school performance; common cognitive problems include deficits in attention, short-term memory, and visuospatial functioning; and common mood problems include affective lability and new-onset anxiety disorders. Among children with Lyme disease and headaches, a lumbar puncture may reveal elevated intracranial pressure (also called *pseudotumor cerebri*), which, in extreme cases, may result in damage to the optic nerves. Other, less common neuropsychiatric aspects associated with Lyme disease include panic-like attacks associated with spontaneous palpitations, transient paranoia, illusions or hallucinations (visual, olfactory, and auditory), anorexia, depersonalization, OCD, agitated mania, and what appears to be personality change. Because of the multisystem involvement in Lyme disease and the frequent concurrence of anxiety, depression, or both, patients may be mistakenly diagnosed as having a primary psychiatric or a somatoform disorder before Lyme disease is even considered. If Lyme disease is considered, but serological tests are equivocal despite the presence of a clinical profile typical of Lyme disease, the somatoform label may once again be mistakenly applied.

Consider the following case:

A 30-year-old, previously healthy landscaper in a Lyme endemic area developed intermittent paranoid delusions followed, over the next few months, by progressive short-term memory loss. After not appearing at work, he was found collapsed on the front lawn of his house, calling the sky green and the grass blue. After an extensive medical workup revealed elevated Lyme antibodies in his cerebrospinal fluid (CSF) and serum, he was treated with 3 weeks of intravenous (IV) ceftriaxone (Rocephin) with marked improvement in his mental status. Two weeks after discharge, he developed painful knees and elbows and worsening verbal fluency, short-term memory, and processing speed. Reevaluation by the infectious disease specialist revealed a reduction in the CSF Lyme antibody levels, although the CSF was not yet normal. Because of the improved CSF, and because 3 weeks of IV antibiotic therapy were believed to be curative, the specialist denied additional antibiotic therapy. The family persisted in their concern, the doctor relented, and the patient received 2 more weeks of IV therapy without improvement. A team of mental health professionals then evaluated the patient and, based on the absence of a definite medical diagnosis and the presence of profound memory loss, diagnosed the patient as having a dissociative disorder and recommended inpatient psychiatric treatment. Contrary to medical advice, the patient's family removed him from the hospital's care and found a community doctor who agreed to treat the patient medically. After 4 months of IV cephalosporin therapy, the patient was able to feed himself but was not able to recall any event from the prior year. A brain single photon emission computed tomography (SPECT) scan revealed multiple areas of marked hypoperfusion in a patchy pattern. Faced with an inadequate response to the IV cephalosporin, the private physician switched to oral minocycline

(Minocin), which resulted in rapid improvement in mental status that has been sustained, with intermittent antibiotic therapy for presumed relapses, over a 4-year interval.

The previous case highlights several points: (1) Psychiatric symptoms may be the initial features of Lyme neuroborreliosis; (2) more typical Lyme symptoms (arthralgias) may not be present initially but may emerge later; (3) if IV cephalosporins are no longer helpful, antibiotics with different modes of action should be considered; (4) mental health professionals may mistakenly diagnose a patient as having a primary psychiatric disorder when faced with an atypical presentation of Lyme disease; and (5) SPECT imaging may be helpful in identifying a vasculitic-like hypoperfusion pattern among patients with Lyme disease. This case also highlights the uncertainty among physicians about how to treat patients with relapsing symptoms; some, who consider 3 weeks to be curative, deny additional antibiotic therapy, whereas others, who consider the return of symptoms to be a sign of reactivated infection, recommend extended courses of treatment.

Tests for CNS Lyme Disease Examination of the CSF is critical to rule out other possible causes of CNS disease and to identify the presence of Lyme meningitis or encephalitis. In the latter conditions, a spinal tap may reveal lymphocytic pleocytosis, mildly increased protein, and, in some cases, an elevated immunoglobulin (Ig) G index or the presence of oligoclonal bands. In later stage neurologic Lyme disease, however, the CSF may appear normal. Magnetic resonance imaging (MRI) studies may reveal punctate white matter lesions on T2-weighted images, suggestive of a demyelinating disorder, such as MS. Electroencephalogram (EEG) studies are generally normal, although diffuse slowing or epileptiform discharges may be seen. SPECT and positron emission tomography (PET) studies may be particularly helpful in late-stage CNS Lyme disease, demonstrating a pattern of diffuse, heterogeneous hypoperfusion which, in some cases, improves after antibiotic treatment (Fig. 2.9–1). Given the difficulties facing the clinician attempting to determine whether fatigue, mood lability, and cognitive tracking problems are due to primary depression or to an underlying systemic disease, functional imaging studies provide a valuable tool to assist in the differential diagnosis.

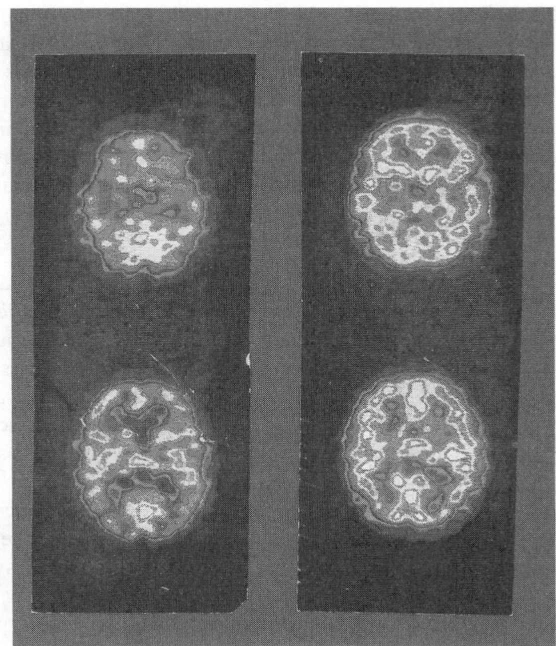

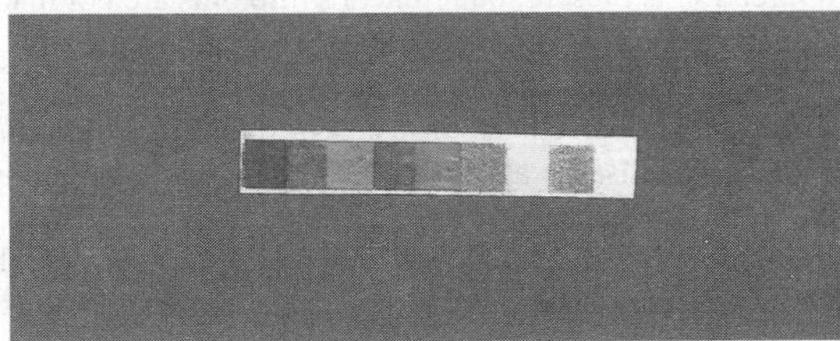

FIGURE 2.9–1 Single photon emission computed tomography scan image demonstrating multiple areas of decreased blood flow in a Lyme disease patient compared to a healthy control. (See Color Plate.)

Differential Diagnosis In considering the diagnosis of Lyme disease, it is critical to ask about exposure to a Lyme endemic area, history of a tick bite or unusual rash, and the presence of multisystemic involvement. Called the "new great imitator" (after the original great imitator, syphilis), the broad spectrum of atypical neurological manifestations of Lyme disease includes strokes, Guillain-Barré syndrome, cerebellar syndromes, seizures, pseudotumor-like syndrome in children, spastic paraparesis, MS-like illnesses, and progressive dementias. Similarly, other diseases that may look like neuropsychiatric Lyme disease need to be excluded, such as major depression with somatic preoccupation, panic disorder, systemic lupus erythematosus or other connective tissue diseases, chronic fatigue syndrome, endocrinological disorders, vitamin deficiencies, other infectious illnesses, multiinfarct dementias, and other neurodegenerative disorders.

Treatment For early Lyme disease without CNS involvement, 3 to 4 weeks of oral doxycycline (Doryx) (100 mg b.i.d.), amoxicillin (Amoxil) (500 mg t.i.d.), cefuroxime (Ceftin) (500 mg b.i.d.) is recommended. For Lyme disease with CNS involvement, an initial course of 4 to 6 weeks of IV ceftriaxone (2 g per day) or cefotaxime (Claforan) (2 g every 8 hours) is recommended. Symptoms may worsen during the first week of antibiotic treatment, much like the Jarisch-Herxheimer reaction during the treatment of syphilis. For patients who relapse, longer and repeated courses of antibiotics may be helpful. Failure to treat Lyme disease early in its course or for a sufficiently long duration may lead to a chronic illness characterized by persistent waxing and waning neuropsychiatric disturbances, arthralgias, myalgias, sensory hyperacuities, or severe fatigue, or a combination of these. In some patients, these symptoms reflect the effects of persistent infection, whereas, in others, the symptoms may reflect a residual postinfectious syndrome. Because the laboratory tests for chronic Lyme disease are not sufficiently reliable to document the presence or absence of persistent infection, decisions regarding treatment should be based primarily on the physician's clinical judgment. Research indicates that *B. burgdorferi* is capable of remarkable persistence in the host, despite standard courses of antibiotic treatment, and clinical reports document improvement in chronic Lyme disease among some patients treated with long courses of antibiotics. Two well-controlled trials provide conflicting results on the efficacy of repeated courses of IV antibiotic therapy for patients with chronic Lyme disease symptoms after having previously received the standard recommended treatment, with one showing no benefit in functional ability and the other showing significant improvement in the primary outcome measure of fatigue. At this point, some physicians treat their patients who have relapses with additional courses of antibiotic therapy in the hope of improvement, whereas others, wary of the risks associated with long-term antibiotic treatment, choose not to treat. Until additional, well-controlled clinical trials are published, much debate will remain about the proper antibiotic treatment for chronic Lyme disease.

Neurosyphilis The cause of syphilis, *T. pallidum*, was identified in 1905. Because of the cognitive loss and neuropsychiatric disturbances associated with tertiary neurosyphilis, these patients accounted for 5 to 15 percent of psychiatric hospital admissions, labeled as *general paresis*, *general paralysis of the insane*, or *dementia paralytica*. With penicillin treatment of primary and secondary syphilis, neurosyphilis is now an uncommon cause of hospital admissions.

Primary syphilis is manifest by a syphilitic ulcer, the chancre, at the site of inoculation. Secondary syphilis, a result of hematogenous dissemination of the spirochete, is characterized by flu-like symptoms followed by a skin rash, generalized lymphadenopathy, and mucosal lesions. Left untreated, primary and secondary syphilis resolve on their own, after which the patient enters a latent period wherein infection is present, but clinical symptoms are not manifest. After months to years, approximately one-third of patients with untreated latent syphilis develop tertiary syphilis affecting the brain or heart. As in neuroborreliosis, invasion of the CNS by *T. pallidum* occurs early in the disease and may be asymptomatic for months to years before clinical expression.

Clinical neurosyphilis can be divided into four types: syphilitic meningitis, meningovascular syphilis, parenchymatous neurosyphilis, and gummatous neurosyphilis. Syphilitic meningitis, the result of direct meningeal inflammation, rarely has focal findings. Meningovascular syphilis results from the ischemic changes caused by proliferative endarteritis, causing permanent CNS damage. In parenchymatous neurosyphilis (general paresis or tabes dorsalis), which generally starts 10 to 20 years after infection, there is direct neural destruction resulting in diminished neuron concentration, demyelination, and gliosis. In gummatous neurosyphilis, the mass effect causes neurological symptoms.

General paresis, peaking in incidence 10 to 20 years after infection, often starts with subtle cognitive and emotional changes, such as problems with concentration and irritability, and, if untreated, can lead to memory loss, confabulation, anomia, apraxia, or pseudobulbar palsy. The disease may mimic any psychiatric disorder, as well. One-half of the patients with neurosyphilis manifest dementia, of whom one-fourth of patients have prominent psychiatric manifestations, such as depression, paranoia, psychosis, or mania. A worsening of symptoms during the first 24 hours after the initiation of antibiotic treatment has been termed the Jarisch-Herxheimer reaction; in rare cases, psychosis may emerge shortly after antibiotics are started. With disease progression, there is loss of muscle tone, fine motor control, seizures, spasticity, and, eventually, paralysis and death. Focal neurological findings are rare, consistent with the generalized pathophysiology. Tabes dorsalis, on the other hand, develops somewhat later than general paresis, 15 to 20 years after infection, and causes a more characteristic clinical picture of lancinating pains, abdominal pain attacks, and paresthesias. Because of progressive loss of proprioception and sensation, patients compensate by a broad-based shuffling gait. Unlike general paresis, not all patients with tabes have CSF abnormalities.

Tests *T. pallidum* is difficult to demonstrate in the CSF and is difficult to culture. Although PCR techniques are being developed to detect the genetic material of the spirochete, this method is currently only available in research laboratories. Clinicians must rely on serological tests in the context of a careful history and physical examination. Serological tests for syphilis include the nontreponemal Venereal Disease Research Laboratory (VDRL) or rapid plasma reagin (RPR) tests and, for confirmatory purposes, the fluorescent treponemal antibody absorption (FTA-ABS) test. CSF studies are useful to confirm the diagnosis of neurosyphilis, if clinical findings are suggestive; to diagnose asymptomatic involvement, so that treatment can be started; and to follow treatment efficacy. These CSF studies are limited by the low specificity of the typical abnormalities of elevated protein, γ-globulin, and leukocyte count and the low sensitivity (but high specificity) of the VDRL. The CSF FTA-ABS, on the other hand, is thought to have excellent sensitivity but less specificity than the CSF VDRL. A positive CSF VDRL or CSF RPR result from a patient with appropriate clinical history establishes the diagnosis of neurosyphilis. Neuroradiological studies of neurosyphilis report cortical atrophy, most commonly affecting the frontal and temporal lobes.

Treatment The goal in clinical neurosyphilis is to reverse the manifestations or to arrest the disease progression, although, in some patients, antibiotic therapy may not be able to achieve these goals. Standard courses consist of IV aqueous penicillin G (Permapen), 12 to 24 million U daily in divided doses at 4-hour intervals for 2 weeks, or, alternatively, intramuscular (IM) weekly injections of 2.4 to 4.8 million U of benzathine penicillin for 3 weeks or IM injections of 2.4 million U of procaine penicillin four times daily for 2 weeks. The likelihood of marked improvement for patients with general paresis is less than that for patients with syphilitic meningitis or meningovascular syphilis, reflecting the pathological process that, in the former, is irreversible neuron damage and, in the latter, is CNS inflammation. During the first year after treatment, the serum and CSF should be regularly monitored for the reemergence of reactivity, so that treatment can be reinitiated if necessary. Certain conditions, such as comorbid HIV infection, may place patients at greater risk for persistence of treponemal infection after antibiotic treatment. Most neurosyphilis patients, however, with treatment show improvement in the cognitive, psychiatric, and functional domains.

NON-HIV VIRAL INFECTIONS OF THE CENTRAL NERVOUS SYSTEM

Numerous viruses are invasive and neurotropic, with the extent of consequent neuronal dysfunction varying widely depending on the virulence of the virus and the immunological response of the host. This section focuses on agents known to cause striking neuropsychiatric diseases: herpes simplex virus (HSV), rabies, measles, and subacute sclerosing panencephalitis (see Table 2.9–1 for other viruses).

Herpes Viruses Included under the spectrum of herpesviruses are herpesvirus type 1 (HSV-1), herpesvirus type 2 (HSV-2), varicella-zoster virus, Epstein-Barr virus (EBV), cytomegalovirus (CMV), human herpesvirus 6, human herpesvirus 7, and Kaposi's sarcoma–associated herpesvirus.

Herpes Simplex HSV encephalitis is a dramatic disorder, characterized by abrupt onset of fever, personality change, and headaches, followed by cognitive changes and focal neurological signs, such as aphasia, visual field deficits, hemiparesis, or partial seizures. Although focality is an important feature of HSV encephalitis, other viruses may also have focal signs, such as the La Crosse virus or the nonpolio enteroviruses. Neurobehavioral aspects of HSV encephalitis, such as hallucinations, memory loss, or behavioral disturbances, may be the presenting features, a consequence of the predilection of the virus for the temporal lobes. Although the course of illness is typically rapidly progressive, resulting in refractory seizures, coma, and death within 2 weeks, occasionally, the progression may be slower with varied neuropsychiatric features.

HSV-1 is usually transmitted orally, entering the CNS through sensory nerves, particularly the trigeminal ganglia. HSV-2 is transmitted genitally and may seed the sacral ganglia or disseminate hematogenously. HSV typically produces a lytic infection with neuronal necrosis and tissue destruction and intranuclear inclusion bodies in the neurons and glia. Patients who survive HSV encephalitis may exhibit postencephalitic symptoms, such as amnesia, aphasia, and, less commonly, Klüver-Bucy syndrome or dementia.

Routine serological studies are of little value in suspected HSV encephalitis. The CSF usually demonstrates leukocytosis (approximately 100 cells per mm^3), a moderate protein elevation, and a normal or depressed glucose content. PCR analysis of the CSF to detect HSV DNA is, at present, the diagnostic procedure of choice, as the PCR assay has high sensitivity and specificity. Recent studies indicate that approximately 80 percent of patients with biopsy-proven HSV encephalitis have focal EEG abnormalities consisting of slowing or repetitive epileptiform discharges in the frontotemporal area. MRI studies in early stages of HSV encephalitis may reveal T2 relaxation time prolongation in the insular cortex and cingulate gyrus. SPECT or PET imaging may show reduced blood flow in the orbitofrontal and temporal regions. Brain biopsy can be helpful in difficult to diagnose cases, although the complication rate is approximately 3 percent.

If untreated, 40 to 70 percent of patients with HSV encephalitis die. Antiviral therapies include acyclovir (Zovirax) and vidarabine (Vira-A); however, even with acyclovir treatment, fewer than 40 percent of patients survive with minimal or no sequelae.

Epstein-Barr Virus

Most adults have evidence of past exposure to EBV, with approximately 50 percent seropositivity among children older than 5 years of age. Infection in childhood is generally mild, whereas, in adolescence and young adulthood, it may result in infectious mononucleosis or, rarely, a fulminant life-threatening disease. EBV enters the body by infecting oral mucosal epithelial cells. The clinical symptoms of infectious mononucleosis of sore throat, headache, malaise, and fatigue are largely a result of the vigorous cellular immune response to EBV infection rather than direct cytotoxic effects. Significant neurological complications of EBV infection are rare, occurring in less than 0.5 percent of cases of infectious mononucleosis.

EBV encephalitis occurs usually within 1 to 3 weeks after the onset of clinical infectious mononucleosis. Patients with EBV encephalitis may present with cerebellar ataxia, personality changes, psychosis, transient global amnesia, perceptual distortions of size and space, focal neurological findings, seizures, or coma. EEG usually reveals generalized slowing with occasional sharp wave activity. The diagnosis of an EBV neuropsychiatric syndrome requires an appropriate clinical history in the setting of serological evidence of acute or, rarely, chronic active infection. In cases of EBV encephalitis, commonly, there is a lymphocytic pleocytosis (atypical lymphocytes are particularly suggestive) with elevated protein. In most cases, EBV encephalitis is self-limited, with recovery occurring within weeks to months. Rarely, acute EBV infection may result in a relapsing or chronic encephalitis. Treatment is generally supportive.

Other Herpes Viruses

With herpes zoster, neuropsychiatric complications occur most frequently in immunocompromised patients, resulting in encephalitis, myelitis, or leukoencephalitis. With CMV infection, encephalitis may also occur, as CMV is tropic for the CNS; however, only in rare exceptions has CMV encephalitis occurred in non-HIV–infected immunocompromised individuals.

Rabies

Although most cases of human rabies occur after animal bites, other sources of rabies virus infection include aerosols (risk for spelunkers) and person-to-person transmission after corneal transplants. The rabies virus is a negatively stranded ribonucleic acid (RNA) virus that replicates locally at the site of inoculation and subsequently spreads to the CNS by retrograde axonal transport, infecting the lower areas of the brain most prominently, particularly the limbic system, hippocampus, brainstem, and cerebellum. Limbic system involvement may result in aberrant sexual behavior and behavioral dyscontrol, whereas brainstem involvement typically results in alterations of body temperature and respiratory control. The site and amount of inoculation are associated with morbidity. For example, multiple dog bites to the face may result in a 60 percent mortality rate without prophylactic intervention, whereas multiple bites to the hand are associated with lower mortality rates of approximately 15 percent. The incubation period before symptomatic expression ranges from a few days to several years. Once symptoms emerge, the course is rapidly fatal. Most patients get the furious form characterized by agitation, hallucinations, odd behaviors, extreme excitability, and, in some cases, hydrophobia. Diagnosis is based on the history of an animal bite in a patient with unexplained encephalitis that has been confirmed by the demonstration of rabies antigen on a skin biopsy of the patient or from a putatively infected animal. There is no treatment for rabies virus infection. Disease prevention is critical, aided by preexposure vaccination in high-risk individuals and postexposure prophylaxis with rabies immunoglobulin and rabies vaccine.

Rubella

The rubella virus, a member of the *Togaviridae* family, causes an acute exanthematous viral infection, characterized by rash, fever, and lymphadenopathy. Because postnatal rubella exposure causes only a mild illness, the main concern is with prenatal exposure, which can cause fetal death and severe congenital defects. Prenatal exposure to rubella virus has also been associated with a much higher risk of the emergence of other diseases in childhood and young adulthood, such as diabetes mellitus, progressive encephalopathy resembling subacute sclerosing panencephalitis, and, as suggested by recent studies, schizophrenia. Since the development of the live attenuated rubella vaccine in 1969, there have been no large rubella epidemics in countries in which the vaccine is widely used.

Subacute Sclerosing Panencephalitis

Subacute sclerosing panencephalitis is a rare, slow infection with measles virus that causes progressive inflammation and sclerosis of the brain. Primarily affecting children and young adults, the rate of subacute sclerosing panencephalitis decreased markedly after 1960 as a result of widespread measles vaccination, with a current rate in the United States of only one per 100 million people per year. The onset generally occurs 7 to 12 years after measles and is subtle, characterized by gradual changes in behavior and school performance. Neuropsychological testing may demonstrate reduced overall intelligence and problems with reading, writing, and visuospatial processing. Neuropsychiatric symptoms may include hallucinations, apraxia, agnosia, and Balint's syndrome (optic ataxia, simultanagnosia, and sticky fixation). Repetitive myoclonic jerks are common, at times accompanied by movement disorders and cerebellar ataxia. In advanced stages, dementia, mutism, cortical blindness, optic atrophy, stupor, coma, and death occur. The usual course of illness is 1 to 3 years, with rare patients surviving for as long as 10 years.

Serological testing may reveal unusually high titers of antibodies to measles virus. CSF studies typically show high measles antibody titers and a greatly elevated γ-globulin fraction with oligoclonal bands in a CSF with slightly elevated protein levels. EEG studies are essential, particularly in the myoclonic stage, revealing high-amplitude bilateral and stereotyped complexes that repeat every 3 to 5 seconds. MRI studies may reveal enlarged ventricles and diffuse brain atrophy, with multifocal low-density white matter lesions and lucent areas in the basal ganglia. PET and SPECT studies may reveal early subcortical hypermetabolism followed by global cortical and subcortical hypometabolism.

No treatments are known to reverse the disease, although slightly prolonged survival has been associated with inosiplex and with intraventricular injections of interferon-γ.

Progressive Multifocal Leukoencephalopathy

Progressive multifocal leukoencephalopathy, affecting immunocompromised subjects, is a progressive infection of oligodendroglial cells with the JC virus. Typically, the onset is abrupt, with focal neurological or neuropsychological signs, and the course is almost invariably fatal within 2 to 4 months. Definitive diagnosis requires a brain biopsy. Neuroimaging studies reveal multifocal areas of high signal intensity in the white matter. Functional imaging with PET or SPECT may reveal a heterogeneous pattern of reduced metabolic activity and perfusion.

SUBACUTE SPONGIFORM ENCEPHALOPATHIES

Included in this group of transmissible neurodegenerative diseases, the subacute spongiform encephalopathies, are Creutzfeldt-Jakob disease (CJD); kuru, a dementing disease of three New Guinea tribes most likely spread by ritual cannibalism; Gerstmann-Sträussler syndrome, a familial disorder characterized by dementia and ataxia; fatal familial insomnia, a disorder causing disturbances of sleep and of motor, autonomic, and endocrine function; and, in cattle, bovine spongiform encephalopathy (also known as *mad cow disease*). These are all fatal neurodegenerative disorders caused by prions. A *prion* is a small infectious pathogen-containing protein that is resistant to procedures that modify or hydrolyze nucleic acids. Human prion diseases share several features: (1) Pathology is almost exclusively confined to the CNS; (2) the diseases typically have long incubation times; (3) the course is progressive and fatal; (4) the neuropathological hallmarks include a reactive astrocytosis with little inflammation and, typically, neuronal vacuolation leading to spongy degeneration of the cerebral cortical gray matter; and (5) each of the diseases appears to result in accumulation of the prion protein (PrP). In prion diseases, there is a posttranslational conversion of a normal host-encoded PrP to an abnormal form (PrP^{Sc}).

Creutzfeldt-Jakob Disease

Invariably fatal, this transmissible, rapidly progressive disorder occurs mainly in middle aged or older patients and is manifested early on by fatigue, flu-like symptoms, mild cognitive impairment, or focal findings, such as aphasia or apraxia. Psychiatric manifestations may then emerge, including mood lability, anxiety, euphoria, depression, delusions, hallucinations, or marked personality changes. Progression of disease occurs over months, leading to dementia, akinetic mutism, coma, and death. Other common neurological findings are generalized startle myoclonus, cortical blindness, and extrapyramidal and cerebellar signs.

Worldwide, the rates of CJD range from 0.25 to 2.0 cases per one million per year. The infectious agent self-replicates and can be transmitted to humans by inoculation with infected tissues and, sometimes, by ingestion in food. Iatrogenic transmission has been reported via transplantation of contaminated cornea or to children via contaminated supplies of human growth hormone. Household contacts are not at greater risk than the general population, unless there is direct inoculation.

Because of an epidemic of a newly recognized prion disease, bovine spongiform encephalopathy (also known as *mad cow disease*), among cattle in the United Kingdom in 1986, and because of the unexpected emergence in 1995 of cases of a new variant form of CJD among teenagers in the United Kingdom, fears emerged that transmission to humans may have occurred as a result of eating infected beef. Strong evidence now supports a causal relationship between bovine spongiform encephalopathy and variant CJD. Since 1995, more than 125 human cases of variant CJD (vCJD) have been reported, the overwhelming majority (>95 percent) from the United Kingdom. Patients with vCJD disease compared to typical sporadic CJD are considerably younger at age of onset (29 years of age vs. 65 years of age), experience a longer duration of illness (14 months vs. 4.5 months), and more frequently present with sensory disturbances and psychiatric manifestations, including psychosis, depression, personality change, and anxiety. As disease progresses, patients with vCJD disease develop pyramidal signs, myoclonus, rigidity, cerebellar signs, and akinetic mutism. Neuropathologically, the main distinction between vCJD disease and sporadic CJD appears to be the prominent involvement of the cerebellum in nearly all cases of vCJD with prominent PrP^{Sc+} amyloid plaques distributed throughout the cerebrum and cerebellum.

Diagnosis of CJD requires pathological examination of the cortex, which reveals the classical triad of spongiform vacuolation, loss of neurons, and glial cell proliferation. Genetic susceptibility is a factor in disease risk, indicated by a common polymorphism of the human PrP. The presence of the 14-3-3 protein in the CSF may serve as a sensitive and specific diagnostic test for sporadic CJD; its sensitivity in vCJD appears lower. EEG abnormalities, although not specific for CJD, are present in nearly all patients with sporadic CJD: a slow and irregular background rhythm with periodic sharp wave complexes. CT and MRI studies may reveal cortical atrophy later in the course of disease. SPECT and PET reveal heterogeneously decreased uptake throughout the cortex. There is no known treatment for CJD.

OTHER INFECTIOUS CAUSES OF NEUROPSYCHIATRIC DISORDERS

A variety of bacterial, mycoplasmal, fungal, and parasitic infections can cause neuropsychiatric disturbances as a result of a chronic meningitis or sequelae from an acute infection (Table 2.9–1).

EMERGING AREAS OF INVESTIGATION

Chronic Fatigue Syndrome

Chronic fatigue syndrome, more commonly referred to as *myalgic encephalomyelitis* in the United Kingdom and Canada, is a multisystem syndrome characterized by 6 months or more of severe, debilitating fatigue, often

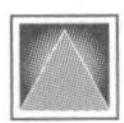

Table 2.9–1
Selected Infectious Causes of Neuropsychiatric Disorders

Bacterial infections
- Acute: *Haemophilus*, meningococcus, pneumococcus
- Subacute: brucellosis, leptospirosis, Lyme disease, syphilis, tuberculosis, Whipple's disease

Fungal infections
- Coccidioidomycosis, cryptococcosis, histoplasmosis, *Candida*

Parasitic infections
- Cysticercosis, malaria, toxoplasmosis

Prions
- Creutzfeldt-Jakob disease, fatal familial insomnia, kuru

Viral infections
- Arbovirus, coxsackievirus, cytomegalovirus, enterovirus, Epstein-Barr virus, flavivirus, herpes simplex virus, human immunodeficiency virus, influenza virus, lymphocytic choriomeningitis virus, measles virus, mumps, papovavirus, poliovirus, rabies virus, rubella, togavirus

accompanied by myalgia, headaches, pharyngitis, low-grade fever, sleep disturbance, cognitive complaints, gastrointestinal (GI) symptoms, postexertional malaise, and tender lymph nodes. The search for an infectious cause of chronic fatigue syndrome has been active because of the high percentage of patients who report abrupt onset after a severe flu-like illness. In the mid-1980s, the etiology of chronic fatigue syndrome was linked to infection with EBV. After EBV was shown, in controlled studies, to have no specific role in the etiology of chronic fatigue syndrome, reports have linked chronic fatigue syndrome to a variety of other agents, including enteroviruses, retroviruses, and new lymphotropic herpesviruses. These reports have not been consistently replicated in well-designed studies. Certain organisms, however, can result in a chronic fatigue syndrome–like picture, such as infection with *B. burgdorferi*, which causes Lyme disease, or infection with *Babesia microti*, which causes babesiosis; however, most cases of chronic fatigue syndrome are not linked to these agents. Evidence of immune dysregulation has been frequently reported among patients with chronic fatigue syndrome, but the data are not consistent across studies nor are they reflective of illness severity. Some patients with chronic fatigue syndrome–like symptoms may have neurally mediated hypotension (NMH), a dysfunction of the autonomic nervous system. Checking for NMH through a tilt-table test among patients with chronic fatigue syndrome is important, as recent research indicates that medications effective for NMH may lead to relief from chronic fatigue syndrome. Various studies have found high rates of depressive disorders among patients with chronic fatigue syndrome, ranging from 15 to 54 percent. In addition, recent research has shown that patients who are most likely to be plagued by persistent fatigue after an acute viral illness are patients with preexisting or comorbid psychiatric problems. However, other research has shown that the cognitive impairment in chronic fatigue syndrome exists even in the absence of preexisting or comorbid psychiatric disorders, thus leading to the conclusion that psychiatric disorders alone cannot account for chronic fatigue syndrome. At present, chronic fatigue syndrome is best conceptualized as a heterogenous syndrome of uncertain etiology, most likely involving an interplay of psychiatric, infectious, neuroendocrine, and immunological factors. Controlled clinical trials among patients with chronic fatigue syndrome do not support the use of antidepressants, corticosteroids, or evening primrose oil. Although limited benefit has been observed in small controlled trials of IgG, the most convincing clinical trial results have come from nonpharmacological therapies. The results from numerous well-designed studies now support the use of cognitive behavior therapy and graded aerobic exercise programs to help alleviate the symptomatology and to reduce the disability associated with chronic fatigue syndrome.

Group A β-Hemolytic Streptococcus Poststreptococcal autoimmunity has been postulated to be a cause of certain types of childhood-onset OCD and Tourette's syndrome based on the observation that children who develop Sydenham's chorea are often observed to have tics or obsessive-compulsive symptoms before the onset of the chorea. Designated by the acronym PANDAS (*p*ediatric *a*utoimmune *n*europsychiatric *d*isorders *a*ssociated with *s*treptococcal infections), these disorders are characterized by abrupt and dramatic symptom exacerbations that are temporally related to group A β-hemolytic streptococcal infections. Affected children also are more likely to have attentional disorders and subtle neurological soft signs, such as mild choreiform movements or tics. Recent research has identified a genetic marker in PANDAS that has previously been shown to be highly specific and sensitive in identifying individuals with rheumatic fever. In one study, 85 percent of children who developed streptococcal-related OCD or tics, or both, and 89 percent of the children with Sydenham's chorea carried the D8/17 monoclonal antibody marker on DR^+ cells in the peripheral circulation, whereas only 17 percent of healthy controls carried this marker. Some neuroimaging studies have revealed increased basal ganglia volumes, a finding consistent with the hypothesis that infection with β-hemolytic streptococci triggers antistreptococcal antibodies, which, by the process of molecular mimicry, cross-react with epitopes on the basal ganglia of susceptible hosts, resulting in acute inflammation. A controlled trial suggests that immunosuppressive treatments can be helpful; IV immunoglobulin therapy resulted in a reduction in obsessive-compulsive symptoms, whereas plasmapheresis resulted in improved OCD and fewer tics. Despite anecdotal reports of efficacy for oral penicillin prophylaxis, the one controlled study did not find that prophylaxis with penicillin was beneficial in preventing symptom exacerbations. Because this negative result may have been due to the failure of oral penicillin to prevent group A streptococcus infection (14 of the 35 infections occurred during the penicillin phase), prophylaxis studies using other antimicrobial agents are needed.

Borna Disease Virus Borna disease virus (BDV) is a small neurotropic RNA virus that infects various domestic animal species, causing disturbances in behavior and cognition and, rarely, fatal outcome. In animals, BDV targets cells of the limbic system and compromises their neuronal function without causing direct damage. Serological and molecular studies on human patients have been performed to determine whether BDV may also cause neuropsychiatric disease in humans. Some studies have found elevated levels of antibodies recognizing BDV antigens in the blood of psychiatric patients. Other studies have reported the presence of BDV RNA or BDV antigens in the peripheral blood samples, as well as in autopsied brains of psychiatric patients. These data support the possibility of human infection with BDV. Other research groups, however, have been unable to replicate these findings, reporting a complete absence of such BDV markers from their samples. The hypothesis of BDV infection in humans therefore remains a controversial area of investigation. The serological studies that supported infection were questioned based on poor interlaboratory reliability using identical blinded specimens and based on Western blot analyses using recombinant BDV proteins that indicated that reactive human sera usually recognized only one of the two major BDV antigens. The detection of BDV-derived nucleic acid and infectious virus in peripheral blood of psychiatric patients has yielded divergent results, with prevalence rates between 0 and 60 percent in patients and between 0 and 57 percent in controls. Although methodological problems (such as accidental contamination of specimens or different environmental risk) may explain divergent or positive findings, methodological problems cannot explain why all groups who reported positive results found that BDV-specific RNA was more often present in the blood of patients than controls. At present, the most cautious conclusion would be that there is insufficient cumulative evidence to conclusively confirm that BDV infects humans or causes human psychiatric disorders.

Retroviruses Endogenous retroviruses, well-known to cause a variety of diseases, including neoplasia, autoimmunity, and encephalitis, have also been reported to be expressed to a significantly greater extent in the brains of individuals affected with schizophrenia and other neuropsychiatric disorders compared to the brains of unaffected individuals. Evidence consists of the identification of viral sequences in affected brains and the increased activity of virally encoded reverse transcriptase. Because retroviruses are capable of cellular infection and integration into the host genome, the activation of these viral sequences in cells within the CNS can then lead to the transcription of adjacent genes and to alterations in neural functioning. Although viral triggers or causes for neuropsychiatric disorders are compelling in their ability to help explain seasonal birth effects, the impact of perinatal complications, and discordance among monozygotic twins, much more investigation in this area is needed before conclusions can be drawn.

Antimicrobial Effect of Psychiatric Medications

That antimicrobial medications may have therapeutic effects for primary psychiatric disorders was first described in the 1950s when astute clinicians observed that when depressed tubercular patients were treated with the antibiotic iproniazid (Marsilid), a monoamine oxidase inhibitor (MAOI), the depression often improved; based on this observation, a class of effective antidepressants was identified. More recently, emerging data raise questions regarding whether the reverse may also be true—that certain psychiatric medications may have an antimicrobial effect. Antipsychotics, for example, have demonstrated inhibitory effect on several neurotropic viruses, including herpes simplex, and on several protozoans, including *Leishmania*, *Trypanosoma*, and *Toxoplasma gondii*. In vitro research now indicates that several antipsychotics (in particular, haloperidol [Haldol]) and the mood stabilizer valproic acid (Depakene) are capable of inhibiting the growth of *T. gondii*, an intracellular protozoan that can cause neuropsychiatric disorders. Because recent studies have reported increased levels of *T. gondii* antibodies in the serum of individuals with schizophrenia and mood disorders, the possible antimicrobial role of certain antipsychotics and mood stabilizers is of particular interest. This line of research, although still highly exploratory, demonstrates the increasingly fruitful interdisciplinary investigations linking infectious disease, neurology, and psychiatry.

SUGGESTED CROSS-REFERENCES

Acquired immunodeficiency syndrome is discussed in Section 2.8. Interactions of the immune system and the CNS are discussed in Section 1.12; neuropsychological testing is discussed in Chapter 7. Neuroimaging is discussed in Sections 1.15 and 1.16. Schizophrenia is discussed in Chapter 12.

REFERENCES

Ackerman R, Rehse-Kupper B, Gollmer E, Schmidt R: Chronic neurologic manifestations of erythema migrans borreliosis. *Ann N Y Acad Sci.* 1988;64:506–512.

Bates DW, Buchwald D, Lee J, Kith P, Doolittle T, Rutherford C, Churchill H, Schur P, Wener M, Wybenga D, Winkelman J, Komaroff AL: Clinical laboratory test findings in patients with chronic fatigue syndrome. *Arch Intern Med.* 1995;155:97–103.

Bloom BJ, Wyckoff PM, Meissner HC, Steere AC: Neurocognitive abnormalities in children after classic manifestations of Lyme disease. *Pediatr Infect Dis J.* 1998;17:189–196.

Bode L, Zimmermann W, Ferszt R, Steinbach F, Ludwig H: Borna disease virus genome transcribed and expressed in psychiatric patients. *Nat Med.* 1995;1:232–236.

*Brown AS, Susser ES: In utero infection and adult schizophrenia. *Ment Retard Dev Disabil Res Rev.* 2002;8:51–57.

Brown P, Cathala F, Castaigne P, Gajdusek DC: Creutzfeldt-Jakob disease: Clinical analysis of a consecutive series of 230 neuropathologically verified cases. *Ann Neurol.* 1986;20:597.

Burrascano JJ. Lyme disease. In: Rakel RE, ed. *Conn's Current Therapy.* Philadelphia: WB Saunders; 1997:140–143.

Collinge J: New diagnostic tests for prion diseases. *N Engl J Med.* 1996;335:963–965.

Conejero-Goldberg C, Torrey EF, Yolken RH: Herpes viruses and *Toxoplasma gondii* in orbital frontal cortex of psychiatric patients. *Schizophr Res.* 2003;60:65–69.

Coyle PK: Neurologic Lyme disease. *Semin Neurol.* 1992;12:200–208.

Coyle PK, Schutzer SE, Deng Z, Krupp LB, Belman AL, Benach JL, Luft BJ: Detection of *Borrelia burgdorferi* specific antigen in antibody-negative cerebrospinal fluid in neurologic Lyme disease. *Neurology.* 1995;45:2010–2015.

DeLuca J, Johnson SK, Ellis SP, Natelson BH: Cognitive functioning is impaired in patients with chronic fatigue syndrome devoid of psychiatric disease. *J Neurol Neurosurg Psychiatry.* 1997;62:151–155.

*Demitrack MA, Abbey SE, eds. *Chronic Fatigue Syndrome.* New York: Guilford Publications; 1996.

Fallon BA, Das S, Plutchok JJ, Tager F, Liegner K, Van Heertum R: Functional brain imaging and neuropsychological testing in Lyme disease. *Clin Infect Dis.* 1997.

*Fallon BA, Nields JA: Lyme disease: A neuropsychiatric illness. *Am J Psychiatry.* 1994;151:1571–1583.

Fallon BA, Nields JA, Burrascano JJ, Liegner K, DelBene D, Liebowitz MR: The neuropsychiatric manifestations of Lyme borreliosis. *Psychiatr Q.* 1992;63:95–117.

Garvey MA, Perlmutter SJ, Allen AJ, Hamburger S, Lougee L, Leonard HL, Witowski E, Dubbert B, Swedo SE: A pilot study of penicillin prophylaxis for neuropsychiatric exacerbations triggered by streptococcal infections. *Biol Psychiatry.* 1999;45:1564–1571.

Hajek T: Higher prevalence of antibodies to *Borrelia burgdorferi* in psychiatric patients than in healthy subjects. *Am J Psychiatry.* 2002;159.

Heegaard ED, Hornsleth A: Parvovirus: The expanding spectrum of disease. *Acta Paediatr.* 1995;84:109–117.

Hendler N, Leahy W: Psychiatric and neurologic sequelae of infectious mononucleosis. *Am J Psychiatry.* 1978;135:842–844.

Hooshmand H, Escobar MR, Kopf SW: Neurosyphilis: A study of 241 patients. *JAMA.* 1972;219:726–729.

*Ikuta K, Ibrahim MS, Kobayashi T, Tomonaga K: Borna disease virus and infection in humans. *Front Biosci.* 2002;7:470–495.

Jackson GS, Collinge J: The molecular pathology of CJD: Old and new variants. *J Clin Pathol.* 2001;54:393–399.

Jones-Brando L, Torrey EF, Yolken R: Drugs used in the treatment of schizophrenia and bipolar disorder inhibit the replication of *Toxoplasma gondii. Schizophr Res.* 2002.

Kamitani W, Ono E, Yoshino S, Kobayashi T, Taharaguchi S, Lee BJ, Yamashita M, Okamaot M, Taniyama H, Tomonaga K, Ikuta K: Glial expression of Borna disease virus phosphoprotein induces behavioral and neurological abnormalities in transgenic mice. *Proc Natl Acad Sci U S A.* 2003;100:8969–8974.

Krupp LB, Masur D, Schwartz J, Coyle PK, Langenbach LJ, Fernquist SK, Jandorf L, Halperin JJ: Cognitive functioning in late Lyme borreliosis. *Arch Neurol.* 1991;48:1125–1129.

Lawrence C, Lipton RB, Lowy FD, Coyle PK: Seronegative chronic relapsing neuroborreliosis. *Eur Neurol.* 1995;35:113–117.

Lecour H, Miranda M, Magro C, Rocha A, Goncalves V: Human leptospirosis: A review of 50 cases. *Infection.* 1989;17:10–14.

Lieb K, Staeheli P: Borna disease virus: Does it infect humans and cause psychiatric disorders? *J Clin Virol.* 2001;21:119–127.

Limosin F, Rouillon F, Payan C, Cohen JM, Strub N: Prenatal exposure to influenza as a risk factor for adult schizophrenia. *Acta Psychiatr Scand.* 2003;107:331–335.

Logigian EL, Kaplan R, Steere AC: Chronic neurologic manifestations of Lyme disease. *N Engl J Med.* 1990;323:1438–1444.

Oksi J, Kalimo H, Marttila RJ, Marjamaki M, Sonninen P, Nikoskelainen, Viljanen MK: Inflammatory brain changes in Lyme borreliosis. *Brain.* 1996;119:2143–2154.

Pachner AR: *Borrelia burgdorferi* in the nervous system: The new "great imitator." *Ann N Y Acad Sci.* 1988;539:56–64.

Sauder C, Muller A, Cubitt B, Mayer J, Steinmetz J, Trabert W, Ziegler, Wanke K, Mueller-Lantzsch N, de la Torre JC, Grasser FA: Detection of Borna disease virus (BDV) antibodies and BDV RNA in psychiatric patients: Evidence for high sequence conservation of human blood-derived BDV RNA. *J Virol.* 1996;70:7713–7724.

Scheld WM, Whitley RJ, Durack DT, eds. *Infections of the Central Nervous System.* New York: Lippincott–Raven Publishers; 1997.

Swedo SE: Sydenham's chorea: A model for childhood autoimmune neuropsychiatric disorders. *JAMA.* 1994;272:1788–1791.

*Swedo SE: Pediatric autoimmune neuropsychiatric disorders associated with streptococcal infections (PANDAS). *Mol Psychiatry.* 2002;7:S24–S25.

Swedo SE, Leonard HL, Mittleman BB, Allen AJ, Rapoport JL, Dow SP, Kanter ME, Chapman F, Zabriskie J: Identification of children with pediatric autoimmune neuropsychiatric disorders associated with streptococcal infections by a marker associated with rheumatic fever. *Am J Psychiatry.* 1997;154:110–112.

Thomas EW. *Syphilis: Its Course and Management.* New York: Macmillan; 1949.

Waltrip RW, Buchanan RW, Summerflet A, Breier A, Carpenter WT, Bryant NL, Rubin SA, Carbone KM: Borna disease virus and schizophrenia. *Psychiatry Res.* 1995;56:33–44.

Weed MR, Hienz RD, Brady JV, Adams RJ, Mankowski JL, Clements JE, Zink MC: Central nervous system correlates of behavioral deficits following simian immunodeficiency virus infection. *J Neurovirol.* 2003;9:452–464.

Wessely S, Chalder T, Hirsch S, Pawlikowska T, Wallace P, Wright DJM: Postinfectious fatigue: Prospective cohort study in primary care. *Lancet.* 1995;345:1333–1338.

Yolken RH, Torrey EF: Viruses, schizophrenia, and bipolar disorder. *Clin Microbiol Rev.* 1995;8:131–145.

▲ 2.10 Neuropsychiatric Aspects of Prion Disease

KIMBRA KENNEY, M.D.

The complex but fascinating field of prion disorders received little public, media, or even medical attention until 1996 when it was announced that ten young people in the United Kingdom had a fatal disease etiologically linked to bovine spongiform encephalopathy (commonly referred to as *mad cow disease*). Since then, interest has exploded in this exotic family of disorders, as the public health implications of a potentially large epidemic of variant Creutzfeldt-Jakob disease (vCJD) have emerged. Its "interest factor," measured by the number of publications divided by the incidence of the disease, yields a factor more than ten times that of any other medical condition and more than 100 times that of many illnesses.

This once obscure human disease has a long history in veterinary medicine, dating back to the 18th century when scrapie, a naturally occurring prion disease of sheep and goats, was first described in England. Scrapie is prevalent in many countries around the world. Introduced into the United States in the 1940s from the United Kingdom, scrapie was shown to be experimentally transmissible in 1936. Initially, it was presumed to have a viral etiology. Discrete epidemics of transmissible mink encephalopathy, another prion disease of animals, have occurred in captive mink ranches in the United States, Europe, and Russia, with most episodes attributable to a single-source contaminant. Chronic wasting disease of mule deer and elk, a form of spongiform encephalopathy unique to the United States, was first described in 1967 and appears to be spreading both west of the Continental Divide and east of the Mississippi River from its central origin in Colorado and Wyoming by the migration of affected wild deer and elk. And, of course, bovine spongiform encephalopathy, first reported in the United Kingdom in 1985 and the largest prion epidemic to date, has afflicted more than 185,000 cattle, principally in the United Kingdom but also in native cattle in several continental European countries and Japan. The U.K. bovine spongiform encephalopathy agent has crossed the species barrier to infect domestic cats, zoo felines, and exotic ungulates in addition to humans. The consequences of this disease have expanded well beyond the medical community, with major economic, political, and public health effects (Table 2.10–1).

Prion diseases were first described in humans in the 1920s when Drs. Hans Creutzfeldt and Alfons Jakob separately described five patients with a degenerative neurological syndrome. Interestingly, only two of these five patients would fulfill current clinical diagnostic criteria for CJD. Walter Spielmeyer introduced the term *Creutzfeldt-Jakob disease* in 1922. A separate familial, neurodegenerative disorder, now known as *Gerstmann-Sträussler syndrome*, a prion disease with prominent ataxia, was described by Austrian neurologists of the same names in 1936.

A major breakthrough in understanding prion diseases occurred in 1957 when D. Carleton Gajdusek and Vincent Zigas first described kuru, a fatal neurological disease of epidemic proportions within an isolated, primitive people in the highlands of Papua New Guinea. Based on neuropathological similarities between scrapie and kuru, William Hadlow, an American veterinarian, suggested in 1959 that kuru may have an infectious etiology akin to that of scrapie. In 1966, Gajdusek and C. Joe Gibbs experimentally transmitted kuru to primates after a 2-year incubation period, followed shortly thereafter in 1968 by the experimental transmission of CJD to primates. This discovery paved the way for the intense scientific interest that has ensued and the birth of a new family of diseases. Presciently, John Griffith, a mathematician intrigued by these disorders, suggested in 1967 that the transmissible agent may be a protein capable of self-replication and infectious on that basis alone. Since then, prion diseases have convened multiple scientific disciplines, including neurology, veterinary medicine, microbiology, genetics, biochemistry, epidemiology, molecular biology, immunology, and neuropathology, to name a few, in a quest to resolve some of the most basic questions of biology. To date, two Nobel Prizes have been awarded in this field, and many speculate that a third is due when the nature of the infectious agent of these diseases is finally conclusively established.

An attempt to comprehensively review these diseases must be laid on a few ground rules. First and foremost, the terminology has evolved as the science was discovered, oftentimes in parallel in human and animal forms, before the realization of shared common properties. Consequently, there is marked redundancy within the nomenclature. An example of this is the discovery and naming of the sinc (scrapie incubation) gene in sheep and the PRNP (prion protein) gene; they were subsequently shown to be identical despite their different names. This has cloaked an already complex field in an additional layer of confusion. These disorders have collectively been called *prion diseases* based on Stanley Prusiner's prion hypothesis as well as *transmissible spongiform encephalopathies*, a nomenclature describing the essential features of experimental transmissibility, microscopic spongiform pathology, and clinical dementia coupled with extensive neurological dysfunction. Nonetheless, the nomenclature should not detract from the basic hypothesis that the prion disorders question the fundamental property of an infectious agent—that is, that a protein alone can carry all the information required for its replication in a host without the benefit of genetic information. Furthermore, that same infectious agent can simultaneously be both familial and infectious, a feature unique to these diseases.

NORMAL PRION PROTEIN

From the discovery that kuru and CJD were transmissible diseases, the race was on to identify the infectious agent, a presumed virus with the unique feature of long latency from inoculation until clinical disease and death. Over the next few decades, properties of the

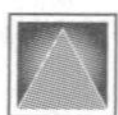

Table 2.10–1
Human and Animal Transmissible Spongiform Encephalopathy Overview

Disease	Distribution	Cause	Comment
CJD	Worldwide	Unknown	~1/million/yr
Gerstmann-Sträussler syndrome	Familial	Genetic	Very rare
Fatal familial insomnia	Familial	Genetic	Extremely rare
Kuru	Papua New Guinea	Ritual cannibalism	Vanishing; 0–1 cases/yr
Variant CJD	Countries affected by BSE, especially the United Kingdom	Exposure to BSE agent	~150 cases to date; all cases associated with methionine homozygosity at codon 129 of PRNP gene
Scrapie	Sheep, goats, moufflon	Unknown	Worldwide (with a few exceptions)
BSE	United Kingdom[a], Europe[b], Japan, Oman, Falkland Islands, Canada, Israel	Initial common source epidemic by contamination of MBM with BSE agent	Large epidemic in the United Kingdom due to recycling and amplification of contaminated materials through rendering process
Related BSE	Feline (domestic cats, ocelot, puma, cheetah, tiger) and exotic ungulates (nyala, gemsbok, Arabian oryx, greater kudu, eland, ankole)	Feeding of MBM contaminated by BSE or, in the case of zoo felines, BSE-infected carcasses	Isolated cases except >100 cases of feline spongiform encephalopathy in domestic cats
Chronic wasting disease	Captive mule deer and elk in the United States and Canada; wild white-tailed deer	Unknown	Recent recognition of the disease east of the Mississippi River and west of the Continental Divide
Transmissible mink encephalopathy	Ranch-bred mink	Contaminated feed; in one case, mink were fed only U.S. "downer cattle"	United States, Europe, and Russia

BSE, bovine spongiform encephalopathy; CJD, Creutzfeldt-Jakob disease; MBM, meat and bone meal.
[a]To date, more than 97 percent of the more than 187,000 cases of BSE worldwide occurred in the United Kingdom.
[b]As of November 2003, this includes Austria, Belgium, Czech Republic, Denmark, Finland, France, Germany, Greece, Ireland, Italy, Liechtenstein, Luxembourg, Netherlands, Portugal, Spain, Slovakia, Slovenia, Switzerland.

infectious agent were described and cataloged, and multiple attempts were made to isolate the infectious agent from both experimentally and naturally acquired cases of animal and human disease. But this infectious agent proved to be a particularly elusive and unconventional one. Early on, the infectious agent was noted to be resistant to many physicochemical treatments that inactivate nucleic acids (arguing against a viral etiology) but exhibited other properties typical of viral agents (supporting a viral etiology). Ultrastructurally, no infectious agent could be identified by light or electron microscopy (EM) nor was any immune reaction to the infectious agent ever seen pathologically.

In 1981, by EM, Patricia Merz described aggregates she called *scrapie-associated fibrils* that were present in the brains of sheep with scrapie but absent in those of normal sheep (Fig. 2.10–1). In 1982, David Bolton isolated and partially purified particles from infected brain homogenates. These were found to be a protease-resistant sialoglycoprotein and the major constituent of the brain homogenate fraction containing infectivity. This enriched, infectious material proved to be the same material as that seen by EM by Merz in scrapie. Prusiner coined them *proteinaceous infectious particles* or *prions*; more important, he hypothesized that these prion proteins (PrP) were the infectious agents capable of replication without the benefit of nucleic acid, reiterating the theory of John Griffin. All together, three hypotheses have been proposed to explain these disorders—the prion, viral, and virino theories (Table 2.10–2)—and supporters of each theory persist within the scientific community researching these diseases, although the prion hypothesis by far enjoys the strongest support.

In the 1980s, PrP was still widely believed to have a viral origin. And so, by molecular biological techniques, complementary deoxyribonucleic acid (cDNA) for PrP was obtained, and Bruno Oesch and colleagues (1985) discovered that the gene encoding PrP was a host one (Fig. 2.10–2), not that of a virus (with its nucleic acid shielded and surrounded by the enriched infectious PrP fraction as formerly believed to be the case). In fact, there was no amino acid sequence difference between noninfectious PrP and the pathogenic form (Table 2.10–3). This supported Prusiner's hypothesis that the prion protein alone was capable of self-replication and transmission. But how did a normally occurring protein become the infectious agent of these fatal neurological diseases?

Although much has been discovered regarding PrP^{C} and PrP^{Res}, even more remains to be uncovered. PrP^{C} is a highly conserved pro-

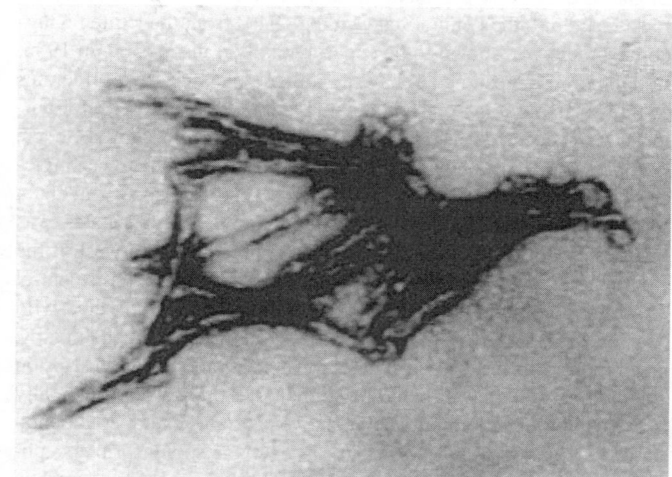

FIGURE 2.10–1 Electron micrograph of scrapie-associated fibrils extracted from a scrapie hamster brain.

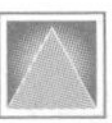

Table 2.10–2
Transmissible Spongiform Encephalopathy Hypotheses

Type	Hypothesis
Prion	Conformational change of normal host protein confers infectivity.[a]
Viral	Infection-specific informational molecule that is closely associated with and protected by abnormal PrP.[b]
Virino	Unusual but conventional virus.[c]

[a]Prusiner S: Novel proteinaceous infectious particles cause scrapie. *Science.* 1982;216:136–144.
[b]Dickinson AG, Outram GW: Genetic aspects of unconventional virus infections: The basis of the virino hypothesis. *Ciba Foundation Symposium 135: Novel Infectious Agents and the Central Nervous System.* 1988.
[c]Rohrer RG: The scrapie agent: "A virus by any other name." *Curr Top Microbiol Immunol.* 1991.

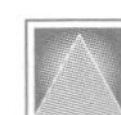

Table 2.10–3
Prion Protein Terminology

Term	Definition
Prion	A small *pro*teinaceous *in*fectious particle that resists inactivation by procedures that modify nucleic acids
PrP^{c}	Normal cellular isoform of the prion protein
PrP^{33-35}	Normal cellular isoform of the prion protein that weighs 33–35 kDa
PrP^{Inf}	Infectious isoform of prion protein
PrP^{Res}	Infectious isoform of prion protein that resists proteinase K digestion
PrP^{27-30}	Infectious isoform of PrP that yields a molecule of 27–30 kDa when incompletely digested with proteinase K
PrP^{Sc}	Isoform of the prion protein isolated from scrapie-infected brains
PrP^{CJD}	Isoform of the prion protein isolated from CJD-infected brains
PrP^{GSS}	Isoform of the prion protein isolated from Gerstmann-Sträussler syndrome–infected brains
PrP^{vCJD}	Isoform of the prion protein isolated from variant CJD–infected brains
Prion rod	Aggregate of prions comprised largely, if not entirely, of PrP^{Sc} or PrP^{27-30} molecules; created by detergent extraction of membranes; morphologically and histochemically indistinguishable from many amyloids

CJD, Creutzfeldt-Jakob disease.

tein that is present in all mammalian species and possibly in all vertebrates. It is highly expressed during fetal development and initially was believed to be essential for development and possibly lethal if absent. However, genetically engineered null mice ($PrP^{0/0}$, or knockout mice lacking the PRNP gene and thereby any functioning PrP^{C}) develop normally and have a normal lifespan, with only subtle differences measured on performance tests (electrophysiologically with abnormalities of synaptic transmission and grossly with disturbed circadian rhythms).

Recently, research has again focused on the function of normal host PrP^{C}. Information has been gleaned regarding its cellular life cycle from translation to degradation. The open reading frame of the PRNP gene is contained within a single exon on the short arm of chromosome 20. PrP^{C} is a small glycolipid anchored membrane protein of 250 amino acids (Fig. 2.10–3) with an amino-terminal signal peptide and a hydrophobic carboxy terminal for membrane attachment. There are five polymorphisms recognized within the normal PrP proteins expressed in the general population (most important, a Met-Val polymorphism at codon 129). Although PrP^{C} and PrP^{Sc} have identical primary structures, their secondary structures differ: PrP^{C} has a high α-helical (approximately 42 percent) and almost no β-sheet (3 percent) structure. With respect to its tertiary structure, the normal protein contains three α-helical domains, two β-strands, and five random N-terminal octapeptide repeats within codons 51 to 91 (Fig. 2.10–4). Two oligosaccharide side chains determine three different glycoforms of the normal protein and mono-, di-, and unglycosylated isoforms of different molecular weights (MWs; 30 to 35 kDa). PrP^{C} is translated from messenger ribonucleic acid (mRNA) in the endoplasmic reticula, processed in the Golgi apparatus, and then exocytosed where it is attached to the outer membrane of the cell by its glycolipid anchor. It is then internalized and processed through the acidic lysosomal cellular compartments and degraded, with a rapid turnover rate and transit time of approximately 1 hour and complete degradation within 6 hours. This life cycle is typical of a protein involved in receptor or cell-signaling functions (Fig. 2.10–5).

PrP^{C} is expressed by nearly all adult tissues, but its highest level of expression is in the central nervous system (CNS), particularly within neurons. Peripherally, it is also relatively highly expressed in cells of the immune system. It may be a metalloprotein and has been

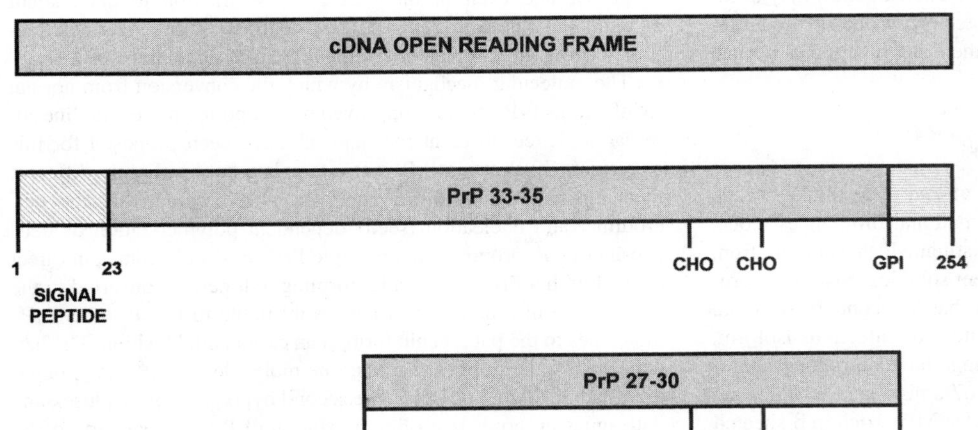

FIGURE 2.10–2 Illustration of the open reading frame of the human PRNP gene on chromosome 21. Cellular prion protein is translated from a single exon. It is comprised of 254 amino acids with a 23–amino acid signal peptide that is cleaved during processing. The infectious isoform of the prion protein is a truncated form, weighing 27 to 30 kDa, and is insoluble in detergent and resistant to proteinase K digestion. cDNA, complementary DNA; CHO, carbohydrate moiety; GPI, glycolipid anchor.

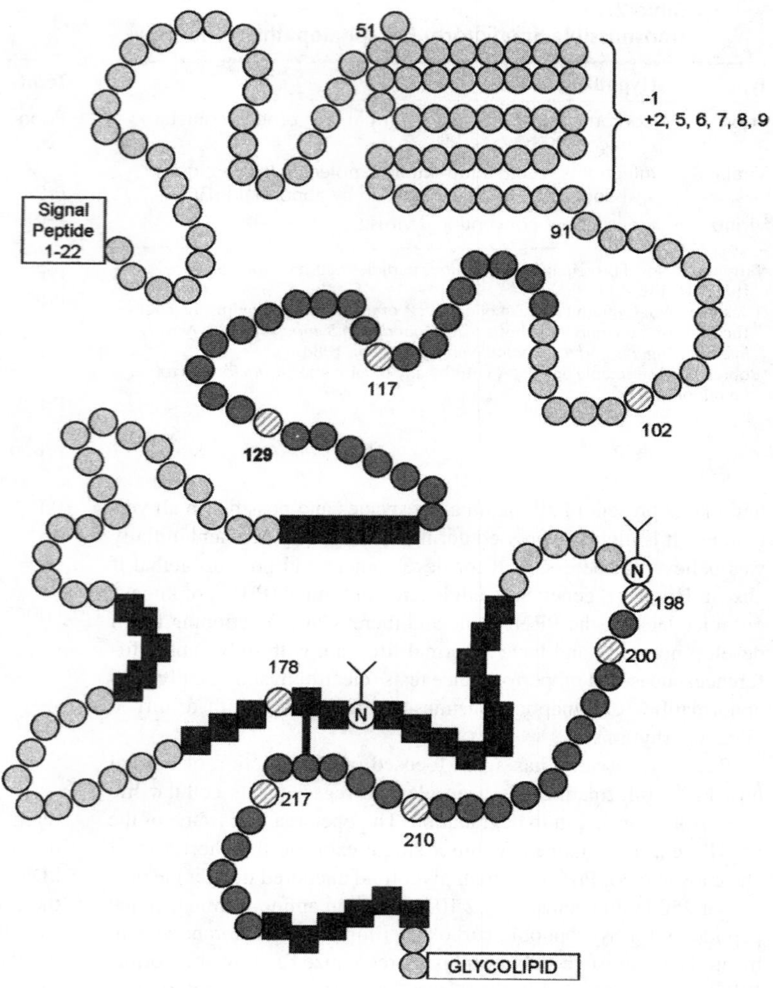

FIGURE 2.10–3 This is an illustration of the human PrP molecule showing the signal peptide, five octapeptide repeat regions, the polymorphism at codon 129, and several common point and insertion mutations associated with familial Creutzfeldt-Jakob disease. (Courtesy of Paul Brown.)

shown to bind copper and possess superoxide dismutase activity in the presence of high concentrations of copper chloride, thus supporting a role in copper homeostasis. Other studies have implicated other possible cellular functions such as promotion of neurite outgrowth, modulation of synaptic transmissions, cell protection as an antioxidant, or regulation of apoptosis. A very recent study has suggested that the codon 129 Met-Val PrP polymorphism may influence human cognitive abilities in a gene dose–dependent manner. The mechanism of its influence in human cognition is unclear, but it may occur through its proposed role as a neuroprotector by one of the aforementioned pathways. However, to date, the exact function of normal cellular PrP remains unknown.

INFECTIOUS PRION PROTEIN

The differences between PrP^{C} and PrP^{Sc} appear to be the key to the disease's infectivity and rely on conformational differences alone. There are several characteristics that distinguish the normal from abnormal PrP molecules: PrP^{C} is detergent soluble, sensitive to proteinase K (PK) with complete digestion, has a secondary structure rich in α-helices, and does not accumulate. The infectious isoform, PrP^{Res}, is detergent insoluble (assembling into amorphous aggregates of prion rods), PK resistant (only 67 amino acid residues are removed, yielding a protein of 27 to 30 kDa MW), rich in β-sheeted pleats in its secondary structure, an amyloid based on its Congo red affinity, and accumulates in affected animals. Finally, within the limits of current technology, when highly purified, PrP^{Res} is the only fraction from infected brain homogenates containing infectivity, leading many to assert that it is the infectious particle itself. However, a single infectious unit corresponds to approximately 10^5 PrP molecules, leaving the possibility that an as-yet-undetected agent, embedded within the highly insoluble PrP^{Res}, may be the true culprit responsible for infectivity. Moreover, the agent is extremely difficult to purify, and even in the best PrP^{Res} extraction to date, small amounts of nucleic acids can still be identified in the infectious fraction, leaving the exact nature of the infectious agent unresolved.

The molecular mechanism by which the conversion from normal to infectious PrP occurs is unproven but supported by several lines of research. Three different mechanisms have been proposed for this conversion, each using PrP^{Res} as a template but by slightly different mechanisms (Fig. 2.10–6). The two most common are the heterodimer and nucleation (seed)–dependent polymerization models. Prusiner et al. proposes that a single PrP^{C} molecule comes in direct contact with a PrP^{Res} molecule, forming a dimer; is converted to the abnormal conformation; and then is available to recruit other PrP^{C} molecules to the pathogenic form in an exponential fashion. The heterodimer model implies that just one molecule of PrP^{Res} is required to initiate the lethal process. The second hypothesis of Gajdusek and colleagues proposes that oligomerization of PrP is necessary to stabilize PrP^{Res} so that rare small seeds of PrP^{Res} occur and become sta-

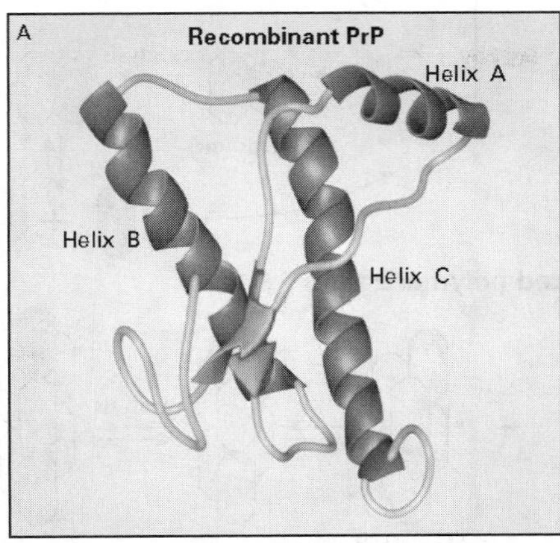

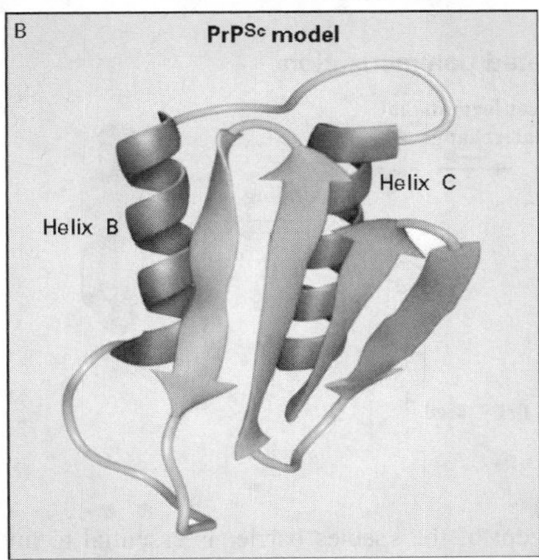

FIGURE 2.10–4 Conformational changes between normal PrP and infectious PrP. **A:** An illustration of the structure of recombinant PrP. **B:** The three-dimensional structure of PrP^{Sc} based on nuclear magnetic resonance studies. The thin tube represents loops of protein, the coils represent α-helices, and the flat ribbons represent β-pleated sheets. Note the loss of α-helices and the increase of β-pleated sheets from one form to the other. (Courtesy of Stanley Prusiner.)

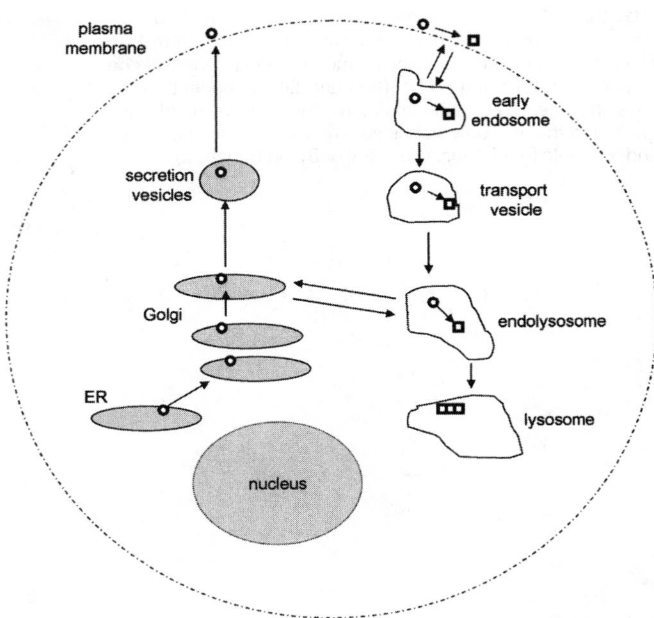

FIGURE 2.10–5 The life cycle of cellular PrP. This illustration depicts the cell trafficking of normal cellular PrP from the endoplasmic reticula (ER) through the Golgi apparatus into secretory vesicles and externally attached to the cell membrane. It is then endocytosed and processed through the lysosomal degradatory system, where the conversion from PrP^{C} to PrP^{Inf} is hypothesized to occur.

bilized as they recruit, increasing molecules of PrP^{C} into their abnormal conformation. Thus, a "seed" of PrP^{Res}, rather than a single molecule of PrP^{Res}, is necessary to initiate infection. A third model does not rely on direct physical contact between PrP^{C} and PrP^{Res}. It proposes that PrP can rapidly alternate between the normal and abnormal conformations but that it is only stabilized and sustained when there are other like conformations available for binding. These mechanisms all remain hypothetical.

Several lines of research support the prion hypothesis, but none conclusively proves it. First and foremost, despite multiple sophisticated attempts, no other infectious agent has ever been identified. In the early 1990s, Karen Hsiao developed transgenic mice bearing multiple copies of the mouse equivalent to the codon 102 PRNP gene mutation associated with Gerstmann-Sträussler syndrome. These mice, as in the human familial form of the disease, developed spontaneous disease in adulthood. Most convincing of all the molecular genetic studies are those in knock-out mice in which the PRNP gene has been removed from the mouse through genetic engineering. As stated before, these mice develop and breed normally. In addition, these animals are completely resistant to prion infection. If the null ($PrP^{0/0}$) mice are then back bred with wild-type ($PrP^{+/+}$) mice (thus producing mice heterozygous for PrP or $PrP^{+/0}$), susceptibility reappears. If fetal brain tissue with normal PrP^{C} function ($PrP^{+/+}$) is transplanted into null mice ($PrP^{0/0}$) and the mice are then experimentally inoculated with PrP^{Res}, the transplants become infected (showing typical spongiform change with gliosis microscopically), but the surrounding "null" $PrP^{0/0}$ brain remains unaffected, and the mouse stays clinically well, living a normal life despite some accumulation of PrP^{Res} in the $PrP^{0/0}$ portion of its brain. This accumulation has no associated pathological changes such as astrogliosis, neuronal loss, or spongiform change.

The final proof of the prion hypothesis may rely on producing infectivity in vitro by showing that pure noninfectious PrP^{C} can be chemically or physically manipulated to produce infectious PrP^{Res} that is transmissible when experimentally inoculated into laboratory animals. The recent experiments of Byron Caughey et al. are tantalizing and may form the basis for the experimental establishment of the prion hypothesis. Caughey and colleagues developed a cell-free conversion experiment in which purified PrP^{Res} induces conversion of PrP^{C} to PrP^{Res}. In their experiment, PrP^{Res} was incubated with radioactively labeled PrP^{C}. All PrP^{C} was then removed by digestion with PK, and the remaining PrP^{Res} fraction was shown to have newly incorporated radioactive labeling, demonstrating that PrP^{C} was converted from the normal to the infectious form in vitro. However, within this system, no new infectivity has been shown.

One of the problems with their in vitro system was the fact that, although small amounts of newly formed and radioactive PrP^{Res} could be measured in their experimental design, it took so much initial PrP^{Res} to drive the system that no *new* infectivity could be detected. So, while new PrP^{Res} could be detected, the amounts produced were manyfold less than the amount produced when cellular elements are present. Nathan Deleault and colleagues designed new studies to determine which cellular elements were essential or most facilitated conversion of PrP^{C} to PrP^{Res}. Their elegantly designed and

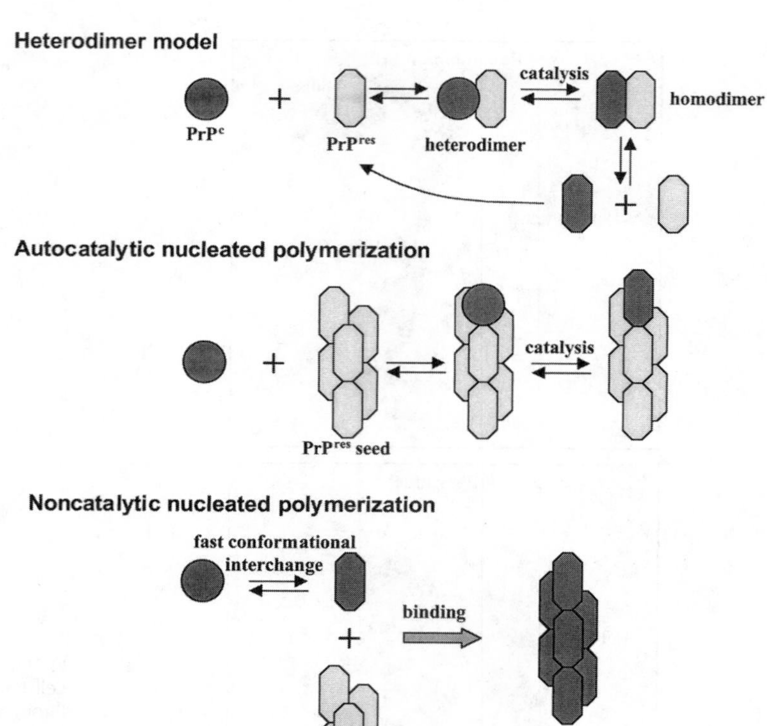

FIGURE 2.10–6 The heterodimer, autocatalytic, and noncatalytic polymerization models for formation of PrP^{Res} from PrP^{C}. The heterodimer and autocatalytic models require physical contact between PrP^{C} and PrP^{Res}. The noncatalytic model hypothesizes that there is a rapid interconversion between PrP^{C} and PrP^{Res}, but that it is only stabilized when a PrP^{Res} seed is present and available for binding. (Courtesy of Byron Caughey.)

recently published study demonstrated that cellular RNA (and possibly ribosomal RNA) was necessary to amplify PrP^{Res} in vitro and may do so by stabilizing the pathogenic configuration of PrP as it is generated. Both prion hypothesis advocates and skeptics have heralded these recent findings to support their argument for the etiology of these diseases. Prion hypothesis skeptics emphasize that nucleic acids are necessary to catalyze the configurational change from PrP^{C} to PrP^{Res}. Prion hypothesis supporters counterargue that the necessary RNA is a normal host element. Further RNA is a nuclear and cellular component and is not normally found in the cellular lysosomes where the conversion is thought to take place. Although research has moved closer to the final proof, it has not yet arrived.

One of the more long-standing arguments against the prion hypothesis has been the issue of transmissible spongiform encephalopathy strains. Strains are defined by the incubation time, different clinical symptoms produced, region and severity of brain affected, and electrophoretic properties of the PrP^{Res} extracted when brain homogenates are inoculated into a particular species of inbred mice. To date, more than 30 strains of scrapie and six strains of CJD have been identified. It is difficult to explain the multiple strains reported based on conformational differences alone in PrP. In other words, the existence of multiple strains argues that there must be some other source of information conferring so many distinctions among the numerous types of scrapie so far identified. However, adherents to the prion hypothesis counterargue that infectious PrP can have many conformations (even 30 or more) as long as it retains the essential properties associated with infectivity so that the mere existence of strains does not disprove the hypothesis. To support this contention, they refer to the recent studies describing four different types of sporadic CJD distinguished by relative amounts of de-, mono-, and diglycosylated PrP seen by Western blot analysis from PrP extraction from infected brain (Fig. 2.10–7).

The concept of the species barrier is essential to understanding the transmissibility of the prion diseases. The first experimental transmissions were from sheep to sheep with scrapie and from kuru and CJD patients to other primates. When attempting to produce a laboratory animal model of the disease, the species barrier became apparent. The species barrier is defined by the presence of a longer incubation time for the initial transmission of a prion disease from one species to a second than the incubation time for any subsequent passage once the disease is established in the new species. This shortening between initial and subsequent incubation periods defines the barrier. Its molecular basis is unknown but is hypothesized to reflect the amount of homology between the PrP sequences of the inoculum and the recipient, particularly at key sites in the PrP molecule that are associated with conformational changes. There are still many unexplained features of the species barrier, and a clearer understanding of the biochemical basis for the species barrier may help explain the pathogenesis of various human and animal prion diseases.

PATHOGENESIS

The mechanism of neuronal death in prion diseases is still unknown. In accordance with the prion hypothesis, PrP^{Res} could be harmful to neurons through three mechanisms: loss of normal PrP^{C} function, PrP^{Res} toxicity, or some combination of the two. There is evidence to both support and refute each of these hypotheses. Most recent research has focused on the toxicity of PrP^{Res} rather than loss of PrP^{C} function. This is supported by the fact that in experimentally infected animals, areas of the brain that are affected the most by neuronal loss and spongiform change frequently also have the highest concentrations of PrP^{Res}. By immunocytochemistry, PrP^{Res} is shown to accumulate before the development of the hallmark pathological

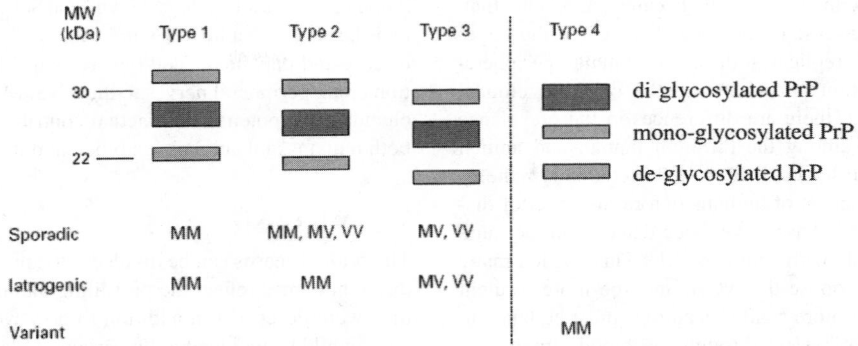

FIGURE 2.10–7 Molecular strain types of Creutzfeldt-Jakob disease (CJD). This is an illustration of the Western blot extraction of PrP^{CJD} from different forms of CJD. After proteinase K (PK) digestion, a PK-resistant protein is visualized on the immunoblot. The extract from each brain comprises three different PrP molecules based on how many glycosyl side chains there are (zero, one, or two). The four different types shown are based on the slight variations in molecular weight (MW; probably due to different clipping sites by PK) as well as the relative amounts of di- versus mono- versus deglycosylated PrP. All variant CJD cases to date have electrophoretically shown the type 4 pattern, as do PrP extracts from cattle with bovine spongiform encephalopathy. MM, homozygous methionine; MV, heterozygous methionine/valine; VV, homozygous valine. (Courtesy of John Collinge.)

features (i.e., gliosis, neuronal loss, and spongiform change), but this relationship is not absolute, and there have been recent laboratory examples of PrP^{Res} accumulation in the absence of clinical disease and pathological changes. Further support of PrP^{Res} toxicity comes from studies with synthetic PrP peptides (corresponding to amino acids 106 to 126 of PrP^{C}, regions associated with PK resistance and amyloid formation in PrP) in cell culture, wherein the peptides induce neuronal death through apoptosis. Some propose that PrP^{C}'s normal function is to regulate apoptosis, and with the accumulation of PrP^{Res} and loss of PrP^{C}, apoptosis proceeds unchecked. The most convincing evidence supporting a toxic effect of PrP^{Res} relies on the fact that PrP-null mice develop normally and have a normal life span despite the lack of any PrP^{C}. However, the situation is not completely resolved because PrP^{Res} is toxic only when PrP^{C} is present. In knock-out mice with wild-type brain transplants, the transplant becomes infected and shows pathology. This is as expected, but in addition, a small amount of PrP^{Res} accumulates in the host brain of the null mouse. If the pathology of transmissible spongiform encephalopathies was a result of PrP^{Res} toxicity, there should be some deleterious effects in both the host and transplanted parts of the brain, but there is none in these neurons that do not express PrP^{C}. What may be important in determining prion neurotoxicity is the cellular location of the abnormal PrP^{Res}. John Collinge and colleagues recently reported that depleting endogenous neuronal PrP^{C} reversed spongiform change and prevented neuronal loss in mice with an established prion infection. Interestingly, extraneuronal PrP^{Res} continued to accumulate unabated; this suggests that halting the ongoing conversion of PrP^{C} to PrP^{Res} intracellularly prevents neurotoxicity. This may have therapeutic implications for both animal and human forms of the disease.

Experimentally, prion diseases can be transmitted by multiple routes, through intracerebral, intraperitoneal, intravenous (IV), oral, or even intradermal routes. In human and animal diseases, the route(s) of the various forms of the disease is in many cases unknown. The pathway from the peripheral sites to the CNS is still uncertain. Elucidating these pathways will have major implications in both disease prevention and therapy. However, it appears that there are multiple routes from the periphery to the CNS, and any effective therapy must block all possible routes, thus magnifying the challenge for those developing therapeutic agents (Fig. 2.10–8).

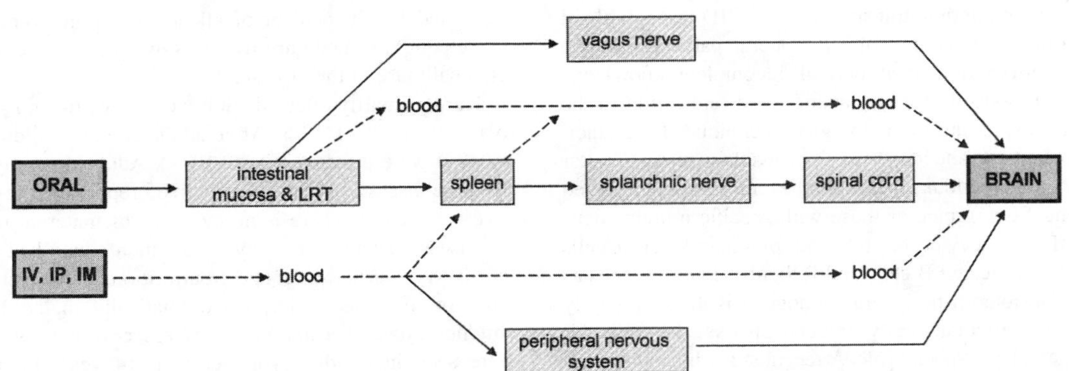

FIGURE 2.10–8 This schematic depicts the multiple routes that PrP, when peripherally introduced, can use to gain entrance to the central nervous system. The routes through the vagus nerve (n.) and splanchnic nerve have been thoroughly evaluated in experimental scrapie in sheep. The role of blood and blood components is still being researched; particularly, its ability to transmit disease in Creutzfeldt-Jakob disease and variant Creutzfeldt-Jakob disease. LRT, lymphoreticular tissue. (Courtesy of Paul Brown.)

From early studies with scrapie, it became apparent that, although the brunt of the disease takes place in the CNS, the infectious agent is found and replicates throughout many peripheral organs during the incubation period before the onset of clinical symptoms. More important, there are differences in the prevalence of PrP^{Sc} in the periphery among the different human and animal forms of the diseases. For instance, PrP^{vCJD} is detected in lymphoreticular tissues, including tonsils, of humans before the onset of disease in vCJD, whereas PrP^{CJD} has not yet been detected in the same peripheral tissues of patients with sporadic CJD. This has led many public health officials to propose that vCJD may be more virulent than sporadic CJD and that more rigid precautions must be taken to prevent iatrogenic spread of vCJD through the blood supply and contaminated surgical instruments.

The earliest and most complete studies of the pathogenesis of prion diseases were reported in scrapie, followed by studies of mouse-adapted scrapie strains, and demonstrated that there are multiple routes to the CNS by oral inoculation. Time course studies of orally infected animals showed that the infectious agent was first detected in the gastrointestinal (GI) tract, including the tonsils and Peyer's patches, then in the spleen, where significant replication took place, followed by neuroinvasion of the splanchnic nerves until infectivity was detected in the thoracic spinal cord. Infection then spread rostrocaudally within the CNS, first infecting the basal part of the brain but ultimately the cerebrum. The spleen is particularly important in the preclinical phase of orally transmitted disease, and splenectomy before transmission prolongs the incubation period but, unfortunately, does not block disease transmission. Direct axonal neurotransmission can occur experimentally via optic, vagal, and sciatic nerves. In fact, it has been demonstrated that PrP^{Sc} can spread both centripetally and centrifugally along peripheral nerves and possibly first travels centripetally to the CNS, then up and down the spinal cord, and finally centrifugally to other peripheral nerves and ganglia.

Using a recently developed method of PrP^{CJD} detection that, to date, is the most sensitive, Adriano Aguzzi and colleagues revisited the peripheral distribution of PrP^{CJD} in sporadic CJD. In addition to the abundant amounts of PrP^{CJD} in the brain, at autopsy they found the pathological protein in approximately one-third of spleens and one-fourth of skeletal muscles tested. The presence of extraneuronal PrP seemed to correlate with a longer disease duration. This recent finding may have implications for the possible iatrogenic spread of sporadic CJD and even the pathogenesis of cases of sporadic CJD for which there is currently no known etiology.

The recent issue of possible transmission of vCJD through blood has sparked further research into the peripheral pathways of the infectious agent with more elegant, but still incomplete, knowledge of the cell types responsible for propagation and replication in the periphery. Studies exploiting immunological techniques have elucidated factors, receptors, and cell types involved in replication or propagation of the infectious agent. Studies in severe combined immune-deficient (SCID) mice or those with specific immune deficiencies of B or T lymphocytes, or both, and follicular dendritic cells have alternatively implicated B cells and follicular dendritic cells as the cell type responsible for peripheral pathogenesis. In peripherally inoculated and, in particular, orally induced disease, the follicular dendritic cells may play a special role. A recent study by Aguzzi and colleagues showed that the splenic follicular dendritic cells that are in close proximity to splenic sympathetic nerves may play a critical role in the transfer of PrP^{Res} from the periphery to the CNS. Most recent studies have implicated macrophage subsets as candidates of pathogenesis in the absence of follicular dendritic cells and B cells. Another recent study has shown that Schwann's cells express PrP^{C} and that PrP^{Res} replicates within this cell type during experimental disease and may be the cell type responsible for centripetal propagation along peripheral nerves to the CNS. More research is required to elucidate the potential and actual contributions to disease burden in both humans and animals via blood and its precise pathways.

CLASSIFICATION

The prion diseases can be divided into animal and human forms. The different names reflect the prevailing naming convention at the time they were described in addition to how well it was recognized that they should be included in this group of diseases (Table 2.10–1). The prototypical human disease is kuru, an epidemic disease that has now almost completely disappeared. CJD can be subcategorized into three distinct forms: sporadic, familial, and iatrogenic. Both Gerstmann-Sträussler syndrome and fatal familial insomnia can be included under familial CJD. vCJD is grouped separately from other forms of CJD, although, arguably, it could be included as a form of iatrogenic CJD.

Sporadic CJD accounts for 85 to 90 percent of all CJD cases and was named because it occurred sporadically throughout the world without any obvious cause. In this author's opinion, it is better called *idiopathic CJD,* as this more accurately describes the understanding of how this form of the disease occurs. Despite being the most frequent form of the disease, it is still a rare disease, occurring at a rate of one to two cases per million population per year in all developed countries where good epidemiological surveys have been performed. Familial CJD accounts for 10 to 15 percent of CJD cases and is associated with nearly 30 different mutations in the PRNP gene. Iatrogenic CJD, in less than 1 to 5 percent of CJD cases, is the rarest form of prion disease, but more research on the pathogenesis must be performed to confirm this statistic and further minimize accidental transmission of disease. vCJD, although worldwide a very rare disease, has accounted for 12 to 35 percent of all CJD cases in the United Kingdom from 1996 to 2003. Each form of the human prion diseases has unique features and is considered individually.

Kuru Kuru first came to the attention of Western medicine in the 1950s when Gajdusek and Zigas reported the endemic disease among the Fore people of the Eastern Highlands of Papua New Guinea, an isolated, rugged region populated by approximately 17,000 people. The origin of the disease is uncertain, but it had been prevalent since at least the 1940s and at the peak of the epidemic accounted for 50 percent of all deaths within some villages. The native people named kuru for its "shivering" or "trembling" character, a hallmark of the disease.

Kuru primarily affected adult women, with—at its peak—a male to female ratio of 1:25. After adult women, children (both sexes equally) were affected (Fig. 2.10–9). Adult men only rarely developed the disease. The youngest person reported to be affected was a 4-year-old child. There is no evidence of maternal transmission of the disease despite the many kuru patients who had and died from the disease during pregnancy, parturition, or lactation. The prevalence of the disease dropped dramatically in the 1960s, and the childhood onset became gradually older so that, by 1967, no cases were seen in children younger than 14 years of age. It is now believed that the disease was transmitted via ritual cannibalism, a funeral practice of the Fore people. Women prepared the bodies; men consumed the "prime" tissues, such as skeletal muscle, and the women and children ate the less desirable and highly infectious tissues such as the CNS. Today, zero or one case occurs annually in

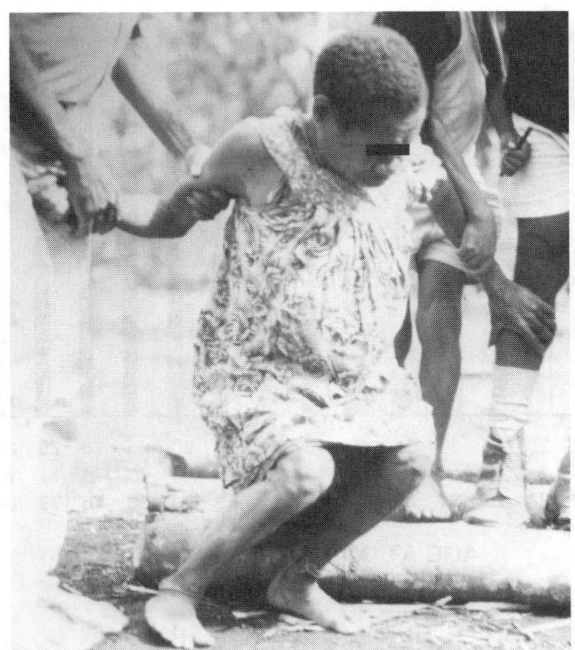
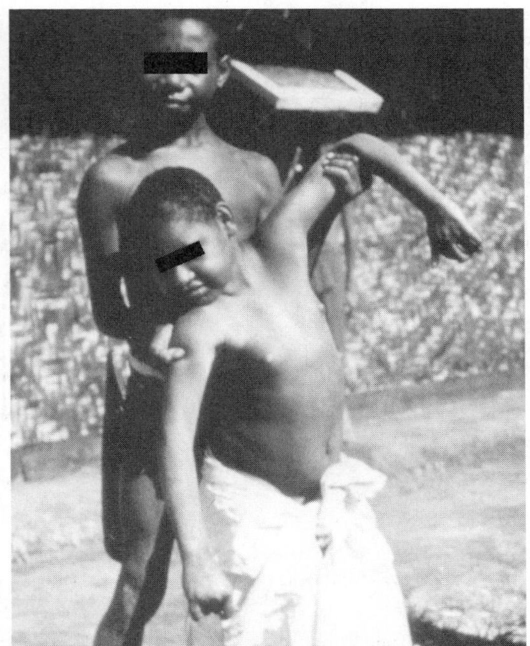

A B

FIGURE 2.10–9 Two kuru patients. These figures show a young woman **(A)** and a child **(B)** in the late ambulatory phases of kuru.

New Guinea, but now all cases are in people who are older than 40 years of age and who participated in a cannibalistic funeral before the practice ceased in the late 1950s.

The disease begins insidiously and culminates in death, usually within 6 to 9 months. There may be a prodrome of arthralgias, headache, or malaise. The disease begins with a subtle, progressive gait ataxia with unsteady walking requiring ambulatory aids as months pass. The gait is broad based and lurching, and incoordination of the upper limbs, eye movements, and speech may also occur. Irregular, coarse intention tremors, sometimes resembling shivers, soon follow and may become quite large in amplitude. Other involuntary movements (such as clonus, chorea, or athetosis as well as hyperreflexia and convergent strabismus) may appear, but rigidity and muscle weakness are not usually present. Cognition is relatively spared until late in the course of the disease when assessment becomes difficult because of anarthria and almost constant tremulousness. However, euphoria, emotional lability, and a pseudobulbar affect are commonly described in kuru patients during the ambulatory phase. By the time the patient enters the second sedentary phase of illness, the patient's predominant mood is apathetic and withdrawn. Finally, dysphagia develops, and the patient becomes completely dependent for care, with death usually resulting from aspiration pneumonia or sepsis from decubitus ulcers.

All routine laboratory tests of kuru patients have been normal. However, there is an association between earlier onset and shorter duration of disease and homozygosity at the polymorphic codon 129 of the PRNP gene, particularly with homozygosity for methionine at this site. This may have epidemiological significance for estimates of the vCJD epidemic, as there are numerous similarities between the two diseases: possible oral transmission, younger age at onset, and presence of amyloid plaques. Microscopically, the disease is characterized by spongiform vacuolation of the neuropil, astrocytic gliosis, and kuru plaques. The spongiform change is widespread and maximal in the cerebral cortex but also usually affects the striatum, midbrain, and cerebellum and less so the thalamus, pons, medulla, and spinal cord. Kuru plaques are seen in 50 to 70 percent of cases, and their likelihood increases with longer duration of clinical illness. They are most commonly seen in the granular layer of the cerebellum. Kuru plaques stain immunocytochemically for PrP and with Congo red and periodic acid-Schiff for amyloid. Florid plaques—that is, plaques ringed by spongiform vacuolation like the petals on a flower—are not seen in kuru. The disease is uniformly fatal, and isolated reports of recoveries probably occurred in patients with conversion disorders rather than kuru.

Sporadic CJD Although a rare disease, this is by far the most common human prion disease. Recent epidemiological surveys have shown a slightly higher incidence than that of 10 to 20 years ago, but this apparent increase probably reflects better case ascertainment than a true increase in disease incidence. Sporadic CJD affects men and women equally and is a disease of late middle age, with peak age of death at 68 years. The graph of the age incidence of disease is a bell-shaped curve with a long tail toward a younger age and, inexplicably, a marked drop of incidence among people older than 75 years of age (Fig. 2.10–10). The disease has been reported in people as young as 16 years of age and as old as 84 years of age. However, with a U.S. incidence of one case per million population per year overall, the incidence among those younger than 30 years of age is five cases per billion per year in the United States.

The cause of this form of the disease remains unknown and, according to the prion hypothesis, occurs as a random, one in a million misfolding of host PrP^C within the CNS itself without any exogenous stimulus. A random chance somatic mutation in the PRNP gene in an adult neuron that changes the protein from the normal to the pathogenic conformation has been hypothesized to explain the disease onset in later life. Keeping in mind that small numbers and consequent lack of statistical power hamper epidemiological studies of rare diseases, numerous such studies have been performed in the United States and Europe to search for predisposing factors. Despite isolated studies showing various factors (physical injury, surgery, ocular tonometry, and employment as clergy to

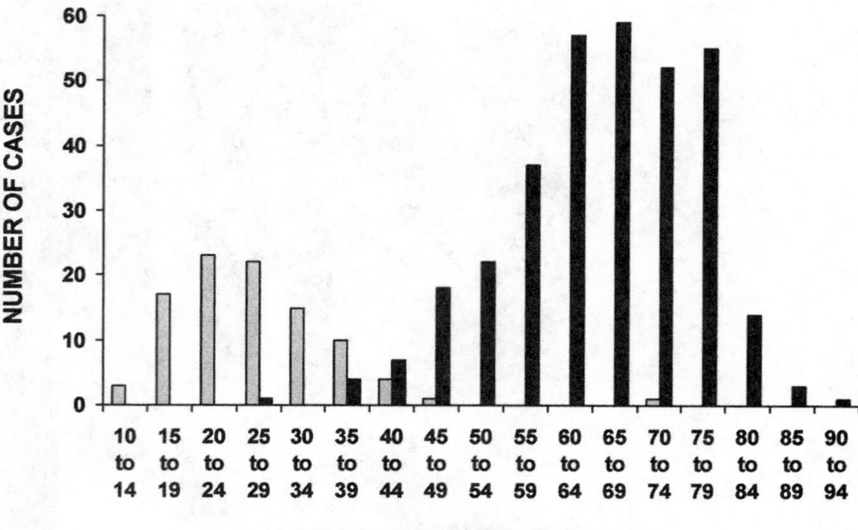

FIGURE 2.10–10 Age of onset of sporadic Creutzfeldt-Jakob disease (CJD) versus variant CJD. This graph shows the age of onset in more than 350 cases of sporadic CJD in dark gray versus the ages of onset for the first 100 variant CJD cases in light gray. (Courtesy of Paul Brown.)

name a few) as relative risk factors, no entity has repeatedly or consistently been associated with disease. No link has ever been shown with scrapie; countries with and without scrapie (e.g., the United Kingdom and Australia, respectively) have similar disease incidence. There is no evidence for case clustering (after careful study, all apparent clusters have represented familial disease) or direct case-to-case transmission (there is a single, published case of conjugal CJD). There is no epidemiological evidence for disease transmission through blood transfusion, and case-control studies have failed to show any link to diet or occupational exposure, including the consumption of different animal products and those occupations that involve exposure to scrapie or bovine spongiform encephalopathy. As with kuru, the only risk factor that has consistently been demonstrated is homozygosity for methionine at the polymorphic codon 129 of the PRNP gene so that 80 percent of sporadic cases of CJD are homozygous methionine (MM), whereas the normal distribution of the gene is MM (40 percent), homozygous valine (VV; 10 percent), and heterozygous methionine/valine (MV; 50 percent) among the U.K. population.

Various prodromal symptoms have been described in one-fourth of patients in the weeks to months preceding neurological signs. These include headache, fatigue, anorexia, or depression. There is often a vague complaint of visual difficulty, enough to prompt an eye examination, but abnormalities are rarely found on ophthalmological examination. Patients or their concerned families seek medical attention because of mental deterioration, cerebellar dysfunction, or both (Table 2.10–4). The onset is usually gradual over a period of weeks to months and can be associated with behavioral changes such as apathy, self-neglect, anorexia, emotional lability, confusion, disorientation, or hallucinations. In approximately 15 percent of cases, the onset is more precipitous, with symptoms appearing over a few days. The disease can even have a stroke-like presentation, with symptoms appearing in a matter of hours. Visual symptoms, such as diplopia, blurred vision, or visual agnosias, occur early in the course of illness. Dementia or ataxia is quickly followed by a constellation of neurological symptoms and signs reflecting the extensive, but patchy, gray matter involvement of the disease. The dementia rapidly progresses, and the patient becomes globally demented, often culminating in an akinetic mute state followed by coma and death. CJD is a dramatic disease with frequently obvious daily progression and loss of neurological function. Other pyramidal and extrapyramidal symptoms and signs, including parkinsonism, hyperreflexia, and, particularly, myoclonus, appear. A distinctive feature of CJD is startle myoclonus—that is, myoclonus precipitated by a variety of sensory stimuli such as touching or loud noises. Seizures occur in 10 percent of CJD patients, and lower motor neuron signs may occur but are less common than pyramidal and extrapyramidal signs. Sensory symptoms and signs are absent from the disease. The patient becomes obtunded, and death occurs in 70 percent of patients within 2 to 4 months of onset of disease. Sporadic CJD has a mean duration of illness of 6 months, but approximately 10 percent of patients with sporadic CJD survive for 1 year or more. Sporadic CJD is suspected when the triad of rapidly progressing dementia, ataxia, and myoclonus present. However, myoclonus is rare at the onset of disease but eventually appears in 80 percent of cases (Table 2.10–4). In addition, myoclonus can occur in other dementing illnesses, including Alzheimer's disease, the most common disease from which CJD must be distinguished.

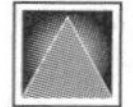

Table 2.10–4
Symptoms and Signs of Sporadic Creutzfeldt-Jakob Disease among a Cohort of 350 Patients

Symptom/Sign	At Onset (%)	During Course (%)
Dementia	70	100
Cerebellar	33	71
Visual or oculomotor	19	42
Vertigo or dizziness	13	19
Headache	11	18
Sensory	6	11
Abnormal movements[a]	4	91
Pyramidal	2	62
Extrapyramidal	1	56
Lower motor neuron	1	12
Pseudobulbar	1	7
Akinetic mutism	0	81
Seizures	0	19

[a]Includes myoclonus, tremor, and chorea.

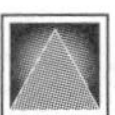

Table 2.10–5
World Health Organization Clinical Diagnostic Criteria for Sporadic Creutzfeldt-Jakob Disease

Diagnosis	Criteria
Definite	1. Routine neuropathology showing neuronal loss, spongiform change, and astrocytic gliosis **OR**
	2. Immunocytochemical or Western immunoblot, or both, presence of protease-resistant PrP **OR**
	3. Presence of scrapie-associated fibrils by electron microscopy
Probable	1. Progressive dementia **AND**
	2. At least two of the four following clinical features
	Myoclonus
	Visual or cerebellar disturbance
	Pyramidal/extrapyramidal dysfunction
	Akinetic mutism
	3. Typical EEG or positive cerebrospinal fluid 14-3-3 assay, or both
	4. Clinical duration <2 yrs
	5. Routine investigations do not suggest an alternative diagnosis
Possible	1. Progressive dementia **AND**
	2. Two of the four clinical features listed above
	3. No EEG or atypical EEG
	4. Duration <2 yrs
	5. Routine investigations do not suggest an alternative diagnosis

EEG, electroencephalogram.

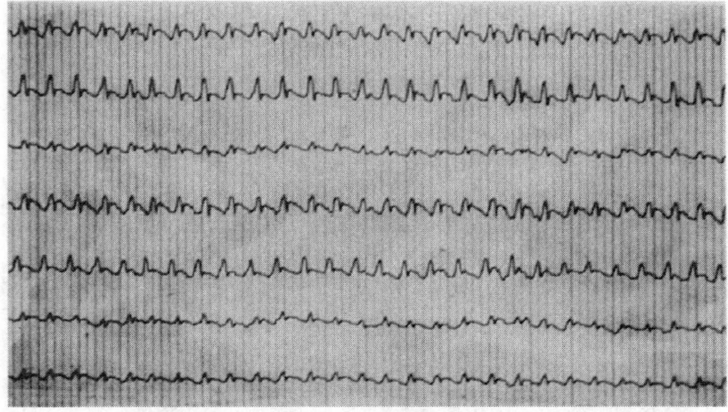

FIGURE 2.10–11 Typical triphasic periodic electroencephalogram of sporadic Creutzfeldt-Jakob disease. This shows the typical 1- to 2-Hz periodic electroencephalogram with triphasic waves that is seen diffusely in 70 percent of sporadic Creutzfeldt-Jakob disease patients in the later stages of illness. (Courtesy of Paul Brown.)

Among patients with sporadic CJD, several variants have been identified. The most frequent is Heidenhain's variant, characterized by prominent visual symptoms, including early cortical blindness, followed by dementia and other pyramidal and extrapyramidal signs. On neuropathological examination, there is extensive spongiform change, neuronal loss, and gliosis in the occipital lobes. Less common is the Brownell-Oppenheimer variant, a pure cerebellar syndrome. A panencephalopathic form has been described, particularly in Asia, in which there is extensive degeneration of the cerebral white matter in addition to the typical pathological findings in the gray matter. The amyotrophic form with dementia and motor neuron disease is controversial. Cases were reported in the early medical literature, but this form has not transmitted to laboratory animals. These probably represent cases of amyotrophic lateral sclerosis (ALS) with associated dementia rather than a prion disease.

International clinical diagnostic criteria have been established and are routinely used by surveillance centers and clinical research studies, but they have been less frequently used by clinicians (Table 2.10–5). Patients fulfilling clinical criteria for probable CJD prove to have CJD at autopsy more than 90 percent of the time. Patients fulfilling clinical criteria for possible CJD have autopsy confirmation of disease in only 60 to 70 percent of cases.

The differential diagnosis of CJD can be divided into two categories: treatable diseases that can present similarly to CJD and other degenerative diseases that need to be distinguished from CJD. It is critical to diagnose and treat the first group, and it is helpful to the patient and family to distinguish CJD from the latter group because of prognostic differences among the diseases. Reversible, treatable diseases that have been confused with CJD include acute intoxications (lithium, bismuth, cyclical antidepressants), Hashimoto's thyroiditis, encephalitides (viral, cryptococcal), CNS vasculitis, multiple cerebral abscesses, strokes, neoplasms, normal pressure hydrocephalus, hyperparathyroidism, Wernicke-Korsakoff syndrome, vitamin B_{12} deficiency, and paraneoplastic syndromes. Other neurodegenerative diseases that may have a more rapid course than usual and may be confused with sporadic CJD include Alzheimer's disease, multiinfarct dementia, corticobasal ganglionic degeneration, diffuse Lewy body disease, human immunodeficiency virus (HIV) dementia, Pick's disease, Parkinson's disease with dementia, progressive supranuclear palsy, olivopontocerebellar atrophy, Huntington's disease, and Ramsay Hunt syndrome.

In sporadic CJD, routine hematological and biochemical tests are usually normal except for occasional mild elevations of serum transaminases or alkaline phosphatase. Likewise, cerebrospinal fluid (CSF) studies are also normal except for a nonspecific mildly elevated protein and occasionally a mild leukocytosis. Three laboratory tests have become quite helpful in supporting a diagnosis of CJD in patients who fulfill clinical criteria for possible CJD.

The first test is the electroencephalogram (EEG), in which a tracing of 1- to 2-Hz periodic sharp wave (simple biphasic, triphasic, or more complex polyspike) complexes (PSWCs) on a slow background with loss of alpha rhythm is considered diagnostic of the condition (Fig. 2.10–11). However, this classic EEG pattern does not develop until late in the course of the illness and then only in 70 percent of cases. Further, it has also been described in treatable diseases such as lithium toxicity and Hashimoto's thyroiditis, both of which can have similar clinical presentations. Early in the course of illness, the EEG usually shows nonspecific abnormalities, such as background slowing, and, terminally, it may have a burst-suppression pattern with short runs of high-voltage spikes followed by periods of flat, electrical silence. Because the characteristic EEG pattern is transient during the disease course, it is generally recommended that serial EEGs be performed in suspected CJD patients. Other abnormalities in electrophysiological tests, such as visual evoked responses and electroretinograms, have been reported, and further study may be warranted to determine their diagnostic usefulness.

Detection of 14-3-3 proteins in the CSF is the most sensitive and specific surrogate marker of sporadic CJD. The 14-3-3 proteins are a group of cytoplasmic neuronal proteins, and their presence in the CSF probably reflects the massive neuronal destruction that is a hallmark of the disease. When applied to a population that fulfills clinical criteria

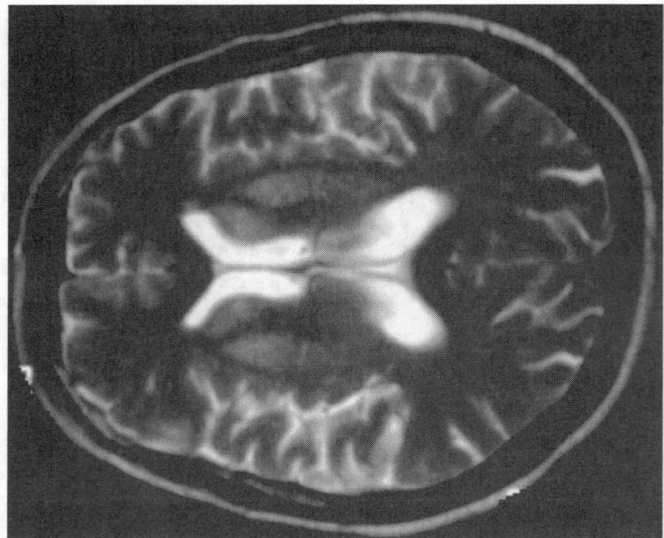

FIGURE 2.10–12 Magnetic resonance imaging in sporadic Creutzfeldt-Jakob disease. This is a T2-weighted magnetic resonance image of a patient with sporadic Creutzfeldt-Jakob disease. There is hyperintense signal in the caudate nuclei and putamen. (Courtesy of Donald Collie.)

for possible CJD, the test has more than 90 percent sensitivity and specificity. Other CSF markers have been evaluated, including neuron-specific enolase, S-100, tau protein, ubiquitin, lactic acid, and inflammatory cytokines among others, but these markers have not proved as sensitive or specific as the 14-3-3 assay in diagnosing CJD. It may be that a combination of the CSF tests may yield a more accurate antemortem test. Many researchers have assayed for the diagnostic protein PrP^{Res} in both peripheral blood and CSF without success to date. There is an urgent need for a rapid, reliable, premortem test, and currently there is intense research in this area.

Most recently, magnetic resonance imaging (MRI) has emerged as a useful diagnostic aid for sporadic CJD. Besides nonspecific atrophy, abnormalities are not seen by computed tomography (CT) scans, and initial reports suggested likewise that MRI in sporadic CJD was only nonspecifically abnormal. However, after characteristic MRI changes were identified in vCJD, review of sporadic CJD MRIs revealed subtle, but consistent, changes. On T2-weighted imaging, symmetrical, high signals are seen in the putamen and caudate nuclei of 67 percent of sporadic CJD cases. Fortunately, this can be seen early in the course of illness (Fig. 2.10–12). These changes are subtle and can be easily overlooked. Less frequently, high-intensity changes can be seen in the cortex, globus pallidus, thalamus, or periaqueductal gray matter. These changes can be visualized more easily on proton density–weighted images (DWI) or with fluid-attenuated inversion recovery (FLAIR) sequences, and, in correlation studies, the changes seen reflect the areas with the most spongiform vacuolation and neuronal loss rather than gliosis. Positron emission tomography (PET) and single photon emission computed tomography (SPECT) have not shown consistent, specific abnormalities in sporadic CJD.

A 74-year-old woman developed visual agnosia, depression, and visual hallucinations, followed by ataxia, dementia, and myoclonus. CT showed atrophy, and the patient's EEG tracing was slow and disorganized. She developed seizures, and her dementia rapidly progressed so that she became mute and nonambulatory and then unresponsive. 14-3-3 Proteins were detected in her CSF, and she died 6 months after the onset of her symptoms. Autopsy confirmed sporadic CJD.

This is a classic case of sporadic CJD.

A 28-year-old woman complained of weakness and unsteady gait. She then developed progressive ataxia and marked dysarthria. She was admitted 2 months later with dementia, lethargy, choreoathetosis, constant lip smacking, diffusely increased muscle tone, and hallucinations. In the hospital, she developed focal motor seizures. Her EEG was abnormal with diffuse, slow triphasic waves. An MRI was normal. A brain biopsy was performed and showed only gliosis. She died 4 months after the onset of her illness. Autopsy confirmed the diagnosis of CJD. There were no PrP plaques, and genetic analysis revealed no pathogenic mutations associated with familial CJD.

This is a rare example of sporadic CJD in a young person.

A 66-year-old woman complained of decreasing memory and headache. Over several months, she developed episodic involuntary movements with rhythmic jerking and right versive head movements. On one occasion, a generalized tonic-clonic seizure was witnessed in the emergency department of a local hospital. She demonstrated behavioral problems, with hyperphagia, hypersexuality, and social withdrawal. On examination, she had marked memory difficulties with confabulation as well as impaired word fluency. She had decreased upgaze, normal strength, increased tone and deep tendon reflexes, and intermittent myoclonus. She had gait unsteadiness but no clear ataxia. Her dementia progressed so that she was unable to care for herself, including toilet and bathing care. Her CSF 14-3-3 was positive, and an EEG was "suggestive" of CJD. She died 12 months after the onset of illness. There was no family history of neurological disease. Autopsy revealed senile plaques and neurofibrillary tangles without spongiform change, astrocytic gliosis, or PrP plaques.

This is an unusual case of rapidly progressive Alzheimer's disease. This case emphasizes the need for pathological confirmation of clinical disease.

A 49-year-old woman developed acute lower back pain and had lower extremity weakness on examination. She then developed a "total body" tremor and proximal weakness, resulting in a gait abnormality, and then progressive ataxia. She was diagnosed with "atypical multiple sclerosis" (MS). Five months into her disease, she complained of diplopia, dysphagia, and urinary frequency. A videofluoroscopic swallowing study was normal. It was believed that her symptoms had a psychiatric component, and she was referred to a psychiatrist. She had no evidence of dementia, and her neurological examination was completely normal despite her symptomatic complaints of a waxing and waning nature. She was diagnosed with depression and conversion disorder and treated with fluoxetine (Prozac) and buspirone (BuSpar). She was discharged to a residential psychiatric facility where, under hypnosis, her symptoms improved; however, she complained of symptom progression and became wheelchair bound and completely dependent for all activities of daily living. She was again hospitalized and scored 24 out of 30 on the Mini-Mental State Examination (MMSE). Her tremors waxed and waned on examination, and she was diagnosed with conversion disorder and major depression. Two months later, she developed intermittent primitive reflexes and disinhibited behavior such as throwing food or smearing it on herself. She also developed an exaggerated startle response. MRI and EEG were normal. One evening, she was found in cardiopulmonary arrest; suction performed during cardiopulmonary resuscitation (CPR) revealed small bits of food in her airways. She was successfully resuscitated but declared brain dead 36 hours later. An autopsy revealed CJD.

This is an atypical presentation for sporadic CJD but a reminder that psychiatric features are not unique to vCJD!

The diagnosis of sporadic CJD, as with all prion diseases, relies on pathological confirmation of disease despite the overall reduction in autopsy rate in the United States and reluctance to perform autopsies on suspect CJD cases. Brain biopsies are also less frequently performed but, with its inherent risks to both the patient (5 percent mortality among CJD patients) and the medical staff, are not warranted unless an alternative treatable disease is a diagnostic possibility. Because the disease can have an irregular distribution throughout the cortices, brain biopsies are falsely negative in 5 to 10 percent of cases in which it is performed.

At autopsy, the brain grossly often shows focal or diffuse atrophy. The routine neuropathological hallmarks of CJD are neuronal loss, spongiform vacuolation, and reactive astrogliosis (Fig. 2.10–13). If extensive, the spongiform change may coalesce to form status spongiosis with cystic collapse of the cortex. Neuronal loss is variable and frequently overshadowed by the striking astrogliosis. Each of these changes can be seen in other diseases, and spongiform vacuolation may even occur as an artifact of handling and processing. Amyloid plaques are seen in 10 percent of sporadic CJD cases, primarily in the cerebellum, and are comprised of PrP^{CJD}; their presence is associated with longer duration of illness and the presence of one or more valine alleles at codon 129 of the PRNP gene. Transmissibility is no longer required to confirm the diagnosis of a transmissible spongiform encephalopathy. However, replacing transmissibility is the reliance on the demonstration, through various immunological means, of the presence of PrP^{Res} within affected brain tissue. This can be performed on either fresh frozen or fixed tissues. PrP^{CJD} can be extracted from brain homogenate (as little as 200 mg) to diagnose the disease. Alternatively, it can be visualized immunocytochemically on fixed tissue sections after PrP^{C} has been digested by PK treatment. Immunohistochemical staining is positive in nearly all cases of sporadic CJD, and there are several distinct patterns of staining that have been described: perivacuolar, neuronal, synaptic, and plaque-like. These different patterns have been correlated with different forms of the disease (e.g., sporadic CJD vs. vCJD). CJD has also been categorized into four different types based on the differences among the relative amounts of glycosylated PrP from Western blot conformations (Fig. 2.10–7).

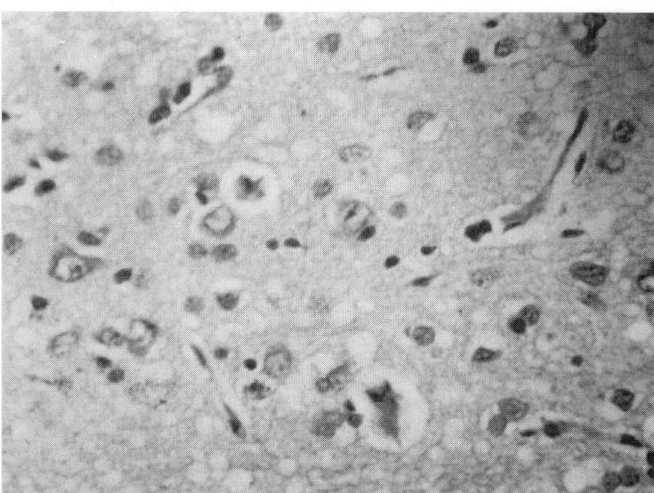

FIGURE 2.10–13 Photomicrograph of the cortex of a patient with sporadic Creutzfeldt-Jakob disease. This is a hematoxylin and eosin stain of the cortex showing spongiform degeneration of the neuropil with neuronal loss, characteristic of Creutzfeldt-Jakob disease. Magnification ×200 before reduction.

Familial Prion Diseases

Approximately 10 to 15 percent of human spongiform encephalopathy cases are familial and associated with, to date, nearly 30 point and insert mutations in the PRNP gene on chromosome 20 (Fig. 2.10–14). These various syndromes are unique in that they are genetically based and passed vertically from one family member to the next and yet, at the same time, are transmissible to laboratory animals and, by definition, infectious. One study suggested that familial forms of the disease may be underdiagnosed because point or insert mutations had been found in 25 percent of cases of apparent sporadic CJD (those without any associated family history of neurological disease). Whether these represented new mutations within the family, incomplete family histories, or incomplete penetrance remains to be determined. Familial prion diseases can have several clinical manifestations and are usually named before the recognition that they belonged to this family of disorders. They include familial CJD, Gerstmann-Sträussler syndrome, and fatal familial insomnia. All familial forms are transmitted in an autosomal dominant fashion with varying degrees of penetrance. Thus, they affect males and females equally. As noted above, all apparent case clusters of CJD have proven to be familial, including the clusters in Slovakia, Libya, and Chile.

The oldest disease of this group is Gerstmann-Sträussler syndrome, which was recognized to be familial in 1936 when a cohort of eight family members was reported. It was originally categorized as a cerebellar degeneration because of the prominent cerebellar ataxia and the degenerative changes seen in the cerebellum pathologically. The disease is associated with pyramidal symptoms and signs as well as dementia, but the dementia usually occurs later in the course of illness after the motor symptoms are well established. Gerstmann-Sträussler syndrome usually has a much longer duration than sporadic CJD, with a mean of 5 years, as well as an earlier onset, usually in the third or fourth decade of life. Myoclonus and PSWCs on EEG occur only occasionally. CSF protein 14-3-3 is present in a small percentage of Gerstmann-Sträussler syndrome patients; however, the clinical presentation can be quite heterogeneous. Recently, it has become apparent that, within a family, there can be clinical phenotypes indistinguishable from sporadic CJD with prominent and rapid dementia, little or no ataxia, and death within 2 to 3 months of onset in addition to other family members with the classic cerebellar phenotype. Pathologically, Gerstmann-Sträussler syndrome is distinguished from sporadic CJD by the presence of amyloid plaques with a multicentric configuration within the cerebellum (Fig. 2.10–15). Otherwise, it is characterized by the diagnostic hallmarks of spongiform change, neuronal loss, and astrogliosis.

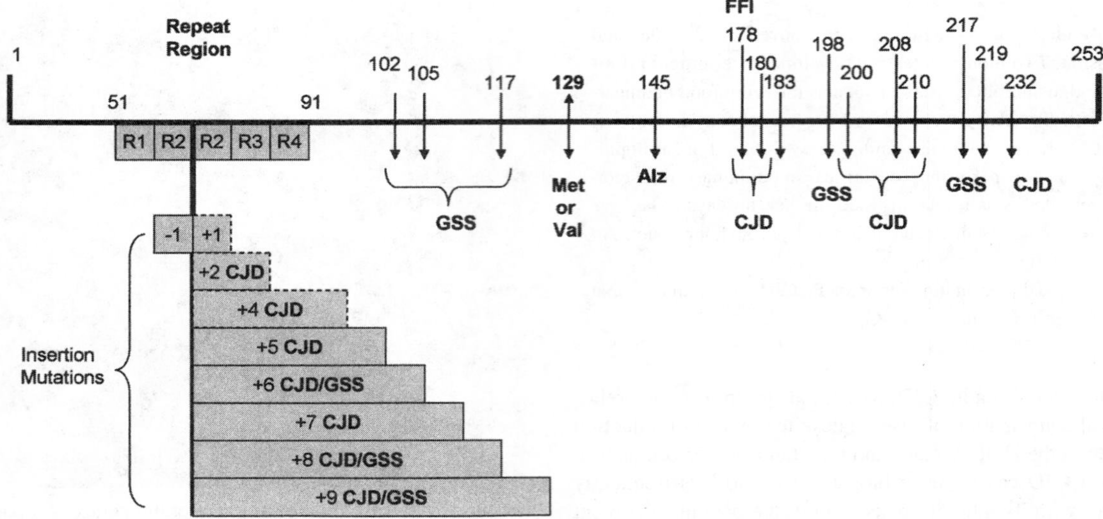

FIGURE 2.10–14 PrP mutations associated with familial prion disease. This illustration shows the mutations commonly associated with familial prion disease. The numbers indicate the codon at which the mutation occurs. The polymorphic site 129 is also indicated. The codon 178 mutation is associated with both familial Creutzfeldt-Jakob disease (CJD) and fatal familial insomnia (FFI). GSS, Gerstmann-Sträussler syndrome. (Courtesy of Paul Brown.)

Classic Gerstmann-Sträussler syndrome is associated with a point mutation at codon 102 (P102L, proline substituted for leucine at codon 102) of the PRNP gene on chromosome 20. This is the most common mutation associated with the disease, including the original Austrian family, and has been transmitted to laboratory animals, although only in 40 percent of inoculations with brain homogenate from P102L cases. However, Gerstmann-Sträussler syndrome is also associated with several other point mutations (A117V, P105L, F198S, D202N, Q217R, Q212P, G131V, H187R), a stop mutation (Y145STOP), and one insert mutation (three different patterns of an eight-octapeptide repeat). There have also been isolated reports of sporadic Gerstmann-Sträussler syndrome in which a mutation could not be found. Recently, Gerstmann-Sträussler syndrome has become a heterogeneous group of clinical syndromes. There is an American kindred, associated with the F198S point mutation, in which the clinical syndrome includes prominent parkinsonism and pathologically cortical neurofibrillary tangles. The amber stop mutation, causing termination of PRNP translation and resulting in a truncated PrP protein, was associated with a dementing illness of at least 20 years' duration in a patient who at autopsy had pathological changes of Alzheimer's disease as well as PrP^{GSS} plaques in the cerebellum by immunocytochemistry. The P105L mutation has been associated with a syndrome characterized by familial spastic paraparesis with dementia and prominent pathological changes in the motor cortex and pyramidal tracts with little or no abnormalities in the cerebellum.

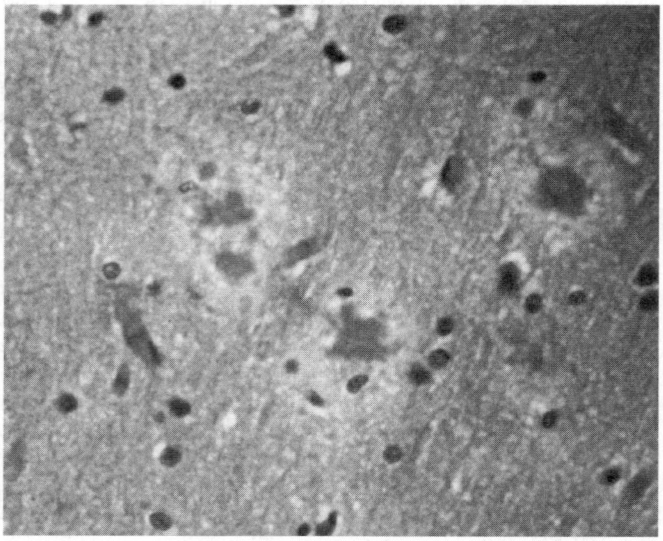

FIGURE 2.10–15 Polycentric PrP plaques in Gerstmann-Sträussler syndrome. This hematoxylin and eosin stain photomicrograph shows the densely eosinophilic cores of the PrP plaques seen in the cerebellum of patients with Gerstmann-Sträussler syndrome. Magnification ×250.

A 64-year-old man became apathetic and withdrawn and 9 months later rapidly became confused, losing his way driving near his house. He was irritable and had generalized motor weakness. Over the next few days, his dementia became apparent and rapidly progressed with aphasia, dysarthria, dyscalculia, decreased memory, and disorientation. He recognized but could not name family members. MRI showed mild to moderate atrophy without any focal lesions. His CSF was positive for 14-3-3 proteins. Within 2 months, he was mute and nonambulatory. He had a disorder of upgaze, occasional myoclonic jerks, left hemiparesis, bilateral Babinski signs, and diffusely increased tone. He lapsed into a coma and died at home 3 months after the onset of his dementia. An autopsy confirmed a prion disease with frequent cerebellar PrP plaques, typical of Gerstmann-Sträussler syndrome.

There was a family history of a degenerative cerebellar disease. Several family members had a progressive cerebellar ataxia of several years' duration culminating in death in their 40s or 50s. A first cousin died of pathologically confirmed Gerstmann-Sträussler syndrome.

Genetic testing confirmed the P102L mutation, the most common mutation associated with Gerstmann-Sträussler syndrome.

This is a large family with many affected members and marked phenotypic heterogeneity. The patient had a clinical course indistinguishable from sporadic CJD, whereas others had phenotypes more like classic Gerstmann-Sträussler syndrome, and even another family member carrying the P102L mutation has had a long, slowly progressing dementia of nearly 10 years' duration with onset in her late 20s.

Familial CJD is most commonly associated with one of two point mutations, D178N and E200K, the latter representing the most common of all mutations associated with familial prion disorders. The E200K mutation has incomplete penetrance, so approximately 50 percent of mutation-bearing individuals develop the disease during their lifetime. It is very similar to sporadic CJD in all respects—clinically, pathologically, and experimentally. One distinguishing feature is that it may have an earlier onset of disease (mean, 55 years), sometimes as early as the third decade of life. Unlike the other familial forms, the EEG is frequently periodic, and 14-3-3 proteins are present in the CSF during the disease at the same rate as in sporadic CJD. The second most common mutation is D178N, a point mutation of particular interest to prion researchers because the clinical phenotype associated with this mutation is determined by the amino acid present at the polymorphic codon 129. The less common valine allele is associated with familial CJD. However, when the point mutation is present with a methionine at codon 129, phenotypically, the patient develops fatal familial insomnia. The PrP^{Res} extracted from these two forms has slightly different MWs and supports the hypothesis that different strains can be determined by slightly different PrP^{Res} conformations. Familial CJD has also been associated with V180I, H208A, V210I, and M232R mutations. However, insufficient family data are available to adequately characterize these syndromes, particularly with respect to phenotype and penetrance.

A 39-year-old woman complained of progressive blindness of 1 month's duration. She then developed dysarthria, gait ataxia, dementia, incontinence, and occasional myoclonus. An MRI showed increased signal in the left caudate and putamen with small areas of increased signal in the right parietal cortex. CSF studies revealed a total protein of 51 g/dL, and the assay for 14-3-3 proteins was strongly positive. She died 3 months after the onset of her symptoms. Family history revealed that her mother had died of CJD. Genetic testing showed the E200K mutation associated with familial CJD. Autopsy confirmed the diagnosis of CJD.

This is a typical case of familial CJD in which the patients have clinical courses indistinguishable from sporadic CJD, harbor the E200K mutation, but can develop disease earlier in life than in sporadic CJD.

Fatal familial insomnia was first described in 1986 when five members of an Italian family developed a fatal disease characterized by prominent insomnia and mild gliosis in the thalamus and hypothalamus. In 1992, it was proposed that this syndrome represented a familial prion disease when a point mutation was discovered in the PRNP gene among family members with the disease. This was further corroborated as a prion disease when very small amounts of PrP^{Res} were detected in cortical and subcortical areas of brain. Subsequently, fatal familial insomnia transmitted to laboratory animals in 1995. Fatal familial insomnia is associated with a point mutation (D178N, substitution of asparagine for aspartic acid at codon 178) of the PRNP gene. Interestingly, fatal familial insomnia clinically presents when the D178N mutation is present on an allele with methionine at the polymorphic codon 129 (D178N-129M); otherwise, when the mutation is associated with valine at codon 129 (D178N-129V), the phenotype is that of familial CJD. There have also been reports of "sporadic" fatal familial insomnia, cases in which the clinical and pathological syndromes are present but lack the pathogenic gene mutation. Retrospectively, it appears that many families previously diagnosed with "selective thalamic degeneration" harbor this point mutation. Currently, there are nearly 30 fatal familial insomnia pedigrees in Europe, the United States, Australia, Japan, and China, and it is the third most common hereditary prion disease.

Clinically, fatal familial insomnia is an autosomal dominant disease with incomplete penetrance. Onset usually occurs in the fifth decade of life but can range from 20 to 70 years of age (average, 50 years of age). Fatal familial insomnia has a mean disease duration of 1 to 2 years. Like CJD, there can be a nonspecific prodrome of lethargy, anorexia with weight loss, and fatigue. The prominent feature for which the disease is named is a profound disruption of the normal sleep–wake cycle, with accompanying disorganization of the sleep EEG pattern, sympathetic overactivity, endocrine abnormalities, and impaired attention. The dysfunction of the mediodorsal nucleus of the thalamus is believed to underlie the sleep disorder, and the disconnection between the limbic cortex and the hypothalamus is believed to determine the autonomic and endocrine abnormalities. The most prominent clinical feature is nocturnal insomnia, often with excessive daytime sleepiness (in sleep studies, loss of sleep spindles and slow-wave sleep and enacted dreams during rapid eye movement [REM] sleep). However, this is progressive, and often over weeks to months, no normal sleep occurs, leaving the patient in a stupor accompanied often by vivid dreams and frequently by visual, tactile, and auditory hallucinations. Dysautonomia, usually an early finding, can be characterized by impotence, sphincteric dysfunction, hypersalivation, rhinorrhea, lacrimation, hyperthermia, hyperhidrosis, tachycardia, tachypnea, and hypertension. The sleep and autonomic disturbances are joined by pyramidal and cerebellar signs, including limb, gait, and bulbar abnormalities as well as hyperreflexia, Babinski signs, and myoclonus. Dementia usually occurs late, if at all, although inattention and insomnia may make neuropsychological testing very difficult. As with other forms of the disease, fatal familial insomnia culminates in stupor and coma and terminates with sepsis from various sources.

Sleep studies confirm reduced sleep time with EEG disorganization and virtual absence of REM periods. Routine biochemical and hematological serum and CSF studies are usually normal. CSF 14-3-3 protein is usually absent in this disorder. The diagnostic EEG of sporadic CJD is rarely seen in fatal familial insomnia but may be seen in family members who, with the same genotype, phenotypically resemble a CJD patient. PET shows pronounced thalamic and limbic hypometabolism. Neuropathologically, the abnormalities are usually restricted to the anterior ventral and dorsomedial nuclei of the thalami, with almost complete neuronal loss and marked astrocytic gliosis. Spongiform change is not a feature of fatal familial insomnia. Very low levels of PrP^{Res} can be detected by PrP extraction from brain homogenates of the subcortical gray matter (especially the thalamus) and brainstem, but none is usually visualized by PrP immunocytochemistry.

Insertion mutations compose the last group of mutations causing familial prion disorders. The normal PrP^{C} protein carries five-octapeptide base pair repeats between codons 51 and 91 (Fig. 2.10–14). Several prion disease phenotypes have been associated with octapeptide repeat insertions of varying lengths (one through nine octapeptide repeats). These include CJD, Gerstmann-Sträussler syndrome, and atypical dementia phenotypes. Many of these patients present at an early age, as early as the third or fourth decade of life. The length of disease can be quite variable, with durations of a few months as in sporadic CJD but also with very long durations of 15 years or more. Experimental transmission has been successful with some mutations but not with all.

Iatrogenic CJD The first iatrogenic CJD case occurred in 1974 when a cornea transplant recipient developed CJD from a donor who had died of a dementing illness that was subsequently pathologically confirmed as CJD. A rare disease, more than 300 cases of iatrogenic CJD have been recognized worldwide as results of accidental inoculation of infected tissues, tissue extracts, or instruments. The majority of cases have occurred from either infected human growth hormone injections (as of June 2002, 161 cases, principally in France, the United Kingdom, and the United States) or dura mater grafts (136 cases, with 88 of the cases in Japan). But iatrogenic CJD has also been documented as a result of contaminated neurosurgical instruments (five cases), depth electrode stereotactic EEG needles (two cases), human-derived gonadotropin (four cases), and cornea transplants (four cases).

There are two distinct clinical phenotypes associated with iatrogenic CJD dependent on the mode of transmission. With cases in which the infectious agent is inoculated directly into or adjacent to the CNS (stereotactic EEG depth electrodes, contaminated neurosurgical instruments, dura mater grafts, corneal transplants), there is a short (1.5 to 4.0 years) incubation period and a clinical syndrome identical to sporadic CJD with a rapidly progressing dementia. With peripherally inoculated cases (contaminated pituitary derived, cadaveric growth, and gonadotropin hormone injections), there is a long incubation period (5 to 15 years and, in some recent cases, up to 30 years) and a clinical syndrome akin to that of kuru, with early and prominent ataxia and no or late dementia. As with sporadic CJD, there appears to be a genetic susceptibility to iatrogenic CJD with an excess of homozygosity for both methionine and valine at codon 129 among all iatrogenic CJD patients, irrespective of the route of inoculation, compared with the general population. Periodic EEG recordings have been seen in approximately one-half of all iatrogenic cases, and CSF 14-3-3 protein is present in most patients with iatrogenic CJD, especially those with a rapidly progressing dementia.

A 45-year-old woman presented with severe ataxia and dysarthria. In a few months, she rapidly demented. She then became mute and developed bilateral spontaneous and startle myoclonus with rigidity and increased obtundation. Her EEG showed generalized slow activity with periodic biphasic and triphasic waves. The CSF contained high levels of neuron-specific enolase, and genetic testing revealed no pathogenic mutations associated with CJD and methionine homozygosity at codon 129. She died 8 months after her disease onset. Thirty years earlier, the patient had undergone corneal transplantation. Review of the organ donor's records showed that the donor died of CJD confirmed at autopsy.

Despite the very long incubation period, this is a case of iatrogenic CJD.

An important aspect of iatrogenic CJD is prevention. Neurosurgical instruments formerly were subjected to standard steam autoclaving, and EEG electrode needles were disinfected with benzene, ethanol, or formaldehyde. New regulations increase the temperature requirement for steam autoclaving of neurosurgical instruments to 134°C and mandate the use of disposable EEG needles, and pituitary hormones are now derived from recombinant nonhuman sources. However, renewed attention has been placed on limiting other potential routes of iatrogenic prion disease, particularly in light of vCJD.

Variant CJD The first ten cases of vCJD in the United Kingdom were reported in March 1996, and as of November 2003, there have been more than 150 cases of vCJD worldwide (143 in the United Kingdom, six in France, one each in Hong Kong, Ireland, Italy, Canada, and the United States; the Hong Kong, Canadian, and U.S. cases were all individuals who had lived for many years in the United Kingdom and only recently immigrated to the countries where they became ill). The first ten cases came to medical attention because of concern that bovine spongiform encephalopathy could have crossed the species barrier and infected humans, particularly after the realization that bovine spongiform encephalopathy had crossed the species barrier and infected other mammalian species—that is, domestic cats and exotic ungulates and felids. With a bovine spongiform encephalopathy threat in mind, a CJD surveillance center was reestablished in Edinburgh, Scotland, in 1990 to determine the incidence and prevalence of CJD in the United Kingdom as well as any new patterns of disease. In the early 1990s, they found an increase of CJD among dairy farmers, but these proved to be sporadic CJD cases occurring at the same rate among U.K. farmers as among farmers in other European countries without a bovine spongiform encephalopathy epidemic. In 1995, they reported two cases of CJD in people 16 and 18 years of age, an extremely rare chance occurrence. This followed with the report of a cohort of ten young patients with a prion disease with clinical and pathological features that distinguished these cases from the established forms of CJD.

Bovine spongiform encephalopathy was first reported in 1985 and, despite being diagnosed in many other countries outside the United Kingdom since then, has only occurred at epidemic proportions in the United Kingdom (of the more than 187,000 cases diagnosed to date, more than 97 percent have occurred in the United Kingdom). The origins of bovine spongiform encephalopathy are disputed. The two prevailing hypotheses are (1) naturally occurring sheep scrapie crossed the species barrier and infected cattle; and (2) bovine spongiform encephalopathy is a naturally occurring cattle disease that arose on a sporadic one-in-a-million basis in accord with the prion hypothesis. Regardless of its precise origins, the bovine spongiform encephalopathy epidemic within dairy herds in the United Kingdom is generally believed to have resulted from the feeding of contaminated meat and bone meal (MBM) protein supplements to dairy cattle, followed by the recycling and amplification of contaminated materials through the rendering process. MBM is a protein dietary supplement that is produced from the rendering of animal carcasses after butchering. In response to economic pressures from the energy crisis of the late 1970s and early 1980s, the rendering industry changed its procedures; in particular, it lowered temperatures and used fewer solvents. These changes may have allowed a transmissible spongiform encephalopathy infectious agent present (either scrapie or naturally occurring rare bovine spongiform encephalopathy material) to survive the rendering process. Unchecked, cattle infected with bovine spongiform encephalopathy entered the rendering process, were processed into MBM, and then fed back to healthy cattle, amplifying the epidemic with each rendering cycle. The disease was first reported in 1985, studied, and found to represent a common-source illness epidemiologically, and regulatory laws were introduced to curb the disease. In 1988, the ruminant protein feed ban was introduced to eliminate the recycling of infectious material through the rendering process. The feed ban prohibited the use of any ruminant animal parts in the production of MBM. In 1990, the ban on the human consumption of specified bovine offals (SBO, specifically brain, spinal cord, thymus, tonsil, spleen, and intestines) was imposed to protect

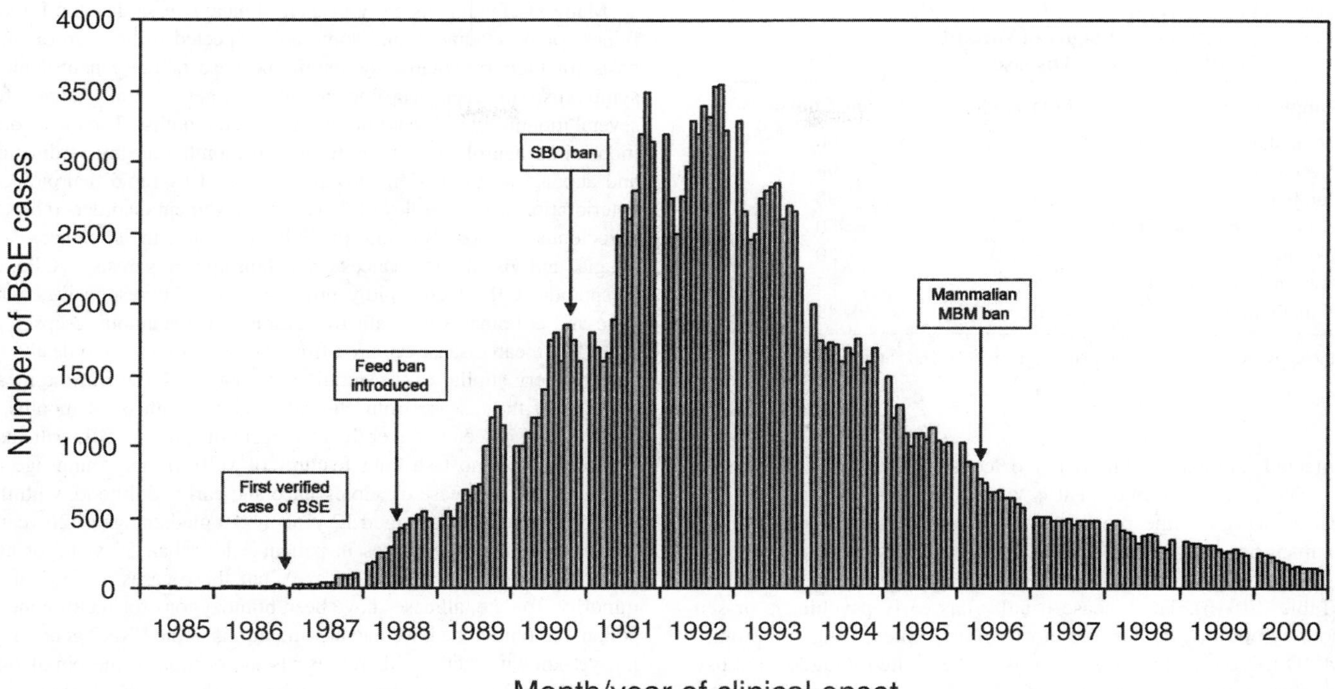

FIGURE 2.10–16 The bovine spongiform encephalopathy (BSE) epidemic. This graph depicts the total number of cases of bovine spongiform encephalopathy per quarter from 1985 until 2001 in the United Kingdom. The epidemic peaked in 1992 and has had a long tail to the right of slowly diminishing cases. The graph shows the regulations that were imposed, in particular the ruminant-to-ruminant meat and bone meal (MBM) ban that was introduced in 1988 so that the recycling of infectious material was interrupted. The epidemic peaked 4 years later and has been diminishing ever since, supporting the claim that the epidemic resulted from contaminated MBM protein supplements. The specified bovine offals (SBO) ban was put in place in 1990 to protect humans from accidental consumption of infectious material from bovine spongiform encephalopathy–infected cattle. (Courtesy of Paul Brown.)

humans from the transmission of bovine spongiform encephalopathy by the consumption of bovine organs known to harbor the bovine spongiform encephalopathy infectious agent. By 1992, the epidemic had peaked and has slowly been disappearing from the United Kingdom (Fig. 2.10–16). These bans, as well as the public response to the vCJD cases, have significantly economically impacted the cattle industry in the United Kingdom. Besides the 180,000 cattle that have had the disease, more than 4.5 million asymptomatic cattle have been slaughtered and incinerated as precautionary measures in the United Kingdom.

Bovine spongiform encephalopathy has an incubation period of 5 years and presents as a neurological disease with ataxia, abnormal and frequently aggressive behavior, recumbency, and death. Unlike scrapie, to date there is only one strain of bovine spongiform encephalopathy, although there are very recent data suggesting multiple strains of bovine spongiform encephalopathy in native cattle in both Japan and Italy. Strain typing experiments have shown that the spongiform encephalopathies in domestic cats (feline spongiform encephalopathy [FSE]), exotic ungulates and felids, and humans (vCJD) are identical to that in cattle. Bovine spongiform encephalopathy is not restricted to the United Kingdom; early reports found cases among imported cattle in nearby countries. However, with increased surveillance, more cases among native cattle have been diagnosed throughout Europe and, most recently, in Canada and Japan. The United Kingdom exported MBM throughout Europe during the height of the bovine spongiform encephalopathy epidemic, and it is believed that contaminated MBM infected native cattle in other countries. Bovine spongiform encephalopathy was recently identified in Japan, Canada (May 2003), and the United States (December 2003).

vCJD differs from other forms of CJD by numerous features and is a unique form because of the following features: (1) clinical presentation; (2) neuropathology; (3) the lack of any mutations in the PRNP gene and occurrence exclusively in those with methionine homozygosity at codon 129; (4) temporospatial linkage with bovine spongiform encephalopathy—that is, it appeared in the United Kingdom 10 years after bovine spongiform encephalopathy was first diagnosed and 4 years after the bovine spongiform encephalopathy epidemic had peaked; and (5) unique characteristics of the PrP^{Res} recovered from vCJD patients (strain-typing experiments of material have shown by two different methods that the agent of vCJD is identical to the bovine spongiform encephalopathy agent in cattle and other animals infected with the bovine spongiform encephalopathy agent). It is now hypothesized that vCJD occurred as a result of the consumption of meat or meat products that were contaminated with the bovine spongiform encephalopathy infectious agent, particularly those that make up the SBO (*vide supra*). Skeletal muscle has never been shown to transmit disease in any form of prion disease (recently, Prusiner et al. demonstrated the presence of PrP^{Sc} in hindlimb skeletal muscles of laboratory mice, and Aguzzi et al. showed the presence of PrP^{CJD} in the muscle and spleen of some cases of sporadic CJD, thereby reopening the possibility that skeletal muscle can transmit prion diseases). Meat products made from mechanically recovered meat have been proposed as the route by which humans were most likely infected with the bovine spongiform encephalopathy agent. Mechanically recovered meat is produced by a harsh method using high pressures to mechanically separate meat from carcasses; the pressures used can fracture bones and contaminate the product with spinal cord or dorsal root ganglia, tissues known to harbor large amounts of the bovine spongiform encephalopathy agent in

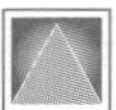

Table 2.10–6
Symptoms and Signs of Variant Creutzfeldt-Jakob Disease

Symptom/Sign	At Onset (%)	During Course (%)
Dementia	17	100
Psychiatric	66	98
Cerebellar	9	98
Visual/oculomotor	0	>50
Sensory	19	70
Abnormal movements[a]	4	94
Akinetic mutism	0	49

[a]Includes myoclonus, chorea, tremors, jumpiness, and "fidgeting."

infected animals. Although the consumption of contaminated mechanically recovered meat is widely accepted as the most likely cause of vCJD, the precise mode of transmission from cattle to humans has not yet been proven.

Clinically, vCJD is characterized by several unique features (Table 2.10–6). The disease usually has early psychiatric or sensory symptoms. By far, the most common presenting symptom in vCJD (32 out of the first 33 cases in the United Kingdom) is psychiatric. Among the first 100 vCJD patients, 63 percent presented with psychiatric symptoms, 22 percent with simultaneous psychiatric and neurological symptoms, and 15 percent with neurological symptoms alone. Common initial psychiatric symptoms (present in more than 50 percent of the cases) include dysphoria, withdrawal, anxiety, insomnia, and loss of interest. Depression or depression secondary to organic disease is the most common initial diagnosis (diagnosed in approximately one-half of the cases to date). Less common (less than 50 percent of cases), patients present with anergia and behavioral changes and rarely with obsessive features, panic attacks, and suicidal ideation. Four to 6 months into the disease course, further psychiatric features develop. These frequently include poor memory, impaired concentration, and aggression but also tearfulness, weight loss, hypersomnia, and confusion. Rarely, patients develop psychomotor retardation and loss of confidence. As other neurological symptoms appear, the psychiatric features evolve, and prominent symptoms after 6 months among vCJD patients are disorientation and agitation. Up to 50 percent of patients develop auditory or visual hallucinations, paranoid delusions, thought insertion and thought withdrawal, and inappropriate affect late in the course of their illness. Delusional symptoms are usually intermittent and have included such ideas as a missing child, microscopic people being inside a patient's body, snipers in the kitchen, and possession by the devil. Like delusions, suicidal ideation, when present, is generally fleeting and not persistent. The prominent psychiatric symptoms are unique to vCJD; they were present in the oldest vCJD patient to date (74 years of age), are not characteristic of familial CJD with early onset, and, thus, are a unique feature of this disease. There are also early changes on neuropsychological testing. In particular, there are deficits in verbal fluency, digit-symbol substitution, and face recognition memory with relative preservation of basic vocabulary, digit span, and verbal reasoning skills. Overall, there is a strikingly low performance IQ, usually less than 90 in the patients tested to date. In addition, in approximately one-half of the cases, there are sensory symptoms. These consist of painful limb syndromes and are believed to reflect a central thalamic pain syndrome (physiological tests of peripheral nerves have been normal).

Many vCJD patients early in their clinical course develop forgetfulness or unsteadiness, and some are suspected to have an organic basis for their psychiatric symptoms because of these neurological symptoms. However, neurological signs do not generally appear for several months after disease onset (median, 6 months). The most common initial neurological signs (at 4 to 6 months) are incoordination and ataxia, and these signs are then followed by rapid neurological deterioration with a medley of dementia, movement disorders (chorea, myoclonus, tremor, dystonia, or "fidgety" state), incontinence, dysphagia, and visual disturbances (including upgaze paresis). vCJD, as in sporadic CJD, then rapidly progresses to an unresponsive, mute state and culminates in death from aspiration pneumonia, sepsis, or both. The mean disease duration from the onset of ataxia to death is 5 months, very similar to the duration of sporadic CJD. But the mean duration of the disease from clinical onset to death is 14 months, a duration that is seen in fewer than 5 percent of sporadic CJD patients.

One of the most striking features of vCJD is its young age of onset. This is a disease of adolescence and early adulthood, with the youngest patient to date aged 12 years and a median age of 26 years. There have been eight cases in patients older than 50 years of age (with the oldest at 74 years of age), but these cases are a distinct minority. To date, all cases have been homozygous for methionine at codon 129 (and none have had any mutations in the PRNP gene). It is not yet known whether this represents the portion of the population most susceptible to the disease or with the shortest incubation time, or both, so that patients with valine homozygosity or methionine/valine heterozygosity, or both, may follow (predicting a large epidemic of cases ultimately). Conversely, this group (with MM homozygosity at codon 129) could represent the only subgroup susceptible to the disease (predicting a smaller number of vCJD cases). Analyses have been drawn between vCJD and kuru because both are hypothesized to represent orally transmitted disease. Kuru occurred in people with all three polymorphisms at codon 129, but methionine homozygosity was overrepresented among kuru patients. The different susceptibilities to the disease are only one factor confounding epidemiologists trying to predict the total number of vCJD cases that will ensue. Another unknown factor is the incubation period of vCJD, a critical bit of knowledge when predicting disease epidemics.

None of the vCJD patients have had periodic EEGs, and only approximately one-half to two-thirds have had 14-3-3 protein present in their CSF. The most helpful diagnostic aid to date has been neuroimaging. Initially, no abnormalities were reported, but on careful review, abnormalities have been seen on MRI. These include increased signal in the posterior thalamus, particularly within the pulvinar nuclei (Fig. 2.10–17). As in other forms of CJD, high signal can be seen in the basal ganglia, and this has led to the "hockey puck" sign in the diagnosis of vCJD. FLAIR sequences are more sensitive than other MRI sequencing methods. Clinical diagnostic criteria have been established for definite, probable, and possible vCJD (Table 2.10–7).

A 26-year-old man became depressed, emotional, and irritable and complained of burning pain in his back. Six months later, he complained of the inability to taste and extension of the burning back pain into his lower limbs. Six months later and 1 year after the onset of his depression, he showed intellectual deterioration and slowing of pursuit eye movements. Five months later, he became obtunded with dysphagia and dystonic extensor posturing and died shortly thereafter. An MRI showed mild cortical atrophy and slightly increased intensity in the posterior thalamus and cerebral peduncles on T2-weighted imaging. He carried no mutation in his PRNP gene, and he was homozygous for methionine at codon 129. A cerebral biopsy showed spongiform change with florid plaques, and the autopsy confirmed the diagnosis of vCJD.

Confirmation of a clinical diagnosis of vCJD is dependent on the presence of pathological features that distinguish it from other forms of CJD. The essential diagnostic feature of vCJD is the presence of multiple florid amyloid plaques in the cerebral and cerebellar cortices, particularly in the occipital cortex. Like other forms of CJD, the plaques are made up of PrP^{CJD}, but the plaques are unique because they are large, fibrillary, and surrounded by a ring of spongiform vacuoles that have been likened to a daisy (Fig. 2.10–18). Florid plaques, initially described in murine scrapie, have been seen in naturally occurring chronic wasting disease of deer and elk but have not been seen in any other human prion disease except in a single case of iatrogenic CJD from infected dura mater. Neuropathologically, vCJD is also characterized by the usual triad of neuronal loss, astrocytic gliosis, and spongiform change. The spongiform vacuolation is generally most prominent in the basal ganglia, and the astrogliosis is most prominent in the thalamus, especially the pulvinar nuclei of the thalamus. Immunocytochemically, PrP^{Res} is detected as multiple small plaques (in addition to the florid plaques) and as perivascular and pericellular deposits throughout the cortices. There is a massive amount of PrP^{Res} detected in the brains of vCJD patients far more than in the brains from other human forms (Fig. 2.10–19). Unique to vCJD patients, PrP^{Res} can be detected in peripheral lymphoreticular tissues (tonsils, lymph nodes, spleen, and Peyer's patches) as well as in dorsal root and trigeminal ganglia. Some have advocated the use of tonsillar biopsies for diagnosis in suspected vCJD cases, particularly as brain biopsies are not recommended unless a treatable condition is considered a diagnostic possibility. The widespread detection of infectious PrP outside the CNS in vCJD patients has led to the fear that this form of the disease may be more easily transmitted through the blood supply, reuse of surgical instruments, and other

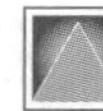

Table 2.10–7
World Health Organization Clinical Diagnostic Criteria for Variant Creutzfeldt-Jakob Disease (vCJD)

Diagnosis	Criteria
I	1. Progressive neuropsychiatric disorder
	2. Duration of illness >6 mos
	3. Routine investigations do not suggest any alternative diagnosis
	4. No history of potential iatrogenic exposure
II	1. Early psychiatric symptoms (depression, apathy, withdrawal, delusions)
	2. Persistent, painful sensory symptoms (pain ± dysesthesia)
	3. Ataxia
	4. Myoclonus, chorea, or dystonia
	5. Dementia
III	1. EEG that does not show the typical appearance of sporadic CJD (or no EEG obtained)
	2. Bilateral pulvinar high signal on magnetic resonance imaging scan
IV	1. Positive tonsil biopsy
Definite	1. Progressive neuropsychiatric disorder
	2. Neuropathological confirmation of vCJD (spongiform change with extensive PrP deposition with florid plaques throughout the cerebrum and cerebellum)
Probable	1. I **AND** four of five of II **AND** III-1 **AND** III-2
	2. I and IV

EEG, electroencephalogram.

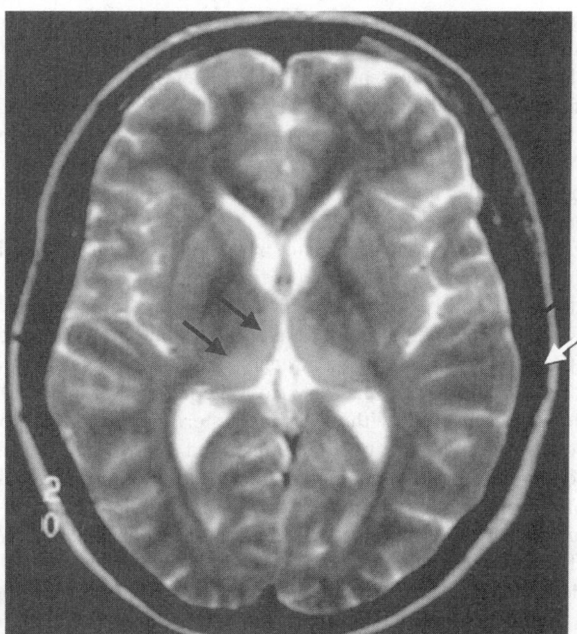

FIGURE 2.10–17 This is a T2-weighted magnetic resonance image from a patient with variant Creutzfeldt-Jakob disease. There is hyperintensity (*black arrows*) of the pulvinar nuclei extending into the more anterior thalamus, leading to the "hockey-stick" sign of variant Creutzfeldt-Jakob disease, as the hyperintense regions take the shape of a hockey stick. (Courtesy of Donald Collie.)

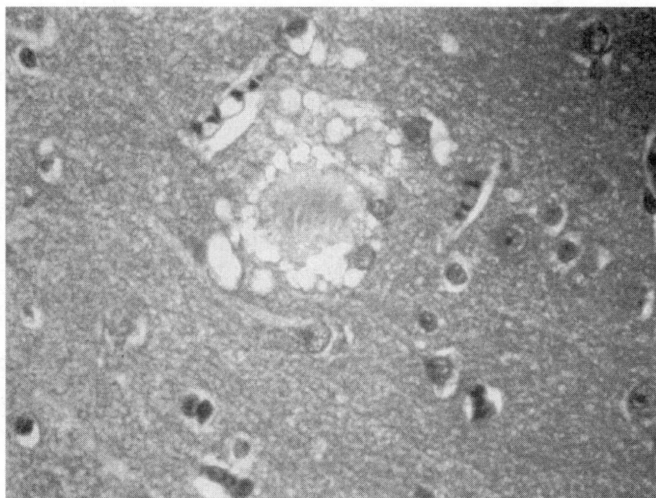

FIGURE 2.10–18 Florid plaques of variant Creutzfeldt-Jakob disease. This is a photomicrograph from a patient with variant Creutzfeldt-Jakob disease. At the center is a PrP plaque with a surrounding halo spongiform vacuolation in the shape of a "daisy." To the right of the largest PrP plaque is a daughter plaque with its own associated spongiform vacuolation. Hematoxylin and eosin stain ×300 magnification.

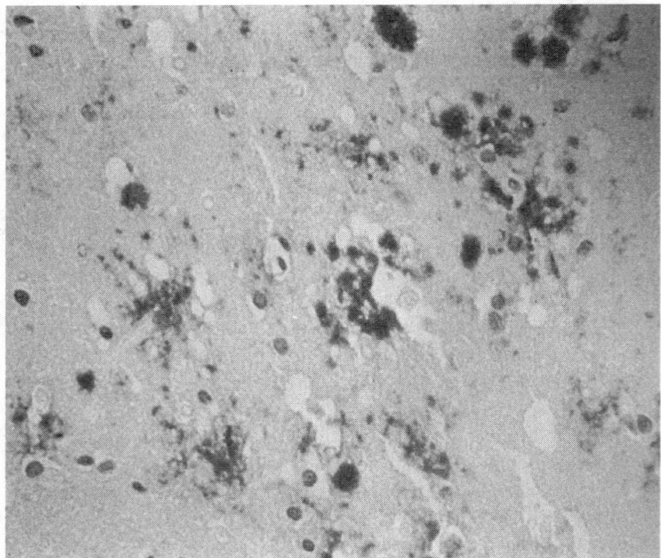

FIGURE 2.10–19 This is an immunocytochemical stain (×200 magnification) for PrP in the cortex of a patient with variant Creutzfeldt-Jakob disease. There are numerous PrP plaques as well as extensive pericellular and perivascular deposits of PrP.

yet-to-be-established means. Finally, a most important difference between vCJD and other forms of CJD is the pattern of PrP^{Res} detected by Western blot analysis (Fig. 2.10–7). This has formed the basis for establishing the disease as a separate variant and currently is also used for diagnosis.

To date, no clear epidemiological link has been shown between vCJD and occupational or dietary habits, including the consumption of food prepared from mechanically recovered meat (sausages, burgers, and meat pies). The incidence of vCJD is higher in the north of Great Britain than in the south. A single cluster of five cases of vCJD has been identified in the Leicestershire region in the United Kingdom. Currently, the transmission of the disease there has been linked to contaminated butcher instruments. Nonetheless, the link between bovine spongiform encephalopathy and vCJD is presumed because of the temporospatial association, strain-typing experiments, and molecular strain typing. Further, bovine spongiform encephalopathy has been transmitted orally to primates with as little as 0.5 g of tissue, and these primates have developed disease neuropathologically identical to vCJD.

As with other forms of disease, vCJD is uniformly fatal. Recently, biological agents shown to eliminate PrP^{Res} from cell culture have been tried in vCJD patients. No reports have been published to date, but the first vCJD patient to receive the medication was initially reported by family members to show clinical improvement. However, even with treatment, the disease progressed, and the patient died. Clinical trials with quinacrine are currently in progress. In 2003, a Belfast patient with vCJD sued in the courts to receive a novel treatment of intraventricular pentosan sulfate. Before his treatment, it was not known whether the drug delivery method would be harmful, but the drug has been known to eliminate PrP^{Res} in vitro for some time. With the very recent stabilization of the teenager's neurological condition with even a suggestion of improvement, along with his survival well beyond that which was expected, plans are currently under way for a small clinical trial in medicine. Finally, precautions must be taken to avoid accidental transmission of disease. No special precautions need to be taken by family members and caretakers other than universal precautions, but medical workers and surgeons should take special care with instruments used on these patients.

PROGNOSIS, TREATMENT, AND PREVENTION

Although the different forms of human prion diseases have varying ages of onset, clinical courses, and disease durations, they are all uniformly fatal. Furthermore, no treatment has ever slowed down, reversed, or halted the disease in humans or animals. Historically, many agents have been assayed based on the prevailing understanding of the pathogenesis of the disease at the time. The list of failed treatment protocols is long but has included antiviral, antifungal, and antibacterial agents, among many others, as well as agents that are known to bind PrP^{Res} (Congo red, anthracycline, dextran sulphate, pentosan polysulfate, and other polyanions). Some of the agents that bind PrP^{Res} have prolonged the incubation period if given before inoculation in laboratory animals and experimental transmission of disease. But no agent has been able to halt or reverse the disease once the infectious agent has reached the CNS. Recently, research has focused on agents that have been shown to clear cultured cell lines infected with PrP^{Res} in vitro, including a current human clinical trial with an old malaria drug, quinacrine. Results are pending, but the two patients who have received the drug and been followed by the news media have both died of their disease.

Until effective treatments are developed, caretakers can only provide prevention of disease transmission and palliative care of the troubling symptoms of the disease. As described in the section Sporadic CJD, medical treatment should be used to ameliorate problematic symptoms, such as myoclonus, seizures, movement disorders, and spasticity, to minimize suffering. The dementia, frequently so rapidly progressive, does not respond to agents that show modest benefit in Alzheimer's patients. Likewise, the depression of vCJD is usually unresponsive to antidepressants. Once the patient becomes immobile and unable to protect his or her airway, the mainstay of treatment includes prevention of infections from aspiration, decubitus, and urosepsis.

When handling routine bedside medical procedures, caretakers should practice universal precautions; there is no evidence for infectivity in bodily secretions, including tears, saliva, urine, or feces. Family members and caretakers can have normal contact with the patient without risk of transmission of the disease. Likewise, soiled clothing and laundry from the patient can be handled in the usual fashion without special sterilization or disposal methods. Infectivity has been demonstrated in CSF and possibly in blood; therefore, an accidental penetrating injury from used spinal tap and venipuncture needles or scalpel blades should be encouraged to bleed, soaked in bleach, and then washed thoroughly with soap and water. Unnecessary surgeries should be avoided. Disposable instruments should be used as much as possible, and if not possible, instruments should be sterilized as directed by the World Health Organization (WHO) (http://www.who.int/emc-documents/tse/whocdscsraph2003c.html). Likewise, patients who die of a prion disease can be autopsied or cremated according to published protocols and safety guidelines (see WHO Web site above).

Because the infectious agent is more widespread in vCJD patients than in other prion diseases, concern regarding the possibility of iatrogenic transmission of vCJD through surgical instruments or blood products has been raised. Public health organizations have reviewed the evidence, weighed the risks, and recommended restrictions (e.g., leukodepletion of the blood supply in the United Kingdom, restrictions on blood donors in the United States eliminating those who have lived 6 months or longer in Europe between 1980 and 1996 or who have a family history of CJD). Practical precautions, such as scheduling surgeries at the end of the day in patients with or suspected of having a prion disorder, can minimize risk to others via contaminated surgical instruments. Whenever possible, surgeries should be performed using disposable instruments. Concerns recently have been raised regarding dental and ophthalmic procedures and their potential to spread disease. These recommendations are reviewed and updated regularly. The most current restrictions can be found on Web sites of the U.S. Food and Drug Administration (FDA) (http://www.cfsan.fda.gov/~mow/prion.html) and the United Kingdom Department of Health (http://www.archive.official-documents.co.uk/document/doh/spongifm/contents.htm for a complete list of procedures or http://www.archive.official-documents.co.uk/document/doh/spongifm/part-4.htm#p-4.10). The latter includes guidelines for postmortem care, as does the previously referenced WHO Web site.

Familial CJD presents a unique opportunity to prevent transmission of the disease via prenatal genetic testing and selective therapeutic abortion when the lethal mutation is present. This preventive measure is controversial and should be discussed by a trained genetic counselor to guide the family through the medical and ethical decisions that must be considered. Likewise, there are special preventive measures that should be undertaken to prevent iatrogenic spread of prion diseases. First and foremost, the pathogenesis of sporadic CJD must be determined to eliminate any possible as-yet-unrecognized means of iatrogenic CJD transmission. Donors for organ transplants must be carefully screened to eliminate the possibility of iatrogenic transmission of CJD. For instance, cornea banks must ensure that CJD has been ruled out in any donor who dies with a dementing illness before harvesting organs for donation. Patients with dementias who may have a prion disease must be identified before surgical procedures, particularly neurosurgical ones, to minimize iatrogenic transmission via contaminated surgical instruments. Finally, research needs to be completed to definitely answer whether blood and blood products are capable and, in fact, have transmitted disease. If there is evidence for disease transmission by blood products, effective preventive measures need to be imposed.

FUTURE RESEARCH

Although the science of prion diseases has come a long way since Creutzfeldt and Jakob described the clinical and pathological syndromes in their patients, there is still much to be learned in this field before a treatment or cure can be attained. First, the exact nature of the infectious agent must be fully elucidated and its biochemistry completely unraveled. Then, the pathogenesis of all forms of CJD needs to be precisely determined. Diagnostic tests that reliably identify the infectious agent before the accumulation of debilitating neurological loss must be developed so that treatments targeting each or all pathway(s) of each variant's pathogenesis can halt and ultimately reverse the disease. Finally, procedures and regulations must be implemented to avoid any iatrogenic modes of disease transmission to protect the general public. This is a tough order for researchers in the field.

There are promising avenues of research. As noted, when peripherally inoculated, the infectious agents have three potential routes to the CNS: directly via the vagus nerve; indirectly via the spleen, splanchnic nerve, and spinal cord; and possibly via blood components. Variants of the disease that develop from peripheral exposure and subsequent CNS infection can be treated or prevented by blocking entrance of the infectious agent into the CNS. Drugs are being designed and tested for their ability to block the formation of or clear PrP^{Res} from infected cell cultures, and a clinical trial is already under way with one of the most promising drugs in vitro, quinacrine. A second clinical trial with the intraventricular administration of pentosan sulfate is being designed, and the United Kingdom is planning to establish clinical trial centers for patients with CJD. Eliminating PrP^{Res} is one approach to treating transmissible spongiform encephalopathies. Another is to deplete neuronal PrP^{C} so that there is no fuel for the pathological conversion of normal host PrP to the infectious and possibly neurotoxic infectious form. However, if the prion hypothesis is true and sporadic CJD represents a process that occurs randomly and by chance in the CNS initially in those affected, treatments will be effective only if they are able to prevent, halt, or reverse changes within the brain itself. This is a more daunting challenge. Furthermore, diagnostic tests will have to reliably predict disease at the initial misfolding of the host PrP^{C} within the CNS so that therapies can be implemented before extensive neurological destruction. Other promising avenues of research are the use of drugs that block the neurotoxic effects of PrP^{Res}. For example, if the damage of prion diseases occurs through apoptosis, then agents that halt this process may slow down or halt the disease even though the infectious agent accumulates unabated. This accentuates the need for a clearer understanding of the pathogenesis of these diseases. More creative strategies, such as vaccines, so that the immune system recognizes PrP^{CJD} as foreign and removes it before its exponential accumulation, are being explored. Finally, through genetic engineering, it may be possible to eliminate or turn off mutant genes from family members with PRNP mutations or even partially inactivate PrP^{C} in patients with sporadic CJD so that there is no fuel for the conversion of the host PrP^{C} into PrP^{CJD}. The hope is that effective treatments will be in place in the not-too-distant future.

SUGGESTED CROSS-REFERENCES

For further information about the neuroanatomical areas discussed in this section, see Section 1.2 on functional neuroanatomy and Section 1.3 on developmental neuroanatomy. The biology of memory is covered in Section 3.4. See Chapter 10 for a discussion of the cognitive disorders, including delirium and dementia.

REFERENCES

Aguzzi A: Peripheral prion pursuit. *J Clin Invest.* 2001;108:661.

Aguzzi A, Glatzel M, Montrasio F, Prinz M, Heppner FL: Interventional strategies against prion diseases. *Nat Rev Neurosci.* 2001;2:745.

Belay ED, Gambetti P, Schonberger LB, Parchi P, Lyon DR, Capellari S, McQuiston JH, Bradley K, Dowdle G, Crutcher JM, Nichols CR: Creutzfeldt-Jakob disease in unusually young patients who consumed venison. *Arch Neurol.* 2001;58:1673.

Bosque PJ, Ryou C, Telling G, Peretz D, Legname G, DeArmond SJ, Prusiner SB: Prions in skeletal muscle. *Proc Natl Acad Sci U S A.* 2002;99:3812.

Brown P: The pathogenesis of transmissible spongiform encephalopathy: Routes to the brain and the erection of therapeutic barricades. *Cell Mol Life Sci.* 2001;58:259.

*Brown P. Transmissible spongiform encephalopathies. In: Hodges JR, ed. *Early-Onset Dementia, A Multidisciplinary Approach.* New York: Oxford University Press; 2001.

Brown P, Will RG, Bradley R, Asher DM, Detwiler L: Bovine spongiform encephalopathy and variant Creutzfeldt-Jakob disease: Background, evolution, and current concerns. *Emerg Infect Dis.* 2001;7:6.

*Caughey B: Interactions between prion protein isoforms: The kiss of death? *Trends Biochem Sci.* 2001;26:235.

Caughey B, Chesebro B: Transmissible spongiform encephalopathies and prion protein interconversions. *Adv Virus Res.* 2001;56:277.

Chiesa R, Harris DA: Prion diseases: What is the neurotoxic molecule? *Neurobiol Dis.* 2001;8:743.

Collie DA, Sellar RJ, Zeidler M, Colchester ACF, Knight R, Will RG: MRI of Creutzfeldt-Jakob disease: Imaging features and recommended MRI protocol. *Clin Radiol.* 2001;56:726.

*Collinge J: Prion diseases of humans and animals: Their causes and molecular basis. *Annu Rev Neurosci.* 2001;24:519.

*Collins S, McLean CA, Masters CL: Gerstmann-Sträussler-Scheinker syndrome, fatal familial insomnia, and kuru: A review of these less common human transmissible spongiform encephalopathies. *J Clin Neurosci.* 2001;8:387.

Coulthart MB, Cashman NR: Variant Creutzfeldt-Jakob disease: A summary of current scientific knowledge in relation to public health. *CMAJ.* 2001;165:51.

Cousens S, Smith PG, Ward H, Everington D, Knight RSG, Zeidler M, Stewart G, Smith-Bathgate EAB, Macleod MA, Mackenzie J, Will R: Geographical distribution of variant Creutzfeldt-Jakob disease in Great Britain, 1994–2000. *Lancet.* 2001;357:1002.

Deleault NR, Lucassen RW, Supattapone S: RNA molecules stimulate prion protein conversion. *Nature.* 2003;425:717.

Foster JD, Parnham DW, Hunter N, Bruce M: Distribution of the prion protein in sheep terminally affected with BSE following experimental oral transmission. *J Gen Virol.* 2001;82:2319.

Glatzel M, Abela E, Maissen M, Aguzzi A: Extraneural pathologic prion protein in sporadic Creutzfeldt-Jakob disease. *N Engl J Med.* 2003;34:1812.

Heckmann JG, Lang CJG, Petruch F, Druschky A, Erb C, Brown P, Neundörfer B: Transmission of Creutzfeldt-Jakob disease via a corneal transplant. *J Neurol Neurosurg Psychiatry.* 1997;63:388.

Heppner FL, Musahi C, Arrighi I, Klein MA, Rülicke T, Oesch B, Zinkernagel RM, Kalinke U, Aguzzi A: Prevention of scrapie pathogenesis by transgenic expression of anti-prion protein antibodies. *Science.* 2001;294:178.

Irani D: The classic and variant forms of Creutzfeldt-Jakob disease. *Semin Clin Neuropsych.* 2003;8:71.

Jackson GS, Collinge J: The molecular pathology of CJD: Old and new variants. *J Clin Pathol Mol Pathol.* 2001;54:393.

Kapur N, Abbott P, Lowman A, Will RG: The neuropsychological prolife associated with variant Creutzfeldt-Jakob disease. *Brain.* 2003;126:2693.

Korth C, May BCH, Cohen FE, Prusiner SB: Acridine and phenothiazine derivatives as pharmacotherapeutics for prion disease. *Proc Natl Acad Sci U S A.* 2001;98:9836.

Lantos PL, Cairns NJ. Neuropathology. In: Hodges JR, ed. *Early-Onset Dementia, A Multidisciplinary Approach.* New York: Oxford University Press; 2001.

Lueck CJ, McIlwaine GG, Zeidler M: Creutzfeldt-Jakob disease and the eye. I. Background and patient management. *Eye.* 2000;14:263.

Mallucci G, Dickinson A, Linehan J, Klöhn P-C, Brandner S, Collinge J: Depleting neuronal PrP in prion infection prevents disease and reverses spongiosis. *Science.* 2003;302:871.

McKintosh E, Tabrizi SJ, Collinge J: Prion diseases. *J Neurovirol.* 2003;9:183.

McLean CA, Beyreuther K, Masters CL. Molecular pathology of early onset dementia. In: Hodges JR, ed. *Early-Onset Dementia: A Multidisciplinary Approach.* New York: Oxford University Press; 2001.

Müller WEG, Laplanche J-L, Ushijima H, Schröder HC: Novel approaches in diagnosis and therapy of Creutzfeldt-Jakob disease. *Mech Ageing Dev.* 2000;116:193.

Parchi P, Gambetti P: Human prion diseases. *Curr Opin Neurol.* 1995;8:286.

Prusiner SB: Shattuck lecture—neurodegenerative diseases and prions. *N Engl J Med.* 2001;344:1516.

Rujescu D, Hartmann AM, Gonnermann C, Möller H-J, Giegling I: M129V variation in the prion protein may influence cognitive performance. *Mol Psychiatry.* 2003;8:937.

Spencer MD, Knight RSG, Will RG: First hundred cases of variant Creutzfeldt-Jakob disease: Retrospective case note review of early psychiatric and neurological features. *BMJ.* 2002;324:1479.

*Zeidler M, Ironside JW: The new variant of Creutzfeldt-Jakob disease. *Rev Sci Tech.* 2000;19:98.

Zeidler M, Johnstone EC, Bamber RWK, Dickens CM, Fisher CJ, Francis AF, Goldbeck R, Higgo R, Johnson-Sabine EC, Lodge GJ, McGarry P, Mitchell S, Tarlo L, Turner M, Gyley P, Will RG: New variant Creutzfeldt-Jakob disease: Psychiatric features. *Lancet.* 1997;350:908.

Zeidler M, Stewart GE, Barraclough CR, Bateman DE, Bates D, Burn DJ, Colchester AC, Durward W, Fletcher NA, Hawkins SA, Mackenzie JM, Will RG: New variant Creutzfeldt-Jakob disease: Neurological features and diagnostic tests. *Lancet.* 1997;350:903.

Zerr I, Brandel JP, Masullo C, Wientjens D, de Silva R, Zeidler M, Granieri E, Sampaolo S, van Duijn C, Delasnerie-Laupretre N, Will R, Poser S: European surveillance on Creutzfeldt-Jakob disease: A case-control study for medical risk factors. *J Clin Epidemiol.* 2000;53:747.

▲ 2.11 Neuropsychiatric Aspects of Headache

Kathleen Ries Merikangas, Ph.D., and
James R. Merikangas, M.D.

Headache is one of the most common human afflictions. Although it is the condition that most often leads people to seek medical advice, many headache sufferers do not seek professional treatment. Nevertheless, more than one-half of those with migraine report that headache leads to impairment in their daily lives. The substantial disability associated with migraine is grossly underestimated. The percent lifetime disability attributable to migraine of 0.5 in terms of disability-adjusted life years (DALYs) is equal to or exceeds that of several other major chronic human diseases, including hypertension, breast cancer, and rheumatoid arthritis. With advances in neuroscience, there is increased knowledge of the etiology of headache. Because headache is commonly associated with psychiatric syndromes, the psychiatrist is often consulted for the evaluation and treatment of people suffering from headache. The goals of this chapter are to (1) provide an overview of the current diagnostic nomenclature for headache syndromes; (2) describe the magnitude, risk factors, and patterns of comorbidity in migraine; (3) summarize the clinical and laboratory examination necessary for making a diagnosis of headache and the neuropsychiatric manifestations of migraine and other headache syndromes; and (4) review current acute and prophylactic treatment strategies for the major headache syndromes.

DEFINITIONS

The International Headache Society (IHS) recently introduced an updated edition of their headache classification system, which was first published in 1988 (Table 2.11–1) to provide specific operational criteria for the major headache syndromes and to facilitate international standardization of the diagnostic nomenclature of headache syndromes. The IHS classification system provides a classification scheme and diagnostic criteria as well as guidelines for differential diagnosis. The criteria are intended to be applied to classify headache subtypes based on information obtained from a history, a physical and neurological examination, and appropriate laboratory investigations. The second edition of the IHS classification system now includes a category for *headache attributed to psychiatric disorder.* The IHS recommends that labeling be generally used for headaches that resolve or greatly improve only after effective treatment or spontaneous remission of a psychiatric disorder. This category is controversial because of the lack of objective evidence regarding what constitutes a true somatic manifestation of a psychiatric disorder. The most frequent primary headache syndromes are migraine, tension-type headache, and cluster headache. The remainder of the headache subtypes described in the IHS are secondary to a variety of acute and chronic conditions. For a thorough clinical evaluation of headache, it is essential to perform a differential diagnosis of the multiple causes of headache. The IHS has recently developed a new version of the diagnostic criteria for headache syndromes based on accumulating empirical evidence during the past decade. This updated edition can be reviewed at the IHS Web site (http://www.i-h-s.org/).

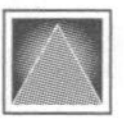

Table 2.11–1
Headache Classification System of the International Headache Society

1. Migraine
2. Tension-type headache
3. Cluster headache and other trigeminal autonomic cephalalgias
4. Other primary headaches
5. Headache attributed to head and/or neck trauma
6. Headache attributed to cranial or cervical vascular disorder
7. Headache attributed to nonvascular intracranial disorder
8. Headache attributed to substance or its withdrawal
9. Headache attributed to infection
10. Headache attributed to disorder of homeostasis
11. Headache or facial pain attributed to disorder of cranium, neck, eyes, ears, nose, sinuses, teeth, mouth, or other facial or cranial structures
12. Headache attributed to psychiatric disorder
13. Cranial neuralgias and central causes of facial pain
14. Other headache, cranial neuralgia, central or primary facial pain

From Olesen J: The International Classification of Headache Disorders, 2nd ed. *Cephalalgia.* 2004;24(Suppl 1), with permission.

Migraine

Migraine is a complex, debilitating condition characterized by either the presence or absence of aura symptoms. Migraine presentation is multifaceted, with symptoms emanating from multiple systems, including vascular, neurological, gastrointestinal (GI), endocrine, and visual. These symptoms may be accompanied by a variety of changes in behavior and cognition, including mood alterations and confusion. Historically, the usual definitions of migraine included the presence of cyclic headaches associated with a variety of GI and neurological symptoms. There is general agreement that a thorough neuropsychiatric evaluation is required for all patients presenting with headache complaints.

The IHS criteria for migraine without and with aura are presented in Tables 2.11–2 and 2.11–3, respectively. The core features of most definitions of migraine include recurrent headache accompanied by GI symptoms, such as nausea or vomiting, and hyperesthesia manifested by photophobia or phonophobia. The headache generally has a pulsatile or throbbing quality, often unilateral, and therefore is exacerbated by routine physical activity involving movement of the head. The IHS criteria operationalize these features of headache to draw common thresholds and distinctions between migraine and other types of headache. Migraine was formerly divided into two major subtypes, common and classic, with the latter being distinguished by the presence of neurological symptoms that precede the onset of the headache. The new classification of migraine by the IHS no longer includes the common–classic distinction; instead, migraine is subtyped according to the presence or absence of aura symptoms (reversible neurological dysfunction). Approximately 20 percent of people with migraines experience aura.

Aura typically occurs between 5 and 30 minutes before the onset of migraine and is characterized by several symptoms, including numbness or a pins-and-needles sensation in the head, and alterations in auditory, olfactory, speech, or visual senses, with the latter producing effects such as tunnel vision, blind spots, and the appearance of flashing lights or wavy or jagged lines.

Despite recent progress in the standardization of the classification of migraine by the IHS, the diagnostic criteria have not been subjected to intensive investigation with respect to reliability or validity. There are still several features unique to the headache syndromes that constitute impediments to developing a valid set of diagnostic criteria for headache syndromes that need to be addressed. These include the co-occurrence of multiple headache syndromes within individual persons, the tendency for headache characteristics to change across the life span, the effects of professional and self-treatment of headache in obscuring the manifestations of the underlying headache syndrome(s), and the lack of generalizability of treated samples from which the diagnostic criteria were derived. Specific areas of the classification system have also been identified as requiring additional clarification, notably the specification of procedures for ensuring standardized methodology for the ascertainment of the diagnostic criteria, methods for assessing and coding multiple headache syndromes within individuals, and the development of standardized methods for discriminating between primary headache syndromes and those for which the etiology is known (e.g., secondary headaches). A recent study suggests a higher risk of cerebral infarction among migraine sufferers than in controls.

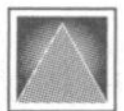

Table 2.11–2
International Headache Society Criteria: Migraine without Aura

A. At least five attacks fulfilling criteria B–D
B. Headache attacks lasting 4–72 hrs (untreated or unsuccessfully treated)
C. Headache has at least two of the following characteristics:
   1. Unilateral location
   2. Pulsating quality
   3. Moderate or severe pain intensity
   4. Aggravation by or causing avoidance of routine physical activity (walking or climbing stairs)
D. During headache, at least one of the following:
   1. Nausea and/or vomiting
   2. Photophobia and phonophobia
E. Not attributed to another disorder

From Olesen J: The International Classification of Headache Disorders, 2nd ed. *Cephalalgia.* 2004;24(Suppl 1), with permission.

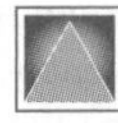

Table 2.11–3
International Headache Society Criteria: Migraine with Aura

A. At least two attacks fulfilling criteria B–D
B. Aura consisting of at least one of the following but no motor weakness:
   1. Fully reversible visual symptoms, including positive features (e.g., flickering lights, spots, or lines) and/or negative features (i.e., loss of vision)
   2. Fully reversible sensory symptoms, including positive features (i.e., pins and needles) and/or negative features (i.e., numbness)
   3. Fully reversible dysphasic speech disturbance
C. At least two of the following:
   1. Homonymous visual symptoms and/or unilateral sensory symptoms
   2. At least one aura symptom develops gradually over 5 or more mins and/or different aura symptoms occur in succession over 5 or more mins
   3. Each symptom lasts 5 or more mins and less than or equal to 60 mins
D. Headache fulfilling criteria B–D for migraine without aura begins during the aura or follows the aura within 60 mins
E. Not attributed to another disorder

From Olesen J: The International Classification of Headache Disorders, 2nd ed. *Cephalalgia.* 2004;24(Suppl 1), with permission.

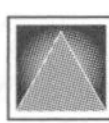

Table 2.11–4
International Headache Society Diagnostic Criteria for Tension-Type Headache

Frequent episodic tension-type headache
- A. At least ten episodes occurring on ≥1 but <15 days per mo for at least 3 mos (≥12 and >180 days per yr) and fulfilling criteria B–D
- B. Headache lasting from 30 mins to 7 days
- C. Headache that has at least two of the following characteristics:
  1. Bilateral location
  2. Pressing/tightening (nonpulsating) quality
  3. Mild or moderate intensity
  4. Not aggravated by routine physical activity such as walking or climbing stairs
- D. Both of the following:
  1. No nausea or vomiting (anorexia may occur)
  2. Absence of photophobia and phonophobia

Chronic tension-type headache
- A. Headache occurring on ≥15 days per mo on average for more than 3 mos (≥180 days/yr) and fulfilling criteria B–D
- B. Headache that lasts hrs and may be continuous
- C. Headache that has at least two of the following characteristics:
  1. Bilateral location
  2. Pressing/tightening (nonpulsating) quality
  3. Mild or moderate intensity
  4. Not aggravated by routine physical activity such as walking or climbing stairs
- D. Both of the following
  1. No more than one of photophobia, phonophobia, or mild nausea
  2. Neither moderate or severe nausea nor vomiting
- E. Not attributed to another disorder

From Olesen J: The International Classification of Headache Disorders, 2nd ed. *Cephalalgia.* 2004;24(Suppl 1), with permission.

Tension-Type Headache The definition of tension-type headache according to IHS criteria is presented in Table 2.11–4. Briefly, *tension-type headache* is characterized by episodes of stable bilateral pain lasting several days at a time, often with frequent recurrences. It is distinguished from migraine headache by its generally longer duration, the lack of pulsating quality of the pain, the lack of worsening with physical activity, and the absence of GI concomitants. However, migraine and tension-type headache may often coexist, either simultaneously or alternating over time. It is no longer believed that tension-type headache results from muscle tension. Indeed, neck pain may result from head movement to reduce headache pain.

Cluster Headache *Cluster headache* is a distinct syndrome characterized by frequent, extreme attacks (often several per day) over a 1- to 2-month period, separated by headache-free intervals for as long as 1 or 2 years. Although it is commonly grouped with migraine, current evidence, including epidemiological data, treatment response, and clinical features, suggests that cluster headache may comprise a distinct syndrome. Table 2.11–5 shows the IHS diagnostic criteria for cluster headache.

Cluster refers to a "clustering in time," with the headache bouts occurring every day to several times a day over a period of days to weeks, followed by a lengthy headache-free interval. Cluster headache is generally retro-orbital in location and is accompanied by autonomic changes such as lacrimation, rhinorrhea, erythema of the eye, and agitation. Males tend to have more cluster headache than females. Patients with cluster headache do not retire to dark rooms and lie down to avoid the stimulation but may in fact do quite the opposite, appearing almost manic in their agitation. The pain can be so intense that the patient may appear to be psychotic because of the screaming and thrashing that may be associated with the pain. Prior smoking and alcohol use have been associated with cluster headache, with alcohol often triggering the onset of the headache.

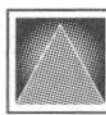

Table 2.11–5
International Headache Society Criteria: Cluster Headache

- A. At least five attacks fulfilling criteria B–D
- B. Severe or very severe unilateral orbital, supraorbital, and/or temporal pain lasting 15–180 mins if untreated
- C. Headache is accompanied by at least one of the following:
  1. Ipsilateral conjunctival injection and/or lacrimation
  2. Ipsilateral nasal congestion and/or rhinorrhea
  3. Ipsilateral eyelid edema
  4. Ipsilateral forehead and facial sweating
  5. Ipsilateral miosis and/or ptosis
  6. A sense of restlessness or agitation
- D. Attacks have a frequency from one every other day to eight per day
- E. Not attributed to another disorder

From Olesen J: The International Classification of Headache Disorders, 2nd ed. *Cephalalgia.* 2004;24(Suppl 1), with permission.

Chronic paroxysmal hemicrania is a type of cluster headache specifically responsive to treatment with indomethacin and characterized by many daily focal attacks of pain lasting for short periods, generally approximately 15 or 20 minutes per attack.

Posttraumatic Headache *Posttraumatic headache* is variable in symptom presentation, severity, and duration. The diagnostic criteria are presented in Table 2.11–6. The key symptoms include a headache after head trauma, which may or may not have been accompanied by a loss of consciousness, posttraumatic amnesia, and abnormal laboratory tests.

Although headache after a traumatic head injury has often been attributed to emotional factors, empirical evidence suggests that emotional factors are more likely to be a sequela rather than a cause of posttraumatic headache. Nevertheless, the pathogenesis of posttrau-

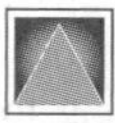

Table 2.11–6
International Headache Society Criteria: Chronic Posttraumatic Headache

- A. Headache, no typical characteristics known, fulfill criteria C and D
- B. Head trauma with at least one of the following:
  1. Loss of consciousness for >30 mins
  2. Glasgow Coma Scale <13
  3. Posttraumatic amnesia for >48 hrs
  4. Imaging demonstration of a traumatic brain lesion (cerebral hematoma, intracerebral and/or subarachnoid hemorrhage, brain contusion and/or skull fracture)
- C. Headache develops within 7 days after head trauma or after regaining consciousness after head trauma
- D. Headache persists for more than 3 mos after head trauma

From Olesen J: The International Classification of Headache Disorders, 2nd ed. *Cephalalgia.* 2004;24(Suppl 1), with permission.

matic headache is unknown. The major hypotheses include cerebral edema, cortical spreading depression, innate vulnerability to cerebral vasospasm, and transient elevation of intracranial pressure. There is no direct relationship between the prevalence or chronicity of posttraumatic headache and several indicators of severity of head injury, including duration of unconsciousness, posttraumatic amnesia, electroencephalographic abnormalities, presence of skull fracture, or the presence of blood in the cerebrospinal fluid (CSF). There appears to be an inverse relationship between the severity of the head injury and the development of post–head injury headache; posttraumatic headache is more common after injuries that do not result in skull fracture.

The onset of typical migraine attacks after acute head trauma occurs so frequently that it has been hypothesized that head trauma serves as a trigger for migraine in people with underlying susceptibility to migraine or with a personal or family history of migraine. Moreover, relatives of posttraumatic migraine subjects have an increased prevalence of neurological symptoms, suggesting a propensity to neurological manifestations of migraine.

EPIDEMIOLOGY AND COURSE

Community studies have shown that approximately 60 percent of people in the general population report a history of severe headaches. Milder headaches are reported by approximately 80 percent of the general population. Migraine without aura and tension-type headache are the most common headache syndromes in the general population.

The lifetime prevalence of migraine derived from systematic population surveys ranges from 9 to 13 percent. The severity of migraine ranges from mild to nearly total disability. More than 80 percent of those with migraine report some degree of disability. Recent community studies have underscored the enormous personal and social burden of migraine in terms of both direct and indirect costs. Although there is an increasing proportion of those with headaches seeking professional treatment, only approximately one-half of those individuals who suffer from debilitating migraine seek professional help.

Migraine is more common among women and people between the ages of 20 and 45 years, with the incidence decreasing after the fourth decade of life. Migraine may often begin in childhood when boys and girls are equally likely to suffer from migraine headache. Migraine in childhood is more likely to be associated with GI complaints, particularly episodic bouts of stomach pain, vomiting, or diarrhea, and the duration is shorter than that commonly observed in adults. Children with migraine are often misdiagnosed as having "psychosomatic headaches" or school refusal. In women, migraine is strongly associated with reproductive system function, with increased incidence during puberty and the first trimester of pregnancy, and is associated with exogenous hormone use. After menopause, the frequency of migraine attacks generally decreases dramatically, unless estrogen replacement therapy is administered.

Aside from sex and age, a family history of migraine is one of the most potent and consistent risk factors for migraine. The results of twin studies implicate genetic factors underlying approximately one-third of the familial clustering of migraine, but the mode of inheritance is clearly complex. The most fruitful searches for the role of genetic factors in the etiology of migraine have focused on the use of the disease model of familial hemiplegic migraine—a rare, highly penetrant, autosomal dominant form of migraine. Loci on chromosomes 19p and 1q have been linked to this form. Genes underlying the more common forms of migraine, including migraine with aura and migraine without aura, have also been reported. As with the findings from genetic studies of other complex diseases, these findings await replication. It is likely that there will be both phenotypic and genotypic heterogeneity, as well as multiple genes underlying susceptibility to migraine and other headache subtypes.

Migraine is strongly associated with a variety of medical disorders, especially asthma, eczema, allergies, epilepsy, cardiovascular disease, cerebrovascular disease, and, particularly, ischemic stroke. Comorbid psychiatric disorders include depression, particularly the bipolar subtype, and phobic and panic states. Prospective data from community studies of youth reveal that depression in childhood is associated with the subsequent development of headache in young adulthood. This suggests that childhood psychopathology may be used to identify risk factors for the development of headache in adulthood.

The course of migraine is highly variable. In general, both the frequency and duration of migraine decrease at midlife in both men and women, and the symptomatic manifestations may change substantially over time. There are numerous precipitants of migraine attacks that have been consistently implicated as precipitants of acute headache attacks (including hormonal changes, stress or its cessation, fasting, fatigue, oversleeping, particular foods and beverages, drug intake, chemical additives, bright light, weather changes, and exercise), but these agents/situations vary dramatically within and among individuals in prospective research.

Compared with studies of migraine, far fewer studies have been conducted that have investigated the epidemiology and risk factors associated with tension-type headache. The prevalence of tension-type headache has been estimated to range from approximately 30 to 80 percent depending on the definitions used. It is difficult to arrive at true estimates of the prevalence of tension-type headache, given that migraine and tension-type headaches may co-occur in the same individual. Tension-type headaches are also more common in women and young adults, but there is a less steep decrement in prevalence with age.

Although posttraumatic headache is quite rare in the general population (i.e., approximately 1 percent lifetime prevalence), it is not uncommon among those with a history of concussion or head injury. The estimates of the prevalence of severe and chronic headache after severe head injury based on retrospective data range from 28 to 62 percent. Children and young adults appear to be particularly susceptible to the development of headache after head trauma. The results of prospective studies of the incidence of headache after severe head injury, usually defined as postconcussion headache, reveal that approximately 50 percent of each series of admissions continue to have headache at the time of discharge from the index admission, with a gradual dissipation to 20 percent at 1 year. Persistence of headache has been related to female sex; age older than 45 years; the presence of dizziness; lack of skull fracture; intracranial hematoma; disorders of smell, hearing, or vision; depression; and impaired concentration.

Cluster headache has a very low population prevalence (less than 1 percent of the general population) and occurs nearly exclusively in males. The age at onset of cluster headache is somewhat later than that of migraine and tension-type headache; the first attack of cluster headache usually begins in the late 20s or 30s and may recur intermittently throughout life. Risk factors include smoking and heavy alcohol use. There are family studies and twin research demonstrating the role of genetic factors in the etiology of cluster headache.

ETIOLOGY

Although the etiology of the major types of headaches is still unknown, the application of neuroimaging techniques has begun to shed light on the neuroanatomical and physiological basis of headache. The most important finding from this research is evidence that migraine and cluster are primary brain disorders comprised of neurovascular headache in which vascular changes result from neural events. Peter J. Goadsby and colleagues propose that migraine is a dysfunction of an ion channel in the aminergic brainstem nuclei that normally modulates sensory input and exerts neural influences on cranial vessels. Dysfunction in the hypothalamus may be involved in the prodrome, or first phase of migraine, which may be characterized by fatigue, sleep disturbance, food cravings, depression, irritability, and other symptoms. Recent neuroimaging research also suggests activation of the midbrain and pons in migraine and the hypothalamic gray in cluster headache. Positron emission tomography (PET) has shown vasodilatation of the major basal arteries during the acute pain attack in cluster headache, representing the first convincing activation of neuronal vasodilator mechanisms in humans. Current theory of the etiology of cluster headache posits that hypothalamic and central pain control regions trigger a cascade of events in the brainstem comprising afferent pain and efferent parasympathetic pathways. Far less is known about the etiology of tension-type headache. It is clear, however, that tension-type headache is a misnomer because there is no evidence that muscle tension is the underlying cause of this headache subtype.

DIFFERENTIAL DIAGNOSIS AND CLINICAL EVALUATION

A very skillful workup is essential because headache is such a nonspecific complaint with an enormous number of etiologies ranging from the trivial to the acutely life-threatening. A thorough examination should include a description of the type and location of pain, timing, precipitants, prodromal events, and associated symptoms. Patients should be encouraged to keep a headache diary. The following factors are important to determine whether the headache is migrainous: (1) onset; (2) frequency; (3) location; (4) duration; (5) quality; (6) severity; (7) precipitants; (8) precursors; (9) triggers; (10) phenomena that worsen or relieve the pain; (11) warning signs; (12) prodromal events; (13) specific symptoms, including visual changes, GI symptoms, or neurological symptoms; (14) sensitivity to light, noise, sounds, or touch; mood changes; and (15) cognitive changes. In addition, it is important to obtain a detailed family history, description of course, and a history of previous evaluation and treatment. Differential diagnosis of headache is based on a neurological examination to rule out pathognomonic signs that might indicate other brain disorders.

Migraine is more than a headache. There are a variety of manifestations of migraine that may mimic a number of neurological or psychiatric disorders, including epilepsy, psychosis, and "conversion." Visual and auditory hallucinations may occur, especially in children. Migraine may have autonomic manifestations suggesting cardiac disease, irritable bowel syndrome, or even acute abdominal emergency. Migraine may be associated with irritability, mood swings, and, in some cases, impulsive temper outbursts. In a sense, migraine may be considered as lying on a continuum between the rapid neurophysiological changes of epilepsy and the less rapid state changes of bipolar disorder. Basilar artery migraine, defined by a particular vascular distribution, may produce stupor and coma or paralysis, blindness, ataxia, dysarthria, or perceptual abnormalities. The extent to which such manifestations may be attributed to comorbid disorders has not been established.

In addition to a history and physical examination, laboratory studies are critical. Even if the results are negative and do not uncover a metabolic, endocrine, or autoimmune etiology, this information may serve as a baseline for subsequent drug therapy. Application of the IHS requires that all of the potential causes of headache shown in Table 2.11–1 be considered. The diagnosis of headache requires the exclusion of other conditions, including structural lesion, vascular malformation, viral or bacterial meningitis or encephalitis, intracranial abscess or hemorrhage, cerebral contusion, metabolic disorders (urea cycle disorders, aminoacidopathies, mitochondrial disorders), pseudotumor cerebri, vasculitis, brain tumors, or sinusitis or ocular disorders, any of which may be concurrent rather than causal. One of the most important findings of the past decade is the converging evidence that there is an increased risk of ischemic (but not hemorrhagic) stroke among young women with migraine. This finding supports the importance of reduction of other stroke risk factors, including oral contraceptive use, hypertension, and smoking among young women with migraine.

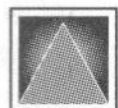

Table 2.11–7
Headache Symptoms Indicating Further Diagnostic Workup

First headache
Worst headache
Gradual worsening over days or weeks
Vomiting before headache onset
Abnormal neurological examination
Ongoing systemic illness
Onset after age 50 yrs
Accompanied by fever
Sleep onset

Based on the low frequency of detection of lesions, such as arteriovenous malformation or brain tumors, the American Academy of Neurology has recently issued a practice parameter discouraging the routine use of neuroimaging procedures in patients with headaches who have normal neurological examinations. However, headache experts who often serve as tertiary referral sources may often ignore this recommendation because of the lack of diagnostic certainty in headache, lack of curative properties of current treatment, and unacceptable medical and legal risks of any missed diagnosis. Table 2.11–7 lists the headache symptoms that indicate further diagnostic workup.

Although imaging procedures may not be considered necessary in the evaluation of primary headache syndromes, an image of the brain is mandatory for the evaluation of patients with severe or persistent headache, the "first" or "worst" headache, or when a subdural hematoma is suspected. A computer-assisted tomography (CAT) scan is indicated to rule out acute hemorrhage, whereas magnetic resonance imaging (MRI) is indicated when hydrocephalus, brain tumor, pseudotumor cerebri, sinusitis, vasculitis, or posterior fossa lesions are suspected. X-rays of the jaw and cervical spine are useful to rule out malocclusions and degenerative changes of arthritis. Pseudotumor cerebri is an important consideration in the differential diagnosis of tension headache. Usually affecting overweight young women, pseudotumor is often associated with hormonal treatment or abnormalities. The patients may have papilledema or extraocular nerve abnormalities resulting in diplopia. MRI or computed tomographic (CT) imaging of the brain may be mistaken for normal because the ventricles are symmetrically smaller than normal (slit-like lateral ventricles), and it may be overlooked by radiologists who are unaware of this condition. Lumbar puncture reveals elevated CSF pressure with low protein count and no cells on analysis.

MIGRAINE COMORBIDITY

Somatic Conditions

Several factors complicate the investigation of the comorbidity of migraine and other conditions. These include the difficulty in discriminating from "migraine equivalents," or alternate manifestations of migraine that occur in an "attack-like" fashion, including abdominal pain, dizziness or vertigo, or visual symptoms; the lack of specificity of symptom expression or constellations within individuals over time; and the involvement of multiple symptoms, including cardiovascular, gastrointestinal, and sensory organs, as well as both the peripheral and central nervous systems (CNS). There is also significant variability in the methodology of studies of migraine comorbidity, which limits the conclusiveness of the findings. Studies of comorbidity require valid definitions and reliable assessment of each of the disorders under consideration. Despite these challenges, it is nonetheless essential for clinicians to consider migraine in the context of other possible comorbid conditions.

Cardiovascular conditions, such as hypertension, several manifestations of heart disease, and stroke, have been the most widely studied of all classes of comorbid conditions associated with migraine. It is likely that the focus on these conditions is the result of concern about migraine-induced stroke and the role of underlying vascular disease in the triggering of migraine attacks. Although well studied, the negative results of studies conducted in large-scale community surveys have prevented researchers from firmly establishing an association between migraine and hypertension. Likewise, there is little evidence for an association between heart disease and migraine, after considering the effects of other cardiovascular factors, including hypertension and smoking. A review of clinical and case control studies supports an association between migraine and stroke, although findings vary according to sex and age group in which the risk of stroke is elevated.

The relationship between migraine and seizures was first investigated by Paskind in 1934, and, although there have been many systematic, controlled studies since then, there have been no large-scale, community-based population studies of this association. The lack of consistency with respect to the definitions and subtypes of epilepsy across studies precludes an accurate estimate of risk based on aggregate findings. Additional research is necessary to further investigate the association between migraine and epilepsy.

There has been much research on the association of migraine and several allergic conditions, including food allergies, asthma, hay fever, and bronchitis. Studies have noted a relationship between migraine and many of these conditions, as well as eczema, rhinitis, obstructive pulmonary disease, and respiratory symptoms. The only negative study was an uncontrolled series of asthma patients, in whom there was no increased risk of migraine when compared with rates from the general community. Despite this finding, a review of the literature on migraine comorbidity supports a strong and consistent association between allergic conditions and migraine in clinical studies of both adults and children.

Although several gastrointestinal conditions have been linked with migraine, it is difficult to discriminate whether these conditions are truly independent or whether they represent manifestations of the gastrointestinal component of migraine. Particularly in children, distinguishing recurrent abdominal pain and undiagnosed abdominal migraine often presents problems when studying the relationship between migraine and abdominal pain. Given the variability of findings in this area, there have been no clearly established associations between migraine and specific gastrointestinal disorders.

Psychiatric Conditions

Among the psychiatric illnesses, mood and anxiety disorders have been shown to be most strongly associated with migraine. The majority of studies investigating comorbid depression and migraine have found a higher prevalence of both disorders. An analysis of study findings discourages the idea of a causal mechanism in explaining the relationship between depression and migraine. Instead, a shared, common risk factor likely increases the risk for either condition.

The prevalence of migraine in people with bipolar disorder is also clearly elevated. Studies have shown an increased prevalence of migraine in people with panic disorder, generalized anxiety disorder, obsessive-compulsive disorder (OCD), and social and specific phobias.

As described below, it is essential to consider comorbid medical and psychiatric disorders in determining appropriate treatment strategies.

TREATMENT OF HEADACHE SYNDROMES

Migraine

The mainstay of migraine treatment is pharmacological intervention. Treatment of migraine can be prophylactic, with medication taken daily; abortive, with medication taken at the onset of an attack; or palliative, with medication taken after the pain has begun. Prophylactic treatments for migraine are of varying effectiveness. Clinical trials of migraine treatment are complicated by the high placebo response rate among subjects with migraine, the heterogeneity of diagnostic subtypes of headache, the intermittent nature of the condition, and the frequent use of additional analgesics to treat headache pain. The treatment of migraine chosen for an individual depends not only on the diagnosis of migraine headache but also on related factors specific to the patient. The U.S. Headache Consortium has identified the following goals of long-term migraine treatment:

- reduce attack frequency and severity
- reduce disability
- improve quality of life
- prevent headache
- avoid headache medication escalation
- educate and enable patients to manage their disease

Excellent reviews of acute and prophylactic treatments of migraine are available. There are also a variety of nonpharmacological approaches to reduce headache. These include eliminating triggers of attacks; maximizing the regularity of daily schedule, particularly with respect to sleeping and eating habits; biofeedback; regular exercise; and relaxation treatment. Nonetheless, patients should be made aware of the potential limitations of, delayed effect of, or need for an escalating dosage associated with drug therapies.

Symptomatic Relief

The nonsteroidal antiinflammatory drugs (NSAIDs), including ibuprofen (Motrin), naproxen sodium (Naprosyn), and indomethacin and the analgesics acetylsalicylic acid (ASA) and acetaminophen (Tylenol) are commonly used as the first-line treatment of mild to moderate migraine. The acetaminophen-aspirin-caffeine formulation Excedrin is approved for migraine, as are the ibuprofen drugs Advil and Motrin. Other classes of drugs that are commonly prescribed for more severe attacks include ergot derivatives (ergotamine [Ergomar] and dihydroergotamine [DHE]), serotonin agonists, and narcotics. Ergotamine tartrate and dihydroergotamine are two of the most commonly prescribed ergot derivatives for moderate to severe attacks of migraine. To counterbalance the common side effect of nausea, metoclopramide (Reglan) or prochlorperazine (Compazine) is recommended. Combination agents generally comprising barbiturates, analgesics, and caffeine are also highly effective in the treatment of migraine episodes. Clinicians should be particularly alert to the dangers of abusing drugs such as ergotamine and narcotics. In general, narcotics should be restricted to severe attacks that are not responsive to other agents. Although oral narcotic agents, such as Percocet and Percodan, do not produce addiction when used infrequently for acute attacks, physicians should be cautioned about their use in people with preexisting addictions. However, chronic narcotic treatment is not appropriate for headache.

The triptans are 5-hydroxytryptamine type 1D (5-HT_{1D}) agonists that have been used for the acute treatment of migraine since sumatriptan was first introduced in 1991. They act through vasoconstriction to reduce the acute migraine attack. Although they were originally self-administered subcutaneously, other modes of administration, including oral preparations, nasal spray, and patch, are now available for some of the triptans. Triptans in current use include sumatriptan, zolmitriptan (Zomig), naratriptan (Amerge), rizatriptan (Maxalt), almotriptan (Axert), eletriptan (Relpax), and frovatriptan (Frova). In general, the triptan compounds are quite safe, but, because of coronary vasoconstriction, they should be avoided in individuals with vascular disease. Factors to consider when choosing a triptan for an acute migraine attack include the time it takes for the medication to begin working, its duration, the likelihood of a headache recurrence, and potential side effects of the medication. Recent research has shown that frovatriptan, for example, is effective in prolonged attacks as well as in migraine with a high probability of recurrence and migraine related to the menstrual cycle. Topiramate is also effective for migraine prophylaxis, with a side effect of weight loss. Coadministration of serotonergic drugs with triptan compounds is particularly dangerous because of the risk of serotonin syndrome.

Migraine Prophylaxis Prophylactic treatment of migraine should be considered in patients who experience frequent, debilitating attacks on less than a monthly basis, particularly if attacks occur more than twice a week. Patients who miss a substantial amount of work or school due to headache (i.e., more than 3 days per month) are also candidates for migraine prophylaxis, as are those with comorbid disorders such as depression, anxiety, or epilepsy; those who have not had success with acute treatments; and those with less common afflictions, including hemiplegic migraine, basilar migraine, migraine with prolonged aura, or migrainous infarction.

However, the goal of complete prevention of migraine on a long-term basis has not yet been achieved. Most of the migraine prophylaxis trials have shown that no agent has succeeded in reducing migraine attacks or severity by more than 50 percent. Headache scientists believe that the disappointing results in migraine prevention are due to the lack of animal models and poor understanding of etiology of specific headache subtypes. Nevertheless, there are numerous drugs and combinations of drugs that do reduce the frequency and duration of migraine at the level of the individual case. Therefore, careful clinical management on a regular basis remains the best strategy to reduce the burden of headache.

There are several major classes of drugs that have been investigated in the prophylaxis of migraine headaches. These include the β-adrenergic–blocking agents, antidepressants, calcium channel blockers, and anticonvulsants. Table 2.11–8 presents the classes of drugs used in migraine prophylaxis and a range of recommended daily doses. β-Adrenergic blockers and calcium channel blockers have also been widely used to prevent migraine.

The β-blockers are currently the most popular treatment choice in migraine prophylaxis. However, the effect of this class of drugs is moderate at best. No study has reported complete elimination of migraine; however, the average duration and severity are reduced by 50 percent in most subjects. Clinicians should be particularly cautious in prescribing this class of drugs to individuals with a history of depression because the β-blockers are associated with the development of anhedonia, irritability, and lassitude, which may occur

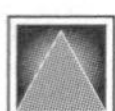

Table 2.11–8
Prophylactic Treatment of Migraine

Substance	Daily Dose (mg)
β-Blocking agents	
Metoprolol	50–200
Propranolol	40–200
Atenolol	50–200
Timolol	20–60
Calcium channel blockers	
Flunarizine	5–15
Other pain relief agents	
Antisalicylic acid	300
Nonsteroidal antiinflammatory agents	400–600
Diclofen potassium	50–100
Naproxen	750
Antidepressants	
Amitriptyline	10–150
Doxepin	10–150
Nortriptyline	50–150
Desipramine	100–300
Anticonvulsants	
Sodium valproate	500–600

after many months on any of these agents. Patients with high levels of autonomic anxiety may actually benefit from this class of drugs. Recent studies suggest that the angiotensin-converting enzyme (ACE) inhibitors captopril (Capoten) or enalapril (Vasotec) are also effective in the prevention of migraine. Several drugs used for the treatment of acute headache, such as aspirin and NSAIDs, may also be effective when used on a regular basis.

Given the overlap of symptoms of the actual migraine episode, including acute changes in energy, appetite, mood, and level of anxiety as well as those that occur between attacks and those on the anxiety/depression spectrum, it is not surprising that similar pharmacological agents have been successfully used in the treatment of migraine and anxiety/depression. However, the antidepressant drugs, particularly those of the tricyclic class, have also been shown to be superior to the above-cited "first-line" agents of migraine treatment regardless of comorbid depression or anxiety, although patients often report excessive sedation from tricyclic agents as well as dry mouth, constipation, and weight gain. Combinations of the above classes of drugs have also been used for patients who do not respond to first-line treatments. Tricyclics plus β-blockers and tricyclics plus monoamine oxidase inhibitors (MAOIs) have been used concomitantly in the preventive treatment of severe migraine. Use of tricyclic antidepressants other than amitriptyline (Elavil) should be encouraged because this agent is the most sedating of all of the drugs in this class. The secondary amines (e.g., nortriptyline [Aventil] and desipramine [Norpramin]) appear to be equally efficacious in the treatment of depression but have fewer side effects than do the parent tertiary amines (e.g., amitriptyline, imipramine [Tofranil]). However, the relative efficacy of the various tricyclic antidepressants in migraine prevention has not been examined. The selective serotonin reuptake inhibitors (SSRIs) do have not demonstrated efficacy in migraine. In fact, many patients complain of headache as a secondary effect of the latter class of drugs.

The MAOIs have also been reported to be efficacious in the treatment of migraine headache, particularly in patients who have been unresponsive to first-line prophylactic treatment. Phenelzine (Nardil) is considered to be one of the most efficacious antimigraine agents.

However, clinicians have generally been reluctant to prescribe MAOIs because of the possibility of a hypertensive reaction to dietary tyramine and the other side effects of these agents (e.g., orthostatic hypotension, weight gain, and excessive stimulation). The use of oral calcium channel blockers to treat the hypertensive crisis associated with MAOIs may reduce clinicians' reservations about prescribing these agents.

During the past few years, antiepileptic agents have been used to prevent migraine. Valproate (Depakene), which is a first-line treatment for bipolar affective disorder, has been approved for the treatment of migraine. Valproate may be particularly useful in the presence of comorbid affective disorder. Other antiepileptic agents that have been assessed in their efficacy for migraine include gabapentin (Neurontin) and topiramate (Topamax).

The strong association between migraine with both depression and anxiety should be considered in the treatment of individuals with migraine. Systematic evaluation of the lifetime history of both depression and anxiety is necessary for determining optimal treatment strategies. If there is a subtype of migraine associated with anxiety and depression, it is critical to treat the entire syndrome rather than limiting the treatment goal to headache cessation. In general, comorbid depression and anxiety are more important in the selection of migraine prophylaxis than is the treatment of an acute attack of migraine. The use of prophylactic medications with side effects of lassitude, fatigue, or depression should be avoided, if possible. If not, careful clinical evaluation of the above-cited manifestations of depression, including anergia, hypersomnia, and irritability, should be monitored. When nonpharmacological approaches have failed and the frequency and severity of migraine attacks lead to impairment in functioning, preventative treatment is indicated.

Tension-Type Headache Treatment of tension-type headache may be either pharmacological or nonpharmacological, depending on the frequency and severity of headaches. Nonpharmacological approaches, such as biofeedback, massage, relaxation, cervical traction, chiropractic manipulation, hot packs, and cold packs, all have been reported to be effective, although there are no convincing guidelines to recommend one modality over another.

Similar to the acute treatment of migraine, analgesics and NSAIDs are the first-line treatment for tension-type headache. Aspirin is the most commonly used agent, followed by ibuprofen and naproxen sodium. It is important to note that symptoms of tension-type headache may arise iatrogenically from drugs, such as ergotamine, used to treat migraine, often as a result of overuse of the drug. Up to 40 percent of chronic headache cases are associated with overuse of drugs intended to alleviate headache. Fiorinal, which is a mixture of butalbital (a short-acting barbiturate), aspirin, and caffeine, is frequently used by nonneurologists for treatment of headache. However, tolerance or drug dependence may occur. The treatment of chronic tension-type headache is similar to that of migraine; the most commonly used drug treatment for chronic tension-type headache is the tricyclic antidepressant amitriptyline (dosage ranging from 100 to 150 mg per day).

Cluster Headache Prophylactic medicine is almost always indicated for treating cluster headache because of the extreme severity of pain induced by an acute attack, which often occurs at night. Inhaled oxygen and subcutaneous and nasal sumatriptan are the most commonly used agents for the treatment of acute attacks. Medications that have been shown to be effective in preventing attacks of cluster headache are lithium (Eskalith), corticosteroids, and methysergide (Sansert). Side effects can be severe, and combinations of these agents are often necessary to achieve success. Some may benefit from adjuvant valproic acid (Depakote) or topiramate. Histamine desensitization and surgical intervention are options on exhaustion of traditional agents.

Posttraumatic Headache Posttraumatic headache is often treated on an emergency basis, but chronic posttraumatic headache is commonly encountered in psychiatry. Steroids are often given immediately after the acute injury, and diagnostic imaging reveals the presence of skull fracture or subdural hematoma. NSAIDs are the most commonly prescribed agents for headache that persists beyond the acute injury. Thereafter, the prophylactic approaches to migraine and treatment strategies for the primary headaches can be applied.

SUGGESTED CROSS-REFERENCES

Sections 2.2, 2.3, 2.4, and 2.5 cover the neuropsychiatric aspects of cerebrovascular disorders, brain tumors, epilepsy, and traumatic brain injury, respectively. Psychosomatic disorders are covered in Chapter 24. Drugs used in psychiatry (including antidepressants and benzodiazepines) are discussed and organized pharmacologically in Chapter 31.

References

Chang CL, Donaghy M, Poulter N: Migraine and stroke in young women: Case-control study. The World Health Organisation Collaborative Study of Cardiovascular Disease and Steroid Hormone Contraception. *BMJ.* 1999;318:13–18.

Diener H-Ch: Pharmacological approaches to migraine. *J Neural Transm Suppl.* 2003;64:35–63.

Dodick DW, Capobianco DJ: Treatment and management of cluster headache. *Curr Pain Headache Rep.* 2001;5:83–91.

Ekbom K, Hardebo JE: Cluster headache: Aetiology, diagnosis and management. *Drugs.* 2002;62:61–69.

Fasmer OB: The prevalence of migraine in patients with bipolar and unipolar affective disorders. *Cephalalgia.* 2001;21:894–899.

*Ferrari MD, Roon KI, Lipton RB, Goadsby P: Oral triptans (serotonin 5-$HT_{1B/1D}$ agonists) in acute migraine treatment: A meta analysis of 53 trials. *Lancet.* 2001;358:1668–1675.

*Goadsby PJ: Neuroimaging in headache. *Microsc Res Tech.* 2001;53:179–187.

*Goadsby PJ, Lipton RB, Ferrari MD: Migraine—current understanding and treatment. *N Engl J Med.* 2002;346:4, 257–270.

Haas DC, Lourie H: Trauma-triggered migraine: An explanation for common neurological attacks after mild head injury: Review of the literature. *J Neurosurg.* 1988;68:181.

*International Headache Society: Classification and diagnostic criteria for headache disorders, cranial neuralgias, and facial pain. *Cephalalgia.* 1988;[Suppl 7]:1.

Kearney JM, Holm JE, Kearney ML: Chronic tension-type headache: An investigation of the appraisal process. *Headache.* 1994;34:351.

Lipton R, Pan J: Is migraine a progressive brain disease? *JAMA.* 2004;291:443–494.

Lipton RB, Scher AI, Kolodner K, Liberman J, Steiner TJ, Stewart WF: Migraine in the United States: Epidemiology and patterns of health care use. *Neurology.* 2002;58: 885–894.

Low NCP, Galbaud du Fort G, Cervantes P: Prevalence, clinical correlates, and treatment of migraine in bipolar disorder. *Headache.* 2003;43:940–949.

Low NCP, Merikangas KR: Comorbidity of migraine. *CNS Spectrums.* 2003;8:433–445.

May A, Leone M: Update on cluster headache. *Curr Opin Neurol.* 2003;16:333–340.

Merikangas KR: Association between psychopathology and headache syndromes. *Curr Opin Neurol.* 1995;8:248–251.

Merikangas KR: Genetics of migraine and other headache. *Curr Opin Neurol.* 1996;9:202–205.

Merikangas KR, Merikangas JR: Combination monoamine oxidase inhibitor and beta-blocker treatment of migraine, with anxiety and depression. *Biol Psychiatry.* 1995;38:603–610.

National Headache Foundation (NHF). Advances in migraine prophylaxis. *NHF Continuing Education Monograph.* 2003:1–7.

Olesen J, Tfelt-Hansen P, Welch KMA, eds. *The Headaches.* 2nd ed. New York: Lippincott Williams & Wilkins; 2000.

Packard RC. Epidemiology and pathogenesis of posttraumatic headache. *J Head Trauma Rehabil* 1999;14:9–21.

Pryse-Phillips WEM, Dodick DW, Edmeads JG, Gawel MJ, Nelson RF, Purdy RA, Robinson G, Stirling D, Worthington I: Guidelines for the diagnosis and management of migraine in clinical practice. *CMAJ.* 1997;156:1273–1287.

Pryse-Phillips WEM, Dodick DW, Edmeads, JG, Gawel MJ, Nelson RF, Purdy RA, Robinson G, Stirling D, Worthington I: Guidelines for the nonpharmacologic management of migraine in clinical practice. *CMAJ.* 1998;159:47–54.

Report of the Quality Standards Subcommittee of the American Academy of Neurology: Practice parameter: The utility of neuroimaging in the evaluation of headache in

patients with normal neurological examinations [summary statement]. *Neurology*. 1994;44:1353.
Russell MG, Olesen J: Increased familial risk and evidence of genetic factor in migraine *BMJ*. 1995;311:541–544.
*Silberstein SD, for the US Headache Consortium: Practice parameter: Evidence-based guidelines for migraine headache (an evidence-based review): Report of the Quality Standards Subcommittee of the American Academy of Neurology. *Neurology*. 2000;55:754–763.
Stewart WF, Staffa J, Lipton RB, Ottman R: Familial risk of migraine: A population-based study. *Ann Neurol*. 1997;41:166–172.
Stillman MJ: Pharmacotherapy of tension-type headaches. *Curr Pain Headache Rep*. 2002;6:408–413.
Tepper SJ: Safety and rational use of the triptans. *Med Clin North Am*. 2001;85:959–970.
Tepper SJ, Millson D: Safety profile of the triptans. *Expert Opin Drug Saf*. 2003;2:123–132.
U.S. Headache Consortium. Evidence-based guidelines for migraine, 2001. Available at http://www.aan.com. Accessed 11/2003.

▲ 2.12 Neuropsychiatric Aspects of Neuromuscular Disease

JAMES C. EDMONDSON, M.D., PH.D.

The language of psychiatry often invokes the language of neuromuscular neurology. For example, the psychoanalyst's question, "And how do you feel about that?" seems to guide one's associations gently to the level of somatosensory and visceral perception. Moreover, other emotionally evocative words, such as warm, cool, hot, cold, tight, loose, heavy, light, tough, soft, sharp, dull, painful, smooth, rough, and numb, are common parlance in both psychiatry and neuromuscular neurology. Not surprisingly, the language of emotional feelings borrows much from that of somatosensory and kinesthetic experience.

Patients with neuropathic or neuromuscular disorders commonly complain of pain, numbness, tingling, and, perhaps, weakness. Indeed, a large number of depressed and anxious patients who may choose to avoid mental health services are referred instead to neurologists because of pain, numbness, tingling, or weakness.

The brain's pain circuitry is intimately interwoven with the affective systems. There are more serotonergic neurons in the pain pathways of the spinal cord than in the widely projecting brainstem raphe nuclei, fibers of which are believed to be a major target of serotonergic antidepressant and antianxiety drugs. In this light, it is of no small interest that depression and anxiety may markedly intensify neuromuscular symptoms.

Many depressed and anxious people accept the suggestion that they have depression or anxiety, but hypochondriacal patients insist that their suffering cannot possibly have a psychological cause. Repeated medical and neurological evaluations are routinely indicated for patients with neuropathic or neuromuscular symptoms because the differential diagnosis of neuromuscular conditions is broad. Although these evaluations may initially fail to uncover a treatable medical condition, additional evaluations may eventually yield a novel insight. A complicated patient may need neurological and psychiatric evaluations in parallel, with active dialogues between the patient and the providers as well as among the providers directly. An awareness of the main classes of neuromuscular diseases and of the methods of neuromuscular evaluation may help mental health providers to interpret neuromuscular symptoms in their patients.

ORGANIZATION OF THE NEUROMUSCULAR SYSTEM

The neuromuscular system includes all nerves outside of the central nervous system (CNS) together with the skeletal muscles. Specifically, this refers to two broad functional systems: the sensory apparati and the motor systems. The brain contains numerous representations of the body with which to model and predict all bodily functions, only a minority of which, however, are accessible to the conscious mind. As with any processor, the quality of the input (the senses) directly determines the quality of the output (awareness and action). The neuromuscular system, which transmits and receives all human communications, helps define personality, character, mood, and thought. Biochemical and structural defects in the neuromuscular system can therefore have a profound influence on all aspects of the human condition.

Sensory Apparati The sensory fibers of the peripheral nervous system transmit somatic and visceral sensory information from all parts of the body to the spinal cord and the brain. The extraction of relevant sensory features from the totality of sensory experience begins in the peripheral sensory organs and is refined at all levels of the sensory pathway, most importantly in the brain. The peripheral somatic sensory fibers can be viewed as accurate point-to-point transmitters of data from the skin to the spinal cord, with the visceral sensory fibers being less precise in their localizations. Under ideal circumstances, the peripheral fibers should color the perception of touch as little as possible and should therefore afford the CNS as faithful an internal image of the external world as possible. However, peripheral fibers may be susceptible to physical compression and metabolic insult, conditions that can compromise the quality of their transmissions. In the most common example, diabetes often eliminates peripheral sensory fibers and reduces sensory acuity, in the process causing aberrant sensations to be transmitted to the brain. How the mind handles inaccurate sensory information is complex and is influenced by a person's psychological state.

Motor Systems The CNS contains a nested hierarchy of phylogenetically ancient motor systems. The most ancient, "reptilian," descending motor systems are contained entirely within the brainstem and spinal cord and are under continuous modulation by the more recently evolved corticospinal system. Minor damage to a motor nerve may cause little functional disruption, whereas a comparable amount of damage in a sensory nerve may cause distressing early symptoms.

EVOLUTIONARY CONSIDERATIONS

Specialized nerves and muscles are, conceptually, modifications and adaptations of sensory and motile organelles of unicellular animals originating over the past 3.5 billion years. Nerves and muscles are among the most ancient organ systems of multicellular animals, first appearing in the fossil record approximately 600 million years ago. Sixty-five million years ago, as the dinosaurs vanished, mammals appeared and diversified. All mammalian species conformed to an archetypal quadrupedal body plan containing a flexible backbone supporting a cranium at one pole. Six million years ago, the bipedal human body appeared, consisting of further evolutionary modifications of the basic quadrupedal mammalian body plan.

The evolution of the human body occurred through two mechanisms of selection, as defined by Charles Darwin: natural selection and sexual selection. Natural selection is the better known of the two and is sometimes referred to as the *survival of the fittest* in the struggle for existence. Well-known selective pressures in natural selection include predators, extremes of climate, limitations in food supply, limitations in the availability of shelter, parasites, and natural disasters such as floods, volcanos, storms, or even meteorites. Natural selection favors genetic variants that are best adapted to life in a particular ecological niche. Natural selection thus promotes the acquisition of those niche-specific survival and defense traits required for basic survival of the species. Because a single niche may support the existence of numerous diverse species, however, natural selection alone cannot explain what makes humans unique.

Sexual selection was also a force behind mammalian speciation, including the divergence of humans from other apes during the last 7 million years. Assortative mating over hundreds of thousands of generations fixed favorable genetic variations into the human genome step by step. By analogy, animal breeders may create a lineage displaying specific morphological or behavioral traits in a few generations by exerting tightly controlled sexual selection for only those traits.

In adopting a bipedal posture by essentially taking the horizontal mammalian body plan and tipping it onto its end, the early bipedal ancestors gained communication abilities, improved their distance vision, and fundamentally altered the use of their forelimbs. In contrast to the huge period over which the horizontal body plan evolved, the upending of the horizontal body plan to create the vertical human body plan occurred in the evolutionary blink of an eye. The current fossil record suggests that the basic horizontal vertebrate body plan was slowly perfected over at least 500 million years, long before the appearance of hominids. In contrast, early hominids adapted the horizontal body plan into a vertical body plan within a period of probably considerably less than 2 million years. This extremely hasty evolution of a radically different mammalian chassis from any seen before, however, left a number of unintended consequences that continue to plague the human condition.

The industrial revolution in the 18th century triggered a massive sixfold increase in the world's population into the 21st century and bonded humans inextricably to technology. Yet, life for most people in today's world causes chronic neuromuscular stresses and produces a steady stream of pain signals from the neuromuscular system to the brain. Neural "gates" closely regulate which pain messages reach consciousness. These gates function best in mentally healthy individuals. For example, there is a strong inverse correlation between indices of mental health and pain scales: The intensity of subjective pain correlates closely with the severity of depression or anxiety.

Neck

The frailty of the human neck, handicapped by having to balance the huge head on its very tip, necessitates constant use of the neck muscles even in deepest sleep. This causes chronic headaches, lower back pain, neck pain, and other types of upper body pains that are endemic in the human species. Humans' long, narrow necks, stuffed with muscular, vascular, and ventilatory support structures for the immense head, also require cautious positioning during swallowing to avoid choking and aspiration of food into the lungs.

Spine

The outcome of human vertical posture is that the body elegantly and acrobatically supports greatly enlarged heads containing weighty brains. The unintended internal consequence, however, has been that a structurally weak sigmoidal spinal column is balanced precariously on the pelvis. This, in turn, has placed a huge weight on the wedge-shaped vertebrae and the semirigid intervertebral discs that has caused muscle and ligament strains and disc herniations. The emphasis on manual work has focused a constant tension on the spine, especially on the neck and the lower back—common sites of chronic pains.

Carpal Tunnel Syndrome

A common current etiology for pain is carpal tunnel syndrome. Manual dexterity is part of the livelihood of a huge segment of the population. The remarkable human hand is one of the major defining features of the human species. The evolution of the thumb into an indispensable multipurpose tool is the most striking difference between nonhuman ape hands and the human hand. The nonhuman ape thumb can only move within the plane of the hand and can be directly opposed only to the first two fingers. The critical human modification is the ability to abduct the thumb—in other words, to move it perpendicular to the plane of the hand. This permitted the thumb to be directly opposed to all four fingers, which allowed a previously unattainable and very precise manipulation. Inside the hand, however, the nerve that controlled the new thumb abductor muscle, and thus made the hand human, appears to the modern eye to have a major design flaw: The branch of the median nerve that innervates the thumb abductor is highly vulnerable to compression at the carpal tunnel, formed by the bones and ligaments of the wrist. In the carpal tunnel, the delicate median nerve lies in direct contact with the nine tough finger flexor tendons, causing inevitable traumatic injury to the median nerve with any use of the fingers. This nerve trauma can weaken the thumb abductor muscles and elicit the aberrant sensations of pain, numbness, and tingling that compose CTS.

The CTS may, in turn, trigger a cascade of muscle strains and sensory symptoms. When the weakened thumb muscle is used, it may start to ache, so the subconscious utilitarian brain tends to replace the pincer grasp with a clumsier four-fingered claw grip. To compensate for the loss of dexterity due to CTS, inefficient twists and turns of the wrists, forearms, arms, shoulders, and neck are necessary. The chronic overuse of these secondary muscles creates spasms throughout the entire upper body. For some people, this unrelenting muscle tension triggers back pains, chest pains, all types of headaches, blurry vision, ringing sounds in the ears, numbness of the face and tongue, floating sensations, loss of balance, and mild to severe dizzy spells.

ANATOMY

The peripheral nervous system contains motor and sensory fibers. Sensory fibers carry information from the peripheral receptors to the CNS. Motor fibers conduct action potentials from the CNS to the muscles, where they trigger the contraction of muscle fibers. In cross section, a peripheral nerve consists of fibers of various diameter, some of which are wrapped in a myelin sheath and others of which are unmyelinated. The fibers are grouped into fascicles and are enmeshed in connective tissue layers called *endoneurium*, *perineurium*, and *epineurium*. Nerves also contain blood vessels and small amounts of adipose tissue (Fig. 2.12–1). The functional unit is the nerve axon and its myelin sheath (Fig. 2.12–2). Without myelin, an action potential can be propagated along the nerve fiber at a rate of only 1 m per second, whereas large myelinated fibers can conduct impulses at a rate of up to 70 m per second. Peripheral nerve disease can affect the myelin, in which case conduction velocity is slowed, or the axon, in which case the amplitude of the action potential is reduced, or both.

Each peripheral nerve corresponds to one or a few spinal segments. There are eight cervical spinal segments, 12 thoracic seg-

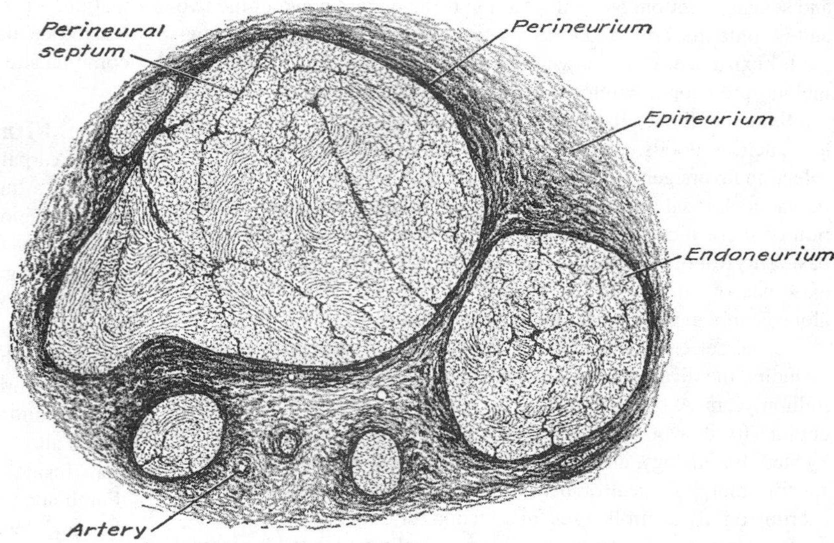

FIGURE 2.12–1 Cross section of the sciatic nerve. Fascicles of myelinated and unmyelinated nerve fibers are enmeshed in endoneurium and are separated from other fascicles by perineurium. The outer layer of connective tissue is the epineurium, in which are embedded blood vessels and adipose tissue. (From Parent A. *Carpenter's Human Neuroanatomy.* 9th ed. Baltimore: Williams & Wilkins; 1996:269, with permission.)

ments, five lumbar segments, and five sacral segments. The skin innervated by nerves that converge on a particular spinal segment is called a *dermatome*, and the muscles innervated by nerves exiting in a particular segment compose a *myotome*. The posterior pattern of sensory dermatomes is shown in Figure 2.12–3. Once nerve roots in the cervical and lumbar regions leave the spinal canal, they converge and diverge in a plexus and emerge as the named peripheral nerves. The organization of the brachial plexus is shown in Figure 2.12–4, and a comparison of the innervation of the skin according to dermatome or named nerve is shown in Figure 2.12–5. It is usually possible to localize a lesion in the peripheral nervous system quite accurately by physical examination, noting the particular combination of sensory and motor defects produced by the lesion.

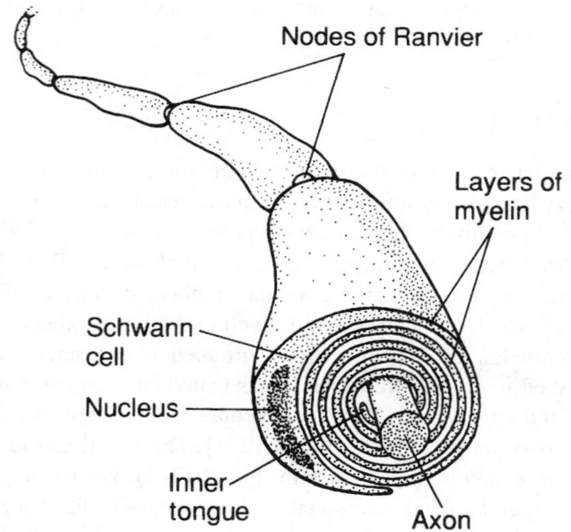

FIGURE 2.12–2 Representation of the axon and its myelin sheath. The inner tongue of Schwann cells wraps layers of hydrophobic myelin around the axon. Individual Schwann cells are separated approximately every 1 mm by a bare section of axon called the *node of Ranvier.* Action potentials jump from one node to the next, which increases the rate of propagation of the action potential. (From Kandel ER. Nerve cells and behavior. In: Kandel ER, Schwartz JH, Jessell TM, eds. *Principles of Neural Science.* 3rd ed. New York: Elsevier; 1991:23, with permission.)

Motor fibers terminate on muscle fibers, forming the neuromuscular junction. At the nerve terminus, the action potential triggers the influx of calcium ions, which cause the release of acetylcholine from vesicular stores. Acetylcholine enters the synaptic cleft and binds to receptors on the muscle cell that trigger release of intracellular calcium and initiate contraction of the muscle fiber (Fig. 2.12–6). Acetylcholine is degraded and inactivated in the synaptic cleft by acetylcholinesterase, and the resulting acetic acid and choline are taken up by the nerve terminus and recombined into acetylcholine for storage in vesicles. Neuromuscular transmission is usually highly efficient, but it may be compromised in myasthenia gravis and other disorders of neuromuscular transmission.

Each motor nerve branches within the muscle and innervates a handful of muscle fibers. If a nerve ending dies, the resulting denervated muscle fibers initially exhibit spontaneous activity, then eventually are reinnervated by collateral sprouts of neighboring nerves. This forms motor units covering an unusually large volume (Fig. 2.12–7).

PHYSIOLOGY

Nerve impulses are called *action potentials*. In the resting state, the intracellular compartment of the neuron is negatively charged at a potential of –70 to –80 mV, but during an action potential, the inside of the neuron becomes positively charged. For an action potential to be generated by a neuron, ion channels open, and sodium ions begin to enter the cell and gradually make the inside of the neuron less negatively charged relative to the outside. The point at which the interior of the neuron is sufficiently less negatively charged to initiate an action potential is called the *spike threshold* and is characteristically approximately –60 mV. The action potential itself is a brief (0.1- to 2.0-msec) wave of reversal of membrane potential that moves along an axon (Fig. 2.12–8). During an action potential, the interior of the neuron is positively charged in comparison to the outside of the neuron. The initial ion channel involved in the action potential is the Na^+ channel, which, when opened, allows positively charged sodium ions to enter the neuron. The Ca^{2+} channels are next to open, thus allowing the positively charged calcium ions to enter the neuron and further contribute to the spike of the action potential. Entry of the calcium ions activates ion channels that carry an outgoing flow of potassium ions that are involved in arresting the action potential. The activation of these K^+ channels results in the afterhy-

C2
C3
C4
C5
C6
C7
C8
T1
T2
3
4
5
6
7
8
9
10
11
12
L1
L2
L3
L4
L5
S1
S2
S3
S5
Co

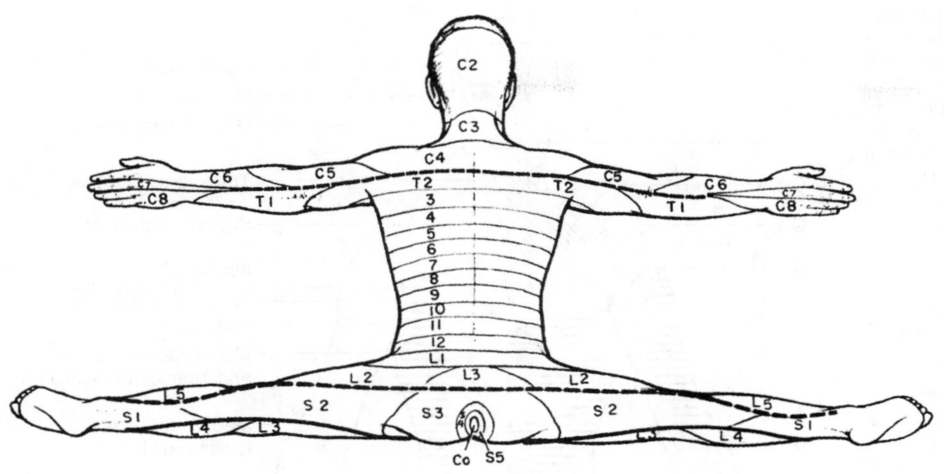

FIGURE 2.12–3 Posterior distribution of dermatomes. The arms expand the cervical dermatomes, and the legs expand the lumbosacral dermatomes. (From Parent A. *Carpenter's Human Neuroanatomy*. 9th ed. Baltimore: Williams & Wilkins; 1996:270, with permission.)

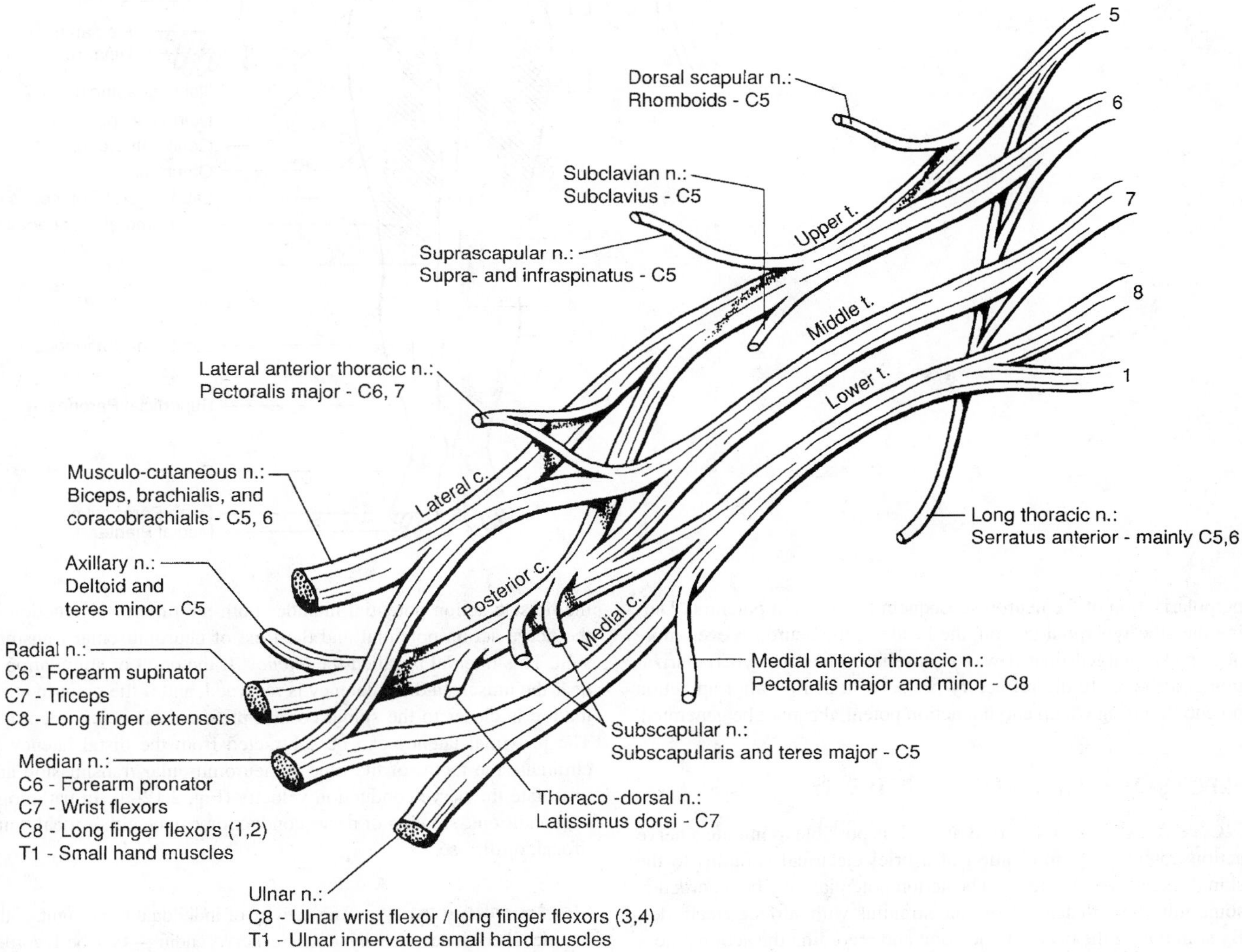

5
6
7
8
1
Dorsal scapular n.:
Rhomboids - C5
Subclavian n.:
Subclavius - C5
Suprascapular n.:
Supra- and infraspinatus - C5
Upper t.
Middle t.
Lower t.
Lateral anterior thoracic n.:
Pectoralis major - C6, 7
Musculo-cutaneous n.:
Biceps, brachialis, and
coracobrachialis - C5, 6
Lateral c.
Posterior c.
Medial c.
Long thoracic n.:
Serratus anterior - mainly C5,6
Axillary n.:
Deltoid and
teres minor - C5
Radial n.:
C6 - Forearm supinator
C7 - Triceps
C8 - Long finger extensors
Medial anterior thoracic n.:
Pectoralis major and minor - C8
Subscapular n.:
Subscapularis and teres major - C5
Median n.:
C6 - Forearm pronator
C7 - Wrist flexors
C8 - Long finger flexors (1,2)
T1 - Small hand muscles
Thoraco -dorsal n.:
Latissimus dorsi - C7
Ulnar n.:
C8 - Ulnar wrist flexor / long finger flexors (3,4)
T1 - Ulnar innervated small hand muscles

FIGURE 2.12–4 The brachial plexus. The cervical spinal roots are at the upper right. They first fuse to form three trunks (t.). Each trunk splits into an anterior and a posterior division, and these then fuse to form three cords (c.). The main named nerves (n.) of the arm emerge from various segments of the brachial plexus. Each muscle is therefore innervated by a named nerve carrying fibers from a particular set of spinal roots. (From Oh SI. *Clinical Electromyography Nerve Conduction Studies*. 2nd ed. Baltimore: Williams & Wilkins; 1993:57, with permission.)

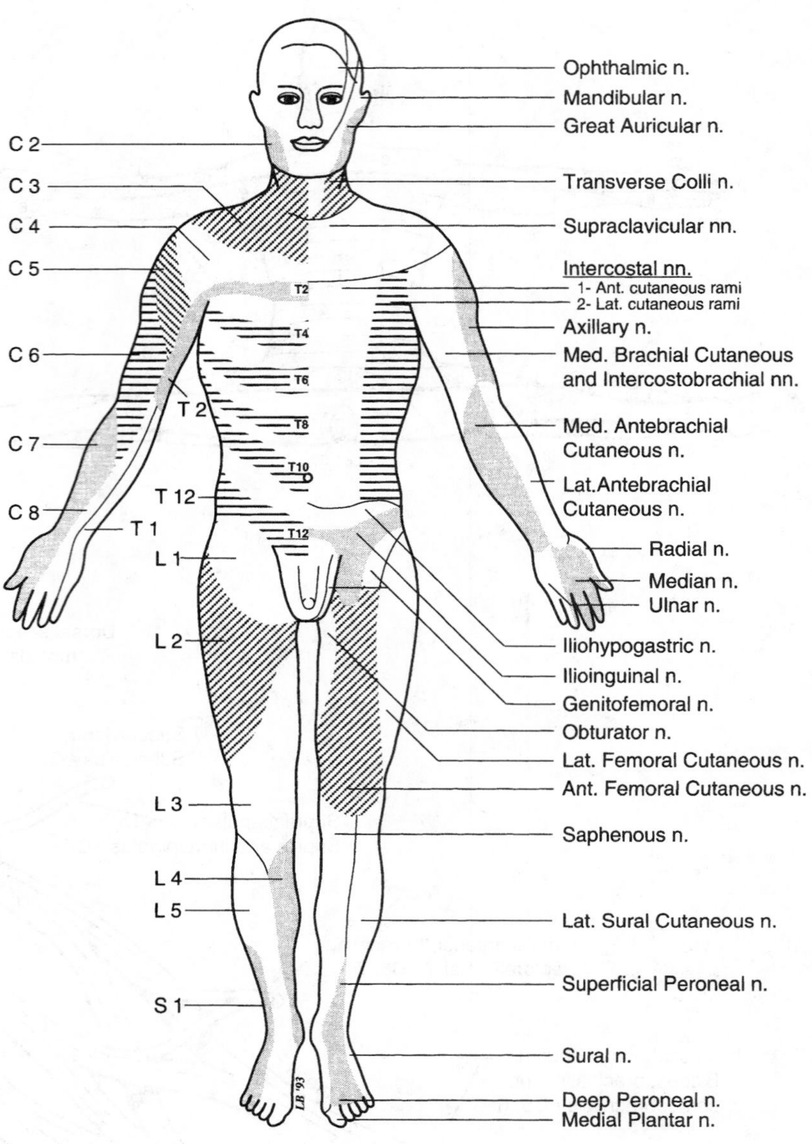

FIGURE 2.12–5 Anterior (ant.) distribution of the dermatomes (*left*) and cutaneous areas supplied by named peripheral nerves (n.; *right*). Dermatomal patches overlap considerably with their neighboring dermatomes, whereas the distributions of peripheral nerves are sharply demarcated on the skin. lat., lateral; med., medial. (From Parent A. *Carpenter's Human Neuroanatomy*. 9th ed. Baltimore: Williams & Wilkins; 1996:271, with permission.)

perpolarization of the neuron subsequent to an action potential. During the afterhyperpolarization, the inside of the neuron is even more negatively charged than it was at baseline. The afterhyperpolarization contributes to the refractory period of a neuron after an action potential, during which another action potential cannot be generated.

ELECTRODIAGNOSTIC STUDIES

Nerve Conduction Studies It is possible to initiate a nerve action potential by application of a brief electrical stimulus to the skin directly over the nerve. The action potential may be recorded at some minimum distance from the stimulus with surface electrodes. By stimulating the nerve at one point and recording the action potential at another point at a defined distance away, a nerve conduction velocity can be calculated. Extensive studies have established reference values for each of the measurable nerves against which patient values can be compared. In the case of motor nerves, the recording is usually made over the muscle, which has a much larger action potential amplitude than the nerve and, thus, is easier to detect electronically. In this case, the time interval between the nerve stimulus and the muscle action potential includes both the time of conduction of the nerve action potential and the time of neuromuscular transmission. This interval is called the *latency*. If the point of stimulation is near the muscle, a distal latency is recorded, and if the point of stimulation is closer to the spinal cord, a proximal latency is recorded. The proximal latency can be subtracted from the distal latency to eliminate the factor of the time of neuromuscular transmission and to isolate the nerve conduction velocity (Fig. 2.12–9). In pathological conditions, slowing of nerve conduction can be either focal, multifocal, or diffuse.

Electromyography The activity of individual motor units—the muscle fibers innervated by a single nerve ending—can be recorded with an electrode placed directly into the muscle. The morphology, amplitude, and duration of the muscle action potential are noted and compared to normal values. After nerve injury, the first abnormal activity, noted at 2 to 3 weeks, is spontaneous firing of denervated muscle fibers. Over the following weeks to months, nerve endings sprout and reinnervate these muscle fibers, and spontaneous activity is replaced by motor unit potentials of very large amplitude and duration. In contrast,

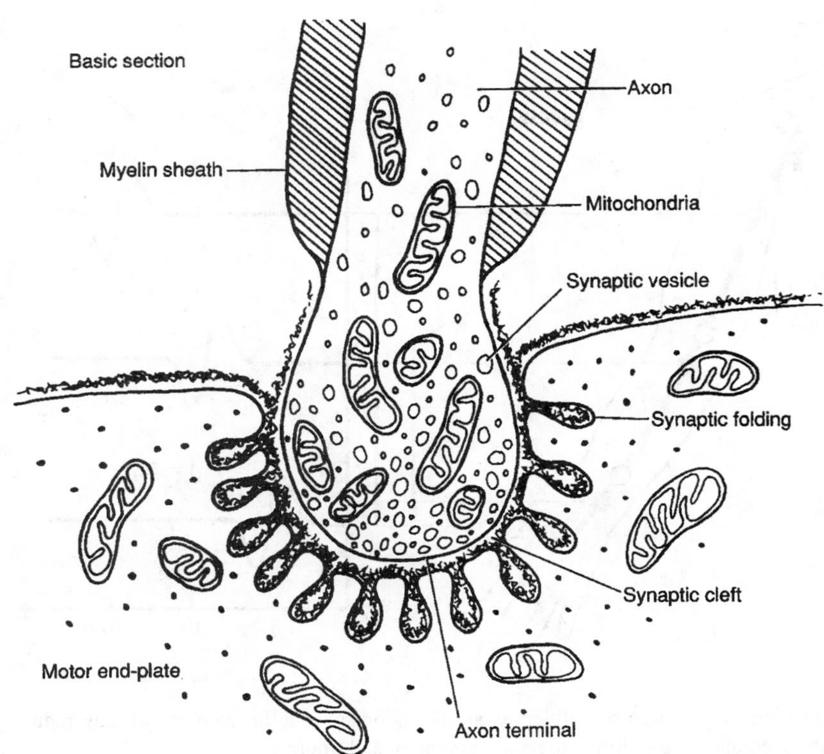

FIGURE 2.12–6 The neuromuscular junction in cross section. The nerve fiber terminus enters from the top and releases acetylcholine from synaptic vesicles. Acetylcholine diffuses through the matrix of the synaptic cleft to activate muscle contraction. (From Oh SJ. *Clinical Electromyography Nerve Conduction Studies*. 2nd ed. Baltimore: Williams & Wilkins; 1993:10, with permission.)

injury to muscle fibers themselves produces brief, low-amplitude motor potentials (Fig. 2.12–10). Examination of 20 or more individual muscle fibers in a muscle with known innervation can detect whether there is an injury to the nerve at some point along its pathway, even if the nerve conduction velocity is normal. Electromyography (EMG) therefore complements the nerve conduction velocity studies, and the combination of the two techniques may, in some cases, permit a more exact localization and quantification of neuromuscular disease than is possible with physical examination alone.

COMMON NERVE COMPRESSION SYNDROMES

Carpal Tunnel Syndrome The median nerve travels from the distal arm into the hand through the carpal tunnel, which is a fascia-lined passage in the ventral wrist. Compression of the nerve at the carpal tunnel produces a characteristic set of symptoms and signs in the hands and arms. Carpal tunnel syndrome is more common among people who perform repetitive hand movements, such as typing, sorting mail, playing a keyboard instrument, or lifting heavy weights, but it may also occur in the absence of such repetitive

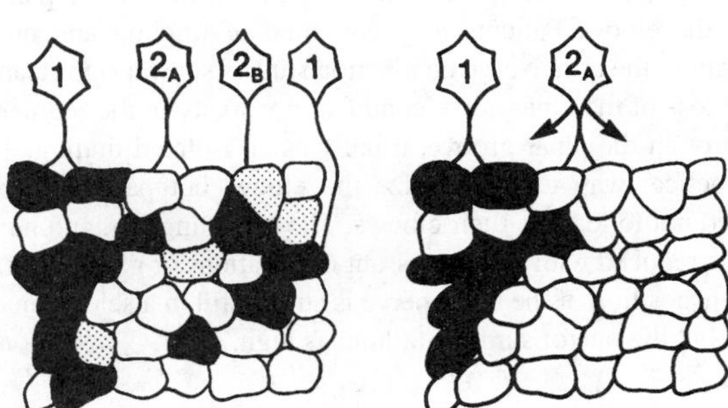

FIGURE 2.12–7 **A:** Normal muscle fibers have a mosaic pattern of innervation: In this figure, four individual nerve endings (1, 2_A, 2_B) each branch to innervate a small subset of muscle fibers. A contiguous set of fibers constitutes a motor unit. **B:** After loss of nerve fibers, remaining nerve fibers sprout to create unusually large motor units. (From Poirier J, Gray F, Escourolle R. *Manual of Basic Neuropathology*. 3rd ed. Philadelphia: W.B. Saunders; 1990:217, with permission.)

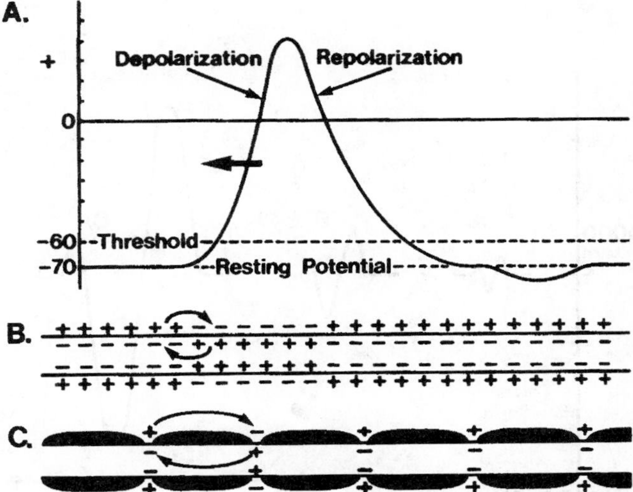

FIGURE 2.12–8 Phases of the action potential during its propagation. **A:** Changes in the membrane potential as the action potential moves from right to left. **B:** In unmyelinated fibers, an action potential triggers changes in the immediately adjacent membrane, called *local circuit conduction*. **C:** In myelinated fibers, the action potential jumps from one node of Ranvier to the next, called *saltatory conduction*. (From Oh SJ. *Clinical Electromyography Nerve Conduction Studies*. 2nd ed. Baltimore: Williams & Wilkins; 1993:7, with permission.)

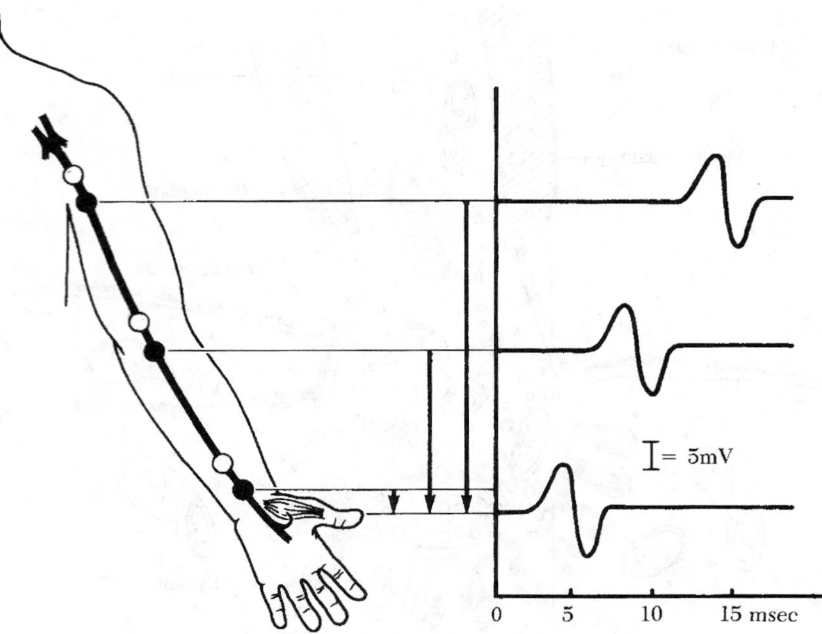

FIGURE 2.12–9 Motor nerve conduction study in the median nerve. The nerve is stimulated at the axilla (*top waveform*), elbow (*middle waveform*), and wrist (*bottom waveform*). Each waveform shows the muscle action potential recorded from the abductor pollicis brevis muscle as a function of time after nerve stimulation. The delay from the time of stimulation to the onset of the muscle action potential is the latency. Subtraction of the proximal latency from the distal latency isolates the time of nerve conduction; division of this value by the distance between the two points of stimulation gives the nerve conduction velocity. (From Oh SJ. *Clinical Electromyography Nerve Conduction Studies.* 2nd ed. Baltimore: Williams & Wilkins; 1993:17, with permission.)

stresses. Physical examination may show decreased light touch in the median nerve distribution in the hand, weakness of the median-innervated APB muscle, or positive Tinel's sign (tingling in the fingers caused by percussion over the carpal tunnel) or Phalen's sign (reproduction of the symptoms of carpal tunnel syndrome by sustained palmar flexion of the wrist). Nerve conduction studies first reveal slowing and loss of amplitude of the sensory fibers, then, in more advanced cases, slowing and, occasionally, loss of amplitude of the motor fibers. EMG of the APB muscle may be normal or may show signs of acute or chronic denervation. Conservative treatment consists of wearing splints that prevent palmar flexion of the wrist, especially at night, and specific stretching exercises. If these measures alone do not alleviate the symptoms after 3 months, then addition of antidepressant drugs or gabapentin (Neurontin) may reduce or eliminate pain, numbness, and tingling.

For those patients whose symptoms do not improve and who are eager to have surgery, surgical release of the trapped median nerve is reported to be beneficial in approximately 80 percent of cases. Because carpal tunnel surgery has not been compared to nonsurgical treatments in randomized trials, the possibility of a large placebo effect of surgery cannot be ruled out. A systematic psychological evaluation of the pain behavior of people with chronic pain commonly reveals a surprisingly high incidence of secondary gain dynamics. Unless the psychodynamic reinforcers of the illness in such cases are adequately addressed, any treatments of carpal tunnel syndrome may not be successful.

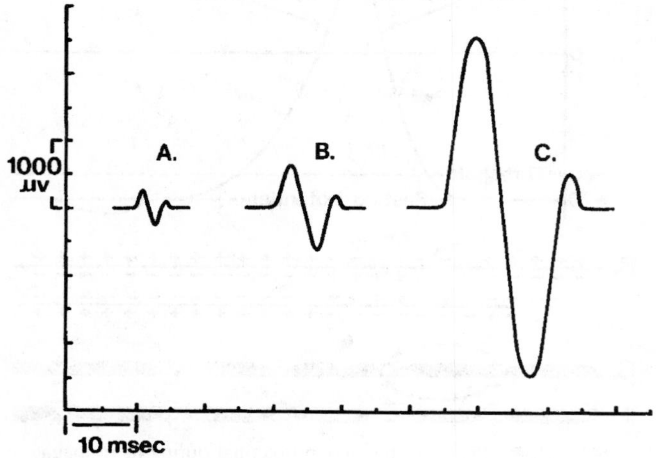

A. B. C.
1000 μV
10 msec

FIGURE 2.12–10 Motor unit potentials. **A:** Small-amplitude and -duration motor unit potential in myopathy. **B:** Normal motor unit potential. **C:** Large-amplitude and -duration motor unit in neuropathy as a result of denervation, collateral sprouting, and reinnervation. (From Oh SJ. *Clinical Electromyography Nerve Conduction Studies.* 2nd ed. Baltimore: Williams & Wilkins; 1993:6, with permission.)

Compression of the Ulnar Nerve at the Elbow (Cubital Tunnel Syndrome) The ulnar nerve is prone to compression in the ulnar groove between the olecranon process of the ulna and the medial epicondyle of the humerus. The clinical symptoms and signs of ulnar neuropathy at the elbow are generally less well defined than in carpal tunnel syndrome, ranging from asymptomatic to sensory loss and, rarely, weakness in the ulnar-innervated pattern distal to the elbow. Patients may complain of tingling and numbness throughout the arm. Nerve conduction studies show a significant slowing or loss of the ulnar nerve conduction velocity in the segment passing through the ulnar groove, usually as an isolated finding. There is no practical way to immobilize the elbow, but patients should be advised not to lean on their elbows. The pain, tingling, and numbness may be reduced with antidepressant medications or gabapentin. Surgical transposition of the ulnar nerve is successful in a select minority of cases, but the rate of surgical failures is high.

Peroneal Palsy The peroneal nerve is vulnerable to compression as it passes over the head of the fibula, just distal and lateral to the knee. It may be injured because of pressure of the opposite leg when the legs are crossed above the knee or during improper positioning during surgery or during immobilization of the leg in a cast. Sensory loss extends down the anterolateral surface of the leg and foot, and there may be complete or partial weakness of foot elevation and eversion. Nerve conduction studies show slowing or loss of conduction across the fibular head, and EMG may show evidence of denervation of the peroneal-innervated muscles. Patients with peroneal palsy should wear an ankle–foot orthosis to prevent the toes from dragging as the leg swings forward. Recovery may take as long as 2 years and is often incomplete. Antidepressant medications and gabapentin often reduce neuropathic pain significantly, whereas nonsteroidal antiinflammatory drugs (NSAIDs) are generally of little benefit. Physical therapy can assist the patient in adapting to the difficulties of ambulation.

Meralgia Paresthetica The lateral cutaneous nerve of the thigh may be compressed under the inguinal ligament, just before it reaches the skin, by prolonged wearing of a heavy belt such as a carpenter's belt. It may also arise spontaneously, particularly in obese individuals. Meralgia paresthetica—literally "tingling pain in the thigh"—describes the resulting sensations in a sharply delineated patch of skin on the lateral surface of the thigh extending down to the knee. Management begins with removal of the heavy belt or loss of weight. Antidepressant medications and gabapentin offer relief in most cases.

Radiculopathy Commonly invoked as a "pinched nerve in the neck or back" to explain what are in fact musculoskeletal pains, true spinal radiculopathies are a relatively rare cause of neck or back pain. The sensory or motor root, or both, may be compressed as it exits the spinal cord by a herniated intervertebral disc or as it leaves the vertebral column by bony prominences formed by degenerative changes of the bones. Sensory loss is in a dermatomal distribution with vague borders due to overlapping of neighboring dermatomes. Weakness occurs in a myotomal pattern, and there may be loss of characteristic deep tendon reflexes. Nerve conduction studies are usually normal, and EMG may show signs of denervation and reinnervation in the first 3 to 4 months of compression. Neuroimaging, either magnetic resonance imaging (MRI) or myelography with computed tomography (CT), is essential. Conservative management is always indicated first, consisting of rest; muscle relaxers, such as benzodiazepines or cyclobenzaprine (Flexeril); effective analgesia; heating pads; and nonstrenuous exercises. If conservative management does not relieve the pain and neurological deficits persist, referral to a neurosurgeon is indicated. In carefully selected cases in which a nerve root is clearly compressed, surgical removal of the dislocated structures can provide definitive relief. It should be noted, however, that arthritic pain and, above all, muscle pain are far more common causes of low back pain than are true radiculopathies. In the opinion of the noted physiatrist John Sarno, 95 percent of low back pain is psychosomatic. The first approach to such uncomplicated low back pain is conservative management. When surgery is not appropriate, several techniques that have been developed for injection of steroids or local anesthetics in the epidural space may be attempted, but the pain relief afforded by these methods is usually temporary, lasting sometimes just for a few hours and only for weeks to months in the most favorable of situations. Invasive pain management techniques all carry a risk of infections and bleeding. Patients who develop chronic low back pain in the absence of demonstrable radiculopathy may benefit from weight loss, physical therapy, psychiatric support, and antidepressant medications.

ACQUIRED NEUROPATHIES

Peripheral nerves are vulnerable to several metabolic and infectious conditions. Prevention is the best approach to acquired neuropathies, as the ability of the nerves to regenerate is best in cases of trauma and worst in cases of metabolic injury.

Diabetes Mellitus Diabetes promotes thrombus formation in the tiniest capillaries, and it slowly eliminates peripheral nerve endings, usually over several years. Approximately 15 percent of diabetic patients have symptoms and signs of peripheral neuropathy, but 50 percent have either neuropathic symptoms or slowing of nerve conduction velocity. The longest nerves are the most vulnerable, and symptoms usually begin in the toes. Several clinical forms are seen: (1) a distal, symmetrical, predominantly sensory painful neuropathy; (2) autonomic neuropathy; (3) painful, asymmetrical multiple neuropathy, also called *mononeuropathy multiplex*; (4) acute mononeuropathies; and (5) diabetic ophthalmoplegia. The burning pain of the sensory neuropathy may respond to antidepressant or anticonvulsant medications. Tight control of plasma blood sugar can slow the progression of the neuropathy and reduce the symptoms.

Other Acquired Metabolic Neuropathies Medical conditions producing diffuse damage to peripheral nerves include vitamin deficiency states, heavy metal poisoning, drug intoxications (including chronic use of lithium), uremia, collagen-vascular disorders, and paraneoplastic syndromes. The principal neuropathic syndromes are listed in Table 2.12–1.

Postherpetic Neuralgia Herpes zoster can infect and remain dormant in dorsal root ganglion cells for as long as decades and then may be reactivated under conditions of emotional stress or immune compromise. Reactivation of herpes zoster causes several days of burning, itching, and tingling, followed by the emergence of very painful blisters in a dermatomal distribution. These resolve in 1 to 4 weeks in most patients, but up to one-third of patients may have pain for months and sometimes for years. Antiviral agents, such as acyclovir (Zovirax), famciclovir (Famvir), or valacyclovir (Valtrex), may shorten the acute course. Antidepressant medications and gabapentin are most effective for chronic postherpetic neuralgia, and carbamazepine (Tegretol) may be useful for lancinating pains.

Guillain-Barré Syndrome *Acute inflammatory demyelinating polyneuropathy*, or Guillain-Barré syndrome, is a postinfectious, autoimmune condition in which antibodies elicited by a usually unidentifiable infectious agent cross-react with the myelin sheaths of the peripheral nerves. In some cases of Guillain-Barré syndrome preceded by diarrhea, antibodies to *Campylobacter jejuni* can be identified and are believed to be pathogenic. Inflammatory loss of myelin results in slowing and blockade of nerve conduction. Initially, there is tingling in the toes, followed by loss of deep tendon reflexes and motor weakness affecting the longest nerves first. The weakness thus begins in the toes and appears to ascend over the course of a few days. Once a patient cannot walk, he or she should be admitted to an intensive care unit, closely monitored for respiratory distress, and mechanically ventilated if necessary. Recovery usually begins by the fourth week and may not be completed for months. Intensive inpatient rehabilitation may be necessary. Patients may need continuous psychiatric support during the recovery. Tingling, pain, and numbness may be treated with antidepressant medications or gabapentin.

Autonomic Neuropathies Hereditary and acquired damage to the autonomic nervous system may produce fluctuations in blood pressure, heart rate, temperature control, bowel and bladder function, or sexual function, which may resemble the effects of emo-

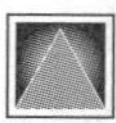

Table 2.12–1
Principal Neuropathic Syndromes

Syndrome of acute motor paralysis with variable disturbance of sensory and autonomic function
- Guillain-Barré syndrome (acute inflammatory polyneuropathy, acute autoimmune neuropathy)
- Acute axonal form of Guillain-Barré syndrome
- Infectious mononucleosis and polyneuritis
- Hepatitis and polyneuritis
- Acute sensory neuropathy syndrome
- Diphtheritic polyneuropathy
- Porphyric polyneuropathy
- Certain toxic polyneuropathies (triorthocresyl phosphate, thallium)
- Rarely, paraneoplastic, vaccinogenic (smallpox, rabies), serogenic, polyarteritic, or lupus polyneuropathy
- Acute panautonomic neuropathy

Syndrome of subacute sensorimotor paralysis
- Symmetrical polyneuropathies
  - Deficiency states: alcoholism (beriberi), pellagra, vitamin B_{12} deficiency, chronic gastrointestinal disease
  - Poisoning with heavy metals and solvents: arsenic, lead, mercury, thallium, methyl-*N*-butyl ketone, *N*-hexane, methylbromide, ethylene oxide, organophosphates (e.g., triorthocresyl phosphate), acrylamide
  - Drug intoxications: ethionamide, hydralazine, nitrofurantoin and related nitrofurazones, disulfiram, carbon disulfide, vincristine, cisplatin, chloramphenicol, phenytoin, amitriptyline, dapsone, stilbamidine, trichloroethylene, thalidomide, clioquinol
  - Uremic polyneuropathy
- Asymmetrical neuropathies (mononeuropathy multiplex)
  - Diabetes
  - Polyarteritis nodosa and other inflammatory angiopathic neuropathies
  - Sicca syndrome
  - Subacute idiopathic polyneuropathies
  - Sarcoidosis
  - Ischemic neuropathy with peripheral vascular disease

Syndrome of chronic sensorimotor polyneuropathy
- Less chronic, acquired forms
  - Carcinoma, myeloma, and other malignancies
  - Chronic inflammatory demyelinating polyneuropathy
  - Paraproteinemias
  - Uremia (occasionally subacute)
  - Beriberi (usually subacute)
  - Diabetes
  - Connective tissue diseases
  - Amyloidosis
  - Leprosy
  - Hypothyroidism
  - Benign form in the elderly
  - Sepsis and chronic illness

Syndrome of more chronic polyneuropathy, genetically determined forms
- Inherited polyneuropathies of predominantly sensory type
  - Dominant mutilating sensory neuropathy in adults
  - Recessive mutilating sensory neuropathy of childhood
  - Congenital insensitivity to pain
  - Other inherited sensory neuropathies, including those associated with spinocerebellar degenerations, Riley-Day syndrome, and universal anesthesia syndrome
- Inherited polyneuropathies of mixed sensorimotor-autonomic types
  - Idiopathic group
    - Peroneal muscular atrophy (Charcot-Marie-Tooth: hereditary motor-sensory neuropathy, types I and II)
    - Hypertrophic polyneuropathy of Dejerine-Sottas, adult and childhood forms
    - Roussy-Lévy polyneuropathy
    - Polyneuropathy with optic atrophy, spastic paraplegia, spinocerebellar degeneration, mental retardation, and dementia
  - Inherited polyneuropathies with a recognized metabolic disorder
    - Refsum's disease
    - Metachromatic leukodystrophy
    - Globoid body leukodystrophy (Krabbe's disease)
    - Adrenoleukodystrophy
    - Amyloid polyneuropathy
    - Porphyric polyneuropathy
    - Anderson-Fabry disease
    - Abetalipoproteinemia and Tangier disease

Syndrome of muscular dystrophy with neuropathy (with mitochondrial diseases)

Syndrome of recurrent or relapsing polyneuropathy
- Guillain-Barré syndrome
- Porphyria
- Chronic inflammatory demyelinating polyneuropathy
- Certain forms of mononeuritis multiplex
- Beriberi or intoxications
- Refsum's disease, Tangier disease

Syndrome of mononeuropathy or plexopathy
- Brachial plexus neuropathies
- Brachial mononeuropathies
- Causalgia
- Lumbosacral plexopathies
- Crural mononeuropathies
- Migrant sensory neuropathy
- Entrapment neuropathies

From Adams RD, Victor M. *Principles of Neurology.* 5th ed. New York: McGraw-Hill; 1996, with permission.

tional instability. Patients may develop orthostatic hypotension on rising from a seated or lying position and complain of persistent dizziness. At other times, blood pressure may increase excessively in response to emotional stress such as visits to the doctor (the "white coat syndrome"). Patients with these symptoms may be assumed incorrectly to have hysteria, anorexia nervosa, or hypochondriasis. Careful medical evaluation of somatic and visceral complaints, including autonomic electrophysiological evaluation, should be performed before a strictly psychiatric condition is diagnosed. Electrical evidence of autonomic neuropathy includes decreased beat-to-beat variability of the heart rate and absence of a sympathetic skin response.

CORRELATION OF COMPLAINTS AND ELECTRODIAGNOSTIC FINDINGS

Patients are referred for electrodiagnostic evaluation because of suspicion that their complaints of pain, numbness, tingling, or weakness may be caused by injury to the peripheral nerves. The most common reason for referral is to determine whether a patient's signs and symptoms of carpal tunnel syndrome, which is a clinical diagnosis, correlate with electrodiagnostic evidence of nerve injury. The majority of patients with convincing signs of carpal tunnel syndrome on examination have at least some electrodiagnostic abnormalities, usually prolongation of the distal sensory latency and reduction of the sensory amplitude. Some patients who are asymptomatic or barely symptomatic nevertheless have very advanced sensory and motor nerve injury on electrodiagnostic studies. Conversely, some patients with prominent complaints and classic signs of carpal tunnel syndrome have electrodiagnostic values completely within the normal range. Questioning of the latter patients often reveals high levels of anxiety and depression, which appear to amplify the symptoms of even minor nerve compression. Such patients often respond very satisfactorily to antidepressant medications.

MANAGEMENT

Diagnostic Workup History should emphasize the location and quality of the pain, whether it is constant or intermittent; how long it has been present; and whether it is improving, remaining steady, or worsening. Medical history should cover diabetes, thyroid disease, autoimmune disease, cancer, and infections and a thorough history of medication use. Physical examination should test muscle bulk and strength, all sensory modalities (light touch, pain, temperature, vibration, and position sense), and deep tendon reflexes, with particular attention to patterns of abnormalities that suggest a dermatome or the distribution of a particular named nerve. Electrodiagnostic studies can corroborate the clinical suspicion of neuropathy and quantitate the abnormalities. If a metabolic disorder is suspected, appropriate blood and urine tests should be ordered. If a radiculopathy that may be amenable to surgery is suspected, then high–field-strength MRI scanning of the spine is indicated.

Medical Treatments If an underlying medical condition, such as diabetes or thyroid disease, is present, it must be vigorously treated. In some cases, the neuropathic symptoms and signs resolve on adequate management of the underlying medical problem.

Surgical Options Surgical release of entrapped nerves is most effective for carpal tunnel syndrome and certain radiculopathies and is less uniformly effective for ulnar neuropathies. Nerve ablation has been of benefit in trigeminal neuralgia but should be avoided for other chronic pain syndromes. Although nerve ablation may temporarily cut off sensation to a painful area, secondary sensory routes often emerge, and painful sensations often return.

Adjunctive Medications Regardless of the cause of neuropathic symptoms, the distressing pain, numbness, and tingling can be reduced or eliminated by antidepressant medications or gabapentin. Neurologists have traditionally relied on low doses of tricyclic drugs, especially amitriptyline (Elavil) and nortriptyline (Aventyl, Pamelor). However, data show no therapeutic advantage of tricyclic drugs over the newer antidepressant medications. The selective serotonin reuptake inhibitors (SSRIs) (e.g., fluoxetine [Prozac], sertraline [Zoloft], paroxetine [Paxil], and fluvoxamine [Luvox]), bupropion (Wellbutrin), nefazodone (Serzone), trazodone (Desyrel), venlafaxine (Effexor), and mirtazapine (Remeron) are probably all equally effective for neuropathic symptoms. Low doses usually suffice, but higher doses may be needed. Lancinating pain, seen in some types of postherpetic neuralgia, may respond to the anticonvulsants carbamazepine or phenytoin (Dilantin). Controlled trials have shown that gabapentin reduces neuropathic pain. Psychotherapy for underlying depression and anxiety may be beneficial. Vitamin therapies have been widely discussed, particularly vitamins B_6 and B_{12}, but true vitamin deficiency states are quite rare in developed countries. Massive quantities of vitamin B_6 should be avoided because it can cause a sensory neuropathy. Alternative therapies, such as herbal medicines, meditation, or acupuncture, work to the extent that they elicit the placebo effect, which may be a powerful therapeutic modality in suggestible individuals.

SUGGESTED CROSS-REFERENCES

Psychosomatic disorders are covered in Chapter 24. Drugs used in psychiatry (including antidepressants and benzodiazepines) are discussed and organized pharmacologically in Chapter 31.

REFERENCES

*Aminoff MJ. *Electrodiagnosis in Clinical Neurology.* 4th ed. Churchill Livingstone; 1999.

Becker D, Sadowsky CL, McDonald JW: Restoring function after spinal cord injury. *Neurology*. 2003;9:1–15.

*Butler S. *Conquering Carpal Tunnel Syndrome and Other Repetitive Strain Injuries.* New Harbinger Publications; 1996.

Chiodo A, Haig AJ: Lumbosacral radiculopathies: Conservative approaches to management. *Phys Med Rehabil Clin N Am.* 2002;13:609–621.

Cros D. *Peripheral Neuropathy: A Practical Approach to Diagnosis and Management.* Lippincott Williams & Wilkins; 2001.

Daffner SD, Hilibrand AS, Hanscom BS, Brislin BT, Vaccaro AR, Albert TJ: Impact of neck and arm pain on overall health status. *Spine.* 2003;28:2030–2035.

Davies A, De Souza LH, Frank AO: Changes in the quality of life in severely disabled people following provision of powered indoor/outdoor chairs. *Disabil Rehabil.* 2003;25:286–290.

Dawson S, Kristjanson LJ: Mapping the journey: Family carers' perceptions of issues related to end-stage care of individuals with muscular dystrophy or motor neurone disease. *J Palliat Care.* 2003;19:36–42.

Dillingham TR, Dasher KJ: The lumbosacral electromyographic screen: Revisiting a classic paper. *Clin Neurophysiol.* 2000;111:2219–2222.

Emmons RA, McCullough ME: Counting blessings versus burdens: An experimental investigation of gratitude and subjective well-being in daily life. *J Pers Soc Psychol.* 2003;84:377–389.

Fisher MA: Electrophysiology of radiculopathies. *Clin Neurophysiol.* 2002;113:317–335. Review.

Geiringer SR: Evaluation and reporting requirements of the disability examiner. *Phys Med Rehabil Clin N Am.* 2001;12:543–557.

Hara Y: Dorsal wrist joint pain in tetraplegic patients during and after rehabilitation. *J Rehabil Med.* 2003;35:57–61.

Hecht MJ, Graesel E, Tigges S, Hillemacher T, Winterholler M, Hilz MJ, Heuss D, Neundorfer B: Burden of care in amyotrophic lateral sclerosis. *Palliat Med.* 2003;17:327–333.

Iannaccone ST, Hynan LS: American Spinal Muscular Atrophy Randomized Trials (AmSMART) Group. Reliability of 4 outcome measures in pediatric spinal muscular atrophy. *Arch Neurol.* 2003;60:1130–1136.

Kandel ER, Schwartz JH, Jessell TM. *Principles of Neural Science.* 4th ed. New York: Appleton & Lange; 2000.

*Kimura J. *Electrodiagnosis in Diseases of Nerve and Muscle.* 2nd ed. Philadelphia: F. A. Davis; 1989.

Kostova V, Koleva M: Back disorders (low back pain, cervicobrachial and lumbosacral radicular syndromes) and some related risk factors. *J Neurol Sci.* 2001;192:17–25.

Meyer-Rosberg K, Kvarnstrom A, Kinnman E, Gordh T, Nordfors LO, Kristofferson A: Peripheral neuropathic pain—a multidimensional burden for patients. *Eur J Pain.* 2001;5:379–389.

Moraru E, Schnider P, Wimmer A, Wenzel T, Birner P, Griengl H, Auff E. Relation between depression and anxiety in dystonic patients: Implications for clinical management. *Depress Anxiety.* 2002;16:100–103.

*Oh SJ. *Clinical Electromyography. Nerve Conduction Studies.* 3rd ed. Baltimore: Williams & Wilkins; 2002.

Parent A. *Carpenter's Human Neuroanatomy.* 9th ed. Baltimore: Williams & Wilkins; 1996.

Pascarelli EF, Hsu YP: Understanding work-related upper extremity disorders: clinical findings in 485 computer users, musicians, and others. *J Occup Rehabil.* 2001;11:1–21.

Patel B, Buschbacher R, Crawford J: National variability in permanent partial impairment ratings. *Am J Phys Med Rehabil.* 2003;82:302–306.
Persson LC, Lilja A: Pain, coping, emotional state and physical function in patients with chronic radicular neck pain. A comparison between patients treated with surgery, physiotherapy or neck collar—a blinded, prospective randomized study. *Disabil Rehabil.* 2001;23:325–335.
Poirier J, Gray F, Escourolle R. *Manual of Basic Neuropathology.* 3rd ed. Philadelphia: W. B. Saunders; 1990.
Tralongo P, Respini D, Ferrau F: Fatigue and aging. *Crit Rev Oncol Hematol.* 2003;48 (Suppl):S57–S64.
*Victor M, Ropper AH. *Adams and Victor's Principles of Neurology.* 7th ed. New York: McGraw Hill; 2000.
White PD, Henderson M, Pearson RM, Coldrick AR, White AG, Kidd BL: Illness behavior and psychosocial factors in diffuse upper limb pain disorder: A case-control study. *J Rheumatol.* 2003;30:139–145.

▲ 2.13 Psychiatric Aspects of Child Neurology

JAMES C. EDMONDSON, M.D., PH.D.

The traditional view that childhood behavior is mainly influenced by caregivers has given way compellingly, in recent years, to a view that human behaviors are genetically encoded adaptations to life in this increasingly complex society. That behavior is more often than not genetically determined has been shown in studies of identical twins separated at infancy and raised in different environments who meet again as adults: The adult twins invariably show higher correlations of behavioral measures with each other than with the families that raised them. Other evidence that specific behaviors are genetically determined comes from the multigenerational pedigrees showing mendelian inheritance of unusual behavioral tendencies or isolated mental deficits in an otherwise normal background. In this view, the neurological substrate of behavior, the brain, is all important, whereas caregivers, in contrast, are reduced to mere facilitators and weak modulators of the expression of innate behaviors. Mental health providers should therefore be keenly interested in the systematic pediatric neurological approach to diseases of the developing brain.

The image of a brain-damaged child is one of the most powerfully disturbing in the human experience, evoking a complex combination of not only pity and charity, but also revulsion, rejection, and guilt. Neurological disorders during infancy, childhood, and adolescence may adversely affect the acquisition of cognitive and emotional milestones. Developmental delays may profoundly influence the psychological state of the affected individuals and their caregivers. Many of the neurological conditions discussed in earlier sections of this chapter also appear in infantile and childhood forms. In addition, a large number of rarer genetic disorders appearing only in infants and children have specific effects on behavior. The diagnosis and treatment of biochemical and physiological disorders of the developing nervous system—the province of child neurology—aim to provide patients and caregivers with an understanding of and a sense of control over often overwhelming fears of suffering and anxiety.

The clinical neurological approach to infants and children, like the approach to adults, includes localization and identification of the lesion. Additionally, child neurologists are intensely concerned with determining whether a disorder is of genetic origin or is acquired, or both. As in all of medicine, the diagnosis in child neurology is made from history, physical examination, imaging, and laboratory tests. The rules of neurological localization that have been finely determined for adults generally apply with equal accuracy to children, but a clinical approach relying more on play and nonverbal cues is often used with infants and children, depending on the developmental stage.

PRINCIPLES OF BRAIN DEVELOPMENT

The adult brain consists of approximately 100 billion neurons, each of which receives, on average, 1,000 to 10,000 synapses from 1,000 other neurons. The study of the development of the nervous system is an actively evolving body of knowledge. In the brain, the life cycle of a neuron consists of cell birth in circumscribed proliferative zones, migration to the adult location, extension of an axon, elaboration of dendrites, synaptogenesis, and, finally, onset of chemical neurotransmission. At the peak of neuronal proliferation in the middle of the second trimester of gestation, 250,000 neurons are born each minute. Postmitotic neurons migrate to their adult locations in the cortex, guided by glial fibers (Fig. 2.13–1). Glial-guided neuronal migration in the cerebral cortex occupies much of the first 6 months of gestation. In the cerebellum, glial-guided neuronal migration continues through the second postnatal year. For some neurons in the prefrontal cortex, migration occurs over a distance that is 5,000 times the diameter of the neuronal cell body. Radial migration forms cortical columns that function as a unit in processing tasks (Fig. 2.13–2). Neuronal migration requires a complex set of cell–cell interactions, and it is susceptible to errors, in which neurons fail to reach the cortex and instead reside in ectopic positions. A group of such incorrectly placed neurons is called a *heterotopia* (Fig. 2.13–3). Neuronal heterotopias have been shown to cause epilepsy and are highly associated with mental retardation. In a classical neuropathological study of four patients with dyslexia, for example, heterotopias were a common finding. Heterotopias in the frontal lobe have been postulated to play a causal role in some cases of schizophrenia. Cortical neuronal migration abnormalities have been found in some people with autism, smaller cortical structures have been found in people with Down syndrome, larger basal ganglia have been found in people with schizophrenia, hypoplastic basal ganglia have been found in people with Tourette's syndrome, and hypoplastic cerebellar structures have been found in numerous developmental disorders. Normal cerebral asymmetries appear to be disrupted in a number of disorders, including schizophrenia, Tourette's syndrome, attention-deficit/hyperactivity disorder (ADHD), and dyslexia. Table 2.13–1 relates developmental events to severe malformations.

Many neurons lay an axon down as they migrate, whereas others do not initiate axon outgrowth until they have reached their cortical targets. Elaboration of a characteristic branched dendritic tree occurs once the neuron has completed migration (Fig. 2.13–4). Synaptogenesis occurs at an astounding rate from the second trimester through the first 10 years or so of life. The peak of synaptogenesis occurs in the first 2 postnatal years, when as many as 30 million synapses form each second. Ensheathing of axons by myelin begins prenatally, proceeds most rapidly in early childhood, and reaches its full extent late in the third decade of life (Fig. 2.13–5). Glucose use, protein synthesis, and cellular metabolic rates in the brain reach their highest levels in the first decade of life, as the brain forms its adult intercellular connections (Fig. 2.13–6).

The effect of experience on the formation of brain circuitry in the first years of life has generated a tremendous interest among neurologists. There are clear examples of the impact of early sensory experience on the wiring of cortical sensory processing areas. Similarly, early movement patterns are known to reinforce neural connections in the supplemental motor area. A common mechanism has emerged in which axons are guided by positional cues to the general target

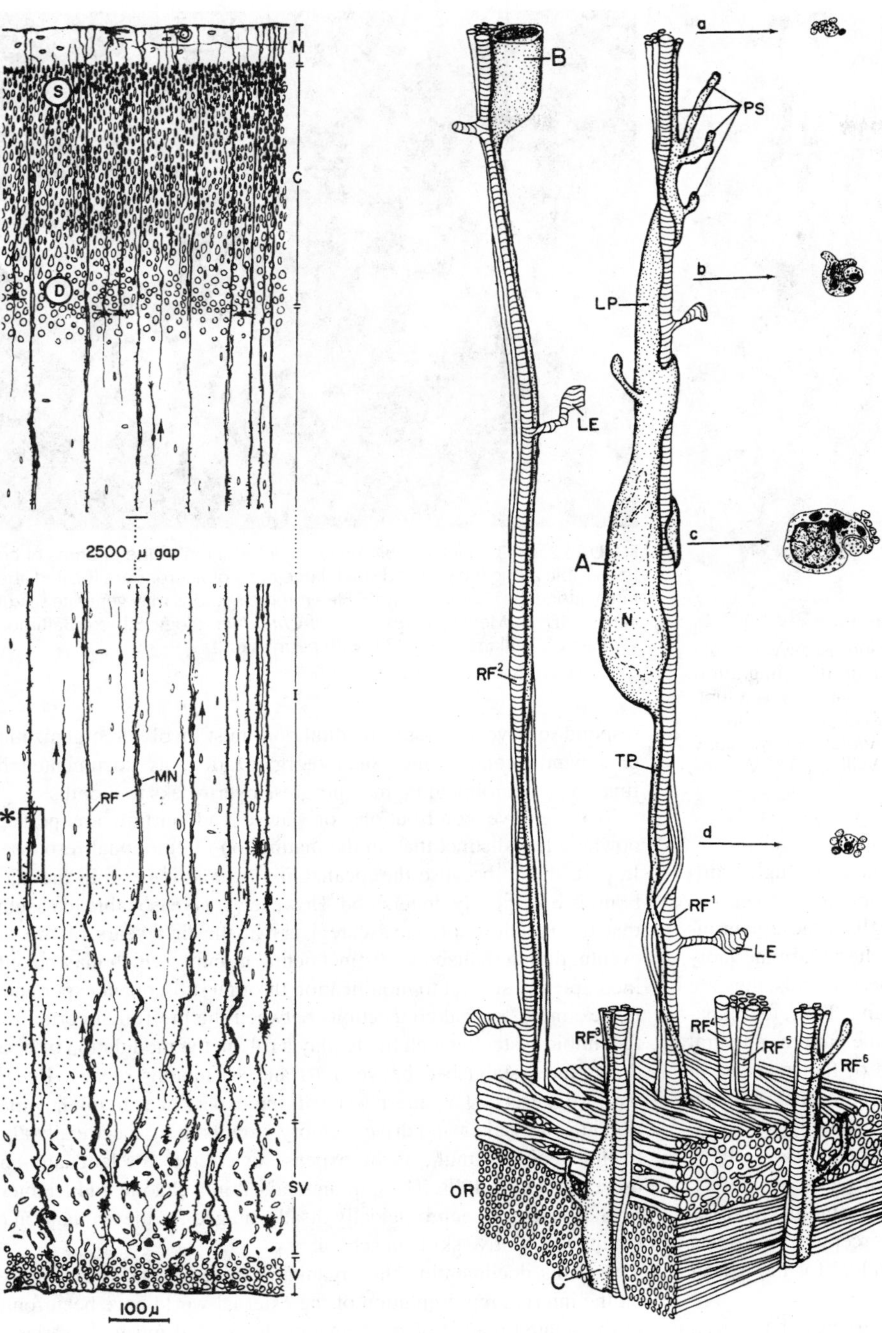

FIGURE 2.13–1 Left: Diagram of the cerebral cortex at mid-gestation. Radially oriented glial fibers guide the migration of neurons from the proliferative zones to the cortical plate. The rectangle marked with an asterisk shows a migrating neuron that is shown enlarged on the right. C, cortical plate; D, deep; I, intermediate zone; M, molecular layer; MN, migrating neuron; RF, radial fiber; S, superficial; SV, subventricular zone; V, ventricular zone. **Right:** Enlarged view of neurons migrating along glial fibers. A leading process (LP) precedes the nucleus as the neuron inches its way up the fiber, laying down a trailing process (TP). A, migrating neuron; B, migrating neuron; C, migrating neuron; LE, lamellate expansion; N, nucleus; OR, optic radiations; PS, pseudopodia; RF, radial fiber. (From Rakic P. Development of the cerebral cortex in human and nonhuman primates. In: Lewis M, ed. *Child and Adolescent Psychiatry: A Comprehensive Textbook.* 2nd ed. Baltimore: Williams & Wilkins; 1996:14, with permission.)

area and then use activity-dependent mechanisms to refine final connections. Arriving axons rapidly form a several-fold excess of synaptic connections, then, through a process of elimination, only those synapses persist that serve a relevant function. Synaptic pruning appears to preserve input in which the presynaptic cell fires in synchrony with the postsynaptic cell. This serves to reinforce neural circuits that are activated repeatedly. Neuroscientists assume that, as demonstrated experimentally in sensory and motor areas, experience plays a critical role in the modulation of the synaptic connectivity of cognitive and emotional association areas. However, the relative contributions of genetic and experiential influences on the connectivity of higher order processing and associational areas remain virtually unknown.

An emerging concept of great significance to child and adult psychiatry is the existence of early windows of time during which the brain adapts the basic circuitry for language, emotion, logic, mathematics, movements, and music to the environment. These windows open within the first few months of life and may close, in some cases, by 1 year of age. For example, a *perceptual map* of phonemes, the building blocks of language, is formed within the higher auditory processing areas of Wernicke's area during the first 12 months of life. The significance of this perceptual map is illustrated by the fact that there are certain sounds used by non–English-speaking peoples that are not found in English. Studies have shown that American babies younger than 6 months of age can be taught to discriminate these non-English sounds, but babies older than 6 months are no

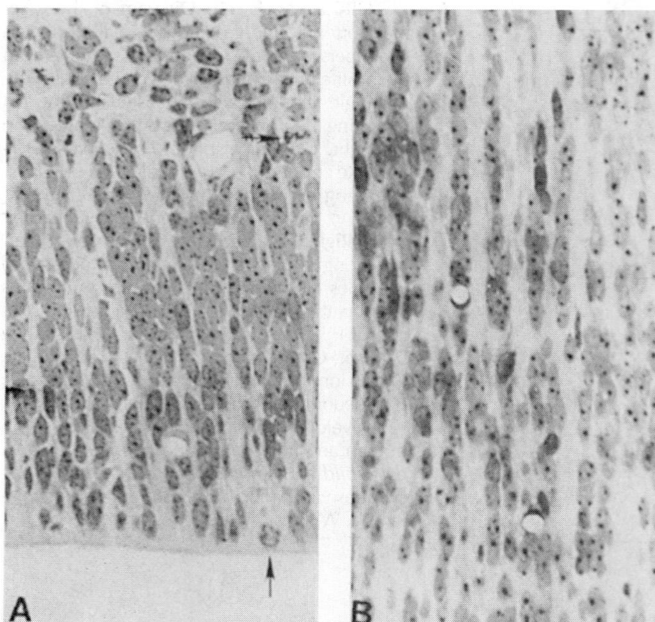

FIGURE 2.13–2 Radial organization of cortical columns. **A:** Ventricular proliferative zone, where neurons are born and begin their migration. **B:** Cortical plate. Each column responds to a specific stimulus as a functional unit. (From Rakic P. Development of the cerebral cortex in human and nonhuman primates. In: Lewis M, ed. *Child and Adolescent Psychiatry: A Comprehensive Textbook.* 2nd ed. Baltimore: Williams & Wilkins; 1996:13, with permission.)

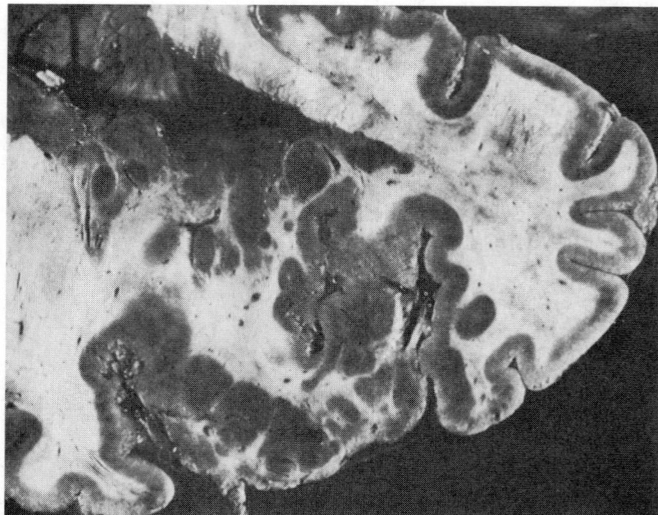

FIGURE 2.13–3 Heterotopic neurons. In addition to the neurons of cortex, visible along the gyri and sulci, large nests of neurons are located aberrantly along the ventricular wall. Heterotopic neurons may generate seizure activity. (From Menkes J. *Textbook of Child Neurology.* 5th ed. Baltimore: Williams & Wilkins; 1995:282, with permission.)

longer capable of hearing them. Moreover, the map for English differs from that for Japanese, for example, in the location of neurons that respond to the sounds "ra" and "la." In English, these neurons are located far apart within the auditory cortex, whereas, in the Japanese brain, which has difficulty distinguishing these sounds, they are so closely intertwined as to be virtually overlapping. Thus, to a Japanese individual, "la" and "ra" elicit nearly the same pattern of neural activity, a fact that may underlie the difficulties of the Japanese in distinguishing these sounds. Indistinct cortical representations can be segregated with practice, however. In the English language, studies have shown that babies of mothers who spoke loquaciously to them acquired a larger vocabulary than babies of taciturn mothers. These findings suggest that early experiences may establish the density and fidelity of neural circuits for specific perceptual functions, the consequences of which may affect the individual for the rest of his or her life.

In the realm of emotion, early childhood experiences have been suspected to be at the root of psychopathology since the earliest theories of Sigmund Freud. Franz Alexander's psychoanalytic method aimed to trace the threads of the earliest childhood memories to allow the patient to relive them in a less pathological environment, a process he termed a *corrective emotional experience.* Although neuroscientists have no data yet to bring this method down to the level of neurons and circuits, results are emerging that demonstrate a profound effect of the reactions of early caregivers on an adult individual's emotional repertoire. For example, the concept of *attunement* is defined as the process by which caregivers "play back a child's inner feelings." If a baby's emotional expressions are reciprocated in a consistent and sensitive manner, then certain emotional circuits are reinforced. These circuits likely include the limbic system and, in particular, the amygdala, which serves as a gate to the hippocampal memory circuits for emotional stimuli. The ability to learn and to respond to psychotherapy in adulthood must involve reorganization of synaptic connections. Such reorganization, as documented by functional neuroimaging, may progress over weeks to months.

The relative contributions of nature and nurture are perhaps nowhere less distinct than in the maturation of emotional responses. In part, this is because the localization of emotion within the adult brain is only poorly understood. However, it is reasonable to assume that the reactions of one's caregivers in the first years of life are eventually internalized as distinct neural circuits, which may be only incompletely subject to modification through subsequent experience. For example, axonal connections between the prefrontal cortex and the limbic system, which likely play a role in the modulation of basic drives, are established between 10 and 18 months of age. Recent work suggests that a pattern of terrifying experiences in infancy may flood the amygdala and drive memory circuits to be specifically alert to threatening stimuli, at the expense of circuits for language and other academic skills. Thus, infants raised in a chaotic and frightening home may be neurologically disadvantaged for the acquisition of complex cognitive skills in school.

Results documenting the organizing effect of early experiences on the internal representation of the external world have been found in the related realms of mathematics, logic, and music. A series of recent studies has shown that groups of children who were given 8 months of intensive classical music lessons in the preschool years subsequently showed significantly improved spatial and mathematical reasoning compared to a control group. In grade school, nonmusical tasks such as navigating mazes, drawing geometric figures, and copying patterns of two-color blocks were performed significantly more skillfully by the musical children. Early exposure to music may thus be an ideal preparation for later acquisition of complex mathematical and engineering skills.

These observations suggest a neurological basis for the developmental theories of Jean Piaget, Erik Erikson, Margaret Mahler, John Bowlby, Sigmund Freud, and others. Erikson's epigenetic theory states that normal adult behavior results from the successful, sequential completion of each of several infantile and childhood stages. According to the epigenetic model, the failure to complete an early

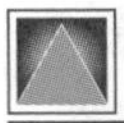

Table 2.13–1
Timetable of Human Central Nervous System Ontogenesis

Gestation Period	Event	Effect of Toxic Stimulus
0–18 days	Three germ layers elaborate, and early neural plate forms	No effect or death
18 days	Neural plate and groove develop	Anterior midline defects (18 to 23 days)
22–23 days	Optic vesicles appear	"Induction" hydrocephalus (18 to 60 days)
24–26 days	Anterior neuropore closed	Anencephaly (after 23 days to ?)
26–28 days	Posterior neuropore closed; ventral horns form	Cranium bifidum, spina bifida cystica; spina bifida occult (after 26 days to ?)
28–32 days	Anterior and posterior nerve roots form	—
32 days	Cerebellar primordium; vascular circulation	Microcephaly (30 to 130 days); cellular proliferation syndromes (30 to 175 days), migration anomalies (30 days to complete development of each brain subdivision)
33–35 days	Prosencephalon cleaves to form paired telencephalon; five cerebral vesicles; choroid plexi and dorsal root ganglion develop	Holoprosencephaly
41 days	Region of olfactory bulb appears in forebrain	Arrhinencephaly
56 days	Differentiation of cerebral cortex; meninges, ventricular foramina; cerebrospinal fluid circulation	Dandy-Walker syndrome
70–100 days	Corpus callosum	Agenesis of corpus callosum
70–150 days	Primary fissures of cerebral cortex; spinal cord ends at L3 level	Lissencephaly; pachygyria
140–175 days	Neuronal proliferation in cerebral cortex ends	Defects of cellular architectonics, myelin defects (175 days to 4 years postnatally)
7–9 mos	Secondary and tertiary sulci	Destructive pathological changes first noted
175 days to 4 yrs postnatally	Neuronal migration; glial cell production; myelin formation; axosomatic and axodendritic synaptic connections; spinal cord ends at L1 to L2 level	—

From Menkes J. *Textbook of Child Neurology.* 5th ed. Baltimore: Williams & Wilkins; 1995, with permission.

stage is reflected in subsequent physical, cognitive, social, or emotional maladjustment. By analogy, the experimental data discussed previously suggest that early experience, particularly during the critical window of opportunity for establishment of neural connections, primes the basic circuitry for language, emotions, and other advanced behaviors. Clearly, miswiring of the brain in infancy may later lead to severe handicaps when the individual attempts to relate to the world at an adult level. On the other hand, genetic determinants and peer interactions are probably at least as important factors in the emergence of the adult personality. Brain development is achieved through the molecular interactions of thousands of gene products. Neurological disorders of infancy and childhood resulting from genetic mutations or from influences external to the brain may thus hinder the proper emergence of mature emotional reactions.

CLASSIFICATION OF DISORDERS IN CHILD NEUROLOGY

An abnormality of mental function due to a neurological condition is called an *encephalopathy*. Encephalopathies are broadly defined as *static* or *progressive*. Children with static encephalopathies gain developmental milestones at a slower rate than healthy age-matched controls but do not lose abilities that they have acquired. Progressive encephalopathies, in contrast, are characterized by a loss of milestones and are prognostically much worse. Either type of encephalopathy may be due to a genetic defect or to an acquired condition, such as infection, trauma, asphyxia, or tumor. In progressive encephalopathies, genetic variants that encode defective versions of crucial organellar proteins may prevent the proper maintenance of cellular homeostasis and may lead to accumulation of toxic molecules on a time scale of days, months, or years. Examples of these disorders include lysosomal storage diseases, mitochondrial disorders, peroxisomal disorders, and metal transport disorders. Compromise of the vascular supply to the brain caused by stroke or hypotension can interfere with cellular metabolism and can produce permanent neuronal damage. Infectious agents can injure neurons directly or indirectly, as a result of an excessive immune response. Space-occupying lesions can disrupt neuronal activity by interrupting intercellular pathways or by compromising the blood supply.

Disorders of the gray matter are called *poliodystrophies* and are characterized by dementia and seizures. Disorders of the white matter are called *leukodystrophies* and are characterized by spasticity, ataxia, and optic atrophy. Many progressive encephalopathies contain features of gray and white matter diseases. Storage diseases consist of accumulations of unmetabolized waste products, which may be found in any of a large number of cell types. The combination of specific cell types in which storage products accumulate determines the neurological deficits.

The age of the patient at the time of an acquired insult and the extent of the insult are the main determinants of the prognosis of an acquired encephalopathy. Younger patients are more susceptible to infection and metabolic stress, but they are also more resilient than older patients in that they generally can recover a larger degree of previous function after a comparable insult. Premature birth is a major cause of static encephalopathy, and there is a strong correlation between low birth weight (LBW) and delays in cognitive and emotional development.

NEUROLOGICAL ASSESSMENT IN INFANTS AND CHILDREN

The neurological assessment in infants and children consists of a thorough history, beginning with conception and proceeding through pregnancy, birth, early neonatal course, subsequent hospitalizations,

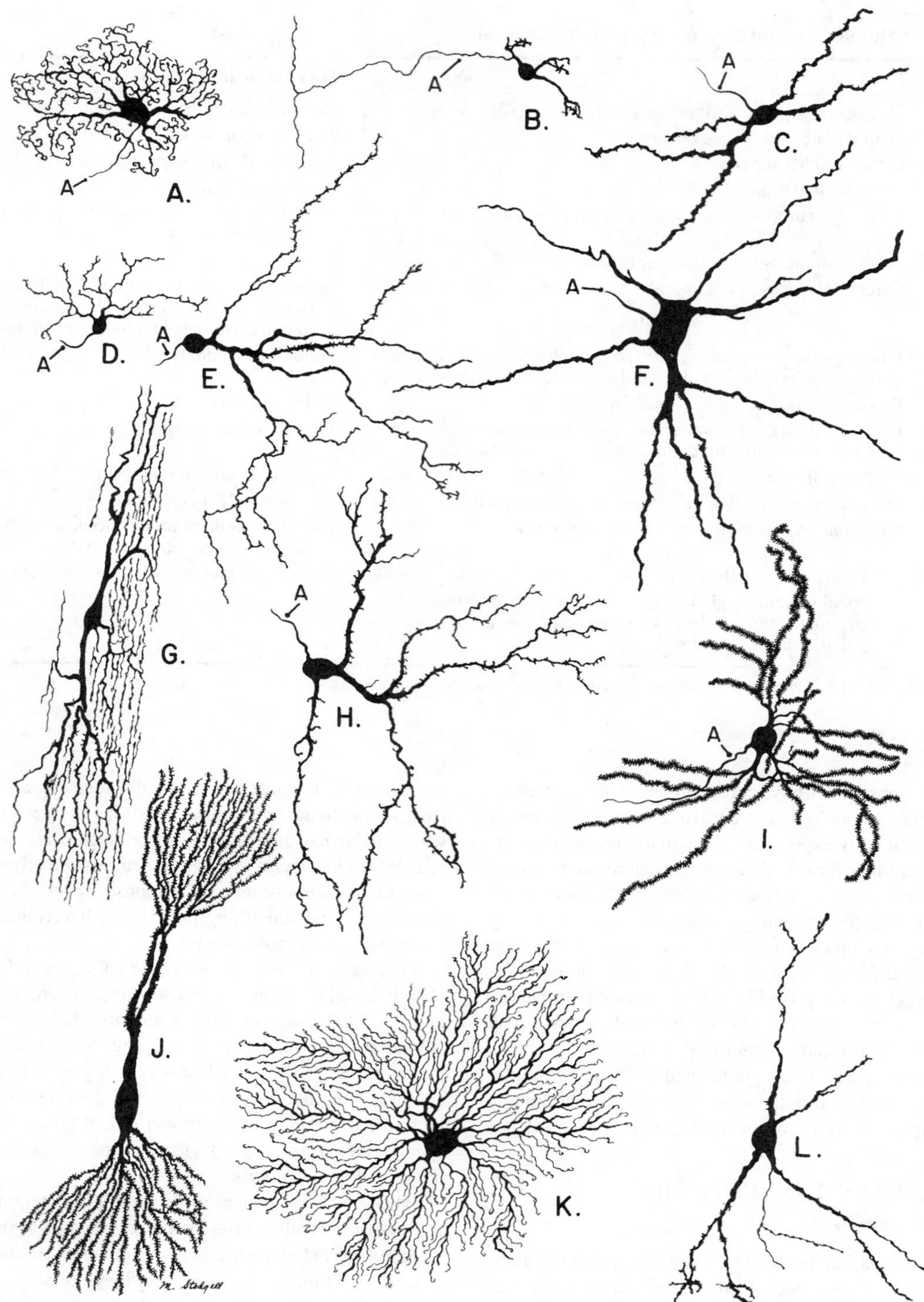

FIGURE 2.13–4 Characteristic neurons whose axons (A) and dendrites remain within the central nervous system. **A:** Neuron of the inferior olivary nucleus. **B:** Granule cell of the cerebellar cortex. **C:** Small cell of the reticular formation. **D:** Small gelatinosa cell of the spinal trigeminal nucleus. **E:** Ovoid cell of the nucleus tractus solitarius. **F:** Large cell of the reticular formation. **G:** Spindle-shaped cell of the substantia gelatinosa of the spinal cord. **H:** Large cell of the spinal trigeminal nucleus. **I:** Neuron of the putamen. **J:** Double pyramidal cell in the horn of Ammon of the hippocampal formation. **K:** Cell from the thalamus. **L:** Cell from the globus pallidus. (From Parent A. *Carpenter's Human Neuroanatomy.* 9th ed. Baltimore: Williams & Wilkins; 1996:143, with permission.)

chronic medical conditions, acquisition of milestones in each category of normal development, medications, allergies, and family history, including consanguinity, social history, and a review of systems (Table 2.13–2). Neurological examination includes mental status examination, cranial nerves, motor system, associated motor system (coordination), sensory system, and reflexes. The neurological examination must be tailored to the age and abilities of the infant or child. Normal development is assessed in the categories of gross motor, fine motor, speech and language, and social and adaptive abilities. In younger patients, assessments often rely more on observa-

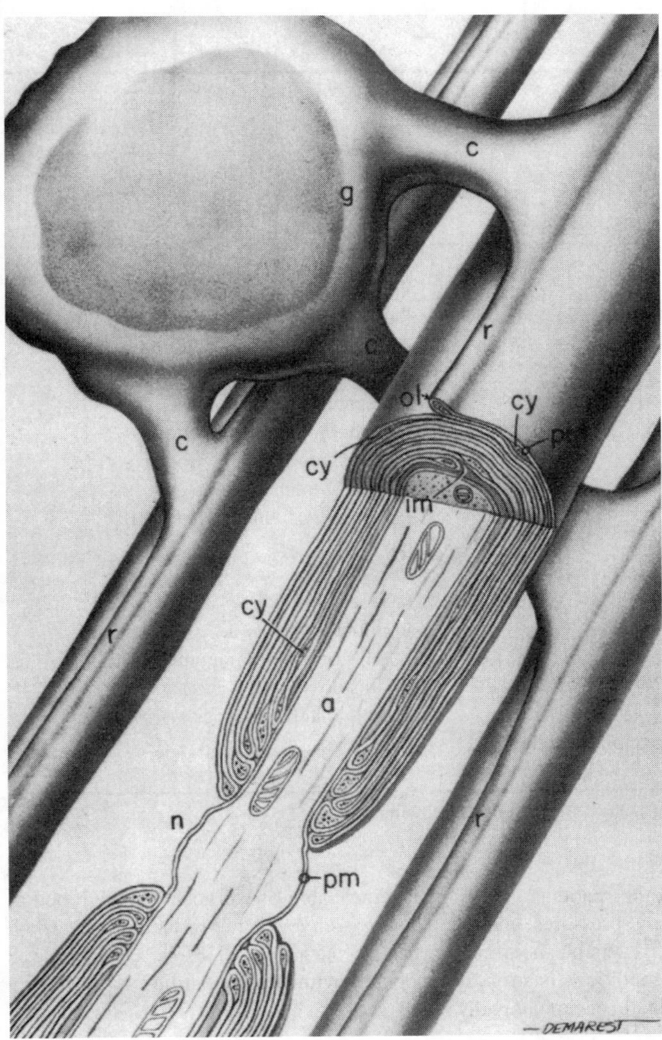

FIGURE 2.13–5 Relationship of the oligodendrocyte (g) and the central myelin sheath to the axon (a). c, cytoplasmic process; cy, glial cell cytoplasm trapped among the layers of myelin; im, inner mesaxon; n, node of Ranvier; ol, outer lamina; pm, plasma membrane; r, ridge. (From Parent A. *Carpenter's Human Neuroanatomy.* 9th ed. Baltimore: Williams & Wilkins; 1996:213, with permission.)

tion and play interactions than on direct questioning. Subtle adaptive deficiencies may be missed in young children, even with detailed testing, and may only become apparent as the age-appropriate context becomes more complex.

Standardized tests of neuropsychological functions may be useful in discriminating between adaptive disorders and primary psychiatric conditions. Parents are the best sources of information about a child's behavior, and confirmatory assessment by teachers or other caregivers may yield important clues to a child's behavioral repertoire.

STATIC ENCEPHALOPATHIES

Static encephalopathies are the sequelae of acute insults to the developing brain that damage brain cells or the result of a genetic deficiency that renders information processing abnormally inefficient but that does not result in storage of metabolic products or ongoing cellular damage. Static encephalopathies are much more common than progressive encephalopathies, yet they are much less likely to

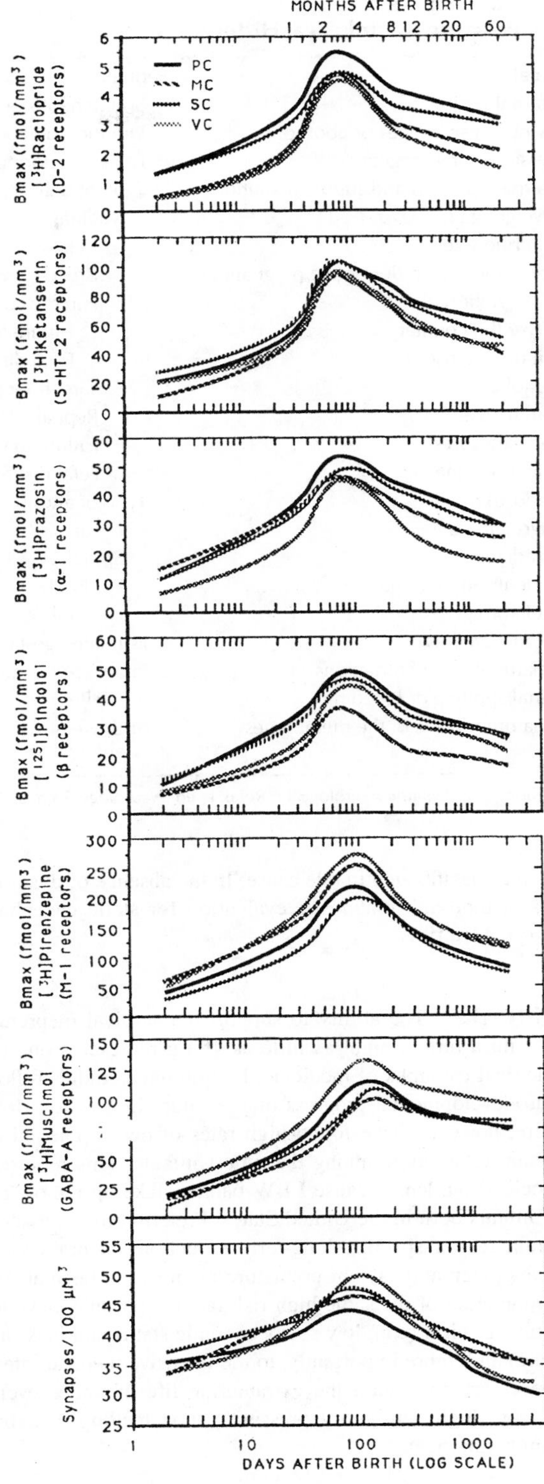

FIGURE 2.13–6 Developmental changes in the density of synapses and receptors in the prefrontal (PC), primary motor (MC), somatosensory (SC), and primary visual (VC) cortical regions. Age is presented in postnatal days on a logarithmic scale. Density of synapses is greatest at 2 to 4 months of age, then it declines as functionally irrelevant synapses are pruned according to experience. Bmax, maximum binding; D_2, dopamine type 2; $GABA_A$, γ-aminobutyric acid type A; ^3H, hydrogen-3; 5-HT_2, serotonin type 2; ^{125}I, iodine-125; M_1, muscarinic acetylcholine type 1. (From Rakic P. Development of the cerebral cortex in human and nonhuman primates. In: Lewis M, ed. *Child and Adolescent Psychiatry: A Comprehensive Textbook.* 2nd ed. Baltimore: Williams & Wilkins; 1996:22, with permission.)

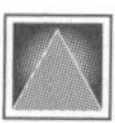

Table 2.13–2
Pediatric Neurological History

- Antenatal
  - Maternal parity
  - Previous miscarriages or abortions
  - Illnesses during pregnancy
  - Maternal nutrition and supplementation
    - Weight gain
    - Uterine size
  - Medications taken during the pregnancy
    - Prescription
    - Over the counter
  - Illicit drug abuse
  - Alcohol use
  - Cigarette use
  - Toxic exposures
    - Occupational
    - Industrial
    - Agricultural
    - Irradiation
  - Accidents and trauma
  - Travel abroad
  - Fetal movements
  - Premature labor contractions
  - Vaginal spotting or bleeding
  - Premature rupture of the membranes
- Perinatal
  - Spontaneous or induced labor
  - Duration of labor
  - Fetal monitoring during labor
  - Type of delivery
    - Vaginal
      - Vertex
      - Breech
      - Forceps- or vacuum-assisted
        - Failure to progress
        - Fetal distress
    - Cesarean section
      - Repeat
      - Failure to progress
      - Fetal distress
  - Type of anesthesia, if any
    - Local
    - Spinal
    - Epidural
    - General
  - Estimated gestational age at time of delivery
  - Infant's appearance at birth and need for resuscitation—Apgar score, if recalled
  - Birth weight, length, frontooccipital circumference
- Neonatal complications
  - Jaundice
  - Temperature
  - Breathing
  - Feeding: breast, bottle, tube
  - Length of time in hospital until released home
- Neurodevelopment
  - Progressing or regressing
  - Development of handedness
  - Attainment of major milestones
  - Academic performance in school
- Immunizations
  - Diphtheria-pertussis-tetanus
  - Measles, mumps, and rubella
  - Bacille Calmette-Guérin
  - *Haemophilus influenzae* type B
- Behavior
  - Peer relations
  - Interpersonal skills
  - Conduct
- Family history—consanguinity
- Social history
  - Intrafamilial psychosocial stressors
  - Pets

From Wilfong AA. Pediatric neurology. In: Rolak L, ed. *Neurology Secrets.* Philadelphia: Hanley & Belfus; 1993, with permission.

be due to a specific identifiable cause. In the absence of dysmorphic features, a thorough diagnostic evaluation for static encephalopathies is often fruitless.

Prematurity The ability to support the survival of premature infants with a birth weight as little as 450 g represents one of the technological triumphs of medicine. Longitudinal studies following the neurodevelopmental progress of premature infants for 10 years and more, however, have found high rates of developmental delay and mental retardation among the tiniest infants. This represents a large societal burden, because LBW babies make up almost 8 percent of infants born in the United States. Preterm birth is associated with brain region–specific, long-term reductions in brain volume. The developmental delays of premature infants have been attributed to a combination of the same high-risk factors that may have led to the premature birth (e.g., low socioeconomic status and lack of prenatal care) and, more importantly, to the intensive medical interventions necessary to sustain the extrauterine life of underdeveloped babies (e.g., high ventilatory pressures, tube feeding, and broad-spectrum antibiotics).

Classification *LBW* is defined as less than 2,500 g, *very low birth weight* (VLBW) is defined as less than 1,500 g, and *extremely low birth weight* (ELBW) is defined as less than 1,000 g. The main factor determining the morbidity and mortality of premature infants is their pulmonary status: Immature lungs are capable of sufficiently oxygenating the blood only when ventilated at high pressures. These pressures increase the intrathoracic pressure and, in turn, increase the intracranial venous pressure, which may cause hemorrhage of blood from the capillaries of the germinal matrix of the brain. In other patients, the lungs are incapable of oxygenating the blood at any pressures, and the blood oxygen levels fall to the point at which irreversible neuronal damage occurs (Fig. 2.13–7). Each of these conditions is strongly associated with subsequent development of a static encephalopathy.

Intracranial Hemorrhage Four grades of intracranial hemorrhage in the premature infant are recognized. Grade I consists of hemorrhage due to high venous pressures limited to the germinal matrix. In grade II, blood also bursts into the adjacent lateral ventricle but does not cause ventricular dilatation. Grade III occurs when the ventricles dilate because the intraventricular blood clogs the drainage of cerebrospinal fluid (CSF). Grade IV, in a contrasting mechanism, results from hypoxic-ischemic injury to cerebral blood vessels in states of very low blood oxygen tension and low blood pressure. When blood at normal pressures subsequently reperfuses damaged vessels, it leaks into the brain in several areas. In extreme cases, large regions of cortex are destroyed, leaving CSF-filled cysts.

Neurodevelopmental Outcome LBW babies are one-fourth to one-half as likely to graduate from high school by 19 years of age as their normal-birth-weight siblings. VLBW babies are eight times more likely to have mental retardation and 24 times more likely to have movement disorders, known as *cerebral palsy*, than are full-term babies. The types of cerebral palsy are spastic quadriparetic, spastic diplegic, hemiplegic, pseudobulbar, and choreoathetotic. Several longitudinal studies have documented an average lowering of IQ scores of 6 to 14 points in cohorts of VLBW infants. Among ELBW infants, as many as 50 to 80 percent required some level of special education by 10 years of age, as compared to 15 percent of full-term infants by the same age. In infants who had intra-

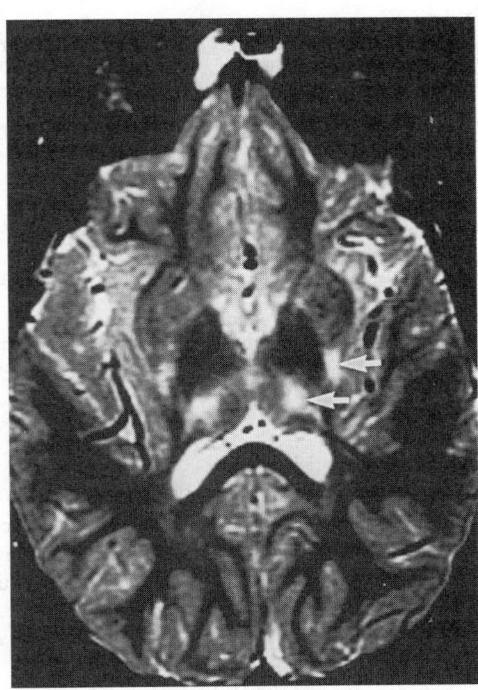

FIGURE 2.13–7 Axial T2-weighted magnetic resonance image at the level of the thalamus, illustrating bilaterally symmetrical hyperintensities in the thalamus (*arrows*). These scars are the result of severe hypoxic-ischemic injury due to birth asphyxia. At 6 years of age, this child had predominantly choreoathetotic cerebral palsy and below normal intelligence. (From Menkes J. *Textbook of Child Neurology.* 5th ed. Baltimore: Williams & Wilkins; 1995:355, with permission.)

cranial hemorrhage, grades I and II generally were not associated with additional cognitive delays, but grade III and, especially, grade IV hemorrhages posed a considerable increased risk of scholastic underachievement during childhood.

Ex-premature infants register higher scores on scales of childhood anxiety, depression, social isolation, conduct disorder, and aggression. The best predictors of these outcomes is the degree of prematurity, whereas neurological evaluations or cranial ultrasonograms in the neonatal period were not predictive of emotional outcome. In general, premature infants are rated as less temperamental as young toddlers, but, as late toddlers, they are rated as more withdrawn and more prone to tantrums. In childhood, 5 to 35 percent of ex-premature infants fit the diagnostic criteria for ADHD, compared to 3 to 15 percent of ex–full-term infants. Particular reasons for this increased risk of ADHD among ex-premature infants may include the fact that low socioeconomic status (SES) is associated with prematurity and ADHD. Another possible reason is that the germinal matrix in which hemorrhages occur in premature infants later gives rise to the caudate nucleus, which has been increasingly implicated in the pathogenesis of ADHD in neurobiological studies.

Strokes Prenatal strokes most commonly occur in the distribution of the middle cerebral artery (MCA) and therefore damage the frontal and parietal lobes. The most common presenting features are seizures and hemiparesis. In longitudinal follow-up studies, mean IQ was in the normal range, but the laterality of the lesion did correlate with lower scores on specific subtests: Left MCA infarctions reduced verbal IQ scores, whereas right MCA infarctions lowered nonverbal IQ scores. Studies of hemispherically injured infants have suggested, with variable consistency, that the adult model of hemispherical localization of emotional responses, in which activation of the left frontal lobe raises mood and activation of the right frontal lobe depresses mood, is evident even at younger than 1 year of age. Other data appear to contradict this model: Lesions that inactivate the right frontal lobe in children unexpectedly elicit more negative behavior. The frontal cortex has various specialized regions that play largely unknown roles in the expression of emotions, and the clinically documented lesions have not yet been systematically characterized to allow a specific correlation between site of lesion and behavioral manifestation, even in adults. At this time, no generalizations can be made from longitudinal studies regarding the emotional consequences of prenatal and childhood ischemic injuries. Children with cognitive and motor disabilities caused by strokes use special education resources much more than children who have not had strokes, and they are more susceptible to a range of psychiatric symptoms, especially depression.

Chromosomal Anomalies The genetic basis of behavior is only beginning to be understood. Epidemiological studies have suggested a significant heritable component to all major psychiatric disorders. The majority of static encephalopathies are due to spontaneous genetic variations. Most children with static encephalopathies do not have characteristic dysmorphic features, and there are, at present, no genetic screening tests available to determine the etiology of their delays. There is reason to believe that such diagnostic tools may emerge in the coming decades, but the inherent variability of clinical expression of current well-characterized genetic variants must temper enthusiasm for the establishment of a genetic explanation for behavior. At the same time, the isolation of genes even partially responsible for specific cognitive functions and emotional repertoires is a high priority. Three chromosomal syndromes have characteristic neuropsychiatric manifestations other than simple mental retardation: fragile X syndrome, Williams syndrome, and Down syndrome.

Fragile X Syndrome Fragile X syndrome is characterized by mental retardation (IQ ranges from 35 to 70), hyperlexia without comprehension, deficits in executive function and visuospatial attention, autism, aggressivity, impulsivity, and depression. Dysmorphic features include macroorchidism, large head, elongated palpebral fissures, and large ears. There are no characteristic abnormalities in brain structure. After Down syndrome, it is the second most common identified genetic cause of mental retardation (1 in 4,000 people), affecting boys almost exclusively. The genetic defect is the expansion of a trinucleotide deoxyribonucleic acid (DNA) repeat in the gene *FMR-1* on the X chromosome. This expansion causes fragility of the chromosome when cells are grown in a folate-deficient medium. The mutation silences expression of the gene, resulting in absence of the FMR proteins, a series of ribosome-associated ribonucleic acid (RNA)–binding proteins generated by alternative splicing of *FMR-1* transcripts. Recently, a highly accurate polymerase chain reaction (PCR) test has become available to identify affected individuals and female carriers. It is reasonable to screen mildly to moderately retarded male children with the PCR test, if the family wishes to exhaust the diagnostic possibilities. It should be emphasized, however, that fragile X syndrome accounts for less than 4 percent of people with mental retardation and is not a cause of academic difficulties in the absence of mental retardation. There is no specific treatment for fragile X syndrome, other than special education and psychiatric care.

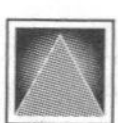

Table 2.13–3
Classification of Traumatic Intracranial Lesions

Primary lesions
Intraaxial
Diffuse axonal injury
Cortical contusion
Subcortical matter injury
Primary brainstem injury
Extraaxial hematomas
Extradural
Subdural
Diffuse hemorrhage
Subarachnoid
Intraventricular
Primary vascular injuries
Secondary lesions
Pressure necrosis (secondary to brain displacement and herniations)
Tentorial arterial infarction
Diffuse hypoxic injury
Diffuse brain swelling
Boundary and terminal zone infarction
Others
Fatty embolism
Secondary hemorrhage
Infection

From Menkes J. *Textbook of Child Neurology.* 5th ed. Baltimore: Williams & Wilkins; 1995, with permission.

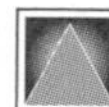

Table 2.13–4
Major Complications Seen in 71 Children after Recovery from Meningitis

Complication	Number of Cases
Mental retardation	3
Seizures	3
Hemiparesis or quadriparesis	1
Bilateral deafness	4
Vestibular disturbance	1
Hydrocephalus	1
Total	13 (18%)

From Menkes J. *Textbook of Child Neurology.* 5th ed. Baltimore: Williams & Wilkins; 1995, with permission.

Williams Syndrome Children with Williams syndrome exhibit a relative preservation of language abilities and may have an unusually large vocabulary. In marked contrast, their visuospatial abilities are severely impaired. For example, they may be able to describe the parts of a house in great detail but cannot draw a recognizable image of a house. They are capable of recognizing individual details but cannot recognize overall patterns in an image. The deficient functions are those usually ascribed to the right hemisphere, although the correlation is not complete. Neuropathological studies show small parietal lobes, narrowing of the corpus callosum, and abnormal proportions of the cortical layers. Genetic studies have implicated a mutation in the LIM–kinase I gene as the cause of the perceptual disturbance. The function of this gene is unknown. The relationship between the genotype and the phenotype is not understood, but further study promises to yield interesting insights into the biological basis of perception.

Down Syndrome In contrast to children with Williams syndrome, children with Down syndrome have relatively preserved visuospatial skills and more impaired verbal skills. Down syndrome children are generally docile and cheerful, but they may have outbursts of anger and hyperactivity. Children with the full Down syndrome phenotype harbor a third chromosome 21, whereas parts of the Down phenotype are seen if only part of an extra chromosome 21 is present. There are several genes in the extra segment, and efforts to correlate specific gene triplications with specific cognitive skills are ongoing.

Head Trauma The neuropsychiatric consequences of head trauma are directly related to the nature and severity of the impact. Mild injuries may or may not cause loss of consciousness, and, if no bleeding occurs, such injuries are called *concussions.* A postconcussive syndrome consisting variously of headache, somnolence, vomiting, syncope, dizziness, irritability, and amnesia for the event may last for days, weeks, or, in some cases, months. A longer duration of symptoms is associated with pretrauma depression and anxiety. The vast majority of children with mild head trauma have complete recovery.

Severe injuries are associated with intracranial hemorrhage, intracranial swelling, or both, and children who regain consciousness after such injuries have a high incidence of long-term behavioral changes (Table 2.13–3). Cognitive and learning disabilities are common, and willful, aggressive outbursts of behavior are characteristic, especially of frontal lobe damage. A multidisciplinary approach to the physical and mental handicaps caused by severe head trauma, including pharmacological and behavioral therapies, is available at specialized rehabilitation units.

Acute Infections Meningitis consists of an infection in the CSF, and encephalitis consists of an infection in the brain itself. The principal organisms are viruses and bacteria and, less commonly, fungi and tuberculosis. When aggressively treated with antibiotics and supportive care, the majority of children recover fully. The most common neurological sequela of bacterial meningitis is hearing loss (Table 2.13–4). A minority of patients with acute meningitis or encephalitis, or both, especially those with hypoxic-ischemic injury, exhibit long-term cognitive deficits and may become depressed or anxious.

PROGRESSIVE ENCEPHALOPATHIES

The neuropsychiatric consequences of progressive encephalopathies initially affect the child, but, as the child's mental functions progressively deteriorate, the caregivers increasingly demonstrate psychiatric symptoms. The stresses of watching a beloved child gradually lose skills, become vegetative, and eventually die are extremely burdensome and try even the strongest families. A thorough neurological evaluation is always indicated when a child begins to lose developmental milestones or ceases to gain milestones at his or her usual rate, suggesting a progressive impairment of functioning. The history and physical examination are often sufficient to narrow the differential diagnosis significantly, and focused neuroimaging and laboratory evaluations frequently indicate the diagnosis. It is of paramount importance to consider potentially treatable diseases and to offer prompt treatment to counteract the biochemical abnormality. Establishment of a diagnosis, even in untreatable conditions, is of value to the family to help them accept their situation and to permit genetic testing for future pregnancies, when applicable. For a small but increasing number of diseases, presymptomatic or even prenatal treatment is available.

Poliodystrophies *Poliodystrophy* refers to a disorder of the neuronal cell bodies, generally those in the cerebral cortex. The main presenting symptoms are seizures and loss of cognitive functions. Major psychiatric symptoms include loss of verbal communication, oppositional behavior, irritability, and inattentiveness. The poliodystrophies include the lipidoses, such as Tay-Sachs disease, Sandhoff's disease, Niemann-Pick disease, Gaucher's disease, Fabry's disease, and neuronal ceroid lipofuscinosis; the mucopolysaccharidoses, such as Hunter's syndrome, Hurler's syndrome, and Sanfilippo's syndrome; Alpers' disease; the mitochondrial encephalomyopathies, such as mitochondrial encephalopathy with lactic acidoses and stroke-like episodes (MELAS), Kearns-Sayre syndrome, myoclonic epilepsy with ataxia and ragged red fibers (MERRF), and Leigh disease; the epileptic encephalopathies, such as West's syndrome (infantile spasms), Lennox-Gastaut syndrome, and Rett's syndrome; and the hereditary movement disorders with dementia, such as Huntington's disease, ataxia-telangiectasia, Wilson's disease, and Lesch-Nyhan syndrome.

Leukodystrophies *Leukodystrophy* refers to a disorder of white matter, which consists of myelinated fiber tracts. The main presenting symptoms are spasticity, ataxia, and optic atrophy. Major psychiatric symptoms include disinhibition, impulsivity, poor judgment, and emotional lability. The leukodystrophies include metachromatic leukodystrophy, globoid cell leukodystrophy, adrenoleukodystrophy, Pelizaeus-Merzbacher disease, Canavan's disease, and Alexander's disease.

Treatment Recent experimental bone marrow replacement protocols have prevented progression and even reversed disease in metachromatic leukodystrophy, globoid cell leukodystrophy, adrenoleukodystrophy, and Hurler's syndrome. Gaucher's disease has been successfully treated with enzyme replacement therapy. Several dietary restrictions or supplements have been tried with varying success for leukodystrophies.

Chronic Infections

Acquired Immune Deficiency Syndrome (AIDS) Pediatric acquired immune deficiency syndrome (AIDS) is most frequently transmitted transplacentally. This transmission can be greatly reduced if the human immunodeficiency virus (HIV)–positive mother takes zidovudine (Retrovir) (also known as *azidothymidine* [AZT]) in the second half of pregnancy. Despite concerns that HIV-positive women would not seek prenatal care because they may not wish their HIV status to be entered in their medical records, it is clearly indefensible for prenatal clinics not to seek such women actively for testing and, if HIV-positive, to offer treatment with AZT. The fear of being identified as HIV-positive has been rendered moot by the recent institution of mandatory HIV testing for all newborns, the positive results of which immediately identify HIV-positive mothers, albeit too late for AZT treatment. Perinatal transmission via breast milk or blood transfusion is much less common and tends to cause milder neuropsychiatric symptoms. Survival in congenitally or perinatally acquired HIV infection is rare beyond 10 years of age.

Neurological symptoms, consisting of progressive motor dysfunction and loss of developmental milestones, and signs, particularly, deceleration of head growth, are the presenting features of AIDS in as much as 18 percent of children and adolescents. Unlike the psychiatric symptoms in HIV-positive adults, which frequently include acute psychosis, the main psychiatric symptoms in HIV-positive children more often are inattentiveness, impulsivity, depression, anxiety, and adjustment disorders. HIV-positive adolescents may also develop acute psychotic symptoms. Any acute change in mental status in an HIV-positive patient of any age requires a thorough neurological evaluation, possibly including neuroimaging, serologies, CSF examination, and brain biopsy. Nutritional status, especially thiamine levels, electrolyte homeostasis, thyroid function, and other metabolic or endocrine indicators should also be checked.

Any chronic infection in children may elicit a reactive depression, especially if family members are ill. The organic effects of HIV tend to exacerbate depression. The best therapeutic approach is to maintain a high level of activity for as long as possible, including schooling and peer activities.

Other Slowly Progressive Infections Other viral infections that may have minimal acute effects on the nervous system but that may produce a slowly progressive encephalopathy include progressive multifocal leukoencephalopathy, caused by the JC virus; subacute sclerosing panencephalitis, caused by the measles or rubella viruses; and chronic enteroviral infections. Spongiform encephalopathies, such as Creutzfeldt-Jakob disease, which is thought to be caused by a prion agent, may affect children, causing anxiety, impaired judgment, and rapid cognitive decline.

Inborn Errors of Metabolism Genetic defects in cellular metabolism may affect the functioning of specific regions of the brain. Wilson's disease, a treatable disorder of copper transport, if left untreated, may cause personality changes, impulsivity, social withdrawal, and flapping movements of the arms. Copper accumulates in the globus pallidus and putamen, cell loss is also seen in the substantia nigra and dentate nucleus, and astrocytes proliferate in the cerebral cortex, basal ganglia, brainstem nuclei, and cerebellum. Chelation therapy may reverse the symptoms, but the initial mobilization of copper by chelators may transiently increase neurological toxicity, sometimes for as long as several years. Infantile nephropathic cystinosis may cause visuospatial deficiencies due to loss of volume in the parietal and occipital regions before the initiation of therapy. Disorders of fatty acid oxidation may selectively affect verbal skills. Acute intermittent porphyria may cause panic attacks, depression, and agitated psychosis. Galactosemia, phenylketonuria, and ornithine transcarbamylase deficiency may cause mental retardation.

Acquired Metabolic Disorders Systemic metabolic disorders may affect behavior. Congenital hypothyroidism may cause severe retardation, which may be only partially reversed by postnatal thyroid replacement therapy. Acquired hypothyroidism in infants and children may cause disorders of spatial orientation, as well as general learning delays. Hyperthyroidism in children may cause hyperactivity, restlessness, and inattentiveness. Chronic hepatic and renal failure may cause deficits in visual learning and in memory.

Brain Tumors Brain tumors have been associated with the entire spectrum of behavioral disorders. The particular behavioral manifestations of a brain tumor are determined by its location, histological type, and size. Posterior fossa tumors may cause cerebellar and brainstem signs and may cause hydrocephalus. Supratentorial infiltrative glial tumors may penetrate nerve fiber tracts and may produce

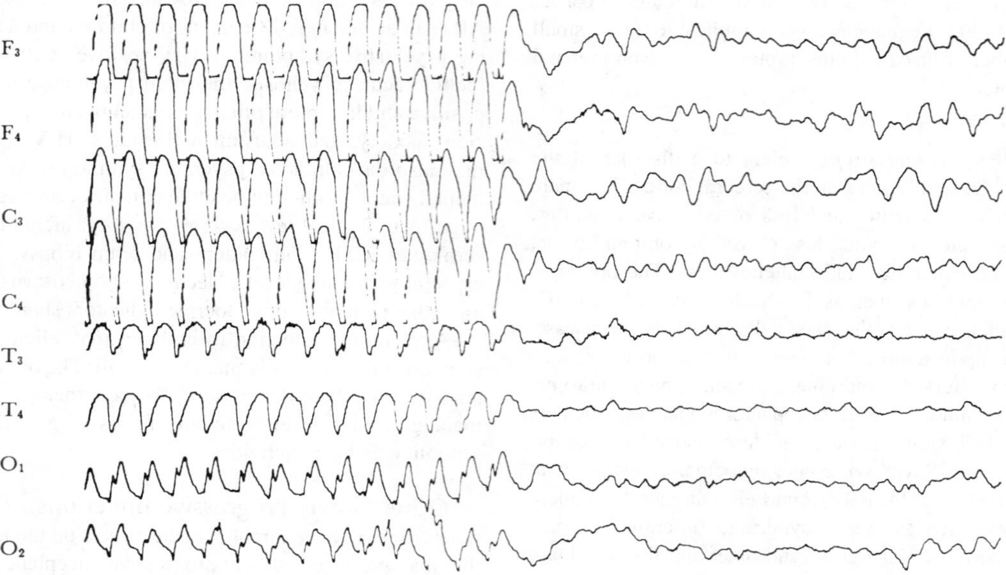

FIGURE 2.13–8 Three-per-second spike-wave discharges in an 11-year-old girl with frequent absence seizures induced by hyperventilation. C_3, left central; C_4, right central; F_3, left frontal; F_4, right frontal; O_1, left occipital; O_2, right occipital; T_3, left temporal; T_4, right temporal. (From Menkes J. *Textbook of Child Neurology.* 5th ed. Baltimore: Williams & Wilkins; 1995:738, with permission.)

dementia. In addition to the effects of the tumor itself, which may be seriously disabling or even deadly, a second risk factor for intellectual decline in survivors is cranial irradiation, which damages all cell types of the nervous system. For example, cystic cerebellar astrocytoma is a posterior fossa tumor typically treated with surgical resection but no irradiation, whereas surgical resection of another posterior fossa tumor, medulloblastoma, is usually followed by irradiation. In one long-term follow-up study, 62 percent of patients with cerebellar astrocytoma so treated had IQs greater than 90, whereas only 11 percent of patients with medulloblastoma treated with irradiation had IQs greater than 90, and 30 percent were in the retarded range. The IQ discrepancy widened over time. The addition of chemotherapy compounded the radiation-induced cognitive deficits.

The most common psychiatric disturbances in patients with brain tumors include reactive depression, oppositional behavior, anxiety disorders, and thought disorders. In some cases, treatment of the tumor improved these conditions, but, in others, new symptoms emerged during treatment. Family members may also be severely affected, especially siblings of the patient, some of whom may view the patient as no longer part of the family. Treatment should include cognitive interventions for the patient and psychiatric support for the patient and the family.

SEIZURE DISORDERS

Much of the neuropsychiatric aspect of epilepsy applies to children, although fewer detailed studies have been done in children. Several types of epilepsy are only seen in infancy and childhood, including infantile spasms, benign rolandic epilepsy, idiopathic generalized epilepsy of childhood, idiopathic absence epilepsy, and febrile seizures (Fig. 2.13–8). Focal seizures are relatively rarer in children than in adults, but they may produce a wide range of behavioral manifestations (Table 2.13–5).

Seventy to 80 percent of patients with seizures can expect good control with anticonvulsant medications. At a minimum, most

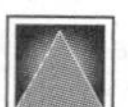
Table 2.13–5
Clinical Manifestations of Complex Partial Seizures in Childhood

	Number of Patients with Manifestations (Total, 25)		
Seizure Manifestation	**1–6 Yrs of Age**	**7–16 Yrs of Age**	**Total**
Aura	6	10	16
Altered consciousness	12	13	25
Change in position of body or limbs	10	11	21
Integrated, but confused, activity	8	11	19
Staring or dazed expression	10	8	18
Epigastric sensation, nausea, and vomiting	9	5	14
Oral movements and drooling	8	5	13
Muttering, mumbling, and hissing	5	5	10
Walking and wandering	4	6	10
Pallor or flushing	5	4	9
Rubbing or fumbling	4	5	9
Speech (usually irrelevant or incoherent)	3	5	8
Affective disturbance (fear and anger)	5	3	8
Stiffening of body or limbs	5	3	8
Falling	4	3	7
Aggressive activity	4	3	7
Dreamy state	2	3	5
Forced thinking or ideational blocking	1	4	5
Searching or orienting movements	1	3	4
Abdominal pain	3	1	4
Incontinence (urinary)	2	1	3
Perceptual disturbance (visual and auditory)	0	3	3

From Menkes J. *Textbook of Child Neurology.* 5th ed. Baltimore: Williams & Wilkins; 1995, with permission.

patients with seizures must take daily medication. Patients in whom seizure control is inadequate live with the specter that a seizure may strike them at any time. Thus, an event lasting, in some cases, 0.001 percent of the person's lifetime nevertheless exerts a pervasive influence on the person's activities. This may lead to parental overprotection, teasing from peers, and disruption of social adjustment. If seizures have been controlled for at least 6 months, and serum levels are in the therapeutic range, then activity restrictions usually may be liberalized to include all activities except climbing, horseback riding, diving into deep water, unsupervised swimming, or using dangerous equipment.

There is no single behavioral disorder found in all patients with epilepsy. Children with childhood absence epilepsy tend to be passive and dependent. Children with temporal lobe focal epilepsy, in contrast, have variously been observed to be irritable, excitable, compulsive, stubborn, hyperactive, aggressive, depressed, or moody. As in adults, children with temporal lobe epilepsy are at increased risk for development of psychosis. Among children who have attempted suicide, there is a 15-fold increased appearance of children with epilepsy, especially those taking phenobarbital (Luminal), compared to that in the general population.

One-third of children with epilepsy have psychiatric disorders, compared with 6.6 percent of healthy children and 11.6 percent of children with physical illnesses not involving the brain. Anticonvulsant medications, especially phenobarbital, may cause hyperactivity and irritability, whereas phenytoin (Dilantin) and carbamazepine (Tegretol) may cause sedation.

Pseudoseizures

Pseudoseizures, also called *nonepileptic seizures*, are psychiatric fugue states caused by an unacceptable emotional conflict. They often occur in patients who have epilepsy or a family member with epilepsy. Nonepileptic seizures usually do not result in physical harm and are typically precipitated by a situation from which the patient would like to escape. Patients with nonepileptic seizures often have a history of physical or sexual abuse. Electroencephalograms (EEGs) are normal, unless there is a concurrent epileptic seizure disorder. The events can sometimes be induced by suggestion. Once the nonepileptic nature of the events is determined, coordination of neurological and psychiatric care is important in the management of the disorder.

HEADACHE

Migraine

Children may have migraine with aura (classic migraine) or migraine without aura (common migraine). Associations with vomiting, true vertigo, visual aura, menstrual cycle, or certain foods and relief with sleep permit the distinction of migraine from tension-type headache. True migraine headaches rarely occur more than once per week. In some extreme cases, amnesia, confusion, and psychosis may result from migraine headaches. There is frequently a family history of migraine. Each patient with headaches, particularly of recent onset, should have a neuroimaging study. Migraines must be managed with patient education regarding avoidance of risk factors and with prompt treatment, including sleeping. Acute migraine treatments include almotriptan (Axert); sumatriptan (Imitrex); rizatriptan (Maxalt); zolmitriptan (Zomig); naratriptan (Amerge); frovatriptan (Frova); caffeine and ergotamine (Cafergot, Wigraine); butalbital, caffeine, and acetaminophen (Fioricet, Esgic); dihydroergotamine (D.H.E. 45); phenothiazines; and opioid analgesics. Migraine prophylactic drugs include serotonin agonists (e.g., cyproheptadine [Periactin]), serotonin antagonists, antidepressants, antihistamines, anticonvulsants (e.g., divalproex [Depakote]), calcium channel blockers, β-adrenergic receptor antagonists, and hormones. Several flawed, double-blind, controlled trials have shown benefit of each of these agents, although the response in the placebo arm of many of the studies was unexpectedly low. It has been difficult to separate the placebo effect from true migraine prophylaxis.

Chronic Tension-Type Headaches

Tension-type headaches may be frequent and are sometimes associated with dizziness, nausea, and scotomata during the headache. Periods of daily headache may be interspersed with headache-free periods lasting days to weeks. The severity of an individual headache waxes and wanes over the course of the day. Migraine and tension-type headaches may coexist in a patient, who usually can describe distinct patterns of pain. The specter of a brain tumor looms in the minds of even young children, and a thorough history and neurological examination followed by an imaging study, which is usually normal, may allay anxieties and may allow the headache to remit fully. An ophthalmological examination to rule out visual refractive errors, particularly astigmatism, is essential. Once structural causes of headache have been ruled out, psychological issues should be explored. Family conflicts, particularly parental conflicts or parental divorce, are at the root of tension-type headaches in a large number of children. Other factors to be addressed are difficulties meeting expected school performance, violence in the school, illness in other family members, and psychiatric conditions, such as depression, anxiety, and ADHD. The affected child and the parents should be interviewed.

Treatment begins with reassurance that the headache does not reflect a serious medical condition. Patients should be instructed to keep a log of each headache, including what triggered it, what was done to treat it, and, in adolescent girls, whether it is associated with menstrual periods. This serves to focus attention on the headaches as a valid medical condition, rather than an inevitable nuisance for which there is no cure. Occasionally, an identifiable trigger can be identified and avoided. Patients should take an adequate dose of over-the-counter analgesics at the earliest opportunity once a headache begins. Such medicines are much more effective at aborting a mild headache than at reversing a fully developed headache. If the headaches persist despite the previously mentioned interventions, prophylaxis often may be achieved with antidepressant drugs. All available antidepressants have equivalent efficacy, and the choice of drug should be based on side-effect profiles. Relaxation exercises or biofeedback may be effective.

Other Causes of Headache

Fatigue or excessive exertion may cause an acute tension-type headache, which responds to analgesics and rest. Sinusitis may cause facial pain in the context of fever and nasal congestion. Headache may be the sole manifestation of an acute viral syndrome. Dental pain, injury to the temporomandibular joint, or malocclusion that forces a child to chew on only one side of his or her mouth may strain one masseter muscle and may produce unilateral headache. Neck or head injury may cause muscle strain that can persist for weeks to months, especially if there is an ongoing legal action based on the presence of disability. Occipital headache may be caused by carpal tunnel syndrome, which can appear in adolescence. Headaches may be associated with epileptiform discharges even in the absence of clinical seizures. A 24-hour ambulatory EEG may be necessary to demonstrate that spike and wave activity correlates with the duration of the headache. Headache may be the presenting symptom of collagen-vascular disease, hypersensitivity

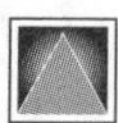

Table 2.13–6
Major Causes of Chorea

- Onset before 3 years of age
  - Physiological chorea of infancy
  - Perinatal asphyxia
  - Kernicterus
  - Postcardiopulmonary bypass
- Onset in childhood
  - "Minimal brain dysfunction"
  - Genetic
    - Disorders of intermediary metabolism
      - Glutaric acidemia type I
      - δ-Glyceric acidemia
      - Sulfite oxidase deficiency
      - GM_1 gangliosidosis
      - GM_2 gangliosidosis
      - Lesch-Nyhan syndrome
      - Leigh disease
    - Heredodegenerative disorders
      - Ataxia-telangiectasia
      - Familial nonprogressive choreoathetosis
      - Paroxysmal dyskinesia
  - Toxic
    - Neuroleptics (tardive dyskinesia)
    - Anticonvulsants (phenytoin [Dilantin], carbamazepine [Tegretol])
    - Metals (thallium, manganese)
    - Isoniazid (Laniazid), reserpine (Serpalan)
  - Metabolic
    - Hepatic encephalopathy
    - Renal encephalopathy
    - Hypoparathyroidism
    - Pseudohypoparathyroidism
    - Hyponatremia and hypernatremia
    - Post protein-calorie malnutrition
  - Infectious
    - Viral encephalitis
    - Behçet's syndrome
  - Immunologic
    - Systemic lupus erythematosus
    - Sydenham's chorea
  - Trauma
- Onset in adolescence
  - Heredodegenerative diseases
    - Wilson's disease
    - Huntington's disease
    - Hallervorden-Spatz disease
    - Pelizaeus-Merzbacher disease
  - Toxic
  - Metabolic
  - Infectious
  - Immunologic
  - Trauma

From Menkes J. *Textbook of Child Neurology.* 5th ed. Baltimore: Williams & Wilkins; 1995, with permission.

reaction, hypertension, or nervous system infection. Drugs and toxins with vasodilating properties may cause headaches. Headaches are especially associated with alcohol, caffeine withdrawal, nitrites, monosodium glutamate, and marijuana.

MOVEMENT DISORDERS

Involuntary movements are usually a sign of dysfunction of the basal ganglia. They may cause a disproportionate amount of anxiety and distress in children, who may be subject to teasing by their peers. Involuntary movements may be distinguished from seizures by their persistence with preservation of consciousness, their disappearance during sleep, and the absence of EEG abnormalities during the involuntary movements.

Classification

Chorea is a rapid, random, dance-like movement of a limb. Persons with choreiform movements may attempt to incorporate them into what appear to be voluntary movements to avoid attention. *Athetosis* is a slow, writhing movement of the limbs. Athetosis may be a sequela of perinatal brain injury, such as hypoxic-ischemic injury, or kernicterus. *Ballismus* is a high-amplitude, violent shooting of the limb from the shoulder or pelvis. It is probably an extreme version of chorea and may be seen in Sydenham's chorea and lupus erythematosus. *Dystonia* is a persistent, simultaneous contraction of agonist and antagonist muscles. Tardive dyskinesia, dystonia, and tremor may be induced by medications in children as well as adults. *Myoclonus* is a sudden jerk of a body part that is not stereotyped, cannot be suppressed, and is nonrhythmic. *Tremor* is a continuous to-and-fro movement. *Tics* are instantaneous, stereotyped, low-amplitude movements. All movement disorders may involve one body part (focal), two or more contiguous body parts (segmental), one side of the body (hemispherical), or the entire body (generalized).

Diagnosis and Treatment

Movement disorders may be primary (idiopathic) or secondary (symptomatic) (Table 2.13–6). A thorough evaluation should be done, including history, especially of perinatal course, drug use, and systemic diseases; physical examination to characterize the movements, which may be difficult even for experts; neuroimaging, including magnetic resonance imaging (MRI) with contrast and, possibly, angiography; and laboratory examination, including toxicology screens, electrolytes, antinuclear antibodies, antistreptolysin O titer, thyroid studies, pregnancy tests, and screens for specific genetic disorders. Among the genetic disorders that may cause movement disorders in children are Tourette's syndrome, Hallervorden-Spatz disease, glutaric aciduria, hepatolenticular degeneration (Wilson's disease), Huntington's disease, abetalipoproteinemia, ataxia-telangiectasia, benign familial chorea, familial paroxysmal choreoathetosis, Lesch-Nyhan syndrome, ceroid lipofuscinosis, dopa-responsive dystonia, and myotonic dystrophy. Each disease has a specific treatment.

SUGGESTED CROSS-REFERENCES

Developmental neuroanatomy is described in Section 1.3. Adult manifestations of each of the conditions described in this section are discussed in the previous sections of Chapter 2. Narcolepsy is discussed in Chapter 20. Genetic counseling is discussed in Section 28.3. Normal child and adolescent development are described in Chapter 32. Mental retardation is discussed in Chapter 34. Tic disorders are discussed in Chapter 42. Psychiatric sequelae of HIV and AIDS are discussed in Section 49.5.

REFERENCES

*Aicardi J. *Diseases of the Nervous System in Childhood.* 2nd ed. Cambridge, UK: Cambridge University Press; 1998.

Al-Twaijri WA, Shevell MI: Pediatric migraine equivalents: Occurrence and clinical features in practice. *Pediatr Neurol.* 2002;26:365–368.

Antunes NL: The spectrum of neurologic disease in children with systemic cancer. *Pediatr Neurol.* 2001;25:227–235.

Avard DM, Knoppers BM: Ethical dimensions of genetics in pediatric neurology: A look into the future. *Semin Pediatr Neurol.* 2002;9:53–61.

Aydin K, Okuyaz C, Serdaroglu A, Gucuyener K: Utility of electroencephalography in the evaluation of common neurologic conditions in children. *J Child Neurol.* 2003;18:394–396.

*Berg BO, ed. *Principles of Child Neurology.* New York: McGraw-Hill; 1996.

Challman TD, Barbaresi WJ, Katusic SK, Weaver A: The yield of the medical evaluation of children with pervasive developmental disorders. *J Autism Dev Disord.* 2003;33:187–192.

Dlugos DJ, Sammel MD, Strom BL, Farrar IT: Response to first drug trial predicts outcome in childhood temporal lobe epilepsy. *Neurology.* 2001;57:2259–2264.

*Fenichel GM: *Clinical Pediatric Neurology.* 4th ed. Philadelphia: WB Saunders; 2001.

*Frank Y, ed. *Pediatric Behavioral Neurology.* Boca Raton, FL: CRC Press; 1996.

Frare M, Axia G, Battistella PA: Quality of life, coping strategies, and family routines in children with headache. *Headache.* 2002;42:953–962.

Gert B: The relevance of moral theory to pediatric neurology. *Semin Pediatr Neurol.* 2002;9:2–9.

Glasscock R: A phenomenological study of the experience of being a mother of a child with cerebral palsy. *Pediatr Nurs.* 2000;26:407–410.

Haydel MJ, Shembekar AD: Prediction of intracranial injury in children aged five years and older with loss of consciousness after minor head injury due to nontrivial mechanisms. *Ann Emerg Med.* 2003;42:507–514.

*Menkes JH, Sarnat HB. *Child Neurology.* 6th ed. Baltimore: Williams & Wilkins; 2000.

Miller V, Palermo TM, Grewe SD: Quality of life in pediatric epilepsy: Demographic and disease-related predictors and comparison with healthy controls. *Epilepsy Behav.* 2003;4:36–42.

Miller VA, Palermo TM, Powers SW, Scher MS, Hershey AD: Migraine headaches and sleep disturbances in children. *Headache.* 2003;43:362–368.

Ott D, Siddarth P, Gurbani S, Koh S, Tournay A, Shields WD, Caplan R: Behavioral disorders in pediatric epilepsy: Unmet psychiatric need. *Epilepsia.* 2003;44:591–597.

Parent A. *Carpenter's Human Neuroanatomy.* 9th ed. Baltimore: Williams & Wilkins; 1996.

Plioplys S: Depression in children and adolescents with epilepsy. *Epilepsy Behav.* 2003;4[Suppl 3]:39–45.

Powers SW, Patton SR, Hommel KA, Hershey AD: Quality of life in childhood migraines: Clinical impact and comparison to other chronic illnesses. *Pediatrics.* 2003;112:e1–e5.

Rolak LA. *Neurology Secrets.* 3rd ed. Baltimore: Lippincott Williams & Wilkins; 2001.

Shevell MI, Majnemer A, Rosenbaum P, Abrahamowicz M: Etiologic yield of autistic spectrum disorders: A prospective study. *J Child Neurol.* 2001;16:509–512.

Shevell MI, Majnemer A, Rosenbaum P, Abrahamowicz M: Profile of referrals for early childhood developmental delay to ambulatory subspecialty clinics. *J Child Neurol.* 2001;16:645–650.

Spencer TI: Attention-deficit/hyperactivity disorder. *Arch Neurol.* 2002;59:314–316.

Swaiman KF, Ashwal S. *Pediatric Neurology: Principles and Practice.* 3rd ed. St. Louis: Mosby; 1999.

Williams J, Griebel ML, Sharp GB, Lange B, Phillips T, DelosReyes E, Bates S, Schulz EG, Simpson P: Differentiating between seizures and attention deficit hyperactivity disorder (ADHD) in a pediatric population. *Clin Pediatr (Phila).* 2002;41:565–568.

Williams J, Steel C, Sharp GB, DelosReyes E, Phillips T, Bates S, Lange B, Griebel ML: Parental anxiety and quality of life in children with epilepsy. *Epilepsy Behav.* 2003;4:483–486.

3 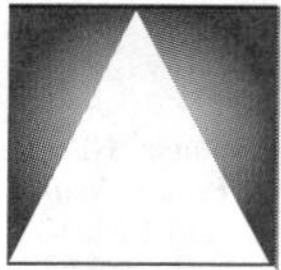

Contributions of the Psychological Sciences

▲ 3.1 Sensation, Perception, and Cognition

LOUIS J. COZOLINO, PH.D., AND DANIEL J. SIEGEL, M.D.

Sensation, *perception*, and *cognition* refer to three broadening tiers of human information processing. *Sensation* is usually defined as the immediate result of stimulation of sensory neurons, whereas *perception* involves the organization and evaluation of these sensations to obtain information about the inner or outer environments. *Cognition* refers to a set of vastly complex processes, such as language, problem solving, and thinking, that apply plans and strategies to sensations and perceptions. Although distinguishing between sensation, perception, and cognition has a long history, the accuracy and value of separating them are increasingly unclear in light of growing knowledge of nervous system functioning.

Most information processing depends on the brain. Because the brain is built and maintained through the interaction of biological, psychological, and social forces, the study of sensation, perception, and cognition is necessarily broad and far reaching. The rapid increase of knowledge of neuroanatomy and the development of new hypothetical models to understand its functioning makes this an exciting time in the cognitive sciences. This chapter reflects the juxtaposition of many new and old models, containing much of the excitement and uncertainty that emerge as researchers strive to understand how humans perceive and understand the world.

COGNITIVE SCIENCE

The fields relevant to this overview are a part of the interdisciplinary studies of cognitive science, which includes cognitive psychology, developmental psychology, psycholinguistics, computational science, and the emerging field of interpersonal neurobiology. Each of these disciplines provides an important and unique perspective on the human psyche. Biological, psychodynamic, and social psychiatry find a common home within cognitive science in which the usual divisions of nature versus nurture and biology versus psychology disappear in an examination of the building of the brain and the origins of mental processes.

In recent years, discoveries in the neurosciences have revealed a wide range of findings relevant to psychiatry. One of the major discoveries was that the brain's structure and function are a result of the transaction of several factors, including genetic, physiological, and experiential variables. In particular, brain development requires specific forms of experience to foster the growth of neural circuits involved in a wide array of mental processes, including attention, memory, emotion, attachment, and self-reflection. Thus, experiences shape the unfolding of genetically programmed development of the central nervous system (CNS). Genes function as a template of information and as a mediator of transcription of the proteins that determine neural structure. Experience directly shapes the selection and timing of how the activity of genes influences the structure of the brain.

The human brain, especially the cerebral cortex, is immature at birth. This immaturity requires that the child's brain use the caregiver's brain to grow and to organize. Findings from developmental neuroscience point to the centrality of interpersonal relationships in the development of the brain. The cooperative communication of infant–caregiver attachments is thought to provide the infrastructure not only for emotional development, but also for abstract reasoning and cognitive abilities. The patterns of interaction between child and caregiver have a direct impact on the way that the brain develops and the mind of the child functions. Thus, cognitive processes need to be considered as the way in which the mind emerges from within the genetic, physiological, and experiential factors that shape the development and maintenance of mental function.

Hot and Cold Cognition Traditionally, cognition was studied by experimental psychologists in university laboratories, whereas emotions were explored by psychoanalysts in consulting rooms. Cognitive psychologists, striving to avoid the subjective and imprecise nature of emotions, devised flowcharts and algorithms similar to those used to describe processes within organizations or, later, in programming computers. Input was calibrated, output was measured, and theories were generated describing what happened within the "black box" of the brain. The increasing complexity of these models did not seem to improve their explanatory power, and words such as motivation and emotion would invariably arise.

As knowledge of brain functioning has increased, it is becoming increasingly clear that neural networks involved in sensation, perception, and cognition are inextricably interwoven with other networks processing survival value, emotion, motivation, and somatic states. The myth of *cold cognition*, that is, cognitive processes devoid of affective influence, is gradually fading. Flow charts and other diagrams depicting linear input-output processes are being replaced with more sophisticated models relevant to the complex neural systems that psychologists are attempting to describe. Not all cognition is "hot," such as traumatic memories or scanning the environment for dangerous or sexually attractive others. Some cognition may be cool, such as adding rows of figures or balancing a checkbook. These same tasks, for someone with math anxiety, during an examination, or before an Internal Revenue Service audit, may become warm or even hot. The fundamental principle, however, is that sensation, perception, and cognition occur in the context of feed-forward and feedback networks, interwoven with and guided by complex (and largely unconscious) emotional determinants.

Emotion What is an emotion? The answer to this question is as complex as the mind itself. Although the lack of clear definitions and good animal models has hindered empirical research, it is clear that emotions play a central role in perceptual and cognitive processes.

One view considers emotion as a primary value system of the brain, allowing activations to be selectively reinforced. For example, emotionally charged experiences may be more readily recalled than uneventful ones. According to this view, the most fundamental aspect of emotion is the arousal-appraisal system in which the brain responds to a given stimulus with the signal of "this is important—take note and pay attention now!" Emotion thus gives value to a representation by arousing attentional mechanisms and by focusing a spotlight of attention on the stimulus. The second stage would then appraise the meaning of such emotional arousal by assessing its hedonic tone: "Is this good or is this bad? Should this be approached or avoided?" Emotion thus directs the flow of energy—the activations within specific circuits of the brain—as the arousal-appraisal system focuses cognitive processes on elements of the internal and external environment. A third level of emotional processing is the elaboration of this appraisal into a more specific form, called a *categorical emotion*, such as joy, interest, surprise, fear, anger, sadness, or shame. These categorical emotions have universal facial expressions of affect found in all cultures, which may have distinct psychophysiological manifestations.

An additional view examines the way in which the changes in the body's state are represented in the brain in the form of what Antonio Damasio has called a *somatic marker*. According to this view, the energizing or deenergizing bodily responses let the brain know how the individual feels about an experience. Such a somatic marker can then be used in future emotional assessments, or gut reactions, to an experience.

A part of the brain called the *orbitofrontal cortex* has been implicated as the site of somatic marker processing or what is called *intuition*. Allan Schore has also noted the importance of early experiences with caregivers in the maturation of this region and also its central role in coordinating self-regulatory functions early in development with basic emotional reactions and social functioning. The orbitofrontal cortex has been implicated not only in monitoring, but also in regulating bodily states and may possibly be involved in psychiatric disturbances ranging from autism to mood disorders. Disorders in self-organization and social functioning may be better understood by examining the central role of emotion and, perhaps, the orbitofrontal cortex and related regions in the development and maintenance of dysfunctional mental states. Studies also suggest that this region is responsible for the capacity for self-knowledge and the subjective experience enabling the mind to reflect on the self in the past, present, and the potential future. Inborn and experiential factors may play important roles in allowing this region to develop the capacity to integrate a wide range of important functions of the mind, including the appraisal of meaning, emotional regulation, social cognition, and autobiographical consciousness.

NEURAL NETWORK GROWTH AND INTEGRATION

The growth and selective connectivity of neurons is the basic mechanism of all learning and adaptation. Learning can be reflected in neural changes in a number of ways, including (1) the growth of new neurons, (2) the expansion of existing neurons, and (3) the changes in the connectivity between existing neurons. All of these changes are expressions of plasticity, or the ability of the nervous system to change. The birth of new neurons, or neurogenesis, is a controversial field of study. Some recent research suggests that new neurons are generated in different areas of primate and human brains, especially in regions involved with new learning, such as the hippocampus, the amygdala, and the frontal and temporal lobes.

Existing neurons grow through the expansion and branching of the dendrites they project to other neurons. There is now sufficient evidence for the fact that neurons demonstrate growth and changes in reaction to new experiences and learning. Although neurons interconnect to form neural networks, neural networks, in turn, integrate with one another to perform increasingly complex tasks. The brain is modular, that is, different networks have evolved to perform diverse tasks. Neural networks converge and coordinate to perform increasingly higher level tasks. For example, networks that participate in language, emotion, and memory interact and integrate for humans to recall and to tell an emotionally meaningful story with the proper affect, correct details, and appropriate words.

Association areas within the brain serve the role of bridging, coordinating, and directing the multiple neural circuits to which they are connected. Executive networks within association areas, like a switchboard operator, have the capability to interconnect different neural networks. Although the actual mechanisms of this integration are not yet known, they are likely to include some combination of changes in (1) the biochemical processing within neurons, (2) the synaptic connections between neurons, (3) the relationships between local neuronal circuits, and (4) the interactions between functional brain systems. Changes in the synchrony of activation of multiple neural networks may also play a role in the coordination of their activity.

If everything humans experience is represented within neural networks, then psychopathology of all kinds, from the mildest neurotic symptoms to the most severe psychosis, must be represented within and between neural networks. Healthy functioning requires proper development and functioning of neural networks organizing conscious awareness, behavior, emotion, and sensation. Psychopathology correlates with the suboptimal integration and coordination of neural networks. Patterns of dysregulation of brain activation in specific disorders support the theory of a brain-based explanation for the symptoms of psychopathology.

In general, psychological integration suggests that the cognitive functions of the executive brain have increasing access to information across networks of sensation, behavior, and emotion. Dissociation among these processes can occur when biochemical changes caused by high levels of stress inhibit or disrupt the brain's integrative abilities. Physical trauma, disease processes, or genetic predispositions that disrupt the development and functioning of neural networks can all result in neural dysregulation and psychiatric symptomatology.

Applying this model to treatment, psychotherapy, psychopharmacology, and psychosurgery can be seen as ways of creating or restoring integration and coordination between various neural networks. For example, research has demonstrated that successful psychotherapy correlates with changes in activation in areas of the brain hypothesized to be involved in disorders, such as obsessive-compulsive disorder (OCD) and depression. The return to normal levels of activation results in reestablishing positive reciprocal control between relevant neural structures and networks.

MIND AND BRAIN

A generally accepted view of the mind is that it emanates from a portion of the activity of the brain. What is this activity of the brain,

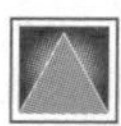

Table 3.1–1
Basic Ideas of the Mind

The mind is a processor of energy and information.
Energy is contained within the activations of neural circuits.
Information is contained within the patterns of activation, termed a *neural net profile* or *mental representation.*
These representations serve as symbols that cause further effects in the mind, leading to the processing of information.

and how does it give rise to such mental processes as perception and cognition? How do the human experiences of sensation, thought, emotion, attention, self-reflection, and memory emerge from neural processes?

The brain is composed of approximately 10 to 20 billion neurons. An average neuron is connected to approximately 10,000 other neurons at synaptic junctions. With hundreds of trillions of connections within and among thousands of web-like neural networks, there are countless combinations of possible activation profiles. The term *neural net profile* is used to describe a certain pattern of activation of the complex layers of neural circuits. The neural net profile is the fundamental way in which mental processes are created. These activations can lead to further neural processes in a cascade of dynamic interactions that produce a range of internal events and external behaviors. The essential components of the mind come directly from how these neural events create the flow of energy and information.

ENERGY AND INFORMATION

The mind is a processor of patterns in the flow of energy and information within the brain (Table 3.1–1). Activations of individual neurons, groups of neurons, circuits, or networks of neurons all involve the flow of energy through the complex system of the brain. This energy reflects the flow of ions across membranes, the consumption of oxygen and nutrients by neural cells, and the active transport of molecules into and out of nervous tissue. However, the mind is much more than some outcome of energy flow—the function and purpose of this flow of energy are to process information.

Information is created within the brain by a process of representation. For example, when an individual sees the Eiffel Tower, the brain responds in particular regions of the visual system with the activation of a neural net profile. When the Eiffel Tower is recalled at a later time, the visual cortex activates a similar neural net pattern, and the Eiffel Tower is visualized. The activation of a particular pattern of neural firing thus contains within it information about something (the Eiffel Tower). Examples of representational forms include perceptual, sensory, linguistic, and more abstract representations of concepts and categories.

INFORMATION PROCESSING

Several elements of the brain's function as an information processor can be described (Fig. 3.1–1). At the most basic level (Fig. 3.1–1A), energy leads to neural responses. This energy can be in the external form of light on the retina or sound waves vibrating the tympanic membrane. It may also take an internal form in which the flow of energy within neural activations themselves produces subsequent neural responses.

A second level of understanding information processing (Fig. 3.1–1B) is in the idea that an input (internal or external) leads to a representational response (a neural net profile of activation), which, in turn, produces a downstream effect or output. This output can be internal, such as the generation of other representations, or external, in the form of observable behavior. Information processing becomes even more complex when the effects themselves carry information. Within cognitive psychology, these information-processing events can be seen as the contrasting, comparing, generalizing, chunking, clustering, differentiating, and extracting processes that lead to interwoven sets of increasingly complex mental representations.

A third level of viewing information processing in the mind (Fig. 3.1–1C) is the conceptualization of forms of sensation, perception, attention, and memory. According to this view, external energy is sensed by the peripheral nervous system and is registered as sensation within the brain. The selective processing of aspects of these sensations, called *filtering*, leads to the production of perception. These perceptions are themselves subject to further filtering in which only a select few are placed within working memory. This is sometimes called the "chalkboard of the mind." It is within working memory that representations can be consciously manipulated, contrasted, clustered, and reassembled. Thus, consciousness may be intimately related to this aspect of mental functioning.

Sensation refers to the initial stages of the basic information-processing model (Fig. 3.1–1). In traditional experimental paradigms, sensory memory is conceptualized as lasting for approximately 0.25 seconds. Items in sensory memory are then filtered into working or short-term memory, where they last for approximately 0.5 minutes. When humans attempt to consciously learn new information, working memory is able to handle approximately seven items, unless further processing creates linkages to other items within longer-term memory. Rehearsal allows these representations to remain for longer periods of time. Cognitive processes that can group bits of information into large chunks (*chunking*) can increase the capacity of working memory by making each unit more information rich. Representations are then processed and placed within long-term memory from which they can be retrieved for future use.

ATTENTION

Attention is the process that controls the focus and flow of information processing. There are many aspects to attention that may derive from

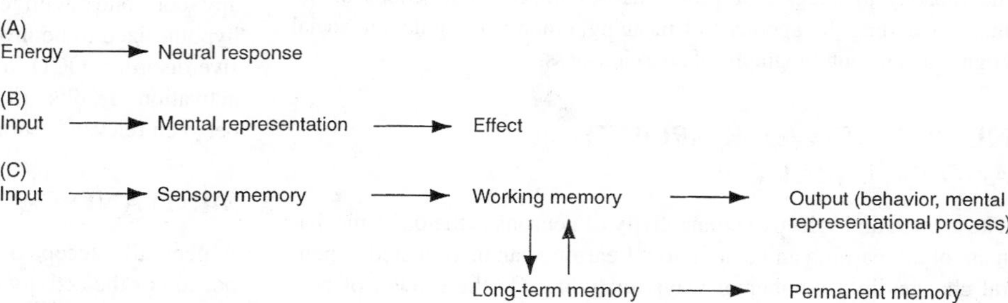

FIGURE 3.1–1 Information-processing models.

their neuroanatomical localization. Three components of attention (selectivity, capacity, and sustained concentration) have traditionally been used to describe cognitive deficits in psychiatric disorders such as schizophrenia and attention-deficit/hyperactivity disorder (ADHD). All aspects of attention in normal and patient populations are influenced by the emotional or motivational value of the stimulus.

Early conceptualizations of attention were based on Donald Broadbent's idea of a filter that selects a limited amount of incoming stimuli to be further processed. Limited capacity of attention was thus attributable to the inability to process the overwhelming amount of incoming stimuli. An attention bottleneck was described as occurring early in the sensory process (automatic) or late in the perceptual processing stage (identification and classification).

Selective Attention One aspect of attention is that it focuses a metaphorical spotlight on external stimuli or internal mental representations. In Broadbent's conceptualization, selectivity has three dimensions: (1) filtering, focusing on specific attributes (e.g., large squares vs. small squares); (2) categorizing, based on stimulus class (e.g., attending to letters in whatever script they are written); and (3) pigeonholing, reducing perceptual information needed to place a stimulus into a specified category (e.g., using only long hair to classify individuals as female). Each of these aspects of attention acts on incoming stimuli to make a determination of fit for the sought-after characteristic. Schizophrenic patients, for example, show greater difficulty with pigeonholing than with filtering when they are symptomatic.

Another conceptualization of selective attention distinguishes between two interactive ways of processing sensory input. *Preattentive processing* (a parallel function) assesses global, holistic patterns and appears to be an early component of the perceptual process. *Focal attention* (a serial process) follows preattentive processing and involves a detailed analysis of stimuli characteristics. Focal attention can be directed at one stimulus form only and is thus limited in its capacity. In contrast, parallel (preattentive) attention processes do not appear to have limited capacity and can detect gestalt aspects of environmental stimuli from numerous sources. The ability to hear one's name called out by a nonattended voice in a crowded, noisy room is an example of an ongoing parallel process with the ability to detect gestalt features and extremely familiar (and thus automatically processed) stimuli.

Attention Capacity The concept of processing capacity involves the idea that a given task makes a demand on a limited pool of resources. A task with a high processing load draws more resources from the finite pool than does a task with a low processing load, thus inhibiting the accessibility of resources for other simultaneous functions drawing from the same pool. Focal attention requires cognitive effort and thus has a high–processing load demand. Cognitive models describing several resource pools suggest an executive process that distributes resources to various cognitive functions. Serial processes that demand processing capacity inhibit the simultaneous action of other serial high-load processes. In contrast, parallel processes have low or no processing capacity demands and can function simultaneously with numerous other functions without inhibiting them.

Optimal performance is attained with moderate levels of arousal that allow for the establishment of task goals and feedback from the performance of the task, leading to appropriate resource allocation. Low levels of arousal impair those processes and lead to inadequate resource allocation. High levels of arousal may be detrimental to the performance because of poor discrimination of stimuli and diminished efficiency of allocation, resulting in poor attention functioning.

Sustained Attention The ability to sustain attention is called *vigilance* and can be tested with task demands for alertness and concentration over a period of a few minutes to an hour. The tests usually involve detection requirements for target stimuli that occur infrequently at random intervals. An example of such a test is the Continuous Performance Test, which has been used to study various psychiatric disorders. Important aspects of the tests are derived from signal detection theory and include the factors of sensitivity and response criterion. Sensitivity is the distinguishing of target stimuli from nontarget stimuli. The response criterion is the amount of perceptual evidence required to support the decision regarding a target item versus a nontarget item.

FORMS OF REPRESENTATIONS

The essential feature of information processing in the brain is that the patterns of activation of neural circuits (the neural net profile) contain information. These mental representations, in turn, produce further neural events. The location and pattern of neural activations determine the nature of what the neural net profile represents. For example, activity in the optic nerve in response to light leads to a cascade of neural responses within the visual cortex generating a visual sensation. Future activation of those layers in the visual cortex in that general pattern is the experience or recollection of the visual image. Pattern and localization determine the kind of representation and the information that it specifically contains.

SENSATION AND PERCEPTION

Forms of representations include sensory and perceptual ones that derive from input from the external world via the peripheral sensory nervous system. The initial stage of encoding a visual representation is called an *iconic image* and is held within sensory memory for a brief period. Features of the initial stimulus, such as its size, direction, and color, are the information held within this sensory representation. Sensory representations are the least processed of mental representations and are thought to be as close as the brain can get to representing the world as it is. This is a form of processing termed *bottom-up processing* and is in contrast to more elaborately processed representations that are directly influenced by more abstract aspects of prior experience, called *top-down processing*. As the initial sensory activations are processed (classified, compared, and linked to representations from prior experience) they become influenced by higher-order processes and become organized as perceptual representations.

Attentional processes at the level of sensory memory act on the initial image with higher cognitive functions, such as classifications and chunking. In their essence, these top-down processes compare, contrast, and transform the initial representation to create new perceptual images within working memory. Studies of patients with schizophrenia reveal specific deficits at this early stage of perceptual processing.

Perception is created by the top-down transformations of sensory images but does not necessarily involve the experience of consciousness. This has important clinical implications in that patients may be influenced by events and stimuli that they cannot consciously recall. However, if conscious, focal attention is involved in perception, then the representations are processed differently. The involvement of focal attention appears to be necessary for the activation of the hippocampus in memory processing, which allows for the encoding of explicit, consciously accessible, autobiographical memory. Posttraumatic dissociative states may involve the blockage of focal processing of perceptual representations, thereby leading to a disconnection among conscious and nonconscious elements of experience.

Imagery involves the activation of brain circuits responsible for perceptual processing. Representations (neural net profile activation patterns) can thus be created by external or internal means. Mental imagery can involve the generation, inspection, retention, and transformation of perceptual images. This processing involves similar effort and timing as when the object is perceived from an external source. Thus, complex visual images require more effort and time to rotate in internal and external reality. The ability of the mind to generate mental images is used in various forms of psychotherapy and may also be an important mechanism in the pathological production of hallucinations and illusions seen in several disorders.

MEMORY SYSTEMS

The neural networks of the brain are capable of responding to experience by the activation of particular patterns of distributed activation. Donald Hebb described a basic principle of memory that has been repeatedly supported by research: "Neurons that fire together, wire together." Neurons that are activated in a particular pattern at one time tend to fire together in a similar pattern in the future—this is the essence of memory.

The brain has various forms of circuits responsible for different systems of memory (Table 3.1–2). The form of memory most commonly thought of as *memory* is termed *explicit* or *declarative memory.* This form involves the conscious sensation of something being recalled at the time of retrieval and allows for the awareness of the autobiographical or factual knowledge to be shared, often verbally, with others and the self. This explicit memory system requires the involvement of focal attention and the activation of the hippocampus for encoding and retrieval. Items focally attended to are placed in working memory, processed further, and then placed in long-term memory. After a period of weeks to months, items are thought to undergo a process called *cortical consolidation* that places them in permanent memory, where their retrieval no longer requires the hippocampus. Cortical consolidation helps to explain the phenomenon of retrograde amnesia after head trauma.

Before explicit autobiographical memory processing becomes available after the first years of life (during which time the hippocampus and cerebral cortex are maturing), a form of memory called *implicit* or *nondeclarative memory* is already in place and remains active throughout the life span. Implicit memory involves a wide range of systems, including behavioral, emotional, and perceptual memory. When these circuits are activated in retrieval, they do not include the conscious sensation of something being recalled. For example, when riding a bicycle, a person may not recall having learned to ride and may not even feel that anything is being recalled. Similarly, a person with a fear of dogs may be unable to explicitly recall (consciously) any event that may explain such an emotional response. The existence of intact implicit recollection in the absence of explicit memory is found in various conditions, including surgical anesthesia; the adverse effects of some benzodiazepines; neurological conditions, such as Korsakoff's syndrome and bilateral hippocampal strokes; and childhood amnesia. Such dissociation may also occur in response to trauma. Thus, patients with posttraumatic stress disorder (PTSD) may have an inability to explicitly recall a traumatic event and yet may avoid contextual stimuli similar to the initial trauma, may evidence startle response and anxiety, and may have intrusive perceptual images for the event. These latter symptoms may reflect the conscious awareness of implicit memory retrieval that lacks the subjective sensation that something is being recalled.

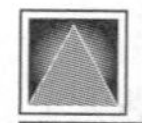

Table 3.1–2
Memory Systems

Implicit

A behavioral, emotional, and perceptual form of memory devoid of the subjective internal experience of recalling of self, or of past. Can include schema or mental models that are summations of representations from numerous experiences.

Also known as *early, procedural, nondeclarative memory*. Cannot be expressed in words.

Present from birth. Does not involve the hippocampus or require focal, conscious attention. Probably involves various circuits, including those of the basal ganglia, limbic system (amygdala, anterior cingulate, and orbitofrontal cortex), and perceptual cortices.

Explicit

A form of memory requiring conscious awareness and involving the subjective sense of recollection and, if autobiographical, of self and past.

Also known as *late, episodic* or *semantic*, or *declarative memory*. Can be expressed in words or drawings.

The autobiographical component of explicit memory does not fully develop until past the first 2 years of life, as the hippocampus and orbitofrontal cortex on which it depends are maturing.

CONSCIOUSNESS

The vast majority of mental processes are outside of conscious awareness. Conscious awareness is a specialized aspect of some cognitive processes. In general, many authors' views converge on the idea that there exist two fundamental forms of consciousness: a *here-and-now* and a *past-present-future* form of awareness. These two processes are likely mediated via the integration of different neural circuits in the brain.

Two hypotheses focus on the way in which representational processes are linked or bound together during the flow of informational transformations within the mind. One hypothesis suggests that a 60-cycle-per-second sweeping process extends from the thalamus to the neocortex. This sweep may serve to bind representational processes together in the internal experience of consciousness. Processes that are active at the time of the sweep thus become linked within consciousness. Another view implicates the role of the lateral prefrontal cortex and its role in working memory. Working memory serves as the chalkboard of the mind, and representational processes that become linked to the activity in this region are then a part of the attentional spotlight of conscious awareness.

Based on a biological assessment of brain function, Gerald Edelman's theory describes two forms of consciousness that derive from the resonant interactions between groups of neurons. In his model, primary consciousness stems from the interaction between perceptual categorizations and conceptual categorizations. This form of consciousness, called the *remembered present*, is also found in higher animals and is unable to transcend momentary awareness. It is embedded in the present but is influenced by categorizations from the past. In human beings, the capacity for lexical or language processing enables a secondary or higher-order consciousness to exist and stems from the resonance between those processes and conceptual categories. Higher-order consciousness frees inner experience from the prison of the present and allows for views of the past and plans for the future. Included in these forms of consciousness is a scene of the present situation in which the self is placed in a temporospatial context.

Cortically blind patients state that they cannot see visual stimuli, but they respond behaviorally as if they were fully sighted. They describe being unaware of visual perception, but they make eye and hand movements that reflect the processing of information about stimulus location, shape, orientation, and direction of motion. In information-processing terms, behavioral tests reveal that blind-sighted patients do sense and perceive visual stimuli but do not have conscious awareness of the perceptual process, an example of a dissociation of the normally associated processes of perception and consciousness or awareness of phenomena.

Misidentification syndromes are other examples of subjective, conscious experience disturbances. In prosopagnosia, patients are unable to consciously access memories regarding persons familiar to them. Capgras syndrome patients are able to recognize a familiar person's face but feel that it is not really that person. Being certain, as in recognition, is one aspect of consciousness as a cognitive process. The pathological uncertainty of patients with OCD theoretically can be viewed as a disturbance in that aspect of conscious functioning.

Consciousness provides a sense of continuity. Many psychiatric patients experience a profound sense of discontinuity and confusion that may be related to a dysfunction in the sense-making, continuity-creating process of consciousness. Some psychiatric symptoms, including derealization and depersonalization, may be understood in terms of alterations in conscious functioning (as seen in some patients with schizophrenia, mood disorders, anxiety disorders, dissociative disorders, PTSD, and some personality disorders), distorted body image (as in eating disorders or mood disorders), intrusive memories and flashback phenomena (as in PTSD), and hallucinations (as in psychotic states).

Mental Models and Schemata Studies of perception and memory support the view that the mind has organizational structures that influence the interpretation of sensory data, shape the encoding of information into long-term memory, bias the retrieval of items stored in memory, and help determine the behavioral response. Those organizing cognitive functions are called *mental models* or *schemata.*

Mental models are unconscious, highly organized, structural processes derived from past experiences that guide in interpreting present stimuli and influence the direction of behavior. Mental models exist for various situations. When a situation activates a given mental model, that model, in turn, guides subsequent information processing and behavior. The adaptational value of a given mental model depends on an accurate reading of the survival demands of the situation. The downside of these models is seen when their unconscious and automatic activation occurs in situations in which they are inappropriate. Aaron Beck's theory of depression is based on the idea that mental models or schemata can produce depressive thinking and depressed moods. John Bowlby used the concept of internal working models to describe the development of early forms of schemata for attachment relationships. Difficulties in intimate relationships and related behavioral dysregulation can be seen as derivatives of models of inadequate early attachment and the presence of multiple, conflictual models. The *inner objects* of psychodynamic theory are examples of mental models. Mardi Horowitz's view of certain personality disorders and maladaptive interpersonal behavior also includes the role of mental models or person schemata. Some psychiatric signs and symptoms can be seen as derivatives of conflicted schemata and situations. Classic descriptions of interpersonal patterns in some patients with personality disorders, such as idealization and devaluation, can be seen as maladaptive schema functions.

Thought, Language, and Cognition There is no universally accepted definition of *thought.* Suggested basic elements include propositions (functions containing meaning), images, and lexical and semantic symbols. Cognitive processes can be carried out in parallel, simultaneously, and without consciousness. Cognitive processes, such as thoughts, are often directly known only through translation into consciousness and language. As in the study of mental models, clinical observation and experimental paradigms can infer the nature of thought processes only through indirect measures. These concepts are important in defining the term *thought disorder.*

Thinking involves the mental representation of some aspect of the world or of the self and the manipulation of those representations. Thinking depends on explicit and implicit memory of prior experiences. In addition, thought processes are influenced by a person's emotional state, mental models, and other unconscious determinants. The basic components of the conscious components of thinking include categorization, judgment, decision making, and general problem solving. The assignment of representations of events or objects to categories is important to subsequent thought processing, because thoughts can act on the general class to which an item belongs rather than on individual representations; this is another example of top-down processing influences.

Rational thought contributes to the ability to judge the probability of uncertain events and the decision to choose among various options. These processes contribute to problem solving in which data are assessed, classified, transformed, and compared on the basis of logical rules to produce a choice that solves a problem. Failures in these steps can result in limitations and distortions in normal thought processes. Psycholinguistics focuses on the cognitive process of language formation and semantic analysis. Cognitive science has traditionally viewed language as a dominant influence on subjective experience. It is the medium that dominates human social communication and is one of the major features distinguishing *Homo sapiens* from other species. Language shapes the ways in which the world is perceived, the manner in which desires are communicated and satiated, and the way in which society responds.

Modes of Processing and Laterality The mind is capable of distinct modes of processing mental representations. A serial mode uses sequential processing in a linear fashion, which is said to be slow and energy-consuming, because only a few items can be processed serially at a time. Focal, conscious attention is believed to occur in serial fashion. A parallel mode involves the simultaneous manipulation of large numbers of representations in a nonlinear fashion. Pattern recognition is an example of such a rapid, low-energy consuming process that can deal with a wide array of stimuli at the same time.

Another distinction in contrasting modes of processing has been identified in the type of mental processes primarily attributed to the right or left cerebral hemisphere. Studies drawing on the findings in patients whose corpus callosum has been surgically severed, who have unilateral neurological lesions, or in subjects undergoing brain-imaging protocols have found a remarkable consistency in trends of left-hemisphere functioning versus right-hemisphere functioning. Some general principles from this array of studies suggest that many processes involve both hemispheres; however, there are distinct patterns primarily originating from each side of the brain.

The following generalizations relate to right-handed individuals and to most left-handed people as well. In the right hemisphere are fast-acting, parallel, holistic processes, including visuospatial perception. The right side specializes in representations, such as images and sensations, and the nonverbal meaning of words, sometimes referred to as *analogic representations.* The right hemisphere is thought to work as a pattern recognition center, capable of assessing the gestalt context of a scene and providing a synthetic interpretation. On the left side are primarily more slowly acting, linear, time-dependent, serial processes. Left-hemispheric processes manipulate the verbal meaning of words in a logical analytical mode of processing. A generalization from a number of studies is that the right hemisphere tends to note the patterns in the world and creates contextual meaning; the left hemisphere can only make a rationalization of the details of what it perceives to create a sense of meaning from a logical view that lacks context and thus may actually seem like a discontinuous and irrational set of data.

The processing of emotion also appears to have a lateralized distribution. The expression of emotion appears to be mediated primarily by the right hemisphere. Facial recognition of the affective expression of others also appears to be a specialty of the right hemisphere. Of note is that the right hemisphere appears to have a more integrated representation of the body's status, information that may be essential for individuals to know how they feel.

Jerome Bruner has described the distinction between the earlier mode of thought, called *narrative cognition*, versus the later mode, called *scientific*, *logical*, or *paradigmatic cognition*. Narrative thinking is a context-dependent form of processing that incorporates the internal experiences of the teller and the perceived expectations of the listener in the production of a story. Stories also involve the subjective experiences of the characters involved in the unfolding sequence of events. Logicoscientific paradigmatic processing is said to occur in a context-independent manner that focuses on abstract concepts and their logical, cause-and-effect relationships. Children develop narrative thinking by 2 years of age, and the co-construction of stories between parent and child is a primary mode of communication in all cultures throughout the world.

Metacognition and Self-Reflective Capacity

Metacognition concerns conscious processes that act on cognitive processes—thinking about thinking. Awareness of cognition appears to develop by approximately 6 years of age; this knowledge takes various forms, including what is known as the *appearance-reality distinction* (things may not be as they appear). Two components of this awareness are representational diversity (the same object may appear to be different to different people) and representational change (thoughts today are different from those of yesterday and may be different again tomorrow). This form of knowledge about the person-specific meaning of cognitive representation requires some sense of the person's awareness of the separateness of minds, a theoretical domain in developmental cognitive psychology called the *theory of mind.*

The regulation of cognition, also called *metacognitive monitoring*, includes such processes as planning activities, monitoring activities, and checking outcomes. Metacognitive monitoring may involve the assessment of thinking sequences for fallacious logic, factual errors, and contradictions in the content of speech. Peter Fonagy and colleagues explored the development of reflective function, or an *internal observer* of mental life. Parents teach children how to be self-reflective by including their own internal state in interactions and by encouraging children to share their own. Children who have been taught to tell stories that include mental states demonstrate a greater frequency of secure attachment. Being able to understand and to consider the mental states of self and others has also been shown to decrease dependency on defensive strategies. Research suggests that what is created in parent–child narratives about experience is not just a story. Embedded within the storytelling is the selection of information to be included, how it is processed and understood, and if it is egocentric or has multiple subjective centers (empathic capacity).

Social Cognition

Bridging the fields of social psychology and cognitive psychology, the study of social cognition focuses on the mental processes involved in social interactions. The domains include the study of empathy, interpersonal communication (verbal and nonverbal), person perception, relationship scripts, and group processes. Other related areas include studies of attribution bias, memory for social interactions, stereotyping, mental control of social cognitive processes, and cognitive origins of a sense of self. Social cognition can be seen as a domain of social psychology that uses information-processing theory to assess the components of attention, perception, encoding, memory, retrieval, and schemata. A dominant theme in social cognition research has been that top-down, theory-driven processing influences interpretations of social situations and actions in such situations. Developmental psychologists have focused on the origins of social cognitive functioning and its deviations. For example, children with autistic disorder have significant deficits in empathic capacity and in the ability to interpret social cues. Social cognitive deficits may be present in different domains in other psychiatric disorders.

Discourse and Narrative

Discourse is communication from one person to another; it is thought to involve a sense of intention or plan. Normal discourse follows a set of rules that ensures the coherence and effectiveness of communication: What is intended to be stated by the sender is understood by the listener or receiver. Some researchers support the idea that discourse is a cognitive function that follows the basic principles of information processing, including a schema for effective communication, and of social cognition, such as taking into account the listener's perspective. Incoherent discourse can be noted by analyzing unlicensed violations of the primary maxims of discourse. Another technique is that of discourse analysis, which examines the ways in which discourse deviates from an assumed discourse plan. The exact method to quantify abnormalities in discourse remains controversial, but clinical impressions of incoherence remain important for assessing deficits in social communication. The deficits may result from learned behavior, inherent cognitive abnormalities in thought or language, or deviations in social cognitive functioning. Deviations from normal discourse can be a general finding in need of further assessment. Abnormal discourse is clinically evident in psychosis, specifically in schizophrenia.

Narrative is a broad domain ranging from the literary study of fiction to the developmental psychology investigations of the origin of autobiographical accounts. From a cognitive point of view, narrative is important in understanding the relations of language, memory, consciousness, mental models, self-schemata, and social cognition. *Narrative* can be generally defined as the way in which a person creates a verbal account of a sequence of events in the world and the internal subjective experience of the characters of the story.

Autobiographical narrative begins early in life as the capacity for language develops. Studies of early monologues find that young children interpret and assign meaning to events in their world from an early age. Narrative helps record and make sense of the past, interpret the present, and anticipate the future. The brain has been called an "anticipation machine," and mental models, prospective memory, and narrative are the major ways in which top-down processing attempts to prepare for the possible future. The enactment of narrative themes directly affects the way in which individuals live out the story of their lives.

Anthropologists who study psycholinguistic development across cultures have described a phenomenon called *co-construction,* in which family members collaboratively create a story of daily events in their lives. How those family behaviors influence the child's emerging capacity to organize experiences and to encode them into long-term memory to be retrieved later in the production of autobiographical narrative is a fundamental question for many disciplines in cognitive science as well as a primary focus of psychodynamic forms of psychotherapy. Specific deficits in early family experiences and in innate cognitive capacities may theoretically impact the child's narrative capacity. These differences can be seen in how different individuals tell the stories of their lives and the way that they make decisions in life.

Cognitive Development Developmental theories and research can be divided into several views. Stage theories (Jean Piaget, neopiagetian, and the sociocultural school of Alexander Luria and Lev Vygotsky) describe discontinuous periods of development, with times of stability and consolidation alternating with instability and transition. Information-processing models have not been explored in as much detail with regard to child development, but the models postulate a nonstage theory, in which the emergence of cognitive capacity is a continuous process that does not require a set of invariant sequences. Stage and nonstage views embrace the idea that a hierarchical integration and an ongoing differentiation are fundamental aspects of cognitive development.

Another distinguishing feature is the degree to which the theories view the contributing role of innate, biological factors and the role of culturally determined social learning experiences. Do cognitive capacities emerge from a genetically determined plan, as in the Piagetian view, or do they develop in response to experience, as in the sociocultural view? Developmental psychologists have found features of both views, supporting the idea of a transaction between innate factors and environmental experiences. More recent conceptualizations have drawn on the functioning of complex systems to conceptualize development as the continual emergence of ever more complex capacities.

Psychiatric disturbances in cognition may reflect arrested patterns of normal cognition (as in mental retardation), deviant developmental pathways (e.g., social cognitive functioning in persons with autistic disorder), and specific cognitive impairments (e.g., schizophrenia) that may have been present early on or only became evident as life requirements, such as school, became demanding (some cases of ADHD). Investigations into the developmental features of these disorders is a major focus of the field of developmental psychopathology.

Self-Organizational Processes An understanding of the development and subjective experience of cognitive processes has been greatly informed by the insights from the fields of evolutionary neurobiology and the nonlinear dynamics of complex systems, otherwise known as *chaos theory.* With billions of neurons, each with an average of 10,000 synaptic connections with other neurons, the brain is capable of organizing an incomprehensible number of possible activation patterns. In selectionist theory, the billions of neurons become clustered into groups that have similar functions and, when activated, become reinforced. Neuronal groups that are not activated die off; those that are activated survive. In other words, the brain generates a diversity of activity that can then be selected by interaction with the environment. In addition, the brain has value systems that selectively reinforce the activity of neuronal groups that enhance survival. In this way the brain's neuronal groups compete and differentiate within the brain and create an ongoing and evolving adaptational system.

Chaos theory suggests that complex systems adhere to a specific set of principles. Three principles—nonlinearity, self-organizational processes, and movement toward complexity—are especially relevant to psychiatry. *Nonlinear* refers to the finding that small changes in input (or initial conditions) can lead to large and unpredictable changes in output. Complex systems function on the rules of probability, which predict that certain combinations of activity within the system are more likely than others and tend to move the system toward self-organization. This probability also predicts that the system moves itself toward increasingly complex states of functioning.

The state of activation of the various parts of the system can cluster into repeated patterns called *states.* In the brain, a *state of mind* or *mental state* describes the way in which various neuronal groups may become activated at a given time. Repeated patterns of neuronal group activation, a neural net profile, can become reinforced if they occur frequently or if the value system of the brain ingrains their profile. These ingrained patterns of activation are called *attractor states*; those states that are least likely to occur are called *repellor states.* The mental states are determined by the constraints on the system. Modification of constraints allows the nature of attractor and repellor states to be altered. Constraints are external and internal. Thus, features of the external environment, such as the way other people behave and relate to an individual, can directly affect which mental state is more likely to be activated within the person. Internal constraints include the synaptic strengths of association, as determined by constitutional features and genetics, and those learned from experience, as encoded within memory processes.

Daniel J. Siegel has proposed that complexity theory may offer a useful working definition of mental health applicable to individuals, families, and larger social systems. In complex systems, self-organizational processes that move the system's states toward maximal complexity are mathematically shown to be the most stable, adaptive, and flexible. These features may be useful in defining *healthy* systems. The movement toward complexity is between the extremes of sameness, with rigidity and order on the one side and change, randomness, and chaos on the other. Complexity is achieved when the components of the system achieve a balance in the two fundamental processes of differentiation (specialization in function) and integration (coming together as a functional whole). For a single individual, such a balance can be achieved as the genetically and experientially influenced growth of neural circuits combines differentiation of specialized regions with their functional integration via neural fibers that connect widely distributed areas into a functional whole. A similar balance would be seen in larger systems as well. Disorder can be seen in this view as occurring when a system is stressed in its flow toward complexity, as revealed in movement toward either extreme: rigidity or chaos. Trauma may impair integration in an individual, as revealed in the finding of negative effects on the integrative regions of the corpus callosum and hippocampus in abused and neglected individuals. A dysfunctional family system would be conceptualized as occurring when the individuals are excessively differentiated (without emotional connections) or integrated (enmeshing that inhibits individuality from being expressed). Such stressed systems are limited in their movement toward complexity and, hence, their stability, flexibility, and adaptability.

Psychiatric disturbances may be conceptualized as disturbances in self-organizational processes. Inherited and experiential internal determinants and ongoing external, environmental, and social influences on the constraints of the system can thus directly affect the development and effective use of self-regulatory mechanisms. Clinical interventions may function at the level of external constraints (psychotherapy) or internal constraints (pharmacological treatments) that alter the ways in which the individual's mind is able to achieve healthy forms of self-organization. Viewing psychiatric disturbances in this way allows for a synthesis of the views of psychodynamic, biological, and social psychiatry.

States of Mind One way of describing the brain's self-organizational process is in the concept of states of mind. Repeatedly reinforced patterns of neuronal group firing link the cognitive processes of attention, perceptual bias, memory, mental models, behavioral response patterns, and emotional tone and regulation. These states of mind result in the patterns of cognitive, emotional, and behavioral symptoms seen in various psychiatric disorders. For example, in a depressed state of mind, one may pay conscious attention to negative aspects of experience, may interpret incoming stimuli in a pessimistic manner, may have greater access to depressing past experiences, may have the activation or instantiation of a mental model of the self and others as bad or guilty, may have the behavioral pattern of withdrawal, and may have a depressed mood with difficulty regulating intense affect.

Healthy mental functioning may depend on a flow of states of mind through time, allowing for flexible adaptation to an ever-changing environment. Chaos theory suggests that nonlinear complex systems must move continually toward maximizing complexity. Achieving such a goal requires a balance between predictability and novelty. Dysfunctional mental states may be conceptualized as a disruption toward either end of this balance: with excessive rigidity, as in the case of character pathology, or excessive fluidity, as in the case of disorders of thought or of mood.

SENSATION, PERCEPTION, AND COGNITION IN PSYCHIATRIC DISORDERS

Since the time of Emil Kraepelin and Eugen Bleuler, psychiatrists have known that certain disorders include profound disturbances in cognitive functioning. Since the 1950s, researchers have attempted to determine the exact nature of such deficits. With advances in computer technology and an increasing technical ability to analyze stimulus presentation and response times on the order of tens of milliseconds, cognitive psychologists have been able to devise research paradigms capable of testing the presence of increasingly subtle aspects of cognitive processing.

Processing research has focused on all three domains of sensation, perception, and cognition. Sensory-processing studies focus on poststimulus events for as long as a maximum of 1 second, using simple stimuli. Perceptual studies examine processing after a period of as long as approximately 5 seconds after a slightly more complex stimulus. Cognitive processing experiments can examine the early aspects of processing (e.g., phenomena occurring within the first 30 seconds) of complex, as well as long-term, processes that occur over hours, days, or years. Recent attempts have been made to correlate complex cognitive findings with clinical presentations.

A general problem correlating cognitive processes with clinical populations is the diversity of patients falling under the same syndrome classification. Schizophrenia, ADHD, major depressive disorder, and PTSD are all characterized by symptomatic heterogeneity. Thus, the array of cognitive dysfunctions identified for certain syndromes must be interpreted in light of the diversity of patient populations.

A related problem is the distinction between general and specific deficits. Care must be taken in interpreting experimental data that show differences among normal controls and patient groups. Do psychiatrically ill patients perform less well on a given paradigm because they are ill or because of a deficit specific to the disorder? For example, psychomotor slowing, as measured by reaction time and response rate, is seen in schizophrenia, depression, and other psychiatric and neurobehavioral disorders. The side effects of medications can also influence processing and response speed. Researchers rely on the creative design of experimental tasks to help distinguish between general and specific deficits. A comparison of target patient populations with matched healthy persons and other psychiatric patients can help to determine disorder-specific cognitive dysfunction.

Another general issue is that of state markers versus trait markers. For example, a patient with schizophrenia may have a cognitive deficit when actively psychotic (state) and also when asymptomatic (trait). These abnormal results have been found in certain cognitive tests of attention that correlate with improvement on medications; some abnormal results are also found in the non-ill first-degree relatives of schizophrenic patients. Is the marker of genetic vulnerability a coincidental finding or part of the core deficit in schizophrenia? An exploration of the implications of these cognitive abnormalities for the daily life of the patient is an important application of the research findings to clinical psychiatry.

Schizophrenia In the late 1890s, Kraepelin described a primary attention deficit in his elaborate clinical description of patients with schizophrenia. Numerous investigators have since attempted to define the nature of the cognitive deficits in schizophrenia. A general approach is that an early perceptual processing deficit leads to problems in perceptual organization and cognition. In general, information-processing models note that two things are processed: energy (in the form of external stimuli impinging on the senses) and information (a stimulus that carries a signal value based on significance derived from the prior processing of similar energy configurations). Schizophrenia patients appear to have deficits in the processing of energy as well as information.

Some cognitive tasks have been identified as trait-linked markers of schizophrenia: reaction time crossover, backward masking, dichotic listening, serial recall tasks, vigilance (sustained attention) tasks requiring high processing loads, and span-of-apprehension tests with large visual arrays. Deficits in those areas have been explored through many studies examining various aspects of processing.

Reaction Time Crossover and Modality Shift Effects These paradigms examine the general finding that schizophrenic patients have a slower than usual response on tasks that require rapid reaction times. A stimulus is presented with varied combinations of warning signals and preparatory intervals. Schizophrenic patients show an advantage only with short preparatory intervals and long response times with regularly spaced stimuli, a pattern distinct from that of normal controls (crossover effect). In a related paradigm, when the modality of the stimulus is varied (e.g., light is interspersed with tone), the latency (delay) of the response in schizophrenic patients, when compared with controls, is longer if the preceding stimulus was of a different modality. That is termed the *modality shift effect*, revealing a greater degree of cross-modal retardation in schizophrenic patients than in controls.

A number of theories have been proposed to explain these effects. They may be quantitative rather than qualitative distinctions from normal control groups. However, the crossover and modality shift effects support the idea that schizophrenic patients are overly influenced by stimuli that occurred immediately before the effect. The information-processing stages that explain the persistence of prior stimulus effects are under investigation.

Visual Backward Masking, Sensorimotor Gating, and Habituation In visual backward masking, a stimulus is followed by an interval of time, and then a subsequent stimulus is presented.

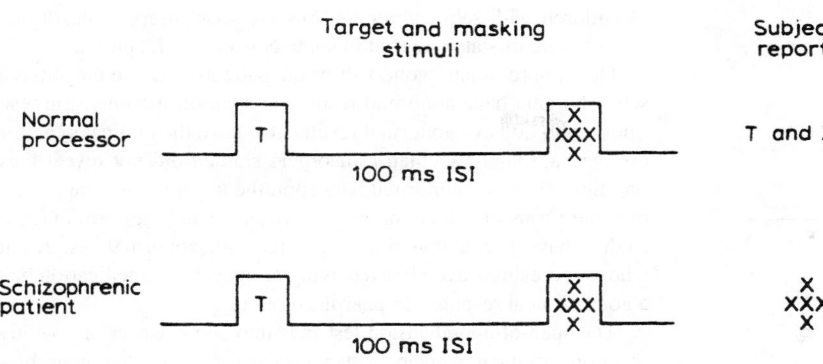

FIGURE 3.1–2 Diagram showing the difference in the verbal reports of normal versus schizophrenic subjects presented with a single backward masking trial with a 100-millisecond interstimulus interval (ISI). The T represents the target stimulus, and the Xs represent the masking stimulus. (From Braff DL, Saccuzzo DT, Geyer MA. Information processing dysfunctions in schizophrenia: Studies of visual backward masking, sensory motor gating and habituation. In: Steinhauer SR, Gruzelier JH, Zubin J, eds. *Handbook of Schizophrenia.* Vol 5. *Neuropsychology and Information Processing.* New York: Elsevier Science; 1991, with permission.)

Figure 3.1–2 shows a typical masking experiment. The presentation of the secondary stimulus leads the schizophrenic patient not to report (or mask) the initial stimulus. Lengthening of the interstimulus interval beyond 500 milliseconds can lead to normalization, with no masking present. Thus, the rapidity of presentation of the secondary stimulus is the factor determining whether it influences the perception or at least the reporting of the initial stimulus. Some studies find that the impairment improves with treatment by medication and can be induced in normal patients given catecholaminergic agents. Other studies find that the impairment may be a marker of increased vulnerability to schizophrenia.

Sensorimotor gating and habituation are the processes by which the reaction to stimuli decreases with repeated presentation. Sensory gating and habituation are believed to involve automatic preattentive processing, whereas visual masking requires higher cognitive functions. Schizophrenic patients show a markedly diminished capacity to habituate. One common study examines the persistent acoustic startle reflex as the person continues to blink with repetitive tones. Lysergic acid diethylamide (LSD) administration and the intracerebral injection of dopaminergic agents in rats lead to similar findings, supporting the idea that excessive dopamine activity, thought to be central in schizophrenia, can induce those deficits.

In general, deficits in habituation and visual backward masking lend support to the idea that schizophrenic patients have a diminished capacity to regulate the flow of rapidly presented information. They experience being inundated by stimuli that are filtered out in the brain of a normal person. Deficits in processing externally derived stimuli, as demonstrated in experimental paradigms, may also occur with internally generated stimuli.

Selective Attention In general, selective attention paradigms present the person with a target stimulus and distracters. In dichotic listening tasks, the subject is asked to attend to messages presented to one ear and to ignore messages presented to the other ear. Studies of schizophrenic patients have revealed consistent deficits in their ability to repeat the message they were asked to focus on. Analysis of these findings suggests that schizophrenic patients have an impairment in their ability to avoid distracting stimuli (to filter) and to pigeonhole (to use category features to reduce stimulus qualities needed to respond). The studies suggest that distractibility is a core cognitive deficit, supported by its high incidence in genetically vulnerable persons, its worsening in acutely psychotic states, and its improvement with medications.

These findings were explained by using the framework of an impaired filtering structure and pigeonholing process, but recent conceptualizations have examined a generalized impairment of the information-processing capacity in schizophrenia. The capacity model examines the way in which a pool or pools of attention capacity can be allocated across mental activities. Two components are quantity of resources available (capacity) and executive allocation policy. Other areas of deficit may involve an impaired response selection process, leading to abnormal results on tasks.

Several possibilities have been proposed to explain attention deficits in schizophrenic patients on the basis of the capacity model: (1) deautomatization of normally automatic preattentive processes, (2) disproportionate allocation of attention to schema-relevant (idiosyncratic) but task-irrelevant information, (3) inability to sustain controlled processes needed to maintain attention allocation without shifting, (4) inability to shift allocation biases to correct wandering attention, and (5) disorganized response selection because of heightened arousal under distracting conditions. Studies of selective attention may begin to examine these possibilities in a capacity model rather than in the previously explored structural framework.

Sustained Attention Sustained attention, or *vigilance*, is required to process stimuli of long duration. The most common research paradigm used to examine sustained attention is the *Continuous Performance Test.* The test consists of a rapidly presented set of tasks with varied spacing and timing of target and nontarget stimuli. The processing load for a Continuous Performance Test can be varied by blurring the stimuli presented or by changing the pace of presentation.

Vigilance tests, such as the Continuous Performance Test, require analysis of response features on the basis of the signal detection theory. The two elements distinguished are sensitivity and the response criterion. Diminished sensitivity is a sign of decreased vigilance and results in a high miss rate (errors of omission). The response criterion can be diminished, leading to a high false-positive rate (error of commission). The analysis is important in the interpretation of results. The vigilance studies using the Continuous Performance Test reveal that schizophrenic patients have a deficit in their ability to distinguish target stimuli from nontarget stimuli when the stimuli are presented as brief signals at a rapid pace.

Schizophrenic patients also appear to have a specific diminishment in sensitivity but not a lowering of the response criterion for verbal and spatial stimuli. The impaired responses were significantly associated with specific clinical features in patients and their first-degree relatives. Test abnormalities, although present in other disorders, appear to be most robust in schizophrenia. Positron emission tomography (PET) in schizophrenic patients performing a Continuous Performance Test found lower metabolic activity than in normal persons in the prefrontal cortex bilaterally but normal or elevated activation in the occipital region. That finding is consistent with other findings supporting the idea of impaired frontal functioning in schizophrenia.

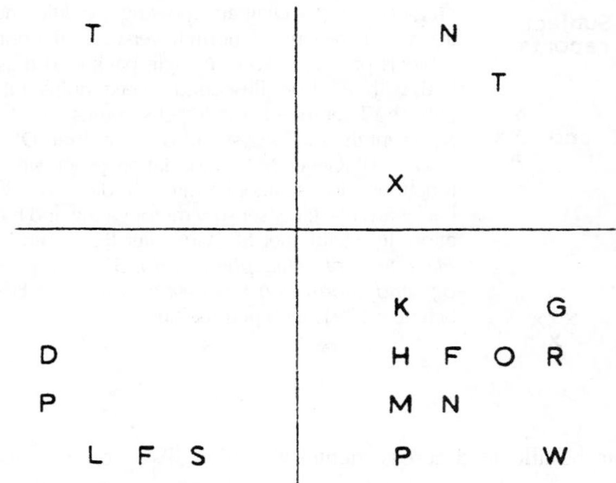

FIGURE 3.1–3 Sample arrays used in the wide–visual-angle version of the partial report span-of-apprehension task. (Courtesy of Robert F. Asarnow, Ph.D.)

Language and Discourse Assessments of language dysfunction in schizophrenia have focused on the basic question of whether the abnormalities in speech are reflections of a core disorder of thought or an abnormality in speech production. The search for a schizophrenic language has yielded negative conclusions. Discourse analyses of conversations with schizophrenic patients suggest that they may have significant difficulties in the maintenance of a specific topic (derailment) and in the lack of a discourse plan directing speech (disorganization).

Other investigators have argued that schizophrenic patients have impaired capacities to perceive the needs of others and may be schema driven in the direction of their speech, rather than intending to communicate effectively. One study showed that delusion-consistent material presented in the nonattended channel in a dichotic listening task leads to diminished attention to the target channel. A clinical implication of this experimental finding is the possibility that schema-driven processing during speech production may be diverting attention to internal stimuli and away from the potentially confusing social demands of conversation.

Span of Apprehension In the span-of-apprehension test, an array of letters is displayed for a brief period (from 50 to 100 milliseconds in most studies). One of the letters is a T or an F, and the person must detect which letter is present. The number of nontarget letters is increased, and significant differences in detection are found for displays of ten or more letters. Figure 3.1–3 provides an example of a visual display for the span-of-apprehension test.

The serial scanning process is an element of focal attention. Parallel processing in the search involves increased aspects of assessment of figure-ground and textual segregation and is thought to be an automatic process. Studies have shown that the sequential scanning of the attention spotlight is directly affected by increasing the complexity of certain display characteristics, leading to increased errors in detection. This is logical, because the iconic image has a limited display time, and the scanning of the image may be incomplete by the time it decays from such an ultrabrief form of memory.

Schizophrenic patients show significantly increased errors in the span-of-apprehension test under conditions of increased complexity of display. Their scores are also worse in psychotic conditions and are improved with symptomatic improvement while taking medications. Increased errors are also found in nonschizophrenic mothers of children with schizophrenia. Thus the span-of-apprehension test is a measure of state and trait in some cases of schizophrenia.

Only approximately one-half of the patients with the diagnosis of schizophrenia have abnormal results on span-of-apprehension tests. Those who do have abnormal results also have the clinical symptom of anergia. Other psychiatric disorders studied did not reveal these findings. Thus, the abnormal results on the test appear to be specific to some forms of schizophrenia. Short-term and long-term outcome studies have found that those patients with abnormal test results whose scores improve after receiving antipsychotic medication have a good clinical response to pharmacotherapy.

The span-of-apprehension test taps into some aspect of cognitive function specific to some patients with schizophrenia, their nonschizophrenic relatives, and persons at risk for developing the symptoms of schizophrenia. To scan the iconic image, the person must (1) engage attention to the iconic register, (2) move the focus of attention, and (3) disengage the focus of attention. Impairments in performing any one of those tasks can explain the test-result abnormalities. Another cause of the deficiency may be that, with each fixation of attention, less information is processed. Thus, although the individual steps of iconic scanning may be intact, less visual information is processed, and more errors occur. A third possibility is that the initiation of the attention process is delayed; this possibility is consistent with the increased reaction times revealed on numerous other tasks. The delay in the face of a rapid decay rate of sensory memory places the patients at a disadvantage when rapid responses are required; this possibility is also consistent with the other forms of attention deficit described previously. Schizophrenic patients may have a number of structural and capacity deficiencies, and these hypotheses are not mutually exclusive. Further studies are needed to elucidate the nature of the cognitive state-trait marker for schizophrenic patients and persons vulnerable to the disorder.

Attention-Deficit/Hyperactivity Disorder

In the revised fourth edition of the *Diagnostic and Statistical Manual of Mental Disorders* (DSM-IV-TR), ADHD integrates two categories from the revised third edition of the *Diagnostic and Statistical Manual of Mental Disorders* (DSM-III-TR): ADHD and undifferentiated attention-deficit disorder. Diagnostic criteria embrace a number of forms of the syndrome, and research into the cognitive deficits has outlined a wide array of tasks in which attention capacity is abnormal. The pervasive findings of cognitive impairment in the setting of numerous intact cognitive functions have left the research field with no clearly accepted view of a core deficit in the disorder. Clinically, child and adolescent patients present with problems in school, with peers, and at home that reflect academic and behavioral dysfunctions. Many studies suggest that the cognitive and behavioral dysfunctions in the disorder may be independent processes with different neurophysiological bases. For example, the finding that children with ADHD are impulsive may be true behaviorally but cannot be stated as a generalization about their cognitive functioning.

Researchers have attempted to find clear-cut diagnostic criteria to help clarify the disorder, but individuals classified as meeting diagnostic criteria at this point appear be quite heterogeneous. There is no definitive test for the disorder nor is a positive response to psychopharmacological intervention pathognomonic. Biochemical studies have found abnormal urinary catecholamine metabolites that normalize as the patient's behavior improves when taking psychostimulants. Those findings and PET scan data suggest abnormal brain functions in patients with ADHD.

Data from numerous studies show that the patients with ADHD have dysfunctions on a variety of tasks ranging from those involving monitoring, perception, memory, and motor control. Intact performance has been found on a number of memory tasks requiring verbal processes (e.g., digit span, word tests, and story recall) and nonverbal processes (e.g., recall, visual arrays, and block series).

A number of theories have been elaborated to explain those differences between patients with the disorder and normal persons. Each theory has strengths, weaknesses, and varied support from the data, but each highlights the complexity of the cognitive dimensions of the disorder. In general, patients with the disorder evidence behavior that has been compared to that of patients with frontal lobe damage: deficits in the control of motor responses, in the execution of fine-motor movements, and in the inhibition of ongoing response patterns. Memory tasks and basic aspects of information processing are intact, but the patients have impaired performance across modalities (auditory, visual, motor, and perceptual-motor), suggesting some global deficit. The patients also appear to be unusually susceptible to boredom when the required tasks are long and repetitive.

Another view examines two proposed systems—an underactive behavioral inhibition system and an impaired behavioral reward system—to explain the behavioral problems that children with the disorder often have. A related view is that the rule-governed behavioral system is not intact; patients with the disorder appear to do especially poorly in a system with delayed or nonexistent rewards, as in tasks that require sustained attention, accuracy, or task-directed activity governed by another person's direction or rules. Under those conditions, the patient's poor regulation and inability to meet functional demands are revealed. A related issue is a diminished motivational drive and, possibly, a diminished arousal regulation system.

Yet another approach supported by research data is that the patients have metacognitive deficits. According to this perspective, metacognitive processes that help plan, monitor, and regulate performance are impaired. The patient's ability to assess the task and to determine strategies also has deficits. That is an example of top-down aspects of attention, with impairment of the higher cognitive processes that regulate information flow. Additional bottom-up deficiencies involve basic aspects of attention focus because of abnormalities in arousal, selectivity, and capacity.

The finding that numerous factors can influence the appearance of deficits led Virginia Douglas to the hypothesis that ADHD is a self-regulatory disorder with pervasive effects. The impairments affect each of four domains—attention, inhibition, reinforcement, and arousal—resulting in deficits in several aspects of self-regulation: (1) the organization of information processing, including planning, metacognition, executive functions, adapting appropriate cognitive sets for a given task, regulating arousal levels and alertness, and self-monitoring and self-correction; (2) the mobilization of attention, including the deployment and the maintenance of adequate attention; and (3) the inhibition of inappropriate responses, such as withholding responses to extraneous stimuli and reinforcers. These deficits in self-regulation imply that increased processing demands would lead to a diffusion of attention processes and to a subsequent impairment of the in-depth, coherent acquisition of knowledge and understanding.

One line of research has been based on the additive factor method, in which experimenters attempt to isolate the stage of the deficit. The model for that approach entails four stages: encoding (the identification of a stimulus), serial comparison (of the stimulus with elements related to the category in long-term memory), decision (pertaining to the category into which the stimulus is stored), and translation and response organization. Studies using evoked potentials suggest that deficits are found after the search and decision stages (the first three stages). The response preparation and execution processes appear to be impaired. Features that increase the processing load—such as speed demands, complexity of stimuli, distractors leading to divided attention, and increased duration of task—reveal different areas of deficit. This fact may explain the diversity of methods and research data supporting various theories. The variables affecting outcome include information-processing demands, the availability of alternate stimuli to which to attend, and the presence of an external regulator.

The diversity of research findings and theoretical explanations is paralleled by the clinical finding that children who are severely impaired in the classroom may have no attention problems in the confined, one-on-one setting of the psychiatrist's or psychoeducational examiner's office. Such children may also be able to attend for indefinite periods to video games and yet be unable to follow complex conceptual information. The important principle is that cognitive dysfunction in psychopathological conditions may be task specific as a function of the nature of the cognitive impairment. The patient's clinical history and evaluation must consider potentially hidden domains of abnormal cognition.

Autistic Disorder Early descriptions of autism delineated the social-functioning deficits that impair normal functioning. Autistic children were seen as having difficulties in normal emotional contact. Cognitive dysfunctions in autistic disorder were described later and were found to involve a number of areas, including abstraction, sequencing, language, and comprehension. Researchers are now focusing on the nature of the core deficit in the disorder. Issues of specificity and universality of areas of dysfunction in the disorder are important. How the cognitive domains relate to the social-affective deficits is of particular interest.

Seventy-five percent of patients with autistic disorder are also mentally retarded. Mental retardation involves global cognitive and language impairments that may make it difficult to distinguish autistic disorder features. General cognitive impairments may be especially difficult to assess if language functioning is severely limited. Studies of high-functioning patients with autistic disorder have permitted various deficits to be determined.

Studies of the cognitive deficits in autistic disorder have distinguished an array of dysfunctional areas, including numerous language problems, excessive or impaired responsiveness to stimuli of various modalities, different encoding of auditory stimuli, and impairment in the ability to extract important features from incoming information. This range of deficits is thought to require the transformation of symbolic representations. In contrast, some patients with autistic disorder have relatively intact visuospatial and gestalt functions, musical abilities, and rote memory. Performances on standardized tests reveal relatively good results in object assembly and block design but poor results in comprehension.

Language deficits vary and include syntactic and phonological domains. These findings initially suggested a left-hemisphere deficit, but other findings, including deficits in prosodic and pragmatic language functions, suggested right-hemisphere involvement as well. The findings can be interpreted as deviations from normal language functioning as well as delays in language functioning. The wide array of dysfunctions in autistic disorder may be due to a number of subtypes, with characteristic deficits and possibly different brain loci of dysfunction.

Other studies have focused on the social cognition of patients with autistic disorder. They have examined the nature of the patient's emo-

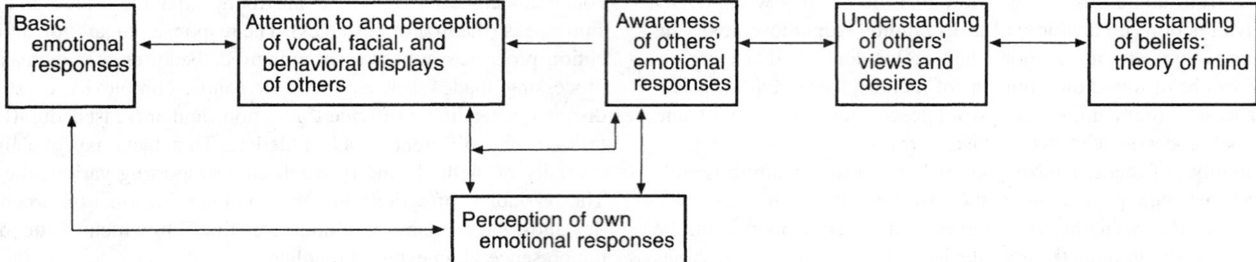

FIGURE 3.1–4 Sigman's model for the development of socioemotional understanding. (Courtesy of M. Sigman.)

tional behavior and understanding to assess the earliest clinical descriptions of an abnormal emotional connection between autistic children and their parents. Recent work in neurobiology suggests a role of the orbitofrontal cortex and the cerebellum in mediating some of these deficits. Two findings support the initial impressions: Autistic children are much less likely than usual to imitate adult vocalizations and gestures, and they show much less sophisticated representational play with objects than do normal children. These findings led to the suggestion that a core deficit in autistic disorder is the representation of representations (metarepresentations), leading to deficits in symbolic play and the inability to understand the mental states of others. The inability to transfer cognitive representations into language symbols may also be a related metarepresentation deficit.

A series of studies explored the relation of these possible cognitive impairments to socioemotional behavior. In contrast to clinical lore, children with autistic disorder were found to look at their parents; they had eye contact with their parents when social interactions were parentally elicited, and they revealed normal behavioral patterns of attachment. The studies found a marked lack of social referencing (looking to parents for emotional cues in ambiguous situations) and protodeclarative gestures (pointing to objects and showing objects to familiar adults). Three domains have been proposed to explain these findings: (1) Autistic children may not have the capacity to have a representation of another person as having ideas, perspectives, or emotions that can be shared. This proposal is consistent with a theory-of-mind hypothesis, in which the core deficit is believed to be the inability to have a sense of another's mind. (2) Autistic patients may have an impaired ability to perceive or to comprehend the emotional (usually facial) signals of others. (3) The core deficit may involve a lack of interest in others or an aversion to responding to others. Studies have found that although children with autistic disorder do express emotions, they have less positive affects in response to their (relatively infrequent) periods of joint attention. Furthermore, they have an impairment in their responsivity to the display of strong emotion by another, whether of distress or of pleasure.

Tests of high-functioning autism patients reveal poor performance on emotion-recognition tasks, little comprehension of and empathy with depictions of social situations, and difficulty in talking about socially derived emotions, such as pride and embarrassment. Autistic patients with relatively high intelligence use adaptive cognitive strategies to interpret social stimuli to compensate for impaired emotion-processing abilities. The development of social cognition and socioemotional understanding requires complex interactions among the cognitive, perceptual, and emotional processes. A series of interactive elements essential to the development of social understanding has been proposed (Fig. 3.1–4). This model describes the basic precursors of emotional responsiveness: the ability to attend to, to encode, and to interpret verbal and nonverbal social stimuli; the awareness of one's own and others' emotional responses; and the ability to contrast oneself with others. Out of that matrix develops the ability to understand others' views, desires, and beliefs. Accordingly, a deficit in any of those basic elements may explain the characteristic deficits observed in the social understanding of persons with autistic disorder.

Mood Disorders

In contrast to schizophrenia, ADHD, and autistic disorder, the mood disorders do not appear to have core cognitive deficits that are diagnosis specific. Instead, cognitive abnormalities appear to be related to the degree of psychopathology and to the severity of the mood disturbance. Most studies have examined patients with depression; only a few studies have assessed cognitive functioning in patients with bipolar I disorder in a manic state. In depressed patients, the severity of the depression has ranged from mild depression in students to severe illness in hospitalized patients with major depressive disorders. The studies have primarily examined attention and memory for neutral and emotionally toned stimuli. For the majority of these studies, the concept of self-organizational processes and state regulation has not been the primary focus of attention. These recent conceptualizations of the brain's functioning as a nonlinear complex system capable of self-organization may aid in the future investigation of the primary deregulatory aspect of disorders of mood.

Depressive Disorders

Depressed patients often complain of difficulties with concentrating, learning, and remembering. Studies have documented that such patients perform poorly on tasks that require sustained attention or effortful and elaborate rehearsal. Thus, controlled limited-capacity processes appear to be impaired in major depressive disorder. This limitation on access to capacity-demanding resources appears to be directly related to the severity of the depression and normalizes with remission from a depressive episode.

Depressed patients have also been found to have an increased response criterion; they require increased supportive data from the presented stimuli to respond in a test situation. Whether this need to be certain before responding is a psychological response to being depressed or a specific feature of the depression itself has not yet been determined. The reluctance to respond needs to be considered in interpreting research data and clinical interview findings.

The attention and memory findings have suggested several theoretical frameworks that are clinically useful. A schema theory of depression outlines a positive feedback loop in which negative self-schemata prime persons to have negative thoughts, to recall negative events in their lives, and to interpret present events with a negative bias. Whether as a cause or as a maintaining influence, these depressogenic schemata are thought to create a series of cognitive functions that produce and maintain a depressed mood.

A network theory of memory and emotion has been supported by research on depressed and nondepressed persons in which mood leads to a spreading activation of items in memory that are congruent with the mood. Thus, emotion directly influences retrieval by a process of state-dependent learning and memory. While depressed, patients are likely to encode items in a form that makes them readily accessible when retrieved in a depressed state; depressed mood thus becomes an internal context cue that accesses depression-related memories.

The network and schemata theories of depression are consonant with research findings but do not explain all the cognitive and clinical findings in depression. They provide a framework for understanding how emotions and moods influence cognitive processing, such as memory retrieval and mental models. The conceptualization may be applicable to transient mood states and severe mood episodes. Thus, emotions in health and illness can shape the mental state instantiated at a given time and thus act as a context cue, leading to the activation of previously formed schemata for oneself and others. The activated schemata, in turn, can produce retrieval biasing and behavioral responses, fundamental to a mental state, that can further elicit a negative emotional response. A reinforcing loop is established to support the continuation of the depressed mood and depressive cognition.

Some patients may be especially prone to marked cognitive alterations because of an emotional state that may be a fundamental part of a clinical presentation. Thus, rapid shifts in state of mind may be a learned or constitutional feature of the individual. From the nonlinear dynamics view, these rapid shifts in mental state can be conceptualized as sudden and intense changes in the constraints on the system, which determine the flow of states of mind across time. Activating a set of constraints that establish and maintain a depressed state can then lead to the persistence of the factors that created the shift in probabilities of that state being active. The depressed state becomes a deeply ingrained attractor state that becomes difficult to alter. Pharmacological interventions may directly alter the synaptic constraints maintaining such a state. Psychotherapeutic interventions, such as cognitive-behavioral and interpersonal therapy, can be proposed to produce changes in the internal processing of constraints and in external social constraints, respectively.

Bipolar I Disorder Patients with manic episodes present with a spectrum of cognitive dysfunctions that appear to be related to the severity of their mood episode and that normalize with remission. The disturbances have been described clinically as rapidly paced thinking and speech, quick associations to self-generated or other-generated stimuli, grandiosity, and increased distractibility.

Formal studies of patients with bipolar I disorder are technically difficult to carry out because of the patient's lack of cooperation and restlessness, and because such patients are few in number. The studies have suggested a high rate of combinatory thinking, the inclusion of loosely associated but related intrusions, and increased distractibility. The clinical impression of humor (even in the face of an underlying dysphoria) in some patients with bipolar I disorder is corroborated by playful, extravagant, or flippant elaborations and intrusions in speech. These findings seem to indicate primarily state-dependent symptoms that improve on recovery. Thus, forced-choice span-of-apprehension and backward masking tasks reveal impairments similar to those seen in actively schizophrenic patients but unlike those seen in schizophrenic patients who have persistent deficits in the remitted state. Bipolar I disorder patients who are not actively ill reveal normal information processing. Thus, bipolar disorders can also be viewed as a disorder of self-organization in which the system fluctuates between the extremes of highly activated manic and highly deactivated depressed states of mind.

Posttraumatic Stress Disorder Studies of PTSD have extended the findings of information-processing abnormalities in anxiety disorders: attention biases toward fear-related and threat-related stimuli. Many of the studies were hampered by poorly defined clinical populations and control groups. However, some general trends, noted especially in the well-controlled paradigms, are promising and provide important insights into the psychopathological cognitive mechanisms in PTSD.

Cognitive studies of patients with anxiety disorders have focused primarily on attention or memory. Various research paradigms have been applied to assess attention bias and memory retrieval for neutral and emotionally activating stimuli. Studies find that anxious patients have an increased tendency to attend to fear-related and threat-related words. One research approach includes a dichotic listening task in which an anxious patient is more easily distracted than are controls by fear-related stimuli in the nonattended channel. This finding suggests that the patients have automatic, parallel attention processes that are primed to detect certain types of stimuli. Another approach uses the Stroop paradigm, in which words are presented in different-colored inks, and the person's task is to look at the word and state the color of the ink. Anxious patients have a significant delay in their response times for fear-related words, a finding that suggests that increased attention capacity or cognitive processing is necessary when those words are perceived and the color of the ink is determined.

One theory that explains these findings is the idea of a fear network that encodes fear-related information in a memory structure that is readily accessible and able to influence cognitive, motor, and psychophysiological responses. The theoretical fear networks, which may be similar to mental models, are thought to contain three related forms of information: fear-eliciting stimulus cues, specific response patterns, and the meaning of the cues and the responses for that particular person. According to this theory, patients with anxiety disorders are believed to have fear networks that are especially coherent and stable and that require few environmental cues to become activated.

Patients with PTSD have been found to have attention biases toward threat-related stimuli specific to the experienced traumatic event. Many of the patients studied were combat veterans, and further work is needed to establish the generalization of those findings to other forms of PTSD. The disorder is clinically characterized by intrusive processes (memories, images, emotions, and thoughts) and avoidance elements (psychic and emotional numbing, amnesia, behavioral avoidance of environmental cues resembling the initial trauma). The patients are thought to have a unique configuration of fear networks with stimulus cues (environmental stimuli), response components (cognitive, motoric, and psychophysiological), and meaning elements (e.g., the moral implications of the trauma, survivor guilt, and the meaning of intentional trauma vs. accidental trauma).

Some theories argue that states of excessive arousal during trauma impair attention capacity and memory encoding during the event. Emotional processing during and after the traumatic experience may also be hampered by the states of psychophysiological arousal and altered memory storage. The part of the brain necessary for explicit memory processing, the hippocampus, has been shown to be abnormal in individuals experiencing chronic PTSD. The subsequent clinical syndrome may have some aspects that are adaptive: Cognitive attention biases that are primed to detect fear-related stimuli may permit the early detection of threatening situations that, if not avoided, would produce incapacitating psychophysiological arousal. Automatic, nonconscious behavioral avoidance response patterns, embedded in the proposed fear networks or mental models, allow the patients to minimize excessive arousal by avoiding trauma-related situations. Patients who used dissociative mechanisms during and after a traumatic experience appear to be at far greater risk for developing PTSD. Dissociation is a complex process that essentially involves the disassociation of usually associated processes, such as attention, perception, memory, consciousness, and sense of self.

The psychopathological aspects of PTSD can be cognitively exemplified as follows: A combat veteran with chronic PTSD may have no direct recall (impaired explicit memory) of a helicopter crash in which his best friend, who was seated next to him, was killed. Years later, continued avoidance of airports, amnesia for combat, general apathy, and social withdrawal (avoidance elements) combined with startle response, panic attacks, intrusive images, and nightmares (intrusive components) all suggest intact implicit memory for the combat trauma. The veteran is emotionally, behaviorally, and cognitively impaired.

Speechless Terror Scott L. Rauch and colleagues explored the neurobiology of intense fear using patients with PTSD. They took eight patients with PTSD and exposed them to two audiotapes: One was emotionally neutral, and the other was a script of a traumatic experience. While they were listening to these tapes, measures of their heart rate and regional cerebral blood flow (rCBF) were measured via PET scans. rCBF was greater during traumatic audio tapes in right-sided structures, including the amygdala; the posterior medial, orbitofrontal, insular, anterior, and medial temporal lobes; and the anterior cingulate cortex. These are the areas thought to be involved with intense emotion.

An extremely interesting and potentially important clinical finding was a decrease in rCBF in Broca's area (left inferior frontal and middle temporal cortex). These findings suggest a potential active inhibition of language centers during trauma. Based on these results, speechless terror, often reported by victims of trauma, may have neurobiological correlates consistent with what is known about brain architecture and brain–behavior relationships. This inhibitory effect on Broca's area impairs the encoding of conscious memory for traumatic events at the time that they occur. It then naturally interferes with the development of narratives that serve to process the experience and lead to neural network integration and psychological healing. Activating Broca's area and left cortical networks of explicit episodic memory may be essential in psychotherapy with patients experiencing PTSD and other anxiety-based disorders.

The evaluation and treatment of patients can be greatly enhanced by an understanding of development, dissociation, and cognitive processes (including memory) and its careful application to the assessment of presenting symptoms and signs. Several areas that have interested clinicians for decades have become of great societal concern. Two topics that inspire intense controversy are the delayed recall of repressed memories of traumatic events and the suggestibility of patients influenced by clinicians, society, or friends to believe that they are the victims of childhood trauma.

Delayed Recall Many scientists and clinicians believe in the cognitive capacity of patients to be unaware for years or decades of severely traumatic experiences that took place in their childhoods. Other researchers disagree and emphasize the paucity of studies of corroborated cases of childhood trauma that have been followed prospectively into adulthood with documentation of impaired access of consciousness to events presumably stored in memory. A cognitive science view of delayed recall can examine the role of memory processes and development and the effect of trauma on the processing of information to describe a theoretically coherent but yet-to-be-proved set of mechanisms.

A repressed memory can be thought of as originating from the active, intentional suppression of memory from consciousness. The mechanisms underlying the process then may become automatic, and the contents of memory may be inhibited from retrieval into consciousness. The blockage may exist to avoid flooding the person's awareness with information that is associated with excessive anxiety or fear that would impair normal functioning. This is an example of knowledge isolation in which information may be layered in the nervous system and certain aspects may be kept from conscious awareness.

In contrast, a traumatic event may be so overwhelming that normal processing may be impaired. If focal attention is divided, the nonfocally attended (traumatic) material is only processed implicitly. Thus, to adapt to a traumatic event, some persons may have the capacity to focus their attention on a nonthreatening aspect of the environment or on their imagination during the trauma; this may be an underlying mechanism in a process called *dissociation.* Traumatic memory that has been only implicitly encoded affects behavior and emotions and possibly contains intrusive images and bodily sensations that are devoid of a sense of past, of self, or of something being recalled. This may partly explain the findings of PTSD with amnesia (blocked conscious access to a memory or its origin) in the setting of avoidance behaviors, hyperarousal, intrusive images, and flashbacks.

Thus, two distinct mechanisms that may explain delayed recall of childhood trauma are the concepts of repressed memories and dissociated memories. A person may use both mechanisms for different aspects of a traumatic event. Recollection of the traumatic memory may take different forms. Repressed memories may have been processed to some degree in narrative form, whereas dissociated memories probably lack that more integrative processing. The latter form thus may be experienced as nonpast and nonself, making the intrusive retrieval of dissociated memories a confusing and frightening experience.

Studies of the development of memory in children suggest that the shared construction of narratives about experienced events is often crucial in making the events accessible to long-term retrieval. The establishment of a personal memory system appears to be a function of such memory talk in which parents discuss with children the contents of their memory. In children who have been forced to keep traumatic events a secret, as may occur with childhood abuse, the normal developmental process of narration may be blocked. This may be an additional cognitive mechanism underlying the inaccessibility of some forms of childhood trauma to consciousness in adult patients.

Suggestibility Knowledge isolation, such as in dissociation and repression, provides a theoretical scientific explanation for the underlying mechanisms that may lead to delayed recall of childhood trauma, but clinicians must also be aware of other cognitive processes that influence memory. Numerous studies have demonstrated that the human mind is easily influenced. Human suggestibility can be used to the benefit or detriment of others. Suggestibility is adaptive for a social being that relies on the experiences of others to inform its knowledge of the world and thus to increase its chance for survival. Thus, listening to the stories of others, reading a textbook, and being coached in athletics all require the receiver to accept data from the sender. The learner (listener) needs to trust the reliability of the teacher (teller) to accept the incoming information. Critical analysis of the data received is an important component of learning. The metacognitive function of assessing the accuracy or usefulness of newly acquired information may be suspended under certain conditions, including hypnosis, drug-altered states, and conditions of severe threat.

Studies of human suggestibility indicate that postevent questioning can bias the metamemory processes that help determine the source and accuracy of a retrieved memory. The verbal and nonverbal cues given by the interviewer may influence a person to believe that aspects of an event or an entire event that may have never happened actually took place. A person can be convinced of the accuracy of an event despite its lack of correspondence with actual experience. Factors that may influence the biasing of interviewees include a belief in the trustworthiness and authority of the interviewer, not being aware that "I don't know" is a permissible response, repetition of a question that already has been answered, and the interviewer's beliefs as communicated through emotional tone and nonverbal gestures.

It is crucial for clinicians to be aware of human suggestibility to avoid iatrogenic distortions. Similarly, it is important for persons who experienced severe trauma early in life to receive informed and empathetic evaluations and treatment. There is a delicate balance between supportive neutrality and active advocacy in assessment and intervention. Awareness of these fundamental cognitive processes may help guide the clinician toward achieving that goal.

Approaches to the treatment of patients with PTSD need careful evaluation but generally include the view that the impaired emotional processing of the traumatic event requires the active recollection, in explicit terms, of the details of the experience. The process of effectively treating unresolved trauma usually involves the active cognitive processing of specific memories, including emotional responses, derived belief systems, and the psychophysiological arousal at the time of the traumatic event. The provision of new cognitive information in the course of psychotherapy can, in theory, alter the configuration of the fear networks and can allow previously inaccessible information to be explicitly processed and made available to consciousness for incorporation into an ongoing autobiographical narrative. Specific techniques, such as those which facilitate such cognitive processing of previously dissociated or in other ways isolated cognitions, such as beliefs, images, and sensations, may be useful in alleviating the symptoms and dysfunction after acute or chronic trauma. Such therapy and changes in mental processing may diminish the avoidant and intrusive components of the clinical syndrome of PTSD and may improve social, emotional, and cognitive functioning.

Complex PTSD Complex PTSD occurs in the context of prolonged and inescapable stress and trauma. It is complex because of its extensive physiological effects and its impact on all areas of development and functioning, especially if it occurs during early childhood. Enduring personality traits and coping strategies evolving from traumatic states tend to increase the individual's vulnerability to future trauma. This manifests in a traumatic resonance through engagement in abusive relationships, poor judgment, and a lack of self protection. Long-term PTSD has been shown to correlate with the presence of what are called *neurological soft signs*, pointing to subtle neurological impairments. These neurological signs could suggest a vulnerability to the development of PTSD or reflect the impact of the long-term physiological dysregulation caused by PTSD.

When confronted with threat under normal circumstances, the processes related to arousal and the fight-or-flight response become activated; the threat is dealt with and soon passes. For obvious reasons, children are not well equipped to cope with threat in this way. Fighting and fleeing may actually decrease their chances for survival, because their survival depends on dependency. When a child first cries for help, but no help arrives, or when trauma is being inflicted by a caretaker, he or she may shift from hyperarousal to dissociation. Traumatized children who are agitated may be misdiagnosed as having attention-deficit disorder, whereas the numbing response in infants can be misinterpreted as a lack of sensitivity to pain. This may also be true for women who are often unable to outrun or outfight male attackers.

Until recently, surgery was performed on infants without anesthesia, because their gradual lack of protest was mistakenly interpreted as insensitivity to pain, as opposed to a traumatic reaction to it. Recent survey research suggests that less than 25 percent of physicians performing circumcision on newborns use any form of analgesia, despite physiological indications that neonates are experiencing stress and pain during and after the procedure. These practices appear to be a holdover of beliefs that newborns do not experience or do not remember pain. It makes sense that an appreciation for the possibility of PTSD reactions in neonates and young children has lagged behind other areas.

Dissociation allows the traumatized individual to escape the trauma via a number of biological and psychological processes. Increased levels of endogenous opioids create a sense of well-being, pain reduction, and a decrease in explicit processing of the overwhelming traumatic situation. Psychological processes, such as derealization and depersonalization, allow the victim to avoid the reality of his or her situation or to watch it as an observer. These processes provide the experience of leaving the body, traveling to other worlds, or immersing oneself into other objects in the environment. Hyperarousal and dissociation in childhood establish an inner biopsychological environment primed to establish boundaries between different emotional states and experiences for a lifetime. If it is too painful to experience the world from inside one's body, self-identity can become organized outside the physical self.

Early traumatic experiences determine biochemical levels and neuroanatomical networking, impacting experience and adaptation throughout development. The tendency to dissociate and disconnect various tracks of processing creates a bias toward unintegrated information processing across conscious awareness, sensation, affect, and behavior. General dissociative defenses resulting in an aberrant organization of networks of memory, fear, and the social brain contribute to deficits of affect regulation, attachment, and executive functioning. The malformation of these interdependent systems results in many disorders resulting from extreme early stress. Compulsive disorders related to eating or gambling and somatization disorders in which emotions are converted into physical symptoms can all be understood in this way. PTSD, borderline personality disorder, and self-harm can all reflect complex adaptation to early trauma.

FUTURE DIRECTIONS

Cognitive science offers a breadth of conceptualizations for understanding the way in which the mind functions in health and disease. The broad interdisciplinary field provides numerous research paradigms that are helpful in further elucidating the nature of psychopathology through techniques from the neurosciences to computer models of brain functioning and biological applications of chaos theory. The cognitive understanding of emotions and consciousness may also expand psychiatry's framework for knowing about human subjective experience. Clinical tools, from medications to in-depth psychotherapy, may also find wider application as the processes of self-organization and psychological change are better understood.

Psychiatry, in turn, has much to offer the field of cognitive science. The long history of descriptive psychopathology and the attempt to synthesize views of the mind and the brain can provide nonclinical cognitive scientists with unique data and relevant questions. Psychiatry is invited to join in the search for understanding the cognitive processes of the human mind.

SUGGESTED CROSS-REFERENCES

Piaget and emotional development are discussed in Section 3.2, memory is discussed in Section 3.4, cognitive disorders are discussed in Chapter 10, schizophrenia is discussed in Chapter 12, mood disorders are discussed in Chapter 13, and anxiety disorders are discussed in Chapter 14. Dissociative disorders are discussed in Chapter 17, and personality disorders are discussed in Chapter 23. Behavior therapy is discussed in Section 30.2, hypnosis is discussed in Section 30.3, and cognitive therapy is discussed in Section 30.6. Mental retardation is discussed in Chapter 34, learning disorders are discussed in Chapter 35, pervasive developmental disorders are discussed in Chapter 38, and ADHD is discussed in Chapter 39.

REFERENCES

Andreasen NC: Linking mind and brain in the study of mental illnesses: A project for a scientific psychopathology. *Science.* 1997;275:1586.

Baddeley A: Working memory: Looking back and looking forward. *Nature.* 2003;4:829.

*Cozolino LC. *The Neuroscience of Psychotherapy: Building and Rebuilding the Human Brain.* New York: W.W. Norton; 2002.

Damasio AR. *Descartes' Error: Emotion, Reason and the Human Brain.* New York: Putnam; 1994.

Douglas VI. Cognitive deficits in children with attention deficit disorder with hyperactivity. In: Bloomingdale LM, Sergeant JA, eds. *Attention Deficit Disorder: Criteria, Cognition, Intervention.* Oxford, UK: Pergamon Press; 1988.

Fonagy P, Steele M, Steele H, Moran GS, Higgitt AC: The capacity to understand mental states: The reflective self in parent and child and its significance for security of attachment. *Infant Ment Health J.* 1991;12:201–218.

Johnson MH, Magaro PA: Effects of mood and severity on memory processes in depression and mania. *Psychol Bull.* 1987;101:28.

Johnson-Laird PN. *Mental Models: Towards a Cognitive Science of Language, Inference and Consciousness.* Cambridge, MA: Harvard University Press; 1983.

Kandel ER: A new intellectual framework for psychiatry. *Am J Psychiatry.* 1998;155:457.

Kosslyn SM. *Image and Brain: The Resolution of the Imagery Debate.* Cambridge, MA: MIT Press; 1994.

Le Doux J. *The Synaptic Self.* New York: Viking Press; 2002.

Lewis MD: Self-organizing cognitive appraisals. *Cogn Emotion.* 1996;10:1.

MacLeod C. Mood disorders and cognition. In: Eysenck MW, ed. *Cognitive Psychology: An International Review.* Chichester, England: Wiley; 1990.

Main M. Metacognitive knowledge, metacognitive monitoring, and singular (coherent) vs. multiple (incoherent) models of attachment: Findings and directions for future research. In: Marris P, Stevenson-Hinde J, Parkes C, eds. *Attachment across the Life Cycle.* New York: Routledge & Kegan Paul; 1991.

Mesulam MM: Review article: From sensation to cognition. *Brain.* 1998;121:1013.

*Metcalfe J, Shimamura AP. *Metacognition: Knowing about Knowing.* Cambridge, MA: MIT Press; 1994.

Milner B, Squire LR, Kandel ER: Cognitive neuroscience and the study of memory. *Neuron.* 1998;20:445.

Morris RGM, ed. *Parallel Distributed Processing: Implications for Psychology and Neurobiology.* Oxford, UK: Clarendon; 1989.

Osherson DN, Smith EE, eds. *Thinking: An Invitation to Cognitive Science.* Vol 3. Cambridge, MA: MIT Press; 1990.

*Posner MI, ed. *Foundations of Cognitive Science.* Cambridge, MA: MIT Press; 1989.

Rauch SL, van der Kolk BA, Fisler RE, Alpert NM, Orr SP, Savage CR, Fischman AJ, Jenike MA, Pitman RK: A symptom provocation study of PTSD using PET and script driven imagery. *Arch Gen Psychiatry.* 1996;53:380–387.

*Schore AN. *Affect Dysregulation and the Damage to the Self.* New York: Norton; 2002.

Siegel DJ: Toward an interpersonal neurobiology of the developing mind: Attachment, "mindsight" and neural integration. *Infant Ment Health J.* 22:67–96.

Siegel DJ. An interpersonal neurobiology of psychotherapy: The developing mind and the resolution of trauma. In: Solomon M, Siegel DJ, eds. *Healing Trauma.* New York: Norton; 2003:1–55.

*Siegel DJ. *The Developing Mind: Toward a Neurobiology of Interpersonal Experience.* New York: Guilford; 1999.

Sigman M. What are the core deficits in autism? In: Broman SH, Grafman J, eds. *Atypical Cognitive Deficits in Developmental Disorders: Implications for Brain Function.* Hillsdale, NJ: Erlbaum; 1994.

Springer SP, Deutsch G. *Left Brain, Right Brain.* 5th ed. New York: WH Freeman; 1998.

Steinhauer SR, Gruzelier JH, Zubin J, eds. *Handbook of Schizophrenia.* Vol 5. *Neuropsychology and Information Processing.* New York: Elsevier Science; 1991.

Taber K, Rausch S, Lanius R, Hurley R: Functional magnetic resonance imaging: Application to posttraumatic stress disorder. *J Neuropsychiatry Clin Neurosci.* 2003;15:125.

van der Kolk BA: The neurobiology of childhood trauma and abuse. *Child Adolesc Psychiatr Clin N Am.* 2003;12:293.

Watts FN, ed. *Neuropsychological Perspectives on Emotion.* Vol 7. *Cognition and Emotion.* Hillsdale, NJ: Erlbaum; 1993.

Wheeler MA, Stuss DT, Tulving E: Toward a theory of episodic memory: The frontal lobes and autonoetic consciousness. *Psychol Bull.* 1997;121:331.

▲ 3.2 Extending Jean Piaget's Approach to Intellectual Functioning

STANLEY I. GREENSPAN, M.D., AND JOHN F. CURRY, PH.D.

Jean Piaget (1896 to 1980) was born in Neuchatel, Switzerland. Building on the work of the German philosopher Immanuel Kant, Piaget explored how intelligence develops from a child's actions on his or her world. Although Piaget focused predominantly on the development of impersonal cognition, he recognized that affect also had an important role. Lev Semenovich Vygotsky and Reuven Feuerstein further explored the social context of learning. More recently, the authors have developed a model to understand how affect and cognition unfold as integral parts of the same developmental process.

GENETIC EPISTEMOLOGY

Widely renowned as a child (or developmental) psychologist, Piaget referred to himself primarily as a *genetic epistemologist.* That self-designation reveals at once that Piaget's central project was not the articulation of a child psychology, as this term is generally understood, but rather an account of the progressive development of human knowledge.

On the classic question of the origins of knowledge, Piaget was neither a nativist nor an empiricist; however, his position should not be considered an amorphous form of interactionism. Piaget stated in detail the interactionist position to which he ascribed. It is, in his words, a "constructivist structuralism," according to which the origin of mental structures is to be sought in the actions of the subject (the child) on objects as the subject strives to adapt to his or her environment. Structures are constructed within the subject as a consequence of interactions between subject and object. What Piaget judged to be innate is an intelligent functioning that makes possible the production of progressively more adequate structures of knowledge on the basis of abstraction from actions performed during the stages of development.

For example, the concept of space is a fundamental mental structure developed in the earliest period of children's lives. In earliest infancy, the child is aware of not one homogeneous space but several heterogeneous spaces, each centered on a certain part of the child's body (e.g., visual space and tactile space). As children act on objects that may traverse these various spaces (e.g., a rattle occupying visual, tactile, and auditory spaces), they come to coordinate these individual spaces. Eventually, actions representing displacements in space are organized mentally into the general concept of space. That concept is a structure that can be described in logicomathematical terms.

EQUILIBRATION

For Piaget, the general criterion for intelligent functioning is *equilibration,* briefly defined as "a compensation for an external disturbance." Hans Furth described equilibration as "the factor that internally structures the developing intelligence. It provides the self-regulation by which intelligence develops in adapting to external and internal changes." At every level of development, the equilibration mechanism operates to further adaptation, but, as development proceeds toward the highest level of cognitive functioning, equilibration becomes progressively more adequate in enabling the organism to adapt to a wider range of internal and external disturbances. Piaget's notion of intelligence as adaptation is therefore essentially bound to an equilibration model of intelligent functioning.

ASSIMILATION AND ACCOMMODATION

To explicate the equilibration model further requires introducing Piaget's concepts of the assimilation and accommodation processes. The biological foundation of Piaget's developmental theory is nowhere more clearly evident; these processes are considered functional invariants of all intelligent behavior. At every level of intellectual development, from infancy to adulthood, the processes operate in adaptation.

The assimilation-accommodation account of development stresses the interaction between organism and environment. A certain readiness within the organism is postulated to be necessary for change or development to occur. In Piaget's view, associationism (empiricism) in psychology has committed the fallacy of crediting only one-half of those conditions necessary for learning with all explanatory power. A full account of human development must include not only the influence of stimuli on respondents (S → R) but also the influence of the responding organism on incoming stimuli (S ← R). Such an account is provided by Piaget's assimilation-accommodation viewpoint: "From a biological point of view, assimilation is the integration of external elements into evolving or completed structures of an organism. In its usual connotation, the assimilation of food consists of a chemical transformation that incorporates it into the substance of the organism."

Furth referred to assimilation as "an inward-directed tendency of a structure to draw environmental events towards itself." Assimilation is the conservative side of intellectual development, ensuring continuity and coherence by incorporating new aliments into existing mental structures. However, assimilation alone cannot account for growth or change within those structures.

Accommodation occurs during the developmental periods when new data cannot be wholly assimilated into the child's existing mental structures, and yet the data are not so foreign to those structures that they can be ignored. Furth referred to accommodation as "an organism-outward tendency of the inner structure to adapt itself to a particular environmental event." Read Tuddenham pointed out the variations in accommodation relative to levels of intellectual development as follows: "At the lowest psychological level, accommodation refers to the gradual adaptation of the reflexes to new stimulus conditions: what others have called conditioning or stimulus generalization. At higher levels it refers to the coordination of thought patterns to one another and to external reality."

This line of thought reveals in what sense *intelligence* is defined by Piaget in terms of equilibration. His equilibration is not a static, balanced system, but a dynamic, or mobile, equilibration between assimilation and accommodation as the child responds to the environment.

STRUCTURALISM

Intelligence has been discussed in terms of an equilibration process involving assimilation of aliments to structures and accommodation of structures to new, somewhat different aliments. Before the stages of intellectual development through which that process passes can be analyzed, one must more fully understand Piaget's notion of intellectual structure and must take a more fundamental look at the origins and developmental forms of the cognitive structures.

The term Piaget used for a cognitive structure is *scheme* (*schema*): "A scheme is the structure or organization of actions as they are transferred or generalized by repetition in similar or analogous circumstances." Schemata exist in the infant as perceptual-motor behavior patterns (e.g., the grasping reflex). They also exist in mature intelligence, although, as Furth pointed out, *schema* is more commonly used to refer to an early mental structure, whereas general schemata resulting from use of higher intelligence are referred to as *operations*.

The abstraction process that leads to the formation of cognitive structures is called *reflective* or *formal abstraction*. It is an abstraction from *actions*, according to which, the similarities inherent in various behavioral acts are dissociated from their particularized contexts (for example, the earlier example of the rattle in space). According to Furth and colleagues, "More precisely, reflective abstractions are an enriching feedback into the structures of the organism from the most general coordinations of actions."

THEORY OF STAGES

An integral part of Piaget's theory on genetic epistemology is a psychology of cognition that seeks to describe how knowledge develops and changes. The genetic framework for that and the process of intellectual adaptation during the major early periods of life are provided in Piaget's theory of the stages of cognitive development.

The stages of cognitive development that Piaget and his associates delineated empirically are not defined merely by the dominance of some aspect that remains present but less dominant throughout development. Rather, each stage constitutes a structured whole that can be defined by a set of criteria.

Piaget was not entirely consistent concerning his stages of cognitive development, but the only possible source of confusion in his later writings is whether the so-called preoperational period is to be considered apart from the period of concrete operations in which it culminates. John Flavell's 1963 study and Piaget's 1983 summary define three major periods and one subperiod of intellectual development (Table 3.2–1). These periods contain subdivisions called *stages*. The major developmental periods are as follows:

1. The sensorimotor period, which extends from birth until approximately 1.5 years of age. The period is divided into six stages, which are described in general in the following discussion with reference to the development of the concept of the permanent object.
2. A period of preparation for, and acquisition of, concrete operations. This period extends from the appearance (at approximately 2 years of age) of the symbolic (semiotic) function to the beginning (at approximately 7 years of age) of higher mental operations applied to concrete objects.
3. The period of formal operations, which begins at approximately 11 years of age. During this period, full adult intelligence develops as the operations are extended to apply to propositional, or hypothetical, thinking.

Sensorimotor Period

The *sensorimotor period* of intelligence is so named because the child's construction of mental schemata is in no way aided by representations, symbols, or thoughts. Rather, schemata depend totally on perceptions and bodily movements.

Stage 1 of sensorimotor development is marked by a relatively few organized reflexes that stand out from the spontaneous general activity of the neonate. Among those early reflexes are the sucking reflex and the palmar reflex. These primitive reflexes take on the nature of the first schema through three types of assimilation: (1) reproductive

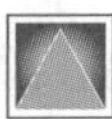

Table 3.2–1
Stages of Intellectual Development Postulated by Piaget

Age (Yrs)	Period	Cognitive Developmental Characteristics
0–1.5 (to 2)	Sensorimotor	Divided into six stages, characterized by: (1) Inborn motor and sensory reflexes (2) Primary circular reaction (3) Secondary circular reaction (4) Use of familiar means to obtain ends (5) Tertiary circular reaction and discovery through active experimentation (6) Insight and object permanence
2–7	Preoperations subperiod[a]	Deferred imitation, symbolic play, graphic imagery (drawing), mental imagery, and language
7–11	Concrete operations	Conservation of quantity, weight, volume, length, and time based on reversibility by inversion or reciprocity; operations; class inclusion and seriation
11 through the end of adolescence	Formal operations	Combinatorial system, whereby variables are isolated and all possible combinations are examined; hypothetical-deductive thinking

[a]This subperiod is considered by some authors to be a separate developmental period.

(repeating the actions); (2) generalizing (repeating the actions on new objects); and (3) recognitory (performing different varieties of the actions on different objects).

Stage 2 contains the first habit and the primary circular reaction. The first habits develop out of the original schemata as they are applied to objects in the environment or parts of the infant's body without any differentiation between means and end. In a primitive state of consciousness, the infant is aware only of action sequences and is not even aware of self. Primary circular reactions occur when, by chance, the infant experiences a new consequence of a motor act and tries to repeat the act.

In stage 3 of the sensorimotor period, an initial distinction between means and end becomes apparent, but in a primitive sense. The infant repeats a particular action pattern that achieved one end for the purpose of achieving other (unrelated) ends. For example, a baby who succeeds in shaking a rattle by pulling a string may repeatedly pull the string in an attempt to effect other sounds or results.

In stages 4 and 5, infants use a variety of available means to obtain particular goals. The distinction between stages 4 and 5 lies in the relative creativity or newness of the means. Stage 4 is marked by use of already familiar means. Stage 5 is marked by a search for new means based on further differentiations of already known schemata and by the tertiary circular reaction. The latter differs from a secondary circular action in that the child no longer produces schemata that were effective in one situation to produce magically efficacious results in every situation. Instead, the child explores the environment and varies means to test for effectiveness. Discovery is a hallmark of stage 5. For example, a child may use a stick to move an object not within reach.

Stage 6 is transitional, leading into the preoperational subperiod. In stage 6, the child becomes capable of inventing new means, not by direct actions on objects but by mental combination. Whereas discovery marked stage 5, insight is a characteristic of stage 6. For example, a child who has seen the father bang on a drawer to loosen it may bang on a toy box to make it easier to open.

During the sensorimotor period, a number of significant concepts are developed, including the child's concepts of space, time, and causality. These categorical concepts develop in a process parallel to the sequence of the six stages outlined in the previous discussion. Most important, during the sensorimotor phase, the child develops the schema of object permanence, the first major victory of conservation and the foundation of all future knowledge.

Schema of Object Permanence The knowledge that objects in the external world have an existence independent of the child's actions on them or interactions with them is a major accomplishment of the sensorimotor period. Flavell has outlined Piaget's observations and interpretations of infants' reactions to the disappearance of interesting objects, which are the foundation for the theory of development of object permanence. In stages 1 and 2, for example, a child simply continues to look at the place where the object was last seen. In stage 3, if an object such as a spoon drops to the floor, the infant will look for it (e.g., by leaning over and looking at the floor). In stage 4 if an object is repeatedly hidden at point A (in sight of the child) and then hidden at point B (also in sight of the child), the child searches for it at the original, rather than the current, hiding place (i.e., at A, not B). Stages 5 and 6 mark the child's increasing understanding of object permanence; the infant is able to follow multiple displacements of the object through points in space, even if the object is hidden within another object.

Preoperational Subperiod and Semiotic Function

The advent of the preoperational subperiod is marked by the appearance of what Piaget called the *semiotic function.* This new ability was defined by Piaget and Bärbel Inhelder as follows: "It consists in the ability to represent something (a signified object, event, conceptual scheme, etc.) by means of a signifier which is differentiated and which serves only a representative purpose: language, mental image, symbolic gesture and so on."

During the sensorimotor period, a thing could be represented in a limited sense by a part of itself (e.g., the mother's voice might represent the presence of the mother in the room). However, such signifiers are indexes undifferentiated from their significants (the voice is part of the mother). Symbols and signs are signifiers that are differentiated from their significants. They become available to the child only with the appearance of the semiotic function, which makes representational thought possible. As Furth pointed out, representation has first of all an active meaning in Piaget's theory. The child becomes capable of summoning up a symbol or sign to stand for a given significant. For Piaget, representation is not at the essence of thought; it has an auxiliary function.

Characteristic Behavior Patterns The semiotic function is heralded by five characteristic behavior patterns in evidence during the second year of life: (1) deferred imitation or imitation that starts after the disappearance of the model; (2) symbolic play or the game of pretending; (3) drawing or graphic imagery; (4) mental image, which appears as an internalized imitation and not as a function of perception; and (5) verbal evocation of events not occurring at the time. Each behavior pattern shows the origins of representational thought as the preoperational subperiod of cognitive development begins. For Piaget, the semiotic function, which so enlarges the children's worlds—liberating them from the bonds of immediate space and time and enabling them to begin to manipulate symbols and to think rather than just to act on immediately present objects—is rooted in imitation.

IMITATION One can follow the development of imitation through the same six sensorimotor stages delineated for the concept of object permanence. Piaget did this in his volume *Play, Dreams* *and Imitation in Childhood.* A radically new form of imitation occurs during the second year of life: deferred imitation. For example, a child may put on father's hat and walk as father does, even hours after father has gone off to work.

For Piaget, intelligence is an equilibration process in which assimilation and accommodation are in balance. However, in imitation, accommodation outweighs assimilation. According to Piaget, imitation is behavior in which "the subject's schemes of action are modified by the external world without his utilizing this external world." In imitation, the child's cognitive structures undergo temporary change without simultaneously incorporating new aliment.

SYMBOLIC PLAY A second new behavior pattern that now appears is symbolic play. In imitation, the imbalance between assimilation and accommodation is weighted in favor of accommodation; however, the opposite is true in symbolic play, which is a lessening of the demand of the adaptive process.

Development of play can also be followed through the six stages of sensorimotor intelligence, but symbols are used in play only after the sensorimotor period, in the type of play characterized by games of pretending. For example, a little girl may pretend that she is asleep, that a box is her pet cat, or that she herself is a church. In each instance, symbols are generated "to express everything in the child's life experience that cannot be formulated and assimilated by means of language alone."

According to Piaget's theory, these symbols are created by the same process of imitation that gives rise to deferred imitation at this time. In fact, Piaget views imitation as the process underlying the development of the entire semiotic function. In symbolic play, then, symbols are generated by a process in which accommodation outweighs assimilation. But instead of being used accurately (i.e., to represent that from which they are derived), they are used in a process in which a liberating assimilation outweighs accommodation.

DRAWING A third behavior pattern associated with the rise of the semiotic function is drawing, or graphic imagery. Piaget sees elements of play and imitation in this activity. In developmental terms, he considers drawing "halfway between symbolic play and the mental image," appearing at approximately 2 or 2.5 years of age. Drawing is playful activity, an end in itself characterized by reproductive assimilation; in other words, the child enjoys producing drawings for their own sake. However, graphic play also has accommodative elements, especially as the child grows older and attempts to draw not just formless scribble but something.

MENTAL IMAGE Closely related to drawing is the mental image. Piaget tied the genesis of mental imagery to accommodation and imitation. He explicitly denies that mental images can be the product of perception; they are a construction, something the child creates. The mental image is not directly given by perceptual input; it is constructed by the process of accommodation.

VERBAL EVOCATION OF EVENTS The fifth behavior pattern associated with the rise of the semiotic function concerns language, the verbal evocation of events that are not present. Piaget gave the example of a little girl saying "Anpa, bye-bye" (Grandpa went away) while pointing to the path he had taken when he left. The parallel with deferred imitation is clear, but the new representational ability is supported by the social system of language.

Concrete Operations

A crucial difference between preoperational and concrete-operational thought is the presence within operative thinking of concepts of conservation. When concrete operations have been organized into a system, the child can conserve, that is, "discover what values do remain invariant . . . in the course of any given kind of change or transformation." The progressive and continual structure building that occurs in the concrete operational period is evident in the increase, with development and age, in the scope of such concepts, such as conservation of quantity, substance, and number.

Conservation of Quantity

The clearest sign that a child remains in the preoperational subperiod is the absence of the concept of conservation. For example, if liquid is poured from a short, wide glass into a tall, narrow one, the child in the preoperational stage thinks the amount of liquid has changed. At the level of concrete operations, however, children are no longer overwhelmed by the perceptual discrepancy between the two configurations. They begin to reason about the transformation, and their correct judgments regarding the conservation of quantity of liquid are accompanied by explanations grounded in logical properties. It is assumed that children are not aware of the logic they use. When problems of conservation begin to be solved, the child passes from the preoperational subperiod into the period of concrete operations, for which the former was a long time of transition and preparation.

Conservation of Substance

At (on average) approximately 7 or 8 years of age, the child can solve the conservation-of-quantity problem and can perform similar judgments of conservation when, for example, a lump of clay is transformed in shape. Between 9 and 10 years of age, the child discovers that the weight of a given object is also conserved, even when its shape is transformed. However, not until approximately 11 or 12 years of age do children have a logical comprehension that the volume displaced by a given object is conserved even after transformation of the object's shape. Conservation entails the logical certainty that one characteristic of an object remains invariant while the object itself undergoes some type of perceived transformation.

Concept of Cardinal Numbers

The concept of cardinal numbers also develops from an initially nonconserving to a conserving stage. Children in the preoperational subperiod can be presented with two horizontal rows of colored dots in one-to-one correspondence (i.e., imaginary vertical lines could be constructed between each red dot and its corresponding blue dot). When the experimenter destroys this optical correspondence by spreading out one of the rows of dots, the child in the preoperational period thinks the larger row contains more dots. Only after conservation of cardinal number has been established as a logical necessity does the child maintain the numerical equivalence of the spread-out row. Clearly, preoperational concepts of number provide inadequate bases for arithmetic skills. It is possible that a lag in the development of number conservation could underlie certain types of arithmetic-related learning disabilities. Again, that points to the importance of children's active experience as a foundation for subsequent concept formation.

Operations

Notions of conservation are the mark of well-established concrete operational thinking; thus, one must understand the meaning of *operation* in Piaget's thought. Operations, themselves, constitute essential thinking. For Piaget, an operation is an action that is (1) interiorized, (2) reversible, and (3) part of an organized system of such actions.

The operations that form this system are interiorized actions. In the sensorimotor period, external behavior patterns give rise through a process of abstraction to the construction of sensorimotor schemata. In a similar fashion, internal thinking patterns later give rise to operations. According to Furth, the possibly generalized aspects of actions, "those which can be found in any coordination of action," enter into the construction of operations. Saying that the crucial aspect of actions in this regard is their ability to be generalized explains the importance of interiorization in the construction of operations. *Interiorization* refers to "the increasing dissociation of general form from particular content." In other words, the notions of generalization and interiorization merely point out the process of abstraction that is occurring. For example, a child adds two apples and three apples to obtain five apples. In another instance, a child adds seven blocks and one block to obtain eight blocks. In a third instance, a child combines the category of fathers with that of mothers to obtain the category of parents. The operation abstracted from these three mental actions is addition or combining, without reference to the particular content of numbers, objects, or categories.

Not only must an operation be interiorized action, it must also be reversible. The action of combining (addition) is not an operation until its relationship to the action of separating (subtraction) is comprehended. To understand reversibility is to understand the third criterion of an operation, its inclusion in a system.

The reversibility essential to operatory thought may be inversion or reciprocity. In reversibility by inversion, an action +A is reversed by –A. For example, in the above conservation-of-quantity example, pouring liquid into container 2 (+A) may be mentally reversed, that is, by mentally pouring it back into container 1 (–A). In reversibility by reciprocity, a relation $A < B$ is reversed by a relation $B < A$. Referring again to the conservation-of-quantity example, let A stand for container 1, and B stand for container 2. The rising height of liquid in container 2 ($A < B$) is offset by its narrower width ($B < A$).

Corresponding to these two types of reversibility are the two major categories of concrete operations: those pertaining to classes and those pertaining to relations. In the system of operations performed on classes, reversibility is by inversion; in those performed on relations, it is by reciprocity. For example, subtraction and addition relate to inversion; comparing sticks of different sizes relates to reciprocity.

Class Inclusion The concrete operation demonstrating understanding of classes is the class inclusion task. In this task, a child is shown, for example, an array of pets (superordinate class) consisting of dogs and cats (subordinate classes). After counting the number of dogs, cats, and pets, the child is asked whether there are more dogs or more pets. Children in the preoperational subperiod cannot keep in mind the superordinate class while perceiving only the subordinate classes. Thus, they fail the task frequently over a series of such arrays.

Relations The concrete operation that demonstrates an understanding of relations is seriation. Children are asked, for example, to arrange a set of rods in order of increasing size. Children in the preoperational subperiod may subgroup the rods but have difficulty completing an entire array along the required dimension. They may understand the concept of smaller versus larger but have difficulty comprehending the gradual nature of change.

Formal Operations In the third and final stage in Piaget's conception of the intellectual development in the child, the logical structures of concrete operations are superseded by structures referred to as formal operations. The relationship between the real and the possible that characterizes adolescent thinking represents a reversal of that relationship in the thinking of the concrete operational child. Inhelder and Piaget note that the *real* has priority for the younger child and that *possibility* is conceived of merely as a prolongation or extension of real operations, "as, for example, when, after having ordered several objects in a series, the subject knows that he could do the same with others." For the adolescent, however, the possible has priority, and the real is seen as a particular instance of it. "Henceforth, they conceive of the given facts as that sector of a set of possible transformations that has actually come about." This immediately presupposes that the adolescent can take a given empirical event (such as, "the long, thin rod bends") and categorize it within a system of possible combinations of events (e.g., long rods or short rods, thin rods or thick rods, bending or not bending). Three characteristics follow from this fundamental reorientation in thought: (1) Adolescent thought is hypothetical-deductive; (2) It deals in propositions rather than in concrete events; and (3) It can isolate variables and examine all possible combinations of variables.

Hypothetical-Deductive Thought As a hypothetical-deductive form of thought, formal operational intelligence proceeds from the possible to the real. In this sense, it mirrors scientific reasoning. The implications of a propositional statement are drawn and then tested against reality. Rather than building up a proposition by induction from disparate concrete examples to a loose generalization, formal intelligence operates systematically from general statement to particular instance by means of testable hypotheses. In Flavell's words, "To try to discover the real among the possible implies that one first entertains the possible as a set of hypotheses to be successively confirmed or infirmed. Hypotheses which the facts infirm can then be discarded; those which the data confirm then go to join the reality sector."

Propositional Thought Saying that formal operations deal in propositions, rather than in concrete events, implies increased freedom from immediate content, with a correspondingly greater intellectual mobility. At one level, this freedom implies the ability to manipulate abstractions that have been tied to concrete examples or events. The adolescent, for example, can perform a transitive inference ($A < B$, $B < C$; therefore, $A < C$) without any empirical demonstration of referents for the terms A and B. At another level, this freedom implies that having performed a concrete operation, the adolescent can abstract the results of that operation and can perform further operations on them. For example, an adolescent can perform the concrete operation of combining two liquids to observe the color of the resultant mix and then take the result of this operation and systematically relate it to results of all other combinations of available liquids.

Isolating Variables and Examining Combinations The example that follows helps explain the third characteristic of adolescent thought mentioned by Flavell, the isolation of variables and the examination of all possible combinations. Instead of dealing with disparate concrete experiments, hypothetical-deductive adolescents can organize their investigations into a coherent pattern a priori and then can perform all relevant combinations of variables to test their hypotheses, thus isolating causal factors. Piaget's theory of formal operational cognition focused on scientific thinking. For example, the weight, speed, shape, and size of an object may all be seen to contribute to the size of a hole the object makes when hitting the ground.

Children in the preoperational substage merely describe what they see, and causal thinking is expressed in an undifferentiated form (e.g., "It has to"). The child with concrete operational thinking can categorize and order the relevant variables independently but has difficulty integrating the system of all relevant variables. The adolescent, however, can generate all possible combinations of relevant variables and then systematically tests the importance of each variable.

A complete combinatorial system appears only during the period of formal operations. Instead of focusing on empirical givens, as a child in the concrete operational stage does, the adolescent using formal operational thinking constructs a hypothetical system comprising the empirical givens. Whereas the younger child could classify events according to various categories, such as length, width, and weight, the adolescent uses that classification as a basis for abstracting all possible combinations of variables. Having done this, the adolescent can then test hypotheses derived from the combinatorial system. The result of this new ability is the capacity to test the causal significance of each individual factor in succession by holding all other factors constant.

Piaget interprets the rise of formal operational thought in the context of his equilibrium model of cognitive development. Thus, he considers neurological maturation and experience of the object and interpersonal world as necessary but not sufficient to explain this qualitative improvement in thinking. In essence, the equilibration explanation is as follows: During the stage of concrete operations, a number of qualitatively heterogeneous factors are constructed by the child, resulting in the achievement of conservation of the factor in question even in the face of perceptual transformations. Such factors include quantity, weight, volume, time, and length. Eventually, the child discovers that, in many concrete instances, the operation of these factors is interrelated. Thus, although the factors have been constructed mentally in relative isolation from one another, their presence in real objects is mixed. Through experience with impersonal and interpersonal objects, the child's concrete operational understanding of these factors is shown to be insufficient, and a more comprehensive, more intelligent understanding is stimulated.

EGOCENTRISM

Each major period of cognitive development is characterized by a qualitative shift toward more comprehensive and more adaptive cognitive structures. In this sense, the adolescent is more intelligent than the infant. However, each transition to a higher level of cognitive organization is initially accompanied by a lack of full differentiation between self and object. Each period has an early organizational phase that is followed by the phase of accomplishment of cognitive developmental tasks. During the early organizational phase, the child's failure to differentiate fully the self from objects is manifested in behavior reflecting stage-specific forms of egocentrism. David Elkind has summarized the process. Each developmental period has characteristic forms of egocentrism.

In the sensorimotor period, *egocentrism* refers literally to a lack of differentiation between self and object, as perceived in the lack of object permanence. The existence of objects independent of action patterns of the self is not acknowledged. In the preoperational subperiod, the capacity to engage in symbolic thinking is accompanied by initial failure to differentiate fully between symbols and their referents. That may be manifested, for example, in the failure to differentiate such mental images as dreams from real objects. In the concrete operational period the capacity to engage in logical operations is accompanied by an unrealistic certainty in which probability is not appreciated and mental construction of the self (self-definition) is not differentiated from facts. Finally, at adolescence the capacity to engage in hypothetical thinking and to understand others' points of view is accompanied by characteristic patterns of thought in which others are unrealistically presumed to be focusing on the self. As Elkind has pointed out, adolescent egocentrism is a "belief that others are preoccupied with (the adolescent's) appearance and behavior," when, in fact, the adolescent is preoccupied with these topics.

INTELLIGENCE: PIAGETIAN MODEL AND ITS ALTERNATIVES

For Piaget, intelligence is adaptation. As the human organism develops over time, progressively more adequate cognitive structures ensue. As noted previously, this development is an active process of construction, based not only on biological maturation, but also on the actions of the subject in the experiential world. Because the cognitive structures of the adolescent are better equipped to adapt to internal and external disturbances than are those of the preschool child, it is accurate to say that the former is more intelligent than the latter.

The Piagetian view of intelligence can be further understood by contrasting it with other contemporary models of intelligence. In the European and American traditions of clinical and educational psychology, intelligence had first of all a pragmatic meaning. Alfred Binet's work in Paris was intended to determine which children were delayed in learning and thus in need of special educational assistance. With Théodore Simon, he developed the first *intelligence test* by choosing a variety of tasks and arranging them in order according to the age at which most children master them. This enabled the clinician to assess at what mental age the child was functioning. Further developments in this tradition involved dividing the mental age by the chronological age to determine the child's intelligence quotient (IQ). This age-corrected notion of intelligence emphasized individual differences through comparisons of children with their peers, instead of emphasizing the most general and progressively adaptive competencies of the individual during childhood and adolescence, as Piaget had done. Age-corrected intelligence came to be viewed as a trait, with some children ahead of or behind their age mates in what was thought to be a basic capacity for learning.

Psychologists who espouse a trait model of intelligence differ among themselves on such key issues as to what extent the trait is heritable and whether there is a single general trait or numerous specific traits (types) of intelligence. Nevertheless, all trait theorists differ from Piaget by focusing on individual differences rather than on the most general aspects of cognitive adaptation.

As Lauren B. Resnick and Sharon Nelson-LeGall recently described, Piagetian and trait models of intelligence also differ from Vygotsky's social model. In the latter, intelligence is viewed chiefly as the outcome of a social interaction process through which children internalize the cultural tools and practices represented in their social context. The contrast between Piaget and Vygotsky may at least superficially appear as one between a theorist who emphasizes the most general cognitive processes and a theorist who emphasizes the most culturally specific cognitive content.

Finally, Piaget's construct of intelligence is contrasted with the cognitive social learning construct of competencies. Although both constructs involve active, developing processes rather than fixed knowledge, the former pertains to the most general structures of logic derived from coordination of actions, and the latter refers to more specific, concrete sets of skills, including social and problem-solving skills. As is discussed in the following sections, contemporary extensions of Piaget's work include attempts to integrate Piagetian notions of intelligence with Vygotsky's social model, on the one hand, or with cognitive social learning theory, on the other.

CRITICISMS OF PIAGET'S THEORY

The previously mentioned contrasts between Piaget's theory of intelligence and alternative theories provide a context in which to understand some of the major criticisms of his theory. As Gerard Duveen has pointed out, the *epistemic subject* that serves as the primary focus of Piaget's study is neither an individual psychological subject nor a socially contextualized subject, but rather a general representative of all psychological subjects at the same level of development. Thus, the epistemic subject may be seen as unaffected by emotions, social pressures, or cultural content.

It is not surprising, then, that Piaget has been criticized for failure to account for individual differences among children in their intellectual development and for failure to account for the effects of cultural setting on the cognitive content of children's intelligence. Educators and clinicians may find Piaget's work of invaluable interest for its broad depiction of developmental stages and processes and yet frustrating because of its failure to provide guidance for interventions that would facilitate learning or correct deficiencies in individual children.

Cross-cultural research has called into question the generality or universality of Piaget's proposed stages. Different tasks appear to be mastered at different ages across cultures. Even within Western culture, there is evidence that modifications in training paradigms or in the way in which cognitive structures are operationalized can lead to significantly different results than those obtained by Piaget regarding children's abilities at different ages. More specifically, the criticism has been made that Piaget relied too heavily on the child's verbalizations to document understanding of a cognitive task. In fact, mastery of concrete and formal operational schema was only acknowledged in Piagetian research if the child could explain verbally why the correct answer was logically necessary.

Moreover, the notion of a developmental stage that may last as long as 7 years or more, during which schemas of conservation are sequentially developed across areas as divergent as quantity and volume, may simply be too broad to represent a cohesive period. Empirical psychologists have also questioned the notion of cognitive structures by noting the low magnitude of correlations that are purported to measure the same underlying intellectual structure. Of course, similar criticisms have been made of proposed traits and of purportedly related functions in nonPiagetian areas of psychology as diverse as personality trait psychology and the neuropsychology of executive functions.

NEOPIAGETIAN RESPONSES TO SELECTED CRITICISMS

It is beyond the scope of the present chapter to offer a thorough defense of Piaget's theory. Instead, several key responses by neopiagetian theorists are mentioned and then several important extensions of Piaget's theory are illustrated. In general, as pointed out by Peter Sutherland, neopiagetian psychologists have integrated information-processing components into a stage theory of development. They retain a Piagetian view that increased cognitive structures are general, rather than totally domain specific. However, they have modified the theory of stages to include more substages, and these are dependent on increases in information-processing capacity. This neopiagetian view is more consistent than traditional Piagetian psychology with other branches of cognitive neuroscience.

Juan Pascual-Leone, for example, has studied the processes involved in moving from a lower-level to a higher-level cognitive structure and has emphasized that inhibition, attention deployment, and sustained attention are necessary for such a change to occur. The child must inhibit the application of an older, lower-level structure in response to a new stimulus. Then, through a process involving active effort, the child must attend to new aspects of the stimulus and coordinate a new schematic response. A type of memory that enables the child to store instructions and an ability to scan relevant cues are notions derived from information processing models of cognition and integrated by Pascual-Leone into his neopiagetian model. By focusing on such variables as inhibition, attention deployment, and sustained attention, Pascual-Leone has brought neopiagetian cognitive psychology into contact with the psychology of executive functions, as these are studied by cognitive psychologists and neuropsychologists.

Robbie Case, who also investigates the transition from lower-level to higher-level cognitive structures, places emphasis on exploration and problem solving in the active, developing child. He also takes from information processing models a notion of short-term or working memory. By so doing, he has brought neopiagetian psychology into contact with contemporary cognitive social learning theory, in which problem solving is a key competence for intellectual and personality development, essential for adequate adjustment, and into contact with cognitive neuropsychology. In cognitive social learning theory, *problem solving* refers to the process of identifying a challenge or problem, generating alternative possible solutions to the problem, evaluating the likely outcomes of any implemented solution, and choosing the optimal alternative. In Piagetian psychology, the internalization of optimal solutions would occur through the process of accommodation of earlier structures.

EXTENSIONS OF PIAGET'S THEORY

By extensions of Piaget's theory, the various attempts that implement a Piagetian model of development beyond the realm of logicomathematical reasoning into forms of cognition that pertain to social constructs or interpersonal schemas are now described. The first and, perhaps, best-known attempt to extend Piaget's theory in this way was made by Lawrence Kohlberg, who studied the moral reasoning of children.

Piaget, himself, wrote *The Moral Judgment of the Child,* but, in subsequent work, he focused much more on logicomathematical reasoning than on social or interpersonal cognition. Kohlberg developed a stage model of moral reasoning in which the child's stage of moral reasoning depended on his stage of (Piagetian) cognitive development. For instance, to demonstrate moral reasoning at the conventional level, the child must have already entered the concrete operational stage of cognitive development. Likewise, principled moral reasoning demanded a foundation in formal operational thought.

Kohlberg described three major stages of moral reasoning, each divided into two substages. The three major stages included the morality of the preschool period (based on notions of avoiding punishment and striving for reward), conventional morality (based on notions of authority or mutual benefit), and principled morality (based on general internalized moral principles). As was the case for Piagetian stages, Kohlberg's stages were proposed as progressively more adequate and more highly structured, that is, a child would move only in a forward direction through the stages. However, it was not proposed that all or even most people would necessarily attain the highest level of moral reasoning. Kohlberg investigated the moral reasoning of individuals by presenting them with moral dilemmas and then observing their thinking as they attempted to resolve the dilemmas. The theory of development pertained to the form of their thinking and not to the content of their solution. The best known of the dilemmas involved a husband who needed to obtain a rare medication to save the life of his wife. The druggist who had the medication was charging an exorbitant price for it. The question is whether the husband would be justified in stealing it. In addressing this dilemma, the research participant might have recourse to such considerations as fear of punishment (preconventional), concerns for social order (conventional), or relative values of life and property (principled). Kohlberg was not concerned with the participant's final choice, but only with the methods of reasoning used to reach that choice.

Kohlberg's extension of Piaget's work was subject to some of the same criticisms that faced Piaget. The moral epistemic subject was criticized as detached from moral content: Individual differences in the predominant forms of moral reasoning did not seem to correlate highly or consistently with individual differences in actual moral behavior. The research methodology was highly verbal, so that intelligence and verbal sophistication could be confounded with moral reasoning. Finally, because his theory was originally developed from research with an entirely male sample, Kohlberg was criticized by Carol Gilligan for having proposed, in general, a theory that was gender biased. Gilligan argued that women's moral reasoning proceeds from a principal concern with relationships, whereas men's moral reasoning proceeds from a principal concern with justice. However, subsequent empirical research has demonstrated that women score as high on Kohlberg's stages of moral reasoning as do men.

Subsequent to Kohlberg's theory, other attempts were made to relate Piaget's model to social cognition. Initial efforts followed Kohlberg's lead, that is, stages of social cognition were proposed as dependent on stages of intellectual development. Interpersonal perspective taking was hypothesized to be dependent on perceptual and cognitive perspective taking. However, it became clear that children's concepts about other people did not always follow such a *layered* structural design. James Youniss then developed a theory of children's concepts of other people that appropriated a different key element from Piaget's work. Rather than attempting to layer stages of social cognition on stages of intellectual development, Youniss proposed that social cognition has its own process of development, but that these are based on abstractions from interpersonal interactions. Integrating Piagetian psychology with the interpersonal psychiatric theory of Harry Stack Sullivan, Youniss proposed two major categories of children's social cognition: schemas about peers and schemas about authority figures. Each of these develops as a function of repeated interactions with peers or elders. As can be seen in this example, the second type of extension of Piaget's work into the interpersonal domain abandoned the position that stages of social cognition depended on broad structures of intellectual development in favor of the position that the active abstracting processes discovered by Piaget were operative across both types of cognition.

A third type of extension of Piaget's work is less direct but also involves his key concepts of egocentrism and perspective taking. In Piaget's theory, egocentrism is opposed by and eventually superseded by perspective taking, or decentering. At the simplest perceptual level, perspective taking involves the child's awareness that two children looking at the same display from different sides of a table have two different views of the display. Later in development, perceptual perspective taking is enhanced by cognitive and emotional perspective taking, as the child comes to realize that other people have thoughts and feelings that can differ from one's own. Considerable research in cognitive and developmental psychology has focused on these or closely related topics. Perspective taking implies a certain degree of *thinking about thinking*, in that the perceptions, thoughts, and emotions of the self are seen as only one among two or more possible perceptions, thoughts, and emotions. Implicit in this process is what contemporary psychologists term a *theory of mind*, an awareness that others have internal states and mental representations.

Thinking about thinking and *theory of mind* have been subjects of considerable recent research. To begin with the latter, an elementary theory of mind appears to develop by 4 years of age. However, in children with autistic disorder, a deficiency in this basic process is noted. Thinking about thinking is often referred to more broadly as *metacognition*. Metacognition includes the awareness of one's own thinking processes, strategies for deployment of attention, the use of feedback to modify thoughts or plans, and the ability to deliberately shift perceptual or cognitive sets. Metacognition is similar to what neuropsychologists refer to as *executive functions* and appears to be relatively underdeveloped in children with attention disorders.

Finally, increased attention is now being directed toward the child's acquisition of social knowledge. Again, the Piagetian roots of this extension are to be found in *The Moral Judgment of the Child*. A recent symposium addressed this topic by way of comparing the developmental psychologies of Piaget and Vygotsky. Where Piaget has been caricatured as a psychologist of the *epistemic subject*, an individual, asocial, acultural entity, Vygotsky's psychology is manifestly social. However, Duveen has argued that, in *The Moral Judgment of the Child*, Piaget actually depicted two methods by which the child acquires knowledge of social and cultural content. The first is through social transmission, based on learning from an authority figure. The second is through processes of argumentation and debate with peers. Piaget's first process is quite similar to Vygotsky's notion that the child internalizes from elders a system of symbols that represents a social or collective product.

However, Anne-Nelley Perret-Clermont has pointed out that Piaget emphasized the second process much more than the first over the course of his career, and that there was a definite sense in which he viewed social transmission as constricting. Indeed, it appeared to him to be based on authority but was lacking in the stimulation to new learning that characterized debate with peers and the social construction of knowledge. By contrast, Vygotsky saw social knowledge as an internalized system of symbols that is, itself, a social product, and authority, in the form of adults or peers with greater knowledge, as facilitating this process of internalization.

To the extent that Piaget neglected or underemphasized the acquisition of knowledge through social transmission, his theory would be deficient in accounting for children's knowledge of social and cultural material that is passed on rather than actively constructed by the individual. Such material would range from the obvious (socially and culturally acceptable behavior) to the subtle (mathematical inventions, such as the current number system). The implications for education are significant. Discovery methods of education, including experimentation and peer discussion, may be more appropriate when the goal is to assist children in formulating the most general principles of reasoning, but other methods, including lecture, assigned reading, and modeling, may be more appropriate when the goal is to convey specific socially constructed content.

NEW CONCEPTS OF INTELLIGENCE: EMOTIONAL BASIS OF INTELLIGENCE

Human emotions have traditionally been viewed as somewhat separate from cognition and as a minor concern to overall development. New clinical observations and theoretical formulations by Stanley Greenspan and emerging findings from a number of recent studies suggest that emotions are central to cognition and may actually regulate and orchestrate cognitive capacities. They may also be critical to development of cognitive capacities. It is suggested that babies' emotional exchanges with their caregivers, rather than their ability to complete cognitive tasks, should become the primary measure of developmental and intellectual competence.

Twelve-month-old Cara sits in her mother's lap at a table, eyes locked onto the psychologist, who tries to get her to follow the bean he is putting under the cup and search for it. Cara knocks over the cup. Is this little girl, as her mother fears, cognitively delayed? Does a 1-year-old child who never babbles like other children her age and who violently flings food and toys away from her show signs of a significant intellectual deficit? After a battery of similarly frustrating tests, the evaluator concludes that cognitive delay is the likely diagnosis in Cara's case.

For 50 years, developmental testers have expected babies to sit still in their mothers' laps, to pay attention, and to perform prescribed tasks while adults assess their basic intelligence. Traditional wisdom has long insisted that carefully scoring how well a tiny child fits pegs into boards, sorts cards by shape, or hunts beans under cups can reveal an accurate measure of intelligence and developmental competence. However, recent results from research and clinical practice by Stanley Greenspan and others suggest that this entire approach to assessing children's capacities rests on false premises and has inadvertently led to mistaken diagnoses that can stigmatize children throughout their school years.

When an evaluator schooled in this new thinking assessed Cara, he focused on her spontaneous interactions with her caregiver. He looked at each of Cara's intentional behaviors as a sign of her emotional interests. For instance, he observed her delight in yanking her mother's nose. At the assessor's suggestion, the mother permitted the tugging on her nose to continue and playfully responded, "Toot, toot." Cara smiled and pulled again. The baby was rewarded with another "Toot, toot" and a big smile from her mother. Cara soon began to copy her mother's gestures and eagerly thrust her nose towards Mom. When the mother squeezed Cara's nose, the 1-year-old girl chirped, "Mo, mo," her first words.

Cara showed that she could initiate social interactions and could comprehend their consequences. That demonstrated degree of understanding put Cara at least at the 12-month level of cognitive development. Further observation revealed an extremely energetic, active, highly physical toddler who liked to have her way and to control her surroundings. With the consultant's help, Cara's mother later altered her parenting style. She learned to follow Cara's behavioral lead, then enthusiastically engaged her daughter in creative interactions while simultaneously setting firm limits. Cara's energy quickly became more focused; her babbling became richer. Before long, she was saying real words and actively cooperating with her parents.

If a series of such simple, pleasurable interactions with her mother could reveal and foster Cara's language development and organizational ability, then any conception of intellect that marked her as cognitively delayed because of an inability to search for a bean has serious flaws. Those flaws are based on a long-standing mistaken belief that the intellect is superior to and supervises the passions. Clearly, as Cara's linguistic debut demonstrates, analysis of a child's early relationships and sensory and emotional experiences is a vital key to accurate assessment of intelligence and developmental competence.

Until now, however, no one has offered an explanation of how emotions give birth to intelligence. In fact, a baby's earliest feelings play a pivotal role in all later intellectual development. Unlikely as the connection between feeling states and intelligence may seem, the emotions orchestrate a vast array of cognitive operations throughout an individual's life span. Indeed, they make possible all creative thought.

Results from four distinct lines of inquiry have recently shed new light on the importance of emotions for intelligence. In work with Arnold Sameroff, Stanley Greenspan has found that children with four or more family emotional risk factors had 24 times the chance of scoring an IQ of less than 80 than children without those risks. Stephen Porges and Stanley Greenspan have shown that measurements in 8-month-old infants of a part of the brain that regulates emotions correlate with these same children's IQ scores at 4 years of age.

Stanley Greenspan's work with a group of children with autistic disorder, who experience some of the most severe thinking and language problems imaginable, has also confirmed the inextricable linkage of emotional and cognitive development. Therapeutic programs for these severely challenged children have traditionally concentrated on trying to stimulate their cognition and to teach them language. However, a program based on emotional cueing (like the one that revealed Cara's true abilities) proved to be more effective for a number of these children in fostering empathy, warmth, and creative thinking.

One young patient, Ashley, neither spoke nor made any response or eye contact with those around her. The 2-year-old child spent hours staring into space, rubbing persistently at the same patch of rug. Her abnormal repetition was viewed by the clinician observing her as more than just a distressing symptom of her autism. That symptom revealed an underlying interest and motivation that could be harnessed and redirected toward interacting with others. To initiate her cognitive progress, the clinician first had to motivate her to communicate with the simplest of emotional gestures—a smile, smirk, or purposeful hand movements. He suggested that her mother place her hand next to Ashley, on the favorite stretch of rug. When Ashley pushed it away, the mother gently put her hand back. Each time the child pushed, the mother's hand would return. A cat-and-mouse game ensued, and, after three sessions of these rudimentary interactions, Ashley was looking, smiling, and anticipating.

From that tiny beginning, through a comprehensive therapeutic program, grew a bridge to emotional relationships and eventual verbal exchanges. For example, as therapy progressed, the therapist helped Ashley use her imagination by repeatedly initiating pretend play. He recognized that each time Ashley repeatedly flung herself on her mother, the child was deriving sensory-based simple pleasure from her behavior. He instructed the mother to whinny like a horse each time Ashley lunged at her. Soon Ashley imitated mother's sounds and then started initiating her own sounds and words. In that way, the therapist helped the mother stretch a pleasant sensation for Ashley into a richer, more complex interaction. Over time, mother and child pretended to be neighing horses, mooing cows, and barking dogs. Their social and emotional interchange grew increasingly complex, passing through the same series of developmental stages identified in children without difficulties. At 7 years of age, Ashley now enjoys warm friendships, argues as well as her lawyer father, and scores in the low-superior IQ range.

A fourth line of inquiry, microscopic clinical observations of children's thinking, further clarifies the relationships between emotion and reason by revealing two necessary elements of thinking. The first process—creating a new idea—stems from the ability to use one's own emotional experience to assign meaning and significance to daily events or concepts. The second process—reflection and logical analysis—examines the newly created idea according to whatever principles of logic the person possesses and places it in a wider frame of reference.

To understand those processes in action, the authors put a simple question to two young boys seen in therapy not long ago. When asked by the clinician, "What do you think about people who act bossy to you?" Chris replied, "Well, teachers are bosses, baby-sitters are bosses, policemen are bosses." That articulate 7-year-old child lacked the emotional pathways that permit creative and intuitive thought. He could provide a formal classification of different types of bosses but could not relate these categories to his own life. However, 7-year-old Josh had no such difficulties. In response to the same question about bosses, he announced, "Most of the time I don't like being bossed, especially when my parents try to tell me when I can watch TV and when I have to go to sleep. I'm big enough to decide for myself. Sometimes when I'm being bad, I guess I need bossing, though. Maybe bosses are okay some of the time, and some of the time they're not." Josh finds his answer in his own, apparently generally irritating, brushes with bosses. Rather than simply listing categories or incidents, he can abstract a principle from the emotional core of those incidents.

How exactly did Josh's ability to think and to abstract develop? A baby's experience begins with sensations like touch and sound. Each sensation, however, also gives rise to an emotion. A toy may feel interesting or boring; a voice may feel soothing or jarring. Even young infants react to sensations emotionally. They prefer the sound or smell of their mother, for example, to any others and, by 4 months of age, can react to certain persons with fear. Furthermore, contrary to long-held assumptions, basic sensations, such as touch and sound, can be perceived differently by different people, giving rise to emotional differences.

Emotional meaning also adheres to early concepts like *big* and *little*, *more* and *less*, *near* and *far*, and *now* and *later*. *A lot* is a bit more than makes a child happy. *Near* is snuggled next to a child in bed. *Later* is a frustrating stretch of waiting. For a child without an intuitive sense of *few* and *many*, numbers have no meaning. Furthermore, a young child's experience of any sensation always occurs within the context of a relationship that gives it broader meaning. Playing with mother's hair, for example, may evoke smiles and hugs or an angry scolding.

Each sensory experience has such a dual aspect and is labeled by its physical properties and its emotional qualities. This double coding helps the child place the memory or experience in a catalogue of experience and retrieve or reconstruct it when needed. As the child grows, emotional reactions come to operate as a sixth sense that allows the child to recognize and to understand situations.

Emotion orchestrates complex judgments as well. One of modern psychology's main enigmas is how children learn to discriminate among situations ("When can I yell and kick") and to generalize from one to another ("Should I behave at school like I do at home?"). Consider how a child makes a seemingly simple judgment about when to say "hello." He or she does not learn a set of cognitive rules like greeting only those who live on his or her street or only those who wave at him or her. Rather, from countless specific encounters she abstracts an emotional pattern; there is a feeling of warmth and friendliness in situations that rate "hello." The child's interactions create an emotional signaling system that tells him or her when to say "hello" and that it is okay to punt the football but not to kick Sarah or Charlie in the shins. That emotional signaling system, which acts like an orchestra leader for the vast array of cognitive instruments, is a quintessentially human process. No computer, for all its apparent so-called brainpower, can ever get beyond limited elements of logical analysis and think like a person. Advocates of artificial intelligence may claim that current computational capacity limits creative, human-like thought, but the real limit is a machine's inherent inability to engage the world emotionally. No collection of microchips can ever have a child's lived emotional experience of "hello," of noses and hugs. None, therefore, can ever create the emotionally based meaning from which creative thought grows and on which it depends.

Looking at Piaget's theory from this perspective reveals the limitations of a cognitive theory that did not adequately deal with the central role of emotions. Piaget's experiments focused on how children comprehend the relationship between physical objects, developing the ability to classify them by such parameters as shape or size, but most children can classify their emotions and emotionally relevant relationships far earlier than they can classify physical objects. For example, they know members of their families from those who are not members, classifying the family as a unit. Some of Piaget's observations are limited, because he depended so heavily on children's perceptual and motor performance to signal cognitive advances, even though motor skills often lag behind other skills.

More important, however, is Piaget's relative lack of focus on the role of emotions. He emphasized learning through doing but did not realize that the doing generates formative emotional reactions as well as perceptual, motor, and cognitive ones. Consider how a child learns what an apple is. You can have the child handle an apple and determine it is something red and round, bigger than a peanut and smaller than a watermelon. Alternatively, the child can observe the aspects mentioned previously, experience more satisfaction eating an apple when he or she is hungry than when he or she is full, and know the pleasure of giving one to his or her favorite teacher.

The child can also imagine how the teacher feels when he or she gives the teacher the apple. The child may catalogue how he or she feels when the child throws one at his or her younger brother and gets him on the shoulder, as well as the child's disgust when another one rots or when the child discovers one-half of a worm inside. If you ask creative adults to write an essay on apples, they will probably bring an enormous amount of personal affective experience to their reflections.

Piaget did emphasize how children's thinking comes to incorporate multiple perspectives as they grow older. A classic Piagetian experiment shows how school-age children learn to solve a problem involving weights on a seesaw. Assessing the heaviness of the weights and noticing where they are placed, they are able to figure out how a seesaw works. But what was not appreciated by Piaget was that the children's postulated perspectives incorporated the additional almost infinite number of perceptions afforded by affective experiences. To neglect this element is therefore to fail to appreciate the rich array of experiences that contribute to forming abstract concepts.

TOWARD A GENERAL DEVELOPMENTAL MODEL

The diagnosis and treatment of emotional and developmental disorders in infants and young children requires that clinicians take into account all facets of the child's experience. Thus, one needs a model with which to look at how constitutional-maturational (regulatory), family, and interactive factors work together as the child progresses through each developmental phase, and each phase must be viewed from affective and cognitive perspectives.

A developmental, structuralist model formulated by Stanley Greenspan integrates cognitive and affective development and applies the types of structure Piaget described to a range of experience. Most importantly, the model also considers individual differences in terms of biology and interaction. New findings suggest that early interaction can alter the structure and wiring of the central nervous system (CNS). In this model, the biological differences express themselves in the unique way an infant processes sensations and organizes motor patterns. Interactions harness and change these basic processes. The model can be visualized with the infant's constitutional-maturational patterns on one side and the infant's environment, including caregivers, family, community, and culture, on the other side. Both sets of factors operate through the infant–caregiver relationship, which can be pictured in the middle. Those factors and the infant–caregiver relationship in turn contribute to the organization of experience at each of six developmental levels (consistent with cognitive and affective milestones), which may be pictured just beneath the infant–caregiver relationship.

This particular clinical and research model enables the user to look at the back-and-forth influence of highly specific, verifiable constitutional-maturational factors on interactive and family patterns and vice versa, in relationship to specific developmental processes (and to relate these processes to later developmental and psychopathological disorders).

Developmental Levels The model contains six developmental levels, which include the infant's and child's ability to accomplish the following:

1. Attend to multisensory affective experience and, at the same time, organize a calm, regulated state and experience pleasure.
2. Engage with and show affective preference and pleasure for a caregiver.
3. Initiate and respond to two-way presymbolic gestural communication.
4. Organize chains of two-way communication (opening and closing many circles of communication in a row), maintain communication across space, integrate affective polarities, and synthesize an emerging prerepresentational organization of self and others.
5. Represent (symbolize) affective experience (e.g., pretend play and functional use of language), which calls for higher-level auditory and verbal sequencing ability.
6. Create representational (symbolic) categories and gradually build conceptual bridges between these categories. This ability creates the foundation for such basic personality functions as reality testing, impulse control, self–other representational differentiation, affect labeling and discrimination, stable mood, and a sense of time and space that allows logical planning. This ability rests not only on complex auditory and verbal processing abilities, but also on visual-spatial abstracting.

At each level, one looks at the range of emotional themes organized (e.g., can the child play out [symbolize] only dependency themes and not aggressive ones? Is aggression behaved out and dealt with presymbolically?). One also looks at the stability of each level. Does a minor stress lead a child to lose the ability to represent, to interact, to engage, or to attend?

In their use in day-to-day clinical work, the six developmental levels can be collapsed into four essential processes that characterize development in infants and young children. These processes concern how an infant and the parents or caregivers negotiate the various phases of their early interactions, and they serve as a basis for diagnosis and treatment.

A 12-month-old infant's mother worried that, "he cries any time I try to leave him, even for a second. If I'm not standing right next to him when he is sitting on the floor, he cries and I have to pick him up. He's a tyrant. He's waking up four times at night and is a fussy eater. He eats for short bursts (breast-feeding) and then stops eating. I'm feeding him all the time."

The mother was feeling cornered, controlled, manipulated, and bossed around. Her baby was like a "fearful dictator" (therapist's term). She said, "that's the perfect way to describe him." The father was impatient with the mother; he felt that she indulged the baby too much. He was getting "fed up" because she had no time for him.

The baby was interactive and sensitive to every emotional nuance. As he came into the room, he immediately caught the clinician's eye. They exchanged smiles and motor gestures. He interacted with his parents with smiles, coos, and motor movements. Father intruded somewhat. He would roughhouse until the baby would cry, put the baby down, and then roughhouse again. Mother, in contrast, was ever so gentle, but long silences passed between her vocalizations. During her long silences, the baby would rev up, get more irritable, and start whining. He whined with his mother and cried fearfully with his father. Even before he could finish his motor gestures or vocalizations, his mother moved in and picked him up, gave him a rattle, or spoke for him. In this way, she undermined his initiative. Even while whining, however, he was interactive and contingent.

On physical examination, this baby was sensitive to loud noises and light touch on the arms, legs, abdomen, and back. He had a mild degree of low motor tone and was posturally insecure. He was not yet ready to crawl.

His constitutional and maturational patterns did not compromise his mastering the first developmental challenge of shared attention and engagement. He was an attentive, engaged baby. However, at the second developmental stage, intentional communication and assertiveness, he was a passive reactor. He was not learning to initiate two-way communication, to be assertive, and to take charge of his interactions. His low motor tone was compromising his ability to control his motor movements. His sensory hyperreactivity was compromising his ability to regulate sensation. He was frequently overloaded by just the basic sensations of touch and sound, and he was not receiving support from his mother through the nurturing and rhythmic care taking that would foster self-initiative.

This family required therapeutic work on a number of tasks simultaneously. The infant's special constitutional-maturational patterns were discussed. Hands-on practice helped the parents help their baby be attentive and calm. Those tasks included helping the mother be more patient, wait for the baby to finish what he started, and support his initiative (e.g., putting something in front of him while he was on his tummy, to motivate him to crawl and to reach); getting the mother to put more affect into her voice and to increase the rhythm and speed of her vocalizations; and getting the father to be more gentle. The parents' own feelings about the interactions were explored: the father's tough-guy background, the mother's fear of her own assertiveness, her fear of her baby being injured, and their own associated family patterns.

Gradually, the baby began to sleep through the night, and he became more assertive and less clinging and fearful. He also became happier. He was slow to reach his motor milestones, so an occupational therapist worked with him and gave the parents advice on motor development and normalizing his sensory overreactivity. In 4 months, this infant was functioning in an age-appropriate manner with a tendency toward a cautious, but happy and assertive, approach to life's developmental challenges.

As developmental clinicians and researchers build on Piaget's findings and formulations, the developmental model serves as a basis for understanding social and emotional development and provides a framework for clinical and educational intervention.

Implications for Psychotherapy Piaget was not an applied psychologist and did not develop the implications of his cognitive model for psychotherapeutic intervention. Nevertheless, his work formed one of the foundations of the *cognitive revolution* in psychology. One aspect of this revolution was an increasing emphasis on the cognitive components of the therapeutic endeavor. In contrast to classical psychodynamic therapy, which focused primarily on drives and affects, and in contrast to behavior therapy, which focused on overt actions, cognitive approaches to therapy focused on thoughts, including automatic assumptions, beliefs, plans, and intentions.

Cognitive theory, including Piaget's, has influenced psychotherapeutic approaches in multiple ways. Some therapists have taken developmental notions from Piaget's work and developed intervention techniques. Others have developed cognitive models of treatment independent of Piaget but with heavy reliance on the role of cognition. Others have included Piaget's concepts in a broader set of constructs to undergird new developmental approaches to psychotherapy.

Some psychotherapists applied Piagetian notions directly to child interventions. Susan Harter, for example, discussed techniques for helping young children become aware of divergent or contradictory emotions and integrate these complex emotions within a more abstract or higher class of emotions. One of Harter's techniques is to ask the young child to draw different and conflicting feelings in one person. This technique represents an application of the concrete operation of class inclusion to the realm of the emotions. Harter's work applied Piagetian findings to the common therapeutic problem of helping children recognize, tolerate, and integrate mixed or ambivalent affects within stable object relations. As such, it drew on cognitive theory and psychodynamic theory.

Other psychotherapists developed treatment models that, although not directly dependent on Piagetian psychology, emphasized core ideas quite similar to those Piaget discovered in his naturalistic observations of cognitive development. Aaron Beck, for example, developed an entire school of cognitive therapy that focuses on the role of cognitions in causing or maintaining psychopathology. Cognitive therapy has been shown to be an effective treatment for problems as diverse as depression, anxiety disorders, and substance abuse.

A core idea in cognitive therapy is that the patient can be assisted to identify the negative automatic thoughts and underlying dysfunctional attitudes or beliefs that contribute to emotional distress or addictive behavior. The cognitive component of the therapy begins with identification of automatic thoughts, so designated because they are rapid, overlearned responses that instantaneously mediate between an event and an affective reaction. The key therapeutic process after identification of the maladaptive thoughts is to help the patient view these thoughts more objectively, not take them in an unquestioning manner as veridical.

In helping patients take an objective or distanced perspective on their own thoughts, cognitive therapists are enhancing the patient's cognitive role-taking ability. In the realm of emotional health and personality development, they are contributing to what Piaget might have referred to as *increased emotional intelligence* on the part of the patient. What the cognitive therapist accomplishes through such techniques as Socratic questioning and asking if there are other ways to look at the same event is similar to what the talented teacher does in guiding children to more adequate, more intelligent understanding of operational tasks. The notion of equilibration is relevant in both instances. By helping the individual see that previous cognitive structures are in some ways inadequate, the therapist or teacher disturbs the old cognitive structure, and the patient or student experiences a disruption that leads to the search for more adequate structures. The compensation for external disturbance is what Piaget termed *equilibration.* New structures can only be constructed through a process of accommodation, enabling the subject to assimilate a wider array of data, a new perspective, or more complex information.

Because it requires *thinking about thinking*, cognitive therapy seems to require formal operational thinking, although this has not been empirically tested. At the least, it requires the ability to recognize and to articulate affects, to recognize and to label events that give rise to affects, and to translate into a thought the mediating process that occurs rapidly between the event and the affect. Cognitive-behavioral models of psychotherapy include cognitive techniques and more behavioral, interactive techniques, such as increasing pleasant activities and improving communication and problem-solving skills. Gregory Clarke and his colleagues have shown that cognitive-behavioral treatment is effective in reducing adolescent depression. It is not clear which components of the treatment are responsible for the overall positive effects, however.

It may be that adolescence is the earliest developmental stage in which a person could benefit from cognitive therapy. Even among adolescents and some adults, such therapy is difficult to conduct. In working with depressed, substance-abusing adolescents, John Curry and his colleagues have found that the cognitive components of the treatment are too difficult for adolescents who lack ready access to their own emotional states or the ability to label affects. Similar findings were reported by Stanley Greenspan regarding the cognitive aspects of psychodynamic therapy with some adults.

Such findings have contributed to the third approach to using Piagetian insights in psychotherapy, namely, integrating Piaget's findings into a broader model. Stanley Greenspan, for example, has articulated a developmentally based psychotherapy that takes account of earlier, presymbolic levels of functioning that precede the ability to recognize, to label, and to articulate affects and their mediating cognitions.

Developmentally Based Psychotherapy Developmentally based psychotherapy, developed by Stanley Greenspan, integrates cognitive, affective, drive, and relationship-based approaches with new understanding of the stages of human development. Different therapies look at different aspects of the proverbial elephant, whether from a psychodynamic, object relation, self-psychology, behavioral, or cognitive-behavioral point of view. A comprehensive, cohesive developmental framework integrates elements from these approaches with a broader understanding of the developmental processes essential for emotional or mental health. It formulates series of principles that an understanding of human development says are prerequisite for emotional growth.

Developmentally based psychotherapy constructs its therapeutic strategies from these principles of human development and growth. The clinician first determines the level of the patient's ego or personality development and the presence or absence of deficits or constrictions. For example, can the person regulate activity and sensations, relate to others, read nonverbal affective symbols, represent experience, build bridges between representations, integrate emotional polarities, abstract feelings, and reflect on internal wishes and feelings?

After determining the developmental level, the clinician looks for constitutional and maturational contributions and difficulties with sensory processing, modulation, or motor planning. The clinician looks for interactive and family contributions. Each of these is explored in the present, the past, and the anticipated future. The patient's fantasies, sense of self and others, and conflicts are understood in the context of all these influences. These are how patients make sense of their ego structure, physical makeup, family patterns, and interactions with others. Developmentally oriented therapists do not permit themselves the luxury of overfocusing on one set of variables, such as inner fantasies, family dynamics, biological proclivities, or prior experience. Similarly, the formulated therapeutic strategy cannot deal only with one or two factors. It must deal with all critical factors that influence the developmental process. As collaborators in the construction of experience, therapists use their understanding of the patient's development to help the patient construct interactions that provide growth and overcome difficulties.

Often, it is assumed that critical aspects of development occur through the maturation of the nervous system along with routine, expectable experiences. It is also assumed that, from these routine, expectable maturational sequences and experiences, certain psychological structures having to do with the ability to regulate, to engage, to interact, to represent (symbolize) experience, and to reflect and to compare experiences are present in most people. With these capacities in place, it is believed that the therapeutic process can focus on conflicts and anxieties and selected maladaptive behaviors or thoughts. The authors have observed, however, that only a small percentage of individuals have these core capacities. For most, such capacities must be learned as part of the therapeutic process.

The developmental perspective shows how one learns these capacities during development. It suggests strategies that can be used in the psychotherapeutic process, so that adults and children who have not achieved these capacities can learn them. From a developmental point of view, the integral parts of the therapeutic process include learning how to regulate experience; to engage more fully and deeply in relationships; to read and respond to boundary-defining behaviors and affects; to perceive, to comprehend, and to respond to complex self- and object-defining affects, behaviors, and interactive patterns; to represent experience; to differentiate represented experience; and to form higher-level differentiations, including the capacity to engage in the ever-changing opportunities, tasks, and challenges during the course of life (e.g., adulthood and aging) and, throughout, to observe and reflect on one's own and others' experiences. Mastering these core developmental processes makes dealing with conflicts, anxieties, maladaptive behaviors, and thoughts possible.

These processes are the foundation of the ego and, more broadly, the personality. Their presence constitutes emotional health, and their absence constitutes emotional disorder. The developmental approach describes how to harness these core processes and so assist the patients in mobilizing their own growth.

SUGGESTED CROSS-REFERENCES

Perception and cognition are discussed in Section 3.1, learning theory is discussed in Section 3.3, biology of memory is discussed in Section 3.4, and brain models of mind are discussed in Section 3.5. Chapter 39 addresses attention-deficit disorders. Chapters 35 through 37 focus on learning disorders, motor skills disorder, and communication disorders, respectively. Feeding and eating disorders in children are the subject of Chapter 41, and mental retardation is covered in Chapter 34.

REFERENCES

Brainerd CJ. Jean Piaget, learning research, and American education. In: Zimmerman BJ, ed. *Educational Psychology: A Century of Contributions.* Mahwah, NJ: L. Erlbaum Associates; 2003:251–287.

Duveen G. Psychological development as a social process. In: Smith L, Dockrell J, Tomlinson P, eds. *Piaget, Vygotsky, and Beyond: Future Issues for Developmental Psychology and Education.* London: Routledge; 1997:67–90.

Finn G. Piaget, Vygotsky and the social dimension. In: Smith L, Dockrell J, Tomlinson P, eds. *Piaget, Vygotsky, and Beyond: Future Issues for Developmental Psychology and Education.* London: Routledge; 1997:121–128.

Gilligan C. *In a Different Voice: Psychological Theory and Women's Development.* Cambridge, MA: Harvard University Press; 1982.

Greenspan SI. *The Clinical Interview of the Child.* New York: McGraw-Hill; 1981.

Greenspan SI. *The Development of the Ego: Implications for Personality Theory, Psychopathology, and the Psychotherapeutic Process.* Madison, CT: International Universities Press; 1989.

*Greenspan SI. *Infancy and Early Childhood: The Practice of Clinical Assessment and Intervention with Emotional and Developmental Challenges.* Madison, CT: International Universities Press; 1992.

Greenspan SI. *Developmentally Based Psychotherapy.* Madison, CT: International Universities Press; 1997.

Greenspan SI. *The Growth of the Mind and the Endangered Origins of Intelligence.* Reading, MA: Addison Wesley Longman; 1997.

Greenspan SI, Shanker S. *The Evolution of Intelligence: How Language, Consciousness, and Social Groups Come about.* Reading, MA: Perseus Books; 2003.

Hamlett KW, Pellegrini DS, Conners CK: An investigation of executive processes in the problem-solving of attention deficit-hyperactive children. *J Pediatr Psychol.* 1987;12:227.

Harter S: A cognitive-developmental approach to children's expression of conflicting feelings and a technique to facilitate such expression in play therapy. *J Consult Clin Psychol.* 1977;45:417.

Inhelder B, Piaget J. *The Growth of Logical Thinking from Childhood to Adolescence.* New York: Basic Books; 1958.

Kant I. *The Critique of Pure Reason.* London: Macmillan; 1963.

Kohlberg L: The development of children's orientations toward a moral order: I. Sequence in the development of moral thought. *Vita Humana* 1963;6:11–33.

Lochman JE, Dodge K: Social cognitive processes of severely violent, moderately aggressive, and nonaggressive boys. *J Consult Clin Psychol.* 1994;62:366.

*Nicolopoulou A. Play, cognitive development, and the social world: Piaget, Vygotsky, and beyond. In: Lloyd P, Ferynhough C, eds. *Lev Vygotsky: Critical Assessments: Thought and Language.* Vol 2. New York: Routledge; 1999.

Ortega R. Play, activity, and thought: Reflections on Piaget's and Vygotsky's theories. In: Lytle DE, ed. *Play and Educational Theory and Practice.* Play and Culture Studies, Vol 5. Westport, CT: Praeger Publishers; 2003:99–115.

Perret-Clermont A. Revisiting young Jean Piaget in Neuchatel among his partners in learning. In: Smith L, Dockrell J, Tomlinson P, eds. *Piaget, Vygotsky, and Beyond: Future Issues for Developmental Psychology and Education.* London: Routledge; 1997:91–120.

Piaget J. *Play, Dreams and Imitation in Childhood.* New York: Norton; 1951.

Piaget J: The stages of the intellectual development of the child. *Bull Menninger Clin.* 1962;26:120.

*Piaget J. *The Early Growth of Logic in the Child.* New York: Norton; 1969.

Piaget J. *Structuralism.* New York: Basic Books; 1970.

Piaget J. Piaget's theory. In: Mussen P, ed. *Manual of Child Psychology.* New York: Wiley; 1983.

*Piaget J, Inhelder B. *The Psychology of the Child.* New York: Basic Books; 1969.

Piaget J, Inhelder B. *The Origin of the Idea of Chance in Children.* New York: Norton; 1975.

Pinard A, Laurendeau M. Stage in Piaget's cognitive-developmental theory: Exegesis of a concept. In: Elkind D, Flavell JH, eds. *Studies in Cognitive Development: Essays in Honor of Piaget.* New York: Oxford University Press; 1969.

Resnick LB, Nelson-LeGall S. Socializing intelligence. In: Smith L, Dockrell J, Tomlinson P, eds. *Piaget, Vygotsky, and Beyond: Future Issues for Developmental Psychology and Education.* London: Routledge; 1997:145–158.

Sameroff A, Seifer R, Barocas R, Zax M, Greenspan SI: IQ scores of 4-year-old children: Social-environmental risk factors. *Pediatrics.* 1986;29:343.

Shayer M: Not just Piaget, not just Vygotsky, and certainly not Vygotsky as alternative to Piaget. *Learn Instruct.* 2003;13:465–485.

Smith L, Dockrell J, Tomlinson P, eds. *Piaget, Vygotsky, and Beyond: Future Issues for Developmental Psychology and Education.* London: Routledge; 1997.

Sternberg RJ, Berg C, eds. *Intellectual Development.* Cambridge, UK: Cambridge University Press; 1992.

Sutherland P. *Cognitive Development Today.* London: Chapman Publishing; 1992.

*Tudge J, Rogoff B. Peer influences on cognitive development: Piagetian and Vygotskian perspectives. In: Lloyd P, Fernyhough C, eds. *Lev Vygotsky: Critical Assessments: The Zone of Proximal Development.* Vol 3. New York: Routledge; 1999.

Youniss J. *Parent and Peers in Social Development: A Sullivan-Piaget Perspective.* Chicago: University of Chicago Press; 1980.

▲ 3.3 Learning Theory

W. STEWART AGRAS, M.D., F.R.C.P.(C), AND
G. TERENCE WILSON, PH.D.

Learning plays a central role in the development of human behavior, including voluntary and involuntary motor behaviors, thinking, and emotion. The effects of the environment on the development and maintenance of disordered behaviors are, with the exception of effects such as injury, malnutrition, or infection, translated through learning; hence, learning plays an important role in the development and maintenance of psychopathology. Conversely, the basis of psychological change by means of psychotherapy depends on learning new and more adaptive behaviors. The theoretical basis for psychotherapy and its practical use depends on a grasp of the principles of learning.

In Russia, at the end of the 19th century, Ivan Petrovich Pavlov (Fig. 3.3–1), a Nobel Laureate in physiology, established the foundations of classical conditioning. At roughly the same time in the United States, pioneering research on animal learning by Edwin Thorndike showed the influence of consequences (rewarding and punishing events) on behavior. Beginning in the late 1930s, this process of instrumental learning was elaborated on by B. F. Skinner in his research on operant conditioning. Research on conditioning and learning principles, conducted largely in the animal laboratory, became a dominant part of experimental psychology in the United States after World War II. In the tradition of Pavlov and Skinner, workers in this area were committed to the scientific analysis of behavior by using the laboratory rat and the pigeon as their subjects. During the first half of the 20th century, isolated attempts were made to apply conditioning principles to a variety of problem behaviors. John B. Watson and Rosalie Rayner experimentally induced a phobic reaction in the famous case of Albert by using a simple classical conditioning procedure, and Mary Cover Jones antedated later investigations by describing the use of several procedures for overcoming children's fears. Researchers O. Hobart Mowrer reported the successful treatment of enuresis by direct conditioning procedures.

These early applications had no impact on the practice of psychotherapy, in part, because conditioning principles, which had been demonstrated with animals, were rejected as too simplistic and irrelevant to the treatment of complex human problems. Nevertheless, some attempts were made to integrate conditioning principles with psychodynamic theories of abnormal behavior, but these eclectic formulations had little effect and only obscured crucial differences between the respective behavioral and psychodynamic approaches. John Dollard and Neal Miller, for example, translated psychodynamic theory but with little consequence for any clinical innovation, because they were reinterpreting psychotherapy rather than advocating different concepts and procedures.

The emergence of behavior therapy as an alternative system of assessment and treatment to psychoanalysis in the late 1950s marked the first systematic extension of the principles of learning to clinical practice. *Behavior therapy* was originally defined as the application of *modern learning theory* to the treatment of psychiatric disorders. At that time, the phrase *modern learning theory* referred to the theories and procedures of classical and operant conditioning. In the 1950s and early 1960s, learning theory (i.e., classical and operant conditioning)

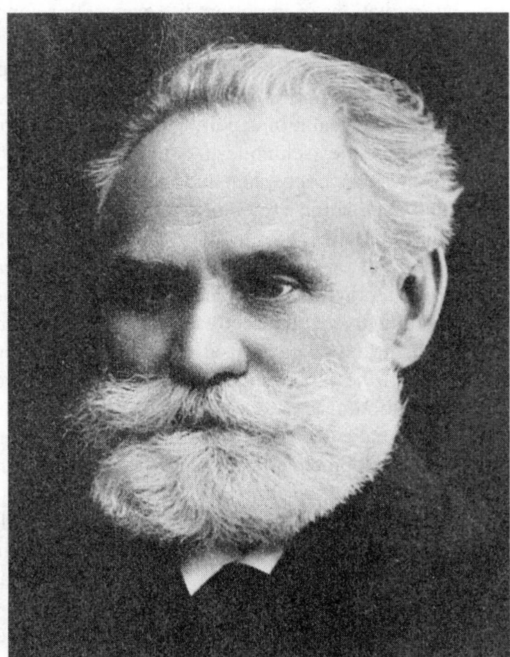

FIGURE 3.3–1 Ivan Pavlov. (Courtesy of the National Library of Medicine.)

was the obvious choice as a body of knowledge within experimental psychology on which to build an applied clinical science.

In the 1970s, experimental research on cognition (e.g., information processing) supplanted classical and operant conditioning as the major focus of theory development and research in experimental psychology. Throughout the 1970s, behavior therapists increasingly incorporated cognitive processes and procedures within their clinical practice, and social-cognitive learning theory emerged as the most influential conceptual framework guiding the clinical application of learning principles and procedures. Social-cognitive theory embraces classical, as well as operant, conditioning procedures. However, in this approach, the influence of environmental events on behavior is largely determined by cognitive processes that govern how environmental influences are perceived and how the individual interprets them. According to this view, psychological functioning involves a reciprocal interaction among three interlocking sets of influences: behavior, cognitive processes, and environmental factors. In the opinion of Albert Bandura, personal and environmental factors do not function as independent determinants; rather, they determine each other. Persons cannot be considered causes independent of their behavior. It is largely through their actions that individuals produce the environmental conditions that affect their behavior in a reciprocal fashion. The experiences generated by behavior also partly determine what individuals think, expect, and can do, which in turn affects their subsequent behavior.

In social-cognitive learning theory, the person is the agent of change. The theory emphasizes the human capacity for self-directed behavior change. Strongly influenced by the social-cognitive learning model, the clinical practice of behavior therapy has increasingly included cognitive methods. A primary focus of cognitive and behavioral techniques is to change the cognitive processes that are viewed as essential to therapeutic success. This theory assumes that it is not so much experience itself but rather the person's interpretation of that experience that produces psychological disturbance. Cognitive and behavioral methods are used to modify misperceptions and misinterpretations of important life events; this approach is called *cognitive-behavioral therapy.*

The principles of classical and operant conditioning applied to individuals with a wide range of psychopathology have been successful in stimulating a wealth of experimental and clinical research and innovative therapeutic techniques. A fundamental contribution of learning theory was the conceptual and methodological emphasis that the study and application of conditioning principles brought to clinical research and practice. The detailed specification of therapeutic techniques; the focus on behavior per se in assessment, treatment, and evaluation of therapy outcome; and the advances in measurement and methodology were all directly associated with the methodological behaviorism that characterized the conditioning approach. Moreover, because of the experimental, hypothesis-testing emphasis deriving from conditioning and social-cognitive theories, cognitive behavioral therapies have become the mainstream of psychotherapy research. These developments have helped to narrow the gap between the laboratory and the clinic.

Every psychotherapy session knowingly or unknowingly contains some of the procedures derived from learning theory. The most effective psychotherapies are targeted to alter a specific behavior or cluster of associated behaviors, are based on a model of factors maintaining the disorder, use a well-designed sequence of behavior change strategies sensitive to the individual problems presented by a particular patient, and are time limited. Most of these psychotherapies now appear in detailed manuals and have been rigorously tested in controlled outcome studies.

BIOLOGY OF LEARNING

Learning leads to neurochemical changes in the central nervous system (CNS). Research with simple organisms has, for example, revealed that the learning of avoidance behavior alters the chemical structure of cells in the nervous system; when the avoidance is unlearned, the chemical changes are reversed. Research conducted by Eric Kandel and his colleagues at Columbia University with *Aplysia californica* has been particularly well covered in the psychiatric literature. *Aplysia*, a sea mollusk, is a useful animal to study because of the simplicity of its nervous system, which contains approximately 20,000 neurons, many of which are large and readily identifiable. The specific avoidance behavior studied is a defensive reflex involving withdrawal of the snail's siphon when the animal is tactually stimulated. When the mollusk is touched repeatedly, it learns not to withdraw its siphon and gill, a process known as *habituation.* However, if the mollusk then receives a strong stimulus, such as an electric shock, it becomes sensitized, such that even a previously subthreshold tactile stimulation causes the animal to withdraw its gill and siphon. Furthermore, the snail can be classically conditioned, so that it withdraws its siphon and gill to a conditioned stimulus. Habituation, sensitization, and classical conditioning of the reflex in the snail can be considered forms of learning and memory. In learning, a short-term stimulus has to be translated into long-lasting changes that involve a series of biochemical changes that are functionally interlinked and operate in overlapping time ranges.

Many of the neuronal anatomical and chemical bases for the learning processes have been worked out in this animal model. Sensory neurons receiving tactile information form excitatory synapses with the gill and siphon motor neurons that cause the withdrawal activity. Habituation, sensitization, and classical conditioning all involve neurochemical changes in the sensory neuron, resulting in alterations in the amount of excitatory neurotransmitter released. The neurochemical basis of habituation is that, after repeated stimulation of the sensory neuron (e.g., repeated tactile stimulation), less calcium than usual enters the presynaptic nerve terminal, resulting in less neurotransmitter being released and, thus, less activity by the motor neurons. Sensitization requires the presence of additional neurons, called *facilitator interneurons*, that synapse onto the sensory neurons. The sensitizing stimulus, such as an electric shock, causes the facilitator interneuron to release serotonin that binds to serotonin receptors on the sensory neuron. Activation of the serotonin receptors activates adenylate cyclase, producing cyclic adenosine monophosphate (cAMP), thereby activating a cAMP-dependent protein kinase, which is believed to phosphorylate an S-type potassium channel. Phosphorylation of the potassium channel results in increased calcium influx during the action potential and increased neurotransmitter release.

The effects of neurotransmitters have now been directly studied in *Aplysia*. For example, stimulation of the esophageal nerve leads to biting, an aspect of the feeding response. Training animals by repeated stimulation alters the biophysical properties of the B51 sensory neuron that seems to be the focal point for the interaction between the behavior (biting response) and reinforcement (in this case repeated stimulation). In an in vitro examination of the B51 neuron, dopamine was applied directly to the neuron. The application of dopamine to the cultured neurons resulted in a firing pattern similar to that seen in the whole animal when feeding occurs. Moreover, after repeated reinforcements with dopamine, the neuron became more excitable with a resultant increase in ingestion-like firing patterns. In this experiment, the neurochemistry underlying the phenomenon of reinforcement was defined.

Because psychotherapy is best viewed as a learning process, and because learning produces changes in neuronal architecture, the behavior changes associated with therapy should produce anatomical changes in the CNS. As Eric Kandel notes, such changes should be detectable by imaging methods. In an interesting study of patients with obsessive-compulsive disorder (OCD), positron emission tomography (PET) was used to investigate changes in cerebral metabolic rates for glucose before and after treatment. The effects of two treatments were compared: fluoxetine (Prozac) and behavior therapy consisting of exposure and response prevention. Although the study involved nine patients per group, glucose metabolic rates in the right head of the caudate nucleus changed when the OCD was successfully treated with fluoxetine or behavioral therapy. These changes did not occur in patients who did not respond to treatment, which suggests that the changes in brain metabolism consequent on learning-based changes in behavior therapy may be similar to those induced by pharmacotherapy. These results underline the reciprocal interaction between learning and the CNS.

In the following sections, classical conditioning, operant conditioning, and social learning theory are reviewed. Some common terms used in learning theory are listed and defined in Table 3.3–1.

CLASSICAL CONDITIONING

History The idea that learning takes place when two events occur closely together in time has a long history, stemming from association theory developed by the British school of philosophical empiricism. Pavlov, the Russian physiologist, and his coworkers documented the parameters of this form of learning in carefully conceived experiments. Traditional accounts of classical conditioning state that learning occurs when an initially neutral stimulus, the conditional stimulus, is paired with a stimulus that naturally elicits a response, the *unconditioned stimulus*. The response elicited by the unconditioned stimulus is the *unconditioned response*. After repeated and continuous pairing of the two stimuli, the conditional stimulus elicits the unconditioned response, which is then called the *conditioned response*. Put

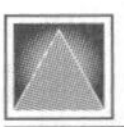

Table 3.3–1
Common Terms Used in Learning Theory

Aversive conditioning: a procedure in which punishment or aversive stimulation is used to reduce the frequency of a target behavior

Avoidance learning: a form of operant learning in which an organism learns to avoid certain responses or situations

Classical conditioning: the association of a neutral stimulus with an unconditioned stimulus, such that the neutral stimulus comes to bring about a response similar to that originally elicited by the unconditioned stimulus

Conditioned response: in classical conditioning, the response elicited by the conditioned stimulus

Conditioned stimulus: in classical conditioning, the originally neutral stimulus that comes to be associated with the unconditioned stimulus and eventually elicits a conditioned response

Continuous reinforcement: a schedule of reinforcement in which a reward is administered every time a response is emitted

Covert reinforcement: a method of increasing behavioral frequency by using the imagination of pleasant events as a reinforcement

Covert sensitization: a method of reducing the frequency of behavior by associating it with the imagination of unpleasant consequences

Discrimination learning: a process in which the tendency toward stimulus generalization is counteracted and responses are made only to specific stimuli

Experimental neurosis: an abnormal behavior pattern produced in animals through the application of classical or operant conditioning techniques

Extinction: the reduction of frequency of a learned response as a result of the cessation of reinforcement

Fixed-interval schedule: a reinforcement schedule in which a reward is given after a specific amount of time has passed

Fixed-ratio schedule: a reinforcement schedule in which a reward is given after a specific number of responses have been emitted

Habituation: a simple form of learning in which the response to a repeated stimulus lessens over time

Higher-order conditioning: in classical conditioning, the establishment of a new conditioned stimulus through association with an established conditioned stimulus

Instrumental learning: operant conditioning

Law of effect: the principle that behaviors followed by pleasant consequences are strengthened and that those followed by negative consequences are weakened

Modeling: observational learning

Negative practice: a method for reducing the frequency of a behavior by the intense repetition of the response

Observational learning: learning new behaviors by observing others responding and receiving some form of consequence; vicarious learning

Operant conditioning: a form of learning in which behavioral frequency is altered through the application of positive and negative consequences

Partial reinforcement: a schedule of reinforcement in which rewards are not given each time a response is made, rendering a learned response highly resistant to extinction

Primary reinforcer: a stimulus affecting a biological process (e.g., food that increases the probability of behaviors it follows)

Reinforcer: a stimulus that increases the frequency of responses it follows

Respondent learning: classical conditioning

Secondary reinforcers: stimuli that gain the power to reinforce a behavior through association with primary reinforcers

Shaping: an operant procedure in which a desirable behavior pattern is learned by the successive reinforcement of approximations to that behavior

Spontaneous recovery: the increase in the strength of an extinguished behavior after the passage of a period of time

Successive approximation: see the term *shaping*

Unconditioned response: in classical conditioning, a response that occurs spontaneously to the unconditioned stimulus

Unconditioned stimulus: a stimulus that, without any training, produces a specific response

Variable-interval schedule: a reinforcement schedule in which a reward is given after varying periods of time have passed

Variable-ratio schedule: a reinforcement schedule in which a reward is given after a varying number of responses have been emitted

Courtesy of Marshall P. Duke, Ph.D., and Stephen Nowicki, Jr., Ph.D.

another way, animals or humans learn that certain environmental cues predict events of importance to the organism.

Pavlov's work was enthusiastically espoused by American psychologists, such as Watson, who demonstrated that classical conditioning can give rise to phobia-like behavior. The subject of the experiment was Albert B., who was 11 months old. Watson demonstrated that a few pairings of a loud noise (unconditioned stimulus) with the sight of a white rat (conditional stimulus) led Albert to avoid not only the rat, which had not caused fear before, but also similar objects, such as cotton wool and sealskin, an example of *stimulus generalization*, in which stimuli similar to the original conditioned stimulus may elicit the conditioned response, although usually with a weakened response. According to that view, which is still widely held by psychologists and psychiatrists, classical conditioning was a rather simple, limited, and automatic form of learning. Current thinking, however, differs substantially from that traditional account.

Current Views Temporal contiguity between two stimuli is neither necessary nor sufficient for classical conditioning to take place. Two examples illustrate the point. In the first example, a rat is exposed to five pairings of a tone and an electric shock in one situation. In another situation, the tone is presented ten additional times in the absence of shock. The contiguity of tone and shock is the same in both situations, but classical conditioning occurs only in the first situation, because only in that situation does the tone predict or provide information about the unconditioned stimulus. In the other situation, the unconditioned stimulus is equally likely whether or not the tone is sounded. Contiguity is not necessary for conditioning to occur. If the presentation of the tone and the shock is arranged so that shocks never occur in the presence of the tone, the tone comes to predict the nonoccurrence of the shock, a phenomenon called *conditioned inhibition*.

In the second example, two groups of animals are exposed to a compound stimulus (tone plus light) that signals a shock. One group has a history of learning in which the light predicts a shock; the other group does not. Both groups have the same contiguous exposure to the tone-light compound stimulus, but, for the group with pretraining, the tone is redundant. When both groups are tested for their conditioning to the tone, the group with pretraining with the light stimulus shows significantly worse conditioning than the other group, because, despite equivalent contiguity, the tone conveys different information to the two groups.

Classical conditioning is not necessarily a slow process dependent on repeated pairings of stimuli. Learning is often rapid and efficient. As Robert Rescorla noted:

> Pavlovian conditioning is not a process by which the organism willy-nilly forms associations between any two stimuli that happen to co-occur. Rather the organism is better seen as an

information seeker using logical and perceptual relations among events, along with its own preconceptions to form a sophisticated representation of the world. An analogy between animals showing pavlovian conditioning and scientists identifying the cause of a phenomenon is useful. If one thinks of pavlovian conditioning as developing between a conditional stimulus and an unconditioned stimulus under just those circumstances that would lead a scientist to conclude that the conditioned stimulus causes the unconditioned stimulus, one has a surprisingly successful heuristic for remembering the facts of what it takes to produce pavlovian associative learning.

Classical conditioning has been viewed as (1) learning that, in humans, at least requires conscious processing and awareness of the relations between events or (2) an automatic process that occurs similarly in the mollusk and the human being, requiring little or no conscious processing or awareness. A good deal of evidence shows that awareness of a relation between events is often necessary for conditioning to occur and greatly facilitates learning. It seems reasonable to conclude that classical conditioning in humans occurs through hierarchically organized neural systems. The operation of some of these systems may predispose to automatic processing, whereas other systems are not so predisposed. On the other hand, evidence indicates that classical conditioning can occur in the absence of intention to learn, without awareness, even if it is resisted. For example, animals and humans acquire conditioned aversions to specific smells and tastes (the conditional stimulus) if they are associated with drug-induced or illness-induced nausea (the unconditioned stimulus–unconditioned response). People develop highly specific aversions to food that they may have eaten at the onset of seasickness or of gastrointestinal (GI) illness. The food becomes a conditioned stimulus for them, despite their knowledge that it did not cause their nausea. In those instances, people seem to be biologically prepared to develop some conditioned responses and not others. For example, nausea is readily conditioned to smell and taste but not to sight and sound. Some phobic reactions in humans may provide similar examples of prepared learning (e.g., fears of animals and heights). The hypothesis is that people are biologically predisposed to learn certain fears as a result of their evolutionary past, when it was adaptive to do so. That explains the fact that people have phobias only to selected situations and objects, which presumably were once associated with threats to survival.

Classical conditioning may affect the responsiveness of the immune system. For example, animals were conditioned by pairing saccharin-flavored water with injections of cyclophosphamide (Cytoxan), an immunosuppressive drug. After a single trial, animals showed immunosuppression and aversion to the taste of saccharin, phenomena not shown by the control group that received saccharin-flavored water paired with a placebo injection. It is well known that humans undergoing immunosuppressive therapy develop nausea that comes to be elicited by hospital cues; indeed, sometimes even the thought of the hospital elicits nausea. Women undergoing treatment with cytotoxic drugs for the treatment of ovarian cancer demonstrated nausea on return to the hospital combined with decreased immune function. This appears to replicate the work with animals and suggests that similar conditioning of immune function is found in humans. Clearly, the person is unaware of such conditioning.

Clinical Applications

Classical conditioning has influenced the way in which clinical disorders have been conceptualized and has generated methods for their treatment. It has, for example, played a prominent role in the analysis and treatment of anxiety disorders. Exposure to a traumatic event is a necessary, but insufficient, condition for the development of posttraumatic stress disorder (PTSD). Classical conditioning explains how stimuli associated with a severe trauma (the unconditioned stimulus) come to elicit stress responses that were part of the original trauma. As with phobic disorders, not everyone who experiences a traumatic event displays the stress response; predisposing genetic factors, adverse early learning experiences, and perception of the traumatic event are determinants of PTSD.

Another area of application has been in the treatment of substance abuse. Cues associated with repeated alcohol and drug use come to elicit conditioned responses. Some of the conditioned responses are opposite in nature to the unconditioned effects of the substance. They are known as *classically conditioned compensatory reactions*, which are believed to reflect homeostatic mechanisms. This conditioning process contributes to the development of behavioral tolerance to alcohol and drugs. In alcohol- or drug-dependent persons, the conditioned responses are believed to be subjectively experienced as craving or anticipatory withdrawal reactions. An alternative view is that the conditioned stimulus triggers craving, because it comes to signal the positively rewarding consequences of alcohol or drug use. In either case, it follows that cues associated with substance abuse need to be addressed in treatment. Cue exposure treatment for alcoholic persons and drug addicts is based on the principle of *extinction*—the procedure of presenting the conditioned stimulus in the absence of the unconditioned stimulus. Doing so results in the elimination of the conditioned response when the conditioned stimulus no longer predicts its occurrence. For example, patients with alcohol dependence are presented with alcohol-related cues (e.g., the sight and the smell of alcohol, which reliably elicit craving, without being allowed to drink alcohol [the unconditioned stimulus]). Because negative emotional states can function as conditioned stimuli, cue-exposure treatment also involves the induction of relevant mood states.

Classical conditioning is no longer necessarily linked to the philosophy of behaviorism, with which it was once associated. Its concepts and methods lend themselves to current perspectives on human behavior, and they continue to play an important role in contemporary behavioral therapy, which itself has become more eclectic and theoretically broader than it was during its early origins in behaviorism.

OPERANT CONDITIONING

The notion that learning occurs as a consequence of action was espoused in the pioneering work of Edward Lee Thorndike, whose learning theory dominated the field of psychology in the United States for the first half of the 20th century. A typical experiment devised by Thorndike consisted of placing a hungry cat in a cage with a latching device that, when correctly manipulated, allowed the cat access to a second cage for a bite of food. Thorndike noted that the cat became efficient at opening the lock, a sequence of events termed *trial-and-error learning*, and he hypothesized that the appropriate behaviors were strengthened by the cat's experiences of success and failure. Following up on Thorndike's work, Skinner and his colleagues made the effects of environment on behavior a central aspect of learning.

The principles and procedures of operant conditioning are the product of Skinner's philosophy of radical behaviorism, according to which overt behavior is the only acceptable target of scientific investigation. Skinner argued that subjective experience (private events) should be included in the experimental analysis of behavior, but their role has always been restricted. Thoughts and feelings are epiphenomena in operant conditioning; they cannot exert a causal influence on behavior. Strictly speaking, apart from biological determinants (which have always been minimized), it is assumed that human behavior is exclusively a function of environmental events that are ultimately beyond personal control. Another hallmark of operant conditioning has been its emphasis on the study of the individual organism. The repeated measurement of the behavior of a person under controlled conditions is the methodological contribution of operant conditioning. Skinner rejected statistical comparisons between groups of subjects, claiming that group averages obscure what is important—the behavior of individuals. The application of the principles and the procedures of operant conditioning to human problems is known as *applied behavior analysis*.

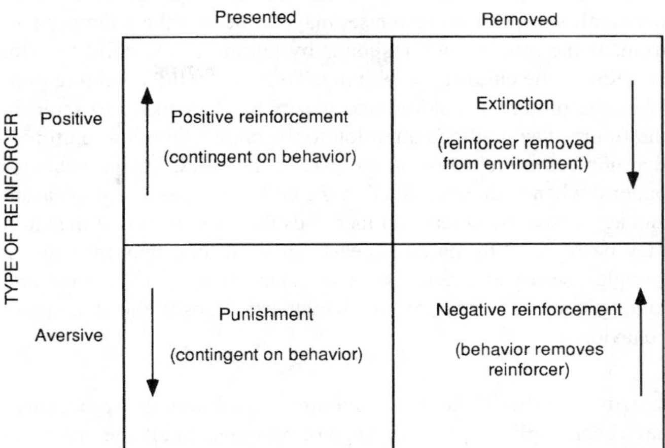

FIGURE 3.3–2 The principal procedures of operant conditioning, depending on whether a positive or negative reinforcer is applied or removed after the behavior is performed. The arrows show the direction of the behavior change.

Positive Reinforcement

The best known learning principle contributed by operant conditioning is the principle of *positive reinforcement*, the process by which certain consequences of behavior raise the probability that the behavior will occur again. On the whole, positive reinforcers are viewed as pleasant (e.g., attention, praise, and money). Reinforcers that affect biological processes, such as food, may be defined as *primary reinforcers*. However, events viewed as aversive by some individuals may be reinforcing for others. For example, the behavior of some children is reinforced by scolding, which, after all, is a form of attention. Many drugs, including opioids, barbiturates, and such stimulants as amphetamine and cocaine, appear to be positive reinforcers. Animals and humans self-administer the substances, reliably discriminating between the active drug and a placebo. Complex patterns of behavior can be shaped in animals by using such drugs as reinforcers.

Traditional textbook descriptions state that reinforcement of a response must be immediate. However, as with classical conditioning, temporal contiguity is not necessary for learning to occur in operant conditioning. Recent research shows that the behavior of a simple organism, such as a laboratory rat, can be controlled by the aggregate consequences of a series of reinforcements of multiple responses over time. Revision of the requirement that reinforcement be immediate if it is to control behavior greatly extends the explanatory power of operant conditioning, but the mechanism by which the organism is able to integrate reinforcing consequences over time is never specified. Critics of operant conditioning point out that the delayed effect of reinforcement contingencies must be mediated by cognitive processes.

The neural mechanism underlying the delayed effect of reinforcement appears to be located in the anterior cingulate cortex. In one experiment, monkeys received a reward when they completed a prolonged behavioral schedule. The schedule included a variable number of trials. However, the number of trials was cued by a light that gradually increased in brightness. Hence, the animals could tell when the reward was due. As the time for the reward grew nearer, the animals demonstrated fewer errors, thus responding to the imminence of the reward. Electrophysiological recording of neurons in the anterior cingulate cortex found that firing increased as the time for the reward grew nearer. Moreover, the firing rate was proportional to the nearness of the reward time. If the relation between the light cue and reward time was made random, no such firing occurred. Hence, there appears to be a neural mechanism facilitating the degree of anticipation of a reward, accounting for the persistence of behavior despite delays in reward.

Negative Reinforcement

Reinforcement increases the probability of behavior. *Negative reinforcement* is the process by which behavior leading to the removal of an aversive event strengthens that behavior. *Negative reinforcers* tend to be aversive events; for example, avoidance behavior, such as phobic reactions and compulsive rituals, is negatively reinforced, because it forestalls actual or perceived aversive outcomes. Research shows that, when patients with anorexia nervosa are placed in a restricted hospital environment to facilitate the use of positive reinforcement for eating and gaining weight, they work (eat and gain weight) to get out of the aversive environment, adding negative reinforcement effects to the positive reinforcement effects.

Punishment

Punishment is the presentation of an aversive stimulus contingent on the occurrence of a particular response. The removal of a positive consequence contingent on behavior, known as *time out* from reinforcement, can also be viewed as punishment. The procedure is commonly used as a means of disciplining children with behavior problems; for example, sending a child to his or her room because of misbehavior. It is necessary to distinguish punishment from negative reinforcement. Punishment decreases the probability that the behavior will occur, whereas negative reinforcement increases the probability. One must also distinguish between the usual use of the term *punishment* and the technical use of the term as meant here. In the punishment paradigm, the punishing event is always delivered contingent on performance and demonstrably reduces the frequency of the behavior being punished. This is considerably different from the use of the term to denote imprisonment, for example, because the prison sentence follows long after the crime and may not affect future criminal behavior. Figure 3.3–2 summarizes the major principles of operant conditioning and the effects that they have on behavior.

Reciprocal Influences

Because much human behavior occurs within an interpersonal context, reciprocal influences occur. An example of this is afforded by the study of predelinquent behavior. Family studies suggest that predelinquent behavior patterns are set in motion by the excessive and inconsistent use of punishment on the part of parents. A mother may severely scold her small son, who, in response, may whine or have a temper tantrum. If the mother then responds by talking to the child to calm him down, the child stops whining. Thus, the child's whining punishes the mother's scolding and makes her less likely to scold in the future. The mother's attention to the child's whining reinforces that unpleasant behavior on the part of the child. Such a behavior pattern, when well established in the child, is viewed as unpleasant and aggressive by others and increases the likelihood that the child may be rejected by parents, peers, and teachers, thus initiating a complex series of events, such as poor school performance and joining a deviant peer group, which predisposes the delinquent behavior.

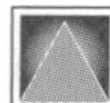

Table 3.3–2
Examples of Reinforcement Schedules in Operant Conditioning

Fixed-ratio (FR) schedule
Reinforcement occurs after a fixed number of responses (e.g., every ten responses—10:1 ratio; ten bar presses release a food pellet; workers are paid for every ten items they make). There is a rapid rate of response to obtain the greatest number of rewards. The animal knows that the next reinforcement depends on a certain number of responses being made.

Variable-ratio (VR) schedule
Reinforcement occurs at random intervals (e.g., after the third, sixth, and then second response, and so on). This generates a fairly constant rate of response, because the probability of reinforcement at any given time remains relatively stable.

Fixed-interval (FI) schedule
Reinforcement occurs at regular intervals (e.g., every 10 minutes or every third hour). The animal keeps track of time. The rate of responding drops to near zero after reinforcement and then increases at approximately the expected time of reward. This is known as *scalloping* and is seen in humans checking their mailboxes.

Variable-interval (VI) schedule
Reinforcement occurs at random intervals, similar to variable ratio, resulting in consistent responding. The response rate does not change between reinforcement. The animal responds at a steady rate to get the reward when it is available; this is common in trout fishermen and in the use of slot machines.

Clinical Applications

Operant conditioning procedures have been applied to a wide range of problems in all age groups in psychiatry, education, rehabilitation, and medicine. In general, the procedures are most commonly used today to change the behavior of young children, persons with mental retardation, and institutionalized populations, such as chronically mentally ill patients. Behavior therapists in clinical practice, particularly with adult outpatient disorders, rarely describe themselves as applied behavior analysts, and they draw on broad theoretical perspectives. Reinforcement procedures may be used alone as applications of operant conditioning, or such procedures may be combined with techniques, such as extinction and punishment. However, reinforcement occurs in any form of psychotherapy, because the therapist differentially attends to the verbal behavior of the patient. Moreover, most behavior therapists today combine the use of reinforcement procedures with many other procedures derived from learning theory.

Positive Reinforcement Much is known about various *schedules of reinforcement,* defined as the pattern or frequency with which a reward is delivered as a consequence of behavior. The most frequently used schedules are listed in Table 3.3–2. One of the most used schedules in clinical practice is *partial reinforcement,* in which reinforcement only occasionally results from a particular behavior. Such a pattern of reinforcement maintains the behavior at full strength. Moreover, partially reinforced behavior may be particularly resistant to extinction. Because many deviant behaviors provoke attention from others, they are maintained by the social environment. Observational and experimental work, for example, has shown that hospital staff members tend to reinforce their patients' abnormal behaviors by attending to them. When the staff members learn to stop giving such attention and attend more frequently to adaptive behaviors, patient behavior improves. Similar findings have been made in school. Teacher attention reinforces disruptive behavior in the classroom; when such attention is withdrawn, the disruptive behavior decreases. The most used reinforcement procedure is a *shaping* paradigm, in which a behavior is changed in form by reinforcing components of the final behavior sequentially. For example, in teaching a mute patient with schizophrenia to talk, the first behavior to be reinforced may be simply looking at the therapist, followed by any mouthing movement, followed by any vocalization (perhaps in imitation of the therapist) and, finally, simple words and sentences. A *continuous reinforcement* schedule may first be used; in it, reinforcement is delivered for every appropriate response. This schedule may be followed by partial reinforcement; each component behavior is first developed with continuous reinforcement and then strengthened with partial reinforcement. If speech is reinforced only in the presence of one therapist, the patient may remain mute with others, which is an example of *discriminative learning.* Similar behavior is seen in everyday life when a motorist stops at a red light and proceeds when the light changes to green—behaviors that are highly reinforced in this society. To overcome discriminative learning, the therapist first establishes the beginnings of speech and then has several therapists reinforce speech to ensure generalization of the new behavior. When speech is fully developed, artificial reinforcement can be phased out, because speaking should be more reinforcing than being mute. This is also an example of chaining of behaviors and reinforcement, because all the initial behavioral sequences are necessary for the final behavior of talking, and a complex sequence of behaviors is gradually built up and reinforced. Many problem behaviors seen in humans have been developed in animals by using various schedules of reinforcement. Thus, head banging, a behavior seen frequently in retarded and autistic children, has been developed in monkeys with the use of reinforcement, such that the monkeys actually injure themselves to obtain reinforcement. Although such experiments do not prove that similar behaviors seen in humans are learned, they do call attention to the powerful effect of reinforcement in developing and maintaining deviant behavior.

Often given in the form of attention and praise contingent on certain behaviors, reinforcement is a basic ingredient of most therapists' repertoire. Skilled therapists of most persuasions use *contingent verbal reinforcement,* as has been shown even in nondirective psychotherapy, so that certain therapeutic themes are strengthened. Other methods used in reinforcement paradigms include tokens exchangeable for goods or activities that cannot be bought or engaged in otherwise. What is reinforcing for one person may not be reinforcing for another, therefore, when reinforcement is used, the clinician must observe and measure the behavior being reinforced to make sure that it is being strengthened. The data from a

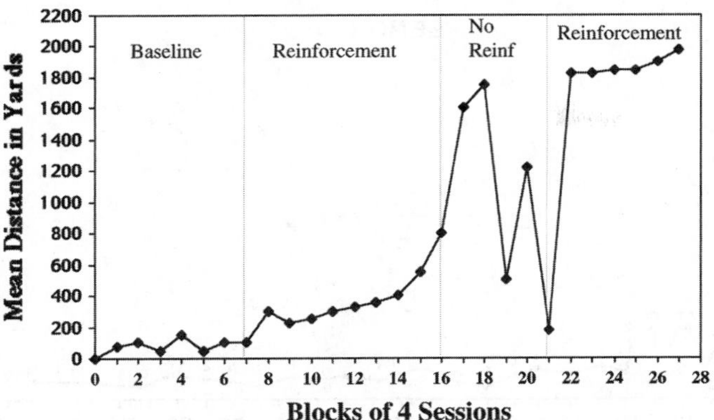

FIGURE 3.3–3 An example of the use of positive reinforcement for the treatment of an agoraphobic patient, with experimental demonstration of the use of such reinforcement.

clinical example of the use of verbal reinforcement to diminish agoraphobic behavior are shown in Figure 3.3–3.

This young woman had developed agoraphobia during adolescence. Agoraphobic avoidance had progressed over the subsequent decade until she was essentially housebound. She could only leave home accompanied by her mother or husband and, even in that circumstance, with considerable anxiety. Leaving home alone had, in the past, often precipitated a panic attack. She had been treated with various medications and with psychotherapy without significant improvement. She was admitted to a clinical research center as part of a study examining the use of social reinforcement in various phobic conditions. A therapist with whom she had developed a good relationship delivered reinforcement in the form of praise contingent on progress. In the baseline period, the patient was encouraged to walk as far away from the clinical research unit as she could. As can be seen in Figure 3.3–3, reinforcement for staying outside the unit resulted in only a small increase in distance walked away from the unit. Positive reinforcement was then introduced. In this phase, praise for progress was given on a shaping schedule. For example, if the patient had been reinforced at a criterion of 100-yd distance on one trial and walked 150 yd on the next trial, the criterion would become 125 yd. She would be praised on the next trial only if she walked 125 yd or more. In this phase, distance walked began to increase. When reinforcement was stopped, distance walked increased dramatically and then decreased, an example of an *extinction burst*. This phenomenon is well known in animal experiments. Finally, when reinforcement was reintroduced, the patient was able to walk long distances away from the unit. This was then generalized to the patient's home environment. In theory, further natural reinforcement would continue to strengthen the patient's new freedom, because being free to move around allows contact with many reinforcing activities.

Extinction Disordered behavior is often developed and maintained by reinforcement in the form of attention from others. In such cases, the clinician must identify the reinforcer and remove it from the patient's environment, a procedure known as *extinction*. A simple example of the use of extinction is the case of a young child who cries interminably before going to sleep. When the mother puts the child to bed, the crying begins after a few minutes, and the mother returns to find out what the problem is. She then reads to the child or engages in some other activity. When she leaves, the pattern is repeated. Clearly, maternal attention is reinforcing the crying. The treatment is to persuade the mother not to return to the child's bedroom once the child is settled for the night. However, as noted in the case described previously, she needs to be warned that the amount of crying may increase for two or three nights (in an *extinction burst*) before it diminishes.

Punishment Punishment is less useful as a therapeutic procedure than reinforcement or extinction, because it may produce unwanted effects, such as aggressive behavior, and the possibility of inflicting physical damage is always present. For the most part, punishment is used only in situations in which the behavior to be changed is injurious to the patient.

A clinical example of such a condition is rumination disorder in which infants regurgitate their food mouthful by mouthful, which leads to malnutrition and dehydration and is frequently life threatening. One treatment is to use the principle of punishment, making an unpleasant event contingent on each episode of regurgitation. In the case illustrated in Figure 3.3–4, a drop of lemon juice applied to the infant's tongue was used as the unpleasant event. During the baseline period before treatment, the infant ruminated between 40 and 70 percent of the time that he was awake. Once lemon juice was presented contingent on spitting up food, the frequency of rumination steadily declined. Punishment was then briefly removed, and rumination returned to baseline levels, demonstrating the efficacy of punishment. The reintroduction of punishment eventually led to the virtual elimination of the behavior and a return to normal weight, with no relapse at 1-year follow-up.

The use of punishment in a clinical situation should be carefully supervised and should follow certain rules. The behavior to be addressed should have been resistant to appropriate behavior-change procedures involving the use of positive reinforcement. Behaviors incompatible with the problem behavior can often be reinforced, and the problem thus can be eliminated. In addition, the behavior to be changed should be severely incapacitating and should threaten physical integrity (e.g., the self-injurious behavior of some children with autistic disorders). Punishment procedures that cause tissue damage should not be used. The behavior to be changed should be observed, measured, and recorded (as shown in Fig. 3.3–4), so that the effects of punishment and the amount of punishment used can be seen. If effectively used, punishment rapidly brings a behavior under control, and behaviors can then be built up with the use of positive reinforcement.

SOCIAL-COGNITIVE LEARNING THEORY

Modes of Learning The psychologist Albert Bandura has integrated traditional classical and operant conditioning principles into a theoretically rich account of behavior and behavior change. A primary tenet of his approach is that the influence of environmental events on the acquisition and the regulation of behavior is primarily a function of cognitive processes. These processes are based on prior experience and determine what environmental influences are attended to, how they are perceived, whether they are remembered, and how they may affect future action. Reinforcement is regarded not as an automatic strengthener of behavior but as a source of guidance for behavior by anticipated outcomes. By observing the consequences of behavior, the person learns what action is appropriate in what situation.

By symbolic representation of anticipated outcomes of behavior, the person generates the motivation to initiate and maintain behavior.

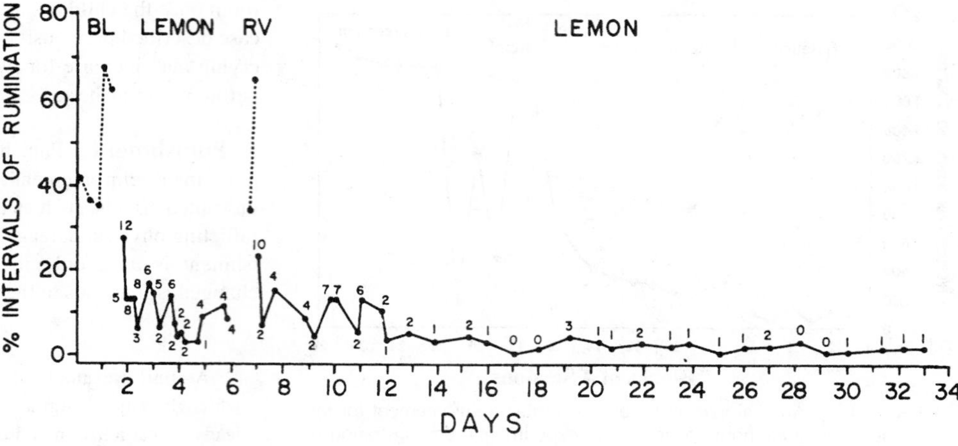

FIGURE 3.3–4 The effects of punishment in an experiment in which lemon juice was delivered contingent on ruminative vomiting in an infant. The frequency of rumination was rapidly reduced from the baseline (BL) and was increased only when punishment was withdrawn during the reversal phase (RV). The number of applications of punishment (lemon juice) is shown by the number above each data point.

Classical conditioning and operant conditioning are viewed as sources of learning about predictive relations among events. A third mode of learning is *modeling* (vicarious learning). In modeling, learning occurs through observation. The person need not exhibit any behavior or be directly reinforced for behavior. Modeling expands the scope and the complexity of learning influences on behavior. For example, it helps explain how phobic reactions may be acquired in the absence of any direct traumatic experience. Young monkeys acquire a severe and lasting fear of snakes after observing their wild-reared parents act fearfully in the presence of a snake. Modeling has many therapeutic applications. For example, children can be prepared for pending surgery by having them observe a film in which a child successfully copes with the novel and frightening events associated with the preparation for and recovery from surgery.

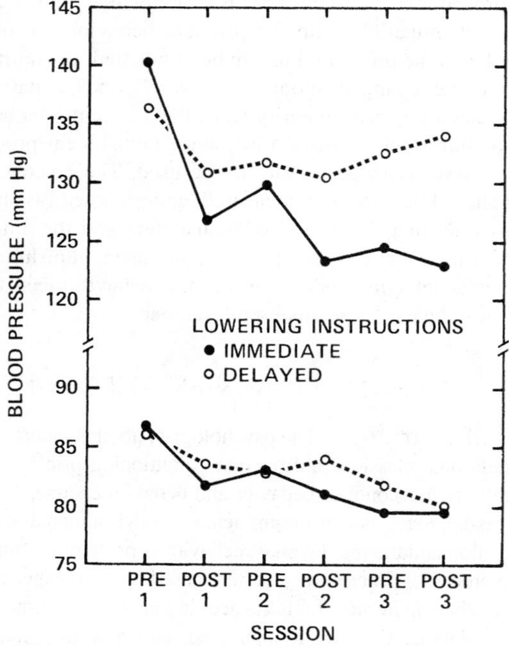

FIGURE 3.3–5 The effects of two expectancies on systolic (*top lines*) and diastolic (*bottom lines*) pressures of hypertensive persons. Systolic blood pressure was markedly reduced in the group that was told that relaxation training would lower blood pressure after one or two training sessions. In comparison, the group that was told that blood pressure lowering would occur only after prolonged practice showed only slight reductions in systolic pressure.

The traditional emphasis on conditioning principles gives short shrift to verbal instruction as a mode of learning. The potential therapeutic effects of verbal instructions are illustrated by a study of hypertensive patients. All participants in the experiment were told that relaxation training would help to lower their blood pressure. One-half of the participants were also told that their blood pressure would show reductions after three sessions of relaxation training given in one morning; the other one-half of the participants were told that they could expect reductions only after prolonged relaxation practice. As shown in Figure 3.3–5, the groups showed no difference in diastolic blood pressure readings. For systolic blood pressure, however, large and significant differences are shown for the group receiving immediate lowering instructions The mechanism underlying this effect is unknown. However, an expectancy of blood pressure lowering may be needed to induce the biochemical changes necessary to lower blood pressure. This is an example of the complex interactions that occur between environmental events, in this case, the instructions given to the patient, the patient's cognitive appraisal of the instructions, and the neurochemical processes. Therapists tend to neglect the effect of therapeutic instructions, but experimental work suggests that the therapist should do everything to enhance the development of realistic outcome and efficacy expectations.

Self-Efficacy Theory A component of social-cognitive learning theory with ramifications for the treatment of clinical problems is *self-efficacy* theory. *Efficacy expectations* are the degree of confidence that a person feels about coping effectively with a particular situation. *Outcome expectations* are defined as beliefs that particular actions produce a certain outcome. *Self-efficacy* is the end product of different cognitive processes. To alter self-efficacy, people must actively appraise a specific experience and attribute successful coping to themselves as opposed to attributing it to some transient factor outside their control. Self-efficacy theory and cognitive-social learning theory, in general, draw heavily on the principles of attribution theory, a cognitive approach concerned with how people perceive the causes of behavior.

Self-efficacy theory predicts that the more people feel capable of predicting and controlling threatening events, the less vulnerable they are to anxiety and stress disorders in response to traumatic experiences. Research with primates supports this prediction: Infant monkeys were reared in an environment in which they exercised control over food, water, and special treats (the masters) or received reinforcers that were administered automatically and independent of their behavior (the controls). Months later, the masters were significantly less fearful in response to a threatening situation than were the controls.

The theory also predicts that psychological treatments, such as exposure to phobic conditions, are effective, because they enhance self-efficacy for coping with threatening events. Behavioral performance is the most powerful means of increasing self-efficacy, but self-efficacy is also influenced by sources of information derived from vicarious learning and verbal persuasion. Numerous studies have established that exposure treatment is one of the most effective methods for eliminating phobias. Exposure also produces greater increases in self-efficacy than do other methods. The greater the increase in self-efficacy, the greater the change in phobic behavior, regardless of the type of treatment. Outcome expectations (i.e., self-reports of anticipated anxiety about entering a phobic situation) tend to be correlated with efficacy expectations. If the correlation with efficacy expectations is eliminated statistically, outcome expectations fail to predict outcome, suggesting that change in self-efficacy is the important variable underlying behavior change.

Critics have charged that self-efficacy is only correlated with treatment-induced changes in phobic behavior and does not cause the behavior change. Bandura, however, points to the systematic covariation of experimentally induced levels of efficacy expectations and phobic behavior as evidence of their causal nature. Self-efficacy is related to measures of fear arousal. Increases in self-efficacy in phobic patients are associated with reductions in autonomic nervous system reactivity and neuroendocrine responses to phobic stimuli. The theory also suggests an explanation of the apparent resistance to the extinction of phobic behavior. Whether phobic reactions are eliminated by exposure to feared situations depends on the nature of the information that people derive from such experiences and not simply on the quantity of exposure. If people conclude that they can cope effectively, they no longer avoid the feared situations. But no change occurs if people conclude that they are unable to cope and hence experience unnerving anxiety. By strengthening patients' expectations that they cannot cope, exposure may even enhance their phobic sensitivity. Treatment should be aimed at increasing the patient's sense of predictability and controllability through enhanced self-efficacy. Treatment of patients with phobias along these lines produces results superior to treatment that passively exposes patients to feared stimuli without fostering coping skills, even if the length of the exposure is greater in the latter therapy. Beyond furthering the analysis and the treatment of phobic disorders (panic disorder with agoraphobia, agoraphobia without a history of panic disorder, specific phobia, and social phobia), self-efficacy has proved fruitful in the experimental analysis of a wide range of clinical problems, including pain management, the effects of stress on behavior and the immune system, and the prevention of relapse in substance abusers.

Self-Regulation In marked contrast to operant conditioning and radical behaviorism, social-cognitive learning theory emphasizes a capacity for self-regulation of behavior. Cognition is more than a passive conduit of external influences; it serves a generative function, allowing people to initiate thought, affect, and action to influence their circumstances, which, in turn, affect their cognition. People are neither driven inexorably by internal forces nor are they passive reactors to environmental pressure; rather, they are both the agents and the objects of external influences. Self-control strategies have become important components of most therapeutic interventions in behavior therapy. Among the most important elements of self-regulation of behavior are goal setting and feedback, self-monitoring, self-evaluation, and self-reinforcement.

Goal Setting and Feedback People set long-term and short-term goals for themselves. The setting of sequential short-term goals leads to better performance than setting a distant goal. This is presumably related to the reinforcing qualities of goal attainment because reinforcing successive small steps is better than reinforcing the final behavior, at least until the behavior is well established. Goal definition is also important because the attainment of well-specified goals is more easily recognized than is the attainment of poorly defined goals. In general, the higher the goal set, the better the performance. At the highest levels of goal setting, performance begins to decline, underlining the fact that unrealistic goals undermine performance. Goal attainment enhances self-efficacy and affects future performance.

From a therapeutic viewpoint, the therapist should help the patient define and set realistic, well-specified goals that signal small steps along the way to the overall goal so that demoralization can be kept at bay by success. Patients should set their own goals, because self-determined goals lead to better performance than goals imposed by others. Teaching patients problem-solving strategies that they can use in many situations is a useful aspect of most therapies.

Goal attainment is not the only indicator of improvement in performance. Behavior change itself, if observed by the patient, can provide information regarding progress toward a particular goal. The process, known as *informational feedback*, enhances performance in a wide variety of tasks, such as learning to shoot accurately at a target, driving an automobile, and self-regulating autonomic processes. Removing informational feedback leads, at least temporarily, to setbacks. Information regarding therapeutic progress can be fed back to the patient in several ways. Patients can observe their own progress when the desired behavior change is relatively linear, such as approaching a phobic object or situation. Many behaviors, however, are complex. In such cases, self-monitoring the behavior can enhance feedback. In addition, patients can plot the results of such feedback in graph form to examine their progress over long periods. Enhancement of information regarding progress is the central focus of biofeedback. In the typical biofeedback paradigm, processes that are not easily observed (e.g., blood pressure, small muscle contractions, and skin temperature) are made available for inspection by amplification. With sensitive and continuous feedback, the patient has the opportunity to learn to regulate invisible behaviors.

Self-Monitoring The basis of all self-control strategies is self-monitoring, which is the identification and recording of target problems and the conditions under which they occur. Typically, patients are asked to complete daily written records. For example, patients with panic disorder track all panic attacks and record the thoughts, feelings, and actions that preceded and accompanied the attacks. The goal is to identify the proximal determinants of the problem. Self-monitoring not only provides patients with an awareness of how their behavior affects or is affected by their social environment, it also prompts behavior change as patients identify specific influences on their behavior.

Self-Evaluation and Self-Reinforcement People who adopt certain standards and monitor their performances evaluate their success or failure in achieving those standards. Such an evaluation is the basis for self-reinforcement. Performances that match or exceed the standards serve as cues for rewards, and people deny themselves rewards for substandard performance. The essence of self-reinforcement is that people make freely available rewards contingent on behavior that meets preset standards. Common clinical problems, such as depression, involve the adoption of unrealistic or perfectionistic standards or excessively harsh and judgmental self-evaluation, regardless of objective performance.

Theories of Relapse One of the major problems facing therapists of all persuasions is that of patient relapse. Some instances of relapse can be easily understood; for example, the original environmental influences reinforcing symptomatic behavior may not have altered, and the patient's behavior is brought under their control once treatment has ended. This is an example of insufficient treatment; for example, perhaps the patient's family should have been brought into therapy. Sometimes, however, relapse denotes an impossible situation for the therapist, who is unable to alter a noxious psychological environment. Less is known about the process of relapse than about the acquisition of behavior. For the most part, relapse has been studied in the addictive disorders, such as alcoholism and opiate addiction, and in related disorders, such as cigarette smoking and obesity. The basic theory concerning relapse involves situations that pose a high risk for engaging in the problem behavior, situations in which the behavior has occurred at a high frequency in the past. According to social-cognitive learning theory, if such a situation is coped with successfully, the person experiences an increase in self-efficacy, which leads to a low probability of relapse. The assumption is that the person has been taught or has developed usable coping skills. However, a former substance abuser who is deficient in coping with the high-risk situation develops a positive expectancy regarding the beneficial effects of the substance and starts using the substance again. This practice results in an abstinence violation effect, defined as the breaking of a self-imposed rule, leading to a diminished sense of self-efficacy.

FROM LEARNING THEORY TO PSYCHOTHERAPY

As a broad-based framework that emphasizes the multidimensional nature of psychological functioning, social-cognitive learning theory provides a flexible guide for the design of treatments for particular conditions. Treatment programs typically combine several principles and procedures. In formulating a therapy for a particular disorder, it is first necessary to develop a model, however simple, of the factors maintaining the symptoms of the particular disorder. Similarly, for the purposes of prevention, a model containing remediable risk factors for the development of the disorder is needed. The factors contained in a particular model and their relation to one another derive from a variety of sources, such as clinical observations, epidemiological studies, naturalistic observations, and laboratory experiments. The models developed at any one time may be updated when new findings concerning the disorder are made or when controlled treatment studies suggest that additional factors need to be taken into account.

For example, the models of factors maintaining bulimia nervosa and depression differ in their details, but both include behavioral antecedents and cognitive mediators of those antecedent behaviors. The treatments themselves share common elements derived from learning principles. The therapy sessions are structured to maximize learning, beginning with a review of self-monitoring, including homework assignments. Based on this information and depending on the stage of therapy, the therapist sets an agenda for the session, which may include information on new procedures to be introduced in that session, followed by behavior

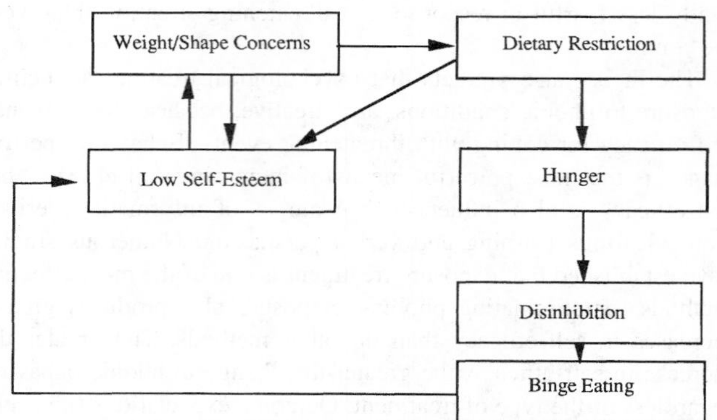

FIGURE 3.3–6 A hypothetical model of psychosocial factors maintaining bulimic behaviors.

change procedures deriving from the information gained from the self-monitoring records. This is followed by a summary of the session and the setting of homework. Within the therapy itself, an array of procedures are used, including setting realistic outcome expectancies, strengthening efficacy expectancies, information and educational strategies, data collection, feedback regarding progress, reinforcement of adaptive behaviors, and cognitive change procedures.

Bulimia Nervosa Clinical, naturalistic, and laboratory studies all suggest that excessive dietary restriction leads to hunger and disinhibition of eating whereby individuals with bulimia nervosa develop a sense of loss of control over eating that leads to binge eating. Dietary restriction appears to be driven by overconcern about shape and weight. Hence, dieting (when it fails) is followed by various methods of purging to compensate for the actual or perceived excessive caloric intake. In addition, low self-esteem deriving from a multiplicity of developmental causes appears to enhance concerns about weight and shape. These considerations led to the development of the relatively simple model of factors that maintain bulimic behavior, illustrated in Figure 3.3–6. One pathway to binge eating is excessive dieting in response to weight and shape concerns. A second pathway involves disinhibition of eating under the influence of negative affect. Such negative affect often stems from faulty interpersonal interactions. It is likely that the effects of negative affect leading to binge eating are stronger when the individual is hungry from dieting.

Learning theory suggests that the antecedent events closest to the primary problem behavior should be addressed first. Hence, the first aim of cognitive-behavioral therapy for bulimia nervosa is to reduce the dietary restriction that leads to hunger and binge eating. To do this, several learning principles are used. First, an educational approach is taken, presenting information concerning the factors maintaining binge eating and purging, together with a rationale for the procedures stemming from the model. This is aimed at developing an expectation on the patient's behalf that reducing dieting helps reduce the sense of loss of control and the consequent binge eating. Once the patient has accepted the rationale, the first phase of therapy begins. In this phase, several additional principles are used. The patient is asked to monitor his or her eating behavior (i.e., meal content, binges, and circumstances surrounding binge eating and purging) on self-monitoring forms. This crucial aid to self-regulation provides information to the therapist and the patient about the details of the problem and, in later sessions, about progress in changing the problem behaviors. Restrictive dieting is directly addressed by helping the patient eat three meals and two snacks each day followed by increasing the amount eaten on each occasion. Here, a process of shaping is used to allow gradual behavior change. Appropriate changes are reinforced by selective therapist attention and praise, and problems are discussed until a new solution is found. Such a solution is then tried out by the patient between sessions as homework.

Once a more stable pattern of eating has been attained, other factors that drive dietary restriction, such as overconcern about weight and shape and faulty interpersonal interactions leading to low mood and to binge eating, are addressed. One of the learning procedures used is data gathering on the problem, including the hoped-for, but unrealistic, outcomes the patient believes he or she can attain by maintaining a thin body shape. Such outcome expectancies can be challenged regarding their reality, and alternative ways of achieving more reasonable outcome expectancies can be considered. Similarly, the antecedent events leading to negative affect are self-monitored, and problem solving procedures used to deal with such events proactively.

In the final phase of therapy, relapse prevention strategies are implemented. First, behavior change strategies that have proved successful in treatment are reviewed. Lapses occurring during this phase of treatment, for example, a small binge or even an urge to binge, are examined in detail. The events leading up to the lapse are reviewed and alternative coping strategies are considered for their potential effectiveness in preventing relapses. More generally, situations specific to the patient that are likely to precipitate relapse are identified, and potential coping strategies are also identified. A case example in which cognitive-behavioral therapy was used to treat a patient with bulimia nervosa illustrates the use of these principles.

The patient was a 29-year-old married woman who, because of concerns about her weight, had begun to diet in early adolescence. Although she was within the normal limits of weight for her height, her mother's concern about her own weight and remarks about the patient's "plumpness" apparently drove her to ever-stricter dieting. This was followed later in adolescence by the occurrence of binge eating with a consequent weight gain of several pounds. To combat this weight gain, the patient began to purge by inducing vomiting with her fingers after binges; later, she was able to induce vomiting at will. When first seen at the clinic, she was binge eating and purging almost 15 times each week. Physical examination and electrolytes were normal, except for a raised serum amylase, a finding not uncommon in patients with bulimia nervosa.

Therapy began by elaborating on her history, exploring in more detail the links between feelings of low self-esteem engendered by childhood experiences and the importance of weight and shape to her morale, which led her to dieting and binge eating. The patient was able to perceive these links and to accept the model outlined in Figure 3.3–6. She accepted the possibility that reducing dieting would lessen binge eating and purging; however, she feared gaining weight if she gave up dieting. She was not particularly reassured by the findings from controlled trials that the average patient does not gain weight but was willing to take an experimental approach to the problem. She was advised to weigh herself no more than once each week to reduce overreaction to natural weight fluctuations and was taught how to monitor and record her food intake, binge eating and purging, and the circumstances under which such behaviors occurred.

At the next session, the food records were examined in detail, with the therapist pointing out her pattern of eating little or no breakfast, a small salad for lunch, and then binge eating at least once during the evening. The link between dieting, hunger, and binge eating was again pointed out, and the therapist suggested that she alter her food intake toward eating three meals and two snacks by the clock, rather than relying on her own hunger sensations, which were disrupted by her chaotic eating patterns. During the next three or four sessions the therapist and patient collaborated to gradually achieve this goal by using the principle of shaping and reinforcing positive changes by therapist praise and attention. By the fifth session, the patient was eating three meals and two snacks on many days. The patient recognized from her food record that she was more likely to binge on days when the desired meal pattern was not maintained. This reinforced her adherence to eating three meals and two snacks daily and also allowed her to experiment with consuming somewhat larger meals with continuing diminution of binge eating and purging. By the eighth therapy session, she completed her first week free of binge eating and purging, without any noticeable weight gain. Such progress during the first half of therapy has been shown to be a good prognostic indicator.

The next phase of treatment involved broadening food choices. The therapist recommended a behavioral task, namely, that the patient visit a supermarket and make a list of all the foods that she would not buy because she feared eating them. The patient compiled the list and was asked to add some of the lesser-feared foods to her diet. With these additions continuing over the next few sessions, the bulk of the work then shifted to an examination of her distorted thinking about weight and shape. The patient was particularly prone to blame her appearance for any rejection she perceived. Such incidents were explored in detail and usually led her to accept an alternative conclusion regarding the perceived rejection. She then began to practice these exercises on her own when such thoughts arose. She was also convinced that her body was less perfect than the bodies of other women. Hence, she was given the task of looking at other women's bodies and considering their imperfections. She gradually became persuaded that she was not as overweight as she had thought. Although the patient occasionally lapsed into binge eating and purging, for most of the time during this phase of therapy, she had been eating normally.

In the final few sessions, the patient was asked to review the procedures that had helped her most to develop a written maintenance plan. Among the essential elements, she listed eating regularly and not avoiding foods, giving up dieting, and being somewhat more accepting about her weight and shape. Circumstances that might lead to further lapses were also explored, focusing on the few lapses that had occurred during the past weeks; this allowed the patient to plan to cope better with such situations. For example, she reported being tempted to binge when she was made angry by an interpersonal interchange, particularly if she returned home alone after such an incident. She developed several alternative coping strategies, such as talking the incident over with a friend or planning to eat out or go to a movie to ensure that she would not be alone under such circumstances. The systematic application of these cognitive and behavioral strategies illustrates the clinical use of relapse prevention strategies based on social-cognitive learning theory. The patient was monitored at 3-month intervals to check up on her progress and to deal with any residual problems. One year after the end of treatment, she had continued to abstain from binge eating and purging, and treatment ended. Not everyone does as well as this patient. Improvements in the therapeutic procedures will be made only if further factors maintaining the disorder are identified and if methods are devised to remove them.

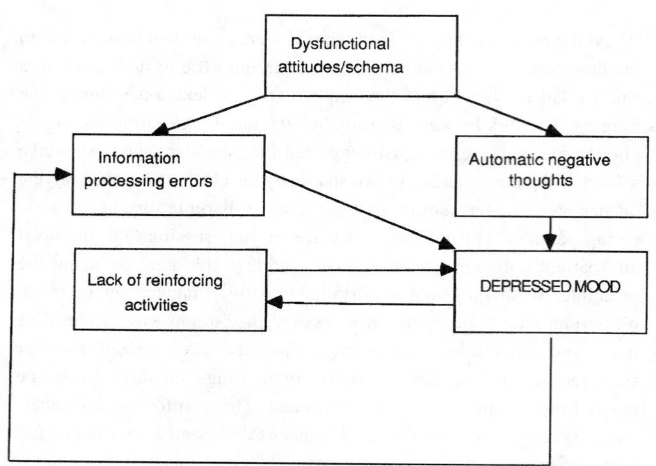

FIGURE 3.3–7 A hypothetical model of psychosocial factors maintaining depression.

Depression There are various models of the factors that maintain a depressed mood. One such model is shown in Figure 3.3–7. Distorted cognitive processes and a lack of reinforcing behavior, particularly of interpersonal behavior, are believed to maintain a depressed mood. A triad of cognitive dysfunctions is postulated; the most proximal to depressed mood are automatic negative thoughts. Errors in information processing, which are state dependent, occurring only in the presence of a depressed mood, are the second element in the cognitive triad. Events are perceived and processed mistakenly to suggest a potentially negative outcome, thus amplifying negative moods. At a deeper level, usually not easily accessible to the patient, are more general distorted attitudes and beliefs that give rise to the automatic negative thoughts and to errors in information processing. Also, the interpersonal world of the patient is often inherently nonreinforcing, which leads to a decline in interpersonal activities that further cuts the patient off from potential reinforcers, with the potential to spiral into a deep withdrawal and a seriously depressed mood.

Cognitive-behavioral therapy for depression begins by clarifying the patient's expectations regarding the outcome of treatment by engendering positive but realistic expectations. The relationship with the patient is described as collaborative—the patient gathers data and, with the help of the therapist, formulates behavior changes that are likely to ameliorate depression. Therapy usually begins with self-monitoring of mood states and the events surrounding them and with encouragement and reinforcement of proactive behaviors that the patient finds reinforcing. The aim is to gradually shape a wider repertoire of behaviors leading to an enhanced frequency of reinforcement in the patient's life by the identification of behaviors associated with depressed or normal mood states, the provision of feedback regarding progress derived from further self-monitoring, and the reinforcement of progress by the therapist. Feedback is also sought from the patient regarding the relevance and effectiveness of the procedures used in each therapy session. As the patient begins to make progress, automatic negative thoughts are examined in detail. Socratic questioning is used to teach the patient to evaluate the accuracy of the outcome expectancies involved in such thoughts. Self-monitoring is now focused on maladaptive thinking. As therapy continues, underlying attitudes and deeper cognitive schemas are gradually uncovered and clarified in similar ways. It appears that, as the examination of disordered cognitions continues, many patients are able to take a less personalized view of their negative thinking, viewing such thoughts as passing phenomenon that may or may not have some truth in them. This process is known as *metacognition*. Recent work suggests that this process can be taught directly to patients without attention to the content of the thought and that this procedure appears to be as effective as the more usual approach involving the content of thoughts.

In the final phase of treatment, relapse-prevention procedures are used, often attempting to identify broad behavior patterns associated with depressive thinking and helping patients better cope with such problems. Research suggests that cognitive-behavioral therapy for depression is associated with a decreased tendency for the patient to relapse. This may be because patients are able to immediately deal with negative thinking: By considering the reality of the thought, or by the process of metacognition, one of the main triggers for relapse is dealt with in a more positive manner.

Recent research has confirmed the efficacy of cognitive-behavioral therapy for depression but has also raised questions about the necessary and sufficient conditions of therapeutic change. As summarized previously, the first phase of cognitive-behavioral therapy is primarily behavioral. The focus is on increasing behaviors that result in positive reinforcement and on reducing avoidance behaviors that deprive patients of access to reinforcing events in their natural environments. No attention is given to the content of negative thoughts or beliefs. This application of the principles of operant conditioning to the treatment of depression is known as *behavioral activation* or *functional analytic therapy*. For example, a patient might hold the belief that everyone at his or her workplace dislikes him or her. Instead of addressing the accuracy or validity of this specific belief, behavioral activation focuses on the impact or consequences of the belief that "everyone dislikes me." It is designed to teach the patient to act differently in this situation so as to increase the probability of reinforcing social interactions.

A component analysis of cognitive-behavioral therapy has shown that behavioral activation alone might be as effective as the full treatment package that additionally includes a detailed analysis of negative thoughts and core depressive beliefs. Behavioral activation appears to be as effective as the full cognitive-behavioral treatment at posttreatment and at 2-year follow-up. Consistent with this finding is other research indicating that patients show an early response to cognitive-behavioral therapy. Most of the eventual improvement produced by this treatment is evident in the early stages of therapy before an explicit focus on cognitive factors, such as core depressive beliefs.

These intriguing findings need to be replicated, but they underscore the importance of focusing on the functional consequences of behavior and call into question the need to address cognitive factors directly. It is well-documented that behavior change can lead to cognitive change. From a practical point of view, the apparent efficacy of behavioral activation is important because it may well prove to be simpler to teach and easier to learn, thereby making it more amenable to dissemination.

SUGGESTED CROSS-REFERENCES

Applications of the principles and procedures discussed in this section, together with an assessment of the effectiveness of therapeutic applications to various conditions, can be found in Section 30.2 on behavior therapy and Section 30.6 on cognitive therapy. Issues basic to learning are discussed in Chapter 1 on neural sciences and in Section 3.1 on perception and cognition. Derivations from the principles and procedures exemplified in this section are discussed in Chapter 6 on theories of personality and psychopathology that are derived from psychology and philosophy.

References

Ader R, Cohen N: CNS-immune system interactions: Conditioning phenomena. *Behav Brain Sci.* 1994;8:379.

Agras WS: Helping people improve their lives with behavior therapy. *Behav Ther.* 1997;28:375.

*Bandura A. *Principles of Behavior Modification.* New York: Holt, Rinehart & Winston; 1969.

Bandura A. *Self-efficacy: The Exercise of Control.* New York: Freeman; 1997.

Beck AT. *Cognitive Therapy of Depression: A Treatment Manual.* New York: Guilford Press; 1979.

Beck AT, Rush AJ, Shaw BF, Emery G. *Cognitive Therapy of Depression.* New York: Guilford Press; 1979.

Bovbjerg DH, Redd WH, Maier LA, Holland JC: Anticipatory immune suppression and nausea in women receiving cyclic chemotherapy for ovarian cancer. *J Consult Clin Psychol.* 1990;58:153.

Brembs B, Lorenzetti FD, Reyes FD, Baxter DA, Byrne JH: Operant reward learning in Aplysia: Neuronal correlates and mechanisms. *Science.* 2002;296:1706.

Brownell KD, Marlatt GA, Lichenstein E, Wilson GT: Understanding and preventing relapse. *Am Psychol.* 1986;41:764.

Buehner MJ, May J: Rethinking temporal contiguity and the judgement of causality: Effects of prior knowledge, experience, and reinforcement. *J Exp Psychol.* 2003;56:865.

Clark A, Hawkins RD, Kandel ER. Cell biological perspectives on learning. In: Ashury AK, McKhann M, MacDonald WH, eds. *Diseases of the Nervous System.* Philadelphia: WB Saunders; 1986.

*Clark DM, Fairburn CG. *Science and the Practice of Cognitive Behaviour Therapy.* New York: Oxford University Press; 1997.

Clark RE, Squire LR: Classical conditioning and brain systems: The role of awareness. *Science.* 1998;280:77.

Dadds MR, Salmon K: Punishment insensitivity and parenting: Temperament and learning as interacting risks for antisocial behavior. *Clin Child Fam Psychol Rev.* 2003;6:69.

Dollard J, Miller NE. *Personality and Psychotherapy.* New York: McGraw-Hill; 1950.

Havermans RC, Jansen AT: Increasing the efficacy of cue exposure treatment in preventing relapse of addictive behavior. *Addict Behav.* 2003;28:989.

Hilgard ER, Bower G. *Theories of Learning.* 4th ed. Englewood Cliffs, NJ: Prentice-Hall; 1975.

Hollon SD: What is cognitive-behavioral therapy and how does it work? *Curr Opin Neurobiol.* 1998;8:289.

Ilardi SS, Craighead WE: The role of nonspecific factors in cognitive-behavior therapy for depression. *Clin Psychol Sci Pract.* 1994;1:138–156.

Jones MB: Two early studies of learning theory and genetics. *Behav Genet.* 2003;33:669.

Kandel ER: The molecular basis of memory storage: A dialogue between genes and synapses. *Science.* 2001;294:1030.

Lidz J, Waxman S, Freedman J: What infants know about syntax but couldn't have learned: Experimental evidence for syntactic structure at 18 months. *Cognition.* 2003;89:65.

Martell CR, Addis ME, Jacobson NS. *Depression in Context: Strategies for Guided Action.* New York: Norton; 2001.

Mineka S, Davidson M, Cook M, Keir R: Observational conditioning of snake fear in rhesus monkeys. *J Abnorm Psychol.* 1984;93:335.

Mischel W, Shoda Y: A cognitive-affective theory of personality: Reconceptualizing situations, dispositions, dynamics, and invariance in personality structure. *Psychol Rev.* 1995;102:206.

Peoples LL: Will, anterior cingulate cortex, and addiction. *Science.* 2002;296:1623.

Pavlov IP. *Conditioned Reflexes.* London: Clarendon Press; 1927.

*Rauhut AS, McPhee JE, Ayres JJB: Blocked and overshadowed stimuli are weakened in their ability to serve as blockers and second-order reinforcers in Pavlovian fear conditioning. *J Exp Psychol Anim Behav Process.* 1999;25:45.

*Rescorla RA: Pavlovian conditioning. It's not what you think. *Am Psychol.* 1988;43:151.

Schwartz JM: Neuroanatomical aspects of cognitive-behavioral therapy response in obsessive-compulsive disorder: An evolving perspective on brain and behavior. *Br J Psychiatry.* 1998;173[Suppl]:38.

Segal ZV, Williams JM, Teadale JD, Gemar M: A cognitive science perspective on kindling and episodic sensitization in recurrent affective disorder. *Psychol Med.* 1996;26:371.

Seligman MEP: Phobias and preparedness. *Behav Ther.* 1971;2:107.

*Skinner BF. *Science and Human Behavior.* New York: Macmillan; 1951.

Teasdale JD, Moore RG, Hayhurst H, Pope M, Williams S, Segal ZV: Metacognitive awareness and prevention of relapse in depression: Empirical evidence. *J Consult Clin Psychol.* 2002;70:275.

Watson JB, Rayner R: Conditioned emotional reactions. *J Exp Psychol.* 1920;3:1.

▲ 3.4 Biology of Memory

Ken A. Paller, Ph.D., and Larry R. Squire, Ph.D.

The topic of memory is fundamental to the discipline of psychiatry. Memory connects the present moment to what came before and is the basis for the formation of one's life story. Personality is, in part, a set of acquired habits that have been learned, many early in life, that create dispositions and determine how people behave. In the same way, the neuroses can be products of learning—anxieties, phobias, and maladaptive behaviors that result largely from experience. Psychotherapy itself is a process by which new habits and skills are acquired through the accumulation of new experiences. In this sense, memory is at the theoretical heart of psychiatry's concern with personality, the consequences of early experience, and the possibility of growth and change.

Memory is also of clinical interest because disorders of memory and complaints about memory are common in neurological and psychiatric illness. Furthermore, memory problems occur in association with certain treatments, notably electroconvulsive therapy (ECT). Accordingly, the effective clinician needs to understand the psychological and neurological foundations of memory, the varieties of memory dysfunction, and how memory can be evaluated.

FROM SYNAPSES TO MEMORY

Memory is a special case of the general biological phenomenon of neural plasticity. Neurons can show history-dependent behavior by responding differently as a function of prior input, and this plasticity of nerve cells and synapses is the basis of memory. In the last decade of the 19th century, researchers proposed that the persistence of memory could be accounted for by nerve cell growth. This idea has been restated many times since, and it is now understood that the synapse is a critical site of change, based on experimental studies in animals with simple nervous systems. Experience leads to structural change at the synapse, including alterations in the number of synaptic contacts along specific pathways and alternations in the strength of existing contacts.

Plasticity

Neurobiological evidence supports two basic conclusions. First, short-lasting plasticity, which may last for seconds or minutes, depends on specific synaptic events, including an increase in neurotransmitter release. Second, long-lasting memory depends on new protein synthesis, physical growth of neural processes, and an increase in the number of synaptic connections.

A major source of information about memory has come from extended study of the marine mollusk *Aplysia californica.* A sufficient number of individual neurons and connections between neurons have been identified to allow the wiring diagram of some simple behaviors to be specified. *Aplysia* is capable of associative learning (including classic conditioning and operant conditioning) and nonassociative learning (habituation and sensitization). *Sensitization* had been studied using the gill-withdrawal reflex, a defensive reaction whereby tactile stimulation causes the gill and siphon to retract. When tactile stimulation is preceded by sensory stimulation to the head or tail, gill withdrawal is facilitated. The cellular changes underlying this sensitization begin when a sensory neuron activates a modulatory interneuron, which enhances the strength of synapses within the circuitry responsible for the reflex. This modulation depends on a second-messenger system whereby intracellular molecules (including cyclic adenosine monophosphate [cAMP] and cAMP-dependent protein kinase) lead to enhanced transmitter release lasting for minutes in the reflex pathway. Short- and long-lasting plasticity within this circuitry are based on enhanced transmitter release, although the long-lasting change uniquely requires the expression of genes and the synthesis of proteins. Synaptic tagging mechanisms allow gene products that are delivered throughout a neuron to increase synaptic strength selectively at recently active synapses. In addition, the long-term change, but not the short-term change, is accompanied by growth of neural processes of neurons within the reflex circuit.

In vertebrates, behavioral manipulations can also result in measurable changes in the brain's architecture. For example, rats reared in enriched environments show an increase in the number of synapses ending on individual neurons in neocortex. These changes are accompanied by small increases in cortical thickness, in the diameter of neuronal cell bodies, and in the number and length of dendritic branches. Behavioral experience thus exerts powerful effects on the wiring of the brain.

Many of these same structural changes have been found in adult rats exposed to an enriched environment, as well as in adult rats given extensive maze training. For example, increases have been observed after training in the size of dendritic fields of pyramidal neurons of occipital cortex. In this case, vision was restricted to one eye, and the corpus callosum was transected to prevent information received by one hemisphere from reaching the other hemisphere. The result was that the structural changes were observed only in the trained hemisphere. This rules out a number of nonspecific influences, including motor activity, indirect effects of hormones, and overall level of arousal. Although more direct data are needed, it seems likely that long-term memory in vertebrates is generally based on morphological growth and change.

Long-Term Potentiation The phenomenon of *long-term potentiation* (LTP) is a candidate mechanism for mammalian long-term memory. LTP is observed when a postsynaptic neuron is persistently depolarized after a brief burst of high-frequency presynaptic stimulation. LTP has a number of properties that make it suitable as a physiological substrate of memory. First, it is established quickly and then lasts for a long time. Second, it is associative in that it depends on the cooccurrence of presynaptic activity and postsynaptic depolarization. Third, it occurs only at the potentiated synapses, not at all the synapses terminating on the postsynaptic cell. Finally, LTP occurs prominently in the hippocampus, a structure with important memory functions, as described in the following discussion. The induction of LTP is known to be mediated postsynaptically and to involve activation of the *N*-methyl-D-aspartate (NMDA) receptor, which permits the influx of calcium into the postsynaptic cell. The mechanism whereby LTP is maintained is not clearly established, but evidence has been presented in favor of a presynaptic locus of change (increased transmitter release) and a postsynaptic locus of change (increased numbers of receptors).

A promising method for elucidating molecular mechanisms of memory relies on introducing specific mutations into the genome. By deleting a single gene, mice can be produced with specific receptors or cell signaling molecules inactivated or altered. For example, in mice with a selective deletion of NMDA receptors in the CA1 field of the hippocampus, many aspects of CA1 physiology remain intact, but the CA1 neurons do not exhibit LTP, and memory impairment is observed in behavioral tasks. Genetic manipulations introduced in the adult are particularly advantageous in that specific molecular changes can be induced in developmentally normal animals.

Associative Learning Additional insights into memory have come from the study of the neural circuitry underlying the *classical conditioning* of the eye blink–nictitating membrane response in rabbits. Repeated pairings of a tone (conditioned stimulus) and an air puff to the eye (unconditioned stimulus) lead to a conditioned eye blink in response to the tone. Reversible lesions of the deep nuclei of the cerebellum eliminate the conditioned response without affecting the unconditioned response. These lesions also prevent initial learning from occurring, and, when the lesion is reversed, rabbits learn normally. Thus, the cerebellum contains essential circuitry for the learned association. The relevant plasticity appears to be distributed between the cerebellar cortex and the deep nuclei. An analogous pattern of plasticity is thought to underlie motor learning in the vestibuloocular reflex and, perhaps, associative learning of motor responses in general. Based on the idea that learned motor responses depend on coordinated control of changes in timing and strength of response, it has been suggested that synaptic changes in the cerebellar cortex are critical for learned timing, whereas synaptic changes in the deep nuclei are critical for forming an association between a conditioned and an unconditioned stimulus (Fig. 3.4–1).

CORTICAL ORGANIZATION OF MEMORY

The biology of memory involves more than understanding the synaptic events that store memory. It is also essential to understand how and where synaptic events are organized in the brain. Many levels of analysis can be identified between synaptic change and behavioral memory. The rich repertoire of memory abilities that humans display results from the complex organization of networks of neurons in the brain.

One pervasive question concerns where memories are stored in the brain. In the 1920s, Karl Lashley carried out a series of experiments that were directed at this problem. Lashley recorded the number of trials that rats needed to relearn a preoperatively learned maze problem after removal of different amounts of cerebral cortex. The deficit was proportional to the amount of cortex removed, and, furthermore, it seemed to be qualitatively similar regardless of the region of cortex that was removed. Lashley concluded that memory for the maze habit was not localized in any one part of the brain but instead was distributed equivalently over the entire cortex. Subsequent work has led to a revision of this idea. Maze learning in rats depends on many forms of information, including visual, tactual, spatial, and olfactory information. These various forms of information are processed and stored in different areas. Thus, the correlation between retention score and lesion size that Lashley observed reflected the progressive encroachment of the lesion on specialized cortical areas serving the many components of cognition important to maze learning.

The specialized cortical areas responsible for processing and storing visual information have been studied most extensively in nonhuman primates. Nearly one-half of the primate neocortex is specialized for visual functions. Cortical pathways for visual information processing (Fig. 3.4–2) begin in primary visual cortex (V1) and proceed from there along parallel pathways or streams. One stream projects ventrally to inferotemporal cortex (also referred to as area TE in the monkey) and processes information about the quality of visual percepts. Another stream projects dorsally to parietal cortex and processes

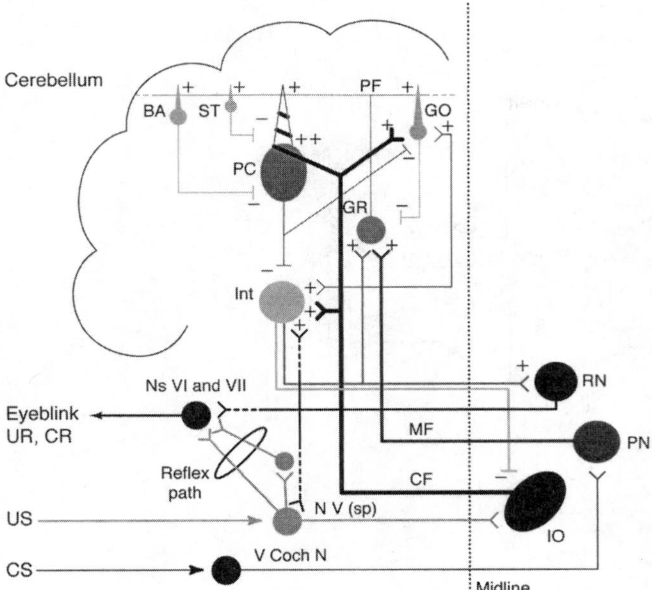

FIGURE 3.4–1 A putative circuit for classical conditioning of the eye blink reflex. The conditioned stimulus (CS) pathway consists of excitatory (+) mossy fiber (MF) projections from the pontine nuclei (PN) to the interpositus nucleus (Int) and to the cerebellar cortex. In the cortex, MFs form synapses with granule cells (GRs) that, in turn, send excitatory parallel fibers (PFs) to Purkinje cells (PCs). The PCs are the exclusive output neurons from the cortex, and they send inhibitory (–) fibers to deep nuclei, such as the Int. The unconditioned stimulus (US) pathway consists of excitatory climbing fiber (CF) projections from the inferior olive (IO) to the Int and to the PCs in the cerebellar cortex. Within the cerebellar cortex, Golgi (GO), stellate (ST), and basket (BA) cells exert inhibitory actions on their respective target neurons. The efferent conditioned response (CR) pathway projects from the Int to the red nucleus (RN) and via the descending rubra pathway to act ultimately on the eye blink reflex path. N V (sp), spinal fifth cranial nucleus; N VI, sixth cranial nucleus; N VII, seventh cranial nucleus; UR, unconditioned response; V Coch N, ventral cochlear nucleus. (From Kim JJ, Thompson RF: Cerebellar circuits and synaptic mechanisms involved in classical eye blink conditioning. *Trends Neurosci.* 1997;20:177, with permission from Elsevier.)

information about spatial location. Electrophysiological studies in the monkey show that neurons in area TE register specific and complex features of visual stimuli, such as shape, and can respond selectively to patterns and objects. Specific visual processing areas in the dorsal and ventral streams, together with areas in prefrontal cortex, register the immediate experience of perceptual processing, which has been called *immediate memory*. Immediate memory can be extended in time by attention or rehearsal to become what has been termed *working memory*. Regions of higher visual cortex also serve as the ultimate repositories of visual memories. Thus, inferotemporal lesions lead to impairments in visual perception as well as in visual learning and memory, although elementary visual functions, such as acuity, remain intact. Inferotemporal cortex can thus be thought of as a higher-order visual processing system and a storehouse of the visual memories that result from that processing.

Memory is distributed and localized in the nervous system. Memory is distributed in the sense that, as Lashley concluded, there is no single cortical center dedicated solely to the storage of memories. Yet, memory is localized in the sense that different aspects or dimensions of events are stored at specific cortical sites—the same regions that are specialized to analyze and process those particular aspects or dimensions of information.

MEMORY AND AMNESIA

The idea that the functional specialization of cortical regions determines the locus of information processing as well as the locus of information storage is important, but it does not provide a complete account of the organization of memory in the brain. If it did, then particular cortical injuries would disrupt only particular domains of learning and memory (i.e., visual memory or spatial memory). In other words, a global disruption of memory would never occur. Brain injury would always produce a difficulty in memory for a restricted type of information along with a loss of some abilities to process information of that same type. Yet, the characteristics of neurological memory impairment (*amnesia*) contradict this expectation.

The hallmark of neurological memory impairment is a profound loss of new learning ability, or *anterograde amnesia*, that extends across all sensory modalities. Typically, this occurs together with *retrograde amnesia*, a memory loss of some knowledge acquired before the onset of amnesia. The retrograde deficit often has a temporal gradient, such that memory for recent events is impaired, but memory for remote events is intact. Other cognitive functions are preserved, including linguistic abilities, attention, immediate memory, personality, and social skills.

This selectivity of the memory deficit in amnesia implies that the brain has, to some extent, separated its intellectual and perceptual functions from the capacity to lay down in memory the records that ordinarily result from intellectual and perceptual work. The fact that impaired new learning (anterograde amnesia) can occur together with intact remote memory indicates that retrieval mechanisms are intact and that the brain structures damaged in amnesia are not the ultimate repositories of memory. Detailed studies of amnesic patients and models of amnesia in nonhuman animals have illuminated these issues considerably.

Specialized Memory Function

Amnesia results from damage to either of two brain regions: the medial temporal lobe or the midline diencephalon. Seminal studies of a severely amnesic patient known as HM have stimulated intensive investigation of the role of the medial temporal lobe in memory.

H. M. became amnesic in 1953, at 27 years of age, when he sustained a bilateral resection of the medial temporal lobe to relieve severe epilepsy. The removal included approximately one-half of the hippocampus, most of the amygdala, and the neighboring entorhinal and perirhinal cortices (Fig. 3.4–3). After the surgery, H. M.'s seizure condition was much improved, but he experienced profound forgetfulness. Yet, his intellectual functions were generally preserved. For example, H. M. exhibited normal immediate memory, and he could maintain his attention during conversation. After an interruption, however, it would become clear that H. M. could not remember what had recently transpired. In H. M.'s words, he felt as if he were just waking from a dream, because he had no recollection of what had just occurred. This memory deficit has persisted for more than 40 years.

Findings from human amnesia stimulated the development of models of amnesia in experimental animals. For example, many parallels have been demonstrated between human amnesia and memory impairment in monkeys with surgical damage to anatomical components of the medial temporal lobe, and cumulative work with the monkey eventually identified the crucial structures and connections within the medial temporal lobe that are important for memory.

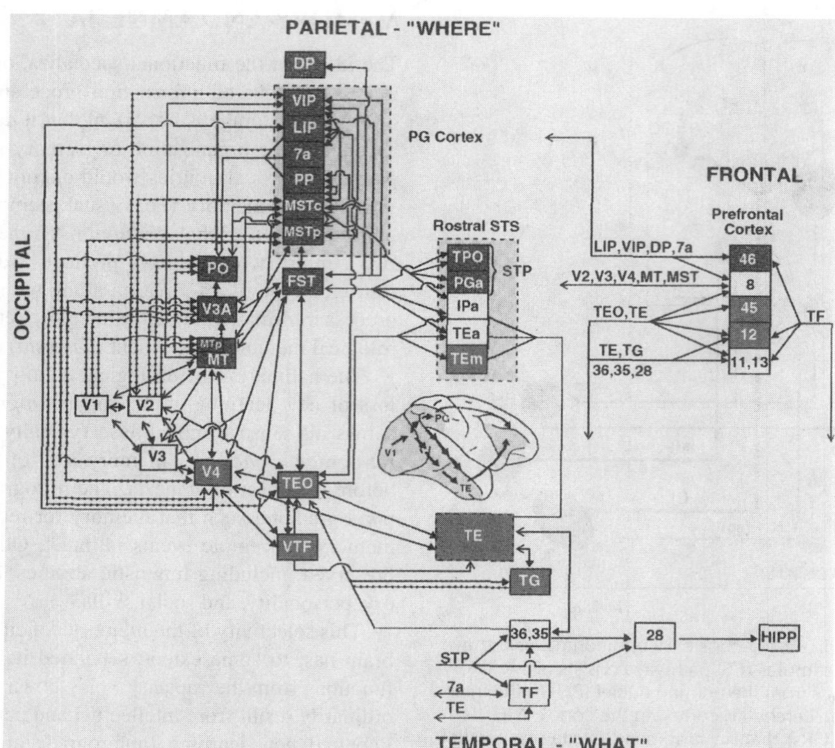

FIGURE 3.4–2 Summary of cortical visual areas and some of their connections. There are two major pathways from striate cortex (primary visual cortex [V1]). The processing stream for object vision follows a ventral route into the temporal lobe, and the processing stream for spatial vision follows a dorsal route into the parietal lobe. Solid lines indicate connections arising from central and peripheral visual field representations; dotted lines indicate connection restricted to peripheral field representations. The shaded region on the lateral view of the brain represents the extent of the cortex included in the diagram. The inferior temporal areas are identified by *TEO* and *TE*, the parahippocampal area by *TF*, temporal pole area by *TG*, and the inferior parietal area by *PG* from Von Bonin and Bailey. The perirhinal areas are identified by *35* and *36*, the entorhinal area by *28*, the inferior parietal area by *7a*, and the prefrontal areas by *8, 11, 12, 13, 45*, and *46* from Brodmann. The rostral superior temporal sulcal (STS) areas are identified by *TPO, PGa, STP, IPa, TEa*, and *TEm* from Seltzer and Pandya. DP, dorsal prelunate area; FST, fundus of superior temporal area; HIPP, hippocampus; LIP, lateral intraparietal area; MSTc, medial superior temporal area, central visual field representation; MSTp, medial superior temporal area, peripheral visual field representation; MT, middle temporal area; MTp, middle temporal area, peripheral visual field representation; PO, parietooccipital area; PP, posterior parietal sulcal zone; STP, superior temporal polysensory area; V2, visual area 2; V3, visual area 3; V3A, visual area 3 part A; V4, visual area 4; VIP, ventral intraparietal area; VTF, visual responsive portion of TF. (From Ungerleider LG: Functional brain imaging studies of cortical mechanisms for memory. *Science.* 1995;270:769, with permission.)

These include the hippocampus proper (CA fields, dentate gyrus, and subiculum) and the adjacent entorhinal, perirhinal, and parahippocampal cortices.

Another important structure within the medial temporal lobe is the amygdala. In 1937, Heinrich Kluver and Paul Bucy showed that monkeys with bilateral temporal lobectomy became tame, approached animals and objects without reluctance, examined objects by mouth instead of by hand, and exhibited abnormal sexual behavior. Subsequent studies indicated that much of emotional behavior is normally regulated by the amygdala. The storage of emotional events engages the amygdala. Moreover, the fact that humans remember emotional, arousing events better than neutral events depends on the modulatory effect of the amygdala. In the rodent, a considerable amount has been learned about the amygdala by studying the neural circuitry for fear conditioning.

Detailed investigations of amnesic patients continue to shed light on the nature of memory. One series of informative studies has described the memory impairment of patient E.P.

E. P. was diagnosed with herpes simplex encephalitis at 72 years of age. Damage to the medial temporal region (Fig. 3.4–3) produced a persistent and profound amnesia. During testing sessions, E. P. is cordial and talks about his experiences, but relies exclusively on stories from his childhood and early adulthood. He often repeats the same story multiple times. Strikingly, his performance on tests of recognition memory is no better than would be produced by guessing (Fig. 3.4–4A). Tests involving facts about his life and autobiographical experiences (Fig. 3.4–4B) revealed poor memory for the recent time period since his illness, reduced memory for his adult years, and normal memory for his childhood. E. P. also has good spatial knowledge about the town in which he lived as a child, but he has been unable to learn the layout of the neighborhood to which he moved after he became amnesic (Fig. 3.4–4C). Given the severity of E. P.'s memory problems, it has been particularly informative that E. P. performs normally on certain kinds of memory tests (examples of which are described in the following discussion).

In another patient, R. B., an episode of global ischemia after cardiac surgery led to moderately severe anterograde amnesia and minimal retrograde amnesia, less severe than in patients H. M. and E. P. After his death 5 years later, detailed histological study of his brain revealed a circumscribed bilateral lesion of hippocampal field CA1. Similar histological evidence of hippocampal damage has also been obtained in other patients with amnesia due to ischemia or other causes (Fig. 3.4–5).

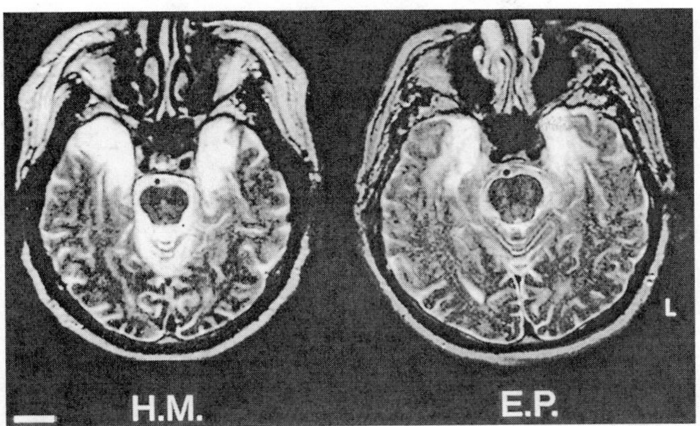

FIGURE 3.4–3 Structural magnetic resonance images of the brains of patients H. M. and E. P. through the level of the temporal lobe. Damaged tissue is indicated by bright signal in these T2-weighted axial images. Both patients sustained extensive damage to medial temporal structures, as the result of surgery for epilepsy in H. M., and as the result of viral encephalitis in E. P. Scale bar: 2 cm. L, left side of the brain. (From Corkin S, Amaral EG, Gonzalez RG, et al.: H. M.'s medial temporal lobe lesion: Findings from magnetic resonance imaging. *J Neurosci.* 1997;17:3964; and Stefanacci L, Buffalo EA, Schmolck H, Squire LR: Profound amnesia after damage to the medial temporal lobe: A neuroanatomical and neuropsychological profile of patient E. P. *J Neurosci.* 2000;20:7024.)

Hippocampal pathology in patients with amnesia has also been revealed using high-resolution magnetic resonance imaging (MRI). Several conclusions about the anatomy of amnesia follow from these studies. First, damage limited to the hippocampus results in a clinically significant memory impairment. Furthermore, several regions of the medial temporal lobe in addition to hippocampal field CA1 also make a critical contribution to memory. Whereas the memory impairment associated with CA1 is only moderately severe, medial temporal damage that includes the hippocampus as well as adjacent cortex (as in patients H. M. and E. P.) results in a severe and disabling memory impairment. Memory impairment and medial temporal lobe damage are also typically observed in early Alzheimer's disease, although the pathology eventually affects many cortical regions as well and produces corresponding cognitive deficits in addition to amnesia.

Amnesia can also result from damage to structures of the medial diencephalon. Which structures are important in diencephalic amnesia is not fully understood, but critical regions likely include the mammillary nuclei, the dorsomedial nucleus of the thalamus, the anterior nucleus, the internal medullary lamina, and the mammillothalamic tract. *Korsakoff's syndrome* is the best-studied example of diencephalic amnesia. Patients with alcoholic Korsakoff's syndrome typically have frontal lobe pathology in addition to diencephalic damage. Thus, in these patients, memory impairment occurs together with signs of frontal lobe dysfunction (Table 3.4–1).

One complication in identifying the anatomy of memory impairment is that structural brain damage in one region may lead indirectly to disrupted functioning in other regions. Therefore, functional neuroimaging, in addition to structural data from neuroimaging or postmortem histology, can be useful for characterizing the neural dysfunction responsible for amnesia. In Korsakoff's syndrome, for example, positron emission tomography (PET) has revealed functional changes in widespread cortical regions. Accordingly, amnesia after diencephalic damage may result indirectly from disrupted thalamocortical connections that are critical for memory storage. In summary, memory depends on the integrity of medial temporal and diencephalic brain areas, which work in concert with widespread areas of neocortex to form and to store memory (Fig. 3.4–6).

Retrograde Amnesia Memory loss in amnesia typically affects recent memories more than remote memories (Fig. 3.4–7). Temporally graded amnesia has been demonstrated retrospectively in studies of amnesic patients and prospectively in studies of monkeys, rats, mice, and rabbits. These findings have important implications for understanding the nature of the memory storage process. Memories are dynamic not static. As time passes after learning, some memories are forgotten, whereas others become stronger due to a process of *consolidation* that depends on cortical, medial temporal, and diencephalic structures. The contribution of these medial temporal and diencephalic regions diminishes over time after initial encoding, such that the neocortex ultimately can support memory storage on its own. Medial temporal and diencephalic structures are critical at the time of learning and during this gradual consolidation process. Thus, distributed neocortical regions are the permanent repositories of enduring memories.

Other (atypical) patterns of memory impairment can also be observed. For example, patients have been described with substantial retrograde memory impairments together with only moderately impaired new learning ability, a pattern termed *focal retrograde amnesia.* Focal retrograde amnesia can result from damage to anterolateral temporal lobes, regions thought to be important for long-term memory storage. Some capacity for new learning remains, presumably because medial temporal lobe structures are able to communicate with undamaged areas of lateral temporal cortex.

MULTIPLE TYPES OF MEMORY

Memory is not a single faculty of the mind but is composed of several types that depend on different brain systems. Amnesia affects only one kind of memory, which is termed *declarative memory.* Declarative memory is what is ordinarily meant by the term *memory* in everyday language. Declarative memory supports the conscious recollection of facts and events, and impaired declarative memory (that is, amnesia) presents itself as a memory impairment for routes, lists, faces, melodies, objects, and other verbal and nonverbal material, regardless of the sensory modality in which the material is presented. Despite this broad impairment, a number of memory abilities are preserved. This heterogeneous set of preserved abilities is collectively termed *nondeclarative memory.* Nondeclarative memory includes skill learning, habit learning, simple forms of conditioning, and the phenomenon of priming. For these types of learning and memory, amnesic patients can perform normally. Thus, a variety of skills, including perceptual, perceptuomotor, and cognitive skills, can be acquired by amnesic patients and healthy individuals at equivalent rates. For example, amnesic patients can learn to read mirror-reversed text normally, they exhibit the normal facilitation in reading speed with successive readings of normal prose, and they improve as rapidly as healthy individuals at speeded reading of repeating nonwords. In addition, amnesic patients can, after seeing strings of letters generated by a finite-state rule system, classify novel strings of letters as rule-based or not rule-based. Classification performance is normal despite the fact that amnesic patients are impaired at remembering the events of training or the specific items they have studied. Amnesic patients can also learn about categories by abstracting prototype information, even though they cannot recognize the specific examples from which their knowledge of the category was built.

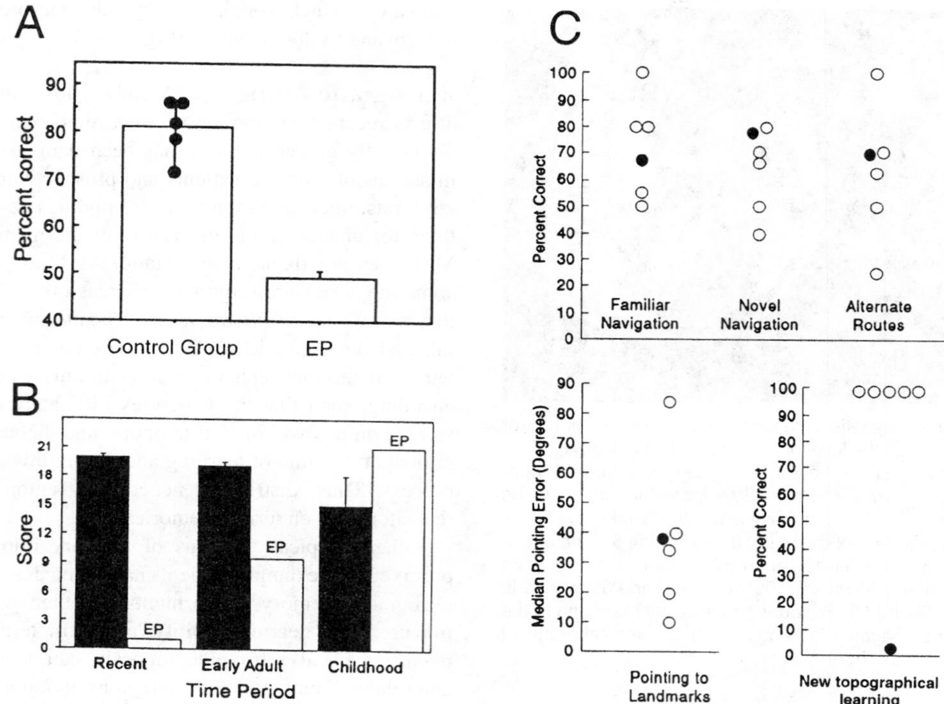

FIGURE 3.4–4 Formal test results from patient E. P. show severe anterograde and retrograde deficits, with intact remote memory. **A:** Scores were combined from 42 different tests of recognition memory for words given to patient E. P. and a group of five healthy control subjects. Some of the tests were two-alternative forced choice, and some were yes–no recognition. Brackets for E. P. indicate standard error of the mean. Data points for the control group indicate each participant's mean score across all 42 recognition memory tests. E. P.'s average performance (49.3 percent correct) was not different from chance and was approximately five standard deviations (SDs) below the average performance of control subjects (81.1 percent correct; SD, 6.3). **B:** Autobiographical remembering was quantified by using a structured interview known as the *Autobiographical Memory Interview.* Items assessed personal semantic knowledge (maximum score: 21 for each time period). Performance for the recent time period reflects poor memory for information that could have been acquired only subsequent to the onset of his amnesia. For E. P., performance for the early adult period reflects retrograde memory deficits. Performance for the childhood period reflects good remote memory. Similar results for semantic and episodic remembering were obtained from these time periods. (Data from Kopelman MD, Wilson BA, Baddeley AD: The autobiographical memory interview: A new assessment of autobiographical and personal semantic memory in amnesic patients. *J Clin Exp Neuropsychol.* 1989;5:724 and Reed JM, Squire LR: Retrograde amnesia for facts and events: Findings from four new cases. *J Neurosci.* 1998;18:3943). **C:** Assessments of spatial memory demonstrated E. P.'s good memory for spatial knowledge from his childhood along with extremely poor new learning of spatial information. Performance was compared to that of five individuals (*empty circles*) who attended E. P.'s high school at the same time as he did, lived in the region over approximately the same time period, and, like E. P. (*filled circle*), moved away as young adults. Normal performance was found for navigating from home to different locations in the area (familiar navigation), between different locations in the area (novel navigation), and between these same locations when a main street was blocked (alternative routes). Subjects were also asked to point to particular locations while imagining themselves in a particular location (pointing to landmarks), or they were asked about locations in the neighborhoods in which they currently lived (new topographical learning). E. P. showed difficulty only in this last test, because he moved to his current residence after he became amnesic. (Data from Teng E, Squire LR: Memory for places learned long ago is intact after hippocampal damage. *Nature.* 1999;400:675.) (Adapted from Stefanacci L, Buffalo EA, Schmolck H, Squire LR: Profound amnesia after damage to the medial temporal lobe: A neuroanatomical and neuropsychological profile of patient E. P. *J Neurosci.* 2000;20:7024.)

Priming *Priming* refers to a facilitation of the ability to detect or to identify a particular stimulus based on recent experience with the same stimulus. Priming is intact in amnesia. In one test, patients named pictures of previously presented objects reliably faster than they named pictures of new objects, even after a delay of a week. This facilitation occurred at normal levels, despite the fact that the patients were markedly impaired at recognizing which pictures had been presented previously. A striking example of preserved priming comes from studies of patient E. P. (Fig. 3.4–8), who exhibited intact priming for words but performed at chance levels when asked to recognize which words had been presented for study. This form of memory, termed *perceptual priming*, is thus a distinct class of memory that is independent of the medial temporal regions typically damaged in amnesia.

Memory Systems One organizational scheme for the multiple types of memory appears in Figure 3.4–9. Declarative memory depends on medial temporal and midline diencephalic structures along with extensive portions of the neocortex. This system provides for the rapid learning of facts (*semantic memory*) and events (*episodic memory*). Nondeclarative memory depends on several different brain systems. Habits likely depend on the neocortex and the neostriatum, the cerebellum is important for conditioning of skeletal musculature, the amygdala for emotional learning, and the neocortex for priming. Declarative and nondeclarative memory differ in important ways. Declarative memory is phylogenetically more recent than nondeclarative memory. In addition, declarative memories are available to conscious recollection. The flexibility of declarative memory permits the retrieved information to be available to multiple response systems.

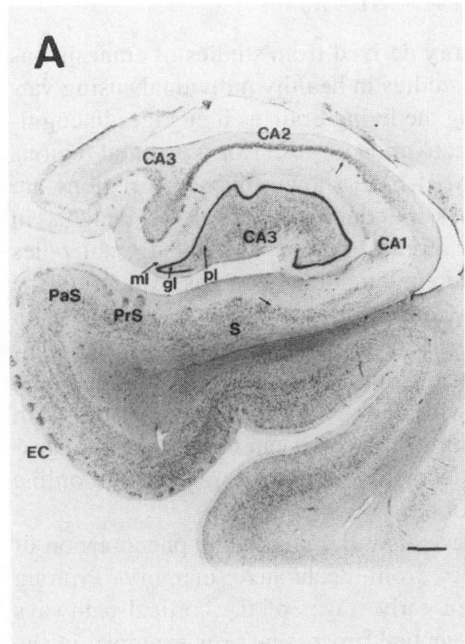

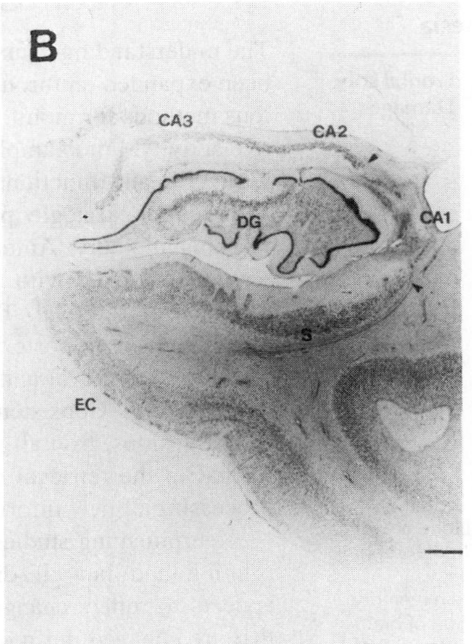

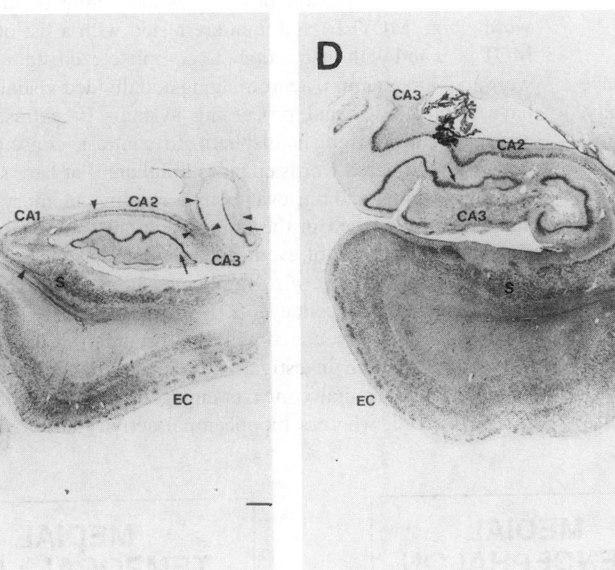

FIGURE 3.4–5 Coronal sections through the hippocampal region stained with thionin in a healthy individual **(A)** and three amnesic patients with bilateral damage to the hippocampal formation, patients G. D., L. M., and W. H. **(B–D)**. The hippocampus proper can be divided into three distinct fields, designated *CA1, CA2,* and *CA3*. The CA1 field extends to the subiculum (S). Other structures include the dentate gyrus (DG), presubiculum (PrS), parasubiculum (PaS), and entorhinal cortex (EC). In **B**, damage included CA1, marked by arrowheads. In **C**, damage included CA1, CA2, CA3, DG, and EC. Arrowheads indicate the borders of the CA fields. Arrows indicate loss of polymorphic cells in DG. In **D**, damage included CA1, CA2, CA3, DG, S, and EC. Arrow indicates abnormal dispersion of granule cells. gl, granular layer; ml, molecular layer; pl, polymorphic layer. (For additional details, see Rempel-Clower N, Zola SM, Squire LR, Amaral DG: Three cases of enduring memory impairment following bilateral damage limited to the hippocampal formation. *J Neurosci.* 1996;16:5233.) (From Squire LR, Zola SM. Memory, memory impairment, and the medial temporal lobe. In: *Cold Spring Harbor Symposia on Quantitative Biology.* Vol LXI. Plainview, NY: Cold Spring Harbor Laboratory Press; 1996:185.)

Nondeclarative memory is inaccessible to awareness and tends to be inflexible, as it is expressed only by engaging specific processing systems. Nondeclarative memories are stored as changes within these processing systems, changes that are encapsulated such that the stored information has limited accessibility to other processing systems.

General knowledge of the world (semantic memory) has often been categorized as a separate form of memory, because facts that are committed to memory typically become independent of the original episodes in which the facts were learned. Although memory for facts is a form of declarative memory, it has been proposed that amnesic patients might be able to adopt special strategies to succeed at learning facts. This possibility was examined in a recent study of patient E. P., who has no detectable capacity for declarative memory. He was given training over the course of 12 weeks to learn novel factual information in the form of three-word sentences (e.g., shark killed octopus). Opportunities to make recall errors were strictly limited during training, because such errors tend to lower performance in patients with memory impairments. Some learning occurred, but it was exceedingly gradual, rigidly organized, unavailable as conscious knowledge, and much weaker than the learning demonstrated in healthy individuals after even less training. Indeed, E. P. did not acquire knowledge in the ordinary sense of the term, but appeared to use nondeclarative memory to change his performance. One possibility is that E. P.'s learning depended on a process akin to perceptual learning that occurs in neocortex. In those cases when patients can acquire factual information as consciously accessible declarative knowledge, the structures that remain intact within the medial temporal lobe presumably support learning. In contrast, when factual information is acquired as nondeclarative knowledge, as in the case of E. P., the learning likely occurs directly within the neocortex.

Frontal Contributions to Memory Although amnesia does not occur after limited frontal damage, the frontal lobes are fundamentally important for declarative memory. Patients with frontal lesions have poor memory for the context in which information was

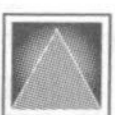

Table 3.4–1
Associated and Dissociated Deficits in Amnesia

Test	Amnesia	Korsakoff's Syndrome	Frontal Lobe Damage
Delayed recall	+	+	–
Dementia rating scale: memory index	+	+	–
Dementia rating scale: initiation and perseveration index	–	+	+
Wisconsin Card Sorting Test	–	+	+
Temporal order memory	+	++	++
Metamemory	–	+	+
Release from proactive interference	–	+	–

Note: Pattern of cognitive impairment associated with amnesia (e.g., after medial temporal lobe damage), Korsakoff's syndrome, and frontal lobe pathology without amnesia. Korsakoff's syndrome is associated with both diencephalic lesions (which produce amnesia) and with frontal lobe pathology.
+, deficit; –, no deficit; ++, disproportionately impaired relative to item memory.
From Squire LR, Zola-Morgan S, Cave CB, et al.: Memory, organization of brain systems and cognition. In: *Cold Spring Harbor Symposia on Quantitative Biology.* Vol LV. Plainview, NY: Cold Spring Harbor Laboratory Press; 1990.

acquired, they have difficulty in free recall, and they may even have some mild difficulty on tests of item recognition. More generally, frontal patients have difficulty implementing memory retrieval strategies and evaluating and monitoring their memory performance.

Patient B. G. suffered an infarction restricted to the right frontal lobe, resulting in substantial false remembering. He had an abnormal tendency to claim that some stimuli were familiar, even though they had not been presented for study. His false responses probably arose because he relied on a general feeling of familiarity for the kind of stimuli that had been presented, rather than on specific memories for the stimuli.

NEUROIMAGING AND MEMORY

The understanding of memory derived from studies of amnesia has been expanded on through studies in healthy individuals using various methods for monitoring the living brain as it engages in cognitive activity. For example, activation of posterior prefrontal regions with PET and functional MRI have shown that these regions are involved in strategic processing during retrieval, as well as in working memory. Anterior frontal regions near the frontal poles have been linked with different functions, such as evaluating the products of retrieval. The frontal lobes function in concert with connections with posterior neocortical regions to support the organization of retrieval and the manipulation of information in working memory. Consistent with the evidence from patients with frontal lesions, frontal-posterior networks can be viewed as instrumental in the retrieval of declarative memories and in the online processing of new information.

Neuroimaging studies have also illuminated the phenomenon of priming and how it differs from declarative memory. Priming appears to reflect changes in early stages of the cortical pathways that are engaged during perceptual processing. For example, in the case of stem-completion priming, where subjects study a list of words (e.g., MOTEL) and then are tested with a list of stems (e.g., MOT___) and with instructions to complete each stem with the first word to come to mind, neuroimaging and divided visual-field studies have implicated visual processing systems in extrastriate cortex, especially in the right hemisphere. In contrast, conscious recollection of remembered words engages brain areas at later stages of processing. Priming and retrieval from declarative memory retrieval can also be distinguished in the brain electrical activity recorded from the scalp in the form of event-related potentials (Fig. 3.4–10). Neuroimaging results have also implicated hippocampal processing in the recollection of recent events (Fig. 3.4–11).

Brain activity associated with the formation of declarative memories has also been investigated with neuroimaging. For example, left inferior prefrontal cortex is engaged as a result of attempts to encode a word, whereas hippocampal activity at encoding is more

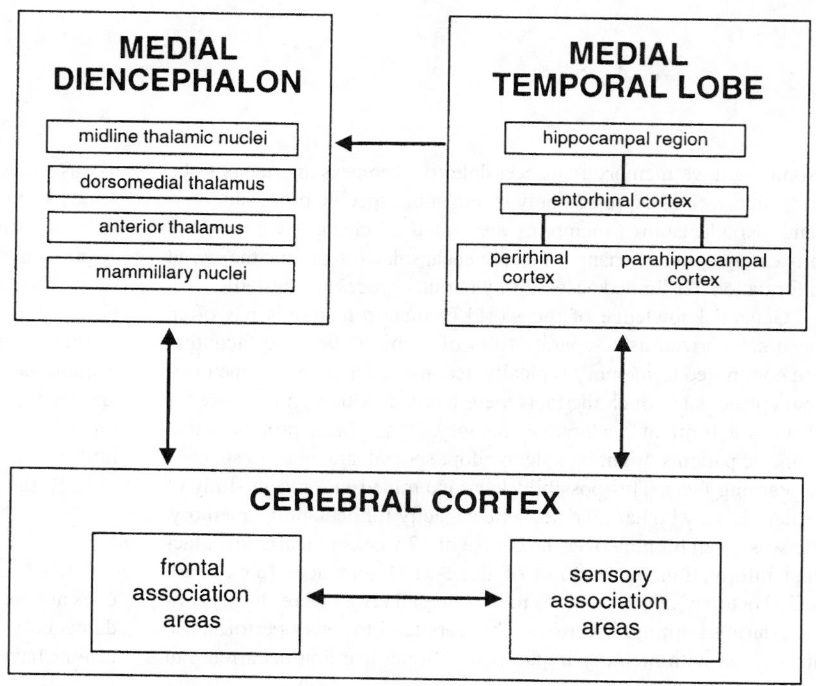

FIGURE 3.4–6 A schematic view of brain regions thought to be critical for the formation and storage of declarative memory. The entorhinal cortex is the major source of projections to the hippocampus, and nearly two-thirds of the cortical input to the entorhinal cortex originates in the perirhinal and parahippocampal cortex. The entorhinal cortex also receives direct connections from the cingulate, insula, orbitofrontal, and superior temporal cortices.

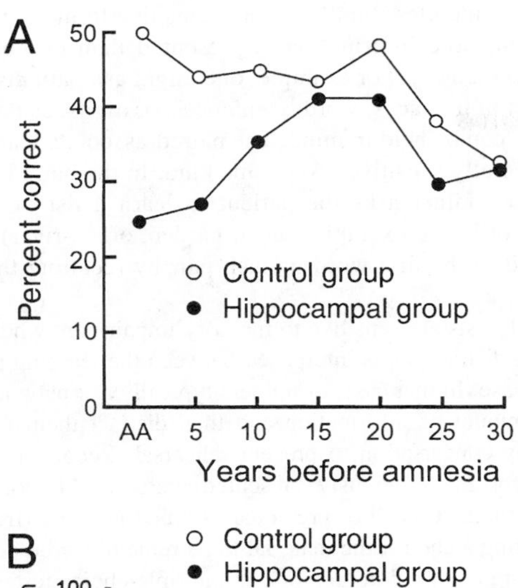

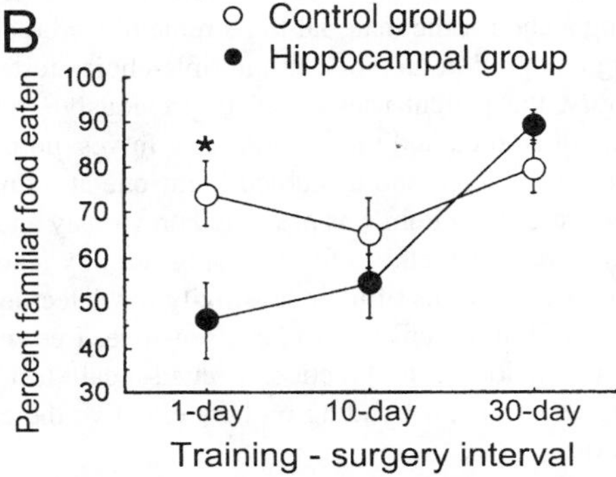

FIGURE 3.4–7 **A:** Temporally limited retrograde amnesia for free recall of 251 news events. Scores were aligned relative to the onset of amnesia in patients (N = 6) and to a corresponding time point in age- and education-matched healthy individuals (N = 12). The time period after the onset of amnesia is labeled *AA* (anterograde amnesia) to designate that this time point assessed memory for events that occurred after the onset of amnesia. Standard errors ranged from 2 to 10 percent. Brain damage in the patient group was limited primarily to the hippocampal region. **B:** Temporally limited retrograde amnesia in rats with lesions of hippocampus and subiculum. Rats learned to prefer an odorous food as the result of an encounter with another rat with that odor on its breath. Percent preference for the familiar food was observed for three training-surgery intervals. At 1 day after learning, the control group performed significantly better than the rats with lesions ($P < .05$). At 30 days, the two groups performed similarly, and both groups performed well above chance. Error bars show standard errors of the mean. (Adapted from Manns JR, Hopkins RO, Squire LR. Semantic memory and the human hippocampus. *Neuron.* 2003;38:127; and Clark RE, Broadbent NJ, Zola SM, Squire LR: Anterograde amnesia and temporally graded retrograde amnesia for a nonspatial memory task after lesions of hippocampus and subiculum. *J Neurosci.* 2002;22:4663.)

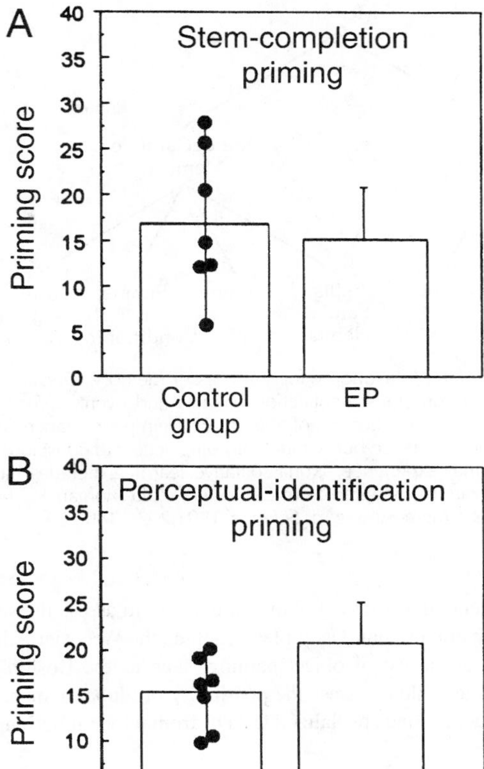

FIGURE 3.4–8 Preserved priming in patient E. P. relative to seven control subjects. **A:** Stem-completion priming on six separate tests. Priming reflected a tendency for subjects to complete three-letter stems with previously encountered words when they were instructed to produce the first word to come to mind (e.g., MOT___ completed to form MOTEL). Priming scores were calculated as percent correct for studied words minus percent correct for baseline words (guessing). **B:** Perceptual-identification priming on 12 separate tests. Subjects attempted to read 48 words that were visually degraded. Priming scores were calculated as percent correct identification of previously studied words minus percent correct identification of nonstudied words. Brackets indicate standard error of the mean. (Data from Hamann SB, Squire LR: Intact perceptual memory in the absence of conscious memory. *Behav Neurosci.* 1997;111:850.) (From Stefanacci L, Buffalo EA, Schmolck H, Squire LR: Profound amnesia after damage to the medial temporal lobe: A neuroanatomical and neuropsychological profile of patient E. P. *J Neurosci.* 2000;20:7024.)

closely associated with whether encoding leads to a stable memory that can later be retrieved (Fig. 3.4–12). These findings confirm and extend the idea that medial temporal and frontal regions are important for memory storage but that they make different contributions.

ASSESSMENT OF MEMORY FUNCTIONS

A variety of quantitative methods are available to assess memory functions in neurological and psychiatric patients. Quantitative methods are useful for evaluating and following patients longitudinally as well as for carrying out a one-time examination to determine the status of memory function. It is desirable to obtain information about the severity of memory dysfunction, as well as to determine whether memory is selectively affected or whether memory problems are occurring, as they often do, against a background of additional intellectual deficits. The following section presents a rationale for evaluating memory and identifies areas of memory function that should be evaluated in any comprehensive assessment. Although some widely available tests, such as the Wechsler Memory Scale, provide useful measures of memory, most single tests assess memory rather narrowly. Even general-purpose neuropsychological batteries provide for only limited testing of memory functions. A complete assessment of memory usually involves a number of specialized tests that sample intellectual functions, new learning capacity, remote memory, and memory self-report.

The assessment of general intellectual functions is fundamental to any neuropsychological examination. In the case of memory testing, information about intellectual functions provides information about a

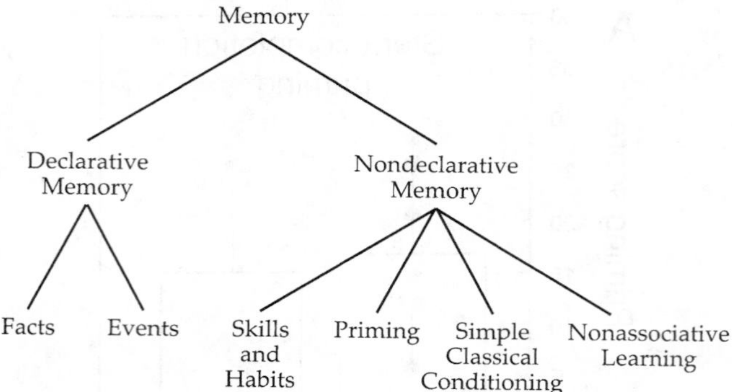

FIGURE 3.4–9 A taxonomy for subtypes of memory. *Declarative memory* refers to conscious recollection of facts and events. *Nondeclarative memory* refers to a collection of abilities wherein performance changes as the result of experience but without affording access to conscious memory of the original experience. Nonassociative learning includes habituation and sensitization. (Adapted from Squire LR, Zola-Morgan S: The medial temporal lobe memory system. *Science.* 1991;253:1380.)

patient's general test-taking ability and a way to assess the selectivity of memory impairment. Useful tests include the Wechsler Adult Intelligence Scale; a test of object naming, such as the Boston Naming Test; a rating scale to assess the possibility of global dementia; a test of word fluency; and specialized tests of frontal lobe function.

New Learning Capacity Memory tests are sensitive to impaired new learning ability when they adhere to either of two important principles. First, tests are sensitive to memory impairment when more information is presented than can be held in immediate memory. For example, one might ask patients to memorize a list of ten faces, words, sentences, or digits, as ten items is more than can be held in mind. The paired-associate learning task is an especially sensitive test of this kind. In the paired-associate task, the examiner asks the patient to learn a list of unrelated pairs of words (for example, queen-garden, office-river) and then to respond to the first word in each pair by recalling the second word.

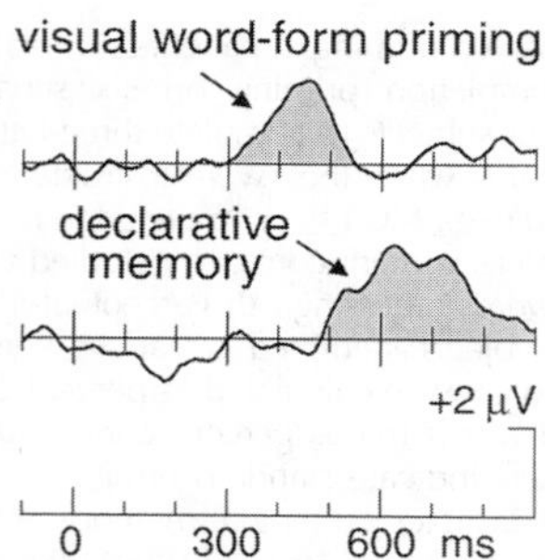

FIGURE 3.4–10 Brain potentials specifically associated with priming and declarative memory. The upper waveform was computed by subtracting brain potentials elicited by words grouped separately according to whether the word was printed forward or backward when the same word was viewed approximately 22 seconds earlier. Priming was greater in the former compared to the latter condition, although recognition scores were similar. The different waveform thus isolated differential priming-related processing and provided an electrophysiological correlate of visual word-form priming. The lower waveform was computed by subtracting brain potentials elicited by words previously studied deeply (using visual imagery) versus words that were studied only shallowly (by focusing on the syllables that made up the word). Recollection was stronger in the former compared to the latter condition, but priming did not differ. This different waveform thus isolated an electrophysiological correlate of recollecting declarative memories for the previously presented words. (Data from Paller KA, Gross M: Brain potentials associated with perceptual priming versus explicit remembering during the repetition of visual word-form. *Neuropsychologia.* 1988;36:559; and Paller KA, Kutas M, McIsaac HK: Monitoring conscious recollection via the electrical activity of the brain. *Psychol Sci.* 1995;6:107. From Paller KA. Cross-cortical consolidation as the core defect in amnesia: Prospects for hypothesis-testing with neuropsychology and neuroimaging. In: Squire LR, Schacter DL, eds. *The Neuropsychology of Memory.* 3rd ed. New York: Guilford Press; 2002:73–87, with permission.)

Second, tests are sensitive to memory impairment when a delay, filled with distraction, is interposed between the learning phase and the test phase. In that case, examiners typically ask patients to learn a small amount of information and then distract them for several minutes by conversation to prevent rehearsal. Recollection is then assessed for the previously presented material. Memory can be tested by unaided recall of previously studied material (free recall), by presenting a cue for the material to be remembered (cued recall), or by testing recognition memory. In multiple-choice tests of recognition memory, the patient tries to select previously studied items from a group of studied and unstudied items. In yes–no recognition tests, patients see studied and unstudied items one at a time and are asked to say "yes" if the item was presented previously and "no" if it was not. These various methods for assessing recently learned material can be ranked in terms of their sensitivity for detecting memory impairment (from most sensitive to least sensitive: free recall, cued recall, and recognition). In practice, a cued-recall test can vary widely in its sensitivity, depending on how effective the cues are at aiding retrieval.

The specialization of function of the two cerebral hemispheres in humans means that left and right unilateral damage is associated with different kinds of memory problems. Accordingly, different kinds of memory tests must be used when unilateral damage is a possibility. Damage to medial temporal or diencephalic structures in the left cerebral hemisphere causes difficulty remembering verbal material, such as word lists and stories. Damage to medial temporal or diencephalic structures in the right cerebral hemisphere impairs memory for faces, spatial layouts, and other nonverbal material that is typically encoded without verbal labels. For example, left medial temporal lobe damage impairs memory for spoken and written text. Right medial temporal lobe damage impairs the learning of spatial arrays, whether the layouts are examined visually or by touch. A useful way to test for memory for nonverbal material is to ask a patient to copy a complex geometric figure and then, without forewarning, to reproduce it after a delay of several minutes.

Remote Memory Disorders of memory are frequently accompanied by *retrograde amnesia*, that is, memory loss for events that occurred before the amnesia began. Evaluations of retrograde memory loss should attempt to determine the severity of the loss and the time period that it covers. Most quantitative tests of remote memory are composed of material in the public domain that can be corroborated. For example, tests have involved questions about former one-season television programs, news events, or photographs of famous persons. An advantage of these methods is that one can sample large numbers of events and can often target particular time periods. A disadvantage is that these tests are not so useful for detecting memory loss for information learned during the weeks or months immediately before the onset of amnesia. Most remote memory tests sample time periods rather coarsely and cannot detect a retrograde memory impairment that covers only a few months.

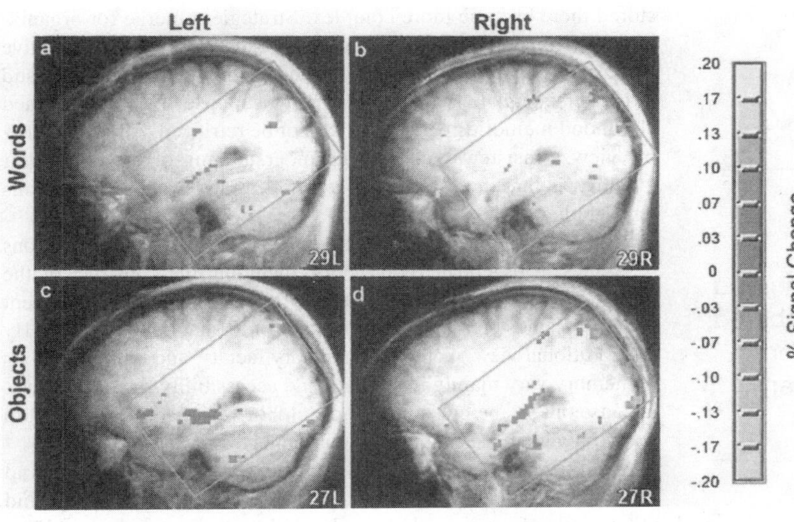

FIGURE 3.4–11 Activity in the left and right hippocampal regions measured with functional magnetic resonance imaging (fMRI) during declarative memory retrieval. Data were collected from 11 participants who saw words at study and test and from 11 different participants who saw pictures of namable objects at study and test. Recognition memory accuracy was 80.2 percent correct for words and 89.9 percent correct for objects. Areas of significant fMRI signal change (targets vs. foils) are shown in sagittal sections as color overlays on averaged structural images. The green box indicates the area in which reliable data were available for all subjects. With words, retrieval-related activity was observed in the hippocampus on the left side **(a)** but not on the right side **(b)**. With namable objects, retrieval-related activity was observed in the hippocampus on the left side **(c)** and the right side **(d)**. (See Color Plate.) [From Stark CE, Squire LR: Functional magnetic resonance imaging (fMRI) activity in the hippocampal region during recognition memory. *J Neurosci.* 2000;20:7776.]

In contrast, autobiographical memory tests can potentially provide fine-grained information about a patient's retrograde memory. In the word-probe task, first used by Francis Galton in 1879, patients are asked to recollect specific episodes from their past in response to single word cues (for example, bird and ticket) and to date the episodes. When normal subjects take the test, the number of episodes recalled is lawfully related to the time period from which the episode is taken. Most of the memories come from recent time periods (the past one or two months). Patients with amnesia often exhibit temporally graded retrograde amnesia, drawing few episodic memories from the recent past, but producing as many remote autobiographical memories as normal subjects.

Memory Self-Reports

Patients can often supply descriptions of their memory problems that are extremely useful for understanding the nature of their impairment. Tests of the ability to judge one's own memory abilities are called tests of *metamemory*. Self-rating scales are available that yield quantitative and qualitative information about memory impairment. As a result, it is possible to distinguish memory complaints associated with depression from memory complaints associated with amnesia. Depressed patients tend to rate their memory as poor in a rather undifferentiated way, endorsing equally all the items on a self-rating form. By contrast, amnesic patients tend to endorse some items more than others; that is, there is a pattern to their memory complaints. Amnesic patients do not report difficulty in remembering very remote events or in following what is being said to them, but they do report having difficulty remembering an event a few minutes after it happens. Indeed, self-reports can match rather closely the description of memory dysfunction that emerges from objective tests. Specifically, new learning capacity is affected, immediate memory is intact, and very remote memory is intact. Some amnesic patients, however, tend to markedly underestimate their memory impairment. In patients with Korsakoff's syndrome, for example, poor metamemory may stem from their frontal lobe dysfunction. In any case, querying patients in some detail about their own sense of impairment and administering self-rating scales are valuable and informative adjuncts to more formal memory testing.

Psychogenic Amnesia

Differentiating psychogenic (or dissociative) amnesia from a memory disorder that results from neurological injury or disease is often straightforward, given that the two kinds of amnesia have markedly different characteristics. Psychogenic amnesias typically do not affect new learning capacity. Patients enter the hospital able to record a continuing procession of daily events. By contrast, new learning problems tend to be at the core of neurological amnesia. The main positive symptom in psychogenic amnesia is extensive and severe retrograde amnesia. Patients may be unable to recall their own name or to recollect pertinent information from childhood or from some part of their past. By contrast, patients with neurological amnesia never forget their names, and their remote memories for the events of childhood and adolescence are typically normal, unless there is brain damage in the lateral temporal or frontal lobes, or both.

Some patients with psychogenic amnesia have circumscribed retrograde memory loss that covers a particular time period or that covers only autobiographical memories. One patient was reported to be able to answer questions about past public events but not questions about past personal events. Another patient scored close to zero on a test of famous photographs, far worse than any neurological amnesic patient would score, and was also unable to identify proper names, such as Los Angeles and Pontiac. Often the challenge for the clinician is not in distinguishing psychogenic amnesia from neurological amnesia but in distinguishing psychogenic amnesia from conscious malingering. Indeed, the diagnosis of psychogenic amnesia can be difficult to substantiate and may be met with skepticism by hospital staff. In some cases, psychogenic amnesia has been observed to clear after a period of days, but, in other cases, it has persisted as a potentially permanent feature of the personality.

IMPLICATIONS

Current understanding of the biology of memory has significant implications for several fundamental issues in psychiatry. One example is the phenomenon of infantile amnesia, the apparent absence of conscious memory for experiences from approximately the first 3 years of life. Traditional views of infantile amnesia have emphasized repression (psychoanalytic theory) and retrieval failure (developmental psychology). A common assumption has been that adults retain memories of early events but cannot bring them into consciousness. However, another possibility is that the capacity for declarative memory does not become fully available until approxi-

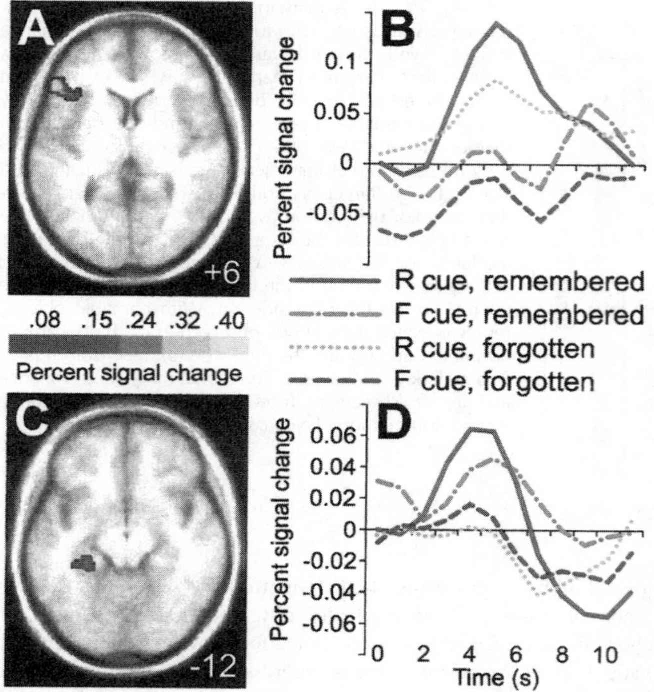

FIGURE 3.4–12 Functional activations of prefrontal and medial temporal regions that were predictive of later memory performance. Single words were presented visually, each followed by an instruction to remember (R cue) or to forget (F cue). Trials were sorted based on the remember or forget instruction and on subsequent recognition performance. Activity in left inferior prefrontal cortex and left hippocampus was predictive of subsequent recognition but for different reasons. Left inferior prefrontal activation **(A)** was associated with the encoding attempt, in that responses were largest for trials with a cue to remember, whether or not the word was actually recognized later. The time course of activity in this region **(B)** was computed based on responses that were time locked to word onset (time 0). Left inferior prefrontal activity increased for words that were later remembered, but there was a stronger association with encoding attempt, as responses were larger for words followed by an R cue that were later forgotten than for words followed by an F cue that were later remembered. In contrast, left parahippocampal and posterior hippocampal activation **(C)** was associated with encoding success. As shown by the time course of activity in this region **(D)**, responses were largest for words that were subsequently remembered, whether the cue was to remember or to forget. (See Color Plate.) (From Reber PJ, Siwiec RM, Gitelman DR, et al.: Neural correlates of successful encoding identified using functional magnetic resonance imaging. *J Neurosci.* 2002;22:9541, with permission. Copyright 2002 by the Society for Neuroscience.)

mately the third year of life, whereas nondeclarative memory emerges early in infancy (e.g., classical conditioning and skill learning). By this view, infantile amnesia results not from the adult's failure to retrieve early memories, but from the child's failure to store them adequately in the first place.

Studies in young infants suggest that a rudimentary capacity for declarative memory is present during the first months of life. As development proceeds, memory can be retained across increasingly long intervals, and what is represented becomes correspondingly richer and full of detail. There is little evidence in humans that the medial temporal lobe or diencephalic region is slow to develop. Rather, what limits the developing capacity for declarative memory is likely the gradual development and differentiation of neocortex. As the neocortex develops, memories supported and stored there become more complex. Strategies emerge for organizing incoming information, language develops, and declarative memories become more richly encoded and interconnected, and more persistent. It is not necessary to suppose that fully formed childhood memories persist but cannot be retrieved. A more plausible view, consistent with current understanding of the biology of memory, is that the capacity to store declarative memory develops only gradually.

The existence of multiple memory systems also has implications for issues in psychoanalytic theory, including the construct of the *unconscious.* How past experience is thought to influence present actions depends on what view one takes of the nature of memory. By the traditional view, memory is a unitary faculty, and representations in memory vary mainly in strength and accessibility. Material that is unconscious is below some threshold of accessibility, but could potentially be made available to consciousness.

An alternative view begins with the distinction between a kind of memory that can be brought to mind (declarative memory) and other kinds of memory that are, by their nature, unconscious. The knowledge is expressed through performance without affording any conscious memory content. In this view, one's behavior might be affected by early events in life, but the effects of that experience can persist without necessarily including a record of the events. Learned behavior can be expressed through altered dispositions, preferences, conditioned responses, habits, and skills, but exhibiting such behavior need not be accompanied by awareness that behavior is being influenced by past experience, nor is there a necessity that any particular past experience has been recorded.

Behavioral change can occur by acquiring new habits that supersede old ones or by becoming sufficiently aware of a habit that one can to some extent isolate it, countermand it, or limit the stimuli that elicit it. However, one need not become aware of the original habits in the same sense that one knows the content of a declarative memory. In this sense, the unconscious does not become conscious. Various forms of nondeclarative memory simply influence behavior without providing the additional capacity for these influences to be accessible to conscious awareness.

A better understanding of the biology of memory has also shed light on memory distortion and the imperfect nature of memory retrieval. It is quite possible to remember events that never happened. For example, it is possible to confuse an event that was only imagined, or dreamed about, with an event that actually occurred, probably because the same brain regions important for visual imagery are also important for long-term storage of visual memories (Fig. 3.4–13). The reconstructive nature of recollection highlights the difficulty in interpreting eyewitness testimony and memories of traumatic events that are apparently brought back to mind after many years. Studies in adults and in children document that illusory memories can be created and that children are particularly susceptible to these effects.

Finally, a biological understanding of declarative memory may have implications for understanding consciousness. Declarative memory provides enduring influences of prior experiences, along with the awareness of remembering. This awareness is not a part of nondeclarative memory. To the extent that memory with and without awareness can be compared and contrasted at a brain systems level of analysis, it may be possible to identify which combinations of neocortical processing, corticodiencephalic interactions, and medial temporal lobe contributions are responsible for the experience of conscious remembering.

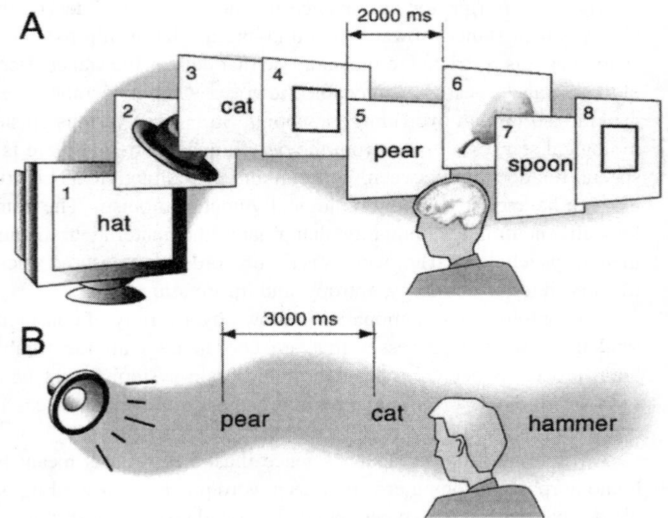

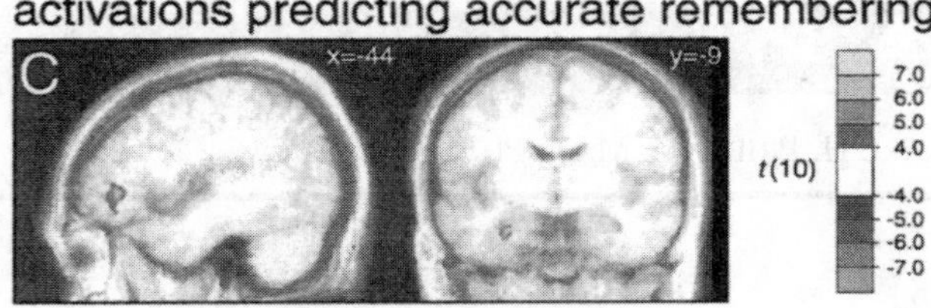

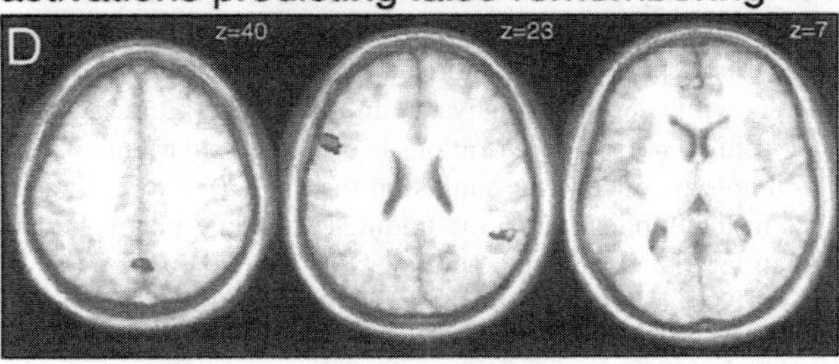

FIGURE 3.4–13 Neural substrates of false memories. **A:** Functional magnetic resonance imaging data were acquired in a learning phase, when subjects read names of objects and visualized the referents. One-half of the names were followed 2 seconds later by a picture of the object. **B:** In a surprise memory test given outside the scanner, subjects listened to object names and decided whether they had seen a picture of the corresponding object. On some trials, subjects claimed to have seen a picture of an object that they had only imagined. **C:** Results showed that left inferior prefrontal cortex and left anterior hippocampus were more active during learning in response to pictures later remembered compared to pictures later forgotten. **D:** Several different brain areas showed a greater response to words in the learning phase that were later falsely remembered as pictures, compared to words not misremembered. Activations that predicted false remembering were found in a brain network important for the generation of visual imagery in response to object names (precuneus, inferior parietal cortex, and anterior cingulate, shown in **left**, **middle**, and **right** images, respectively). (See Color Plate.) (From Gonsalves B, Reber PJ, Gitelman DR, et al.: Event-related fMRI reveals brain activity at encoding that predicts true and false memory for visual objects. *Soc Neurosci Abstr.* 2001, with permission.)

SUGGESTED CROSS-REFERENCES

Functional neuroanatomy is discussed in Section 1.2, delirium, dementia, and amnestic and other cognitive disorders are discussed in Chapter 10; dissociative disorders, including dissociative amnesia, are discussed in Chapter 17; and the broad issue of neuropsychological and intellectual assessment of cognitive functions is discussed in Chapter 7.

REFERENCES

Baddeley AD, Wilson BA, Watts N, eds. *Handbook of Memory Disorders.* 2nd ed. New York: John Wiley and Sons; 2002.

Baddeley A, Aggleton JP, Conway MA, eds. *Episodic Memory: New Directions in Research. Originating from a Discussion Meeting of the Royal Society.* Oxford: Oxford University Press; 2002.

Bayley PJ, Hopkins RO, Squire LR: Successful recollection of remote autobiographical memories by amnesic patients with medial temporal lobe lesions. *Neuron.* 2003;38:135.

Bayley PJ, Squire LR: Medial temporal lobe amnesia: Gradual acquisition of factual information by nondeclarative memory. *J Neurosci.* 2002;22:5741.

Buckner RL, Wheeler ME: The cognitive neuroscience of remembering. *Nat Rev Neurosci.* 2001;2:624.

*Clark RE, Manns JR, Squire LR: Classical conditioning, awareness, and brain systems. *Trends Cogn Sci.* 2002;6:524.

Desimone R: Neural mechanisms for visual memory and their role in attention. *Proc Natl Acad Sci U S A.* 1996;93:13494.

Fuster JM. *Memory in the Cerebral Cortex: An Empirical Approach to Neural Networks in the Human and Nonhuman Primate.* Cambridge, MA: MIT Press; 1995.

Kandel ER: The molecular biology of memory storage: A dialogue between genes and synapses. *Science.* 2001;294:1030.

Kandel ER: Biology and the future of psychoanalysis: A new intellectual framework for psychiatry revisited. *Am J Psychiatry.* 1998;155:457.

Kapur N: Focal retrograde amnesia in neurological disease: A critical review. *Cortex.* 1993;29:217.

Kopelman MD: Disorders of memory. *Brain.* 2002;125:2152.

Lashley KS. *Brain Mechanisms and Intelligence: A Quantitative Study of Injuries to the Brain.* Chicago: Chicago University Press; 1929.

LeDoux JE. *The Emotional Brain.* New York: Simon & Schuster; 1996.

Levy DA, Stark CEL, Squire LR: Intact conceptual priming in the absence of declarative memory. *Psychol Sci.* (*in press*).

Lezak MD. *Neuropsychological Assessment.* 2nd ed. New York: Oxford University Press; 1983.

Manns JR, Hopkins RO, Reed JM, Kitchener EG, Squire LR: Recognition memory and the human hippocampus. *Neuron.* 2003;37:171.

Manns JR, Hopkins RO, Squire LR: Semantic memory and the human hippocampus. *Neuron.* 2003;38:127.

Paller KA: Consolidating dispersed neocortical memories: The missing link in amnesia. *Memory.* 1997;5:73.

Paller KA: Electrical signals of memory and of the awareness of remembering. *Curr Dir Psychol Sci.* (*in press*).

Paller KA, Acharya A, Richardson BC, Plaisant O, Shimamura AP, Reed BR, Jagust WJ: Functional neuroimaging of cortical dysfunction in alcoholic Korsakoff's syndrome. *J Cogn Neurosci.* 1997;9:277.

Paller KA, Hutson CA, Miller BB, Boehm SG: Neural manifestations of memory with and without awareness. *Neuron.* 2003;38:507.

Paller KA, Ranganath C, Gonsalves B, LaBar KS, Parrish TB, Gitelman DR, Mesulam MM, Reber PJ: Neural correlates of person recognition. *Learn Mem.* 2003;10:253.

*Paller KA, Wagner AD: Monitoring the transformation of experience into memory. *Trends Cogn Sci.* 2002;6:93.

Schacter DL, ed. *Memory Distortion: How Minds, Brains, and Societies Reconstruct the Past.* Cambridge, MA: Harvard University Press; 1995.

*Schacter DL. *Searching for Memory.* New York: Basic Books; 1996.

Shimamura AP. Memory and frontal lobe function. In: Gazzaniga MS, ed. *The Cognitive Neurosciences.* Cambridge, MA: MIT Press; 1995:803.

Squire LR: *Memory and Brain.* New York: Oxford University Press; 1987.

Squire LR: Memory and the hippocampus: A synthesis of findings with rats, monkeys, and humans. *Psychol Rev.* 1992;99:195.

*Squire LR, Kandel E. *Memory: From Mind to Molecules.* New York: Scientific American Library; 1999.

*Squire LR, Schacter DL, eds. *Neuropsychology of Memory.* 3rd ed. New York: Guilford; 2002.

Squire LR, Zola SM: Structure and function of declarative and nondeclarative memory systems. *Proc Natl Acad Sci U S A.* 1996;93:13515.

Squire LR, Zouzounis JA: Self-ratings of memory dysfunction: Different findings in depression and amnesia. *J Clin Exp Neuropsychol.* 1988;10:727.

Stickgold R, Hobson JA, Fosse R, Fosse M: Sleep, learning, and dreams: Off-line memory reprocessing. *Science.* 2001;294:1052.

Tulving E: Episodic memory: From mind to brain. *Annu Rev Psychol.* 2002;53:1.

Tulving E, Craik FIM. *The Oxford Handbook of Memory.* Oxford: Oxford University Press; 2000.

Zola-Morgan S, Squire LR: The primate hippocampal formation: Evidence for a time-limited role in memory storage. *Science.* 1990;250:288.

▲ 3.5 Brain Models of Mind

KARL H. PRIBRAM, M.D., PH.D.

For two centuries, brain models of mind have fascinated scientists and the lay public alike. This intense interest began with the pioneering discovery of correlations between brain pathology and characteristic personality histories of patients studied by Francis J. Gall. As with every major advance in understanding the mind/brain relationship, Gall's demonstrations became a popular fad in the form of *phrenology*, or reading bumps on the skull. Today, a similar fad exists in the application of the findings regarding hemispheric specialization: Educators and politicians alike recommend using the right brain more lest the human race fall forever into damnation.

Brain models of mind have shown a remarkable coherence over the 19th and 20th centuries despite the often acrimonious debate regarding emphasis on this or that phenomenon to the exclusion of a comprehensive analysis. Further, when carefully considered, each of the often opposing views captures important aspects of the issues; reconciliation often depends on making distinctive definitions and reading the proposals in their original form with these definitions in mind.

A useful definition of mind was provided by Gilbert Ryle: *mind* comes from minding, or paying attention. In old English, the word is *gemynd*, akin to remind and was derived from terms indicating *to warn* and *to intend*. The Sanskrit word *mynas* means to think.

As a whole, the human brain is critical to minding. One case history highlights the obvious.

> While in the practice of neurosurgery, I was called about a 14-year-old girl who had fallen out of a rapidly moving automobile and sustained a head injury with multiple scalp lacerations. She was several hundred miles away and transporting her to our hospital, although considered, was thought too risky for an already traumatized head. Her head was swathed in bandages through which some blood had oozed, making them appear bright red. By contrast, the girl looked green. When addressed, "Hello Cathy, you look like a Christmas package all dolled up in your bandages," she smiled and said, "Hello Doctor." It was clear that her brain was intact. She minded appreciatively and with a sense of humor. Thorough examination revealed a broken rib with a puncture to one lung, which explained her green color. Bandages and a brief time in an oxygen tent quickly allowed healing to commence.

The diagnosis rested on the truism that scrambled brains result in scrambled minds. This truism, however, because of its pervasive validity, can obscure the more subtle aspects of the mind–brain relationship. For instance, the close association of mind to brain might lead to the assumptions that mind and brain are the same, which would be as absurd as stating that the islands of Langerhans of the pancreas are the same as glucose metabolism. Just as glucose metabolism is a function of the organism metabolizing environmentally derived nutrients, *minding* is a function of the entire organism interacting with its environment.

Thus, although the special relation between the brain and minding is widely acknowledged, the inherent nature of the relationship continues to be debated. In this respect, apparently no progress has been made in the past two millennia.

The time is ripe for an advance in understanding. Each of the philosophical stances toward the mind–brain relationship has merit as long as it is restricted to the database that defines the stance. Each of these stances becomes untenable, however, when it becomes overgeneralized into an overriding viewpoint. Still, these various epistemological stances all stem from the overriding truism that there is a special relationship between the brain and mental activity. This truism can be anchored in an ontologically neutral monism. The ontologically neutral commonality that relates the material brain and mental (psychological) processes is *order*—order as measured scientifically in terms of energy, entropy, and information.

This ontological commonality is shown by a variety of conscious (and unconscious) processes that are coordinate with identifiable brain processes occurring in identifiable brain systems—that is, at some level, the descriptions of brain processes and mental processes become homomorphic.

An example from computer science illustrates what is meant by homomorphic: A computer is used as a word processor when English words and sentences are typed into it. The word processing system, by virtue of an operating system (e.g., assembler, ASCII, octal, or hexadecimal), converts the keyboard input to binary, which is the "language" of the computer. There is nothing in the description of English that appears to be similar to that of binary machine language. Despite this, by virtue of the transformations produced in the encoding and decoding operations of the various stages leading from typescript to binary, the information of the typescript is preserved in the binary language of the operation of the computing machine.

In a similar fashion, there is little in conscious experience that resembles the operations of the neural apparatus with which it has such a special relationship. However, when the transformations, or *transfer functions*, the codes that intervene between experience and neural operations, are sufficiently detailed, a level of description is reached in which the *transformations* of experience are homomorphic with the language used by the brain. As will be reviewed in this section, this language is the language of the operations of a microprocess taking place in synaptodendritic fields, a mathematical language similar to that which describes processes in micro (i.e., subatomic) physics.

At this microprocessing level, an identity describes the relationship between the brain and mental processes. At more remote processing levels, encompassing larger event structures (assemblers, operating systems, or their counterparts in brain systems), pluralism and, eventually, (at the natural language level) dualism characterize the relationship. The special relationship between the brain and mental processes is, thus, not an identity, except in implementation at the microprocessing level. At the neuronal and neural system levels, several types of relationship (codes or languages) with psychological processes can be discerned.

First, there are neurochemical states operating in the synaptodendritic processing web that determine states of consciousness. The very active field of psychoneuropharmacology is replete with evidence of relationships between catecholamines and indolamines acting in specified brain locations to produce states of consciousness, such as wakefulness and sleep, depression and elation, and perhaps even the production of dissociated states, such as those seen in schizophrenia. The relationships between relative concentrations of blood glucose and hunger, between osmolarity and thirst, between sex hormones and sexually characteristic behaviors, and between peptides, such as endorphins and enkephalins, and the experiences of pain and stress are all well documented.

Second, there are detailed descriptions of the relations between the sensory systems of the brain and the sensory aspects of perception: the *contents of consciousness*. Great strides in understanding the brain's contribution to sensory perception were made during the latter half of the 20th century by tracing with microelectrodes the effects of visual, auditory, tactile, and olfactory inputs from receptor to cortex.

States of consciousness often determine contents and, as often, are determined by them. When hungry, one tends to notice restaurant signs; the fresh aromas emanating from a bakery tend to whet the appetite. This connection between states and the contents of consciousness is mediated by the minding process, which is made up of processes ordinarily termed *attention* (the control of sensory input), *intention* (the control of motor output), and *thought* (the control of remembering). Understanding the brain organizations involved in the processes of minding clarifies the relationship between states and contents of experience.

VARIETIES OF BRAIN ORGANIZATION

Localization and Distribution of Function There are some models of brain organization that are crucial for determining the organization of minding. First is the issue of localization of function. Gall brought this issue to the foreground by correlating different local brain pathologies to the histories of the cadavers he autopsied. Though often wrong in detail and naïve in delineating the faculties of mind for which he sought localization, Gall was correct in his methods. However, systematic classification of mental functions continues to be elusive despite a century of operational behaviorism. Today it is popular to discuss the modularity of mind and the component systems of the brain and relate them both in the clinic and in the laboratory by crafting experimental designs and behavioral and verbal testing procedures. The use of these techniques traces its heritage directly to Gall's enterprise.

The excesses of localization, as expressed in phrenology, brought reaction. First, the question was raised as to which brain system brought together the various faculties into a single conscious self. Breaking mentation into a mere collection of faculties challenged the unity of being, the soul of humankind. Furthermore, experimental evidence accrued to demonstrate a relationship between impairments in complex behaviors and the amount of brain tissue destroyed irrespective of location. In the recent past, Karl Lashley became the exponent of this mass action view.

However, upon reading Lashley carefully, the seeds of conciliation can be found. In a letter to Fred Mettler, Lashley once stated his exasperation with being misinterpreted: "Of course I know the front of the brain does something different from the back end. The visual sensory input terminates in the occipital lobes. Electrical stimulations of the pre-Rolandic areas elicit movements and the front parts are more enigmatic in their functions. But this is not the issue." Elsewhere he stated the issue clearly: "certain coordinated activities, known to be dependent upon definite cortical areas, can be carried out by any part (within undefined limits) of the whole area."

Lashley emphasized that certain selected mental functions appeared to be related to brain processes that are distributed. For instance, he pointed out that sensory and motor equivalences could not be accounted for, even by a duplication of brain pathways: "Once an associated reaction has been established (e.g., a positive reaction to a visual pattern), the same reaction will be elicited by the excitation of sensory cells which were never stimulated in that way during training. Similarly, motor acts (e.g., opening a latch box) once acquired, may be executed immediately with motor organs which were not associated with the act during training."

The following is an example of motor equivalence: A dog was conditioned to raise his right hind leg to the sound of a tone. After this conditional response was well established, his right motor cortex (which controls the left side of the body) was exposed. Then, during the performance of the conditioned reaction, a patty of strychninized filter paper (which chemically excited the cortical tissue) was placed on the area that controls the left forepaw. Immediately, the dog switched the responding leg and now raised his left forepaw to the conditional signal. A temporary dominant focus of excitation had been established in the cortex by the chemical stimulation. E. Roy John summarizes the experiments that demonstrate such shifts in cerebral dominant foci in Figure 3.5–1.

The distributed aspect of brain function becomes most evident in memory storage. Even with large deletions of brain tissue, such as those resulting from strokes or tumor resections, specific memories, or *engrams*, are seldom lost. When amnesias do occur, they are apt to be spotty and difficult to classify. This suggests that memory is stored deep within the synaptodendritic interstices of the brain's connective structures in a distributed fashion. The storage process dismembers the input, which is then remembered on the occasions necessitating recognition and recall. The retrieval processes, in contrast to storage, are localized within systems composed of neural circuits that form a surface structure that can address the deeper distributed store. When such systems are damaged, sensory-specific and even category-specific agnosias result. Thus, with regard to memory, both a distributed deep structure and a localized surface structure can be identified, depending on which property of the process is being considered. This principle of analyzing a mental process to identify specific aspects is basic to understanding the pluralistic epistemology and ontological unity that characterize the mind–brain relationship.

Systems in the Control of Attention, Intention, and Thought Minding, or consciousness, comprises processes usually referred to as attention, intention (or volition), and thought. Controls on attention determine the span of sensory processing, those on intention determine the span over which action becomes effective, and those controlling thought determine the span of memories being considered.

Two decades of investigation into the neural processes involved in the control of attention discerned three such mechanisms: one deals with the short phasic response to an unfamiliar input (*arousal*); a second relates to the prolonged tonic readiness of the organism to respond selectively (*activation*); and a third (*effort*) acts to coordinate the phasic and tonic processes. Separate neural and neurochemical systems are involved in the phasic and tonic processes: the phasic centers on the amygdala, and the tonic centers on the basal ganglia of the forebrain. The coordinating system critically involves the hippocampus, a phylogenetically ancient part of the neural apparatus.

Evidence from the analysis of changes in the electrical activity of the brain evoked by brief sensory stimulation has shown that the phasic and tonic systems operate on a more basic process centered on the dorsal thalamus, the way station of sensory input to the cerebral cortex. Brain electrical activity evoked by sensory stimulation can be separated into components. Early components reflect processing via systems that directly (via the thalamus) connect sensory surfaces with cortical surfaces. Later components reflect processes initiated in the thalamocortical and related basal ganglia systems that operate downward onto the brainstem (tectal region), which, in turn, influence a thalamic "gate" that modulates activity in the direct sensory pathways. It is the activity reflected in these later components of the brain's electrical activity that constitutes activation. The tha-

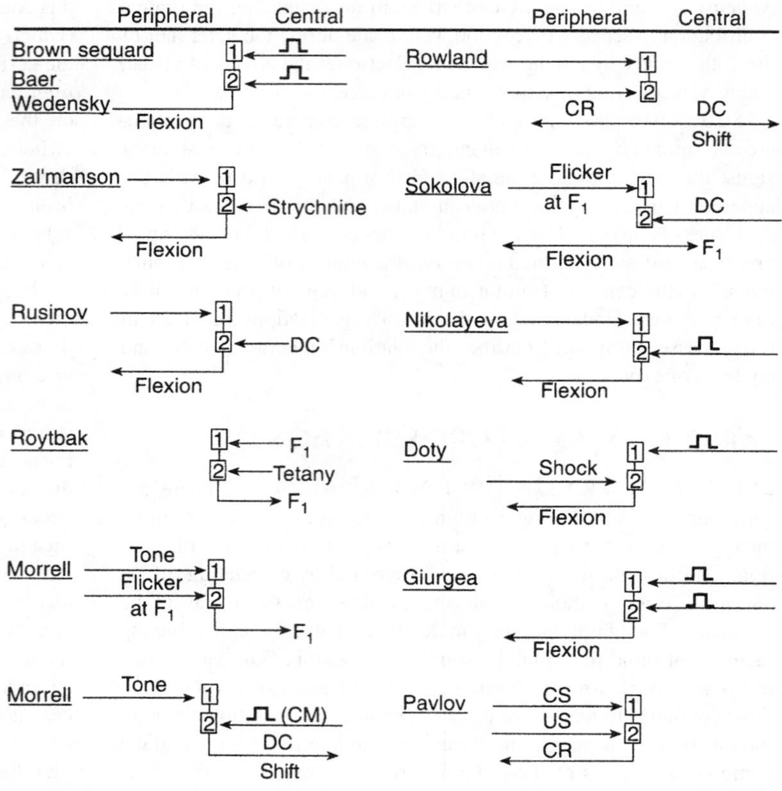

FIGURE 3.5–1. Methods of conditioning that have been used by various investigators to establish and produce shifts in cerebral dominant foci. The example in the text refers to Zal'manson's experiment. CR, conditioned response; CS, conditioned stimulus; US, unconditioned stimulus. (Reprinted with permission from Pribram K: *Languages of the Brain: Experimental Paradoxes and Principles in Neuropsychology.* New York: Random House; 1971.)

lamic gate, however, is also regulated by input from the system centered on the amygdala—the *arousal system.* This system, when stimulated, produces an effect on the thalamic gate opposite that of the activation system.

Evidence also indicates that the coordination of phasic and tonic attentional processes often demands effort. When attention must be paid, the hippocampal system becomes involved, influencing the arousal system rostrally through frontal connections with the amygdala system and the activation system caudally via connections in the brainstem.

William James once proposed that the responses of body organs to a perceived input resulted in the feelings that accompany the perception. Beginning with Walter Cannon's experimentally based critique of James, which was followed by Lashley's critique of Cannon, the anatomically based suggestions of James Papez, and their more current versions by Paul MacLean, brain scientists gradually shifted the locus of the processes that organize emotional and motivational experience and expression. Two major discoveries have added considerably to these earlier accounts. One discovery is the role of the reticular formation of the brainstem and its chemical systems of brain amines that regulate states of alertness and mood. Donald Lindsley proposed an activation mechanism of emotion and motivation on the basis of this discovery and has more recently detailed the pathways by which such activation can exert control over the brain processes. The other discovery, made by James Olds and Peter Milner, is the system of brain tracts that, when electrically excited, results in reinforcement (i.e., increase in probability of recurrence of the behavior that has produced the electrical brain stimulation) or deterrence (i.e., decrease in probability that such behavior will recur).

These discoveries make it necessary to distinguish clearly between those data that refer to experience (feelings) and those that refer to expression and, further, to distinguish emotion from motivation. Feelings encompass both emotional and motivational experience, emotional as affective and motivation as readiness to act. The affective processes of emotion are based on arousal—that is, phasic responses to unfamiliar input that "stop" the motivational processes of activation that maintain readiness.

This wealth of new data makes it fruitful to reexamine the Jamesian position with regard to his visceral theory of emotions. James is almost universally misinterpreted as holding a peripheral theory of emotion. Although he emphasized stimuli of visceral origin, he noted that these stimuli exert their effects via their input to the brain. Nowhere does he identify emotions with bodily processes. Emotions are always the resultant effect of these processes on the brain. What James failed to take into account is the role of expectations (the states of familiarity) against which unfamiliar inputs are matched to control neuronal models of experience that entail the functions of the basal ganglia, including the amygdala. Nonetheless, James is explicit when he discusses the nature of the input to the brain from the viscera. He points out two possibilities: feelings are processed by either a separate brain system or the same systems that process perceptions. Today, it is known that both possibilities are realized: parts of the frontolimbic forebrain (especially the amygdala and related systems) process visceroautonomic bodily inputs, and the results of processing become distributed via brainstem systems that diffusely influence perceptual systems. James perhaps overemphasized the visceral determination of emotional experience, but he did occasionally include attitudinal factors (as did Papez) as depending on sensory feedback from the somatic musculature.

The distinction between the brain mechanisms of motivation and will are less clearly enunciated by James. Motivations (which James called *instincts*) were distinguished from emotions in that motivations reach out to produce practical relations with the environment, whereas emotional processes remain within the skin. Volition was distinguished from motivation, but no precise neural distinction was proposed. James grappled with the problem and established the questions that must be answered. These questions remained unanswered until the late 1960s, when several theorists began to point out the difference between homeostatic feedback processes and homeorhetic feedforward programs. Feedback mechanisms depend on error processing and are therefore sensitive to perturbations. Feedforward programs, however, unless completely stopped, run to completion, regardless of obstacles placed in their way.

Clinical neurology had classically distinguished the mechanisms involved in voluntary behavior from those involved in involuntary behavior. The distinction rests on the observation that lesions of the cerebellar hemispheres impair voluntary behavior, whereas basal ganglia lesions result in disturbances of involuntary movements. Damage to the cerebellar circuits is involved in a feedforward rather than a feedback mechanism. Recent microelectrode analyses indicate that the cerebellar hemispheres perform calculations in fast-time—that is, they extrapolate where a particular movement would end were it to be continued and send the results of such a calculation to the cerebral motor cortex, where they are matched to a target to which the movement is directed. Experimental analysis of the functions of the motor cortex have shown that such targets are composed of "images of achievement" constructed from experience.

Just as the cerebellar circuit has been shown to serve intentional behavior, the basal ganglia have been shown to be important to involuntary processes. As noted, these structures control activation, or the readiness of organisms to respond. Lesions in the basal ganglia grossly amplify tremors at rest and markedly restrict expressions of motivational feelings. Neurological theory has long held that these disturbances are due to obstruction by the lesion of the normal feedback relationships between the basal ganglia and the cerebral cortex. In fact, surgical removals of the motor cortex have been performed on patients with basal ganglia lesions to redress the imbalance produced by the initial pathology. Such resections have proved remarkably successful in alleviating the often distressing disturbances of involuntary movement that characterize disorders of the basal ganglia.

Massively Parallel Distributed Processes Two closely related issues concerning the organization of brain function are often confounded: (1) localization versus distribution of function within each system and (2) whether processing proceeds among different localizable systems in a hierarchical fashion or in a parallel fashion and, thus, heterarchically.

The fact that a temporary dominant focus in the cerebral cortex can take control of the expression of a learned behavior indicates that hierarchical control undoubtedly operates in the central nervous system (CNS). Equally persuasive is the evidence for control over spinal cord activity by the brainstem and the forebrain. Neuronal activity in the spinal cord displays an extremely high rate of spontaneous impulse generation. These generators are modulated by inhibitory local circuit neurons in such a way that the resultant activity can be modeled in terms of coupled ensembles of limit cycle oscillatory processes.

In turn, these ensembles of oscillators become organized by brainstem systems that consist of cholinergic and adrenergic neurons. The cholinergic set regulates the frequency of a wide range of tonic rhythmic activities, such as those involved in locomotion, respiration, cardiovascular responses, and sleep. This cholinergic system is coupled to an adrenergic set of neurons that segment the rhythmic activities into episodes. Both systems are subject to further hierarchical control by the dopaminergic system of the basal ganglia.

Clinically, loss of this hierarchical control becomes manifest in an exaggeration of the normally present, almost subliminal tremors, which, under extreme conditions, lead to spastic paralysis, hyperreflexia, and uncontrollable fits of oscillatory muscular spasm.

However, the evidence from experiments that demonstrated temporary dominant foci can be viewed from another perspective: The flexibility demonstrated by the shift from one controlling locus to another shows the organization of the cortical system to be heterarchical. Any locus within the system can become dominant if sufficiently excited. The following story attributed to Warren McCulloch illustrates the nature of heterarchical organization:

> After the battle of Jutland in which the British Navy took a beating, both the British and American navies reorganized to change from hierarchical to heterarchical control. Thus, battleships no longer had to await orders from a central command source to engage in defensive maneuvers. During World War II, the American Fifth Fleet was stationed in a slightly dispersed mode of operation somewhere in the Pacific Ocean when it was attacked from two directions by separate air squadrons. Sightings of the attackers were made from different locations in the fleet by observers on the ships closest to one or the other of the attacking planes. Thus, the sailor who made the sighting became a dominant focus, and his ship and those in his proximity took off to defend against the attackers. However, because the attack came from two different directions, two dominant foci were created, each commanding parts of the fleet to steam away in different directions. This left the ship at the center of the fleet, which housed its admiral, haplessly unprotected and, because no sightings were made by his ship, at a momentary loss as to what to do. Fortunately, both attacking squadrons were defeated and turned back without any damage accruing to the Fifth Fleet.

There is, thus, a possible penalty to be paid for the flexibility achieved by temporary dominance, as any person who has ever been of two minds knows well.

Ordinarily, hierarchical control is thought to be a serial process, because there is a causal connection between the controller and the controlled when control is direct. Causality implies that the origination of the control signal precedes its effect on the system being controlled. Seriality remains when there are feedback loops. However, when feedforward operations are inserted into the process, seriality is no longer as clear-cut. For example, lower the temperature on a thermostat or blood sugar on a glucostat, and the sensor responds and closes a circuit, and then the effector responds; this is a serial process. However, if a control dial or other bias becomes involved in the process, there are two (or more) ways for the sensor to be adjusted. The temperature falls, but because the heating bill was too high last month, the dial is reset, and warmer clothes are worn. In this example, there are parallel inputs to the sensor. Herman von Helmholtz is credited with pointing out that voluntary processes, such as those that move the eyes, are constituted of such parallel feedforward corollary discharges, this time to the effectors. Control can be hierarchical yet dependent on a parallel process.

Processing in the cerebral cortex is massively parallel. Simulations of these parallel cortical processes have, during the past decades, become implemented on personal computers to such an extent that the endeavors have been dubbed a cottage industry.

These simulations of neural networks are capable of pattern recognition, language learning, and decision making, all remarkably true to life. Single-layered simulations have given way to three-layered computations that involve an input layer, an output layer, and a hidden layer. All the elements of the network are interconnected. In several such simulations, the input is fed forward through the net, and the output is compared with one that is desired, and the difference between the actual output and the desired output is fed back to the network. The process is repeated until the desired output is achieved. Variations on this theme abound, each variation better adapted for a particular purpose than its alternates.

One of the most fascinating attributes of these neural networks is the fact that the information contained in the input becomes fragmented and distributed in the elements of the layers. Thus, the simulations are said to be massively parallel distributed processes (PDP), which makes them akin to optical information processing systems, such as holography and tomography, from which they were in fact derived.

Perspectives on Reality Surrounding the major fissures of the primate cerebral cortex are the terminations of the sensory and motor projection systems. These systems have been termed *extrinsic* because of their close ties (by way of a few synapses) with peripheral structures. The sensory surface and muscle arrangements are mapped more or less isomorphically onto the perifissural cortical surface by way of discrete, practically parallel lines of connecting fiber tracts. When a local injury occurs within these systems, a sensory scotoma, or a scotoma of action, ensues. A *scotoma* is a spatially circumscribed hole in the field of interaction between organism and environment: a blind spot, a hearing defect limited to a frequency range, a location of the skin where tactile stimuli fail to provoke a response. These are the systems in which what Henry Head called *epicritic processing* takes place. These extrinsic, massively parallel sensory-motor projection systems are so organized that the results of processing are projected away from the sensory surfaces where interactions with the environment take place and out into the world external to the organism. The process is akin to that which projects sound in a stereo audio system away from the speakers and into the space in front and between them. Thus, processing within these extrinsic systems constructs an objective reality for the organism.

Each major sensory apparatus (with the exception of olfaction) has a fairly direct input to areas in the cortex. Immediately surrounding these areas are others that, when electrically stimulated, originate movements of the musculature associated with each of the sense organs (for example, eye muscles for vision, ear muscles for hearing, and body muscles for somatic sensations). Both the sensory and motor areas are extrinsically connected—that is, connected to organs in the periphery of the body—and, therefore, relate the body to the outside world.

Surrounding these extrinsic areas are sensory-specific areas that are primarily connected intrinsically, that is, to other brain structures. These areas provide perspectives (e.g., egocentric, allocentric, and object-centered) that are intrinsic to the entities perceived. These perspectives are provided by constancies constructed by segmenting and then grouping segments of the sensory input by movement. Thus, constancies are achieved by operations of the intrinsic cortical process on the extrinsic process—a top-down operation. In addition, there are areas that coordinate inputs from a variety of senses that relate their perspectives to each other. All of these areas and the brain systems that they represent are involved in organizing phenomenal perceptions of reality. In today's terminology, they are called the *sensory-driven aspects of perception*. Finally, a totally different set of systems more noumenal in function is located frontally and on the limbic medial border of the brain's hemispheres. These systems monitor and, under certain circumstances, such as ambiguity in the sensory input, control the more posterior systems.

Cerebral Dominance and the Unity of Conscious Experience Three important discoveries have fueled the interest in hemispheric specialization with regard to the processing of perspectives on reality. One of these was actually a rediscovery during the latter half of the 19th century of the fact that, in most right-handed individuals, speech is controlled, for the most part, by the left hemisphere. Hippocrates already knew this, and he may well have learned it from the Egyptians. Running from back to front, comprehension, grammar, and fluency (*semantics*, *syntactics*, and *pragmatics* in Charles S. Peirce's and A. Morris' terms) are affected by lesions centering on the sylvian fissure. However, dominance is not as complete in women as it is in men or as pervasive in cultures that do not use phonemic writing.

What is newer in the appreciation of hemispheric specialization is the realization that the non–speech-dominant hemisphere has its own characteristic modes of processing. Because the left hemispheres of right-handed persons are taken over by an aural–oral dimension, the right hemisphere is free to process visual–spatial relations.

The third and most pervasive and persistent focus of interest has been a theme that also organized debate regarding localization of function in the 19th century: the unity of consciousness. When the corpus callosum was severed in patients who had experienced severe unilateral epileptic seizures to prevent involvement of the healthy hemisphere, testing revealed that what was sensed by the right hemisphere could only be expressed nonverbally. The left verbal hemisphere appeared to be ignorant of what had transpired. It seemed as if consciousness had been split when the hemispheres were sundered. The assumption that there is ordinarily a unity to consciousness received support in that this unity had been ruptured.

Taken together with the facts of hemispheric specialization and the dominance of the left hemisphere in language, it was but a step to generalize these observations into the conception that civilization suffered from left brain dominance and that training for greater brain balance would restore balance to civilization. Innumerable studies have demonstrated, however, that all but the most rudimentary processing involves both hemispheres. Even in language, the appreciation and expression of emotional communication (*prosody*) involves the right hemisphere, and extreme specialization is limited to right-handed men raised in a phonemic literary environment.

Although the popular overgeneralization is to be deplored, it did renew interest in the question as to whether consciousness could be divided. Sir John Eccles argued that consciousness is tied to language, an argument also made by Sigmund Freud, and that, therefore, the speechless right hemisphere was, for all intents and purposes, essentially unconscious. However, the right hemisphere clearly communicates by way of left-handed, nonverbal, instrumental responses to inputs presented to it. The nonverbal hemisphere obviously has a mind of its own. Thus, conscious minding is of two sorts: objective and narrative. Objective experience is largely controlled by the posterior convexity of the brain, and narrative is largely controlled by the frontolimbic forebrain. In humans, however, with the development of language, additional hemispheric specialization has occurred.

VARIETIES OF CONSCIOUS EXPERIENCE

The Brain, the Me, and the I The reciprocity between subject and object and some causal connection between them is inherent in language once it emerges from simple naming to predication. Eric Neumann and Julian Jaynes suggested that a change in consciousness (i.e., in distinguishing an aware self from what the self is aware of) occurred somewhere during the 8th century BC between the time of the *Iliad* and the *Odyssey*, which links it to the invention and promulgation of phonemically based writing. Prehistory was transmitted orally and aurally; written history is visual and verbal. In an oral and aural culture, a greater share of objective reality is carried subjectively in memory and is, thus, personal; once writing becomes a ready means of recording events, these events become a part of extrapersonal objective reality. The shift described is especially manifest in a clearer externalization of the sources of conscience—the gods no longer speak personally to guide individual man.

This process of ever-clearer distinctions between personal and extrapersonal objective realities culminates in Franz Brentano's *intentional inexistence*, which was shortened by Edmund Husserl to *intentionality*.

A case history illuminates this distinction. During a seminar a few years ago, the left arm of a graduate student was moving somewhat awkwardly as she arranged papers on a table. When asked if she was all right, the student, Ms. C., replied, "Oh, that's just Alice; Alice doesn't live here anymore." At the end of the semester, Ms. C. presented a detailed account of her experiences with Alice:

I was doing laundry about mid-morning when I had a migraine. I felt a sharp pain in my left temple, and my left arm felt funny. I finished my laundry towards mid-afternoon and called my neurologist. He told me to go to the emergency department. I packed a few things and drove about 85 miles to the hospital where he is on staff (the nearest was 15 minutes away). In the emergency department, the same thing happened again. And again the morning after I was hospitalized, only it was worse. The diagnosis of a stroke came as a complete surprise to me because I felt fine, and I didn't notice anything different about myself. I remember having no emotional response to the news. I felt annoyed and more concerned about getting home, because I was in the process of moving.

Not until several days later, while I was in rehabilitation, did I notice strange things happening to me. I was not frightened, angry, or annoyed. I didn't feel anything—nothing at all. Fourteen days after I was admitted to the hospital, I became extremely dizzy, and I felt I was falling out of my wheelchair. The floor was tilting to my left and the wheelchair was sliding off the floor. Any stimulus on my left side or repetitive movement with my left arm caused a disturbance in my relationship with my environment. For instance, the room would tilt down to the left, and I felt my wheelchair sliding downhill off the floor, and I was falling out of my chair. I would become disoriented, could hardly speak, and my whole being seemed to enter a new dimension. When my left side was placed next to a wall or away from any stimuli, this disturbance would gradually disappear. During this period, the left hand would contract, and the arm would draw up next to my body. It didn't feel or look like it belonged to me. Harrison moved the left arm repeatedly with the same movement, and a similar behavior occurred, except I started crying. He asked mewhat was I feeling, and I said anger. In another test, he started giving me a hard time until the same episode began to occur, and I began to cry. He asked me what I was feeling, and I said anger. Actually, I didn't feel the anger inside, but in my head when I began to cry. Not until I went back to school did I become aware of having no internal physical feelings.

I call that arm *Alice* (Alice doesn't live here anymore)—the arm I don't like. It doesn't look like my arm and doesn't feel like my arm. I think it's ugly, and I wish it would go away. Whenever things go wrong, I'll slap it and say, "Bad Alice" or "It's Alice's fault." I never know what it's doing or where it is in space unless I am looking at it. I can use it, but I never do consciously because I'm unaware of having a left arm. I don't neglect my left side, just Alice. Whatever it does, it does on its own, and, most of the time, I don't know it's doing it. I'll be doing homework, and then I'll take a sip of coffee. The cup will be empty. I was drinking coffee with that hand and didn't know it. Yet, I take classical guitar lessons. I don't feel the strings or frets. I don't know where my fingers are nor what they are doing, but still I play.

How do I live with an illness I'm not aware of having? How do I function when I'm not aware that I have deficits? How do I stay safe when I'm not aware of being in danger?

Ms. C. is a widowed woman in her mid-50s, enrolled in adult education and majoring in clinical psychology. She is obviously intelligent, understanding lecture material and asking interesting questions. She gets around splendidly despite Alice and despite a history of a temporary left hemiparesis. The diagnosis was damage of the right temporal-parietal cortex confirmed by an abnormal electroencephalogram (EEG) recorded from that location. The damage was not sufficiently extensive to show in a positron emission tomography (PET) scan.

There is, however, an entirely different sort of conscious experience, a way of experiencing oneself that is completely intact in Ms. C. Contrast Ms. C.'s story with the following observations of an 8-year-old boy, which were made by Chuck Ahern as part of his doctoral research:

T. J. had an agenesis of the corpus callosum with a midline cyst at birth. During the first 6 months of his life, two surgical procedures were carried out to drain the cyst. Recently performed magnetic resonance imaging (MRI) showed considerable enlargement of the frontal horns of the lateral ventricle—somewhat more pronounced on the right. The orbital part of the frontal lobes appeared shrunken, as did the medial surface of the temporal pole.

T. J. appears to have no ability for quantifying the passage of time and no experiential appreciation of the meaning of time units. For example, a few minutes after tutoring begins, he cannot say, even remotely, how long it has been since the session started. He is as apt to answer this question in years as in minutes. He does always use one of seven terms of time quantification (seconds, minutes, hours, days, weeks, months, or years) when asked to estimate the duration of an episode but uses them randomly. He can put these terms in order but does not have any sense of their meaning or their numerical relationships to one another.

When T. J. returned from a trip to the Bahamas, he did recall that he had been on the trip; however, the details he could recount about the trip numbered fewer than five. His estimates of how long it had been since his trip were typical in that they were inaccurate and wildly inconsistent on repeated trials. Also, the first five times back at tutoring, he stated that he had not been at tutoring since his trip. It appears that he is unable to place in sequence those few past events that he can recall. Nonetheless, he can answer questions correctly based on his application of general knowledge about development (e.g., he knows he was a baby before he could talk because "everyone starts as a baby"). One day, however, he asked his tutor if he knew him when he was a kid, indicating his incomprehension of the duration of each of these developmental periods and his unawareness of what events constituted such a period for him.

T. J. is aware that he has a past, that events have happened to him, but he cannot recollect those events. He also spontaneously speaks of events in his future, such as driving an automobile, dating, and growing a beard. He has play-acted on separate occasions his own old age and death. T. J. is capable of excitement about the immediate future. On the very day that he was going to the Bahamas, he was very excited as he exclaimed repeatedly, "I'm going to the Bahamas." But when his tutor asked him when, he said blankly, "I don't know." He also displayed keen anticipation when he saw a helicopter preparing to take off from the hospital. The helicopter engines revved approximately 13 minutes before it took off, and T. J. became increasingly more vocal and motorically active, laughing as he repeated, "When's it going to take off?" He also anticipates future punishment when he is "bad." He is aware, on some level, of the immediate future in his constant question "What's next?" which he asks his mother at the end of each activity.

There are a variety of other occasions on which he demonstrated this capacity regarding tempo (as opposed to evaluating the duration of an experience). There have been several breaks in his usual thrice-weekly tutoring schedule. Each of the four times this schedule has been interrupted, he has run to meet his tutor rather than waiting inside as he usually does. Also, on these occasions, he has typically asked if his tutor missed him. However, he states he does not know how long it has been since his last session, and there was no evidence that he knew it had been longer than usual.

T. J. can compare who walks faster and who draws faster. He has at least a basic sense of sequencing as when he says "I'll take a turn and then you take a turn." He also uses terms like "soon" and "quick" correctly in conversation. For example, when he wanted to do a drawing at the beginning of a session and his tutor said that they needed begin to work, he countered, "This will be quick." Unsurprisingly, he finished his drawing at his normal pace. He somehow seems to use such terms correctly without any experiential appreciation of them.

These two case histories illuminate two very important dimensions of self. One dimension, portrayed by Ms. C., *locates* an objective "me" in the world with respect to the body's configural integrity. The other dimension, highlighted by T. J., *monitors* experience. Without such monitoring, the events that constitute the experience fail to become relevant and are not evaluated with respect to an autobiographical self, a narrative "I." Hubert Hermans, Kempen, and van Loon provide an excellent review of the history of differentiating an objective "me" from a hermeneutic "I."

The locational dimension includes *clock time*, what the Greeks called *chronos* and Hermann Minkowski and Albert Einstein related to space. Locating begets space–time for a moving organism. Monitoring entails experiencing not only the duration, but also the decisive moment, what the Greeks referred to as *kairos*.

Unconscious Processing Freud had training in both medical practice and philosophy. When he emphasized the importance of unconscious processes, was he implying the medical definition or the philosophical definition? Most interpretations of Freud suggest that unconscious processes operate without awareness in the sense that they operate automatically, much like respiratory and gastrointestinal processes in someone who is stuporous or comatose. Freud himself seems to have promulgated this view by suggesting a horizontal split between conscious, preconscious, and unconscious processes, with repression operating to push memory-motive structures into deeper layers, where they no longer access awareness. Nevertheless, in the "Project for a Scientific Psychology," memory-motive structures are neural programs that are located in the core portions of the brain. These programs access awareness by their connections to cortex, which determine whether a memory-motivated wish comes to consciousness. When the neural program becomes a secondary process, it comes under voluntary control, which involves reality testing and, thus, consciousness. For example, it is possible to know two languages but, at any one time, "connect only one to cortex," and, thus, the other remains unconscious and unexpressed.

The thrust of most recent psychoanalytical thinking, as well as that of experimentalists, such as Jack Hilgard, is in the direction of interpreting the conscious–unconscious distinction in the philosophical sense. For instance, Matte Blanco proposes that consciousness be defined by the ability to make clear distinctions, to identify alternatives. Making clear distinctions would include being able to tell personal from extrapersonal reality. By contrast, unconscious processes would be composed of infinite sets "where paradox reigns and opposites merge into sameness." When infinities are being computed, the ordinary rules of logic do not hold. Thus, dividing a line of infinite length results in two lines of infinite length, that is, one equals two. Being deeply involved allows love and ecstasy, but also suffering and anger. In keeping with this paradoxical nature of unconscious processes, Carl Jung defined them as archetypical.

To bring the wellsprings of behavior and experience to consciousness is to make distinctions, provide alternatives, make choices, and become informed in Claude Shannon's sense of reduction of uncertainty. Clarity regarding the details of how such distinctions are achieved did not come until the late 1960s, when several theorists began to point out the difference between homeostatic feedback processes and homeorhetic feedforward programs. Feedback mechanisms depend on error processing and are therefore sensitive to perturbations. Feedfoward programs, like oral language, unless completely stopped, run to completion irrespective of obstacles placed in their way. A classic example of this tendency appears at conferences, when speakers are difficult to stop despite warnings by the chairman.

Of course, unconscious processes as defined by psychoanalysis are not completely submerged and unavailable to experience. Rather, unconscious processes produce feelings that are difficult to localize in time or space and difficult to identify correctly. Unconscious processes construct the emotional dispositions and motivational context within which extrapersonal and personal realities are constructed. Feelings are, to a large extent, undifferentiated, and humans tend to cognize and label them according to the circumstances in which they are manifest.

It is in this sense that behavior is under the control of the unconscious processes. During angry outbursts, individuals are certainly aware of their actions and the effects their anger has on others. Despite this awareness, however, the anger may be uncontrolled. Only when the events leading to the anger become clearly separated into alternative distinctions (alternative response possibilities) is unconscious control converted into conscious control. A person with an obsession or compulsion is not unaware, in the instrumental sense, of his experience or behavior. The patient is very aware of it and feels awful; however, without help, he or she cannot differentiate the necessary controls on the behavior.

Consequential Processing As is well known, frontal lesions were once produced to relieve intractable suffering, compulsions, obsessions, and endogenous depressions. When effective in relieving pain and depression, these psychosurgical procedures portrayed in humans the well-established relationship in nonhuman primates between the far frontal cortex and the limbic forebrain. Further, frontal lesions can lead either to perseverative, compulsive behavior or to distractibility in both monkeys and humans. Failure to be guided by the consequences of the behavior accounts for this effect; the opposite—the alleviation of obsessive-compulsive behavior—can also occur. Extreme forms of distractibility and obsession are due to a lack of sensitivity to feedback from consequences. The results of experiments with monkeys as well as clinical observations attest to the fact that subjects with frontal lesions, whether surgical, traumatic, or neoplastic, fail to be guided by consequences.

Consequences are the outcomes of behavior. In the tradition of the experimental analysis of behavior, consequences are reinforcers that influence the recurrence of the behavior. Consequences are, thus, a series of events (Latin *ex-venire*, meaning *outcome*), outcomes that guide action and thereby attain predictive value (as determined by confidence estimates). Such consequences self-organize to form their own confidence levels. These confidence levels, in turn, provide contexts that, in humans, become envisioned eventualities.

Confidence implies familiarity. Experiments on both monkeys and humans have shown that repeated arousal to an orienting stimulus habituates, that is, the orienting reaction gives way to familiarization. Limbic (amygdala) and frontal lesions disrupt familiarization. Ordinarily, familiarization allows continued activation of readiness; disruption of familiarization (repetitious orienting) leads to repeated distraction and, thus, a failure to allow consequences to form. Even when the process of familiarization is intact, it is still segmented (by occasional orienting reactions) into episodes within which confidence values can be established.

In such an episodic process, the development of confidence is a function of coherences and correlations among the events being processed. When coherence and correlation span multiple episodes, the organism becomes *committed* to a course of action (a prior intention, a strategy), which then guides further action, and is resistant to perturbation by particular orienting reactions (arousals). The organism is now *competent* to carry out the action (intention-in-action; tactic). Because particular outcomes now guide competent performance, orienting reactions are no longer produced.

This cascade, which characterizes episodic processing, leads ultimately to considerable autonomy of committed competence. Envisioned events are woven into a coherent story, a narrative, the myth by which the "I" lives. This narrative composes and is composed of an intention, a strategy that works for the individual in practice, a practical guide to action in achieving (temporary) stability in the face of a staggering range of options.

Consciousness is manifest (by verbal report) when familiarization is perturbed and an episode is updated and incorporated into a larger contextual scheme (the narrative) that includes both the familiar and novel episodes. Consciousness becomes attenuated when actions adhere to their guides and become skilled, graceful, and automatic.

Transcendental Consciousness—The Spiritual Nature of Humankind The contents of consciousness are not exhaustively described by the qualia of feelings of familiarity and novelty that are the basis for episodic and narrative consciousness, nor by those of allocentric and egocentric consciousness. The esoteric tradition in Western culture and the mystical traditions of the Far East are replete with instances of uncommon states that produce uncommon contents. These states are achieved by a variety of techniques, such as meditation, yoga, and Zen. The contents of processing in such states appear to differ from ordinary feelings and perceptions. Experiences are described as oceanic, a merging of corporeal and extracorporeal reality, or as out-of-body—that is, corporeal and extracorporeal realities continue to be clearly distinguished but are experienced by still another reality: "a meta-me." Alternatively, the "I" becomes transparent, a throughput experiencing everything everywhere; there is no longer the segmentation into episodes, nor are events enmeshed in a narrative structure.

All of these experiences have in common a transcendental relationship between ordinary experience and some more encompassing organizing principle. This relationship is ordinarily termed *spiritual.* The spiritual contents of consciousness can be accounted for by the effect of excessive excitation of the frontolimbic forebrain (ordinarily involved in narrative construction) on cortical receptive fields in the sensory extrinsic systems (ordinarily involved in the construction of objective reality).

In addition to the gross topological correspondence between cortical receptive fields and the organization of sensory surfaces that gives rise to the overall characteristics of processing in the extrinsic systems, a microprocess that depends on the internal organization of each receptive field comes into play. This internal organization of receptive fields embodies, among other characteristics, a spectral domain: Receptive fields of neurons in the extrinsic cortex are tuned to limited bandwidths of frequencies of radiant energy (vision), sound, and tactile vibration.

The most dramatic of these data are those that pertain to vision. The cortical neurons of the visual system are arranged, as they are in the other sensory systems, more or less isomorphically with the arrangement of the receptor surfaces to which they are connected (thus, the "homunculi" that Wilder Penfield and others have mapped onto the cortical surface of the extrinsic projection systems). However, within this gross arrangement lie the receptive fields of each of the neurons—a receptive field being determined by the dendritic arborization of the neuron that makes contact with the more peripheral parts of the system. Thus, the receptive field of a neuron is the part of the environment that is processed by the part of the system to which the neuron is connected. Each receptive field is sensitive to approximately an octave (range from $1/2$ to $1\,1/2$ octaves) of spatial frequency. This frequency-selective microprocess operates in a holographic-like manner.

Processing can thus be conceived to operate somewhat like the production of music by means of a piano. The sensory surface is analogous to a keyboard. Keyboard and strings are isomorphically related to provide the overall organization of the process. When individual strings are activated, they resonate over a limited bandwidth of frequency. It is the combination of the spatial arrangement and the frequency-specific resonance of the strings that makes the production of music possible.

The gross organization and microorganization of the cortical neurons in the extrinsic systems resemble the organization of the piano in that an overall spatial arrangement is supplemented by resonances specific to the strings that become activated. In the case of the sensory cortex, the "strings" are the dendritic fields of the neurons. Mathematically, the resonances of these dendritic receptive fields can be described by a Gabor wavelet, which David Gabor called a *quantum of information.* A gaussian envelope constrains the otherwise unlimited sinusoid described by a Fourier transform to make up the Gabor wavelet. Experiments have shown that electrical excitation of frontal and limbic structures relaxes the gaussian constraints that are manifest as inhibitory surrounds or flanks in the receptive field architecture. There is neuropsychological evidence that indicates that when the constraints relax during ordinary excitation of the frontolimbic systems, processing leads to narrative construction. When frontolimbic excitation becomes overwhelming, experience is determined by an unconstrained holistic, holographic-like process.

The mathematical descriptions of holographic-like processes of the type involved in brain function are composed by converting (e.g., via Fourier transformations) successive sensory images (e.g., frames of a movie film) into their spectral representations and patching these microrepresentations into orderly spatial arrangements that represent the original temporal order. The spectral domain is peculiar in that information (in the Gabor sense) becomes both distributed over the extent of each receptive field (each *quantum*) and enfolded within it. Thus, sensory image reconstruction can occur from any part of the total aggregate of receptive fields. This is what gives the aggregate its holographic, holistic aspect. All input becomes distributed and enfolded, including the dimensions of space and time and, therefore, causality. It is this apparently timeless/spaceless/causeless aspect of processing, instigated by overwhelming frontolimbic excitation, that is responsible for the extrasensory dimensions of experience that characterize the esoteric traditions. Because of their enfolded property, these processes tend to swamp distinctions, such as corporeal and extracorporeal reality.

An intriguing and related development (because it deals with the specification of a more encompassing "cosmic" order) has occurred in quantum physics. Over the past 50 years, it has become clear that there is a limit to the accuracy with which certain measurements can be made when others are being taken. This limit is expressed as an indeterminacy. Gabor, in his description of a quantum of information, showed that a similar indeterminacy holds for communication: The Gabor wavelet describes a limit to the amount of information that can be compressed for processing. Thus, the understanding of the microstructure of communication converges with observation of the microstructure of matter. This need to specify the observations that lead to the inference of the properties of matter has led noted physicists to write a representation of the observer into the description of the observable. Some physicists have noted the similarity of this specification to some of the esoteric descriptions of consciousness.

The scientific and esoteric traditions have clearly been at odds since the time of Galileo. Each new scientific discovery and the theory developed from it has, until recently, resulted in widening the rift between objective science and the hermeneutic spiritual aspects of human nature. The rift reached a maximum toward the end of the 19th century: Humankind was asked to choose between God and Darwin; Freud proposed that heaven and hell resided within the individual and not in his or her relationship to the natural universe. The discoveries of 20th century science, however, do no fit this mold. For once, the recent findings of science and the spiritual experiences of humankind are consonant. This augurs well for the new millennium—a science that comes to terms with the spiritual nature of humankind may well outstrip the technological science of the immediate past in its contribution to human welfare.

The brain models of mind have a consistent history. However, this consistency has been obscured by controversy. Controversy, however, can be resolved in each instance by carefully defining concepts and referring to the original descriptions of data.

In this section, defining *mind* and *minding* related brain states to the contents of conscious experience. States of consciousness were shown to coordinate with neurochemical states. The relationship of state to content, or minding, was shown to devolve on attention, volition, and thought. Brain systems coordinate with emotion, motivation, and effort were shown to control the mental processes of attention, intention, and thought. Finally, the contents of consciousness were shown to fall into three major categories: (1) the construction of egocentric and allocentric reality by virtue of processing by systems of the posterior cerebral convexity; (2) the construction of an autobiographical narrative composed of episodes and eventualities as processed by the frontolimbic forebrain; and (3) a transcendental holistic category that releases a quantum-like cortical dendritic microprocess from the spatiotemporal constraints essential to the construction of an objective "me" embedded in an objective world and a narrative "I," with its multiple hermeneutic possibilities for expression.

SUGGESTED CROSS-REFERENCES

Sections 1.2 and 1.3 discuss neuroanatomy, Section 1.9 discusses electrophysiology; Section 3.1 discusses perception and cognition; Section 6.1 discusses psychoanalysis; and Section 31.31 discusses psychosurgery.

References

Ashby WR. *Design for a Brain: The Origin of Adaptive Behavior.* 2nd ed. New York: Wiley; 1960.

*Avi G, Amir B: Brain organization and psychodynamics. *J Psychother Pract Res.* 1999;8:24.

Bekesy Von G. *Sensory Inhibition.* New Jersey: Princeton University Press; 1967.

Bogen JE, Bogen GM: The other side of the brain III: The corpus callosum and creativity. *Bull Los Angeles Neurol Soc.* 1969;34:191.

Bracewell RN. The Fourier transform. *Sci Am.* 1989;260:86.

Brentano F. *Psychologie vom empirischen Standpunki.* Vol. 3. In: Mayer-Hillebrand F, ed. *Vom sinnlichen und noetischen Bewusfstsein.* 2nd ed. Hamburg: Felix Meiner; 1968.

Bucy PC. *The Precentral Motor Cortex.* Chicago: University of Illinois Press, 1944.

Cannon WB. The James-Lange theory of emotions: a critical examination and an alternative theory. *Am J Psychol.* 1927;32:106.

Efron R. *The Decline and Fall of Hemispheric Specialization.* New York: Erlbaum; 1989.

Gabor D: Theory of communication. *J Inst Elect Eng.* 1946;93:429.

Gall FJ, Spurtzheim G. Research on the nervous system in general and on that of the brain in particular. In: KH Pribram, ed. *Brain and Behavior.* Middlesex, England: Penguin; 1969.

Gazzaniga MS. *The Social Brain: Discovering the Network of the Mind.* New York: Basic Books; 1985.

Hermans HJM, Kempen HJG, van Loon RJP: The dialogical self: beyond individualism and rationalism. *Am Psychol.* 1992;47:23.

Hilgard ER. *Divided Consciousness: Multiple Controls in Human Thought and Action.* New York: Wiley; 1977.

Hinton GE, Anderson JA. *Parallel Models of Associative Memory.* Hillsdale, NJ: Erlbaum; 1981.

Jaynes J. *The Origin of Consciousness in the Breakdown of the Bicameral Mind.* Boston: Houghton-Mifflin; 1990.

John ER. *Mechanisms of Memory.* New York: Academic; 1967.

Kelso JAS, Saltzman EL: Motor control: Which themes do we orchestrate? *Behav Brain Sci.* 1982;5:554.

Lashley D. The thalamus and emotion. In: Beach FA, Hebb DO, Morgan CT, Nissen HW, eds. *The Neuropsychology of Lashley.* New York: McGraw-Hill, 1960.

Llinás R. *I of the Vortex.* Cambridge, MA: MIT Press; 2001.

Matte Blanco I. *The Unconscious as Infinite Sets.* London: Gerald Duckworth Ltd; 1975.

McFarland DJ. *Feedback Mechanisms in Animal Behavior.* London: Academic Press; 1971.

Miller GA, Galanter A, Pribram KH. *Plans and the Structure of Behavior.* New York: Henry Holt; 1960.

Neumann E. *The Origins and History of Consciousness.* Princeton, NJ: Princeton University Press; 1954.

Olds J, Milner P: Positive reinforcement produced by electrical stimulation of septal area and other regions of rat brain. *J Comp Physiol Psychol.* 1954;47:419.

Peirce CS. *Pragmatism and Pragmaticism: Collected Papers.* Vol. 5. Cambridge, MA: Harvard University Press; 1934.

Pribram KH. The intrinsic systems of the forebrain. In: Field, Mogoan HW, Hall VE, eds. *Handbook of Physiology, Neurophysiology*. Washington, DC: American Psychological Society; 1960.

Pribram KH. Limbic system. In: Sheer DE, ed. *Electrical Stimulation of the Brain*. Austin, TX: University of Texas Press; 1961.

Pribram KH. *Languages of the Brain: Experimental Paradoxes and Principles in Neuropsychology*. Englewood Cliffs, NJ: Prentice-Hall; 1971.

Pribram KH. How is it that sensing so much we can do so little? In: Schmitt FO, Worden FLG, eds. *Central Processing of Sensory Input*, MIT Press, Cambridge, MA, 1974.

Pribram KH, Gill M. *Freud's "Project" Reassessed*. New York: Basic Books; 1976.

Pribram KH. Localization and distribution of function in the brain. In: Orbach J, ed. *Neuropsychology after Lashley*. Hillsdale, NJ: Erlbaum Associates; 1982.

Pribram KH. *Brain and Perception: Holonomy and Structure in Figural Processing*. New York: Erlbaum; 1991.

Pribram KH. The deep and surface structure of memory and conscious learning: toward a 21st century model. In: Solso RL, ed. *Mind and Brain Sciences in the 21st Century*. Cambridge, MA: MIT Press; 1997.

Pribram KH. What is mind that the brain may order it. In: Mandreka V, Masani PR, eds. *Proceedings of the Norbert Weiner Centenary Congress, 1994*. Providence, RI: American Mathematical Society; 1997.

*Pribram KH: The composition of conscious experience. *J Conscious Studies*. 1999;6:20.

*Pribram KH. The primary of conscious experience. In: Amoroso RL, Antunes R, Coelho C, Farias M, Leite A, Soares P, eds. *Science and the Primacy of Consciousness*. Orinda, CA: Noetic; 1999.

Pribram KH: Forebrain psychophysiology of feelings: Interest and involvement. *Int J Psychophysiol*. 2003;48:115–131.

Pribram KH. Consciousness reassessed. *Mind and Matter (in press)*.

Pribram KH, McGuinness D: Arousal activation and effort in the control of attention. *Psychol Rev*. 1975;82:116.

Pribram KH, Reitz S, McNeil M, Spevack AA: The effect of amygdalectomy on orienting and classical conditioning in monkeys. *Pavlov J Biol Sci*. 1979;14:203.

Rumelhart DE, McClelland JL, and the PDP Research Group. *Parallel Distributed Processing*. Vols. 1 and 2. Cambridge, MA: MIT Press; 1986.

Schachter S, Singer TE: Cognitive, social and physiological determinants of emotional state. *Psychol Rev*. 1962;69:379.

Searle JR. *The Mystery of Consciousness*. New York: New York Review of Books; 1997.

Thatcher RW, John ER. *Functional Neuroscience*. Vol. 1. Hillsdale, NJ: Erlbaum; 1977.

Weiskrantz L. *Blindsight: A Case Study and Implications*. Oxford: Clarendon Press; 1986.

▲ 3.6 Neuroscientific Bases of Consciousness and Dreaming

RODOLFO R. LLINÁS, M.D., PH.D.

Attempting to understand how the brain, as a whole, might be organized has now become a topic of inquiry that is addressable from a neuronal viewpoint. One aspect of the brain's neuronal organization that seems particularly central to global function is the rich thalamocortical interconnectivity and, most particularly, the reciprocal nature of the thalamocortical neuronal loop. Moreover, the interaction between the specific and nonspecific thalamic loops suggests that, rather than a simple gate into the brain, the thalamus represents a hub from which any site in the cortex can communicate with any other cortical site or sites. The goals of this chapter are to explore (1) the basic assumption that large-scale, temporal coincidence of specific and nonspecific thalamic activity generates, via temporal binding, the functional states that characterize human cognition and (2) the possible relation of such binding to some neuropsychiatric conditions.

COGNITION AS AN INTRINSIC FUNCTIONAL STATE OF THE BRAIN

It was suggested more than a decade ago that consciousness is an oneiric-like functional state that is modulated, rather than generated, by the senses. According to this view, the internal events, such as thinking, imagining, or remembering, are strictly confined to intrinsic neuronal activity looping continuously through the brain's neuronal circuits. This proposal is supported by the fact that a large percentage of the brain's connectivity is recurrent and is not necessarily driven by sensory input but rather by intrinsic neuronal activity.

Thus, consciousness (i.e., being awake and able to feel, to judge, to respond, and to remember) is but one functional state of the brain. Other conditions, such as being in one of the many dreamless sleep states, do not support consciousness or even the feeling of self-awareness. Perhaps the most spectacular difference concerning global brain states is that between wakefulness and dreamless delta sleep. It is recognized that there are no gross morphological changes in the brain during sleep that could explain the enormous disparity between sleep and wakefulness. The difference, of necessity, is functional. If a strong sensory stimulus occurs during sleep (e.g., the havoc wrought by an alarm clock), a person can awaken extraordinarily fast. It is also clear that, given the large number of neuronal elements involved, the only substrate capable of supporting the speed of these changes from one state to the other must be electrical and time coherent in nature. That is, the globally organized electrical activity of neurons and their synaptic interactions comprise the only mechanism that is fast enough to initiate or terminate abruptly wakefulness from the dream state. These, together with the speed with which humans can perceive and respond to their environment, are among the most important clues concerning the nature of consciousness.

Concerning the localization of such activity, it is known from classical neurology that damage to the cerebral cortex in mammals can cause a variety of well-defined dysfunctional conditions that modify or curtail consciousness. Visual cortex damage is accompanied by blindness that can be of different types depending on the precise location of the cortical insult. Similar findings are also encountered in other cortical structures. Thus, injuries to the auditory, somatosensory, motor, or premotor cortices are accompanied by well-defined conditions. In fact, the first such neurological lesion to be described in the terms used previously was that after damage of Broca' s area, generating dysarthria.

Given the previous statement, it has been historically accepted that consciousness can be equated with cortical function, more or less exclusively. However, this view ignores the fact that the nervous system is deeply cursive in its connectivity. As such, a dynamically recurrent corticosubcortical organization is more likely than a strictly hierarchical organization.

There are several other problems with the hierarchical proposal relating to the categorization of cortical activity into ever increasing functional specialization. This hierarchy converges into the famous grandmother neuron concept (i.e., the idea that specialized neurons represent each object in cognition, for example, the image of a person's grandmother). Among the problems with the hierarchical proposal are (1) The number of possible percepts is much larger than the total number of neurons in the cortical mantle. To make the matter worse, given the proposed hierarchical architecture, the number of such neurons would have to be a small percentage of all cortical neurons. (2) Another difficulty with a hierarchical model is that of sampling size. Indeed, the number of specialized neurons, each representing a component of reality, would be so exorbitantly large that addressing specific neuronal elements would make the retrieval problem immense. Thus, even considering that neuronal elements integrate and transmit signals at a millisecond rate from the onset of sensory primitives, exhausting all sequential combinations of all grandmother cells would be awkwardly time intensive. This is, however, not the case concerning cognition. It takes roughly the same amount of time to recognize that a face is familiar as it takes to recognize that it is not. Yet, in any sequential strategy, it would take much longer to conclude no familiarity (as it would require comparing it with "all known faces") than it would to conclude familiarity (the search would proceed for only as long as necessary to "find" the match). From a different perspective, the grandmother neuron hypothesis fails to explain how the unique perceptual insights of such neurons (the specific elements in a given category) are communicated to the rest of the nervous system. How do grandmother cells tell the rest of the neurons what they know, given their unique position at the top of a hierarchy?

Alternatively, if categories are generated by spatiotemporal mapping in the thalamocortical system, a dynamic representation based on temporal coherence would have the necessary speed to support cognition time constants. Thus, a simultaneity mapping may be envisioned that takes advantage of the parallel and synchronous organization of brain networks to generate cognition.

THALAMOCORTICAL GAMMA-BAND RESONANT COLUMNS

The hypotheses to be discussed in the following section are derived from two areas of research: (1) single neuron and network electrophysiological recordings made in vivo and in vitro in animals and (2) measurements made using noninvasive imaging of human brain function, in particular, present day magnetoencephalography (MEG). The central issue to be discussed is the assumption that the intrinsic electrical properties of neurons, and the dynamic events resulting from their connectivity, result in global resonant states known as *consciousness*.

Given this approach, two related views are presently considered in the literature regarding the actual mechanism for this functional condition. One view is that coherent events occur at the cortical level and that such cortical events are the primary binding substrate. A second view proposes that the binding event must be thalamocortical rather than purely cortical. Some of the reasons for supporting the latter view are sketched in the following discussion.

Even though the cortex receives a large number of nonthalamic inputs, damage to the thalamus is cognitively equivalent to damage to the cortex to which it projects. Experimental results from studies using noninvasive techniques, such as MEG in humans, as well as animal research using extracellular and intracellular recordings in vivo, indicate that cognition is supported by resonant recurrent electrical activity between thalamic and cortical structures at gamma-band frequencies (i.e., having a 25- to 50-Hz oscillatory frequency), often centered close to 40 Hz. Such findings favor the hypothesis that cognitive events depend on activity involving thalamocortical resonant columns. Indeed, the neuronal mechanisms responsible for the high-frequency thalamic oscillations that support thalamocortical synchronization and coherence are beginning to be understood.

OSCILLATORY PROPERTIES OF THALAMIC CELLS

In the early 1980s, it was suggested that the presence of neuronal elements with intrinsic oscillatory or resonant properties in a network would facilitate coherence between interconnected elements. Moreover, in a recent series of in vitro studies, the intrinsic electrical properties of thalamic neurons that support gamma-band frequencies (25 to 50 Hz) have been characterized. These proved to be subthreshold oscillations that were generated at the dendritic level (see the following discussion) when thalamic neurons were depolarized beyond –45 mV (Fig. 3.6–1B). Indeed, the neuronal mechanism underlying the generation of gamma oscillations has been studied at

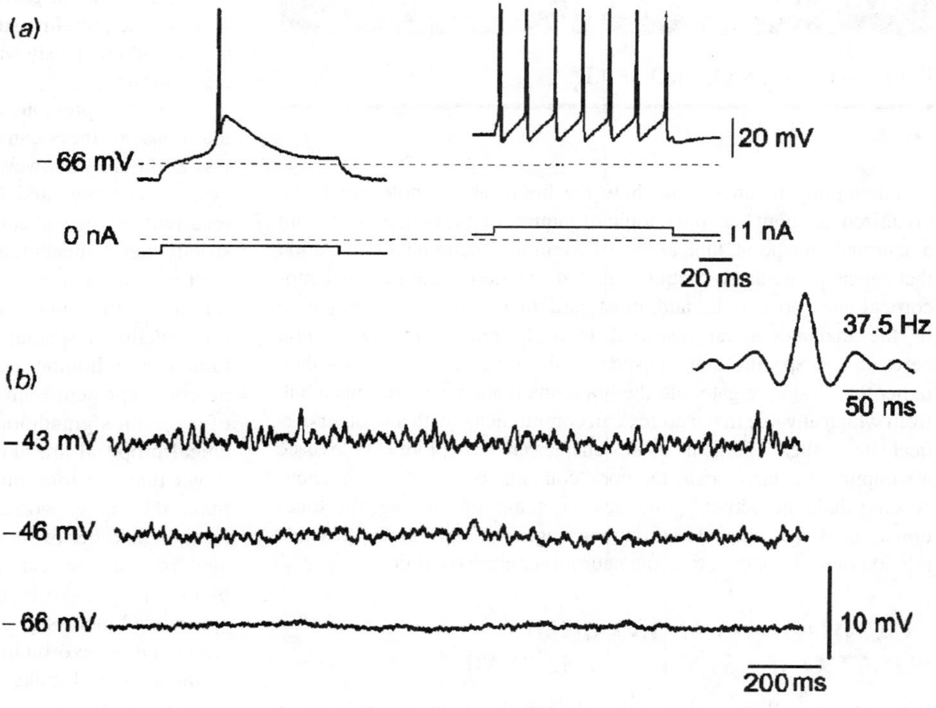

FIGURE 3.6–1 Oscillatory properties of thalamic neurons. In vitro intracellular recording from a thalamic neuron. **A:** Direct activation of a thalamic cell from a resting potential of –66 mV **(left panel)** evoked a short burst of spikes triggered by the activation of a low-threshold calcium conductance. The same amplitude direct activation at a resting potential near –40 mV **(right panel)** evoked tonic repetitive firing. **B:** High-frequency subthreshold oscillations were evoked by protracted outward direct current injection through the recording microelectrode (bringing the membrane to –46 mV and –43 mV). The autocorrelogram in the inset corresponds to the –43-mV trace. (Modified from Pedroarena C, Llinás R: Dendritic calcium conductances generate high-frequency oscillation in thalamocortical neurons. *Proc Natl Acad Sci U S A.* 1997;94:724–728, with permission.)

the level of single neurons and of neuronal circuits at sites other than the thalamus. For example, it has been shown that the membrane potential of sparsely spiny inhibitory neurons in cortical layer IV supports gamma-frequency membrane voltage oscillations (Fig. 3.6–1). The mechanism for the oscillation, in this case, is the sequential activation of a persistent low-threshold sodium current. In contrast, fast oscillations in thalamocortical cells depend on the activation of voltage-gated calcium channels.

Dendritic oscillations are functionally significant because the return input from the cortex to thalamic neurons terminates in distal dendritic segments, providing a unique opportunity for resonance between intrinsic dendritic oscillation and thalamic synaptic inputs. This issue is of further significance because waking and rapid eye movement (REM) sleep states are associated with thalamic neuron depolarization, whereas slow wave sleep is associated with thalamic hyperpolarization. The two levels of membrane potential each elicit a different intrinsic oscillatory property in thalamic cells. Given the previous statement, it can be concluded that coherence of fast rhythms in thalamocortical loops depends on the pattern of synaptic inputs and on the responsive state of the neurons as modulated by their intrinsic properties.

Because sensory inputs generate but a fractured representation of universals, the issue of perceptual unity concerns the mechanisms that allow these different sensory components to be gathered into one global image. In recent years, this has been described as *binding*, and one of the mechanisms proposed for such implementation is known as *temporal conjunction*.

Synchronous neuronal activation during sensory input has been studied in mammalian visual cortical cells as light bars of optimal orientation and displacement rate are presented. The components of a visual stimulus that correspond to a singular cognitive object, for example, a line in a visual field, yield coherent gamma-band oscillations in regions of the cortex that may be as far as 7 mm apart or that may even be in the contralateral cortex. Moreover, gamma-band oscillatory activity between related cortical columns is highly correlated under such circumstances. In addition, MEG recordings demonstrated coherent 40-Hz thalamocortical oscillations in an awake human in the early 1990s. These oscillations could be reset by sensory stimuli and displayed a high degree of spatial organization. This geometrical peculiarity makes such an oscillatory frequency particularly apt to support the temporal conjunction of rhythmic activity over a large ensemble of neurons, while conserving a high degree of spatial differentiation.

The possibility of coherent temporal-spatial conjunction in thalamocortical circuits has been supported by the direct imaging of the spatiotemporal distribution of afferent activity using voltage-sensitive dye imaging in rodent visual cortex in vitro. Indeed, the delivery of two cortical afferent inputs repeated at low frequency (10 Hz or less) gave rise to two waves of excitation (Fig. 3.6–2, upper left quadrant) that moved horizontally and summed over a wide cortical area (Fig. 3.6–2, upper right quadrant) with a time course of 10 milliseconds. This spatial distribution of activity lacks the high granularity required for a rich cognitive discrimination and does not conform with the specific columnarity observed in the somatosensory and visual cortices. In contrast, when stimuli were delivered at a higher frequency (40 Hz), the geometry of activation was rapidly restricted to submillimeter areas, that is, to cortical column size (Fig. 3.6–2A, lower right panel), rather than the wider geometry observed with low-frequency activation.

These results agree with data showing that slow frequency brain rhythms (less than 15 Hz), such as those characteristic of slow wave sleep (e.g., sleep spindles and slow oscillations), demonstrate long-range cortical coherence sometimes spanning the entire neocortex. In contrast, during activated states, such as walking or REM sleep, high-frequency oscillations (20 to 50 Hz) show a pattern of coherence that is restricted to its immediate vicinity or occurs between distant discrete areas. More fundamentally, however, a pharmacological examination of the mechanism by which the granularity of activation is engendered indicates that the areas of silence between patches of activity at 40 Hz are generated by active inhibition. Thus, in the presence of γ-aminobutyric acid (GABA) blockers, the spatial filtering of cortical activity described previously disappears. These results clearly agree with the findings that cortical inhibitory neurons are capable of high-frequency oscillation and with the view that, if such neurons are synaptically coupled and fire in synchrony, they might be formative in generating cortical gamma-band activity.

Such in vivo findings suggest yet another function for coherent inhibition at the cortical level: that of generating the *thalamocortical resonant column*. From this point of view, the thalamocortical resonant column would comprise a basic functional unit in the generation of consciousness. Thus, these columns may be viewed as a permissive network endowed with frequency-gated spatial filter properties. Accordingly, frequency forges activity into a well-specified cortical activation geometry by increasing the encoding contrast, as the activity areas are intensified and focused by gamma-band oscillation. By increasing the contrast between activation and inhibition, such an organization may underlie the columnar organization observed in vivo during visual stimulation of the cortical mantle. This would have the added advantage of a thalamocortical resonance that might link this expanded columnar activation into the binding patterns required for consciousness.

When the interconnectivity of the thalamic nuclei is combined with the intrinsic properties of the individual neurons, a network for resonant neuronal oscillation emerges in which specific cortico-thalamocortical circuits would tend to resonate at gamma frequency. According to this hypothesis, neurons at different levels, most particularly, those in the reticular nucleus, would be responsible for the synchronization of gamma oscillation at distant thalamic and cortical sites, especially because it has been shown that neighboring reticular nucleus cells may be electrotonically coupled.

BINDING OF SPECIFIC AND NONSPECIFIC GAMMA-BAND ACTIVITY

Coherent Gamma-Band Thalamocortical Activity and Temporal Binding Given the spatially fractured nature of sensory representation over the cortex, activity such as that described previously addresses fundamental issues concerning the mechanism responsible for the unity of perception. As stated previously, one possibility is that such binding occurs via temporal coincidence of specific and nonspecific thalamocortical synaptic activation of the apical dendrites of pyramidal cells. This activation would result in the generation of outgoing pyramidal action potentials that would return to the thalamus and establish a resonant thalamocortical reactivation loop. Because many such loops are activated simultaneously, coherent function can be supported in brain areas remote from each other. These large sets of isochronous events, supported by the oscillatory properties of thalamic neurons, can conjoin all sensory inputs on the basis of temporal coincidence. For this mechanism to be useful,

FIGURE 3.6–2 ▶ **A:** Voltage imaging of cortical brain activity in a rodent slice. **Upper left panel:** Averaged snapshots at 5 and 10 milliseconds to stimulation at 10 Hz. **Lower left and right panels:** Averaged snapshots at 5 and 10 milliseconds in response to stimulation at 40 Hz. The color of the image represents membrane potential of the stained neurons, depolarized (*red*) and hyperpolarized (*purple*) (see color bar to the right). Dotted lines indicated the upper and lower cortical borders in the slice. White dots represent the position of the bipolar stimulating electrodes at the subcortical white matter. Note that, at 10 milliseconds after the start of 10-Hz stimulation, the cortical activity covered most of the cortex in the slice **(upper left)**, whereas, at 40 Hz, the activation became columnar, demonstrating that the geometry of cortical activation is frequency dependent. (Adapted from Llinás R, Ribary U, Contreras D, Pedroarena C: The neuronal basis for consciousness. *Philos Trans R Soc Lond.* 1998;353:1841–1849.) **B:** Voltage imaging of thalamocortical activation in the rodent brain slice. Average of a set of single pulse stimulation of thalamic nuclei. Centrolateral (CL) **(left panel)** and ventrobasal (VB) **(right panel)**. The spread of activity after CL and VB stimulation is superimposed on the Nissl's method–stained brain slice. CL and VB stimulation activated reticular nucleus followed by striatum. A different set of patterns of cortical activation was observed for each stimulation site. Although VB stimulation activated layers 4, 2/3, and 5, CL stimulation activated layers 6, 7, and 1. Left and right insets correspond to individual pixel profiles at reticular thalamic nucleus (RTN) (*white lines*), striatum-putamen (Str/Pu) (*blue lines*), layer 5 (*green lines*), and layer 1 (*red lines*) after CL and VB stimulation, respectively, illustrating differences in the latencies. The average delay between the site of stimulation and the point of recording (measured as time between the stimulus and the beginning of the individual pixel responses) is shown in the table under each slice. (Adapted from Llinás R, Leznik E, Urbano IF: Temporal binding via coincidence detection of specific and non-specific thalamocortical inputs: A voltage dependent dye imaging study in mouse brain slices. *Proc Natl Acad Sci U S A.* 2002;99:449–454.) **C:** Voltage imaging of thalamocortical temporal binding in the rodent brain slice. Optically recorded in response to gamma-frequency stimulation in the somatosensory cortex, in response to ten stimuli to CL **(upper panel)**, VB **(middle panel)**, and VB and CL thalamic nuclei simultaneously **(lower panel)**. The response to the fifth stimulus was imaged in each case. Note the marked summation of the response when CL and VB stimuli are presented simultaneously. On the right, the profiles of a single pixel taken from layer 5 are shown for the three different stimulation conditions. Summation was supralinear. (Adapted from Llinás R, Leznik E, Urbano IF: Temporal binding via coincidence detection of specific and non-specific thalamocortical inputs: A voltage dependent dye imaging study in mouse brain slices. *Proc Natl Acad Sci U S A.* 2002;99:449–454.) **D:** Diagram of two thalamocortical systems. Specific sensory or motor nuclei project to cortex layer 4, producing cortical oscillation by direct activation and feedforward inhibition via 40-Hz inhibitory interneurons. Collaterals of these projections produce thalamic feedback inhibition via the reticular nucleus. The return pathway (*circular arrow on the right*) returns this oscillation to specific- and reticularis-thalamic nuclei via pyramidal cells in layer 6 (*blue*). The second loop shows nonspecific intralaminar nuclei projecting to the most superficial layer of the cortex and giving collaterals to the reticular nucleus. Pyramidal cells in layer 5 return the oscillation to the reticular and the nonspecific thalamic nuclei, establishing a second resonant loop. The conjunction of the specific and nonspecific loops is proposed to generate temporal cognitive binding. (Adapted from Llinás R, Leznik E, Urbano IF: Temporal binding via coincidence detection of specific and non-specific thalamocortical inputs: A voltage dependent dye imaging study in mouse brain slices. *Proc Natl Acad Sci U S A.* 2002;99:449–454.) **E:** Magnetoencephalography data from a thalamocortical dysrhythmia (TCD) patient. Power spectra **(upper panels)** and coherence plots **(lower panels)** are displayed. **Top left panel:** Averaged power spectra from control subjects (*blue*) and a TCD patient (*red*). A peak shift into the theta domain and power increase in the theta and beta bands are demonstrated for TCD patients in comparison to controls. **Top right panel:** Power spectrum of a schizoaffective patient presurgery (*red*) and after microsurgery (*blue*). **Bottom panels:** Coherence determined by cross-correlation analysis of the variation along time of the spectral power for frequencies between 0 and 40 Hz. Left panel shows results from a control subject. The middle and right panels illustrate pre- and postsurgical coherence results for the power spectrum shown in the upper right panel. (Adapted from Llinás R, Ribary U, Jeanmonod D, et al.: Thalamocortical dysrhythmia I: Functional and imaging aspects. *Thalamus Related Syst.* 2001;1:237–244.) **F:** Magnetoencephalography source localization for a schizoaffective patient before and after selective miniablation. Projection of 4- to 10-Hz activity onto a magnetic resonance image of the whole brain, before **(top images)** and after **(bottom images)** surgery. The TCD of this patient was localized in the right-sided paralimbic domain comprising the temporopolar, anterior parahippocampal, orbitofrontal, and basal medial prefrontal areas. This low-frequency focus disappears postsurgically. (Adapted from Jeanmonod D, Schulman J, Ramirez R, et al.: Neuropsychiatric thalamocortical dysrythmia: Surgical implications. *Thalamus Related Syst.* 2003;2:103–113.) (See Color Plate to follow color directions in legend.)

the specific thalamic inputs must constantly update cortical structures about external events (content), whereas the nonspecific thalamic inputs serve to bind content information on the basis of internal significance (context) arising from association cortices. According to this hypothesis, the activation of the thalamus via corticothalamic recurrent activity would serve to maintain a self-supporting feedback activity loop that is continuously modified by the incoming sensory information. The hypothesis that specific and nonspecific thalamocortical inputs can sum in pyramidal cell dendrites was tested experimentally using voltage-sensitive dye imaging in an in vitro thalamocortical slice preparation. In these experiments, specific (ventrobasal [VB]) and nonspecific (centrolateral [CL]) thalamic nuclei were stimulated at gamma-band frequency. The spread of activity from VB and CL nuclei into the cortex and the interaction of their activity at the cortex were imaged directly.

A representative spread of activity for VB and CL stimulation is superimposed on a Nissl's method–stained thalamocortical slice in Figure 3.6–2B. VB stimulation was followed by synaptic activation of reticular nucleus, striatum-putamen, and the somatosensory cortex. In the cortex, layer 4 activation was continued by the radial spread of activity to layers 2/3 and 5. By contrast, although CL stimulation was also followed by the activation of reticular nucleus and striatum-putamen, it activated different cortical layers at the cortical level, and the activity within cortical layers 5, 6, and 1 was more widespread. These results show that, in thalamocortical slices, there is specific and nonspecific thalamic nuclei connectivity to the somatosensory primary cortex, thus, supporting the hypothesis that temporal binding occurs between specific and nonspecific thalamic inputs at gamma-band frequency.

Temporal Binding of CL and VB Nuclear Activity at Cortical Level

The last set of experiments in this series investigated whether the gamma-band temporal binding of specific and nonspecific thalamic nuclei activity could be visualized using voltage-dependent dye imaging. The distribution of the activity during 40-Hz stimulation of the VB and CL nuclei demonstrated a supralinear summation of the individual VB and CL responses. Indeed, at gamma-band frequency, the focus of cortical activity increases for the duration of the train (Fig. 3.6–2C), as previously demonstrated for subcortical white matter stimulation.

Thus, specific and nonspecific thalamocortical inputs sum supralinearly in cortex in a time sensitive fashion, where coincidence of layers 1 and 4 activation is integrated at the cortex, most probably over the apical dendrite of layers 5 and 6 pyramidal cells. This is a central issue, because these two layers represent the return output to thalamus (via layer 6) and the main output to the rest of the nervous system (via layer 5). Concerning the thalamocortical projections, the fact that the nonspecific system activates cortical layer 1 is in agreement with the anatomical distributions of these terminal axons and addresses the importance of synaptic inputs to the tuft of pyramidal cell apical dendrites in that layer.

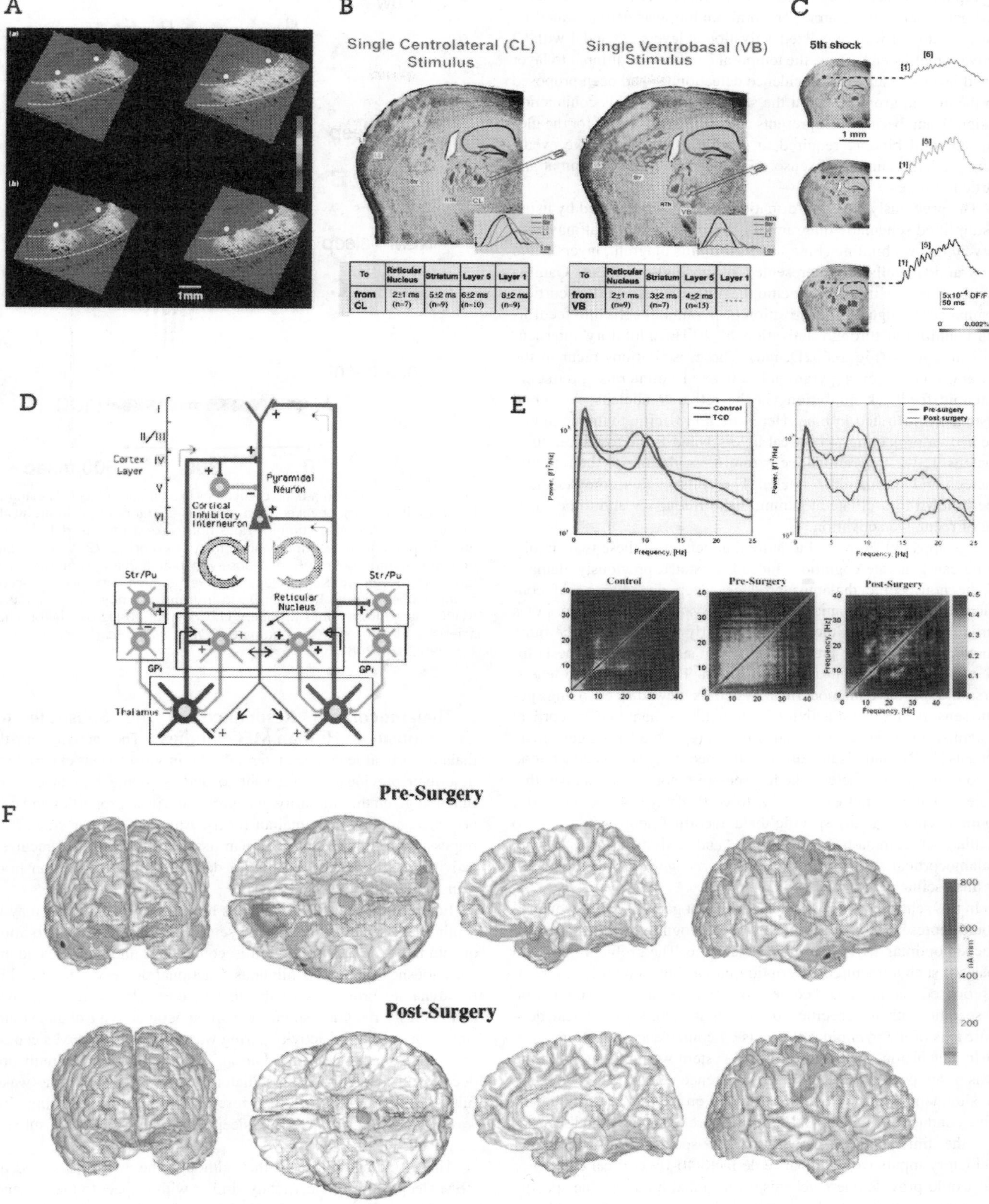
A
(a)
(b)
1mm
B
Single Centrolateral (CL) Stimulus
Single Ventrobasal (VB) Stimulus
RTN
CL
VB
To | Reticular Nucleus | Striatum | Layer 5 | Layer 1
from CL | 2±1 ms (n=7) | 5±2 ms (n=9) | 6±2 ms (n=10) | 8±2 ms (n=9)
To | Reticular Nucleus | Striatum | Layer 5 | Layer 1
from VB | 2±1 ms (n=9) | 3±2 ms (n=7) | 4±2 ms (n=15) | ----
C
5th shock
[1]
[6]
1 mm
[5]
50 ms
0.002%
D
I
II/III
Cortex Layer
IV
V
VI
Pyramidal Neuron
Cortical Inhibitory Interneuron
Str/Pu
GPi
Reticular Nucleus
Thalamus
E
Control
TCD
Pre-surgery
Post-surgery
Frequency, [Hz]
Control
Pre-Surgery
Post-Surgery
F
Pre-Surgery
Post-Surgery
800
600
400
200

Input to the dendritic tuft has been shown experimentally to serve as a coincidence integrator. Temporal binding was demonstrated by the summing of well organized activation at layers 2/3 and 4 with Cl activation of layer 1. Thus, the temporal conjunction of input to layer 1 and layer 4 results in coincidence detection, as had been proposed on theoretical grounds and at the single cell level. This conjunction is significant, because it represents a possible mechanism for the global temporal binding required to generate single cognitive events from the large number of sensory inputs arriving at the brain at any particular time.

The previously stated information may be summarized by using a simplified schematic diagram of a neuronal circuit that may subserve temporal binding (Fig. 3.6–2D). In this diagram, layers 5 and 6 pyramidal cells are represented by a single element. Gamma oscillations in neurons in specific thalamic nuclei establish cortical resonance through direct activation of pyramidal cells and feedforward inhibition through activation of 40-Hz inhibitory interneurons in layer 4 (Fig. 3.6–2D, red). These oscillations recur in the thalamus via layer 4 pyramidal cell axon collaterals, producing thalamic feedback inhibition via the reticular nucleus. A second system is illustrated in blue. Here, the nonspecific thalamic nuclei are shown projecting to cortical layers 1 and 5 and to the reticular nucleus. Layer 5 pyramidal cells return oscillations to the reticular nucleus and intralaminar nuclei. The cells in this complex have been shown to oscillate at gamma-band frequency and to be capable of recursive activation.

It is apparent from the literature that neither of these two circuits alone can generate cognition. Indeed, as stated previously, damage of the nonspecific thalamus produces deep disturbances of consciousness, whereas damage of specific systems produces loss of a particular modality. Although, at this early stage, it must be quite simple in its form, the previous statement suggests a hypothesis for the overall organization of brain function. This rests on two tenets: First, the *specific* thalamocortical system is viewed as encoding specific sensory and motor activity through the resonant thalamocortical system specialized to receive such inputs (e.g., the lateral geniculate nucleus [LGN] and visual cortex). The specific system is understood to comprise those nuclei, whether sensorimotor or associative, that project mainly, if not exclusively, to cortical layer 4. Second, after optimal activation, any specific thalamocortical loop would tend to oscillate at gamma-band frequency, and activity in the *specific* thalamocortical system would be easily *recognized* over the cortex by this oscillatory characteristic.

In this scheme, areas of cortex peaking at gamma-band frequency would represent those components of the cognitive world that have reached optimal activity at a particular time. The problem now is to coalesce such a fractured description into a single cognitive event. It is proposed that this could come about by the concurrent summation of specific with nonspecific 40-Hz activity along the radical dendritic axis of the pyramidal elements by coincidence detection.

In conclusion, the thalamocortical system would function on the basis of temporal coherence. Such coherence would be embodied by the simultaneity of neuronal firing based on passive and active dendritic conduction along apical dendritic core conductors. In this fashion, the time-coherent activity of the specific and nonspecific oscillatory inputs would enhance de facto 40-Hz cortical coherence and would provide one mechanism for global binding. The specific system would thus provide the content from the external world, and the nonspecific system would give rise to the temporal conjunction or the context (not the basis of a more interoceptive context) concerned with alertness. These would together generate a single cognitive experience.

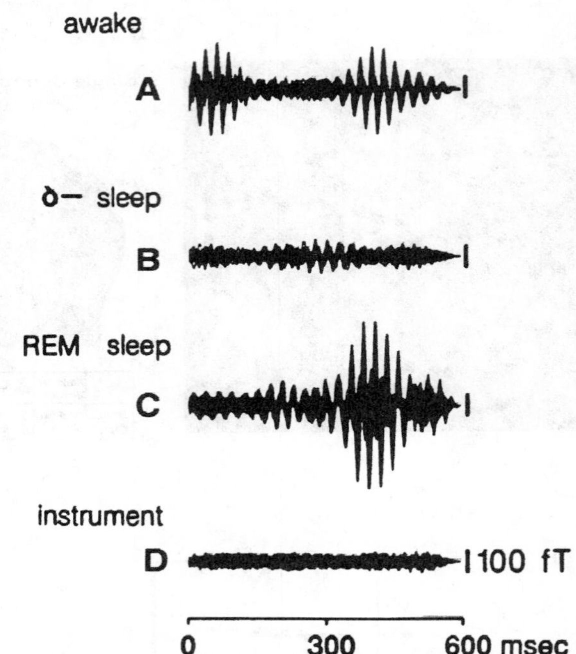

FIGURE 3.6–3 Gamma-band oscillations in a human subject. **A:** Gamma-band oscillation reset evoked by a stimulus (auditory click) in an awake individual. **B:** A similar stimulus does not evoke a reset in delta sleep, and no spontaneous gamma-band activity is observed. **C:** A similar lack of gamma-band reset response is observed to an auditory stimulus during rapid eye movement (REM) sleep. However, gamma-band activity occurs spontaneously during REM. **D:** Basic instrumental noise in femptotesla (fT). (Adapted from Llinás R, Ribary U: Coherent 40-Hz oscillation characterizes dream state in humans. *Proc Natl Acad Sci U S A.* 1993;90:2078–2081.)

Thalamocortical Resonance as the Substrate for Consciousness: Human MEG Studies The activity at the thalamocortical level encountered in the in vitro rodent experiments described previously is relevant to understanding human cerebral function given the similarity in neuronal intrinsic properties and connectivity amongst mammalian forms. Although similar studies are impossible to implement in human tissue, thalamocortical recurrent activity was demonstrated over a decade ago in the human brain using MEG.

Furthermore, such MEG studies have indicated that they may be a minimal temporal interval for sensory discrimination, a binding quantum, on the order of 15 milliseconds. This finding indicated that consciousness is a noncontinuous functional process determined by the dynamic properties of the thalamocortical system. Moreover, continuously recorded spontaneous magnetic activity demonstrated similar gamma-band activity during wakefulness and REM sleep but not during delta sleep. In addition, although auditory stimuli produced well-defined 40-Hz oscillatory reset responses during wakefulness (Fig. 3.6–3A), no such resetting was observed during slow wave (Fig. 3.6–3B) or REM sleep (Fig. 3.6–3C) in all subjects examined.

These findings indicated that, although the awake state and the REM sleep state are electrically similar with respect to the presence of 40-Hz oscillations, a central difference remains: the inability of the sensory input to reset 40-Hz activity during REM sleep. In contrast, during slow wave sleep, no gamma-band activity was observed, and, as in REM sleep, no 40-Hz sensory response could be evoked. Indeed, stimuli from the external world (below a certain level) are not perceived during REM sleep, as they are out of context with the functional state being generated by the brain at that time. Putting it another way, the dreaming condition is a state of hyperattentiveness to intrinsic activity in which sensory input cannot easily access the machinery that generates conscious experience. This may also be the case in hallucinatory psychiatric conditions.

An interesting possibility in considering a morphophysiological substrate is that the nonspecific thalamic system, particularly the intralaminar complex, has an important role in coincidence generation. Indeed, neurons in this complex project in a spatially continuous manner to the most superficial layers of all cortical areas, including the primary sensory cortices. This possibility is particularly attractive, given that single neurons burst at 30 to 40 Hz, especially during REM sleep. This finding is consistent with the macroscopic magnetic records observed in this study (Fig. 3.6–3) and with the fact that damage to the intralaminar system results in lethargy or coma.

Introspection, Reality Emulation, and Cognition

As reviewed previously, several lines of research suggest that the brain is fundamentally a closed system capable of self-generated activity based on the intrinsic electrical properties of its component neurons and their connectivity. According to this hypothesis, the central nervous system (CNS) is viewed as a reality-emulating system. The parameters of such a reality are determined by sensory input, but thalamocortical iterative activity provides the mechanism for the setting of such input into a coherent context resulting in consciousness. This is also in keeping with the observation that the thalamic input from the cortex is larger than that from the peripheral sensory system.

In addition, neurons with intrinsic oscillatory capabilities that reside in the complex thalamocortical synaptic network allow the brain to generate dynamic oscillatory states that shape the functional events elicited by sensory stimuli. In this context, functional states, such as wakefulness, REM sleep, and other sleep stages, are prominent examples of the multiple states that brain activity can support. This hypothesis assumes that, for the most part, the connectivity of the human brain is present at birth and is fine-tuned during normal maturation. This neurological a priori was suggested by early neurological research. It includes the identification by Pierre Paul Broca of a cortical speech center and the discovery of point-to-point somatotopic maps in the motor and sensory cortices and in the thalamus.

A second organizing principle may be equally important—one that is based on the temporal, rather than the spatial, relationships among neurons. This temporal mapping may be viewed as a type of functional geometry.

Thalamocortical Dysrhythmic Syndrome Neuropsychiatric conditions have long been associated with paralimbic cortical areas and the mediodorsal thalamic nucleus. Indeed, studies of patients have revealed low-frequency oscillatory activity, histopathological abnormalities, and hypometabolism, as well as magnetic resonance (MR) changes, in these brain areas.

Recent MEG studies of patients with neurological or psychiatric conditions have suggested a significant correlation between these disorders and the thalamocortical dialogue hypothesis concerning the genesis of consciousness. Spontaneous MEG activity recorded from patients with neurogenic pain, tinnitus, Parkinson's disease, depression, obsessive-compulsive disorder (OCD), or schizoaffective syndrome shows increased low-frequency theta rhythmicity (Fig. 3.6–2E, upper panels) in conjunction with a widespread and marked increase of coherence among high- and low-frequency oscillations (Fig. 3.6–2E, lower central panel). That is, a thalamocortical dysrhythmia (TCD), characterized by a continuous abnormal oscillatory state and by hypercoherence, is present in patients with the previously mentioned conditions.

The coherent theta activity, the result of a resonant interaction between thalamus and cortex, is clearly correlated with the generation of low-threshold calcium spike bursts by thalamic cells. The presence of these bursts is directly related to thalamic cell hyperpolarization brought about by excess inhibition or by disfacilitation. The emergence of positive clinical symptoms is viewed as resulting from ectopic gamma-band activation, which is referred to as the *edge effect*. This effect is seen as increased coherence between low- and high-frequency oscillations and probably results from inhibitory asymmetry between high- and low-frequency thalamocortical modules at the cortical level.

That the neuropsychiatric ailments discussed previously correspond to the TCD syndrome is supported by finding low-threshold thalamic spike activity during neurosurgical procedures and the characteristic MEG patterns described previously in such patients.

The TCD syndrome is characterized by the following sequence of events:

1. Hyperpolarization of thalamic relay or reticular thalamic nucleus (RTN) cells, or both, due to disfacilitation or overinhibition, or both.
2. This hyperpolarized state is the source of T-type calcium channel deinactivation, causing the production of low-threshold spike (LTS) bursts in thalamic (Fig. 3.6–1) or reticular neurons, or both.
3. Neurons in such a state impose a slow rhythmicity on their thalamocortical loops and are locked in the theta low-frequency domain by their membrane conductances. Recurrent corticothalamic and RTN projections back to the projection thalamus provide the necessary coherent diffusion of these frequencies to various related cortical areas. MEG and electroencephalogram (EEG) recordings demonstrate increased theta power under these conditions, which may be directly correlated with cortical and thalamic hypometabolism seen in positron emission tomography (PET) results. In psychotic disorders, the disease source may be found in the paralimbic cortical domain or in the paralimbic striatum, leading to corticothalamic low-frequency activation.
4. The final step in the description of this syndrome is the proposed existence of the activation of gamma-frequency cortical domains due to an asymmetrical corticocortical GABAergic lateral inhibition. The proposed mechanism, named the *edge effect* (analogous to the edge effect observed in the retina due to lateral inhibition), would result from the asymmetrical inhibition between a low-frequency cortical area and neighboring high-frequency domains, providing an area of disinhibition that results in the activation of the cortex surrounding the low-frequency area. This is not unlike the visual imagery encountered in migraine. MEG studies support the postulation of such an edge effect, as evidenced by a large multifrequency coherence between theta and gamma domains—an event absent in the normal brain. This activation of high-frequency areas might express itself through abnormal EEG spiking activity, as seen in psychotic patients.

The characteristics of the TCD syndrome suggests the basis for a possible treatment that goes beyond the neuroleptics now used. A promising approach will be the development of T-type calcium channel blockers that would specifically address particular thalamic groups. Such agents would control the low-frequency intrinsic thalamic activity seen in the type of patient described previously.

Although these specific drugs are being developed, procedures that have been used quite favorably in patients with Parkinson's disease may be implemented in these patients. These include deep brain stimulation (DBS) or selective miniablation (SMA) of unspecific thalamic or prethalamic structures.

An example is illustrated here.

Male patient, born in 1957, presented with a 20-year history of a schizoaffective disorder characterized by delusional, hallucinatory, and affective bipolar manifestations, with a few ICD elements. Over a few weeks after the second centrolateral thalamic and anterior media pallidal stereotaxic microlesion, the patient experienced progressive and then complete relief of all thesedisease signs. Three years after surgery, he enjoys a complete improvement in stability. Initially, he experienced two episodes of agitation, anxiety, and confusion, followed by a reactive depressive phase. These were apparently based on internal stressors related to personal and interactive family factors, with activation of powerful guilt and self-insufficiency feelings. These initial events were followed by the recovery from symptoms described above. Drug reduction is being processed very slowly, however, in view of the 20-year-long intake. Figure 3.6–2 describes MEG power spectrum and coherence plot (Fig. 3.6–2E) and localization (Fig. 3.6–2F) of theta-band MEG activity before and 3 months after surgery.

FUTURE DIRECTIONS

The basic assumption concerning the genesis of this syndrome is that TCD is a CNS intrinsic property brought about by changes in intrinsic voltage-gated ionic conductances at the level of thalamic relay cells, namely, the deinactivation of T-type calcium channels by cell membrane hyperpolarization. Low-threshold spike bursts are thus produced, which lock the affected portion of thalamocortical circuits in a low-frequency resonance attractor. Low-frequency loops disfacilitate anatomically related cortical circuits giving rise to gamma-band activity, the *edge effect*, and to the generation of a positive symptoms, such as those seen in tinnitus, neurogenic pain, Parkinson's disease, and some neuropsychiatric disorders. In these cases, the dysrhythmic mechanism originates in a bottom-up fashion, that is, from the thalamus toward the cortex. In other situations, such as epilepsy, neuropsychiatric conditions of cortical origin, and central cortical neurogenic pain, a top-down mechanism may be at work. This would be triggered by a reduction of the corticothalamic input. Bottom-up and top-down situations result in excess inhibition at the thalamic level or in disfacilitation, generating thalamic cell membrane hyperpolarization and low-frequency oscillations. The proposal, then, is that the same mechanism that is responsible for the genesis of consciousness can generate neuropsychiatric conditions when its organization and timing are altered.

In conclusion then, cognition, a property of thalamocortical cycling, would function on the basis of temporal coherence. Such coherence would be embodied by the simultaneity of neuronal firing based on passive and active dendritic conduction along the apical dendritic core conductors. In this fashion, the time-coherent activity of the specific and nonspecific oscillatory inputs, by summing distal and proximal activity in given dendritic elements, would enhance de facto 40-Hz cortical coherence by their multimodal character and, in this way, would provide one mechanism for global binding. The *specific* system would provide the *content* that relates to the external world, and the *nonspecific* system would give rise to the temporal conjunction, or the *context* (on the basis of a more interoceptive context concerned with alertness), that would together generate a single cognitive experience. Furthermore, when this rhythmicity is altered in particular ways, neurological and psychiatric conditions ensue.

REFERENCES

Castaigne P: Ramollissement pédonculaire median, tegmento-thalamique avec ophtalmoplegie et hypersomnie. *Rev Neurol.* 1962;106:357–367.

Crick F, Koch C: Some reflections on visual awareness. *Cold Spring Harbor Symp Quant Biol.* 1990;55:953–962.

Edelman GM. *Neuronal Darwinism: The Theory of Neuronal Group Selection.* New York: Basic Books; 1987.

Facon E, Steriade M, Wertheim N: Hypersomnie prolongée engendree par des lesions bilatérales due system activateur medial le syndrome thrombotique de la biffurcation du tronc basilaire. *Rev Neurol.* 1958;98:117–133.

*Gray CM, Singer W: Stimulus-specific neuronal oscillations in orientation columns of cat visual cortex. *Proc Natl Acad Sci U S A.* 1989;86:1698–1702.

*Hubel DH, Wiesel TN: Sequence regularity and geometry of orientation columns in the monkey striate cortex. *J Comp Neurol.* 1974;158:267–294.

Jeanmonod D: Thalamocortical dysrhythmia II. Clinical and surgical aspects. *Thalamus Relat Sys.* 2001;1:245–254.

Jeanmonod D: Neuropsychiatric thalamocortical dysrhythmia: Surgical implications. *Thalamus Relat Sys.* 2003;2:103–113.

Joliot M, Ribary U, Llinás R: Neuromagnetic oscillatory activity in the vicinity of Hz coexists with cognitive temporal binding in the human brain. *Proc Natl Acad Sci U S A.* 1994;91:11748–11751.

Landisman CE, Long MA, Bierelein M, Deans MR, Paul DL, Connors BW: Electrical synapses in the thalamic reticular nucleus. *J Neurosci.* 2002;22:1002–1009.

Larkum ME, Zhu JJ, Sakmann B: A new cellular mechanism for coupling inputs arriving at different cortical layers. *Nature.* 1999;398:338–341.

*Llinás R: The intrinsic electrophysiological properties of mammalian neurons: Insight into central nervous system function. *Science.* 1988;242:1654–1664.

Llinás R. Content and context in temporal thalamocortical binding. In: Buzsaki G, ed. *Temporal Coding in the Brain.* Berlin: Springer-Verlag; 1994.

Llinás R. *I of the Vortex; from Neurons to Self.* Cambridge, MA: MIT Press; 2001.

Llinás R: Thalamocortical dysrhythmia I. Functional and imaging aspects. *Thalamus Relat Sys.* 2001;1:237–244.

Llinás R, Jahnsen H: Electrophysiology of mammalian thalamic neurones in vitro. *Nature.* 1982;297:406–408.

Llinás R, Leznik E, Urbano IF: Temporal binding via coincidence detection of specific and non-specific thalamocortical inputs: A voltage dependent dye imaging study in mouse brain slices. *Proc Natl Acad Sci U S A.* 2002;99:449–454.

Llinás R, Pare D: Of dreaming and wakefulness. *Neuroscience.* 1991;44:521–535.

Llinás R, Ribary U: Coherent 40-Hz oscillation characterizes dream state in humans. *Proc Natl Acad Sci U S A.* 1993;90:2078–2081.

Llinás R, Ribary U, Contreras D, Pedroarena C: The neuronal basis for consciousness. *Philos Trans R Soc Lond.* 1998;353:1841–1849.

*Llinás R, Ribary U, Jeanmonod D, Kronberg E, Mitra PP: Thalamo-cortical dysrhythmia: A neurological and neuropsychiatric syndrome characterized by magnetoencephalography. *Proc Natl Acad Sci U S A.* 1999;96:15222–15227.

*Mounteastle VB: The columnar organization of the neocortex. *Brain.* 1997;120:701–722.

Pedroarena C, Llinás R: Dendritic calcium conductances generate high-frequency oscillation in thalamocortical neurons. *Proc Natl Acad Sci U S A.* 1997;94:724–728.

Rhodes PA. Functional implications of active currents in the dendrites of pyramidal neurons. In: Ribary U, ed.: Magnetic field tomography of coherent thalamocortical 40-Hz oscillations in humans. *Proc Natl Acad Sci U S A.* 1991;88:11037–11040.

Steriade M, Curró-Dossi R, Contreras D: Electrophysiological properties of intralaminar thalamocortical cells discharging rhythms (40 Hz) spike-bursts at 1000 Hz during waking and rapid eye movement sleep. *Neuroscience.* 1993;56:1–9.

Steriade M, Jones EG, McCormick DA. *Thalamus.* Elsevier Science; 1997.

Ulinski PS, Jones EG, Peters A, eds. *Cerebral Cortex.* Vol 13. New York: Plenum Press; 1984:139–200.

Zonenshayn M, Mogilner AY, Rezai AR: Neurostimulation and functional brain imaging. *Neurol Res.* 2000;22:318–325.

▲ 3.7 Normality and Mental Health

George E. Vaillant, M.D., and
Caroline O. Vaillant, M.S.S.W.

Too often, psychiatry has been only preoccupied with mental illness. To paraphrase Mark Twain's quip about the weather, psychiatry is always talking about mental health, but nobody ever does anything about it. Science has conceptualized the building blocks of nuclear fission more readily than the building blocks of mental health. Thus, with the notable exception of the chapter by Daniel Offer and Melvin Sabshin in the early editions of this textbook, a review of recent major psychiatric textbooks reveals virtually no serious discussion of mental health. One reason for this lack of attention is that the study of positive mental health is a new field. Only since the 1970s has mental health per se been addressed empirically instead of platonically.

There has been an implicit assumption that mental health could be defined as the antonym of mental illness. In other words, mental health was the absence of psychopathology and was synonymous with *normal*. Achieving mental health through the alleviation of gross pathological signs and symptoms of illness is also the definition of a mental health model strongly advocated by third-party payers. Indeed, viewing mental health as simply the absence of mental illness is at the heart of much of the debate concerning mental health policies. The great epidemiological studies of the past half-century have also focused on who was mentally ill and not who was well. Only the Sterling County Studies by Alexander Leighton came close to defining positive mental health operationally. *Mental illness*, after all, is a condition that is easy to define reliably, and its limits are relatively clear. As a result, it has been argued that achieving above average mental or physical health is not the province of medicine but of education. Such a definition ignores concepts of positive health, such as physical fitness and cardiac reserve.

Like physical fitness, however, positive mental health is too important to be ignored. To believe that mental health is merely a global assessment of functioning (GAF) of 70 on Axis V of the revised fourth edition of the *Diagnostic and Statistical Manual of Mental Disorders* (DSM-IV-TR) is to underestimate human potential. Sports medicine does more than mend a skier's broken legs; sports medicine rehabilitates the skier to ski advanced trails once more. Starting in the early 1900s, internists began studying physiology at high altitude and devised measures of positive physical health for athletes, pilots, and, finally, astronauts. In 1929 and 1930, at the University of California at Berkeley, the Institute of Human Development was founded by Howard Jones, Nancy Bayley, and Jean McFarlane. Originally founded to study healthy child development, the Institute was to provide a seminal influence on Erik Erikson's model of healthy adult development. A decade later, in the late 1930s, Arlie Bock, an internist trained in high-altitude physiology and interested in positive physical health, began, at the Harvard University Health Services, the Study of Adult Development. The study was designed as an interdisciplinary study of mental and physical health. Results from that study, lasting for 60 years, have informed many facets of this chapter.

Although above average mental health is more difficult to define than physical fitness, it is important for psychiatrists to emulate sports medicine to provide precise definitions and measures of positive mental health. Psychologists have already learned to quantify not only normal, but also better-than-normal intelligence. Thus, the antonym of mental retardation is regarded not as an intelligence quotient (IQ) of 100 but as an IQ greater than 130. Psychiatry must follow suit.

Certainly, over the last 50 years, psychiatrists have become increasingly involved in mental health consultations to agencies. Rather than merely deciding who is too sick for a job, they are called on to make decisions about who is mentally healthy enough for certain positions—such as air traffic controllers and submariners. Analogous to cardiac reserve, the measurement of resilience and of the capacity to withstand adversity are on psychiatry's psychometric wish list. In addition, interest in the empirical evaluation of psychiatric therapy outcome has also brought the issue of positive mental health into focus. Indeed, one of the weaknesses of much existing work on psychotherapy assessment has been a lack of clarity regarding outcome definitions. *For health is not the absence of negatives but the presence of positives.*

The definition of positive mental health, however, is not easy. Several cautionary steps are necessary. The first step in discussing mental health is to note that *average* is not healthy; it always includes mixing in with the healthy the prevalent amount of psychopathology. For example, in the general population, *average* weight or eyesight is unhealthy, and, if all sources of biopsychosocial pathology were excluded from the population, the average IQ would be significantly greater than 100. As with Garrison Keillor's description of Lake Wobegon youth, mentally healthy children "are all above average." Being at the center of a normal bell curve of distribution may not be healthy. In the case of red blood count, body temperature, or mood, the middle of the bell curve *is* healthy. In the case of eyesight, exercise tolerance, or empathy, only the upper end of the bell curve is healthy; in the case of serum cholesterol, bilirubin, and narcissism, only the low end of the curve is healthy.

The second cautionary step in discussing mental health is to appreciate the caveat that what is healthy sometimes depends on geography, culture, and historical moment. Sickle cell trait is unhealthy in New York City, but, in the tropics, where malaria is endemic, the sickling of red blood cells may be lifesaving. Punctuality is a virtue in Germany and a failing in Brazil. General George Patton's competitive temperament was a psychological liability in a time of peace but a virtue in two world wars. In the 1940s, paranoid personalities made poor submariners but excellent airplane spotters.

A third cautionary step is to make clear whether one is discussing *trait* or *state*. Who is physically healthier: an Olympic miler disabled by a simple but temporary (state) ankle fracture or a type I diabetic (trait) with a temporarily normal blood sugar? In cross-cultural studies, such differences become especially important. Temporarily, an Indian mystic in a state of trance resembles a catatonic schizophrenic but does not resemble this same condition over time.

In defining mental health, the fourth and most important cautionary step is to appreciate the twofold danger of *contamination by values*. On the one hand, cultural anthropology shows how fallacious any definition of mental health can be. Competitiveness and scrupulous neatness may be healthy in one culture and may be regarded as personality disorder in another. Furthermore, if mental health is good, what is it good for? The self or the society? For fitting in or for creativity? For happiness or survival? And who should be the judge? Because every culture differs in its diet, the World Health Organization (WHO) should never be called on to design restaurant menus.

On the other hand, common sense must prevail. Biology trumps anthropology. It is true that cultural anthropology shows that almost no form of behavior is considered abnormal in all cultures, but that does not mean that the tolerated behavior is mentally healthy. The WHO would be in error to ignore the universal importance to diet of vitamins and of the four basic food groups. Just because Portugal does not recognize alcoholism as an illness does not reduce the contribution of alcoholism to Lisbon morbidity. Just because the American Constitution protected the right to own slaves as inalienable did not make slavery mentally healthy for slave or for slave owner. The best way to enrich the understanding of what constitutes mental health is to study a variety of healthy populations from different perspectives in different cultures for a long period of time.

This chapter contrasts six different empirical approaches to mental health. Significantly, the empirical underpinnings of all six models have emerged only in the past 30 years. First, mental health can be conceptualized as *above normal* and as a mental state that is objectively desirable—as in Sigmund Freud's alleged definition of mental health as the capacity to work and to love. Second, mental health can be conceptualized as *positive psychology*—as epitomized by the presence of multiple human strengths. Third, from the viewpoint of healthy adult development, mental health can be conceptualized as *maturity*. Fourth, mental health can be conceptualized as *emotional intelligence*. Fifth, mental health can be conceptualized as *subjective well-being*—a mental state that is subjectively experienced as happy, contented, and desired. Sixth, mental health can be conceptualized as *resilience*, as the capacity for successful adaptation and homeostasis. In such a view, mental health, analogous to a competent immune system, allows the individual to function well despite stressful or dangerous environments.

MODEL A: MENTAL HEALTH AS ABOVE NORMAL

The first perspective is the traditional medical approach to health and illness. No manifestation of psychopathology equals mental health. In this model, if one were to put all individuals on a continuum, normality would encompass the major portion of the young adults, and abnormality would be the small remainder. This definition of health correlates with the traditional role model of the doctor who attempts to free his patient from grossly observable signs of illness. In other words, in this context, *health* refers to a reasonable, rather than an optimal, state of functioning.

Yet, as already pointed out, mental health is not normal, it is above average. Some believe that mental health is the exception not the rule. Certainly, the absence of illness and the presence of health overlap but do not always coincide. In the military, the mental health for a jet pilot must exceed the draft board's 1-A. In primary school teachers, and in Supreme Court justices, employers look for more than simply freedom from symptoms or for Freud's capacity to work and to love. However, to avoid quibbling over what traits characterize mental health, it is helpful to adopt the analogy of a decathlon champion. What constitutes a track star? Is it muscle strength, speed, endurance, grace, or competitive grit? Does not the definition differ from nation to nation and from century to century? Not really. The salience of given facets of track or of mental health may vary from culture to culture, but all are important. A high score on the decathlon has conveyed behavioral skill in track for millennia and in every country of the world—even as the hair splitters argue over the right words with which to describe a track athlete.

As with excellence in the decathlon, no single measure defines mental health, but all measures are highly intercorrelated. Table 3.7–1 illustrates how multifaceted and unique each model of positive mental health can be and how different can be the semantics. The familial resemblance of each definition to each other, however, is unmistakable.

In 1835, Adolphe Quetelet published the first important book on normality ever written. Rather than focus on pathology, he tried "to approach more closely to what is good and beautiful," and his goal was the statistical analysis of healthy humans. He challenged generations of future investigators with his introductory sentence: "Man is born, grows up, and dies, according to certain laws which have never been properly investigated."

Until World War II, however, Quetelet's challenge to mental health workers went largely unnoticed. When, in 1941, John Clausen and his coworkers were commissioned to assess mental health for the draft board, they were embarking on a novel task. As a way of assessing mental health of recruits they focused on the absence of psychosomatic symptoms. Although limited, their approach was not abandoned until the 1970s, and questions about psychosomatic symptoms still form an important part of the Hopkins SCL-90 and of scales assessing neuroticism.

After World War II, influential works on normal adaptive behavior began to be published—Roy Grinker's and John Paul Spiegel's *Men under Stress*, Robert White's *Lives in Progress*, Leo Srole's *Mental Health in the Metropolis*, and Dorothea and Alexander Leighton's *Cove and Woodlot* were four of the more important works. Although all four studies concentrated on the adaptation of nonpatient or normal populations, they still put their emphasis on *not pathological* rather than on *above normal mental health.*

Besides, many postwar psychiatrists continued to agree with Freud, who had dismissed mental health as "an ideal fiction." In the late 1950s, two of the world's most distinguished psychiatrists could dismiss the term entirely. Sir Aubrey Lewis wrote in 1958: "Mental health is an invincibly obscure concept." In 1957, Fritz Redlich asserted: "We do not possess any general definition of normality and mental health from either a statistical or a clinical viewpoint."

Then, in 1958, Marie Jahoda's report to the Joint Commission on Mental Illness and Health led to a psychiatric sea of change regarding the existence of mental health. As illustrated in Table 3.7–1, Jahoda suggested that mentally healthy individuals should (1) be in touch with their own identity and their own feelings. (2) They should be oriented toward the future, and, over time, they should remain fruitfully invested in life. (3) Their psyches should be integrated and should provide them resistance to stress. (4) They should possess autonomy and should recognize what suits their needs. (5) They should perceive reality without distortion and yet should possess empathy. (6) They should be masters of their environment—able to work, to love, to play, and to be efficient in problem solving. Instead of emphasizing the absence of negative symptoms, Jahoda underscored a number of positive traits. Nevertheless, although the purpose of Jahoda's report was to rid the term *mental health* of "vague, elusive and ambiguous connotation," at the time she published her criteria, there was still no evidence to prove that her plausible definition was more than mere platitudes that reflected her own culture-bound values.

Thus, it was with Roy Grinker's 1962 studies of *homoclites* that investigators began the empirical study of positive mental health. Grinker's homoclites were physical education majors selected for normality and followed up 32 years later by Jerry Westermeyer. A second, more longitudinal study was the elimination process by which, out of 130 healthy jet pilots already selected for mental health, the seven original astronauts were selected. The process underscored the importance and the commonsensical nature of mental health. The final seven astronauts not only enjoyed exem-

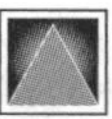

Table 3.7–1
Three Contrasting Definitions of Mental Health

Model A: Mental Health or Normality	Model B: Positive Psychology	Model C: Maturity
Marie Jahoda, as summarized by Daniel Offer and Melvin Sabshin	Christopher Peterson and Martin Seligman	William Menninger
Ability to love, to work, and to play	Love	The capacity for love
Possesses empathy	Intimacy and reciprocal attachment	The capacity for a variety of mutually fulfilling and lasting relationships
Adequacy in interpersonal relations	Kindness, generosity, and nurturance	
	Social intelligence and emotional intelligence	The need to seek a major source of fulfillment in productive work
Efficient in problem solving	Temperance	Free of stereotyped and nonproductive patterns of problem solving
Perceives reality	Forgiveness and mercy	
Resistance to stress	Modesty and humility	Ability to discharge hostility without harming others or oneself
Environmental mastery	Prudence and caution	
	Self-control and self-regulation	The capacity to adapt to change and to endure frustration and loss
Invested in life	Wisdom and knowledge	A realistic acceptance of the destiny imposed by one's time and place in the world
Self-actualization	Curiosity and interest	
Oriented toward future	Love of learning	
	Judgment and open-mindedness	
	Perspective	
	Creativity, originality, and ingenuity	
Autonomy	Courage	Appropriate expectations and goals for oneself
Recognition of needs	Valor	Ability to respond to the uncertainties of reality in a manner consistently free of domination by one's wishes or peers
In touch with own identity and feelings	Honesty and authenticity	
	Industry and perseverance	
	Zest and enthusiasm	
	Justice	
	Citizenship, loyalty, and teamwork	
	Equity and fairness	
	Leadership	
	Transcendence	Having the capacity for hope
	Awe and wonder	An altruistic concern for other human beings outside one's own group and beyond one's own time and place
	Gratitude	
	Hope and future-mindedness	The capacity to suspend one's adult identity and to engage in childish play at appropriate times
	Spirituality and faith	
	Playfulness and humor	

plary work records but also were competent at loving. All came from intact, happy, small-town families; they all were married with children. Although venturesome test pilots, they all had few accidents during their years of flying or even earlier. They could tolerate close interdependent association and extreme isolation. They trusted others and were uncomplaining under discomfort. They manifested great capacity for withstanding frustration; nevertheless, emotions, negative and positive, were strongly experienced. Not introspective, the astronauts seldom dwelt on their inner emotions, but they were sensitive to their emotions and could describe them when asked. They were aware of the feelings of others, and they avoided interpersonal difficulties. Unlike most people, their performance improved under stress (e.g., working at a simulated altitude of 65,000 feet in a poorly functioning pressure suit). Their group neuroticism (Maudsley Personality Inventory) score was the lowest of any group reported in the literature. Although each of the astronauts was different, they all would have starred in a mental health "decathlon."

A still more influential study of mental health was the Menninger Psychotherapy Project. To cut through the hair splitting of projective tests and the subjectivity of pencil and paper tests, Menninger psychologist Lester Luborsky devised a behavioral guide (Health-Sickness Rating Scale [HSRS]) to assess psychological functioning on a scale of 0 to 100. In 1976, because Luborsky's scale had been designed to evaluate candidates for psychotherapy rather than for general epidemiological studies, two of the architects of the third edition of the *Diagnostic and Statistical Manual of Mental Disorders* developed a revision of the HSRS called the *Global Assessment Scale* (GAS). Rater reliabilities for both instruments and between the two instruments were approximately 0.85 to 0.95. In cross-cultural comparison, investigators noted that "the usefulness of HSRS as an international thermometer of mental health is strongly supported." A modified version of the GAS was introduced in the revised third edition of the *Diagnostic and Statistical Manual of Mental Disorders* as the GAF (see Table 7.9–2).

On Luborsky's scale, a score of 95 to 100 reflected "an ideal state of complete functioning integration, of resiliency in the face of stress, of happiness and social effectiveness." On the GAF, a score of 95 to 100 equaled "no symptoms, superior functioning in a wide range of activities; life's problems never seem to get out of hand; patient is sought out by others because of his warmth and integrity." The words differ, but the melody is the same.

By 1978, *The Report to the President* by the President's Commission on Mental Health forcefully reiterated the importance of defining clearly what is meant by *mental health*. Nevertheless, it was not until 15 years later, when evidence emerged to support the validity of Axis V DSM-IV-TR, that psychiatry finally possessed a metric for the measurement of *above average* mental health.

To identify mental health empirically, behavioral data are needed, and a longitudinal biopsychosocial perspective must be maintained. Two different life histories from Harvard's Study of Adult Development illustrate what is meant by *above normal mental health.* One man, "Alfred Paine," received an *average* score for mental health (GAF = 72); he never sought psychiatric care. In contrast, "Richard Luckey" received an above normal score for mental health (GAF = 95). These two (disguised) case histories help underscore that objective and subjective mental health are not merely value ridden "ideal fictions." Both men had been selected at 18 years of age for mental health and were prospectively observed for a lifetime. Confounding variables, such as gender, education, social class, ethnicity, age, and birth cohort, are held constant. Neither man had ever sought psychiatric help for nor been diagnosed with mental illness, but there is no question regarding who was the healthier individual.

Alfred Paine was a master of cheerful denial. On questionnaires, he described himself as a social drinker, in quite good physical health, and close to his children. It was only by interviewing him personally, talking with his wife, examining his medical record, reading the disappointed questionnaires from his children—and then, finally, by reading his obituary—that Alfred Paine's misery could be fully appreciated.

The ancestors of Alfred Paine had been successful New England clipper ship captains. All his grandparents had graduated from high school. One grandfather became a merchant banker, and the other became the president of a Stock Exchange. Paine's father had graduated from Harvard, and his mother graduated from a fashionable boarding school. When Alfred Paine was 2 weeks old, his mother died from the complications of childbirth. When he was 2 years old, his father died. Paine was bottle-fed by a variety of surrogates and raised by his grandmother. As a young boy, Paine was a head-banger; in adolescence, he was a "lone wolf."

In college, Alfred Paine was often in love. However, for Paine, being in love meant having someone to care for him. His three marriages were all unhappy—in part, because of the alcohol abuse that he maintained that he did not have and, in part, because he was frightened of intimacy. At 50 years of age, Paine answered "true" to the statements "sexually, most people are animals" and "I would have preferred an asexual marriage."

At 47 years of age, Paine recalled the years from 1 to 13 years of age as the unhappiest in his life. At 70 years of age, he believed that the years from 20 to 30 years of age were the unhappiest. However, there had never been a time that Paine was happy. Nevertheless, on a pencil and paper test of depression, Paine achieved one of the best scores in the study. He had never sought psychotherapy, and none of his doctors ever called him mentally ill. His alcohol abuse never led to an arrest or to missed days of work. At 70 years of age, Paine wrote that his own physical health was "excellent," but, in fact, he was seriously overweight, had hypertension and gout, and had obstructive pulmonary disease—the result of lifelong smoking. By 75 years of age, he lost all his teeth; both his kidneys and his liver were failing, and he was cursed with a mild dementia, the result of a drunken fall.

Although he had made a good living over the years at a job he disliked, by 75 years of age, Paine's trust fund and his pension had been eroded through multiple divorces and self-inflicted tax troubles. His house looked as if furnished from yard sales, and little other than television now absorbed him. On his age-75 questionnaire, Paine refused to answer the part that dealt with life enjoyment. Thus, his subjective lack of joy in life had to be inferred from the fact that, over the past 20 years, there was no area of his life other than his religious activities in which he had expressed satisfaction. On average, he saw his three children once every 2 years, and he grumbled that "they hardly let me see my grandchildren." Although Paine's third wife was protective and quite loving toward him, he was quite disrespectful and uncaring toward her. Asked how he and his wife collaborated, he replied: "We don't. We lead parallel lives." Since 50 years of age, he had engaged in no pastimes with friends, and, at 73 years of age, when asked to describe his oldest friend, he growled, "I don't have any." Often, in his life, Paine had found love, but he could not let it inside.

In contrast, Richard Luckey was a well-loved child who took excellent care of himself. Unlike Alfred Paine, Luckey had come from more modest beginnings. None of his four grandparents had gone beyond grade school. His father graduated from high school and went on to become a successful businessman. After college, Luckey became head of two successful businesses (one of which he created)—at the same time. He loved his work.

At 70 years of age, when looked at through the eyes of his internist, Richard Luckey's objective physical health had seemed actually worse than Alfred Paine's. Luckey had high blood pressure, atrial fibrillation, a cardiac pacemaker, and pancreatitis. He was even more overweight than Paine. However, if Luckey was ill, he certainly did not feel sick. Over the next 10 years, Paine sickened unto death, and Luckey's health got steadily better. Thus, by 76 years of age, Luckey had completely recovered from his pancreatitis. He still wore a pacemaker, and his blood pressure remained high, but, in his doctor's words—not just his own—"Mr. Luckey continues to enjoy relatively good health . . . he continues to be active physically and also mentally." As Luckey, himself, expressed it: "I have done less chain sawing, but I still split wood." At 76 years of age, Luckey spent 2 months downhill skiing in Austria.

Another crucial difference was that Luckey had never smoked, and he had used alcohol in moderation. "Almost everything we do," Luckey explained, "is family oriented." His wife amplified, "We rarely go out, but we will have groups for supper such as the church fellowship group or the basketball team for a weekend of skiing, or a vestry meeting at the house." Luckey was also commodore of his yacht club, and he had friends with whom he exercised regularly.

Richard Luckey described not only his hobbies, his religion, and his income-producing work as "very satisfying," but also, more importantly, he experienced his relationships with his wife and with his children as "very satisfying." His wife and children's questionnaires revealed a similar satisfaction with him. Luckey's daughter had described her parent's marriage as "better than my friends;" then, for good measure, she had added two pluses. Luckey's wife gave her marriage a 9 out of 9, and, on her questionnaire, she wrote the study, "My husband is my best friend; I like looking after him. We have grown closer and fonder every year." Asked how his marriage had lasted for 40 years, Luckey replied, "I really love Chrissie and she loves me. I really respect her, highly esteem her, and she is a real person." Luckey was close to his brother with whom he fished regularly in the summer. He stayed in touch with and took great pleasure from his children and his grandchildren. It was so easy for Luckey to take in, to "metabolize," any love that he was offered.

Asked about his retirement, Richard Luckey replied, "I think it is all pretty nice. I don't have a day when I don't have something to do that I want to do . . . creativity is absolutely necessary for someone to be healthy. With painting," he added dreamily, "you forget everything, and that is why it is so very relaxing." In church, Luckey sang solo and in the choir. Despite an indifferent college scholastic record, at 75 years of age, Luckey was making a serious effort to master the technology of a research institute of which he had become a trustee.

Health is the activity of a living body in accordance with its specific excellencies.

> "What, for example, is a healthy squirrel?" asked Leo Kass, a research professor in bioethics and neurology. "Not a picture of a squirrel, not really or fully the sleeping squirrel, not even the aggregate of his normal blood pressure, serum calcium, total body zinc, normal digestion, fertility, and the like. Rather, the healthy squirrel is a bushy-tailed fellow, who looks and acts like a squirrel; who leaps through the trees with great daring, who gathers, buries, and covers but later uncovers and recovers his acorns; who perches out on a limb cracking his nuts, sniffing the air for smells of danger, alert, cautious, with his tail beating rhythmically; who chatters and plays and courts and mates and rears his young in large improbable looking homes at the tops of trees; who fights with vigor and forages with cunning; who shows spiritedness, even anger, and more prudence than many human beings . . . Health is a natural standard or norm—not a moral norm, not a 'value' as opposed to a 'fact,' not an obligation but a state of being that reveals itself in activity."

In other words, health is based on an active, joyous, energetic engagement with the world. Such a naturalistic model of health is congruent with the increasing attention to *flow*, a concept recently elaborated and empirically studied by psychologist Mihaly Csikszentmihalyi and his students. Flow involves the focused attention and psychic absorption that is characteristic of meditation, but, unlike meditation, with flow, the clutch is engaged, and skilled behavior takes place. With flow, the participant feels alive and in the world. In the flow experience, the emotions are not just contained and channeled, they are energized and aligned with consciousness of the task at hand. Action, cognition, and feeling are merged into one. Often, when manifested in intense experiences, such as advanced tennis, technical rock climbing, or violin playing, the flow experience has required hours of prior practice until much of the effort involved has become second nature.

Csikszenmihalyi's concept of flow is distinct from Freud's libido. Flow occurs when a task is challenging and requires skill and concentration, when there are clear goals and immediate involvement, when time seems to stop and sense of self vanishes, and when one finds oneself deeply involved and in control. A species does not survive just by reproducing; it also has to produce and face new challenges.

MODEL B: MENTAL HEALTH AS POSITIVE PSYCHOLOGY

The fact that psychologists have approached mental health somewhat differently from psychiatry has led to the second model. Psychologists, like physiologists, look at continua (traits) rather than categories, whereas, in medicine, a person has an illness or does not have an illness. In psychology, interventions to improve adequate intelligence or social skills are common, whereas, in medicine, to meddle with adequate thyroid function, a healthy hematocrit, or a normal mood is only to cause trouble. In the healthy rested individual, virtually all psychopharmacological interventions, over time, make the brain function worse; in contrast, many psychological interventions (e.g., literacy training and stress management) make the brain function better. Thus, the medical goal of using medication to remove pathology is different from the psychologists' goal of fostering joy, enthusiasm, curiosity, and love for others in an educative model. As a result, physicians and psychologists draw attention to quite different—if complementary—approaches to mental health.

The second model conceives of mental health as the *best possible* and has provided the basis for the positive psychology movement. In the 19th century, mental health was deemed related to morality, and the psychiatrists wrote of "moral insanity" and "good character." However, in the 20th century, medicine became concerned more with concrete pathology, whereas psychology remained interested in education and in platonic and utopian virtue.

The last century witnessed not only psychologist John Dewey's idealism regarding education, but also the work of Carl Jung and William James (physicians by training, but psychologists in spirit) concerning the search for and discovery of deeper meanings in life. In the last 50 years, Abraham Maslow's concept of self-actualization and his emphasis on humanistic psychology have drawn attention to "full use and exploitation of talents, capacities, potentialities." However, until most recently, humanistic psychology has not undertaken empirical research and has ignored predictive validity and follow-up. Humanistic psychology has emphasized *happiness* and the *self* at the expense of collective well-being and has spawned myriad self-help movements that have benefited clients more through placebo effect than from controlled and replicated therapeutic interventions. As early as 1925, psychiatrist Adolf Meyer was already warning of the need to stop "moralizing" about utopian mental health. Mental health, he suggested, should be studied through "conscientious and impartial study" and "constructive experimentation."

Recently, two popular books by distinguished psychologist Martin Seligman, *Learned Optimism* and *Authentic Happiness*, have served notice that positive psychology is beginning to follow Meyer's rules of conscientious and impartial study and constructive experimentation. Seligman's concepts of *learned optimism* and positive psychology incorporate the empirical advances in cognitive psychology that have taken place since the 1970s. Creating a positive attributional style not only serves as a cognitive behavioral treatment for depression, but also can lead to positive mental states.

Positive psychology wishes to learn how to build the qualities that help individuals and communities not just to endure and survive but also to flourish. Formally introduced in the January 2000 issue of *American Psychologist*, positive psychology hopes to render the psychology of strength and well-being amenable to scientific study and intervention. In that issue, Seligman and Csikszentmihalyi wrote:

> At the individual level, it is about positive individual traits; the capacity for love and vocation, courage, interpersonal skill, aesthetic sensibility, perseverance, forgiveness, originality, future mindedness, spirituality, high talent, and wisdom . . . Psychology is not just a branch of medicine concerned with illness or health; it is much larger. It is about work, education, insight, love, growth, and play. And in this quest for what is best, positive psychology does not rely on wishful thinking, faith, self-deception, fads, or hand waving; it tries to adapt what is best in the scientific method to the unique problems that human behavior presents to those who wish to understand it in all its complexity.

Over the past 30 years, cognitive therapists have demonstrated that altered cognition can not only change behavior, it can also alter brain function. If pessimism is the dominant cognition of the depressed, optimism appears to be the dominant cognition of the mentally healthy. If learned helplessness leads to depression, learned optimism and self-efficacy lead to mental health. Even if the depressed often appear to view reality more realistically, such accurate reality testing avails depressed individuals nothing.

In part, the importance of optimism to positive mental health depends on an attributional cognitive style that asserts that the good things that happen to a person last forever and are pervasive. The bad things that happen to a person are limited and unlikely to happen again. In addition, optimism includes hope, a facet of mental health as old as the Greek myth of Pandora, yet hope is a topic to which psychiatry, up to now, has given little formal consideration. In contrast, the explanatory style of many chronically depressed individuals is that bad events, for which a person may be responsible, last forever and generalize, whereas this same person bears no responsibility for good events that occur by chance but are limited and fleeting.

Longitudinal studies reveal that an optimistic attributional style improves physical health and wards off depression, rather than merely "prolonging human suffering," as Friedrich Nietzsche feared. In addition, the so-called illusion of optimism permits one to contemplate and plan for rather than to deny the future. As longitudinal studies have repeatedly shown, future-mindedness is a critical ingredient of mental health. In addition, in major depression, the hopeful illusion of placebo effect accounts for roughly 50 percent of the variance between the effect size produced by selective serotonin reuptake inhibitors (SSRIs) and no treatment. Thus, experimentally and longitudinally, optimism has been linked to positive mood and good morale, to perseverance and effective problem solving, to longevity, and to success in a wide spectrum of activities.

A critical distinction, of course, is the degree to which optimism distorts and to which pessimism accurately perceives reality. The pessimism of psychotic depression, like the psychotic optimism of acute mania, involves reality-defying delusion. The comforting illusions of the optimists, however, do not interfere with learning that stoves are hot, whereas the pessimistic perceptions of the dysthymic, although often accurate, can still inhibit future efforts to cook. In the prevention of future mental illness, one of psychiatry's most powerful tools may be the inculcation in the young of optimism, hope, and future-mindedness.

Recently, advocates of positive psychology have divided positive mental health into four components: *talents*, *enablers*, *strengths*, and *outcomes*. *Talents* are inborn and genetic and are not much effected by intervention (e.g., high IQ or being an easy baby). *Enablers* reflect benign social conditions, interventions, and environmental good luck (e.g., a strong family, a good school system, and living in a democratic meritocracy); enablers can be experimentally modified to enhance strengths. *Strengths* (Table 3.7–1) are character traits such as curiosity and openness that reflect facets of mental health that are amenable to change. *Outcomes* reflect dependent variables (improved GAF, social relationships, and subjective well-being) that can be used to provide evidence for the predictive validity that efforts by clinicians to enhance *strengths* are not just wishful thinking.

Admittedly, which so-called strengths are most associated with mental health is open to debate. Wisdom, kindness, and the capacity to love and be loved are strengths with which few would argue. However, should courage be included as a strength, and why are intelligence, perfect musical pitch, and punctuality excluded? The answer is that the 24 strengths listed in Table 3.7–1 may be subjected to a variety of tests. First, they have been recurrent positive values across cultures and across centuries. Second, they may be valued in their own right and not just as a means to ends.

There are several pitfalls with positive psychology. First, the perspective of mental health as utopia is one of the bogey men of national health policymakers. They are afraid, without directly expressing it, that this perspective will put a backbreaking burden on health insurance. Indeed, many psychotherapists do believe that the alleviation of signs and symptoms of psychopathology is only the first step in intensive, long-term individual psychotherapy. Thus, there is considerable debate within the mental health professions about whether helping people become happier with themselves is a process that any insurance program should reasonably be expected to cover. Helping people achieve their potential for community participation is perhaps a more laudable goal. However, that, too, is highly value laden and culture bound. Over time, society will have to decide who should pay for positive mental health: the individual, the educational system, third-party payers, religious organizations, or a combination of all four.

A second caution to positive psychology is the danger of culturally insensitive prescription of parochial virtues. The dangers of value judgments are enormous. *Virtues*, even aristotelian virtues, need to be distinguished from health. Keeping wounds clean is healthy but is not a virtue. Body hygiene in public places is a virtue but is not necessarily healthy.

A third controversial facet of positive psychology is its emphasis on optimism. Since the late 19th century, many social scientists, especially those in Europe, have mistrusted optimistic cognition, especially religious optimism, as a maladaptive, so-called American illusion interfering with accurate perception of reality. Nietzsche, Freud, Karl Marx, and Charles Darwin all perceived optimism as evidence of an ingenuous cultural adolescence, not of mature mental health. It was healthier to face the hard facts of life. In addition, for most of the 20th century, investigators like Ivan Petrovich Pavlov and B. F. Skinner have viewed the study of cognitions of all kinds, of which optimism is one, as inferior to the study of behavior. Only since the 1980s has this position been seriously challenged.

MODEL C: MENTAL HEALTH AS MATURITY

Unlike other organs of the body that are designed to stay the same, the brain is designed to be plastic. Therefore, just as optimal brain development requires almost a lifetime, so does assessment of positive mental health. A 10-year-old child's lungs and kidneys are more likely to reflect optimal function than are those of a 60-year-old adult, but that is not true of their central nervous systems (CNSs). To some extent, then, adult mental health reflects a continuing process of maturational unfolding. Statistically, physically healthy 70-year-old adults are mentally healthier than they were at 30 years old, and prospective studies reveal that individuals are less depressed and show greater emotional modulation at 70 years of age than they did at 30 years of age.

However, if prospective studies of adult development reveal that the immature brain functions less well than the mature brain, does that mean that adolescents are mentally healthier than toddlers? Are the middle-aged mentally healthier than adolescents? The answer is both yes and no, but the question illustrates why, to understand mental health, physicians must understand what is meant by maturity.

In some respects, in 1950, Erikson anticipated Jahoda and Grinker when he provided the first model of adult social development. He viewed each of his well-known eight "stages" of human development as a "criterion of mental health." Subsequently, Jane Loevinger provided a model of adult ego development. Lawrence Kohlberg has provided a model of adult moral development, and, most recently, James Fowler has provided a model of spiritual development. Implicit in all these models is the assumption that greater maturity reflected greater mental health. Arguably, the best definition of mental health that exists today is William Menninger's definition of maturity depicted in Table 3.7–1. In his model, maturity is not

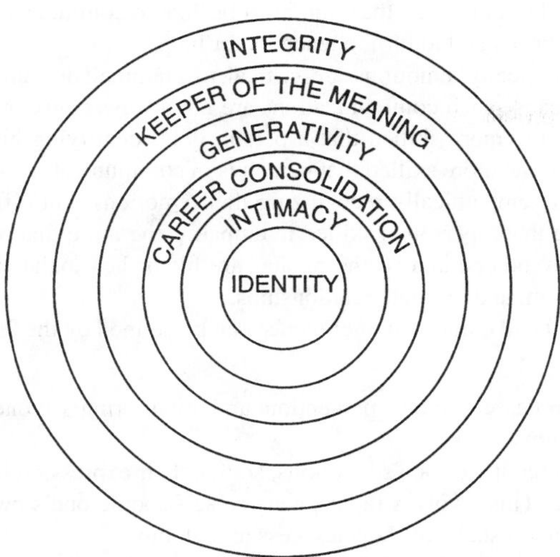

FIGURE 3.7–1 A schematic model of the expanding social radius of maturing individuals during adulthood.

only the antonym of narcissism, but it is quite congruent with other models of mental health.

To confirm the hypothesis that maturity and positive mental health are almost synonymous, the study of the behavior and feeling states of persons studied over a lifetime becomes necessary. Although such longitudinal studies have come to fruition only recently, all illustrate the association of maturity with increasing mental health. After 50 years of age, of course, the association between mental health and maturity is contingent on a healthy CNS. The ravages of brain trauma, major depression, arteriosclerosis, Alzheimer's disease, alcoholism, and schizophrenia must all be avoided.

The association of mental health to maturity is probably mediated not only by progressive brain myelinization into the sixth decade of life, but also by the evolution of emotional and social intelligence through experience. Erikson conceptualized that such development produced a "widening social radius." In such a view, life after 50 years of age was no longer to be a staircase leading downward, as in the Pennsylvania Dutch cartoons of life-span development, but a path leading outward. In Erikson's model, the adult social radius expanded over time through the mastery of the four tasks of "identity versus identity diffusion," "intimacy versus isolation," "generativity versus stagnation," and "integrity versus despair." On the basis of empirical data from Harvard's Study of Adult Development, Vaillant has added two more tasks—career consolidation and keeper of the meaning—to Erikson's four (Fig. 3.7–1). The mastery of such tasks appears relatively independent of education, gender, social class, and, probably, culture.

In such a model, the social radius of each adult developmental task fits inside the next. First, adolescents must achieve an *identity* that allows them to become separate from their parents, for mental health and adult development cannot evolve through a false self. The task of *identity* requires mastering the last task of childhood: sustained separation from social, residential, economic, and ideological dependence on family of origin. Identity is not just a product of egocentricity, running away from home, or marrying to get out of a dysfunctional family, for there is a world of difference between the instrumental act of running away from home and the developmental task of knowing where one's family values end and one's own values begin. Such separation derives as much from the identification and internalization of important adolescent friends and nonfamily mentors as it does from simple biological maturation. For example, individuals' accents become relatively fixed by 16 years of age and reflect those of their adolescent peer group rather than the accents of their parents.

Next, young adults should develop *intimacy*, which permits them to become reciprocally, and not selfishly, involved with a partner. However, living with just one other person in an interdependent, reciprocal, committed, and contented fashion for years and years may seem neither desirable nor possible to a young adult. Once achieved, however, the capacity for intimacy may seem as effortless and desirable as riding a bicycle. Sometimes, the relationship is with a person of the same gender; sometimes, it is completely asexual; and sometimes, as in religious orders, the interdependence is with a community. Superficially, mastery of intimacy may take different guises in different cultures and epochs, but *mating for life* and *marriage-type love* are developmental tasks that are built into the developmental repertoires of many warm-blooded species, including humans.

Career consolidation is a task that is usually mastered together with intimacy or that follows the mastery of intimacy. Mastery of this task permits adults to find a career as valuable as they once found play. On a desert island, one can have a hobby, but not a career, for careers involve being of value to other people. There are four crucial developmental criteria that transform a *job* or hobby into a *career*: contentment, compensation, competence, and commitment. Obviously, such a career can be *wife* and *mother*—or, in more recent times, *husband* and *father*. To the outsider, the process of *career consolidation* often appears selfish, but, without such selfishness, one becomes selfless and has no self to give away in the next stage of *generativity*. Not only schizophrenics, but also individuals with severe personality disorder often manifest a lifelong inability to achieve intimacy or sustained, gratifying employment.

Mastery of the fourth task, *generativity*, involves the demonstration of a clear capacity to care for and guide the next generation. Existing research reveals that, sometime between 35 years of age and 55 years of age, the need for achievement declines and the need for community and affiliation increases. Depending on the opportunities that the society makes available, generativity can mean serving as a consultant, guide, mentor, or coach to young adults in the larger society. Like leadership, *generativity* means to be in a caring relationship in which one gives up much of the control that parents retain over young children. Good mentors learn to hold loosely and to share responsibility. Generativity reflects the capacity to give the self—finally completed through mastery of the first three tasks of adult development—away. Its mastery is strongly correlated with successful adaptation to old age. This is because, in old age, there are inevitable losses, and these may be overwhelming if a person has not continued to grow beyond his or her immediate family.

The penultimate life task is to become a *keeper of the meaning*. Like grandparenthood, this task involves passing on the traditions of the past to the future. Generativity and its virtue, *care*, requires taking care of one person rather than another, whereas keeper of the meaning and its virtues of *wisdom* and *justice* are less selective, for justice, unlike care, means not taking sides. Indeed, mastery of this fifth task is epitomized by the role of the wise judge. The focus of a keeper of the meaning is with conservation and preservation of the collective products of mankind—the culture in which one lives and its institutions—rather than with just the development of its children.

Just as selfless coaches play a different role from selfish athletes, the organizers, judges, and guardians of the Olympic Games play different roles from the Olympic Games' more generative, but still parochial, coaches. Clearly, caretakers and grandparents are not mentally healthier than caregivers and parents. The distinction is only that grandparents are usually better at the tasks of keepers of the meaning than are 30-year-old adults.

Finally, in old age, it is common to feel that some life exists after death and that one is part of something greater than one's self. Thus, the last life task, in Erikson's words, is *integrity*, the task of achieving some sense of peace and unity with respect to one's own life and to the whole world. Erikson described integrity as "an experience which conveys some world order and spiritual sense. No matter how dearly paid for, it is the acceptance of one's one and only life cycle as something that had to be and that, by necessity, permitted of no substitutions."

Admittedly, healthy adult development does not follow rigid rules. Some individuals, often due to great stress, tackle developmental tasks out of order or all at once. On the one hand, Alexander the Great, General Lafayette, Napoleon Bonaparte, and Joan of Arc were inspirational and generative leaders in their 20s. On the other hand, William Osler, one of the most generative physicians of all time, did not confront the task of intimacy until he married at 40 years of age—well after he had established his career as a brilliant professor of medicine. Ludwig van Beethoven enjoyed a brilliant, committed career but never enjoyed intimacy.

Finally, it must be kept in mind that mastery of one life task is not necessarily healthier than mastery of another, for adult development is neither a foot race nor a moral imperative. Rather, these six sequential tasks are offered as a road map to help physicians make sense of where they are and where their patients might be located. One can be a mature 20-year-old adult that is healthy. One can be an immature 50-year-old adult that may be unhealthy. Nevertheless, acquiring a social radius that extends beyond the self, by definition, allows more flexibility and thus is usually healthier than self-preoccupation.

MODEL D: MENTAL HEALTH AS SOCIOEMOTIONAL INTELLIGENCE

High socioemotional intelligence reflects above average mental health in the same way that a high IQ reflects above average intellectual aptitude. Such emotional intelligence lies at the heart of positive mental health. In *Nicomachean Ethics*, Aristotle defined *socioemotional intelligence* as follows: "Anyone can become angry—that is easy. But to be angry with the right person, to the right degree, at the right time, for the right purpose, and in the right way—that is not easy." Nevertheless, as recently as the 1960s, a textbook on intelligence dismissed the concept of such aristotelian social intelligence as "useless." Indeed, only in the 1970s did the modulation of "object relations" become more important to psychoanalysis than the modulation of "instinct." By definition, a model of socioemotional intelligence suggests that instinct and object relations are equal partners.

All emotions exist to assist basic survival. Although the exact number of primary emotions is arguable, seven emotions are currently distinguished by characteristic facial expressions connoting anger, fear, excitement, interest, surprise, disgust, and sadness. The capacity to identify these different emotions in ourselves and in others plays an important role in mental health. The benefits of being able to read feelings from nonverbal cues have been demonstrated in almost a score of countries. These benefits included being better emotionally adjusted, more popular, and more responsive to others. Empathic children, without being more intelligent, do better in school and are more popular than their peers. Head Start found that early school success was achieved not by intelligence but by knowing what kind of behavior is expected, how to rein in the impulse to misbehave, being able to wait, and how to get along with other children. At the same time, the child must be able to communicate his or her own needs and to turn to teachers for help.

Ethologically, emotions are critical to mammalian communication. Because such communications are not always consciously recognized, the more skilled that a person is in identifying his or her emotions, the more skilled that person is in communicating with others and in empathically recognizing their emotions. Put differently, the more that a person is skilled in empathy, the more that person is valued by others, and so the greater are his or her social supports, self-esteem, and intimate relationships.

Social and emotional intelligence can be defined by the following criteria:

- Accurate, conscious perception and monitoring of one's own emotions.
- Modification of one's emotions, so that their expression is appropriate. This involves the capacity to self-soothe one's own anxiety and to shake off hopelessness and gloom.
- Accurate recognition of and response to emotions in others.
- Skill in negotiating close relationships with others.
- Capacity for focusing emotions (motivation) toward a desired goal. This involves delayed gratification and adaptively displacing and channeling impulse.

Some behavioral scientists divide emotions into positive and negative, as if negative emotions were unhealthy. This is probably an error. As with pus, fever, and cough, so the negative emotions of sadness, fear, and anger are also important to healthy self-preservation. Positive emotions, such as joy, love, interest, and excitement, are associated with subjective contentment. Although negative emotions interfere with contentment, their expression can be equally healthy.

Since the late 1980s, three important empirical steps have been taken in the understanding of the relationship of socioemotional intelligence to positive mental health. The first step is that functional magnetic resonance imaging (MRI) and ingenious neurophysiological experimentation have led to advances in the understanding of the integration of prefrontal cortex with the limbic system, especially with the amygdyla and its connections. These research advances have brought researchers closer to understanding emotions as neurophysiological phenomena rather than as platonic abstractions. It has been learned that the prefrontal cortex is the region of the brain responsible for working memory and that the frontal lobes, through their connections to the amygdyla, hippocampus, and other limbic structures, encode emotional learning in a manner quite distinct from conventional conditioning and declarative memory.

The second step forward has been the slow but steady progress in the conceptualizing and even the measuring of *emotional intelligence*. Since the 1990s, measures of emotional intelligence are evolving rapidly.

The third advance is the use of videotape to chart emotional interaction. Videos of sustained family interactions reveal that the most important aspect of healthy infant development, adolescent development, and marital harmony is how partners or parents respond to emotion in others. To ignore, to punish, and to be intimidated or contemptuous of how another feels spells disaster. Children of emotionally attuned parents are better at handling their own emotions and are more effective at soothing themselves when upset. Such children even manifest lower levels of stress hormones and other physiological indicators of emotional arousal.

Where the passive study of positive mental health ends and active primary prevention begins is unclear, but, like the model of positive psychology, the model of socioemotional intelligence is potentially interventionist. Just as an individual can have above average musical skill or physical coordination and yet can train these strengths to be even higher, so can an individual learn to enhance emotional modulation. Until late in the Cold War, empirically researched techniques for "getting to yes" in negotiations were not in any academic curricula.

There are now many exercises in handling relationships that help couples, business executives, and diplomats become more skilled at conflict resolution and negotiation. In the 1990s, there has also been an increasing effort to teach schoolchildren core emotional and social competencies, sometimes called *emotional literacy*. The relevance of these advances in psychology to psychiatry includes teaching emotion recognition and differentiation in the eating disorders and teaching anger modulation and finding creative solutions to social predicaments for behavior disorders.

MODEL E: MENTAL HEALTH AS SUBJECTIVE WELL-BEING

Is it better to meet some expert's definition of mental health, or is it better to feel subjectively fulfilled? The answer is both. Positive mental health does not just involve being a joy to others; one must also experience subjective well-being. Long before humankind considered definitions of mental health, they pondered criteria for subjective happiness. For example, objective social support accomplishes little if, subjectively, the individual cannot feel loved. Thus, the capacity for subjective well-being becomes an important model of mental health.

Subjective well-being is never categorical. Healthy blood pressure is the objective absence of hypotension and hypertension, but happiness is less neutral. Subjective well-being is not just the absence of misery but the presence of positive contentment. Nevertheless, if happiness is an inescapable dimension of mental health, happiness is often regarded with ambivalence. If, through the centuries, philosophers have sometimes regarded happiness as the highest good, psychologists and psychiatrists have tended to ignore it. An electronic search of psychological abstracts since 1987 turned up 57,800 articles on anxiety and 70,856 on depression, but only 5,701 mentioned life satisfaction, and only 851 mentioned joy.

On the one hand, "no man is happy who does not think himself so." Happiness that comes from joy or that comes from unselfish love (agape), happiness that comes from self-control and self-efficacy, or happiness that comes from play and flow (deep but effortless involvement) reflects health. Happiness that comes from spiritual discipline and concentration, that comes from humor, or that comes from being relieved of narcissistic focus on shame, resentments, and self-pity is a blessing. The subjective gratification derived from the *strengths* described in Model B: Mental Health as Positive Psychology is hard won and has sticking power. Authentic happiness depends on achieving autonomy, forgiveness, close relationships, and self-efficacy.

On the other hand, subjective happiness can have maladaptive, as well as adaptive, facets. The search for happiness can appear selfish, narcissistic, superficial, and banal. Pleasures can come easily and can be soon gone. Happiness is often based on illusion or on dissociative states. Illusory happiness is seen in the character structure associated with bipolar and dissociative disorders, with the maladaptive denial of Pollyanna and Voltaire's Dr. Pangloss, and with the exaltation of "me" advocated by much pop psychology. Examples of maladaptive so-called happiness can be the excitement of risk taking, from being high on drugs, and from turning on to any unmodulated but gratifying primitive need, such as binge eating, tantrums, promiscuity, and revenge. Such maladaptive happiness can bring temporary bliss but has no sticking power. It is because of such ambiguity of meaning that, throughout this section, the term *subjective well-being* is substituted for happiness.

The mental health issues involved in subjective well-being are complicated and clouded by historical relativism, value judgment, and illusion. Europeans have always been skeptical of the American concern with happiness. Only in the 1990s have investigators like Barbara Fredrickson, Seligman, and David Snowdon pointed out that a primary function of positive emotional states and optimism is that they facilitate self-care. Subjective well-being makes available personal resources that can be directed toward innovation and creativity in thought and action. Thus, subjective well-being, like optimism, becomes an antidote to learned helplessness. Again, controlling for income, education, weight, smoking, alcohol abuse, and disease, happy people are only one-half as likely as unhappy people to die at an early age or to become disabled.

A distinction can be made between *pleasure* and *gratification*. Pleasure is in the moment, is closely allied with happiness, and involves satisfaction of impulse and of biological needs. Pleasure is highly susceptible to habituation and satiety. In contrast, gratification can be equated with what Aristotle called *eudaimania* and Csikszentmihalyi terms *flow*. In such a distinction, if pleasure involves satisfaction of the senses and emotions, gratification involves joy, the satisfaction of "being the best you can be" and of meeting aesthetic and spiritual needs. This can be manifested by a child lost in play, a mountaineer transported by rock climbing, or a father marveling at his daughter's first solo on a bicycle.

However, once again, the role of value judgment clouds the view of whether any given form of happiness is good or bad. Is the happiness of helping others better than the happiness of gratifying creative play? The jury is still out. In addition, all emotions exist to promote survival as well as to communicate with others. Subjective (unhappy) distress can be healthy. As ethologically minded investigators have long pointed out, subjective negative affects (e.g., fear, anger, and sadness) can be healthy reminders to seek environmental safety and not to wallow in subjective well-being. If positive emotions facilitate faith, hope, optimism, and contentment, fear is the first protection against external threat, sadness protests against loss and summons replacement, and anger signals trespass.

Positive emotion generates exploration and promotes mastery. Unlike negative emotions, which generate zero-sum, win–lose situations, positive emotions generate win–win situations. However, tolerance of negative emotions may characterize some periods of the life cycle more than others. The relative absence of depression and anxiety over time is healthy in grammar school children from 8 to 10 years of age and in young submariners in their 20s. Increasing capacity to tolerate and to bear subjective depression and anxiety distinguishes healthy adolescents from healthy fifth graders and healthy (generative) submarine skippers from healthy enlisted men. There is a time to hope and a time to fear. Human development is complex.

Until recently, the scientific parameters of subjective well-being were as vague as those for objective mental health. A 1967 definition suggested that a happy person is "*young, healthy, well-educated, well paid,* extroverted, optimistic, *worry free,* religious and married with high self esteem, a good job, morals, and *modest aspirations*." Since the 1970s, however, research has shown that such a vacuous generalization is only partly correct and that the italicized adjectives are untrue or true only with qualifications.

The Nun Study by Snowdon provides perhaps the most convincing link between subjective happiness and health. In their 20s, 180 nuns were asked to write a two- to three-page autobiography. Of those who expressed the most positive emotion, only 24 percent had died by 80 years of age. In contrast, by 80 years of age, 54 percent of those who expressed the least positive emotion had died.

Only since the 1970s have investigators, especially Edward Diener, made a serious effort to attend to definitional and causal parameters of subjective well-being and thereby address important questions. One such question is the following: Is subjective well-being more a function of environmental good fortune, or is it more a function of an inborn, genetically based temperament? Put differently, does subjective well-being reflect trait or state? If subjective well-being reflects a safe environment and the absence of stress, it should fluctuate over time, and those individuals who are happy in one domain or time in their lives might not be happy in another.

A second question, but one related to the first, is what is cause and what is effect. Are happy people more likely to achieve enjoyable jobs and good marriages or does conjugal stability and career contentment lead to subjective well-being? Or are such positive associations the result of still a third factor? For example, the absence of a genetic tendency for alcoholism, major depression, trait neuroticism, and even the presence of a chronic wish to give socially desirable answers (impression management) might facilitate subjective well-being and reports of good marriage and career contentment.

Research since the 1970s has provided a tentative answer to the first question. Modern research has confirmed the aphorism of Duke La Roche-Foucauld: "Happiness and misery depend as much on temperament as on fortune." Subjective well-being is highly heritable and relatively independent of demographic variables. Subjective well-being is due more to *top-down* processes—temperamental factors governing subjective well-being—rather than due to *bottom-up* factors—for example, the fulfillment of universal human needs leading to subjective well-being.

As with physiological homeostasis, evolution has prepared humans to make subjective adjustments to environmental conditions. Thus, a person can adapt to good and bad events so that he or she does not remain in a state of elation or despair. Humans have a harder time, however, adjusting to their genes. Studies of adopted-away twins have demonstrated that one-half of the variance in subjective well-being is due to heritability. The subjective well-being of monozygous twins raised apart is more similar than the subjective well-being of heterozygous twins raised together. Among the heritable factors making a significant contribution to high subjective well-being are low trait neuroticism, high trait extraversion, absence of alcoholism, and absence of major depression. In contrast to tested intelligence, when heritable variables are controlled, subjective well-being is not affected by environmental factors, such as income, parental social class, age, and education.

For example, investigators have been startled that a significant number of acquired immune deficiency syndrome (AIDS) victims perceive that their illness has enhanced the quality of their subjective lives. Paraplegic victims of spinal injuries adapt so that, within 2 months after injury, their subjective well-being returns to a state in which positive emotion exceeds negative emotion. Similarly, after a few weeks of temporary elation, lottery winners also return to baseline. Some of the homeostatic mental mechanisms underlying such adaptation are elaborated in the next section.

If subjective well-being were due largely to the meeting of basic needs, then there should be a relatively low correlation between subjective well-being in work settings and subjective well-being in recreational settings or between subjective well-being in social settings versus subjective well-being in solitary settings. However, in most studies, the correlations between subjective well-being in different facets of life are high—higher than the correlation between height and weight. People who are satisfied with their lives at one point in time are more likely to be satisfied with their jobs in the future, and people with high job satisfaction are more likely to report satisfaction with retirement. Admittedly, a few studies exist in which correlations are low between satisfaction with different facets of life. Again, more work is needed.

Because women experience more objective clinical depression than men do, the fact that gender is not a determining factor in subjective well-being is interesting. One explanation is that women appear to report positive and negative affects more vividly than men. In one such study, gender accounted for only 1 percent of the variance in happiness but 13 percent of the variance of the intensity of reported emotional experiences.

Consistently, relationships are more important to subjective well-being than money. In a representative study of 800 college alumni, respondents who preferred high income, occupational success, and prestige to having close friends and a close marriage were twice as likely to describe themselves as "fairly" or "very" unhappy. Since the 1980s, the doubling of net disposable income (controlling for inflation) in the Western world (Fig. 3.7–2) did not affect subjective well-being. Additional evidence that environmental events are much

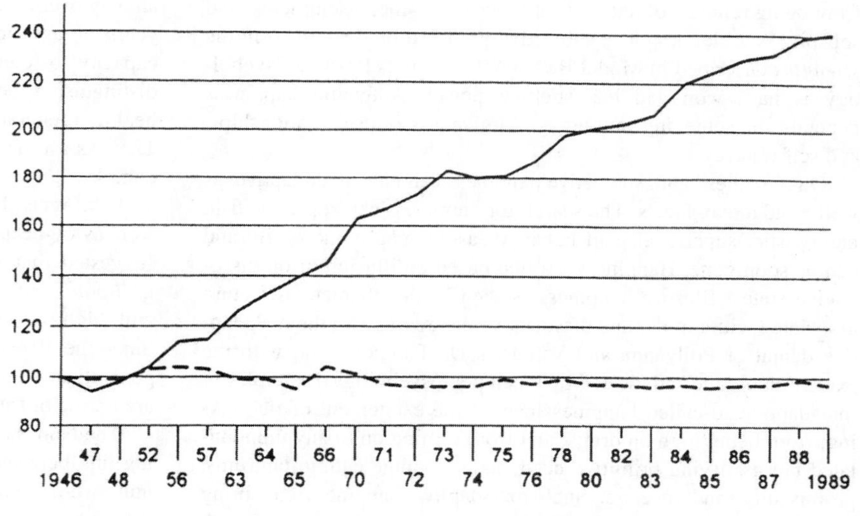

FIGURE 3.7–2 The independence of a 240 percent increase in U.S. individual income (adjusted for inflation) from subjective well-being (SWB) over 40 years.

less important to subjective well-being than might be expected come from cross-cultural studies. Mean life satisfaction in socioeconomically challenged Brazil and China is higher than in socioeconomically blessed Japan and Germany.

In some instances, environment *can* be important to subjective well-being. Young widows remain subjectively depressed for years. Even though their poverty has been endured for centuries, respondents in poor nations, like India and Nigeria, report lower subjective well-being than do more prosperous nations. The loss of a child never stops aching. Although the achievement of concrete goals, such as money and fame, does not lead to a sustained increase in subjective well-being, social comparison, such as watching one's next door neighbor become richer than you, does exert a negative effect on subjective well-being.

The maintenance of self-efficacy, -agency, and -autonomy makes additional environmental contributions to subjective well-being. For example, surprisingly, elders use discretionary income to live independently, even though this means living alone rather than with relatives. Subjective well-being is usually higher in democracies than in dictatorships. Assuming responsibility for favorable or unfavorable outcomes (internalization) is another major factor leading to subjective well-being. Placing the blame elsewhere (externalization) significantly reduces subjective well-being. In other words, the mental mechanisms of paranoia and projection make people feel worse rather than better.

Religiosity is consistently and positively correlated with well-being, but there may be a chicken-and-egg relationship between social support and religious observance. For example, among church-goers, it is difficult to disentangle where spiritual faith ends and community support begins. Nevertheless, it makes sense that positive faith should enhance subjective well-being. Heightened spirituality provides hope that bad events will diminish and lends wonder and joy to ordinary events.

Since the 1970s, methodological solutions have accelerated the understanding of subjective well-being, just as they have accelerated the understanding of objective mental health. Longitudinal studies, multivariate analysis, and causal modeling have each done much to free investigators from correlational reasoning. Nevertheless, efforts to measure subjective well-being have been quite varied and lack a gold standard. Some investigators measure subjective well-being as simply global life satisfaction; other investigators assess more specific domains, such as work, marital satisfaction, and positive affect. The question "How do you feel about your life as a whole?" answered on a simple seven-point scale ranging from "delighted" to "terrible" works surprisingly well.

More refined methods of measurement of subjective states of mind have included the Positive and Negative Affect Scale (PANAS), which assesses positive and negative affect each with ten affect items. The *Satisfaction with Life Scale* represents the most recent evolution of a general life satisfaction scale. Most recently, the widely validated SF-36 has allowed clinicians to assess the subjective cost benefits of clinical interventions. Because short-lived environmental variables can distort subjective well-being, consensus is emerging that naturalistic experience-sampling methods are the most valid ways to assess subjective well-being. With such sampling methods, research subjects are contacted by beeper at random times during the day for days or weeks and, at each interval, are asked to assess their subjective well-being. This method provides a more stable report of subjective well-being. Finally, to tease verbal self-report from actual subjective experience, physiological measures of stress (for example, measures of galvanic skin response, salivary cortisol, and filming facial expression by concealed cameras) have also proven useful.

MODEL F: MENTAL HEALTH AS RESILIENCE

In 1856, Claude Bernard, a French physiologist and a founder of experimental medicine, started the understanding of positive health when he wrote, "We shall never have a science of medicine as long as we separate the explanation of the pathological from the explanation of normal, vital phenomena." For example, coughing and pus in response to infection seemed pathological but, in fact, were often healing. In other words, it is not stress that kills individuals but the healthy mastery of stress that permits individuals to survive.

In 1925, Meyer, a founder of modern American psychiatry, started the understanding of mental health when he asserted that there were no mental diseases; there were only characteristic reaction patterns to stress. Meyer's point was that although adaptive mental *reaction patterns*, such as denial, phobias, and even projections, can appear to reflect illness, they may, in fact, be "normal, vital phenomena" related to healing. Just as immune mechanisms, clotting mechanisms, and callus formation heal by distorting bodily equilibrium, so do equally involuntary coping mechanisms heal by distorting mental processes.

Of course, the symptoms of organic brain damage usually reflect disease and not adaptation. Manic-depressive psychosis is due to genetic defect, the mental devastation produced by alcoholism is due to poisoning, and the negative symptoms of schizophrenia reflect brain defect and not adaptation. Nevertheless, much so-called mental illness is more like the healthy, but red and tender, swelling that immobilizes a fracture, so that it may heal. Much of what is called *mental illness* in diagnostic nomenclature—the symptoms of many anxiety disorders, some depressions, and most personality disorders—are the outward manifestations of homeostatic struggles to adapt to life. Admittedly, analogous to acne and autoimmune disease, such reaction patterns often reflect rigid, poorly modulated, and pathological efforts at adaptation.

To set the stage, there are three broad classes of coping mechanisms that humans use to overcome stressful situations. First, there are the ways in which an individual elicits help from appropriate others: namely, *consciously seeking social support*. Second, there are *conscious cognitive strategies* that individuals intentionally use to master stress. Third, there are *adaptive involuntary coping mechanisms* (often called *defense mechanisms*) that distort an individual's perception of internal and external reality to reduce subjective distress, anxiety, and depression.

By 1970, the term *defense mechanisms*, like many psychoanalytic metaphors, had been largely discarded by empirical social scientists. Consistency of definition and rater reliability was lacking. However, since the 1970s, the idea of involuntary coping has entered the literature of empirical cognitive psychology under such rubrics as *hardiness*, *self-deception* and *emotional coping*, and *illusion*. In recent years, experimental strategies for assessing such mechanisms, especially with videotape and the q-sort, have also improved reliability. Several empirical studies, well-reviewed by Andrew Skodol and Christopher Perry, have clarified the understanding of healthy and unhealthy defenses. By offering a tentative hierarchy and glossary of consensually validated definitions, the axis of defense mechanisms in DSM-IV-TR has set the stage for further progress in the understanding of positive mental health (Table 3.7–2). Nevertheless, no one has yet developed a method for assessing defenses that meets conventional standards for psychometric reliability.

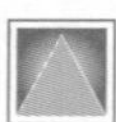

Table 3.7–2
Defense Levels and Individual Defense Mechanisms

I. Level of defensive deregulation: This level is characterized by failure of defensive regulation to contain the individual's reaction to stressors, leading to a pronounced break with objective reality. Examples are
- Delusional projection (e.g., psychotic delusions)
- Psychotic denial of external reality
- Psychotic distortion (e.g., hallucinations)

II. Action level: This level is characterized by defensive functioning that deals with internal or external stressors by action or withdrawal. Examples are
- Acting out
- Passive aggression
- Apathetic withdrawal
- Help-rejecting complaining

III. Major image-distorting level: This level is characterized by gross distortion or misattribution of the image of self or others. Examples are
- Autistic fantasy (e.g., imaginary relationships)
- Splitting of self-image or image of others (e.g., making people all good or all bad)

IV. Disavowal level: This level is characterized by keeping unpleasant or unacceptable stressors, impulses, ideas, affects, or responsibility out of awareness, with or without a misattribution of these to external causes. Examples are
- Denial
- Projection
- Rationalization

V. Minor image-distorting level: This level is characterized by distortions in the image of the self, body, or others that may be used to regulate self-esteem. Examples are
- Devaluation
- Idealization
- Omnipotence

VI. Mental inhibitions (compromise formation) level: Defensive functioning at this level keeps potentially threatening ideas, feelings, memories, wishes, or fears out of awareness. Examples are
- Displacement
- Reaction formation
- Dissociation
- Repression
- Intellectualization
- Undoing
- Isolation of affect

VII. High adaptive level: This level of defensive functioning results in optimal adaptation in the handling of stressors. These defenses usually maximize gratification and allow the conscious awareness of feelings, ideas, and their consequences. They also promote an optimum balance among conflicting motives. Examples of defenses at this level are
- **Anticipation**
- Self-assertion
- Affiliation
- Self-observation
- **Altruism**
- **Sublimation**
- **Humor**
- **Suppression**

Adapted from American Psychiatric Association. Defense levels and individual defense mechanisms. In: *Diagnostic and Statistical Manual of Mental Disorders*. 4th ed. Washington, DC: American Psychiatric Association Press; 1994:752.

This third class of adaptive involuntary coping mechanisms reduces conflict and cognitive dissonance during sudden *changes* in internal and external reality. If such changes in reality are not "distorted" and "denied," they can result in disabling anxiety or depression, or both. In summary, such homeostatic mental defenses shield individuals from sudden changes in the four lodestars of conflict: affect, reality, relationships, and conscience (Fig. 3.7–3).

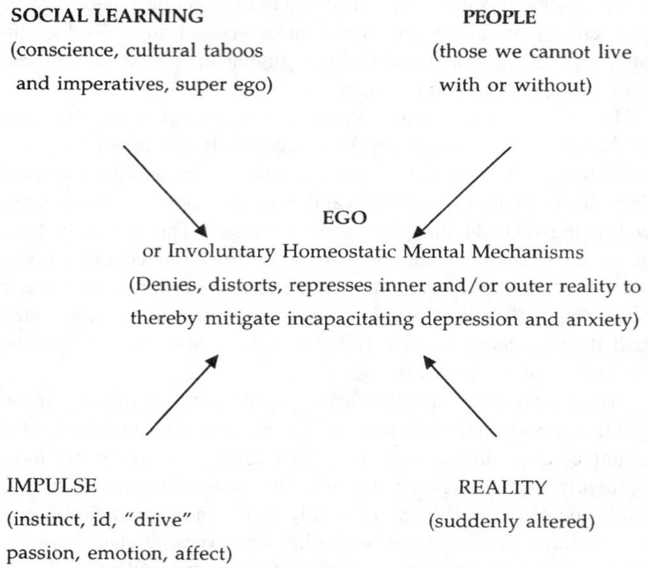

SOCIAL LEARNING
(conscience, cultural taboos
and imperatives, super ego)

PEOPLE
(those we cannot live
with or without)

EGO
or Involuntary Homeostatic Mental Mechanisms
(Denies, distorts, represses inner and/or outer reality to
thereby mitigate incapacitating depression and anxiety)

IMPULSE
(instinct, id, "drive"
passion, emotion, affect)

REALITY
(suddenly altered)

FIGURE 3.7–3 The four lodestars of human conflict.

First, such involuntary mental mechanisms can restore psychological homeostasis by ignoring or deflecting sudden increases in the lodestar of impulse, affect, and emotion. (The emotions of grief, longing, and dependency loom just as important as sources of conflict as do lust, fear, and rage.) Psychoanalysts call this lodestar *id*, fundamentalists call it *sin*, cognitive psychologists call it *hot cognition*, and neuroanatomists relate it to the hypothalamic and limbic regions of brain.

Second, such involuntary mental mechanisms can provide a mental time out to adjust to sudden changes in *reality* and self-image, which cannot be immediately integrated. Individuals who initially responded to the television images of the sudden destruction of New York's World Trade Center as if it were a movie provide a vivid example of denial of an external reality that was changing too fast for voluntary adaptation. Sudden good news—the instant transition from student to physician or winning the lottery—can evoke involuntary mental mechanisms as often as can an unexpected accident or diagnosis of leukemia.

Third, involuntary mental mechanisms can mitigate sudden unresolvable conflict with important *people*, living or dead. People become a lodestar of conflict when an individual cannot live with a person and yet cannot live without him or her. Death is such an example; another is an unexpected proposal of marriage. Because people exist within an individual as well as without, internal representations of important people may continue to haunt a person and to cause conflict for decades after a person has ceased to live with them and thus evoke involuntary mental response.

Finally, the fourth source of conflict or anxious depression is social learning or conscience. Psychoanalysts call it *superego*, anthropologists call it *taboo*, behaviorists call it *conditioning*, and neuroanatomists relate it to the associative cortex and the amygdala. This lodestar is not just the result of admonitions from an individual's parents that are absorbed before 5 years of age but is formed by an individual's whole identification, with an individual's culture, and sometimes by irreversible learning resulting from overwhelming trauma.

There are many ways that individuals can ignore or distort one or more of these four lodestars to mitigate intrapsychic conflict. For semantic consistency, the Defensive Function Scale of *DSM-IV-TR* has labeled these involuntary mental mechanisms *defenses* (Table 3.7–2). These coping mechanisms, or *defenses*, can abolish impulse (e.g., by reaction formation), social learning (e.g., by acting out), other people (e.g., by schizoid fantasy), or reality (e.g., by psychotic denial). They can abolish the conscious recognition of the subject (e.g., by projection), the object of a conflict (e.g., by turning against the self), the awareness of the idea (e.g., by repression), or the affect associated with the idea (e.g., isolation of affect).

All classes of defenses in Table 3.7–2 are effective in *denying*, or defusing, conflict and in *repressing*, or minimizing, stress, but they differ greatly in the psychiatric diagnoses assigned to their users and in their consequences for long-term biopsychosocial adaptation. In level I, the most pathological category, are found denial and distortion of external reality. These mechanisms are common in young children, in dreams, and in psychosis. To breach them requires altering the brain by neuroleptics or waking the dreamer.

More common to everyday life are the relatively maladaptive defenses found in levels II through V. Defenses in these categories are common in adolescents, in immature adults, and in individuals with personality disorders. They often make others more uncomfortable than the user. Such defenses are consistently and negatively correlated with global assessment of mental health, and they profoundly distort the affective component of interpersonal relationships.

The third class of defenses, those in level VI, are often associated with what DSM-IV-TR calls *Axis I anxiety disorders* and with the psychopathology of everyday life. These include mechanisms like repression, intellectualization, reaction formation (i.e., turning the other cheek), and displacement (i.e., directing affect at a more neutral object). In contrast to the *immature* defenses, these intermediate defenses are manifested clinically by phobias, compulsions, obsessions, somatizations, and amnesias. Such users often seek psychological help, and such "compromise formations" respond more readily to interpretation. Such defenses usually cause more conscious suffering to the user than to other people. They are common to everyone from 5 years of age until death. They are neither healthy nor unhealthy.

The mechanisms at level VII still distort and alter feelings, conscience, relationships, and reality, but they achieve these alterations gracefully and flexibly. These mechanisms allow the individual consciously to experience the affective component of interpersonal relationships, but in a tempered fashion. Thus, the beholder regards level VII adaptive defenses as virtues, just as the beholder may regard the prejudice of projection and the tantrums of acting out as sins.

Doing as one would be done by (altruism), keeping a stiff upper lip (suppression), keeping future pain in awareness (anticipation), the ability not to take one's self too seriously (humor), and turning lemons into lemonade (sublimation) are the very stuff from which positive mental health is made. Unfortunately, like tightrope walking, without months of practice, mature mechanisms cannot easily be deployed voluntarily and only then by those with innate balance.

Identification of defenses is difficult. Rarely can individuals identify their defenses, and individuals often fail to recognize them in others or, still worse, "project" their own defenses onto them. To identify a defense, an objective observer needs to triangulate past truth with present behavior and subjective report. For example, one woman wins community praise for founding a shelter for battered women (altruism), but she dismisses her behavior as "a need to rent my house." Another woman is imprisoned for breaking her toddler daughter's arm in a tantrum (acting out), but she dismisses her behavior as an accident. In fact, social agency records from 30 years before reveal that both women had been taken at 2 years of age from the care of physically abusive alcoholic mothers. Whether another's coping response is ultimately viewed as healthy or psychopathic depends on the results of their involuntary efforts. Ultimately, like other facets of mental health, the reliable identification of healthy, but involuntary, coping mechanisms requires longitudinal study.

Healthy Involuntary Mental Mechanisms Longitudinal studies from Berkeley's Institute of Human Development and Harvard's Study of Adult Development have illustrated the importance of the mature defenses to mental health.

Humor It is largely recognized that humor makes life easier. As Freud suggested, "humor can be regarded as the highest of these defensive processes," for humor "scorns to withdraw the ideational content bearing the distressing affect from conscious attention, as repression does, and thus surmounts the automatism of defense." With humor, individuals see all and feel much but do not act. Humor permits the discharge of emotion without individual discomfort and without unpleasant effects on others. Mature humor allows the individual to look directly at what is painful, whereas dissociation and slapstick distract the individual to look somewhere else. Yet, like the other mature defenses, humor requires the same delicacy as building a house of cards—timing is everything.

Altruism When used to master conflict, altruism involves getting pleasure from giving to others what an individual himself or herself would have liked to receive. For example, using reaction formation, a former alcohol abuser works to ban the sale of alcohol in his town and annoys his social drinking friends. Using altruism, the same former alcoholic serves as an Alcoholics Anonymous sponsor to a new member—achieving a transformative process that may be lifesaving to giver and receiver. Obviously, many acts of altruism involve free will, but others involuntarily soothe unmet needs.

Sublimation The sign of a successful sublimation is neither careful cost accounting nor shrewd compromise, but rather psychic alchemy. By analogy, sublimation permits the oyster to transform an irritating grain of sand into a pearl. In writing his *Ninth Symphony*, the deaf, angry, and lonely Beethoven transformed his pain into triumph by putting Schiller's *Ode to Joy* to music.

Suppression Suppression is a defense that modulates emotional conflict or internal and external stressors through stoicism. Suppression minimizes and postpones, but does not ignore, gratification. Empirically, this is the defense most highly associated with other facets of mental health. Used effectively, suppression is analogous to a well-trimmed sail; every restriction is precisely calculated to exploit, not to hide, the winds of passion. Evidence that suppression is not simply a conscious "cognitive strategy" is provided by the fact that jails would empty if delinquents could learn to just say "no."

Anticipation If suppression reflects the capacity to keep current impulse in mind and to control it, anticipation is the capacity to keep affective response to an unbearable future event in mind in manageable doses. The defense of anticipation reflects the capacity to perceive future danger affectively, as well as cognitively, and, by this means, to master conflict in small steps. Examples would be the fact that moderate amounts of anxiety before surgery promote postsurgical adaptation and that anticipatory mourning facilitates the adaptation of parents of children with leukemia.

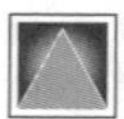

Table 3.7–3
Cross Correlation between Four Different Models of Mental Health at Midlife (47 Years of Age), Their Positive Prediction of Late-Life (65 Years of Age) Mental Health, and Their Independence from Parental Social Class and Childhood Environment

	A	C	D	F
Model A: Axis V	—			
Model C: Maturity	0.61	—		
Model D: Social intelligence	0.57	0.50	—	
Model F: Resilience	0.81	0.57	0.51	—
Subjective well-being at 65 years of age	0.44	0.32	0.42	0.35
Mental health at 65 years of age	0.52	0.38	0.43	0.50
Parental social class	0.08	0.05	0.12	0.06
Warm childhood environment	0.19	0.12	0.16	0.13

Note: N = 160. Correlations greater than 0.25 are significant at $P<.001$, n = 137–143. Correlations greater than 0.15 are significant at $P<.05$.

As with the use of altruism and suppression, the use of anticipation can often be voluntary and independent of conflict. However, it is in cases of "hot cognition" that these defenses can become involuntary and lifesaving.

Just as psychiatry needs to understand how a GAF of 75 might become 90, so does psychiatry need to understand how best to facilitate the transmutation of less adaptive defenses into more adaptive defenses. One suggestion has been, first, to increase social supports and interpersonal safety and, second, to facilitate the intactness of the CNS (e.g., rest, nutrition, and sobriety). The newer forms of integrative psychotherapies using videotape can also catalyze such change by allowing patients to see their involuntary coping style.

FUTURE DIRECTIONS

This chapter has suggested six conceptually distinct ways to assess a single construct—mental health. It would be a terrible mistake to believe that any one of these six models is superior to the others. From different vantage points, they all measure the same thing. For example, in the case example, Richard Luckey not only had a GAF of 95, but another independent rater also saw him as highly generative, and a third rater saw him using defenses largely from level VII. He radiated subjective well-being. The contrasting case example, Alfred Paine, had a GAF of 72, was not generative, used largely level II through V defenses, and was chronically dissatisfied with his life.

Table 3.7–3 (from the Study of Adult Development at Harvard) provides an empirical illustration of the interrelationship of these different models in a 50-year prospective study of nondelinquent inner-city men. Not only was each of four models (measured by independent raters) significantly correlated with the other three, but each model predicted objective global mental health and subjective well-being assessed 20 years later. Significantly, none of the four models was well predicted by parental social class or a warm childhood environment.

In Table 3.7–3, Axis V was assessed by Luborsky's HSRS. Maturity was determined by an assessment of presence or absence of generativity. Subjective well-being at 55 years of age was quantified by summing each man's report of satisfaction over the past 20 years (on a five-point scale) in four life areas (marriage, children, job, and friends) and then by adding his best score from one of four additional areas (hobbies, sports, community activities, and religion). Social intelligence was assessed by objective evidence of good relations with friends, work mates, wife, children, and siblings. Resilience was measured by the relative frequency with which men deployed the five, bolded, level VII defenses in Table 3.7–2 against the relative frequency with which they used levels II through V defenses. Mental health at 65 years of age reflected success at work, relationships, play, and not using psychiatrists. Parental social class used the method of Hollinshead and Redlich (parental residence, education, and occupation). Warm childhood environment reflected good relations with mother, father, and siblings and a cohesive home at 14 years of age.

Currently, four of this chapter's models are capable of being assessed psychometrically—above average normality by the GAF (Axis V), maturity by the presence or absence of generativity, subjective well-being by self-report, and resilience by defense level on the optional DSM-IV-TR axis. As already noted, measures to assess psychometrically the other two models—the strengths of positive psychology and socioemotional intelligence—are under way.

The concept of mental health also raises the issue of therapeutic interventions to achieve it. What facets of mental health are fixed and which are susceptible to change? With clozapine (Clozaril) or with cognitive-behavioral therapy a GAF can be raised from 40 to 70, but how would a GAF be raised from 70 to 90? Chemicals can alleviate mental illness but do not improve healthy brain function. Mental health can be enhanced only through cognitive, behavioral, and psychodynamic education.

Some facets of brain function can be changed better than others. By analogy, the most intensive educational intervention in individuals who are not severely deprived raises their IQ only by approximately seven points, but sustained therapeutic intervention can change individuals utterly illiterate in Italian into fluent Italian conversationalists. Admittedly, a correct accent to go with the words is harder to teach.

In concluding this chapter, it seems important to review some of the safeguards for a study of positive mental health. First, mental health must be broadly defined in terms that are culturally sensitive and inclusive. Second, the criteria for mental health must be empirically and longitudinally validated. Third, validation means paying special attention to cross-cultural studies. In somatic medicine, criteria have been developed so that people of widely varying backgrounds and beliefs can agree on what constitutes rational therapy for disease. The same criteria need to be developed for mental health. Fourth, although mental health is one of humanity's important values, it should not be regarded as an ultimate good in itself. Efforts must proceed toward trying to improve mental health while maintaining due respect for individual autonomy. Finally, any student of health must remember that there are differences between real mental health and value-ridden morality, between human adaptation and mere preoccupation with darwinian survival of the fittest, and between real success at living and mere questing after the bitch goddess success.

There is no logically perfect method of analysis by which private bias and culturally determined value judgment can be distinguished from a culturally universal and scientifically valuable definition of mental health. Predictive validity remains the best guide. A parable offered by the protagonist in Gotthold Lessing's great 18th century play, *Nathan the Wise*, helps illustrate why mental health can only be identified by longitudinal study. In Lessing's play, an angry sultan had asked Nathan, a Jew, on pain of death, to identify the one true religion—Christianity, Islam, or Judaism. Nathan gently pointed out the need to maintain a longitudinal perspective.

A man lived in the East,
Who owned a ring of marvelous worth,
Given to him by a hand beloved.
The stone was opal, and possessed the secret power
To make the owner loved of God and man,
If he but wore it in this faith and confidence . . .

The ring was sought as an inheritance by each of Nathan's three sons. Because he loved them all equally, the doting father gave each son an identical ring. After their father's death, the three sons hurried off to a judge and demanded that the judge identify the lucky owner of the one true ring. The judge exclaimed,

But stop! I've just been told that the right ring,
Contains the wondrous gift to make its wearer loved,
Agreeable alike to God and man.
That must decide, for the false rings will not have this power . . .
Let each one strive to gain the prize of proving by results
The virtue of his ring and aid its power
With gentleness and heartiest friendliness . . .
The virtue of the ring will then
Have proved itself among your children's children.

In the future, it is incumbent on psychiatry to understand the implications of each of these six models of mental health. In conducting research on positive mental health, it is important for psychiatrists to recognize which model they use. Equally important, in the area of national health policy, a clear understanding is needed of not only what constitutes positive mental health, but also of who is responsible for intervention and who is responsible for paying for it.

Primary prevention is clearly superior to treating disease once it has occurred. Thus, individuals with positive mental health need to be studied in the way that agronomists study wheat that is resistant to drought and blight. Measurements and records of mental health also need to be enabled. Although room exists for improvement, Axis V, the GAF, provides the same reliability and has much greater predictive validity than the presence or absence of most Axis I and II designations. No psychiatric chart should be without Axis V. The capacities to work and to love over time are extremely important indices of mental health. They are far more important than the cross-sectional presence or absence of anxiety, depression, or illegal drug use. However, such capacities must be assessed longitudinally. "How many years since 21 years of age have you spent employed?" is more useful than "what is your present job?" Again, "Tell me about your longest intimate relationship" is more useful than "are you married?"

Finally, assessment of maturational development provides the best prediction of future clinical course. Thus, the mental status and diagnostic formulation should reflect an assessment of social maturation and coping style. If the person is 35 years of age, has he or she mastered Erikson's task of intimacy? If he or she is 40 years of age, has he or she achieved competence in, commitment to, contentment with, and compensation from a career? If he or she is older than 50 years of age, has he or she mastered generativity and learned to care less about him- or herself and more about his or her children? Again, when the going gets tough, does he or she eschew less mature mental mechanisms, such as projection, passive-aggression, and dissociation (being in denial), and does he or she use level VII involuntary coping mechanisms, such as stoicism, humor, altruism, and sublimation?

SUGGESTED CROSS-REFERENCES

Other aspects of normality are covered in Section 32.2 on normal child development and in Section 18.1a on normal human sexuality. Psychological changes in aging are covered in Section 51.2c. Chapter 6, on theories of personality and psychotherapy, contains relevant information on normality and mental health.

References

American Psychiatric Association. Global assessment at functioning (GAF) scale. In: *Diagnostic and Statistical Manual of Mental Disorders.* 4th ed. Washington, DC: American Psychiatric Association Press; 1994:32.

American Psychiatric Association. Defense levels and individual defense mechanisms. In: *Diagnostic and Statistical Manual of Mental Disorders.* 4th ed. Washington, DC: American Psychiatric Association Press; 1994:752.

Csikszentmihalyi M. *Flow: The Psychology of Optimal Experience.* New York: Harper & Row; 1990.

*Diener E, Suh EM, Lucas RE, Smith HL: Subjective well being: Three decades of progress. *Psychol Bull.* 1999;125:276–302.

Erikson E. *Childhood and Society.* New York: Norton; 1950.

Frederickson BL: What good are positive emotions? *Rev Gen Psychol.* 1998;2:300–319.

*Goleman D. *Emotional Intelligence.* New York: Bantam Books; 1995.

Grinker RR Sr, Grinker RR Jr, Timberlake J: Mentally healthy young males (homoclites). *Arch Gen Psychiatry.* 1962;6:405–453.

Jahoda M. *Current Concepts of Positive Mental Health.* New York: Basic Books; 1958.

Jones CJ, Meredith W: Developmental paths of psychological health from early adolescence to later adulthood. *Psychol Aging.* 2000;15:351–360.

Kohlberg L. *Essays on Moral Development. Vol 2: The Nature and Validity of Moral Stages.* San Francisco: Harper & Row; 1984.

Korchin SJ, Ruff GF. Personality characteristics of the Mercury astronauts. In: The Massachusetts Institute of Technology, ed. *The Threat of Impending Disaster.* Boston: MIT Press; 1964.

Ledoux J. *The Emotional Brain.* New York: Simon and Schuster; 1996.

Loevinger J. *Ego Development.* San Francisco: Jossey Bass; 1976.

Luborsky L: Clinicians' judgment of mental health: A proposed scale. *Arch Gen Psychiatry.* 1962;7:407–417.

Maslow AH. *The Farthest Reaches of Human Nature.* New York: Viking; 1971.

Mayer JD, Caruso D, Salovey P: Emotional intelligence meets traditional standards for an intelligence. *Intelligence.* 1999;27:267–298.

Menninger WC. *A Psychiatrist for a Troubled World: Selected Papers of William C. Menninger, M. D.* New York: The Viking Press; 1967:788–804.

Oden MH: The fulfillment of promise: 40-Year follow-up of the Terman gifted group. *Genet Psychol Monogr.* 1968;77:3-93.

Offer D, Sabshin M. *Normality: Theoretical and Clinical Concepts of Mental Health.* New York: Basic Books; 1966.

Offer D, Sabshin M. Normality. In: Kaplan HI, Freedman AM, Sadock BJ, eds. *Textbook of Psychiatry III.* Baltimore: Williams & Wilkins; 1980:608–613.

*Peterson C, Seligman MEP. *The VIA Classification of Strengths.* Cincinnati, OH: Values in Action Institute; 2003.

Salovey P, Sluyter DJ, eds. *Emotional Development and Emotional Intelligence.* New York: Basic Books; 1997.

Seligman MEP. *Authentic Happiness.* New York: Free Press; 2002.

Seligman MEP, Csikszentmihalyi M: Positive psychology. *Am Psychol.* 2000;55:5–14.

Skodol AE, Perry JC: Should an axis for defense mechanisms be included in DSM-IV? *Compr Psychiatry.* 1993;34:108–119.

Snowdon D. *Aging with Grace.* New York: Doubleday; 2001.

Tellegen A, Lykken DT, Bouchard TJ, Wilcox KJ, Segal NL, Rich, S: Personality similarity in twins reared apart and together. *J Pers Soc Psychol.* 1988;54:1031–1039.

Tseng WS: *Handbook of Cultural Psychiatry.* San Diego: Academic Press; 2001.

*Vaillant GE. *Ego Mechanisms of Defense: A Guide for Clinicians and Researchers.* Washington DC: American Psychiatric Association Press; 1992.

Vaillant GE. *Aging Well.* New York: Little, Brown and Company; 2002.

*Vaillant GE, Milofsky ES: Natural history of male psychological health: IX. Empirical evidence for Erikson's model of the life cycle. *Am J Psychol.* 1980;137:1348–1359.

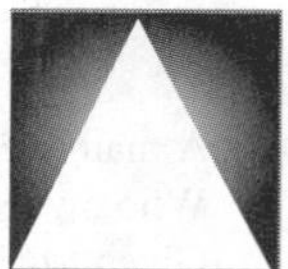

4 Contributions of the Sociocultural Sciences

▲ 4.1 The Psychiatric Scientist and the Psychoanalyst

Armando Favazza, M.D., M.P.H.

Behavior is determined by the interplay among a person's environment, life experiences, and biological endowment. Culture is the matrix within which these psychological, social, and biological forces operate and become meaningful to humans; it is important for psychiatry, because it affects not only patients' experiences of mental illness, but also lay and professional theories of etiology, diagnostic procedures, and therapeutic approaches. Culture is not a thing that a person has, but rather is an ongoing process created by shared interpersonal experiences that reverberate throughout a society and affect its institutions and the daily life of its members. Matter is neutral; molecules and energies are meaningless until they are personally interpreted, explained, and accepted as reality through the cultural process.

Health and illness are cultural categories based on universal biological events and culturally diverse bodily experiences that may be interpreted and acted on differently. Suppose, for example, that a woman somewhere in the world experiences an enduring and difficult-to-control sense of apprehensive expectations, tense muscles, irritability, and difficulty falling asleep. Her reaction to this complex of experiences depends greatly on her culture. Does her culture provide a word or a construct to identify and to explain what she is experiencing? Should her experiences be construed as normal suffering or as evidence of a moral flaw, a disharmony of inner energies, an existential crisis, deflected rage, nerves, or generalized anxiety disorder? What is the culturally accepted limit that she must reach before disclosing her experiences? Whom does her culture sanction to receive her disclosures? God, perhaps, or a priest, a congregation, a local healer, a televangelist, a self-help group, a friend, a family member, a counselor, a family physician, or a psychiatrist? The remedies she may be offered—prayer, acts of contrition, increased group participation, change of diet, exercise, interesting hobbies, changing jobs, going on a vacation, family or marital counseling, individual therapy, meditation, medication—are culturally determined, as are the criteria used to judge the efficacy of the remedy.

CULTURE

Culture is a vast, complex concept that is used to encompass the behavior patterns and lifestyle of a society—a group of persons sharing a self-sufficient system of action that is capable of existing longer than the life span of an individual and whose adherents are recruited, at least in part, by the sexual reproduction of the group members. Culture consists of shared symbols, artifacts, beliefs, values, and attitudes. It is manifested in rituals, customs, and laws and is perpetuated and reflected in shared sayings, legends, literature, art, diet, costume, religion, mating preferences, child rearing practices, entertainment, recreation, philosophical thought, and government. Culture serves many purposes. It provides an overall consistency to a society's patterns and components over the generations. It helps organize diversity and mediate between the forces of stability and conformity and those of new ideas and actions. By classifying phenomena into good and bad, right and wrong, healthy and sick, desirable and undesirable, people are provided with behavioral guidelines and an interpretation of life's events. Because cultural components change at varying speed (for example, technological advances may outpace a society's capacity to deal with new ethical issues), cultural systems attempt to minimize stress. Culture is learned through contact with family, friends, classmates, teachers, significant persons, and the media; the term for this process is *enculturation.* It results in a personal sense of belonging to one's own society and in a native identity.

Except, perhaps, for a few totally isolated, small social groups, there are no pure cultures. Societies are not static. Access to printed media, radio, telephone, television, and easy travel, as well as geopolitical changes, has resulted in a great deal of cultural blending. Adults such as migrants or refugees who only in part adopt the culture of a host society are said to be *assimilated,* whereas those who assume a new cultural identity consonant with that of the host culture are said to be *acculturated.* Persons who, voluntarily or by force, abandon their native culture but fail to be assimilated or acculturated usually lose their sense of identity or purpose in life and are at high risk for suicide, substance abuse, and alcoholism.

The holistic and functional concept of culture also allows for the existence of smaller subcultural groups and patterns within the larger society. Native Americans, for example, have distinct cultures, especially in tribal groups that live on reservations. On a smaller, less comprehensive scale, there are many subcultural groups and units in which there are shared feelings, ideas, and behaviors, for example, cults, neighborhood associations, institutional inmates, athletic teams, students and teachers at a school, and unions. Many subcultural patterns serve to preserve and to integrate the general society, but some may be socially disruptive (organized criminal groups) or truly destructive (terrorist organizations). Each family may be said to have its own microculture. Although the term *culture* is a grand abstraction that implies stability, homogeneity, and coherence, social life is often replete with change, heterogeneity, and inconsistencies.

Anthropologists traditionally have been the major professional group to study culture, whereas sociologists have studied social class. A culture is not the same as a social class. Within every society, one may find the five levels usually described for social stratification ranging from class I, characterized by high financial income, prestigious occupations, and possession of desiderata, to class V, characterized by just the opposite. In a geographical area, one or more differing cultural systems may be present, each containing members of the five social classes. Terms such as *the culture of poverty* and *mental health of the poor* are misleading, because they imply that all members of the lowest social class share a common culture. It may be true that impoverished areas outwardly appear similar and that slum dwellers share some common attitudes and behavior patterns, but these socioeconomic phenomena should not be confused with culture.

Anthropologists and sociologists have separate traditions, methodologies, and points of view. Anthropologists, for example, study acculturation, whereas sociologists study migration. Both of these processes share identical referents in many instances. Acculturation studies typically emphasize small-scale, non-Western populations, direct contact between investigators and their subjects, and a focus on behavior itself; however, migration studies typically emphasize sociodemographic variables, psychiatric use rates, large Western populations, and little or no direct contact between investigators and their subjects. Sociologists do not have museums; anthropologists do—this reflects the anthropological concern for biology and artifacts, as well as for concepts. Both sciences are pertinent to medicine, in general, and to psychiatry, in particular.

Medical anthropologists study the impact of sociocultural processes on health and on people's experiences of illness, especially by using cross-cultural comparisons. Their studies on the lives of patients in mental hospitals and then, after deinstitutionalization, in the community have had direct clinical impact. More than any other medical specialist, psychiatrists have developed expertise in understanding sociocultural processes and in using this understanding clinically. American psychiatric interest in culture began in the mid-1800s when mental hospitals admitted a large number of Irish and German immigrants. Toward the end of that century, European psychiatrists in African, Asian, and Caribbean colonies described a number of unusual syndromes such as *latah*, *amok*, and *koro*. W. H. R. Rivers, a British psychiatrist renowned for developing the field of social anthropology, did research on religious healing and on the perception of pain in South Pacific Islanders that he then used in treating mentally traumatized soldiers in World War I. At the turn of the 20th century, Emil Kraeplin traveled from Europe to Southeast Asia, described differences in symptomatology among patients, and developed the field of comparative psychiatry.

Sigmund Freud's psychoanalytic office was filled with archeological relics, and, as he dug through the layers of his patients' neurotic minds, he believed that he could reconstruct past epochs of human behavior and thought. Among the conclusions of his widely read books written between 1913 and 1938, *Totem and Taboo*, *The Future of an Illusion*, *Civilization and its Discontents*, and *Moses and Monotheism*, are that culture and repression are reciprocally related and that the superego was socially created to control the dangerous human destructive instinct. Many psychoanalysts, including Otto Rank, Theodor Reik, and Carl Jung, published studies of rituals and myth. Geza Roheim, Erik Erikson, and George Devereux were psychoanalyst anthropologists with actual field experience. Roheim founded the series known as *The Psychoanalytic Study of Society*. He used his vast knowledge of arcane cultural details to support his extreme psychoanalytical theories and then to twit his anthropological colleagues, whom he accused of rejecting obvious proof of the oedipal complex because of their own repressed conflicts. Erikson wrote psychocultural studies of Mahatma Gandhi and Martin Luther. His experiences with Dakota and Yurok Indians inspired *Childhood and Society*, written in 1950, in which he linked the intrinsic wisdom and unconscious "planfulness" of cultural conditioning with the ongoing processes of individual psychosocial development. Devereux, working with American Plains Indians, believed that shamans caused a social remission in patients by repatterning ethnopsychologically suitable defense mechanisms. In treating Mohawk Indian patients, he explicated problems such as dream interpretation and transference-countertransference, which are encountered in clinical work with ethnically diverse populations. Because psychoanalysis developed from the study of the individual, its application to cultural phenomena is at least one step removed and is open to question. Also, the psychoanalytic concepts of mind and mental processes may not be applicable or meaningful when applied to non-Western groups. The trend among some ethnopsychoanalysts to attend to informants' explanations of their behavior and to synthesize psychological and sociocultural observations is exemplified in Robert LeVine's work and in articles published in the *Journal of Psychoanalytic Anthropology* and in *Psychiatry*, a journal founded by Harry Stack Sullivan with the assistance of Edward Sapir, a cultural anthropologist.

Modern cultural psychiatry began in 1955, when a Transcultural Psychiatry Division was started at McGill University in Montreal with the leadership of Erick Wittkower and H. B. M. Murphy. Raymond Prince and, more recently, Laurence Kirmayer have continued leading the Division, including publication of the journal *Transcultural Psychiatry*. In 1971, a Transcultural Psychiatry section was established in the World Psychiatric Association; recent directors include Wen-Shing Tseng, a Chinese-American who wrote the first truly comprehensive *Handbook of Cultural Psychiatry* in 2001; Wolfgang Jilek, an Austrian-Canadian with extensive experience in working with refugees in Southeast Asia and Africa; and Goffredo Bartocci, an Italian who has vitalized European cultural psychiatry and who has published in the area of religion. In the United States, the journal *Culture, Medicine and Psychiatry* was established in 1976 by Arthur Kleinman, a prominent cultural psychiatric researcher, and Byron Good, a medical anthropologist. The Society for the Study of Psychiatry and Culture was founded in 1979 by Armando Favazza, Edward Foulks, John Spiegel, Joseph Westermeyer, and Ronald Wintrob. Similar organizations exist in China, Germany, Italy, Japan, and the United Kingdom.

CULTURE AND THE HUMAN BODY

Western science now locates the construct of mind in the brain; in past times, it was linked with the heart, the liver, and other organs. Just as some body parts can be modified through use patterns—for example, physical exercise affects muscle strength and size—so too can the brain's neural network be modified. Repetitive thoughts, sights, sounds, smells, tastes, and touches tend to increase specific neuronal dendritic connections and to intensify neurotransmitters, so that certain sensations and thoughts become physically patterned in the brain. The ability to speak a particular language, for example, depends on a culture-specific neural organization that influences cognitive processing and creation of cognitive schema so as to structure a person's perception and experience of the world. Culture exerts a great influence on the birth, development, and death of the human body. Two New Guinean tribes, the Enga and the Fore, provide an example of how culture may affect fertility. The Enga, who live in a state of chronic overpopulation and have reached the upper limits of survival for their territory, have cultural patterns that serve to limit population growth. Premarital sex is forbidden, celibacy is highly valued, and incest taboos are broad; a woman cannot marry any man related through men to her paternal grandfather. Men cannot marry until they are 30 years of age; on the death of a man, his widow is shunned or strangled to death. Infanticide is practiced, and death is not a cause for anguish. In contrast, the Fore live in an underpopulated area, and their cultural practices serve to increase population growth. Sexual experimentation and early marriage are encouraged, widows are inherited by the dead husband's male relatives, tribal ceremonies have erotic elements, and death causes great communal anguish. In large, complex societies, fertility rates are often affected by monetary incentives, for example, taxation to encourage or to discourage large families. In China, government policies to lower population growth reportedly have included forced abortion and even infanticide. In Italy, the exceedingly low birth rate reflects a secular culture shift away from the Catholic church's traditional stance that birth control is sinful.

Culture also affects the ways in which the body is treated. Hunger could be eliminated if all food sources were used, but the people of Western nations are unwilling to eat cats, dogs, rats, beetles, and grubs. Dietary preferences and food processing may affect mental status; pellagra and its associated dementia are caused by a niacin-deficient diet. In 1912, Joseph Goldberger discovered that pellagra in the American South was caused by the removal of niacin from corn during the milling process. Corn is currently at the center of a great social debate over genetically modified foods; proponents argue that genetically modified corn is safe to eat and produces prodigious crop yields, whereas opponents refer to it as *Frankencorn* and call for more testing before it is allowed into the marketplace. Beyond its scientific merit, this debate reflects the cultural conflict between traditionalism and progressivism and mirrors other contemporary cultural clashes over such disparate topics as homosexuality, abortion, global warming, and creationism.

Problems associated with the drinking of alcohol depend greatly on culture. The Chinese have a low rate of alcoholism, whereas the Japanese have a high rate of alcoholism. Both groups contain many persons who have an unpleasant "flush" reaction to alcohol, but the low alcoholism rate in China appears to be the result of a cultural emphasis on moderation and self-control, low respect for problem drinkers, the association of drinking and eating, and a traditional belief in the medicinal value of alcohol.

Deviant and culturally sanctioned behaviors that alter or destroy body tissue are found in all social groups. Most body modification practices are performed to promote beauty and to enhance sexuality, to signify membership in a particular group, or to express rebelliousness and individuality; examples of these behaviors are earlobe piercing to affix jewelry, insertion of nipple rings, tattoos to identify gang members, and a simple tattoo on the ankle. The widespread fad of body piercing and tattooing in Western nations has no particularly significant meaning other than, perhaps, a dissatisfaction with an increasingly bureaucratic and computer-driven society in which people are identified by numbers and in which artificial products are replacing "the real thing," for example, chemical organic substitutes and vitamins in pill form. Although a group of persons who have modified their bodies (excluding single earlobe piercing) probably would exhibit more psychopathology than a control group, a psychiatric diagnosis cannot be inferred simply by the presence of tattoos or piercings.

Body modification rituals, unlike fads and practices, are socially functional, integrative, adaptive, and enduring cultural components. Participants believe that the rituals promote health, heal pathological conditions, maintain social stability, enhance spirituality, and provide for religious salvation.

Body modification rituals for promoting health and curing illness often focus on the importance of blood. Many native tribes in Papua New Guinea, for example, consider womb blood to be a pathological substance that persists in the circulatory system of adults. Menstruation allows women to purify themselves naturally, but men must resort to periodic penis cutting, tongue abrasion, or nasal hemorrhages. Thrusting sharp, stiff grass into the nostrils once a month induces copious nasal bleeding, thus supposedly eliminating womb blood. Members of the Hamadsha, a Moroccan Sufi healing sect, believe that healers possess a sacred force known as *baraka* that can promote health and cure mental and physical illnesses caused by *jinn* spirits. Afflicted patients gather in a circle, and the healers enter into an ecstatic trance induced by rhythmic music and wild dancing. The healers then slash open their heads. Patients acquire the healer's *baraka* by eating sugar cubes or bread bits dipped into the flowing blood or by smearing themselves with the blood.

Body modification rituals frequently also serve to maintain social stability; they may help to define group membership and adult status, to control gender-linked behaviors, and to solidify social bonds. Elaborate patterns are carved on the flesh of Tiv (Nigeria) females on reaching puberty. The scars represent the Tiv family, heritage, land, traditions, genealogy, and myth, and they duplicate the decorations on sacred objects. This scarification ritual transforms the girl into a woman and into a sacred object on whom the group's fertility depends. In some cultures in which female sexuality is considered problematic, body modification rituals have been established to control women's behavior. In an analogy to a psychodynamic formulation in which a morbid symptom serves to bind conflict-caused anxiety in an individual, these rituals with their consequent physical, psychological, and social morbidity serve to bind communal anxiety in societies in which sexual conflicts have the potential to disrupt the male–female relationship. Through the practice of foot-binding, for example, Chinese men literally prevented their women from "running around" by crippling them. Girls' feet were tightly bound with bandages to keep them from growing; the flesh often became infected, and, sometimes, one or more toes sloughed off. The pain lasted for almost 1 year and then diminished when the feet became numb. Men extolled the beauty of the "lotus foot" and considered it erotic. Because women with bound feet could not walk any distance without the help of attendants, men could be sure of their whereabouts. The practice existed for a millennium and ended in the 1920s. A more direct approach to the control of female sexuality involves genital modification of young girls in Sudan and Somalia and parts of Ethiopia, Egypt, Kenya, and Nigeria. Simple circumcision involves cutting off the clitoral prepuce; excision involves also removing the tip of the clitoris. Infibulation involves removal of the clitoris, the labia, and mon veneris; the vagina is then sewn shut except for a small opening. Immediate or early medical complications include infection, urinary retention, urethral and anal damage, and hemorrhagic shock or death. Long-term morbidity includes chronic pelvic sepsis, urinary tract infections, dermoid cysts and abscesses, dyspareunia, and complicated childbirth. An infibulated woman is marriageable, because she is a guaranteed virgin. Excision of the sensitive clitoral area is done to attenuate the woman's sexual desires and to free her from personal lust. Uncircumcised women are regarded as unclean and not worthy of being a wife and a mother; the Arabic word *tahur* refers to purity, cleanliness, and circumcision.

The rituals are perpetuated, in part, because marriage and motherhood are often the only social roles available to women; attempts to ban them have been modestly successful. Circumcised women who move to cultural settings in which the experience of pleasure in females is considered desirable may become clinically depressed when they realize that an important part of their sexuality has been cut away. In many cultures, especially patriarchal ones, discomfort with female sexuality is evident; a rationalization for this discomfort is that untamed female sexuality causes men to act irrationally.

The path to enhanced spirituality and religious salvation often involves body modification. In the index ritual of the Plains (American Midwest) Indians, the strongest of the braves, while tethered to a rope affixed to skewers in their chests, danced, gazed at the sun, and ripped through their muscles in a struggle to be free from the snares of the flesh. Severe self-flagellation occurs in Shia Islam and Christianity. The Catholic church has canonized many saints who zealously mortified their flesh; some became "holy" anorectics. In the Eastern Orthodox mystical tradition, the beardless, corpulent 18th and 19th Skoptsi castrated themselves to achieve the purity of the first man, Adam, before he ate the forbidden fruit, which God then supposedly grafted onto his body as testicles. In ancient Rome and the Middle East, the self-emasculation of Attis who was unfaithful to the Great Mother Goddess, Cybele, was memorialized annually in the ritual of the Day of Blood when cult priests flagellated themselves and cut off their genitals; the emperor Julian called it "a holy harvest." In the Hindu Thaipusum festival, many persons pierce their bodies with replicas of Lord Murugan's magic trident.

An appreciation of the purposes served by culturally sanctioned body modification rituals helps demystify the seeming senseless deviant self-mutilation of the mentally ill. As stated by Edward Podvoll:

> The self-mutilator can incorporate into his actions patterns which, to a greater or lesser degree, remain unarticulated in most of us. That is, such patterns already exist in muted intensities within the patient's social field. . . . Still the patterns involved are those which elicit silent levels of admiration and envy. The history of these images reaches as far back as the passion of the cross and has prevailed among some of the most respected members of our culture.

Body modification rituals and deviant self-mutilation are not alien to the human condition; rather, they are culturally and psychologically embedded in the profound, elemental experiences of healing, social stability, and religion. These acts acknowledge disruptions within the individual and the collective social body and provide a mechanism for the reestablishment, however brief, of harmony and equilibrium. The self-inflicted cuts of Western adolescents are not so different from those experienced during the rite of passage by aboriginal initiates, blood brothers desperate to achieve social acceptance and integration into the adult world.

CULTURAL IDENTITIES

This section deals with three types of identity that persons assume or have thrust on them, namely, race, ethnicity, and charismatic group membership. Among the many other identities that are greatly influenced by culture are those associated with age and gender.

Race and Racism In standard medical case presentations, psychiatrists identify patients by age, gender, marital status, occupation, race, and, sometimes, ethnicity. Recipients of such information immediately process it, consciously and unconsciously, and make certain assumptions. Of special concern to cultural psychiatry are assumptions based on race or ethnicity, because both of these constructs are so emotionally evocative that they may distort the diagnostic and therapeutic process.

A characteristic of human beings is to compare themselves to other persons for reasons of enhancing self-esteem and for setting behavioral boundaries. The comparative group is usually found lacking in one regard or another. The ability of a group to perceive flaws in a different group is so prodigious as to encompass every aspect of existence, such as political systems, skin color, religious beliefs, sexual practices, and gender. Relationships between so-called superior and inferior groups range from friendly rivalry to enslavement, from covert hostility to mass murder. Depending on the place and time, men have disparaged women, whites have disparaged blacks, free persons have disparaged slaves, the rich have disparaged the poor, and heterosexuals have disparaged homosexuals; the complete list of superior-inferior polarities is discouragingly long. When cultural patterns based on perceived superiority and inferiority continue over several generations, their persistence may be thought to reflect a natural order that culture then serves to protect. Inventive rationalizations, as well as political expediency, are often used to perpetuate polarities, for example, men have denied suffrage to women in the belief that they should tend to cooking, children, and church activities rather than deal with political issues that are far too complicated for them to understand. The Founding Fathers of the United States wrote a Constitution and Bill of Rights proclaiming that all men are created equal and have a right to pursue happiness, yet slavery was common at the time in the northern and southern states. Healthy cultures have the capacity to change their social patterns in response to new ideas, desires, and technologies; change may come gradually, especially when many of the perceived inferior group members come to believe that they are truly inferior, or it may come rapidly with forceful rebellion and civil war.

The notion that persons can be categorized meaningfully by race has been abandoned by most scholars but persists universally in the general public. Physical traits, especially skin color, are the most common lay markers of basic divisions into white, black, red, and yellow races. Through the 1950s, some anthropologists classified the races as Caucasian with Nordic, Alpine, and Mediterranean groups; Mongoloids with Mongolian, Chinese, Japanese, Korean, Vietnamese, and Tibetan groups; Malaysian and Indonesian; Native Americans; Negroids with Negro, Melanesian, Negrito, Bushman, and Hottentot groups; and Australoids. Deoxyribonucleic acid (DNA) testing demonstrates the fallacy of racial divisions, because the great majority of human alleles are present in all population groups, although their frequencies vary; genetic variability within populations is greater than the variability between them. Moreover, skin color, hair type, nose shape, and other physical traits are independently inherited and are not linked one to another.

The saving grace of ancient beliefs about different groups was the provision of methods for overcoming alleged faults. Barbarians could gain acceptance from Greeks by learning to speak and to write the Greek language. By religious conversion, Romans and Jews could join the Christian community. Modern forms of differentiation, especially those based on the flawed biological construct of race, however, rarely permit the inferior group to rise to the status of the superior one.

Modern racism began in 15th century Spain, where Christians were divided into old and new groups. Old Christians had "purity of blood," whereas the new group—converted Jews—was hounded by the Inquisition. On biological grounds, Jews, and later Muslims, were declared incorrigibly inferior and therefore were excluded from mainstream Spanish society. In the New World, Spanish conquerors brutalized and enslaved the local populations to mine for gold; their justification came from some theologians who declared that Indians lacked rationality and morality and therefore were, in Aristotelian terms, "natural slaves." Also, the famous physician, Paracelsus, determined that Indians were soulless, inferior beings because they had not descended from the biblical Adam. A great debate ensued, and, in 1537, Pope Paul III ruled that "the Indians are truly men." However, economic interests prevailed, the papal declaration was ignored, and harsh slavery continued for several hundred years.

Before the 17th century, there was no tradition of whiteness among Europeans or of blackness among Africans. Distinctions among groups of people in the Bible, in Greek and Roman histories, and in the writings of Marco Polo who traveled from Italy to China were made on the basis of food preference, costume, political systems, and rituals; skin color was not mentioned. White and black became cultural categories in the 17th century when the transatlantic slave trade was developed to stock European colonies in the New World.

Europeans and Americans exploited local populations and participated in the slave trade for economic profit. Rationalizations for these practices came from religious, philosophical, and then-current scientific theories. Blacks (many British referred to all nonwhite persons as *blacks*) supposedly were cursed by God as descendents of Ham, an Old Testament biblical figure who saw his father naked. The Scottish utilitarian philosopher, Dave Hume, wrote that only white persons were capable of creating civilized nations and of producing ingenious manufacture, art, and science. During the Enlightenment, the English physician-philosopher John Locke supported the degeneracy theory, namely, that the normal natural state of human beings was typified by the white European and that other races of men developed through biological and psychological degeneration. Scientists noted that white was the true color of nature and that the degenerative process found in persons of different colors might be reversed through exposure to European culture. Nonwhites were deemed to be psychologically flawed and unable to rule themselves as demonstrated by the ease with which European colonialists subjugated vast areas of the world. Even as late as 1963, a noted British historian took the position that, although black Africans have darkness, only Europeans have a history in Africa.

In the United States, a 19th century professor of anatomy named Samuel Morton measured the cranial capacity of various skulls by filling them with peppercorns. He claimed that the cranial capacity was unchanged for at least 3,000 years and was largest for whites, followed by Asians, Native Americans, and Africans. This finding was confirmed in 1906 by Robert Bean, Professor of Anatomy at The Johns Hopkins University in Baltimore; based on brain size, Bean reported that Negroes have well-developed lower mental faculties, such as smell and melody, whereas whites had well-developed higher faculties, such as self-control and reason. In 1856, a Southern psychiatrist coined the diagnostic term *drapetomania*, which was applicable to slaves and cats who had an irrestrainable propensity to run away from their masters. Another diagnosis given to black slaves was *dysoesthesia oethiopica*; symptoms included idleness, sloth, carelessness when driven to work by the compulsive power of white masters, breaking tools, and not paying attention to the rights of others. A 19th century scientific theory that became institutionalized in the laws of southern states was based on the transmission of heredity in blood from parents to offspring. Parental blood supposedly blended in the offspring; thus, children received one-half of their nature from each parent, one-fourth from each grandparent, and so on. This belief gave rise to such words as *half-breeds*, *quadroons*, and *octoroons*. Black blood was considered to be more potent than white blood; a person with even one drop of black blood was classified as negro. The blood theory is scientifically baseless. Genes undergo neither blending nor contamination.

At the turn of the 20th century, American psychiatrists published articles in prestigious journals supposedly demonstrating that the lower rate of mental illness among slaves, as compared to blacks in the free states, proved that slavery protected the mental health of blacks because of the supervision they received. One study in 1914 concluded that the negro mind is irresponsible, unthinking, easily aroused to happiness, and rarely experiences depression.

A World Health Organization (WHO) monograph published in 1953 perpetuated the myth that black persons rarely experience depression; the same author noted that Africans are like leukotomized Europeans, thereby "proving" that Africans did not use the frontal lobes of their brains. In his writings on the collective unconscious, Carl Jung noted that the brains of blacks probably have a whole historical layer less than Europeans; he also warned that "racial infection" exercised a tremendous pull on white persons who are exposed to blacks. Some educational psychologists, namely Lewis Terman, in 1916, and Arthur Jensen, in 1969, claimed that racial genetic factors accounted for low scores by blacks on intelligence tests. Frantz Fanon, a black psychiatrist from Martinique who studied in France and then actively participated in the 1950s' Algerian revolution against France, angrily concluded that the color black symbolizes evil, sin, wretchedness, death, war, and famine in the collective unconscious of Western thought.

A trend in many Western societies is the replacement of biologically based racism by social theories and political policies that often are meant to attenuate racism but that actually may worsen it. A psychodynamic study of 25 American blacks in 1951 considered the legacy of slavery to be family disorganization, low self-esteem, passivity, and a wretched internal life. Other studies negatively point out the matriarchal structure of black families in the United States and Britain, as well as the psychological emasculation of black males. Suman Fernando, a leading British cultural psychiatrist, notes:

> The arguments are based on a naive view of human development where negative experiences are assumed to lead to personality defects. The lack of cohesion of black family life and the passivity of black people are clearly the deductions made by whites. Black experience is looked at from the outside; the fact that oppression may uplift as well as depress self-worth and may promote as well as destroy communal cohesion is not considered. After all, if this argument is applied to the Jewish people, generations of prosecution should have left them incapable of any leadership quite apart from being able to establish a political state.

In studying American immigrants, Franz Boas, the founder of modern anthropology, found that the head shapes of second-generation children were more like those of dominant, established Anglo-Saxon Americans. For Boas, this proof of the plasticity of physical traits clearly contradicted biological theories that claimed that racial groups had fixed physical and, by extrapolation, fixed psychological and personality characteristics. Despite this and other evidence debunking the scientific validity of race, racial prejudice exists throughout the world. In the West, it is usually directed against persons of color. Pigmentation supposedly indicates deficiencies ranging from intellectual capacity to morality to the capability for experiencing normal emotions. Racism is so culturally embedded in social structures that even rational, well-meaning persons are not only affected by it, but also are often amazed and taken aback when the racial undercurrents of their behaviors are pointed out to them.

Psychiatrists are probably less racist than most subcultural groups, but they are not immune from biases. Studies show that white psychiatrists dealing with black patients are more apt to diagnose schizophrenia, to prescribe higher doses of tranquilizing medications, to fail to recognize depression, to use involuntary commitment more frequently, to extend hospital stays, and to underuse psychotherapeutic treatment. The Surgeon General's 2001 supplemental report, *Mental Health: Culture, Race and Ethnicity*, concluded that the rates of mental illness are similar for African Americans and whites who live in a community; rates are much higher in vulnerable populations in which African Americans are overrepresented, such as the homeless, prisoners, and children placed in foster care. Mentally ill African Americans are less likely than whites to receive psychiatric treatment. They tend to seek help in primary care and, because they often delay seeking treatment until their symptoms are more severe, in emergency rooms and psychiatric hospitals. Even African Americans with adequate insurance coverage are less inclined to seek psychiatric treatment. The report notes that the legacy of slavery, racism, and discrimination continues to influence African Americans' social status, economic standing, and health-related behavior; additionally, there is a lack of African-American mental health specialists. In practice, patients are customarily identified as black or white; those with other skin colors typically are identified by ethnicity. In European-American societies, the revelation that a patient is white is relatively meaningless and, in fact, usually is processed as meaning that the patient is not black. On learning that a patient is black, psychiatrists can infer that the patient has been victimized to some extent by institutional and personal racism. However, the emergence of a substantial black middle class, as well as high-profile leaders in the past several decades, along with sociopolitical changes, has challenged the concept of a typical black cultural experience. White psychiatrists, in dealing with black patients, must confront their own countertransference and must be attuned to the actual perceived, and unperceived, impact of racial prejudice on patients' lives, symptomatology, and prognosis.

Ethnic Identity Every person assumes multiple roles in the course of a lifetime. Infants, for example, mature through childhood, adulthood, and old age. People also develop personal, family, and group identities that change with circumstances, such as remarriage, relocation to a different region, religious conversion, or switching vocations. Ethnicity is a type of group identity based on cultural heritage, including place of origin, cuisine, costume, language, and rituals. Unlike the pseudoscientific biological concept of race, ethnicity is a purely cultural self-identification that denotes connectedness to other persons who claim the same identification. The intensity of feelings of connectedness may fluctuate widely as people and their social context change. In times of extreme duress, for example, people may deny a certain ethnicity, or they may embrace it fervently, depending on whichever is more psychologically and socially advantageous. Governmental and other programs may reward or punish persons who select a certain ethnicity. Ethnicity is a fluid phenomenon. It may be a cause of great stress in immigrant families, especially when parents cling to the "old ways" while their children come to identify more with host cultural groups. Barriers to interethnic marriages are decreasing, especially in Western countries; a person may marry into an ethnic group and adopt its identity. The children of parents who are Mexican and American may decide to identify themselves initially as Mexican, American, Mestizo, Chicano, Latino, or Mexican American; these self-identifications may change over time.

The concepts of race and ethnicity may be confounded. Adolf Hitler combined German ethnicity with a fabricated Aryan race to promote a Nazi society. He selected two ethnic groups, Jews and gypsies, for extermination. The history of the world is filled with examples of demagogues who have exploited ethnic passions, even to the point of genocide. Some persons, because of their skin color and physiognomy, may be stuck with a racial designation that makes it difficult, if not impossible, to change their ethnicity.

Joseph Westermeyer studied American Indian mental patients reared in non–American Indian foster, adoptive, and group homes in Minnesota. As children they developed ethnic identities, such as rural, Norwegian-American, Lutheran, small-town German-American Catholic, or urban Scotch-American Presbyterian. They referred to American Indian people as *they* instead of *we*. Problems arose during adolescence when society refused to accept their non–American Indian ethnicity. Repeated rejections by the same ethnic groups with whom they shared values, attitudes, and behaviors gave rise to anger and attempts to reject their ethnicity. They were red on the outside and white on the inside. The psychiatric symptoms they developed—the *apple syndrome*—included alcoholism, drug abuse, suicide attempts, chronic anxiety, panic attacks, depression, and legal and behavioral problems. All these symptoms were far in excess of what might be expected in persons reared in foster, adoptive, or group homes. Most of the syndromic patients tried to assume an American Indian ethnic identity by wearing traditional clothes, adopting American Indian drinking behaviors, and marrying American Indian spouses. These attempts usually resulted in failure, and their psychiatric symptoms became chronic.

Sensitivity to ethnicity facilitates accuracy in evaluation and success in treatment. However, it is possible to be overly sensitive and to misinterpret psychopathology as some sort of ethnic quirk. In uncertain situations, the assistance of persons familiar with the patient's sociocultural status should be obtained.

Culture and Personality The culture and personality school of anthropology, influenced by psychoanalysis and influential in the early mid-20th century, attempted to link individual personality with various identifications, especially ethnicity. Ruth Benedict's popular book, *Patterns of Culture*, written in 1934, held that cultures were really the summation of individual psychologies over a long time span. She thought that persons with *normal* personality types are those who conform to a society's dominant cultural configuration, whereas *deviants* do not, although some deviants might be considered normal in a different, more congenial cultural setting. This formulation is applicable to homosexuals who can lead normal lives in many large American cities but who might be tormented and considered deviant in rural towns.

In the mid-20th century, anthropologists and some psychiatrists developed the concept of national character. The personality of Russian peasants was supposedly characterized by depressive and manic traits that resulted from the practice of fairly severe swaddling of infants by farm-worker mothers; the arms were tied close to the body with tight crisscross lashing, and the infant was wrapped in a blanket, so that only its face was visible. Depression was linked to the impotence experienced in struggling against the swaddling bandages; mania was linked to orgiastic Russian feasts and drinking bouts that exemplified the feeding and love that accompanied the removal of these bonds. The rage caused by swaddling led to later guilt feelings, such as those expressed in Dostoevsky's novels. The celebrated expressivity of Russian eyes was the result of restricted infant mobility that perforce emphasized vision as a means of contact with the world. Such "destiny in the nursery" studies were criticized for their reductionism. It also became apparent that findings often were biased, as is evident when the American military commissioned national character studies of enemies in World War II. Japanese brutality was said to result from severe toilet training practices, German culture was described as paranoid and neurotic, and the harsh-sounding German language was seen as the manifestation of a crude mentality. A 1997 study grouped the continuity of the American national character into six clusters: self-reliance, autonomy, and independence; communal action, volunteerism, and neighborly cooperation; confidence in the trustworthiness of others; openness to new experiences; antiauthoritarianism; and the equality of justice for everyone. The American national character doubtlessly would be delineated differently from a Middle Eastern or Asian perspective.

Although national stereotypes may contain a kernel of truth, there is more personality variability within a national group than there is among different groups. Traits perceived to be peculiarly

German, French, or Italian turn out, in reality, to be generally human, Occidental, or continental European. The current consensus is that a clinically meaningful prediction about an individual's personality cannot be made on the basis of nationality alone.

Charismatic Groups The process of conversion—the destruction of the old self and the construction of a new self with new cognitive frameworks and behaviors—can take many pathways. In naturalistic settings, the process usually involves periods of incubation, steps forward, and backsliding. Artists, saints, and others have written about their conversion after enduring "a dark night of the soul."

In 1934, Bill Wilson, an alcoholic stockbroker and a cofounder of Alcoholics Anonymous (AA), was hospitalized for depression. He was not a spiritual person but cried out in despair for God to show himself. Suddenly, the room lit up with a great white light, and he was caught up in an indescribable ecstasy. He pictured himself on a mountain in a spiritual windstorm and realized that he had become a free man. As the ecstasy subsided, he experienced a new world or consciousness. All about him and through him there was a wonderful feeling of the presence of God. A great peace came over him, and he thought that, no matter how wrong things seem to be, they are all right. He was reassured by his psychiatrist, William Silkworth, that his experience was not the result of a brain damaged by alcohol.

Wilson's life changed for good when he discovered William James' book, *The Varieties of Religious Experience*. In it, he learned about the ecstasy that accompanies religious conversion and the hopelessness that often precedes that change. The book presented many case histories, including that of a homeless, friendless, dying drunkard who became an active and useful rescuer of alcoholics after his conversion. James described the special features of the state of assurance that accompany conversion; a sense that all is ultimately well, a sense of perceiving truths not known before, and an internal and external sense of clear and beautiful newness. Wilson talked about the hopelessness of his condition and his subsequent conversion with a friend. From these talks, he imagined a chain reaction among alcoholics in which the message about the possibility of change would be spread.

Of special concern to society, in general, and to psychiatrists, in particular, are those conversions of identity that occur when young adults, usually between the ages of 15 and 30, are indoctrinated into charismatic groups that use duplicitous methods, have a totalistic philosophy, and are associated with psychological and social morbidity. What distinguishes charismatic groups from other groups, clubs, and associations is their strict control over members' behavior and the belief that their leaders or mission possesses a transcendent power. Classification of these groups is problematic, because they may overlap with benign, fringe groups, and because they may be perceived as progressive in certain cultural settings. Mark Galanter includes among these groups cults, zealous religious sects, some highly cohesive self-improvement groups, some political action movements, and terrorist groups. Charismatic groups may be small (the Symbionese Liberation Army of the 1960s had less than a dozen members) or large (Reverend Sun Myung Moon's neo-Christian Unification church has thousands of members).

Recruiters for these groups cast a wide net in the hope of gaining a few new members. There is no way of profiling a personality type who responds to the bait, although a study of recruits to the Divine Light Mission (Hare Krishna) cult found that 30 percent had previously sought psychiatric help. Many recruits seem to be psychologically quite normal albeit naively idealistic and trusting. Some may be disillusioned with life, frustrated by romantic failures, and unhappy with school. Other vulnerabilities include loneliness and a sense of disorientation that may be apparent in newly arrived college students, foreigners, and runaways. They often feel flattered when approached by a recruiter, often of the opposite sex, who offers friendship, conversation about social injustices and life's meaning, and an invitation to attend a meeting or study group. Persons usually do not know that they are being recruited or the name and purposes of the group. They are greeted warmly by the group and only hear vague generalities. They are then invited to intense workshops or retreats that may last several days, during which they are overwhelmed with attention, exposure to nonspecific but laudable generalities on the need for more self-awareness and self-improvement in the world, and joyful expressions of the love and acceptance that group members have for one another. The emotionality of those few days may be so powerful that the recruits may experience a conversion, although they are still unclear about to what they are converting; may accept new beliefs; express high levels of commitment; and develop a sense of well-being that often follows a brief dissociative episode.

Fascination turns to reliance as recruits continue their indoctrination and slowly learn the nature and purposes of the group to which they now belong. Any potential resistance is prevented by a number of techniques, including decreased and eventual total lack of contact with family and friends, participation in many group activities so as to leave no free time and to create fatigue, the confession of doubts to the group in "struggle sessions," and the induction of altered consciousness through meditation, chanting prayer sessions, or drugs. Louis J. West described a cult indoctrination syndrome that includes the following features:

- Drastic alteration of the victim's value hierarchy, including abandonment of previous academic or career goals. The changes are often sudden and catastrophic, rather than the gradual changes that might result from maturation or education.
- Redirection of cognitive flexibility and adaptability. Victims answer questions mechanically, substituting cult-specific responses for what their own previously reasoned answers might have been.
- Narrowing, blunting, or artificiality of affect. The victim may appear emotionally flat and lifeless or almost frantically cheerful and ebullient.
- Regression. Victims become childishly dependent on the cult leaders, who are expected to make decisions for them.
- Sometimes there are physical changes, such as pallor or weight loss, with deterioration in the victim's physical appearance, strange or mask-like faces, blank stares, or darting, evasive eyes.
- Clear-cut psychopathological changes may appear, including depression, dissociative phenomena, anxiety states, obsessional ruminations, delusional thinking, hallucinations, and various other psychiatric signs and symptoms.

The disconnection between the "everything's fine" self-perceptions of group members and the perceptions of them by their family members and friends is striking and a testament to the power of the group. Members surrender their autonomy and their worldly possessions in exchange for a sense of being protected. They abandon their independence and conform to the group's behavioral norms in return for a sense of well-being and exclusivity. Galanter has described the relief effect that motivates persons to remain with the group: The relief of neurotic distress depends on the affiliated commitment of the group members. Attempts to leave the group result in increased distress. This can even be seen in committed members of AA who become irritable and uncomfortable when they miss some meetings. The group fosters dependency and group identity, because it then becomes the agent of relief. This effect can be seen in what is called the *Stockholm syndrome*: Hostages whose lives are in deadly peril for a period of time become so dependent on their captors that they then may identify with them, come to support their cause, and even attempt to thwart rescue attempts.

The leaders of charismatic groups often lie to members to maintain group morale and to negate unfavorable comments made by outsiders. They solidify the group's boundaries when they feel threatened; techniques include staring vacantly as a response to outsiders' questions or aggressively counterattacking perceived enemies. When the xenophobia of a leader turns to full-blown paranoia, the group members may share the leader's delusions; the result may be catastrophic.

In the 1970s, Jim Jones, the charismatic, African-American leader of a neo-Christian apocalyptic sect, moved with 900 followers from San Francisco to the remote jungles of Guyana, South America. In this captive society, he was called *Dad* by the members. He demanded total allegiance and constant vigilance, preaching about persecution by enemies and the extermination of all blacks. He whipped members who committed crimes, such as smoking, and even forced a celibate woman to have intercourse with a man whom she disliked in front of the entire community. As Jones' persecutory and grandiose delusions escalated, he repeatedly drilled his followers in preparation for the final battle by arming them with rifles and giving them a red, supposedly fatal liquid to drink. In 1978, he announced that anarchy was rampant in the United States, that drought had forced the evacuation of Los Angeles, and that the Ku Klux Klan was marching through the sect's former city, San Francisco. A month later, a U.S. Congressman violated the borders of Jonestown by coming to inspect it. When four group members decided to leave with the Congressman, Jones attacked him and then drilled his group for the true final battle; this time, however, the liquid that they drank was real poison. He succeeded in encouraging more than 900 persons, including 216 children, to die by telling them that they were committing a revolutionary act and not suicide.

Noxious charismatic groups appeal to various human interests, such as religion (Universal Church of Christ), outer space (the Heaven's Gate group practiced castration; all of its small membership committed suicide in 1997 with the expectation of being transported to a spaceship near the Hale-Bopp comet), and science (the Church of Scientology is violently antipsychiatry, antimedication, and litigious).

Persons who eventually leave charismatic groups do so because of disgust at the group's behavior and because of strong ties to family and friends. Some ex–cult members are hired as exit counselors by desperate families to persuade their children to leave the group; elaborate ruses may be used to achieve this goal. The process is usually difficult and protracted. Psychiatrists called on to treat rescued cult members should collaborate with reentry counselors who have knowledge of, and often firsthand experience with, the specific groups. Victims typically display symptoms of what the West terms a *pseudoidentity* disorder characterized by doubts about their "true" identity, along with depression and feelings of loneliness and ambivalence about the entire process of recruitment, indoctrination, group membership, and rescue. Among the therapeutic issues that need to be addressed are victims' guilt over abandoning their family at the onset and their group at the end, the reestablishment of independent behaviors, and the forging of a new sense of self and direction in life. The prognosis depends on a victim's premorbid personality, the severity of psychopathological symptoms, family support, the use of reentry counseling, and, if necessary, psychiatric care.

CULTURE CHANGE

In the broadest sense, persons experience culture change when moving into a different culture or by staying put while their own culture changes around them. Acute and wide-sweeping change may overwhelm the adaptive mechanisms of individuals and of their social support systems. Distortions in parenting and in life experiences may occur, and cultural landmarks may become unreliable and difficult to interpret; the result may be individual and sociocultural disintegration. The four categories for situations that necessitate coping with marked culture change are (1) sojourning, (2) settling, (3) segregation, and (4) changes in society. In a more narrow sense, the status changes that result from events such as retirement, entry into a profession, marriage, and adoption may be considered subcultural mobility; these changes require coping skills that, when deficient, may result in adjustment disorders, as well as more enduring psychopathology.

Sojourning Sojourners are persons who have a brief, usually voluntary, exposure to a new culture; examples include tourists; business representatives; scientific field workers; technical consultants and aid workers, such as Peace Corps volunteers; military personnel; and limited contract workers. Swiss mercenaries in the 16th century were described as having the prototypical sojourner's syndrome; physicians referred to it as *nostalgia* and recorded its symptoms as fever, diarrhea, delusions, and convulsions. Later, nostalgia was described as a psychosomatic condition. Napoleon's troops reportedly were devastated by nostalgia, and it was considered to be a mild form of insanity among troops in the American Civil War. The name was changed to *homesickness* and was a diagnostic entity in military psychiatry during World War II; it was the most common maladjustment reaction experienced by American soldiers. Adjustment disorders can be prevented in sojourners by a process of learning about the new culture before arrival, by providing access to telephone and e-mail communication with supportive persons back home, and by shortening the lengths of stay in the new culture. Exposure to intense trauma or to unanticipated environmental toxins in the new culture, especially during wartime, may result in delayed medical and psychiatric symptoms.

Settling Settling involves a more permanent, forced, or voluntary move to a new culture, for example, a change made by refugees and international or internal immigrants. Settling can be a relatively easy process or a dramatically difficult one. In general, the stress of settling may be associated with adjustment disorders, panic, anxiety, depression, alcohol and substance abuse, suicidal behaviors, the triggering of mania, and transient psychotic episodes. In 1932, Odegaard concluded that a higher rate of state hospital admission for schizophrenia in Norwegian immigrants to Minnesota than in the native-born Minnesotans or in the population of Norway was best explained by selective migration. Some subsequent studies have supported this explanation, but others have not. Early African and Asian immigrants to the new country of Israel were far more likely to be admitted to a mental hospital than were European immigrants whose hospitalization rate paralleled that of the local population. Selective migration may play a minor role, but current evidence demonstrates that enduring psychotic disorders may be exacerbated, but not caused, by settling. Among the factors that affect psychopathology in settlers are premorbid mental and physical health status, characteristics of the host society and locale of settlement, and conditions necessitating the move. In an ideal immigration scenario, a mentally and physically healthy, intact, multigenerational family voluntarily resettles in a new area in which all the family members are welcomed warmly, in which decent housing and jobs are readily available, in which the language is the same as the country of origin, in which an established core of settlers from the same region already lives, and in which public and private programs are in place to provide social, legal, and financial aid.

Refugees are typically involuntarily displaced because of warfare and natural disasters. Those who have witnessed and have been the victims of horrific atrocities are at high risk for posttraumatic stress disorder (PTSD), panic, and depression. Even after real danger is over, refugees who are placed in camps often project their fear of their persecutors onto neutral personnel and continue to experience anxiety. The struggle for self-preservation and access to food and shelter may lead to a deterioration in moral behaviors; recognition of this deterioration and of the inability to adhere to the values of their lost homeland may result in demoralization and depression. Refugees who are resettled to a foreign land may initially overvalue their country of asylum and may develop savior fantasies about persons of authority. However, psychopathological symptoms may emerge among refugees after the realizations that they may never return to their country of origin and that they had been forced to decide among unattractive alternatives in their new place of resettlement.

Most international migration stems from a desire for upward economic mobility. Premigration mental illness tends to worsen with the stress of moving to a new culture; this situation may be encountered when mentally healthy immigrants bring mentally ill family members with them. Children usually adapt better to immigration than do elderly persons who may be fixed in their ways and unable to learn a new language or to find meaningfulness in new customs. Middle-class persons with ordinary occupations usually handle the migration experience better than upper– and lower–social class persons, because employment may be easier to find. Women who are confined to their homes may become socially isolated and depressed. Elderly family members may lose the prestige they once had in their country of origin as their children adopt the mentality of the host culture, thus creating intergenerational stresses.

Access to support systems depends on personal family preferences, traditional patterns, and host country practices and programs, such as welfare and legal aid. Immigrants often do better when they live in areas populated by others from the same country of origin. Such a situation can provide comfort and ease of transition at first but, in the long run, may delay acculturation and may even foster resentment in some segments of the host society. Marital conflicts among immigrants often center on differences between gender-appropriate behaviors in their old and new countries. Intergenerational conflicts may arise over communications, because children learn the language of their new culture more rapidly than their parents and tend to lose interest in their original language; in addition, children are more rapidly acculturated than their parents because of the knowledge gained through socialization experiences in school. It is not uncommon for immigrants, especially those from third world countries, to develop acute psychotic episodes with persecutory delusions (the so-called aliens' paranoid reaction syndrome). These episodes usually have clear-cut precipitants, may recur several times, and do not necessarily progress to chronic mental illness.

In a 1998 major study of 3,012 adult Mexican Americans living in Fresno County, California, those born in Mexico had a prevalence rate for any mental disorder of 24.9 percent, compared to a rate of 48.1 percent among those born in the United States. Substance abuse and dependency rates were seven times higher in native-born women than in immigrant women; the ratio for men was 2:1. Another California study of 1,500 users of primary care medical services found that immigrants, one-half of whom were born in Mexico and Central America, had a significantly lower prevalence of depression and PTSD, despite their lower socioeconomic status, than Latinos born in the United States. Other studies indicate that immigrant Mexican women, in comparison to Mexican women born and living in the United States, have lower infant mortality rates, much better nutritional intake, and are significantly less likely to test positive for drugs at time of delivery. These somewhat shocking findings may, in part, be due to the migration of the fittest, healthiest, and most resilient Mexicans; a more powerful explanation is that the immigrants are buffered by their closeness to a traditional culture characterized by close-knit, extended families that offer social support, low rates of divorce, and healthier eating habits. The generalization and sustainability of these negative findings on the effects of acculturation to other cultural situations remain to be seen. A typical pattern is that each succeeding generation of immigrants over time more closely approximates the behavioral patterns and physical characteristics of the majority of persons in the host country.

Segregation Persons may be removed from the community and placed in more-or-less total care institutions. Erving Goffman lists five types of segregated institutions: (1) those that care for incapable harmless persons (orphanages and old-age homes), (2) those that care for ill persons who pose an unintended threat to society (mental hospitals and leprosaria), (3) those that protect the community from persons who pose intentional threats (prisons and concentration camps), (4) those established to pursue work-like tasks (boarding schools and military barracks), and (5) those designed as retreats from the world (monasteries and convents). Institutional inmates conduct all their activities in the same place and are regulated by the same authority. This situation, incompatible with family life and the basic work-payment structure of society, is reinforced by a strongly enforced split between inmates and staff with restrictions against social mobility between the two.

Until the 1950s, large state mental hospitals were considered to be a static setting within which psychiatrists treated patients. These neatly landscaped, tightly ordered, and tranquil hospitals were thought to instill a beneficial sense of neatness, order, and tranquility to the patients. The impact of these hospitals' sociocultural environment on patient care became evident in 1954, when Alfred Stanton and Morris Schwartz published their study on Chestnut Lodge, demonstrating that patients usually improved during periods of effective collaboration among personnel and deteriorated during periods when staff disagreements were not discussed openly. This important link between a hospital's administrative process and the patient–staff therapeutic process was also demonstrated by William Candill, an anthropologist influenced by Maxwell Jones' work in establishing therapeutic communities on mental hospital wards, who admitted himself as a patient to the Yale Psychiatric Institute to make around-the-clock observations about life on a ward. These and other studies, combined with the growth of the community mental health movement in the 1960s and the development of effective medications, have led to the demise of large state hospitals and to the placement of patients in the least restrictive environment, that is, the community. The deinstitutionalization process has been fraught with difficulties, but there now exists a number of residential facilities, supervised apartments, day hospitals, and other placements for patients with severe and persistent mental illnesses. Unfortunately, because of the shortage and inadequacy of facilities, a major proportion of those patients who have been unable to live successfully in the community now reside inappropriately in jails and prisons.

Changes in Society Human beings have always had to deal with social change induced by natural disasters, warfare, colonization, revolutions, and new technology. However, in the past two centuries, the rapidity and extent of change have been more vast than the total previous accumulative experience of human existence. Many benefits, such as improved public health, better communications, and ease of transportation, have resulted, but some of the costs include degradation of the environment, homelessness, and the increased lethality of weapons. Change increases the number of stressful events in people's lives; these events range from annoying traffic jams to disastrous losses of jobs. Persons whose mental health is already marginal may decompensate when confronted by rapid change. Eugene Brody examined rural to urban migration resulting from industrialization in Brazil. He identified many persons, "the lost ones," who needed psychiatric care. They had feelings of rootlessness from the loss of familiar cultural guideposts, from sadness and inadequacy due to alienation from work and separation from families, and from suspicion and distrust of the unknown. Illiteracy was a major factor in determining the mental health of "the lost ones," because it decisively limited their capacity to understand and to manipulate symbols, to receive and to integrate information, and to form relationships with the more dominant members of society.

Cultural adaptation always lags behind rapid social change; the more resilient the culture, the briefer the lag. Societies whose culture is unprepared for rapid change may disintegrate. Some overwhelmed Native American tribes, for example, have died off. The native Alaskan population in newly discovered oil-rich areas experienced rapid social upheaval. A report on the Inupiat in Barrow found that (1) 72 percent of an adult sample scored in the definite or suggestive alcoholic range on the Michigan Alcoholism Screening Test; (2) 42 percent had been detained or arrested for alcoholism at least once; (3) areas that had been almost free of suicide and homicide showed marked increase; and (4) when the only liquor store was closed, widespread bootlegging ensued as an extension of the social relationships among family and friends. These problematic behaviors have diminished somewhat over a generation as Inupiat culture has adjusted to the intrusion on its traditional way of life.

RELIGION AND SPIRITUALITY

The practice of medicine, including psychiatry, is experiencing major changes as a result of rapid biotechnological advances. Diagnostic machines are replacing hands-on examinations, robots are already performing some surgical procedures, computerized psychotherapy programs are being perfected, medications are replacing dialogue, and doctor–patient relationships are giving way to provider–client interactions that are overseen by economically driven and faceless organizations. One reaction to the impersonality fostered by these changes has been the newfound respectability of alternative medicine, an approach that emphasizes traditional, folksy remedies and encourages persons to take a more active role in their health care. Another reaction is increasing interest in the importance of personal religion and spirituality in medicine. In 1995, instruction in religious and spiritual issues was made mandatory for accredited psychiatric residency programs in the United States.

This section focuses on religion and spirituality. It presents information on religious and spiritual problems and on an objective understanding of the human experience of God. Basic material about sacred texts, especially the Bible and the Qur'an, is presented because they are at the core of the two most widespread religions, Christianity and Islam. The reconfiguration of sin, once a central force in Western life, into mental illness and criminality is discussed, as is the influence of religion on problematic behaviors related to sexuality, gender, the drinking of alcohol, and healing. The relationship between religion and mental health is examined, as are differences between religion and spirituality and the psychiatrist's role in dealing with these issues.

Religion Throughout history, human beings have held religious beliefs and have engaged in religious practices. However, the diversity of these beliefs and practices is so vast that it is impossible to define the word *religion* succinctly. It generally refers to belief in a supernatural, creative God and in the practice of rituals meant to appease, to glorify, to obey, or to relate better with this God. For some persons, religion is an ongoing, self-actualizing quest for holiness, whereas, for others, it is an achievable destination. Religions serve the mythopoetic yearnings of humankind and provide a stable orientation and moral compass. Religious systems have greatly influenced human behavior for millennia and often underlie a society's political, legal, medical, and educational practices. The three great monotheistic religions—Judaism, Christianity, and Islam—believe in a single omnipotent God and in a book, the Bible or the Qur'an, that reveals God's plan for believers. Buddhism, a religion prevalent in China, Japan, Korea, Sri Lanka, and South Asia, has differing traditions; Therovada Buddhism emphasizes a spiritual quest for wisdom, whereas Mahayana Buddhism stresses compassion, the divine power of the Savior Buddha, and spiritual rituals. Hinduism, prevalent on the Indian subcontinent, emphasizes the many manifestations of God, reincarnation, a divine power that sustains life, a dazzling array of religious symbols, yoga, and meditation.

The revised fourth edition of the *Diagnostic and Statistical Manual of Mental Disorders* (DSM-IV-TR) now includes *religious or spiritual problem* as an Axis I condition that may be a focus of clinical attention. Examples include distress over the loss or questioning of faith, problems associated with converting to a different faith and questioning of spiritual values, and the sense of damnation that may be experienced by persons with PTSD. Modern times have seen jolting crises of faith; many Christians, especially Catholics, are shocked by the revelation of pederasty among clergy, whereas many Muslims feel that extremists have replaced traditional Islamic values with intolerance and militarism. DSM-IV-TR has also reduced the use of religious examples to illustrate psychopathology.

Religious problems have long been part of the human experience. Some problems are due to the fact that the faith required for a belief in the supernatural can be fragile. In the face of horrific individual tragedies, such as the death of a child or the accidental disfigurement of a guiltless person, as well as large-scale disasters, such as world wars, concentration camps, ethnic cleansing, and famine, some people rely on their faith for strength and turn to God and to religion for consolation, whereas others may abandon their faith and adopt the belief that human beings are responsible for their own fate.

None of the major religions is monolithic, but rather they are comprised of numerous subdivisions that may share some core beliefs but disagree dramatically in their interpretation of sacred texts and in their rituals and practices. Christianity alone has hundreds of subdivisions; examples include Roman and Eastern Rite Catholic, Eastern Orthodox, Baptist, Pentecostal, Presbyterian, Methodist, Coptic, Maronite, Christian Science, Jehovah's Witnesses, and Church of

Jesus Christ of Latter-Day Saints. Among Christians who claim to be "born again in the Holy Spirit" and to be "alive in Christ," Evangelicals recognize the authority of the Bible and a duty to share their faith with others in addition to having a personal experience with God; Fundamentalists are like Evangelicals but insist on the absolute inerrancy of every word in the Bible; Pentecostals are like Evangelicals but place a major emphasis on an immediate encounter with the Holy Spirit and on an exuberant style of worship; Charismatics are persons in mainstream Catholic and protestant churches who practice a Pentecostal form of worship. A growing number of Christians belong to nondenominational churches in which the ministers and congregation as a group agree on their beliefs and practices; extension of this trend is the formation of small groups in which members do not attend any church but rather meet in individual homes to study the Bible and attempt to relate it to their lives.

The subdivisions of the major religions often have other subdivisions based on the degree of orthodoxy and the adoption of local customs. Orthodox Jews, for example, conform their behavior to a strict interpretation of Levitical laws, whereas "cultural" Jews may practice their religion predominantly by taking part in selected rituals. In Islam, the injunction that women must dress modestly in public may have differing interpretations; Orthodox women may fully cover their bodies except for eye slits, whereas others may simply wear a head scarf, and still other women may disregard any special dress code. Religious problems for believers may arise out of discord between major religious groups, such as Hindus and Muslims in India, and between subdivisions, such as conservative and liberal Baptists in the United States. Even among groups that share the same beliefs and practices, there is a uniqueness to every church, temple, mosque, and synagogue, based on the characteristics of the clergy and the congregation.

Religious problems may arise when there is discord among members of a congregation or when the institutional leaders behave inappropriately. Neither religious institutions nor religious leaders, like their secular counterparts, are immune from petty politics and from sexual, financial, and other scandals. Religion may stir deep feelings of altruism, forgiveness, tolerance, charity, creativity, and, most of all, hope. However, it may be problematic when used to rationalize hatred, intolerance, irresponsible behavior, and bodily mortification: examples include anti-Semitism because Jews were implicated in the crucifixion of Christ, prejudice against blacks because they are supposedly cursed in the Bible, indulging in compulsive behaviors because of supposed demonic oppression, and severe fasting.

The intensity of feelings aroused by religion is so prodigious as to produce a wide variety of reactions. A well-known quote from Edward Gibbon's *The Decline and Fall of the Roman Empire* states that "the various modes of worship which prevailed in the Roman World were all considered by the people as equally true; by the philosopher as equally false; and by the magistrate as equally useful." The 16th century conflict in which Galileo was forced by church authorities to recant his discovery that the earth moved around the sun set the stage for the modern conflict between naturalistic and supernaturalistic explanations of events and behavior that began with the Age of Reason in 18th century Europe.

Most anthropologists regard religion, or sacred culture, as a projection of human wishes that serve to cope with anxieties. Westin La Barre, for example, describes religion as a group dream that originates in the visionary mental state of the shaman-originator, for example, in dreams, trances, episodes of spirit possession, epileptic seizures, and periods of sensory deprivation. In another theory, sound is a link to religion; infrasonic sound waves in the low hertz range can produce a high-intensity sound pressure in the absence of audible sound. Sound waves are perceived and processed in the brain, but, because they cannot be heard or their source identified (commonly distant thunder), they have a mystifying, uncanny, anxiety-provoking effect on a person who then labels the experience as religious. Drumbeats and chants facilitate religious experience not by what can be heard but rather by what cannot be heard, namely subauditory, infrasonic sound waves. This theory involves processing of the waves in the temporal lobe, a portion of the brain in which lesions are associated with symptoms such as hallucinations, delusions, illusions, déjà vu experiences, hyperreligiosity, feelings of ecstasy, intense philosophical and cosmological concerns, postseizure psychosis with a religious content, and mystical states.

There is a long Western medical tradition of conflict with cooperation and religion. Once Hippocrates declared epilepsy to be a biological and not a divine illness, physicians have continued to provide naturalistic explanations for illnesses once thought to be caused or influenced by the supernatural. The struggle to rescue mental illness from demonology, although still ongoing in many third world countries and some Western groups, generally has been successful. Perhaps this struggle has played a role in antipathy toward religion sometimes expressed by psychiatrists. Studies have shown consistently that psychiatrists are not as religious as the general public; in surveys done in 1975 to 1976, belief in God was endorsed by 90 percent of Americans but only by 43 percent of psychiatrists and 5 percent of psychologists; only 27 percent of psychiatrists surveyed in London in 1993 reported a belief in God. A study of articles in major psychiatric journals from 1977 to 1982 found that only 59 out of 2,348 articles contained a religious variable, usually a simple listing of a patient's denomination.

Freud regarded religion as an infantalizing, neurosis-producing, tyrannical force, and most psychoanalysts followed his critique with the prominent exception of Carl Jung. Even when they said something positive about religion, they often managed to find a rankling counterbalance. Ernest Jones, for example, wrote about the "enormous civilizing influence of Christianity" and "sublimated homosexuality" in the same sentence. Even Henry Maudsley, the most influential English psychiatrist of his time and certainly not a Freudian, wrote in 1918 that, "the corporeal or the material is the fundamental fact—the mental or the spiritual only its effect." In 1975, the outspoken psychologist, Albert Ellis, declared that religion itself is a self-depreciating, dehumanizing mental illness. However, at approximately that time, psychiatrists began a turnaround in their thinking about religion. More and more, psychiatrists are treating patients with severe mental illnesses by using new and better medications and spending less time talking with patients. In such an environment, psychiatrists have come to realize the importance of programs and personnel such as case managers, sheltered workshops, supervised apartment living, and self-help groups in helping patients survive and, occasionally, prosper in the community. Ministers, priests, and rabbis are now regarded as allies in dealing with the mentally ill, and church congregations are seen as a potentially healing resource. Ezra Griffith, for example, has demonstrated the psychological benefits of rituals in African-American churches. Most clergy now accept the usefulness of psychiatric treatment, although a minority of fundamentalists still regard psychiatrists as agents of the devil and mental illness as a moral flaw.

God and the Sacred Throughout history, people have sought an understanding about the purpose and meaning of life, the world, and the cosmos. This quest invariably has led to a belief in some sort of divine power or process that is called God, the Holy, or the Sacred. In 1917, the theologian, Rudolph Otto, published an influential study in which he considered the Holy to be so special a category that neither it nor the human experience of it can be denied. In the presence of the Holy, a person is filled with emotions that Otto labeled in Latin *mysterium tremendum et fascinosum*, that is, eerie, sublime, numinous, astounding feelings of wonder and dread. He regarded these feelings as primary, unique, underived from anything else, and the basic factor and impulse underlying the entire process of human thought.

Paul Tillich, one of the most influential 20th century theologians, asserted that the sense of the numinous presence of the Holy is really an awareness of the ultimate reality of God who is being itself and not *a* being. He claimed that it is just as atheistic to affirm the existence of God as to deny it. Apart from being and existence, there is nothing and nonexistence; psychiatrists can treat neurotic anxiety, but existential anxiety can be dealt with only by encountering God, the ground of being. For Tillich, true wisdom demands a religious experience that is a saving transformation and an illuminating revelation not of a personal god but rather of a God on whom everything is dependent.

A leading Catholic theologian, Karl Rahner, asserts that God and self come together in the mysticism of everyday life, the discovery of God in all things, and the sober intoxication of the Holy Spirit. In addition to *everyday mysticism*, persons may experience mystical states during which consciousness is briefly altered and all things are experienced as interrelated. In religious conversions or illuminations, the mystical state may be perceived as extraordinarily meaningful and coherent; the personal self expands to a close contact with God. Inner peace prevails and may give rise to a vision or special message.

Behavioral scientists have offered mundane explanations of religion and mystical states. In 1923, Freud wrote that individuals form the idea of God by merging the image of an exalted childhood father with the inherited memory traces of the primal father; thus, God is a type of father substitute. Romain Rolland, the French humanist, then chided Freud for not appreciating the eternal, richly energetic, beneficent, real core of religion that produced an oceanic-like experience. In *Civilization and Its Discontents*, written in 1930, Freud considered the oceanic experience as the essence of mystical states and explained it as an adult regression to the earliest undifferentiated state of infantile life in which there is a communal unity between infant and mother. This unity recedes as the self emerges, but many persons retain a connection to this primal unity, which may be experienced more commonly as awe, wonderment, and creative insight. The importance of the earliest stages of being, when infants record their first experience of mother as a "process" rather than an "object," is found in the psychoanalytic work of Christopher Bollas. He theorizes that these primal experiences are not processed through language or mental representation but rather as bodily sensations and emotions. An infant first knows mother existentially as a recurrent experience of being. The infant eventually transforms into a self, and mother is experienced as a process of this transformation. Adults carry the memory of this process as evidenced by their search for a person, place, event, or ideology that promises to transform the self. Humans revere objects that may transform us and may consider them to be sacred. Humans are religious beings because they carry with them the potential to be transformed and recreated. From this perspective, the experience of God is ultimately based on the transformative potential of creating the self, but this act of creation depends on a relationship with another human being. Although Bollas' configuration is wholly human, it is possible to imagine a broader dependency and relationship on what Tillich called *the ground of being itself*, namely God.

Psychiatrists William Meissner and Ana-Maria Rizzuto have each proposed a nontheological understanding of the human experience of God through the life cycle. A child's initial image of God is based primarily on the image of its parents. The child's God may be loving and protective, as well as fearsome, cruel, and not always available to gratify the child's wishes. A positive mother–child experience at this stage results in a basic sense of trust that, in later years, may lead to a trusting faith in God, whereas a negative, insecure experience may distort the experience of God. As the child begins the process of separation and of becoming an individual with some independence, it hears about something called God but lacks the capacity to understand what a spirit or transcendent force is. The child hears that God has made the world and, thus, likens God to the most powerful person that is known, namely both parents but especially father, who tends to be the more forceful or aggressive parent. Over the next few years, as the child comes to recognize that its parents neither know everything nor are all powerful, a romantic view of a perfect, heavenly father may emerge, as well as a distorted view of the family. God and parents may be idealized as totally protecting, or there may be a split into a good God and mean parents or into good parents and a mean God. Between 6 and 11 years of age, the child begins to appreciate symbols. The concept of God shifts from that of a flesh and blood person to a still imperfectly understood spirit whose power must be revered and feared, because God exacts punishment for every misdeed. In this stage, an immature obsessional religiosity may emerge in conjunction with ritualistic behaviors.

During adolescence, God becomes more personalized as "my Savior" or "my Father" and is more connected to emotions and to subjective attitudes, such as love, obedience, trust, and fear. God is experienced as the ideal leader and advisor who patiently and kindly listens to one's innermost problems and desires. When not tempered by some maturity of judgment, this realization of God may lead to fanatical tendencies. As adolescents become moralists, the burden of sinfulness emerges, and they may engage in the extremes of loose or puritanical behavior. Rebellion against parental authority may carry over to the parent's religion as well as to the God whom the parents symbolically represent.

As adolescents step into adulthood, they must decide to follow the religion of their parents, to seek a different religion, or to avoid religion altogether. A true religious faith that is based less on conflict and more on mature understanding probably is not acquired until 30 years of age. For some, the inner representation of God remains solid; for others, it may change; and for still others, it may be rejected or replaced. Thoughts about and the memory of God usually return in old age, especially when death nears. A person may decide to embrace God gracefully or grudgingly, for reasons that include mature acceptance of the cycle of life, hope of entering a heavenly afterlife, avoidance of eternal damnation, and neurotic fear, or to spurn God's ultimate encroachment; a person's last breath may be an inspiration or an expiration.

Freud regarded belief in God to be an illusion that softens fears about the dangers of life; the moral world order that God promises instills hope that justice will be served, and belief in an afterlife creates an ultimate setting for the fulfillment of wishes. For Freud, this illusion was noxious, because it distorted reality and promoted a state of psychic infantilism. However, in some modern thought, God is a benevolent illusion necessary for the growth and nourishment of mental and spiritual health. God is like the baby blanket or teddy bear that is special to the infant who endows it with a unique quality, cuddles it lovingly, and sometimes hates it. As the child matures, these transitional objects are neither mourned nor forgotten but rather simply lose meaning. They are the stuff of illusion and exist mentally somewhere between subjective and objective reality. In this formulation, God is a special transitional object who does not lose meaning totally and who is always available in religion. Rizzuto concludes that a person's humanity depends on illusion; the type of illusion selected, be it science, religion, or something else, "reveals our personal history and the transitional space each of us has created between his objects and himself to find a resting place to live in."

Sacred Texts Some, especially tribal, religions have only an oral history and tradition, whereas others have books considered to be authoritative; examples include the four Hindu *Vedas*, the Tibetan Buddhist *Great Liberation through Hearing in the Bardo*, and the Taoist *Tao Te Ching* (The Way and its Power). This section discusses the two most globally influential sacred texts, the Judeo-Christian Bible and the Muslim Qur'an.

The Bible The Bible is a compilation of papyrus or parchment scrolls into two books: Hebrew Scripture (relabeled as the Old Testament by Christians) and the New Testament. Hebrew Scripture, written in a language that belonged to Israel and never really spread geographically, presents the stories of creation; the selection of the Jews by the one, true God as the chosen people; and the suffering of the Jews in their quest for holiness. It contains a lengthy catalogue of laws, rituals, and commandments for the faithful to obey, as well as a variety of historical recollections, psalms, wise sayings, and prayers. The book of the prophet Isaiah refers to Israel as a suffering servant, a man of sorrow who was despised and rejected yet who "carried our sorrows, was wounded for our transgressions, was bruised for our iniquities . . . by his wounds we are healed" (53:3–5).

Christians claim that their New Testament completes and fulfills the Old Testament. The suffering servant, for example, is identified as Jesus Christ, the Son of God who allowed himself to be crucified to save humankind. The New Testament also speaks of the problems associated with starting a new religion, of healing miracles, of the resurrection of Jesus, of the power of the Holy Spirit, and of an impending apocalypse. It was written in koiné Greek, a language known throughout the cultures of the Mediterranean area and of the ancient Near East.

Jesus Christ was born and reared as a Jew and many of his early followers were converted Jews, but the religion founded in his name spread to include converts from many religions. A Jew named Paul, who was a persecutor of Christians, had a profound religious experience on the road to Damascus, claimed that he directly came to know Jesus and God the Father as a result of this experience, and equated himself with the 12 apostles who had personally known Christ. His genius and hard work were greatly responsible for the development and growth of the new religion, Christianity, which superseded the Levitical laws of Hebrew Scripture and promised believers tribulations and eventual resurrection.

Hebrew Scripture was written from approximately 900 BC to 165 BC; all the scrolls were edited over the centuries and, in approximately 150 AD, reached a form that approximates what appears in modern Bibles. There were many scrolls, each somewhat different, so that there never was a unique set of original scrolls. Hebrew Scripture is divided into the 22 Books of Law (also known as the Books of Moses, the Pentateuch, and the Torah), the Prophets, and the Writings.

Between 150 BC and 50 AD, no religious material was written that entered into the Bible. The Christian Church began to compile revered written documents in the second century. In 367 AD, Athanasius, the bishop of Alexandria, elected 27 books that he considered sacred; by and large, this list, which contained four Gospels, 13 of Paul's letters, and other writings, was accepted by the Christian community and came to be known as the *New Testament*. In 50 AD, the first entry was written, probably Paul's Letter to the Galatians; the last entry, II Peter, was written in approximately 150 AD None of the Gospel writers, with the possible exception of John, knew Jesus personally.

Modern versions of Hebrew Scripture are approximations of an idealized text and are based on an unsatisfactory 3rd century translation of the text into Greek (the Septuagint Bible), St. Jerome's 4th century updated translation of the Septuagint into Latin (the Vulgate Bible), and portions from scrolls found in the 20th century in the Dead Sea area. The oldest existing complete copy of Hebrew Scripture was written in 1009 AD (the Masoretic Bible). Knowledge about the New Testament text comes from a few inscribed pottery remnants; fewer than 100 fragmentary 2nd, 3rd, and 4th century Egyptian papyrus manuscripts; 250 incomplete 4th to 9th century parchments called *uncials*; 2,500 manuscripts, called *miniscules*, written from the 9th to 18th centuries; 85,000 quotations from the early Church Fathers; nearly 5,000 Greek manuscripts, each one different than the other; and translations, such as the Vulgate, from the Greek (there are no existing translations of a manuscript before the 4th century). Variants in every New Testament sentence can be found in the manuscript tradition. In 1966, the United Biblical Societies issued a "standard" text but noted that more than 2,000 choices had to be made concerning significant alternative readings of manuscripts; in 1975 a new, improved, "standard" edition was published. Textual problems have been compounded by the difficulty of translations into nearly all the languages of the world. Hundreds of English language translations of the Bible are available; these range from the magisterial King James version to a Basic English version that limits its vocabulary to 1,000 words to a politically correct inclusive version in which, for example, the opening line of the Lord's Prayer is translated as "Our Mother-Father in heaven."

In addition to varying and sometimes confusing accounts of events presented in the Bible, textual and translational differences have influenced the interpretations and practices of believers, some of whom hold that everything in the Bible is literally true. Such fundamentalists believe, for example, that Adam and Eve were actual persons from whom all human beings have descended, that the sun moves around the earth, that Noah's ark really contained a pair of every animal, and that the earth itself was created at 9 AM on October 23, 4004 BC However, most believers hold that the Bible was inspired by God but written by men who compiled their narratives in their own style; that the Bible is truthful on significant spiritual matters, such as faith and salvation, but is not necessarily accurate in scientific matters, such as astronomy, animal husbandry, and botany; and that many biblical accounts are best understood as meaningful allegories. Although there have always been skeptics about supernatural events recorded in the Bible, such as the resurrection of Jesus, the historical truth about fundamental facts is being questioned by many scholars. There is no good evidence outside of the Bible itself, for example, that Moses and Jesus were actual persons or, if they did exist, that their lives were recorded accurately. The effects of these reports on believers have undoubtedly played some role in the marked decline of religious attendance and influence in Europe; the Catholic Archdiocese of Dublin, Ireland's largest archdiocese, for example, ordained only one priest in 2001. The United States presents a mixed picture in that, although most people profess a belief in God, church attendance is sporadic, and the number of persons adopting a religious vocation has fallen dramatically. However, Christianity is blossoming in third world countries.

Al-Qur'an Al-Qur'an is a compilation of poetical verses divided into 114 chapters; it is the sacred text of Islam. Muslims believe that, in 610 AD, the angel Gabriel confronted Mohammed in a cave atop a mountain near Mecca, proclaimed him the messenger of the one true God, Allah, and ordered him to read the verses from written Scriptures that existed in heaven. After experiencing doubts about this experience, Mohammed consulted a man familiar with Jewish and Christian Scripture who convinced him that Moses had seen the same angel. When Mohammed realized that he was, indeed, a prophet, he followed the angel's instructions and, over the next 23 years, while in trance-like states and in many geographic locations, read and spoke aloud the heavenly verses (Al-Qur'an means *the Reading*).

His utterances were written down by various scribes. Four varying collections of the verses were collected that included material from persons who claimed to have memorized some of Mohammed's words that had not been written down. Within a generation, the Caliph Uthman issued a standard version that is still used today, although there are some variations because the original Arabic script neither noted vowels nor contained diacritical dots, thus complicating the parsing of a verb as active or passive. The Qur'an has no story line; the chapters begin with the longest passages and end with the shortest passages. Translations have been pedestrian and invariably fail to convey its august and lofty language.

The content of the book focuses on the necessity of professing faith in the unity of one God who was known to the Jews and Christians. They were the original proto-Muslims, but then they supposedly turned from the true path. They must become Muslims again by now embracing Islam (submission to God). Abraham, Ishmael, and Jesus were true prophets, and Muslims anticipate the return of Jesus in an apocalyptic time. The book establishes the duty of Muslims to pray several times daily, to give alms to the poor, to fast during the month of Ramadan, to make a pilgrimage to Mecca, and to obey certain commandments, seven of which are similar to the Ten Commandments found in the Bible.

In the 8th century, Muslims solidified a belief that their behaviors and laws should parallel those of Mohammed, his Companions, and followers. Thus, collections of sayings were gathered into books of tradition called *hadith*. The literature on hadith is enormous; out of several hundred thousand hadith that have been proposed, only several hundred are generally regarded as absolutely authentic, whereas the others are classified into numerous categories based on the strength of the evidence that they can be traced back to Mohammed's time. Two other forces that have influenced Muslim behaviors and laws are analogous reasoning applied to similar cases and consensus by learned persons. Consideration of all these factors has resulted in a classification of behaviors into five categories: obligatory, recommended, indifferent, disapproved but not forbidden, and prohibited. A combined system of secular and religious law emerged, the *shari'a*. In situations not covered by the *shari'a*, highly esteemed judges may issue an opinion called a *fatwa*. Shi'ite Muslims, second only to the Sunnis in number, have replaced the concept of consensus by a belief that God selects an infallible, authoritative leader, or Imam, who is descended from Mohammed to lead the faithful of each generation.

There are many Sunni, Shi'ite, and other Muslim groups and subdivisions with differing interpretations of history, sacred texts, and *shari'a*. Local customs, the establishment of political states based on Islamic principles, the struggle among fundamentalists, moderates, and liberals, and the encroachment of Western ideas and attitudes have influenced behaviors and caused religious problems. The homicide-suicide bomb attacks on Israeli civilians have been both denounced by a majority and praised by a minority of differing interpreters of Islamic principles and *shari'a*. Turkey exemplifies a Muslim nation that has adopted a secular, democratic constitution. Saudi Arabia exemplifies a kingdom caught up in the battle between modernization and adherence to fundamentalist principles: Non-Muslims are not allowed to enter the city of Mecca, nor are they allowed to display their own religious symbols or to be buried in Saudi soil, yet Western clothes, fast food, and television shows are widely available.

Sin One of the most profound accomplishments of the Bible was the moral delineation of sin as a rebellion against the one true God and its characterization as wicked, evil, and guilt evoking. Hebrew Scripture notes that wicked persons are estranged from the womb and go astray as soon as they are born, following the dictates of an evil heart. First century BC Jewish theologians believed that, from the moment of his creation, Adam, the first human, had a grain of evil seed that all subsequent humans possess. The penalties for transgressing God's laws included death by stoning, horrible diseases, financial failure, severe humiliation, and chronic sadness. However, most modern Jews are not Orthodox and, rather than referring to notions of innate badness or goodness, teach about personal responsibility for one's actions.

Christianity claims that Adam's misuse of free will—he ate forbidden fruit—is the original sin that affects humankind and that it can be removed only by baptism in the Holy Spirit and belief in Jesus Christ, the Redemptor. Christianity rejected a majority of Jewish laws and teaches that, through confession and repentance, it is possible for sins to be forgiven and unrighteousness to be cleansed. A list of seven capital sins based on the Ten Commandments, Jesus' Sermon on the Mount, and St. Paul's writings was completed by Pope Gregory (1540 to 1604) and endures to the present: pride (from which all the others derive), avarice, envy, wrath, lust, gluttony, and sloth. Christianity elevated the role of Satan, a rebellious evil spirit, and a host of lesser demons who enticed humans to sin. It perfected a concept of heaven and hell after death and predicted a cosmic apocalyptic conflict in which God will vanquish Satan and then usher in a new blessed age for the faithful.

Although apocalyptic seminars and "fire and brimstone" sermons persist, in modern times, the notions of sin, Satan, and hell have gradually withdrawn into the recesses of Western consciousness. In 1973, William Menninger noted in the popular press that sin had dropped out of daily conversation and debate. No longer were people accused of being sinners, nor were they expected to display public remorse for their sins. Indeed, attempts by some high profile politicians, as well as common prisoners, to explain their problematic behaviors as sinful are nowadays usually met with cynicism and derision. Current social morality has reconfigured sin into criminal behavior, defective character, or a symptom of mental disorder, and mind has replaced soul in psychiatry. Free will, a necessary ingredient of sin, has become less meaningful as evidence accumulates demonstrating that much of human behavior is determined by genetic factors, neuronal functioning, learned responses, peer pressure, childhood experiences, and a host of other naturalistic forces.

Sexuality and Gender The major monotheistic religions reflect the patriarchal cultures in which they were founded. God and his priests are masculine. Women traditionally were valued for their roles as mothers and house keepers and were duty bound to obey their husbands and to remain silent on most matters. Jewish Scripture contains many references to prostitutes and adulteresses; the phrase "to play the harlot" is used to describe the act of abandoning one's faith. Distrust and fear of women's sexuality are common: The book of Proverbs states that "the mouth of an immoral woman is a deep pit; he who is abhorred by the Lord will fall there." Menstruating women were shunned as impure.

Jesus elevated the status of women somewhat when he healed a woman with chronic vaginal bleeding who had touched his robe, talked with women on the street, allowed women to accompany him and his male disciples, and absolutely forbade divorce (scholars believe that, in a later addition to the Bible, Jesus supposedly made an exception in the case of an adulterous wife). Despite several New Testament letters encouraging husbands to love their wives, St. Paul and many of the Church fathers tolerated marriage only if a person could not exercise sexual self-control. With Eve as a model, women were perceived as seducers who stimulated men's lustful appetites; to St. Bernard (1109 to 1153) was attributed the sentiment that "a beautiful woman is like a temple built over a sewer." Female virginity became a pathway to heaven, and, in 649, Pope Martin I officially declared the perpetual virginity of Mary, the mother of Jesus, a required belief of the Church. Devotion to Mary has remained a hallmark of Catholicism, especially among women for whom she is a model of comportment. The incompatibility between virginity and motherhood has been a cause of sexual confusion for some believers who dichotomize women into two types, the so-called Madonna-whore complex, in which "good" women are like the asexual Virgin Mary, whereas "bad" women are like the biblical prostitute, Mary Magdalen. The church's recent rehabilitation of Mary Magdalen, who is no longer considered a harlot but rather is revered as the first person to see the resurrected Jesus, reflects a slowly changing attitude toward women. Catholicism holds that all sexual acts should not limit the possibility of achieving pregnancy, therefore prohibiting the use of birth control devices. The defiance of the prohibition by Catholics represents the growing challenge to ecclesiastical authority seen among many Christian groups; in a 1995 survey, 75 percent of sexually active Catholic women used contraceptives.

By reference to their sacred texts, Jews, Christians, and Muslims traditionally have cited the social superiority of men over women. However, from a historical perspective, the 20th century may be best remembered as the era in which Western women achieved a great measure of equality with men. This revolution in gender relationships began in earnest in 1878, when the American National Women Suffrage Association passed resolutions declaring that religion had been used to subjugate women, that female self-sacrifice and obedience were self-defeating, and that women should claim the right of individual conscience and judgment that men alone claimed. Elizabeth Cady Stanton gathered together 20 learned women in the 1890s to publish the first real document of the revolution, *The Women's Bible*. Feminist biblical scholarship has blossomed since the social ferment of the 1960s in an attempt to liberate the Bible from its masculine orientation and its use by political religious groups to deny women's rights and freedoms. Feminist scholars believe that they are continuing the tradition of the biblical prophets who expressed God's will by passing judgment on injustices and on the perversion of religion.

Islamic societies generally limit the freedoms of women in comparison to Western societies, although change is slowly becoming apparent. Men are still legally allowed four wives, although each must be treated like the others; in fact, most Muslims today have only one wife. Some Shi'ite Muslims recognize *mut'a* marriages in which a man pays a woman for her sexual services for a day or so, after which the marriage automatically is dissolved. In a few areas, Muslim women can get a divorce somewhat easier than in the past, whereas men cannot get a divorce without incurring the same sort of civil liabilities as in the West. In areas under Fundamentalist control, women may not travel alone without getting a permit, and adulterers may be stoned to death (it is easier to convict a woman, especially if she becomes pregnant, than a man). There is little, if any, feminist quranic scholarship. Resistance to change in gender relationships stems from the endurance of patriarchal attitudes in Islamic societies with high levels of poverty and low levels of education, from the inward looking nature of Islamic intellectual life over the past few centuries, and from a strong belief in a literal and unchanging interpretation of the Qur'an.

Condemnation of homosexuality, a socially divisive issue, is often based on several biblical citations. The Book of Leviticus contains myriad laws, such as prohibitions against trimming one's beard, eating shellfish or pork, and wearing garments made of a mixture of linen and wool; in addition, crops must not be planted every seventh year, and adulterers, fortune tellers, and male homosexuals should be put to death. Although Christians are not obligated to follow the Levitical laws, most groups have selectively chosen to uphold the prohibition again homosexual behavior.

The book of Genesis tells the story of two angels dressed as men who came to the city of Sodom, where a man named Lot allowed them to stay in his home. A group of townsmen surrounded the home and asked about the two men, saying "bring them out to us that we may know them." Frightened, Lot told them to leave his guests alone and offered his virginal daughters in their place. The townsmen failed to break down the door and left. The next day, God rained fire and brimstone on the city, killing all its inhabitants, although Lot and his children escaped. The earliest interpretations of this story focused on the Sodomites' arrogance and rudeness to strangers; God killed them for incivility to his angels. The theme of sexuality emerged full force in the 1st century BC in the writings of Philo of Alexandria, a Jewish historian. Rabbinical writings about Sodom in the Talmud and the Midrashim (commentaries) generally did not mention homosexuality. Although some Church fathers agreed with Philo, others did not, pointing to a parallel story in Chapter 19 of the Book of Judges in which homosexuality was not implicated. The Sodomite townsmen wanted "to know" the men; the verb "to know" is used 943 times in Jewish Scripture, and in only 10 places does it clearly refer to sexual intercourse. However, over time, the homosexual interpretation won out: the King James Bible translates the townsmen's request, "that we may know them carnally," whereas the New English Bible says, "so that we can have sexual intercourse with them." Some scholars refute these translations and note that Lot was not a full citizen of Sodom. The townsmen were suspicious because he had allowed two strangers to stay in the city at night without asking permission of the proper officials and, thus, they wanted "to know" who the two men were.

Jesus does not mention homosexuality. However, he did link Sodom with the inhospitality that his disciples might encounter when preaching (Matthew 10:14–15). St. Paul, who barely tolerated marital sexuality, seems to have disapproved of homosexual behavior, but the exact meaning of the specific words he used is unclear. In I Corinthians 5:11, for example, he includes in his list of the unrighteous who will not go to heaven people who are *malakoi* and *arsenokoitai*. The translations of these words vary widely and include effeminate, child molesters, homosexual, masturbators, immoral, sexually immoral, depraved, and male prostitutes. In fact, sacred, cultic male and female prostitution associated with the god Baal and the goddess Ishtar are condemned in Jewish Scripture. Although homosexual behavior was practiced throughout the ancient world, the designation of a person as a *homosexual* did not become prevalent until the 11th century AD when St. Peter Damian coined the word *sodomia*, thus establishing an abstract essence: Persons who indulged in *sodomia* were thereafter sodomites (homosexuals).

Alcohol Despite the Qur'an's clear prohibition of alcohol, many cultural Muslims drink. Although the total quantity consumed in Muslim countries is small, problem drinking is prevalent, because alcohol is feared and is not integrated into daily life. Jews have drunk alcohol for thousands of years with minimal disruptive consequences. The basis of Jewish sobriety was established during the 200-year period after the return to Israel in 537 BC of the Jews who were held captive in Babylon. Before this, the Bible contained many references to drunkenness, but none afterwards, even though Jews continued to make wine, to drink it ritually and for pleasure, and to pour sacrificial libations. In addition to the banishment of pagan gods whose rituals demanded heavy drinking, alcohol was positively integrated into religiously oriented ceremonies in the home and synagogue. Drunkenness disappeared as a social problem once wine came to be regarded as a substance that should be drunk in moderation and only in conjunction with food and holy rituals. Even the fear of drunkenness vanished, as evidenced by a scientifically unsound medieval rabbinical ruling that European wine was not as potent as the wine produced in biblical times and therefore could be drunk undiluted. Drunkenness and alcoholism became alien to Jewish identity; the Yiddish expression *skikker vi a goy* means "drunk as a Gentile." However, with the increasing loss of Orthodoxy, Jewish alcoholism rates are rising.

No Christian religious group condones drunkenness, but there are variations in attitudes to alcohol. The official stance of Catholicism, reflecting the view of St. Thomas Aquinas, is that drinking wine is lawful, except if a person takes a vow not to drink, if a person gets drunk easily, or if drinking scandalizes others. Protestants leave decisions about drinking to individual discretion, but groups such as the Lutherans and Methodists preach moderation, whereas Pentecostals and Baptists preach abstinence and regard alcohol as an invariably destructive substance. These variations stem from conflicting biblical passages.

The clearest negative comments on drinking are found in the book of Proverbs 23:29–33: "Who has woe? Who has sorrow? Who has complaining? Who has redness of eyes? Do not look at wine when it is red, when it sparkles in the cup, and goes down smoothly. At the last it bites like a serpent and stings like an adder. You will see strange things, and your mind utter perverse things."

Among the Hebrew prophets, Isaiah described Egypt as akin to a drunken man who staggers in his vomit and Israel's leaders as irresponsible, because they devote themselves to intoxicating drinks. Hosea warned that harlotry and wine enslave the heart. Jesus warned against being drunk at the time of his second coming. Several lists in the New Testament cite drunkenness among the vices of those persons who do not walk with Christ, who will not inherit the kingdom of God, and who live doing the work of the Gentiles instead of God.

Other biblical passages consider wine as a staple of life and a blessing from God. Isaac asked God to give his son, Jacob, the dew of heaven, the fatness of the land, and the plenty of grain and wine. In the book of Amos, God promised to return the Jewish captives to Israel, where they shall plant vineyards and drink their wine. Zechariah notes that when the people of Judea and Israel are restored, then their hearts will rejoice as if with wine. Judges 9:13 refers to wine "which cheers both God and men." Proverbs advocates giving wine to persons who are bitter of heart, so that they can forget their misery and poverty. I Timothy 5:23 encourages the use of wine "for the sake of your stomach and your frequent ailments."

In the United States, alcohol and religion have a unique, linked history. The consumption of alcohol was quite high after the Revolutionary War. Americans felt patriotic about drinking liquor distilled from healthful, native corn and regarded intoxication as a freedom consonant with their hard-won independence. Benjamin Rush, one of the founders of the American Psychiatric Association, considered whiskey and rum as the ruination of the new nation, although wine and beer in moderation were fine. In the 1780s, Methodists and Quakers were like-minded in forbidding the drinking of hard liquor, the former because it interfered with religious practices and the latter because it interfered with self-control. In 1826, a Presbyterian minister in Connecticut delivered six sermons on the evils of liquor that became a basic text of the American Temperance Society. Local temperance societies grew from 222 in 1827 to 8,500 in 1834, and antidrinking laws became popular. New towns were established to advance temperance values, the best known being Palo Alto, California, the site of Stanford University. In 1874, the Women's Christian Temperance Union was founded and demanded the worldwide prohibition of alcohol, prostitution, child marriages, foot binding in China, the Japanese geisha system, and the sale of opium. Evangelical frontier churches held that temperance was not enough to claim salvation; only total abstinence would do so.

In 1893, a minister from Ohio founded the Anti-Saloon League and successfully delivered votes for politicians who supported prohibition. James Cannon, a Methodist bishop from Virginia, pushed through the prohibition amendment to the U.S. Constitution in 1917 by demonizing alcohol as the major cause of the nation's ills. Although alcoholism rates declined, prohibition resulted in widespread lawlessness and the creation of a vast criminal underclass. Instead of prosperity, the nation experienced a great economic depression. Bishop Cannon was disgraced by charges of war profiteering, illegal stock deals, adultery, and corrupt political practices. Tired of austerity and naysayers, Americans repealed prohibition in 1933.

Healing In the earliest days of humankind, spiritually powerful men and women known as *shamans* healed disease and reversed misery by retrieving lost souls, by pacifying and exorcising malign spirits, and by providing counter-magic. Their legacy continues today in "faith healers" that exist in all cultures, although, especially in Western nations, many are impostors.

Hebrew Scripture attributes most disease to God's retribution against disobedient believers; Exodus 15:17 is the definitive statement on God the healer: "If you diligently heed the voice of the Lord your God and do what is right in his sight, give ear to his commandments, and keep all his statutes, I will put none of the diseases on you which I have brought on the Egyptians. For I am the Lord who heals you." The early Hebrews disdained formal medical practice, because it diminished God's position. However, by 180 BC, the book of Ecclesiastes noted that sick persons should pray to the Lord for healing but should also consult physicians who can provide medicines that heal and take away pain.

The approach of Jesus to the sick, many of whom had been disenfranchised from full participation in temple activities, was revolutionary. He welcomed the sick and did not blame them for their illnesses. Almost 20 percent of the Gospels are devoted to Jesus' 41 healing encounters with individuals and groups. He healed medical and spiritual and psychological disorders; his most common technique was to say a few words and to touch the sick person. A disproportionate number of his healings involved the exorcism of demons, and he passed on this power to his 12 disciples and all of his followers. The classic healing text is found in the book of James 5:13–16 in which sick people were enjoined to call the Church elders to their bedside, to be anointed with oil in the name of the Lord, to confess their sins, and to pray for one another, and "they will be healed." In approximately 400 AD, St. Jerome translated the Bible into Latin; instead of "they will be healed," Jerome wrote, "they will be saved." By this alteration, spiritual salvation displaced the healing of illness as the central focus of the text and resulted in a neglect of physical healing for almost 1,500 years. In fact, physical suffering became a Christian avocation that allowed a person to share in Jesus' suffering on the cross. When God refused to cure Paul (he may have been epileptic) on three occasions, the Bible notes that God's grace was sufficient and that his power was made perfect in weakness. Thus, defects were no longer liabilities but rather were opportunities to receive the power of Jesus. This formulation enhanced the self-worth of disabled and ill persons, but it also contained the potential for persons to accept their infirmities with passivity or even to mortify themselves in pursuit of a higher, spiritual goal.

Medicine was devalued, physicians ridiculed, and religious healing forgotten (except for occasional exorcisms), so sick people turned to dead saints for help. A cult of relics, namely, the preserved body parts of saints who supposedly had performed miracles, prospered for over a millennium from the 4th century. The church assigned saints to specific diseases; St. Vitus was the patron of persons with chorea, St. Lucy was the patron of persons with eye disease, and St. Dympna was the patron of the mentally ill. The many shrines that held the healing relics faded into obscurity when medical practice became more effective. A major exception is the relatively new shrine of Lourdes in France, where St. Bernadette had her vision of "the lady" in 1858. Local enthusiasts identified "the lady" as the Virgin Mary. Although St. Bernadette died of tuberculosis at 35 years of age and never stated that "the lady" would cure anything, the shrine at Lourdes was promoted by merchants as a place for healing. Several million visitors from around the world travel there yearly, including many desperate persons whose illnesses have not responded to medical treatment. Lourdes has an official medical bureau for the certification of miraculous healing; less than 100 have been issued. The ceremonies at Lourdes are emotionally charged and spiritually uplifting, so that temporary functional improvement in some cases does occur despite the lack of organic changes.

Interest in religious healing in the form of "mind cures" emerged at the end of the 19th century in New England. Mary Baker Eddy, for example, wrote *Science and Health* in 1875; she declared that sickness is a fearful belief made manifest on the human body and that it can be annihilated by the divine mind. The real rebirth of Christian healing occurred in Topeka, Kansas, when a preacher rediscovered glossolalia, linked it to healing, and started a Pentecostal revival that relied on the verses found in the Gospel of Mark 16:16–18: "He who believes and is baptized will be saved; but he who does not believe will be condemned. And these signs will follow those who believe: In my name they will cast out demons; they will speak with tongues; they will take up serpents; and if they drink anything deadly, it will by no means hurt them; they will lay hands on the sick, and they will recover."

The American Midwest proved to be a congenial cultural setting for Pentecostal faith healing. From its humble beginnings in small churches, faith healing ceremonies have progressed to radio and large scale television presentations that raise millions of dollars throughout North and South America, Europe, and Africa. The presentations usually are spectacular extravaganzas replete with extremely large and expectant crowds, high-tech lighting, fast-paced music, and continual choruses of praise. The healers have celebrity status and are skilled performers. The healings often consist of the dramatic exorcism of illness—demons who have supposedly possessed the sick person. Some sophisticated healers speak more about demonic oppression rather than possession, especially in persons with impulsivity problems, such as compulsive gamblers, alcoholics, substance abusers, and self-cutters.

Even mainstream Christian churches have turned to healing, although in a less spectacular and calmer manner, in a charismatic renewal that includes speaking in tongues, uttering prophecies, and prayers for healing. After a lapse of 1,600 years, the Catholic Church rediscovered healing during the Vatican Council II in the 1960s. The sacrament of Extreme Unction, for example, was renamed Anointing of the Sick and is no longer reserved for the dying in private but is given publicly as soon as any of the faithful begins to be in danger of dying from sickness or old age.

Many flamboyant faith healers have been exposed as charlatans, whereas others probably believe they are doing God's work. Follow-up studies have consistently found no evidence of cures, although many persons may feel better briefly. A study of 71 Pentecostal Christians who experienced hands-on faith healing for conditions ranging from leukemia to peptic ulcer to warts found that all the subjects reported an instantaneous or gradual healing, despite the fact that the original symptoms were unchanged. They proclaimed themselves to be healed because their belief in God increased, as did their conviction that they were leading a proper, righteous life.

Studies of attempts to heal persons by prayers offered at a distant site, so that subjects have no knowledge of the prayer attempts, have shown no great advantage to prayed-for versus control groups. An often-cited study of coronary care patients did show a slightly better hospital course among prayed-for patients, but a flawed methodology casts doubts on the results: No information was provided about the psychological characteristics of the subjects or the treatment practices of the various health care plans; the coordinator of the study not only knew which patients were in the prayed-for and control groups, but also was responsible for record keeping on all subjects; and, when the study was returned by a journal editor with a revision request, the author reconstructed the criteria about what established a good or bad hospital course after he knew which group each patient was in.

Especially in times of crisis, prayers offer hope. Christians may point to the New Testament, which states, "whatever things you ask in prayer, believing, you will receive" (Matthew 21:22), and, "whatever you ask the Father in My name, He will give you" (John 16:23). However, when a petitioner's prayers are not answered, as is usually the case, theologians turn to the biblical example of Jesus in the garden of Gethsemane before his betrayal and capture when he prayed to God the Father, "not what I will, but what You will" (Matthew 31:39). Any interpretation of a supernatural intervention, such as intercessory prayer for a sick person, depends on the mind-set of the participants. If a prayed-for person is cured, the skeptical scientist may posit a natural, but not yet understood, mechanism; if the person is not cured, the skeptical theologian may contend that the wrong prayer or not enough prayer was offered, that God was angry at being tested, or that the result was God's will.

Religion and Mental Health

The complicated relationship between religion and mental health is due, in part, to definitions. Is mental health, for example, merely the absence of psychopathological symptoms or does it imply happiness, contentment, tranquility, spontaneity, the capacity to love and to work, the maintenance of a right relationship with God, and the fulfillment of one's intellectual potential? Is it mentally healthier to criticize or to submit to authority, to be independent or to be dependent on family and friends? Is it religiously healthier to focus on self-realization or to accept dogma that demands obedience? Good data on the relationship between religion and mental health are hard to come by, especially in non-Western countries in which so-called official statistics are often misleading

Psychiatry has a formal list of psychopathological signs and symptoms, but there is no such list for religion. Also, because at least 21 variables have been identified as components of religiosity, the selection of appropriate variables to include in scientific studies is problematic. The most useful delineation of religiosity is probably Gordon Allport's and J. Michael Ross' intrinsic and extrinsic types: The former implies a sincere commitment to one's beliefs, which are internalized and serve as a guiding motivation of behavior, whereas the latter implies the use of religion to obtain status, security, self-justification, and sociability.

Psychiatric studies on the relationship between religion and mental health have generally treated religiosity superficially. Religious studies, although numerous, tend to rely on self-reports, overrepresent churchgoers and college students, usually exclude nonbelievers, emphasize church attendance as a variable, and lack longitudinal data. Most studies are correlated: A consistent finding that elderly persons who attend church demonstrate better mental health than those who do not, for example, may simply mean that elderly churchgoers are in good enough physical health to make the trip to church. Because there is a positive relationship between physical and mental health, church attendance in this group may signify good physical health and may have little to do with mental health.

No meaningful general conclusions can be made at this time about the impact of religion on mental health. A conceptually sound study of 1,902 female twins over a 6-year period found that, except for a lower use of tobacco and alcohol and a possibly lower level of depression, there was little evidence overall for a relationship between current psychiatric symptoms, lifetime psychopathology, and religiosity. A survey of 14,000 youths found that any sort of religious commitment was related to a decreased likelihood of substance abuse. Studies of religious coping measures in persons who had experienced stressful life events within the past year found that religious rituals in times of crisis were helpful in 40 percent of cases and harmful in 23 percent. These coping measures were more helpful to religious persons who had less access to material resources and power, such as the elderly, the poor, the less educated, African Americans, the widowed, and women.

Religious beliefs may affect the expression of psychopathology. Some psychotic and manic patients may proclaim themselves to be a god, a prophet, a messiah, or a saint. Paranoia may focus on satanic plots. Hallucinations may be interpreted as supernatural events. Depression is a special case in that its psychological torments have, until recently, often been considered an authentic part of the religious experience; for Christians, it is a sharing of the sufferings of the martyrs and of Jesus on the cross, whereas many Shi'ite Muslims, during the ritual remembrance of the martyrdoms of religious heroes, flagellate themselves frenetically and recall the words of Husain: "Trial, affliction and pains, the thicker they fall on man, the better do they prepare him of his journey heavenward." The tribulations of Moses are an important component of Jewish identity. Buddhism acknowledges the Noble Truth that suffering is universal and that birth, aging, and death are suffering produced by a craving for and repulsion of sense pleasure, for existence and nonexistence, and for becoming and self-annihilation. Indeed, the calmness and seeming passivity of some Buddhists in dealing with their suffering may test the patience of Western psychiatrists who are accustomed to patients seeking rapid symptomatic relief with medication. Guilt, another component of depression, and sin are reported by fewer patients nowadays. Even though obsessive-compulsive disorder (OCD) mimics the precisely calculated rituals of some religions, fewer patients today ruminate about right and wrong and good and evil. These shifts indicate a decrease in religiosity and an increase in naturalistic, scientific beliefs and modes of expression.

Although conversion disorders are still prevalent in third world countries, their decline in Western nations has been attributed to the transparency of the symptoms in the light of widespread, public understanding of psychological principles. In fact, persons with conversion disorders may be overrepresented in the throngs of unsophisticated attendees at faith healing revivals and crusades, some of which may attract 100,000 participants, as well as a vast television audience. Attraction to these spectacles represents a disappointment that modern medicine, despite its technological advances, still cannot cure all diseases. The rapid growth of Christian groups that emphasize unabashed emotionality, music, singing, glossolalia, and a quest to attain spiritual joy may reflect a response to what seems to be a worldwide increase in depression. Glossolalia or speaking in tongues is a poorly understood, nonpathological phenomenon in which a person utters a series of words that are totally unintelligible to the speaker and to listeners. It can occur in quiet or in highly emotional settings, in groups or in solitary privacy, in children as well as adults, and in upper– and lower–social class persons. It usually is not associated with an altered state of consciousness. It rarely is a negative experience; most of the time, it is mildly positive and sometimes very positive. It possibly benefits depressed and anxious persons a little bit. The practice is mentioned in the New Testament as a minor gift of the Holy Spirit, ranking below wisdom, faith, healing, miracles, and prophecy.

Spirituality Spirituality is a somewhat nebulous concept. In 1990, David Elkins, a psychologist, outlined the values of spiritual persons as belief in a "greater self" or personal God, a sense of purpose in life and quest for meaning, acceptance of the sacredness of nature and of all human experience, knowledge that ultimate fulfillment is found in spirituality and not in material things, altruism, idealism, awareness of suffering and death, and leading a life that has a positive effect on people, nature, and whatever they consider to be ultimate, transcendent reality. Spiritual and religious values overlap, but a person with extrinsic religiosity may be lacking in spirituality, whereas a nonchurchgoer who volunteers at a homeless shelter and is active in environmental causes may be spiritual but lacking in religiosity.

The spectrum of spirituality is exceedingly broad. At one end is religious spirituality as exemplified by the quiet prayerful practices of monks and nuns and by the enthusiastic, highly motoric practices of Sufi Muslims and Pentecostal Christians. At the other end is *New Age* spirituality, which includes ethereal music, cosmic vibrations, abductions by aliens from outer space, psychic readings, past-life regressions, being touched by angels, and near-death experiences that occur when persons are in a state of what appears to be death but then are revived. Some persons later report that they were out of their bodies during the near-death period, looked down at themselves, and felt themselves moving through a dark tunnel peacefully. They reviewed their lives as in a panorama. They saw a glowing light with a human shape, cities of lights, and a border from which there is no return. They met deceased relatives and friends. They heard doctors or spectators who pronounced them dead, but they were rescued from death by a spirit. Remarkable similarities exist between the reports of near-death survivors and by users of hallucinogenic or other drugs. It is likely that, when a person approaches death, there is a decrease in response to external stimuli, a turning inward of attention, the release of old memories, reminiscence, and a fear of death that triggers hallucinations, dreams, and fantasies of God, heaven, and rescue. Should the person survive, then the near-death experience may be interpreted as a valued spiritual phenomenon, although, in various studies, as much as 22 percent of such experiences have been described as hellish and terrifying.

It is not surprising that the therapeutic approach of AA centers on spirituality because of the nature of alcohol. In *The Varieties of Religious Experience*, written in 1902, James commented on alcohol's power to stimulate the mystical faculties of human nature, to bring drinkers to the radiant core of life, and to make them, for the moment, one with truth. Distilled spirits were originally called *aqua vitae*—the water of life. The ancient Greeks worshiped the god Dionysus, who supposedly invented wine. At his chaste orgies, women were intoxicated with wine, danced ecstatically in the darkness of the mountains, and then ripped apart wild animals and devoured them in the belief that each morsel contained a bit of Dionysus himself. He was also revered as the Lord of Souls, his likeness, leading drunken revelers to a happy afterlife, painted on numerous sarcophagi. The Bible calls wine "the blood of the grape," and, in Christian thought, Jesus instituted the Eucharistic sacrifice at the Last Supper, when he offered his disciples bread and wine that he declared to be his body and blood. By eating the bread-flesh and drinking the wine-blood, the disciples ingested their God, and his immortality became theirs, an immortality available forevermore to believers who partake of this sacrament of Holy Communion. Elvin Jellinek, one of the greatest alcohol researchers, believed that alcoholics used drunkenness as a type of shortcut to a higher life and higher mental state without an emotional or intellectual effort. To be "high" is to be closer to heaven.

AA is not a religion, although some critics have described it as a religion in denial. Its roots are Christian; its famous 12 steps and traditions unconsciously recall the 12 tribes of Israel and the 12 disciples of Jesus. To fulfill the steps, members must believe in a power greater than themselves, turn their lives over to God as they understand him, improve their conscious contact with God through prayer and meditation, and experience a spiritual awakening. The most detailed study of AA dynamics is Ernest Kurtz's book, *Not God: A History of Alcoholics Anonymous*. The curious title refers to the fundamental message of AA, namely, that each alcoholic must reject any claim to be more than human. Religion's aspiration for perfection and absolute truths was too grandiose for the founders of AA, who broke away from the Christian Oxford Group and established AA's mission of saving "drunks" and not the world. One of the founders noted that, before AA, he was trying to find God in a bottle. For many alcoholics, the spiritual approach of AA is undoubtedly effective, although the organization's commitment to remain forever nonprofessional has hampered impartial research.

Psychiatrist's Role Psychiatrists should ask all patients about the importance of religion and spirituality in their lives, the frequency and intensity of their participation in religious and spiritual practices, and the leadership style and members' behaviors of the religious and spiritual groups in which they are involved. General familiarity with the beliefs and behaviors of certain groups in which patients are involved must be joined with knowledge about specific local groups. Some patients may eschew participation in congregational life—they may lack transportation, have health problems, feel embarrassed by their shabby clothes, or get panic attacks in crowded churches—and watch televangelists in the comfort of their homes. Many pray, put their trust in guardian angels, and read sacred texts daily; although their level of understanding may be unsophisticated, the mere presence of the sacred text and their reading of it suffice to provide a sense of security and purpose, feelings of hope and solace, and reaffirmation in a God who personally cares for them.

Psychiatrists should assess patients' religious and spiritual involvement in terms of mental health and social benefits and must be alert to the misuse of religion; an example is the citation of sacred texts by some Christians, Jews, and Muslims to justify the humiliation and physical abuse of wives. By using passionately pious appeals, abusers may gain the support of their in-laws and local groups. Psychiatrists who treat the wives of such persons may be portrayed as evil doers who subvert the will of God, unless they endorse the status quo. However, if therapeutic efforts to ameliorate the abusive situation fail, then divorce must be considered, even though the patient may find herself estranged from her family, her congregation, and maybe even her religion.

It is improper for a psychiatrist to proselytize or to dispense specific spiritual advice or to pray with patients other than to remain respectfully silent if a patient does pray. It is proper to suggest to appropriate patients that participation in religious and spiritual activities may have some psychosocial benefits and to respect and to encourage those religious and spiritual beliefs and practices being used by patients to cope with their illness. However, it is important to know that religious organizations are not mental health providers, although the promotion of mental health may be provided through such activities as caring human contacts, forums for the open discussion of values and behaviors, and material help, prayers, and moral support in times of crisis. The ultimate purposes of religion are not mental health and euthymia but rather salvation and the quest for holiness. Psychiatrists should warn patients about membership in cultic groups and should refer patients to mental health chaplains when issues such as salvation and dogma arise. "Born-again" Christians usually seek out psychiatrists and therapists who belong to their congregation or who publicly identify themselves as Christians, may pray with their patients, may use biblical examples in treatment, may regard homosexuality as a sin, and may be loathe to consider divorce as an option. However, most Christian psychiatrists are aware of the tendency of some patients to disguise psychological problems by a religious presentation. In a study of Christian-oriented cognitive-behavior psychotherapy, religious and nonreligious therapists were equally effective.

CULTURE AND MENTAL ILLNESS

Mental illness is the result of a complicated chain of events that implicate flawed biological, psychological, social, and cultural processes. Sometimes, the proximal causes of psychopathology are clear cut; examples include thyroid storm, drug intoxication, and the experience of a traumatic event. However, in most cases, psychopathology emerges slowly in ways not fully understood over the course of a lifetime. Scientific explanations of psychopathology are based on naturalistic, material findings, although the observation, determination, and interpretation of these findings may be incorrect and based on cultural biases; at various times, psychiatrists have believed that female masturbation may result in mania and epilepsy, that faulty mothering may cause children to be schizophrenic, that homosexuality in itself is pathological, and that one or two exposures to heroin invariably result in addiction.

Culture influences mental illness in many ways. The content of people's delusions, auditory hallucinations, obsessional thoughts, and phobias often reflects what is significant in their culture; examples include the grandiose delusion of being Jesus, Mohammed, or Buddha; the delusion of being persecuted by terrorists, the Central Intelligence Agency (CIA), or space aliens; and phobias of contamination by germs, nuclear waste, and environmental toxins. Social phobia, as it is known in the West, may be shaped by Japanese culture into a condition known as *taijin-kyofu-shio*, an excessive concern about interpersonal relations, body odor, and eye contact, along with flushing. The Japanese psychiatrist, Shoma Morita, developed a special therapy rooted in Zen Buddhism for this condition in which patients undergo rest and isolation followed by participation in simple tasks, make entries in a diary for written comments by the therapist, learn to appreciate and to accept things as they are, and change their attitudes toward life.

Culture can elaborate normal behaviors, such as the startle reflex and sleep paralysis. In Malaysia and Indonesia, hyperstartling persons, called *latahs*, may be gleefully goaded by onlookers until they are so flustered that they utter obscene words, obey forceful commands, and imitate the onlookers' behaviors. In Newfoundland, Canada, the experience of sleep paralysis, which occurs when falling asleep or awakening and may be associated with hallucinations, has been elaborated into an "old hag" syndrome. Culture can facilitate the prevalence of disorders such as substance abuse and suicide, whose rates differ depending on social attitudes. The cultural acceptance of technological advances has contributed to global obesity; the replacement of bicycles by motorized vehicles and of shovels and saws by mechanized tools has resulted in sedentary lifestyles. In some areas of Africa, obesity has come to be valued as an indicator that a person is not infected with human immunodeficiency virus (HIV). Cultural mating patterns may influence the prevalence of psychopathological genes; intermarriage on the small island of Belau, Micronesia, has resulted in a high schizophrenia rate, whereas the effects of female infanticide in China, which has caused a surplus of 50 million single men and the rise of cousin-marriages in "incest villages," remain to be seen. Cultural attitudes resulting in stigmatization affect the prognosis of mental disorders; a positive effect of the current, albeit oversimplified, notion that major mental illness is the result of a "chemical imbalance" has led to greater acceptance of the mentally ill by family, friends, and society and greater access to treatment resources.

Culture-Related Syndromes There is extreme diversity among the peoples of the world concerning the recognition, classification, and understanding of mental behavior symptoms. Western psychiatrists classify mental diseases according to the DSM-IV-TR and the International Classification of Diseases (ICD), which are thought to reflect scientific categories. People living in Western countries, in part because of economic might and military prowess, have assumed that their world view is basic and true, whereas the world views of others are variations on what is natural. However, the lack of biological markers and the differing interpretations of behavior contribute to the ethnocentricity of these classifications. The DSM-IV-TR and ICD are not universally applicable; psychopathological syndromes exist, especially in non-Western cultures that do not fit the scientific nomenclature unless they are placed into the "atypical" category. These syndromes are perceived to be more influenced by culture than are most Western syndromes and, therefore, have been labeled *culture-bound*, although *culture-related* is a better term. Some syndromes are found in distinct cultural groups, whereas others are found in large cultural regions. *Malgri*, or intruder sickness, is a syndrome of some Australian aborigines in which an offended spirit attacks persons who enter the sea or a foreign territory without performing a proper ceremony and causes fatigue, headaches, and painful distended abdomens. *Family suicide* is a Japanese behavior pattern in which disgraced parents kill themselves rather than live with shame; they also may kill their children for fear that their orphans would be social outcasts. *Koro* in Malaysia and *suoyang* in China are disorders in which men become panicked and fearful of death, because they believe that their penis is shrinking into their abdomen. Western patients with *koro*-like symptoms tend to be schizophrenic, brain damaged, or intoxicated with alcohol or drugs, such as amphetamines. *Amok* runners are Malaysian men who, after a period of brooding, erupt into a state of frenzied violence and indiscriminate homicidal attacks that end with exhaustion and amnesia. Often amok runners are killed by the police, although attempts are made to subdue them. Most surviving amok runners have been diagnosed as schizophrenic. Indiscriminate mass homicidal behaviors have been increasing in Western cultures, especially in the United States, in schools and workplaces, such as factories and post offices. These behaviors differ from terrorist attacks in that they are less driven by political and religious motivations. Psychiatric diagnoses have rarely been made in Western cases, although, on autopsy, a small pineal tumor was found in a man who climbed a tower at the University of Texas and shot at a passersby. Fear-of-becoming-fat anorexia nervosa appears to be a culture-related syndrome in Western countries, as is dissociative identity disorder, which seems to derive from a lingering notion of demon possession; a well-publicized case in France in 1611 involved a girl, who, after being seduced by a priest, was sent to convent at which she and a young nun were found to be possessed by more than 6,000 demons after developing convulsions, visions of demons, and lewd behaviors with a crucifix.

FOLK BELIEFS ABOUT MENTAL ILLNESS

The distinction between cultural explanations of symptoms and true syndromes is often problematic. Folk beliefs about mental illness are rarely found in written form, fall outside of the scientific tradition, and are often magical, integrative, and definitive. Although scientifically irrational, they offer explanations for life's vagaries and make the seeming capriciousness of pathology more acceptable. Scientific and folk beliefs are ritualistic and, in regard to mental illness, have successes and failures. Both systems may function simultaneously within a culture and within a person. A mentally disturbed person may seek psychiatric help and, at the same time, indulge in folk therapies.

Folk beliefs about the causation of mental illness may refer to naturalistic and supernatural forces. Examples of natural causation include heart distress in Iran and renal deficiency and nervous system exhaustion (neurasthenia) in China. Mystical theories include fate, astronomical influences, predestination, bad luck, ominous sensations, nightmares, contact with menstrual blood or a corpse, violation of taboos, speaking forbidden words, trespassing, and improper conduct toward kinsmen, strangers, social superiors, or spirits. Animistic theories include soul loss and aggressive acts by spirits. Magical theories ascribe illness to the use of sorcery or witchcraft; sorcerers acquire their power by such means as apprenticeship, purchase, or theft, whereas witches possess inherent powers. Magical techniques include spells; hexes; prayers; curses; the supposed intrusion of objects into a person's body; rites performed over portions of a person's body (e.g., nail clippings and hair), excreta, or possessions; administration of poisons that are usually inert pharmacologically; theft or capture of a victim's soul; sending alien spirits to posses a victim; and rites performed over pictures and dolls thought to resemble the victim.

Scientific beliefs hold that disharmonies in the environment and in society may be linked with mental and physical disorders in individuals, whereas folk beliefs often include spiritual and supernatural disharmonies. In traditional Chinese medicine, pathology of the human body and of emotional expression reflects imbalances of cosmic forces; epilepsy and *koro* result from excessive *yin*, a female negative force, whereas mania results from excess *yang*, a masculine, positive force. In this system, specific emotions are linked to five visceral organs that are linked to five elements and that are affected by humidity, wind, heat, dryness, and cold. Vitality and health in this system also depend on *jing* (vital energy) and *qi* (vital air). Western psychological concepts have little place in Chinese medicine in which the focus is on a holistic balance of internal and external forces and on the prescription of herbal remedies, medications, diet, and acupuncture. Traditional Indian medicine, Ayurveda, has some similarities with Chinese medicine, although it pays more attention to mental disorders, is somewhat more psychologically minded, allows for sorcery, and has a broader pharmacopeia. Western alternative medicine practitioners, especially those who practice in luxurious health-spa settings, often claim to use traditional Chinese and Indian practices; patients are usually told to stop smoking, to eat a nutritious diet, to drink green tea, to relax, to meditate, to get massages, to practice yoga, and to take some herbal "medications" (one well-known physician has sold an expensive herbal mix that he described as "pure knowledge compressed into herbal form").

Folk beliefs about mental illness are too numerous to report; however, three examples—nerves, hexing, and spirit possession—are presented.

Nerves The English-language terms *nervous*, *a case of the nerves*, and *nervous breakdown* are used commonly to express mental disturbances ranging from mild anxiety to a psychotic episode. Among Latinos, the word *nervios* has similar general meaning but is more frequently used and has been elevated by cultural psychiatrists to an idiom of distress. It is usually associated with feeling frustrated in a stressful situation. *Ataque de nervios* (nervous attack), prevalent among Puerto Ricans, is characterized by sudden, dramatic, loss-of-control, anger-discharging behaviors, such as falling on the floor, flailing limbs, grinding teeth, and clinching fists. It may involve aggression toward others, in which case, it often is associated with amnesia. Attacks have been likened to adult temper tantrums and epileptic seizures. Some persons may appear to be in a dissociative state during the attack but are not unconscious. Attacks always occur when in the presence of observers, and, unlike true seizures, there is no incontinence or tongue biting. They are attention getting and may be used for secondary gain, such as family control; persons may instill fear and guilt in family members by threatening to have an attack if they are angered.

Hexing: The Evil Eye More than one-third of world cultures hold a belief in the evil eye hex. It is widespread throughout Europe, the Near East, Hispanic America, the Indian subcontinent, and Africa. It is called *mal occhio* (Italian) and *mal de ojo* (Spanish).

The evil eye is generally considered to be a sudden, destructive power—sometimes unknown even to the persons who possess it—from the eye of a human being or an animal. The victim who is hexed may develop headaches, sleepiness or fitful sleep, exhaustion, depression, hypochondriasis, spirit possession, impotence, failure to thrive, anorexia, listlessness, diarrhea, vomiting, disrupted social relationships, and sudden death. The hex supposedly can cause the death of animals, the spoilage of food, and the wilting of crops; in centuries past, Jews in Germany were forbidden to look at crops for fear that their glance (*Judenblick*) would be damaging. Persons who are thought most likely to possess the evil eye are those with a physical deformity (especially a hunchback), strangers, jealous kin or neighbors, marginal members of society, barren women, the poor and hungry, persons dissatisfied with their lot in life, children who return to their mother's breast after weaning (seen among Slovak-Americans), and, most importantly, anyone who utters a word of praise or compliment. The evil eye can strike anyone, but most susceptible are wealthy, handsome, and weak persons; children; and women, especially when pregnant. A case has been reported of a 27-year-old Italian-American male, living in Philadelphia, who thought himself hexed (others in his community agreed with him) and subsequently murdered six people whom he believed were sorcerers responsible for striking him with the evil eye.

Diagnosis of the *mal occhio* in southern Italy reflects practices found in other cultures. A female specialist puts three drops of oil into a bowl of water, crosses herself, and recites ritual words, calling on God to remove the evil eye. If the oil and water mix, the patient's sickness is considered to be organic. Coagulation of the mixture is evidence of the evil eye. Symbolically, the water represents holiness, and the oil represents evil. The force of the Holy Trinity counterbalances the evil eye, thought, and desire. Many techniques are used to ward off evil eye attacks; examples include building high, solid fences or walls around one's home, avoiding the display of one's wealth, smudging the face of an infant with dirt to make it appear unattractive, invoking God's name immediately after one receives a compliment, and possessing amulets in the shape of chili horn or of a hunchback holding a horseshoe.

Root Work Probably derived from hoodoo, root work is a hexing belief found among some African Americans, especially those with lower social class, rural, Southern backgrounds. The hex is administered by tampering with a victim's food or drink or by a touch or an evil glance. Other techniques include sprinkling sand, salt, or pepper on a victim's door step; burying a knife with its point towards a victim's house; and magically manipulating various items—household goods, blood, excreta, and hair—in conjunction with special times, such as sunrise or the dark of the moon, and special days, such as Fridays, and the 13th day of the month.

Persons who believe themselves to be hexed may come to emergency rooms with symptoms such as chest and abdominal pain, unresponsiveness, fainting spells, lip smacking, and epileptic seizures or pseudoseizures. Psychiatrists may encounter such patients because of severe anxiety, hallucinations, and persecutory or grandiose delusions. Because they think that psychiatrists might be ignorant about or disparaging of the notion of hexes, victims rarely report their belief that they have been hexed. It is important to ask specifically about the possibility of root work or hoodoo.

Spirit Possession Altered states of consciousness can be induced pharmacologically, psychologically, and physiologically and are experienced in many ways, such as sleep, concussion, a reaction to drugs, delirium, depersonalization and other dissociative states, and deep meditation. Depersonalization is a fairly common experience and becomes pathological only when associated with marked distress and impaired functioning. Some of the features seen in dissociative disorders, in general, and depersonalization, in particular, may be interpreted in various cultures as pathological (examples include the frenetic excitement and seizures known as *pibloktoq* among Arctic native peoples and some forms of *amok*), but they may also be regarded as purposeful and even desirable. Trance is the most common socially institutionalized altered state of consciousness, and spirit possession is the most common cultural explanation for trance. In some belief systems, spirits are thought to reside permanently within a person and may even serve as an explanation for a variety of scientifically defined disorders, such as epileptic seizures, schizophrenia, and slow-growing viral encephalopathy. It is more usual for spirits to stay within a person for brief periods of time. Western expressions such as "What got into you?" and "What possessed you to do that?" reflect this old belief. In fact, the spirit possession belief probably is the most ancient prototype of many medical disorders, such as an axis I psychiatric disorder, in which people theoretically can be dispossessed of a disease which comes on them. In some situations, possessed persons may be diagnosed as ill in their own culture, as is the case in some culture-related syndromes.

A world view that allows for spirit possession can be understood fully only on its own terms and not scientifically; within a given culture, spirit possession may be quite logical, and the pantheon of consensually validated spirits is unlike a projected paranoid pseudocommunity. Cultural settings conducive to the occurrence of spirit possession are those in which an oppressive social structure stifles personal protest and weakens trust in the efficacy of social institutions and in direct actions to resolve social conflicts. Some healers make diagnoses and perform therapeutic acts while under the influence of spirits; examples include Christian televangelists who are "moved" by the Holy Spirit and male Sufis (Muslim), known in Morocco as the *Hamadsha*, who must tame the she-demon spirit of 'A'isha Qandisha. However, most possessed persons have a low social status and are female. By watching others, they typically learn how to react to the spirits within them; some spirits have a specific name and agenda, whereas others may be ambiguous in their character and demands.

Possessed persons become spirit carriers and are not personally responsible for what the spirits force them to do or say, although there always are some social constraints on their behaviors. Malevolent spirits may demean, chastise, and cause their carriers mental, bodily, and interpersonal harm. During positive experiences, carriers may improve their own social situation as well as make astute diagnoses and prescribe treatments for persons seeking help. The spirits are usually judgmental and can speak openly about social injustice, abusive relationships, and flawed family dynamics. They may call on onlookers to esteem the carriers and to fulfill the carrier's desires for certain possessions and for improved relationships. When men possessed by female spirits act like women, and when women possessed by male spirits act like men, the construct of sexual identity is publicly examined. The intricate dynamics of spirit possession vary greatly among cultures, and attempts to reduce and to explain them fully by using Western psychiatric concepts are invariably unsuccessful. Although some spirit carriers may, indeed, be paranoid, psychotic, or hysterical, the process is not pathological. Analogously, the psychiatric process would not be invalidated just because some psychiatrists are mentally ill.

FOLK HEALING

The number of persons who, to some extent, fall into the category of folk healer is large, and they range from the ludicrous to the sublime; examples include palm and Tarot card readers, astrologers, channelers, herbalists, New Age counselors, psychic surgeons, and shamans. Shamans are persons who follow a diverse call to healing and who receive and communicate instructions from spirits. Different types of shamans exist in almost all cultural groups, such as Haitian hungans, West Indian Obeah men, Puerto Rican spiritists, and Christian faith healers. Psychosocial profiles of shamans show that some are impostors, some are mentally ill, and some are mentally healthy, mature individuals. True shamans have an unusual ability to recognize and to organize unconscious needs and concerns, in themselves and in their cultural group. Those aspiring to be shamans typically undergo an initiation that includes formal didactic training and recovery from a frightening, culturally-formulated, illness-like experience. Some Western observers have mistakenly regarded this experience as evidence of psychopathology—"the crazy witch-doctor."

Shamanic therapy usually takes place in a group context. It is a public drama in which the patient and the shaman are given strong support by the group. Shamans often present themselves as extraordinary persons, because entering the supernatural world and negotiating with spirits is harrowing, even dangerous, work. Hallucinogens may be taken to facilitate contact with spirits; an almost instantaneous contact may be achieved when hallucinogenic snuff is blasted up the shaman's nose through a blowpipe, a practice of the Yamomomo Indians in South America. The shaman's tasks include the retrieval of lost souls, the pacification and exorcism of demons, and the provision of counter-magic, often by supposedly sucking out harmful stones and animal parts from a person's body. By demonstrating objectively that disease has been dispelled, the shaman may effect cures through suggestion. Other shamanic treatments that may be therapeutic include herbal and other medications, minor surgery, bandaging, and chiropractics. Finally, shamans prescribe steps through which patients can stabilize their cure and demonstrate their healthy state. Patients may be told to perform acts of atonement and to adopt a new name or a new manner of dress.

The varieties and contexts of folk healing rituals are so vast that it is impossible to generalize about them all, but shared commonalities can be delineated:

- Folk healing often is a group phenomenon, even when a single person is identified as sick; healer–patient relationships are not emphasized.
- Healing groups are often ongoing rather than time limited. They occur with some regularity, and persons may drop in or drop out of the groups whenever they desire.
- Healing groups may be quite large, sometimes involving hundreds of persons, thus enhancing group support for participation, the magnificence of the ritual, and, through contagion, the manifestation of desired effects, such as trance states and abreaction.
- Healing rituals are public events. Attendees include not only identified patients or troubled persons, but also family, friends, community members, and cult devotees.
- Persons who are healed and prove to be adept at healing others may rise through the ranks to become assistant and then primary healers with a personal following.
- Alterations in consciousness are central to many healing experiences. When in a trance, healers or patients may express thoughts and emotions that otherwise might be repressed or suppressed. This expression may be therapeutic in itself, but it also often serves to call attention to interpersonal and social conflicts that are troubling the entire group. These conflicts have a better chance of resolution when they are brought out in the context of a controlled healing ritual, rather than in private confrontations. Also, because suggestibility increases during altered states of consciousness, patients may respond positively to the suggestion that their experience clearly indicates successful therapy.
- The concept of insight, as usually understood by psychiatrists, does not play a role in folk healing rituals.

Perhaps the most psychiatrically detailed study of a folk-healing ritual is that of the Pacific Northwest Coast Salish Guardian Spirit ceremonial described by Wolfgang Jilek in 1982. The ceremonial appears to be therapeutic for Salish society as a whole, as well as for depressed, alcoholic, and aggressive persons. Initiates are reduced to a state of infantile dependency during 10 days of seclusion in the quasi-uterine shelter of the dark longhouse. Personality depatterning and reorientation are accomplished through 4 days of alternating sensory overload and deprivation, which result in rapidly alternating states of consciousness; techniques include sleep deprivation, fasting to the point of dehydration and hypoglycemia, rhythmic drumming and chants, blindfolding, restricted mobility, forced runs in the woods, and sudden grabbing of initiates to stage a symbolic clubbing to death of their diseased, faulty selves. Initiates then go through a phase of physical training, such as swimming in ice-cold water and dancing to the point of exhaustion. This is accompanied by intense indoctrination and instruction in tribal lore. The mythic theme of the ceremonial is death and rebirth. Initiates are "reborn" when they fully accept the wisdom of their culture, when they see the Guardian Spirit in a dream or vision, and when they are given new clothes and a new identity. A large number of tribal group members participate in the ritual. Successful initiates who straighten out their lives may be invited to return as leaders in subsequent ceremonials.

A number of Native American tribes have institutionalized the ingestion of peyote and other consciousness-altering hallucinogens to achieve a religious and healing experience. However, the Navajo, perhaps the most therapeutically oriented of all cultures, focus instead on mind-numbing, ritual, group sings that may last as long as

1 week to treat illnesses. Patients first undergo self-purification by bathing, sweating, and emesis. The gods are invoked through specific songs and prayers, and their healing powers are channeled onto a symbolic design and then onto the patient, while tribal members work to reharmonize the patient's natural, supernatural, and human environments. Ancient, relevant myths are recalled, and the gods are compelled to help, provided that the ceremony is performed sincerely and accurately.

Analogous to the Christian belief in demons is the Muslim belief in *jnun* (masculine singular: *jinn*), whimsical but potentially malevolent spirits. When insulted or angered, they may possess a person and cause depression, chronic psychosis, sudden blindness, seizures, anorexia, or paralysis of the face and limbs. Treatment may dispossess the spirit, but sometimes, when the spirit resides permanently within a person, treatment is aimed at placating it by following its orders and by joining therapeutic cults. Similar spirits, as well as a healing ritual, are termed *zar* in northeast Africa and the Arabian peninsula. *Zar* illness often is diagnosed when usual herbal, medical, and magical treatments fail to cure a person. Victims, who are usually frustrated women, attend elaborate healing rituals with their families, friends, and *zar* cult devotees. When a spirit's special song is played, the entranced victim must dance and tell everyone what gifts and favors her spirit wants to be appeased with to stop the symptoms. This thinly veiled attempt to get attention and desirable things usually is effective, at least temporarily. Victims may attend fairly regular *zar* rituals not only for ongoing therapy, but also as a form of entertainment.

Clinical Psychiatric Practice

The history of modern American psychiatry reveals that various schools, each fairly certain, at the time, that they held the key to understanding and treating mental illness, have arisen, made contributions, and eventually have been found lacking. Thus, in one period, intrapsychic conflict and the need for accurate interpretations were paramount. This was followed by an emphasis on interpersonal relationships, replete with schizophrenogenic mothers, double binds, and catch 22s. Next came social approaches embodied by the community mental health movement. The current new school is biologically oriented and uses a guilt-relieving, politically savvy, and financially reimbursable brain disease metaphor for mental illness.

Opposite to reductionism is synthesis, the core of the cultural psychiatric approach. This approach demands consideration of all the biological, psychological, and social forces that impinge on mentally ill persons and their treatment. It broadens the biopsychosocial model by pointing out that culture overarches and provides meanings for biological, psychological, and social constructs, such as brain disease, insight, and trance. However, the use of this approach in everyday clinical practice is quite difficult; it is easier to go with the flow of one's culture, because it feels right and natural, and because there are incentives to do so.

The role of culture often becomes apparent only when psychiatrists assess and treat patients whose cultural backgrounds differ from theirs. The special problems that arise in such situations can be resolved only if psychiatrists are able to adapt their standard procedures. This need for adaptability in clinical practice may be regarded with skepticism by those psychiatrists who have embraced a certain theory or approach that they apply to all patients. However, from a cultural perspective, no one biological, psychological, or social approach can fulfill the needs of all patients. DSM-IV-TR provides an outline for a cultural formulation designed to assist in the systematic evolution and treatment of patients. The formulation calls for data on (1) the cultural identity of the patients, including ethnicity, involvement with original and host cultures, and language abilities; (2) the cultural explanations and idioms of distress used by patients and their community concerning their illness or situation; (3) the cultural factors impacting patients' social situations, including work, religion, and kin networks; (4) the cultural and social status differences between the patient and clinician that may affect assessment and treatment, including problems with communicating, negotiating a patient–clinician relationship, and distinguishing between normal and pathological behaviors; and (5) the formulation of an overall cultural assessment for diagnosis and care.

Assessment

Ethnic stereotyping is a problem not only for the clinician, but also for the patient and for society as a whole. This practice is insidiously fostered in scientific and popular articles, books, and polls that lump groups of people together in one category, such as African Americans, whites, or Catholics, and make generalizations. Clinicians need to know about the various ethnic identities of patients as well as their current importance. One cannot assume that all Hispanics are alike; Mexican-Americans and Puerto Rican Americans, for example, share as many cultural differences as they do commonalities. Social class is a major variable. This basic information may be required through direct questioning and by observation of the patient's language, dress, knowledge of social customs, and interpersonal style.

Clinicians should not jump to conclusions based on partial knowledge of a patient's culture. Having visited a patient's homeland or community, having read a book about it, or having a personal friend whose cultural heritage is similar to that of the patient does not make one an expert, although it may help clinicians to ask appropriate questions and alert them to possibilities, for example, that a Puerto Rican may engage in spiritism or that a Greek immigrant may believe in the evil eye hex. It is better to approach ethnic patients without preconceived notions in even the most basic areas; in some cultures, for example, a sibling may include a person other than those regarded as brothers or sisters in the West. Attitudes and relationships with authority figures should be determined. An upper-class Anglo patient is apt to react negatively to an authoritarian stance by a psychiatrist, but a patient from another culture may regard such a stance as appropriate and helpful. Similar attention should be given to attitudes toward sex-related roles; male patients from a culture that emphasizes machismo may have difficulty in working with a female clinician and so may distort their complaints and history.

Clinicians must determine whether patients' reluctance to discuss certain topics is the result of personal shyness, psychopathology, or adherence to their social group's customs and etiquette. Frank and detailed questions about sexuality, especially in the initial evaluation, may be perceived as inappropriate and even offensive by persons from cultures in which sexuality is considered a private matter. Ethnic patients may be touchy about many topics, such as immigration status, family relationships, and finances.

An Algerian man with a long history of panic disorder was evaluated in an American clinic with a chief complaint of, "I need medicine." He told the psychiatrist that he had been unable to find a job in 6 months and that he depended on the charity of several people at the local mosque at which he was allowed to sleep. He planned to return home for a week, to get married, and to return to his current situation. When asked how he planned to support himself and a wife, he became angry and said, "that is none of your business." He refused any more conversation and demanded medication. The psychiatrist explained that the question he had asked was routine and that he was concerned about the patient's welfare. The patient was given a 1-month supply of medication but did not keep his return appointment. The case also typifies many Muslim patients who expect only medications from psychiatrists; in Pakistan, psychiatric patients usually refuse therapy but rather demand intravenous (IV) fluids, in part to demonstrate to family and friends that their illness is medical. In contrast, some Hindu patients may regard the psychiatrist as a type of guru and accept advice and guidance, especially if family members can be drawn into the process.

Mainstream Americans may talk about depression, anxiety, hallucinations, and conflicts, but persons from other cultures may talk about somatic pains, liver problems, heavenly or satanic visions, brain ache, and shadowy figures. The use of psychological terms and constructs to express distress is a relatively recent phenomenon in the course of human history; it is neither superior nor inferior to somatic presentations. However, psychiatrists may be befuddled by patients reared in cultures in which Western psychologizing seems to be an odd way of self-expression. In fact, somatic presentations may be advantageous in that they avoid the stigma of mental illness. Also, they may serve to elicit help and social support without directly confronting persons or institutions who might retaliate against the patient. It is true that administration of medications labeled as antidepressants is often useful in treating patients with somatic presentations, but the complex possibilities associated with somatization may be completely missed if they are regarded *merely* as depressive equivalents.

Verbal and nonverbal communication patterns vary greatly among cultural groups. Tseng and John F. McDermott provide the following examples:

> The Japanese patient nods his head and keeps saying *hai* (yes).... The *hai* and the nod probably show only polite participation in the conversation. The Hawaiian may avoid your eyes because he was brought up by a grandmother who taught that eye contact is rude and has an aggressive meaning.... The Samoan's missed appointment may mean no more than a cultural-social casualness toward fixed dates and arrangements.... The Chinese client who says, "My mother is always kind," when the mother has been dead for some time is not necessarily suffering from unrealized, incomplete grief. The Chinese language has no past tense verb forms.... People of Oriental background tend to smile and laugh when they are embarrassed, anxious, or sad.

Assessment of emotionality and motor behavior is influenced by the cultural norms of the psychiatrist and the patient. Reserved Anglo psychiatrists may interpret the flamboyant or seemingly oversincere behavior of some Mediterranean area and Middle Eastern patients as histrionic, whereas the patients may judge the psychiatrist to be uncaring. The diagnosis of hyperactivity in children often depends on the tolerance levels of family, teachers, and psychiatrists. A study involving psychiatrists from five Asian countries who were shown videotapes of active children demonstrated great national differences in thresholds for diagnosing hyperactivity.

Hallucinations may be a symptom of psychosis, but, among some Hispanic groups, they may be associated with milder psychopathology or may even be considered normal. A teenage girl who has visions of the Virgin Mary may simply be indicating her own purity. When stressed, persons may experience positive hallucinations in which they receive advice and support from a dead parent. The assessment of delusions can be tricky, because, by definition, a delusion is a belief considered false by most members of a society. The existence of the devil cannot be verified scientifically, yet so many people believe in the devil that such a belief cannot per se be considered delusional. Although there is no such entity as the Aryan race, belief in it among Germans in the Nazi era was so widespread that it could not be regarded as delusional. Various subcultural religious cults, political groups, and organizations, such as the white supremacist Aryan Brotherhood, may hold beliefs considered false by most persons in society at large, but they are probably not delusional in a traditional psychiatric sense; exceptions include odd beliefs that may result in suicide pacts or other truly harmful behaviors. Cases involving established religions, such as Jehovah's Witnesses and Christian Science, in which persons may refuse certain medical treatments when severe bodily harm and even death may ensue, are usually handled by the legal system; courts generally have upheld the rights of adults to withhold necessary medical treatment for themselves but not for minors under their control.

Behaviors that may appear psychotic may, in fact, be normal when understood in their cultural context; a traditional Chinese treatment for kidney deficiency disorder requires an adult to drink the first morning urine of a young boy. Conversely, some behaviors that may appear normal may be pathological. Among the Amish, for example, symptoms of mania may include racing one's horse and buggy, driving a car, using illegal drugs, flirting with a married person, excessively using a public telephone, and treating livestock too roughly. However, in recent years, the "English" (outside) world has intruded on Amish society, so that teenagers engaging in the previously listed behaviors may be acting out as opposed to manic. Psychiatrists must not only assess patients vis-à-vis their particular cultural groups but also must assess each patient's group vis-à-vis the mainstream culture of which the group is a part. When in doubt, the psychiatrist should ask members of the patient's social group if they consider the patient's beliefs and behaviors to be normal. This process also allows the psychiatrist to assess, even if superficially, the social group itself.

Patients experience and describe their illnesses, whereas psychiatrists diagnose and treat diseases. Each has his or her own way of comprehending the patient's condition. It is extremely important for the psychiatrist to elucidate the patient's explanatory model of the illness. What does the patient think caused the illness? How is the illness affecting the patient's mind and body? Through what mechanisms does the illness work? Does the illness have a name? What does the patient think will happen if the illness goes untreated? What treatment does the patient think may be effective? What treatments have already been tried? If the patient's explanatory model differs from that of the psychiatrist, then assessment and treatment become problematic.

Special problems arise when the psychiatrist and the patient do not speak the same language. There is a tendency to diagnose more psychopathology when bilingual patients are interviewed in English rather than their native tongue, for example, slow speech may suggest depression and grammatical errors, a thought disorder. Interpreters function best when they have some familiarity with and training in mental health. Westermeyer has described three models in which interpreters may serve: (1) as an assistant to the psychiatrist who conducts the interview, (2) as a partner to the psychiatrist in a triangular interaction with the patient, (3) as a primary interviewer in the presence of and under the direct supervision of the psychiatrist. Interpreters must be taught when to provide translations that are word-for-word summaries or elaborations of what the patient presents. It is helpful for the psychiatrist to inquire about the translator's feelings about and identification with the patient, the patient's cultural group, and social class or caste differences that might distort the accuracy of the translation. Similarly, patients should be asked about their level of comfort with and confidence in the translator. Family members acting as interpreters pose special problems in that they may skew their translations to achieve a specific goal, such as ensuring hospitalization or special treatment.

Finally, great caution should be used in interpreting the results of psychological tests and rating scales unless they have been validated for the cultural group under consideration. More and more, such tests and scales, suitable for use in specific groups, have become available. Clinicians should not attempt to use their own translations, because the results may be quite misleading. In a recent study of 1,005 adult, low-income, primary care patients in New York City, the typical profile of a person among the 20.9 percent of those who endorsed psychotic symptoms was a separate or divorced Hispanic who spoke Spanish as a primary language. Although the rating instruments were translated from English to Spanish and then back-translated to identify and to correct translational difficulties, they were not validated for the mainly immigrant Dominican and Puerto Rican groups under study. It is likely that many of the so-called psychotic symptoms were really misperceptions of stimuli associated with depression and anxiety, a well-known phenomenon in Caribbean cultures.

Therapy Psychiatrists are trained in what anthropologists call an *etic* approach in which scientific and presumably valid constructs apply to all patients, although there is a place for atypicality. The *emic* approach eschews preconceived constructs and, instead, attempts to discover patients' understandings of their illnesses as experienced within the context of their cultures. The culturally sensitive psychiatrist balances the etic and emic approaches and, in some cases, may attempt to "convert" patients to accept the psychiatric perspective of their condition. However, some patients' explanatory models for mental illness may be embedded within a cultural world view that is resistant to change by negotiation or education. In such cases, psychiatrists must be flexible in their therapeutic approach and must respect the patients' beliefs. If psychotic patients, for example, inflexibly attribute their symptoms to a root-work hex, psychiatrists may support family efforts to obtain folk antidotes or protective amulets and may also attribute specific antihex properties to the medicine that they prescribe. This is not trickery on the part of psychiatrists (patients will detect insincerity quickly) but an adaptation of scientific therapy to make it acceptable to patients. The better the psychiatrists' understanding of patients' explanatory models, the better they are able to develop an adaptive strategy. In some cultures, even the color of the medication may alter its effectiveness for the patient. Possible medication side effects, even relatively minor ones, must be explained in great detail, because some ethnic patients may become noncompliant at the first inkling of a side effect, although, out of respect or deference to the psychiatrist, they may state that they are still taking their medication. The field of ethnopsychopharmacology, pioneered by Ken-Ming Lin, is showing that genetic and dietary ethnic differences may alter responses to medication. Many Asian patients, for example, metabolize benzodiazepines slowly and respond to lower doses of lithium (Eskalith) and haloperidol (Haldol) than do Caucasians.

Mainstream psychotherapy often focuses on the achievement of independence as a result of working through conflicts. The goal and the process used to reach it may be inappropriate for patients from many cultural groups. Therapy with a Hindu in India, for example, may focus on restoration of the patient within a family and a social group that values dependence and the suppression of angry thoughts; therapy with a Hindu Indian immigrant to the United States, however, may have a different focus. Immigrant patients may be torn between maintaining the values of their homeland and adopting those of their new country. The process of acculturation may be painful, but therapeutic attempts to hasten the process may exacerbate the situation with resultant depression, anxiety, and even acute psychotic episodes. Immigrants often do best when they are able to retain some of their old values and behavior patterns and to participate in institutions and rituals that have been transplanted from their homeland. Immigrant children through their participation in schools tend to acculturate rapidly and to act as socialization agents for adult family members; however, the process may be a cause of intergenerational strife.

Psychotherapy with patients from different ethnic and social backgrounds may require much flexibility and awareness of stated and unstated issues that must be addressed. Trust is an issue in a white therapist–black patient relationship, whereas status contradiction is an issue when the situation is reversed, and identity is an issue when the patient and psychiatrist are black. Patients from groups who believe themselves to be victims of discrimination may be unwilling to engage in self-disclosure unless the psychiatrists answer questions about themselves. Some patients may present gifts or may bring their families to sessions. Psychiatrists must be able, in these instances, to distinguish between psychologically and culturally motivated disorders.

Sometimes, it is desirable to collaborate with folk healers. In 1978, the World Health Association and United Nations Children's Fund (UNICEF) issued a joint declaration on primary health care which called on clinicians to support folk healing practices that were proven or considered by the community to be helpful. Collaboration is feasible only when the psychiatrist and the folk healer are ethical practitioners who respect each other's skills and wisdom. A patient, for example, may accept medication and hospitalization from a psychiatrist and psychological and social help from a folk healer. It is not uncommon for a patient independently to seek help from psychiatrists and folk healers at the same time.

Recognition of the importance of culture in assessing and treating patients is evidenced by a 2002 report of the Group for the Advancement of Psychiatry. It provides up-to-date, helpful examples of cultural formulations and of culturally informed therapy on six patients: a middle aged, depressed, alcoholic, sexually troubled Irish American man whose symptoms subsided after he was reintroduced to spirituality through AA and who then entered a seminary to pursue a religious vocation; a middle aged, devout Muslim, Pakistani housewife with severe depression and acculturation and personality problems who believed she had been hexed and was helped during a 5-year course of individual and couples therapy; a Filipino-American medical student with social phobia and academic problems whose culturally mediated distorted thoughts were helped with cognitive-behavioral therapy; a 30-year-old black, Kenyan immigrant with major depression, alcohol and cocaine dependence, and religious and spiritual problems who was helped by an inpatient interdisciplinary team that he likened to a traditional, African, tribal "Council of Elders"; a 30-year-old, single, dysthymic "good Catholic girl" who resolved her oedipal and rage issues with psychodynamic psychotherapy; and a 56-year-old Ecuadorian, Baptist minister with many personality problems who finally trusted a Spanish-speaking therapist with whom he could discuss personal issues without fear of being criticized, denounced, or stigmatized.

Just as culture strives to organize a society into a logically integrated, functional, sense-making whole, so too does cultural psychiatry strive to make clinical psychiatry more logically integrated, functional, and sense making. Many insights from cultural psychiatry are applicable to the entire spectrum of psychiatric practice, from psychoanalysis to psychopharmacology.

SUGGESTED CROSS-REFERENCES

Section 4.2 covers sociology and psychiatry. An expanded review of socioeconomic aspects of health care is contained in Sections 51.5a and 52.2. Also relevant to sociocultural issues in psychiatry is the discussion of public psychiatry (in Section 52.1).

REFERENCES

Alarcon RD, Foulks EF, Vakkur M. *Personality Disorders and Culture.* New York: Wiley; 1998.

*Al-Issa I, ed. *Handbook of Culture and Mental Illness: An International Perspective.* Madison, CT: International Universities Press; 1995.

Berry JW, Poortinga YH, Pandey J, eds. *Handbook of Cross Cultural Psychology.* 2nd ed. Boston: Allyn and Bacon; 1996.

Bolhenlein JK, ed. *Psychiatry and Religion.* Washington, DC: American Psychiatric Press; 2000.

Boswell J. *Christianity, Social Tolerance, and Homosexuality.* Chicago: University of Chicago Press; 1980.

Brown LB. *The Psychology of Religious Beliefs.* London: Academic Press; 1987.

Comas-Diaz L, Griffith EEH. *Clinical Guidelines in Cross-Cultural Mental Health.* New York: Wiley; 1988.

Crapanzano V, Garrison V, eds. *Case Studies in Spirit Possession.* New York: Wiley Interscience; 1977.

Desjarlais R, Eisenberg L, Good B, Kleinman A. *World Mental Health: Problems in Low Income Countries.* New York: Oxford University Press; 1995.

*Favazza A. *Bodies Under Siege: Self-Mutilation and Body Modification in Culture and Psychiatry.* 2nd ed. Baltimore: Johns Hopkins University Press; 1996.

Favazza A. *PsychoBible: Behavior, Religion, and the Holy Book.* Charlottesville, VA: Pitchstone Publishing; 2004.

Fernando S. *Mental Health, Race, and Culture.* New York: St. Martin's Press; 1991.

*Galanter M. *Cults: Faith, Healing, and Coercion.* 2nd ed. New York: Oxford University Press; 1999.

*Group for the Advancement of Psychiatry. *Cultural Assessment in Clinical Psychiatry (Formulated by the Committee on Cultural Psychiatry, Report No. 145).* Washington, DC: American Psychiatric Publishing; 2002.

Hollifield M, Geppert C, Johnson Y, Fryer C: A Vietnamese man with selective mutism: The relevance of multiple interacting "cultures" in clinical psychiatry. *Transcult Psychiatry.* 2003;40:329.

Jelek WG. *Indian Healing: Shamanic Ceremonialism in the Pacific Northwest.* Surrey, Canada: Hancock House; 1982.

Jones JW. *Contemporary Psychoanalysis and Religion.* New Haven, CT: Yale University Press; 1991.

Kirmayer LJ: Asklepian dreams: The ethos of the wounded healer in the clinical encounter. *Transcult Psychiatry.* 2003;40:248–277.

Kleinman A. *Rethinking Psychiatry: From Cultural Category to Personal Experience.* New York: Free Press; 1988.

Koenig HC, ed. *Handbook of Religion and Mental Health.* San Diego: Academic Press; 1998.

Kurtz E. *Not God: A History of Alcoholics Anonymous.* Wayzeta, MN: Hazeldon Educational Services; 1979.

Littlewood R. *The Butterfly and the Serpent: Essays in Psychiatry, Race, and Religion.* London: Free Association Books; 2000.

Mezzich JE, Kleinman A, Fabrega H, Parron DL. *Culture and Psychiatric Diagnosis.* Washington, DC: American Psychiatric Press; 1996.

Parament KI. *The Psychology of Religion and Coping.* New York: Guilford Press; 1997.

Pedersen PB, Iraguns JG, Lonner WJ, Trimble JE, eds. *Counseling Across Cultures.* 4th ed. Thousand Oaks, CA: Sage; 1996.

Podvoll EM: Self-mutilation within a hospital setting. *Br J Med Psychol.* 1969;42:213–221.

Randi J. *The Faith Healers.* Buffalo, NY: Prometheus Books; 1989.

Rizzuto AM. *The Birth of the Living God.* Chicago: University of Chicago Press; 1979.

Satcher D. *Surgeon Generals' Report on Mental Health: Culture, Race, and Ethnicity.* Rockville, MD: U. S. Department of Health and Human Services; 2001.

Simons RC. *Boo! Culture, Experience, and the Startle Reflex.* New York: Oxford University Press; 1996.

*Tseng WS. *Handbook of Cultural Psychiatry.* San Diego: Academic Press; 2001.

Tseng WS, McDermott JF. *Culture, Mind and Therapy.* New York: Brunner, Mazel; 1981.

Ward D, ed. *Culture and Altered States of Consciousness.* Beverly Hills, CA: Sage; 1989.

Warner M. *Alone of All Her Sex: The Myth and Cult of the Virgin Mary.* New York: Landon House; 1976.

Westermeyer J. *Psychiatric Care of Migrants.* Washington, DC: American Psychiatric Press; 1989.

▲ 4.2 Sociology and Psychiatry

RONALD C. KESSLER, PH.D.

Sociology is the study of human groups and population based on analysis of patterns and structural determinants of social organization. Sociologists carry out their work based on the assumption that social life is governed by underlying principles that influence organizational and individual actions. The work of sociologists consists largely of attempting to uncover these principles by systematic observation and to trace out the effects of social structures on human behavior at the group and individual levels. Contemporary sociology has largely been concerned with three broadly defined aspects of mental illness: the social construction of definitions of mental illness, the structural determinants of mental illness, and the social consequences of and responses to mental illness. The last of these three has been the subject of particular interest, with separate areas of investigation concerned with social factors in help seeking, attitudes toward the mentally ill, and mental health service organization.

SOCIAL CONSTRUCTION OF DEFINITIONS OF MENTAL ILLNESS

Cultures provide organizing principles for their members that function to make sense of otherwise confusing experiences. Although the existence of abnormal cognitions, emotions, and behaviors is beyond question, the designation of these things as mental illness is a social construction. This construction is increasingly grounded in scientific evidence, but this is not the way in which ideas about mental illness first came into being or evolved over most of the time they have existed. Sociologists are interested in the social processes that shape the ways in which cultural conceptions of mental illness form and change over time and the ways in which they continue to influence decisions about the behaviors that are defined as mental illness and those that are not considered mental illness. The thresholds used to define cut-points to indicate the existence of mental illness on syndromes that are continuously distributed in a population are also the subjects of sociological interest.

There are many important examples of cases in which social factors have played a role in the definition of mental illness. A few examples include the rapid expansion of the diagnosis of attention-deficit/hyperactivity disorder (ADHD), the debate regarding whether homosexuality is a mental illness, and the continued failure of mental health professionals to consider anger and hostility as having less clinical significance than anxiety and depression. Sociologists use examples such as these as case studies of the ways in which social processes influence attributions of mental illness. Sociologists also use the knowledge gained in these investigations to pinpoint potential problems that occur inadvertently because of mismatches between social constructions of reality and genuine needs for treatment.

One example of the latter concerns the diagnosis of ADHD. The rapid spread of diagnosis and treatment of ADHD after the development of methylphenidate (Ritalin) came about, at least in part, because of a massive public relations campaign by the pharmaceutical industry aimed at teachers (e.g., heavy advertisements in educational journals and magazines). The diagnosis and treatment of a great many children in need of treatment make this a good thing. However, there is also evidence of overuse of the diagnosis, especially in inner-city schools in low-income neighborhoods and of use of the designation and treatment of children for ADHD as a social control strategy for the benefit of the teacher in an overcrowded classroom rather than as a treatment strategy for the benefit of the student.

This example shows that sociological investigations and critiques of social construction processes can be valuable in helping clinicians take a step back and recognize that treatment decisions are sometimes partly based on considerations that should not play a part in these processes. This is perhaps clearest in the observation that attributions of mental illness for a specific type of behavior vary considerably based on the setting and characteristics of the person under consideration. The same behaviors that might be considered eccentric, for example, in an artist would be considered signs of mental illness in a secretary. Symptoms that would be considered indicative of anxious agitation in a person from the same racial-ethnic background as the clinician might be misinterpreted as indicative of psychosis when expressed in the culturally equivalent way by a patient from a different racial-ethnic background. In some instances such as these, definitional distortions can work to the disadvantage of a person with a clinically significant disorder who is kept out of treatment because of social constructions that define their behaviors in ways that do not lead to an illness label. Religious or moral constructions, for example, can dramatically reduce the probability that a person in need of mental health treatment will receive that treatment. At other times, as illustrated previously with the ADHD example, social constructions can lead to inappropriate treatment, sometimes involving social control processes (e.g., involuntary sedation, incarceration, or hospitalization) of people who do not need treatment.

STRUCTURAL DETERMINANTS OF MENTAL ILLNESS

Sociological research on social and cultural determinants of psychopathology is varied. One line of research investigates the effects of stressful life experiences on the onset and course of psychiatric disorders. A related line of research studies the extent to which reactivity to environmental stress is mediated or modified by social and cultural forces. Both of these lines of research are investigated in this section of the chapter.

Stress and Mental Health: Effects of Life Events

Although the hypothesis that stress can cause mental disorder is an old one, definitively documenting causal effects of this sort in representative community surveys of people who have been exposed to varied stressors is difficult. Most such work focused on the putative effects of commonly occurring life events, such as job loss and divorce, or ongoing stressful situations, such as financial strain and marital difficulty. Although these studies have consistently documented significant associations between these stressful experiences and mental illness, the interpretation is ambiguous, because this association could reflect an influence of the illness on the stresses. No certain way exists of discounting this possibility in the nonexperimental studies that are the mainstays of stress research.

Nonetheless, the strength and consistency of the associations documented in this literature are striking. In addition, carefully matched studies that focus on a sample of people who all were exposed to a single event or who were spared exposure to this event for reasons independent of their background characteristics have provided important information about stress processes. For example, studies of job loss because of plant closings (i.e., excluding job loss due to firing because of individual job performance problems that might indicate preexisting psychopathology) have documented rates of clinically significant anxiety and depression among unemployed workers that are two to three times higher than those found among the stably employed who were fortunate enough to work in plants in the same geographic areas that did not close. Furthermore, in a few cases, these studies have collected preevent data that document associations between exposure to stress and the onset of psychiatric disorders, arguing against the possibility of the involvement of selection processes and in favor of the interpretation that stress is a cause of the ill health outcomes.

Elaboration of the stress–illness relationship in focused studies of exposure to specific stressful life events provides information that is consistent with a causal interpretation. This can be seen in studies that attempt to unpack the effects of life events into the dimensions that make them stressful. For example, job loss seems to promote anxiety and depression by increasing financial strain and heightening reactivity to unrelated stresses. As a result, the most serious psychiatric outcomes associated with job loss are found among people who lack financial reserves and who experience some other major crisis (for example, their child develops a life-threatening illness) during the period of unemployment. Widowhood, in comparison, seems to promote anxiety and depression among elderly women by increasing concerns about safety (living alone) and social interaction. As a result, the most serious psychiatric outcomes associated with widowhood in this population are found among physically and socially isolated women. Research by sociologists and others is ongoing to unpack stressful life events into component parts, to delineate contextual features that account for variation in effects, and to consider intervention opportunities that focus on stress components (such as social isolation) and stress modifiers.

A related line of research involves the determinants of posttraumatic stress disorder (PTSD) after such highly stressful events as rape or combat. Although a substantial proportion of people exposed to such events develop PTSD or some related anxiety or mood disorder, they typically represent only a minority of those exposed to the traumas. This is true even for extraordinary events, such as the September 11th terrorist attack on the World Trade Center in 2001, as documented by several community surveys carried out in the weeks and months after that event that showed PTSD to be a response of only a minority of people exposed to that traumatic event. Much higher proportions of people develop PTSD when exposed to chronic traumatic experiences, but, even here, the proportions that do not develop PTSD are nontrivial, even among people exposed to the most horrific traumas. This observation prompted an interest in the protective factors that allow some trauma victims to avoid mental disorders, an issue discussed later in this chapter.

Another related line of research examines the long-term effects of earlier life adversities in the context of a developmental perspective on psychopathology. Clinical studies clearly suggest that early adversities, such as parental death and family violence, have lifelong effects on mental health. However, a relatively new development is the systematic investigation of these effects in representative community samples of adults who are asked retrospectively about childhood experiences. Studies through the late 1980s largely focused on only one type of childhood adversity, such as death of a parent, childhood family violence, or early sexual abuse, and one clinical outcome (usually major depression). These studies consistently found significant effects of early adversities on adult disorders. Beginning in the 1990s, these studies began to be concerned with the long-term effects of multiple childhood adversities on a range of mental health outcomes. These studies showed that it is much more difficult than previously realized to pinpoint any one particular early adversity as a central risk factor for adult disorders. Instead, it appears that many early adversities cluster in the lives of particular youngsters and that these clusters, rather than the individual adversities that compose the clusters, are the most important determinants of psychopathology and that these clusters have nonspecific effects on a wide range of mental health outcomes. It is likely that future work in this area will examine more closely the differential effects of various isolated early adversities and commonly occurring adversity clusters. An important observation in the newest of these studies is that the long-term effects of childhood adversity are largely confined to child-adolescent onsets of mental disorders. There is little evidence that childhood adversities have effects on adult-onset mental disorders or on the course of mental disorders. This means that efforts to address the mental health effects of childhood adversity need to focus on primary prevention during the child and adolescent years.

The most recent development in this area of research is interdisciplinary collaborative investigation in which biological psychiatrists work with sociologists to embed neurological studies within large-scale community surveys of stress and mental disorder. This innovation is based on the results of recent laboratory studies that document distinctive patterns of neurological structure and function among adult patients who retrospectively reported exposure to extreme childhood adversity. The next logical question is whether similar patterns can be found in community surveys of adults. If so, community surveys of children could then replicate this result and could follow youngsters with these abnormalities plus controls into adulthood to investigate patterns and predictors of the onset recurrence of stress-related disorders (e.g., reactive depression and recurrence of PTSD associated with exposure to adult traumas) in adulthood. Both of these lines of interdisciplinary investigation—cross-sectional studies of adults and baseline investigations of children who will be followed into adulthood—are currently underway in a team that includes sociologists who are carrying out large community surveys and working with biological psychiatrists who are carrying out laboratory studies with targeted subsamples of respondents who report exposure to childhood traumas.

Despite incomplete knowledge of the processes that lead to their effects, there is considerable interest among sociologists and other behavioral scientists in the design of social policy interventions aimed at preventing mental disorders by reducing childhood adversity. The largest body of research along these lines focuses on the effects of the various state-level welfare reform programs established in the United States during the 1990s. A number of innovative experiments associated with these programs have shown that the provision of adult education, health insurance guarantees, residential relocation, and housing allowances to families making the transition from welfare to work have powerful effects in reducing childhood adversities and in reducing the prevalence of child mental disorders.

A related series of studies evaluates the effects of model foster care programs. The foster care system, originally established precisely to reduce exposure to the extreme forms of childhood adversity, has declined sharply in the United States since the expansion of the public welfare system in the 1960s. The reason for this is that the financial guarantees provided by the public welfare system made it possible for the vast majority of low-income families to maintain their children at home as well as to provide a financial incentive to do so. With the introduction of welfare reform, however, foster care has begun to increase as welfare mothers who do not make successful transitions from welfare to work start to lose their benefits and become unable to care for their children. This new expansion of foster care raises serious questions about the best ways to promote healthy development among children exposed to extreme adversities that include not only poverty, but also neglect and abuse. A lively debate is currently underway about the possibility that high-quality orphanages might promote better mental health outcomes among children exposed to extreme adversity than the currently fragmented and poorly controlled foster care system. Research by sociologists and other behavioral scientists is currently underway to evaluate existing foster care programs, including conventional programs and model programs, in an effort to shed some light on their relative effects on child development.

Research on Chronic Stress It is easier to study the effects of stressful life events than the effects of ongoing chronic stress situations owing to the facts that the time an event occurred can be dated and that before-after comparisons of mental disorder rates to sort out cause and effect can be made much more easily in the case of life events than in the case of chronic stresses. Research on the effects of life events is consequently much more developed than research on chronic stresses. This does not imply, however, that life events are more important than chronic stresses. Indeed, chronic stresses are often more predictive of mental disorders than stressor events in community surveys. Methodological research is consequently needed to expand the understanding of stress processes that involve chronic stresses.

The most advanced work on chronic stress is concerned with job stress. This is due to the greater ease of measurement of job stress than other types of chronic stress. This research shows that such indicators as time pressure, closeness of supervision, and job insecurity are all associated with depression, anxiety, and substance abuse. Based on these results, more focused studies of such high-risk occupations as assembly-line workers and air-traffic controllers have been undertaken. Those studies describe particular constellations of job conditions associated with emotional disability. For example, several large studies link the combination of high job demands (for example, a job in which workers must rush to meet important deadlines) with low decision latitude (for example, low control over the pace or organization of work) to emotional disability and cardiovascular disease. A number of corporations redesigned jobs to modify some of these health-damaging job conditions. Those efforts, motivated partly by a desire to increase worker productivity, provide an unparalleled opportunity to study the effects of chronic stress. Such experiments should yield important new knowledge about the determinants of chronic job stress and about effective strategies for changing work environments to reduce the most pernicious kinds of stress.

Parallel research on the effects of chronic marital difficulties, economic pressures, family burdens, and other commonly occurring chronic stresses is desperately needed. In some cases, as with marital difficulties, these studies need to focus on the determinants of initial exposure (e.g., the premarital predictors of getting into a violent marriage) and the determinants of continued exposure (e.g., the predictors of remaining in a violent marriage rather than separating), in addition to the effects of chronic stress exposure. The greatest opportunity for rapid expansion of knowledge in this area is to focus on chronic stresses in which exposure is largely random, and selection out of exposure after its occurrence is unlikely, such as the family burden of having a child with a seriously impairing chronic illness that occurred for reasons unrelated to the prior behaviors of the parents. Several such studies, focused on such things as childhood cancer, are currently under way.

Research on Vulnerability Factors As noted earlier in the chapter, only a minority of the people who are exposed to stress develop stress-related disorders. Much research on the determinants of this variation in stress reactivity exists, and a number of determinants have been identified. The focus has been on the ability of the putative vulnerability factors to exacerbate the impact of stress on health. These studies considered three broad classes of vulnerability factors—biological, intrapsychic, and environmental. Environmental vulnerability factors have most concerned sociologists, particularly potentially modifiable environmental vulnerability factors that intervention efforts could target, such as income maintenance, housing, access to neighborhood resources, and social supports.

Recent research on vulnerability factors emphasizes the fact that vulnerability is multidimensional and is nested within social structures that constrain coping options. Family, school, work, neighborhood, and community structures are all relevant in this regard. Vulnerabilities at one level can sometimes be neutralized by counteracting resources at the same level or a different level of social ecology. Simultaneous analysis of vulnerabilities at these different levels requires interdisciplinary collaboration. Because of the great complexity of this conceptual framework, sorting out potentially important causes and consequences is difficult. In the case of vulnerability factors associated with self-selected environments, furthermore, one cannot, in a naturalistic study, rule out the possibility that some predisposition to become mentally ill accounts for the presumed exacerbating effects of vulnerability factors. For example, individuals predisposed to becoming depressed under conditions of stress may also, for reasons related to this predisposition or its personality correlates, be less likely than others to form close, confiding personal relationships. As a result of this uncertainty, recent research on vulnerability factors has focused on experimental studies.

Experimental Interventions As researchers recognize the methodological shortcomings of naturalistic studies of vulnerability factors, experimental interventions become more popular. Most experimental interventions examine the effects of attempting to remove vulnerability factors on such outcomes as preoperative anxiety, recovery from surgery, and compliance with medical regimens. The institution of related interventions also facilitates coping with such life crises as widowhood, rape, and job loss. The vulnerability factors manipulated in these experiments have included various types of cognitions, coping strategies, and objective environmental coping resources. The evidence from these studies suggests that a number of vulnerability factors play an important part in protecting against the onset of health problems and serious illness progression and that sociocultural factors are critical determinants of many of these vulnerability factors. A clearer understanding of those influences requires research advances in conceptualization and measurement, as well as the development of more powerful interventions aimed at modifying vulnerability factors.

As noted previously, one coping resource of special interest to sociologists is *social support*. *Social support* is generally defined as access to networks of friends and relatives who are available to provide aid and comfort during times of crisis. A great many naturalistic studies document that access to social support is related to low rates of mental disorder and that the impact of life events in provoking anxiety and depression is substantially reduced among individuals who have an intimate, confiding relationship with a friend or relative. In one study, nearly 40 percent of the stressed women without a confidant became depressed compared to only 4 percent of those women with access to a confidant. Several community surveys and case-control studies replicated this result.

However, few experimental studies have attempted to manipulate access to social support to evaluate its effects on mental health. The most promising of these interventions are a series of experiments that randomly assigned a neighborhood volunteer to provide informational and emotional support to socially isolated inner-city women. An interesting variant was an intervention that created peer-to-peer telephone-based social support interventions for the homebound elderly. These experimental support interventions consistently document statistically significant reductions in depression.

A problem with these experimental social support interventions is that they are artificial and, as such, are unlikely to persist in the absence of expensive research recruitment and retention protocols that are not feasible for large-scale implementation. Recognition of this problem has led to a good deal of theorizing among sociologists about ways in which the widespread disseminations of health-promoting social support interventions might be carried out inexpensively by manipulating various aspects of naturally occurring neighborhood social structures. The next generation of social support interventions is likely to feature interventions of this type.

Another class of interventions that has been the subject of considerable recent sociological interest focuses on neighborhoods. As noted earlier in this chapter, childhood adversities are known to occur often in clusters, and intervention strategies are needed that deal with the clusters as wholes. Many of these clusters occur because of neighborhood factors related to concentrated economic disadvantage, violence, and instability. Single-component interventions (e.g., interventions that provide access to social support without addressing any of the many other vulnerabilities found among people with clusters of multiple adversity) have been shown not to be effective in such situations. As a result, interest now exists in multicomponent interventions aimed at creating healthy communities. These interventions require interdisciplinary collaborations of child psychiatrists with psychologists and social scientists who are sensitive to the requirements of conforming interventions to community contexts. Several successful interventions of this type have been conducted. Researchers continue to follow initial treatment cohorts as well as to provide treatment to new cohorts. Continued analysis of these interventions will inevitably lead to refinements and wider dissemination.

Group Differences in Mental Disorder A large part of sociological research on psychopathology traditionally showed concern with structural correlates of psychiatric illness, such as social class, gender, and age. As shown in Table 4.2–1, the associations between these variables and the prevalence of psychiatric disorders are substantial. The most obvious hypothesis to test in examining such associations is that differential exposure to stress explains group differences in mental illness. It is now clear that this hypothesis can be rejected. Although it is true that people in comparatively disadvantaged positions in society (for example, women, lower-class persons, and nonwhites) are exposed to more stress than their advantaged counterparts, differential exposure cannot totally explain their higher rates of anxiety, depression, and nonspecific distress in general population samples. As a result, vulnerability factors have taken center stage in research on group differences. That research shows consistently that there are group differences in vulnerability to stress and that this plays an important part in explaining group differences in rates of psychiatric disorder. Current research on group differences is centrally concerned with the processes that promote vulnerability to stress.

A good example of this new work can be seen in research on the relationship between social class and mental illness. This is one of the oldest and most firmly established associations in psychiatric epidemiology. People in socially disadvantaged positions have higher rates of psychiatric disorder than do their more advantaged counterparts, as measured by treatment statistics, nonspecific distress in community surveys, and clinically significant psychiatric disorders in epidemiological studies. Early work on social class and psychopathology documents that lower-class people have a significantly higher probability of hospitalization and remain hospitalized longer than their middle-class counterparts. Subsequent work shows that socioeconomic status is also related to psychopathology in community samples.

Until the early 1970s, the dominant line of thinking in the literature on class and mental illness was that lower-class people had

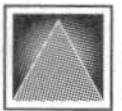

Table 4.2–1
Demographic Correlates of 12-Month DSM-III-R Psychiatric Disorders in a Nationally Representative U.S. Epidemiological Survey

	Any Mood Disorder		Any Anxiety Disorder		Any Substance Use Disorder		Any Disorder	
	OR	(95% CI)	OR	(95% CI)	OR	(95% CI)	OR	(95% CI)
Gender								
Male	1.0[a]	—	1.0	—	1.0	—	1.0	—
Female	1.8[b]	(1.4, 2.2)	2.2[b]	(1.9, 2.6)	0.4[b]	(0.3, 0.4)	1.2[b]	(1.1, 1.3)
Age (Yrs)								
15–24	1.7[b]	(1.1, 2.4)	1.4[b]	(1.1, 1.8)	3.6[b]	(2.3, 5.8)	2.1[b]	(1.7, 2.6)
25–34	1.3	(0.9, 2.0)	1.1	(0.8, 1.5)	2.6[b]	(1.7, 4.1)	1.5[b]	(1.2, 1.9)
35–44	1.4	(0.9, 2.0)	1.0	(0.8, 1.3)	2[b]	(1.3, 3.0)	1.2	(1.0, 1.6)
45–54	1.0	—	1.0	—	1.0	—	1.0	—
Education (Yrs)								
0–11	1.8[b]	(1.3, 2.4)	2.8[b]	(2.3, 3.5)	2.1[b]	(1.6, 2.8)	2.3[b]	(1.9, 2.8)
12	1.4[b]	(1.0, 1.9)	2.1[b]	(1.7, 2.7)	1.8[b]	(1.4, 2.3)	1.8[b]	(1.5, 2.2)
13–15	1.4[b]	(1.0, 1.8)	1.6[b]	(1.2, 2.2)	1.7[b]	(1.2, 2.4)	1.6[b]	(1.3, 2.0)
≥16	1.0	—	1.0	—	1.0	—	1.0	—

CI, confidence interval; OR, odds ratio.
[a]Categories with an OR of 1 and omitted 95 percent CI are the reference categories used to compute the ORs.
[b]Significant OR at the 0.05 level, two-tailed test.
From Kessler RC, McGonagle KA, Zhao S, Nelson CB, Hughes M, Eshleman S, Wittchen H-U, Kendler KS: Lifetime and 12-month prevalence of DSM-III-R psychiatric disorders in the United States: Results from the National Comorbidity Survey. *Arch Gen Psychiatry.* 1994;51:8, with permission.

greater exposure to more stressful life experiences than had those of more advantaged social status and that this differential exposure accounted for the negative relationship between class and mental illness. The Midtown Manhattan Study challenged this view for the first time and attempted to demonstrate empirically that greater exposure to stressful life experiences could account for the excess of lower-class mental health problems. Although this attempt failed, this study documented a more complex association: The capacity for stressful life experiences to provoke mental health problems is greater in the lower class than it is in the middle class.

Subsequent work shows that this class-linked vulnerability to stress accounts for the major part of the association between social class and depression and between social class and nonspecific distress. Differential vulnerability might arise in several ways. One of the most plausible ways is that some type of selection or "drift" of people with incompetent coping to the lower class might lead to the relationship between class and vulnerability. Another explanation is that one's experience as a member of a particular class leads to the development of individual differences in coping capacity, as well as to differences in access to interpersonal coping resources. The available evidence supports both hypotheses. Most of the evidence for the drift hypothesis comes from studies of major mental illnesses, primarily schizophrenia. Those studies show that the early onset of a disorder can reduce one's chances of socioeconomic achievement, a fact that seems true primarily for people who become ill before establishing a career. Recent longitudinal studies carried out by sociologists clearly show, however, that less severe disorders do not interfere with socioeconomic achievement, indirectly suggesting that the environmental resources associated with social class are the main determinants of differential vulnerability to stress based on social class.

Evidence of a linkage between environmental vulnerability factors and social class is widespread. Lower-class people are disadvantaged in their access to supportive social relationships. Evidence also indicates that personality characteristics associated with vulnerability to stress, such as low self-esteem, fatalism, and intellectual inflexibility, are more common among lower-class people. As of 2003, the major efforts in this area have been confined to the study of social support. The most influential work in this area has been that of the English sociologist George Brown. Brown documented that lower-class people have fewer confidants than those in the middle class and that this increases their vulnerability to undesirable life events. Several investigations replicate this finding, but more work needs to be done to assess in parallel fashion the importance of coping strategies and personality characteristics. Also, as most investigations of class and stress focus on life events, a more serious consideration of ongoing stressful situations may help develop a more complete understanding of the relationship between class and psychopathology.

A related series of studies have concerned gender differences in anxiety and mood disorders. Community surveys show that adult women are twice as likely as men to report extreme levels of psychiatric distress and mood disorders. Although other types of psychopathology are as common among men as among women and still others are more prevalent among men, most research emphasizes affective disorders and nonspecific distress in community samples. There are several lines of research to pursue on gender differences in nonspecific distress and affective disorders. The first is based on indirect assessments of role-related stress. The dominant perspective in sociology since the 1980s holds that women are disadvantaged relative to men, because their adult roles expose them to more chronic stress. Because of the difficulties in measuring chronic stress objectively, empirical analysis uses indirect assessments based on measures of objectively defined role characteristics or constellations of multiple roles to document the relation. More recent research, however, shows that this explanation is inadequate, owing to the fact that the gender differences in mental illness begin to appear in adolescence, well before the age when gender role differentiation occurs.

Another line of research on gender differences examines stressful events. Studies show that there is a significant interaction between gender and undesirable events in predicting depression and PTSD, with women appearing more vulnerable than men to the effects of a number of stressful events. There are several different hypotheses advanced to account for female vulnerability to stress, including the arguments that women are disadvantaged in access to social support, in the use of effective coping strategies, and in personality characteristics. An important piece of the puzzle is that, although aggregate analyses of live event inventories show that women are, on average, more vulnerable than men, this is not true for some events. Research on widows, for example, shows that women adjust to spousal death better than men. Women also adjust as well as or better than men to divorce. Furthermore, financial difficulties do not affect women as much as they do men.

A challenge for future research will be to reconcile the discrepancy between these studies of particular life events and aggregate life event surveys. The only such attempt to date, a metaanalysis of several large-scale community surveys that separately assessed the effects of different types of events, found no evidence that women are more distressed than men by such major life crises as job loss, divorce, or widowhood. Their greater vulnerability primarily concerned events that happen to people close to them—death of a loved one other than a spouse being the most commonly reported event in this regard. The greater impact of network events on women can be interpreted in several ways. One component of the difference is probably linked to the fact that women provide more support to others than men do, creating stresses and demands that can lead to psychological impairment. Another interpretation is that women might be more empathic than men or might extend their concern to a wider range of people. Those and other possibilities need to be investigated in the future, because the role played by network events appears to account for a substantial part of the overall gender-distress relation.

An exciting addition to the investigation of role stress and life event studies of gender difference recently occurred as part of the larger interest in prior history of disorder. Survey research on the different predictors of onset and recurrence of depression shows clearly that, although adult women are twice as likely as men to report a recent episode of depression, there is no significant gender difference in risk of recurrence. The fact that women are twice as likely as men to have a lifetime history of depression explains this seeming anomaly. Among men and women with such a history, there is no gender difference in recurrence risk. The observation means that an understanding of gender differences requires an understanding of the determinants of first onset. Analysis of gender-specific age of onset curves shows that the 2:1 female to male ratio of lifetime depression occurs by the mid 20s and that rates of first onset after that age are similar for men and women. This means that the focus of attention in studies of gender differences in depression needs to be redirected from the mid-life period, where most of the current research on gender roles is concerned, to the late adolescent and early adult periods.

Recent community epidemiological studies of adolescents attempted to expand the understanding of the emergence of gender differences in mental disorder during this period of the life cycle by including sex hormone assays. These studies consistently showed that sex hormones are associated with the rise of female depression in adolescence, a result interpreted as refuting the gender-role hypothesis. However, these studies are at fault for not controlling social factors that might interact with biological factors. A critical sociological study relevant to this issue is a classic study by Morris Rosenberg that showed that a gender difference in self-esteem favoring boys over girls emerges in 9th grade among adolescents who live in a community with a K–8 elementary school system but in the first year of junior high school in communities that have a junior high system. Rosenberg argued that this variation reflects the interaction between emerging biological differences and gender-specific role stresses that arise when adolescent girls first encounter older boys. New epidemiological research carried out by an interdisciplinary team of sociologists, psychologists, and child psychiatrists is currently underway to tease out the separate and joint effects of sex hormones and gender-specific role stresses on gender differences in the emergence of depression during adolescence.

SOCIAL CONSEQUENCES OF AND RESPONSES TO MENTAL ILLNESS

Sociologists have traditionally shown much more concern with the social determinants than the social consequences of ill health. However, interest in the consequences of psychiatric disorders increased in the 1990s in response to the changing position of mental health treatment in managed care. Specifically, managed care plans impose more severe restrictions on the treatment of psychiatric disorders than physical disorders and call for the use of evidence-based decision making in the allocation of funds for treatment. These demands make it important to investigate the adverse social consequences of psychiatric disorders as well as to determine whether treatment can ameliorate these consequences.

Part of this investigation uses the methods of social demography, a branch of sociology, to study the effects of early-onset psychiatric disorders on subsequent role transitions. This work shows that early-onset disorders are powerful predictors of a wide range of adverse social consequences: school failure, teen childbearing, early marriage, marital instability, job instability, and financial adversity. Importantly, these sociological studies show that history of mental illness is associated with high rates of marital distress, low rates of employment, and low earnings among the employed throughout life, even when the mental disorder has remitted. There is an interpretation of these enduring effects of mental disorders that attributes them to channeling effects of early-onset mental disorders on adverse life trajectories that take on a life of their own once they are set in place.

Recent community surveys also found active mental disorders to affect sickness absence and work performance in recent community surveys. As shown in Table 4.2–2, a recent national survey estimated three mental disorders—major depression, panic disorder, and generalized anxiety disorder—to be among the top ten most influential of all commonly occurring chronic conditions in causing sickness absence among working people in the United States. Importantly, major depression, as measured in the screening scale used in that survey, was also one of the most commonly occurring of the conditions included in that survey. This prevalence estimate is an overestimate of the true prevalence of major depression according to the revised fourth edition of the *Diagnostic and Statistical Manual of Mental Disorders* (DSM-IV-TR) criteria. However, it is nonetheless striking that this definition, which included respondents whom a rigorous clinical assessment would classify as having subthreshold depression, was associated with quite a high number of work-impairment days. This number of days would presumably be even higher if the analysis included only those respondents who met all criteria for major depression.

Importantly, community surveys such as this one also show that remitted mental disorders are not associated with work performance decrements, a result that is consistent with the possibility that successful treatment of workers with mental disorders leads to a recovery of impaired work performance. Such reversal effects of treatment, if they exist, could be of great interest to employers owing to the fact that the costs of workplace performance decrements are substantial. For example, a recent analysis of the economic burden

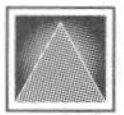

Table 4.2–2
Prevalences and 30-Day Work Impairments Associated with the Ten Most Impairing Common Chronic Health Problems in the U.S. Labor Force

	Conditions		Mean Impairment Days	
Types of Conditions	**Percent**	**(se)**	**Days**	**(se)**
Cancer	0.5	(0.2)	10.9	(3.2)
Heart disease	3.4	(0.4)	6.6	(1.2)
Ulcer	4.4	(0.5)	5.8	(1.0)
Generalized anxiety disorder	4.0	(0.4)	5.5	(0.9)
Panic	7.9	(0.6)	5.1	(0.6)
Major depression	16.5	(0.8)	4.3	(0.4)
Arthritis	12.6	(0.7)	4.0	(0.5)
High blood pressure	12.4	(0.7)	3.9	(0.5)
Diabetes	3.7	(0.4)	3.6	(0.8)
Autoimmune disease	4.3	(0.4)	3.2	(0.7)

se, standard error.
Adapted from Kessler RC, Greenberg PE, Mickelson KD, Meneades LM, Wang PS: The effects of chronic medical conditions on work loss and work cutback. *J Occup Environ Med.* 2001;43:220.

of depression, the mental disorder thought to be associated with the largest amount of sickness absence, estimated that this disorder causes an annual $17 billion in salary-equivalent work absenteeism in the United States.

Results such as these led social policy analysts and employee benefits managers to urge employers to reconceptualize treatment of the mental disorders of their workers as investment opportunities rather than as workplace costs. Several primary care depression treatment effectiveness trials included measures of work performance as secondary outcomes and showed consistently that treatment can reduce work impairment. Based on these results, a new workplace-based depression screening and treatment effectiveness trial is currently being carried out by an interdisciplinary team of sociologists and psychiatrists. The primary outcome in this new trial is the return on investment of screening, outreach, and treatment of depressed workers from the perspective of the employer.

Social Factors in Help Seeking

Needs assessment surveys show that only a minority of people with current mental disorders are in current professional treatment. Those surveys also document a number of consistent attitudinal, demographic, and system-dependent determinants of help seeking. The system-dependent determinants particularly interest sociologists. The strongest and most consistent of these is social class. A positive correlation between social class and help seeking for mental health problems persists in the United States, even though community mental health centers and other inexpensive treatment facilities have reduced the financial barriers to care. In the most recent surveys, education emerged as a stronger predictor of help seeking than income, which suggests that some cultural facilitating factors are more important than financial resources in accounting for the influence of social class.

Importantly, the social class gradient in help seeking varies cross-nationally. A comparison between the United States and Canada is especially instructive. This kind of comparison is possible because these two jurisdictions recently carried out parallel community surveys of help seeking for mental disorders. The results indicated that the overall rate of help seeking among people with mental disorders was higher in the United States than Ontario, but this was entirely due to the fact that middle-income people with not-seriously impairing mental disorders in the United States had a substantially higher rate of treatment than their counterparts in Ontario. People with seriously impairing mental disorders, in comparison, more often obtained treatment in Ontario than the United States, independent of socioeconomic status. These results suggest that the U.S. approach to rationing health care on the basis of ability to pay rather than need leads to comparative overuse of services by insured people with low need at the expense of uninsured people with higher need.

Help-seeking surveys show that the determinants of use of mental health services differ markedly from one community to another, a fact suggesting that local alternatives and barriers play a major part in determining who seeks treatment. Interestingly, most of the careful retrospective case studies that traced out pathways to mental health help seeking document that the critical point in the process is the decision that help is needed. The difficulty is that most people do not have any conception of when a personal problem is big enough to warrant professional care.

Differences in perceived need appear to play a critical role in the fact that women are much more likely than men with the same objective emotional problems to seek mental health care. Research shows that women are more likely to recognize their emotional problems than men and that this recognition is critical in the decision-making process that discriminates men and women. Once men or women recognize that they have a problem, they do not differ in their likelihood of obtaining professional help. The subject of why women are more likely to recognize their problems is currently under study.

The results of the recent comparative general population survey of the United States and Ontario mentioned previously document that perceived need explains a substantial part of the cross-national differences in seeking help for emotional problems. A higher level of perceived need for help in the United States than Ontario among the subsample of respondents with low need for services accounts for the significant between-country difference in the probability of obtaining treatment found in people with low objective, among whom more than twice as many sought help in the United States as sought help in Ontario. This difference was especially pronounced among middle-class people with insurance, raising the possibility that the demand-side controls used to limit access to mental health services in the United States are less effective in controlling unnecessary use of services than the supply-side controls used in Ontario. Clearly, this possibility needs more detailed investigation.

Another issue of considerable current interest in mental health services research is that persons with comorbid conditions are more likely than those with only a single disorder to seek professional help for psychiatric difficulties. This result is consistent with the more general finding that the likelihood of seeking help is positively related to severity. However, a complication here is that people with comorbid conditions often have alcohol or drug problems, or both, superimposed on mental disorders. The help-seeking patterns of these people often result in their treatment in substance use programs that often overlook and undertreat underlying mental disorders.

Recent commentators noted that intervention efforts aimed at attracting mentally ill people into treatment before they develop secondary disorders might conceivably address the problems associated with comorbid diagnoses. The thinking is that these early interventions might effectively prevent the onset of secondary comorbid conditions. The difficulty in implementing this approach is that the motivation to seek help often occurs only in the context of the severe role impairments associated with comorbid conditions. Devising strategies to attract patients into treatment at an earlier stage in their illness, before they develop secondary comorbid disorders, is a future challenge. Given recent evidence that the vast majority of adults with serious comorbid mental disorders had first onsets in childhood or adolescence, this interest in early intervention will likely grow in the future.

An obvious strategy in finding early-onset cases of mental illness is classroom screening of school-aged samples. Some schools have implemented screening efforts of this sort in conjunction with the establishment of school-based mental health clinics. However, these programs face formidable challenges involving funding, community resistance, and competing needs of school officials for student activities during the school day and for school classroom space after school hours. Evaluations of school-based screening, outreach, and treatment programs are few in number and focus largely on short-term effects. Sociological theorizing about the diffusion of innovations, as well as about community organization to embrace collaborative school-community innovations, could be of great value in tracking the dissemination of school-based early intervention programs and in facilitating this dissemination.

Another consistent finding in mental health needs assessment surveys is that a high proportion of patients drop out of treatment before they receive a therapeutic course of care. Analyses of self-reported reasons for drop out show that financial factors are not paramount. Indeed, the vast majority of people with health insurance who receive treatment for mental disorders end treatment well before they exceed the number of visits for which their insurance pays. The more commonly reported reasons include wanting to handle the problem oneself and not feeling that treatment helps.

In the same way that perceived need for treatment is now recognized to play a pivotal role in initial help seeking, other cognitions are now seen to be equally important in treatment drop out. Lay theories used by patients to make sense of their symptoms appear to be of special importance. These theories include lay accounts of the cause, course, symptoms, and prophylaxis for various illnesses. Research shows that a number of different lay theories of this sort exist and that characteristics of the theories held by a particular person provide important insights into help seeking and compliance habits. Interventions aimed at manipulating these lay theories are successful in improving compliance with treatment regimens for physical disorders. Patients with mental disorders need parallel efforts.

Social Factors Influencing Treatment Adequacy

Recent research shows that only a minority of people who seek treatment for commonly occurring mental disorders in the United States receive even minimally adequate treatment. This is illustrated in Table 4.2–3, which presents evidence from a recent national survey that judged that only approximately one-third of the people in treatment for major depression, generalized anxiety disorder, or panic disorder receive minimally adequate care. This is partly true, because, as shown in the table, many people receive treatment for mental health problems from self-help groups or from religious counselors and other human services professionals who are untrained in treating mental illness. It is also true, however, that people who seek mental health treatment from primary care physicians and even from mental health professionals do not always receive adequate treatment.

Adequacy of treatment is not randomly distributed. Low-income people, for example, are less likely to receive adequate treatment than middle-income people with the same disorders.

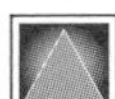

Table 4.2–3
Prevalences of 12-Month Treatment for DSM-III-R Major Depression, Generalized Anxiety Disorder, and Panic Disorder in the United States

	Major Depression (%)	Generalized Anxiety Disorder (%)	Panic Disorder (%)
Sectors of treatment			
Health care sector[a]	50.4	66.9	43.2
General medical sector	38.6	56.3	34.1
Nonpsychiatrist MHS[b] sector	20.7	30.5	17.3
Psychiatrist MHS[b] sector	16.3	21.1	12.2
Self-help sector	12.3	11.2	11.4
Human services sector	11.0	9.8	10.0
Overall treatment			
Any treatment	57.7	70.2	48.6
Guideline-concordant treatment[c]	16.9	24.6	16.0

MHS, mental health specialty.
[a]*Health care sector* is defined as the general medical, nonpsychiatrist MHS and psychiatrist sectors.
[b]*MHS sector* is defined as treatment by a psychiatrist or nonpsychiatrist mental health specialist.
[c]*Guideline-concordant treatment* is defined as receiving medication from a general medical doctor or psychiatrist plus greater than or equal to 4 visits to the same type of provider or receiving greater than or equal to 8 visits to a psychiatrist or mental health specialist in the absence of medication.
Adapted from Wang PS, Berglund PA, Kessler RC: Recent care of common mental disorders in the United States: Prevalence and conformance with evidence-based recommendations. *J Gen Intern Med.* 2000;15:288.

This is not true because low-income people are less likely to receive treatment, but because the treatment received by low-income people is less likely to be adequate than the treatment received by middle-income people. This lower treatment adequacy is due largely to the fact that low-income patients are more likely than middle-income patients to receive treatment in the human services or self-help sectors and, if treated in the medical sector, are more likely than middle-income patients to see a primary care doctor or non–Doctor of Medicine mental health professional than a psychiatrist. However, some evidence also suggests that low-income patients receive less adequate care than middle-income patients, even in the same treatment sector.

As sector of treatment plays such a large part in the probability of treatment adequacy, the selection of treatment sector is a topic of considerable research. A wide variety of personal and situational determinants of sector of treatment are documented. Differential availability and access are, of course, important situational determinants. These become increasingly complex due to the proliferation of alternative therapies (e.g., St. John's Wort), the growth of self-help groups, the creation of financial incentives for primary care doctors in some managed health care plans to treat people with common mental disorders rather than to refer them to specialists, and the recent rise of managed behavioral health care carve-outs.

As noted previously in the chapter, cultural conceptions aimed at making sense of emotional problems are also important determinants of help-seeking pathways. Sociologists who study determinants of help-seeking pathways actively investigate the joint effects of changes in availability and cultural conceptions on trends in help-seeking patterns.

Community Responses to the Mentally Ill

Attitudes Public opinion surveys since the 1950s have charted attitudes about the mentally ill. Dislike and fear of the mentally ill remain high in these surveys. Negative attitudes are particularly pronounced among the poorly educated and among elderly people. Men consistently report more negative attitudes toward the mentally ill than do women. The core concerns about mentally ill people revolve around their presumed unpredictability and dangerousness. These concerns have some basis in reality, as patients released from state psychiatric hospitals evidence comparatively high arrest rates. However, most crimes committed by released patients are property crimes that do not involve violence. Unfortunately, the mass media typically emphasize cases in which people with a history of emotional problems commit violent crimes, thus exacerbating the problem of public misperception.

Intensely negative attitudes about the mentally ill sometimes appear to be part of a larger cluster of beliefs, attitudes, and values characterized by an absence of sympathy for people who need help, a deep-seated distrust of people and institutions who are different, and a rigid outlook on what is right and wrong. Rational arguments to change their views cannot easily sway people with this orientation. Fortunately, however, most people have much less intense negative feelings about the mentally ill. There is good reason to believe that experience and increased knowledge of kinds of mental illness and treatment can modify these feelings. Visits to a psychotherapist, for example, appear much less stigmatized in public opinions than hospitalization for a mental illness. Private hospitalization seems less stigmatizing than public hospitalization. The perception that drug therapies are evidence of greater disorder than talk therapies provokes more fear and distrust of these patients. For a similar reason, treatment by a psychiatrist involves more negative attitudes than consultation with a psychologist, social worker, or member of the clergy.

Survey data suggest that contact with mentally ill people can influence attitudes of community members. In general, survey respondents who report knowing someone with a history of mental illness are less negative than people who report no personal contact. It is difficult, however, to sort out cause and effect here, because negative attitudes might relate to failure to report the mental illness of a close relative. In addition, family studies and studies of the reintegration of former patients into their old work roles show that contact with former coworkers and associates promotes positive attitudes about the mentally ill. Seeing a former patient perform adequately in a normal role is particularly important in this regard. Self-disclosure by the former patient about what having a mental illness and being hospitalized was like also helps promote normalization and acceptance by reducing the aura of mystery that otherwise surrounds the illness.

Much less is known about how to change negative attitudes about mental illness in general as opposed to attitudes about particular individuals known to have a history of mental illness, although that is the focus of much empirical research and theorizing by sociologists involved in this area of investigation. Studies of the mass media show that the stereotyped depictions of former patients that commonly appear on television and in movies reinforce negative public perceptions about the mentally ill. Whether sympathetic treatments of mentally ill people in the mass media might change these negative attitudes or whether informational campaigns making use of the mass media could increase public knowledge about mental illness is less understood.

This last issue attracts considerable interest because of the launch of several large mass media campaigns designed to increase public awareness, recognition, and treatment of mental illness. The National Institute of Mental Health developed one such campaign to increase knowledge about anxiety and depression and to encourage increased voluntary help seeking for these disorders. Unfortunately, this campaign did not include an evaluation, so the kinds of message strategies and information channels that led most effectively to attitude and behavior changes among persons with these disorders can only be inferred. Gauging from the experiences of health educators in conducting campaigns aimed at other public health problems, information of this sort is vitally important to successful campaign design and implementation.

A more recent related campaign instituted an annual national depression awareness day in which mass media around the country mobilized to encourage possibly depressed people to seek treatment. Local screening sites and a toll-free number facilitated screening and encouraged people who screen positive to seek treatment. Evaluations show that this growing campaign succeeded in bringing tens of thousands of people into treatment. Comparable programs were established to create annual national anxiety disorder, eating disorder, and substance abuse screening days. Refining the messages and referral strategies of these campaigns to increase their reach and effectiveness needs interdisciplinary research that takes into consideration the importance of social and personal barriers.

Community Reactions to Sheltered Care Homes

Negative attitudes about the mentally ill are important for a number of reasons, including the fact that they inhibit help seeking for personal problems and interfere with the recovery and reintegration of mentally ill people into normal social roles. Another way in which these negative attitudes interfere with the treatment of mentally ill people involves attempts to establish group homes for the mentally ill. Sociologists have done a great deal of research on collective action. Community opposition to group homes is one of the mobilization activities studied by those working in this tradition. This research shows clearly that middle-class neighborhoods are much more resistant to having group homes in their midst than are working-class neighborhoods. This greater resistance is traceable to effective mobilization efforts. In particular, efforts to meet and organize local opposition come off much more quickly in middle-class neighborhoods in which selection of a person or a committee to act on the neighborhood's behalf and multipronged political actions are more likely to occur.

Attitudes also play an important role in the success of group homes in fostering readjustment among deinstitutionalized patients. Ethnographic research shows clearly that patients are aware of the accepting or rejecting attitude climates in their neighborhoods and that this influences their social functioning. The ease with which the residents of these homes adjust to life in the community depends largely on community acceptance. The conflict that can attend the creation of the home does not make a good foundation on which to build such acceptance. In general, public opinion surveys show that contact with former patients who are strangers exacerbates whatever fears and uncertainties community residents already have, particularly in cases in which conflict previously arose about the establishment of the group home.

Most sociological studies of community opposition to group homes neglect these issues and generally concentrate on structural determinants of neighborhood mobilization and on strategies available to agencies for diffusing this opposition. Research is urgently needed on what happens after the home opens and the residents must live in the neighborhood. There is evidence that contact with a former mental patient known before hospitalization can foster positive attitude changes, especially when the former patient performs adequately in normal roles. One future challenge is the creation of structured situations that facilitate contact between residents of sheltered care homes and their neighbors in such a way that these kinds of positive attitude changes can occur.

ORGANIZATION OF MENTAL HEALTH SERVICES

Research on Interorganizational Coordination

Research on complex organizations is one of the liveliest areas in sociology today as a result of the enormous changes in the delivery and financing of health care services in the 1990s. Indeed, the mental health care delivery system is a favorite example used by social theorists to test new ideas about interorganizational linkage, because it provides unique opportunities to study a decentralized system consisting of many overlapping organizations with complex coordinating functions.

One focus of this research is the continuing diminution of state mental hospitals and the impact of this downsizing on general hospitals and community-based programs. Although there is a general perception that most of the reductions in state mental hospital systems throughout the country occurred in the 1950s and 1960s, as much as a 50 percent decrease in the number of inpatients occurred in many state mental health systems during the 1980s. The result is an increased burden on general hospitals and a *revolving-door policy* whereby patients receive treatment during periods of crisis and are largely ignored between admissions.

Case studies of community responses to these changes document enormous coordination problems and inconsistencies in organizational rationalities. Historical analyses show that these problems result from the accumulation over many years of decisions that lack any overall plan or purpose. The challenge for researchers is to synthesize these case studies to discover mechanisms that facilitate rationality in the relations among community organizations. Such work is currently the subject of intense interest among organizational sociologists.

A related series of studies attempts to trace the influence of state and national policy initiatives on community-based organizations and systems. Studies exist on how considerations concerning the future actions of state and national funding agencies affect strategic decision making in local organizations. The studies show that inability of state and national initiatives to develop community-based programs leads to local processes of adaptation that the policy makers who developed the programs did not intend. Current research is moving in the direction of comparative studies aimed at isolating characteristics of particular community systems that determine the directions of local responses.

There is also a great deal of interest in designing and evaluating organizational innovations that might improve the quality of care for the chronically mentally ill, particularly for that segment of patients unable to afford private care. Capitation programs, managed care programs, and programs that mainstream the mentally ill into existing health maintenance organizations (HMOs) created exclusively for persons with chronic mental illness are among the organizational innovations that are currently under discussion. Notions of treatment success must broaden for this population to include fundamental quality-of-life issues, such as adequacy of housing, nutrition, employment, social integration, and other issues of central concern to sociologists.

As noted earlier in the chapter, new models are evolving to integrate child and adolescent mental health clinics into schools. Interdisciplinary collaborations are also developing between social welfare and mental health professionals to provide mental health treatment in coordination with welfare reform. Collaborations between criminal justice and mental health workers are also expanding. Barriers to these different kinds of collaboration include competition for funds and inconsistent institutional demands. Organizational sociologists study all of these interorganizational relationships in the hope of pinpointing structural changes that can reduce barriers to collaboration.

An area of interorganizational coordination that is the subject of particularly intense debate involves coordinated versus integrated public treatment of patients with dual diagnoses of mental and substance use disorders. The treatment literature is quite clear in showing that patients with serious mental disorders and co-occurring substance use disorders receive much more successful and cost-effective care when provided with integrated treatment of both disorders by cross-trained professionals than with separate treatment of the two types of disorders by two separate treatment providers. This is true even with coordination of the separate treatments. However, legislatively mandated prohibitions on blending state block grant funds for mental disorders and substance use disorders make it extremely difficult to sustain integrated treatment programs. Substance abuse treatment professionals also actively fought against integrated treatment based on a concern that integration would substantially reduce the funds available for substance abuse treatment. The basis of this concern is the fact that block grants account for the majority of public substance abuse treatment funds in many states. New incentives to integrate services for patients with dual diagnoses are currently in development by the Substance Abuse and Mental Health Services Administration in an effort to resolve this controversy in a way that protects funds for substance treatment and increases access to integrated treatment.

Organizational Factors in Service Delivery

Another kind of organizational research extends the work on job stress by studying the influence of organizational structure on the health, well-being, and productivity of its members. Some of this work studies the structural components of mental health care organizations that affect staff satisfaction with their work. A few studies also examined the impact of organizational structure on patient outcomes. All of this work, as of 2003, is naturalistic rather than experimental and comparative rather than based on case studies of individual treatment settings.

Findings include the fact that staff satisfaction and productivity are positively associated with decision latitude. Patient functioning in long-term mental hospitals is also positively associated with the decision latitude of lower-level staff. Other correlates of good patient functioning include high staff job satisfaction and high staff participation in treatment decisions. Patient functioning in acute-care inpatient settings is positively associated with an active management style. Patient functioning in community-based shelter care homes is likely to be better when the homes are small, have flexible rules, and require patients to take some responsibility for the activities of daily living.

As these results suggest, there is, as yet, no overarching theoretical framework that integrates the specific findings into a coherent model of organizational influence on staff and patient functioning. Job redesign experiments in industrial settings will facilitate integrative work of this type. Similar experiments in treatment meetings are much less common, although innovative experiments are now underway to change the structures of community-based shelter care homes in an effort to reduce the problems of staff burnout and turnover. The success of organizational redesign efforts likely will determine whether similar experiments are carried out in a wider range of treatment settings.

Evaluation of Community Mental Health Services

The development and maintenance of an effective community-based system require a cyclical process of service planning, implementation, evaluation, and feedback. The first step in this process is usually a needs assessment that identifies patterns of unmet need for treatment in the community and establishes priorities for the creation of services to address these problems. Such an assessment is vitally important to organizational success by monitoring demand for services and pinpointing needs not recognized by community residents.

The most direct way to conduct such an assessment is by means of a large-scale community survey. However, such surveys are expensive, and most local service organizations are unable to afford them. There are a number of innovative approaches devised to obtain more indirect information about need at a lower cost. These techniques include systematic interviews with key informants, the establishment of citizen advisory councils, the use of national statistics on need profiles in conjunction with small-area social indicators on community demographics, and extrapolation from data on demand for services to estimates about need for services.

After the development of programs, research can also be important in evaluating effectiveness and targeting areas that need to be changed. Program effectiveness relies on at least two levels of research. The first focuses on success in attracting participants to the program; the second focuses on success in helping people with their problems. Behavioral scientists have been more active in the first research area than in the second area.

Research on success in attracting program participants emphasizes *acceptability*, *accessibility*, and *awareness*. *Acceptability* refers to how willing community residents are to use the new service. *Accessibility* involves how easy the program is to reach. Time, distance, transportation, and financial barriers are all important to consider here. *Awareness* relates to community knowledge that the service exists and that it is appropriate for particular needs. To develop programs that are sensitive to these issues requires an understanding of local culture. Sociological research using ethnographic research or other qualitative strategies can increase the sensitivity of program staff to local norms and customs.

Research that evaluates the effectiveness of programs is much less common for several reasons: the substantial costs of implementing a carefully controlled study of treatment effectiveness, the high level of methodological sophistication required to carry out such an investigation, and the potential threat to clinicians and program administrators of openly studying the therapeutic value of their services. Although sociologists and other behavioral scientists have the expertise to do such work, this remains an underdeveloped area of investigation.

Social Context of Professional Activity The medical profession is undergoing enormous changes, engendered by such things as diagnosis-related groups (DRGs) and other new payment arrangements, the shifting of care from inpatient to ambulatory settings, the diversification of the medical care industry, the increasingly overt competition among providers, the growing importance of third-party payers, the use of evidence-based guidelines to control quality of care in ways that many professionals see as constraining their autonomy, and the growth of demand management programs that empower patients to renegotiate doctor–patient relationships. Those changes are part of broader societal forces that include the aging of the population and cohort shifts that have led to massive expansion in the plant facilities of the medical care industry and a marked increase in the number of physicians in the marketplace.

Sociologists are keenly interested in the implications of these trends for the future of medicine. One perspective holds that physician domination of the health care system is so firmly established that it cannot be shaken by the changes in social context that are taking place. The legal subordination of nurses, pharmacists, and other medical care professionals to the physician is critical in this regard, as are the exclusive licensing powers granted to physicians as gatekeepers of the medical care system. An opposing view, however, is that the medical profession is in a period of declining power as a result of the resurgence of consumerism in medicine. The greater number of medical patients who experience chronic rather than acute conditions leads to the creation of interest groups. These groups consist of lay people who acquire considerable technical knowledge about their own afflictions and tend to challenge their providers. The technical diversification of medical procedures and the increasingly important contributions to health care by technician-specialists who are not physicians also play a part. With changes in the organization of professional care, new systems of ownership and management promote competition among physicians, which inevitably brings with it increased consumer control. Finally, the more dominant position of large insurers consolidates the bargaining position of consumers in a novel way. These views are particularly relevant to psychiatrists, because the existence of auxiliary mental health specialists, such as clinical psychologists and psychiatric social workers, has no counterpart among other medical specialties.

Another perspective on the changing nature of medical practice involves the proletarianization of medical work. More and more physicians work as salaried employees in large, bureaucratically managed organizations. As those organizations institute managerial styles orchestrated by the graduates of business schools rather than of medical schools, changes in procedures for professional control invariably will occur. Formal review procedures now apply to a wider range of professional behaviors. Within particular institutions, mechanisms are in development to monitor and to control the technical decisions of clinicians. All of these trends will result in increasing external control of the domain of professional practice.

The future shape of psychiatric practice is difficult to forecast in light of these many different forces. Sociologists who specialize in this area of research have conflicting notions, although they all share a concern that the likely changes may adversely affect the quality of care provided to patients with emotional problems. Carrying out programmatic sociological research that monitors these changes and provides clear evidence regarding the effects on quality of care is important. Despite disagreements about specifics of likely changes, it is agreed that primary care doctors rather than psychiatrists treat more and more patients with mental health problems. This shift coincides with a trend away from psychotherapy to pharmacotherapy as the dominant treatment for mental disorders. The development of psychopharmacological agents that are much easier to administer than earlier medications and the cost-cutting pressures imposed by managed care systems drive this trend. Another important trend is to deliver combined pharmacotherapy and psychotherapy more and more by a team made up of a primary care doctor and a nonpsychiatrist mental health professional than by a psychiatrist. All of these changes point to the likelihood that psychiatry will, in the future, become more similar to other medical specialties in focusing largely on complicated cases that primary care doctors cannot manage and in working closely in a consultative role with primary care doctors to provide expert advice regarding the management of more routine cases. The specific decision rules for sorting cases between general and specialty care, however, remain unclear, as does the quality of care that patients with mental disorders who are treated in the primary care system will receive.

SUGGESTED CROSS-REFERENCES

Other discussions of sociocultural influences on psychiatry may be found in Section 4.1 (anthropology and cultural psychiatry), Section

4.3 (sociobiology and psychiatry), and Section 4.4 (sociopolitical aspects of psychiatry). Social influences on the onset and course of mental disorders are discussed in Section 5.1 (epidemiology), as well as in the epidemiology sections dealing with schizophrenia (Sections 12.3 and 12.4), mood disorders (Section 13.2), anxiety disorders (Section 14.2), and geriatric psychiatry (Section 51.1b). Social influences on help seeking are discussed in Section 5.3 (mental health services research).

References

Aneshensel CS, Phelan JC, eds. *Handbook of the Sociology of Mental Health.* New York: Kluwer Academic Publishers; 1999.

Angermeyer MC, Matschinger H: Public beliefs about schizophrenia and depression: Similarities and differences. *Soc Psychiatry Psychiatr Epidemiol.* 2003;38:526.

Brown G, Harris T, eds. *Social Origins of Depression: A Study of Psychiatric Disorder in Women.* London: Tavistock Publications; 1978.

Cockerham WC. *Sociology of Mental Disorder.* Upper Saddle River, NJ: Prentice Hall; 1999.

Earls F: Community factors supporting child mental health. *Child Adolesc Psychiatr Clin North Am.* 2001;10:693.

*Earls F, Carlson M: The social ecology of child health and well-being. *Annu Rev Public Health.* 2001;22:143.

Eaton WW. *The Sociology of Mental Disorders.* Westport, CT: Praeger; 2001.

Eaton WW, Muntaner C, Bovasso G, Smith C: Socioeconomic status and depressive syndrome: The role of inter- and intra-generational mobility, government assistance, and work environment. *J Health Soc Behav.* 2001;42:277.

Gallagher BJ III. *The Sociology of Mental Illness.* Upper Saddle River, NJ: Prentice-Hall; 2002.

Harris T, Brown GW, Robinson R: Befriending as an intervention for chronic depression among women in an inner city. 1: Randomised controlled trial. *Br J Psychiatry.* 1999;174:219.

*Horwitz AV. *The Social Control of Mental Illness.* Clinton Corners, NY: Eliot Werner Publications; 2002.

Horwitz AV, Scheid TL, eds. *A Handbook for the Study of Mental Health: Social Contexts, Theories, and Systems.* New York: Cambridge University Press; 1999.

Kessler RC: The effects of stressful life events on depression. *Annu Rev Psychol.* 1997;48:191.

Kessler RC, Davis CG, Kendler KS: Childhood adversity and adult psychiatric disorder in the U.S. National Comorbidity Survey. *Psychol Med.* 1997;27:1101.

Kessler RC, Greenberg PE, Mickelson KD, Meneades LM, Wang PS: The effects of chronic medical conditions on work loss and work cutback. *J Occup Environ Med.* 2001;43:218.

Link BG, Phalen JC, Bresnahan M, Stueve A, Pescosolido BA: Public conceptions of mental illness: Labels, causes, dangerousness, and social distances. *Am J Public Health.* 1999;89:1328.

*Link BG, Struening EL, Neese-Todd S, Asmussen S, Phelan JC: Stigma as a barrier to recovery: The consequences of stigma for the self-esteem of people with mental illnesses. *Psychiatr Serv.* 2001;52:1621.

Lynch SM, George LK: Interlocking trajectories of loss-related events and depressive symptoms among elders. *J Gerontol B Psychol Sci Soc Sci.* 2002;57:S117.

Mechanic D. *Improving Inpatient Treatment in an Era of Managed Care: New Directions in Mental Health Services.* San Francisco: Jossey-Bass; 1997.

Mechanic D. Organization of care and quality of life of persons with serious and persistent mental illness. In: Katschnig H, Freeman H, Sartorius N, eds. *Quality of Life in Mental Disorders.* Chichester, England: John Wiley and Sons; 1997:305–317.

*Mechanic D: Removing barriers to care among persons with psychiatric symptoms. *Health Aff.* 2002;21:137.

Mojtabai R, Olfson M, Mechanic D: Perceived need and help-seeking in adults with mood, anxiety, or substance use disorders. *Arch Gen Psychiatry.* 2002;59:77.

Mulatu MS, Schooler C: Causal connections between SES and health: Reciprocal effects and mediating mechanisms. *J Health Soc Behav.* 2002;43:22.

Pescosolido BA, Monahan J, Link BG, Stueve A, Kikuzawa S: The public's perception of the competence, dangerousness, and need for legal coercion of persons with mental health problems. *Am J Public Health.* 1999;89:1339.

Pilgrim D, Rogers A. *A Sociology of Mental Health and Illness.* Philadelphia: Open University Press; 2002.

Rosenberg M. *Society and the Adolescent Self-image.* Princeton, NJ: Princeton University Press; 1965.

Rosenberg M, Simmons R. *Black and White Self-esteem: The Urban School Child. Rose Monograph Series.* American Sociological Association; 1971.

*Wang PS, Demler O, Kessler RC: The adequacy of treatment for serious mental illness in the United States. *Am J Public Health.* 2002;92:92.

Wang PS, Gilman SE, Guardino M, Christiana JM, Morselli PL, Mickelson K, Kessler RC: Initiation of and adherence to treatment for mental disorders: Examination of patient advocate group members in 11 countries. *Med Care.* 2000;38:926.

Wang PS, Simon G, Kessler RC: The economic burden of depression and the cost-effectiveness of treatment. *Int J Methods Psychiatr Res.* 2003;12:22.

Woodward CA, Abelson J, Tedford S, Hutchison B: What is important to continuity in home care? Perspectives of key stakeholders. *Soc Sci Med.* 2004;58:177.

▲ 4.3 Sociobiology

Judith Eve Lipton, M.D., and David P. Barash, Ph.D.

After four billion years, natural selection has created a creature that can look at itself, understand its origins, and even dare to tinker with the mechanics of evolution itself. That creature is *Homo sapiens*; the implications are staggering.

Given that evolution by natural selection has "created" human anatomy and physiology, it seems logical that evolution impacts human behavior as well. The search for genes for psychiatric disorders is moving rapidly, and no one doubts that evolution created the nerves, neurotransmitters, and receptors that comprise the central nervous system (CNS) of human beings. Yet for some, it is harder to accept that evolution has created natural human behavior—including instinctual drives, such as lust, parental love, and sexual jealousy—than it is to accept that evolution has created disease states. The goal of Darwinian psychiatry is to explore human nature and normal emotions as well as psychopathology within the context of evolutionary biology.

Charles Darwin's *The Origin of Species* appeared in 1859, and his work was well known to psychiatric theoreticians at the turn of the 20th century. Sigmund Freud especially admired Darwin and adopted some evolutionary language into psychoanalytical vernacular. However, any attempt to reconcile natural selection with human behavior would have been premature in 1900, given that the concept of evolution by natural selection had yet to be joined to Gregor Mendel's discovery of genes; thus, there was no known mechanism by which natural selection could occur. In addition, the very notion of biological continuity between *Homo sapiens* and other living creatures offended many people, based alternatively on theological considerations or the presumably unique power of human social and cultural traditions. Politicians misappropriated Darwin's description of "survival of the fittest" to justify everything from British imperialism to Nazi eugenics. No wonder evolutionary theory was ignored, criticized, and misunderstood by philosophers, psychologists, and social scientists of the later 20th century. Meanwhile, biologists increasingly embraced evolution by natural selection as the new general field theory of life.

By the early 20th century, the "modern synthesis" of Darwinism with Mendelian genetics had given rise to an explosion of interest in evolutionary biology. Classic comparative psychology with rats and pigeons in laboratory experiments yielded ethology, the study of animal behavior in natural environments. Yet, a significant gap remained between naturalistic observations of behavior and an understanding of the means by which such behavior evolved.

A second "synthesis"—sociobiology—was born in the late 1960s and early 1970s, uniting ethology, population biology, ecology, anthropology, game theory, and genetics. The word itself became controversial, however—largely because of its presumed political implications—such that some have taken to using phrases such as *evolutionary psychology* or *evolutionary biology* instead. There is, however, essentially no difference between these disciplines and approaches. To honor the early pioneers who braved vicious ideological criticism for merely suggesting that human behavior could have genetic underpinnings, this chapter uses "sociobiology" because it possesses the dual merits of priority and brevity.

Ironically, the derision that many sociobiologists endured was similar to that endured by Darwin, and for many of the same reasons.

Despite 150 years of scientific progress, the certainty of genes, and genetic homologies between *Homo sapiens* and other species, society was nonetheless shocked by the revelation that human beings and other animals evolved by natural selection without divine engineering. Due to persisting social trends, such as unyielding beliefs in special creation and postmodern concepts of contextual reality, psychiatry has yet to fully use the powerful concepts and techniques that sociobiologists take for granted. To the modern biologist, evolutionary theory is as solid as relativity is to the physicist. The power of natural selection is no more in doubt than the power of the covalent bond.

A third evolutionary synthesis is rapidly approaching: As the human genome is unraveled, the dichotomous "nature/nurture" controversy evaporates, and molecular biology joins sociobiology to extend knowledge of human behavior. It is now known that 60 percent to 80 percent of disease-causing genes in human beings have orthologs in the fruit fly genome; the vertebrate zebrafish seems to have a gene counterpart for almost *every* genetic disease in humans. The continuity of life is not in dispute. Human beings are neither the sole products of culture and experience, John Locke's *tabula rasa* on which experience writes, nor genetically determined robots forced by their deoxyribonucleic acid (DNA) into automatic behaviors and, thus, devoid of free will. Rather, René Descartes' famous maxim, "I think, therefore I am," becomes inverted: "I am, therefore I think (and feel)." Human beings are able to function mentally because their DNA interacts seamlessly with the cultural contingencies of everyday life.

Having breached the 21st century, the developing field of evolutionary psychiatry has abundant seeds and some healthy roots, but it has yet to fully flourish. A mature evolutionary perspective would help its practitioners to understand human nature—normalcy as well as pathology—and also to make sense of new developments in law, economics, politics, and even computer science. This chapter summarizes existing findings and theory and makes suggestions for future research.

BASICS AND DEFINITIONS

Many misunderstandings about sociobiology derive from its specialized jargon, which uses common phrases and words to mean precise mathematical constructs. The central theorem of sociobiology can be summarized as follows: Insofar as genetics influence behavior, individuals will behave so as to maximize their inclusive fitness. "Fitness" is a measure of success in projecting genes into the future. Thus, it refers to reproductive success, not physical robustness; individuals can be in excellent cardiovascular condition and still be evolutionarily unfit if they do not reproduce. In more recent usage, fitness is also seen as a measure of the reproductive success of genes such that individual organisms (including human beings) are merely the mechanism whereby genes replicate themselves. The central concept of sociobiology is deceptively simple and mathematical: Successful genes pass from generation to generation and increase in frequency, whereas less successful ones die out. Genes that increase the reproductive success of their bodies (via their impact on structure, physiology, behavior, and so forth) prosper at the expense of alternative alleles.

A useful tool in sociobiological analysis has been the recognition that natural selection acts by sifting and winnowing various alternative phenotypes—including behavior—and that as a result, all behavior has some adaptive significance—that is, it has consequences for the fitness of the individuals (and genes) concerned. Behavior is essentially another phenotype no less susceptible to evolutionary pressure than any other biological trait. Thus, behavior—just as anatomy and physiology—is likely to have some adaptive significance under existing constraints of history, development, and so forth, at least within the environments in which it evolved.

Natural selection operates by differential reproduction, and individuals behaving in a particular way, by virtue of their behavior, leave either somewhat fewer or somewhat more descendants. If the former, the behavior in question is "selected against"; if the latter, it is "selected for." It is also possible for behavior to be neutral—that is, to have no fitness consequences—but for most traits, given a large enough population and sufficient time, this is considered unlikely. Most behavior is therefore assumed to reflect "fitness maximization," at least to some degree.

Differential reproduction does not in itself produce evolutionary change or an adaptive change in behavior unless there is at least some correlation between genotype and phenotype. The field of behavior genetics has expanded rapidly, revealing numerous examples of such correlations, and it seems likely that additional ones will be elucidated in the future. Importantly, it is not necessary for the genetic influence on behavior to be precise for evolutionary principles to come into play.

Thus, for example, "risk-taking" behavior has been found to be strongly associated with the presence of a dopamine subtype allele. People who enjoy riding roller coasters or climbing mountains may well be disproportionately likely to possess this allele, compared with those more inclined to stay home or to buy sedans with reliable airbags. This is *not* to suggest, however, that there is a gene "for" roller coasters or Volvos. Rather, the substitution of one allele for another likely has a ramifying effect on behavior that goes beyond narrowly defined specifics. Moreover, any such substitution has a mean arithmetic effect on fitness, as a result of which evolution favors those genes that maximize fitness under prevailing conditions.

A key consequence is that genes can influence behavior in myriad ways without there necessarily being genes "for" a given activity. Natural selection thereby has the opportunity to select for genetically influenced behavior traits without those traits being genetically "determined" in the sense of being rigidly fixed. For example, there probably exist genes for glucose or fructose receptors. Most people agree that sugary foods are "sweet," and there is a cross-cultural bias toward sweetness, suggesting that its perception has genetic underpinnings. However, there is probably no specific allele for candy bars; moreover, people can decide not to consume sweets. Genes influence behavior, but in most cases, they whisper, rather than shout.

Sex and Mating Systems

In the sociobiological perspective, sex is important to human beings, not merely because of its symbolic or emotional salience, its hormonal underpinnings, its connection to early childhood experiences, or its sociocultural elaboration, but also as a result of its direct connection to the crucial evolutionary process of reproduction.

Among the insights provided by sociobiology, those relating to sex and sex differences are especially cogent. A key concept is "parental investment," defined as any expenditure of time, energy, or risk provided by a parent on behalf of its offspring, which increases the probability of that offspring surviving and eventually reproducing but at the cost of the parent's ability to invest similarly in other offspring. The patterning of parental investment differs substantially between men and women because men—as makers of sperm—produce a very large number of small gametes, each of which involves a small amount of parental investment, whereas women—egg makers, by definition—produce a comparatively small number of large gametes, each of which necessitates a large amount of parental investment. Furthermore, male and female gametes are not only dramatically different in metabolic content but also in the subsequent parental investment that they necessitate.

In the case of mammals (including, of course, human beings), even though eggs are small compared with those of reptiles or birds, they dwarf the size of sperm. Moreover, a fertilized egg obligates its producer to massive amounts of subsequent investment via pregnancy and lactation. Sperm makers, by contrast, are not biologically obligated to a comparable degree of reproductive follow-through. Although human beings are unusual among mammals in the degree of parental investment provided by fathers, they nonetheless are characteristic mammals in that females provide the overwhelming bulk of such investment.

Consider, similarly, that men are capable of impregnating many different women; their reproductive success is, thus, limited by the number of inseminations they achieve. By contrast, the reproductive success of women is typically limited not by their ability to be inseminated but by the rearing of successful offspring. As a general biological principle, men tend to have a higher variance in reproductive success than do women, and this, in turn, inclines men to be competitive with other men because the fitness of each man is to some extent negatively impacted by that of any other. By contrast, competition among women, although genuine, typically involves social undermining rather than overt violence.

Across the animal kingdom, sperm makers and egg makers mate in a huge variety of different patterns. Plants and some marine invertebrates often disperse their sex cells into the environment without aiming, whereas most animals engage in some sort of courtship and in a characteristic mating system. *Polygamy* refers to any general system in which one individual is reproductively bonded to more than one individual of the opposite sex; *polygyny* means that one male associates with multiple females, and *polyandry* is one female associating with many males. A relatively new term, *polyamory*, refers to multiple lovers for both sexes. Polygyny is the most common mammalian pattern, predisposed by the gametic differences described above, because, whereas male reproductive success is enhanced by having multiple mates, that of women is less dramatically affected, and adding extra males to a female's "harem" is likely to diminish the fitness of males already present. Accordingly, most mammals are polygynous, whereas a relatively few species are socially monogamous but sexually promiscuous.

The evidence is overwhelming that human beings are mildly polygynous by nature. First, men are, on average, larger than women and are also more inclined toward physically competitive, sometimes violent behavior. When found among other mammals, this tendency in itself is strongly correlated with polygyny because "sexual dimorphism" of this sort is typically selected when male fitness is enhanced by success in male–male competition, an arena in which size and aggressive physical attributes often convey an advantage.

Second, women become sexually mature somewhat earlier than men, a pattern of "sexual bimaturism" that in other species signals the existence of more intense competition in the later-maturing sex. Thus, among highly aggressive, harem-forming species, females become sexually mature considerably earlier than do males; their fitness is maximized by reproducing early and often, whereas that of males depends on success in social competition with other males, which in turn makes it advantageous for them to delay maturity until they are older, larger, and possibly wiser, and, hence, better able to succeed in the competitive reproductive fray.

Finally, before the cultural homogenization that followed Western colonial expansion, 85 percent of human societies were preferentially polygynous. Nearly all women were mated and reproductive, whereas some men were nonreproductive bachelors, and others were highly successful harem masters. Putting these observations together, the biological polygyny of human beings can be considered proven, although serial monogamy (with departures by both men and women) remains the social norm in Judeo-Christian cultures. Even polyandry—the mating of one woman with multiple males—although extremely rare and very much contrary to evolutionary inclination, has occasionally been reported, but in these instances, the men are often brothers (consistent with the expectations of kin selection; see the section Altruism, Kin Selection, and Inclusive Fitness).

Monogamy and Adultery

The evidence is undeniable that human beings are not "naturally" monogamous. However, people are clearly capable of monogamy and, moreover, are more inclined toward monogamy than are most mammals. This is presumably because of the biological payoff of biparental care in a species whose young are helpless at birth, grow slowly, and require substantial postnatal parental investment, often lasting several decades. Monogamy is also strongly encouraged by the world's dominant religious and social traditions.

At the same time, human beings are susceptible to sexual infidelity. In this regard, they are not alone. DNA fingerprinting has revealed that among many species, including numerous birds that had long been believed to be strictly monogamous, 10 percent to 80 percent of the offspring are not fathered by the social partner of the female. Biologists had long known that males are inclined to seek extra-pair copulations (EPCs), a pattern consistent with the male–female difference in parental investment discussed earlier. However, it is now clear that females of many species are far more sexually active outside the pair bond than had been believed. Female EPCs with distant males directly increased hybrid vigor and survival rates in their offspring compared to their half-siblings fathered by their social father in blue tit songbirds in a 2003 study. This was the first study to demonstrate a clear-cut genetic advantage to infidelity in monogamous songbirds.

Whereas a male propensity for multiple partners is easy to explain biologically, its existence among females is more problematic, given that such behavior is potentially risky in view of the well-documented potential of males to react violently to evidence of infidelity by their mates. In addition, males of many other animals—and presumably, human beings as well—are prone to abandon their mates or at least to refrain from investing parentally in their mates' offspring on indications of infidelity. Compensating benefits of EPCs for females may include increasing the probability of fertilization, improving the genetic quality or sexual desirability of their offspring, obtaining additional resources from EPC partners, and, occasionally, making a "bridge" to an alternative mateship.

Males who form harems must first win them in competition with other males and then guard them from poachers. Maintaining a harem (of either sex) is expensive and time consuming. Rather than forming real harems and instead of organizing a group of contentious males, females form virtual harems within their reproductive tracts, allowing sperm to compete with other sperm directly. Sperm competition has been studied extensively in animals and is being explored in human beings. Recent DNA evidence suggests that approximately 10 percent of human infants are sired by someone other than the wife's husband, and this figure is cross-cultural. In any event, it is clear that female sexuality is neither passive nor resignedly domestic.

Departures from monogamy are the norm for both sexes in most cultures despite social proscription in Judeo-Christian cultures. A typical marital history in the United States includes several marriages—serial monogamy—with dating and adultery interspersed. Both men and women are sexual opportunists, often using different means toward the same end (maximizing their fitness). Males typically provide resources to obtain sexual opportunities, whereas females provide sex to obtain resources. Patterns of adulterous behavior in human societies are in agreement with sociobiological predictions: Males are more likely to stray given the opportunity, whereas females use sex as a means to move up in social strata, to obtain better genes, or to increase resources. Also consistent with sociobiological prediction is the observation that men are more susceptible to pornography, prostitution, and paraphilias, as expected of the sex that provides less parental investment and, hence, has a lower threshold for sexual activity.

Mate Selection Human beings are especially expert in sexual selection, the choice of one mate over another based on physical and behavioral traits. Given the substantial disparity in male–female parental investment and the fact that females are a limiting resource for the reproductive success of males, whereas access to males is not typically limiting for female fitness, it is expected that males generally are the aggressive sexual advertisers, and females are relatively coy comparison shoppers. Sperm makers, producing hundreds of millions of gametes, compete among themselves for egg makers, who offer a few large gametes and the biobehavioral resources to rear the young. Thus, females possess something that males want (access to their promised parental investment); accordingly, they are positioned to choose among males, who are in turn selected to demonstrate their desirability.

Freud asked, "What do women want?" Sociobiology gives an answer: good genes (pleasing appearance, adequate size, evidence of basic health), good resources (money; the ability to obtain food, clothing, and territory as well as willingness to dispense the above during courtship), and good behavior (indications of one's quality as a protector and caregiver). Females generally, and human females to a large degree, select mates based on their wealth, behavior, and appearance, not necessarily in that order.

Compared to females, males tend to have a lower threshold for sexual excitement; greater willingness to engage in sex with a partner they do not know; greater concern about a prospective partner's physical attributes; less concern about a prospective partner's intellectual qualities, personality, or wealth; and more likelihood of being agitated by any indication that an existing partner may be sexually involved with someone else.

Because human beings are unusual among mammals in the degree to which men provide parental investment, they can also be expected to be unusual in the degree to which they are choosy in selecting women. Moreover, although sperm are inexpensive and abundant compared with eggs, they are not free, and socially imposed obligations often limit the extramarital opportunities of even the most desirable men. As a result, men, too, are likely to be somewhat selective in their choice of mates, although generally less discriminating than women. An important new social development is the advent of DNA fingerprinting, which allows for accurate paternity determination. In the future, one might, therefore, expect men to be more choosy about casual sexual partners.

Although studies have consistently found that women are especially influenced by male access to resources, men are significantly more attuned to sexual opportunity and appeal, which in turn is highly correlated with likely reproductive success. Thus, cross-culturally, men are attracted to women who offer signs of basic health such as youth, symmetrical features, clear skin, and a low waist-to-hip ratio, indicating that they are not already pregnant. The mechanism for these choices is largely unconscious: In exercising a preference for partners who are, for example, youthful and healthy, people are not usually intentionally evaluating their reproductive success and then behaving accordingly. It is rare even for a sociobiologist to marry based on a rational calculation of the cost-to-benefit ratio of a particular partner versus another. Rather, individuals who preferentially mated with those who were especially fertile, healthy, inclined to take good care of their children, and able to be good providers have been more fit and therefore have left more genetic representation for such tendencies in future generations. The archetypes for "sexiness" belie an underlying calculation of reproductive potential, even in those with absolutely no intention to have children or no understanding of their motivation.

Violence It is a cross-cultural universal that men are more violent than women. This, in turn, is consistent with the sociobiology of male–female differences and the biology of polygyny, because in every known polygynous species, males are more violence prone than are females; moreover, the greater the degree of polygyny, the greater this male–female disparity. This correlation likely arises because polygyny conveys an adaptive advantage on males who succeed in overt competition with other males, whereas equivalent female–female competition—although important—is more subtle and less tied to violence.

It seems undeniable that inclinations toward violence are influenced by cultural expectations, insofar as boys and men are taught that aggressiveness and violence are akin to "manliness," whereas girls and women are taught that similar behavior is "unfeminine"; such learning in itself contributes importantly to male–female differences. However, if these differences are solely due to the arbitrary influence of culture, then there should be as many societies in which women are arbitrarily taught that femininity requires aggression and violence, and men are taught that masculinity demands restraint and nonviolence. The absence of such societies strongly suggests that cultural promptings as to male–female differences in violence themselves derive, at least in part, from an underlying degree of male–female difference.

Although homicide rates vary substantially among different societies—being, for example, approximately ten times higher in the United States than in Canada and approximately ten times higher in Canada than in Iceland—as well as across historical periods, it is notable that the difference between male and female homicide rates remains remarkably constant regardless of the society. Also worth noting is that homicide rates tend to be especially high among people of low socioeconomic status, a finding that is also consistent with sociobiological theory, because in a polygynous species, low-ranking males are more likely to be evolutionary failures; as a result of which, they can be predicted to engage in riskier behavior.

Sexual Violence: Rape Some feminists insist that rape is solely an act of physical aggression, reflecting violence against women and girls as a component of domination. By contrast, a sociobiological view—although fully recognizing the social unacceptability of rape—emphasizes the sexual and evolutionary component of this violent behavior. Although it is sometimes claimed that rape is unique to human beings, behavior exactly analogous has been reported for numerous animal species; moreover, the perpetrators are often, although not always, males that are otherwise socially and sexually unsuccessful. This suggests that, at least to some degree, human rape may be an unconscious strategy on the part of males who are otherwise sexually unsuccessful and less likely to succeed in traditional patterns of both male–male competition and attractiveness to females.

Certain observations are consistent with this interpretation: Rape is more frequent when men are required to pay a "bride price" and are unable to do so; rapists tend to be young men rather than those who are older and typically more successful; and rape victims are overwhelmingly drawn from the population of young, reproductively competent females, whereas the "domination" hypothesis suggests that victims are at least as likely to be middle aged or older because such individuals—although less sexually attractive and also less likely to contribute to the fitness of rapists—are more likely to possess social power.

Parenting An important evolutionary principle states that—all things being equal—individuals are disinclined to provide parental care when they are not genetically related to the recipients or when there is a substantial probability that they are unrelated. This is because genes that predispose their bodies to invest indiscriminately in other genes leave fewer copies of themselves than do alternative alleles that preferentially enhance the fitness of their own identical copies. Parental care, accordingly, is not randomly distributed to juveniles generally; rather, it is preferentially directed toward one's genetic offspring. Among fish and amphibians that practice external fertilization, the two sexes are comparable in their (lack of) confidence of relatedness to the next generation, and, consequently, females and males are on average equally likely to perform the primary parenting duties.

By contrast, among mammals, females are overwhelmingly the primary parent. Human beings, like other mammals, experience internal fertilization. As a result, women are assured that they are genetically related to their offspring; men are not (at least without DNA testing, which is a very recent innovation). Among mammals, of course, females are also specialized to provide nourishment after parturition, but there is no physiological reason why males could not be similarly capable; they even possess nipples. The likelihood, therefore, is that female mammals lactate, whereas males do not, because females—unlike males—are guaranteed genetic relationship to their offspring.

Consistent with the significance of mother–father differences in confidence of genetic relatedness to their offspring, mothering is more intense than fathering in every human society. It has also been found that immediately after a birth, the mother's family (confident of their relative's relationship to the newborn) is significantly more likely to comment on physical resemblance between the father and the newborn, presumably in an effort to reassure the less confident parent. Insofar as fathers are less assured of paternity than mothers are of maternity, it can be predicted that a cross-generational father link introduces a degree of uncertainty not paralleled by mother links; accordingly, it was therefore predicted that grandparents connected to grandchildren via father–father links are less solicitous than grandparents connected via mother–father or father–mother links, which in turn are less solicitous than grandparents connected via mother–mother links. This prediction has also received cross-cultural support.

Altruism, Kin Selection, and Inclusive Fitness *Altruism* is defined by sociobiologists as a behavior that reduces the personal reproductive success of the initiator while increasing that of the recipient. It thus differs from conventional use of the word, which implies conscious intent to "do good." Biologists are strictly concerned with the evolutionary effect of seemingly altruistic acts, not with their motivation. According to traditional Darwinian theory, altruism should not occur in nature because, by definition, selection acts against any trait whose effect is to decrease its representation in future generations; and yet, an array of altruistic behaviors occurs among free-living animals as well as human beings.

This paradox was largely resolved by an important insight that also clarified a fundamental issue in evolutionary theory generally. According to "inclusive fitness theory," the key unit of selection is actually genes rather than individuals because it is genes that are capable of replicating themselves across generations. Selection, operating at this level, can generate behavior that appears altruistic among individuals so long as it is actually "selfish" at the level of the gene—specifically, those genes responsible for the seemingly altruistic behavior. The general principle is that selection favors altruism whenever B is greater than rC, when B equals benefit of the altruistic act, C equals its cost, and r equals the coefficient of genetic relationship between altruist and beneficiary. In the above case, B and C are measured in units of fitness, and r is a probability ranging from 1.0 in the case of identical twins, 0.5 for full siblings, and 0 for unrelated individuals.

This insight galvanized much of sociobiology, emphasizing, as it did, the behavioral significance of natural selection acting at the genetic level and suggesting a view whereby organisms are essentially devices created by their genes, serving the genes' perpetuation. It resolved the paradox of altruistic behavior by revealing that phenotypic altruism is actually genotypic selfishness and, thus, not an evolutionary conundrum. It also initiated an important modification of traditional Darwinian theory, which had equated fitness with reproductive success. Under the newer, gene-oriented conception, organisms tend to maximize their "inclusive fitness," which includes not only Darwinian fitness but also the effect of a given behavior on the reproductive success of other relatives, with the importance of each relative devalued in proportion as he or she is more distantly related and therefore less likely to share a given gene by virtue of common descent. Because of the importance of genetic kin, this process is also frequently called *kin selection.*

Confidence in inclusive fitness theory has been enhanced not only by its elegant logic and mathematical consistency but also by its effectiveness in explaining hitherto mysterious patterns of altruism in animals ranging from the social insects to lions. It also has received confirmation in studies of human behavior, including patterns of inheritance, risk taking, and numerous aspects of family structure. Nepotism, a cross-cultural universal, is also consistent with the expectations of inclusive fitness theory.

Stepfamilies, Child Abuse, and Infanticide It is widely known that stepfamilies are often emotionally conflicted. Traditional social science theory attributes this to confusing and contradictory social pressures. Sociobiological theory looks instead to instincts rooted in evolutionary genetics. Thus, insofar as natural selection tends to discourage parental patterns of solicitude directed toward nonrelatives, it can be predicted that nonbiological "parents" feel torn between a socially generated responsibility and obligation toward unrelated children and a biologically generated disinclination to invest substantially in them. At minimum, even in emotionally healthy stepfamilies, conflict can be predicted between unrelated adults and children and, derivatively, between husband and wife.

Stepfamilies are unusual among free-living animals, as expected. When created experimentally, nonbiological "parents" typically behave nonparentally. This is most often manifested as neglect, but it can involve violent rejection or even murder. An extreme example occurs in many polygynous species when a previously bachelor male periodically succeeds in replacing the harem master. At this point, the newly ascendant male often proceeds to kill any newborns who had been fathered by the previous male and are therefore "stepchildren" to the new harem master. This commonly induces the children's mothers to resume ovulation, whereon they mate with the infanticidal male whose fitness is thus enhanced by the grisly affair.

Infanticide is rare among human beings, although stepparenting is increasingly common. Clearly, most stepparents are quite capable of being good parents, or at least they refrain from infanticide. But significantly, stepparenting is a highly significant risk factor for infanticide and child abuse and neglect—more predictive than age, socioeconomic status, or any other identifiable correlate.

Parent–Offspring Conflict

A naïve view of evolutionary theory suggests that parent–offspring dynamics are conflict free because both parents and offspring have a shared interest in the eventual success of the offspring. This perspective is valid insofar as shared genes predispose individuals generally toward a degree of beneficence. However, an important sociobiological insight—one that has not yet received the attention from the psychiatric community that it warrants—reveals the existence of substantial and predictable patterns of parent–offspring conflict. The key point is that parents and offspring share a coefficient of genetic relationship of 0.5, not perfect identity. Hence, parents and offspring can each be expected to devalue the other's fitness by a factor of one-half. Put another way, offspring are likely to be only one-half as concerned about the costs to a parent of a given behavior as the parent is and vice versa.

Consider, for example, the temporal progression of nursing and weaning. Early postpartum, both mother and infant are likely to agree on the desirability of nursing, which enhances the fitness of both while imposing very little cost on either. At a certain point, however, the mother's fitness is maximized if she discontinued further investment in the infant and turned her attention instead to producing—or otherwise investing in—another child. This point is reached whenever the cost to the mother of continuing to nurse is greater than the benefit she derives by discontinuing that aspect of their relationship. The nursing infant, however, does not necessarily agree; he or she seeks to continue nursing until the cost to the mother is twice the benefit she would otherwise derive. Accordingly, there is a predicted zone of parent–offspring conflict, with the offspring seeking to obtain more parental investment than the parent (mother, in this case) is selected to provide. This might explain much of the near-universal phenomenon of "weaning conflict" as well as possibly the case of many "terrible 2-year-olds." Eventually, this conflict is resolved at the point when the interests of parent and offspring once again coincide because the cost of continued nursing for the offspring ultimately exceeds its benefit for both offspring and parent, even with the offspring's 50 percent devaluing of parental costs.

A similar analysis applies to parent–offspring conflict over the amount of parental investment, as well as to parent–offspring conflict regarding offspring inclinations toward other family members. For example, a child can be expected to behave altruistically toward its full sibling whenever the cost of doing so is less than one-half the benefit derived by the sibling. The parental perspective, however, is different, since parents are equally related to each offspring; hence, parental fitness is maximized if offspring behave altruistically toward each other whenever the benefit derived by the recipient exceeds the altruist's cost. The result, once again, is a potential zone of conflict, with parents likely to urge their children to "play more nicely" than the children—intent on maximizing their own fitness rather than that of their parents—are inclined to do.

Of course, parents and offspring are not equally empowered; parents are stronger, more experienced, and presumably wiser. As pointed out by Robert L. Trivers, who first identified the evolutionary biology of parent–offspring conflict, offspring cannot fling their mothers to the ground and nurse at will! On the other hand, parents and offspring have substantial shared interests, with the former especially predisposed to invest appropriately in the latter. Moreover, offspring can take advantage of the fact that they have information on which parents are expected to act: informing their parents when they are hungry, cold, wet, tired, and so forth. This, in turn, gives offspring the opportunity to manipulate their parents by sending signals of distress that exceed their genuine need and which, in turn, could select for parental ability to discriminate honest from manipulative signaling. It might also help explain aspects of "infantile regression" as well as the typical adult assertion that they know better than their children what is in the latter's best interests!

Certain traditional constructs of psychoanalysis, such as oedipal rivalry, may also be revisited in the light of parent–offspring conflict theory. Thus, insofar as children are unconsciously motivated to attempt to garner parental investment beyond the inclinations of their parents, they might be expected to take advantage of opportunities to do just this, in part by competing with their same-sex parent while interacting somewhat seductively toward the opposite-sex parent. An added role of male–male competition may also be relevant here because in many animal species, juvenile males are intimidated by their fathers and must disperse from the natal herd to find breeding opportunities. This was probably true in ancient human tribes as well. In any event, future elaboration of parent–offspring conflict theory may well shed new light on developmental dynamics by replacing traditional focus on the "parent–child nexus" with investigation into the tactics likely to be used by parents and children, treated as separate (although related) individuals, each with his or her distinct evolutionary agenda.

Menopause and the "Grandmother Hypothesis"

Human beings are unusual—although not quite unique—in experiencing menopause: Virtually all other mammals remain reproductively competent until extreme old age. The sociobiology of inclusive fitness theory provides an explanation for why women undergo a prolonged anovulatory stage when several decades of life still remain. Pregnancy, birth, and lactation are physically rigorous, with the demands enhanced by the prolonged dependence of human juveniles plus the fact that upright posture combined with the large brain size of neonates has made parturition itself more problematic than in other mammals. It is thus possible that the costs of reproduction for women are sufficiently high that selection has favored a shutting down of reproduction at an age when a woman's earlier offspring are themselves becoming reproductively competent. At this point, the inclusive fitness of a middle-aged woman could be maximized by investing in her grandchildren rather than by seeking to produce another offspring, with its attendant (and increasing) risks. Consistent with this interpretation is the fact that, whereas middle-aged and elderly men experience a decline in reproductive competence, they do not undergo an equivalent "male menopause"; whereas grandfathers are as capable, theoretically, of enhancing their inclusive fitness by "grandfathering," they do not experience costs comparable to those of women in their 50s, 60s, or 70s who attempt to reproduce.

Cooperation, Conflict, Reciprocity, and Reputation

An evolutionary perspective on human behavior suggests that normal people are naturally predisposed toward neither cooperation nor nastiness; they are no more inherently altruistic than inherently competitive. Rather, they are potentially inclined to be either, as a function of situation and circumstance. Thus, the same individuals who participate in aggressive sexual and dominance-oriented competition are also likely to be "selfless" altruists when interacting with close relatives. Sociobiological theory has also developed the following analyses of interpersonal relations.

Benevolent interactions between individuals need not be based solely on the probability of shared genes (i.e., inclusive fitness theory). They may also be selected—even if in the process each participant incurs short-term costs—so long as the "bottom line" of such behavior results in a net positive fitness consequence for the individuals and their genes. One series of such interactions involves "reciprocity," whereby individuals essentially exchange favors—for example, if individual #1 gives food to individual #2 in the expectation that #2 will return the favor at some time in the future. Such behavior appears to be altruistic in that individual #1 experiences an immediate fitness cost because of his or her action, whereas #2 benefits. However, if there is a sufficient probability that the situation will be reversed in the future, whereon #2 reciprocates his or her "debt" to #1, then both participants will have enhanced their fitness, so long as the cost of the assistance to each donor is less than the benefit derived by the recipient. Under such circumstances, the exchange results in increased personal fitness for each participant; hence, it is not strictly "altruistic." Moreover, the participants need not be genetically related; in theory, they could even be members of different species.

Examples of such reciprocity have been adduced for animals, although they have proved less common than might be expected. The clearest case, involving vampire bats, may be especially instructive. These animals live in small social groups and forage at night for blood. Success is unpredictable, and their metabolic rate is such that individuals cannot survive if they do not obtain a blood meal for three consecutive nights; a well-fed vampire bat, on the other hand, has more nourishment than needed. Hungry individuals beg food from those with full stomachs, and the latter typically oblige. Subsequently, individuals who receive such assistance are especially likely to reciprocate when they are well fed and their previous benefactors are needy. It may also be significant that, as bats go, vampires have unusually large brains, which facilitates identification of individuals to which reciprocity is owed as well as those who did not meet their social obligations.

Reciprocal systems are highly vulnerable to "cheaters," individuals who receive a benefit but do not return the favor when the opportunity arises. This may help explain the relative rarity of reciprocity among animals as well as its prominence among human beings, among whom there is typically great sensitivity to matters of fairness and reliability. Much of human friendship may also be attributed to reciprocity as well as, to some extent, the great elaboration of the brain, part of which is occupied with cataloging past interactions, recalling "who owes what to whom" and even, perhaps, calculating the extent to which one might be able to get away with nonreciprocity. On the positive side, reciprocity evidently works for human beings, evidenced by the universality of systems of exchange as well as the strongly felt obligation that follows the receipt of assistance.

Just as failure to reciprocate leads to a decrement in social reputation, reliable reciprocation typically generates an increase. Moreover, it also appears to help select for seemingly "generalized altruism," whereby individuals may be inclined to behave benevolently toward others—even those who may be unrelated or who are unable or unlikely to reciprocate in the future—insofar as by doing so, such individuals are perceived by others as upright and worthy, which in turn is likely to enhance their eventual fitness.

Prisoner's Dilemma and Other Games

The vulnerability of reciprocating systems to cheating is modeled by a much-studied example of game theory known as the *prisoner's dilemma*. In this situation, two individuals are faced with the choice of behaving in two ways—cooperate or defect—with the payoffs determined as follows: The highest payoff is received if an individual defects and the other cooperates; the next highest, if both cooperate; third best, when both defect; and lowest, when an individual cooperates and the other defects. As a result, each individual is forced to defect because of the temptation that by doing so, he or she will receive the highest payoff (if the other cooperates) as well as fear of obtaining the lowest payoff of all if he or she cooperates and the other defects. The dilemma is that when both defect—each following a rational calculus of maximizing his or her payoff—both receive a relatively poor return, whereas they could have done substantially better had they figured out a means of mutual cooperation.

Prisoner's dilemma has been used to elucidate the difficulty of generating cooperation in a world of independently acting egoists. Moreover, simple mathematical techniques have been developed whereby players in repeated games—otherwise inadvertently stuck in a spiral of mutual defection—can enjoy the benefits of mutual cooperation. It is also possible, for example, that prisoner's dilemma provides a model for the evolution of paranoia because individuals who are predisposed to defect predictably evoke defection by other players, which in turn could produce yet more defection along with the expectation of further noncooperation; paranoia, in short, could then become a self-fulfilling prophecy, likely with some initial impetus provided by biochemical imbalance or predisposing early experience.

Game theory has a long history of application to military affairs, economics, and experimental social psychology; more recently, it has been widely applied in sociobiological studies of animal behavior, and its potential value in understanding human interactions is being actively explored. Game theory applies most cogently to encounters between pairs of "players," when each must choose—independent of the other—among a limited number of options, with the payoffs determined by what both players do. Each is assumed to maximize his or her payoff analogous to fitness returns over evolutionary time; as a result, game theoretical analyses may well use the same pathways as those actually followed by natural selection. It remains to be seen to what degree various well-studied games, such as prisoner's dilemma or the game of "chicken," will cast light on human behavior.

Communication: Truth and Lies

Sociobiology promotes a novel and, in some ways, cynical view of communication. Communication is traditionally seen as an interaction in which a minimum of two participants—a sender and a receiver—share the same goal: the exchange of accurate information. Ethologists, for example, have long focused on the role of postures and other nonverbal signals to convey information about the internal state of the sender: whether aggressive, subordinate, sexually motivated, and so forth. Although shared interest in accurate communication remains valid in some domains of animal signaling—notably such well-documented cases as the "dance of the bees," whereby foragers inform other workers about the location of food sources—a more selfish and, in the case of social interaction, more accurate model of animal communication has largely replaced this conception.

Sociobiological analyses of communication emphasize that because individuals are genetically distinct, their evolutionary interests are similarly distinct, although admittedly with significant fitness overlap, especially among kin, reciprocators, parents and offspring, and mated pairs. However, such overlaps are rarely 100 percent; hence, individuals do not enjoy a complete correspondence of interest in communication. Senders are motivated to convey information that induces the receivers to behave in a manner that enhances the senders' fitness. Receivers, similarly, are interested in responding to communication only insofar as such response enhances their fitness. In such cases, "truth" is incidental and of importance only insofar as it might influence the probability that the information is likely to be believed and, thus, acted on. Communication accordingly involves attempted manipulation of receivers by senders and corresponding selection on recipients for the ability to discriminate messages of value to themselves from those involving attempts at manipulation.

Deceptive communication is rife in the natural world, with examples including camouflage, mimicry, or instances of intraspecies aggressive communication, in which individuals seek to appear larger, fiercer, and more determined than they actually are. At the same time, despite the expected tendency of individuals to send misleading information, there should also be selection in favor of reliable signaling, when it is mutually advantageous for the sender to be believed. One important way to enhance reliability is to make the signal itself costly; for example, an animal could reliably indicate its physical fitness, freedom from parasites and other pathogens, and possibly its genetic quality as well by growing elaborate and metabolically expensive secondary sexual characteristics such as the oversized tail of a peacock. Human beings, similarly, can signal their wealth by conspicuous consumption. This approach, known as the *handicap principle*, suggests that effective communication may require that the signaler engage in especially costly behavior to ensure success. Initially questioned, the handicap principle has received both theoretical and empirical support in animal studies; its potential for offering insight into human behavior remains to be elaborated.

Self-Esteem Self-esteem may be considered an economic analysis of one's place in the social milieu and sexual marketplace and, thus, of one's fitness. Similarly, self-esteem may be an unconscious calculation of "resource holding potential," defined by sociobiologists as an individual's ability to compete for resources with others of the same species. Males, especially, compete with others to obtain resources, including females. Rather than actually fight repetitively, individuals often know their rank in a dominance hierarchy and choose contests they might win based on their self-assessment. Females compete with other females for access to desirable males and resources, and again, individuals are more fit if they can assess the outcome of potential conflicts without actually engaging in combat. High self-esteem can thus be considered a calculation of one's capacity to hold resources and obtain mates. Low self-esteem, then, is an anticipated losing outcome in social competition.

It is adaptive to assess one's self-worth accurately, so as to avoid unnecessary losses with further erosion of resources or danger to self. Many psychiatric disorders may be disorders of risk–benefit calculations in social circumstances and poor appraisals of personal market value.

Emotions Sociobiology is generally concerned more with observations of behavioral patterns than inner dynamics because most animals cannot speak, much less describe dreams or write poetry. The novel contributions awaiting further developments in Darwinian psychiatry will likely include the role of emotions in self-conscious, verbally expressive creatures. From an evolutionary perspective, emotions appear to be strategic decisions dealing directly with primordial concerns such as sex, parenting, betrayal, loss, and competition. Human beings are perfectly good mammals, endowed with a repertoire of inherited strategies to be used in a complicated social universe. Each individual is equipped by nature to recognize kin, to compete for access to resources, to optimize social rank or signs of social rank, and to seek sexual gratification. An important point is that humans, as other animals, have the innate capacity to evaluate complex cost–benefit calculations without knowing that they are doing differential equations and probability statistics. These strategic analyses happen every day, and emotions are their physiological manifestation.

Lust, for example, is a desire to mate, which at a deep level involves a fitness calculation. Happiness, similarly, appears to be the sense of self-gratification that results from meeting one's biological requirements. Emotions are also signals to others, efficient mechanisms for communication that bypass self-conscious assessment. However, it is clear that the capacity for deception is not unique to human beings, nor is it rare in human interactions. Emotions communicate, but they can be false indicators, although not beyond the reach of evolution. Thus, sometimes the best liar is one who believes his or her own falsehoods, leading to the possibility that emotions can be a way of manipulating oneself and thereby others.

Darwinian Psychiatry Familiar psychiatric concepts can be translated into sociobiological terms. For example, Freud's concept of eros, the sexual instinct, is not unlike the underlying potency of genes seeking to replicate themselves in new bodies. Sexual propensities are largely hardwired into sexually reproducing species, if only because abstemiousness would quickly die out under selective pressure from successful breeders. However, Freud's concept of thanatos, the death instinct, can have no direct biological basis because any instinct for suicide before breeding is selected against relative to genes that inclined their carriers to survive and rear successful offspring. One could, however, imagine several variations on thanatos—for example, genes for aggression, competition, and violence. There is no conflict between the concept of a Freudian instinct for bloodthirstiness and an evolutionary drive for violence toward others in the service of reproductive success. A key insight of sociobiology involves the recognition that even altruistic self-sacrifice could be positively selected, if the altruists contribute to the ultimate success of altruistic genes, in the bodies of beneficiaries.

Friedrich Nietzsche's "will to power" might be an adaptive instinct to obtain rank and resources. The insights of Alfred Adler are no longer prominent in the standard psychiatric curriculum but may warrant renewed attention because they are compatible with a sociobiological perspective on the role of social hierarchy in human emotional illness. Thus, Adler's "inferiority complex" recurs in new research on the neurophysiology of subordination stress. Animals, including human beings, that lose in social competition or fall in dominance suffer serious psychophysiological consequences, including cortisol elevation and immune and hormonal suppression, particularly testosterone. These animal models mimic the human state of depression and may be isomorphic.

John Bowlby's seminal work on infant–maternal attachment was a direct outgrowth of ethology, influenced particularly by the work of Niko Tinbergen. Further studies of attachment and social bonding have focused, for example, on cooperation and reconciliation in primates and on the role of oxytocin in promoting maternal behavior and other forms of attachment. Finally, Carl Jung's idea of the archetype may have directly prefigured the concept of inborn strategies encrypted by DNA into a repertoire of behavioral options:

> The archetype is not meant to denote an inherited idea but rather an inherited mode of functioning, corresponding to the inborn way in which the chick emerges from the egg, the bird builds its nest, a certain kind of wasp stings the motor ganglion of the caterpillar, and eels find their way to the Bermudas. In other words, it is a "pattern of behavior." This aspect of the archetype, the purely biological one, is the proper concern of scientific psychology.

Whether one thinks of inherited behavior as traits, susceptibility, archetypes, algorithms, instincts, or drives, certain patterns are clearly universal in human beings throughout time and in every culture; for example, people enjoy sex, nurture babies, recognize kin, form hierarchical social groups, cooperate on some occasions and compete in others, and mourn the dead. Emotions, as discussed, may be considered unconscious strategies for analyzing and communicating social situations, especially potent when dealing with basic patterns of social behavior. They involve deeply personal calculations with coefficients derived from both heredity and experience. Emotional health and appropriate logical processing are likely to be adaptive and selected for, contributing to social and biological success; failures of either constitute pathology.

PSYCHOPATHOLOGY

It is unlikely that "emotional disorders" evolved directly under natural selection unless they conferred some type of inclusive fitness benefit for self or close relatives. In all likelihood, either these traits are adaptive strategies or were adaptive in the early environment in which humanity evolved but are outmoded in the contemporary environment, or they represent malfunctions of otherwise adaptive components. Such malfunctions can result from disease or as a consequence of the statistical properties of large populations. Thus, insofar as "carefulness," for example, is likely to be adaptive, manifested as caution with regard to potential injury, a normal distribution of such carefulness reflected across millions of individuals presumably generates some people at either tail of the curve who are diagnosable as having anxiety on the one hand and impulsiveness on the other.

It is generally acknowledged that human beings evolved on the Pleistocene savannas of Africa approximately 150,000 years ago, living in social groups of several dozen individuals. There were no domesticated animals or farms, no cities, no armies, and only rudimentary culture and technology. Tribes of relatives, reciprocators, and competitors moved about Eurasia as hunter-gatherers in a rich ecosystem. Social evolution proceeded rapidly, whereas genetic changes have been comparatively slow; thus, there may well be a disconnect between emotions and behaviors that were adaptive then and now.

Many theories of the adaptive significance of traits that may induce psychiatric disorders have been proposed. Depression has been seen as a strategy that inhibits futile efforts so that resources may be conserved. An individual who is depressed acts subordinately, feels unlovable, and may endure subordination stress, including cortisol nonsuppression, reduced immunity, and testosterone suppression. Depressed males are especially vulnerable to suicide, perhaps because, given their higher-stakes situation, they perceive no fitness-enhancing opportunities beyond their own death, which might at least conserve resources for kin. On the other hand, depression in women is more likely a conservative strategy to delay reproduction and induce relatives to bestow resources. Mania may usefully be seen as a self-deceptive increase in status, with hypersexuality and impulsivity, a particularly good strategy for males to increase rates of copulation. Seasonal affective disorder results in more sleep and reduced activity during winter months; this could be, to some extent, an extreme manifestation of a basically adaptive tendency to downregulate in the winter, especially adaptive in Northern climates; interestingly, this disorder is more common in people of northern European descent.

There is some evidence that relative fitness is higher in families with a tendency toward psychotic disorders, suggesting some adaptive benefit. Although reproductive success is low in individuals with schizophrenia and other psychoses, studies have found greater-than-average fertility rates in the parents and siblings of schizophrenics. It could be that the gene or genes that confer susceptibility to these diseases produce enhanced fitness when heterozygous, similar to the sickle cell gene. Another theory is that mania and schizophrenia were maintained by reproductive success on the part of charismatic leaders, shamans, and other "possessed" individuals who hear voices, exhibit paranoid traits, and have episodes of sustained excitement.

Anxiety, a state of wariness and watchfulness, occurs in many animals, with some species or even artificial breeds more susceptible than others. Thoroughbred horses, for example, are exceptionally prone to panic reactions and sudden flight, whereas quarter horses show more equanimity. Similarly, jitteriness and watchfulness may be familial traits displayed over a vast continuum. Phobias to natural situations, such as heights, closed spaces, snakes, and spiders, are much more common than phobias of black toilet seats or telephones, suggesting an adaptive biological substrate. Human ancestors who avoided snakes were more likely to reproduce than those who were indifferent, whereas selection has not had time to act on fears of human-made articles.

Personality disorders are stable traits over time. They may be interpreted as consistent social strategies used by individuals who lack other repertoire. Sociopaths specialize in deceit to obtain resources and are therefore freeloaders in society; they are nonreciprocators who take without giving, faking signals of cooperation. Hysteria may be a female form of sociopathy, deceptive hypersexuality used by low-status females to obtain resources from multiple males.

It has been suggested that drugs of abuse generate signals in the brain that indicate, falsely, the arrival of a huge fitness benefit. This could be seen as an adaptive strategy whereby plant genes induce humans to conserve and propagate those organisms. In other words, plants such as coffee, tobacco, marijuana, opium, and coca may stimulate a false sense of a fitness bonanza, which benefits them rather than their consumers.

CAUTIONS AND QUIBBLES

The chapter concludes with some objections that have been raised to sociobiology along with brief responses.

Sociobiology assumes, falsely, that most of human behavior is genetic. No characteristic of any living thing—whether structure, physiological mechanism, or behavior—is produced by either genes or environment acting alone. If a woman, for example, is 5 ft 6 in., it is absurd to assert that 3 ft of her height is due to genes and 2 ft 6 in. to her nutrition or any other comparable breakdown. Every inch of her stature is attributable to her genes and her experiences acting together, and the same with behavior. To be sure, a sociobiological approach focuses especially on the "nature" side of the "nature/nurture" interaction, but this does not deny the importance of culture and social learning, which are typically the concern of traditional social science.

Human behavior, especially in its more complex manifestations, is overwhelmingly determined by learning, culture, and social traditions. Thus, human specialness derives from what humans teach each other and themselves, especially their complex symbolic systems, including, but not limited to, language. Sociobiologists mislead by deemphasizing these traits. Even renowned evolutionary biologist Julian Huxley warned against "nothing butism," the erroneous notion that just because human beings are animals, they are nothing but animals. Huxley's point is well taken; human beings are indeed the product of their learning, their culture, their social norms, and their penchant for symbols, complex language, and elaborate thought processes. But the sociobiological perspective also turns Huxley's argument around, pointing out that even though human beings are all of the above, it is equally erroneous to presume that they are *nothing but* the product of their learning, their culture, their social norms, and so forth. People are also the product of evolution by natural selection, perfectly good mammals whose biological nature is revealed in their behavior no less than their fossils, physiology, or physique. For sociobiologists, in short, there is also such a thing as human nature, just as there is harvest mouse nature or hyacinth nature.

Sociobiology is a doctrine of genetic determinism that deprives people of their free will. First, no science can deprive people of their free will or indeed of anything else, although applications (rather, misapplications) of science can sometimes do so. If people possess free will, sociobiology cannot take it away; if they lack it, sociobiology cannot provide it. Second, genetic *determinism* is not at the heart of sociobiology; genetic *influence* is. The two are quite different: Whereas blood type, for example, is genetically determined, tendencies to behave aggressively, parentally, romantically, and so forth appear to be genetically influenced, which simply means that certain genetic combinations predispose people to behave in one direction or another. And a predisposition, inclination, or tendency is a far cry from a fixed action pattern from which there is no escape. Finally, it may be even more erosive of freedom and dignity if human behavior was entirely a function of learning, cultural traditions, social norms, and so forth, as social science traditionalists often claim, because in that case, people are simply a pale reflection of what they have experienced instead of bringing something (their "nature," derived from evolution) to the encounter.

Sociobiology is a political and social doctrine that is conservative, if not downright reactionary, because it supports the status quo as the way things naturally are and, thus, how they ought to be. This confuses *explaining* something with *excusing* it. To be sure, there is something appealing about the "natural" and the "organic" such as organic foods, natural environments, and so forth. But some of the most natural things are also among the most unpleasant: gangrene, for example, or syphilis. When virologists study human immunodeficiency virus (HIV), they are not justifying acquired immune deficiency syndrome (AIDS). And when sociobiologists seek to unravel the underlying basis of male violence, polygyny, female-biased parental care, and so forth, they are seeking insight, not moral authority. As to the supposed conservatism of evolution, Karl Marx was so impressed with *The Origin of Species* that he proposed dedicating his first edition of *Das Kapital* to Darwin! After all, evolution is a doctrine of change, even of revolution, demonstrating that the living world is in flux, as opposed to the special creation of an unvarying natural or social order. When *The Origin of Species* first appeared, it was not seen as conservative or supporting the status quo—far from it. The royal houses of Europe, recently shaken by the revolutions of 1848, were, in fact, terribly frightened that evolution—by demonstrating the naturalness of change—might provide ammunition for social revolution. Either way, however, there is no necessary connection between how things are (a statement of physical and biological fact) and how they ought to be (an ethical judgment).

Sociobiology is racist and thus dangerous. Given the terrible history of misused and misunderstood genetic theorizing—from the hijacking of racial theory by the Nazis to the excesses of the eugenics movement in the United States—this worry is understandable but nonetheless misplaced. Thus, sociobiology says virtually nothing about the differences between human groups but a lot about their underlying similarities. A sociobiological view of human behavior focuses on cross-cultural universals, those behavioral traits that people share by virtue of the biological commonality, regardless of such superficial differences as cultural tradition, language, or skin color that might appear to separate them. If anything, then, sociobiology offers a powerful antidote to racism.

Sociobiology is sexist. If sexism means the identification of male–female differences, then sociobiology is indeed sexist, but so are anatomy, physiology, embryology, biochemical genetics, and so forth. Some of the most cogent insights from sociobiology are those that explain why men and women and boys and girls are different. This is a far cry, however, from valuing the two sexes differently or suggesting social policy; rather, it aims to help illuminate the biology that underlies human reality. Interestingly, the "sexism" of sociobiology is compatible with an increasingly influential approach, known as *difference feminism*, which extols certain male–female differences, such as the purported female penchant for social relationships over hierarchy and for nurturance over violence. Sociobiology promises to shed light on some of these differences. What—if anything—people choose to do about them is the realm of ethics and social policy, not science.

Sociobiology cannot be tested. Sociobiological predictions are being tested constantly. As a result, the field has moved from what Thomas Kuhn called "revolutionary science" to the more mundane "puzzle solving," in which hypotheses are generated and quantitatively tested. Indeed, the approach has been so successful that several new journals have been founded, such as *Behavioral Ecology and Sociobiology* and *Human Behavior and Evolution*. In a sense, the immense diversity of human cultures and social systems is itself a huge, ongoing scientific experiment. One thing is held constant—the biological nature of *Homo sapiens*—whereas something else is varied, namely, social and cultural rules, languages, and so forth. Insofar as universal patterns emerge, it is only reasonable to attribute these commonalities to the biological constant; namely, the nature of human beings. The existence of consistent, shared behavior patterns among all people is itself, therefore, prima facie evidence for a consistent, shared biology. This interpretation is reinforced when the shared behavior patterns are in directions predicted by evolutionary biology.

Sociobiology ignores mechanisms, concerning itself with matters of function that are unscientific. The physical sciences are typically unconcerned with "why" questions. They devote themselves exclusively, instead, to questions of "how." Physicists, for example, don't ask *why* there are negative and positive charges but *how* they function. Nor do physicists usually ask *why* light travels at 186,000 miles per second but rather *how* this impacts the material world. Medical researchers, too, are largely concerned with answering *how* questions: how viruses cause disease, how neurons function, how energy is processed, and so forth. On the other hand, sociobiology usually functions at a different explanatory level, a departure that may be confusing to those accustomed to *how* centeredness. Its focus is on *why*. Why are males typically more aggressive than females? Why does altruism occur? Why is stepparenting so difficult? To be sure, these questions can be answered in "how" terms, with reference to hormones, physiological or anatomical mechanisms, experience, and so forth. But this ignores an underlying question: Why does the body respond to, say, testosterone in a particular way rather than in another way? For example, it is not sufficient to say that males are more aggressive than females "because of" testosterone, when, in many species, testosterone increases female aggression as well. The question then becomes: Why are males, on balance, more aggressive than females?

Sociobiology is largely driven by attempts to answer this sort of question, which introduces an evolutionary bias: Namely, what is the adaptive significance of the phenomenon at issue? Thus, when sociobiologists pose *why* questions about such things as male versus female aggressiveness, they are less concerned with the immediate mechanisms that generate an effect than with the underlying evolutionary reason for its existence in the first place. When confronted with a sociobiological explanation for something, it is therefore quite reasonable to ask, "But *how* is this achieved?" At the same time, the fact that sociobiologists are more concerned with *why* than with *how* is not a weakness but simply a description of their science's primary concern. Ideally, a complete explanation of any biomedical phenomenon includes both how ("proximal causation") and why (evolutionary or "ultimate" causation).

Sociobiology is based on unjustified extrapolations from animals to human beings. Sociobiology began with the study of nonhuman animals, but it is not limited to them. Moreover, human beings are also animals; witness the value of animal models for the study of physiology, development, genetics, and even anatomy. Sociobiological extrapolations are no more egregious, and every bit as justifiable, as using mice to investigate cancer drugs or *Drosophila* to study biochemical genetics. Just as animal-based research is suggestive with respect to human implications, sociobiological insights derived from the study of social insects, birds, or mammals often point to parallel patterns among human beings. In no cases do sociobiologists argue that because species X engages in a particular behavior that it is necessarily characteristic of *Homo sapiens*. Rather, as in other research fields, animal findings—especially when confirmed in diverse species—can lead to useful generalizations that may well be applicable to human beings.

America was shocked by Freud's theory of sexuality and the unconscious, and yet, 100 years after publication, these ideas are mainstream. It is curious that Darwin's theory, 50 years older than Freud's, is still provocative and unacceptable to many, despite having become the cornerstone of modern biology. Both Freud and Darwin challenged basic human narcissism, the notion that human beings are so special that they are separate from the rest of the biological world. In the concluding paragraph of *The Origin of Species*, Darwin noted that "there is grandeur in this view of life." Darwinian psychiatry holds out the hope that there will also be grandeur—or at minimum, insight—in similarly viewing the mental life of *Homo sapiens*.

SUGGESTED CROSS-REFERENCES

The neural sciences are covered in Chapter 1 and genetics in Sections 1.17 and 1.18. Other relevant discussions are covered in Section 26.2, Adult Antisocial Behavior and Criminality, and in Section 5.4, Animal Research and Its Relevance to Psychiatry. Mood disorders are described in Chapter 13, anxiety disorders in Chapter 14, and personality disorders in Chapter 23.

References

Alcock J. *The Triumph of Sociobiology*. New York: Oxford University Press; 2001.

Alexander RD. *The Biology of Moral Systems*. Hawthorne, NY: Aldine de Gruyter; 1987.

Aureli F, de Waal FBM, eds. *Natural Conflict Resolution*. Berkeley, CA: University of California Press; 2000.

Axelrod, R. *The Evolution of Cooperation*. New York: Basic Books; 1984.

*Barash DP. *Revolutionary Biology, the New, Gene-Centered View of Life*. New Brunswick, NJ: Transaction Publishers; 2001.

Barash DP. *The Survival Game: How Game Theory Explains the Biology of Cooperation and Competition*. New York: Times/Holt; 2003.

Barash DP, Lipton JE. *Gender Gap: The Biology of Male-Female Differences*. New Brunswick, NJ: Transaction Publishers; 2001.

Barash DP, Lipton JE. *The Myth of Monogamy: Fidelity and Infidelity in Animals and People*. New York: Henry Holt; 2002.

*Barkow JH, Tooby J, Cosmides L, eds. *The Adapted Mind: Evolutionary Psychology and the Generation of Culture*. New York: Oxford University Press; 1992.

Birkhead TR, Möller AP, eds. *Sperm Competition and Sexual Selection*. San Diego: Academic Press; 1998.

*Buss DM. *Evolutionary Psychology*. Boston: Allyn & Bacon; 1999.

Daly, M, Wilson M. *Homicide*. Hawthorne, NY: Aldine de Gruyter; 1988.

*Dawkins R. *The Selfish Gene*. New York: Oxford University Press; 1989.

Ehrlich, PR. *Human Natures: Genes, Cultures, and the Human Prospect*. Washington, DC: Island Press; 2001.

Foerster K, Delhey K, Johnsen A, Lifjeld JT, Kempenaers B: Females increase offspring heterozygosity and fitness through extra-pair matings. *Nature*. 2003;425:714.

Hamilton WD: The genetical evolution of social behavior. I and II. *J Theor Biol*. 1964;7:1h.

Hariharan IK, Haber DA: Yeast, flies, worms, and fish in the study of human disease. *N Engl J Med*. 2003;348:2457.

Hrdy SB. *Mother Nature: Maternal Instincts and How They Shape the Human Species*. New York: Pantheon; 1999.

Konner M. *The Tangled Wing: Biological Constraints on the Human Spirit*. New York: Times Books; 2002.

Miller GF. *The Mating Mind*. New York: Doubleday; 2000.

Nesse, RM, Williams G. *Why We Get Sick: The New Science of Darwinian Medicine*. New York: Times Books; 1994.

Pinker S. *How the Mind Works*. New York: W. W. Norton & Co; 1997.

Pinker S. *The Blank Slate*. New York: Viking; 2002.

Ridley M. *The Red Queen: Sex and the Evolution of Human Nature*. New York: Macmillan; 1993.

Stevens A, Price J. *Evolutionary Psychiatry: A New Beginning*. London: Routledge; 1996.

Thornhill R, Palmer CT. *The Natural History of Rape*. Cambridge, MA: MIT Press; 2000.

Trivers RL: The evolution of reciprocal altruism. *Quart Rev Biol*. 1971;46:35.

Trivers RL. Parental investment and sexual selection. In: Campbell B, ed. *Sexual Selection and the Descent of Man*. Chicago: Aldine; 1972.

Trivers RL: Parent-offspring conflict. *Am Zool*. 1974;14:249.

Williams GC. *Adaptation and Natural Selection*. Princeton, NJ: Princeton University Press; 1964.

Wilson EO. *Sociobiology*. Cambridge, MA: Harvard University Press; 1975.

*Wilson EO. *On Human Nature*. Cambridge, MA: Harvard University Press; 1978.

Zahavi A, Zahavi A. *The Handicap Principle: A Missing Piece of Darwin's Puzzle*. New York: Oxford University Press; 1997.

▲ 4.4 Sociopolitical Trends in Mental Health Care: The Consumer/Survivor Movement and Multiculturalism

Sally L. Satel, M.D., and
Richard E. Redding, J.D., Ph.D.

Since the 1990s, two sociopolitical developments have left a substantial mark on mental health care: the "consumer/survivor" movement and multiculturalism. Consumer/survivors claim that psychiatrists make them sick, and their advocacy, funded in part by the federal government and state mental health agencies, has resulted in legal and policy initiatives that restrict the work of psychiatrists and care for the seriously mentally ill, including laws restricting involuntary treatment and electroconvulsive therapy (ECT). While consumer/survivors see themselves as the "last minority," women, sexual minorities, and ethnic minorities are the focus of multicultural therapy, which makes identity politics the central theme of therapy. The goal of these therapies is to foster the patient's understanding of how his or her psychological distress is due to oppression and social injustice.

This chapter provides an overview of these two influential developments in mental health care and illustrates the practical implications of these developments for psychiatric care and the mental health care system generally.

ORIGINS OF RADICAL CONSUMERISM

At the outset, it is important to distinguish between the mental health "consumer movement," which has been positive through empowering patients, increasing patients' involvement in their own health care (e.g., through consumer-run self-help groups and supportive services), reducing the perceived shame of mental illness, and lobbying efforts to achieve parity for mental health care, and the "consumer/survivor" movement, which has advanced a radical reform agenda aimed at reducing the availability of psychiatric care for the seriously mentally ill. Despite its modest head count, the consumer/survivor movement has exerted a significant sociopolitical influence on the mental health care system.

The radical consumer/survivor movement grew out of the 1960s liberationist ethos, which saw mental patients as a class of social dissidents and psychiatry as an agent of social control. In the words of Marxist social critic Herbert Marcuse, psychiatry was seen as "one of the most effective engines of suppression." Explanations for the origins of psychosis abounded. Some implicated psychiatry itself. According to Erving Goffman, author of the influential *Asylums* (1961), the mental hospital itself imposed "abasements, degradation, humiliation and profanations of the self," reinforcing the psychopathology it was meant to cure. Ronald David Laing, a Scottish psychiatrist, thought of psychosis as a rational adaptation to an insane world. In popular culture, films, such as *King of Hearts* (1966), and books, such as Ken Kesey's *One Flew over the Cuckoo's Nest* (1962), sentimentalized the insane as embodying truth, spontaneity, and innocence, their souls crushed by stone-hearted authoritarians. "Every psychotic is a potential sage or healer," wrote the physician Andrew Weil, later to become famous as an alternative medicine guru, in his 1972 book *The Natural Mind.* Although he eschewed mainstream psychiatry, Thomas Szasz, author of the 1960 classic *The Myth of Mental Illness*, is not an important figure in the consumer/survivor movement. Like Goffman, Laing, and Weil, all of whom acknowledge the reality of mental illness, Szasz does not even believe that severe mental illness exists. He views virtually all abnormal behaviors and cognitions as products of the will.

By 1974, the number of patients in psychiatric hospitals had been cut in half, from slightly more than 500,000 in the mid-1950s. Once released, many of these ex-patients understandably gravitated to one another. However, "in daily life they were shunned and stigmatized," wrote Rael Jean Isaac and Virginia Armat in *Madness in the Streets.* They found solace in "an ideology that cast them as romantic figures combating oppression, individuals whose perceptions of the world had equal if not greater validity than those of 'sane' society." The Insane Liberation Front was founded in 1970 in Portland, Oregon. In 1971, the Mental Patients Liberation Project and the Mental Patients Liberation Front appeared in New York and Boston, respectively. The next year, former patients in San Francisco organized the Network Against Psychiatric Assault and the Madness News Network. The first Conference on Human Rights and Psychiatric Oppression was held in Detroit in 1973. Today, the most vocal antipsychiatry consumer/survivor groups are the National Empowerment Center near Boston, the National Association for Rights Protection and Advocacy in Rapid City, South Dakota, and the Support Coalition in Eugene, Oregon.

Working with civil liberties lawyers and patients' rights groups, such as the Mental Health Law Project (which changed its name to the Bazelon Center for Mental Health Law in 1993), activists have lobbied to scale back commitment laws and block involuntary treatment laws from being passed or implemented. They have championed the right of severely ill patients to refuse treatment (representing the expressed wishes of their client/patients even when they are delusional) and campaigned against ECT. They have succeeded in getting lawmakers in a number of states, including California, Massachusetts, Tennessee, and Texas, to collaborate in writing and, in some cases, passing legislation restricting the availability of ECT. ECT has a bad public image, crystallized in many minds by the horrific scene in the 1975 film version of *One Flew over the Cuckoo's Nest.* In fact, ECT is one of the most effective treatments available for severe depression, yet some major public hospitals have stopped performing ECT, in large part because of pressure from consumer groups. When the first-ever surgeon general's report on mental health, issued in 1999, gave a clean bill of health to ECT, the consumer/survivor community was livid, the *New York Times* reported. "Your lies threaten to re-traumatize these survivors," wrote David Oaks in a letter to the surgeon general.

Consumer/survivor ideology has found expression in the protection and advocacy for the mentally ill programs created by Congress in 1986. Like so many other consumer/survivor–friendly enterprises, it is funded by the Center for Mental Health Services (CMHS). The 50 protection and advocacy programs, one for each state, were created to investigate allegations of abuse and neglect of mental patients in hospitals and group homes. Federal regulations required that protection and advocacy programs establish a mental health advisory council and that 60 percent of the council membership be current or former psychiatric patients or their family members—a good many of whom, no doubt, offer useful suggestions.

Indeed, many protection and advocacy programs have scored important victories, uncovering serious cases of mistreatment and enacting some valuable reforms. The New York State program, for example, was responsible for making Clozaril (clozapine), a highly effective but expensive antipsychotic drug, available to patients on Medicaid. But in some other states, the protection and advocacy programs have collaborated with civil liberties lawyers to obstruct patients' access to care. In late 1999, for example, Vermont's protection and advocacy program managed to overturn a law making it easier to medicate psychotic individuals.

A tragic example occurred in Texas in 1987. Despite a mother's warning to the protection and advocacy agency that her hospitalized and suicidal daughter wanted to leave the San Antonio state hospital, a protection and advocacy lawyer went to the daughter, ascertained her desire to leave, and then represented her. After her discharge was secured, the daughter killed herself. This story was reported to the authors of *Madness in the Streets* by Carmen Johnson, one of the few members of the Texas protection and advocacy advisory board who was not a recovering mentally ill person. What surprised Johnson even more than the girl's release and subsequent suicide was the board's reaction: They reported it as a "successfully closed case."

The American Psychiatric Association (APA) has also objected to the priorities of many protection and advocacy lawyers. "We are deeply concerned," the association wrote in a letter to Bernard Arons, director of CMHS, "that the critical element of protecting patients has been seriously under-emphasized." Little has changed, however. An item in the newsletter of the National Association of Protection and Advocacy Systems, *Protection and Advocacy Systems News,* rhetorically asks whether outpatient commitment is "prescription or persecution?" and answers, implicitly, that it is the latter. When protection and advocacy agencies have been unable to derail commitment policies, they adopt the useful role of watchdog, making sure the policies are fairly and efficiently applied. It is this kind of oversight that Congress intended as their mission all along.

Politicians are vulnerable to pressure from consumer/survivor groups. Budget-conscious politicians who want to save money are sympathetic to advocates who want to dismantle the expensive state institutions. Legislators get understandably nervous when told that their constituents' rights are being trampled, but they rarely know enough about the management of severe mental illness to evaluate the consumer/survivors' claims of having been abused through involuntary treatment policies. Such claims make them quick to grant concessions. In instances in which actual abuse or neglect has been uncovered, politicians are again quick to take the advice of vocal consumer/survivor groups, not realizing that their recommendations may only create more problems.

A less obvious dynamic contributing to the rise of the consumer/survivor movement is the behavior of psychiatrists themselves. One element to consider is the origin of CMHS. The agency had a modest $3.5 million beginning in 1977 as the Community Support Program within the National Institute of Mental Health (NIMH; part of the National Institutes of Health). It was created because of the widely appreciated inability of NIMH's Community Health Centers program to address the problems of the increasing numbers of severely mentally ill individuals being discharged from state psychiatric hospitals. The mandate of the Community Support Program, according to a 1978 report, was to coordinate services "for one particularly vulnerable population—adult psychiatric patients whose disabilities are severe and persistent." This mandate, which focused on severe mental illness, was quickly forgotten as the Community Support Program expanded to encompass all mental health issues.

In 1992, the Community Support Program and related activities of NIMH were transferred to the newly created CMHS when NIMH was reincorporated into the National Institutes of Health. CMHS, in turn, became a component of the Substance Abuse and Mental Health Services Administration, and its investment in social issues and patient rights continued, in many ways, to overshadow the clinical and administrative responsibilities of quality care for the extremely mentally ill.

Indeed, as Seymour Halleck observed in 1971, "[Many] envision community psychiatry as a political movement, as an effort to change the distribution of power . . . provid[ing] the psychiatrist with the opportunity to directly confront and perhaps change the oppressive institutions." More recently, Michael Fox, a community psychologist, urged: "The prevention of mental disorder must begin with widespread and expansive social reform in order to prevent the emotional distress and mental disturbance in our society that is due to dehumanizing social influences such as oppression, meaningless work, racism and sexism." Community psychiatrists and psychologists criticize "the hegemony exercised by the medical model and its concomitant conservatism." Traditional therapeutic approaches, such as psychodynamic or cognitive-behavioral therapy, are seen as blaming the patient and ignoring societal causes and solutions for mental illness.

Psychiatrists, and especially other mental health professionals, such as social workers, may be receptive to the consumer/survivor movement because of their personal ideologies. A number of surveys indicate that mental health professionals tend to have liberal sociopolitical values and beliefs. Many university psychology and psychiatry departments, for example, have no conservatives among the faculty or graduate student bodies. Liberal professionals are also vastly overrepresented among practicing clinicians.

Perhaps one's sociopolitical view is less likely to color the way he or she makes *Diagnostic and Statistical Manual of Mental Disorders* (DSM) diagnoses, prescribes medications, or conducts practical therapies such as cognitive-behavioral psychotherapy. After all, these activities are (or at least should be) driven by relatively objective guidelines, but attitudes about the nature of the clinician–patient relationship, the role of the individual in affecting his or her circumstances, and other dimensions that contribute to mental health do vary with one's position on the political spectrum. For example, political preferences have been linked to individual differences in early family experiences, personality style, foundational views about human nature, and self-identifications, with liberals tending to favor egalitarian–nurturing models of parenting and family life versus authoritarian–paternalistic models. Liberals tend to favor an egalitarian versus meritocratic social order, identify with the marginalized rather than the privileged, prioritize empathy over cost–benefit analyses, and ascribe causes of individual and social problems as much to environmental and social forces as to endogenous causes.

The liberal political orientation of mental health professionals has consequences. Liberal sociopolitical trends in American culture, such as identity politics, ideologies of oppression, and victimology—all embodied in the consumer/survivor movement—have gained wide currency in the mental health professions.

CONSUMER/SURVIVOR MOVEMENT TODAY

Midday on October 5, 1998, 46-year-old Margaret Mary Ray set her backpack and purse down by the railroad tracks in a small Colorado town. She then knelt in front of an oncoming coal train and was instantly killed. Ray, who had schizophrenia, had become infamous for stalking David Letterman, the television personality; she harbored the delusion that she was having a love affair with him. Ray's history of mental illness had been long and troubled. Since her 20s, she had been in and out of psychiatric hospitals and jails. On antipsychotic medication, she did well, but eventually, she stopped taking the medicine and quickly deteriorated. Two months before her suicide, she was arrested for the last time. At the hearing at which she was freed, the *New York Times* reported: "A judge openly lamented the absence of any legal mechanism to make sure she received medical help."

In fact, such a mechanism does exist. In a form of involuntary treatment called *outpatient commitment*, a court may order a regimen of therapy and medication, and the patient may be rehospitalized if he or she does not comply. Because of activism by a small but vocal group of former psychiatric patients, however, supported by civil liberties lawyers, thousands of people like Ray are not receiving the treatment they need to get well or at least to be safe. These activists call themselves "consumer/survivors" or "psychiatric survivors." The term *consumer* denotes a user of mental health services, and *survivor* refers to one who has endured psychiatric care. "Survivor" is not used in the same sense as "cancer survivor," says the psychiatrist and researcher E. Fuller Torrey. "Rather, it is being used like 'Holocaust survivor,' an individual who has been unjustly imprisoned and even tortured." Some consumer/survivors have requested that the mental health profession "make an apology to consumers for past abuses of power."

Some consumer/survivors go so far as to claim that psychiatrists make them sick. As Coni Kalinowski, a psychiatrist herself, and the consumer/survivor Darby Penney put it: "Ex-patients came to learn that their feelings of isolation, inadequacy, and powerlessness were the result of real practices within the mental health system—not products of their illnesses." They point to the deplorable history of the mental health system earlier in the 20th century, when negligence and even brutality were common in state psychiatric hospitals, but ignore the reforms that have virtually eliminated such abuses. The National Association of Consumer-Survivor Mental Health Administrators—a subcommittee of a group called *MadNation*—wants "an oversight board including consumers and survivors to inspect treatment facilities and mechanisms for grievances" and laws "to limit the powers of psychiatry by making consumers full partners in diagnosing and treatment."

But Jackie Parrish, a nurse who formerly served as director of community support programs at the federal CMHS, sees this type of partnership as merely a transitional phase. Consumer/survivor involvement in developing state mental health plans is good, Parrish believes, but it "is only an interim step to being totally consumer driven." Optimally, she says, the patients should become "the managers, and administrators—that is what will bring real change."

Parrish envisions peer-run services. Based on relationships of equality between peers, these services are a postmodern alternative to the traditional psychiatrist–patient relationship, which is condemned for perpetuating a power differential between the healthy, dominant doctor and the ill, dependent patient. MadNation sponsored an online referendum asking respondents to vote yes or no on the question: "Is the demonization of people diagnosed with mental illness a hate crime?" Cecilia Vergaretti of the Mental Health Association of Oregon extends the battle against power differentials beyond the mental health system, which, to her, is merely a microcosm of the larger universe of societal injustice. "This is not about reforming an ailing [mental] health care system," she says, "it's about reforming society."

Have some mentally ill people been treated insensitively, even maltreated, by psychiatrists and hospitals? Not for a minute. The authors would readily join with consumer/survivors if they worked toward weeding out incompetent clinicians or promoting more vocational rehabilitation, supported housing, and so forth. But the prospects of severely mentally ill people, such as Ray, should not be compromised by allowing consumer/survivors to be in charge of others' treatment.

FEDERAL FUNDING FOR THE CONSUMER MOVEMENT

The federal government and state mental health agencies across the country are giving moral and financial support to the consumer/survivor movement. Precisely how much money the CMHS has given to antipsychiatry efforts is difficult to determine. According to Torrey, as much as two-thirds of its $230 million or so annual discretionary funds (in fiscal year [FY] 2003) were being used to support such groups.

One of the biggest boosters is Arons, director of CMHS. Under him, CMHS funds the National Empowerment Center, an advocacy organization firmly opposed to psychiatric treatment. "Our primary physicians must be ourselves," writes Scott Snedecor, program manager of a consumer-operated drop-in center in Portland, Oregon, who claims that "medication can be worse than psychosis." Pat Deegan, a consumer activist and Snedecor's colleague at the Portland center, is interested in "rehabilitating mental health workers." She produced a project called "Spirit Breaking: How the Helping Professions Hurt." Paolo Del Vecchio, a CMHS consumer affairs specialist, explained why he and his colleagues oppose involuntary treatment: It reminds patients of "their own personal Holocaust and leaves them feeling hopeless, believing they will never recover."

Clearly, not all "consumer/survivors" are hostile to psychiatry, and many of their efforts are to be applauded.

> Ken Steele, a 52-year-old New York City man with schizophrenia who was profiled in a front-page story in the *New York Times* and who was writing a book about his life, sadly died in 2000, but his efforts are worth reporting. Steele simply wanted to see consumers more actively involved in the system. (Steele himself served on the boards of several mental health professional organizations.) He saw a psychiatrist and took the antipsychotic medication risperidone (Risperdal). When he began the medication in 1995, 1 year after it came on the market, the unseen voices that he had heard since the age of 14 years finally ceased. Steele published *New York City Voices,* a newspaper about mental health issues, and he counseled and hosted groups for people with schizophrenia to prevent them from lapsing into social isolation. As a self-identified consumer/survivor, Steele was an asset. He was not part of the radical element that denies the reality of mental illness, rejects medication, and will not acknowledge the need to intervene when individuals are seriously mentally ill and in need of treatment. Steele did not want to take over the system.

But the National Mental Health Consumers' Self-Help Clearinghouse, funded largely by the federal CMHS, promotes the work of the *radical* consumer/survivors. In the summer of 1999, the clearinghouse organized the National Summit of Mental Health Consumers and Survivors in Portland, Oregon. Among the major topics were seclusion and restraint and outpatient commitment. Both practices were deemed intolerable by the summit leadership.

Consumer/survivors have been spreading the word to other countries as well. In 1999, a group flew to Santiago, Chile, to attend the biannual meeting of the World Federation for Mental Health (an otherwise mainstream conference), courtesy of travel scholarships funded by CMHS.

> Among the scholarship recipients was David Oaks, director of the National Support Coalition International, based in Eugene, Oregon. Oaks, a Harvard graduate who experienced a psychotic episode as a young man, is staunchly opposed to psychiatry. He talks about having been a "guinea pig" for doctors and psychiatric drugs ("a hundred times worse than a bad acid trip") and vows to lead a "guinea pigs' rebellion." Oaks insists that mentally ill people can recover through diet, exercise, meditation, writing, and peer support. Most dramatically, he claims to have organized what coalition members call an "underground railroad" to help patients cross state lines to "escape forced outpatient psychiatric drugging." One month before the Santiago conference, he helped defeat several involuntary treatment bills under consideration by the Oregon legislature.

CMHS also publishes the *Consumer Affairs Bulletin,* in which the mental health system (the very system that the Center's block grants sustain) is portrayed as heartless and repressive. Here is an excerpt from an item by a consumer/survivor who calls herself Niyyah:

> I would like to share with you what life has been like for myself, my children, and my grandchildren as a consumer/survivor/patient. How race, sex, and disability have hurt us. I believe that racism, stigma, mentalism, poverty, victimization, homelessness, and institutionalization have contributed to a continued intergenerational cycle of needs and dependency. I am a woman who has survived every form of violence known to man, sexual incest, ritual abuse, neglect, and system abuse. I've also survived what many of us call re-traumatization. This happens when you try to get help and the doctors hurt you again. I've been misdiagnosed, beaten, battered, raped repeatedly, held hostage.

Federal tax money was also spent to get the consumer/survivor message to Congress and the president via the National Disability Council, an independent federal agency with 15 presidentially appointed and Senate-confirmed members. The council's recommendations for mental health services, released in early 2000, had on them the fingerprints of the radical consumer/survivors. This was not surprising because the public hearing at which the council listened to testimony was held onsite at the 1998 annual meeting of the National Association of Rights, Protection, and Advocacy, a vigorously antipsychiatry organization.

The title of the council report embodies the ethos of the consumer/survivor movement: "From Privileges to Rights: People Labeled with Psychiatric Disabilities Speak for Themselves." Yet, in other council documents, there is no reference to people *labeled* with physical disabilities. That is because physical disabilities can be seen; it is hard for any observer to dispute the reality of a wheelchair. But many psychiatric diagnoses, consumer/survivors argue, do not exist as fixed and defined entities. They are socially constructed and exist merely in the eyes of the beholders—namely, psychiatrists and other members of the dominant culture.

In a letter to former President Clinton, the council tried to portray involuntary treatment as a violation of the Americans with Disabilities Act. "All policies that restrict the rights of people with psychiatric disabilities simply because of their disabilities are inharmonious with basic principles of law and justice, as well as with such landmark civil rights laws as the Americans with Disabilities Act," wrote Marca Bristo, chairperson of the council. The council missed the vital point that psychosis itself, the very justification for involuntary interventions in the first place, can be "inharmonious" with the basic human impulse toward self-preservation. In its zeal to promote alternatives to medical and biochemical approaches, the council denounced ECT and insurance coverage for involuntary hospitalizations.

When President George W. Bush announced in 2002 the composition of the year-long New Freedom Commission on Mental Health, one of its 16 members was Daniel Fisher, director of the National Empowerment Center in Lawrence, Massachusetts. Fisher is a psychiatrist and says he is a recovered schizophrenic; the center he runs is considered one of the most radical in its outright discouragement of pharmaceuticals and promotion of herbal and other natural remedies for psychosis. He told a reporter for *U.S. News and World Report* that there is little evidence for a genetic or biochemical basis for severe mental illness. The charge of the New Freedom Commission is to advise the administration on improving the public mental health system.

"ALTERNATIVES" CONFERENCE

Since 1985, CMHS has funded an annual consumer/survivors' conference called *Alternatives*. At one conference, psychologist Al Siebert presented a talk entitled "Successful Schizophrenia: The Survivor Personality," advertised in the conference program as a discussion of "how schizophrenia is a healthy, valid, desirable condition, not a disorder." According to Siebert: "Schizophrenia has never been proven to be an illness or disease. What is called schizophrenia in young people appears to be a healthy transformational process that should be facilitated instead of treated." How ironical that CMHS is supporting a movement that minimizes the severity of mental illness and discourages the treatments and programs for which CMHS itself, in its role as the government's administrator of public funds for mental health treatment, is paying.

During the Alternatives 1999 conference, for instance, there were seminars on grassroots organizing and on creating openings for consumer/survivors on the boards of managed care organizations and other social services agencies. Consumer/survivors were given ample instruction on how to lobby congresspeople, stop involuntary commitment bills, and get more funding from the federal government. Everyone seemed to agree that the state-level success of the consumer/survivor movement had to be replicated at the national level.

There were dozens of personal testimonials about the abuses of the "system" and the triumphs of self-help. The "Memorial Wall" was meant to be a palpable reminder of the failure of organized psychiatry. Mounted on huge poster boards were scores of 3-in. × 5-in. cards, each a remembrance of someone who had died. It was a sad and touching display, yet one wonders how many of these people would still be alive if involuntary treatment laws were more widely in use.

To concede that involuntary treatment is sometimes necessary, however, was beyond the capacity of these consumer/survivors, who already felt so subjugated and powerless. A major theme of the meeting was that consumer/survivors are the "last minority." "I've always been struck by the similarities between our struggles and those of women, minorities, and homosexuals," said Jean Campbell, a consumer/survivor who is on the faculty of the University of Missouri School of Medicine in Columbia, Missouri. "We are all disempowered, stigmatized, discriminated against, denied our humanity."

Sally Zinman, of the state-funded California Network of Mental Health Clients, documented the experience of being a member of the last minority. In her study, funded by the state of California, Zinman discovered a "consumer/survivor culture" as recognizable as any ethnic culture. After interviewing 135 consumer/survivors in focus group settings, Zinman found that the most frequent self-descriptions were "second-class citizen," "stereotyped," and member of "another civil rights movement." Some spoke of being "celebrated" as mental health clients and others about the importance of "identify[ing] with their consumer culture."

Zinman works with ethnic diversity trainers teaching the personnel in managed care organizations about the consumer culture. A few months before the Alternatives 1999 conference, Zinman was one of a group of psychiatric "survivors" invited by Tipper Gore to participate in the White House Conference on Mental Health. Zinman had wanted to engage the vice president's wife in a candid discussion about consumer/survivors and offer her "critiques of a system that often does harm," as she wrote in an op-ed article, but she did not get the opportunity.

STATE-LEVEL CONSUMER MOVEMENTS

Currently, more than one-half of states have at least one paid position for a consumer in the central office of the state mental health department. So sympathetic to the consumer/survivors was Eileen Elias that, during her tenure as Massachusetts commissioner of mental health during the mid-1990s, she sent a memorandum to state hospital staff members instructing them to allow themselves to be put in restraints as an educational exercise. Subsequently, advisers to the National Association for State Mental Health Program Directors suggested that training for physicians, nurses, and social workers "might also include such first hand experiences as being admitted to an inpatient facility." Rodney E. Copeland, a psychologist and Vermont's commissioner of mental health, issued a mea culpa to the citizenry in which he said that the mental health profession was guilty of "over-emphasis on power, control, and paternalism."

State-employed consumer/survivors have access to high-level meetings. Their ability to use the political clout of their departments gives them considerable power over the administration of mental health services. Approximately 30 state mental health authorities have established offices of consumer affairs. These are generally staffed by consumer/survivors whose job, according to CMHS, is to "support consumer empowerment and self-help in their particular states." Federal block grants to states require the establishment of a mental health planning council in each state to monitor the allocation and adequacy of mental health services. At least one-half of the council staff members must be "adults with serious mental illness who are receiving (or have received) mental services" or family members of such people. At the federal level, CMHS created the Consumer/Survivor Subcommittee to assist its own National Advisory Council. "The creation of this subcommittee is a landmark occasion," said CMHS Director Arons. "[It] continues our efforts to promote consumer/survivor participation at every level of the mental health system."

Those committed to the radical consumer/survivor ethos are sometimes put in charge of state offices of patient affairs. Penney, the director of recipient affairs of the New York State Office of Mental Health and a member of MadNation's steering committee, is one. In 1992, she was appointed by the commissioner of mental health, Richard C. Surles, to advise him on the perspectives of consumer/survivors in policymaking. By all reports, she has consistently used her position to thwart compulsory treatment.

This was the experience of Paul F. Stavis, a lawyer who served as chief counsel of the New York State Commission on the Quality of Care for the Mentally Disabled. In 1995, Stavis was asked by Governor George Pataki to head an investigation of a high-profile killing by Ruben Harris, a 42-year-old man with a long history of schizophrenia and violence. He had run away from the Manhattan Psychiatric Center, stopped his medication, and started using drugs. Ten days later, he pushed Soon Sin, a Korean grandmother, into the path of a subway train.

"We did our review and advised the Office of Mental Health to compel high-risk patients to stay on the treatment regimens," Stavis said. His recommendation was straightforward: Simply revive the law on "conditional release," which had been on the books since 1919. This would allow a director of a psychiatric facility to release a psychotic patient, once successfully treated, on the condition that he or she complied with medication and other necessary treatment. The conditions often included abstaining from illicit drugs and alcohol as well. If the patient violated the agreement, he or she would be returned to the facility. "Penney fought us all the way," Stavis recalls, "And in the end, she prevailed upon the commissioner to disregard our proposal."

The authors affirm their conviction that individuals who have been very ill in the past with psychotic or severe mood disorders can do much that is positive. Steele, for example, lectured to patient groups, family members, and the public on the importance of medication compliance. Others occupy advisory spots with local mental health agencies; there is a group called *Schizophrenics Anonymous*. The difference between these consumers and members of the *radical* consumer/survivor movement is that they want to make the current system function better, not tear it down. Toward that end, they use public funds to sponsor drop-in centers, clubhouses, employment services, and peer-support and self-help groups, which can provide desperately needed opportunities for socialization and morale building.

Consumer-run organizations vary greatly in quality. "When government agencies first started to involve former patients in the early eighties in order to help in planning community services, I thought it was a good idea," says Torrey. "The tragedy is that the effort got hijacked by bureaucrats who were antipsychiatry and naturally gave funding to activist patients." Mentally ill individuals take a considerable risk if they mistakenly join one of the organizations that puts victim politics before their own clinical best interests. For example, some actively discourage patients from cooperating with the conventional mental health system and from taking medication. It is certainly true that some of the older antipsychotic medications, such as Thorazine (chlorpromazine), Mellaril (thioridazine), and Haldol (haloperidol), were once given in doses considered too high by today's standards. Psychiatrists used to increase doses abruptly; now they are increased more gradually. The side effects experienced by many patients, such as oversedation, "cotton headedness," muscle stiffness, and tardive dyskinesia spasms with the potential for uncontrollable movements, made them understandably leery of those medications. Now, dosing schedules are more refined, and the new antipsychotics produce fewer disabling side effects. But many consumer/survivors who had bad experiences with medication in the 1970s and 1980s are fighting an image of pharmacotherapy that no longer applies. Perhaps they do not realize how much things have changed.

DENYING THE REALITY OF MENTAL ILLNESS

The vast majority of severely mentally ill people can lead safe and comfortable lives in the community as long as they continue to take medication to control their psychotic symptoms. Without medication, however, some risk the fate of Ray, which is why outpatient commitment was developed. Such intervention can also interrupt the downward spiral into violence. True, only a small percentage of psychotic individuals ever inflict serious bodily harm, and when they do, it is mostly on other family members—but the assaults and killings that do occur are tragedies that often could have been avoided.

The potential for violence is a reality of mental illness that is not heard about very much. But 30 years of data show that psychotic individuals not taking medication are indeed more prone to violence. A study of 300 patients discharged from California's Napa State Hospital between 1972 and 1975 showed that their arrest rate for violent crimes was ten times higher than that of the general population. According to the Department of Justice, approximately one-fourth of all offspring who kill their parents have a history of serious mental illness. As University of Virginia School of Law professor John Monahan, the leading expert in violence risk assessment, summed it up:

> The data that have recently become available, fairly read, suggest the one conclusion I did not want to reach: Whether the measure is the prevalence of violence among the disordered or the prevalence of disorder among the violent, whether the sample is people who are selected for treatment as inmates or patients in institutions or people randomly chosen from the open community, and no matter how many social and demographic factors are statistically taken into account, there appears to be a relationship between mental disorder and violent behavior.

To be sure, the relationship between mental disorder and violence is relatively modest, and most severely mentally ill individuals are not violent. But after years of denying the association between untreated mental illness and aggression, the National Alliance for the Mentally Ill (NAMI) has come full circle. Carla Jacobs, an alliance board member from California, became an activist for involuntary commitment after her mother-in-law was fatally stabbed and shot by a mentally ill relative. "We used to think it was stigmatizing to acknowledge violence. Now we recognize that violence by the minority tars the majority and makes communities less likely to welcome the community-based housing that can facilitate treatment and reduce violence. Too many of our relatives are hurting others and winding up in jail," she laments. "The first step to helping the mentally ill lies in admitting there is a problem."

The connection between certain types of severe mental illness and violence seems to be a matter of common sense. But before the 1960s, when deinstitutionalization began in earnest, most of the severest cases were kept out of sight, and the public forgot how volatile some psychotic people can be. In the 1970s, patients' rights activists tried to reduce the stigma of mental illness, and rightfully so, but they downplayed the risk of violence. As they became better organized and more influential, the old commonsense view became increasingly controversial.

Reinstitutionalization on a grand scale certainly is not to be recommended. But more states need to enact laws that protect the person who is not yet helpless or dangerous but, as his or her family, doctors, or local police know from experience, is likely to deteriorate unless treated. A number of states allow authorities to hospitalize such people against their will, but judges are reluctant to do so.

States should uniformly require judges to consider past violence when deciding about commitment.

Obviously, treatment and specialized social services are of profound importance. There are still gaping holes in the treatment network in most states, and there desperately needs to be more community-based housing and case-worker programs. Insurance companies and the public hospital system, for example, routinely refuse to let patients stay in the hospital long enough to recover from a crisis. Even fixing such holes in the system, however, would not eliminate the need for involuntary treatment policies. The better the mental health system, the less the need for coercion, but that need will never go away entirely. Approximately one-half of people who are actively psychotic have minimal insight into their condition. Others know they need help but are too paranoid to seek it. Even when medicated, some remain unaware of their illness (although they feel much calmer and are less symptomatic). These people are not avoiding treatment because of the embarrassment of the "stigma" of schizophrenia, as is the popular belief among even mainstream mental health advocacy groups such as the National Mental Health Association. The truth is that they do not even know they are ill.

In 1989, Jonathan Stanley found himself standing naked on a milk crate in the middle of a Manhattan delicatessen. As he tells it: "Secret agents had been chasing me through the streets of New York for 3 straight days and nights. They had finally cornered me. Only the plastic milk crate insulated me from the deadly radiation aimed at the deli from the satellite dish across the street." Stanley was diagnosed with bipolar illness. With treatment, he was able to go to law school and graduate. "Without treatment, my world would be one of psychosis and delusion," he says. "I would most likely be homeless, in jail, or dead."

Frederick Frese, diagnosed with schizophrenia, tells this story:

I was first diagnosed with paranoid schizophrenia at the age of 25 years and experienced a series of some ten inpatient stays during the following decade. All but one admission was voluntary. I personally feel that I greatly benefited from being forced to accept treatment during periods in which I was incapable of understanding that I needed it. In fact, sometimes I wonder what would have become of me had someone not given me the treatment I so desperately needed but was so opposed to accepting.

Frese's recovery was so spectacular that he went on to earn a doctorate in clinical psychology and now works in a state hospital.

Data suggest that most patients who are coerced into the hospital later acknowledge that they needed the care. One recent study in the *American Journal of Psychiatry* interviewed patients 2 days after admission and then again several weeks later. At 2 days, almost one-half of all patients admitted involuntarily said that they had needed to be admitted. Only 5 percent had changed their minds when interviewed again several weeks later. Of the patients who initially felt that they did not need to be admitted (approximately 52 percent), approximately one-half had changed their minds a few weeks after admission, saying that the decision to hospitalize them against their will was justified. Thus, more than three-fourths of the study sample ultimately believed that their treatment had been warranted, although few expressed gratitude as effusively as Stanley and Frese.

NOT REALLY ALL THAT SICK?

One might reasonably ask: Could someone like Ray, David Letterman's stalker, hold a responsible position in a government agency? Of course not. The leaders of the radical consumer/survivor movement are relatively well functioning for those with serious mental illness. There apparently is no systematic survey of the diagnoses or current symptom profile of the movement's most active members, but it is safe to say that their activities require the energy, focus, and coherence that elude people who are hallucinating, incoherent, clinically paranoid, or unable to concentrate.

The radical consumer/survivors spend much of their time speaking to audiences, mobilizing activists, applying for grant money, organizing and attending conferences, lobbying politicians, and advising state and federal agencies involved with treatment and disability rights. In 2002, when the New Freedom Commission (appointed by President George W. Bush to help him "transform" the public mental health system) had public hearings, the radical consumers were there to testify. The commission prided itself on soliciting testimony from these individuals: "nearly every consumer . . . expressed the need to fully participate in his or her plan for recovery," said the commission report. When patients are able to participate in developing treatment goals, psychiatrists should indeed welcome it. But at least half of all patients with chronic psychosis do not acknowledge even needing treatment in the first place. These are among the sickest; the silent minority that is languishing in back bedrooms, jail cells, and homeless shelters—that is too paranoid, oblivious, or lost in madness to attend hearings, never mind testify.

Radicals fight to preserve the right of psychotic people to refuse medication, to ensure that hospitals abandon the use of restraints, and to overturn outpatient commitment laws. In doing so, they work against the best interests of those who are the most seriously ill, those too psychotic to competently refuse medication, too aggressive or confused to be safe without restraint, and too unreliable to take the medications that keep them from lapsing back into psychosis.

The point of imposing treatment is to help patients attain autonomy, to help them break out of the figurative straitjacket binding thought and will. So many people with untreated schizophrenia become incapable of facing even the modest challenges of ordinary life, much less exercising their rights as individuals. Being required to take medication is hardly a violation of the civil rights of a person who is too ill to exercise free will in the first place. The freedom to be psychotic is not freedom.

More effective treatments, both social and pharmacological, are available now than ever before in the history of psychiatry, and it is a shame when ill people are denied them. By supporting consumer/survivor activities or by simply saying nothing when they are given funding or administrative control, mental health professionals and administrators are promoting a movement that may have disastrous consequences for people with severe psychiatric illness.

Bernard Zuber, for one, is appalled by the rhetoric of activists who presume to speak for him. In 1952, when he was 19 years of age and living in Paris, he tried to commit suicide by hurling himself backward into the path of a taxi. He spent 8 years, from 1982 to 1989, in and out of psychiatric hospitals and jails, setting small fires, homeless and filthy on the street. ("I looked like Anthony Hopkins in the movie *Instinct*.") Then Zuber was admitted to the West Los Angeles Veterans' Hospital. He had cellulitis and was malnourished; he stayed mute and curled in a fetal position, refusing to eat. He denied wanting to kill himself because, as he told psychiatrists, "I'm already dead," convinced he had been killed years before under the wheels of that Parisian taxi. Clearly, he was in no position to give informed consent for treatment and would have died had his psychiatrists not petitioned the court to authorize surgery for an intestinal blockage that developed during the hospitalization. It was not until 1990 that the doctors diagnosed bipolar disorder; before then, his diagnosis had been depression.

Today, Zuber works as a clerk for a state agency. As an active member of the California NAMI, he also supports involuntary treatment, which he credits for saving his life. He is dismayed by the efforts of Ron Schraiber, the director of the Office of Consumer Affairs of the Los Angeles County Department of Mental Health. Zuber says that Schraiber is supposed to be advising the state's mental health director about helping people like him but instead is fighting against involuntary care. "Schraiber and the other consumer/survivors portray a medical issue as a civil rights issue," Zuber said. "Some even say they don't believe in the 'medical model' of mental illness. So what was happening to me? There wasn't something wrong with my brain? I just decided to live a certain way? Oh, please."

Another instance follows.

Moe Armstrong, a 54-year-old resident of Cambridge, Massachusetts, with schizophrenia, agrees with Zuber on the issue of compulsory care. Armstrong spent approximately 12 years in mental facilities. Many "professional consumers," as he calls them, really "don't have enough contact with sick people, and so they are not a true voice for us." Some people simply need to live in state hospitals, he insists, or should be highly supervised in programs like outpatient commitment.

Consumer/survivors, on the other hand, maintain that anyone can live independently with proper community supports that are individualized to the patient. Robert E. Nikkei, a social worker, and his colleagues describe this mind-set in an article in *Psychiatric Services*: "Living in the community is viewed as a civil right and a necessary antidote to the victimization, subtle and not-so-subtle, that has accompanied the status of mental patients in most Western industrialized cultures." As Fisher, the physician and former psychiatric patient, proclaims: "We are not cases, and we do not want to be managed. Instead we seek to work with personal care attendants like people with other disabilities." The state of Massachusetts shows how far accommodation can go: It bought a patient a house and supplied him with attendants 24 hours a day. He needed around-the-clock monitoring because one manifestation of his mental condition was habitual fire setting. The psychiatrist Jeffrey L. Geller, then medical director of the county adjacent to the one in which this patient resided, calculated that the arrangement cost $150,000 a year—more than three times the cost of supervising and caring for this individual in the state hospital.

Independent living proved deadly for Shirley Mattos of Modesto, California. In 1993, the 38-year-old Mattos was placed in a board and care home where she was to be under constant observation by case workers. A few months earlier, Mattos was admitted to Napa State Hospital because she had an odd habit of swallowing objects, such as pens and pencils, when she became angry or frustrated. Having undergone more than 50 operations to remove these objects, she still wanted to live independently. Approximately 1 year after Mattos and her lawyer secured her discharge from Napa State (over the objections of her psychiatrists), she swallowed a pencil and died soon after having surgery to remove it. "That year," said Dan Pone, Mattos's lawyer, "was probably one of the best, if not the best year, of her life. She was able to live out her dream."

Even for patients who do not require protection from themselves, independent living is not always the best approach. "It can be devastatingly lonely and isolated," Armstrong says. "Some people actually prefer a sanctuary—not all, but some." He thinks the mental health system needs "more humanity," but he does not want it dismantled. "I'll need medication and supervision for the rest of my life; I freely admit it. I wish others would."

State agencies and politicians may be erroneously assuming that those who claim to represent consumers are actually representative of them, explains D. J. Jaffe, a founder of the Treatment Advisory Center, which advocates the benefits of involuntary treatment for the severely mentally ill. "The people I most worry about are the ones who are too psychotic to even know they are ill," Jaffe says.

Jaffe's statement describes approximately one-half of all individuals with schizophrenia. The condition of being unaware of one's illness and impairment is called *anosognosia* and is strongly linked to poor medication compliance. But the radical consumer/survivors would let people like Larry Hogue live on the streets. Dubbed the "Wild Man of Ninety-Sixth Street," Hogue terrorized the Upper West Side of Manhattan in the early 1990s by screaming at people, lunging out at them from between parked cars, and destroying property. Homeless and mentally ill, he became violent when he used crack cocaine, but local judges released him to the streets as soon as he was not overtly dangerous. On release, he stopped his medication, used cocaine, and ended up back in jail or in the psychiatric emergency department in a cycle that went on for years.

Or consider the case of Joyce Brown, who, in 1987, became a test case for civil liberties. Homeless and wildly psychotic, screaming obscenities and smeared with her own excrement, Brown was taken against her will to New York's Bellevue Hospital. In the legal battle over whether Brown, 40 years of age at the time, could be released, the presiding judge, Robert Lippman, sided with Brown, who called herself a political prisoner and was represented by the New York Civil Liberties Union (NYCLU). Society, not Brown, was sick, Judge Lippman insisted, declaring that "the blame and shame must attach to us." After her discharge, the NYCLU employed her for a while as a receptionist. It also helped arrange a speaking engagement for her at Harvard Law School; the title of her talk was "The Homeless Crisis: A Street View."

Soon, however, Brown was back living over the steam grate she called home. For a while in the early 1990s, her family had no idea where she was, but acquaintances told the *New York Times* that she lived in a group home. She was back at Bellevue at least once, but as of the spring of 2000, she was not in an institution, according to Norman Siegel of the NYCLU. As he had promised Brown, he did not give out details about whether she was working or living in a group home. Some have wondered whether she suffered from her brush with fame. "All the exposure, going to Harvard and all, in the end was very detrimental in terms of coming to terms with who she really is," says Joan Olson, director of an agency that once provided housing for Brown. Robert Gould, Brown's former psychiatrist, agrees. "In retrospect, it was too much."

The sickest patients are likely oblivious to or uninterested in consumer/survivor politics, but other patients are very much aware of it and feel excluded from the universe of CMHS-funded consumers. According to "Susan," who functions reasonably well on medication, drop-in centers are sometimes run by radical consumers who treat the "lesser clients," referring to people like herself, no better than psychiatrists have supposedly treated them—with imperiousness and disrespect. Susan's description of one radical consumer-run operation invokes an arrangement organized, unconsciously, of course, around the Freudian principle of identification with the aggressor. Susan writes:

> I do not want to be warehoused in one of their drop-ins while they get federal money to attend conferences, sit on boards to declare they represent me, and they become head staff of drop-ins while the lesser clients mop the floors and mow the neighbors' lawns. They offer the lesser clients donuts and coffee and free bus rides to state capitals to scream in protest, but you are only bussed if you parrot their cause . . . . Instead of going out into the market to get an education or a job, they dominate the system with demands; it is a business to them . . . the true clients do not run the drop-in center. They become the slaves, mopping floors, doing dishes while the power-hungry sit on boards telling us they represent us . . . . They tell me my therapist is trying to poison me [with medication] which is not true . . . she is very nice.

VOICES AGAINST CONSUMER/SURVIVORISM: THE FAMILY MOVEMENT

One of the voices against the antipsychiatry extremism of consumer/survivors is the so-called family movement led by the NAMI. Begun in 1978 by parents seeking services for their severely mentally ill children, NAMI and the consumer/survivors have clashed bitterly over the virtues of involuntary treatment. The alliance lobbies for treatment services and research into diseases, such as schizophrenia and bipolar illness, and is vocal about tightening involuntary treatment laws. As of 2001, it had 195,000 members, 70 percent of whom have adult children with schizophrenia or bipolar illness.

Consumer/survivors paint NAMI as parents seeking to control their children and, in part, to alleviate their own guilt at having raised a child who developed a mental illness. Sylvia Caras, a disability rights advocate and former psychiatric patient in Santa Cruz, California, says that families find "exoneration" when medications are prescribed for their children. Pharmacology then becomes the parents' way to "medicate social disarray." Caras has felt "their shunning since I started publicly to reformulate what I thought about my own experiences with the mental health system." She condemns families who commit family members to treatment as intent on silencing them. Because these parents acknowledge the occasional need for restraints, sedation, or seclusion, Caras accuses them of endorsing practices that have a "chilling effect on civil rights." Today's mental health approaches, she declares, "will be remembered along with the Salem witchcraft trials as a dishonorable scapegoating of transformative experiences."

Consumer/survivors also lobby strenuously against extending insurance coverage, including Medicare and Medicaid, to hospitals that care for involuntarily committed patients. The Anti-Psychiatry Coalition, a Midwestern volunteer group of "people who feel we have been harmed by psychiatry," goes a step further. The group lobbied hard in Massachusetts to defeat a bill that would have required that psychiatric services be covered on the same basis as other medical and surgical care. As the coalition proclaimed

> Mental health parity [coverage] will encourage more human rights violations: unnecessary psychiatric incarceration ("hospitalization"), harmful psychiatric drugs unnecessarily imposed on people against their will, more brain-damaged people by psychiatry's drugs and electroshock, more people with unjustified psychiatric stigma for the remainder of their lifetimes. Contrary to popular belief, psychiatry is not health care. It is a form of social control.

Radical consumer/survivors can be counted on to reject proposals that NAMI favors. Mental health courts are one such innovation. The first one was started in Broward County, Florida, in 1997. The courts are a diversionary program for mentally ill nonviolent offenders; instead of going to jail, they are "sentenced" to treatment, and the judge keeps a close eye on the patient/offender to make sure he or she complies.

With approximately 10 to 15 percent of jail inmates nationwide known to be mentally ill individuals who were arrested for disruptive behaviors that could have been controlled with medication or supervision, these courts could make a real impact. Patient/offenders could be ushered into supervised treatment and kept out of jail (where they are often brutalized by other patients). Meanwhile, jail crowding would be relieved—and the crowding can be extreme. "The nation's largest mental institution," is how the *New York Times* referred to the Los Angeles County Jail. On any given day in the spring of 2000, it held more than 2,000 inmates who had severe mental illness. The largest mental institution in California, Patton State Hospital in San Bernardino County, has approximately 1,200 patients.

Mental health courts are gaining popularity. There were plans in Congress to offer grants through the U.S. Attorney General's office to set up and evaluate 25 of the courts between 2000 and 2005. King County in Washington unveiled its mental health court in the winter of 1999, and the NAMI of Multnomah County, Oregon, has proposed establishing one. The Oregon proposal immediately sparked panic in the state's consumer/survivor community. "What's next," asked Pat Risser, a consumer/survivor, "'African-American' courts, or maybe 'gay and lesbian courts'?" Judi Chamberlin of the National Empowerment Center nominated "apartheid courts." These sentiments reflect the consumer/survivors' collective self-image as "the last minority."

To be sure, not all psychiatric patients oppose involuntary treatment, reject psychiatric medication, or regard mental illness as a transformative experience.

"You get excommunicated from the consumer/survivor movement if you speak against the status quo," says Eve, a former psychiatric patient who works with a visiting nurse service in New York City. Most of her patients have schizophrenia or bipolar illness. Thirty-eight years of age, married, and the mother of a 7-year-old daughter, Eve spent much of her late adolescence institutionalized. After her daughter was born, her post-partum depression was treated with ECT. Several years later, she had another bout of depression and agreed to have ECT again. Now she takes an antidepressant and a mood stabilizer and is doing well. Eve was once active with the radical consumer/survivor movement but is reluctant to disagree openly lest she be frozen out altogether. She departs from the consumer/survivor party line in two ways. She favors involuntary commitment (approximately one-half of her patients are under court order to receive treatment and take medications), and she sees value in ECT. Eve tells of a tenant of a housing program who stopped his antipsychotic medication, began hallucinating, and went back to using crack cocaine. Psychotic and aggressive, he got into a fight and broke his arm—a stroke of luck because it landed him in the hospital. Otherwise, Eve says, the housing director would have "just let him deteriorate, because that was what her politics said she should do."

It is at this level of day-to-day management that ideology overrides clinical judgment with frightening consequences. Many clinicians report similar stories: Patients stop taking their medication and then become too psychotic to remain in supervised housing. The "compassionate" response of the consumer-friendly management has been to *evict* these patients rather than obtain court orders for treatment. Consumer/survivor advocacy groups, such as the Bazelon Center for Mental Health Law, insist that treatment not be required as a condition of residence, and they are quite adept at creating legal and political obstacles for facilities that do not comply.

In their essay "Housing as a Tool of Coercion," Henry Korman and his colleagues at Cambridge and Somerville Legal Services in Massachusetts denounce residence contracts that require treatment. Although they properly stress that treatment plans must be flexible enough to accommodate changes in a person's clinical status, they do not realize that individuals sometimes require involuntary treatment to remain stable. "The only real means of ending compelled acquiescence to treatment in [residential facilities] is to separate housing from receipt of services," they write. "Principles of equal treatment forbid intrusion into the zone of privacy defined by the home."

Thus, Korman effectively undercuts the value of specialized housing for the mentally ill. His rights-based solution would return us to the days when the mental health system was hopelessly fractured (more so than it is today), and thousands of sick people dropped through the cracks and onto the streets. Furthermore, a lax housing scheme spells disaster for public relations. For example, when the consumer-run Collaborative Support Programs Inc. tried to establish a residence in a Clifton, New Jersey, neighborhood in 1998, the townspeople refused to allow it. They knew that program housing did not have a treatment requirement, and they had visions of unmedicated patients wandering the neighborhood or, worse, becoming aggressive—a scenario that might well have come to pass had Korman's vision been realized.

MULTICULTURAL THERAPIES

Consumer/survivors may see themselves as the "last minority," but women and ethnic groups have also had a significant sociopolitical influence in mental health care. Multicultural and feminist therapies have made identity politics the central theme of therapy. One goal of these therapies is to foster the patient's understanding of how his or her psychological distress is due in large part to oppression and social injustice. Feminist approaches, for instance, variously espouse raising patients' consciousness that patriarchal society and sex-role stereotyping are responsible for their psychological distress and encouraging the development of a feminist or lesbian ideology.

The feminist therapist is also an activist. "We are aware of the limitations that racism, sexism, classism, anti-Semitism, ageism, heterosexism, ablebodiedism, and other oppressions impose on groups and individuals," reads a statement of the Feminist Therapy Institute in Portland, Oregon. To "ally ourselves with those who are dedicated to building a society free from oppression," the institute urges therapists to get involved in "public education—lobbying for legislative action and other appropriate activities." Some feminist therapists encourage patients to take political action. "How would you encourage [your patients] to take social and political action?" asks a textbook written for students studying feminist therapy. One article on ethical issues in feminist and multicultural therapies states that "essential for the success of such therapies is the demand by psychologists for changes not only from clients, but from the general society." Ultimately unsuccessful, feminist therapists had even proposed to the DSM-IV-TR Revisions Task Force a new diagnostic category called "delusional dominating personality disorder" to describe a dysfunctional form of male personality.

Feminist therapy is becoming increasingly popular. Graduate training programs in clinical psychology offer specialty tracks in "feminist practice," and university-run student health centers routinely hire feminist therapists to counsel undergraduates. Fledgling clinical psychologists taking the licensing examination are expected to study feminist therapy. The board review preparatory manual of the Association for Advanced Training in the Behavioral Sciences devotes an entire section to it. The American Psychological Association features feminist therapy along with more traditional techniques in its information to the public on the kinds of psychotherapies conducted by psychologists.

Just as feminist therapists may think of their patients as battling the patriarchy, multicultural counselors may assume that their patients are struggling against racism. Multicultural counseling grew out of the civil rights–era efforts to integrate black men into the workforce. A 1950 article published in the *Journal of Clinical Psychology* introduced the topic of psychotherapy for minority patients. Titled "The Negro Patient in Psychotherapy," it raised two important questions: What is the nature of the relationship between a minority patient and a white therapist he perceives as racist? And can a white therapist respond to a minority patient as an individual rather than as a member of a minority group?

The goal in 1950 was to move beyond race and treat all patients as individuals and to appreciate the role of race in personal identity and interpersonal relationships. Today's multicultural counseling, in contrast, frequently goes a step further and argues for treating minority patients as members of a group. Elaine Pinderhughes nicely captures this perspective in her book *Understanding Race, Ethnicity and Power.* A psychiatric social worker, Pinderhughes condemns psychotherapists who practice what she calls a "white, middle-class model of therapy" that "has valued individual responsibility, looking inward, self-understanding and insight, personal growth and change, resolution of dependency needs, verbal and emotional expressiveness, and thinking problems through." According to Pinderhughes, "Non-white, non-middle-class cultures" may be more likely to benefit from hands-on approaches, advice giving, and "change efforts directed toward the environment." Her recommended approach has merits, but advice giving aimed at making practical changes in the patient's environment is often helpful regardless of the patient's race.

Like feminist therapy, multicultural counseling promotes activism. At the American Counseling Association (ACA) 1999 world conference in San Diego, many members voiced approval of the move to incorporate social activism into the formal role of the professional counselor. A new division called *Counselors for Social Justice* recently joined the ACA with the goal of "eradicating oppressive systems of power and privilege [and] the implementation of social action strategies." In 1998, the association published a book, *Social Action: A Mandate for Counselors.*

Before counselors can become activists, they should undergo sensitivity training. The "Multicultural Counseling Competencies" devised by the Association for Multicultural Counseling and Development focus on race and ethnicity, stating that "white counselors [must] understand how they may have directly or indirectly benefited from individual, institutional and cultural racism." Some multicultural practitioners are pessimistic that counselors can help patients unless the counselors themselves undergo these soul-searching exercises. At the 1998 ACA world conference, Robbie J. Steward and her colleagues at Michigan State University in East Lansing, Michigan, focused on the experiences and attitudes of counselor trainees. They puzzled over "white trainees who, for reasons we do not quite understand at this time, are perceived as multiculturally competent by minority clients before receiving multicultural counseling training or course work."

The textbooks, too, assume that trainees may be racist. *Counseling the Culturally Different* asks the reader: "As a member of the White group, what responsibility do you hold for the racist, oppressive, and discriminating manner by which you personally and professionally deal with minorities?" The textbook's authors insist that "without a strong anti-racism training component, trainees (especially Whites) will continue to deny responsibility for the racist system that oppresses their minority clients."

This may encourage impressionable trainees to expect that minority patients may be hostile. It may also inculcate the kind of guilt-ridden attitude manifested by "Paul," a subscriber to the multicultural counseling mailing list server: "While it remains important to bring experiences of oppressed people to the fore, I believe this must be balanced by engaging members of privileged groups in a conversation about their roles and responsibilities regarding [homophobia and heterosexism] . . . . I, as a white person . . . must identify racism as my disease as I am part of an institution that gains power by it."

This is the kind of sentiment that prompted Robert E. Wubbolding, professor of counseling at Xavier University in Ohio, to remark: "I am convinced that the multicultural movement is largely negative. I suggest graduate students ask their professors to spend at least as much time on the positive aspects of society as they do on racism, bigotry, and prejudice." How can counselors help their patients overcome outlooks that are bleak and hopeless, Wubbolding wonders, if young counselors are being trained to see patients as set on by such dark societal forces? "I can't think of a better way to hold minorities back than to teach that everyone is biased, prejudiced, racist, and bigoted. It engenders an 'I can't' worldview in clients," he says.

Another potential problem with multicultural counseling is that it may reify ethnic stereotypes. Consider the following examples from textbooks on multicultural counseling:

The worldview of the culturally different client boils down to one important question: "What makes you any different from all the others out there who have oppressed and discriminated against me?"

The Asian American's "greater social awareness causes him/her to be somewhat more sensitive to racism and to often react with overt anger or militance."

"Time is not a fundamental variable [for Hispanics]; do not ask a [Hispanic] client reasons for being late to therapy."

"Avoid linking mental problems [of African Americans] to parents' behaviors; these problems result from environmental conflicts in society."

To be sure, a multicultural perspective has many benefits. Culture has a considerable influence on personal identity, and here multicultural and feminist therapies play an important and valuable role in considering the role of racial, ethnic, or gender issues in therapy, mental health, and interpersonal and psychological functioning. But race and gender are only several influences among a multitude, and they do not predictably determine the nature of one's distress nor the formula for its amelioration. By evaluating cultural influences the same way they evaluate every other influence—individually, one patient at a time—therapists can avoid the confusion that is the byproduct of the group stereotyping found in various textbooks. To some degree, of course, all counseling relationships are "cross-cultural" relationships. No person can fully "know" the reality of another's life, no matter how similar their lives may be in outward appearance.

A student named Regina innocently succumbed to that confusion. Here is the message she posted on the diversity counseling mailing list server:

> I am a graduate student in a counseling program . . . . Is it difficult to work with [a patient] whose values and beliefs may be unknown or completely different from yours? I have a dilemma. I have lived long enough in the Middle East, Italy, Belgium, Poland, and other countries so that I consider myself an individual with a multicultural background. Every client in my caseload will be an individual with a different background from my own. Do you think it will be possible for me to be an effective counselor with such a background?

Regina's query epitomizes the downside of multiculturalism in therapy. Here we have a dedicated student with a wonderful breadth of cultural and linguistic experiences. *There must be some counseling formula I can memorize,* she is thinking, *that will tell me what to do if my ethnic background is A and my client's ethnic background is B.* If so, Regina is doomed. After all, every client belongs to numerous groups. "It does not take much imagination to recognize that the number of combinations and permutations of these groups is staggering," notes C. H. Patterson, emeritus professor of counseling at the University of Illinois.

Indeed, as Patterson points out, attempting to develop different theories, methods, and techniques for each of these groups would be an insurmountable task. Have Regina's professors taught her that the individual, with his or her unique emotions, cognitions, actions, and spirituality, is the focus of counseling? Has she learned that a keen interest in her patients and her kindness to them may transcend the specifics of culture? How helpful is the multicultural perspective when it obscures the true purpose of therapy: to help patients observe themselves, understand and take responsibility for their choices, and appreciate how they unwittingly get in the way of their own happiness and accomplishment? Critics of multicultural therapy have questioned the assumption that a minority client's presenting problems are linked to his or her ethnicity or that race, ethnicity, and gender are the most relevant aspects of cultural diversity for informing clinical case conceptualization and treatment. As Kenneth Thomas and Stephen Weinrach observe, the focus on race and ethnicity only perpetuates stereotyping and "is too limiting a notion with which to conceptualize what any given human being is all about" and that the "within-group differences among clients having similar gender, ethnic, and social characteristics are almost always more variable than between-group differences."

WHAT MULTICULTURAL THERAPY OVERLOOKS: SOCIOPOLITICAL DIVERSITY

"The clinical is political" for these therapists. But is it ethical? There are myriad ethical and legal concerns raised by therapies that promote sociopolitical agendas. In some cases, patients are not explicitly informed of the therapist's political agenda, raising the problem of informed consent. The patient's uniqueness may be subordinated to his or her racial, gender, or sexual identity, thus treating the patient as a member of a victimized or oppressed class rather than as an individual with unique strengths and abilities.

As studies have shown, therapists' sociopolitical values influence clinical assessment and diagnosis, treatment goals, therapeutic interventions, relationships with patients, and assessments of treatment progress. One of the most robust findings in social psychology is that people tend to have affinity for those who share their values and may be resistant to those whose values differ substantially from their own. Thus, the therapeutic relationship—a dyadic interaction between two value systems—may be adversely affected when the therapist fails to understand and appreciate the sociopolitical values of the patient. Research on treatment effectiveness has consistently shown that the therapeutic bond between patient and therapist is a central determinant of treatment success—understanding, appreciating, and empathizing with patient values is critical. Therapists who share or appreciate their patients' basic values are more likely to understand and empathize with the patient and, when appropriate, enlist the patients' values as agents for therapeutic change. One study found that the ideological match between the therapist and patient significantly affected the therapist's empathy for the patient, with politically liberal therapists having less empathy for conservative patients and vice versa. A common frame of reference, trust, and mutual liking between patient and therapist is more likely to develop when there is a basic congruence in values. Yet, if, as multicultural therapists believe, human identity is culture dependent, then sociopolitical values are an important aspect of culture and identity that they often overlook.

Multiculturalists have not yet embraced differing political values (including conservative values) under the rubric of "diversity." But studies suggest that sociopolitical values may be far more important than race, gender, or socioeconomic status. As Edward Shafranske and H. Newton Maloney observe: "Belief in a common vision of reality, or rather a shared, social construction of reality, may be a far more potent social glue than the color of one's skin, cultural heritage, or gender."

Finally, clinical training is adversely affected when therapists are inappropriately molded or evaluated on political grounds. Because many issues (e.g., spousal abuse, unwanted pregnancy, childrearing, substance abuse, lifestyle choices, gender relations, and sexual harassment, to name only a few) discussed in therapy implicate moral and sociopolitical values, becoming a psychotherapist necessarily entails critical introspection about one's own values and how those may be played out as a therapist through transference, countertransference, clinical judgment, and relationships with patients. The lack of diverse sociopolitical views among clinical educators and supervisors, along with the exclusion or marginalization of conservatives and their views, makes it difficult or uncomfortable for students to explore or express conservative views and to experiment with conservative paradigms. This chilling effect interferes with learning and creativity and may reduce therapists' self-efficiency or make them reluctant to participate in multicultural training. Without question, it leaves therapists less prepared for work with patients of diverse sociopolitical values.

SUGGESTED CROSS-REFERENCES

Cultural psychiatry is discussed in Section 4.1 and sociology in Section 4.2. Mental health services research is covered in Section 5.3. Some of the major disorders discussed in this section are covered in Chapter 12, Schizophrenia and Other Pyschotic Disorders; Chapter 13, Mood Disorders; and Chapter 15, Anxiety Disorders.

REFERENCES

Cuellar I, Paniagua FA, eds. *Handbook of Multicultural Mental Health.* San Diego: Academic Press; 2000.

Gardner W, Lidz CW, Hoge SK: Patients' revision of their beliefs about the need for hospitalization. *Am J Psychiatry.* 1999;156:1385.

Gibson-Leek M: Client vs. client. *Psychiatr Serv.* 2003;54:1101–1102.

Halleck SL. *The Politics of Therapy.* New York: Science House; 1971.

*Isaac RJ, Armat VC. *Madness in the Streets: How Psychiatry and the Law Abandoned the Mentally Ill.* New York: Free Press; 1990.

Kaufman CL. An Introduction to the Mental Health Consumer Movement. In: Horowitz AV, Scheid TL, eds. *A Handbook for the Study of Mental Health: Social Contexts, Theories, and Systems.* New York: Cambridge University Press; 1999.

Korman H, Engster D, Milstein BM. Housing as a Tool of Coercion. In: Dennis DL, Monahan J, eds. *Coercion and Aggressive Community Treatment.* New York: Plenum Press; 1996.

Lakin M: Some ethical issues in feminist-oriented therapeutic groups for women. *Int J Group Psychother.* 1991;41:199.

Monahan J: Mental disorder and violent behavior. *Am Psychologist.* 1992;47:511.

Monahan J, Swartz M, Bonnie J: Mandatory community treatment: pros and cons. *Health Affairs.* 2003;22:28–38.

Negy C: A critical examination of selected perspectives in multicultural therapy and psychology. *Psychology.* 1999;36:2.

New Freedom Commission on Mental Health: Achieving the promise: transforming mental health care in America. July, 2003. Available at: http://www.mentalhealthcommission.gov. Accessed November 4, 2003.

Nikkei RE, Smith G, Edwards D: A consumer-oriented case management project. *Psychiatric Serv.* 1992;43:577.

Paniagua FA. *Assessing and Treating Culturally Diverse Clients: A Practical Guide.* Thousand Oaks, CA: Sage Publications; 1994.

Prilleltensky I: The politics of abnormal psychology: Past, present, and future. *Pol Psycho.* 1990;11:767.

*Redding RE: Sociopolitical diversity in psychology: The case for pluralism. *Am Psychologist.* 2001;56:205.

Richards PS, Rector JM, Tjeltveit AC. Values, spirituality, and psychotherapy. In: Miller WR, ed. *Integrating Spirituality Into Treatment: Resources for Practitioners.* Washington, DC: American Psychological Association; 1999.

Rodis PT, Strehorn KC: Ethical issues for psychology in the postmodern era: Feminist psychology and multicultural therapy. *J Theoret Philos Psychol.* 1997;17:13.

*Satel S. *PC, M.D.: How Political Correctness Is Corrupting Medicine.* New York: Basic Books; 2000.

Shafranske EP, Maloney HN. Religion and the Clinical Practice of Psychology. In: *Religion and the Clinical Practice of Psychology.* Washington, DC: American Psychological Association; 1996.

Steadman HJ, Mulvey EP, Monahan J, Robbins PC, Appelbaum PS, Grisso T, Roth LH, Silver E: Violence by people discharged from acute psychiatric inpatient facilities and by others in the same neighborhoods. *Arch Gen Psychiatry.* 1998;55:393.

*Sue GW, Sue D. *Counseling the Culturally Different: Theory and Practice.* 3rd ed. New York: John Wiley and Sons; 1999.

Szegedy-Maszak M. Consuming passion: The mentally ill are taking charge of their own recovery. But they disagree on what that means. *US News & World Report.* 2002;Jun 3.

Thomas KR, Weinrach SG: Multiculturalism in counseling and applied psychology: A critical perspective. *Ed Child Psychol.* 1999;16:470.

*Torrey EF. Hippie healthcare policy. *Washingtonian Monthly.* 2002;Apr.

Weinrach SG, Thomas KR: Diversity-sensitive counseling today: A postmodern clash of values. *J Counsel Dev.* 1998;76:115.

Weinrach SG, Thomas KR: A critical analysis of the multicultural counseling competencies: Implications for the practice of mental health counseling. *J Mental Health Counsel.* 2002;24:20.

Wester SR, Vogel DL: The emperor's new clothes: Sociopolitical diversity in psychology. *Am Psychol.* 2002;57:295.

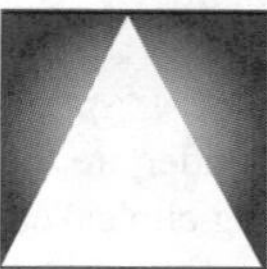

5 Quantitative and Experimental Methods in Psychiatry

▲ 5.1 Epidemiology

Juan E. Mezzich, M.D., Ph.D., and
Tevfik Bedirhan Üstün, M.D., Ph.D.

GENERAL CONCEPTS

Epidemiology is one of the fundamental sciences of public health and a major approach to the understanding and advancement of medicine and health care. Epidemiology is a useful tool for clinicians to link their work to populations and complete the clinical picture. It provides a perspective about the health of the general population, including the causes and courses of these illnesses. As the concept of health is undergoing discernible expansion, the subject and methods of epidemiology require growing differentiation and refinement. Consequently, it is important that epidemiology be understood and discussed in a comprehensive manner so as to potentiate the fulfillment of its mission and broad objectives.

In line with the above perspectives, this chapter on psychiatric epidemiology, although concise, attempts to take a broad look at its subject matter. It starts with an examination of its definition, evolution, and context, striving for a capsular understanding of the fundamentals of this burgeoning field, as well as of its historical and cross-sectional contextualization. It proceeds to review the methods of epidemiology, including its key constructs and variables, the design of epidemiological studies (issues and types), and the properties, forms, and validation of epidemiological instrumentation. Next, some important epidemiological findings are presented and commented on as they deal with the distribution of mental disorders and its related factors, of disability and the burden of disease, and of the positive aspects of health (functioning, social supports, and quality of life), as well as findings concerning the application of epidemiological methods to health care and the formulation and evaluation of health policies. The final section explores future perspectives, including the integration of genetic and environmental analyses, a fuller consideration of the social matrix and cultural frameworks, and the more active use of innovative informational, and communication technologies, all these contributing to the broadly based development of international classification and diagnostic systems for health and their effective use for health restoration and health promotion at clinical and population levels.

Definitions of Epidemiology and Psychiatric Epidemiology The etymological roots of epidemiology include *epidemics* (diseases visiting a community) and *logos* (their study). This and the consideration of the origins of epidemiology within the medical field seem to have led the *Random House Dictionary of the English Language* to define epidemiology narrowly as "the branch of medicine dealing with epidemic diseases."

The evolving broadening of the range of diseases relevant to epidemiology and an incipient interest for its contextualization contributed in recent decades to definitions such as that in *Mausner & Bahn's Epidemiology*: "the study of the distribution and determinants of diseases and injuries in human populations." This notion is still quite prevalent.

An emerging new concept of epidemiology presents this discipline as the study of health and disease as a full spectrum across the human life span with a population approach, including etiological factors, phenomenology, comorbidities, and uses and outcomes of clinical care. In line with this, Mervyn Susser proposes cogently that epidemiology is the study of the occurrence, causes, and control of health events in human populations. Furthermore, the last 2001 edition of the *Dictionary of Epidemiology*, fourth edition, defines epidemiology as the study of the distribution of health-related states or events in specified populations and the application of this study to the control of health problems.

To arrive at a reasonable definition of the specific field of psychiatric epidemiology, it should be helpful to be consistent with the emerging concept of epidemiology outlined above—concerned with both ill and positive aspects of health—as well as with a modern concept of psychiatry involving the diagnosis and treatment of mental disorders and the promotion of mental health. Thus, *psychiatric epidemiology* may be defined as the study of the distribution of mental illness and positive mental health and related factors in human populations. Among the principal positive mental health variables to be considered are individual strengths, social functioning and participation, social supports, and quality of life. These positive health aspects are, of course, not only relevant to mental health, but also to general health. Among related factors, one could include contributing etiological factors, associated general health conditions, phenomenological and course characteristics, mental health services, and mental health policies. Evidence-based medicine enhanced by experience and wisdom is a basic methodological approach for epidemiological study.

Evolution of the Concepts of Epidemiology and Psychiatric Epidemiology The intricacies of epidemiology in its goals and methods can be organized paradigmatically across recent centuries in ways reflective of the prevailing cultural framework and social matrix. In effect, Ezra and Mervyn Susser have proposed an elegant schema formulating the evolution of modern epidemiology in terms of the following eras and symbols:

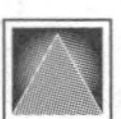

Table 5.1–1
Four Eras in the Evolution of Modern Epidemiology

Era	Paradigm	Analytical Approach	Preventive Approach
Sanitary statistics (first half of 19th century)	Miasma: poisoning by foul emanations from soil, air, and water	Demonstrate clustering of morbidity and mortality	Draining, sewage, sanitation
Infectious disease epidemiology (late 19th century through first half of 20th century)	Germ theory: single agents relate one to one to specific diseases	Laboratory isolation and culture from disease sites, experimental transmission, and reproduction of lesions	Interrupt transmission (vaccines, isolation of the affected through quarantine and fever hospitals, and, ultimately, antibiotics)
Chronic disease epidemiology (second half of 20th century)	Black box: exposure related to outcome without necessity for intervening factors or pathogenesis	Risk ratio of exposure to outcome at individual level in populations	Control risk factors by modifying lifestyle (diet, exercise, etc.) or agent (guns, food, etc.) or environment (pollution, passive smoking, etc.)
Ecological epidemiology (emerging)	Chinese boxes: relations within and between localized structures organized in a hierarchy of levels	Analysis of determinants and outcomes at different levels of organization: within and across contexts (using new information systems) and in depth (using new biomedical techniques)	Apply both information and biomedical technology to find leverage at efficacious levels, from contextual to molecular

From Susser M, Susser E: Choosing a future for epidemiology. II. From black box to Chinese boxes and eco-epidemiology. *Am J Public Health.* 1996;86:674–677, with permission.

1. The era of sanitary statistics (first half of the 19th century), emblematized by the concept of *miasma*, and focused on foul and toxic environmental conditions.
2. The era of infectious disease epidemiology (late 19th century through the first half of the 20th century), emblematized by germ theory.
3. The era of chronic disease epidemiology (second half of the 20th century), allegorized with a black box, and involved with a myriad of risk factors.
4. An emerging era of ecological epidemiology, allegorized with Chinese boxes, and concerned with gene–environment interactions and the different layers of the social matrix.

Further delineation of these paradigms is provided in Table 5.1–1, which also includes features of the analytical and preventive approaches characteristic of each era. This schema is valuable not only to organize and explain the complex history of epidemiology, but also to point out the importance of public health as an ultimate goal in each era, transcending variations in social circumstances and instrumental methodology.

The above schema is also applicable to psychiatric epidemiology, although the history of this specialized field started in full force in the course of the 20th century—especially in its second half—and has now entered energetically into the 21st century. Thus, psychiatric epidemiology as a recognized discipline today largely corresponds to the chronic disease era and, at a stage to walk into more tentatively, to the era of ecological epidemiology, the general schema outlined earlier.

It would be useful now to examine briefly the various phases or generations of psychiatric epidemiology that correspond principally to the types of design and instrumentation used for epidemiological investigation.

First-Generation Studies First-generation studies, which tended to be relatively unsystematic inquiries, often dealing with treated populations, extended typically through the mid-20th century. Some illustrative examples follow.

In 1838, Jean Etienne Esquirol documented that the number of individuals admitted to hospitals in Paris because of insanity had increased fourfold in 15 years (from 1786 to 1801).

A study of the prevalence of mental derangement and retardation in Massachusetts using key informants (general practitioners, clergy) and hospital records found 2,632 "lunatics" and 1,087 "idiots" that needed care.

Joseph Goldberger et al. determined in the 1920s, through case-control methods, that pellagra was connected to nutritional deficiency. Without specifying specific nutrients, dietary changes led to drastic reductions of pellagra in institutionalized populations.

Brugger's study in 1929 attempted to estimate the prevalence of mental disorders in a defined population (Thuringia, Germany), using a census method.

Robert Faris and Warren Dunham investigated the geographical distribution of all patients hospitalized for the first time between 1922 and 1934 in Chicago. They found that the rate of schizophrenia decreased progressively with distance away from the center of the city (from 46 to 13 percent of all admissions), leading to the formulation of a number of explanatory proposals.

Second-Generation Studies Second-generation studies were conducted after World War II, taking advantage of the extensive interest generated by the perceived frequency of mental disorders in war settings and information and instrumentation emerging from professional work with such cases and situations. They established *community surveys* as a major tool in psychiatric epidemiology. They used either symptom checklists or relatively unstructured interviews as basic information-gathering methodology. Some key studies of this type follow.

The Midtown Manhattan Study engaged specially trained social workers to conduct interviews of community residents and collect symptom and other checklist data. The study assumed that mental illness was distributed fundamentally as a continuum from normality and that it was anchored adequately by psychosocial impairment (i.e., dysfunctioning). On the basis of psychiatrists' review of the collected data, it was found that 23 percent of the sample was severely psychiatrically impaired.

The Stirling County Study in New York assessed 1,010 adult individuals in the community via lay interviewers using a questionnaire. Additional information was obtained from general practitioners and psychiatrists in the area. Research psychiatrists then reviewed the obtained data using the American Psychiatric Association's first edition of the *Diagnostic and Statistical Manual of Mental Disorders* (DSM) as a reference and concluded that prevalence of mental disorders was 20 percent.

A study of social class and mental illness in a treated population in New Haven, Connecticut, was conducted by August Hollingshead and Frederick Redlich. They found a higher prevalence of mental disorders in individuals of lower socioeconomic classes. They also found that people in lower socioeconomic classes tended to be treated with electroconvulsive treatment (ECT) and medication, whereas those in higher classes tended to be treated with psychotherapy.

Third-Generation Studies Third-generation studies have characteristically used more structured interview data aimed at identifying specific psychiatric disorders, as well as more sophisticated statistical techniques. Fundamental to the implementation of survey interviews that were not only more structured, but actually specific in the list of questions to be covered and scheduled in the order in which they were formulated, was the establishment of psychiatric nosologies with explicit inclusion and exclusion diagnostic criteria (assignment rules to particular categories of psychiatric disorders).

The use of operational or explicit diagnostic criteria for the diagnosis of mental disorders was first proposed by Edward Stengel in his international review of psychiatric classifications. The earliest set of explicit diagnostic criteria reported in the scientific psychiatric literature was that published by José Horwitz and Juan Marconi in 1966 in Latin America for alcohol abuse and those by Berner in Austria for psychotic disorders. However, the diagnostic criteria sets first used for the development of fully structured and scheduled survey interviews were those included in DSM-III, which were based on the earlier efforts of John P. Feighner et al. and Robert Spitzer et al. In due course, the value of psychiatric nosology developments for a new generation of epidemiological findings was reciprocated by the use of population epidemiological results for the refinement of psychiatric nosologies. This has articulated a promising relationship between clinical diagnosis and population epidemiology.

Illustratively, four major epidemiological studies corresponding to this third generation are outlined below from a methodological perspective.

The Epidemiological Catchment Area (ECA) study used trained lay workers to administer the Diagnostic Interview Schedule (DIS), a fully structured and scheduled instrument aimed at identifying a set of DSM-III diagnostic categories, to individuals in several institutional and community samples in available U.S. sites.

The National Comorbidity Survey (NCS) was aimed at appraising the prevalence of a set of psychiatric disorders, in association or not with substance use disorders, in a representative U.S. national household sample. It also investigated risk factors for mental illness. Given its national scope, this study was able to explore several contrasts of interests, such as that between urban and rural areas. This study, as did the preceding one, used trained lay interviewers to administer, in this case, the Composite International Interview Schedule (CIDI), a fully structured and scheduled interview. This instrument was focused in identifying DSM-III-R, as well as some DSM-IV-TR and tenth revision of the *International Statistical Classification of Diseases and Related Health Problems* (ICD-10), mental disorders.

Fourth-Generation Studies The first three generations of psychiatric epidemiological studies outlined above have been characterized and differentiated from each other by design and instrumentation variables, but are all similar in their focus on mental disorders. It is possible now to elucidate a fourth generation in psychiatric epidemiology investigations, which is characterized by a broader focus that certainly includes mental disorders but uses more comprehensive frameworks, such as both ill and positive health, and deals with meaning, culture, and other interpretative analyses. The emergence of these broader studies has, in part, been heralded by what Arthur Kleinman has termed *the new wave of ethnographies.* Also discernible in this array of epidemiological studies is their substantial interest and involvement in the development and formulation of health policies. For illustrative purposes, three recent studies follow.

The Brazilian Multicentric Study of Psychiatric Morbidity combined a highly structured epidemiological cross-sectional design with an anthropological interpretation of the meaning of risk factors. A representative sample of 6,470 adults was screened for the presence of psychopathology, with a subsample selected for diagnostic psychiatric interviews with a Brazilian version of DSM-III. This evolved into a nested case-control study in which all subjects positively diagnosed as having a nonpsychotic disorder were considered cases and compared to a random sample of those not having evidence of any disorder. The results suggested that gender (and related social processes and roles) has to be taken as a fundamental dimension. They further concluded that any theoretical interpretation of the findings should consider the fundamental issue of meaning with a sociocultural matrix.

The National Survey of Mental Health and Well-Being in Australia engaged a national population sample assessed with the CIDI to elicit ICD-10 mental disorders. Of particular relevance to its consideration as fourth generation is that this Australian study also investigated years of life lost, quality of life, and use of mental and general health services. Its impact on the development of national health policies seems to have been considerable.

The World Mental Health Survey (WMH) is a collaborative World Health Organization (WHO) initiative that aims to examine the form and frequency, severity, associated disability, and treatment of mental disorders in more than 14 countries. The novelty of this study is not only the simultaneous application of similar instruments in different countries, but also the assessment of social consequences, burden of disease, and service delivery in a comprehensive manner. The initial report of the study edited by Ronald C. Kessler and Tevfik Bedirhan Üstün, covered a total of 60,559 community adult respondents from general population samples in 14 countries (six less developed, eight developed) in different world regions. The assessments were carried out within the WMH version of the WHO Composite International Diagnostic Interview. The estimated lifetime prevalence of having any WMH-CIDI disorder (according to DSM-IV criteria) ranged widely from 8.6 percent in Shanghai to 47.3 percent in the United States. At least one-third of the lifetime cases had a 12-month episode. In the United States, 33.7 percent of the cases were mild, whereas, in Nigeria, 81.6 percent of the cases were mild. Serious disorders were associated in most countries with substantial disabilities, such as being out-of-usual-role in the past year. Although severity of a disorder is strongly related to treatment in all countries, 30 to 53 percent in developed countries and 72 to 83 percent in less developed countries received no health care treatment. This is not merely a matter of limited treatment resources, as the number of treated mild and subthreshold cases seem to exceed the number of untreated serious cases in all countries. These findings put in perspective many pieces regarding the need and utilization of services and illness impact on the lives of people and provide many useful insights about the organization of mental health services. For example, many mental disorders seem to start in late childhood and adolescence and progress into more serious disorders with significant social consequences, which appears to reinforce the need for early clinical interventions.

Purposes and Uses of Epidemiology In a classic paper written in 1955, the British epidemiologist Jeremy N. Morris proposed a number of uses for epidemiology. Despite their relatively early formulation, they are widely acknowledged as still relevant. They are summarized and briefly commented on below.

Historical studies: This refers to the importance of having a chronological perspective in the study of health and illness in human populations. The preceding section on the evolution of general and psychiatric epidemiology illustrates the value of these appraisals. Also relevant here is the longitudinal depiction of changes in patterns of disease distribution in human populations.

Community diagnosis: It has long been acknowledged that epidemiology furnishes crucial information on the health of a community (i.e., on its diagnosis in a fundamental sense). Efforts to conceive community health indices are relevant here (e.g., D. F. Sullivan, 1966). This application of epidemiology also has direct implications for clinical care in terms of situational and contextualized clinical diagnosis and of the identification of high-morbidity areas.

Appraisal of an individual's health prospects: This is based on relevant population studies and inferences made on the likelihood of life or death of an individual as a member of the researched population. Such inferences may refer to risk factors, as well as to life expectation and life lived with disabilities.

Health services and operational research: Scientific investigations on the organization and performance of health services are becoming an area of active research. For this, epidemiological methods can be quite helpful—from prevalence studies to the assessment of need for care to the evaluation of treatment coverage and outcomes.

Completing the clinical picture: When initially proposed by Morris, this use of epidemiology was best illustrated by determining gender and age factors associated with a disease. In mental health, this epidemiological purpose is exemplified, in particular, by the refinement of a nosological profile afforded by community surveys, which have been used for development of psychiatric classifications in ICD-10 and DSM-IV, as discussed by Tim Slade.

Identification of syndromes: The use of epidemiology for the elucidation of different types of "peptic ulcer" and for distinguishing Alzheimer's disease from multiinfarct dementias is illustrative here. Models could be built to associate risk and other contributory factors to signs, symptoms, and course to generate nosological hypotheses. More recently, opportunities to use ethnographical approaches along with epidemiological methods for elucidating new syndromes, such as *ataque de nervios* and *chi-gong* psychosis, that before were neglected as exotic, culture-bound syndromes have begun to emerge.

Clues to causes: There are substantial indicators for the use of epidemiology in clarifying the etiology of clinical problems. Examples include the investigations of nutritional deficiencies, industrial cancers, linkage of smoking to lung cancer, and occupational accidents. The searching for causes of disease and protective factors for health may lead to better prevention efforts. Within the emerging multilevel paradigm, epidemiology is not a "head-counting" activity. It is a systemic scientific activity that answers clinical and public health questions with proper analyses of risk factors, outcomes, and other associated variables. It also offers a broader perspective of overall population health and health care provision in a society. Health policy makers and other health stakeholders can use epidemiological information as a strategic input for decision making on priorities and resource allocation. As epidemiology enters a new "ecological" era, concerned with understanding internal and external connections, investigations formed by a multilevel framework and considering a wide array of contributors may become increasingly frequent.

Each of the uses outlined above is applicable to psychiatric epidemiology. It should be mentioned, however, that, in addition to these seven uses—which rather explicitly refer to work with illness or pathology—the emerging expansion of the concept of health to include pointedly positive health aspects (i.e., social participation and supports, quality of life) suggests that the investigation of these aspects will become a significant new use of epidemiology.

METHODS IN PSYCHIATRIC EPIDEMIOLOGY

This section reviews the conceptual and procedural tools that are used in epidemiology to fulfill its purposes and goals. First, the basic constructs and parameters in epidemiology and health are considered. Key categorical and dimensional measures and prototypical designs of epidemiological studies are examined next. The last subsection outlines the types of instruments used in psychiatric epidemiology.

Basic Constructs and Study Parameters in Epidemiology

Disease, Illness, Disorder, and Syndrome The terms *disease*, *illness*, *disorder*, and *syndrome* refer to recognized forms of pathology. *Disease* and *illness* represent crystallized or established entities of significant severity and with definite implications for the individual and for public health. *Disease* is often used with biomedical connotations, referring to a condition with specific etiopathogenesis, whereas *illness* is often used with experiencial and sociocultural connotations. There is, however, no wide agreement on these distinctions. *Syndrome* represents a condition characterized by a particular symptom profile, the etiology, clinical significance or severity of which is variable. *Disorder* is a term midway between a disease or illness and a syndrome, in terms of consistency, correlates, and significance. Given the complexity, intricacy, and variable significance of the psychiatric conditions included in standard mental and behavioral nosologies, *disorder* is the term that has gained preference at the current stage in nosological formulations.

Important features of diseases or disorders of epidemiological interest include (1) *course of illness*. This refers to the age and mode of onset, the episodic or continuous presentation of illness, and the stable, improving, or worsening progression of the illness. (2) *Comorbidity*. This is a complex and intricate term that refers to the cooccurrence or copresentation of two disorders. It has been argued that comorbidity may sometimes involve two faces of the same basic clinical condition or constitute artifactual consequences of a particular nosological architecture. Comorbidity may take place within the domain of mental disorders (e.g., depression and alcoholism) and across chapters of the ICD (e.g., depression and arterial hypertension).

Disability *Functioning* is an umbrella term that encompasses the bodily functions and personal activities of an individual. *Disability* refers to limitations in functioning that may take place at the following different levels.

- Body level: e.g., brain and nervous system impairments
- Personal level: e.g., limitations in personal care and daily activities
- Societal level: e.g., restrictions in social participation and in available social supports

Other Health Problems *Other health problems* is the term used in the current ICD-10 to refer to conditions of clinical interest that are not diseases *senso stricto* and may explain presentation to health services for evaluation and care. Examples include *accentuated personality, hazardous use of substances*, and *burn-out syndrome*.

Risk Factors *Risk factors* are characteristics, variables, and hazards that make it more likely that a given individual will develop a disorder. They can reside within the individual (e.g., personality and temperament), with his or her family or community (e.g., life events), and with the environment (e.g., certain chemicals). Usually, there is an assumed and plausible causal association between the risk factor and a disorder or health problem.

Positive Health Positive health is the counterpart of ill health, which, as listed above, includes disease, illness, disorder, syndrome, and related health problems. Positive health reflects growing interest in a more comprehensive concept of health. Such a concept was already enshrined as "a state of complete physical, social and emotional well-being and not merely the absence of illness" in the constitution of the WHO. Presently, positive health encompasses concepts such as effective personal care, good interpersonal and occupational functioning, social supports, and quality of life.

Clinical Care *Clinical care* refers to the array of actions or interventions taking place in health services. Broad categories of clinical care include the following:

Diagnosis: This is an evaluative process and formulation conducted by health professionals in collaboration with the patient (or consulting person), family, and pertinent members of the community. Illustrative of modern diagnostic concepts and procedures are the recent World Psychiatric Association's International Guidelines for Diagnostic Assessment (IGDA).

Treatment: This refers to the array of professional interventions—in cooperation with the consulting person and family—aimed at improving the disorders presented and restoring health.

Health promotion: This refers to a set of actions aimed at empowering the consulting person to raise the level of his or her health. As such, health promotion can be regarded as relevant to both public health and clinical care.

Context of Epidemiology Critical aspects of the context of epidemiology include the following domains:

Social environment: This includes human aspects of the environment at various levels of aggregation (i.e., family, community, nations, and humankind). Cultural diversity and political considerations also play a major role in this domain.

Physical environment: This includes climate, housing, finances, transportation, and other material resources.

Genetic endowment: This includes the genetic bases for illness and health. Recent analyses of the human genome have pointed out that the expression of genetic factors is largely influenced by environmental factors.

These concepts and factors are, of course, interrelated. Robert Evans and Greg Stoddart offer a modern perspective on these interrelations through an integrative schema presented in Figure 5.1–1. It reflects the complexity of the field and outlines the interactive influences of various individual and social factors, as well as health care, on the various faces of health. The latter involves disease or illness, health and function, and a sense of well-being.

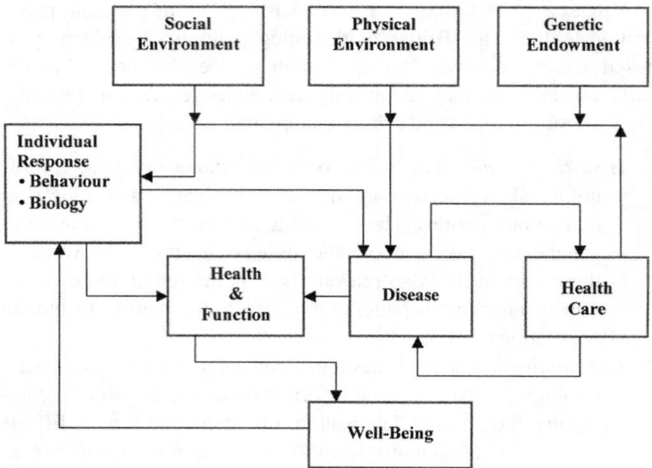

FIGURE 5.1–1 Relationships among social and individual factors, health care, and the various aspects of health. (From Evans RG, Stoddart GL. Producing health, consuming health care. In: Evans RG, Barer ML, Marmor TR, eds. *Why Are Some People Healthy and Others Not? The Determinants of Health of Populations.* New York: Aldine de Gruyter; 1994, with permission.)

Key Categorical and Dimensional Measures in Epidemiology

The measurement of key variables in epidemiology is guided by the scaling requirements of the type of variables involved (categorical versus dimensional), as well as by historical and customary considerations.

Measures for Categorical Variables Variables that are structured in terms of discrete categories or types (e.g., disorders, inpatient versus outpatient care) are measured through nominal scaling arrangements, such as a standardized typology or classification of disorders. Some of the most frequently used measures in this domain follow:

Proportion or *percentage*: This is a widely used measure of frequency for all categorical variables—for example, percentage of emergency psychiatric evaluations that result in inpatient admissions (as opposed to outpatient referrals).

Prevalence: This indicates the proportion of individuals in a given population who have a disorder at a particular point or period in time. It is usually expressed in percentages. For point prevalence, the time of measurement is to be specified—for example, percentage of a village's inhabitants who presented manifestations of generalized anxiety disorder on July 1, 2003. Period prevalence is often measured by 1-month, 6-month, and 1-year intervals—for example, percentage of a village's inhabitants who experienced a schizophrenic disorder during calendar year 2003.

Incidence: This indicates the proportion of new cases of a disorder that emerge in a population during a specified time interval (usually 1 year). An approximate estimation of incidence may be obtained through anamnestic means, whereas a careful appraisal requires two surveys of the population involved—one at the beginning and another at the end of the period of interest. A refined index, described by Olli Miettinen, is *incidence density*, which deals with possible changes over time and loss at follow-up of individuals in the at-risk population and is defined as an average incidence rate over the period of interest.

Odds ratio: This index involves a comparison of the presence of a risk factor for disease in a sample of diseased subjects and nondiseased controls. In other words, it compares the proportion of cases to noncases in a sample exposed to a given risk to the proportion of cases to noncases in a nonexposed sample.

Measures for Dimensional Variables Variables that are measurable with dimensional scales are informationally more powerful (convey more detailed structured information) and mathematically and statistically more tractable than yes or no categorical variables. In other words, although categorical variables are measured in terms of the presence or absence of the variable, dimensional variables are measured in reference to the extent of their presence—for example, a score of 75 in a 100-point scale.

Many variables of epidemiological interest, particularly those corresponding to positive health (e.g., functioning and quality of life), are measured with dimensional variables.

Measures of Association Indices of intervariable association or relationships depend on the scaling of the variables involved. Contingency tables are used to appraise the interrelation between categorical variables, and their statistical significance is expressed through the chi-square statistic.

Product–moment correlation coefficients convey the degree of association between dimensional variables. They can vary from –1, indicating perfectly negative or inverse association, to +1, indicating full same-directional association, with 0 expressing no association at all between the investigated variables.

Point biserial correlation coefficient is an adjusted correlation index designed to measure the association between a binomial variable (e.g., presence versus absence of a given disorder) and a dimensional one (e.g., level of occupational functioning).

Multivariate Analyses Complex situations involving several variables as potential contributors or predictors call for multivariate analyses. Such analyses are facilitated when the predictor and predicted variables are dimensionally measured. Stepwise procedures allow the identification of the smallest and most efficient set of predictors. When the predicted variable is categorical, reducible to binomial, it is possible to use a logistic regression model to elucidate a multivariate predictor.

Design of Epidemiological Studies

The most important issue in designing epidemiological studies involves its *population setting*—that is, a clinic or treated population versus a community or general population. Traditionally, a general population was regarded as always the proper setting for epidemiology. Clinical populations have begun to emerge as an additional proper focus of epidemiological studies. This is in line with the enormous significance and cost of health care in today's world and with the opportunity that medical centers offer to investigate the relationship between environmental and biological factors of illness.

Cross-Sectional versus Longitudinal Perspectives Cross-sectional versus longitudinal perspectives constitute another crucial design issue in psychiatric epidemiology. Most studies have been cross-sectional in design, reflecting the fact that many descriptive research questions call for such designs and that this type of study is simpler and less expensive to conduct. Other research questions, including those involving etiological hypotheses, the elucidation of a chain of events, and developmental considerations, call for longitudinal designs.

Longitudinal designs include cohort and case-control studies and usually involve a time interval between cause and effect. *Cohort studies* characteristically engage a sample (cohort) from a well-defined population (typically with a particular exposure or nonexposure status), which is followed up for a specified time to determine whether a particular health outcome emerges. Cohort studies may be divided into prospective studies and retrospective studies. In the prospective type, exposure status is determined at the initiation of the longitudinal study; in the retrospective type, exposures are determined at a past point. *Case-control studies* engage identified cases of a particular disorder and control subjects (those without the disorder) and follows them up. This design is particularly suited for the study of rare disorders and for the exploration of possible risk factors. Case-control studies are attractive because of their convenience and relatively low cost. A major limitation is recall bias, especially when corroborating information cannot be obtained.

Family Studies Family studies represent a significant type of epidemiological study stimulated by the interest arising about genetic contributions to the development of mental disorders. These studies examine aggregation of disease in families that may be due to heredity or shared exposure to environmental risk factors. Family studies may use general population samples or samples of cases ascertained through probands, including family case-control studies.

Health Services Research Health services research has become a major area of investigation, stimulated by the complexity of the organization of clinical services and the magnitude and intricacy of its financing. Characteristic of this type of study is a naturalistic approach, which involves appraising the process and outcome of services in their regular settings. Epidemiological methods, including descriptions of the types and extent of services provided and the levels of unmet need for service, are applicable to this field. Illustratively, health services research deals with questions such as the following: (1) Need: Who comes to care? (2) Coverage of service: Who gets care? (3) How much resources are required to meet the need for care? (4) What are the outcomes of health care?

Life Span Stages Research Life span stages research addresses the complexity of human development by dividing it into three categories—childhood and adolescence, adult development, and old age. Studies on the distribution of mental disorders in childhood and adolescence are challenged by the intricacy and instability of psychopathology during these years. Most epidemiological studies have been conducted with adult samples. Attention must be paid to basic features of adult development, such as resilience as a protective factor and levers for health promotion. Old age brings new challenges to the methodology of epidemiological research—from measurement of nosological comorbidity to late-life risk factors to the role and needs of caregivers.

Cultural and International Frameworks Cultural and international frameworks are emerging as fundamental for health studies in general and epidemiology in particular. Culture pervades experience and understanding of life and health (both ill and positive aspects). The vitality of new research in cultural psychiatry has led to the development of practical tools, such as the cultural formulation, which may be helpful for clinical care and may also enhance epidemiological descriptions. The interactive nature of today's world makes it compelling to consider international perspectives in health at all its organizational levels—governmental (e.g., WHO) and nongovernmental (e.g., World Psychiatric Association).

Evidence-Based Approaches Evidence-based approaches to medicine and epidemiology have attracted wide attention as efforts to upgrade the solidity and quality of information on which health care and public health are based. It is important to place in proper perspective such efforts, given the complexity of the health field. As indicated by some of their most authoritative proponents, evidence-based medicine is about integrating individual clinical expertise and the best external evidence. The need for balancing hard data with informed wisdom is extensible to public health policy development.

Instruments for Epidemiological Studies

Instrument Properties The appraisal of the quality and relevance of instruments for measuring the variables of interest in epidemiology is usually conducted in terms of their reliability, their validity or usefulness, and their feasibility or administrability.

RELIABILITY *Reliability* refers to the quality of an instrument to yield similar or consistent results across various circumstances, such as time (test–retest reliability) and evaluators (interrater reliability). For categorical variables, such as the identification of psychiatric disorders, the most accepted reliability index is the *kappa coefficient* (κ), the formula of which follows:

$$\kappa = p_o - p_c/1 - p_c$$

where p_o is the proportion of observed agreement and p_c is the proportion of chance agreement.

For the not infrequent case of multiple raters formulating multiple categorical diagnoses, an extension of the κ has been designed and operationalized. For the assessment of reliability or agreement among raters using dimensional scales, the most frequently used statistical index is the intraclass correlation coefficient.

VALIDITY *Validity* refers to the quality or strength of an instrument to measure the variable or construct it is supposed to measure. In line with this, validity is thought to correspond to the faithfulness, relevance, and usefulness of the instrument to reflect the reality of interest. Consequently, validity is regarded as the most fundamental quality of an instrument. However, it is not always simple to appraise validity directly. The following represent common approaches to the estimation of an instrument's validity:

Criterion validity: According to this approach, the validity of a new instrument is determined by comparing the results or measurements it yields to those obtained with an instrument of widely accepted relevance and value. For example, the validity of a new depression scale could be estimated by correlating its results to those of the Hamilton Depression Scale.

Face or content validity: This is assessed by having experts in the field determine the extent to which a new instrument is relevant to its intended purpose and covers the informational areas pertinent to that purpose.

Discriminant validity: Here, an attempt is made to determine if a new instrument is well able to distinguish between samples of populations presumed to be quite different from each other in the instrument's domain or field of application. Illustratively, the discriminant validity of a new depression scale could be indicated by the extent to which it yields higher scores in a sample of depressed people than in another sample of healthy individuals.

Construct validity: This corresponds to the theoretical validity of an instrument (i.e., to the extent that it yields results consistent with the theory underlying its domain and design. For example, if it is properly assumed that an anxiety disorder is substantially caused by environmental stress, a new scale designed to measure the presence of that anxiety disorder would be expected to yield high scores among people recently exposed to a serious disaster.

FEASIBILITY OR ADMINISTRABILITY This evaluative parameter refers to the case of use of an instrument, as well as low cost and accessibility.

Instruments for Psychopathological Assessment There is a large number and variety of instruments for the evaluation of psychopathology and mental disorders. Some are of a screening nature. These include, first, instruments for detecting the likelihood of an individual having mental disorders (which are usually based on affective symptoms and, in some cases, other indicators, such as social dysfunction). This type of screening instrument may be used as the first of a two-stage design, in which they are followed by a second in-depth instrument. Second, screening instruments may also represent a preliminary attempt at detecting the likelihood of a particular disorder, such as a depressive or anxiety disorder. For the full evaluation of mental disorders, including the identification of specific forms of them, fully structured or semistructured interviews—often administered by trained nonclinicians—have become standard in epidemiological studies. Well-trained clinicians or psychiatrists, using adequate nosologies and diagnostic criteria, can also represent an adequate approach to full psychopathological evaluation in epidemiology, although the cost of such professional services and the lower explicitness of the proceedings may represent significant limitations and are usually restricted to validation studies.

A selection of instruments for general psychopathological screening and full identification of a substantial set of mental disorders are presented below.

INSTRUMENTS FOR GENERAL PSYCHOPATHOLOGICAL SCREENING

General Health Questionnaire (GHQ): This is one of the earliest screening instruments to have received wide acceptance in a variety of settings. It was developed by David Goldberg and collaborators. Its complete version is composed of 60 items, mostly affective symptoms. Shorter versions of 28 and 12 items also exist. Adequate reliability and validity have been documented.

Self-Reporting Questionnaire (SRQ): This instrument was designed as part of a WHO project to screen for mental disorders in primary health care settings. It includes 30 items—20 on depressive and anxiety symptoms, four on psychotic phenomena, one on epilepsy, and five related to alcohol abuse—and has been adjusted in length for use in different world settings.

Personal Health Scale: This instrument, developed by Juan Mezzich and associates, is based on an empirical prototypical model for the definition of psychiatric illness and includes 10 items (six affective psychological and somatic symptoms, three reflecting social dysfunction, and one on global self-evaluation of illness and need for clinical care). It can be completed in 2 to 4 minutes and has several language versions with documented reliability and discriminant validity.

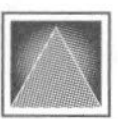

Table 5.1–2
An Overview of the International Classification of Functioning, Disabilities, and Health (ICF)

	Part 1: Functioning and Disability		Part 2: Contextual Factors	
Components	Body functions and structures	Activities and participation	Environmental factors	Personal factors
Domains	Body functions and structures	Life areas (tasks, actions)	External influences on functioning and disability	Internal influences on functioning and disability
Constructs	Change in body functions (physiological) Change in body structures (anatomical)	Capacity, executing tasks in a standard environment Performance, executing tasks in the current environment	Facilitating or hindering impact of features of the physical, social, and attitudinal world	Impact of attributes of the individual
Positive aspect	Functional and structural integrity (function)	Activities, participation	Facilitators	Not applicable
Negative aspect	Impairment (disability)	Activity limitation Participation restriction	Barriers/hindrances	Not applicable

From World Health Organization. *International Classification of Functioning, Disability and Health (ICF)*. Geneva: World Health Organization; 2001, with permission.

INSTRUMENTS FOR FULL ASSESSMENT OF PSYCHIATRIC DISORDERS

DIS: This fully structured and scheduled diagnostic interview was originally designed to identify a set of DSM-III mental disorders through interviews conducted by lay interviewers. It was most prominently applied in the ECA study in five U.S. sites.

CIDI: This structured interview was built on the DIS approach and was extended to identify sets of mental disorders in DSM-IV and ICD-10. It has been applied in a number of studies, including the U.S. NCS and the WMH.

Standardized Clinical Assessment for Neuropsychiatry (SCAN): This modular instrument was built on the tenth edition of the Present State Examination (a structured interview for psychiatric symptoms) and a categorical diagnostic algorithm (CATEGO). It has been used in a national survey of psychiatric morbidity in Great Britain. Both PSE and SCAN were used in WHO Longitudinal Studies of Schizophrenia.

Mini-International Neuropsychiatric Interview (MINI): This brief structured diagnostic interview, recently developed by David Sheehan and collaborators, aimed at the identification of a set of DSM-IV and ICD-10 mental disorders in multicenter clinical trials and epidemiological studies. It can usually be completed in less than 30 minutes. It has been validated against the CIDI and the Structured Clinical Interview for DSM-IV.

Instruments for the Assessment of Disability and Functioning

WHO PSYCHIATRIC DISABILITY ASSESSMENT SCHEDULE The WHO developed a new version of the Disability Assessment Schedule (WHO-DAS II) as a general measure of functioning and disability that reflects major life domains and is sensitive to change. This endeavor builds on the development of the revision of the International Classification of Functioning, Disability, and Health and aims to develop a common metric tool that is culturally applicable, psychometrically reliable and valid, and useful for health services research, such as the evaluation of needs and outcomes. WHO-DAS II was conceived as a general health state assessment measure that can be used for multiple purposes, such as epidemiological surveys, clinical use, or as a potential description system to contribute to summary measure of population health. It gives a general score as well as different profiles on cognition, mobility, self-care, interpersonal relations, and participation in the community.

INTERNATIONAL CLASSIFICATION OF FUNCTIONING, DISABILITIES AND HEALTH (ICF) The International Classification of Functioning, Disabilities and Health (ICF) is a major revision of the International Classification of Impairments, Disabilities, and Handicaps (ICIDH). The first edition assumed that disabilities result exclusively from illnesses. The second considered that disabilities might result from the interaction among illnesses, the person, and the social environment. In effect, disability is conceptualized here as involving dysfunctions at body, personal, and social levels—impairments, activity limitations, and participation restrictions. An outline of the ICF is presented in Table 5.1–2. A checklist assesses the presence and severity of various functional limitations. Figure 5.1–2 displays the interactions between the components of the ICF.

GLOBAL ASSESSMENT OF FUNCTIONING SCALE The Global Assessment of Functioning Scale appraises, in combination, social dysfunction and psychopathological severity using a 100-point scale. It is used to assess Axis V of DSM-IV and DSM-IV-TR.

Instruments to Assess Contextual Factors: Life Events, Stressors, Social Supports

MEASURING LIFE EVENTS The appraisal of stressors and life experiences as potential contributors to the emergence of mental disorders represents an intricate challenge. Interesting here is the approach of George Brown, which addresses the definitions of life events, stress, and contextual threat. A practical and simple proposal to evaluate the presence of frequent threatening experiences was offered by Terry Brugha et al.

APPRAISAL OF A STANDARD SET OF CONTEXTUAL FACTORS This may be attempted using the *Z*-coded categories of Chapter XXI of ICD-10. As part of the development of the multiaxial system for ICD-10, a schema was designed for the reporting of contextual factors that may influence the diagnosis, treatment, and prognosis of mental disorders.

Instruments to Assess Quality of Life

Quality of life as a notion has become increasingly popular with the recognition that the impacts on health conditions and health care–seeking behavior are often determined not just by symptoms and signs, disorders, or functioning, but also by subjective global appraisals of health. This is especially important for health conditions that are either recurrent or of a long duration (as is the case with a larger number of mental

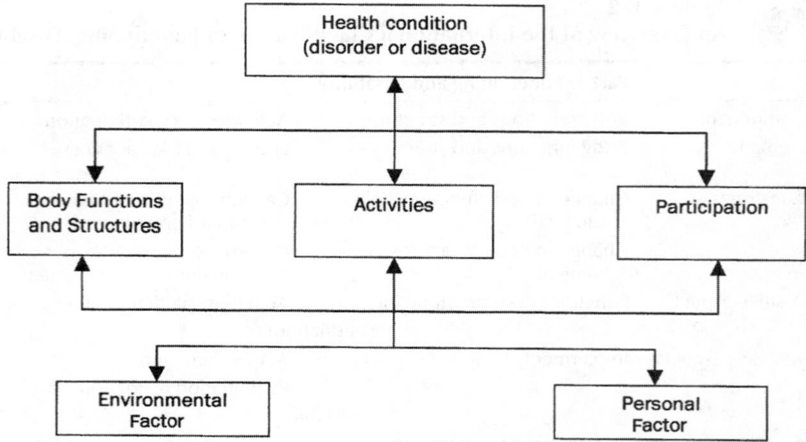

FIGURE 5.1–2 Interactions among the components of the International Classification of Functioning, Disability and Health. (From World Health Organization. *International Classification of Functioning, Disability and Health (ICF)*. Geneva: World Health Organization; 2001, with permission.)

health conditions). The concept has also gained currency in the pharmacoeconomic literature. Quality of life can thus be considered an operational measure of overall health and well-being.

There are a growing number of procedures and tools to assess health-related quality of life. Some were designed for the evaluation of individuals experiencing specific illnesses, psychiatric and nonpsychiatric. Others appraise quality of life generically and are most appropriate as part of a comprehensive assessment of health status. The WHO Quality of Life Instrument (WHOQoL) is noteworthy for its broad international anchorage, careful development, and wide range of content. The WHOQoL was developed through an international cross-cultural collaborative effort to measure people's self-perception of their position in life in the context of the culture and value systems in which they live and in relation to their goals, expectations, standards, and concerns. It has been extensively used and is being currently revised to reflect new frameworks for measuring health and health-related outcomes. The 10-item Quality of Life Index, developed by Juan Mezzich and collaborators, is also wide in content (physical and emotional well-being, personal and social functioning, social supports, and personal and spiritual fulfillment) and also quite efficient, using a culture-informed rating system, and validated in terms of several language versions.

EPIDEMIOLOGICAL FINDINGS ON ILLNESS AND HEALTH

This section presents selected recent findings on distribution and patterns of mental disorders, disabilities, positive aspects of health, clinical care, and health policy. These epidemiological results are presented principally in tabular form.

Findings on Mental Disorders As an illustration of findings on distribution of mental disorders in a broad population, Ronald Kessler et al. reported on the lifetime and 12-month prevalence of DSM-III-R disorders in a U.S. national household sample (Table 5.1–3). The lifetime prevalence of any NCS disorder was found to be 48.0 percent. Of the broad categories of disorders, substance use disorder (26.6 percent) was the most common, followed by any anxiety disorder (24.9 percent) and any mood disorder (19.3 percent). Of the specific disorders, major depression was most common (17.1 percent), followed by alcohol dependence (14.1 percent).

Also of high interest, the NCS found that 79 percent of all psychiatrically ill people presented with comorbidity involving two or more psychiatric disorders. More than half of all lifetime disorders occurred in 14 percent of the population.

The figures obtained in the NCS were higher than those obtained in the ECA study. Furthermore, lifetime prevalence of "any mental disorder" with the CIDI was found to vary greatly, from more than 40 percent in the U.S. and the Netherlands to 20 percent in Mexico and 12 percent in Turkey.

Complementing the above-mentioned National Comorbidity Study in the United States, findings from a recent study conducted as part of the WHO World Mental Health Survey in 12 different settings are presented in Table 5.1–4. Considerable variations can be noted across countries. Quite consistently, the results obtained in the United States tended to be highest (e.g., 47.3 percent as lifetime prevalence of any disorder investigated, and 26.1 percent as 12-month prevalence), whereas those obtained in Shanghai, China, tended to be the lowest (e.g., 8.6 percent as lifetime prevalence of any disorder investigated, and 4.5 percent as 12-month prevalence).

One of the most important settings for appraising the prevalence of mental disorders is primary health care. David Goldberg and Yves Lecrubier studied such prevalence with the CIDI in 15 cities across all continents and found that the prevalence of all mental disorders varies from 53 percent in Santiago, Chile, to 7.3 percent in Shanghai, China, with an average across sites of 24 percent. Likewise, depressive disorder ranged from 30 percent in Santiago to 2.6 percent in Nagasaki, Japan. Some interesting contrasts across continents are apparent (Table 5.1–5).

As an example of international work with specific psychiatric disorders, Ezra Susser et al. reported on the delineation of acute and transient psychotic disorders in Chandigarh, India. On examining the distribution of duration of illness for 46 cases of nonaffective acute psychosis, they found a bimodal distribution of this variable, with 80 percent of the cases lasting less than 28 weeks and 20 percent lasting more than a year. This supports the nosological separation of acute transient psychosis from schizophrenia.

The distribution of mental disorders in children and adolescents in North Carolina was recently reported on by E. Jane Costello et al. Using the Child and Adolescent Psychiatric Assessment (CAPA) as a structured interview, they found that by age 16, one in three adolescents gave indications of having a mental disorder. A similar finding (30 percent) was obtained by Kessler et al. for 15-year-olds in the NCS.

More broadly, the prevalence of child and adolescence disorders in recent studies across the world are presented comparatively in Table 5.1–6. This prevalence varied from 23 percent in Switzerland to 13 percent in India.

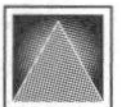

Table 5.1–3
Lifetime and 12-Month Prevalence of DSM-III-R Disorders

	Male				Female				Total			
	Lifetime		12-Mo		Lifetime		12-Mo		Lifetime		12-Mo	
Disorders	%	(SE)	%	(SE)	%	(SE)	%	(SE)	%	(SE)	%	(SE)
Mood disorders												
Mania	1.6	0.3	1.4	0.3	1.7	0.3	1.3	0.3	1.6	0.3	1.3	0.2
Major depression	12.7	0.9	7.7	0.8	21.3	0.9	12.9	0.8	17.1	0.7	10.3	0.6
Dysthymia	4.8	0.4	2.1	0.3	8.0	0.6	3.0	0.4	6.4	0.4	2.5	0.2
Any mood disorders	14.7	0.8	8.5	0.8	23.9	0.9	14.1	0.9	19.3	0.7	11.3	0.7
Anxiety disorders												
Generalized anxiety disorder	3.6	0.5	2.0	0.3	6.6	0.5	4.3	0.4	5.1	0.3	3.1	0.3
Panic disorder	2.0	0.3	1.3	0.3	5.0	1.4	3.2	0.4	3.5	0.3	2.3	0.3
Social phobia	11.1	0.8	6.6	0.4	15.5	1.0	9.1	0.7	13.3	0.7	7.9	0.4
Simple phobia	6.7	0.5	4.4	0.5	15.7	1.1	13.2	0.9	11.3	0.6	8.8	0.5
Agoraphobia without panic	3.5	0.4	1.7	0.3	7.0	0.6	3.8	0.4	5.3	0.4	2.8	0.3
Any anxiety disorder	19.2	0.9	11.8	0.6	30.5	1.2	22.6	0.1	24.9	0.8	17.2	0.7
Substance use disorders												
Alcohol abuse	12.5	0.8	3.4	0.4	6.4	0.6	1.6	0.2	9.4	0.5	2.5	0.2
Alcohol dependence	20.1	1.0	10.7	0.9	8.2	0.7	3.7	0.4	14.1	0.7	7.2	0.5
Drug abuse	5.4	0.5	1.3	0.2	3.5	0.4	0.3	0.1	4.4	0.3	0.8	0.1
Drug dependence	9.2	0.7	3.8	0.4	5.9	0.5	1.9	0.3	7.5	0.4	2.8	0.3
Any substance use disorder	35.4	1.2	16.1	0.7	17.9	1.1	6.6	0.4	26.6	1.0	11.3	0.5
Other disorders												
Antisocial personality[a]	4.8	0.5	—	—	1.0	0.2	—	—	2.8	0.2	—	—
Nonaffective psychosis[b]	0.3	0.1	0.2	0.1	0.7	0.2	0.4	0.1	0.5	0.1	0.3	0.1
Any NCS disorder	48.7	0.2	27.7	0.9	47.3	1.5	31.2	1.3	48.0	1.1	29.5	1.0

NCS, National Comorbidity Study; SE, standard error.
[a]Antisocial personality was only assessed on a lifetime basis.
[b]Nonaffective psychosis: schizophrenia, schizophreniform disorder, schizoaffective disorder, delusional disorder, and atypical psychosis.
From Kessler RC, McGonagle KA, Zhao S, et al.: Lifetime and 12-month prevalence of DSM-III-R psychiatric disorders in the United States: results from the National Comorbidity Survey. *Arch Gen Psychiatry.* 1994;51:8–19, with permission.

Findings on Disabilities The proportion of all disability-adjusted life years attributed to neuropsychiatric disorders has been found to be 12 percent in the Global Burden of Disease Study. Table 5.1–7 lists the leading causes of disability-adjusted life years in all ages and both sexes—unipolar depressive disorders is in fourth place, and two other behavioral conditions (self-inflicted injuries and alcohol use disorders) are included among the top 20 health conditions.

Neuropsychiatric conditions account for 31 percent of years of life lived with disability. Table 5.1–8 identifies the leading causes of years of life lived with disability in all ages and both sexes. Five of the top 20 health conditions are mental—unipolar depressive disorder, alcohol use disorders, schizophrenia, bipolar affective disorder, and Alzheimer's disease and other dementias. T. B. Üstün and associates have prepared an update of the initial Global Burden of Disease Study, confirming and extending the importance of depression as a public health problem.

Further illustration of significant epidemiological findings on disabilities is furnished by the National Survey of Mental Health and Well-Being in Australia. Figure 5.1–3 lists health conditions in Australia and their associated overall disability, expressed as years of life lost through disability. Mental disorders exceeded all the other major health categories in this regard.

Findings on Positive Aspects of Health The National Survey of Mental Health and Well-Being in Australia included measurement of well-being at the strong request of consumers and caregivers. Well-being was appraised with the single-item Life Satisfaction Scale, with 0 percent indicating "terrible" and 100 percent representing "delighted." The mean score for the Australian adult population was 70.4 percent. Men and women had very similar mean scores. Well-being was higher in people with tertiary education and in those owning or purchasing their homes. It was lower in individuals with physical or mental disorders, particularly depression. It was higher in mild users of alcohol than it was in abstainers and heavy users. Of particular interest was the existence of a few individuals with current anxiety or depressive disorders who reported high life satisfaction.

Quality of life, using the Spanish version of the Quality of Life Index (QLI-Sp), was studied in a Spanish community sample by Esther Lorente et al. The mean scores of the ten items of the QLI-Sp and the average score in this community sample composed of 489 men and women—70 percent university students and 30 percent having other occupations—is presented in Table 5.1–9. Within the framework of this 0- to 10-point scale, the average score obtained in this community sample was 6.98 (quite consistent with the findings of Keith Dear et al. in Australia). There was not a significant difference in the average scores of men and women. The scale item presenting the highest loading on the single factor underlying the scale was "personal fulfillment." More recently, Saavedra and associates studied an adapted version of the QLI-Sp on a statistical sample of 2,418 households in Lima, Peru, and found a mean average score of 7.64, with no highly significant differences among age or gender groups.

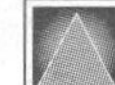

Table 5.1–4
Lifetime (LT) and 12-Month Prevalence of World Mental Health Survey–Composite International Diagnostic Interview/DSM-IV Disorders[a]

	Anxiety				Mood[b]				Impulse Control[c]				Substance[d]				Any			
	LT		12-Mo		LT		12-Mo		LT		12-Mo		LT		12-Mo		LT		12-Mo	
	%	SE	%	SE	%	SE	%	SE	%	SE	%	SE	%	SE	%	SE	%	SE	%	SE
Americas																				
Colombia	19.5	1.2	9.9	0.8	13.2	0.7	6.2	0.4	9.3	0.7	3.8	0.4	9.4	0.8	2.6	0.4	36.1	1.4	17.7	0.9
Mexico	11.9	0.7	6.9	0.5	10.0	0.7	5.1	0.4	5.0	0.5	1.3	0.3	8.0	0.6	2.6	0.4	25.3	1.1	12.5	0.9
United States	28.6	0.9	18.2	0.7	21.4	0.8	9.8	0.4	17.8	0.7	5.8	0.4	14.6	0.6	3.8	0.3	47.3	1.1	26.1	0.9
Europe																				
Belgium	13.3	1.9	6.2	1.1	14.4	1.1	5.0	0.5	3.4	0.8	0.8	0.3	8.7	1.5	1.0	0.3	28.7	2.3	10.4	1.1
France	22.0	1.5	9.7	0.9	23.3	1.3	6.4	0.7	3.4	0.5	0.5	0.2	5.6	0.8	0.7	0.2	37.9	2.0	14.3	1.2
Germany	14.1	1.3	5.9	0.8	10.9	0.8	3.4	0.4	2.3	0.7	0.2	0.1	6.2	0.8	1.1	0.4	25.2	1.6	8.6	0.9
Italy	10.9	0.9	5.0	0.6	10.2	0.6	3.1	0.2	1.1	0.3	0.2	0.1	1.2	0.3	0.1	0.1	18.1	1.1	7.2	0.7
Netherlands	15.2	1.0	7.2	0.9	17.5	1.4	4.8	0.6	4.3	1.1	0.7	0.3	7.7	1.0	1.5	0.4	31.2	2.1	11.4	0.9
Spain	10.0	1.0	5.2	0.6	11.6	0.6	4.4	0.3	1.2	0.3	0.4	0.2	2.9	0.7	0.3	0.1	19.7	1.4	8.4	0.6
Ukraine	11.3	1.0	7.4	0.8	16.1	1.2	8.8	0.8	6.0	0.7	3.3	0.4	12.3	1.1	4.8	0.6	33.4	1.7	19.1	1.3
Middle East and Africa																				
Lebanon	13.3	1.3	10.9	1.2	11.7	1.0	6.3	0.7	2.4	0.5	1.3	0.3	1.5	0.5	0.8	0.4	22.0	1.6	15.9	1.3
Nigeria	5.8	0.7	3.3	0.4	3.2	0.3	1.0	0.2	0.2	0.1	0.0	0.0	4.2	0.5	0.8	0.2	11.8	0.7	4.9	0.5
Asia																				
Japan	8.4	0.9	4.7	0.8	8.5	0.7	3.0	0.5	3.2	0.7	1.0	0.3	4.9	0.9	1.4	0.5	19.8	1.7	8.3	1.1
PRC Beijing	5.9	1.2	3.4	0.7	4.6	0.6	2.7	0.6	4.1	1.2	2.4	0.6	7.5	1.2	2.6	0.7	17.4	2.4	9.3	1.6
PRC Shanghai	3.9	1.0	2.6	0.8	3.7	0.8	1.8	0.6	0.9	0.3	0.7	0.2	1.9	0.4	0.5	0.1	8.6	1.3	4.5	0.9

PRC, People's Republic of China; SE, standard error.

[a]Anxiety disorders include agoraphobia, generalized anxiety disorder, obsessive-compulsive disorder, panic disorder, posttraumatic stress disorder, social phobia, and specific phobia. Mood disorders include bipolar I and II disorders, dysthymia, and major depressive disorder. Impulse-control disorders include bulimia, intermittent explosive disorder, pathological gambling disorder, and reported persistence in the past 12 months of symptoms of three child-adolescent disorders (attention-deficit hyperactivity disorder, conduct disorder, and oppositional defiant disorder). Substance disorders include alcohol or drug abuse or dependence. In the case of substance dependence, respondents who met full criteria at some time in their life and who continue to have any symptoms are considered to have 12-month dependence even if they currently do not meet full criteria for the disorder. Organic exclusions were made as specified in the DSM-IV, but diagnostic hierarchy rules were not used.

[b]Bipolar disorders were not assessed in the European Study of the Epidemiology of Mental Disorders (ESEMeD) surveys (Belgium, France, Germany, Italy, the Netherlands, and Spain).

[c]Intermittent explosive disorder was not assessed in the ESEMeD surveys.

[d]Drug abuse and dependence were not assessed in the ESEMeD surveys.

From World Mental Health Survey Consortium: Prevalence, severity and unmet need for treatment of mental disorders in the World Health Organization World Mental Health (WMH) Surveys. *JAMA*. (*in press*.), with permission.

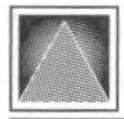

Table 5.1–5
Prevalence of Major Psychiatric Disorders in Primary Health Care

Cities	Current Depression (%)	Generalized Anxiety (%)	Alcohol Dependence (%)	All Mental Disorders (According to the Composite International Diagnostic Interview) (%)
Ankara, Turkey	11.6	0.9	1.0	16.4
Athens, Greece	6.4	14.9	1.0	19.2
Bangalore, India	9.1	8.5	1.4	22.4
Berlin, Germany	6.1	9.0	5.3	18.3
Groningen, the Netherlands	15.9	6.4	3.4	23.9
Ibadan, Nigeria	4.2	2.9	0.4	9.5
Mainz, Germany	11.2	7.9	7.2	23.6
Manchester, UK	16.9	7.1	2.2	24.8
Nagasaki, Japan	2.6	5.0	3.7	9.4
Paris, France	13.7	11.9	4.3	26.3
Rio de Janeiro, Brazil	15.8	22.6	4.1	35.5
Santiago, Chile	29.5	18.7	2.5	52.5
Seattle, USA	6.3	2.1	1.5	11.9
Shanghai, China	4.0	1.9	1.1	7.3
Verona, Italy	4.7	3.7	0.5	9.8
Total	10.4	7.9	2.7	24.0

From Goldberg DP, Lecrubier Y. Form and frequency of mental disorders across centres. In: Üstün TB, Sartorius N, eds. *Mental Illness in General Health Care: An International Study*. Chichester, U.K.: John Wiley; 1995, with permission.

A study of sociodemographics, self-rated health, and mortality in the United States was conducted by P. Franks et al., who analyzed data from the 1987 National Medical Expenditure Survey on a representative sample of U.S. civilians. Self-reported health was measured with the Medical Outcome 20-Item Short Form (SF-20) subscales (health perceptions, physical function, role function, and mental health). Physical function showed the greatest decline with age, whereas mental health increased slightly. Women reported lower health for all scales except role function. Greater income was associated with better health, least marked for mental health. Com-

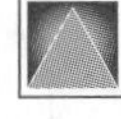

Table 5.1–6
Prevalence of Child and Adolescent Disorders, Selected Studies

Country	Age (Yrs)	Prevalence (%)
Ethiopia[a]	1–15	17.7
Germany[b]	12–15	20.7
India[c]	1–16	12.8
Japan[d]	12–15	15.0
Spain[e]	8, 11, 15	21.7
Switzerland[f]	1–15	22.5
USA[g]	1–15	21.0

[a]Tadesse B, et al.: Childhood behavioural disorders in Ambo district, Western Ethiopia: I. Prevalence estimates. *Acta Psychiatr Scand.* 1999;100(Suppl):92–97.
[b]Weyerer S, Castell R, Biener A, et al.: Prevalence and treatment of psychiatric disorders in 3–14-year-old children; results of a representative field study in the small rural town region of Traunstein, Upper Bavaria. *Acta Psychiatr Scand.* 1988;77:290–296.
[c]Indian Council of Medical Research (ICMR). *Epidemiological Study of Child and Adolescent Psychiatric Disorders in Urban and Rural Areas.* New Delhi: ICMR; 2001.
[d]Morita H, Suzuki M, Suzuki S, et al.: Psychiatric disorders in Japanese secondary school children. *J Child Psychol Psychiatry.* 1993;34:317–322.
[e]Gomez-Beneyto M, Bonet A, Catala MA, et al.: Prevalence of mental disorders among children in Valencia, Spain. *Acta Psychiatr Scand.* 1994;89:352–357.
[f]Steinhausen HC, Metzke CW, Meier M, et al.: Prevalence of child and adolescent psychiatric disorders: the Zurich Epidemiological Study. *Acta Psychiatr Scand.* 1998;98:262–271.
[g]Shaffer D, Fisher P, Dulcan MK, et al.: The NIMH Diagnostic Interview Schedule for Children version 2.3 (DISC-2.3): description acceptability, prevalence rates, and performance in the MECA study. *J Am Acad Child Adolesc Psychiatry.* 1996;35:865–877.

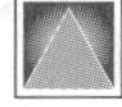

Table 5.1–7
Leading Causes of Disability-Adjusted Life Years in All Ages, Both Sexes

	Health Conditions	Percent of Total
1.	Lower respiratory infections	6.4
2.	Perinatal conditions	6.2
3.	Human immunodeficiency virus/acquired immunodeficiency syndrome	6.1
4.	Unipolar depressive disorders	4.4
5.	Diarrheal diseases	4.2
6.	Ischemic heart disease	3.8
7.	Cerebrovascular disease	3.1
8.	Road traffic accidents	2.8
9.	Malaria	2.7
10.	Tuberculosis	2.4
11.	Chronic obstructive pulmonary disease	2.3
12.	Congenital abnormalities	2.2
13.	Measles	1.9
14.	Iron-deficiency anemia	1.8
15.	Hearing loss, adult-onset	1.7
16.	Falls	1.3
17.	Self-inflicted injuries	1.3
18.	Alcohol use disorders	1.3
19.	Protein-energy malnutrition	1.1
20.	Osteoarthritis	1.1

From Murray CJL, Lopez AD, eds. *The Global Burden of Disease.* Boston: Harvard University Press; 1996, with permission.

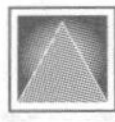

Table 5.1–8
Leading Causes of Years of Life Lived with Disability in All Ages, Both Sexes

	Health Conditions	Percent of Total
1.	Unipolar depressive disorders	11.9
2.	Hearing loss, adult-onset	4.6
3.	Iron-deficiency anemia	4.5
4.	Chronic obstructive pulmonary disease	3.3
5.	Alcohol use disorders	3.1
6.	Osteoarthritis	3.0
7.	Schizophrenia	2.8
8.	Falls	2.8
9.	Bipolar affective disorder	2.5
10.	Asthma	2.1
11.	Congenital abnormalities	2.1
12.	Perinatal conditions	2.0
13.	Alzheimer's disease and other dementia	2.0
14.	Cataracts	1.9
15.	Road traffic accidents	1.8
16.	Protein-energy malnutrition	1.7
17.	Cerebrovascular disease	1.7
18.	Human immunodeficiency virus/acquired immunodeficiency syndrome	1.5
19.	Migraine	1.4
20.	Diabetes mellitus	1.4

From Murray CJL, Lopez AD, eds. *The Global Burden of Disease*. Boston: Harvard University Press; 1996, with permission.

pared with whites, blacks reported lower health, whereas Latinos reported higher health. Lower socioeconomic status and being black were factors associated with lower reported health status and higher mortality, women reported lower health status but exhibited lower mortality, and Latinos reported higher health status and exhibited lower mortality.

Findings on Clinical Care

There is a trend worldwide to diversify the settings for mental health care. The extent and patterns of this process are being investigated by the WHO Atlas Survey on Mental Health Resources by asking governments to complete questionnaires about mental health resources. The distribution of psychiatric beds per 10,000 population by WHO regions is presented in Figure 5.1–4. It shows that bed availability rates are highest in Europe (9.3) and the Americas (3.6) (which includes North America and Latin America) and are quite low (under 1.0) in the rest of the world.

According to the previously mentioned Atlas Survey, the median numbers of psychiatrists per 100,000 population are 1.0 worldwide, 9.0 in Europe, 1.6 in the Americas, 0.95 in the Eastern Mediterranean, and under 0.28 in the rest of the world. The median numbers of psychiatric nurses per 100,000 population are 2.0 worldwide, 27.5 in Europe, 2.7 in the Americas, 1.1 in the Western Pacific, and under 0.5 in the rest of the world. The median rates of psychologists working in mental health are 0.4 worldwide, 3.0 in Europe, 2.8 in the Americas, and under 0.2 in the rest of the world. Finally, the median rates of social workers in mental health care are 0.3 worldwide, 2.35 in Europe, 1.9 in the Americas, and under 0.4 in the rest of the world.

Focusing attention on Australia, Gavin Andrews et al. have ascertained the use of the services of different types of health professionals for mental problems. This study documented the predominant roles of general practitioners and even other health professionals (including nurses, pharmacists, and welfare counselors) above that of psychiatrists, for the care of people experiencing mental disorders (even a large number of these) (Table 5.1–10).

Jyrki Korkeila et al. investigated the factors predicting readmission to psychiatric hospitals in Finland during the early 1990s. The most prominent factors were previous admissions, long lengths of stay, and identification of psychotic or personality disorders. These

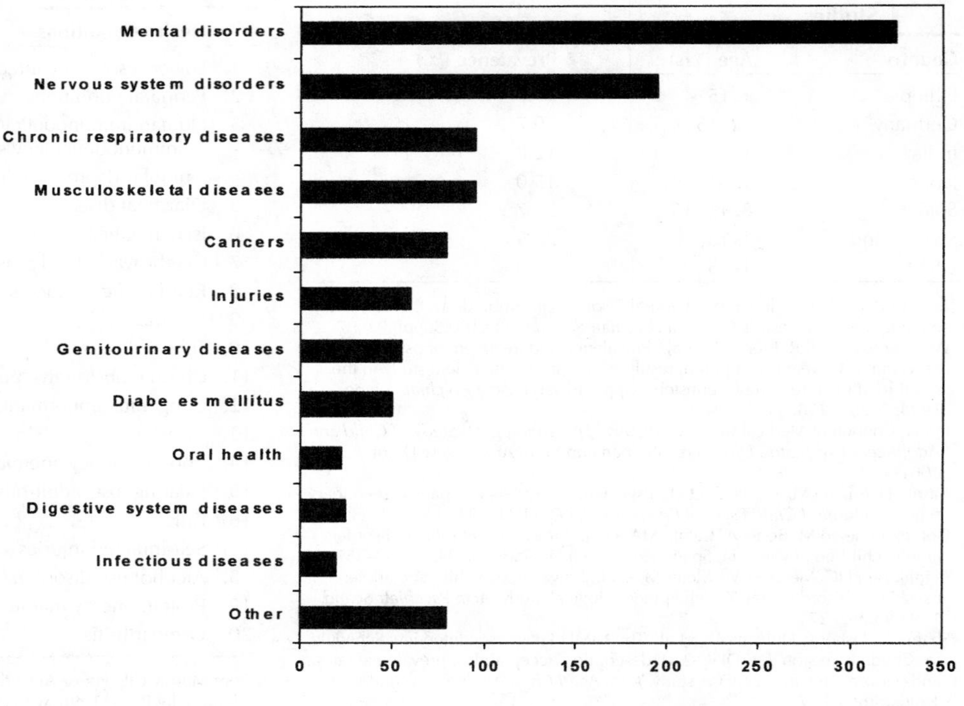

FIGURE 5.1–3 Years of life lost through disability (YLD), Australia, 1996. (From Mathers C, Vos T, Stevenson C. *The Burden of Disease and Injury in Australia*. Canberra: Australian Institute of Health and Welfare; 1999, with permission.)

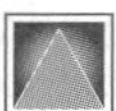

Table 5.1–9
Quality of Life Findings in a Spanish Community Sample (489 Men and Women)

Quality of Life Index[a] Items	Mean	Standard Deviation
1. Physical well-being	6.58	1.65
2. Psychological/emotional well-being	6.48	1.74
3. Self-care/independent functioning	7.31	1.48
4. Occupational functioning	7.48	1.56
5. Interpersonal functioning	7.68	1.56
6. Social emotional support	7.46	1.81
7. Community instrumental support	6.67	1.54
8. Personal fulfillment	6.78	1.76
9. Spiritual fulfillment	6.04	1.95
10. Global perception of quality of life	7.27	1.65
Average	6.98	1.11

[a]Score range: 0 (bad) to 10 (excellent).
From Lorente E, Ibáñez MI, Moro M, et al.: Indice de calidad de vida: estandarización y características psicométricas en una muestra española. *Psiquiatría y Salud Integral.* 2002;2:45–50, with permission.

findings pointed out that, despite recent emphasis on community care, a continuing need for inpatient facilities for some psychiatric patients seems to exist.

Illustrating the importance of primary health care for people presenting mental disorders, M. G. Rowe et al. found that one in five women and one in ten men seeing their primary physicians have been recently depressed. Bernardo Ng et al., surveying nonpsychiatrist physicians in rural California, documented the need for enhanced postgraduate training on depression for primary care physicians.

Findings on Mental Health Policy

The WHO Atlas Survey Ministries of Health revealed that 40 percent of countries in the world have no mental health policies, 30 percent have no national mental health programs, 25 percent have no mental health legislation, 28 percent have no specific budget for mental health, and 41 percent have no regular mental health training for primary care personnel. These figures are preliminary, and the survey is now being enhanced in collaboration with the World Psychiatric Association.

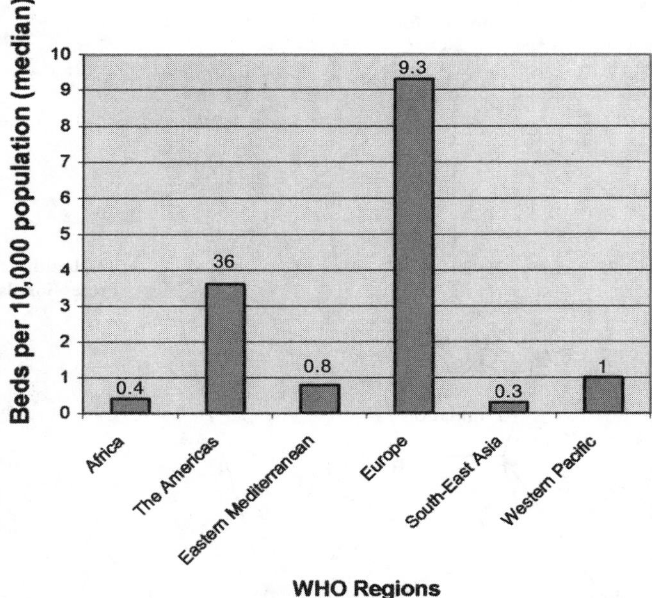

FIGURE 5.1–4 Psychiatric beds per 10,000 population by World Health Organization (WHO) regions. (From World Health Organization. *Atlas of Mental Health Resources in the World 2001.* Geneva: World Health Organization; 2001, with permission.)

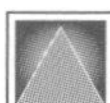

Table 5.1–10
Use of Professional Services for Mental Problems in Australia, 1997

Consultations for Mental Problems	No Disorder (%)	Any Disorder (%)	>3 Disorders (%)
General practitioner only[a]	2.2	13.2	18.1
Mental health professional only[b]	0.5	2.4	3.9
Other health professional only[c]	1.0	4.0	5.7
Combination of health professionals	1.0	15.0	36.4
Any health professional[d]	4.6	34.6	64.0

[a]Refers to individuals who had at least one consultation with a general practitioner in the previous 12 months but did not consult any other type of health professional.
[b]Refers to individuals who had at least one consultation with a mental health professional (psychiatrist, psychologist, mental health team) in the previous 12 months but did not consult any other type of health professional.
[c]Refers to persons who had at least one consultation with another health professional (nurse, nonpsychiatric medical specialist, pharmacist, ambulance officer, welfare worker, or counselor) in the previous 12 months but did not consult any other type of health professional.
[d]Refers to persons who had at least one consultation with any health professional in the previous 12 months.
From Andrews G, Henderson S, Hall W: Prevalence, comorbidity, disability and service utilization: overview of the Australian National Mental Health Survey. *Br J Psychiatry.* 2001;178:145–153, with permission.

Illustrating the value of pointed investigations in the complex mental health field to upgrade health and social policies, Table 5.1–11 displays the relationship between women experiencing domestic violence and then contemplating suicide in eight developing countries in Latin America, Africa, and Asia. In all the study sites, more than twice the percentages of women ever experiencing physical violence by an intimate partner contemplate committing suicide, as compared to women never experiencing such domestic violence.

With reference to instrumentation for mental health care, the use of standard diagnostic systems is of significant relevance. Darrel Regier et al. have highlighted discrepancies in mental disorder rates obtained through different interviews and surveys and discussed their implications for determining treatment need. T. B. Üstün et al. have further examined the intricacy of need for treatment. Dealing more broadly with diagnostic systems, a survey of leading psychiatrists across the world (205 respondents from 66 different countries) conducted by Juan E. Mezzich documented that ICD-10 is now the most frequently used and valued classification system for clinical diagnosis and training, and DSM-IV is more valued for research purposes. Accessibility to diagnostic manuals and training appeared limited, particularly for the research criteria, primary care, and multiaxial versions of ICD-10.

FUTURE DIRECTIONS

In line with the perspectives for a multidimensional, ecological, and culturally informed epidemiology enunciated by Susser and Susser and Naomar Almeida-Filho, it appears that, for the continuous development of the field both as a solid scientific and professional disci-

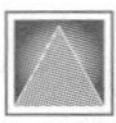

Table 5.1–11
Relationship between Domestic Violence and Contemplation of Suicide

	Percentage of Women Who Have Ever Thought of Committing Suicide ($P < .001$)	
Country of Study	**Never Experienced Physical Violence by Intimate Partner**	**Ever Experienced Physical Violence by Intimate Partner**
Brazil[a] (N = 940)	21	48
Chile[b] (N = 422)	11	36
Egypt[b] (N = 631)	7	61
India[b] (N = 6,327)	15	64
Indonesia[c] (N = 765)	1	11
Philippines[b] (N = 1,001)	8	28
Peru[a] (N = 1,088)	17	40
Thailand[a] (N = 2,073)	18	41

[a]World Health Organization. *WHO Study on Women's Health and Domestic Violence.* Geneva: World Health Organization; 2001.
[b]International Network of Clinical Epidemiologists. *World Studies of Abuse in Family Environments.* Manila: International Network of Clinical Epidemiologists; 2001.
[c]Hakimi M, Hayati EN, Marlinawatie VU, et al. Silence for the Sake of Harmony: Domestic Violence and Women's Health in Central Java. Yogyakarta, Indonesia: Program for Appropriate Technology in Health; 2001.

pline and a rich contributor to public health, the following considerations are pertinent.

A multilevel architecture would be valuable for understanding the complexity of an epidemiology of illness and health, an epidemiology helpful to advance the life goals of the culturally diverse population of today's world. Such an architecture would involve the integration of biological, psychological, and social factors, of objective and subjective approaches, and of statistical and anthropological information.

Even less intricate fields than epidemiology, now more than ever, require alliances and partnerships based on joint commitment to agreed objectives. Figure 5.1–5 articulates the contributions of a number of stakeholder groups (health professionals, policy makers, health services, health financing, and proactive communities) toward the promotion of healthy individuals and populations. As pointed out by Lowell Levin, public participation is essential for health care quality. He argued for the value of expanding and deepening the dialogue among public interest groups and the health professions, a dialogue that is honest, courageous, and respectful.

The enormous and intriguing findings emerging from genetics and the neurosciences must be incorporated into the discussions and formulations of psychiatric epidemiology. The deciphering of the human genome is leading us to recognize the crucial role of the environment to activate the expression of genetic influences. In the exploration of new biologically based nosologies, the role of endophenotypes as intermediary between genotypes and phenotypes may be helpful here (Fig. 5.1–6).

Also crucial for the conceptual and methodological advancement of epidemiology—in interaction with multiple groups across the world—will be the optimal use of the new informational and communicational technologies. This would include the development of Internet knowledge-base platforms, establishment of pertinent intranets, design of institutional Web sites, and organization of electronic journals.

Illustrative of the challenges and opportunities ahead is the upcoming development of a new international classification and diagnostic system of value for clinical care and public health. It will require the best scientific efforts to refine the epistemological bases of a sound and useful diagnostic system, include emerging findings of etiological pertinence, resolve current controversies on comorbidity, incorporate essential aspects of positive health, and adopt more effective models of measurement and formulation. It must also integrate mental health classification more fully within general health

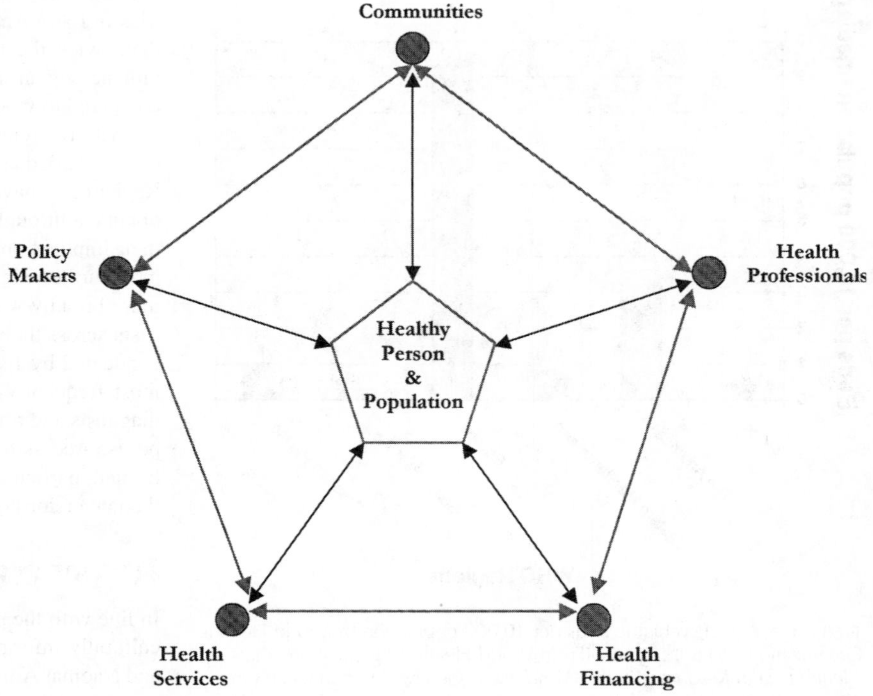

FIGURE 5.1–5 Integrating stakeholders' perspectives and commitment toward a healthy person and a healthy population.

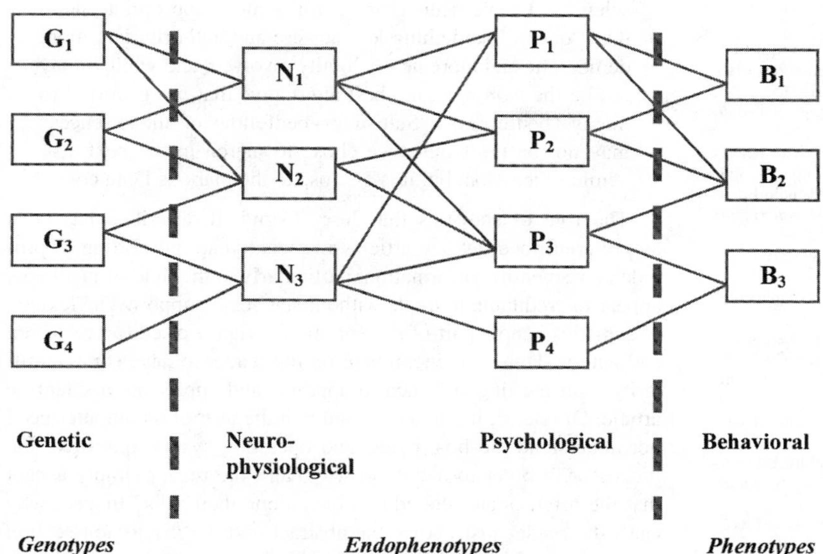

FIGURE 5.1–6 Gene-to-behavior pathways prototype. (From Üstün TB: Toward a clinical epistemology of mental disorders. Paper presented at the WPA-WHO Forum on Integrating Concepts and Partners towards a New ICD. WPA International Congress of Psychiatry, Caracas, October 3, 2003.)

classification and engage research groups and stakeholder representatives from across the world actively and respectfully.

One hopes that through the exercise of scientific dedication and professional wisdom and a perspective that attends creatively to patterns of illness and health, psychiatric epidemiology, as allegorized by Diego Rivera's painting (Fig. 5.1–7) (evocatively titled as both *History of Medicine* and *People in Demand of Health*), will increasingly be a helpful contributor to the advancement of clinical care and public health for all peoples in the world.

SUGGESTED CROSS-REFERENCES

Other quantitative and experimental methods in psychiatry are discussed in Chapter 5. The classification of mental disorders is discussed in Section 9.1, and international psychiatric diagnoses in Section 9.2. Schizophrenia is the subject of Chapter 12; mood disorders are covered in Chapter 13; anxiety disorders are the focus of Chapter 14; substance-related disorders are discussed in Chapter 11; somatization disorder is discussed in Chapter 15; and personality disorders are the subject of Chapter 23.

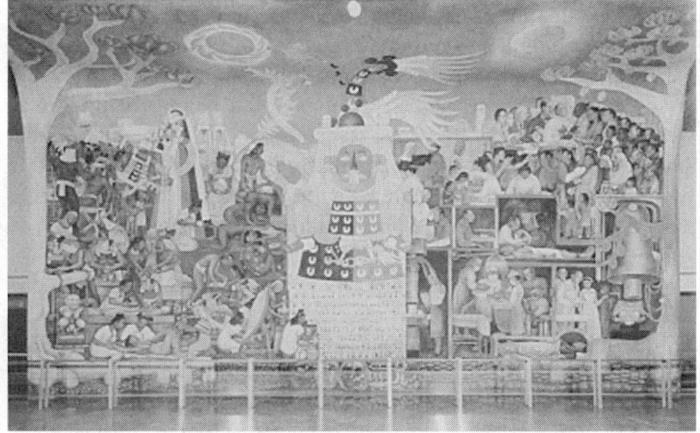

FIGURE 5.1–7 Diego Rivera's *History of Medicine*, or *People in Demand of Health*.

REFERENCES

Almeida-Filho N, Mari J, Coutinho E, França J, Fernandez J, Andreoli S, Busnello E: Brazilian multicentric study of psychiatric morbidity: methodological features and prevalence estimates. *Br J Psychiatry*. 1997;171:524–529.

Andrews G, Henderson S, Hall W: Prevalence, comorbidity, disability and service utilization: overview of the Australian National Mental Health Survey. *Br J Psychiatry*. 2001;178:145–153.

Aspinwall LG, Staudinger UM, eds. *A Psychology of Human Strengths: Fundamental Questions and Future Directions for a Positive Psychology*. Washington, D.C.: American Psychological Association; 2002.

Berganza CE: Broadening the international base for the development of an integrated diagnostic system in psychiatry. *World Psychiatry*. 2003;1:38–40.

Costello EJ, Mustillo S, Erkanli A, Keeler G, Angold A: Prevalence and development of psychiatric disorders in childhood and adolescence. *Arch Gen Psychiatry*. 2003;60:837–844.

Dear K, Henderson S, Korten A: Well-being in Australia—findings from the National Survey of Mental Health and Well-being. *Soc Psychiatry Psychiatr Epidemiol*. 2002;37:503–509.

Goldberg DP, Lecrubier Y. Form and frequency of mental disorders across centres. In: Üstün TB, Sartorius N, eds. *Mental Illness in General Health Care: An International Study*. Chichester, U.K.: John Wiley; 1995.

Henderson S: The national survey of mental health and well-being in Australia: impact on policy. *Can J Psychiatry*. 2002;47:819–824.

Horwitz J, Marconi J: El problema de las definiciones en el campo de la salud mental. Definiciones aplicables en estudios epidemiológicos. *Bol Oficina Sanit Panam*. 1966;60:300–309.

Hyman SE: Neuroscience, genetics, and the future of psychiatric diagnosis. *Psychopathology*. 2002;35:139–144.

Jenkins R, Bebbington P, Brugha TS, Farrell M, Lewis G, Meltzer H: British psychiatric morbidity survey. *Br J Psychiatry*. 1998;173:4–7.

Kessler RC: The World Health Organization International Consortium in Psychiatric Epidemiology (ICPE): Initial work and future directions—the NAPE Lecture 1998. *Acta Psychiatr Scand*. 1999;99:2–9.

*Kessler RC, Üstün TB: Initial report from the WHO World Mental Health Survey. *JAMA*. (*in press*.)

Kirmayer LJ, Minas IH: The future of cultural psychiatry: an international perspective. *Can J Psychiatr*. 2000;45:438–446.

Kuyken W, Orley J: WHO Quality of Life Assessment. *Soc Sci Med*. 1995;41:1403–1409.

Mezzich JE: An empirical prototypical approach to the definition of psychiatric illness. *Br J Psychiatry*. 1989;154:42–46.

Mezzich JE: International surveys on the use of ICD-10 and related diagnostic systems. *Psychopathology*. 2002;35:72–75.

Mezzich JE: From financial analysis to policy development in mental health care: the need for broader conceptual models and partnerships. *J Ment Health Policy Econ*. 2003;6:156–158.

Mezzich JE, Berganza CE, von Cranach M, Jorge MR, Kastrup MC, Murthy RS, Okasha A, Pull C, Sartorius N, Skodol A, Zaudig M, eds.: Essentials of the World Psychiatric Association's International Guidelines for Diagnostic Assessment (IGDA). *Br J Psychiatry*. 2003;182(Suppl 45):S37–S66.

Mezzich JE, Cohen NL, Ruipérez MA, Pérez C, Yoon G, Liu J, Mahmud S: The Spanish version of the Quality of Life Index: presentation and validation. *J Nerv Ment Dis*. 2000;138:301–305.

Mezzich JE, Fabrega H, eds. Cultural Psychiatry: International Perspectives. *Psychiatr Clin North Am*. September, 2001.

Mezzich JE, Kraemer HC, Worthington DR, Coffman GA: Assessment of agreement among several raters formulating multiple diagnoses. *J Psychiatr Res*. 1981;16:29–39.

Murray CJL, Lopez AD, eds. *The Global Burden of Disease*. Boston: Harvard University Press; 1996.
Regier DA, Kaelbert CT, Rae DS, Farmer ME, Knauper B, Kessler RC, Norquist GS: Limitations for diagnostic criteria and assessment instruments for mental disorders: Implications for research and policy. *Arch Gen Psychiatry*. 1998;55:109–115.
Robins LN, Helzer JE, Croughan J, Ratcliff KS: NIMH Diagnostic Interview Schedule: its history, characteristics, and validity. *Arch Gen Psychiatry*. 1981;38:381–389.
Saavedra JE, Malpartida C, Nizama M, Vasquez F, Matos L, Huaman J, Arrelano C, Pomalima M, Guerra M, Paz V, Robles Y, Gonzalez S, Sagastegui A, Vargas H, Stucchi S, Chirinos R, Diaz R (Instituto Especializado de Salud Mental): Estudio Epidemiologico Metropolitano en Salud Mental 2002. *Anales de Salud Mental (Lima)*. 2002;18(1,2).
Sackett DL, Rosenberg WMC, Gray JAM, Haynes RB, Richardson WS: Evidence based medicine: what it is and what it isn't. *BMJ*. 1996;312:71–72.
Schmolke MM, Lecic-Tosevski D, eds.: Health promotion as an integral component of clinical care. *Dynamic Psychiatry*. 2003;36(special issue).
Sheehan DV, Lecrubier Y, Sheehan KH, Amorim P, Janavs J, Weiller E, Hergueta T, Baker R, Dunbar GC: The Mini-International Neuropsychiatric Interview (M.I.N.I.): the development and validation of a structured diagnostic psychiatric interview for DSM-IV and ICD-10. *J Clin Psychiatry*. 1998;59(Suppl 20):22–57.
Slade T. *Using Epidemiology to Inform Classification in Psychiatry* [dissertation]. Australia: School of Psychiatry, University of New South Wales; 2002.
Spitzer RL, Williams JBW, Gibbon M, First MB: The Structured Clinical Interview for DSM-III-R (SCID). I. History, rationale, and description. *Arch Gen Psychiatry*. 1992;49:624–629.
Stengel E: Classification of mental disorders. *Bull World Health Organ*. 1950;21:601–663.
Sullivan DF. Conceptual problems in developing an index of health. U.S. Department of Health, Education & Welfare. USPH Publication No. 1000, Series 2, No. 17. Washington, DC: U.S. Government Printing Office; 1966.
*Susser M, Susser E: Choosing a future for epidemiology. I. Eras and paradigms. *Am J Public Health*. 1996;86:668–673.
Üstün TB: Mainstreaming mental health. *Bull World Health Organ*. 2000;78:412.
Üstün TB, Ayuso-Mateos JL, Chatterji S, Mathers C, Murray CJR: Global burden of depressive disorders in the year 2000. *Br J Psychiatry*. 2004;184:386–392.
*Üstün TB, Chatterji S, Bickenbach J, Kostanjsek N, Schneider M: The international classification of functioning, disability and health: a new tool for understanding disability and health. *Disabil Rehabil*. 2003;25:565–571.
Üstün TB, Chatterji S, Rehm J: Limitations of diagnostic paradigm: It doesn't explain "need." *Arch Gen Psychiatry*. 1998;55:1145–1146.
Üstün TB, Chisholm D: Global "burden of disease"—study for psychiatric disorders. *Psychiatr Prax*. 2001;28(Suppl 1):S7–S11.
*Üstün TB, Mezzich JE: Epilogue of international classification and diagnosis: critical experience and future directions. *Psychopathology*. 2002;35:199–201.
Wing JK, Babor T, Brugha T, Burke J, Cooper JE, Giel R, Jablenski A, Regier D, Sartorious N: SCAN. Schedules for Clinical Assessment in Neuropsychiatry. *Arch Gen Psychiatry*. 1990;47:589–593.
Wing JK, Cooper JE, Sartorius N: Measure and Classification of Psychiatric Symptoms: An Instructional Manual for the PSE and CATEGO Programs. Cambridge: Cambridge University Press; 1974.
World Health Organization. *Tenth Revision of the International Classification of Diseases and Related Health Problems (ICD-10)*. Geneva: World Health Organization; 1992.
World Health Organization. *International Classification of Functioning, Disability and Health (ICF)*. Geneva: World Health Organization; 2001.
WHO International Consortium in Psychiatric Epidemiology: Cross-national comparisons of the prevalences and correlates of mental disorders. *Bull World Health Organ*. 2000;78:413–426.
*WHO World Mental Health Survey Consortium: Prevalence, severity, and unmet need for treatment of mental disorders in the World Health Organization. World Mental Health (WMH) Surveys. *JAMA*. (*in press*.)

▲ 5.2 Statistics and Experimental Design

EUGENE M. LASKA, PH.D., MORRIS MEISNER, PH.D., AND CAROLE SIEGEL, PH.D.

In his presidential address to the American Statistical Association in 1974 entitled "A Statistician's Apology," Jerry Cornfield reflected on what statistics is and where it is going as a field. He wrote

> no one has ever claimed that statistics was the queen of the sciences—a claim which, even for mathematics, was dependent on a somewhat restricted view of what constituted the sciences. I have been groping for a more appropriate noun than "queen," something less austere and authoritarian, more democratic and more nearly totally involved, and while it may not be the *mot juste*, the best alternative that has occurred to me is "bedfellow." "Statistics—bedfellow of the sciences" may not be the banner we chose to march in the next academic procession, but it is as close to the mark as I can come.

The role of statistics that Jerry Cornfield described has been amply confirmed, as few articles in recent years purporting to provide new scientific information, particularly in the field of medicine, appear in creditable journals without statistical support. The lexicon of statistics is now part of the common parlance of editor, reviewer, and author. Thus, it is incumbent on the reader to have some familiarity with the lingua franca to appraise and appreciate a scientific article. Of course, it may be argued that the user of a computer need not understand the bits, bytes, and operating system that drive the processor in order to use it, so why can't the reader simply accept that the referees and the editors have done their jobs? Indeed, why can't the reader just peruse the abstract and the discussion section and be done with it? Well, truth be told, they can. An individual with limited computer skills can successfully use a word processor. Likewise, an individual without an appreciation of the nuances of the methods used can skim a scientific report to obtain the essence of its message. However, this strategy will not enable an independent view of the strength of the evidence nor of the credibility of the findings. The reputations of the author and the journal may provide some comfort, and, perhaps, in reports related only peripherally to the reader's interests, that is all that is required. In one's own field of expertise, however, a full understanding of the techniques used to obtain the results and reach the conclusions ought to be accessible. If the reader wants to really understand the material, then at least a rudimentary understanding of statistical concepts is necessary.

What, then, are the must-know elements of statistics? It is hard to say. It depends on the area of science or therapeutics that is of interest. The discipline of statistics has become so vast that few, if any, professionals can pretend to be an expert in all of its parts, but a psychiatrist should have at least a basic understanding of the rudiments. The contents of countless articles, books, and abbreviated introductory courses will not be replicated in this chapter. In many elementary texts and chapters, the basic ideas are described without any assumptions about the mathematical skill level of the reader. This chapter assumes, however, that the reader already has some familiarity with the basic concepts but, nevertheless, begins with a very brief review of some elementary statistical ideas. The remainder of this chapter discusses just some of the many topics in statistics, selected in the hope that they will enlarge the capacity of the reader to make independent judgments and interpretations of the articles they read. Necessarily, the presentations are not complete, the choice of topics is somewhat arbitrary, and many topics that belong in this essay were left out. Hopefully, this presentation will stimulate further study of statistical methods, particularly by individuals interested in psychiatric research. Although the authors have strived to keep technical details to a minimum, some complexities are unavoidable.

BASIC IDEAS

This section reviews the notions of elementary probability theory and introduces the concepts of *random variable*, *measures of central tendency*, and *measure of dispersion*. To describe the joint behavior of two random variables, the ideas of statistical independence, covariance, and correlation are necessary and enable the introduction of multivariate density.

Probability Theory The mathematical foundation on which statistical methods are built is probability theory. This theory considers an experimental situation in which the outcomes are random events. The set of all possible simple outcomes of the experiment is called the *sample space*. For example, throwing a die once gives rise to a sample space containing six elements: 1, 2, 3, 4, 5, and 6. A *random variable* is a mapping of the sample space onto the real line. It is usually denoted by an uppercase Latin letter, such as X, and an actual outcome is usually denoted by its corresponding lowercase letter. Thus, X is the random outcome of the face value resulting from the roll of the die, and $x = 6$ is an observed outcome. Assigned to each simple outcome is a positive number corresponding to the probability of that outcome. The sum of these probabilities over all simple outcomes in the sample space is 1. The assignment of a probability to a simple outcome automatically determines the probability of all subsets of the sample space. For example, the probability that the outcome of the roll of the die is an odd number is the probability that $X = 1$ plus the probability that $X = 3$ plus the probability that $X = 5$.

Probability Density Functions The random nature of an experiment is characterized by the chance of observing a particular value x. If there are only a finite number of possible outcomes, the probability of each event x, $P(X = x)$, can be positive, and, as a function of x, it is called a *probability density function* (PDF). If the range of outcome values includes all values in an interval, sometimes called the *continuous case*, the PDF, generically denoted by $f(x)$, has a different meaning. This is because the probability of observing any particular single value x, possibly with a finite (countable) number of exceptions, is zero. In this case, the integral of $f(x)$ over the interval is equal to the probability that an outcome falls in that interval. The *cumulative distribution function*, frequently represented by $F(x)$, is the probability that the random variable takes a value less than or equal to x. It is obtained in the discrete case by summing the probabilities of all possible outcomes that are less than or equal to x and, in the continuous case, by integrating the PDF from minus infinity to x. All probabilities must be nonnegative, and their sum over all possible events—or, in the continuous case, the integral over the sample space—must be one. Therefore, as x goes to infinity, $F(x)$ goes to 1. The frequentist interpretation of probability is that, in the long run, the fraction of times that the outcome x is observed (or that x falls in a specific interval $[a,b]$ of the sample space) in N replications of the experiment, tends to $f(x)$ (or to the integral of the PDF from a to b) as N tends to infinity.

Conditional Probability and Independence Many compound events can be defined from the simple outcomes in an experiment. In the roll of the dice experiment, the event that an odd number occurs and the event that either a 1 or a 5 occurs are two examples. In some cases, knowing that one event has occurred can impact the likelihood of another event occurring. For example, if the faces of the die are equally likely (all have a probability of 1 out of 6), then the probability of a 1 or 5 occurring, given that an odd number has occurred, is 2 out of 3, whereas the probability of a 1 or 5 occurring, with no other event information, is 1 out of 3. The random variable X that takes the value 1 if the dice falls on face 1 or 5, and 0 otherwise, and the random variable Y that takes the value 1 if the dice falls on an odd-numbered face are said to be dependent. Two random variables, X and Y, are said to be independent if $P(X = x|Y = y) = P(X = x)$. The notation $P(X = x|Y = y)$ is read "the probability that $X = x$ given (or conditional on) $Y = y$." It is the probability that the event $X = x$ occurs, calculated in the outcome space defined by the event $Y = y$. Formally, $P(X = x|Y = y) = P(X = x \text{ and } Y = y)/P(Y = y)$. Also, two random variables are independent if the probability of the joint event $X = x$ and $Y = y$ is equal to the product of the probabilities of the two events, i.e., $P(X = x \text{ and } Y = y) = P(X = x)P(Y = y)$. Independence and conditional probabilities play a major role in statistical thinking. For example, suppose treatment assignment and degree of improvement on a five-level clinical global improvement scale (CGI) are reported in a table with five rows (CGI) and two columns (treatment or placebo.) A chi-square statistic is used to analyze such contingency tables for testing the independence of two random variables that define the rows and columns. If the statistic is significant, the data suggest that the variables are dependent and the distribution of CGI outcomes conditioned on a value of treatment assignment differs depending on the value of the conditioning variable. If treatment and placebo improvement rates differ, then one would expect a chi-square test to be significant because the distribution of CGI conditional on receiving the treatment is not the same as the distribution conditional on receiving placebo.

Parametric Forms In parametric analyses, the *form* of the PDF is assumed known, with the exception of the value of one or more parameters, which, once specified, completely determines the distribution. The most commonly assumed parametric form is the so-called gaussian, or normal, distribution. The shape of the normal PDF is the familiar bell-shaped curve, whose peak (mode), mean, and median occur at the same value. In fact, the curve merely translates to the right or left, retaining the same form as the mean is respectively increased or decreased. Distributions with this property are called *translation parameter families*, and they have the mathematical form $f(x - \phi)$, where ϕ is the mean of the random variable X. Greek letters, such as ϕ, are often used to represent parameters of the PDF to distinguish them from random variables. The logistic, beta, exponential, F, and t, for continuous random variables, and the binomial, multinomial, and Poisson, for discrete random variables, are PDFs that frequently appear in the scientific literature.

Mean, Median, and Variance A variety of measures that help characterize the nature of a random variable have been defined. Among the most important are the mean, median, and variance. The *mean* is the average of all of the possible outcomes, weighted by the probability of the outcome. The mean is thought of as a measure of central tendency of the random variable. It is also called the *expected value*, and if X is the random variable, then it is usually denoted by $E(X)$. The value m is the median if the probability that the random variable X is less than m equals the probability that X is greater than m. The variance is the average of the square of the difference between each outcome x and the mean, weighted by the probability of the outcome. The *variance*, usually denoted by σ^2, and its square root, σ, the standard deviation, are thought of as measures of the spread of the observations about the mean.

Multivariate Random Variables Most serious investigations of scientific phenomena cannot be described by the outcome of a single random variable. A *multivariate probability distribution* describes the chance of various outcomes of an experiment in which k events are observed in each unit in a sample. Typically, in trials in mental health, a *unit* is a patient, and observations are made on one measure collected over time, many measures collected at one point in time, or many measures collected at multiple times. Two random variables, X_1 and X_2, may be independent or dependent. As discussed above, they are independent if and only if their joint (simultaneous) probability function, $f(x_1, x_2)$, is always equal to $f_1(x_1) \times f_2(x_2)$. The PDFs $f_1(x_1)$ and $f_2(x_2)$ are called the *marginal distributions* of X_1 and X_2.

Covariance and Correlation One important measure of the relationship between dependent pairs of random variables X_1 and X_2 is the *covariance*, or the average of the product of the difference between each outcome x_1 and its mean and the difference between each outcome x_2 and its mean, weighted by the probability of the joint outcome x_1, x_2. Closely related is the *correlation*, usually denoted by ρ, which is defined to be the covariance divided by the product of the standard deviation of X_1 and the standard deviation of X_2. The distribution most widely used in multivariate applications is, by far, the multivariate normal. If the mean and variance of each of the random variables and the covariance between all pairs of random variables are known, then the multivariate normal distribution is completely specified.

USING DATA TO ESTIMATE PARAMETERS

The scientific question under consideration must be represented by a statistical model, which at least approximately characterizes the set of outcomes that can be observed after the data collection is complete. If the model, represented in parametric form as the PDF f(x, ϕ), is fully known, there is little left to do. Neither an experiment nor statistical inference is needed. The probability distribution is the answer to the question: If the experiment is performed, what can be expected with what probability? However, the true value of the distribution is rarely known, and the reason for the experiment is to collect data so that something can be said about the nature of the PDF and the value of the parameters that specify it. This section discusses the problem of parameter estimation, beginning with a description of the method of maximum likelihood. Some of the properties that are used to appraise the merits of an estimator are described. Confidence interval estimators and their interpretations are introduced.

Point Estimators

In many application areas, the general form of the parametric distribution that describes the collected data is well established. After an experiment is performed, the first question an investigator should attempt to answer is what values of the unknown parameters within the assumed PDF form best represent the data. This is the setting of the theory of statistical estimation, which has a rich and long history. Of course, the principal goal is to come as close to the true value of the parameter as possible. Estimation theory is concerned with the problem of how to obtain an estimator and appraise its worth, not in an individual case but over all possible outcomes, weighted by the probability of the outcome. Perhaps the premier approach, introduced by Sir Ronald Fisher, is *maximum likelihood estimation*. The idea is both intuitive and simple. Suppose that the parameter ϕ is unknown and f(x, ϕ) is the probability of observing the event x. The likelihood is just f(x^*, ϕ), where x^* is the value of the observed outcome. Here, x^* is fixed and f is thought of as a function that depends only on ϕ. For any given ϕ, the likelihood is a measure of how "likely" the observation x^* is if the outcome had been selected randomly from the probability distribution f with parameter ϕ. If the observed random variables are independent, then the likelihood is the product of the likelihoods of each observation. It is a measure of the probability of the joint occurrence of $x_1^*, x_2^*, \ldots$, and maximum likelihood theory posits that ϕ should be chosen so that the probability of the event that was actually observed is as large as possible. Any other choice of parameters would make the observed data set less likely to have been observed. For example, if a coin is tossed 20 times and lands heads 10 of the times, setting the probability of a head, P, equal to 10 out of 20, or .5, is perfectly sensible. In fact, under the assumption that the distribution of the random variable (the number of heads) is binomial, it makes the chance of 10 heads in 20 tosses maximal. Setting it equal to a lower or higher number makes the estimator less consonant with the data. In many cases, the properties of the maximum likelihood estimation are very desirable.

Properties of Estimators

Because an estimator is itself the result of a random experiment, it is a random variable and, thus, has a mean, or expected, value. The theoretical calculation of its mean involves the use of the density f(x, ϕ), where the true value of ϕ is unknown. We refer to the estimator as *unbiased* if, for each value of the parameter ϕ, the mean of the estimator is ϕ. Such estimators exhibit a kind of impartiality that is usually desirable. Another property of an estimator concerns its behavior as the sample size of the experiment increases. Imagine a sequence of estimators in which the ith estimator is based on a sample of size i. For example, the ith estimator in the sequence could be the sample mean based on a sample of size i. An estimator is said to be *consistent* if, for any true value ϕ, the sequence converges to ϕ. Another property of an estimator concerns its precision, as measured by its variance. An estimator is said to be *efficient* if it is unbiased and its variance is as small as it can possibly be. In some situations, a lower bound for the variance of an estimator can be determined. In this circumstance, the *efficiency* of an estimator can be determined by comparing its variance to the theoretical minimum variance. Consistency suggests that as the sample size increases, the variance decreases and the estimator approaches ϕ.

Confidence Interval Estimation

Even if an estimator has all of the most desirable properties, it is not likely that it will be exactly right. To leave a little room for error, an interval estimate, in addition to a point estimate, is desirable. These are termed *confidence interval* (CI) *estimators*. The amount of confidence placed on the estimator, in the sense that the parameter being estimated lies within the interval, is called the *confidence level*, or *confidence coefficient*. The usual form of a CI is $P[a \leq \phi \leq b] = c$. If $c = .95$, this is read: $[a,b]$ is a 95 percent confidence interval for the parameter ϕ, or $[a,b]$ is a confidence interval for ϕ, with a confidence coefficient of .95. Typically, for a fixed sample size, as the confidence coefficient increases, so does the length of the interval. An interval from minus infinity to plus infinity, with a confidence coefficient of 1, always covers the unknown parameter, but it is completely uninformative.

Interpretation of a Confidence Interval

It is important to understand how to interpret a confidence interval. From a frequentist point of view, the probability of an event is characterized by the frequency with which the event occurs in infinitely many replications of the experiment. The form of the interval before the experiment is conducted is usually given in terms of some not-yet-observed random variable. For a normal random variable with a mean of ϕ and a variance of 1, the probability statement $P[\bar{X} - 1.96/\sqrt{N} \leq \phi \leq \bar{X} + 1.96/\sqrt{N}] = .95$, where $\bar{X}$ is the arithmetic mean of N observations, has a clear and unambiguous meaning. Suppose that a random sample of $N = 100$ observations is repeatedly drawn from a population governed by a normal distribution with a mean of ϕ and a variance of 1. As the number of repeated draws becomes very large, regardless of the true value of ϕ, the proportion of times that the interval $[X - 1.96/\sqrt{N} \leq \phi \leq \bar{X} + 1.96/\sqrt{N}] = [\bar{X} - .196, \bar{X} + .196]$ covers ϕ approaches .95. Once data are collected, however, the game has changed. The statement $P[.304 \leq \phi \leq .696]$ can only take the value 1 or 0, depending on whether or not the true value of ϕ falls in the interval. So, from a frequentist point of view, it is incorrect to think of the confidence coefficient of a confidence interval estimate as the probability that the observed interval includes the true value of the parameter. Rather, it is a statement about the joint probability that the random variable that defines the lower limit falls below ϕ and the random variable that defines the upper limit of the interval falls above ϕ (before data are collected) for any true value of ϕ.

USING DATA TO TEST HYPOTHESES

A statistical hypothesis is a statement about the possible values of the parameters of a probability distribution. In this section, test statistics are introduced and the potential errors that may arise in testing a statistical hypothesis are discussed. The roles of power and the ubiquitous *P* value in hypothesis testing are presented.

Hypothesis Testing Sometimes interest is focused on answering a scientific question about a random variable with a (qualified) yes or no (e.g., Is drug 1 more effective than drug 2?). In such cases, the goal often is to determine whether the mean of one distribution is larger than the mean of another. Many scientific questions can be framed in statistical terms as a hypothesis test about the parameters of a probability distribution. Suppose a clinical trial is designed to test the null hypothesis that two treatments have the same mean effect. Formally, the treatments have true mean effects, denoted respectively by parameters ϕ_1 and ϕ_2, and our interest lies in testing whether the difference of the parameters of the two treatments, $\phi = \phi_1 - \phi_2$, is 0. The null hypothesis, then, is H_o: $\phi = 0$. Many alternative hypotheses are possible. The two most common in this setting are the two-sided alternative, H_1: $\phi \neq 0$ and the one-sided alternative, H_1: $\phi > 0$ (or H_1: $\phi < 0$). A test statistic must be chosen to test the null hypothesis against the alternative. Notably, different alternative hypotheses often lead to different rejection regions for the same test statistic. If the data from both treatments are assumed to follow a normal distribution and both have the same, albeit unknown, variance, then the test statistic usually used is a Student's *t* statistic, which is of the form.

$$t = (\bar{x}_1 - \bar{x}_2) / \sqrt{\frac{s_1^2}{n_1} + \frac{s_2^2}{n_2}}$$

Here, $\bar{x}_1$ and s_1, and $\bar{x}_2$ and s_2 are estimates of the mean and standard deviation based on samples of size n_1 and n_2 from the two respective populations. The *t* distribution depends on the expected value of $\bar{x}_1 - \bar{x}_2$, which is equal to $\phi_1 - \phi_2$, the variance of the random variable, and sample sizes, n_1 and n_2.

Type 1 and Type 2 Errors The decision as to whether to accept or reject the null hypothesis is determined by the value of the test statistic, which, of course, is a random variable whose value is unknown before the data are analyzed. If the value of the statistic falls in a prespecified *rejection*, or *critical*, region *R*, the null hypothesis is rejected. Even if the null hypothesis is true, there is still a chance that the statistic will lie in *R*, in which case a type 1 error has occurred—that is, a true null hypothesis has been erroneously rejected. Alternatively, the test statistic may not fall in *R*, even though H_o is not true, in which case a type 2 error has occurred—that is, a false hypothesis has not been rejected. Each of these types of error must be considered in choosing *R*. Usually, the choice is made so as to ensure that the probability of a type 1 error, usually denoted by the Greek letter α, is small. In most clinical trials, *R* is chosen so that α is .05, although, in some applications, choosing a type 1 error rate of .10 may be reasonable. This value is called the *level* of the test. For the comparison of two means, the calculation of this probability is performed under the assumption that $\phi = 0$, a *point*, or *simple*, null hypothesis. If the alternative hypothesis is H_1: $\phi \neq 0$, the sample sizes are large, and the *t* statistic is either less than −1.64 or greater than 1.64, the hypothesis is rejected. These are the *large sample critical values* of a *t* distribution with $n_1 + n_2 - 2$ degrees of freedom, with α set equal to .05. This is the so-called two-tailed test. If the alternative hypothesis is H_1: $\phi > 0$ and the *t* statistic is greater than 1.96, the null hypothesis is rejected.

If there are only two parameter values under study (i.e., two simple hypotheses), which one should be labeled the null and which the alternative? The null hypothesis should be the one whose false rejection would be considered to be the more serious error. This is because the testing paradigm that selects α, the level of the test, controls the probability of this error.

Power of a Test One minus the probability of a type 2 error is called the *power* of the test. Because the alternative hypothesis contains many values of ϕ, it is called a *composite* hypothesis—power is a function of the possible values of ϕ in H_1. In the example, power is an increasing function of ϕ and the sample size and a decreasing function of σ^2. During the design phase of a study, the sample size is chosen so that the power to reject a false null is relatively large, perhaps 0.8 or greater, for a value of ϕ that is sufficiently large to be clinically meaningful. The calculation is often performed under an assumed value of σ^2 that is based on data from other similar clinical trials. Suppose that the estimated value of ϕ turns out to be a number that is smaller than the clinically meaningful value chosen when the power calculation was performed and that the test statistic falls in the critical region. There is no difference in the statistical interpretation of the results of the trial. The hypothesis is still rejected at the designated level of the test.

***P* Values** Even a casual reader of the psychiatric literature will encounter a study in which *P* values are reported. Unfortunately, in some articles, only *P* values appear, without estimates of the parameters themselves or the variance of the estimators. All too often, both the author and the reader misinterpret the *P* values. Does a very small *P* value mean that one of the treatments is much better than the other?

First, the meaning of the *P* value should be explained. Before the analysis of data commences, the value of the test statistic is, of course, random, and, in the example comparing two treatments, it follows a *t* distribution. Suppose that the null hypothesis being tested is true, so the expected value of $\bar{x}_1 - \bar{x}_2 = 0$. In this case, the distribution of the statistic is completely specified. It follows a *t* distribution with $n_1 + n_2 - 2$ degrees of freedom. So, for every possible value of the test statistic, the chance of obtaining a value more extreme can be computed or found in a table. If t^* is the value of the test statistic observed in the trial, then the corresponding chance of observing a more extreme value is defined to be the *P* value. Alternatively, it may be regarded as the smallest level (had it been chosen in advance) for which the hypothesis would be rejected. However, a small *P* value and a true null hypothesis are inconsistent, for were the trial repeated over and over again, obtaining the observed value of the test statistic or a value more extreme would be very rare. This compellingly argues against the null hypothesis and suggests that it should be rejected. Scientific tradition, or, perhaps, convention, usually defines *rare* as an occurrence whose frequency is less than or equal to 1 time out of 20. Note that the fact that the null hypothesis is rejected does not mean that the magnitude of the difference has any clinical or scientific relevance. The sample size could be so large that even small trivial differences achieve statistical, but not practical, significance. Also, the inference that a large *P* value implies that the mean values of the two treatments are equal cannot be made. A calculation of the power of the test would help to rule out the possibility that the sample size was not adequate to detect a meaningful difference. More helpful still would be a confidence interval for the parameter whose upper limit falls below any values that would be scientifically or clinically meaningful. Finally, it is necessary to emphasize that in the frequentist tradition of statistical inference, the *P* value cannot be interpreted as the probability that the null hypothesis is true. The hypothesis is not a random event, so it is either true or it is false. In the next section, the Bayesian approach will be introduced. In this framework, a method for forming the probability or, perhaps, the degree of belief in the truth of a null hypothesis modified by the collected data will be described.

BAYESIAN APPROACH

The formal setting for incorporating former beliefs into a statistical analysis in which the data modify such beliefs is the essence of the method presented below.

Bayes' Theorem One of the most important results that emanates from elementary probability theory is Bayes' theorem, which states

$$P(A|B) = P(B|A)P(A)/P(B)$$

Bayesian inference played a major role in statistical thinking until the early part of the 20th century. Although the hypothesis-testing ideas of Jersey Neyman, Karl Pearson, and Sir Ronald Fisher played the dominant role in the rest of the century, in the last 25 years, the tide has begun to turn. The methodology and intuitive logic of the Bayesian approach, made more feasible by high-speed computers, is now pervasive in the literature of modern science and statistics.

Bayesian Inference Bayes' theorem is the basis on which Bayesian inference is built. Suppose that ϕ is a parameter and that $\phi = 0$ represents the event that the null hypothesis is true. Then, according to Bayes' theorem,

$$P(\phi|\text{data}) = P(\text{data}|\phi)P(\phi)/P(\text{data})$$

The parameter ϕ may be thought of as a representation of the scientific theory under investigation. The left side of the equation is a quantification of the probability, or, perhaps, degree of belief of the truth of the proposition that ϕ represents the true state of nature, given the observed data. In this setting, the unknown parameters are viewed as random variables, and, as such, they follow a probabilistic law. Remarkably, if the right side can be evaluated, a numerical value for the probability can be determined for this quantity, which is arguably the main issue once data collection is complete. It reflects the current belief, given the data, about the veracity of any value of ϕ and is called the *posterior distribution*. The first term on the right is just the likelihood of the observed data, evaluated at the parameter value ϕ. It is the next term that has made Bayesian inference controversial. What is the value of $P(\phi)$? This quantity is a function of all of the possible values of the unknown parameter ϕ, and it is called the *prior probability distribution*, or just *prior* for short. A prior distribution that has the same functional form as the posterior distributions is called a *conjugate prior*. This is a particularly desirable situation, for it permits efficient sequential updating of the posterior distribution as more data are collected. The posterior distribution at one stage is used as the prior in the next.

Note that the result of applying the Bayesian method is an entire posterior distribution and not a single estimate of the unknown parameter. The posterior summarizes all of the information, past and present, about the unknown parameter value. In the Bayesian framework, issues such as estimation and hypothesis testing are all based on the posterior distribution. For example, sensible estimators of a parameter are the mean or median of the posterior distribution. For hypothesis testing, the posterior distribution can be used to calculate the probabilities that the null and the alternative hypotheses are true. One possible rule is to accept the null as true only if the ratio of the posterior probability of the null divided by the posterior probability of the alternative exceeds some constant. The interpretation of a P value in this context is more natural than it is in the frequentist paradigm. The value of P is, in fact, the probability that the null hypothesis has been erroneously rejected. Contrast this with the frequentist interpretation that P is the chance of obtaining a data set that is more extreme.

The controversy about the use of Bayesian inference hinges on the problem of objectively choosing a prior. In many, if not most, cases, knowledge gleaned from previous experiments and, perhaps, scientific theory can guide the mathematical specification of $P(\phi)$. However, in situations in which little is known or there is controversy about prior experience or relevant theory, the choice of the prior is subjective. There are two schools of thought about choosing the prior. In one approach, the prior reflects the individuals' real-world experience and insights. An alternative approach is mechanistic or objective. The prior is chosen to satisfy some property (e.g., it is noninformative, or it is the conjugate distribution).

What price is paid for introducing subjectivity into the scientific process? Supporters of the Bayesian approach argue that Bayes' theorem mathematically demonstrates the inevitability of a subjective component to scientific inquiry. Scientists are the first to admit that insight, intuition, judgment, and beliefs are part of the process that drives their practice. Regulatory bodies are less convinced, but even in such scientifically driven agencies as the U.S. Food and Drug Administration (FDA), Bayesian approaches frequently appear. A full discussion of how the *a priori* distribution can be specified and the dependence of the final *a posteriori* distribution on this choice is somewhat technical. It is needless to say that there is a wide array of formal *a priori* distributions, including a noninformative prior (i.e., one in which values of the parameter are equally likely), that can be used. A commonly used approach is to specify a range of priors and examine the degree to which conclusions are sensitive to the choice. The more robust the finding under different priors, the more believable they are.

RANDOMIZED CLINICAL TRIALS

There are many kinds of research projects in mental health that require the use of statistical methods to appraise the results. Here, the discussion is focused on randomized clinical trials, because they are important, ubiquitous, and many of the issues apply in other research contexts. The methods discussed are neither exhaustive in the range of topics covered nor complete in the detail that is required to appreciate the nuances fully. The goal of many mental health studies is to conclude causality—that is, some observed effect is the result of an intervention. The discussion begins with a model that leads to conditions under which causality may validly be concluded. This may be accomplished by randomization or by using matched subjects. In the situation in which matching is practically difficult, an alternate approach, the propensity score, is introduced. The section concludes by introducing randomization tests that are valid, regardless of the underlying distribution of the random variable of interest.

Causality The principal reason for carrying out clinical research is to demonstrate the causal effect of the treatments being studied. Donald B. Rubin described an approach by which causality can be demonstrated in a clinical trial. Suppose that a putative antidepressant is given to a well-diagnosed patient with depression. If the patient does poorly, assuming the agent does no harm, no evidence is adduced about its effectiveness. Suppose that the patient does well and there is considerable reduction in symptoms. How can it be concluded that the treatment was the causal agent? If the clock could be turned back and the same patient with the same symptoms did not benefit from placebo treatment, it would be reasonable to conclude that the administration of the test agent caused clinical improvement in this patient. Each patient has two hypothetical outcomes, O_T and O_P, that would result from being treated with T (treatment) or P (placebo), respectively. If this hypothetical thought experiment were repeated a large number of times and the average effect of an individual receiving the treatment is larger than the average effect produced by placebo in the same individual, then the frequentist would conclude causality. In statistical terms, we write $E(O_T - O_P) > 0$ and recognize that the concept is the same whether the hypothetical experiment is repeated over and over with the same patient each time or with different patients. However, the generalizability of the conclusion is not the same in the two cases, and, from a statistical perspective, it is necessary to examine population causality rather than individual causality. Of course, the clock cannot be turned back. So what other possibilities are there? If each of the patients has an identical twin with the same genetic makeup and identical clinical symptom profiles, then one of each pair could be given the test treatment and the other given placebo. If the former improved and the latter did not, a causal relationship has been demonstrated. That is, it has been demonstrated that $E(O_T) - E(O_P) > 0$. Unfortunately, in the real world, each subject has only one outcome, O. If the treatment assignment is T, then the outcome is O_T, and, if it is P, the outcome is O_P. In this case, $E(O|T) - E(O|P) = E(O_T) - E(O_P) = E(O_T - O_P)$. What is necessary to be able to conclude causality is a mechanism that would enable the conclusion that $E(O_T - O_P) = E(O_T|T) - E(O_P|P) > 0$, where the expectation on the left side indicates that each individual received both treatments and the expectation on right side indicates that each individual received only one of the treatments. The notation beyond the vertical bar indicates which treatment was assigned to the patient, and the expectation, the computation of the average over the population, is restricted to those receiving the indicated treatment. Suppose that the treatment assignment is a random variable determined by some mechanism that is independent of the outcome, O. For example, suppose a patient is assigned to the test treatment if a fair coin (one whose probability of each of the two outcomes is .5) lands heads and to placebo otherwise. Then the treatment assignment is independent of the outcome, random variable O. Then, however, $E(O|T) - E(O|P) = E(O_T) - E(O_P) = E(O_T - O_P)$. So, use of a random assignment mechanism enables conclusions of causality.

The coin did not have to be a fair coin for the treatment assignment to be random. The same conclusion on causality would be reached were the probability of assignment to the treatment group equal to, say, .6. This is called a *biased coin random allocation.* The only difference is that the result of such a randomization process would be that more individuals would tend to be assigned to the treatment group (approximately 60 percent) than to the control group (approximately 40 percent). This fact is important for application of propensity score methods, which are discussed below.

In fact, the idea extends to situations in which treatments are assigned to subjects based on factors, z, that are observed. For example, z might be severity at baseline or some other stratification factor. Even *response adaptive designs,* where the probability that the next subject is assigned to the test treatment depends on outcomes observed on patients studied earlier in the trial, can demonstrate causal effects, so long as response to treatment and assignment to treatment are independent and conditional on z.

Matching and Randomization

Suppose that a clinical trial is to be conducted to establish a causal relationship between receipt of a treatment believed to be an active drug and clinical improvement, the effect produced. The treatment is to be allocated to one group of patients and a control treatment, a placebo, is to be allocated to another. As discussed earlier, if the control group is composed of one member from each set of twins and the test treatment group is composed of the remaining twins, causal conclusions can be reached. Although such a design can only rarely be realized, matching two groups on all variables that are prognostic indicators of the outcome may be feasible. Subjects can be matched on the basis of characteristics such as age, weight, severity, prior episodes, genetic factors, family factors, and so forth. However, in psychiatric research, it will be a rare study indeed in which the investigator and, more importantly, the target audience of the research believe that the two groups are truly matched. However, there are some circumstances in which this will be the best approach and such cases should be appraised individually. In the idealized twin case, treatment assignment need not be random. In this case, however, because there is no guarantee that paired subjects are truly identical, the assignment mechanism within the pair must be random for causal inference.

Randomization helps to avoid systematic bias (for example, evaluating one treatment in older or more severely ill patients and the other in younger or less severely ill patients). It has no effect on selection bias, which chooses individuals to participate in the study who are not representative of the target population. For example, in most drug comparison studies, the various eligibility requirements, both inclusion and exclusion, as well as the option candidates have of declining to participate in the trial, bias the sample. However, this does not compromise the validity of the treatment contrasts so long as treatments are randomly assigned to participants.

The very mechanism of assigning treatments to subjects in the clinical trial provides the probabilistic basis for computing, under the null hypothesis, valid probabilities of the various possible experimental outcomes. However, this is exactly what is needed to assess the likelihood that the null hypothesis is true. In particular, it enables calculation of a rejection region corresponding to a chosen type 1 error, which is the basis of hypothesis testing. Further, because randomization guarantees that outcomes for different subjects are independent, a valid estimate of the experimental error can be obtained. This quantity is required for obtaining valid confidence interval estimates of treatment effects and for parametric testing of a null hypothesis. Also, given a sufficiently large sample size, all of the possible known and unknown confounding effects that might possibly affect outcome are, with high probability, eliminated in the sense that they are averaged out. Finally, the objectivity and repeatability of randomized assignment to treatment must be pointed out.

There is no point in conducting a clinical trial whose results will not be creditable. The ability to describe exactly how candidate patients were placed into the various treatment groups makes the process transparent and gives credence to the conclusions reached.

Randomization Tests

Randomization tests make no assumptions as to the distribution of the random variables and, thus, are considered to be distribution-free. The results of the test depend only on the data actually collected. Suppose there are two groups of patients whose group assignment is determined by a randomization procedure, with one group receiving the test treatment and the other receiving a placebo. After a suitable period of time, an outcome is obtained on each subject. The quantity of interest is the difference between the mean outcomes of the two groups. The first step in a randomization test is to compute the statistic, the difference between means, from the sample. The second step is to re-randomize and recalculate the value of the mean difference for the new treatment assignments. Under the null hypothesis, there is no difference between the groups; so reassigning some patients from one group to the other should not change any probabilistic properties of the distribution of treatment differences. Reassigning treatments to patients by re-randomization (or, for small numbers of subjects, by exhausting all possible permutations of possible treatment assignments) and recalculating the mean differences induces a probability distribution of mean differences. The percentile in the randomization-induced probability distribution of the actual mean difference observed in the trial is informative regarding the plausibility of the null hypothesis. If the observed mean difference lies near the middle of the distribution, the null distribution seems likely to be true. If, on the other hand, the observed mean difference falls into one of the extremes of the randomization distribution, say, less than .05 (alpha) of the values are larger, then the null hypothesis seems unlikely to be true. The mean values of the two treatments are likely to be different. The randomization *P* value is the proportion of re-randomizations in which the value of the statistic is more extreme than the value obtained from the original treatment assignment. Randomization tests produce valid significance levels (probability of a type 1 error) regardless of the usually unknown underlying probability distribution of the outcome measures.

Rank randomization tests are similar to randomization tests. First, however, the observations are converted to ranks. That is, the two groups are merged and put in numerical order. The largest is assigned rank one, the second largest is assigned rank two, and so on. Next, the two groups are separated into their original configuration and a randomization test is computed on the ranks. This is a particularly useful approach when the scale used to measure patient response has some nonlinear properties and when outliers in the data might skew estimates of mean effects. The disadvantage is that some information is lost when the actual observed values are converted to ranks. Although rank randomization tests may be somewhat less powerful than randomization tests based on the original data, the loss in power may be a small price to pay to purge the potential contamination caused by exceptional large or small outcomes.

Propensity Scores In efforts to understand the properties of a new treatment or intervention, it is often impossible or too expensive to conduct a randomized clinical trial. On the other hand, there may be data available on the new treatment, as well as on standard practice that has been collected under naturalistic conditions. In earlier sections, considerable attention was paid to the merits of randomization and the benefits that accrue from its use. Randomization of persons to treatment or control groups allows statements of causality to be made, and systematic differences in characteristics between the groups are not likely to occur if the sample size is sufficiently large. Is it possible to nevertheless obtain valid estimates of effect size from data on patients who were not randomly assigned to treatment? Many standard statistical methods of analysis are not appropriate, because they implicitly (at least for the purpose of causal inference) assume that the groups were formed by random assignment.

Suppose that background characteristics, some known, such as severity of illness and age, and others that may be unknown are markers for the assignment of patients to a new treatment or to a control or usual practice group. This might occur as part of usual care procedures or by unconscious hunches designed to individualize and optimize treatment outcome. If the two groups are compared without regard to the treatment assignment mechanism, the results can be biased, particularly if there is an imbalance across groups in variables that influence outcome.

If there are only a few confounding variables and they are known, it may be possible to form stratum in which the treatment and control groups look alike. For example, suppose there is a difference in the proportion of men receiving treatments in the two groups. Then, a group containing only men and a group containing only women can be formed. The treatments can be compared within groups, and, if they are similar, the results can be pooled.

If there are two known confounding variables, such as age (young, middle-aged, and old) and gender, then age/gender groups can be formed, yielding six strata in which to make comparisons. However, as the number of confounding variables grows, it becomes increasingly difficult to form the multiple stratum that would be required. Sample sizes in each stratum would considerably diminish, resulting in a loss of power to detect differences when they truly exist.

Propensity score methods are used to control for a collection of confounding covariates. The propensity score is a probability of treatment group membership based on patient covariates. An estimate of the propensity score for each individual in the study is usually obtained by first fitting a logistic regression and then substituting his or her covariates into the resulting model. Naturally, persons who are actually in the treatment group will tend to have higher propensity scores than those in the control group. If the range of propensity score values in the two groups overlap, then it is possible to match individuals in one group with those in the other group who have similar scores. Rather than one-to-one matching, usually the propensity scores for the combined groups are ordered, and five strata (i.e., quintiles) are formed. Within a stratum, all individuals have approximately the same estimated likelihood of being assigned to the treatment group, and the multivariate distribution of the covariates used to estimate the propensity score in the two groups does not differ statistically. Across strata, the likelihood of being assigned to the treatment group differs. Within each stratum, some individuals were assigned to treatment and some to the control, so biased coin randomization has, in essence, been mimicked. If all subjects have a propensity score of approximately one-half, then treatment assignment appears to have been determined by a fair coin randomization process. Treatment effects are estimated within propensity score strata, and if the results are similar, they can be combined to obtain an estimate of the overall effect size. As Philip Lavori put it, within each observational study there lives a randomized study that can be found with the help of propensity scores.

Missing or Incomplete Data In the conduct of research in mental health settings, missing data are inevitable. Such data sets are said to be incomplete, and the problem of parameter estimation or hypothesis testing is regarded as an incomplete-data problem. Missing data problems occur in both clinical trials and studies that are survey- or field-based, and the data can be missing for many reasons. In a clinical trial in which data are collected at multiple time points, subjects may not be available for all interviews. Some may drop out of the trial before it is completed, because of adverse events or death; or they may move to another home, hospital, or jail or to the streets; or they may just perceive continuing in the trial to be a nuisance. In surveys, respondents may refuse to answer particular questions, because of the sensitive nature of the inquiry, or they just may not know the answer.

There is no single approach to handling all missing data situations, but ignoring holes in the data when performing a statistical analysis can have an enormous effect on the results. The possibility of substantial structural biases that might have led to the data losses can lead to analyses that may even be so fatally flawed as to nullify the results. Conceptually, the complete data consist of two parts, only one of which is observed. The missing part can only be inferred from the observed part. The steps to take depend on the mechanisms that led to the missing data. This is often referred to as the *missingness* of the data. Roderick Little and Donald Rubin have defined three kinds of missing data mechanisms: missing completely at random, missing at random, and nonignorable missing.

A very simple probabilistic model can be used to conceptualize data that are missing completely at random. Suppose that a random variable taking the value 1 or 0, with respective probabilities of P and $1 - P$, was observed for each observation of the variable Y. Assume further that the value of the observation on Y is independent of the binomial random variable. Such a random variable is obtained by tossing a coin whose probability of landing heads is P. If the coin toss corresponding to a particular observation of Y lands heads, the data are lost. The remaining observations are a random subsample of the original sample, thus, the data remains a random sample. An example of missing at random can be obtained in a similar fashion. Suppose Z is gender and a coin is tossed for men with probability P_1 of landing heads and a second coin is tossed for women with probability P_2 of landing heads. For each observed Y, one or another coin is tossed, depending on the gender as captured by Z. If the coin lands heads, the data are lost. The remaining data in each subsample are still random samples. As an example of nonignorable missing data, suppose that the observations on Y have been sorted into good and bad outcomes, and two coins are tossed with respective probabilities of heads P_1 and P_2 for the two types of outcomes for each observation. If either coin lands heads, then the corresponding observation is lost. The remaining data no longer arise from the same underlying probability distribution that gave rise to the original sample. If $P_1 = P_2$, then the effect of sorting on outcome no longer matters, and the subsample is a random subsample of the original sample. In this case, the data would be missing at random.

There are several methods used to handle the situation when data are missing completely at random or missing at random. Certainly the simplest strategy is to delete from the study those records with missing data on the primary variable of interest. If the sample size is sufficiently large, this may be a viable approach. However, if the amount of information lost diminishes the ability of the study to reach confident conclusions, then this method is not recommended. If the data are multivariate and only some of the variables in a record are missing, it would be rather wasteful to dispose of the entire record. Some analysts retain those parts that have data that are present and use them in marginal analyses not involving the variables with missing data. This approach can also be problematic. For example, suppose a clinical trial is designed to compare an active treatment with a placebo. Those individuals who respond to the placebo remain in the trial, whereas the others drop out. For a self-limiting illness, the placebo responders and the treatment responders are not likely to differ toward the end of the trial. Ignoring the early dropouts and limiting the analysis to those who remain in the trial could lead to the erroneous conclusion that the drug loses its efficacy after a while. Filling in or imputing the missing data with a conservative estimate of its value is the current favored approach. However, this strategy can also lead to erroneous conclusions if there are too many records with missing data. Neither strategy is completely satisfactory, nor is there a satisfactory rule of thumb as to how much missing data is too much for imputation. Individual variations among studies require critical appraisal in each particular case as to what is an appropriate analytical approach.

Imputation of missing data can be done in several ways. One simple imputation procedure, called *mean/median substitution*, substitutes the mean or median value of the observed data for the missing value. This approach tends to reduce the estimated variance, which thereby provides more comfort to the researcher than may be warranted. Several methods rely on a matching strategy. Records with missing data are matched with records of subjects with similar demographics whose outcomes are present. The data from the matched records are used to impute the missing value. In *hot deck imputation*, cases with missing data are matched with similar cases with complete data, based on defined background variables (e.g., age and gender). A critical issue is how to choose the variables that define "similar." Matching criteria variables are chosen because they are prognostic indicators of the missing data variables. The value substituted for the missing value is randomly selected from data present in the set of matched cases. *Multiple imputation* uses an imputation method, such as hot deck, to repeatedly generate estimates for the missing data values. For each replication, the full data set, actual and imputed, is analyzed. The results from these multiple analyses are combined into one overall analysis. This approach gives an idea of the variability of the results among the various possible imputations that could have been randomly selected.

For data collected longitudinally, many researchers have used the last observed value carried forward approach to fill in the missing value. If values are available before and after the missing time point, many interpolate a value. These approaches also tend to reduce the estimated variance, which can lead to a greater chance of reporting an effect when there really is none. Hierarchical linear modeling provides a more satisfactory approach for analyzing longitudinal data. In these models, a time curve is estimated for each individual in the study from the available data without imputation, which works well as a substitute for interpolation. If many patients have missing observations in the later stages of a study, there may be a considerable degree of extrapolation. In this case, the method must be used with caution.

More sophisticated methods for imputing missing values are model based. For example, regression models have been used when the variable with missing data is the dependent variable. Parameters in the regression equation are estimated based on data from complete records. The predicted value from the model is used as an estimate of the missing data value. Another approach relies on maximizing a likelihood function using the available data values, while taking into account the nature of the missingness. Here, great care must be taken in specifying the underlying distribution function of the random variables.

Perhaps the most widely used method of imputation is the expected/maximization, or EM, algorithm. It was originally conceptualized as a method for finding maximum likelihood estimators for incomplete data. The algorithm starts by choosing initial estimates of the values of the unknown parameters. The estimates are improved iteratively by first computing the conditional probability distribution of the missing data, given the observed data and the current estimate of the parameters. The expectation of the log likelihood over the previously calculated distribution of missing values is obtained. This is called the *E step* of the algorithm. A new or updated estimate of the unknown parameters may be obtained by maximizing this expectation. This step is called the *maximization step* (M step), after which the E step is repeated. An important feature of the EM algorithm is that it gives the complete probability distribution for the missing data and point estimates for the model parameters. Under some reasonably general conditions, the EM estimates obtained in the iteration procedure converge locally to the maximum likelihood estimates.

The methods described above handle missing data under the missing at random assumption. Pattern-mixture models have been proposed for nonignorable missing data. Records are stratified into groups with different expected patterns of response and missingness. The group then becomes a predictor variable in a method of analysis (e.g., hierarchical linear models) that allows subjects to have incomplete data across time. In this way, the degree to which missingness influences outcomes can be assessed. Group membership can also be used in an interaction term in the model. This allows the assessment of the degree to which missingness patterns interact with key effect variables, such as treatment group.

In sum, there is no one simple recipe for handling missing data. An understanding of the reason for the missingness is necessary, and a critical eye must be kept on the question of whether the missing at random assumption is plausible. Whatever technique is used, some form of sensitivity analysis should be used to see how the imputation carried out in different ways affects the results. The choice of technique used to handle the missingness must be made on a case-by-case approach.

SPECIFIC STATISTICAL METHODS

In this section, a variety of commonly used analytical techniques are introduced. These include linear regression and logistic regression, contingency tables, the general linear model, and survival analysis. In mental health research, outcomes are typically observed over time, and a discussion of longitudinal methods to address such situations is given.

Regression Models Regression models quantify a relationship between a dependent variable and one or more independent, explanatory variables. A statistical model is complete only if both its functional and probabilistic form and its parameters are determined. The procedure for estimating the unknown parameters is known as *model fitting*. Historically, the dependent variable, for example Y, is assumed to follow a normal distribution, and the hypothesized model relates its mean or expected value and a function of the independent variables, for example, $x_1, x_2, \ldots, x_k$. The data consist of an observation on independent and dependent variables on each of N subjects. The most common model assumes that the normal mean is a linear function of the explanatory variables. That is, it is of the form

$$E(Y) = \alpha + \beta_1 x_1 + \beta_2 x_2 + \ldots + \beta_k x_k,$$

where the $k + 1$ Greek letters, $\alpha, \beta_1, \beta_2, \ldots, \beta_k$ are unknown parameters to be determined from the data. In terms of the actual observations, rather than the expected value of Y, the form of the model is assumed to be

$$Y = \alpha + \beta_1 x_1 + \beta_2 x_2 + \ldots + \beta_k x_k + \varepsilon.$$

Here, ε represents a random error term that accounts for the deviations among the observations from their mean value. For each subject, the difference between the observation Y and the model fit evaluated at his or her specific value of the independent variables is called the *residual error*. If Y follows a normal distribution with mean $\alpha + \beta_1 x_1 + \beta_2 x_2 + \ldots + \beta_k x_k$ and variance σ^2, then the error term is also normal with the same variance but with mean 0. In a regression analysis, estimates of the coefficients are obtained by maximizing the likelihood of the observations. Elementary calculus is used to find the value of the estimates, which are the solutions of a set of simultaneous equations referred to as the *normal equations*. An alternative strategy for finding estimates of the parameters is to minimize the sum of the squared errors as a criterion for the goodness of the fit of the model to the data. The errors, or the *residuals*, are the differences between the observed values and the predicted values, the latter obtained by substituting the values of the x's into the regression equation. The *ordinary least squares* approach makes no assumption as to the distribution of the error term. The method of ordinary least squares was developed at the turn of the 18th century by the mathematician Karl Friedrich Gauss working in Germany (some historians say it was developed by others, including Adrien Marie Legendre, Pierre-Simon Laplace, and [possibly] Robert Adrain, in France and America, respectively). The least squares solution and the maximum likelihood solution are identical if the dependent variable is normally distributed.

Because specification of the set of explanatory variables is somewhat subjective, regression analyses include tests of whether each coefficient is equal to 0. If the null hypothesis is rejected, then the explanatory variable is included in the model. Stepwise procedures for choosing the variables to include in the model are also commonly used. Goodness of fit may be ascertained in a variety of ways, and model validation is a critical step in building a creditable model. At a bare minimum, the value of an R^2 statistic, which is the fraction of the total variability in the response that is accounted for by the model, should be obtained. However, a high value of R^2 is not a guarantee that the model fits the data well, so it is wise to examine the residuals as well. Different types of plots of the residuals provide information on the adequacy of different aspects of the model. If the model fits well, a plot of the residuals will appear to behave randomly. This approximates the random errors that explain the difference between the independent variables and the response variable. If nonrandom structure is evident, then the model does not fit the data well.

There is, of course, no reason to limit the function on the right side of the regression equation to linear forms. Many applications use rather complex nonlinear functions to represent the hypothesized relationships. In these cases, numerical methods are the only practical means for obtaining the estimates, and hypothesis tests are usually valid for large samples only. In the last quarter century, statisticians have generalized regression models in many directions, and applications incorporating these extensions appear frequently in the psychiatric literature.

Logistic Regression Many research studies deal with outcome variables that are discrete. The simplest and most common case is of dichotomous or binary random variables. A binary variable is often used to define the occurrence of an event, such as a treatment success, a treatment-emergent side effect from a study medication, the disappearance of a symptom, or death. If the event occurs, the random variable Y takes the value 1 with probability P, otherwise, Y takes the value 0 with probability $1 - P$. This is called a *Bernoulli random variable*, and an experiment in which many Bernoulli random variables are observed is called a *Bernoulli trial*.

An investigator may want to know how other explanatory variables (covariates or risk factors) affect the frequency of the occurrence of the event. If the dependent variable is continuous and approximately normally distributed, multiple linear regression would likely be used to explore its relationship to the covariates. Here, linear regression is not appropriate. An applicable model for a dichotomous variable is *logistic regression*. In this approach, the model assumes that the log of the odds ratio of the event occurring is linear in the covariates. These independent variables may be continuous variables, categorical variables, or both. The *odds ratio* is the ratio of the probability that the event occurs to the probability that it does not occur. Odds are commonly used in gambling contexts. If the odds that a team will win are three to one, then one would expect the team to win approximately three times more often than it loses. In this case, the probability of winning is .75. Suppose q is the probability of the occurrence of the event. Then odds $= q/(1 - q)$ and $q =$ odds/(1 + odds).

The logistic model is

$$\log q/(1 - q) = \alpha + \beta_1 x_1 + \beta_2 x_2 + \ldots + \beta_k x_k.$$

The left side of the equation is called a *logit*. The covariates on the right side of the equation can be continuous, dichotomous, nominal, or ordinal. Tests of the null hypothesis that each parameter is 0 may be made. Interpretations of the coefficients are made in a manner similar to ordinary linear regression. However, logistic regression calculates changes in the log odds of the dependent variable, not changes in the dependent variable itself as in linear regression. For plotting and interpreting results from logistic regression, it is usually more convenient to express fitted values on the scale of probabilities. The inverse transformation of the model equations yields the logistic function for the probability of the event q,

$$q = \exp\,[\alpha + \beta_1 x_1 + \beta_2 x_2 + \ldots + \beta_k x_k]/(1 + \exp[\alpha + \beta_1 x_1 + \beta_2 x_2 + \ldots + \beta_k x_k]).$$

The fit of a logistic regression can be assessed by looking at a classification table, which displays whether the model has correctly classified each of the observed outcomes of Y. Goodness-of-fit tests are available as indicators of model appropriateness. One method begins by dividing the subjects into ten groups, in increasing order of estimated probability of occurrence of the event. The first group corresponds to those subjects who have the lowest predicted probability, the next group corresponds to those with the next lowest predicted probability, and so on. A chi-square statistic is used to examine whether the observed counts in each group are close to the expected count under linearity. If they are, the chi-square statistic will be small and the corresponding P value will be large.

Logistic regression can be extended beyond dichotomous response variables to ordered polychotomous (more than two) categories.

Contingency Tables and Log Linear Models

Many research studies involve discrete random variables. Frequency distributions of two discrete variables tabulated simultaneously are called *contingency tables*. The levels of one variable are listed in the rows of a table, the levels of the other variables are listed in the columns, and the joint frequency is entered in each cell. The sums of the cell frequencies across both the rows and columns are placed in the margins. The lower right corner of the table displays the sum of the row marginal frequencies, which is equal to the sum of the column marginal frequencies, which is equal to the sample size.

Reports of many research studies begin with a description of the sample population, including the distribution of patient characteristics, such as treatment and baseline severity of illness. If there are two treatment groups being compared, then it is important to assess whether the groups were comparable at baseline. Define a treatment group indicator variable for the columns and a severity level variable for the rows. The question, then, is, Are the two variables independent, or is there an association? Effects in a contingency table are relationships between the row and column variables in which levels of the row variable are differentially distributed over levels of the column variables. If the two variables are not independent, the two treatment groups have different distributions of baseline severity level, and the row variable will need to be controlled in any subsequent treatment comparisons in the analyses. Failure to reject the null means that there is not enough evidence to conclude that the variables are dependent; observed differences in cell frequencies are likely due to chance. (Nevertheless, even if the test failed to reject the independence hypothesis, it may still be necessary to adjust for imbalances in baseline variables. Important prognostic variables may be sufficiently imbalanced to alter inference and cause statistical errors.)

Hypothesis tests of association are often based on a chi-square statistic. The test statistic examines the difference between the observed counts in the table and those counts that would be expected if the variables were independent. The statistic sums the ratio of the squared difference between the actual count and the expected count to the expected count under the assumption of independence. If the differences are small, the data support the hypothesis that the variables are independent. In the 2×2 table, the difference of proportions, the relative risk, and the odds ratio are measures of the strength of association.

Contingency tables can involve more than two variables. One of the most common situations is the $2 \times 2 \times K$ table. For example, one variable may be treatment assignment to a drug or a placebo, the second may be a variable that measures success or failure, and the third may represent a control variable, such as research sites, gender, or initial severity. There are three test statistics commonly used to analyze such tables. The Cochran-Mantel-Haenszel statistic assumes a common odds ratio and tests the null hypothesis that two of the variables are conditionally independent, while controlling for the possible confounding factors of the rest of the variables. The odds ratio is a measure of the increase in odds of success for those given the drug relative to those given a placebo. If the odds ratio is 1, the drug has no effect. The Cochran-Mantel-Haenszel tests whether the response is conditionally independent of the explanatory variable (treatment assignment), while adjusting for the control variable (site). If the directions in some strata are opposite to the direction of those in other strata, the Cochran-Mantel-Haenszel statistic has low power for detecting an association. The Mantel-Haenszel procedure first estimates a common odds ratio across the K strata and tests whether it is equal to 1. The Breslow-Day statistic tests the null hypothesis of homogeneous odds ratios. That is, it tests whether the odds ratio between the assignment and outcome variables are the same for the K levels of the third control variable.

Higher-level multidimensional contingency tables and more complex hypotheses are often analyzed using an approach known as *log linear models*. These models are used when two or more variables are measures of response rather than explanatory or control variables. The log linear model is one of the specialized cases of the generalized linear model, discussed below, for Poisson-distributed data.

General Linear Model

The restriction to a normally distributed dependent random variable in regression theory was removed with the introduction of the general linear model by John Nelder and Robert Wedderburn. This model assumes that the dependent random variable has a distribution in what is called a *parametric exponential family*. This family includes not only normally distributed and other continuous random variables, but also many discrete random variables such as the binomial and the Poisson. The latter distributions are used for modeling count data. The classic regression approach that models a normal mean as a linear function of the explanatory variables is generalized in the general linear model to a regression between a function of the mean and the explanatory variables. The function is called the *link function*. Although there are many possible link functions, a natural or *canonical link function*, which enables efficient estimation of the coefficients, is associated with each particular parametric distribution. Here, too, estimation is accomplished by maximizing the likelihood of the observations under the assumed parametric exponential family distribution via the link function. For example, in the case of a Bernoulli response variable with mean p, the canonical link function is $\log[p/(1 - p)]$, the log of the odds. Here, the general linear model assumes that the error term follows a logistic distribution, which is a member of the exponential family of distributions. However, this is exactly what is done in logistic regression, which is, therefore, a special case of the general linear model. As in ordinary linear regression, tests of the hypotheses that coefficients of the explanatory variables do not differ from zero are used to determine which ones have an effect on the mean. Similarly, if count data are distributed as Poisson variables and the link function is the log of the counts, then the general linear model analysis is equivalent to a log linear model analysis of a contingency table.

Longitudinal Models In the general linear model and regression context, a single dependent random variable for each subject is considered. Subjects are usually observed at multiple time points or occasions, especially in studies of mental and other chronic illnesses. A typical hypothesis in such situations is that the means at all T time points are equal. This corresponds to the statement that there is no change over time. Conceptually, data in this situation may be described as a rectangular array, comprised of N rows and T columns. The rows correspond to the N subjects, and the entries in the columns are the subjects' responses at the T time points. In a pre–postmedication trial with N subjects, there are $T = 2$ columns. In the simplest case, the question is whether the mean effects of the pre- and postmedication responses are the same. A paired t, based on the difference between the pre- and postmedication responses, is the usual statistic for this comparison.

Until fairly recently, the most common approach to analyzing longitudinal data was based on a repeated measures model. The statistical assumption for this model requires that the T random responses of each subject follow a multivariate normal distribution in which the covariance structure is completely symmetrical. That is, the variances at each time point are equal and the covariance between any two responses, irrespective of their time difference, are equal. Clearly, these are rather demanding assumptions. Also, missing observations presented a significant problem, and, in many trials, all data on some subjects have been omitted. More recently, methods such as the EM algorithm enabled incomplete repeated measures data sets to be analyzed. However, hierarchical multivariate linear models, a generalization of repeated measures model, have become more popular.

In a longitudinal study, despite the best of intentions, the occasions when subjects are observed, as well as the number of time points that subjects are observed, may vary widely from patient to patient. Hierarchical linear models allow such deviations, which overcomes the missingness problem when the data are missing at random. While still retaining the multivariate normal distribution assumption for each subject, these models do not restrict the structure of the covariance matrix. The name *hierarchical* refers to the view that, conceptually, the analysis proceeds on different levels. Time is nested within subjects, subjects may be nested within sites, sites may be nested within countries, and so on. The model posits that the random normal observation is a sum of three terms: the first is itself a sum of the form $\alpha + \beta_1 x_1 + \beta_2 x_2 + \ldots + \beta_k x_k$, the second is a sum of random effects, and the third is an independent error term. The first sum is referred to as the *fixed effects* term. Although the random effects comprising the second sum are not observed, they enter the model by contributing to the variances and covariances of the observations. Because subjects are independent, the form of the likelihood is a product, which leads to a set of extended normal equations for estimating the parameters. Parameters may also be estimated using a least squares approach, although, within this model, a generalized least squares criterion that weights the residuals in terms of variances and covariances is used.

In a still more recent development, the multivariate normal assumption has been relaxed through the introduction of a *semiparametric regression* method that incorporates elements of the general linear model. The method of generalized estimating equations, introduced by Kung-Yee Liang and Scott Zeger, focuses on the means at each time point through link functions. In this way, each marginal mean response at each observed occasion is modeled. In many psychiatric studies, hypotheses are concerned with the behavior of marginal means. In lieu of modeling the entire joint distribution of the observations over time, the generalized estimating equations method models only the variance and covariances of the observations over time. The variance at a given occasion is modeled as a function of the marginal mean at that occasion. The method allows missing data, provided they are missing completely at random—that is, they are missing at random conditional on the covariates. Although the likelihood function cannot be formed because the parametric form of the distribution is not specified, estimators can be obtained by solving an analog of the normal equations. The resulting estimators are consistent. That is, as the number of subjects increases, the estimators converge to their true values. Consistency holds even if the structure of the correlation matrix has been misspecified. Also, asymptotically, the distribution of the estimators are normal so that testing whether the coefficients of the independent variables differ from 0 can be accomplished.

Survival Analysis Many psychiatric issues are related to events in the time domain (e.g., time to onset of effect of a treatment, time in hospital, and time to remission of symptoms of depression). These are generically called *time-to-event*, or *survival, variables*. The first survival variable that was studied was time-to-death. *Life table methods* were originally devised for actuarial and insurance uses to describe expected survival time. For a particular group of persons (e.g., men) and selected age intervals (e.g., decades), life tables usually exhibit the number of persons entering the age interval alive, the proportion of these who die in the interval, and the proportion for whom data became unavailable during the interval. The proportion that die in the interval is called the *hazard rate*. Other useful statistics that can be derived from such tables include the *conditional survival rate* (among those who enter the interval, the proportion surviving beyond the interval) and the *survival function* (the cumulative proportion of individuals surviving to the end of the interval). The *survival distribution* is defined to be one minus the cumulative distribution function, $1 - F(x)$. The time at which the survival function is equal to .5, the *median survival time*, is the statistic most often used to characterize the distribution. Other percentiles are, of course, of interest as well. Although life tables provide a great deal of information, they are of little use for predictive purposes or for assessing the impact of other variables on survival.

Sophisticated statistical methods for estimating survival time distributions were developed primarily to model data from clinical trials of cancer treatments, and even more sophisticated methods have emerged in association with the study of acquired immunodeficiency syndrome. Survival time methods are widely used in most of the medical and biological sciences, as well as in engineering (where the method is called *failure time analysis*) and in the social and economic sciences. The methods for estimating survival time frequency distributions from sample data have been developed to take into account the possibility that persons may still be alive at the end of the study period. Such individuals, in essence, have missing data as to the time of their death, but it would be folly to exclude them from the analysis. Observations on these individuals, as well as the times of those who dropped out of the study before the signal event occurred (e.g., a subject has moved and contact is lost), are called *censored observations*. If a new treatment is designed to study recurrence of depression and the study lasts 2 years, a censored observation at study completion or at loss to follow-up indicates that the treatment has been successful, at least for that period of time. As in the missing data situation, analysis of this latter type of censored observations is facilitated if the data are missing completely at random and are, therefore, noninformative as to the distribution of the time to the event being studied. Nonignorable missingness, such as systematic censoring, if erroneously assumed to be missing completely at random, may greatly bias the estimation of the survival time distribution.

The Kaplan-Meier survival function estimation technique is nonparametric because it makes no assumption as to the underlying shape of the distribution. Based on the observed survival times and censoring times, it defines time intervals that contain exactly one observed case (except if there are ties). This is in sharp contrast with life table methods that count the number of deaths in fixed time intervals. The probability of surviving beyond time T is the product of the probability of being alive in each interval up to time T. If a case is censored at some time point, it is used in the calculation of the estimated probabilities up to the time of censoring and not used in subsequent calculations. Survival distributions generated from two samples, such as two treatment groups, can be compared statistically. The most commonly used tests are nonparametric, including Gehan's test, the generalized Wilcoxon test, and the log rank test.

Parametric survival methods assume an underlying shape of the survival distribution, for example, exponential, Weibull, or Gompertz. Techniques such as maximum likelihood estimation or least squares to fit the parameters of the model from the observed data are used to estimate the value of unknown parameters.

Many research projects entail an investigation of the influence that covariates have on survival time. Cox proportional hazard models were introduced to enable regression-type analyses to be conducted on time-to-event data. No assumptions are made concerning the underlying form of the survival distribution, so the method is called *semiparametric*. The model assumes that the hazard rate, the probability of dying at time T, given that one is still alive up to that time, is equal to a fixed population, or *underlying hazard rate*, multiplied by the exponential of a linear function of the covariates. The log of the exponential multiplier is a linear sum of the covariates. The multiplicative form of the model implies that the hazards are proportional. This is called the *proportionality assumption*, which explains the name of the method.

Proportional hazard models are frequently used to test the null hypothesis of equality of the survival distributions of two treatments. If there is reason to believe that there is a common underlying hazard function for the two groups, a treatment group assignment term is used as a covariate and the null hypothesis that the corresponding parameter is 0 is tested. If there is reason to believe that each group has its own underlying hazard, a stratified analysis may be used to test the null hypothesis that the same regression model applies to the two groups.

Cure models have been proposed to account for situations in which the event being studied cannot occur for some part of the population. Cure models were introduced in cancer studies in which time-to-death was the principle outcome variable, but some fraction of the population were cured. In essence, there are two populations: those who, when given the test treatment, will be cured and those who will die from the disease. In a genetics context, these are the susceptible and nonsusceptible groups. In psychiatry, the study of onset of treatment effect parallels this situation. In a study of the effectiveness of an antidepressant, an important parameter is the time for the treatment to take effect. However, some in the population may not respond to the treatment and will never have onset. This group is analogous to the cured group in the disease model. The quantities of interest in this model are the proportion cured (proportion of nonresponders) and, among the group not cured (responders), the conditional probability of surviving (having onset). The estimation of these quantities needs to be made with care. A subject may survive beyond the end of the study either because he or she is cured or because he or she has a true survival time that exceeds the time at which observations cease. The proportion not cured may be estimated nonparametrically by the proportion still surviving at the end of the trial, as estimated in the Kaplan-Meier approach. The Kaplan-Meier curve can also be used to solve for the conditional survival distribution of the population not cured. If two or more groups are being compared, parametric and nonparametric models can be used to test for the equality of the cure fraction and for the equality of the conditional survival distribution. The advantage of parametric cure models is that they can include covariates that affect either the proportion not cured or the conditional survival distribution, or both. Thus, one can learn about treatment effects, as well as the characteristics of a group that predict cure, as well as those that predict shorter or longer survival time.

STUDY DESIGN

Usually, in the pursuit of a research question, there are many ways to design a study to estimate parameters and to test hypotheses. In all fields of inquiry, but particularly in medical research, an experiment must be designed so as to produce the most accurate possible estimates of treatment effect within the limitations of sample size and personal safety. To use a design that is less than optimal is certainly inefficient but also may be unethical. The study of the design of experiments is a field of inquiry in statistics that searches for designs that are as efficient as possible. In this section, we will discuss only one issue, the design of a crossover trial, as an illustration of the kind of considerations that enter the search for optimality.

Crossover Designs There has been much interest and, indeed, controversy about the use of crossover designs. In a crossover trial, the comparison of t study treatments is accomplished by observing N subjects on several occasions, usually called *periods*. A subject may receive a different treatment in each period or one or more treatments may be repeated, so a subject acts as his or her own control. The best known crossover design is a two-treatment, two-period, two-sequence trial in which each subject receives both treatments, some in the order AB and the rest in the order BA. Experimental designs in which subjects are crossed over to other treatments have long been recognized as having considerable potential for achieving greater precision than can be obtained from parallel groups (also called *completely randomized*) designs. This is because between-subject variation is eliminated from the error term. Another advantage is that a crossover design requires fewer subjects to obtain the same number of observations. In a two-period design, each subject contributes two observations. For some types of studies, it is expensive to recruit participants, and once one has been trained in the details of the study procedure, there may be high motivation to continue to obtain observations on the response to other treatments. Although they have not been used frequently in psychopharmacology, their use may well increase as the value of crossover designs is more widely appreciated by psychopharmacologists.

The negative aspect of crossover designs is the possibility that carryover or residual effects (i.e., the effects of the previous treatment, whether pharmacological or psychological), may alter subsequent responses. The standard analysis of a two-period, two-treatment, two-sequence design (AB, BA) is rife with problems. An FDA advisory committee compared this simplest of crossover designs, in terms of precision and cost, to the completely randomized one-period design. Byron Brown, a member of the committee, concluded, "the crossover experiment can yield great savings in cost if the assumption of no carryover effect is valid, but the design should not be used if this assumption is in doubt." In many cases, the sample size needed to test whether carryover is present exceeds the sample size needed for a similarly powered parallel groups trial. For many years, the crossover design (AB, BA) was in disfavor, particularly by researchers in the pharmaceutical industry, as a result of Brown's analysis and the presumed concurrence of FDA statisticians. However, enlarging the number of sequences to four so that the two-period design is (AB, BA, AA, BB) avoids the carryover problems of the (AB, BA) design, albeit with diminished efficiency to separate treatments. However, expanding the number of periods results in designs without the inefficiency of the two-period designs. These results have led to considerable renewed interest in finding ways to capitalize on the known advantages of crossover designs with three or more periods without falling prey to the problem of carryover. However, there are many sequences possible. Even for a three-period, two-treatment design, there are eight possible sequences: (AAA, AAB, ABB, BBB, BBA, BAA, ABA, BAB). If there are to be N participants in the trial, how should they be allocated to each sequence to achieve the maximum possible efficiency in estimating the parameters that characterize the treatment effects?

In a p period crossover design, there are p responses from each subject, which, naturally, are correlated. If the $p \times p$ covariance matrix of the responses is known, then the optimal design can be exactly determined. However, this is hardly ever the case, and ignorance of the covariance matrix greatly complicates the problem of specifying an optimal design. There are two practical approaches to solving the design dilemma: (1) Based on information from similar studies, the researcher can assume that the correlation structure is of some specified form from which an optimal design may be determined. Almost all medical research involving crossover designs has been conducted under some assumption as to the form of the covariance matrix. In this case, the design is called *fixed*, because the entire design is specified before the clinical trial begins. (2) A clinical trial with p periods can commence, and, as data accumulate, the information on the first few of the N subjects to be studied can be used to estimate the covariance matrix. Treating the estimate as if it were the true covariance matrix, the optimal sequences to which the next few subjects will be allocated are determined. Their data are added to the first set of data, and a new estimate of the covariance matrix is obtained. The process continues until all N subjects are studied. For reasonable sample sizes, simulated experiments suggest that the resulting trials are nearly as efficient as the optimal design that would have been used had the covariance matrix been known. Designs in which no specific form of the covariance matrix is assumed are called *response-adaptive*, because the subsequent course of the design is specified only after prior responses are obtained.

Notably, the controversy over the use of crossover designs has not subsided. Optimality results are based not only on the assumed covariance matrix, but also on the assumed response model (i.e., the set of assumptions as to how carryover and response are related). Different models may yield entirely different results. For example, some authors maintain that the carryover effect that occurs if two consecutive treatments are identical (e.g., AA) is not the same as the carryover effect that arises from two consecutive treatments that are different (e.g., AB). Recently, statisticians have begun to consider response models that reflect this and other views, and designs that are optimal under some of these models have been found.

EVALUATING TREATMENTS UNDER CONTROLLED CONDITIONS IN THE REAL WORLD AND UNDER FINANCIAL CONSTRAINTS

Efficacy studies, designed to determine whether a treatment has an effect, are usually carried out under relatively pristine laboratory-like conditions, with rigid adherence to detailed protocols. In contrast, *effectiveness studies* attempt to evaluate how and if a treatment works under real-world conditions. Invariably, treatment choices must involve their costs. Statistical cost-effectiveness analysis provides information to help support the decision maker.

Efficacy Studies Randomized, double-blind, controlled clinical trials are the gold standard for efficacy studies, enabling, theoretically at least, an unbiased assessment of the relative merits of the study treatments and causal inference. In an efficacy study, extraneous variables that might have an impact on outcome and therefore confound the results and their interpretation are controlled to the greatest extent possible. However, when experimental trials are conducted under the best of laboratory-like conditions, it must be kept in mind that the ability to generalize the findings are limited. Such trials provide little evidence as to how the study treatments will work under usual care conditions in the real world. Efficacy studies are usually conducted in a limited number of well-circumscribed patient populations, and many of the patients most likely to receive the treatment if the FDA approves it are excluded. Trial eligibility criteria may exclude, for example, patients with comorbidities, those whose symptoms are too severe or not severe enough, those suspected or known to be noncompliant, or those who have a history of violence. The trials may involve care conditions that are quite specialized, delivered by highly trained staff that provide individual attention far in excess of the norm. A positive finding does prove that the experimental treatment works, but the issue of efficacy beyond the well-defined populations on whom it has been tested in the well-defined environments in which the studies were conducted remains open.

Effectiveness Studies These studies examine how well a treatment works under real-world conditions. Many studies designed as randomized clinical trials should actually be considered to be effectiveness studies, and the environmental deviations from controlled conditions should be taken into account. For example, clinical trials of psychotropic agents are rarely conducted under pristine experimental conditions. They may take place for a short time in hospitals, but follow-up is usually in an outpatient setting. They may be based in outpatient clinics or in multiple practitioners' offices, so subjects come and go from their homes. They may have multiple exposures to various unreported risk factors that impact the conditions for which they are being treated. Such conditions cannot be completely controlled. Over the course of the study, treatment groups may be differentially affected in ways that can influence outcome to such a degree that the effect of the treatment they receive is overwhelmed.

Although randomization is preferred, this may not always be possible; many studies are conducted in which patients have been assigned to treatments in the naturalistic course of their care. Although methods for mimicking randomization (e.g., propensity scores) can be used, findings from these studies are often affected by environmental factors unrelated to the study treatment. Sometimes study treatment and the locus of care are confounded because of the nature of the intervention. This is almost always true in trials that test nonpharmaceutical treatments, such as new clinical programs, screening models, or complex approaches, such as supported housing. In such trials, blind treatment assignment is essentially impossible, and, therefore, unbiased assessment of outcomes may be questionable.

Such situations create studies in which analysis of the data and, more importantly, their interpretation are substantially more complex than analyses of the traditional randomized, double-blind, controlled clinical trial. Nevertheless, the value of these studies can be enormous. Besides having the potential to provide information on efficacy, a well-designed effectiveness study can discover the way to maximize the yield on use of an efficacious agent under real-world conditions. These studies test acceptability to both consumers and the health professionals who deliver the treatment. Outcomes of interest include measures of the treatment's acceptability to recipients and to caregivers, its impact on quality of life, and its costs. Compliance issues need to be examined with respect to events in the clients' world and to the biological or structural elements of the intervention itself. To understand the factors that affect compliance, data should be collected on basic demographic descriptors and on substance use, work and housing conditions, social relations, and environmental conditions, including those of the caregiver and the treatment setting. Such data items need to be collected at baseline and also over the course of the study.

From a statistical perspective, multiple analyses of multiple outcomes are required. In the comparison of treatment groups based on an *intent-to-treat analysis,* all subjects, including noncompliers, treatment crossovers, and dropouts, remain members of the group to which they were originally assigned. This analysis provides a view of how well the "policy" of assigning the study treatments works in the real world, blemishes and all. An efficacy analysis can be conducted using the same data set by identifying matched persons from each group based on predicted treatment assignment, compliance, or crossover behavior patterns. Treatment outcomes are compared within matched groups. Propensity score methods can be used to accomplish the matching. A third set of analyses might examine the impact of environmental factors on treatment acceptability and compliance.

Cost-Effectiveness The high cost of health care provides a compelling reason to examine the costs of interventions, not just their effectiveness. Cost-effectiveness analysis is an economic technique for guiding choices among alternative treatments, policies, or program-level interventions so as to maximize effectiveness under a constrained budget. In a cost-effectiveness study, alternative interventions are compared in terms of the costs required to provide a particular level of effect.

For cost-effectiveness purposes, a program P is characterized by an ordered pair of positive values (ε, γ), representing, respectively, its mean effectiveness and its mean cost. Programs are *mutually exclusive* if only one of them may be used at one time in one patient. However, a mixture occurs when two or more mutually exclusive treatments are given to a collection of subjects. For example, if 100 patients are to receive medication treatment A or B and no person can receive both treatments because they are incompatible, then if 80 percent receive drug A and 20 percent receive drug B, a mixture of programs has occurred. Programs are independent if any number of them may be used at one time and neither the cost nor effectiveness of any program is affected by a decision to use or not to use any other program(s) in the set. A program is *dominated* if there is another program with greater or equal effectiveness and less cost. A *weakly dominated* program is one that is dominated by a mixture of programs. Within a class of mutually exclusive programs, in most cases only those that are neither dominated nor weakly dominated (the admissible class) should be considered for use. The cost-effectiveness ratio of a program, the price per unit of effectiveness, is the ratio γ:ε. If two programs are ranked in order of increasing cost, the incremental cost-effectiveness ratio of the program with higher cost compared to the program with lower cost, the additional price per additional unit of effectiveness, is the incremental cost divided by the incremental effectiveness.

Subject to conditions of independence and mutual exclusivity among specified programs and given the values of their mean cost and mean effectiveness, the deterministic resource allocation problem of cost-effectiveness analysis is the selection of a set of programs for funding whose effectiveness is the maximum that can be achieved without incurring a cost greater than a specified fixed budget, C^*. For independent programs, resources are allocated sequentially in order of increasing cost-effectiveness ratios until the budget is exhausted. For mutually exclusive programs, dominated programs are eliminated and the remaining programs ranked in order of increasing effectiveness, incremental cost-effectiveness ratios are computed, weakly dominated programs are eliminated, incremental cost-effectiveness ratios are recalculated, and the process continues until all remaining programs are admissible. The remaining programs form the *frontier*, the piecewise line segments connecting adjacent admissible programs. Given a budget constraint, the program that should be funded is the one on the frontier with that budget; if the budget lies between the budgets of two frontier programs, a mixture of these two is funded.

When analyzing cost-effectiveness from the societal perspective, the above fixed budget approach is replaced by a fixed price approach. Economists have shown that the greatest feasible health gain is achieved by implementing within each independent set of mutually exclusive programs that program whose incremental cost-effectiveness ratio is largest among those programs that do not exceed a specified threshold value. This value, denoted by λ, is interpreted as the amount society is willing to pay for an additional unit of health gain. Programs with incremental cost-effectiveness ratios above the threshold value are not implemented. The fixed budget and fixed price approaches prescribe the same allocation, except that the latter does not allow partial or mixture implementations of programs.

Statistical methods, specifically for cost-effectiveness analysis, began to emerge in the mid-90s, centered around methods for obtaining CIs for incremental cost-effectiveness ratios. The inherent difficulty of dealing with a random ratio whose denominator may assume the value zero compounded the difficulties of this approach. Recently, the value of net health benefit (NHB) for statistical cost-effectiveness analysis has become widely accepted. The NHB of program k is defined as $NHB_k(\lambda) = \varepsilon_k - \gamma_k / \lambda$, $k = 1, 2, \ldots, K$. At each willing-to-pay value λ, the optimal NHB rule for mutually exclusive programs funds the program with the largest positive NHB. For resource allocation, both the standard ratio-based allocation rules of cost-effectiveness analysis and the new NHB-based rule lead essentially to the same optimal solution.

The NHB rule requires neither rank ordering of programs nor elimination of inadmissible programs, which enables statistical methods that control errors and that emulate the optimal deterministic rules of cost-effectiveness analysis. For bivariate normally distributed cost and effectiveness variables and a specified willing-to-pay λ, the statistical procedure is based on the method of constrained multiple comparisons with the best for determining the program with the largest NHB. This method both controls the pointwise error rate at each λ and provides a confidence set for the programs that are either best or comparable to the best. The statistical frontier, plotted in the λ-NHB plane, displays the program, or, possibly, the set of programs, with the largest NHB at each willing-to-pay value. Bayesian methods for performing a cost-effectiveness analysis have also been developed.

SUGGESTED CROSS-REFERENCES

Section 5.1 discusses epidemiology, and Section 5.3 discusses mental health services research.

References

Agresti A. *Categorical Data Analysis*. New York: Wiley; 1990.

Bluman AG. *Elementary Statistics: A Step By Step Approach*. New York: McGraw-Hill; 1995.

Brown BW: The crossover experiment for clinical trials. *Biometrics*. 1980;36:69–79.

*Cornfield J: A statistician's apology. *JASA*. 1975;70:7–14.

Dempster AP, Laird NM, Rubin DB: Maximum likelihood from incomplete data via the EM algorithm. *JRSS Series B*. 1977;39:1–38.

Draper NR, Smith H. *Applied Regression Analysis*. New York: Wiley; 1998.

Fliess JL. *The Design and Analysis of Clinical Experiments*. New York: John Wiley & Sons; 1986.

Gehan EH, Lemak N. *Statistics in Medical Research: Developments in Clinical Trials*. London: Plenum Pub Corp; 1994.

*Gelman A. *Bayesian Data Analysis*. London: Chapman & Hall; 1995.

Hedeker D, Gibbons R: A random-effects ordinal regression model for multilevel analysis. *Biometrics*. 1994;933–944.

Holland PW: Statistics and causal inference. *JASA*. 1986;81:945–970.

Hsu JC. *Multiple Comparisons, Theory and Methods*. London: Chapman & Hall; 1996.

Jones B, Kenward M. *Design and Analysis of Cross-Over Trials*. Monographs on Statistics and Applied Probability 34. London: Chapman and Hall; 1989.

*Kleinbaum DG. *Survival Analysis: A Self Learning Text*. New York: Springer Verlag; 1996.

*Kotz S, Read CB, Banks DL. *Encyclopedia of Statistical Sciences*. New York: Wiley; 1997.

Kushner HB: Optimality and efficiency of two-treatment repeated measurements designs. *Biometrika*. 1997;84:455–468.

Laska EM, Klein DF, Lavori PW, Levine J, Robinson DS. Design issues for the clinical evaluation of psychotropic drugs. In: Prien RF, Robinson DS. *Clinical Evaluation of Psychotropic Drugs*. New York: Raven Press; 1994.

Laska EM, Meisner M, Siegel C, Wanderling J. Statistical determination of cost-effectiveness frontier based on net health benefits. *Health Econ*. 2002;11:249–264.

Lavori PW, Laska EM, Uhlenhuth EH. Statistical issues for the clinical evaluation of psychiatric drugs. In: Prien RF, Robinson DS. *Clinical Evaluation of Psychotropic Drugs*. New York: Raven Press; 1994.

Lehmann EL. *Nonparametrics: Statistical Methods Based on Ranks*. San Francisco: Holden-Day; 1975.

Liang KY, Zeger S: Longitudinal data analysis using general linear models. *Biometrika*. 1986;73:13–22.

Little R, Rubin D. *Statistical Analysis with Missing Data*. New York: Wiley; 1987.

McCullagh P, Nelder JA. *Generalized Linear Models*. London: Chapman & Hall; 1989.

Piantadosi S. *Clinical Trials: A Methodologic Perspective*. New York: Wiley; 1997.

Rosenbaum PR. *Observational Studies*. New York: Springer Verlag; 2002.

Rosenbaum PR, Rubin DB: The central role of the propensity score in observational studies for causal effects. *Biometrika*. 1983;70:41–55.

*Rosenberger WF, Lachin JM. *Randomization in Clinical Trials: Theory and Practice*. New York: Wiley; 2002.

Rubin D. *Multiple Imputation for Nonresponse in Surveys*. New York: Wiley; 1987.

Rubin DB: Estimating causal effects of treatment in randomized and nonrandomized studies. *J Educ Psychol*. 1974;66:688–701.

Whitehead A. *Meta-Analysis of Controlled Clinical Trials*. New York: Wiley; 2002.

Zeger S, Liang KY, Albert P: Models for longitudinal data: a generalized estimating equation approach. *Biometrics*. 1988;44:1049–1060.

▲ 5.3 Mental Health Services

Mark Olfson, M.D., M.P.H.

Mental health services research is a broad multidisciplinary field that draws on a variety of methods and approaches to understand and improve the operation of the mental health services system. Mental health services researchers are interested in defining not only who receives, provides, and pays for care, but also the extent to which service provision meets the health care needs of the population, and the mix and combinations of policies, programs, and interventions that are most effective and cost-effective.

Mental health services research can be loosely classified into five broad perspectives: service delivery, service utilization, service finance, quality of care, and outcomes research. The service delivery perspective seeks to define the structures of the mental health service system by measuring the number and variety of mental health service organizations, their clinical operation, and the volume and characteristics of the patients they serve. Service utilization research examines the delivery of care from the patient's perspective. It includes measuring unmet need for treatment in the community, the flow of patients into treatment, and processes governing use of different services. Research on the financing of mental health services addresses the effects of economic incentives on patients, professionals, and organizations, and the cost-effectiveness of alternative ways of organizing, financing, and delivering services. A clinical quality of care perspective focuses on the extent to which available services increase the likelihood of desired health outcomes and are consistent with current professional knowledge. Finally, outcomes research focuses on the effects of service utilization on a range of health and health-related outcomes. Individual mental services research efforts commonly span two or more research perspectives.

SERVICE DELIVERY RESEARCH

Policy makers and program planners seek an understanding of mental health organizations and providers, including the types of services they provide and the patients they treat. A variety of research approaches are used to collect and analyze these data ranging from large-scale surveys of mental health care organizations to detailed studies of individual clinical encounters.

National Perspective A national perspective on mental health service delivery helps define general trends in health care delivery. Nationally representative service delivery data describe broad patterns and trends in practice. Examples of recent important national trends include an increase in privatization of publicly financed mental health services, growth in the use of antidepressants by adults and children, increased use of stimulants by children, continuing decline in the number and length of inpatient psychiatric hospital stays, and growing popularity of involuntary outpatient programs.

In the United States, the most extensive national provider-based surveys of mental health services are conducted by the Survey and Analysis Branch of the Center for Mental Health Services (CMHS). These surveys provide a complete enumeration of specialty mental health organizations and psychiatric services of general hospitals. They offer estimates of the volume, diagnostic composition, demographic characteristics, and payment profile of patients treated in various types of mental health organizations. The findings allow policy makers and program planners to examine patterns of mental health services received by special patient groups (e.g., children, adolescents, and persons with severe and persistent mental illness) at a specific point in time.

The CMHS surveys do not capture mental health services provided in office-based practice or general medical settings. It has been evident for many years that primary care physicians and other non–mental health professionals treat a substantial proportion of child and adult patients with mood and anxiety disorders. Nationally representative information concerning these patients and providers can be gleaned from surveys conducted by the National Center for Health Statistics. Population-based surveys conducted by the Agency for Healthcare Research and Quality (AHRQ) also provide information on the full spectrum of health care settings and professionals. For example, AHRQ surveys have revealed that during the period from 1987 to 1997, the percentage of Americans who received treatment for depression more than tripled. During the same period, the proportion who were treated for depression with an antidepressant medication increased from 37 to 74 percent. Such findings help shape program development priorities for meeting the service needs of rapidly growing patient groups.

Regional Perspective A regional perspective on service delivery emphasizes the composition, range, frequency, and coordination of mental health services provided to patients in a defined region such as a state, county, or catchment area. There is particular interest in measuring the extent to which specific changes in health care policy affect service delivery in well-defined regions.

If a change in policy is planned in advance, such as the closing of a state mental hospital, data collection can begin before the policy change occurs and can continue after the change in policy. More commonly, mental health services researchers seek to understand the implications of a regional policy change by retrospectively examining treatment patterns and patient outcomes before and after a change in the organization or financing of care. For example, an analysis of changes in treatment patterns and costs of care for children after the implementation of the Massachusetts Medicaid carve-out managed care plan revealed a decrease in per-child expenditures, especially for disabled children, and evidence of declining continuity of care. This study illustrates an interrupted time series design. Secular change, events that occur separate from the policy change under study, may confound attribution of temporal trends to the policy change.

New policies may have the intended effects on service delivery, but these effects may not be sufficient to result in meaningful change in clinical outcomes. An illustration of the importance of studying patient outcomes together with service delivery variables is provided by the Robert Wood Johnson Foundation Program on Mental Illness. This project examined the hypothesis that by strengthening the role of local mental health authorities it would be possible to promote the development of comprehensive mental health care and social welfare services. Greater coordination in service delivery would, in turn, improve the health outcomes of patients with severe and persistent psychiatric illness. Nine cities were selected for the project. Although the project succeeded in creating structural change through the creation of centralized mental health authorities, these changes were not sufficient to promote improved patient outcomes in such critical areas as symptomatic distress or quality of life. These findings suggest that structural change in service delivery without a complementary focus on clinical and social service processes may not be sufficient to achieve meaningful improvement in patient outcomes.

There is also interest in studying unintended effects of policy change. An example of unintended policy effects followed the enactment Tennessee's Medicaid managed mental health and substance abuse program, TennCare Partners. This policy sought to lower Medicaid expenditures through privatization of mental health and substance abuse services. However, an analysis revealed that many patients did not receive care or lost continuity of existing services. The problems were related to a design flaw that spread funds previously allocated to patients with severe mental disorders over the entire Medicaid population.

Program Perspective A programmatic perspective on service delivery considers patterns of service provision from the vantage point of individual mental health programs. Researchers are interested to learn about the nature, frequency, and range of specific treatments provided by different programs. There is also keen interest in experimental studies of the effects of innovative programs on patient outcomes. Recent research on the treatment of depression in primary care provides illustrations of a program-level mental health services research.

Studies of physician education or training programs have not found large or enduring effects on the quality of mental health treatment or outcomes of primary care patients with depression. Randomized trials of physician reminders or feedback systems have also yielded unimpressive results. In one study of elderly primary care patients, providing primary care physicians with the results of depression screening data with management recommendations resulted in a small increase in treatment initiation but no improvement in patient outcomes. In contrast, programs that involve specialty mental health care professional consultations with primary care physicians or nurse support of patients have yielded more promising results.

One randomized controlled trial that involved primary care patients who were initiating antidepressant therapy examined the effects of two to four patient visits with a consultation psychiatrist. Patients who received the intervention experienced significantly higher levels of medication adherence, satisfaction with treatment, and superior clinical outcomes than control patients who received treatment exclusively from their primary care physicians. Telephone contacts with trained primary care nurses have also been shown to improve the early course of treatment of primary care patients starting antidepressant treatment. Similar results were achieved in a second study of psychiatrist consultations to depressed primary care patients who had persistent symptoms despite 6 to 8 weeks of antidepressant treatment.

Clinical Encounter Perspective The most microscopic service delivery research perspective examines specific aspects of individual clinical encounters. One important goal is to define variations in clinician behaviors and link them to patient outcomes. There is a long tradition in psychotherapy research of seeking to relate specific therapeutic approaches to favorable clinical outcomes.

Clinical encounter research methods have been used to examine the assessment and diagnosis of mental disorders by primary care clinicians. Scales have been developed to score videotaped patient visits for clinical techniques and behaviors associated with appropriate recognition of mental disorders. One study found that only a small proportion of primary care visits with depressed patients include the necessary questions to establish a depressive disorder diagnosis. Another study revealed that accurate recognition of the mental disorder was increased by establishing eye contact with the patient at the outset of the interview, clarifying the presenting complaint, responding to verbal and nonverbal cues of psychological distress, and effectively eliciting cues from the patient that indicate distress. A study that was limited to visits that included psychotropic medication prescriptions revealed that, whereas higher-income patients usually request these medications from their physicians, it is the physicians who usually initiate the discussion of psychotropic medications in visits with lower-income patients. Such findings highlight areas of quality concern, identify promising strategies to improve care, and suggest potential biases in service delivery.

SERVICE UTILIZATION RESEARCH

Health Care Seeking Service utilization research considers service provision from the perspective of the patient rather than the provider. Common service utilization research themes include describing the extent to which individuals in need of care receive treatment and describing the processes involved in entering and moving within the mental health services system.

An important public health goal is to provide services that meet the mental health care needs of the population. Assessing this issue requires epidemiological sampling and measures of psychopathology, service utilization, and socioeconomic characteristics. One well-known such study is the National Comorbidity Survey (NCS) that surveyed a nationally representative sample of 8,098 persons aged 15 to 55 between 1990 and 1992. The results revealed that, across several sociodemographic strata and a wide range of mental disorders, most individuals do not receive treatment for their disorders in any given year. From the NCS and other epidemiological studies, it is evident that groups with the highest rates of unmet need for clinical care include socioeconomically disadvantaged groups, including poor persons, uninsured individuals, blacks, Hispanics, and adults with lower levels of formal education, as well as children, adolescents, and elderly persons.

For people seeking mental health services, self-report of mental health symptoms tends to be fairly accurate. However, because a great majority of individuals in epidemiological surveys have not sought mental health treatment, concern about underreporting of symptoms exists. Self-report information regarding mental disorders, especially substance use disorders, is highly sensitive to subtle variations in survey context and the mode of questioning. In addition to concerns about validity, concerns exist over response bias, especially in the measurement of relatively rare disorders that may interfere with survey participation (e.g., psychotic disorders). Measurement issues further complicate the measurement of some disorders in community surveys, including problems distinguishing psychotic symptoms from momentary cognitive misperceptions, culturally sanctioned religious experiences, or simple misunderstandings that do not represent mental illness. These technical concerns limit the accuracy of assessing unmet need for treatment of persons with the most serious and persistent mental illnesses.

An appreciation of the extent of unmet need for mental health services has led to the study of service access. Numerous factors are thought to facilitate or impede use of mental health services for well-defined disorders. The main steps of the mental health care–seeking process are recognition of a mental health problem, contact with a general medical provider, and referral to a mental health specialist. In the United States, these steps do not necessarily proceed in an orderly or a sequential manner, as many individuals bypass general medical care and present directly for specialized mental health care, sometimes on an emergency basis.

Individual determinants of health care–seeking processes are commonly conceptualized as involving interactions between health needs, predisposing factors, and enabling resources. Health needs include objective and subjective aspects of mental and physical health status. The assessment of health needs typically includes measures of the type, severity, frequency, and duration of symptoms or distress. Subjective appraisal of mental health is another important dimension of the health assessment. Health beliefs, including perceived need for treatment, perceived efficacy of treatment, and barriers to seeking treatment, are believed to play important roles.

Predisposing factors relate to the willingness to seek care. Norms and beliefs, role obligations, and demographic characteristics are important predisposing factors. Enabling or restrictive influences, on the other hand, reflect the availability of resources that facilitate or impede service utilization. Health insurance, disposable income, and local availability of services are key enabling influences. The operation of predisposing and enabling factors is generally considered to be contingent on the presence of some underlying clinical need for care.

Beyond individual determinants of health care seeking, health care utilization patterns are determined by provider variables such as the skill, training, attitudes, orientation, knowledge, and behavior of the health care professional. Administrative controls over service access are another important set of determinants of health care access and utilization.

Epidemiological data indicate that greater objective illness severity is associated with higher rates of treatment. Among those who receive mental health care, individuals with more severe conditions are disproportionately served by psychiatrists and other mental health specialists as opposed to primary care physicians or other general medical professionals.

Specific aspects of psychopathology influence treatment-seeking behavior. Symptom pattern and severity play important roles in determining the timing of treatment seeking and the pathway to mental health care. In one community study of depression, depressed mood and weight loss, but not sadness or agitation, predicted mental health care from a primary care physician. In another study, chest pain, but not palpitations, during a panic attack was associated with seeking mental health treatment from a primary care physician. Similarly, retrospective research reveals that in the first year after disorder onset, a far greater proportion of individuals receive treatment for panic disorder, which typically has a sudden and dramatic onset, than receive treatment for depression, substance use disorders, or other anxiety disorders.

The basis for the observed lower rates of mental health treatment among racial and ethnic minorities remains an important and poorly understood aspect of service utilization. Although some researchers have suggested that interethnic differences in mental health utilization are largely attributable to socioeconomic differences, research demonstrates that, even within privately and publicly insured populations, blacks and Hispanics have substantially lower rates of outpatient mental health service utilization than whites.

Cultural and attitudinal factors may help to explain the lower rates of professional mental health service utilization by blacks and Hispanics in relation to whites. Some members of ethnic minorities may be reluctant to use specialized services provided by English-speaking whites, whereas others may prefer to rely on traditional, nonmedical care providers. Some racial minorities, for example, have been found to have a stronger belief than whites in the effectiveness of the clergy as providers of mental health care.

Treatment Nonadherence Treatment nonadherence poses a major challenge to the delivery of mental health services. High rates of treatment nonadherence have been observed in a variety of service settings. After hospitalization, up to one-third of psychiatric patients fail to make their first scheduled outpatient visit. Treatment nonadherence is also common after referral from emergency departments and primary care practices to outpatient psychiatric services. Up to one-third of patients who enter psychotherapy terminate after one or two sessions. In many treatment contexts, active substance use, lack of insight into the need for treatment, and a history of treatment nonadherence predispose toward premature treatment termination.

A failure to take antipsychotic drugs as prescribed is one of the most important and well-studied aspects of nonadherence with mental health services. In one report, almost one-half of outpatients with schizophrenia stopped taking antipsychotic medications during the first year after hospital discharge. By 2 years after discharge, approximately three out of four patients had stopped taking antipsychotic medications. The clinical and public health implications of such widespread medication nonadherence are underscored by the high rates of relapse after experimental withdrawal of antipsychotic medications and by the close association of antipsychotic medication nonadherence with rehospitalization.

Adherence with mental health treatment is a joint function of the patient's personal characteristics, psychiatric symptoms, prescribed treatment, social context, and access to relevant services. Patient characteristics, including demographic, financial, cultural, social, geographic, and attitudinal factors, all influence treatment adherence. Psychiatric symptoms such as pessimism, hopelessness, grandiosity, paranoia, and cognitive impairment may also interfere with appropriate adherence to prescribed treatments. In one study of schizophrenia, for example, greater conceptual disorganization, emotional withdrawal, hostility, and grandiosity, but not anxiety or depression, were associated with rejection of antipsychotic medications.

Aspects of the treatment intervention, such as its availability, effectiveness, associated side effects, complexity, and characteristics of the patient–provider relationship have all been found to influence treatment adherence in schizophrenia. An increased risk of nonadherence or drop-out has been related to long clinic scheduling delays, restrictive admission and discharge policies, and inadequate development of outreach or emergency services.

In the management of medication nonadherence in schizophrenia and other psychotic disorders, psychoeducational programs without behavioral components and supportive services are unlikely to be effective. Clinical interventions that integrate principles of motivational interviewing and problem-solving strategies, such as reminders, self-monitoring tools, and reinforcements, appear to be more useful in improving medication adherence.

Inappropriate Service Utilization Growth of prepaid and capitated care has increased efforts to control the costs of care. There has been a particular focus on seeking to reduce care that is deemed unnecessary or inappropriate. This area is marked by considerable controversy as managed care organizations, third-party payers, service providers, and symptomatic individuals often have very different perceptions as to what constitutes inappropriate and appropriate care.

Primary care patients who use very high levels of general medical services have been studied from the standpoint of inappropriate service utilization. Accumulating evidence suggests that these patients also have high rates of psychiatric disorder. In one study of distressed high utilizers of primary care, nearly one-fourth of the patients met criteria for current major depression.

It has been hypothesized that appropriate provision of psychiatric care to distressed high utilizers of general medical care will save treatment costs by reducing unnecessary and poorly focused medical expenditures. Thus far, however, this effect has not been convincingly demonstrated in a well-controlled study. However, a cost-offset effect has been shown after the provision of psychiatric consultation services to inpatients with general medical disorders and medical outpatients with somatization disorder. The psychiatric consultation–primary care physician collaboration model has been shown to improve the treatment of primary patients with depression.

FINANCING OF MENTAL HEALTH SERVICES

Early mental health economic research focused on the effects of insurance and copayments on the demand for mental health services. Because cost sharing and service limits are more common in mental health than in general health care, mental health economists sought to understand the effects of cost containment mechanisms on total expenditures and service access. Economists subsequently examined the spread of private prepaid mental health care plans to populations that had been previously covered by traditional private fee-for-service plans. More recently, there has been interest in understanding the economics of publicly financed care, especially the Medicaid program.

State Medicaid agencies have turned in increasing numbers to companies that provide managed mental health services. In most states, a majority of Medicaid patients are now managed under prepaid plans. The wide appeal of these financing arrangements is that they promise access to needed mental health services, containment or reductions of treatment costs, and improvements in the quality of care by integrating the financing and delivery of treatment. Several techniques are used to control access to care as well as the types, amounts, and costs of care. These techniques include authorizing only selected clinicians to provide care, reviewing decisions concerning service utilization, closely monitoring high-cost cases, and using financial incentives. These cost-containment mechanisms are thought to have their greatest impact on patients who are the most severely ill and are therefore the most vulnerable to service reductions.

There is general agreement that managed care has been effective in reducing or at least slowing the growth of the costs of providing mental health services. However, there is much less consensus over the effects of managed care, especially managed Medicaid on the quality of mental health services. Critics assert that managed care has jeopardized the quality of mental health services by underfunding services, excluding patients with more severe disorders, threatening confidentiality, and relying too extensively on less highly trained health professionals.

The debate surrounding the growth of managed mental health care has been conducted in the near absence of systematic empirical data on its actual clinical effects. Most of the empirical research on managed care has focused on cost-containment issues from the perspective of the payer, insurer, or managed care organization. Considerably less work has been done on the effects of managed behavioral health care on the quality and effectiveness of clinical services.

In one study, Medicaid patients with chronic mental illness were randomly assigned to prepaid care and followed for 1 year. All patients rejoined fee-for-service arrangements after the demonstration project. As expected, patients assigned to prepaid care had lower rates of service utilization in several areas. There were no significant differences between the groups in clinical outcomes. In multivariate analyses, however, patients with schizophrenia in the prepaid group had significantly poorer global functioning once they returned to fee-for-service care. Some indication of longer-term effects of Medicaid managed care can be gleaned from retrospective analyses of claims data. This research suggests that Medicaid managed care for severely ill psychiatric patients is associated with slight decreases in the rate and length of inpatient admissions but an increase in the rate of rapid rehospitalization after hospital discharge.

QUALITY OF CARE RESEARCH

Quality of care is the degree to which treatment conforms with predefined standards of appropriate or acceptable care. Research on quality of care requires the existence of standards of care or treatment guidelines that can be operationally defined and reliably measured. Quality standards are typically developed by experimental or quasi-experimental observation, systematic review of the research literature, or expert consensus. A distinguishing characteristic of quality of care outcomes research is that it does not involve experimental manipulation of service delivery. Instead, quality of care research studies the degree, extent, and determinants of naturally occurring variation in the organization, financing, and delivery of mental health services as it relates to adherence or departure from established quality standards.

Investigators may use existing treatment outcome studies or well-established treatment guidelines to assess quality of care by measuring variations in clinical practice. Findings of widespread departures from quality standards suggest priority areas for quality improvement initiatives. For example, research indicates that, despite a strong empirical support for the value of family interventions in reducing early relapse after hospital discharge in schizophrenia, these services are only rarely available to patients and their families in the public sector.

Psychotropic medication prescribing practices are particularly amenable to quality of care research. There is accumulating evidence and concern that substantial numbers of patients with schizophrenia are prescribed antipsychotic medication regimens that are inconsistent with evidence-based treatment recommendations, including inadequate or excessive dosing, insufficient use of depot preparations in patients with a history of medication nonadherence, and failure to appropriately move patients who are treatment resistant on to newer-generation antipsychotics. Several factors are believed to contribute to these departures from guideline consistent practice.

Physicians who practice alone have been shown to be less likely to be aware of new information regarding patient care, to adopt new procedures, or to conform with practice guidelines. Clinicians who are not involved in education or research have been found to have higher rates of inappropriate treatment provision. In one study, excessive antipsychotic medication dosing was more common at hospital clinics without teaching affiliations than at others with such affiliations.

Formulary restrictions and other cost-containment practices may limit expenditures for the newer and more expensive antipsychotic medications to patients who have the greatest probability of achieving reductions in direct treatment costs. As compared with fee-for-service reimbursement, prepaid care has been associated with lower use of the more effective, but costly, newer antipsychotic agents and with increased risk of suboptimal dosing of antipsychotic medications.

Lack of provider knowledge is widely believed to be an important cause of serious problems in quality of care. It has been argued that if physicians knew the latest scientific evidence regarding the effectiveness of specific interventions, the quality of their clinical decisions would improve. According to a review of 46 quality studies, an average of 54.5 percent of providers identified lack of knowledge as a barrier to guideline adherence.

Patient characteristics have been shown to influence the quality of medication management in schizophrenia. Specifically, African Americans and patients with comorbid substance use disorders may be especially likely to receive antipsychotic dosages above the recommended therapeutic range. Patients with a history of violence, severe agitation, or an inability to care for themselves are also at increased risk of receiving exceedingly high doses of antipsychotic medication.

Quality concerns extend to the management of bipolar disorder. A study of lithium (Eskalith) prescribing revealed that, despite persuasive evidence that lithium has prophylactic mood-stabilizing properties in bipolar disorder, the median period of continuous lithium use in bipolar was less than 3 months in one health maintenance organization. This is far shorter than the duration of mood-stabilization prophylaxis recommended by treatment guidelines. In a second study, an analysis of Medicaid data demonstrated that more than one-third of patients prescribed lithium or other mood stabilizers did not receive therapeutic drug level testing of their medications during a 12-month period. In a British study that compared the management of bipolar disorder by general practitioners and psychiatrists, general practitioners less frequently obtained serum lithium levels of their patients, and patients were more likely to experience lithium levels above the therapeutic range. One-third of the general practitioners made no change in the dosing regimen during the 6-week period after high serum lithium levels. These findings point to areas of clinical concern and suggest the need for targeted provider educational interventions.

OUTCOMES RESEARCH

Experimental Outcomes Research

Outcomes research involves studying the health and health-related consequences of service use. The hallmark of experimental outcomes research is the systematic manipulation of the independent variable. Random assignment to treatment reliably overcomes important shortcomings of observational studies, including biases in selection to treatment and confounding of treatment exposure with patient characteristics and changes in the clinical environment. For these reasons, randomized clinical trials remain the most internally valid experimental design in outcomes research.

Prospective randomized designs have been used to study various mental health interventions and treatments. These investigations exist along a continuum from pure efficacy studies to applied effectiveness research. The continuum spans several related dimensions: stringency of patient selection, complexity of the interventions, and breadth of the outcome measures.

Efficacy studies typically select a narrow band of patients who possess characteristics that make them particularly responsive to the treatment and who lack characteristics that limit their responsiveness. The treatments studied in efficacy research tend to be relatively simple, time-limited, and capable of being administered in a highly reliable fashion (e.g., psychotropic medications). Outcome assessment in efficacy research tends to be narrowly focused on specific target symptoms.

Effectiveness research typically uses far less restrictive patient selection criteria. In this type of research, there is an overriding interest in studying patients who are representative of broader patient populations. The interventions tend to be more complex and studied for longer periods. Given the complex nature of the interventions studied in effectiveness research, it may be difficult to ascertain which aspects of the intervention in effectiveness research are responsible for observed outcomes. In effectiveness research, outcome assessments are typically broad and may extend beyond clinical symptoms to include social functioning, social relations, treatment and societal costs, work or school performance, family burden, quality of life, satisfaction with care, and other aspects of well being.

Experimental outcomes studies often mix elements of efficacy and effectiveness research. In one recent primary care study, for example, patients with panic disorder were randomly assigned to receive either a multifaceted collaborative care intervention, including antidepressant therapy, patient educational material, coordinated psychiatric consultation, and follow-up monitoring, or usual care from their primary care physician. Compared with patients who received usual care, those who received the collaborative care significantly improved in several clinical and functional outcomes over 1 year. This study included aspects typical of an efficacy trial, such as exclusion of patients with substance use disorder or those in treatment, and features of an effectiveness trial, including subject ascertainment by screening patients in the waiting room, a complex intervention, a relatively long follow-up period, and a broad range of outcome measures.

A variety of innovative models of continuous mental health service delivery have been studied in randomized, controlled effectiveness studies. The most well-studied such model is assertive community treatment. This intervention for patients with severe and persistent mental illness involves using an interdisciplinary treatment team to provide a broad, individualized, aggressive, and continuous mix of outpatient rehabilitative and psychiatric services. Assertive community treatment staff assume ultimate responsibility for ensuring that patients receive food, shelter, clothing, and medical services, and they help patients locate appropriate work and develop recreational interests.

Outcomes research indicates that assertive community treatment consistently increases patient satisfaction with care, usually reduces use of inpatient services, and sometimes reduces clinical symptoms and improves role functioning in relation to traditional outpatient care. The selective use of assertive community treatment has also been associated with savings in total costs. The impressive experimental research of assertive community treatment is widely credited as contributing to the dissemination of this treatment model throughout the United States.

Quasi-Experimental Outcomes Research Quasi-experimental designs exploit naturally occurring changes and variations in service delivery. In before–after designs, for example, each individual or group of individuals serves as his or her own control surrounding a discrete or sentinel event. Comparison groups are typically matched to experimental groups on characteristics thought to influence the outcomes of interest. In one recent quasi-experimental study, employee work records and health care claims data from a large corporation were used to study the effects of cutbacks in mental health coverage. Claims were available for more than 20,000 employees, billing and work loss data were reliably measured, there was little employee turnover, and the reduction in mental health coverage provided a discrete sentinel event. The results revealed that the mental health coverage cutbacks were accompanied by a significant increase in general medical (non–mental health) care utilization and an increase in sick time.

Information routinely collected for billing purposes is often used in quasi-experimental designs to study relationships between naturally occurring variations in specific clinical treatments and patient outcomes. In one study, Medicaid claims records were used to study whether adherence to antidepressant treatment guidelines helps to prevent relapse and recurrence in depression. Patients with four or more prescriptions of antidepressant medications were less likely to relapse than those with fewer prescriptions. In this study, statistical adjustments were made for group differences in comorbid medical diagnoses and sociodemographic characteristics.

One important limitation of administrative data is that available information is typically limited to data elements required for billing, such as basic demographic data, diagnostic and procedures codes, length of treatment episodes, and discharge status. This limits the extent to which researchers are able to adjust for confounding by treatment indication. Such confounding occurs when a variable other than the service and outcome variables under study is independently related to the service and outcome variables. Confounding can create an apparent association between service delivery and outcomes or mask an association that actually exists. Findings from the landmark Medical Outcomes Study (MOS) illustrate the importance of adjusting for confounding by treatment selection effects.

The MOS was a large practice-based observational study that examined differences in the costs, treatment, and outcome of depression by provider specialty and payment system. More than 600 depressed patients of psychiatrists, psychologists, other therapists, and general medical clinicians were followed for 2 years at three urban sites. In unadjusted analyses, antidepressant medication and counseling were associated with poorer depression outcomes than no treatment. After controlling for baseline background health characteristics, treated and untreated patients had similar outcomes. In analyses limited to severe depression, antidepressant medications and counseling were associated with superior outcomes. Through multivariate adjustment and stratification, clinical insights were gained into the effectiveness of commonly available treatments for depression.

Sometimes, statistical adjustments result in the appropriate loss of apparent associations between treatment and outcome. In one evaluation, veterans with war-related posttraumatic stress disorder (PTSD) who participated in an innovative compensated work program were compared with veterans who received usual care. Patients and controls were matched using a propensity scoring that weighted characteristics including baseline PTSD symptom scores associated with participation in the work program. The adjusted findings revealed that the compensated work program had no effect on the clinical and cost measures.

OVERVIEW

Much remains to be learned about the delivery and effectiveness of mental health services. There are methodological difficulties in defining and measuring the wide variety of financial arrangements, service interventions, and patient outcomes that characterize routine clinical practice. Few randomized controlled effectiveness studies have been conducted on innovative programs and emerging forms of service delivery. In several areas, however, observational and quasi-experimental research provide a rational basis for informing efforts to improve service delivery through public mental health promotion, patient and clinician educational programs, and health care system and policy reform.

In many areas, a wide gap separates research from clinical practice. Patients seldom have easy access to state-of-the art care, and clinicians often find it difficult to implement evidence-based practices. Although advances in pharmacological management are far easier to disseminate than new psychosocial interventions, large numbers of mentally ill patients do not receive optimal pharmacological management. The development of effective strategies to disseminate research findings into practice remains a leading public mental health objective. Meaningful progress is likely to require clear priorities; adequate financial support, including health insurance reform; and the discovery and implementation of effective strategies for disseminating evidence-based treatment into practice. Mental health services have a key role to play in this vital process.

SUGGESTED CROSS-REFERENCES

Medicare is discussed in Section 51.5a and managed care is discussed in Sections 51.5b and 52.2. Public psychiatry is covered in Section 52.1; emergency psychiatry is covered in Chapter 29; and consultation–liaison psychiatry is covered in Section 24.11. Section 5.1 discusses epidemiology in psychiatry and Section 5.2 discusses statistics. Chapter 11 presents substance-related disorders, and Chapter 12 presents schizophrenia. Discussion of various classes of antipsychotics are found in Sections 12.12, 31.16, 31.25, and 51.4d, and benzodiazepines are covered in Sections 14.9, 31.11, and 51.4c; lithium is discussed in Sections 13.7 and 31.17.

REFERENCES

Badger LW, DeGruy FV, Hartman J, Plant MA, Leeper J, Anderson R, Tietze R: Patient presentation, interview content, and the detection of depression by primary care physicians. *Psychosom Med.* 1994;56:128–135.

*Cabana MD, Rand CS, Powe NR, Wu AW, Wilson MH, Abboud PA, Rubin HR: Why don't physicians follow clinical practice guidelines? *JAMA.* 1999;282:1458–1465.

Chang CF, Kiser LJ, Bailey JE, Martins M, Gibson WC, Schaberg KA, Mirvis DM, Applegate WB: Tennessee's failed managed care program for mental health and substance abuse services. *JAMA.* 1998;280:864–869.

*Cooper LA, Gonzales JJ, Gallo JJ, Rost KM, Meredith LS, Rubenstein LV, Wang NY, Ford DE: The acceptability of treatment for depression among African-American, Hispanic, and white primary care patients. *Medical Care.* 2003;41:479–489.

Corrigan PW, Bodenhausen G, Markowitz F, Newman L, Rasinski K, Watson A: Demonstrating translational research for mental health services: an example from stigma research. *Ment Health Serv Res.* 2003;5:79–88.

Dickey B, Normand SL, Norton EC, Rupp A, Azeni H: Managed care and children's behavioral health services in Massachusetts. *Psychiatr Serv.* 2001;52:183–188.

Gilbody SM, House AO, Sheldon TA: Outcomes research in mental health: systematic review. *Br J Psychiatry.* 2002:181:8–16.

Goldberg D, Jenkins R, Millar T, Faragher EB: The ability of trainee general practitioners to identify psychological distress among their patients. *Psychol Med.* 1994;23:185–193.

Goldman HH, Morrissey JP, Ridgely MS: Evaluating the Robert Wood Johnson Foundation Program on Chronic Mental Illness. *Milbank Q*. 1994;72:37–47.

Hunkeler E, Meresman HJ, Hargreaves W, Fireman B, Berman WH, Kirsch AJ, Groebe J, Hurt SQ, Braden P, Getzell M, Feigenbaum PA, Peng T, Salzer M: Efficacy of nurse telehealth care and peer support in augmenting treatment of depression in primary care. *Arch Fam Med*. 2000;9:700–708.

Johnson RE, McFarland BH: Lithium use and discontinuation in a health maintenance organization. *Am J Psychiatry*. 1996;153:993–1000.

Katon W, Robinson P, VonKorff M, Lin E, Bush T, Ludman E, Simon G, Walker E: A multifaceted intervention to improve treatment of depression in primary care. *Arch Gen Psychiatry*. 1996;53:924–932.

Katon W, Von Korff M, Lin E, Bush T, Russo J, Lipscomb P, Wagner E: A randomized trial of psychiatric consultation with distressed high utilizers. *Gen Hosp Psychiatry*. 1992;14:86–98.

Kehoe RF, Mander AJ: Lithium treatment: prescribing and monitoring habits in hospital and general practice. *BMJ*. 1992;304:1178–1179.

Kessler RC, McGonagle KA, Zhao S, Nelson CB, Hughes M, Eshlmean S, Wittchen HU, Kendler KS: Lifetime and 12-month prevalence of DSM-III-R psychiatric disorders in the United States: results from the National Comorbidity Survey. *Arch Gen Psychiatry*. 1994;51:8–19.

Lurie N, Moscovice IS, Finch M, Christianson JB, Popkin MK: Does capitation affect the health of the chronically mentally ill? Results from a randomized trial. *JAMA*. 1992;267:3300–3304.

*Mechanic D: Is the prevalence of mental disorders a good measure of the need for services? *Health Aff*. 2003;22:8–20.

*Melfi C, Chawla A, Croghan T, Hanna MP, Kennedy S, Sredl K: The effects of adherence to antidepressant treatment guidelines on relapse and recurrence of depression. *Arch Gen Psychiatry*. 1998;55:1128–1132.

Nichol MB, Stimmel GL, Lange SC: Factors predicting the use of multiple psychotropic medications. *J Clin Psychiatry*. 1995;56:60–66.

Olfson M, Marcus SC, Druss B, Elinson L, Tanielian T, Pincus HA: National trends in the outpatient treatment of depression. *JAMA*. 2002:287:203–209.

Rosenheck RA, Druss B, Stolar M, Leslie D, Sledge W: Effect of declining mental health service use on employees of a large corporation. *Health Affairs*. 1999;18:193–203.

Rosenheck RA, Stolar M, Fontana A: Outcomes monitoring and the testing of new psychiatric treatments: work therapy in the treatment of chronic post-traumatic stress disorder. *Health Serv Research*. 2000:35:133–152.

Roy-Byrne PP, Katon W, Cowley DS, Russo J: A randomized effectiveness trial of collaborative care for patients with panic disorder in primary care. *Arch Gen Psychiatry*. 2001;58:869–876.

Soumerai SB, McLaughlin TJ, Ross-Degnan DR, Casteris CS, Bollini P: Effects of limiting Medicaid drug-reimbursement benefits on the use of psychotropic agents and acute mental health services by patients with schizophrenia. *N Engl J Med*. 1994;331:650–655.

Valenstein M, Copeland LA, Blow FC, McCarthy JF, Zeber JE, Gillon L, Bingham CR, Stavenger T: Pharmacy data identify poorly adherent patients with schizophrenia at increased risk for admission. *Medical Care*. 2002;40:630–639.

*Wells KB: Cost containment and mental health outcomes: experiences from US studies. *Br J Psychiatry*. 1995:166(S):43–51.

▲ 5.4 Animal Research and Its Relevance to Psychiatry

Stephen J. Suomi, Ph.D.

Research with animals, especially the use of animal models, has long played a prominent role in medical science and practice. *Animal models*, in general, can be defined as experimental efforts to reproduce in nonhuman subjects the essential features of various human disorders. Such models have been widely used since the dawn of medical research. Indeed, it can be persuasively argued that the overwhelming majority of fundamental advances in knowledge about human diseases and disorders over at least the past century have involved some form of research with animals at some point or points in the discovery process leading to each major advance.

Animal models of human psychopathology can be traced at least as far back in time as Ivan Pavlov's studies of *experimental neurosis* at the beginning of the 20th century, followed by the efforts of J. Horsley Gantt and Jules Massermann, among others. Yet, for many years, mainstream psychiatry largely lagged behind most other medical specialties and biomedical disciplines in the development and general use of animal models as important tools for research and practice. Indeed, nearly a half century after Pavlov's initial experiments, Lawrence S. Kubie summed up the views of many of his colleagues when he argued that animal models were unlikely to be of much use in advancing knowledge in psychiatry, because most, if not all, major psychiatric disorders were considered to be uniquely human—at that time animals, given their so-called subhuman brains, were simply viewed as incapable of experiencing those human-like complex feelings, emotions, or intrapsychic conflicts thought to underlie the human disorders. This once-common view has changed considerably since Kubie's exhortation, and, as a result, animal models of human psychopathology have been gaining increasing respectability and use in recent years. The change has been not only the product of striking improvements in the sophistication and empirical validity of these animal models, but also, in large part, the result of changing views among clinical researchers and practitioners regarding the role of biological process in most (if not all) major human psychiatric disorders.

An important impetus for this change came from Harry Harlow's pioneering experiments with rhesus monkeys in the 1950s, 1960s, and early 1970s. In these studies, Harlow demonstrated not only that rhesus monkeys were capable of developing and using complex cognitive problem-solving strategies, but also that they were inherently curious, highly social in their daily activities, and emotionally involved in the numerous and diverse social relationships that they inevitably developed throughout their lives. More importantly for psychiatry, Harlow showed in dramatic fashion that these basic cognitive, social, and emotional propensities could be altered significantly by the social environments in which his rhesus monkeys grew up, with some environments consistently producing profound and long-lasting psychopathology.

Another force behind the change in attitude regarding animal models in psychiatric research, also beginning in the 1950s and dramatically expanding thereafter, involved the increasing use of pharmacological compounds in the treatment of major psychiatric disorders. Extensive research and testing with animals before any human clinical trials was (and still is) a legally mandated requirement for any new drug to be approved for use in psychiatric treatment, and, as a result, there was a marked increase in the number of pharmacologically based studies using animal subjects in the 1960s and 1970s. During the same period, biological psychiatry emerged as a major force in psychiatric theory, research, and practice, a role that continues to this day. Acknowledging that clinical symptoms were most likely reflecting certain abnormalities in some underlying biological systems provided powerful incentives for experimental efforts to learn more about the nature and operation of those systems, at least some of which were largely shared by other species, especially nonhuman primates. As a result, the 1980s witnessed a virtual explosion of neuroscience-based research using animals and animal preparations, culminating with the designation of the 1990s as the *decade of the brain*.

Finally, the complete mapping of the entire human genome with the advent of the 21st century has resulted in burgeoning efforts to link various aspects of certain psychiatric disorders to the actions of specific genes or gene products. Because mammals, especially nonhuman primates, share many of the same genes that humans possess and, in some cases, the same or functionally equivalent polymorphisms, it is now possible to study the effects of manipulating those *candidate* genes in a variety of animal preparations. Indeed, a major research tool in the rapidly expanding field of molecular psychiatry involves the use of transgenic organisms, such as mice, in which specific genes can be deleted, added, or otherwise modified, inserted into the animal, and then studied extensively throughout its lifetime.

Thus, whereas in the 1950s, research with animals was largely ignored or explicitly rejected as irrelevant or inappropriate by all but a handful of psychiatrists and psychiatric researchers, some animal models now arguably stand at the cutting edge of research in the field. This chapter focuses on two developmentally based models that use rhesus monkeys as subjects. The chapter begins by outlining the basic rationale for developing animal models in general and providing some criteria by which they can be evaluated with respect to their relevance for the diagnosis and treatment of human psychopathology. One possible strategy for developing models that are ethologically based, are focused on developmental processes, and use nonhuman primates, such as rhesus monkeys, as subjects is then presented. Next, the basic pattern of biobehavioral development typically exhibited by rhesus monkeys growing up in natural habitats is characterized and then contrasted with that of two different subgroups of monkeys, the first of whom appear to be overly fearful and at risk for developing anxiety- and depressive-like symptoms and the second of whom are overly impulsive and excessively aggressive in their social interactions. Both subgroups exhibit significant abnormalities in certain biological functions apparently linked to their aberrant patterns of behavior, and these functions can clearly be influenced by genetic and environmental factors. Indeed, some of these abnormalities appear to be largely the product of specific gene–environment *interactions*. The section concludes with a discussion of the possible relevance of these findings from studies of rhesus monkeys for advancing understanding of human psychopathology.

BASIC RATIONALE AND EVALUATIVE CRITERIA FOR ANIMAL MODELS

Why would any researcher interested in learning more about a particular human disorder try to reproduce its essential features in a different species when presumably plenty of affected humans exist for detailed study? Perhaps the most powerful rationale for developing animal models stems from the many problems inherent in carrying out research involving human subjects or patients. Virtually all studies of any human psychopathology in which a particular disorder might be deliberately induced and then studied prospectively are strictly prohibited by strict and appropriate ethical constraints; consequently, in most cases, specific etiologies must be largely inferred from retrospective data. Additionally, there are usually substantial limitations on the range and amount of data characterizing any disorder that can be collected from any one subject or patient. Moreover, it is often difficult to assess the long-term effects of any planned intervention or treatment in acceptably rigorous scientific fashion, not only because of inevitably confounding treatment factors and the frequent lack of appropriate control subjects, but also because of the practical difficulties and often prohibitive expenses involved in accumulating extensive long-term follow-up data.

Faced with the difficulties outlined previously, some investigators have turned to animal models to address basic questions about the origins, development, expression, and possible treatment or prevention of human psychopathologies. Research with animals is generally not subject to the same limitations and restrictions that are mandated for research with human subjects and patients. Although there presently exist numerous legal regulations and formal ethical standards governing animal research—and they are now far more rigorous than they were in the 1980s—such regulations and standards nevertheless allow for manipulations and measurements with animals that are simply not ethically permissible or, in many cases, practically possible with human subjects or patients.

For example, animals can be selectively bred or genetically manipulated (e.g., via *knock-out* gene procedures) to possess genetic features that put them at risk to develop biological or behavioral anomalies, or both. Animal subjects can be placed in prospective studies specifically designed to induce psychopathology via experimental manipulations, such as brain lesions or intraventricular drug injections. They can be reared, maintained, and observed in well-controlled laboratory environments literally every day of their lives, and, in these settings, a variety of measures of biological and behavioral functioning too extensive or obtrusive to be readily collected from human subjects or patients can be routinely gathered on a daily or even more frequent basis. Various pharmacological treatments or therapeutic interventions can be systematically administered to animal subjects, and their effects can be objectively determined via careful comparisons with scientifically appropriate controls. Finally, and perhaps most significantly, from a developmental perspective, because most animals used in laboratory studies grow up far more rapidly and have shorter natural life spans than humans, the long-term and even intergenerational consequences of a particular pathology or the effectiveness of specific treatments can be assessed in a fraction of the time that it would take to obtain comparable longitudinal human developmental data.

Animal models, of course, are theoretically meaningful and clinically useful only to the extent that they *generalize* to the human phenomenon or condition being modeled. Several authors have posited specific criteria by which the validity of any animal model can be objectively judged. In general, animal models are considered more valid to the extent that they are able to reproduce (or at least to simulate) the presumed etiology, behavioral symptomology, biological underpinnings or correlates, and effective treatments or preventive strategies, or both, for the human disorder under study. Of course, in most cases, not all of these factors are particularly well established or fully understood at the human level.

Generality is further enhanced when the phenomena in question follow the same or similar patterns and sequences of change throughout development. In addition, for cases of pathology per se, assertions of generality between humans and animals seem more compelling when there exist *naturally occurring* analogs (or, better yet, homologs) of the human disorder in at least some nonhuman species, independent of any phenomena produced in a laboratory setting. In many fields of medicine, fundamental advances in understanding the basis for specific diseases and disorders have often followed the discovery that certain individuals from another species readily develop some form of the pathology in question in an apparently spontaneous fashion in nature. It would seem that finding and characterizing specific cases of naturally occurring, *ethologically relevant* patterns of obvious psychopathological behavior could likewise prove to be of considerable value for psychiatry, especially for the biological and molecular branches of the field.

For many phenomena, pathological or otherwise, the most compelling parallels between animals and humans are often found when the animal data come from humans' closest evolutionary relatives—nonhuman simian primates. Monkeys and apes share most of their genes with humans; for example, the genetic overlap between humans and Old World monkeys ranges between 90 and 95 percent, depending on the monkey species, whereas the genetic overlap between humans and chimpanzees approaches 99 percent. As a result, many features of their morphology and physiology are essentially homologous with human features. The basic patterns and sequences of brain growth and development are also highly conserved across the primate order, especially among Old World monkeys, apes, and humans. Moreover, the rich behavioral repertoires, emotional expressiveness, advanced cognitive capabilities, and complex social relationships characteristic of most monkey and ape species provide opportunities for modeling many aspects of human behavior—normal and pathological—that simply do not exist for rodents or other nonprimate animals. Indeed, these behavioral, cognitive, and socioemotional patterns provide a face validity for primate models that simply cannot be matched by models using any other animal species.

Over the past 25 years, researchers have used nonhuman primates to develop models for many different forms of major human psychopathological disorders, including anxiety, depression, obsessive-compulsive disorder (OCD), phobia, alcoholism, drug abuse, self-injurious behavior, child abuse, impulsivity, and violent aggression, among others. Rather than attempting to provide a comprehensive review of the relevant research in each of these areas, the rest of this section focuses instead on two models of psychopathology that have used rhesus monkeys in captive and naturalistic settings, that have involved naturally occurring patterns of behavioral and biological dysfunction exhibited by a subset of individuals that place them at risk for displaying far more extreme psychopathology under certain environmental conditions, and that have followed the development of the patterns in question from infancy to adulthood in these at-risk individuals. One subgroup, comprising perhaps 15 to 20 percent of captive and wild populations, appears to be excessively fearful in novel and mildly challenging circumstances. Monkeys in the other subgroup, accounting for 5 to 10 percent of the population, are behaviorally impulsive and inappropriately and excessively aggressive. The ways in which their respective developmental trajectories differ from those exhibited by most other rhesus monkeys as they grow up are summarized in the following discussion.

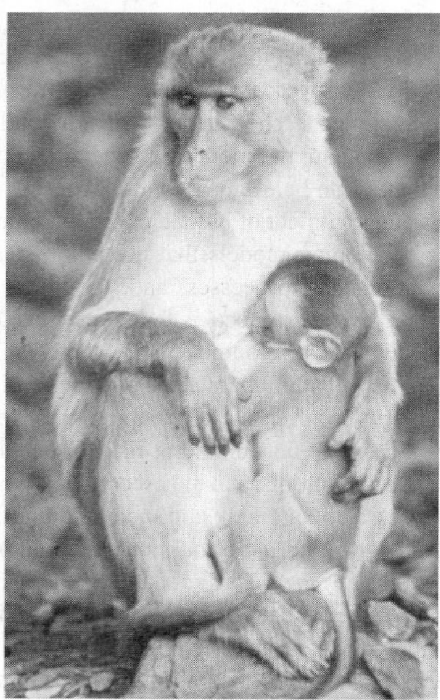

FIGURE 5.4–1 Rhesus monkey mother and infant.

INDIVIDUAL DIFFERENCES IN RHESUS MONKEY BIOBEHAVIORAL DEVELOPMENT

Rhesus monkeys typically live in large social groups (troops), each comprised of several different female monkey–headed families (matrilines) spanning several generations of kin, plus numerous immigrant male monkeys. This pattern of social organization derives from the fact that female rhesus monkey stay in their natal troop for their entire lives, whereas virtually all male rhesus monkey emigrate from their natal troop around the time of puberty, usually in their fourth or fifth year of life, and then join other troops. These troops are also characterized by multiple social dominance relationships, including distinctive hierarchies between and within families, as well as a hierarchy among the immigrant adult male monkeys. Among those male monkeys, relative status seems to be largely a function of one's ability to join and to maintain coalitions, especially with high-ranking female monkeys. In sum, the dominance status of any particular rhesus monkey within its troop depends not so much on how big and strong it is but rather who its family and friends are—and the latter is clearly dependent on the development of complex social skills during ontogeny.

Rhesus monkey infants begin life completely dependent on their mother for all of their essential needs, receiving from her nourishment, physical warmth and other basic biological support, and psychological comfort derived from tactile contact, as well as protection from the elements, potential predators, and even other troop members. Infants spend virtually all of their first month of life in physical contact with or within arm's reach of their mother (Fig. 5.4–1), and mothers typically limit any other social contact of their infants to female members of their immediate family. During this time, a strong and enduring social bond inevitably develops between mother and infant, recognized by John Bowlby to be basically homologous with the mother–infant attachment relationship universally seen in all human cultures.

Once infants have established an attachment bond with their mother, they quickly learn to use her as a secure base from which to start exploring their environment, beginning as early as their second month of life. Shortly thereafter, they begin engaging in social interactions with other troop members, especially peers, and, by 6 months of age, most youngsters typically are spending many hours each week in peer-directed activities. Interactions with peers continue to increase in frequency and complexity throughout the rest of the young monkeys' first year of life, and they remain at high and essentially stable rates throughout the second and third year of life. During this time, peer play becomes increasingly gender specific and sex segregated (i.e., male monkeys tend to play more with male monkeys, and female monkeys tend to play more with female monkeys) and involves behavioral sequences that appear to simulate virtually all adult social activities, including courtship and reproductive behaviors, as well as dominance–aggression interactions (Fig. 5.4–2). The importance of these play bouts with peers for the socialization of aggression becomes apparent when one considers that rhesus monkey infants reared in laboratory environments that deny them regular access to peers during their initial months inevitably exhibit excessive and socially inappropriate aggression later in life.

The onset of puberty, which usually begins at the end of the third year for female monkeys and at the start of the fourth year of life for male monkeys, is associated with major life transitions for male and

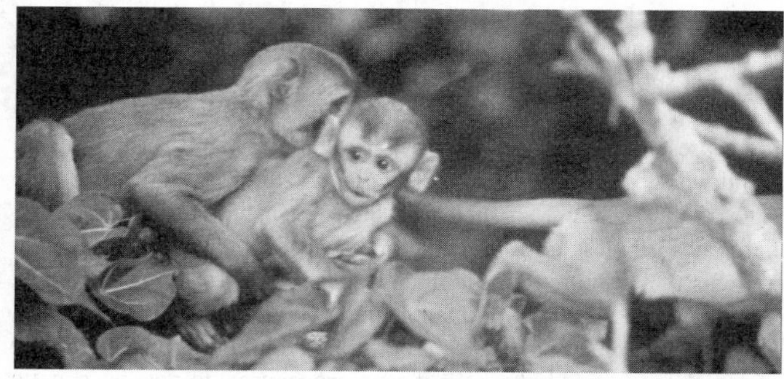

FIGURE 5.4–2 Peer play among rhesus monkey juveniles.

female monkeys, involving not only major hormonal alterations, pronounced growth spurts, and other obvious physical changes, but also major social changes for both sexes. Although female monkeys remain in their natal troop throughout adolescence and thereafter, their interactions with peers decline substantially from prepubertal levels as they redirect many of their social activities toward matrilineal kin, including their mothers and the offspring that they subsequently bear and rear. Pubertal male monkeys, in contrast, leave their family and their natal troop permanently, typically joining all-male gangs for varying periods before attempting to enter a different troop. Once a male monkey has joined a new troop, he must not only establish new relationships with the various members, but also learn about the specific kinship relationships and multiple dominance hierarchies to become successfully integrated within that troop. Not surprisingly, this period of transition represents a time of major stress and potential danger for adolescent and young adult male monkeys—indeed, the mortality rate for male monkeys during the process of natal troop emigration and subsequent immigration approaches 50 percent in some wild monkey populations. Some surviving male monkeys remain in their new troop for the rest of their lives, whereas other male monkeys may transfer from one troop to another several times during their adult years, but they never return to their natal troop.

Developmental Trajectories for Fearful Monkeys

Although virtually all rhesus monkeys growing up in naturalistic settings go through the same basic developmental sequences described previously, there are substantial differences among individual troop members in the precise timing and relative ease with which they make major developmental transitions, as well as how they manage the day-to-day challenges and stresses that are an inevitable consequence of complex social group life. In particular, as mentioned previously, recent research has identified two subgroups of monkeys who exhibit specific biobehavioral proclivities throughout development that can result in increased long-term risk for behavioral pathology and even mortality. Members of one subgroup, comprising approximately 15 to 20 percent of wild and captive populations, seem excessively fearful. These monkeys consistently respond to novel or mildly challenging situations with extreme behavioral disruption and pronounced physiological arousal (Fig. 5.4–3). Highly fearful monkeys can usually be identified during their initial weeks and months of life. Most begin leaving their mothers later chronologically and explore their physical and social environment less than other infants in their birth cohort. Highly fearful youngsters also tend to be shy and withdrawn in their initial encounters with peers—laboratory studies have shown that they exhibit significantly higher and more stable heart rates and greater secretion of cortisol in such interactions than do their less reactive age-mates. However, when these fearful monkeys are in familiar and stable social settings, they are virtually indistinguishable, behaviorally and physiologically, from their peers. In contrast, when fearful monkeys encounter extreme or prolonged stress, their behavioral and physiological differences from others in their social group usually become exaggerated.

For example, young rhesus monkeys typically experience functional maternal separations during the 2-month–long annual breeding season, when their mothers repeatedly leave the troop for brief periods to consort with selected male monkeys. The sudden loss of access to its mother is a major social stressor for any young monkey, and, not surprisingly, virtually all youngsters initially react to their mother's departure with short-term behavioral agitation and physiological arousal, much as Bowlby described for human infants experiencing involuntary maternal separation. However, whereas most young monkeys soon begin to adapt to the separation and readily seek out the company of others in their social group until their mother returns, highly fearful individuals typically lapse into a behavioral depression characterized by increasing lethargy, lack of apparent interest in social stimuli, eating and sleeping difficulties, and a characteristic, hunched-over, fetal-like posture. Laboratory studies simulating these naturalistic maternal separations have shown that, relative to their similarly reared peers, highly fearful monkeys not only are more likely to exhibit depressive-like behavioral reactions to short-term social separation, but also tend to show greater and more prolonged hypothalamic-pituitary-adrenal (HPA) activation, more dramatic sympathetic arousal, more rapid central noradrenergic turnover, and greater immunosuppression (Fig. 5.4–4). Most of these symptoms can be reversed via treatment with tricyclic or selective serotonin reuptake inhibitor (SSRI) antidepressant medications.

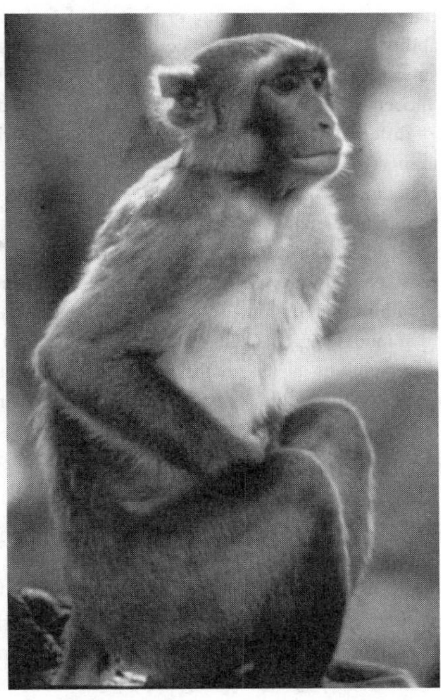

FIGURE 5.4–3 Example of excessively fearful rhesus monkey.

A monkey's characteristic pattern of biobehavioral response to separation, whether mild or extreme, tends to remain remarkably stable throughout prepubertal development and may be maintained during adolescence and

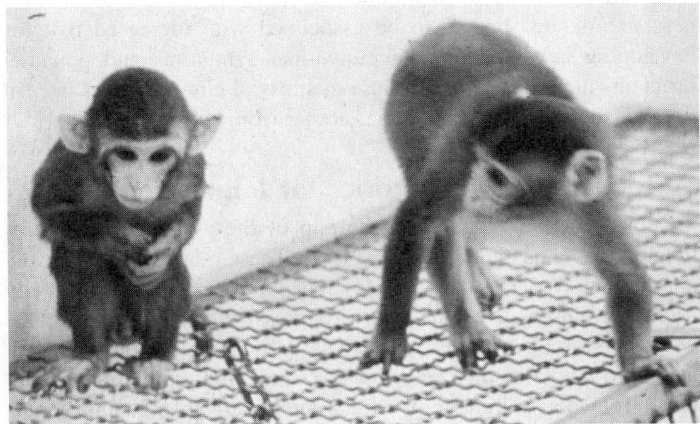

FIGURE 5.4–4 Depressive-like reaction to social separation in a fearful rhesus monkey juvenile.

even into adulthood. An increasing body of evidence has demonstrated significant heritability for at least some components of these differential responses to stress. Recent research has also demonstrated that individual differences in biobehavioral measures of fearfulness obtained during infancy are predictive of differential responses to other situations experienced later in life. One of the most striking of these involves differences in the propensity to consume alcohol in a "happy hour" situation, an experimental paradigm in which group-living rhesus monkeys are given the opportunity to consume an aspartame-flavored 9-percent ethanol beverage, a nonalcoholic aspartame-flavored beverage, or plain tap water, or a combination of these, for daily 1-hour periods within their familiar social group. Claudia Fahlke and colleagues found that monkey infants who exhibited high levels of plasma cortisol after brief separations at 6 months of age subsequently consumed significantly more alcohol in this "happy hour" situation when they were 5 years of age than did monkeys whose 6-month cortisol responses were more moderate, independent of gender or rearing background. These monkeys appeared to be self-medicating in that particular situation.

In the wild, highly fearful male monkeys usually emigrate from their natal troop at significantly older ages than the rest of their male birth cohort, and, when they do finally leave, they typically use much more conservative strategies for entering a new troop than do their less fearful peers. This pattern of delayed emigration may actually be adaptive, in that the physically larger and heavier a male monkey is at the time that he emigrates from his natal trop, the greater the likelihood that he will survive and successfully join another troop. Therefore, if a male monkey is able to postpone emigration until he has largely finished his adolescent growth spurt, he appears to be better able to make the transition to adult male life than if he leaves home before or during the growth spurt. Because fearful adolescent male monkeys pose little apparent threat to adult female monkeys and their offspring, they tend to be tolerated by other troop members at ages when the other male monkeys in their birth cohort have left voluntarily or have been forcibly driven away. Thus, even though excessive fearfulness apparently puts an individual male monkey at increased risk for adverse biobehavioral reactions to stress throughout development, there may be some circumstances in which this characteristic can actually be adaptive.

A parallel situation exists for female monkeys: Highly fearful young mothers in the wild tend to reject and punish their infants at higher rates around the time of weaning than do other mothers in their troop, and, in the absence of social support, they appear to be at increased risk for infant neglect or abuse, or both. Yet, under stable social circumstances, these fearful female monkeys may not only turn out to be highly competent mothers, but also often achieve relatively high positions of social dominance. In sum, excessive fearfulness in infancy appears to be associated with increased risk for developing anxious- and depressive-like symptoms and potential problems in parenting in response to stressful circumstances later in life, but such long-term outcomes are far from inevitable.

Developmental Trajectories for Impulsively Aggressive Monkeys Another subgroup of rhesus monkeys appears to have problems regulating aggression. These monkeys, comprising approximately 5 to 10 percent of the population, seem unusually impulsive, insensitive, and overly aggressive in their interactions with other troop members. Impulsive young male monkeys seem unable to moderate their responses to rough-and-tumble play initiations from peers, frequently escalating initially benign play bouts into full-blown aggressive exchanges that may result in actual wounding. Not surprisingly, most of these individuals tend to be avoided by peers, and, as a result, they become increasingly isolated

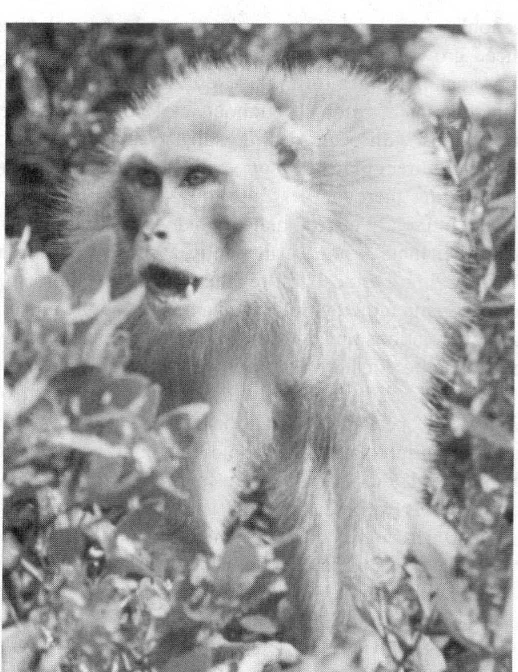

FIGURE 5.4–5 Example of an impulsively aggressive male rhesus monkey.

within their natal troop. In addition, many of these juvenile male monkeys often appear unwilling (or unable) to follow the rules that are inherent in rhesus monkey social dominance hierarchies (Fig. 5.4–5). For example, they may directly challenge a dominant adult male monkey, a foolhardy act that can result in serious injury, especially when the juvenile refuses to back away or to exhibit submissive behavior once defeat becomes obvious. Impulsive male monkeys also show a propensity for making dangerous leaps from treetop to treetop, sometimes with injurious or even fatal outcomes.

Overly impulsive monkeys of both genders consistently exhibit chronic deficits in central serotonin metabolism, as reflected by unusually low cerebrospinal fluid (CSF) concentrations of the primary central serotonin metabolite 5-hydroxyindoleacetic acid (5-HIAA). Laboratory studies have shown that these deficits in serotonin metabolism appear early in life and tend to persist throughout development, as was the case for HPA responsiveness among highly fearful monkeys. Monkeys who exhibit such deficits are also likely to show poor state control and visual orienting capabilities during early infancy, poor performance on delay-of-gratification tasks as juveniles, and sleep disturbances as adults. Moreover, individual differences in 5-HIAA concentrations appear to be highly heritable among monkeys of similar age and comparable rearing background. As was the case for excessively fearful monkeys, overly impulsive and aggressive individuals tend to consume excessive amounts of alcohol when placed in the aforementioned "happy hour" experimental paradigm. Interestingly, their pattern of alcohol consumption during the 1-hour sessions appears to be more like binge-drinking than the self-medication pattern typically exhibited by excessively fearful individuals.

Recent field studies have found that the timing of natal troop emigration that is typical for impulsive male monkeys is seemingly the reverse of that for fearful male monkeys, often with deadly consequences. Ostracized by their peers and frequently attacked by adults of both sexes, most of these excessively aggressive young male monkeys are physically driven out of their natal troop before 3 years of age, well before the onset of puberty and long before most of their male cohort begin the normal emigration process. These male monkeys tend to be grossly incompetent socially and, lacking the requisite social skills necessary for successful entrance into another troop or even into an all-male gang, most of them become solitary and typically perish within 1 year. Young female monkeys who have chronically low CSF levels of 5-HIAA also tend to be impulsive, aggressive, and generally rather incompetent socially. However, unlike the male monkeys, they are not expelled from their natal troop but instead remain with their family throughout their lifetime, although studies of captive rhesus monkey groups suggest that these female monkeys likely remain at the bottom of their respective dominance hierarchies. Although most become mothers, their maternal behavior often leaves much to be desired. In sum, rhesus monkeys who exhibit poor regulation of impulsive and aggressive behavior and low central serotonin metabolism early in life tend to follow developmental trajectories that often result in premature death for male monkeys and chronically low social dominance and poor parenting for female monkeys.

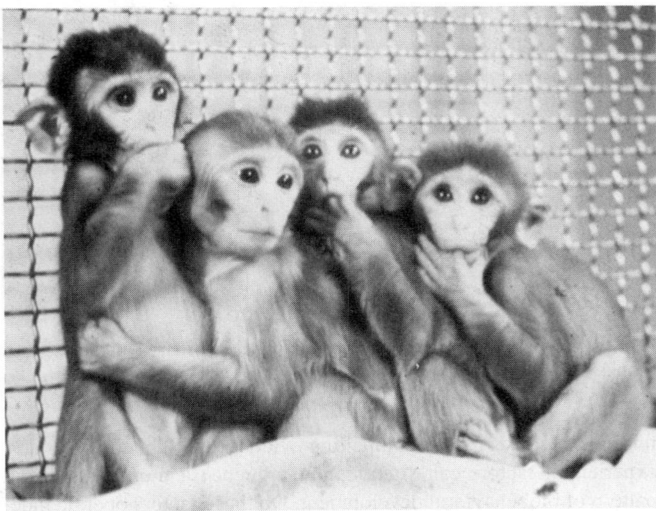

FIGURE 5.4–6 Mutual clinging by peer-reared juvenile monkeys. Attachment relationships of these infants are almost always anxious in nature. (See Color Plate.) (Courtesy of Stephen Suomi, Ph.D.)

BIOBEHAVIORAL CONSEQUENCES OF EARLY PEER REARING

Although the findings from the field and the laboratory studies reviewed previously have shown that individual differences in expressions of fear and aggression tend to be quite stable from infancy to adulthood and are, at least in part, heritable, this does not mean that they are necessarily fixed at birth, immune to subsequent environmental influence. To the contrary, an increasing body of evidence from laboratory studies has demonstrated that patterns of socioemotional development, neuroendocrine responsiveness, and neurotransmitter metabolism alike can be modified substantially by certain early social experiences, especially those involving early attachment relationships.

Some of the most compelling evidence comes from laboratory studies of rhesus monkey infants reared exclusively with peers rather than raised by their biological mothers. During their initial weeks of life, peer-reared infants readily establish strong social bonds with each other, much as mother-reared infants develop attachments to their own mothers. However, because peers are not nearly as effective as typical monkey mothers in reducing fear in the face of novelty or in providing secure bases for environmental exploration, the attachment relationships that these peer-reared infants develop are almost always anxious in nature (Fig. 5.4–6).

As a result, although peer-reared monkeys show completely normal physical and motor development, most appear to be excessively fearful—their early exploratory behavior tends to be somewhat limited, they seem reluctant to approach novel objects, and they tend to be shy in initial encounters with unfamiliar peers.

Social play among peer-reared monkeys occurs less frequently and tends to be less complex with respect to the duration, the diversity of specific behaviors incorporated, and the number of partners involved in most play episodes than is typically shown by their mother-reared counterparts. One explanation for their relatively poor play performance is that their partners have to serve as attachment figures and playmates, dual roles that neither mothers nor mother-reared peers have to fulfill. Another obstacle faced by peer-reared monkeys to developing sophisticated play repertoires is that all of their early play bouts involve partners who are basically as incompetent socially as themselves. Perhaps as a result of these factors, peer-reared youngsters typically drop to the bottom of their respective dominance hierarchies when they are subsequently housed with mother-reared monkeys of their own age.

Several prospective longitudinal studies have found that peer-reared monkeys consistently exhibit more extreme behavioral, adrenocortical, and noradrenergic reactions to social separations than do their mother-reared cohorts, even after they have been living in the same social groups for extended periods. Such differences in prototypical biobehavioral reactions to separation persist from infancy to adolescence, if not beyond. Interestingly, the general nature of the separation reactions exhibited by peer-reared monkeys seems to mirror that shown by naturally occurring highly fearful mother-reared subjects. In this sense, early rearing with peers appears to have the effect of making rhesus monkey infants generally more fearful than they might have been if reared by their biological mothers.

Early peer rearing has another long-term developmental consequence for rhesus monkeys: It tends to make them more impulsive, especially if they are males. Like the previously described impulsive monkeys growing up in the wild, peer-reared male monkeys initially exhibit overly aggressive tendencies in the context of juvenile play; as they approach puberty, the frequency and severity of their aggressive episodes typically exceed those of mother-reared group members of similar age (Fig. 5.4–7). Peer-reared female monkeys tend to groom (and be groomed by) others in their social group less frequently and for shorter durations than their mother-reared counterparts, and they usually stay at the bottom of their respective dominance hierarchies. These differences between peer-reared and mother-reared age-mates in aggression, grooming, and dominance remain relatively robust throughout the preadolescent and adolescent years. Peer-reared monkeys also consistently show lower CSF concentrations of 5-HIAA than their mother-reared counterparts. These group differences in 5-HIAA concentrations appear well before 6 months of age, and they remain stable at least throughout adolescence and into early adulthood. Thus, peer-reared monkeys exhibit the same general tendencies that characterize excessively impulsive wild-living (and mother-reared) rhesus monkeys, not only behaviorally, but also in terms of decreased serotoninergic functioning.

SPECIFIC GENE–ENVIRONMENT INTERACTIONS

Studies examining the effects of peer rearing and other variations in early rearing history, along with the previously cited heritability

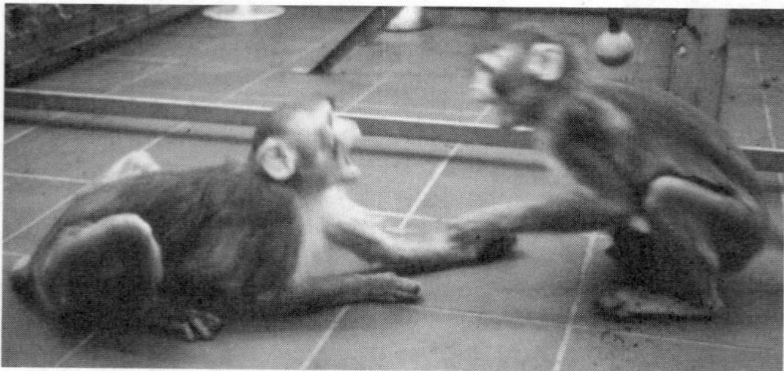

FIGURE 5.4–7 Aggressive exchange between peer-reared juvenile rhesus monkeys.

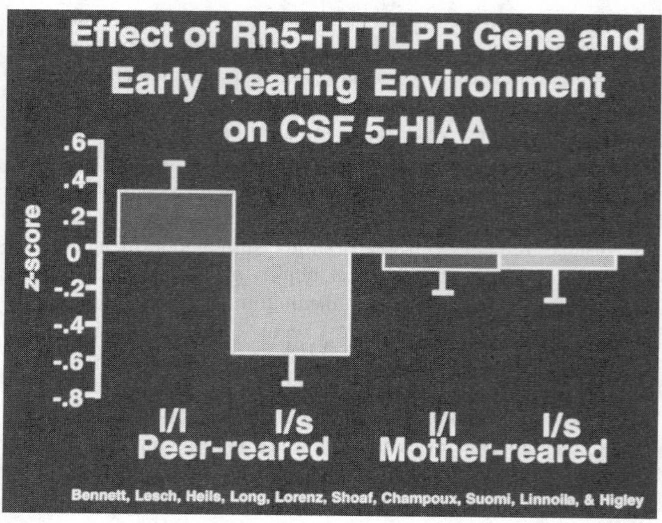

FIGURE 5.4–8 Cerebrospinal fluid (CSF) concentrations of 5-hydroxyindoleacetic acid (5-HIAA) in peer-reared l/l, peer-reared l/s, mother-reared l/l, and mother-reared l/s subjects. The gene X rearing environment interaction is the result of significantly lower CSF 5-HIAA concentrations in the peer-reared l/s monkeys than the other three subject groups. (From Bennett AJ, Lesch KP, Heils A, et al.: Early experience and serotonin transporter gene variation interact to influence primate CNS function. *Mol Psychiatry.* 2002;17:118–122, with permission.)

findings, clearly provide compelling evidence that genetic *and* early experiential factors can significantly influence a monkey's overall pattern of biobehavioral development. Do these factors operate independently, or do they interact in some fashion in shaping individual developmental trajectories? Ongoing research capitalizing on the discovery of polymorphisms in one specific gene—the serotonin transporter gene (5-HTT)—suggests that gene–environment interactions not only occur, but also can be expressed in multiple forms.

5-HTT, considered by biological psychiatrists to be a candidate gene for impaired serotoninergic function, has length variation in its promoter region that results in allelic variation in serotonin expression. A heterozygous *short* allele (LS) confers low transcriptional efficiency to the 5-HTT promoter relative to the homozygous *long* allele (LL), raising the possibility that low 5-HTT expression may result in decreased serotoninergic functioning, although evidence in support of this hypothesis in humans has been decidedly mixed to date. The 5-HTT polymorphism was first characterized in humans, but it also appears in a largely homologous form in rhesus monkeys—but, interestingly, *not* in many other species of primates and not in any other mammals studied to date.

In a series of recent analyses, polymerase chain reaction (PCR) techniques were used to characterize the 5-HTT allelic status of monkeys used in some of the studies comparing peer-reared monkeys with mother-reared subjects described previously. Because extensive observational data and biological samples had been previously collected from these monkeys throughout development, it was possible to examine a wide range of behavioral and physiological measures for potential 5-HTT polymorphism interactions with early rearing history. Analyses completed to date suggest that such interactions are widespread and diverse.

For example, Allyson J. Bennett and colleagues found that CSF 5-HIAA concentrations did not differ as a function of 5-HTT status for mother-reared subjects, whereas, among peer-reared monkeys, individuals with the LS allele had significantly lower CSF 5-HIAA concentrations than those with the LL allele (Fig. 5.4–8). One interpretation of this interaction is that mother-rearing appeared to buffer any potentially deleterious effects of the LS allele on serotonin metabolism. A similar buffering effect was found with respect to aggression: High levels of aggression were found in peer-reared monkeys with the LS allele, whereas mother-reared LS monkeys exhibited low levels that were comparable to those of mother- and peer-reared LL monkeys. Additionally, Christina S. Barr and colleagues found a parallel pattern of maternal buffering with respect to HPA activity in response to social separation: LS peer-reared juveniles had significantly higher adrenocorticotropic hormone (ACTH) concentrations than LS mother-reared, LL mother-reared, and LL peer-reared juveniles. Finally, Maribeth Champoux and colleagues examined the relationship between early rearing history and 5-HTT polymorphic status on measures of neonatal neurobehavioral development during the first month of life and found further evidence of maternal buffering. Specifically, infants possessing the LS allele who were being reared in the laboratory neonatal nursery showed significant deficits in measures of attention, activity, and motor maturity relative to nursery-reared infants possessing the LL allele, whereas LS and LL infants who were being reared by competent mothers exhibited normal values for each of these measures.

In sum, the consequences of having the LS allele differed dramatically for peer-reared and mother-reared monkeys. Peer-reared monkeys with the LS allele exhibited deficits in measures of neurobehavioral functioning during their initial weeks of life, increased HPA activity and high levels of aggression as juveniles, and reduced serotonin metabolism as adolescents. Mother-reared subjects with the exact same allele developed normal early neurobehavioral functioning, HPA activity, regulation of aggression, and serotonin metabolism. Indeed, it could be argued on the basis of these findings that having the LS allele may well lead to psychopathology among monkeys with poor early rearing histories but might actually be adaptive for monkeys who develop secure early attachment relationship with their mothers.

SUMMARY AND RELEVANCE FOR PSYCHIATRY

At the beginning of this section, it was pointed out that, although research with animals has always played a prominent role throughout the history of medical research, it was largely ignored by mainstream psychiatry until biological and molecular psychiatry came into vogue. Animal research clearly provides investigators with opportunities for manipulating genetic and experiential backgrounds, collecting multiple levels of biological and behavioral measures under rigorously controlled conditions and obtaining long-term follow-up data that, in most cases, are simply not ethically permissible or practically feasible in studies involving human subjects and patients. On the other hand, animal models are conceptually meaningful and clinically useful only to the extent that they generalize to the human condition being modeled, including the degree to which they share common etiologies, behavioral symptoms, underlying biological and genetic mechanisms, and effective treatments. Of course, it is unlikely that *any* animal model could ever reproduce every feature of any particular human psychopathological disorder at all levels of analysis—genetic, biological, behavioral, or otherwise—if for no other reason than the fact that humans possess mental capabilities of representation and self-reflection that are not shared by any other species, as Kubie noted in 1953.

On the other hand, there are some phenomena observed in animals that provide compelling analogs, if not actual homologs, to specific features of at least some human psychopathologies. Rhesus monkeys who are excessively fearful clearly resemble human children who are *behaviorally inhibited* with respect to adrenocortical, psychophysiological, and behavioral responses to novelty, stability over developmental time, and risk for exhibiting anxiety- and depressive-like symptoms in the face of prolonged stress, whereas monkeys who are excessively impulsive and aggressive appear to have many biological and behavioral features in common with children and adolescents with severe conduct disorders. How relevant are these findings from studies of rhesus monkeys for advancing understanding of human anxiety, depressive, and conduct disorders per se? To be sure, rhesus monkeys are not furry little humans with tails, and direct translation of the monkey data to the human condition can be problematic in a number of respects. Nevertheless, there are some general principles for which cross-species generalizations may not only be appropriate but also incisive.

First, many of the behavioral tendencies and biological characteristics that differentiate excessively fearful and excessively aggressive monkeys from other monkeys in their social groups appear early in life and tend to be quite stable throughout development. Some of these characteristics have been shown to be highly heritable. The fact that they can be observed in monkeys growing up in naturalistic settings strongly suggests that they are not merely the product of life in an artificial laboratory environment but rather represent capacities or potentials that have evolved and have been preserved during the natural history of the species. To the extent that whatever genes or biological systems, or both, that might be involved in the expression of these characteristics in rhesus monkeys are shared by humans, it could be argued that the capability or potential to develop psychopathology is also a product of human evolution.

Second, findings from laboratory studies have demonstrated that heritable characteristics, even those that are biological in nature, can be significantly influenced by environmental factors, particularly those involving early social attachment relationships. Thus, the manner in which a rhesus monkey has been reared can markedly affect its pattern of neonatal reflex development, its propensity to activate its HPA axis and to exhibit fear in the face of novelty, its likelihood of escalating play bouts into aggressive episodes, and its chronic CSF concentrations of 5-HIAA, respectively, no matter how many genes might be involved in each instance. Moreover, the effects of an early environmental manipulation, such as peer-rearing, are not limited to a single domain but rather are reflected in a variety of different biological and behavioral systems, not only during the period of the actual manipulation, but also often throughout the whole of development. Thus, adverse early rearing conditions appear to increase the risk for developing not one but several patterns of aberrant behavior and biological dysfunction. For example, peer rearing clearly elevates the risk for displaying depressive-like symptoms, excessive and inappropriate aggression, and high rates of alcohol consumption for rhesus monkeys. Given these findings, it seems reasonable to expect that adverse early rearing experiences in humans could also result in a range of comorbid disorders, at least for some individuals.

Finally, the recent findings regarding significant gene–environment interactions involving differential effects of specific polymorphisms in the 5-HTT gene as a function of early rearing history lend additional credence to the view that neither genes nor environments operate in a vacuum but instead interact in ubiquitous and likely complex ways. A recent demonstration of a similar pattern of gene–environment interaction involving 5-HTT allelic status and early life stress associated with a significant increase in risk for developing depression in a large New Zealand cohort suggests that such interactions may be as ubiquitous and complex in humans as in other primates. In addition, the consistent finding that good mothering can protect monkeys whose genetic status puts them at risk for developing behavioral pathologies or biological dysfunction, or both, in less benign rearing environments suggests that environmental factors not only can influence behavioral and biological functioning, but also can perhaps even regulate specific gene expression at the molecular level. Indeed, Michael J. Meaney and his colleagues have recently demonstrated actual regulation of specific genes by differential maternal behavior in rats, with lifelong and even transgenerational behavioral and biological consequences, and research in this and several other laboratories is currently directed toward elucidating the actual mechanisms through which such regulation takes place. If the general principle that specific genes can be regulated at the molecular level by certain environmental factors generalizes not only to monkeys, but also to humans, then the potential implications for developing therapeutic and preventative strategies targeted toward individuals whose family history or other factors indicate increased risk for developing psychopathology become substantial. All in all, it seems likely that research with animals is now and will continue to be relevant for psychiatry in the 21st century.

SUGGESTED CROSS-REFERENCES

Section 1.5 is a discussion of amino acid neurotransmitters. Section 1.9 covers basic electrophysiology. Learning theory is the subject of Section 3.3. Normal child development is covered in Section 32.2. Chapter 12 focuses on schizophrenia. Chapter 13 covers mood disorders, and sleep disorders are reviewed in Chapter 20. Biological therapies are the subject of Chapter 31.

REFERENCES

Barr CS, Newman TK, Becker ML, Parker CC, Champoux M, Lesch KP, Goldman D, Suomi SJ, Higley JD: The utility of the non-human primate model for studying gene by environment interactions in behavioral research. *Genes Brain Behav.* 2003;2:336–340.

*Barr CS, Newman TK, Becker ML, Parker CC, Champoux M, Lesch KP, Goldman D, Suomi SJ, Higley JD: Early experience and rh5-HTTPLR genotype interact to influence social behavior and aggression in nonhuman primates. *Genes Brain Behav. (in press).*

Barr CS, Newman TK, Shannon C, Parker C, Dvoskin RL, Becker ML, Schwandt M, Champoux M, Lesch KP, Goldman DA, Suomi SJ, Higley JD: Rearing condition and rh5-HTTLPR interact to influence LHPA axis response to stress in infant monkeys. *Biol Psychiatry.* 2004;55:733–738.

Bennett AJ, Lesch KP, Heils A, Long J, Lorenz J, Shoaf SE, Champoux M, Suomi SJ, Linnoila M, Higley JD: Early experience and serotonin transporter gene variation interact to influence primate CNS function. *Mol Psychiatry.* 2002;17:118–122.

Berard J: Male life histories. *Puerto Rican Health Sci J.* 1989;8:47–58.

*Berman CM, Rasmussen KLR, Suomi SJ: Responses of free-ranging rhesus monkeys to a natural form of maternal separation: I. Parallels with mother-infant separation in captivity. *Child Dev.* 1994;65;1028–1041.

Blum D. *Love at Goon Park: Harry Harlow and the Science of Affection.* Cambridge, MA: Perseus Publishing; 2002.

Bowlby J. *Attachment.* New York: Basic Books; 1969.

Caspi A, Sugden K, Moffitt TE, Taylor A, Craig IW, Harrington H, McClay J, Mill J, Martin J, Baithwaite A, Poulton R: Influence of life stress on depression: Moderation by a polymorphism in the 5-HTT gene. *Science.* 2003;301:386–389.

Champoux M, Bennett AJ, Lesch KP, Heils A, Nielson DA, Higley JD, Suomi SJ: Serotonin transporter gene polymorphism and neurobehavioral development in rhesus monkey neonates. *Mol Psychiatry.* 2002;7:1058–1063.

*Fahlke C, Lorenz JG, Long J, Champoux M, Suomi SJ, Higley JD: Rearing experiences and stress-induced plasma cortisol as early risk factors for excessive alcohol consumption in nonhuman primates. *Alcohol Clin Exp Res.* 2000;24:644–650.

Harlow HF, Harlow MK. Effects of various mother-infant relationships on rhesus monkey behaviors. In: Foss BM, ed. *Determinants of Infant Behaviour.* Vol 4. London: Metheun; 1969:15–36.

Heils A, Teufel A, Petri S, Stober G, Riederer P, Bengel B, Lesch KP: Allelic variation of human serotonin transporter gene expression. *J Neurochem.* 1996;6:2621–2624.

Higley JD, King ST, Hasert MF, Champoux M, Suomi SJ, Linnoila M: Stability of individual differences in serotonin function and its relationship to severe aggression and competent social behavior in rhesus macaque females. *Neuropsychopharmacology.* 1996;14:67–76.

Higley JD, Mehlman PT, Taub DM, Higley S, Fernald B, Vickers JH, Suomi SJ, Linnoila M: Excessive mortality in young free-ranging male nonhuman primates with low CSF 5-HIAA concentrations. *Arch Gen Psychiatry.* 1996;53:537–543.

Higley JD, Mehlman PT, Taub DM, Higley SB, Vickers JH, Suomi SJ, Linnoila M: Cerebrospinal fluid monoamine and adrenal correlates of aggression in free-ranging rhesus monkeys. *Arch Gen Psychiatry.* 1992;49:436–444.

Higley JD, Suomi SJ, Linnoila M: A nonhuman primate model of Type II alcoholism?: Part 2: Diminished social competence and excessive aggression correlates with low CSF 5-HIAA concentrations. *Alcohol Clin Exp Res.* 1996;20:643–650.

Higley JD, Thompson WT, Champoux M, Goldman D, Hasert MF, Kraemer GW, Scanlan JM, Suomi SJ, Linnoila M: Paternal and maternal genetic and environmental contributions to CSF monoamine metabolites in rhesus monkeys (Macaca mulatta). *Arch Gen Psychiatry.* 1993;50:615–623.

*Kagan J, Rezinck JS, Clark S, Snideman N, Garcia-Coll C: Behavioral inhibition to the unfamiliar. *Child Dev.* 1984;55:2212–2225.

Kubie LS. The concept of normality and neurosis. In: Heiman H, ed. *Psychoanalysis and Social Work.* New York: International Universities Press; 1953:31–84.

Lesch LP, Meyer J, Glatz K, Flugge G, Hinney A, Hebebrand J, Klauck SM, Poustka A, Poustka F, Bengel D, Mossner R, Riederer P, Heils A: The 5-HT transporter gene-linked polymorphic region (5-HTTLPR) in evolutionary perspective: Alternative biallelic variation in rhesus monkeys. *J Neural Transm.* 1997;104:1259–1266.

Lindburg DG. The rhesus monkey in north India: An ecological and behavioral study. In: Rosenblum LA, ed. *Primate Behavior: Developments in Field and Laboratory Research.* Vol 2. New York: Academic Press; 1971:1–106.

Lovejoy CO: The origins of man. *Science.* 1981;211:341–350.

McKinney WT, Bunney WE: Animal models of depression. *Arch Gen Psychol.* 1969;21:240–248.

Meaney MJ: Maternal care, gene expression, and the transmission of individual differences in stress reactivity across generations. *Annu Rev Neurosci.* 2001;24:1161–1192.

Mehlman PT, Higley JD, Faucher I, Lilly AA, Taub DM, Vickers JH, Suomi SJ, Linnoila M: Low cerebrospinal fluid 5-hydroxyindoleacetic acid concentrations are correlated with severe aggression and reduced impulse control in free-ranging primates. *Am J Psychiatry.* 1994;151:1485–1491.

Mehlman PT, Higley JD, Faucher I, Lilly AA, Taub DM, Vickers JH, Suomi SJ, Linnoila M: CSF 5-HIAA concentrations are correlated with sociality and the timing of emigration in free-ranging primates. *Am J Psychiatry.* 1995;152:901–913.

Pavlov IP. *Conditioned Reflexes.* London: Oxford University Press; 1927.

Rasmussen KLR, Timme A, Suomi SJ: Comparison of physiological measures of Cayo Santiago rhesus monkey females within and between social groups. *Primate Rep.* 1997;47:49–55.

Sibley CG, Comstock JA, Alquist JE: DNA hybridization evidence of hominid phylogeny: A reanalysis of the data. *J Mol Evol.* 1990;30:202–236.

Suomi SJ. Up-tight and laid-back monkeys: Individual differences in the response to social challenges. In: Brauth S, Hall W, Dooling R, eds. *Plasticity of Development.* Cambridge, MA: MIT Press; 1991:27–56.

Suomi SJ. A biobehavioral perspective on developmental psychopathology: Excessive aggression and serotonergic dysfunction in monkeys. In: Sameroff AJ, Lewis M, Miller S, eds. *Handbook of Developmental Psychopathology.* New York: Plenum Press; 2000:237–256.

*Suomi SJ. Behavioral inhibition and impulsive aggressiveness: Insights from studies with rhesus monkeys. In: Balter L, Tamis-Lamode C, eds. *Child Psychology: A Handbook of Contemporary Issues.* New York: Taylor & Francis; 2000:510–525.

Suomi SJ: How gene-environment interactions can influence emotional development in rhesus monkeys. In: Garcia-Coll C, Bearer EL, Lerner RM, eds. *Nature and Nurture: The Complex Interplay of Genetic and Environmental Influences on Human Development.* Mahwah, NJ: Lawrence Erlbaum Assoc.; 2004:35–51.

Suomi SJ, Ripp C. A history of motherless mother monkey mothering at the University of Wisconsin Primate Laboratory. In: Reite M, Caine N, eds. *Child Abuse: The Nonhuman Primate Data.* New York: Alan R. Liss; 1983:49–77.

Williamson DE, Coleman K, Bacanu S, Devlin BJ, Rogers J, Ryan ND, Cameron JL: Heritability of fearful-anxious endophenotypes in infant rhesus macaques: A preliminary report. *Biol Psychiatry.* 2003;53:284–291.

6 Theories of Personality and Psychopathology

▲ 6.1 Classic Psychoanalysis

W. W. MEISSNER, M.D., S.J.

Psychoanalysis has existed since before the turn of the 20th century and, in that span of years, has established itself as one of the fundamental disciplines within psychiatry. The science of psychoanalysis is the bedrock of psychodynamic understanding and forms the fundamental theoretical frame of reference for a variety of forms of therapeutic intervention, embracing not only psychoanalysis itself but also various forms of psychoanalytically oriented psychotherapy and related forms of therapy using psychodynamic concepts. Likewise, current efforts are being directed to connecting psychoanalytic understandings of human behavior and emotional experience with emerging findings of neuroscientific research. Consequently, an informed and clear understanding of the fundamental facets of psychoanalytic theory and orientation is essential for the student's grasp of a large and significant segment of current psychiatric thinking.

One of the difficulties in presenting such a synthetic account is that it must draw its material from more than a century of thinking and theoretical development. Although there is more than one way to approach the diversity of such material, the material in this chapter is organized along historical lines, tracing the emergence of analytical theory or theories over time but with a good deal of overlap and some redundancy. But there is an overall pattern of gradual emergence, progressing from early drive theory to structural theory to ego psychology to object relations and on to self-psychology, intersubjectivism, and relational approaches.

ROOTS OF PREPSYCHOANALYTICAL THINKING

Psychoanalysis was the child of Sigmund Freud's genius. He put his stamp on it from the very beginning, and it can be fairly said that, although the science of psychoanalysis has advanced far beyond Freud's wildest dreams, his influence is still strong and pervasive. In understanding the origins of psychoanalytic thinking, it is useful to keep in mind that Freud himself was an outstanding product of the scientific training and thinking of his era.

Scientific Orientation Freud was a convinced empirical scientist whose early training in medicine and neurology had been in the most progressive scientific centers of his time. He shared the conviction of most of the scientists of his day that scientific law and order and the systematic study of physical and neurological processes would ultimately yield an understanding of the apparent chaos of mental processes. When he began his study of hysteria, he believed that brain physiology was the definitive scientific approach and that it alone would yield a truly scientific understanding.

With his own increasing clinical experience, Freud was forced to modify that basic scientific credo, but it is significant nonetheless that he maintained it in one or another form throughout the whole of his long career. His own efforts to elaborate a scientific physiology of mental phenomena were, in the end, to prove frustrating and disappointing. After abandoning that attempt, contained in the long-lost pages of the *Project for a Scientific Psychology* (1895), he continued to believe that, although the clinical material he dealt with forced him to work on a level of psychological reflection, there was a close and intimate connection between physical and psychical processes.

On Aphasia Although a good deal of attention has been paid to Freud's *Project* as expressing his early model of the mind, more recent attention has been drawn to his important neurological work *On Aphasia* (1891), in which Freud advanced his earliest views of the relation between structure and function in the brain. Following John Hughlings Jackson's emphasis on the complex relations between thought and language, Freud challenged the prevailing notions of brain localization of function advanced by Pierre Broca, Karl Wernicke, Theodor Meynert, and others. Rather than thinking in terms of brain centers, à la Broca's speech center, Freud related the functions of speech to functional capacities in a widespread network of visual, acoustic, tactile, and even kinesthetic associations reflecting generalized changes in the functioning of the brain as a whole. Thus, he viewed simple psychological functions, such as perception or memory, as physiologically complex and involving multiple brain systems. In his view, it was the disruption in the associative network that was responsible for various forms of aphasia rather than destruction of specific centers.

Following Jackson's differentiation between mind and brain and his concept of functional retrogression from higher levels of organization to lower, Freud regarded aphasia as reflecting retrogression to earlier developmental states of speech development. He attributed speech functions to a "zone of language" that was independent of anatomical location, a position that resonated with his later stipulations regarding hysteria in which symptoms were not related to anatomical lesions but had to do with meaning and symbolization related to a network of associations. In any case, the concepts he developed in his study of aphasia later reemerged in his psychological theory, specifically, concepts of association, mental representation, cathexis, symbol formation, and word and object representation. The view of retrogression from higher to lower levels of functioning seems to foreshadow his later doctrine of regression, and his comments on forms of paraphasia read like a preliminary draft of the psychopathology of everyday life.

The *Project* The effort to bridge the chasm between psychological processes and neurological mechanisms reached a peak of intensity in Freud's attempt to construct a "scientific psychology"—that is, a psychology based on neurological principles. Earnestly dedicated to the scientific ideals of Hermann Helmholtz's approach to physiology and psychology, he conceived the scheme of elaborating a complete psychology that would be based on the physicalistic supposition of the Helmholtz school. For nearly 2 years, from 1895 to 1897, Freud struggled with these ideas. Finally, in the white heat of intense inspiration in a period of no more than 3 weeks, he wrote out what is known today as the *Project*. When the intensity of his inspiration had begun to wane, Freud became increasingly discouraged with what he had written and finally, in disgust, threw it into a desk drawer where it was to remain for years. In 1898, he wrote in discouragement and despair to his friend Wilhelm Fliess that he was "not at all inclined to leave the psychology hanging in the air without an organic basis. But apart from this conviction [that there must be such a basis] I do not know how to go on, neither theoretically nor therapeutically, and therefore must behave as if only the psychological were under consideration." It was his intention that the *Project* should be destroyed, but after his death, his papers came into the hands of those who recognized its importance, and it was finally published posthumously. If it brought Freud's neurological period to a brilliant close, it also opened the way to the broad vistas of psychoanalysis and, in extremely important and significant ways, determined the shape that psychoanalytic principles were to take.

Freud's understanding of the principles of mental functioning traditionally formed the core of explanations of how the mental apparatus works and functions, but within the last half century, the central position of these principles has come into question. The *Project* was based on two principal theorems: first, the idea that the nervous system was comprised exclusively of neurons, separated by "contact barriers" (Freud's expression for synapses); and second, a quantitative concept of neural excitation (Qn) transmitted from cell to cell in the nervous system and either stored or discharged, thus accounting for various forms of nervous activity. The energy in this early model was simply a form of quantitative excitation within an open-system neuronal reflex model, but it quickly acquired surplus meaning as a hypothetical substance with hydrostatic properties. Out of these simple elements, in combination with a set of regulatory principles, Freud elaborated his complex and ingenious account of mental functioning. The basic model used in the *Project* centered on a reflex apparatus whose function was withdrawal from stimuli, particularly excessive stimuli, and discharge of accumulated excitation as governed by the *constancy principle* and the necessity of withdrawing from excessive stimulation in accordance with the *unpleasure principle*.

When Freud finally surrendered his effort to formulate his psychology in terms of a physical model, he was forced to shift to a more specifically psychological model of the mental apparatus but without completely abandoning the ideas in the *Project*. His thinking remained tied to the physicalistic model of energy systems and their distribution. Surrender of his objective of explaining mental life in terms of physiological and neurological processes was more a compromise than a surrender. In his view, the mind possessed certain dynamic properties so that the psychological model had to be constructed according to the dynamic laws and principles inherent in current physical theories of the distribution and regulation of the flow of energy. Nonetheless, psychic energy was clearly distinct and different from the metabolic energy of the brain and referred specifically to purposeful striving.

Psychic energy became the central concept around which Freud erected his economic model of mental functioning. *Psychic energy* was that energy, assumed to be operating in the mental apparatus deriving from instinctual drives, related to affective experience, especially anxiety, and modified in various ways by psychic structures, always with a tendency toward discharge. Although it derived from instinctual drives, it had no specified relationship to physical energies assumed to be operating in corresponding neural structures.

In any case, the concept prevailed that psychic energy represented a purely quantitative and nonqualitative capacity for work, which the psychic apparatus carried out by the transformation, storage, discharge, or delay of discharge of psychic energy. In the classic theory, the instinctual drives impose this demand for work on the mind. Not only does the concept of energy as work potential divorce it from the hydrostatic model, but separating the economic principle from connections with psychic energy removes it from the line of causal efficacy; in other words, economic principles are not principles of efficiency—they are principles of quantitative regulation. Efficiency (causality, work) belongs to energic factors. However, the regulatory principles, as essential to the economic perspective, were originally formulated in terms of the regulation of psychic energies and have been viewed almost exclusively in such terms ever since. They may retain some validity in economic rather than energic terms as regulatory principles of how the mental system works (Table 6.1–1). Other questions remain regarding the place of the drives in relation to the capacity for work or force and whether the drives are the only guarantee of connection between the mind and the physical organism.

Freud used psychic energy both as a device to describe observable phenomena and as a construct in his model of the mind. People have only begun to appreciate the extent to which Freud used the neurological and energic terminology of Helmholtz and Gustav Fechner as metaphorical devices to express his psychological constructs. The use of such metaphors may have usefulness, especially in expressing issues of conflict and development dealt with by psychoanalysis—phenomena that lend themselves readily to verbal metaphorical hypotheses and less readily to mathematical quantification. As Freud's viewpoint became increasingly psychological, his use of concepts of drive and energy became increasingly metaphorical, as in *Three Essays* (1905). Probably after 1900, Freud became increasingly aware of the limitations of his theory, especially the closed-system and hydraulic aspects of his model, which prompted further revisions. After his abandonment of the *Project*, he preferred to think of his theories as purely psychological, but even so, the energic assumptions carried over into structural theory.

Criticisms of Psychic Energy All these uncertainties and ambiguities come to roost in contemporary criticisms of psychic energy. The following statements summarize the objections and the reasons why critics conclude that the classic notion of psychic energy can no longer be tolerated in a contemporary psychoanalytic theory:

Psychic energy is not measurable, so we are unable to test any quantitative assumptions of the theory.

The relationship between neural energies in the brain and psychic energy remains vague and poorly understood, and therefore any laws for the transformation of one to the other remain elusive.

The hydraulic analogy is outmoded, and the view of psychic energy was based on a simplified view of causality and a misleading equation of psychic energy with physiological energy as an explanatory principle. The model is internally contradictory

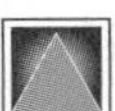

Table 6.1–1
Energic Principles Based on the *Project* Revised

Principle	Explanation
Entropy	Sigmund Freud: Tendency for energy in any physical system to flow from a region of high energy to regions of lower energy; tendency of system toward homogeneity; tendency of system to spontaneously diminish the amount of energy available for work.
	Revised: A revised schema rejects the physical model for psychic processes in favor of a psychological model based on motivation and the tendency of psychic systems to seek and achieve purposeful goals.
Conservation	Freud: The sum of forces (energy) in any isolated (closed) system remains constant.
	Revised: The psychic apparatus is not a closed system, but open, and does not operate on the basis of closed-system dynamics.
Neuronic inertia	Freud: Neurons tend to divest themselves of quantities of excitation. Application of entropy and conservation to neuronal activity.
	Revised: General psychic tendency to resolve situations of conflict, tension, affective imbalance (including anxiety, fear, guilt, shame, depression) in favor of greater balance and more harmonious integration with other psychic systems.
Constancy	Freud: The nervous system tends to maintain itself in a state of constant tension or level of excitation. Return to a level of constant excitation is achieved by a tendency to immediate energic discharge (through the path of least resistance).
	Revised: Tendency of psychic functions to return to a state of resting potential as contextual stimulus conditions and the balance of feedback-regulated conditions in the same and related psychic systems allow.
Nirvana	Freud: The dominant tendency to reduce, keep constant, or remove the internal psychic tension due to the excitation of stimuli; the tendency to reduce the level of excitation to a minimum; extension of constancy principle; expressed in pleasure principle, ultimately in death instinct.
	Revised: This principle has no place in an economically revised schema but is replaced by an opposite tendency to seek stimulation, even to seek complex rather than simple stimulation.
Pleasure-unpleasure	Freud: Tendency of mental apparatus to seek pleasure and avoid unpleasure. Unpleasure is due to the increase of tension or level of excitation, whereas pleasure is due to the release of tension or discharge of excitation. The pleasure principle thus follows the economic requirements of constancy.
	Revised: Indicates the degree of functional satisfaction/dissatisfaction and efficacy derived from effective/ineffective operation of psychic systems; pleasure reflects successful transition from potential to actual operation of the psychic function(s) and achievement of purposeful and wished-for goals.
Reality	Freud: Modification or delay of energic discharge adapting pleasurable discharge according to the demands of reality.
	Revised: Modification or delay of psychic functioning as mutually conditioned by the internal context of intra- and intersystemic functions within the mental apparatus; limiting conditions for specific functions outside the mind are determined by reality factors.
Repetition	Freud: Tendency of instinctual forces, as a result of inertial tendencies, to repeat patterns of discharge even when resulting in unpleasure.
	Revised: Rather than resulting from inertial energic dynamics, repetition may relate to stabilization of psychic functions and structural integrations, thus contributing to development and the continual process of assimilating and accommodating to reality.

and lacks consistency; it presents a logically closed system that misinterprets metaphor as fact; it involves tautological renaming of observable psychological phenomena in energic terms, which masquerades as explanation; it is unable to explain all the relevant data; it tends to lead to a false sense of explanation, particularly to the extent that it offers pseudoexplanations that are inconsistent with current knowledge of neurophysiology. Rather than serving as a bridge between psychoanalysis and physiology, especially neurophysiology, it becomes a barrier to interdisciplinary communication and integration.

The human organism is in some degree tension seeking and maintaining, whereas the energic model is based on the principle of tension reduction.

Psychic energy comes in multiple forms, such as libidinal, aggressive, narcissistic, and various degrees of neutralized energies, bound energies, and fused energies. The difficulty here has not so much to do with the varying manifestation of energies in different forms but, rather, with the idea that the differences are inherent in the energies themselves. This objection focuses on the differentiation of the energy itself, as opposed to the idea that various manifestations of psychic energy may be determined by the structures through which they are expressed—qualitative differences would be due to the patterned control, channeling, and mediation of intervening structures. In the analogous case of physical energy, the differences of the various forms, such as heat and light, are not attributed directly to energy as such but, rather, to the physical channels through which the energy is expressed. By implication, qualitative energic differences undercut the idea of the id as unstructured chaos consisting only of energy and its modes of discharge.

There are also problems with the energic metaphor itself. Freud did not clearly distinguish drive and energy as biological, physiological, or psychological and connected them almost exclusively with the sexual drive. The terms share both physical and psychological reference: Cathexis is both an electrochemical charge and a wish. This opened the door not only to conceptual errors but also to the use of an essentially nonanalytical model to explain analytical material.

If energy serves as a metaphor for experience, it is merely descriptive and not explanatory; if it stands for some neurophysiological function, any explanatory value rests on dualistic mind–brain assumptions.

The notion of psychic energy does not meet minimal criteria of accepted scientific method. Specifically, it is internally contradictory and lacks consistency; it presents a logically closed system that misinterprets metaphor as fact; it involves a tautological renaming of observable and experienced psychological phenomena in energic terms that masquerade as explanations; it is unable to explain all of the relevant data, especially the phenomena of pleasurable tension, exploratory behavior, and stimulus hunger; it tends to lead to a false sense of explanation, particularly insofar as it offers pseudoexplanations that are inconsistent with current knowledge of neurophysiology; and it promotes a form of mind–body dualism—dualistic interactionism—that prevents integration of psychoanalytic concepts with related sciences of the mind and behavior. The metaphor is given surplus meaning, which elevates it to an objective phenomenon and introduces circularity, vitiating any verification of drive–energy concepts.

The energic metaphor is inconsistent with current neurophysiological understanding based on principles of selective inhibition rather than energy depletion or the all-or-none nature of the nervous impulse rather than fluid dynamics.

The usefulness of the energic model for clinical purposes has been questioned. Using a quantitative model for qualitative events limits both the range and depth of explanation. Such quantitative translation persists in the name of presumed objectivity and in the belief that it offers a more scientific view of clinical conceptions. The drive-discharge model interprets aim in terms of discharge, thus blurring any distinction between drive and motive. But in the clinical context, libido and sexuality do assume significant connotations of meaning and motive. Even if meaning and motive do not exclude quantitative dimensions, the quantitative cannot substitute for the qualitative.

On the basis of such slender postulates, Freud elaborated a complex and ingenious account of mental functions. He was unable, however, to provide a satisfactory account of either defense or consciousness. In both cases, he became embroiled in a continuing regress in which he seemed unable to stop. Despite a variety of ingenious feedback loops that he built into the system—Freud was many decades ahead of his time in envisioning informational servomechanisms—he was unable to complete the functioning of his system without violating the demands of his mechanical principles. He thus introduced into his system a major concession to vitalism, an observing ego. This observing ego was able to see danger for the mobilization of defenses and was able to sense the indication of quality in conscious experiences. The ego remained as a sort of primary "willer" and ultimate "knower," a personal center within the theory that could not be reduced to the physicalistic terms of Helmholtzian postulates and that consequently enjoyed a significant degree of autonomy.

One of the persistent difficulties inherent in the discussion of psychic energy is that, because of the original mode in which Freud expressed his economic views, the economic hypothesis has become overidentified with the hypothesis of psychic energy. There is little doubt that psychoanalytic theory cannot do without a principle of economics. It is impossible to express or understand matters of quantitative variation, degrees of intensity, levels and intensity of motivation, or informational communication or to explain how individual subjects are able to make choices among conflicting motivations and goals to bring about the resolution of conflict—or, for that matter, to explain the whole range of affective, motivational, and structural concepts that form the backbone of psychoanalytic understanding—without invoking the very concepts and issues of quantity and intensity that led Freud from the very beginning to postulate an economic point of view. The shifting focus on informational- and communication-based concepts does not escape the need for economic governing principles.

BEGINNINGS OF PSYCHOANALYSIS

In the decade from 1887 to 1897, Freud turned his attention to the serious study of the disturbances of his hysterical patients, and, in this period, the beginnings of psychoanalysis took root. These slender beginnings had a threefold aspect: emergence of psychoanalysis as a method of investigation, as a therapeutic technique, and as a body of scientific knowledge based on an increasing fund of information and basic theoretical propositions. These early researches flowed out of Freud's initial collaboration with Joseph Breuer and then, increasingly, from his own independent investigations and theoretical developments.

The Case of Anna O.

Breuer was an older physician, a distinguished and well-established medical practitioner in the Viennese community. Knowing Freud's interests in hysterical pathology, Breuer told him about the unusual case of a woman he had treated for approximately 1.5 years, from December 1880 to June 1882. This woman became famous under the pseudonym Fräulein Anna O., and study of her difficulties proved to be one of the important stimuli in the development of psychoanalysis.

Anna O. was, in reality, Bertha Pappenheim, who later became independently famous as a founder of the social work movement in Germany. At the time she began to see Breuer, she was an intelligent and strong-minded woman of approximately 21 years of age who had developed a number of hysterical symptoms in connection with the illness and death of her father. These symptoms included paralysis of the limbs, contractures, anesthesias, visual disturbances, disturbances of speech, anorexia, and a distressing nervous cough. Her illness was also characterized by two distinct phases of consciousness: one relatively normal, but the other reflecting a second and more pathological personality.

Anna was very fond of and close to her father and shared with her mother the duties of nursing him on his deathbed. During her altered states of consciousness, Anna was able to recall the vivid fantasies and intense emotions she had experienced while caring for her father. It was with considerable amazement, both to Anna and Breuer, that when she was able to recall, with the associated expression of affect, the scenes or circumstances under which her symptoms had arisen, the symptoms could be made to disappear. She vividly described this process as the "talking cure" and as "chimney sweeping."

Once the connection between talking through the circumstances of the symptoms and the disappearance of the symptoms themselves had been established, Anna proceeded to deal with each of her many symptoms one after another. She was able to recall that, on one occasion, when her mother had been absent, she had been sitting at her father's bedside and had had a fantasy or daydream in which she imagined that a snake was crawling toward her father and was about to bite him. She struggled forward to try to ward off the snake, but her arm, which had been draped over the back of the chair, had gone to sleep. She was unable to move it. The paralysis persisted, and she was unable to move the arm until, under hypnosis, she was able to recall this scene. It is easy to see how this kind of material must have made a profound impression on Freud. It provided convincing demonstration of the power of unconscious memories and suppressed affects in producing hysterical symptoms.

In the course of the somewhat lengthy treatment, Breuer had become increasingly preoccupied with his fascinating and unusual patient and, consequently, spent more and more time with her. In the meanwhile, his wife had grown increasingly jealous and resentful. As soon as Breuer began to realize this, the sexual connotations of it frightened him, and he abruptly terminated the treatment. Only a few hours later, however, he was recalled urgently to Anna's bedside. She had never alluded to the forbidden topic of sex during the course of her treatment, but she was now experiencing hysterical childbirth. Freud saw that the phantom pregnancy was the logical termination of the sexual feelings she had developed toward Breuer in response to his therapeutic efforts. Breuer had been quite unaware of this development, and the experience was quite unnerving. He was able to calm Anna down by hypnotizing her, but then he left the house in a cold sweat and immediately set out with his wife for Venice on a second honeymoon.

According to a version that comes from Freud through Ernest Jones, the patient was far from cured and later had to be hospitalized after Breuer's departure. It seems ironical that the prototype of a cathartic cure was, in fact, far from successful. Nevertheless, the case of Anna O. provided an important starting point for Freud's thinking and a crucial juncture in the development of psychoanalysis.

Studies on Hysteria The collaboration with Breuer brought about publication of "Preliminary Communication" in 1893. Essentially, Freud and Breuer extended Jean Charcot's concept of traumatic hysteria to a general doctrine of hysteria. Hysterical symptoms were related to psychic traumata, sometimes clearly and directly but also sometimes in a symbolic disguise. Observations based on these later cases established a connection between pathogenesis of common hysteria and that of traumatic neurosis; in both cases, trauma is not followed by sufficient reaction and is thus kept out of consciousness.

They observed that individual hysterical symptoms seemed to disappear when the event provoking them was clearly brought to life, with the patient describing the event in great detail and putting accompanying affect into words. Fading of a memory or loss of its associated affect depends on various factors, including whether there has been an energetic reaction to the event that provoked the affect. Thus, memories can be regarded as traumata that have not been sufficiently abreacted. They noted that the splitting of consciousness, so striking in classic cases of hysteria as "double consciousness," is present to at least a rudimentary degree in every hysteria. They described the basis of hysteria as a hypnoid state—that is, a state of dissociated consciousness. They believed psychotherapy achieved its curative effect on hysterical symptoms by bringing to an end the emotional force of the idea that had not been sufficiently abreacted in the first instance. It does this by allowing strangulated affect to gain discharge through speech, thus subjecting it to associative correction, integrating it with normal consciousness.

"Preliminary Communication" created considerable interest and was followed in 1895 by *Studies on Hysteria* in which Breuer and Freud reported on their clinical experience in the treatment of hysteria and proposed a theory of hysterical phenomena. Freud's case discussions proved to be extremely significant because they formed the original basis for much of his psychoanalytic thinking.

Freud concluded from these observations that an experience that had played an important pathogenic role, together with its subsidiary emotional concomitants, was accurately retained in the patient's memory even when apparently forgotten and unrecoverable by voluntary recall. He postulated that repression of an idea from consciousness and exclusion from any modification by association with other ideas was an essential condition for development of hysteria. At this early stage, Freud regarded repression as intentional and believed it served as the basis for conversion of a sum of neural excitation. When cut off from more normal paths of psychic association, this sum of excitation would find its way all the more easily along a deviant path leading to somatic innervation. The basis for such repression, he argued, must be a feeling of unpleasure derived from the incompatibility between the idea to be repressed and the dominant mass of ideas constituting the ego.

Moreover, as one symptom was removed, another often developed to take its place. The illness could be acquired even by a person of sound heredity as the result of appropriate traumatic experiences. It should be noted that Freud's view was quite different from Breuer's, ascribing the origin of hysteria to hypnoid states. In Freud's view, in the actual traumatic moment, the incompatibility of ideas forces itself on the ego so that the ego repudiates the incompatible idea. This reaction brings into being a nucleus for crystallization of a separate psychic group somehow divorced from the ego. This process results in the splitting of consciousness characteristic of acquired hysteria. The therapeutic process consists in compelling this split-off psychical group to unite once more with the main mass of conscious ego ideas. In every case of hysteria based on sexual traumas, Freud believed that impressions from the presexual period, which produce little or no effect on the child, can attain traumatic power at a later date as memories when the girl or married woman begins to acquire an understanding of and exposure to adult sexual life.

On the basis of these cases, Freud reconstructed the following sequence of steps in the development of hysteria: (1) The patient had undergone a traumatic experience, by which Freud meant an experience that stirred up intense emotion and excitation and that was intensely painful or disagreeable to the individual; (2) the traumatic experience represented to the patient some idea or ideas incompatible with the "dominant mass of ideas constituting the ego"; (3) this incompatible idea was intentionally dissociated or repressed from consciousness; (4) the excitation associated with the incompatible idea was converted into somatic pathways, resulting in hysterical manifestations and symptoms; (5) what was left in consciousness was merely a mnemonic symbol only connected with the traumatic event by associative links that are frequently enough disguised; and (6) if the memory of the traumatic experience can be brought into consciousness and if the patient is able to release the strangulated affect associated with it, then the affect is discharged, and symptoms disappear.

Freud's Technical Evolution One interesting aspect of the *Studies on Hysteria* is the evolution in Freud's development of technical approaches to the treatment of hysteria. Resulting from his early interest in hypnosis, as well as his exposure to hypnotic techniques both in Charcot's clinic and later at Nancy, Freud began using hypnosis extensively in treating his patients when he opened his own practice in 1887. In the beginning, he used hypnotic suggestion to enable patients to rid themselves of their symptoms. It became quickly obvious, however, that, although patients responded to hypnotic suggestion and tried to treat the symptoms as if they did not exist, the symptoms nonetheless reasserted themselves again during the patient's waking experience.

By 1889, then, Freud was sufficiently intrigued by Breuer's cathartic method to use it in conjunction with hypnotic techniques as a means of retracing the histories of neurotic symptoms. In his early efforts, he stayed quite close to the notion of the traumatic origins of hysterical symptoms. Consequently, the goal of treatment was restricted to removal of symptoms through recovery and verbalization of suppressed feelings with which symptoms were associated. This procedure has since been described as "abreaction." However, as in the case of hypnotic suggestion, Freud was still somewhat dissatisfied with the results of this treatment approach. The beneficial effects of hypnotic treatment seemed to be transitory; they tended to last, or seemed effective, only as long as the patient remained in contact with the physician. Freud suspected that alleviation of symptoms was in fact dependent in some manner on the personal relationship between patient and physician.

From Hypnosis to Analysis Freud had begun to feel that inhibited sexuality may have a role to play in production of the patient's symptoms. His suspicion of a sexual aspect in the treatment of such patients was amply confirmed one day when a female patient awoke from a hypnotic sleep and suddenly threw her arms around his neck. Freud suddenly found himself in the same position in which Breuer had found himself during his earlier treatment of Anna O. Perhaps bolstered by Breuer's experience and apparently able to learn from it, Freud did not panic or retreat in the face of this sexual advance. Rather, the peculiar observant quality of his mind was able to disengage itself sufficiently so that this experience could be treated as a scientific observation.

From this point on, Freud began to understand that the therapeutic effectiveness of the patient–physician relationship, which had seemed so mystifying and problematic to him until this time, could be attributed in fact to its erotic basis. These observations were to become the basis of the theory of transference that he developed later into an explicit theory of treatment. In any event, these experiences reinforced his dissatisfaction with hypnotic techniques. He became aware that hypnosis was masking and concealing a number of important manifestations that seemed to be related to the process of cure or, in some cases, to the inability of the patient to achieve a definitive resolution of the neurosis. Later, his dissatisfaction with hypnosis became more specific in that he could see that continued use of hypnosis precluded further investigation of transference and resistance phenomena.

Freud had also discovered that many of the patients in his private practice were in fact refractory to hypnosis. Only gradually did he come to recognize that what seemed to be his inability to hypnotize a patient might often enough be due to a patient's reluctance to remember traumatic events. He was able later to identify this reluctance as resistance. The vagaries of the hypnotic method did not satisfy Freud, and he believed it necessary to develop an approach to treatment that could be usefully applied regardless of whether the patient was hypnotizable. Consequently, although Freud continued to use hypnotic techniques as a basic approach to treatment of hysteria, he began to experiment with it and gradually succeeded in modifying the technique.

CONCENTRATION METHOD One of the patients whom Freud found to be refractory to hypnotic technique was Elizabeth von R. For the first time, in this case, Freud decided to abandon hypnosis as his primary therapeutic tool. He based his decision to alter his technique on the observation of Hippolyte Bernheim that, although certain experiences appeared to be forgotten, they could be recalled under hypnosis and then subsequently recalled consciously if the physician were to ask the patient leading questions urging reproduction of these critical memories. Freud thus evolved his method of concentration.

The patient was asked to lie on a couch and close her eyes. She was then instructed to concentrate on a particular symptom and to recall any memories associated with it. The method was substantially a modification of the technique of hypnotic suggestion. Freud pressed his hand on the patient's forehead and urged her to recall the unavailable memories. Freud's graphic descriptions of this technique carry with them the unavoidable impression that he was struggling against a force he sensed in the patient and against which he found himself battling, as though in hand-to-hand combat. He came slowly, by dint of this laborious experience, to realize that the isolation of certain memory contents was a matter of the operation of mental forces generating considerable power that kept the complex of pathogenic ideas separate from the mass of conscious ideation. This substantially provided him both with the empirical notion of resistance and with the basic metapsychological perspective of the mind as operating in terms of psychic forces.

FREE ASSOCIATION The material presented in such graphic detail in *Studies on Hysteria* reflects dramatically the evolution of Freud's technique in the direction of his more definitive approach to psychoanalysis. He became increasingly convinced by the late 1890s that the process of urging, pressing, questioning, and trying to defeat the resistance offered by the patient—all of which were part and parcel of the "concentration" method—rather than facilitating overcoming of the patient's resistances, actually interfered with the free flow of the patient's thoughts. Piece by piece, then, Freud gave up the concentration method. Through this progressive evolution, the basic principle of psychoanalysis—free association—was focused and articulated. Gradually, Freud surrendered his technique of forehead pressure as well as the requirement that patients close their eyes while lying on the couch. The only remnant of this earlier procedure persisting in the practice of psychoanalysis is the use of the couch. The emergence of the central principle of psychoanalysis was the essential product of Freud's evolution.

The evolution of Freud's associative technique continued to progress until it had been perfected. The modification continued with increasing reliance on the patient's capacity to freely manifest mental contents without suggestive interference on the part of the therapist. By the end of the 19th century, Freud had more or less established his associative technique. He described it in the following terms:

> This [technique] involves some psychological preparation of the patient. We must aim at bringing about two changes in him: an increase in the attention he pays to his own psychical perceptions and the elimination of the criticism by which he normally sifts the thoughts that occur to him. In order that he may be able to concentrate his attention on his self-observation it is an advantage for him to lie in a restful attitude and to shut his eyes. It is necessary to insist explicitly on his renouncing all criticism of the thoughts that he perceives. We therefore tell him that the success of the psychoanalysis depends on his noticing and reporting whatever comes into his head and not being misled, for instance, into suppressing an idea because it strikes him as unimportant or irrelevant or because it seems to him meaningless. He must adopt a completely impartial attitude to what occurs to him, since it is precisely his critical attitude which is responsible for his being unable, in the ordinary course of things, to achieve the desired unraveling of his dream or obsessional idea or whatever it may be.

In just a few years more, closing of the eyes was also abandoned. Thus, free association became the definitive technique of psychoanalysis. In fact, it was development of this technique that opened the door to exploration of dreams, which became one of the primary sources of data bolstering the nascent psychoanalytic point of view.

Theoretical Innovations The theoretical point of view in *Studies on Hysteria* was relatively complex. Breuer adopted the point of view that hysterical phenomena were not altogether ideogenic—that is, that they were not determined simply by ideas. In fact, the phenomena of hysteria may be determined by a variety of causes, some brought about by an explicitly psychical mechanism but others without it. Although so-called hysterical phenomena were not necessarily caused by ideas alone, their ideogenic aspects were specifically described as hysterical. The contribution of Freud and Breuer was that they focused on investigation of these ideogenic aspects and discovered some of their psychic origins. Particularly, the concept of neuronal excitation, conceived of as subject to processes of hydraulic flow and discharge as in the *Project*, was of fundamental importance in understanding hysteria as well as neurosis in general.

A careful reading of Breuer's theoretical section in *Studies of Hysteria* makes it abundantly clear that what he proposed was a reworking of the ingenious ideas of Freud's *Project*, with specific application to the explanation of hysterical phenomena. Breuer described two extreme conditions of central nervous system (CNS) excitation, namely, a clear waking state and the state of dreamless sleep. When the brain performs actual work, greater consumption of energy is required than when it is merely prepared to do work. The phenomenon of spontaneous awakening could take place in conditions of complete quiet and darkness without any external stimulus. This demonstrates that development of psychic energy is based on vital processes of neural elements themselves.

Breuer also provided an explanation of hysterical conversion. His basic explanatory concept—originally proposed by French psychiatrists, particularly Pierre Janet—was the notion of hypnoid states. Such states were believed to resemble the basic condition of dissociation obtaining in hypnosis. Their importance lay in the amnesia that accompanied them and in their power to bring about splitting of the mind. The spontaneous origin of such states through autohypnosis was identifiable relatively frequently in a number of fully developed hysterics. These states often alternated rapidly with normal waking states. Experience of the autohypnotic state was found to be subjected to a more or less total amnesia while the patient was in the waking state. Hysterical conversion seemed to take place more easily in such autohypnotic states than in waking states, similar to more facile realization of suggested ideas in states of artificial hypnosis.

Neither hypnoid states during periods of energetic work nor unemotional twilight states were pathogenic. The reveries, however, filled with emotion and states of fatigue arising from protracted affects did seem to be pathogenic. Occurrence of such hypnoid states was important in the genesis of hysterical phenomena because they somehow made conversion easier and prevented, by way of resulting amnesia, the converted ideas from wearing away and losing their intensity.

It must be said that Freud was not sympathetic to Breuer's concept of hypnoid states, although, at this stage, Freud had not been able to bring himself to reject it. The concept, in fact, did not explain very much. The hypnoid state was used as an explanation for hysterical states, but the occurrence and function of hypnoid states themselves were in no way explained or supported—they were merely postulated. The only explanatory attempt made was in terms of a hereditary disposition to such states. This unproven postulate was one that Freud's scientific attitude could not accept.

The spirit of Freud's treatment of the psychotherapy of hysteria was quite different from that embodied in Breuer's theoretical treatment. His discussion of the treatment of hysteria in *Studies of Hysteria* gives one a good sense of the extent to which Freud had moved away in his own thinking from the somewhat restrictive formulations of the *Project*. He pointed out that each individual hysterical symptom seemed to disappear more or less permanently when the memory of the traumatic event provoking it was brought into conscious awareness along with its accompanying affect. It was necessary that the patient describe such traumatic events in the greatest possible detail and be able to express verbally the affective experience connected with it.

Freud believed that the basic etiology of the acquisition of neurosis had to be located in sexual factors. Different sexual influences operated to produce different pictures of neurotic disorders. Usually, the neurotic picture was mixed, and purer forms of either hysterical or obsessional neurosis were relatively rare. Freud did not regard all hysterical symptoms as psychogenic in origin so that they could not all be effectively treated by a psychotherapeutic procedure. In the context of his theory and technique at that time, he found that a significant number of patients could not be hypnotized despite an apparently certain diagnosis of hysteria. In these patients, Freud believed that he had to overcome a certain psychic force in the patient, a force that was set in opposition to any attempt to bring the pathogenic idea into consciousness. In the therapy, he experienced himself engaging in sometimes forceful psychic work to overcome this intense counterforce.

The pathogenic idea, however, despite the force of resistance, was always close at hand and could be reached by relatively easily accessible associations. The patient seemed to be able to rid himself or herself of such ideas by turning them into words and describing them. Nevertheless, Freud's experience was that, even in cases in which he was able to surmise the manner in which things were connected and could tell the patient before the patient had actually uncovered it, he could not force anything on the patient about matters in which the patient was essentially ignorant nor could the therapist influence the product of the analysis by arousing the patient's expectations.

Resistance The basic question that confronted Freud and Breuer had to do with the mechanism that made pathogenic memories unconscious. The divergence in their points of view was not simply a matter of theoretical differences. Freud's own thinking underwent a definite transition, and the transition seemed to be based primarily on his experience in dealing with his patients. In the beginning, he and Breuer had agreed that their hysterical patients had undergone traumatic sexual experiences. These traumatic experiences were not available to conscious recollection. They had also agreed, at least for a time, that recovery of these forgotten experiences during an induced hypnotic state resulted in abreaction and consequent symptomatic improvement.

Freud discovered that his patients were often quite unwilling or unable to recall the traumatic memories. He defined this reluctance of his patients as *resistance*. As his clinical experience expanded, he found that, in the majority of patients he treated, resistance was not a matter of reluctance to cooperate—that is, the patients willingly engaged in the treatment process and were willing to obey the fundamental rule of free association. The patients generally seemed to be well motivated for treatment, but frequently enough, it was particularly patients who were most distressed by their symptoms who seemed most hampered in treatment by resistance. Freud's conclusion was that resistance was a matter of the operation of active forces in the mind, of which the patients themselves were often quite unaware, that maintained the exclusion from consciousness of painful or distressing material. Freud described the active force that worked to exclude particular mental contents from conscious awareness as *repression*, one of the fundamental ideas of psychoanalytic theory.

Repression The concept of repression, together with its related notion of defense, came to be the basic explanation for hysterical phenomena in Freud's thinking. The notion of repression reflects one of the basic hypotheses of psychoanalytic theory, namely, that the human mind includes in its operation basic dynamic forces that can be set in opposition and that serve as the source of powerful motivation and defense. Freud described the mechanism of repression in the following terms: A traumatic experience or a series of experiences, usually of a sexual nature and often occurring in childhood, had been "forgotten" or "repressed" because of their painful or disagreeable nature; but the excitation involved in sexual stimulation was not extinguished, and traces of it persisted in the unconscious in the form of repressed memories. These memories could remain without pathogenic effect until some contemporary event, for example, a disturbing love affair, revived them. At this juncture, the strength of the repressive counterforce was diminished, and the patient experienced what Freud termed *the return of the repressed*. The original sexual excitement was revived and found its way by a new path, allowing it to manifest itself in the form of a neurotic symptom. Thus, the symptom results from a compromise between repressed desire and the "dominant mass of ideas constituting the ego." The whole process of repression and the return of the repressed was thus conceived of as involving conflicting forces—that is, the force of the repressed idea struggling to express itself against the counterforce of the ego seeking to keep the repressed idea out of consciousness.

Freud's development of the notions of repression and resistance was based primarily on his studies of cases of conversion hysteria. Specifically, in such cases, he believed that impulses that were not allowed access to consciousness were diverted into paths of somatic innervation, resulting in such hysterical symptoms as paralysis, blindness, disturbances of sensations, and other manifestations. Despite this early emphasis on conversion hysteria as the prototype of repression, Freud believed that the basic proposition that symptoms resulted from compromise between a repressed impulse and other repressing forces could be applied to obsessive-compulsive phenomena and even to paranoid ideation. The logical consequence of this hypothesis was that the treatment process during this period focused primarily on enabling the patient to recall repressed sexual experiences, so that the accompanying excitation could be allowed to find its way into consciousness and be discharged along with the revivified and previously dammed-up affects.

Seduction Hypothesis and Infantile Sexuality One additional aspect of psychoanalytic theory emerged with striking clarity from these early researches into hysteria. Invariably, when inquiring into the histories of his hysterical patients, Freud found that the repressed traumatic memories that seemed to lay at the root of the pathology had to do with sexual experiences. His attention became increasingly focused on the importance of these early sexual experiences, usually recalled in the form of a sexual seduction occurring before puberty and often rather early in the child's experience. Freud began to feel that these seduction experiences were of central importance for understanding the etiology of psychoneurosis. Over a period of several years, he continued to collect clinical material that seemed to reinforce this important hypothesis. He even went so far as to distinguish between the nature of the seductive experiences involved in hysterical manifestations and those involved in obsessional neurosis. In the case of hysteria, he believed that the seduction experience had been primarily passive—that is, the child had been the passive object of seductive activity on the part of an adult or older child. In obsessive-compulsive neurosis, however, he believed the seduction experience had been active on the part of the child. Thus, the child would have actively and aggressively pursued a precocious sexual experience.

What was significant in all of this development was that Freud had taken literally the accounts his patients had given him in the form of forgotten but revived memories of such sexual involvement. The patients provided him with "tales of outrage" committed by such relatives or caretakers as fathers, nursemaids, or uncles. Freud had devoted little attention to the role of the child's own psychological experience in the elaboration of these tales. But, little by little, he began to have some second thoughts about these so-called memories. Several factors contributed to his doubt. First, he had gained additional insight into the nature of pathological processes from his clinical experience and his increasing awareness of the role of fantasy in childhood. Second, he simply found it hard to believe that there could be so many wicked and seductive adults in Viennese society. The third influence, however, which undoubtedly was of major significance in this reconsideration, was his own self-analysis.

As this important process of self-analysis progressed, Freud began to have more and more reason to call the seduction hypothesis into question. During this time, from 1893 to 1897, Freud was still using the combined technique of pressure and suggestion with relatively great assurance. Often, he insisted that patients recall the seduction scene so that much of the evidence on which the seduction hypothesis was based was open to the charge of suggestion. Consequently, as Freud became more aware of the role of suggestion in his technique, his doubts about the seduction hypothesis grew apace. In September 1897, his doubts came to a focus, and he wrote to his good friend Fliess as follows:

> And now I want to confide in you immediately the great secret that has been slowly dawning on me in the last few months. I no longer believe in my *neurotica* [theory of the neuroses]. This is probably not intelligible without an explanation, after all, you yourself found credible what I was able to tell you. So I will begin historically [and tell you] where the reasons for disbelief came from. The continual disappointment in my efforts to bring a single analysis to a real conclusion; the running away of people who for a period of time had been most gripped [by analysis]; the absence of the complete successes on which I had counted; the possibility of explaining to myself the partial successes in other ways, in the usual fashion—this was the first group. Then the surprise that in all cases, the *father*, not excluding my own, had to be accused of being perverse—the realization of the unexpected frequency of hysteria, with precisely the same conditions prevailing in each, whereas surely such widespread perversions against children are not very probable. . . . Then, third, the certain insight that there are no indications of reality in the unconscious, so that one cannot distinguish between truth and fiction that has been cathected with affect. [Accordingly, there would remain the solution that the sexual fantasy invariably seizes upon the theme of the parents.] Fourth, the consideration that in the most deep-reaching psychoses the unconscious memory does not break through, so that the secret of childhood experiences is not disclosed even in the most confused delirium. If one thus sees that the unconscious never overcomes the resistance of the conscious, the expectation that in treatment the opposite is bound to happen, to the point where the unconscious is completely tamed by the conscious, also diminishes.

It is obvious that at this period Freud was struggling with his own great reluctance to abandon the seduction hypothesis. The doubts and the clarifying realization that he expressed to Fliess were depressing. After all, he had put in years of effort and had compiled a significant amount of evidence to bolster this seduction hypothesis. It was only with reluctance that he could surrender it. He also sensed, however, that, in surrendering the seduction hypothesis, new possibilities for psychological exploration were opened up. In fact, this juncture in the development of Freud's thinking was crucial. The abandonment of the seduction hypothesis, with its reliance on actual physical seduction, forced Freud to turn with new realization to the inner fantasy life of the child.

It can be said, in the real sense, that this shift from an emphasis on reality factors to an attention to and an understanding of the influence of inner motivations and fantasy products marks the real beginning of the psychoanalytic movement. In this attempt to distinguish psychic reality and fantasy from actual external events and psychoneurosis from perversion, psychoanalysis itself took on a new and highly significant dimension. What inevitably emerged from this shift in direction was a dynamic theory of infantile sexuality in which the child's own psychosexual life played the significant and dominant role. This notion replaced the more static point of view in which the child represented an innocent victim whose eroticism was prematurely disrupted at the hands of unscrupulous adults.

The turning point was one of extreme significance for Freud himself. Increasingly, he turned his attention to his own self-analysis and put increasing reliance on it. He wrote to Fliess, "My self-analysis is in fact the most essential thing I have at present and promises to become of the greatest value to me if it reaches its end." More and more, he became involved in the study of dreams, all the more so as he developed the technique of free association, which provided him with a tool for exploring the associative content underlying the dream experience. He concerned himself ever more so with the nature of infantile sexuality and with the inner sources of fantasy and dream content, namely, the unconscious instinctual drives. In recent years, this so-called abandonment of the seduction hypothesis has been subjected to severe criticism on the grounds that it tended to minimize the role of actual seduction, which looms as a pervasive problem in our contemporary society. But in Freud's defense, it should be said that he never denied that seduction was a problem; he knew well enough that it existed, but it was not for him a path to deeper understanding of the dynamic aspects of instinctual infantile sexual life.

By 1897, when the hypothesis of actual seduction had fallen in the dust at Freud's feet, he could look to a number of significant accomplishments. The fundamental concepts of psychic determinism and the operation of a dynamic unconscious were established, and concomitantly, a theory of psychoneurosis based on the idea of psychic conflict and the repression of disturbing childhood experiences had become clearly established. Sexuality, particularly in the form of childhood sexuality, had been unveiled as playing a significant but previously underemphasized or ignored role in the production of psychological symptoms. More significantly, perhaps, Freud had arrived at a technique, a method of investigation, that could be exploited as a means of exploring a wide range of mental phenomena that had previously been poorly understood. Moreover, the horizons of psychoanalytic interest had begun to expand rapidly. Freud's attention was no longer focused on certain limited forms of psychopathology. It had begun to reach out, reflecting the wide-ranging curiosity and interests of Freud's mind and to embrace the understanding of dreams, creativity, wit, and humor, the psychopathology of everyday experience, and a host of other normal and culturally significant mental phenomena. Psychoanalysis had indeed come to life.

INTERPRETATION OF DREAMS

Currently, the whole area of sleep and dream activity is one of the most exciting and intensely studied aspects of psychological functioning. The discovery of rapid eye movement (REM) cycles and the definition of the various stages of the sleep cycle have stimulated an intense and extremely productive flurry of research activity into the neurobiology of dreaming. A whole new realm of fresh and important questions has been opened as a result of this activity, and psychoanalysts are drawing much closer to a more comprehensive understanding of the links between patterns of dream activity and underlying neurophysiological and psychodynamic variables. As more is learned about this fascinating and complex question, one comes much closer to understanding the nature of the dream process and the dream experience itself.

In this context, it is difficult to look back and to appreciate the uniqueness and originality of Freud's immersion in the dream experience. Only when Freud's attention had been refocused to the significance of inner fantasy experiences, by reason of abandonment of the seduction hypothesis and in the context of his developing the technique of free association, did the significance and value of the investigation of dreams impress on him. Freud became aware of the significance of dreams in his experience with his patients when he realized that, in the process of free association, his patients frequently reported their dreams along with the associative material that seemed connected with them. He discovered little by little that dreams had a definite meaning, although that meaning was often quite hidden and disguised. Moreover, when he encouraged his patients to associate freely to the dream fragments, he found that what they frequently reported was more closely connected with repressed material than associations to the events of their waking experience. Somehow, the dream content seemed to be closer to the unconscious memories and fantasies of the repressed material, and associations to dream material seemed to facilitate disclosure of this content.

Theory of Dreaming

The rich complex of data derived from Freud's clinical exploration of his patients' dreams and the profound insights derived from his associated investigation of his own dreams were distilled into the landmark publication in 1900 of *The Interpretation of Dreams*. Basing his analysis on these data, Freud presented a theory of the dream that paralleled his analysis of psychoneurotic symptoms. He viewed the dream experience as a conscious expression of an unconscious fantasy or wish not readily accessible to conscious waking experience. Thus, dream activity was considered one of the normal manifestations of unconscious processes.

The dream images represented unconscious wishes or thoughts disguised through a process of symbolization and other distorting mechanisms. This reworking of unconscious contents constituted the dream work. Freud postulated the existence of a "censor," pictured as guarding the border between the unconscious part of the mind and the preconscious level. The censor functioned to exclude unconscious wishes during conscious states but, during regressive relaxation of sleep, allowed certain unconscious contents to pass the border, yet only after transformation of unconscious wishes into disguised forms experienced in the dream contents by the sleeping subject. Freud assumed that the censor worked in the service of the ego—that is, as serving the self-preservative objectives of the ego. Although he was aware of the unconscious nature of the processes, he tended to regard the ego at this point in the development of his theory more restrictively as the source of conscious processes of reasonable control and volition. It should not be forgotten that, even in *Studies on Hysteria*, repression was still envisioned in intentional and volitional terms. Freud's deepened appreciation of the unconscious dimension of these processes led him to view the ego as in some part unconscious, one of the reasons for his formulation of the structural theory in 1923.

Analysis of Dream Content

Freud's view of dream material was that it contained content that has been repressed or excluded from consciousness by defensive activities of the ego. The dream material, as consciously recalled by the dreamer, is simply the end result of unconscious mental activity taking place during sleep. Freud believed that the upsurge of unconscious material was so intense that it threatened to interrupt sleep itself so that he envisioned one function of the censor was to act as a guardian of sleep. Instead of being awakened by these ideas, the sleeper dreams.

From a more contemporary viewpoint, it is known that cognitive activity during sleep has a great deal of variety. Some cognitive activity follows the description that Freud provided of dream activity, but much of it is considerably more realistic and more consistently organized along logical lines. The dreaming activity that Freud analyzed and described is probably more or less associated with the stage 1 REM periods of the sleep–dream cycle. The so-called manifest dream that embodies the experienced content of the dream, which the sleeper may or may not be able to recall after waking, is the product of dream activity. Unconscious thoughts and wishes that in Freud's view threatened to awaken the sleeper were described as "latent dream content."

Freud referred to unconscious mental operations by which latent dream content was transformed into the manifest dream as the *dream work*. In the process of dream interpretation, he was able to move from the manifest content of the dream by way of associative exploration to arrive at the latent dream content that lay behind the manifest dream and that provided it with its core meaning.

In Freud's view, there were a variety of stimuli that initiated dreaming activity. The contemporary understanding of the dream process, however, suggests that dreaming activity takes place more or less in conjunction with the psychic patterns of central nervous activation that characterize certain phases of the sleep cycle. What Freud believed to be initiating stimuli may in fact not be initiating at all but may be merely incorporated into the dream content, and determine to that extent the material in the dream thoughts. Stimuli could arise from various sources.

NOCTURNAL SENSORY STIMULI A variety of sensory impressions, such as pain, hunger, thirst, or urinary urgency, may play a role in determining dream content. Thus, instead of disturbing one's sleep and leaving a warm bed, a sleeper who is in a cold room and who urgently needs to urinate may dream of awakening, voiding, and returning to bed. Freud's view would have been that the activity of dreaming preserved and safeguarded the continuity of sleep. It is known now, however, that the function of dreaming is considerably more complex and cannot be regarded simply as preserving sleep, although there is still room for this process to be counted among the dream functions.

DAY RESIDUES One of the important elements contributing to shaping the dream thoughts is the residue of thoughts and ideas and feelings left over from experiences of the preceding day. These residues remain active in the unconscious and, like sensory stimuli, can be incorporated by the sleeper into thought content of the manifest dream. Thus, day residues could be amalgamated with unconscious infantile drives and wishes deriving from the level of unconscious instincts. The amalgamation of infantile drives with elements of the day's residues effectively disguises the infantile impulse and allows it to remain effective as the driving force behind the dream. Day residues may in themselves be quite superficial or trivial, but they acquire significance as dream instigators through unconscious connections with deeply repressed instinctual drives and wishes.

REPRESSED INFANTILE DRIVES Although these various elements may be determining aspects of the thought content of the dream experience, the essential elements of the latent dream content derive from one or several impulses emanating from the repressed part of the unconscious. In Freud's schema, the ultimate driving forces behind dream activity and dream formation were the wishes, originating in drives, stemming from an infantile level of psychic development. These drives took their content specifically from oedipal and pre-oedipal levels of psychic integration. Thus, nocturnal sensations and day residues played only an indirect role in determining dream content. A nocturnal stimulus, however intense, had to be associated with and connected with one or more repressed wishes from the unconscious to give rise to the dream content. This point of view needs some revision because it seems that, in some phases of nighttime cognitive activity, the mind is able to process residues of daytime experience without much indication of connection with unconscious repressed content. However, in phases of cognitive activity during sleep that bear the stamp of dreaming activity as Freud described and defined it, this essential link to the repressed probably still retains some validity.

Significance of Dreams

Once Freud's attention had definitively shifted to the study of inner processes of fantasy and dream formation, the study of dreams and the process of their formation became the primary route by which he gained access to understanding unconscious processes and their operation. In *The Interpretation of Dreams*, he maintained that every dream somehow represents a wish fulfillment. He bolstered this hypothesis with a considerable amount of documentation, including exhaustive analysis of his own dreams.

There is a more general tendency today to view the dream activity as expressing a broader spectrum of psychological processes, keeping the aspect of wish fulfillment as one among the dimensions of dream activity but not as an absolute principle, as it seemed to be in Freud's thinking. The manifest dream content may represent imaginary fulfillment of a wish or impulse from early childhood, before such wishes have undergone repression. In later childhood, and even later in adulthood, however, the ego acts to defend itself against unacceptable instinctual demands of the unconscious. Wish fulfillment in the dream process is usually quite obscured by the extensive distortions and disguises brought about by the dream work so that it often cannot be readily identified on a superficial examination of the manifest content.

Dream Work

The theory of the nature of dream work became the fundamental description of the operation of unconscious processes—the basic mechanisms and the manner of their operating—that stands even today as an unsurpassed and foundational account of unconscious mental functioning. The focus of Freud's analysis was on the process by which unconscious latent dream thoughts were disguised and distorted in such a fashion as to permit their expression and translation into conscious manifest content of the dream. However, these unconscious processes, part of the fruit of his investigation, found ready application and extrapolation not only to understanding the formation of neurotic symptoms but also, more broadly, to a whole range of unconscious productivity. The theory of dream work consequently became the basis for a wide-ranging analysis of unconscious operations that found expression in Freud's study of everyday experiences, as well as artistic creativity, jokes, and humor, and a variety of culturally based activities of the human mind. Aspects of the dream work are as follows.

Representability

The basic problem of dream formation is to determine how it is that latent dream content can find a means of representation in the manifest content. As Freud saw it, the state of sleep brought with it relaxation of repression, and, concomitantly, latent unconscious wishes and impulses were permitted to press for discharge and gratification. Because the pathway to motor expression was blocked in the sleep state, these repressed wishes and impulses had to find other means of representation by way of mechanisms of thought and fantasy. Activity of the dream censor provided continual resistance to discharge of these impulses, with the result that the impulses had to be attached to more neutral or "innocent" images to be able to pass the scrutiny of censorship and be allowed into conscious expression. This displacement was made possible by selecting apparently trivial or insignificant images from residues of the individual's current psychological experience and linking these trivial images dynamically with latent unconscious images, presumably on the basis of some resemblance that allowed associative links to be established. In the process of facilitating economic expression of latent unconscious contents and, at the same time, maintaining the distortion that was essential for unconscious contents to escape the repressing action of the censor, the dream work used a variety of mechanisms, making it possible for more neutral images to represent repressed infantile components. These mechanisms included symbolism, displacement, condensation, projection, and secondary revision.

SYMBOLISM *Symbolism* is a complex process of indirect representation that in the psychoanalytic usage has the following connotations:

A *symbol* is representative of or substitute for some other idea from which it derives a secondary significance that it does not possess itself.

A symbol represents this primary element by reason of a common element that these ideas share.

A symbol is characteristically sensory and concrete in nature, as opposed to the idea it represents, which may be relatively abstract and complex. A symbol thus provides a more condensed expression of the idea represented.

Symbolic modes of thought are more primitive, both ontogenetically and phylogenetically, and represent forms of regression to earlier stages of mental development. Consequently, symbolic representations tend to function in more primary process or relatively regressed conditions: in the thinking of primitive peoples, in myths, in states of poetic inspiration, and, particularly, in dreaming.

A symbol is thus a manifest expression of an idea that is more or less hidden or secret. Typically, the use of the symbol and its meaning are unconscious. Thus, symbols tend to be used spontaneously, automatically, and unconsciously. The use of symbols is a sort of secret language in which instinctually determined content can be reexpressed as other images; for example, money can symbolize feces, or windows can symbolize the female genitals.

Many questions still persist about the origins of symbolic processes; the stage of development in which they become organized; the extent to which they require altered states of consciousness, such as the sleep state, for their implementation; and the degree to which symbolic expression is related to underlying conflicts. Current formulations regard the symbolic function as a uniquely human trait involved in all forms of human mental activity, from the most primitive expression of infantile wishes to the most complex creative processes of literary, artistic, religious, and scientific thinking.

DISPLACEMENT The mechanism of *displacement* refers to the transfer of amounts of energy (cathexis) from an original object to a substitute or symbolic representation of the object. Because the substitute object is relatively neutral—that is, less invested with affective energy—it is more acceptable to the dream censor and can pass the borders of repression more easily. Thus, whereas symbolism can be taken to refer to the substitution of one object for another, displacement facilitates distortion of unconscious wishes through transfer of affective energy from one object to another. Despite the transfer of cathectic energy, the aim of the unconscious impulse remains unchanged. For example, in a dream, the mother may be represented visually by an unknown female figure (at least one who has less emotional significance for the dreamer), but the naked content of the dream nonetheless continues to derive from the dreamer's unconscious instinctual impulses toward the mother.

CONDENSATION *Condensation* is the mechanism by which several unconscious wishes, impulses, or attitudes can be combined into a single image in the manifest dream content. Thus, in a child's nightmare, an attacking monster may come to represent not only the dreamer's father but may also represent some aspects of the mother and even some of the child's own primitive hostile impulses as well. The converse of condensation can also occur in the dream work, namely, an irradiation or diffusion of a single latent wish or impulse that is distributed through multiple representations in the manifest dream content. The combination of mechanisms of condensation and diffusion provides the dreamer with a highly flexible and economic device for facilitating, compressing, and diffusing or expanding the manifest dream content, which is derived from latent or unconscious wishes and impulses.

PROJECTION The process of *projection* allows dreamers to rid themselves of their own unacceptable wishes or impulses and experience them as emanating in the dream from other people or independent sources. Not surprisingly, the figures to whom these unacceptable impulses are ascribed in the dream often turn out to be those toward whom the subject's own unconscious impulses are directed. For example, the individual who has a strong repressed wish to be unfaithful to his wife may dream that his wife has been unfaithful to him; or a patient may dream that she has been sexually approached by her analyst, although she is reluctant to acknowledge her own repressed wishes toward the analyst. Similarly, the child who dreams of a destructive monster may be unable to acknowledge his or her own destructive impulses and the fear of the father's power to hurt the child. The figure of the monster consequently is a result of both projection and displacement.

SECONDARY REVISION The mechanisms of symbolism, displacement, condensation, and projection are all characteristic of relatively early modes of cognitive organization in a developmental sense. They reflect and express the operation of the primary process. In the organization of the manifest dream content, however, primary-process forms of organization are supplemented by a final process that organizes the absurd, illogical, and bizarre aspects of the dream thoughts into a more logical and coherent form. The distorting effects of symbolism, displacement, and condensation thus acquire a coherence and rationality that are necessary for acceptance on the part of the subject's more mature and reasonable ego through a process of secondary revision. Secondary revision thus uses intellectual processes that more closely resemble organized thought processes governing rational states of consciousness. It is through secondary revision, then, that the logical mental operations characteristic of the secondary process are introduced into and modify dream work.

AFFECTS IN THE DREAM WORK In the process of displacement, condensation, symbolism, or projection, as Freud hypothesized, the energic component of the instinctual impulses is separated from its representational component and follows an independent path of expression in the form of affects or emotions. The repressed emotion may not appear in the manifest dream content at all, or it may be experienced in a considerably altered form. Thus, for example, repressed hostility or hatred toward another individual may be modified into a feeling of annoyance or mild irritation in the manifest dream expression, or it may even be represented by an awareness of not being annoyed—that is, a conversion of the affect into its absence. The latent affect may possibly be directly transformed into an opposite in the manifest content, for example, as when a repressed longing might be represented by a manifest repugnance or vice versa. Thus, the vicissitudes of affect and the transformation by which latent affects are disguised introduce another dimension of distortion into the content of the manifest dream. The vicissitudes of affect, then, take place in addition to and in parallel with processes of indirect representation that characterize the vicissitudes of dream content.

Regression In the seventh theoretical chapter of *The Interpretation of Dreams*, Freud provided a model of the psychic apparatus as he understood it at the turn of the 20th century. Not only was the model a description of the functioning of the dreaming mind, but it also represented a broader conceptualization of the psychic apparatus as it functioned in both pathological and normal human experience, as he had formulated previously in the *Project*. It seems clear that the economic model, on which Freud had expended such intense effort in the 1890s and had seemingly abandoned in frustration, had come back to reassert itself, now in a new language and in a different setting. The lines of continuity and parallels between the model of the mind in the *Project* and the model of the seventh chapter could not be appreciated until the manuscript of the *Project* was rediscovered after Freud's death.

The model was an elaborate construction based on a basic notion of a stimulus–response mechanism. In normal waking experience, sensory input is taken into the receptor end of the apparatus and then processed in a number of mnemonic systems of increasing degrees of elaborateness and complexity. After varying degrees of processing, the impulse is subsequently discharged through the motor effector apparatus. In the dream state, motor effector pathways are blocked so that, instead of discharge through motor systems, excitation is forced to move in a backward or regressive direction through the mnemonic systems and back toward sensory systems.

During waking hours, the path leading from unconscious levels of the apparatus through preconscious to conscious levels is barred to the dream thoughts by activity of the censor. In sleep, however, this pathway is again made more available because resistance of the censor is diminished in sleep. Consequently, unconscious memories and their instinctual determinants could press to discharge through the perceptual apparatus, as is particularly the case in hallucinatory dream experiences. Thus, dreams could be described as having a regressive character. Consisting specifically of the turning back of an idea into the sensory image from which it was originally derived, regression is an effect of the resistance opposing discharge of psychic energy associated with the thought into consciousness along the normal path. Regression is also contributed to by simultaneous attraction exercised on the thought by the presence of associated memories in the unconscious.

In dreams, regression is further facilitated by diminution of the progressive current flowing from continuing sensory input during waking hours. Regression, as Freud viewed it, is essentially a regression to the originating source of an impression in the reversal he describes within the mental apparatus, but it also is a regression in time. Freud thus distinguished several forms of regression, namely, a topographical regression involving a regression in conscious to unconscious systems within the mental model; a temporal regression according to which the mental process refers back to older psychical structures, particularly those deriving from an infantile level of development; and formal regression, in which more primitive methods of expression and representation take the place of the more normal ones. "All these three kinds of regression," Freud commented, "are, however, one at bottom and occur together as a rule; for what is older in time is more primitive in form and in psychical topography lies nearer to the perceptual end."

Primary and Secondary Process Perhaps the most central aspect of the functioning of this mental model, closely related to the formulations of the *Project*, has to do with Freud's notions of the primary and secondary processes. To begin with, the impulses and instinctual wishes originating in infancy serve as the indispensable nodal force for dream formation. The energic conception of these drives follows the basic economic principles laid down by the *Project* (Table 6.1–1). They are elevated states of psychic tension in which the energy is constantly seeking discharge according to the constancy principle and the pleasure principle.

The tendency to discharge, however, is opposed by other psychic systems. Thus, Freud envisioned two fundamentally different kinds of psychic processes involved in the formation of dreams. One of these processes tends to produce a rational organization of dream thoughts, which was of no less validity in terms of contact with reality than normal thinking. However, another system—the first psychic system in Freud's schema—treats the dream thoughts in a bewildering and irrational manner. He believed that a more normal train of thought could only be submitted to abnormal psychic treatment if an unconscious wish, derived from infancy and in a state of repression, had been transferred to it. As a result of the operation of the pleasure principle, the first psychic system is incapable of bringing anything disagreeable into the context of the dream thoughts. It is unable to do anything but wish. Operating in conjunction with the demands of this primary system, the secondary system can only cathect an unconscious idea if it can inhibit any development of unpleasure that may have proceeded from the coming to awareness of that idea. Anything that may evade that inhibition is equivalently inaccessible to the second system, as well as to the first, because it is promptly eliminated in accordance with the unpleasure principle.

The psychic process derived from the operation of the first system is referred to as *primary process*. The process resulting from the inhibition imposed by the second system is referred to as the *secondary process*, and it reflects the operation of the system of inhibition and delay sketched in the *Project*. The secondary system thus corrects and regulates the primary system in accordance with principles of logic, rationality, and reality. Among the wishful impulses derived from infantile impulses, there are some whose fulfillment is a contradiction of the purposes and ideas of secondary process thinking. The fulfillment of these wishes can no longer generate an affect of pleasure but is unpleasurable. This formulation, it should be noted, forms the basis for Freud's later elaboration of the pleasure principle, as opposed to the reality principle. The secondary process organization of preconscious thinking is aimed at avoiding unpleasure, at delaying instinctual discharge, and at binding mental energy in accordance with the demands of external reality and the subject's moral principles or values. Thus, functioning of the secondary process is closely connected with the reality principle and is governed, for the most part, by the dictates of the reality principle.

TOPOGRAPHICAL THEORY

Beginning with abandonment of the seduction hypothesis, with the concomitant turning of Freud's interests to inner processes of fantasy and dream formation, and ending with publication of *The Ego and the Id* in 1923, in which Freud propounded his structural model of the psychic apparatus, Freud's thinking was cast largely in terms of the topographical theory.

Basic Assumptions There were a number of assumptions underlying Freud's thinking that served as lines of continuity between various stages of his investigations and helped him to organize his thinking in terms of successive models of the mental apparatus. The first assumption was that of "psychological determinism," according to which all psychological events, including behaviors, feelings, thoughts, and actions, are caused by—that is, are the end result of—a preceding sequence of causal events. This assumption derived from Freud's Helmholtzian convictions and represented application of a basic natural science principle to psychological understanding; but it was also reinforced by Freud's clinical observation that apparently meaningless hysterical symptoms, which had been previously attributed to somatic etiology, could be relieved by relating them to past, apparently repressed, experiences. Thus, apparently arbitrary pathological behavior could be tied to a causal psychological network.

The second assumption is that of "unconscious psychological processes." This assumption derived from a considerable amount of evidence gathered through the use of hypnosis, but it was also consolidated by Freud's experience of the free associating of his patients bringing past experiences to awareness. The unconscious material, which survived and was able to influence present experience, was found to be governed by specific regulatory principles, for example, the pleasure principle and the mechanisms of primary process that differed radically from those of conscious behavior and thought processes. Thus, the unconscious processes were brought within the realm of psychological understanding and explanation.

The third assumption was that "unconscious psychological conflicts" between and among psychic forces formed the basic elements at the root of psychoneurotic difficulties. This assumption related to Freud's experience of resistance and the drive to repression in his patients. The full realization of this aspect of psychic functioning came only with awareness that the reports of patients represented not memories of actual experiences but, rather, unconscious fantasies. The assumption of unconscious forces accounted for the process that created those fantasies and brought them into consciousness during free association. It also accounted for the agency that opposed the coming to consciousness of such fantasies. This counterforce that clashed with the sexual drives and diverted them into fantasies or symptoms was related to the function of censorship as developed in the dream theory and, later, to the operation of ego instincts that were set in opposition to the sexual instincts.

The final assumption of the topographical theory was that there existed "psychological energies" that originated in instinctual drives. This assumption was derived from the observation that recall of traumatic experiences and their accompanying affect resulted in disappearance of symptoms and anxiety. This suggested, therefore, that a displaceable and transformable quantity of energy was involved in the psychological processes responsible for symptom formation. Freud originally assumed that this quantity was equivalent to the affect, which became dammed up or strangulated when it was not appropriately expressed and, thus, was transformed into anxiety or conversion symptoms. After he had developed his notion of instinctual drives, this quantitative factor was conceived of as drive energy (cathexis). As noted previously in the discussion of the *Project*, the assumption of psychic energies served Freud as an important heuristic metaphor. The usefulness of the metaphor and its necessity as a basic assumption of analytical theory have been questioned and found wanting.

Topographical Model Freud's thinking about the mental apparatus at this time was based on the classification of mental operations and contents according to regions or systems in the mind. These systems were described neither in anatomical nor spatial terms but, rather, were specified according to their relationship to consciousness. The topographical model has essentially fallen into disfavor because of its limited usefulness as a working model of psychoanalytic processes largely because it has been surpassed and supplanted by the structural theory. The topographical viewpoint, however, is still useful for classifying mental events descriptively by quality and degree of awareness. There is a tendency currently to revive aspects of the topographical model of the mind in viewing mental processes as descriptively more or less conscious or unconscious, rather than as reflecting operation of a mental structure as in the systemic unconscious of classic metapsychology.

Consciousness The conscious system is that region of the mind in which perceptions coming from the outside world or from within the body or mind are brought into awareness. Internal perceptions can include introspective observations of thought processes or affective states of various kinds. Consciousness is, by and large, a subjective phenomenon, the content of which can only be communicated by language or behavior. It has also been regarded psychoanalytically as a sort of superordinate sense organ, which can be stimulated by perceptual data impinging on the CNS. It was assumed that the function of consciousness used a form of neutralized psychic energy called *attention cathexis*.

The nature of consciousness was described in less detail in Freud's early theories, and certain aspects of consciousness are not yet completely understood and are actively debated by psychoanalysts. Freud regarded the conscious system as operating in close association with the preconscious. Through attention, the subject can become conscious of perceptual stimuli from the outside world. From within the organism, however, only elements in the preconscious are allowed to enter consciousness. The rest of the mind lies outside awareness in the unconscious. Before 1923, however, Freud also believed that consciousness controlled motor activity and regulated the qualitative distribution of psychic energy.

Preconscious The preconscious system consists of those mental events, processes, and contents that are, for the most part, capable of reaching or being brought into conscious awareness by the act of focusing attention. The quality of preconscious organizations may range from reality-oriented thought sequences or problem-solving analysis with highly elaborated secondary process schemata all the way to more primitive fantasies, daydreams, or dream-like images, which reflect a more primary process organization. Thus, it stands over and against unconscious processes in which the transformation to consciousness is accomplished only with great difficulty and by dint of the expenditure of considerable energy in overcoming the barrier of repression.

The preconscious has been amplified by recent findings in neuroscientific study of memory. An essential distinction is between episodic memory and procedural memory. Episodic memory deals with past events in the individual's experience that are usually autobiographical or semantic in content. Other memories, however, have more to do with skills and habitual patterns of behavior, as, for example, riding a bike, driving a car, playing the piano, grammatical rules, social norms of politeness and etiquette, and so forth. These are aspects of normal daily living and behavior that people rarely, if ever, think about—people just do them, but the procedures are embedded in our memories and are readily applied without any effort to recall them. In fact, any effort to recall them more than likely only interferes with their usefulness. These memory systems, along with others that can be differentiated, are apparently served by different neural circuits and have different connections with consciousness and behavior.

Unconscious Unconscious mental events, namely, those not within conscious awareness, can be described from several viewpoints. One can think of the unconscious descriptively, that is, as referring to the sum total of all mental contents and processes at any given moment outside the range of conscious awareness, including the preconscious.

One can also think of the unconscious dynamically, that is, as referring to those mental contents and processes that are incapable of achieving consciousness because of the operation of a counterforce of censorship or repression. This repressive force or "countercathexis" manifests itself in psychoanalytic treatment as resistance to remembering. The unconscious mental contents in this dynamic sense consist of drive representations or wishes that are in some measure unacceptable, threatening, or abhorrent to the intellectual or ethical standpoint of the individual. This results in intrapsychic conflict between the repressed forces and the repressing forces of the mind. When repressive countercathexis weakens, this may result in formation of neurotic symptoms. The symptom is thus viewed as essentially a compromise between conflicting forces. These unconscious mental contents are also organized on the basis of infantile wishes or drives and strive for immediate discharge, regardless of the reality conditions. Consequently, the dynamic unconscious is believed to be regulated by the demands of primary process and the pleasure principle.

Finally, there is a systemic sense of the unconscious referring to a region or system within the organization of the mental apparatus that embraces the dynamic unconscious and within which memory traces are organized by primitive modes of association, as dictated by the primary process. This systemic view of the unconscious is considered, in a specifically topographical sense, as a component subsystem within the topographical model and in the structural theory is attributed to the id. Consequently, the systemic unconscious can be described in terms of the following characteristics in Freud's view:

Ordinarily, elements of the systemic unconscious are inaccessible to consciousness and can only become conscious through access to the preconscious, which excludes them by means of censorship or repression. Repressed ideas, consequently, may only reach consciousness when the censor is overpowered (as in psychoneurotic symptom formation), relaxes (as in dream states), or is fooled (in jokes).

The unconscious system is exclusively associated with primary process thinking. The primary process has as its principal aim facilitation of wish fulfillments and instinctual discharge. Consequently, it is intimately associated with—and functions in terms of—the pleasure principle. As such, it disregards logical connections, permits contradictions to coexist simultaneously, recognizes no negatives, has no conception of time, and represents wishes as fulfillments. The unconscious system also uses those primitive mental operations that Freud identified in the operation of the dream process. Moreover, the quality of motility, characteristic of primary process thinking and of unconscious energy, is also frequently linked to the capacity for creative thinking.

Memories in the unconscious have been divorced from their connection with verbal symbols. Freud discovered in the course of his clinical work that repression of a childhood memory could occur if the energy was withdrawn from it and, especially, if the verbal energy was removed. When the words are reconnected to the forgotten memory traits (as during psychoanalytic treatment), it becomes recathected and can thus reach consciousness once more.

The content of the unconscious is limited to wishes seeking fulfillment. These wishes provide the motive force for dreams and neurotic symptom formation. It has already been noted that this view may be oversimplified.

The unconscious is closely related to the instincts. At this level of theory development, the instincts are considered to consist of sexual and self-preservative (ego) drives. The unconscious is believed to contain mental representatives and derivatives, particularly of the sexual instincts.

Dynamics of Mental Functioning Freud conceived of the psychic apparatus, in the context of the topographical model, as a kind of reflex arc in which the various segments have a spatial relationship. The arc consists of a perceptual or sensory end through which impressions are received; an intermediate region, consisting of a storehouse of unconscious memories; and a motor end, closely associated with the preconscious, through which instinctual discharge can occur. In early childhood, perceptions are modified and stored in the form of memories.

According to this theory, in ordinary waking life, the mental energy associated with unconscious ideas seeks discharge through thought or motor activity, moving from the perceptual end to the motor end of the apparatus. Under certain conditions, such as external frustration or sleep, the direction in which energy travels along the arc is reversed, and it moves from the motor end to the perceptual end instead of the other way around. It thereby tends to reanimate earlier childhood impressions in their earlier perceptual forms and results in dreams during sleep or hallucinations in mental disorders. This reversal of the normal flow of energy in the psychic apparatus is the "topographical regression" discussed previously. Although Freud subsequently abandoned this model of the mind as a reflex arc, he retained the central concept of regression and applied it later in somewhat modified form in the theory of neurosis. The theory states that libidinal frustration results in reversion to earlier modes of instinctual discharge or levels of fixation, which had been previously determined by childhood frustrations or excessive erotic stimulations. Freud called this kind of reversion to instinctual levels of fixation *libidinal* or *instinctual regression*.

Framework of Psychoanalytic Theory: Repressed versus Repressing Throughout his long lifetime and in the course of many twistings and turnings of the theoretical developments in his thinking, Freud's mind was dominated by a tendency to describe many aspects of mental functioning in terms of contrasting polarities; some of the primary polarities are that of subject (ego) versus object (outer world), pleasure versus unpleasure, and activity versus passivity. The fundamental and dominant dualism is between the forces and contents of the mind viewed as repressed and unconscious and those forces and mental agencies responsible for the act of repressing. Although the persistence of such basic dualism in psychoanalytic thinking has clear advantages and undoubtedly helps one understand some fundamental aspects of the mind, one should not forget that such paradigms may prove to be overly restrictive. There is real question in the current state of psychoanalysis as to whether some of these assumed basic dimensions may not, in fact, be limiting the capacity of psychoanalytic theory to grow apace with the expanding horizons of both clinical experience and experimental, especially neuroscientific, exploration. The historical role and the present vitality of the basic psychoanalytic dualism, however, should not be undervalued because they provide a powerful tool for understanding and treating clinical pathology.

INSTINCTUAL THEORY

All human beings have similar instincts. The actual discharge of these instinctual impulses is organized, directed, regulated, or even repressed by functions of the individual ego, which mediates between the organism and the external world. Historically, Freud's exploration of instincts in psychoanalysis preceded his development of a structural theory and his concern with psychology of the ego.

Concepts of Instincts One of the first problems to be dealt with in considering the theory of instincts is what is meant by the term "instinct." The problem is made more complex by the variation in usage between a primarily biological meaning and Freud's primarily psychological concept. The difficulties are also compounded by the complexities in Freud's own use of the term. The term "instinct" was introduced primarily by students of animal behavior, referring generally to a pattern of species-specific behavior based mainly on potentialities determined by heredity and was therefore considered to be relatively independent of learning. The term was applied to a great variety of behavior patterns, including patterns described in such terms as a maternal instinct, a nesting instinct, or a migrational instinct. Such usage resisted successful physiological explanation and tended to introduce a strong teleological connotation, thus implying some sense of purposefulness, as in the concept of a self-preservation instinct. Freud adopted this usage unquestioningly, but its validity has been questioned even by strong proponents of instinctual theory among animal behaviorists, for whom the line between instinctual and learned behavior has become increasingly more complex and debatable. The dichotomy of nature/nurture can no longer be simplistically or rigidly maintained. Thus, instinctually derived patterns of behavior are seen to be increasingly modifiable in the interests of adaptation. Ethologists consequently prefer to speak simply of species-typical behavior patterns that are based on innate equipment but that mature and develop or are elicited through a certain degree of environmental interaction.

Freud, of course, took as the basis of his thinking the older concept of instinct, but in adopting it for his purposes, he transformed it. Actually, Freud's own formulation of the notion of instinct underwent contextual modification so that he actually offered a variety of definitions. Perhaps the most cogent was the following: "An 'instinct' appears to us as a concept on the frontier between the mental and the somatic, as the psychical representative of the stimuli originating from within the organism and reaching the mind, as a measure of the demand made upon the mind for work in consequence of its connection with the body." It is immediately evident that the basic ambiguity in the concept of instinct between biological and psychological aspects continued to influence Freud's thinking about instinctual drives and remains latent in subsequent psychoanalytic usage of the term. Freud himself varied in the emphasis he placed on one or another aspect of the concept so that subsequent discussions of the concept of instinct in psychoanalysis have varied similarly between emphasis on biological aspects and emphasis on psychological aspects.

Theory of the Instincts

When Freud began his investigation into the nature of unconscious drives, he strove consistently to base psychoanalytic theory on a firm biological foundation. One of the most important of his attempts to link psychological and biological phenomena came when he based his theory of motivation on instincts. Freud viewed instincts as a class of borderline concepts that functioned between the mental and organic spheres. Consequently, his use of the term "instinct" is not always consistent because it emphasizes either the psychic or biological aspect of the term in varying degrees in varying contexts. Sometimes, then, *libido* refers to the somatic process underlying the sexual instinct, and at other times, it refers to the psychological representation itself. Thus, Freud's usage is quite divergent from the Darwinian implications of the term "instinct," which imply innate, inherited, unlearned, and biologically adaptive behavior. The clearest formulation of the notion of instinct is as a concept of functions between the mental and the somatic realms as a psychic representative of stimuli, which come from the organism and exercise their influence on the mind. Thus, they are a measure of the demand made on the mind for work as a result of its connection with the body.

Characteristics of the Instincts

Freud ascribed to instinctual drives four principal characteristics: source, impetus, aim, and object. In general, the *source* of an instinct refers to the part of the body from which it arises, the biological substratum that gives rise to the organismic stimuli. The source, then, refers to a somatic process that gives rise to stimuli, which are represented in the mental life as drive representations or affects. In the case of libido, the *stimulus* refers to the process or factors that excite a specific erotogenic zone. The *impetus* or *pressure behind the drive* is a quantitative economic concept referring to the amount of force or energy or demand for work made by the instinctual stimulus. The *aim* is any action directed toward satisfaction or tension release. The aim in every instinct is satisfaction, which can only be obtained by reducing the state of stimulation at the source of the instinct. The *object* is the person or thing that is the target for this satisfaction-seeking action and that enables the instinct to gain satisfaction or discharge the tension and thus gain the instinctual aim of pleasure.

Freud commented that the object was the most variable characteristic of the instinct because it is only appropriate to the extent that its characteristics make satisfaction possible—a view that has been significantly revised in light of object relations. At times, the subject's own body may serve as an object of an instinct as, for example, in masturbatory activity. Although this early view of the instinctual object long held sway in psychoanalytic thinking, it has come under some serious criticism recently. Considerably more weight is put on the significance of the objects of libidinal attachment, particularly by object relations theorists. Increasingly, it has become apparent that the psychoanalytic concept of instincts is meaningless unless it includes and derives from a context of object relatedness. Moreover, it cannot be said simply that the objects of infantile drives are the most variable characteristic of the instinct because attachment to the primary objects, particularly the mothering object, is of the utmost significance developmentally.

CONCEPT OF LIBIDO The ambiguity in the term *instinctual drive* is reflected also in use of the term *libido*. Briefly, Freud regarded the sexual instinct as a psychophysiological process that had both mental and physiological manifestations. Essentially, he used the term *libido* to refer to "the force by which the sexual instinct is represented in the mind." Thus, in its accepted sense, *libido* refers specifically to the mental manifestations of the sexual instinct. Freud recognized early that the sexual instinct did not originate in a finished or final form, as represented by the stage of genital primacy. Rather, it underwent a complex process of development at each phase of which the libido had specific aims and objects that diverged in varying degrees from the simple aim of genital union. The libido theory thus came to include all of these manifestations and the complicated paths they followed in the course of psychosexual development.

INFANT SEXUALITY It had long been supposed, as one of the favored myths of analytical lore, that Freud's belief on infantile sexuality constituted an assault on the cherished ideas of 19th-century and Victorian thinking and that he was violently attacked for his views of the erotic life of young children. It seems, however, that his significant contribution, the 1905 *Three Essays on the Theory of Sexuality*, came to light not as a revolutionary work but as part of a flood of literature dealing with sexual problems.

Freud had become convinced of the relationship between sexual trauma, in both childhood traumata and the genesis of psychoneurosis, and disturbances of sexual functioning as related to the so-called actual neuroses—that is, hypochondriasis, neurasthenia, and anxiety neuroses. Freud originally viewed these conditions as related to misuse of sexual function. Thus, for example, he believed anxiety neurosis to be due to inadequate discharge of sexual products, leading to the damming up of libido that was then converted into anxiety. Also, he attributed neurasthenia to excessive masturbation and a diminution in available libidinal energy. In any case, these studies led Freud to an awareness of the importance of sexual factors in the etiology of psychoneurotic states.

PART INSTINCTS Freud described the erotic impulses arising from the pregenital zone as *component* or *part instincts*. Thus, kissing, stimulation of the area surrounding the anus, or even biting the love object in the course of lovemaking are examples of activities associated with these part instincts. The activity of component instincts or early genital excitement may undergo displacement, as, for example, to the eyes in looking and being looked at (scoptophilia), and may consequently be a source of pleasure. Ordinarily, these component instincts undergo repression or persist in a restricted fashion in sexual foreplay. More specifically, young children are characterized by a polymorphous perverse sexual disposition. Their total sexuality is relatively undifferentiated and encompasses all of the part instincts. In the normal course of development to adult genital maturity, however, these part instincts are presumed to become subordinate to the primacy of the genital region.

Aggression and Ego Instincts The aggressive drives hold a peculiar place in Freud's theory. His thinking about aggression underwent a gradual evolution. Early in his thinking, his attention had been preoccupied by the problems posed by libidinal drives. He was quite aware of the aggressive components often expressed in the operation of libidinal factors, but he could not long avoid taking explicit account of the more destructive aspects of instinctual functioning. Undoubtedly, also, the horrors and destructiveness of World War I made a significant impression on him so that he began to realize more profoundly the significance of destructive urges in human behavior.

By 1915, Freud arrived at a dualistic conception of the instincts as divided into sexual instincts and ego instincts. He recognized a sadistic component of the sexual instincts, but this still lacked a sound theoretical basis. Oral, anal, and phallic levels of development all had their sadistic components. Devoid of any manifest eroticism and covering a wide range from sexual perversions to impulses of cruelty and destructiveness, the sadistic aspects certainly had different aims from the more strictly libidinal.

Increasingly, Freud saw the sadistic component as independent of the libidinal and gradually segregated it from the libidinal drives. Moreover, impulses to control, tendencies toward the acquisition and exercise of power, and defensive trends toward attacking and destroying all manifested a strong element of aggressiveness. It seemed, then, that there was sadism associated with the ego instincts as well as with the libidinal instincts. Freud once again followed the dualistic bent of his mind and postulated two groups of instinctual impulses, two qualitatively different and independent sources of instinctual impulses with different aims and modalities. With the publication of *The Ego and the Id* in 1923, Freud gave aggression a separate status as an instinct with a separate source, which he postulated to be largely the skeletomuscular system, and a separate aim of its own, namely, destruction. Aggression was no longer a component instinct nor was it a characteristic of the ego instincts; it was an independently functioning instinctual system with aims of its own.

The elevation of aggression to the status of a separate instinct, on a par with sexual instincts, dealt a severe blow to any lingering romantic notions of the essentially or exclusively benign nature of man. Aggression and destructiveness were seen as inherent qualities of human nature such that aggressive impulses were elicited whenever an individual was sufficiently thwarted or abused. Freud's new formulation also drew attention to the specific role of aggression in forms of psychopathology as well as to understanding of the developmental processes through which aggression could be normally integrated and controlled.

It should be noted that aggression remains a problem for psychoanalytic thinking even today. Although a great deal has been learned about the operation and vicissitudes of aggression since Freud originally struggled with it, there is still a great deal that remains to be learned about its nature, its origins, and the conditions that produce and unleash it as well as the developmental factors that contribute to its pathological deviations and to its more constructive integration in the realm of human functioning. Some more recent revisions of aggression see it less in terms of destructive or sadistic aims but more broadly as a capacity for effective action in the face of obstacles or opposition-embracing capacities for mastery and self-assertion and as related to patterns of motivation rather than as a biologically determined drive force.

Life and Death Instincts When Freud introduced his final theory of life and death instincts in *Beyond the Pleasure Principle* in 1920, he took what can now be seen as an inevitable and logical next step in the evolution of the instinct theory he had been developing. It was nonetheless a highly speculative attempt to extrapolate the directions in which his instinct theory was taking shape to the broad realm of biological principles. One can recall that Freud's thinking about the instincts always casts its shadow in a dual modality. In the beginning, he had distinguished sexual and ego instincts. This distinction provided the basic dichotomy for the explanation of psychological conflict and the understanding of psychoneurosis.

The introduction of the life and death instincts must be seen in the course of this development and as extending the inherent duality of instinctual theory to the level of ultimate and final biological principle. Freud had not divorced his notion from the underlying economic principles derived from principles of entropy and constancy. The constancy principle was extended to the Nirvana principle, the objective of which was cessation of all stimuli or a state of total rest. It was only a small, subsequent step that led Freud from the formulation of a Nirvana principle to the death instinct, or Thanatos. Freud postulated that the death instinct was a tendency of all organisms and their component cells to return to a state of total quiescence—that is, to an inanimate state.

In opposition to this instinct, he set the life instinct, or Eros, referring to tendencies of organic particles to reunite and of parts to bind to one another to form greater unities, as in sexual reproduction. In Freud's view, the ultimate destiny of all biological matter, driven by the inexorable tendencies of all life to follow principles of entropy and constancy (with the exception of the germ plasm), was to return to an inanimate state. He believed that the dominant force in biological organisms had to be the death instinct. In this final formulation of life and death instincts, the instincts were considered to represent abstract biological principles, which transcended the operation of libidinal and aggressive drives. The life and death instincts represented the forces underlying sexual and aggressive instincts. Consequently, they represented a general trend in all biological organisms.

Needless to say, Freud's extravagant speculation has been subjected to severe criticism. It is impossible to argue that a general biological principle exists merely on the basis of clinical observation. If the inherent destructiveness of some states of psychopathology can permit the inference of destructive forces operating in the individual psyche, it by no means points to the existence of inherent and biologically determined forces of self-destructive potential. However one regards the argument as a biological speculation, for these thinkers, it has little relevance as a psychological speculation. On the contrary, the life and death instincts are alive and flourishing in Kleinian and French analytical circles. The school of analysts following the lead of Melanie Klein constitute the most significant group of psychoanalytic theorists who embrace the death instinct. Kleinian analysis bases a considerable portion of its understanding of intrapsychic processes on the operation of the life and death instincts. In Klein's work with severely disturbed children, she ascribed the manifestations of aggressive instincts in such children to the operation of the death instinct. This point of view seems to collapse the intervening steps in the organization of instinctual theory and makes almost any manifestation of destructive aggression a direct expression of the death instinct. Although contributions of Klein and her followers to the psychopathology of childhood disturbances are significant, other schools of analytical thinking have not followed their lead in this conceptualization of the primary instincts.

NARCISSISM AND THE DUAL INSTINCT THEORY

The concept of narcissism holds a pivotal position in the development of psychoanalytic theory. It was Freud's dawning realization of the importance of narcissism that led him to important modifications in his understanding of libido and his instinct theory. At the same time, Freud's examination of narcissism and its related clinical phenomena led to an increasing concern with the origins and functions of the ego. It must be said that the introduction of and focus on narcissism have had broad implications and reverberations in psychoanalytic thinking since Freud's day. The whole problem of narcissism remains difficult and problematic for psychoanalysis. The problem of pathological narcissism remains a focus of active interest, thinking, and clinical concern even today. The problem has special relevance with regard to certain forms of character pathology, which are relatively resistant to therapeutic intervention.

Freud observed that in cases of dementia praecox (schizophrenia), libido appeared to have been withdrawn from other people and objects and turned inward. He concluded that this detachment of libido from external objects might account for the loss of reality contact so typical of these patients. He speculated that the detached libido had then been reinvested and attached to the patient's own ego, resulting in megalomaniacal delusions and suggesting that this libidinal reinvestment found expression in their grandiosity and omnipotence.

Freud also became aware at the same time that narcissism was not limited to these psychotic manifestations. It might also occur in neurotic and, to a certain extent, even in "normal" individuals under certain conditions. He noted, for example, that in states of physical illness and hypochondriasis, libidinal cathexis was frequently withdrawn from outside objects and from external activities and interests. Similarly, he speculated that, in sleep, libido was withdrawn from outside objects and reinvested in the person's own body. Thus, he believed it could be that the hallucinatory intensity of the dream experience and the intensity of the emotional quality of the dream might result from the libidinal cathexis of fantasy representations of the people who composed the dream images. Freud also appealed to the basically narcissistic form of object choice in perversions, particularly homosexuality.

The introduction of narcissism into his theory played a significant role because it required that he reconcile his theory of libido with what now seemed to be a libidinal force operating within the ego. Freud originally thought of the reinvestment of libido as directed to the ego as such. This formulation has given rise to a considerable confusion in the understanding of narcissistic libido. A decisive reorganization of the concept of narcissism was provided by Heinz Hartmann when he pointed out that it was more accurate to regard narcissistic libido as attached not to the ego as such but to the self. The ego, as an intrapsychic construct, is opposed to the self as related to external objects extrapsychically. The proper opposition, then, between object libido and narcissistic libido is that the former is attached to object representations, whereas the latter is attached to self-representations. This important shift in the understanding of narcissism has opened an area of theoretical reconsideration that is still very much in flux and has introduced into psychoanalytic thinking the concept of self as an important, albeit as-yet-ill-defined, intrapsychic structural component.

Narcissism and the Choice of Love Object Reference was made earlier to the crucial role of early object relationships in later choice of love objects. Freud found that a deepened understanding of the vicissitudes of narcissism made it easier to understand the basis for choice of certain love objects in adult life. A love object might be chosen, as Freud put it, "according to the narcissistic type," that is, because the object resembles the subject's idealized self-image (or fantasized self-image). Possibly the choice of object might be an "anaclitic type," in which case the object might resemble someone who took care of the subject during the early years of life.

In summary, the concept of narcissism occupies a central and pivotal position in psychoanalytic theory. With the introduction of the concept of narcissism, it became obvious that the concept of the "individual" and the individual's "body" and "ego" could no longer be used interchangeably. It became clear that further understanding and advances in psychoanalytic theory depended on a clearer definition of the concept of self and its more adequate delineation from the concept of ego. Attempts to implement such understanding have brought into focus the ambiguities in the concept of the ego and have underscored the need for the systematic study of its development, structure, and functions. Attention to narcissistic phenomena has also enlarged the understanding of a variety of mental disorders as well as various normal psychological phenomena. These issues are discussed in relation to treatment issues.

STRUCTURAL THEORY AND EGO PSYCHOLOGY

The topographical theory was essentially a transitional model in the development of Freud's thinking and served an important function in providing a framework for development of his basic instinct theory. However, the problems inherent in the topographical theory underscore, once again, the need for a more systematic concept of psychic structure. The main deficiency of the topographical model lies in its inability to account for two extremely important characteristics of mental conflict.

The first important problem was that many of the defense mechanisms that Freud's patients used to avoid pain or unpleasure and that appeared in the form of unconscious resistances during psychoanalytic treatment were themselves not initially accessible to consciousness. He drew the obvious conclusion that the agency of repression, therefore, could not be identical with the preconscious because this region of the mind was, by definition, easily accessible to consciousness. The second problem was that he found that his patients frequently exhibited an unconscious need for punishment or an unconscious sense of guilt. According to the topographical model, however, the moral agency making this demand was allied with the antiinstinctual forces available to consciousness in the preconscious level of the mind.

From Topographical to Structural Perspective The germination of the shifting currents of Freud's thinking finally came to fruition in his abandoning the topographical model and replacing it with the structural model of the psychic apparatus in *The Ego and the Id*. The introduction of the structural hypothesis initiated a new era in psychoanalytic thinking. The structural model of the mind, or the "tripartite theory" as it is often called, is comprised of three distinct entities or organizations within the psychic apparatus—the id, the ego, and the superego.

The terms have become so familiar and the tendency to hypostasize them so great that it is well to bear in mind their nature as scientific constructs. The terms are theoretical constructs that have as their primary referents the specific groups of mental functions and operations that they are intended to organize and integrate into higher-order systems. Each refers to a particular aspect of mental functioning, and none of them expresses or represents the sum total of mental functioning at any one time. Although they are often spoken of as though they functioned as quasiindependent systems, they are, nonetheless, ultimately coordinated aspects of the operation of the mental apparatus representing mental actions of the person. Attribution of agency to any one of them is a form of misplaced concreteness because their actions and functions are basically those of the persons themselves. Moreover, unlike such phenomena as infantile sexuality or object relations, id, ego, and superego are not empirically demonstrable phenomena in themselves but must be inferred from the observable effects of the operations of specific psychic functions.

Historical Development of Ego Psychology The evolution of the concept of ego within the framework of the historical development of psychoanalytic theory parallels to a large extent the shifts in Freud's view of the instincts and can be divided into four phases. The first phase ended in 1897 and coincided with the development of the early psychoanalytic formulations. The second phase extended from 1897 to 1923, thus spanning the development of psychoanalysis proper. The third phase, from 1923 to 1937, saw development of Freud's theory of the ego and the gradual emergence to prominence of the ego in the overall context of the theory. Parallel to this development was the evolution of Freud's thinking about anxiety. Finally, the fourth phase, coming after Freud's death, saw the emergence and systematic development of a general psychology of the ego as well as a shifting of focus from the operation of ego functions themselves to the broader social and cultural contexts within which the ego developed and functioned.

First Phase: Early Concepts of the Ego In the initial phase, the ego was not always precisely defined. Rather, it referred to the dominant mass of conscious ideas and moral values that were distinct from impulses and wishes of the repressed unconscious. The ego was concerned primarily with defense, a term Freud soon replaced with the notion of repression, so that repression and defense were regarded as synonymous. In the neurophysiological jargon of the *Project*, the ego was described as "an organization . . . whose presence interferes with passages of quantity (of excitation)." Translating this into the language of psychology, the ego was regarded as an agent defending against certain ideas that were unacceptable to consciousness. These ideas were found to be primarily sexual in nature and were initially believed to have been engendered by premature sexual trauma and real seduction. Presumably, because memory of such trauma led to arousal of unpleasant and painful affects, they evoked a defensive response and repression of the original thought content. This repression, however, led to a damming up of energy and the consequent production of anxiety. Functioning of this "early ego" was contradictory to a degree because its primary purpose was to reduce tension and thus avoid unpleasant affects connected with sexual thoughts, but in the process of repression, it seemed to evoke an equally unpleasant affect state, that of anxiety.

Second Phase: Historical Roots of Ego Psychology During the years preceding publication of *The Ego and the Id,* analysis of the ego as such received little direct attention because Freud was concerned primarily with the instinctual drives—their representatives and transformations. Consequently, references to defense or defensive functions were much less frequent. The clarification of these concepts required further elucidation of the ego, its functions, and the nature of its organization. It was during this second phase that Freud grappled with these problems and gradually approached the more definitive resolution provided by the structural theory.

The ego's relationship to reality is particularly relevant in this connection. As noted earlier, the concept of a secondary process implies the ability to delay discharge of instinctual drives in accordance with demands of external reality. The capacity for delay was later to be ascribed to the ego. The progression from pleasure principle to reality principle in childhood involves a similar capacity to "postpone gratification" and thereby conform to the requirements of the outside world.

Finally, if neither the preconscious nor the ego instincts were solely responsible for repression or censorship, how was repression to be achieved? Freud tried to answer this question by postulating that ideas are maintained in the unconscious by a withdrawal of libido or energy (cathexis). In the manner characteristic of unconscious ideas, however, they constantly renew their attempt to become attached to libido and thus reach consciousness. Consequently, the withdrawal of libido must be constantly repeated. Freud described this process as "anticathexis" or "countercathexis." Again, however, if such countercathexis is to be consistently effective against unconscious ideas, it must be permanent and must itself operate on an unconscious basis. Understanding of psychic structure, specifically of the ego, which could perform this complicated function, was clearly called for and constituted still another indication of the need for the development of ego psychology. Thus, the way was pointed toward the third phase, wherein the ego was delineated as a structural entity and separated definitively from the instinctual drives.

Third Phase: Freud's Ego Psychology With publication of *The Ego and the Id*, the phase of introduction and development of Freud's own theory of the ego was accomplished. The ego was presented as a structural entity, a coherent organization of mental processes and functions, primarily organized around the perceptual-conscious system, but it also included structures responsible for resistance and unconscious defense. The ego at this stage was relatively passive and weak. Its functioning was still a result of pressures deriving from id, superego, and reality. The ego was the helpless rider on the id's horse, more or less obliged to go where the id wished to go. The assumption remained that the ego was not only dependent on forces of the id but was somehow genetically derived and differentiated out of the id. Freud had yet to recognize any real development of the ego comparable to the phases of libidinal development.

During this period, the view of the ego underwent radical transformation. Some of the details of this development took place in connection with Freud's theory of anxiety. In *Inhibitions, Symptoms, and Anxiety* in 1926, Freud repudiated the conception of ego as subservient to the id. Signal anxiety became an autonomous function for initiating defense, and the capacity of the ego to turn passively experienced anxiety into active anticipation was underlined. Here, too, the relatively rudimentary conception of the defensive capacity of the ego was enlarged to include a variety of defenses that the ego had at its disposal and could use in the control and direction of id impulses. Moreover, elaboration of Freud's conception of the reality principle introduced a function of adaptation that allowed the ego to curb instinctual drives when action prompted by them led to real danger.

The effect of this transformation of his theory of the ego was threefold. First, it brought the ego into prominence as a powerful regulatory force responsible for integration and control of behavioral responses. Second, the role of reality was brought to center stage in the theory of ego functioning. It had been banished to the wings in the preceding quarter century, but concern with the adaptive function of the ego again brought it back to prominence. Even so, the conception of adaptation here was rudimentary and limited to the ego's capacity to avoid danger. The notions that Freud was evolving during this phase provided the foundation for the later concept of the autonomy of the ego, as developed by later theorists. Finally, it was toward the end of this period that Freud finally made explicit the assumption of independently inherited roots of the ego that were quite independent of the inherited roots of the instinctual drives. This formulation was taken over by Hartmann and served as the basis for his notion of primary ego autonomy, which consequently stimulated the developments of the fourth phase.

Fourth Phase: Systematization of Ego Psychology If the third phase can be thought of as culminating in Anna Freud's work on the defense mechanisms of the ego, the fourth phase can be seen as taking its initiation from the publication of Hartmann's work on the ego and adaptation. Hartmann's work primarily focused on two aspects of Freud's later notions of the ego, namely, the autonomy of the ego and the problem of adaptation. Discussion of the apparatuses of primary autonomy was the basis for a doctrine of the genetic roots of the ego and a development of the notion of epigenetic maturation. Hartmann's treatment of adaptation also brought the adaptational point of view into focus in such a way that it has become generally acceptable as one of the basic metapsychological assumptions of psychoanalytic theory.

Although this development of thinking about the ego was an important advance, many psychoanalysts began to feel that it created an imbalance in the theory and that, by increasingly focusing on the mechanical and quantitative aspects of ego functioning, it left a picture of personality functioning and dysfunctioning that seemed relatively mechanistic and inhuman. Moreover, there developed a widening split between the id, the vital stratum of the mind and the dynamic source of psychic energies, and the noninstinctual, nondynamic structural apparatuses of the ego. Consequently, the id increasingly came to be seen as the source of instinctual energies—the image of the seething cauldron—without the representational or directional qualities that so long characterized Freud's views of the instincts and their functions.

The other extremely important aspect of the fourth phase is reemergence of the importance of reality in its broadest and most profound meanings as a significant dimension of psychoanalytic thinking. This is in many ways a direct extrapolation of Hartmann's thinking about adaptation because the adaptive functioning of the organism has directly to do with fitting in with the requirements of external reality and adaptively interacting with the environment, not only the inanimate but also the personal and social environment.

Structure of the Psychic Apparatus From a structural viewpoint, the psychic apparatus is divided into three groups of functions designated as id, ego, and superego and distinguished by their different functions. The id is the locus of the instinctual drives and is under domination of primary process. It operates according to dictates of the pleasure principle, without regard for the limiting demands of reality. The ego, however, represents a coherent organization of functions whose task is to avoid unpleasure or pain by opposing or regulating the discharge of instinctual drives to conform to demands of the external world. The regulation of id discharges is also contributed to by the third structural component of the psychic apparatus, the superego, which contains the internalized moral values, prohibitions, and standards of the parental imagoes.

Id Freud separated the instinctual drives in his tripartite theory into a separate compartment, the vital stratum of the mind, and in so doing reached the culminating point of the evolution of his theory of instincts. In contrast to his concept of the ego as an organized, problem-solving capacity, Freud conceived of the id as a completely unorganized, primordial reservoir of energy, derived from the instincts, and under the domination of primary process. It was not, however, synonymous with the unconscious because the structural viewpoint was unique in that it demonstrated that certain functions of the ego, specifically certain defenses against unconscious instinctual pressures, were unconscious; for the most part, the superego also operated on an unconscious level.

Ego The conscious and preconscious functions typically associated with the ego—for example, words, ideas, or logic—do not account entirely for its role in mental functioning. The discovery that certain phenomena that emerge most clearly in the psychoanalytic treatment setting, specifically repression and resistance, both associated with the ego, could themselves be unconscious pointed out the need for an expanded concept of the ego as an organization retaining original close relationship to consciousness and to external reality and yet performing a variety of unconscious operations in relationship to drives and their regulation. Once the scope of the ego had been thus broadened, consciousness was redefined as a mental quality that, although exclusive to the ego, constitutes only one of its qualities or functional aspects rather than a separate mental system itself, as in the topographical model.

No more comprehensive definition of the ego is available than the one Freud himself provided toward the end of his career in *Outline of Psychoanalysis*:

> *Here are the principal characteristics of the ego.* In consequence of the pre-established connection between sense and perception and muscular action, the ego has voluntary movement at its command. It has the task of self-preservation. As regards external events, it performs that task by becoming aware of stimuli, by storing up experiences about them (in the memory), by avoiding excessively strong stimuli (through flight), by dealing with moderate stimuli (through adaptation) and finally by learning to bring about expedient changes in the external world to its own advantage (through activity). As regards internal events, in relation to the id, it performs that task by gaining control over the demands of the instinct, by deciding whether they are to be allowed satisfaction, by postponing that satisfaction to times and circumstances favourable in the external world or by suppressing their excitations entirely. It is guided in its activity by consideration of the tension produced by stimuli, whether these tensions are present in it or introduced into it.

Thus, the ego controls the apparatuses of motility and perception, contact with reality, and, through mechanisms of defense, inhibition of primary instinctual drives.

ORIGINS OF THE EGO If the ego is defined as a coherent system of functions for mediating between instincts and the outside world, one must concede that the newly born infant has no ego or, at best, the most rudimentary of egos. Nonetheless, the neonate certainly has a rather complex array of intact capacities and both sensory and motor functions. There is, however, little coherent organization of these so that one must say that the ego is at best rudimentary. Developmental ego psychology is then faced with the problem of explaining the processes that permit modification of the id and the concomitant genesis of the ego.

Freud believed that the modification of the id occurs as a result of the impact of the external world on the drives. Pressures of external reality enable the ego to appropriate energies of the id to do its work. In the process of formation, the ego seeks to bring the influences of the external world to bear on the id, substitute the reality principle for the pleasure principle, and thereby contribute to its own further development. In summary, Freud emphasized the role of instincts in ego development and, particularly, the role of conflict. At first, this conflict is between the id and the outside world, but later, it is between the id and the ego itself.

DEVELOPMENT OF THE EGO The processes by which the internal world is built up and by which structure is consolidated within the self are referred to under the heading of *internalization*. Forms of internalization—incorporation, introjection, and identification—are variously connected with development of the ego.

Incorporation was originally conceived of as an instinctual activity derived from and based developmentally on the oral phase and was considered as a genetic precursor of identification. However, even though incorporation fantasies are often associated with internalizing processes, they are by no means identical and may be quite independent. Some authors envision incorporation as the mechanism of primary identification, aimed at a primary union between oneself and the maternal object. Incorporation as a mechanism of internalization seems to involve a primitive oral wish for union with an object. The union has a quality of totality and globalization so that in the internalization of the object, the object loses all distinction and function as object. The external object is completely assumed into the person's inner world. Incorporation is thus operative in infantile or relatively regressive conditions.

Introjection is perhaps the most central process in development of the structural apparatus involving ego and superego. Introjection was originally described by Freud in *Mourning and Melancholia* as a process of narcissistic identification in which the lost object is introjected and thus retained as a part of the internal structure of the psyche. Freud later applied this mechanism to the genesis of superego, making introjection the primary internalizing mechanism by which parental imagoes were internalized at the close of the oedipal phase. The child tried to retain gratifications derived from these object relationships, at least in fantasy, through the process of introjection. By this mechanism, qualities of the person who was the center of the gratifying relationship are internalized and reestablished as part of the organization of the self. Freud referred to this internalized product as a *precipitate of abandoned object cathexis*.

Identification has often been confused with introjection, partially because the two processes were treated in an overlapping and somewhat interchangeable fashion by Freud. There are, nonetheless, grounds for maintaining a distinction between them. *Identification* is, properly speaking, an active structuralizing process that takes place within the self by which the self constructs the inner constituents of regulatory control on the basis of selected elements derived from the model. What constitutes the model of identification can vary considerably and can include introjects, structural aspects of real objects, or even value components of group structures and group cultures. The process of identification is specifically an intrasystemic structuralizing activity attributed to the ego functions of the self, related to its synthetic function, and affecting structural integration in all parts of the psychic apparatus, including superego.

FUNCTIONS OF THE EGO The ego comprises an organization of functions that share in common the task of mediating between instincts and the outside world. Thus, the ego is a subsystem of the personality and is not synonymous with the self, the personality, or character. Any attempt to compile a complete list of ego functions has to be relatively arbitrary. Invariably, the list of basic ego functions suggested by various authors differs in varying degrees. This discussion is limited to several functions generally conceded to be fundamental to ego operation.

Control and Regulation of Instinctual Drives Development of the capacity to delay immediate discharge of urgent wishes and impulses is essential if the ego is to assure the integrity of the individual and fulfill its role as mediator between id and outside world. Development of the capacity to delay or postpone instinctual discharge, like the capacity to test reality, is closely related to the progression in early childhood from pleasure principle to reality principle.

Relation to Reality Freud always regarded the ego's capacity for maintaining relationship to the external world among its principal functions. The character of its relationship to the external world may be divided into three components: (1) the sense of reality, (2) reality testing, and (3) the adaptation to reality.

Sense of Reality The sense of reality originates simultaneously with the development of the ego. Infants first become aware of the reality of their own bodily sensations. Only gradually do they develop the capacity to distinguish a reality outside of their own bodies.

Reality Testing *Reality testing* refers to the ego's capacity for objective evaluation and judgment of the external world, which depends first on primary autonomous functions of the ego, such as memory and perception, but then also on the relative integrity of internal structures of secondary autonomy. Under conditions of internal stress, in which regressive pulls are effectively operating, introjective aspects of inner psychic structure can tend to dominate and, thus, become susceptible to projective distortions that color the individual's perception and interpretation of the outside world. Because of the fundamental importance of reality testing for "negotiating" with the outside world, its impairment may be associated with severe mental disorder.

Adaptation to Reality *Adaptation to reality* refers to the capacity of the ego to use the individual's resources to form adequate solutions based on previously tested judgments of reality. It is possible for the ego to develop not only good reality testing, with perception and grasp, but also to develop an adequate capacity to accommodate the individual's resources to the situation thus perceived. Adaptation is closely allied to the concept of mastery, both in respect to external tasks and to the instincts. It should be distinguished from adjustment, which may entail accommodation to reality at the expense of certain resources or potentialities of the individual. The function of adaptation to reality is closely related to the defensive functions of the ego. The mechanism that may serve defensive purposes from one point of view may simultaneously serve adaptive purposes when viewed from another perspective. Thus, in the obsessive-compulsive person, intellectualization may serve important inner needs to control drive impulses, but by the same token, from another perspective, the intellectual activity itself may serve highly adaptive functions in dealing with the complexities of external reality.

Object Relationships The capacity for mutually satisfying relationships is one of the fundamental functions to which the ego contributes, although self–other relationships are more properly a function of the whole person, the self, of which the ego is a functional component. Significance of object relationships and their disturbance—for normal psychological development and a variety of psychopathological states—were fully appreciated relatively late in the development of classic psychoanalysis. The evolution in the child's capacity for relationships with others, progressing from narcissism to social relationships within the family and then to relationships within the larger community, is related to this capacity. Development of object relationship may be disturbed by retarded development, regression, or conceivably by inherent genetic defects or limitations in the capacity to develop object relationships or impairments and deficiencies in early caretaking relationships. The development of object relationships is closely related to the concomitant evolution of drive components and the phase-appropriate defenses that accompany them.

Defensive Functions of the Ego As was pointed out previously, in his initial psychoanalytic formulations and for a long time thereafter, Freud considered repression to be virtually synonymous with defense. More specifically, repression was directed primarily against the impulses, drives, or drive representations and, particularly, against direct expression of the sexual instinct. Defense was thus mobilized to bring instinctual demands into conformity with demands of external reality. With development of the structural view of the mind, the function of defense was ascribed to the ego. Only after Freud had formulated his final theory of anxiety, however, was it possible to study the operation of the various defense mechanisms in light of their mobilization in response to danger signals.

Thus, a systematic and comprehensive study of ego defenses was only presented for the first time by Anna Freud. In her classic monograph *The Ego and the Mechanisms of Defense*, she maintained that everyone, whether normal or neurotic, uses a characteristic repertoire of defense mechanisms but to varying degrees. On the basis of her extensive clinical studies of children, she described their essential inability to tolerate excessive instinctual stimulation and discussed processes whereby the primacy of such drives at various developmental stages evoked anxiety in the ego. This anxiety, in turn, produced a variety of defenses. With regard to adults, her psychoanalytic investigations led her to conclude that, although resistance was an obstacle to progress in treatment to the extent that it impeded the emergence of unconscious material, it also constituted a useful source of information concerning the ego's defensive operations.

Genesis of Defense Mechanisms In the early stages of development, defenses emerge as a result of the ego's struggles to mediate pressures of the id and the requirements and strictures of outside reality. At each phase of libidinal development, associated drive components evoke characteristic ego defenses. Thus, for example, introjection, denial, and projection are defense mechanisms associated with oral-incorporative or oral-sadistic impulses, whereas reaction formations, such as shame and disgust, usually develop in relation to anal impulses and pleasures. Defense mechanisms from earlier phases of development persist side by side with those of later periods. When defenses associated with pregenital phases of development tend to predominate in adult life over more mature mechanisms, such as sublimation and repression, the personality retains an infantile cast.

Classification of Defenses The defenses used by the ego can be categorized according to a variety of classifications, none of which is all inclusive or takes into account all of the relevant factors. Defenses may be classified developmentally, for example, in terms of the libidinal phase in which they arise. Thus, denial, projection, and distortion are assigned to the oral stage of development and to the correlative narcissistic stage of object relationships. Certain defenses, however, such as magical thinking and regression, cannot be categorized in this way. Moreover, certain basic developmental processes, such as introjection and projection, may also serve defensive functions under certain specifiable conditions.

The defenses have also been classified on the basis of the particular form of psychopathology with which they are commonly associated. Thus, the obsessional defenses include isolation, rationalization, intellectualization, and denial; however, defensive operations are not limited to pathological conditions. Finally, the defenses have been classified as to whether they are simple mechanisms or complex, in which a single defense involves a combination or composite of simple mechanisms. Table 6.1–2 gives a brief classification and description of some of the basic defense mechanisms most frequently used and most thoroughly investigated by psychoanalysts.

Synthetic Function The *synthetic function* of the ego refers to the ego's capacity to integrate various aspects of its functioning. It involves the capacity of the ego to unite, organize, and bind together various drives, tendencies, and functions within the personality, enabling the individual to think, feel, and act in an organized and directed manner. Briefly, the synthetic function is concerned with the overall organization and functioning of the ego in the self-system and consequently must enlist the cooperation of other ego and nonego functions in its operation.

Although the synthetic function subserves adaptive functioning in the ego, it may also bring together various forces in a way that, although not completely adaptive, is an optimal solution for the individual in a particular state at a given moment or period of time. Thus, the formation of a symptom that represents a compromise of opposing tendencies, although unpleasant in some degree, is nonetheless preferable to yielding to a dangerous instinctual impulse or, conversely, trying to stifle the impulse completely. Hysterical conversion, for example, combines a forbidden wish and the punishment for it into a physical symptom. On examination, the symptom often turns out to be the only possible compromise under the circumstances.

Autonomy of the Ego Although Freud only referred to "primal, congenital ego variations" as early as 1937, this concept was greatly expanded and clarified by Hartmann. Hartmann advanced a basic formulation about development that the ego and id differentiate from a common matrix, the so-called undifferentiated phase, in which the ego's precursors are inborn apparatuses of primary autonomy. These apparatuses are rudimentary in nature, present at birth, and develop outside the area of conflict with the id. This area Hartmann referred to as a "conflict-free" area of ego functioning. He included perception, intuition, comprehension, thinking, language, certain phases of motor development, learning, and intelligence among the functions in this conflict-free sphere. Each of these func-

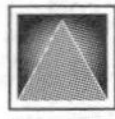

Table 6.1–2
Classification of Defense Mechanisms

	Narcissistic Defenses
Projection	Perceiving and reacting to unacceptable inner impulses and their derivatives as though they were outside the self. On a psychotic level, this takes the form of frank delusions about external reality, usually persecutory, and includes both perception of one's own feelings in another with subsequent acting on the perception (psychotic paranoid delusions). Impulses may derive from id or superego (hallucinated recriminations).
Denial	Psychotic denial of external reality, unlike repression, affects perception of external reality more than perception of internal reality. Seeing, but refusing to acknowledge what one sees, or hearing, and negating what is actually heard, are examples of denial and exemplify the close relationship of denial to sensory experience. Not all denial, however, is necessarily psychotic. Like projection, denial may function in the service of more neurotic or even adaptive objectives. Denial avoids becoming aware of some painful aspect of reality. At the psychotic level, the denied reality may be replaced by a fantasy or delusion.
Distortion	Grossly reshaping external reality to suit inner needs, including unrealistic megalomaniacal beliefs, hallucinations, wish-fulfilling delusions, and using sustained feelings of delusional superiority or entitlement.
	Immature Defenses
Acting out	The direct expression of an unconscious wish or impulse in action to avoid being conscious of the accompanying affect. The unconscious fantasy, involving objects, is lived out impulsively in behavior, thus gratifying the impulse more than the prohibition against it. On a chronic level, acting out involves giving in to impulses to avoid the tension that results from postponement of expression.
Blocking	An inhibition, usually temporary in nature, of affects especially, but possibly also of thinking and impulses. It is close to repression in its effects but has a component of tension arising from the inhibition of the impulse, affect, or thought.
Hypochondriasis	Transformation of reproach toward others arising from bereavement, loneliness, or unacceptable aggressive impulses into self-reproach and somatic complaints of pain, illness, and so forth. Real illness may also be overemphasized or exaggerated for its evasive and regressive possibilities. Thus, responsibility may be avoided, guilt may be circumvented, instinctual impulses may be warded off.
Introjection	In addition to the developmental functions of the process of introjection, it also serves specific defensive functions. The introjection of a loved object involves the internalization of characteristics of the object with the goal of closeness to and constant presence of the object. Anxiety consequent to separation or tension arising out of ambivalence toward the object is thus diminished. If the object is a lost object, introjection nullifies or negates the loss by taking on characteristics of the object, thus, in a sense, internally preserving the object. Even if the object is not lost, the internalization usually involves a shift of cathexis, reflecting a significant alteration in the object relationships. Introjection of a feared object serves to avoid anxiety through internalizing the aggressive characteristic of the object and thereby putting the aggression under one's own control. The aggression is no longer felt as coming from outside but is taken within and used defensively, thus turning the subject's weak, passive position into an active, strong one. The classic example is "identification with the aggressor." Introjection can also be out of a sense of guilt in which the self-punishing introject is attributable to the hostile, destructive component of an ambivalent tie to an object. Thus, the self-punitive qualities of the object are taken over and established within one's self as a symptom or character trait, which effectively represents both the destruction and the preservation of the object. This is also called *identification with the victim.*
Passive-aggressive behavior	Aggression toward an object expressed indirectly and ineffectively through passivity, masochism, and turning against the self.
Projection	Attributing one's own unacknowledged feelings to others; it includes severe prejudice, rejection of intimacy through suspiciousness, hypervigilance to external danger, and injustice collecting. Projection operates correlatively to introjection, such that the material of the projection is derived from the internalized configuration of the introjects. At higher levels of function, projection may take the form of misattributing or misinterpreting motives, attitudes, feelings, or intentions of others.
Regression	A return to a previous stage of development or functioning to avoid the anxieties or hostilities involved in later stages. A return to earlier points of fixation embodying modes of behavior previously given up. This is often the result of a disruption of equilibrium at a later phase of development. This reflects a basic tendency to achieve instinctual gratification or to escape instinctual tension by returning to earlier modes and levels of gratification when later and more differentiated modes fail.
Schizoid fantasy	The tendency to use fantasy and to indulge in autistic retreat for the purpose of conflict resolution and gratification.
Somatization	The defensive conversion of psychic derivatives into bodily symptoms; tendency to react with somatic rather than psychic manifestations. Infantile somatic responses are replaced by thought and affect during development (desomatization); regression to earlier somatic forms or response (resomatization) may result from unresolved conflicts and may play an important role in psychophysiological reactions.
	Neurotic Defenses
Controlling	The excessive attempt to manage or regulate events or objects in the environment in the interest of minimizing anxiety and solving internal conflicts.
Displacement	Involves a purposeful, unconscious shifting from one object to another in the interest of solving a conflict. Although the object is changed, the instinctual nature of the impulse and its aim remain unchanged.
Dissociation	A temporary but drastic modification of character or sense of personal identity to avoid emotional distress; it includes fugue states and hysterical conversion reactions.
Externalization	A general term, correlative to internalization, referring to the tendency to perceive in the external world and in external objects components of one's own personality, including instinctual impulses, conflicts, moods, attitudes, and styles of thinking. It is a more general term than projection, which is defined by its derivation from and correlation with specific introjects.
Inhibition	The unconsciously determined limitation or renunciation of specific ego functions, singly or in combination, to avoid anxiety arising out of conflict with instinctual impulses, superego, or environmental forces or figures.

(*continued*)

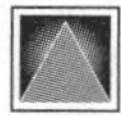

Table 6.1–2 (*continued*)

Intellectualization	The control of affects and impulses by way of thinking about them instead of experiencing them. It is a systematic excess of thinking, deprived of its affect, to defend against anxiety caused by unacceptable impulses.
Isolation	The intrapsychic splitting or separation of affect from content resulting in repression of either idea or affect or the displacement of affect to a different or substitute content.
Rationalization	A justification of attitudes, beliefs, or behavior that might otherwise be unacceptable by an incorrect application of justifying reasons or the invention of a convincing fallacy.
Reaction formation	The management of unacceptable impulses by permitting expression of the impulse in antithetical form. This is equivalently an expression of the impulse in the negative. Where instinctual conflict is persistent, reaction formation can become a character trait on a permanent basis, usually as an aspect of obsessional character.
Repression	Consists of the expelling and withholding from conscious awareness of an idea or feeling. It may operate either by excluding from awareness what was once experienced on a conscious level (secondary repression) or by curbing ideas and feelings before they have reached consciousness (primary repression). The "forgetting" of repression is unique in that it is often accompanied by highly symbolic behavior, which suggests that the repressed is not really forgotten. The important discrimination between repression and the more general concept of defense has been discussed.
Sexualization	The endowing of an object or function with sexual significance that it did not previously have, or possesses to a lesser degree, to ward off anxieties connected with prohibited impulses.
Mature Defenses	
Altruism	The vicarious but constructive and instinctually gratifying service to others. This must be distinguished from altruistic surrender, which involves a surrender of direct gratification or of instinctual needs in favor of fulfilling the needs of others to the detriment of the self, with vicarious satisfaction only being gained through introjection.
Anticipation	The realistic anticipation of or planning for future inner discomfort: implies overly concerned planning, worrying, and anticipation of dire and dreadful possible outcomes.
Asceticism	The elimination of directly pleasurable affects attributable to an experience. The moral element is implicit in setting values on specific pleasures. Asceticism is directed against all "base" pleasures perceived consciously, and gratification is derived from the renunciation.
Humor	The overt expression of feelings without personal discomfort or immobilization and without unpleasant effect on others. Humor allows one to bear, and yet focus on, what is too terrible to be borne, in contrast to wit, which always involves distraction or displacement away from the affective issue.
Sublimation	The gratification of an impulse whose goal is retained but whose aim or object is changed from a socially objectionable one to a socially valued one. Libidinal sublimation involves a desexualization of drive impulses and the placing of a value judgment that substitutes what is valued by the superego or society. Sublimation of aggressive impulses takes place through pleasurable games and sports. Unlike neurotic defenses, sublimation allows instincts to be channeled rather than dammed up or diverted. Thus, in sublimation, feelings are acknowledged, modified, and directed toward a relatively significant person or goal so that modest instinctual satisfaction results.
Suppression	The conscious or semiconscious decision to postpone attention to a conscious impulse or conflict.

Adapted from Vaillant GE. *Adaptation to Life.* Boston: Little, Brown; 1977; Semrad E. The operation of ego defenses in object loss. In: Moriarity DM, ed. *The Loss of Loved Ones.* Springfield, IL: Charles C. Thomas; 1967; and Bibring GL, Dwyer TF, Huntington DS, Valenstein AA: A study of the psychological principles in pregnancy and of the earliest mother-child relationship: Methodological considerations. *Psychoanal Stud Child.* 1961;16:25.

tions, however, might also become involved in conflict secondarily in the course of development. For example, if aggressive, competitive impulses intrude on the impulse to learn, they may evoke inhibitory defensive reactions on the part of the ego, thus interfering with the conflict-free operation of these functions.

Primary Autonomy With the introduction of the primary autonomous functions, Hartmann provided an independent genetic derivation for at least part of the ego, thus establishing it as an independent realm of psychic organization that was not totally dependent on and derived from the instincts. This was an insight of major importance because it laid the foundations for the emerging doctrine of ego autonomy and meant that the analysis of ego development would have to consider an entirely new set of variables quite separate from those involved in instinctual development.

Secondary Autonomy Hartmann observed that the conflict-free sphere derived from structures of primary autonomy can be enlarged and that further functions could be withdrawn from the domination of drive influences. This was Hartmann's concept of secondary autonomy. Thus, a mechanism that arose originally in the service of defense against instinctual drives may in time become an independent structure, such that the drive impulse merely triggers the automatized apparatus. Thus, the apparatus may come to serve other functions than the original defensive function, for example, adaptation or synthesis. Hartmann referred to this removal of specific mechanisms from drive influences as a process of change of function.

Superego The origins and functions of the superego are related to those of the ego, but they reflect different developmental vicissitudes. Briefly, the superego is the last of the structural components to develop, resulting in Freud's analysis from resolution of the oedipal complex. It is concerned with moral behavior based on unconscious behavioral patterns learned at early pregenital stages of development. Frequently, the superego participates in neurotic conflict by allying itself with the ego and thus imposing demands in the form of conscience or guilt feelings. Occasionally, however, the superego may be allied with the id against the ego. This happens in cases of severely regressed reaction, in which functions of the superego may become sexualized once more or may become permeated by aggression, taking on a quality of primitive (usually anal) destructiveness.

HISTORICAL DEVELOPMENT In a paper written in 1896, Freud described obsessional ideas as "*self-reproaches* which have re-emerged from *repression* and which always relate to some *sexual* act that was performed with pleasure in *childhood*." The activity of a self-criticizing agency was also implicit in Freud's early discussions of dreams, which postulated existence of a "censor" that did not permit unacceptable ideas to enter consciousness on moral grounds. He first discussed the concept of a special self-critical agency in 1914, suggesting that a hypothetical state of narcissistic perfection existed in early childhood; at this stage, the child was his or her own ideal. As the child grew up, admonitions of others and self-criticism combined to destroy this perfect image. To compensate for this lost narcissism or to recover it, the child "projects before him" a new ideal or ego-ideal. It was at this point that Freud suggested that the psychic apparatus might have still another structural component, a special agency whose task it was to watch over the ego, to make sure it was measuring up to the ego-ideal. The concept of the superego evolved from these formulations of an ego-ideal and a second monitoring agency to ensure its preservation.

Again in 1917, in *Mourning and Melancholia*, Freud spoke of "one part of the ego" that "judges it critically and, as it were, takes it as its object." He suggested that this agency, which is split off from the rest of the ego, was what is commonly called *conscience*. He further stated that this self-evaluating agency could act independently, could become "diseased" on its own account, and should be regarded as a major institution of the self. In 1921, Freud referred to this self-critical agency as the *ego-ideal* and held it responsible for the sense of guilt and for the self-reproaches typical in melancholia and depression. At that point, he had dropped his earlier distinction between the ego-ideal, or ideal self, and a self-critical agency, or conscience.

In 1923, however, in *The Ego and the Id*, Freud's concept of the superego again included both these functions—that is, the superego represented the ego-ideal as well as conscience. He also demonstrated that operations of the superego were mainly unconscious. Thus, patients who were dominated by a deep sense of guilt lacerated themselves far more harshly on an unconscious level than they did consciously. The fact that guilt engendered by the superego might be eased by suffering or punishment was apparent in the case of neurotics who demonstrated an unconscious need for punishment. In later works, Freud elaborated on the relationship between ego and superego. Guilt feelings were ascribed to tension between these two agencies, and the need for punishment was an expression of this tension.

ORIGINS OF THE SUPEREGO In Freud's view, the superego comes into being with resolution of the Oedipus complex. During the oedipal period, the little boy wishes to possess his mother, and the little girl wishes to possess her father. Each must, however, contend with a substantial rival, the parent of the same sex. The frustration of the child's positive oedipal wishes by this parent evokes intense hostility, which finds expression not only in overt antagonistic behavior but also in thoughts of killing the parent who stands in the way along with any brothers or sisters who may also compete for the love of the desired parent.

Quite understandably, this hostility on the part of the child is unacceptable to parents and, in fact, eventually becomes unacceptable to the child as well. In addition, the boy's sexual explorations and masturbatory activities may themselves meet with parental disfavor, which may even be underscored by real or implied threats of castration. These threats and, above all, the boy's observations that women and girls lack a penis convince him of the reality of castration. Consequently, he turns away from the oedipal situation and its emotional involvements and enters the latency period of psychosexual development. He renounces the sexual expressions of the infantile phase.

Girls, when they become aware of the fact that they lack a penis (in Freud's terms, they have "come off badly"), seek to redeem the loss by obtaining a penis or a baby from the father. Freud pointed out that, although the anxiety surrounding castration brings the Oedipus complex to an end in boys, in girls it is the major precipitating factor. Girls renounce their oedipal strivings, first, because they fear the loss of the mother's love and, second, because of their disappointment over the father's failure to gratify their wish. The latency phase, however, is not so well defined in girls as it is in boys, and their persistent interest in family relations is expressed in their play; throughout grade school, for example, girls "act out" the roles of wife and mother in games that boys scrupulously avoid. This was the basic outline of Freud's theory of the superego.

EVOLUTION OF THE SUPEREGO What, indeed, is the fate of the object attachments given up with resolution of the Oedipus complex? Freud's formulation of the mechanism of introjection came into play here. During the oral phase, the child is entirely dependent on the parents. Advancing beyond this stage, the child must abandon these earliest symbiotic ties with the parents and form initial introjections of them, which, however, follow the anaclitic model—that is, they are characterized by dependence on the parents. Thus, dissolution of the Oedipus complex and the concomitant abandonment of object ties led to rapid acceleration of the introjection process.

These introjections from both parents became united and formed a kind of precipitate within the self, which then confronted other contents of the psyche as the superego. This identification with the parents was based on the child's struggles to repress instinctual aims that were directed toward them, and it was this effort of renunciation that gave the superego its prohibiting character. It is for this reason, too, that the superego results, to such a great extent, from introjection of the parents' own superegos. Yet, because the superego evolved as a result of repression of instinctual desires, it had a closer relation to the id than did the ego itself. Its origins were more internal; the ego originated to a greater extent in relation to the external world and was its internal representative.

Finally, throughout the latency period and thereafter, the child (and later the adult) continues to build on these early identifications through contact with teachers, heroic figures, and admired people, who form the sources of the child's moral standards, values, and ultimate aspirations and ideals. The child moves into the latency period endowed with a superego that is, as Freud put it, "the heir to the Oedipus complex." Its structures at first might be compared to the imperative nature of demands of the id before it developed. The child's conflicts with the parents continue, of course, but now they are largely internal, between his or her own ego and superego. In other words, the standards, restrictions, commands, and punishments imposed previously by the parents from without are internalized in the child's superego, which now judges and guides behavior from within, even in the absence of the parents.

CURRENT INVESTIGATIONS OF THE SUPEREGO Exploration of the superego and its functions did not end with Freud, and such studies remain of current active interest. Recent interest has focused on the differentiating between superego and ego-ideal, a distinction that Freud periodically revived and abandoned. At present, the term *superego* refers primarily to a self-critical, prohibiting agency bearing a close relationship to aggression and aggressive identifications. The ego-ideal, however, is a kinder function, based on a transformation of the abandoned perfect state of narcissism, or self-love, which existed in early childhood and has been integrated with positive elements of identifications with the parents. In addition, the concept of an ideal object—that is, the idealized object choice—has been advanced as distinct from the ideal self. Many theorists regard the ego-ideal as an aspect of superego organization derived from good parental imagoes.

A second focus of recent interest has been the contribution of the drives and object attachments formed in the pre-oedipal period to the development of the superego. These pregenital (especially anal) precursors of the superego are generally believed to provide some of the very rigid, strict, and aggressive qualities of the superego. These qualities stem from projection of the child's own sadistic drives and primitive concept of justice based on retaliation, which is attributed to the parents during this period. The harsh emphasis on absolute cleanliness and propriety that is sometimes found in very rigid individuals and in obsessional neurotics is based to some extent on this sphincter morality of the anal period. One result of these developments is that the connections between oedipal dynamics and superego development have been significantly diluted in the sense that pre-oedipal superego precursors and pre-oedipal superego functions are better understood on one hand, and postoedipal adaptive integrations, especially with ego functions, on the other hand, have modified the understanding of superego functions.

PSYCHIC DEVELOPMENT—INTEGRATION OF PSYCHOSEXUAL PHASES AND OBJECT RELATIONS

As his clinical experience increased, Freud was able to reconstruct to a certain degree the early sexual experiences and fantasies of his patients. These data provided the framework for a developmental theory of childhood sexuality, which, in the subsequent course of psychoanalytic developmental exploration based on direct observation of childhood behavior, has been widely corroborated, accepted, and elaborated by developmental theorists. These views have been subjected to considerable revision and development, as well as criticism and rejection, in ensuing years. Perhaps an even more important source of information that contributed to Freud's thinking about infantile sexuality was his own self-analysis, begun in 1897. He was gradually able to recover memories of his own erotic longings in childhood and his conflicts in relationship to his parents, related specifically to his oedipal involvement. Realization of the operation of such infantile sexual longings in his own experience suggested to Freud that these phenomena might not be restricted only to the pathological development of neuroses, but that essentially normal individuals might undergo similar developmental experiences. The progressive integration of psychosexual developments and object relations has been further elaborated in Freud's phases of instinctual development, Margaret Mahler's separation-individuation process, and Erik Erikson's epigenetic sequence.

Phases of Psychosexual Development

The earliest manifestations of infantile sexuality arose in relation to bodily functions that were basically nonsexual, such as feeding and development of bowel and bladder control. Therefore, Freud divided these stages of psychosexual development into a succession of developmental phases, each of which was believed to build on and subsume accomplishments of the preceding phases—namely, the oral, anal, and phallic phases. The oral phase occupied the first 12 to 18 months of the infant's life; next, the anal phase, until approximately 3 years of age; and, finally, the phallic phase, from approximately 3 to 5 years of age.

Freud postulated that, in boys, phallic erotic activity was essentially a preliminary stage for adult genital activity. In contrast to the male, whose principal sexual organ remained the penis throughout the course of psychosexual development, the female had two leading erotogenic zones, the clitoris and the vagina. Freud believed that the clitoris was preeminent during the infantile genital period but that erotic primacy after puberty was transposed to the vagina. Recent sexual investigations have cast some doubt on a supposed transition from clitoral to vaginal primacy, but many analysts retain this view on the basis of their clinical experience. The question for the time being remains unresolved.

Freud's basic schema of the psychosexual stages was modified and refined by Karl Abraham, who further subdivided the phases of libido development, dividing the oral period into a sucking and biting phase and the anal phase into a destructive-expulsive (anal sadistic) and a mastering-retaining (anal erotic) phase. Finally, he hypothesized that the phallic period consisted of an earlier phase of partial genital love, which was designated as the true phallic phase, and a later, more mature genital phase. For each of the stages of psychosexual development, Freud delineated specific erotogenic zones that gave rise to erotic gratification. Table 6.1–3 provides an overview of current, more or less tentative, views on psychosexual development.

Development and Object Relations

Current theories in psychoanalytic psychiatry have focused increasingly on the importance for later psychopathology of early disturbances in object relationships—that is, a disturbance in the relationship between the child's affect and the significant objects in the environment, particularly the mothering object. From the very beginning of the child's development, Freud regarded the sexual instinct as "anaclitic" in the sense that the child's attachment to the feeding and mothering figure was based on the child's utter physiological dependence on the object. This view of the child's earliest attachment seems consistent with Freud's understanding of infantile libido developed on the basis of his insight, acquired early in his clinical experience, that sexual fantasies of even adult patients typically centered on early relationships with their parents. In any event, throughout his descriptions of libidinal phases of development, Freud made constant reference to the significance of children's relationships with crucial figures in their environment. Specifically, he postulated that the choice of a love object in adult life, the love relationship itself, and object relationships in other spheres of interest and activity depend largely on the nature and quality of the child's object relationships during the earliest years of life.

Object Relations during Pregenital Phases

At birth, the infant's responses to external stimulation are relatively diffuse and disorganized. Even so, as recent experimental research on neonates has indicated, the infant is quite responsive to external stimulation, and the patterns of response are quite complex and relatively organized, even shortly after birth. Even neonates of a few hours of age respond selectively to novel stimuli and demonstrate remarkable preferences for complex, as compared with simple, patterns of stimulation. The infant's responses to noxious and pleasurable stimuli are also relatively undifferentiated. Even so, sensations of hunger, cold, and pain give rise to tension and a corresponding need to seek relief from painful stimuli. At the beginning of life, however, the infant does not respond specifically to objects as objects. A certain degree of development of perceptual and cognitive apparatuses is required, as well as a greater degree of differentiation of sensory

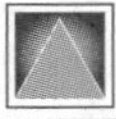

Table 6.1–3
Stages of Psychosexual Development

	Oral Stage
Definition	Earliest stage of development in which the infant's needs, perceptions, and modes of expression are primarily centered in mouth, lips, tongue, and other organs related to the oral zone.
Description	Oral zone maintains dominance in psychic organization through approximately the first 18 mos of life. Oral sensations include thirst, hunger, pleasurable tactile stimulations evoked by the nipple or its substitute, and sensations related to swallowing and satiation. Oral drives consist of two components: libidinal and aggressive. States of oral tension lead to seeking for oral gratification, as in quiescence at end of nursing. Oral triad consists of wish to eat, sleep, and reach that relaxation that occurs at the end of sucking just before onset of sleep. Libidinal needs (oral erotism) predominate in early oral phase, whereas they are mixed with more aggressive components later (oral sadism). Oral aggression expressed in biting, chewing, spitting, or crying. Oral aggression connected with primitive wishes and fantasies of biting, devouring, and destroying.
Objectives	Establish a trusting dependence on nursing and sustaining objects, establish comfortable expression and gratification of oral libidinal needs without excessive conflict or ambivalence from oral sadistic wishes.
Pathological traits	Excessive oral gratifications or deprivation can result in libidinal fixations contributing to pathological traits. Such traits can include excessive optimism, narcissism, pessimism (as in depressive states), or demandingness. Envy and jealousy often associated with oral traits.
Character traits	Successful resolution of oral phase results in capacities to give to and receive from others without excessive dependence or envy, capacity to rely on others with a sense of trust as well as with a sense of self-reliance and self-trust. Oral characters are often excessively dependent and require others to give to them and look after them and are often extremely dependent on others for maintaining self-esteem.
	Anal Stage
Definition	Stage of psychosexual development prompted by maturation of neuromuscular control over sphincters, particularly anal sphincters, permitting more voluntary control over retention or expulsion of feces.
Description	Period extends roughly from 1–3 yrs of age, marked by recognizable intensification of aggressive drives mixed with libidinal components in sadistic impulses. Acquisition of voluntary sphincter control associated with increasing shift from passivity to activity. Conflicts over anal control and struggles with parents over retaining or expelling feces in toilet training give rise to increased ambivalence together with struggle over separation, individuation, and independence. *Anal erotism* refers to sexual pleasure in anal functioning, both in retaining precious feces and presenting them as a precious gift to the parent. *Anal sadism* refers to expression of aggressive wishes connected with discharging feces as powerful and destructive weapons. These wishes often displayed in fantasies of bombing or explosions.
Objectives	Anal period is marked by striving for independence and separation from dependence on and control of parents. Objectives of sphincter control without overcontrol (fecal retention) or loss of control (messing) are matched by attempts to achieve autonomy and independence without excessive shame or self-doubt from loss of control.
Pathological traits	Maladaptive character traits, often apparently inconsistent, derive from anal erotism and defenses against it. Orderliness, obstinacy, stubbornness, willfulness, frugality, and parsimony are features of anal character. When defenses against anal traits are less effective, anal character reveals traits of heightened ambivalence, lack of tidiness, messiness, defiance, rage, and sadomasochistic tendencies. Anal characteristics and defenses are typically seen in obsessive-compulsive neuroses.
Character traits	Successful resolution of anal phase provides basis for development of personal autonomy, a capacity for independence and personal initiative without guilt, a capacity for self-determining behavior without a sense of shame or self-doubt, a lack of ambivalence and a capacity for willing cooperation without either excessive willfulness or self-diminution or defeat.
	Urethral Stage
Definition	This stage not explicitly treated by Sigmund Freud but serves as transitional stage between anal and phallic stages. It shares some characteristics of anal phase and some from subsequent phallic phase.
Description	Characteristics of the urethral phase often subsumed under phallic phase. *Urethral erotism*, however, refers to pleasure in urination as well as pleasure in urethral retention analogous to anal retention. Similar issues of performance and control are related to urethral functioning. Urethral functioning may also have sadistic quality, often reflecting persistence of anal sadistic urges. Loss of urethral control, as in enuresis, may frequently have regressive significance that reactivates anal conflicts.
Objectives	Issues of control and urethral performance and loss of control. Not clear whether or to what extent objectives of urethral functioning differ from those of anal period.
Pathological traits	Predominant urethral trait is competitiveness and ambition, probably related to compensation for shame due to loss of urethral control. This may be start for development of penis envy, related to feminine sense of shame and inadequacy in being unable to match male urethral performance. Also related to issues of control and shaming.
Character traits	Besides healthy effects analogous to those from anal period, urethral competence provides sense of pride and self-competence based on performance. Urethral performance is area in which small boy can imitate and try to match his father's more adult performance. Resolution of urethral conflicts sets stage for budding gender identity and subsequent identifications.
	Phallic Stage
Definition	Phallic stage begins sometime during 3rd yr and continues until approximately end of 5th yr.
Description	Phallic phase characterized by primary focus of sexual interests, stimulation, and excitement in genital area. Penis becomes organ of principal interest to children of both sexes, with lack of penis in females being considered as evidence of castration. Phallic phase associated with increase in genital masturbation accompanied by predominantly unconscious fantasies of sexual involvement with opposite-sex parent. Threat of castration and related anxiety connected with guilt over masturbation and oedipal wishes. During this phase, oedipal involvement and conflict are established and consolidated.

(*continued*)

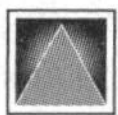

Table 6.1–3 (*continued*)

Objectives	To focus erotic interest in genital area and genital functions. This lays foundation for gender identity and serves to integrate residues of previous stages into predominantly genital-sexual orientation. Establishing oedipal situation essential for furtherance of subsequent identifications serving as basis for important and enduring dimensions of character organization.
Pathological traits	Derivation of pathological traits from phallic-oedipal involvement are sufficiently complex and subject to such a variety of modifications so that it encompasses nearly the whole of neurotic development. Issues, however, focus on castration in males and penis envy in females. Patterns of identification developed from resolution of oedipal complex provide another important focus of developmental distortions. Influence of castration anxiety and penis envy, defenses against them, and patterns of identification are primary determinants of the development of human character. They also subsume and integrate residues of previous psychosexual stages so that fixations or conflicts deriving from preceding stages can contaminate and modify oedipal resolution.
Character traits	Phallic stage provides foundations for emerging sense of sexual identity, of a sense of curiosity without embarrassment, of initiative without guilt, as well as a sense of mastery not only over objects and people in environment but also over internal processes and impulses. Resolution of the oedipal conflict gives rise to internal structural capacities for regulation of drive impulses and their direction to constructive ends. This internal source of regulation is the superego, based on identifications derived primarily from parental figures.
	Latency Stage
Definition	Stage of instinctual relative quiescence or inactivity of sexual drive during period from resolution of the Oedipus complex until pubescence (from approximately 5–6 yrs of age until approximately 11–13 yrs of age).
Description	Institution of superego at close of oedipal period and further maturation of ego functions allow for considerably greater degree of control of instinctual impulses. Sexual interests generally believed to be quiescent. Period of primarily homosexual affiliations for both boys and girls as well as a sublimation of libidinal and aggressive energies into energetic learning and play activities, exploring environment, and becoming more proficient in dealing with world of things and people around them. Period for development of important skills. Relative strength of regulatory elements often gives rise to patterns of behavior that are somewhat obsessive and hypercontrolling.
Objectives	Primary objective is further integration of oedipal identifications and consolidation of sex-role identity and sex roles. Relative quiescence and control of instinctual impulses allow for development of ego apparatuses and mastery of skills. Further identificatory components may be added to the oedipal ones on basis of broadening contacts with other significant figures outside family (e.g., teachers, coaches, and other adult figures).
Pathological traits	Danger in latency period can arise either from lack of development of inner controls or excess of them. Lack of control can lead to inability to sufficiently sublimate energies in interest of learning and development of skills; excess of inner control, however, can lead to premature closure of personality development and precocious elaboration of obsessive character traits.
Character traits	Latency period frequently regarded as period of relatively unimportant inactivity in the developmental schema. More recently, greater respect has been gained for developmental processes in this period. Important consolidations and additions are made to basic post-oedipal identifications and to processes of integrating and consolidating previous attainments in psychosexual development and establishing decisive patterns of adaptive functioning. The child can develop a sense of industry and capacity for mastery of objects and concepts that allows autonomous function and a sense of initiative without risk of failure or defeat or a sense of inferiority. These are all important attainments that need to be further integrated, ultimately as the essential basis for a mature adult life of satisfaction in work and love.
	Genital Stage
Definition	Genital or adolescent phase extends from onset of puberty from 11–13 yrs of age until young adulthood. Current thinking tends to subdivide this stage into preadolescent, early adolescent, middle adolescent, late adolescent, and even postadolescent periods.
Description	Physiological maturation of systems of genital (sexual) functioning and attendant hormonal systems leads to intensification of drives, particularly libidinal drives. This produces a regression in personality organization, which reopens conflicts of previous stages of psychosexual development and provides opportunity for reresolution of these conflicts in context of achieving a mature sexual and adult identity. Often referred to as a *second individuation*.
Objectives	Primary objectives are ultimate separation from dependence on and attachment to parents and establishment of mature, nonincestuous, heterosexual object relations. Related are achievement of mature sense of personal identity and acceptance and integration of adult roles and functions that permit new adaptive integrations with social expectations and cultural values.
Pathological traits	Pathological deviations due to inability to achieve successful resolution of this stage of development are multiple and complex. Defects can arise from whole spectrum of psychosexual residues because developmental task of adolescence is in a sense a partial reopening and reworking and reintegrating of all of these aspects of development. Previous unsuccessful resolutions and fixations in various phases or aspects of psychosexual development produce pathological defects in the emerging adult personality.
Character traits	Successful resolution and reintegration of previous psychosexual stages in adolescent genital phase set stage normally for fully mature personality with capacity for full and satisfying genital potency and a self-integrated and consistent sense of identity. This provides basis for capacity for self-realization and meaningful participation in areas of work, love, and in creative and productive application to satisfying and meaningful goals and values.

impressions and integration of cognitive patterns, before babies are able to differentiate between impressions belonging to themselves and those derived from external objects. Consequently, observations and inferences based on data derived from the first 6 months of life must be interpreted in the context of the child's cognitive functioning before self–object differentiation.

In these first months of life, human infants are considerably more helpless than any other young mammals. Their helplessness continues for a longer period than in any other species. They cannot survive unless they are cared for, and they cannot achieve relief from the painful disequilibrium of inner physiological states without help of external caretaking objects. Object relationships of the most primitive kind only begin to be established when an infant first begins to grasp this fact of experience. In the beginning, an infant cannot distinguish between its own lips and its mother's breasts, nor does an infant initially associate satiation of painful hunger pangs with presentation of the extrinsic breast. Because the infant is aware only of its own inner tension and relaxation and is unaware of the external object, longing for the object exists only to the degree that the disturbing stimuli persist, and longing for satiation remains unsatisfied in the absence of the object. When the satisfying object finally appears, and the infant's needs are gratified, longing also disappears. Gradually, but also rather quickly, the infant becomes aware of the mother herself, in addition to her breast, as a need-satisfying object.

ORAL PHASE AND OBJECTS This experience of unsatisfied need, together with the experience of frustration in the absence of the breast and need-satisfying release of tension in the presence of the breast, forms the basis of the infant's first awareness of external objects. This first awareness of an object, then, in the psychological sense, comes from longing for something that is already familiar and for something that actually gratified needs in the past but is not immediately available in the present. Thus, it is basically the infant's hunger in this view that in the beginning compels recognition of the outside world. The first primitive reflex reaction to objects, putting them into the mouth, then becomes understandable. This reaction is consistent with the modality of the infant's first recognition of reality, judging reality by oral gratification, that is, whether something will provide relaxation of inner tension and satisfaction (and should thereby be incorporated, swallowed) or whether it will create inner tension and dissatisfaction (and consequently should be spit out).

Early in this interaction, the mother serves an important function, that of empathically responding to the infant's inner needs in such a manner as to become involved in a process of mutual regulation, which maintains the homeostatic balance of the infant's physiological needs and processes within tolerable limits. Not only does this process keep the child alive, but it sets a rudimentary pattern of experience within which the child can build elements of a basic trust that promote reliance on the benevolence and availability of caretaking objects. Consequently, the mother's administrations and responsiveness to the child help to lay the most rudimentary and essential foundation for subsequent development of object relations and the capacity for entering the community of human beings.

As differentiation between the limits of self and object is gradually established in the child's experience, the mother becomes acknowledged and recognized as the source of gratifying nourishment and, in addition, as source of the erotogenic pleasure the infant derives from sucking on the breast. In this sense, she becomes the first love object. The quality of the child's attachment to this primary object is of the utmost importance, as developmental and attachment theorists have demonstrated. From the oral phase onward, the whole progression in psychosexual development, with its focus on successive erotogenic zones and emergence of associated component instincts, reflects the quality of the child's attachment to the crucial figures in the environment as well as the strength of feelings of love or hate, or both, toward these important people. If a fundamentally warm, trusting, secure, and affectionate relationship has been established between mother and child during the earliest stages of the child's career, then at least theoretically, the stage is set for development of trusting and affectionate relationships with other human objects during the course of life.

ANAL PHASE AND OBJECTS During the oral stage of development, the infant's role is not altogether passive because, caught up as it is in a process of mutual interaction, the infant makes its own contribution to eliciting certain responses from the mother. The activity, however, is more or less automatic and dependent on such physiological factors as level of activity, irritability, or responsiveness to stimuli. Generally speaking, however, the infant's control over the mother's feeding responses is relatively limited. Consequently, the primary onus remains on the mother to gratify or frustrate the demands of the infant.

In the transition to the anal period, however, this picture changes significantly. The child acquires a greater degree of control over behavior and particularly over sphincter function. Moreover, for the first time during this period, demands are placed on the child to relinquish some aspect of freedom by reason of expectations to accede to parental demands to use the toilet for evacuation of feces and urine. However, the primary aim of anal eroticism is enjoyment of the pleasurable sensations of excretion. Somewhat later, stimulation of the anal mucosa through retention of the fecal mass may become a source of even more intense pleasure. Nonetheless, at this stage of development, the demand is placed on the child to regulate gratification, to surrender some portion of the gratification at the parent's wish, or to delay gratification according to a schedule established by the parent's wishes. It can be readily seen that one of the important aspects of the anal period, therefore, is that it sets the stage for a contest of wills over when, how, and on what terms the child achieves gratification.

PHALLIC PHASE AND OBJECTS The passage from anal to phallic phase marks not only the transition from pre-oedipal to beginnings of the oedipal level of development but also marks completion of the work of separation individuation and, in the normal course of development, achievement of object constancy. The oedipal situation evolves during the period extending from the third to the fifth year in children of both sexes.

Oedipus Complex In the normal course of development, the so-called pregenital phases are regarded as primarily autoerotic. Primary gratification derives from stimulation of erotogenic zones, whereas the object serves a significant, although secondary and instrumental, role. A fundamental shift begins to take place in the phallic phase in which the phallus becomes the primary erotogenous zone for both sexes, thus laying a foundation for and initiating a shift of libidinal motivation and intention in the direction of objects. The phallic phase sets the stage for the fundamental task of finding a love object, a dynamic that moves to another level of progression in establishing love relations of the oedipal period and beyond to more mature adult object choices and love relationships. The phallic period is also a critical phase of development for the budding formation of the child's own sense of gender identity—as decisively male or female—based on the child's discovery and realization of the significance of anatomical sexual differences. The events associated with the phallic phase also set the stage for the developmental predisposition to later psychoneuroses. Freud used the term *Oedipus complex* to refer to the intense love relationships, together with their associated rivalries, hostilities, and emerging identifications, formed during this period between the child and parents.

Castration Complex There is some differentiation between the sexes in the pattern of development. Freud explained the nature of this discrepancy in terms of genital differences. Under normal circumstances, he believed that, for boys, the oedipal situation was resolved by the castration complex. Specifically, the boy had to give up his strivings for his mother because of the threat of castration—castration anxiety. In contrast, the Oedipus complex in girls was also evoked by reason of the castration complex, but unlike the boy, the little girl was already castrated, and as a result, she turned to her father as bearer of the penis out of a sense of disappointment over her own lack of a penis. The little girl was thus more threatened by a loss of love than by actual castration fears.

The Boy's Situation

In boys, development of object relations is relatively less complex than for girls because the boy remains attached to his first love object, the mother. The primitive object choice of the primary love object, which develops in response to the mother's gratification of the infant's basic needs, takes the same direction as the pattern of object choice in response to opposite-sex objects in later life experience. In the phallic period, in addition to the child's attachment to and interest in the mother as a source of nourishment, he develops a strong erotic interest in her and a concomitant desire to possess her exclusively and sexually. These feelings usually become manifest at approximately 3 years of age and reach a climax at 4 or 5 years of age.

With appearance of the oedipal involvement, the boy begins to show his loving attachment to his mother almost as a little lover might—wanting to touch her, trying to get in bed with her, proposing marriage, expressing wishes to replace his father, and devising opportunities to see her naked or undressed. Competition from siblings for mother's affection and attention is intolerable. Above all, however, the little lover wants to eliminate his arch rival—mother's husband. His wishes may involve not merely displacing or superseding father in mother's affection but eliminating him altogether. The child understandably anticipates retaliation for his aggressive wishes toward his father, and these expectations in turn give rise to a severe anxiety in the form of the "castration complex."

This somewhat simplified picture of the resolution of the Oedipus complex is considerably more complex in the actual course of development. Usually, the boy's love for his mother remains a dominant force during the period of infantile sexual development. It is known, however, that love is not free of some admixture of hostility and that the child's relationship with both parents is to some degree ambivalent. The boy also loves his father, and at times when he has been frustrated by his mother, he may hate her and turn from her to seek affection from his father. Undoubtedly, to some degree, he loves and hates both his parents at the same time. In addition, Freud's postulation of an essentially bisexual basis of the nature of the libido complicates matters further. On the one hand, the boy wants to possess his mother and kill the hated father rival. On the other hand, he also loves his father and seeks approval and affection from him, whereas he often reacts to his mother with hostility, particularly when her demands on her husband interfere with the exclusiveness of the father–son relationship. The *negative Oedipus complex* refers to those situations in which the boy's love for his father predominates over the love for the mother, and the mother is relatively hated as a disturbing element in this relationship.

The Girl's Situation

Understanding of the little girl's more complex oedipal involvement was a later development. Because it could not be regarded as equivalent to the boy's development, it raised a number of questions that proved to be more difficult. Freud could not get beyond viewing female sexual development as a variant of male development. Similar to the little boy, the little girl forms an initial attachment to the mother as a primary love object and source of fulfillment for vital needs. For the little boy, the mother remains the love object throughout his development, but the little girl is faced with the task of shifting this primary attachment from the mother to the father to prepare herself for her future sexual role. Freud was basically concerned with elucidating the factors that influenced the little girl to give up her pre-oedipal attachment to the mother and to form the normal oedipal attachment to the father. A secondary question had to do with the factors that led to the dissolution and resolution of the Oedipus complex in the girl so that paternal attachment and maternal identification would be the basis for adult sexual adjustment.

The girl's renunciation of her pre-oedipal attachment to the mother could not be satisfactorily explained as resulting from ambivalent or aggressive characteristics of the mother–child relationship, for similar elements influenced the relationship between boys and the mother figure. Freud attributed the crucial precipitating factor to anatomical differences between the sexes—specifically the girl's discovery of her lack of a penis during the phallic period. Up to this point, exclusive of constitutional differences and depending on variations in parental attitudes in relating to a daughter in comparison to a son, the little girl's development parallels that of the little boy.

Fundamental differences, however, emerge when she discovers during the phallic period that her clitoris is inferior to the male counterpart, the penis. The typical reaction of the little girl to this discovery is an intense sense of loss, narcissistic injury, and envy of the male penis. At this point, the little girl's attitude to the mother changes. The mother had previously been the object of love, but now she is held responsible for bringing the little girl into the world with inferior genital equipment. The hostility can be so intense that it may persist and color her future relationship to the mother. With the further discovery that the mother also lacks the vital penis, the child's hatred and devaluation of the mother becomes even more profound. In a desperate attempt to compensate for her "inadequacy," the little girl then turns to her father in the vain hope that he will give her a penis or a baby in place of the missing penis.

Obviously, the Freudian model of feminine psychosexual development has undergone, and is currently undergoing, considerable revision. The charge has been made, and justifiably so, that masculine phallic-oedipal development was the primary model in Freud's thinking and that feminine development was viewed as defective by comparison. Freud saw women as basically masochistic, weak, dependent, and lacking in conviction, strength of character, and moral fiber. He believed these defects were the result of failure in the oedipal identification with the phallic father because of female castration. The resulting internalization of aggression was both constitutionally determined and culturally reinforced.

These concepts must now be regarded as obsolete. Freud's hypotheses of a passive female libido, arrest in ego development, incapacity for sublimation, and superego deficiencies in women are outdated and inadequate. Differences in male and female ego and superego development may be defined, but there are no grounds for judging one to be superior or inferior to the other. They are simply different. As Harold Blum observed: "Female development cannot be described in a simple reductionism and overgeneralization. Femininity cannot be predominantly derived from a primary masculinity, disappointed maleness, masochistic resignation to fantasied inferiority, or compensation for fantasied castration and narcissistic injury. Castration reactions and penis envy contribute to feminine character, but penis envy is not the major determinant of femininity."

The adequate conceptualization and understanding of feminine psychology and its development are still very much in process. There is much that is poorly understood and much more that is hardly understood at all. Current research has given partial support to and convincing refutation of Freud's ideas. Current views emphasize the role of primary femininity and conflicts in identification with the mother as determining the course of development of feminine gender identity rather than the outmoded views of castration anxiety and penis envy. It is clear in all this that Freud was simply wrong about much of this whole area, but much of what he described may have simply expressed what he was able to observe in the women of his time and reflected the influence of attitudes toward women in his society and culture. Times change, however, and the culture and the place of women in it have changed and are changing. To that extent, women are different, and much of their psychology is different, too. Psychoanalytic understanding must inevitably lag behind these changing patterns of psychological experience, but a new view of feminine development and functioning is gradually emerging.

Mahler's Separation–Individuation Process

Autistic Phase

Mahler has conceptualized the process of development in terms of phases of separation and individuation. The first phase of development she describes is the autistic phase:

"During the first few weeks of extrauterine life, a stage of absolute primary narcissism, marked by the infant's lack of awareness of a mothering agent, prevails. This is the stage we have termed normal autism. It is followed by a stage of dim awareness that need satisfaction cannot be provided by oneself, but comes from somewhere outside the self. . . . The task of the autistic phase is the achievement of homeostatic equilibrium of the organism within the new extramural environment, by predominantly somatopsychic physiological mechanisms."

To the external observer, newborn infants seem to relate to their mothers in a condition of unique dependence and responsiveness. This relationship is, however, at least at first, purely biological based on physiological reflexes and ordered to the fulfillment of basic biological needs. It is only as babies' egos begin to develop, along with the organization of perceptual capacities and memory traces, which allow for the initial differentiation of self and object, that infants can be said to experience something outside of themselves, to which they can relate, as satisfying their inner needs. This dawning awareness of the external object is a most significant state in the psychological development of children and involves not only cognitive and perceptual developments but also goes hand in hand with the organization of rudimentary infantile drives and affects in relation to emerging object experiences.

The emergence of the psychological need-satisfying relationship to the object or part-object occurs during the oral phase of libidinal development. It should be noted, however, that the notion of the oral phase of development and the concepts of need-satisfying relationships are not equivalent. The oral phase is primarily concerned with libidinal development and stresses predominance of the oral zone as the main erotogenic zone. The concept of the need-satisfying relationship, however, is not concerned directly with issues of drive development but, rather, with the characteristics of object involvement and object relationship.

Symbiotic Phase This awareness signals the beginning of normal symbiosis "in which the infant behaves and functions as though he and his mother were an omnipotent system—a dual unity within one common boundary." The symbiotic phase is described as a "hallucinatory or delusional somatopsychic omnipotent fusion with the representation of the mother and, in particular, the delusion of a common boundary between two physically separate individuals." These boundaries become temporarily differentiated only in the state of "affect hunger" but disappear again as a result of need gratification. Only gradually does the child form more stable part-images of the mother such as breasts, face, or hands. Consequently, the object is recognized as separate from the self only at moments of need so that, once the need is satisfied, the object ceases to exist—from the infant's (subjective) point of view—until a need again arises. Moreover, from the infant's perspective, the relationship is not to a specific object (or part-object) but rather to a function of the object satisfying the need and to the pleasure accompanying that function. It is only when the specific object—that is, the whole object—becomes as important to the child as the need-satisfying function that it performs that one can regard the child's development as moving beyond the level of need-satisfying relationships toward the attainment of object constancy.

Thus, it is useful to distinguish between need satisfaction as a stage of development in object relationships, related to but not synonymous with the oral phase of libidinal development, and need satisfaction as a determinant in object relationships at every level of development. The satisfaction of various kinds of psychological needs continues to play a role at all levels of object relatedness, but the satisfaction of such needs cannot be used as a distinguishing characteristic of the specific stage of need-satisfying object relationships. As objects become increasingly differentiated in the child's experience, their representations achieve increasing psychological complexity and value in a context of increasingly complex and subtle needs for a variety of input from objects. Development of object constancy implies a constant relationship to a specific object, but within that relationship, the wish for satisfaction of needs and the actual satisfaction of those needs may still be a significant component of the object relationship.

Separation and Individuation

HATCHING During this period, the child with effort gradually differentiates out of the symbiotic matrix. The first behavioral signs of such differentiation seem to arise at approximately 4 or 5 months of age at the high point of the symbiotic period. The first stage of this process of differentiation is described as "hatching" from the symbiotic orbit:

> In other words, the infant's attention, which during the first months of symbiosis was in large part inwardly directed, or focused in a coenesthetic vague way within the symbiotic orbit, gradually expands through the coming into being of outwardly directed perceptual activity during the child's increasing periods of wakefulness. This is a change of degree rather than of kind, for during the symbiotic stage the child has certainly been highly attentive to the mothering figure. But gradually that attention is combined with a growing store of memories of mother's comings and goings, of "good" and "bad" experiences; the latter were altogether unrelievable by the self, but could be "confidently expected" to be relieved by mother's ministrations.

PRACTICING As the child's differentiation and separation from the mother gradually increase, there is a move to the second or "practicing" subphase of separation–individuation. The practicing period can be usefully divided into an early practicing period and a practicing period proper. The early practicing phase begins with the infant's earliest ability to move physically away from the mother by locomotion, that is, crawling, creeping, climbing, and assuming an upright sitting position. Moving away from the safe protective orbit of the mother has its risks and uncertainties, however. In the early practicing phase, there is frequently a pattern of visually "checking back to mother" or even crawling or paddling back to her to touch or hold on as a form of "emotional refueling."

The practicing period proper is characterized by the attainment of free upright locomotion. It is marked by three interrelated developments that contribute to the continuing process of separation and individuation. These are (1) rapid bodily differentiation from the mother, (2) establishment of a specific bond with her, and (3) growth and functioning of autonomous ego-apparatuses in close connection and dependence on the mothering figure.

RAPPROCHEMENT As this testing of the freedom of individuation proceeds, by approximately the middle of the second year of life, the child enters the third subphase of rapprochement:

> He now becomes more and more aware, and makes greater and greater use, of his physical separateness. However, side by side with the growth of his cognitive faculties and the increasing differentiation of his emotional life, there is also a noticeable waning of his previous imperviousness to frustration, as well as a diminution of what has been a relative obliviousness to his mother's presence. Increased separation anxiety can be observed: at first this consists mainly of fear of object loss, which is to be inferred from many of the child's

behaviors. The relative lack of concern about the mother's presence that was characteristic of the practicing subphase is now replaced by seemingly constant concern with the mother's whereabouts, as well as by active approach behavior. As the toddler's awareness of separateness grows—stimulated by his maturationally acquired ability to move away physically from his mother and by his cognitive growth—he seems to have an increased need, a wish for mother to share with him every one of his new skills and experiences, as well as a great need for the object's love.

The crisis in the rapprochement phase is particularly that of separation anxiety. The child's wishes and desires to be separate, autonomous, and omnipotent are tempered by an increasing awareness of the need for and dependence on the mother. Ambivalence is characteristic of the middle phase of the rapprochement subphase. There is a tension between the child's need to use the mother as a personal extension, as having her magically fulfill wishes, and the realization that, with the child's increasing separateness, the mother becomes less available and more distant. Thus, the mother's availability and the reassurance of her continuing love and support become all the more important.

OBJECT CONSTANCY As developments of the rapprochement phase are gradually realized, the child enters the fourth and final phase of separation and individuation, namely, the phase of consolidation of individuality and the beginnings of emotional object constancy. At this stage, there are significant developments in the structuralization and integration of the ego as well as definite signs of internalization of parental demands reflecting the development of superego precursors.

Attainment of object constancy marks a transition from the stage of need-satisfying relationships to a more mature psychological involvement with objects. Object constancy implies a capacity to differentiate between objects and to maintain a meaningful relationship with one specific object regardless of whether needs are being satisfied. Such object constancy also implies stability of object cathexis and, specifically, the capacity to maintain positive emotional attachments to a particular object in the face of frustration of needs and wishes in regard to that object. This achievement also implies the capacity to tolerate ambivalent feelings toward the object and the capacity to value that object for qualities that it possesses over and beyond the functions that it may serve in satisfying needs and in gratifying drives.

To summarize, it can be said that the notion of object constancy implies involvement of a number of specific elements that are central to further emergence of the meaningful capacity for relationships with objects. These elements include perceptual object constancy; the capacity to maintain drive attachment to a specific object regardless of whether it is present; the capacity to tolerate both loving and hostile feelings toward the same object or to maintain a loving relationship with the object in the face of hostile and destructive impulses; the capacity to maintain significant emotional attachment to a single specific object; and, finally, the capacity to value the object for qualities and attributes that it possesses in itself, in virtue of its own uniqueness as individually and separately existing, and as independent of any need-satisfying function it may serve.

Erikson's Epigenetic Sequence: Instinctual Zones and Modes of Ego Development Erikson made a major contribution to the psychoanalytic concept of development in his study of the relationship between instinctual zones and the development of specific modalities of ego functioning. Erikson's theory ingeniously links aspects of ego development with the epigenetic timetable of instinctual psychosexual development by postulating a parallel relationship between specific phases of ego or psychosocial development and specific phases of libidinal development. During libidinal development, particular erotogenic zones become loci of stimulation for development of particular modalities of ego functioning. The relationship between zones of instinctual stimulation and their corresponding modalities of ego functioning is easily specifiable in pregenital levels of development, but Erikson projects this basic modality of relationship, extending it to the limits of the life cycle.

The first modality of development is related to the oral phase, specifically to stimulus qualities of the oral zone. This early stage is called the *oral-respiratory-sensory stage*, and it is dominated by the first oral-incorporative mode, which involves the modality of "taking in." Other auxiliary modes are also operative, including a second oral-incorporative (biting) mode, an oral-retentive mode, an oral-eliminative mode, and, finally, an oral-intrusive mode. These modes become variably important according to individual temperament but remain subordinated to the first incorporative mode unless the mutual regulation of the oral zone with the providing breast of the mother is disturbed, either by a loss of inner control in the infant or a defect in reciprocal and responsive nurturing behavior on the part of the mother. The emphasis in this stage of development is placed on the modalities of "getting" and "getting what is given," thus laying the necessary ego groundwork for eventually "getting to be a giver." The second stage, also focused on the oral zone, is marked by a biting modality because of the development of teeth. This phase is marked by development of interpersonal patterns, centered in the social modality of "taking" and "holding" onto things.

Similarly, with the advent of the anal-urethral-muscular stage, the "retentive" and "eliminative" modes become established. Extension and generalization of these modes over the whole of the developing muscular system enable the 18- to 24-month-old child to gain some form of self-control in the matter of conflicting impulses such as "letting go" and "holding on." When this control is disturbed by developmental defects in the anal-urethral sphere, a fixation on modalities of retention or elimination can be established that can lead to a variety of disturbances in the zone itself (spastic), in the muscle system (flabbiness or rigidity), in obsessional fantasy (paranoid fears), and in social spheres (attempts at controlling the environment by compulsive routinization).

Erikson laid out a program of ego development that reached from birth to death: The individual passes through the phases of the life cycle by meeting and resolving a series of developmental psychosocial crises.

These phases of the life cycle and their respective crises accomplish several things. First, they make it clear that ego development is open ended and never finished. The child's capacity to successfully resolve any one developmental crisis depends on the degree of resolution of the preceding crises. One can form a mature and integral sense of identity only to the extent that one has achieved a meaningful sense of trust, autonomy, initiative, and industry. Successful resolution at any level lays the foundation for engaging in the next developmental crisis. Second, they clarify the relation between the various phases of development and earlier phases of libidinal development. The latter had been the basic contribution of earlier efforts of psychoanalysis, but Erikson's developmental schema gave a better understanding of the way in which earlier libidinal developmental residues were carried along in the course of growth and were built into later developmental efforts of the ego. Psychoanalysis had not previously had the conceptual tools to deal with this problem, particularly in regard to the postadolescent phases of the life cycle. Finally, Erikson's treatment of these crises as specifically psychosocial brought into focus the fact that the development of the ego was not merely a matter of intrapsychic vicissitudes dealing with the economics of inner psychic energies. It was that, certainly, but it was also a matter of the interaction and "mutual regulation" between the developing human organism and significant people in its environment. Even more strikingly, it is a matter of mutual regulation evolving between the growing child and the culture and traditions of society. Erikson has made the sociocultural influence an integral part of the developmental matrix out of which the personality emerges.

Trust versus Mistrust The crisis of trust versus mistrust is the first psychosocial crisis the infant must face. It takes place in the context of the intimate relationship between infant and mother. The infant's primary orientation to reality is erotic and centers on the mouth. The primary locus for significant contact with reality, therefore, is oral. The typical situation in which the infant experiences oral eroticism is the feeding relationship. Depending on the quality of experience with feeding contacts, the child learns to accept what is given by the warm and loving mother, to depend on that mother, and to expect that what she provides will be satisfying. The importance of the child–mother interaction here should not be underestimated. The child's basically oral orientation is largely biologically determined; the mother's feeding orientation is not only a product of biological factors but also of a complex process of personal development in which her sense of identity as a female and as a mother plays a vital part. Any defect in her identity, thus, has important consequences for the quality of the interaction between herself and her child.

Successful resolution of this initial phase of interaction entails a disposition to trust others, basic trust in oneself, a capacity to receive from others and to depend on them (to entrust oneself), and a sense of self-confidence. Unsuccessful resolution of this crisis results in the defect of these same qualities and relative dominance of such opposite qualities as mistrust and lack of confidence. Consequently, the designations "basic trust" and "basic mistrust" stand for a complex of personality factors characterizing successful or unsuccessful resolution of this first crisis.

Autonomy versus Shame and Self-Doubt The second stage of psychosexual development is anal eroticism. Biologically, this stage is marked by formation of a fuller stool and maturation of the neuromuscular system to a point sufficient to allow control of sphincter muscles governing retention and release of waste materials. Likewise, the anal zone becomes a source of erotic stimulation through pleasurable sensations of retaining or releasing. Psychosocially, this period is marked by emergence in the child of self-awareness as a separate and independent unit. Growing muscular control is accompanied by increasing capacity for autonomous expression and self-regulation, which typically centers on problems of sphincter control of the so-called anal period. The ego thus enters into interactions of assertiveness with other wills in the social environment, particularly with the parents. Successfully resolved, the crisis of autonomy lays the foundation for a mature capacity for self-assertion and self-expression, a capacity to respect the autonomy of others, an ability to maintain self-control without loss of self-esteem, and a capacity for rewarding and effective cooperation with others. The corresponding defect lays the foundation of false autonomy that must feed on the autonomy of others by domination and excessive demands or of an excessive rigidity that can be identified in the fragile autonomy of the compulsive (anal) personality. Inability to achieve basic autonomy implies the lack of self-esteem reflected in a sense of shame and the lack of self-confidence implied in self-doubt.

Initiative versus Guilt When the child enters the play age, the maturing organism reaches a developmental stage in which the subsystems serving functions of locomotion and language are sufficiently organized to permit facile use. The motor equipment has reached a sufficient level of development to permit not merely performance of motions but a wide-ranging experimentation in locomotion. The child begins to "test the limits" of this new-found capability. The child's activity becomes vigorous and intrusive. A similar crystallization of function occurs in the use of language, which becomes an exciting new toy calling for experimentation and the satisfaction of curiosity. The child's mode of activity is marked by intrusion: intrusion into other bodies by physical attack, into other's attention by activity and aggressive talking, into space by vigorous locomotion, and into the unknown by active curiosity. All this activity is accompanied by a growing sexual curiosity and a development of the prerequisites of specifically masculine or feminine initiative, which are conditioned by development of a phallic eroticism.

If the crisis of initiative is successfully resolved, positive residues are provided for development of conscience, a sense of responsibility and dependability, self-discipline, and a certain independence in the mature personality. This stage is therefore crucial for the formation of the superego based on the introjection of authoritative, and especially parental, prohibitions. The unsuccessful resolution provides the basis for the harsh, rigid, moralistic, and self-punishing superego that serves as the dynamic source of a basic sense of guilt.

Industry versus Inferiority The period of infantile (phallic) sexuality and the period of adult sexuality (puberty) are separated by the so-called latency period in which the child's interest is generally diverted to other matters. The child takes a step up from the level of imaginative exploration and play to a level in which participation in the adult world is foreshadowed. In Western culture, children are sent to school, where they begin to learn skills that will equip them to take their places one day in adult society. Their interests turn to doing and making things; in general, they become involved in developing the necessary technology for adult living. They are drawn away from home and its close associations and plunged into the matrix of the school system. They learn the reward systems of the school society and assimilate the values of application and diligence. They also assimilate the implicit cultural values of work and productivity. They achieve a sense of the pleasure of work, of the satisfaction of a task accomplished, and of the merit of perseverance in difficult enterprises. In other words, normally developing children add to their evolving personality a sense of industry. The danger at this stage is that a lack of success in meeting demands of the school society and inability to resolve this psychosocial crisis produce a sense of inadequacy and inferiority.

Identity versus Identity Confusion The passage to adolescent years is marked by an intense period of physiological growth and sudden maturation of genital organs. The psychosexual phase of puberty is accompanied on the psychosocial level by a kind of organization or crystallization of the residues of the preceding formative phases. The developmental preparations for participation in adult life must now begin to take a more or less definitive shape, so the adolescent must begin to experiment with establishing a future role and function within adult society. The adolescent must develop a confident sense of self-awareness predicated on the ability to maintain inner sameness and continuity and on the confidence that this awareness is matched by the sameness and continuity of his or her meaning to others. This particular psychosocial crisis is therefore peculiarly vulnerable and sensitive to social and cultural influences. The context of the crisis is specifically interpersonal, and as such, its successful resolution becomes all the more tenuous and problematic. In a special sense, achieving a sense of personal identity requires an awareness of the context of relations to reality within which the self forms and maintains its own proper identity.

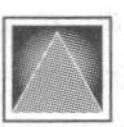

Table 6.1–4
Parallel Lines of Development

Instinctual Phases	Separation–Individuation	Object Relations	Psychosocial Crises
Oral	Autism, symbiosis	Primary narcissism, need-satisfying	Trust/mistrust
Anal	Differentiation, practicing, rapprochement	Need-satisfying, object constancy	Autonomy/shame, self-doubt
Phallic	Object constancy, Oedipal complex	Object constancy, ambivalence	Initiative/guilt
Latency	—	—	Industry/inferiority
Adolescence	Genitality, secondary individuation	Object love	Identity/identity confusion
Adulthood	Mature genitality	—	Intimacy/isolation, generativity/stagnation, integrity/despair

Intimacy versus Isolation The status of adulthood is marked on the psychosexual level by achievement of genital maturity. On the psychosocial level, this development is paralleled by the establishment of significant interpersonal relationships that complement the previously formed identity in the social sphere. Typically, the emerging sexual drive focuses on another individual of the opposite sex as its object. The elements of sexual identification, which are essential aspects of personal identity, are naturally expressed as established by the standards of intersex behavior of the society and culture. The intimate association of male and female in a close interpersonal union is thus an extension of their own identities as well as a culturally approved institution (marriage). This fact does not mean that the sexual act is the only path to a sense of intimacy. From the point of view of personality development, the crucial element is the capacity to relate intimately and meaningfully with others in mutually satisfying and productive interactions. The pattern of such self-fulfilling relations depends in large measure on the identity one has accepted as his or her own.

The inability to achieve a successful resolution of this psychosocial crisis results in a sense of personal isolation. The incapacity to establish warm and rewarding relationships with others is but a reflection of the inability to realize a secure and mature self-acceptance. Interpersonal relationships become strained, stiff, or formal. Even if a façade of personal warmth can be erected, there is a rigidly maintained inner wall that is never breached, a wall defended by intellectualization, distancing, and self-absorption.

Generativity versus Stagnation "Generativity" points to a primary concern with establishing and guiding the succeeding generation (through genes and genitality). In Erikson's terms, "Generativity, as the instinctual power behind various forms of selfless 'caring,' potentially extends to whatever a man generates and leaves behind, creates and produces (or helps to produce)." It must also be recognized, however, that other areas of altruistic effort cannot be excluded. Perhaps "productivity" or "creativity" are better terms.

Such creativity can assume a myriad of forms, depending on the native endowment of the person; but realized generativity is also determined to a large extent by the identity the individual has accepted and by the extent to which one is capable of interacting maturely and cooperatively with others. Consequently, successful resolution of this crisis depends closely on the degree of success achieved in the resolution of the preceding phases of identity and intimacy. Moreover, true generativity has as its goal enrichment of the lives of others; it involves a direct concern with the welfare of others, exclusive of any concern over self-interest.

Integrity versus Despair Integrity marks the culmination of development of the personality in Erikson's schema. It means acceptance of oneself and all aspects of life and integration of these elements into a stable pattern of living. It implies the experience of and adjustment to the trials and troubles of life as well as to its rewards and joys. Consequently, existence holds no fear; the ego has resigned itself to acceptance of life itself and to acceptance of the end of that life in death. Integrity thus represents the fully developed personality in its most mature self-realization. The inability to achieve ego integration results often in a kind of despair and an unconscious fear of death: The one life cycle, given to every human as his or her own, has not been accepted. The person who does not achieve integrity is doomed to live in basic self-contempt.

The parallel lines of development and their interrelation are indicated in Table 6.1–4.

Current Considerations

In recent years, a fresh current has entered the mainstream of analytical developmental theory. In some degree reacting to the work of Freud and Mahler, on the basis of observational studies of very young infants, the view of the infant emerged as active, surprisingly well organized even at the very beginning of life, and as attuned to and interactive with the mothering figure in complicated and quite sophisticated ways. Particular objections to Mahler's approach to separation–individuation focused on her use of pathological terms (autism, symbiosis) to describe the developmental phases of normal infants and the fact that her extensive observations were often too overlaid with metapsychological terms that obscured the boundary between fact and theory. The work of Daniel Stern particularly presented a different view of the infant and focused attention on other important aspects of development that had been treated only tangentially in previous studies.

Stern's observations brought into clearer focus the intense affective and interactional matrix between mother and child and directed attention more specifically to the emergence of a sense of self than had previously been available. To begin with, Stern's baby was calm, alert, cognitively well organized, and highly responsive to and interactive with the mother. The extent to which the infant was preadapted to stimuli from the mother and active in eliciting certain responses from the mother, whether caretaking or affective, cast a different light on early stages of development. The relation between mother and child proved to be more active and interactive than had previously been appreciated. Also following in the wake of Heinz Kohut's self–selfobject views and the intersubjective developments that arose from them, much of the analysis of mother–child interaction was cast in terms of the relational and intersubjective models of relating. Stern centered his interest on study of a subjective sense of self separately from study of the ego, which had held center stage in Mahler's view. Whether such a separate self is necessary or whether the separation–individuation process and object relations theory already covered this ground remain debatable questions. Certainly, Mahler's concentration on the sense of identity and self-constancy cannot be discounted, but Stern emphasized intersubjective relatedness, suggesting "a deliberately sought sharing of experiences about events and things." All these interactions, including the highly intimate bodily interchanges between mother and child, are steeped in affective resonances. Stern carefully traced the emergence of a core sense of self out of increasingly complex bodily and self–other experiences, especially with the mother, all taking place within an intensely affective ambiance leading to development of an affective core in emerging self-experience. This process leads ultimately to establishing a degree of libidinal self-constancy involving a sense of self as relatively integrated and independent, as relatively durable and stable, as differentiated from others but involved in complex relationships, and as an active agent capable of causing effects and influencing the surrounding environment.

Whether and to what extent this approach to development of the self and its affective resonances is contradictory to the Mahlerian schema or is open to eventual integration remains a subject of debate. Despite the at times oppositional stance that advocates of one or the other view assume, the potential exists for combining these perspectives in the hope of deepening the understanding of the complexities of human psychological development. Critics have pointed out that these different approaches may be looking at children in different contexts of observation—the Stern baby in periods of relatively calm and unconflicted interaction with the mother, Mahler's baby in contexts of greater conflict and separation. It may be that the observations of both groups are valid enough and need to be brought together to accomplish a more complete view of the developing infant. Certainly Stern's focus on the emergence of the self adds a fresh direction of inquiry more congruent with evolving theoretical concepts of the self in psychoanalysis.

OBJECT RELATIONS THEORY

One of the important developments in psychoanalysis, which emerged more or less in parallel to the evolution of psychoanalytic ego psychology, is object relations theory. Only gradually over the years have these parallel and somewhat independent courses of theoretical development converged into complementary rather than oppositional perspectives. The development of classic psychoanalytic theory through elaboration of a systemic ego psychology has led inexorably in the direction of better understanding of the adaptive functions of the ego, particularly the close involvement between the ego and reality in its functioning and development. One important dimension of the problem of reality in psychoanalytic theory is the whole question of object relations. The integration of these complementary currents of analytical thinking provides a more comprehensive basis for thinking about the mind as it functions not only intrapsychically but interpersonally in its relation to others as important sources of the social environment of the human person.

Origins The origins of the object relations view can best be traced from the contribution of Klein. Klein's theorizing based itself on Freud's later instinct theory, primarily on the death instinct as the main theoretical prop of her metapsychology. Working primarily with very young children, she described instinctual dynamics in the first years of life. Driven by the death instinct, the child was compelled to rid him- or herself of intolerable, destructive impulses (predominantly oral) and to project them externally. The earliest recipient of these projected impulses was the mother's breast, which provided need-satisfying nourishment and satiation (good breast) but also often deprived and did not satisfy (bad breast). At this stage, the images of the breast are part-objects that the infant had yet to combine into a single whole object, the mother. Early frustration of oral needs, even in the first year of life, reinforced these trends so that the bad breast became a persecutory object that was hated, feared, and envied.

Experience of the bad breast and its associated persecutory anxiety formed the earliest developmental stage in Klein's theory: the paranoid-schizoid position. The bad breast withheld gratification and thus stimulated the child's primitive oral envy, provoking sadistic wishes to penetrate and destroy the mother's breasts and body. In boys, these primitive destructive impulses gave rise to the fear of retaliation (based in part on projection) in the form of castration anxiety; in girls, the primitive envy was expressed in envy of the mother's breast during the oral developmental phase and later was transformed into penis envy during the genital phase. Klein held that by the time of weaning, the child was capable of recognizing the mother as a whole object possessing good and bad qualities. But the combination of good and bad qualities in a single object—previously separated in part-objects—created a dilemma: Destructive attacks on the bad object also destroyed the good and needed object. This prevented the child from unleashing aggressive impulses against the object and lay the basis for the depressive position, in which aggression was turned against the self rather than against the object. The guilt associated with destructive wishes against the object was the precursor of conscience.

Klein's emphasis in the child's developmental experience fell on the processes of introjection and projection, derived from basic instinctual drives, and their interactions with the important and primary objects of the child's early experience. Projection of destructive superego elements permitted acceptance of good introjects (internalization of good objects), thus alleviating the underlying paranoid anxiety. The projected superego elements were later reintrojected to become the agency of guilt and early forms of obsessional behavior. The Kleinian emphasis on good and bad introjects concentrated on vital relationships to objects at the earliest level of child development, and the delineation of the internal structuring of the child's inner fantasy world in terms of the vicissitudes of these introjects, or internal objects, provided the basis and the rudimentary content for an object relations view of development.

Thus Klein's "inner world" was peopled by internal objects that were either good or bad and with whom the individual was involved in intrapsychic interactions and struggles that were in many ways as real as those carried on with the real objects outside the person. In fact, Klein saw external object relations as derived from and influenced by projective content derived from the internal object relations. Klein has been generously criticized for her almost blind interpretation of all forms of aggressive or destructive intent as manifestations of the death instinct, for her inability to distinguish among the various kinds of intrapsychic content (lumping object representations, self-representations, internal objects, fantasies, and psychic structures of various kinds together indiscriminately and treating them in a unitary fashion), for her tendency to substitute theoretical inferences for observations, and, finally, for her marked tendency to predate the emergence of intrapsychic organizations that are generally thought by other theorists to be achieved only in later developmental stages, for example, locating the origin of the superego in the first year of life rather than in resolution of the oedipal situation in latency.

In any case, Klein's observations and formulations had a tremendous impact, particularly in bringing into prominence the role of aggression in pathological development, in making theorists of development much more aware of the early developmental precursors of later structural entities, and particularly in providing the basic rudiments and foundations for an emergent theory of object relations.

Wilfred Bion extended and applied Klein's ideas, especially developing the ramifications of the notion of projective identification—a process, originally described by Klein, by which a subject displaces a part of the self into an object and then identifies with that object or elicits a response in the object corresponding to qualities of the projection. Bion applied this notion to a wide range of psychotic and cognitive operations. He developed the metaphor of the "container" and the "contained" to express the manner in which projective identification occurs, especially in the contexts of mother–child and analyst–patient interaction. The child/patient projects toxic or destructive contents onto the mother/analyst, who, in turn, absorbs, modifies, or "contains" it so that it becomes available in more benign form for subsequent reinternalization by the child/patient, resulting in a healthier modification of the child/patient's pathogenic introjects. Bion also contributed significantly to the understanding of group processes by demonstrating the "basic assumptions" that operate on an unconscious emotional level in therapeutic groups and are expressed in patterns of fight-flight, pairing, and dependence.

EGO AND OBJECTS

Beginning around 1931, Ronald Fairbairn shifted the emphasis in his thinking specifically to the problem of ego analysis. Fairbairn's contribution was to bring personal object relations into the center of the theory. Whereas the ego in Freudian theory had been regarded as a superficial modification of the id, developed specifically for the purpose of impulse control and adaptation to the demands of reality, Fairbairn conceived of the ego as the core phenomenon of the psyche. Rather than an organization of functions, he conceived of it more specifically as embodying a real self—that is, as the dynamic center or core of the personality. Instead of basing his theory on the instinctual drives as the basic concept, Fairbairn shifted the emphasis to the ego and saw everything in human psychology as specifically an effect of ego functioning.

With this reorientation, there came a parallel reformulation of the instinctual perspective. The libido or instincts in general, rather than mechanisms for energic discharge, were regarded as essentially object seeking. Erotogenic zones were not the primary determinants of libidinal aims but, rather, channels that mediated the primary relationships with objects, particularly with relationships with objects that had been internalized during early life under the pressure of deprivation and frustration. Ego development itself was characterized by a process whereby an original state of infantile dependence, based on a symbiotic union with the maternal object, was abandoned in favor of a state of adult or mature dependence based on differentiation between self and object. Thus, Fairbairn conceptualized the developmental process in terms of the vicissitudes of relations with objects rather than the vicissitudes of instinctual dynamics.

The basis for much of Fairbairn's theorizing is his experience with schizoid patients. He contrasted the basic dilemma of the schizoid with that of neurotic patients on whom he felt classic psychoanalytic theory was based. He saw that the schizoid was not primarily concerned with control of threatening impulses toward significant objects, but that the issue for this kind of patient was essentially that of having an ego capable of forming object relations at all. The relationship to objects presented a difficulty, not because of dangerous impulses arising in connection with them, but because the ego was weak, undeveloped, infantile, and fragile. In the struggle to overcome this inner weakness, the schizoid's impulses became antisocial.

Thus, object relations theory in its bare essentials contains a number of basic points that differentiate it from classic theory. First, the ego is conceived of as whole or total at birth, becoming split or losing inner unity as a result of early bad experiences in object relationships, particularly in relation to the mothering object. This point differs quite radically from the classic theory, according to which the ego begins as undifferentiated and unintegrated and only achieves unity through the course of development. Second, libido is regarded as a primary life drive of the psyche, the energic source of the ego's search for relatedness with good objects, which is essential for ego growth. Third, aggression is regarded as a natural defensive reaction to frustration of the libidinal drive rather than specifically as an independent instinct. Fourth, the structural ego pattern that emerges when the pristine ego unity is lost involves a pattern of ego splitting and the formation of internal ego–object relations.

The shift in emphasis toward the primacy of the external environment and the influence of objects on the course of development has established a definite trend in psychoanalytic thinking and has been advanced primarily in the work of British theorists, among whom the work of Michael Balint and Donald Winnicott stands out. Winnicott particularly has emphasized the importance of early interactions between mother and child as determining factors in the laying down of important components of ego development. Currently, there is ample room for overlap and integration in the approaches and formulations of both object relations theorists and more classic psychoanalytic ego theorists. Such integration has advanced to the point that they are generally regarded as forming at least complementary aspects of a common theory, if not a more comprehensive and unified theory as such.

Both Balint and Winnicott were concerned with levels of early developmental failure that were essentially pre-oedipal, were manifested in forms of personality disorder that are more primitive and more difficult to treat than the usual neurotic disorders, and seemed to involve critical aspects of the relationships with objects early in the course of development and correspondingly do not fit well with classic psychoanalytic structural theory with its basic focus on issues of intrapsychic conflict.

Balint envisioned several layers of psychological functioning in analysis. The first is the familiar genital level, centering on triadic relationships and concerned specifically with intrapsychic conflicts. These conflicts and quality of relationships were usual and familiar material in most analytical processes and could be treated by use of adult language in verbal interpretations. There was, however, a second, deeper level in which the conventional meaning of words no longer had the same impact, and interpretations were no longer perceived as meaningful by the patient. This was the level of preverbal experience. He referred to this level of impairment in object relations as the *basic fault*. Balint recognized that at this level of preverbal experience any attempt to address or describe the child's experience in adult language is bound to fail. Problems arose in analysis when efforts were made to interpret events from this preverbal level in adult or secondary process terms.

Balint distinguished between forms of regression that he described as benign and malignant. The benign regression was more or less an extension of the basic notion of the usual analytic regression to a level of primitive relationship with primary objects. Such a regression was gradual, tempered, and modulated according to the patient's capacity to tolerate and productively integrate the resulting anxiety. During this regression, the analyst's empathic responsiveness and recognition made it possible for the patient to withstand this unstructured experience and to keep the anxiety within manageable limits. At the level of the basic fault, the lost infantile objects can be mourned, and the quality of the relationship with them was open to reworking so that the patient's basic assumptions governing his or her interaction with the internal and external object world could be reformed.

During phases of benign regression to this preverbal and pregenital level of object relationship in the analysis, the analyst could usually provide an adequate degree of empathic acceptance and recognition, rather than verbalized interpretations, of this level of the patient's unstructured and regressive experience, without anxiety or any need to escape or subvert this level of experience through interpretation. Balint felt that the dynamics at this level are more primitive than can be adequately expressed in terms of conflict because they derive from the basic form of dual relationship involved in early mother–child interaction—that is, the basic fault.

In contrast, malignant regression tends to be precipitous and extreme; the ego is prematurely overwhelmed by traumatic and unmanageable anxiety.

This anxiety prevented any effective reworking of fundamental disturbances in object relationships, re-creating and reinforcing the basic fault, rather than creating the conditions for its therapeutic revision. At an even deeper level, beyond the reach of analytic resources, lay the area of creativity; that is, an idiosyncratic, uncommunicable, and objectless area that lies beyond conventional expression.

Regression to the level of the basic fault was a quite different and distinct phenomenon than the more usual oedipal regressions experienced in the analysis of adult neurotics. In the oedipal regression, the aim was gratification of infantile instinctual wishes. Regression to the level of the basic fault, however, sought a basic recognition by the therapist, as well as protective support and consent to express the inner core of creativity that lies at the heart of the patient's being and accounts for the capacity to become ill or well. Balint used the notion of primary love at this deepest level to describe withdrawal of libido from a frustrating object in the effort to reestablish a certain inner harmony in which it becomes possible to recover the conditions of early care and tranquility. He referred to a "harmonious interpenetrating mix-up" to describe this early, almost undifferentiated interaction of the infant and environment. The analogy he used was that of breathing air; the organism cannot exist without air, so air and the organism are seemingly inseparable, but cutting off the supply of air reveals both the organism's need for it and the distinction between air and the organism. In terms of primary love as it came to bear in analysis, then, the patient would seek a basic form of recognition from the analyst, as he had from significant objects in the patient's early life experience.

Winnicott also was concerned with the earliest phase of the mother–child relationship and the importance of what he described as "good-enough mothering" for the child's personality development. The course of development involved movement from an early stage of total or absolute dependence toward a more adult phase of relative independence. As he saw it, the inherited native potential for growth was strongly influenced by the quality of maternal care. This potential for development is affected even from the moment of conception. Even before birth, the child becomes invested by a strong narcissistic cathexis that allows the mother to identify with the child and to become empathically attuned to the child's inner needs, as if the child were—and indeed is—an extension of her own self. Winnicott called this early prenatal involvement of mother and child in the womb a *primary maternal preoccupation*. This set the stage for development of a holding relationship in which the mother becomes sensitively attuned to the infant's needs and sensitivities and is both physically and emotionally responsive to them, thus providing a physical, physiological, and emotional ambiance, protection, and security for the absolutely dependent infant.

As the infant moves from this early stage of absolute dependence toward a more relative dependence, awareness of personal needs and of the existence of the mother as a caretaking object grows. The optimal relationship at this stage involves a continuation of protective holding, along with an optimal titration of gratification and frustration. As a result of this optimally attuned relationship between the patterning of infantile drives and initiatives and their harmonious fitting in with maternal sensitivities and responsiveness, there is a developing sense of reliable expectation that the infant's needs will be satisfied without the threat of excessive withdrawal of the mothering object and without the threatening, overwhelming, and short-circuiting of the infant's initiatives as a result of excessive maternal impingements.

In the course of normal development, this allowed for emergence of a certain omnipotence from which the child gradually retreats with the experiences of tolerable degrees of frustration by and separateness of the maternal object. Although the mother continues her holding at this phase, she must yet allow enough separation between herself and the developing infant to permit expression of the baby's needs and initiatives that form the rudiments of an emerging sense of self. If she is too distant, too unresponsive, or not sufficiently present, anxiety arises and is accompanied by the fading of the infant's internal representations of her.

The transition from a phase of absolute dependence to one of relative dependence represents a crucial development in the capacity for object relations. It is accompanied by a critical transition from total subjectivity to the capacity for objectivity in the perception of and relation to objects. The transition from subjectivity to objectivity is accomplished by development of Winnicott's transitional phenomenon, expressed in the first instance in the emergence of transitional objects. These objects are the child's first object possessions that are perceived as separate from the emerging self—the first "not me" possessions. From the study of infant behavior, Winnicott argued that the transitional object was a substitute for the maternal breast, the first and most significant object in the environment to which the infant related. The transitional object exists in an intermediate realm contributed to both by the external reality of the object (the mother's breast) and by the child's own subjectivity. This intermediate realm is at once both subjective and objective without being exclusively either.

Winnicott referred to this realm as the *realm of illusion*, an intermediate area of experience that embraced both inner and external reality and may be retained in areas of adult functioning having to do with such imaginative capacities as creativity, religious experience, and art. In its primitive form, however, the transitional object commonly experienced in childhood development may take the form of a particular object, a blanket, a pillow, or a favorite toy or teddy bear to which the child becomes intensely attached and from which it cannot be separated without stirring up severe anxiety and distress. Attachment to this object is an immediate displacement from the figure of the mother and represented an important developmental step, insofar as it allows the child to tolerate increasing degrees of separation from the mother, using the transitional object as a substitute.

The mother participates in this intermediate transitional realm of illusion by her responsiveness to the infant's need to continually create her as a good mother. In her sensitivity and responsiveness, she functions as a good-enough mother. However, her inability to provide such adequate mothering, either by excessive withdrawal or by excessive intrusion and control, may result in emergence of a false self in the child based on compliance with the demands of the external environment, a condition that reflects a developmental failure and results in a variety of often severe character pathologies.

When such patients are seen as adults, they are neither neurotic nor psychotic but seem to relate to the world through a compliant shell that is not quite real to them or to the analyst. They are often mistrustful without being specifically paranoid, they appear withdrawn and disengaged and seem able to relate only by means of the protective shell, which seems apparently obsessive and compliant but which separates and isolates them from meaningful contacts with their fellows, even as it provides their only basis for relationship. These disturbed personality types reflect a basic impairment in very early object relations, particularly in the mutuality and responsiveness of very early mother–child interaction.

Infants who developed in the direction of a false self mode have not experienced the security and mutual satisfaction of such a relationship. Such mothers are empathically out of contact with the child and react largely on the basis of their own inner fantasies, narcissistic needs, or neurotic conflicts. The child's survival depends on the capacity to adapt to this pattern of the mother's response, which is so grossly out of phase with the child's needs. This established a pattern of gradual training in compliance with whatever the mother was capable of offering, rather than seeking out and finding what is needed and wanted. Consequently, the child's needs, instinctual impulses, wishes, and initiatives, instead of becoming a meaningful guide to satisfying growth experiences and enlarging capacities to interact meaningfully with objects, become from the very beginning a threat to the harmony of the relationship with the mother, who remains unresponsive to effective feedback from the child.

Winnicott's attempts to formulate principles of treatment for such basically impaired patients built on the model of good-enough mothering. This called for a capacity for holding, for empathic responsiveness, and for a capacity for creatively playful exchange that allowed the patient's capacities for growth to emerge and flourish, permitting expansion of the patient's authentic sense of self, which remains hidden behind the external facade of false-self compliance.

ATTACHMENT THEORY

Another more recent development in the study of relationships with objects has taken the form of attachment theory. Attachment theory takes its origin in the work of John Bowlby. In his studies of infant attachment and separation, Bowlby pointed out that attachment constituted a central motivational force and that mother–child attachment was an essential medium of human interaction that had important consequences for later development and personality functioning. Attachment theorists have studied patterns of early infant attachment and related them to patterns of adult interaction with significant objects. Using the Adult Attachment Interview (AAI), developed by Mary Main and others, they document the nature of internal working models of early attachment relations. Both attachment theorists and object relations theorists emphasize the significance of the mother's empathic responsivity to infant needs for self-development and relatedness, the importance of the mother–child involvement for personality development, and the role of the mother as catalyst for age-appropriate development.

Study of infant responses in the Stranger Situation, an arrangement for observing the quality of parent–child interaction and the effects of separation, led to definition of four categories of infant behavior: secure, avoidant, resistant, and disorganized-disoriented. These patterns could be related to attachment attitudes in adults on the basis of the AAI. Secure infants were related to secure and relatively autonomous patterns of attachment and interaction in adults, avoidant infants were associated with an adult pattern of dismissing relationships as important or significant, resistant infants connected with a preoccupied adult stance in which subjects were preoccupied with past attachments often with angry or fearful emotions, and the disorganized-disoriented pattern related to an unresolved and disorganized pattern in adults suggesting more severe disturbance in self–object relations. These findings provide an extension and specification of an object relations approach as well as providing specific empirical and observational methods for more detailed study of the development of object relations from childhood to adulthood.

PSYCHOLOGY OF THE SELF

Over the last two score and more of years, the concept of the self has been emerging with increasing emphasis and definition as a central notion in the deepening psychoanalytic understanding of the organization and functioning of the human psyche. Although the concepts regarding the understanding of the self are still very much in flux, and the place of the notion of the self in psychoanalytic theory remains tentative and uncertain, the issues addressed by the psychology of the self seem to be of sufficient significance and to have gained a more or less permanent place in psychoanalytic thinking so that a consideration of these issues is warranted in this presentation.

The issues to which a self-psychology addresses itself are by no means new to psychoanalysis. Part of the problem stems from the ambiguity in Freud's use of the term *Ich*, standing ambiguously both for the ego as part of the mental apparatus, a structural agency, and for the more experiential subjective and personal sense of self. The decision of the editors of the English *Standard Edition* to translate *Ich* to the term "ego" tended to shift the meaning of the term toward the more impersonal structural sense of agency and away from the more subjective experiential implications. There are passages where it is quite clear that Freud uses the German term *selbst* as synonymous with the term *Ich*, referring to the subjectively experienced self—the person as such.

This unresolved ambiguity and the progressive shift in implications of the term *ego* have left a certain vacuum in psychoanalytic metapsychology. This deficit has been attacked by a number of thinkers as reflecting a lack of personal ego or a sense of self-as-agent in psychoanalytic theory. Partly in an attempt to deal with this issue, the notion of the self has been focused by various analytic thinkers in a variety of contexts. Kohut's development of self psychology has been a major stimulus to renewed interest in the self.

The self psychology movement came into prominence largely as the result of Kohut's efforts in the late 1960s, but there was a history of development of a self-concept in psychoanalysis well before that. Development of a concept of the self in the context of the structural theory was stimulated by Hartmann's distinction between ego and self, terms that had been left ambiguous by Freud: The ego was an intrapsychic organization of functions, whereas the self was cast in terms of a self-representation that then became the object of narcissistic libido but also was specifically connected with object relations. In these terms, the ego was related to and interactive with other intrapsychic structures, for example, superego, and the self was concerned with object relations and self–object interactions. This distinction also clarified the differentiation of object-libido and narcissistic libido because the self was the repository for secondary narcissism and, as such, distinct from the ego.

Hartmann's distinction between the ego and the self cast the self in representational terms. The self was conceptualized either as a complex representation, organized and synthesized as a function of the ego or, by later theorists, in structural terms as a more complex and supraordinate integration of the tripartite structures (that is, embracing the tripartite entities as subordinate substructures). The former view regarded the self as part of the representational world, whereas the latter assigned it to the realm of internal psychic structure. The differences of emphasis and formulation regarding these two perspectives remain a persistent problem in developing a consistent concept of the self.

Kohutian Self Psychology Self psychology, as a separate movement within psychoanalysis, takes its origin from contributions of Kohut and his followers. Kohut linked the origin of the self to narcissism, viewing the self as the result of a separate line of narcissistic development that progresses through a series of archaic narcissistic structures toward establishing a mature and cohesive self-organization.

Kohut argued that narcissism went through a separate line of development independent from object libido and object relations. In his view, the original primary narcissism differentiates in the course of development and in response to lapses in parental empathy into two archaic configurations, the grandiose self and the idealized parental imago. The *grandiose self* involves an exaggerated and exhibitionistic image of the self that becomes the repository for infantile perfection; the *idealized parental imago*, in contrast, transfers the previous perfection to an admired omnipotent object or objects. Further normal development of the grandiose self leads to more mature forms of ambition, self-esteem, self-confidence, and pleasure in accomplishment. The idealized parental imago likewise becomes integrated into the ego ideal with the mature values, ideals, and standards it represents. Pathological persistence of the grandiose self results in intensification of grandiosity, exhibitionism, shame, envy, depression, hypochondriacal concerns, and undermining of self-esteem. Loss of the idealized object or the idealized object's love can result in narcissistic imbalance, leaving the individual vulnerable to depression, depletion, poor self-esteem, failure of ideals and values, and even fragmentation.

Kohut bases his self psychology on the need, both during the course of development and during the course of life, for empathic interaction with *selfobjects*. The original selfobject is the mother or caretaking person who provides empathic response to selfobject needs in the infant in the form of love, admiration, acceptance, joyful participation, warmth, and responsiveness, communicating a sense of valued and cherished existence to the child. Human beings continue to seek objects to fulfill these basic selfobject needs throughout life. Failures to fulfill such needs can result in the formation of pathological psychic structures and patterns of behavior during development and pathological character structures during adult life. (This analysis comes close to Winnicott's views on good-enough mothering.)

Evolving Concepts of the Self The direct line of development of the notion of the self in psychoanalysis, as previously discussed, is best traced back to Hartmann's effort to clarify the ambiguity latent in Freud's use of the term *Ich*. Hartmann distinguished ego from the self by assigning the respective terms to different frames of explanatory reference. The ego referred to the specific intrapsychic agency whose frame of reference and action was within the intrapsychic structure and in relation to other intrapsychic entities, for example, superego and id. The self, in contrast, had its proper frame of reference in relationship to objects. Thus formulated, the notion of the self came to be regarded as roughly equivalent to the concept of the person as such.

In an effort to clarify the theoretical implications of the self, early thinkers, following Hartmann's lead, came to define the self in representational terms—that is, as referring to the self-representation, which was then regarded as a subordinate function of the ego. Another point of view, however, sees the self as a structural organization, either envisioned as a fourth focus of organization in addition to the tripartite entities or as a supraordinate organization, including the tripartite structures and perhaps additional structural aspects.

Part of the difficulty is that the notion of the self can be looked at from a variety of perspectives. The self can be seen as agent, or as object, or even in locational terms with respect to questions of what is inside or outside of the mind or the psychic structure and what it might mean for parts of the self to be internalized or externalized. The representational view of the self seems to lend itself most clearly to a view of the self as object, that is, as what can be cognitively and experientially grasped of the self as an object of inner experience. Such an experienced self-as-object must have representational qualities to be cognitively relevant. By the same token, the structural perspective seems to be most congruent with the view of the self-as-agent, as a source of psychic integration and activity, and as synonymous with the originating source of personal action and awareness. The structural aspect of the self-as-agent, with particular reference to its function of conscious subjectivity, comes closest to satisfying the demand for a "personal ego" in the theory.

The theory of the self remains at this juncture uncertain and very much in flux. However the ultimate conceptualization may be resolved, it seems apparent that the psychology of the self will continue to gain a permanent place in psychoanalytic thinking and theory. It is possible to specify some of the theoretical gains of the emerging role of the self-concept:

The self as a theoretical construct provides a focus for formulating and understanding the complex integrations of functional processes that involve combinations of functions of the respective component agencies. This has specific application to such complex activities as affects, in which all of the psychic systems seem to be in one way or other represented; complex superego integrations reflected in such formations as value systems; and other complex interactions of psychic systems that involve fantasy production, drive-motor integration, or cognitive-affective processes. There is room here for considerable reworking and refocusing of traditional psychoanalytic ways of looking at and understanding psychic phenomena in terms of the self as a referent system.

The self-concept provides a more specific and less ambiguous frame of reference for the articulation of self–object interrelationships and interactions, including the complex areas of object relations and internalizations.

The emergence of a self-concept provides a locus in the theory for articulating the experience of the personal self, either as grasped introspectively and reflectively or experienced as the originating source of personal activity. This sense of the self-as-subject provides a place within the theory for an account of subjectivity and subjective meaning.

This approach raises an important metapsychological issue; namely, the relationship between the experienced organization of the self and the tripartite entities. The organization of the self and the organization of structural tripartite entities cannot be simply identified. The self-organization operates at a different level of psychic organization than do the structural entities; moreover, the structural entities in the strict theoretical sense are understood to be organizations of specific functions. This concept applies not only to the ego as such but also to the superego and the id. Although the theory at various points attributes more or less personalized, anthropomorphized metaphors to the operation of these structures, their strict theoretical intelligibility is nonetheless given in terms of the organization of specific functions attributed to the respective structures.

Relational and Intersubjective Approaches These more recent approaches to understanding the analytical interaction derive from a form of constructionist epistemology in which transference was regarded as resulting from the interaction of analyst and patient. This constructivist view contrasts with the more objectivist view of ego psychology and object relations. The analyst's attention is focused on the here-and-now interaction with the patient rather than on the inner dynamics of the patient's mental life and experience. This effects a shift from a one-person to a two-person psychology in which the ongoing interactions, whether conscious or unconscious, between the participants are central, and transference and countertransference are regarded as mutually cocreated by both.

This approach was further developed into a view of analytical interaction in intersubjective and relational terms. The self psychological emphasis on self–selfobject transference has encouraged movement away from considerations of the analyst's stance as neutral or observational, questioning the analyst's subjectivity, authority, and capacity to know any objective reality about the patient. On these terms, personality development is dependent on the interpersonal field insofar as psychic life is continually being remodeled in terms of both past and present relationships and not determined by fixed patterns deriving from past unconscious conflicts. The concept of personality as developing within a relational matrix calls for a central focus on the intersubjective field within the relationship between analyst and patient. It is this aspect of the analytical situation that is explored and interpreted in the interest of bringing about personal growth in the patient. The analyst's technical neutrality and objectivity are rejected in this approach as illusory and little more than expressions of the analyst's authoritarian position. Within a self–selfobject or intersubjective relation, neutrality is precluded as potentially traumatizing and destructive to potential consolidation of the self. An inevitable consequence of these approaches is that they do away with the traditional notion of the unconscious and undercut any sense of transference as reflecting unconscious aspects of the patient's inner psychic life because transference is created anew in the present analytical interaction.

Psychology of Character

The development of the concept of character in psychoanalysis has drawn increasingly closer to the issues that are latent in a psychology of the self. Character has come to stand for a unique combination of the components of the individual's psychic organization that reflects the basic elements of that person's personality organization and style. The implications of the concept of character, then, lie much closer to the framework of the personality functioning as a whole, rather than to specific psychic agencies.

The concept of character can vary widely in meaning, depending on whether it is used in a moralistic, sociological, or general sense. Application of the concept in psychoanalysis has remained restrictive despite the fact that theoretical propositions concerning the meaning of character have undergone an evolution that parallels the evolution in psychoanalytic theory, particularly in the theory of the ego. During the period when Freud was developing his ego theory, he noted the relationship between certain character traits and particular psychosexual components. For example, he recognized that obstinacy, orderliness, and parsimoniousness were associated with anality. He noted that ambition was related to urethral eroticism and that generosity was related to orality. He concluded, in his paper on "Character and Anal Eroticism," that permanent character traits represented "unchanged prolongations of the original instincts, or sublimation of those instincts, or reaction-formations against them."

In 1913, Freud made an important distinction between neurotic symptoms and character traits: Neurotic symptoms come into being as a result of failure of repression, the return of the repressed; character traits owe their existence to the success of repression or, more accurately, of the defense system, which achieves its aim through a persistent pattern of reaction formation and sublimation. Later, in 1923, with increased understanding of the phenomenon of identification and the formulation of the ego as a coherent system of functions, the relationship of character to ego development came into sharper focus. At this point, Freud observed that the replacement of object attachment by identification (introjection), which set up the lost object inside the ego, also made a significant contribution to character formation. A decade later, in 1932, Freud emphasized the particular importance of identification (introjection) with the parents for the construction of character, particularly with reference to superego formation.

Several of Freud's disciples made important contributions to the concept of character during this period. A major share of Karl Abraham's efforts were devoted to the investigation and elucidation of the relationship between oral, anal, and genital eroticism and various character traits. Wilhelm Reich made an important contribution to the psychoanalytic understanding of character when he described the intimate relationship between resistance in treatment and character traits of the patient's personality. Reich's observation that resistance typically appeared in the form of these specific traits anticipated Anna Freud's later formulation concerning the relationship between resistances and typical ego defenses.

The development of psychoanalytic ego psychology has led to an increasing tendency to include character traits among the properties of the ego, superego, and ego-ideal. It should be noted, however, that character is not synonymous with any of these properties. Concomitantly, the emphasis has been extended from an interest in specific character traits to a consideration of character and its formation in general. Psychoanalysis has come to regard character as the pattern of adaptation to instinctual and environmental forces, which is typical or habitual for a given individual. The character of a person is distinguished from the ego by virtue of the fact that it refers largely to directly observable behavior and styles of defense, as well as of acting, thinking, and feeling. The clinical value of the concept of character has been recognized by psychiatrists and psychoanalysts and has become a meeting ground for the two disciplines.

The formation of character and character traits results from the interplay of multiple factors. Innate biological predispositions play a role in character formation in both its instinctual and ego fundaments. The interactions of id forces with early ego defenses and with environmental influences, particularly the parents, constitute the major determinants in the development of character. Various early identifications and imitations of objects leave their lasting stamp on character formation.

The degree to which the ego has developed a capacity to tolerate delay in drive discharge and to neutralize instinctual energies, as a result of early identifications and defense formation, determines the later emergence of such character traits as impulsiveness. Finally, a number of authors have stressed the particularly close association between character traits and the development of the ego-ideal. The development of the ego-ideal must be understood in the context of the developmental vicissitudes of narcissism. It is in this respect that the psychoanalytic concept of character begins to parallel the more common use of the term *character* in a somewhat moral sense. The exaggerated development of certain character traits at the expense of others may lead to character disorders later in life. At other times, such distortions in the development of character traits can produce a vulnerability in personality organization or a predisposition to psychotic decompensation.

CLASSIC PSYCHOANALYTIC TREATMENT

Certain aspects of the therapeutic technique that Freud developed and that were later expanded by his followers are closely related with psychoanalytic theory. One of the distinctive aspects of the psychoanalytic approach to treatment in general is its consistent attempt to integrate therapeutic usages and approaches with the understanding of psychic functioning available from psychoanalytic theory. In its origins and clinical application, psychoanalysis is uniquely a theory of therapy.

Analysis versus Analytical Psychotherapy

One of the chronically recurring issues among analysts is whether and to what extent psychoanalysis is distinguishable from psychotherapy. There are distinguishing features between them as more or less pure forms: the use of couch in analysis, not in therapy; free association as a primary method in analysis, not in therapy; intensive and long-term scheduling in analysis, not in therapy; emphasis on neutrality, abstinence, and interpretation on the part of the analyst in analysis, not in therapy; and the central focus on transference and countertransference in analysis, not in therapy. Over the years, however, forms of psychotherapy have evolved modifying all of these criteria and resulting in a spectrum of psychotherapeutic interventions, ranging from psychoanalysis at one end to diluted forms of supportive psychotherapy at the other. The distinction between explorative versus supportive therapy parallels this continuum so that many variants of the analytical process have arisen in which both components are used in varying degrees. Some of this variation has come about by reason of the expansion of analytical techniques to the widening scope of psychopathology and the corresponding challenge of adapting analytical techniques to these patient needs. Another factor, however, has been the rejection of traditional analytical approaches and methods accompanying rejection of more traditional analytical theories. One conclusion is that better means for determining what patients are better served by what forms of therapy needs to be developed.

Analytical Process Some of the origins of Freud's approach to treatment have been considered, particularly in the development of his basic techniques of free association and in his growing awareness and interpretation of the transference. In essence, modern psychoanalytic treatment procedures differ from those that Freud originally developed in one fundamental respect. Early in his approach to therapy, Freud believed that recognition by the physician of the patient's unconscious motivations, the communication of this knowledge to the patient, and its comprehension by the patient would of itself effect a cure. This was his basic doctrine of therapeutic insight. Further clinical experience, however, has demonstrated the fallacy of these expectations.

Specifically, Freud found that his discovery of the patient's unconscious wishes and his ability to impart these findings to the patient so that they were accepted and understood were insufficient. Such insight might permit clarification of the patient's intellectual appraisal of problems, but the emotional tensions for which the patient sought treatment were not effectively alleviated in this way. This discovery led to a significant breakthrough. Freud began to realize that the success of treatment depended on the patient's ability to understand the emotional significance of an experience on an emotional level and depended on the patient's capacity to retain and use that insight. In that event, if the experience recurred, it elicited another reaction; it was longer repressed, and the patient would have undergone a psychic economic change. Freud's formula for this process was: "Where id was, there ego shall be."

Freud thus elaborated a treatment method that attached minimal importance to the immediate relief of symptoms, to moral support from the therapist, or to guidance. The goal of psychoanalysis was to pull the neurosis out by its roots, rather than to prune off the top. To accomplish this, it was necessary to break down the pregenital, deep crystallization of id, ego, and superego and bring underlying material near enough to the surface of consciousness so that it could be modified and reevaluated in light of reality. This method distinguishes the classic psychological treatment from more psychodynamic forms of psychotherapy.

The patient is unaware of the repression of the forces of conflict and the psychic mechanisms of defense the mind uses. By isolating the basic problem, the patient has protected her- or himself against what seems, from the patient's view, to be unbearable suffering. No matter how it may impair functioning, the neurosis seems somehow preferable to the emergence of unacceptable wishes and ideas. All the forces that permitted the original repression are thus mobilized once again in the analysis as a resistance to this threatened encroachment on dangerous territory. No matter how much the patient may cooperate consciously with the therapist in the analysis, and no matter how painful the neurotic symptoms may be, the patient automatically defends against reopening of old wounds with every subtle resource of defense and resistance available.

In discussing the analytical process, one must clarify the basic distinction between the analytical process and the analytical situation. The *analytical process* refers to the regressive emergence, working through, interpretation, and resolution of the transference neurosis. The *analytical situation*, however, refers to the setting in which the analytical process takes place, specifically the collaborative relationship between patient and analyst based on the therapeutic alliance.

The regression induced by the analytical situation (instinctual regression) allows for a reemergence of infantile conflicts and thus induces formation of a transference neurosis. In the classic transference neurosis, the original infantile conflicts and wishes become focused on the person of the analyst and are thus reexperienced and relived. In the analytical regression, earlier infantile conflicts are revived and can be seen as a manifestation of the repetition compulsion. Regression has a dual aspect; from one point of view, it is an attempt to return to an earlier state of real or fantasy gratification, but from another point of view, it can be seen as an attempt to master previous traumatic experience. The regression in the analytical situation and the development of transference are preliminary conditions for the mastery of unresolved conflicts. They can also represent regressive and unconscious wishes to return to an earlier state of narcissistic gratification. The analytical process must work itself out in the face of this dual potentiality and tension.

If the analytical regression has a destructive potentiality (ego regression) that must be recognized and guarded against, it also has a progressive potentiality for reopening and reworking infantile conflicts and for achieving a reorganization and consolidation of the personality on a more mature and healthier level. As in any developmental crisis, the risk of regressive deterioration must be balanced against the promise of progressive growth and mastery. The therapeutic importance of the criteria of analyzability can be easily recognized because patients who are unable to achieve the progressive potentiality of the analytical regression cannot be expected to realize a good therapeutic result. The determining element within the analytical situation against which the regression must be balanced and by which the destructive or constructive potential of the regression can be measured is the therapeutic alliance. A firm and stable alliance offers a buffer against excessive (ego) regression and also offers a basis for positive growth.

The Analytical Relation The analytical or therapeutic relation is compounded of at least three components that are coexistent, mutually interacting and influencing, and intermingled at all points in the analytical process. Although constantly interacting to influence the patterns of interaction between analyst and patient and determining the course of the analytical process, they can be usefully distinguished in that they point to differentiable issues and aspects of the therapeutic process and call for different therapeutic responses and interventions. They are the transference and countertransference, the therapeutic alliance, and the real relation.

TRANSFERENCE Through free association, hidden patterns of the patient's mental organization that may be fixated at immature levels and refer to events or fantasies in the patient's private experience are brought to life and activated in the relation with the analyst. In the simplest model of transference, the analyst is gradually invested with emotions usually associated with significant figures in the past. The patient displaces or projects feelings originally directed toward these earlier objects onto the analyst, who then becomes alternately a friend or enemy, one who is nice or frustrates needs and punishes, or one who is loved or hated as the original objects were loved or hated. Moreover, this tendency persists so that, to an increasing extent, the patient's feelings toward the analyst replicate feelings toward the specific people being talked about or, more accurately, those about whom the patient's unconscious is talking. This transference object acts as a lens through which the patient views the analyst, seeing him or her in the image of the transference representation.

As unresolved childhood attitudes and feelings emerge and begin to function as fantasized projections toward the analyst, he or she becomes for the patient a phantom composite figure representing various important people in the patient's early environment or objects represented in his or her inner world. Those earlier relationships are reactivated with some of their original affective vigor, thus exposing in some degree the roots of the patient's disturbance. The concept of transference has undergone considerable elaboration over time, resulting in multiple variants, broadening its connotations to include every emotional connection to the analyst, and extending the transference model to encompass the widening range of psychopathology addressed by psychoanalysis. Variations in transference and their descriptions are contained in Table 6.1–5. Understanding transferences requires some exploration of mechanisms involved in their formation and their dynamic interactions. The basic mechanisms by which transferences are effected—displacement, projection, and projective identification—are described in Table 6.1–6.

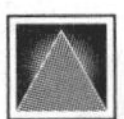

Table 6.1–5
Transference Variants

Libidinal transferences

Follow the classic model and usually in milder forms as positive *transference reactions* but can take the form of more intense and disturbing *erotic transferences.* They are derivatives of phallic-oedipal, libidinal impulses and may be permeated variously by pregenital influences. They may occur with varying degrees of intensity and in mild forms may not even require interpretation if they contribute to and support the therapeutic relation. Sigmund Freud recommended that they call for interpretation only when they begin to serve as a resistance.

Aggressive transferences

Take the form either of negative or more pathological paranoid transferences. *Negative transferences* are seen at all levels of psychopathology but may predominate in some borderline patients who tend to see the therapeutic relationship in terms of power and victimization, regarding the therapist as omnipotent and powerful, whereas the patient experiences him- or herself as helpless, weak, and vulnerable. However, negative transferences are identifiable in varying degrees in all analyses and usually require specific intervention and interpretation.

Transferences of defense

Opposed to *transferences of impulse*; defense against impulses finds its way into the transference rather than the impulses themselves. In this form of transference, attention shifts from drives to the ego's defensive functioning so that transference is no longer merely repetition of instinctual cathexes but includes aspects of ego functioning as well.

Transference neurosis

Involves the re-creation or more ample expression of the patient's neurosis enacted anew within the analytical relation and at least theoretically mirroring aspects of the infantile neurosis. The transference neurosis usually develops in the middle phase of analysis, when the patient, at first eager for improved mental health, no longer consistently displays such motivation but engages in a continuing battle with the analyst over the desire to attain some kind of emotional satisfaction from the analyst so that this becomes the most compelling reason for continuing analysis. At this point of the treatment, the transference emotions become more important to the patient than alleviation of distress sought initially, and the major, unresolved, unconscious problems of childhood begin to dominate the patient's behavior. They are now reproduced in the transference, with all their pent-up emotion.

The transference neurosis is governed by three outstanding characteristics of instinctual life in early childhood: the pleasure principle (before effective reality testing), ambivalence, and repetition compulsion. Emergence of the transference neurosis is usually a slow and gradual process, although in certain patients with a propensity for *transference regression*, particularly more hysterical patients, elements of transference and transference neurosis may manifest themselves relatively early in the analytical process. One situation after another in the life of the patient is analyzed and progressively interpreted until the original infantile conflict is sufficiently revealed. Only then does the transference neurosis begin to subside. At that point, termination begins to emerge as a more central concern.

Contemporary opinion is divided as to its importance and centrality, whether it forms to the extent Freud believed, and whether it is necessary for successful analysis—for some, it remains an essential vehicle for analytical interpretation and therapeutic effectiveness; for others, it may never develop or, to the extent that it does, may play a less central role in the process of cure.

Transference psychosis

Occurs when failure of reality testing leads to loss of self–object differentiation and diffusion of self and object boundaries. This may reflect an attempt to re-fuse with an omnipotent object, investing the self with omnipotent powers as defense against underlying fears of vulnerability and powerlessness. Transference psychosis may also include negative transference elements in which fusion carries the threat of engulfment and loss of self that may precipitate a *paranoid transference reaction.*

Narcissistic transferences

Clarified by Heinz Kohut (1971) as variations of patterns of projection of archaic narcissistic configurations onto the therapist. They are based on projections of narcissistic introjective configurations, both superior and inferior—the superior form reflecting narcissistic superiority, grandiosity, and enhanced self-esteem, and the inferior opposite qualities of inferiority, self-depletion, and diminished self-esteem. The therapist comes to represent, in Kohut's terms, either the grandiose self in *mirror transferences* or the idealized parental imago in *idealizing transferences.* In idealizing transferences, all power and strength are attributed to the idealized object, leaving the subject feeling empty and powerless when separated from that object. Union with the idealized object enables the subject to regain narcissistic equilibrium. Idealizing transferences may reflect developmental disturbances in the idealized parent imago, particularly at the time of formation of the ego ideal by introjection of the idealized object. In some individuals, narcissistic fixation leads to development of the grandiose self. Reactivation in analysis of the grandiose self provides the basis for formation of mirror transferences, which occur in three forms: *archaic merger transference,* a less archaic *alter-ego* or *twinship transference,* and *mirror transference in the narrow sense.* In the most primitive merger transference, the analyst is experienced only as an extension of the subject's grandiose self and, thus, becomes the repository of the patient's grandiosity and exhibitionism. In the alter-ego or twinship transference, activation of the grandiose self leads to experience of the narcissistic object as similar to the grandiose self. In the most mature form of mirror transference, the analyst is experienced as a separate person but, nonetheless, one who becomes important to the patient and is accepted by him or her only to the degree that he or she is responsive to the narcissistic needs of the reactivated grandiose self.

Selfobject transferences

Represent extensions of the self-psychology paradigm beyond merely narcissistic configurations. The selfobject involves investment of the self in the object so that the object comes to serve a self-sustaining function that the self cannot perform for itself—either in maintaining fragile self-cohesion or in regulating self-esteem. The other is, thus, not experienced as an autonomous and separate object or agency in its own right but as present only to serve the needs of the self. Transference in this sense reflects a continuing developmental need that seeks satisfaction in the analytical relation.

(*continued*)

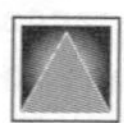

Table 6.1–5 (*continued*)

Selfobject transferences reflect the underlying need structure the patient brings to the therapeutic relationship based on the predominant pattern of selfobject deprivation or frustration and the corresponding seeking for the appropriate form of selfobject involvement. These configurations have been described as the *understimulated self*, the *overstimulated self*, the *overburdened self*, and the *fragmenting self*. Other descriptions of selfobject need translate patterns of transference interaction based on narcissistic dynamics into the perspective of the relationship between self and selfobject, as in mirror-hungry personalities and ideal-hungry personalities. Variations on the mirroring transference theme include the alter-ego–hungry personality, the merger-hungry personality, and, in contrast, the contact-shunning personality. In transferences derived from such personality configurations, the classic meaning of transference has undergone radical modification. Rather than displacements or projections from earlier object relational contexts, the patient brings to bear a need based in his or her own currently deficient capacity and defective character structure—a need to involve the object in a dependent relationship to complete or stabilize his or her own psychic integration.

Transitional relatedness

This transference model is based on Donald Winnicott's notion of the transitional object. Transference in more primitive character structures is regarded as a form of *transitional object relation* in which the therapist is perceived as outside the self but is invested with qualities from the patient's own archaic self-image. The transference field in this view is envisioned as a transitional space in which the transference illusion is allowed to play itself out.

Transference as psychic reality

Reflects the need of each participant in analysis to draw the other into a stance corresponding to his or her own intrapsychic configuration and needs as a reflection of the individual subject's psychic reality. This regards the classic view of transference, based on displacement or projection from past objects, as inadequate, resulting in further diffusion of meaning of transference as equivalent to the individual's capacity to create a meaningful world or to inform the world with meaning. In this rendition, transference becomes equivalent to the patient's psychic reality so that any distinction between the meanings given to reality and the meanings inherent in transference are lost. Transference in these terms becomes all-encompassing, and whatever distinguishing and dynamic significance it may have had fades into obscurity. In this form of transference, there does not seem to be any definable mechanism at work other than whatever is involved in the subject's psychic reality. The subject's view of his or her environment and his or her impression of objects of his or her experience, including the analytical object, are indistinguishable from ordinary cognitive and affective processes characterizing his or her involvement and responsiveness to the world about him or her.

Transference as relational or intersubjective

The relational or intersubjective view of transference as emerging from or cocreated by the subjective interaction between analyst and analysand transforms transference into an interactive phenomenon in which individual intrapsychic contributions from either participant are obscured. Transference in this sense is not anything individual to or intrapsychically derived from the patient but is based on the present ongoing interaction between analyst and patient coconstructing transference. On these terms, analysis of transference has little to do with past derivatives and everything to do with the ongoing relation with the analyst, primarily in the form of interpersonal enactments. Transference in this sense is no longer a one-person phenomenon but reflects a two-person transference–countertransference interaction. The supposition is that there is no such thing as transference without countertransference and no such thing as countertransference without transference. The patient is thus relieved of any burden of a personal dynamic unconscious reflecting developmental vicissitudes and residues of a life history. Transference is created anew in the immediacy of present analytical interaction as the product of mutual influence and communication between analyst and analysand, probably relying on some form of mutual projective identification to sustain the interactive connotation.

COUNTERTRANSFERENCE If the patient is capable of transference in the analytical interaction, the analyst is correspondingly capable of countertransference, meaning that the analyst engages in the interaction with his or her own burden of elements coming from his or her own developmental past or elements that may be activated in the course of his or her interaction with the patient, especially in response to the patient's transference. Originally, countertransference was a matter of a response in the analyst's unconscious affecting his or her view of and reaction to the patient, but recent views tend to see it as encompassing the total affective response of the analyst to the patient, whether conscious or unconscious, and as reflecting more responses aroused in the present interaction with the patient than influences coming from the analyst's past experience or unconscious.

When patient transference and analyst countertransference are caught up in an interaction, the result is a transference–countertransference interaction. Early views of countertransference saw it as interfering in the work of the analysis, as it may often do, but recent revisions have emphasized the contributions to more effective analytical work arising from attention to and use of countertransference responses in the course of an analysis. Countertransference has thus become regarded as inevitable and not necessarily destructive to the analytical process. The author's opinion is that it is useful insofar as it reveals unconscious factors that would otherwise remain hidden but that therapeutic application and effect cannot be achieved through countertransference as such but only through the effective use made of it from the vantage point provided through the therapeutic alliance. If the therapist finds him- or herself annoyed at a patient, it is not therapeutically useful to express or act out the annoyance on the patient. Rather, it is useful to analyze the sources of the anger in his or her past experience and find a constructive way to deal with it in relation to the patient.

THERAPEUTIC ALLIANCE The therapeutic alliance is based on the one-to-one collaborative relationship that the patient establishes in interaction with the analyst. This interaction deals with those aspects of the therapeutic relation that enable patient and analyst to engage meaningfully and productively in the analytical process with the objective of achieving therapeutic benefit for the patient. The terms of the alliance are negotiated between analyst and patient; obviously, not any terms of their working together do but only those that can predictably contribute to or set the stage for their effectively working together. The alliance on these terms includes at least the following elements: empathy, trust, autonomy, responsibility, authority, freedom, honesty, and neutrality. All these elements are as pertinent to the role of the patient in analysis as to the analyst.

The therapeutic alliance allows a split to take place in the patient's ego—that is, the observing part of the patient's ego can ally itself with the analyst in a working relationship, which allows it to gradually identify positively with the analyst in analyzing and modifying pathological defenses put up by the defensive ego against internal danger situations. Maintenance of this therapeutic split, as well as the relationship to the analyst involved in the therapeutic alliance, requires maintenance of self–object differentiation, tolerance and mastery of ambivalence, and the capacity to distinguish fantasy from reality in the relationship. In many analyses, consequently, the alliance requires work and effort to establish and can thus serve as one of the objectives of the analytical work. In no case can the alliance be taken for granted

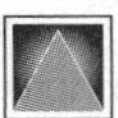

Table 6.1–6
Transference Mechanisms

Displacement

The basic mechanism of classic transference paradigms in which an object representation derived from any level or combination of levels of the subject's developmental experience is displaced to the representation of the new object, namely, the analyst, in the therapeutic relationship. Displacement is the basic mechanism for libidinally based transferences, both positive and erotic, as well as for aggressive and especially negative transferences. By and large, displacement transferences tend to play a more dominant role in neurotic disorders in which phallic-oedipal (and to a lesser degree pre-oedipal) dynamics tend to play a dominant, although not exclusive, role.

Projection

Process by which qualities or characteristics of the self-as-object, usually involving introjections or self-representations, are attributed to an external object, and the subsequent interaction with the object is determined by the projected characteristics. Thus, the analyst/object may be seen as sadistic—that is, as possessing the sadistic character of the analysand/subject, an aspect of the subject's self that is denied or disowned by the subject. Projection tends to play a more prominent, although again not exclusive, role in formation of transferences in more primitive character disorders but can be found in variously modified forms throughout the spectrum of neuroses. Because projections derive primarily from the configuration of introjects constituting the patient's self-as-object, the effect of projective or externalizing transferences is that the image of the therapist comes to represent part of the patient's own self-organization rather than simply an object representation.

Projections derived from destructive introjects can provide the basis for both negative and paranoid transference reactions. Those based on the victim/introject result in the patient relating to the therapist as his or her victim and him- or herself assuming a hostile or sadistic position as a destructive aggressor or victimizer to the therapist's victim. Then again, projection based on the aggressor/introject results in the patient relating to the therapist as an aggressor and him- or herself assuming a weak, vulnerable, or masochistic position in which he or she becomes a passive and vulnerable victim to the therapist's destructive aggression. Similar patterns can take place around narcissistic issues involving introjective configurations of narcissistic superiority and inferiority.

However, projective dynamics in selfobject transferences seem to involve more than narcissistic projections because these forms of transference tend to draw the analyst into meeting the pathological needs of the self. If anything is projected, it is an infantile wished-for imago, one lacking earlier in the patient's experience, as, for example, an empathic and idealized parental figure. On the other hand, transitional transferences, despite their considerable overlap with selfobject phenomena, tend to involve a more explicit projective element as the self-related contribution to the transitional experience.

Projective identification

The concept of projective identification was first proposed by Melanie Klein, arguing that the projection of impulses or feelings into another person brought about an identification with that person based on attribution of one's own qualities to that other. This attribution served as the basis for a sense of empathy and connection with the other. On these terms, projective identification was a fantasy taking place solely in the mind of the one projecting.

Projective identification is often appealed to as a mechanism of transference, or more exactly transference–countertransference interactions, particularly in Kleinian usage. Confusion arises from the failure to clearly distinguish between projection and projective identification. The notion of projective identification added to the basic concept of projection the notes of diffusion of ego boundaries, a loss or diminishing of self–object differentiation, and inclusion of the object as part of the self.

Later elaborations of the notion of projective identification transformed it from a one-body to a two-body phenomenon, describing interaction between two subjects, one of whom projects something onto or into the other, whereon the other introjects or internalizes what has been projected. Instead of the projection and introjection taking place in the same subject, the projection now takes place in one and the internalization in the other. This latter usage has led to extensive extrapolation of the concept of projective identification to apply to object relations of all sorts, including transference. The emphasis in Kleinian transference is less on the influence of the past on the present but rather the influence of the internal world on the external in the here-and-now interaction with the analyst.

or assumed because the propensity of all patients to create various subtle forms of misalliance is pervasive. If they are not carefully looked for and attuned to, such misalliances can easily distort the course of an analysis and only become apparent when they reach a point of crisis or impasse. In more severely disturbed personalities, there is a greater tendency to disruptions of the alliance rather than misalliances, which can destroy an analytical process and often require extreme efforts to salvage the therapy.

Maintenance of the therapeutic alliance requires that the patient be able to differentiate between the more mature and the more infantile aspects of the experience in relationship to the analyst. The therapeutic alliance serves a double function. On one hand, it acts as a significant barrier to excessive regression of the ego in the analytical process; on the other hand, it serves as a fundamental aspect of the analytical situation, against which the wishes, feelings, and fantasies evoked by the transference neurosis can be evaluated, measured, and interpreted. In many pathological conditions—some character neuroses, borderline personalities, and more severe neurotic disorders—it may be difficult to maintain a clinical distinction between therapeutic alliance and the transference neurosis.

The therapeutic alliance derives from the mobilization of specific ego resources relating to the capacity for object relations and reality testing. The analyst must direct attention toward eliciting the patient's capacity to establish such a relationship that is able to withstand the inevitable distortions and regressive aspects of the transference neurosis. It is inevitable that the fundamental features of the therapeutic alliance be carefully evaluated and understood and ultimately integrated with the analysis of the transference neurosis. This point is particularly and graphically displayed in the analysis of hysterical patients. The initial transference neurosis of such patients tends to present primarily oedipal material, but analysts have learned to appreciate the importance of underlying oral factors in the genesis of many hysterical disorders. In the terminal stages of analysis of these patients, it becomes increasingly clear that resolution of oedipal conflicts depends on the successful analysis of earlier conflicts stemming from the pregenital level of development. Specifically involved are conflicts, usually on an oral level, that are related to achieving early object relations and the acceptance of reality and its limitations. These elements, however, are specifically those that form the developmental basis of the therapeutic alliance.

REAL RELATION Reality pervades the analytical relationship. On one hand, there is the reality of the personalities and characteristics of analyst and analysand; on the other, there are the realities of time, place, and circumstance external to the analytical setting but constantly influencing the course of the analytical relation. These include realities of the location of the analyst's office, the physical surroundings, the furniture and decorations in the room, the geographical location itself, and even how the analyst dresses; they all have their effects in the analytical situation and influence how the patient experiences the person of the analyst. The surrounding circumstances that create the framework for the analytical effort—the patient's financial situation, marital status, and job demands; arrangements for payment of the fee; whether the patient has insurance and what kind; what kinds of pressures are pushing the patient into treatment; accidental factors such as illness, interfering obligations—are reality factors extrinsic to the analysis but exercising significant influence on the analytical relationship and how it is established and maintained.

The most important and central reality for the patient is the person of the analyst. Every analyst has his or her own constellation of personal characteristics, including mannerisms, style of behavior and speech, habits of dress, gender, way of going about the task of managing the therapeutic situation, attitudes toward the patient as a human being, prejudices, moral and political views, and personal beliefs and values. These are all relevant aspects of one's real existence and personality as a human being. They are realities that play a role in the therapeutic relationship and are entirely distinct from transference and countertransference. In terms of the analytical process, none of this is lost on the patient who is comprehensively observant of and sensitive to the smallest details of the analyst's real person. The same considerations operate from the side of the analyst in relation to the patient.

Technical Aspects The analytical technique is always adapted to the idiosyncrasies of the patient's developmental capacities, needs, and defensive constellation. Analytical techniques do not stand in isolation but are part of a living, dynamic process that is intended to induce and achieve significant internal psychic growth.

FREE ASSOCIATION The cornerstone of the psychoanalytic technique is free association. The patient is encouraged to use this method as far as possible throughout the treatment. The primary function of free association, besides obviously providing content for the analysis, is to help to induce the necessary regression and relatively passive dependence connected with establishing and working through the transference neurosis. Thus, free association is conjoined with the other techniques that induce such regression, namely, lying on the couch, not being able to see the analyst, and conducting the analysis in an atmosphere of quiet and restful tranquility.

One also cannot simply regard the process of free association as something that takes place in isolation in the patient. In fact, the process is more complex, more difficult to conceptualize, and increasingly must be seen in the context of and in reference to the more fundamental relationship between analyst and patient. The patient's free associating is a function of the more basic relationship. Moreover, it is increasingly clear from a contemporary perspective that much more is required of a patient than simply free associating. It is not enough for the patient to lay back and allow self-surrender to a position of passive dependency within the analytical relationship without at the same time being able to mobilize basic ego resources in the service of mastery, gaining insight, mobilizing executive and synthetic capacities, and, ultimately, being able to assume a less passive and more active and autonomous function within the analytical relationship. Obviously, there is a gradation in the mobilization of these capacities in the patient, which varies from phase to phase of the analytical process.

RESISTANCE The most conscientious efforts on the part of the patient to say everything that comes to mind are never completely successful. No matter how willing and cooperative the patient may be in attempting to free associate, the signs of resistance are apparent throughout the course of every analysis. The patient pauses abruptly, corrects him- or herself, makes a slip of the tongue, stammers, remains silent, fidgets with some part of clothing, asks irrelevant questions, intellectualizes, arrives late for appointments, finds excuses for not keeping them, offers critical evaluations of the rationale underlying the treatment method, simply cannot think of anything to say, or even censors thoughts that do occur and decides that they are banal or uninteresting or irrelevant and not worth mentioning.

The development of resistance in the analysis is quite as automatic and independent of the patient's will as the development of the transference itself. The sources of resistance are just as unconscious as sources of transference. The emotional forces, however, that give rise to resistance usually are defending against those producing the transference. Thus, resistances tend to emerge more in the middle phase of the analysis, in which regressive emergence of the transference is a central concern. The analysis becomes a recurring field of conflict between the tendencies toward transference and those toward resistance, manifested by the involuntary inhibition of the patient's efforts to associate freely. This inhibition may last for moments or days or may persist through the whole course of the analysis.

Resistance may take place in all phases of the analysis, but its quality and significance are different depending on the analytical task at hand. In any case, the patient's resistance enables the analyst to evaluate and become familiar with the defensive organization of the patient's ego. In this way, the pattern of resistance not only offers valuable information to the analyst but also offers a channel by which the patient can be approached therapeutically.

The significance of this basic conflict is clear. It is a repetition of the very same sexuality–guilt conflict that originally produced the neurosis itself. Transference itself may be a form of resistance, in that the wish for immediate gratification in the analysis can circumvent and postpone essential goals of treatment. Consequently, the analysis of resistance, particularly transference resistance, is one of the analyst's primary functions. It also accounts in many cases for the extended time period required for successful psychoanalytic treatment. No matter how skillful the analyst, resistance is never absent.

In the light of relational and intersubjective perspectives on the analytical process, the concept of resistance has fallen out of favor in that any such phenomenon is a byproduct of the interaction between analyst and patient. There is, then, no resistance coming from the patient but rather is contributed by both participants. Resistance can only be dealt with by examining the interaction causing it and not by interpretation of the patient's defenses. This point of view remains highly controversial.

INTERPRETATION Interpretation is the chief tool of the analyst in efforts to reduce unconscious resistance. As mentioned earlier, in the early stages of the development of psychoanalytic therapeutic techniques, the sole purpose of interpretation was to inform the patient of his or her unconscious wishes. Later, it was designed to help the patient understand the resistance to spontaneous self-awareness. In current psychoanalytic practice, the analyst's function as interpreter is not limited to simply paraphrasing the patient's verbal reports but, rather, to indicating at appropriate moments what is not reported or is implicit in what is reported. Consequently, as a general rule, analytical interpretation does not produce immediate symptomatic relief. On the contrary, there may be a heightening of anxiety and an emergence of further resistance.

If a correct interpretation is given at the proper time (mutative interpretation), the patient may react either immediately or after a period of emotional struggle during which new associations are offered. These new associations often confirm the validity of previous interpretations and add significant additional data, thus disclosing motivations and experiences of the patient of which the analyst could not previously have been aware. Generally speaking, it is not so much the analyst's insight into the patient's psychodynamics that produces progress in the analysis as it is the patient's ability to gain this insight independently; the analyst can facilitate this process by reducing unconscious resistance to such self-awareness through appropriate, carefully timed interpretation. The most effective interpretation is timed so that it is given by the analyst in such a way as to meet the emerging, if hesitant and half formed, awareness of the patient. Thus, the analyst must gauge the capacity of the patient at any given moment to hear, assimilate, and integrate the content of a given interpretation.

Another important aspect of interpretations is that they cannot be seen in isolation from the total context of the analytic situation and the analytic process. An interpretation, both as given by the analyst and as received by the patient—and that includes elements of both transference neurosis and therapeutic alliance—takes place within the context of the therapeutic relationship. Thus, the giving and receiving of interpretations are cloaked with a series of meanings that unavoidably influence both the capacity of the patient to accept and integrate interpretations and the analyst's sense of offering and providing such interpretations. Experience has shown that, at best, the therapeutic benefits produced by virtue of the analyst's exhortations or unilaterally provided insights are only temporary. Those interpretations are most effective and of lasting therapeutic value that are arrived at by the delicate dialectic arising from the mutually facilitated and growing awareness of both patient and analyst.

MODIFICATIONS IN TECHNIQUES There are no shortcuts in psychoanalytic treatment. Psychoanalytic treatment typically extends over a period of years and requires interminable patience on the part of both analyst and patient. Rigid adherence, however, to the fundamental principles of psychoanalytic technique is an impossibility. For example, the immediate environmental situation may be so serious for the patient that the analyst must pay commonsense attention to its practical implications. Those patients whose early childhood was extraordinarily deficient in love and affection so that they have a basic developmental defect in their capacity for one-to-one relationship and, consequently, in their capacity to sustain a therapeutic alliance must be given more support and encouragement than usually advocated by strict psychoanalytic technique.

The analyst's role in the early stages of analysis in helping to establish the therapeutic alliance is of particular importance. As noted, with the primitive patients, the establishing of a therapeutic alliance can be the more significant aspect of the treatment process and can even persist as a problem through most of the analysis. Even so, establishing the therapeutic alliance for most patients is a significant aspect of the analytic process.

The nature and the degree of the analyst's active intervention in the opening hours of analysis are still matters of considerable discussion and controversy. The transference neurosis usually develops only gradually, so that attempts at premature interpretation in the early hours may not be productive and may even be counterproductive. This has tended to foster the use of prolonged silences, lack of responsiveness, rigidity, and relative lack of participation in the analysis on the part of the analyst, as if any reference to the analytic situation or to the person of the analyst or to the patient's feelings about the analyst was to be taken as contrary to developing a transference interpretation and, thus, to be avoided. Often, however, serious problems in the subsequent stages of analysis of the transference can be due to a failure to establish a meaningful alliance in the initial stages of treatment. Thus, suitable interventions of the analyst in the early stages of treatment can help the patient in establishing such a meaningful therapeutic alliance.

Patients who are more borderline or very narcissistic must establish a strong personal tie and strong feelings of attachment and relationship with the analyst before they can develop sufficient interest and motivation for treatment. Moreover, such a strong object tie with the analyst for these more primitive patients is an absolute necessity if the destructive effects of excessive regression are to be avoided. Development of sufficient trust is also essential for these patients if they are to establish any meaningful alliance. These are difficult problems, however, because experience also suggests that every deviation from analytic technique that such special conditions compel tends to prolong the length of treatment and to considerably increase its vicissitudes and problems.

Such modifications in analytical technique usually go under the heading of "parameters," and they remain a considerable source of discussion and controversy among analytical therapists. A significant trend today is the increasing tendency of analysts to treat more difficult and complex cases; thus, the necessity for introducing modifications in various aspects of the treatment process correspondingly increases. As a result, what might previously have been thought of as parameters are increasingly accepted as valid technical practices. The resolution of such difficulties in assessing and exploring modifications of techniques must ultimately rest on the basis of clinical experience.

Results of Treatment The therapeutic effectiveness of psychoanalysis presents problems in its evaluation. Impartial and objective critics are handicapped in attempts to appraise therapeutic results by the fact that so many patients state that they have been analyzed when no such procedure was, in fact, undertaken or when it was undertaken by someone who used the title of analyst and who had little understanding of analytical science and technique. Other patients have been in analysis only for a very short time and then discontinued treatment on their own initiative or were advised that they were not suitable candidates for analytical treatment. Except for psychoanalysts themselves, professionals, as well as lay people, demonstrate varying degrees of confusion as to what psychoanalysis is and what it is not.

No analyst can ever eliminate all the personality defects and neurotic factors in a given patient, no matter how thorough or successful the treatment. Mitigation of the rigors of a punitive superego, however, is an essential criterion of the effectiveness of treatment. Psychoanalysts do not usually regard alleviation of symptoms as the most significant aspect in evaluating therapeutic change. The absence of a recurrence of the illness or a further need for psychotherapy is perhaps a more important index of the value of psychoanalysis. The chief basis of evaluation, however, remains the patient's general adjustment to life—that is, the capacity for attaining reasonable happiness, for contributing to the happiness of others, the ability to deal adequately with the normal vicissitudes and stresses of life, and the capacity to enter into and sustain mutually gratifying and rewarding relationships with other people in the patient's life.

More specific criteria of the effectiveness of treatment include the reduction of the patient's unconscious; neurotic need for suffering; reduction of neurotic inhibitions; decrease of infantile dependency needs; and an increased capacity for responsibility and for successful relationships in marriage, work, and social relations. Other important criteria are the capacity for pleasurable and rewarding sublimation and for creative and adaptive application of the patient's own potentialities. The most important criterion of the success of treatment, however, is the release of the patient's normal potentiality, which had been blocked by neurotic conflicts, for further internal growth, development, and maturation to mature personality functioning.

Despite the methodological difficulties and complexities of outcome studies, extensive empirical evaluations from a number of centers have demonstrated the effectiveness and relative success of psychoanalysis and psychoanalytic therapy for appropriately selected cases in the psychoneurotic conditions, personality disorders, and forms of self-pathology. Therapeutic outcomes have been more guarded in cases of psychosomatic illness, more primitive levels of personality disorder, and psychoses.

SUGGESTED CROSS-REFERENCES

The psychoanalytic perspective is relevant to virtually every chapter of this book. Of particular interest are the discussion of Erikson in Section 6.2, other psychodynamic schools in Section 6.3, and approaches derived from psychology and philosophy in Section 6.4. Neurodevelopmental theory of schizophrenia is covered in Section 12.5. Psychological treatments of mood disorders are covered in Section 13.9; anxiety disorders in Chapter 14; personality disorders in Chapter 23; psychoanalysis and psychoanalytic psychotherapy in Section 30.1; evaluation of psychotherapy in Section 30.11; and psychotherapy with the elderly in Section 51.4h.

References

Balint M. *Primary Love and Psycho-Analytic Technique.* New York: Liveright; 1965.

Blum HP: Masochism, the ego ideal, and the psychology of women. *J Am Psychoanal Assoc.* 1976;24[Suppl]:157.

Diamond D, Blatt SJ: Attachment research and psychoanalysis. 1. Theoretical considerations. 2. Clinical implications. *Psychoanal Inquiry.* 1999;19:4–5.

Diamond D, Blatt SJ, Lichtenberg J: Attachment research and psychoanalysis. 3. Further reflections on theory and clinical experience. *Psychoanal Inquiry.* 2003; 23(1).

Erikson EH. *Childhood and Society.* New York: Norton; 1963.

Erle JB, Goldberg DA: The course of 253 analyses from selection to outcome. *J Am Psychoanal Assoc.* 2003;51:257.

Fairbairn WRD. *Psychoanalytic Studies of the Personality.* London: Routledge and Kegan Paul; 1972.

*Fenichel O. *The Psychoanalytic Theory of Neurosis.* New York: Norton; 1945.

Freud A. The ego and the mechanisms of defense. In: *The Writings of Anna Freud.* Vol II. 1936. New York: International Universities Press; 1975.

Freud S. *On Aphasia: A Critical Study.* New York: International Universities Press; 1953.

*Freud S. *The Standard Edition of the Complete Psychological Works of Sigmund Freud.* 24 Vols. London: Hogarth Press; 1953–1974.

*Greenberg JR, Mitchell SA. *Object Relations in Psychoanalytic Theory.* Cambridge, MA: Harvard University Press; 1983.

Hartmann H. *Essays on Ego Psychology.* New York: International Universities Press; 1954.

Hartmann H. *Ego Psychology and the Problem of Adaptation.* New York: International Universities Press; 1958.

Hinshelwood RD. *A Dictionary of Kleinian Thought.* London: Free Association Books; 1991.

Kohut HS. *The Analysis of the Self.* New York: International Universities Press; 1971.

Kohut HS. *The Restoration of the Self.* New York: International Universities Press; 1977.

Kohut HS. *How Does Analysis Cure?* Chicago: University of Chicago Press; 1984.

Levin FM. *Psyche and Brain: The Biology of Talking Cures.* Madison, CT: International Universities Press; 2003.

Loewald HW. *Papers on Psychoanalysis.* New Haven, CT: Yale University Press; 1980.

Mahler MS, Pine F, Bergman A. *The Psychological Birth of the Human Infant.* New York: Basic Books; 1975.

Masson JM. *The Complete Letters of Sigmund Freud to Wilhelm Fliess 1887–1904.* Cambridge, MA: Harvard University Press; 1985.

Meissner WW. *Internalization in Psychoanalysis.* New York: International Universities Press; 1981.

*Meissner WW. *The Therapeutic Alliance.* New Haven, CT: Yale University Press; 1996.

Meissner WW. *The Ethical Dilemma of Psychoanalysis—A Dialogue.* Albany, NY: State University of New York Press; 2003.

Mitchell SA. *Relational Concepts in Psychoanalysis.* Cambridge, MA: Harvard University Press; 1988.

*Moore BE, Fine BD. *Psychoanalysis: The Major Concepts.* New Haven, CT: Yale University Press; 1995.

Richards AD, Tyson P: The psychology of women: Psychoanalytic perspectives. *J Am Psychoanal Assoc.* 1996;44.

Rizzuto AM, Meissner WW, Buie DH. *The Dynamics of Human Aggression: Theoretical Foundations, Clinical Applications.* New York: Brunner-Routledge; 2004.

Schafer R. *Aspects of Internalization.* New York: International Universities Press; 1968.

Shapiro T, Emde RN: Research in psychoanalysis: Process, development, outcome. *J Am Psychoanal Assoc.* 1993;41[Suppl].

Stern D. *The Interpersonal World of the Infant.* New York: Basic Books; 1985.

Stolorow R, Atwood G. *Contexts of Being: The Intersubjective Foundations of Psychological Life.* Hillsdale, NJ: Analytic Press; 1992.

Tyson P, Tyson RL. *Psychoanalytic Theories of Development.* New Haven, CT: Yale University Press; 1990.

Winnicott DW. *Playing and Reality.* New York: Basic Books; 1971.

▲ 6.2 Erik H. Erikson

DORIAN S. NEWTON, PH.D.

Erik Erikson was a psychoanalyst who created an original and highly influential theory of psychological development and crisis occurring in periods that extended across the entire life cycle. His theory grew out of his work first as a teacher, then as a child psychoanalyst, next as an anthropological field worker, and, finally, as a biographer. Rather than starting within the nervous system of the individual, as Sigmund Freud had done, Erikson focused on the boundary between the child and the environment and then graphed the evolution of the maturing ego's relations with an expanding social world. Erikson identified dilemmas or polarities in the ego's relations with the family and larger social institutions at nodal points in childhood, adolescence, and early, middle, and late adulthood.

Of Erikson's many works, three are already firmly established as classics. *Childhood and Society* set forth his theory of the life cycle. *Young Man Luther* reconstructed and analyzed the developmental crisis of identity in a young man and its creative resolution in his 30s. *Gandhi's Truth* showed the coming together of authentic identity and calling in a man at midlife. In his psychological biographies of these world historical leaders, Erikson demonstrated the interrelations between individual psychodynamics and development, on the one hand, and social structure and history, on the other, gracefully avoiding a reductionism in a psychodynamic or sociological direction. Erikson showed in complex, intricate detail how great leaders solve the problem of their own identities by creating solutions for crises in their cultures.

LIFE AND WORK

Erik Homburger Erikson was born on June 15, 1902, in Karlsruhe, Germany, an old capital of a Lutheran principality. His father was Protestant, and his mother was Jewish. His parents, both Danish, had separated before his birth; his mother was visiting friends in Germany when the baby was born. She stayed in Karlsruhe and, a few years later, married her child's pediatrician, a well-to-do Jewish doctor, Theodor Homburger, in whose house young Erik grew up. During an alienated adolescence, the tall, blond boy found himself regarded as a gentile in his father's Jewish milieu and as a Jew at school. He remembered his mother as sad, bookish, and artistic, his adoptive father as professionally respected, and both parents as loving. The boy's adoption by his stepfather was the formative occasion of what became a lifelong pattern of getting himself adopted by kind men. His last name remained Homburger until he was 37 years of age, when he changed it to Erikson.

Erikson attended the *Humanistiche Gymnasium* in Karlsruhe where he studied Greek, Latin, philosophy, literature, ancient history, art, and science. By 18 years of age, he had the educational attainments of all but a few American college graduates and a stronger base than many. His primary interest was art; impatient with formal study and possessed by a restlessness he never lost, Erikson chose not to go to a university, preferring to travel about the countryside reading, drawing, and making wood carvings. Back home after a year, he tried formal art study with some success, first in Karlsruhe at the Badische Landeskunstschule and then in Munich at the Kunst-Akademie but in neither case with decisive commitment.

This sort of wandering about was not uncommon among German youth of the period, so Erikson was permitted, as his biographer Robert Coles sagely wrote, "To go through his own years of discontent and confusion without being especially singled out and thereby forced to defend behavior often best granted the limits of its own momentum." As Erikson confided to Coles, "If ever an identity crisis was central and long drawn out in somebody's life it was so in mine." Erikson was having what he would later term a *psychosocial moratorium*; in so doing, he was also mitigating the asperity of an *identity crisis*. At approximately 21 years of age, Erikson went to live in Florence, where he continued his art studies informally. There he enjoyed the friendship of his old *Gymnasium* chum Peter Blos, a writer who later became a famous American child psychoanalyst.

Becoming a Child Psychoanalyst When Erikson was 25 years of age, Peter Blos invited him to become a faculty member in a progressive grammar school in Vienna, where Blos taught language and science. Erikson's difficult transition from adolescence to early adulthood was over. The year was 1927; Sigmund Freud was 71 years of age, and his youngest child, Anna, an educator and psychoanalyst, had started a psychoanalytically enlightened school for children with an American friend named Dorothy Burlingham. Erikson joined Blos and later recalled Blos's determination to turn him into a disciplined worker: "To make a teacher of me . . . the highly disciplined Peter first had to teach me to keep regular work hours, a task which was initiated every morning, no matter what time of year, by a cold shower, then the preferred shock treatment for identity confusion." At the school, "Herr Erik" taught his students art and history; together, they studied different cultures and illustrated what they learned with drawings, essays, toys, tools, and exhibits.

Before long, Erikson found himself not only a teacher of children, but also an *analysand*, what is now called a *candidate*, at the Vienna Psychoanalytic Institute, in treatment with Anna Freud. Any sort of psychoanalytic approach to treating or educating children was then a radical idea, even an approach as cautious as Freud's. Educationally and clinically, Freud's group was sufficiently deviant such that a person with Erikson's diverse identity was able to fit in. There was, in 1927, a *configurational affinity* between Erikson's personal history and the history of psychoanalysis as a profession. Still, there was the worry: What was a fledgling artist without a university education to do among those high-powered theorists and intellectuals at the Vienna Psychoanalytic Institute?

Erikson recalled this epiphanic exchange with his analyst, Anna Freud: "When I declared once more that I could not see a place for my artistic inclinations in such high intellectual endeavors, she said quietly: 'You might help to make them see.'" Dreams had been Sigmund Freud's royal road to the unconscious; observing children's play (and later, anthropological field studies in the role of participant observer) would be Erikson's path to understanding the ego and its development. Looking back, Erikson thought that it was Anna Freud's "simple mandate" that enabled him to succeed in combining the artistic and the theoretical in *Childhood and Society*.

Erikson remained in Vienna for 6 years, until 1933. In those years between 25 and 31 years of age, he turned his artist's eye from the observation of nature to the analysis of children; he learned about psychoanalysis by studying children's play and his own free associations as a patient, and he learned fundamental clinical skills in the supervised treatment of others. As he explained to Coles, Erikson related art to psychoanalysis in this way: "I began to perceive how important visual configurations were, how they actually preceded words and formulations: certainly dreams are visual data, and so is children's play, not to speak of the 'free associations' which often are a series of images, pure and simple—only later put into words." Erikson trained with a Montessori group in Vienna, graduating from the Montessori teachers' association, the Lehrerinnenverein. He studied psychoanalysis with August Aichhorn, Edward Bibring, Helene Deutsche, and Ernst Kris. He formed mentor relationships with Anna Freud and Heinz Hartmann and a more distant, admiring-inspirational relationship with Freud's sick, aging, but still-productive father.

During his own late adulthood, Sigmund Freud had moved beyond clinical problems more narrowly conceived to problems of the ego, society, and history in works such as *Beyond the Pleasure Principle* (written at 64 years of age), *Group Psychology and the Analysis of the Ego* (at 65 years of age), and *The Ego and the Id* (at 66 years of age); during Erikson's years in Vienna, Freud was working on *The Future of an Illusion* (at 71 years of age) and *Civilization and Its Discontents* (at 73 years of age). Erikson seemed to identify with both Freuds, internalizing them as mentors, and they provided him with a strong, inner basis for a lifetime of psychoanalytic treatment and psychosocial research.

In 1929, Erikson met Joan Serson, a woman of mixed Canadian and American background. She had a Master's degree in sociology and a special interest in the history and social origins of modern dance and in psychoanalysis. They married, and Serson joined the faculty of Burlingham's school, where she taught English, literature, and American history. Serson's unusual combination of interests and skills—education, psychoanalysis, and sociology—coupled with her ability as a writer, gave Erikson a skilled coworker for a lifetime of intellectual work. Several articles were coauthored, Joan Erikson helped with most of the others, and the endowed chair at Harvard that was named after Erikson carried both of their first names.

With the birth of their sons, Kai and Jon (their daughter, Sue, was to be born 5 years later), Erikson had, by 31 years of age, become a husband, a father, and a child psychoanalyst. He had come a long way from the aimless youth of his early 20s and was productively engaged in the stage of ego development that he later characterized by the polarity *intimacy versus isolation*. He continued to work on that ego stage, but changes were now required in the life that Erikson had begun to build at 25 years of age.

Emigrating to America By 1933, the Fascist menace in Europe was growing. When Erikson graduated that year from the Vienna Psychoanalytic Institute, he and his family prepared to leave. They considered repatriating to Denmark but encountered problems because Erikson had lost his Danish citizenship when he had been adopted and had become a naturalized German. A serendipitous meeting between Erikson and Freud's disciple Hanns Sachs in which Sachs enthusiastically invited Erikson to come to Boston settled the matter. In 1933, the Eriksons emigrated to the United States. At 31 years of age, Erikson became Boston's first child psychoanalyst and a member of the faculty of the Harvard Medical School. He took a job as a consultant at Judge Baker Guidance Center, where he helped to diagnose and to treat poor and delinquent children with emotional disorders. In Cambridge, Erikson met Margaret Mead, Gregory Bateson, Ruth Benedict, and Kurt Lewin, each of whom influenced his intellectual development in important ways.

Erikson joined a group of personality researchers working under the leadership of Henry Murray, who was Director of the Harvard Psychological Clinic. Murray's book *Explorations in Personality: A Clinical and Experimental Study of Fifty Men of College Age* was published in 1938. It is one of the few integrative masterpieces in American psychology—experimental and biographical, psychological and sociological, Freudian and Jungian, developmental and diagnostic. Murray's example proved seminal when Erikson later turned his hand to the biographical study of the world historical figures Sigmund Freud, Martin Luther, and Mohandas Gandhi.

Listed on the title page of Murray's book, among other research associates, was "Erik Homburger." The next year, at 37 years of age, Homburger renamed himself Erikson, retaining Homburger as his middle name. With characteristically bold creativity, Erikson solved the problem of his paternity by adopting himself.

Psychoanalytic Anthropology In 1936, Erikson hit the road again, this time to the Institute of Human Relations of the department of psychiatry at Yale University. The interdisciplinary work of the institute further shaped Erikson's interest in cross-cultural research, and, in 1938, he joined a colleague on a research expedition to the Sioux Indians in South Dakota. On the Pine Ridge reservation, he observed children, interviewed adults, and noted the impact of economic, geographical, and historical factors on child-rearing practices. Based on this research, Erikson published his paper, "Observations on Sioux Education," in 1939.

In the same year, the peregrinating Eriksons moved to California, where he joined the faculty at the University of California at Berkeley. Erikson affiliated himself with Mount Zion Hospital and the San Francisco Psychoanalytic Institute and, ultimately, became a U.S. citizen. At Berkeley, Erikson continued his cross-cultural research, this time with the Yurok Indians of northern California. He also lent his research skills to the war effort in articles on submarine habitation, the interrogation of prisoners of war, and difficulties encountered by veterans in returning to civilian life.

Erikson remained at U. C. Berkeley for a decade, the longest period that he had spent in one place since his preadulthood years in Karlsruhe. During that time, he became his own man, visible first in the outward signs of changing his name and later in refusing to sign the university's loyalty oath of anti-Communist purity. To Erikson, the contract was "an empty gesture toward meeting the danger of infiltration into academic life of indoctrinators, conspirators, and spies." In 1950, after the dismissal of some of his peers for refusing to declare themselves noncommunist, Erikson resigned his position as professor of psychology. He wrote a protest that was subsequently read at a meeting of the American Psychoanalytic Association. In that statement, he asserted,

> Young people are rightfully suspicious and embarrassingly discerning. I do not believe they can remain unimpressed by the fact that the men who are to teach them to think and to act judiciously and spontaneously must undergo a political test; must sign a statement which implicitly questions the validity of their own oath of office; must abrogate "commitments" so undefined that they must forever suspect themselves and one another; and must confess to an "objective truth" which they know only too well is elusive.

He continued, "if the universities themselves become the puppets of public hysteria, if their own regents are expressly suspicious of their faculties, if the professors themselves tacitly admit that they need to deny perjury, year after year—will that allay public hysteria?"

At Harvard, Erikson had studied "normal" students and their use of toys and dramatic scenes to enact and to illustrate internal conflicts. At the Institute of Child Welfare at the University of California, Erikson continued his research and found important gender-related differences in the use of toys and play space by normal adolescents. As Coles noted, "psychological themes—what the child says he is up to, what he can be seen doing and experiencing—are related to 'spatial configurations,' namely, objects and forms that exist in a world outside the mind. The mind in turn uses those objects or forms to express and reveal its wishes, fears, and conflicts." In research that had its roots in his work at Burlinghams's experimental school, Erikson had once again combined his artistic and psychoanalytic sensibilities in the study of human behavior.

At 40 years of age, as Erikson was entering middle age, he was becoming more biographical and more interested in the adult years of the life cycle. Like others who manage to continue developing, he found a way to pursue his development through the strictures of exigent reality. World War II was under way, and Erikson was deeply concerned about it. After his initial narrowly framed attempts at scholarly patriotism, he began writing his first psychobiographical essays on Adolf Hitler and the psychosocial dynamics of his appeal to young Germans—"Hitler's Imagery and German Youth" was published in 1942. It united Erikson's interests in political science, history, and anthropology. As Coles stated, "Very little that Erikson would do for the next two decades was not in some respects foreshadowed by this paper."

Midlife Transition *Childhood and Society* was the creative product of Erikson's transition to midlife. He had intended it to be a contribution to the psychiatric education of clinicians from various disciplines, but the book outgrew its author's intentions and found its way into every corner of the academy and beyond.

Erikson began work on the book when he was 42 years of age and largely completed work on it by 46 years of age. Published in 1950, it is at once a product of early research, a prospectus of what was to come, and an initial integration of both. In it, he presented clinical cases in which individual psychodynamics, society, and history are interwoven with a skill not seen before or since; analyses of children's play and development in various cultures; a theoretical sketch of the entire human life cycle; pieces on the problem of identity; and biographical essays on Hitler and the Russian writer Maxim Gorky.

As in Karl Abraham's and Freud's psychosexual stages, most of Erikson's stages in ego development occur in childhood and adolescence. Unlike the Abraham-Freud conception, however, Erikson's stages are psychosocial, describing crucial steps in the maturing ego's relations with the social world rather than a biological unfolding of neurophysiological capacities for excitation. Also, whereas Freud's developmental theory falls back on itself after adolescence, Erikson's continued with characterizations of developmental tasks during youth, middle age, and old age.

Erikson's emphasis, like Freud's, was cross-cultural and universal. Erikson's eight stages were ineluctable parts of the human life cycle, yet each person traversed them in distinct ways determined by culture, concrete circumstance, and personality. With *Childhood and Society*, Erikson became and remained an ego psychologist, shifting the traditional psychoanalytic focus on the drives to adaptation and growth. In so doing, he was furthering the work of his analyst-mentor, Anna Freud, who, in 1936, had written ego psychology's basic theoretical treatise, *The Ego and the Mechanisms of Defense.*

Eight Stages of the Life Cycle Erikson's conceptualization of psychosocial development across the life cycle is the centerpiece of his life's work, and he elaborated the conception throughout his subsequent writings. It takes as its model the epigenetic principle of organismic growth in utero. In Erikson's view, psychosocial growth occurs in phases, with individual aspects of development proceeding according to a predetermined timetable. Elements of each phase are present from birth and differentiate over time. Every phase has its own period of quiescence and critical ascendancy, and each is dependent on the proper development of the other phases in the proper sequence. Work on any particular phase, Erikson theorized, is never complete, and old developmental conflicts can be activated by critical life events.

The eight stages of the life cycle represent points along a continuum of development in which physical, cognitive, instinctual, and sexual changes combine to trigger an internal crisis whose resolution results in psychosocial regression or growth and the development of specific *virtues*. In *Insight and Responsibility*, Erikson defined virtue as "inherent strength," as in the active quality of a medicine or a liquor. He wrote in *Identity: Youth and Crisis* that "crisis" refers not to a "threat of catastrophe, but to a turning point, a crucial period of increased vulnerability and heightened potential, and therefore, the ontogenetic source of generational strength and maladjustment." Elsewhere, Erikson averred, "We do not consider all development a series of crises: we claim only that psychosocial development proceeds by critical steps—'critical' being a characteristic of turning points, of moments of decision between progress and regression, integration and retardation." A child's experience of each crisis or critical turning point is affected by the attitudes of the child's parents and the values and customs of the child's culture.

Trust versus Mistrust (Birth to Approximately 18 Months) In *Identity: Youth and Crisis*, Erikson noted that the infant "lives through and loves with" its mouth. Indeed, the mouth forms the basis of its first *mode* or pattern of behavior, that of incorporation. The infant is taking the world in through the mouth, eyes, ears, and sense of touch. The baby is learning a cultural modality that Erikson termed *to get*, that is, to receive what is offered and to elicit what is desired. As the infant's teeth develop, and it discovers the pleasure of biting, it enters the second oral stage, the active-incorporative mode. The infant is no longer passively receptive to stimuli; it reaches out for sensation and grasps at its surroundings. The social modality shifts to that of *taking and holding on* to things.

The infant's development of basic trust in the world stems from its earliest experiences with its mother or primary caretaker. In *Childhood and Society*, Erikson asserts that trust depends not on "absolute quantities of food or demonstrations of love, but rather on the quality of maternal relationship." A baby whose mother is able to anticipate and to respond to its needs in a consistent and timely manner, despite its oral aggression, learns to tolerate the inevitable moments of frustration and deprivation. The defense mechanisms of introjection and projection provide the infant with the means to internalize pleasure and to externalize pain, such that "consistency, continuity, and sameness of experience provide a rudimentary sense of ego identity." Trust predominates over mistrust, and hope crystallizes. For Erikson, the element of society corresponding to this stage of ego identity is religion, as both are founded on "trust born of care."

In keeping with his emphasis on the epigenetic character of psychosocial change, Erikson conceived of many forms of psychopathology as examples of what he termed *aggravated development crisis*, development that, having gone awry at one point, affects subsequent psychosocial change. A person who, as a result of severe disturbances in the earliest dyadic relationships, fails to develop a basic sense of trust or the virtue of hope may be predisposed as an adult to the profound withdrawal and regression characteristic of schizophrenia. Erikson hypothesized that the depressed patient's experience of being empty and worthless is an outgrowth of a developmental derailment that causes oral pessimism to predominate. Addictions may also be traced to the mode of oral incorporation.

Autonomy versus Shame and Doubt (Approximately 18 Months to Approximately 3 Years) In the development of speech and sphincter and muscular control, the toddler practices the social modalities of *holding on and letting go* and experiences the first stirrings of the virtue that Erikson termed *will*. Much depends on the amount and the type of control exercised by adults over the child. Control that is exerted too rigidly or too early defeats the toddler's attempts to develop its own internal controls, and regression or false progression results. Parental control that fails to protect the toddler from the consequences of his or her own lack of self-control or judgment can be equally disastrous to the child's development of a healthy sense of autonomy. In *Identity: Youth and Crisis*, Erikson asserted: "This stage, therefore, becomes decisive for the ratio between cooperation and willfulness, and between self-expression and compulsive self-restraint or meek compliance."

Where that ratio is favorable, the child develops an appropriate sense of autonomy and the capacity to "have and to hold"; where it is unfavorable, doubt and shame undermine free will. According to Erikson, the principle of law and order has at its roots this early preoccupation with the protection and regulation of will. In *Childhood and Society*, he concluded that "[t]he sense of autonomy, fostered in the child and modified as life progresses, serves (and is served by) the preservation in economic and political life of a sense of justice."

An individual who becomes fixated at the transition between the development of hope and autonomous will, with its residue of mistrust and doubt, may develop paranoiac fears of persecution. When psychosocial development is derailed in the second stage, delinquency and others forms of pathology may emerge. The perfectionism, inflexibility, and stinginess of the person with an obsessive-compulsive personality disorder may stem from conflicting tendencies to hold on and to let go. The ruminative and ritualistic behavior of the person who has an obsessive-compulsive disorder (OCD) may be an outcome of the triumph of doubt over autonomy and the subsequent development and retention of a primitively harsh conscience.

Initiative versus Guilt (Approximately 3 Years to Approximately 5 Years) The child's increasing mastery of locomotor and language skills expands its participation in the outside world and stimulates omnipotent fantasies of wider exploration and conquest. Here, the youngster's mode of participation is active and intrusive; the child's social modality is that of *being on the make*. The intrusiveness is manifested in the child's fervent curiosity and genital preoccupations, competitiveness, and physical aggression. The Oedipus complex is in ascendance as the child competes with the same-sex parent for the fantasized possession of the other parent. In *Identity: Youth and Crisis*, Erikson wrote that "jealousy and rivalry . . . now come to climax in a final contest for a favored position with one of the parents: the inevitable and necessary failure leads to guilt and anxiety."

Guilt over the drive for conquest and anxiety over the anticipated punishment are both assuaged in the child through repression of the forbidden wishes and the development of a superego to regulate its initiative. This conscience, the faculty of self-observation, self-regulation, and self-punishment, is an internalized version of parental and societal authority. Initially, the conscience is harsh and uncompromising; however, it constitutes the foundation for the subsequent development of morality. Having renounced oedipal ambitions, the child begins to look outside the family for arenas in which it can compete with less conflict and guilt. This is the stage that highlights the child's expanding initiative and forms the basis for the subsequent development of realistic ambition and the virtue of *purpose*. As Erikson noted in *Childhood and Society*, "[t]he 'oedipal' stage . . . sets the direction toward the possible and the tangible which permits the dreams of early childhood to be attached to the goals of an active adult life." Toward this end, social institutions provide the youngster with an economic ethos in the form of adult heroes who begin to take the place of their storybook counterparts.

When there has been an inadequate resolution of the conflict between initiative and guilt, the individual may ultimately develop a conversion disorder, inhibition, or phobia. Those who overcompensate for the conflict by driving themselves too hard may experience so much stress as to produce psychosomatic symptoms.

Industry versus Inferiority (Approximately 5 Years to Approximately 13 Years) With the onset of latency, the child discovers the pleasures of production. He or she develops industry by learning new skills and takes pride in the things made. Erikson wrote in *Childhood and Society* that the child's "ego boundaries include his tools and skills: the work principle . . . teaches him the pleasure of work completion by steady attention and persevering diligence." Across cultures, this is a time when the child receives systematic instruction and learns the fundamentals of technology as they pertain to the use of basic utensils and tools. As children work, they identify with their teachers and imagine themselves in various occupational roles.

If the child is unprepared for this stage of psychosocial development, through insufficient resolution of previous stages or by current interference, the child may develop a sense of inferiority and inadequacy. Teachers and other role models help transmit social values and become crucially important in the child's ability to overcome a sense of inferiority and to achieve the virtue known as *competence*. In *Identity: Youth and Crisis*, Erikson noted: "[T]his is socially a most decisive stage. Since industry involves doing things beside and with others, a first sense of division of labor and of differential opportunity, that is, a sense of the technological ethos of a culture, develops at this time."

The pathological outcome of a poorly navigated stage of *industry versus inferiority* is less well defined than in previous stages, but it may concern the emergence of a conformist immersion into the world of production in which creativity is stifled, identity is subsumed under the worker's role, and feelings of inferiority are warded off through a defensive preoccupation with status and compensation.

Identity versus Role Confusion (Approximately 13 Years to Approximately 21 Years) With the onset of puberty and its myriad social and physiological changes, the adolescent becomes preoccupied with the question of identity. Erikson noted in *Childhood and Society* that youth are now "primarily concerned with what they appear to be in the eyes of others as compared to what they feel they are, and with the question of how to connect the roles and skills cultivated earlier with the occupational prototypes of the day." Childhood roles and fantasies are no longer appropriate, yet the adolescent is far from equipped to become an adult. In *Childhood and Society*, Erikson writes that the integration that occurs in the formation of ego identity encompasses far more than the summation of childhood identifications: "It is the accrued experience of the ego's ability to integrate these identifications with the vicissitudes of the libido, with the aptitudes developed out of endowment, and with the opportunities offered in social roles." Coles explains that ego identity is an "accrued confidence" that develops over time and crystallizes in early adulthood—or does not. It is the confidence that "somehow in the midst of change one *is*; that is, one has an 'inner sameness and continuity' which others can recognize and which is so certain that it can unselfconsciously be taken for granted."

The formation of cliques and the intolerance of individual differences are ways in which the young person attempts to ward off a sense of identity confusion. In *Childhood and Society*, Erikson noted:

> For adolescents not only help one another temporarily through much discomfort by forming cliques and by stereotyping themselves, their ideals, and their enemies; they also perversely test each other's capacity to pledge fidelity. The readiness for such testing also explains the appeal which simple and cruel totalitarian doctrines have on the minds of the youth of such countries and classes as have lost or are losing their group identities (feudal, agrarian, tribal, national) and face world-wide industrialization, emancipation, and wider communication.

Falling in love, a process by which the adolescent may clarify a sense of identity by projecting a diffused self-image onto the partner and seeing it gradually assume a more distinctive shape, and an overidentification with idealized figures are means by which the adolescent seeks self-definition. With the attainment of a more sharply focused identity, the youth develops the virtue of *fidelity*—a faithfulness not only to the nascent self-definition but to an ideology that provides a version of self in world. As Erikson, Joan Erikson, and Helen Kivnick wrote in *Vital Involvement in Old Age*, "[f]idelity is the ability to sustain loyalties freely pledged in spite of the inevitable contradictions of value systems. It is the cornerstone of identity and receives inspiration from confirming ideologies and affirming companionships."

Role confusion ensues when the youth is unable to formulate a sense of identity and belonging. Coles explains,

> In a state of "acute identity diffusion" the young individual may feel isolated, empty, anxious, and unable to make any number of choices or decisions that he himself (let alone his parents or teachers) feels pending. He feels threatened by what he senses to be close at hand: the possibility of intimacy, the chance at last to choose a career or find a job, the presence of others who are seen as competitors, as somehow "better" or less "troubled." He finds himself at a loss, and he fears that the world is breathing hard down his back—ready to restrict him, type him, define him, and thus close him off from any number of possibilities he still finds attractive. He wants "out," he wants to be away, he wants "time" to think and decide and only later act.

Erikson held that delinquency, gender-related identity disorders, and borderline psychotic episodes can result from such confusion.

Intimacy versus Isolation (Approximately 21 Years to Approximately 40 Years) Freud's famous response to the question of what a normal person should be able to do well, "Lieben und arbeiten" (to love and to work), is one that Erikson often cited in his discussion of this psychosocial stage, and it emphasizes the importance he placed on the virtue of *love* within a balanced identity. Erikson asserted in *Identity: Youth and Crisis* that Freud's use of the term *love* referred to "the generosity of intimacy as well as genital love; when he said love and work he meant a general work productivity which would not preoccupy the individual to the extent that he might lose his right or capacity to be a sexual and a loving being."

Intimacy in the young adult is closely tied to fidelity; it is the ability to make and honor commitments to concrete affiliations and partnerships even when that requires sacrifice and compromise. The person who cannot tolerate the fear of ego loss arising out of experiences of self-abandonment (e.g., sexual orgasm, moments of intensity in friendships, aggression, inspiration, and intuition) is apt to become deeply isolated and self-absorbed. *Distantiation*, an awkward term coined by Erikson to mean "the readiness to repudiate, isolate, and, if necessary, destroy those forces and people whose essence seems dangerous to one's own," is the pathological outcome of conflicts surrounding intimacy and, in the absence of an ethical sense in which intimate, competitive, and combative relationships are differentiated, forms the basis for various forms of prejudice, persecution, and psychopathology.

Erikson's separation of the psychosocial task of achieving identity from that of achieving intimacy and his assertion that substantial progress on the former task must precede development on the latter have engendered much criticism and debate. Critics have argued that Erikson's emphasis on separation and occupationally based identity formation fails to take into account the importance for women of continued attachment and the formation of an identity based on relationships.

Generativity versus Stagnation (Approximately 40 Years to Approximately 60 Years) Erikson asserted in *Identity: Youth and Crisis* that "generativity . . . is primarily the concern for establishing and guiding the next generation." The term *generativity* applies not so much to rearing and teaching one's offspring as to a protective concern for all the generations and for social institutions. It encompasses productivity and creativity as well. Having previously achieved the capacity to form intimate relationships, the person now broadens the investment of ego and libidinal energy to include groups, organizations, and society. *Care* is the virtue that coalesces at this stage. In *Childhood and Society*, Erikson emphasized the importance to the mature person of feeling needed: "[M]aturity needs guidance as well as encouragement from what has been produced and must be taken care of." Through generative behavior, the individual is able to pass on knowledge and skills while obtaining a measure of satisfaction in having achieved a role with senior authority and responsibility in the tribe.

When people are unable to develop true generativity, they may settle for pseudoengagement in occupation. Often, such people restrict their focus to the technical aspects of their roles at which they may now have become highly skilled, eschewing larger responsibility for the organization or profession. This failure of generativity can lead to profound personal stagnation, masked by a variety of escapisms, such as alcohol and drug abuse and sexual and other infidelities. Midlife crisis or premature invalidism (physical and psychological) may occur. In this case, pathology appears not only in middle-aged persons, but also in the organizations that depend on them for leadership. Thus, the failure to develop at midlife can lead to sick, withered, or destructive organizations that spread the effects of failed generativity throughout society; examples of such failures have become so common as to constitute a defining feature of modernity.

Integrity versus Despair (Approximately 60 Years to Death) In *Identity: Youth and Crisis*, Erikson defined integrity as "the acceptance of one's one and only life cycle and of the people who have become significant to it as something that had to be and that, by necessity, permitted of no substitutions." From the vantage point of this stage of psychosocial development, the individual relinquishes the wish that important people in his life had been different and is able to love in a more meaningful way—one that reflects an acceptance of responsibility for one's own life. The individual in possession of the virtue of *wisdom* and a sense of integrity has room to tolerate the proximity of death and to achieve what Erikson termed in *Identity: Youth and Crisis* a "detached yet active concern with life." Despair may be present, but it does not predominate.

Erikson underlined the social context for this final stage of growth. In *Childhood and Society*, he wrote: "The style of integrity developed by his culture or civilization thus becomes the 'patrimony' of his soul. . . . In such final consolidation, death loses its sting."

When the attempt to attain integrity has failed, the individual may become deeply disgusted with the external world and contemptuous of persons as well as institutions. Erikson wrote in *Childhood and Society* that such disgust masks a fear of death and a sense of despair that "time is now short, too short for the attempt to start another life and to try out alternate roads to integrity." In thinking about the relationship between adult integrity and infantile trust, Erikson observed, "[h]ealthy children will not fear life if their elders have integrity enough not to fear death."

Becoming a Biographer of Youth

In 1949, as *Childhood and Society* was going to press, Erikson's stand on the University of California loyalty oath had rendered his position at the university untenable. News of his availability spread east, and other institutions vied to capitalize on Berkeley's mistake. Erikson was well known at the Menninger Clinic in Topeka, Kansas, where he had lectured, so, when Robert Knight left Menninger to become the director of the Austen Riggs Center in Stockbridge, Massachusetts, he took Erikson with him. The Austen Riggs Center was devoted to psychoanalytic research and to the treatment of severely disturbed adolescents and young adults—Erikson had been happily adopted once again.

Erikson stayed at Austen Riggs from 1950 to 1960, from 48 to 58 years of age, when he returned to the faculty of Harvard University. During those years, Erikson completed the transition to biographer, forming more fully the approach foreshadowed in his incomplete essays on Hitler, Gorky, and George Bernard Shaw. The transition was not easy; Coles describes that time as constituting a second "identity crisis." Erikson had been a clinician and a theorist of youth; he was now old enough to enact the program promised in *Childhood and Society* and to become a biographer and theorist of the whole life cycle. However, before he wrote *Young Man Luther*, he once again returned to Freud and the origins of his own professional identity. The way to the future was through the past.

In his early 50s, Erikson wrote three biographical essays on Freud: "The Dream Specimen of Psychoanalysis," "Freud's 'The Origins of Psychoanalysis,'" and "The First Psychoanalyst." These essays all concern themselves with the crisis Freud experienced during his own midlife transition as he struggled to leave neuropathology and to define a new professional identity as a psychoanalyst. Strengthened by that reexamination of Freud's successful transition (and perhaps having reassured himself of Freud's blessing), Erikson began writing one of the genuine masterworks of psychoanalysis, *Young Man Luther*.

As always, Erikson's clinical work and observations enriched his theorizing about the life cycle. He acknowledged his debt to Austen Riggs and the Western Psychiatric Institute at the University of Pittsburgh in his preface to *Young Man Luther*. His work there had allowed him to "study the afflictions of young patients as variations on one theme, namely, a life crisis, aggravated in patients, yet in some form normal for all youth. I could identify those acute life tasks that would bring young people to a state of tension in which some would become patients."

However, Erikson would neither make Martin Luther a patient nor reify the psychopathology of the young people who were his patients. Instead, he asserted that comparisons between Martin Luther and his patients were "not restricted to psychiatric diagnosis . . . but . . . oriented toward those moments when young patients, like young beings anywhere, prove resourceful and insightful beyond all professional and personal expectation. We will concentrate on the powers of recovery inherent in the young ego."

Working with the young patients at Austen Riggs helped Erikson hone his understanding of identity formation. As he later put it in "The Problem of Ego Identity," "[i]dentity . . . is gradually established by successive ego syntheses and re-syntheses throughout childhood. It is a configuration gradually integrating *constitutional givens, idiosyncratic libidinal needs, favored capacities, significant identifications, effective defenses, successful sublimations, and consistent roles*."

These "ego syntheses and re-syntheses" were about to receive great attention as Erikson attempted his biography of Luther. To do that work, however, Erikson the biographer had to move further away from his own professional origins as a child psychoanalyst. He had criticized psychoanalysis for its contention that something has been explained by finding an analogy to its earliest manifestations. Yet his own conception of the life cycle, with most of its stages occurring within the preadult era, left him still heavily rooted in childhood. In his study of Luther, Erikson was trying to understand a life, not just a personality; from that perspective, childhood and adolescence had to be introductory rather than the story itself.

Seeing that a child-centered view was not adequate for the tasks of biography, without formally changing the imbalance in his theory or neglecting childhood determinants, Erikson deftly devoted the greatest attention to an explication of development in the adult years. So successful was he in interrelating Luther's adult problems with those of his early development that *Young Man Luther* provided the seminal inspiration for the next generation of life-cycle investigators. Some of those investigators, such as Daniel Levinson, formally redressed in their own theories the originological bias vestigial in Erikson's theories.

In Luther's early or mid-20s, according to some of his contemporaries, the young monk had fallen to the floor of the choir of his monastery in a fit and shouted, "Ich bin's nit!" or "Non Sum!"—"It isn't me," or "I am not." Erikson's task as a psychological biographer was to explain how Luther got from the identity crisis of his 20s to nailing his 95 theses to the door of the church in Wittenberg at 32 years of age. Yet *Young Man Luther* is also, as it is subtitled, "a study in psychoanalysis and history." Because it is not a psychoanalysis of history, some nonreductionist connecting concepts between the individual and the collectivity were needed. One of Erikson's connecting concepts was *ideology*, which he defined as "an unconscious tendency underlying religious and scientific as well as political thought: the tendency at a given time to make facts amenable to ideas, and ideas to facts, in order to create a world image convincing enough to support the collective and the individual sense of identity."

Luther had personal and psychiatric problems, but, in his defiance of Catholic orthodoxy, he created a new religious ideology that not only supported his own identity, but also the identities of emerging generations of Europeans as well. "Ich bin's nit" expressed the young monk's identity crisis as he found himself "fatally overcommitted" to what he was not, a young man authentically embarking on a future as an orthodox Catholic priest. "In some periods of history," Erikson asserted, "and in some phases of his life cycle, man needs . . . a new ideological orientation as surely and as sorely as he must have air and food." As such a man, Luther commanded Erikson's "sympathy and empathy" as he "faced the problems of human existence in the most forward terms of his era."

The reception of the book cemented Erikson's international reputation, initially won by *Childhood and Society*, as a leader in original, humane thought about psychological development. In no other biography have the dynamics of individual conflict and development been so seamlessly interwoven with those of society and history. With *Young Man Luther*, Erikson, in his late 50s, ascended from the first rank of developmental psychoanalysts to that of a cultural seer.

Becoming a Biographer of Middle Age As Erikson moved through the transition from middle to old age, he abandoned clinical work with patients to turn his attention fully to the study of the life cycle and the survival of the species. His emphasis, emergent in *Young Man Luther* and implicit in all his earlier work, was on the ego virtues that permit a person to live in a constructively critical relationship with the social institutions of his time. Earlier, Erikson had described the stages in the development of the ego across the life cycle. In 1964, he wrote more about the ego virtues in *Insight and Responsibility*. He was getting ready amidst the American moral and political crises of the mid-1960s to embark on his last major work, a study of the great moral leader Mohandas Gandhi. In the end, he dedicated it, *in memoriam*, to Martin Luther King, Jr.

Young Man Luther had been a story of personal choice and historical change wrought by a young man establishing and revising an initial identity and life structure as an adult. In his mid-60s, Erikson had gained sufficient perspective on the life cycle to analyze a case of decisive crisis and change in a man who was going through a midlife transition and solving it by creating a vital life structure for middle age. Gandhi did that, as he himself put it, by realizing "his vocation in life," leading *Satyagraha* truth force campaigns in his nation, in his family, and in his own soul. Gandhi was entering the stage of the life cycle in which Erikson's ego polarity of *generativity versus stagnation* becomes active; from his developmental work on this polarity, Gandhi was learning the ego virtue of *care*.

Erikson saw that Gandhi, like Luther, was a leader and a "religious actualist." As a leader, he succeeded in articulating inner concerns in a way that struck a collective chord. Self-rule and home rule were inextricably combined in Gandhi's program. He would have endorsed in his own terms, Erikson believed, Luther's assertions: "Christ comes today; God's way is what makes us move; we must always be reborn, renewed, regenerated; to do enough means nothing else than always to begin again."

Gandhi had begun and successfully completed his political novitiate as an Oxford-trained barrister in South Africa during his 20s and 30s. By his late 30s, he had developed passive resistance as a political strategy to defeat the Black Act, a law that required all Indians in the Transvaal to register with the government and to carry identification papers on their persons. At 40 years of age, Gandhi staked out his claim for leadership in his Indian Home Rule Manifesto, and, during the next few years of his midlife transition, he developed the device of the Satyagraha campaign, culminating in the Great March of striking mine workers in South Africa when he was 44 years of age.

When Gandhi returned to India in 1915 at 45 years of age, he did so, Erikson wrote, "like a man who knew the nature and the extent of India's calamity and that of his own fundamental mission." As a mature, middle-aged man, he was, in Erikson's view, a person who has determined what "he does and does not *care for*" as well as "what he *will* and *can* take *care of*. He takes as his baseline what he irreducibly is and reaches out for what only he can, and therefore, *must* do."

What Gandhi had to do was lead a labor strike at the mills in Ahmedabad and, the next year, at 50 years of age, a national strike for independence from Britain. Erikson contended that Gandhi's emergence at that time as the "father of his country" underlined "the fact that the middle span of life is under the dominance of the universal human need and strength which I have come to subsume under the term *generativity*." Erikson refers here not merely to the generativity that a parent at 20 or 30 years of age may feel for a child. Erikson's concept of generativity is often mistakenly taken to apply to the child-rearing work of young adults. Instead, he is describing the protective concern for the generations and their retarding-facilitating social institutions, whose leadership is the essential responsibility of the middle-aged individual.

In the early 1970s, Erikson returned to the San Francisco Bay Area to live and to begin again. The Eriksons relocated to Cambridge, Massachusetts, some 10 years later. In 1981, the Eriksons and psychologist Helen Kivnick undertook an intensive study of 29 octogenarian parents of children whose lives had been meticulously scrutinized in the Guidance Study begun in 1928 at the Institute of Human Development at the University of California at Berkeley. The results of their research were published in *Vital Involvement in Old Age*.

In this work, Erikson, Erikson, and Kivnick revisit the eight stages of psychosocial development and their attendant virtues or strengths. They emphasize the opportunities that exist at the end of life to integrate "maturing forms of hope, will, purpose, competence, fidelity, love, and care into a comprehensive sense of wisdom." A successful integration results from a final reworking of the earlier polarities of basic trust versus mistrust; autonomy versus shame and doubt; initiative versus guilt; industry versus inferiority; identity versus confusion; intimacy versus isolation; generativity versus self-absorption; and integrity versus despair. The authors use the term *vital involvement* to identify an involvement with the environment that is characterized by "actuality" and "mutuality." The elder who is able to maintain a vital involvement with his world—no matter how small its scope—is better able to tolerate the depredations of aging: loss of sensory acuity, physical mobility, and stamina; changes in intimate relationships as children marry and move away and friends and partners sicken and die; loss of social status, financial security, and sources of pride in professional competence; and realization that relatively little time remains.

Developed in infancy, hope is the basis on which the senescent individual attempts to integrate faith in the universe and the relative predictability of its laws with a realistic mistrust about that which is unpredictable and unreliable. The elder may experience a need to affirm a basic faith—in religion or nature—and to understand more deeply his own place in a generational progression.

Late in life, the individual must struggle to redefine a sphere of autonomy even as he becomes increasingly dependent on others. Living independently, residing in familiar surroundings, and following established routines can be crucial symbols of autonomy and the means by which signs of impairment (e.g., a walker) may be accepted without undue shame. An individual's lifelong experience of autonomy influences his or her capacity to adjust to restrictions on freedom. The ability to allow others to help supports the generative impulses of younger adults and reinforces for both the sense of a generational cycle.

The polarities of initiative versus guilt, first evident in the youngster's exploration and play and subsequently evident in adult work and recreation, must be balanced anew in old age. With the passage of time, the person faces a diminution of opportunities for the exercise of initiative and must regret those instances in which he or she failed to act decisively or with sufficient concern for others. Successful adaptation to the limitations of old age must draw on the strength of purposefulness developed in childhood and tempered by maturity.

With the natural decline in physical strength and sensory acuity, the senescent individual increasingly depends on a lifelong sense of effectiveness. External rewards are usually not as numerous as they were in young adulthood or middle age. The feeling of competence and mastery must be sustained internally. An old person may cope with growing physical limitations by changing the criteria for a sense of accomplishment, pursuing new hobbies or modifying old ones, developing new avenues of involvement with former professions, or living vicariously through the accomplishments of children and grandchildren.

Old age provides the individual with the chance to review a lifetime of beliefs, to come to terms with choices made and opportunities lost, and to make and act on any final commitments, which now most clearly reflect what Erikson termed "the 'I' in the totality of life." In striking a final balance between identity and identity confusion, the elder concerns himself with an external image and a personal image. The external image is the way that the individual may expect to be remembered; the personal image reconciles the sense of who he or she has been with an evolving sense of who he or she may yet become. Identification with the successes of younger generations and satisfaction in one's own part in the transmission of values helps the senescent stave off feelings of insignificance or obsolescence in the face of technological and sociological changes.

The sense of love that can emerge at the end of life is one that is built on a foundation of love, expressed and unexpressed, throughout the life cycle. A new balance may be forged between intimacy and isolation in the face of decline. Intimate relationships may be recast in more positive terms; reminiscences provide the elder with the opportunity to draw on and to reintegrate earlier experiences of tenderness and sexuality.

To reconcile feelings of integrity and despair, the individual must make peace with previous choices, acknowledging what was gained and lost and accepting that it is too late to change. Relationships and values may be reviewed with more room to consider alternate points of view. In balancing the dispositions toward generativity and stagnation, the elderly person may be able to build on years of experiences as a parent, worker, and creatively productive person from middle age, which themselves were shaped by childhood experiences of caring or its absence. Grandparenthood offers another chance at generativity and a way to undertake it more robustly and less ambivalently. Erikson coined the term *grand-generativity* to distinguish the generativity of old age in which the person, freed from the direct responsibility for family, institution, and community, is better able to incorporate care for the present with concern for the future. Such concern may be expressed through advice or financial assistance to family members or, on a larger scale, through commitment to religious beliefs, political involvement, or community action. Grand-generativity contributes to a feeling of immortality; in caring for the younger generation and allowing oneself to be taken care of, the senescent secures a personal place in a generational history.

The "joint reflections of old age" contained in the book are an effort to elucidate the psychosocial process of vital involvement and to extend Erikson's observations to the outer limits of the life cycle. The book also brought Erikson back full circle to his professional beginnings, having made almost 40 years earlier, play observations on the Guidance Study children.

Application of Erikson's Concepts to Clinical Work

Erikson's view of individual experience as inexorably embedded in developmental, familial, societal, and historical contexts crucially shaped his ideas concerning mental illness and psychiatric treatment. As noted previously, Erikson was reluctant to pathologize behavior or to rush to judgment about the meaning of any given symptom. He asserted, "Perhaps there are certain stages in the life cycle when even seemingly malignant disturbances are more profitably treated as *aggravated life crises* rather than as diseases subject to routine psychiatric diagnosis."

To understand the meaning of such "disturbances," Erikson drew on his training in classical drive theory (with its concepts of the unconscious; id, ego, and superego conflicts; and repression, regression, and repetition compulsion) but emphasized the adaptive and synthesizing capacities of the ego in brokering relations between internal drives and external reality. When Erikson listened to his patients, he thought about their symptoms not simply as compromise formations between libidinal drive and superego prohibition, but also as expressions of arrested or derailed psychosocial development. Toward this end, Erikson examined many aspects of his patients' current lives (e.g., skills, talents, and aspirations; religious and political commitments; social and intimate relationships; and roles as worker, partner or spouse, and parent) and located them within a larger social, cultural, and historical context. His focus was on the entire life cycle, the development of specific virtues, and those factors that facilitated or retarded psychosocial growth. As Edward R. Shapiro and M. Gerard Fromm point out,

> He paid attention to the whole life context of any immediate situation. He asked a number of questions. What is the immediate stimulus for the patient's reaction? What is the acute life conflict, the current developmental stage, the issues that are manifest? In what developmental context did the patient's reaction first occur? Is it now manifest in the relationship to the therapist, in a repetitive conflict, in a characteristic way that the individual solved earlier developmental struggles? In what social context is the individual embedded, what roles are available? . . . What defenses does the individual use? What are the individual's deepest psychological investments?

Erikson conceived of these psychological investments in broad terms. He used concepts of attachment, separation, and mutuality (defined as "a relationship in which partners depend on each other for the development of their respective strengths") to illustrate ways in which the individual is essentially a social being. He recognized that psychological crises often occurred at times of developmental separation or individuation and that fears regarding dependency and abandonment were frequently the catalyst for such crises. Although Erikson acknowledged the influence of early childhood conflict or trauma on an individual's progress in negotiating developmental tasks in adolescence and adulthood, he did not think that the issues being played out were simply reiterations of infantile conflict.

Erikson's belief that psychosocial development continues throughout the life cycle led him to caution psychotherapists against a theoretical reductionism in which symptomatic behavior was attributed to a traumatic past and in which insufficient attention was paid to contemporary conflicts in the ego's relations with the world. He was particularly critical of the "originology" in psychoanalytic thought. "I mean by it a habit of thinking which reduces every human situation to an analogy with an earlier one, and most of all to that earliest, simplest and most infantile precursor which is assumed to be its 'origin.'" Erikson was wary of other theoretical blind spots within his profession. As Coles noted, "Psychiatric and psychoanalytic concepts emerge from and become very much suited to a particular society—which exerts its (moral and puritanical) influence on everything, even the most complicated, rarefied, and 'objective' of abstractions."

In his article, "The Nature of Clinical Evidence," Erikson outlined the relationship between patient and therapist. He described the "clinical core of medical work" as the "encounter of two people, one in need of help, the other in the possession of professional methods. Their *contract* is a therapeutic one: in exchange for a fee, and for information revealed in confidence, the therapist promises to act for the benefit of the individual patient, within the ethos of the profession." Although he acknowledged certain parallels between medical and psychiatric consultations (e.g., the patient presents with a list of symptoms, the physician or psychiatrist asks questions designed to elucidate the problems, arrives at a tentative diagnosis, and proposes a treatment plan), Erikson departed from a traditional medical model in important ways. Although according the therapist the respect and authority appropriate to his special training and expertise, Erikson envisioned the patient as an active participant in a collaborative endeavor. Within the limitations imposed by treatment setting (e.g., inpatient vs. outpatient) and degree of psychological impairment, the patient was expected to take significant responsibility for his treatment. Erikson noted a natural transformation that occurs in the patient: "'Under observation,' he becomes self-observant. As a patient he is inclined, and as a client often encouraged, to historicize his own position by thinking back to the onset of the disturbance, and to ponder what world order (magic, scientific, ethical) was violated and must be restored before his self-regulation can be reassumed."

How does the patient participate in his own "cure"? He is invited to free associate. Erikson noted that "[w]e consider a patient's 'associations' our best leads to the meaning of an as yet obscure item brought up in a clinical encounter, whether it is a strong affect, a stubborn memory, an intensive or recurring dream, or a transitory symptom." The associations consist of whatever thoughts, feelings, sensations, or images occur to the patient during and after the mention of that item. Erikson continued,

> Except in cases of stark disorganization of thought, we can assume that what we call the synthesizing function of the ego will tend to associate what "belongs together," be the associated items ever so remote in history, separate in space, and contradictory in logical terms. . . . It is . . . this basic synthesizing trend in clinical material itself which permits the clinician to observe with "free-floating attention," to refrain from undue interference, and to expect sooner or later a confluence of the patient's search for curative clarification and his own endeavor to recognize and to name what is most relevant, that is, to give an *interpretation*.

Free-floating attention "turns inward to the observer's ruminations even as it attends the patient's 'free associations' and which, far from focusing on any item too intentionally, rather waits to be impressed by recurring themes." A message represented by a patient's memory, dream image, or symptom can be overdetermined—"a condensed code transmitting a number of other messages, from other life situations, seemingly removed from the therapy. This we call 'transference.'"

As for the therapist's role in working with the patient's free associations, Erikson averred, "I have to assume that the patient is (to varying degrees) unconscious of the meaning which I discern in his communications, and that I am helping him by making fully conscious what may be totally repressed, barely conscious, or simply cut off from communication. . . . I take for granted an effective wish on his part (with my help) to see, feel and speak more clearly." Erikson felt that a "therapeutic" interpretation was one which was clear and concise, yet presented the patient with a "unitary" theme, "a theme common at the same time to a dominant trend in the patient's relation to the therapist, to a significant portion of his symptomatology, to an important conflict of his childhood, and to corresponding facets of his work and love life." How would the therapist determine if an interpretation was "right"? Erikson believed that "[t]he proof lies in the way in which the communication between therapist and patient 'keeps moving,' leading to new and surprising insights and to the patient's greater assumption of responsibility for himself."

Erikson acknowledged that there was a great deal of subjectivity involved in the patient's complaints and the therapist's interpretations. He cautioned that "even while facing most intimate and emotional matters, [the therapist] must maintain intellectual inner contact with his conceptual models, however crude they may be." He must evince "a *specific self-awareness* in the very act of perceiving his patient's actions and reactions." Erikson wrote that "there is a core of *disciplined subjectivity* in clinical work—and this both on the side of the therapist and of the patient—which it is neither desirable nor possible to replace altogether with seemingly more objective methods." The therapist was advised to undergo a personal psychoanalysis to reduce or to eliminate potential blind spots that might compromise this disciplined subjectivity.

Erikson noted "the power of the transference, i.e., the patient's transfer to me of significant problems in his past dealings with the central people in his life" but also conceived of what would now be called a "real" relationship between himself and his patient. In "The Nature of Clinical Evidence," Erikson provided a lengthy clinical vignette illustrating dream analysis and his use of his emotional reactions in his interpretations to his patient. Because he did not conceive of clinical work as primarily oriented toward the development and interpretation of the transference, Erikson accorded himself and other clinicians the freedom to cultivate "real" aspects of the relationship with the patient. He believed it important and necessary at times that the therapist educate and guide his patient. Erikson averred that "only by playing my role as a new person in his present stage of life can I clarify the inappropriateness of his transferences from the past."

A psychotherapy informed by Eriksonian principles is essentially optimistic in nature, for it takes as a given the notion that psychosocial development is universal and continues throughout the life cycle. Natural forces propel the individual forward. Psychiatric symptoms are often best understood as manifestations of aggravated developmental crises—development that has been blocked or derailed. In such cases, the therapeutic task is to release or to redirect those built-in forces for growth and adaptation.

As Erikson noted in *Identity: Youth and Crisis*, the object of psychotherapy is not to head off future conflict but to assist the patient in emerging from each crisis "with an increased sense of inner unity, with an increase of good judgment, and an increase in the capacity 'to do well' according to his own standards and to the standards of those who are significant to him."

SUGGESTED CROSS-REFERENCES

Sigmund Freud's theories are discussed most fully in Section 6.1. Other theories of personality and psychopathology are discussed in Sections 6.3 and 6.4. Schizophrenia is discussed in Chapter 12, personality disorders are discussed in Chapter 23, and psychosomatic disorders are discussed in Chapter 24. Normal child development and adolescent development are discussed in Sections 32.2 and 32.3, respectively; adulthood is discussed in Chapter 50; normal human sexuality is discussed in Section 18.1a; and normal aging is discussed in Section 51.2c. Psychoanalysis and psychoanalytic psychotherapy are discussed in Section 30.1. Another perspective on Erikson's work is given in Section 30.9.

REFERENCES

Capps D: John Nash's predelusional phase: A case of acute identity confusion. *Pastoral Psychol.* 2003;51:361.
*Coles R. *Erik H. Erikson: The Growth of His Work.* Boston: Little, Brown and Company; 1970.
*Erikson EH. *Childhood and Society.* New York: Norton; 1950.
Erikson EH: The dream specimen of psychoanalysis. *J Am Psychoanal Assoc.* 1954;2:5.
Erikson EH: The first psychoanalyst. *Yale Rev.* 1956;46:40.
Erikson EH: Freud's "The Origins of Psychoanalysis." *Int J Psychoanal.* 1955;36:1.
*Erikson EH. *Gandhi's Truth.* New York: Norton; 1969.
Erikson EH: Hitler's imagery and German youth. *Psychiatry.* 1942;5:475.
Erikson EH. *Identity: Youth and Crisis.* New York: Norton; 1968.
Erikson EH. *Insight and Responsibility.* New York: Norton; 1964.
Erikson EH. The nature of clinical evidence. In: *Insight and Responsibility.* New York: Norton; 1964.
Erikson EH: Observations on Sioux education. *J Psychol.* 1939;7:101.
Erikson EH: The problem of ego identity. *Psychol Issues.* 1959;1:379.
*Erikson EH. *Young Man Luther.* New York: Norton; 1962.
*Erikson EH, Erikson J, Kivnick H. *Vital Involvement in Old Age.* New York: Norton; 1986.
Evans R. *Dialogue with Erik Erikson.* New York: Harper and Row; 1967.
Freud A. *The Ego and Mechanisms of Defense.* New York: International Universities Press; 1966.
Freud S. Beyond the pleasure principle. In: *Standard Edition of the Complete Psychological Works of Sigmund Freud.* Vol 18. London: Hogarth Press; 1955.
Freud S. Civilization and its discontents. In: *Standard Edition of the Complete Psychological Works of Sigmund Freud.* Vol 21. London: Hogarth Press; 1961.
Freud S. The ego and the id. In: *Standard Edition of the Complete Psychological Works of Sigmund Freud.* Vol 19. London: Hogarth Press; 1961.
Freud S. The future of an illusion. In: *Standard Edition of the Complete Psychological Works of Sigmund Freud.* Vol 20. London: Hogarth Press; 1961.
Freud S. Group psychology and the analysis of the ego. In: *Standard Edition of the Complete Works of Sigmund Freud.* Vol 18. London: Hogarth Press; 1955.
Friedman LJ: Erik Erikson on identity, generativity, and pseudospeciation: A biographer's perspective. *Psychoanal Hist.* 2001;3:179.
Friedman LJ. *Identity's Architect: A Biography of Erik Erikson.* New York: Scribner; 1999.
Gilligan C: Woman's place in man's life cycle. *Harv Educ Rev.* 1979;49:431.
Kivnick H. Through the life cycle: Psychosocial thoughts on old age. In: Pollock G, Greenspan S, eds. *The Course of Life: Completing the Journey.* Vol 7. Madison, CT: International Universities Press; 1998.
Levinson D, Darrow C, Klein E, Levinson M, McKee B. *The Seasons of a Man's Life.* New York: Knopf; 1978.
Murray H. *Explorations in Personality: A Clinical and Experimental Study of 50 Men of College Age.* New York: Oxford University Press; 1938.
Newton P: Samuel Johnson's breakdown and recovery in middle-age: A lifespan developmental approach to mental illness and its cure. *Int J Psychoanal.* 1984;11:93.
Newton P, Levinson D. Crises in adult development. In: Lazare A, ed. *Outpatient Psychiatry.* Baltimore: Williams & Wilkins; 1979.
Pietikainen P, Ihanus J: On the origins of psychoanalytic psychohistory. *Hist Psychol.* 2003;6:171.
Schein S, ed. *Erik Erikson: A Way of Looking at Things.* New York: Norton; 1987.
Shapiro ER, Fromm MG. Eriksonian clinical theory and psychiatric treatment. In: Sadock BJ, Sadock VA, eds. *Comprehensive Textbook of Psychiatry.* Vol 7. New York: Lippincott Williams & Wilkins; 2000.
Slater C: Generativity versus stagnation: An elaboration of Erikson's adult stage of human development. *J Adult Dev.* 2003;10:53.
Wallerstein R, Goldberger L, eds: *Ideas and Identities: The Life and Work of Erik Erikson.* Madison, CT: International Universities Press; 1998.
Wulff D: Freud and Freudians on religion: A reader. *Int J Psychol Rel.* 2003;13:223.

▲ 6.3 Other Psychodynamic Schools

PAUL C. MOHL, M.D.

The 11 men and women presented in this chapter—Adolf Meyer, Alfred Adler, Carl Gustav Jung, Sandor Rado, Otto Rank, Karen Horney, Franz Alexander, Harry Stack Sullivan, Wilhelm Reich, Erich Fromm, and Eric Berne—made their contributions in the early and middle years of the 20th century. At that time, with knowledge of the neurosciences very primitive, the ethos of psychiatry was to use clinical observation to search for an overarching theory that would encompass not only psychopathology but all of human behavior. None of these individuals doubted that the mind has a biological basis, but they all were aware of Sigmund Freud's woeful failure in his *Project for a Scientific Psychology* to develop a theory of how experience, thoughts, and feelings are transduced to and from material states. Because of this, they were forced to stand back from the physical organism and view humans strictly as psychological entities. Many doubted that biology would ever be capable of explaining human experience, and respected philosophical positions of the time buttressed their opinion.

A question, then, can legitimately be asked: What is the relevance of these theories to 21st-century psychiatry? Are these theories (and others included in this textbook, for that matter) of merely historical interest, or do they hold some wisdom for current clinical practice? Thirty years ago, psychiatrists spent great time and energy comparing and contrasting various theorists and arguing the pros and cons of various formulations. Great implications for the conduct of treatment were seen in the differences between theories. Now, these differences between the theories are of little interest and are seen as having minimal relevance to clinical practice.

These theories themselves continue to be relevant in several important ways. First, regardless of what is learned about neurobiology, psychiatry is and will remain concerned with disordered and diseased behavior, thoughts, emotions, and relationships. Inevitably, these disorders will be communicated through words and nonverbal signals. Psychiatrists will always need some organizing cognitive templates at the behavioral and verbal communicational levels (psychological theories, if you will) to help order and interpret their observations. A sad, pensive, tearful expression does not automatically translate into a serotonin or norepinephrine deficiency. It must first transmute through the psychological constructs of loss, depression, grief, and so forth. Second, these theorists spent enormous time listening to patients, and all were careful observers. Their theorizing was not devoid of empirical data. The problem was the replicability of their data. As such, their observations remain helpful in defining key dimensions for psychiatrists to consider in understanding the inner experiences patients attempt to communicate. As these theories are reviewed, the author was struck by the cogency of many aspects of the formulations that the reader finds in this chapter. Finally, all of these theorists were well versed in something modern psychiatrists are not familiar with: philosophical rules regarding theory construction. Every human being has a "theory of personality," acknowledged or otherwise. This theory, often intuitive and unrigorous, based on a mixture of reading, personal values, and unsystematic observation, influences much of the way people interact with one another. In the clinical situation, when a psychiatrist mixes supportive management and medication, he or she is using a personal theory of personality. The advantage of knowing these 11 theories is that models of intellectual rigor can be brought to personal intuitions.

The problem so many of these theories pose for the modern psychiatrist stems from the fact that, in the absence of empirical or neurobiological data, each theorist seems inevitably tempted to explain as much as possible. Thus, the 21st-century psychiatrist must master these theories while sorting through which observations and inferences remain valid in light of modern information. It is in this spirit that each theory is presented in a sympathetic light, attempting to perform some of that sorting through, retaining what seem to be enduringly accurate observations, inferences, and formulations.

To illustrate the different understandings and therapeutic approaches of each theorist, the following case is used as a basis for formulation according to each theorist.

Mr. A. was a 26-year-old white man who had a history of bipolar I disorder. He was brought in for treatment after not completing the last required course for his advanced degree and being arrested for disturbing the peace. He had consistently lied to his family about where he stood with his coursework and about having skipped an examination that would have qualified him to use his professional degree. He had also not told them that he had been using marijuana almost daily for a number of years and occasionally used hallucinogens. His arrest for disorderly conduct was for swimming naked in an apartment complex in the middle of the night while under the influence of hallucinogens.

Mr. A.'s use of marijuana began early in college but became daily during graduate school. He was diagnosed as having bipolar I disorder early in his senior year at college after a clear episode of mania. His mood disorder was well controlled on lithium (Eskalith). During graduate school, he was episodically compliant with medications, preferring to try to maintain a state of hypomania. He saw a psychiatrist every 3 to 6 months for medication checks. During his 4 years in graduate school, he had two clear episodes of depression and began taking sertraline (Zoloft), 100 mg a day, with questionable benefit. Mr. A. believed that he could be a great writer. He spent most of his time reading and trying to write. He dreamed of going to New York and becoming part of a group of avant-garde writers that would parallel the Algonquin Club of the 1930s or the Beat poets of the late 1940s. This aspiration and his marijuana abuse predated his development of bipolar I disorder. He attended class episodically, nonetheless performing adequately. His last class had no final examination but required a paper. He planned to write this paper in the form of a play, involving a dialogue between two thinkers from different times and cultures. His professor was very excited about this idea, but Mr. A. kept postponing the task until he was forced to extend his schooling by a year. His other major interest during this time involved growing and photographing flowers.

Mr. A. was born and raised in a large city. His father had been very successful in commercial real estate, and his mother, after raising the children, used the substantial real-estate holdings she inherited from her father to set up a business to manage them. Most of the money was placed in a trust for the patient and his siblings. His mother had total financial control of the trusts and doled out the proceeds to the children as they needed them. There was no family history of any psychiatric disorders.

The patient described his mother as very loving and caring but to the point of being intrusive and controlling. For example, the mother arranged the initial treatment but then was angry that the psychiatrist had not called her regularly to report on her adult son's progress. She was also critical of various aspects of the treatment as reported to her by her son. The patient's two older siblings had attended prestigious colleges and graduate schools but had returned home to work in the mother's real-estate management company. The 30-year-old sister was living in the parents' home. The 35-year-old brother had lived at home for a time but then moved out to a location a few blocks away. There was a younger brother, still in college, who also smoked marijuana excessively. He tried to minimize the patient's problems to the family and tried to protect the patient, who desperately had not wanted to return home. Of note is that none of the children were married, although the two older ones had each had a couple of serious relationships.

The children seemed to regard the mother with affectionate amusement and bemusement. The father was seen as a very caring but undemonstrative man who put much energy into keeping the mother from becoming too upset and encouraged the children to do the same. The children often wanted to provoke the mother for her judgmental, detail-oriented intrusiveness. The father discouraged them but occasionally found their provocations amusing.

The family viewed itself as very close, with strong values oriented toward community service and family loyalty. The family belonged to a religious community but expressed their involvement primarily in social service and social action volunteer work, accompanied by very generous financial contributions.

The patient had been a very successful debater in high school and recalled his development as very positive but provided few details. He tended to place himself in the role of the outsider, an observer of humanity, which he saw as consonant with the role of a writer. He was proud to have bipolar I disorder and tried to regulate his medications so that he would be hypomanic much of the time, seeing this as enhancing his creativity. He viewed his use of marijuana in the same vein. One of the most distressing aspects to him of his depressive episodes was that marijuana no longer created a feeling of well-being but made him feel worse. His current depressive episode involved no neurovegetative symptoms. Rather, he presented as flat, numb, apathetic, ashamed, anhedonic, and anergic. He was particularly ashamed of being back in his hometown and of living with his parents.

The patient ostensibly understood and accepted his illness well and had read much about it. However, the family had responded to the information "with proper treatment, bipolars can live normal lives" as meaning that the information should be kept secret so that he should be treated normally. Mr. A., on the other hand, was very open with friends at graduate school about his illness and his pride in it and the creativity he associated with it.

The patient had two long-standing recurrent dreams. One involved him flying. The narrative line varied, but the flying theme recurred. Often, he had other magical powers in his dreams such as the ability to heal, to not be killed by bullets, to save the world or some group of people from mortal danger, and so on. The other recurrent dream was of a hotel lobby. These dreams regularly began with him entering a hotel lobby to meet a group of people, accompanied by a feeling of dread.

ADOLF MEYER

Meyer (1866 to 1950) immigrated to the United States after having trained as a neuropathologist in Switzerland (Fig. 6.3–1). Not interested in metapsychology, he espoused a commonsense psychobiological methodology for the study of mental disorder, emphasizing the interrelationship of symptoms and individual psychological and biological functioning. His approach to the study of personality was biographical; he attempted to bring psychiatric patients and their treatment out of isolated state hospitals and into communities and was also a strong advocate of social action for mental health. He began his career as a clinically oriented state hospital pathologist, becoming the second head of the Pathological Institute (later, the New York Psychiatric Institute, whose affiliation with the Columbia College of Physicians and Surgeons he created). He later became the president of the American Psychiatric Association and had a 32-year tenure as chairman of psychiatry at Johns Hopkins. His major social contribution was helping to found the National Committee on Mental Hygiene.

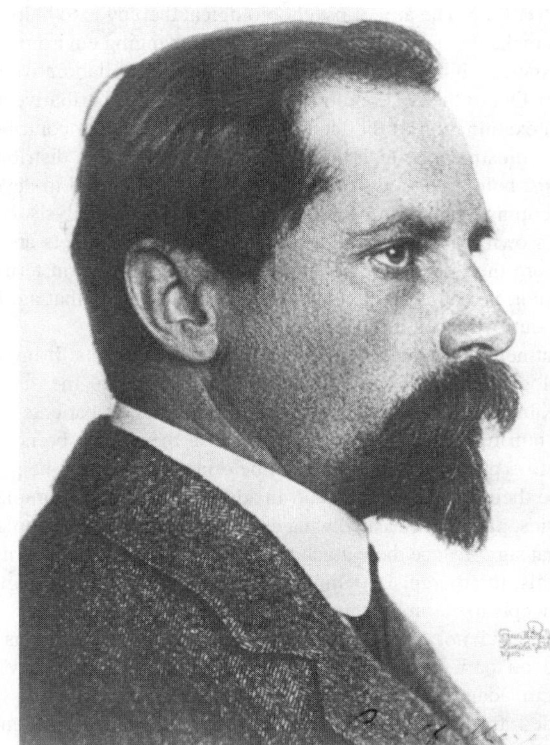

FIGURE 6.3–1 Adolf Meyer. (Courtesy of National Library of Medicine, Bethesda, MD.)

Psychobiology Despite his background as a neuropathologist, which was common among European psychiatrists of his generation, Meyer strongly opposed the Kraepelinian view of mental illness as having a predetermined course based on phenomenologically identified syndromes. Instead, he believed that individuals' habitual reaction patterns made them more susceptible to specific types of breakdown. Meyer used biographical study, strongly encouraging psychiatrists to take a thorough, detailed life history of the patient to understand each individual's reaction patterns. He saw development as lifelong, thus viewing the data from adolescence onward as equally important as that from childhood in understanding the patient's narrative.

He observed reaction patterns, attempted to predict the conditions under which they might occur, and tested and validated methods for their modification. He acknowledged the contributions of Freud and Jung but believed they were too narrow. A thoroughgoing pragmatist, he preferred common sense to metapsychological constructs as the means to understand and deal with psychopathology.

Theories of Personality and Psychopathology

Meyer believed that, through a basic tendency toward integration, multiple biological, social, and psychological forces contribute to personality development. The vulnerable person uses poorly planned, ill-suited means of adaptation. Meyer used the biographical approach as a practical guide to elicit information about personality development, to organize the information, and to check and reevaluate the information obtained under different circumstances. His clinical examination assessed each patient's life history; physical, neurological, genetic, and social status; and the relationship between those factors and personality factors. A diagnosis and an individual treatment plan were based on this assessment.

Treatment The aim of psychobiological therapy is to help individuals make the best possible adaptation to changing environmental circumstances. It began with the development of a collaborative relationship. Out of the collaborative relationship came distributive analysis, an examination of the factors in patients' lives that contributed to their adjustment or lack thereof, and concluded with distributive synthesis, helping patients to understand themselves and to develop better coping skills. The first step in distributive analysis is the patient's own exposition of the presenting problem. Assets and liabilities are then determined by eliciting the life history in terms of the memories that are immediately available and those that are later fleshed out by reconstructing past experiences.

Treatment is initiated by focusing on patients' assets. It involves psychological, chemical, physical, and environmental measures as needed. In more severe cases, attention is paid first to patients' sleep habits, nutrition, and daily routines because these must be normalized before psychological work can be done. Patients are helped to describe their difficulties in detail. In addition to eliciting complaints or worries, patients are asked what eases or worsens their complaints and what significance they attach to their symptoms and concerns. In doing this, the therapist attempts to use the patient's own language and concepts to communicate suggestions and advice.

Meyer did not pay attention to unconscious mechanisms but focused on patients' functioning in reality. Both present-day and long-term adaptive patterns are considered. Therapeutic sessions proceeded from immediate, obvious problems in the present to longer-term issues and historical data. With guidance, patients investigate their own personality problems, ascertain the origin of their conflicts, and work to develop more useful behavior patterns. Meyer called this *habit training*, a term he may or may not have borrowed from behavioral tradition. When unhealthy adaptive patterns are modified, proper adjustment and personal satisfaction result.

Meyerians would focus first on the adequate treatment of Mr. A.'s mental illness. Because he is still dependent on his parents, they are included in the treatment plan and might be seen separately by a social worker. Both Mr. A. and his parents are told that failure to control the symptoms of his mental illness could cost him his life and any satisfaction that he might derive from it. Mr. A.'s mood swings are stabilized on an appropriate medication, and he is observed closely for restoration of normal sleeping and eating habits. He is asked to discontinue his habit of marijuana use because of its tendency to aggravate the symptoms of his mental illness and its clouding of the assessment of treatment efficacy. Random urine screening might be recommended. Mr. A. is helped to develop a daily schedule, including time for work, social interaction, and recreation. He is not encouraged to return to school because of his tendency to use school as an escape from responsibility. He is encouraged to develop his photography as a hobby after a period of stable work performance. Later, he would begin the distributive analysis phase of his treatment and would be asked to reflect on the impact of his bipolar I disorder and his avoidance of responsibility in his life. In the distributive synthesis phase of treatment, he is helped to realize that his avoidance of responsibility keeps him from achieving independence and the pleasure of attaining any realistic goal. He is asked to develop a plan for achieving both appropriate independence and for remaining within the family structure. Mr. A.'s parents are seen periodically for a progress report and to urge them to push Mr. A. toward appropriate self-care, toward making use of his own resources. They might be asked to place Mr. A. on an allowance and to hold him to it strictly to reinforce his accountability for his actions. Over time, his parents are asked to slowly withdraw financial support and to give Mr. A. more independence. They might be asked to place his inheritance in a trust designed so that he could not impulsively misspend it.

ALFRED ADLER

Adler (1870 to 1937) was born in Vienna, Austria, and spent most of his life there (Fig. 6.3–2). A general physician, he became one of the original four members of Freud's circle in 1902. Adler never accepted the primacy of the libido theory, the sexual origin of neurosis, or the importance of infantile wishes. In 1911, he resigned as president of the Vienna Psychoanalytic Society and continued the development of his own socially and interpersonally focused theory of development. He posited a striving for self-esteem through overcoming a sense of inferiority, which he saw as an inevitable presence in the human condition as a result of its extended childhood. He equated psychological health with constructive social consciousness, developing a system that he called *individual psychology*, which is still vigorous in many countries. His major social contribution was the establishment of child guidance centers in Vienna that served as a model for the rest of the world.

Personality Theory If Meyer's system is captured in a phrase, that phrase is common sense. Adler's system might be described similarly as *Menschenkenntnis,* which is the concrete, practical knowledge of humankind. Adler saw individuals as unique, unified biological entities whose psychological processes fit together into an individual lifestyle (*lebensstil*). He also postulated a principle of dynamism, which in every individual is future directed and moves toward a goal. Once the goal is established, the psychic apparatus shapes itself toward attainment of that goal. Life goals are chosen and are thus subject to change. Changes require modification of

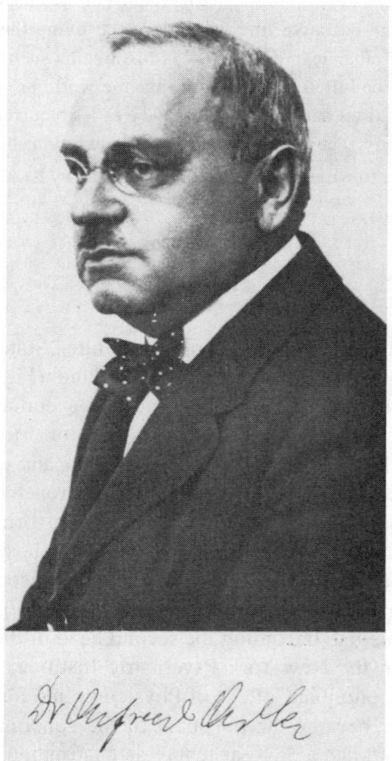

FIGURE 6.3–2 Alfred Adler (print includes signature). (Courtesy of Alexandra Adler.)

memories, dreams, and perceptions to fit the accomplishment of the new goal. Adler also emphasized the interface between individuals and their social environment: the primacy of action in the real world over fantasy. Community mindedness, acceptance of the need to conform to the legitimate demands of society, is an important precept, but Adler also recognized a dialectic that occurs between individuals and their interpersonal environment, each constantly reacting to and shaping the other. Thus, Adler anticipated some of the modifications of Freud's theories introduced by Heinz Hartmann as well as some of Sullivan's thinking.

Normal Personality and Adaptation The cornerstone of Adler's personality theory is the concept of moving from a sense of inferiority to a sense of mastery. Early in life, everyone has a sense of inferiority resulting from realistic comparison with adults' size and abilities. Moving from this sense of inferiority to a sense of adequacy is the important motivational motif in life. Thus, the ideal person strives for superiority and does so through high social interest and activity; the emotionally handicapped person continues to feel inferior and reinforces that position through lack of striving and social interest.

There are many obstacles to the development of self-esteem and social interest. Prominent among them are poorly developed or "inferior" organs or systems (such as poor eyesight or poor eye–hand coordination), childhood diseases, pampering, and neglect. Physical handicaps and childhood diseases may promote self-centeredness and loss of social interest; birth order is another factor. According to Adler, first-born children, having lost their position of only child, tend not to share and become conservative. Later children change and become social activists. Youngest children feel secure because they have *never* been displaced. These theoretical thoughts and clinical observations by Adler anticipated recent psychological research on the importance of birth order in human behavior.

Theory of Psychopathology

Emotional disorders result from mistaken lifestyles that are subject to change by will and by self-understanding. Individuals subject to emotional disorders have false ideas about themselves and the world and inappropriate goals that lead them away from constructive social interest. Individuals with a pampered lifestyle, for example, expect and demand from others, avoid responsibility, and blame others for their failures, but they feel incompetent and insecure because their well-being depends on pressing others into service. If life poses no challenge, a mistaken lifestyle may have no consequences. When a mistaken lifestyle is ineffective, symptoms develop that protect self-esteem while helping the individual to avoid dealing realistically with the problem being confronted. The difference between neurosis and psychosis is that neurotic individuals maintain social interest but are blocked from life goals by symptoms, whereas psychotic individuals lose social interest and retreat into their own world.

Psychotherapy

Because his theory emphasized the mismatch of lifestyles with the demands of the real world, Adler focused on blocks to living productively in the real world, not on exploring unconscious conflict. His aim was to point out mistaken self-views and mistaken views of the world and then, by mobilizing will, make the needed changes, including a change in life goals.

Therapeutic Process Starting with three sessions per week and tapering off to one per week, a positive relationship with patients is established and used to lead patients to awareness of their lifestyle, how it is discordant with the demands of social reality, and ways in which it may be reoriented. Instead of striving for goals of no social value that falsely increase self-esteem, they are pushed to work toward ameliorating their own situation. Having become aware of the obstacles they have placed in their own path and of the consequences of these self-defeating behaviors, they are now helped to develop constructive interests in themselves and others. As they become less self-engaged, they find themselves better accepted by others, which reinforces their constructive efforts. People who have dedicated themselves to symbolically defeating others learn to cooperate and advance toward useful goals. Any endeavor in which patients can develop real competence is encouraged, whether social, work, artistic, or musical.

Patients are encouraged to remove the concrete obstacles to developing a useful lifestyle, including reading instruction for slow readers or contact lenses for people who are self-conscious about their appearance. Early recollections, birth order, dreams, daydreams, and present-day interactions are all used to help patients see the inappropriateness or falseness of their ideas and life goals. Actual life events or memories of events are less important than individuals' reactions to those events or memories. Because memories are likely to be retrospective falsifications justifying an erroneous lifestyle, there is little need to verify them. There is also no need to look for latent content in dreams; they are merely an expression of present-day concerns. Nor is it necessary that therapists' interpretations be correct because they need only to help patients build a useful conception of themselves and the world. This perspective anticipated what has come to be called the *hermeneutic approach* to psychotherapy.

Several of Adler's techniques, including reframing and paradoxical communication, now enjoy wide popularity. *Reframing* is viewing the same data from a different point of view. Indecision, for example, was reframed from a product of mixed feelings to a wish to maintain the status quo. Failure to act keeps everything the same, which is the self-fulfilling prophecy of the discouraged person. After this reframing statement, patients are pushed to act constructively. Paradoxical communication is instructing patients to do the opposite of what the therapist wishes them to do. In dealing with an indecisive person, for example, Adler might caution against doing anything rash. Adler also paid attention to the impact of his patients on their environment and recognized that individuals do much to create their own interpersonal worlds. In response to complaints about being treated unfairly by others, Adler asked patients how they dealt with the people about whom they complained. Above all, Adler treated his patients as rational and as able to learn more productive ways of living. In his emphasis on practical, constructive solutions; misconstrued goals; and misperceived views of the world and the self, Adler also anticipated important elements of cognitive therapy.

As seen from the Adlerian point of view, Mr. A. has developed a mistaken lifestyle and an inappropriate life goal. He maintains himself in fantasy as a writer while failing at the accomplishments that would enable him to become a writer. Thus, he has been attempting to make the normal step of moving from inferiority to mastery in fantasy instead of through realistic achievement. Blocks to his development include pampering and his concomitant denial and abuse of his bipolar I disorder, the latter representing his organ inferiority. He has lost the social interest he had earlier in life and become extremely self-centered, unconcerned with others or with the consequences of his actions. He uses drugs and hypomania to avoid the pain of defeat. An Adlerian therapist encourages Mr. A. to develop a realistic self-view. He has a mental illness that requires lifelong treatment. Grandiose dreams and intoxication with drugs cannot substitute for accomplishments in the real world and always lead to defeat. He is asked to set and to strive to accomplish small, realistic goals for himself such as holding a steady job while enjoying photography as a hobby. His mental illness is reframed as a challenge to his creativity and his use of marijuana as an obstacle to mobilizing his creativity. He might initially be encouraged to accept his dependency on his family and later, as he stabilizes, to reduce his dependency on his family as a means to heighten his self-esteem and to make a transition into adulthood. He is encouraged to join the Depressive and Manic Depressive Association or other available support and educational groups as a means to better understand and accept his illness, to develop a social conscience, and to stimulate his altruism. His dream about flying is interpreted as his wish to achieve mastery; his dream about the hotel lobby is recast as awareness that he has been trying to substitute fantasy for reality.

CARL GUSTAV JUNG

Jung (1875 to 1961) was a lifelong resident of Switzerland (Fig. 6.3–3). He trained in psychiatry under Eugen Bleuler at the Burgholzli Mental Hospital in Zurich and was strongly involved with Freud and the psychoanalytic movement from 1906 to 1914, when he resigned as president of the International Psychoanalytic Association. After a "creative illness" that lasted from 1914 to 1918, Jung became an advocate of active introspection as the means to intrapsychic change. This episode and Jung's subsequent interpretation of it, as well as that of his disciples, form the focus of much of the recent controversy about him and his ideas. Although Jung rejected Freud's notion of libido as sexual energy and the Oedipus complex as a universal developmental stage, he believed not only in the unconscious mind but in a shared racial and species unconscious. Jung, an intuitive introvert, was not interested in the practical aspects of living in the world; his focus was instead on individuation through becoming aware of the unconscious.

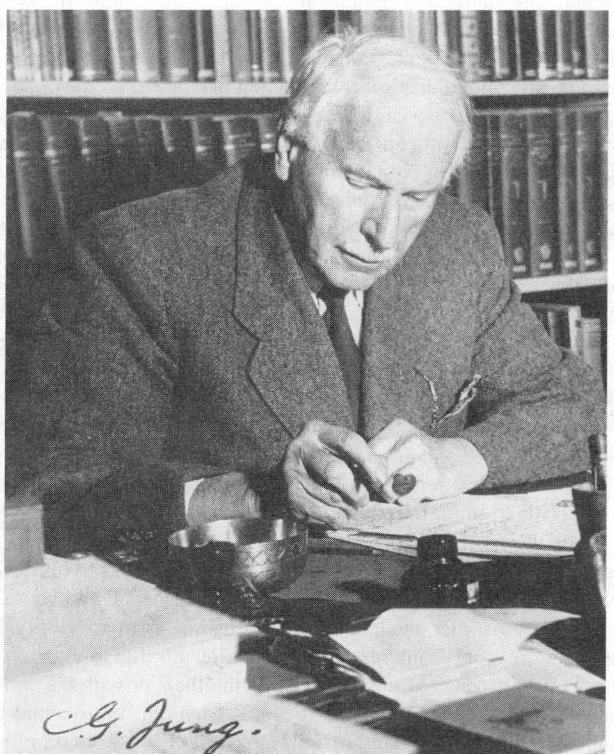

FIGURE 6.3–3 Carl Gustav Jung (print includes signature). (Courtesy of National Library of Medicine, Bethesda, MD.)

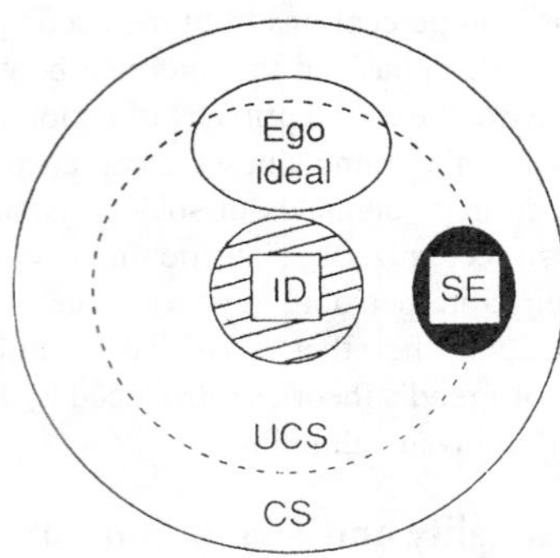

FIGURE 6.3–4 The Freudian topology of the psychic apparatus. CS, conscious; SE, superego; UCS, unconscious.

Personality Theory

Jung developed an elaborate metapsychology that was every bit as detailed and formalized as Freud's. In addition, his theories most clearly identify most of the important fault lines in classic psychoanalysis. His construct of the psychic apparatus differs from the Freudian structure of ego, superego, id, and ego ideal (Fig. 6.3–4). Below an outer rim of consciousness is the personal unconscious, which contains the complexes. Contained within the personal unconscious and connected to the complexes are the archetypes, the elements of the self, which in turn connect to the surface of the personality as the ego.

Complexes

Complexes are groups of unconscious ideas associated with particular emotionally toned events or experiences. Jung inferred them from his early word-association studies, when he noted that certain words provoked intense reactions or produced less reaction than expected. Complexes are built around genetically determined intrinsic psychic structures known as *archetypes.* Complexes are also reinforced by environmental events and by selective attention or inattention and are thus self-perpetuating. They are endowed with psychic energy from their affective tone: positive, negative, mild, or strong; the more intense the complex, the greater the emotion, imagery, and tendency to action. Complexes are often stimulated by interactions with others. A father complex can be stimulated by a person who symbolizes a father (such as an older friend) or by a stimulus, such as music or art, that evokes father memories. The complex, formerly dormant in the unconscious, comes to the fore and tends to dominate consciousness and to displace other complexes, which then sink into the unconscious. As the father-related external stimuli diminish, the father complex, including what was thought, felt, and expressed during its ascendancy, also ebbs. This is a very different model of the dynamic unconscious from Freud's. The boundary between the conscious and unconscious is far more permeable, and there is no emphasis on forces that maintain ideas and feelings in one place or another. Movement between conscious and unconscious experience is triggered by experience. Similarly, Jung's conceptualization of interpersonal boundaries was far more permeable than Freud's; Jung also placed much more emphasis on nonverbal stimulation (music, art, spiritual life) in this process than did Freud, who was the archetypal Enlightenment rationalist.

Some complexes are more conscious, better developed, and more ego-syntonic; others are less conscious, poorly developed, and ego-alien. The latter are projected onto the environment, especially by the immature psyche of children, and from this, projective and introjective processes evolve. One person may introject and identify with a complex being projected by another person. Thus, therapists may become psychologically infected by their patients. It is also possible to project a complex that is not integrated within oneself onto another person and then develop a relationship with that projected complex. One can envision an interpersonal environment charged with mutual projections available for introjection, thus offering endless potential for mutating perceptions and misperceptions. Thus, for Jung, the psychological boundary between individuals was far less clear than for Freud or Adler. In addition, one can see that Jung was much less concerned with an ultimate, objective, rational reality to be determined and compared with the individual's complexes of projections and introjections. Jung also had a parallel appreciation for the process of projective identification that Melanie Klein was developing at approximately the same time.

In another insight that paralleled Klein's observations, an important aspect of complexes is their bipolarity. Each complex has a positive and negative pole such as good father and bad father or rewarding father and punishing father. One pole of a complex can be projected onto another person, who in turn introjects it and acts on it in a relationship. In this way, the theory of complexes is a theory of interpersonal as well as intrapsychic relationships.

In Jungian theory, the ego is also a complex. It serves the same function as the Freudian ego, controlling conscious life and bridging the intrapsychic and external world. The other complexes that also make up the psyche may align with or lie in opposition to the ego. For example, emotionally charged primitive complexes have a great tendency to become autonomous and may behave like partial personalities that oppose or control the ego. These personalities appear as images in dreams, as hallucinations, and as separate personalities in dissociative identity disorder. They also appear in séances when mediums bring forth so-called personalities from the dead. For Jung, this phenomenon also explained animism and states of possession.

Jung had a great interest in mystical experience, which Freud saw as the persistence of infantile, magical thinking; primary process; or wish fulfillment. This is another of the clear divisions in their thinking. For Freud and Freudians, the world is a harsh, demanding place that forces one to give up primitive wishes for magical experiences. For Jung and Jungians, magic is alive and well in the inner world and is to be embraced.

Archetypes Complexes are connected to structures embedded more deeply in the psychic apparatus, the archetypes. Complexes, the more superficial aspect of the complex–archetype continuum, are related to events, feelings, and memories from individual lives. They are the means by which archetypes express themselves in the personal psyche. *Archetypes* are the inherited capacity to initiate and carry out behaviors typical of all human beings, regardless of race or culture, such as nurturing and accepting nurturance and being aggressive or dealing with aggression by others. These predispositions are analogous to the organization of the cerebral cortex into the anlage for perception of visual or auditory stimuli that become the capacity to see and hear but that require particular environmental stimulation for their development. Just as vision cannot develop without visual input during physiologically critical stages, so archetypes require interactional stimulation for their elaboration into complexes. Thus, the human infant's psyche is not amorphous energy awaiting organization by the environment; it is instead a complex and organized set of potentials whose fulfillment and expression depend on the appropriate environmental stimuli. There are as many archetypes as there are prototypical human situations. In positing the archetypes based on anthropological data, Jung was remarkably prescient of current understanding of the brain's organization.

The mother complex archetype illustrates the interrelationship of complex and archetype. All humans are born with a poorly formed but relatively clear model of an all-nurturing caretaker, which Jung referred to as the *earth mother archetype*. The mother complex emerges from this based on experiences with mothers or mother surrogates: their attitudes, personalities, and relationship to the particular individual. The mother archetype is found in dreams or fantasies, often as a huge woman or an animal with many breasts. The motif of a many-breasted animal, found in many cultures, is that of unlimited nurturance.

Unconscious The Jungian unconscious has two layers, the more superficial being the personal unconscious and the deeper layer the collective unconscious. The complexes exist in the personal unconscious, the archetypes in the collective unconscious or *objective psyche*. The *personal unconscious* is the equivalent of the Freudian unconscious, a repository of individual memories that have been repressed. The *collective unconscious* is the residue of what has been learned in humankind's evolution and ancestral past, much as human deoxyribonucleic acid (DNA) is an aggregate of the past. In this portion of the psyche reside instincts, potential for creativity, and the spiritual heritage of humankind. The potent synthesis of Darwinian natural selection theories with Mendelian genetics, which has had such a profound impact on all of biology, occurred in the 1920s. It is not clear whether Jung was aware of this intellectual thrust, but his understanding of the collective unconscious and of the archetypes is remarkably consonant in form, if not in detail, with the modern understanding of hereditary and developmental neurobiology as applied by cognitive science.

The psyche, like all other living systems, attempts to stay in balance. Jung's term for homeostasis in the relationship of conscious to unconscious life is the *law of compensation*. For any conscious attitude or experience that is overly intense, there is an unconscious compensation. A person experiencing neglect might fantasize or dream about a huge, many-breasted mother. When interpreting dreams, Jung asked himself what conscious attitude the dream compensated for.

Symbols Although Jung accepted that certain symbols are universal, he suggested that, in dealing with patients, it is wisest to view symbols as expressions of content not yet consciously recognized or conceptually formulated. A tall, cylindrical object might symbolize a penis, but it could also stand for creativity or healing. Symbols are often attempts to unite and strike a balance between images from the collective unconscious with the personal unconscious. A tall, cylindrical object that symbolizes a penis in the personal unconscious might symbolize the phallic principle of creativity or fertility in the collective unconscious.

Personality Structure At the center of the conscious personality is the complex called the *ego*. Several universal complexes attend the ego. The *persona* (named after the mask worn by ancient Greek actors), or public personality, mediates between the ego and the real world. The *shadow,* a reverse image of the persona, contains traits that are unacceptable to the persona, whether they are positive or negative. A brave persona, for example, has its fearful shadow. The archetype of the shadow is the enemy or feared intruder. The *anima* is a residue of all the experiences of woman in a man's psychic heritage; the *animus*, the residue of all the experiences of man in a woman's psychic heritage. The anima or animus connects the ego to the inner world of the psyche and is projected onto others in day-to-day or intimate relationships. When connected with the shadow, a man, for example, might see attributes of woman as undesirable and might experience guilt encountering such qualities in himself.

SELF The *self* is the archetype of the ego; it is the innate potential for wholeness, an unconscious ordering principle directing overall psychic life that gives rise to the ego, which compromises with and is partly shaped by external reality. In Jungian metapsychology, the unconscious gives rise to integration, order, and individuation. The self appears from the unconscious in dreams, fantasies, and altered states of consciousness to give direction. In the first half of life, the ego attempts to identify with the self and to appropriate the power of the self in the service of the ego's growth and differentiation. During this time, the ego may become inflated with an unrealistic sense of power: the arrogance of youth. If cut off from the self, there may be a sense of alienation and depression.

INDIVIDUATION In the second half of life, the ego begins to attend more to the self than to the conscious realm of life. Jung called this developmental process *individuation*, the drive for individuals to become unique and to fulfill the spiritual propensities common to all humanity. Often, this process requires withdrawing from earlier identities and conventional definitions of success and seeking new paths. This change often has the paradoxical effect of leading to broader and more mature relationships in addition to greater creativity.

PSYCHOLOGICAL TYPES Jung's theory of psychological types has three axes (Fig. 6.3–5). The *extroversion–introversion* polarity refers to the two basic types of object relatedness. Extroverts are oriented to others and to the world of consciousness. Their energy flows outward first, then inward. Introverts are oriented to their inner world, their energy flowing first inward and then to outer reality. Introverts might therefore be seen as selfish and unadaptable because they attend first to their inner world and then determine how the outer world can fit them. Extreme extroverts, on the other hand, can seem insensitive to themselves and to the inner lives of others.

The *sensation–intuition* polarity concerns perception. The perceptive type that Jung called *sensation oriented* is stimulus bound and attuned to the specifics of here-and-now reality, external reality as perceived by the senses. The intuitive type blurs the details but apprehends the overall picture. The sensation type comes to understand a situation by assembling the details; the intuitive type grasps the overall situation before attempting to assimilate its parts. The sensation type sees the trees first; the intuitive type sees the forest first.

The *thinking–feeling* polarity deals with information processing and judgment. In the *thinking* mode, data are evaluated according to logical principle. *Feeling*, at the opposite pole, is making judgments through nonlogical processes having to do with values and understanding relationships. In social relationships, the thinking type deals with people according to their social rank or according to the tradition of etiquette; a feeling type deals with others in terms of their present social relationship or perceived emotional state. The thinking type asks of an event, "What is it?"; the feeling type, "Is it good or bad?"

Each individual has a preferred mode on each of these three polarities. By placing an individual on each of the three axes indicated in Figure 6.3–6, each individual can be identified as a type. An extroverted-sensation-thinking type is oriented to the real world, tends to perceive external details, and organizes them into a logical structure. An introverted-intuition-feeling type is self-oriented, grasps situations as a whole, and is sensitive to their emotional implications.

Everyone's psyche contains all of the types. However, each person has a superior set of functions: types that are evolved from early life and that are shaped strongly by constitutional factors. In the second half of life, adults who continue the process of individuation attempt to integrate or broaden and deepen their understanding of their inferior functions. Thinking types become more aware of feelings, sensation types allow themselves to rely more on intuition, and extroverts become more interested in their own inner lives. The Myers-Briggs Type Indicator, a simple paper-and-pencil test consisting of approximately 40 questions, reliably places individuals on

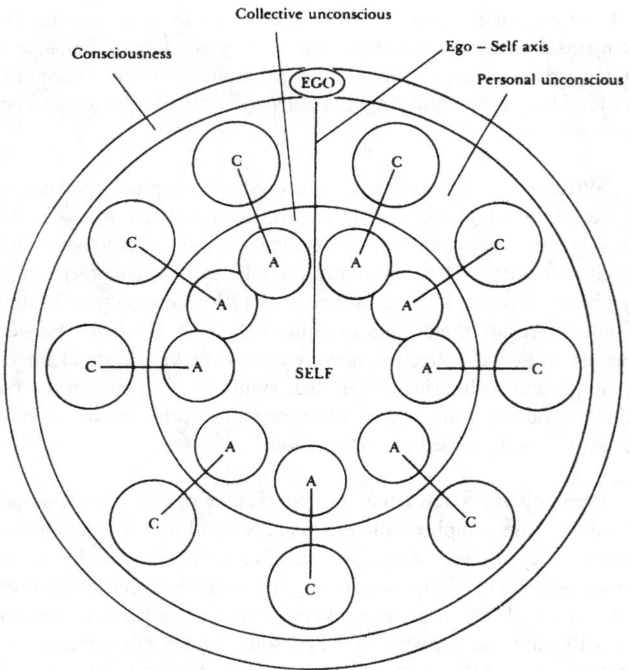

FIGURE 6.3–5 The Jungian psychic apparatus. A, archetype; C, complex. (From Stevens A. *On Jung*. London: Routledge; 1990, with permission.)

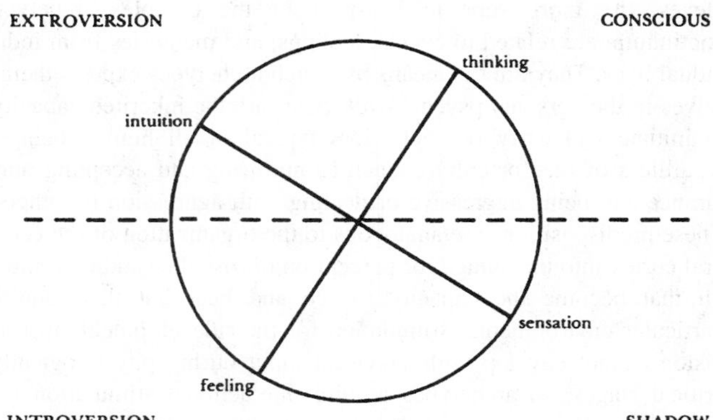

FIGURE 6.3–6 The three personality axes: extroversion–introversion, thinking–feeling, and intuition–sensation. (From Stevens A. *On Jung*. London: Routledge; 1990, with permission.)

these dimensions. It has become a very popular instrument among popular psychology, management consulting, counseling, and self-improvement organizations for quickly identifying the qualities of individual participants. The typology may be the most widely known and accepted aspect of Jung's theories, although it is often used independently of its original context.

Psychopathology When another complex becomes incompatible with the ego complex, anxiety is experienced. To contain the anxiety, the incompatible complex splits off from the ego and moves unconsciously against the ego or other complexes identified with the ego. This splitting enables individuals to live out the two incompatible complexes, one more ego-identified and the other more ego-alien. The latter is often experienced as being inflicted by the outer world ("I am being mistreated" rather than "I have inner conflict"). This splitting and dissociation of consciousness is particularly evident in hysteria and is an especially good explanation of the phenomenon of multiple personalities (dissociative identity disorder). Within the psyche, ego or part personalities or complexes operate along with shadow personalities that are antithetical to them. In addition, the anima and animus and archetypal images of the self attempt to integrate and to control the chaos. The various personalities that appear in dissociative identity disorder are manifestations of the complexes and the self.

Extroverts tend to develop hysterical or antisocial traits, whereas introverts become dysthymic, anxious, and obsessional. The symptoms are often related to the attempted emergence of inferior functions. Viewed in this way, pathological conditions may contain within them the struggle toward wholeness or health, attempts by inferior functions to become integrated instead of dissociated from consciousness. The integration of these inferior functions often requires emotionally painful rearrangements of conscious thoughts, attitudes, and lifestyle. Thus, Jung saw all psychopathology as an attempt at healthy adaptation, a point of view that did not enter Freudian psychoanalysis until the time of the ego psychologists.

The attempted expression of inferior functions need not result in psychopathology. People with highly developed thinking functions may find themselves wishing to experience life more fully and may involve themselves in highly emotional extramarital relationships. On exploration, one may find the unresolved loss of a mothering person with the resultant inability to achieve intimacy with a woman. The process of reaching for intimacy is enacted outside the marital relationship because the wife has been assigned the role of the cold, abandoning mother. This is an example of how Jungian theory can arrive at a fairly typical Freudian formulation by a rather different route.

Application Jung suggested that therapy begin with four visits per week and then be spaced out to one or two per week. Present-day Jungian practitioners work with their analysands once a week, face to face. Jung placed great emphasis on the human relationship between analyst and analysand and noted that both parties change in the course of analysis. He defined *transference* as the patient's attempt to develop psychological rapport with the doctor and held that without rapport and object relationship, the technical operations of the analyst were of no value. With its emphasis on reintegration, symbolism, and dreams, Jungian analysis seems well suited to helping educated people deal with the developmental problems of midlife. Having achieved a professional identity, material success, and established a firm family role, they often begin to ask, "Who is the real me?" "What is most meaningful to me?" and "What is my relationship to humankind and human history?" Often given strongly to self-criticism in the service of self-improvement, such individuals may be relieved to find themselves described as trying to become fully themselves instead of as being neurotic. However, the complicated, often blurred intrapsychic relationships described, the interest in mystical experience with its potential shading into magical thinking, and the blurring of boundaries between therapist and patient have made analytical psychology particularly attractive to those who are drawn to or inclined toward cults or exploitative relationships with patients. The break between Freud and Jung, which had for decades been ascribed to Freud's rigidity and authoritarianism, now appears to have had a contribution from Jung: Freud disapproved of a complicated, dependent relationship Jung is believed to have had with a former patient.

Jungians see Mr. A.'s bipolar I disorder and use of marijuana as having unleashed conflicting archetypes, all attacking the ego complex he had grown up with. This could be seen as an opportunity for Mr. A. to claim a fuller definition of the self. Mr. A.'s aspirations to be a great writer are taken as potentially healthy, and even the content of his psychotic and substance-induced states is analyzed so as to incorporate their meanings into his ego complex. Mr. A.'s previous psychological type is described as extroverted-sensation-thinking—an observer of life but not a full participant. The type emerging in his psychotic and intoxicated states is described as introverted-feeling-intuitive—the self-absorbed, self-experiencing lover of beauty and ideas. The dreams about flying suggest an expression of the hero archetype; the anxiety dream suggests some emergence of his shadow in association with his aspirations to be a writer. His love of flowers and creativity during his periods of psychosis and intoxication suggests that the shadow is connected to his anima. The task of therapy is to assist Mr. A. in accepting these alien parts of himself and integrating them into his ego complex. Relatively little emphasis is placed on education or specific treatment of his bipolar I disorder, except insofar as it prevented a good therapeutic alliance. His fantasies, dreams, and psychotic experiences are investigated, discussed, and analyzed in terms of the psychological functions used and the archetypes expressed. His interpersonal issues with his family are seen primarily as projections by him of other unacceptable archetypes that need identification, analysis, acceptance, and integration. For example, his relationship with his mother is seen as a projection and fear of the earth mother archetype. The overall goal is to harness the unleashed unconscious material to allow Mr. A. to pursue his ambitious and creative goals.

SANDOR RADO

Hungarian-born and trained in psychiatry, Rado (1890 to 1972) emigrated to the United States in 1931 after helping to organize the Hungarian Psychoanalytic Society and being an active member of the Berlin Psychoanalytic Institute (Fig. 6.3–7). In 1945 at Columbia University, he was the director of the first psychoanalytic institute within a university medical school. Rado believed that learning and cultural and parental influences were of greater importance than instinctual factors as causes of emotional or behavioral disorder but also believed strongly that an underlying genetically determined biochemical abnormality was present in schizophrenia. His work fit in with the development of ego psychology, influenced by Anna Freud, Hartmann, and David Rappoport.

Adaptational Psychodynamics Rado viewed the psychic apparatus as an organ of adaptation. Effective adaptation is psychological health. Psychological illness or maladaptive behavior is a failure

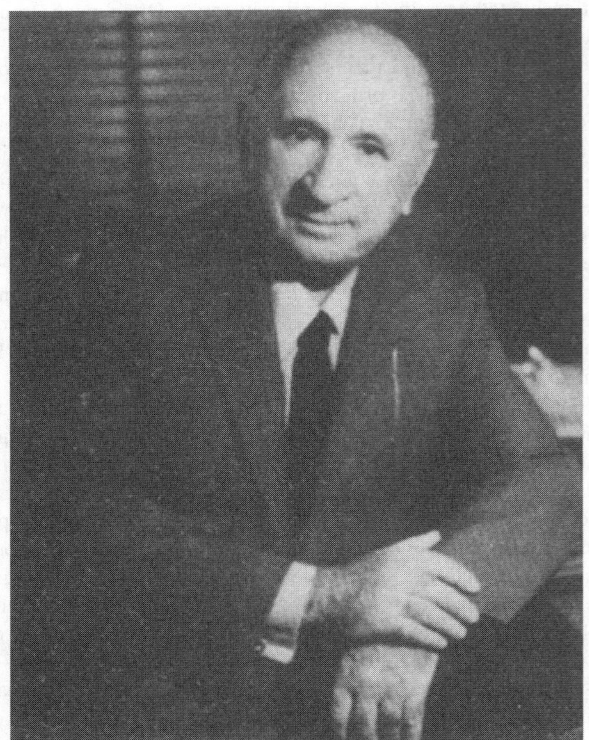

FIGURE 6.3–7 Sandor Rado. (Courtesy of New York Academy of Medicine.)

of this adaptive mechanism. There are hierarchical levels of human mental integration: hedonic, emotional, emotional thought, and unemotional thought. These levels parallel the phylogenetic and ontogenetic evolution of the brain with the gradually increasing influence of the neocortex over the more primitive parts of the brain. The hedonic level is the realm of pain and pleasure. Pain signals impending damage and causes flight. Pleasure indicates benefit and elicits clinging or moving toward. Persistent pain has the secondary effect of reducing self-esteem through a sense of failure; pleasure has the secondary effect of enhancing self-esteem through a sense of success. More than most other psychoanalysts, Rado stayed true to Freud's belief that a neurobiological basis for the psychic apparatus would be discovered. He integrated Walter B. Cannon's theory of emotions with James Papez's identification of the limbic system as the neuroanatomical locus of emotional and hedonic mechanisms. He also anticipated the recognition by modern evolutionary biology and neuropsychology of hedonic mechanisms being the keys to memory.

The emotional level of psychic integration consists of the emergency emotions (fear, rage) and the tender or welfare emotions (love, pride). The *emergency emotions* are responses to real or anticipated pain and result in flight or fight. The *welfare emotions* are responses to actual or anticipated pleasure or benefit and prepare the organism to embrace the pleasurable stimulus. Rado's observation that ordinary human mental activity is primarily at the hedonic and emotional levels represents the kind of astute thinking that these early personality theorists were capable of, anticipating the modern evolutionary neurobiological understanding that the brain has evolved as an adaptation to maximize hedonic behavior.

Emotional thought justifies and reinforces the emotions from which it springs and is not reality based; it corresponds to Freud's primary process. Examples of emotional thought include dreams, fantasies, delusions, and the hallucinations of psychiatric illness. Rational or unemotional thought operates on Freud's reality principle, making it possible to delay action and gratification, to forgo present pleasure for future gain, and to control emotional responses. Rado concluded that much effort is required by ordinary adults to combat emotional thinking and that the emergency emotions are far stronger than the welfare emotions.

Conscience

Conscience is the part of the mature psychic apparatus, operating unconsciously, that rewards good behavior, increasing self-esteem, and punishes bad behavior by guilt, thus lowering self-esteem. Unlike Freud's conception of the superego, conscience is seen as primarily constructive and adaptive. It facilitates cooperation with others and reduces destructive forms of competition. Although conscience stimulates adaptive behavior, it can also produce pathological behavior.

Anticipating the work of Lawrence Kohlberg on the developmental stages of moral thought in both children and adults, Rado described the development of conscience as originating in the dependent child's wish and need to remain in his or her parents' good graces. Initially, the child projects his or her own omnipotent feelings onto the parents. Believing that parents see and know all causes the child to fear punishment that he or she believes is inescapable. A child who misbehaves experiences guilty fear, which has the positive effect of stimulating restitutive behavior. The child admits wrongdoing and accepts punishment to restore the parents' positive feelings. This relieves the painful guilty fear and restores the child's self-esteem. Pain-dependent or masochistic behavior is a form of restitutive behavior based on guilty fear. Fear motivates the person to seek punishment in advance, which may at times permit satisfaction of a formerly proscribed desire. Although not a complete explanation of masochistic behavior, Rado provided an important link in its understanding.

Both discipline and conscience formation are complicated by the buildup of rage that occurs when the child obeys or submits to his or her parents. The rage, which is repressed, constantly seeks discharge and is a potentially serious problem for both the individual and society.

Treatment

According to Rado, *psychological health* is a predominance of welfare emotions in a reasonably independent, self-reliant person. Such a person creates a self-reinforcing interpersonal field by stimulating pleasurable feelings in others. By recognizing the interpersonal field within which emotions occur, Rado reflects the influence of Sullivan and Kurt Lewin. The emergency responses are still active but are released nondestructively through various types of play or constructive activity and through dreaming.

The aim of psychotherapy is to increase the influence of the welfare emotions on behavior and to reduce the influence of the emergency emotions. Patients are encouraged to relinquish the dependency that causes and results from maladaptive behavior and to become reasonably self-reliant. The past is explored in therapy primarily to increase understanding of the present rather than to reconstruct the past. Rado focused more on examining patients' present-day behavior than on the recovery and analysis of memories and the development of insight based on those reconstructions. He preferred to educate patients directly instead of developing and analyzing the transference, as was done in classic analysis.

Rado would have framed Mr. A.'s difficulties as failures of adaptation to his mental illness and adult life and as a regression to the hedonic level of adaptation in which pleasure is sought and pain avoided. As Mr. A.'s self-esteem was reduced through his inability to face his obligations; he avoided the resultant pain through flight into mania and the use of drugs. Activation of his emergency emotions led him to behave and to fail in ways that provoked punishment. He failed at graduate school and was arrested for disturbing the peace. Rado would have emphasized reducing the self-defeating behaviors that alienated Mr. A. from others and increasing behaviors that would result in support and positive input from others. Rado would have encouraged Mr. A. to examine his dependence on his family and to decide if he wanted to continue in this dependent role. Mr. A. would have been helped to uncover his welfare emotions and to relate to his family in a positive way that would allow him to reduce his rage toward his parents for being controlling of him, reduce his acting out against them, and enable him to develop into his own person.

FRANZ ALEXANDER

Alexander (1891 to 1964) was one of the second generation of psychoanalysts. He was born in Budapest and attended medical school there, graduating in 1912 (Fig. 6.3–8). He conducted research at the Institute for Experimental Pathology in bacteriology until World War I, when he practiced clinical microbiology on the Italian front, primarily combating malaria. After the war, he joined the department of psychiatry at the University of Budapest Medical School as a brain researcher. This led to an encounter with Freud's work, and, in 1919, he became the first student of the Berlin Psychoanalytic Institute. In 1930, Alexander became a visiting professor of psychoanalysis at the University of Chicago and, in 1932, founded the Chicago Psychoanalytic Institute. He established the Institute independent of the psychoanalytic societies, leading the Chicago Institute to be one of the most creative sources of psychoanalytic thought. During the same time, he began his interest in psychosomatic illnesses, helping to found the journal *Psychosomatic Medicine.* A guiding principle of his work was to make psychoanalysis an integral part of medicine.

In 1946, Alexander became professor of psychoanalysis at the University of Southern California, where he continued his work on psychosomatic medicine and became interested in the interface of learning theory, the psychophysiology of stress, and psychoanalysis.

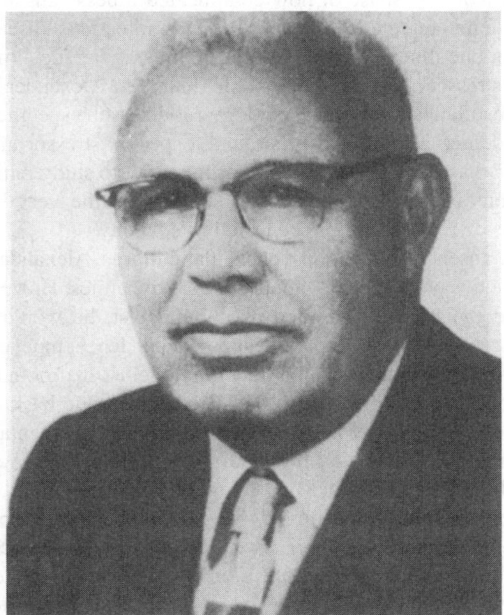

FIGURE 6.3–8 Franz Alexander. (Courtesy of Franz Alexander.)

Theory of Personality

Alexander did not develop a unique overarching theory of personality; his contribution was his application of psychoanalytic thought to pathophysiological processes. In this, he laid the groundwork for the burgeoning fields of psychosomatic medicine, behavioral medicine, and psychophysiology. Alexander created the basis for the biopsychosocial model and studied the mind and body at a time when American psychiatry, despite Freud's original ideas, had become purely psychological in its orientation. In studying and treating many patients with serious physical illnesses, he was also forced to consider creative modifications of therapeutic technique.

Alexander and his group began by intensively studying, by means of clinical interviews, patients who had one of seven illnesses that had been identified by general practitioners as having strong psychological components. Out of these clinical studies emerged the specificity hypothesis, which proposed that certain illnesses are the product of a complex interaction of specific constitutional predispositions, specific unconscious conflicts, and specific types of stressors that activate such conflicts. The group then tested these hypotheses in a series of clinical studies of patient populations. The independent variable was usually the ability of skilled clinicians to predict a patient's illness from disguised case reports. The model he proposed remains the fundamental psychosomatic conceptualization; a variety of illness situations are now studied by controlling for genetic influences while measuring and modifying intrapsychic conflict and external stressors.

In the field of psychotherapy, Alexander was one of many who sought to shorten the analytical process. He hypothesized that intellectual insight was not the central curative factor in therapy, a radical and revolutionary proposal at the time. Rather, he emphasized the role of *corrective emotional experience*. This led him to experiment with variations in technique that might facilitate such experiences. This, his most controversial stand, nearly ruptured his relations with the psychoanalytic movement.

Theory of Psychopathology

The seven diseases that Alexander studied were peptic ulcer disease, ulcerative colitis, essential hypertension, Graves' disease, neurodermatitis, rheumatoid arthritis, and bronchial asthma. Alexander and his group identified what they believed to be the single, specific core conflict that, in interaction with constitutional predispositions and in the circumstance of a particular stressor, would activate the disease.

The core conflict identified in peptic ulcer disease is hyperindependence as a defense against unacceptable dependency needs. The stressor that results in an acute attack can be any situation that demands that the individual openly acknowledge or ask that dependency needs be met. Ordinarily, patients use dominance and control to intimidate others into meeting their dependency needs. Thus, Alexander was the first to describe the "little boy" business executive prone to peptic ulcers. The groundwork was laid for John J. Brady's executive monkey experiments. This particular illness model has received more confirmatory evidence than any of the others, especially from a study of army inductees in whom psychological profiles as described by Alexander, in combination with measurements of serum pepsinogen, were extraordinarily successful in predicting the development of duodenal ulcer. It is not clear what the impact of the recent recognition of a specific pathogen means for this particular hypothesis. On the one hand, there is ample evidence that Alexander was right. Perhaps the identified pathogen, *Helicobacter pylori*, is merely the constitutional factor that had previously been believed to be serum pepsinogen concentration, or perhaps

Alexander's hypothesis applies to some subgroup of patients with duodenal ulcer. However, today, peptic ulcer disease is treated primarily as an infectious ailment.

Alexander's theory of ulcerative colitis also implicated dependency conflicts; however, rage at unmet needs was seen as the defining feature. This rage provokes guilt and the urge to make restitution toward the object of anger by means of gifts of achievements and successes. The model here is clearly the angry child seeking to placate a parent by means of performance. The precipitating event for reactivation of the illness is the perception that the efforts at placation will be unsuccessful. Alexander claimed that this resulted in excess parasympathetic activity, leading to diarrhea. Alexander's own study, in which skilled internists and psychiatrists reviewed case descriptions in which each case had one of the seven identified psychosomatic illnesses and then predicted which illness each patient had, resulted in correct identification of more than one-half of the patients with ulcerative colitis from their dynamics alone—well beyond chance. However, most clinicians now regard George Engel's object relations–based formulation to be the more accurate.

Alexander's hypothesis about essential hypertension focused on inhibited anger and suspiciousness in an outwardly compliant, cooperative individual. A hypertensive patient often goes for long periods with blood pressure under good control and then, seemingly inexplicably, experiences a dramatic increase in blood pressure. Alexander attributed these episodes to incidents when the chronic anger is exacerbated, and intense defenses must be used, causing chronic sympathetic fight-or-flight activation. Several psychophysiological studies have suggested that this theory has some validity at least in terms of short-term changes in the blood pressure of a subset of hypertensives. Labile hypertensive patients appear to fit this model best.

The proposed specific conflict for rheumatoid arthritis postulates conflicts over rebellion against overprotective parents. A compromise formation in which the conflict is discharged via physical activity, especially sports, works for a time, but the anger eventually is expressed in self-sacrifice designed to control others. Failure of this pattern results in increased ambivalent tension, directly expressed via muscular contractions that lead to joint degeneration. A remarkable amount of confirmatory evidence for this constellation appeared in a series of psychological test studies; however, more recent research has failed to replicate much of this and has implicated more general stress issues, life change, and psychoneuroimmunological mechanisms.

Alexander proposed that the wheeze of bronchial asthma represented a symbolic cry. The specific conflict, according to him, was the wish for protection versus the fear of envelopment. This conflict leads to sensitization to separation issues, which become the events that provoke the suppressed cry of the asthma attack. In recent years, it has become clear that the population with asthma is far more heterogeneous both psychologically and physiologically (in terms of vulnerability to allergens) than was recognized in Alexander's time. The role of a vicious physiological–psychological cycle in which asthma stimulates panic, which in turn triggers pathological pulmonary psychophysiological responses, has been a focus of more recent research.

Although the role of conflicts in neurodermatitis remains widely accepted by clinicians, the specific conflict proposed by Alexander, that early deprivation leads to wishes for closeness that are opposed by a fear of it, is no longer accepted. Finally, Graves' disease (thyrotoxicosis) is no longer widely accepted as a psychosomatic illness. Alexander's hypothesis was that premature responsibility led to a martyr-like denial of dependency.

Treatment The specificity hypothesis led Alexander to focus his psychotherapeutic efforts in a way that other analysts of his time did not. He reasoned that if he could help patients to resolve their core-specific conflict without necessarily addressing other parts of their personality structure, the medical illness would improve. Indeed, he published numerous case studies suggesting just this kind of success. In addition, he was among the first to question the value of intellectual insight as the curative agent in psychotherapy. He proposed that a corrective emotional experience is the central agent of change. A corrective emotional experience involved disconfirmation within the transference relationship of previous assumptions and projections.

Thus, Alexander felt justified in introducing a variety of techniques that would initially induce and heighten the emotional experience of the transference and, subsequently, challenge the underlying unconscious assumptions. These techniques included manipulating the frequency and length of sessions, making direct suggestions about the patient's life, self-conscious alteration of the therapist's behavior according to the patient's conflict, and behavior therapy techniques. In many ways, this was the most controversial aspect of Alexander's work. Serious questions about the validity of his suppositions and the ethics of his "manipulative stance" were raised. He was impatient with the slow, methodical process of convincing his colleagues; his intellectual energy led him to embark on ever-newer experiments while other analysts were still struggling to digest his previous suggestions. Yet today, few quarrel with the concept that emotional learning is at least as important as intellectual insight in psychotherapeutic success. Alexander's efforts to modify and shorten the analytical process have come closer to the norm in psychiatric practice than has classic analysis. Indeed, his emphasis on a specific focal conflict that could be addressed in brief therapy by modifying techniques anticipated the later work of Peter Sifneos, David Malan, Habib Davanloo, and James Mann, who systematically developed broad-based models of brief psychodynamic psychotherapy.

Ironically, although Alexander's therapeutic innovations seem prescient today, his specificity hypothesis, which was in his time far less controversial, seems simplistic, naïve, and forced. He did not have available the sense of how complicated illness causation truly is. The dominant model of the time was infectious disease: one organism, one illness. In addition, the complexity of social phenomena and stressors was unknown in his time. Yet, Alexander was the first to postulate a multicausal etiology for disease: a specific constitutional defect, a specific conflict, and a specific stressor all necessary for a disease to occur. He was also the first to study mind–body interactions in a systematic way. Thus, he laid the very basis on which his own formulations seem so limited today.

In the absence of a clear psychosomatic illness, Alexander would have little to say specifically about Mr. A.'s dynamics. However, like any good dynamically oriented psychotherapist, he would readily recognize Mr. A.'s core conflict about dependence–independence. Mr. A. would be understood as rebelling against his mother's nurturant control, although secretly desiring to continue basking in it. He has serendipitously found that illicit drugs and his mental illness can be harnessed such that his mother has to rescue him and take over, although he can avoid becoming aware of the conflict. Alexander's unique contribution to Mr. A.'s case would be to propose that he could be treated with 40 or fewer sessions, focusing exclusively on this conflict (and ignoring others such as oedipal components and issues with his father). Further, Alexander's agenda would be to structure the therapeutic relationship to intensify Mr. A.'s experiencing of this conflict. He might do this by taking a somewhat intrusive, directive stance, thus creating the opportunity for a rapidly intense transference around this issue. Alexander might then spread out the sessions to elicit expression of the patient's yearning for that control. The key therapeutic effort is then to respond constructively to attempts by Mr. A. to assert himself appropriately and take over control of his life—for example, by learning more about his illness and taking responsibility for his treatment.

WILHELM REICH

Reich (1897 to 1957) was one of Freud's most controversial disciples; his latter years were marred by mental illness (Fig. 6.3–9). Reich fixed on and elaborated Freud's early, but later discarded, view that neurosis results from the damming up of sexual energy. Blockage of normal orgasm can lead to partial conversion of sexual energy into aggression, but residual tension manifests in the form of characteristic physical tensions that reflect the underlying character armor of each individual. In so doing, Reich laid the groundwork for a psychoanalytic theory of personality. Before Reich, the focus was on symptoms and psychopathology. There was occasional mention of "character" in psychoanalytic work, but there was no focus on personality as an entity unto itself. This shift is of great importance because, as neurobiology has come to explain more and more Axis I mental disorders, it has become clear that psychodynamic theories' enduring strengths involve understanding and treating personality traits and disorders. Together with Anna Freud and Hartmann, Reich is regarded as the originator of ego psychology.

Personality Theory

Reich did not disagree with Freud's notions concerning personality development, including character types based on fixation at specific levels of psychosexual maturation. Reich elaborated the interpersonal and physical behavior of these personality types. Specific behavioral traits constitute character armor that defends against internal and external dangers. Character armor is comprised of involuntary, repetitive, ego-syntonic behaviors that prevent the emergence of repressed impulses. For instance, the trait of ingratiation frequently defends against hostile impulses, just as the traits of hostility or self-assertion may defend against wishes to be dependent and passive. These traits manifest physically in the voluntary musculature as characteristic postures (clenched jaw or fist, rigid or bowed back) or in excessive stiffness or fluidity of movement. Although Reich's ideas of the behavioral and postural components being central features of character armor are no longer accepted, his ideas successfully transformed the focus of psychodynamic thought from individual wishes defended against by individual defenses, expressed in specific transferential forms into an emphasis on patterns, organization, and intertwining of all of these elements. He also added substantially to the attention paid to nonverbal cues and their implications.

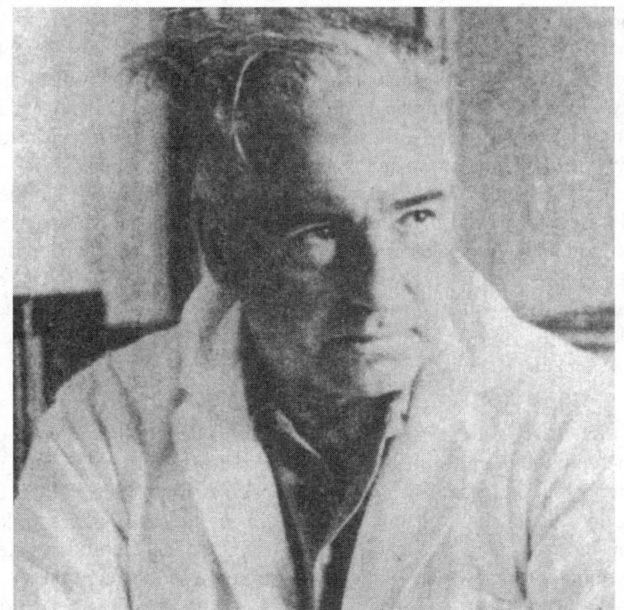

FIGURE 6.3–9 Wilhelm Reich. (Courtesy of New York Academy of Medicine.)

Hysterical Character

The hysterical character has the least body armoring, hence the most lability of function. Body movements tend to be soft, rolling, and sexually suggestive. These individuals are superficial, excitable, flighty, fearful, highly suggestible, and easily disappointed. Their armor helps to defend against easy sexual arousability by flushing out potential sexual stimuli in the environment and then reacting to them with anger.

Compulsive Character

These individuals are tense and restrained, walk stiffly, and sit rigidly. They are overconcerned about orderliness, tend to ruminate, and are indecisive and distrusting. They experience a blockage between their thoughts and feelings. Because they have little access to their feelings, they have little ability to prioritize their actions, to make decisions, or to sense others' reactions to them. The compulsive character avoids expression of repressed impulses by rigid overcontrol. Because of this, these individuals are very threatened by trivial changes in routine.

Phallic-Narcissistic Character

Phallic-narcissistic people appear cold, reserved, and prickly. They are outspoken, provocative, and seek positions of power. Frustrated at the genital-exhibitionist stage of development, the men are identified with the penis and the women with the fantasy of having a penis. The men have strong erective potency but little capacity for intimacy; the women actively dominate men.

Masochistic Character

Masochistic individuals suffer, complain, and damage and deprecate themselves in ways that provoke and torture others. Reich differed with the analytical interpretation that these people enjoy suffering. He believed the opposite—that pleasure is painful for the masochist because of an enormous need, excessive guilt, and the resultant low tolerance for love or pleasure. Suffering allows the masochist to then indulge in a certain amount of self-gratification. Sexual intercourse can be enjoyed, for example, if the partner is inconsiderate or if intercourse is accompanied by the fantasy of rape.

Treatment

Reich's major contribution was in the realm of treatment. He was the first to recognize the need to deal with character resistances before attempting to recover repressed material and that interpersonal resistances need to be dealt with before free association is possible. He did this by analyzing patients' character armor—their characteristic behaviors (including tone of voice, posture, and physical movements)—in the analytical setting before proceeding to an analysis of the unconscious. Reich worked face to face with patients and sought to relax their character armor by physical manipulation. This type of therapy, called *vegetotherapy* by Reich, is still practiced by Reich's followers as *bioenergetics*.

A Reichian analyst might see Mr. A.'s seeming rebellion against conformity as a defense against his fear of being away from his mother's protection and domination. The Reichian might point out that the more Mr. A. rebels, the more tightly he binds himself to his mother. The therapist might also suggest that the behaviors that seem so much under Mr. A.'s control are in fact compulsive behaviors; his prolongation of his manic states and use of drugs are being dictated by forces outside of his awareness to protect him from internal and external dangers—among them, the internal danger of recognizing his rage at his parents for their overprotection and the external danger of not dealing with a world with which he is poorly equipped to deal. As these behaviors become more ego-alien, the Reichian begins a classic analysis of the conflicting unconscious forces involved, including the patient's fear of engulfment by his mother and his wish to be engulfed, fear of his attachment and the wish to be attached, and the harshness of his own superego. The patient's identification with his father as one who superficially placates, but with contempt, is explored. The analysis includes Mr. A.'s dreams. His dream of flying might be interpreted as his fear that to separate from his mother he needs to become invulnerable to all life's potential injuries, a superhuman. His lobby dream might be interpreted as his wish to return to the womb as a defense against the injuries he might experience away from his mother.

OTTO RANK

Rank (1884 to 1939) was a 21-year-old student when he met Freud (Fig. 6.3–10). Rank later earned a doctorate in psychology and eventually became a peer of Freud's before ultimately breaking from him. Rank saw each person as an artist whose ultimate task is the creation of an individual personality. In Rank's view, the neurotic was an *artiste manqué,* a person whose strong creative urge was stultified by the negative use of will.

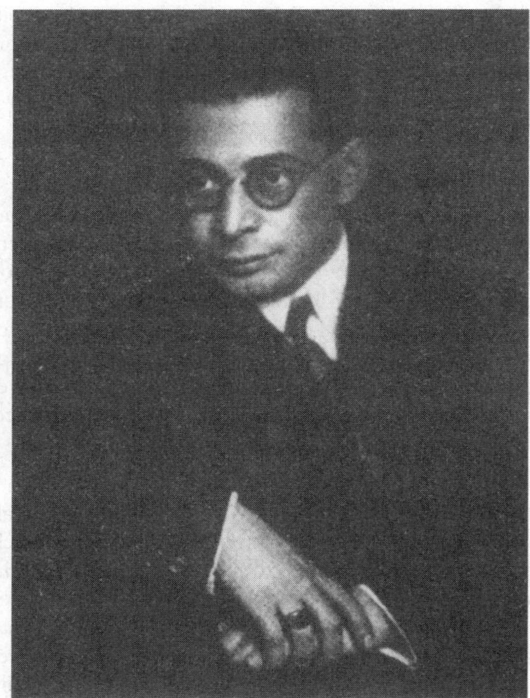

FIGURE 6.3–10 Otto Rank. (Courtesy of New York Academy of Medicine.)

Rankian Dialectic

The basis for his break from Freud was Rank's view that the birth trauma was more important than the oedipal conflict. According to Rank, the physical and psychological experience of birth gives rise to a primal anxiety that is dealt with by primal repression. The crucial intrapsychic conflict that occurs in all developmental phases is the conflict between maintaining the primal bliss of attachment and experiencing the excitement and fear associated with separation. Union stands in contrast to separation; likeness stands in contrast to difference. In adulthood, movement toward another person is possible only if one knows who one is, which can come about only through having experienced separation. Movement toward autonomy is possible only after having established the sense of belonging and self-worth that derive from the experience of fitting in or belonging.

Moving toward union or separation is not an innate biological process but an act of will. In moving toward and engaging with another person, all individuals experience their need for belonging. Moving away from others allows individuals to experience their uniqueness. Maturity is the triumph of will over the forces that inhibit movement both toward and away from others—guilt, death fear, and life fear.

Rank saw guilt as the price to be paid for any act of will. Moving toward union causes guilt over being needy; moving away causes the guilt of abandoning another person. *Death fear* is the fear of losing one's identity by fusing with another person. The weaker one's personal identity, the stronger the death fear. *Life fear*, by contrast, is fear of losing all ties in the process of becoming separate. Every person experiences the cycle of movement from union to separation and back again as part of the life process. This movement takes place at various levels: family, societal, artistic, and spiritual. At each level, there is one or more movement toward union and rebirth. Each person, for example, usually yields to a love experience in which personal differences are set aside to experience unity with another, to experience self-worth, and to be relieved of the sense of difference. The yielding to another ends when the will asserts its separateness, and a new affirmation of individuality occurs.

Will, the prime mover in the Rankian dialectic, is an irreducible creative force. It is not solely an agency for the expression of Freudian sexual or aggressive impulses nor is it the will to power in the Adlerian sense. The beginning of will is in the child's "no," an assertion of what the child will not do. In maturation, will becomes a positive force. Neurotic people, however, deny will because of guilt over what they will. They deal with that guilt by using defense mechanisms such as projection and rationalization. Viewed from this perspective, neurotics are strong-willed people who cannot acknowledge what they will or even that they will. As a result, they cannot use their will constructively in the service of their greatest potential artistic creation, their own personalities.

Treatment

Rankian psychotherapy is a here-and-now interaction with the therapist that mobilizes the patient's will and results in a rebirth experience. The treatment, which is time limited, focuses on the relationship with the therapist. In the therapist–patient relationship are reenacted earlier life struggles, especially struggles involving intimacy. After patients are strengthened through the therapist's acceptance, they begin a process of negative will assertion that is seen as resistance in classic analysis. Rank regarded this negative will assertion as indicative of growth and supported it. Now able to provide self-affirmation on their own, patients free themselves of the therapist and begin to individuate. They overcome the life fear by living up to their fullest potential. Therapy is not aimed at reconstructing personal history, it is a struggle in the here and now between the therapist as a representative of transference objects and reality.

The therapeutic process parallels the process of personality growth. At first, the therapeutic relationship recapitulates prototypical early relationships. The first rebirth experience for patients is claiming their own individual personalities and their uniqueness as human beings. The second phase is their discovery of the physical universe and their likeness to it. Later, they claim their distinctness as creators of themselves. With the emergence of the self, individuals unite with ideological, philosophical, and spiritual reality and experience the final birth of the ideal person, a self-fulfilled person who no longer needs to create to justify his or her existence. In Rank's theories, the beginning of the shift to what is now called *pregenital issues* in psychoanalytic thought can be seen. Very early on, many of Freud's associates sensed that something was missing from the theory. Klein, Rank, and others searched for this understanding in the earliest phases of development. Although rarely cited these days, Rank's work clearly anticipated that of the object-relations therapists and the self psychologists.

A Rankian therapist sees Mr. A. as attempting to achieve separation from his family of origin but as lacking the will to achieve real separation. The prolongation of his manic episodes and his use of drugs help him to avoid the pain of separation and individuation, and his inability to complete graduate school allows him to maintain his dependence on his family. Initially, the Rankian therapist might approve of Mr. A.'s attempts to sustain his manic episodes and his marijuana use as a negative assertion of will against his mother's efforts to run his life. The therapist then would suggest that developing more constructive and positive means might enable Mr. A. to become more free in reality. The Rankian therapist might challenge Mr. A. to develop attachments outside his family and to develop skills to help free himself. Resistance to the development of these skills is interpreted as fear of separation and aloneness. Mr. A. is then encouraged to develop his will in a positive direction, following a path of action that he desires instead of rebelling against a path of action seemingly dictated by others. Finally, Mr. A. would work toward separation from the therapist as a prototypical separation-individuation experience.

KAREN HORNEY

Physician–psychoanalyst Horney (1885 to 1952), who emphasized the preeminence of social and cultural influences on psychosexual development, focused her attention on the differing psychology of men and women and explored the vicissitudes of marital relationships (Fig. 6.3–11). She was one of three women whom Freud trained specifically to have female analysts who would contribute their unique perspective to the psychoanalytic theory about women; the other two were Anna Freud and Helene Deutsch. Horney's view that repression and sublimation of biological drives are not the primary determinants of personality development led to her removal as an instructor in the New York Psychoanalytic Institute and her founding, in 1941, of the American Psychoanalytic Institute.

Personality Theory

Horney believed that personality development results from the interaction of biological and psychosocial forces that are unique for each individual. At the core of each personality is an enduring real self. Partially equivalent to the Freudian

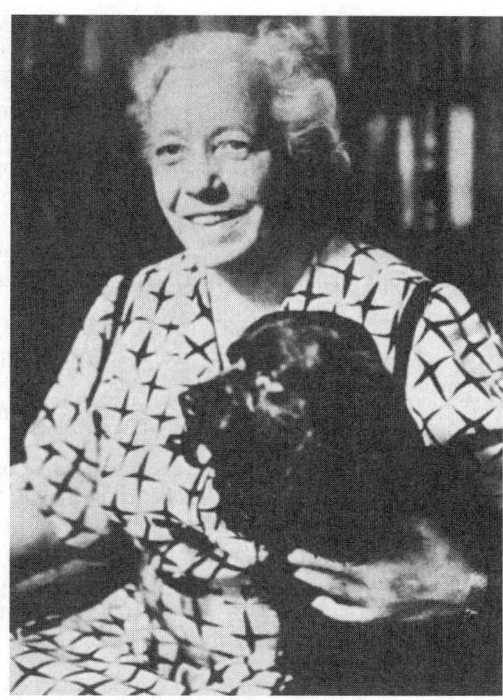

FIGURE 6.3–11 Karen Horney. (Courtesy of the Association for the Advancement of Psychoanalysis, New York.)

ego and similar to Donald Winnicott's focus on selfhood and partly to Berne's child ego state, the real self combines choice, will, responsibility, and identity with spontaneity and aliveness. A natural unfolding process of self-realization leads to the development of human potential in three basic directions: toward others, to express love and trust; against others, to express healthy opposition; and away from others toward self-sufficiency.

Although conditions during childhood may block psychological development, healthy growth is always possible if the internal blockages can be removed. Children whose family situation leads them to feel endangered concentrate on psychological survival and may do so at the cost of developing stereotyped coping mechanisms. All human beings have basic anxiety, which Horney saw as the normal response to the infant's helplessness and separateness. How families respond to this fundamental situation, guided by cultural norms, determines whether individuals spend their lives struggling with basic anxiety or pursuing self-realization. Horney believed that the attributes of passivity and suffering were not biologically specific to women, as taught by the analysts of her day, and that male and female personalities are in fact culturally determined.

Theory of Neurosis

Horney defined neurosis in both intrapsychic and interpersonal terms. She noted that her patients complained not of the symptomatic neuroses, such as phobias and compulsions, but of unhappiness, blockage, lack of fulfillment in their work, and inability to establish or maintain relationships. She saw these individuals as having a complex system of self-perpetuating defensive patterns against basic anxiety—character neuroses.

Safety-seeking children move psychologically in three directions to relieve their anxiety, make life safe and predictable, and achieve satisfaction. They seek affection and approval, become hostile, or withdraw. Children eventually use the coping strategy that best meets their needs, but if only one basic strategy is used, children become limited in their coping repertoire and in their experience of themselves and their world. Their sense of safety is tenuous because there is now danger from within, from suppressed or repressed feelings and impulses. Given continued unfavorable environmental conditions, conflicting feelings are driven into the unconscious, and such children are left with a sense of discomfort, anxiety, apprehension, and an insecure sense of self. At this juncture, their point of reference is externalized; patterns of behavior rigidify, and increase blockages to growth develop. Horney designates these complex, relatively fixed attitudes toward self and others as *neurotic trends.*

Character Types Horney's three main character types are based on the predominant mode of relating to others. The *compliant, self-effacing type* results from the defensive operation of clinging to others. These individuals try to curry the favor of others, subordinate themselves to others, and are reluctant to disagree for fear of losing favor. The *aggressive, expansive type* results from moving against others and relies heavily on power and mastery as a means to achieve security. The *detached, resigned type* results from moving away from others in an attempt to avoid both dependency and conflict. These are very private individuals who, although refusing to compete openly, see themselves as rising above others.

Supplemental Means to Relieve Inner Tension The overdevelopment of any one of the three basic interpersonal styles suppresses the two others. In a manner analogous to Jung's complexes, repressed impulses continue to be active and to produce conflict. An artificial harmony is achieved by the use of mental mechanisms such as blind spots, compartmentalization, rationalization, and coping techniques such as excessive self-control, arbitrariness, elusiveness, cynicism, and externalization.

Idealized Image As teenagers, individuals who grow up to be neurotic create an ideal image that, if achieved, promises to end their painful feelings and provide self-fulfillment. The idealized image counterbalances the alienation from their core selves that developing neurotic individuals undergo because the survival techniques they adopted earlier force them to override their genuine wishes, feelings, and thoughts. The idealized image covers over all the contradictions, conceals the defensive nature of their behavior, and restores a sense of wholeness. Energy formerly available for self-realization is now used in efforts to become like the idealized image. For example, an individual who has adopted the strategy of moving toward others and is consequently dependent on others for affection and approval experiences the fear of reasonable self-assertion as saintly humility and considerateness of others.

Because the ideal self is imaginary, neurotic people are readily bruised by confrontation with reality and work excessively to prove they are in fact their ideal selves. This results in a type of perfectionism that insists on flawless excellence in which "I should" replaces "I want" or "I need." It also results in the neurotic ambition to be first and in a strong drive for revenge against those perceived as having interfered with their efforts to match the ideal self. This aspect of Horney's theories anticipates some of Heinz Kohut's ideas on the origins of narcissism.

Claims, "Shoulds," and Self-Hatred Despite their frequent self-disparagement, neurotic individuals expect to be treated as though they were their ideal selves. These claims to special treatment, when frustrated, produce anger, righteous indignation, and resentment. The "shoulds," or self-imposed demands that they live up to their idealized selves, are irrational and unrelated to the realities of daily life. They are projected, experienced as demands made by others, and are also demanded of others. This results in neurotic people being critical of others and very sensitive to criticism themselves. Self-hatred results when the threat arises that neurotic individuals may be unable to achieve their idealized selves. If support is not needed for the idealized self, claims, shoulds, and self-hatred are not such important parts of the psychic apparatus.

Neurotic Pride and the Pride System Glorifying aspects of the idealized self, *neurotic pride*, substitute for healthy self-confidence. Thus, when their pride is injured by others, neurotic individuals become enraged and seek to avenge their injury and to conceal their self-deception by achieving a vindictive victory over the offending person. Together with supporting claims and shoulds, neurotic pride and self-hatred form a defensive network or pride system that protects the idealized self. Any attempt to reduce elements of the pride system is experienced as an attack on the person. Despite the armoring of their defensive network, such individuals are not at peace because they are in inner conflict with the forces that protect them. The conflict between the forces driving toward healthy self-realization and the pride system is the *central inner conflict.*

There is also conflict within the pride system itself. Neurotic pride and claims are associated with the glorified idealized image; self-hatred and shoulds are associated with the unacceptable aspects of the self. When attempts are made to satisfy both forces simultaneously, conflict arises. Attempts to avoid these conflicts involve further alienation from the real self.

Alienation Alienation from self is one of the most serious consequences of neurotic development. It results from the combination of repeated denial of external reality and the repression of genuine thought, feelings, and impulses. As the process of alienation continues, neurotic individuals lose touch with the core of their being and can no longer determine or act on what is right for them. Their feelings may range from uncertainty and confusion to inner deadness and emptiness.

Analytical Treatment Horney did not regard adult neurotic people as recapitulating childhood experiences and thus did not focus on the recovery of childhood memories; she dealt instead with the self-perpetuating neurotic process. She stressed the importance of dreams in analysis and, later, the exploration of the patient–analyst relationship. She was one of the earliest analysts to recognize and make constructive use of her own feelings toward patients. To Horney, psychoanalysis was a cooperative venture that enabled patients to free themselves from their neurotic structures and mobilize themselves toward self-realization. The analyst's responsibility was to assist in liberating patients from *blockages,* the forces that impede healthy growth.

Early in therapy, termed the *disillusioning process*, the two types of blockages are identified and examined. The first group of safety-oriented blockages, *protective blockages,* helps to avoid the anxiety caused by self-awareness. They include silence, lateness, depreciating the analyst, the use of drugs, and even the use of self-accusation as a means to avoid further exploration.

Positive-value blockages reinforce patients' satisfaction with themselves and support their idealized selves. In the disillusioning process, the analyst identifies both types of blockages, exposing the protective blockages before exposing the blockages that defend the idealized image. Analyzing the positive-value blockages first arouses too much fear.

Qualities of the Analyst These qualities, later described by Carl Rogers as therapist-offered conditions, include maturity, belief in constructive conflict resolution, and the ability to communicate hope and respect. Analysts listen, clarify, provide directions, and suggest alternative resolutions to conflicts. Horney emphasized the need for the analyst to help move patients out of their alienation and suggested that therapists be flexible, tailoring their interventions to patients' present needs. She did not recommend using the couch or a fixed number of sessions per week.

Therapeutic Process Horney believed that fundamental attitudinal changes were the best means to change self-defeating, self-alienating behaviors. She created a setting in which patients were able to assess themselves as individuals, free to discover and choose personal values that fit with their real self. This type of reorientation begins after the disillusioning phase of treatment. As patients begin to question their present values, and their idealizing process abates, they can revise their values and develop more flexible values consonant with their inner self. Dreams are used in all phases of treatment to bring patients into better contact with their real self. As unconscious attempts to solve conflicts, dreams can show constructive forces at work that are not yet discernible in patients' conscious thoughts and behavior. As patients mobilize their constructive forces, they experience the struggle between the pride system and the real self. In the process, they experience uncertainty, psychic pain, and self-hatred. As the central conflict is resolved successfully, patients move into the final phase of treatment: the discovery and use of their real inner self.

From the standpoint of Horney, Mr. A.'s process of self-realization has been blocked in all three directions. He has not developed the ability to love and to trust; he expresses opposition in an unhealthy way, and he has made self-defeating moves toward independence. He is seen as having developed a detached style of relating to others, having substituted hypomania and the use of drugs for real relatedness. He justifies his illness by taking pride in it. His goal of becoming a writer is part of the development of an ideal self that is a detached observer. He supports his ideal self by having fantasies of involvement with other writers, by convincing his professor that he was able to write a play as his term paper, and by procrastination. He has become more and more isolated from his real self by denying the reality of the facts that his mental illness and cannabis abuse pose a danger to him and that he was failing in school.

A therapist in the Horney tradition begins by pointing out that Mr. A.'s drug use and his sustaining of manic episodes are blocking his ability to learn about himself and works with Mr. A. toward abstinence from substances of abuse and appropriate use of mood-stabilizing agents. The therapist later begins to point out that Mr. A.'s pride in his manic episodes serves the purpose of sustaining a false self of boundless energy and creativity. Mr. A. is encouraged to decide whom he really wants to be—a writer in fantasy or a person able to obtain real satisfaction from real accomplishments and real relationships. His dreams are examined and their themes explored. His omnipotent, messianic dreams are interpreted as evidence of his ideal self and viewed in the light of reality. His dreams of being exposed are interpreted as the fear engendered by his ideal self as a means of defending itself against exposure: "If you expose me, you will be embarrassed and humiliated." Mr. A. is supported through his fear of humiliation and the pain of realizing that he has been deceiving himself. His self-loathing is interpreted as the activity of the pride system in defending his ideal self. As he begins to relinquish his ideal self, he will begin to discover and to mobilize his real inner self in directions that might not have been predictable at the beginning of treatment.

ERICH FROMM

Psychoanalyst Fromm (1900 to 1980) was often thought of as the archetypical neo-Freudian, the leader among those who emphasized that culture and social setting influence an individual's dynamics as much as instincts do (Fig. 6.3–12). Neither physician nor biologist, Fromm, a native German, received his doctorate in philosophy, sociology, and psychology from the University of Heidelberg in 1922. There he was exposed to a Marxist emphasis on how history shapes societies and how societies, in turn, shape individuals according to economic needs. He was trained as a psychoanalyst at the Berlin Psychoanalytic Institute and then founded, with his wife, Frieda Fromm-Reichmann, the Frankfurt Psychoanalytic Institute. In 1933, he immigrated to the United States and in 1949 he moved to Mexico City to found another psychoanalytic institute. In 1974, he moved to Switzerland, where he died in 1980. As much a social critic as a personality theorist, he was later claimed by the existential and humanistic psychoanalysts. Fromm's intellectual agenda was the integration of Freud's theory of a dynamic unconscious with Karl Marx's theory of history and social criticism.

Personality Theory For Fromm, two central facts dominate human behavior: the inevitability of separateness and the historical and social moment into which each person is born. He argued that every person struggles to recapture the state of blissful union that existed prenatally. From the moment the baby begins to recognize itself as a separate human being, a titanic struggle begins, pitting the desperate anxiety of loneliness against the urge to fully express and actualize oneself, ultimately transcending the self. Most individuals find the loneliness too painful to bear, and they suppress their striving for individuation in the service of maintaining the illusion of connectedness. They are socialized by their parents into the roles defined by the society into which they are born. Fromm actually used the term

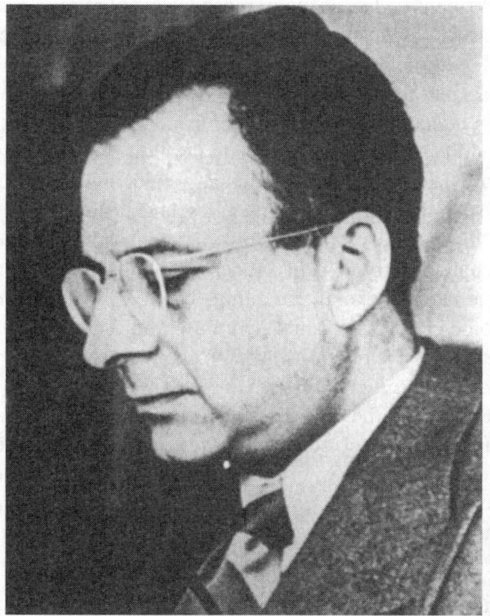

FIGURE 6.3–12 Erich Fromm. (Courtesy of Erich Fromm.)

symbiosis years before Margaret Mahler used it to describe the universal human yearning for fusion, safety, and security.

Facing aloneness and choosing individuation lead to freedom and a productive life. However, true freedom is too terrifying for many people, who instead construct a series of illusions that engender a feeling of safety and security. They create a pseudoself, think pseudothoughts, and experience pseudofeelings in support of these illusions, thereby cutting themselves off from the fullness of their own inner lives. Fromm saw Freud's theory as a special case of his own more general ideas. The illusions that Victorian society offered involved sublimation of sexuality and aggression in the service of social respectability. Social respectability, in turn, provided the illusion of acceptance and security. In other places and at other times, different solutions might be offered. Early in World War II, shortly after his escape from Nazi Germany, Fromm wrote about the willingness of people to give up their freedom to serve an authoritarian society. In the 1950s, he wrote of the pursuit of material acquisitions in the service of postwar productivity, leading to self-satisfied conformity. Fromm's most direct application of Marxism was in his hypothesis that individual development has paralleled historical development since the time that humankind freed itself from symbiosis with nature and embarked on a unique path, evolving inevitably toward the Marxist utopia: the end of history in the universally humane society. However, Fromm departed from other Marxists who saw revolution as the only healthy response to an inevitably repressive society. He believed that even within an imperfect culture, individuals could face their terror, give up their pseudoselves and pseudothoughts, and choose to become themselves, encountering others who had made similar choices with love and mutuality. To achieve this, Fromm said four basic human needs must be met: relatedness, transcendence, identity, and a frame of orientation. *Relatedness* is the need to feel connected to other humans. *Transcendence* refers to rising above basic instincts. *Identity* is the need to feel accepted yet unique. Emphasis on the need for a frame of orientation led Fromm late in his career to an exploration of the constructive and destructive roles that religion may play in individual lives.

Theory of Psychopathology

As a social philosopher and critic, Fromm did not really develop a systematic theory of psychopathology. He identified three major mechanisms of retreat from individuation. Some individuals, he said, may seek an authoritarian solution, trying to live through someone or something external to themselves, relying on that for their sense of adequacy. Others may become destructive, attacking anything that confronts them with their separateness and aloneness. Most individuals develop a conformist attitude, warding off the anxiety of experiencing their own intentionality by accepting socially offered thoughts, roles, and attitudes.

These mechanisms result in four different unproductive orientations or characters typical of modern capitalist society: receptive, exploitative, hoarding, and marketing. The *receptive character* often appears to be cooperative and open; however, the primary agenda is to establish a passive relationship with a leader who solves problems magically. *Exploitative characters* are likewise interested in filling themselves up from the outside; however, they aggressively manipulate and usurp whatever reduces their terror. *Hoarders* collect, store, and close in on themselves, often being cold and aloof in their efforts to feel secure. *Marketers* treat themselves as a plastic commodity to be manipulated as needed to achieve externally validated success.

Treatment

Fromm wrote nothing at all on the practice of psychotherapy; therefore, what is known is derived from anecdotal reports by those who studied with him or were treated by him. They report his emphasis on a tender and empathic inquiry into the self-deceptions and illusions created by patients in their efforts to ward off the anxiety of separateness and to maintain some sense of connectedness to significant others. He placed great emphasis on the tendency of unloved children to identify intensely with parental values to capture the magical safety they seem to offer. At a time when most psychoanalysts were preoccupied with detailed examinations of the instincts and defenses, Fromm contributed a sense of the range and richness of inner experience that underlies superficial adaptation. He contributed the sense that a new authenticity could be found by those willing to confront the truth about themselves with all its terror of aloneness.

In some respects, Fromm's ideas are uniquely applicable to Mr. A., who is clearly maintaining the illusion of his separateness by conforming to the socially sanctioned role of rebellious artist. His bipolar I disorder becomes an unexpected weapon in his battle with his terror of aloneness. The dread in the hotel lobby dream is probably the closest this fear comes to consciousness. Fromm would gently probe this dream and Mr. A.'s self-image. He would point out the chains created by Mr. A.'s seemingly rebellious independence. The self-destructive quality of the patient's lifestyle would also be confronted and investigated. Ultimately, Mr. A. has to experience his own loneliness and face his terror of it to find true freedom, true intimacy, and an authentic self-definition.

HARRY STACK SULLIVAN

Sullivan (1892 to 1949) is generally acknowledged as the most original and distinctive American-born theorist in dynamic psychiatry (Fig. 6.3–13). Although rarely acknowledged explicitly since the late 1970s, most American psychiatrists make significant use of concepts and approaches that he developed. For many years, the primary theoretical dispute within dynamic psychiatry circles was between the classic Freudians and the Sullivanians (or interpersonal psychoanalysts). When psychiatrists use the term *parataxic distortion*, apply the concept of self-esteem, consider the importance of preadolescent peer groups in development, or view a patient's behavior as an interpersonal manipulation, they are applying concepts Sullivan first proposed.

Sullivan graduated from medical school in Chicago in 1917. He spent from 1921 to 1930 in the Washington, D.C. area working with schizophrenia patients at St. Elizabeth's and then Sheppard and Enoch Pratt Hospitals, where he developed a reputation as a remarkable clinician with an uncanny ability to communicate with floridly psychotic patients. He initiated the first of what is now called *therapeutic communities*. Later, he entered private practice in New York and eventually returned to the Washington area, where he was involved in clinical, consulting, and teaching activities. In the 1920s and 1930s, he wrote a number of papers on schizophrenia, later collected in *Schizophrenia as a Human Process*. His other books were compiled from his lectures by his students; most were published posthumously, which explains some of the density and seeming disorganization of his written work.

Personality Theory

Sullivan rejected the Kraepelinian dogma of his day that dominated psychiatric thinking about schizophrenia. Sullivan elucidated the meaning of passages of patient speech that Emil Kraepelin presented as nonsensical. In searching for alternative understandings of psychosis, he turned initially to Freud but rejected his theories as increasingly rigid and dogmatic. Thus, he developed his own working theory of personality, psychopathology, and therapy.

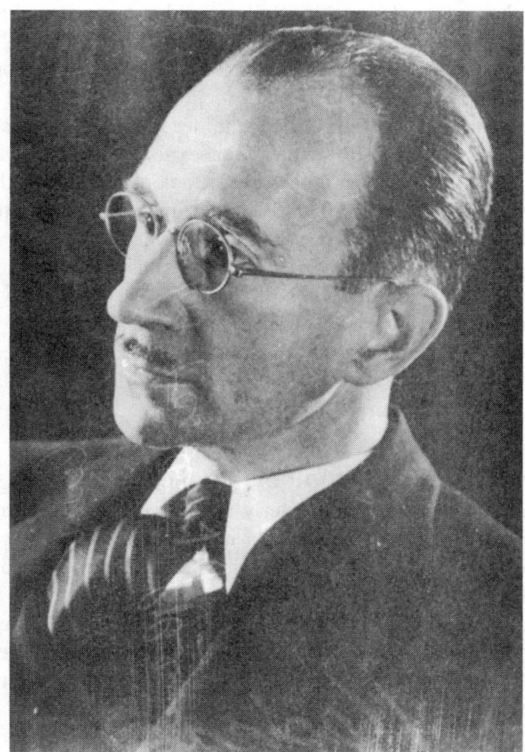

FIGURE 6.3–13 Harry Stack Sullivan. (Courtesy of the New York Academy of Medicine.)

Sullivan was very concerned that language could be misleading. He was very wary of self-reifying conceptualizations that led to rigid theories and tried to emphasize the psychiatrist as participant/observer in the clinical situation. By emphasizing this aspect of the role, he sought to keep observations as objective as possible, although he recognized the difficulty this presented in dealing with private emotional experience. What can be observed is the social interaction of patients; thus, he defined *personality* as the "relatively enduring pattern of interpersonal relations which characterize a human life." From the outset, his focus was very different from the intrapsychic emphasis of psychoanalysis. By approaching psychopathology in this way, he necessarily created a field theory rather than a structural theory, characterized by temporal and interactive processes. Sullivan defined a "dynamism" as "the relatively enduring pattern of energy transformations," that is, recurrent interpersonal behavior patterns.

Sullivan's theory is fundamentally one of needs and anxiety. *Needs* are defined as needs for satisfaction and needs for security. Anxiety occurs when fundamental needs are in danger of not being met and is the primary motivator of human behavior. Needs for satisfaction include physical needs (e.g., air, water, food, warmth), and emotional needs include needs especially for human contact and for expressing one's talents and capacities. Because infants are utterly unable to meet their own needs, interpersonal relationships are a central concern. Decades before Mahler wrote of a symbiotic stage in infant development, Sullivan spoke of the "empathic linkage" between caretaker and infant and described the complicated interaction of infants communicating tension and anxiety, arousing anxiety in the caretaker, leading to tender responses to the infant's needs. Failure to meet these needs results in loneliness and anxiety.

Sullivan defined *security* as the absence of anxiety. Thus, *needs for security* are defined as the need to avoid, prevent, or reduce anxiety. Because there is no such thing as a perfect mother or parent, anxiety is inevitable and becomes the primary driver for personality development. The *self-system* is defined by Sullivan as the dynamism that is responsible for avoiding or reducing anxiety. Sullivan equated the self, identity, or ego with the individual's developed patterns for avoiding the discomforts that arise from the inability of others to meet one's fundamental needs. It exists, like all else, purely within an interpersonal framework. The self-system develops a set of mechanisms, called *security operations,* which affect this goal.

Security operations function within Sullivan's theory much as defense mechanisms do within psychoanalytic theory. The specific security operations, however, were defined interpersonally, and Sullivan tried to link them closely to actual observation or experience. Some bore the same labels and definitions as Anna Freud's, but Sullivan is best known for three contributions that bore his distinct stamp: apathy, somnolent detachment, and selective inattention. These were drawn from observing the way infants and young children react to painful interactions, such as scolding, with their parents.

The self-system accrues from ever-evolving interpersonal experiences—that is, fulfillment of needs for satisfaction as a result of the empathic linkage with the mother. The most difficult experiences are not necessarily those involving the inability to meet the child's needs, but the child's sensing of the caretaker's anxiety in the process of responding to those needs. This arouses anxiety in the child, promotes the need to establish a sense of security, and leads to evolution of the self-system and the development of security operations. The self-system is divided into three parts. The "good me" is a set of images, experiences, and behaviors associated with an unanxious, tender, empathic, and approving or accepting response from the environment. The "bad me" comes to be associated with ideas, actions, and perceptions that provoke anxiety and disapproval from caretakers. Some situations, however, provoke such intense anxiety that they are entirely disavowed and disowned; they become part of the "not me." Eventually, the empathic linkage becomes unnecessary and the self-system operates autonomously within the individual, developing ever more subtle and complex ways to manage the person's anxiety.

Developmental Theories Sullivan had two theories of development, one cognitive, the other social. He postulated three developmental cognitive modes of experience whose degree of persistence into adulthood is important in understanding psychopathology. The *prototaxic* mode, characteristic of infancy and early childhood, involves a series of disconnected, brief states experienced as totalities with no temporal relationship. In later life, mystical experiences and schizophrenic fusion represent persistent prototaxic experiences. *Parataxic* experience begins early in childhood as the self-system begins its more independent functioning. It, too, involves a series of momentary experiences; however, they are now recorded in sequence and with apparent connection to one another. They may be given symbolic meanings, but rules of logic are absent, and coincidence plays a major role in how the world is perceived. The self-system uses this mode to seek effective anxiety-reducing behaviors and to repeat them, seeking sameness and predictability. Sullivan used this mode to explain transference, slips of the tongue, and paranoid ideation. The *syntactic* mode of experiencing is based on the development of language and consensual validation. The world and the self are perceived within rules of logic, temporal sequencing, external validity, and internal consistency. Thinking about oneself as well as others becomes testable and modifiable based on rigorous analysis of experiences in a variety of different situations. *Maturity* may be defined as extensive predominance of the syntactic mode of experiencing.

Social development is somewhat based on these evolving cognitive modes. However, disturbed interpersonal relationships may cause persistence of the more primitive (prototaxic or parataxic) ways of experiencing the world. Social development is characterized by the satisfaction needs, which are predominant, and the interpersonal sphere in which these and their resulting security needs are sought to be fulfilled. Each stage is also characterized by the primary "zone of interaction"—bodily areas through which the individual channels needs, anxiety, and relief—in interactions with the environment. These aspects of Sullivan's theory bear a superficial resemblance to Freud's genetic theory; however, Sullivan accorded them far less importance; they are mere conduits when compared with psychoanalytic libido theory.

Infancy spans birth to the onset of language and is characterized by the primary need for bodily contact and tenderness. The prototaxic mode predominates, and the primary zones of interaction are oral and, to some extent, anal. Insofar as needs are fulfilled with a minimum of anxiety, the infant experiences euphoria and a sense of well-being. To the extent that some anxiety is commonly present in the caretakers, apathy and somnolent detachment are regularly used as security operations, persisting into adult life as a basic detached and passive stance. If anxiety and inconsistency are severe, intense experiences of dread persist, presenting in later life as the eerie, uncanny, bizarrely disruptive internal states seen in individuals with schizophrenia.

Childhood begins with the onset of usable language, continues until the beginning of school, and is characterized by the child's focus on the parents as other from whom praise and acceptance are sought. The primary mode of experience shifts to the parataxic, and the most common zone of interaction is anal. The child needs an approving adult audience. This leads to a variety of learning of language, behavior, self-control, and so on. It can also be observed in a variety of trial-and-error efforts by the child to find what pleases them. Gratification leads to an expansive self-system with many facets of life associated with the "good me" and positive self-esteem. Moderate anxiety leads to chronic anxiety, uncertainty, and insecurity. Extreme anxiety results in giving up known successful behavior in favor of self-defeating patterns that fulfill others' expectations.

The juvenile era covers ages 5 to 8 years. The shift to syntactic cognitive modes begins, and the interpersonal focus spreads to the peer group and outside authority figures. Peers and teachers have the opportunity to approve and accept behavior previously frowned on within the family (e.g., talking dirty with one's friends). Interpersonal cooperation, competition, play, and compromise become the gratifying experiences. Juveniles learn to negotiate their own needs with a legitimate social concern without sacrificing their self-esteem in the process. The risks of excessive anxiety are either too great a need to control and dominate social situations or internalization of restrictive, prejudicial social attitudes.

Preadolescence, ages 8 to 12 years, marks the child's movement from peer group cooperation and competition based on roles toward genuine intimacy with a chum. Sullivan saw this phase as a particularly important stage in which the give and take of the special friend could repair and undo distortions that resulted from excessive anxiety at earlier stages. This is the point at which the individual truly moves outside the family and engages in a free give and take with another person unfettered by the same dynamics. During this stage, the major shift toward syntactic thinking takes place, although some distortions may persist into adolescence. The preteen years see the initiation of a capacity for attachment, love, and collaboration or their inability to develop in the face of excessive anxiety. Although sexual exploration may be a part of the chum relationship, Sullivan did not see sexuality as a central element in this developmental phase.

Adolescents, beginning at puberty, are seen to have concerns similar to those of preadolescents, except that lust is added to the interpersonal equation. Thus, the same needs for a special sharing relationship persist but shift to the other sex for their outlet, whereon a major opportunity for learning or severe anxiety begins. As the person faces culturally defined stereotyping, many new opportunities for social experimentation may lead to consolidation of self-esteem or self-ridicule. The struggle to integrate lust with intimacy is accomplished by painful trial and error. If this is completed with the self-system relatively intact, the later years of adolescence are an opportunity to expand the syntactic mode to such areas as a consensual view of interpersonal relations, values and ideals, career decisions, and social concerns.

Theory of Psychopathology Sullivan abhorred diagnostic labeling for being unhelpful, overly restrictive, dehumanizing, and used primarily to impress patients and colleagues. In discussing schizophrenia, he said, "We are all much more simply human than otherwise." Thus, he sought to understand the fundamental human process within his patients, especially his sickest ones. He saw psychopathology as resulting from excessive anxiety arresting development of the self-system and thereby limiting both opportunities for interpersonal satisfaction and available security operations. He viewed psychiatric patients as struggling to maintain their self-esteem with very limited means. To understand them, the developmental phase at which they operate has to be gauged, and the interpersonal needs they express have to be understood.

Sullivan believed that several different factors could play a role in the particular form that these disturbances might take. The level of anxiety at particular developmental stages can lay the groundwork for a developmental arrest. Basic cognitive capacity might play a role in the choice of security operations relied on or retained. The degree of success achieved interpersonally combined with whatever capacities are used affects later success. Finally, the chance occurrence of stresses encountered during life is deemed a factor. Thus, Sullivan theorized that anyone might develop schizophrenia, even people with relatively successful developmental histories, should their chosen defenses fail dramatically and their life stresses mount in the extreme. However, it was more likely that schizophrenic patients would be highly vulnerable along all four dimensions, whereas others with greater developmental strengths might become obsessive, hysteroid, schizoid, or paranoid.

Interpersonal Psychotherapy Sullivan emphasized that the psychiatrist is a participant–observer in all interactions with patients. He thought deeply and extensively about the nuances and opportunities involved in this unique situation. By interacting actively with patients, verbal and nonverbal expressions of recurrent interpersonal patterns become apparent. These observations then inform the therapist's further behavior, thereby creating the opportunity for change. This process occurs over seconds and over months and years as the psychotherapy unfolds. Sullivan saw this perspective as an antidote to what he perceived as the wrongheaded emphasis on objective neutrality embodied by the "blank screen" model of psychotherapist behavior. He argued that parataxic distortions emerge in all interactions, not only in the classic analytical situation. This differing view of transference and of it being a universal human process was among the core debates for decades between classic analysts and interpersonal analysts.

Sullivan saw therapy as elucidating the patient's interpersonal patterns, exploring their usefulness in the service of the patient's needs, and considering alternative, more favorable possibilities. Thus, he shared the ego psychologists' understanding that even the sickest behavior was the best adaptation available at a given moment to the patient. He emphasized the experiencing of the distortions, the needs, the patterns, and the potential changes within the ongoing interaction with the therapist. He saw great power in the very entanglement of the therapist with the patient and recognized the ability of a skilled therapist to manage the interpersonal process to reveal patterns and to shape the patient's emotional experience. However, he constantly emphasized and respected the ultimate autonomy of his patients, who could still, in the end, choose not to reshape their approach to the world.

Sullivan viewed psychotherapy as divided into four distinct stages: inception, reconnaissance, detailed inquiry, and termination. Inception involves the very beginning, often only a part of the first interview, during which the contract and roles are stipulated. Reconnaissance might go on for as many as 10 to 15 sessions, during which the therapist identifies the patient's recurring patterns and assesses their adaptive and maladaptive qualities. The detailed inquiry is a very lengthy process of exploring the patient's thoughts, feelings, and memories and evaluating and reevaluating data from earlier stages, seeking to recognize, clarify, and change persistent parataxic distortions. The recurrent patterns are discussed within the context of the person's developmental history, needs, anxieties, failures, and successes. There is often much ongoing interchange between patient and psychiatrist as feelings and perceptions are validated or questioned within the context of mutual emotional interchange within each session. Termination is a product of the evolving contract and understanding between the patient and therapist and may reflect either extensive or limited goals. Sullivan emphasized the constant reassessing of goals by the therapist and the power of the ongoing negotiation and renegotiation of the therapeutic contract as a means to reveal and change parataxic distortions. The ultimate goal of psychotherapy is to experience as much as possible within the syntactic mode and to broaden the repertoire of the self-system. To the extent that this is achieved, individuals are in a position to become responsible for their ongoing growth through subsequent interpersonal interactions.

Sullivan would see Mr. A. as probably arrested in childhood, when his fear of displeasing his mother led him to give up healthy self-esteem strivings for independence in favor of a distant yet dependent position. He uses drugs and psychosis as escapes to maintain some degree of self-esteem. His "good me" consists of his debating and his intelligence. His "bad me" is expressed in his rebelliousness, whereas the "not me" seems to encompass issues of closeness, independence, and constructive engagement with others and with life's tasks. In therapy, the reconnaissance phase is extremely important, identifying the moment-to-moment interactions through which Mr. A.'s security operations interfere with his attempts at constructive independence. His bemusement and detachment are identified, as is his escape into prototaxic thought through drugs and noncompliance with medications. His acceptance of his mother's management of his trust fund is noted as well. A Sullivanian therapist actively interacts, empathically identifying and confronting Mr. A.'s ways of avoiding authenticity and constructive interaction. Once identified, their meanings are gently probed, as are the feelings associated with them. The terror of displeasing his mother and its effects on Mr. A.'s ongoing interactions with the therapist are addressed. Interactions are examined for their consequences, with the assumption that the outcome has bearing on the motivation. Finally, Mr. A. is encouraged to try out different ways of relating to the therapist as a prelude to restructuring his outside relationships. He is encouraged to think rationally about his circumstances, to seek a good peer group, develop close friendships, and gradually move away from his near-exclusive focus on his immediate family for all of his interpersonal needs.

ERIC BERNE

Berne (1910 to 1970) was an American original in both style and substance. He worked in the San Francisco area most of his career, breaking with psychoanalysis in the mid-1950s but never becoming antianalytical as did many of his followers (Fig. 6.3–14). Like many others, he felt the need to develop briefer treatments than were offered at the time.

A group gathered around him that came to be known as the *San Francisco Transactional Analysis Seminars.* Through weekly discussions of clinical cases and social and political issues, Berne gradually refined his theory. Berne was wry and provocative in his approach to human behavior. His approach contributed much to what is now called "pop psychology," although his particular popularity and faddishness have long since faded. Few clinicians now call themselves transactional analysis therapists; nonetheless, Berne's ideas remain useful in grasping hidden agendas in human interactions.

Personality Theory

For Berne, the primary motivator of all human behavior is the need for "strokes"—attention, recognition, and response from others. Early survival depends on adequate physical contact, stimulation, and nurturance. This need remains strong but later becomes more symbolic and interpersonal. Children learn rapidly what works within their family and practice it extensively. This led to one of Berne's more widely quoted observations: "Negative strokes are better than no strokes at all." People evolve ways of interacting with their world to obtain regular strokes in whatever way possible and in whatever way they have been taught to define a stroke (e.g.,

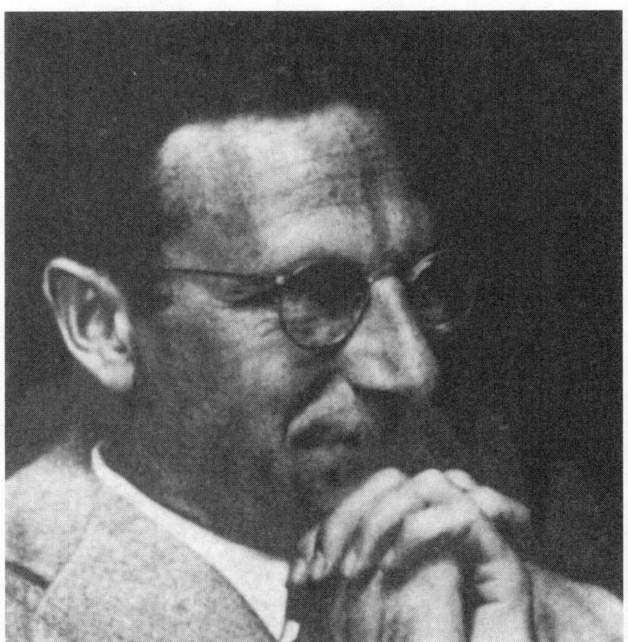

FIGURE 6.3–14 Eric Berne. (Courtesy of Wide World Photos.)

sympathy in response to chronic depression may provide such gratifying attention that the depression cannot be given up). So great is the need for regular stroking that blatantly destructive actions persist in the face of insight, recognition, and enduring psychological or physical pain. Like Adler and Sullivan, Berne suggested that hidden social needs motivate human behavior to the extent that, with rare exceptions, there is an interpersonal hidden agenda in all human activity. For Berne, the unit of observation was the transaction, the short-term process of individuals interacting with each other. He spent much energy analyzing transactions to try to discover patients' definitions of strokes and their preferred mechanism for obtaining them. He noted that most people engage in very predictable, stereotyped, repetitive transactions. The content may vary from situation to situation, but the form tends to be quite rigid. He called these transactions "games," and his bestseller, *Games People Play*, captured the imagination of the American public in 1964. Some games are harmless, some are socially encouraged; many have destructive elements or at least limit opportunities for more gratifying relationships (intimacy), and some are highly destructive. A common, socially accepted game is cocktail party flirtation, which is ordinarily pleasant and harmless but, depending on the intensity, frequency, and seriousness with which it is played, may result in inability to experience intimacy, disrupted marriages, or even physical harm.

Berne divided the human psyche into three primary parts: *child*, *parent*, and *adult*, with two of those further subdivided (Fig. 6.3–15). He called these *ego states*. An ego state consists of characteristic body language, voice qualities, verbal productions, and affective experience. The child represents the persistence of child-like experience and expression in all people. It is divided into the *natural child*, the ego state in which the spontaneity, joy, and intuitive perceptiveness of young children persists in all adults; the *adapted child*, the part that is compliant and cooperative; and the *rebellious child*, the repository of that part of each person prone to fight authority, challenge accepted wisdom, and struggle for autonomy. The parent is the residue of internalized parental messages and injunctions. It is divided into two parts, the *critical parent* and the *nurturing parent*. The critical parent bears some resemblance to Freud's superego, embodying rules, values, instruction, criticism, and restrictions. The nurturing parent is the internalization of positive caring experience, the memory of loving interactions. The adult is a purely rational, data-processing element that is objective, calculating, and weighs options and estimates probabilities.

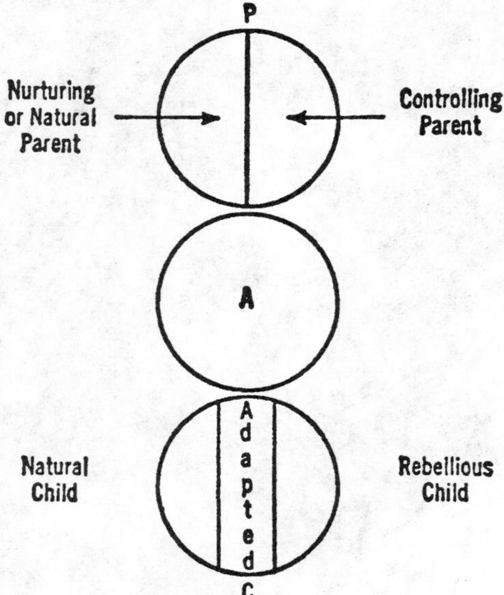

FIGURE 6.3–15 Eric Berne's descriptive model of the personality. A, adult; C, child; P, parent. (From Berne E. *What Do You Say After You Say Hello? The Psychology of Human Destiny.* New York: Bantam; 1972, with permission.)

Mental health is the flexible availability of all ego states with no one predominating. Excess critical parent produces guilt and depression, but insufficient critical parent produces sociopathy. Excess nurturing parent produces a narcissistic laziness, whereas insufficient nurturing parent causes an inability to soothe oneself and to maintain self-esteem. Excess adult results in a cold, overly rational person, but insufficient adult leaves individuals unable to balance the various internal forces in their lives. Too much natural child may result in irresponsible behavior, but not enough depletes the ability to experience joy in living. An overabundance of rebellious child results in self-destructive battles with no constructive purpose; however, insufficient rebellious child may result in an overly conformist stance. Excess adapted child prevents appropriate striving toward autonomy; insufficient adapted child prevents participation in group or hierarchical efforts.

Berne placed great emphasis on the child's ability to intuit parental messages and instructions, especially those communicated nonverbally and unconsciously. In this way, the growing child might encode a conscious verbal instruction in the critical parent (e.g., be strong, be perfect, be smart), whereas internalizing a more powerful, unconscious message in the child (don't grow up, don't leave me, don't surpass me). Usually, a model for carrying out the instruction is preserved in the adult (be passive, drink alcohol, run around with women, act crazy). Together, these make a script. Berne emphasized the active role of the child in searching for the messages and in accepting them. This was crucial for him because it emphasized the individual's responsibility in deciding to follow the script, even though this might have occurred at a very young age. The entire basis for psychological change lies within the person's capacity, having once accepted the script, to later reject it. However, Berne was impressed by the intensity and persistence with which individuals play out the script throughout their lives. Scripts come in all varieties, ranging from the successful to the utterly self-destructive. Thus, for Berne, the business of human living involved carrying out one's script according to the transactions learned as a child.

Theory of Psychopathology Given this view of human nature, Berne's understanding of psychopathology is based on the adaptiveness of a person's games and script and the capacity for adaptive use of all ego states. Written at a time when American psychiatry rejected phenomenological diagnosis, Berne's theories are difficult to accept. However, he did describe numerous clinical situations and case histories that are familiar to all psychiatrists, and he analyzed them according to their scripts. He was very impressed with the role of fantasy and fairy tales in children's development and often asked patients what their favorite story was as a child. He then searched for the hidden identifications and messages within the story to help discern the patient's script. Insofar as he developed a nosology, it lay in the scripts encouraged by culturally sanctioned fairy tales. For example, Cinderella is about a young girl waiting to be rescued by a fairy godmother or a charming prince and unwilling to assert herself against unjust authority. Little Red Riding Hood is about a girl who likes to chat with wolves and gets into trouble trying to please everybody. Men, he found, identified with the wolf or Prince Charming and were unable to regard women as real people.

A separate nosology of games was also developed and catalogued by Berne. Examples from this nosology include cocktail party flirtation (Rapo I), which concludes with the man and woman having experienced the stroke of feeling attractive and attracted, moving on to other conversations, seeking other people to attract. Rapo II usually ends with a line like, "What kind of girl do you think I am?" and Rapo III ends up with a painful, destructive love affair. Another game is "Why Don't You . . . Yes, But." In its mild, socially acceptable form, one person presents a problem, successfully enlisting the advice of many others; however, for every preferred solution the person has a ready explanation of why it will not work. The stroke (or payoff) is the attention and the feeling of superiority achieved by defeating others. The second-degree version of this game produces a chronic, helpless depression; the third-degree version may lead to the back wards of a state hospital.

There was no rigid mapping of his nosology of games and of scripts, and Berne never claimed that either was exhaustive. They were intended as clinical examples to guide the psychotherapist's thinking in evaluating each patient who presented unique script and transactional issues. Individuals were assessed according to the straightness of their transactions (Were there hidden communication and invitations emanating from different ego states?), the adaptiveness of their scripts, and the predominant ego state and its effects. Thus, Berne might describe a compulsive person as having too much critical parent or a histrionic person as having too much natural child. In the final analysis, however, he saw his catalogues and nosology as poor substitutes for careful, clinical study of individual patients.

Treatment Having been trained in psychoanalysis, Berne used many psychoanalytic techniques, but he applied them very differently from traditional psychoanalytic methods. Much of his clinical work was done in groups, with the therapist being very active in confronting and interpreting the interpersonal behavior of the patient. He emphasized the initial contract with the patient and the setting of clear, concrete goals. He encouraged therapists to inquire very early on in therapy, "How will we know when our work is finished?" If a clear and specific answer was not forthcoming, he would inform the patient that therapy had not yet begun. The focus would then be on the patient's difficulty in defining a recognizable end point for the work. Berne's approach was heavily informed by the psychoanalytic concept of resistance, but he applied it in a very different manner. Berne examined any treatment goal defined by patients for evidence that it was a way to continue playing games or pursuing scripts more effectively rather than giving them up entirely.

Like Sullivan, Berne regarded the ongoing interaction between patient and therapist as the key ingredient of psychotherapy. The therapist's job was to interact actively with the patient; recognize the ego states, games, and scripts being enacted; and to counter them using confrontation, interpretation, or various other interpersonal maneuvers that were designed to thwart the enactment and to confront the patient with a choice and an opportunity to relate differently. He emphasized simple direct statements using everyday words to stimulate affective experience and interaction. Commonly, interactions began with his inquiry, "What do you want to work on today?" Observers sometimes described his work as individual therapy within a group context because the other patients, who were silent observers, often responded emotionally to the interaction.

Berne placed great emphasis on the role of individual responsibility for one's life and experience, which he believed had been obscured by the emphasis on psychic determinism. He constantly communicated the opportunity for choosing to continue or discontinue the patterns or habits encouraged as a child. He also showed patients how they invite others to behave in various ways, thereby creating their own interpersonal reality. Health lies in recognizing one's option for deciding which invitations to offer to others and which to accept from others, even though these invitations may be communicated unconsciously and nonverbally.

Mr. A. is clearly playing a very destructive game and living out a particularly unproductive script. The script seems to contain the messages: "Don't ever leave me" and "act crazy." The message "you must be special" may also exist. The games used might be called "I'm out of control," "Helpless," "Artiste," and "I'm better than you are." A transactional analyst places Mr. A. in a group and works with him on these games and scripts. Many such therapists have productively combined Berne's theories with Fritz Perls' empty chair technique. Mr. A. might be asked to carry on imaginary dialogues with his mother, professor, his illness, marijuana, and admired writers of fiction, with Mr. A. assuming both sides of the dialogue. The transactions he uses are elucidated in this way, and he is invited to re-create the transaction more constructively. His internalization of his mother as an excessively critical parent is identified, and the fantasy dialogues are used to enable more internalization of both his mother's and father's nurturing qualities, which contain other script messages such as "grow up" or "be successful." Similarly, his excess rebellious child is demonstrated, and efforts to bring it under more adult control are made.

In looking at the formulations and treatment plans each of these theorists might propose for Mr. A., significant, even contradictory, interpretations become apparent. Commonalities exist but are expressed in different words and concepts. Each of these great thinkers has contributed to the overall understanding of the psychodynamics of psychopathology and treatment.

SUGGESTED CROSS-REFERENCES

Many sections of this textbook refer to the theorists described in this section. Some are included in Section 55.1 on the history of psychiatry. Others are referred to in Section 6.1 on psychoanalysis; Section 6.4 on theories of personality and psychopathology: schools derived from philosophy and psychology; and Section 24.1 on the history and current theoretical concepts in psychosomatic medicine.

References

*Adler A. In: Ansbacher HL, Ansbacher RR, eds. *The Individual Psychology of Alfred Adler: A Systematic Presentation in Selections from His Writings.* New York: Basic Books; 1956.

Adler A. In: Mairet P, ed. *Problems of Neurosis: A Book of Case Histories.* New York: Harper & Row; 1964.

Alexander F. *Psychosomatic Medicine.* New York: Norton; 1950.

Alexander F, French T, Pollack GH. *Psychosomatic Specificity.* Chicago: University of Chicago Press; 1968.

Berne E. *Games People Play.* New York: Grove; 1964.

*Berne E. *What Do You Say After You Say Hello? The Psychology of Human Destiny.* New York: Bantam; 1972.

Boeree CG. Karen Horney Web site. Available at: http://www.ship.edu/~cgboeree/horney.html. Accessed 11/12/2003.

Freud S. *Project for a Scientific Psychology.* Standard ed. Vol 1. 283–397.

Fromm E. *Escape From Freedom.* New York: Avon Books; 1965.

*Greenberg JR, Mitchell SA. *Object Relations in Psychoanalytic Theory.* Cambridge, MA: Harvard University Press; 1983.

Horney K. *The Neurotic Personality of Our Time.* New York: WW Norton; 1937.

Horney K. *Neurosis and Human Growth.* New York: Norton; 1950.

International Transactional Analysis Association Web site. Available at http://www.itaa-net.org/. Accessed 11/12/2003.

Jung CG. *Two Essays on Analytic Psychology.* Princeton, NJ: Princeton University Press; 1966.

Jung CG. *The Practice of Psychotherapy.* 2nd ed. Princeton, NJ: Princeton University Press; 1966.

Lieberman E. *Acts of Will: The Life and Work of Otto Rank.* New York: Free Press; 1985.

Lieberman EJ. Otto Rank Web site. Available at: http://www.ottorank.com. Accessed 11/12/2003.

McGuire W, ed. *Analytical Psychology: Notes of the Seminar Given in 1925 by C.G. Jung.* Princeton, NJ: Princeton University Press; 1989.

McLynn F. *Carl Gustaf Jung.* New York: St. Martin's Press; 1997.

Meyer A. *Collected Papers of Adolph Meyer.* Baltimore: Johns Hopkins University Press; 1948–1952.

Meyer A. *Psychobiology: A Science of Man.* Springfield, IL: Charles C Thomas; 1957.
*Mulahy P. *Psychoanalysis and Interpersonal Psychiatry: The Contributions of Harry Stock Sullivan.* New York: Science House; 1970.
Noll R. *Aryan Christ: The Secret Life of C.G. Jung.* New York: Random House; 1997.
Rado S. *Psychoanalytic Theory of Behavior.* New York: Gone & Sumner; 1962.
Rank O. *The Trauma of Birth.* New York: Harper & Row; 1973.
*Reich W. *Character Analysis.* New York: Fount, Stores & Young; 1949.
Sharaf M. *Fury on Earth: A Biography of Wilhelm Reich.* New York: St. Martin's Press/Marek; 1983.
Sullivan HS. *The Interpersonal Theory of Psychiatry.* New York: W.W. Norton; 1953.
Stevens A. *On Jung.* London: Routledge; 1990.
Wagner J. *USA TAA Articles: Violence in America.* Available at: http:usataa.org/articles_violence.html. Accessed 07/15/1999.
Williams D. CG Jung Web site. Available at: http://www.cgjungpage.org/. Accessed 11/12/2003.

▲ 6.4 Approaches Derived from Philosophy and Psychology

PAUL T. COSTA, JR., PH.D., AND ROBERT R. MCCRAE, PH.D.

This chapter is concerned with attempts to understand human nature. Historically, systematic thought on this topic was offered by philosophers; in modern times, personality theorists—psychologists, psychiatrists, and, occasionally, anthropologists—have taken on the task. Perspectives on human nature provide the most fundamental bases for theories of psychopathology and psychotherapy, and clinicians, such as Sigmund Freud, Carl Rogers, and George Kelly, continue to be taught in courses on personality theory. Increasingly, however, views on human nature are being shaped by empirical research, sometimes with startling results.

It is, of course, impossible to do justice to the full scope of philosophic thought on human nature. Here, a few important examples are selected, and their relation to the empirical tradition that is central to modern psychology and psychiatry is especially considered. The remainder of the chapter provides an overview of psychological theories, grouped under the traditional rubrics of behavioral, humanistic, and trait approaches. Because of its importance in contemporary personality research, special attention is given to the trait perspective.

PHILOSOPHY

The recognition of individual differences is probably as old as human culture, but differences in personality were long confounded with differences in status, class, or caste. Individuals from a higher status were assumed to be superior human beings, more sensitive, honorable, and wise. They were endowed with these characteristics by education, by bloodline, or—in the view of Indian philosophy—by moral behavior in a previous life.

Plato The first major account of personality in Western thought was provided by Plato (circa 428 to 348 BC). In *The Republic,* he made extended comparisons between the constitutions of different states and the constitution of the soul. Just as every state must have peasants, artisans, soldiers, and rulers, so must each individual have appetites (for food, sex, and so on), passions (for honor and advancement), and reason. The relative strength of these three determines character, as well as fitness for a particular place in society. Intelligent and thoughtful people ought to rule, and passionate people should be chosen to defend the state, whereas dull and spiritless individuals, lacking reason and passion, should be given the menial chores of agriculture and industry.

Plato assumed that these psychological characteristics, like physical strength or musical talent, were largely inborn, but he regarded them as a property of the individual, not the individual's social status. Although he assumed that high status citizens would normally bear children of the greatest potential, he specifically acknowledged that there would be exceptions, and, in his ideal state, children of the lower classes would be promoted, and those of the higher classes would be demoted on the basis of their own merit. Here, personality would be the basis of the social order, not vice versa. His most radical extension of this idea was to argue that women should be given social equality and allowed to become soldiers and rulers if they possessed the necessary mental and physical qualifications.

One of the recurring questions in personality theory has been the relative importance of nature versus nurture. Trait psychologists—particularly those interested in the study of temperament—have frequently pointed to innate differences in personality, whereas behaviorists and psychoanalysts have laid great stress on the formative influences of the environment and early childhood experiences. Ready as he was to acknowledge the importance of inborn potential, Plato was also keenly aware of the influence of education. Much of *The Republic* is devoted to his views on the effects of physical exercise, mental instruction, and poetry and music on the development of personality. Present-day concerns about the influences of television and rock music on children follow in this tradition.

Like most philosophers, Plato was more concerned with understanding virtue and vice than psychopathology, but, because he considered vice to be the result of weak or corrupted nature rather than free but evil choice, his discussions of character can be viewed as early descriptions of what might now be viewed as personality disorders. Just as there are better and worse forms of government for states, so are there also better and worse configurations of reason, passion, and appetite. Plato described five types, corresponding to five forms of government. The ideal of mental health, corresponding to government by wise rulers, is one in which reason holds in check passions and appetites. In the arrogant and ambitious type, there is an excess of passion or pride; in the avaricious type, there is an excess of appetite. However, in both of these types, reason still retains some authority; for example, avaricious individuals can control most of their appetites to indulge their desire for money. In the fourth, self-indulgent type, appetites are undisciplined, and, in the debauched, fifth type (corresponding to a government by despot), reason is completely disregarded, and a clearly psychopathological state is reached: "Thus, when nature or habit or both have combined the traits of drunkenness, lust, and lunacy, then you have the perfect specimen of the despotic man."

Aristotle Plato's vivid but rough typology was succeeded by Aristotle's (384 to 322 BC) detailed analysis of human character in the *Nicomachean Ethics.* Courage, temperance, generosity, pride, ambition, irascibility, friendliness, boastfulness, and shame were all defined and distinguished. Aristotle attributed pathological variations on these traits to innate defects or to disease processes: "Among all the excesses of foolishness, cowardice, intemperance and irritability some are bestial, some diseased. If, for example, someone's natural character makes him afraid of everything, even the noise of a mouse, he is a coward with a bestial sort of cowardice." He considered variation within the normal range to be the result of training and habit and thus to be subject to praise or blame.

Aristotle's basic moral precept is the *golden mean*: He argued that extreme standing on either end of a trait dimension should be avoided. Thus, stinginess and extravagance are vices, whereas generosity is a virtue; similarly, vanity and humility represent excessive or insufficient self-esteem. This conception continues to influence some modern notions of psychopathology, in which marked deviation from the norm in either direction is considered pathological. Individuals excessively concerned with social attention may be regarded as having a histrionic personality disorder; those insufficiently concerned with social attachments may have a schizoid disorder.

Aristotle carried conceptual analysis to a level that has seldom been surpassed, distinguishing, for example, between the superficially similar qualities of temperance and self-control: Individuals are temperate if they have healthy and moderate impulses that require little control, whereas individuals have self-control only if they have immoderate appetites that are nevertheless held in check. Such considerations allowed him to form rational taxonomies of traits that anticipate the empirical taxonomies proposed by 20th century factor analysts.

Immanuel Kant and Arthur Schopenhauer The last great period of the Western philosophical tradition begun by Plato and Aristotle was inaugurated at the end of the 18th century by Immanuel Kant (1724 to 1804), whose critical philosophy forms a transition between purely rational approaches to human nature and the empirical sciences that followed. One of Kant's last works, *Anthropology from a Pragmatic Point of View,* considered natural and moral variations in character and reintroduced the Roman physician Galen's taxonomy of choleric, phlegmatic, sanguine, and melancholic types to modern psychology.

Sciences are usually distinguished from philosophy by their reliance on empirical data, but it should not be imagined that philosophers made no use of experience. On the contrary, like many of the clinicians who offered psychological theories of personality, philosophers based their ideas heavily on their observations of human nature. A striking instance of this is provided by Arthur Schopenhauer (1788 to 1860), a 19th century follower of Kant whose dark view of the world as a place of purposeless striving had an extraordinary influence on early personality theorists, including Freud and Jung.

One of the central beliefs of Western thought has been that human happiness or misery is the result of external conditions—what is now called *quality of life*. However, Schopenhauer's acute observations, reported in *The World as Will and Representation,* led him to propose "the paradoxical but not absurd hypothesis that in every individual the measure of pain essential to him has been determined once and for all by his nature. . . . His suffering and well-being would not be determined at all from without, but only by . . . what is called his temperament."

In support of this view, he noted that wealth and power do not make people happy, "for we come across at least as many cheerful faces among the poor as among the rich." He also argued that the effects of great misfortunes or successes are short lived and that, for the most part, evaluations of the external causes of state of mind are illusory attributions: "We often see our pain result only from a definite external [cause] and . . . believe that, if only this were removed, the greatest contentment would necessarily ensue. But this is a delusion. . . . [The pain] would appear in the form of a hundred little annoyances and worries over things that we now entirely overlook."

Recent scientific research on psychological well-being has confirmed this account in every detail: Well-being is chiefly a function of enduring personality dispositions; wealth, social class, and other markers of the objective quality of life are virtually unrelated to subjective happiness; and processes of adaptation quickly return individuals to their own characteristic baseline of happiness after favorable or unfavorable life events. Schopenhauer's observations are also consistent with recent evidence on the heritability and lifelong stability of many mental disorders.

Yet, reason and insight are not enough. On the basis of his own experience and the examples of history, Schopenhauer also concluded that "man inherits his moral nature, his character, his inclinations, his heart from the father, but the degree, quality, and tendency of his intelligence from the mother"—a conclusion not supported by the findings of modern behavior genetics. Psychology broke from philosophy over precisely this need to seek empirical verification of hypotheses, but it carried with it concepts and insights accumulated over two millennia of profound thought about human nature.

Jacques Derrida and Postmodernism Throughout much of the 20th century, philosophers tried to support empiricism by examining the conceptual foundations of the scientific method and inductive inference. Concepts such as operationalism, theory falsification, and construct validity are products of the philosophy of science that have been widely adopted in scientific practice. The most influential philosophical movement of recent years, however, has often been seen as antiscientific. Deconstructionism and its intellectual descendants have provided a radical critique of conventional scientific thinking that has had a marked impact, for good or ill, on the humanities and social sciences.

Jacques Derrida (1930 to present) is a French philosopher who is usually identified as the founder of deconstructionism. Through analyses of literature, history, and psychoanalysis, he questioned the basic tenets of Western thought. He drew attention away from the ostensible subject of any writing, pointing to the writing itself as the object of investigation. Following this lead, social constructionists argued that there is no objective reality for science to study; instead, reality is constructed as a product of language and culture.

Derrida has had an enormous impact on the humanities, which is seen in the scholarly journals that abound with references to *discourse, text,* and *narrative*. In combination with other influences, such as feminism, social constructionism, and multiculturalism, deconstructionism has led to postmodernism, a stance that is critical of conventional empirical science on several accounts. Postmodernists argue that science is a set of cultural conventions revered in the West but is ultimately no more valid than any other belief system. The evidence that a darwinian offers in favor of evolution is no more convincing than the evidence that a Fundamentalist offers in favor of creationism. Both are discourses that have their own justification. Postmodernists are also critical of the claim that science is value neutral. They argue that the enterprise of science is inextricably bound to value judgments, and they have pointed out numerous ways in which science has contributed to the oppression of women, minorities, and non-Western cultures.

Postmodernism has been embraced by many psychoanalysts, humanistic psychologists, and anthropologists. Within psychiatry, one of the pioneers of postmodern thinking is Thomas Szasz, who argued that mental illnesses are not objective medical conditions, but questionable value judgments. Kenneth Gergen has urged psychologists to adopt a postmodern perspective to liberate their science from orthodox methods and theories and to make psychology more relevant outside Western culture. Mainstream psychologists, like most psychiatrists, tend to view postmodernism skeptically; indeed, many reject it outright.

However, the criticisms and alternatives offered by postmodernists can be useful to empirical scientists, even if the radical premises are not accepted. Some of the qualitative methods that they advocate, such as content analysis, can provide a valuable supplement to quantitative methods. It is useful to be reminded that the constructs of science, such as the categories of the revised fourth edition of the *Diagnostic and Statistical Manual of Mental Disorders* (DSM-IV-TR), are not direct representations of reality, but rather imperfect maps always in need of revision. Therapists are well advised to be sensitive to the cultural background of their patients, and, surely, all scientists need to be mindful of the social consequences of their work. This is particularly true in psychiatry, which has so much power over the lives and well-being of its patients.

BEHAVIORAL AND SOCIAL LEARNING APPROACHES

Theories of Personality

Behaviorism as a school of psychology grew up in reaction to the prevailing mentalistic model, in which introspection was used to determine the contents and operations of consciousness. John B. Watson (1878 to 1958) proposed that a scientific psychology should confine itself to an examination of observable behavior and should explain all human conduct in terms of stimuli and learned responses. Ivan Petrovich Pavlov's experiments with conditioned responses offered hope that such a science could be successful, and theorists such as Clark L. Hull (1884 to 1952) provided elaborate mathematical models of learning.

Radical Behaviorism Certainly, the most influential behaviorist and, perhaps, the most influential psychologist of the century was B. F. Skinner (1904 to 1990). Skinner's basic concept was *operant conditioning,* in which behaviors are viewed as a function of the organism's history of reinforcement. The observation that animals can be taught tricks by giving them rewards and punishments is nothing new. However, behaviorists, such as Skinner, refined and systematized this idea, using elegant experimental designs to tease apart the effects of the amount and schedule of reinforcements, the use of reinforcers and punishers, and the difficulty of the discriminations required. Behaviors could be shaped, maintained, or eliminated by the judicious use of these principles.

Skinner was a radical behaviorist, a purist who denied not only the scientific value, but also even the existence of mind. Furthermore, he avoided any neurophysiological or psychophysiological theorizing, preferring to study the *empty organism.* Individual differences were ignored in understanding basic phenomena and were explained in individuals as the result of different histories of reinforcement. Even differences between species were neglected: Skinner believed that the pigeon provided an adequate model for the study of learning in all organisms, and he and his followers were, in fact, able to replicate many of their animal findings by using human subjects. Much of Skinner's success can be attributed to his single-minded pursuit of a highly circumscribed set of variables.

Skinner's view of personality was, predictably, a reductionistic one. As he stated in *About Behaviorism*, "a self or personality is at best a repertoire of behavior imparted by an organized set of contingencies. The behavior a young person acquires in the bosom of his family composes one self; the behavior he acquires in, say, the armed services composes another." This position is rejected by humanistic psychologists, who attribute more choice and control to the individual, and by trait psychologists, who see consistencies of behavior that appear to transcend the consistencies of the reinforcing environment. Many personality psychologists have argued that controlled laboratory experimentation is a poor basis for theories of personality, because individuals play a large role in selecting and shaping their own environments. Skinner's radical behaviorism was rejected or modified by many later learning theorists who acknowledged the power of conditioning but also recognized differences among species and among individuals within a species.

Social Learning Theory One of the most distinctive features of human organisms is their use of speech, which makes possible elaborate thinking and planning and complex social interactions. In recent decades, learning theorists have increasingly emphasized social and cognitive processes. Among the most important have been Julian Rotter and Albert Bandura, both of whom have offered versions of social learning theory.

Rotter's theory proposes that human behavior is guided not only by the actual history of reinforcement, but also by plans, goals, and expectations of success. Individuals perform a behavior if they believe it is likely to lead to a valued goal, based on their past experiences in general and in similar situations. Individuals with a history of success are likely to have a generalized expectancy that they can control their lives; they are described as having an *internal locus of control.* At the opposite extreme are those whose prior efforts have been generally unsuccessful; they come to believe that rewards and punishments are a matter of luck or the arbitrary decisions of powerful others. Such individuals are said to have an *external locus of control.* Locus of control has been one of the most popular variables in personality research, used in numerous studies that generally are consistent with Rotter's theory.

Bandura's version of social learning theory also acknowledges the importance of internal cognitive processes. Individuals learn not only on the basis of their own experience, but also through vicarious reinforcement from observation of others. Bandura's demonstration of modeling effects in experiments conducted in the 1960s gave scientific legitimacy to the social learning perspective.

Rotter's and Bandura's theories are general theories of behavior, not specific theories of personality. However, for them, personality is something more than a collection of learned behaviors. The total pattern of experience leads to a generalized expectation of reinforcement or to a general sense of self-efficacy that can be considered the central individual difference variable. People are to be characterized primarily on the basis of their beliefs in their own ability to control their lives, because these beliefs powerfully determine the effort they make to adapt to their surroundings.

Social-cognitive approaches to personality are among the most influential for current research in personality. These approaches focus on the individual's understanding of himself or herself and how these self-appraisals shape goals, plans, and behaviors. Because of their origins in social learning theory, they tend to emphasize the role of the environment, pointing out that an individual's sense of self varies from setting to setting. Because of their ties to social theory, they usually explain personality in terms of the effects of social interactions. For example, Hazel Markus has suggested that individuals have a number of *possible selves*: conceptions of what one is or could be, which result from the messages significant others provide. For such theorists, concern has moved beyond the social learning of specific behaviors to the learning of entire identities.

Theories of Psychopathology

Psychoanalytic theories of personality grew out of attempts to understand psychopathology, and there are thus intimate connections between the two. By contrast, behavioral approaches have focused on the general principles by which behavior is acquired and maintained, and psychopathology, where it is considered at all, is usually treated as an area of application. Learning theories have had much more influence on methods of psychotherapy than on theories of psychopathology itself.

Behavioral approaches might suggest two different classes of explanations for psychopathology: Psychopathology might be related to the mechanisms of learning themselves, or it might be considered the result of learning behaviors that are maladaptive or socially unacceptable.

In the 1950s, Hans Eysenck (1916 to 1997), a psychologist who has figured prominently in learning and trait schools of personality, proposed that individual differences in the dimension of introversion-extroversion determined the ease with which individuals could acquire conditioned responses, which in turn determined the form of psychopathology to which they were prone. Extremely introverted individuals, he proposed, were easily conditioned and thus acquired many inhibitions. They were predisposed to the development of depressive, anxious, and obsessive-compulsive disorders (OCDs). By contrast, extreme extroverts were considered to be resistant to conditioning and were likely to develop hysterical and psychopathic disorders. (In later versions of Eysenck's theory, psychopathic disorders were grouped with psychotic disorders and linked to a different dimension of personality, *psychoticism.*)

Most behaviorists have viewed the laws of learning as universal processes and considered psychopathology to be the result of normal learning processes. In the 1920s, Irena Shenger-Krestounika taught a dog to discriminate between a circle and an ellipse as a cue for food. When the ellipse was made increasingly circular, the dog's ability to discriminate between them was taxed, and the dog began to struggle, to squeal, and to bite. Pavlov dubbed this an *experimental neurosis* and proposed that human neuroses might have parallel causes.

Probably the most famous attempt to explain psychopathology in learning theory terms was provided by John Dollard and Neal Miller. Dollard, an anthropologist, and Miller, an experimental psychologist, shared an interest in psychoanalysis. Their goal was to translate psychoanalytic concepts into the more testable terminology of learning theory. Consider, for example, the central psychoanalytic notion of *repression.* Sexual behaviors in the child might be punished by parents, and the child might learn to associate the behaviors with pain. By stimulus generalization, even the thought of the behaviors would elicit anxiety, and cognitive processes that blocked those thoughts would lessen anxiety and thus would be reinforced. Eventually, the thoughts would be effectively barred from consciousness.

Many behaviorists who did not share Dollard and Miller's enthusiasm for psychoanalysis followed their lead in attempting to explain psychopathology in terms of principles of learning. Phobias, in particular, were easily explained as conditioned responses reinforced by avoidant behavior. Similarly, compulsions could be understood as a kind of self-reinforcing behavior: Each time the compulsive act is performed, the anxiety associated with not performing the act is reduced, increasing the probability that the behavior will be repeated.

Social learning theorists have also noted the self-perpetuating nature of some maladaptive behavior. Individuals who lack a strong sense of self-efficacy in social situations may avoid them. As a consequence, they fail to learn the social skills that would enhance their self-confidence. Self-defeating behaviors, which may appear irrational from an outside perspective, are often understandable in terms of the dynamics of learning.

Application of Theory to Therapy

Behaviorists have a rather rudimentary view of personality, seeing it as an assemblage of learned behaviors. They also tend to see psychopathology in superficial terms. Psychological maladjustment is considered to be the result of learned behaviors, which are called *symptoms*, but there is no underlying disorder of which they are symptomatic. Curing the symptoms cures the disorder. At worst, this position is naïve and simplistic, equating the patient's presenting problem with the real source of difficulty. At best, however, it focuses attention on a specific problem that can be concretely addressed.

A large number of techniques for behavior modification have been used with considerable success in treating symptoms of psychopathology. Joseph Wolpe developed *systematic desensitization* as a treatment for phobias. Patients were instructed to relax and were then presented with increasingly vivid cues of the phobic object. Eventually, they were able to face the object itself without anxiety. A more dramatic technique is *implosive therapy*, in which the individual is confronted directly with the feared object (e.g., a room full of snakes) without an opportunity to escape. Because the object itself is harmless, and because avoidant behavior cannot be performed and is therefore not reinforced, the phobic reaction is swiftly extinguished.

Therapeutic interventions may be based on eliminating the reinforcements that sustain behavior, punishing unwanted behaviors, modeling or shaping more desirable behaviors, and so on. Any variable known to affect the acquisition or extinction of behaviors may provide an opportunity for behavior change, and behavioral techniques have been applied to physiological responses, as well as voluntary behaviors, through techniques of biofeedback. Behavior therapies have been used extensively in treating phobias, controlling addictive behavior, reducing the self-destructive behavior of autistic children, and improving classroom discipline—for the behaviorist, the distinction between psychopathology and bad behavior is generally unimportant. Behavior therapies are most effective when the problem can be clearly traced to a particular set of behaviors or conditioned responses; they are much less effective in dealing with vague complaints of confusion and distress, although these are frequently the problems that the patient presents to the clinician.

HUMANISTIC APPROACHES

Theories of Personality

Psychoanalysis and behaviorism are mechanistic theories that trace human behavior and experience to the gratification of instinctual impulses or to the acquisition of learned responses. Many of the most influential personality theorists of this century have defined themselves in terms of their opposition to these two approaches. Although they vary widely in terms of the explanations they offer of personality, humanistic approaches share a positive evaluation of human nature and emphasize its unique and distinctively human aspects. Personality produces and reflects organization, rationality, consistency, future orientation, planfulness, self-expression, cognitive complexity, and adaptability. Human reason and freedom of will, the capacity for growth and change, the need for love, and self-transcendence are prized by most of these humanistic theorists.

Social learning theories might be seen as a humanized form of behaviorism, because they recognize the role of complex symbolization and language in human learning. In a similar way, many now-classic humanistic theories were intended as modifications of psychoanalysis. Indeed, the first major psychoanalytic revisionist was Carl G. Jung, who argued that human beings had spiritual, as well as sexual, needs. Henry Murray also made major modifications to psychoanalysis in his view of personality. For example, he credited the mature ego with much more autonomy than Freud granted it, and he argued that the individual's sense of morality was not fixed by the superego instilled in childhood but could continue to develop into more rational and altruistic forms. Erich Fromm and Karen Horney minimized the instinctual origin of personality development and suggested that culture played a large role in shaping the individual. Erik Erikson proposed stages of psychosocial development to parallel Freud's psychosexual development, emphasizing such distinctly human characteristics as identity, intimacy, and generativity. He also theorized that personality development continued throughout the life span, giving encouragement to research on aging and personality.

Gordon Allport Although he is usually classified as a trait psychologist, in his general orientation to theorizing, Gordon Allport (1897 to 1967) was clearly a humanist. For him, man's behavior is proactive, reflecting internal, self-initiating characteristics more than situational forces. In his view, human personality possesses psychological coherence and momentary (cross sectional) and long-term (longitudinal) organization. Allport considered personality functioning to be characteristically rational, organized, and influenced by such conscious characteristics as long-range goals, plans of action, and philosophies of life.

Perhaps the most salient and controversial feature of his approach was the extreme emphasis that he put on the uniqueness of the individual personality. Allport viewed the major task of *personology* (or personality psychology) as the understanding and prediction of the individual case. To grasp the real personality, personal dispositions must be assessed, and this requires intensive study of an individual's past, present, and anticipated future functioning through the use of such techniques as the case history and content analysis of personal documents. In *Becoming: Basic Considerations for a Psychology of Personality,* Allport championed the view that concepts and laws must be developed to fit the individual case, creating the terms *idiographic* and *morphogenic* to symbolize his conviction that "each person is an idiom unto himself, an apparent violation of the syntax of the species."

Allport was deeply concerned with identifying personality functions, which he discussed under the concept of the *proprium,* the superordinate concept in his system. Propriate functioning not only organized and integrated actions and experience, but also provided the impetus to psychological growth. Allport described the functions of the proprium as *sense of body*, *self-identity*, *self-esteem*, *self-extension*, *rational coping*, *self-image*, and *propriate striving*. These propriate functions were vital to personality, and, although they were ongoing, they were by no means considered unchanging. Allport theorized that the propriate functions are modified throughout life, predominantly in the direction of greater differentiation and integration, or growth. The development of selfhood, away from the undifferentiated, opportunistic functioning of infancy and early childhood toward propriate functioning and striving is part of human nature for Allport. The person guides or directs his or her life by attempting to fulfill his or her sense of self or proprium. Development continues into adulthood, with increasing signs of maturity and personal lifestyle.

Abraham Maslow Abraham Maslow (1908 to 1970) interpreted personality in motivational terms. The individual's whole life—his or her perceptions, values, strivings, and goals—is focused on the satisfaction of a set of needs, and the needs themselves are arranged in a universal hierarchy. Maslow's needs serve an organizing and integrating role in life and are not to be understood as a simple and invariant set of responses to environmental pressures. They organize and create action possibilities and external reality.

At the lowest level of the motivational hierarchy are physiological needs for food, water, sex, and sleep. The second level consists of safety needs, needs for protection and security. The third level consists of needs for love and belongingness, and the fourth level consists of needs for self-respect and esteem from others. Above these lie the higher needs—for beauty, truth, justice, and *self-actualization*, the development of one's full potential as a unique human being.

Individuals live at the lowest level of motivation that is problematic for them. That is, if needs for food and shelter are not routinely met, they become the overriding concern in life: The hungry individual risks danger and social ostracism to find food. Those who have always been well-fed, however, learn to take the satisfaction of physiological needs for granted, and their attention is dominated by higher needs. Instead of examining specific behaviors and their reinforcements, Maslow's theory concerns the long-term satisfaction of broad classes of needs and thus gives a much broader depiction of the individual.

Maslow devoted much of his writing to a characterization of higher needs, including self-actualization, a drive to fulfill one's unique potential. He believed that personality psychology had become obsessed with psychopathology and that a corrective emphasis on positive mental health was needed. His biographical studies of such exemplary people as Eleanor Roosevelt and Abraham Lincoln suggested a number of distinctive characteristics of self-actualizers, including accurate perception of reality, creativity, a need for privacy, and the frequent experience of mystical or *peak* experiences. As an exception to his general theory of motivation, he also noted that such individuals often skip the lower levels and proceed directly to self-actualization. The most creative artists and musicians never seemed to care about poverty or lack of social acceptance.

George Kelly One of the most unconventional theories of personality was offered by George Kelly (1905 to 1967). It is, in some respects, a purely cognitive approach, but one with few ties to traditional learning theory. Instead of seeing them as organisms that are conditioned by their environment, Kelly argues that human beings should be seen as scientists trying to make sense of their world. In *The Psychology of Personal Constructs*, he states the fundamental postulate of his theory: "A person's processes are psychologically channelized by the ways in which he anticipates events."

The basic unit for understanding personality is the *personal construct*, a schema for classifying and interpreting experiences. For example, an individual might construe other people in terms of the contrast *strong* versus *weak*. Each new acquaintance would be categorized as a strong or weak person, and subsequent interactions with this person would be guided by the original construal. In the course of experience, it would probably be necessary to reclassify some individuals initially thought to be strong as weak, and vice versa; more importantly, some people might act in ways that were neither strong nor weak, leading the individual to develop new constructs (say, *friendly* versus *hostile*) that were more useful in predicting other people's behavior.

This rather abstract and bloodless theory is made relevant to psychopathology by Kelly's ingenious reconstruals of some basic emotional reactions. *Anxiety* is defined by him as the awareness that one's construct system is inadequate for construing important events. *Guilt* is the recognition that one's behavior is inconsistent with the ways in which one construes oneself. *Hostility* is viewed as the attempt to force experience to fit one's existing constructs. Such definitions are remote from common sense and clinical notions of anxiety, guilt, and hostility, but, precisely for that reason, they offer the prospect of novel ways of treating them.

Carl Rogers Carl Rogers (1902 to 1987) is probably the most influential humanistic personality theorist. He articulated a formal theory of personality; pioneered a major school of therapy, *client-centered therapy*; and encouraged rigorous research on his theory and therapy. Rogers held that all organisms tend toward their own actualization—that mental health and personal growth are the natural condition of humankind. Psychopathology is a defensive distortion of this actualization process, and psychotherapy consists of creating conditions in which defense is unnecessary. Given these conditions, patients (or *clients*, as Rogers called them) essentially cure themselves.

Under ideal conditions, people's needs, desires, and goals emerge naturally as part of self-actualization and are recognized as part of the self; individuals are fully open to experience. In real life, however, one person's needs and desires often conflict with others' needs and desires; in particular, children find themselves in conflict with their parents, who withhold love when the child (from their perspective) misbehaves. Because love is so essential, children internalize these *conditions of worth* and believe that they are good and worthwhile individuals only when their self is consistent with the ideals imposed by significant others. To maintain their sense of worth, they may distort their experience; this leads to anxiety and self-defeating behavior.

In some respects, Rogers' theory is much like Freud's: Both see psychopathology as the result of defensive distortions and see the ideal state as one in which individuals can accept conflicts and deal with them rationally. Rogers is a humanistic theorist, because he assumes that human nature is essentially good and that defenses are ultimately unnecessary. For Freud, the impulses of the id are eternally primitive and selfish, and their full actualization would be socially catastrophic.

Dan McAdams In the past decade, a number of scholars in the humanities and social sciences have turned their attention to the *life narrative* as a focus of research. These writers argue that the consciousness of self that distinguishes human beings from other animals is not a static list of personal characteristics; it takes the form of a story. In telling their life stories, people explain themselves in the context of their history and their significant relationships. Life narratives are not objective life histories; they are subjective interpretations that give personal meaning to past, present, and future events.

The personality psychologist who is most closely associated with this perspective is Dan McAdams. McAdams has postulated that personality can be understood on three levels: Level 1 consists of *traits*, abstract and enduring tendencies seen in general styles of action and experience; level 2 is defined by *personal concerns*, the goals, plans, and strategies that preoccupy the individual at a certain time and place; and level 3 is the *life narrative*, the story the person tells to himself or herself and to others in an effort to give a sense of unity and purpose to life.

Psychiatrists and psychotherapists have, of course, been listening to patients' life stories for many decades, usually seeking clues to the origins of current problems. McAdams' approach is different; he wishes to understand the narratives as stories. Stories can be analyzed in terms of such features as narrative tone (e.g., tragic, comic, and ironic), imagery, theme (what goals the characters pursue), ideological setting, and nuclear episodes (crises and turning points). From this perspective, key life events are not construed as causes of development but as symbols of identity. A patient's vivid recollection of a childhood humiliation may be important chiefly because it conveys the patient's sense of being a victim to whom fate has always been, and always will be, unfair.

Much of the scholarship on life narratives has been in a humanistic tradition that eschewed empirical rigor: A narrative reduced to a set of numbers is no longer a narrative. McAdams and his colleagues, however, have begun to conduct psychometric studies on such basic issues as the interrater reliability and temporal stability of life story variables. These studies will form the basis for a scientific evaluation of narrative perspectives on personality.

Theories of Psychopathology

In general, humanistic theories of personality stress positive aspects of human nature and discuss maladjustment in terms of failures of and blocks to the full growth and development of the individual. It is of some interest to note that Rogers and Kelly formulated their theories in the context of counseling students—individuals who presumably had relatively minor maladjustments and considerable personality strengths. The applicability of humanistic theories to patients experiencing schizophrenia or dementia is certainly questionable, but the theories have had a profound effect on routine clinical practice, in which clearly diagnosable psychiatric disorders seldom account for all of the patient's problems in living.

Humanistic psychologists differ tremendously in their views on the origins of maladjustment. Rogers pointed to internalized conditions of worth acquired chiefly during childhood. Erich Fromm, who was influenced by Marx, blamed society as a whole for instilling nonproductive orientations in individuals, such as *hoarding* or *marketing* orientations. Kelly said little about the origins of maladjustment but thought its essence was an ineffective construct system too rigid to be corrected by experience.

Other personality theorists, such as Rollo May, have been influenced by existential philosophy and have argued that the essential characteristic of human nature is freedom. Freedom, however, implies responsibility, and it is what Fromm called the attempted *escape from freedom* that often leads to psychopathology. In this view, the individual is the ultimate source of his or her own problems. The debate about responsibility and mental illness continues today, perhaps most conspicuously in questions about whether alcoholism should be considered a disease or a failure of self-discipline.

Application of Theory to Therapy

Some humanistic theories of personality—for example, Allport's—have had little impact on psychotherapy; others, such as Rogers', have been tremendously influential. It is helpful to recall that, for decades, the dominant form of therapy was psychoanalysis, a process that might require years and in which treatment was focused on dreams, childhood memories, and the ongoing relation with the therapist (the transference) rather than on the immediate problems of the patient. Many of the standard techniques of contemporary counseling, clinical psychology, and psychiatry rest on a very different set of assumptions about human nature made scientifically respectable by the work of humanistic psychologists.

Brief psychotherapies often consist of opportunities for individuals to express their feelings and to rethink their problems in a supportive atmosphere. The therapist may provide advice and guidance or at least may offer new ways in which patients can think about their problems. (This general approach is used by many psychiatrists as an adjunct to medication even in the treatment of serious mental disorders.) This process implicitly assumes that individuals, even those requiring psychotherapy, are basically rational and able, with some help, to solve their own problems; it also assumes that, given the right conditions, they move toward mental health: Patients are seen as scientists and self-actualizers.

Noting that Freud's "psychoanalytic cure" was based on a conscious understanding of one's life experiences, McAdams has argued that having a satisfying life narrative is a requirement for complete mental health. A good life story has coherence, credibility, a capacity for growth and change, and a generative orientation toward the world. One goal of psychotherapy, then, may be to help the patient rewrite his or her life narrative along these lines. James Pennebaker has claimed that writing about traumatic experiences has beneficial effects on mental and physical health, perhaps because the exercise of writing allows a rethinking of one's life narrative.

Modifying a patient's life story is a modest but, perhaps, realistic goal. Psychotherapists cannot easily alter patients' personality traits nor can they undo traumatic events of the past. They may, however, be able to help patients make sense of their dispositions and their life histories. Human tragedy can bring great suffering, but, in the hands of an artist, it can also be the source of great beauty.

The humanistic emphasis on freedom and responsibility has often clashed with the psychiatric tradition of regarding mental disorders as diseases. Labeling individuals as *schizophrenics* or *phobics* is held by some to be dehumanizing, and critics such as Thomas Szasz have argued that mental disorders are social and ethical judgments, not matters of medical fact. There is, of course, abundant evidence that some mental disorders have a biological basis, but the criticisms of humanistic psychologists make the point that the disorder occurs in a human being who, in many respects, may be like any other person. There may be normal and abnormal behaviors, experiences, or relationships, but there are not normal and abnormal people.

TRAIT AND FACTOR MODELS

Individual differences are peripheral concerns in many social learning and humanistic theories of personality; they are the central focus of trait theories. The study of variations in human character and temperament goes back at least to Theophrastus, a Greek, whose *Characters* depicted 30 different types. The morose type, for example, he described as follows:

> A malignant temper sometimes vents itself chiefly in ferocity of language. The man whose tongue is thus at war with all the world, cannot reply to the simplest inquiry except by some such rejoinder as—"Trouble not me with your questions": nor will he return a civil salutation. . . . He has no pardon for those who may unwittingly shove or jostle him, or tread upon his toe. . . . He will neither wait for, nor stay with anyone long: nor will he sing, or recite verses, or dance in company. It is a man of this spirit who dares to live without offering supplications to heaven.

Theories of Personality The scientific study of individual differences in personality can be traced to Sir Francis Galton in England, who laid the foundations of psychometrics, and to Gerard Heymans in the Netherlands, who undertook the first large-scale study of rated personality traits. The first major trait theorist in the United States was Allport, whose 1937 volume, *Personality: A Psychological Interpretation,* spelled out the basic issues in trait psychology. He defined a *trait* as "a neuropsychic structure having the capacity to render many stimuli functionally equivalent, and to initiate and guide equivalent (meaningfully consistent) forms of adaptive and expressive behavior." In this view, something in the brain of the morose man makes him see even simple questions or greetings as a personal affront, and his sullen attitude is expressed in a variety of social situations.

Allport believed that traits were concrete features of individuals that uniquely described them and that might be understood by a case study of a single individual. A contrasting view is that traits are dimensions of individual difference that can only be discovered by comparing and contrasting different individuals; individuals are then described in terms of their standing on a set of common traits. The two definitions are closely related; people who are more anxious than 99 percent of the population presumably have a neuropsychic structure that makes them so anxious.

Characteristics of Traits Although there are many different trait theories, there is general agreement on several key features of traits: (1) Traits are tendencies to show consistent patterns of thoughts, feelings, and actions. Behaviors that are specific to a single setting or situation may better be considered habits than traits; some evidence of cross-situational consistency is necessary to infer a trait. However, concrete instances of behavior have many determinants, including learned habits, aroused needs, social contexts, role requirements, and the influence of many different and potentially conflicting traits, so the influence of a specific trait on any particular behavior may be quite modest. It is usually only by viewing behavior across many different situations that a consistent pattern can be detected. (2) Traits are relatively enduring features that characterize the individual. In this respect, they are to be distinguished from transient moods or episodes of mental disorder that affect the individual. The fact that traits are relatively enduring does not mean that they cannot change; traits are not immutable, even if they are durable. (3) Traits are continuously distributed, usually approximating a normal or bell curve. Although it is convenient to speak about *introverts* and *extroverts*, in fact, most individuals are *ambiverts*, showing some of the characteristics of introverts and some of the characteristics of extroverts. With the possible exception of masculinity and femininity, there is no consistent evidence of discrete personality *types*.

From time to time, there has been controversy over the reality of traits, fueled by the fact that human beings easily and readily ascribe traits to others on the basis of little or no information, with correspondingly limited accuracy. These personality ascriptions may be triggered by stereotypes of age or physical appearance or may be quite idiosyncratic. Demonstrations of this fact in laboratory experiments by social psychologists, together with the relatively loose cross-situational consistency of most traits, led a generation of psychologists in the 1970s to conclude that traits were cognitive fictions. Subsequent work—particularly, demonstrations that judges who knew the individual well agreed with each other and with the self-reports of the individual about his or her standing on a variety of traits—restored faith in the consensual validity of traits. However, the controversy does make the crucial point that some trait ascriptions are more accurate than others and that first impressions may be quite misleading. Psychiatrists ought not to assume that their clinical judgments of a patient's personality are correct; validated personality questionnaires and rating forms completed by knowledgeable others may be needed to portray and to understand personality accurately.

Personality Structure and Factor Analysis The most important differences among trait theorists are in the specific traits that they have conceptualized and measured. Jung identified introversion and extroversion as basic personality variables, Bandura emphasized self-efficacy, and Rogers was concerned with openness to experience. Over the years, literally thousands of scales have been developed to measure traits that psychologists considered important in understanding personality. As early as 1936, Allport pointed to another source for identifying personality traits: the natural language. In a monograph he published with Henry Odbert, he listed some 18,000 terms extracted from an unabridged dictionary that could be used to describe people; some of them were mere evaluations (e.g., *swell* and *awful*), but he regarded approximately 4,000 as legitimate trait terms.

The problem for trait psychologists was how to choose a manageable set of traits from among the many possible constructs. It was obvious that trait terms were highly redundant—for example, *anxious*, *worrying*, *nervous*, *apprehensive*, and *fearful* reflect similar, if not identical, characteristics—so what was needed was a procedure for identifying major groups of traits that covaried. Factor analysis, a statistical technique that reduces the complexity of a set of correlations among variables, was first used in personality research by J. P. Guilford and has remained one of its basic tools. The factors, or dimensions, identified in this process correspond to groups of closely related traits; the set of basic dimensions identified by the factor analysis constitutes a model of the structure of personality traits.

Raymond Cattell developed one of the first and most influential factor models. He reasoned that, in the course of cultural evolution, any personality trait important in human social interaction would have been noticed and named; the 4,000 trait terms identified by Allport and Odbert could thus be assumed to represent an exhaustive listing of personality characteristics (this has become known as the *lexical hypothesis*). Cattell grouped synonyms and near-synonyms together to obtain a set of 35 personality variables and asked respondents to rate acquaintances on each of these sets of terms. He intercorrelated the ratings and factored the correlations, identifying 12 factors. Together with four more factors found in research using self-report questionnaires, these became the basis for the 16 Personality Factor Questionnaire (16PF), a self-report instrument that has been widely used in personality research and clinical psychology for more than 40 years.

It was originally hoped that factor analysis would provide an objective solution to the question of personality structure, but, for many years, there was little agreement among factor analysts. Eysenck believed that Cattell's model could not be replicated and was needlessly complex. He proposed a simple and powerful two-dimensional model that identified extroversion–introversion (E) and neuroticism–emotional stability (N) as superfactors and showed that, if the scales of the 16PF were themselves factored, the two largest factors resembled his E and N. He and his wife, Sybil Eysenck, developed a series of instruments to measure these factors (and, later, a third superfactor called *psychoticism*) that have also been widely used, particularly in Great Britain. Eysenck's stature as a learning theorist and a critic of psychoanalysis contributed to the importance of these dimensions in psychiatric contexts.

Five-Factor Model Eysenck's two factors were widely replicated, but they seemed to omit many important characteristics, such as curiosity, aggression, and achievement striving. An alternative solution was offered in 1961 by two U.S. Air Force psychologists, Ernest Tupes and Raymond Christal. They began with the 35 clusters of traits identified by Cattell and obtained ratings on these clusters in eight different samples. They found that a five-factor solution fit the data in all eight samples. Two of the factors resembled Eysenck's E and N, but three other factors were new.

A small group of lexical researchers, including Warren Norman and Lewis R. Goldberg, continued to study personality structure as represented by natural language trait adjectives, and, after 20 years, they came to the conclusion that the five-factor structure proposed by Tupes and Christal was essentially correct. Renewed interest in this model showed that the five factors could be recovered in analyses of self-reports and observer ratings; in ratings of children, college students, and older adults; and in several different languages, including non–Indo-European languages, such as Chinese, Hebrew, and Filipino. The factors appeared in analyses of trait adjectives, descriptive phrases, and questionnaire scales. Contemporary five-factor theorists differ somewhat on their conceptualizations of the factors and consequently give them somewhat different labels. The terms *neuroticism* (N), *extroversion* (E), *openness to experience* (O), *agreeableness* (A), and *conscientiousness* (C) are used here. The five factors and some of the traits, or facets, that define them are given in Table 6.4–1, along with associated adjectives.

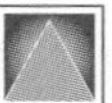

Table 6.4–1
Five Factors of Personality, Defining Traits, and Empirically Associated Adjectives

Factor	Trait	Adjectives
Neuroticism (N)	Anxiety	Anxious, fearful, worrying, tense
	Angry hostility	Irritable, impatient, moody, not gentle
	Depression	Pessimistic, worrying, not contented, moody
	Self-consciousness	Shy, not self-confident, timid, inhibited
	Impulsiveness	Hasty, self-centered, excitable, loud
	Vulnerability	Not confident, not efficient, not clear-thinking, anxious
Extroversion (E)	Warmth	Friendly, warm, sociable, not aloof
	Gregariousness	Sociable, outgoing, talkative, not withdrawn
	Assertiveness	Assertive, forceful, aggressive, confident
	Activity	Energetic, hurried, quick, active
	Excitement seeking	Pleasure-seeking, adventurous, daring, spunky
	Positive emotions	Enthusiastic, humorous, optimistic, jolly
Openness (O)	Fantasy	Dreamy, imaginative, artistic, complicated
	Aesthetics	Artistic, original, inventive, idealistic
	Feelings	Excitable, spontaneous, affectionate, insightful
	Actions	Wide interests, versatile, adventurous, imaginative
	Ideas	Curious, original, insightful, inventive
	Values	Not conservative, not cautious, flirtatious, unconventional
Agreeableness (A)	Trust	Trusting, not suspicious, forgiving, not wary
	Straightforwardness	Not shrewd, not autocratic, not charming, not demanding
	Altruism	Soft-hearted, gentle, generous, kind
	Compliance	Not stubborn, not demanding, not headstrong, not impatient
	Modesty	Not a show-off, not clever, not argumentative, not self-confident
	Tender-mindedness	Sympathetic, soft-hearted, warm, kind
Conscientiousness (C)	Competence	Efficient, thorough, resourceful, intelligent
	Order	Organized, precise, methodical, thorough
	Dutifulness	Thorough, not careless, not distractible, not lazy
	Achievement striving	Ambitious, industrious, enterprising, persistent
	Self-discipline	Energetic, not lazy, organized, not absent-minded
	Deliberation	Not hasty, not impulsive, not careless, not immature

Note: Adjectives are significantly correlated with traits, N = 305, *P* <.001. Adapted from McCrae RR, Costa PT Jr: Discriminant validity of NEO-PI-R facet scales. *Ed Psychol Measurement.* 1992;52:229.

Many psychologists were skeptical of the lexical hypothesis that had led to the five-factor model. These critics believed that personality theory and clinical experience would lead to the identification of important traits for which no lay terms existed, and they continued to offer alternative models. Katharine Briggs and Isabel Myers operationalized Jung's psychological functions in the Myers-Briggs Type Indicator, which classifies individuals in terms of the dichotomies of introversion versus extroversion, intuition versus sensing, thinking versus feeling, and judging versus perceiving. Timothy Leary argued that the traits that influence social interactions were better represented in a circular order than as a set of factors, and many instruments have been developed to measure this model.

A particularly important system was suggested by Theodore Millon, who was interested in personality traits associated with psychiatric disorders. His reviews of clinical literature led to a theory of personality and psychopathology that specified 11 personality disorders as extreme variants of normal traits. For example, the histrionic personality disorder is supposed to be related to the trait of gregariousness; the schizoid personality disorder is related to the trait of detachment. Millon's theory had a profound impact on the formulation of Axis II in the third edition of the *Diagnostic and Statistical Manual of Mental Disorders* (DSM-III) and in subsequent editions. His instrument, the Millon Clinical Multiaxial Inventory, has been widely used by psychiatrists and clinical psychologists.

The fact that trait theories of personality are usually tied to assessment inventories makes it relatively easy to make empirical comparisons, and, in the past decade, researchers in several countries have undertaken the task of relating different trait models. There is a growing consensus among these researchers that virtually all the traits measured by theory-based personality questionnaires—including those derived from psychodynamic, behavioral, and humanistic theories—are related to one or more of the five factors of Tupes and Christal. However, instruments vary in comprehensiveness. For example, the four scales of the Myers-Briggs Type Indicator correspond to four of the five factors, whereas measures of the interpersonal circumplex represent only two factors (extroversion and agreeableness).

These comparisons of instruments can lead to significant reconceptualizations. For example, Cloninger's Temperament and Character Inventory (TCI) consists of four factors that are intended to assess temperament and three that assess character. However, joint analysis with a measure of the five-factor model shows that the Harm Avoidance temperament scales and the Self-Directedness character scales are really opposite poles of a single neuroticism factor, whereas the Reward Dependence temperament scales and the Cooperation character scales are both measures of agreeableness. From the perspective of the five-factor model, the TCI's distinction between temperament and character appears not to be supported.

At the broadest level, then, the problem of personality structure appears to have been resolved: Personality is described by five basic factors. This does not mean that personality can be exhaustively described by standing on five dimensions. Most trait psychologists adopt hierarchical models of trait structure. They assume that the broadest factors are composed of more specific traits, which, in turn, are defined by subtraits that correspond to individual items in a questionnaire. In the Revised NEO Personality Inventory (NEO-PI-R), for example, six specific traits or facets are measured for each of the five factors (or domains) of personality. The facet scales are listed in Table 6.4–1; the hierarchical organization is illustrated in Figure 6.4–1. Assessment on the level of specific facets provides a more detailed and personalized portrait of the individual.

Origin and Development of Personality Traits Psychoanalytic, learning, and humanistic theories have usually offered causal explanations for individual differences. Thus, differences in self-efficacy are supposed to be caused by different histories of success in pursuing goals; variations in openness to experience might be the result of differences in the conditions of worth imposed by parents. The factor analysts who scoured the dictionary for trait terms usually bypassed this issue, being content to describe the personality

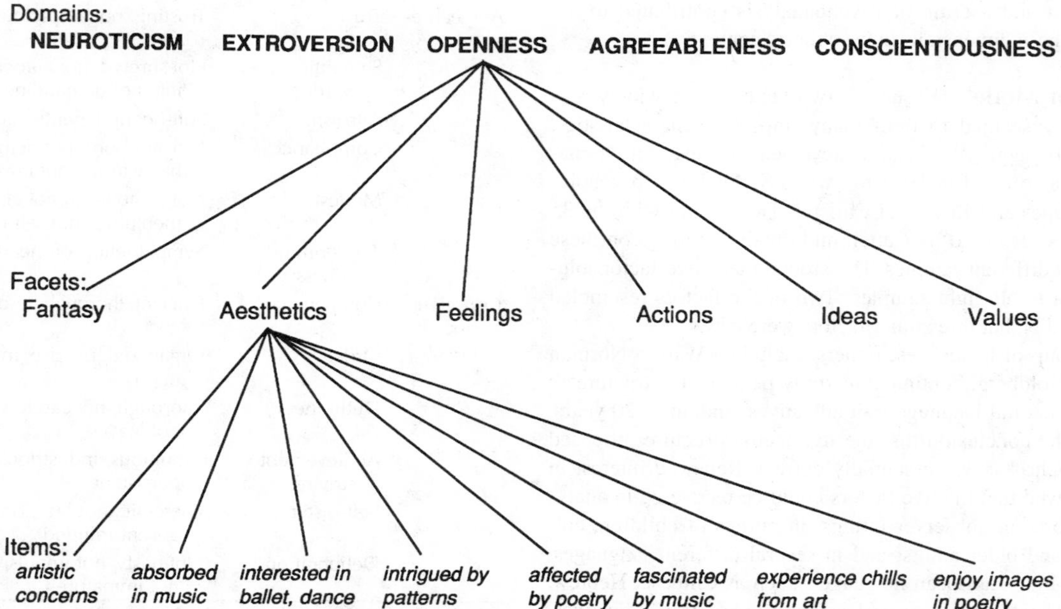

FIGURE 6.4–1 An example of hierarchical organization in the Revised NEO Personality Inventory: domains, facets of openness, and items measuring openness to aesthetics.

differences they found in adults. In principle, some traits might be inherited, some might be instilled by parents, and some might be learned from experience; whatever their origin, they could be measured and used to predict important life criteria.

Until recently, it was generally assumed that personality was shaped primarily by a variety of environmental influences, including parental love and discipline, social and economic opportunities, and life experiences through childhood and adolescence. Surprisingly, this assumption has rarely been tested: There has been little prospective longitudinal research documenting links between early childhood experiences and subsequent adult personality. A different research design, using the techniques of behavior genetics, can answer these questions by comparing personality measures in adults with different degrees of genetic and environmental similarity. For example, similarity between identical twins reared apart can be attributed to genetic influences, whereas similarity between adopted siblings reared together must be due to environmental influences.

Since the early 1980s, behavior genetics studies using many different samples, personality measures, and methods of data analysis have converged on the surprising conclusion that personality traits are, to a considerable extent, heritable, and, to a considerable extent, due to unknown and idiosyncratic causes. The molecular genetics underlying trait heritability have been a topic of great interest in the past few years, but research approaches are still being refined. Early studies claiming to find single genes for major traits are giving way to newer paradigms. These more sophisticated approaches use combinations of traits to define personality styles or patterns that better define the personality phenotypes for genetic linkage and association studies. In addition, gene–environment and gene–gene interactions are leading to new insights into the role that genotypes can play in moderating environmental substrates.

Genes involved in regulation of serotonin function have been logical candidates to evaluate in attempts to identify genes that affect personality dimensions associated with mental and physical illness. Much attention has focused on a 44-bp insertion/deletion polymorphism of the serotonin transporter gene promoter (5HTTLPR) and an upstream VNTR polymorphism of the MAOA gene promoter (MAOA-uVNTR). Avshalom Caspi and colleagues have shown that a genotype that confers low levels of MAOA expression—MAOA-uVNTR 2/3/5 repeat alleles—is associated with development of antisocial and violent behavior in men who had been abused in childhood, and the 5HTTLPR allele is associated with increased depression in adults who experienced high levels of life stress or childhood abuse. Interactions between these two genes as they affect complex personality phenotypes or personality styles are areas of active research. Preliminary findings by Redford Williams and colleagues link a resilient or directed personality style (a pattern of low neuroticism and high conscientiousness) to the MAOA-uVNTR genotypes that produce less MAOA protein and 5HTTLPR genotypes that produce less serotonin transporter protein. Williams and colleagues hypothesize that the less active variants of these genes interact to produce this personality pattern (or profile) via increased serotonergic function that results in reduced enzymatic degradation and clearance of released serotonin.

Less success has been found in identifying environmental origins of personality traits. In fact, they are hardly attributable to shared environmental causes at all. Socioeconomic status, family diet, religious training, parental modeling, and all the other influences that children growing up in the same household would normally share seem to have little or no influence on adult personality. This conclusion applies as much to character traits, such as achievement striving and modesty, as to temperament traits, such as anxiety and energy level. This dramatic and counterintuitive finding will doubtless reshape theories of personality. As Sandra Scarr commented, "psychology [currently] has no adequate theories to account for individual variation in behavior because our theories address the wrong sources of variation."

One new theory that does begin to address the "right" sources of variation is five-factor theory (FFT). This theory attempts to provide a conceptual framework in which the body of research on the five-factor model can be interpreted. FFT is a systems theory, represented schematically in Figure 6.4–2. The central components are *basic tendencies* (including personality traits and intelligence and other abilities) and *characteristic adaptations* (such as skills, attitudes, values, and roles). In this model, as suggested by behavioral genetics, the only input to basic tendencies is from biological bases. However, personality traits and *external influences* are important in shaping characteristic adaptations. For example, an individual who is temperamentally high in self-consciousness and who repeatedly experienced ridicule as a child might develop an *avoidant personality disorder*, which is a *characteristic (mal)adaptation*.

For many years, developmental psychologists assumed that personality development ended with adolescence. A 21-year-old is legally an adult and is unlikely to grow much in physical height or intellectual capacity, but recent research has shown consistent changes in personality between college age and middle adulthood. There is a dramatic decline in excitement seeking over that interval, but, in addition, cross-sectional and longitudinal studies of American college students have shown that the five-factor traits N, E, and O decline during the decade of the 20s, whereas A and C increase. As a result, 30-year-olds are less emotional and better socialized than 20-year-olds.

There is reason to believe that these changes are not the product of the relatively indulgent American experience of adolescence. The same pattern of age differences is seen in less affluent countries, such as Croatia, and in non-Western countries, such as Korea. Such cross-cultural studies suggest that there may be intrinsic maturational processes in personality development, which is consistent with the biological basis of personality traits hypothesized by FFT.

There have also been important developments in understanding personality change in individuals older than 30 years of age. Traits are defined as relatively enduring patterns of behavior, but most psychologists assumed that traits would be modified by life experiences. Jung postulated that the process of individuation required each individual to express all of his or her potentials, and, thus, the young introvert would normally become an extrovert in old age, and vice versa. Lay stereotypes of aging held that, as they age, people become cranky, conservative, and depressed. Gerontologists rebutted these myths of aging, arguing that old age was more likely to bring maturity, wisdom, or detachment. Theories of adult development, popularized in Gail Sheehy's best-selling *Passages*, suggested that personality changed in stages and, in particular, that men (and perhaps women) went through a midlife crisis in their 30s or 40s.

In sharp contrast to all these theories are the findings from a number of independent longitudinal studies of personality in adulthood. These studies present a clear picture of predominant stability of the full range of personality traits. That is, the average levels of most traits neither increase nor decline much with age, and individuals tend to maintain the same rank order. The 30-year-old who is outgoing, curious, and hardworking is likely to become an outgoing, curious, and hardworking 80-year-old. This conclusion has been supported by studies using self-reports and observer ratings of all five factors of personality and appears to apply to men and women. Of course, there are often dramatic changes in personality as a result of dementing disorders in old age, but normal life experience seems to have little impact on personality in individuals older than 30 years of age.

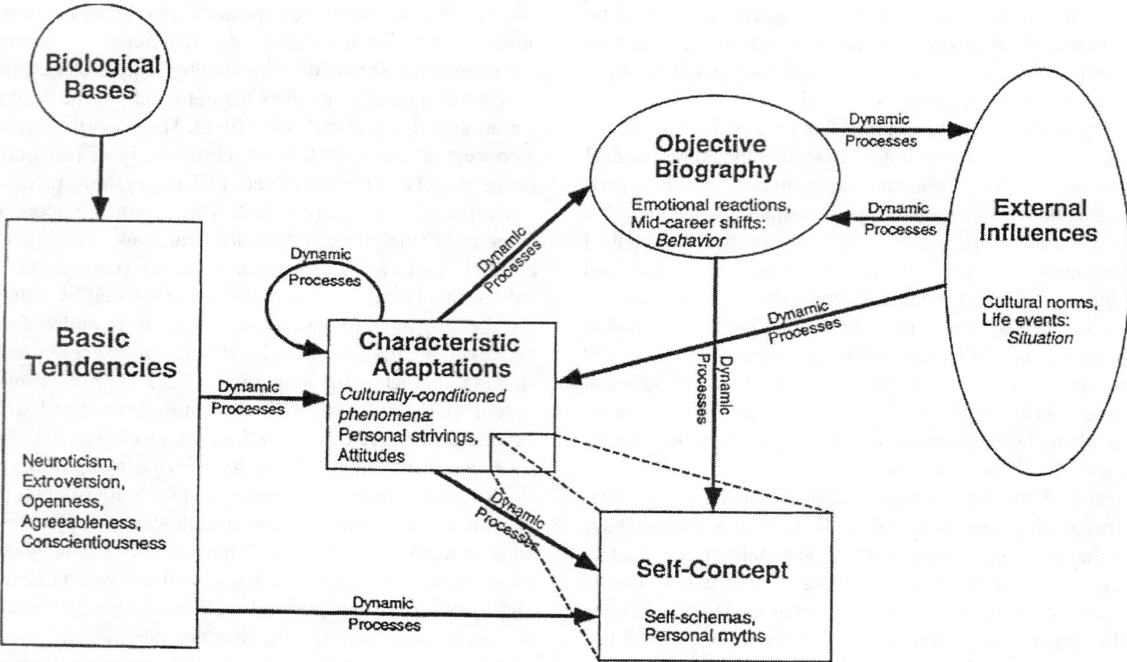

FIGURE 6.4–2 A representation of the personality system as depicted by the five-factor theory. The ellipses represent peripheral elements, and the rectangles represent central elements. Examples of content are given in each. Arrows indicate the direction of causal influences. (Adapted from McCrae RR, Costa PT Jr. A Five-Factor Theory of personality. In: LA Pervin, OP John, eds.: *Handbook of Personality: Theory and Research.* 2nd ed. New York: Guilford; 1999:139.)

There are distressingly few data on the long-term effects of psychopathology on personality. Individuals in recovery from an episode of *major depressive disorder* generally score high on measures of the five-factor trait N, and it is sometimes argued that this is a result of the experience of depression. However, the few prospective studies of the first onset of major depression typically show that these individuals scored high on N before the first episode, suggesting that high N may be an enduring feature of people prone to clinical depression.

Theories of Psychopathology The links between psychopathology and trait psychology are at once intimate and complex. For decades, psychiatrists and clinical psychologists have administered psychological tests such as the Minnesota Multiphasic Personality Inventory (MMPI) and Cattell's measure of personality, the 16PF, to inform the diagnosis of mental disorders; these same tests have been used routinely by trait psychologists to examine relations between personality and such criteria as vocational preference, creative potential, and coping with life stress. The dividing line between normal variations in personality dispositions and psychopathology is frequently unclear.

This poses more of a problem to psychiatric nosology than it does to trait theories of personality. Psychiatric diagnoses are supposed to represent the presence of a discrete disorder, and the DSM-IV-TR specifies the criteria that must be met to confer each diagnosis. This categorical model is appropriate for some disorders but not others. It may be difficult to separate social phobia, for example, from extreme shyness and self-consciousness or a schizoid personality disorder from marked introversion. This is entirely consistent with trait models of personality, which regard individual differences as continuously distributed variables.

Neuroticism and Psychopathology One theory of psychopathology, therefore, is that some psychiatric disorders reflect extreme standing on personality traits, particularly those related to the five-factor trait N. Among the traits that covary in normal populations to define this factor are predispositions to experience chronic levels of negative affects, such as fear, anger, shame, and sadness. Individuals with high standing on these traits may qualify for a diagnosis of generalized anxiety disorder, borderline personality disorder, social phobia, or dysthymia.

The five-factor trait N may also be considered a risk factor for the development of psychiatric disorders that are not themselves trait-like. Several recent studies have demonstrated that individuals scoring high on measures of N are at increased risk of subsequently receiving a diagnosis of major depressive disorder. Poor control of urges and impulses and excessive concern with physical functioning are also characteristics associated with N, and it might be hypothesized that individuals high in N are predisposed to develop eating disorders and hypochondriasis. N is, in essence, a generalized disposition to experience psychological distress, and individuals seeking psychiatric treatment are almost always distressed. It is therefore not surprising that virtually all clinical populations, from drug abusers to schizophrenics, score high on measures of N.

Historically, the term *neurosis* or *psychoneurosis* was coined to identify psychiatric disorders of functional origin that were closely related to anxiety and its control. It survived in the revised third edition of DSM (DSM-III-R) in many secondary labels (dysthymia, for example, was also called *depressive neurosis*) but is not used in DSM-IV-TR. Many personality psychologists object to the term *neuroticism* as a label for a dimension of normal personality because of its suggestion of psychopathology. Many psychiatrists object to the term because it appears tied to an outdated psychiatric nosology. However, the term serves a useful purpose: It is a reminder to clinicians that patients with a wide variety of diagnoses share many features related to chronic psychological distress and is a reminder to personality psychologists that the difference between normal and abnormal functioning is often only one of degree. The cliché that people are all more or less neurotic has some scientific basis.

Personality Traits and Personality Disorders Axis II of the DSM-IV-TR is used for the diagnosis of personality disorders, which are defined as inflexible and maladaptive personality traits. It is reasonable to ask whether these traits are the same as or different from those encountered in nonpsychiatric populations. Several recent studies on this question have concurred in finding strong and replicable links between scales measuring personality disorders and the five factors in normal and clinical populations.

In the case of N, only high scores are associated with psychiatric impairment, but both poles of the other factors appear to be associated with specific forms of psychopathology. Individuals high in E tend to have histrionic and narcissistic personality disorders; those who are low in E have avoidant and schizoid disorders. High C is associated with obsessive-compulsive personality disorder; low C is associated with antisocial personality disorder. Low A, or antagonism, is characteristic of individuals with paranoid, antisocial, and narcissistic personality disorders. High A is associated with dependent personality disorder.

The hypothesized relations between facet-level personality traits and DSM-IV-TR personality disorders are presented in Table 6.4–2. These associations show some of the ways in which disorders can be conceptually distinguished. For example, avoidant and schizoid personality disorders are characterized by low gregariousness, but only the former shows associations with high anxiety, depression, self-consciousness, and vulnerability. Research in several countries has generally supported this mapping of disorders onto personality traits, although the conceptual distinctions highlighted in Table 6.4–2 are usually blurred in real data because of the pervasive comorbidity of personality disorders.

It is a matter of current controversy just how these personality traits are related to the disorders: Are normal personality traits carried to an extreme inherently maladaptive, or do these traits merely predispose individuals to develop disorders under certain circumstances? Some research has also called into question the meaningfulness of the syndromes recognized by DSM-IV-TR by showing that the symptoms used to define the disorders, when separately assessed, do not covary in ways that match the DSM-IV-TR syndromes. Instead, the symptom clusters that do emerge are interpretable in terms of the five-factor model. As a result of such evidence, proposals have been made to replace the current categorical model by dimensional models that relate problems in adjustment to standing on basic dimensions of personality. This would appear to be a logical extension of trait theories of psychopathology.

Thomas Widiger and colleagues have proposed that DSM-IV-TR Axis II diagnosis should be replaced by a four-step process. In the first step, domains and facets of personality would be assessed, providing all the benefits of trait assessment described in the following discussion. In the second step, clinicians would identify specific problems in living associated with salient traits. For example, it might be noted that a patient high in self-consciousness experiences intense embarrassment when around strangers. In the third step, the clinician would evaluate the degree of impairment that the problems caused, to determine if they are clinically significant. Does the patient's embarrassment interfere with holding a job or finding a mate? Finally, in an optional fourth step, the clinician could interpret the full personality profile to see if it matched the prototype for an identified personality disorder. For example, if the patient was high in anxiety, depression, and vulnerability, as well as self-consciousness, and low in gregariousness, assertiveness, and excitement seeking, he or she could be considered to have an avoidant personality disorder (Table 6.4–2). A major advantage of this system is that patients who did not meet full criteria for any recognized personality disorder could still be treated for personality-related problems in living.

Application of Theory to Therapy

Psychodynamic, behavioral, and humanistic theories all specify the causal mechanisms by which psychopathology is created and maintained and thus imply points of intervention. If maladjustment is caused by rigidly internalized conditions of worth, then unconditional positive regard in the therapeutic setting may provide a cure; if the problem is a learned behavior, then altering reinforcements may extinguish it. Trait models do not emphasize causal or developmental explanations and thus may seem to have no implications for psychotherapy. In fact, they have many.

Recent evidence on the substantial heritability of most personality traits clearly indicates that Allport was right: Traits do have some underlying neuropsychic structure. Research on the psychophysiology of traits is a topic of growing interest and parallels the extensive work done on the neurophysiological basis of many forms of psychopathology. In this broad sense, then, psychopharmacological approaches to psychotherapy are, in principle, consistent with trait theories of personality: If personality traits and disorders reflect brain processes, drugs that affect the brain may offer useful instruments for psychotherapy. In practice, there is still much to learn. For example, individuals with dysthymia, who score high on measures of trait depression, often do not respond to antidepressant medication.

Personality Assessment Historically, the chief role of trait psychology in psychotherapy has been in diagnosis and assessment. A number of self-report measures, such as the MMPI and the Millon Clinical Multiaxial Inventory, were designed specifically to measure psychopathology and to include primarily items that tap psychiatric symptoms. They can be regarded as measuring psychopathological traits and states (although they have often been used in college and volunteer samples as measures of personality per se). These instruments are chiefly of value as aids to psychodiagnosis. General personality questionnaires, including the 16PF, the Guilford-Zimmerman Temperament Survey, and the Edwards Personal Preference Schedule, have also been used for decades in clinical psychology and psychiatry as part of a complete psychological assessment. Several measures of the five-factor model have recently appeared, including the Hogan Personality Inventory and the NEO Personality Inventory, and there has been considerable interest in the clinical application of the five-factor model. The primary advantage of this model is its comprehensiveness. By assessing traits from all five dimensions, the clinician can efficiently obtain a full portrait of the individual.

Some psychiatrists are concerned that personality scores obtained from acutely depressed patients are invalid. This concern is based on the empirical finding that scores, particularly on scales related to the five-factor trait N, change with remission and on the belief that personality traits cannot change. If the latter belief were true, it would be necessary to conclude that depression distorts self-reports of personality. However, as Figure 6.4–2 suggests, personality traits may change if their biological basis is altered, and acute major depression has demonstrated effects on brain functioning. Controlled studies and clinical experience suggest that trait scores obtained from acutely depressed patients are indeed informative in most cases.

Personality psychologists and psychometricians have devoted years to the development of self-report inventories, and the usefulness of this approach to assessment is beyond doubt. Self-reports,

Table 6.4–2
Hypothesized Relations between DSM-IV-TR Personality Disorders and Five-Factor Model Personality Traits

Personality Trait	Paranoid	Schizoid	Schizotypal	Antisocial	Borderline	Histrionic	Narcissistic	Avoidant	Dependent	Obsessive-Compulsive
Neuroticism										
Anxiety			H		H			H	H	
Angry hostility	H			H	H		H			
Depression					H	H		H		
Self-consciousness			H			H	H	H	H	
Impulsiveness					H					
Vulnerability					H			H	H	
Extroversion										
Warmth		L	L			H			H	
Gregariousness		L	L			H		L		
Assertiveness								L	L	H
Activity										
Excitement seeking				H		H		L		
Positive emotions		L	L			H				
Openness to experience										
Fantasy			H			H	H			
Aesthetics										
Feelings		L				H				
Actions			H							
Ideas			H							
Values										L
Agreeableness										
Trust	L		L		L	H			H	
Straightforwardness	L			L						
Altruism				L			L		H	
Compliance	L			L	L				H	L
Modesty							L		H	
Tender-mindedness				L			L			
Conscientiousness										
Competence					L					H
Order										H
Dutifulness				L						H
Achievement striving							H			H
Self-discipline				L						
Deliberation				L						

Note: High and low ratings are based on revised fourth edition of the *Diagnostic and Statistical Manual of Mental Disorders* diagnostic criteria.
H, high; L, low.
Adapted from Costa PT Jr, Widiger TA, eds. *Personality Disorders and the Five-Factor Model of Personality.* 2nd ed. Washington, DC: American Psychological Association; 2002.

however, are by no means infallible. Patients may not understand their own personalities or may deliberately misrepresent themselves. Concerns about defensiveness and socially desirable responding have led to the use of projective tests, the development of special validity scales to detect and to correct for distorted responses, and reliance on the clinical judgment of the psychiatrist. Each of these possible solutions introduces problems of its own, however, and most clinicians rely on multiple sources of information.

One source of information that has been underused in clinical settings is informant ratings. Research in the past decade has confirmed that ratings on standardized instruments by significant others—usually spouses or parents—can provide reliable and valid assessments of personality. These findings appear to hold for clinical, as well as volunteer, samples. Personality ratings may be particularly valuable when patients are incapacitated or are strongly motivated to present an overly favorable or unfavorable picture of themselves.

Uses of Trait Profiles Traits are enduring and stable features of the patient's behavior and experience, so assessing a broad range of traits gives the clinician a sense of what the person is like that can be useful for many purposes beyond the formulation of a diagnosis. A complete personality profile can point to the patient's strengths as well as weaknesses, can help predict the course of therapy, and can aid in the selection of an optimal mode of treatment.

Humanistic theories of personality stress human potentials for altruism, creativity, and commitment and argue that psychotherapy must use these assets. Trait theorists would qualify that stance: They believe that some people are altruistic, creative, or committed, but others are not. Assessing traits allows the clinician to identify and to capitalize on the particular strengths that characterize each individual patient.

Standing on trait dimensions can also give clues to the probable course of therapy. Patients who are low on the five-factor trait A are distrustful and uncooperative, and it may prove difficult to form a therapeutic alliance with them; by contrast, patients who are extremely high on A may be excessively compliant and become dependent on the therapist. The five-factor trait C involves commitment and self-discipline. Patients high in C will probably adhere to treatment recommendations and work hard to solve their problems; those low in C are less persistent and dedicated, and the therapist may have to work to motivate them.

Finally, a few controlled studies and a good deal of clinical experience suggest that personality traits influence the effectiveness of various kinds of treatment interventions. Interpersonal therapies, in which patients are required to speak a great deal about themselves, appear to be most effective for extroverts; pharmacological management may be superior for introverts. Similarly, individuals who are high in the five-factor trait O benefit from such techniques as guided imagery, whereas those who are low in O prefer biofeedback. Ideally, the choice of therapies should be guided not only by the nature of the disorder, but also by the enduring characteristics of the patient.

An excellent in-depth case study incorporating trait data with other assessment perspectives is provided in Jerry Wiggins's recent volume on *Paradigms of Personality Assessment.* As a briefer illustration of profile interpretation, Figure 6.4–3 provides data on a

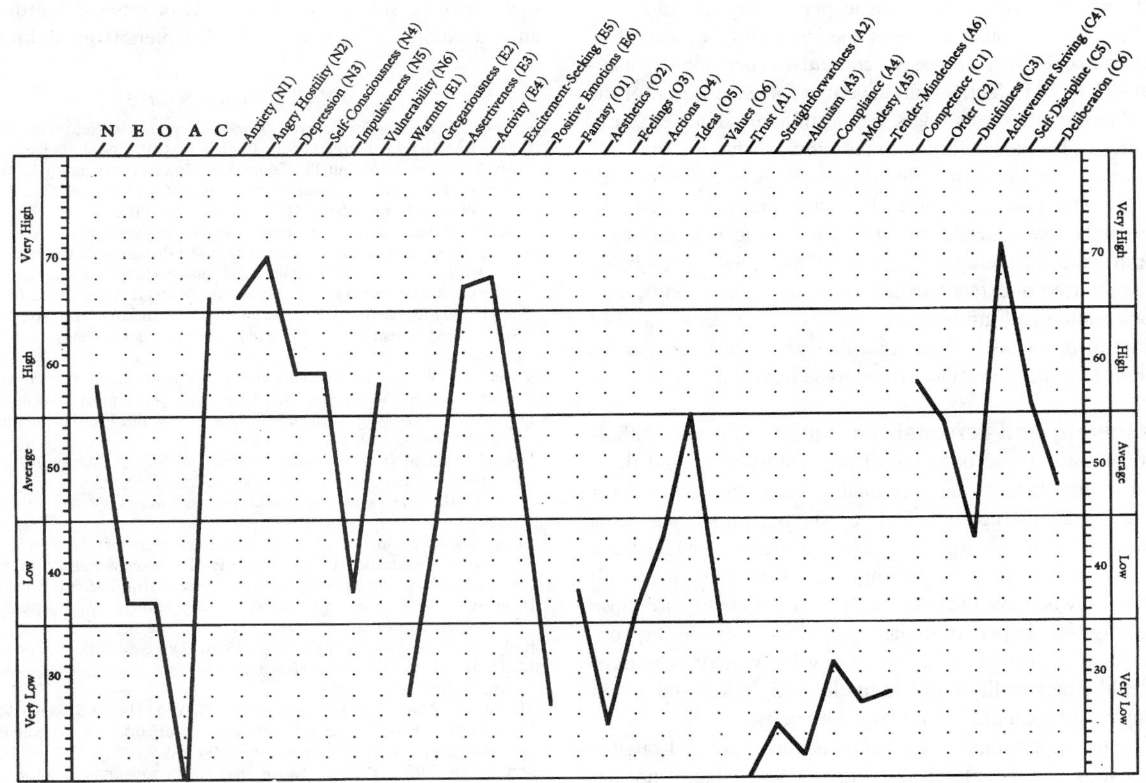

FIGURE 6.4–3 Revised NEO Personality Inventory profile for Richard M. Nixon, based on combined ratings from two experts. A, agreeableness; C, conscientiousness; E, extroversion; N, neuroticism; O, openness. (Data provided courtesy of Rubenzer T, Faschingbauer D. Ones, from Personality and the Presidency: A Scientific Inquiry. Presented at: Annual Convention of the American Psychological Association; August, 1996; Toronto. Profile form reproduced from Costa PT Jr, McCrae RR. *Revised NEO Personality Inventory.* Lutz, FL: Psychological Assessment Resources, Inc.; 1992, with permission.)

well-known public figure, Richard M. Nixon. As part of a project on personality traits of U.S. Presidents, two experts independently described Nixon using the observer rating form of the NEO-PI-R. Agreement between the two experts was high, and their ratings were averaged in the figure.

The left side of the profile sheet shows Nixon's standing on the five factors: high on N, low on E and O, very low on A, and very high on C. Specific traits, grouped by domain, are given toward the right of the profile sheet. Among the most notable features are Nixon's very high N1 (anxiety) and N2 (angry hostility) and his very low scores on all six facets of A, reflecting both his personal distress and his antagonism toward others. However, the profile also shows some clear strengths, such as very high levels of E3 (assertiveness), E4 (activity), and C4 (achievement striving), which help explain his political successes. Combinations of factors also give insight into Nixon's personality. The pairs of factors in the five-factor model can be crossed to assess ten different styles. For example, neuroticism and agreeableness jointly define style of anger control. The combinations of high and low scores on these two factors point to timid, easy-going, cold-blooded, and temperamental styles. Nixon has a temperamental style; according to the NEO-PI-R style graphs, such individuals "may fly into a rage over a minor irritant, and they can seethe with anger for long periods of time. They are deeply involved in themselves and take offense readily."

Table 6.4–2 suggests traits that are likely to be associated with each of the DSM-IV-TR personality disorders, and computer interpretations can compare observed profiles with these patterns. For example, Nixon's high scores on N2 (angry hostility) and N4 (self-consciousness) and his low scores on A2 (straightforwardness), A4 (compliance), A5 (modesty), and A6 (tender-mindedness) are consistent with the diagnosis of narcissistic personality disorder. The profile in Figure 6.4–3 also suggests the possibility of paranoid, schizotypal, antisocial, and obsessive-compulsive personality disorders. Whether Nixon, in fact, would have met formal criteria for the diagnosis of any of these disorders is questionable, but he clearly shared features of his personality with individuals who do.

In addition to suggesting possible diagnoses, personality profiles can be used to anticipate the course of psychotherapy. For example, Nixon's generally low O scores mean that he would probably have been uncomfortable in therapy, and, among therapies, he probably would have preferred directive techniques and behavior modification over free association and guided imagery. His low A scores suggest the likelihood of problems in forming a therapeutic alliance, but his high C scores mean that he would have worked hard at assigned tasks.

Psychotherapy and Personality Change If psychopathology is an expression or an outcome of personality traits and if, as longitudinal studies demonstrate, personality traits change little over time, how can psychotherapy be effective? The pessimistic answer is that it cannot. Many psychiatric disorders are lifelong or recurrent, and treatment consists of management rather than cure. It is well known that those who have the best prognosis for recovery are those who are initially least impaired. In these cases, the disorder may represent a transient adjustment reaction among individuals who have relatively healthy personality traits. Individuals high in N and low in A and C may be poor candidates for psychotherapy.

However, such a pessimistic conclusion is unwarranted. Longitudinal studies show that people change little in the course of normal experience, but they do not rule out the possibility that direct interventions can make changes. It is unlikely that psychotherapy makes dramatic and lasting changes in basic personality traits, but more modest improvements may be enough to allow the patient to function adequately in daily life. Interventions may be particularly effective in early adulthood, when traits are not yet fully developed. Even without changing personality, therapy may help individuals to adapt to their own nature. The chronically anxious person may learn techniques of relaxation; the disagreeable individual may learn social skills that improve interpersonal relationships.

In some sense, most forms of psychotherapy can be seen as learning experiences. Psychoanalysts promote insight into unconscious conflicts; behaviorists help their clients understand the contingencies that reinforce troubling behavior; humanistic psychologists encourage patients to discover their true potential. Trait psychology can also be a source of insight. All human beings are, in some respects, alike, and it is often comforting to learn that one is not alone in one's suffering. In other respects, however, people are different from one another, and it can also be a therapeutic experience to learn this fact. Helping patients understand their own enduring dispositions can prepare them for some of the problems that they face in life.

SUGGESTED CROSS-REFERENCES

Psychodynamic perspectives on personality and psychopathology are treated extensively in Section 6.1 on psychoanalysis and Section 6.3 on other psychodynamic schools. Chapter 23 discusses personality disorders. Chapter 7, on diagnosis and psychiatry, deals with issues of assessment; Section 7.6, on personality assessment, is particularly relevant. Section 3.3, on learning theory, provides technical background for the discussion of behavioral approaches to personality, and Chapter 30 on psychotherapies—particularly Section 30.2 on behavior therapy, Section 30.6 on cognitive therapy, and Section 30.9 on brief psychotherapy—gives details about the application of theories of personality to therapeutic processes. A different view of adult development is explained in Chapter 50 on adulthood.

REFERENCES

Allport GW. *Personality: A Psychological Interpretation.* New York: Holt; 1937.

Bandura A. *Social Learning Theory.* Englewood Cliffs, NJ: Prentice-Hall; 1977.

Caspi A, Sugden K, Moffitt TE, Taylor A, Craig IW, Harrington HL, McClay J, Mill J, Martin J, Braithwaite A, Poulton R: Influence of life stress on depression: Moderation by a polymorphism in the 5-HTT gene. *Science.* 2003;301:386.

Costa PT Jr, McCrae R: Influence of extraversion and neuroticism on subjective well-being: Happy and unhappy people. *J Pers Soc Psychol.* 1980;38:668.

Costa PT Jr, McCrae RR: Domains and facets: Hierarchical personality assessment using the Revised NEO Personality Inventory. *J Pers Assess.* 1995;64:21.

Costa PT Jr, McCrae RR. A Five-Factor Model perspective on personality disorders. In: Strack S, ed. *Handbook of Personology and Psychopathology.* New York: Wiley (*in press*).

*Costa PT Jr, Widiger TA, eds. *Personality Disorders and the Five-Factor Model of Personality.* 2nd ed. Washington, DC: American Psychological Association; 2002.

Digman JM: Personality structure: Emergence of the Five-Factor Model. *Annu Rev Psychol.* 1990;41:417.

Dollard J, Miller NE. *Personality and Psychotherapy: An Analysis in Terms of Learning, Thinking, and Culture.* New York: McGraw-Hill; 1950.

Eysenck HJ, Eysenck M. *Personality and Individual Differences.* London: Plenum; 1985.

Gergen KJ: Psychological science in a postmodern context. *Am Psychol.* 2001;56:803.

Halverson CF, Kohnstamm GA, Martin RP, eds. *The Developing Structure of Temperament and Personality from Infancy to Adulthood.* Hillsdale, NJ: Erlbaum; 1994.

Heatherton TF, Weinberger J. *Can Personality Change?* Washington, DC: American Psychological Association; 1994.

Kelly GA. *The Psychology of Personal Constructs.* New York: Norton; 1955.

*Maddi SR, Costa PT Jr. *Humanism in Personology: Allport, Maslow and Murray.* Chicago: Aldine; 1972.

Maslow AH. *Motivation and Personality.* New York: Harper & Row; 1954.

McAdams DP: Personality, modernity, and the storied self: A contemporary framework for studying persons. *Psychol Inquiry.* 1996;7:295.

McCrae RR, Allik J. *The Five-Factor Model of Personality Across Cultures.* New York: Kluwer Academic Publishers; 2002.

*McCrae RR, Costa PT Jr. *Personality in Adulthood: A Five-Factor Theory Perspective.* New York: Guilford; 2003.

McCrae RR, Costa PT Jr. A Five-Factor Theory of personality. In: Pervin LA, John OP, eds. *Handbook of Personality: Theory and Research.* 2nd ed. New York: Guilford; 1999.

McCrae RR, Costa PT Jr, Martin TA, Oryol VE, Rukavishnikov AA, Senin IG, Hřebíčková M, Urbánek T: Consensual validation of personality traits across cultures. *J Res Pers*. (*in press*).

McCrae RR, Herbst JH, Costa PT Jr. Effects of acquiescence on personality factor structures. In: Riemann R, Spinath FM, Ostendorf F, eds. *Personality and Temperament: Genetics, Evolution, and Structure.* Berlin: Pabst Science Publishers; 2001:217.

McCrae RR, John OP: An introduction to the Five-Factor Model and its applications. *J Pers.* 1992;60:175.

*Miller T: The psychotherapeutic utility of the Five-Factor Model of personality: A clinician's experience. *J Pers Assess.* 1991;57:415.

Ozer DJ, Reise SP: Personality assessment. *Annu Rev Psychol.* 1994;45:357.

Pervin LA: A critical analysis of current trait theory. *Psychol Inquiry.* 1994;5:103.

*Phares EJ. *Introduction to Personality.* 2nd ed. Glenview, IL: Scott, Foresman; 1988.

Rogers CR. *On Becoming a Person: A Therapist's View of Psychotherapy.* Boston: Houghton Mifflin; 1961.

Scarr S: Distinctive environments depend on genotypes. *Brain Behav Sci.* 1987;10:38.

Schopenhauer A. *The World as Will and Representation.* 3rd ed. New York: Dover; 1969.

Skinner BF. *About Behaviorism.* New York: Knopf; 1974.

Watson D, Clark LA. Special issue on personality psychopathology. *J Abnorm Psychol.* 1994;130:1.

Widiger TA, Costa PT Jr, McCrae RR. A proposal for Axis II: Diagnosing personality disorders using the Five-Factor Model. In: Costa PT Jr, Widiger TA, eds. *Personality Disorders and the Five-Factor Model of Personality.* 2nd ed. Washington, DC: American Psychological Association; 2002:431.

Wiggins JS. *Paradigms of Personality Assessment.* New York: Guildford; 2003.

Wiggins JS, Pincus AL: Conceptions of personality disorders and dimensions of personality. *Psychol Assess.* 1989;1:305.

7 Diagnosis and Psychiatry: Examination of the Psychiatric Patient

▲ 7.1 Psychiatric Interview, History, and Mental Status Examination

EKKEHARD OTHMER, M.D., PH.D.,
SIEGLINDE C. OTHMER, PH.D., AND
JOHANN PHILIPP OTHMER, M.D.

INTRODUCTION

Goal of the Clinical Psychiatric Interview The goal of the initial diagnostic clinical psychiatric interview is to collect specific, detailed information about 15 topics. These topics constitute the psychiatric evaluation. Acquiring the database of information for these 15 topics enables the interviewer to make diagnoses compatible with the revised fourth edition of *Diagnostic and Statistical Manual of Mental Disorders* (DSM-IV-TR) on five axes and to develop a treatment plan acceptable to the patient:

I. Identifying data. The patient's name, sex, age, race, marital status, and vital signs.

II. Chief complaint. The chief complaint in the patient's own words. Alternatively, signs of disordered functioning observed by the interviewer.

III. Informants. A list of all informants, their reliability, and level of cooperation; also previous hospital records, if available. Such informants are essential in circumstances that prevent the patient from providing adequate information. Choosing the right set of informants is more important than having a great number of informants.

IV. Reason for admission or consultation. The referral source; in case of hospitalization, statement of legal status—voluntary versus involuntary—and the reason why hospitalization is the safest and least restrictive environment for treatment.

V. History of present illness. Early manifestations and recent exacerbations of all psychiatric disorders present (Axis I and II); review of diagnoses and treatments given by other providers.

VI. Psychiatric disorders in remission. Psychiatric disorders presently in remission, especially substance abuse disorders; psychiatric disorders first diagnosed in childhood and adolescence and their treatments.

VII. Medical history. All medical disorders past and present and their treatments and childhood disorders that involve the central nervous system (CNS). For females, pregnancy status—especially if on psychotropics or expecting the use of psychotropics and precautions against pregnancy and concomitant pharmacological treatment. On all patients, but particularly in consult-liaison work, the medical history includes the interrelation of medical and psychiatric conditions.

VIII. Social history and premorbid personality. Early developmental history. Description of premorbid personality as baseline for patient's best level of functioning. Impact of Axis I and II disorders on patient's life. The patient's psychosocial and environmental conditions predisposing to, precipitating, perpetuating, and protecting against psychiatric disorders. Premorbid versus morbid functioning. Present support system.

IX. Family history. Psychiatric history of first-degree relatives, including treatment response as a possible genetic predisposition for the patient.

X. Mental status examination. Appearance, consciousness, psychomotor functions, speech, thinking, affect, mood, suggestibility, and thought content; cognitive functions, such as orientation, memory, intelligence, and executive functions; insight and judgment.

XI. Diagnostic formulation. Summary of biological, psychological, and social factors contributing to the patient's psychiatric disorder.

XII. Differential diagnosis. Discussion of diagnostic options based on overlapping symptomatology.

XIII. Multiaxial psychiatric diagnosis. Information on all five axes.

XIV. Assets and strengths. Inventory of patient's knowledge, interests, aptitudes, education, and employment status to be used in the treatment plan.

XV. Treatment plan and prognosis. Account of psychopharmacological, psychological, and social treatment modalities planned, frequency of visits, and list of providers; discharge criteria if inpatient.

How does the interviewer get comprehensive, clinically significant, reliable, and valid information to cover these points in a restricted time frame of 20 to 90 minutes? To acquire the communication skills needed for this task, the interviewer has to master the range between disorder-centered and patient-centered interviewing styles and apply them to the four components of the interview: rapport, techniques, mental status, and diagnosing.

Disorder-Centered versus Patient-Centered Interviewing Styles Psychiatric interviewing is a special form of human communication. The interviewer asks the patient to disclose complaints, share problems, and reveal suffering. According to the difficulties that the patient experiences with this request, the interviewer shifts the focus between disorder-centered and patient-centered interviewing. Disorder-centered interviewing is based on a descriptive, atheoretical model of psychiatric disorders called the *medical* *model*, which is the official model supported by the American Psychiatric Association (APA) and the World Health Organization (WHO) codified in DSM-IV-TR (2000) and the International Classification of Diseases (ICD-10). This framework views psychiatric disorders as similar to medical disorders, using criteria for diagnosis as identifiable clusters of occurrences from a restricted menu of symptoms, signs, and behaviors that cause morbidity and mortality. Each disorder can be differentiated from other psychiatric disorders; each has a typical natural history, often occurs in increased frequency in first-degree relatives, with specific comorbidities, and with somewhat predictable treatment responses. Whereas the diagnosis of an infectious disorder is established by tests that determine the presence or absence of a specific etiological agent, tests confirming the etiology of a diagnosis in psychiatric disorders are not available. Except for the presence of established or suspected genetic dispositions, etiology is incomplete. Specific genetic lesions or triggered susceptibilities, perhaps arising through multifactorial genetic factors, which form the basis of the current paradigm of the etiology of psychiatric disorders, remain to be determined. The triggers for psychiatric disorders remain a mystery, as do the triggers for the onset of many infectious diseases and medical conditions. Risk factors are present in more people than actually develop the illness.

To establish a psychiatric diagnosis based on this descriptive medical model, the interviewer chooses proven, symptom-oriented, open-ended questions with a relatively narrow scope followed up by closed-ended, nonleading questions centering on the disorder. Prerequisites for this style are the knowledge of the DSM-IV-TR criteria and the 15 topics to be covered. This disorder-centered interview style works for most cooperative patients, patients whose communication skills are not impaired by their Axis I and II disorders or their defense mechanisms. Disorder-centered interviewing is driven by the patient's help-seeking behavior. Proficiency for disorder-centered interviewing can be acquired during the first few years of training.

In contrast, patient-centered interviewing is based on the introspective model, which emphasizes the individuality of the patient's experience. This model attends to the intrapsychic battle of conflicts. It is sensitive to the patient's educational, emotional, intellectual, and social background, the personality, and the individual symptom constellations tracing their arrival to individual circumstances and the individual's unique response (cognitive-behavioral model). One example of the introspective model is the psychodynamic model. Interviewing based on the psychodynamic model uses nonstructured, open-ended questions with a broad scope, encouraging free association. The psychodynamic model posits the etiology of psychiatric symptoms as responses to often unconscious inter- and intrapersonal conflicts. It explores and interprets behaviors and sequences of answers. In this model, the interviewer strives to help the patient overcome self-defeating intra- and interpersonal conflicts. The prerequisite for such an interview is the interviewer's experience and understanding of coping styles, the knowledge of how Axis I and II disorders interfere with the doctor–patient interaction (transference), and how to manage such interference. Switching to the patient-centered style may become necessary if the patient puts up resistance and defenses and becomes difficult to interview. To acquire proficiency in patient-centered interviewing is a lifelong endeavor, like training for excellence in most sports.

The disorder-centered and patient-centered interviewing styles do not exclude each other. They are end points of a continuum. The interviewer's mobility and flexibility in gliding between the two extremes determine the efficiency, reliability, validity, and quality of data collection. The degree of the patient's impairment determines to which extent the disorder-centered interview has to be augmented by patient-centered strategies.

Five Phases of the Psychiatric Interview and Four Components

The psychiatric interview progresses over time, which can be arbitrarily subdivided into five phases. These phases cover sequentially the 15 (I to XV) topics of the psychiatric evaluation.

Phase 1: Warm-up and Chief Complaint (I to IV)
Phase 2: The Diagnostic Decision Loop (V)
Phase 3: History and Database (VI to X)
Phase 4: Diagnosing and Feedback (XI to XIV)
Phase 5: Treatment Plan and Prognosis (XV)

The five phases divide the psychiatric interview longitudinally. Cross-sectionally, the interview consists of four components, which the interviewer must continuously monitor and propel throughout.

Rapport focuses on the doctor–patient relationship; a good rapport is a prerequisite for an effective interview. Rapport is established in the opening; with a cooperative and insightful patient, there is often little problem in establishing and maintaining a good rapport. However, in patients who are uncooperative or show poor insight, establishing a workable rapport with the patient becomes a central issue.

Technique refers to the approaches the interviewer uses to keep an interview "on track." It includes skills to appropriately select questions to arrive at a diagnosis. Good technique is necessary to therapeutically engage and work with difficult patients.

Mental status assessment captures the patient's experiences, symptoms, signs, behaviors, thought content, cognitive level of functioning, insight, and judgment during the actual time of the interview. Formal testing of mental status may take place late in the interview; however, in a patient with a significantly altered mental status—whether it be a boisterous, irritable, and uninterruptible manic patient, a minimally responsive depressed patient, or a paranoid patient—his or her mental status plays a significant role in the interview.

Diagnosing pursues a progression in the diagnostic decision process from chief complaint to final diagnosis.

RAPPORT

Interviewing relies on rapport, from the French verb *rapporter*, to bring back—that is, to bring back the response to the sender. Creating this feedback between interviewer and patient is the essence of communication. It is rooted in a stream of nonverbal signals. Language adds precision and complexity. If the patient's mental status interferes with this interaction, the interviewer shifts from assessing a disorder to managing the patient's mental status—that is, the disorder-centered interview becomes patient centered.

Disorder-Centered versus Patient-Centered Interviewing and Rapport

With a cooperative patient, the interviewer starts out in a disorder-centered mode, checking whether DSM-IV-TR criteria for psychiatric disorders are met. He or she assumes that the patient seeks help voluntarily and will answer all questions. As the interviewer acts in a professional manner; does not

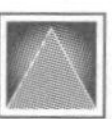

Table 7.1–1
Rapport in Disorder-Centered and Patient-Centered Interviewing Styles

Elements of Relationship	Disorder-Centered Interview	Patient-Centered Interview
Perspective	The interviewer is in charge, knows diagnostic criteria of the disorder.	Patient holds the key to the symptoms; without the patient's genuine contributions, a valid diagnosis cannot be made.
Comfort	Most patients quickly become comfortable with the interview situation; no special attention needed. Minor discomfort by the patient may be disregarded.	The patient and interviewer need to experience comfort. The interviewer has to address tension, especially with anxious and suspicious patients.
Empathy	The interviewer assesses symptoms and expresses understanding.	The interviewer assesses suffering and expresses empathy.
Insight	Most patients know they have a disorder.	The patient may not accept having a disorder. The interviewer has to decrease the distance between the patient's and the interviewer's view of the patient's psychiatric problems.
Alliance	The interviewer cannot diagnose or treat the illness if the patient does not tell what is wrong. If the patient becomes uncooperative, the interviewer may remind the patient of that fact.	Striving for alliance sets the tone of the interview. The interviewer identifies the patient's illness as the common enemy using the patient's level of insight.
Expertise	The interviewer uses a set of DSM-IV-TR–derived generic questions to assess psychiatric disorders.	The interviewer individualizes questions about the specific manifestations of the patient's disorders. The patient contributes the knowledge about his or her problems. The interviewer contributes his or her knowledge about psychiatric disorders and their treatment.
Guidance	Usually at the end of the interview, the interviewer discusses the treatment plan and obtains verbal acceptance from the patient.	Throughout, the interviewer defines the cooperative roles of interviewer and patient in the treatment process.
Trust	Expected byproduct of thorough, detailed interviewing.	Result of purposeful development of several levels of relating, i.e., providing comfort, empathy, insight, alliance, expertise, and guidance.

insult or offend the patient; and asks clear, understandable, and relevant questions; the interviewer expects the patient will respond. Rapport follows.

In contrast, with a difficult patient, the interviewer shifts to a patient-centered mode. To obtain a comprehensive diagnosis and to judge the patient's capacity for staying in treatment, the interviewer explicitly focuses on establishing a cooperative relationship with the patient. Eight elements determine the quality of this relationship (Table 7.1–1).

Perspective Depending on the patient's behavior, the interviewer focuses his or her attention either on the diagnostic process (i.e., the disorders to be explored) or on the patient's immediate emotions and needs without allowing the interview to turn into an ad hoc psychotherapy session. Although the knowledge of the diagnostic criteria is essential for the interviewer, their implementation requires that the patient provide genuine, detailed answers. A patient who states, "You are the doctor, you decide," tries to skirt his or her part. Recognizing possible dependency needs, the interviewer corrects the patient's view by making him or her aware of the expected input.

Comfort Many patients quickly become comfortable with the interview situation. However, if the patient appears anxious, is trembling, or has a moist handshake or a racing pulse, the interviewer may address such discomfort indirectly: "Have you seen a psychiatrist or counselor before?" or directly: "Your pulse is over 100. Is there any problem with your heart?" The interviewer may give the patient time to calm down by offering something to drink or by assessing demographics: "Do you live in this neighborhood?" The interviewer also should pay attention to his or her own comfort if the patient is intimidatingly aggressive or demanding, offensively flirtatious, or anxious and address this problem.

A 42-year-old, red-faced, married Irishman who was accused by his wife of drinking too much entered the office accompanied by his dog, a mixed breed of wolf and German shepherd. The dog circled through the interviewer's office incessantly.

Interviewer (I): Mr. M., your dog distracts me from working with you. Can you have the dog sit?

Patient (P): (Gleaming) Are you scared?

I: (The dog keeps circling in the room and staring at the interviewer) I know neither you nor your dog. Would you like me to be scared?

P: It depends what you will tell me.

I: What are you scared of that I would tell you?

P: That I'm an alcoholic and should stop drinking.

I: (Laughing) And if I don't, you have the wolf eat me?

P: (Also laughing)

I: But you really have to tell me. Do you want to stop drinking?

P: No. I don't.

I: What did you want to accomplish when you came here?

P: My wife says she'll divorce me if I don't stop.

I: So you don't want to stop? You just want to hide your drinking better?

P: I guess that's right.

I: I appreciate your honesty. Most people who are criticized for drinking too much and get threatened with divorce or job loss try to con me and possibly themselves by saying they want to stop. You don't. If you ever want to stop, I believe you can do it because you are honest with yourself.

P: (To the dog who is still circling the room) Molly, come here. Sit! (Molly obeys)

I: Thank you.

Empathy For a symptom to be counted, it has to cause the patient impairment or distress. When a patient describes his or her symptoms, the interviewer can follow up by getting a precise description of duration and frequency of symptoms or, alternatively, especially if the interviewer encounters denial ("otherwise, I'm healthy"), by asking about the impairment and distress that the symptom causes and expressing empathy.

A 74-year-old, white, married, former chief executive officer of a large company.

P: I can't sleep. Otherwise, I'm healthy. I wake up at 4 AM and can't go back to sleep.

I: Do you also have problems falling asleep?

P: Off and on. But I can handle that.

I: What about waking up in the middle of the night?

P: Once or twice. I may have to go to the bathroom.

I: Besides your early morning insomnia, do you have any other problems?

P: No. I'm really pretty healthy.

I: Do you feel depressed?

P: No.

I: Do you have any hobbies?

P: I do volunteer work.

I: Can you still do it?

P: Yes. I think it serves a good purpose. I help young entrepreneurs through the ZZZ foundation.

Alternative:

P: I can't sleep. Otherwise I'm healthy. I wake up at 4 AM and can't go back to sleep.

I: What does your insomnia do to you?

P: It wrecks my life. I toss and turn in my bed. I'm tired during the day and worried about my sleep. When friends come over, I'm bored. They sound so trivial.

I: (Mirroring the patient's facial expression, frowning, tight lips, then bending forward) We have to put our heads together and find a way to get rid of your problem.

The empathic, patient-centered approach invites the patient to express his or her thoughts and feelings about his or her symptoms and describe his or her actions. This approach breaks through the patient's denial of being depressed, which the descriptive, strictly symptom-gathering approach does not do. The interviewer's response reflects the patient's affect and proposes a counteraction more convincing and genuine than a statement such as, "I understand your suffering." The empathic response follows the golden rule: Imagine thinking and feeling from the patient's level of insight. Let the patient know that you can understand his or her point of view and initiate caring.

Insight A conflict about the nature of psychiatric symptoms and disorders can arise between the interviewer and the patient. Undetected or unresolved, such a conflict of view may lead to a breakup of the doctor–patient relationship. Therefore, the interviewer has to be aware of such differences and strive for congruency. If the patient agrees with the interviewer's view, the therapist calls this congruency *full insight.* With respect to the acute hallucinations, delusions, and manic symptoms, experts agree that the patient has very limited insight into the pathological nature of these perceptions, beliefs, and behaviors. To change the patient's view, confrontation and logical arguments are ineffective. Initially, the interviewer has to emulate the patient's view and intervene at the level of the patient's understanding.

A 38-year-old, divorced, male railroad worker.

P: It's coming up again, even after 20 years. They can't let go of it.

I: Of what?

P: You know what, [expletive]!

I: Can you help me out?

P: (With a suspicious look) That I jacked off in the woods on that hunting trip. At work, they are making digs again.

I: What are you doing about it?

P: I try to ignore it but it's getting hard.

I: Well, you are doing the right thing. Don't do or say anything. Don't let them know that they get to you. I will give you some medication that will make it easier to get over it.

P: Okay.

Rather than taking a disorder-centered view and telling the patient that he has a persecutory delusion, which has to be treated with medication, the interviewer addresses the delusion from the patient's viewpoint that something "real" is happening to him. This patient-centered approach does not challenge the patient's false fixed perception but works on his level of insight, still providing effective therapeutic intervention, a neuroleptic, and support for his behavior—namely, to keep his persecutory perceptions to himself.

Patients with a personality disorder may recognize that certain behaviors cause distress to family members but feel the family should change and be more tolerant rather than having to change.

A 46-year-old, male, fundamental Lutheran minister.

P: My wife wants a legal separation and that tears me up. As a minister, I should be able to set an example for my congregation. I can't have that separation.

I: Why does she want that separation?

P: She says I get so angry and critical with her and the kids. She can't take my anger outbursts any more.

I: Do you think you get angry as she says?

P: Yes. It's my job. If I feel I get excuses or my kids or my wife violate commandments of Christian conduct, I become like God's hot sword cutting into butter.

I: Do you feel your anger is too much and out of proportion?

P: No. I think it's justified.

I: Can you not get angry if you wanted to?

P: That's hard to do. Maybe I carry my profession too much into my family.

I: Would it be of advantage to you if you had more of a choice to become angry or not? If you increased your degree of freedom?

P: I probably could live with that.

I: We both have to put our minds to work on increasing the power of free will.

The interviewer discusses the patient's anger outbursts not as a result of a narcissistic perfectionistic personality disorder but as a challenge congruent with the patient's needs. Successful anger control can increase the patient's narcissistic pride and his choices while helping the marital relationship at the same time. Rapport is strengthened by identifying the patient's level of insight and interviewing him from the patient's perspective.

Alliance After the interviewer understands which symptoms, signs, and behaviors the patient identifies as disordered, he or she can explicitly split this part off as sick. The interviewer can explore with the patient what both can contribute to repair the sick. Because the patient guards the treasure box of his or her broken functions, he or she has to be willing to open it so that the interviewer can examine the contents and discuss with the patient options for repair. The interviewer stresses the need for an alliance. Thus, if the patient says, "You are the doctor, I do what you say," the interviewer may reply: "You are the patient, and we both have to put our heads together to come up with the best plan to succeed. I need your input and consent."

Expertise Some patients feel they can receive empathy and alliance from family members and friends. So what is the interviewer's edge? The interviewer can provide at least four things for the patient and may make him or her aware of that fact implicitly or explicitly. The psychiatrist can acknowledge that he or she understands the disorder. He or she can emphasize that the patient is not alone, that others share the same disorder. The interviewer can point out that the patient's personality to deal with the disorder is unique and can contribute to improve the disordered functions. He or she can appreciate the symptoms and signs of the disorder and the distress that it causes. He or she may demonstrate such knowledge by asking for specific symptoms that the patient tried to keep a secret, such as:

I: Whom in your family have you trusted enough to share your obsessions?

P: Nobody. How do you know that I feel embarrassed to talk about it to my family?

The interviewer may give the patient feedback about what is known about the disorder. Patients who read about their condition in books and on the Internet may evaluate the interviewer more in terms of how much he or she knows than by how much he or she cares. If the interviewer does not know the answer to a patient's question, he or she may clearly state that he or she does not know but, "Let's find out."

Some patients are suspicious about the interviewer's expertise but do not want to offend him or her with their distrust. If the interviewer senses reluctance, he or she may explore the nature of the doubts rather than ignoring them and hoping that the patient learns to trust him or her. The interviewer may pass over positive feedback from the patient but, as a rule, should address negative signals, even though he or she may feel uncomfortable in doing so.

The interviewer instills hope. Related to providing a perspective and giving an outlook is the interviewer's ability to emphasize the positive factors regarding the patient's disorder, such as treatability, and the patient's personality, such as intelligence, resilience, and ability to self-criticize.

Guidance Patients rank the therapist's leadership third after expertise and empathy. From the beginning of the interview, the interviewer sets milestones for the progression of the encounter. The interviewer can reach subgoals, such as establishing rapport and collecting information for the diagnostic process with the patient's agreement and cooperation. Thus, if the interviewer reads the patient's expectations for the interview and makes his or her goals congruent to these expectations, he or she steers the interview with an invisible hand. The more the interviewer is willing to explain his or her questions and suggestions and their rationale and give options, the easier it usually is to guide the patient through the interview with little conflict. Special situations may arise. Dependent patients may shy from responsibility and desire to be nurtured by the "strong, all-powerful protector." The oppositional patient or the patient with persecutory feelings may get irritated by any hint of rule setting and may rebel against the interviewer.

P: What do you ask me for? I'm paying you to solve my problems. It really does not make me feel good that you always have to ask me for my view. Don't you know enough that you can do it on your own? Or is this one of those psychobabble tricks to pretend that you need my input?

With such a difficult patient, the interviewer may have to test different approaches to secure cooperation.

I: It's your problem that we are discussing. It's your desire to get help. It's your information that we need to make a plan. So you are part of the solution. I can't do anything without having you on my side so that we can both face your problems and find out what works best to resolve them. Right now your problem is that you can't come to an agreement with me on how to tackle your problems. Let's discuss why that is and what your thinking is.

A patient's negative response to the interviewer's cooperative approach may have deep-rooted resentments of becoming dependent. Such fear may reach far beyond the present interview situation. Not all interpersonal conflicts, such as negative transference and countertransference, can be solved in a time-efficient manner. The patient may need medication or referral to a different provider.

Trust From the beginning, the interviewer shows sensitivity to the patient's needs and comforts the patient. If the patient accepts such caring, the interviewer can forge a therapeutic alliance. Building on it, the interviewer's targeted questions prove his or her understanding and expertise, which qualify him or her as a guide for the patient's care. The interviewer's respect for the patient's dignity allows the patient to trust him or her. Trust is rapport's summit.

TECHNIQUE

The patient interacts on one of three levels with the interviewer: First, the patient cooperates. He or she complains about different areas of malfunctioning and suffering and seeks help. Second, he or she resists, being cautious, anxious, or suspicious and holding back embarrassing, painful information. Third, he or she uses defensive strategies and obstructs the interviewing process.

Interviewing Techniques for the Cooperative Patient The majority of outpatients and voluntarily admitted inpatients cooperate. As a general principle, even with cooperative patients, the interviewer should formulate questions from the patient's vantage point and use familiar language. The interviewer relies on five techniques to achieve a crisp, well-flowing dialogue: openers, clarifications, covering a topic, steering, and transitions.

Openers To initiate the interview or to explore a new topic, the interviewer chooses questions of specific target and scope. The patient's responses shape the follow-up questions. Opening questions or statements target a problem of varying scope. Narrow scope: "What troubles bring you here to see me?" The interviewer expects a prioritized brief list of difficulties. Problem: The patient rambles.

Solution: The interviewer narrows the scope of the question or curbs the response. For instance:

P: (Responds with a long list of events that went wrong in his or her life).

I: Just tell me what problem has troubled you most during the last 3 days.

P: That I can't sleep.

Broad scope: "Give me a sense of how your life is going."

The interviewer expects the patient to put problems and symptoms into a life perspective. Such a broad question works well for an intelligent, educated patient who can condense, abstract, and prioritize his or her life experiences. It fails with a patient with obsessive-compulsive disorder (OCD) by confusing the patient and increasing indecisiveness and anxiety. It puts a patient with bipolar disorder into overdrive. He or she may flood the interviewer with circumstantial details and loosely connected thoughts. Broad questions also fail for a patient who gives literal answers.

A 23-year-old, white, single medical student.

I: What brought you here?

P: My mother's car.

A patient with psychotic symptoms or low intelligence may give such concrete answers. Inability of the interviewer to adjust the scope of the questions can disrupt the flow of the interview and threaten rapport.

A supervised interview (supervisor [S]) by a resident (R) with a white, newlywed woman (P) in her early thirties.

(1) R: What's going on in your life?

P: (Looking around helplessly, shrugging shoulders, blushing) I don't know.

(2) R: Well, for instance, have you felt depressed?

P: Is that what you think?

(3) R: No. This is just an example. I wanted to know how I could help you.

P: I don't know whether you can help me.

(4) R: Why don't you tell me what has been happening lately in your life.

P: (Hunching down in her chair) My husband got promoted. We bought a new house.

(5) R: That's not really what I meant.

P: (After a pause) I don't really know what you mean.

The supervisor intervenes:

(6) S: Well, you just said your husband got promoted and you are moving into a new house. Has that caused any stress for you?

P: Oh yes.

(7) S: Help me understand what stresses you out about the move into a new house.

P: I can't help him enough. I feel so bad.

(8) S: What kind of help can you not give him?

P: I should be able to go out and buy things for the new house. But I can't. I get all choked up when I go to a store.

(9) S: I can sense your frustration. What bothers you about the stores?

P: There are so many people.

When the interviewer noticed that question 1 (Q1) was too broad, he or she went to the opposite extreme and asked a closed-ended question (Q2). Noticing the confusion, the interviewer returned to an open-ended approach (Q3), but the patient became so anxious that she could not read the intent of the question. The interviewer noticed her distress and reformulated Q1 but missed her clue in A4. After the resident voiced his frustration (Q5), she responded with a frustration of her own (A5). The supervisor intervened by linking the content the patient had provided (A4) to her stress—that is, her anxiety level. The patient's response showed the effectiveness of this intervention.

An experienced interviewer monitors the effectiveness of his or her questions by how closely the answers match the intent of the questions and adjusts the scope of the questions.

Clarification

To clarify an answer, the interviewer usually asks for specifics, probes the patient's reasoning, or offers some leads.

SPECIFICATION Problem: The patient's complaint is vague. Solution: The interviewer uses specifying questions that focus on the five Ws of interviewing: What? When? Where? Who? Why?

Alternatively, the interviewer may ask for general or typical examples or focus on the latest specific occurrence and then generalize the occurrence.

A 26-year-old, white, unemployed, single woman.

(1) I: What kind of problems make you seek my help?

P: I have many problems.

(2) I: Is there any one problem that has troubled you lately?

P: (After a long hesitation) I wake up in the middle of the night.

(3) I: How does that trouble you?

P: I really don't know. I can't explain.

(4) I: What do you feel like when you wake up?

P: Kind of leery.

(5) I: Did you wake up last night?

P: Yes.

(6) I: What time was that?

P: 3:30 AM

(7) I: What did you feel?

P: I don't know. Just leery.

(8) I: Did you see anything?

P: (Puzzled) My cat's hair stood up straight.

(9) I: What did you hear?

P: A noise in the kitchen.

(10) I: What is making that noise?

P: I don't know.

(11) I: What did you feel?

P: A breeze.

(12) I: Does this happen every night?

P: Just about.

(13) I: You wake up and the cat's fur stands up on end, you hear the noise in the kitchen, and you feel a breeze?

P: That's right.

(14) I: Something that makes you leery is going on and that means (raising his voice) there is . . . ?

P: A spirit. A spirit lives in my place.

The set of specifying questions adds up to a composite, which the interviewer summarizes in Q13. When the patient accepts that summary (A13), the interviewer induces the patient to complete a sentence designed to capture the patient's interpretation of her leeriness.

PROBING Problem: The patient denies recurrence of past problems and stresses emphatically that he or she is healthy. This emphasis alerts the interviewer to the presence of denial. Solution: The interviewer asks for recent changes—not problems—and for the patient's interpretation.

A 47-year-old, white, married woman who had recently moved to town reports that she has been treated in the past for major depression. She emphasizes that she is doing just fine and that she only wants check-ups because of her past problems. She works in her husband's law office answering the phone, filing, and typing.

I: Is there anything new going on in your life since you moved here?

P: You know, I'm glad that you asked. I've always had problems getting up. But now I'm wide awake at 5:30 AM

I: Why do you think that is?

P: My sister is a nun, and at that time, she goes to mass in New Orleans. And that's when she communicates with me.

I: How does she do that? Does she call you?

P: Oh no. We've been close. It's with telepathy.

The patient's strong intention was to be certified as healthy and asymptomatic. This emphasis alerted the interviewer to scrutinize the patient's recent history, discovering a delusion that, as the interviewer learned later, was an early indicator of relapse for this patient.

LEADING Problem: A male patient, when asked how he feels, answers: I don't know. Solution: (1) The interviewer asks how the patient dealt with others last week. Thus, reported behaviors may have to take the place of a mood symptom. (2) The interviewer asks the patient to try to remember how he recently felt. While the patient tries to remember, his posture and facial expression may change. The interviewer reads that emotion and feeds his or her reading back to the patient for his confirmation. This technique, however, is suggestive and leads the patient's response. The interviewer has to remain cognizant of possibly distorting input.

A 28-year-old, white, married man knocks holes in the wall of his kitchen with his fists. He also reports problems sleeping.

I: Can you tell me how you feel most of the time?

P: I don't know.

I: Try to remember how you felt yesterday.

P: (Looks down, closes his eyes, makes a fist, then grins)

I: You get a frown on your face. Your knuckles turn white. You appear tense . . . angry . . . anxious.

P: Angry! Yeah.

I: Then a brief grin ran over your face. What were you thinking just now?

P: These Mexicans . . . when they buy one tire from me, they bring their kids . . . they come with all their family. Like 20 of them.

I: You get angry . . . then you smile . . . your feelings change quickly.

P: (Puzzled) I guess.

I: Mixed up . . . up and down . . . bouncing around?

P: My wife says I'm up and down.

The patient can reexperience some feelings but cannot read and express them himself.

Covering a Topic

After opening a topic and clarifying the answers, the interviewer collects information linked to this topic to draw the big picture. Helpful techniques include asking for events that are associated in time or are logically interrelated. The interviewer may finally summarize what he or she has learned.

ASSOCIATING When assessing clinical symptomatology, the interviewer usually encounters one major symptom (i.e., the chief complaint). However, psychiatric disorders occur as syndromes rather than single symptoms. Therefore, the interviewer asks what other symptoms concurred in time with the chief complaint: "What else happened during the time of your crying spells?" or "What else happened when your crying spells were worst?" or "What else happened when you had your spell the last time?" If the patient lists only a few symptoms, the interviewer may actively ask for disturbances in sleep, appetite, sex drive, ability to work, or ability to relate to others.

INTERRELATING The interviewer uses interrelating when referring to the same theme, such as medical history, psychiatric family history, or work or marital history. Such interrelating represents logical connections. Problem: A patient offers an illogical interrelationship. Solution: The interviewer addresses the illogical connection.

A 38-year-old, married, black, male airline engineer.

I: What brought you here?

P: My wife wanted me to have a second opinion.

I: About what?

P: About Alicia and the television. The pain in my groin should have stopped by now.

I: Fill me in. What do Alicia and the television have to do with your groin pain?

P: Man, don't you understand? I felt it most when I watched television.

I: What does that have to do with Alicia?

P: Alicia knows about witchcraft. She's a medium. She said my new television set is bewitched. I have to bring it over to her house.

I: Did you take it over there?

P: Of course. But my pain is still there.

I: Besides your groin pain, was the television doing anything else to you?

P: It gave me messages.

I: What kind?

P: I noticed it mainly with politicians. They hold their hands with the fingers pointing down, and I understand immediately what they mean.

I: What do they mean?

P: Isn't it obvious? That my life is going down.

I: What does your wife think about all that?

P: Oh, she's mad with me. She thinks that Alicia ripped me off and that I need to see a psychiatrist.

SUMMARIZING Summarization should be informal, supportive, and interactive. Problem: The patient gets easily sidetracked. While the interviewer assesses the history of present illness, the patient mentions that her mother had similar problems. When talking about the medical history, the patient adds that her only sibling, her older brother, was admitted for detoxification. When reviewing the social history, the patient mentions that her father is the only person in the immediate family who did not have any psychiatric problems. To give closure to the topic of family history, the interviewer pulls together and summarizes informally the data that belong to this topic but were collected at different parts of the interview: "Let me make sure I'm keeping up with what you told me about your family history."

Problem: The patient's answers are vague, and it takes the interviewer several specifying questions to collect relevant information. Solution: The interviewer supportively summarizes the topic intermittently, "We are getting there," to nudge the patient to complete the topic. Problem: A patient describes a good relationship but his or her facial expression contradicts the words. Solution: The interviewer gives an interactive summary and confronts the patient with inconsistencies to provoke his or her protest and to probe his or her true convictions.

A 19-year-old, single, white woman.

I: You described to me some of the conflicts that you have with your stepfather, right? (Patient nods.) But you said they were really minor. You learned to tolerate each other, did I catch that? (Patient looks down.) But while you were saying "tolerate," some spit came out of your mouth.

P: (Throwing her head back and rolling up her eyes) I try to be understanding because of my mother. He really bugs me a lot.

Steering

Inside a topic and between topics, the interviewer steers the flow of information. The main choices are to encourage the patient to continue or to redirect the focus of attention.

CONTINUATION The interviewer tends to the patient's talk by raising eyebrows or uttering *hmmms* to signal to the patient nonverbally to continue. He or she may use short tracking phrases, such as "And?" "Then what?" "How is that?" if his or her nonverbal signals get ignored. The interviewer may also use phrases such as "That's interesting," "What a surprise!" "Really?" "Oh, no!" to reward the patient with his or her attention and to encourage the patient to continue.

ECHOING The interviewer may echo a part of what the patient has said. He or she may intend to prod the patient to continue or to shift the emphasis.

REDIRECTION Problem: The patient introduces a new productive topic. Solution: The interviewer follows the new lead. Alternatively, the interviewer may delay the transition: "What you are saying is very important. We will come back to this topic. But before we do, let's finish up on . . . (old topic)." Problem: The patient introduces all irrelevant topics, such as the problems of other people or political opinions about current events. Solution: The interviewer uses redirection. He or she interrupts the patient and asks to return to the previous topic. If the patient repeatedly gets distracted by irrelevant subjects, the interviewer may overtly educate the patient, saying: "We have to cover several topics. Let's not get distracted. Let's continue what we were talking about before." If the patient remains overtalkative, a request to make the patient just answer a series of yes-or-no questions or multiple-choice questions may help. If the interviewer is not versatile and skillful in using redirection, the entire interview may derail.

Transitions

To cover the 15 sections of the clinical interview, the interviewer has to transition from a completed topic to a new one. These transitions can be smooth, accentuated, or abrupt.

SMOOTH TRANSITIONS Smooth transitions connect topics without the seam becoming apparent. Problem: The patient startles when new topics get introduced. Solution: (1) The patient introduces a change in topic and the interviewer follows the new lead. (2) The interviewer portrays different topics as part of a larger theme. For example:

I: Both of your parents had problems with drinking. How did this affect your relationship with them?

P: Well, it was rough. There was a lot of fighting going on.

Thus, the interviewer has transitioned effectively from the topic of family history to social history.

The interviewer addresses a cause-and-effect relationship that also leads to smooth transition. (3) The interviewer references a point in time to smoothly link events that occurred together. Interviewers often have problems in transitioning to the testing of orientation and recent memory. They may introduce this topic with a statement such as, "Psychiatrists routinely ask some strange questions, such as what is today's date?"

To create a smooth transition, the interviewer may link questions about orientation to the problems that the patient has reported.

I: You said you have felt down in the dumps and could not sleep well for the last 3 weeks. Such moods can affect memory and sometimes the ability to track time. Have you encountered those problems?

P: I don't think so.

I: So you had no problems with tracking time?

P: Hmmm. Not really.

I: Can we test it?

P: Go right ahead.

I: What's the date today?

ACCENTUATED TRANSITIONS An accentuated transition emphasizes the start of a new topic. Problem: The patient loses attention and interest in the interview. Solution: The interviewer announces a new topic and freshens the patient's interest.

ABRUPT TRANSITIONS The interviewer jumps into a new topic without preparing the patient. Problem: The patient's history shows many contradictions. The patient seems to be lying. Solution: The interviewer jumps back and forth among different elements of the patient's story. The patient cannot replace quickly enough the true events of his or her story with invented ones.

Interviewing the Resisting Patient

For the initial interview, a patient may decide not to talk about certain subjects. He or she may overtly express his or her refusal: "I don't want to talk about this." Alternatively, the patient may divert his or her answer to a different topic. The reason for such refusal is often a fear of loss of face. Six techniques help to overcome resistance.

Sharing Concern

Problem: The patient refuses to disclose details of an event because he or she is not certain about legal consequences. Solution: The interviewer shares the patient's concern but points out the negative consequences that secrecy may have for the understanding of the problem.

A 57-year-old, white, retired man has a problem with road rage.

P: I've done some bad things in my life.

I: Such as . . . ?

P: (Pause) Such as bumping off two people. Do you have to report that if I tell you?

I: We could discuss the circumstances in general terms. But I have to document it. If you talk about it, it would help us to understand your rage attacks better. I understand your concern. You may want to consult your lawyer.

Expressing Acceptance Problem: A patient with OCD fears that the interviewer may think he or she is "crazy" and therefore gives vague and misleading answers. Solution: Reassuring the patient and showing understanding and acceptance of his or her symptoms help to reveal the "ridiculous" symptoms. Accepting certain symptoms as normal often reduces the patient's embarrassment.

Confrontation Problem: By the patient's behavior and open refusal, a patient resists discussing a topic. Solution: Confronting the patient repeatedly with his or her refusal or pointing out his or her evasive strategies or exploring the reasons for the resistance and describing the consequences for diagnosis and treatment may convince the patient to be more open.

Shifting Focus Problem: A patient resists a particular line of questions that he or she dreads. Solution: Shifting the approach without losing sight of the topic, the interviewer often secures the answers that he or she desires. The interviewer may shift to neutral ground or to a different angle to find a new entry point.

A 57-year-old white man.

I: When did you start having problems with your mental health?

P: Oh that's all a thing of the past. I've forgotten most of it. And I'd rather talk about my future.

I: Okay. You are divorced now. Would you like to get married again?

P: Oh, yes.

I: What went wrong with your first marriage?

P: My wife got mean with me when I first got sick when I was 23 years old.

I: I'm sorry to hear that. So she did not really support you? She did not believe in the phrase "for better, for worse?"

P: That's right.

I: What was it that bothered her?

P: That I asked the same questions over and over again, that I felt so bad, checked things, and washed my hands. She said I leave 30 dirty towels a day. She dumped me when I was 28.

The patient did not want to recall the symptoms that gave him so much trouble in the past but was ready to discuss his past history in connection with his still unresolved, painful divorce.

Exaggeration Problem: A patient experiences a minor failure as a major infraction and feels that he or she will lose the interviewer's support if he or she admits to it. Solution: The interviewer exaggerates the patient's actions to make them fit such inflated guilt feelings. Such exaggeration may help the patient to regain perspective and give up his or her resistance.

A 49-year-old man refused to discuss his shortcomings as a bank teller.

I: So you must have cleaned out the vault and got away with it.

P: (With a thin smile) No, not quite that bad.

I: Not that bad? But you said it is so bad that you could not talk about it.

P: I made a private long-distance call without reporting it. And I've worried about it ever since. Do you think I should still report it?

Induction to Bragging Problem: A patient hides his or her true motives for request of a sick leave to remain in good standing with the interviewer. Solution: The interviewer challenges the patient's cleverness and induces bragging to uncover the patient's motives.

A 47-year-old man, 290 lbs, requesting sick leave from his job because of stress on his delivery service job.

I: So you deliver all these advertising brochures.

P: (With a broad grin) Yes, and I'm doing a good job with that, but I'm stressed out now. That's the first time I try this route getting disability.

I: You look quite content to me. Maybe you need a vacation rather than a sick leave.

P: I've used up all my vacation at the beginning of the year. Now I need short-term disability.

I: You said this is the first time you tried this route. Why don't you tell me why you really want the sick leave?

P: I'm telling you. These 7 years at the job have really taken a toll on me. I feel I need time off.

I: I wonder whether you have learned how to work the system.

P: I've been at it for 7 years. (With a grin) I should be good at it.

I: How is that? What do you mean being good at it?

P: I have that quiet spot close to the cemetery where I can look at a lake. That's where I take a break from all that driving. (Sheepishly) I just dump some of the printings.

I: You wouldn't have enough miles on your car if you did that.

P: Don't you think I know that? I run out to my place and grab some lunch. That gives me the miles.

Induction to bragging revealed the patient's antisocial features behind his request for stress relief and sick leave.

Interviewing the Defensive Patient

Defense mechanisms may disrupt the interviewing process. Nevertheless, the interviewer has to deal with them. The DSM-IV-TR groups 31 defense mechanisms in seven levels of adaptation.

The interviewer can spot a defense mechanism by its observable, characteristic behavior (Table 7.1–2). The interviewer may identify the emotional conflicts, stressors, and the processes that activate the defense if the defense interferes with the interview. If the interviewer identifies a defense mechanism, he or she may determine its adaptive levels. For each of the levels, a general strategy is outlined that may help the interviewer to address the defense.

High Adaptive Level These eight defense mechanisms can be viewed as assets for the patient.

I: I admire your sense of humor. It will help you to deal better with your depression. You are able to take the Viennese approach and say, "The situation is hopeless but not serious."

Mental Inhibitions Level The seven defense mechanisms on this level deprive the patient of some degrees of freedom in

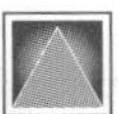

Table 7.1–2
Defense Mechanisms on Seven Levels (DSM-IV-TR)

Defense Mechanism	Observable Behavior or Symptom	Emotional Conflict and Stressors	Process
High adaptive level			
Affiliation	Formation of work and troubleshooting teams; striving for cooperation	Isolation, imperfection, responsibility	Sharing of anxiety and rewards
Altruism	Unconditional offer of help	Defeat in competition	Replacing aggression and competition by support
Anticipation	Predicting probable events and planning countermeasures	Sudden, overwhelming threats	Projecting events and coping strategies
Humor	Highlighting amusing aspects of threat	Failure, loss, or destruction	Converting anxiety of threat to comedy or irony
Self-assertion	Expression of impulses in socially acceptable form	Fear, anxiety, and anger	Transformation of fear, anxiety, and aggression into socially acceptable expressions
Self-observation	Reflection on own feelings, impulses, and thoughts	Fear, anxiety, failures, aggression	Enhancing awareness of feelings, impulses, and thoughts
Sublimation	Socially acceptable behavior	Unacceptable feelings or impulses	Rechanneling of impulses into socially acceptable expressions
Suppression	Avoidance of discussing painful problems, wishes, or feelings	Painful event, sadistic or sexual impulse	Intentional blocking of recall
Mental inhibitions level			
Displacement	Phobias	Fear and threat by an object or love and hate for an object	Transferring a feeling from its actual object to a substitute
Dissociation	Multiple personality, fugue, amnesia	Promiscuous, hostile, or irresponsible behavior, painful events	Temporary alteration of consciousness, memory, perception, and identity
Intellectualization	Abstract thinking, doubting, indecisiveness, generalizations	Disturbing feelings and thoughts	Removal of the emotional and personal components of an event
Isolation of affect	Obsessions, talking about emotional events without feeling	Painful emotions and memories	Separation of content and affect, removal of affect
Reaction formation	Devotion, self-sacrificing behavior, correctness, cleanliness	Feelings of hostility and disinterest	Substitution by wishes or feelings opposite of the true feelings
Repression	Gaps in memory	Threatening memories, feelings, fears, wishes	Banning thoughts and feelings from recall
Undoing	Compulsive behavior	Sadistic wishes, unacceptable impulses	Symbolic negating of an impulse
Minor image distortion level			
Devaluation	Derogatory statements about others or self, "sour grapes" about a goal	Positive qualities of others, unattainable goal	Ignoring of positive and exaggeration of negative qualities of self, others, or object
Idealization	Exaggerated praising of self or others	Negative qualities of self or significant others	Ignoring of negative and exaggeration of positive qualities of self or others
Omnipotence	Self-glorification, presumption, entitlement	Inferiority feelings, failure, low self-esteem	Converting inferiority into superiority feelings and actions
Disavowal level			
Denial	Stubborn and angry negation of some reality obvious to others	Painful reality	Refusal to acknowledge the awareness of some reality
Projection	Ideas of reference, prejudice, suspiciousness, injustice	Hostility, other unacceptable attitudes, wishes, desires	Attributing one's own feelings to others
Rationalization	Self-serving explanations and justification of behavior	Socially unacceptable impulses, low self-esteem	Giving false but socially acceptable explanations for behavior
Major image distortion level			
Autistic fantasy	Daydreaming	Unsatisfied impulses and wishes	Imagined wish fulfillment
Projective identification	Accusing others of causing distress, hostility, and anger	Hate, anger, and hostility	Converting own hostile impulses into justifiable reactions to other people's aggression
Splitting of self-image or image of others	Idealization alternating with devaluation of self or others	Experience of negative and positive qualities of self or others	Stripping off either all positive or all negative qualities of self or others
Action level			
Acting out	Violent acts, stealing, lying, rape	Sexual and aggressive impulses	Nonreflective, uncontrolled wish fulfillment
Apathetic withdrawal	Decreased emotions, activity, and social interactions	Needs, impulses, wishes	Responding to needs with increasing passivity
Help-rejecting complaining	Depicting oneself with self-pity as unsavable victim	Hostility and reproach toward others	Converting hostility into victimization
Passive aggression	Procrastination, lack of follow-through	Aggressive, hostile impulses, resentment	Expression through inactivity
Level of defensive dysregulation			
Delusional projection	Persecutory delusions	Overpowering, unacceptable and uncontrollable impulses	Attributing own impulses to others in spite of contradicting reality
Psychotic denial	Negation of obvious reality	Overpowering, painful reality	Profound annulment of obvious reality
Psychotic distortion	Obviously unrealistic statements and claims and irrational actions	Overpowering, unacceptable impulses and reality	Profound misperception and misinterpretation of external reality and feelings

From Othmer E, Othmer SC. *The Clinical Interview Using DSM-IV-TR.* Vol 1. American Psychiatric Press; 2002:82–85, with permission.

decision making. Usually, the patient has insight into the pathological nature of phobias, obsessive-compulsive behavior, and dissociative identity disorders without being aware of the underlying process. In the case of intellectualization, isolation of affect, reaction formation, and repression, the patient misses that a defense mechanism inhibits his or her ability to recognize his or her true feelings. Confrontation with the observable behavior may allow the patient to recognize his or her true feelings.

> I: What value do you attach to life?
>
> P: I feel as a Christian it is a sin to even think about suicide. God gave us our life and he is the one who should take it.
>
> I: You mentioned suicide when I just wanted to know what you think about life.
>
> P: Don't you think suicide is a sin?
>
> I: I'm more concerned about your generic answer. It hides your feelings. What are your feelings about your present life?
>
> P: (Starts crying) It's awful. I would not care if I didn't wake up in the morning.

Minor Image Distortion Level A patient may idealize an interviewer at the beginning of the interview and subsequently devaluate the interviewer because of a minor perceived failure, such as asking an embarrassing question. When idealization, devaluation, or omnipotence interfere with the interview, the overt behavior itself may have to be addressed.

> I: How quickly I end up in the doghouse! Let's find out what got me there.

Disavowal Level From the three defense mechanisms on the disavowal level, projection is the most disruptive during an interview.

> A patient accuses the interviewer of not liking her. When asked whether she herself dislikes the interviewer, she answers, "How could I like you if you don't like me?" When he asks her whether there is anything that she does not like about him she answers: "The way how you make me feel. I don't like sex." Solution: The interviewer has to make the patient aware that her feelings and not his actions cause her difficulties. He may accept her feelings as normal and repeatedly discuss them with her to neutralize them.

Major Image Distortion Level The three defense mechanisms on this level have to be identified and addressed but not interpreted.

> A 45-year-old, white, married truck driver avoided his mother for several years because he believed she made him sick. He then quit his job because his coworkers rejected him. He felt hate and anger toward them. In the interview, he told his psychiatrist that his questions were making him sick. The interviewer pointed out to him that he had felt the same way about his mother and later about his coworkers. Avoiding his mother and quitting his job did not give him peace of mind. Therefore, he and the interviewer had to find new ways of dealing with the patient's social discomfort other than accusing people next to him. "Let's work on your anger and distrust of me and others. With your help, we can find out what actions and medications make you less sensitive to other people's remarks."

The interviewer recognized the accusations as projective identification. Instead of an interpretation that is usually not effective, the interviewer offered support and medication.

Action Level Problem: A patient acts out his or her anger. Solution: The interviewer sets limits rather than trying to interpret the behavior. The diagnosis helps to decide which combination of behavioral and medical intervention is necessary to manage this patient.

Level of Defensive Dysregulation The three defense mechanisms on this level produce all psychotic symptoms. If, for instance, the interviewer challenges a delusion as nonsensical, the patient may get angry and distrustful and break off the interview. Therefore, the interviewer has to adopt the patient's vantage point and offer support accordingly.

> A 43-year-old, white, single farmer claims that spacemen at night cause his headaches.
>
> I: I will protect you against these spacemen. I'll put you in the hospital, and I will give you medication that will make you immune to their attacks.
>
> P: So you believe me that spacemen cause my headaches?
>
> I: I can't tell you that. But I know that you feel this, and I know that the medication may help.

Recognizing the behaviors that, according to a psychodynamic view, represent an unconscious defense mechanism is in the realm of descriptive psychiatry. However, descriptively oriented psychiatrists doubt the validity of the underlying psychological mechanisms and therefore prefer behavioral and medical management over interpretation.

MENTAL STATUS

The third component of psychiatric interviewing is the online monitoring of the patient's mental status. The interviewer screens the mental status to detect signs and symptoms of mental disorders (Tables 7.1–3 and 7.1–4) with four assessment methods: observation, conversation, exploration, and testing.

Observation For observation, the interviewer does not need the patient's cooperation. Besides sex and race, the interviewer observes appearance, level of consciousness, psychomotor functions, body language, and affect. Through the power of observation, Sherlock Holmes could deduce a person's life history and occupation. Similarly, for the astute interviewer, observation can give clues to diagnosis.

Conversation Even if the patient refuses to speak about him- or herself or his or her symptoms or suffering, the interviewer can draw conclusions from conversation about the patient's speech, thinking, affect, thought content, concentration, memory, intelligence, insight, and judgment.

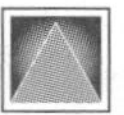

Table 7.1–3
Quantitative Changes in Frequency, Duration, and Intensity of Mental Status Functions Secondary to Some Axis I and II Disorders

Function and Assessment Method	Category	Increased In	Decreased In
Appearance (O)	Apparent vs. stated age	AD, MDD, Schiz with chronic course, SRD, precocious puberty	MA, HistrPD
	Grooming and clothing	OC-PD, HistrPD, narcissistic PD (mint condition), MA	AD, MDD, SRD, Schiz
	Eye contact	DelD (hostile)	GAD, DelD, MA, ADHD
	Nutritional status	SRD (antihistamine use), MDD atypical, SD; use of medication: olanzapine, valproic sodium, clozapine, lithium, mirtazapine	SRD (stimulants), AN, MDD (cachectic)
Attitude toward interviewer (C, E, T)	Cooperation	Dependent PD, HistrPD, MA	Ds with psychotic features, MA, intoxication, MDD, AD, AsPD, conduct D
Consciousness (O, C, T)	Alertness	SRD (stimulants), GAD, posttraumatic stress disorder, paranoid D	SRD (alcohol, sedatives)
Psychomotor (O, C, T)	Posture	MA	MDD, dementia
	Movements		
	Reactive	MA, GAD, SRD	MDD, Schiz (catalepsy)
	Grooming	SocPh, ADHD, GAD	MDD
	Symbolic	MA, cluster B PD	MDD, Schiz (catalepsy)
	Illustrative	MA, SD	MDD, Schiz (catalepsy)
	Expressive	MA, GAD, SD, HistrPD	MDD, Schiz (catalepsy)
	Goal directed	MA, ADD	MDD, Schiz
Speech (C, E, T)	Articulation	—	SRD, neurological Ds
	Flow	MA	PD, MDD
	Speed	MA, GAD	PD, MDD
	Volume	MA	MDD
	Latency of response	MDD	MA, ADHD
	Inflection	MA	MDD
Thinking (C, E, T)	Speed	MA, SRD	MDD, SRD, AD, OCD, Parkinson's disease
	Abstraction	—	Mental retardation, Schiz, AD, frontal lobe dementia
	Tightness of association	OCD, OC-PD	MA, Schiz, SRD
	Goal directedness	—	MA, Schiz, OCD, AD, SRD
Affect (O, C, E, T)	Quality	MA	MDD, AnxD, AN, bulimia nervosa, intermittent explosive D
	Reactivity	MA, SD, SRD, AD, retarded MDD, OCD MA, SD, HistrPD	AD, MDD, OCD MDD, OCD, Schiz
	Intensity	MA, AnxD, EatD	MDD
	Range	MA	Schiz, MA, GAD, SocPh
	Appropriateness	—	Schiz, D with psychotic features
Mood (E, T)	Quality	MA, SRD	MDD, AnxD, EatD, SRD
	Stability	MDD	AsPD, BID mixed, SRD, SD
	Intensity	MA, OCD	MDD
	Duration	OCD, OC-PD, MDD	BID rapid cycling, SRD
Thought content (C, E)	Congruency of delusions and hallucinations to mood; pathological content (see Table 7.1–4)	Schizoaffective D (see Table 7.1–4)	—
Cognition (C, E, T)	See Tables 7.1–4 and 7.1–6	—	See Tables 7.1–4 and 7.1–6
Insight (C, E)	Being sick, needing help	—	AD, SRD, MA, Schiz, Pick's
Judgment (C, E)	Future plans, dealing with friends and money	—	MA, MDD, Schiz, AD, Pick's, SRD

AD, dementia of Alzheimer's type; ADHD, attention-deficit/hyperactivity disorder; AN, anorexia nervosa; AnxD, anxiety disorder; AsPD, antisocial personality disorder; BID, bipolar disorder; C, conversation; D, disorder; DelD, delusional disorder; E, exploration; EatD, eating disorders; GAD, generalized anxiety disorder; HistrPD, histrionic personality disorder; MA, mania; MDD, major depressive disorder and depression; O, observation; OCD, obsessive-compulsive disorder; OC-PD, obsessive-compulsive personality disorder; PD, personality disorder; Pick's, Pick's disease; Schiz, schizophrenia; SD, somatization disorder; SocPh, social phobia; SRD, substance-related disorders; T, testing.

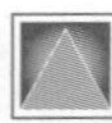

Table 7.1–4
Qualitative Changes in Mental Status Functions Secondary to Some Axis I and II Psychiatric Disorders and Syndromes

Function and Assessment Method	Symptom, Sign	Disorder, Syndrome
Appearance (O)	Needle marks	SRD
	Scars on forearm and wrist	MDD, BID, borderline PD, Cl B PD
	Inappropriate attire	MA, PsychD
	Missing eyelashes, eyebrows, hair	ID, trichotillomania
	Bitten-off nails	ID, AnxD, PsychD
	Reddened, chapped hands	OCD
	Excessive piercing or tattoos	Cl B PD
Consciousness (O, T)	Hyperalertness	SRD (sedative withdrawal or stimulant Intox)
	Lethargy, stupor, coma	SRD sedation (Intox), psychiatric D due to a medical condition
Psychomotor (O, C, T)	Rigidity	ParkD, neuroleptic malignant syndrome, extrapyramidal symptoms
	Tremor	Idiopathic, S induced, S withdrawal, ParkD
	Tics (motor, vocal)	TOUR, other tic D
	Restless fidgeting, squirming, overflow	ADHD
	Choreatic, athetotic movements	TD
	Buccolingual movements	TD
	Catalepsy	Schiz, D with psychotic features, AD, FLD
	Gegenhalten (opposing movement)	Schiz
	Echopraxia	Schiz
	Pseudoaphonia, pseudoparalysis, pseudoseizures	Conversion D
	Avoidance of touching	OCD
	Apraxia	FLD, AD, NeurolD
	Seizures	SRD (sedative withdrawal)
	Cataplexy	Narcolepsy
	Micrographia	ParkD
	Stereotypical movements	Pervasive developmental D
Speech (C, E, T)	Stuttering, stammering	AnxD, generalized anxiety D, NeurolD
	Vocal tics	TOUR
	Aphasias	FLD, AD, NeurolD
	Push of speech	MA
Thinking (C, E, T)	Blocking and derailment	PsychD
	Circumstantiality	OCD
	Flight of ideas	MA
	Loose associations	MA, PsychD, Schiz
	Perseveration	FLD
	Verbigeration	PsychD (catatonia), NeurolD
	Palilalia	NeurolD
	Clang association	Schiz, MA
	Nonsequitur	Schiz
	Fragmentation	Schiz
	Rambling	Delirium, SRD
	Driveling	Aphasia (Wernicke's), Schiz
	Word salad	PsychD, Aphasia (global)
	Tangentiality	Schiz, NeurolD, D with psychotic features
Affect (O, C, E, T)	Lability	BID, SRD, MDD
	Inappropriateness	D with psychotic features
Thought content (C, E)	Suicidality, homicidality	MDD, SRD, Schiz, BID
	Hallucinations, delusions	BID, MDD, Schiz, SRD, AD
	Obsessions, compulsions	OCD
	Panic attacks	MDD, panic D
	Medically unexplained pain	Somatization D
	Derealization, depersonalization	DissD
Cognition (C, E, T; see Table 7.1–6)	Confabulation	Amnestic D
	Dissociative amnesia	DissD

AD, dementia of Alzheimer's type; ADHD, attention-deficit/hyperactivity disorder; AnxD, anxiety disorder; BID, bipolar disorder; BPD, borderline personality disorder; C, conversation; Cl, cluster; ConvD, conversion disorder; D, disorder; DissD, dissociative disorder; E, exploration; FLD, frontal lobe dementia; ID, impulse-control disorder; Intox, intoxication; MA, mania; MDD, major depressive disorder and depression; NeurolD, neurological disorders; O, observation; OCD, obsessive-compulsive disorder; ParkD, Parkinson's disease; PD, personality disorder; PsychD, psychotic disorders; S, substance; Schiz, schizophrenia; SRD, substance-related disorders; T, testing; TD, tardive dyskinesia; TOUR, Tourette's disorder.

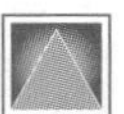

Table 7.1–5
Change in Emotional Response as an Indicator of Some Psychiatric Axis I and II Disorders

Emotion	Event	Action	Increase	Decrease
Surprise	Unexpected stimulus	Evaluation, integration	PTSD, MDD, MA, GAD, PanD, SocPH	MDD, Schiz
Interest	Need reducing stimulus	Exploration	MA, ADHD	MDD, Schiz PD, MDD, dementia of Alzheimer's type, frontal lobe dementia
Elation	Expected satisfaction of need	Satisfaction of need	MA	MDD, ADHD, GAD
Contentment	Completed need satisfaction	Relaxation	—	SocPH, PTSD
Anger	Obstacle	Destruction of obstacle	MA, delusional disorder, ADHD MDD, cluster B PD, intermittent explosive disorder, substance-related disorder, PanD, AsPD	Schizoid PD?
Disgust	Intrusion	Expulsion or withdrawal	Anorexia nervosa, bulimia nervosa, OCD, SpecPH, SocPH	Paraphilias
Anxiety	Threat	Avoidance	SocPH, agoraphobia, SpecPH, PTSD, OCD	MA
Sadness	Loss	Undoing, replacement	MDD, PTSD, histrionic PD	MA, AsPD
Guilt	Violation of code	Remorse, self-punishment	MDD, borderline PD	AsPD, MA, ID

ADHD, attention-deficit/hyperactivity disorder; AsPD, antisocial personality disorder; GAD, generalized anxiety disorder; ID, impulse-control disorder; MA, mania; MDD, major depressive disorder and depression; OCD, obsessive-compulsive disorder; PanD, panic disorder; PD, personality disorder; PTSD, posttraumatic stress disorder; Schiz, schizophrenia; SocPH, social phobia; SpecPH, specific phobia.

Exploration Exploration requires the patient's willingness to disclose information about mood; content of thinking, such as obsessions, compulsions, suicidal ideation, delusions, hallucinations, panic attacks, avoidance behaviors, and "spells;" amnesias; personality changes; and pain sensations. To verify his or her impression, the interviewer may feed back to the patient his or her reading of symptoms and signs assessed during the interview. Thus, the patient's mental status becomes the object of exploration.

Testing Testing of the patient's mental functions, whether intact or impaired, demands the highest degree of cooperation. Testing adds a quantitative component to the interview.

Combining observation, conversation, exploration, and testing, the interviewer screens at least 12 mental status functions often affected by psychiatric disorders. Table 7.1–3 lists the mental status function and the method of its assessment, the categories that are assessed for the individual functions, the mental disorders that may show an increase, and the mental disorders that may show a decrease in the specific category. The interviewer identifies signs and symptoms of disorders in these mental status functions. Table 7.1–4 lists mental status functions and assessment methods, symptoms and signs, and the disorders and syndromes in which the symptoms and signs are frequently encountered. The mental status functions of Tables 7.1–3 and 7.1–4 are discussed subsequently.

In Tables 7.1–3, 7.1–4, 7.1–5, and 7.1–6 the term *MDD* is used to designate major depressive disorder as well as depression due to other disorders, such as dysthymia, bereavement, or adjustment disorder, substance use, or a general medical condition.

Appearance Table 7.1–3 lists quantitative and Table 7.1–4 qualitative changes in appearance that may be due to a psychiatric disorder. The onset of some disorders is age related (Table 7.1–3). Gender is associated with certain diagnoses. For instance, anorexia and bulimia nervosa, somatization disorder, and major depression are more common in women, whereas antisocial personality disorder and alcohol abuse predominate in men.

Race and ethnic background are important: First, rapport across racial and ethnic boundaries may be impeded. Second, the attitude toward mental illness varies from culture to culture and may delay consultation. Third, race and ethnicity affect the incidence of some psychiatric disorders.

Attitude The patient's attitude reflects his or her disorder and his or her evaluation of the doctor–patient relationship. A patient may hide his or her uncooperative attitude behind vagueness, memory loss, or one-word answers or express it openly. He or she may refuse to answer questions or refuse to be tested.

Consciousness Most common disturbances of consciousness are due to intoxication or substance withdrawal resulting in increased or decreased reactivity. More severe disturbances of consciousness (Table 7.1–4) can be assessed by bedside tests (Table 7.1–6).

Psychomotor Function Besides posture, humans display types of movements that differ in their purpose (Table 7.1–3). Reactive movements are directed toward a new stimulus, such as responses to phone ringing or door knocking. Grooming movements control appearance, such as straightening out clothes, hair, or mustache. Such movements frequently indicate discomfort with the situation. Symbolic movements are culture specific and can replace language. Instead of saying, "We will win," a presidential candidate, for instance, may form a V with his or her arms. During an interview, a patient may sometimes make an unintended symbolic gesture that reveals hidden thoughts. Illustrative movements duplicate what is said—they are redundant. Expressive movements reflect in a rudimentary form the motor action that a patient would like to undertake in response to an emotion-provoking stimulus; for instance, an angry patient who says he or she will take on his or her employer assumes an erect posture and makes a fist as if anticipating a fight. Goal-directed movements occur as a part of a physical action, such as reaching for a coffee cup. Psychiatric disorders can affect frequency

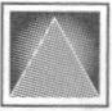

Table 7.1–6
Brief Tests for Selected Mental Status Functions at the Bedside or Office

Function	Test	Pathological Response	Evaluation	Disorder
Consciousness	Ask questions in normal voice once.	Prompt exaggerated response.	Hyperalert	SRD
	Ask question in loud voice repetitively.	Delayed incomplete response.	Lethargic	SRD, PsychD due to a medical condition
	Apply painful squeeze to chest.	Moaning, groaning, restless.	Stuporous	SRD, PsychD due to a medical condition
	Apply painful squeeze to chest.	No response.	Comatose	SRD, PsychD due to a medical condition
Nonresponsiveness	Ask pt. to recall what was said when pt. was nonresponsive.	Pt. does not know.	Comatose	Coma, malingering, catatonic state, cataleptic attack, dizziness
		Pt. recalls detail.	Catatonic stupor, conversion	Schiz, catatonic state, conduct D, pseudoseizure
Attention	Repeat up to 7 digits forward (1 digit/sec).	Pt. recalls <5 digits.	Inattention	ADHD, mania, MDD, AD
	Repeat up to 7 digits backward.	Pt. recalls <4 digits.	Inattention	SRD, PsychD due to medical condition, MR, DissD not otherwise specified (Ganser)
Vigilance	Tap when you hear an A in a sequence of letters: K, D, A, M, G, N, T, X, O, A, and so forth for 10 mins.	Taps after each letter.	Perseveration	FLD
		<90% correct.	Decreased concentration	ADHD, MDD psychomotor retarded, SRD
Perseverance	Subtract 7 from 100 or 3 from 30 if IQ <80.	Commits errors.	Impersistence	MDD, MR, LD mathematics
	Name as many words as you can in 1 min that start with F. Repeat with A and S.	<12 words per letter; <36 words for all 3 letters.	Impersistence	AD, FLD, MDD psychomotor retarded
	Copy these figures.		Visual perseveration	FLD
	Count letters of the alphabet: A1, B2, C3.	A1, B2, C3, D3, E3, F3.	Auditory perseveration	FLD
Memory	Copy visual designs after exposure of 5 secs.	Unrecognizable or distorted reproduction.	Decreased immediate visual memory	Damage to nondominant temporal lobe
	Repeat figures after >5-min latency.	Incomplete reconstruction.	Decreased short-term visual memory	AD, AmnD
	Repeat: brown, honesty, tulip, eyedropper.	Incomplete immediate recall.	Inattention, aphasia	Central aphasias
		Incomplete recall after 5 mins.	Decreased short-term auditory memory	AD, AmnD, late FLD, intact in dissociated amnesia
	Recall historical events.	Incomplete recall.	Disturbed remote memory	Late stages of AD, FLD
Orientation	Tell your name, date, and present location.	Errors.	Disorientation	AD, SRD, PsychD due to medical condition
Language	Write a sentence.	Failure.	Aphasia suspected	AD, FLD, PsychD due to medical condition, illiteracy
	Spontaneous speech.	Lack of correct grammar, nouns, verbs, telegram style, nonfluent speech.	Expressive aphasia	AD, NeurolD
		Fluent incomprehensible speech filled with articles, conjunctions, abnormal words (neologisms).	Receptive aphasia	AD, NeurolD
Ability to know (gnosia)	Trace letter or number on skin; "Tell me what coin I put in your hand."	Unable to identify.	Agnosia	AD, PsychD due to medical condition, FLD
Ability to perform (praxia)	Show me how to ride a bike.	Unable to do.	Apraxia, whole body	AD, PsychD due to medical condition, FLD
Pathological reflexes	Scratch alongside of outside margin of sole.	Big toe moves up.	Babinski's reflex present	PsychD due to medical condition
	Tap repetitively above bridge of nose.	Repeated eye blinking.	Positive Glabellar tap	ParkD
	Stroke with index finger pt.'s palm between thumb and index finger.	Pt. grasps interviewer's index finger.	Positive grasp reflex	AD, FLD, NeurolD, Pick's

(continued)

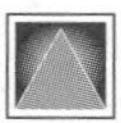

Table 7.1–6 (*continued*)

Function	Test	Pathological Response	Evaluation	Disorder
	Scratch surface of hand vigorously.	Ipsilateral angle of mouth twitches downward.	Positive palmomental reflex	AD, FLD, NeurolD, Pick's
	Scratch below angle of pt.'s mouth.	Ipsilateral downward twitch.	Positive rooting reflex	AD, FLD, NeurolD, Pick's
	Tap upper lip.	Pt.'s mouth forms a snout.	Snout reflex positive	AD, FLD, NeurolD, Pick's
	Strike lightly upper lip.	Sucking movement.	Sucking reflex positive	AD, FLD, NeurolD, Pick's
Pathological motor response	Stick out tongue (give a pin prick on the tongue).	Repeatedly sticks out tongue.	Pathological obedience	AD, PsychD, Schiz (catatonia)
	Bend pt. in awkward body position.	Pt. remains in the body position.	Waxy flexibility	AD, PsychD, Schiz (catatonia)
	I: Sit down!	Pt. repeatedly sits down and rises up again.	Ambitendency	AD, PsychD, Schiz (catatonia)
	I: Resist me moving your arm.	Pt.'s arms can be easily moved.	Pathological cooperation (*mitmachen*)	—
	I: Let me move your limbs.	Pt. resists all movements.	Pathological opposition (*gegenhalten*)	—
Affect	I: Say and enact each of the following emotions: I feel surprised, interested in new things, happy, content; I feel angry, disgusted, scared, sad, guilty.	Lacks changes in one or more; rate: tone of voice, 0–1; facial expression, 0–1; gestures, postures, 0–1; inflection in voice, 0–1.	<4 points for each affect may indicate restriction	Mood Ds, AnxDs, Schiz, AD
Suggestibility	I: Put your feet together. Close your eyes. Imagine you stand at the end of a 6-ft-long board; somebody slowly raises the board on the other side. You start falling backwards . . . you fall, you fall . . . I'll catch you.	Pt. loses balance and falls backward.	Positive sway test	ConvD, DissD, SD
	I: Look up at my index finger above your forehead without moving your head. Your eyelids get heavy . . . get tired . . . they close . . .	Eyelids close while pupils turn upward; white sclera shows below pupils that eyelids cover.	Positive eyelid test	ConvD, DissD, SD
	I: Fold your hands and clasp fingers tightly together in front of your chest. Imagine that a force from above and below presses your fingers together. Imagine it. Now you can't pull your hands apart.	Pt.'s fingers stick together. Pt. cannot pull them apart no matter how hard he or she pulls.	Positive finger sticking test	ConvD, DissD, SD
	Interviewer gives the pt. a pendulum made of a string and a ring. I: Hold the string between your fingers. Now imagine that it swings in a circle. The circle gets larger and larger.	The pendulum swings in a circle.	Positive pendulum test	ConvD, DissD, SD
Abnormal perception	How do you respond to your voices? (similar for delusions)	I obey them.	Action level	D with psychotic features
		I just talk about them.	No insight	D with psychotic features
		I ignore them.	Confusion about reality	D with psychotic features
		They are in my past.	Confusion	D with psychotic features
		I was sick.	Full insight	D with psychotic features
Abstract thinking	What do the following proverbs mean: Don't cry over spilled milk; a stitch in time saves nine; people who live in glass houses should not throw stones	Pt. gives a concrete answer missing the abstract meaning of the proverb.	Concreteness of thinking	AD, MR, Pick's, Schiz, unfamiliarity with culture
	What do the following objects have in common: an apple and an orange; a table and a chair; a bicycle and a plane?	Pt. misses to name the abstract category—fruits, furniture, and means of transportation.	Concreteness of thinking	AD, MR, Pick's, Schiz, unfamiliarity with culture
Intelligence	Why does the moon look larger than the stars?	Pt. misses that closer objects look larger than farther objects.	Possible borderline IQ	Possible borderline intelligence
	What is 2 × 48?	Pt. cannot calculate.	Possible borderline IQ	Possible borderline intelligence
Complex cognitive functions	Mini-Mental State Examination, full scale: 30 points.	Scores <25.	Mild cognitive impairment	MDD

(*continued*)

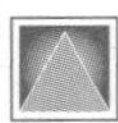

Table 7.1–6 (*continued*)

Function	Test	Pathological Response	Evaluation	Disorder
		Scores <10.	Severe cognitive impairment	AD
	Executive interview.	0	Normal	—
		0–10	Independent living	AD, Pick's, FLD <0
		18–23	Residential care	Same
		24–32	Skilled nursing	Same
		33–50	Special care unit	Same
	Qualitative Evaluation of Dementia.	0	Subcortical impairment	Pure subcortical dementia, e.g., Parkinson's
		30	Cortical impairment	Pure cortical dementia, e.g., AD, Pick's, FLD
		15	Normal	Normal

AD, dementia of Alzheimer's type; ADHD, attention-deficit/hyperactivity disorder; AmnD, amnestic disorder; AnxD, anxiety disorder; ConvD, conversion disorder; D, disorder; DissD, dissociative disorder; FLD, frontal lobe dementia; I, interviewer; IQ, intelligence quotient; LD, learning disorder; MDD, major depressive disorder and depression; MR, mental retardation; NeurolD, neurological disorders; Park D, Parkinson's disease; Pick's, Pick's disease; PsychD, psychotic disorders; pt., patient; Schiz, schizophrenia; SD, somatization disorder; SRD, substance-related disorders.

and intensity of such movements (Table 7.1–3), but they can also induce qualitative changes, such as pathological movements specific to psychiatric or neurological disorders (Table 7.1–4).

Speech *Speech* is a motor function driven by the patient's thought processes. Therefore, most disorders that affect motor functions in frequency and intensity affect speech as well. Rapid speech is seen in mania and in anxiety disorders (Table 7.1–3). A constant rapid flow of speech that can be interrupted is called *push of speech*. If it is difficult to interrupt, it is called *pressure of speech*. Both forms are seen in mania (Table 7.1–4). Qualitative changes of speech are usually of diagnostic significance (Table 7.1–4). If speech centers in the brain are damaged, specific forms of aphasia (inability to speak) occur. Bedside tests help to determine which type of aphasia is present (Table 7.1–6). Developmental disorders affect speech. Speech is noticeably impaired in patients with low intelligence quotient (IQ) or with dementias.

Thinking The interviewer judges thinking according to the categories listed in Table 7.1–3. The interviewer's impression and a patient's report may conflict. Some patients report racing thoughts but talk with a normal rate or even slowly. Such a mismatch may be more common in anxiety disorders, psychotic disorders, or hypomania; in mania, racing thoughts are usually accompanied by increased rate of speech. The ability to understand the abstract meaning of words varies with the level of intelligence and is not pathognomonic for schizophrenia. The ability to abstract can be tested by asking for communality of categories and proverb interpretation (Table 7.1–6). Concreteness of thinking in first-episode psychosis may be associated with lack of insight.

Association between sentences can be loosened by several psychiatric disorders (Tables 7.1–3 and 7.1–4). Thoughts seem to jump from topic to topic and their goal gets lost, a phenomenon called *flight of ideas* (Table 7.1–4). The associations between thoughts can become very close, and the patient may be unable to omit irrelevant details, making his or her thinking circumstantial. Some patients lose the goal of their answer but touch on the general topic, called *tangential thinking* (Table 7.1–4).

Affect Affect communicates to the interviewer the emotional value that the patient puts on his or her experience. The interviewer sees affect expressed in the patient's posture, face, and body movements. He or she hears it in the patient's voice. External events and internal experiences, such as thoughts, ideas, and memory, evoke affect. The interviewer has to explore to what extent immediate circumstances, such as being pressured by a family member to see a psychiatrist, contribute to the present affect. The nine basic emotions that Carroll Izard and others have identified are transcultural, innate expressions (Table 7.1–5). Each is triggered by a specific event and urges the individual to take a specific action (Table 7.1–5). The quality of the first four emotions—surprise, interest, elation, and contentment—is positive; the last five have a negative quality—anger, disgust, anxiety, sadness, and guilt.

Most psychiatric disorders influence affect and mood (Table 7.1–5). They shift a patient's emotional response toward a dominating affect and mood, thus increasing the intensity of that specific affect but at the same time restricting the range of responsiveness. For instance, in mania and some substance-related disorders, elation dominates. In depression, sadness and guilt are prominent. In eating disorders, disgust is prominent, and in anxiety disorders, anxiousness is of course prevalent. Therefore, the interviewer gets significant clues about psychiatric disorders by noticing the shift in quality and intensity of affect (Tables 7.1–3 and 7.1–5). Furthermore, psychiatric disorders influence the reactivity of affect. For instance, patients with bipolar disorder may display dramatic, rapid changes in quality and intensity of affect in response to changing thought content (Table 7.1–3). The interviewer then observes a labile affect (Table 7.1–4). Psychiatric disorders with psychotic features often affect the appropriateness of affect to thought content. A patient may report and show elation but have delusions of being forced to commit suicide, thus showing thought content incongruent to mood. For instance, a patient may giggle while describing her mother's funeral (Table 7.1–4). Without being sad or depressed, some patients may lack an affective response, which is often described as flat or bland affect in contrast to full affect. To evaluate affect, the interviewer may explore the patient's response to events listed in Table 7.1–5. For instance, he or she may ask a salesman, "How does it make you feel when you meet a representative of a competing company in your territory?" The mixture of anger about the obstacle, disgust about the intrusion, and anxiety about the threat may give valuable clues of the patient's emotional responsiveness. A second method to assess mood is by brief tests (Table 7.1–6). With respect to affect, the interviewer can ask the patient to enact the nine basic affects (Table 7.1–6). As in all these areas, patients may exhibit situationally driven responses due to recent stressors or external circumstances of the interview.

Mood *Mood* refers to the predominant, longer-lasting quality of experienced emotion. Therefore, if the interviewer wants to evaluate the patient's mood, he or she has to ask. The interviewer can judge to what extent the observed affect and the reported mood correspond to each other. A patient with high social skills can often display an affect inconsistent with the mood. This apparent discrepancy between affect and mood occurs more frequently when the patient speaks. When the patient listens and feels unobserved, the happy mask may drop. Prolonged periods of depression, as seen in major depressive disorder, show a pathological stability and duration of mood. A patient with OCD or obsessive-compulsive personality disorder may also report that his or her dysphoric mood lasts for a long time, yet it may be unstable because of his or her anger outbursts. Depending on the severity of a psychiatric disorder, the predominant mood can be intense.

Thought Content During exploration, the interviewer searches the patient's past for the occurrence of pathological thought content (Table 7.1–4). To assess suicidality, the interviewer may discuss the patient's quality of life, thus getting a better reading of suicide risk than with direct questioning. Follow-up questions for suicide risk include past attempts, immediate intent, lethal plan, availability of means, family history of suicide, and perceived outcome. Concurrent presence of psychotic features, such as command hallucinations, as well as depression, substance abuse, recent loss of social support, male gender, white race, and middle age or older, may increase the risk of suicide. The comorbidity of major depression and substance use disorder leads to the highest risk of suicide. A mnemonic for risk factors of suicide is helpful: SAD PERSONS.

Sex: Women are more likely to be attempters, men more likely to be committers.
Age: Highest rate of suicide is in teenagers and the elderly.
Depression: 15 percent commit suicide.
Previous attempts: 10 percent of previous attempters finally succeed.
Ethanol abuse: 15 percent of alcoholics commit suicide.
Rational thinking loss, psychosis. 10 percent of chronic schizophrenics commit suicide.
Social support is lacking.
Organized plan increases the suicide risk.
No spouse increases the suicide risk.
Sickness. Chronic illness increases the risk.

Homicidality may become apparent if the interviewer discusses the patient's enemies. As in the assessment of suicidality, previous homicidal attempts or completions, intent, lethality of plan, and available means have to be assessed. Patients at risk for homicide are those with persecutory delusions, antisocial personality disorder, and substance-related disorders. To increase the likelihood that a patient admits to homicidal ideas or plans, use the golden rule: Approach the subject from the patient's point of view as understandable. Use questions such as "Are there people in your life who have harmed you and who deserve to die for what they have done?" "Are there people whom you wish to be dead?" If the patient voices an intent to harm such foes, introduce the subject of safe management, including warning of identified victims, which is the interviewer's duty. Contrary to expectation, to tell the patient about the duty to warn has only minimal impact on the alliance with the patient.

When asked about experiences with extrasensory perception (ESP), the patient may report hallucinations and delusions. Hallucinations and delusions can be staged according to the patient's level of insight (Table 7.1–6). Hallucinations and delusions are also evaluated by their mood congruency. Because the patient usually has good insight into obsessions, compulsions, panic attacks, unexplained pain, derealization, and depersonalization, the interviewer can explore these thought contents and experiences with targeted questions. However, the patient may consider some obsessions and compulsions as embarrassing and may attempt to hide them.

Cognition The interviewer judges cognition by the patient's ability to comprehend questions and express the responses. Even if the interviewer finds no evidence of a cognitive disturbance during conversation and exploration, he or she still may select a few brief tests that assess orientation, attention, recent memory, remote memory, abstraction, and intelligence (Table 7.1–6).

Insight The interviewer asks the patient to what extent he or she feels sick. Usually, a patient with schizophrenia, mania, dementia, or substance-related disorders may deny being sick, yet some such patients have partial insight. They may acknowledge being depressed but explain that the depression is a response to the scolding voices. A patient may acknowledge that he or she needs help but deny being sick. Such a patient may accuse other people and factors—the employer, the spouse, the lack of resources—as being the cause of his or her problems. Insight is often reported as being good, fair, or poor. A more informative technique is to describe to what extent the patient recognizes being sick.

Judgment Review of significant life events, money management, and personal relationships reflects a history of the patient's judgment. Judgment often varies in accordance with the patient's state of illness. In patients with bipolar disorder, judgment may deteriorate during mania but may be fully intact during euthymic or even depressed states. Assessing a patient's current judgment in comparison with his or her historical judgment may provide a measure of the impact of a disorder. If a patient's judgment is not apparent or inconsistent with the diagnosis, judgment can be more formally assessed. Some psychiatrists use questions from the Wechsler Intelligence Test to assess judgment. Example: What do you do when you first detect a fire in a crowded theater? Such questions do not involve the patient's affect, mood, and motivation and, therefore, may fail to measure the appropriateness of judgment. A more powerful question is to ask about future plans. If these plans appear consistent with the educational background and resources, the patient appears to have appropriate judgment.

Testing Testing is a highly structured form of exploration. To get valid results, the patient has to be fully compliant. The majority of the brief tests that a psychiatric interviewer uses at the bedside or office measure some aspect of cognitive function (Table 7.1–6). Interviewers select bedside tests according to the patient's complaints or demonstrated cognitive deficits apparent during the interview. Table 7.1–6 shows the function to be tested, the test, the description of abnormal response, the clinical evaluation, and key examples of disorders that may test positive. Table 7.1–6 covers 15 cognitive and three noncognitive functions—affect, suggestibility, and abnormal perception. The testing of two of the noncognitive functions and the staging of hallucinations as part of abnormal perception are discussed above. Suggestibility may be tested if the patient shows dissociative symptoms. A high degree of suggestibility need not be a weakness but can be a strength used for therapeutic purposes. Thus, suggestibility is not a symptom of a psychiatric disorder. However, high suggestibility is a prerequisite for dissociative disorders and conversion disorder, in which a patient nearly automatically convinces him- or herself of being amnestic of a particular traumatic event (dissociative amnesia) or feels, for instance, that he or she is paralyzed (conversion disorder).

The interviewer uses some of the cognitive tests in most diagnostic interviews—that is, vigilance or concentration, short- and long-term memory, orientation, abstract thinking, and intelligence. Severe anxiety, major depression with psychomotor retardation, and attention-deficit/hyperactivity disorder (ADHD) may interfere with concentration and lead to the impression of an impaired recent memory. If the interviewer evidences poor concentration, he or she should make an effort to obtain error-free immediate recall. Major depression and other noncognitive psychiatric disorders may interfere only with retrieval of information and not with storage. Hints or multiple-choice options may help to overcome the retrieval block. If storage of information is impaired, such as in dementia of Alzheimer's type, this help fails. The interviewer may focus on evaluating abstract thinking (Table 7.1–6) and intelligence testing if the quality of the patient's answers during the interview suggests that concentration, orientation, and memory are intact. The interviewer selects any one of the other tests in Table 7.1–6 when he or she believes that a particular function may be impaired and needs documentation.

If not already assessed, at the end of the mental status examination, the interviewer evaluates four risk factors for the patient's and others' safety, summarized by the acronym SOAP. The interviewer explores which of the major psychiatric disorders is responsible for these key risk factors and makes plans for their immediate management.

Suicidality, homicidality, physically assaultive, unpredictable, explosive, and self-injurious behaviors and implied or overt threats.

Organic disturbances of cognitive functions: disorientation, memory disturbances, decline of executive functions, aphasias and apraxias that prevent the patient from exercising the activities of daily living (ADL).

Alcohol and other substance abuse, ranging from occasional social use to uncontrollable addictive behavior and dependency that may endanger the patient's and others' safety on the road and in legal, marital, occupational, and financial status.

Psychotic features, such as delusions, especially delusions of control, and hallucinations, especially command hallucinations, and their dangerousness and the patient's obedience to these experiences. Included here are illogical thinking and speech and catatonic behavior.

The interviewer compares the patient's psychiatric history with the patient's mental status to confirm the diagnostic impression. Inconsistencies have to be explored. Such inconsistencies may raise the possibility of incomplete assessment by the interviewer or of factitious intentions, lying, or malingering on the patient's part.

DIAGNOSIS

For the treatment plan, the interviewer verifies one or more Axis I or II, or both, psychiatric diagnoses and excludes others. The interviewing style matches the patient's responses. Usually, a strategy that strikes a balance between a disorder- and a patient-centered approach is appropriate. The diagnostic process can be arbitrarily divided into five phases.

Phase 1: Assessing the Chief Complaint

To choose an opening for the chief complaint is the beginning of a chain of eight decisions (A to H) in a diagnostic loop (Fig. 7.1–1). The interviewer may link these decisions in an order suggested by the clues that the patient offers.

Openings for Chief Complaint

The interviewer selects one out of several possible openings that leads to the patient's genuine chief complaint (Box A in Fig. 7.1–1). Below are some options.

DIRECT QUESTIONING "What brought you here?" "What kind of problems do you have?" "What's going on in your life?"

Such questions target the patient's chief complaint and may lead to the history of the present illness.

CONFRONTATION WITH A SIGN The interviewer confronts the patient with a possible sign of a mental illness, such as wearing dark glasses indoors, walking with a cane, exuding the smell of alcohol, or having slurred speech, cold and clammy hands, ataxic gait, or bruises on the face.

I: I notice you are wearing dark glasses.

P: (Looking behind the interviewer at the door, whispering) Yes, I don't like people to see my eyes. They can look right through me and read my mind.

I: Is this fear the reason why you came?

P: My colleagues at work really look at me. They want to get into my head, but I won't let them.

Such an entry leads the interviewer to the chief complaint, the history of present illness, and the mental status evaluation.

MEDICAL HISTORY

P: (Obviously anxious; her hands make wet imprints on the interviewer's desk)

I: Have you ever been to a psychiatrist's office before?

P: Never. I'm so ashamed. Why do you have "Psychiatric Center" written above your door? I had a hard time coming because of that.

I: Well, have you had the same feeling at your family doctor's office?

P: Of course not.

I: What did you see the general practitioner for?

P: Oh, I have a thyroid condition. I'm on Synthroid.

I: Any other medicines you take?

Here, the interviewer shows sensitivity to the patient's anxiety. To give the patient time to calm down, the interviewer assesses the

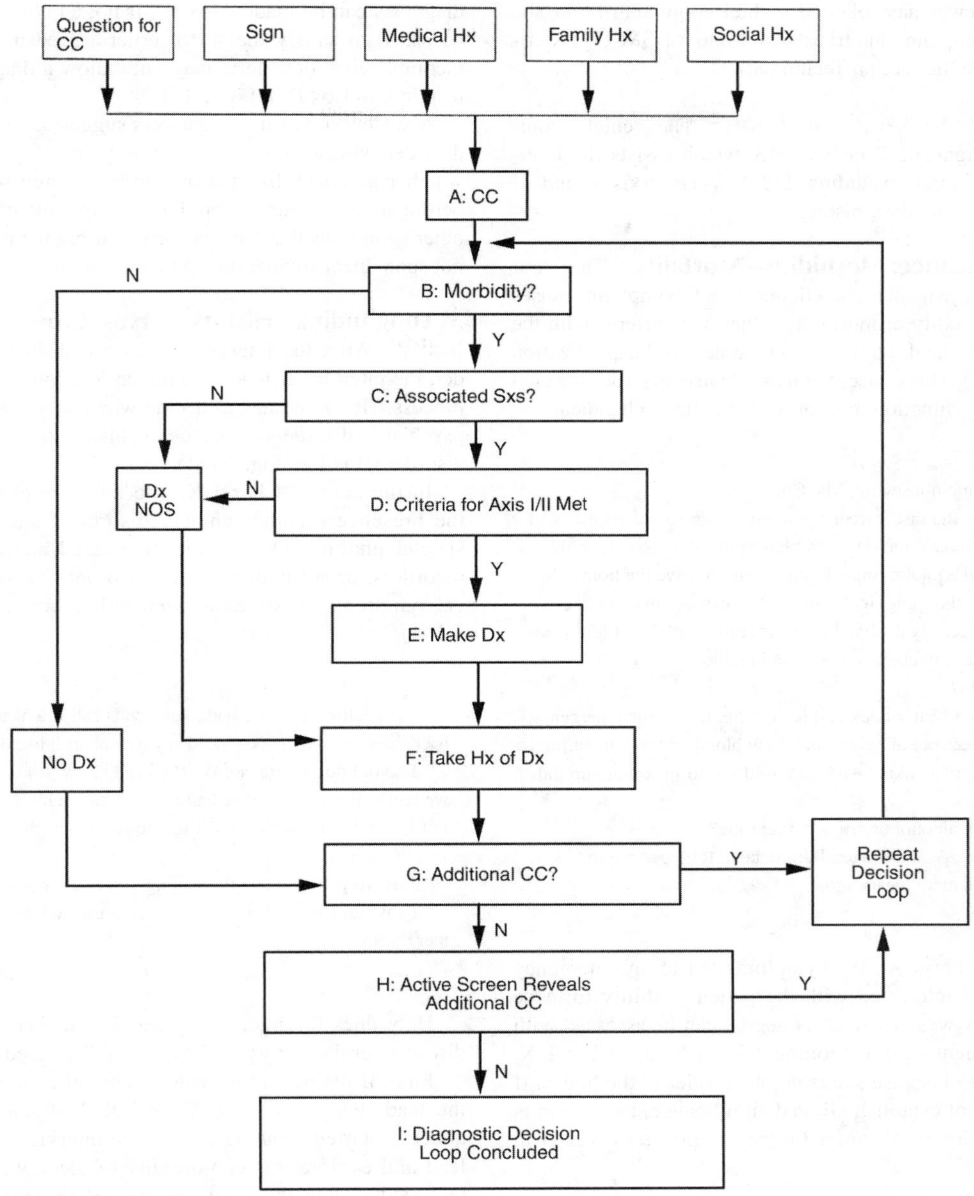

FIGURE 7.1–1 Diagnostic decision loop for psychiatric disorders. CC, chief complaint; Dx, diagnosis; Hx, history; N, no; NOS, not otherwise specified; Sxs, symptoms; Y, yes.

medical history first before returning to the psychiatric chief complaint, which may center on anxiety and persecutory thoughts.

FAMILY HISTORY

P: (After the greeting ceremony) I never thought I would have to see a psychiatrist myself.

I: Oh? Who had to see a psychiatrist before you?

P: My mother did. She was in and out of psychiatric hospitals.

I: Tell me about it. It may give us some clues about your own problem.

Family history provides a link to the chief complaint.

SOCIAL HISTORY

P: (Looking around, anxious) I didn't expect Monet and Degas prints at a doctor's office.

I: Do you have any art background?

P: Well, not really, but I'm a professional fundraiser, and sometimes we run into some interesting pieces. I have developed an eye for it. And art really interests me.

I: How long have you been into fundraising?

P: For 12 years now. And it hasn't always been easy.

The interviewer picks up on the patient's clue and starts with the social history, which leads to stressors in the patient's life and offers an entry for the chief complaint.

After the interviewer has solicited a chief complaint, he or she clarifies the chief complaint and translates it into a DSM-IV-TR criterion if possible (see the section Technique).

Phase 2: Diagnostic Decision Loop The chief complaint leads to a diagnostic decision loop, which assists the interviewer in including and excluding DSM-IV-TR Axis I and II disorders and in assessing their history.

Clinical Significance: Morbidity—Mortality The first step is to determine whether the elicited chief complaint causes increased risk of mortality or morbidity—that is, interferes with the patient's life, work, or health or requires treatment or hospitalization (Box B in Fig. 7.1–1). This concept of a psychiatric disorder is based on the presence of dysfunction that causes the patient a handicap.

A 27-year-old white housewife, Ms. Cheryl X.

I: You say that for the last 3 weeks you have been so scared that you cannot go to the mailbox. What other problems have you experienced?

P: I startle when the phone rings. I don't want to leave the house. My husband has to do the shopping. It all started 3 weeks ago in church. I had to run out of the service. My husband came after me, and then I felt like a knife was rammed into my chest. I could not breathe.

I: What did you do?

P: I thought I had a heart attack and had to die. But in the emergency room, they took an electrocardiogram and drew blood and told me after a few hours that my heart is okay. And they told me to make an appointment with you.

I: Did you use any alcohol or drugs at that time?

P: No. Drugs never. As a teenager, I drank beer. It helped me to talk to the boys. But that was many years ago.

In the case of Cheryl X., the symptoms led to an emergency department visit and interfered with the patient's ability to leave the house. Morbidity was obvious. Its degree can be assessed with the Global Assessment of Functioning (GAF) Scale. Cheryl X. may be rated GAF 35 because she is not able to leave the house. If the interviewer cannot establish clinical significance, the option is to diagnose no psychiatric disorder (a "no" response to Box B in Fig. 7.1–1).

Symptoms Associated and Not Associated with the Chief Complaint The interviewer gathers symptoms that occur approximately at the same time as the chief complaint (Box C in Fig. 7.1–1). Excluded should be symptoms, signs, or laboratory results that the chief complaint suggests but cannot be verified.

In the case of Cheryl X., the interviewer found psychiatric symptoms associated with the chief complaint. At the same time, the interviewer excluded cardiac disorders and drug and alcohol abuse as associated conditions. Infrequently, the interviewer may elicit a chief complaint without being able to identify associated symptoms. In this case, he or she considers a psychiatric disorder not otherwise specified (NOS), or, if clinical significance is lacking, he or she may not diagnose a psychiatric disorder at all (a "no" response to Box C in Fig. 7.1–1).

Criteria for Axis I or II Met? After the interviewer has elicited with open-ended questions a list of symptoms associated with the chief complaint, he or she checks whether sufficient criteria for an Axis I or II disorder are met (Box D in Fig. 7.1–1). If yes, the diagnosis can be made (Box E). If no, additional questions have to be asked to satisfy the set of criteria needed for a diagnosis. An incomplete set of criteria may only allow a diagnosis NOS (a "no" response to Box D in Fig. 7.1–1).

Ms. Cheryl X.'s initial answers suggest the onset of Axis I panic disorder with agoraphobia. At this point, the interviewer may ask whether an attack like the one during church service had occurred before and, if so, how often. Furthermore, the interviewer may elicit other symptoms that have occurred during the panic attack but were not spontaneously mentioned by the patient.

Longitudinal History versus Cross-Sectional Comorbidity After the interviewer has established a psychiatric disorder, the interviewer reaches a major decision point in the diagnostic process. He or she has to decide whether to assess other comorbid psychiatric disorders or pursue the history of the already established disorder (Box F in Fig. 7.1–1).

In the case of Cheryl X., the interviewer could either assess the presence of other anxiety disorders, such as social phobia, special phobias, OCD, and generalized anxiety disorder, mood disorders, or substance-related disorders or follow up on historical symptoms of panic disorder with agoraphobia (Box F in Fig. 7.1–1).

I: The attack that you had in church is called a panic attack. If you think back, have you ever experienced any type of spell like this?

P: No. I don't think so. Wait . . . You know, when I was in high school, we had to jog, and then we had to work on the high bar. All of a sudden, I felt I could not breathe, and I had to lie down. But I never had anything like that again.

I: Have you ever had the feeling you could not leave the house?

P: When I was 12, I did not want to go back to school after the summer vacation.

How does the interviewer decide whether to pursue comorbid disorders or the history of the already diagnosed disorder?

First, if the patient provides a clue, the interviewer may follow the lead. For instance, if Cheryl X. had said, "Since I had the attack, I started drinking again," the interviewer would follow this lead and explore this comorbidity of alcohol abuse. If Cheryl X. had said, "Now that you ask me all these questions about my attack, I think I've had some mild ones before," the interviewer would take the history of the panic disorder.

Second, the interviewer may follow up on comorbidity if the chief complaint or associated symptoms suggest the presence of a more serious psychiatric disorder. For instance, if Cheryl X. mentions she cannot go to the mailbox because the neighbors do not like her, the interviewer may want to explore the presence of ideas of reference or persecutory delusions. Such exploration may lead to disorders with psychotic features and reveal possible homicidal and suicidal tendencies.

Third, the clinical significance of the disorder may guide the interviewer: If the disorder is severe, the interviewer may pursue its history; if the disorder is mild, the interviewer may explore comorbidity to exclude a more severe disorder.

Fourth, if the patient is circumstantial or has difficulties in focusing or abstracting, the interviewer may complete the history of the disorder already diagnosed to avoid confusing the patient.

Finally, if leads are lacking, the interviewer is left with an arbitrary decision.

Search for an Additional Chief Complaint If the interviewer screens for comorbidity (a "yes" response to Box E in Fig. 7.1–1), he or she searches for an additional chief complaint.

> Ms. Cheryl X.
> I: Besides your panic attacks and your difficulty with leaving your home, do you have any other problems?

If Cheryl X. mentions a second chief complaint, the interviewer loops back to Box B, assessing clinical significance and associated symptoms (Box C), followed by the decision whether the symptoms fulfill sufficient criteria for an Axis I or II psychiatric disorder (Box D).

Depending on the symptomatology, the interviewer may complete the diagnostic decision loop B through H several times. With each newly made diagnosis, the interviewer lengthens the list of established Axis I and II disorders, shortens the list of unexplored disorders, and may add to the list of excluded disorders.

Screening for Additional Diagnoses If the interviewer runs dry of new chief complaints or significant psychiatric symptoms, he or she may switch from open-ended to closed-ended questions and actively screen for all those psychiatric disorders that have not been covered yet (Box H in Fig. 7.1–1). Closed-ended screening questions, most well researched, are reproduced in Table 7.1–7. For each positive answer, the interviewer may establish clinical significance. The Standardized Assessment of Personality–Abbreviated Scale (SAPAS) for example, may be a helpful screening tool for personality disorders.

If the patient endorses any of the symptoms targeted by the screening questions, the interviewer loops back in the diagnostic decision loop

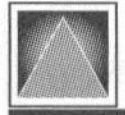

Table 7.1–7
Screen for Psychiatric Disorders (Axis I and II)

Disorder	Questions
Cognitive disorders	Use tests of memory, orientation, aphasia, and apraxia in Table 7.1–6.
Mental retardation	While you were in school, did anyone ever say that you were a very slow learner?
	Did you ever have to go into a special education class when you were in school?
Substance-related disorders	Has heavy drug or alcohol use ever caused you problems in your life?
	Have you ever used pot, speed, crack, heroin, ice, or any other drugs to make yourself feel good?
Psychosis	Have you ever heard voices or seen things that no one else could hear or see?
	Have you ever felt your mind or body was being secretly controlled or controlled somehow against your will?
	Have you ever felt others wanted to hurt you or really get you for some special reason, maybe because you had secrets or special powers of some sort?
	Have you ever had any other strange, odd, or very peculiar things happen to you?
	If yes to any of the above: Did this happen even when you were not drinking or taking drugs?
Bipolar disorder, manic episode	Have there ever been times when you felt unusually high, charged up, excited, or restless for 1 week at a time?
	Have there ever been times when other people said that you were too high, too charged up, too excited, or too talkative?
	Have these high, excitable moods ever stayed with you most of the time for at least 1 week?
Major depressive disorder	Have there ever been times when you felt unusually depressed, empty, sad, or hopeless for several days or weeks at a time?
	Have there ever been times when you felt very irritable or tired most of the time for hardly any reason at all?
	Have these feelings ever stayed with you most of the time for as long as 2 weeks?
Panic disorder	Have you ever had sudden spells or attacks of nervousness, panic, or a strong fear that just seems to come over you all of a sudden, out of the blue, for no particular reason?
	If yes: Did you have these attacks even though a doctor said that there was nothing seriously wrong with your heart?
Phobic disorders	Have you ever been much more afraid of things the average person is not afraid of? Like flying, heights, animals, needles, thunder, lightning, the sight of blood, or things like that?
	Have you ever been so afraid to leave home by yourself that you would not go out, even though you knew it was really safe?
	Have you ever been afraid to go into places like supermarkets, tunnels, or elevators because you were afraid of not getting out?
	Have you ever been so afraid of embarrassing yourself in public that you would not do certain things most people do? Like eating in a restaurant, using a public restroom, or speaking out in a room full of people?
	If yes to any of the above: When your fears were the strongest, did you try to avoid or stay away from (name feared stimulus) whenever you could?
Obsessive-compulsive disorder	Have you ever been bothered by certain embarrassing, scary, or ridiculous thoughts that came into your mind over and over even though you tried to ignore or stop them?
	If yes: Please describe them.
	Have you ever felt you had to repeat a certain act over and over even though it did not make much sense? Like checking or counting something over and over or washing your hands over and over again, although you knew they were clean?
Posttraumatic stress disorder	Have you ever experienced flashbacks when you found yourself reliving some terrible experience over and over again?

(*continued*)

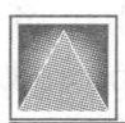

Table 7.1–7 (*continued*)

Disorder	Questions
Generalized anxiety disorder	Have there ever been days at a time when you felt extremely nervous, anxious, or tense for no special reason?
	If yes: Have you sometimes felt this way even when you were at home with nothing special to do?
	If yes: Have these nervous or anxious feelings ever bothered you off and on for as long as 6 months or more at a time?
Somatization disorder	Have you had a lot of physical problems in your life that forced you to see different doctors?
	If yes: Have doctors had trouble finding what caused these physical problems?
	Did you start having any of these problems before you were 30 years of age?
Dissociative disorder	Do you experience at times a loss of memory for hours or longer without being under the influence of a drug?
	If yes: Do you travel during such periods?
	Have you felt not yourself, or have you been told that you use a name other than your own?
Sexual disorders	Do you have problems with your sex life?
	Do you get sexually aroused by exposing yourself, by female undergarments, by rubbing against nonconsenting people, or by children?
	Do you intensely wish to be a member of the opposite sex?
Anorexia nervosa	Have you ever deliberately lost so much weight on a diet that people started to seriously worry about your health?
	If yes: Were you afraid of getting fat even when other people said you were thin enough?
Bulimia nervosa	Did you ever have a problem with binge eating, when you would eat so much food so fast that it made you feel sick?
	If yes: When you were doing this, did you feel your eating binges were not really normal?
	If yes: Was the urge to binge sometimes so strong that you could not stop, even though you wanted to?
	If yes: After you had binged, did you often feel depressed, ashamed, and disgusted with yourself?
	If yes: Did you ever vomit after eating, use laxatives, or excessively exercise?
Adjustment disorder	In the last 3 months, have you been very worried or upset about something that happened to you? Like the death of a loved one, loss of a job, separation, divorce, an accident, serious illness, or that sort of thing?
	If yes: Do you feel that you had more trouble handling this situation than most people would have had?
Sleep disorders	Do you have insomnia or inability to fall asleep or wake up at a desired time?
	Do you have sleep attacks during the day, or do you feel always tired?
	Do you snore or wake up gasping for air?
	Do you have nightmares, wake up in terror, or do you sleepwalk?
Personality disorders	
Cluster A	Are you a person who usually is suspicious of other people, who does not care much about the company of other people, or who realizes that things have a second meaning beneath the surface?
Cluster B	Are you a person who feels that if you want to be paid attention to and be respected you have to really put it on, express yourself loudly, and make your point?
	Do you feel you are denied what you are entitled to?
Cluster C	Are you a person who, to feel less anxious, tries to be perfect, gives in to others, does what they want to do, or tries to avoid public exposure?

Adapted from Othmer E, Penick EC, Powell BJ. *Psychiatric Diagnostic Interview-Revised (PDI-R). Manual and Administration Booklet.* Los Angeles: Western Psychological Services; 1989.

to search for clinical significance (Box B) and associated symptoms (Box C in Fig. 7.1–1). This active process often yields psychiatric disorders in remission, especially substance-related disorders, and disorders that start during childhood, such as learning disabilities, attention-deficit disorder with and without hyperactivity, conduct disorder, and personality disorders. Active screening for the disorders (Box H in Fig. 7.1–1) assures their inclusion in the multiaxial diagnoses and their effect as predisposing factors for current psychiatric disorders (Table 7.1–8). Instruments such as the Psychiatric Diagnostic Interview (PDI) or the Structured Clinical Interview for DSM-IV may ensure diagnostic thoroughness. The interviewer may also keep track of all disorders excluded by negative answers to the screen, thus lengthening the list of excluded psychiatric disorders.

Taking the Psychiatric History After the interviewer has established the presence of one or more psychiatric Axis I and II disorders, he or she establishes their history if not already done during the diagnostic looping. The interviewer may follow a timeline, going either backward from the present (e.g., when did it happen last before this time) or forward, starting with childhood. Important points of the history are onset, course, and treatment responses.

The onset can be assessed with a double question: When did you first notice a symptom of your present psychiatric disorder? Up to which age do you feel you were at your best and had no psychiatric problems?

Often, patients give different ages for the end of their healthy, premorbid state and the beginning of their psychiatric disorder.

> I: When did you first experience any problems with depression?
>
> P: During the seventh grade, I had a time where I did not want to get out of bed, felt tired and sad all the time, and did not even want to talk to my friends on the phone.
>
> I: For how long did this last?
>
> P: Two or 3 months.

I: If you look back on your life, when was the last time that you felt at your best and did not have any problems?

P: Maybe when I was 8 years old. I remember in the second or third grade, I was often tearful for no reason. It did not last very long. My mother told me that I was very sensitive.

The answers to these two questions indicate that the patient had either a preexisting personality disorder or a prolonged prodromal state to the onset of his or her major depressive disorder. This dual questioning is a powerful tool to identify premorbid states, personality disorders, and prodromal states to Axis I psychiatric disorders.

The onset of personality disorders can be traced back by focusing on a symptom or behavior of which the patient is aware, such as shyness or problems with authority figures. For example: When did you first notice that you were shy? When did you first notice that you rebelled against authority figures?

An alternate approach is to identify a present conflict that the interviewer judges to be due to a personality disorder and search the patient's past for similar conflicts. The interviewer should be able to trace personality disorders back to at least teenage years because they represent lifelong patterns of maladjusted behaviors. The course of the psychiatric disorder can help to confirm the presence of the Axis I disorders.

To draw a profile of the course of a psychiatric disorder gives an idea about exacerbations and remissions. Of importance are the intervals in which the disorder appears to be in remission. These intervals can identify the patient's capacity of functioning when relatively well and can help to define the goal of treatment. Patients often have difficulties in relating their psychiatric history to calendar years. The interviewer should introduce anchors of memorable events, such as getting married, moving, or job changes.

History of treatment responses provides information about what treatments have led to improvement, remission, failure, or adverse effects. Treatment response may be judged as being consistent or not consistent with the diagnosis.

Psychiatric Disorders in Full or Partial Remission The diagnostic decision loop also helps to detect psychiatric disorders in full or partial remission. They can be listed according to the developmental stages before adulthood such as disorders diagnosed in infancy, childhood, and adolescence.

Phase 3: History and Database Diagnosing psychiatric disorders may arouse the patient's sensitivities and activate defenses. Such responses are mostly absent when family, medical, and even social history and routine mental status items are assessed. Therefore, the interviewer can take a disorder-centered approach.

Medical History (Axis III) The medical history is of importance to the psychiatric interviewer for three reasons: (1) Medical disorders can cause symptoms of panic, anxiety, depression, and delusional thinking diagnosed as "psychiatric disorder due to a medical condition;" (2) side effects of medications prescribed for medical disorders may mimic psychiatric symptoms and disorders; and (3) any medical disorder and its treatment can complicate course and treatment of psychiatric disorders and vice versa. Drug–drug interactions can range from mild to severe.

Biopsychosocially, a chronic medical disorder may be a predisposing and perpetuating factor of a psychiatric disorder. The onset of a severe medical disorder may precipitate a psychiatric disorder (Table 7.1–7).

A 51-year-old farmer without a family or personal history of any psychiatric disorder developed a severe depression after he had a myocardial infarction. He feared that his physical incapacity to work might prevent him from paying off his expensive equipment.

The absence of a medical disorder in combination with good health maintenance is a protective factor in the fight against psychiatric disorders. A dual approach helps to detect medical disorders, asking open endedly for the patient's medical health and reviewing all systems as usually done in general medicine. The open-ended questions may be followed by a request to list all medical disorders that the patient presently is treated for, by what specialist, and with which medications. A history of surgeries and medication allergies rounds up this first approach. The review of systems covers all medical specialties.

Family History Psychiatric Axis I and II disorders are familial. Monozygotic twin and adoption studies suggest that the familial occurrence is not merely learned but follows a genetic disposition. The familial occurrence in first-degree relatives and their treatment response can therefore confirm the patient's diagnosis and predict

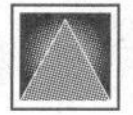

Table 7.1–8
Biopsychosocial Conditions Presenting as Predisposing, Precipitating, Perpetuating, and Protective Factors of Psychiatric Axis I Disorders

Factor	Bio	Psycho	Social
Predisposing	Positive psychiatric family history; delay in reaching developmental milestones; psychiatric disorders first diagnosed in infancy, childhood, or adolescence; medical history (head injury, central nervous system disorders Axis III)	Impaired premorbid personality, isolation, suspiciousness, poor impulse control, anxiousness, perfectionism, presence of personality disorders (Axis II), low adaptive defense mechanisms	Neglect, abuse, low education, poor parental role models, antisocial behavior, substance use, poverty
Precipitating	Onset of severe medical disorders	Stress intolerance, poor impulse control, self-pity, blaming (projection)	Trauma, loss of job or partner, increased stress (Axis IV)
Perpetuating	Chronic medical illness	Poor insight, judgment, and impulse control; low IQ; noncompliance with Rx.	Social isolation, unemployment, poverty
Protective	Good health maintenance, absence of chronic medical disorders	Good insight, judgment, and impulse control; high IQ; compliance with Rx. (high ego strength, high adaptive defense mechanisms)	Extended support system; well-paying, satisfying job

IQ, intelligence quotient; Rx., prescription.

the treatment response. Furthermore, the parental natural history may provide a prognostic look into the patient's course. Therefore, family history is the most important predisposing factor of the biological part of the patient's biopsychosocial condition. The drawing of a pedigree with men as squares and women as circles is an effective way to assess the family history with the patient's collaboration. Psychiatrically affected members are represented by blackened shapes, questionable members are striped. Names, ages, type of disorder, and treatment all fit into the genogram.

Developmental History Even if a psychiatric diagnosis during childhood or adolescence is not made, the interviewer should consider five important areas:

Developmental milestones: delayed psychomotor and speech development and toilet training may point to early developmental problems.

Ability to learn in school: slow learning or repetition of the first grade may point to mental retardation; circumscribed deficits, such as dyslexia or acalculia, may indicate a learning disorder.

Attention problems with hyperactivity and poor impulse control may contribute to substance abuse and to the development of a personality disorder, such as antisocial personality disorder.

Disciplinary problems may cover a broad range. Arguments with teachers, objections to rules, temper tantrums, resentfulness, and vindictiveness point to oppositional defiant disorder. Fighting, stealing, vandalism, and school discipline problems characterize males; lying, truancy, running away from home, substance use, and prostitution characterize females with conduct disorder. Furthermore, symptoms such as violent behavior toward superiors, peers, or animals and fire setting also suggest conduct disorder, which, in later adolescence, may progress to antisocial personality disorder. The earlier the onset of conduct disorder, the worse the prognosis and the greater the risk for later mood, anxiety, somatoform, and substance-related disorders.

During childhood and adolescence, social withdrawal with decline in hygiene, truancy, and anger outbursts may herald schizophrenia; phobias, obsessions, compulsions, and depressive symptoms may precede adulthood psychiatric disorders.

Social History A biographical, detailed social history of key life events may be informative but may not serve the assessment of social factors in the patient's psychiatric disorders. The relationship between social factors and psychiatric disorders is reciprocal. To tease out this reciprocal relationship is the interviewer's task in addition to sociodemographic fact finding. The interviewer should target four topics:

Premorbid versus postmorbid psychosocial functioning. Premorbid functioning represents the highest level of patient performance measurable by the social component of the GAF. The difference between the present and the past GAF scores measures the morbidity caused by the psychiatric disorder. The return to the premorbid level of functioning is a goal of psychosocial rehabilitation. Therefore, the interviewer wants to clarify the patient's premorbid versus postmorbid level of functioning with respect to family life and work, including school and military, friends, and community functions such as church and social organizations.

Social factors as risks for psychiatric disorders. Social factors can predispose to a psychiatric disorder, precipitate its onset, perpetuate its course, or protect the patient against morbid influences (Table 7.1–7). A history of physical, sexual, and emotional abuse, rejection and neglect during upbringing, and provision of poor role models can become a predisposing factor for the development of psychiatric disorders. For instance, patients with dissociative disorders, including dissociative identity disorder, often report a history of physical and sexual abuse, especially during childhood. Barring memory distortions, the presence of abuse can often be confirmed by outside evidence. Severe life-threatening trauma can predispose and precipitate the onset of posttraumatic stress disorder (PTSD). Acute or chronic stressors, single or multiple, can predispose, precipitate, and perpetuate adjustment disorders with symptoms of depression, anxiety, or disturbances in conduct. These factors are listed on Axis IV as psychosocial and environmental problems.

Social support. In contrast, the absence of abuse, rejection, and neglect and the presence of strong, positive role models and an extensive support system in the past and present that secured adequate childrearing and education can be strong protective factors against exacerbations of psychiatric disorders. Social support can improve prognosis. It can motivate the patient to comply with treatment.

Negative impact of psychiatric disorders on social advancement. Psychiatric disorders can impede the patient's social development and can lead to demotion, job loss, and divorce.

Mental Status Exploration and Testing The interviewer monitors the patient's mental status throughout the interview. Toward the end, the interviewer usually addresses some mental status areas directly, especially by exploration (Tables 7.1–3, 7.1–4, and 7.1–5) and testing (Table 7.1–6). If not previously assessed, the interviewer explores risk factors such as suicidality, homicidality, cognitive impairment, substance abuse, and psychotic symptomatology, including command hallucinations.

Phase 4: Diagnosing and Feedback

Throughout the session, the interviewer collects data that he or she organizes in a biopsychosocial formulation—assets and strengths, differential diagnoses, if applicable, and multiaxial diagnosis. He or she feeds this information back to the patient when the interviewer discusses the evaluation of the patient. The interviewer also uses this information in phase 5 when he or she proposes the treatment plan and discusses the prognostic outcome.

Biopsychosocial Formulation The interviewer may summarize the findings of the session in the form of a biopsychosocial formulation. The biopsychosocial conditions that contribute to the development, onset, and course of a psychiatric disorder can be classified according to their impact as predisposing, precipitating, perpetuating, or protective factors (Table 7.1–8).

Assets and Strengths The interviewer also assesses the patient's assets and strengths. This evaluation should be made in descriptive terms. It includes the patient's knowledge, interest, skills, aptitude, experience, education, and employment status, all items that are closely related to the protective factors of Table 7.1–8.

Differential Diagnosis Initial psychiatric diagnostic interviews may yield incomplete, vague, and contradictory information so that the interviewer believes he or she cannot make a diagnosis with confidence. A differential diagnosis that weighs the pros and cons for a group of Axis I and II psychiatric disorders may then take the place of a specific diagnosis. The advantage of the differential diagnosis is that it comprehensively captures the perimeter of psychopathology that the interviewer takes into account.

Multiaxial Diagnosis DSM-IV-TR encourages multiple diagnoses on Axis I and II. The more pervasive disorder receives priority over the less pervasive one. For instance, a patient who has the diagnosis of schizophrenia may not receive the additional diagnosis of dysthymic disorder because dysthymic disorder is believed to be an associated feature of schizophrenia. If a psychiatric disorder is judged to be due to a medical condition, such as reserpine-induced depressive disorder, the interviewer should not make the additional diagnosis of major depressive disorder. DSM-IV-TR uses a host of specifiers to increase the precision of the diagnosis. Their discussion exceeds the frame of this chapter. However, some determinations are particularly useful:

Principal diagnosis. The interviewer assigns this determination to the psychiatric disorder that most reliably and comprehensively explains the present symptomatology and is the focus of treatment.

Provisional diagnosis. The interviewer believes a patient fulfills sufficient criteria for a particular psychiatric diagnosis; however, the interviewer lacks documentation for some of the criteria.

Psychiatric disorder NOS. The patient does not have sufficient symptoms to fulfill criteria for a specific diagnosis, even though the information appears accurate and complete.

Past psychiatric diagnosis. This widespread term is replaced in DSM-IV-TR by specifiers such as "in full remission, partial remission, or residual state."

Axis III Disorders These are the medical disorders. If a medical disorder is considered as the cause of the psychiatric disorder, it is listed on Axis I as a mental disorder due to a general medical condition and on Axis III as medical disorder.

Axis IV On Axis IV, the interviewer lists psychosocial and environmental problems that were present during the preceding year of the diagnosis and that may affect diagnosis, treatment, course, and prognosis. However, stressors that clearly relate to the present psychiatric disorder, such as a life-threatening trauma in PTSD, may also be included even if they fall outside the 1-year time frame. DSM-IV-TR lists nine categories that usually qualify as stressors: problems with primary support group, social environment, education, occupation, housing, economics, health care access, legal system, and psychosocial and environmental.

Axis V: Global Assessment of Functioning The GAF scale is a dual scale. It measures two aspects of psychiatric disorders: severity of symptoms and level of psychosocial functioning. It ranges from 100 (superior functioning, no symptoms) to 1 (persistent danger to others and self with inability to maintain minimal personal hygiene). The interviewer assigns a score that reflects the lowest level of either of the two. This score can be assessed through key points of the patient's psychiatric history, and it can trace the course of the illness. Usually, the interviewer measures the present level of functioning and the highest level of functioning during the last year.

Phase 5: Treatment Plan and Prognosis In phase 5, the roles of interviewer and patient stay reversed: The interviewer answers the patient's asked or unasked questions. The interviewer decides first which level of care the patient requires. He or she discusses with the patient the diverse treatment options and their possible adverse effects. The interviewer may identify the immediate targets of treatment and tell the patient what to expect if he or she cooperates. The interviewer's interventions are most effective if he or she has been able to forge an alliance with the patient. If the patient is severely disabled, such as being suicidal, homicidal, violent, or psychotic, or has lost impulse control, is disoriented, or intoxicated, the patient may need hospitalization. Most patients can be treated as outpatients without interruption of their work schedule. Some need temporary disability or home supervision.

The interviewer designs a biopsychosocial treatment plan. To improve the biological condition, the interviewer may use medication. Most psychotropic medications have a delayed onset of action, as, for example, the selective serotonin reuptake inhibitors (SSRIs) and mood stabilizers. Therefore, the interviewer may, for the immediate temporary effect, combine substances with delayed onset of action with those with an immediate onset, such as anxiolytics, low dosages of atypical neuroleptics, and, in rarer cases, stimulants.

A woman who has a major depression with psychomotor retardation and no history of substance abuse who in 3 days wants to attend her daughter's wedding may be prescribed a stimulant for the day of the festivity. Furthermore, she may design strategies to manage key symptoms of the disorders behaviorally or cognitively. For the psychological dimension, the interviewer may design psychotherapeutic interventions used in cognitive therapy that increase insight, correct perceptual distortions and maladjusted behaviors, and support psychological functioning.

Social conditions may be improved, for instance, by activating family support, with short-term relief of stress by sick leave, by arranging vocational rehabilitation, or by facilitating the ventilation of traumatic events. Strategies used in interpersonal psychotherapy may help. Referral to a psychologist or social worker as case manager may be considered. The interviewer may contrast the natural history of the untreated disorder with the course that may be achieved if the patient cooperates fully and the treatment is effective. The patient's clear understanding of the difference can be a strong motivating factor for the patient's compliance.

PSYCHIATRIC INTERVIEW: A SAMPLE

The four components of interviewing are integrated and run simultaneously. Their course can be divided into five phases, illustrated in the sample interview below.

Phase 1: Warm-up and Chief Complaint The interviewer puts the patient and him- or herself at ease (rapport). The interviewer sets the scope of the open-ended screening questions (technique); observes the patient's appearance, movements, speech, and affect (mental status); and notices clues and the chief complaint (diagnosis).

Phase 2: Diagnostic Decision Loop Interviewer and patient forge an alliance (rapport). The interviewer progresses from questions with broader to narrower scope. In case of an acute trauma, such as in cases of bereavement, divorce, rape, or recently diagnosed cancer, the interviewer reduces anxiety by addressing the emotions evoked by the trauma (technique). He or she explores the thought content, such as hallucinations, delusions, obsessions, compulsions, avoidance behavior, panic attacks, and dangerousness to others and self (mental status). He or she relates the chief complaint to concurring symptoms, signs, precipitating events, and stressors. He or she verifies and excludes specific diagnoses (diagnosis).

Phase 3: History and Database The interviewer demonstrates expertise in handling the patient's problems and offers guidance (rapport). He or she transitions from topic to topic to fill in gaps, follow clues, and reconcile inconsistencies (technique). He or she probes judgment and insight and tests cognition and suggestibility (mental status). The interviewer assesses the patient's social, family, and medical history (diagnosis).

Phase 4: Diagnosing and Feedback The interviewer discusses the diagnosis with the patient and secures the patient's acceptance (rapport). He or she explains the nature of the disorder and the treatment options (technique). He or she reflects on the patient's behavior during the interview (mental status) and summarizes the diagnostic findings on five axes (diagnosis).

Phase 5: Treatment Plan and Prognosis The interviewer outlines the future therapeutic relationship, his or her availability, and the need for compliance (rapport) and obtains consent for the treatment plan (technique) using the patient's language and level of insight (mental status). The interviewer shares the prognostic outlook with the patient (diagnosis).

Sample Interview Ms. Lorraine R. is a 56-year-old, white, mildly obese female with puffy, red eyes, and washed out mascara who is tearful and shaking.

Phase 1: Warm-Up and Chief Complaint

(1) I: Hello, Ms. R. I'm Dr. O. Please come in and take a seat.

P: (Walking slowly into office, with a quivering voice) Hi. Please call me Lorraine. (slumping into the chair)

(2) I: What's going on? (Pause) You are all tears . . . .

P: (Looking up, sobbing, breathing rapidly, and pumping her shoulders) I cried all night. I heard my gynecologist's voice again and again: "Sorry, Ms. R. It's stage 1 breast cancer."

(3) I: Your friend Joan called me yesterday. She told me I really had to see you today.

P: Yeah. It hit me yesterday afternoon. (Crying) I called Joan because she went through the same thing.

(4) I: So that's why Joan called me.

P: Yes, she said you had helped her. (wipes her nose, stops crying)

(5) I: (Looking at her with concern) Hmm. I'm glad she feels this way.

P: (Wiping her eyes but with a firmer voice) I had the biopsy yesterday morning.

(6) I: When did he first suspect it?

P: (Even more collected) A week ago. I had a mammogram, and he told me he felt a lump.

(7) I: How did that strike you?

P: Like an out-of-body experience. I heard it without hearing it.

(8) I: And yesterday?

P: It hit me right here. (grabbing her chest) I couldn't stop crying. (her eyes fill with tears again)

RAPPORT The patient requested to be called by her first name, expressing her need to have a personal, close, possibly dependent relationship to the interviewer (answer 1 [A1]). The interviewer addressed the patient's tearful affect, thus immediately shifting toward a patient-centered interviewing mode. When the patient reported that she cried all night (A2), the interviewer avoided empathizing with her (Q3) by saying something such as, "You must have really been torn up." Instead of catharsis, the interviewer put her emotional pain into a social framework to remind her of her support system and steered her toward a cognitive management of her emotions. Referring to Joan, he introduced her relationship to the interviewer as a model of alliance.

TECHNIQUE The interviewer opens by addressing the patient's mental status. The patient responds by describing her chief complaint (Q2, A2). As a continuation technique, the interviewer points to the urgency of the patient's problems (Q3), which results in the description of the trauma and the patient's emotional response (A3 to A8) aided by specifiers (Q6 to Q8).

MENTAL STATUS The patient displayed a sad affect, which intensified when she reported the gynecologist's telephone call. However, this affect reacted to the interviewer's neutralizing remark (Q4, 5), excluding a melancholic depression. The patient's initial emotion to the gynecologist's telephone call indicated a dissociative traumatic response (A7), which raised the possibility that the patient is suggestible. The patient's emotional responsiveness confirmed her reactivity (A8) noted above (A4, 5), excluding the possibility that her affect was frozen into a depressive state but reacted according to thought content.

DIAGNOSIS In the dual opening approach, by asking for the chief complaint and by confronting the patient with her affect, the interviewer found an economic, individualized pathway to her chief complaint (Q2; Box A in Fig. 7.1–1). Clarifying her emotions (Q7), the interviewer found a dissociative traumatic response (A7), suggesting the onset of an acute stress disorder, which may turn into an acute PTSD if untreated. Alternatively, an adjustment disorder with mixed anxiety and depressed mood could be considered.

Phase 2: Diagnostic Decision Loop

(9) I: Could you sleep?

P: (Wiping her eyes again, even though she is not crying) Not at all. All night I heard the gynecologist's voice: (coldly) "Sorry, Ms. R., it's stage 1 breast cancer."

(10) I: So you relived the bad news . . .

P: (Interrupting) Over and over again. His voice stirred me up. (Sitting up erect) Like from a bad dream. After the mammogram, I was, like, in a daze. Nothing sank in. (Closes her eyes)

(11) I: So it really shook you up.

P: (Looking past the interviewer) Yeah. I forgot to make a new appointment. I didn't even fix my breakfast this morning. Felt, like, paralyzed. No appetite. (Bites her lower lip) Instead, I started smoking again. Five cigarettes yesterday and one this morning.

(12) I: Has anything like this ever happened to you before?

P: Not really . . . . when my husband asked me for a divorce I felt numbed at first, but we had problems for a long time.

(13) I: Ever felt down like you feel now?

P: (Tilting her head left to right) During the last 5 years, I felt down most of the time. I never felt really normal, but work kept me busy.

(14) I: Did you get any treatment for depression lately?

P: Not recently. Only for smoking. But 15 years ago, I was treated for depression with Prozac and then again 10 years ago before I got divorced.

(15) I: When you were depressed in the past, what changed in your life?

P: I stayed away from people (with a sigh), even from my own family. But I wanted them to tell me that that they love me. I did not want to do anything. I was so tired all the time, couldn't fall asleep but overslept in the mornings. I ate a lot of junk food and gained weight.

(16) I: How did you value your life then?

P: I dropped to an all-time low.

(17) I: Did you ever want to die?

P: I wished I wouldn't wake up in the morning.

(18) I: Ever tried to do anything to hurt or kill yourself?

P: (With a frown) I thought about it, but I have my children.

(19) I: Did you get down when you had your children?

P: No.

(20) I: The baby blues?

P: (With an open smile) No. I felt good.

(21) I: Did those suicidal thoughts come back since yesterday?

P: (Firmly) No. I want to live.

(22) I: When you felt down and depressed, did you ever feel that people were against you?

P: I was hiding from them.

(23) I: Did you ever get so down that your thoughts became loud?

P: I thought I was worthless.

(24) I: Did you hear voices telling you that?

P: No, just my thoughts.

(25) I: Ever heard any voices when nobody was around?

P: No. (Frowning) I don't think I was crazy. (Shaking her head)

(26) I: So your depression was never so severe that you heard voices or that you were serious about killing yourself?

P: I thought I was losing it, but I didn't hear or see things. And then I would smoke more and that helped my mood.

(27) I: Did your mood ever become so good that you were full of energy or didn't seem to need much sleep?

P: (With a laugh) I don't think so.

(28) I: Ever become hypersexual . . . . have affairs . . . . (patient frowns and shakes her head), or go on buying sprees?

P: Sometimes when I was depressed, I liked to buy things, but it didn't make me feel better. (The corners of her mouth drop)

(29) I: Have cleaning sprees?

P: (With a sour smile) No, just chain-smoking sprees.

(30) I: Were you a heavy smoker?

P: Two and a half packs a day. (Looking down) But I quit 3 months ago. (Looking the interviewer in the eye)

(31) I: What helped you quit?

P: (Fast, with a firm voice and nodding) The patches and Zyban. I took them for 2 months.

(32) I: How did that help you?

P: (Smiling) It lifted my mood, too.

(33) I: You felt depressed?

P: I think I have always been somewhat unhappy—for the last 4 or 5 years, or more. Did not want to do much, was irritable and anxious, and cried easily. (Swallows)

(34) I: Did you ever feel better in between?

P: (Shaking her head) Maybe for a few weeks, but it never lasted.

(35) I: How did Zyban help?

P: I started to do more things and felt better. I could stop smoking.

(36) I: Did you drink also?

P: (With disgust) I hate alcohol. It makes me woozy.

(37) I: Do you drink coffee?

P: No. I drink soda pop with caffeine.

RAPPORT Rapport remained intact. The patient actively participated in the interview, interrupting the interviewer (A10) and volunteering details in answering the interviewer's expert questions, thus engaging in a cooperative alliance (A9 to 11, 14, 15, 26, 28, 30, 33). Her answers portrayed good insight into the pathological nature of her mood symptoms. The interviewer worded the empathic statement (Q11) in a manner that elicited a description of her traumatic symptoms. Because the patient showed her emotions freely, the interviewer believed that the patient was comfortable with him (A9 to 11, 13, 15, 18, 20, 21, 27 to 34, 36), making interventions to improve rapport unnecessary.

TECHNIQUE The interviewer completed the coverage of the topic of her recent traumatic response (Q9 to 12). She followed the interviewer's smooth transition when the interviewer screened for depression (Q13 to 15), suicidal tendencies (Q16 to 18), postpartum depression (Q19, 20), psychotic symptoms (Q22 to 26), mania (Q27 to 29), nicotine addiction (Q30 to 32), dysthymia (Q33 to 35), and alcohol (Q36) and caffeine use (Q37). The interviewer overcame the patient's evasive answers (A22, 23, 26) by more direct questions for hallucinations (Q24, 25) and by summarizing the patient's responses (Q26). The patient agreed with all the interviewer's summaries, documenting good verbal understanding (Q10, 11, 26).

MENTAL STATUS The patient responded with relevant details to closed-ended questions or statements (Q9 to 14, 17 to 30, 33, 34, 36, 37), showing that she remained verbally productive in spite of her depressed affect. She handled open-ended questions in an appropriate, goal-directed manner (Q15, 16, 31, 32, 35), showing her ability to focus and to interpret questions accurately. Her affect remained reactive and was appropriate to the content of her answers (A9 to 11, 13, 15, 18, 20, 21, 25, 27 to 32, 36) but showed a depressive quality (A9, 11, 15, 18).

DIAGNOSIS The interviewer assessed symptoms associated with the chief complaint (Q9 to 11; Box C in Fig. 7.1–1), reliving the traumatic experience, derealization (A10), and impaired functioning (A10, 11; Box B in Fig. 7.1–1), confirming the initial impression of a first-time acute traumatic disorder (A12; Box D in Fig. 7.1–1). With Q13, the interviewer searched for a second chief complaint (a "yes" response to Box G in Fig. 7.1–1) and found 5 years of anhedonia (A13, 33 to 35) with only short remissions of a few weeks (A34), suggesting dysthymic disorder, which the interviewer did not pursue any further. The interviewer also established clinical significance for a third chief complaint, depression (A14; a "yes" response to Box G in Fig. 7.1–1). This chief complaint was associated with several symptoms (Box C in Fig. 7.1–1): social withdrawal, loss of initiative, tiredness and insomnia (A15), death wish (A17), suicidal ideation, feelings of worthlessness (A23), and losing her mind (A26). A history of suicide attempts (A18) or present suicidal thoughts (A21) were missing. These findings confirmed the diagnosis of major depressive disorder currently in remission (A14; Box D in Fig. 7.1–1). The patient denied persecutory delusions (A23) or hallucinations (A23 to 26), excluding a major depression, severe, with psychotic features (Box D in Fig. 7.1–1).

Actively, the interviewer screened for essential symptoms of other psychiatric disorders (Box H in Fig. 7.1–1). The interviewer excluded mania (A27 to 29) and alcohol abuse (A36; Box H in Fig. 7.1–1) but found evidence for nicotine dependence in early partial remission (A29 to 33). The reported depressed, irritable, and anxious feelings (A33) may have been related to nicotine dependence and intermittent withdrawal because smoking relieved the depressed feelings (A26). Alternatively, the depressive symptoms could be part of a dysthymic disorder with late onset (A33, 34) that, besides smoking, was improved by Zyban (bupropion) (A35).

Phase 3: History and Database

MEDICAL HISTORY

(38) I: What prescription medications or over-the-counter medicines do you take?

P: No prescriptions any more. My gynecologist stopped my hormones when he felt the lump. But I have a chronic cough, and I take some cough drops.

(39) I: Do you have any other medical problems? (Speaking slowly) Such as thyroid problems? Diabetes? High blood pressure? A head injury? Allergies?

P: (Shaking her head) No, not that I know of.

FAMILY HISTORY

(40) I: Who in your family had problems with mood like you?

P: My three kids are okay, but I'm adopted (her voice cracking). I don't know my biological parents or siblings.

(41) I: Your voice changed when you said adopted.

P: Yeah. My adoptive parents always told me I was special. (With sad contempt) Yes, special. I always fought rejection.

DEVELOPMENTAL HISTORY

(42) I: How did you feel in school?

P: I felt I had to prove myself, but I was a good student.

(43) I: And in front of a class? . . . or in front of strangers? Any spells of anxiety?

P: I got a lump in my throat and butterflies in my stomach, but it excited me. I could do it.

SOCIAL HISTORY AND SUPPORT

(44) I: How do you feel about rejection now?

P: That's the worst. I feel my daughter will stay away from me. She will reject me because of my cancer.

(45) I: Stay away from you? How's that?

P: Well . . . I stayed away from my cousin for her last year when she had breast cancer. I panicked when I saw her. I did not know how to deal with it. Now I feel I'll lose my daughter over this. And I don't know what to do.

(46) I: Do you have other children?

P: Yes. I also have two sons, all are from my ex.

(47) I: How is their support?

P: Good. But my daughter is my friend, and I hate to lose her. I couldn't bear it. None of my children know what depression is. They are all so healthy.

(48) I: What about your ex?

P: What's left of him is a big settlement. He divorced me to marry his secretary. He rejected me, too, when I went through the changes.

(49) I: So you experienced rejection. What images come to mind?

P: My cousin. (With expression of fear and disgust) How she shriveled away when she had cancer. How I could not take it when she shriveled away.

(50) I: So you can't shrivel away yourself.

P: You're right. But how do I do that?

(51) I: By rejecting yourself. Reject your cancer! Stay strong! Fear and depression may weaken your immune system.

P: Everybody tells me I can do it. My friends say I can fight it. (With a thin smile and frown) I heard it over and over again since yesterday.

(52) I: They don't want you to shrivel away.

P: That's right. They don't want me to shrivel away. (With a sigh of relief) They say it for their own sake.

(53) I: That's right. They don't want to see you shrivel away like your cousin. (With emphasis) Your friends and your daughter look at you as an example. They want you strong for their own sake. Do you have any ties to religion?

P: No. I'm not going to mass, but I believe in a higher power.

(54) I: Do you pray?

P: No.

(55) I: You told me you see your cousin shrivel away. Do you work through your eyes?

P: Yes. I'm an interior designer.

(56) I: Oh? How did that start?

P: I have a college degree in design. Decorating became my profession. I still enjoy my work and my colleagues.

MENTAL STATUS EXPLORATION AND TESTING

(57) I: So you can image things. We will use imagining to fight your fears and your depressions and teach you to imagine your cancer shriveling.

P: (Smiles)

(58) I: Let's see how strong your imagining is. Please pass me your ring. (The patient hands the interviewer her wedding band). I'm going to attach a string to your ring (interviewer does). Let me show you how one can move the ring with imagining. (The interviewer swivels his chair around away from his desk and sits now in front of the patient. The interviewer holds the string in his right hand and unsupported arm with the ring hanging 1 in. above the floor.) Now I can swing the ring around like this (swings the ring). I do this with my will power like we do many things. But I can also move the ring without swinging it voluntarily. (He brings the ring to a standstill.) I can just let it hang down and start imagining. I imagine now that the ring starts to swing . . . swing in a circle . . . swing in a circle (the ring moves slightly back and forth, not in a circle). Now I imagine that the ring swings in a circle, the circle gets rounder and rounder, the circle becomes bigger and bigger (the ring actually swings in a circle of a 5-in. diameter). You can train yourself in imagining. (The interviewer offers the string to the patient.) Now you try.

P: (Takes the string with the ring)

(59) I: Swing the ring around in a circle.

P: (Complies)

(60) I: That's what we don't want to do. We want to use our imagination. Hold the swinging.

P: (Complies)

(61) I: Now let the ring hang down still and start imagining that the ring starts moving. (The ring swings back and forth in a 1-in. swing). Now imagine that the ring starts to go in a circle, rounder and rounder, in a circle, bigger

and bigger. (The ring starts to move in a 3-in. circle). You can train yourself to do this. It's called the pendulum test. It tests your imagination.

In addition to the ring test, the interviewer also uses the sway test, the Spiegel Eye Test, and the finger sticking test (see X. Mental Status Examination). The four tests show the patient's moderate ability to follow images with motor action.

61. P: (Smiling and shaking her head as in disbelief) I can use my imagination to help me.

Because the interviewer is in a testing mode, he also examines orientation, recent memory, and abstraction by interpreting proverbs and identifying the common category of bicycle and airplane and finds the patient to be fully oriented and have intact cognitive functioning. Furthermore, the patient has at least average intelligence because she could multiply 2 × 192 on the Wilson Approximate Intelligence Test and by her responses to the Kent Test.

(62) I: We need your fighting spirit. Can you believe?

P: I don't trust easily.

(63) I: Can you believe in science?

P: I'm not sure.

(64) I: Do you believe in medical science?

P: I'm not sure, but I will do what they tell me.

(65) I: I'm so glad that your cancer was detected at an early stage and that you got your diagnosis 24 hours after the biopsy. That means treatment can start soon. Have you met the oncologist?

P: No. But I've heard of him. My friends recommend him.

(66) I: So you don't plan to go out of state to the X Institute?

P: No. I'll stay with the doctors here.

RAPPORT Reviewing the medical history signaled to the patient thoroughness and concern about her general health (Q38, 39). The interviewer addressed the cracking in her voice, showing sensitivity to her affect about her adoption (Q41). The interviewer used her fear of rejection (A41 to 45) to explore her own rejecting of the cousin. The interviewer channeled the patient's tendency to reject toward her cancer rather than toward herself (A51). The interviewer built up her confidence in her ability to imagine her cancer to shrivel (Q57) and to turn her imagination into action (Q58 to 61). This approach initiated her positive outlook and cognitive restructuring, including imagining. With these interventions, the interviewer added to the diagnosis-centered interview a patient-centered therapeutic intervention. Such ad hoc crisis intervention activated the therapeutic alliance and put guidance into action.

TECHNIQUE Using a smooth transition (Q38), the interviewer attempted to complete the database, opening up medical, family, developmental, and social history with open-ended questions (Q38, 40, 42, 44), followed by closed-ended questions and some open-ended ones (Q47 to 49). When the interviewer noticed a sign of fear and sadness in the patient's voice (A40), the interviewer clarified this sign (Q41) and searched for associated symptoms to be able to fit the sign into a possible diagnosis. Because the patient expressed fear and disgust (A49), the interviewer decided to make an immediate therapeutic intervention against her harmful self-image of shriveling away. The interviewer reverted the patient's tendency to project on herself to projecting on her cancer (Q51). This reversal fed into the supportive statements of the patient's friends (Q51 to 53) and initiated training in image control (Q55 to 61).

MENTAL STATUS The patient showed fear of abandonment (A40, 44), possibly based on her phobia of physically crippling disease, which she projects on her daughter. Tests of suggestibility (A58 to 61), orientation, recent memory, and abstraction are within the normal range. Suggestibility is tested for two reasons: (1) to examine whether increased suggestibility can lead to pathological autosuggestions (i.e., dissociative and conversion symptoms), and (2) to increase the patient's control over imaging directing it against her cancer.

DIAGNOSIS The medical history is positive for chronic cough (Q38, 39). The patient's fear of abandonment encountered during the assessment of the family history adds an additional chief complaint and reopens the diagnostic decision process (A40; Box F in Fig. 7.1–1). The interviewer screens the patient's developmental history for associated symptoms of fear of rejection. Social phobia and learning disability (A42) are excluded, but the patient's response suggests the possibility of generalized anxiety ("butterflies in my stomach"), somatization, or conversion symptoms ("lump in my throat;" A43). Obsessions and compulsions are not assessed. The fear of rejection (Q44) signifies a special phobia of physical decay (A49) also projected onto her daughter (A44, 45, 47), which intensifies her phobia of cancer. She fears less premature death than abandonment because of her physical decay. This specific phobia of a terminal, crippling disease (A45, Q49) is based on the defenses of suppression and repression operating on a high adaptive and mental inhibition level, respectively. Her projection operated on the disavowal level and not at the level of defensive dysregulation, as is the case in delusional projection. The coding of defenses on a sixth axis, the defensive functioning axis, is under consideration in the DSM-IV-TR.

The patient's average level of suggestibility may lower the risk that her acute stress disorder progresses to a PTSD with pathological dissociation (A61) as a result of negative autosuggestion. The interviewer limited the assessment of predisposing, precipitating, perpetuating, and protective factors for the social history taking to the extent that it may be relevant for Axis IV. For time reasons, the interviewer omitted exploration of relationships to parents, coworkers, and friends other than Joan. Besides her children, the patient did not seem to have support from her church or self-support from prayers (A53, 54) or confidence in medical science (Axis IV).

Phase 4: Diagnosis and Feedback

(67) I: Let me tell you what I have learned from our meeting today. You were overwhelmed when you learned that you have stage 1 breast cancer. You felt numbed and had flashbacks of the gynecologist's message. Such response may mark the onset of an acute stress disorder. You fear your friends, especially your daughter, will avoid you as you avoided your cousin, so they don't have to deal with your wasting away. You are sensitive to such abandonment because lifelong you fought with the rejection that you imagined occurred from your biological parents.

P: (Emphatically) Yes, yes, yes! What can I do about it?

(68) I: Believe in your daughter. She does not have your anxiety of shriveling away. She will not avoid you. With her, we want to fight the progression of your traumatic stress response and prevent recurrence of depression.

P: How?

RAPPORT The interviewer shows his or her expertise in addressing the patient's dependency needs from the patient's point of insight, namely, as sensitivity to abandonment (Q67). The patient accepts the diagnosis (A67) and shows interest in the interviewer's approach to her treatment (Q68).

TECHNIQUE With an accentuated transition, the interviewer prepares the patient for the diagnostic feedback, a role reversal. Now the interviewer and not the patient provides the bulk of information (Q67).

MENTAL STATUS The patient's affect has dramatically changed since the beginning of the interview. She had switched from sadness, anxiety, and despair to an emphatic approval of the interviewer's feedback, expressing openness and interest in the interviewer's treatment plan showing her affective reactivity (A67).

DIAGNOSIS The interviewer initiates the diagnostic feedback based on biopsychosocial information, including the patient's assets and strengths, and multiaxial diagnoses.

Phase 5: Treatment Plan and Prognosis

(69) I: Well, you have conquered your addiction to nicotine with your determination and with the help of Zyban or Wellbutrin, which is an antidepressant. You had depression in the past and Wellbutrin has helped you. So did Prozac. Since you started smoking again, I think Zyban can become our Old Faithful again. We should start it now. Do you recall its major risk?

P: What do you mean?

(70) I: The potential for a seizure.

P: Yes, I know.

(71) I: Did you ever have a seizure in your life? Like as a child?

P: No.

(72) I: Did you have one when you took the Zyban?

P: No.

(73) I: You told me you don't drink much. Alcohol withdrawal could possibly make you more sensitive to the seizure risk by Zyban.

P: I'm somewhat afraid of that. But Zyban made me feel well before.

(74) I: If you wake up and have soiled your clothes or bitten your tongue, stop Zyban and call me immediately. Now, your ability to tolerate the medication in the past gives us an edge.

P: I understand the risk, and I will take it again.

(75) I: Psychologically, you have strong feelings about rejection. This feeling can hurt you, but it also can help you.

P: How's that?

(76) I: (With emphasis) It's you who rejects rather than you being rejected.

P: I can never do that.

(77) I: You've done it before. You rejected the cigarettes. Your determination against cigarettes helped you. Taking Zyban would not have made you stop smoking. It's you who make the drug work. You noticed how it lifted your spirits. You have to use this spirit to tell yourself you will do everything you can to fight the cancer. See the physicians, stay with the treatment, and have the image of strength. You said yourself others want you to be strong for their sake. Your cancer will shrivel away, (with emphasis) not you. You think in images. We will work to implant the image in your mind how the cancer is shriveling under the therapy.

P: But my cousin's . . .

(78) I: (Interrupting her) Purge that image like you purged the cigarettes. Purge it like you'll purge your cancer. That image of your wasting cousin is a cancer of the mind.

P: But how do I fight it?

(79) I: Whenever your cousin's image pops up in your mind, straighten your posture, take a deep breath, and envision how your own body rejects cancer cells after removal of the small lump in your breast.

P: (With a questioning expression in her face and straightening her posture)

(80) I: As homework to strengthen your imagination, use the pendulum as often as you can but at least three times a day. I will see you weekly at the beginning and work with you on other imagining exercises, on positive thoughts, and I'll check the effects of the Zyban and the need for additional medication to control anxiety and depression. But I need your help. We have to put our heads together to make it work. And we may ask your daughter to come in with you and maybe even Joan.

P: I will take my medication and try to work on the exercise. I will also talk to my daughter and to Joan.

(81) I: Our success depends on how well we can control depression and anxiety. You had success in overcoming smoking and depression in the past and that bodes well for the future.

P: (With a broad smile) I feel so much better now. I'll call Joan and thank her for getting me here.

RAPPORT Because the patient has accepted the interviewer as an expert, the interviewer continues this role as a guide for a biopsychosocial treatment plan: Biologically, the interviewer refers to the patient's positive experiences with Zyban and Prozac and emphasizes the concern about the safety of treatment (Q69 to 74). Psychologically, the interviewer uses the patient's thinking in images to combat her self-destructive vision. Socially, the interviewer uses the patient's desire to be supported by her daughter, which rounds out the interviewer's role as a trustworthy guide.

TECHNIQUE The interviewer summarizes the patient's positive experiences and strengths that she had shown in the interview as a basis for the treatment plan.

MENTAL STATUS The prominent feature (Q,A69 to 81) is the patient's change from an anxious and doubtful to a confident affect.

DIAGNOSIS The patient's emotional reactivity to the interviewer's input added to a favorable prognosis of the patient's traumatic stress reaction.

Case Summary

I. IDENTIFYING DATA Ms. Lorraine R. is a 56-year-old, white, divorced, mildly obese, Catholic woman and the mother of three children who had an acute stress response to a recent diagnosis of breast cancer.

II. CHIEF COMPLAINT "I cried all night. I heard my gynecologist's voice again and again: Sorry, Ms. R. It's stage 1 breast cancer."

III. INFORMANTS The patient and her friend, a former patient, who requested that the patient had to be seen immediately.

IV. REASON FOR CONSULTATION Acute stress response to a recent diagnosis of breast cancer.

V. HISTORY OF PRESENT ILLNESS The day before the interview, the patient was diagnosed with stage 1 breast cancer. She cried all night and replayed in her mind the gynecologist's telephone message of having breast cancer. Two days ago, she had been forewarned of such a diagnosis. She felt "numb" and avoided discussing it with her family and friends. She never had experienced a life-threatening trauma before. The patient reported concurrent depressive symptoms with anhedonia and ruminations of being abandoned because of her crippling disease, as she had avoided her cousin dying of cancer. These chronic, continuous depressive feelings were present over the last 5 years. The patient had two periods of acute depressive episodes with social withdrawal, loss of energy and initiative, oversleeping, overeating, weight gain, sensitivity to rejection, and suicidal ideation but no attempts lasting for several months.

Her depression had responded to fluoxetine (Prozac). However, she had no evidence of any mood elation, overactivity, excessive spending sprees, reduced need of sleep, hypersexuality, or other symptoms of mania or hypomania. She had no history of alcoholism or substance abuse except for nicotine abuse for which she was treated successfully with Zyban 5 months ago but had relapsed for 1 day. She reported avoidance behavior regarding a female cousin in her adopting family who became physically emaciated due to treatment-resistant progressive breast cancer. The patient gave no evidence of generalized anxiety disorder, panic disorder, or social phobia. OCD was not assessed. She denied ever having had any psychotic symptoms.

VI. PSYCHIATRIC DISORDERS IN REMISSION A major depressive disorder, recurrent, was in remission for the last 10 years. Her nicotine abuse was in early partial remission, but she had a relapse for 1 day.

VII. MEDICAL HISTORY Positive for a recent diagnosis of breast cancer stage 1 and chronic cough; menopause; no allergies.

VIII. SOCIAL HISTORY AND PREMORBID PERSONALITY The patient has been divorced for the last 10 years. She has three children by the same man, works as an interior decorator, and is financially well off due to her divorce settlement and her present income. Premorbid personality: The patient has a college education and had functioned well before her first major depressive episode and intermittently between two episodes.

IX. FAMILY HISTORY A psychiatric family history of parents and siblings is unknown because of patient's adoption. However, her children show no evidence of psychiatric disorder.

X. MENTAL STATUS EXAMINATION

Appearance The patient is a 56-year-old, mildly obese, white, Catholic woman who is alert, has good eye contact, and is cooperative during the interview. She wore makeup, but the tears had washed out some of the mascara.

Movements Appropriate reactive movements when addressed. Grooming movements were limited to wiping her eyes even when not crying. Goal-directed movements were appropriate but showed some slowing when she entered the office and when sitting down. No illustrative movements but appropriate expressive movements when she discussed how she avoided her cousin.

Speech Voice was quivering at the beginning of the interview. She talked with normal rate and appropriate modulation. Initially, she breathed rapidly with pumping of shoulders. Comprehended questions well and answered in a goal-directed, precise, mildly dramatic manner, volunteering appropriate details.

Mood and Affect Mood was depressed and anxious. Affect was sad, labile, and anxious but became brighter and hopeful toward the end of the interview, showing reactivity.

Thought Content Denied any psychotic symptoms in the past or present. She had decreased interest in living during her two depressed episodes but expressed a strong will to live now. No evidence of panic attacks. Obsessions or compulsions not assessed. Fearful of being emotionally abandoned like she felt about her being given up for adoption. Brief dissociative experience during the last 48 hours. Suggestibility approximately average.

Cognition Oriented to place, time, and person. Recent memory is intact. Spelling backward and serial sevens are normal. She was able to interpret proverbs and to abstract the commonalties of categories. Her IQ is at least average according to the Wilson Approximate Intelligence Test and the Kent Test.

Insight Aware that she has a depressive disorder and nicotine addiction but less insight into the pathological nature of her response to the cancer diagnosis. Limited insight that her fear of abandonment is not based on facts but on projection of her own behavior toward her cousin.

Judgment Affected by her recent trauma. Expected a terminal course of cancer and abandonment not based on facts of her prognosis or her daughter's behavior.

XI. DIAGNOSTIC FORMULATION

Biological

Predisposing factors: Except for three healthy children, family history of psychiatric disorders is unknown. No history of head injury. History of major depression and possibly dysthymic disorder. Both may negatively impact on her traumatic stress response.

Precipitating: Concurrent cancer, future pain, and the side effects of cancer therapy may worsen the course of her acute stress disorder, major depression, and nicotine addiction.

Perpetuating: History of intermittent smoking may lead to dysphoric withdrawal reaction. Concurrent stage 1 breast cancer.

Protective: Good response to antidepressant medication to both depression and smoking.

Psychological

Predisposing: Phobic response to crippling disorders with avoidance and projection. Both mechanisms operate on a level below mature adjustment. Her ability to emotionally support herself is limited.

Precipitating: The patient fears a terminal cancer course and abandonment.

Perpetuating: Cancer therapy will be a steady reminder of her cancer risk.

Protective: Past success with therapy for her depression and smoking, cooperation with treatments. She avoided a possible conflict between local physicians and out-of-town experts. The patient was receptive to controlling her images of the course of her cancer.

Social

Predisposing: Interpreted her adoption as a rejection by her biological parents. Avoided a cousin who had cancer. Interpreted her divorce as rejection by her husband. Assumed the victim role.

Precipitating: Experiences the gynecologist's voice as cold, replays his message repeatedly in her mind.

Perpetuating: The memory of the crippling and fatal course of the cousin's cancer.

Protective: Has strong support from her friend who had a positive response to therapy; support from friends who have expressed confidence in her ability to fight the cancer. The patient is still working as an interior decorator. She enjoys her work and her colleagues, which distract her from her illness.

XII. DIFFERENTIAL DIAGNOSIS

Risk for an acute stress disorder progressing to a PTSD
Adjustment disorder with anxious and depressed mood
Onset of a third major depressive episode precipitated by acute stress
Special phobia of crippling terminal illness

The patient developed a special phobia but not an acute stress disorder to the terminal course of cancer in a cousin. She responded with a major depression to her divorce. Therefore, a recurrence of major depression is likely. An adjustment disorder may be an initial response but could progress to a major depressive episode. Early intervention may reduce the risks for all three disorders.

XIII. MULTIAXIAL PSYCHIATRIC DIAGNOSIS

Axis I:
- Acute stress disorder (308.3)
- Major depressive disorder with atypical features, recurrent, in full remission (296.36)
- Specific phobia (300.29)
- Rule out dysthymic disorder (300.4)

Axis II: features of dependent and histrionic personality

Axis III:
- Breast cancer, stage 1
- Rule out chronic bronchitis
- Rule out asthma
- Rule out pulmonary cancer

Axis IV:
- Traumatic response to recent diagnosis of breast cancer
- Fear of loss of support

Axis V: current GAF equals 35, highest last year was 70

XIV. ASSETS AND STRENGTHS The protective factors discussed in the section XI. Diagnostic Formulation are identical with the patient's assets and strengths.

XV. TREATMENT PLAN AND PROGNOSIS

Biological

Bupropion (Wellbutrin/ Zyban) has helped her in the past with both smoking and depression: bupropion, 150 mg #1 AM, in 1 week #1 twice a day (BID).

In case of incomplete response, consider combining bupropion with fluoxetine (Prozac).

Pursue cancer therapy and make an appointment immediately.

Psychological

Patient to take control and actively reject the cancer. Visualize the cancer as shriveling.

Instill hope by telling the patient that her cancer has been detected early and that early detection has excellent prognosis to respond to therapy.

Include her daughter in some of the upcoming therapy sessions.

Social

Reframe the fact that the patient has been selected by her adoptive parents as acceptance.

Discuss her criticism of the husband, helping her to overcome the victim role and appreciate her own contribution to the divorce.

Emphasize the expediency of cancer diagnosis in 24 hours, which allows timely treatment.

Point out support by her friend Joan.

Prognosis Cooperated with treatment in the past with good response. Psychiatric symptoms appear to be manageable with therapy, thus preventing disability. Psychiatric prognosis appears good. The main risk factor for psychiatric well-being is a poor response to cancer therapy.

SUGGESTED CROSS-REFERENCES

Section 7.4 deals with the typical signs and symptoms of psychiatric illness, Section 7.5 deals with neuropsychological and intellectual assessment of adults, and Section 7.9 deals with psychiatric rating scales. Similarly, Chapter 8, on the clinical manifestations of psychiatric disorders, is an essential correlate to interviewing and examining the patient. Section 2.1 deals with the clinical assessment and approach to diagnosis in neuropsychiatry. Section 3.1 on perception and cognition and Section 3.4 on the biology of memory amplify points made in this section. Section 29.1 includes more detailed information on suicide, and Section 29.2 includes information on other psychiatric emergencies. Chapter 45 deals with mood disorders and suicide in children and adolescents. Aspects of normal and abnormal development are found in Section 6.2 on Erik H. Erikson; Chapter 32 deals extensively with normal development in children and adolescents; adult development is covered at great length in Chapter 50; and normal aging is the focus of Section 51.2c.

REFERENCES

Ayd FJ. *Lexicon of Psychiatry, Neurology and the Neurosciences.* 2nd ed. Philadelphia: Lippincott Williams & Wilkins; 2000.

Beck AT. *The Integrated Power of Cognitive Therapy.* New York: Guilford; 1997.

Bennett MJ. *The Empathic Healer: An Endangered Species?* San Diego: Academic Press; 2001.

Carlat DJ. *The Psychiatric Interview.* Philadelphia: Lippincott Williams & Wilkins; 1999.

Cheng AT: Mental illness and suicide. *Arch Gen Psychiatry.* 1995;52:594–603.

Chochinov HM: Dignity—conserving care. A new model for palliative care. Helping the patient feel valued. *JAMA.* 2002;287:2253–2260.

Cox A, Rutter M, Holbrook D: Psychiatric interviewing techniques. A second experimental study: Eliciting feelings. *Br J Psychiatry.* 1988;152:64–72.

*First MB, Frances A, Pincus HA. *DSM-IV-TR Handbook of Differential Diagnosis.* Washington DC: American Psychiatric Publishing, Inc.; 2002.

Fish F. *Clinical Psychopathology.* Bristol, UK: John Wright and Sons; 1967.

Goodwin DW, Guze SB. *Psychiatric Diagnosis.* 5th ed. New York: Oxford University Press; 1996.

Hill CJ: Factors influencing physician choice. *Hospital and Health Services Administration.* 1991;36:491–503.

International Guidelines for Diagnostic Assessment (IGDA): Workgroup, WPA (World Psychiatric Association). *Br J Psychiatry.* 2003;182(Suppl 45):S40–S59.

Izard C. *Human Emotions.* New York: Plenum; 1977.

Izard C. *Emotions in Personality and Psychopathology.* New York: Plenum; 1979.

Keller MB, McCullough JP, Klein DN, Arnow B, Dunner DL, Gelenberg AJ, Markowitz JC, Nemeroff CB, Russell JM, Thase ME, Trivedi MH, Zajecka J: A comparison of nefazodone, the cognitive behavioral-analysis system of psychotherapy, and their combination for the treatment of chronic depression. *N Engl J Med.* 2000;342:1462–1470.

Kendell RE: Five criteria for an improved taxonomy of mental disorders. In: Helzer JE, Hudziak JJ, eds. *Defining Psychopathology in the 21st Century. DSM-V and Beyond.* Washington DC: American Psychiatric Publishing, Inc.; 2002:3–17.

Keshavan MS, Rabinowitz G, De Smedt G, Radomsky E, Schooler N: Correlates of insight in first episode psychosis. *Biol Psychiatry.* 2002; 51:115S–116S.

Klerman GL, Weissman MM, eds. *New Applications of Interpersonal Psychotherapy.* Washington DC: American Psychiatric Press; 1993.

Kraemer HC, Measelle JR, Ablow JC, Essex MJ, Boyce T, Kupfer DJ: A new approach to integrating data from multiple informants in psychiatric assessment and research: mixing and matching contexts and perspectives. *Am J Psychiatry.* 2003;160:1566–1577.

Ludwig AM, Othmer E: The medical basis of psychiatry. *Am J Psychiatry.* 1977;134:1087–1092.

Moran P, Leese M, Lee T, Walters P, Thornicroft G, Mann A: Standardised Assessment of Personality—Abbreviated Scale (SAPAS): preliminary validation of a brief screen for personality disorder. *Br J Psychiatry.* 2003;183:228–232.

*Othmer E, Othmer SC. *The Clinical Interview Using DSM-IV-TR. Vol 1: Fundamentals.* Washington DC: American Psychiatric Publishing, Inc.; 2002.

*Othmer E, Othmer SC. *The Clinical Interview Using DSM-IV-TR. Vol 2: The Difficult Patient.* Washington DC: American Psychiatric Publishing, Inc.; 2002.

Othmer E, Othmer SC, Othmer JP: Brain functions and psychiatric disorders. A clinical view. In: Diagnostic dilemmas, part I. *Psychiatr Clin North Am.* 1998;21:517–566.

Othmer E, Penick EC, Powell BJ, Read MR, Othmer SC. *Psychiatric Diagnostic Interview-Revised (PDI-R). Manual and Administration Booklet.* Los Angeles: Western Psychological Services; 1989.

Patterson WM, Dohn HH, Bird J, Patterson G: Evaluation of suicidal patients: The SAD PERSONS scale. *Psychosomatics.* 1983;24:343–349.

Payne RW, Hewlett JHG. Thought Disorder in Psychotic Patients. In: Eysenck HJ, ed. *Experiments in Personality, Vol. 2, Psychodiagnostics and Psychodynamics.* New York: Humanities Press; 1960.

*Shea SC. *Psychiatric Interviewing. The Art of Understanding.* 2nd ed. Philadelphia: WB Saunders Co.; 1998.

*Sommers-Flanahan R, Sommers-Flanahan J. *Clinical Interviewing.* New York: John Wiley & Sons; 1999.

Tasman A, Riba MB, Silk KR. *The Doctor-Patient Relationship in Pharmacotherapy. Improving Treatment Effectiveness.* New York: Guilford Publications; 2000.

Tatro DS, ed. *Drug Interaction Facts 2002. Facts and Comparisons.* St. Louis: A Wolters Kluwer Company; 2002.

Warnock JK: Tips on taking the psychiatry and neurology oral exam. *Resid Staff Physician.* 1991;15:121–123.

Zimmerman M: What should the standard of care for psychiatric diagnostic evaluations be? *J Nerv Ment Disord.* 2003;191:281–286.

▲ 7.2 Interviewing Techniques with the Difficult Patient

MYRL MANLEY, M.D.

In 1978, James Groves published in the *New England Journal of Medicine* a seminal paper titled "Taking Care of the Hateful Patient." He described four patterns of behavior and personal interactions that make some patients not only unlikable, but also difficult to treat: dependent clinging, entitled demanding, manipulative help-rejecting, and self-destructive denying. The paper provoked an immediate response of recognition, and it continues to be one of the most cited sources in the literature on the doctor–patient relationship. In "Taking Care of the Hateful Patient," Groves explicitly acknowledged what clinicians had known for generations—not all patients are likable, and their unlikability gets in the way of good medical treatment. More importantly, he argued that, when physicians recognize their own negative reactions to patients and attempt to examine and understand them (as opposed to denying them), medical care improves.

Groves was a psychiatrist at Harvard, but he was writing for a general medical audience. He focused his attention on behavioral interactions between doctor and patient and drew heavily on the psychoanalytic concepts of transference and countertransference. Since the paper first appeared, his four typologies have been much discussed, reexamined, and modified. It is now recognized that a multiplicity of factors, such as social, economic, and cultural, can make some patients more difficult, in addition to interpersonal behavior and personality style. The issue is especially pertinent for psychiatrists, because the underlying pathology of their patients may manifest as behavioral interactions that themselves provoke negative responses. The principle that difficult patients need acknowledgment, understanding, and special skills remains unchallenged. Whether patients are likable or not, there are a number of circumstances in psychiatry that require a modified approach.

PERSONALITY TRAITS AND DISORDERS

Almost all physicians treat patients who are difficult, not because of their medical illness, but because they engage in power struggles, are demanding, or are uncooperative. Psychiatrists recognize that these difficulties are often the manifestation of underlying personality traits or disorders and are therefore fixed, largely inflexible habits of behavior that cannot be reasoned away. It is a natural human quality to feel anger and resentment toward difficult patients, to try to limit the amount of time spent with them, and to hope secretly (or explicitly) that they move on to another physician. Although these reactions are understandable, they are likely to make a bad situation worse and to interfere with the doctor's primary mission—providing the best possible medical care. Understanding some of the hidden fears and conflicts shaping the behavior of difficult patients helps the physician develop patience and greater compassion and makes it easier to provide medically sound interventions. In special situations, interview techniques need to be varied according to the personality features of the patient. Varying degrees of permissiveness and direction may be used. Table 7.2–1 lists some of the common personality patterns that can interfere with good medical care and that call for special understanding.

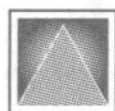

Table 7.2–1
Personality Styles That Interfere with Good Medical Care

Dependent patients	Some patients seem to need an inordinate amount of attention and yet never seem reassured. They are the patients who are likely to make repeated urgent calls between scheduled appointments and to demand special consideration. The doctor needs to be firm in establishing limits while reassuring the patient that his or her needs are taken seriously and are treated professionally.
Demanding patients	Some patients have a difficult time delaying gratification and demand that their discomfort be eliminated immediately. They are easily frustrated and can become petulant or even angry and hostile if they do not get what they want when they want it. They may impulsively do something self-destructive if they feel thwarted, and they appear manipulative and attention seeking. Beneath their surface behavior, they may fear that they will never get what they need from others and thus must act in that inappropriately aggressive way. The doctor must be firm with these patients from the outset and must clearly define acceptable and unacceptable behavior. These patients must be treated with respect and care, but they must also be confronted with their behavior.
Narcissistic patients	Narcissistic patients act as though they are superior to everyone around them, including the doctor. They have a tremendous need to appear perfect and are contemptuous of others whom they perceive to be imperfect. They may be rude, abrupt, arrogant, and demanding. They may initially idealize a doctor out of a need to have their doctor be as perfect as they are, but the idealization can quickly turn to disdain when they realize that the doctor is only human after all. Underneath their surface arrogance, narcissistic patients feel desperately inadequate and fear that others will see through them.
Isolated patients	Isolated and solitary patients do not appear to need or to want much contact with other people. Intimate contact with the doctor is viewed with distaste, and such patients would prefer to take care of themselves entirely without the doctor's help if it were possible. Some isolated patients would receive a diagnosis of schizoid personality disorder. They are withdrawn, absorbed in a world of fantasy, and are unable to talk about their feelings. The doctor should treat these patients with as much respect for their privacy as possible and should not expect them to respond to the doctor's concern in kind.
Obsessive patients	Obsessive patients are orderly, punctual, and so concerned with detail that they often don't see the larger picture. They may appear unemotional, even aloof, especially when confronted with anything disturbing or frightening. They have a strong need to be in control of everything in their lives and may struggle with their doctor whenever they feel that decisions are being imposed. Underneath, obsessive patients are often frightened of losing control and of becoming helpless and dependent. Their physicians should try to include them in their own care and treatment as much as possible. Doctors should explain in detail what is going on and what is being planned, allowing the patient to make choices on his or her own behalf.

PSYCHOTIC PATIENTS

Patients with psychotic symptoms have difficulty thinking clearly and reasoning logically. Their ability to concentrate may be impaired, and they may be distracted by hallucinations and delusional beliefs. Psychotic patients are often frightened and may be quite guarded. Quite often, the evaluation of a patient with psychotic symptoms needs to be more focused and structured than that of other patients. Open-ended questions and long periods of silence are apt to be disorganizing. Short questions are easier to follow than long ones. Questions calling for abstract responses or hypothetical conjectures may be unanswerable.

Hallucinations For patients with hallucinations, the full phenomenology of the hallucination should be explored. The patient is asked to describe the sensory misperception as fully as possible. For auditory hallucinations, this includes content, volume, clarity, and circumstances; for visual hallucinations, this includes content, intensity, the situations in which they occur, and the patient's response. The evaluator should distinguish between true hallucinations, on the one hand, and illusions, hypnagogic and hypnopompic hallucinations, and vivid imaginings, on the other. Hallucinations are perceived as real sensory stimuli and should not be dismissed as fanciful; however, the psychiatrist should ask questions about their fixity and the patient's level of insight: "Does it ever seem that the voices are coming from your own thoughts?" or "What do you think is causing the voices?"

Delusions *Delusions*, by definition, are fixed, false beliefs. Delusional patients often come to psychiatric evaluation having had their beliefs dismissed or belittled by friends and family. They are on guard for similar reactions from the examiner. It is possible to ask questions about delusions without revealing belief or disbelief (e.g., "Does it seem that people are intent on hurting you?" rather than "Is there a plot to hurt you?"). Careless use of psychiatric jargon should be avoided, particularly in evaluating delusions. Words such as *grandiose* and *paranoid* and, indeed, the word *delusion* itself seem harsh and judgmental and are unlikely to be helpful in eliciting information. Many psychiatrists have found that patients can speak more freely when asked to talk about the accompanying emotions rather than the belief itself ("It must be frightening to think there are people you don't know who are plotting against you"). Although the psychiatrist does not attempt to reason them away, a gentle probe may determine how tenaciously the beliefs are held ("Do you ever wonder whether those things might not be true?").

Paranoid Thinking Patients with paranoid delusions (and patients with high levels of nondelusional suspiciousness) are best evaluated with a respectful, but somewhat distant, formality and with scrupulous honesty. Efforts to reassure or to ingratiate often increase suspicion. The psychiatrist must keep in mind the possibility of being incorporated into a delusional belief and should ask about it directly ("Are you concerned that I might try to hurt you?").

Thought Disorders Disorders of thought form can seriously impair effective communications. The evaluating psychiatrist should note formal thought disorders while minimizing their adverse impact on the interview. When derailment is evident, the psychiatrist typically proceeds with questions calling for short responses. For a patient experiencing thought blocking, the psychiatrist needs to repeat questions, to remind the patient of what was already said, and, in general, to provide an organization for thinking that the patient is unable to provide.

DEPRESSED AND POTENTIALLY SUICIDAL PATIENTS

Severely depressed patients may also have difficulty concentrating, thinking clearly, and speaking spontaneously. The intensity of mood disturbance can seem all-consuming and may well lead to distortions in thinking and perception. Some depressed patients have psychotic symptoms in addition to cognitive difficulties. The psychiatrist evaluating a depressed patient may need to be more forceful and directive than usual. It sometimes seems that the examiner must provide all the emotional and intellectual energy for both participants. Although depressed patients should not be badgered, long silences are seldom useful, and the examiner may need to repeat questions more than once. Ruminative patients—for example, those who continually repeat how worthless or guilty they are—need to be interrupted and redirected.

All patients must be asked about suicidal thoughts; however, depressed patients may need to be questioned more fully. A thorough assessment of suicide potential addresses intent, plans, means, and perceived consequences, as well as history of attempts and family history of suicide. Many patients mention their thoughts of suicide spontaneously. If not, the examiner can begin with a somewhat general question, such as "Do you ever have thoughts of hurting yourself?" or "Does it ever seem that life isn't worth living?" These questions can then be followed up with more specific questions. The examiner must feel comfortable enough to ask simple, straightforward, noneuphemistic questions. Asking about suicide does not increase the risk. The psychiatrist is not raising a topic that the patient has not already contemplated. Specific, detailed questions are essential for prevention.

Intent The examiner must determine the seriousness of the wish to die. Some patients report that they wish that they were dead but would never intentionally do anything to take their own lives. This level of intent is sometimes referred to as *passive suicidal ideation.* Other patients express greater degrees of determination. Near the other end of the spectrum of intent is the patient who says, "I've decided that I have to kill myself and nothing you can say or do will change that." At the most extreme level of determination are the patients who are the most difficult to help, those who tell no one about their suicidal plans and proceed in a deliberate, systematic manner. It is also useful to ask about restraining influences, internal and external (e.g., "Do you worry that you might not be able to resist those impulses?" or "How have you been able to keep from hurting yourself so far?"). Patients with auditory hallucinations commanding them to kill themselves often describe the hallucinations as irresistible despite any real desire to die.

Plans Patients with well-formulated plans are generally at greater risk than patients who do not know what they would do, but the method of suicide is not always a reliable indication of the risk. Even though some actions, such as jumping or shooting, are much more likely to be fatal than others, patients make mistakes. A pill overdose taken at the time at which a spouse is expected to arrive home may become deadly if the spouse is delayed in traffic. The psychiatrist should also ask about preparatory actions, such as giving away goods and putting one's estate in order.

Means Asking patients about the intended means of suicide is helpful in two ways. First, it clarifies the urgency of the situation; persons wanting to shoot themselves who own a loaded gun are more dangerous than those who have no idea where to find a gun. Second, the understanding of intent is sharpened by knowing whether a patient has thought through the steps necessary to carry out the action.

Perceived Consequences Patients who see something desirable resulting from their deaths are at increased risk for suicide.

A reunion fantasy, the belief that a person will be reunited with a deceased loved one, may be a powerful motivating force toward suicide. On the other hand, some potentially suicidal patients are restrained by what they see as negative consequences (e.g., "My children need me too much; they'd never be able to get along without me," or "I couldn't hurt myself. My parents would never get over their grief."). The psychiatric history and the family history for all patients, even those not currently suicidal, should mention any previous suicide attempt or suicides by family members. Both circumstances are recognized to increase the current risk, even if previous attempts were thought to be superficial.

At times, treatment must take precedence over evaluation. In rare circumstances, the threat of suicide is so imminent that immediate action must be taken to hospitalize the patient. Even during a first evaluation session, the psychiatrist must be prepared to make whatever professional response is necessary to safeguard the well-being of the patient.

A summary of questions that may be helpful in establishing suicidal patients is provided in Table 7.2–2.

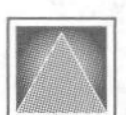

Table 7.2–2
Questions That May Be Helpful in Inquiring about Specific Aspects of Suicidal Thoughts, Plans, and Behaviors

Begin with questions that address the patient's feelings about living:
- Have you ever felt that life was not worth living?
- Did you ever wish that you could go to sleep and just not wake up?

Follow up with specific questions that ask about thoughts of death, self-harm, or suicide:
- Is death something that you have thought about recently?
- Have things ever reached the point at which you have thought of harming yourself?

For individuals who have thoughts of self-harm or suicide:
- When did you first notice such thoughts?
- What led up to the thoughts (e.g., interpersonal and psychosocial precipitants, including real or imagined losses; specific symptoms, such as mood changes, anhedonia, hopelessness, anxiety, agitation, psychosis)?
- How often have those thoughts occurred (including frequency, obsessional quality, and controllability)?
- How close have you come to acting on those thoughts?
- How likely do you think it is that you will act on them in the future?
- Have you ever started to harm (or kill) yourself but stopped before doing something (e.g., holding knife or gun to your body but stopping before acting or going to the edge of bridge but not jumping)?
- What do you envision happening if you actually killed yourself (e.g., escape, reunion with significant other, rebirth, or reactions of others)?
- Have you made a specific plan to harm or kill yourself? (If so, what does the plan include?)
- Do you have guns or other weapons available to you?
- Have you made any particular preparations (e.g., purchasing specific items, writing a note or a will, making financial arrangements, taking steps to avoid discovery, or rehearsing the plan)?
- Have you spoken to anyone about your plans?
- How does the future look to you?
- What things would lead you to feel more (or less) hopeful about the future (e.g., treatment, reconciliation of relationship, or resolution of stressors)?
- What things would make it more (or less) likely that you would try to kill yourself?
- What things in your life would lead you to want to escape from life or be dead?
- What things in your life make you want to go on living?
- If you began to have thoughts of harming or killing yourself again, what would you do?

For individuals who have attempted suicide or have engaged in self-damaging actions, parallel questions to those in the previous section can address the prior attempts. Additional questions can be asked in general terms or can refer to the specific method used and may include:
- Can you describe what happened (e.g., circumstances, precipitants, view of future, use of alcohol or other substances, method, intent, and seriousness of injury)?
- What thoughts were you having beforehand that led up to the attempt?
- What did you think would happen (e.g., going to sleep versus dying or getting a reaction out of a particular person)?
- Were other people present at the time?
- Did you seek help afterward yourself, or did someone get help for you?
- Had you planned to be discovered, or were you found accidentally?
- How did you feel afterward (e.g., relief versus regret at being alive)?
- Did you receive treatment afterward (e.g., medical versus psychiatric, emergency department versus inpatient versus outpatient)?
- Has your view of things changed, or is anything different for you since the attempt?
- Are there other times in the past when you have tried to harm (or kill) yourself?

For individuals with repeated suicidal thoughts or attempts:
- Approximately how often have you tried to harm (or kill) yourself?
- When was the most recent time?
- Can you describe your thoughts at the time that you were thinking most seriously about suicide?
- When was your most serious attempt at harming or killing yourself?
- What led up to it, and what happened afterward?

For individuals with psychosis, ask specifically about hallucinations and delusions:
- Can you describe the voices (e.g., single versus multiple, male versus female, internal versus external, recognizable versus unrecognizable)?
- What do the voices say (e.g., positive remarks versus negative remarks versus threats)? (If the remarks are commands, determine if they are for harmless versus harmful acts; ask for examples.)
- How do you cope with (or respond to) the voices?
- Have you ever done what the voices ask you to do? (What led you to obey the voices? If you tried to resist them, what made it difficult?)
- Have there been times when the voices told you to hurt or to kill yourself? (How often? What happened?)
- Are you worried about having a serious illness or that your body is rotting?
- Are you concerned about your financial situation even when others tell you there's nothing to worry about?
- Are there things that you've been feeling guilty about or blaming yourself for?

Consider assessing the patient's potential to harm others in addition to himself or herself:
- Are there others who you think may be responsible for what you're experiencing (e.g., persecutory ideas or passivity experiences)? Are you having any thoughts of harming them?
- Are there other people whom you would want to die with you?
- Are there others whom you think would be unable to go on without you?

From *Practice Guideline for the Assessment and Treatment of Patients with Suicidal Behaviors, Work Group on Suicidal Behaviors. American Psychiatric Association Practice Guidelines.* Washington, DC; American Psychiatric Association; 2003:160, with permission.

SOMATIZING PATIENTS

Some patients experience and describe emotional distress in terms of physical symptoms. This is certainly true for the group of somatoform disorders, but it also occurs in some mood and anxiety disorders and adjustment disorders and as a component of personality style or personality disorder. Somatizing patients pose a number of difficulties for the consulting and the treating psychiatrist. They are often referred by an internist or primary care physician, and the referral itself may be experienced as dismissive. Somatizing patients may be reluctant to engage in self-reflection and psychological exploration. Moreover, somatic distress without physical findings can lead to diagnostic uncertainty, which, in turn, makes treatment less certain. Antidepressant or anxiolytic medications may be helpful, but side effects are often less tolerable to individuals who are already highly attuned to small changes in body sensations.

Many somatizing patients live with the fear that their symptoms are not taken seriously and the parallel fear that something medically serious may be overlooked. Psychiatrists' main task in dealing with these patients is to acknowledge the suffering conveyed by the symptoms without necessarily accepting the patient's explanation for the symptoms. Clinicians should be curious about not only the nature of the physical complaints, but also the impact of those complaints on the patient's life (e.g., "It must be very difficult to keep on working with such severe headaches," or "It sounds as though your illness has crowded everything else out of your life.").

It is essential that somatizing patients feel that their physical complaints are not being dismissed. Rather than limiting the scope of inquiry to psychological issues, the psychiatrist wants to expand discussion to include all aspects of the patient's well-being, emotional health, and physical health. Many patients become more willing to discuss personal issues, such as job-related stress or relationship difficulties, when they believe the psychiatrist will not automatically assume that those issues are the cause of physical symptoms. It is often helpful for the physician to propose a purely pragmatic approach—one that stresses a willingness to use whatever works to relieve the patient's suffering without causing harm. At times, this may include nonstandard approaches, such as meditation, yoga, or acupuncture, in addition to psychotherapy.

It is especially important for the psychiatrist working with a somatizing patient to form a collaborative relationship with the primary medical doctor and to obtain thorough copies of medical records and evaluations and for them to consult freely with one another about the patient's health and symptoms. An important goal of treatment is to minimize the harm caused by aggressive and unwarranted medical interventions. These patients often do better with frequent, short medical consultations that are scheduled in advance, rather than urgent visits prompted by new symptoms or an intensification of old symptoms, in which case high levels of anxiety make a sober assessment more difficult. In addition, the momentary relief of medical reassurance after negative tests may behaviorally condition the patient and may increase the likelihood of future crises.

A degree of humility and flexibility is always desirable in working with psychiatric patients, and this is certainly true with somatizing patients. It is foolhardy for the psychiatrist to assume with absolute conviction that a patient's physical complaints have no real medical basis. Knowledge of medicine is constantly expanding but still incomplete. New disorders are described, and the range of symptoms recognized for known disorders changes. Meanwhile, the ability to detect and to diagnose accurately physical disease may lag behind. For example, it is almost certain that some patients with Lyme disease—presenting with vague, shifting, ill-defined physical complaints, fatigue and lethargy—were misdiagnosed as having a somatoform disorder before the disease was well-described and diagnostic markers were identified. The psychiatrist's task is not to close the door on medical investigation, but to invite patients to consider an even larger range of factors, including emotional and psychological issues, all of which may affect their health.

A 45-year-old man was convinced he had acquired immune deficiency syndrome (AIDS), despite having no risk factors. He repeatedly sought out human immunodeficiency virus (HIV) testing and blood cell counts. When tests reported that he was not HIV positive, he felt considerable, but short-lived, relief. He soon began to doubt the accuracy of the tests and reporting. "Can you tell me with certainty, that there is 100 percent no chance of error?" he asked his medical doctor. Over several months, his anxiety and depression increased, and he accepted referral to a psychiatrist.

The psychiatrist reframed the issue by saying that the major cause of the patient's distress was not AIDS, but the fear of AIDS. He observed that frequent testing had not provided reassurance but, in fact, had increased the patient's anxiety. The psychiatrist stressed that he would not ignore the patient's physical health. The patient agreed to scheduled medical consultations every 6 months and, in the course of psychotherapy, became more open in discussing considerable nonsomatic concerns. He also benefited from antidepressant medication.

AGITATED AND POTENTIALLY VIOLENT PATIENTS

Whether in a private office or a psychiatric emergency department, psychiatrists sometimes find themselves interviewing potentially violent patients. In these circumstances, the task is twofold: to conduct an assessment and also to contain behavior and to limit the potential for harm.

Most unpremeditated violence is preceded by a prodrome of accelerating psychomotor agitation. The patient may begin pacing and pounding the fist in a hand. Speech may become loud, abusive, obscene, and threatening. The temporal arteries may begin to throb. Researchers and clinicians in emergency psychiatry suggest that the prodrome lasts from 30 to 60 minutes before erupting into physical violence. Thus, the psychiatric evaluator has early signals of impending violence and a period of time in which the agitation may be quieted.

Several steps can be taken to minimize the agitation and potential risk. The interview should be conducted in a quiet, nonstimulating environment. There should be enough space for the comfort of the patient and the psychiatrist, with no physical barrier to leaving the examination room for either of them. During the interview, the psychiatrist should avoid any behavior that could be misconstrued as menacing: standing over the patient, staring, or touching.

The psychiatrist must ask the questions that are necessary to complete an adequate evaluation but must attempt not to be provocative. It is certainly appropriate to allow the patient to drink water, to use a bathroom and, for extended evaluations in an emergency room, to eat food. However, these should never be offered as bargaining chips ("I'll let you get a drink of water if you'll tell me what happened just before the police brought you here"). The examiner must also avoid promising outcome in exchange for cooperation ("If you'll just talk with me for another 30 minutes, I'll make sure you don't have to go into the hospital").

The psychiatrist should ask whether the patient is carrying weapons and may ask the patient to leave the weapon with a guard or in a holding area. The psychiatrist should not request that the patient hand over any weapons. Dangerous mishaps can occur during the transfer; moreover, the sudden shift in power created by an armed psychiatrist may feel extremely threatening to paranoid patients. If the patient's agitation continues to increase, the psychiatrist may need to terminate the interview. Depending on the setting, assistance from security personnel or physical or chemical restraints may be appropriate. The physician's own subjective sense of comfort or fear should be heeded. A frightened, intimidated examiner may be incapable of an accurate professional evaluation.

SEDUCTIVE PATIENTS

The warmth, openness, acceptance, and understanding that are helpful to most psychiatric interviews may engender feelings of romantic longing in some patients, especially (but not exclusively) those who are lonely and socially isolated. Other patients behave in flirtatious and seductive ways as their habitual style of relating with other people. Seductiveness may be manifested in a patient's dress, behavior, and speech. It runs the gamut from gentle suggestion to explicit proposition. A young man may sit with his legs spread wide apart, a young woman may wear a low-cut, revealing dress, or a middle-aged woman, when shaking hands, may hold the psychiatrist's hand a few seconds longer than is appropriate for the situation.

Of course, sex is not the only enticement with which psychiatrists can be seduced. Patients may offer insider information for profitable trading in the stock market, may promise an introduction to a movie star friend, or may suggest that they will dedicate their next novel to the psychiatrist. Although it is easy to understand that some offers by patients, such as the possibility of a sexual involvement, cannot be accepted without considerable harm to the patient, others may seem more innocuous. However, because they nearly always introduce a different agenda into the therapy than that originally contracted for, and because they create additional, more ambiguous levels of obligation between therapist and patient, any psychiatric work is inevitably contaminated, and the ability to help the patient is compromised. Consequently, gaining any material or social benefit from the patient other than the agreed-on fee is unethical.

Whether to offers of sex, money, or celebrity, the psychiatrist's response is the same. In the course of ongoing psychotherapy and in the context of an established relationship, seductive behavior is discussed and examined in an effort to understand its meaning. Is it, for example, a way of distancing, gaining control, or compensating for feelings of vulnerability and inferiority? To what extent are the feelings being expressed by the patient part of the transference? The psychiatrist should make it clear that what is being offered will not be accepted, in a way that preserves good rapport and does not unnecessarily assault the patient's self-esteem.

Seductive behavior during an initial psychiatric assessment must be handled somewhat differently. When the behavior is mild and indirect, it may be best to ignore it: Commenting on a woman's exposed cleavage only makes it clear that the psychiatrist picks up sexual cues, and it is most unlikely to facilitate the interview. More explicit propositions call for more direct responses and may afford the psychiatrist the chance to explain the nature of the therapeutic relationship and the need to establish boundaries. The psychiatrist should also make clear that it is the violation of those boundaries that is being rejected and not the patient. For example, to the patient who offers a celebrity introduction, the interviewer might reply, "That's very nice of you to propose, but I think I will best be able to help you if we pretty much stick to the issues that brought you in to see me."

A woman who was pregnant and in her late trimester began acting seductively toward her obstetrician. She would rub against him whenever possible and constantly asked him questions about his personal life. Recognizing this behavior as unusual, the obstetrician decided to explore the possible underlying reasons for the change. He began by asking what prompted her husband to have a child at this time and how each of them was feeling about becoming a parent. The patient quickly told how difficult it was to think about becoming a mother, because she was afraid that her husband would no longer find her sexually attractive. Further discussions about her past history revealed that the patient's parents did not seem interested in each other as a husband and wife once they became parents. There was even a strong suspicion that, after the birth of the patient's younger sister, the patient's father had an affair. She now began to recognize that she was afraid that her husband would react in exactly the same way as her father did. In this transference reaction, the patient was responding to her husband as though he were her father. After discussing the problem further, the obstetrician suggested to the patient that she share her concerns with her husband. As she did, the marital relationship improved considerably, and the patient's sexual interest in her obstetrician disappeared.

PATIENTS WHO LIE

A fundamental stance in psychiatric interviewing is recognizing that what is being heard may not be the literal truth. The unreliability of memory and the vagaries of psychopathology through which a patient's narrative is processed distort and falsify. The interviewer understands that what is historically untrue may nevertheless be emotionally true and is therefore a meaningful part of the diagnostic assessment or psychotherapy. At times, patients lie consciously with the explicit intent of deceiving the therapist. The purpose may be secondary gain (e.g., exemption from jury duty, a supply of psychoactive drugs, or leave of absence from graduate school), in which case the person is malingering. Malingering is not a mental disorder in the revised fourth edition of the *Diagnostic and Statistical Manual of Mental Disorders* (DSM-IV-TR). More rarely, a patient explicitly lies not for any obvious external advantage, but simply for whatever psychological advantage is conferred by assuming the sick role, in which case the person has a factitious disorder that is a DSM-IV-TR diagnosis.

Because psychiatrists do not have recourse to biological markers or other external validating criteria, the patient's report must be accepted as an honest statement of experience. There is no way to establish whether a person is experiencing auditory hallucinations other than through self-report. Nevertheless, an experienced clinician may detect subtle discrepancies, internal inconsistencies, or suspiciously atypical symptoms; these can certainly be queried without necessarily assuming that the patient is lying.

A 29-year-old woman describes an almost unremitting migraine headache and is asking for narcotic pain medication.

Patient: I really need your help. The pain is unbearable. I can't do anything anymore. I just want to lie in bed in a dark room with the cover pulled up over my head.

Doctor: That does sound miserable. I'm struck by the fact that you obviously care about your appearance and have given some time and attention to your hair, makeup, and the way you are dressed. Was that despite the pain that you have been describing?

Of course, the examiner is more likely to be deceived during the initial diagnostic assessment than in an ongoing psychotherapy in which the therapist has much more knowledge of a patient's background, thinking, and functioning over time. It may be difficult to catch a practiced liar in an initial session. Arguably, the interviewer should not try to do so. Being lied to angers most people, certainly no less psychiatrists who must depend on trust to perform their work. However, believing a patient's lies is not a professional failure. Psychiatrists are trained to detect, to understand, and to treat psychopathology, not to function as lie detectors. Although a certain level of suspicion is essential to the practice of psychiatry, the clinician determined never to be taken in by deceitful patients approaches patients with such exaggerated suspiciousness that therapeutic work is not possible.

Finally, not all patients' untruths are conscious lies. Patients with somatoform disorders, such as conversion disorder or pain disorder, are presumably unaware of the emotional bases of their physical complaints. In describing their somatic symptoms, they are stating psychological reality, not attempting to deceive the interviewer.

PATIENTS WHO DO NOT COOPERATE

Lack of patient cooperation can take many forms: failure to keep appointments, refusal to talk or to take the session seriously, failure to pay for services. Causes of noncooperation include manifestations of the patient's underlying pathology, anger at the psychiatrist, feelings of being coerced into an evaluation or treatment against one's will, or manifestations of transference. How the psychiatrist responds depends on the setting and context.

The evaluation of an uncooperative patient during an emergency necessarily proceeds differently from that during nonemergencies; an emergency psychiatric evaluation must often proceed without full cooperation or even against the patient's will. Neuroleptic malignant syndrome and delirium tremens, for example, are life-threatening emergencies, and an evaluation must be conducted as quickly as possible, with or without the patient's cooperation. Similarly, the assessment of an agitated psychotic patient with paranoid delusions who is brought to an emergency department by police after threatening to harm others cannot be deferred because of patient noncooperation. In these situations, sedation or restraint is sometimes necessary to complete even a basic triage assessment. The patient's refusal to cooperate is superseded by concern for the patient's life and the safety of others.

The evaluation of an uncooperative patient is different in a nonemergency outpatient setting. The patient who has been engaged in a meaningful therapy for some time and then becomes uncooperative is sending a powerful signal to the psychiatrist, the meaning of which must be explored. The change in behavior may be a manifestation of resistance to upsetting material that is beginning to emerge in therapy or of transference. Not every emotional reaction of a patient toward the psychiatrist, however, is transference; it may be in response to real life interactions between doctor and patient.

> A 52-year-old man who had been in psychotherapy for 1.5 years following difficulties in his marriage began missing sessions and arriving late. This followed several last-minute cancellations by the psychiatrist who offered neither explanation nor apology.
>
> When asked about his absences, the man quickly acknowledged how angry he was at the therapist for standing him up. "I see no reason why I should have to be more responsible than you," he said. The lateness and absences in therapy were motivated by anger at the psychiatrist's unprofessional behavior.

Pursuing transferential meaning while ignoring real interactions between physician and patient is unbeneficial and may worsen the situation if the patient believes that the psychiatrist is using therapeutic techniques to avoid responsibility for his or her own behavior. It should also be borne in mind that, although transference and countertransference are important concepts in psychoanalytic psychotherapies, their use in other modalities, such as cognitive-behavioral therapy, may be inappropriate and counterproductive.

The situation is different during an initial nonemergency assessment. There is little basis for pursuing the meaning of uncooperative behavior when a psychiatrist is meeting with a patient for the first time. Here, the psychiatrist's task is not to accept uncritically any and all behavior, but rather to guarantee a setting in which an honest evaluation or productive therapy can take place. The psychiatrist may need to insist on change in the patient's behavior as a precondition for proceeding. This can be done in a nonjudgmental and nonpunitive manner. In the same way that a surgeon is obligated and justified to say, "These are the conditions I must have to perform a safe and successful surgery," the psychiatrist must be willing to say "These are the conditions that are necessary for me to do my work." For patients who cannot or will not cooperate, the treatment contract may need to be renegotiated, for example, by changing the frequency of sessions, switching to a different psychotherapeutic modality, or focusing on medication management rather than psychotherapy. There are circumstances however, in which the initial assessment or therapy has to be terminated because of a patient's uncooperative behavior. This does not represent a therapeutic failure. On the contrary, failing to recognize and to respond to the limitations imposed by patient noncooperation may itself be an error of clinical judgment.

> A third-year psychiatry resident working in the outpatient clinic of a large hospital was assigned, for twice-a-week psychodynamic psychotherapy, a 26-year-old man with mild anxiety and depression and career difficulties. From the start of treatment, however, the patient came no more than three or four times per month, usually calling in advance to cancel, but sometimes simply not showing up. The resident struggled to build a treatment alliance and to interpret the man's behavior by using the little that she knew about him, but the pattern of noninvolvement continued. After 3 months, a new supervisor pointed out to the resident that therapy had never really started and that her first task was to create a situation in which therapy could occur. The resident explained to her patient that meaningful therapy was possible only with his full cooperation and that they needed to decide what level of involvement he could commit to. The patient agreed to come once a week. He was able to keep that schedule for the most part and, over the next 6 months, engaged in a beneficial supportive therapy.

Compliance versus Noncompliance One of the most common forms of noncooperation is noncompliance with medication. This can be especially frustrating for the psychiatrist when medication is clearly effective in controlling symptoms, and noncompliance results in relapse. Anger on the part of the physician may be understandable, but it is never helpful. Rather than assuming that noncompliance is due to a patient's perversity or character defect, an honest effort must be made to understand the reasons for noncompliance. Some of the common reasons are listed in Table 7.2–3. Understanding what is motivating the patient to stop medication makes intervention to improve compliance much more possible. Compliance can be increased when physicians explain to patients the value of a particular treatment outcome and emphasize that following the recommendation produces this outcome. Compliance can also

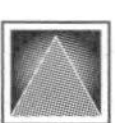

Table 7.2–3
Common Reasons for Noncompliance with Medication

The instructions are poorly given or the patient incompletely understands them.

Example: A 34-year-old woman with a first episode of major depression is prescribed paroxetine (Paxil) 20 mg per day. She responds well with full resolution of all symptoms within 4 weeks. Two weeks later, feeling back to normal, she stops taking the medication. Three weeks later, she has a relapse.

Comment: The woman did not understand (perhaps it was not well explained) that it would be necessary to continue the medication for several months after full recovery to minimize the risk of a relapse.

The patient may find side effects intolerable.

Example: A 20-year-old man is given a provisional diagnosis of schizophrenia when he begins to experience auditory hallucinations. He is treated with haloperidol (Haldol) 5 mg twice a day. The hallucinations resolve, but he begins to experience erectile dysfunction and stops the medication without telling anyone.

Comment: Common potential side effects and toxicities should always be reviewed with patients before they start medication. It is equally important to encourage the patient to discuss with the physician any adverse experiences and to reassure the patient that it is not necessary to put up with intolerable side effects, because there are alternative medications that can be tried.

Psychiatric symptoms interfere with treatment.

Example: A 41-year-old woman with a diagnosis of paranoid schizophrenia is admitted to an inpatient service with the delusion that she is being poisoned by an alien force. She is treated with risperidone (Risperdal) 2 mg per day and discharged after 1 week. She stops taking medication on the day of her discharge, believing it also to be poison and part of the plot to hurt her.

Comment: The clinician must be alert to the possibility that symptoms may interfere with treatment, must establish a trusting rapport as best as possible, and must inquire about the possibility that the patient distrusts the clinician ("Are you sometimes frightened that I might want to hurt you too?"). If medications are prescribed, they must be in doses that are sufficient to provide benefit.

Patients like their symptoms and don't want them treated.

Example: A 37-year-old man with bipolar disorder, well controlled with lithium (Eskalith) for 2 years, begins to feel mildly euphoric, more energetic, and more gregarious than usual. He stops taking lithium, because he feels it slows him down. Within 2 weeks, he is in a full manic episode.

Comment: Psychoeducation is part of the ongoing therapeutic process and may take time to be fully accomplished. Compliance is more easily achieved when a solid collaborative relationship has been established, when the physician is receptive to the patient's subjective experience of illness and treatment, and when the patient fully understands that mildly pleasant symptoms can become destructive and unpleasant if they are inadequately treated.

The lives of some patients are so chaotic and disorganized that good compliance is difficult without close monitoring and follow-up.

Example: A 47-year-old homeless woman with a diagnosis of chronic undifferentiated schizophrenia was treated in an emergency room, was given a prescription for a 1-month supply of an antipsychotic, and was told to come back to the outpatient clinic in 1 month. After discharge, the woman lived in a series of shelters and church refuges. Her bags containing her Medicaid and Medicare cards, prescription, and appointment card were stolen. She could not remember the date or place of follow-up and did not attend.

Comment: Failure to provide close, structured follow-up for this patient almost guaranteed treatment failure. Individual case managers help, although sometimes the number of cases that they are assigned to follow is overwhelming.

Patients stop taking medications because they cannot afford them.

Example: An elderly man living on a modest fixed income consulted his internist because of fatigue. She diagnosed depression and prescribed a relatively new selective serotonin reuptake inhibitor. When the man went to fill the prescription at his pharmacy, he was told a 1-month supply would cost $300. He did not fill the prescription and was embarrassed to tell his internist why he did not fill it.

Comment: The cost of medications is too seldom factored into prescribing decisions. This is particularly important for patients relying on Medicare, because Medicare currently has no outpatient prescription benefits. Generic drugs are always cheaper than brand-name equivalents. However, when a drug is new and still under patent, there may be no low-cost alternative. Many pharmaceutical companies have patient assistance programs, in which a physician can apply for substantially reduced-cost brand-name prescription medication for patients with limited resources.

increase if patients know the names and effects of each drug they are taking.

PATIENTS FROM DIFFERENT CULTURES AND BACKGROUNDS

Differences in race, nationality, and religion and other significant cultural differences between patient and interviewer can impair communication and can lead to misunderstandings. Despite its widespread use throughout the world, the possible cultural biases of DSM-IV-TR are still being debated; for example, the distinctions between mood disorders and somatoform disorders appear less valid in some countries than in the United States.

In addition, it may be difficult for a culturally naïve psychiatrist to evaluate symptoms that are relative rather than absolute. There is usually no difficulty in documenting the presence of auditory hallucinations regardless of cultural differences. However, assessing whether a delusion is *bizarre* (as required by DSM-IV-TR for delusional disorder) is more difficult, because the term *bizarre* has meaning only in reference to cultural norms. The belief by East Africans in the direct intervention of ancestral spirits in the day-to-day life of individuals is commonplace. The chief executive officer of an American corporation who announces that he will divest the company of two subsidiaries because of signals he received that morning from ancestral spirits will be thought exceedingly bizarre by colleagues and shareholders. Personality disorders, whose criteria are preponderantly relative rather than absolute (e.g., "shows arrogant, haughty behaviors or attitudes"), are notoriously difficult to diagnose cross-culturally.

Apart from diagnostic categories, the vocabulary used to describe emotional distress varies from culture to culture. European Americans commonly describe symptoms in terms of named emotions ("I've been feeling anxious and depressed all week"). Hispanic Americans are more likely to describe physical symptoms ("I've had a headache all week, and I'm so tired I can hardly move"). Sometimes symptoms that are commonplace within a culture are unheard of to outsiders. Residents of Anglophone countries in East and West Africa often describe the sensation of a snake crawling under their skin, moving from one part of the body to another. This appears to be a symptom of general emotional distress without particular diagnostic significance. Heard by a Western physician, the symptom may be misinterpreted as a somatic delusion or may be ignored altogether, because it does not register in the examiner's conceptual understanding of disorders.

Additional problems are encountered when doctor and patient speak different languages. When an interpreter is needed, the person should be a disinterested third party, unknown to the patient. Using family or friends to translate inevitably invites distortions in what the patient is said to report. Translators must be instructed to translate verbatim what the patient says—a difficult task for even the most experienced professional translators. Some words and expressions are simply untranslatable. It may be impossible to convey a formal thought disorder through translation.

An additional difficulty may arise in establishing rapport between doctor and patient of different ethnic or cultural groups. The use of honorifics, the extent of direct eye contact considered appropriate, and whether it is acceptable for men and women to shake hands all vary considerably among different groups. Patients from minority groups may be quite guarded in speaking with a doctor from the majority group. Some groups, such as traditional Chinese Americans, strongly believe that family problems should not be discussed outside the family, including with physicians. The evaluating psychiatrist must proceed with humility and respect. Rather than offer reassurances of understanding and acceptance, it is usually better to ask, "Have I understood this in the way that you meant it?"

EMPATHY

A diagnostic interview often provides considerable relief to patients. Puzzling and sometimes frightening symptoms are framed in the context of medical understanding. Bizarre experiences can be rationally understood and intelligently organized in meaningful ways that allow informed predictions about treatment response and recovery to be made. Of equal importance to an intellectual understanding is the capacity to understand emotionally the experiences of patients.

Empathy is an essential characteristic of psychiatrists, but it is not a universal human capacity. An incapacity for normal understanding of what other people are feeling appears to be central to certain personality disturbances, such as antisocial and narcissistic personality disorders. Although empathy can probably not be created, it can be focused and deepened through training, observation, and self-reflection. It manifests in clinical work in a variety of ways. An empathic psychiatrist may anticipate what is felt before it is spoken and can often help patients articulate what they are feeling. Nonverbal cues, such as body posture and facial expression, are noted. Patients' reactions to the psychiatrist can be understood and clarified.

Patients sometimes say, "How can you understand me if you haven't gone through what I'm going through?" but clinical psychiatry is predicated on the belief that it is not necessary to have other people's literal experiences to understand them. The shared experience of being human is often enough. Whether in an initial diagnostic setting or in an ongoing therapy, patients draw comfort from knowing that psychiatrists are not mystified by their suffering.

SUGGESTED CROSS-REFERENCES

An understanding of transference and countertransference is found in Section 6.1 on psychoanalysis. Clinical manifestations of mental disorders are covered in Chapter 8. Psychotic disorders, mood disorders, and anxiety disorders are discussed in Chapters 12, 13, and 14, respectively. Culture-bound syndromes appear in Chapter 27. The suicidal patient is discussed in Section 29.1. Further information on medication noncompliance is covered in Section 30.12 on combined psychotherapy and pharmacology.

REFERENCES

Alarcon RD: Culture and psychiatric diagnosis: Impact on DSM-IV and ICD-10. *Psychiatr Clin North Am.* 1995;18:449.

*Andreasen N, Black D. *Introductory Textbook of Psychiatry.* 3rd ed. Washington, DC: American Psychiatric Association Press; 2001.

Chikara F, Manley MRS: Psychiatry in Zimbabwe. *Hosp Community Psychiatry.* 1991;42:943.

Cohen BJ. *Theory and Practice of Psychiatry.* New York: Oxford University Press; 2003.

Dewar MJ, Pies R. *The Difficult to Treat Patient.* Washington, DC: American Psychiatric Association Press; 2001.

Fadem B. *Behavioral Science Medicine.* Philadelphia: Lippincott Williams & Wilkins; 2004.

*Franks RD. The angry and seductive patient. In: Simons RC, ed. *Understanding Human Behavior in Health and Illness.* 3rd ed. Baltimore: Williams & Wilkins; 1985.

Groves JE: Taking care of the hateful patient. *N Engl J Med.* 1978;298:883.

Kay J, Tasman A, Lieberman JA. *Psychiatry: Behavioral Science and Clinical Essentials.* New York: WB Saunders; 2000.

Kirk HW, Weisbrod JA, Ericson KA. *Psychosocial and Behavioral Aspects of Medicine.* Philadelphia: Lippincott Williams & Wilkins; 2003.

*Lewis JM: For better or worse: Interpersonal relationships and individual outcome. *Am J Psychiatry.* 1998;155:582.

Manley M. The psychiatric interview, history, and mental status examination. In: Sadock BJ, Sadock VA, eds. *Comprehensive Textbook of Psychiatry.* 7th ed. Baltimore: Lippincott Williams & Wilkins; 2000.

Manley M. *Psychiatry Clerkship Guide.* New York: Elsevier; 2003.

Othner E, Othner S. *The Clinical Interview Using DSM-IV-TR: The Difficult Patient.* Vol 2. Washington, DC: American Psychiatric Association Press; 2002.

*Sadock BJ, Sadock VA. *Kaplan and Sadock's Synopsis of Psychiatry.* 9th ed. Baltimore: Lippincott Williams & Wilkins; 2003.

*Simon RI. *Assessing and Managing Suicide Risk.* Washington, DC: American Psychiatric Publishing, Inc.; 2004.

Stoudemire A. *Human Behavior: An Introduction for Medical Students.* Philadelphia: Lippincott–Raven Publishers; 1998.

▲ 7.3 Psychiatric Report, Medical Record, and Medical Error

BENJAMIN J. SADOCK, M.D.

PSYCHIATRIC REPORT

The psychiatric report is a written document that details the findings obtained from the psychiatric history and mental status examination. The report may follow the outline described in Section 7.1, Psychiatric Interview, History, and Mental Status; however, it may also be formatted in other ways, provided that all of the pertinent data are recorded.

The psychiatric report includes a summary of positive and negative findings and an interpretation of the data. It has more than descriptive value; it has meaning that helps provide an understanding of the case. The examiner addresses critical questions in the report: Are future diagnostic studies needed, and, if so, which ones? Is a consultant needed? Is a comprehensive neurological workup, including an electroencephalogram (EEG) or computed tomography (CT) scan, needed? Are psychological tests indicated? Are psychodynamic factors relevant? The report includes a diagnosis made according to the revised fourth edition of the *Diagnostic and Statistical Manual of Mental Disorders* (DSM-IV-TR), which uses a multiaxial classification scheme consisting of five axes, each of which should be covered (Table 7.3–1). A prognosis is also discussed in the report, with good and bad prognostic factors listed. Finally, a treatment plan discusses and makes firm recommendations about management issues.

A detailed outline of the psychiatric report follows. It is one of the most comprehensive available, developed jointly by the author and Harold I. Kaplan, M.D.

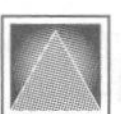

Table 7.3–1
DSM-IV-TR Multiaxial Classification of Diagnoses

Axis I: Clinical syndromes—list the mental disorder here (e.g., schizophrenia and bipolar I disorder). Other conditions that may be a focus of clinical attention (except borderline intellectual functioning) are also listed on Axis I. These are problems that are not sufficiently severe to warrant a psychiatric diagnosis (e.g., relational problems and bereavement).

Axis II: Personality disorders and mental retardation are listed here. Defense mechanisms and personality traits may be listed here. Diagnoses on Axis I and Axis II can coexist. The Axis I and Axis II condition that is responsible for bringing the patient to the psychiatrist or hospital is called the *principal* or *main diagnosis*.

Axis III: Physical disorders or conditions—if the patient has a physical disorder (e.g., cirrhosis), list that here.

Axis IV: Psychosocial and environmental problems—describe current stress in the patient's life (e.g., divorce, injury, or death of a loved one).

Axis V: GAF—rate the highest level of social, occupational, and psychological functioning of the patient according to the GAF scale (Table 7.9–2). Use the 12 months before the current evaluation as a reference point. Rate from 1 (lowest) to 100 (highest) or 0 (inadequate information).

GAF, global assessment of functioning.

I. Psychiatric history

A. *Identification:* name; age; marital status; sex; occupation; language, if other than English; race; nationality; religion, if pertinent; previous admissions to a hospital for the same or a different condition; and persons with whom the patient lives.

B. *Chief complaint:* exactly why the patient came to the psychiatrist, preferably in the patient's own words; if that information does not come from the patient, note who supplied it.

C. *History of present illness:* chronological background and development of the symptoms or behavioral changes that culminated in the patient's seeking assistance; patient's life circumstances at the time of onset; personality when well; how illness has affected life activities and personal relations—changes in personality, interests, mood, attitudes toward others, dress, habits, level of tenseness, irritability, activity, attention, concentration, memory, speech; psychophysiological symptoms—nature and details of dysfunction; pain—location, intensity, fluctuation; level of anxiety—generalized and nonspecific (free floating) or specifically related to particular situations, activities, or objects; how anxieties are handled—avoidance, repetition of feared situation, use of drugs or other activities for alleviation.

D. *Past psychiatric and medical history:* (1) emotional or mental disturbances—extent of incapacity, type of treatment, names of hospitals, length of illness, effect of treatment; (2) psychosomatic disorders: hay fever, arthritis, colitis, chronic fatigue, recurrent colds, skin conditions; (3) medical conditions—customary review of systems, sexually transmitted diseases, alcohol or other substance abuse, at risk for acquired immune deficiency syndrome (AIDS); (4) neurological disorders—headache, craniocerebral trauma, loss of consciousness, seizures or tumors.

E. *Family history:* elicited from patient and from someone else, because quite different descriptions may be given of the same people and events; ethnic, national, and religious traditions; other people in the home, descriptions of them—personality and intelligence—and what has become of them since the patient's childhood; descriptions of different households lived in; present relationships between the patient and those who are in the patient's family; role of illness in the family; family history of mental illness; where does the patient live—neighborhood and particular residence of the patient; is the home crowded; privacy of family members from each other and from other families; sources of family income and difficulties in obtaining it; public assistance (if any) and attitudes about it; will the patient lose his or her job or apartment by remaining in the hospital; who is caring for the patient's children.

F. *Personal history (anamnesis):* history of the patient's life from infancy to the present to the extent it can be recalled; gaps in history as spontaneously related by the patient; emotions associated with different life periods (painful, stressful, and conflictual) or with phases of the life cycle.

1. Early childhood (through 3 years of age).
   a. Prenatal history and mother's pregnancy and delivery: length of pregnancy, spontaneity and normality of delivery, birth trauma, whether the patient was planned and wanted, birth defects.
   b. Feeding habits: breast fed or bottle fed, eating problems.
   c. Early development: maternal deprivation, language development, motor development, signs of unmet needs, sleep pattern, object constancy, stranger anxiety, separation anxiety.
   d. Toilet training: age, attitude of parents, feelings about it.
   e. Symptoms of behavior problems: thumb sucking, temper tantrums, tics, head bumping, rocking, night terrors, fears, bed wetting or bed soiling, nail biting, masturbation.
   f. Personality and temperament as a child: shy, restless, overactive, withdrawn, studious, outgoing, timid, athletic, friendly patterns of play, reactions to siblings.
   g. Early or recurrent dreams or fantasies.
2. Middle childhood (3 to 11 years of age): early school history—feelings about going to school, early adjustment, gender identification, conscience development, punishment; social relationships and attitudes toward siblings and playmates.
3. Later childhood (prepuberty through adolescence).
   a. Peer relationships: number and closeness of friends, leader or follower, social popularity, participation in group or gang activities, idealized figures; patterns of aggression, passivity, anxiety, antisocial behavior.
   b. School history: how far the patient went in school; adjustment to school; relationships with teachers—teacher's pet or rebellious; favorite studies or interests; particular abilities or assets; extracurricular activities; sports; hobbies; relationships of problems or symptoms to any school period.
   c. Cognitive and motor development: learning to read and other intellectual and motor skills, minimal cerebral dysfunction, learning disabilities—their management and effects on the child.
   d. Particular adolescent emotional or physical problems: nightmares, phobias, bed wetting, running

away, delinquency, smoking, drug or alcohol use, weight problems, feeling of inferiority.

e. Psychosexual history.
   i. Early curiosity, infantile masturbation, sex play.
   ii. Acquiring of sexual knowledge, attitude of parents toward sex, sexual abuse.
   iii. Onset of puberty, feelings about it, kind of preparation, feelings about menstruation, development of secondary sexual characteristics.
   iv. Adolescent sexual activity: crushes, parties, dating, petting, masturbation, wet dreams (nocturnal emissions), and attitudes toward them.
   v. Attitudes toward same and opposite sex: timid, shy, aggressive, need to impress, seductive, sexual conquests, anxiety.
   vi. Sexual practices: sexual problems, homosexual and heterosexual experiences, paraphilias, promiscuity.

f. Religious background: strict, liberal, mixed (possible conflicts), relationship of background to current religious practices.

4. Adulthood.
   a. Occupational history: choice of occupation, training, ambitions, and conflicts; relations with authority, peers, and subordinates; number of jobs and duration; changes in job status; current job and feelings about it.
   b. Social activity: whether patient has friends; whether he or she is withdrawn or socializing well; social, intellectual, and physical interests; relationships with same sex and opposite sex; depth, duration, and quality of human relations.
   c. Adult sexuality.
      i. Premarital sexual relationships, age of first coitus, sexual orientation.
      ii. Marital history: common-law marriages; legal marriages; description of courtship and role played by each partner; age at marriage; family planning and contraception; names and ages of children; attitudes toward raising children; problems of any family members; housing difficulties, if important to the marriage; sexual adjustment; extramarital affairs; areas of agreement and disagreement; management of money; role of in-laws.
      iii. Sexual symptoms: anorgasmia, impotence (erectile disorder), premature ejaculation, lack of desire.
      iv. Attitudes toward pregnancy and having children; contraceptive practices and feelings about them.
      v. Sexual practices: paraphilias, such as sadism, fetishes, voyeurism; attitude toward fellatio, cunnilingus; coital techniques, frequency.
   d. Military history: general adjustment, combat, injuries, referral to psychiatrists, type of discharge, veteran status.
   e. Value systems: whether children are seen as a burden or a joy; whether work is seen as a necessary evil, an avoidable chore, or an opportunity; current attitude about religion; belief in heaven and hell.

II. Mental status

Sum total of the examiner's observations and impressions derived from the initial interview.

A. *Appearance.*
   1. Personal identification: may include a brief nontechnical description of the patient's appearance and behavior as a novelist might write it. Attitude toward examiner can be described here: cooperative, attentive, interested, frank, seductive, defensive, hostile, playful, ingratiating, evasive, or guarded.
   2. Behavior and psychomotor activity: gait, mannerisms, tics, gestures, twitches, stereotypes, picking, touching examiner, echopraxia, clumsy, agile, limp, rigid, retarded, hyperactive, agitated, combative, or waxy.
   3. General description: posture, bearing, clothes, grooming, hair, nails; healthy, sickly, angry, frightened, apathetic, perplexed, contemptuous, ill at ease, poised, old looking, young looking, effeminate, masculine; signs of anxiety—moist hands, perspiring forehead, restlessness, tense posture, strained voice, wide eyes; shifts in level of anxiety during interview or with particular topic; eye contact (50 percent is normal).

B. *Speech:* rapid, slow, pressured, hesitant, emotional, monotonous, loud, whispered, slurred, mumbled, stuttering, echolalia, intensity, pitch, ease, spontaneity, productivity, manner, reaction time, vocabulary, prosody.

C. *Mood and affect.*
   1. Mood (a pervasive and sustained emotion that colors the person's perception of the world): how does patient say he or she feels; depth, intensity, duration, and fluctuations of mood—depressed, despairing, irritable, anxious, terrified, angry, expansive, euphoric, empty, guilty, awed, futile, self-contemptuous, anhedonic, alexithymic.
   2. Affect (the outward expression of the patient's inner experiences): how the examiner evaluates the patient's affects—broad, restricted, blunted or flat, shallow, amount and range of expression; difficulty in initiating, sustaining, or terminating an emotional response; whether the emotional expression is appropriate to the thought content, culture, and setting of the examination; examples should be given if emotional expression is not appropriate.

D. *Thinking and perception.*
   1. Form of thinking.
      a. Productivity: overabundance of ideas, paucity of ideas, flight of ideas, rapid thinking, slow thinking, hesitant thinking; whether the patient speaks spontaneously or only when questions are asked; stream of thought, quotations from patient.
      b. Continuity of thought: whether the patient's replies really answer questions and are goal directed, relevant, or irrelevant; loose associations; lack of cause-and-effect relationships in the patient's explanations; illogical, tangential, circumstantial, rambling, evasive, persevering statements, blocking or distractibility.
      c. Language impairments: impairments that reflect disordered mentation, such as incoherent or incomprehensible speech (word salad), clang associations, neologisms.
   2. Content of thinking.
      a. Preoccupations: about the illness, environmental problems; obsessions, compulsions, phobias; obsessions or plans about suicide, homicide; hypochondriacal symptoms, specific antisocial urges or impulses.

3. Thought disturbances.
   a. Delusions: content of any delusional system, its organization, the patient's convictions as to its validity, how it affects his or her life; persecutory delusions—isolated or associated with pervasive suspiciousness; mood-congruent or mood-incongruent; thought insertion.
   b. Ideas of reference and ideas of influence: how ideas began, their content, and the meaning that the patient attributes to them.
4. Perceptual disturbances.
   a. Hallucinations and illusions: whether the patient hears voices or sees visions; content, sensory system involvement, circumstances of the occurrence; hypnagogic or hypnopompic hallucinations; thought broadcasting.
   b. Depersonalization and derealization: extreme feelings of detachment from self or from the environment.
5. Dreams and fantasies.
   a. Dreams: prominent ones, if the patient will tell them; nightmares.
   b. Fantasies: recurrent, favorite, or unshakable daydreams.

E. *Sensorium.*

1. Alertness: awareness of environment, attention span, clouding of consciousness, fluctuations in levels of awareness, somnolence, stupor, lethargy, fugue state, coma.
2. Orientation.
   a. Time: whether the patient identifies the day or the approximate date and the time of day correctly; if in a hospital, whether the patient knows how long he or she has been there; whether the patient behaves as though oriented to the present.
   b. Place: whether patient knows where he or she is.
   c. Person: whether patient knows who the examiner is and the roles or names of the persons with whom the patient is in contact.
3. Concentration and calculation: whether the patient can subtract 7 from 100 and keep subtracting 7s; if the patient cannot subtract 7s, whether easier tasks can be accomplished, such as 4×9 and 5×4; whether the patient can calculate how many nickels are in $1.35; whether anxiety or some disturbance of mood or concentration seems to be responsible for difficulty.
4. Memory: impairment, efforts made to cope with impairment—denial, confabulation, catastrophic reaction, circumstantiality used to conceal deficit; whether the process of registration, retention, or recollection of material is involved.
   a. Remote memory: childhood data, important events known to have occurred when the patient was younger or free of illness, personal matters, neutral material.
   b. Recent past memory: past few months.
   c. Recent memory: past few days, what did the patient do yesterday and the day before, what did the patient have for breakfast, lunch, and dinner.
   d. Immediate retention and recall: ability to repeat six figures after the examiner dictates them—first forward, then backward, then after a few minutes' interruption; other test questions; whether the same questions, if repeated, called forth different answers at different times.
   e. Effect of defect on patient: mechanisms the patient has developed to cope with the defect.
5. Fund of knowledge: level of formal education and self-education; estimate of the patient's intellectual capability and whether the patient is capable of functioning at the level of his or her basic endowment; counting, calculation, general knowledge; questions should have relevance to the patient's educational and cultural background.
6. Abstract thinking: disturbances in concept formation; manner in which the patient conceptualizes or handles his or her ideas; similarities (e.g., between apples and pears), differences, absurdities; meanings of simple proverbs, such as "a rolling stone gathers no moss"; answers may be concrete (giving specific examples to illustrate the meaning) or overly abstract (giving generalized explanation); appropriateness of answers.
7. Insight: degree of personal awareness and understanding of illness.
   a. Complete denial of illness.
   b. Slight awareness of being sick and needing help but denying it at the same time.
   c. Awareness of being sick but blaming it on others, external factors, or medical or unknown organic factors.
   d. Intellectual insight: admission of illness and recognition that symptoms or failures in social adjustment are due to irrational feelings or disturbances, without applying that knowledge to future experiences.
   e. True emotional insight: emotional awareness of the motives and feelings within and of the underlying meaning of symptoms; whether the awareness leads to changes in personality and future behavior; openness to new ideas and concepts about self and the important people in the patient's life.
8. Judgment.
   a. Social judgment: subtle manifestations of behavior that are harmful to the patient and contrary to acceptable behavior in the culture; whether the patient understands the likely outcome of personal behavior and is influenced by that understanding; examples of impairment.
   b. Test judgment: the patient's prediction of what he or she would do in imaginary situations; for instance, what patient would do with a stamped, addressed letter found in the street.

III. Further diagnostic studies

A. Physical examination.
B. Neurological examination.
C. Additional psychiatric diagnostic interviews.
D. Interviews with family members, friends, or neighbors by a social worker.
E. Psychological, neurological, or laboratory tests, as indicated: EEG, CT scan, magnetic resonance imaging (MRI), tests of other medical conditions (e.g., human immunodeficiency virus [HIV]), reading comprehension and writing tests, test for aphasia, projective or objective psychological tests, dexamethasone-suppression test (DST), 24-hour urine test for heavy metal intoxication, urine screen for drugs of abuse, sleep studies in chronic insomnia.

IV. Summary of findings

Mental symptoms, medical and laboratory findings, and psychological and neurological test results, if available, are summarized. Include the medications that the patient has been taking, their dosage, their duration.

Clarity of thinking is reflected in clarity of writing. When summarizing the mental status, for example, the phrase "patient denies hallucinations and delusions" is not as precise as "patient denies hearing voices or thinking that he is being followed." The latter indicates the specific question asked and the specific response given. Similarly, in the conclusion of the report, one would write, "Hallucinations and delusions were not elicited."

V. Diagnosis

Diagnostic classification is made according to DSM-IV-TR, which uses a multiaxial classification scheme consisting of five axes, each of which should be covered in the diagnosis (Table 7.3–1).

VI. Prognosis

Opinion about the probable future course, extent, and outcome of the disorder; good and bad prognostic factors; specific goals of therapy.

VII. Psychodynamic formulation

Causes of the patient's psychodynamic breakdown—influences in the patient's life that contributed to the present disorder, environmental, genetic, and personality factors relevant to determining the patient's symptoms; primary and secondary gains; outline of the major defense mechanism used by the patient (Table 7.3–2).

VIII. Comprehensive treatment plan

Modalities of treatment recommended, role of medication, inpatient or outpatient treatment, frequency of sessions, probable duration of therapy; type of psychotherapy; individual, group, or cognitive-behavioral family therapy; symptoms or problems to be treated. Initially, treatment must be directed toward any life-threatening situations, such as suicidal risk or risk of danger to others, which require psychiatric hospitalization. Danger to self or others is an acceptable reason (legally and medically) for involuntary hospitalization. In the absence of the need for confinement, a variety of outpatient treatment alternatives are available: day hospitals, supervised residences, outpatient psychotherapy, or pharmacotherapy, among others. In some cases, treatment planning must attend to vocational and psychosocial skills training and even legal or forensic issues. Comprehensive treatment planning requires a therapeutic team approach using the skills of psychologists, social workers, nurses, activity and occupational therapists, and a variety of other mental health professionals, with referral to self-help groups (e.g., Alcoholics Anonymous [AA]) if needed. If the patient or family members are unwilling to accept the recommendations of treatment, and the clinician thinks that the refusal of the recommendations may have serious consequences, the patient, parent, or guardian should sign a statement to the effect that the recommended treatment was refused.

MEDICAL RECORD

The psychiatric report is a part of the medical record; however, the medical record is more than the psychiatric report. It is a narrative that documents all events that occur during the course of treatment, most often referring to the patient's stay in the hospital. Progress notes record every interaction between doctor and patient; reports of all special studies, including laboratory tests; and prescriptions and orders for all medications. Nurses' notes help describe the patient's course: Is the patient beginning to respond to treatment? Are there times during the day or night when symptoms get worse or remit? Are there adverse effects or complaints by the patient about prescribed medication? Are there signs of agitation, violence, or mention of suicide? If the patient requires restraints or seclusion, are the proper supervisory procedures being followed? Taken as a whole, the medical record tells what happened to the patient since first making contact with the health care system. It concludes with a discharge summary that provides a concise overview of the patient's course with recommendations for future treatment, if necessary. Evidence of contact with a referral agency should be documented in the medical record to establish continuity of care if further intervention is necessary.

Use of the Record

The medical record is not only used by physicians, but is also used by regulatory agencies and managed care companies to determine length of stay, quality of care, and reimbursement to doctors and hospitals. In theory, the inpatient medical record is accessible to authorized persons only and is safeguarded for confidentiality. In practice, however, absolute confidentiality cannot be guaranteed. Guidelines for what material needs to be incorporated into the medical record are given in Table 7.3–3.

The medical record is also crucial in malpractice litigation. Robert I. Simon summarized the liability issues as follows:

> Properly kept medical records can be the psychiatrist's best ally in malpractice litigation. If no record is kept, numerous questions will be raised regarding the psychiatrist's competence and credibility. This failure to keep medical records may also violate state statutes or licensing provisions. Failure to keep medical records may arise out of the psychiatrist's concern that patient treatment information be totally protected. Although this is an admirable ideal, in real life the psychiatrist may be legally compelled under certain circumstances to testify directly about confidential treatment matters.

Outpatient records are also subject to scrutiny by third parties under certain circumstances, and psychiatrists in private practice are under the same obligation to maintain a record of the patient in treatment as the hospital psychiatrist. Table 7.3–4 lists documentation issues of concern to third-party payers.

Personal Notes and Observations

According to laws relating to access to medical records, some jurisdictions (such as in the Public Health Law of New York State) have a provision that applies to a physician's personal notes and observations. *Personal notes* are defined as "a practitioner's speculations, impressions (other than tentative or actual diagnosis) and reminders." The data are maintained only by the clinician and cannot be disclosed to any other person, including the patient. Psychiatrists concerned about material that may prove damaging or otherwise hurtful to the patient if released to a third party may consider using this provision to maintain doctor–patient confidentiality.

Psychotherapy Notes

Psychotherapy notes include details of transference, fantasies, dreams, personal information about per-

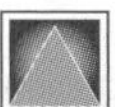

Table 7.3–2
Glossary of Specific Defense Mechanisms

Acting out: The individual deals with emotional conflict or internal or external stressors by actions rather than reflections or feelings. This definition is broader than the original concept of the acting out of transference feelings or wishes during psychotherapy and is intended to include behavior arising both within and outside the transference relationship. Defensive acting out is not synonymous with "bad behavior" because it requires evidence that the behavior is related to emotional conflicts.

Altruism: The individual deals with emotional conflict or internal or external stressors by dedication to meeting the needs of others. Altruism differs from the self-sacrifice sometimes characteristic of reaction formation in that the individual receives gratification either vicariously or from the response of others.

Anticipation: The individual deals with emotional conflict or internal or external stressors by experiencing emotional reactions in advance of, or anticipating consequences of, possible future events and considering realistic, alternative responses or solutions.

Denial: The individual deals with emotional conflict or internal or external stressors by refusing to acknowledge some painful aspect of external reality or subjective experience that would be apparent to others. The term *psychotic denial* is used when gross impairment in reality testing is present.

Displacement: The individual deals with emotional conflict or internal or external stressors by transferring a feeling about, or a response to, one object onto another (usually less threatening) substitute object.

Dissociation: The individual deals with emotional conflict or internal or external stressors with a breakdown in the usually integrated functions of consciousness, memory, perception of self or the environment, or sensory/motor behavior.

Humor: The individual deals with emotional conflict or external stressors by emphasizing the amusing or ironic aspects of the conflict or stressor.

Idealization: The individual deals with emotional conflict or internal or external stressors by attributing exaggerated positive qualities to others.

Intellectualization: The individual deals with emotional conflict or internal or external stressors by the excessive use of abstract thinking or the making of generalizations to control or minimize disturbing feelings.

Isolation of affect: The individual deals with emotional conflict or internal or external stressors by the separation of ideas from the feelings originally associated with them. The individual loses touch with the feelings associated with a given idea (e.g., a traumatic event) while remaining aware of the cognitive elements of it (e.g., descriptive details).

Omnipotence: The individual deals with emotional conflict or internal or external stressors by feeling or acting as if he or she possesses special powers or abilities and is superior to others.

Projection: The individual deals with emotional conflict or internal or external stressors by falsely attributing to another his or her own unacceptable feelings, impulses, or thoughts.

Projective identification: As in projection, the individual deals with emotional conflict or internal or external stressors by falsely attributing to another his or her own unacceptable feelings, impulses, or thoughts. However, the individual does not fully disavow what is projected, as in simple projection. Instead, the individual remains aware of his or her own affects or impulses but misattributes them as justifiable reactions to the other person. Not infrequently, the individual induces the very feelings in others that were first mistakenly believed to be there, making it difficult to clarify who did what to whom first.

Rationalization: The individual deals with emotional conflict or internal or external stressors by concealing the true motivations for his or her own thoughts, actions, or feelings through the elaboration of reassuring or self-serving but incorrect explanations.

Reaction formation: The individual deals with emotional conflict or internal or external stressors by substituting behavior, thoughts, or feelings that are diametrically opposed to his or her own unacceptable thoughts or feelings (this usually occurs in conjunction with his or her repression).

Repression: The individual deals with emotional conflict or internal or external stressors by expelling disturbing wishes, thoughts, or experiences from conscious awareness. The feeling component may remain conscious, detached from its associated ideas.

Splitting: The individual deals with emotional conflict or internal or external stressors by compartmentalizing opposite affect states and failing to integrate the positive and negative qualities of the self or others into cohesive images. Because ambivalent affects cannot be experienced simultaneously, more balanced views and expectations of self or others are excluded from emotional awareness. Self and object images tend to alternate between polar opposites: exclusively loving, powerful, worthy, nurturing, and kind—or exclusively bad, hateful, angry, destructive, rejecting, or worthless.

Sublimation: The individual deals with emotional conflict or internal or external stressors by channeling potentially maladaptive feelings or impulses into socially acceptable behavior (e.g., contact sports to channel angry impulses).

Suppression: The individual deals with emotional conflict or internal or external stressors by intentionally avoiding thinking about disturbing problems, wishes, feelings, or experiences.

Undoing: The individual deals with emotional conflict or internal or external stressors by words or behavior designed to negate or to make amends symbolically for unacceptable thoughts, feelings, or actions.

From American Psychiatric Association. *Diagnostic and Statistical Manual of Mental Disorders,* 4th ed. Text rev. Washington, DC: American Psychiatric Association, 2000, with permission.

sons with whom the patient interacts, and other intimate details of the patient's life. They may also include the psychiatrist's comments on his or her countertransference and feelings toward the patient. Psychotherapy notes should be kept separate from the rest of the medical records.

Patient Access to Records

Patients have a legal right to access their medical records. This right represents society's belief that the responsibility for medical care has become a collaborative process between doctor and patient. Patients see many different physicians, and they can be more effective historians and coordinators of their own care with such information.

Psychiatrists must be careful in releasing their records to the patient if, in their judgment, the patient can be harmed emotionally as a result. Under these circumstances, the psychiatrist may choose to prepare a summary of the patient's course of treatment, holding back material that might be hurtful—especially if it were to get into the hands of third parties. In malpractice cases, however, it may not be possible to do so.

When litigation occurs, the entire medical record is subject to discovery. Psychotherapy notes are usually protected, but not

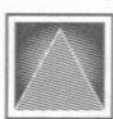

Table 7.3–3
Medical Record

There shall be an individual record for each person admitted to the psychiatric inpatient unit. Patient records shall be safeguarded for confidentiality and should be accessible only to authorized persons. Each case record shall include

- Legal admission documents
- Identifying information on the individual and family
- Source of referral, date of commencement of service, and name of staff member carrying overall responsibility for treatment and care
- Initial, intercurrent, and final diagnoses, including psychiatric or mental retardation diagnoses in official terminology
- Reports of all diagnostic examinations and evaluations, including findings and conclusions
- Reports of all special studies performed, including X-rays, clinical laboratory tests, clinical psychological testing, electroencephalograms, and psychometric tests
- The individual written plan of care, treatment, and rehabilitation
- Progress notes written and signed by all staff members having significant participation in the program of treatment and care
- Summaries of case conferences and special consultations
- Dated and signed prescriptions or orders for all medications, with notation of termination dates
- Closing summary of the course of treatment and care
- Documentation of any referrals to another agency

Adapted from the 1995 guidelines of the New York State Office of Mental Health.

always. If psychotherapy notes are ordered to be produced, the judge would probably review them privately and select what is relevant to the case in question.

E-Mail E-mail is increasingly being used by physicians as a quick and efficient way to communicate not only with patients but with other doctors about their patients; however, it is a public document and should be treated as such. The dictum of not diagnosing or prescribing medication over the telephone to a patient one has not examined should also apply to e-mail. It is not only dangerous but also unethical. All e-mail messages should be printed out for the paper chart unless electronic archives are regularly backed up and secure.

Problem-Oriented Medical Record In 1969, Lawrence L. Weed published *Medical Records, Medical Education and Patient Care* in which he described the problem-oriented medical record. The problem-oriented medical record lists all health problems discovered in the initial workup. Problem areas are added to and corrected over time. Active problems are listed in one column, and, as they are resolved, they are transferred to an inactive column. Progress notes are dated, titled, and numbered according to the problem list. As a final check, the record is audited for thoroughness, reliability, efficiency, and standards of treatment and outcome.

Problem-Oriented Record in Medical Education Many medical schools are using educational techniques based on the problem-oriented medical record. Teaching and testing organizations such as the United States Medical Licensing Examination (USMLE) are relying on the ability of a student to deal with a problem-oriented medical record as an evaluation tool. In such exercises, students are provided with general patient information, which may include a summary of the physical examination and positive elements in the psychiatric report. Students must delineate the problem areas that need attention, determine preventive or treatment options for each problem, and understand the patient from biological, social, and psychological points of view.

Although the problem-oriented medical record is not the standard format used by psychiatrists, it has influenced how patients are viewed. For example, in DSM-IV-TR, specific psychosocial and environmental problems that may affect diagnosis of mental disorders are recorded on Axis IV. The problems are divided into nine categories that can each affect the person adversely: (1) problems with primary support group (e.g., death of family member), (2) problems related to the social environment (e.g., absence of friends), (3) educational problems (e.g., discord with teachers or classmates), (4) occupational problems (e.g., stress at work), (5) housing problems (e.g., unsafe neighborhood), (6) economic problems (e.g., excess debt), (7) problems with access to health care services (e.g., no health insurance), (8) problems with the legal system (e.g., litigation), and (9) other problems (e.g., floods, earthquakes).

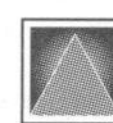

Table 7.3–4
Documentation Issues

- Are patient's areas of dysfunction described? From the biological, psychological, and social points of view?
- Is alcohol or substance abuse addressed?
- Do clinical activities happen at the expected time? If too late or never, why?
- Are issues identified in the treatment plan and followed in progress notes?
- When there is a variance in the patient's outcome, is there a note in the progress notes to that effect? Is there also a note in the progress notes reflecting the clinical strategies recommended to overcome the impediments to the patient's improvement?
- If new clinical strategies are implemented, how is their impact evaluated? When?
- Is there a sense of multidisciplinary input and coordination of treatment in the progress notes?
- Do progress notes indicate the patient's functioning in the therapeutic community and its relationship to their discharge criteria?
- Can one extrapolate from the patient's behavior in the therapeutic community how he or she will function in the community at large?
- Are there notes depicting the patient's understanding of his or her discharge planning? Family participation in discharge planning must be entered in the progress notes with their reaction to the plan.
- Do attending progress notes bridge the differences in thinking of other disciplines?
- Are the patient's needs addressed in the treatment plan?
- Are the patient's family needs evaluated and implemented?
- Is patient and family satisfaction evaluated in any way?
- Is alcohol and substance abuse addressed as a possible contributor to readmission?
- If the patient was readmitted, are there indications that previous records were reviewed, and, if the patient is on medication other than that prescribed on discharge, is there a rationale for this change?
- Do the progress notes identify the type of medication used and the rationale for increase, decrease, discontinuation, or augmentation of medication.
- Are medication effects documented, including dosages, response, and adverse or other side effects?

Note: Documentation issues are of concern to third-party payers, such as insurance companies and health maintenance organizations who examine patients' charts to see if the areas listed above are covered. In many cases, however, the review is conducted by persons with little or no background in psychiatry or psychology who do not recognize the complexities of psychiatric diagnosis and treatment. Payments to hospitals, doctors, and patients are often denied because of what such reviewers consider to be so-called inadequate documentation.

A 55-year-old married man complains of being fearful that he will be forced to resign from an administrative job because his company is being downsized. He complains of anxiety, insomnia, and irritability and gives no history of previous dysphoric states. After a thorough evaluation, it becomes apparent that the proximate cause of his symptoms is the probability of losing his job. Symptom removal is relatively simple with the aid of anxiolytic or hypnotic drugs; however, a more comprehensive approach is required. The therapist has to attend to the occupational problem, which might include having the patient confront his superiors, applying for reassignment to another area within the company, seeking other employment, evaluating his assets for early retirement, job retraining, or other approaches directed toward the vocational crisis.

Ethical Issues and the Medical Record Psychiatrists continually make judgments about what is appropriate material to include in the psychiatric report, the medical record, the case report, and other written communications about the patient. Such judgments often involve ethical issues. In a case report, for example, the patient should not be identifiable, a position made clear in the American Psychiatric Association's (APA's) *Principles of Medical Ethics with Annotations Especially Applicable to Psychiatry*, which states that published case reports must be suitably disguised to safeguard patient confidentiality without altering material to provide a less-than-complete portrayal of the patient's actual condition. In some instances, obtaining a written release from the patient that allows the psychiatrist to publish the case may also be advisable, even if the patient is appropriately disguised.

Psychiatrists sometimes include material in the medical record that is specifically directed toward warding off future culpability if liability issues are ever raised. This may include having advised the patient about specific adverse effects of medication to be prescribed.

Military Psychiatry Psychiatrists in the military face unique ethical problems, because confidentiality does not exist under the military code of conduct.

A 19-year-old, white, single man, new to military service, presented with a history of periodic episodes of anxiety when taking showers in groups with other men. He identified himself as gay and recognized that his anxiety was related to his fear of acting out his sexual impulses, thus risking court-martial and dishonorable discharge, should he ever be discovered. The psychiatrist was on the horns of a dilemma: whether to report the soldier to his commanding officer (as he was obliged to do under the military code) or to protect the soldier from acting on his impulses that would place him in danger (in keeping with the medical ethic to do no harm). After discussing various options, he and the patient agreed on the latter option. A diagnosis of anxiety disorder was made, which allowed the patient to receive an honorable discharge on medical grounds, based on a recognized psychiatric disorder. No record of his homosexual orientation was made.

Managed Care With the advent of managed care and the need to send periodic progress reports and documentation of signs and symptoms to third-party reviewers to pay for treatment, some psychiatrists may diminish or exaggerate symptomatology. The following case report and discussion illustrates the ethical difficulties psychiatrists face in dealing with managed care.

Mrs. P. admitted herself to the hospital because she was afraid she might kill herself. She was experiencing a major depressive episode, but she improved markedly during the first weeks on Dr. A.'s ward. Although Dr. A. believed that Mrs. P. was no longer suicidal, he thought she would benefit greatly from continued hospitalization. Because he knew that Mrs. P. could not afford to pay for hospitalization and that the insurance company would pay only if the patient was suicidally depressed, he decided not to document Mrs. P.'s improvement. He noted in the chart that "the patient continues to have a risk of suicide."

Does Dr. A. engage in a form of deception? Yes, he intentionally misleads by what he writes and what he omits writing in the chart. Although what he writes is true in some literal sense, his statement is misleading in the context of treatment. Mrs. P. is not suicidally depressed in the way that she was.

What Dr. A. omits from the chart is also deceptive. Whether a particular omission is deceptive depends, in part, on the roles and expectations of the people involved. Not telling a colleague that one dislikes his tie is not a deception. It is simply tact, unless the role or relationship involves the expectation that one offers a candid opinion. Dr. A.'s case is different. His professional role is to document the patient's course, and the expectation is that he will note any significant improvement. Thus, his failure to document Mrs. P.'s progress accurately is a kind of deception.

The second and more difficult question is whether deception is justified in this instance. The answer to that question depends on the reasons for the deception, the reasons against it, and the alternatives available.

The reasons for this deception are obvious. Dr. A.'s aim and primary obligation is to help the patient. He believes that Mrs. P. would benefit greatly from continued hospitalization that she cannot afford. He may also believe that it is unfair for the insurance company to refuse to pay for inpatient treatment of nonsuicidal depression and that his deception rectifies that unfair practice.

There are also important reasons against this deception. The first reason concerns honesty and social trust. It is a good thing if people can rely on what others say and write. Without some honesty and trust, many social exchanges and practices would be impossible. Deception, even for beneficent purposes, has real potential to damage social trust. A risk exists that deception may damage people's trust in the profession of psychiatry and even patients' trust in their psychiatrists. Damage to trust may, in turn, compromise treatment.

The second reason concerns future medical treatment. If Mrs. P. seeks medical treatment in the future, the physicians who attend her will read the misleading notes. If they believe that the notes are an accurate account of the previous treatment, they may suggest an inappropriate treatment for the present problem. Even if they have doubts about the accuracy of the notes in her chart, they are deprived of an accurate history and report. In either case, the prior deception can hinder treatment.

The third reason concerns obligations and coverage policies. Dr. A. seems to ignore the obligation that he has to the population that is covered by the insurance policy. He shifts a burden onto this population by forcing the insurance company to pay for treatment that it did not agree to cover. Perhaps the insurance company should pay for inpatient treatment in cases like Mrs. P.'s; perhaps its policies are unreasonable and unfair. However, Dr. A.'s deception does not challenge the insurance company and pressure it to change its policy, nor does his deception encourage patients and their families to contest the company's policies. The use of deception simply circumvents, in an ad hoc way, a policy that should be challenged and discussed.

Dr. A. also seems to ignore his obligation to future patients. By introducing an inaccuracy into the chart, he compromises the value of medical records research. His deception works, in a small way, to deprive future patients of the benefit of research that relies on medical records.

Whether the deception is justified depends not only on the weight of the reasons for and against the deception but also on the available alternatives. One alternative is to tailor the chart. Another alternative is to describe Mrs. P.'s response accurately and to discharge her to outpatient care. However, a third alternative exists. Dr. A. can accurately document the patient's course and can recommend continued hospitalization. He can petition the insurance company for coverage. If the insurance company decides not to approve further inpatient care for the patient, Dr. A. can appeal that decision. This alternative is more time consuming, and there is no guarantee that it will succeed, but it avoids all the problems associated with the use of deception.

Health Insurance Portability and Accountability Act (HIPAA) The Health Insurance Portability and Accountability Act (HIPAA) was passed in 1996 to address the medical delivery system's mounting complexity and its rising dependence on electronic communication. The act orders that the federal Department of Health and Human Services (HHS) develop rules protecting the transmission and confidentiality of patient information, and all units under HIPAA must comply with such rules.

Two rules were finalized in February, 2003: the Transaction Rule and the Privacy Rule. The Transaction Rule facilitates transferring health information effectively and efficiently by means of regulations created by the HHS that established a uniform set of formats, code sets, and data requirements. The Privacy Rule, administered by the Office of Civil Rights (OCR) at HHS, protects the confidentiality of patient information. This means that a patient's medical information belongs to the patient and that the patient has the right to access it, with the exception of psychotherapy notes, which are deemed as property of the psychotherapist who wrote them.

In 2002, the Transaction Rule was implemented, meaning that all entities covered under HIPAA must comply. The health care information involved and code sets are listed in Table 7.3–5. In 2003, the Privacy Rule was executed. Under this rule, patients have new statutory rights (Table 7.3–6).

Under the Privacy Rule, there are certain guidelines by which every practice must abide:

1. Every practice must establish written privacy procedures. These include administrative, physical, and technical safeguards that establish who has access to the patient's information, how this information is used within the facility, and when the information will and will not be disclosed to others.
2. Every practice must take steps to make sure that its business associates protect the privacy of medical records and other health information.
3. Every practice must train employees to comply with the rule.
4. Every practice must have a designated person to serve as a privacy officer. If it is an individual practice or private practice, this person can be the physician.
5. Every practice must establish complaint procedures for patients who wish to ask or to complain about the privacy of their records.

The OCR at HHS is responsible for making sure that the Privacy Rule is enforced; however, it is not clear as to how it will be done. One method expressed by the government is a *complaint-driven* system in which the OCR will respond to complaints made by patients concerning confidentiality violations or denied access to records, all of which are covered under HIPAA. In such cases, OCR may follow up and audit compliance.

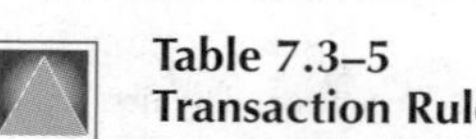

Table 7.3–5
Transaction Rule Code Sets

Health care information: The Transactions Rule defines standards and establishes code sets and forms to be used for electronic transaction that involve the following health care information:
- Claims or equivalent encounter information
- Eligibility inquiries
- Referral certification and authorization
- Claims status inquiries
- Enrollment and disenrollment information
- Payment and remittance advice
- Health plan premium payments
- Coordination of benefits

Code sets: Under the Transaction Rule, the following code sets are required for filing claims with Medicare:
- Procedure codes
  - American Medical Association Current Procedural Terminology codes
  - Healthcare Common Procedure Coding System codes
- Diagnosis codes
  - *International Classification of Disease*, ninth edition, clinical modification, codes
  - Note: Revised fourth edition of the *Diagnostic and Statistical Manual of Mental Disorders* codes are not used
- Drugs and biologicals
  - National Drug Codes
- Dental codes
  - Code on dental procedures
  - Nomenclature for dental services

Adapted from Jaffe E: HIPAA Basics for psychiatrists. *Psych Pract Manage Care.* 2002;8:15.

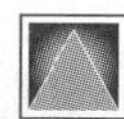

Table 7.3–6
Patient's Rights under the Privacy Rule

Physician must give the patient a written notice of his or her privacy rights, the privacy policies of the practice, and how patient information is used, kept, and disclosed. A written acknowledgment should be taken from the patient verifying that they have seen such notice.

Patients should be able to obtain copies of their medical records and to request revisions to those records within a stated amount of time (usually 30 days). Patients do not have the right to see psychotherapy notes.

Physicians must provide the patient with a history of most disclosures of their medical history on request. There are some exceptions. The APA Committee on Confidentiality has developed a model document for this requirement.

Physicians must obtain authorization from the patient for disclosure of information other than for treatment, payment, and health care operations (these three are considered to be routine uses, for which consent is not required). The APA Committee on Confidentiality has developed a model document for this requirement.

Patients may request another means of communication of their protected information (i.e., request that the physician contact them at a specific phone number or address).

Physicians cannot generally limit treatment to obtaining patient authorization for disclosure of their information for nonroutine uses.

Patients have the right to complain about Privacy Rule violations to the physician, their health plan, or to the Secretary of HHS.

APA, American Psychiatric Association; HHS, Department of Health and Human Services.
Adapted from Jaffe E: HIPAA Basics for psychiatrists. *Psych Pract Manage Care.* 2002;8:15.

The APA's Committee on Confidentiality, along with legal experts, has developed a set of sample forms. They are part of the APA's HIPAA educational packet, which can be obtained on the APA web site (http://www.psych.org/). On the site, there are also recommendations for enabling physicians to comply with HIPAA.

MEDICAL ERROR

In 2000, the public was warned about medical errors as a significant cause of patient mortality by the Institute of Medicine, which reported that more than 50,000 Americans may die each year as a result of such mistakes. A number of congressional actions followed that led eventually to legislation requiring mandatory national or state reporting by hospitals of medical errors. The result of such documentation is, as yet, unknown: Issues to contend with are the need to protect doctors and hospitals from frivolous lawsuits resulting from public disclosure and failure to maintain confidential information about patients. Additionally, a clear description of what constitutes a medical error is needed. Did the error occur because the physician departed from an accepted standard of treatment? Was the error avoidable, or the result of poor training? Or, was it unintentional—an accident—and better considered a close call or a borderline case?

By definition, medical errors require that there be a component of negligence. This is especially important in order to distinguish them from adverse events or outcomes. The latter are related to a particular disease process and are most often predictable or, if not predictable, are known risks. Medical errors usually lead to adverse events and may harm the patient temporarily or permanently, may increase the time for recovery from disease, or may result in patient death. Distinction between the two terms—*medical error* and *adverse event*—is essential to ensure rational thinking about this topic. Adverse events may occur in the absence of medical errors, and medical errors may not be associated with an adverse event.

At Johns Hopkins University, the term *medical mistake* is used instead of *medical error* and is defined as follows:

> A medical mistake is a commission or an omission with potentially negative consequences for the patient that would have been judged wrong by skilled and knowledgeable peers at the time it occurred, independent of whether there were any negative consequences. This definition excludes the natural history of disease that does not respond to treatment and the foreseeable complications of a correctly performed procedure, as well as cases in which there is reasonable disagreement over whether a mistake occurred.

Types of Error Errors may be systemic or individual. Systemic errors are caused by flaws in the hospital system or in the transfer of information from one unit of the hospital or from one group of doctors to another. In general, no one person is to blame. An example would be the unavailability or inability to retrieve a patient's medical records or a mismatched blood transfusion. The failure is in the health care delivery system as a whole rather than in the individual.

Individual errors are attributed to a particular physician or to a specific member of the treatment team. Examples include prescribing the wrong medicine or operating on the wrong leg. The physician bears the responsibility, even if the error is made by a person under his or her supervision. In one study of individual errors by medical house officers in several U.S. academic centers, the most frequently reported mistake was a missed diagnosis.

In this same study, the next most common error was related to prescribing the wrong drug or the wrong dose of the drug. Other errors had to do with procedural complications (e.g., placing a feeding tube in the trachea instead of the esophagus) or faulty communication (e.g., failure to obtain informed consent or to document do-not-resuscitate [DNR] orders).

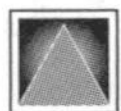

Table 7.3–7
Examples of Drug Name Confusion

Psychoactive Medication	Confused with
Metadate CD (methylphenidate)	Methadone (Dolophine)
Levoxine[a] (levothyroxine) (thyroid preparation)	Lanoxin (digoxin)
Serzone (nefazodone)	Seroquel (quetiapine)
Lamictal (lamotrigine)	Lamisil (terbinafine) (for nail infection)
Zyprexa (olanzapine)	Zyrtec (cetirizine) (for allergies)
Celexa (citalopram)	Celebrex (celecoxib) (for arthritis)

[a]Name changed to Levoxyl after U.S. Food and Drug Administration report in 1994.

Psychiatric Errors

Medication Most mistakes in psychiatry occur in two major areas: medication errors and suicide. A wrong prescription may be written, for example, the wrong medication for a disorder or the wrong dosage of a drug. A common cause of medication error is poor handwriting by physicians, which is then misread by a pharmacist or nurse. A remedy is to insist that all prescriptions be typed or transmitted via computer. Similar-sounding drug names have also been to blame for medication mistakes, for example, citalopram (Celexa) and celecoxib (Celebrex) and buspirone (BuSpar) and bupropion (Wellbutrin) (Table 7.3–7). Drugs with similar phonemes lend themselves to miscommunication in writing or in speech. Not to be confused with error are the side effects and possible adverse reactions to psychotropic or other medications. In general, most drug side effects are annoying and do not lead to serious complications, but patients must be advised if and when to expect them. Generally, litigation is rare even if the drug effect was severe, provided that informed consent is obtained beforehand, a legal requirement. A medication error would be to prescribe drugs that should not be given concomitantly, for example, imipramine (Tofranil) and meperidine (Demerol), which may be fatal.

Suicide Unlike most physicians, psychiatrists rarely have to deal with the death of patients. Exceptions may be made for geriatric psychiatrists who deal with the aged or for consultation-liaison psychiatrists who deal with the seriously medically ill; however, when death occurs in those instances, it is often expected and part of the disease progress.

Suicide is unexpected. It is also viewed by many persons as preventable. Based on that expectation, family members may sue for malpractice after the event. Suicide is not always preventable, however. Some persons who have a strong desire to kill themselves will do so despite the many advances that have been made in the treatment and management of suicidal patients. When mistakes occur, they are usually the result of the psychiatrist having underestimated the suicidal risk or, if the psychiatrist has appraised it accurately, the nurses and attendants not taking the necessary steps to ensure the patient's safety (e.g., constant observation). Litigation is more common for suicides that occur in a hospital than for those that occur in an outpatient setting, presumably because one-to-one coverage is the standard of care in the actively suicidal hospitalized patient.

Courts have not penalized psychiatrists for honest errors of judgment in clinical practice. One court stated: "The accurate predication of dangerous behavior, and particularly suicide and homicide, are almost never possible. Thus, an error of prediction or even of judgment does not necessarily establish negligence." In spite of this, however, psychiatrists are expected to evaluate patients properly for suicide risk and to establish a rational treatment plan to ensure that the risk of a patient successfully killing himself or herself is minimized as much as possible.

In the following case, the psychiatrist and hospital were held to be guilty of negligence at trial and the patient's family was awarded $950,000.

A 33-year-old woman was admitted to the hospital for suicidal risk and psychosis. When she was admitted, the locked ward had no empty beds. To lower her risk of suicide, she was sedated but placed in an open ward with no special suicidal precautions. On awakening, she jumped to her death.

Cause of Medical Error Causes of medical error are multifactorial. In most instances, they correlate with inexperience. For example, first-year house officers make more errors than do second- and third-year residents. Junior attendings make more errors than senior attendings. Clearly, the aphorism of experience being the best teacher seems to apply in these instances, but experience or the lack thereof is not the only factor. Job overload in which doctors are required to care for too many patients is a major contributor to medical errors. In the hospital setting, interns are assigned too many patients with too few supervisors. In the outpatient setting, too many patients are cared for by too few doctors. Private practitioners are under pressure by managed care companies who often reward doctors financially for productivity, which translates into a high caseload of patients that leads to overwork. Similarly, some managed care and insurance companies reward doctors who order few laboratory tests, thus lowering cost; however, this may result in misdiagnosis, especially in complex cases with atypical presentations. Finally, there is the element of fatigue, which interferes with judgment and may lead to mistakes.

Preventing Medical Error

Practice Guidelines Practice guidelines have been developed by the APA for a variety of disorders. These include delirium, dementia, substance use disorder, depressive disorder, panic disorder, borderline personality disorder, suicide, and schizophrenia. Guidelines for other psychiatric disorders will be forthcoming. According to the APA, the term *practice guideline* refers to a "set of patient care strategies developed to assist physicians in clinical decisions." They are careful to point out that guidelines are not meant to be standards of care:

> The APA Practice Guidelines are not intended to be construed or to serve as a standard of medical care. Standards of medical care are determined on the basis of all clinical data available for an individual case and are subject to change as scientific knowledge and technology advance and patterns evolve. These parameters of practice should be considered guidelines only. Adherence to them will not ensure a successful outcome in every case, nor should they be construed as including all proper methods of care or excluding other acceptable methods of care aimed at the same results. The ultimate judgment regarding a particular clinical procedure or treatment plan must be made by the psychiatrist in light of the clinical data presented by the patient and the diagnosis and treatment options available.

Although no studies have been done, common sense indicates that guidelines will improve quality of care and diminish medical errors in psychiatry. They are works in progress, however. As new methods of treatment develop, they will have to be revised and updated, lest they become fossilized and irrelevant. Other risks are their possible misuse by third parties such as managed care companies and health maintenance organizations (HMOs). Many guidelines are prepared by third-party payers and may be compromised by conflicts of interest of cost versus quality of care. Some HMOs pay bonuses to their doctors based on high scores on how closely they adhere to a set of guidelines in the treatment of a specific disorder. This may influence psychiatrists in the choice of therapy or the length of the patient's hospital stay if they are not in keeping with the set of guidelines being used. The APA practice guidelines are not the only ones that relate to psychiatry. There is a Web-based resource in a National Guideline Clearinghouse (NGC) that lists more than 500 practice guidelines with some relevance to psychiatry (http://www.guideline.gov).

There is no indication that there has been an increase in malpractice suits against psychiatrists since their introduction; however, published guidelines are often brought forward in litigation as standards of care. Psychiatrists and other physicians should not be intimidated by this practice. Psychiatrists may legally and ethically deviate from guidelines; however, the decision to do so and its rationale should be documented in the chart.

As mentioned previously, the APA guidelines do not include all proper methods of care for a particular disorder, nor do they allow for ambiguity, controversy, or dissent. For this, the practitioner must turn to a textbook, such as the *Comprehensive Textbook of Psychiatry*, in which such differences are discussed.

Regulating Working Hours of Interns and Residents Teaching hospitals often rely on interns and residents to perform services such as phlebotomies and intravenous (IV) therapy and to serve as messengers and transporters, tasks that are more appropriately performed by ancillary personnel. In addition, house staff are often required to work long hours, and sleep deprivation can impair their judgment and clinical skills. The average resident works more than 80 hours per week, with a shift of 30 hours every third or fourth night. Because of this, in 1988, a limit on the number of hours interns and residents may work was set forth by the U.S. Health Care Financing Administration (HCFA), now officially known as the Center for Medicare and Medicaid Services (CMS). Their work rules are (1) residents are limited to no more than 12 consecutive hours per assignment in emergency services, (2) residents may not work more than 80 hours per week over a 4-week period and cannot be scheduled to work more than 24 consecutive hours, and (3) scheduled rotations must be separated by not less than 8 hours of nonworking time, provided for each week. Nonworking time is time away from training and patient care activities. In 2000, 8 percent of residency training programs nationwide were cited by the Accreditation Council for Graduate Medical Education for violating the CMS work hour requirements.

In response to the death of a patient at a New York hospital in 1989, the New York state legislature enacted the Bell Commission

Report, which implied that resident work hours contributed in part to that accidental death. The state responded by establishing rules for resident work hours, including 80-hour week limits and 24-hour consecutive call limits. The impact of these limits on the continuity and quality of care remains to be seen.

In an effort to eliminate mistakes that might occur in medical schools, the CMS defined medical student responsibilities as follows: (1) Students can take histories and perform physical examinations with the approval of the patient's attending physicians; (2) they may write in the patient's chart, but all entries must be countersigned by the attending physicians; and (3) medical or surgical procedures may be performed if they are under direct inpatient supervision.

Many medical educators believe that the current CMS rules do not go far enough and that interns and residents are not used properly by many teaching hospitals. It is not uncommon for a resident in cardiac surgery to assist at an operation for 14 hours and then to stay on duty for an additional 10 hours. Similarly, a pediatric resident may be in the emergency room for 24 hours without sleep. Even though their hours fall within the CMS guidelines, they are not conducive to the resident's education in view of the inevitable fatigue when a person is without sleep for 24 hours. For residents with families, especially those who are mothers, current work schedules disrupt marital harmony and child rearing. This added stress interferes with optimal functioning. It has been suggested that chronic sleep deprivation may put residents at increased risk for motor vehicle crashes, medication errors, and decreased mental clarity. There are no easy answers to these problems, but the current situation clearly requires resolution.

Coping with Medical Errors and Adverse Events

Doctors have a long tradition of examining adverse events and of learning from their mistakes. The case presentation (also called the *clinicopathologic conference* [CPC]) is a group exercise attended by clinicians, researchers, educators, and students who examine all aspects of patient diagnosis, treatment, and outcome. Ideally, CPCs do not attempt to cast blame on a practitioner; however, if negligence has occurred, it becomes evident in the open discussion of those in attendance. In addition, most hospitals have risk management teams whose duty is to identify potential or actual instances of malpractice by physicians in the facility and to approach the patient and to discuss the situation openly and honestly. Also, offices of quality assurance function to assess and to prevent risks to patients in a continuous effort to improve care. An example of how one hospital attempts to document adverse events is provided in Table 7.3–8.

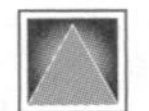

Table 7.3–8
Medical Documentation Requirements for Patient Adverse Events

These guidelines apply to instances of *adverse patient events,* which are defined as follows: *"A significant adverse patient event is an unplanned or unexpected occurrence that results in patient death, harms the patient, temporarily or permanently, or significantly increases the planned length of hospitalization."* These guidelines are applicable, however, to all medical documentation, and should be universally followed.

It is most important that the responsible attending physician (or covering attending) write a note as soon as possible after an adverse event, certainly within 24 hrs. This note should clearly document his or her active participation in the care of the patient. Subsequently, an attending note must be written daily, for as long as appropriate to the patient's status. This is a supplement to the standard Medical Board documentation requirement, especially crucial in the first few days after an adverse event occurs.

All notes must be dated, timed, and signed. If the signature is not legible, the attending should print his or her name.

When correcting or editing a note, a single strikeout line through the words to be corrected should be made; no overwriting, obliteration, whiteout, or erasures should be attempted. The corrections should be initialed along with the time and date of the correction.

The purpose of medical documentation is to promote patient care and safety, not to cast blame on an individual for an adverse patient event. When describing a patient adverse event, extreme care must be exercised to avoid implied blame for such an event by another caregiver. The note should clearly document the attending's participation in the care of the patient, and the discussion should be an objective analysis of the events that transpired, an assessment of the patient status, and a plan for subsequent management. An open disclosure approach to adverse event documentation must be followed.

Courtesy of New York University Medical Center, New York City, NY.

ETHICS OF DISCLOSURE There is an ethical duty on physicians to disclose medical errors, accidents, injury, or bad results to their patients who have an absolute right to understand what occurred during their course of treatment. An explanation is mandatory, and an apology is appropriate if an error was made. If, as a result of disclosure, legal proceedings ensue, the physician has the opportunity to offer an explanation—but appropriate compensation for harm suffered as a result of malpractice is a patient's legal right.

DOCTOR–PATIENT RELATIONSHIP A good doctor–patient relationship is characterized by a sense of trust, respect, and honesty between the two parties. The better the doctor–patient relationship, the less chance for misunderstanding leading to litigation. Studies have shown that, when a medical error or adverse event occurs within the context of a good doctor–patient relationship, litigation is rare. In its absence, however, litigation is likely in as much as 70 percent of cases of medical error, especially if a major mistake was made, regardless of whether or not death ensues. In surveys of patients, almost 100 percent desire that doctors report and discuss medical errors with them. Acknowledging medical error, minor or major, may actually reduce the risk of malpractice action.

THERAPEUTIC PRIVILEGE Therapeutic privilege is the physician's right to withhold information from a patient, if, in his or her opinion, such disclosure would cause irreparable harm to the patient. Some patients do not wish to know the nature of their illness and that right needs to be respected. Others may be so prone to anxiety or panic that even a hint of medical error (especially if no adverse outcome occurred) would be potentially dangerous to the patient's overall sense of well-being.

DUTY TO DISCLOSE There is a patient-consumer movement supported by some members of the legal profession that would require physicians by law to report medical errors. As mentioned previously, disclosure is currently an ethical, not a legal, obligation. Proponents of duty to disclose argue that self-policing by the medical profession is inefficient, and a legal duty to disclose malpractice would provide a remedy. Proponents of such laws would also require that they apply not only to the person committing the error, but also to those who witness the error, for example, nurses and members of the treatment team.

Opponents of the duty to disclose law argue that it would harm the doctor–patient relationship and, in particular, weaken the trust and teamwork among health care professionals who would be required to be informants on one another. Adopting a rule of disclosure also suggests to the public that doctors, as a group, are not to be trusted. Opponents of the law also note that quality assurance and risk management programs that bring negligent acts to light are already in place and that

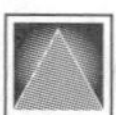

Table 7.3–9
Confusing Medical Notations

Prohibited Abbreviation	Potential Problem	Preferred Term
U (for unit)	Read as a zero (0) or a four (4), causing a tenfold overdose or greater (4 U seen as "40" or 4 u seen as "44").	Write "unit."
IU (for international unit)	Misread as "IV" (intravenous) or 10.	Write "international unit."
Q.D. and Q.O.D. (Latin for once daily and every other day)	Mistaken for each other. Also, the period after the Q can be mistaken for an I and the O can be mistaken for an I.	Write "daily" or "every other day."
Trailing zero (X.0 mg) and lack of leading zero (.X mg)	Decimal point is missed.	Never write a zero by itself after a decimal point (X mg) and always use a zero before a decimal point (0.X mg).
MS, MSO_4, and $MgSO_4$	Confused for one another. Can mean morphine sulfate or magnesium sulfate.	Write "morphine sulfate" or "magnesium sulfate."

further enforcement is unnecessary. Most experts take the position that physicians are the ones who ultimately must decide to disclose errors based on their professional and ethical beliefs.

Regulation of the Quality of Health Care

HOSPITAL STANDARDS AND PERFORMANCE A group of agencies, such as the Joint Commission of Accreditation of Healthcare Organizations (JCAHO) and the Liaison Committee on Medical Education (LCME), influence the standards of hospital care and performance. In addition, hospitals must comply with government regulations (city and state health rules). The JCAHO inspects hospitals every 2 years and is also responsible for determining the requirements for hospital accreditation. Hospital reimbursements from Medicare and Medicaid are contingent on meeting these standards, but the accreditation is done on a voluntary basis. The LCME and the Liaison Committee on Graduate Education are charged with accrediting medical schools and residency training programs, respectively. The two accrediting committees review education and training programs every 4 years; the procedure is voluntary.

The JCAHO is also involved in preventing medical errors and developed guidelines to help surgical teams standardize safety systems. The guidelines, called "The Universal Protocol for Preventing Wrong Site, Wrong Procedure, Wrong Person Surgery," address the verification of documents, marking operative sites, and other issues related to patient safety.

The JCAHO issued a list of dangerous, unapproved abbreviations, acronyms, and symbols that accredited organizations must discontinue using as part of their National Patient Safety Goal requirements. The list of unapproved abbreviations pertains to all handwritten, patient-specific communication (Table 7.3–9).

HOSPITAL UTILIZATION REVIEW This in-house evaluation process was created to make sure that institutions provide efficient, quality health care that meets patients' needs. The members of the utilization review committee consist of hospital administrators, physicians, and nurses. The committee reviews each patient's chart within a specified number of days of admission. The appropriateness of the admission, treatment strategies, and the length of the hospital stay are reviewed to facilitate the patient's discharge. Through this process, the utilization review committee determines whether a particular admission was really indicated and whether the hospital stay was longer than necessary. A hospital must conduct utilization reviews to be eligible for JCAHO accreditation.

PROFESSIONAL STANDARDS REVIEW ORGANIZATION The Professional Standards Review Organization (PSRO) was set up by the federal government to review and to monitor care received by patients whose care is paid for with government funds. PSROs are made up of physicians elected by local medical societies that have been established by local medical associations and serve several functions: They attempt to ensure high-quality care, to control costs, to determine maximum lengths of stay by patients in hospitals, to conduct utilization reviews, and to censure physicians who do not adhere to established guidelines. A PSRO may conduct a medical audit to evaluate the quality of care retrospectively by carefully examining charts.

PEER REVIEW ORGANIZATION In the early 1980s, the peer review organization (PRO) replaced PSROs as the federal review organization for hospitals receiving Medicare funds. To promote compliance with federal guidelines for health and hospital care, PROs conduct independent utilization reviews and quality-of-care studies, validate diagnosis-related group (DRG) assignments, and review hospital admissions and readmissions.

Federally mandated and funded, the PROs have greater authority than the PSROs. PROs can impose sanctions on hospitals for inadequate care; they can even recommend the termination of federal funding to hospitals that consistently violate federal standards. In addition, PROs can adjust or refuse payment for health services that they consider unnecessary.

SUGGESTED CROSS-REFERENCES

Psychiatric rating scales appear in Section 7.9 on psychiatric rating scales and in Section 9.1 on classification of mental disorders. A detailed discussion of DSM-IV-TR's multiaxial system appears in Section 9.1 on the classification of mental disorders. The psychiatric interview, history, and mental status examination are discussed in Section 7.1. Medical assessment and laboratory testing are discussed in Section 7.8. Computer-based testing of the psychiatric patient is covered in Section 7.10.

References

*Ball C: Evidence-based medicine on the wards: report from an evidence-based minion. *ACP J Club.* 1999;130:15.

Callis R, Polmantier PC, Roeber EC. *A Casebook of Counseling.* New York: Appleton-Century-Crofts; 1955.

Coleman M, Gillberg C. *The Schizophrenias: A Biological Approach to the Schizophrenia Spectrum Disorders.* New York: Springer; 1996.

Dwyer J, Shih A: The ethics of tailoring the patient's chart. *Psychiatr Serv.* 1998;49:1309.

Evans J. *Three Men.* New York: Knopf; 1954.

*Fischer CB, Fried AL: Internet-mediated psychological services and the American Psychological Association Ethics Code. *Psychother Theor Res Pract Train.* 2003; 40:103.

*Ginzberg E: The uncertain future of managed care. *N Eng J Med.* 1999;340:144.

Greist H: Computer-based assessment of patients. *J Clin Pharmacol.* 1998;18:359.

Groth-Marnat G. *Handbook of Psychological Assessment.* 4th ed. New York: John Wiley & Sons, Inc.; 2003.
Jeffords JM: Confidentiality of medical information: Protecting privacy in an electronic age. *Prof Psychol Res Pract.* 1999;30:115.
Krauss JB: A matter of privacy. *Arch Pract Nurs.* 2003;17:99.
Lewis ND. *Outline for Psychiatric Exam.* Albany, NY: New York State Department of Mental Hygiene; 1943.
Lysaker PH, Wickett AM, Campbell K, Buck KD: Movement toward coherence in the psychotherapy of schizophrenia: A method for assessing narrative transformation. *J Nerv Ment Dis.* 2003;191:538.
Maio JE: HIPAA and the special status of psychotherapy notes. *Lippincott Case Manage.* 2003;8:24.
*Mark D: Effects of physician awareness of symptom-related expectations and mental disorders: A controlled trial. *Arch Fam Med.* 1999;8:135.
Martin S: Indefinite delay in E & M. *AMA News.* 1998;41:18.
Pierluissi E, Fischer MA, Campbell AR, Landefeld CS: Discussion of medical errors in morbidity and mortality conferences. *JAMA.* 2003;290:2838.
Shea SC. *Psychiatric Interviewing.* 2nd ed. Philadelphia: WB Saunders; 1998.
Simon RI. *Clinical Psychiatry and the Law.* 2nd ed. Washington, DC: American Psychiatric Press; 1992:89.
Stephenson W: Methodology of single case studies. *J Oper Psychiatry.* 1974;5:3.
Weber B, Schneider B, Fritze J, Gille B, Hornung S, Kuehner T, Maurer K: Acceptance of computerized compared to pencil-and-paper assessment in psychiatric inpatients. *Comput Hum Behav.* 2003;19:81.
Wedding D, Corsini RJ. *Case Studies in Psychotherapy.* Itaska, IL: Peacock; 1989.
*Weed LL: Medical records that guide and teach. *N Engl J Med.* 1968;278:593.
Zilboorg G, Henry GB. *A History of Medical Psychology.* New York: Norton; 1941.

▲ 7.4 Signs and Symptoms in Psychiatry

BENJAMIN J. SADOCK, M.D.

Signs are objective; symptoms are subjective. Signs are the clinician's observations, such as noting a patient's agitation; symptoms are subjective experiences, such as a person's complaint of feeling depressed. In psychiatry, signs and symptoms are not so clearly demarcated as in other fields of medicine; they often overlap. Because of this, disorders in psychiatry are often described as syndromes—a constellation of signs and symptoms that together make up a recognizable condition. Schizophrenia, for example, is more often viewed as a syndrome than as a specific disorder. This concept is expressed in the use of the terms *schizophrenic spectrum* or *the group of schizophrenias.*

RELATIONSHIP OF PSYCHIATRIC SIGNS AND SYMPTOMS TO NORMALITY

Normality and mental health are central issues in psychiatric theory and practice but are difficult to define. For example, *normality* has been defined as patterns of behavior or personality traits that are typical or that conform to some standard of proper and acceptable ways of behaving and being. The use of terms such as *typical* or *acceptable*, however, has been criticized, because they are ambiguous, involve value judgments, and vary from one culture to another. To overcome this objection, psychiatrist and historian George Mora devised a system to describe behavioral manifestations that are normal in one context but not in another, depending on how the person is viewed by the society (Table 7.4–1). This paradigm, however, may give too much weight to peer group observations and judgments. The World Health Organization (WHO) defines *normality* as a state of complete physical, mental, and social well-being, but, again, this definition is limited, because it defines *physical* and *mental health* simply as the absence of physical or mental disease.

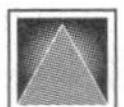

Table 7.4–1
Normality in Context

Term	Concept
Autonormal	Person seen as normal by his or her own society
Autopathological	Person seen as abnormal by his or her own society
Heteronormal	Person seen as normal by members of another society observing him or her
Heteropathological	Person seen as unusual or pathological by members of another society observing him or her

Data courtesy of George Mora, M.D.

The text revision of the fourth edition of the *Diagnostic and Statistical Manual of Mental Disorders* (DSM-IV-TR) offers no definition of *normality* or *mental health*, although a definition of *mental disorder* is presented. According to DSM-IV-TR, a mental disorder is conceptualized as a behavioral or psychological syndrome or pattern that is associated with distress (e.g., a painful symptom) or disability (i.e., impairment in one or more important areas of functioning). In addition, the syndrome or pattern must not be merely an expected and culturally sanctioned response to a particular event, such as the death of a loved one. DSM-IV-TR emphasizes that neither deviant behavior (e.g., political, religious, or sexual) nor conflicts that are primarily between the individual and society are mental disorders.

In *Mental Health: A Report of the Surgeon General*, *mental health* is defined as "the successful performance of mental functions, in terms of thought, mood, and behavior, that results in productive activities, fulfilling relationships with others, and the ability to adapt to change and to cope with adversity." A controversial view is held by the psychiatrist Thomas Szasz, who believes that the concept of mental illness should be abandoned entirely. In his book *The Myth of Mental Illness*, Szasz states that normality can be measured only in terms of what persons do or do not do and that defining normality is beyond the realm of psychiatry.

Finally, psychiatry has been criticized over the years by certain groups for its portrayal of normality. The psychology of women, for example, has been criticized as sexist, because it was formulated initially by men; similar criticism comes from other groups who believe that the portrayal of their psychological issues is biased by placing undue emphasis on psychopathology rather than healthy attributes. A much discussed issue is the change in psychiatry's view of homosexuality from abnormal to normal that took place in the 1970s, an evolution shaped by cultural norms, society's expectations and values, professional biases, individual differences, and the political climate of the time.

FUNCTIONAL PERSPECTIVES OF NORMALITY

The many theoretical and clinical concepts of normality seem to fall into four functional perspectives. Although each perspective is unique and has its own definition and description, the perspectives complement each other, and, together, they represent the totality of the behavioral science and social science approaches to the subject. The four perspectives of normality as described by Daniel Offer and Melvin Sabshin are (1) normality as health, (2) normality as utopia, (3) normality as average, and (4) normality as process.

Normality As Health The first perspective is basically the traditional medical psychiatric approach to health and illness. Most physicians equate normality with health and view health as an almost universal phenomenon. As a result, behavior is assumed to be within normal limits when no manifest psychopathology is present. If all behavior were to be put on a scale, normality would encompass the major portion of the continuum, and abnormality would be the small remainder.

This definition of normality correlates with the traditional model of the doctor who attempts to free his or her patient from grossly observable signs and symptoms. To this physician, the lack of signs or symptoms indicates health. *Health*, in this context, refers to a reasonable, rather than an optimal, state of functioning. In its simplest form, this perspective, as described by John Romano, views a healthy person as one who is reasonably free of undue pain, discomfort, and disability.

Normality As Utopia The second perspective conceives of normality as that harmonious and optimal blending of the diverse elements of the mental apparatus that culminates in optimal functioning. Such a definition emerges when psychiatrists or psychoanalysts talk about the ideal person, when they grapple with a complex problem, or when they discuss their criteria for a successful treatment. This approach can be traced back to Sigmund Freud, who, when discussing normality, stated, "A normal ego is like normality in general, an ideal fiction."

Although this approach is characteristic of many psychoanalysts, it is by no means unique to them. It can also be found among other psychotherapists in the field of psychiatry and among psychologists of quite different persuasions.

Normality As Average The third perspective is commonly used in normative studies of behavior and is based on a mathematical principle of the bell-shaped curve. This approach considers the middle range to be normal and the extremes to be deviant. The normative approach based on this statistical principle describes each individual in terms of general assessment and total score. Variability is described only within the context of groups, not within the context of the individual.

Although this approach is more commonly used in psychology than in psychiatry, psychiatrists have been relying on normative pencil-and-paper tests to a much larger extent than in the past. Not only do psychiatrists use instruments such as the Minnesota Multiphasic Personality Inventory (MMPI), they also construct their own tests and questionnaires.

Normality As Process The fourth perspective stresses that normal behavior is the end result of interacting systems. Based on this definition, temporal changes are essential to a complete definition of normality. In other words, the normality-as-process perspective stresses changes or processes rather than a cross-sectional definition of normality.

Investigators who subscribe to this approach can be found in all of the behavioral and social sciences. A typical example of the concepts in this perspective is Erik Erikson's conceptualization of the epigenesis of personality development and the seven development stages essential in the attainment of mature adult functioning.

PSYCHOANALYTIC THEORIES OF NORMALITY

Some psychoanalysts base their concepts of normality on the absence of symptoms, but, although the disappearance of symptoms is necessary for cure or improvement, the absence of symptoms alone does not suffice for a comprehensive definition of normality. Accordingly, most psychoanalysts view a capacity for work and enjoyment as indicating normality or, as Freud put it, the ability "to love and to work."

The psychoanalyst Heinz Hartmann conceptualized normality by describing the "autonomous functions of the ego." These are psychological capacities present at birth that are conflict free, that is, uninfluenced by the internal psychic world. They include perception, intuition, comprehension, thinking, language, certain aspects of motor development, learning, and intelligence. The concept of autonomous and conflict-free functions of the ego helps explain the mechanisms whereby some persons lead relatively normal lives in the presence of extraordinary external experiential traumas—the so-called invulnerable child, that is, a child who is invulnerable to the "slings and arrows of outrageous fortune" by virtue of autonomous ego strengths. A summary of some psychoanalytic views of normality is given in Table 7.4–2.

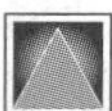
Table 7.4–2
Concepts of Normality

Theorist	Concept
Sigmund Freud	Normality is an ideal fiction.
Kurt Eissler	Absolute normality cannot be obtained, because the normal person must be totally aware of his or her thoughts and feelings.
Melanie Klein	Normality is characterized by strength of character, the capacity to deal with conflicting emotions, the ability to experience pleasure without conflict, and the ability to love.
Erik Erikson	Normality is the ability to master the periods of life: trust vs. mistrust, autonomy vs. shame and doubt, initiative vs. guilt, industry vs. inferiority, identity vs. role confusion, intimacy vs. isolation, generativity vs. stagnation, and ego integrity vs. despair.
Laurence Kubie	Normality is the ability to learn by experience, to be flexible, and to adapt to a changing environment.
Heinz Hartmann	Conflict-free ego functions represent the person's potential for normality; the degree to which the ego can adapt to reality and be autonomous is related to mental health.
Karl Menninger	Normality is the ability to adjust to the external world with contentment and to master the task of acculturation.
Alfred Adler	The person's capacity to develop social feeling and to be productive is related to mental health; the ability to work heightens self-esteem and makes one capable of adaptation.
R. E. Money-Kryle	Normality is the ability to achieve insight into one's self, an ability that is never fully accomplished.
Otto Rank	Normality is the capacity to live without fear, guilt, or anxiety and to take responsibility for one's own actions.
John Romano	Normality is to be free of pain, discomfort, and disability.

Karl Jaspers Karl Jaspers (1883 to 1969), the German psychiatrist and philosopher, described a "personal world"—the way a person thinks or feels—that could be normal or abnormal. According to Jaspers, the personal world is abnormal when it (1) springs from a condition that is recognized universally as abnormal, such as schizophrenia; (2) when it separates the person from others emotionally;

and (3) when it does not provide the person with a sense of "spiritual and material" security.

Jaspers was a proponent of phenomenology, in which the clinician studies psychological signs and symptoms with the goal of understanding the internal experience of the patient. By listening carefully to the patient, the psychiatrist temporarily enters the mental life of the patient. Jaspers believed that, to fully understand the signs and symptoms observed in the patient, the clinician must have no prior assumptions. A person who reports a hallucinatory experience, for example, must not be judged thereby as being abnormal or psychotic. To be used diagnostically, the phenomenon must occur repeatedly and must be characteristic of a known disorder.

Some investigators are developing a research strategy that defines normality by examining a person's mental state at various times during the day in different life settings. What is abnormal in one setting or at one time of day may be normal in another.

Robert Campbell Finally, there is the commonly accepted and widely used definition of mental health adapted from Robert Campbell's *Psychiatric Dictionary*: Psychically normal persons are those who are in harmony with themselves and with their environment. They conform with the cultural requirements or injunctions of their community. They may possess medical deviation or disease, but, as long as this does not impair their reasoning, judgment, intellectual capacity, and ability to make a harmonious personal and social adaptation, they may be regarded as psychically sound or normal.

Many psychiatric signs and symptoms can be understood as various points on a spectrum of behavior ranging from normal to pathological. It is extremely rare to have a pathognomonic sign or symptom in psychiatry, although, in some cases, the disturbance is specific to a neurological deficit. As John Nemiah wrote: "Psychiatry is a science of inexhaustible complexity. It is as infinite as the range of human emotions and behavior. One cannot possibly learn it all." Because of that, psychiatry still remains as much art as science.

GLOSSARY OF SIGNS AND SYMPTOMS

abreaction A process by which repressed material, particularly a painful experience or a conflict, is brought back to consciousness; in this process, the person not only recalls, but also relives the repressed material, which is accompanied by the appropriate affective response.

abstract thinking Thinking characterized by the ability to grasp the essentials of a whole, to break a whole into its parts, and to discern common properties. To think symbolically.

abulia Reduced impulse to act and to think, associated with indifference about consequences of action. Occurs as a result of neurological deficit, depression, and schizophrenia.

acalculia Loss of ability to do calculations; not caused by anxiety or impairment in concentration. Occurs with neurological deficit and learning disorder.

acataphasia Disordered speech in which statements are incorrectly formulated. Patients may express themselves with words that sound like the ones intended but are not appropriate to the thoughts, or they may use totally inappropriate expressions.

acathexis Lack of feeling associated with an ordinarily emotionally charged subject; in psychoanalysis, it denotes the patient's detaching or transferring of emotion from thoughts and ideas. Also called *decathexis.* Occurs in anxiety, dissociative, schizophrenic, and bipolar disorders.

acenesthesia Loss of sensation of physical existence.

acrophobia Dread of high places.

acting out Behavioral response to an unconscious drive or impulse that brings about temporary partial relief of inner tension; relief is attained by reacting to a present situation as if it were the situation that originally gave rise to the drive or impulse. Common in borderline states.

aculalia Nonsense speech associated with marked impairment of comprehension. Occurs in mania, schizophrenia, and neurological deficit.

adiadochokinesia Inability to perform rapid alternating movements. Occurs with neurological deficit and cerebellar lesions.

adynamia Weakness and fatigability, characteristic of neurasthenia and depression.

aerophagia Excessive swallowing of air. Seen in anxiety disorder.

affect The subjective and immediate experience of emotion attached to ideas or mental representations of objects. Affect has outward manifestations that may be classified as restricted, blunted, flattened, broad, labile, appropriate, or inappropriate. *See also* **mood.**

ageusia Lack or impairment of the sense of taste. Seen in depression and neurological deficit.

aggression Forceful, goal-directed action that may be verbal or physical; the motor counterpart of the affect of rage, anger, or hostility. Seen in neurological deficit, temporal lobe disorder, impulse-control disorders, mania, and schizophrenia.

agitation Severe anxiety associated with motor restlessness.

agnosia Inability to understand the import or significance of sensory stimuli; cannot be explained by a defect in sensory pathways or cerebral lesion; the term has also been used to refer to the selective loss or disuse of knowledge of specific objects because of emotional circumstances, as seen in certain schizophrenic, anxious, and depressed patients. Occurs with neurological deficit. For types of agnosia, see the specific term.

agoraphobia Morbid fear of open places or leaving the familiar setting of the home. May be present with or without panic attacks.

agraphia Loss or impairment of a previously possessed ability to write.

ailurophobia Dread of cats.

akathisia Subjective feeling of motor restlessness manifested by a compelling need to be in constant movement; may be seen as an extrapyramidal adverse effect of antipsychotic medication. May be mistaken for psychotic agitation.

akinesia Lack of physical movement, as in the extreme immobility of catatonic schizophrenia; may also occur as an extrapyramidal effect of antipsychotic medication.

akinetic mutism Absence of voluntary motor movement or speech in a patient who is apparently alert (as evidenced by eye movements). Seen in psychotic depression and catatonic states.

alexia Loss of a previously possessed reading facility; not explained by defective visual acuity. *Compare with* **dyslexia.**

alexithymia Inability or difficulty in describing or being aware of one's emotions or moods; elaboration of fantasies associated with depression, substance abuse, and posttraumatic stress disorder (PTSD).

algophobia Dread of pain.

alogia Inability to speak because of a mental deficiency or an episode of dementia.

ambivalence Coexistence of two opposing impulses toward the same thing in the same person at the same time. Seen in schizophrenia, borderline states, and obsessive-compulsive disorders (OCDs).

amimia Lack of the ability to make gestures or to comprehend those made by others.

amnesia Partial or total inability to recall past experiences; may be organic (*amnestic disorder*) or emotional (*dissociative amnesia*) in origin.

amnestic aphasia Disturbed capacity to name objects, even though they are known to the patient. Also called *anomic aphasia.*

anaclitic Depending on others, especially as the infant on the mother; anaclitic depression in children results from an absence of mothering.

analgesia State in which one feels little or no pain. Can occur under hypnosis and in dissociative disorder.

anancasm Repetitious or stereotyped behavior or thought usually used as a tension-relieving device; used as a synonym for obsession and seen in obsessive-compulsive (anankastic) personality.

androgyny Combination of culturally determined female and male characteristics in one person.

anergia Lack of energy.

anhedonia Loss of interest in and withdrawal from all regular and pleasurable activities. Often associated with depression.

anomia Inability to recall the names of objects.

anorexia Loss or decrease in appetite. In *anorexia nervosa*, appetite may be preserved, but the patient refuses to eat.

anosognosia Inability to recognize a physical deficit in oneself (e.g., patient denies paralyzed limb).

anterograde amnesia Loss of memory for events subsequent to the onset of the amnesia; common after trauma. *Compare with* **retrograde amnesia.**

anxiety Feeling of apprehension caused by anticipation of danger, which may be internal or external.

apathy Dulled emotional tone associated with detachment or indifference; observed in certain types of schizophrenia and depression.

aphasia Any disturbance in the comprehension or expression of language caused by a brain lesion. For types of aphasia, see the specific term.

aphonia Loss of voice. Seen in conversion disorder.

apperception Awareness of the meaning and significance of a particular sensory stimulus as modified by one's own experiences, knowledge, thoughts, and emotions. *See also* **perception.**

appropriate affect Emotional tone in harmony with the accompanying idea, thought, or speech.

apraxia Inability to perform a voluntary purposeful motor activity; cannot be explained by paralysis or other motor or sensory impairment. In *constructional apraxia*, a patient cannot draw two- or three-dimensional forms.

astasia abasia Inability to stand or to walk in a normal manner, even though normal leg movements can be performed in a sitting or lying down position. Seen in conversion disorder.

astereognosis Inability to identify familiar objects by touch. Seen with neurological deficit. *See also* **neurological amnesia.**

asyndesis Disorder of language in which the patient combines unconnected ideas and images. Commonly seen in schizophrenia.

ataxia Lack of coordination, physical or mental. (1) In neurology, refers to loss of muscular coordination. (2) In psychiatry, the term *intrapsychic ataxia* refers to lack of coordination between feelings and thoughts; seen in schizophrenia and in severe OCD.

atonia Lack of muscle tone. *See* **waxy flexibility.**

attention Concentration; the aspect of consciousness that relates to the amount of effort exerted in focusing on certain aspects of an experience, activity, or task. Usually impaired in anxiety and depressive disorders.

auditory hallucination False perception of sound, usually voices, but also other noises, such as music. Most common hallucination in psychiatric disorders.

aura (1) Warning sensations, such as automatisms, fullness in the stomach, blushing, and changes in respiration, cognitive sensations, and mood states usually experienced before a seizure. (2) A sensory prodrome that precedes a classic migraine headache.

autistic thinking Thinking in which the thoughts are largely narcissistic and egocentric, with emphasis on subjectivity rather than objectivity, and without regard for reality; used interchangeably with autism and dereism. Seen in schizophrenia and autistic disorder.

behavior Sum total of the psyche that includes impulses, motivations, wishes, drives, instincts, and cravings, as expressed by a person's behavior or motor activity. Also called *conation.*

bereavement Feeling of grief or desolation, especially at the death or loss of a loved one.

bizarre delusion False belief that is patently absurd or fantastic (e.g., invaders from space have implanted electrodes in a person's brain). Common in schizophrenia. In nonbizarre delusion, content is usually within the range of possibility.

blackout Amnesia experienced by alcoholics about behavior during drinking bouts; usually indicates reversible brain damage.

blocking Abrupt interruption in train of thinking before a thought or idea is finished; after a brief pause, the person indicates no recall of what was being said or was going to be said (also known as *thought deprivation* or *increased thought latency*). Common in schizophrenia and severe anxiety.

blunted affect Disturbance of affect manifested by a severe reduction in the intensity of externalized feeling tone; one of the fundamental symptoms of schizophrenia, as outlined by Eugen Bleuler.

bradykinesia Slowness of motor activity, with a decrease in normal spontaneous movement.

bradylalia Abnormally slow speech. Common in depression.

bradylexia Inability to read at normal speed.

bruxism Grinding or gnashing of the teeth, typically occurring during sleep. Seen in anxiety disorder.

carebaria Sensation of discomfort or pressure in the head.

catalepsy Condition in which persons maintain the body position into which they are placed; observed in severe cases of catatonic schizophrenia. Also called *waxy flexibility* and *cerea flexibilitas. See also* **command automatism.**

cataplexy Temporary sudden loss of muscle tone, causing weakness and immobilization; can be precipitated by a variety of emotional states and is often followed by sleep. Commonly seen in narcolepsy.

catatonic excitement Excited, uncontrolled motor activity seen in catatonic schizophrenia. Patients in catatonic state may suddenly erupt into an excited state and may be violent.

catatonic posturing Voluntary assumption of an inappropriate or bizarre posture, generally maintained for long periods of time. May switch unexpectedly with catatonic excitement.

catatonic rigidity Fixed and sustained motoric position that is resistant to change.

catatonic stupor Stupor in which patients ordinarily are well aware of their surroundings.

cathexis In psychoanalysis, a conscious or unconscious investment of psychic energy in an idea, concept, object, or person. *Compare with* **acathexis.**

causalgia Burning pain that may be organic or psychic in origin.

cenesthesia Change in the normal quality of feeling tone in a part of the body.

cephalagia Headache.

cerea flexibilitas Condition of a person who can be molded into a position that is then maintained; when an examiner moves the person's limb, the limb feels as if it were made of wax. Also called *catalepsy* or *waxy flexibility.* Seen in schizophrenia.

chorea Movement disorder characterized by random and involuntary quick, jerky, purposeless movements. Seen in Huntington's disease.

circumstantiality Disturbance in the associative thought and speech processes in which a patient digresses into unnecessary details and inappropriate thoughts before communicating the central idea. Observed in schizophrenia, obsessional disturbances, and certain cases of dementia. *See also* **tangentiality.**

clang association Association or speech directed by the sound of a word rather than by its meaning; words have no logical connection; punning and rhyming may dominate the verbal behavior. Seen most frequently in schizophrenia or mania.

claustrophobia Abnormal fear of closed or confining spaces.

clonic convulsion An involuntary, violent muscular contraction or spasm in which the muscles alternately contract and relax. Characteristic phase in grand mal epileptic seizure.

clouding of consciousness Any disturbance of consciousness in which the person is not fully awake, alert, and oriented. Occurs in delirium, dementia, and cognitive disorder.

cluttering Disturbance of fluency involving an abnormally rapid rate and erratic rhythm of speech that impedes intelligibility; the affected individual is usually unaware of communicative impairment.

cognition Mental process of knowing and becoming aware; function is closely associated with judgment.

coma State of profound unconsciousness from which a person cannot be roused, with minimal or no detectable responsiveness to stimuli; seen in injury or disease of the brain, in systemic conditions such as diabetic ketoacidosis and uremia, and in intoxications with alcohol and other drugs. Coma may also occur in severe catatonic states and in conversion disorder.

coma vigil Coma in which a patient appears to be asleep but can be aroused (also known as *akinetic mutism*).

command automatism Condition associated with catalepsy in which suggestions are followed automatically.

command hallucination False perception of orders that a person may feel obliged to obey or unable to resist.

complex A feeling-toned idea.

complex partial seizure A seizure characterized by alterations in consciousness that may be accompanied by complex hallucinations (sometimes olfactory) or illusions. During the seizure, a state of impaired consciousness resembling a dream-like state may occur, and the patient may exhibit repetitive, automatic, or semipurposeful behavior.

compulsion Pathological need to act on an impulse that, if resisted, produces anxiety; repetitive behavior in response to an obsession or performed according to certain rules, with no true end in itself other than to prevent something from occurring in the future.

conation That part of a person's mental life concerned with cravings, strivings, motivations, drives, and wishes as expressed through behavior or motor activity.

concrete thinking Thinking characterized by actual things, events, and immediate experience, rather than by abstractions; seen in young children, in those who have lost or never developed the ability to generalize (as in certain cognitive mental disorders), and in schizophrenic persons. *Compare with* **abstract thinking.**

condensation Mental process in which one symbol stands for a number of components.

confabulation Unconscious filling of gaps in memory by imagining experiences or events that have no basis in fact, commonly seen in amnestic syndromes; should be differentiated from lying. *See also* **paramnesia.**

confusion Disturbances of consciousness manifested by a disordered orientation in relation to time, place, or person.

consciousness State of awareness, with response to external stimuli.

constipation Inability to defecate or difficulty in defecating.

constricted affect Reduction in intensity of feeling tone that is less severe than that of blunted affect.

constructional apraxia Inability to copy a drawing, such as a cube, clock, or pentagon, as a result of a brain lesion.

conversion phenomena The development of symbolic physical symptoms and distortions involving the voluntary muscles or special sense organs; not under voluntary control and not explained by any physical disorder. Most common in conversion disorder, but also seen in a variety of mental disorders.

convulsion An involuntary, violent muscular contraction or spasm. *See also* **clonic convulsion** *and* **tonic convulsion.**

coprolalia Involuntary use of vulgar or obscene language. Observed in some cases of schizophrenia and in Tourette's syndrome.

coprophagia Eating of filth or feces.

cryptographia A private written language.

cryptolalia A private spoken language.

cycloplegia Paralysis of the muscles of accommodation in the eye; observed, at times, as an autonomic adverse effect (anticholinergic effect) of antipsychotic or antidepressant medication.

decompensation Deterioration of psychic functioning caused by a breakdown of defense mechanisms. Seen in psychotic states.

déjà entendu Illusion that what one is hearing one has heard previously. *See also* **paramnesia.**

déjà pensé Condition in which a thought never entertained before is incorrectly regarded as a repetition of a previous thought. *See also* **paramnesia.**

déjà vu Illusion of visual recognition in which a new situation is incorrectly regarded as a repetition of a previous experience. *See also* **paramnesia.**

delirium Acute reversible mental disorder characterized by confusion and some impairment of consciousness; generally associated with emotional lability, hallucinations or illusions, and inappropriate, impulsive, irrational, or violent behavior.

delirium tremens Acute and sometimes fatal reaction to withdrawal from alcohol, usually occurring 72 to 96 hours after the cessation of heavy drinking; distinctive characteristics are marked autonomic hyperactivity (tachycardia, fever, hyperhidrosis, and dilated pupils), usually accompanied by tremulousness, hallucinations, illusions, and delusions. Called *alcohol withdrawal delirium* in DSM-IV-TR. *See also* **formication.**

delusion False belief, based on incorrect inference about external reality, that is firmly held despite objective and obvious contradictory proof or evidence and despite the fact that other members of the culture do not share the belief.

delusion of control False belief that a person's will, thoughts, or feelings are being controlled by external forces.

delusion of grandeur Exaggerated conception of one's importance, power, or identity.

delusion of infidelity False belief that one's lover is unfaithful. Sometimes called *pathological jealousy.*

delusion of persecution False belief of being harassed or persecuted; often found in litigious patients who have a pathological tendency to take legal action because of imagined mistreatment. Most common delusion.

delusion of poverty False belief that one is bereft or will be deprived of all material possessions.

delusion of reference False belief that the behavior of others refers to oneself or that events, objects, or other people have a particular and unusual significance, usually of a negative nature; derived from idea of reference, in which persons falsely feel that others are talking about them (e.g., belief that people on television or radio are talking to or about the person). *See also* **thought broadcasting.**

delusion of self-accusation False feeling of remorse and guilt. Seen in depression with psychotic features.

dementia Mental disorder characterized by general impairment in intellectual functioning without clouding of consciousness; characterized by failing memory, difficulty with calculations, distractibility, alterations in mood and affect, impaired judgment and abstraction, reduced facility with language, and disturbance of orientation. Although irreversible because of underlying progressive degenerative brain disease, dementia may be reversible if the cause can be treated.

denial Defense mechanism in which the existence of unpleasant realities is disavowed; refers to keeping out of conscious awareness any aspects of external reality that, if acknowledged, would produce anxiety.

depersonalization Sensation of unreality concerning oneself, parts of oneself, or one's environment that occurs under extreme stress or fatigue. Seen in schizophrenia, depersonalization disorder, and schizotypal personality disorder.

depression Mental state characterized by feelings of sadness, loneliness, despair, low self-esteem, and self-reproach; accompanying signs include psychomotor retardation or, at times, agitation, withdrawal from interpersonal contact, and vegetative symptoms, such as insomnia and anorexia. The term refers to a mood that is so characterized or a mood disorder.

derailment Gradual or sudden deviation in train of thought without blocking; sometimes used synonymously with *loosening of association.*

derealization Sensation of changed reality or that one's surroundings have altered. Usually seen in schizophrenia, panic attacks, and dissociative disorders.

dereism Mental activity that follows a totally subjective and idiosyncratic system of logic and fails to take the facts of reality or experience into consideration. Characteristic of schizophrenia. *See also* **autistic thinking.**

detachment Characterized by distant interpersonal relationships and lack of emotional involvement.

devaluation Defense mechanism in which a person attributes excessively negative qualities to self or others. Seen in depression and paranoid personality disorder.

diminished libido Decreased sexual interest and drive. (Increased libido is often associated with mania.)

dipsomania Compulsion to drink alcoholic beverages.

disinhibition (1) Removal of an inhibitory effect, as in the reduction of the inhibitory function of the cerebral cortex by alcohol. (2) In psychiatry, a greater freedom to act in accordance with inner drives or feelings and with less regard for restraints dictated by cultural norms or one's superego.

disorientation Confusion; impairment of awareness of time, place, and person (the position of the self in relation to other persons). Characteristic of cognitive disorders.

displacement Unconscious defense mechanism by which the emotional component of an unacceptable idea or object is transferred to a more acceptable one. Seen in phobias.

dissociation Unconscious defense mechanism involving the segregation of any group of mental or behavioral processes from the rest of the person's psychic activity; may entail the separation of an idea from its accompanying emotional tone, as seen in dissociative and conversion disorders. Seen in dissociative disorders.

distractibility Inability to focus one's attention; the patient does not respond to the task at hand but attends to irrelevant phenomena in the environment.

dread Massive or pervasive anxiety, usually related to a specific danger.

dreamy state Altered state of consciousness, likened to a dream situation, that develops suddenly and usually lasts a few minutes; accompanied by visual, auditory, and olfactory hallucinations. Commonly associated with temporal lobe lesions.

drowsiness State of impaired awareness associated with a desire or inclination to sleep.

dysarthria Difficulty in articulation, the motor activity of shaping phonated sounds into speech, not in word finding or in grammar.

dyscalculia Difficulty in performing calculations.

dysgeusia Impaired sense of taste.

dysgraphia Difficulty in writing.

dyskinesia Difficulty in performing movements. Seen in extrapyramidal disorders.

dyslalia Faulty articulation caused by structural abnormalities of the articulatory organs or impaired hearing.

dyslexia Specific learning disability syndrome involving an impairment of the previously acquired ability to read; unrelated to the person's intelligence. *Compare with* **alexia.**

dysmetria Impaired ability to gauge distance relative to movements. Seen in neurological deficit.

dysmnesia Impaired memory.

dyspareunia Physical pain in sexual intercourse, usually emotionally caused and more commonly experienced by women; may also result from cystitis, urethritis, or other medical conditions.

dysphagia Difficulty in swallowing.

dysphasia Difficulty in comprehending oral language (*reception dysphasia*) or in trying to express verbal language (*expressive dysphasia*).

dysphonia Difficulty or pain in speaking.

dysphoria Feeling of unpleasantness or discomfort; a mood of general dissatisfaction and restlessness. Occurs in depression and anxiety.

dysprosody Loss of normal speech melody (*prosody*). Common in depression.

dystonia Extrapyramidal motor disturbance consisting of slow, sustained contractions of the axial or appendicular musculature; one movement often predominates, leading to relatively sustained postural deviations; acute dystonic reactions (facial grimacing and torticollis) are occasionally seen with the initiation of antipsychotic drug therapy.

echolalia Psychopathological repeating of words or phrases of one person by another; tends to be repetitive and persistent. Seen in certain kinds of schizophrenia, particularly the catatonic types.

ego-alien Denoting aspects of a person's personality that are viewed as repugnant, unacceptable, or inconsistent with the rest of the personality. Also called *ego-dystonia. Compare with* **ego-syntonic.**

egocentric Self-centered; selfishly preoccupied with one's own needs; lacking interest in others.

ego-dystonic *See* **ego-alien.**

egomania Morbid self-preoccupation or self-centeredness. *See also* **narcissism.**

ego-syntonic Denoting aspects of a personality that are viewed as acceptable and consistent with that person's total personality. Personality traits are usually ego-syntonic. *Compare with* **ego-alien.**

eidetic image Unusually vivid or exact mental image of objects previously seen or imagined.

elation Mood consisting of feelings of joy, euphoria, triumph, and intense self-satisfaction or optimism. Occurs in mania when not grounded in reality.

elevated mood Air of confidence and enjoyment; a mood more cheerful than normal but not necessarily pathological.

emotion Complex feeling state with psychic, somatic, and behavioral components; external manifestation of emotion is *affect.*

emotional insight A level of understanding or awareness that one has emotional problems. It facilitates positive changes in personality and behavior when present.

emotional lability Excessive emotional responsiveness characterized by unstable and rapidly changing emotions.

encopresis Involuntary passage of feces, usually occurring at night or during sleep.

enuresis Incontinence of urine during sleep.

erotomania Delusional belief, more common in women than in men, that someone is deeply in love with them (also known as *de Clérambault syndrome*).

erythrophobia Abnormal fear of blushing.

euphoria Exaggerated feeling of well-being that is inappropriate to real events. Can occur with drugs such as opiates, amphetamines, and alcohol.

euthymia Normal range of mood, implying absence of depressed or elevated mood.

evasion Act of not facing up to, or strategically eluding, something; consists of suppressing an idea that is next in a thought series and replacing it with another idea closely related to it. Also called *paralogia* and *perverted logic.*

exaltation Feeling of intense elation and grandeur.

excited Agitated, purposeless motor activity uninfluenced by external stimuli.

expansive mood Expression of feelings without restraint, frequently with an overestimation of their significance or importance. Seen in mania and grandiose delusional disorder.

expressive aphasia Disturbance of speech in which understanding remains, but ability to speak is grossly impaired; halting, laborious, and inaccurate speech (also known as *Broca's*, *nonfluent*, and *motor aphasias*).

expressive dysphasia Difficulty in expressing verbal language; the ability to understand language is intact.

externalization More general term than *projection* that refers to the tendency to perceive in the external world and in external objects elements of one's own personality, including instinctual impulses, conflicts, moods, attitudes, and styles of thinking.

extroversion State of one's energies being directed outside oneself. *Compare with* **introversion.**

false memory A person's recollection and belief by the patient of an event that did not actually occur. In *false memory syndrome*, persons erroneously believe that they sustained an emotional or physical (e.g., sexual) trauma in early life.

fantasy Daydream; fabricated mental picture of a situation or chain of events. A normal form of thinking dominated by unconsciousness material that seeks wish fulfillment and solutions to conflicts; may serve as the matrix for creativity. The content of the fantasy may indicate mental illness.

fatigue A feeling of weariness, sleepiness, or irritability after a period of mental or bodily activity. Seen in depression, anxiety, neurasthenia, and somatoform disorders.

fausse reconnaissance False recognition, a feature of paramnesia. Can occur in delusional disorders.

fear Unpleasurable emotional state consisting of psychophysiological changes in response to a realistic threat or danger. *Compare with* **anxiety.**

flat affect Absence or near absence of any signs of affective expression.

flight of ideas Rapid succession of fragmentary thoughts or speech in which content changes abruptly and speech may be incoherent. Seen in mania.

floccillation Aimless plucking or picking, usually at bedclothes or clothing, commonly seen in dementia and delirium.

fluent aphasia Aphasia characterized by inability to understand the spoken word; fluent but incoherent speech is present. Also called *Wernicke's*, *sensory*, and *receptive aphasias.*

folie à deux Mental illness shared by two persons, usually involving a common delusional system; if it involves three persons, it is referred to as *folie à trois*, etc. Also called *shared psychotic disorder.*

formal thought disorder Disturbance in the form of thought rather than the content of thought; thinking characterized by loosened associations, neologisms, and illogical constructs; thought process is disordered, and the person is defined as psychotic. Characteristic of schizophrenia.

formication Tactile hallucination involving the sensation that tiny insects are crawling over the skin. Seen in cocaine addiction and delirium tremens.

free-floating anxiety Severe, pervasive, generalized anxiety that is not attached to any particular idea, object, or event. Observed particularly in anxiety disorders, although it may be seen in some cases of schizophrenia.

fugue Dissociative disorder characterized by a period of almost complete amnesia, during which a person actually flees from an immediate life situation and begins a different life pattern; apart from the amnesia, mental faculties and skills are usually unimpaired.

galactorrhea Abnormal discharge of milk from the breast; may result from the endocrine influence (e.g., prolactin) of dopamine receptor antagonists, such as phenothiazines.

generalized tonic-clonic seizure Generalized onset of tonic-clonic movements of the limbs, tongue biting, and incontinence followed by slow, gradual recovery of consciousness and cognition; also called *grand mal seizure.*

global aphasia Combination of grossly nonfluent aphasia and severe fluent aphasia.

glossolalia Unintelligible jargon that has meaning to the speaker but not to the listener. Occurs in schizophrenia.

grandiosity Exaggerated feelings of one's importance, power, knowledge, or identity. Occurs in delusional disorder and manic states.

grief Alteration in mood and affect consisting of sadness appropriate to a real loss; normally, it is self limited. *See also* **depression** *and* **mourning.**

guilt Emotional state associated with self-reproach and the need for punishment. In psychoanalysis, refers to a feeling of culpability that stems from a conflict between the ego and the superego (conscience). Guilt has normal psychological and social functions, but special intensity or absence of guilt characterizes many mental disorders, such as depression and antisocial personality disorder, respectively. Psychiatrists distinguish shame as a less internalized form of guilt that relates more to others than to the self. *See also* **shame.**

gustatory hallucination Hallucination primarily involving taste.

gynecomastia Female-like development of the male breasts; may occur as an adverse effect of antipsychotic and antidepressant drugs because of increased prolactin levels or anabolic-androgenic steroid abuse.

hallucination False sensory perception occurring in the absence of any relevant external stimulation of the sensory modality involved. For types of hallucinations, see the specific term.

hallucinosis State in which a person experiences hallucinations without any impairment of consciousness.

haptic hallucination Hallucination of touch.

hebephrenia Complex of symptoms, considered a form of schizophrenia, characterized by wild or silly behavior or mannerisms, inappropriate affect, and delusions and hallucinations that are transient and unsystematized. Hebephrenic schizophrenia is now called *disorganized schizophrenia.*

holophrastic Using a single word to express a combination of ideas. Seen in schizophrenia.

hyperactivity Increased muscular activity. The term is commonly used to describe a disturbance found in children that is manifested by constant restlessness, overactivity, distractibility, and difficulties in learning. Seen in *attention-deficit/hyperactivity disorder* (ADHD).

hyperalgesia Excessive sensitivity to pain. Seen in somatoform disorder.

hyperesthesia Increased sensitivity to tactile stimulation.

hypermnesia Exaggerated degree of retention and recall. It can be elicited by hypnosis and may be seen in certain prodigies; also may be a feature of OCD, some cases of schizophrenia, and manic episodes of bipolar I disorder.

hyperphagia Increase in appetite and intake of food.

hyperpragia Excessive thinking and mental activity. Generally associated with manic episodes of bipolar I disorder.

hypersomnia Excessive time spent asleep. May be associated with underlying medical or psychiatric disorder or narcolepsy, may be part of the Kleine-Levin syndrome, or may be primary.

hyperventilation Excessive breathing, generally associated with anxiety, which can reduce blood carbon dioxide concentration and can produce lightheadedness, palpitations, numbness, tingling periorally and in the extremities, and, occasionally, syncope.

hypervigilance Excessive attention to and focus on all internal and external stimuli; usually seen in delusional or paranoid states.

hypesthesia Diminished sensitivity to tactile stimulation.

hypnagogic hallucination Hallucination occurring while falling asleep, not ordinarily considered pathological.

hypnopompic hallucination Hallucination occurring while awakening from sleep, not ordinarily considered pathological.

hypnosis Artificially induced alteration of consciousness characterized by increased suggestibility and receptivity to direction.

hypoactivity Decreased motor and cognitive activity, as in psychomotor retardation; visible slowing of thought, speech, and movements. Also called *hypokinesis.*

hypochondria Exaggerated concern about health that is based not on real medical pathology, but on unrealistic interpretations of physical signs or sensations as abnormal.

hypomania Mood abnormality with the qualitative characteristics of mania but somewhat less intense. Seen in cyclothymic disorder.

idea of reference Misinterpretation of incidents and events in the outside world as having direct personal reference to oneself; occasionally observed in normal persons, but frequently seen in paranoid patients. If present with sufficient frequency or intensity or if organized and systematized, they constitute delusions of reference.

illogical thinking Thinking containing erroneous conclusions or internal contradictions; psychopathological only when it is marked and not caused by cultural values or intellectual deficit.

illusion Perceptual misinterpretation of a real external stimulus. *Compare with* **hallucination.**

immediate memory Reproduction, recognition, or recall of perceived material within seconds after presentation. *Compare with* **long-term memory** *and* **short-term memory.**

impaired insight Diminished ability to understand the objective reality of a situation.

impaired judgment Diminished ability to understand a situation correctly and to act appropriately.

impulse control Ability to resist an impulse, drive, or temptation to perform some action.

inappropriate affect Emotional tone out of harmony with the idea, thought, or speech accompanying it. Seen in schizophrenia.

incoherence Communication that is disconnected, disorganized, or incomprehensible. *See also* **word salad**.

incorporation Primitive unconscious defense mechanism in which the psychic representation of another person or aspects of another person are assimilated into oneself through a figurative process of symbolic oral ingestion; represents a special form of introjection and is the earliest mechanism of identification.

increased libido Increase in sexual interest and drive.

ineffability Ecstatic state in which persons insist that their experience is inexpressible and indescribable and that it is impossible to convey what it is like to one who never experienced it.

initial insomnia Falling asleep with difficulty; usually seen in anxiety disorder. *Compare with* **middle insomnia** *and* **terminal insomnia.**

insight Conscious recognition of one's own condition. In psychiatry, it refers to the conscious awareness and understanding of one's own psychodynamics and symptoms of maladaptive behavior; highly important in effecting changes in the personality and behavior of a person.

insomnia Difficulty in falling asleep or difficulty in staying asleep. It can be related to a mental disorder, can be related to a physical disorder or an adverse effect of medication, or can be primary (not related to a known medical factor or another mental disorder). *See also* **initial insomnia, middle insomnia,** *and* **terminal insomnia.**

intellectual insight Knowledge of the reality of a situation without the ability to use that knowledge successfully to effect an adaptive change in behavior or to master the situation. *Compare with* **true insight.**

intelligence Capacity for learning and ability to recall, to integrate constructively, and to apply what one has learned; the capacity to understand and to think rationally.

intoxication Mental disorder caused by recent ingestion or presence in the body of an exogenous substance producing maladaptive behavior by virtue of its effects on the central nervous system (CNS). The most common psychiatric changes involve disturbances of perception, wakefulness, attention, thinking, judgment, emotional control, and psychomotor behavior; the specific clinical picture depends on the substance ingested.

intropunitive Turning anger inward toward oneself. Commonly observed in depressed patients.

introspection Contemplating one's own mental processes to achieve insight.

introversion State in which a person's energies are directed inward toward the self, with little or no interest in the external world.

irrelevant answer Answer that is not responsive to the question.

irritability Abnormal or excessive excitability, with easily triggered anger, annoyance, or impatience.

irritable mood State in which one is easily annoyed and provoked to anger. *See also* **irritability.**

jamais vu Paramnestic phenomenon characterized by a false feeling of unfamiliarity with a real situation that one has previously experienced.

jargon aphasia Aphasia in which the words produced are neologistic; that is, nonsense words created by the patient.

judgment Mental act of comparing or evaluating choices within the framework of a given set of values for the purpose of electing a course of action. If the course of action chosen is consonant with reality or with mature adult standards of behavior, judgment is said to be *intact* or *normal*; judgment is said to be *impaired* if the chosen course of action is frankly maladaptive, results from impulsive decisions based on the need for immediate gratification, or is otherwise not consistent with reality as measured by mature adult standards.

kleptomania Pathological compulsion to steal.

la belle indifférence Inappropriate attitude of calm or lack of concern about one's disability. May be seen in patients with conversion disorder.

labile affect Affective expression characterized by rapid and abrupt changes, unrelated to external stimuli.

labile mood Oscillations in mood between euphoria and depression or anxiety.

laconic speech Condition characterized by a reduction in the quantity of spontaneous speech; replies to questions are brief and unelaborated, and little or no unprompted additional information is provided. Occurs in major depression, schizophrenia, and organic mental disorders. Also called *poverty of speech.*

lethologica Momentary forgetting of a name or proper noun. *See* **blocking.**

lilliputian hallucination Visual sensation that persons or objects are reduced in size; more properly regarded as an illusion. *See also* **micropsia.**

localized amnesia Partial loss of memory; amnesia restricted to specific or isolated experiences. Also called *lacunar amnesia* and *patch amnesia.*

logorrhea Copious, pressured, coherent speech; uncontrollable, excessive talking; observed in manic episodes of bipolar disorder. Also called *tachylogia*, *verbomania*, and *volubility.*

long-term memory Reproduction, recognition, or recall of experiences or information that was experienced in the distant past. Also called *remote memory. Compare with* **immediate memory** and **short-term memory.**

loosening of associations Characteristic schizophrenic thinking or speech disturbance involving a disorder in the logical progression of thoughts, manifested as a failure to communicate verbally adequately; unrelated and unconnected ideas shift from one subject to another. *See also* **tangentiality.**

macropsia False perception that objects are larger than they really are. *Compare with* **micropsia.**

magical thinking A form of dereistic thought; thinking similar to that of the preoperational phase in children (Jean Piaget), in which thoughts, words, or actions assume power (e.g., to cause or to prevent events).

malingering Feigning disease to achieve a specific goal, for example, to avoid an unpleasant responsibility.

mania Mood state characterized by elation, agitation, hyperactivity, hypersexuality, and accelerated thinking and speaking (flight of ideas). Seen in bipolar I disorder. *See also* **hypomania.**

manipulation Maneuvering by patients to get their own way, characteristic of antisocial personalities.

mannerism Ingrained, habitual involuntary movement.

melancholia Severe depressive state. Used in the term *involutional melancholia* as a descriptive term and also in reference to a distinct diagnostic entity.

memory Process whereby what is experienced or learned is established as a record in the CNS (registration), where it persists with a variable degree of permanence (retention) and can be recollected or retrieved from storage at will (recall). For types of memory, see **immediate memory, long-term memory,** and **short-term memory.**

mental disorder Psychiatric illness or disease whose manifestations are primarily characterized by behavioral or psychological impairment of function, measured in terms of deviation from some normative concept; associated with distress or disease, not just an expected response to a particular event or limited to relations between a person and society.

mental retardation Subaverage general intellectual functioning that originates in the developmental period and is associated with impaired maturation and learning, and social maladjustment. Retardation is commonly defined in terms of IQ: mild (between 50 and 55 to 70), moderate (between 35 and 40 to between 50 and 55), severe (between 20 and 25 to between 35 and 40), and profound (below 20 to 25).

metonymy Speech disturbance common in schizophrenia in which the affected person uses a word or phrase that is related to the proper one but is not the one ordinarily used; for example, the patient speaks of consuming a *menu* rather than a *meal*, or refers to losing the *piece of string* of the conversation, rather than the *thread* of the conversation. *See also* **paraphasia** *and* **word approximation.**

microcephaly Condition in which the head is unusually small as a result of defective brain development and premature ossification of the skull.

micropsia False perception that objects are smaller than they really are. Sometimes called *lilliputian hallucination. Compare with* **macropsia.**

middle insomnia Waking up after falling asleep without difficulty and then having difficulty in falling asleep again. *Compare with* **initial insomnia** *and* **terminal insomnia.**

mimicry Simple, imitative motion activity of childhood.

monomania Mental state characterized by preoccupation with one subject.

mood Pervasive and sustained feeling tone that is experienced internally and that, in the extreme, can markedly influence virtually all aspects of a person's behavior and perception of the world. Distinguished from affect, the external expression of the internal feeling tone. For types of mood, see the specific term.

mood-congruent delusion Delusion with content that is mood appropriate (e.g., depressed patients who believe that they are responsible for the destruction of the world).

mood-congruent hallucination Hallucination with content that is consistent with a depressed or manic mood (e.g., depressed patients hearing voices telling them that they are bad persons and manic patients hearing voices telling them that they have inflated worth, power, or knowledge).

mood-incongruent delusion Delusion based on incorrect reference about external reality, with content that has no association to mood or is mood inappropriate (e.g., depressed patients who believe that they are the new Messiah).

mood-incongruent hallucination Hallucination not associated with real external stimuli, with content that is not consistent with depressed or manic mood (e.g., in depression, hallucinations not involving such themes as guilt, deserved punishment, or inadequacy; in mania, not involving such themes as inflated worth or power).

mood swings Oscillation of a person's emotional feeling tone between periods of elation and periods of depression.

motor aphasia Aphasia in which understanding is intact, but the ability to speak is lost. Also called *Broca's, expressive,* or *nonfluent aphasias.*

mourning Syndrome following loss of a loved one, consisting of preoccupation with the lost individual, weeping, sadness, and repeated reliving of memories. *See also* **bereavement** *and* **grief.**

muscle rigidity State in which the muscles remain immovable; seen in schizophrenia.

mutism Organic or functional absence of the faculty of speech. *See also* **stupor.**

mydriasis Dilation of the pupil; sometimes occurs as an autonomic (anticholinergic) or atropine-like adverse effect of some antipsychotic and antidepressant drugs.

narcissism In psychoanalytic theory, divided into primary and secondary types: primary narcissism, the early infantile phase of object relationship development, when the child has not differentiated the self from the outside world, and all sources of pleasure are unrealistically recognized as coming from within the self, giving the child a false sense of omnipotence; secondary narcissim, when the libido, once attached to external love objects, is redirected back to the self. *See also* **autistic thinking.**

needle phobia The persistent, intense, pathological fear of receiving an injection.

negative signs In schizophrenia: flat affect, alogia, abulia, and apathy.

negativism Verbal or nonverbal opposition or resistance to outside suggestions and advice; commonly seen in catatonic schizophrenia in which the patient resists any effort to be moved or does the opposite of what is asked.

neologism New word or phrase whose derivation cannot be understood; often seen in schizophrenia. It has also been used to mean a word that has been incorrectly constructed but whose origins are nonetheless understandable (e.g., *headshoe* to mean *hat*), but such constructions are more properly referred to as *word approximations.*

neurological amnesia (1) Auditory amnesia: loss of ability to comprehend sounds or speech. (2) Tactile amnesia: loss of ability to judge the shape of objects by touch. *See also* **astereognosis**. (3) Verbal amnesia: loss of ability to remember words. (4) Visual amnesia: loss of ability to recall or to recognize familiar objects or printed words.

nihilism Delusion of the nonexistence of the self or part of the self; also refers to an attitude of total rejection of established values or extreme skepticism regarding moral and value judgments.

nihilistic delusion Depressive delusion that the world and everything related to it have ceased to exist.

noeisis Revelation in which immense illumination occurs in association with a sense that one has been chosen to lead and command. Can occur in manic or dissociative states.

nominal aphasia Aphasia characterized by difficulty in giving the correct name of an object. *See also* **anomia** *and* **amnestic aphasia.**

nymphomania Abnormal, excessive, insatiable desire in a woman for sexual intercourse. *Compare with* **satyriasis.**

obsession Persistent and recurrent idea, thought, or impulse that cannot be eliminated from consciousness by logic or reasoning; obsessions are involuntary and ego-dystonic. *See also* **compulsion.**

olfactory hallucination Hallucination primarily involving smell or odors; most common in medical disorders, especially in the temporal lobe.

orientation State of awareness of oneself and one's surroundings in terms of time, place, and person.

overactivity Abnormality in motor behavior that can manifest itself as psychomotor agitation, hyperactivity (hyperkinesis), tics, sleepwalking, or compulsions.

overvalued idea False or unreasonable belief or idea that is sustained beyond the bounds of reason. It is held with less intensity or duration than a delusion but is usually associated with mental illness.

panic Acute, intense attack of anxiety associated with personality disorganization; the anxiety is overwhelming and accompanied by feelings of impending doom.

panphobia Overwhelming fear of everything.

pantomime Gesticulation; psychodrama without the use of words.

paramnesia Disturbance of memory in which reality and fantasy are confused. It is observed in dreams and in certain types of schizophrenia and organic mental disorders; it includes phenomena such as *déjà vu* and *déjà entendu*, which may occur occasionally in normal persons.

paranoia Rare psychiatric syndrome marked by the gradual development of a highly elaborate and complex delusional system, generally involving persecutory or grandiose delusions, with few other signs of personality disorganization or thought disorder.

paranoid delusions Includes persecutory delusions and delusions of reference, control, and grandeur.

paranoid ideation Thinking dominated by suspicious, persecutory, or grandiose content of less than delusional proportions.

paraphasia Abnormal speech in which one word is substituted for another, the irrelevant word generally resembling the required one in morphology, meaning, or phonetic composition; the inappropriate word may be a legitimate one used incorrectly, such as *clover* instead of *hand*, or a bizarre nonsense expression, such as *treen* instead of *train*. Paraphasic speech may be seen in organic aphasias and in mental disorders such as schizophrenia. *See also* **metonymy** *and* **word approximation.**

parapraxis Faulty act, such as a slip of the tongue or the misplacement of an article. Freud ascribed parapraxes to unconscious motives.

paresis Weakness or partial paralysis of organic origin.

paresthesia Abnormal spontaneous tactile sensation, such as a burning, tingling, or pins-and-needles sensation.

perception Conscious awareness of elements in the environment by the mental processing of sensory stimuli; sometimes used in a broader sense to refer to the mental process by which all kinds of data, intellectual, emotional, and sensory, are meaningfully organized. *See also* **apperception.**

perseveration (1) Pathological repetition of the same response to different stimuli, as in a repetition of the same verbal response to different questions. (2) Persistent repetition of specific words or concepts in the process of speaking. Seen in cognitive disorders, schizophrenia, and other mental illness. *See also* **verbigeration.**

phantom limb False sensation that an extremity that has been lost is, in fact, present.

phobia Persistent, pathological, unrealistic, intense fear of an object or situation; the phobic person may realize that the fear is irrational but, nonetheless, cannot dispel it. For types of phobias, see the specific term.

pica Craving and eating of nonfood substances, such as paint and clay.

polyphagia Pathological overeating.

positive signs In schizophrenia: hallucinations, delusions, and thought disorder.

posturing Strange, fixed, and bizarre bodily positions held by a patient for an extended time. *See also* **catatonia.**

poverty of content of speech Speech that is adequate in amount but conveys little information because of vagueness, emptiness, or stereotyped phrases.

poverty of speech Restriction in the amount of speech used; replies may be monosyllabic. *See also* **laconic speech.**

preoccupation of thought Centering of thought content on a particular idea, associated with a strong affective tone, such as a paranoid trend or a suicidal or homicidal preoccupation.

pressured speech Increase in the amount of spontaneous speech; rapid, loud, accelerated speech, as occurs in mania, schizophrenia, and cognitive disorders.

primary process thinking In psychoanalysis, the mental activity directly related to the functions of the id and characteristic of unconscious mental processes; marked by primitive, prelogical thinking and by the tendency to seek immediate discharge and gratification of instinctual demands. Includes thinking that is dereistic, illogical, magical; normally found in dreams, abnormally in psychosis. *Compare with* **secondary process thinking.**

projection Unconscious defense mechanism in which persons attribute to another those generally unconscious ideas, thoughts, feelings, and impulses that are in themselves undesirable or unacceptable as a form of protection from anxiety arising from an inner conflict; by externalizing whatever is unacceptable, they deal with it as a situation apart from themselves.

prosopagnosia Inability to recognize familiar faces that is not due to impaired visual acuity or level of consciousness.

pseudocyesis Rare condition in which a nonpregnant patient has the signs and symptoms of pregnancy, such as abdominal distention, breast enlargement, pigmentation, cessation of menses, and morning sickness.

pseudodementia (1) Dementia-like disorder that can be reversed by appropriate treatment and is not caused by organic brain disease. (2) Condition in which patients show exaggerated indifference to their surroundings in the absence of a mental disorder; also occurs in depression and factitious disorders.

pseudologia phantastica Disorder characterized by uncontrollable lying in which patients elaborate extensive fantasies that they freely communicate and act on.

psychomotor agitation Physical and mental overactivity that is usually nonproductive and is associated with a feeling of inner turmoil, as seen in agitated depression.

psychosis Mental disorder in which the thoughts, affective response, ability to recognize reality, and ability to communicate and relate to others are sufficiently impaired to interfere grossly with the capacity to deal with reality; the classical characteristics of psychosis are impaired reality testing, hallucinations, delusions, and illusions.

psychotic (1) Person experiencing psychosis. (2) Denoting or characteristic of psychosis.

rationalization An unconscious defense mechanism in which irrational or unacceptable behavior, motives, or feelings are logically justified or made consciously tolerable by plausible means.

reaction formation Unconscious defense mechanism in which a person develops a socialized attitude or interest that is the direct antithesis of some infantile wish or impulse that is harbored consciously or unconsciously. One of the earliest and most unstable defense mechanisms, closely related to repression; both are defenses against impulses or urges that are unacceptable to the ego.

reality testing Fundamental ego function that consists of tentative actions that test and objectively evaluate the nature and limits of the environment; includes the ability to differentiate between the external world and the internal world and to accurately judge the relation between the self and the environment.

recall Process of bringing stored memories into consciousness. *See also* **memory.**

recent memory Recall of events over the past few days.

recent past memory Recall of events over the past few months.

receptive aphasia Organic loss of ability to comprehend the meaning of words; fluid and spontaneous, but incoherent and nonsensical, speech. *See also* **fluent aphasia** *and* **sensory aphasia.**

receptive dysphasia Difficulty in comprehending oral language; the impairment involves comprehension and production of language.

regression Unconscious defense mechanism in which a person undergoes a partial or total return to earlier patterns of adaptation; observed in many psychiatric conditions, particularly schizophrenia.

remote memory Recall of events in the distant past.

repression Freud's term for an unconscious defense mechanism in which unacceptable mental contents are banished or kept out of consciousness; important in normal psychological development and in neurotic and psychotic symptom formation. Freud recognized two kinds of repression: (1) repression proper, in which the repressed material was once in the conscious domain, and (2) primal repression, in which the repressed material was never in the conscious realm. *Compare with* **suppression.**

restricted affect Reduction in intensity of feeling tone that is less severe than in blunted affect but clearly reduced. *See also* **constricted affect.**

retrograde amnesia Loss of memory for events preceding the onset of the amnesia. *Compare with* **anterograde amnesia.**

retrospective falsification Memory becomes unintentionally (unconsciously) distorted by being filtered through a person's present emotional, cognitive, and experiential state.

rigidity In psychiatry, a person's resistance to change, a personality trait.

ritual (1) Formalized activity practiced by a person to reduce anxiety, as in OCD. (2) Ceremonial activity of cultural origin.

rumination Constant preoccupation with thinking about a single idea or theme, as in OCD.

satyriasis Morbid, insatiable sexual need or desire in a man. *Compare with* **nymphomania.**

scotoma (1) In psychiatry, a figurative blind spot in a person's psychological awareness. (2) In neurology, a localized visual field defect.

secondary process thinking In psychoanalysis, the form of thinking that is logical, organized, reality oriented, and influenced by the demands of the environment; characterizes the mental activity of the ego. *Compare with* **primary process thinking.**

seizure An attack or sudden onset of certain symptoms, such as convulsions, loss of consciousness, and psychic or sensory disturbances; seen in epilepsy and can be substance induced. For types of seizures, see the specific term.

sensorium Hypothetical sensory center in the brain that is involved with clarity of awareness about oneself and one's surroundings, including the ability to perceive and to process ongoing events in light of past experiences, future options, and current circumstances; sometimes used interchangeably with *consciousness.*

sensory aphasia Organic loss of ability to comprehend the meaning of words; fluid and spontaneous, but incoherent and nonsensical, speech. *See also* **fluent aphasia** *and* **receptive aphasia.**

sensory extinction Neurological sign operationally defined as failure to report one of two simultaneously presented sensory stimuli, despite the fact that either stimulus alone is correctly reported. Also called *sensory inattention.*

shame Failure to live up to self-expectations; often associated with fantasy of how person will be seen by others. *See also* **guilt.**

short-term memory Reproduction, recognition, or recall of perceived material within minutes after the initial presentation. *Compare with* **immediate memory** and **long-term memory.**

simultanagnosia Impairment in the perception or integration of visual stimuli appearing simultaneously.

somatic delusion Delusion pertaining to the functioning of one's body.

somatic hallucination Hallucination involving the perception of a physical experience localized within the body.

somatopagnosia Inability to recognize a part of one's body as one's own (also called *ignorance of the body* and *autotopagnosia*).

somnolence Pathological sleepiness or drowsiness from which one can be aroused to a normal state of consciousness.

spatial agnosia Inability to recognize spatial relations.

speaking in tongues Expression of a revelatory message through unintelligible words; not considered a disorder of thought if associated with practices of specific Pentecostal religions. *See also* **glossolalia.**

stereotypy Continuous mechanical repetition of speech or physical activities; observed in catatonic schizophrenia.

stupor (1) State of decreased reactivity to stimuli and less than full awareness of one's surroundings; as a disturbance of consciousness, it indicates a condition of partial coma or semicoma. (2) In psychiatry, used synonymously with *mutism* and does not necessarily imply a disturbance of consciousness; in *catatonic stupor,* patients are ordinarily aware of their surroundings.

stuttering Frequent repetition or prolongation of a sound or syllable, leading to markedly impaired speech fluency.

sublimation Unconscious defense mechanism in which the energy associated with unacceptable impulses or drives is diverted into personally and socially acceptable channels; unlike other defense mechanisms, it offers some minimal gratification of the instinctual drive or impulse.

substitution Unconscious defense mechanism in which a person replaces an unacceptable wish, drive, emotion, or goal with one that is more acceptable.

suggestibility State of uncritical compliance with influence or of uncritical acceptance of an idea, belief, or attitude; commonly observed among persons with hysterical traits.

suicidal ideation Thoughts or act of taking one's own life.

suppression Conscious act of controlling and inhibiting an unacceptable impulse, emotion, or idea; differentiated from repression in that repression is an unconscious process.

symbolization Unconscious defense mechanism in which one idea or object comes to stand for another because of some common aspect or quality in both; based on similarity and association; the symbols formed protect the person from the anxiety that may be attached to the original idea or object.

synesthesia Condition in which the stimulation of one sensory modality is perceived as sensation in a different modality, as when a sound produces a sensation of color.

syntactical aphasia Aphasia characterized by difficulty in understanding spoken speech, associated with gross disorder of thought and expression.

systematized delusion Group of elaborate delusions related to a single event or theme.

tactile hallucination Hallucination primarily involving the sense of touch. Also called *haptic hallucination.*

tangentiality Oblique, digressive, or even irrelevant manner of speech in which the central idea is not communicated.

tension Physiological or psychic arousal, uneasiness, or pressure toward action; an unpleasurable alteration in mental or physical state that seeks relief through action.

terminal insomnia Early morning awakening or waking up at least 2 hours before planning to wake up. *Compare with* **initial insomnia** *and* **middle insomnia.**

thought broadcasting Feeling that one's thoughts are being broadcast or projected into the environment. *See also* **thought withdrawal.**

thought disorder Any disturbance of thinking that affects language, communication, or thought content; the hallmark feature of schizophrenia. Manifestations range from simple blocking and mild circumstantiality to profound loosening of associations, incoherence, and delusions; characterized by a failure to follow semantic and syntactic rules that is inconsistent with the person's education, intelligence, or cultural background.

thought insertion Delusion that thoughts are being implanted in one's mind by other people or forces.

thought latency The period of time between a thought and its verbal expression. Increased in schizophrenia (*see* **blocking**) and decreased in mania (*see* **pressured speech**).

thought withdrawal Delusion that one's thoughts are being removed from one's mind by other people or forces. *See also* **thought broadcasting.**

tic disorders Predominantly psychogenic disorders characterized by involuntary, spasmodic, stereotyped movement of small groups of muscles; seen most predominantly in moments of stress or anxiety, rarely as a result of organic disease.

tinnitus Noises in one or both ears, such as ringing, buzzing, or clicking; an adverse effect of some psychotropic drugs.

tonic convulsion Convulsion in which the muscle contraction is sustained.

trailing phenomenon Perceptual abnormality associated with hallucinogenic drugs in which moving objects are seen as a series of discrete and discontinuous images.

trance Sleep-like state of reduced consciousness and activity.

tremor Rhythmical alteration in movement, which is usually faster than one beat a second; typically, tremors decrease during periods of relaxation and sleep and increase during periods of anger and increased tension.

true insight Understanding of the objective reality of a situation coupled with the motivational and emotional impetus to master the situation or change behavior.

twilight state Disturbed consciousness with hallucinations.

twirling Sign present in autistic children who continually rotate in the direction in which their head is turned.

unconscious (1) One of three divisions of Freud's topographic theory of the mind (the others being the conscious and the preconscious) in which the psychic material is not readily accessible to conscious awareness by ordinary means; its existence may be manifest in symptom formation, in dreams, or under the influence of drugs. (2) In popular (but more ambiguous) usage, any mental material not in the immediate field of awareness. (3) Denoting a state of unawareness, with lack of response to external stimuli, as in a coma.

undoing Unconscious primitive defense mechanism, repetitive in nature, by which a person symbolically acts out in reverse something unacceptable that has already been done or against which the ego must defend itself; a form of magical expiatory action, commonly observed in OCD.

unio mystica Feeling of mystic unity with an infinite power.

vegetative signs In depression, denoting characteristic symptoms such as sleep disturbance (especially early morning awakening), decreased appetite, constipation, weight loss, and loss of sexual response.

verbigeration Meaningless and stereotyped repetition of words or phrases, as seen in schizophrenia. Also called *cataphasia. See also* **perseveration.**

vertigo Sensation that one or the world around one is spinning or revolving; a hallmark of vestibular dysfunction, not to be confused with dizziness.

visual agnosia Inability to recognize objects or persons.

visual amnesia *See* **neurological amnesia.**

visual hallucination Hallucination primarily involving the sense of sight.

waxy flexibility Condition in which a person maintains the body position into which they are placed. Also called *catalepsy*.

word approximation Use of conventional words in an unconventional or inappropriate way (metonymy or of new words that are developed by conventional rules of word formation) (e.g., *handshoes* for *gloves* and *time measure* for *clock*); distinguished from a *neologism,* which is a new word whose derivation cannot be understood. *See also* **paraphasia.**

word salad Incoherent, essentially incomprehensible, mixture of words and phrases commonly seen in far-advanced cases of schizophrenia. *See also* **incoherence.**

xenophobia Abnormal fear of strangers.

zoophobia Abnormal fear of animals.

FUTURE DIRECTIONS

Descriptions of signs and symptoms in psychiatry have remained fairly constant over the years; however, some terms fall in and out of favor. In the various editions of the *Diagnostic and Statistical Manual of Mental Disorders* (DSM), for example, some terms have been retained and others omitted, and some terms are not common to DSM and the *International Classification of Diseases* (ICD).

DSM-IV eliminated the diagnosis of organic mental disorder in an attempt to indicate that all mental disorders may have a biological basis or medical cause. The diagnosis of organic mental disorder is called *delirium, dementia, and amnestic and other cognitive disorders* in DSM-IV. The tenth edition of the *International Statistical Classification of Diseases and Related Health Problems* (ICD-10), however, retains the diagnostic category of organic mental disorders.

Neurasthenia is omitted from DSM-IV but is retained in ICD-10. Although a significant number of patients diagnosed with neurasthenia can also be classified as having a depressive or anxiety disorder, many patients cannot, and ICD-10 reflects that fact.

DSM-IV eschews the term *psychogenic*. Nevertheless, it appears in ICD-10 to refer to the fact that life events or difficulties play an important role in the genesis of many psychiatric disorders. Similarly, DSM-IV has eliminated the term *neurosis*, which is used in ICD-10. The author regards both as useful terms that should be retained.

The grouping of signs and symptoms with diseases, disorders, or syndromes may be influenced by social traditions, prevalent customs or philosophies, and even unconscious determinants, such as the classifier's view of the world. In 1963, Karl Menninger anticipated the structure of the mathematical device currently in use in DSM-IV-TR. He wrote: "If the patient has, let us say, five symptoms, one can look up each of these symptoms and find which disease is so characterized under all five headings. Then, *voila*! the diagnosis!" Menninger suggested that the trend toward tabulating disease states was antithetical to understanding the person experiencing the illness and deemphasized the compassionate approach toward the patient that is the hallmark of psychiatry. That mathematical approach is reflected in the algorithms and decision trees used in DSM-IV-TR and in the various computer programs that record signs and symptoms to provide a diagnosis.

A description of a sign and symptom is a fact that can be validated by a group of observers. It is not emotive. A description of signs and symptoms is the science of psychiatry; the skill of the observers and their creative imagination and ability to empathize is the art of psychiatry.

Finally, as the physician-philosopher William Osler (1898 to 1919) said of medicine in general, "It is learned only by experience; it is not an inheritance; it cannot be revealed. Learn to see, learn to hear, learn to feel, learn to smell, and know that by practice alone can you become expert." So it is with psychiatry. One sees the posture of depression, hears the neologisms in schizophrenia, smells the odor of alcoholism, and feels the violent patient's anger. Eventually, with practice, the psychiatrist learns the full range of signs and symptoms. It is the rare psychiatrist, however, who encounters them all.

SUGGESTED CROSS-REFERENCES

Section 7.3 describes the psychiatric report and medical record. Chapter 8 on clinical manifestations of mental disorders provides examples of signs and symptoms in psychiatric disorders. Section 9.1 describes the classification of mental disorders. Normality is covered in Section 3.7.

References

*Andreasen NC: The clinical assessment of thought, language, and communication disorders: I. The definition of terms and evaluation of their reliability. *Arch Gen Psychiatry.* 1979;36:1315.

*Ayd FJ. *Lexicon of Psychiatry, Neurology, and the Neurosciences.* Baltimore: Williams & Wilkins; 1995.

Baethge C, Salvatore P, Baldessarini RJ: "On cyclic insanity" by Karl Ludwig Kahlbaum, MD: A translation and commentary. *Harv Rev Psychiatry.* 2003;11:78.

Bruno FJ. *Psychological Symptoms.* New York: Wiley; 1993.

*Campbell RJ. *Psychiatric Dictionary.* 7th ed. New York: Oxford University Press; 1995.

de Vries MW: Recontextualizing psychiatry: Toward ecologically valid mental health research. *Transcult Psychiatry.* 1997;34:185.

*Etter HS: Doctor discontent. *N Engl J Med.* 1999;340:649.

Gonzalez-Pinto A, Ballesteros J, Aldama A, Perez de Heredia JL, Gutierrez M, Mosquera F: Principal components of mania. *J Affect Disord.* 2003;76:95.

Hammond EC: Some preliminary findings on physical complaints from a prospective study of 1,064,004 men and women. *Am J Public Health.* 1964;54:11.

Jaspers K. *General Psychopathology.* Baltimore: The Johns Hopkins University Press; 1997.

Kaplan HI, Sadock BJ. *Comprehensive Glossary of Psychiatry and Psychology.* Baltimore: Williams & Wilkins; 1991.

Kaplan HI, Sadock BJ. Typical signs and symptoms of psychiatric illness. In: Kaplan HI, Sadock BJ, eds. *Comprehensive Textbook of Psychiatry.* 6th ed. Baltimore: Williams & Wilkins; 1995.

Kutchins H, Stuart KA. *Making Us Crazy—DSM: The Psychiatric Bible and the Creation of Mental Disorders.* New York: Free Press; 1997.

Luhrmann TM. *Of Two Minds: The Growing Disorder in American Psychiatry.* New York: Knopf; 2000.

Meninger K. *The Vital Balance.* New York: Viking; 1963.

Satel S. *PCMD How Political Correctness is Corrupting Medicine.* New York: Basic Books; 2000.

Segal DL, Coolidge FL. Structured interviewing and DSM classification. In: Hersen M, Turner SM, eds. *Adult Psychopathology and Diagnosis.* 4th ed. New York: John Wiley & Sons, Inc.; 2003:72.

*Woods BT: Utility of soft and hard signs in psychiatric research. *Psychiatr Ann.* 2003;33:181.

World Health Organization. *Lexicon of Psychiatric and Mental Health Terms.* 2nd ed. Geneva: World Health Organization; 1994.

▲ 7.5 Clinical Neuropsychology and Intellectual Assessment of Adults

REX M. SWANDA, PH.D., AND
KATHLEEN Y. HAALAND, PH.D.

ROLE OF CLINICAL NEUROPSYCHOLOGY

Clinical neuropsychology is a specialty in psychology that examines the relationship between behavior and brain functioning in the realms of cognitive, motor, sensory, and emotional functioning. In general, the clinical neuropsychologist integrates the medical and psychosocial history with the reported complaints and the pattern of performance on neuropsychological procedures to determine whether results are consistent with a particular area of brain damage or a particular diagnosis. Although neurological syndromes are often the focus of referrals, the neuropsychological examination also has a valuable place in diagnosing and treating behavioral symptoms that are associated with other medical, psychological, and psychiatric conditions.

Relationship to Other Disciplines

The unique contributions of neuropsychology can be clarified by examining its relationship to the closely allied disciplines of clinical psychology, behavioral neurology, and neuropsychiatry.

Clinical Psychology Clinical neuropsychology is recognized by the American Psychological Association as a distinct specialty area, with board certification through the American Board of Clinical Neuropsychology under the auspices of the American Board of Professional Psychology. It is primarily differentiated from general clinical psychology by its focus on thorough and extensive evaluation of a broad range of cognitive and emotional factors and their potential relationship to brain damage. There is considerable overlap between the two areas in the approach to assessment, chiefly characterized by reliance on the psychometric foundations of reliability, validity, and normative standards to objectively define behavioral symptoms and complaints. Emotional factors are the province of both. Both evaluate cognition, although the clinical psychologist generally focuses on issues involving general intellectual, academic, and vocational skills, rather than neurological factors. Clinical psychologists and neuropsychologists are involved in treatment, which can include psychotherapy, as well as cognitive retraining to remediate deficits. Pychoeducational functions are also served by both fields in discussing symptoms, assessment results, and their implications with patient, caregivers, and other health professionals.

Behavioral Neurology and Neuropsychiatry The medical specialties of behavioral neurology and neuropsychiatry overlap considerably with clinical neuropsychology. However, the neuropsychologist's unique contribution to the assessment of cognitive deficits lies in the theoretical background in cognitive psychology, as well as psychometrically-based methods, which use standardized instruments with age- and education-based normative data whenever possible. In contrast, the behavioral neurologist and the neuropsychiatrist are more likely to use a mental status examination approach for identifying cognitive deficits, relying on *internal norms*, which are based on the individual clinician's extensive experience with the examination procedures or pathognomonic signs (e.g., dysfluent speech or visual neglect). The behavioral neurologist is trained to diagnose a broad spectrum of neurological disorders, the neuropsychiatrist's focus lies in diagnosing neurological features of psychiatric patients, and the neuropsychologist focuses on the cognitive and behavioral manifestations of a broad range of disorders that can produce cognitive impairment. Ideally, all three work together to provide complementary perspectives to a patient's workup.

HISTORICAL INFLUENCES

Clinical neuropsychology has its roots in psychology, neurology, and psychiatry. The groundbreaking work of Pierre Paul Broca and Karl Wernicke in the 19th century first suggested that complex functions, such as speech and auditory comprehension, could be localized to particular areas in the left hemisphere. In 1909, Korbinian Brodmann published a *cytoarchitectonic* map of the cerebral cortex (Fig. 7.5–1), based on different histological patterns of cells in various parts of the cortex. Over the years, this representational map has proved to have value in identifying functional differences across distinctive cortical regions and has become a standard reference for identifying cortical areas. Views of functional localization were repopularized in the 1960s by Norman Geschwind, who emphasized the importance of connections among different parts of the brain in producing complex behavior. Arthur Benton's Iowa School developed a series of carefully constructed psychometric tests, based on concepts that had originally been identified by behavioral neurology to assess specific deficits relative to the normal population. At approximately the same time, Hans-Lukas Teuber defined the concept of *double dissociation*, which is regarded as the strongest evidence for localization of a particular function. This notion is based on observations of mutually exclusive brain–behavior relationships, such that damage affecting region 1 produces performance deficits in test A but not in test B, whereas damage affecting region 2 produces performance deficits in test B but not in test A. Aleksandr Luria, the Russian neuropsychologist, also developed notions of functional localization but used a theoretical framework that associated component cognitive processes with complex skills and their neuroanatomical correlates. In the United States, Ralph Reitan applied the psychometric standards of North America to a number of instruments for the express purpose of assessing brain damage, resulting in the widely used *Halstead-Reitan Neuropsychological Test Battery*.

NEUROANATOMICAL CORRELATES

The early history of neuropsychology was driven in large part by the goal of linking behavioral deficits to specific neuroanatomical areas of dysfunction or damage. Although this emphasis helped validate neuropsychological tests that are commonly used today, the localizing function of neuropsychological assessment is now less important in light of recent advances in neuroimaging techniques. Increasing knowledge in the neurosciences has also led to a more sophisticated view, in which complex cognitive, perceptual, and motor activities are controlled by neural systems rather than single structures within the brain. An understanding of these brain–behavior relationships is particularly helpful when evaluating patients with focal damage, to ensure that the neuropsychological evaluation adequately assesses relevant behavior that is likely to be associated with that area and its interconnecting pathways. The following section briefly reviews some of the basic concepts of brain–behavior relationships that are

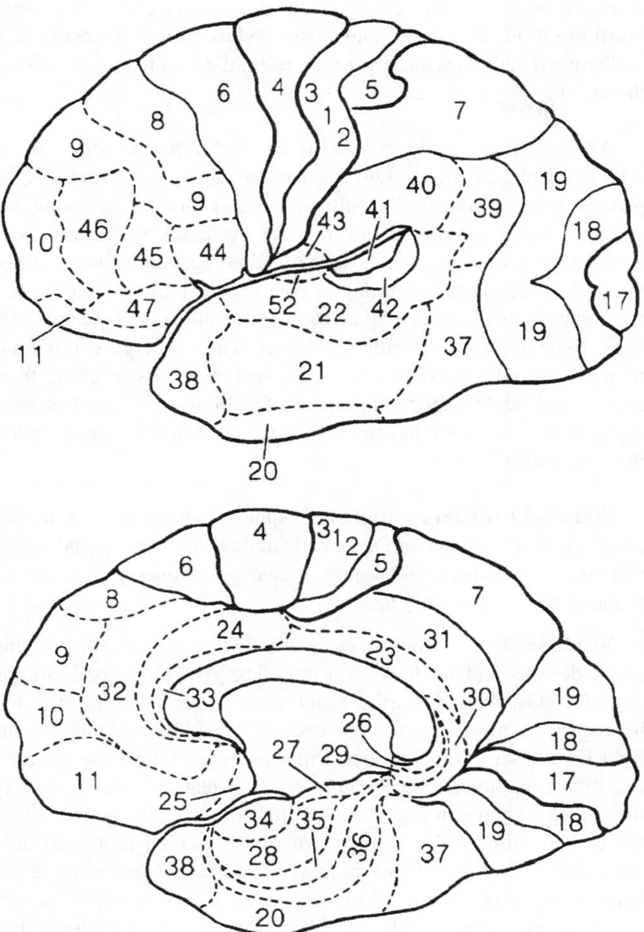

FIGURE 7.5–1 Brodmann's areas of the human cortex, showing convex surface **(top)** and medial surface **(bottom)**. (From Elliott HC. *Textbook of Neuroanatomy*. Philadelphia: Lippincott; 1969, with permission.)

used routinely by the neuropsychologist in interpreting neuropsychological results.

Hemispheric Dominance and Intrahemispheric Localization

Many functions are mediated by the right and left hemispheres. However, important qualitative differences between the two hemispheres can be demonstrated in the presence of lateralized brain injury. Various cognitive skills that have been linked to the left or right hemisphere in right-handed people are listed in Table 7.5–1. Although language is the most obvious area that is largely controlled by the left hemisphere, the left hemisphere is also generally considered to be dominant for limb praxis (i.e., performing complex movements, such as brushing teeth, to command or imitation) and has been associated with the cluster of deficits identified as Gerstmann's syndrome (i.e., finger agnosia, dyscalculia, dysgraphia, and right–left disorientation). In contrast, the right hemisphere is thought to play a more important role in controlling visuospatial abilities and hemispatial attention, which are associated with the clinical presentations of constructional apraxia and neglect, respectively.

Although lateralized deficits such as these are typically characterized in terms of *damage* to the right or left hemisphere, it is important to keep in mind that the patient's performance can also be characterized in terms of *preserved* brain functions. In other words, it is the remaining intact brain tissue—not only the absence of critical brain tissue—that drives many behavioral responses after injury to the brain.

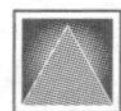

Table 7.5–1
Selected Neuropsychological Deficits Associated with Left or Right Hemisphere Damage

Left Hemisphere	Right Hemisphere
Aphasia	Visuospatial deficits
Right–left disorientation	Impaired visual perception
Finger agnosia	Neglect
Dysgraphia (aphasic)	Dysgraphia (spatial, neglect)
Dyscalculia (number alexia)	Dyscalculia (spatial)
Constructional apraxia (details)	Constructional apraxia (gestalt)
Limb apraxia	Dressing apraxia
	Anosognosia

Language Disorders Appreciation for the special role of the left hemisphere in the control of language functions in most right-handed individuals has been validated in many studies. These include the results of amobarbital (Amytal) testing in epilepsy surgery patients, as well as the incidence of aphasia after unilateral stroke to the left, versus the right, hemisphere. Although it is rare for right-handed people to be right hemisphere dominant for language, it does occur in approximately 1 percent of the cases. Hemispheric dominance for language in left-handed people is less predictable. Approximately two-thirds of left-handers are actually left hemisphere dominant for language, whereas approximately 20 percent each are right hemisphere dominant or bilaterally dominant.

A number of classification systems have been developed over the years for describing various patterns of language breakdown. A common method takes into account the presence or absence of three key features: (1) fluency, (2) comprehension, and (3) repetition (i.e., intact ability to repeat verbally presented words or phrases).

BROCA'S APHASIA Broca's aphasia (also called *nonfluent* or *expressive aphasia*) has traditionally been characterized by impaired verbal fluency, intact auditory comprehension, and somewhat impaired repetition. It has long been thought to be associated with damage to Broca's area (i.e., left inferior frontal convolution) or Brodmann's area 44 (Fig. 7.5–1). However, more recent neuroimaging data in stroke patients have shown that the full syndrome of Broca's aphasia, including agrammatism (telegraphic speech), is found only in the presence of more extensive damage, which encompasses the suprasylvian area from Broca's area to the posterior extent of the sylvian fissure.

WERNICKE'S APHASIA Wernicke's aphasia (also called *fluent* or *receptive aphasia*) is characterized by intact verbal fluency, impaired comprehension, and somewhat impaired repetition. It has been associated with damage to Wernicke's area in the region of the superior temporal gyrus. The impaired ability to comprehend language directly impacts on the individual's ability to self-monitor language output and may be related to a breakdown of the syntactic structure of language. It would not be unusual for an affected patient to produce fluently unintelligible strings of utterances that might potentially be confused with the so-called jargon aphasia, which is associated with schizophrenia.

CONDUCTION APHASIA Patients with conduction aphasia demonstrate relatively intact auditory comprehension and spontaneous speech, owing to the preservation of Wernicke's and Broca's

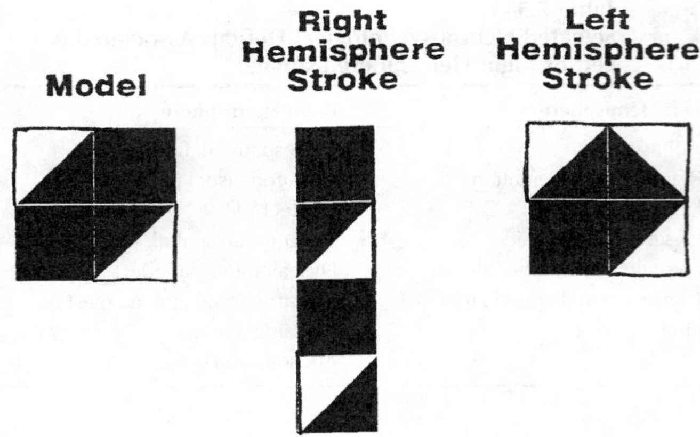

FIGURE 7.5–2 Examples of block design constructions seen in a right hemisphere stroke patient and a left hemisphere stroke patient.

areas. However, the ability to repeat words and phrases is specifically impaired and has traditionally been attributed to damage to the arcuate fasciculus, which interconnects Wernicke's and Broca's areas.

GLOBAL APHASIA Another common classification, global aphasia, is characterized by impairment in all three dimensions of fluency, comprehension, and repetition. In reality, many aphasic patients cannot be neatly classified within a specific system, because the pattern of deficits does not exactly fit clear descriptive categories. In fact, detailed language assessment of most aphasic patients typically demonstrates deficits in all three areas, although the degree of deficit among the three areas varies.

Limb Apraxia Limb apraxia and other cognitive–motor skills deficits are more commonly seen with left hemisphere damage than with right hemisphere damage. However, Kathleen Haaland and Deborah Harrington reviewed data showing that the difference in the incidence of limb apraxia after left or right hemisphere damage is not as great as with language, suggesting that left hemisphere dominance for disorders of complex movement is not as strong as for language. Although limb apraxia has not traditionally been considered to be of substantial functional importance, recent data reviewed by Leslie Rothi and Kenneth Heilman also suggest that limb apraxia significantly affects rehabilitation outcome. For instance, ideomotor limb apraxia can be associated with impaired spatiotemporal execution of complex movements, which results in orientation errors, such as carving a turkey by moving the knife up and down rather than back and forth. Conceptual apraxia might result in using the wrong object to perform a movement, such as attempting to use a toothbrush to eat. Finally, sequencing errors and ideational errors can lead to disrupted activities, such as trying to light a candle before striking the match.

Arithmetic Arithmetic skills can be impaired after left or right hemisphere damage. Left hemisphere damage, especially of the parietal lobe, produces difficulty in reading and appreciating the symbolic meaning of numbers (number dyslexia). Left hemisphere damage can also be associated with impaired conceptual understanding of the problem (anarithmia). In contrast, the deficits in arithmetic computation that can accompany right hemisphere damage are more likely to be observed in written problems. These emerge as problems with the spatial aspects of arithmetic, such as errors resulting from hemispatial neglect, poor alignment of columns, or visual misperceptions and rotations that can result in confusion of signs for addition and multiplication.

Spatial Disorders Right hemisphere damage in right-handed people is frequently associated with deficits in visuospatial skills. Common assessment techniques include drawings and constructional or spatial assembly tasks.

VISUOSPATIAL Distinctive qualitative errors in constructing block designs and in drawing a complex geometric configuration (e.g., Rey-Osterreith Complex Figure) can be seen with right or left hemisphere damage. In the presence of lateralized damage to the right hemisphere, impaired performances often reflect the patient's inability to appreciate the *gestalt* or global features of a design. In the example shown in Figure 7.5–2, this is seen in the patient's failure to maintain the 2 × 2 matrix of blocks, which is instead converted into a column of four blocks. In contrast, damage to the left hemisphere commonly results in inaccurate reproduction of internal details of the design, including improper orientation of individual blocks, but the 2 × 2 matrix (i.e., the gestalt) is more likely to be preserved. Similar differences can be seen with drawings, as in the example of the Rey-Osterreith Complex Figure shown in Figure 7.5–3. The patient with right parietal damage draws isolated details of the design, while failing to convey the interrelationship of the details in the overall design configuration. In contrast, the patient with left hemisphere damage tends to maintain the global framework, or gestalt, of the design but to lose the details. Therefore, many neuropsychologists emphasize that a neuropsychological understanding of the impairment depends not just on a set of test scores, but also on a qualitative description of the *type* of error. This often allows the impairment to be linked to a specific neuroanatomical region, as well as enables a better understanding of the mechanisms of the deficit for rehabilitation purposes.

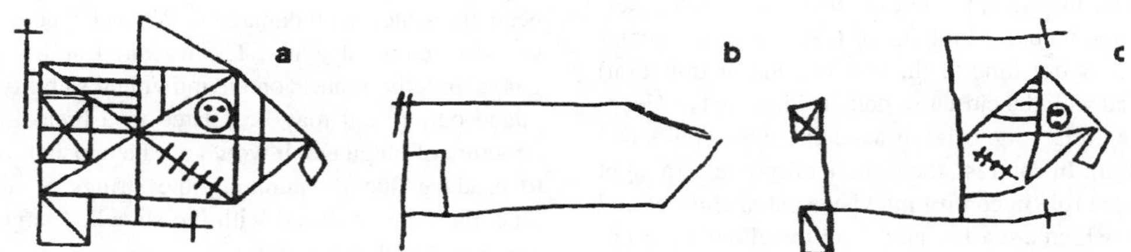

FIGURE 7.5–3 **a:** Rey-Osterreith Complex Figure model. **b:** Drawings from memory in a patient with left hemisphere injury. **c:** Drawings from memory in a patient with right hemisphere injury. (From Robertson LC, Lamb MR: Neuropsychological contributions to part/whole organization. *Cognit Psychol.* 1991;23:300, with permission from Elsevier Science.)

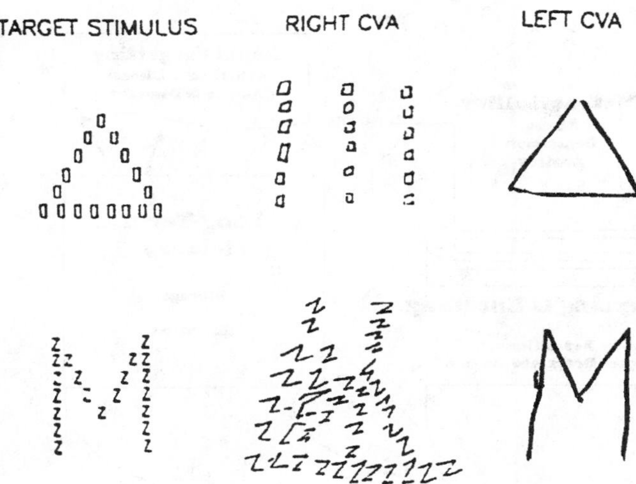

FIGURE 7.5–4 Global local target stimuli with drawings from memory by a patient with right hemisphere cerebrovascular accident (CVA) and by a patient with left hemisphere CVA. (From Robertson LC, Lamb MR: Neuropsychological contributions to part/whole organization. *Cognit Psychol.* 1991;23:325, with permission from Elsevier Science.)

In another example, damage to the right hemisphere tends to be associated with decreased appreciation of *global* features of visual stimuli, whereas left hemisphere damage tends to be associated with decreased analysis of *local* features and detail. This notion is illustrated in Figure 7.5–4, in which a left hemisphere–damaged patient reproduces ambiguous figures as a simple triangle or the letter M with no regard for the internal characters that actually make up the designs. In contrast, the local approach of a patient with right hemisphere damage emphasizes the internal details (small rectangles or the letter Z) without appreciation for the gestalt that is formed by the internal details. This example also illustrates the important point that behavioral responses (including errors) are driven as much by preserved regions of intact brain functioning as by the loss of other regions of brain functioning.

NEGLECT Failure to detect visual or tactile stimuli or to move the limb in the contralateral hemispace is most commonly associated with right hemisphere damage. Visual neglect can be assessed at bedside with line cancellation and line bisection tasks, in which the paper is placed at the patient's midline, and he or she is asked to cross out all the lines on the page or to bisect the single line presented. The method of double simultaneous stimulation is another standard procedure for demonstrating the deficit. Neglect has devastating functional effects and should be taken into account as a standard consideration in the evaluation process. It is most frequently associated with right parietal damage, but damage to other areas within the cerebral cortex and subcortical areas can also produce this problem.

DRESSING APRAXIA This syndrome tends to arise in association with spatial deficits after right hemisphere damage. The resulting difficulty in coordinating the spatial and proprioceptive demands of dressing can be seen in the patient's difficulty in identifying the top or bottom of a garment, as well as right–left confusion in inserting their limbs into the garment. As a result, dressing time can be painfully protracted, and the patient may actually present with a greater level of functional dependence than might otherwise be expected from assessment of simple motor or spatial skills alone.

Memory Disorders Memory complaints constitute the most common referral to neuropsychology. Thorough neuropsychological examination of memory considers the modality (e.g., verbal versus spatial) in which the material is presented and uses presentation formats that systematically assess different aspects of the information processing and storage system that forms the basis for memory. Accumulated research indicates that specialized processing of verbal and spatial memory material tends to be differentially mediated by the left and right hemispheres, respectively. In addition to interhemispheric differences in functional localization, specific memory problems can be associated with breakdown at any stage in the information processing model of memory (Fig. 7.5–5). These stages include (1) registration of the material through *attention*, (2) initial processing of the material within *short-term memory*, (3) encoding and storage of material in *long-term memory*, and (4) *retrieval* processes, in which material moves from long-term memory storage back into consciousness. A great advantage of neuropsychological assessment is that these various types of memory problems can be readily isolated and described in the course of the examination procedures. Once identified, the specific nature of the deficit can then have important implications for diagnosis, treatment, and prognosis.

ENCODING The initial encoding of material can be influenced by a variety of factors, including deficits in attention, language, and spatial processing abilities. It is usually measured by immediate recall of information (e.g., narrative stories and designs) or by demonstrating learning of new material across multiple trials (e.g., word lists). Because attention itself can be affected by many factors, including neurologically based disorders (e.g., head injury and acute confusional state) and psychiatric disorders (e.g., depression and anxiety), this is a particularly important aspect of a proper assessment of memory.

RETRIEVAL AND STORAGE Deficits in recall can be associated with impaired retrieval, in which case the material is still present but not readily accessible, or it can be due to impaired storage of information. The best way of differentiating these problems is to assess *recognition*, typically by using test conditions that offer some version of a multiple choice format. If the patient is able to demonstrate intact recognition, the problem lies in poor retrieval, but, if recognition is impaired, the problem is better attributed to impaired storage of new information. This distinction is important, because the functions of retrieval and storage are subserved by different neuroanatomical structures. Impaired storage is associated with dysfunction of the medial temporal lobe–diencephalic systems, whereas impaired retrieval can be associated with a variety of structures, including the frontal lobes. Because it is always easier to recognize than to recall memory material, these techniques also offer a reasonable basis for assessing the possibility of malingering.

Executive Function The prefrontal lobes and their interconnections are thought to play an important role in controlling executive functions. As conceptualized by Muriel Lezak, these executive functions include volition (i.e., formulation of a goal, motivation to achieve the goal, and awareness of one's own ability to achieve the goal), planning, purposive action (response initiation, maintenance, switching and stopping), and execution, which requires self-monitoring, and self-correction, as well as control of the spatiotemporal aspects of the response. Damage to the frontal lobes has also been associated with personality changes, as was historically exemplified by the famous 19th century case of Phineas Gage, who became irresponsible, socially inappropriate, and unable to carry out plans after a tamping iron was blown through his frontal lobes. Although hemi-

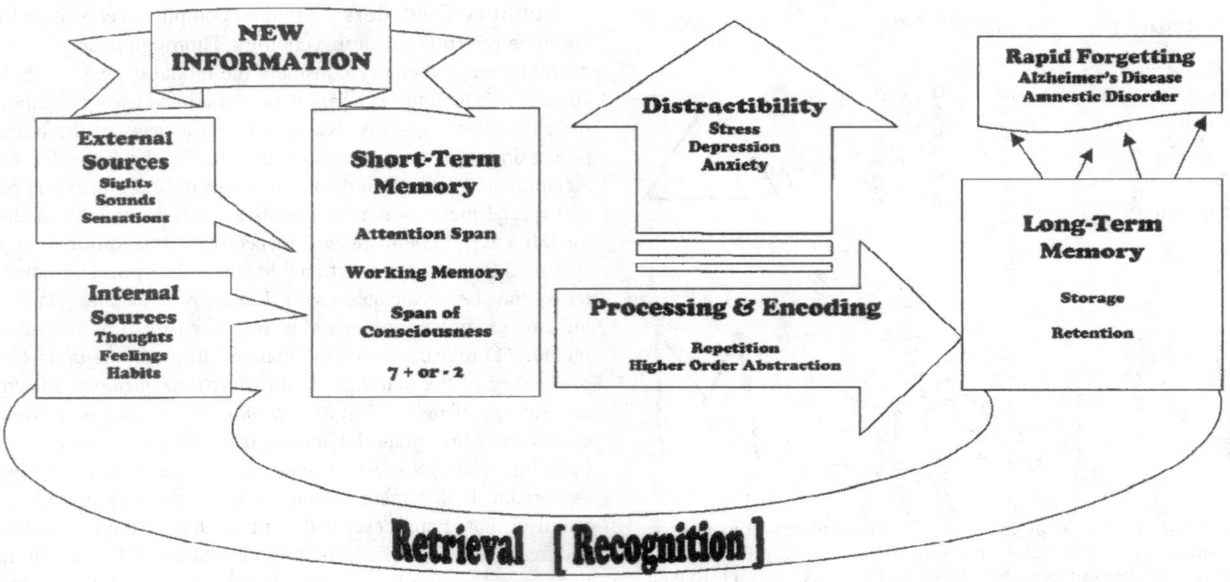

FIGURE 7.5–5 Information processing model of memory.

spheric differences in the control of executive functions by the frontal lobes have not been as well documented as in the parietal and temporal lobes, the Montreal Neuropsychology Group led by Brenda Milner has identified asymmetry in the control of verbal and design fluency.

The prefrontal lobes and their interconnections have been separated into the dorsolateral, orbitofrontal, and anterior cingulate divisions. Jeffrey Cummings has identified neurobehavioral roles for each of these divisions and has linked them to differential neuroanatomical relationships between cortical and subcortical areas. Although this conceptual organization has not been examined in great detail, it provides a useful working model. All of these syndromes are associated with specific corticostriate circuits and are identified here by their cortical sites.

The *dorsolateral* prefrontal lobe circuit is associated with higher cognitive functions, such as working memory, hypothesis generation, retrieval and initiation of unique words and designs, organization of information (e.g., clustering word lists on the basis of semantic category), and development of alternating and sequential motor programs. The *orbitofrontal* syndrome is characterized by marked personality changes, such as instability, lability, and impulsivity. The *anterior cingulate* circuit is associated with impaired response initiation (i.e., akinetic mutism in the most extreme case) and response inhibition. These patients have difficulty inhibiting prepotent responses on "go–no go" tests (e.g., "when I say red, squeeze my hand; when I say green, do nothing").

PSYCHOMETRIC ISSUES

One of the strengths of neuropsychological assessment lies in the detailed quantitative record it provides for different areas of cognitive performance, as well as the foundation of normative standards on which interpretations are based. The normative database for any given test is particularly important to consider to ensure that deficits seen on individual test performances cannot be explained by demographic characteristics of the patient, such as age, education, or cultural considerations. Of course, this approach is also dependent on the care that has been expended in the development and validation of specific testing techniques. Ethical guidelines for psychological assessment established by the American Psychological Association require that tests have demonstrated validity and reliability for the particular clinical application in which they are used. These guidelines serve as the basis for valid judgments to be made about change over time, based on a given individual's performance over successive examinations. This foundation also ensures that test scores can be regarded as comparable even when administered by different examiners and in different settings.

Validity

Validity refers to a test's ability to measure what it purports to measure. Validity can be ascertained by (1) correlating scores from a particular test with other, well-established measures of the same skill, (2) relating test scores to diagnostic classifications or to measures of brain structure and function, or (3) relating test outcomes to aspects of everyday functions that are thought to be dependent on that skill (e.g., comparing pencil-and-paper tests of visuospatial skill with the ability to find one's way around a shopping center). Historically, neuropsychological tests have been validated by examining their ability to differentiate brain-damaged patients from non–brain-damaged patients. More recently, they have been validated against neuroradiological or neurosurgical data and diagnostic categories (e.g., patients with multiple sclerosis [MS] versus medical controls). Less attention has been paid to relationships between neuropsychological test outcomes and everyday function, although modest correlations have been documented between test outcomes, self-care activities, and selected complex skills.

Reliability

Reliability refers to the consistency of test scores. Tests are judged by (1) their internal consistency (i.e., the extent to which all items appear to be measuring the same thing), (2) their ability to yield similar scores across multiple test occasions in normal individuals, and (3) the consistency in scores that is obtained when different persons administer and score a test. Individual cognitive measures often have lower reliabilities than composite scores that are derived from several measures. Within a particular ability domain, some measures exhibit higher reliabilities than do others. For example, within the Wechsler Memory Scale–Revised, some tests of attention or concentration and delayed recall have fairly low test–retest reliabilities (e.g., $r = 0.68$ and 0.45 for digits backward and delayed recall of word pairs, respectively), but the composite index scores for attention or concentration and delayed recall have acceptably high test–retest stability ($r = 0.93$ and 0.84, respectively). This underscores the importance of using more than one test to measure each type of ability in a thorough neuropsychological evaluation.

Predictive Usefulness

In selecting tests for diagnostic applications, it is important to estimate in advance the predictive usefulness of particular tests for particular diagnostic discriminations. An estimation of predictive usefulness takes into consideration the sensitivity, specificity, and positive and negative predictive values of a test. A test that yields positive findings for most persons with disease and negative outcomes for most persons without disease has high sensitivity and specificity. Often, published values for sensitivity and specificity are based on ideal comparisons (e.g., clear cases of Alzheimer's disease versus carefully screened normal controls) and do not permit a clinician to estimate how useful a test is in a general clinical population.

Base Rates

Computation of positive and negative predictive values addresses different and potentially more practical questions: Given a positive test outcome, what is the probability of having disease? Given a negative test outcome, what is the probability of not having disease? Positive and negative predictive values are computed as the ratio of accurate positive findings to total positive outcomes and the ratio of accurate negative findings to total negative outcomes, respectively. Predictive values are judged relative to estimated base rates of illness within the referral setting. For example, if the base rate of dementia among older adults referred for psychiatric assessment is 50 percent, then any test that purports to ascertain dementia must have a predictive value of greater than 50 percent to warrant its application.

Another aspect of base rate is related to the frequency with which abnormal neuropsychological findings are obtained in normal individuals. Figure 7.5–6 illustrates the importance of appreciating the fact that non–brain-damaged individuals without psychiatric problems may perform in the impaired range. In fact, important normative standards developed by Robert Heaton, Igor Grant, and Charles Matthews indicate that few healthy individuals complete a neuropsychological protocol without any impaired scores, whereas as many as 38 percent of normals perform in the impaired range on six or more discrete scores in a 40-score battery. Given these data, a naïve approach to neuropsychology that considers an individual to be impaired by simply counting the number of test scores in the impaired range would be misleading. This information is particularly important when considering whether subtle deficits are present in the evaluation of mild head injury. These data also underscore the importance of basing conclusions on a *pattern* of deficits. In other words, the strongest evidence of brain injury would be based on a pattern of consistent impairment on several measures within the same cognitive domain, as opposed to impairment on isolated tasks that represent several different cognitive domains.

The predictive value of neuropsychological tests varies considerably for different diagnostic questions. As discussed in the section Neuroanatomical Correlates, certain performance impairments are highly specific to deficits in specific brain regions. However, in many neurological diagnoses, multiple brain systems can be affected, and there is overlap in affected systems across disease entities. In testing for dementia, for example, neuropsychological outcomes are more sensitive than they are specific and must be used in combination with other medical and historical data to arrive at a more specific diagnosis. This underscores the importance of interpreting neuropsychological data in the context of the patient's history.

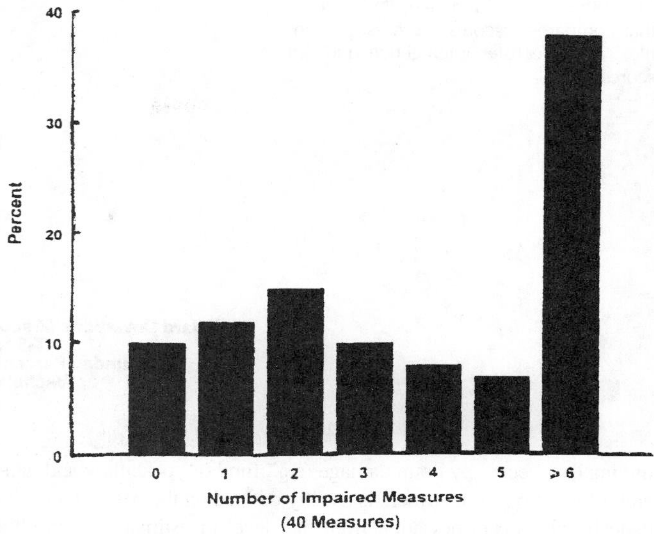

FIGURE 7.5–6 Graph showing percentages of normal individuals who score in the impaired range of 0 to 6 or more neuropsychological measures in a battery of 40 measures. (Adapted from Heaton RK, Grant I, Matthews CG. *Comprehensive Norms for an Expanded Halstead-Reitan Battery.* Odessa, FL: Psychological Assessment Resources; 1991.)

Normative Data

Considerable research in recent years has been directed toward expanding the normative database for clinical neuropsychological tests with respect to important demographic factors. Normative data are now available for many cognitive measures across a broad age range. On the average, persons in their early 70s score approximately one standard deviation lower than those in their 20s on tasks that combine cognitive processing demands with requirements for speed of performance, so it is important to compare a given individual's performance on these tasks with that of age peers. *Education* can have an even stronger effect on many aspects of cognitive performance. For subtests of the Wechsler Adult Intelligence Scale–Revised, for example, education accounts for an average of 26 percent of the variance in performance, compared to just less than 9 percent of the variance that is attributable to age. *Cultural factors* and linguistic background can affect familiarity with particular stimuli, such as the use of clocks to tell time, or can influence the manner in which common tasks are routinely performed, such as remembering telephone numbers. *Gender* differences are relatively small on most clinical neuropsychological tests, but there are a few types of tasks, such as those measuring motor speed and strength, for which it is important to consider gender. Among healthy individuals, the combined effects of age, education, and gender account for approximately 45 percent of the variability in intelligence test performance and for approximately 64 percent of the variance in the average impairment rating from the Halstead-Reitan Neuropsychological Battery (HRNB).

Estimates of Premorbid Functioning

For the neuropsychologist to conclude that deficits are present, premorbid levels of functioning must be estimated, usually based on educational and occupational history, as well as performance on tests that are usually

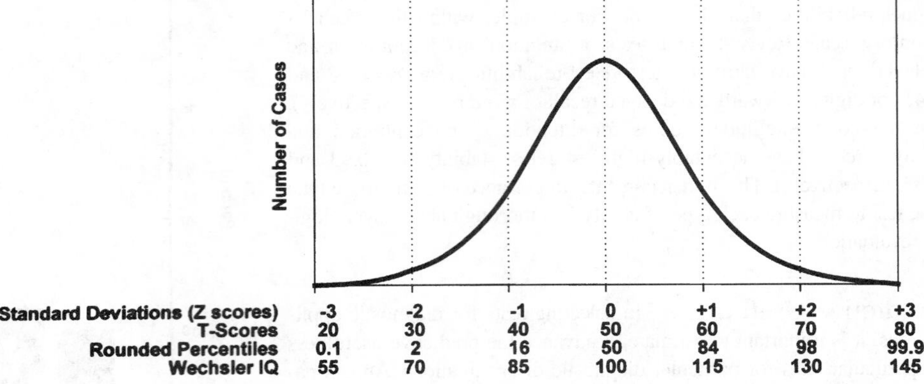

FIGURE 7.5–7 Normative (bell) curve that compares *z* scores, *t* scores, percentiles, and Wechsler intelligence quotient scores.

minimally affected by brain damage (e.g., fund of vocabulary and general information). Impairment is usually defined on the basis of any statistically significant deviation from that level of estimated premorbid ability. As illustrated in the normal *bell curve* that is shown in Figure 7.5–7, statistically significant findings on any given set of tests would be at least one standard deviation above or below the *mean* (or average) performance that is established for that individual in comparison to established normative standards or in relation to his or her performance across the other tests. For example, if a 32-year-old white patient from the Midwest has only 4 years of education and has worked as a laborer, his or her premorbid level functioning might well be estimated to lie in the borderline to low-average range, which represents the population that performs at least one standard deviation below average. Therefore, most test scores would be expected to hover around that level. To identify the likely presence of brain injury in such a patient, they would have to demonstrate test scores that were at least two standard deviations below average, or pathognomic signs of definite impairment that would be consistent with the medical history, such as signs of lateralized neglect or aphasia. This example provides another example of the importance of considering the context of other demographic and cultural factors in the interpretation of neuropsychological evaluation.

Moderating Factors Performance on neuropsychological tests can be influenced by transient or situational factors. *Alcohol and drug use* can impair attention, memory, and speed of cognitive processing, as can many *prescription medications*, especially in the elderly and the brain injured. *Psychiatric disorders* such as mania, severe depression, or psychosis can undermine cognitive performance, rendering formal testing invalid in severe conditions or reducing scores below expected levels in milder cases. For many clinical neuropsychological tests, the impact of drug use and psychiatric state on neuropsychological performance has been documented through research. However, the entire performance profile, combined with clinical observation and input from the patient and collaterals, must be considered in interpreting the impact of these moderating variables. An experienced neuropsychologist should be expected to explicitly identify relevant factors that could be expected to undermine or to contribute to lower than expected performance, such as impaired vision or hearing loss, acute illness, or recent significant stressors.

GENERAL REFERRAL ISSUES

Most neuropsychological referrals are made for diagnostic purposes to ascertain if brain impairment is present or to differentiate among different neurological or psychiatric disorders. Other important uses of testing include establishment of a baseline of performance for assessing future change and planning for rehabilitation or management of behaviors that are affected by brain impairment. The specific methods of neuropsychological assessment reflect the individual's unique presentation of symptoms and complaints, history and development, the perspective of the neuropsychologist, and the referral question.

Level of Functioning A common referral issue involves documentation of level of functioning for a variety of purposes, including assessment of change or competence, especially in the presence of diagnoses such as dementia, stroke, and head injury.

Differential Diagnosis Like any other diagnostic procedure, the results of a neuropsychological examination must be interpreted in light of all available information, including the history and any associated medical factors that are documented or reported for the individual. Many neurological and psychiatric disorders have similar clusters of symptoms in common, with complaints of concentration or memory problems being among the most frequently reported problems. For example, impaired attention and concentration are commonly found among patients who present with a history of mild closed head injury, psychiatric issues (e.g., depression, posttraumatic stress disorder [PTSD], and anxiety), or any of several types of neurological disorders that are associated with subcortical involvement (e.g., Parkinson's disease, MS, human immunodeficiency virus [HIV]–related cognitive decline). Therefore, a pattern of cognitive impairment across several critical areas of functioning does not necessarily provide a sufficient basis for a specific diagnostic conclusion but must be integrated with the medical and relevant psychosocial factors to arrive at a specific differential diagnosis. The following discussion reflects some common clinical syndromes in which psychiatrists and neuropsychologists share an interest and may work together in the assessment and treatment of patients.

Age- or Stress-Related Cognitive Change Many middle-aged and older adults have concerns about everyday concentration and memory failures, and, with heightened public awareness about conditions such as Alzheimer's disease, an increasing number of these individuals seek evaluations for these concerns. Neuropsychological testing provides a detailed, objective picture of different aspects of memory and attention, which can be helpful in reassuring healthy persons about their abilities. It also provides an opportunity for assessing undetected mood or anxiety disorders that may be reflected in cognitive concerns and for offering suggestions about mnemonic strategies that can sharpen everyday function.

A 77-year-old, left-handed man with a high school education was referred for neuropsychological assessment by his primary physician after the patient mentioned a recent episode of getting turned around while driving. He reported a 25-year work history with the postal service and current part-time work as a cashier in a community recreation facility. He also reported an active social life. Medical history was stable despite past treatment history for cataracts and prostate cancer, and magnetic resonance imaging (MRI) scan of the head was unremarkable. In interview, the patient and his wife complained that the referring physician had "made a mountain out of a molehill." They agreed that he had always had a poor sense of direction and gave several humorous examples of "getting turned around" when driving over the years.

Results of neuropsychological assessment indicated variable performance on tests of attention and concentration. His performance was excellent on tests of memory, language, and executive problem solving abilities, but visuospatial and constructional abilities were moderately impaired. Mild levels of grief-related depression were indicated on self-report. Follow-up discussion of the results provided an opportunity to discuss the significant visuospatial problems that were identified. Neither the patient nor his wife was surprised to hear this, and they good-naturedly pointed out that they had tried to tell the referring physician that he had always had such problems. The evaluation concluded that the findings were most consistent with a probable developmental history of visuospatial learning disability. However, the couple was advised to seek follow-up if significant changes become apparent in the future, to compare to the objective baseline established by this examination.

Mild Traumatic Brain Injury A significant proportion of persons who have had a mild traumatic brain injury complain of problems with attention, memory, and mood, in addition to headache or other forms of pain, for many months after the injury. In many of these cases, there is no clear evidence of brain injury on MRI or other neuroradiological tests. Neuropsychological testing can be a crucial method for determining the extent of objective cognitive deficit, examining the role of psychological factors in perpetuating cognitive problems, and assessing for possible residual brain impairment. Many such patients receive medications for mood or anxiety problems, possibly in combination with pain medications, and many could benefit from psychological help in managing chronic pain and psychological distress. In addition, many of these patients are in litigation, which can complicate the neuropsychologist's ability to identify the causes for impairment. Although outright malingering represents a relatively infrequent complication, more subtle presentations of chronic illness behavior must be a prominent consideration when potential legal settlements or disability benefits are in question. This is a particularly important factor in the case of mild head injury, when subjective complaints may be disproportionate to the objectively reported circumstances of the injury, especially because most follow-up studies of mild head injury indicate return to neuropsychological baseline with no objective evidence of significant cognitive sequelae 3 to 12 months after injury.

Poststroke Syndromes After the acute phase of recovery from stroke, patients may be left with residual deficits, which can affect memory, language, spatial skills, reasoning, or mood. Neuropsychological testing can help identify areas of strength, which can be used in planning additional rehabilitation and can provide feedback on the functional implications (e.g., for work or complex activities of daily living) of residual deficits. Such assessment of functional skills can also be helpful to a psychiatrist who is managing mood and behavioral symptoms or dealing with family caregivers.

Detecting Early Dementia Conditions that particularly warrant neuropsychological assessment for early detection and potential treatment include HIV-related cognitive deficits and normal pressure hydrocephalus. When concerns about a person's memory functioning are expressed by relatives instead of the patient, there is a higher probability of a neurological basis for the functional problems. Neuropsychological testing, combined with a good clinical history and other medical screening tests, is highly effective in distinguishing early dementia from the mild changes in memory and executive functioning that can be seen with normal aging. Neuropsychological evaluation is particularly helpful in documenting cognitive deterioration and differentiating among different forms of dementia. An additional incentive for early diagnosis of dementia now lies in the fact that a portion of patients with early dementia may be candidates for memory-enhancing therapies (e.g., acetylcholinesterase inhibitors), and testing can provide an objective means of monitoring treatment efficacy.

Neuropsychological profiles have been used in recent studies to identify patients who do not meet the full criteria for Alzheimer's disease but who demonstrate memory deficits with normal performance in other cognitive domains. This pattern, termed *mild cognitive impairment* (MCI), may represent prodromal Alzheimer's disease, in that such patients show a higher incidence of conversion to Alzheimer's disease than individuals with no such cognitive impairment. Annual rates of conversion to Alzheimer's disease among MCI patients have been found to range from 6 percent for persons who are 65 to 69 years of age to 25 percent for persons who are 85 to 89 years of age, as compared to persons without cognitive impairment (only 0.2 and 3.9 percent, respectively). This diagnosis must be made cautiously owing to the possible negative emotional repercussions of such information, the fact that not all MCI patients convert to Alzheimer's disease, and the fact that current medications based on acetylcholinesterase inhibitors produce only mild improvement even in Alzheimer's disease patients. However, because research data suggest that the greatest benefit of these medications (in terms of slowed progression) is found among patients with mild Alzheimer's disease, there is hope that the same medications may provide optimal effects in MCI patients. In reality, many clinicians currently routinely prescribe cholinesterase inhibitors to patients diagnosed with MCI. In the future, the combination of genetic information, neuroimaging, and neuropsychological results is likely to improve the ability to diagnose dementia at an earlier stage, which will be important as new treatments are developed.

Distinguishing Dementia and Depression A substantial minority of patients with severe depression exhibit serious generalized impairment of cognitive functioning. In addition to problems with attention and slowing of thought and action, there may be significant forgetfulness and problems with reasoning. By examining the pattern of cognitive impairments, neuropsychological testing can help identify dementia syndrome of depression or *pseudodementia*. Perhaps more common is a mixed presentation, in which depression coexists with various forms of cognitive decline, increasing the severity of cognitive dysfunction beyond what would be expected from the neurological impairment alone. Neuropsychological testing can provide a baseline for measuring the effectiveness of antidepressant therapy in alleviating cognitive and mood symptoms.

A 75-year-old gentleman with a Ph.D. in the social sciences sought neuropsychological reexamination for ongoing memory complaints, stating that "several of my friends have Alzheimer's." In an initial examination 1 year before, he had performed in the expected range (above average) for most procedures, despite variable performance on measures of attention and concentration. His medical history was unremarkable, with no known family history of dementia, but he continued to be treated for chronic depression. Results of the follow-up examination again clustered in the expected above-average range, with variable performance on measures of attention. On list learning tests of memory, his initial learning of a word list was lower than expected, but delayed retention of the material was above average, with excellent discrimination of target items on a recognition subtest. He also endorsed a large number of symptoms of depression on a self-report inventory.

In follow-up discussion of these results, when asked to evaluate his own performance, the gentleman was convinced that the results would verify evidence of dementia. Rather than directly refuting the gentleman's belief, the examiner adopted a psychoeducational therapeutic approach, using an information processing model of memory to explain how memory complaints can result from several common causes (Fig. 7.5–5). He was shown how the pattern of his performance was most similar to attention-based memory problems that interfere with initial encoding of new information. He was also shown how his intact retention of material over time contrasted with the expected pattern for Alzheimer's disease. The examination results were used to validate this gentleman's experience of so-called memory problems and to reinforce appropriate treatment for depression, while moving him away from an inappropriate interpretation of his problems and unrealistic expectations for his own performance.

Change in Functioning over Time In many cases, it may be most productive and clinically essential to reexamine a given patient with follow-up neuropsychological assessment after 6 months to 1 year, because many neurological diagnoses carry clear expectations regarding normal rates of recovery and decline over time. This is illustrated by the population of patients who complain of cognitive sequelae after mild head trauma, for whom the current literature indicates that the greatest proportion of recovery of function is likely to occur over the initial 6 months to 1 year postinjury. Although continuing subtle signs of recovery can continue after that period, failure to improve after the injury—or worsening of complaints—would clearly indicate the probability of contributing psychological factors; the existence of a preexisting condition, such as dementia; or outright malingering.

Assessment of Decision-Making Capacity Neuropsychologists are often asked to consult in determining individuals' capacity to make decisions or to manage personal affairs. Neuropsychological testing can be useful in these cases by documenting areas of clear and significant impairment and by identifying areas of strength and well-preserved skill. Opinions about decision-making capacity can seldom be based on test findings alone and usually include other more direct observations (e.g., in-home assessment and collateral interviews) of everyday function. Keep in mind that standards for decision-making capacity are generally defined by state statutes and that the final opinion regarding this aspect of competence rests with a presiding judge. However, the neuropsychologist or other health professional can have a powerful impact on the judge's opinion to the extent that the professional opinion is supported by compelling behavioral data. As a general rule of thumb, consideration of decision-making capacity is usually best approached in the narrowest possible sense, so as to infringe as little as possible with the individual's freedom to represent his or her own interests. Therefore, requests for neuropsychological assessment for purposes of evaluating decision-making capacity should identify as specifically as possible those aspects of decision-making and behavior that are of concern. Frequent concerns about decision-making capacity arise with regard to the individual's ability to make decisions in the areas of (1) financial and legal decisions, (2) health care treatment decisions, and (3) decisions regarding living situations or placements, which often require institutional care arrangements. Other issues that involve higher standards of competence include the ability to drive or the ability to work or practice in a given profession (e.g., air traffic controller, surgeon, or financial advisor). Although decisions regarding competence in any of the previously mentioned areas must ultimately be made by judicial or legislatively empowered bodies (e.g., state licensing boards), the behaviorally based recommendations from a neuropsychological examination can provide crucial data on which decisions of competency are likely to be based.

Forensic Evaluation Neuropsychological evaluation of individuals in matters pertaining to criminal or civil law requires specialized knowledge beyond expertise in neuropsychology. Although neuropsychological evidence may be pertinent in criminal cases, the involvement of neuropsychologists is frequently called on in matters involving head injury, especially in the case of mild head injury associated with motor vehicle accident. As a distinct subspecialty, this area of practice requires integration of knowledge of statutes, laws, precedents, and legal procedures, as well as expertise in identifying and describing the impact of an injury or event on cognitive, emotional, and behavioral functioning.

COGNITIVE SCREENING BY OTHER HEALTH CARE PROFESSIONALS

A wide range of health care professionals are involved in the assessment of cognitive and emotional status. Although many informally estimate a patient's cognitive state, research has shown that systematic use of a structured mental status examination greatly increases the accuracy of detecting cognitive impairment, much as depression rating scales increase the accurate identification of mood disturbance. One of the most widely used screening instruments for documenting gross changes in mental status is the Mini-Mental State Examination (MMSE). It is widely used in general medical and geriatric settings as an initial assessment of mental status and can serve, along with a careful history, as an indicator for more precise neuropsychological evaluation. This is particularly true if performance on the MMSE deteriorates over time. Although the MMSE is likely to underestimate the prevalence of cognitive deficits in well-educated older persons with early Alzheimer's disease or in younger adults with focal brain injury, it probably overestimates the presence of cognitive deficits in persons with little education. Therefore, cut-off scores for concluding that impairment is present must be adjusted for age and education.

Although cognitive mental status examinations can be useful in screening for gross signs of cognitive impairment, they do not provide a sufficient foundation for diagnosing specific etiologies of cognitive impairment and are not interchangeable with neuropsychological testing. The in-depth analysis and standardized testing approach that is offered by neuropsychological assessment is most useful in cases of questionable or mild impairment, when there is evidence or complaint of persistent focal impairments, or when psychiatric and neurological symptoms coexist.

DOMAINS OF FORMAL NEUROPSYCHOLOGICAL ASSESSMENT

Neuropsychological examination systematically assesses functioning in the realms of attention and concentration, memory, language, spatial skills, sensory and motor abilities, executive functioning, and emotional status. Overall intellectual abilities are described, not only as a reflection of current abilities, but also because subtest variability can be used as an indicator of any differences from documented or estimated levels of intellectual functioning at some earlier point in time. Psychological contributions to performance are also considered with regard to personality and coping style, emotional lability, presence of thought disorder, developmental history, and significant past or current stressors. The expertise of the neuropsychologist lies in integrating findings that are obtained from many diverse sources, including the history, clinical presentation, and several dozen discrete performance scores that make up the neuropsychological data. The overall summary of the examination can be expected to describe distinctive patterns in the individual's ability to process efficiently and to integrate materials that differ in level of structure and complexity as well as modality of presentation and response.

The actual practice and procedures of clinical neuropsychology have developed in two general directions, which are effectively described in greater detail in texts by Lezak or by Igor Grant and Kenneth Adams.

Battery Approach The battery approach, exemplified by the HRNB, grew directly out of the psychometric tradition in psychology. This battery includes a large variety of tests that measure most cognitive domains, as well as sensory and motor skills. Typically, all parts of the test battery are administered regardless of the patient's presenting problem. This approach has the advantage of identifying problems that the patient has not mentioned and that the medical history may not necessarily predict. It has the disadvantage of being time consuming (i.e., 6- to 8-hour examination) and of originally not including a thorough assessment of memory or attention.

Hypothesis Testing Approach The qualitative hypothesis testing approach was best exemplified historically by the work of Luria and was developed more recently as the *Boston Process Approach* by Edith Kaplan and her colleagues. It is characterized by detailed evaluation of areas of functioning that are related to the patient's complaints and predicted areas of impairment, with relatively less emphasis on aspects of functioning that are less likely to be impaired. The hypothesis testing approach has been particularly helpful in illuminating the differential roles of the two hemispheres, as discussed previously. This approach has the advantage of efficiently honing in on areas of impairment and producing a detailed description of the deficits from a cognitive processing standpoint, but it has the shortcoming of potentially overlooking unexpected areas of deficits.

Screening Approaches *Battery* and *hypothesis testing* approaches have increasingly converged since the 1990s in the form of *screening approaches.* These changes in clinical practice are driven by economic factors that make it less practical to evaluate patients for long periods of time, as well as more efficient clinical practice standards that draw on a widening array of well-normed clinical instruments. Neuropsychologists increasingly use screening evaluations as a first step in determining whether a diagnosis can be made with less information or whether additional testing is necessary to identify more subtle problems. Therefore, even those neuropsychologists who emphasize a hypothesis testing approach are likely to begin with a screening protocol that efficiently assesses the major areas of neuropsychological functioning. This may be followed by additional testing in selected areas that might help the neuropsychologist better understand the reasons for the deficits demonstrated on the screening evaluation.

Neuropsychological Examination Techniques The past decade has seen a virtual explosion in the growth of more sophisticated and better standardized tests and procedures for neuropsychological evaluation. A comprehensive listing of tests and techniques is beyond the scope of this section, but standard works that provide excellent reviews of current techniques are found in texts by Lezak as well as Otfried Spreen and Esther Strauss. Asenath LaRue also has published detailed observations about pertinent assessment issues in aging and neuropsychology. A list of examples of common neuropsychological tests and techniques is provided in Table 7.5–2.

Interview The clinical interview provides the single best opportunity for identifying the patient's concerns and questions, eliciting a direct description of current complaints from the patient and providing an understanding of the context of the patient's history and current circumstances. Although the patient typically serves as the primary interview source, it is important to seek corroborating information for the patient's account from interview with caregivers or family members as well as thorough review of relevant records, such as medical and mental health treatment, educational, and employment experiences.

Intellectual Functioning Assessment of intellectual functioning serves as the cornerstone of the neuropsychological examination. The Wechsler Intelligence Scales have represented the traditional gold standard in intellectual assessment for many years, based on carefully developed normative standards. The scope and variety of subtests on which the summary intelligence quotient (IQ) values are based also provide useful benchmarks against which to compare performances on other tests of specific abilities. The latest revision of this instrument, the *Wechsler Adult Intelligence Scale–Third Edition* (WAIS-III), offers the additional advantage of greatly extended age norms (16 to 89 years of age) and direct normative comparisons to performances on the Wechsler Memory Scale III (WMS-III). In general, the Wechsler Intelligence Scales use a broad set of complex verbal and visuospatial tasks that are normatively summarized as verbal IQ (VIQ), performance IQ (PIQ), and full-scale IQ. In the context of a neuropsychological examination, the patient's performance across the procedures provides useful information regarding long-standing abilities, as well as current functioning. Most neuropsychologists recognize that the summary IQ values provide only a ballpark range for characterizing an individual's general level of functioning. Therefore, it is usually more appropriate and meaningful to characterize an individual's intellectual functioning in terms of the range of functioning (i.e., borderline, low average, average, high average, and superior) that is represented by the IQ value rather than the specific value itself.

Careful examination of the individual's performance across the various verbal and performance subtests is crucial for observing the patient's pattern of strengths and weaknesses, as well as the degree

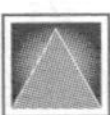

Table 7.5–2
Selected Tests of Neuropsychological Functioning

Area of Function	Comment
Intellectual functioning	
Wechsler Intelligence Scales	Age-stratified normative references; appropriate for adults as old as 89 yrs of age, adolescents, and young children.
Shipley Scale	Brief (20-min) paper-and-pencil measure of multiple-choice vocabulary and open-ended verbal abstraction.
Attention and concentration	
Digit span	Auditory-verbal measure of simple span of attention (*digits forward*) and cognitive manipulation of increasingly longer strings of digits (*digits backward*).
Visual memory span	Visual–spatial measure of ability to reproduce a spatial sequence in forward and reverse order.
Paced Auditory Serial Addition Test	Requires double tracking to add pairs of digits at increasing rates; particularly sensitive to subtle simultaneous processing deficits, especially in head injury.
Memory	
Wechsler Memory Scale III	Comprehensive set of subtests measuring attention and encoding, retrieval, and recognition of various types of verbal and visual material with immediate recall and delayed retention; excellent age-stratified normative comparisons for adults as old as 89 yrs of age with intellectual data for direct comparison.
California Verbal Learning Test II	Documents encoding, recognition, and immediate and 30-min recall; affords examination of possible learning strategies, as well as susceptibility to semantic interference with alternate and short forms available.
Fuld's Object Memory Test	Selective reminding format requires patient to identify objects tactually, then assesses the consistency of retrieval and storage, as well as the ability to benefit from cues; normative reference group is designed for use with older individuals.
Benton Visual Retention Test	Assesses memory for ten geometric designs after 10-sec exposures; requires graphomotor response.
Brief Visuospatial Memory Test–Revised	Serial learning approach used to assess recall and recognition memory for an array of six geometric figures; six alternate forms.
Language	
Boston Diagnostic Aphasia Examination	Comprehensive assessment of expressive and receptive language functions.
Boston Naming Test–Revised	Documents word finding difficulty in a visual confrontation format.
Verbal fluency	Measures ability to fluently generate words within semantic categories (e.g., animals) or phonetic categories (e.g., words beginning with S).
Token Test	Systematically assesses comprehension of complex commands using standard token stimuli that vary in size, shape, and color.
Visuospatial-constructional	
Judgment of line orientation	Ability to judge angles of lines on a page presented in a match-to-sample format.
Facial recognition	Assesses matching and discrimination of unfamiliar faces.
Clock drawing	Useful screening technique is sensitive to organization and planning, as well as constructional ability.
Rey-Osterreith Complex Figure Test	Ability to draw and to recall later a complex geometric configuration; sensitive to visual memory, as well as executive deficits in development of strategies and planning.
Motor	
Finger tapping	Standard measure of simple motor speed; particularly useful for documenting lateralized motor impairment.
Grooved pegboard	Ability to place rapidly notched pegs in slotted holes; measures fine finger dexterity, as well as eye-hand coordination.
Grip strength	Standard measure of lateralizing differences in strength.
Executive functions	
Wisconsin Card Sorting Test	Measure of problem-solving efficiency is particularly sensitive to executive deficits of perseveration and impaired ability to flexibly generate alternative strategies in response to feedback.
Category Test	This measure of problem-solving ability also examines ability to benefit from feedback while flexibly generating alternative response strategies; regarded as one of the most sensitive measures of general brain dysfunction in the Halstead-Reitan Battery.
Trail-Making Test	Requires rapid and efficient integration of attention, visual scanning, and cognitive sequencing.
Delis-Kaplan Executive Function System	Battery of measures that are sensitive to executive functions.
Psychological factors	
Beck Depression Index	Brief (5–10 mins) self-report measure that is sensitive to symptoms of depression. Best for screening depression in adults as old as late middle-age, who can be expected to frankly report symptoms. Available in standard (21 four-choice items) or short (13-item) form.
Geriatric Depression Scale	30-item self-report screen for symptoms of depression. The yes–no format is less cognitively demanding than other scales.
Minnesota Multiphasic Personality Inventory–2	This psychometrically developed self-report instrument remains highly useful for documenting quantitative levels and qualitative features of psychological symptoms. Drawbacks include administration time (567 true-false questions; requires approximately 1–1.5 hrs) for frail individuals, and the emphasis on pathological features for persons who are generally psychologically healthy. Advantages include well-developed validity scales and availability of many symptom-specific subscales that have been identified over the years.
Test of Memory Malingering	Effectively identifies persons who tend to exaggerate impairment by using a forced-choice recognition procedure based on 50 line drawings of common objects.

to which these performance characteristics are consistent with the history and performance on other aspects of the neuropsychological examination. Estimation of long-standing (premorbid) intellectual abilities is as important as the measurement of current functioning to gauge the degree to which an individual may have deteriorated. However, it may be difficult to demonstrate subtle cognitive decline among individuals who fall into either extreme of the intellectual spectrum, with premorbid abilities in the superior or borderline ranges of functioning.

With regard to the question of differential hemispheric representation, the VIQ and PIQ have historically been reported to be associated with left and right hemisphere functioning, respectively, over the past few decades. However, more recent views indicate that, in addition to language and spatial skills, the subtests of the Wechsler Intelligence Scales reflect other contributions, such as speed and sustained concentration. Therefore, experienced neuropsychologists do not simply assume that a discrepancy between VIQ and PIQ is due to unilateral hemispheric damage. Important clues to the nature of the contributing problem can often be gleaned by considering the pattern of performance across other aspects of the examination and by carefully analyzing the types of errors that are observed to occur. As an example, consider the fact that, in addition to visuospatial demands, the PIQ subtests (e.g., Block Design and Picture Arrangement) tend to be timed and are relatively more dependent on novel problem-solving skills than that required in the verbal subtests. Clearly then, lower PIQ relative to higher VIQ might reflect more general executive problem-solving deficits or generalized slowing, perhaps in association with depression or any of a number of neurological syndromes with motor symptoms (e.g., Parkinson's disease and MS). Finally, qualitative analysis of performance patterns on the WAIS-III is further facilitated by the introduction of four additional summary scores, labeled *verbal comprehension index* (VCI), *perceptual organization index* (POI), *working memory index* (WMI), and *processing speed index* (PSI).

Attention Attention underlies performance in virtually all other areas of functioning and should always be considered as a potential contributor to impaired performances on any tests that require vigilance or rapid integration of information. Measures of attention and concentration have traditionally been included in the Wechsler Intelligence and Wechsler Memory Scales to assess orientation and *freedom from distractibility*. These procedures also provide a useful basis for *previewing* the individual's ability to comprehend, to process information, and otherwise to engage in the assessment process. *Digit span* requires patients to repeat increasingly longer strings of digits as a way of assessing ability to process relatively simple information, whereas *digit span backwards* reflects more complex simultaneous processing and cognitive manipulation demands. The *mental control* subtest includes measures that require serial addition and recitation of automatic or overlearned sequences of numbers or letters. More demanding specialized techniques have also been developed that are highly sensitive to subtle deficits in rapid simultaneous processing. For example, Dorothy Gronwall's *Paced Auditory Serial Addition Test* (PASAT) requires patients to successively sum pairs of numbers at increasingly faster rates of presentation, adding each new digit to the immediately preceding digit. Other procedures for assessing attention and sustained concentration can be found in the form of pencil-and-paper measures of digit, letter, or symbol cancellation and various versions of computer-assisted measures of attention and vigilance.

Memory Complaints of memory problems constitute one of the most common reasons for referral to neuropsychology. As described previously, the neuropsychologist uses an information processing approach to assess memory problems that might involve difficulty with encoding, retrieval, or storage of new information. The *WMS-III* is the latest revision of a widely used battery of subtests that uses several measures of attention, memory, and new learning ability. The original version, which was developed by David Wechsler in 1945, was adapted in the 1970s by Elbert Russell to include immediate and delayed recall comparisons and was supplemented by the development of older age norms from several laboratories. A revised version of the battery was published in 1987, which formalized these modifications and added five summary indices, consisting of verbal and visual memory, general memory, attention and concentration, and delayed memory. The current version, published in 1997, offers additional advantages by extending the normative comparisons to 89 years of age, adding procedures for standardized assessment of recognition (to determine if impaired recall performance is due to impaired retrieval or storage) and linking normative comparisons to performances on the WAIS-III.

Many clinicians choose not to administer the entire Wechsler Memory Scale and instead use particular procedures for which standardized normative data are available. For basic assessment of memory encoding and recall, *logical memory* assesses the individual's ability to recall two different narrative stories immediately after presentation and then again after a 30-minute delay interval. The difference between the amount of material recalled immediately and after the delay constitutes a sensitive measure of memory retention. *Visual reproduction* requires immediate and delayed recall of increasingly complex geometric designs, each of which is presented for 10 seconds before being drawn by the patient. Retention of the material after a similar 30-minute delay interval can be measured against standardized normative data. The WMS-III also includes a WMI, which may be useful for further differentiating memory impairment due to problems with encoding versus retention.

A well-standardized example of a verbal list learning technique is the *California Verbal Learning Test II* (CVLT-II). This procedure uses five learning trials of a 16-item word list, which is made up of four exemplars from each of four semantic categories. Aside from measuring several aspects of learning and memory, the CVLT-II also yields rich qualitative data about the patient's use of higher-order conceptual strategies and efficiency of verbal learning. Proactive interference is examined by the use of a single free-recall trial of a second list of words. Free and cued recall of the original list after short and long delays, as well as recognition and forced-choice trials, further examine memory processes of storage, retention, and retrieval. Published norms for this recently revised instrument extend from 16 to 89 years of age for men and women. This revised task also offers advantages of an alternative form and a nine-item short form. Because administration time for the standard form typically requires 15 to 25 minutes (not counting a 20-minute delay interval), the short form can be particularly useful for examining more severely impaired individuals. Recent findings suggest that the CVLT-II might serve as a sensitive early cognitive marker for dementia of the Alzheimer's type.

An alternative list learning procedure to consider for older patients is Paula Fuld's *Object Memory Test*, in which the patient must identify (tactually or visually) ten common objects that are hidden in a bag and then attempt to learn the list over a series of five *selective-reminding* trials. This is a specialized technique for measuring memory retention and storage, in which patients are asked to learn a list of items over five trials. At the end of each recall trial, subjects are selectively reminded of only those words that were omitted. This test is especially useful for patients with hearing impairment, and the normative standards afford limited comparisons to older individuals who are community residing or who live in assisted living arrangements. The WMS-III also includes a list learning task that may be useful for screening purposes, especially in the elderly or for patients whose premorbid functioning is estimated to be below average.

A number of procedures have been standardized over the years for assessing memory for visual material. These include the *Rey-Osterreith Complex Figure Test*, which is illustrated in Figure 7.5–3 and is further discussed as a visuospatial assessment technique in the following discussion. *Benton Visual Retention Test* requires persons to recall a series of ten geometric designs, each of which is presented for only 10 seconds. Three alternate forms are available, and items are scored for errors and classified as omissions, distortions, perseverations, rotations, misplacements, and size errors. The *Brief Visuospatial Memory Test–Revised* offers six alternate forms and uses a three-trial serial learning approach to assess recall and recognition memory for an array of six geometric figures that are presented in a two-by-three array on a single page.

Language Assessment of language examines expressive abilities and comprehension. However, most neuropsychologists screen for language impairment rather than administer an extensive formal language assessment battery, such as the *Boston Diagnostic Aphasia Examination*. Expressive language is commonly assessed by measures of *verbal fluency*, which require the patient to rapidly generate words within semantic (e.g., names of animals) and phonetic categories (e.g., words beginning with specified letters of the alphabet). Another measure of expressive language, the *Boston Naming Test–Revised*, provides a standard 60-item measure of visual confrontation naming ability. Standardized evaluation of comprehension often uses procedures that systematically assess one-, two-, and three-step commands in a format, such as the *token test*, or by examining comprehension of more complex narrative material, as in the complex ideational subtest of the Boston Diagnostic Aphasia Examination.

Visuospatial Functions Complex visuospatial abilities can be assessed through procedures that were developed in Arthur Benton's laboratory, such as *facial recognition* and *judgment of line orientation*. Visual constructional ability is another important aspect of the examination that taps into the person's ability to draw spatial designs or to assemble two- or three-dimensional figures (Figs. 7.5–2 and 7.5–3). In addition to the significant visuospatial component, these tasks reflect contributions of executive planning and organizational abilities. More impaired individuals can be asked to copy simple geometric forms, such as a Greek cross or intersecting pentagons.

The widely used technique of *clock drawing* provides a surprisingly sensitive measure of planning and organization, especially for older individuals suspected of dementia. Although problems involving poor organization, perseveration, and possible neglect are obvious in the drawing that is illustrated in Figure 7.5–8, more subtle difficulties can also be detected, especially when a patient's performance is evaluated in light of premorbid expectations. Like virtually all assessment techniques, it is important to use even this relatively simple procedure in a standard manner. Most neuropsychologists use the same set of instructions each time, offering the patient a single sheet of unlined paper and saying, "Now I would like you to draw a clock. Put all the numbers on the clock, and set the time to 10 after 11." It is best to encourage the patient to use the whole page and to draw a relatively large clock, so that evidence of neglect or executive deficits in organization and planning can be easily seen. Although the rich qualitative information that can be gleaned from this task

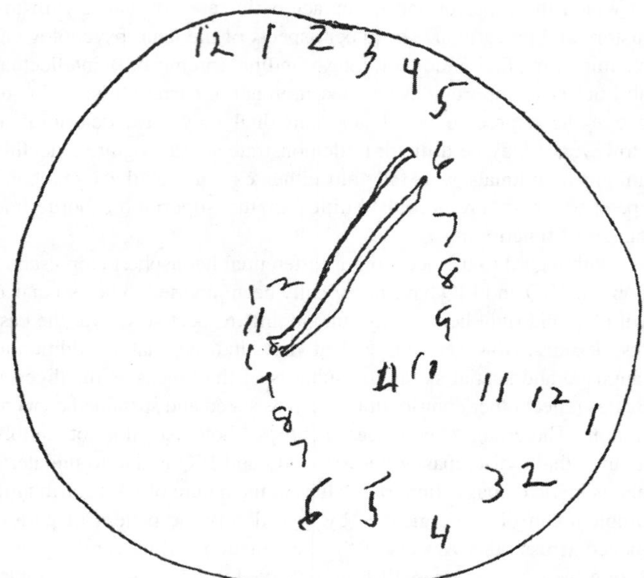

FIGURE 7.5–8 Clock drawing by a patient with vascular dementia, showing poor planning and organization, perseveration, and possible neglect.

may not be sufficient to stand alone for diagnostic purposes, this measure provides a useful screening technique—especially for older or more seriously impaired individuals—and can serve as a basis for deciding whether to refer the patient for more detailed neuropsychological examination.

The *Rey-Osterreith Complex Figure Test* is a more demanding constructional task that requires the individual to copy a highly complex geometric configuration and then to draw the figure from memory. Important qualitative information having to do with problem-solving strategies can be extracted by carefully monitoring and documenting the strategy that is used in drawing the figure. In a prior discussion in this chapter, Figures 7.5–2 and 7.5–3 illustrated different spatial deficits that were seen on the block design and complex figure constructional tasks in the presence of lateralized brain damage in the right or left hemispheres. It should be noted that apparent visuospatial constructional difficulties can also be observed in the presence of frontal executive types of problems with organization, planning, and poor self-monitoring.

Sensory and Motor Functions *Double simultaneous stimulation* in the visual, tactile, and auditory modalities is a standard component of the HRNB and can be useful for assessing the integrity of basic sensory functions. *Grip strength* and rapid *finger tapping* are commonly used measures of motor strength and speed that are sensitive to lateralized brain dysfunction. A related measure, the *grooved pegboard*, assesses the individual's ability to integrate efficiently tactual motor dexterity, motor speed, and eye–hand coordination, but it may be bilaterally impaired after unilateral brain injury owing to its high demands for cognitive integration.

Executive Functions One of the most important aspects of the neuropsychological examination lies in the assessment of higher *executive* functions, which play an important role in the planning and initiation of independent activities, self-monitoring of performance, inhibition of inappropriate responses, switching between tasks, and the planning and control of complex motor and problem-solving responses. Although the prefrontal lobes have long been regarded as an important component in mediating these functions, more recent developments in the neurosciences have also led to an increased appreciation for the essential role that is played by extensive cerebral interconnections between subcortical and cortical regions of the brain.

An underlying executive component is implied to some degree in many of the techniques discussed previously. For example, complex attention, as assessed on a serial addition task, is dependent on the ability to shift focus flexibly and to sustain a cognitive set. Memory functions rely on the ability to process information efficiently, including the use of strategies to organize incoming information (e.g., clustering words in a memory list on the basis of semantic categories). In fact, memory deficits that can be attributed to retrieval failure in the information processing model of memory are often associated with other executive deficits. However, some specific techniques have gained favor over the years as primary measures of executive functions. The *Wisconsin Card Sorting Test* (WCST) requires an individual to sort a long series of cards with designs according to various principles that can only be gleaned by incorporating feedback from the examiner. This measure, then, assesses the individual's ability to generate and to test various solutions and to flexibly respond to changing circumstances, as well as the ability to integrate new information with past experience to respond as efficiently as possible. However, recent data show that deficits on the WCST are not dependent solely on the frontal lobes. The *Category Test* from the Halstead-Reitan Battery is another commonly used technique for assessing the individual's ability to incorporate flexibly feedback into problem-solving responses. Other techniques based largely on the work of Luria are more qualitative in nature and assess the individual's ability to inhibit inappropriate motor responses, as well as the tendency to perseverate when asked to draw a series of repetitive graphomotor sequences. Figure 7.5–9 contains several examples of such sequences. In each case, the sample is presented with instructions for the patient to reproduce the sample and to repeat continuously the segment across a page. Each prior sequence should be covered or removed from the patient's view before going on to the next, so that any tendency to reproduce elements from a prior sequence can properly be interpreted as evidence of perseveration. The *Delis-Kaplan Executive Function System (DKEFS)* is a newly published instrument that is based on a number of other techniques that are associated with executive abilities. These include variations on the *Trail-Making Test*, the *Verbal Fluency Test*, the *Design Fluency Test*, the *Color-Word Interference Test*, the *Sorting Test*, the *20 Questions Test*, the *Word Context Test*, the *Tower Test*, and the *Proverb Test*.

Psychological Factors A key component of any neuropsychological examination involves consideration of the degree to which long-standing personality or other psychological factors (including current stressors) might contribute to the patient's presentation. Common techniques for assessing personality and psychological factors include the *Minnesota Multiphasic Personality Inventory–2* (MMPI-2), and paper-and-pencil techniques, such as the *Beck Depression Index*. Because the results of neuropsychological examinations may eventually be introduced as evidence in litigation or other forensic proceedings, it is important for the neuropsychologist to address any possible concerns about effort and motivation as a routine matter. Several recently developed instruments are based on evaluating the patient's responses to a long series of forced-choice items. Normative research indicates that patients with histories of bona fide brain injury perform close to perfect levels on such instruments, so poor performance may indicate tendencies to exaggerate symptoms. More detailed discussion of psychological tests and techniques can be found elsewhere in this text.

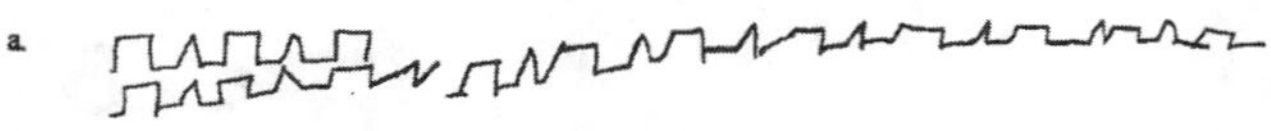

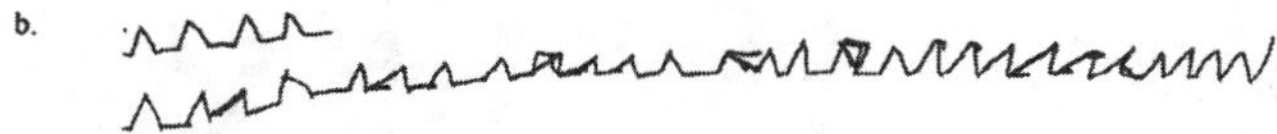

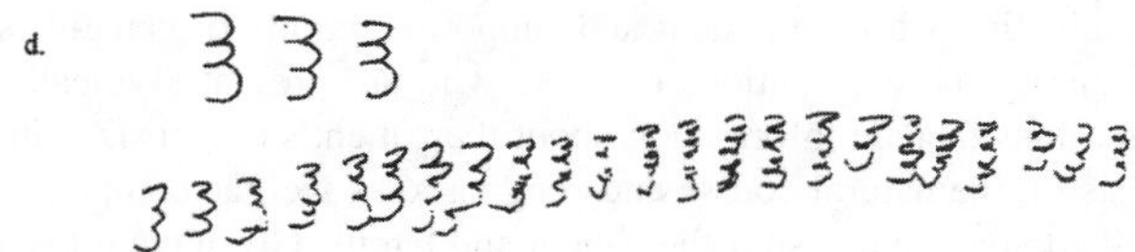

FIGURE 7.5–9 Patient reproductions of repetitive graphomotor sequences, showing perseveration of elements across designs (from **a** to **b**) and within designs (**c** and **d**).

> A 32-year-old woman with 13 years of education was seen for disability evaluation, claiming current "trouble remembering things." Her account of personal history was vague, and she "forgot" information such as her own birth date and her mother's maiden name. Response latencies were extremely long, even for highly familiar information (e.g., count from 1 to 20), she could not repeat more than three digits forward consistently, and, on a word list learning procedure, she was not able to correctly recognize more items (only five) than she could freely recall (also five). Despite otherwise fluent language, she was only able to generate five examples of animals in one minute. She performed far below chance levels (only 12 out of 50 and 11 out of 50 correct on the Test of Memory Malingering [TOMM]) on two presentations of a 50-item forced-choice (only two choices for each item) visual recognition procedure that is sensitive to overt efforts to exaggerate memory complaints. When asked to recall 15 items on a procedure (Rey's Memory Test) that is presented as a challenging task but, in reality, is fairly simple, her performance demonstrated exaggerated errors of commission (Fig. 7.5–10). The evaluation concluded that current levels of cognitive functioning could not be conclusively established, owing to overt symptom exaggeration.

THERAPEUTIC DISCUSSION OF RESULTS

A key component of the neuropsychological examination process is found in the opportunity to discuss results of the examination with the patient and family or other caregivers. This meeting can represent a powerful therapeutic opportunity to educate and to clarify individual and relationship issues, which can impact on the identified patient's functioning. If the patient's active cooperation in the initial examination has been appropriately enlisted, the patient will be optimally prepared to invest value and confidence in the findings of the examination.

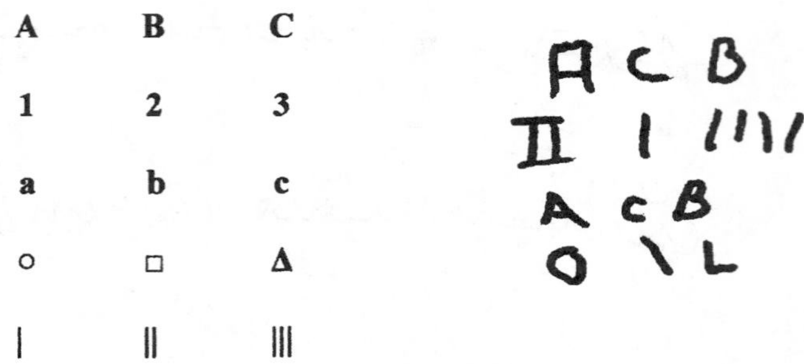

FIGURE 7.5–10 Rey's Memory Test with example of a response that is typical of exaggerated memory problems.

At the time of the results discussion, it is useful to review the goals of the examination with the patient and supportive family or caregivers and to clarify the expectations of those who are present. Typically, these sessions include information about the patient's diagnosis, with emphasis on the natural course and prognosis, as well as compensation and coping strategies for the patient and family. Given the impact of chronic neurological disease on the family system, as well as the patient, explicit discussion of these issues is critical in maximizing adjustment to brain injury. It is equally important to relate the impact of the results to the patient's current living circumstances, future goals, and course of adjustment. It is not unusual for strong emotions and underlying tensions within family relationships to come to light in the context of honest discussion, and so the results discussion can represent an important therapeutic opportunity to model effective communication and problem-solving techniques.

Perhaps the most challenging discussions arise when the objective examination results do not meet the preconceived beliefs of the patient or family members. In such cases, it is helpful to begin the feedback discussion by first asking the patient to describe his or her impression of his or her own performance to explicitly identify the patient's perspective and associated expectations. For those persons who appear to be strongly invested in confirming a pathological diagnosis of memory impairment, it may be particularly helpful to adopt a psychoeducational approach by using materials such as the information processing model of memory that is presented in Figure 7.5–5.

SUGGESTED CROSS-REFERENCES

Neuropsychological and intellectual assessment of children is discussed in Section 7.7, assessment of older adults is reviewed throughout Section 51.2, and Alzheimer's disease and other dementias are addressed in Section 51.3e. Other related material includes the neural sciences (Chapter 1), neuropsychiatry and behavioral neurology (Chapter 2), the biology of memory (Section 3.4), brain models of mind (Section 3.5), and delirium, dementia, and amnestic and other cognitive disorders (Chapter 10). Cholinesterase inhibitors are discussed in Section 31.15, communication disorders are discussed in Chapter 37, and attention-deficit disorders are addressed in Chapter 39.

REFERENCES

American Psychological Association: Ethical principles of psychologists and code of conduct. *Am Psychol.* 2002;57:1060–1073.

Benton AL, Sivan AB, Hamsher KD, Varney NS, Spreen O. *Contributions to Neuropsychological Assessment.* 2nd ed. New York: Oxford University Press; 1983.

Bondi MW: Genetic and brain imaging contributions to neuropsychological functioning in preclinical dementia. *J Intl Neuropsychol Soc.* 2002;8:915.

Crum RM, Anthony JC, Bassett SS, Folstein MF: Population-based norms for the Mini-Mental State Examination by age and educational level. *JAMA.* 1993;269:2389.

Cummings J: Frontal-subcortical circuits and human behavior. *Arch Neurol.* 1993;30:873.

Cummings J, Mega MS. *Neuropsychiatry and Behavioral Neuroscience.* New York: Oxford University Press; 2003.

Cummings J, Trimble MR. *A Concise Guide to Neuropsychiatry and Behavioral Neurology.* 2nd ed. Washington, DC: American Psychiatric Press; 2002.

Devinsky O, D'Esposito M. *Neurology of Cognitive and Behavioral Disorders.* New York: Oxford University Press; 2004.

Doody RS, Stevens JC, Beck C, Dubinsky RM, Kaye JA, Gwyther L, Mohs RC, Thal LJ, Whitehouse PJ, DeKosky ST, Cummings JL: Practice parameters: Management of dementia (an evidence-based review). Report of the quality standards subcommittee of the American Academy of Neurology. *Neurology.* 2001;56:1154.

Goodglass H, Kaplan E. *Assessment of Aphasia and Related Disorders.* Philadelphia: Lea & Febiger; 1972.

*Grant I, Adams KM. *Neuropsychological Assessment of Neuropsychiatric Disorders.* 2nd ed. New York: Oxford University Press; 1996.

Haaland KY, Harrington DL: Hemispheric asymmetry of movement. *Curr Opin Neurobiol.* 1996;6:796.

Heaton RK, Grant I, Matthews CG. *Comprehensive Norms for an Expanded Halstead-Reitan Battery.* Odessa, FL: Psychological Assessment Resources; 1991.

*Heilman KM, Valenstein E. *Clinical Neuropsychology.* 3rd ed. New York: Oxford University Press; 1993.

Heilman KM, Valenstein E. *Clinical Neuropsychology.* 4th ed. New York: Oxford University Press; 2003.

Knight RT, Stuss DT. *Principles of Frontal Lobe Function.* New York: Oxford University Press; 2002.

LaRue A. *Aging and Neuropsychological Assessment.* New York: Plenum Press; 1992.

*Lezak M. *Neuropsychological Assessment.* 3rd ed. New York: Oxford University Press; 1995.

Loring DW, ed. *INS Dictionary of Neuropsychology.* New York: Oxford University Press; 1999.

Luria AR. *Higher Cortical Functions in Man.* Haigh B, trans. New York: Basic Books; 1966.

Mitrushina MN, Boone KB, D'Elia LF. *Handbook of Normative Data for Neuropsychological Assessment.* New York: Oxford University Press; 1999.

Petersen RC. *Mild Cognitive Impairment: Aging to Alzheimer's Disease.* New York: Oxford University Press; 2003.

Petersen RC, Smith GE, Waring SC, Ivnik RJ, Tangalos EG, Kokmen E: Mild cognitive impairment: Clinical characterization and outcome. *Arch Neurol.* 1999;56:303.

Rizzo M, Tranel D. *Head Injury and Post Concussive Syndrome.* New York: Churchill Livingstone; 1996.

Rothi LJG, Heilman KM. *Apraxia: The Neuropsychology of Action.* East Sussex, UK: Psychology Press Publishers; 1997.

*Snyder PJ, Nussbaum PD. *Clinical Neuropsychology: A Pocket Handbook for Assessment.* Washington, DC: American Psychological Association; 1998.

Spar JE, LaRue A. *A Concise Guide to Geriatric Psychiatry.* 3rd ed. Washington, DC: American Psychiatric Press; 2002.

*Spreen O, Strauss E. *A Compendium of Neuropsychological Tests.* 2nd ed. New York: Oxford University Press; 1998.

Stuss DR, Knight RT. *Priniciples of Frontal Lobe Function.* New York: Oxford University Press; 2002.

Wechsler D. *Wechsler Adult Intelligence Scale.* 3rd ed. San Antonio, TX: The Psychological Corporation; 1997.

Yudofsky SC, Hales RE. *The American Psychiatric Press Textbook of Neuropsychiatry.* 2nd ed. Washington, DC: American Psychiatric Press; 1992.

▲ 7.6 Personality Assessment: Adults and Children

RUSSELL L. ADAMS, PH.D., AND JAN L. CULBERTSON, PH.D.

Psychiatry and psychology address concepts that are frequently difficult to quantify. Depression, anxiety, and anger are notable examples. The quantification of these constructs is the purview of personality assessment. Quantification is essential not only to scientific study, but also to clinical applications. For example, to determine if a given treatment is effective in depression, one must establish a baseline of the intensity of the depression, apply the treatment, and conduct a follow-up assessment to determine if a change in the level of the depression has occurred.

Personality assessment tools allow for this quantification. In this chapter, the term *personality* refers to an individual's enduring and pervasive motivation, emotion, interpersonal style, attitude, and traits. *Personality assessment* is a systematic measurement of an individual's personality. This chapter is presented in two major sections—one deals with adult personality assessment and the other deals with child personality assessment. Both of these major sections present objective and projective assessment approaches. Although vast literature exists with respect to personality assessment and many books have been written focusing on one particular personality assessment instrument, the purpose of this chapter is to present an overview of this diverse field. Those interested in a more detailed presentation on this subject can refer to the references listed at the end of this section.

Thousands of personality tests exist, but this chapter does not address each one. Instead, it presents representative samples of the major categories of personality assessment in both narrative and tabular format. The personality assessment instruments discussed in this chapter are those most commonly used in both adult and child personality assessment.

PURPOSES OF PSYCHOLOGICAL TESTING

Personality testing can be an expensive undertaking. A considerable amount of time is required to administer, score, and interpret psychological test results. Personality testing should not be routinely gathered from all psychiatric patients, especially in today's cost-containment environment. Nevertheless, personality testing can be helpful with selective patients from both a clinical and cost–benefit analysis perspective.

Assisting in Differential Diagnosis As any clinician knows, psychiatric diagnosis can be a difficult and, at times, confusing exercise. However, knowing a patient's diagnosis is essential to treatment, as a proper diagnosis can assist in understanding the etiology of the presenting psychiatric problem and the prognosis of the disorder. Consider the diagnostic dilemma in the following example:

> A 49-year-old white man had abruptly resigned from his position as an accountant and decided that he was going to start an oil exploration business. He had never worked in the oil business before and knew nothing about the profession. The patient had received a revelation from an unknown entity through an auditory hallucination. This voice told him he would become quite wealthy in the business if he simply followed the directions given to him. Around this time, the patient had a marked change in personality. Although his grooming was formerly very neat and appropriate, he became disheveled. He began sleeping approximately 3 hours a night. He also became somewhat agitated and talked loudly to those around him.

The differential diagnosis in this case study includes schizophrenia and bipolar disorder. Psychological testing might be helpful in assisting in this differential diagnosis, as well as in formulating a treatment plan.

Aiding Psychotherapy Psychological tests can be useful in psychotherapy. The usefulness of these tests can be even more important for short-term, problem-centered therapy in which understanding the patient and his or her problem must be accomplished quickly. Psychological assessment can be used in pretreatment planning, in assessing progress once therapy begins, and in evaluating the effectiveness of therapy. Patients need to have objective information about themselves at the time of therapy if they are to change themselves productively. Personality tests, particularly objective tests, allow patients to compare themselves to objective norms and evaluate the extent and magnitude of their problem. Testing can also reveal areas of the patient's life that may be problematic but for which the patient may not have a full appreciation. Information about patients' willingness to reveal information about themselves can also be helpful. In some instances, the test report can be the subject of an early treatment session. Psychological tests may reveal considerable information about the patient's inner life, feelings, and images, which may make therapy progress faster. Psychological testing can provide baseline information at the beginning of therapy, and repeat testing can then be used to assess changes that occurred during the course of therapy.

Providing Narrow-Band Assessment Narrow-band personality tests measure a single personality characteristic or a few related characteristics. Broad-band personality tests, on the other hand, are designed to measure a wide spectrum of personality characteristics. A psychiatrist may need answers to specific questions, such as those that arise when assessing the degree of clinical depression, measuring the intensity of the state or trait anxiety, or, possibly, quantifying the amount of a patient's anger. Such quantification can be helpful in measuring severity or in providing a baseline for future assessment.

Psychological tests can often assist with a specific problem area. For example, a young college student may be unsure what to major in. Vocational interest inventories, such as the Strong Vocational Interest Inventory and the Kuder Occupational Interest Survey, may help to better define the student's vocational interest. The Strong Vocational Interest Inventory compares a given individual's responses with those of a large group of successful individuals in a variety of occupations. Test results can show that a student's interests are similar, for example, to those of successful persons in occupations such as social work or public administration and dissimilar to those of engineers or scientists.

PSYCHOMETRIC PROPERTIES OF PERSONALITY ASSESSMENT INSTRUMENTS

The quality of personality tests varies widely. On the one hand, there are well-constructed, empirically validated instruments, and, on the other hand, there are "psychological tests" that one can find in the Sunday supplement of the newspaper or on the Internet. Evaluating the usefulness of particular psychological instruments can be challenging, even to the well informed.

Just as the *Physician's Desk Reference* helps physicians evaluate the usefulness of medications, the *Buros Mental Measurement Yearbook* helps psychologists evaluate the usefulness of personality instruments and other psychological and achievement tests. The *Mental Measurement Yearbook* is a reference source of critical reviews of individual tests. These reviews evaluate the scientific underpinnings of each test by an expert in the field. The reviews generally address such issues as the reliability and validity of the tests, the normative group used in construction, and various empirical studies used to check the reliability and validity of the instrument. The advantages and disadvantages of the test are described. The reviews generally describe situations in which the test can be appropriately used. Practical information concerning the test publisher, length of administration time, and other considerations are also included. The *Buros Mental Measurement Yearbook* is available in most medical school and university libraries and can be ordered through the book's publisher.

Normative Sample To construct a personality test, a representative sample of subjects (normative sample) should be administered the test to establish expected performance. Basic issues, such as the size and representativeness of the sample used to construct the test, must be evaluated. A sample of 30 individuals of a given diagnosis in a single location is seldom appropriate, because there are so many moderating factors impacting results, such as age, education, sex, and racial and ethnic grouping. These factors frequently impact the norms, and appropriate controls must be made for these variables in many cases.

To illustrate this point, the Minnesota Multiphasic Personality Inventory–2 (MMPI-2), a well-constructed instrument, initially tested approximately 2,900 subjects. However, approximately 300 subjects were eliminated because of test invalidity or incompleteness of needed information. The final group was composed of 2,600 community volunteers, including 1,462 women and 1,138 men. The MMPI-2 normative group was selected using census data as a guide and was broadly representative in terms of region of the country, racial composition, age, and formal education. Despite efforts to control for moderating variables, the sample was slightly overrepresentative in higher education levels. Obviously, the cost of obtaining large census-based normative samples is enormous, and few tests are able to meet these challenging criteria. Nevertheless, many tests that fall short of the national sample (and most do) can be useful in the hands of an experienced clinician who is sensitive to the problem and makes appropriate clinical adjustments in interpreting the results.

Test Characteristics To be useful, any psychological test must be completed, in its entirety, by the intended test taker. If the questions are offensive or difficult to understand, the individual taking the test may not complete all items. These omissions can create problems, especially when normative tables are used to interpret results. To be useful, an instrument should be short enough to complete in a relatively short period of time. The Beck Depression Inventory and the Geriatric Depression Scale can each be easily completed in 5 to 10 minutes. Because of its short length, the test can be given repeatedly to a depressed patient in treatment to monitor changes over time. The MMPI-2, on the other hand, takes approximately 1 to 1½ hours to complete. This test is not appropriate for repeat testing over a short period of time. Most tests are easily scored and compared to normative tables.

Validity Issues Perhaps the most important characteristic in evaluating the scientific merit of a given personality test is the validity of the instrument. Does the test measure what it purports to measure? If a test is designed to measure depression, does it indeed measure depression? Although validity may seem like a simple issue to address, it can become complex, especially when attempting to measure such characteristics as self-esteem, assertiveness, hostility, and self-control. The test developer must first operationally define what is meant by the personality characteristic in question. A number of different approaches have been used to measure validity, including face validity, logical content validity, construct validity, criterion validity, and factor validity.

Face Validity *Face validity* refers to the content of the test items themselves. In other words, do the items appear to measure what they purport to measure? For example, does a depression scale ask questions concerning sadness, guilt, sleep disturbance, weight loss, helplessness, hopelessness, or suicidal thoughts? One problem with face validity is that professionals differ in their subjective appraisal of individual items. One psychologist may think a given item does, indeed, measure the concept under consideration, whereas other professionals may not. To address these differences in definition, the test developers may use an approach known as *logical content validity*. Using this approach, the developer will describe in the manual the procedure used to select items for the test that will not depend significantly on the subjective judgment of any one professional. For example, in developing the Taylor Manifest Anxiety Scales, a number of different psychologists were asked to review items from the MMPI that seemed to measure a formal definition of manifest anxiety, and only those items agreed on by this group of psychologists were included. Many creative approaches have been used to demonstrate the logical content validity of various tests.

Criterion and Construct Validity Although face validity refers to the degree that test items appear on the surface to measure what the instrument, as a whole, purports to measure, *criterion validity* uses data outside the test to measure validity. For example, if a test were designed to measure hypochondria, one would expect that a patient with high scores would have more visits to the physician's office, complain of more physical symptoms, and use prescribed and over-the-counter medications more extensively. These criteria are objective and external to the test itself and can be independently measured. Scores on the hypochondria instrument can be statistically correlated with a number of separate objective criteria, such as those mentioned previously, to determine if the test measures the theoretical construct being measured (*construct validity*).

Concurrent and Predictive Validity To determine test's *concurrent validity*, external measures are obtained at the same time the test is given to the sample of subjects. Thus, the concurrent validity of the test reveals that, at a given point in time, high scorers on a test may be more likely than low scorers on a test to manifest the behavior reflected in the criteria (e.g., more physician visits, more medication for a hypochondriac patient). Occasionally, however, a test developer is interested in predicting future events. For example, a test designed to predict marital satisfaction among engaged couples may use the couples' future marital satisfaction and marital status as an external criterion. Thus, the external criterion would have to be obtained a number of years down the road for the test to have this predictive validity. This type of validity is referred to as *predictive validity*. Because it is difficult to obtain such information several years later, predictive validity is seldom available in most personality tests, although such data can be valuable when available.

The *discriminant validity* of a test tells whether the test is able to discriminate between known groups of patients at a given point in time. For example, is a test of depression able to statistically discriminate nondepressed subjects from subjects with independently diagnosed major depression, adjustment disorder with depressed mood, and dysthymia? Is a measure of depression able to statistically discriminate among mild, moderate, and severe major depressive disorder?

Factor Validity Factor validity uses a multivariate statistical technique known as *factor analysis* to determine if certain major groups of items on a given test empirically cluster together. For example, on a personality test measuring depression, do items concerning vegetative symptoms tend to covary together? Are there other clusters of items on the depression test measuring cognitive problems, mood disturbance, and social withdrawal?

Reliability To be useful, a test must not only be valid, but it must also be reliable. *Reliability* refers to the degree that a test measures what it purports to measure, consistently. The key word here is *consistently*. For example, a patient with agoraphobia takes a new agoraphobia test today and takes the same test tomorrow. However, on the second testing, the scores change markedly even though the patient has not received any treatment or undergone any change in his or her underlying agoraphobia. Such a test would not be useful, because it would not consistently measure the trait in question. The test would have poor reliability. There are several means of checking reliability, including test–retest reliability, internal consistency reliability, and parallel form reliability.

Test–Retest Reliability *Test–retest reliability* is obtained by simply administering the same test on two occasions to a group of subjects and statistically correlating the results. To be useful, the correlation coefficient should be at least .80 if the two tests were administered within 2 weeks of each other and if the trait in question is stable.

Internal Consistency Reliability Another approach to determine *internal consistency reliability* is to divide a given test into two equal parts and statistically correlate the two halves of the test with each other. This technique determines the *split-half reliability* of a test. The first half of the test should be highly correlated with the second half of the test if the test is consistently measuring what it purportedly measures. Alternatively, the odd-numbered items could be correlated with the even-numbered items (*odd–even consistency reliability*). When a test is split into two parts and the obtained scores correlate with each other, the resulting correlation coefficients statistically underestimate the true reliability of the test, because the number of items in the test influences the magnitude of the correlation. Hence, if there were only half that number of items in the original test, the results would be underestimated. To correct for this underestimation, the *Spearman-Brown formula* is used. Again, a reliability coefficient of .80 to .85 is needed to demonstrate usefulness in most circumstances. However, the higher the reliability as measured by the correlation coefficient, the better the test instrument. No test is perfectly reliable. The highest possible correlation coefficient is 1.0 and the lowest is 0, assuming no negative correlation.

To determine how internally consistent a given test is, a test developer also may use a statistical technique called *Cronback's coefficient alpha*. With Cronback's coefficient alpha statistic, one can determine the average correlation among all of the items on the test. The higher the average correlation, the better the reliability.

Parallel Form Reliability Sometimes, two separate forms of the same test are needed. For example, if the process of taking a test at one point in time would by itself influence a patient's score the second time that he or she took the same test, then parallel forms of the tests are needed. *Parallel forms* of a test measure the same construct but use different items to do so. To ensure that the test does, in fact, measure the same construct, the correlation coefficient between the two parallel forms of the same test is computed. Such parallel form reliability should be at least .90 or higher.

Use of Standard Error of Measurement to Assess Reliability Another way to assess the usefulness of a given test is to examine the test's standard error of measurement (SEM), which should be included in the test's manual. The SEM is a single statistic that is used to estimate what the score of a given patient would be on the test if the patient took the same test again within a short period of time. Consider the following example: A patient takes a given test today and obtains a score of 90 on that test. The SEM on that test is 3. An SEM value of 3 together with an individual's score of 90 on the test means that if that patient were to take the same test again tomorrow, he or she would score within ± 1 SEM of the original test performance (e.g., ± 3 points) 68 percent of the time. Thus, the patient in question should score between 87 (90 – 3) and 93 (90 + 3) on the second test 68 percent of the time. The same individual would score ± 2 SEM values (e.g., 2 × 3 = 6) on the second test 95 percent of the time.

In the above example, the patient with an original score of 90 on a given test would score between 84 (90 – 6) and 96 (90 + 6) on the second test 95 percent of the time. Other things being equal, the smaller the SEM of the estimate relative to the standard deviation of the tests, the better.

ADULT PSYCHOLOGICAL TESTS

Objective Personality Tests

Objective personality tests are rather straightforward in approach. Patients are usually asked specific and standard questions in a structured written or oral format. Each patient is typically asked the same question. The data obtained from a given patient are compared to similar data obtained from the normative group. The degree to which the patient deviates from the norm is noted and is used in the interpretive process. The patient's responses are scored according to certain agreed-on criteria. The obtained scores are then compared with normative tables and often converted to standardized scores or percentiles, or both. The MMPI-2 is an example of an objective personality test.

There are literally hundreds of different objective personality instruments, and discussing all of these instruments is beyond the scope of this chapter. Table 7.6–1 contains a representative sample of objective personality tests and concise descriptions of each test, along with brief listings of strengths and weaknesses. Because the MMPI-2 is, by far, the most frequently used objective personality test, it is discussed in considerable detail in this section to give the reader an orientation to objective personality assessment, as well as objective personality development.

This focus on MMPI-2 is not meant to imply that the MMPI-2 is the only valid and reliable objective personality instrument or that other objective personality tests are not as useful as the MMPI-2 for a particular purpose. There are many useful objective personality instruments.

Minnesota Multiphasic Personality Inventory–2 (MMPI-2) Two excellent books on the MMPI-2 are James N. Butcher's *The MMPI-2 in Psychological Treatment* and John R. Graham's *MMPI-2: Assessing Personality and Psychopathology*. The following discussion relies heavily on information contained in these two resources. The MMPI-2 consists of 567 true-or-false questions concerning a wide variety of issues. The patient completes the test using a pencil. The MMPI-2 is relatively easy to administer and score and takes approximately 1 to 1½ hours for most patients to complete. It requires only an eighth grade reading comprehension. The test provides a number of internal checks for measuring the patient's degree of cooperation. The patient is simply asked to answer true or false to such questions as "I have a good appetite" and "No one seems to understand me."

Scoring of the MMPI-2 involves adding up the number of responses on numerous scales and comparing the results to certain normative information. Interpretation of the MMPI-2 is more straightforward than with many other tests, because of the vast amount of empirical information available concerning the MMPI-2. More than 12,000 articles and books have been published on this test to date.

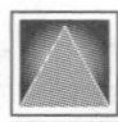

Table 7.6–1
Objective Measures of Personality in Adults

Name	Description	Strengths	Weaknesses
Minnesota Multiphasic Personality Inventory (MMPI)	566 items, true–false; self-report format; 17 primary scales (numerous special scales)	Provides wide range of data on numerous personality variables; strong research base	Tends to emphasize major psychopathology; needs revision with current normative data
MMPI-2	567 items; true–false; self-report format; 20 primary scales	Current revision of MMPI with updated response booklet; revised scaling methods, and new validity scores; new normative data	Preliminary data indicate that the MMPI-2 and the MMPI can provide discrepant results; normative sample biased toward upper socioeconomic status; no normative data for adolescents
Millon Clinical Multiaxial Inventory (MCMI)	175 items; true–false; self-report format; 20 primary scales	Brief administration time; corresponds well with DSM-III diagnostic classifications	Needs more validation research; no information on disorder severity; needs revision for DSM-IV-TR
MCMI-II	175 items; true–false; self-report format; 25 primary scales	Brief administration time; corresponds well with DSM-III-R	High degree of item overlap in various scales; no information on disorder or trait severity
16 Personality Factor Questionnaire (16 PF)	True–false; self-report format; 16 personality dimensions	Sophisticated psychometric instrument with considerable research conducted on nonclinical populations	Limited usefulness with clinical populations
Personality Assessment Inventory (PAI)	344 items; Likert-type format; self-report; 22 scales	Includes measures of psychopathology, personality dimensions, validity scales, and specific concerns to psychotherapeutic treatment	Inventory is new and has not yet generated a supportive research base
California Personality Inventory (CPI)	True–false; self-report format; 17 scales	Well-accepted method of assessing patients who do not exhibit major psychopathology	Limited usefulness with clinical populations
Jackson Personality Inventory (JPI)	True–false; self-report format; 15 personality scales	Constructed in accord with sophisticated psychometric techniques; controls for response sets	Unproved usefulness in clinical settings
Edwards Personal Preference Schedule (EPPS)	Forced choice; self-report format	Follows Murray's theory of personology; accounts for social desirability	Not widely used clinically because restricted information obtained
Psychological Screening Inventory (PSI)	103 items; true–false; self-report format	Yields four scores that can be used as screening measures for the possibility of a need for psychological help	Scales are short and have correspondingly low reliability
Eysenck Personality Questionnaire (EPQ)	True–false; self-report format	Useful as a screening device; test has a theoretical basis with research support	Scales are short, and items are transparent as to purpose; not recommended for other than a screening device
Adjective Checklist (ACL)	True–false; self-report or informant report	Can be used for self-rating or other rating	Scores rarely correlate highly with conventional personality inventories
Comrey Personality Scales (CPS)	True–false; self-report format; eight scales	Factor-analytical techniques used with a high degree of sophistication in test construction	Not widely used; factor-analytical interpretation problems
Tennessee Self-Concept Scale (TSCS)	100 items; true–false; self-report format; 14 scales	Brief administration time yields considerable information	Brevity is also a disadvantage, lowering reliability and validity; useful as a screening device only

Courtesy of Robert W. Butler, Ph.D., and Paul Satz, Ph.D.

There are more than 115 translations of the MMPI-2. The test is also cost-effective, as relatively little professional time is involved in the administration and scoring. The patient is simply given instructions, and then he or she completes the test independently in the professional's office. In certain situations, the MMPI-2 can be administered on a computer. A computer can also plot test profiles and compute various supplemental scales. The number of available specialized scales increases the usefulness of the MMPI-2 with various populations (e.g., patients with posttraumatic stress disorder [PTSD], college students who are maladjusted, and prisoners with violent tendencies).

Questions cover a wide range of areas. When a patient takes the MMPI-2, questions are not grouped in any particular order. To aid in interpretation, various items in the MMPI-2 can be selected, sorted, and analyzed according to various criteria. The most common scales of the MMPI-2, including the validity scales, clinical scales, content scales, supplemental scales, and critical items, are discussed below.

VALIDITY SCALES The patient can approach a mental status interview in a variety of ways. The patient can be painfully honest and straightforward with the interviewer, revealing his or her innermost aspirations and fears. The patient may be somewhat distrusting of the interviewer and try to slant the content of the interview in a certain fashion to manipulate the outcome he or she wants. The patient may be disingenuous or even attempt to be deceitful by malingering. Obviously, the information obtained by psychiatrists or other mental health professionals in an interview may well be colored by the patient's approach to the interview. Some patients are, by nature, reserved and may use denial successfully during a clinical interview. Other patients may have little insight into their feelings and thoughts.

When patients are administered personality tests like the MMPI-2, they approach the test as they would approach an interview. One advantage of the MMPI-2 is that the test has been devised to assess different test-taking attitudes (e.g., fake bad, fake good, social desirability responding). Through use of the validity scales, the clinician gleans information that helps in interpreting the remaining scales of the MMPI-2. Is the patient overly defensive? Is he or she attempting to fake good or fake bad? Does the patient maintain a reasonable balance between self-disclosure and excessive defensiveness?

Lie (L) Scale This scale consists of 15 items designed to measure general frankness. The items include questions about personal characteristics that, although highly desirable in our culture, are, nevertheless, infrequently practiced (e.g., questions such as "I have never failed to tell the truth," "Once in a while I think of things too bad to talk about," and "I do not always tell the truth"). Patients who score high on the lie scale may be psychologically naïve or defensive. They may want to be seen in a positive light or may have difficulty admitting common human frailties.

F-Scale This is one of the longest scales, consisting of 60 items that 10 percent or fewer of the normative samples responded to in the positive direction. This scale includes items such as "Evil spirits possess me at times" and "Most any time I would rather sit and daydream than do anything else."

The items on the F-Scale are quite diverse in content and may be indicative of severe psychopathology, such as hallucinations and delusions. Most people in the normal sample responded to fewer than five of these items. Individuals who obtain exceptionally high scores on this scale are often either extremely pathological or trying to claim mental illness falsely. As with all personality tests, interpretation depends greatly on the setting in which the test was given, as base rates for different settings and circumstances differ. For example, patients who have been seen for court sanity evaluations have different base rates of symptom magnification than do patients seen for adjustment problems in an outpatient clinic.

Backpage Infrequency (Fb) Scale A few patients, particularly those with passive-aggressive tendencies, will start to complete the MMPI-2 but, toward the end of the test, may respond to the items in a random fashion. The patient may simply want to finish the test quickly and leave the testing situation. The Backpage Infrequency (Fb) Scale for the MMPI-2 is designed to pick up this tendency.

Variable Response Inconsistency Scale (VRIN) The VRIN consists of 67 pairs of items. Each question of the pair probes for the same or similar information in a slightly different way, for example: (1) I sleep very poorly at night and (2) I wake up fully refreshed each morning. If the patient responds "true" to question 1, then he or she would normally respond "false" to question 2. Failure to do so would reflect inconsistency.

CLINICAL SCALES The clinical scales are generally considered the meat or substance of MMPI-2 clinical interpretations. The original clinical scales have an empirical base in the sense that the items were selected because they differentiated between specific clinical groups and the normative control group. The control group for the original MMPI, developed in the 1940s, consisted of 1,500 persons who were visitors to the University of Minnesota hospitals and other normal groups. Clinical groups varied in size but, for the most part, contained at least 50 subjects. For example, the schizophrenic scale group was developed with patients with different types of schizophrenia, and the depression scale was developed with a sample of psychiatric patients with depression, including some with manic-depressive illness. Table 7.6–2 presents a brief illustration of the original sample groups. Although most clinical scales were developed using a specific clinically defined group, researchers with the MMPI soon learned that a given patient (such as one with schizophrenia) did not simply score high on the schizophrenia scale and low on all other scales. A schizophrenic might score high on many scales, but his or her highest score may well be on the schizophrenic scale. If one were to diagnose all patients who scored high on the schizophrenic scales as schizophrenic patients, a large number of false-positives would result. To address this confusion, clinicians began to refer to the clinical scales by numbers (0 to 9) rather than by the diagnostic entity that underlies the scale's development.

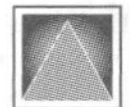

Table 7.6–2
Minnesota Multiphasic Personality Inventory (MMPI) Scale Development

***Scale 1* (Hs: Hypochondriasis):** The clinical group for this scale consisted of patients who had an obsessive overconcern about their physical health. This group had little or no organic basis for these complaints.

***Scale 2* (D: Depression):** This group consisted of a variety of patients with symptomatic depression, including reactive depression and manic depression, among others.

***Scale 3* (Hy: Hysteria):** The hysteria group consisted of patients who had some type of sensory or motor deficit for which no organic basis could be found.

***Scale 4* (Pd: Psychopathic Deviancy):** This patient group had continual run-ins with legal authorities, yet they had normal intelligence and no serious neurotic or psychotic symptomatology. No major criminal types were included. These patients exhibited delinquent acts such as stealing, lying, excessive drinking, and sexual promiscuity.

***Scale 5* (Mf: Masculinity–Femininity):** This scale was originally developed to discriminate homosexual invert men. However, only a small number of items statistically differentiated this group from the controls. As a result, other items were included that differentiated men from women in the normative sample. An attempt to identify sexual inversion in women was unsuccessful.

***Scale 6* (Pa: Paranoia):** Patients in this group consisted of suspicious, mistrusting individuals who often had diagnoses other than paranoia. These persons could have a paranoid personality, paranoid schizophrenia, or an affective disorder. The scale had few false-positives but a rather large number of false-negatives.

***Scale 7* (Pt: Psychasthenia):** This scale was originally developed using a group of patients with psychasthenia. This diagnosis is not used today but does resemble a diagnosis of obsessive-compulsive disorder (OCD). These patients worry excessively; have major fears, compulsions, and rituals; and possess generalized anxiety and distress.

***Scale 8* (Sc: Schizophrenia):** The patient group used for this scale consisted of various types of schizophrenic patients. Efforts to develop separate scales for different subtypes of schizophrenia were not successful.

***Scale 9* (Ma: Mania):** Because many patients who have full-blown mania are not testable, this scale was developed with patients in the earlier stages of manic episodes.

***Scale 0* (Si: Social Introversion):** This scale was not developed on a particular diagnostic group. The items were determined by contrasting selected women who scored in the high or low range on another measure of social introversion, Social Introversion–Extroversion scale of the Minnesota TSE (Thinking–Social–Emotional) Inventory.

Adapted from Graham J. *MMPI-2: Assessing Personality and Psychopathology.* New York: Oxford University Press; 1990.

COMBINING SCALE ELEVATIONS IN THE CODE TYPES As has been illustrated previously, interpreting single-scale evaluations on the MMPI-2 is problematic; thus, most clinicians use a combination of scale elevations in interpretation. This procedure usually involves using the patient's highest two clinical scales that exceed a *t*-score of 65 to provide a configured interpretation that takes into account the relation between the scales. In this approach, for example, a 1-2 or 2-1 code type would be the same. In other words, a patient who scored highest on scale 1 (hypochondriasis [Hs]) and second highest on scale 2 (depression [D]) would be considered to have the same basic profile as an individual who scored highest on scale 2 (D) and second highest on scale 1 (Hs).

A three-point code, likewise, would list the three highest scales, all of which normally would be above a *t*-score of 65. These scales also would usually be significantly higher than all the other clinical scales.

On the MMPI-2, uniform *t*-scores are used on clinical scales, except in scales 5 and 0. *Uniform t-scores*, briefly stated, are standardized scores in which the percentile equivalent and distribution are matched among the various clinical scales in terms of skewness and kurtosis. Thus, a uniform *t*-score of 65 on scale 7 is roughly equivalent to a uniform *t*-score of 65 on scale 9. The use of uniform *t*-score rather than linear *t*-scores was one of the improvements of the MMPI-2 from the original MMPI.

A review of the interpretation of common two- and three-code types can be found in most standard textbooks on the MMPI, some of which are included in the references. Certain MMPI authorities have used slightly more complex means of interpreting the MMPI-2. This approach emphasizes specific relationships about multiple scales. For example, Harold Gilderstadt and Jan Duker described criteria in their book *A Handbook for Clinical and Actuarial MMPI Interpretation* for what is referred to as a *1,2,3,4-type scale* as follows:

1. Hs, D, Hy, and Pd scales greater than *t*-score 70 and higher than all other scales.
2. Si scale less than *t*-score of 70.
3. L, F, and K less than *t*-score 70 unless two or more scales are greater than 100, in which case F, less than *t*-score 80.

The problem in using this complex method is that, in many settings, only a relatively small percentage of patients match these criteria. In other words, if one uses this method rigidly, a substantial number of patients seen in an inpatient unit would not precisely match one of these complex criteria.

CONTENT SCALES FOR MMPI-2 Several efforts have been made to group items according to certain specified dimensions. Using a combination of rational and statistical procedures, Butcher and colleagues developed these 15 narrow-band scales. The 15 scales are internally consistent and relatively independent. Item overlap between scales is minimal. Scales include such content areas as anxiety, anger, cynicism, low self-esteem, fears, obsessiveness, and depression, among many others. Norms for both men and women were simply derived using the same uniform *t*-scores used in the MMPI-2 clinical scale formation. Reliability data on the scales are acceptable given the relatively few items in some of the content scales.

John R. Graham presents scoring guidelines in his book *MMPI-2: Assessing Personality and Psychopathology.* Validity data for the new scales are limited at the current time; however, data are expected to accumulate over the years. Because efforts were made to develop reasonably homogeneous items, interpretation of these scales consists of examining high scores and low scores. For example, patients with high scores on the low self-esteem scale tend to have poor self-concept, anticipate failure, be overly sensitive to criticism, and have trouble making decisions. Low scores, on the other hand, are self-confident and decisive. A given content scale, such as the anger scale, when considered alone, is very similar to the rapid assessment instruments discussed in a later section of this chapter.

HARRIS & LINGOES CONTENT SCALES As previously stated, most of the MMPI clinical scales were developed using empirical key approaches. For example, an item was included in the depression scale because that item discriminated patients in the reference group from individuals in the normal group. Although this method is scientifically sound, the approach results in the inclusion of subtle items that seemingly have little to do with depression. For example, items such as "I sometimes tease animals" (false) and "It takes a lot of argument to convince most people of the truth" (false) are included in the depression scale (D) even though, on the surface, they have little to do with depression. Such items are called *subtle items*. Obvious items are those that have strong face validity, such as "I wish I could be as happy as others" (true) and "I brood a great deal" (true). The depression subscale reflects a heterogeneous item group coming from a variety of aspects of depression, such as subjective depression, psychomotor retardation, and mental dullness. The same total score might reflect a considerably different combination of items. Knowing which items in combination actually contribute to the total score can be helpful in interpretation. The Harris & Lingoes scales can help in that process.

The Harris & Lingoes scales were developed logically by grouping items in a given clinical scale into standard scales that were judged to reflect a more homogeneous trait. Thus, the Harris & Lingoes scales for depression reflect separate scales for subjective depression (D1), psychomotor retardation (D2), physical malfunction (D3), mental dullness (D4), and brooding (D5).

The Harris & Lingoes scales can be used for two major purposes: (1) to see which group of items were elevated for a patient scoring high on a given clinical scale and (2) to see why a marginally elevated scale was elevated. For example, one patient who scored marginally high on the depression scale may be evidencing psychomotor retardation and no subjective depression, whereas another may be just the opposite.

SUPPLEMENTAL SCALES Given that the MMPI contained 566 items, numerous investigators have used the items to develop special-purpose or supplemental scales. By 1972, more than 450 supplemental scales were developed, and the number has kept growing. Scales have been developed to predict success in psychotherapy (ego strength [Es]), to differentiate alcoholic patients from nonalcoholic patients (MacAndrew Revised [MACR]), and to differentiate assaultive prisoners from others not committing a crime (overcontrolled hostility [Oh]). Many a dissertation for doctoral research has been conducted to uncover a new supplemental scale. The success of supplemental scales in accomplishing their stated purpose varies considerably. Many such scales were used for only one study, and others, such as the MacAndrew alcoholism (MAC) scale, have been used in many studies over the years.

COMPUTER SCORING AND INTERPRETATION A computer program can score the MMPI-2. A typical computer scoring program not only scores individual items into validity, clinical, content, and supplemental scales, but also prints out certain positive critical items marked by the patient. These programs save considerable time because the program scores all the material that may take hours to score by hand. Few clinicians have the time or patience to routinely score the vast number of scales found in the output of a typical computer program. The MMPI-2 computer programs can also be used to interpret the test clinically, or at least give clinical hypotheses concerning the patient. These computer-generated reports are in narrative format. Because the report comes from a computer, one may get the impression that the information is more valid or accurate than a clinical interpretation. Although attempts have been made to "validate" narrative statements made by the computer, efforts have only begun in this regard. One problem with computer interpretation of narrative reports is that the algorithms underlying the narrative reports are proprietary information owned by the company producing the program and are not available to the general user.

Rapid Personality-Assessment Instruments Rapid personality-assessment instruments are narrow-spectrum, self-report, objective instruments that measure some unidimensional aspect of personality. The instrument is written in clear, simple language and provides face validity. Typically, these short instruments can be completed in less than 15 minutes. The scoring is simple and straightforward, usually just adding up the number of positive responses. On many instruments, there are cutting scores above which an individual is considered to have a clinically significant problem in that area.

There are literally hundreds of such measures capable of assessing a wide variety of personality states and traits, such as geriatric depression, obsessive-compulsiveness, impulsivity, and state–trait anger. Table 7.6–3 presents a list of such measures. The overall score typically provides an index of the magnitude of the patient's problems. Most of these tests can be used repeatedly to assess change over time. Most of the instruments were developed using relatively small samples and have just been reported in a few studies. There are, however, clear exceptions, as a few instruments are widely used.

Some rapid assessment instruments were developed out of the behavioral assessment tradition. One advantage of short personality-assessment procedures is high face validity for the domain of the behavior in question. Most instruments have standardized instructions and small normative groups. Performances of patients with the psychiatric problem in question (anger dyscontrol or geriatric depression) are frequently reported in terms of mean performance and standard deviation. One can find a rapid assessment instrument

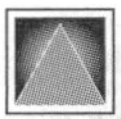

Table 7.6–3
Rapid Personality Instruments

Name	Description	Weaknesses	Strengths
Geriatric Depression Scale	30 items covering depression in the elderly; given orally or written; does not emphasize the vegetative signs of depression	Geriatric patients frequently unwilling to admit depression because of denial; normative data limited	Has reasonably good internal consistency reliability; good concurrent validity with other measures; can distinguish normal, mildly depressed, and severely depressed patients
Beck Depression Inventory II	21 self-administered items for assessing depression in persons having at least a sixth-grade education; originally designed for use with trained interviewers, the test is self-administered; can assess the severity of depression; sensitive to changes due to psychotherapy and medication; measures patient change weekly during therapy; assessed depression during specified period of 1 wk; alpha coefficients were reported to be in the high .80s; effective in discriminating mild, moderate, and severe depression	No validity scales to assess approach to testing; is not specific to depression; patients with other disorders may score high on the test	Large number of studies available in the literature establish both its test–retest reliability and validity
State–Trait Anxiety Inventory	Anxiety is conceptualized as subjective tension and worry along with heightened arousal of the autonomic nervous system; *state anxiety* is the amount of anxiety a person has at a given moment in time; *trait anxiety* refers to the degree of anxiety a person usually experiences; there are two separate but similarly worded instruments, one measuring state anxiety (S Anxiety), the other measuring trait anxiety (T Anxiety); both consist of 20 questions	No validity scales; patients who score high on anxiety also frequently score high on depression and other psychological measure instruments	Large normative sample of more than 5,000 in one study; inventory translated into many languages; excellent internal consistency, reliability, and concurrent validity
State–Trait Anger Scale	Anger is conceptualized as a spectrum ranging from subjective irritation to feelings of annoyance, rage, and associated autonomic arousal; there are separate state and trait instruments available, each with ten items	No validity scales available; individuals who score high on this test also score high on other instruments measuring anxiety and depression	Large normative clinical sample; alpha coefficients are exceptionally high; concurrent validity with other anger instruments is moderate
Michigan Alcoholism Screening Test (MAST)	Designed to screen for alcoholism and problem drinking, presumably in people not manifestly affected by these problems; original scale consists of 25 items that can be completed in 10 mins; several versions of the test available	Extensive norms of population not available; may overdiagnose alcoholism in some cases and produced high false-positive rates, particularly in college students; lack of candor on part of respondent can affect usefulness; high face validity makes it easy to fabricate responses	Most frequently used screening instrument for alcoholism; high internal consistency and good test–retest reliability; discriminates controls from other alcoholic problem groups (hospitalized alcoholics, driving-under-the-influence offenders, persons convicted of drinking and disorderly conduct)
McGill Pain Questionnaire (MPQ)	Designed to assess quantitatively the qualitative characteristics of pain; instrument consists of 78 adjectives that the patient marks concerning the sensory, affective, and evaluative nature of pain, along with other characteristics; a pain-rating index and pain intensity score is calculated	Adjectives can be hard for individuals with low educational background or low IQ to understand; pain complaints can be easily malingered	Used with patients suffering from all types of pain; can be used to assess effectiveness of various pain treatments (medication, biofeedback, relaxation exercise, surgery); also has been used to discriminate between patients who have pain associated with objective physical findings and individuals who have pain without such findings

IQ, intelligence quotient.

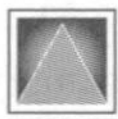

Table 7.6–4
Projective Measures of Personality

Name	Description	Strengths	Weaknesses
Rorschach test	Ten stimulus cards of inkblots, some colored, others achromatic	Most widely used projective device and certainly the best researched; considerable interpretative data available	Some Rorschach interpretive systems have unproved validity
Thematic Apperception Test (TAT)	20 stimulus cards depicting a number of scenes of varying ambiguity	A widely used method that, in the hands of a well-trained person, provides valuable information	No generally accepted scoring system results in poor consistency in interpretation; time-consuming administration
Sentence completion test	A number of different devices available, all sharing the same format with more similarities than differences	Brief administration time; can be a useful adjunct to clinical interviews if supplied beforehand	Stimuli are obvious in intent and subject to easy falsification
Holtzman Inkblot Technique (HIT)	Two parallel forms of inkblot cards with 45 cards per form	Only one response is allowed per card, making research less troublesome	Not widely accepted and rarely used; not directly comparable to Rorschach interpretive strategies
Figure drawing	Typically human forms but can involve houses or other forms	Quick administration	Interpretive strategies have typically been unsupported by research
Make-a-Picture Story (MAPS)	Similar to TAT; however, stimuli can be manipulated by the patient	Provides idiographic personality information through thematic analysis	Minimal research support; not widely used

Courtesy of Robert W. Butler, Ph.D., and Paul Satz, Ph.D.

to assess many of the common psychiatric problems seen today. Another advantage of these instruments is the ease of administration and scoring. The major disadvantage is that these instruments differ greatly in their reliability and validity. Normative groups are frequently small and are obtained in one location. Most do not have national examples. Many of these short instruments have few, if any, studies of their construct validity. Most instruments do not systematically assess response styles such as faking bad, faking good, and social desirability responding. Examples of the hundreds of rapid assessments include measures of bulimia, obsessive-compulsive behavior, sexual functioning, fear and panic, and personal beliefs.

Projective Personality Tests

Projective personality tests, in contrast to objective personality instruments, are more indirect and unstructured. Unlike objective tests in which the patient may simply mark "true" or "false" to given questions, the variety of responses to projective personality tests are almost unlimited. Instructions are usually very general in nature, allowing the patient's fantasies to be expressed. The patient generally does not know how his or her responses will be scored or analyzed. Consequently, trying to feign the test becomes difficult. Projective tests typically do not measure one particular personality characteristic, such as "type A personality" (e.g., narrow-band measurement), but, instead, are designed to assess one's personality as a whole (e.g., broad-band measurement).

Projective tests often focus on "latent" or unconscious aspects of personality. Obviously, psychologists and others differ in the degree to which they rely on "unconscious" information. In many projective techniques, the patient is simply shown a picture of something and asked to tell what the picture reminds them of. An underlying assumption of projective techniques (projective hypothesis) is that, when presented with an ambiguous stimulus, such as an inkblot, for which there are an almost unlimited number of responses, the patient's responses will reflect fundamental aspects of his or her personality. The ambiguous stimulus is a sort of screen on which the individual projects his or her own needs, thoughts, or conflicts. Different persons have different thoughts, needs, and conflicts and, hence, have widely different responses. A schizophrenic's responses often reflect a rather bizarre, idiosyncratic view of the world.

There are literally hundreds of different projective techniques developed—most of which are not widely used today. Table 7.6–4 contains a list of common projective tests and descriptions of the tests. The strengths and weaknesses of the projective tests are also presented. This chapter will focus on more widely used projective instruments, such as the Rorschach test, Thematic Apperception Test (TAT), and sentence completion test.

The literature on projective techniques is vast, and the history of projective techniques goes back for many years. Arthur Carr pointed out in the fourth edition of the *Comprehensive Textbook of Psychiatry* that Shakespeare had an appreciation of the importance of one's association to ambiguous stimuli. In an effort to feign insanity, Hamlet associated to a cloud formation certain images that presumably reflected his personality.

Rorschach Test

Hermann Rorschach, a Swiss psychiatrist, developed the first major use of projective techniques around 1910. The Rorschach test is the most frequently used projective personality instrument (Fig. 7.6–1). The test consists of ten ambiguous, symmetrical inkblots. The inkblot card appears as if a blot of ink was poured onto a piece of paper and folded over—hence, the symmetrical appearance. These $6^1/_2 \times 9^1/_2$–inch inkblot cards are the standard stimuli and, by convention, are referred to by Roman numerals I to X.

Using John E. Exner's Comprehensive System, the examiner, in essence, gives the patient the following instructions: "You'll be given a series of inkblots. Look at each inkblot and tell me what you see." The examiner gives the patient each card and asks, "What might this be?"

Minimal interaction between the examiner and the patient occurs while the Rorschach test is administered, which ensures that standardization procedures are upheld. The examiner writes down verbatim what the patient says during the above-described "free association" or "response-proper" phase. If the patient rotates the card during his or her response, the examiner makes the appropriate notation on the test protocol. After the patient has given responses to all ten cards, an inquiry phase of administration begins. The examiner asks the patient to go through the cards again and help the examiner see the responses he or she gave. The examiner reads the patient's initial response and asks the patient to point out what he or she saw and

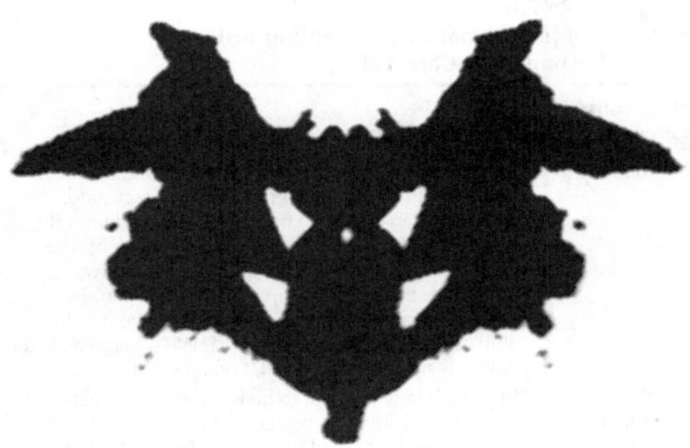

FIGURE 7.6–1 Card I of the Rorschach test. (From Hermann Rorschach, Rorschach®-Test. Copyright © Verlag Hans Huber AG, Bern, Switzerland, 1921, 1948, 1994, with permission.)

explain what made it look like that to him or her. An almost unlimited range of responses is possible with the Rorschach test and most projective tests. Six different scoring and interpretation systems for the Rorschach test are available for the clinician; however, Exner's Comprehensive System is the most widely used and accepted. A structural summary of the various measures derived from the patient's response is usually computed.

Scoring and interpretation of the Rorschach test can be a time-consuming process. Administering and scoring the Rorschach test usually takes approximately 1½ to 2 hours of time. Typically, examiners score the Rorschach responses according to the *location* on the blot where the patient sees the response. The factors that make patients respond the way they do are referred to as the *determinants* (shape of blot, color, and shading). The examiner also scores the actual *content* of the patient's response (e.g., animals, human anatomy). The scoring system is elaborate and can result in dozens of different indices being computed. Although some investigators question the reliability of certain measures, many studies do support the usefulness of the Rorschach test as a personality assessment instrument in the hands of a qualified and experienced psychologist.

The limited scientific support of the Rorschach test, however, has resulted in critical reviews by some psychologists. A number of graduate schools of clinical psychology no longer offer formal coursework in the Rorschach test, although most still do.

Table 7.6–5 gives the sample Rorschach responses of a number of patients to the Rorschach card I. Notice how different the responses are to this same card and how the responses reflect the patients' underlying personality.

Table 7.6–6 shows certain cluster variables derived from Exner's Comprehensive Scoring System. The interpretive utility of these cluster variables is also described in the table.

Thematic Apperception Test (TAT) Although the Rorschach test is clearly the most frequently used projective personality test, the Thematic Apperception Test (TAT) is probably in second place. Many clinicians will include both the TAT and the Rorschach test in a battery of tests for personality assessment. The TAT consists of a series of ten black-and-white pictures that depict individuals of both sexes and of different age groups who are involved in a variety of different activities. For example, on card 1, a young boy is shown sitting at a table, looking at a violin. Card 2 depicts a farm scene in which a young woman is in the foreground carrying books in her hands. A man is working in the fields nearby, and an older woman is seen in the background. Typically, a patient is shown ten TAT cards and is asked to make up stories about them. The patient is asked to tell what is going on in the picture, what was going on before the picture was taken, what the individuals in the picture are thinking and feeling, and what is likely to happen in the future. An example of a TAT card is presented in Figure 7.6–2. Some examples of typical sample responses to the TAT appear in Table 7.6–7.

Henry Murray developed the TAT in 1943 at the Harvard Psychological Clinic. The stories patients make up concerning the pictures, according to the projective hypothesis, reflect the patient's own needs, thoughts, feelings, stresses, wishes, desires, and view of the

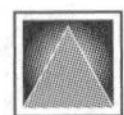

Table 7.6–5
Sample Rorschach Responses and Interpretation to Card I by Diagnostic Category

Diagnostic Category	Patient's Response Proper	Patient's Response on Inquiry	Interpretation
Nonpatient	"Well, the first impression is of a wolf's head, ears here and eyes."	"Overall the head, nose, eyes, ears, the whole thing."	Common response using the white space as the eyes; responding to the whole blot; good attention and response to the task at hand.
Psychotic patient	"Could even be a spider, with the little claw things on top."	"When I was watching horror movies, I remember the spiders having these little dealy things on top. I don't know what you call those things. Maybe that's where the poison is, I don't know. Just the top half of the spider."	The response shows distortion on the percept, inappropriate use of words and logic, and an inability to stay on track with the task.
Depression	"Evil, bad, evil eyes, mouth, someone coming after me, horns."	"Mouth, eyes, it's black, there's horns." (What makes it look evil?) "The shape of the eyes and mouth, nothing is contoured in place, all random, it's dark."	The response shows attention to the shading on the card, a focus on a dangerous view of the world and/or self.
Anxiety	"I don't know, I'd have to think about it. It could be trees."	"Like if you are in the forest, stalks you know, when trees blend together they are nondescript. I'm a real outdoor person, I like to go to the forest and spend time there." (Can you help me see the trees?) "Just this little Christmas tree here and here, the outline."	The response shows discomfort in committing to a response and discomfort in beginning the task; some anxiety is also seen in the rambling personalization used to justify the response, but there is no distortion.

Courtesy of Dana Foley, Ph.D.

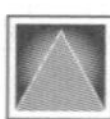

Table 7.6–6
Cluster Variables (Exner System) and Basic Interpretive Utility

Cluster Variable	Interpretive Value
Control stress tolerance	Can assess a person's stress tolerance, ability to control behavior, and responses in the environment; can assess a person's style of processing information
Situation-related stress	Can assess the amount of situational stress affecting a person's capacity for control
Affective features	Can assess how a person manages emotional stimuli, types of emotional features (e.g., depression and anger), and ability to modulate their affect
Self-perception	Can assess how individuals view themselves and their ability to look at themselves
Interpersonal perception	Can assess how individuals view others, how they interact with others, and how they identify with others
Information processing	Can assess how individuals organize information in their world and how they process it
Cognitive mediation	Can assess the conventionality of a person's perceptions and degree of reality distortions
Ideation	Can assess aspects of ideation such as processing style, use of defenses such as fantasy and intellectualization, and whether thoughts proceed in a logical, coherent fashion or have some thought slippage

Courtesy of Dana Foley, Ph.D.

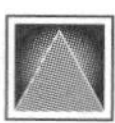

Table 7.6–7
Sample Thematic Apperception Test Responses to Card 12F

Diagnostic Category	Indicated Response
Nonpatient	"This lady has a serious look on her face. She had been talking with the older woman in the background. The older woman had been trying to persuade her to do something that she did not feel was quite right. The younger lady is thinking 'I can't do what she wants.' She is feeling somewhat put upon by this woman. The young lady is frustrated by the request. She is trying to think of a response to the request. What happens in the future is she ignores the old woman's request."
"Schizo" patient	"This young lady is about to be killed by that witch in the background. The witch is getting ready to poison her. You have to be careful nowadays, the witch wants all of her money and her car. I know I have to watch out. Everybody will get you if they can. I don't trust anyone. Better safe than sorry . . . I'm not sorry for what I've done, sorry is not something a person should be. Love means you don't have to say you are sorry."
Depression	"I hate pictures like this, I am not really good at it anyway. The lady in front is thinking about her mother. Her mother was not an evil lady but the young lady feels like her mother didn't care about her, didn't love her and was very selfish. Her mother didn't provide support. The young woman is thinking that she has been deprived and emotionally abused. The young lady will think for a few minutes and will then go into the bedroom to be by herself."
Anxiety	"The young lady is getting ready to go to work but she doesn't want to go. She rented a room from the old lady in the background. The young lady is about to get tired at work. She does not like her job but she needs the money. She doesn't know how she is going to support herself when she loses her job. She goes on to work but has a miserable day. She eventually loses her job and the old landlady kicks her out of her room."

future. According to the theory underlying the test, a patient identifies with a particular individual in each picture. This individual is called the *hero*. The hero is usually close to the age of the patient and frequently of the same sex, although not necessarily so. Theoretically, the patient would attribute his or her own needs, thoughts, and feelings to this hero. The forces present in the hero's environment represent the *press* of the story, and the *outcome* is the resolution of the interaction between the hero's needs and desires and the press of the environment. The TAT, in the hands of a skilled interpreter, can reveal considerable information about the patient's personality that can then be combined with other information obtained from the interview and other testing.

By itself, the TAT is not an effective diagnostic instrument, nor was it designed to be. Moreover, as measured by traditional methods of assessing reliability and validity, the TAT lacks the scientific merit of objective instruments. The fact that it has remained reasonably popular today, however, speaks to the instrument's usefulness in clinical practice.

Sentence Completion Test Although a projective instrument, the sentence completion test is much more direct in soliciting responses from the patient. He or she is simply presented with a series of incomplete sentences and is asked to complete each sentence with the first response that comes to mind. The following are examples of possible incomplete sentences:

My father seldom . . .
Most people don't know that I'm afraid of . . .
When I was a child, I . . .
When encountering frustration, I usually . . .

The purpose of this test is to elicit, in a somewhat indirect manner, information about the patient that cannot be elicited from other measures. Because the patient responds in writing, the examiner's time is limited. The length of time it takes to complete the sentence completion varies greatly depending on the number of incomplete sentences. Tests can range from fewer than ten sentences to more than 75.

There are many variations of sentence completion tests. Some clinicians have developed their own tests. One form of the test, developed by Julian Rotter, has some established validity and reliability, but most sentence completion tests do not. Special-purpose sentence completion tests have been developed to measure different problem areas. For example, there is a sentence completion test that is used with patients who have chronic pain and another that is used to assess issues concerning transsexual patients. The sentence completion test is seldom, if ever, used alone but is combined with other appropriate instruments.

Advantages of the sentence completion test are short administration time, ease of administration, variety of instruments, and ease of construction. Disadvantages are lack of reliability and validity studies and ease of fabrication and deception.

Behavioral Assessment Behavioral assessment involves the direct measurement of a given behavior. Rather than focus primarily on human characteristics, such as repression, ego strength, or self-esteem (vague terms to a behaviorist), strict behavioral measurement concentrates on a direct measurement that can be observed, such as number of temper tantrums per unit of time, duration and intensity and number of hyperventilation episodes, or the number of cigarettes smoked per 24-hour period.

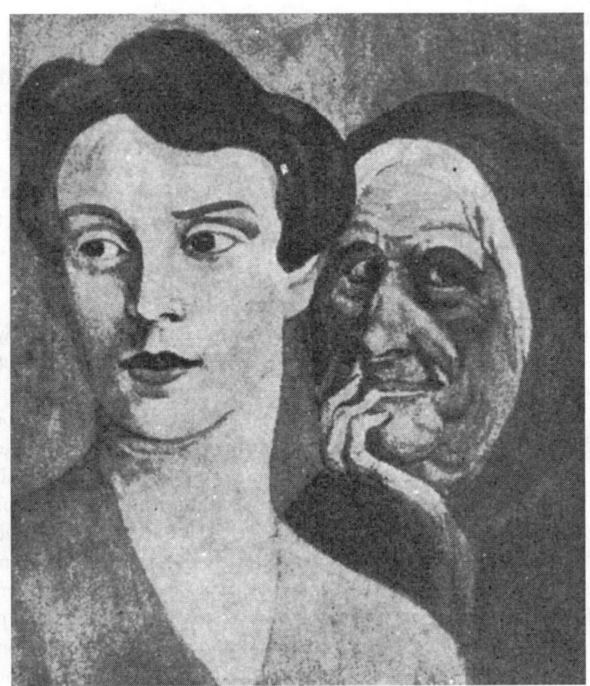

FIGURE 7.6–2 Card 12F of the Thematic Apperception Test. (Reprinted from Henry A. Murray, Thematic Apperception Test, Harvard University Press, Cambridge, MA. Copyright © 1943 President and Fellows of Harvard College, © 1971 Henry A. Murray, with permission.)

Although early strict behaviorists would count only behaviors that were observable, a broader definition of behavior has emerged, under which just about anything people do—whether it is overt, such as crying, swearing, or hand-washing, or covert, such as feeling and thinking—is considered behavior. To measure covert behavior, the patient is typically the informant. For example, to measure dysfunctional thinking, the patient may simply carry a mechanical counter and press it every time he or she has a particular target self-disparaging thought during a given unit of time.

Direct Counting of Behavior Measuring overt behavior is direct and can be done by the patient, a family member, or an impartial observer.

Cognitive-behavioral therapists use these measurements to establish baselines of a given undesirable behavior (i.e., violent thoughts that the patient may wish to reduce). Similarly, therapists can measure behavior that the patient wants to increase (time studying, time out of bed, or distance walked on a treadmill). Follow-up measures of the same behavior monitor progress and quantify improvement.

Different aspects of a target behavior can be counted or measured, such as frequency of behavior (e.g., number of behavioral occurrences), duration of behavior (length of time behavior occurred), and intensity. Occasionally, a behavior may occur so frequently that counting each occurrence becomes problematic. In such instances, simply having the individual indicate whether or not the behavior occurred during a given period of time can be useful.

The advantage of counting specific behavior is that it is direct, objective, easily understood, and quantifies degree of behavioral change. The problem with counting specific behavior is that many patients have so many different symptoms it would not be possible to quantify them all. Sometimes, the process of counting a target behavior may itself alter the behavior. Covert behavior can be measured using a number of different approaches. For example, a patient could be asked to keep a log of the dysfunctional thoughts he or she has concerning her employer during a given 18-hour period.

Rating Scales Rating scales have been developed to detect various aspects of personality. On some of these scales, the patient simply rates her- or himself on a given scale dimension such as sadness: 1 = I am not sad, 7 = I wish I were dead. On other scales, a significant other person is asked to rate the patient: 1 = The individual seldom mentions being sad, 7 = The individual says he or she would be better off dead. Some of the more commonly used rating scales, however, are designed to quantify information obtained by the mental health professional during a mental status interview.

Brief Psychiatric Rating Scale One of the more commonly used interview rating scales is the Brief Psychiatric Rating Scale (BPRS). To use the BPRS, the psychologist or psychiatrist simply completes a mental status interview with the patient. After completing the interview, the interviewer rates the patient on a series of 18 psychiatric symptoms, such as motor retardation, blunted affect, conceptual disorganization, anxiety, and guilt. Expanded definitions of each of these terms are provided to the examiner. The interviewer rates each domain on a seven-point Likert scale from "not present," the lowest rating, to "extremely severe," the highest rating. An experienced interviewer can complete the ratings in 2 or 3 minutes. The BPRS has been used extensively in drug outcome and other studies. The advantage of the BPRS is that the interrater reliability is reasonably high for a rating scale of this nature. A summary article of more than 300 studies using the BPRS found interrater reliability correlative of .80 or higher on the total score in the majority of studies. The first author has used this instrument to teach medical students to be observant of patients' behavior, and relatively inexperienced medical students can establish reasonably good reliability. Other advantages of the BPRS include the ease and speed of rating and the well-defined symptom description.

One disadvantage of this scale is examiner subjectivity. Another disadvantage is that the interviewer can only rate the patient on what he or she personally observes during the interview. Examiners differ greatly in their style of conducting a mental status interview, thus, one examiner might ask many questions on interviews in one given area (i.e., somatic concern) while nearly overlooking another area (i.e., suspiciousness). Another examiner might do just the opposite.

Schedule for Affective Disorders and Schizophrenia (SADS) As stated in the previous section, the BPRS ratings are made on the basis of a mental status interview and do not require the examiner to ask any specific questions of the patient. This approach allows for flexibility but results in considerable variation and interview style. A flexible interview results in different information being gathered by different interviewers. The SADS, on the other hand, is a highly structured interview instrument. The interviewer is required to ask a series of prescribed questions to each patient to ensure that all relevant areas are addressed. The structured interview, however, does vary somewhat from patient to patient because of the branching quality of the interview schedule. For example, a patient is asked a question similar to the following: "Have you ever heard voices or other things that were not there or that other people could not hear or see?" Based on the patient's response, the examiner either asks other detailed prescribed follow-up questions concerning hallucination or, if the response was negative, moves on to the next question in a different area. This approach ensures that all areas are covered in a comprehensive fashion. The SADS is especially helpful for establishing a reliable diagnosis. The SADS can also be used as an index of behavioral severity. Behavioral changes can be determined by repeated administration.

The SADS is very time consuming, mainly because of its comprehensive nature. After an initial evaluation using the complete SADS, a condensed SADS (SADS/C) can be used in those cases that require follow-up.

The advantage of the test is that it is comprehensive and has reasonably good reliability. One disadvantage is its length. Another disadvantage is that the structured interview requires the interviewer to read questions from a lengthy booklet. Such an approach makes it difficult to establish eye contact and rapport with the patient. The SADS has been used for both research and clinical purposes, although it is probably more frequently used for research purposes.

ASSESSMENT OF PERSONALITY IN CHILDREN AND ADOLESCENTS

Assessment of emotional and interpersonal characteristics in children presents many challenges to mental health clinicians, because of the need to place symptoms of concern within both developmental and psychosocial/environmental contexts that are rapidly changing over the years, from infancy through adolescence. Often, symptoms will appear only transiently or in an incomplete or somewhat vague state that is less clear-cut than will be seen at later ages. Many clinicians are reluctant to assign the diagnosis of a personality disorder before the ages of 16 to 18 years, due to rapid changes that occur during childhood. However, assessment of children and adolescents can often reveal antecedent symptoms, behaviors, or traits associated with emotional disorders at an age when these problems are very amenable to intervention. For this reason, facility in assessment of emotional disorders in children and adolescents is important for mental health professionals. This section of the chapter discusses special considerations in assessment of children and adolescents and commonly used measures and procedures available to clinicians.

Special Considerations in Assessment of Children

Children with symptoms of emotional or behavioral disorders are best assessed within developmental and ecological contexts—both of which help interpret the child's symptoms from the perspective of developmental influences on behavior and also with consideration of the risk and protective factors in the child's psychosocial environment. Indeed, the balance of risk and protective factors may often provide important clues as to the etiology of the child's current problems and the prognosis for effective intervention.

Developmental Context Knowledge about the normal sequence and transitions of development forms a fundamental backdrop from which to view the suspected psychopathology of a child. The major developmental theme of infancy is the formation of a secure attachment relationship with significant caregivers, thus, forming the basis for self-esteem, empathy, and confident interpersonal interactions within the social environment. Toddlers who form secure attachment relationships use their caregivers as a secure base of support from which to venture out and explore their world, paving the way for learning, increased independence, and initial social interactions with peers. During the preschool years, children show a desire to master developmental tasks, the most salient of which involve a growing capacity for empathy and self-regulation of emotions and behavior. During the early to middle elementary years, youngsters strive for greater mastery of knowledge and intellectual and academic skills, leading to feelings of productivity and competence. The developmental tasks of adolescence center around identity formation, resolving conflicts with authority figures, peer-group identification, and realistic appraisal and evaluation of self-qualities. Although development does not occur in linear stages, familiarity with the primary developmental themes and transitions of each age period provides an important context from which to view current symptoms.

Decisions about appropriate assessment methods are also based on developmental factors. Before children participate in projective testing procedures, such as story-telling tasks, clinicians must have developmental information about their expressive language, receptive language, and conceptualization abilities. Knowledge of a child's reading proficiency is critical when presenting them with self-report measures. If children are asked to complete projective drawings, information about their visual–motor maturity is important for interpretation. Young children often do not have the motor or language abilities to provide meaningful responses to projective testing procedures, but they may reveal much about their socialization abilities, fears, anxieties, and significant relationships through play. Therefore, play observation techniques can be a useful alternative to more formal projective measures. Likewise, some adolescents may resist providing responses on projective measures that require verbal disclosure to a clinician but may willingly complete objective paper-and-pencil personality measures that require a less direct response. Choosing an approach to assessment with the developmental context in mind enhances the validity of the information obtained.

Ecological Context The ecological perspective assumes that development throughout the lifespan is a function of the interactions between the individual and the changing, multilayered environments in which the individual lives and interacts. These environments include not only the immediate settings of family, school, and friends, but also the larger social contexts in which these settings are embedded, such as the neighborhood, extended family relationships, access to needed services (e.g., health care), cultural values and beliefs, and events in history that influence humankind. The ecological perspective emphasizes the bidirectional influence that multiple levels of the environment have on development. Development is seen as a dynamic process that not only considers biological and genetic influences on the individual, but also takes into account the possible influence of the environment in modifying anatomical structures and physiological processes in the brain during development. The course and outcome of development ultimately reflect the balance between specific risk factors (e.g., genetic, environmental, traumatic) and protective factors (e.g., secure attachment relationship with a primary caregiver who provides consistent nurturance, extended support of family and community systems, cultural values and beliefs that promote resilience) that can influence the individual's positive development in the face of possible adverse conditions. The following cases illustrate the importance of the social/familial context in interpreting the presenting symptoms:

Two 4-year-old girls were referred by their Head Start teacher because of concerns about recent onset of regressive behavior (e.g., enuresis during the school day, immature speech patterns). Both girls were interviewed separately but were reluctant to talk with the clinician. A play interview was set up with each, using dolls and a dollhouse with a variety of furniture. The first girl assumed the role of "mother" and played out the scenario of feeding and diapering the baby doll in a nurturing manner. The second girl was aggressive in her play, with enactment of the "adult" dolls hitting the "child" dolls and making them "die." The child dolls were described as having blood on them. The family context for the first girl revealed that a new baby sibling had been born just before the onset of regressive symptoms; the infant was born prematurely and the mother spent much time with the infant in the hospital. Both the arrival of the new sibling and the mother's separation from her 4-year-old daughter created the social context for the emergence of the child's regressive behavior. In the second case, the girl's mother was interviewed and initially denied any recent stresses in the family.

After the clinician questioned her further and provided a description of her daughter's play, the mother revealed that she had a new boyfriend who had just moved into the house. She ultimately revealed that she had noted her daughter's fear of the boyfriend and her frequent tearfulness at home. She reported a suspicion that her boyfriend might be sexually molesting her daughter and agreed to call Protective Services in the presence of the clinician to make a report.

As these cases illustrate, there can be vastly different explanations for similar presenting symptoms, and, often, the projective assessment procedures only suggest concerns without providing enough specific information about the nature and etiology of the problems. The social context can reveal both risk and protective factors that are important in conceptualizing the child's problems. For instance, in the case of the 4-year-old girl who was sexually abused, the presence of the mother's boyfriend in the home was a risk factor, as was the mother's isolation from her extended family, poverty, and living in a dangerous and violent neighborhood. However, protective factors included the mother's strength in wanting to protect her daughter by admitting the problem, making a report to Protective Services, and forcing the boyfriend to leave the home. Another protective factor was a concerned and observant Head Start teacher who noted the girl's behavioral change and sought help immediately. The ecological approach allows one to examine the possible multiple determinants of emotional psychopathology in children and to better understand the interaction between risk and protective factors that are present in the child's life.

Use of Informant Information Children and adolescents are usually referred for assessment because of the concerns of their parents or caregivers. Teachers may also be the source of specific concerns. For this reason, information relevant to the diagnosis is typically obtained from these significant adults who can provide important information regarding the child's behavior in various settings. Reliance on individuals other than the client as reporters of the primary symptoms represents a fundamental difference between the diagnostic process for children and that for adults.

The validity of the information presented about children's symptoms is often a concern to clinicians. During intake, parents often express feelings of anxiety and frustration regarding their child's problems, and their descriptions of the child may be exaggerated or vague (e.g., "she never minds" or "he always acts like a monster"). It is not uncommon for depressed parents to report an increased number and severity level of symptoms in their children. In cases in which it is suspected that the informant's perceptions may be distorted, collateral information must be obtained from teachers or others familiar with the child's current problems. A primary task is helping informants translate imprecise complaints to specific descriptions of behaviors of concern using methods that help the clinician ascertain the nature, frequency, and severity of symptoms. The behavioral assessment procedures described later are very useful in providing age- and gender-referenced ratings of symptom characteristics.

Specialized Training Clinicians who conduct personality assessment of children need training not only in clinical assessment methods, but also in developmental psychology and child psychopathology. Presentation of many emotional disorders in prelatency years differs from postlatency presentation. For instance, young children with depression may exhibit predominant symptoms of conduct problems, tantrums, oppositional behavior, and hyperirritability rather than the presentation most often associated with older children and adults (depressed mood, diminished interest in activities, vegetative symptoms, anhedonia). Training and experience in assisting the child to meet the demands of the testing situation are also critical. The child's ability to participate in testing depends on his or her attention and concentration ability, anxiety regarding separation from significant others during the testing, fatigue or hunger states, motivation and persistence ability, and the relatively greater influence of familial, cultural, and environmental variables. A clinician with specialized training in working with children will both understand these influences on child test-taking behavior and have the skills to work with children to achieve more valid results.

ASSESSMENT OF CHILDREN AND ADOLESCENTS

Like assessment of adults, personality assessment of children can be accomplished via three primary methods: projective, objective, and behavioral tests and procedures. The projective methods involve direct interaction with the child or adolescent, whereas objective and behavioral methods often involve obtaining information from significant adults in the child's life, as well as direct interaction with the child. With the evolution of more sophisticated statistical methodology and psychometric science in recent years has come the development of new objective and behavioral measures of personality. Improved validity indices and psychometric procedures that take into account informant reporting are now routinely included. Many of the projective procedures have changed less, although improvements in developmental norms for interpretation have increased the diagnostic validity of measures such as the Rorschach test.

Projective Assessment Procedures As stated in the adult section, objective tests of personality present the patient with a structured set of questions and a finite range of answers. Projective tests, on the other hand, present more ambiguous stimuli and ask the adult or child to make up something (i.e., story, percept, or drawing) from the stimulus. The most common projective assessment procedures for children and adolescents are the Rorschach test, various projective story-telling measures (i.e., Roberts Apperception Test for Children [RATC], Children's Apperception Test [CAT]), projective drawings (e.g., human figure and Kinetic Family Drawings), and incomplete sentence procedures (Table 7.6–8).

Rorschach Test Projective instruments such as the Rorschach test allow the clinician to explore dynamics of the child's personality by gathering information on both the child's perceptual–cognitive world and inner fantasy world. Ideally, the Rorschach test is used as part of a more comprehensive battery that includes an interview with the child and significant adults, expressive (play) techniques, and, perhaps, story-telling techniques to allow the child maximum freedom and spontaneity of expression.

The Rorschach test with children has a long research and clinical history of examining developmental norms and symbolic interpretations. Various normative studies have added to its interpretive validity, with the comprehensive studies of Exner and Irving B. Weiner discussed in *Assessment of Children and Adolescents*, the third vol-

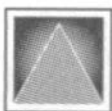

Table 7.6–8
Projective Assessment Procedures for Children

Name	Age Range	Description
Rorschach test	5 yrs–Adulthood	Consists of ten inkblots, some colored and others achromatic, used as basis for eliciting associations that are revealing of disrupted personality development.
Children's Apperception Test (CAT)	3–10 yrs	Two versions of the CAT—animal and human—depict characters in various social situations and are used to elicit stories from children. Younger children are felt to identify more readily with the animal figures, whereas older children are usually presented with the human figures. Scoring and interpretation are based on psychodynamic theory.
Adolescent Apperception Cards	12–19 yrs	Eleven picture cards focus on parent–, peer–, and sibling–adolescent interaction, pulling for themes of physical and sexual abuse, neglect, peer acceptance, loneliness, depression, drug use, and domestic violence. Two versions are available—one depicting white teenagers, the other depicting black teenagers.
Roberts Apperception Test for Children (RATC)	6–15 yrs	Sixteen picture cards—with parallel male and female versions depicting white or black characters—are designed to elicit information about both adaptive and maladaptive functioning. The Interpersonal Matrix links the adaptive and clinical scales to specific people in the child's life and facilitates a better understanding of the nature of interaction with family members, peers, teachers, and others. Has standardized scoring system and normative data to aid interpretation.
Tell-Me-a-Story (TEMAS)	5–18 yrs	Multicultural apperception test with 23 color picture cards (11 of which are sex specific) depicting minority (Hispanic, black) or nonminority characters. Measures ten personality functions (e.g., aggression, interpersonal relations, self-concept), 18 cognitive functions (e.g., time, fluency, inquiries), and seven affective functions (e.g., happy, sad, angry, fearful). Has an objective scoring system and normative data based on a diverse cultural and ethnic sample.
Projective drawings	3–4 yrs–Adolescence	Various versions exist, from individual drawings of human figures, a house, and tree, to kinetic drawings of family. Simple, cost-effective measures that provide information on children's perception of self and relationships with others. Especially useful with children who have difficulty with verbal expression. Objective scoring available for some drawings (e.g., human figures), but interpretation of other types of projective drawings is often subjective.
Sentence- and story-completion tasks	4 or 5 yrs–Adolescence	A number of different formats available, each providing a sentence stem or initiating a story, after which the child is asked to complete the sentence or story. Provides information on such factors as interpersonal relationships and dynamics, self-perception, wishes, and worries.

ume of their book *The Rorschach: A Comprehensive System*, providing the most recent and detailed normative data available for children between the ages of 5 and 16 years. Exner's descriptive statistics for the normative data are provided in tables for each year of age; computerized programs for obtaining the structural summaries in the context of these developmental norms are also available. Clinicians using the Rorschach test for evaluation of children and adolescents must take care to analyze the structural summary within the context of appropriate age norms, as a given result interpreted as normal for a young child could be of concern in an adolescent. Children's Rorschach responses have been examined as a function of their cognitive functioning, academic performance, and behavioral problems within the school setting. The underlying conceptual framework for this work hypothesizes a direct relationship between the degree of secondary process development and school achievement. A published review of projective tests suggests that the child who can deal successfully with drive-laden impulses through play and fantasy is seen as more capable, open, and flexible. According to Exner and Weiner, the Rorschach test is not particularly good at discriminating one specific personality disorder from another, as is, for instance, a structured clinical interview. However, the Rorschach test can provide useful information regarding the way children with personality disorder traits view the world and can shed light on manifestations of flawed or disrupted personality development.

As with adults, there are numerous systems for administering and scoring the Rorschach test with children, but all ask children to say what they see on the blot (i.e., the percept), followed by an inquiry referring back to each response. Whether the inquiry should be done after the child's free association responses to all ten blots or whether the inquiry is best accomplished after each individual blot is controversial. Proponents of the latter approach suggest that young children may have difficulty remembering the reasoning behind the original free associations or may become fatigued by the end of the test, thus limiting their cooperation and responsiveness to the inquiry. Research by Exner and Weiner found the latter approach to inquiry unnecessary in their large child sample, except for a small percentage of children who were seriously disturbed. Of most concern is that inquiry immediately after each free association response may contaminate subsequent responses; thus, reserving inquiry until free association responses have been obtained for all ten blots is preferred. Clinicians must also be aware of state anxiety as a potential confounding variable in children's responses to the Rorschach test. Care in building rapport and an explanation of the purpose and process of testing can ease the situational anxiety.

As with adults, scoring is done on the basis of response characteristics, or determinants, such as form, color, shading, texture, and dimensionality. The content and form quality of the child's responses are also used in scoring and interpretation.

Projective Story-Telling Procedures In projective story-telling approaches, the child is presented with a picture stimulus of human or animal figures in rather ambiguous situations. The child is asked to make up a story about the figures—a story that has a beginning and an end and includes the thinking and feeling of the individuals represented in the pictures. A fantasy response is evoked, and the resulting projective information is a combination of the perceptual and the imaginative. Stories are typically analyzed for repetitive, unique, intense, or problematic themes, beliefs, or affects. This procedure is very similar to the TAT approach used with adults.

Children's Apperception Test The initial CAT, developed in 1949, used animal figures and was developed for children between the ages of 3 and 10 years. Animal figures were thought to be more culture-free than human characters. In 1965, the human figures version (CAT-H) was produced, showing human figures in situations as analogous as possible to those pictured in the animal version. During administration, the cards are presented individually in the numbered order of the card (because certain cards were designed for sequential impact). The child is asked to tell a story about each picture (e.g., what is going on, what happened before, what will happen next). There is some debate about the use of prompts with young children and whether such prompts (e.g., "How did the story end?") may contaminate important projective information. Generally, prompts are often necessary to help the young child understand what is expected. Young children have a tendency to merely describe or label portions of the picture and may not understand the concept of telling a story with a beginning, middle, and conclusion. However, the clinician must always guard against overly intrusive or helpful prompts that guide the child's responses in a particular direction or suggest a specific format for the story. The various scoring protocols for the CAT have focused on analysis of ego functions and evaluating the relative use of various defense mechanisms. However, qualitative interpretation is also made based on recurrent or sequential themes and determination of identification figures, while taking into consideration the child's family and case history information.

Comparisons have been made between the CAT and the Rorschach test as to the types of information obtained and the overlap between them. These tests have been found to complement rather than duplicate each other, as they tap different aspects of personality functioning. The CAT generally can be expected to reflect interpersonal and familial relationships, ego functioning, sources of discomfort, conflicts, and past traumas. In contrast, the Rorschach test, according to M. R. Haworth, explores deeper levels of personality, emotional responsiveness, mechanisms for control, extent of reality contact, and available defenses.

Although the CAT continues to be used, its picture stimuli are quite outdated in appearance and often do not appeal to children today. Further, clinicians are not as apt to be trained formally in psychodynamic theories of interpretation that are used with the CAT. Newer apperception tests, such as RATC, are being used with increasing frequency because of their modern appearance and because they use scoring procedures that are less reliant on psychodynamic theory.

Roberts Apperception Test for Children The manual for the RATC offered several criticisms of existing picture apperception tests as a rationale for the development of the RATC. It reported that most of the previously developed techniques either were not developed specifically for children or were appropriate for a limited age range. Second, the nature of the stimulus characteristics of the cards, rather than the child's unique personality, often was the primary determinant of the child's responses. Finally, the existing tests lacked a standardized system for scoring the thematic content and structural characteristics of the child's responses. Therefore, the interpretation of thematic apperception tests was very subjective and often based on the clinician's own experiences, theoretical orientation, and personality style. The RATC was designed to overcome these limitations by using stimulus cards that (1) depict children and are designed for use with children between the ages of 6 and 15 years, (2) emphasize everyday interpersonal events of contemporary life, (3) are consistent in their presentation, and (4) are easily scored, objective measures that yield high interrater agreement. In addition, the RATC provides normative data for 200 well-adjusted children between the ages of 6 and 15 years to aid in clinical interpretation. Interpretation of the RATC, like that of other projective measures, is based on the assumption that children presented with ambiguous drawings of children and adults in everyday interaction will project their typical thoughts, concerns, conflicts, and coping styles into the stories they create.

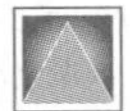

Table 7.5–9
Profile Scales and Indicators for Roberts Apperception Test for Children

Adaptive scales	**Clinical scales**
Reliance on others	Anxiety
Support-other	Aggression
Support-child	Depression
Limit setting	Rejection
Problem identification	Unresolved
Resolution 1	**Indicators**
Resolution 2	Atypical response
Resolution 3	Maladaptive response
	Refusal

The RATC uses 16 stimulus cards, with parallel male and female versions, that represent important interpersonal themes (e.g., parental disagreement and affection, peer conflicts, observation of nudity, and sibling rivalry). A supplemental version of the RATC has African American figures. The responses are scored on a number of scales measuring both adaptive and maladaptive functioning. Table 7.6–9 illustrates the profile scales and indicators.

In addition, the child's responses may be scored on the Interpersonal Matrix, which summarizes the relationships between the scales and indicators and the figures identified in the child's stories. In general, the standardized scoring procedures aid interpretation and clinical use of this scale.

Projective Drawing Techniques Projective drawing techniques are often helpful in establishing rapport and engaging shy or negative children who are reluctant to become involved in more verbal interaction with the clinician. The nondirective nature of the technique allows the child time to adjust to the testing environment and to the clinician without being propositioned for a verbal response. The nonverbal nature of the task also makes it amenable to younger children and those who are cognitively impaired or non-English–speaking.

Two common approaches to projective drawings are the House-Tree-Person and Kinetic Family Drawing. In the former, the child is first asked to draw a person, and, after completing that drawing, is asked to draw a person of the sex opposite to that of the first drawing. When finished, the child is asked to draw a house and then a tree. Interview questions asking the child to identify the humans, tell what they are doing in the picture, and tell how they are feeling can shed light on the child's thoughts about the drawings. With the house, the child may be asked who lives in the house, what they are doing, and so forth. Kinetic Family Drawing is accomplished by telling the child to draw a picture of his or her family doing something. The drawing can elicit verbal comments that concern family cohesiveness or conflict, the perceived role of the child within the family system, relationships with significant others within the family, the degree of interaction versus isolation of various family members, the family structure, and the hierarchy of power.

In addition to the verbal information elicited from the drawings, graphic analysis can include placement of the drawing on the page, overworking or sketchiness of the lines, size and relative placement of the drawings, pencil pressure used, amount of detailing, symmetry, indicators of dissociation (i.e., incongruities between the graphic drawing and the verbal description of it), and use of shading or color.

As with other projective techniques, projective drawings are not meant to be used alone to make interpretations of personality functioning. Corroborating information to support any interpretations of the drawings must be obtained through interview or other test procedures that could shed light on the meaning of the child's performance.

Story and Sentence Completion Techniques A story completion technique often begins with a sentence (or a couple of sentences) that represents the beginning of a story plot to be completed by the child. An illustrative example from the Madeline Thomas Stories follows:

> A boy goes to school. During recess he does not play with the other children. He stays by himself in a corner. Why?

Story completion techniques are useful in adding clinical information about rather focal problems and, possibly, the child's problem-solving skills in addressing these problems. Although there is little research on diagnostic utility and standardized scoring and interpretation schemata, the qualitative information obtained is often worth the time expended in administering the technique.

Sentence completion procedures can be administered in various formats. One approach is to read the sentence stems to the child rapidly while asking him or her to respond with the first information that comes to mind. This approach may reduce response latencies and loosen the child's defenses to response, especially if the items are rather repetitive. Often, information about family dynamics and relationships and the child's self-esteem, wishes, and worries are revealed more directly than with other projective techniques. Valuable clinical information can be obtained by noting the child's response latencies, the positive or negative tone of the responses, and the predominant mood endorsed in the responses. Another administration approach allows children to write the answers to the sentence stems on paper, working at their own pace. This is often the best approach to use with adolescents, who value autonomy. Another advantage of sentence completion techniques is their economy and flexibility of administration.

Objective Personality Measures

Objective approaches to child personality assessment typically have straightforward test stimuli and clear instructions regarding completion of the tests, as opposed to projective approaches, which typically use more unstructured, ambiguous test stimuli. Objective tests typically have good standardization, reliability, and validity, and they often are norm-referenced so as to provide comparisons with a particular criterion group.

The advantages of using objective measures with children are similar to those previously discussed with adults. Disadvantages include the length of the measures (most have several hundred questions to which the informant must respond), the reading level required for completion (which could place children and adolescents at a disadvantage), and the initial expense of purchasing either computer administration or computer scoring software. Despite the disadvantages, objective personality measures remain an important part of a comprehensive personality assessment by providing a broad survey of major areas of psychopathology at the initial stages of the evaluation. Descriptions of some of the major objective personality measures follow, and a more complete listing is provided in Table 7.6–10.

Robert P. Archer states in his book *MMPI-A: Assessing Adolescent Psychotherapy* that the MMPI–Adolescent (MMPI-A) serves two important functions in assessment of adolescents: (1) it provides an objective evaluation and description of an adolescent's level of functioning related to selected standardized dimensions of psychopathology, and (2) repeated administration can provide a means of assessing ongoing changes in psychopathology, perhaps as a result of intervention. The MMPI-A should be administered, in most cases, only to adolescents between the ages of 14 and 18 years. On occasion, 12- and 13-year-old adolescents who meet the administration guidelines can be evaluated with the MMPI-A, but it should not be administered to anyone younger than 12 years of age. Above age 18, the MMPI-2 is the most appropriate version to administer. This lengthy measure demands that an adolescent of any age be able to read and understand the items (which are written at an average seventh-grade level) and tolerate the time and persistence required to complete the measure. Trained personnel must administer the test in a supervised environment. The MMPI-A is geared toward a population at risk for psychopathology, and is not particularly useful for exploring personality styles of nonclinical adolescents.

One concern about the use of the MMPI-A and other objective personality measures during adolescence is the stability of the symptomatology. Most would agree that the MMPI-A is best used to obtain a description of current adolescent psychopathology rather than to make long-term predictions regarding future functioning. The ongoing maturational changes in adolescent personality development most likely account for the lack of stability in predictions of future psychopathology; this underscores the need for the clinician to be sensitive to the developmental issues in this population.

Millon Clinical Multiaxial Inventories Among the most widely used objective measures of child personality is the Millon series of assessment instruments. Two of the scales are specific to adolescents—the Millon Adolescent Personality Inventory (MAPI) and the Millon Adolescent Clinical Inventory (MACI). The original MAPI was designed to be used in both clinical and nonclinical (e.g., vocational, educational) settings to provide an appraisal of adolescent personality and concerns. The goal of Millon and his colleagues was to create a broad instrument that would be valid and reliable in assessing the inherent traits and current state of adolescents. The MAPI is written at a sixth-grade reading level and provides information on eight personality styles that mirror Millon's theory of personality (Table 7.6–10 provides a listing of the MAPI scales). At maladaptive levels, the personality styles correspond to Axis II disorders found in the revised fourth edition of the *Diagnostic and Statistical Manual of Mental Disorders* (DSM-IV-TR). In addition, the MAPI contains 12 additional scales: eight that focus on worries that many teenagers experience and four that address specific behaviors of concern. Because of its nonclinical nomenclature and design, the MAPI can be used successfully to identify personality styles and concerns in a population of normal adolescents. Before the development of the MACI, the MAPI was used with clinical populations as well. However, as Mark Marvish stated in *The Use of Psychological Testing for Treatment Planning and Outcome Assessment*, the MAPI shares the same disadvantage as the MMPI-A in that the stability of prediction based on its scores varies.

The MACI was designed to assess maladaptive levels of the original eight MAPI personality styles. In addition, it added items to correspond to the three new personality disorders added to the DSM-IV-TR, and it identifies those adolescents who have marked tendencies toward borderline functioning. The 12 personality patterns assessed by the MACI are given descriptive rather than diagnostic labels, partly because of the problems of predictive stability within the adolescent population. The MACI also added several new clinically oriented scales to the original MAPI format; whereas the MAPI had four

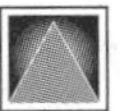

Table 7.6–10
Objective Personality Measures for Children

Name	Age Range	Description
Children's Personality Questionnaire (CPQ)	8–13 yrs	140-item questionnaire that measures 14 basic personality traits useful in predicting school achievement, delinquency, leadership, and potential emotional problems. Can be individually or group administered.
High School Personality Questionnaire (HSPQ)	13–18 yrs	An upward extension of CPQ, this scale can be individually or group administered to junior and senior high school students. Has 142 items measuring 14 personality traits. Useful in predicting school achievement, vocational fitness, delinquency, and leadership, as well as need for clinical assistance.
Millon Adolescent Personality Inventory (MAPI)	Adolescents	An objective, 150-item, true–false, self-report inventory that identifies eight personality styles (introversive, inhibited, cooperative, sociable, confident, forceful, respectful, and sensitive); eight concerns frequently expressed by adolescents (self-concept, personal esteem, body comfort, sexual acceptance, peer security, social tolerance, family rapport, and academic confidence); and four scales that are typically of interest to clinicians (impulse control, societal conformity, scholastic achievement, and attendance consistency).
Millon Adolescent Clinical Inventory (MACI)	Adolescents	Designed to expand the clinical utility of the MAPI, the MACI stresses maladaptive levels of the original eight personality styles on the MAPI. The MACI also incorporates disorders that were added to the DSM-IV-TR. Includes Clinical Indices Scales that tap eating dysfunctions, academic noncompliance, alcoholic predilection, drug proneness, delinquent disposition, impulsivity propensity, anxious feelings, depression affect, and suicidal ideation.
Minnesota Multiphasic Personality Inventory–Adolescent (MMPI-A)	14–18 yrs	This 478-item, true–false, objective measure of psychopathology is specifically designed for use with adolescents. It contains the basic clinical scales of the original MMPI, along with four new validity scales, 15 content scales, 6 supplementary scales, and 28 Harris-Lingoes and 3 Si subscales. Both hand-scoring and computer scoring programs are available. As this version of the MMPI is relatively new, further research is needed to determine its sensitivity and specificity for accurate detection of psychopathology in adolescents.
Personality Inventory for Children–Revised (PIC-R)	Preschool to adolescence	An objective, multidimensional parent-report measure of behavior, affect, ability, and family function. The total scale is quite lengthy, with 420 items that provide scores for 20 scales in their full-length format. There are briefer options available. Parents can respond to the first 280 items, which provide scores for an abbreviated 20 scales; or they can respond to the first 131 items, which provide scores for the Lie scale and four broad-band scales. Although the PIC has excellent psychometric properties, its length and its use of a single-informant (i.e., parent) format are disadvantages.
Personality Inventory for Youth (PIY)	9–19 yrs	270-item, self-report measure that assesses emotional and behavioral adjustment, family interaction, and neurocognitive and attention-related academic functioning. Has nine nonoverlapping clinical scales and 24 subscales. Four validity scales help determine whether the respondent is uncooperative or is exaggerating, malingering, responding defensively, carelessly, or without adequate comprehension. The PIY is written at a third-grade reading level and takes 45 mins to complete. Although the length is a disadvantage, the validity scales, careful standardization, and good reliability and validity make it a good measure of child and adolescent psychopathology.
Adolescent Psychopathology Scale (APS)	12–19 yrs	The APS is a self-report measure that evaluates the presence and severity of symptoms associated with specific DSM-IV-TR clinical and personality disorders. It also assesses other psychological problems that may interfere with an adolescent's psychological adaptation and personal competence, including substance abuse, suicidal behavior, emotional lability, excessive anger, aggression, alienation, and introversion.

scales that address behavioral adjustment problems, the MACI expanded this section to include 11 scales that reflect more extremely maladjusted behaviors (Table 7.6–3).

Given the recent development of the MACI, empirical support for its validity, reliability, and interpretation is needed. However, it is well grounded in theory, and it benefits from the empirical information gained with its predecessor, the MAPI.

Personality Measures for Specific Disorders in Children In contrast to the multidimensional personality measures already discussed, several measures address more specific disorders in children, such as depressive and anxiety disorders. Several of these measures are described in Table 7.6–11.

Often, clinicians use the multidimensional personality measures to obtain a broad overview of risk for psychopathology and then use the narrower-band, more specific measures to explore a particular set of symptoms in greater detail. Neither type of personality inventory is used alone to confirm a diagnosis, but both provide valuable information about the nature and severity of symptoms that can be combined with other approaches to arrive at a diagnosis. Recently developed inventories are especially useful in evaluating the effects of a child's exposure to various types of trauma—an increasingly common reason for referral.

Advantages of the specific personality inventories include their brevity, low cost in terms of time to administer, and ease in scoring and interpreting. However, as with similar adult measures, caution should be taken in reviewing the psychometric qualities of these personality measures, particularly with regard to discriminant validity for the disorder under study versus other disorders versus results for children without disorders. Many of the scales were developed for children in a narrow age range, with a small normative sample that is not representative or stratified, and they have questionable discriminant validity. As long as the clinician uses these measures as part of a more comprehensive approach to making diagnoses of emotional problems and understands their strengths and weaknesses, the measures can be very useful.

Behavioral Assessment Procedures Behavioral assessment procedures offer a highly structured method of obtaining infor-

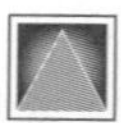

Table 7.6–11
Personality Measures for Specific Disorders in Children

Name	Age Range	Description
Children's Depression Inventory (CDI)	7–17 yrs	Self-report inventory that assesses symptoms of depression. Contains 27 multiple-choice items that cover such depressive symptoms as sadness, anhedonia, suicidal ideation, and sleep and appetite disturbance. Cut-off scores are provided for various levels of severity. Discriminant validity between depressive disorders and other disorders on the CDI has been questionable in some studies.
Reynolds Child Depression Scale (RCDS)	8–12 yrs	Brief, self-report measure of depressive symptomatology in children. Contains 30 items written at a second-grade reading level. May be administered individually or in groups. A cut-off score is provided to designate a clinically relevant level of depressive symptoms.
Reynolds Adolescent Depression Scale, second edition (RADS-2)	11–20 yrs	Brief, self-report measure of clinically relevant levels of depressive symptomatology in adolescents. Contains 30 items rated on a four-point Likert scale along four basic dimensions of depression, including dysphoric mood, anhedonia/negative affect, negative self-evaluation, and somatic complaints. May be administered individually or in groups. RADS-2 Total Score and Cutoff Score can be used to judge severity of depressive symptoms.
Revised Children's Manifest Anxiety Scale (RCMAS)	6–19 yrs	Brief, self-report measure of anxiety symptoms in children and adolescents. The 37-item scale contains 28 Anxiety and 9 Lie Scale items. Results are expressed in three subscales: Physiological Anxiety, Worry and Oversensitivity, and Concentration Anxiety. Normative data are available from a sample of 5,000 children.
Multidimensional Anxiety Scale for Children (MASC)	8–19 yrs	39-item, self-report inventory that assesses anxiety symptoms across clinically significant domains, including physical symptoms, social anxiety, harm avoidance, and separation/panic. The MASC provides an Anxiety Disorders Index and Total Anxiety Index. The MASC is written at a fourth-grade reading level and can be completed in approximately 15 mins.
State–Trait Anxiety Inventory for Children (STAIC)	9–12 yrs	Developed to assess both enduring tendencies to experience anxiety and also temporal and situational variations in levels of perceived anxiety. Normative data, using a nonstratified sample of fourth- through sixth-grade students, are available. Reliability studies for internal consistency are strong, but validity studies have not strongly supported the state–trait distinction in children.
Adolescent Anger Rating Scale	11–19 yrs	41-item, self-report measure that assesses the level and type of adolescent response to anger. Using a four-point Likert scale, individuals rate which behaviors they exhibit when angered and how often each behavior typically occurs. Scores are reported for Total Anger and three subscales measuring aspects of adolescents' typical anger response patterns (instrumental anger, reactive anger, and anger control). Five ethnic groups are represented in the normative sample of 4,187 adolescent boys and girls.
Fear Survey Schedule For Children (FSSC) and FSSC–Revised (FSSC-R)	7–12 yrs	The FSSC is an 80-item scale developed to assess specific fears in children. Categories of items include school, home, social, physical, animal, travel, classic phobia, and miscellaneous. Few data are available regarding psychometric properties of the FSSC. A revised version of the scale (FSSC-R) has shown good internal consistency, and total scores have discriminated between normal and school-phobic children.
Trauma Symptom Checklist for Children (TSSC)	8–16 yrs	54-item, self-report measure that evaluates acute and chronic posttraumatic symptomatology in children and youth. Assesses for traumatic events, such as physical or sexual abuse, major loss, natural disaster, witnessing violence. Has two validity scales (under-response and hyper-response). Well-normed on 3,000 inner city, urban, and suburban children and includes data from trauma and child abuse centers.
Child Sexual Behavior Inventory (CSBI)	2–12 yrs	Parent-report measure that evaluates children who have been sexually abused or who are showing precocious sexual behavior. Nine major content domains include boundary issues, exhibitionism, gender role behavior, self-stimulation, sexual anxiety, sexual interest, sexual intrusiveness, sexual knowledge, and voyeuristic behavior. Has a large normative group of children from diverse socioeconomic backgrounds in the general population and a cohort of 512 children from child abuse centers.
Eating Disorder Inventory 2 (EDI-2)	11 yrs–adult	Brief, self-report inventory that measures the psychological and behavioral dimensions of anorexia nervosa and bulimia. Subscales assess traits that are important to the development of eating disorders, including drive for thinness, body dissatisfaction, maturity fears, ineffectiveness, perfectionism, interpersonal distrust, impulse regulation, social insecurity, and others.

mation about behavioral/emotional functioning and social competencies of children and adolescents. These procedures include direct observations and informant ratings on age- and gender-normed scales. The popularity of these measures has grown in recent years, due in part to their improved psychometric properties, their cost-effectiveness, and their use in multitrait–multimethod diagnostic procedures (see Table 7.6–12 for examples of measures).

Validity of Informant Reports Use of behavioral rating scales raises questions about the validity of informant information. The research on agreement among various raters of child behaviors is consistent in showing greater agreement between raters who interact with a child in similar situations (e.g., between mothers and fathers) than between raters who interact with the child in different situations (e.g., between parents and teachers or between parents and children). Thomas Achenbach and colleagues found that agreement tends to vary across age and types of problems rated: agreement was greater for 6- to 11-year-olds than for adolescents and was greater for externalizing than for internalizing behavior problems. Sex differences are also apparent when the number of reported behavioral problems is examined. Achenbach reports that both parents and teachers observe more behavioral and emotional problems for referred and nonreferred boys than for girls in childhood and adolescence. Achenbach says that studies of youth self-report of problems reveal that 11- to 18-year-old girls report more problems than do boys of the same age. Differences in number of problems reported are also a function of the type of population (inpatient vs. outpatient vs. nonreferred). According to Achenbach, for nonreferred boys and

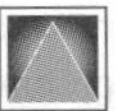

Table 7.6–12
Behavioral Assessment Procedures for Children

Test Name	Age Range	Description
Behavior Assessment System for Children (BASC)	Preschool: 2½–5 yrs; School age: 6–11 yrs; Adolescent: 12–18 yrs	Multidimensional scale, normed by age and gender, that measures behavior, emotions, and self-perceptions. Includes parent and teacher rating scales, a youth self-report scale, and a structured developmental history. Assesses internalizing, externalizing, school problems, atypical behavior, and social/adaptive skills. Has validity scales to elucidate excessively negative or inconsistent responding, as well as omitted and critical items. Both computer- and hand-scored versions available.
Child Behavior Checklist (CBCL), Teacher's Report Form (TRF), and Youth Self Report (YSR)	CBCL: 1½–5 yrs TRF: 1½–5 yrs; CBCL: 6–18 yrs; TRF: 6–18 yrs; YSR: 11–18 yrs	Multiaxial, empirically based scales, normed by age and gender, that assess social competencies and behavioral/emotional problems. The CBCL/6–18, TRF/6–18, and YSR/11–18 were designed to obtain similar types of data in a similar format from parents, teachers, and youth. The behavior problem items on these scales cluster into eight subscales: Anxious/Depressed, Withdrawn/Depressed, Somatic Complaints, Social Problems, Thought Problems, Attention Problems, Rule-Breaking Behavior, and Aggressive Behavior. The analogous CBCL/1½–5 extends the empirically based assessment to younger children. It includes an Emotionally Reactive subscale, but excludes the Social, Thought, and Rule-Breaking subscales.
Direct Observational Form (DOF)	4–18 yrs	Developed as a counterpart to the CBCL/4–18 and TRF, this observational approach is used for assessment of problem behavior in school classrooms or other group settings. Items are designed to capture problem behavior that can be observed in 10-min observational sessions over several occasions.
Semistructured Clinical Interview for Children (SCIC)	6–11 yrs	Developed to accompany the CBCL/4–18 and TRF, this interview format was adapted to the cognitive levels and interactive style of 6- to 11-yr-old children. It provides open-ended questions designed to elicit children's reports on various important areas of their lives, including family, friends, school, activities, concerns, and fantasies. Also includes a Kinetic Family Drawing, brief achievement tests, screening for fine and gross motor abnormalities, and probe questions about problems attributed to the child by others.
Conners Rating Scales–Revised (CRS-R): Parent Rating Scales & Teacher Rating Scales; Conners-Wells' Adolescent Self-Report Scale	3–17 yrs	Factor-analytically derived, age- and gender-normed, behavioral rating scales for parents, teachers, and adolescent self-report. Both long and short forms available. Revised CRS is designed to correspond to DSM-IV-TR criteria for attention-deficit/hyperactivity disorder, as well as other internalizing and externalizing behavioral problems.
Symptom Checklist–90 Revised (SCL-90-R)	13+ yrs	A 90-item, self-report scale that asks respondents to rate the subjective severity of psychological symptoms in nine areas: somatization, obsessive-compulsive behaviors, interpersonal sensitivity, depression, anxiety, hostility, phobic anxiety, paranoid ideation, and psychoticism. It also yields a Global Severity Index of overall symptom severity.
Beck Youth Inventories	7–14 yrs	Five 20-item inventories that assess depression, anxiety, anger, disruptive behavior, and self-concept. It is designed as a self-report inventory that screens for emotional and social difficulties that may impair a child's ability to function in school settings. Children describe how frequently the statement has been true for them during the past 2 wks. Each of the brief inventories can be used separately as screenings to assist in initial diagnosis of emotional/behavioral problems and to monitor treatment progress.
Piers-Harris Children's Self-Concept Scale, second edition (PHCSCS-2)	7–18 yrs	60-item, self-report scale of self-concept and self-esteem in children. It yields a total score, along with subscale scores of self-concept in six areas (behavior adjustment, freedom from anxiety, happiness and satisfaction, intellectual and school status, physical appearance and attributes, anxiety, and popularity). This scale is useful in clinical settings to determine specific areas of conflict, typical coping and defense mechanisms, and appropriate intervention techniques.

girls, children's self-ratings of total problems were higher than parent or teacher ratings. In an inpatient sample, Alan Kazdin and colleagues reported that children rated their own symptoms of depression and aggression lower than their mothers did, but not lower than their fathers. Yet the magnitude of the children's self-ratings relative to those of other children accurately discriminated diagnostic groups. Catherine Stanger and Michael Lewis, in a study of inter-rater (i.e., parent, teacher, youth) agreement with 13-year-old youth, demonstrated that the youth rated themselves significantly higher than all other raters on all scales and that mothers and fathers rated more behavioral concerns than teachers, especially for internalizing problems. Stanger and Lewis say that the research, to date, suggests that it is important to collect information from multiple informants regarding child and adolescent behaviors and that ratings of no one informant can be substituted for another.

Advantages and Disadvantages of Behavioral Approaches There are several advantages of the behavioral approaches to assessment of behavior and emotional functioning in children and youth. These procedures are cost-effective in that they maximize the amount of information obtained with little clinician time. They often have convenient hand-scoring or computer scoring methodology, another cost-effective aspect. Use of behavioral assessment increases the likelihood of obtaining information from multiple sources (e.g., teachers, parents) across multiple settings (e.g., school, home, day care). These sources of information are necessary for some diagnoses, such as attention-deficit/hyperactivity disorder (ADHD). Many of the scales are empirically derived, factor-analytical scales that are normed for age and gender and generally possess good psychometric properties.

Disadvantages of behavioral rating methods in children include questions about the validity of informants' reports and concerns about informant reading level. The behavioral ratings are filtered through the perceptions of the informant, and the degree of frustration, emotional pathology (e.g., depression), and intellectual and academic skills of the informant are critical to understanding the report. There is much debate about how to handle discrepant ratings across informants. Although perfect correlation is not expected, the issue of how to weigh one individual's observations against those of another is an important issue that has not been resolved.

Behavioral Assessment System for Children (BASC) The BASC was developed as a multimethod, multidimensional approach to evaluating the behavior and self-perceptions of children between the ages of 2½ and 18 years. It is *multimethod* in that it has five components that can be used individually or in any combination: a self-report scale on which children or adolescents can describe their own emotions and self-perceptions, two rating scales (one for parents and one for teachers) that gather descriptions of the child's observable behavior, a structured developmental history, and a form for recording and classifying direct observations of the child's classroom behavior. It is *multidimensional* in that it measures many aspects of behavior and personality, including positive and negative dimensions. The BASC allows for comparisons of information from multiple sources and offers various types of validity checks that allow the clinician to interpret the consistency and veracity of the informants. Scales are consistent across age, gender, and forms (i.e., parent, teacher). For the Parent and Teacher Rating Scales, the Externalizing Problems Scale includes subscales of aggression, hyperactivity, and conduct problems; the Internalizing Problems Scale includes subscales of anxiety, depression, and somatization; and the School Problems Scale includes subscales of attention and learning problems. The Other Problems Scale includes two subscales: atypicality and withdrawal. Finally, the Adaptive Skills Scale includes adaptability, leadership, social skills, and study skills. In the Self-Report of Personality (SRP), there are four primary scales that differ from the Parent and Teacher versions. The Clinical Maladjustment Scale includes subscales of anxiety, atypicality, locus of control, social stress, and somatization. The School Maladjustment Scale includes attitude toward school, attitude toward teachers, and sensation seeking. The Other Problems Scale includes depression and sense of inadequacy subscales; and the Personal Adjustment Scale includes subscales of relations with parents, interpersonal relations, self-esteem, and self-reliance. Information obtained on each of the scales can be referenced against national age norms (general, male, and female versions) or clinical norms. Special indexes are incorporated into the BASC to assess the validity of each respondent's responses (F index). Critical items may be interpreted individually on the Parent and Teacher Rating Scales. On the SRP, the youth's responses are also viewed on an L ("fake good") index, and the V index designed to detect invalid responses due to poor reading comprehension, failure to follow directions, or poor contact with reality.

The BASC offers the clinician a psychometrically well-developed behavioral measure that takes only 10 to 20 minutes to complete. An advantage of the BASC, compared to many other rating scales, is the clear distinction between attention and hyperactivity symptoms for children suspected of having ADHD. The BASC thus provides information in a format to support clinical subtyping of ADHD. A disadvantage is the amount of time necessary to score and develop the profiles for each rating scale by hand. Computer scoring is likely the most cost-effective way to make use of this scale without spending undue time on the tedious scoring procedures.

Achenbach Child Behavior Checklists The checklists developed by Achenbach have perhaps been the most widely used behavioral rating scales in child and adolescent clinics in recent years. Similar to the BASC, the Achenbach scales include a parent rating (the Child Behavior Checklist [CBCL]), a teacher rating (Teacher Report Form [TRF]), and a self-report (Youth Self-Report [YSR]). The CBCL is appropriate for children between the ages of 4 and 18 years, the TRF is appropriate for children between the ages of 5 and 18 years, and the YSR is appropriate for those between the ages of 11 and 18 years. Each scale is interpreted in comparison to a large normative sample stratified by age and sex. A cross-informant computerized scoring paradigm is provided to assist with comparisons of the CBCL, TRF, and YSR measures regarding a given client.

A version of the CBCL for toddlers (CBCL/2-3) was developed in 1992 and has gained popularity since that time. It includes five of the subscales from the CBCL but adds a subscale on sleep problems. A separate computerized scoring system is available for this version of the CBCL.

Other Behavioral Personality Approaches Many other behavioral approaches to assessment are available in addition to behavior rating scales, as discussed earlier. Direct observations of child and adolescent behavior can be a useful adjunct to other assessment procedures, whether the observation is unstructured or structured according to a specific format. For instance, Russell Barkley and colleagues developed a structured observational paradigm called the *Restricted Academic Playroom Situation*, designed to provide an analog situation for observing and recording symptoms of ADHD during individual academic work. In this paradigm, the child or adolescent doing independent math problems is observed in a clinic playroom with toys or age-appropriate materials present. The child is told to complete as many math problems as possible, not to leave the chair at the table, and not to touch the toys or materials. Interval ratings are made in five behavioral categories: off-task behavior, fidgeting, being out of seat, vocalizing, and playing with objects. Many structured observational paradigms offer normative data against which to compare the clinical behaviors of interest, thus helping the clinician place the observational information within a broader context.

SUGGESTED CROSS REFERENCES

Chapter 2 discusses clinical assessment and approaches to diagnosis in neuropsychiatry. Section 5.2 presents statistics and experimental design. Chapter 8 discusses theories of personality that are derived from philosophy and psychology. Section 7.1 discusses the psychiatric interview, history, and mental status examination. Sections 7.5 and 7.7 present neuropsychological assessment of adults and children, respectively. Cognitive therapy is presented in Section 30.6.

References

American Psychiatric Association. *Handbook of Psychiatric Measures*. Washington, DC: American Psychiatric Association; 2000.

*Anastasi A. *Psychological Testing*. New York: MacMillan; 1988.

Archer RP. *MMPI-A: Assessing Adolescent Psychopathology*. Hillsdale, NJ: Lawrence Erlbaum Associates; 1992.

Beck JG, Novy DM, Diefenbach GJ, Stanley MA, Averill PM, Swann AC: Differentiating anxiety and depression in older adults with generalized anxiety disorder. *Psychol Assess*. 2003;15:184.

Bleiberg E. *Treating Personality Disorders in Children and Adolescents: A Relational Approach*. New York: Guilford; 2001.

Butcher JN. *The MMPI-2 in Psychological Treatment*. New York: Oxford University Press; 1990.

Butcher JN, Williams CL, Fowler RD. *Essentials of MMPI-2 and MMPI-A Interpretations*. 2nd ed. University of Minnesota Press; 2000.

Butler RW: Personality assessment of adults and children. In: Kaplan HI, Sadock BJ, eds. *Comprehensive Textbook of Psychiatry*. 6th ed. Baltimore: Williams & Wilkins; 1995.

Christophersen ER, Mortweet SL. *Treatments that Work with Children*. Washington, DC: American Psychological Association; 2001.

Conoley MC, Kramer JJ, eds. *The Tenth Mental Measurements Yearbook.* Lincoln, Nebraska: The Buros Institute of Mental Measurements, The University of Nebraska Press; 1989.
Corcoran K, Fischer J. *Measures for Clinical Practice.* New York: The Free Press; 1987.
Cushman LA, Scherer MJ. *Psychological Assessment in Medical Rehabilitation.* Washington, DC: American Psychological Association; 1995.
*Exner JE. *The Rorschach, Basis Foundations and Principles of Interpretation.* 4th ed. New York: John Wiley & Sons; 2002.
Exner JE, Weiner IB. *The Rorschach: A Comprehensive System: Vol. 3: Assessment of Children and Adolescents.* New York: John Wiley; 1995.
Gilberstadt H, Duker J. *A Handbook for Clinical and Actuarial MMPI Interpretation.* Philadelphia: W. B. Saunders Company; 1965.
Gomez R, Burns GL, Walsh JA: Alves de Moura M: A multitrait-multisource confirmatory factor analytic approach to the construct validity of ADHD rating scales. *Psychol Assess.* 2003;15:3.
*Graham JR. *MMPI-2: Assessing Personality and Psychopathology.* 3rd ed. New York: Oxford University Press; 2000.
Green RL. *MMPI-2: An Interpretive Manual.* 2nd ed. Boston: Allyn and Bacon; 1999.
*Groth-Marnot G. *Handbook of Psychological Assessment.* 4th ed. New York: John Wiley & Sons; 2003.
Hunsley J, Meyer GJ: The incremental validity of psychological testing and assessment: conceptual, methodological, and statistical issues. *Psychol Assess.* 2003;15:446.
Lopez SJ, Snyder CR, eds. *Positive Psychological Assessment, A Handbook of Models and Measures.* Washington, DC: American Psychological Association; 2003.
Morrison J, Anders TF. *Interviewing Children and Adolescents: Skills and Strategies for Effective DSM-IV Diagnosis.* New York: Guilford; 1999.
Nichels DS. *Essentials of MMPI-2 Assessment, Essentials of Psychological Assessment Series.* New York: John Wiley & Sons; 2001.
Reid JB, Patterson GR, Snyder JJ. *Antisocial Behavior in Children and Adolescents.* Washington, DC: American Psychological Association; 2002.
*Reynolds CR, Kamphaus RW. *The Clinician's Guide to the Behavior Assessment System for Children (BASC).* New York: Guilford; 2002.
Schroeder CS, Gordon BN. *Assessment and Treatment of Childhood Problems.* New York: Guilford; 2002.
Shaffer D, Lucas CP, Richters JE, eds. *Diagnostic Assessment in Child and Adolescent Psychopathology.* New York: Guilford; 1999.
Shapiro ES, Kratochwill TR. *Conducting School-Based Assessments of Child and Adolescent Behavior.* New York: Guilford; 2000.
Spirito A, Overholser J. *Evaluating and Treating Adolescent Suicide Attempter: From Research to Practice.* San Diego: Elsevier; 2003.
Vittengl JR, Clark LA, Jarrett RB: Interpersonal problems, personality psychopathology, and social adjustment after cognitive therapy for depression. *Psychol Assess.* 2003;15:29.
Zuckerman M. *Vulnerability to Psychopathology: A Biosocial Model.* Washington, DC: American Psychological Association; 1999.

▲ 7.7 Neuropsychological and Cognitive Assessment of Children

MARTHA BATES JURA, PH.D., AND
LORIE A. HUMPHREY, PH.D.

There are times in any mental health practice when psychological testing might help shed light on a child's ability to think and learn. Take, for example, a child who hates school.

> Simon refuses to do his homework and tends to "melt down" into tears if pushed to read. He is able to think creatively about many topics, yet forgets where he has put his backpack, his baseball cap, and his puppy's leash. These issues have gotten worse in the past year, and next year's fifth-grade curriculum is looming. It has been a difficult year in other respects as well. Simon's grandfather died in September, after having lived with the family for the past 5 years. The boy also took a bad spill on his skateboard in October that landed him in the hospital for an overnight observation due to a loss of consciousness for up to 5 minutes. He was referred for evaluation in November of his fourth-grade year.

Where does a psychiatrist begin to tease apart the many issues and risk factors present in this boy's story? Questions running through the psychiatrist's mind would probably include whether Simon has had ongoing learning or attentional problems and whether grief or head injury has contributed to his diagnostic picture and ability to cope. Formal cognitive and neuropsychological assessment would likely be a great help in understanding what primary issues drive Simon's distress and difficulties. The quantitative nature of the results helps the psychiatrist determine where and how a patient's functioning differs from that of other children.

The theoretical basis of psychological testing is fairly simple, although the elaboration on core cognitive principles has become very complex. Basically, psychological testing involves the systematic exploration of what a child sees and hears; how they handle, understand, and remember that information; and how they show their understanding through what they do, write, and say. Attention is the cognitive variable that impacts every aspect of the process, from initial perception through mental manipulation, leading to expression. Based on the pattern seen in psychological testing (supplemented by observations of test behavior and historical data), the clinician can comment on a range of diagnostic possibilities and formulate recommendations.

During this process, clinical psychologists attempt to make connections between thinking and behavior through psychological testing. Neuropsychologists take an additional step by attempting to identify behavioral relationships in brain functioning by using specialized instruments. This chapter describes cognitive and neuropsychological assessment and testing, as well as the testing process, from referral to report. The sections on general cognitive analysis focus on the types of tests used and the reasons for selecting some over others. The sections on specialized neuropsychological testing focus on the kinds of processing assessed and its meaning for central nervous system (CNS) adequacy. Both sections describe the manner in which the evaluation is undertaken and diagnoses and recommendations are made. The section on brain function and assessment describes attempts to relate testing to neurological findings.

GETTING STARTED

In the case of children and adolescents, the concerns of parents and teachers commonly bring students to the offices of psychiatrists and other professionals. In this context, a number of techniques are brought to bear on understanding what the problem is and what to do about it. What characterizes testing from history or observation is the availability of statistical ways of comparing patients to their peers. Because of a number of mathematical devices, a child's scores on psychological tests can be compared to those of others in his or her developmental group and, also, to each other. This allows the clinician to comment not only on the client's absolute scores, but also on the pattern of scores. Observation and understanding of this pattern lead to diagnostic clarification. Thus, discrepancies in scores from separate tests can be compared to each other to detect relative differences or absolute dysfunction in a number of cognitive spheres.

Reasons for Referral There are many reasons for referral for psychological testing. Let us return to Simon. How would a psychologist determine how to proceed in choosing the tests Simon should be given? A quick look at his presenting issues indicates that assessment should probably address questions of learning disabilities (unexpected underachievement), specific processing issues (inattention/executive functioning, memory), and social and emotional functioning (responses to internal states and external stressors), as well as the sequelae of a possible head injury (which could lead to—although there may be only one—cognitive dysfunction). Although, in one way or another, all of these might be considered in any particular case, this section focuses on the cognitive and neuropsychological assessment aspect of an overall workup. In Simon's case, the task of the psychologist would be to tease out the cognitive issues that were present before and after the grandfather's death and the head injury. In his case, the neuropsychological assessment would be a necessary aspect of his overall evaluation, which would also include more general cognitive assessment and social/emotional information.

Although Simon presents with a complex picture, in other simpler situations, a client might be referred directly for assessment due to problems with thinking and behavior. While there are many reasons that children are referred for cognitive assessment (intellectual, achievement, or processing testing), they often involve academic failure or school difficulties. There are other situations, however, in which a more detailed neuropsychological assessment is indicated because the client's problems are particularly severe, there have been drastic changes in functioning, or the situation has gotten particularly complex. While full evaluations include batteries of different kinds of tests, the following are reasons different assessments are undertaken:

Cognitive Evaluation: Cognitive assessment is often pursued when there have been academic and/or adaptive problems, but there is a range of reasons for undertaking cognitive testing. Various aspects of the evaluation include:

Intellectual Testing: Intellectual testing may reveal not only cognitive level (superior to deficient), but also strengths and weaknesses that can impact academic and social functioning.

Achievement Testing: Achievement testing can reveal a pattern of academic strengths and weaknesses that can be associated with school failure or success. Achievement testing is particularly undertaken when there is a discrepancy between performance and expectation.

Processing Assessment: Sometimes, information-processing problems can impact efficiency and accuracy when it comes to understanding the world and can help explain academic or social problems.

Neuropsychological Assessment: The client may present with a variety of developmental or learning issues, where clarification of brain–behavior relationships would help to determine the interventions. Additionally, when medical issues are involved—for example, a medical diagnosis (such as diabetes or seizure disorder) or a change in medical status (such as head injury)—neuropsychological testing is indicated.

Although there are many occasions when testing is appropriate, there are also times when it is not. Occasionally, a child has been tested so extensively or recently on intellectual instruments that a practice effect, particularly among nonverbal tasks, would make the new results invalid. For example, as a general rule, a particular intellectual test should be administered only once a year. In addition, sometimes the child is in no condition to have his or her cognitive functioning evaluated. For instance, when a patient is in the throes of psychosis or significant depression, intellectual testing is sometimes more a measurement of his or her disruption than of the patient's ability.

Testing Process In Simon's case, as in other cases, assessment procedures beyond testing are also indicated. These include examining past records (medical examinations, prior testing, report cards), interviewing Simon and his family (in structured and unstructured formats), obtaining information from home and school (and, sometimes, on-site observations), and getting rating scales filled out by his parents and teachers (regarding developmental, behavioral, emotional, and diagnostic issues). The diagnostic aspect of the process involves an attempt to determine which categories the client meets criteria for. The cognitive and neuropsychological testing are only aspects of an attempt to get a broad view of the way a child solves problems in the world, to describe his functioning in cognitive terms, and to understand his unique interaction with any diagnostic category.

Although psychologists prefer to administer tests with particular psychometric properties (the scores are distributed along a normal curve), they also (like other mental health professionals) supplement the evaluation with inventories and rating scales. Many of those used in cognitive assessments do not involve scores so much as acknowledgments or rankings. There are a wide variety of tools, particularly rating scales, with which it is often very hard to assess these results statistically. Many instruments have their own ways of noting whether symptoms occur at criterion levels. The methods and standards of each instrument should be perused. Some rating scales, such as the Achenbach Child Behavior Checklists (CBCL), allow for statistical or numerical analysis. Some diagnostic scales do not involve scores so much as comments. However, instruments such as the Vineland Adaptive Behavior Scales allow for the numerical comparison of the client to a normative population in several domains. In fact, the Vineland yields a full range of scores, including standard scores, percentile ranks, and age equivalents. There are many types of instruments and measures that are helpful in describing a client's status as compared to others. However, psychological instruments that involve standardized scores facilitate the comparison of scores within and between population members.

Measurements in Testing The point of testing is to create a way of comparing one individual to a population of individuals. The psychologist will select an instrument that is valid (it measures what is intended) and reliable (it measures it consistently). The testing involves establishing a basal (the level at which all items are passed) and a ceiling (the level at which no items are passed). The testing process involves converting a raw score to a standard score that can be compared to other scores along what is thought of as a normal distribution with predictable statistical properties. It is accepted that the measure is an approximation and not exact. This approximation is recognized by the concept of standard error of measurement, which is the naturally occurring error that takes place in the real world as one attempts to measure anything. One question that is often asked is "How good is this measurement?" Because of this question, test scores are often given within a range (confidence interval)—for example, plus or minus a certain number of points. In comparing any two scores, the big question is whether the difference is significant. This question is answered in terms of the likelihood of finding this difference by chance and by taking into account information such as the error of measurement and the distance between the two scores on the normal distribution. This distance is estimated by using a dispersion score, or standard deviation. Therefore, scores that fall further from the mean, or further from each other, are thought to be significantly different. Usually, scores must differ by one standard deviation before they are considered interesting. Scores two standard deviations from the mean, or each other, are considered quite significant. Differences between scores are often accompanied by an estimate of the chance (probability estimate) that the discrepancy would be found by fluke. For example, a discrepancy at the .01 level indicates that there is only one chance in 100 of finding this difference at random.

There are different ways of describing a child's placement in large populations, the most common of which are standard scores and percentiles. It should be noted that there are different kinds of scores and values within the normal distribution, and that they differ by mean and dispersion (see Fig. 7.5–7). In neuropsychology, there are ways of converting percentiles based on research populations (instead of standardized tests) into standard scores. Otherwise, because tests can differ in construction and the way in which the results are reported, or because nontest data is included in a comparison, percentiles themselves are often quoted. This allows results to be compared across disparate instruments or for a child to be described in terms of his or her placement in the normative population. Parents often respond well to the concept of a percentile. The percentile can be explained in terms of place in line. For example, when one says that an individual performs at the 50th percentile, they are indicating that, in a line of 100 children, this child stands in place 50. In addition to percentiles and standard scores, many cognitive tests provide age equivalents or grade equivalents. These measures suggest how the child compares to others of his or her age or grade.

It should be noted that the testing process involves more than scores. Although scores are important, how the patient goes about solving cognitive problems is carefully observed, noted, and analyzed. It makes a difference to the examiner whether the child says "This is easy" as he or she fails, or laments "Oh, this is hard" as he or she succeeds. Both have been seen and give the examiner a very different sense of how the client will experience school and life.

Testing of Children versus Testing of Adults Whether a clinician is doing a general cognitive or more specific neuropsychological assessment, children are often harder to evaluate than adults. For example, the interpretation of the results can be more complicated, in part because children's CNSs are still developing. Also, children are harder to examine, because they have more difficulties with attention (might be distracted by extraneous sounds) and motivation (might not even want to be there). As a result, certain accommodations (brief periods over several days) and reinforcements (stickers for trying) are used with children that are not used with adults. In addition, it is important for the examiner to understand normal development before attempting to diagnose deficits in children. For example, it is crucial for the examiner to know when a behavior has ceased to be developmentally appropriate and, instead, represents a delay, deficit, or deviance.

Diagnostic considerations may also be different for children than they are for adults. Child practitioners must have a thorough understanding of how symptoms of specific maladies present differently in children than they do in adults. For example, children's early symptoms of brain tumor tend to be more generalized than those of adults and can include intermittent headaches, middle or late insomnia, morning nausea, or poor appetite. Also, the role of the diagnosis when testing children goes beyond just naming the disorder. The diagnosis should also describe the child's level of difficulty and suggest appropriate treatment. Neuropsychological, as well as cognitive, testing can be helpful. However, because of greater uncertainty about the relationship between the brain and behavior in children, the greater variability in outcome introduced by this uncertainty, and the role of plasticity in the developing brain, the results are often most useful for identifying interventions rather than for fixing any specific prognosis.

COGNITIVE AND NEUROPSYCHOLOGICAL ASSESSMENT

Both general cognitive assessment and focused neuropsychological assessment are described in this section. Because the purposes of the evaluations tend to differ, so do the instruments used. The general cognitive assessment tends to be a practical event with an eye to the policies and possibilities in the outside world. As a result, the tests used are often "large" instruments with subtests and composite scores. The very factors that make them useful for general assessment limit them when it comes to fine-tuning understanding of neurological functioning. The focused neuropsychological evaluation tends to be a theoretical, as well as practical, event with an eye to the regions and pathways of an inside world. Appropriately, the tests used are "precision" instruments that often address a single cognitive function with, perhaps, one or two scores.

The general cognitive section of this chapter explores intellectual, achievement, and processing tests. The uses of the instruments are exemplified through descriptions of particular well-known instruments. The focused neuropsychological section describes the domains evaluated and the kinds of cognitive processes measured. Although some instruments are identified, they are too numerous to be described individually. The neuropsychological evaluation, in contrast to the cognitive assessment, which may use several tests, uses many procedures. Both the cognitive and neuropsychological sections include figures that are comprehensive but not exhaustive and list the most commonly used tests organized according to their uses. Jerome M. Sattler's book *Assessment of Children: Cognitive Applications* is a good reference for current psychological tests.

It should be noted that tests are constantly updated. This is often undertaken to correct perceived shortcomings, to adjust for cohort changes, and to make instruments more relevant. Because of this, instruments are referred to in "generic form" in this text, without any notation that would identify the edition. However, in real life, it is important to know that the clinician has used the most up-to-date version of the test, unless there is a good reason not to. For example, some clinicians with specialized practices continue to use old editions of tests because they find that a particular instrument best meets the needs of his or her particular population or best answers a type of diagnostic question. Clinicians must select from among the available tests the one that seems to best meet the needs of any particular client. In Tables 7.7–1 and 7.7–2, editions of tests current as of publication are noted.

General Cognitive Assessment General cognitive assessment can include, in addition to tests of intellectual functioning, tests of achievement and processing. The purpose of the evaluation is to shed light on disruptions in adaptive and academic adequacy, as well as in interpersonal functioning. When psychoeducational assessment is discussed, the focus is on the identification of specific learning disabilities, along with the securing of special educational services through the school system under learning disability eligibility. So far, from a practical (operational) standpoint, the federal definition of learning disability has required a severe discrepancy between ability and achievement (which is not accounted for by some other disorder or significant disadvantage) and has implicated the processing problem(s) that might explain the academic shortfall. However, because the federal government has given legal flexibility to the states to further operationalize the category (and, in turn, states have given flexibility to school districts regarding how to assess the designation), there is no uniform way to determine eligibility under learning disabilities. As a result, while learning disability has legal guidelines, the description of the category is subject to variability. Further, because legal guidelines can be modified, the description of the designation is subject to change (see Appendix). There are a number of other ambiguities around the term *learning disability*, and these will also be explored. The assessment of learning issues through intellectual, achievement, and processing testing will also be described.

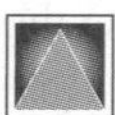

Table 7.7–1
Cognitive Tests

Test	Age Range[a]	Description
Intellectual tests		
Omnibus intellectual and ability tests		
Wechsler Preschool and Primary Scale of Intelligence–Third Edition (WPPSI-III)	2 yrs, 6 mos–7 yrs, 3 mos	The tests consist of several subtests that can be combined in different ways to understand basic intellectual functioning. The Wechsler tests yield a full-scale intelligence quotient (IQ) score, as well as overall scores within the verbal and nonverbal areas. There are ways of grouping subtests of the WISC and WAIS to distinguish between more pure verbal and perceptual reasoning, as well as to measure working memory and processing speed. Because of its age range, the WISC is probably the most familiar of the Wechsler tests to child clinicians. The SB also provides full-scale as well as verbal and nonverbal IQ scores. In addition, it provides factor indexes in fluid reasoning, knowledge, quantitative reasoning, visual–spatial processing, and working memory. The KABC scales and their subtests (which minimize verbal instructions and responses) include measures of sequential and simultaneous processing, fluid reasoning and crystallized ability, and long-term retrieval. Many, if not most, cognitive tests (including intellectual, achievement, and processing) are structured in the same way (mean is 100, standard deviation is 15), and so results can be compared across instruments. This is particularly important in identifying learning problems.
Wechsler Intelligence Scale for Children–Fourth Edition (WISC-IV)	6 yrs–16 yrs, 11 mos	
Wechsler Adult Intelligence Scale–Third Edition (WAIS-III)	16 yrs–89 yrs	
Stanford-Binet Intelligence Scales–Fifth Edition (SB5)	2 yrs–90 yrs	
Kaufman Assessment Battery for Children–Second Edition (KABC-II)	3 yrs–18 yrs	
Infant and child tests		
Revised Gesell Development Schedules	1–72 mos	The Gesell is an "old" test that is still administered by medical professionals, as well as psychologists. Along with the BSID, the Gesell is as useful for its opportunities for observations as it is for its scores. Both can be helpful in the identification of children at risk for developmental delay. The MSEL, with its five scales (Gross Motor, Visual Reception, Fine Motor, Expressive and Receptive Language), is often valued in assessing readiness for school, as well as in identifying specific interventions for children with developmental disabilities. The MSCA consists of six scales (Verbal, Perceptual–Performance, Quantitative, General Cognitive, Memory, and Motor). It is a good instrument for assessing general strengths and weaknesses in young children.
Bayley Scales of Infant Development–Second Edition (BSID-II)	1–42 mos	
Mullen Scales of Early Learning (MSEL)	0–68 mos	
McCarthy Scales of Children's Abilities (MSCA)	2 yrs, 6 mos–8 yrs, 6 mos	
Nonverbal and language-free tests		
Leiter International Performance Scale–Revised (Leiter-R)	2 yrs–20 yrs, 11 mos	Although the nonverbal tests are often seen as language- or culture-free, strictly speaking, this is not always true. For example, items that need to be understood linguistically and conceptually (the solution might be to observe that the pattern is "clothing") are not language- or culture-free. However, some nonverbal tests (such as the TONI-3) depend more on abstract pattern recognition and can make fewer demands on language systems. Tests like Raven's Progressive Matrices (which actually come in several forms) are thought of as "culturally reduced," if not unbiased or unloaded. It requires the client to complete a visual array by identifying a portion/figure that completes a pattern. Nonverbal tests can be useful in assessing individuals with hearing or language problems.
Test of Nonverbal Intelligence–Third Edition (TONI-3)	6 yrs–89 yrs, 11 mos	
Comprehensive Test of Nonverbal Intelligence (CTONI)	6 yrs–89 yrs, 11 mos	
Raven's Progressive Matrices	5 yrs–17+ yrs	
Quick tests		
Kaufman Brief Intelligence Test–Second Edition (KBIT-2)	4 yrs–90 yrs	Although the KBIT and WASI include verbal and nonverbal scores, they do not include as much information as more comprehensive intellectual tests. However, they provide an estimate of intellectual level in a fraction of the time.
Wechsler Abbreviated Scale of Intelligence (WASI)	6 yrs–89 yrs	
Achievement tests		
Wechsler Individual Achievement Test–Second Edition (WIAT-II)	4 yrs–85 yrs	The WRAT3 is sometimes used to screen learning disabilities. However, its usefulness, particularly with older children, is limited. Reading only addresses decoding, not comprehension. Arithmetic addresses calculation but not math reasoning. And the test includes spelling but no other aspect of writing. The PIAT assesses general information, reading recognition and comprehension, written expression, spelling, and mathematics. The KTEA assesses reading (decoding and comprehension), mathematics (applications and calculations), spelling, written expression, and oral language (listening comprehension and oral expression). The WIAT and WJ-ACH also systematically address all the areas that have been identified by code as relevant for learning disability.
Woodcock-Johnson–III Test of Achievement (WJ III ACH)	2 yrs–90+ yrs	
Kaufman Test of Educational Achievement–Second Edition (KTEA-II)	4.5 yrs–25 yrs	
Peabody Individual Achievement Test–Revised (PIAT-R)	5 yrs–22 yrs, 11 mos	
Wide Range Achievement Test–Third Edition (WRAT3)	5 yrs–75 yrs	
Reading tests		
Gray-Oral Reading Tests–Fourth Edition (GORT-4)	6 yrs–18 yrs, 11 mos	The WRMT (which includes a measure of sound–symbol association) and GORT (which includes a measure of fluency) involve systematic approaches to assessing different aspects of reading skills. Because of the importance of phonological awareness in the development of reading skills, tests of phonological processing (such as the CTOPP) are often included in assessments in which reading problems are identified.
Woodcock Reading Mastery Tests–Revised (WRMT-R)	5 yrs–75+ yrs	
Comprehensive Test of Phonological Processing (CTOPP)	5 yrs–24 yrs, 11 mos	

(continued)

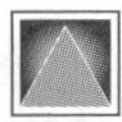

Table 7.7–1 (*continued*)

Test	Age Range[a]	Description
Processing tests		
General processing tests		
Woodcock-Johnson–III Test of Cognitive Abilities (WJ III COG)	2 yrs–90+ yrs	The WJ-COG scores provide information about intellectual ability as well as a variety of processing and clinical areas. The NEPSY provides scores in attention/executive functioning, as well as language, sensorimotor, visuospatial, and memory/learning.
NEPSY (a developmental neuropsychological assessment)	3 yrs–12 yrs, 11 mos	
Visual–motor tests		
Bender Visual–Motor Gestalt Test–Second Edition (Bender Gestalt II)	4 yrs–85+ yrs	Both the Bender and VMI involve copying geometric figures. Because the Bender allows the student to organize the items on the page and the VMI asks the student to copy each figure in its own space, the two can be used together to assess organizational issues, as well as visual–motor integration. Both the current versions of the Bender and VMI provide ways of assessing perceptual separate from motor skills. The TVPS is motor-free and involves making judgments about visual information—for example, a client might be asked to identify an item from a fragmented presentation.
Beery Developmental Test of Visual–Motor Integration–Fifth Edition, Revised (VMI-5)	2 yrs–18 yrs	
Test of Visual–Perceptual Skills–Revised (TVPS-R)	4 yrs–13 yrs	
Test of Visual–Perceptual Skills–Upper Level–Revised (TVPS-UL-R)	12 yrs–17 yrs, 11 mos	
Auditory–vocal tests		
Test of Auditory-Perceptual Skills–Revised (TAPS-R)	4 yrs–13 yrs, 11 mos	The TAPS involves making judgments about auditory information. For example, the student might be asked to discriminate sounds or remember words or numbers under different constraints. The TARPS measures the "quality" and "quantity" of the client's auditory thinking and reasoning.
Test of Auditory-Perceptual Skills–Upper Level (TAPS-UL)	12 yrs–17 yrs, 11 mos	
Test of Auditory Reasoning and Processing Skills (TARPS)	5 yrs–13 yrs, 11 mos	
Memory		
Wide Range Assessment of Memory and Learning–Second Edition (WRAML2)	5 yrs–90 yrs	Memory scales attempt to systematically assess memory skills within different spheres. The WRAML core battery consists of Verbal, Visual, and Attention/Concentration subtests. The CMS allows for the assessment of attention and working memory, verbal and visual memory, short-delay and long-delay memory, recall and recognition, and learning characteristics.
Children's Memory Scale (CMS)	5 yrs–16 yrs	

[a]Please note: Age ranges should be regarded as approximate. Also note that this is not a comprehensive list, but rather a sampling of commonly used instruments. Keep in mind that publishers are constantly updating their tests, and these editions will be superceded by newer and better versions. Even now, there are variations on some instruments that are expanded, integrated, or newly normed.

Intellectual Testing Because of the importance of intellectual functioning as it impacts the ability to learn and adapt in social and academic situations, intellectual testing is often part of a variety of psychological assessment batteries, including psychoeducational and neuropsychological evaluation, as well as developmental and emotional evaluations.

BACKGROUND Intellectual testing is usually undertaken to determine the patient's general intellectual level of functioning. The intelligence quotient (IQ) is valued because of its stability over time in the general population, as well as for the protective aspect of intelligence in a range of potentially disabling situations. It should be noted that, although intellectual level can be measured, it is hard to actually define intelligence.

Definition Different theorists have had their own take on intelligence. Although, theoretically, Sattler sees intelligence as "multifaceted and hierarchically organized," practically, there is no agreement about what intelligence is, and this is reflected in the different ways it is measured. However, a common-sense definition of intelligence would include the ability to learn from and adapt to the environment. It would also include the ability to think abstractly (to use symbols and higher-level concepts) and to recognize patterns in diverse situations (on tests and in life). Although intelligence tests yield one IQ score (or several IQ or index scores), they are, in fact, devices for "sampling" many tasks in a variety of verbal and nonverbal areas. Intelligence tests differ from achievement tests in that they are more process- than content-oriented. That is, for the most part, they put the student in a position to solve verbal or nonverbal problems in the present rather than use specific reading, mathematics, or writing skills learned in the past.

Stability Although there is some disagreement, IQ scores tend to be relatively stable starting as young as 5 to 7 years of age. In general, the older the child is when tested and the smaller the interval between test administrations, the greater the correlation between two IQ scores. Although using an IQ score can be useful as a way of assessing the client's basic trajectory through life, the prudent practitioner must be aware that there are a number of factors that can impact intellectual functioning and, thus, IQ scores. Factors associated with disorder and illness can suppress scores, particularly in psychiatric practice. These can include situational factors, such as lack of motivation, as well as transient factors, including inattention, depression, and psychosis. Some ongoing conditions (for example, those that involve problems with relating, involvement, or cognition) can negatively impact learning and performance and potentially impact intellectual levels as well. In some cases, treatments and interventions implemented to improve cognition and enhance development can improve functioning and, thus, IQ scores.

Protection Despite conceptual and practical complications, high intelligence is associated with better prognosis in a wide range of psychiatric conditions; lower rates for behavior, conduct, and emotional problems in children; and lower rates of referral for psychiatric problems in adults. In the case of any kind of brain damage (neuronal death), intellectual level accounts for a great deal of vari-

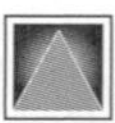

Table 7.7–2
Neuropsychological Test List (Selected)

Memory and learning
- **Verbal**
  - Children's Memory Scale (CMS): Stories, Word Pairs, Wordlists
  - Wide Range Assessment of Memory and Learning (WRAML): Story Memory, Sentence Memory, Verbal Learning
  - California Verbal Learning Test for Children
  - Children's Auditory Verbal Learning Test
  - NEPSY: Memory For Names, Narrative Memory, List Learning
- **Visual**
  - CMS: Dot Locations, Faces, Family Pictures
  - WRAML: Design Memory, Picture Memory, Visual Learning
  - NEPSY: Memory For Faces
  - Rey-Osterrieth Complex Figure
  - Benton Visual Recognition Test

Sensorimotor functions
- **Sensory perceptual**
  - Reitan-Klove Sensory Perceptual Exam
  - Finger recognition
  - NEPSY: Finger Discrimination
  - Assessment of visual fields
- **Motor**
  - Handedness exam
  - Pegboard tests
  - Apraxia exam
  - Hand Dynamometer Test (Grip Strength)
  - NEPSY: Sensorimotor Functions Test
  - Fingertip tapping
  - Manual motor sequencing
  - Large motor assessment

Attention and executive functions
- **Sustained attention**
  - Continuous performance tests (Test of Variables of Attention [TOVA], Conners' Continuous Performance Test [CPT], the AX version of the CPT [CPT AX])
  - Cancellation tests
  - NEPSY: Auditory Attention and Response Set, Knock and Tap
  - Paced Auditory Serial Addition Task (PASAT)
- **Working memory**
  - Wechsler Intelligence Scale for Children (WISC): Digit Span, Arithmetic, Letter-Number Sequencing
  - WRAML: Finger Windows, Number/Letter Memory, Sentence Memory
  - NEPSY: Sentence Repetition
  - CMS: Numbers, Sequences
  - Auditory Consonant Trigrams
- **Problem solving**
  - Children's Category Test
  - Wisconsin Card Sorting Test (WCST)
  - Tower Tests
  - Delis-Kaplan Executive Functions (D-KEFS): Sorting Test
- **Cognitive flexibility**
  - Trailmaking Test A & B
  - Children's Color Trails
  - D-KEFS: "Switching" components of Trailmaking, Verbal Fluency, Design Fluency, Color-Word Interference
- **Inhibition**
  - NEPSY: Statue, Auditory Attention and Response Set, Knock and Tap
  - Stroop Interference Test
  - Go–no go test
  - Matching Familiar Figures Test
  - D-KEFS: Color-Word Interference
- **Fluency**
  - Controlled word association (Word Fluency)
  - NEPSY: Design Fluency, Verbal Fluency
  - Word associations (Clinical Evaluation of Language Fundamentals–Third Edition [CELF-III])
  - D-KEFS: Verbal Fluency, Design Fluency

Language
- **Expressive**
  - NEPSY: Phonological Processing, Speeded Naming, Sentence Repetition
  - Gardner Expressive One Word Picture Vocabulary Test
  - Expressive Vocabulary Test
  - Boston Naming Test
  - Woodcock-Johnson–III: Oral Language, Oral Expression, Listening, Auditory Processing Composites
  - CELF-IV
- **Receptive**
  - Wepman Auditory Discrimination Test
  - Peabody Picture Vocabulary Test
  - Token Test
  - NEPSY: Comprehension of Instructions
  - CELF: Sentence Structure, Concepts and Directions, Word Classes, Semantic Relationships, Listening to Paragraphs

Visuospatial and visuoconstruction
- **Visuospatial**
  - Benton Judgment of Line Orientation
  - Benton Facial Recognition
  - Hooper Visual Organization Test
  - NEPSY: Route Finding, Arrows
  - Test of Visual–Perceptual Skills
  - WRAVMA: Matching
- **Visuoconstruction**
  - WISC: Block Design
  - Beery Buktenica Developmental Test of Visual–Motor Integration
  - Wide Range Assessment of Visual Motor Achievement: (WRAVMA): Drawing
  - Rey-Osterrieth Complex Figure
  - NEPSY: Block Construction, Design Copying

ance in predicting outcome, with lower IQs associated with poorer outcomes and higher IQs associated with better outcomes.

ASSESSMENT Although IQ is what is obtained with an IQ test, there are a variety of intellectual tests, as well as other ways of calculating intellectual level. There are a number of instruments from which to choose, and the psychologist must make his or her selection based on the specific characteristics of each test (for example, normative sample and construction of the instrument) as they relate to the characteristics of the client (for example, age and referral question). Once the test has been administered, the clinician must make interpretations based on the analysis of overall and subtest scores and their pattern in the context of the diagnostic process.

Sometimes, there are misinterpretations of scores at the bottom of the intellectual range. Because of the possibility of confusion, a distinction must be made between terms such as mentally retarded (and intellectually deficient) when they refer to functional intellectual ranges and mentally retarded when it is used as a clinical diagnosis. The diagnosis of mental retardation is reserved for individuals with a pattern of generally low scores (approximately 69 or 70 or below) along with adaptive deficits and onset before age 18 years. In making determinations about low intellectual level, the psychologist must look at the pattern of strengths and weaknesses not only within the instrument, but also within the overall case presentation. For example, some IQ scores can be brought down by specific language disorders or perceptual–motor difficulties.

Sometimes, there is a focus on significant discrepancies between verbal and nonverbal scores. Because of the interest in basic processing issues, clinicians often interpret these data in terms of "crystallized" versus "fluid" thinking or intelligence. Crystallized thinking (based on more stable and factual knowledge) tends to be associated with verbal tasks and information that has been learned in the past and provided in the present. Fluid intelligence (related to more dynamic and kaleidoscopic processing) tends to be associated with nonverbal tasks and responses that are provided as a result of on-the-spot problem solving. These concepts can be applied not only to intellectual test results, but also to other processing test findings. However, these concepts are more complicated than this verbal–nonverbal dichotomy, and the notion of fluid and crystallized thinking can be applied to both verbal and nonverbal tasks.

Comprehensive Intellectual Tests The two best-known intellectual tests are probably the Wechsler Intelligence Scales and the Stanford-Binet Intelligence Scales (SB). The current editions of both are divided into separate subtests, and the data are analyzed in separate spheres. Each test has an overall mean of 100 (50th percentile) and a standard deviation of 15. Subtests have a mean of 10 and a standard deviation of 3. In the case of the Wechsler tests, three separate instruments (Wechsler Preschool and Primary Scale of Intelligence [WPPSI], Wechsler Intelligence Scale for Children [WISC], and Wechsler Adult Intelligence Scale [WAIS]) are designed for three different age groups over the lifespan. In the case of the SB, one instrument covers a lifetime. All instruments include full-scale IQ scores, as well as (broadly speaking) verbal and nonverbal composite scores. Both instruments have made attempts to assist decision making regarding attentional problems. The WISC has made particular attempts to link its findings to memory, adaptive, and giftedness scales. The SB includes a routing system so that the examiner can "adapt" the administration to the functioning level of the examinee. The SB provides an extended score range (at the top and bottom of the scale) that may make it more useful for individuals within the "gifted" and "mentally retarded" ranges. Both the SB and the Wechsler tests have been the "standard" individual intellectual tests for the school-age psychiatric population. They allow for the assessment of overall functioning and verbal and nonverbal reasoning, as well as of some processing. Both instruments have taken care to relate to achievement tests to facilitate the recognition of learning disabilities according to the current "discrepancy model." The WISC is coordinated with the Wechsler Individual Achievement Tests (WIAT), but, of course, its IQ can be compared to any standard score. The new SB provides extensive discrepancy analyses with the current Woodcock-Johnson Tests of Achievement (WJ-ACH) and correlational studies with other tests, such as the current WIAT. Table 7.7–3 provides the intellectual classifications systems for the SB and Wechsler tests. Although these categories are applied to these intellectual tests, they are also relevant to other cognitive results, as long as the test is psychometrically similar to these instruments (mean is 100, standard deviation is 15).

Other Intellectual Tests Sometimes, specific characteristics of clients, such as age, suggest the use of specific instruments.

Infant and Child Tests Although very young clients can be "tested," these administrations are often as useful for their observations as their scores. Because of the emphasis on sensorimotor functioning and development of language skills of very young clients, the

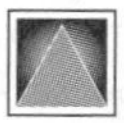

Table 7.7–3
Comparison of Wechsler Intelligence Scales and Stanford-Binet Intelligence Scales–Fifth Edition Intellectual Ranges[a]

Wechsler Intellectual Ranges[b]		SB5 Intellectual Ranges	
IQ/Index Score	Range	IQ/Index Score	Range
		145–160	Very gifted or highly advanced
≥130	Very Superior	130–144	Gifted or very advanced
120–129	Superior	120–129	Superior
110–119	High Average	110–119	High average
90–109	Average	90–109	Average
80–89	Low Average	80–89	Low average
70–79	Borderline	70–79	Borderline impaired or delayed
≤69	Extremely Low	55–69	Mildly impaired or delayed
		40–54	Moderately impaired or delayed

IQ, intelligence quotient.
[a]Both instruments have a mean of 100 and standard deviation of 15.
[b]These ranges apply to the composite scores of all current Wechsler IQ tests (WPPSI-III, WISC-IV, WAIS-III).
Reproduced with permission from *Wechsler Intelligence Scale for Children—Fourth Edition.* Copyright © 2003 by Harcourt Assessment, Inc.; and Roid GH. *Stanford-Binet Intelligence Scales, Fifth Edition, Examiner's Manual.* Itasca, IL: Riverside Publishing. Copyright © 2003 by the Riverside Publishing Company. All rights reserved.

instruments (such as the Bayley Scales of Infant Development) are not as useful for predicting later IQ scores as they are for identifying individuals who are, or are not, at risk. The instruments do not become predictive in a more specific way until children are of school age.

Nonverbal and Language-Free Tests Although some tests seem especially suited for individuals who are hard of hearing or have language issues (such as the Leiter International Performance Scale), the nonverbal tests can have broader applications. Their emphasis is on cognitive problem solving based on visual information. Although these tests are useful, it is important to remember that they may not provide the whole picture, and the significance of these tests for the client's ability and functioning must be carefully assessed.

Quick Tests The commonly used tests in research and clinical practice are the Kaufman Brief Intelligence Test (KBIT) and the Wechsler Abbreviated Scale of Intelligence (WASI). Both the KBIT and the WASI include verbal and nonverbal tasks to assess crystallized and fluid thinking. The original K-BIT and the WASI report good correlations between the composite and full-scale IQs on child and adult Wechsler tests (approximately .75 to .90). These data suggest that the quick tests, in fact, yield very representative IQ scores. Although a clinician might not get all the processing information made available by a full intellectual test, these correlation coefficients suggest that the quick tests can provide a very good estimate of the client's general level of functioning.

General Comment In discussing intellectual testing, it is important to note what IQ tests are and what they are not. Although IQ scores are commonly used as estimates of ability, they are not measures of "native" or "raw" intelligence. Every client brings a long learning history (including opportunities) to the testing situation. The debate over whether tests are culture-free or culture-fair has raged over the years. Although some instruments (such as those that emphasize nonverbal functioning) may seem less biased or loaded, it must be acknowledged that probably no intellectual test is either culture-free or -fair. However, because IQ tests have, in large part, been designed to predict school success, they can be useful in the context of assessing learning capacity. All the same, because of the way tests have been constructed and normed, caution has to be exercised in making conclusions in any case involving an unusual cultural or medical situation. Although IQ scores are useful as estimates of ability, they are, in fact, measures of functioning. There are a variety of transient factors that can be associated with alterations in IQ scores, including problems with involvement, attention, and disorganization. As a result, the clinician has to be prepared for changes in intellectual level based on changes in medical status. For example, in some cases, clinicians have observed increases in IQ scores subsequent to medical treatment for attention-deficit/hyperactivity disorder (ADHD), partly due to increased efficiency on the instrument itself and partly due to increased learning over time in the environment and in school.

Considerations Here are a number of factors professionals should keep in mind when they deal with intellectual test results.

- When scores have a mean of 100 and a standard deviation of 15 (such as the WISC or new SB), the scores are distributed so that 68 percent of the population falls between 85 and 115 (one standard deviation in either direction). Cognitive tests (including achievement tests) tend to be distributed in this way; thus, comparisons can be made from one instrument to another.
- The more variability seen on intellectual testing, the less composite or summary scores mean. For example, on the WISC or SB, when the verbal and nonverbal scores (or other contributing indices or composites) differ significantly, the full-scale IQ is not informative. Similarly, when subtest scores differ significantly within a sphere, the emphasis should be on specific processing issues rather than overall functioning.
- Sometimes a practitioner will ask what a patient's IQ is. It is clear, from the multiplicity of the tests and scores available, that there is no one IQ. Although IQ is what the client gets on an IQ test, it is prudent to be well aware of which test was administered and which IQ is being quoted. The practitioner should be aware of disparities on different tests or in different areas; this pattern is often important in making decisions for a client.
- In the context of a psychoeducational assessment, when scores differ significantly on intellectual testing, the full-scale IQ may not be the best estimate of "ability," and the clinician will make attempts to choose among the possible summary scores on a range of instruments to identify the one that best represents the student's learning potential.
- What can be most helpful about the IQ score is the way it helps the practitioner to be aware of the client's general level of functioning. Each intellectual test uses its own language to indicate relatively low or high functioning. In school or practice, the designations at the higher end of the scale might include mildly gifted (starting at 115), moderately gifted (at 130), highly gifted (at 145), exceptionally gifted (at 160), and profoundly gifted (at 180). However, because of a ceiling effect on most newer intellectual test scores, there is some question about the utility of these traditional ranges, and they (and how to characterize "giftedness") are being reconsidered. In this context, it is worth noting that the "old" Stanford-Binet L-M is useful in detecting these very high IQ scores, and the "new" SB5 has an expansion that also allows for the detection of these very high IQs.
- Practitioners need to know what IQ scores do not measure. They do not measure social intelligence or street smarts, the kind of savvy large portions of the population use every day to keep jobs and raise families, nor do they reflect the creativity that artists of different kinds bring to their art and that entertains and informs us daily.

FURTHER ASSESSMENT The following is a list of patterns that suggest the need for further evaluation:

Significant discrepancies between verbal and nonverbal scores: When the verbal score is significantly lower than the nonverbal score, the possibility of a language disorder should be considered. In the case of a low verbal score, a speech and language assessment, to include measures of receptive and expressive language, as well as pragmatics (the factors impacting successful communication), might be indicated. When the nonverbal score is significantly lower than the verbal score, further assessment regarding a variety of possibilities must be considered. More than the verbal tasks, the performance tasks (which might be timed) are vulnerable to ongoing and transient factors mediated by attention. In the case of particularly large discrepancies, the possibility of nonverbal learning disorder should also be considered. This is a pattern of cognitive assets and deficits that can be associated with social, as well as academic, problems.

When the full or composite score is above the 98th or below the 2nd percentile (130 or 70): At the intellectual extremes, the examiner may consider whether further assessment regarding educational or adaptive needs might be in order. When a client has a very high intellectual level (for example, moderately to profoundly gifted), the professional might refer the family to a psychologist specializing in very bright children or consult http://www.davidsoninstitute.org for information about how to meet the needs of his or her client. In the case of individuals with very low intellectual level, further assessment can be obtained through the school system or the local public agency serving developmentally delayed clients. Professionals and parents may access http://www.aamr.org and http://www.thearc.org or http://www.eparent.com for information about services and products associated with mental retardation and developmental disabilities.

When the intellectual score shifts downward in a significant way: Because it is anticipated that intellectual scores will remain relatively stable over time, the mental health professional is advised to look for an explanation, either psychological or medical, for dramatic score changes. This is a time when the psychologist should look at raw, as well as standard, scores; a drop in a raw score is the test equivalent of losing functioning in everyday life. After some exploration, discussion with the pediatrician and referral to a neuropsychologist might be in order.

Achievement Testing When achievement testing is undertaken along with intellectual and processing testing, the overall evaluation is commonly referred to as a *psychoeducational assessment*. The purpose of the assessment is to identify learning problems. In addition, its purpose has been to establish eligibility for services through the public school system under learning disability, which has been widely established by demonstrating a significant discrepancy between ability and achievement. However, how the discrepancy is measured, and whether or not a processing problem must be cited to explain the discrepancy, can vary greatly by time and place. Because they are subject to legal guidelines, learning disability eligibility criteria can vary and change. This has never been more true than now, with proposed modifications to special education law. As the legal context of learning disabilities changes, the way cognitive instruments are used to explore learning issues will also change.

BACKGROUND Achievement testing is administered to determine a student's level of functioning in basic academic areas, including reading, mathematics, and composition. The factors assessed are more transient and circumscribed than those assessed in intellectual testing. Unlike intellectual testing, achievement testing is not necessarily expected to be stable over time, as it measures the child's success in formal learning and is highly dependent on the home's environment and the school's curriculum.

Learning disability is commonly defined in terms of "unexpected underachievement"—that is, the child has the potential and opportunities to have learned more. The purpose of the achievement testing is often to identify the need for educational services due to a learning disability. As long as parents hope to obtain these services through school (rather than in the community at their own expense), the family is highly dependent on the procedures and policies of the school system, in response to federal and state laws and regulations. At this time, the two federal laws most commonly cited in securing services for students are the Individuals with Disabilities Education Act (IDEA) and the Rehabilitation Act of 1973 (Section 504). The former provides for a formal assessment and administrative procedure (the Individualized Education Program [IEP]) by which students with specific learning disabilities are identified for special educational services. The latter provides for a potentially less formal evaluation and meeting by which students with a substantial handicap affecting learning can receive accommodations and supportive services. Although the legal situation is more complicated than this, under ordinary circumstances, this description characterizes the difference between pursuing services through an IEP and 504.

In the future, it is possible that learning disability will be defined not relative to general intellectual ability, but in terms of more absolute dysfunction in academic areas, along with a pattern of deficits and capabilities within cognitive functioning. It is not impossible that learning rate, as well as disparity of functioning, may become part of the definition or that processing problems may become a more important characteristic of learning disability. Under federal law, IDEA is reauthorized approximately every 5 years, and categorical definitions can be revised at that time to bring them in line with current scientific evidence. The reader should be aware that, with the next IDEA reauthorization, there may be a ripple effect in which changes in the federal operationalization of learning disability will be followed by changes in state and school system codes, rules, and regulations. In addition, the reauthorization of IDEA comes at a time when the No Child Left Behind Act (NCLB) of 2001 and its implementation are being debated. The NCLB initiative focuses attention on accountability regarding reading and mathematics skills. As a result of improvements in teacher qualifications and educational instruction, more children may receive appropriate intervention without any eligibility process and while in regular classrooms. In any case, the point being made is that the term *learning disability* is a legal entity and that how services are provided to students with learning problems can be highly responsive to political forces.

Table 7.7–4 provides further discussion of the federal laws that impact access to special services at the local level for students with learning disability.

ASSESSMENT Because the definition of learning disability is a political, as well as theoretical, issue, any assessment must be in reference to laws at the federal and state level, as well as to the policies of any particular school system. As a result, undertaking psychoeducational assessment requires knowledge of eligibility requirements. In assessing difficulties, the clinician must pay attention to the appropriateness of the overall assessment in addressing eligibility issues, as well as to the utility of each instrument in representing the function it is meant to measure.

When ability has needed to be assessed in the school system, there have been many ways of doing so, including administering a standard IQ test and using alternative methods (such as nonverbal tests or composite scores from processing tests). In some jurisdictions, intellectual testing has not been used to establish potential in assessing learning disabilities because it has been seen as racially biased. Thus, assessing intelligence has often been associated with differences of opinion. However, assessing achievement has been less controversial and has commonly involved standardized tests. Although there might be a variety of ways to concurrently assess incremental academic progress, less frequent assessment has involved complex instruments. In addition, although assessing reading and mathematics disabilities has been fairly straightforward, assessing written expression has been more problematic. Controversy has arisen when spelling alone has been presented as the problem with written expression, and this raises the issue of whether

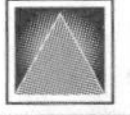

Table 7.7–4
Education and the Law

In trying to meet the needs of students who require services through public schools, mental health professionals should be aware of (1) the federal laws (and their associated regulations) that define populations who are eligible for services, (2) the procedures by which students can obtain services, and (3) the nature of the services available.

The federal government has protected the rights of disabled students since 1975 under a series of public laws. In 1990, the Education of All Handicapped Children Act was renamed the Individuals with Disabilities Education Act (IDEA). Reauthorized in 1997, IDEA establishes the obligation of public school systems to identify and teach students with disabilities who "by reason thereof" (because of them) need special education and related services. Such students exhibit a wide range of disabling conditions, including (in addition to sensory and orthopedic impairments) mental retardation, speech or language impairments, serious emotional disturbance, autism, traumatic brain injury, other health impairments, and, particularly relevant to this discussion, a specific learning disability.

The process by which such students would be identified and served under IDEA is called an Individualized Education Program (IEP). Broadly defined, the IEP refers to an evaluation and group process by which eligibility for special education and related services is determined and a plan specifying goals and interventions is written and periodically reviewed. Although the language used to describe learning disabilities and demonstrate eligibility for services differs depending on the rules referred to, as a practical matter, the student (1) must show a discrepancy between ability and achievement in one of seven academic areas involved in reading, math, writing, and language, and (2) may need to show a disorder in one or more of the basic psychological processes (such as visual and auditory processing or attention). The academic areas for potential disability are identified as basic reading skill, reading comprehension, mathematics calculation, mathematics reasoning, and written expression. Although oral expression and listening comprehension are also included under learning disability, in practice, services for students with receptive or expressive language problems are usually obtained under a speech and language eligibility. There are circumstances in which a learning disability cannot be designated—for example, when the academic problem is primarily due to another problematic condition (such as visual, hearing, or motor handicap, as well as mental retardation or emotional disturbance) or to environmental, cultural, or economic disadvantage. In contrast, in the case of learning disabilities, the underachievement is "unexpected."

(*continued*)

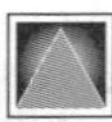

Table 7.7–4 (*continued*)

When a discrepancy model is used, it allows for learning disability to be identified among students who test at the bottom of the intellectual scale (whose intellectual levels fall within the low-normal range, and theoretically, but perhaps not practically, within the below-normal range), as well as students who test at the top of the intellectual scale (whose levels fall within the gifted range). That is, so long as the clinician can demonstrate a significant discrepancy between ability and achievement, along with a processing problem associated with the underachievement, the student can be labeled "learning disabled."

In contrast to a learning disability, a learning disorder requires only that achievement be "substantially below that expected given the person's chronological age, measured intelligence, and age-appropriate education." It is worth reminding psychiatrists that because of the current potential legal importance of a processing problem in identifying a learning disability in school, it would be advisable to comment on any processing problem in diagnosing a learning disorder, even though it is not required according to DSM-IV-TR criteria.

Under IDEA, even if a child meets criteria for a learning disability, or any other eligibility criteria (for example, under autism or emotional disturbance), they are still not eligible for special educational services unless they need them. Special education means "specially designed instruction." As a result, the boundary between special education and a classroom that (without labeling) individualizes instruction based on diverse learning styles or more formal classroom accommodations and modifications under 504 is a growing controversy.

In addition to IDEA and the IEP, there are also Section 504 protections and procedures established under the Rehabilitation Act of 1973, which is a philosophical spin-off of civil rights legislation of 1964 focused on issues of access. The 504 provisions cover individuals with a handicapping condition which "substantially limits" their ability to learn. Although there is potentially some overlap and variability, the 504 procedures are potentially less formal than the IDEA and IEP process. The IEP involves an administrative meeting and is regarded as the most typical avenue for receiving special educational services such as resource help, special class, and specialized interventions. In contrast, the 504 assessment can be very descriptive, and the meeting can be as casual as a conversation between a parent and teacher. However, the 504 process is designed to basically parallel the IEP process in terms of requirements for evaluation and placement, as well as a system of safeguards, for school children. Although it may be unclear that the 504 needs to be written, it would be prudent to do so to keep expectations clear. The interventions specified tend to be accommodations that might benefit the student, such as seating toward the front of the room, extra time on tests, or adjustments in homework. The 504 procedure is a way of intervening with students with learning differences or problems who do not necessarily meet the strict criteria for disability under IDEA and its related regulations. For example, children who have a processing disorder (such as auditory processing problems) but do not demonstrate a severe enough discrepancy to have learning disability might be covered under 504. Although some parents and schools prefer the 504 procedures because they can streamline getting help to a student without labeling them, clinicians often prefer the IEP process because it includes more procedural protections than 504, and students found to be disabled through the IEP process are automatically covered under 504. As a result, clinicians have incentives for evaluating students to determine whether they have learning disability or not and to pursue interventions (special services in addition to accommodations) through the IEP process. Although 504 procedures are thought of as less formal and interventions as less inclusive, like IDEA, 504's implementing regulations guarantee a Free Appropriate Public Education (FAPE) in the Least Restrictive Environment (LRE). An LRE is education that is provided to the maximum extent appropriate with nondisabled students. Affirmative services (such as speech therapy or even special placement) are also technically available through 504 procedures. Misunderstandings about the possible provisions of the 504 procedure may have sometimes blocked services for 504-only students, and perceptions of funding models may have, at times, favored the assignment of services through the IEP process and under IDEA.

Because IDEA is reauthorized and can be amended approximately every 5 years, the way learning disability is operationalized, assessed, and served can change. In addition, federal initiatives under NCLB, as well as ongoing state reform projects, may positively impact reading and math instruction in regular classes, thus decreasing pressure on special services. Although at one level, it may appear that funding needs for IDEA and NCLB are in competition, the climate created during debate regarding educational legislation may result in the improvement of services to all students and ultimately decrease the need to label students to get services. However, although this is the hope, there is also the possibility that if accountability efforts emphasize testing rather than remediation, administrators may respond to financial incentives in ways that worsen the situation of students with special needs.

At the time of this writing in 2004, the reauthorization of IDEA is under way. The passage of HR1350 (2003) and S1248 (2004) provides some information about what may be in store. These bills (and their amendments) need to be reconciled, and a final law actually passed by both houses of Congress. This could occur as early as the end of 2004. Alternatively, if the differences between the two bills cannot be reconciled, the reauthorization may not be completed in 2004, and the reauthorization process will have to start over. However, as the bills stand, the list of various qualifying disabilities (which includes "specific learning disabilities") and the general description of learning disabilities (which includes cognitive "perceptual disabilities") are the same as those in 1997. However, the language actually operationalizing a specific learning disability is different from that in 1997. These bills (HR1350/S1248) provide that the local educational agency (1) is not required to take into consideration whether a child has a severe discrepancy between achievement and intellectual ability in the previously specified seven academic areas, and (2) may use a process that determines if a child responds to scientific, research-based intervention. The current focus of professional discussion and debate around the educational trial as part of the IDEA operational definition of learning disability has been on reading, which is consistent with the focus of educational concern in NCLB. It should be noted that there are a number of uncertainties in all of this. First, until a law passes and federal regulations are framed, it is unclear what states and school systems will be responding to. Second, it will take time for the states and school systems to change their laws and policies in response to federal definitions and mandates. Third, these bills, at least in their current form, would allow educational agencies to choose to keep the discrepancy model or adopt the intervention model. It is also not impossible that some schools would elect a new and different model. However, in all this, it is entirely possible that some school systems would decide to keep the familiar discrepancy model. In the end, whether these bills find their way into law, their language may well frame future debate. However, until federal legislation is actually passed, and until rules and policies trickle down to the states and school systems, the "current" definition may be the "old" definition for some time.

Whatever the definition for learning disability, the *starting point* for obtaining services for any student with school problems is to request an evaluation in writing from their home school. If the client does not feel the IEP evaluation team's recommendations will meet their student's needs, they can appeal the findings through a fair hearing (and opportunity for mediation) process. If they disagree with the district's assessment, they may obtain an independent evaluation (before or after filing for fair hearing), which the district is required to consider and for which the district may be required to pay under certain circumstances. If you want your client to receive services through the public school system, it would help if you knew the current and local guidelines and procedures that might apply to their assessment, eligibility, and services. Parents and professionals may consult the UCLA/Wallis Foundation Learning Disabilities Web site for information on how to obtain services for children with learning disabilities and related disorders: http://www.learningdisabilities.ucla.edu. Readers who want information about this legislation and legal issues may consult http://www.napas.org or http://www.ldanatl.org. This discussion about educational law was prepared with the help of Maureen Graves, Attorney at Law. If you have a client for whom legal issues will probably be important in obtaining special education services through the school district, it would be prudent for them to consult an attorney or advocate. This discussion in no way constitutes legal advice.

spelling in and of itself can constitute a learning disability in writing. Regardless, problems with spelling can reflect serious difficulties with basic phonological skills or visual memory that typically manifest themselves in reading or other aspects of writing. In the context of identifying a learning disability, federal regulations list spelling and writing separately as skills that may be adversely affected by a processing disorder.

Comprehensive Achievement Tests The WIAT and the WJ-ACH allow for the systematic assessment of reading (basic word recognition/decoding and comprehension), mathematics (calculation and reasoning), and writing (brief to extensive composition), as well as spelling and other academic spheres. Each test has its strengths and weaknesses, and, often, most of one and portions of the other are included in an educational assessment. The WIAT has been conveniently divided into subtests that have separately assessed the learning disability areas, and the WJ-ACH also provides the information necessary to recognize learning disabilities. The WJ-ACH is a companion instrument to the Woodcock-Johnson Tests of Cognitive Abilities (WJ-COG), which tests processing skills and includes measures of intellectual ability. As individual achievement tests, both the WIAT and WJ-ACH are widely used in the community and schools. An additional comprehensive test is the Kaufman Test of Educational Achievement (KTEA), which is conormed with the Kaufman Assessment Battery for Children (KABC).

Other Achievement Tests These and additional achievement tests are also available and can involve general or specific assessment.

General Achievement Tests Some instruments focus on screening, such as the basic Wide Range Achievement Test, which includes spelling, arithmetic (calculation), and reading (word recognition). Others, such as the Peabody Individual Achievement Test, assess a range of academic areas in more depth. Some also focus on one area of achievement, usually reading.

Specific Reading Tests Because of the importance of reading in school and in life, particular effort has gone into systematically assessing reading skills and the ability to make symbolic associations between sights and sounds, as well as the ability to decode words and understand text. In addition to reading subtests on major achievement instruments, there are specific reading tests, such as the Gray Oral Reading Tests (GORT) and the Woodcock Reading Mastery Tests (WRMT). These instruments facilitate the pinpointing of the level and nature of the reading problems—for example, by presenting not only common words, but also nonsense words to assess decoding ability. In addition, because of the importance of phonological awareness in reading, tests of phonological strengths and weaknesses, such as the Comprehensive Test of Phonological Processing (CTOPP), are also often given. It is up to the psychologist to select the battery of instruments that best meets the needs of a particular student in any particular situation. It should be noted that, because achievement tests assess academic functioning in slightly different ways, psychologists often administer a combination of achievement tests to any one client. For example, reading comprehension might be assessed by asking a student to read a passage and supply a missing word or by asking a student to answer questions about a paragraph. The format of the test can influence how well a student does. How the student does in different contexts may help explain the nature of their academic problems.

General Comment It should be reiterated that learning "disabilities" are legal entities defined by federal regulations and state codes. In contrast, learning "disorders" are diagnoses made by mental health practitioners. However, any practitioner who wants public services for his or her client should be aware of the assessment procedures required in his or her client's particular case. This can involve who should do the assessment and how it should be done. For example, in the schools, learning disabilities have required the implication (implicitly or explicitly) of the processing problem contributing to the academic shortfall, whereas learning disorders have not. Learning disorders have involved the identification of unexpected underachievement in reading, mathematics, and written expression (or not otherwise specified) but not the specification of any contributing processing problem. In schools, at times the processing problem has been presumed after a process of elimination, but at other times it has needed to be established through evaluation.

Considerations Here are a number of issues mental health professionals should keep in mind in assessing achievement results:

- Although estimates vary greatly, it can be realistically to conservatively estimated that between 15 and 30 percent of children with attention-deficit/hyperactivity disorder (ADHD) have a learning disability and between 20 and 30 percent of children with a learning disability also have ADHD. As a result, when a clinician finds one condition, he or she should look for the other. Although they can cooccur, ADHD and learning disabilities are separate conditions requiring separate and specific interventions, one being potentially medical and the other educational.
- The vast majority of individuals with a learning disability have problems with reading (between 70 and 85 percent). Students who have learning issues in other academic areas commonly also have reading problems. Isolated learning disabilities in mathematics are much less frequent (perhaps 10 to 15 percent).
- There are a variety of reasons why there have been objections to using a discrepancy formula (between ability and achievement) in assessing learning disabilities. An important one is that it has been common for the identification of students with learning disabilities to be delayed into mid-elementary school, when earlier identification might have allowed for more preventive or effective work. But there are other issues. One is whether it makes sense to identify a child with superior intelligence but average achievement as learning disabled, even when there is a processing problem. Another is whether it makes sense to exclude slow learners who might need special supports.
- Although all schools must provide services to individuals identified as disabled, there are other populations who, despite being at an advantage, may still need help but are not protected by federal laws and regulations. Because giftedness is not a disability, it is not defined and covered under IDEA. There is, however, a federal definition of "gifted and talented" referring to high performance/achievement capability students who need services or activities "not ordinarily provided," and the federal government encourages their provision through state enrichment ("GATE") programs.
- If the definition of learning disability sounds complicated and convoluted, that is because it is. Many constituencies seek input into and have impact on descriptions and rules regarding learning disabilities. Relevant laws and policies can vary, for example, regarding the size of the ability–achievement discrepancy and whether an explanatory processing problem must be specified. It is hard to generalize, one can receive contradictory information, and procedures for special education eligibility can be complicated. Also, students can present with unique and pressing needs. Mental health professionals should know that parents can and often do seek legal consultation regarding eligibility and services. While the issue of reimbursement for the expenses of legal consultation and additional assessment is in flux, depending on how the laws are written, under some circumstances it will be possible to continue to receive

some financial relief when disputing eligibility and special educational services with a school system.

FURTHER ASSESSMENT When any academic problem is extreme or does not respond to appropriate intervention, further evaluation of the problem is in order. Reading problems in particular may need very careful evaluation regarding the basic processes that might underlie the difficulty. A language specialist who deals with reading issues or a neuropsychologist who might shed light on the pathways available or impaired in any student can perform this assessment.

Processing Assessment Processing tests are given, or information processing is analyzed, in a range of psychological evaluations. However, processing problems are discussed here primarily as they are related to psychoeducational assessment—that is, the problems are identified to help explain academic problems, to meet criteria for learning disability, or to help identify a student's learning style. In this case, it is a functional assessment. Processing problems can also be assessed from a neuropsychological point of view in which the problems are explored in an attempt to evaluate neurological integrity or to fine-tune understanding of specific domains of cognitive functioning. In this latter case, instruments are chosen and administered in a systematic way so as to evaluate the differential functioning of different systems in the brain. Both the psychoeducational assessment and the neuropsychological assessment are undertaken with a view to making recommendations. The psychoeducational assessment is a broad-band evaluation undertaken to recommend particular educational programs in the context of educational research. The neuropsychological assessment is a fine-tuned evaluation undertaken to describe particular adaptive strategies in the context of neurological research.

BACKGROUND Processing problems or disorders are often evaluated as a supplement to achievement testing. The evaluation is undertaken in an attempt to understand the factors that may be related to academic underachievement. The processing problems that might be evaluated as part of a psychoeducational assessment are diverse and not well defined. Even when schools have required an identified processing problem and specified a number of possibilities, an "other" category has often been included that allows for more descriptive than diagnostic procedures and language.

Processing disorders is the term often used by professionals to designate spheres of difficulty, such as specific perceptual inputs (visual, auditory) and expressive outputs (motor, vocal). The term processing disorder also includes difficulties in integrating information between two or more of these areas—for example, visual–motor dysfunction or sensory integration difficulties. The term processing disorder may also refer to particular functions, such as memory or attention, or other factors, such as organizational issues. Such processing problems can interfere with academic learning and even social interaction.

The term *processing* has been used in different ways in cognitive literature. However, the term is most often used in connection with auditory and visual input, as in "auditory processing disorder" or "visual processing disorder." In these cases, the professional is referring to the student's inability to make sense of the relevant input. These two areas of functioning are focused on because of their importance in the acquisition of basic academic skills.

Information processing can be relevant to not only specific academic performance, but also more general social functioning. Clinicians often distinguish between the child's ability to deal with ambiguous, as opposed to structured, situations or immediate problem solving, as opposed to past learning. Individuals with these kinds of problems often cannot get organized. For example, students who can adequately copy figures in separate boxes may have more difficulty when required to copy and organize several on one page.

ASSESSMENT Assessment of processing variables can be conceptualized in terms of different models using omnibus or specialized tests.

Comprehensive Processing Tests The NEPSY (a developmental neuropsychological assessment) is particularly useful as an instrument that allows for the systematic assessment of cognitive processing across a range of specific areas, including attention and executive, language, sensorimotor, visuospatial, and memory functioning. These are similar to the neuropsychological domains, but, in the context of cognitive or psychoeducational testing, they are handled in a descriptive way. The WJ-COG allows for the extensive assessment of processing across a diverse range of areas. Although it includes composite scores referring to intellectual ability, it is most often thought of as a processing test and is often administered in addition to a comprehensive intellectual test. The data are provided for individual subtests, as well as for informative composite scores.

Other Processing Tests In addition to these more general tests, there are other instruments designed to provide more specific assessments according to different ways of understanding processing.

Spheres Processing understood in terms of spheres refers to an input–output model dealing primarily with visual–motor or auditory–vocal systems. Testing involves the systematic presentation of auditory or visual stimuli, along with vocal or motor output. Such tests include the Test of Auditory-Perceptual Skills (TAPS) and the Test of Visual–Perceptual Skills (TVPS), as well as the Beery Developmental Test of Visual–Motor Integration (VMI).

Functions In addition, there may be other processing problems, perhaps having to do with attention or memory. As mentioned, the NEPSY includes measures of attention. The Wide Range Assessment of Memory and Learning (WRAML) is helpful in the systematic assessment of what children recollect.

Other Clinicians may identify processing problems regarding the integration of information according to an organizational model. In addition to factors such as fluid versus crystallized thinking, this might refer to the ability to process information presented in structured versus unstructured formats or situations. Although there is no real agreement regarding what these terms mean, relevant information is often gleaned from intellectual or more general processing instruments. For example, intellectual tests are often organized into verbal and nonverbal sections, thus affording opportunities to explore crystallized versus fluid thinking (including the WISC). However, a test like the new SB assesses fluid reasoning and crystallized ability in both the verbal and nonverbal spheres. Commonly, several instruments (general and specific) are used in concert to understand processing problems.

General Comment It should be noted that, although assessing processing is commonly part of a psychoeducational assessment, the extent to which the direct remediation of processing problems can benefit learning disabilities varies, and such interventions should be viewed with caution. Some previous research has been very disappointing. For example, according to Forness and colleagues in *Learning Disabilities and Related Disorders*, a review of 180 studies of visual– or perceptual–motor training for students with learning disabilities found the training to have no impact on basic academic skills, such as reading, mathematics, and writing. In fact, in almost half of the outcome measures, the students were worse off in basic skills than they had been before the training, probably due to lack of direct instruction in the areas of need. In addition, there was only a negligible direct effect on their visual– or perceptual–motor skills. Actual treatment (if it does not involve medication for attention) is apt to be linked to the academic area impacted by the processing difficulty. However, in contrast, recent studies linking the teaching of basic auditory processing and phonological skills in the context of reading programs are promising and leading to research-based intervention. In addition, simply describing a student's processing issues and how to work around them often helps teachers instruct students and parents manage and interact with their offspring.

Considerations These are some factors mental health professionals should keep in mind when considering processing problems:

- In the area of learning disability eligibility, whether or not a processing problem has to be specified in addition to an unexpected discrepancy between ability and achievement is subject to some uncertainty and debate. To a certain extent, this has to do with disagreements about whether a processing problem needs to be identified at all, whether it can be regarded as implicit in the academic shortfall, or whether it needs to be made explicit during the assessment. Although some argue that a processing problem is legally "necessary" because the federal definition emphasizes processing disorders as underlying learning disabilities, as a matter of fact, many states have not required a specified processing problem to establish eligibility for learning disability. Even when states have included processing disorder in their definition of learning disability, there has been a lack of classification criteria regarding the establishment of a processing disorder in eligibility determination. (See http://www.nrcld.org/html/research/states/.)
- It should be noted that, although public schools may require the specification of a processing problem to make the designation of a learning "disability," it is not required for the diagnosis of a learning "disorder" in hospitals and clinics. All the same, the revised fourth edition of the *Diagnostic and Statistical Manual of Mental Disorders* (DSM-IV-TR) indicates that there may be "underlying abnormalities in cognitive processing (such as deficits in visual perception, linguistic processes, attention or memory, or combination of these) that often precede or are associated with Learning Disorders." Because schools can require the identification of a processing problem in addition to a discrepancy between ability and achievement, it would be prudent to include comments about the processing issues that might be associated with any learning disorder.
- Problems with attention are commonly associated with learning problems. They can come into play in a variety of ways. They can be seen as the processing problem explaining academic shortfall in the discrepancy model of learning disability, or they can be seen as part of the diagnosis of ADHD, which could allow for eligibility under other health impairment (OHI). In some circumstances, students with attentional problems become qualified for services under emotional disturbance (ED), when they meet eligibility criteria under that category. The involved practitioners need to help the school system select the designation(s) that lead to the most appropriate interventions.
- It should be noted that the term *attentional problems* can be used diagnostically or descriptively. The fact that clinicians detect problems with attention on a student's individual intellectual or processing tests (including computerized instruments) does not mean that the student has ADHD. This is a clinical diagnosis that involves specific criteria, that is described behaviorally (inattention, hyperactivity and impulsivity), and is determined by history (symptoms before age 7 years) and current functioning (seen in two settings). Systematic assessment can help clarify issues around ADHD (and medication), but this will not be done with a single instrument and will require a pattern of responding on a selected group of tools along with interviews, observations, and, usually, rating scales from home and school.
- Commonly, processing problems are identified to help explain the discrepancy between ability and achievement in establishing current criteria for learning disability. However, significant scatter between tests and subtests suggesting perceptual or processing disorder may cast doubt on a composite intellectual score as accurately indicative of ability, suggesting the need for other ways of measuring potential. Or, some may argue (based on the reference to cognitive perceptual disability in the general definition of learning disability) that a child with a perceptual or processing disorder might be eligible for special education under learning disability on this basis alone. It should also be noted that some constituencies—for example, some colleges—may accept a processing disorder in and of itself as evidence of learning disability. In this context, it should be noted that, in public school systems, it is often up to the IEP team's discretion to decide which students might be identified as learning disabled and in need of services.
- Procedurally, in the current discrepancy model, processing problems do not come into play in identifying learning disability until two conditions have been met: (1) There is a severe discrepancy between intellectual ability and academic achievement, and (2) this discrepancy is not accounted for by one of several disabling conditions (such as visual, hearing, or motor impairment; mental retardation; emotional disturbance; or environmental, cultural, or economic disadvantage). Once these factors have been established, in some states, a processing problem is basically presumed (or bypassed) and a learning disability declared "by default." In other states, it is still necessary to identify the actual processing problem associated with the academic shortfall through separate assessment to identify learning disability.

FURTHER ASSESSMENT When processing problems are particularly severe or present a complicated pattern, further assessment may be in order. Neuropsychologists can fine-tune information about processing in a variety of spheres.

Conclusions A wide variety of intellectual, achievement, and processing tests have been explored as they apply to clarifying cognitive functioning in general and describing learning disability in particular. Despite the importance of establishing a learning disability in obtaining special educational services through schools, there are a variety of ambiguities and uncertainties in the whole assessment and identification process. Here, learning disability has been emphasized in terms of unexpected underachievement. In this context, although it is possible that the operational definition of learning disability may change, the notion of discrepancy (between what might have been anticipated and what has been accomplished) seems likely to be a unifying concept in describing learning disabilities over time (see Appendix).

Cognitive assessments tend to be practical events highly related to diagnoses and policies as defined by external groups. Psychoeducational assessment in particular should be pursued with an understanding of legal guidelines. As a result, learning disability has been discussed as it is operationally defined currently and may be defined in the future, along with basic information about how to obtain services (testing and intervention) through the school system. The reader should know, however, that educational assessment and educational therapy can be obtained in the community, but this is costly. In addition, because of the needs of children in school, even independent assessments are usually done with school policies in mind. If psychoeducational assessment involves legalities, neuropsychological assessment emphasizes science. However, all cognitive and neurocognitive applications are in flux—psychoeducational assessment because of shifting social and political forces and neuropsychological assessment because of technological and research advances.

As for Simon, his cognitive battery included the following instruments: an omnibus intellectual instrument and general achievement test, along with selected subtests and other reading tests, after decoding and comprehension problems were identified. The reading instruments included an oral reading test and test of phonological processing, as well as a visual–auditory subtest of a reading instrument. The visual–auditory subtest serves as an example of the kind of assessment done. It teaches the student a language composed of symbols that are then combined to relate a simple narrative; the subtest is an attempt to assess the student's ability to make sound–symbol associations, a capacity that is crucial in reading. In addition, tests of visual processing and visual–motor integration were done. This psychoeducational assessment was separate from the neuropsychological evaluation.

Focused Neuropsychological Assessment The field of neuropsychology was first developed by studying cognitive score patterns of adults with brain damage. Applying adult neuropsychological principles to children has not always been appropriate, however, and must be undertaken cautiously, given maturational differences and the ways in which children's behavior and understanding differ from those of adults. When children are evaluated from a neuropsychological point of view, issues regarding brain development, as well as test interpretation, must be considered.

The adult neuropsychological literature has been able to be quite specific about the organization and location of many functions in right-handed adults. Far less is known about early brain mapping in children. With the recent advent of functional magnetic resonance imaging (fMRI), however, developing behaviors can now be mapped, providing information on how the functional organization seen in most adults evolves. Recent studies have demonstrated that more generalized aspects of brain mapping are true for children and adults, whereas more distinct behaviors that are consistently found in specific cortical regions in adults are located in differing brain regions across children until late in adolescence.

These early studies demonstrate that it is not appropriate to assume that the patterns of brain mapping seen in most adults are also applicable to children. Thus, whereas the adult neuropsychological literature often attempts to answer the question "Where is it?" in describing cognitive impairment, with children, the questions are "How bad is it?" and "What can be done?" These differences between adult and child development affect interpretation of test results, diagnosis, treatment, and prognosis.

Neuropsychologists assess specific *domains* of behavior (such as memory). These domains represent cognitive systems that reflect both brain development (e.g., specific neural pathways or cortical location) and overt behavior. One goal of the neuropsychological examination is to examine the integrity and development of the component parts of a complex behavior. This analysis clarifies the issues driving breakdowns in complex behavior. For example, is a student's difficulty with mathematics due to an inability to do two calculations in his or her head simultaneously (working memory), or due to problems with seeing the differences between geometric designs (visual perception), or, perhaps, due to difficulties working with symbols (such as numbers)? The identification of the core deficits that underlie the larger academic or behavioral problem makes diagnosis and treatment far more clear.

Typically, in addition to assessing IQ, academic achievement, and social and emotional functioning, neuropsychologists assess domains of memory, attention, executive functioning, language, visual perception, and motor development. Tests have been developed to examine specific aspects of these domains in isolation so as to increase diagnostic clarity.

Although these domains are discussed as different constructs in this section, in truth, they overlap with one another in many different ways. For example, the term *working memory* is often conceptualized as being an aspect of attention, as well as a necessary component of good planning (which is part of executive functioning). It is also a component of memory in that, when it is not well developed, it leads to the phenomenon of "forgetfulness." Many of the measures used to discuss one of these constructs will also be used to discuss others. Additionally, neural substrates and pathways supporting their functions are often overlapping or, at least, parallel systems.

Thus, the interdependence of these domains is an assumption of this portion of the chapter. Each section will provide an overview of the theory supporting the conceptualization of the domains, followed by a description of the ways in which a neuropsychologist might assess them. The last section will address questions regarding the mapping of these functions in the brain.

Memory

OVERVIEW To memorize something, a person must, first, pay attention to it. Assuming that this attention is intact, the next step is to "make" the memory, or *encode* it. Once the memory has been made, however, it must be available on demand to be of use. Knowing the name of France's first president is of no benefit if you cannot *retrieve* it during the history examination.

A metaphor for this two-step memory process would be a filing cabinet. *Encoding*, then, is when a person puts information into the "filing drawer." Someone with a true amnestic disorder (such as Alzheimer's disease) never gets the information into the drawer. No amount of cueing or reminders will help the person recall the information, because it never "got into the drawer" in the first place. This type of impairment can be seen in some children, most often those with seizure disorders that adversely affect the temporal lobes. For most children, however, the problem described as "poor memory" is actually a difficulty with retrieval. *Retrieval* is the ability to get information out of the "file drawer" once it has been put in. Poor retrieval is associated with problems of organization (the folders are missing labels) and is more often the issue when children are described as being "forgetful."

To differentiate between encoding and retrieval, children are asked to memorize material and then, 20 to 30 minutes later, to recall it. If they are unable to remember it spontaneously, the examiner does not know if they have not encoded it or are just having problems with retrieval. If the child can remember the material with cueing (e.g., "In the story I read you, was the boy's name Johnny or Sam?"), retrieval is implicated. For the child who cannot encode, however, cueing will not help.

ASSESSMENT In assessing memory, several guidelines should be followed. Both visual and verbal memory tasks should be given. Visual memory tasks (such as learning location of dots or memory of faces) are usually aided by the right hemisphere. In most people, verbal memory tasks (such as memorizing a shopping list or a story) are supported by the left hemisphere. Additionally, material to be memorized should include rote tasks (such as word lists), as well as material that is presented in context (such as stories). Some memory tasks assess learning, or the child's ability to benefit from several presentations of the material. It is expected that, after three exposures to a picture of dots, the child's memory of it will be stronger than it was after the first exposure. If not, encoding may be implicated. A 20- to 30-minute delay should also be part of the memory assessment, and cues should be available to differentiate between encoding and retrieval difficulties.

Other terms in the neuropsychological literature appear to describe memory but are actually probably better classified as part of the attention system. These include *short-term memory* and *working memory*. These terms are discussed in the attention section below.

Attention

OVERVIEW The attention literature is large and includes many different conceptualizations. The following illustration demonstrates some elements of good attention.

Suppose you arrive at a lecture hall, open your notebook, and turn your attention onto the professor who is just beginning to speak rather than scanning the room indiscriminately (*selective attention*). The lecture is mildly interesting, and you are able to pay attention for the full 20-minute presentation (*sustained attention* or *vigilance*). At the same time that you are listening to the professor, you are taking handwritten notes incorporating headings and subheadings. It appears that you are able to simultaneously listen, write, and organize rather effortlessly, although you are probably shifting your attention between these competing tasks (*divided attention*). A fire engine goes by the lecture hall and you look up (*distraction*), but are then able to ignore the dimming noise of the siren (*inhibition*) and continue to listen to the lecture (again, sustained attention). Suddenly, the fire alarm rings, and you smell smoke. These distracters capture your full attention (*disengagement* from lecture), and their importance causes you to change your attention and behavior (*set shifting*) as you hurriedly head for the door.

A breakdown in any one of these areas can lead to a breakdown in attention. Some children are so caught up in their own private thoughts that they have difficulty disengaging from their inner musings, not realizing, for instance, that their babysitter is asking them a question. Or, once they are involved in a task, they have trouble switching to something new, causing them to "get stuck" or perseverate.

Another aspect of attention is *simple attention* (also called *short-term memory*). This is the ability to "hold" discrete items in storage for a brief period. Remembering a telephone number you have just looked up (while reaching for the phone to begin dialing) is an example of short-term memory. Poor short-term memory is a common complaint of people who have recently suffered a closed head injury.

Working memory is the ability to mentally manipulate information that is held in storage. This skill allows the person to hold some kinds of information "on-line" mentally while thinking about something else. Take, for example, the nurse who needs to remember that Johnny has the thermometer in his mouth and that she needs to get back to him and check it as soon as she finishes bandaging another boy's wound. If she moves onto yet another young patient without remembering to get Johnny's temperature, her problem would be with keeping one piece of information "alive" while thinking about something else. Students with poor working memory are the ones who are most often considered "forgetful," although, when cued, it is clear that they remember information, just not when they are supposed to.

The attention literature also discusses divided attention. This is the ability to pay attention to two things at the same time, although, in truth, a shifting of attention between two things is probably occurring. Good divided attention is important in multitasking. Some authors use the terms *divided attention* and *working memory* synonymously.

ASSESSMENT Assessment of attention requires a number of approaches. Children with attention problems exhibit them at home and at school whenever a task becomes less interesting to them. They function better when working one-on-one with a person or when working on a new activity, because it is more stimulating. For this reason, the testing environment may not elicit the inattentive behavior (especially on the first day). To assess the child's attention "in real life" and across settings, attention questionnaires should be completed by both parents and teachers. Many researchers consider this aspect of the assessment of attention to be the most important.

Some neuropsychological measures have been found to be sensitive to attention as well. Computerized measures of sustained attention that are designed to be long and boring can capture the loss of attention described above. Additionally, specific kinds of performance patterns on these measures have been shown to differentiate different types of attention problems.

Assessment of verbal short-term memory might include the repetition of digits or of short sentences. Assessment of visual short-term memory can be achieved by having the child point to dots or circles on the page in the same order in which the examiner has just pointed to them.

Working memory is usually assessed as the second part of a short-term memory test. It requires that the material that has been stored in short-term memory be manipulated in some way. Verbal working memory can be assessed by having the child repeat digits backward or by doing mathematics in his or her head. Saying the months of the year backward can also assess verbal working memory (as long as the child is able to give them in their usual order without difficulty). Having the child point to the dots on the page in the reverse order in which they are shown can assess visual working memory.

Divided attention is often assessed with dot-connecting tasks that require the child to "switch" between two competing demands (e.g., draw a line connecting 1 to A to 2 to B to 3, and so on). The ability to manage both the alphabet and the number system simultaneously requires divided attention.

Executive Functioning

OVERVIEW Executive functioning could be considered to be the mature product of good attention. Although not developed in earnest until children reach early adolescence, many aspects of executive functioning begin to appear when children are younger and, thus, can be measured. *Executive functioning* refers to the person's ability to organize his or her behaviors to perform a specific goal. Good executive functioning allows a person to identify problems, generate solutions, choose among them, follow through on the chosen strategy, and evaluate its effectiveness as the work progresses. Without good executive functioning, children who are bright have difficulty demonstrating their abilities. Their parents often report school underachievement that cannot be explained by learning problems. The issue is not about "knowledge," but rather the application of that knowledge to everyday functioning.

Martha Denckla attempts to illustrate this concept by describing a cook whose executive functioning is poor. She writes,

> Imagine an individual who is setting out to cook a certain dish, who has a well-equipped kitchen, including shelves stocked with all necessary ingredients, and who can even read the recipe in the cookbook. Now imagine, however, that this individual does not take from the shelves all the ingredients relevant to the recipe, does not turn on the oven in a timely fashion so as to have it at the proper heat when called for in the recipe, and has not defrosted the central ingredient. This individual can be observed dashing to shelves, searching for the spice next mentioned in the recipe, hurrying to defrost the meat and heat the oven out of sequence, and so forth. Despite possession of all equipment, ingredients, and recipe, this motivated but disheveled cook is unlikely to get dinner on the table at the appointed hour. This is the picture of the patient with "pure" [executive functioning] impairment: "a day late and a dollar short" in most of life's undertakings.

Several neuropsychologists are working to identify the factors that support good executive functioning. One model, put forth by Joaquín

Fuster, conceptualizes a two-component model. He suggests that the combination of inhibition and working memory are needed. Inhibition controls the amount of information that the working memory system (which is limited) must manage. In this model, irrelevant bits of information are ignored, thereby reserving the valuable space of the working memory ("temporary storage") system for more pertinent issues. This two-part model is assessed in measures of "planning."

Fuster's elegant model explains many behaviors associated with executive functioning, but other factors have also been proposed. For example, fluency, or the ability to generate many strategies, is necessary for good problem solving. Similarly, cognitive flexibility (e.g., set shifting) allows a person to switch strategies when one is not working. Perseveration on a wrong response keeps many children from reaching their goals.

ASSESSMENT Assessment of executive functioning requires several tests, given its many facets. Good attention and working memory, already discussed, are crucial to goal-directed behavior. Inhibition can be tested by giving the child a task in which he or she must control an automatic response. For example, on tests using the Stroop paradigm, the child is shown a color word printed in ink of a different color (e.g., the word "BLUE" written in red ink). The automatic response is to just read the word "BLUE," but this task requires that the child, instead, name the color of the ink. After several items, inhibition appears to tire, and children with poor impulse control perform worse than their peers do.

Fluency can be assessed by having the child generate category words under a time limit. For example, a child might be asked to name as many articles of clothing as he or she can in one minute. A variant of this task requires the child to create as many designs as he or she can in a 1-minute period, according to strict guidelines.

Cognitive flexibility is often tested with the Wisconsin Card Sorting Test (WCST), a measure of problem solving. On this test, the child is not told how to solve the puzzles; rather, he of she must use feedback that his or her attempts are "right" or "wrong" and is then expected to use this information to generate strategies. During the course of this test, the rules often change without warning, requiring that the child "regroup" and develop a new strategy. This measure generates information about the child's ability to initially figure out the task, his or her tendency to perseverate on wrong responses, and his or her ability to use feedback to generate new responses.

Planning is another aspect of executive functioning. Variants of a "tower" test are often used to assess this ability. On a tower test, the child is shown a picture with colored balls or disks stacked on top of one another on wooden pegs in a specific configuration. The child is told to move the balls or disks on the pegs to match the model. The child is instructed to move only one ball or disk at a time and to use as few moves as possible. To perform the task well, the child must first "hold back" and not make impulsive moves (thereby wasting moves). The child must also visualize the first few steps of the problem. Thus, both impulse control and visual working memory are required to exhibit good planning on this rather entertaining test.

Language

OVERVIEW Human language organizes, supports, and communicates knowledge, memories, and ideas. Although traditionally discussed in terms of left hemisphere functioning, much of the human cortex is involved in various aspects of language. Communication includes both *speech*, the rapid and complex motor movements involved in talking, and *language*, the code used to express thoughts and ideas.

Linguists conceptualize language as being composed of four separate parts: *phonemes*, defined as the smallest unit of sound in a language; *morphemes*, the smallest unit of meaning; *syntax* at the level of the sentence (for example, use of direct or indirect pronouns); and *discourse*, the stringing together of sentences to create a narrative.

In considering language, the most common distinction made is between *expressive* and *receptive* language. Expressive language requires the production of language, including articulating clearly, finding the right word, applying grammar and syntax to one's ideas, in addition to vocal fluency and voice tone (prosody). Receptive language involves the ability to comprehend and remember what is said.

Children with expressive language problems may appear to have little to say and are often considered to be shy. In fact, however, their difficulty may be with self-expression. Some children who are very talkative ("fluent") may also have difficulty with finding the word they want or organizing their sentences to make them clear. The paradox of a fluent child with an expressive language disorder may cause his or her problems to be overlooked.

Receptive language, or the ability to understand what is being said, represents another aspect of the language system. Children with poor receptive language have difficulty processing information that is spoken to them and may have difficulty learning in the classroom or appear to be inattentive. Sometimes they appear to be oppositional, because of their difficulty with understanding (and therefore *doing*) what they are told.

Secondary problems of children with language disorders include difficulties with social interactions and processing of emotions. Language is what humans use to interact and communicate their ideas to one another. When this ability is compromised, children may isolate or try to find less language-intense activities to occupy their time. Emotional problems may ensue from the child's difficulty with using language to express and, therefore, process his or her inner world. "Talk therapy" in which the child is provided with a quiet, safe environment to begin to practice speaking about his or her feelings and experiences can help address these issues.

ASSESSMENT Assessment of language should include several measures meant to identify the child's specific language profile. Tests should assess all levels of language, including phonemes, single words, simple phrases, complex sentences, and conversation. Measures of both expressive and receptive language should be included. In the assessment of receptive language, children are asked to distinguish between similar sounds and words, remember and repeat word lists, as well as related strings of words, and point to a picture that depicts a vocabulary word. In the assessment of expressive language, children are asked to perform tasks such as listing as many round objects as they can within a time limit, name a depicted or described item, or define words or concepts. In addition, the psychologist might explore *pragmatics*, which is the child's ability to participate in conversation and use social language. This involves the ability to interpret nonverbal aspects of communication, as well as observe basic social rules, such as turn-taking in conversation. Although neuropsychologists often evaluate pragmatics in addition to receptive and expressive language, they also work in concert with speech and language specialists when additional assessment is indicated.

Visuoperceptual Functioning

OVERVIEW There are several associated constructs in neuropsychology that reflect people's ability to make sense of what they see, to organize it, or to copy it. These abilities are referred to as *visuoperceptual–visuoconstructive abilities*.

Problems with *visuoperception* are distinct from problems with vision. A person with acute eyesight can struggle with perceptual difficulties, such as identifying which of several figures are exactly alike. Some children have difficulty seeing exactly where something is, and these children may have trouble localizing a point in space or judging the direction of a line. *Visuoconstruction* abilities allow a child to join parts to make a whole. These skills require the integration of the motor system with the visual system. Examples include the ability to put together blocks to form a design or to draw three lines to form a triangle.

Problems with visuoperceptual development have academic, as well as social, ramifications. Academic areas, such as mathematics, that are less reliant on verbal support are at risk. Additionally, concepts such as time and monetary values may not be clearly understood. Students with these difficulties often exhibit a poor sense of direction, and problems with integrating complex visual arrays may lead to feelings of being overwhelmed. They may also have difficulty "reading between the lines," thereby making comprehension of less tangible reading concepts (such as theme) more elusive.

Social problems are also often seen in students with these delays. Many elements of good social interactions are nonverbal, including the ability to notice and interpret gestures, facial expression, body posture, and tone of voice. Students with visuoperceptual delays may be overreliant on verbal information and may not understand when people are being sarcastic or when something is said in jest.

ASSESSMENT Assessment of visual processing must address each of the specific elements of this system. The visuoperceptual abilities should be tested using tasks that do not require the child to use his or her hands to produce the response—for example, activities that require the child to identify designs that match or differ from the target, as well as identify measures of mental rotation (which one is the same as the target, only rotated). Visuoconstruction tasks add the demand of integrating the hands and eyes in producing the response—for example, having the child draw copies of designs or use blocks to create a replica of a model.

Motor Functioning

OVERVIEW The motor system is also assessed as part of the neuropsychological examination. Lateralized motor problems suggest neurological problems on the opposite side of the brain and are often correlated with cognitive processes localized to the right or left hemisphere. Tasks requiring the integration of movements (such as shoelace tying or skipping) demonstrate the development of connections between the two hemispheres.

Large and fine motor development, as well as the ability to plan motor responses (praxis), are also assessed. Handedness is another aspect of the motor examination.

ASSESSMENT Both fine and large motor tests are usually assessed on both the right and left sides of the body. Having the child place pegs in holes with the dominant and then the nondominant hand often tests manual dexterity, and having the child demonstrate grip strength with each hand tests fine motor strength. Fingertip tapping is one way of testing motor sequencing, as is having the child repeat a sequence of movements from memory. Finger agnosia is tested by touching a finger when the child's hand is hidden behind a screen and then having them indicate which finger was touched. Handedness is best assessed by having the child do a number of tasks with one hand (e.g., "Show me how you use this spoon," "Hand me the dime," and "Throw me the ball.") in random order. Assessment of difficulties with motor planning can be done using pantomime. Having the child demonstrate gait while walking forward and backward, running, skipping, walking a straight line, and balancing on one foot tests large motor function. In cases in which the findings of this motor screening are significant, the neuropsychologist might refer the child to an occupational or physical therapist for further, more specific, evaluation.

Conclusions Neuropsychological testing is commonly undertaken according to several discrete domains that reflect areas of brain functioning. Typically, these include attention and executive functioning, memory, language, visuoperception, and motor functioning.

As for Simon, several domains needed to be assessed. Simon's attention and executive functioning had to be evaluated, given the vulnerability of these domains in children with ADHD or closed head injury. This assessment included giving behavior checklists to teachers and parents to determine the severity of the behavioral disruptions, in addition to testing and other procedures. A computerized continuous performance test provided information regarding Simon's ability to sustain his attention on a boring task. Measures of working memory evaluated Simon's capacity to hold mental information "on-line" while considering other aspects of the problem. Impulse control was tested with a number of measures that required the child to inhibit an automatic response. Tests of language and visuoperceptual abilities were administered to help lateralize brain-based difficulties, as well as determine underlying issues that might be driving any learning disorders. Language testing included single-word tests, as well as measures of more complex language. Elements of visuoperceptual testing included both a nonmotor, untimed visual matching test and a measure requiring the child to visually organize a figure that is being copied. Memory testing was very important, as a good memory is often how students with learning differences manage complex academic demands. By assessing verbal and visual memory systems separately, the psychologists were able to tell Simon's teachers which modality was the strongest, encouraging them to emphasize that approach when teaching him new concepts. Verbal memory was assessed with a multitrial list-learning test, as well as a test on which Simon had to memorize stories. Visual memory tests included measures requiring recall of spatial information as well as photographs of faces. Testing of right- and left-sided motor development added further information regarding lateralization of functioning, and a drawing test indicated how well Simon was integrating his visual and motor systems. Other motor testing included a pegboard placement test, informal measures of praxis, manual sequencing, and large motor tests. These instruments, together with information from the IQ test, achievement testing, and social–emotional testing, provided information about how Simon's neuropsychological functioning was impacting him intellectually, academically, and emotionally. The findings also provided information about his cognitive strengths and weaknesses that was useful in fine-tuning academic recommendations and identifying recommendations.

Brain Function and Assessment

So far, the emphasis in cognitive and neuropsychological assessment has been on functional description. In the case of general cognitive assessment, this is sufficient because of the emphasis on the practical description of problems and their solutions. However, in the case of neuropsychological assessment, the goal is ultimately to identify brain regions and pathways that might be associated with disruptions and to use this information to fine-tune diagnostic understanding and recommendations.

Cognitive Testing: Whole-Brain Constructs Many constructs evaluated in a psychoeducational assessment, such as intellectual and achievement functioning, are global in nature and, therefore, cannot be attributed to specific pathways or cortical regions in the brain. Something as broad as intelligence and as complex as an intellectual test might instead be seen as reflecting the integrity of a well-functioning CNS. Whereas some component aspects of intelligence have been mapped onto the brain with some reliability in adults, a broad construct such as intelligence is not limited to specific cortical regions. Rather, intelligence may reflect cerebral complexity demonstrated through numbers of synaptic connections, efficient cerebral organization, speed of processing (suggesting well-myelinated pathways), and well-developed supporting structures, such as glial cells. Similarly, constructs such as broad reading, mathematics, and writing also reflect complex neural systems. This level of behavior, which involves past learning and present performance, requires activation of multiple brain connections in concert with one another. In the case of processing tests, the ways they are constructed confounds attempts to relate them to brain functioning. Different subtests may have more relevance for specific neurological functioning than do others. Thus, the processing tests and tasks will vary in their ability to identify particular neuropsychological disruptions.

Neuropsychological Assessment: Mapping of Domains In contrast to more global constructs, the brain mapping of specific neuropsychological tasks is occurring in many laboratories around the world. This process has become far more precise with the addition of functional neuroimaging techniques such as positron emission tomography (PET) scans and fMRI. Functional neuroimaging research in mapping the development of these domains in children, however, has only recently become available. As early findings are reported, it is clear that many aspects of brain mapping occur in a developmental fashion, making the "location" of functions in the child's brain far less predictable than are those in the mature brain. As increased knowledge is gained about this process, however, it appears that more general aspects of adult brain organization (such as language in the left hemisphere, memory in posterior regions) are in place in children from an early age. More specific functions that have been mapped in the adult brain (such as single word processing) are not specifically localized in children, however. Thus, although brain mapping of functions in children is very much a work in progress at the time of this writing, a discussion of the mapping of functions in the adult brain may be helpful for the reader (Table 7.7–5).

Example in Developmental Neuropsychology: Reading The complexity of relating assessment results to brain functioning does not mean, however, that there is no place for neuropsychological investigation or brain mapping of broad cognitive domains, or that adult findings cannot be related to the development of skills in children. Part of the task seems to be to divide complex behaviors into their component parts and analyze the possible relationship between adult and child behavior. For example, researchers are trying to understand the development of reading ability. Poor phonological processing has been identified as the core deficit in most reading disabilities. fMRI with normal adult readers indicates that specific pathways (in the posterior left hemisphere) are involved in this skill. For adults with dyslexia, however, these pathways are minimally activated during reading. The fMRI data suggest that alternate pathways and cortical regions have assumed the task of recognizing words, resulting in less proficient reading skills. Although adults with dyslexia do learn to read, they process the words differently, resulting in more errors and slower speed.

A study using fMRI of two groups of 6- and 7-year-old children ("at risk" for dyslexia and "not at risk") showed that, even at this young age, different activation patterns during a letter-sound pronunciation test could distinguish the two groups. Consistent with findings seen in adult studies, children in the "at-risk" group exhibited reduced activity in the superior temporal gyrus and inferior parietal areas of the left hemisphere, as well as increased activation in the right hemisphere corresponding areas. This research demonstrates that the accessing of alternate (and apparently less efficient) neural pathways for core reading skills is present from a very young age. This finding makes early identification and treatment crucial.

Considerations In considering neuropsychological issues, the following factors should be kept in mind:

- After early brain injury, language and motor functioning are the most likely to benefit from "plasticity." Some research suggests that, with this process of reorganization, other functions (most notably, visuoperceptual abilities) may be "crowded out," yielding scores that are lower than expected.
- Interventions for neurologically driven developmental delays have their most profound effect on younger children. Recent studies have shown that, in children with reading disabilities, bilateral representation of language identified with fMRI before intervention shifted to the left hemisphere by several orders of magnitude in every subject after only 80 hours of reading intervention. These changes in the brain were accompanied by improved reading skills. Thus, the philosophy of delaying intervention until a deficit is fully expressed may keep children from receiving the full benefit that early intervention provides.
- Risk factors for reading disabilities include family history, early language delays, poor articulation, chronic ear infections, poor early rhyming abilities, inability to recite (not sing) the alphabet by the end of kindergarten, and early brain injury.
- "Ambidexterity" (consistently using the right hand for some specific tasks and the left hand for other specific tasks) often runs in families where several members are left-handed. In contrast, "ambiguous handedness" (or the use of either hand for the same task; sometimes writing with right hand, sometimes writing with left hand) can be a pathognomonic sign suggesting poor cerebral organization for specific behaviors.
- ADHD more adversely affects abilities typically associated with right hemisphere functioning (such as fine motor skills and visuoperceptual abilities) and impacts attention and executive functioning. Psychostimulant medication has been shown to improve functioning in all of these domains in children with ADHD.
- Both ADHD and autistic spectrum disorder demonstrate significant delays in executive functioning.

REPORTING RESULTS

Once the testing has been completed, the psychologist will report the results in oral and written form. Exactly how this will be done will be determined by the professionals and clients in any particular case. Particular emphasis is placed on the report, as it is the enduring record of the evaluation.

The report includes a list of instruments given and a description of the testing process and the client's behavior, as well as test results and their analysis. The format of the report depends on a variety of factors, including the reason for doing the testing and the audience likely to read the report. A general cognitive or psychoeducational report is commonly organized according to the types of instruments that are given (intellectual, achievement, processing), in addition to the diagnostic questions posed. A neuropsychological report is commonly organized according to the domains assessed (for example, memory, attention and executive function, and language) and how the result reflects on the referral questions. Given the current state of understanding of neurological functioning in children, both the cognitive and neuropsychological reports are likely to be descriptive. However,

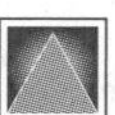

Table 7.7–5
Brain Mapping and Assessment

Although it is unclear how adult findings regarding brain mapping relate to children, the following may be informative.

Memory: There is considerable support for the role of the medial temporal lobe in memory functions. Encoding is thought to be subserved by the hippocampal formations, especially the entorhinal cortex. Other areas involved in memory include the amygdala (for emotional memories) and the mamillary bodies. Organizational aspects of memory, such as retrieval, however, involve circuits between the posterior and frontal regions of the brain.

Attention and Executive Functioning: Various sites in the frontal lobes, as well as in the posterior structures in the brain, activate during tasks of attention and executive functioning. Posner and his colleagues emphasize posterior regions in the initial, "orienting" phase of attention. His work identifies the three steps of orienting as *disengaging* from the current object of interest (superior parietal cortex), *scanning* the visual field for a new point of interest (superior colliculus), and then *amplifying the target* (pulvinar nucleus of the thalamus).

Aspects of executive functioning have been localized in the frontal lobes and, as attentional demands of a task increase, so does the area of involvement of the frontal activation. Orbital frontal regions of the brain are involved in inhibition and fluency. Dorsolateral prefrontal regions activate during tasks of working memory and cognitive set shifting. The anterior cingulate is activated during tasks that involve both perceptual demands and response selection. Posner's theory suggests that the anterior cingulate is the locus of communication for the posterior "orienting" system and the "executive attentional system" served by anterior regions of the brain. Additionally, an emerging body of research implicates the cerebellum in coordinating higher-level tasks.

Language: Most aspects of language are served by left hemisphere structures, but elements such as semantic processing and prosody are, at least in part, supported by the right hemisphere. Traditionally, anterior regions of the left hemisphere (centered by Broca's area) were associated with expressive language, and posterior regions (centered by Wernicke's area) were thought to serve receptive language. Positron emission topography (PET) and lesion studies, however, have corrected some traditional hypotheses and have specified the location of various aspects of language to a far greater degree. In these more recent studies, both cortical and subcortical regions that support language have been identified.

Although anterior regions (including Broca's region and Brodmann's area 22) are active in controlling articulated speech in normal adults, damage to posterior regions of the left hemisphere has a far greater impact on language overall. Additionally, specific left-sided nuclei of the thalamus (left ventrolateral and pulvinar) are associated with arrest of speed, problems with naming, slower speed of talking, and perseveration of speed. These subcortical regions may activate or arouse cortical language centers.

Other sites have been associated with language functioning as well. Expression of the same words on generation tasks activate two different pathways, depending on whether the subject is selecting responses for the first time (inferior frontal and posterior temporal cortex) or whether the word generation has been practiced and is, therefore, "automatic" (insular cortex).

Thus, although large regions of the cortex serve language functioning, some specific functions are represented by fairly precise loci in the brain.

Visuoperceptual Functioning: Visuoperceptual, visuospatial, and visuoconstructive abilities represent distinct domains of functioning, but are related by their reliance on interpretation and manipulation of visual stimuli. "Spatial cognition" is a category of abilities requiring that the spatial properties of a stimulus be manipulated or otherwise processed mentally. Tasks such as map-reading or mental rotation require spatial cognition, which is often assumed to be served by parietal cortex. Although left parietal cortex likely works with the right hemisphere to correctly image the stimulus mentally, right-sided inferior parietal regions are likely accessed to perform operations on this mental image. Thus, this region of the brain is probably involved in tasks such as map reading and navigation.

Visuoconstruction abilities require one to assemble, build, or draw a visually presented design and are likely served by posterior parietal cortex. This same region is involved in visuomotor guidance (such as reaching or grasping). Connections between the parietal lobes and prefrontal cortex also support visuomotor guidance. Additionally, projections from these two regions to paralimbic and temporal cortex (in addition to hippocampal and subcortical areas) illustrate the complexity and varied aspects of spatially guided behavior.

Motor Functioning: Most of the brain is involved in supporting motor functions and includes separate systems that serve whole-body, limb, and skilled hand and digit movements. The spinal cord and brainstem are primary aspects of both simple and complex movements (such as reflexes and sequencing of movement). Cortical areas are also involved, including motor cortex that works with sensory cortex in producing more complex and skilled movements. Subcortical regions, including the basal ganglia and cerebellum, provide appropriate force, timing, and execution of these skilled movements.

Conclusion: Again, the reader must be cautioned that it is not possible to transfer understanding of the adult brain to children. However, over time, through latency and adolescence, the neurological system seems to be sorting itself out into closer and closer approximations to the adult model. Progress is being made in the context of understanding broad constructs by breaking them down into component parts. In addition, progress is being made in relating a number of cognitive processes to brain function in children, as well as in adults.

there are times when a neuropsychologist is in a position to comment on brain function and its implications for prognosis and intervention.

Any report should be easy for the intended reader to understand. In assessing the value of any report, the referring professional should ask the following kinds of questions: Does the testing make sense in view of the referral questions? Do the results help describe the functioning of this particular client? Does the report integrate the test findings with known symptoms or behaviors? Is it clear what to do next?

It is not uncommon for test results to confirm suspicions or seem familiar in view of the way the referent understands the client. However, the results should help clarify diagnostic issues and describe the way this unique individual operates in the world.

Most reports include recommendations. It is the function of these suggestions to steer caretakers in the direction of strategies and specialists beneficial to the child. It is the recommendations that carry the message of hope that things can be different and situations can improve. Most parents are not as interested in what the problem is so much as what to do about it.

As for Simon, it turns out that his difficulties in school started in the fourth grade before the head injury or the loss of his grandfather. The history suggested that, in fact, he had been struggling in school for awhile, but the increasing demands of school in the third and fourth grades had taxed his academic and study skills. It was noted that the school curriculum usually shifts around the third grade from mastery of basic skills to higher academic applications in the fourth grade, such as reading chapter books or writing full (and working up to multiple) paragraphs. Simon had difficulty with this transition and, by November of that year, his struggles had become clear. In December, psychological assessment indicated a significant discrepancy between ability and achievement in basic reading skills and reading comprehension, as well as in written expression. (His mathematics was pretty good.) The assessment also indicated auditory processing problems and disorganization. These findings were consistent with those of the neuropsychological assessment, which had been under way since November.

Describing Simon's difficulties was relatively easy. Determining the etiology for Simon's disorganization and inattention, however, was more complex. Because both ADHD and closed head injury are associated with poor attention and problems with executive function, the questions facing the examiner were: (1) whether these behaviors predated the closed head injury and, thus, were part of an ADHD syndrome, (2) whether they were part of a postconcussive syndrome secondary to the "skateboard spill" and closed head injury alone, or (3) whether both ADHD and closed head injury were present and the head injury was exacerbating the ongoing inattentive symptoms and executive dysfunction. To clarify these diagnostic questions, the clinician needed to go beyond poor scores on tasks of attention and executive functioning found on testing and look to both individual and family history. Distinguishing features of these two disorders (ADHD and closed head injury) include history and course. By history, ADHD symptoms are present before age 7 years and tend to run in families. By course, symptoms of a postconcussive syndrome show rapid improvement just after the injury, whereas symptoms of ADHD are stable for longer periods of time, often gradually ameliorating with maturity. Additionally, other supportive findings (such as low Glasgow Coma Scale score or findings on neuroimaging) may be present if the head injury is of adequate severity to change cognitive functioning.

Examination of Simon's history indicated that symptoms of inattention, hyperactivity, and disorganization had been part of his presentation since he first entered pre-kindergarten and were also present in his brother and father (and paternal aunt). Additionally, retesting of executive functioning and inattention 4 months postinjury yielded similar results to those obtained shortly after his fall. The possibility remained that mild head injury may have exacerbated the attentional problems. However, given the family history and results of retesting, along with the lack of other neurological sequelae, the neuropsychologist's opinion was that Simon's inattentiveness and executive dysfunction were predominantly due to ADHD (which likely contributed to his reckless skateboarding behavior in the first place).

Ultimately, after the full cognitive and neuropsychological assessment, as well as the psychiatric (and in this case neurological) evaluation, Simon's underachievement in reading and writing did not seem to be caused by a head injury (which by itself might have qualified him for "other health impairment"). In addition, it could not be explained by a disabling condition or impairment such as mental retardation or emotional disturbance or attributed to environmental, cultural, or economic disadvantage. The underachievement seemed to be associated with processing problems, including making sense of auditory information in particular and disorganization in general. These data indicated that Simon could be labeled "learning disabled" and found eligible for school services under IDEA (and 504). It should be added that the data also indicated that Simon could be found eligible under "other health impairment" because of his ADHD. In some cases, students can be found eligible for services under more than one criterion. However, whether the student has one or two designations does not ordinarily matter. Once the student is found eligible for special educational services, his or her program should address all the difficulties impacting school performance.

Although these theoretical diagnostic issues might be complex, the recommendations regarding care and interventions were simpler. Part of Simon's management involved being closely followed by a psychiatrist, particularly regarding medication management for ADHD. However, much of his treatment was requested through the school system. At IEP, special services were requested, and he was found eligible under learning disability for resource help with reading and writing skills. Because his academic difficulties were in the area of language (and there was some evidence in the testing and presentation of possible language problems), further speech and language assessment was also recommended. Because of the nature of Simon's basic reading problems, a systematic (explicit) phonologically based program was recommended. In addition, classroom modifications and accommodations for his distractibility and organizational issues were recommended. These included seating Simon close to the front of the room and asking the teacher to cue him when necessary to keep him on task. The teacher was to work with the resource teacher regarding written assignments so that Simon would have extra time in resource room to craft short compositions. It was recommended that he have computer software available to help him outline and produce written work. The teacher was to also work with the parents to create a strategy to support homework completion. In retrospect, Simon's parents realized that the increased academic demands of the fourth grade had taxed Simon, causing him to dread school. The overall plan was to make the academic sphere more manageable and rewarding and to facilitate his learning.

Subsequent to the psychological testing and psychiatric evaluation, Simon's family was relieved that he was responding to the loss of the grandfather in a developmentally appropriate way. The family was especially relieved to learn that, in all probability, he had not been seriously injured in the skateboarding accident (but it did reinforce wearing safety gear!). However, they accepted the need to monitor his developmental progress and psychiatric interventions carefully over time. They read about ADHD and learning disability and felt better prepared to help their son at home. They also joined a parent training program to help them deal with Simon's behavior. Among other things, they learned to give short, clear requests as an adaptation to his problems with auditory processing. The parents were made aware of two other possible interventions they could access in the future if problems persisted. These included a social skills group to help him make friends and educational therapy to teach him organizational skills. They also assisted him in developing organizational strategies at home, including helping him find permanent places for his backpack, his baseball cap, and the puppy's leash.

Conclusions It is the role of all cognitive testing to systematically evaluate how well clients take in information (input) and demonstrate understanding (output), as well as the (invisible) processing in between. Neuropsychological testing attempts to relate behavior to brain function, whereas more general cognitive testing remains more narrative. However, because of uncertainties regarding brain maturation and neurological development in children, all cognitive and neuropsychological testing remains largely descriptive. The hope is that by comparing one child to others or one function to others, professionals have a better sense of the ability of their client to adapt to a complex world.

Because children are constantly changing and growing, cognitive and neuropsychological assessment is often undertaken over time, with measurements being taken on a regular basis. In this case, the professional is not interested in just their level, but also the rate of change. It is factors like this that will help psychiatrists and other mental health professionals get a better sense of their client's prognosis and to formulate successive interventions to maximize the client's potential in life.

SUGGESTED CROSS-REFERENCES

Chapter 2 discusses clinical assessment and approaches to diagnosis in neuropsychiatry. Section 5.2 presents statistics and experimental design. Chapter 8 discusses theories of personality that are derived from philosophy and psychology. Section 7.1 discusses the psychiatric interview, history, and mental status examination. Section 7.5 covers neuropsychological assessment of adults, and Section 7.6 discusses personality assessment of adults and children. Cognitive therapy is presented in Section 30.6. See also Chapter 35 on learning disorders for an extensive description of problems in reading, mathematics, and written expression. Section 49.12 covers school consultation.

References

Aman CJ, Roberts RJ, Pennington BF: A neuropsychological examination of the underlying deficit in attention deficit hyperactivity disorder: frontal lobe versus right parietal lobe theories. *Dev Psychol.* 1998;34:956.

Balsamo LM, Xu B, Grandin CB, Petrella JR, Braniecki SH, Elliott TK, Gaillard WD: A functional magnetic resonance imaging study of left hemisphere language dominance in children. *Arch Neurol.* 2002;59:1168.

Baron IS. *Neuropsychological Evaluation of the Child.* New York: Oxford; 2004.

Baron IS, Fennel EB, Boeller KKS. *Pediatric Neuropsychology in the Medical Setting.* New York: Oxford; 1995.

Denckla MB. A theory and model of executive function: a neuropsychological perspective. In: Lyon GR, Krasnegor NA. *Attention, Memory, and Executive Function.* Baltimore: Paul H Brookes; 1996.

Forness SR, Sinclair E, Jura M, McCracken J, Cadigan J. *Learning Disabilities and Related Disorders.* Los Angeles: UCLA Wallis Foundation; 2002.

Fuster JM. *The Prefrontal Cortex: Anatomy, Physiology, and Neuropsychology of the Frontal Lobe.* Philadelphia: Lippincott-Raven; 1997.

Kavale KA, Forness SR. *The Nature of Learning Disabilities: Critical Elements of Diagnosis and Classification.* Hillsdale, NJ: Erlbaum; 1995.

*Kolb B, Whishaw IQ. *Fundamentals of Human Neuropsychology.* New York: W.H. Freeman; 1996.

LeFever LE. *Adult Attention Deficit Disorder: Brain Mechanisms and Life Outcomes.* New York: New York Academy of Sciences; 2001.

*Lezak, MD, Howieson DB, Loring DW, Hannay HJ, Fischer JS. *Neuropsychological Assessment.* 4th ed. New York: Oxford; 2004.

Mirsky AF, Duncan CC. A nosology of disorders of attention. In: Wasserstein J, Wolf LE, Papanicolau AC, Simos PG, Breier JI, Fletcher JM, Foorman BR, Francis D, Castillo EM, Davis RN: Brain mechanisms for reading in children with and without dyslexia: a review of studies of normal development and plasticity. *Dev Neuropsychol.* 2003;24:593–612.

Pennington BF, Ozonoff S: Executive functions and developmental psychopathology. *J Child Psychol Psychiatry.* 1996;37:51.

Posner MI, Raichle ME. *Images of Mind.* New York: Henry Holt; 1996.

*Sattler JM. *Assessment of Children: Cognitive Applications.* San Diego, CA: Jerome M. Sattler; 2001.

Schlagger BL, Brown TT, Lugar HM, Visscher KM, Miezin FM, Petersen SE: Functional neuroanatomical differences between adults and school-age children in the processing of single words. *Science.* 2002;296(5572):1408.

*Shapiro BK, Accardo PJ, Capute AJ. *Specific Reading Disability: A View of the Spectrum.* Timonium, MD: York; 1998.

Simos PG, Fletcher JM, Foorman BR, Francis DF, Castillo EM, Davis RN, Fitzgerald M, Mathes PG, Denton C, Papanicolau AC: Brain activation profiles during the early stages of reading acquisition. *J Child Neurol.* 2002;17:159–163.

Simos PG, Fletcher JM, Bergman E, Breier JI, Foorman BR, Castillo EM, Davis RN, Fitzgerald M, Papanicolaou AC: Dyslexia-specific brain activation profile becomes normal following successful remedial training. *Neurology.* 2002;58:1203.

Stiles J, Moses P, Passarotti A, Dick FK, Buxton R: Exploring developmental change in the neuronal bases of higher cognitive functions: the promise of functional magnetic resonance imaging. *Dev Neuropsychol.* 2003;24:641–668.

*Yeates KO, Ris MD, Taylor HG. *Pediatric Neuropsychology: Research, Theory, and Practice.* New York: Guilford Press; 2000.

APPENDIX

What Is a Learning Disability?

Despite all the talk about *specific learning disabilities*, the meaning of the term itself is not specific! When a parent says that his or her young child has a learning disability, the parent may as well be talking about attentional problems as academic failure. However, among professionals, *learning disability*, in its simplest form, is defined as unexpected underachievement. While there is some variability and difference of opinion, the concept of *discrepancy* is at the heart of most definitions. Although the legal guidelines operationalizing learning disability are currently being reconsidered, the term will almost certainly include two concepts: (1) the learning disability is specific because it is not explained by overall low intellectual functioning (for example, mental retardation), and (2) the learning disability is not primarily the result of physical or emotional disabilities or other disadvantage (for example, limitations in English proficiency). All the same, although it has been presumed that learning disabilities are due to neurologically based processing problems, currently it is recognized that they involve the interaction of constitutional and environmental factors that are not yet well understood.

In thinking about learning disability, one might consider the following possible discrepancies:

Academic achievement is significantly below estimated ability.

Academic achievement is significantly below national norms.

Significant test scatter suggests perceptual or processing problem or disorder.

A fourth might be considered that is somewhat different but related to the above discrepancies:

There is a notable discrepancy between this child's response (and that of other students) to appropriate scientific research-based intervention in an important area of learning, such as reading.

Especially with the changes in the law, it is difficult to know which of these discrepancies might be important in establishing the diagnosis of a learning disability, but the concept of discrepancy will almost certainly remain implicitly or explicitly in any definition of learning disability.

Currently, especially when making an official diagnosis of learning disability around the issue of eligibility for special educational services, the concept of discrepancy is a necessary but not sufficient condition for the label. There may be inclusionary or exclusionary criteria that would need to be explored. However, even when using the term *learning disability* or *difference* in a less official and more descriptive way, noting a discrepancy is just the starting point in exploring why the student is having learning problems.

Whatever the outcome of national legislation around learning disabilities or school policies around criteria for the diagnosis, different professionals will use the terms *learning disability* and *specific learning disability* to note that the child in question has a discrepancy between his or her actual performance and what one would have predicted based on the child's capacities and experiences—that is, the discrepancy is unexpected and needs to be explained.

Failure in any of the four previously listed categories would require understanding and, possibly, intervention. The legal definition of learning disability and specific learning disability, and a school system's policies, would only determine whether the student would be protected as disabled under the Individuals with Disabilities Education Act (IDEA) and entitled to special educational services through school. However, even students who did not qualify under IDEA might qualify for support under 504.

Keep in mind that, because of the long history in which learning disability has been defined in terms of a discrepancy between ability and achievement (and potentially the processing problem to explain it), much educational research done in this area will have been designed and interpreted in this context. Although, in the future, national legislation may not require a discrepancy between ability and achievement to establish a learning disability, it will be some time before state and local guidelines change. Further, parents and teachers will always think of learning difficulties in the context of a student's reaching his or her academic potential. In addition, whatever the legal definitions of learning disability and specific learning disability, mental health professionals will always want to understand the functioning of any child with school problems as well as possible to determine treatment. This should involve measures of intelligence, achievement, and processing, including neurocognitive functioning in complex cases.

▲ 7.8 Medical Assessment and Laboratory Testing in Psychiatry

BARRY H. GUZE, M.D., AND MARTHA JAMES LOVE, M.D., J.D.

The goal of this section is to outline the basic imaging studies, laboratory tests, and other tools of medical assessment applicable to psychiatric practice and the strategies for using them in an effective manner. In addition to reviewing imaging studies and the role of the electroencephalogram (EEG), various biochemical, hematological, endocrine, immunological, and toxicological assessments are discussed. A logical and systematic approach to the use of these tools by the psychiatrist is vital to achieving the goals of arriving at accurate diagnoses, implementing appropriate treatment, and delivering cost-effective care. Although this section guides the clinician in the use of many relevant tests, some of these tests are designed to diagnose or to manage medical, rather than psychiatric, disease. With respect to the diagnosis or management of medical disease, consultation with colleagues in other specialties is important. Medical specialists also are a useful source of information about test methodology and the proper performance and interpretation of tests. Analogous consultation with appropriate specialists is important when ordering nonlaboratory tests such as the EEG, electrocardiogram (ECG), and neuroimaging. Good clinicians recognize the limits of their expertise and the need for consultation with their nonpsychiatric colleagues.

Physicians are accustomed to ordering tests. Before ordering any test, it is always worthwhile to review how this test will alter patient management. If the test results will not alter management, the test is unlikely to be relevant to the patient's current care.

Despite increasing pressure to deliver cost-effective care, many clinicians still order a large number of screening laboratory and other studies. The lack of consensus regarding optimal patient workup may contribute to this tendency. Increasingly, however, clinicians are becoming more selective in ordering tests. Requested studies are chosen because of clinical hypotheses based on a particular patient's clinical data. This selective approach minimizes the ordering of unnecessary studies and tests. Such an approach often uses a narrow selection of routine screening tests. Later, clinicians order nonroutine, additional tests as necessary or based on the results of screening tests or particular findings on examination. The psychiatric literature contains no consensus regarding the optimal battery of screening laboratory and other studies. Few would disagree that the best screening evaluation includes a good history and physical examination, including a neurological examination and mental status examination. Excessive testing yields unnecessary costs, as well as unnecessary discomfort and inconvenience to the patient. False-positive results may lead to additional unnecessary testing. Yet, ordering an insufficient number of tests is also not without risk: Significant illness may go unrecognized and untreated.

Psychiatrists use diagnostic testing to identify possible nonpsychiatric medical illnesses that may cause or contribute to a patient's clinical presentation. Such testing occurs within the context of the history of the present illness, the physical examination, and the review of systems. Other tests are specific to psychiatry. For example, the measurement of blood levels of psychotropic medications can be useful to determine the adequacy of dosing or to monitor compliance. In addition, many tests, such as liver function tests, white blood cell count (WBC), and serum glucose, are performed to monitor the consequences of treatment of psychiatric illness. Furthermore, psychiatrists often treat patients who abuse illicit substances. Because histories of alcohol and drug use are often unreliable, laboratory detection of substances of abuse is helpful. For patients known to abuse substances, additional testing may be performed to assess the consequences of a patient's substance abuse.

Many medical illnesses produce psychiatric symptoms. Symptoms such as delirium, anxiety, depression, and hallucinations are nonspecific. To be certain that a patient's symptoms are due to a mental illness, potential physical causes must first be excluded. This assessment is not performed in a vacuum but occurs in the context of the patient's medical history and physical examination. Laboratory studies supplement the history and examination. The goal of the assessment is to identify causative factors that contribute to the patient's current symptoms. When psychiatric symptoms are found to be due to a general medical condition, initial efforts are focused on the treatment of the underlying condition. For many patients, treatment of the underlying medical condition results in a resolution of psychiatric symptoms. In addition, the diagnostic criteria for many psychiatric conditions, as listed in the revised fourth edition of the *Diagnostic and Statistical Manual of Mental Disorders* (DSM-IV-TR), exclude symptoms attributable to a general medical condition or substance abuse.

In addition to ordering diagnostic studies, psychiatrists increasingly use laboratory testing to establish that administration of a particular treatment is safe before its initiation and to monitor the ongoing safety of specific treatments. For example, "baseline" laboratory studies may be obtained before the initiation of particular psychotropic medications. Testing may also be used to monitor compliance, measure therapeutic concentrations, and assess toxicity. Many psychotropic medications may have significant effects on physical health. For this reason, a psychiatrist may perform a pretreatment assessment of a patient's general health before initiating treatment. This assessment commonly includes a variety of laboratory tests.

Finally, there is a widely held hope that biological markers for major mental illnesses will be identified in the future and will eventually be of assistance in the diagnosis and selection of treatment. Unfortunately, research has not yet identified such markers. Nonetheless, the ongoing search for biological markers furthers understanding of the pathophysiology of major mental illnesses and continues to enhance clinical psychiatric practice.

ROLE OF THE HISTORY AND PHYSICAL EXAMINATION

A thorough history, including a review of systems, is the basis for a comprehensive patient assessment. The history often guides the clinician in the selection of laboratory studies that are relevant for a specific patient. However, many psychiatric patients, owing to their illnesses, are not capable of providing sufficiently detailed information. Collateral sources of information, including family members and prior clinicians and their medical records, may be particularly helpful in the assessment of such patients.

The history of present illness includes the chief complaint (or the reason the patient seeks assistance), the nature of the current problems, and their current treatments. The past psychiatric history should include information about previous psychiatric problems and a history of prior treatments. It should contain the medications used to treat the patient, the doses prescribed, and the durations of each medication trial. The past psychiatric history should also contain documentation of dates and locations of past psychiatric admissions, the reason for admission, and the treatments provided. If the patient reports an allergy to a specific medication, the nature of the allergic response should be noted.

The patient's medical history is an important component of the history. It should include notation of prior injuries and, in particular, head injuries that resulted in loss of consciousness and other causes of unconsciousness. The patient's medical history also should note pain conditions, ongoing medical problems, prior hospitalizations, and prior surgeries. The history should also include a list of the patient's current medications. Toxic exposures are another important component of the medical history. Such exposures are often workplace related.

The social history contains many of the details relevant to the assessment of character pathology, including risk factors for personality disorders. Commonly, the social history also includes an occupational history. The clinician should take a thorough history of alcohol and substance use. History of the use of substances, illicit and prescribed, should contain information regarding the timing of the initiation of use, the frequency of use, the quantity used, and the date of last use for each substance. A thorough review of symptoms should be performed. Unrecognized medical conditions are often detected during the review of systems.

Although many psychiatrists perform physical examinations on their patients, it is not uncommon in some community and institutional settings for other physicians to perform the physical examination after the psychiatrist obtains the history. Under certain clinical scenarios, it is appropriate to postpone the physical examination. Examples include the agitated or aggressive patient. Examinations should be postponed only after consideration of the risks and benefits to the patient. Such deferments should be for as brief a time as possible. As a general rule, it is often wise to have a chaperone present during the physical examination.

IMAGING OF THE CENTRAL NERVOUS SYSTEM

Imaging of the central nervous system (CNS) can be broadly divided into two domains: structural and functional. Structural imaging provides detailed, noninvasive visualization of the morphology of the brain. Functional imaging provides a visualization of the spatial distribution of specific biochemical processes. Structural imaging includes X-ray computed tomography (CT) and magnetic resonance imaging (MRI). Functional imaging includes positron emission tomography (PET), single photon emission computed tomography (SPECT), functional MRI (fMRI), and magnetic resonance spectroscopy (MRS). With the limited exception of PET scanning, functional imaging techniques are still research tools that are not yet ready for routine clinical use.

A common clinical dilemma involves whether to obtain an MRI or a CT scan. CT scans usually are less expensive and more commonly available. Although CT scans are a relatively inexpensive screening examination, most clinicians have a hypothesis-based approach to the selection of an imaging modality: The question they need answered drives the selection of the scan. The following sections provide some guidance regarding the relative advantages of MRI scans and CT scans.

Currently, the use of structural imaging techniques is limited to the identification of nonpsychiatric disease. Scans are performed when a clinician suspects or seeks to rule out a nonpsychiatric illness. Attempts to use structural imaging techniques to subcategorize various psychiatric illnesses have not yielded data that are useful in clinical practice. Consequently, structural imaging techniques are not useful for making psychiatric diagnoses.

Magnetic Resonance Imaging

MRI scans are used to distinguish structural brain abnormalities that may be associated with a patient's behavioral changes. These studies provide the clinician with images of anatomical structures viewed from cross-sectional, coronal, or oblique perspectives. MRI scans can detect a large variety of structural abnormalities. The MRI is particularly useful in examining the temporal lobes, the cerebellum, and deep subcortical structures. It is unique in its ability to identify periventricular white matter hyperintensities. MRI scans are useful in examining the patient for particular diseases, such as nonmeningeal neoplasms, vascular malformations, seizure foci, demyelinating disorders, neurodegenerative disorders, and infarctions. The advantages of MRI include the absence of ionizing radiation and the absence of iodine-based contrast agents. Contrast agents are based on gadolinium, a rare earth metal, and usually do not provoke an allergic response.

MRI scans are not always obtained with the same parameters. The nature of the scan is modified in a manner that is most likely to help provide data relevant to the clinical hypothesis that generated the request for the scan. For this reason, clinicians should provide the radiologist with clear, concise indications for the scan. Scan parameters include modes referred to as T1 and T2. T1-weighted scans provide detailed visualizations of brain anatomy. Extracellular fluid, such as edema, looks dark. In contrast, T2-weighted scans reveal a white pattern for edema. These scans are useful in examining the patient for white matter disease.

MRI scans are contraindicated when the patient has a pacemaker, aneurysm clips, or ferromagnetic foreign bodies.

Computed Tomography

CT scans are used to identify structural brain abnormalities that may contribute to a patient's behavioral abnormalities. These studies provide the clinician with cross-sectional X-ray images of the brain. CT scans can detect a large variety of structural abnormalities in the cortical and subcortical regions of the brain. Commonly, clinicians who request a CT scan are looking for evidence of a stroke, subdural hematoma, tumor, or abscess. These studies also permit visualization of skull fractures. CT scans are the preferred modality when there is suspicion of a meningeal tumor, calcified lesions, acute subarachnoid or parenchymal hemorrhage, or acute parenchymal infarction. CT scans have some resolution limits in the posterior fossa and the inferior surfaces of the temporal lobes owing to artifacts created by the skull. These scans are not as successful in detecting focal gliosis as the MRI scans.

CT scans may be performed with or without contrast. The purpose of contrast is to enhance the visualization of diseases that alter the blood–brain barrier, such as tumors, strokes, abscesses, and other infections. Contrast is administered intravenously (IV). Allergic reactions to contrast may occur and can include an anaphylactic reaction with cardiovascular collapse. This type of reaction most commonly occurs in patients with asthma or allergies to seafood.

Indications for a CT scan are not agreed upon in the literature. Less controversial indications commonly include focal findings on the neurological examination or abnormalities on an EEG. Slightly more controversial indications include impaired cognition on the mental status examination, the first episode of psychosis (especially if the presentation is atypical), delirium, late-onset (after 50 years of age) personality disorders, psychosis, or affective illness. Prolonged catatonia is also a possible indication.

Positron Emission Tomography

PET is performed predominately at university medical centers. PET scans require a PET tomograph (the scanner) and a cyclotron to create the relevant isotopes. This type of scan involves the detection and measurement of emitted positron radiation after the injection of a compound that has been tagged with an positron emitting isotope. Typically, PET scans use fluorodeoxyglucose (FDG) to measure regional brain glucose metabolism. Glucose is the principal energy source for the brain. These scans can provide information about the relative activation of brain regions, because regional glucose metabolism is directly proportionate to neuronal activity. Brain FDG scans are useful in the differential diagnosis of dementing disease. The most consistent finding in the PET literature is the pattern of temporal-parietal glucose hypometabolism in patients with Alzheimer's type dementia.

Standard laboratory studies commonly assessed in dementia patients include a complete blood count (CBC), serum electrolytes, liver function tests, blood urea nitrogen (BUN), creatinine (Cr), thyroid function tests, serum B_{12} and folate levels, Venereal Disease Research Laboratory (VDRL) test, and a urinalysis. Often, a CT scan is performed if there are focal neurological findings, and an EEG may be performed if there is a delirium.

By using other compounds and, in some cases, other isotopes, it is possible to use PET scanning to measure regional cerebral blood flow, oxygen use, and binding parameters of pharmaceutical agents that attach to specific neurotransmitter receptor sites. The usefulness of PET scans remains limited to use in research studies.

Single Photon Emission Computed Tomography

SPECT is commonly available in most hospitals but is rarely used to study the brain. SPECT is more commonly used to study other organs, such as the heart or liver and spleen. SPECT scans are performed using a dedicated tomographic camera to detect radiation emitted from a patient after the injection of radiolabeled compounds. Some compounds used to measure brain blood flow are commercially available. These compounds have been used with SPECT scanners to measure blood flow in dementia patients in whom a pattern of reduced temporal-parietal blood flow is found.

Functional Magnetic Resonance Imaging

fMRI is a research scan used to measure regional cerebral blood flow. Often, fMRI data are superimposed on conventional MRI images, resulting in detailed brain maps of brain structure and function. The measurement of blood flow involves the clever use of the heme molecule as an endogenous contrast agent. The rate of flow of heme molecules can be measured, resulting in an assessment of regional cerebral metabolism. These scans are performed in high–field strength magnets that are not usually found outside of university research settings.

Magnetic Resonance Spectroscopy

MRS is another research method to measure regional brain metabolism. MRS scans are performed on conventional MRI devices that have had specific upgrades to their hardware and software. The upgrades permit the signal from protons to be suppressed and other compounds to be measured. (Conventional MRI images are, in reality, a map of the spatial distribution of protons found in water and fat.) The abundance of these nonprotonated compounds can be measured, yielding a quantitative assessment of a multitude of neurochemical compounds. MRS is able to measure compounds tagged with nonradioactive isotopes of hydrogen, phosphorus, lithium, sodium, and fluorine.

Magnetic Resonance Angiography

Magnetic resonance angiography (MRA) is a clever method for creating three-dimensional maps of cerebral blood flow. Exogenous contrast agents are not necessary. Instead, the effect of the iron atom in the hemoglobin molecule is used as an endogenous contrast agent. Psychiatrists rarely order this test. Neurologists and neurosurgeons more commonly use it.

ELECTROENCEPHALOGRAM

The EEG is the assessment of regional cerebral cortical electrical activity. Clinical neuroscience has a long history of using the EEG. The EEG can be used in different ways to study specific brain states or activities by modifications to the technique of data collection or to the data itself. EEG data can be displayed on paper tracings in the manner of conventional EEG recordings. Alternatively, the data can be digitized, and the digitized data can be transformed, often using a Fourier transformation, to yield color-coded topographic brain maps of regional activity. The collection periods can be prolonged, and the data can be electronically displayed along with video monitoring of the patient to provide telemetry assessments of patients with epilepsy for whom an attempt is made to correlate behavioral abnormalities with brain electrical activity as part of the workup of seizure disorders. Prolonged periods of EEG recording during sleep, when coupled with recording of a limited lead ECG and facial muscle activity, result in the sleep EEG or polysomnography. EEG also is used by many clinicians to monitor electroconvulsive therapy (ECT) administration.

Clinicians use the EEG to localize seizure foci and to evaluate delirium. The EEG and its topographic descendants have not found a clear role in the diagnostic assessment of psychiatric patients. The EEG is usually used in psychiatry to rule out nonpsychiatric disease, such as seizure disorders or delirium, as a cause of psychiatric symptoms. When the differential diagnosis includes strokes, tumors, subdural hematomas, or dementia, the yield is usually higher with imaging tests. Not surprisingly, the yield is highest in patients with a history of a seizure disorder or a clinical history that is strongly suggestive of a recent seizure or other organic illness. Such clinical features would include a history of altered consciousness, atypical hallucinations (e.g., olfactory), head injury, and automatism. In addition, the EEG is commonly obtained when there is an abnormal CT or MRI. It is important to remember that seizures are a clinical diagnosis; a normal EEG does not rule out the possibility of a seizure disorder.

When a conventional EEG does not demonstrate the dysrhythmia (abnormal bursts of spike, sharp wave, or slow activity) associated with seizures, other measures can be taken to enhance the sensitivity of the evaluation. These measures include sleep deprivation, hyperventilation, and photic stimulation. Detection also can be improved through the use of nasopharyngeal leads, computer-transformed recordings, and evoked potentials (EPs). Sleep deprivation assists in seizure detection by a simple mechanism. Patients are more likely to fall asleep during the EEG after a period of sleep deprivation. It is during the changes in consciousness associated with various stages of sleep that the spike and sharp wave activity associated with seizure disorders is more likely to be detected. Hyperventilation, usually for approximately 3 minutes, may produce slow wave activity or spike waves. Photic stimulation consists of exposing the patient to a flashing strobe light during the EEG. Abnormal wave activity not synchronized to the flashing light is pathological. Studies involving the use of nasopharyngeal leads, although uncomfortable for the patients, may increase the yield of positive findings when there is a suspicion of temporal lobe epilepsy.

Evoked Potential

EP testing is the measurement of the EEG response to specific sensory stimulation. The stimulation may be visual, auditory, or somatosensory. During visual EPs, the patient is exposed to flashing lights or a checkerboard pattern. With auditory EP, the patient hears a specific tone. In somatosensory EP, the patient experiences an electrical stimulation to an extremity. These stimuli occur repeatedly while the patient undergoes a routine EEG. Using a computer, the responses to these stimuli are recorded and averaged. The time frame is measured in milliseconds. These tests are useful in neurology and neurosurgery. For example, they assist in the assessment of demyelinating disorders such as multiple sclerosis (MS). In psychiatry, EP testing may help in the differentiation of organic from functional impairments. A classic example is the use of EP testing to evaluate possible hysterical blindness. The usefulness of these tests in psychiatry is still under investigation.

Computer-transformed EEG data is the creation of color-coded two-dimensional maps of summaries of the EEG data. Such transformations can be done for EPs as well. Currently, EEG maps are research tools without validation for clinical use.

Polysomnography

Polysomnography is used to assess disorders of sleep by concurrently assessing the EEG, ECG, blood oxygen saturation, respirations, body temperature, the electromyogram, and the electrooculogram. Polysomnography has demonstrated an increase in the overall amount of rapid eye movement (REM) sleep and a shortened period before the onset of REM sleep (decreased REM latency) in patients with major depression. These studies may assist in differentiating depression from other conditions that mimic depression. For example, patients who appear depressed from dementia do not have a decreased REM latency or an increase in the amount of REM sleep.

ELECTROCARDIOGRAM

The ECG is a graphic representation of the electrical activity of the heart. Abnormalities in this activity correlate with cardiac pathology. The EEG is most commonly used in psychiatry to assess side effects of psychotropic medications.

Ziprasidone (Geodon) has been associated with a dose-related prolongation of the QTc interval. There is a known association of fatal arrhythmias (e.g., torsades de pointes) with QTc prolongation by some other medications. For this reason, clinicians usually obtain an ECG before initiation of treatment with ziprasidone. Ziprasidone is contraindicated in patients with a known history of QTc prolongation (including congenital long QT syndrome), with recent acute myocardial infarction, or with uncompensated heart failure. Bradycardia, hypokalemia or hypomagnesemia, or the concurrent use of other drugs that prolong the QTc interval all increase the risk for serious arrhythmias. Ziprasidone should be discontinued in patients who have persistent QTc measurements greater than 500 msec.

Like ziprasidone, thioridazine (Mellaril) has been associated with prolongation of the QTc interval in a dose-related manner. Prolongation of QTc interval has been associated with torsades de pointes arrhythmias and sudden death. An ECG should be obtained before initiating treatment with thioridazine to rule out QTc prolongation.

Tricyclic antidepressants (TCAs) are, at times, associated with ECG changes. Anticholinergic effects may increase heart rate. Prolongation of the PR, QT, and QRS intervals, along with ST-segment and T-wave abnormalities, may occur. The TCAs can cause or increase preexisting atrioventricular or bundle branch block. When the QTc exceeds 0.440 second, a patient is at increased risk for sudden death due to cardiac arrhythmias. Many clinicians obtain an ECG before beginning a TCA in a patient older than 40 years of age and in any patient with known cardiovascular disease.

Lithium (Eskalith) therapy can cause benign reversible T-wave changes, can impair SA node function, and can cause heart block. ECGs are often obtained before initiation of treatment with lithium and in cases of lithium toxicity or overdose.

The ECG is also used by psychiatrists when treating patients with certain psychiatric diagnoses. Eating disorder patients commonly have low potassium levels that may result in abnormal ECG recordings. As the serum potassium drops below normal, T waves become flat (or inverted) and U waves may appear.

Holter Monitoring

Holter monitoring is the continuous recording of a patient's ECG activity for a sustained time period (e.g., 24 hours). Patients are ambulatory during this time. It is useful for the evaluation of dizziness, palpitations, and syncope. It is commonly used in the evaluation of patients with panic disorder who manifest cardiac symptoms.

Cardiac Ultrasound

Cardiac ultrasound is the visualization of cardiac anatomy by the use of computer-transformed echoes of ultrasound. It is commonly used in the evaluation of mitral valve prolapse. There is an unclear association between mitral valve prolapse and panic attacks and anxiety disorders.

LABORATORY STUDIES

There is no consensus about standard laboratory tests for psychiatric patients. Laboratory studies are usually ordered based on a clinical hypothesis about the patient's primary diagnoses. However, newly admitted inpatients commonly receive the following tests: BUN, Cr, serum electrolytes, CBC, thyroid-stimulating hormone (TSH), aspartate aminotransferase (AST), alkaline phosphatase, VDRL, a urinalysis, and a serum calcium if the patient is depressed. Test batteries such as this are common, because these laboratory studies screen for illnesses commonly found in newly admitted patients.

Toxicology

Many drugs of abuse and prescribed medications can produce psychotropic effects. Psychiatric symptoms are not uncommon when prescribed medications are at toxic levels. For many psychiatric medications, it is possible to determine therapeutic concentrations. Adverse psychiatric symptoms are more common when the medication levels are toxic. However, in the debilitated and the elderly, pathological symptoms are more common at therapeutic concentrations. Normal reference range varies between laboratories. It is usually best to check with the laboratory performing the test to ascertain the normal reference range for that laboratory. It is reasonable to consider an assessment of medication therapeutic concentration when a patient has recent mental status changes and has recently had adjustments made to his prescribed medication dosages. Many clinicians obtain levels of psychotropic medications after an overdose of psychotropic medication. Levels of psychotropic medications can also be useful in assessing medication compliance.

Drug Abuse Screen

Indications for ordering a drug abuse screen include unexplained behavioral symptoms, a history of illicit drug use or dependence in a new patient evaluation, or a high-risk background (e.g., criminal record, adolescents, and prostitutes). A drug abuse screen is frequently ordered to monitor patient abstinence during treatment of substance abuse. Such tests can be ordered on a scheduled or random basis. Many clinicians believe random testing may be more accurate in the assessment of abstinence. The tests may also help motivate the patient. It is worth remembering that patients are frequently unreliable when reporting their drug abuse history. Drug-induced mental disorders frequently resemble primary psychiatric disorders. Furthermore, substance abuse can exacerbate preexisting mental illness.

Tested Substances

Routine tests are available for phencyclidine (PCP), cocaine, tetrahydrocannabinol (THC) (also known as *marijuana*), benzodiazepines, methamphetamine and its metabolite amphetamine, morphine (Duramorph), codeine, methadone (Dolophine), propoxyphene (Darvon), barbiturates, lysergic acid diethylamide (LSD), and 3,4-methylenedioxymethamphetamine (MDMA) (also known as *ecstasy*). Different laboratories have varying thresholds for detection. What constitutes a positive result varies widely. Some laboratories report a positive finding based only on the results of an initial screening test. Other facilities require a second, confirming test, often by a more sensitive or specific method.

Drug screening tests may have high false-positive rates. This is often due to the interaction of prescribed medication with the test, resulting in false-positive results, and lack of confirmatory testing. False-negative tests are common as well. False-negative results may be due to problems with specimen collection and storage. An unbroken chain of custody of the specimen is important. Patients may attempt to alter a specimen by dilution, by changing the pH (bleach and baking soda), or by using other additives (perfume and salt) that interfere with the test. Allowing a specimen to remain at room temperature too long may result in inaccurate testing.

Testing is most commonly performed on urine, although serum testing is also possible for most agents. Hair and saliva testing are also available in some laboratories. Alcohol can also be detected in the breath (Breathalyzer). With the exception of alcohol, drug levels are not usually determined. Generally, only the presence or absence of the drug is determined. There is usually not a meaningful or useful correlation between the level of the drug and clinical behavior.

The length of time that a substance can be detected in the urine is listed in Table 7.8–1. These are approximate times that are influenced by the frequency and duration of antecedent drug use, and the presence of illnesses that could alter excretion, such as renal or hepatic disease.

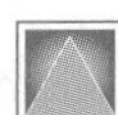

Table 7.8–1
Drugs of Abuse That Can Be Detected in Urine

Drug	Length of Time Detected in Urine
Alcohol	7–12 hrs
Amphetamine	48 hrs
Barbiturate	24 hrs (short acting); 3 wks (long acting)
Benzodiazepine	3 days
Cocaine	6–8 hrs (metabolites, 2–4 days)
Codeine	48 hrs
Heroin	36–72 hrs
Marijuana	36–72 hrs
Methadone (Dolophine)	3 days
Methaqualone	7 days
Morphine (Duramorph)	48–72 hrs
Phencyclidine	8 days
Propoxyphene (Darvon)	6–48 hrs

Alcohol

In patients with acute alcohol intoxication, a blood alcohol level (BAL) may be useful. A high BAL in a patient who clinically does not show significant intoxication is consistent with tolerance. Significant clinical evidence of intoxication with a low BAL should suggest intoxication with additional agents. Intoxication is commonly found with levels between 100 and 300 mg/dL. The degree of alcohol intoxication can also be assessed using the concentration of alcohol in expired respirations (Breathalyzer). Chronic alcohol use is commonly associated with other laboratory abnormalities, including elevation in liver enzymes, such as AST, which is usually greater than serum alanine aminotransferase (ALT). Bilirubin is also often elevated. Total protein and albumin may be low, and prothrombin time (PT) may be increased. Typically, there is a macrocytic anemia. The greater the number of abnormal tests and the greater their degree of abnormality, the more severe the alcoholism. However, some alcoholic patients have such extensive liver disease that they can no longer produce enzyme elevations. Too much of the hepatic parenchyma has been replaced with scar tissue for the liver to function adequately. Serum γ-glutamyltransferase (GGT) may also be elevated in patients with alcohol abuse.

Alcohol withdrawal consists of an elevation in blood pressure and pulse and a tremor. These symptoms commonly occur when serum alcohol levels are low or rapidly declining. Active intervention with benzodiazepines is necessary to prevent the condition progressing to alcohol withdrawal delirium, which is a medical emergency that may be fatal. There is a need to assess the alcohol-using patient for withdrawal when the BAL is low or undetectable to prevent the evolution of withdrawal symptoms.

A common set of laboratory studies to perform in a patient with the diagnosis of alcohol abuse or dependence would include a CBC (check mean corpuscular volume [MCV] and red cell distribution width [RDW] to check for a macrocytic profile), serum electrolytes (check magnesium and potassium, which are commonly low), and liver enzymes (check GGT, which is sensitive for acute alcohol abuse, along with AST and ALT). Commonly, total protein, serum albumin, and PT are assessed as indices of nutritional status and liver function. In the case of possible acute intoxication, the BAL may be assessed. Symptoms of withdrawal can occur with elevated BALs. It is the degree of change and the rate of change that, for many patients, are associated with symptoms of withdrawal. Because it is increasingly uncommon to find patients who only abuse alcohol, especially in younger patients, urine toxicology screens for other drugs of abuse may be helpful in understanding the patient's full clinical picture. Because alcohol and drug use are risk factors for sexually transmitted diseases (STDs), tests such as the VDRL are commonly performed.

Intravenous Drug Use

The IV route is commonly used for many substances of abuse. Most commonly, heroin, amphetamines, and cocaine are used alone or in combination via the IV route. Because needles are commonly contaminated, IV drug users are at risk for bacterial endocarditis, hepatitis, and acquired immune deficiency syndrome (AIDS) from the human immunodeficiency virus (HIV).

CBC and Serum Blood Cultures

Use of contaminated needles or nonsterile injection sites place IV drug users at risk for bacterial infections, including abscesses, bacteremia, and bacterial endocarditis. Findings on physical examination suggestive of endocarditis, possible bacteremia, or abscess necessitate obtaining a CBC to rule out an elevated WBC. Blood cultures should be obtained from at least two different sites if the patient is febrile or if findings are suggestive of bacteremia or endocarditis, and internal medicine consultation should be obtained.

SEXUALLY TRANSMITTED INFECTIOUS DISEASES

STDs include herpes simplex virus types 1 and 2, chlamydia, hepatitis viruses, gonorrhea, syphilis, and HIV.

Chlamydia and gonorrhea screening uses nucleic acid amplification (NAA) tests. These amplification tests are more than 95 percent sensitive and more than 99 percent specific for men and women, using urine or cervical or urethral swabs.

Screening for hepatitis B uses the hepatitis B surface antigen (HBsAg). The HBsAg indicates the carrier state or an active infection. The presence of only hepatitis B surface antibody identifies vaccinated individuals, whereas hepatitis B core antibody identifies individuals with past infection. HIV antibody determination is indicated for high-risk patients.

Screening for syphilis uses the VDRL test, which becomes positive 3 to 6 weeks after infection. False-positive serological reactions are encountered in illnesses such as collagen diseases, infectious mononucleosis, malaria, and many febrile diseases. False-positive reactions may be distinguished from true positives by specific treponemal antibody tests. The fluorescent treponemal antibody absorption (FTA-ABS) test detects antibody against *Treponema* spirochetes and is more sensitive and specific than nontreponemal tests.

Hepatitis

Viruses causing hepatitis are (1) hepatitis A virus (HAV), (2) hepatitis B virus (HBV), (3) hepatitis C virus (HCV), and (4) hepatitis D virus (HDV) (delta agent).

HAV transmission is by the fecal-oral route. Chronic hepatitis A does not occur, and there is no carrier state. Antibodies to HAV (anti-HAVs), specifically immunoglobulin M (IgM) and immunoglobulin G (IgG) anti-HAV, are detectable in serum soon after the onset. Peak titers of IgM anti-HAV occur during the first week of clinical disease and disappear within 3 to 6 months. Detection of IgM anti-HAV is an excellent test for diagnosing acute hepatitis A. Titers of IgG anti-HAV peak after 1 month of the disease and may persist for years.

HBV is usually transmitted by inoculation of infected blood or blood products or by sexual contact and is present in saliva, semen, and vaginal secretions. The incubation period of hepatitis B is 6 weeks to 6 months (with an average of 12 to 14 weeks). After acute hepatitis B, HBV infection persists in 1 to 2 percent of immunocompetent adults. Persons with chronic hepatitis B are at substantial risk of cirrhosis and hepatocellular carcinoma (as much as 25 to 40 percent).

HBV has an inner core protein (hepatitis B core antigen [HBcAg]) and an outer surface coat (HBsAg). The appearance of HBsAg is the first evidence of infection and persists throughout the clinical illness. The detection of HBsAg establishes infection with HBV and implies infectivity.

Specific antibody to HBsAg (anti-HB_s) appears after clearance of HBsAg and after successful vaccination against hepatitis B. Disappearance of HBsAg and the appearance of anti-HB_s signal recovery from HBV infection, noninfectivity, and immunity.

IgM antibody to HBcAg (anti-HB_c) in the setting of acute hepatitis indicates a diagnosis of acute hepatitis B. It fills the serological gap in patients who have cleared HBsAg but do not yet have detectable anti-HB_s. IgM anti-HB_c can persist for 3 to 6 months or more.

IgG anti-HB_c also appears during acute hepatitis B but persists indefinitely, whether the patient recovers or develops chronic hepatitis.

Hepatitis B early antigen (HBeAg) is a soluble protein found only in HBsAg-positive serum. HBeAg indicates viral replication and infectivity. Persistence of HBeAg in serum beyond 3 months indicates an increased likelihood of chronic hepatitis B.

HDV is a defective ribonucleic acid (RNA) virus that causes hepatitis only in association with hepatitis B infection.

More than 50 percent of cases of HCV are transmitted by IV drug use. Clinical illness is often mild, usually asymptomatic, and is characterized by waxing and waning aminotransferase elevations and a high rate (>80 percent) of chronic hepatitis.

Diagnosis of hepatitis C is based on an enzyme immunoassay that detects antibodies to HCV (anti-HCVs). Anti-HCV in patients with hepatitis generally signifies HCV. Limitations of the enzyme immunoassay include moderate sensitivity (false negatives) for the diagnosis of acute hepatitis C early in the course and low specificity (false positives) in some persons with elevated γ-globulin levels. In these situations, a diagnosis of hepatitis C may be confirmed by use of an assay for HCV RNA and, in some cases, a supplemental recombinant immunoblot assay (RIBA) for anti-HCV. Most RIBA-positive persons are potentially infectious, as confirmed by use of polymerase chain reaction–based tests to detect HCV RNA.

The WBC is normal to low, especially in the preicteric phase. Large atypical lymphocytes may occasionally be seen. Rarely, aplastic anemia follows an episode of acute hepatitis not caused by any of the known hepatitis viruses. Mild proteinuria is common, and bilirubinuria often precedes the appearance of jaundice. Acholic stools are often present during the icteric phase. Strikingly elevated AST or ALT occurs early, followed by elevations of bilirubin and alkaline phosphatase; in a minority of patients, the latter persist after aminotransferase levels have normalized. Cholestasis is occasionally marked in acute hepatitis A. Marked prolongation of the PT in severe hepatitis correlates with increased mortality.

Chronic hepatitis, characterized by elevated aminotransferase levels for more than 6 months, develops in 1 to 2 percent of immunocompetent adults with acute hepatitis B. More than 80 percent of all persons with acute hepatitis C develop chronic hepatitis, which, in many cases, progresses slowly. Ultimately, cirrhosis develops in much as 30 percent of those with chronic hepatitis C and 40 percent of those with chronic hepatitis B; the risk of cirrhosis is even higher in patients coinfected with both viruses or with HIV. Patients with cirrhosis are at risk, with a rate of 3 to 5 percent per year, of hepatocellular carcinoma. Even in the absence of cirrhosis, patients with chronic hepatitis B—particularly those with active viral replication—are at increased risk.

Serum Medication Concentrations

Serum concentrations of psychotropic medications are assessed to minimize the risk of toxicity to patients receiving these medications and to ensure the administration of amounts sufficient to produce a therapeutic response. This is particularly true for medications with therapeutic blood levels. Medication levels are often influenced by hepatic metabolism. This metabolism occurs via the action of enzymes in the liver.

Cytochrome P450 (CYP) is significant in hepatic drug oxidations. Some drug substrates induce CYP by enhancing the rate of its synthesis or by reducing its rate of degradation. Induction results in an acceleration of metabolism and, usually, in a decrease in the pharmacological action of the inducer and also of coadministered drugs. However, in the case of drugs metabolically transformed to reactive metabolites, enzyme induction may exacerbate metabolite-mediated toxicity.

Certain drugs may inhibit CYP enzyme activity. Imidazole-containing drugs, such as cimetidine (Tagamet) and ketoconazole (Nizoral), bind tightly to the heme iron of CYP and effectively reduce metabolism through competitive inhibition. However, macrolide antibiotics, such as troleandomycin (TAO), erythromycin (E-Mycin), and other erythromycin derivatives, are metabolized, apparently by CYP 3A, to metabolites that complex the cytochrome heme-iron and render it catalytically inactive. It is noteworthy that CYP 3A4 alone is responsible for more than 60 percent of the clinically prescribed drugs metabolized by the liver.

Acetaminophen

Acetaminophen is a common substance ingested in overdose attempts. Toxic levels are greater than 5 mg/dL (>330 μmol/L). Prompt treatment with acetylcysteine (Mucomyst) is necessary to prevent hepatotoxicity. Such patients are best treated in collaboration with internal medicine.

Acetylcysteine may protect against acetaminophen overdose–induced hepatotoxicity by maintaining or restoring hepatic concentrations of glutathione. Glutathione is required to inactivate an intermediate metabolite of acetaminophen that is thought to be hepatotoxic. In acetaminophen overdose, excessive quantities of this metabolite are formed, because the primary metabolic (glucuronide and sulfate conjugation) pathways become saturated.

Administration of acetylcysteine is only part of an overall regimen for the treatment of acetaminophen overdose. Other measures include emptying the stomach via induction of emesis or gastric lavage; monitoring plasma acetaminophen concentration, liver function, renal function, and fluid and electrolyte balance; and providing supportive treatment. The administration of activated charcoal plus acetylcysteine may be more effective than acetylcysteine alone in preventing hepatotoxicity after an acetaminophen overdose.

Acetylcysteine therapy should be initiated within 24 hours after ingestion of an acetaminophen overdose. The plasma acetaminophen concentration should be determined not less than 4 hours after ingestion of the overdose. If the initial determination shows a high concentration, a full course of acetylcysteine should be administered. If a low plasma concentration is reported, initiation or continuation of acetylcysteine treatment is not necessary.

Liver function tests (serum AST, serum ALT, PT, and bilirubin) should be performed at 24-hour intervals for at least 96 hours postingestion if the plasma acetaminophen concentration indicates potential hepatotoxicity. If no abnormalities are detected within 96 hours, further determinations are not needed.

Salicylate Toxicity Aspirin frequently is ingested in overdoses. Consequently, serum salicylate levels often are obtained in overdose cases. Ingestion of sufficient amounts of aspirin may be fatal. Furthermore, some rheumatic patients chronically may ingest large amounts of salicylates for therapeutic reasons. High salicylate levels are associated with tinnitus and hallucinations.

Antipsychotics Serum concentrations are not routinely obtained for most antipsychotic medications. Management usually consists of titration of the prescribed dose to levels that achieve reasonable symptomatic control and acceptable side effects. However, in some cases, blood levels may be helpful. These situations include suspected medication noncompliance and cases of poor response with prescription of apparently adequate doses. In the latter scenario, the concern may include rapid hepatic metabolism.

CLOZAPINE Clozapine (Clozaril) levels are trough levels determined in the morning before administration of the morning dose of medication. Weekly CBCs are required during the first 6 months of treatment with clozapine because of the risk of agranulocytosis. After the first 6 months of treatment, CBCs are checked every 2 weeks. Results must be sent to a pharmacy for the patient to receive his or her medication. Clozapine should be held for a WBC of less than 3,000 per mm^3 or a neutrophil count of less than 1,500 per mm^3.

A therapeutic range for clozapine has not been established; however, a level of 100 ng/mL is widely considered to be the minimum therapeutic threshold. Although concentrations between 200 and 700 ng/mL correlate more with response, nonresponse does occur within this range. At least 350 ng/mL of clozapine is considered to be necessary to achieve a therapeutic response in patients with refractory schizophrenia. The likelihood of seizures and other side effects increases with clozapine levels greater than 1,200 ng/mL or dosages greater than 600 mg per day, or both.

HALOPERIDOL Haloperidol (Haldol) levels are trough levels determined in the morning before administration of the morning dose of medication.

Mood Stabilizers

LITHIUM Lithium has a narrow therapeutic index. Consequently, blood levels of lithium must be monitored to achieve therapeutic dosing and avoid toxicity. For acute mania, target serum levels of lithium are in the range of 0.8 to 1.2 mEq/L. Many psychiatrists believe optimum maintenance serum levels are greater than 0.8 mEq/L. Side effects are dose dependent. Symptoms of toxicity may begin to manifest with serum levels of greater than 1.2 mEq/L and are common with levels greater than 1.4 mEq/L. Elderly or debilitated patients may show signs of toxicity with levels less than 1.2 mEq/L. With high levels (e.g., >2 mEq/L), consultation with a nephrologist or internist often occurs. In the debilitated patient or in patients with high levels, dialysis may be necessary to remove the lithium. Lithium levels should be carefully monitored during pregnancy and after labor. Rapid shifts in fluid volume can give rise to rapid changes in lithium levels during this time.

Steady-state serum lithium levels are achieved after five half-lives, and lithium levels typically reach steady-state 5 days after a change in dosage in patients with normal renal function. Levels are obtained 12 hours after the last dose and are usually measured using samples obtained in the morning, before administration of the morning dose (trough level). In cases of suspected lithium toxicity, levels are obtained sooner.

Maintenance levels are checked every 3 to 6 months and sometimes more frequently in patients with compromised renal function, general debilitation, or signs of toxicity. Close monitoring is required for patients who take medications that may alter lithium levels, such as diuretics or certain nonsteroidal antiinflammatory drugs (NSAIDs).

Baseline pretreatment studies and periodic follow-up tests for lithium should include monitoring of renal and thyroid function. Renal function is monitored using BUN, serum Cr, and a urinalysis. Because of the lithium's ability to impair the release of thyroid hormone from the thyroid gland, a baseline screening assessment of thyroid function (TSH) is usually obtained. These tests are usually repeated every 6 months to every year. Clinicians also should obtain thyroid studies in patients taking lithium who experience fatigue or asthenia, cold intolerance, or changes in skin, voice, or weight (symptoms of impaired thyroid function).

Before the administration of lithium in women of childbearing age, a screening urine pregnancy test generally should be obtained. Lithium is contraindicated during the first trimester of pregnancy owing to risk of congenital heart disease. Clinicians should advise women taking lithium to use adequate contraception. Because lithium can elevate the WBC, a pretreatment WBC also is usually obtained.

CARBAMAZEPINE Carbamazepine (Tegretol) may produce changes in the levels of white blood cells, platelets, and, under rare circumstances, red blood cells. Anemia, aplastic anemia, leukopenia, and thrombocytopenia may all occur but are rare. For these reasons, pretreatment evaluation typically includes a CBC. Many clinicians monitor the CBC every 2 weeks for the first 2 months of administration. Then, if the counts have been within normal limits, the CBC is monitored every quarter. Patients should be cautioned to watch for petechiae, fever or signs of infection, pallor, or undue weakness. Carbamazepine should be discontinued if the WBC count is less than 3,000 per mm^3, the erythrocyte count is less than 4.0×10^6 per mm^3, hemoglobin is less than 11 mg/dL, the neutrophil count is less than 1,500 per mm^3, and the platelet count is less than 100,000 per mm^3.

Because carbamazepine may produce changes in hepatic enzyme levels, baseline liver function tests also are indicated.

Carbamazepine has a molecular structure similar to TCAs and has the same propensity as TCAs to effect cardiac conduction (QTc and QRS prolongation). Many clinicians obtain pretreatment ECGs before starting carbamazepine. Patients with a QTc of longer than 0.440 second are at an increased risk for serious cardiac arrhythmias with carbamazepine treatment.

Carbamazepine may produce hyponatremia. This hyponatremia is usually mild and does not produce clinical symptoms. However, carbamazepine may cause the syndrome of inappropriate secretion of antidiuretic hormone (SIADH).

Carbamazepine may produce a variety of congenital abnormalities, including spina bifida and anomalies of the fingers. A pretreatment urine pregnancy test is usually obtained in women of childbearing years. Women should be cautioned to use adequate contraception when taking carbamazepine.

When used as an anticonvulsant, target blood levels for carbamazepine are 4 to 12 mg/mL. Levels in this range also should be achieved in mood disorder patients taking carbamazepine before discontinuation of carbamazepine owing to lack of efficacy. Levels should be obtained before the morning dose and after the patient has taken the same total daily dose for a minimum of 5 days.

Carbamazepine levels may be altered by coadministration of medications that inhibit metabolism of carbamazepine. Such agents include erythromycin and related antibiotics, valproic acid (Depakene), cimetidine, propoxyphene, isoniazid (Laniazid), and verapamil (Calan). Carbamazepine has the ability to lower its own serum level through the process of hepatic enzyme autoinduction. Carbamazepine is metabolized primarily by CYP 3A4 enzymes. Because carbamazepine also acts as an inducer of CYP 3A4 enzymes, it induces its own metabolism. Typically, autoinduction of hepatic enzymes occurs several weeks after initiation of carbamazepine treatment. Many clinicians follow levels over time and adjust the administered dose as necessary to maintain a therapeutic concentration. In debilitated patients, it may be advisable to monitor serum albumin levels. A portion of the drug is bound to serum proteins. It is the free (unbound) component that is biologically active. When there are reductions in serum proteins that bind the drug, adjustment in the dose may be necessary, particularly in patients who show signs of toxicity.

VALPROATE Valproate (valproic acid [Depakene] and divalproex [Depakote]) are used to treat acute mania and for the prophylactic treatment of bipolar disorder. Therapeutic levels for acute mania are thought to range from 50 to 120 mg/L. Side effects are more common with levels greater than 100 mg/L. Because of the risk of hepatotoxicity, ranging from mild dysfunction to hepatic necrosis, pretreatment liver function tests are usually obtained. More commonly, valproate may cause a sustained, mild elevation in liver transaminase levels of as much as three times the upper limit of normal. Hepatic necrosis is rare and is more likely to occur in the young (younger than 2 years of age) and in those individuals taking multiple anticonvulsants.

Valproate may also increase the risk of birth defects. A pretreatment urine pregnancy test is usually obtained in women of childbearing years. Women should be cautioned to use adequate contraception.

Hematological abnormalities are also possible and include leukopenia and thrombocytopenia. Acute pancreatitis may also occur.

Antidepressants

TRICYCLIC AND TETRACYCLIC Routine laboratories before initiation of tricyclic or tetracyclic antidepressants (TCAs) typically include a CBC, serum electrolytes, and liver function tests. Because TCAs affect cardiac conduction, clinicians also may obtain an ECG to assess for the presence of abnormal cardiac rhythms and prolonged PR, QRS, and QTc complexes before the initiation of these medications. When the QTc interval is longer than 0.440 second, a patient is at increased risk for potentially fatal cardiac arrhythmias. Heart rate may also be increased from the anticholinergic effects of the medication. Pretreatment ECGs are commonly obtained in patients older than 40 years of age to exclude a QTc interval of longer than 0.440 second, a QRS interval of longer than 0.10 second, or bundle branch block. In an overdose, a QRS interval of longer than 0.10 second appears to be the most reliable predictor of an ultimately fatal cardiac arrhythmia.

Baseline vital signs with orthostatic measurements should be obtained before the initiation of TCAs, especially in the elderly in whom TCA treatment can significantly increase the risk of hip fracture owing to TCA side effects of orthostasis. Subsequent orthostasis measurements should also be obtained to assist with dose titration in this population.

Plasma levels of TCAs may be useful when there is a need to rapidly achieve a therapeutic dose of the medication, when patients need the lowest effective dose (e.g., sensitivity to side effects), when questions exist about a patient's compliance, and when there is a poor response to a standard dose. Other indications for obtaining plasma TCA levels include concomitant administration of medications that may alter TCA blood levels or the reemergence of depression in a patient who had an initial therapeutic response to TCA treatment.

TCA levels are usually obtained 12 hours after the administration of a dose. Typically, this is in the morning, before administration of the morning dose. Levels are most meaningful when steady state has been achieved, at least five half-lives (usually 10 days) after the last change in dose. Meaningful serum levels have been determined only for nortriptyline (Aventyl) (50 to 150 ng/mL), desipramine (Norpramin) (>125 ng/mL) and imipramine (Tofranil) (total of imipramine and desmethylimipramine [desipramine] >200 ng/mL).

MONOAMINE OXIDASE INHIBITORS Treatment with monoamine oxidase inhibitors (MAOIs) can cause orthostasis and, rarely, hypertensive crisis. Baseline blood pressure measurement should be obtained before the initiation of treatment, and blood pressure should be monitored during treatment.

Direct monitoring of blood levels of MAOIs is not clinically indicated. There are no meaningful blood levels for MAOIs. Treatment with MAOIs is occasionally associated with hepatotoxicity. For this reason, liver function tests usually are obtained at the initiation of treatment and periodically thereafter.

Neuroleptic Malignant Syndrome

Neuroleptic malignant syndrome (NMS) is a rare, potentially fatal, consequence of neuroleptic administration. The syndrome consists of autonomic instability, hyperpyrexia, severe extrapyramidal symptoms (i.e., rigidity), and delirium. Sustained muscle contraction results in peripheral heat generation and muscle breakdown. Muscle breakdown contributes to elevated levels of creatine phosphokinase (CPK). Peripheral heat generation with impaired central mechanisms of thermoregulation results in hyperpyrexia. Myoglobinuria and leukocytosis are common. Hepatic and renal failure may occur. Liver enzymes become elevated with liver failure. Patients may die from hyperpyrexia, aspiration pneumonia, renal failure, hepatic failure, respiratory arrest, or cardiovascular collapse. Treatment includes discontinuation of the neuroleptic, hydration, administration of muscle relaxants, and general supportive nursing care.

The diagnosis of NMS is often made when three of the following criteria are present: (1) two or more extrapyramidal side effects (choreiform movements, cogwheeling, dyskinetic movements, dysphagia, festinating gait, flexor-extensor posturing, lead pipe–type muscle oculogyric crisis, opisthotonos, rigidity, retrocollis, sialorrhea, and trismus), (2) a temperature of at least 38°C (oral) without other known cause, and (3) two or more signs of autonomic instability (diaphoresis, hypertension, incontinence, tachycardia, and tachypnea).

A typical laboratory workup of NMS includes a CBC, serum electrolytes, BUN, Cr, and creatine kinase (CK). A urinalysis, including an assessment of urine myoglobin is also usually performed. As part of the differential, blood and urine cultures are performed as part of a fever workup.

Electroconvulsive Therapy

ECT is usually reserved for the most treatment-resistant depressive patients. Typical laboratory tests obtained before the administration of ECT include a CBC, serum electrolytes, urinalysis, and liver function tests. Usually, an ECG is also obtained. A spinal X-ray series is no longer considered a routine indication because of the low risk of spinal injury associated with modern administration techniques that use paralyzing agents.

HEMATOLOGICAL EVALUATIONS

Some psychiatric medications may affect a patient's hematological state. For this reason, some tests are commonly performed before initiation of medication and periodically thereafter.

Complete Blood Count

The CBC typically consists of a WBC, in some cases a differential WBC, and, usually, a red blood cell count, along with assessment of hemoglobin, hematocrit, and red cell indices. A platelet count may also be obtained.

The WBC may be elevated in cases of infection and leukemia and in response to some medications. The conditions of direct relevance to psychiatry are somewhat limited. Lithium commonly produces a mild leukocytosis. More pronounced elevations in the WBC may occur in NMS. In contrast, leukopenia may occur in response to certain medications. Clozapine and carbamazepine are the most significant medication causes of a leukopenia in psychiatry.

The differential WBC is the assessment of the abundance of the various types of white cells. A common occurrence in infection is a *shift to the left* in the granulocyte series. This indicates a shift from segmented neutrophils to band forms (early neutrophilic precursors). Although this usually indicates bacterial infection, it is also commonly seen in NMS.

The red blood cell count is used in the assessment of anemia and polycythemia. Anemia is associated with depression and, rarely, psychosis. Hemoglobin and hematocrit are also helpful in the evaluation of anemia. Carbamazepine treatment, in rare cases, may result in anemia.

Red cell indices include mean corpuscular hemoglobin concentration (MCHC), MCV, RDW, and mean corpuscular hemoglobin (MCH). The MCV is commonly elevated in patients with alcohol abuse, along with folate and vitamin B_{12} deficiencies. It is low in patients with an iron deficiency anemia.

The platelet count may be decreased by certain psychotropic medications, including clozapine and carbamazepine.

Ferritin, a storage protein for iron, is low in iron deficiency states and increased in some inflammatory conditions. Total iron binding capacity (TIBC) is an assessment of the quantity of iron that would be in the plasma if all of the transport protein for iron (transferrin) were saturated with iron.

The reticulocyte count is an estimate of red blood cell production in the bone marrow. It is low in megaloblastic and iron deficiency anemia. When these conditions are treated, it increases. It is also elevated in anemia owing to blood loss.

Folate and vitamin B_{12} deficiencies are associated with dementia; delirium; psychosis, including paranoia; fatigue; and personality change. Folate and vitamin B_{12} can be directly measured. Low folate levels may be found in patients who use contraceptive pills or other forms of estrogen, who drink alcohol, or who take phenytoin (Dilantin).

WEIGHT AND BODY MASS INDEX

Monitoring of weight and body mass index (BMI) is important in the management of many patients with psychiatric illness. A variety of psychiatric illnesses can affect appetite and may cause weight loss or weight gain. Measurement of weight may be useful in assessing response to treatment and recovery.

Many psychotropic drugs, including antidepressants, mood stabilizers, and antipsychotic medications, have weight gain as a potential side effect. Weight gain can lead to obesity, a major risk factor for the development of multiple medical problems such as hypertension, diabetes, cardiovascular disease, cerebrovascular disease, and lipid abnormalities. Weight gain can also contribute to medication noncompliance and poor self-image. Some clinicians advocate regular monitoring of BMI by both patient and clinician for patients with schizophrenia and recommend intervention in the form of nutritional counseling, exercise program, or change in antipsychotic medication when BMI increases by one unit. Waist circumference measuring greater than 35 inches for a woman or 40 inches for a man should also prompt similar intervention. Similar monitoring and intervention techniques also are useful for patients with bipolar disorder and other patient populations.

ENDOCRINE EVALUATIONS

Endocrine disease is of great relevance to psychiatry. Management of psychiatric illness is complicated by comorbid endocrine disease. Endocrine illness frequently has psychiatric manifestations. For these reasons, screening for endocrine disease often is of relevance to the psychiatrist.

Adrenal Disease

Adrenal disease may have psychiatric manifestations, including depression, anxiety, mania, dementia, psychosis, and delirium. However, patients with adrenal disease rarely come to the attention of psychiatrists. Assessment and management of these patients are best done in conjunction with specialists. Low plasma levels of cortisol are found in Addison's disease. Elevated levels of cortisol are seen in Cushing's syndrome. Cortisol levels have not been found to be useful in the assessment or management of primary psychiatric disease. In particular, the dexamethasone-suppression test (DST) remains a research tool in psychiatry that is not used in routine clinical care.

Antidiuretic Hormone

Arginine vasopressin (AVP), also called *antidiuretic hormone* (ADH), is decreased in central diabetes insipidus (DI). DI may be central (due to the pituitary or hypothalamus) or nephrogenic. Nephrogenic DI may be acquired or due to an inherited X-linked condition. Lithium-induced DI is an example of an acquired form of DI. Lithium has been shown to decrease the sensitivity of renal tubules to AVP. Patients with central DI respond to the administration of vasopressin with a decrease in urine output. Secondary central DI may develop in response to head trauma that produces damage in the pituitary or hypothalamus.

Excessive secretion of AVP results in increased retention of fluid in the body. This condition is called *SIADH*. Water retention in SIADH causes hyponatremia. SIADH may develop in response to injury to the brain or from medication administration (including phenothiazines, butyrophenones, and carbamazepine). The hyponatremia associated with this condition may produce delirium. The relationship between AVP and psychogenic polydipsia remains unclear. However, it appears that in a minority of cases with psychogenic polydipsia, AVP levels may be abnormal. SIADH is associated with hyponatremia, low serum osmolality, and high urine osmolality. It should be considered when patients demonstrate hyponatremia and concentrated urine (i.e., high urine osmolality or high specific gravity). This condition should be investigated with the assistance of a specialist.

Fasting Blood Sugar and Glycosylated Hemoglobin

Some atypical antipsychotic agents have been associated with abnormalities in serum glucose levels, including the development of diabetes mellitus. Many clinicians monitor their patients who take atypical antipsychotic agents for the development of hyperglycemia by obtaining fasting blood glucose levels and glycosylated hemoglobin levels on a quarterly or semiannual basis. In addition, extremes in serum glucose concentrations have been associated with delirium. Hypoglycemia has also been associated with agitation and anxiety. Evaluation for diabetes or other abnormalities in glucose metabolism is usually best done by specialists.

Human Chorionic Gonadotropin Human chorionic gonadotropin (HCG) can be assessed in the urine and blood. The urine test for HCG is the basis for the commonly used urine pregnancy test. This test is able to detect pregnancy approximately 2 weeks after an expected menstrual period has passed. Pregnancy tests are commonly obtained before initiating certain psychotropic medications, such as lithium, carbamazepine, and valproic acid, which are associated with congenital anomalies.

Lipids Hyperlipidemia, including elevated cholesterol and triglyceride levels, is associated with cardiovascular and cerebrovascular disease. Certain antipsychotic medications, including clozapine and some of the second-generation antipsychotics, have been associated with hyperlipidemia. Additionally, patients with schizophrenia are at increased risk of cardiovascular disease. Their risk for cardiovascular disease may be further increased by the development of hyperlipidemia. Clinicians treating patients with schizophrenia should obtain lipid panels for their patients at the onset of treatment and then every 5 years or when there is evidence that lipid levels may have increased to the point of requiring treatment. Clinicians treating patients with other psychiatric diagnoses with clozapine or second-generation antipsychotic medications should also consider following lipid levels.

Parathormone Parathormone (parathyroid hormone) modulates serum concentrations of calcium and phosphorus. Dysregulation in this hormone may, via the production in abnormalities in calcium and phosphorus, produce depression or delirium.

Prolactin Prolactin levels may become elevated in response to the administration of antipsychotic agents. Elevations in serum prolactin result from blockade of dopamine receptors in the pituitary. This blockade produces an increase in prolactin synthesis and release. Elevated prolactin levels are associated with galactorrhea, menstrual abnormalities, and alterations in libido and bone calcium concentrations.

Prolactin levels may briefly rise after a seizure. For this reason, prompt measurement of a prolactin level after possible seizure activity may assist in differentiating a seizure from a pseudoseizure.

Thyroid Hormone Disease of the thyroid is associated with many psychiatric manifestations. Thyroid disease is most commonly associated with depression and anxiety but may also give rise to symptoms of panic, dementia, and psychosis. Thyroid studies are commonly assessed in patients with depression. Thyroid disease may mimic depression. In addition, it is difficult to achieve euthymia if a patient is not euthyroid.

Measurements of TSH typically are used as a screening test for thyroid disease. Some clinicians also order serum thyroxine (T_4) and triiodothyronine (T_3) levels. Usually, thyroid function is assessed in psychiatric patients with a history of thyroid disease or those with symptoms suggestive of thyroid illness. Such symptoms may include increased appetite, weight loss, and heat intolerance in patients with hyperthyroidism or weight gain, fatigue, and cold intolerance in hypothyroidism. Alternatively, risk factors for thyroid disease may prompt examination of thyroid function. Risk factors include prior treatment with lithium or iodine-131, a history of irradiation of the neck and chest, or a history of thyroidectomy. Additionally, thyroid function commonly is assessed in patients currently receiving exogenous thyroid hormone replacement to ensure that they are euthyroid.

Interpretation of thyroid function tests may be complex and is often best done with the assistance of a specialist. Interpretation is further complicated by the presence of transient abnormalities of thyroid function in many newly admitted psychiatric patients. These abnormalities normalize over time without treatment and may be related to stress. Thyroid tests have not been found to be useful in the assessment or management of primary psychiatric illness.

Serum Electrolytes Serum electrolytes are a useful component of a screening evaluation for psychiatric patients. They are often abnormal in patients with delirium. Abnormalities may also occur in response to the administration of psychotropic medications.

Low serum chloride levels may occur in eating disorder patients who purge by self-induced vomiting.

Serum bicarbonate levels may be elevated in patients who purge or who abuse laxatives. Bicarbonate levels are commonly low in patients who hyperventilate in response to anxiety.

Hypokalemia may be present in eating disorder patients who purge or abuse laxatives and in psychogenic vomiting. Diuretic abuse by eating disorder patients also may produce hypokalemia. Low levels of potassium are associated with weakness and fatigue. Characteristic ECG changes occur with hypokalemia and consist of cardiac arrhythmias, U waves, flattened T waves, and ST-segment depression.

Eating disorder patients (those with anorexia nervosa or bulimia nervosa) usually receive a fairly standard set of laboratory studies, including serum electrolytes (check potassium and phosphorus), blood glucose, thyroid function tests, liver enzymes, total protein, serum albumin, BUN, Cr, CBC, and ECG. Serum amylase is often assessed in bulimic patients.

Magnesium levels may be low in alcohol-abusing patients. Low magnesium levels are associated with agitation, confusion, and delirium. If untreated, convulsions and coma may follow.

Low levels of serum phosphorus may be present in eating disorder patients with purging behavior. Phosphorus levels may also be low in anxiety patients who hyperventilate. Hyperparathyroidism may produce low serum phosphorus levels. Elevated serum phosphorus levels are seen in hypoparathyroidism.

Hyponatremia is seen in psychogenic polydipsia and SIADH and in response to certain medications, such as carbamazepine. Low sodium levels are associated with delirium.

Serum calcium abnormalities are associated with a variety of behavioral abnormalities. Low serum calcium levels are associated with depression, delirium, and irritability. Elevated levels are associated with depression, psychosis, and weakness. Laxative abuse, common in eating disorder patients, can be associated with hypocalcemia. Hypocalcemia secondary to hypoparathyroidism may occur in patients who have undergone surgery for thyroid disease.

Serum copper levels are low in Wilson's disease, a rare abnormality in copper metabolism. Copper is deposited in the brain and liver, resulting in decreased intellectual functioning, personality changes, psychosis, and a movement disorder. Symptoms are usually present in the second and third decades of life. Laboratory assessment for Wilson's disease includes the measurement of serum ceruloplasmin; the transport protein for copper, which is low; and urine copper, measured in a 24-hour specimen, which is elevated.

Renal Function Tests Tests of renal function commonly include BUN and Cr. Other relevant laboratory studies include the routine urinalysis and Cr clearance. An elevated BUN often results in lethargy or delirium. BUN is commonly elevated with dehydration. Elevations in BUN are often associated with impaired clearance of lithium. A less sensitive index of renal function is Cr. Elevations in Cr may indicate extensive renal impairment. Elevated levels occur when approximately 50 percent of the nephrons are damaged.

Routine urinalysis is a common screening test that includes examination of the general appearance of the sample and measurement of the pH, urine specific gravity, urine bilirubin, and urine glucose. Elevations in urine glucose can be seen in diabetes. Elevated urine bilirubin occurs in biliary disease. A high urine specific gravity may occur in diabetes mellitus, in dehydrated states, or from SIADH. A low urine specific gravity may occur in DI or from excessive water ingestion.

Cr clearance is often assessed in patients taking lithium. It is a sensitive measurement of renal function. The test is performed in a well-hydrated patient by collecting all of the patient's urine for 24 hours. During the midpoint of the 24-hour collection period, a serum Cr level also is obtained. The resulting data are used to calculate the patient's Cr clearance. Usually, the laboratory performs the calculation.

Elevated levels of porphobilinogen are found in the urine of symptomatic patients with acute intermittent porphyria. Symptoms of this disease include psychosis, apathy, or depression, along with intermittent abdominal pain, neuropathy, and autonomic dysfunction. If urine porphobilinogen levels are elevated when the patient is symptomatic, collection of a 24-hour urine specimen for quantitative assessment of porphobilinogen and aminolevulinic acid is indicated.

Liver Function Tests Elevations in AST may occur with diseases of the liver, heart, lungs, kidneys, and skeletal muscle. In patients with alcohol-induced liver disease, AST is commonly more elevated than ALT. In viral and drug-induced liver disease, ALT is often elevated. Serum GGT is elevated in hepatobiliary disease, including alcohol-induced liver disease and cirrhosis.

Alkaline phosphatase elevations occur in many diseases, including diseases of the liver, bone, kidney, and thyroid. Levels of alkaline phosphatase may be elevated in response to some psychiatric medications, most notably the phenothiazines.

Serum ammonia levels are often elevated in patients with hepatic encephalopathy. High levels are associated with the delirium of hepatic encephalopathy.

Serum bilirubin is an index of hepatic and bile duct function. Prehepatic, unconjugated, or indirect bilirubin and posthepatic, conjugated, or direct bilirubin are often assessed to help elucidate the origin of the elevation in bilirubin.

Lactate dehydrogenase (LDH) may be elevated in diseases of the liver, skeletal muscle, heart, and kidney. It is also elevated in pernicious anemia.

Total protein is the measurement of serum albumin and globulins. Many psychiatric medications are protein bound. Low levels of serum total protein result in a high fraction of an ingested drug remaining in the unbound (active) state. High levels of unbound drug increase the active effects and side effects that a patient experiences. Total protein may be low in malnourished states, such as those seen in eating disorder patients. Low total protein and serum albumin in a patient with elevated liver enzymes is an indicator of significant liver disease. Consequently, these levels are often assessed in patients who abuse alcohol.

Pancreatic Function Measurement of serum amylase is used to monitor pancreatic function. Elevations in amylase levels may occur in alcohol-abusing patients who develop pancreatitis. Serum amylase levels may also be fractionated into salivary and pancreatic components. Elevations in salivary levels are commonly seen in eating disorder patients who purge. When pancreatic disease is suspected, serum lipase is also commonly measured. This enzyme is unique to the pancreas. Elevations in amylase and lipase suggest pancreatic disease. Eating disorder patients who purge typically have elevated levels of serum amylase and normal levels of serum lipase.

Muscle Injury Serum CK levels may rise in response to repeated intramuscular (IM) injections, prolonged or agitated periods in restraint, or NMS. Dystonic reactions from neuroleptic administration may also result in elevated levels of CK.

INFECTION

Sexually Transmitted Disease Testing Testing for STDs has become common, given the current frequency of these diseases. Many of these illnesses are directly associated with behavioral symptoms. Some psychiatric illnesses, such as mania, are associated with a higher risk of contracting STDs. In addition, many patients require supportive counseling before and after testing. Counseling consists of allowing patients the opportunity to ask questions, providing patients with educational material, and assessing their emotional response to the process. Inquiring about a patient's motivation for testing often is a helpful way to initiate discussion of other issues. Patients should be informed about the meaning of positive and negative results. Patients who test positive require referral to a specialist who can discuss the implications of the result and future treatment. Patients with high-risk behaviors and a negative test result should be cautioned about the length of time required for conversion and the need, when appropriate, for supplemental testing. It may be beneficial to explore the patient's anticipated emotional response to a positive result. This assessment can be supplemented by an exploration of how they have responded to significant stress in the past. It is useful to evaluate the patient's understanding of ways to reduce the risk of contraction or transmitting the HIV virus and emotional response to the test results. Patients in the positive and negative result categories can benefit from a discussion of high-risk behaviors, and, for patients who test positive, it is particularly important for clinicians to provide the patient with information about how to minimize the risk of transmission. Clinicians should emphasize the need for protected sex with fully informed partners and the avoidance of donating sperm, blood, or organs. Clinicians should warn patients about the risks associated with sharing razors, toothbrushes, and any other objects that could have blood on them.

Syphilis The FTA-ABS is a test for antibodies to the agent that produces syphilis, *Treponema pallidum*. The test is commonly used to confirm positive screening tests for syphilis, such as the rapid plasma reagin (RPR) test and the VDRL test. The FTS-ABS test also is used when neurosyphilis is suspected. Once positive, a patient usually remains so for life. False-positive results may occur in patients with systemic lupus erythematosus (SLE).

The RPR is a common screening test for syphilis. When positive, it is commonly quantified. Quantification enables levels to be followed to assess response to treatment. After a positive RPR test, the more specific FTA-ABS test is used to confirm the positive result. False-positive RPR tests are found in patients with various rheumatic diseases and in some other infections, such as infectious mononucleosis.

The VDRL test also is used to screen patients for syphilis. The VDRL test is most sensitive in secondary syphilis and can be positive or negative in primary syphilis. Titers often are low in tertiary syphilis. When positive, the VDRL test is commonly quantified. Quantification permits the use of subsequent levels to assess response to treatment. A positive VDRL is confirmed with the more specific FTA-ABS test. False-positive VDRL tests are found in patients with various rheumatic diseases and in some other infections, such as infectious mononucleosis. When syphilis of the CNS is suspected, a

VDRL is performed on cerebrospinal fluid (CSF). Patients with neurosyphilis also commonly have abnormalities in protein levels, γ-globulins, and cell counts in CSF.

HIV HIV-infected patients may have CNS manifestations as their predominant symptoms. CNS symptoms may occur even when other symptoms are absent. Behavioral changes in an individual patient may be due to either the direct effect of the virus on the brain or associated conditions such as infection, mass effect, or malnutrition. CNS manifestations of HIV infection include dementia, personality changes, affective symptoms of either mania or depression, and psychosis.

The enzyme-linked immunosorbent assay (ELISA) test and the Western blot test are used in the assessment of a patient's HIV status. Both tests detect the presence of antibodies to the HIV virus. Antibodies to HIV become detectable anywhere from 3 weeks to 3 months after infection. Typically, the ELISA test is used as a screening test, and the Western blot test is used to confirm the result. Other tests are performed to assess the extent of HIV disease burden and the degree to which the virus has affected the immune system. Measurement of viral load is used to assess HIV disease burden. Measurement of T4 cell counts and T4 to T8 cell ratios provide information about the extent of the effects of the virus on the immune system. The T4 to T8 cell ratio commonly is called the *T-cell helper to suppressor ratio*. In patients infected with HIV, the helper to suppressor ratio is decreased. Suppressor T lymphocytes inhibit B-lymphocyte activity. Antigens stimulate T4 cells. This results in an augmented response by B lymphocytes. These cells are low in HIV-infected patients.

HIV testing is indicated in high-risk populations. High-risk groups include men who have had sex with other men; IV drug users; individuals with direct, unprotected, exposure to body fluids from HIV-infected individuals (e.g., those with needle sticks from HIV-positive patients); and those who have had sex with individuals in any of these groups. HIV is usually transmitted via contamination by body fluids. Viral transmission can occur during sexual contact, use of shared implements for IV drug abuse, tattooing and piercing, and needle-stick injuries. It is also common to test individuals who request testing; individuals planning to donate organs, semen, or blood; and individuals from high-risk groups who are pregnant or plan to become pregnant. HIV testing is also frequently performed in patients with early-onset dementia.

Viral Hepatitis Viral hepatitis may be caused by several types of viruses, including type A, type B, and type C. The illness produces an elevation of liver function tests, especially ALT. Symptoms range from mild flu-like manifestations to rapidly progressive and fatal liver failure. Psychiatric manifestations include depression, anxiety, weakness, and psychosis. Viral hepatitis also may impair the metabolism of those psychotropic medications that are metabolized in the liver. Impaired liver metabolism requires an adjustment of the dose or consideration of agents that are less affected by alterations in liver metabolism.

HEPATITIS A Psychiatric manifestations of hepatitis A include fatigue, anorexia, and depression. Generally, this illness has a more benign clinical course than hepatitis B. Hepatitis A is transmitted by the fecal-oral route and is associated with food and water contamination, poor sanitation, and close contact with infected individuals. Many infections are subclinical. Measurement of viral antigens and antibodies to the virus can detect hepatitis A infection.

HAV antigen can be detected during acute infection. Total anti-HAVs include IgG and IgM antibodies to the HAV. The IgG anti-HAV persists for life and confers immunity. Its presence indicates prior exposure to the HAV. The IgM anti-HAV appears soon after infection and is therefore an index of acute infection. It is usually present for only a few weeks after infection.

HEPATITIS B Psychiatric manifestations have been reported during all stages of hepatitis B infection. Hepatitis B is transmitted via contamination by body fluids. Transmission of hepatitis B commonly occurs during sexual contact, by sharing implements for IV drug use, through tattooing and piercing, and as a result of needle-stick injuries. Hepatitis B infection can be detected by measuring viral antigens and antibodies to the virus. There is a common comorbidity between hepatitis B infection and HIV infection, given the shared risk factors for both conditions.

The presence of hepatitis B antigen indicates greater risk of infectivity. When it is present beyond 10 to 12 weeks, there is a greater probability of the disease progressing to the chronic state. HBsAg, when present, indicates active infection with the HBV. The antibody to HBV (anti-HBV) usually can be detected as infectivity diminishes. Anti-HB_s usually is detected after recovery from infection. Anti-HB_s usually remains present for life and implies persistence of immunity to infection.

Anti-HB_c total is an index of anti-HB_c, IgM, and IgG antibodies. This test is usually positive in patients with acute, chronic, and resolved hepatitis B. The IgG anti-HB_c component persists for life in some patients. Anti-HB_c IgM, the antibody to the core antigen, is high in patients with acute hepatitis B and is commonly used as an index of acute hepatitis B infection. Levels in chronic carriers are usually low or undetectable.

HEPATITIS C Hepatitis C is detected with increasing frequency. It is common in individuals who abuse IV drugs. It is associated with an increased risk of liver cancer. Anti-HCV, the test for the hepatitis C antibody, is commonly used for detection.

Epstein-Barr Virus The Epstein-Barr virus (EBV) produces infectious mononucleosis. Mononucleosis is associated with weakness, depression, personality changes, and psychosis. Tests for this condition include tests for EBV-specific antibody and antigen. IgM and IgG antibodies to the viral capsid antigen are measured. IgM is usually elevated during the acute phase. IgG also may be elevated during the acute phase, but high levels of IgG may persist after clinical manifestations of the disease have resolved. Additional tests include the Monospot test and the heterophil antibody test. The Monospot test detects infectious mononucleosis antibodies. The heterophil antibody test is usually positive during acute infection, but it is not specific for infectious mononucleosis. During EBV infection, the WBC is elevated. Liver enzymes (ALT and AST) and bilirubin also commonly are elevated during acute illness.

Controversy remains about the possible existence of a chronic infectious mononucleosis condition, commonly referred to as *chronic fatigue syndrome*. Reports associate the condition with fatigue and depression. Many patients with chronic fatigue syndrome meet diagnostic criteria for other mental illnesses. Not all patients with chronic fatigue syndrome have antibodies to EBV, suggesting that chronic fatigue syndrome may be a heterogenous condition associated with other etiologies, possibly including infection with other viral entities. Patients are commonly comanaged with other specialists, such as infectious disease specialists. Infection with infectious mononucleosis has also been associated with depression. The exact nature of this relationship remains unclear.

Systemic Lupus Erythematosus SLE is an autoimmune disorder. Psychiatric manifestations include depression, dementia, delirium, and psychosis. Tests for SLE are based on detection of antibodies formed as part of the disease. Antinuclear antibodies are found in virtually all patients with SLE. Antibody levels also are used to monitor the severity of the illness. A fluorescent test is used to detect the antinuclear antibodies. This test can be positive in a variety of rheumatic diseases. For this reason, a positive result usually is followed by additional tests, including a test to detect anti–deoxyribonucleic acid (DNA) antibodies. Anti-DNA antibodies, when associated with antinuclear antibodies, are strongly suggestive of a diagnosis of lupus. Anti-DNA antibodies are followed to monitor the response to treatment.

Environmental Toxins Specific toxins are associated with a variety of behavioral abnormalities. Exposure to toxins commonly occurs through occupation or hobbies.

Aluminum intoxication can cause a dementia-like condition. Aluminum can be detected in the urine or blood.

Arsenic intoxication may cause fatigue, loss of consciousness, anemia, and hair loss. Arsenic can be detected in urine, blood, and hair.

Manganese intoxication may present with delirium, confusion, and, commonly, a parkinsonian syndrome. Manganese may be detected in urine, blood, and hair.

Symptoms of mercury intoxication include apathy, poor memory, lability, headache, and fatigue. Mercury can be detected in urine, blood, and hair.

Manifestations of lead intoxication include encephalopathy, irritability, apathy, and anorexia. Lead can be detected in blood or urine. Typically, a lead level is assessed by using a 24-hour urine sample. The free erythrocyte protoporphyrin test is a screening test for chronic lead intoxication. This test is commonly coupled with a blood lead level. The Centers for Disease Control state that a lead level greater than 25 μg/dL is significant for children. The incidence of lead toxicity in children has been falling recently.

Organic Compounds Significant exposure to organic compounds, such as insecticides, may produce behavioral abnormalities. Many insecticides have strong anticholinergic effects. Commonly, it is the cluster of anticholinergic effects such as dry mouth, blurred vision, constipation, and urinary retention that alerts clinicians to the possibility of toxicity. There are no readily available laboratory tests to detect these compounds. Poison control centers may assist in the identification of appropriate testing facilities.

VOLATILE SOLVENT INHALATION Chronic use of volatile solvents is associated with the production of panic attacks and an organic personality disorder. Volatile solvents are used occasionally as drugs of abuse. Chronic abuse of volatile solvents is associated with damage to the brain, liver, kidneys, lung, heart, and blood. Exposure to toluene, which is present in many cleaning solutions, paints, and glues, has been associated with loss of clear gray–white matter differentiation and with brain atrophy on MRI scans. Poison control centers may assist in the identification of appropriate testing facilities.

ANABOLIC STEROID USE Use of anabolic steroids has been associated with irritability, aggression, depression, and psychosis. Athletes and bodybuilders commonly abuse anabolic steroids. Urine specimens can be used to screen for these agents.

SENSITIVITY, SPECIFICITY, AND PREDICTIVE POWER

Not every patient with a particular illness manifests all symptoms, including all laboratory abnormalities. Moreover, some patients may manifest laboratory abnormalities associated with a specific illness without having the illness. Clearly, the presence or absence of a specific laboratory abnormality does not necessarily indicate whether a patient has a particular illness. It is useful to think in terms of the probability of a patient having a particular illness and its associated laboratory abnormalities.

Sensitivity

Sensitivity is the percentage of positive test results found in patients who have a particular disease. In essence, it is the probability of a test being positive in a patient who has the disease. A perfectly sensitive test detects 100 percent of patients who have the illness. The sensitivity can be modified by defining the population that has the illness (e.g., sensitivity in inpatients as opposed to all patients with the disease).

Specificity

Specificity is the percentage of negative results in patients who do not have the disease in question. In essence, it is the probability that an individual who does not have the illness will have a negative test result. A perfectly specific test is negative in 100 percent of the individuals who do not have the illness. Specificity can also be influenced by the population being studied (e.g., carefully screened disease-free individuals as opposed to a random sample of the general population).

Predictive Power

Predictive power is the percentage of results that are accurate. It is the probability that a patient with a positive test result actually has the illness and the probability that a patient with a negative result does not have the illness. A test with perfect predictive power is only positive in those who have the illness. A positive predictive value helps assess the probability that a patient with a positive result actually has the illness. A negative predictive power helps assess the probability that a patient with a negative finding does not have the disease.

SUGGESTED CROSS-REFERENCES

Assessment is also discussed in Section 2.1, the other sections of Chapter 7, Chapters 32 through 49 on child psychiatry, and Chapter 51 on geriatric psychiatry. Neuroimaging is discussed in Sections 1.15 and 1.16. Substance-related disorders are discussed in Chapter 11, schizophrenia is discussed in Chapter 12, mood disorders are discussed in Chapter 13, and anxiety disorders are discussed in Chapter 14. Endocrine and metabolic disorders are discussed in Section 24.6; dementia of the Alzheimer's type is discussed in Chapter 10.

REFERENCES

*American Psychiatric Association Task Force on the Use of Laboratory Tests in Psychiatry: Tricyclic antidepressants—blood level measurements and clinical outcome: An APA Task Force report. *Am J Psychiatry.* 1985;142:155–162.

Aronne LJ, Segal KR: Weight gain in the treatment of mood disorders. *J Clin Psychiatry.* 2003;64[Suppl 8]:22–29.

*Boehnert MT, Lovejoy FH: Value of the QRS duration versus the serum drug level in predicting seizures and ventricular arrhythmias after an acute overdose of tricyclic antidepressants. *N Engl J Med.* 1985:313:474–479.

Chue P, Kovacs CS: Safety and tolerability of atypical antipsychotics in patients with bipolar disorder: Prevalence, monitoring, and management. *Bipolar Disord.* 2003;5[Suppl 2]:62–79.

Foster NL: Validating FDG-PET as a biomarker for frontotemporal dementia. *Exp Neurol.* 2003;184[Suppl 1]:S2–S8.

*Garber HJ, Weinberg JB, Buonanno FS, et al: Use of magnetic resonance imaging in psychiatry. *Am J Psychiatry.* 1988;145:164–171.

Kantarci K, Jack CR Jr: Neuroimaging in Alzheimer's disease: An evidence-based review. *Neuroimaging Clin N Am.* 2003;13:197–209.

Larson EB, Reifler BV, Sumi SM, Canfield CG, Chinn NM: Diagnostic tests in the evaluation of dementia: A prospective study of 200 elderly outpatients. *Arch Intern Med.* 1986;146:1917–1922.

Lambert TJ, Velakoulis D, Pantelis C: Medical comorbidity in schizophrenia. *Med J Aust.* 2003;178[Suppl]:S67–S70.

Lyndenmayer JP, Czobor P, Volavka J, Sheitman B, McEvoy JP, Cooper TB, Chakos M, Lieberman JA: Changes in glucose and cholesterol levels in patients with schizophrenia treated with typical or atypical antipsychotics. *Am J Psychiatry.* 2003;160:290–296.

Marder SR, Essock SM, Miller AL, Buchanan RW, Casey DE, Davis JM, Kane JM, Lieberman J, Schooler NR, Covell N, Stroup S, Weissman EM, Wirshing DA, Hall CS, Pogach L, Xavier P, Bigger JT, Friedman A, Kleinber D, Yevich S, Davis B, Shon S: Health monitoring of patients with schizophrenia. *Am J Psychiatry.* 2004 (*in press*).

*Pope HG, Keck PE, McElroy SL: Frequency and presentation of neuroleptic malignant syndrome in a large psychiatric hospital. *Am J Psychiatry.* 1986;143:1227–1233.

*Post RM. Clinical approaches on the treatment resistant manic and depressive patient. In: *Psychopharmacology in Practice: Clinical and Research Update 1984.* Bethesda, MD: Foundation for Advanced Education in the Sciences; 1984.

Schulte P: What is an adequate trial with clozapine? Therapeutic drug monitoring and time to response in treatment refractory schizophrenia. *Clin Pharmacokinet.* 2003;42:607–618.

▲ 7.9 Psychiatric Rating Scales

DEBORAH BLACKER, M.D., SC.D.

A variety of questionnaires, interviews, checklists, outcome assessments, and other instruments are available to inform psychiatric practice, research, and administration. These instruments, which are grouped here under the term *psychiatric rating scales*, are used with increasing frequency in the practice of psychiatry. Psychiatrists must be aware of rating scales for several reasons. Most critically, many such scales are useful, in practice, for monitoring patients over time or for providing information that is more comprehensive than what is generally obtained in a routine clinical interview. In addition, sometimes scales are required administratively to justify the need for services or to assess quality of care. Last, but equally important, these scales are used in research that informs the practice of psychiatry, so familiarity with them provides a deeper understanding of the results of that research and the degree to which it applies to psychiatric practice.

POTENTIAL BENEFITS AND LIMITATIONS OF RATING SCALES IN PSYCHIATRY

Rating scales in psychiatry serve to standardize the information collected across time and by various observers. This standardization ensures a comprehensive evaluation that may aid treatment planning by establishing a diagnosis, assuring a thorough description of symptoms, identifying comorbid conditions, and characterizing other factors affecting treatment response. In addition, it can establish a baseline for follow-up of the progress of an illness over time or in response to specific interventions. This is particularly useful when several clinicians are involved—for instance, in a group practice or clinical setting or in the conduct of psychiatric research.

In addition to standardization, most rating scales also offer the user the results of a formal evaluation of his or her performance characteristics. This allows the clinician to know to what extent a given scale produces reproducible results (reliability) and how it compares to more definitive or established ways of measuring the same thing (validity).

Rating scales also offer some practical advantages. First, they can save valuable physician time—self-administered rating scales can be completed in the waiting room, or a nurse or technician can administer an interview before a session with the physician. In addition, rating scales may make it easier to obtain information about sensitive areas, such as cognitive decline or sexual side effects, in which direct questioning may sometimes be experienced as more intrusive.

It is important to realize, however, that rating scales are not a panacea. They can provide erroneous measurements due to difficulties in administration or limitations in the underlying construct. In this respect, they are no different than clinical assessments but may appear to provide more definitive information and, thus, a spurious sense of security. At the practical level, they take time that might better be devoted to other pursuits. The critical decision when deciding to use a formal assessment tool in clinical practice is whether, on balance, it contributes useful information in an efficient manner. This decision depends on the specific clinical setting and goal, the practical attributes of the scale, and its psychometric properties.

TYPES OF SCALES AND WHAT THEY MEASURE

Scales are used in psychiatric research and practice to achieve a variety of goals. They also cover a broad range of areas and use a broad range of procedures and formats.

Measurement Goals

Most psychiatric rating scales in common use fall into one or more of the following categories: making a diagnosis (e.g., the Structured Clinical Interview for the revised fourth edition of the *Diagnostic and Statistical Manual of Mental Disorders* [DSM-IV-TR] [SCID] or the Diagnostic Interview Schedule for Children [DISC]); measuring severity and tracking change in specific symptoms (e.g., the Hamilton Anxiety Rating Scale [HAM-A] or the Mini-Mental State Examination [MMSE]), in general functioning (e.g., the Short Form 36 [SF-36]), or in overall outcome (e.g., the Behavior and Symptom Identification Scale [BASIS-32]); and screening for conditions that may or may not be present (e.g., the CAGE).

Constructs Assessed

Psychiatric practitioners and investigators assess a broad range of areas, referred to as *constructs* to underscore the fact that they are not simple, direct observations of nature. These include diagnoses, signs and symptoms, severity, functional impairment, quality of life, and many others. Some of these constructs are fairly complex and are divided into two or more domains (e.g., positive and negative symptoms in schizophrenia, or mood and neurovegetative symptoms in major depression). Many scales yield separate scores, or *subscales*, for each domain. In cases in which these domains are seen as substantially independent, they may be referred to as *dimensions* (e.g., Axis I and Axis II in DSM-IV-TR, multidimensional personality traits).

Categorical versus Continuous Classification

Some constructs are viewed as *categorical* or classifying, whereas others are seen as *continuous* or measuring. Categorical constructs describe the presence or absence of a given attribute (e.g., competency to stand trial) or the category best suited to a given individual among a finite set of options (e.g., assigning a diagnosis). Continuous measures provide a quantitative assessment along a continuum of intensity, frequency, or severity. In addition to symptom severity and functional status, multidimensional personality traits, cognitive status, social support, and many other attributes are generally measured continuously.

The distinction between categorical and continuous measures is by no means absolute. *Ordinal* classification, which uses a finite, ordered set of categories (e.g., unaffected, mild, moderate, severe), stands between the two. In addition, a cutpoint is frequently used with a continuous or ordinal scale to indicate a threshold for membership in a corresponding category. For instance, individuals with MMSE scores below 24 may be considered to have a dementia, or those with Hamilton Rating Scale for Depression (HAM-D) scores above 8 may be considered to have an episode of major depression.

Measurement Procedures

Rating scales differ in measurement methods. Issues to be considered include format, raters, and sources of information.

Format

Rating scales are available in a variety of formats. Some are simply checklists or guides to observation that help the clinician achieve a standardized rating. Others are self-administered questionnaires or tests. Still others are formal interviews that may be *fully structured* (i.e., specifying the exact wording of questions to be asked) or *partly structured* (i.e., providing only some specific wording, along with suggestions for additional questions or probes). Whether fully structured or not, instruments may be written such that all questions are always included, or they may have formal skip-out sections to limit administration time.

Individual items also vary in format. Most commonly, scales use yes–no or multiple-choice questions. Often, answers will be graded on a *Likert* scale, an ordinal scale with three to seven points that measures severity, intensity, frequency, or other attributes. Likert scales are most often partially or fully *anchored*, assigning a meaning to each numeric level. The same anchors can apply to all of the items, or the instrument may provide specific anchors for each. Occasionally, questionnaires include open-ended questions, especially at the beginning, which may be used to help establish rapport. In semistructured or unstructured interviews, this information also serves to guide the rest of the interview and to aid in forming a clinical impression about the patient.

Raters Some instruments are designed to be administered by doctoral-level clinicians only, whereas others may be administered by psychiatric nurses or social workers with more limited clinical experience. Still other instruments are designed primarily for use by lay raters with little or no experience with psychopathology. In general, more training is required to administer less-structured scales. In addition, some scales require extensive training, even for experienced clinicians, to master the appropriate procedures and achieve a good result. Virtually all scales perform better when raters are familiar with their format and specific content.

Source of Information Instruments also vary in the source of information used to make the ratings. Information may be obtained solely from the patient, who generally knows the most about his or her condition. In some instruments, some or all of the information may be obtained from a knowledgeable informant. When the construct involves limited insight (e.g., cognitive disorders or mania) or significant social undesirability (e.g., antisocial personality, substance abuse), other informants may be preferable. Informants may also be helpful when the subject has limited ability to recall or report symptoms (e.g., delirium, dementia, or any disorder in young children). Some rating scales also allow or require information to be included from medical records or from patient observation.

ASSESSMENT OF RATING SCALES

In clinical research, rating scales are mandatory to ensure interpretable and potentially generalizable results and are selected based on coverage of the relevant constructs, expense (based on the nature of the raters, purchase price if any, and necessary training), length and administration time, comprehensibility to the intended audience, and quality of the ratings provided. In clinical practice, one considers these factors and, also, whether a scale would provide more or better information than what would be obtained in ordinary clinical practice or would contribute to the efficiency of obtaining that information. In either case, the assessment of quality is based on *psychometric*, or mind-measuring, properties.

Psychometric Properties

The two principal psychometric properties of a measure are *reliability* and *validity*. Although these words are used almost interchangeably in everyday speech, they are distinct in the context of evaluating rating scales. To be useful, scales should be *reliable*, or consistent and repeatable even if performed by different raters at different times or under different conditions, and they should be *valid*, or accurate in representing the true state of nature.

Relationship between Reliability and Validity Establishing a measure's reliability is generally considered primary, as it is difficult to reach valid judgments without first achieving consistency. However, problems with reliability can be overcome to an extent by combining information from several assessments. Unfortunately, improved reliability does not guarantee improved validity, and some efforts to improve reliability may actually limit validity. For example, a personality disorder instrument might focus on overt behaviors rather than inner thoughts and feelings to achieve higher reliability, but at the cost of losing some of the most valid information about personality. Even with clinically trained raters, it is particularly difficult to achieve reliability on items requiring subjective clinical judgment (e.g., feelings evoked in the examiner). Nonetheless, when used by experienced diagnosticians, such items may contribute substantially to valid diagnoses.

Reliability *Reliability* refers to the consistency or repeatability of ratings and is largely empirical. In the categorical context, it refers to whether there is agreement on the classification of each individual. In the continuous context, it refers to whether there is agreement on the assignment of a given score. It can also be seen as precision (i.e., whether a measure yields a "ballpark" estimate or a finely graded score). An instrument is more likely to be reliable if the instructions and questions are clearly and simply worded and the format is easy to understand and score. There are three standard ways to assess reliability: *internal consistency*, *interrater*, and *test–retest*.

INTERNAL CONSISTENCY Internal consistency assesses agreement among the individual items in a measure. This provides information about reliability, because each item is viewed as a single measurement of the underlying construct. Thus, the coherence of the items suggests that each is measuring the same thing. Internal consistency is measured most often with *coefficient alpha* (also known as *Cronback's coefficient alpha*), which ranges between 0 and 1—values of .75 or higher are considered good. However, it should be noted that the internal consistency of a *measure* depends on the internal consistency of the *construct* that the measure purports to assess and will be higher for unidimensional constructs than for those with two or more relatively independent domains.

INTERRATER AND TEST–RETEST RELIABILITY Interrater (also called *interjudge* or *joint*) reliability is a measure of agreement between two or more observers evaluating the same subjects using the same information. Estimates may vary with assessment conditions—for instance, estimates of interrater reliability–based videotaped interviews tend to be higher than those based on interviews conducted by one of the raters. Interrater reliability tends to be higher than *test–retest reliability*, a measure of agreement between evaluations at two points in time in which there may be differences in the information obtained (e.g., associated with differences in interviewer skill, interviewer mood, room conditions, or subject's attitude). In addition, test–retest evaluations measure reliability only to the extent that the subject's true condition remains stable in the time interval, which is problematic for many conditions but virtually impossible for rapidly fluctuating conditions like state anxiety. However, the test–retest situation more closely reflects the clinical problems associated with serial evaluations by multiple clinicians, so, to the extent that concerns about interval change can be eliminated, it is generally a more useful indicator of reliability in practice.

Interrater reliability and test–retest reliability of continuous constructs are measured with the intraclass correlation coefficient (ICC), whereas those of categorical constructs are measured with the kappa coefficient (κ). A weighted version of κ is available to give greater penalties for large disagreements than for small ones (e.g., between schizophrenia and psychotic depression, as compared to schizophrenia and schizoaffective disorder). Both κ and the ICC are measures of agreement corrected for the agreement expected by chance alone, and both range from 0 to 1. As a rule of thumb, a κ or ICC above 0.8 is considered excellent, those in the 0.7 to 0.8 range are considered good, and those in the 0.5 to 0.7 range are considered fair. However, the degree of reliability required varies with the clinical purpose: extremely reliable ratings are required before administering potentially dangerous treatments, whereas more modest reliability may be satisfactory for estimating rates in a population.

ISSUES IN INTERPRETING RELIABILITY DATA When interpreting reliability data, it is important to bear in mind that reliability estimates published in the literature may not generalize to other settings. Factors to consider are the nature of the sample, the training and experience of the raters, and the test conditions. Issues regarding the sample are especially critical. In particular, reliability tends to be higher in samples with high variability in which it is easier to make discriminations among individuals. Thus, for continuous measures, reliability tends to be higher when the sample includes individuals with a wide range of scores. For categorical measures, reliability tends to be higher when the prevalence of the attribute being measured is fairly high. Reliability estimates also depend on the fraction of difficult cases (e.g., individuals near a diagnostic threshold or those resistant to being interviewed), as large numbers of these tend to diminish observed reliability.

Validity

Validity refers to conformity with truth, or a gold standard that can stand for truth. In the categorical context, it refers to whether an instrument can make correct classifications. In the continuous context, it refers to accuracy, or whether the score assigned can be said to represent the true state of nature. Although reliability is an empirical question, validity is partly theoretical—for many constructs measured in psychiatry, there is no underlying absolute truth. Even so, some measures yield more useful and meaningful data than others do. Validity assessment is generally divided into face and content validity, criterion validity, and construct validity.

FACE AND CONTENT VALIDITY *Face validity* refers to whether the items appear to assess the construct in question. Although a rating scale may purport to measure a construct of interest, a review of the items may reveal that it embodies a very different conceptualization of the construct. For instance, an insight scale may define *insight* in either psychoanalytic or neurological terms. However, items with a transparent relationship to the construct may be a disadvantage when measuring socially undesirable traits, such as substance abuse or malingering. *Content validity* is similar to face validity but describes whether the measure provides good balanced coverage of the construct and is less focused on whether the items give the appearance of validity. Content validity is often assessed with formal procedures such as expert consensus or factor analysis.

CRITERION VALIDITY *Criterion validity* (sometimes called *predictive* or *concurrent validity*) refers to whether or not the measure agrees with a gold standard or criterion of accuracy. Suitable gold standards include the long form of an established instrument for a new, shorter version, a clinician-rated measure for a self-report form, and blood or urine tests for measures of drug use. For diagnostic interviews, the generally accepted gold standard is the *L*ongitudinal, *E*xpert, *A*ll *D*ata (LEAD) standard, which incorporates expert clinical evaluation, longitudinal data, medical records, family history, and any other sources of information.

When comparing continuous measures to a gold standard, a correlation coefficient is the statistic most often reported. For categorical variables, such as diagnoses (or continuous measures with a cutpoint), *sensitivity* and *specificity* are the statistics of choice. *Sensitivity* refers to the test's ability to identify true cases, or its *true-positive rate*. Specificity is the test's accuracy in identifying noncases, or one minus the *false-positive rate*. In general, the more sensitive a test, the less specific it is. If the threshold for diagnosis, for example, is lowered, more cases will be detected, but at the expense of some false positives; if the threshold is raised to decrease the false positives, true cases will inevitably be missed. The optimal threshold depends on the consequences of false positives and false negatives.

CONSTRUCT VALIDITY When an adequate gold standard is not available—a frequent state of affairs in psychiatry—or when additional validity data are desired, construct validity must be assessed. To accomplish this, one can compare the measure to *external validators*, attributes that bear a well-characterized relationship to the construct under study but are not measured directly by the instrument. External validators used to validate psychiatric diagnostic criteria and the diagnostic instruments that aim to operationalize them include course of illness, family history, and treatment response. For example, when compared to schizophrenia measures, mania measures are expected to identify more individuals with a remitting course, a family history of major mood disorders, and a good response to lithium.

Two special cases of assessing validity using external validators have particular relevance for clinical psychiatry. One is *discriminant validity*, which examines a measure's ability to discriminate between populations that are expected to differ on the construct of interest. For example, does a sociopathy measure correctly separate individuals in jails from those living in the community? Although such discriminations are important in clinical practice, it is important to remember that the true test of a measure is its ability to discriminate at the margins. A study of discriminant validity is more clearly relevant if it includes the types of cases encountered in clinical practice (e.g., psychotic depression versus schizoaffective disorder) rather than more easily discriminated populations (e.g., psychotic depression versus normal). Another special case is *sensitivity to change*: the fact that a measure shows expected changes (e.g., an improvement with an efficacious treatment or a decrement with a progressive disease) can be a strong validator.

When assessing validity in areas in which there are few established measures and a gold standard or criterion of accuracy cannot be established, the assessment of the validity of the measure is limited by the validity of the construct itself. Nonetheless, by triangulating between a better definition of the construct, better ways to measure it, and better exploration of how it operates in clinical practice and research, the field moves to greater validity over time.

SELECTION OF PSYCHIATRIC RATING SCALES

In this section, a group of rating scales used in psychiatric practice and research is presented. The scales are grouped by topic, beginning with general issues, including diagnosis, functioning, symptom severity, and side effects, and then proceeding to specific diagnostic groups, organized according to the sections of DSM-IV-TR. Selections were made based on coverage of major areas and common use in clinical research or current (or potential) use in clinical practice. For each area, there is a brief discussion of measurement issues followed by a description of each instrument, its psychometric properties, and its potential uses. In addition, whenever possible, a brief, clinically useful instrument is provided in each area. References for each measure, organized by topic, are listed in Table 7.9–1. These references include more detailed information about each measure and its psychometric properties and may also provide either the measure itself or instructions regarding how to obtain a copy. Access to instruments via the World Wide Web is increasing rapidly, but Internet addresses evolve still more rapidly, so they are not included here. Instead, a quick search using Google or a similar search engine is recommended to locate a Web site that may offer the instrument for purchase or download, an up-to-date list of references, and other information.

Functional Status, Impairment, and General Symptom Severity

This broad area cuts across a variety of diagnoses and is, thus, useful for grading patients by functional status or overall severity without reference to specific symptomatology. Most of the instruments presented here have a strong mental health focus and often include items on psychiatric symptomatology.

Global Assessment of Functioning (GAF) and the Social and Occupational Functioning Assessment Scale (SOFAS)

The GAF (Table 7.9–2) was developed in the early 1990s to rate Axis V of DSM-IV and provides a measure of overall

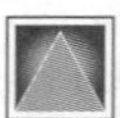

Table 7.9–1
Key References for Measures Included

Rating Scale	Reference
Functional status, impairment, and general symptom severity	
GAF[a]	Patterson DA, Lee MS: Field trial of the Global Assessment of Functioning Scale—Modified. *Am J Psychiatry.* 1995;152:1386.
SOFAS[a]	DSM-IV-TR
GARF[a]	DSM-IV-TR
BASIS-32[a]	Eisen SV, Dill DL, Grob MC: Reliability and validity of a brief patient-report instrument for psychiatric outcome evaluation. *Hosp Community Psychiatry.* 1994;45:242.
SF-36	McHorney CA, Ware JE, Raczek AE: The MOS 36-Item Short Form Health Survey (SF-36), II: psychometric and clinical tests of validity in measuring physical and mental health constructs. *Med Care.* 1993;31:247.
Side effects	
SAFTEE	Levine J, Schooler NR: SAFTEE: a technique for the systematic assessment of side effects in clinical trials. *Psychopharmacol Bull.* 1986;22:343.
AIMS[a]	Lane RD, Glazer WM, Hansen TE, Berman WH, Kramer SI: Assessment of tardive dyskinesia using the Abnormal Involuntary Movement Scale. *J Nerv Ment Dis.* 1985;173:353.
Simpson-Angus Rating Scale for Extrapyramidal Side Effects	Simpson GM, Angus JWS: A rating scale for extrapyramidal side effects. *Acta Psychiatr Scand.* 1970;46(Suppl 212):11.
Psychiatric diagnosis	
SCID	Spitzer RL, Williams JB, Gibbon M, First MB: The Structured Clinical Interview for DSM-III-R (SCID). I: History, rationale, and description. *Arch Gen Psychiatry.* 1992;49: 624.
DIS	Robins LN, Helzer JE, Croughan J, Ratcliff KS: National Institute of Mental Health Diagnostic Interview Schedule. *Arch Gen Psychiatry.* 1981;38:381.
CIDI	Wittchen H-U: Reliability and validity studies of the WHO-Composite International Diagnostic Interview (CIDI): a critical review. *J Psychiatr Res.* 1994;28:57.
PRIME-MD	Spitzer RL, Williams JBW, Kroenke K, Linzer M, deGruy FV, Hahn SR, Brody D, Johnson JG: Utility of a new procedure for diagnosing mental disorders in primary care: the PRIME-MD Study. *JAMA.* 1994;272:1749.
Psychotic disorders	
BPRS[a]	Overall JE, Gorham DR: The Brief Psychiatric Rating Scale (BPRS): a comprehensive review. *J Operational Psychiatry.* 1991;148:472.
PANSS	Kay SR, Fiszbein A, Opler LA: The positive and negative syndrome scale (PANSS) for schizophrenia. *Schizophr Bull.* 1987;13:261.
SAPS/SANS	Andreasen NC, Arndt S, Miller D, Flaum M, Nopoulos P: Correlational studies of the Scale for the Assessment of Negative Symptoms and the Scale for the Assessment of Positive Symptoms: an overview and update. *Psychopathology.* 1995;28:7.
Mood disorders	
HAM-D[a]	Hamilton M: A rating scale for depression. *J Neurol Neurosurg Psychiatr.* 1960;23:56.
BDI	Beck AT, Steer RA, Garbin MG: Psychometric properties of the Beck Depression Inventory: twenty-five years of evaluation. *Clin Psychology Rev.* 1988;8:77.
IDS	Rush AJ, Gullion CM, Basco MR, Jarrett RB, Trivedi MH: The Inventory of Depressive Symptomatology (IDS): psychometric properties. *Psychol Med.* 1996;26:477.
YMRS	Young RC, Biggs JT, Ziegler VE, Meyer DA: A rating scale for mania: reliability, validity and sensitivity. *Br J Psychiatry.* 1978;133:429.
Anxiety disorders	
HAM-A[a]	Hamilton M: The assessment of anxiety scales by rating. *Br J Psychol.* 1959;32:50.
PDSS	Shear MK, Brown TA, Barlow DH, Money R, Sholomskas DE, Woods SW, Gorman JM, Papp LA: Multicenter collaborative Panic Disorder Severity Scale. *Am J Psychiatry.* 1997;154:1571.
CAPS	Blake DD, Weathers FW, Nagy LN, Kaloupe DG, Klauminzer G, Charney DS, Keane TM: A clinician rating scale for assessing current and lifetime PTSD: the CAPS-1. *Behav Therapist.* 1990;18:187.
YBOCS	Goodman WK, Price LH, Rasmussen SA, Mazure C, Fleischman RL, Hill CL, Heninger GR, Charney DS: The Yale-Brown Obsessive Compulsive Scale: I. Development, use, and reliability. *Arch Gen Psychiatry.* 1989;46:1006.
Substance use disorders	
CAGE	Ewing JA: Detecting alcoholism: the CAGE questionnaire. *JAMA.* 1984;252:1905.
AUDIT[a]	Saunders JB, Aasland OG, Babor TF, de le Fuente JR, Grant M: Development of the Alcohol Use Disorders Identification Test (AUDIT): WHO Collaborative Project on Early Detection of Persons with Harmful Alcohol Consumption-II. *Addiction.* 1993;88:791.
DAST	Skinner HA: The Drug Abuse Screening Test. *Addictive Behav.* 1982;7:363.
ASI	McLellan AT, Kushner H, Metzger D, Peters F, Peters R, Smith I, Grissom G, Pettinati H, Argeriou M: The fifth edition of the Addiction Severity Index. *J Subst Abuse Treat.* 1992;9:199.
Eating disorders	
EDE	Cooper Z, Fairburn CG: The Eating Disorder Examination: a semistructured interview for the assessment of the specific psychopathology of eating disorders. *Int J Eat Disord.* 1987;6:1.

(*continued*)

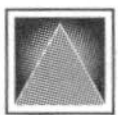

Table 7.9–1 (*continued*)

Rating Scale	Reference
BULIT-R	Thelen MH, Mintz LB, Vander Wal JS: The Bulimia Test 3/4 Revised: validation with DSM-IV criteria for bulimia nervosa. *Psychol Assess.* 1996;8:219.
Cognitive disorders	
MMSE	Folstein MF, Folstein SE, McHugh PR. "Mini-Mental State": a practical method for grading the cognitive state of patients for the clinician. *J Psychiatr Res.* 1975;12:189.
IMC	Blessed G, Tomlinson BE, Roth M: The association between quantitative measures of dementia and of senile change in the cerebral grey matter of elderly subjects. *Br J Psychiatry.* 1968;114:797.
OMC	Katzman R, Brown T, Fuld P, Peck A, Schecter R, Schimmel H: Validation of a Short Orientation-Memory-Concentration Test of cognitive impairment. *Am J Psychiatry.* 1983;140:734.
CDR[a]	Hughes CP, Berg L, Danziger WL, Cohen LA, Martin RL: A new clinical scale for the staging of dementia. *Br J Psychiatry.* 1982;140:566.
Personality disorders	
SCID-II	First MB, Spitzer RL, Gibbon M, Williams JBW: The Structured Clinical Interview for DSM-III-R Personality Disorders (SCID-II): part I: description. *J Personal Disord.* 1995;9:83.
PDQ	Hyler SE, Rieder RO, Williams JBW, Spitzer RL, Hendler J, Lyons M: The Personality Diagnostic Questionnaire: development and preliminary results. *J Personal Disord.* 1988;2:229.
Childhood disorders	
CBCL[a]	Achenbach TM. *Manual for the Child Behavior Checklist/4-18 and 1991 Profile.* Burlington: University of Vermont; 1991.
DISC	King C, Katz S, Ghaziuddin N, Brand E, Hill E, McGovern L: Diagnosis and assessment of depression and suicidality using the NIMH Diagnostic Interview Schedule for Children (DISC-2.3). *J Abnorm Child Psychol.* 1997;25:173.
Conners Rating Scales	Conners CK, Wells KC, Parker JD, Sitarenios G, Diamond JM, Powell JW: A new self-report scale for assessment of adolescent psychopathology: factor structure, reliability, validity, and diagnostic sensitivity. *J Abnorm Child Psychol.* 1997;25:487.

Note: For full name of scales denoted by these abbreviations, please see relevant section of this chapter.
[a]Full text of scale is included in chapter.

functioning related to psychiatric symptoms. The GAF is extremely similar to the Global Assessment Scale (GAS) used for the same purpose in DSM-III and DSM-III-R, from which it was derived. A related instrument is the SOFAS (Table 7.9–3), proposed as a new axis listed in Appendix B of DSM-IV, which focuses only on functioning and not on symptoms and does not try to discriminate between functional changes related to psychiatric and nonpsychiatric causes. Both scales are clinician-rated on a 100-point scale based on all available information, with clear descriptions of each ten-point interval. Ratings are generally made for the past week, but longer intervals (e.g., highest during the past year) can be used. Instructions for rating the GAF and SOFAS are included in DSM-IV-TR; clinician raters do not require additional training to use these scales. The GAS has received more extensive evaluation and shows fair to good reliability and good validity judged against clinician ratings of the degree of impairment. GAF or GAS ratings are often required for billing purposes. In addition, the scales have been used to track change with treatment in inpatient and outpatient practice and in multiple research studies. The major criticism of the GAS and GAF is that they tend to confound symptoms and functioning, causing individuals with significant symptomatology (e.g., fixed delusional system) to score low even when their social and occupational functioning is relatively spared. The SOFAS was designed to overcome this limitation but is generally not as widely used.

Global Assessment of Relational Functioning (GARF) The GARF (Table 7.9–4) was developed in the late 1980s to provide a measure of the quality of functioning in relationships analogous to the measure of individual functioning provided by the GAF or SOFAS. It was subsequently included in Appendix B of DSM-IV as an additional axis for further consideration. It provides a global rating on a 100-point scale based on a review of three major areas: problem-solving, organization, and emotional climate. Anchors are provided for each quintile of each domain. The GARF is focused on the particular needs of family and couple therapists but can be rated by any clinician. Ratings are generally based on the present, but alternate periods (e.g., the past year, or the period after a major stressor) can be implemented. Available psychometric evidence suggests that clinician and even nonclinician raters can achieve good to excellent reliability with only minimal training. The validity of the GARF is supported by expected correlations with other measures of family and couple distress and functioning. The GARF shows promise for rating relational functioning, and it may also be useful in clinical or research practice.

Behavior and Symptom Identification Scale (BASIS-32) The BASIS-32 (Table 7.9–5) was developed in the early 1990s to provide a broad but brief overview of psychiatric symptoms and functional status from the patient's point of view for use in assessing the outcome of psychiatric treatment. The instrument assesses a wide range of areas, including family and work relationships; ability to complete regular tasks at home, work, or school; and symptoms of anxiety, depression, psychosis, and substance abuse. Each item is rated on a five-point scale focused on the degree of difficulty during the preceding week. The BASIS-32 can be completed as a paper-and-pencil test (requiring 5 to 20 minutes), or the questions can be read aloud with the patient selecting the best answer from a laminated card (requiring 15 to 20 minutes). It can be scored readily by hand, but a computerized scoring system is also available. The BASIS-32 generates an overall score and five subscales: relation to self and others, daily living and role functioning, depression and anxiety, impulsive and addictive behavior, and psychosis. Good reli-

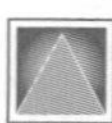

Table 7.9–2
Global Assessment of Functioning (GAF) Scale

Consider psychological, social, and occupational functioning on a hypothetical continuum of mental health–illness. Do not include impairment in functioning due to physical (or environmental) limitations.

Code	(**Note:** Use intermediate codes when appropriate, e.g., 45, 68, 72.)
100–91	Superior functioning in a wide range of activities, life's problems never seem to get out of hand, is sought out by others because of his or her many positive qualities. No symptoms.
90–81	Absent or minimal symptoms (e.g., mild anxiety before an exam), good functioning in all areas, interested and involved in a wide range of activities, socially effective, generally satisfied with life, no more than everyday problems or concerns (e.g., an occasional argument with family members).
80–71	If symptoms are present, they are transient and expectable reactions to psychosocial stressors (e.g., difficulty concentrating after family argument): no more than slight impairment in social, occupational, or school functioning (e.g., temporarily falling behind in schoolwork).
70–61	Some mild symptoms (e.g., depressed mood and mild insomnia) OR some difficulty in social, occupational, or school functioning (e.g., occasional truancy, or theft within the household), but generally functioning pretty well, has some meaningful interpersonal relationships.
60–51	Moderate symptoms (e.g., flat affect and circumstantial speech, occasional panic attacks) OR moderate difficulty in social, occupational, or school functioning (e.g., few friends, conflicts with peers or coworkers).
50–41	Serious symptoms (e.g., suicidal ideation, severe obsessional rituals, frequent shoplifting) OR any serious impairment in social, occupational, or school functioning (e.g., no friends, unable to keep a job).
40–31	Some impairment in reality testing or communication (e.g., speech is at times illogical, obscure, or irrelevant) OR major impairment in several areas, such as work or school, family relations, judgment, thinking, or mood (e.g., depressed man avoids friends, neglects family, and is unable to work; child frequently beats up younger children, is defiant at home, and is failing at school).
30–21	Behavior is considerably influenced by delusions or hallucinations OR serious impairment in communication or judgment (e.g., sometimes incoherent, acts grossly inappropriately, suicidal preoccupation) OR inability to function in almost all areas (e.g., stays in bed all day; no job, home, or friends).
20–11	Some danger of hurting self or others (e.g., suicide attempts without clear expectation of death, frequently violent, manic excitement) OR occasionally fails to maintain minimal personal hygiene (e.g., smears feces) OR gross impairment in communication (e.g., largely incoherent or mute).
10–1	Persistent danger of severely hurting self or others (e.g., recurrent violence) OR persistent inability to maintain minimal personal hygiene OR serious suicidal act with clear expectation of death.
0	Inadequate information.

Note: The rating of overall psychological functioning on a scale of 0 to 100 was operationalized by Luborsky in the Health-Sickness Rating Scale (Luborsky L: Clinicians' judgments of mental health. *Arch Gen Psychiatry.* 1962;7:407). Spitzer and colleagues developed a revision of the Health-Sickness Rating Scale called the Global Assessment Scale (GAS) (Endicott J, Spitzer RL, Fleiss JL, Cohen J: The Global Assessment Scale: a procedure for measuring overall severity of psychiatric disturbance. *Arch Gen Psychiatry.* 1976;33:766). A modified version of the GAS was included in DSM-III-R as the Global Assessment of Functioning (GAF) Scale.

From American Psychiatric Association. *Diagnostic and Statistical Manual of Mental Disorders.* 4th ed. Text rev. Washington, DC: American Psychiatric Association; 2000, with permission.

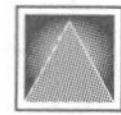

Table 7.9–3
Social and Occupational Functioning Assessment Scale (SOFAS)

Consider social and occupational functioning on a continuum from excellent functioning to grossly impaired functioning. Include impairments in functioning due to physical limitations, as well as those due to mental impairments. To be counted, impairment must be a direct consequence of mental and physical health problems; the effects of lack of opportunity and other environmental limitations are not to be considered.

Code	(**Note:** Use intermediate codes when appropriate, e.g., 45, 68, 72.)
100–91	Superior functioning in a wide range of activities.
90–81	Good functioning in all areas, occupationally and socially effective.
80–71	No more than a slight impairment in social, occupational, or school functioning (e.g., infrequent interpersonal conflict, temporarily falling behind in schoolwork).
70–61	Some difficulty in social, occupational, or school functioning, but generally functioning well, has some meaningful interpersonal relationships.
60–51	Moderate difficulty in social, occupational, or school functioning (e.g., few friends, conflicts with peers or coworkers).
50–41	Serious impairment in social, occupational, or school functioning (e.g., no friends, unable to keep a job).
40–31	Major impairment in several areas, such as work or school, family relations (e.g., depressed man avoids friends, neglects family, and is unable to work; child frequently beats up younger children, is defiant at home, and is failing at school).
30–21	Inability to function in almost all areas (e.g., stays in bed all day; no job, home, or friends).
20–11	Occasionally fails to maintain minimal personal hygiene; unable to function independently.
10–1	Persistent inability to maintain minimal personal hygiene. Unable to function without harming self or others or without considerable external support (e.g., nursing care and supervision).
0	Inadequate information.

Note: The rating of overall psychological functioning on a scale of 0 to 100 was operationalized by Luborsky in the Health-Sickness Rating Scale. (Luborsky L: Clinicians' judgments of mental health. *Arch Gen Psychiatry.* 1962;7:407.) Spitzer and colleagues developed a revision of the Health-Sickness Rating Scale called the Global Assessment Scale (GAS) (Endicott J, Spitzer RL, Fleiss JL, et al: The Global Assessment Scale: a procedure for measuring overall severity of psychiatric disturbance. *Arch Gen Psychiatry.* 1976;33:766). The SOFAS is derived from the GAS and its development is described in Goldman HH, Skodol AE, Lave TR: Revising Axis V for DSM-IV: a review of measures of social functioning. *Am J Psychiatry.* 1992;149:1148.

ability and validity have been demonstrated. Its simple administration, brevity, and broad coverage make it well suited to its original task, and it is frequently used at baseline, during treatment, and after treatment to monitor progress. It is capable of providing valid ratings across a wide range of psychiatric impairment but is not generally suitable for individuals with substantial cognitive impairment. It is also not suitable for children under 14 years of age. Over the past several years, a new version of the instrument, known as the *BASIS-R*, has been developed and tested around the country. The revision, which is expected to be released in the near future, is designed to streamline the instrument and make it more suitable for use with ethnic minorities and a still broader range of psychiatric patients.

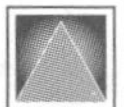

Table 7.9–4
Global Assessment of Relational Functioning (GARF)

INSTRUCTIONS: The GARF Scale can be used to indicate an overall judgment of the functioning of a family or other ongoing relationship on a hypothetical continuum ranging from competent, optimal relational functioning to a disrupted, dysfunctional relationship. It is analogous to Axis V (Global Assessment of Functioning Scale) provided for individuals in DSM-IV. The GARF Scale permits the clinician to rate the degree to which a family or other ongoing relational unit meets the affective and/or instrumental needs of its members in the following areas:

A. *Problem solving*—skills in negotiating goals, rules, and routines; adaptability to stress; communication skills; ability to resolve conflict.

B. *Organization*—maintenance of interpersonal roles and subsystem boundaries; hierarchical functioning, coalitions and distribution of power, control and responsibility.

C. *Emotional climate*—tone and range of feelings; quality of caring, empathy, involvement and attachment/commitment; sharing of values; mutual affective responsiveness, respect, and regard; quality of sexual functioning.

In most instances, the GARF Scale should be used to rate functioning during the current period (i.e., the level of relational functioning at the time of the evaluation). In some settings, the GARF Scale may also be used to rate functioning for other time periods (i.e., the highest level of relational functioning for at least a few months during the past year). **Note:** Use specific, intermediate codes when possible, for example, 45, 68, 72. If detailed information is not adequate to make specific ratings, use midpoints of the five ranges, that is, 90, 70, 50, 30, or 10.

(81–100) Overall: Relational unit is functioning satisfactorily from self-report of participants and from perspectives of observers.

Agreed-on patterns or routines exist that help meet the usual needs of each family/couple member; there is flexibility for change in response to unusual demands or events; occasional conflicts and stressful transitions are resolved through problem-solving communication and negotiation.

There is a shared understanding and agreement about roles and appropriate tasks; decision making is established for each functional area; and there is recognition of the unique characteristics and merit of each subsystem (e.g., parents/spouses, siblings, and individuals).

There is a situationally appropriate, optimistic atmosphere in the family; a wide range of feelings is freely expressed and managed within the family; there is a general atmosphere of warmth, caring, and sharing of values among all family members. Sexual relations of adult members are satisfactory.

(61–80) Overall: Functioning of relational unit is somewhat unsatisfactory. Over a period of time, many but not all difficulties are resolved without complaints.

Daily routines are present but there is some pain and difficulty in responding to the unusual. Some conflicts remain unresolved, but do not disrupt family functioning.

Decision making is usually competent, but efforts at control of one another quite often are greater than necessary or are ineffective. Individuals and relationships are clearly demarcated but sometimes a specific subsystem is depreciated or scapegoated.

A range of feeling is expressed, but instances of emotional blocking or tension are evident. Warmth and caring are present but are marred by a family member's irritability and frustrations. Sexual activity of adult members may be reduced or problematic.

(41–60) Overall: Relational unit has occasional times of satisfying and competent functioning together, but clearly dysfunctional, unsatisfying relationships tend to predominate.

Communication is frequently inhibited by unresolved conflicts that often interfere with daily routines; there is significant difficulty in adapting to family stress and transitional change.

Decision making is only intermittently competent and effective; either excessive rigidity or significant lack of structure is evident at these times. Individual needs are quite often submerged by a partner or coalition.

Pain or ineffective anger or emotional deadness interferes with family enjoyment. Although there is some warmth and support for members, it is usually unequally distributed. Troublesome sexual difficulties between adults are often present.

(21–40) Overall: Relational unit is obviously and seriously dysfunctional; forms and time periods of satisfactory relating are rare.

Family/couple routines do not meet the needs of members; they are grimly adhered to or blithely ignored. Life cycle changes, such as departures or entries into the relational unit, generate painful conflict and obviously frustrating failures of problem solving.

Decision making is tyrannical or quite ineffective. The unique characteristics of individuals are unappreciated or ignored by either rigid or confusingly fluid coalitions.

There are infrequent periods of enjoyment of life together; frequent distancing or open hostility reflect significant conflicts that remain unresolved and quite painful. Sexual dysfunction among adult members is commonplace.

(1–20) Overall: Relational unit has become too dysfunctional to retain continuity of contact and attachment.

Family/couple routines are negligible (e.g., no mealtime, sleeping, or waking schedule); family members often do not know where others are or when they will be in or out; there is little effective communication among family members.

Family/couple members are not organized in such a way that personal or generational responsibilities are recognized. Boundaries of relational unit as a whole and subsystems cannot be identified or agreed upon. Family members are physically endangered or injured or sexually attacked.

Despair and cynicism are pervasive; there is little attention to the emotional needs of others; there is almost no sense of attachment, commitment, or concern about one another's welfare.

0 Inadequate information.

From American Psychiatric Association. *Diagnostic and Statistical Manual of Mental Disorders.* 4th ed. Text rev. Washington, DC: American Psychiatric Association; 2000, with permission.

Short Form 36 (SF-36) The SF-36 was developed in 1993 as a general measure of health status from the patient's point of view that would be independent of specific diseases and equally applicable to medical and psychiatric patients and to the general population. The SF-36 consists of 36 items, a mixture of yes–no questions and short Likert scales. It is focused on the individual's functional status as it relates to physical problems, pain, and emotional difficulties over the last 4 weeks. An acute version, focused on the past week, is also available, as are 8- and 12-item versions; however, the 4-week, 36-item version is the most widely used. The items are used to rate eight separate subscales: physical function, physical role function, pain, general health, vitality, social function, emotional role function, and mental health. Computer programs are available for administration and scoring. It is designed as a self-report instrument but can easily be read by an interviewer in person or over the phone. The instrument can be completed in 10 to 15 minutes. It has been subjected to extensive psychometric testing in clinical and general population samples, with extensive norms available. There is demonstrated high internal consis-

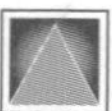

Table 7.9–5
Behavior and Symptom Identification Scale (BASIS-32)

FOR OFFICE USE ONLY Site code ☐☐☐

INSTRUCTIONS TO STAFF: Please write the respondent's Identification Number and Visit Number, one digit in each box. Fill in the Visit Type and Level of Care using the code numbers below.

Identification Number ☐☐☐☐☐☐☐☐☐☐

Visit Number ☐☐☐☐☐☐☐☐

Visit Type ☐

1 = Admission/Intake
2 = Mid-Treatment
3 = Discharge/Termination
4 = Post-Treatment Follow-up

Level of Care ☐

1 = Inpatient
2 = Outpatient
3 = Partial Hospital/Day Treatment

BASIS-32™

BEHAVIOR AND SYMPTOM IDENTIFICATION SCALE

INSTRUCTIONS TO RESPONDENT: Below is a list of problems and areas of life functioning in which some people experience difficulties. Using the scale below, fill in the box with the answer that best describes how much difficulty you have been having in each area during the **PAST WEEK.**

0 = No difficulty
1 = A little difficulty
2 = Moderate difficulty
3 = Quite a bit of difficulty
4 = Extreme difficulty

Please respond to each item. Do not leave any blank. If there is an area that you consider to be inapplicable, indicate that it is ***No Difficulty.***

IN THE PAST WEEK, how much difficulty have you been having in the area of:

1. **Managing day-to-day life.** (For example, getting places on time, handling money, making everyday decisions) . . . . 1 ☐
2. **Household responsibilities.** (For example, shopping, cooking, laundry, cleaning, other chores) . . . . 2 ☐
3. **Work.** (For example, completing tasks, performance level, finding/keeping a job) . . . . 3 ☐
4. **School.** (For example, academic performance, completing assignments, attendance) . . . . 4 ☐
5. **Leisure time or recreational activities.** . . . . 5 ☐
6. **Adjusting to major life stress.** (For example, separation, divorce, moving, new job, new school, a death) . . . . 6 ☐
7. **Relationships with family members.** . . . . 7 ☐
8. **Getting along with people outside of the family.** . . . . 8 ☐
9. **Isolation or feelings of loneliness.** . . . . 9 ☐
10. **Being able to feel close to others.** . . . . 10 ☐
11. **Being realistic about yourself or others.** . . . . 11 ☐
12. **Recognizing and expressing emotions appropriately.** . . . . 12 ☐
13. **Developing independence, autonomy.** . . . . 13 ☐
14. **Goals or direction in life.** . . . . 14 ☐
15. **Lack of self-confidence, feeling bad about yourself.** . . . . 15 ☐
16. **Apathy, lack of interest in things.** . . . . 16 ☐
17. **Depression, hopelessness.** . . . . 17 ☐
18. **Suicidal feelings or behavior.** . . . . 18 ☐
19. **Physical symptoms.** (For example, headaches, aches and pains, sleep disturbance, stomachaches, dizziness) . . . . 19 ☐
20. **Fear, anxiety, or panic.** . . . . 20 ☐
21. **Confusion, concentration, memory.** . . . . 21 ☐
22. **Disturbing or unreal thoughts or beliefs.** . . . . 22 ☐
23. **Hearing voices, seeing things.** . . . . 23 ☐
24. **Manic, bizarre behavior.** . . . . 24 ☐
25. **Mood swings, unstable moods.** . . . . 25 ☐
26. **Uncontrollable, compulsive behavior.** (For example, eating disorder, hand-washing, hurting yourself) . . . . 26 ☐
27. **Sexual activity or preoccupation.** . . . . 27 ☐
28. **Drinking alcoholic beverages.** . . . . 28 ☐
29. **Taking illegal drugs, misusing drugs.** . . . . 29 ☐
30. **Controlling temper, outbursts of anger, violence.** . . . . 30 ☐
31. **Impulsive, illegal or reckless behavior.** . . . . 31 ☐
32. **Feeling satisfaction with your life.** . . . . 32 ☐

For the following questions, please write the response code in the appropriate box.

33. How old were you on your last birthday? . . . . 33 ☐
34. What is your sex? . . . . 34 ☐
    1 = Male
    2 = Female
35. What is your race? . . . . 35 ☐
    1 = Black/African-American
    2 = White/Caucasian
    3 = Asian/Pacific Islander
    4 = American Indian/Alaskan
    5 = Other
36. Are you Hispanic or Latino? . . . . 36 ☐
    1 = Yes
    2 = No
37. What is your marital status? . . . . 37 ☐
    1 = Never married
    2 = Married
    3 = Separated
    4 = Divorced
    5 = Widowed
38. How much school have you completed? . . . . 38 ☐
    1 = 8th grade or less
    2 = Some high school, but did not graduate
    3 = High school graduate or GED
    4 = Some college
    5 = 4-year college graduate
39. In the past 30 days, what were your usual living arrangements? . 39 ☐
    1 = Alone
    2 = Halfway house/group home/hospital
    3 = With family
    4 = With non-relative
    5 = Shelter/Street
    6 = Other
40. In the past 30 days, were you working at a paid job? . . . . 40 ☐
    1 = Yes
    2 = No
41. If yes, how many hours per week? (If no, leave blank) . . . . 41 ☐
    1 = 1–10 hours
    2 = 11–20 hours
    3 = 21–30 hours
    4 = More than 30 hours
42. In the past 30 days, were you a student attending a high school vocational training program, college or graduate degree program? . . . . 42 ☐
    1 = Yes
    2 = No
43. Today's date ☐☐ MONTH ☐☐ DAY ☐☐☐☐ YEAR . . . . 43 ☐

From Department of Mental Health Services Research, McLean Hospital, Belmont, MA, 1985, with permission.

tency for the eight subscales and good test–retest reliability over a 2-week period. Validity has been demonstrated by correlation with other functional scales and with various severity-of-illness and burden-of-care scales. The SF-36 is in wide use around the world, especially in health services research and has special utility for comparing health outcomes across disparate diagnostic groups. It can also be used in clinical and health administration practice to track outcomes for individual patients or health systems and offers the benefit of patient-centered assessment of treatment and its impact.

Side Effects The instruments described below are used to detect and quantify side effects from medications. One is a general interview that is applicable to all medications. The remaining two (the Abnormal Involuntary Movement Scale [AIMS] and the Simpson-Angus Rating Scale for Extrapyramidal Side Effects) are focused on the motor symptoms commonly observed with antipsychotics and, for this reason, include a brief focused physical examination, as well as questions posed to the patient.

Systematic Assessment of Treatment-Emergent Events (SAFTEE) The SAFTEE is a systematic tool developed in 1986 to assess side effects in clinical trials. It has two versions, a general inquiry form (SAFTEE-GI) and a much more detailed specific inquiry form (SAFTEE-SI) that incorporates a formal review of symptoms. The SAFTEE-GI is rated based on three open-ended questions regarding new symptoms experienced in the past week: (1) Have you had any physical or health problems during the past week?, (2) Have you noticed any changes in your physical appearance during the past week?, and (3) Have you cut down on the things you usually do because of not feeling physically well during the past week? To avoid bias on the part of the examiner or patient, the questions are focused on the novelty of the symptoms rather than on any relationship to the drug. The SAFTEE form provides specified terms (listed by organ system) for reporting the answers to the three questions and suggests specific ways to follow up on any positive answers regarding (1) the duration, temporal pattern, severity, and associated functional impairment for each; (2) any contributory factors other than the drug (e.g., other medication changes, intercurrent illness) and any hypothesized relationship of the drug to the event (e.g., dose response, noted in other subjects); and (3) any observed changes in behavior and appearance (e.g., shortness of breath, rash). The SAFTEE takes 5 to 10 minutes to administer if there are few symptoms but could potentially take much longer. The SAFTEE-GI has fair to good reliability in use (somewhat better for the presence of symptoms than for detailed ratings like severity). The SAFTEE-GI has good validity based on a comparison with similar measures and on its ability to detect expected side effects. The SAFTEE-GI is more sensitive to side effects than is typical clinical practice, and the SAFTEE-SI is more sensitive still. Although the SAFTEE-SI is only suitable for use in research settings, the SAFTEE-GI could be used in clinical practice when a new drug is administered as a complement to specific questions about expected side effects of a particular drug.

Abnormal Involuntary Movement Scale (AIMS) The AIMS (Table 7.9–6) is a clinical examination and rating scale developed in the 1970s to measure dyskinetic symptoms in patients taking antipsychotic drugs. The AIMS has 12 items, each of which is rated on an item-specific five-point severity scale ranging from 0 to 4. Total scores are not generally reported. Instead, changes in global severity and individual areas can be monitored over time. Ten items cover the movements themselves, divided in sections rating global severity and those related to specific body regions; two items concern dental factors that can complicate the diagnosis of dyskinesia. In the presence of extended neuroleptic exposure and the absence of other conditions causing dyskinesia, mild dyskinetic movements in two areas or moderate movements in one area suggest a diagnosis of tardive dyskinesia. The AIMS was developed for clinician raters, but lay raters can be trained to use it. It can be completed in less than 10 minutes. Excellent reliability has been demonstrated, especially for experienced raters, and the instrument appears valid. The AIMS is considered standard clinical practice for patients receiving long-term neuroleptic drugs in many clinical settings and is essential in clinical practice and research, both for monitoring patients for the development of tardive dyskinesia and for tracking changes in tardive dyskinesia over time.

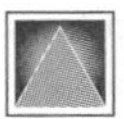

Table 7.9–6
Abnormal Involuntary Movement Scale (AIMS) Examination Procedure

Patient identification:__________________ Date:________
Rated by:__________________

Either before or after completing the examination procedure, observe the patient unobtrusively at rest (e.g., in waiting room).

The chair to be used in this examination should be a hard, firm one without arms.

After observing the patient, he or she may be rated on a scale of 0 (none), 1 (minimal), 2 (mild), 3 (moderate), and 4 (severe) according to the severity of symptoms.

Ask the patient whether there is anything in his/her mouth (i.e., gum, candy, etc.) and if there is to remove it.

Ask patient about the current condition of his/her teeth. Ask patient if he/she wears dentures. Do teeth or dentures bother patient now?

Ask patient whether he/she notices any movement in mouth, face, hands, or feet. If yes, ask to describe and to what extent they currently bother patient or interfere with his/her activities.

Rating	Procedure
0 1 2 3 4	Have patient sit in chair with hands on knees, legs slightly apart, and feet flat on floor. (Look at entire body for movements while in this position.)
0 1 2 3 4	Ask patient to sit with hands hanging unsupported. If male, between legs; if female and wearing a dress, hanging over knees. (Observe hands and other body areas.)
0 1 2 3 4	Ask patient to open mouth. (Observe tongue at rest within mouth.) Do this twice.
0 1 2 3 4	Ask patient to protrude tongue. (Observe abnormalities of tongue movement.) Do this twice.
0 1 2 3 4	Ask the patient to tap thumb, with each finger, as rapidly as possible for 10–15 secs; separately with right hand, then with left hand. (Observe facial and leg movements.)
0 1 2 3 4	Flex and extend patient's left and right arms. (One at a time.)
0 1 2 3 4	Ask patient to stand up. (Observe in profile. Observe all body areas again, hips included.)
0 1 2 3 4	Ask patient to extend both arms outstretched in front with palms down. (Observe trunk, legs, and mouth.)[a]
0 1 2 3 4	Have patient walk a few paces, turn and walk back to chair. (Observe hands and gait.) Do this twice.[a]

[a]Activated movements.

Simpson-Angus Rating Scale for Extrapyramidal Side Effects The Simpson-Angus Rating Scale for Extrapyramidal Side Effects was developed to monitor the effects of antipsychotic drugs. It has ten items, each of which is rated on an item-specific five-point severity scale ranging from 0 to 4. Scores are reported as the mean on all ten items, with 0.3 considered the upper limits of normal. It is strongly focused on parkinsonian symptoms, particularly rigidity, but includes one akathisia item. It is designed for clinician use but can be administered by trained lay raters and takes approximately 10 minutes to administer. Good reliability has been reported, and validity is supported by the correlation of scores with antipsychotic drug dose. The scale is useful in a wide variety of clinical settings to monitor parkinsonian side effects and the impact of interventions to treat these effects.

Psychiatric Diagnosis Instruments assessing psychiatric diagnosis are central to psychiatric research and may be useful in clinical practice as well. However, they tend to be rather long, especially with individuals reporting many symptoms, potentially requiring many follow-up questions. When evaluating such instruments, it is important to be sure that they implement current diagnostic criteria and cover the diagnostic areas of interest. For instance, few cover personality disorders (with the exception in some cases of antisocial personality), and not all cover disorders that typically onset in childhood.

Structured Clinical Interview for DSM-IV-TR (SCID) The SCID was developed in the late early 1990s to provide a standardized DSM-III-R Axis I diagnosis based on an efficient but thorough clinical evaluation. It has since been updated for DSM-IV. The semistructured diagnostic interview begins with a section on demographic information and clinical background. Then there are seven diagnostic modules focused on different diagnostic groups: mood, psychotic, substance abuse, anxiety, somatoform, eating, and adjustment disorders. Both required and optional probes are provided, and skip outs are suggested where no further questioning is warranted. All available information, including that from hospital records, informants, and patient observation, should be used to rate the SCID. The SCID is designed to be administered by experienced clinicians and is generally not recommended for use by lay interviewers. In addition, formal training in the SCID is required, and training books and videos are available to facilitate this. For individuals without symptoms, the interview takes approximately 1 hour to complete but may take up to 3 hours for individuals with extensive symptomatology. Although the primary focus is research with psychiatric patients, a nonpatient version (with no reference to a chief complaint) and a more clinical version (without as much detailed subtyping) are also available. Reliability data on the SCID suggest that it performs better on more severe disorders (e.g., bipolar disorder, alcohol dependence) than on milder ones (e.g., dysthymia). Validity data are limited, as the SCID is more often used as the gold standard against which to judge other instruments. It is considered the standard interview to verify diagnosis in clinical trials and is extensively used in other forms of psychiatric research. It can also be used to assure a systematic evaluation in psychiatric patients—for instance, on admission to an inpatient unit or at intake into an outpatient clinic. It is also used in forensic practice to assure a formal and reproducible examination.

Diagnostic Interview Schedule (DIS) and Composite International Diagnostic Instrument (CIDI) The DIS and CIDI are fully structured diagnostic interviews designed for lay administration. The DIS was developed in the 1980s for use in the Epidemiologic Catchment Area (ECA) study in the United States, which aimed to assess rates of current and lifetime psychiatric illness according to DSM-III in a large and diverse community sample and has since been updated for DSM-III-R and DSM-IV criteria. In 19 diagnostic modules, it covers a broad range of Axis I conditions in adults, plus several childhood disorders and antisocial personality. The most recent version also includes greater information about symptoms, impairment, and treatment. The CIDI was developed from the DIS for international use and covers both ICD and DSM-IV criteria in 11 diagnostic modules: The CIDI does not cover antisocial personality or childhood disorders. The instruments are fairly similar and both involve verbatim reading of questions with little or no rewording allowed; only specified probes may be used for follow-up. The DIS takes 90 minutes to 2 hours to complete; the CIDI may be somewhat shorter. Both can be scored by computer, yielding diagnoses and symptom profiles. A computerized, self-administered version of the CIDI is also available, as are a short form (the DIS-SF) and an even shorter screening version (DIS-S). The instruments are designed for use by lay interviewers with extensive training in their use (formal training is recommended). Reliability appears to be good for both, at least for more severe disorders. Validity appears problematic for the DIS: studies of agreement with clinician diagnoses have been inconsistent, with marked discrepancies often observed for psychotic disorders. Both instruments have been used extensively in psychiatric research, particularly in epidemiologic settings, and provide valuable data. However, some caution is warranted in interpreting these data given concerns about the instruments' validity, particularly for psychotic disorders.

Primary Care Evaluation of Mental Disorders (PRIME-MD) The PRIME-MD was developed in the mid-1990s to provide an efficient screening and evaluation tool for common mental disorders seen in the primary care setting. The instrument has two parts: a 25-item patient questionnaire that screens for a range of symptoms and a structured interview designed to follow up on any symptoms identified in the patient questionnaire or through other means. The interview has five modules covering mood, anxiety, alcohol, somatoform, and eating disorders. The patient questionnaire is very brief and can be completed in less than 5 minutes. If follow-up is required, a primary care practitioner can complete the structured questionnaire in approximately 10 minutes. Training in the use of the instrument or careful review of the instruction manual is recommended. A self-report version of the structured interview is in development. Reliability appears to be fair to good, better for more severe diagnoses. Validity judged against psychiatrist evaluations is quite good. The screening instrument has appropriately high sensitivity, and the follow-up interview provides reasonable specificity. The PRIME-MD appears to be useful for primary care settings and may also be useful in psychiatric practice when a quick screen is desired. However, its usefulness for the latter purpose is limited by its lack of coverage of the more severe psychopathology not typically seen in primary care (e.g., psychotic symptoms, mania).

Psychotic Disorders A variety of instruments are used for patients with psychotic disorders. Those reported here are symptom severity measures. A developing consensus suggests that the distinction between positive and negative symptoms in schizophrenia is worthwhile, and more recently developed instruments implement this distinction. Because patients with psychotic disorders often lack insight and are sometimes agitated, patient observation is required in addition to direct questioning. Thus, most instruments in this domain must be administered by psychiatrists or others with clinical training.

Brief Psychiatric Rating Scale (BPRS) The BPRS (Table 7.9–7) was developed in the late 1960s as a short scale for measuring the severity of psychiatric symptomatology. It was developed primarily to assess change in psychotic inpatients and covers a broad range

Table 7.9–7
Brief Psychiatric Rating Scale

DEPARTMENT OF HEALTH AND HUMAN SERVICES PUBLIC HEALTH SERVICE Alcohol, Drug Abuse, and Mental Health Administration NIMH Treatment Strategies in Schizophrenia Society BRIEF PSYCHIATRIC RATING SCALE—Anchored Overall and Gorham	PATIENT NUMBER — — — —	DATA GROUP bprs	EVALUATION DATE — — — — — — MM DD YY
	PATIENT NAME		
	RATER NAME		

RATER NUMBER	EVALUATION TYPE (*Circle*)			
— — —	1 Baseline	4 Start double-blind	7 Start open meds	10 Early termination
	2	5 Major evaluation	8 During open meds	11 Study completion
	3 4-week minor	6 Other	9 Stop open meds	

Introduce all questions with "During the past week have you . . . "

[a]1. **SOMATIC CONCERN:** Degree of concern over present bodily health. Rate the degree to which physical health is perceived as a problem by the patient, whether complaints have a realistic basis or not. Do not rate mere reporting of somatic symptoms. Rate only concern for (or worrying about) physical problems (real or imagined). **Rate on the basis of reported (i.e., subjective) information pertaining to the past week.**
   1 = Not reported
   2 = Very Mild: occasionally is somewhat concerned about body, symptoms, or physical illness
   3 = Mild: occasionally is moderately concerned, or often is somewhat concerned
   4 = Moderate: occasionally is very concerned, or often is moderately concerned
   5 = Moderately Severe: often is very concerned
   6 = Severe: is very concerned most of the time
   7 = Very Severe: is very concerned nearly all of the time
   9 = Cannot be assessed adequately because of severe formal thought disorder, uncooperativeness, or marked evasiveness/guardedness; or Not assessed

[a]2. **ANXIETY:** Worry, fear, or overconcern for present or future: **Rate solely on the basis of verbal report of patient's own subjective experiences pertaining to the past week.** Do not infer anxiety from physical signs or from neurotic defense mechanisms. Do not rate if restricted to somatic concern.
   1 = Not reported
   2 = Very Mild: occasionally feels somewhat anxious
   3 = Mild: occasionally feels moderately anxious, or often feels somewhat anxious
   4 = Moderate: occasionally feels very anxious, or often feels moderately anxious
   5 = Moderately Severe: often feels very anxious
   6 = Severe: feels very anxious most of the time
   7 = Very Severe: feels very anxious nearly all of the time
   9 = Cannot be assessed adequately because of severe formal thought disorder, uncooperativeness, or marked evasiveness/guardedness; or Not assessed

3. **EMOTIONAL WITHDRAWAL:** Deficiency in relating to the interviewer and to the interview situation. Overt manifestations of this deficiency include poor/absence of eye contact, failure to orient oneself physically toward the interviewer, and a general lack of involvement or engagement in the interview. Distinguish from BLUNTED AFFECT, in which deficits in facial expression, body gesture, and voice pattern are scored. **Rate on the basis of observations made during the interview.**
   1 = Not observed
   2 = Very Mild: e.g., occasionally exhibits poor eye contact
   3 = Mild: e.g., as above, but more frequent
   4 = Moderate: e.g., exhibits little eye contact, but still seems engaged in the interview and is appropriately responsive to all questions
   5 = Moderately Severe: e.g., stares at floor or orients self away from interviewer but still seems moderately engaged
   6 = Severe: e.g., as above, but more persistent or pervasive
   7 = Very Severe: e.g., appears "spacey" or "out of it" (total absence of emotional relatedness) and is disproportionately uninvolved or unengaged in the interview (DO NOT SCORE IF EXPLAINED BY DISORIENTATION)

4. **CONCEPTUAL DISORGANIZATION:** Degree of speech incomprehensibility. Include any type of formal thought disorder (e.g., loose associations, incoherence, flight of ideas, neologisms). DO NOT include mere circumstantiality or pressured speech, even if marked. DO NOT rate on the basis of the patient's subjective impressions (e.g., "my thoughts are racing. I can't hold a thought," "my thinking gets all mixed up"). **Rate ONLY on the basis of observations made during the interview.**
   1 = Not observed
   2 = Very Mild: e.g., somewhat vague, but of doubtful clinical significance
   3 = Mild: e.g., frequently vague, but the interview is able to progress smoothly; occasional loosening of associations
   4 = Moderate: e.g., occasional irrelevant statements, infrequent use of neologisms, or moderate loosening of associations
   5 = Moderately Severe: as above, but more frequent
   6 = Severe: formal thought disorder is present for most of the interview, and the interview is severely strained
   7 = Very Severe: very little coherent information can be obtained

5. **GUILT FEELINGS:** Overconcern or remorse for past behavior. **Rate on the basis of the patient's subjective experiences of guilt as evidenced by verbal report pertaining to the past week.** Do not infer guilt feelings from depression, anxiety or neurotic defenses.
   1 = Not reported
   2 = Very Mild: occasionally feels somewhat guilty
   3 = Mild: occasionally feels moderately guilty, or often feels somewhat guilty
   4 = Moderate: occasionally feels very guilty, or often feels moderately guilty
   5 = Moderately Severe: often feels very guilty
   6 = Severe: feels very guilty most of the time, or encapsulated delusion of guilt
   7 = Very Severe: agonizing constant feelings of guilt, or pervasive delusion(s) of guilt
   9 = Cannot be assessed adequately because of severe formal thought disorder, uncooperativeness, or marked evasiveness/guardedness; or Not assessed

(*continued*)

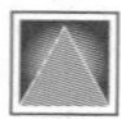

Table 7.9–7 (*continued*)

DEPARTMENT OF HEALTH AND HUMAN SERVICES PUBLIC HEALTH SERVICE Alcohol, Drug Abuse, and Mental Health Administration NIMH Treatment Strategies in Schizophrenia Society BRIEF PSYCHIATRIC RATING SCALE—Anchored Overall and Gorham	PATIENT NUMBER — — — —	DATA GROUP bprs	EVALUATION DATE — — — — — — MM DD YY
	PATIENT NAME		
	RATER NAME		

RATER NUMBER	EVALUATION TYPE (*Circle*)			
— — —	1 Baseline 2 3 4-week minor	4 Start double-blind 5 Major evaluation 6 Other	7 Start open meds 8 During open meds 9 Stop open meds	10 Early termination 11 Study completion

6. **TENSION: Rate motor restlessness (agitation) observed during the interview.** DO NOT rate on the basis of subjective experiences reported by the patient. Disregard suspected pathogenesis (e.g., tardive dyskinesia).
   1 = Not observed
   2 = Very Mild: e.g., occasionally fidgets
   3 = Mild: e.g., frequently fidgets
   4 = Moderate: e.g., constantly fidgets, or frequently fidgets, wrings hands and pulls clothing
   5 = Moderately Severe: e.g., constantly fidgets, wrings hands and pulls clothing
   6 = Severe: e.g., cannot remain seated (i.e., must pace)
   7 = Very Severe: e.g., paces in a frantic manner
7. **MANNERISMS AND POSTURING:** Unusual and unnatural motor behavior. **Rate only abnormality of movements.** Do not rate simple heightened motor activity here. Consider frequency, duration, and degree of bizarreness. Disregard suspected pathogenesis.
   1 = Not observed
   2 = Very Mild: odd behavior but of doubtful clinical significance, e.g., occasional unprompted smiling, infrequent lip movements
   3 = Mild: strange behavior but not obviously bizarre, e.g., infrequent head-tilting (side to side) in a rhythmic fashion, intermittent abnormal finger movements
   4 = Moderate: e.g., assumes unnatural position for a brief period of time, infrequent tongue protrusions, rocking, facial grimacing
   5 = Moderately Severe: e.g., assumes and maintains unnatural position throughout interview, unusual movements in several body areas
   6 = Severe: as above, but more frequent, intense, or pervasive
   7 = Very Severe: e.g., bizarre posturing throughout most of the interview, continuous abnormal movements in several body areas

[a]8. **GRANDIOSITY:** Inflated self-esteem (self-confidence), or inflated appraisal of one's talents, powers, abilities, accomplishments, knowledge, importance, or identity. Do not score mere grandiose *quality* of claims (e.g., "I'm the worst sinner in the world," "The entire country is trying to kill me") unless the guilt/persecution is related to some special, exaggerated attributes of the individual. Also, *the patient* must claim exaggerated attributes: e.g., if patient denies talents, powers, etc., even if he or she states that *others* indicate that he/she has these attributes, this item should not be scored. **Rate on the basis of reported (i.e., subjective) information pertaining to the past week.**
   1 = Not reported
   2 = Very Mild: e.g., is more confident than most people, but of only possible clinical significance
   3 = Mild: e.g., definitely inflated self-esteem or exaggerates talents somewhat out of proportion to the circumstances
   4 = Moderate: e.g., inflated self-esteem clearly out of proportion to the circumstances or suspected grandiose delusion(s)
   5 = Moderately Severe: e.g., a single (definite) encapsulated grandiose delusion, or multiple (definite) encapsulated grandiose delusion, or multiple (definite) fragmentary grandiose delusions
   6 = Severe: e.g., a single (definite) grandiose delusion/delusional system, or multiple (definite) grandiose delusions that the patient seem preoccupied with
   7 = Very Severe: e.g., as above, but nearly all conversation is directed towards the patient's grandiose delusion(s)
   9 = Cannot be assessed adequately because of severe formal thought disorder, uncooperativeness, or marked evasiveness/guardedness; or Not assessed

[a]9. **DEPRESSIVE MOOD:** Subjective report of feeling depressed, blue, "down in the dumps," etc. Rate only degree of reported depression. Do not rate on the basis of inferences concerning depression based upon general retardation and somatic complaints. **Rate on the basis of report (i.e., subjective) information pertaining to the past week.**
   1 = Not reported
   2 = Very Mild: occasionally feels somewhat depressed
   3 = Mild: occasionally feels moderately depressed, or often feels somewhat depressed
   4 = Moderate: occasionally feels very depressed, or often feels moderately depressed
   5 = Moderately Severe: often feels very depressed
   6 = Severe: feels very depressed most of the time
   7 = Very Severe: feels very depressed nearly all of the time
   9 = Cannot be assessed adequately because of severe formal thought disorder, uncooperativeness, or marked evasiveness/guardedness; or Not assessed

[a]10. **HOSTILITY:** Animosity, contempt, belligerence, disdain for other people outside the interview situation. **Rate solely on the basis of the verbal report of feelings and actions of the patient toward others during the past week.** Do not infer hostility from neurotic defenses, anxiety, somatic complaints.
   1 = Not reported
   2 = Very Mild: occasionally feels somewhat angry
   3 = Mild: often feels somewhat angry, or occasionally feels moderately angry
   4 = Moderate: occasionally feels very angry, or often feels moderately angry
   5 = Moderately Severe: often feels very angry
   6 = Severe: has acted on his anger by becoming verbally or physically abusive on one or two occasions
   7 = Very Severe: has acted on his anger on several occasions
   9 = Cannot be assessed adequately because of severe formal thought disorder, uncooperativeness, or marked evasiveness/guardedness; or Not assessed

(*continued*)

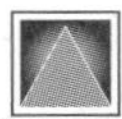

Table 7.9–7 (*continued*)

DEPARTMENT OF HEALTH AND HUMAN SERVICES PUBLIC HEALTH SERVICE Alcohol, Drug Abuse, and Mental Health Administration NIMH Treatment Strategies in Schizophrenia Society	PATIENT NUMBER — — — —	DATA GROUP bprs	EVALUATION DATE — — — — — — MM DD YY
	PATIENT NAME		
BRIEF PSYCHIATRIC RATING SCALE—Anchored Overall and Gorham	RATER NAME		

RATER NUMBER	EVALUATION TYPE (*Circle*)			
— — —	1 Baseline	4 Start double-blind	7 Start open meds	10 Early termination
	2	5 Major evaluation	8 During open meds	11 Study completion
	3 4-week minor	6 Other	9 Stop open meds	

[a]11. **SUSPICIOUSNESS:** Belief (delusional or otherwise) that others have now, or have had in the past, malicious or discriminatory intent toward the patient. On the basis of verbal report, rate only those suspicions which are currently held whether they concern past or present circumstances. **Rate on the basis of reported (i.e., subjective) information pertaining to the past week.**

1 = Not reported
2 = Very Mild: rare instances of distrustfulness which may or may not be warranted by the situation
3 = Mild: occasional instances of suspiciousness that are definitely not warranted by the situation
4 = Moderate: more frequent suspiciousness, or transient ideas of reference
5 = Moderately Severe: pervasive suspiciousness, frequent ideas of reference, or an encapsulated delusion
6 = Severe: definite, delusion(s) of reference or persecution that is (are) not wholly pervasive (e.g., an encapsulated delusion)
7 = Very Severe: as above, but more widespread, frequent, or intense
9 = Cannot be assessed adequately because of severe formal thought disorder, uncooperativeness, or marked evasiveness/guardedness; or Not assessed

[a]12. **HALLUCINATORY BEHAVIOR:** Perceptions (in any sensory modality) in the absence of an identifiable external stimulus. **Rate only those experiences that have occurred during the last week.** DO NOT rate "voices in my head," or "visions in my mind" unless the patient can differentiate between these experiences and his or her thoughts.

1 = Not reported
2 = Very Mild: suspected hallucinations only
3 = Mild: definite hallucinations, but insignificant, infrequent, or transient (e.g., occasional formless visual hallucinations, a voice calling the patient's name)
4 = Moderate: as above, but more frequent or extensive (e.g., frequently sees the devil's face, two voices carry on lengthy conversations)
5 = Moderately Severe: hallucinations are experienced nearly every day, or are a source of extreme distress
6 = Severe: as above, and has had a moderate impact on the patient's behavior (e.g., concentration difficulties leading to impaired work functioning)
7 = Very Severe: as above, and has had a severe impact (e.g., attempts suicide in response to command hallucinations)
9 = Cannot be assessed adequately because of severe formal thought disorder, uncooperativeness, or marked evasiveness/guardedness; or Not assessed

13. **MOTOR RETARDATION:** Reduction in energy level evidenced in slowed movements. **Rate on the basis of observed behavior of the patient only.** Do not rate on the basis of the patient's subjective impression of his or her own energy level.

1 = Not observed
2 = Very Mild and of doubtful clinical significance
3 = Mild: e.g., conversation is somewhat retarded, movements somewhat slowed
4 = Moderate: e.g., conversation is noticeably retarded but not strained
5 = Moderately Severe: e.g., conversation is strained, moves very slowly
6 = Severe: e.g., conversation is difficult to maintain, hardly moves at all
7 = Very Severe: e.g., conversation is almost impossible, does not move at all throughout interview

14. **UNCOOPERATIVENESS:** Evidence of resistance, unfriendliness, resentment, and lack of readiness to cooperate with the interviewer. **Rate only on the basis of the patient's attitude and responses to the interviewer and the interview situation.** Do not rate on the basis of reported resentment or uncooperativeness outside the interview situation.

1 = Not observed
2 = Very Mild: e.g., does not seem motivated
3 = Mild: e.g., seems evasive in certain areas
4 = Moderate: e.g., monosyllabic, fails to elaborate spontaneously, somewhat unfriendly
5 = Moderately Severe: e.g., expresses resentment and is unfriendly throughout the interview
6 = Severe: e.g., refuses to answer a number of questions
7 = Very Severe: e.g., refuses to answer most questions

15. **UNUSUAL THOUGHT CONTENT:** Severity of delusions of any type—consider conviction, and effect on actions. Assume full conviction if patient has acted on his or her beliefs. **Rate on the basis of reported (i.e., subjective) information pertaining to past week.**

1 = Not reported
2 = Very Mild: delusion(s) suspected or likely
3 = Mild: at times, patient questions his or her belief(s) (partial delusion)
4 = Moderate: full delusional conviction, but delusion(s) has little or no influence on behavior
5 = Moderately Severe: full delusional conviction, but delusion(s) has only occasional impact on behavior
6 = Severe: delusion(s) has significant effect, e.g., neglects responsibilities because of preoccupation with belief that he/she is God
7 = Very Severe: delusion(s) has major impact, e.g., stops eating because believes food is poisoned
9 = Cannot be assessed adequately because of severe formal thought disorder, uncooperativeness, or marked evasiveness/guardedness; or Not assessed

(*continued*)

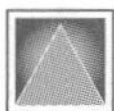

Table 7.9–7 (*continued*)

DEPARTMENT OF HEALTH AND HUMAN SERVICES PUBLIC HEALTH SERVICE Alcohol, Drug Abuse, and Mental Health Administration NIMH Treatment Strategies in Schizophrenia Society	PATIENT NUMBER — — — —	DATA GROUP bprs	EVALUATION DATE __ __ __ MM DD YY
	PATIENT NAME		
BRIEF PSYCHIATRIC RATING SCALE—Anchored Overall and Gorham	RATER NAME		

RATER NUMBER	EVALUATION TYPE (*Circle*)			
— — —	1 Baseline 2 3 4-week minor	4 Start double-blind 5 Major evaluation 6 Other	7 Start open meds 8 During open meds 9 Stop open meds	10 Early termination 11 Study completion

16. **BLUNTED AFFECT:** Diminished affective responsivity, as characterized by deficits in facial expression, body gesture, and voice pattern. Distinguish from EMOTIONAL WITHDRAWAL, in which the focus is on interpersonal impairment rather than affect. Consider degree and consistency of impairment. **Rate based on observations made during interview.**
    - 1 = Not observed
    - 2 = Very Mild: e.g., occasionally seems indifferent to material that is usually accompanied by some show of emotion
    - 3 = Mild: e.g., somewhat diminished facial expression, *or* somewhat monotonous voice *or* somewhat restricted gestures
    - 4 = Moderate: e.g., as above, but more intense, prolonged, or frequent
    - 5 = Moderately Severe: e.g., flattening of affect, including at least two of the three features: severe lack of facial expression, monotonous voice or restricted body gestures
    - 6 = Severe: e.g., profound flattening of affect
    - 7 = Very Severe: e.g., totally monotonous voice, *and* total lack of expressive gestures throughout the evaluation
17. **EXCITEMENT:** Heightened emotional tone, including irritability and expansiveness (hypomanic affect). Do not infer affect from statements of grandiose delusions. **Rate based on observations made during interview.**
    - 1 = Not observed
    - 2 = Very Mild and of doubtful clinical significance
    - 3 = Mild: e.g., irritable or expansive at times
    - 4 = Moderate: e.g., frequently irritable or expansive
    - 5 = Moderately Severe: e.g., constantly irritable or expansive; or, at times, enraged or euphoric
    - 6 = Severe: e.g., enraged or euphoric throughout most of the interview
    - 7 = Very Severe: e.g., as above, but to such a degree that the interview must be terminated prematurely
18. **DISORIENTATION:** Confusion or lack of proper association for person, place or time. **Rate based on observations made during interview.**
    - 1 = Not observed
    - 2 = Very Mild: e.g., seems somewhat confused
    - 3 = Mild: e.g., indicated 1982 when, in fact, it is 1983
    - 4 = Moderate: e.g., indicates 1978
    - 5 = Moderately Severe: e.g., is unsure where he/she is
    - 6 = Severe: e.g., has no idea where he/she is
    - 7 = Very Severe: e.g., does not know who he/she is
    - 9 = Cannot be assessed adequately because of severe formal thought disorder, uncooperativeness, or marked evasiveness/guardedness; or Not assessed
19. **SEVERITY OF ILLNESS:** Considering your total clinical experience with this patient population, how mentally ill is the patient at this time?
    - 1 = Normal, not at all ill
    - 2 = Borderline mentally ill
    - 3 = Mildly ill
    - 4 = Moderately ill
    - 5 = Markedly ill
    - 6 = Severely ill
    - 7 = Among the most severely ill patients
20. **GLOBAL IMPROVEMENT:** Rate total improvement whether or not, in your judgment, it is due to treatment.

At *baseline* assessment, mark "Not assessed" for item 20.

For assessments *up to the start of double-blind* medication, rate Global Improvement compared to *baseline.*

For assessments *following the start of double-blind* medication, rate Global Improvement compared to the *start of double-blind.*

- 1 = Very much improved
- 2 = Much improved
- 3 = Minimally improved
- 4 = No change
- 5 = Minimally worse
- 6 = Much worse
- 7 = Very much worse
- 9 = Not assessed

[a]Ratings based primarily on verbal report.

of areas, including thought disturbance, emotional withdrawal and retardation, anxiety and depression, and hostility and suspiciousness. Its 18 items are rated on a seven-point, item-specific Likert scale from 0 to 6, with the total score ranging from 0 to 108 (in some scoring systems, the lowest level for each item is 1, and the range is 18 to 126). Because the ratings include observations, as well as patient reports of symptoms, the BPRS can be used to rate patients with very severe impairment. It is intended for use by experienced clinicians and can be administered in 30 minutes or less, including patient interview and observation. Reliability of the BPRS is good to excellent when raters are experienced, but this is more difficult to achieve without substantial training; a semistructured interview has been developed to increase reliability. Validity is also good as measured by correlations with other measures of symptom severity, especially those assessing schizophrenia symptomatology. The BPRS has been used extensively for decades as an outcome measure in treatment studies of schizophrenia; it functions well as a measure of change in this context and offers the advantage of comparability with earlier trials. However, it has been largely supplanted in more recent clinical trials by the newer measures described below. In addition, given its focus on psychosis and associated symptoms, it is only suitable for patients with fairly significant impairment. Its use in clinical practice is less well supported, in part because considerable training is required to achieve the necessary reliability.

Positive and Negative Syndrome Scale (PANSS) The PANSS was developed in the late 1980s to remedy perceived deficits in the BPRS in the assessment of positive and negative symptoms of schizophrenia and other psychotic disorders by adding additional items and providing careful anchors for each. The PANSS includes 30 items on three subscales: seven items covering positive symptoms (e.g., hallucinations and delusions), seven covering negative symptoms (e.g., blunted affect), and 16 covering general psychopathology (e.g., guilt, uncooperativeness). In recent years, these three scales have come to be replaced by a finer division of five subscales based on factor analysis. Each item is scored on a seven-point, item-specific Likert scale ranging from 1 to 7; thus, the positive and negative subscales each range from 7 to 49, and the general psychopathology scale ranges from 16 to 112. The PANSS requires a clinician rater because considerable probing and clinical judgment are required. A semistructured interview guide is available. The ratings can be completed in 30 to 40 minutes. Reliability for each scale has been shown to be fairly high, with excellent internal consistency and interrater reliability. Validity also appears good based on correlation with other symptom severity measures and factor analytic validation of the subscales. The PANSS has become the standard tool for assessing clinical outcome in treatment studies of schizophrenia and other psychotic disorders and has been shown to be sensitive to change with treatment. Its high reliability and good coverage of both positive and negative symptoms make it excellent for this purpose. It may also be useful for tracking severity in clinical practice, and its clear anchors make it easy to use in this setting.

Scale for the Assessment of Positive Symptoms (SAPS) and Scale for the Assessment of Negative Symptoms (SANS) The SAPS and SANS were designed to provide a detailed assessment of positive and negative symptoms of schizophrenia and may be used separately or in tandem. The domains assessed include hallucinations, delusions, bizarre behavior, and thought disorder for the SAPS, and affective flattening, poverty of speech, apathy, anhedonia, and inattentiveness for the SANS. Each instrument consists of 30 fully anchored items each scored from 0 to 5; thus, the total score ranges from 0 to 150 for each. Each must be rated by an experienced clinician and requires approximately 30 minutes to complete. Good to excellent interrater reliability has been demonstrated if trained interviewers are used, and each scale has high internal consistency as well. Validity is supported by correlation with other symptom severity instruments. The SANS and SAPS are principally used to monitor treatment effects in clinical research and have also been used to help characterize positive and negative symptoms in studies of schizophrenia phenomenology. The SAPS has been largely supplanted by the PANSS, but the SANS still has a place in studies aimed at negative symptoms. The instruments are generally too detailed for use in clinical practice, although the comprehensive characterization of symptomatology provided might be useful as part of a formal evaluation.

Mood Disorders The domain of mood disorders includes both unipolar and bipolar disorder, and the instruments described here assess depression and mania. For mania, the issues are similar to those for psychotic disorders in that limited insight and agitation may hinder accurate symptom reporting, so clinician ratings including observational data are generally required. Rating depression, on the other hand, depends, to a substantial extent, on subjective assessment of mood states, so interviews and self-report instruments are both common. Because depression is common in the general population and involves significant morbidity and even mortality, screening instruments—especially those using a self-report format—are potentially quite useful in primary care and community settings.

Hamilton Rating Scale for Depression (HAM-D) The HAM-D was developed in the early 1960s to monitor the severity of major depression, with a focus on somatic symptomatology. The version in most common use has 17 items, although versions with different numbers of items, including the 24-item version in Table 7.9–8, have been used in many studies as well. The 17-item version does not include some of the symptoms for depression in DSM-III and its successors, most notably the so-called reverse neurovegetative signs (increased sleep, increased appetite, and psychomotor retardation). Items on the HAM-D are scored from 0 to 2 or from 0 to 4, with total score ranging from 0 to 50. Scores of 7 or less may be considered normal; 8 to 13, mild; 14 to 18, moderate; 19 to 22, severe; and 23 and above, very severe. The HAM-D was designed for clinician raters but has been used by trained lay administrators as well. Ratings are completed by the examiner based on patient interview and observations. A structured interview guide has been developed to improve reliability. The ratings can be completed in 15 to 20 minutes. Reliability is good to excellent, including internal consistency and interrater assessments. Validity appears good based on correlation with other depression symptom measures. The HAM-D has been used extensively to evaluate change in response to pharmacological and other interventions and, thus, offers the advantage of comparability across a broad range of treatment trials. It is more problematic in the elderly and the medically ill, in whom the presence of somatic symptoms may not be indicative of major depression.

Beck Depression Inventory (BDI) The BDI was developed in the early 1960s to rate depression severity, with a focus on behavioral and cognitive dimensions of depression. The current version, the Beck-II, has added more coverage of somatic symptoms to be compatible with DSM-IV and covers the most recent 2 weeks. Earlier versions are focused on the past week or even shorter intervals, which may be preferable for monitoring treatment response. The BDI includes 21 self-report items, each of which has four state-

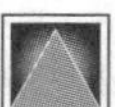

Table 7.9–8
Hamilton Rating Scale for Depression

For each item select the "cue" which best characterizes the patient.

1: Depressed mood (sadness, hopeless, helpless, worthless)
- 0 Absent
- 1 These feeling states indicated only on questioning
- 2 These feeling states spontaneously reported verbally
- 3 Communicates feeling states nonverbally—i.e., through facial expression, posture, voice, and tendency to weep
- 4 Patient reports VIRTUALLY ONLY these feeling states in his spontaneous verbal and nonverbal communication

2: Feelings of guilt
- 0 Absent
- 1 Self-reproach, feels he has let people down
- 2 Ideas of guilt or rumination over past errors or sinful deeds
- 3 Present illness is a punishment. Delusions of guilt
- 4 Hears accusatory or denunciatory voices and/or experiences threatening visual hallucinations

3: Suicide
- 0 Absent
- 1 Feels life is not worth living
- 2 Wishes he were dead or any thoughts of possible death to self
- 3 Suicide ideas or gesture
- 4 Attempts at suicide (any serious attempt rates 4)

4: Insomnia early
- 0 No difficulty falling asleep
- 1 Complains of occasional difficulty falling asleep—i.e., more than 1/4 hour
- 2 Complains of nightly difficulty falling asleep

5: Insomnia middle
- 0 No difficulty
- 1 Patient complains of being restless and disturbed during the night
- 2 Waking during the night—any getting out of bed rates 2 (except for purpose of voiding)

6: Insomnia late
- 0 No difficulty
- 1 Waking in early hours of the morning but goes back to sleep
- 2 Unable to fall asleep again if gets out of bed

7: Work and activities
- 0 No difficulty
- 1 Thoughts and feelings of incapacity, fatigue, or weakness related to activities, work, or hobbies
- 2 Loss of interest in activity, hobbies, or work—either directly reported by patient, or indirect in listlessness, indecision, and vacillation (feels he has to push self to work or activities)
- 3 Decrease in actual time spent in activities or decrease in productivity. In hospital, rate 3 if patient does not spend at least three hours a day in activities (hospital job or hobbies) exclusive of ward chores
- 4 Stopped working because of present illness. In hospital, rate 4 if patient engages in no activities except ward chores, or if patient fails to perform ward chores unassisted

8: Retardation (slowness of thought and speech; impaired ability to concentrate; decreased motor activity)
- 0 Normal speech and thought
- 1 Slight retardation at interview
- 2 Obvious retardation at interview
- 3 Interview difficult
- 4 Complete stupor

9: Agitation
- 0 None
- 1 "Playing with" hands, hair, etc.
- 2 Hand-wringing, nail biting, hair pulling, biting of lips

10: Anxiety psychic
- 0 No difficulty
- 1 Subjective tension and irritability
- 2 Worrying about minor matters
- 3 Apprehensive attitude apparent in face or speech
- 4 Fears expressed without questioning

11: Anxiety somatic
- 0 Absent
- 1 Mild
- 2 Moderate
- 3 Severe
- 4 Incapacitating

Physiological concomitants of anxiety, such as:
Gastrointestinal—dry mouth, wind, indigestion, diarrhea, cramps, belching
Cardiovascular—palpitations, headaches
Respiratory—hyperventilation, sighing
Urinary frequency
Sweating

12: Somatic symptoms gastrointestinal
- 0 None
- 1 Loss of appetite but eating without staff encouragement. Heavy feelings in abdomen
- 2 Difficulty eating without staff urging; requests or requires laxatives or medication for bowels or medication for GI symptoms

13: Somatic symptoms general
- 0 None
- 1 Heaviness in limbs, back or head. Backaches, headache, muscle aches. Loss of energy and fatigability
- 2 Any clear-cut symptom rates 2

14: Genital symptoms
- 0 Absent
- 1 Mild
- 2 Severe

Symptoms such as:
Loss of libido
Menstrual disturbances

15: Hypochondriasis
- 0 Not present
- 1 Self-absorption (bodily)
- 2 Preoccupation with health
- 3 Frequent complaints, requests for help, etc.
- 4 Hypochondriacal delusions

16: Loss of weight
- A: When rating by history
  - 0 No weight loss
  - 1 Probable weight loss associated with present illness
  - 2 Definite (according to patient) weight loss
- B: On weekly ratings by ward psychiatrist, when actual weight changes are measured
  - 0 Less than 1 lb weight loss in week
  - 1 Greater than 1 lb weight loss in week
  - 2 Greater than 2 lb weight loss in week

17: Insight
- 0 Acknowledges being depressed and ill
- 1 Acknowledges illness but attributes cause to bad food, climate, overwork, virus, need for rest, etc.
- 2 Denies being ill at all

18: Diurnal variation

AM	PM		
0	0	Absent	If symptoms are worse in the morning or evening, note which it is and rate severity of variation
1	1	Mild	
2	2	Severe	

19: Depersonalization and derealization
- 0 Absent
- 1 Mild
- 2 Moderate
- 3 Severe
- 4 Incapacitating

Such as:
Feeling of unreality
Nihilistic ideas

20: Paranoid symptoms
- 0 None
- 1, 2 Suspiciousness
- 3 Ideas of reference
- 4 Delusions of reference and persecution

21: Obsessional and compulsive symptoms
- 0 Absent
- 1 Mild
- 2 Severe

(continued)

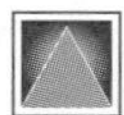

Table 7.9–8 (*continued*)

22: Helplessness
- 0 Not present
- 1 Subjective feelings which are elicited only by inquiry
- 2 Patient volunteers his helpless feelings
- 3 Requires urging, guidance, and reassurance to accomplish ward chores or personal hygiene
- 4 Requires physical assistance for dress, grooming, eating, bedside tasks, or personal hygiene

23: Hopelessness
- 0 Not present
- 1 Intermittently doubts that "things will improve" but can be reassured
- 2 Consistently feels "hopeless" but accepts reassurances
- 3 Expresses feelings of discouragement, despair, pessimism about future, which cannot be dispelled
- 4 Spontaneously and inappropriately perseverates: "I'll never get well" or its equivalent

24: Worthlessness (ranges from mild loss of esteem, feelings of inferiority, self-deprecation to delusional notions of worthlessness)
- 0 Not present
- 1 Indicates feelings of worthlessness (loss of self-esteem) only on questioning
- 2 Spontaneously indicates feelings of worthlessness (loss of self-esteem)
- 3 Different from 2 by degree. Patient volunteers that he is "no good," "inferior," etc.
- 4 Delusional notions of worthlessness—i.e., "I am a heap of garbage" or its equivalent

From Hamilton M: A rating scale for depression. *J Neurol Neurosurg Psychiatry.* 1960;23:56, with permission.

ments describing increasing levels of severity, and the total score ranges from 0 to 84. Scores of 0 to 9 are considered minimal; 10 to 16, mild; 17 to 29, moderate; and 30 to 63, severe. The scale can be completed in 5 to 10 minutes. Internal consistency has been high in numerous studies. Test–retest reliability is not consistently high, but this may reflect changes in underlying symptoms. Validity is supported by correlation with other depression measures. The principal use of the BDI is as an outcome measure in clinical trials of interventions for major depression, including psychotherapeutic interventions. Because it is a self-report instrument, it is sometimes used to screen for major depression. However, in trials of various cutoffs for a diagnosis of major depression, the best seemed to be 9, which had only fair sensitivity, at a cost of considerable nonspecificity, suggesting that the instrument has limited use for screening. The instrument's strength lies in measuring the depth of depression and in its comprehensive coverage of the cognitive dimension of depression.

Inventory of Depressive Symptomatology (IDS) The IDS was developed in 1982 to reflect a broader conceptualization of major depression than the HAM-D and other earlier instruments and to provide a comprehensive assessment of depressed inpatients and outpatients. It has fuller coverage of the full range of DSM-IV symptoms of depression and covers mild, as well as severe, symptoms of depression. Both clinician-rated (IDS-C) and self-report (IDS-SR) versions are available. The clinician version comes with a structured interview guide to improve the reliability of the ratings. The original version had 28 items, but two were subsequently added to cover atypical symptoms. Each item has four to five scaled multiple-choice answers, ranging from no difficulty to significant difficulty in that area. The instrument can be completed in 15 to 20 minutes, and the clinician version can be completed in 30 minutes or less. Although the IDS is a relatively new instrument, it has been subjected to rigorous reliability and validity assessment. It shows good reliability in a variety of paradigms and excellent validity, as judged by comparison with other depression scales. It has also been shown to have good validity in the classification of depressive subtypes. Because of these advantages, the IDS is gaining popularity for following patients in clinical trials and shows promise for the evaluation of depression and response to treatment in clinical practice as well.

Young Mania Rating Scale (YMRS) The YMRS is a checklist developed in the late 1970s to provide a brief but thorough evaluation of the severity of mania that could be used to monitor treatment response or detect relapse. It consists of a checklist of 11 items rated either from 0 to 4 (seven items) or from 0 to 8 (four items). Each item has five item-specific anchors. The total score ranges from 0 to 60. Ratings include clinical observation, so it must be rated by a clinician, but reliable ratings have been obtained by nurses on inpatient units and beginning psychiatric residents. Reliability is good based on interrater reliability and internal consistency studies. Validity also appears good based on correlation with other mania measures. The YMRS is useful for evaluating response to treatment in clinical research, and it has been found to be sensitive to change in this setting. It might also be used to assess treatment response or to monitor for relapse in treated or untreated patients, although extensive experience with this use has not been reported.

Anxiety Disorders

The anxiety disorders addressed by the measures below include panic disorder, generalized anxiety disorder, posttraumatic stress disorder (PTSD), and obsessive-compulsive disorder (OCD). When examining anxiety measures, it is important to be aware that there have been significant changes over time in how they are defined. Both panic and OCD are relatively recently recognized, and the conceptualization of generalized anxiety disorder has shifted over time. Thus, older measures have somewhat less relevance for diagnostic purposes, although they may identify symptoms causing considerable distress. Whether reported during an interview or on a self-report rating scale, virtually all measures in this domain, like the measures of depression discussed above, depend on subjective descriptions of inner states.

Hamilton Anxiety Rating Scale (HAM-A) The HAM-A (Table 7.9–9) was developed in the late 1950s to assess anxiety symptoms, both somatic and cognitive. Because the conceptualization of anxiety has changed considerably, the HAM-A provides limited coverage of "worry" required for DSM-IV diagnosis of generalized anxiety disorder and does not include the episodic anxiety found in panic disorder. There are 14 items, each of which is rated from 0 to 4 on an unanchored severity scale, with the total score ranging from 0 to 56. A score of 14 has been suggested as the threshold for clinically significant anxiety, but scores of 5 or less are typical in individuals in the community. The scale is designed to be administered by a clinician, and formal training or the use of a structured interview guide is required to achieve high reliability. A computer-administered version is also available. Reliability is fairly good based on internal consistency, interrater, and test–retest studies.

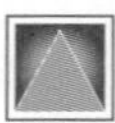

Table 7.9–9
Hamilton Rating Scale for Anxiety

Instructions: This checklist is to assist the physician or psychiatrist in evaluating each patient as to his degree of anxiety and pathological condition. Please fill in the appropriate rating:

NONE = 0 MILD = 1 MODERATE = 2 SEVERE = 3 SEVERE, GROSSLY DISABLING = 4

Item		Rating	Item		Rating
Anxious	Worries, anticipation of the worst, fearful anticipation, irritability	______	Somatic (sensory)	Tinnitus, blurring of vision, hot and cold flushes, feelings of weakness, pricking sensation	______
Tension	Feelings of tension, fatigability, startle response, moved to tears easily, trembling, feelings of restlessness, inability to relax	______	Cardiovascular symptoms	Tachycardia, palpitations, pain in chest, throbbing of vessels, fainting feelings, missing beat	______
Fears	Of dark, of strangers, of being left alone, of animals, of traffic, of crowds	______	Respiratory symptoms	Pressure or constriction in chest, choking feelings, sighing, dyspnea	______
Insomnia	Difficulty in falling asleep, broken sleep, unsatisfying sleep and fatigue on waking, dreams, nightmares, night-terrors	______	Gastrointestinal symptoms	Difficulty in swallowing, wind, abdominal pain, burning sensations, abdominal fullness, nausea, vomiting, borborygmi, looseness of bowels, loss of weight, constipation	______
Intellectual (cognitive)	Difficulty in concentration, poor memory	______	Genitourinary symptoms	Frequency of micturition, urgency of micturition, amenorrhea, menorrhagia, development of frigidity, premature ejaculation, loss of libido, impotence	______
Depressed mood	Loss of interest, lack of pleasure in hobbies, depression, early waking, diurnal swing	______			
Somatic (muscular)	Pains and aches, twitching, stiffness, myoclonic jerks, grinding of teeth, unsteady voice, increased muscular tone	______	Autonomic symptoms	Dry mouth, flushing, pallor, tendency to sweat, giddiness, tension headache, raising of hair	______
			Behavior at interview	Fidgeting, restlessness or pacing, tremor of hands, furrowed brow, strained face, sighing or rapid respiration, facial pallor, swallowing, belching, brisk tendon jerks, dilated pupils, exophthalmos	______

ADDITIONAL COMMENTS:

Investigator's signature:

From Hamilton M: The assessment of anxiety states by rating. *Br J Psychiatry.* 1959;32:50, with permission.

However, given the lack of specific anchors, reliability should not be assumed to be high across different users in the absence of formal training. Validity appears good based on correlation with other anxiety scales but is limited by the relative lack of coverage of domains critical to the modern understanding of anxiety disorders. Even so, the HAM-A has been used extensively to monitor treatment response in studies of generalized anxiety disorder and may also be useful for this purpose in clinical settings.

Panic Disorder Severity Scale (PDSS) The PDSS was developed in the 1990s as a brief rating scale for the severity of panic disorder. It was based on the Yale-Brown Obsessive-Compulsive Scale and has seven items, each of which is rated on an item-specific, five-point Likert scale. The seven items address frequency of attacks, distress associated with attacks, anticipatory anxiety, phobic avoidance, and impairment. The items are scored from 0 to 4, and the total score ranges from 0 to 28. The instrument was designed for use by clinicians, but a patient-scored computerized version is also available. Reliability is excellent based on interrater studies, but, in keeping with the small number of items and multiple dimensions, internal consistency is limited. Validity is supported by correlations with other anxiety measures, both at the total and item level, and lack of correlation with the HAM-D. Growing experience with the PDSS suggests that it is sensitive to change with treatment and is useful as a change measure in clinical trials or other outcome studies for panic disorder, as well as for monitoring panic disorder in clinical practice.

Clinician-Administered PTSD Scale (CAPS) The CAPS was developed in 1990 to operationalize the DSM-III-R diagnosis of PTSD and can easily be modified to obtain a diagnosis by DSM-IV criteria. The interview includes 17 items required to make the diagnosis, covering all four criteria: (1) the event itself, (2) reexperiencing of the event, (3) avoidance, and (4) increased arousal. For each of the 17 items, the interviewer rates both the severity and the intensity on a five-point scale ranging from 0 to 4. The diagnosis requires evidence of a traumatic event, one symptom of reexperiencing, three of avoidance, and two of arousal (typically, an item is counted if frequency is at least 1 and intensity is at least 2). The items can also be used to generate a total PTSD severity score obtained by summing the frequency and intensity scales for each item. The CAPS also includes several global rating scales for the impact of PTSD symptomatology on social and occupational functioning, for general severity, for recent changes, and for the validity of the patient's report. The CAPS must be administered by a trained clinician and requires 45 to 60 minutes to complete, with follow-up examinations somewhat briefer. It has demonstrated reliability and validity in multiple settings and multiple languages, although it has had more limited testing in the setting of sexual and criminal assault. It performs well in the research setting for diagnosis and severity assessment but is generally too lengthy for use in the clinical practice.

Yale-Brown Obsessive-Compulsive Scale (YBOCS) The YBOCS was developed in the late 1980s to measure the severity of symptoms in OCD. It has ten items rated based on a semistructured interview. The first five items concern obsessions: the amount of time they consume, the degree to which they interfere with normal functioning, the distress they cause, the patient's attempts to resist them, and the patient's ability to control them. The remaining five items ask parallel questions about compulsions. Each item has a set of item-specific anchors scored from 0 to 4, so total scores for obsessions and compulsions each range from 0 to 20, and overall total score ranges from 0 to 40. Typical scores for patients with OCD are in the 16 to 30 range, and a threshold of 16 is typically used for inclusion in drug trials. The semistructured interview and ratings can be completed in 15 minutes or less. A self-administered version has recently been developed and can be completed in 10 to 15 minutes. Computerized and telephone use have also been found to provide acceptable ratings. Before the first use of the YBOCS, an associated 64-item checklist is administered to provide a more detailed assessment of the specific content of the patient's obsessions and delusions. Reliability studies of the YBOCS show good internal consistency, interrater reliability, and test–retest reliability over a 1-week interval. Validity appears good, although data are fairly limited in this developing field. The YBOCS has become the standard instrument for assessing OCD severity and is used in virtually every drug trial. It may also be used clinically to monitor treatment response.

Substance Use Disorders Substance use disorders include abuse and dependence on both alcohol and drugs. These disorders, particularly those involving alcohol, are common and debilitating in the general population, so screening instruments are particularly helpful. Because these behaviors are socially undesirable, underreporting of symptoms is a significant problem. Validation against drug tests or other measures is of great value, particularly when working with patients who have known substance abuse.

CAGE The CAGE was developed in the mid-1970s to serve as a very brief screen for significant alcohol problems in a variety of settings, which could then be followed up by clinical inquiry. CAGE is an acronym for the four questions that comprise the instrument: (1) Have you ever felt you should *c*ut down on your drinking?, (2) Have people *a*nnoyed you by criticizing your drinking?, (3) Have you ever felt bad or *g*uilty about your drinking?, and (4) Have you ever had a drink first thing in the morning to steady your nerves or to get rid of a hangover (*e*ye-opener)? Each "yes" answer is scored as 1, and these are summed to generate a total score. Scores of 1 or more warrant follow-up, and scores of 2 or more strongly suggest significant alcohol problems. The instrument can be administered in a minute or less, either orally or on paper. Reliability has not been formally assessed. Validity has been assessed against a clinical diagnosis of alcohol abuse or dependence, and these four questions perform surprisingly well. Using a threshold score of 1, the CAGE achieves excellent sensitivity and fair to good specificity. A threshold of 2 provides still greater specificity, but at the cost of a fall in sensitivity. The CAGE performs well as an extremely brief screening instrument for use in primary care or in psychiatric practice focused on problems unrelated to alcohol. However, it has limited ability to pick up early indicators of problem drinking that might be the focus of preventive efforts.

Alcohol Use Disorders Identification Test (AUDIT) The AUDIT (Table 7.9–10) was developed by the World Health Organization (WHO) in the late 1980s as a brief screening instrument designed for the early detection of hazardous (i.e., involving the risk of harm) and harmful (i.e., involving the presence of harm) alcohol use in a variety of settings. It focuses on both the past year and current drinking. It includes a ten-item core screening instrument covering alcohol consumption, drinking behaviors, and alcohol-related problems. Each item is rated using item-specific anchors scored from 0 to 4 and summed for a total score from 0 to 40. The AUDIT can be administered and scored in less than 5 minutes and does not require professional training. The AUDIT also offers a clinical screening procedure involving a physical examination and blood tests, which adds no more than 5 to 10 minutes to a routine medical examination. Reliability of the AUDIT appears good based on internal consistency data. Validity judged against a clinical diagnosis of alcoholism is also good: using a threshold score of 8 is quite sensitive but somewhat nonspecific. A score of 10 is more specific, but at a cost in specificity. Validity also appears good based on correlation with other alcohol self-report measures and risk factors for alcoholism. The AUDIT provides an excellent brief screen for alcohol problems and is particularly good for detecting problem drinking at a fairly mild stage. However, its focus on early detection of hazardous and harmful drinking makes it less suitable to use as a diagnostic instrument.

Drug Abuse Screening Test (DAST) The DAST was developed in the early 1980s to serve as a screening and assessment instrument for drug abuse. The DAST is an adaptation of the Michigan Alcohol Screening Test (MAST), used to screen for alcoholism. It focuses on lifetime drug use, so it is not designed to measure changes over time. The current version of the DAST has 20 items, all of which are answered yes or no, and can be given orally or as a paper-and-pencil questionnaire. An earlier version had 28 items, so the 20-item version is sometimes called the *Brief DAST*. The positive items can be summed to form a 20-point scale. The DAST can be administered and scored in less than 10 minutes. Reliability is very good based on internal consistency. Validity based on ability to detect drug abuse disorder also appears high, with excellent sensitivity and fairly good specificity using a threshold score of 5. The DAST is useful as a screening device for drug abuse problems in patients with other mental disorders, particularly alcohol abuse. It also provides an overview of problem severity that may be useful to guide treatment choices.

Addiction Severity Index (ASI) The ASI was developed in the early 1980s to serve as a quantitative measure of symptoms and functional impairment due to alcohol or drug disorders. It covers demographics, alcohol use, drug use, psychiatric status, medical status, employment, legal status, and family and social issues. Frequency, duration, and severity are assessed. It has 142 items in varying formats, including yes–no, multiple-choice, and scaled items. It includes both subjective and objective items reported by the patient and observations made by the interviewer. In each area, the ASI yields the rater's global assessment of severity, along with a computer score on a 0 to 1 scale. The 142-item version includes information on the past 30 days and lifetime status, but a shorter version is available for use at follow-up. The instrument is designed for clinician administration but has been used successfully by trained lay raters. Training is recommended, and both manuals and formal training programs are available. A computerized version is also available. The standard ASI requires 45 to 75 minutes to complete, but the follow-up version can be completed in 15 to 20 minutes. Very good to excellent reliability has been demonstrated for the overall composite score, with somewhat lower reliability for severity ratings in each area. Validity has also been demonstrated based on correlation with other measures and discrimination of patient from nonpatient populations. Normative data are available for a range of populations of alcohol and drug abusers, including alcohol clinic patients, drug abusers, homeless persons, and prisoners. The principal use of the ASI is as an aid to treatment planning and the assessment of treatment outcome in clinical and law enforcement settings. It is relatively time consuming to administer but performs well for this purpose. It has also been used in clinical research as a sensitive indicator of baseline severity and change over time, which allows comparison between clinical research and clinical practice.

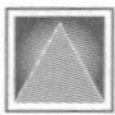

Table 7.9–10
Alcohol Use Disorders Identification Test (AUDIT)

The Alcohol Use Disorders Identification Test: Self-Report Version

PATIENT: Because alcohol use can affect your health and can interfere with certain medications and treatments, it is important that we ask some questions about your use of alcohol. Your answers will remain confidential so please be honest.

Place an X in one box that best describes your answer to each question.

Questions	0	1	2	3	4	
1. How often do you have a drink containing alcohol?	Never	Monthly or less	2–4 times a month	2–3 times a week	4 or more times a week	______
2. How many drinks containing alcohol do you have on a typical day when you are drinking?	1 or 2	3 or 4	5 or 6	7 to 9	10 or more	______
3. How often do you have six or more drinks on one occasion?	Never	Less than monthly	Monthly	Weekly	Daily or almost daily	______
4. How often during the last year have you found that you were not able to stop drinking once you had started?	Never	Less than monthly	Monthly	Weekly	Daily or almost daily	______
5. How often during the last year have you failed to do what was normally expected of you because of drinking?	Never	Less than monthly	Monthly	Weekly	Daily or almost daily	______
6. How often during the last year have you needed a first drink in the morning to get yourself going after a heavy drinking session?	Never	Less than monthly	Monthly	Weekly	Daily or almost daily	______
7. How often during the last year have you had a feeling of guilt or remorse after drinking?	Never	Less than monthly	Monthly	Weekly	Daily or almost daily	______
8. How often during the last year have you been unable to remember what happened the night before because of your drinking?	Never	Less than monthly	Monthly	Weekly	Daily or almost daily	______
9. Have you or someone else been injured because of your drinking?	No		Yes, but not in the last year		Yes, during the last year	______
10. Has a relative, friend, doctor, or other health care worker been concerned about your drinking or suggested you cut down?	No		Yes, but not in the last year		Yes, during the last year	______
					Total	______

Note: The minimum score (for nondrinkers) is 0 and the maximum possible score is 40. A score of 8 or more indicates a strong likelihood of hazardous or harmful alcohol consumption.

From Babor T, Higgins-Biddle JT, Saunders JB, Monteiro MG. *The Alcohol Use Disorders Identification Test: Guidelines for Use in Primary Care.* 2nd ed. Geneva: World Health Organization; 2001, with permission.

Eating Disorders

Eating disorders include anorexia nervosa, bulimia nervosa, and binge-eating disorder, which is included in Appendix B of DSM-IV and is gaining acceptance among eating disorders clinicians and researchers. A wide variety of instruments, particularly self-report scales, are available. Because of the secrecy that may surround dieting, bingeing, purging, and other symptoms, validation against other indicators (e.g., body weight for anorexia, dental examination for bulimia) may be very helpful. Such validation is particularly critical for patients with anorexia, who may lack insight into their difficulties.

Eating Disorders Examination (EDE)

The EDE was developed in 1987 as the first interviewer-based comprehensive assessment of eating disorders. A self-report version (the EDE-Q), as well as an interview for children, has since been developed. The EDE focuses on symptoms during the preceding 4 weeks, although longer-term questions are included to assess diagnostic criteria for eating disorders. Each item on the EDE has a required probe with suggested follow-up questions to judge severity or frequency or both, which are then rated on a seven-point Likert scale. For the self-report version, subjects are asked to make similar ratings of frequency or severity. The instrument provides both global severity ratings and ratings on four subscales: restraint, eating concern, weight concern, and shape concern. The interview, which must be administered by a trained clinician, requires 30 to 60 minutes to complete, whereas the self-report version is somewhat faster. Reliability and validity data for both the EDE and EDE-Q are excellent, although the EDE-Q may have greater sensitivity for binge-eating disorder. The EDE performs well both in the diagnosis and detailed assessment of eating disorders in the research context. It also has the sensitivity to change required for use in clinical trials or monitoring of individual therapy. Even in the research setting, however, the EDE is fairly lengthy for repeated use, and the EDE-Q may be preferable for some purposes. Although the EDE is too lengthy for routine clinical practice, the EDE or EDE-Q might be helpful in providing a comprehensive assessment of a patient with a suspected eating disorder, particularly during an evaluation visit or on entry into an inpatient facility.

Bulimia Test–Revised (BULIT-R)

The BULIT-R was developed in the mid-1980s to provide both a categorical and continuous assessment of bulimia nervosa. The current version, although designed for DSM-III-R criteria, has been validated for DSM-IV as well. The BULIT-R has 36 self-report items, each scored on an item-specific, five-point Likert scale. Of these items, eight provide descriptive information, and the remaining 28 are summed to provide the total score, which ranges from 28 to 140. Young women with bulimia nervosa typically score above 110, whereas young women without disordered eating typically score below 60. The instrument can be completed in approximately 10 minutes. The BULIT-R shows high reliability based on studies of internal consistency and test–retest reliability in multiple studies. Validity is supported by high correlations with other bulimia assessments. The recommended cutoff of 104 suggested to identify probable cases of bulimia shows high sensitivity and specificity for a clinical diagnosis of bulimia nervosa. Using cutoffs between 98 and 104, the BULIT-R has been used successfully to screen for cases of bulimia nervosa. As with any screening procedure, follow-up by clinical examination is indicated for individuals scoring positive; clinical follow-up is particularly critical because the BULIT-R does not distinguish clearly between different types of eating disorders. The BULIT-R may also be useful to track symptoms over time or in response to treatment, in both clinical and research practice, although more detailed measures of the frequency and severity of bingeing and purging may be preferable in research settings.

Cognitive Disorders

This section reviews measures of dementia, which is becoming an increasing focus of psychiatric practice. A wide variety of measures are available. Most involve cognitive testing and provide objective, quantifiable data. However, scores vary by educational level in subjects without dementia, so these instruments tend to be most useful when the patient's own baseline score is known. Other measures focus on functional status, which can be assessed based on a comparison with a description of the subject's baseline function; these types of measures generally require a knowledgeable informant and, thus, may be more cumbersome to administer but tend to be less subject to educational biases.

Mini-Mental State Examination (MMSE)

The MMSE is a 30-point cognitive test developed in the mid-1970s to provide a bedside assessment of a broad array of cognitive function, including orientation, attention, memory, construction, and language. It can be administered in less than 10 minutes by a busy doctor or a technician and scored rapidly by hand. The MMSE has been extensively studied and shows excellent reliability. Validity appears good based on correlations with a wide variety of more comprehensive measures of mental functioning and clinicopathological correlations. One common use of the MMSE is in screening for dementia, both in office practice and epidemiologic or clinical research. For this purpose, a cutoff of 24 for identifying cases of dementia has been suggested, but it is probably more accurate to use age- and education-adjusted norms to interpret the results. For patients with extensive education, who may score 30 out of 30 despite clear evidence of functional decline, a more difficult cognitive test, full neuropsychological battery, or clinical interview about functional change may be required to detect dementia. The other principal use of the MMSE is in following the progression of dementia over time in the clinic or in clinical trials. As a rule of thumb, patients with mild dementia tend to score from 20 to 24, moderate from 11 to 19, and severe from 0 to 10. However, it should be noted that these figures do not take the educational differences noted above into account. In addition, the MMSE does not do as well tracking progression of dementia at later stages; scores of 10 or less are difficult to obtain, as many patients become untestable.

Blessed Information Memory Concentration Test (IMC)

The IMC, sometimes called the *Blessed IMC* after its developer, was developed in the late 1960s for studies of the relationship between dementia severity and neuropathological changes. The original version of the scale, developed in Britain, had 29 items; the current American version has 26. Areas assessed include information (date, time, place, name, age, remote personal information, dates of the world wars, name of governmental leaders), memory (a name and address for 5-minute recall), and concentration (counting forward and backward from 1 to 20). A six-item version, sometimes called the *short form* of the Blessed or the *Orientation Memory Concentration Test* (OMC), is also available. It asks only the time of day, month, year, 5-minute recall of the address, and counting backward from 20 and is highly predictive of total IMC score. IMC scores on individual items are weighted: on the 26-item IMC, scores range from 0 (no errors) to 33; on the six-item version, scores range from 0 to 28. The IMC can be administered in person or over the phone by a trained clinician or lay rater. Based on internal consistency and test–retest studies in demented subjects over a 1- to 6-week interval, reliability of the 26- and 6-item IMCs both appear very good. Validity also appears good based on clinicopathological correlations and correlations with other dementia severity measures. Studies of changes with time in patients with Alzheimer's disease show an average annual increase of 3 to 4 points on the 26-item version and 2.5 points on the 6-item version. The principal use of the IMC is assessing dementia severity over time, either through the natural course of the disease or in response to treatment interventions. The IMC is also sometimes used as a screening instrument in clinical practice or community research studies. A cutoff score of 10 has been recommended for the 6-item version, but no standard cutoff is recommended for the 26-item version. In any case, there is very limited population data, and norms are not available by age or education, which are very likely to affect test results. On the other hand, because of its focus on memory items, the IMC may perform better than the MMSE as a severity or screening measure in patients with very mild Alzheimer's disease.

Clinical Dementia Rating Scale (CDR)

The CDR (Table 7.9–11) was developed in 1982 as a standardized staging system for dementia based on all available information about the patient. Patients are rated in each of six domains (memory, orientation, judgment and problem solving, community affairs, home and hobbies, and personal care) on a six-point scale (0 = no dementia, 0.5 = questionable dementia [approximately equivalent to Minimal Cognitive Impairment or prodromal Alzheimer's disease], 1 = mild dementia, 2 = moderate dementia, 3 = severe dementia, 4 = profound dementia, and 5 = terminal dementia). For levels 0 to 3, detailed descriptions are provided to anchor the ratings in each area. The ratings in each domain are typically combined into an overall CDR rating on the same six-point scale following a weighting system that favors memory. However, they can also be summed to generate a CDR Sum of Boxes score. The staging system can be used on its own or based on the CDR protocol, developed to standardize information obtained for ratings of 3 or below. The protocol includes interviews of the patient and informant, as well as cognitive testing. Ratings can be made relatively quickly by a clinician who is very familiar with the patient, but the full protocol requires 1 hour or more to administer. CDR ratings of 4 and 5 are based on overall status. Stage 4 indicates *profound* dementia, with problems recognizing loved ones, incontinence, and severe impairment in language, mobility, and self-care. Stage 5 refers to *terminal* dementia, when patients are completely uncommunicative, bedridden, vegetative, and incontinent. Whether based on the CDR protocol or on clinical experience with the patient, the CDR must be rated by a trained clinician. Additional training in the use of the scale and protocol are strongly recommended. The reported reliability of CDR scores based on the full protocol is high, but achieving this level of reliability requires extensive training. Validity of the CDR has also been shown to be high, particularly if based on the formal protocol. Although the CDR *protocol* is clearly intended for research, the CDR *scale* is of potential usefulness as a stage marker for clinical communication and charting decline over time. It is also helpful for understanding the dementia research literature, as the CDR is increasingly used as a stage marker for clinical trials and other research. However, the CDR's lack of detail makes it relatively insensitive to change over short periods (the average annual decline is approximately one half-stage per year). The Sum of Boxes, on the other hand, provides a more detailed score that is considerably more sensitive to change and is gaining popularity as a quantitative measure of dementia in a variety of research settings.

Personality Disorders and Personality Traits

Personality may be conceptualized categorically as personality disorders or dimensionally as personality traits, which may be viewed as normal or

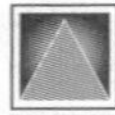

Table 7.9–11
Modified Clinical Dementia Rating (CDR): 0, 0.5, 1, 2, 3

Impairment	None (0)	Questionable (0.5)	Mild (1)	Moderate (2)	Severe (3)
Memory	No memory loss or slight inconstant forgetfulness	Consistent slight forgetfulness; partial recollection of events	Moderate memory loss; more marked for recent events; defect interferes with everyday activities	Severe memory loss; only highly learned material retained; new material rapidly lost	Severe memory loss; only fragments remain
Orientation	Fully oriented	Fully oriented or slight difficulty with time relationships	Moderate difficulty with time relationships; oriented for place at examination; may have geographic disorientation elsewhere	Severe difficulty with time relationships; usually disoriented in time, often to place	Oriented to person only
Judgment and problem	Solves everyday problems and handles business and financial affairs well; judgment good in relation to past performance	Slight impairment to solving problems, similarities, differences	Moderate difficulty in handling problems, similarities, differences; social judgment usually maintained	Severely impaired in handling problems, similarities, differences; social judgment usually impaired	Unable to make judgments or solve problems
Community affairs	Independent function at usual level in job, shopping, volunteer and social groups	Slight impairment in these activities	Unable to function independently at these activities though may still be engaged in some; appears normal to casual inspection	No pretense of independent function outside of home; appears well enough to be taken to functions outside of family home	No pretense of independent function outside of home; appears too ill to be taken to functions outside a family home
Home and hobbies	Life at home, hobbies, intellectual interests well maintained	Life at home, hobbies, intellectual interests slightly impaired	Mild but definite impairment of function at home; more difficult chores abandoned; more complicated hobbies and interests abandoned	Only simple chores preserved; very restricted interests, poorly maintained	No significant function in home
Personal care	Fully capable of self care	Fully capable of self care	Needs prompting	Requires assistance in dressing, hygiene keeping of personal effects	Requires much help with personal care; frequent incontinence

Note: Score only as decline from previous usual level due to cognitive loss, not impairment due to other factors.

pathological. The focus here is on personality disorders and the traits generally viewed as their milder forms. DSM-IV defines ten personality disorders in three clusters, and there are an additional two disorders (passive-aggressive and depressive personality) proposed in Appendix B for further study. Patients tend not to fall neatly into DSM-IV personality categories; instead, most patients who meet criteria for one personality disorder also meet criteria for at least one other, particularly within the same cluster. This and other limitations in the validity of the constructs themselves make it difficult to achieve validity in personality measures. Personality measures include both interviews and self-report instruments. Self-report measures are appealing in that they require less time and may appear less threatening to the patient. However, they tend to overdiagnose personality disorders. Because many of the symptoms suggesting personality problems are socially undesirable and because patients' insight tends to be limited, clinician-administered instruments, which allow for probing and patient observation, may provide more accurate data.

Structured Clinical Interview for DSM-IV-TR Axis II Personality Disorders (SCID-II) The SCID-II is the counterpart of the SCID for making DSM diagnoses of personality disorders. The initial version was developed for DSM-III-R in the mid-1990s, and the current version makes diagnoses according to DSM-IV. The SCID-II is organized by disorder and includes all ten DSM-IV personality disorders, plus the two proposed in Appendix B. A 119-item, self-report screening questionnaire is generally given first to eliminate sections not needing further exploration; each of the items corresponds to a specific criterion for a DSM-IV personality disorder. The SCID-II proper includes one or two yes–no items for each criterion, with each affirmative answer to be followed up by examples from the person's life. Based on these answers, each criterion is scored 1 for false, 2 for subthreshold, and 3 for present, allowing criteria scores to be summed for a dimensional measure of each disorder or combined following the DSM-IV diagnostic rules for a categorical approach. The screening questionnaire can be completed by the patient in approximately 20 minutes; the interview generally requires approximately 1 hour. The SCID-II must be administered by doctoral-level clinicians, and training in the SCID-II is also required. A computerized administration and scoring program is available. Reliability is good for the presence or absence of any disorder but only fair for specific personality disorders; the reliability of dimensional assessment is somewhat better. Validity is somewhat harder to determine, as agreement with clinician assessment tends to be modest. However, given the instrument's comprehensiveness and strict adherence to DSM-IV-TR criteria, the SCID-II may actually be more valid than clinician ratings. The SCID-II is most useful to provide a standardized, comprehensive assessment of personality disorders, whether in research, forensic, or clinical settings.

Personality Disorder Questionnaire (PDQ) The PDQ was developed in the late 1980s as a simple self-report questionnaire designed to provide categorical and dimensional assessment of DSM-III-R personality disorders and was subsequently revised for DSM-IV. An alternate version includes the two disorders in Appendix B as well. Another alternate version allows for ratings within the last few weeks and is designed to serve as a change measure. The current PDQ, the PDQ-IV, includes 85 yes–no items, designed primarily to assess the diagnostic criteria for DSM-IV personality disorders. Within the 85 items, two validity scales are embedded to identify underreporting, lying, or inattention. There is also a brief clinician-administered Clinical Significance Scale to address the impact of any personality disorder identified by the self-report PDQ. The PDQ can provide categorical diagnoses, a scaled score for each, or an overall index of personality disturbance based on the sum of all the diagnostic criteria. Overall scores range from 0 to 79; patients with personality disorders generally score above 30, psychotherapy outpatients without such disorders tend to score in the 20 to 30 range, and normal controls tend to score below 20. The PDQ can be completed in less than 30 minutes. Computerized administration and scoring are available. Reliability is fair to good for dimensional assessment and quite variable for categorical assessment, with good reliability for obsessive-compulsive and antisocial personality disorders and inadequate reliability for many disorders. Validity judged against semistructured clinician-administered interviews is also variable. The PDQ, like other self-report instruments, tends to overdiagnose personality disorders, with many false positives and few false negatives. Its brevity, good sensitivity, and poor specificity make it most useful as a screening device, with follow-up administration of a semistructured interview in patients screening positive.

Childhood Disorders

A wide variety of instruments are available to assess mental disorders in children. Despite this rich array of instruments, however, the evaluation of children remains difficult for several reasons. First, the child psychiatric nosology is at an earlier stage of development, and construct validity is often problematic. Multiple changes in diagnostic criteria from DSM-III to DSM-III-R to DSM-IV complicate the choice of measures. Second, because children change markedly with age, it is virtually impossible to design a measure that covers children of all ages. Last, because children, particularly young children, have limited ability to report their symptoms, other informants are necessary. This often creates problems because there are frequent disagreements among child, parent, and teacher reports of symptoms, and the optimal way to combine information is unclear.

Child Behavior Checklist (CBCL) The CBCL is a family of self-rated instruments that survey a broad range of difficulties encountered in children from preschool through adolescence. One version of the CBCL, designed for completion by parents of children between 4 and 18 years of age, is shown in Table 7.9–12. Another version is available for parents of children between 2 and 3 years of age. The Youth Self-Report is completed by children between 11 and 18 years of age, and the Teacher Report Form is completed by teachers of school-age children. The scale includes not only problem behaviors, but also academic and social strengths. Each version includes approximately 100 items scored on a three-point Likert scale. Scoring can be done by hand or computer, and normative data are available for each of the three subscales: problem behaviors, academic functioning, and adaptive behaviors. A computerized version is also available. The CBCL does not generate diagnoses but, instead, suggests cutoff scores for problems in the "clinical range." Parent, teacher, and child versions all show high reliability on the problem subscale, but the three informants frequently do not agree with one another. The CBCL may be useful in clinical settings as an adjunct to clinical evaluation, as it provides a good overall view of symptomatology and may also be used to track change over time. It is used frequently for similar purposes in research involving children and, thus, can be compared to clinical experience. The instrument does not, however, provide diagnostic information, and its length limits its efficiency for tracking purposes.

Diagnostic Interview Schedule for Children (DISC) The DISC was originally developed in the early 1990s as a fully structured diagnostic interview for making DSM-III diagnoses in children. It has since been revised for DSM-III-R and DSM-IV. The current DISC, the DISC-IV, covers a broad range of DSM-IV diagnoses, both current and lifetime. It has nearly 3,000 questions but is structured with a series of stem questions that serve as gateways to each diagnostic area, with the remainder of each section skipped if the subject answers no. Subjects who enter each section have very few skips, so complete diagnostic and symptom scale information can be obtained. Child, parent, and teacher versions are available. Computer programs are available to implement diagnostic criteria and generate severity scales based on each version or to combine parent and child information. A typical DISC interview may take more than 1 hour for a child, plus an additional hour for a parent. However, because of the stem question structure, the actual time varies widely with the number of symptoms endorsed. The DISC was designed for lay interviewers. It is fairly complicated to administer, and formal training programs are highly recommended. Reliability of the DISC is only fair to good and generally better for the combined child and parent interview. Validity judged against a clinical interview by a child psychiatrist is also fair to good—better for some diagnoses and better for the combined interview. The DISC is well tolerated by parents and children and can be used to supplement a clinical interview to ensure comprehensive diagnostic coverage. Because of its inflexibility, some clinicians find it uncomfortable to use, and its length makes it less than optimal for use in clinical practice. However, it is used frequently in a variety of research settings.

Conners Rating Scales The Conners Rating Scales are a family of instruments designed to measure a range of childhood and adolescent psychopathology but are most commonly used in the assessment of attention-deficit/hyperactivity disorder (ADHD). There are teacher, parent, and self-report (for adolescents) versions and both short (as few as ten items) and long (as many as 80 items, with multiple subscales) forms. Extensive normative data drawn from an ethnically diverse population are available for each sex across a broad age range. Even the longer forms can be completed in 15 to 20 minutes, and scoring can be accomplished rapidly. Training for raters is not required. Reliability data are excellent for the Conners Rating Scales. However, teacher and parent versions tend to show poor agreement. Validity data suggest that the Conners Rating Scales are excellent at discriminating between ADHD patients and normal controls. It has more difficulty separating ADHD from other disruptive behavioral disorders, such as conduct disorder, but this may be, in substantial part, related to the genuine clinical difficulties separating these syndromes. Newer versions of the Conners Rating Scales have been developed that aim to improve these discriminations, but have not yet been subjected to extensive testing. The principal uses of the Conners Rating Scales are in screening for ADHD in school or clinic populations and following changes in symptom severity over time; sensitivity to change in response to specific therapies has been demonstrated for most versions of the Conners Rating Scales.

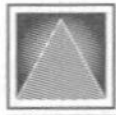

Table 7.9–12
Child Behavior Checklist for Ages 4–18

For office use only
ID #

CHILD'S FULL NAME	FIRST	MIDDLE	LAST	**PARENTS' USUAL TYPE OF WORK, even if not working now.** *(please be specific—for example, auto mechanic, high school teacher, homemaker, laborer, lathe operator, shoe salesman, army sergeant.)*
SEX ❒ Boy ❒ Girl	AGE	ETHNIC GROUP OR RACE		FATHER'S TYPE OF WORK: ____________ MOTHER'S TYPE OF WORK: ____________
TODAY'S DATE Mo. _____ Date _____ Yr. _____		CHILD'S BIRTHDATE Mo. _____ Date _____ Yr. _____		THIS FORM FILLED OUT BY:
GRADE IN SCHOOL _____ NOT ATTENDING SCHOOL ❒	Please fill out this form to reflect *your* view of the child's behavior even if other people might not agree. Feel free to print additional comments beside each item and in the spaces provided on page 2.			Mother (full name) Father (full name) Other—name & relationship to child:

I. Please list the sports your child most likes to take part in. For example: swimming, baseball, skating, skate boarding, bike riding, fishing, etc.
❒ None

	Compared to others of the same age, about how much time does he/she spend in each?				**Compared to others of the same age, how well does he/she do each one?**			
	Don't Know	**Less Than Average**	**Average**	**More Than Average**	**Don't Know**	**Below Average**	**Average**	**Above Average**
a.	❒	❒	❒	❒	❒	❒	❒	❒
b.	❒	❒	❒	❒	❒	❒	❒	❒
c.	❒	❒	❒	❒	❒	❒	❒	❒

II. Please list your child's favorite hobbies, activities, and games, other than sports. For example: stamps, dolls, books, piano, crafts, cars, singing, etc. (Do **not** include listening to radio or TV.)
❒ None

	Compared to others of the same age, about how much time does he/she spend in each?				**Compared to others of the same age, how well does he/she do each one?**			
	Don't Know	**Less Than Average**	**Average**	**More Than Average**	**Don't Know**	**Below Average**	**Average**	**Above Average**
a.	❒	❒	❒	❒	❒	❒	❒	❒
b.	❒	❒	❒	❒	❒	❒	❒	❒
c.	❒	❒	❒	❒	❒	❒	❒	❒

III. Please list any organizations, clubs, teams, or groups your child belongs to.
❒ None

	Compared to others of the same age, how active is he/she in each?			
	Don't Know	**Less Active**	**Average**	**More Active**
a.	❒	❒	❒	❒
b.	❒	❒	❒	❒
c.	❒	❒	❒	❒

IV. Please list any jobs or chores your child has. For example: paper route, babysitting, making bed, working in store, etc. (Include ***both*** paid and unpaid jobs and chores.)
❒ None

	Compared to others of the same age, how well does he/she carry them out?			
	Don't Know	**Below Average**	**Average**	**Above Average**
a.	❒	❒	❒	❒
b.	❒	❒	❒	❒
c.	❒	❒	❒	❒

(*continued*)

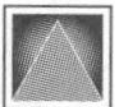

Table 7.9–12 (*continued*)

V. 1. About how many close friends does your child have? ❒ **None** ❒ **1** ❒ **2 or 3** ❒ **4 or more**
(Do *not* include brothers & sisters)

2. About how many times a week does your child do things with any friends outside of regular school hours?
(Do *not* include brothers & sisters) ❒ **Less than 1** ❒ **1 or 2** ❒ **3 or more**

VI. Compared to others of his/her age, how well does your child:

	Worse	About Average	Better	
a. Get along with his/her brothers & sisters?	❒	❒	❒	❒ Has no brothers or sisters
b. Get along with other kids?	❒	❒	❒	
c. Behave with his/her parents?	❒	❒	❒	
d. Play and work alone?	❒	❒	❒	

VII. 1. For ages 6 and older—performance in academic subjects. ❒ **Does not attend school because**

Check a box for each subject that child takes		Failing	Below Average	Average	Above Average
	a. Reading, English, or Language Arts	❒	❒	❒	❒
	b. History or Social Studies	❒	❒	❒	❒
	c. Arithmetic or Math	❒	❒	❒	❒
Other academic subjects—for example: computer courses, foreign language, business. Do **not** include gym, shop, driver's ed., etc.	d. Science	❒	❒	❒	❒
	e.	❒	❒	❒	❒
	f.	❒	❒	❒	❒
	g.	❒	❒	❒	❒

2. Does your child receive special remedial services or attend a special class or special school? ❒ **No** ❒ **Yes—kind of services, class, or school:**

3. Has your child repeated any grades? ❒ **No** ❒ **Yes—grades and reasons:**

4. Has your child had any academic or other problems in school? ❒ **No** ❒ **Yes—please describe:**

When did these problems start?
Have these problems ended? ❒ No ❒ Yes—when?

Does your child have any illness or disability (either physical or mental)? ❒ **No** ❒ **Yes—please describe:**

What concerns you most about your child?

Please describe the best things about your child:

Below is a list of items that describe children and youth. For each item that describes your child **now or within the past 6 months,** please circle the **2** if the item is **very true or often true** of your child. Circle the **1** if the item is **somewhat or sometimes true** of your child. If the item is **not true** of your child, circle the **0.** Please answer all items as well as you can, even if some do not seem to apply to your child.

Please Print

0 = Not True (as far as you know) **1 = Somewhat or Sometimes True** **2 = Very True or Often True**

0 1 2 1. Acts too young for his/her age
0 1 2 2. Allergy (describe): ____________
0 1 2 3. Argues a lot
0 1 2 4. Asthma
0 1 2 5. Behaves like opposite sex
0 1 2 6. Bowel movements outside toilet
0 1 2 7. Bragging, boasting
0 1 2 8. Can't concentrate, can't pay attention for long
0 1 2 9. Can't get his/her mind off certain thoughts; obsessions (describe): ____________
0 1 2 10. Can't sit still, restless, or hyperactive
0 1 2 11. Clings to adults or too dependent
0 1 2 12. Complains of loneliness
0 1 2 13. Confused or seems to be in a fog
0 1 2 14. Cries a lot
0 1 2 15. Cruel to animals
0 1 2 16. Cruelty, bullying, or meanness to others
0 1 2 17. Daydreams or gets lost in his/her thoughts
0 1 2 18. Deliberately harms self or attempts suicide
0 1 2 19. Demands a lot of attention
0 1 2 20. Destroys his/her own things
0 1 2 21. Destroys things belonging to his/her family or others
0 1 2 22. Disobedient at home
0 1 2 23. Disobedient at school
0 1 2 24. Doesn't eat well
0 1 2 25. Doesn't get along with other kids
0 1 2 26. Doesn't seem to feel guilty after misbehaving
0 1 2 27. Easily jealous
0 1 2 28. Eats or drinks things that are not food—**don't** include sweets (describe): ____________

(*continued*)

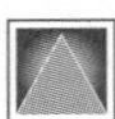

Table 7.9–12 (*continued*)

0 1 2 29. Fears certain animals, situations, or places, other than school (describe): ____________

0 1 2 30. Fears going to school

0 1 2 31. Fears he/she might think or do something bad

0 1 2 32. Feels he/she has to be perfect

0 1 2 33. Feels or complains that no one loves him/her

0 1 2 34. Feels others are out to get him/her

0 1 2 35. Feels worthless or inferior

0 1 2 36. Gets hurt a lot, accident-prone

0 1 2 37. Gets in many fights

0 1 2 38. Gets teased a lot

0 1 2 39. Hangs around with others who get in trouble

0 1 2 40. Hears sounds or voices that aren't there (describe): ____________

0 1 2 41. Impulsive or acts without thinking

0 1 2 42. Would rather be alone than with others

0 1 2 43. Lying or cheating

0 1 2 44. Bites fingernails

0 1 2 45. Nervous, high-strung, or tense

0 1 2 46. Nervous movements or twitching (describe): ____________

0 1 2 47. Nightmares

0 1 2 48. Not liked by other kids

0 1 2 49. Constipated, doesn't move bowels

0 1 2 50. Too fearful or anxious

0 1 2 51. Feels dizzy

0 1 2 52. Feels too guilty

0 1 2 53. Overeating

0 1 2 54. Overtired

0 1 2 55. Overweight

0 1 2 56. Physical problems **without known medical cause:**

0 1 2 a. Aches or pains (**not** stomach or headaches)

0 1 2 b. Headaches

0 1 2 c. Nausea, feels sick

0 1 2 d. Problems with eyes (**not** if corrected by glasses) (describe): ____________

0 1 2 e. Rashes or other skin problems

0 1 2 f. Stomachaches or cramps

0 1 2 g. Vomiting, throwing up

0 1 2 h. Other (describe): ____________

0 1 2 57. Physically attacks people

0 1 2 58. Picks nose, skin, or other parts of body (describe): ____________

0 1 2 59. Plays with own sex parts in public

0 1 2 60. Plays with own sex parts too much

0 1 2 61. Poor school work

0 1 2 62. Poorly coordinated or clumsy

0 1 2 63. Prefers being with older kids

0 1 2 64. Prefers being with younger kids

0 1 2 65. Refuses to talk

0 1 2 66. Repeats certain acts over and over; compulsions (describe): ____________

0 1 2 67. Runs away from home

0 1 2 68. Screams a lot

0 1 2 69. Secretive, keeps things to self

0 1 2 70. Sees things that aren't there (describe): ____________

0 1 2 71. Self-conscious or easily embarrassed

0 1 2 72. Sets fires

0 1 2 73. Sexual problems (describe): ____________

0 1 2 74. Showing off or clowning

0 1 2 75. Shy or timid

0 1 2 76. Sleeps less than most kids

0 1 2 77. Sleeps more than most kids during day and/or night (describe): ____________

0 1 2 78. Smears or plays with bowel movements

0 1 2 79. Speech problem (describe): ____________

0 1 2 80. Stares blankly

0 1 2 81. Steals at home

0 1 2 82. Steals outside the home

0 1 2 83. Stores up things he/she doesn't need (describe): ____________

0 1 2 84. Strange behavior (describe): ____________

0 1 2 85. Strange ideas (describe): ____________

0 1 2 86. Stubborn, sullen, or irritable

0 1 2 87. Sudden changes in mood or feelings

0 1 2 88. Sulks a lot

0 1 2 89. Suspicious

0 1 2 90. Swearing or obscene language

0 1 2 91. Talks about killing self

0 1 2 92. Talks or walks in sleep (describe): ____________

0 1 2 93. Talks too much

0 1 2 94. Teases a lot

0 1 2 95. Temper tantrums or hot temper

0 1 2 96. Thinks about sex too much

0 1 2 97. Threatens people

0 1 2 98. Thumb-sucking

0 1 2 99. Too concerned with neatness or cleanliness

0 1 2 100. Trouble sleeping (describe): ____________

0 1 2 101. Truancy, skips school

0 1 2 102. Underactive, slow moving, or lacks energy

0 1 2 103. Unhappy, sad, or depressed

0 1 2 104. Unusually loud

0 1 2 105. Uses alcohol or drugs for nonmedical purposes (describe): ____________

(*continued*)

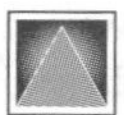

Table 7.9–12 (*continued*)

0 1 2	106. Vandalism	**0 1 2**	111. Withdrawn, doesn't get involved with others
0 1 2	107. Wets self during the day	**0 1 2**	112. Worries
0 1 2	108. Wets the bed	**0 1 2**	113. Please write in any problems your child has that were not listed above:
0 1 2	109. Whining		
0 1 2	110. Wishes to be of opposite sex	**0 1 2**	______________________
		0 1 2	______________________
		0 1 2	______________________
PLEASE BE SURE YOU HAVE ANSWERED ALL ITEMS.		**UNDERLINE ANY YOU ARE CONCERNED ABOUT**	

From Achenbach TM, University of Vermont, 1 S. Prospect St., Burlington, VT 05401. © by T. M. Achenbach, with permission.

SUGGESTED CROSS-REFERENCES

Section 5.1 discusses epidemiology. Section 5.3 covers mental health services research. Section 7.1 discusses the psychiatric interview, history, and mental status examination. The neuropsychology and intellectual assessment of adults is covered in Section 7.5; Sections 7.6 and 7.7 discuss the personality assessment of adults and children and the neuropsychological assessment of children, respectively. Section 9.1 discusses the classification of mental disorders. See also chapters describing specific diagnostic areas.

REFERENCES

*American Psychiatric Association. *Handbook of Psychiatric Measures*. Washington, DC: American Psychiatric Press; 2000.

Buka SL, Monuteaux M, Earls F. Epidemiology of childhood psychiatric disorders. In: Tsuang MT, Tohen M, eds. *Textbook in Psychiatric Epidemiology*. 2nd ed. New York: Wiley; 2002.

*Burt T, Sederer L, Isgak WW, eds. *Outcome Measurement in Psychiatry, A Critical Review*. Washington, DC: American Psychiatric Press; 2002.

Carmines E, Zeller R. *Reliability and Validity Assessment*. Beverly Hills: Sage Publications #17; 1979.

Hulley SB, Cummings SR. Planning the measurements: precision and accuracy. In: Hulley SB, Cummings SR, eds. *Designing Clinical Research: An Epidemiologic Approach*. Baltimore: Williams and Wilkins; 1987.

Kendler KS: Toward a scientific psychiatric nosology: strengths and limitations. *Arch Gen Psychiatry*. 1990;47:969.

Kessler RC: The categorical versus dimensional assessment controversy in the sociology of mental illness. *J Health Soc Behav*. 2002;43:171.

McDowell I, Newell C. *Measuring Health: A Guide to Rating Scales and Questionnaires*. London: Oxford University Press; 1996.

*Murphy J. Diagnostic schedules and rating scales in adult psychiatry. In: Tsuang MT, Tohen M, eds. *Textbook in Psychiatric Epidemiology*. 2nd ed. New York: Wiley; 1995.

Murphy JM, Berwick DM, Weinstein MC, Borus JF, Budman SH, Klerman GL: Performance of screening and diagnostic tests: application of receiver operating characteristic (ROC) analysis. *Arch Gen Psychiatry*. 1987;44:550.

Myers K, Winters NC: Ten-year review of rating scales. I: overview of scale functioning, psychometric properties, and selection. *J Am Acad Child Adolesc Psychiatry*. 2002;41:114–122.

*Regier DA, Kaelber CT, Rae DS, Farmer ME, Knauper B, Kessler RC, Norquist GS: Limitations of diagnostic criteria and assessment instruments for mental disorders: implications for research and policy. *Arch Gen Psychiatry*. 1998;55:109.

*Robins E, Guze SB: Establishment of diagnostic validity in psychiatric illness: its application to schizophrenia. *Am J Psychiatry*. 1990;126:983.

Robins L: Epidemiology: reflections on testing the validity of psychiatric interviews. *Arch Gen Psychiatry*. 1985;42:918.

Schutte NS, Malouff JM. *Sourcebook of Adult Assessment Strategies*. New York: Plenum Press; 1995.

Shrout PE, Spitzer RL, Fleiss JL: Quantification of agreement in psychiatric diagnosis revisited. *Arch Gen Psychiatry*. 1998;744:172.

Spitzer RL: Psychiatric diagnosis: are clinicians still necessary? *Compr Psychiatry*. 1983;24:399.

Spitzer RL, Fleiss JL: A re-analysis of the reliability of psychiatric diagnosis. *Br J Psychiatry*. 1974;125:341.

Sudman S, Bradburn NM, Schwarz N. *Thinking About Answers: The Application of Cognitive Processes to Survey Methodology*. San Francisco: Jossey-Bass; 1996.

Winokur G, Zimmerman M, Cadoret R: 'Cause the Bible tells me so. *Arch Gen Psychiatry*. 1988;45:683.

Zarin DA, Earls F: Diagnostic decision making in psychiatry. *Am J Psychiatry*. 1993;150:197.

▲ 7.10 Telemedicine, Telepsychiatry, and Online Therapy

ZEBULON TAINTOR, M.D.

This chapter describes the use of electronic media in therapy. Words and images are captured and available for both the patient and therapist to examine. Electronic media can be used to provide feedback and communication, sometimes over distance and time, or to present a different reality. Use of electronic media is not a new form of therapy but a different way of carrying out a variety of therapies, some of which lend themselves better to the use of electronic media.

DEFINITIONS

The prefix *tele-*, having to do with transmission over distances, was used to form the word *telegraph*, an early form of e-mail involving transmission of text, *telephone*, which involves the transmission of sounds over distance, and *television*, the transmission of images, usually with sound. *Telemedicine* is the practice of medicine using electronic transmission of images, and *telepsychiatry* is the practice of the medical specialty of psychiatry using electronic transmission of images. The prefix *radio-* is used for radiation, with *wireless* used for transmission of radio waves. *Video*, a potentially more accurate prefix, is used in *videotherapy* to indicate the use of electronic images without transmission to distant points. *E-therapy* is therapy via electronic communication, which, at present, means exchanging text messages, although images can be added with increasing ease. *Online* is the subset of e-therapy done in real time, in which the pauses between messages can be as brief as those between two people in the same room. *Unmet e-therapy* is e-therapy in which the client and therapist have not met. There is no definition of treatment otherwise, and Web sites offering unmet e-therapy uniformly state, probably to reduce malpractice liability, that counseling, rather than therapy, is what is being offered. A *webcam* is a camera used in conjunction with a personal computer for video communication via the Internet.

HISTORY

Therapeutic uses of electronic media have evolved along with the media themselves and the uses of their predecessors.

Letters An e-mail basically is a letter, the most ancient regular form of communication across distance. Various published correspondences often include the writers' agreement that the letters were more important than actual meetings. Numerous examples of correspondences show the process of psychotherapy in traditional letter writing. Sigmund Freud developed several therapeutic correspondences. The first e-mail was the telegraph, first used between cities in 1844. Some case reports mention exchanges of telegrams between patients and therapists, although lack of confidentiality; limitations of word numbers, cost, and so forth; and the development of the telephone cut short the use of telegraphs for psychotherapy. Telegraphic styles survive today in the form of instant messaging.

Telephone Calls Telephone calls have been used to help people feel better since the invention of the telephone in 1885. Telephone calls are immediate and convey nonverbal data through pauses, tone of voice, inflections, and so forth. Usually, costs are computed by time and distance, so telephone calls tend to be brief. However, therapists have routinely scheduled long sessions with patients when one or the other is traveling. Unless recorded, telephone calls are not retrievable, which may or may not be an advantage. Telephone calls need not be part of a patient's chart.

Crisis hotlines are widely used in emergencies and are accepted as one part of the range of patient care services. Medical curricula typically do not include instruction in how to use telephones in patient care, an issue receiving belated attention. There is extensive experience with telephone therapy in the form of suicide prevention centers and other hotlines. Studies showed that suicide prevention centers did not reduce suicide rates in the cities they served, a phenomenon attributed to the likelihood that more seriously suicidal patients did not call before attempting to kill themselves. Generally, callers used hotlines once or twice, from which they received support and were urged to seek out services where they were seen in person and helped. Some suicidal patients called crisis hotlines and visited emergency departments for months or years before getting involved in more regular treatment, and others did not progress beyond use of crisis hotlines. Some proponents of e-therapy argue from the hotline experience that some people in need of therapy will get involved via the Internet because of its convenience and anonymity.

Use of the telephone to transmit images became widely available through facsimile machines, which have been used in published correspondences, but minimally in therapy. Although videophones have been available for decades to transmit moving images in real time, they have yet to become popular, and they serve as an example of a choice not to show one's image spontaneously.

Tape Recording Tape recording of psychotherapy sessions has been used by both patients and physicians since audiotape became available in the 1940s, especially with the development of audiocassettes that allow for playback in automobiles and elsewhere, and lend themselves to easy storage and retrieval.

Television Although television was invented before World War II, its use in therapy did not occur until the arrival of recording media, specifically videotape. Milton Berger demonstrated the use of videotaped group therapy and other psychotherapy sessions to help patients see themselves as others saw them, especially how a patient's body language conveyed unintended messages.

Telemedicine The first recorded use of telepsychiatry was in 1957. Decreasing equipment and transmission (typically by dedicated telephone lines) costs and improved image quality have resulted in more widespread use of telemedicine for particular populations. Telepsychiatry has benefitted from the perception that it is part of telemedicine. Data reduction is less of an issue for other specialties, such as radiology, pathology, and, to a lesser extent, dermatology. A patient visiting a specialist expects the specialist to concentrate on the specialty area of interest, with the general reassurance that the patient has a primary care physician who has performed a comprehensive physical examination. The primary, and essentially the only reimbursable, use of telemedicine is for consultation. The rationale for consultation by television is that something is better than nothing. Medical specialists are unavailable in many areas and in various locations, such as prisons. Second opinions are recognized as contributing to high-quality care and lowering medical costs.

Reimbursement Reimbursement for consultation was provided in Montana and presently is provided by 180 insurance plans and Medicaid in 19 states, with three more states conducting pilot projects. Telemedicine reimbursement for health professions–shortage areas began in 1999 via Medicare. Although there were optimistic predictions of rapid growth, total reimbursements from Medicare totaled only $20,000 in the first 2 years. Coverage was expanded via the Telehealth Improvement and Modernization Act of 2002, for which regulations appeared in 2002. Changes included the requirement that "the physician or provider" at a distant site be paid the same as if the services were provided face-to-face, elimination of fee-sharing requirements, expansion of eligible locations to any county not part of a standard metropolitan statistical area, and expansion of the number of CPT (Current Procedural Terminology) codes that are eligible for Medicare reimbursement. The requirement that the consultation be conducted in real time with interaction between patient and physician was suspended for Alaska and Hawaii, where storage of data for later forwarding is now allowed.

Government Support Government support has been evident nationally through the establishment of the Office of Telehealth in the Department of Health and Human Services and in various laws on rural health care. The World Health Organization (WHO) regularly promotes telemedicine through publications and regional priorities.

Licensure Issues Licensure issues do not arise when the physician and patient are in the same states, as no special training, credentialing, or privileging is required for telemedicine. When the patient and physician are in different states, it is understood that the physician must have a license for the state in which the patient is located. The Federation of State Medical Boards developed a model licensing act in 1996 to ensure that a physician fully licensed in one state could obtain a special license for the states in which patients to be seen in telemedicine encounters would be located. Nine states have authorized such a telemedicine license. Ohio decided on requirements that generally are the same as for a full license. California appears not to be willing to implement a registration system authorized by the legislature.

Internet The Internet was established in 1969 at the University of Southern California as a way of linking computers for national defense uses, with e-mail and civilian use appearing after 1973. Use of e-mail for therapy was documented in the 1980s, and simulated patients were developed (e.g., Eliza and Parry) to demonstrate typical psychopathology to those who signed on to interact with them.

The Internet has five major uses that affect psychiatrists and their patients: (1) a source of information on disease, diagnosis, treatments, and therapists; (2) support and self-help groups (moderated or not); (3) advice, diagnosis, and counseling in situations in which the person being helped has not met the helper, except over the Internet; (4) prescription drug sales; and (5) the opportunity for people to do things that would tend to bring them to the attention of a psychiatrist even if they did not happen to use the Internet (e.g., sex, gambling).

Information The Internet has become a major source of data, presently with approximately 20,000 Web sites offering pages of information on many topics, including health care, psychiatric treatments, and so forth. Web searches yield more pages than can be searched effectively—for example, more than 700,000 Web pages mention diabetes. Although many health information firms attracted investment capital and had large valuations based on share price, many have been sold or are now worth relatively little. Many practitioner-operated Web sites discuss philosophical and practical aspects of treatment and serve as gateways for further contact. Many commercially operated Web sites have been found, frequently in violation of their own privacy policies, to track those who visit the site for follow-up marketing. Enforcement of sanctions against many objectionable uses of the Internet has been problematic, both because of complex technical issues, such as accessing off-shore sites, and because of an apparent lack of will among the enforcers. For example, online gambling is illegal in all states in the United States, but revenues from Americans account for 60 percent of all online gambling revenues globally.

Support and Self-Help Groups Web sites and organizations offer opportunities for people with similar interests to find one another and to begin relationships. The Internet has been very useful as a matchmaker, with millions of people subscribing to dating services. People meet on the Internet, fall in love, and have happy marriages. Occasionally, there is a report of a couple that met to marry only to discover they had not verified crucial details, such as each other's sex. Voluntary associations that develop through chat groups and self-help groups are not subject to regulation and are not considered to be medical practice. Dozens, if not hundreds, of groups—for battered spouses, breast cancer survivors, and so forth—have evolved online and through e-mail. Some groups are hybrid and meet occasionally in person and keep in touch frequently, sometimes daily, by e-mail. If a professional agrees to be "present" online (if the group is conducted in real time) or to review and comment on e-mails, then the group is called a *moderated support group*. Sometimes professional moderation is achieved through a bulletin board format, with professional comments on messages posted by users or messages sent to the professional for posting. Many of these groups are sponsored by health Web sites or commercial firms that make products that members of the group can use. Several hundred mental health professionals moderate such groups, carefully wording terms and conditions of participation to reduce potential liability. Members can group themselves by diagnosis—a recent search yielded dozens of schizophrenia support groups (both moderated and unmoderated)—or by other criteria.

Self-help groups are unmoderated support groups that emphasize traditional self-help mechanisms such as following steps to wellness. These groups offer low-cost, usually available (members often agree to have instant messaging, so anyone online can be reached) support. E-mail technology lends itself to mailing lists, since addressees can be added to a message with ease and without costs, and e-mail programs typically include a "reply to all" option that makes it easy to respond to everyone who received the original message. Variations in format allow for user-friendly "chat rooms," where an e-mail user can sign in and participate in a conversation with others who have signed in for that particular session, which typically lasts minutes or hours, although asynchronous communication could extend it to days or weeks.

E-mail has been increasingly accepted in general medicine, especially for anything a patient may have to write down if told on the telephone, such as test results, written instructions, directions, or phone numbers. Cost per communication is insignificant, usually a monthly charge for Internet usage that provides unlimited e-mail. E-mail use has skyrocketed in this pricing structure, which does not depend on the number of units or distance each unit travels. Increased use has been recommended by the Institute of Medicine's report, "Crossing the Quality Chasm." E-mail messages often are linked to Web sites for patient education.

Advice, Diagnosis, and Therapy (Counseling) in Situations in which the Patient Has Only Met the Helper over the Internet It is estimated that there are approximately 800 mental health professionals (mostly social workers, psychologists, and counselors) who are willing to pick up advice seekers online and work with them only by e-mail. These professionals justify this practice on the grounds that those advice seekers would not otherwise come for therapy for various reasons: geographic isolation, loss of privacy, disability, and so forth. Fortified by an infusion of venture capital, online therapy peaked in popularity in 1997 through 2000, with several well-funded Web sites, numerous articles in the popular press, and presentations at scientific meetings. By 2001, some disillusion was evident, and commercial Web sites largely had disappeared. However, the number of practitioners has increased slightly, with practitioners operating their own inexpensive Web sites. There is scholarly activity in journals and an organization, the International Society for Mental Health Online, but there were few scientific meeting presentations in 2002, suggesting a separation of online therapists from the mainstream of their professions.

The Clinical Social Work Federation opposed online therapy in which the patient and clinician have not met in 2001, citing concerns about efficacy, liability, and jurisdiction. The Federation's press release says, in part,

> This area is totally unregulated and potentially very dangerous for clients and therapists alike. . . This new, very powerful medium blurs all the usual boundaries. Most organizations believe that it cannot or should not be evaluated by well-accepted professional standards. That just is not the case. The standards developed by the U.S. Department of Health and Human Services and Coordinated by the Office for the Advancement of Telehealth, are used by the federal government to assess federal policy on an ongoing basis. . . We have yet to see the first law suits in this area, but we know they're coming. Our concern with establishing a position on the delivery of online therapy services is in absolute alignment with the mission of state licensing boards. . . the protection of the consumer. The standards used to analyze the growing area of text-based counseling include principles related to confidentiality, informed consent, quality of treatment, competence

> of the therapist, and basic ethical and professional requirements. These standards cannot be ensured when the client and therapist know each other only from a text on a screen. Assessment is the first phase of psychotherapy and frequently significant information about the client is based on nonverbal cues. Psychotherapy has at its heart a profoundly human connection, a connection that is, in itself, the major vehicle for change. Healing and restoration occur when the therapist and the client together find the bridge leading back, and forward at the same time, to the true self. Alienation from others and the self will not be healed through a virtual connection in cyberspace, a connection that is fraught with risks and hazards for both clients and clinicians.

As this activity is now defined as not being acceptable in the practice of medicine, it is likely that other professions will follow.

In October 2002, state medical licensing boards began to implement a consensus statement ("Model Guidelines for the Appropriate Use of the Internet in Medical Practice") adopted by the Federation of State Medical Boards earlier in the year. It said, in part, "Treatment and consultation recommendations made in an online setting, including issuing a prescription via electronic means, will be held to the same standards of appropriate practice as those in traditional (face-to-face) settings. Treatment, including issuing a prescription, based solely on an online questionnaire or consultation does not constitute an acceptable standard of care." Actions included Illinois closing down the Web site http://www.MyDoc.com, an online consultation service that offered assessment and prescriptions for "minor illnesses." Online pharmacies banded together to form the Council for Responsible Telemedicine to prevent the online filling of prescriptions for patients who had not been seen by the prescribing physician, and several pharmacies had to pay substantial fines. Thus, the uses of the Internet have been redefined to emphasize that there is no unlicensed practice of medicine. The guidelines recommend use of electronic media "to supplement and enhance" the physician–patient relationship. MyDoc.com's guidelines now clearly state that the online service "is not meant to substitute for establishing a regular physician-patient relationship with a physician in your community."

Thus far, liability issues have not been serious, although the lawsuits that have been filed have been settled rather than decided. Many traditional malpractice carriers will not cover online therapy. Although a few new insurance companies have appeared to fill the gap, a consortium of national medical societies and malpractice carriers (the eRisk Working Group for Healthcare), with the participation of state medical licensing boards, has developed guidelines to limit the liability risks of communicating via e-mail. The guidelines, announced in December 2002, advise that physicians should conduct e-mail consultations only if they have previously established a relationship with a patient (see http://www.medem.com). Suggested principles for providing services online can be found at www.dr-bob.org/psi/suggestions.current.html. The evolving licensing situation may be another deterrent, as well as the positions taken by professional associations, such as the Clinical Social Work Federation's opposition in 2001 to e-therapy in which the patient and clinician have not met.

Prescription Drug Sales The sale of medications over the Internet is relevant to the use of electronic media in psychiatry only in that it is has been a confidentiality concern and an area of increasing regulation. In 2002, patients who previously had fluoxetine (Prozac) prescriptions received unwanted samples of a longer-acting Prozac preparation, with letters mentioning the patients' previous treatment for depression. Online pharmacies were subject to large fines in 2002 for dispensing medications without prescriptions from physicians licensed to practice in the states in which the patients lived.

Pathological Internet Use Approximately 30 percent of those "addicted" to the Internet report using the Internet to escape negative feelings. It is possible to lose real money on the Internet by gambling constantly, without ever being seen. Potential sexual partners have many venues in which they can meet and provide mutual gratification—via e-mail, telephone, or webcams, or by setting up face-to-face meetings. Online connections can take a malignant turn when sexual predators use false identities to deceive victims and exploit and harm the victim when they meet in person. These contacts are unregulated and difficult to detect except by monitoring and checking the computers used.

The combination of anonymity, convenience, and escape (ACE model) promotes the Internet as a focus of psychopathology. "Internet addiction" is mentioned on 20,000 Web pages, with those at risk suffering from depression, bipolar disorder, anxiety, low self-esteem, or being addicted to substances, at least previously. Surveys on Internet users show that 4 to 10 percent of users meet criteria for Internet addiction, defined as having at least five of the following indicators: preoccupation with the Internet; increasing amount of time spent online; failure to cut back use with concomitant restlessness, moodiness, or depression; staying online longer than originally intended; running the risk of losing a job, relationship, or other opportunity because of Internet use; lying to conceal the extent of Internet use; or using the Internet to escape negative feelings. Subgroups of Internet addiction include cybersex addiction (viewing pornography), cyber-relational addiction (online relationships become more important than those in one's physical world), gaming addiction (e.g., gambling, stock trading, shopping), and information overload. Some Web pages offer a chance to evaluate one's Internet use to determine whether it is possibly pathological and offer both education and online counseling, with some Web pages urging face-to-face counseling as a way of becoming less involved with the Internet. A rough idea of the ratio of what is offered to possible sources of help online can be obtained by comparing the number of sites mentioning "cybersex" (approximately 862,000) to those mentioning "cybersex addiction" (approximately 1,600), coupled with universal agreement that more money is made on sex via the Internet than through the sale of anything else. Combinations abound, as evidenced by the 19,900 Web sites mentioning both "cybersex" and "casino."

Virtual Reality Development of large-scale, increasingly cheap computing power enables storage of sounds and images in digital form, leading to compact discs and other formats for music storage and digital video discs (DVDs) for storing movies and television programs. Digital cameras recently have surpassed film in ability to capture data in greater detail and higher image resolution. Construction of images that never existed in reality has become widespread in computer games, movies, and on personal computers. Playback equipment in helmets provides for a sense of total immersion with 360-degree sound and complete occupation of the visual fields. The first use of virtual reality for a psychiatric condition was in 1992 for fear of flying, then agoraphobia, acrophobia, claustrophobia, social phobia, anxiety related to public speaking, and other situations involving anxiety.

THEORETICAL ISSUES

Theoretical issues relate to (1) electronic media per se, (2) selection of data to be recorded, (3) identity and the Internet, and (4) applicability of electronic media to particular diagnoses and treatments.

Electronic Media Although almost everyone has a television set, use of electronic media, especially e-mail and exploration of the Internet, varies widely according to personal reactions to electronic media and preferences for other types of interactions. Some people prefer to work with computers and tend to disclose more facts to impersonal electronic media than they do to interviewers with whom they are face to face. Several dozen studies show that patients give more detailed and accurate substance abuse histories in computer interviews than they do to live interviewers, although patients' feelings about the substances used are not conveyed well. However, many of these studies were conducted before privacy concerns became an issue and computers were perceived as feeding into large databases. On the other hand, many people are put off by junk e-mail, advertising, and an increased centralization of infrequently encountered content.

Safeguards Although the original intent of the Health Insurance Portability and Accountability Act (HIPAA) was to cover electronic records (with some debate about whether e-mails would necessarily be part of the record) only, there were years of delay and protests from many quarters. Gradually, the regulations came to embody the concept of protected health information, which is to be safeguarded in whatever form or location it may be in. Thus, the standards apply to paper and electronic records, despite some initial confusion as to whether they applied only to records involving protected health information that were transmitted electronically. The safeguards to be applied to a record that exists only on paper and is confined to a secure office are simple and likely to be as effective as the safeguarding of any valued object. Use of electronic media and transmission increases the risk because protected health information can be retrieved from multiple locations, usually having been stored along the way. There are two types of risks: (1) organizations that have a commercial interest in patient data and (2) individuals who want data on a particular patient. Organizations with commercial interests typically obtain protected health information by purchasing databases of insurance billings, prescriptions, and so forth. Sales of medical information before HIPAA reached $16 billion per year. Authorities differ on the extent to which they think the regulations will inhibit this traffic, with some maintaining that significant loopholes exist. Aspects of the regulations doubtlessly will be tested in court. Meanwhile, the regulations carry a substantial documentation burden, both for an overall plan for safeguarding protected health information and for documenting informed consent, with additional requirements that each individual practice document how it will safeguard protected health information in electronic media. The more secondary sources of protected health information that exist, the more difficult it is to determine where confidentiality may have been lost. Such secondary sources can be useful to individuals seeking data on a particular patient. Such people may be, for example, criminals or unethical private investigators. These individuals hack into databases and retrieve protected health information that might bear on competence, custody, divorce, and other adversarial situations. They, rather than organizations, may be interested in the content of specific e-mails. In the past, members of this group have broken into offices to get individual patient records. Computer break-ins can be easier, depending on the relative skills of the hacker versus the burglar, and may leave no trace. Although current guidelines for transmission and storage of protected health information recommend password protection, encryption, and other security measures, it would be unwise to expect that such safeguards would prevail against a specific, determined, individual attack. Penalties for criminal acts related to medical records have existed for years.

Selection of Data to be Recorded Any capture of data involves not capturing other data, and no use of electronic media is ever the same as being in the same room with another person. Some data will be lost, even with the capacity to, for example, magnify images and move cameras around. In some ways, this is desirable, as one's attention inevitably focuses on one thing or another. However, some recording setups do not allow for operator choices and some choices may miss the key points. E-therapy captures only words without tone of voice, inflections, and the social cues voices carry. Telephones do not capture facial expressions. Telepsychiatry may focus on the smiling face of an apparently open, cooperative person while missing the squared-off shoulders and rigid posture of controlled hostility. Use of multiple cameras and observers may increase data input, but increased equipment expense and observer time still do not close the gap between being there and dealing with the recorded reality. No one claims that all data can be captured—rather, the decision to use electronic media depends on whether the advantages of such use outweigh the disadvantages of data reduction.

Identity and the Internet Certain people believe that their real identity is the one they present on the Internet and that the identity they present in live social situations is false. Although numerous studies have shown that patients entering treatment tended to be more accurate when filling out questionnaires on a computer than in person, because they perceive the computer to be nonjudgmental, motivation is key—recent studies show that 25 to 40 percent of chat group members may be lying. Opportunities for choosing false, misleading, or incomplete identities abound. Sometimes choosing a false identity is done maliciously for exploitation. Sexual predators use the Internet, often with disastrous results when face-to-face meetings turn out to cause harm. Couples have been known to meet on the Internet, fall in love, and arrange to marry, only to discover they had not verified one another's sex. The movie *You've Got Mail* showed Tom Hanks' character, a cutthroat businessman, able to express kinder, nobler feelings over e-mail than he could in person. However, studies on e-mail show that feelings are more likely to be disinhibited, angry ("flaming"), and paranoid—phenomena thought to be associated with e-mail's ease of response and lack of social cues that more data input would provide.

Virtual reality therapy practitioners note that each person brings his or her own background into a virtual reality experience. Practitioners describe a "virtual presence" that increases as patients spend more time in the virtual environment. Doing so involves giving up some of the sense of presence in the real world. Although, initially, virtual reality therapy was patterned after systematic desensitization as practiced without electronic assistance, some of its practitioners now speculate that it is, in fact, oriented more toward neurophysiological information processing theory. Patients in virtual reality therapy typically would not communicate back to their therapists in the physical world, but, instead, seemed to be reliving their previous anxiety-provoking experiences. Other therapists point to the flight simulator analogy as one in which the evaluation instrument is also the means of remedying the skill deficits it elicits.

Adding Images and Other Data to E-mail The current line between e-mail alone as not acceptable medical practice and telemedicine as licensable and reimbursable probably will be resolved as images are added to e-mails. Increasing use of webcams has resulted in images, voices, and other data being transmissible. Webcams also mean that telemedicine will pass from the control of the telemedicine studio at the referring site to the patient's desktop computer.

TECHNIQUES

Because the use of electronic media is not a therapy per se as much as electronic media is applied to the process of other therapy, techniques vary according to use. However, there are some general considerations.

E-mail Even with encryption, e-mail offers ease of composition by typing or dictating onto a screen, the capability to edit on screen, speed of delivery, ease of retrieval, legibility, ease of response, and storage. Retrieval can be so quick as to allow a conversation in real time, or at one's leisure, which means that the recipient can be in a state of mind favorable for communication.

Recording Techniques All use of electronic media is a production of some sort, requiring attention to whatever is chosen for recording. Issues in microphone placement, lighting, and other production values often are neglected and contribute to fewer data being captured.

Storage Data storage is a function of cost and convenience. E-mail tends to be stored wherever it goes, requiring active steps to limit storage. E-mail messages between doctor and patient are now regarded as part of the patient's record and should be stored with it. Generally, the lower the cost of storing e-mail, the greater the convenience, but with less security. Storage of telemedicine sessions typically is local, using videotape or DVDs.

Transmission Similar considerations apply to transmission of data in that low-cost applications are less secure but more convenient. Wireless transmission is particularly insecure. Data in digital format get stored in ways that promote both encryption and retrieval. Typically, for example, digital data are transmitted through Internet servers in bursts or batches that are stored as they pass through servers. Analog data are not stored as they are transmitted, typically on telephone lines, sometimes by satellite. Analog data can be recorded only in analog terms. Organizations typically are not interested in analog data. These considerations favor telemedicine over e-therapy.

Virtual Reality A person's experience of a situation in a virtual environment tends to be the same as a similar real-world situation. It is possible to add and subtract elements of the virtual environment to determine what specifically causes the anxiety a patient feels. Generally, the patient is sitting rather than standing, even if the patient is standing in virtual reality, and begins with brief sessions, a narrow field of view, and the ability to see one's physical body partially. As tolerance develops, longer sessions with fuller immersion can be used. Use of 360-degree cameras has led to capturing social situations in which, for example, a patient with social phobia can find himself surrounded by people at a party, one of whom may then speak to him. The program can branch in one of several directions depending on the patient's reply.

CLINICAL ISSUES

Indications Indications for e-mail, telepsychiatry, and virtual reality therapy include symptoms, diagnoses, and defense mechanisms. Although e-mail and telepsychiatry share some of the same indications, the mode of initial interaction may vary. With e-mail, the patient and therapist generally have met on their own, either face to face or via the Internet. Telepsychiatry presently consists mostly of consultations, with referrals having been arranged by someone where the patient is located. Both e-mail and telepsychiatry may be useful as ways overcoming limitations of access, distance, and disability. Both are useful as adjuncts to therapy in situations in which the patient and therapist meet face to face but want more frequent contact. E-mail's format lends itself, for example, to the sort of written daily homework expected in cognitive-behavioral therapy. E-mail may be useful as a way of getting patients into treatment that they otherwise would not seek, but which should then progress to more definite involvement via telepsychiatry or face-to-face contact. As webcams come into wider personal use, some patients will find telepsychiatry more convenient and less expensive than traveling to a therapist's office.

Virtual reality experiments showing efficacy in various forms of situational anxiety are convincing. Most phobias and fear-provoking situations can be simulated in virtual reality therapy. Investigations of virtual reality therapy's usefulness in obsessive-compulsive disorder (OCD), attention-deficit disorder, and posttraumatic stress disorder (PTSD) are under way.

Limitations

E-mail The principal limitations of e-mail are related to the data that are not transmitted or available. There are potential problems with identification of both the patient and the therapist—investigations of therapists offering online services found that many did not give their professional credentials or were incomplete (e.g., an M.S. degree used in a context that implies it is in counseling when it may not be). Similarly, potential clients often give themselves fictional names. Although the use of fictional identities is seen as a way of preserving an anonymity without which help might not be sought, therapy cannot progress far without more disclosure. Not all deception is deliberate, however: As noted above, patients may feel that they have a different identity on the Internet, which may lead them to portray problems consistent with that identity rather than with their real-life identity. Although controlled studies show that patients divulge facts more rapidly and completely to computers, most of the studies were done with substance abusers before the Internet and, with it, the rise of confidentiality concerns. Computer-based assessments have not replaced live interviews because communication of facts still does not convey how a person thinks or feels about those facts. On the other hand, the disinhibition of emotion noted in unstructured e-mails is both an indication for therapy where defenses must be overcome and a limitation if the feeling is impulsive or marginally related to the issues for which therapy is sought. These same limitations apply to support and self-help groups. Therapist limitations must also be noted. Extensive use of e-mail is not recommended for therapists who have not mastered expressive writing, typing, use of computers and the Internet, encryption, security of electronic data, and how to deal with computer glitches. Therapists must be aware of how they may seem online, be able to correct miscommunications in both directions, and be able to shift modalities (e.g., to face-to-face) when indicated.

Virtual Reality The limitation of virtual reality is its limited generalization to real life.

Complications

A person may get very good at e-therapy and working on the Internet without this result generalizing to the physical world. Cyborg theory has been invoked to describe the mechanisms whereby the animal–human boundary blurs, along with the human–computer boundary.

E-mail Online therapists report having to refer patients for face-to-face therapy, but often view this as a desirable progression rather than a complication. Self-help groups can be taken over by chat room addicts. Patients and therapists may present false identities. Predators can pick up vulnerable people online and develop private correspondences with them that lead to disaster.

Telepsychiatry There have been no reports of complications from telepsychiatry. It is possible that complications could develop with data that are not conveyed in the consultation, but these usually are averted by the local team of providers.

Virtual Reality No complications have been reported with virtual reality therapy. It is possible that a patient would continue to have anxiety after treatment, especially if subject to flashbacks.

Contraindications

The use of both e-mail and telepsychiatry are contraindicated in situations in which the patient and psychiatrist can meet face to face, although the patient may continue use of a support or self-help group otherwise. Psychiatrists should always be sensitive to the possibility that virtual reality therapy might be contraindicated for patients with serious medical problems and patients taking medications with major physiological or psychological effects. Flickering images, especially at 8 to 12 Hz, may produce symptoms that range from headache to epileptic seizures, and thus no frame replacement speeds that approach these frequencies should be used.

Case Examples

These pairs of case studies illustrate desirable and undesirable applications of each form of electronic media to therapy.

E-mail

A depressed person searches online for "depression + help," finds and takes a self-assessment scale via e-mail, concludes that face-to-face help is needed, and benefits from treatment.

An apparently anxious person seeking help is actually using the Internet's anonymity, convenience, and possibilities for escape by trying out a new identity. Getting involved with online counseling results in the patient spending more and more time online, resulting in confusion and diminution of real-world relationships.

Telepsychiatry

A patient is referred for a second opinion. The consultant elicits new symptoms, substantiates a different diagnosis, and recommends treatment that proves to be effective.

A well-known psychiatrist performs what he considers to be an excellent interview but misses the fact that the patient has been increasingly resentful about the picture-in-picture showing her. Her gestures to get the local crew to tape paper over her image to cover it are performed off-camera, and she continues to smile while the interviewer suggests that her previous head trauma could benefit from a neurological workup, which would reduce her need for 25 mg of diazepam (Valium) a day, but her shoulders square and her posture conveys belligerence. The interviewer's first clue that the interview has gone badly is her response when asked if she had any questions. She says, "Yeah, what do I do the next time I'm feeling suicidal and don't want to call anyone?"

Virtual Reality

A patient with social phobia is treated in her psychiatrist's office with a virtual reality program that provides a series of social stimuli, adding and subtracting as she copes successfully with each. She realizes she has a particular problem with older men and develops skills in dealing with them.

A similar patient has not been able to accept that virtual reality has anything to do with his problems and instead benefits from medication, the need for which has decreased as he develops new skills in handling real-life challenges.

Goals of Treatment

E-mail The goal of any exchange of e-mails should be to develop, supplement, and enhance a real-world therapeutic relationship. If such a relationship is not possible, e-mail should be used for developing a relationship with appropriate safeguards. E-mail can be included as part of treatments that involve correcting cognitive distortions, reporting events, or providing frequent support.

Telepsychiatry The goal of telepsychiatry is the provision of services that otherwise are not available.

Virtual Reality The goal of virtual reality is desensitization, achieved by replicating anxiety-provoking situations and training for unfamiliar, feared challenges.

ETHICAL ISSUES

Ethical issues pertaining to the use of electronic media in therapy abound. The newness of the medium, regulations, and practice ensure that years will pass before standards are generally accepted and followed. The path will be marked by malpractice and anecdotes from which there will be an attempt to draw lessons.

The ethical issues will also depend on theoretical considerations and practicality of maintaining confidentiality. It is likely that the current trend of improving quality and decreasing price will lead to more widespread use of electronic media.

A therapist who refers patients to an online support group will face an added ethical burden to maintain contact with the group and to have some sense of what is occurring in it, as such groups can change rapidly. Ethical issues surrounding identity and disclosure will persist, as patients will want to know what information about them is stored, where it is stored, and how it can be accessed.

In all cases, the therapist is required to explain the procedure in detail, how data are stored and safeguarded and transmitted, and the limitations and potential complications of the treatment. Informed consent must be obtained. It is wise to record the consent both in writing and electronically.

RESEARCH AND EVALUATION

Use of electronic media has progressed with little research and evaluation.

Video feedback has been shown to be helpful in several studies where it is used in the context of an ongoing face-to-face relationship.

There are no comparisons between online and face-to-face therapy, since it is generally accepted that the former excludes observation of body language, facial expressions, eye movement, tone of voice, and other nonverbal cues. Studies confirm the commonsense view that evaluative feedback (not in therapy) is given more effectively in person than by computer. Anecdotal evidence supports the widespread view that online availability and e-mail contact can be helpful in the time between actual meetings in therapeutic sessions.

Published reports on telemedicine generally are brief, with an emphasis on how to conduct telemedicine and a minimization of any differences between the telemedicine experience and the face-to-face experience. Evaluative data describe satisfied patients and savings on travel time and costs. Although it is understood that some data are excluded, there has been no systematic investigation of how missing data can influence outcome. Despite more than four decades of use, a Cochrane review in 2002 comparing telemedicine with face-to-face patient care found only seven randomized, controlled studies, none involving telepsychiatry. It concluded: "Establishing systems for patient care using telecommunications technologies is feasible, but there is little evidence of clinical benefits."

As with most forms of therapy and new treatments, there have been phases of zealotry, exaggeration of possible benefits, some disillusionment, and loss of interest. Annual meeting programs of the American Psychiatric Association, American Psychological Association, and World Psychiatric Association show decreasing reports on the use of electronic media from a peak in 1999. However, the basic decision to use more telepsychiatry has been adopted by those who pay for public and private care. In addition to reimbursement through Medicare and Medicaid, the Office for the Advancement of Telehealth of the Health Resources and Services Administration (part of the Department of Health and Human Services), among many funding sources, provides grants and contracts and published a directory of supported projects. The WHO promotes telemedicine annually in its regional advisory committee meetings, especially for patients in developing countries. The growth in teleconferencing reflects the evaluation of those who pay for it. Rather than being compared to face-to-face therapy, telepsychiatry should be compared to no or inexpert service.

Virtual reality therapy has been evaluated positively versus standard desensitization for phobias, especially fear of flying, using standard outcome measures. There are no studies demonstrating its superiority, although it is likely that clinicians who invest in the equipment and master the technique eventually will attract patients who have not improved with standard desensitization. A few studies dealing with other diagnoses such as body image distortion and eating disorders showed positive outcomes persisting up to a year after treatment.

SUGGESTED CROSS-REFERENCES

Section 3.1 discusses perception and cognition. Brain models of mind are covered in Section 3.5, and anthropology and cultural psychiatry are discussed in Section 4.1. Psychiatric rating scales are presented in Section 7.9. Substance-related disorders are discussed in Chapter 11. Psychological treatments of anxiety disorders are covered in Section 14.10, and Sections 30.4, 30.6, and 54.4i discuss group psychotherapy, cognitive therapy, and cognitive-behavioral therapy, respectively. Other methods of psychotherapy are presented in Section 30.10. Section 39.1 discusses attention-deficit disorders, and Section 52.4 covers psychiatric rehabilitation.

References

Aas IHM: Changes in the job situation due to telemedicine. *J Telemed Telecare.* 2002;8:41.

Alleman JR: Online counseling: the internet and mental health treatment. *Psychotherapy: Theory/Research/Practice/Training.* 2002;39(2):199.

Amichai-Hamburger Y, Ben-Artzi E: Loneliness and internet use. *Comput Human Behav.* 2003;19:71.

Currell R, Urquhart C, Wainwright P, Lewis R: Telemedicine versus face to face patient care: effects on professional practice and health care outcomes. *Cochrane Database Syst Rev.* 2002;Issue 4.

Darkins AW, Cary MA. *Telemedicine and Telehealth: Principles, Policies, Performance, and Pitfalls.* New York: Springer; 2000.

*Dewan NA, Lorenzi NM, Riley RT, Bhattacharya SB. *Behavioral Healthcare Informatics.* New York: Springer-Verlag; 2002.

Emmelkamp PMG, Krijna M, Hulsboscha AM, de Vriesa S, Schuemieb AS, van der Mastb CAPG: Virtual reality treatment versus exposure in vivo: a comparative evaluation in acrophobia. *Behav Res Ther.* 2002;40:509.

Federation of State Medical Boards of the United States, Inc.: A Model Act to Regulate the Practice of Medicine Across State Lines: An Introduction and Rationale. Adopted April 1996.

Federation of State Medical Boards of the United States, Inc.: Model Guidelines for the Appropriate Use of the Internet in Clinical Practice. Dallas, TX., Adopted April 2002.

Frueh BC, Deitsch SE, Santos AB, Gold PB, Johnson MR, Meisler N, Magruder KM, Ballenger JM: Procedural and methodological issues in telepsychiatry research and program development. *Psychiatr Serv.* 2000;51:1522.

*Gackenbach J. *Psychology and the Internet.* London: Academic Press; 1998.

Hebert BG, Jacquie D, Vorauer JD: Seeing through the screen: is evaluative feedback communicated more effectively in face-to-face or computer-mediated exchanges? *Comput Hum Behav.* 2003;19:25.

Hills P, Argyle M: Uses of the Internet and their relationships with individual differences in personality. *Comput Hum Behav.* 2003;19:59.

*Hsiung RC. *E-Therapy: Case Studies, Guiding Principles, and the Clinical Potential of the Internet.* New York: W.W. Norton; 2002.

Hsiung RC: The best of both worlds: an online self-help group hosted by a mental health professional. *Cyberpsychol Behav.* 2001;3:935.

Hyler SE, Gangure DP: A review of the costs of telepsychiatry. *Psychiatr Serv.* 2003;54:976.

*Maheu M, Whitten P, Allen A. *E-Health, Telehealth, and Telemedicine: A Guide to Start-Up and Success.* San Francisco: Jossey Bass; 2001.

Maltby N, Kirsch I, Mayers M, Allen G: Virtual reality therapy for the treatment of fear of flying: a controlled investigation. *J Consult Clin Psychol.* 2002;70:1112.

May C, Gask L, Atkinson T, Ellis N, Main F, Esmail A: Resisting and promoting new technologies in clinical practice: the case of telemedicine. *Soc Sci Med.* 2001;52:1889.

Monnier J, Knapp RG, Frueh BC: Recent advances in telepsychiatry: an updated review. *Psychiatr Serv.* 2003;54:1604.

Riva G, Bacchettaa M, Baruffia M, Rinaldid S, Molinarib E: Virtual reality based experiential cognitive treatment of anorexia nervosa. *J Behav Ther Exp Psychiatry*. 1999;30:221.

Roine R, Ohinmaa A, Hailey D: Assessing telemedicine: a systematic review of the literature. *CMAJ*. 2001;165:765.

Shaw LH, Gant LM: In defense of the Internet: The relationship between Internet communication and depression, loneliness, self-esteem, and perceived social support. *Cyberpsychol Behav*. 2002;5:157.

Smith SD, Reynolds C: CYBER-Psychotherapy. *Ann Am Psychother Assoc*. 2002;5:20.

*Taintor Z, ed. *Computers and the Psychiatric Patient*. Washington, DC: American Psychiatric Press, Inc.; 1997:87. (Available separately bound and as Section 6 of the *Review of Psychiatry Volume 16*, Washington, DC: American Psychiatric Press, Inc.; 1997.)

Taintor Z: Multimedia reviews: multimedia convergence for clinicians. *Psychiatr Serv*. 2003;54:1584.

Werner A, Anderson LE: Rural telepsychiatry is economically unsupportable: the Concorde crashes in a cornfield. *Psychiatr Serv*. 1998;49:1287.

Yoshino A, Shigemura J, Kobayashi Y, Nomura S, Shishikura K, Den R, Wakisaka H, Kamata S, Ashida H: Telepsychiatry: assessment of televideo psychiatric interview reliability with present- and next-generation Internet infrastructures. *Acta Psychiatr Scand*. 2001;104:223.

Young KS, Rogers RC: The relationship between depression and Internet addiction. *Cyberpsychol Behav*. 1998;1:25.

Zaylor C, Nelson EL, Cook DJ: Clinical outcomes in a prison telepsychiatry clinic. *J Telemed Telecare*. 2001;7:47.

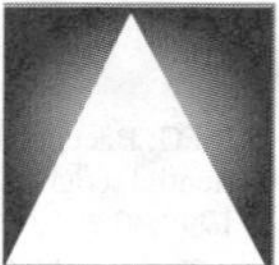

8 Clinical Manifestations of Psychiatric Disorders

JOEL YAGER, M.D., AND MICHAEL J. GITLIN, M.D.

Manifestations of psychiatric disorders express themselves as a variety of alterations, from normal functioning, from subtle to blatant, from intermittent to constant. Some can be recognized by laypeople from a distance. Detecting others may require discerning training and intimate familiarity with an individual over time. Deviations from normal, from mild to severe, may occur in intensity, duration, timing and content of thoughts, emotions, and behaviors and may be highly context dependent. Eliciting the subjective complaints, clinical symptoms, and signs of psychiatric disorders requires history taking and formal examination processes that parallel those of general medicine. Many psychiatric complaints and disorders have to be understood in broad context, requiring a more thorough evaluation and comprehension of the patient's interpersonal world, work role, family life, and culture than is typical in general medical practice. The nature and expression of psychiatric signs and symptoms are profoundly altered by the patient's strengths, coping capacities, psychological defenses, and situational context so that the clinical picture ultimately represents a balance between psychopathology and psychological strengths. The disturbed and disturbing behaviors that observers view as pathological must also be understood as part of the individuals' attempts to cope with the biological, psychological, and environmental challenges they face. When attempts to cope overwhelm individuals' capacities to respond, less adequate, more disorganized, and ineffective thoughts and behaviors emerge, and these comprise the impairments that present in clinical situations.

The most important distinction between typical presentations of medical diseases and those of psychiatric disorders is the greater importance in psychiatric disorders of the patients' sometimes idiosyncratic descriptions of his or her qualitative internal states, subjective experiences that are often difficult to describe in words. Poets and novelists are often more capable than clinicians at characterizing and delineating the precise quality and experience of many psychiatric symptoms. Many patients and clinicians often find it difficult to accurately communicate a fully comprehensible and reliable description of even familiar, somewhat universal feeling states.

A 34-year-old sociology professor was trying to explain the difference in the subjective experience of fatigue from her chronic fatigue syndrome versus the fatigue of her depressive disorder. Whereas she was typically precise and articulate, she stumbled over both translating somatic and psychological feelings into words that would make sense to her doctor. After a few attempts, she gave up, imploring her doctor simply to trust that there was a difference, and she could distinguish the two states.

These subjective descriptions of psychiatric symptoms are inherently less reliable, or at least less objective, than more directly measurable and quantifiable data such as blood pressures, temperatures, and laboratory test results. A great deal of the research in psychiatric diagnosis over the last 25 years has been concerned with increasing the reliability of observer-rated clinical symptom assessments. In many ways, this research has had the desired impact—clinicians and researchers using a variety of structured interviews can come to reasonable agreement on what symptoms patients are experiencing and whether these patients meet criteria for most of the specific psychiatric disorders in the revised fourth edition of the *Diagnostic and Statistical Manual of Mental Disorders* (DSM-IV-TR). However, one of the costs of this increasing reliability has, in many instances, been the narrowing of the field of clinical vision. That is, clinicians who rely predominantly on structured interviews and checklists may become somewhat closed minded and risk ignoring clinical phenomena that are very important but that may not be part of the structured interview framework or mental set. Furthermore, the quest for reliability can lead only so far in describing phenomena for which there are few precise words. An additional related difficulty can be seen in the use of nonclinical research staff who are trained to interview individuals using structured interviews (as in large epidemiological studies). In these instances, the need for interrater reliability is often achieved at the expense of a more nuance-based appreciation of the different meanings of subjective sensations, especially when the interviewer has no clinical experience with which to interpret the subject's descriptions.

Despite these difficulties, a thorough assessment of the clinical history and description of the psychopathology and detailed account of the patient's subjective experiences are important for the following reasons:

1. Significant diagnostic distinctions are made primarily on the basis of the historical information and elicited phenomenology. The more detailed, complete, and correct the diagnosis, the more rational and precise the treatment planning and the more reliable the prognosis. Consider, for example, the importance of accurately distinguishing between neuroleptic-induced akathisia versus anxiety symptoms related to psychotic thinking. Based on which of these diagnoses the clinician selects, the therapeutic strategy might be diametrically opposite.

2. The clinician's capacity to fully hear and communicate a comprehensive understanding of the patient's internal experiences helps diminish the patient's sense of isolation so characteristic of

many of these disorders and fosters the growth of a therapeutic alliance, increasing the likelihood of treatment adherence.

This chapter focuses on (1) predisposing vulnerabilities and stressors in whose context psychiatric signs, symptoms, and other manifestations appear, (2) the nature of psychiatric manifestations, and (3) descriptions of the specific types of disturbances seen in psychiatric disorders.

PREDISPOSING VULNERABILITIES

Genetic and Intrauterine Factors Genetic vulnerabilities play an important role in the expression of many, if not most, psychiatric disorders. Prominent among these are dementias of the Alzheimer's type, schizophrenia, unipolar and bipolar mood disorders, anxiety disorders, alcohol dependence, and some personality traits. For virtually all of these disorders and traits, what is largely unknown at this point is the nature of the inherited vulnerabilities.

Intrauterine processes contribute to many psychiatric disorders. For example, maternal starvation and influenza infections during the second trimester of pregnancy have been implicated in the pathogenesis of schizophrenia. Maternal smoking and low birth weight may be risk factors in the pathogenesis of attention-deficit disorders in children. Maternal alcoholism may lead to fetal alcohol syndrome, a major cause of developmental disability.

Constitutional Factors Considerable research demonstrates that, by birth and shortly afterward, infants differ widely in temperament—in their spontaneous activity levels and thresholds, intensity, and duration of their reactions to external stimuli; the regularity or irregularity of certain biological rhythms such as sleep; tendencies to approach or withdraw from new stimuli; the speed and degree of adaptation; attention span and distractibility; the persistence of behavior; and qualities of mood. Based on such early behaviors, children may be described as having easy or difficult temperaments, quick or slow to warm up. Temperament, however, is not immutable. There are discontinuities over time, and the development of temperament and its lasting impact on personality development is at least, in part, a function of the goodness of fit with a child's family. Nevertheless, these temperamental qualities correlate somewhat with behavioral problems, at least through early childhood.

Aside from temperament, other persistent normal variations in personality development seem to be constitutionally related and may influence subsequent resilience or vulnerability. Traits, such as introversion, extroversion, and neuroticism, appear to be relatively enduring and stable personality dimensions. Other temperamental qualities that endure include novelty seeking, being relatively open to new experiences, and stick-to-it-iveness. Subtypes of intelligence, such as those related to conceptual, mathematical, musical, kinesthetic, and interpersonal abilities, have been postulated as having separate genetic determinants and patterns of development. The type A and B personality patterns, hardy and resilient personalities, high-strung, sensitive, fussy, irritable, and pessimistic characteristics have all been described as generally lifelong qualities that originate in early childhood. Even dimensions of character, referring to concepts about the self in relation to others that develop over time through social learning and maturation of interpersonal behavior, have been shown to have moderate heritability. These include such qualities as self-directedness, the ability to engage cooperatively with others, and the capacity to "transcend" the self by developing a sense of one's place or purpose in the larger social context.

Other characteristics relevant to psychopathology but not diagnostically specific may also be inherited. These include psychosis proneness, cognitive styles (such as obsessionality or detail orientation), and emotional reactivity (which is part of the dimension of neuroticism). The relationship between the inheritance of these traits and the patterns of transmission of specific psychiatric disorders is unknown.

Physiological Stressors Physiological vulnerability may result from long-standing problems or from newly acquired ones. All of the metabolic, toxic, infectious, and other causes of physical illness produce increased vulnerability to psychiatric disturbance. Studies have shown higher use of psychiatric services by those who are physically ill and higher than expected prevalence of physical disease among the psychiatrically impaired.

Some children with prepubertal onset, obsessive-compulsive disorder (OCD), and tic disorders that have an episodic symptom course have been found to have pediatric autoimmune neuropsychiatric disorders associated with streptococcal (group A β-hemolytic streptococcus) infections (PANDAS). Accompanying symptoms during episodes of exacerbation are emotional lability, separation anxiety, nighttime fears and bedtime rituals, cognitive deficits, oppositional behaviors, and motoric hyperactivity. In PANDAS, patients' flare-ups of behavioral problems are commonly associated with documented group A β-hemolytic streptococcus infections or symptoms of pharyngitis and upper respiratory infections.

Human immunodeficiency virus (HIV) infection leading to seropositivity and acquired immune deficiency syndrome (AIDS) vividly illustrates the multiple and complex ways in which stressors can lead to psychiatric disturbances. These patients' psychiatric symptoms may represent organic changes that are the direct effects of the virus on the central nervous system (CNS), producing changes in cognition, personality and mood, expectable psychological adjustment responses of the patients in response to an overwhelming life-threatening disorder, or the emergence of latent or quiescent primary psychiatric problems provoked by the psychological stress of the viral illness. Adding to the complexity, some individuals with cluster B personality traits may engage in excessive risk-taking behaviors, increasing the likelihood of viral exposure; they may then be at higher risk for developing psychiatric symptoms/disorders in response to being HIV positive because of their preexisting cluster B traits.

A 42-year-old physician noticed the onset of decreased stamina, fatigue, disinterest in work, and weight gain without a feeling of increased appetite. Because his wife initially believed he was getting depressed, he consulted a psychiatrist. After the initial interview, the psychiatrist ordered a standard chemistry screening panel that revealed a thyroid-stimulating hormone of 48 mIU/L. He was referred to an endocrinologist and treated for his hypothyroidism, and all of his depressive symptoms disappeared.

Environmental Stressors Complex relationships exist between the occurrence of various life events, particularly threatening, unpredictable, and uncontrollable negative events, and the development of psychiatric symptoms. In general, such undesirable life events predispose individuals to develop psychiatric symptoms, especially if they already have a preexisting psychiatric disorder. After exposure to the same negative stressors, such as a serious accident or act of violence, individuals who previously had anxiety disorders are more prone than those without such histories to subsequently develop symptoms of posttraumatic stress disorder (PTSD). Other factors, such as gender, may also predict risk of developing PTSD, with women more likely to develop the disorder given the same exposure to stress. Although individual responses vary widely, truly catastrophic events, such as incarceration in a concentration camp, cause enduring psychiatric disturbances in a high percentage of survivors regardless of whether they had prior psychiatric problems. Similarly, the stress-related consequences of combat also vary widely, so that some heavily combat-exposed veterans develop long-lasting PTSD, whereas others develop very few persistent symptoms. The death of a parent or spouse, divorce, and major physical injury affect some people profoundly and others hardly at all in the long run. Significant stressors are likely to be more traumatic during early development rather than later or at certain critical developmental periods, compared with other times. For example, the loss of a parent at a very young age is likely to be more traumatic and have more profound and lasting effects than the loss of a parent as an adult.

The combined impact of negative life events and poor emotional and practical social supports is important in predicting the emergence of at least some psychiatric disturbances. One British study found that women who were depressed were much more likely to have lost a parent at an early age, to be relatively housebound with three or more young children, and to lack a good confiding relationship with a spouse or other confidant. In that study, at least, biological vulnerability to depression seemed less important than the accumulation of negative life circumstances in the development of the disorder. People who are ordinarily very competent in all role functions may fall apart completely when a supportive spouse who has bolstered them and taken care of many of their needs suddenly dies. Patients presenting with a major depressive episode have experienced more uncontrollable actual and threatened losses such as the death of a spouse in the year before onset. Nevertheless, not all psychiatric disturbance is attributable to easily identified, provoking negative life events; indeed, some major negative life events that at first glance appear to have preceded the onset of a serious psychiatric disturbance may, in fact, have occurred only after the psychiatric disturbance actually began. For example, someone who attributes the onset of depression to having been fired from a job several months previously may already have been functioning suboptimally at that time and may have been fired as a consequence of a depression-induced decline in role function.

Certain environmental features can counter the effects of environmental stressors and protect against breakdowns. Stable families and friends, good financial circumstances, and supportive churches and communities offer some protection. Research has shown that individuals with psychiatric disturbances have fewer social supports than normal controls. This may be due to friends' and relatives' withdrawal from deviant behaviors or to the disturbed individual's withdrawal from deleterious family and social relationships. In contrast, physically ill people have more social supports than others, perhaps reflecting their ability to recruit help in times of need. Of course, the quality, as well as the quantity, of social supports is important. As has been demonstrated in schizophrenia and mood disorders, for example, negative relationships even in close families may have deleterious effects, both in initiating and in sustaining psychiatric disturbance.

The negative impact of a physiological or environmental stressor is closely related to its personal meaning. For example, the loss of a spouse who has been chronically demented, disabled, and burdensome ordinarily has a very different impact than the loss of a vital, supportive, loving spouse.

Finally, an elegant study has demonstrated the interaction of genetic vulnerabilities with adverse life events. In a study involving several hundred young adults followed prospectively, genetic vulnerability to depression was conferred by certain polymorphisms of the serotonin receptor. Over a period of several years, individuals with one or two copies of the short allele of the 5-hydroxytryptamine T promoter polymorphism exhibited more depressive symptoms, diagnosable depression, and suicidality in relation to stressful life events involving finances, housing, employment, and relationships than individuals homozygous for the long allele. This research provides strong evidence for gene–environment interactions, in which a person's responses to environmental insults are moderated by his or her genetic makeup.

CHARACTERISTICS OF PSYCHIATRIC SIGNS AND SYMPTOMS

Signs and symptoms form the two major categories of clinical phenomena. Classically, for most medical disorders, the distinction between the two is clear. *Symptoms* refer to subjectively experienced disturbances that are not necessarily observable by others. Patients complain of symptoms—chest pain, headache, tingling sensations. *Signs* are abnormalities that are observable by an examiner, including those that are easily evident in the course of a routine encounter with the patient as well as those elicited only through specific physical, mental status, or laboratory examinations.

In psychiatry, the line between symptoms and signs is often blurrier than in general medicine. For instance, many phenomena often considered to be symptoms of psychiatric disorders may not be experienced as psychiatric problems by patients. Hearing an angel's voice may represent a manifestation of a psychotic disorder, yet the patient may vigorously dispute that the experience is a psychopathological symptom. Additionally, auditory hallucinations are often considered to be signs of a psychotic disorder, even though, by their very nature, they are subjective internal experiences (symptoms). Further complicating the distinction, some psychiatric phenomena, such as the classic psychological defense mechanisms, may only be inferred from speech and behaviors but are not directly observable.

Signs and symptoms are said to be present when the limits of normal variability are surpassed. Abnormalities may manifest as alterations in amplitude (e.g., excesses or deficits), duration, intensity, timing, and modifiability of physiological events, perceptions, emotions, thoughts, and motor activities. These limits are often arbitrary. Examples include the number of hours of sleep, the intensity of anger, or the extent of mood lability. However, for other experiences, the distinction between normal and abnormal is qualitative, not quantitative. For some phenomena, "any" is "too much." In mainstream American culture, for instance, any experience of thoughts being broadcast out loud is considered pathological. These signs and symptoms must all be considered in context: Exactly what constitutes normal varies from culture to culture and from situation to situation. A behavior or subjective experience that may be defined as symptomatic in one context may be perfectly acceptable and within normal bounds in another. A phenomenon should be considered abnormal only if it seems deviant within the patient's specific culture after its full physiological and environmental context is taken into account and if it causes personal or interpersonal impairment. Too often, phenomena prematurely mislabeled as psychopathology turn out to be perfectly understandable and nonpathological once the whole situation is appraised. Conversely, some examiners are loath to label certain phenomena as psychopathological even when they clearly are, for fear of stigmatizing the patient.

On the other hand, some relatively normal-appearing behaviors, or behavioral omissions, may signal impairments. For example, individuals may overtly or covertly use so-called safety behaviors to avoid feared outcomes, but these behaviors may in fact perpetuate the very pathological states they are intended to alleviate because they may prevent the individual from facing and directly dealing with their problems or from disconfirming the cognitive distortions that may be underpinning the problems in the first place. Examples of safety behaviors include drinking alcohol to deal with insomnia, consistently talking about traumatic events in an intentionally affectless manner to put off dealing with the associated emotions, and avoiding masturbation to deter delusionally imagined persecutors who go around castrating masturbators. Although, on the surface, these behaviors may not in themselves appear to be pathological, they constitute less-than-satisfactory defense mechanisms and may coincide with those commonly described in the psychoanalytical and psychological literatures, such as reaction formation, dissociation, and others.

Within cultures, most interpersonal interactions are carefully regulated by tight sets of rules and controls and constrained by reasonably well-defined sets of expectations and acceptable limits. Even slight deviations from these acceptable limits are quickly perceived by laypeople, as well as professionals, because behavioral deviances are often experienced as threats. Deviations in amplitude, duration, and intensity can occur in facial expressions, gestures, postures, vocalizations, language, and other expressions of emotion and thought. A small increase in the rate of speech, an intrusion into one person's conversation by another who does not allow proper pauses, a gesture that comes just a bit too close to a face, an excessively rigid or distant stance, or a gaze that is too staring or too avoidant each signals social insensitivity and alerts the observer to deviant behavior.

Reliability Problems Among the core difficulties in psychiatric evaluation has been that multiple observers may note different symptoms or interpret signs differently when interviewing the same patient. These discrepancies may be due to differences in the patient's status or in information imparted by the patient from examination to examination, in the observers' definitions of the symptoms or signs in question, and differences in perceiving and interpreting the patient's responses to general presentation or questions within the interview. These three types of reliability problems are called *information variance*, *criterion variance*, and *observation bias*. A substantial amount of information variance in clinical practice reflects the impossibility of asking all questions within the time available for clinical evaluation. As an example, in one study, the rate of sexual side effects increased from 14 percent when depending on spontaneous patient report to 58 percent when the interviewer directly asked about these side effects.

> A 37-year-old woman, treated with a selective serotonin reuptake inhibitor (SSRI) for the last 2 years, saw a new psychiatrist on relocating to a new city. As part of the initial history, her new psychiatrist asked about sexual side effects from the antidepressant. She acknowledged that she had new-onset anorgasmia for 2 years since she had started the antidepressant. When asked why she had not discussed this with her previous psychiatrist, she said that he had never asked, and she was too embarrassed to spontaneously mention it.

Although good interrater reliability can be achieved for most symptoms of Axis I disorders, this may not hold true for personality disorders or for some specific symptoms. Furthermore, good interrater reliability may occur consistently only under optimal circumstances and may not be as common in clinical practice.

Even when simply responding to direct questions about symptoms, patients may respond differently depending on the interviewer's manner, how the questions are asked, their personal sense of trust or safety, whether they have answered these questions before, the amount of cuing that may signal the "desired" response, their fatigue, or a host of other variables.

Most clinicians still rely heavily on their own clinical intuition and subjective responses to patients as part of a diagnostic assessment. However, these clinical inferences, whether accurate or not, are often based on nonconscious assumptions, comparisons with other patients not well remembered, or distortions based on the clinician's own personal experiences. When the bases for these intuitions can be identified and described clearly, they may prove to be reliable and valid. However, intuitions are often wrong—simple trust in intuition alone is not sufficient. Thus, a clinician's sense that a patient is angry and potentially violent may result from the patient's subtle (but verifiable) body language and tone of voice, or it may represent a countertransference distortion that is not prompted by any observable patient behavior. In this regard, clinicians are becoming more aware of the presence of the so-called intersubjective field in clinical encounters. This term recognizes the fact that clinical phenomena that emerge from the patient are often highly dependent on the nuances of behavior and perception that the clinician brings to the encounter. The clinician's contributions may powerfully shape how the patient behaves and what the patient reveals, in turn potentially seriously distorting what the clinician perceives.

Clinicians often too quickly label behaviors as inappropriate when they do not appreciate and understand contextual or cultural considerations. Appropriateness depends heavily on context, and definitions of what is proper in a given context may also be highly subjective. Appropriate behavior (or dress) in some parts of California may be inappropriate in Boston. A low intensity of emotional expression leading to a clinical description of "constricted affect" may reflect cultural norms or a psychopathological state.

Nonspecific Nature of Signs and Symptoms Until psychiatry discovers reliable diagnostic laboratory tests to define clinical syndromes, the field will continue to construct diagnostic categories based on the clustering of signs and symptoms within specific time frames. However, pathognomically specific signs or symptoms rarely exist in psychiatry; virtually all psychiatric symptoms are nonspecific and are usually seen in many different disorders. Depressed mood, for example, occurs in a wide variety of diagnostic groups, including major depressive disorder, schizophrenia, some personality disorders, organic mood syndromes, and so on. Even the so-called first-rank symptoms of schizophrenia described by Kurt Schneider are diagnostically nonspecific. They are seen with some frequency in otherwise classic depressive and bipolar disorders. Apathy offers another good example of an important nonspecific phenomenon. Although apathy is often part of depression, research has shown this symptom to be a clinically distinct syndrome. Apathy is marked by lack of spontaneity, initiation, and emotionality as well as lack of activity and interest in friends, family, and hobbies. Apathy and the associated symptom of amotivation may exist in their own right without the presence of significant depression, as in initial phases of abstinence from cocaine and in other syndromes characterized by reduction in dopaminergic tone, such as frontotemporal dementias, Parkinson's disease, or progressive supranuclear palsy.

In general medicine, symptoms not recognized as part of a clearly defined syndrome are often described as being of unknown origin. Thus, a fever that cannot be ascribed to a known disorder, such as pneumonia, is described as a fever of unknown origin. Given the nonspecific nature of psychiatric symptoms, it seems wise to use similar conventions, referring to hallucinations of unknown origin or depressed mood of unknown origin when a symptom cannot be clearly linked to a well-described syndrome. However, the dominance of the categorical system of DSM-IV-TR and the demands of a health care and insurance system that requires a specific diagnosis for reimbursement make this type of diagnostic thinking unlikely in the near future.

Even though individual signs and symptoms may be organized into syndromes and disorders, they often have courses of their own. Thus, in the appearance or the resolution of a disorder, certain associated signs and symptoms may appear very early or may persist after all the others have waned. For example, in the restricting form of anorexia nervosa, excessive exercise is often the first symptom to appear and the last to abate even after dieting has stopped. In some cases, certain signs and symptoms that are commonly associated with a given disorder may not appear. Each sign and symptom may have its own pattern and variable response to treatment. In the treatment of schizophrenia, for example, some patients experience rapid resolution of hallucinations but have persistent delusions without ever having any other thinking disorders, whereas others may have no residual hallucinations or delusions but still have prominent thinking disorders.

Sign and Symptom Categories

Signs and symptoms have been categorized in a variety of ways: state versus trait, primary versus secondary, and form versus content. The *state versus trait* distinction refers to whether the sign or symptom is an enduring characteristic of the person ("traits") or time-limited phenomena associated with specific Axis I disorders, which are usually state phenomena. However, some enduring traits may also be symptoms. A person who always worries a great deal, chronically exhibits catastrophic thinking, and feels subjectively nervous in many different circumstances since early childhood may have *trait anxiety*. However, if such symptoms of anxiety are present only during a specific time frame, for example, over a 9-month period in conjunction with a full depressive syndrome, they are best described as state-related symptoms. At times, trait and state symptoms may be one and the same. For instance, in one study, patients who had remission of their depression with treatment still showed relatively high rates of fatigue and sleep disturbances. In these circumstances, long-term symptoms of fatigue and sleep disturbances may be both trait markers of the depressive disorder as well as symptoms of the acute depressive episode. During the acute stages of psychiatric disorders marked by dramatic state characteristics, it is unwise to infer that any of the prominent signs or symptoms are enduring traits, even those usually associated with personality. Thus, a diagnosis of dependent personality traits based on an acutely depressed patient's behavior is often incorrect. Similarly, manipulative behavior in the midst of a hypomanic or manic episode should not be considered evidence for enduring manipulative traits unless these behaviors are also present when the mania has clearly resolved.

Distinctions between primary and secondary symptoms have been confused by varying definitions of these terms. The distinction may refer to causal relationships between what is primary and secondary, temporal sequence between the two symptom sets, or inability to more clearly understand the origin of the various symptoms. Basing the distinction between primary and secondary on causality implies that it is actually understood what is cause and what is effect. In attention-deficit/hyperactivity disorder (ADHD), for instance, the attention deficit is believed to be primary, whereas the hyperactivity is believed to be secondary, caused by the inability to attend. Patients who develop severe dependent personality traits and chronic demoralization only after numbers of incapacitating psychotic mood episodes might be described as having primary mood disorders and secondary personality disorders. Conceptual models of psychopathology in which some signs and symptoms are seen as restitutive, albeit ineffective, attempts to cope with more fundamental psychopathological deficits use a primary–secondary model. To illustrate, Eugen Bleuler viewed thought disorder as a primary symptom in schizophrenia, whereas he viewed hallucinations and delusions as secondary symptoms, formed to help the patient cope with the chaos of the primary symptoms. These models must be viewed as hypothetical constructs only and used with great caution because, in the vast majority of clinical phenomena, little evidence indicates that one symptom is more primary than another.

Temporal sequence in the appearance of certain symptoms is regularly used as the basis for deciding the primacy of certain symptoms, behaviors, or disorders, as in trying to determine what is primary and what is secondary when substance abuse occurs in conjunction with depression or anxiety symptoms. These differences are not trivial but may have treatment implications because, for example, treating a primary mood disorder in a substance-abusing patient (with a long course of medication) may be quite different from simply expecting that, with prolonged sobriety, a secondary mood disorder will resolve on its own. However, the primary–secondary distinction with mood and substance abuse problems, although logical, may not always be consistent with treatment studies. As an example, in one study, patients with primary alcohol abuse and secondary depression (whose depressions should theoretically have responded to simple sobriety) responded better to antidepressants than to placebo. Furthermore, it is becoming increasingly clear that the presence of certain preexisting psychiatric conditions, such as personality disorders, increases one's vulnerability for the subsequent development of other psychiatric disorders such as major depressive disorders.

However, establishing temporal sequence with any certainty is typically difficult. To illustrate, although there is a high comorbidity between bulimia nervosa and major depressive disorder, in excess of 50 percent in some studies, attempts to establish which disorder is primary have been inconclusive. Even with careful historical analysis, major depression precedes bulimia nervosa, bulimia nervosa precedes major depressive episodes, and the two conditions start concurrently in approximately equal percentages.

Ultimately, making simple categorical distinctions between primary and secondary signs, symptoms, and disorders is less important than understanding the contribution of each element as a thread in the evolution and development of a given clinical presentation. From this perspective, each element can be viewed as dynamically affecting the appearance, manifestations, and course of the others, exerting its own influence on the pathogenesis and treatment of the specific syndromes and associated disorders. This view is particularly important because, despite the excellent conceptual contributions made by categorical diagnostic systems, such as the American Psychiatric Association's DSM-IV-TR, in clinical practice distinctions are often fuzzy, and comorbidity among so-called categorically distinct disorders is often the rule rather than the exception. For example, data from the National Comorbidity Study show that 14 percent of the population experience three or more comorbid psychiatric disorders. In such individuals, the dynamic interactions and mutual influences of various signs and symptoms, and their biological underpinnings, become impossible to disentangle.

Furthermore, the categories that currently comprise DSM-IV-TR are not going to be the last word in the evolving history of psychiatric diagnosis. Recent studies show that psychiatric signs and symptoms may be usefully grouped into psychotic syndromes that differ in some respects from current DSM-IV-TR categories. In a large family study of probands with broadly defined schizophrenia and affective illness and their first-degree relatives, using a sophisticated statistical technique called *latent class analysis*, Kenneth Kendler and colleagues found six classes of psychosis, including classic schizophrenia, major depression, schizophreniform disorder, bipolar schizomania, schizodepression, and hebephrenia. Although these classes bore substantial resemblance to current or historical nosological constructs, several of them differed from DSM-IV-TR nosological constructs. In another study, the three factors ordinarily associated with symptoms of schizophrenia, representing positive, negative, and disorganized symptom domains, were found not to be specific to schizophrenia but were found in other schizophrenia-spectrum psychoses and in nonschizophrenia-like psychotic conditions as well.

Additionally, a dimensional view of psychopathology fits much recent data better than the categorical view that is inherent in DSM-IV-TR. Personality disorders fit poorly into a categorical scheme, and the frequent "comorbidity" of these disorders likely reflects the descriptive overlap rather than the patient having two distinct disorders. Similarly, in DSM-IV-TR, dysthymia and major depression are seen as two mood disorders when recent studies indicate that they are more likely manifestations of one disorder that differs in course and intensity.

Context Signs and symptoms are usually not static entities; depending on the context, they often vary in intensity or even in their existence. The depressed mood of a melancholic depression may persist regardless of the external situation, whereas the depressed mood in milder, reactive depression may vanish completely during certain situations—including a psychiatric interview—only to reappear at other times. Signs and symptoms that occur only in specific settings or with certain internal states are referred to as *state dependent*. For example, certain hallucinations or memories may be present only during states of drug or alcohol intoxication; in some patients, hives may erupt as a psychophysiological response only during states of anger. Interpersonal context is also important. Some people become violent only when involved in sadomasochistic relationships or in certain group settings such as adolescent gangs. In gangs, social pressures for conformity and expectations for aggressive behavior may provoke or release pathological behaviors that might otherwise never be expressed by gang members individually.

Problems and Impairments Beyond the classic signs and symptoms of psychiatric disorders, recent attention has focused on the problems and impairments that psychiatric signs, symptoms, and disorders generate in affecting specific role functions and causing social and economic burdens for the patient and others. These problems and impairments often cut across traditional sets of signs and symptoms of which categorical diagnoses are comprised, affecting, for example, basic abilities to care for oneself and one's family, marital functioning, child rearing, wage earning, school performance, and social behavior. They constitute the issues with which patients and families contend, and they need to appear on the problem lists that treatment plans and specific interventions target. Studies reveal, for example, that the impairments imposed by major depression are considerable with regard to physical functioning, role limitations, and social functioning. Problems such as violent temper outbursts, sexual aggression, or lack of job skills, which may impair role functioning in several spheres, must be directly addressed regardless of the associated DSM-IV-TR diagnoses. These impairments enter determinations of ratings for Axis V of the DSM-IV-TR, which addresses the global assessment of functioning, and are of considerable importance in evaluating treatment outcomes. Table 8–1 lists some illustrative critical impairments that have been recognized as often requiring urgent or intensive levels of care.

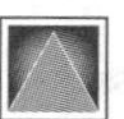

Table 8–1
Illustrative Critical Impairments That May Require Service-Intensive Treatment, More Intensive Treatment Settings, or Acute Care

Anxiety	Medical risk factor
Assaultiveness	Medical treatment noncompliance
Compulsions	Mood lability
Concomitant medical condition	Obsessions
Delusions (nonparanoid)	Phobia
Delusions (paranoid)	Physical abuse perpetrator
Dissociative states	Psychomotor retardation
Dysphoric mood	Psychotic thought/behavior
Eating disorder	Running away
Fire setting	Self-mutilation
Hallucinations	Sexual trauma perpetrator
Homicidal thought/behavior	Substance abuse
Inadequate health care skills	Suicidal thought/behavior
Manic thought/behavior	

Adapted from Goodman M, Brown J, Deitz PM. *Managing Managed Care II. A Handbook for Mental Health Professionals.* 2nd ed. Washington DC: American Psychiatric Press, Inc.; 1996.

Furthermore, the relationship between symptoms and disorders on one hand and functional impairments on the other is not always straightforward. For example, in both bipolar and unipolar mood disorders, many patients recover symptomatically from episodes but achieve premorbid psychosocial function either months later or not at all. In one review of previously published studies on major depression, there was a consistent lag time between symptomatic and functional recovery. Whether this disparity between symptomatic and functional recovery reflects subtle residual symptoms, unrecognized cognitive disturbances, personality difficulties, or a combination of factors is unknown.

A 45-year-old teacher with a relatively severe major depression stopped work because of depressive symptoms. He was treated with a combination of medication and psychotherapy and became asymptomatic, with virtually complete normalization of mood, sleep, appetite, concentration, and energy. Nonetheless, he felt unable to return to work soon after the depression remitted, being unable to explain this other than as simply feeling "not ready" for the stresses of the job he had done consistently for 15 years.

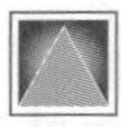

Table 8–2
Common Current Clinical Hypotheses Used to Assess Signs and Symptoms: Ways of Understanding the Patient's Problems

Biologically derived hypotheses
- Related to a brain impairment or organic mental disorder
- Related to mood disorder
- Related to nonaffective functional psychosis
- Related to the abuse of drugs or alcohol
- Related to biologically mediated developmental issues
- As a disorder other than those listed above in the biologically derived hypotheses category

Psychodynamically derived hypotheses
- Related to personality and temperament style
- Related to environmentally mediated developmental issues, such as abuse, neglect, and traumatic events, and more subtle life processes regarding nurture by primary caregivers, interactions with family, peers, and others in both shared and nonshared environments
- Related to precipitating life events and their dynamic meaning
- Related to manifestations of unresolved grief
- Related to a current developmental crisis
- Related to ego functioning and associated psychodynamic issues

Socioculturally derived hypotheses
- Related to the nature and the social effects of stressful life events
- Related to the extent, nature, and accessibility of practical (particularly financial) or emotional social support, or both
- Related to definitions of and responses to breakdown in the sociocultural grouping
- Related to the patient's motivation, treatment goals, and the dynamics of the entry process to help seeking
- Related to practical matters in negotiating and sustaining ongoing relationships with professional caregivers and care-giving systems
- As social communication

Behaviorally derived hypotheses
- As disordered thinking, feeling, or acting resulting from specific antecedent events
- As disordered thinking, feeling, or acting resulting from reinforcing consequences of the behaviors
- As disordered thinking, feeling, or acting in response to sociocultural and biological events
- As a deficit of behaviors (rather than disordered behaviors) in the areas of thinking, feeling, and acting
- As compensatory behaviors used to compensate for behavioral deficits
- By an analysis of areas of effective functioning

Adapted from Lazare A. Hypothesis testing in the clinical interview. In Lazare A, ed. *Outpatient Psychiatry: Diagnosis and Treatment*. Baltimore: Williams & Wilkins; 1979.

Need for a Comprehensive Perspective A psychiatric disorder may be characterized by disturbances involving a wide variety of areas in the patient's life, including the biological, psychological, behavioral, interpersonal, and social spheres. In practice, common psychiatric syndromes often manifest in each of these dimensions (Table 8–2). Viewing the patient from multiple perspectives, using the so-called biopsychosocial model (similar to the multiaxial approach of DSM-IV-TR), enables clinicians to consider psychopathology and its effects on a patient's life in the broadest possible manner. To illustrate, Figure 8–1 lists some clinical hypotheses commonly used by clinicians as they link collections of signs and symptoms into syndromes and consider the treatment options that logically follow.

Because the amount of information gathered in a thorough assessment of a psychiatric disorder is potentially overwhelming, clinicians often tend to limit their fields of vision and appreciate only part of the available information; the clinician's theoretical orientation and other personal and cultural factors also limit what is perceived. Research has demonstrated that clinicians tend to perceive primarily those signs and symptoms that are most in accord with their theoretical points of view and with the tools they have available to treat psychiatric disorders, a phenomenon known as *concept-driven perception*. The theoretical biases of clinicians seem to be related both to the microcultures of their training programs and to their own personality traits. Such differences may lead one clinician to see a major mood disorder to be treated with medication, whereas another sees a pervasive personality problem with depressed mood to be treated with psychotherapy and to use different technical terms to label roughly the same phenomena. A psychodynamic psychiatrist might see psychomotor retardation, whereas a neuropsychiatrist sees bradykinesia; a psychodynamicist might see depressed affect and muted speech, whereas a neuropsychiatrist sees mask-like facies and aprosodic speech; the psychodynamicist might see ruminative thought, whereas a neuropsychiatrist sees forced thinking; a psychodynamicist might see a grimace, whereas a neuropsychiatrist sees a tic. Given the extent to which words themselves shape our concepts of reality, the consequences of using these different labels for very similar phenomena may be significant. Figure 8–1 illustrates concept-driven perception in which each clinician who adheres to a prominent contemporary point of view perceives only some of the potentially available phenomena related to a psychiatric disorder. Although there is overlap, each observer also perceives information not appreciated by the others. At the same time, some information that may be highly relevant to diagnosing or treating the disorder may be missed by all the observers; so clinicians 100 years from now will, no doubt, be able to detect and understand the significance of signs and symptoms not appreciated by anyone today.

The intermittent nature of many psychiatric signs and symptoms; the potential unreliability, selective recall, and false remembering of patients and others in reporting symptoms and events; differing interpretations of elicited information or observations; and subjective theoretically driven biases that influence the clinician's perception of signs and symptoms all contribute to potential errors in data collection. To help guard against misinformation and simplistic understandings and formulations, whenever possible, complete assessment of a psychiatric patient requires consultation with family, friends, coworkers, and other professional observers to enrich the history and to provide supplemental observations of the patient over time.

SOMATIC MANIFESTATIONS OF PSYCHIATRIC DISORDERS

Most psychiatric disorders and virtually all Axis I symptom-based disorders are characterized by disturbances in at least some basic physiological functions. Although frequently nonspecific in nature, the severity of these somatic signs and symptoms provides markers as to the amount of biological disruption seen in the disorders that cause them. Furthermore, somatic symptoms can also cause exacerbations of some disorders. If untreated, these processes can create destructive feedback loops in which the disorder causes symptoms, which then exacerbates the disorder, which causes increases in the symptoms, and so on. As examples, the insomnia of manic or hypomanic states, if untreated, causes a marked worsening of the mania; similarly, the weight loss of anorexia nervosa causes starva-

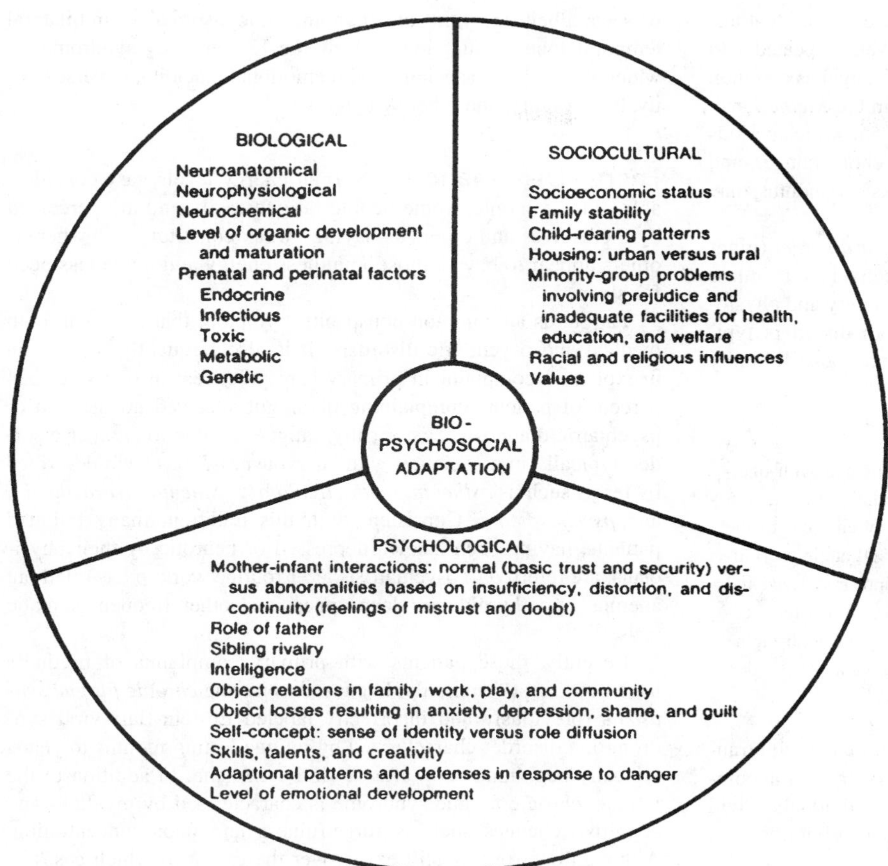

FIGURE 8–1 Biological, psychological, and social forces interact and affect the psychiatric health of a person. (Adapted from Richmond JB, Lustman SL: Total health: A conceptual visual aid. *J Med Educ.* 1954;29:23.)

tion effects, such as a preoccupation with food, thus exacerbating one of the hallmark features of the underlying disorder.

Sleep Disturbances Abnormalities of sleep may manifest in the amount, quality, and timing of sleep as well as by the presence of abnormal events during sleep.

Insomnia is usually defined by its subjective component as the sensation of sleeping poorly. Most, but not all, patients complaining of insomnia demonstrate some sleep abnormality if examined in a sleep laboratory. Insomnia is a common, often chronic symptom or sign of many different psychiatric disorders, including substance abuse, depression, generalized anxiety disorder, panic, mania (in which the diminished sleep does not always provoke a complaint), and acute schizophrenia. It may also occur as a consequence of aging or as a symptom or disorder not associated with other psychopathology. Insomnia may also result from the ingestion of substances that alter the normal sleep–wake cycle, including alcohol or stimulants, and by the discontinuation of sedative-hypnotics. Although much attention is often paid to distinguishing patterns of insomnia, such as difficulty falling asleep versus middle or terminal insomnia (early morning awakening), or linking specific patterns to a specific disorder (for example, melancholic depression with terminal insomnia), the clinical usefulness of these distinctions is unclear.

A 62-year-old woman complained of chronic insomnia, characterized by both initial insomnia and fitful sleep during the night. She had a history of recurrent major depressions in association with marked life stressors but had not had a depressive episode for 10 years. A medical workup, including an extensive medical and psychiatric history, revealed no obvious cause for the insomnia. Her mood was euthymic, and no evidence of sleep apnea or other primary sleep disorder was apparent. She was treated with low-dose trazodone, which was somewhat effective and which she used intermittently for the next few years.

Hypersomnia, characterized by either excessive nighttime sleep or excessive sleepiness during the day, is less common than insomnia. It, too, however, may reflect a number of different pathological states. Some depressed patients, especially those with a history of mania or hypomania, may exhibit hypersomnia. Hypersomnia may also be seen during stimulant withdrawal, with excessive use of sedatives or tranquilizers, or in conjunction with a variety of medical disorders. In *narcolepsy*, the patient has sudden attacks of irresistible sleepiness, a symptom that may be part of a broader syndrome that includes *cataplexy* (sudden attacks of generalized muscle weakness leading to physical collapse in the presence of alert consciousness), *sleep paralysis* (waking from sleep with a sensation of being totally paralyzed that may persist for minutes), and *hypnagogic hallucinations* (vivid visual hallucinations that occur at the point of falling asleep). Narcoleptic attacks are often precipitated by unusual states of arousal (e.g., cataplexy may immediately follow unrestrained laughter or orgasm). Daytime sleepiness may reflect *sleep apnea*. In this disorder, typically middle-aged patients demonstrate severe snoring—often first reported by their bed partners—and periods when breathing stops. The condition results from soft palate abnormalities that cause intermittent airway obstruction throughout the night; patients awake repeatedly to find themselves gasping for air. Associated daytime fatigue is common in sleep apnea. Periodic hypersomnia also occurs in the *Kleine-Levin syndrome*, a condition typically affecting young men in which periods of sleepiness alternate with confusional states, ravenous hunger, and protracted sexual activity. Intervals of days, weeks, or months may pass between these episodes.

Somnambulism, or sleepwalking, and *sleep terror disorder* (night terror) are two sleep disorders characterized, respectively, by aimless wandering with incomplete arousal and by acute anxiety and physiological arousal without awakening. Although both disorders typically begin in childhood, sleepwalking may be also initially precipitated by some psychotropic medications.

A 51-year-old woman with complex PTSD was treated with olanzapine. Within 1 year after starting this medication, she had gained 35 lbs. During this period, her husband noted that she often went to the refrigerator in the middle of the night, sound asleep, and ate indiscriminately. When he woke her during these episodes, she appeared dazed and had no awareness of her purposive behaviors. To the best of her recollection, confirmed by her husband, before treatment with olanzapine (Zyprexa), she had no history of somnambulistic phenomena.

Nightmares are a common complaint, often associated with traumatic events, anxiety disorders, and mood disorders, but not uncommon as an occasional event in otherwise healthy individuals. Vivid dreams and nightmares may also be a medication side effect.

A 32-year-old woman was treated for a mild depression with an SSRI. Her sleep pattern before treatment had been characterized by hypersomnia, sleeping between 10 and 12 hours nightly. Soon after the initiation of her SSRI antidepressant, she noticed that her sleep was not only shorter and more fractured but that she had remarkably intense dreams that she remembered vividly. She made clear that these were not nightmares, just dreams with intense colors and clarity, which she rather enjoyed.

Sensory symptoms during sleep, typically described by patients as peculiar feelings in their legs causing an irresistible need to move around, are characteristic of *restless legs syndrome*. The motor abnormality of repetitive myoclonic jerking of the legs, awakening both patients and their partners, is known as *nocturnal myoclonus*.

Appetite and Weight Disturbances

Aside from the anorexia of medical illnesses, especially in their later stages, loss of appetite is most commonly seen in depressive disorders, grief, some anxiety disorders, and primary anorexia nervosa and as a side effect of some medications. Anorexia is often accompanied by changes in taste (e.g., foods begin to taste different, bitter, or flat or have an unpleasant aroma). In eating disorders, patients may resist hunger to restrict food intake to achieve a physiologically unrealistic low weight. Hyperphagia (increased appetite) occurs in some depressed patients, both with and without a history of mania or hypomania. Binge eating, of up to several thousand calories per episode, may occur as an attempt to self-soothe and emotionally self-regulate during times of increased tension and anxiety and as a key feature of bulimia nervosa or of binge-eating disorder. Increased appetite may be seen, albeit rarely, in some hypothalamic disorders or in bilateral temporal lobe dysfunction such as the Klüver-Bucy syndrome, in which it occurs in association with emotional placidity, hypersexuality, hyperorality, and other symptoms.

Energy Disturbances

Normal energy levels vary considerably among people. Some people fatigue easily and are perceived by themselves and others as having "weak constitutions," whereas others appear to have almost boundless energy and much less need for sleep.

Fatigue is an common nonspecific symptom that occurs in both medical and psychiatric disorders. It is also frequently seen as an unexplained complaint in primary care practices; in one study, 24 percent of patients complaining of fatigue received no medical or psychiatric diagnosis. Historically, fatigue not due to another disorder, typically in association with "nervousness," has been described by terms such as *asthenia*, *neurocirculatory asthenia*, *neurasthenia*, and *psychasthenia*. Consistent with this tradition, many fatigued patients, having been labeled depressed or neurotic by their physicians, are referred to psychiatrists after routine workup has ruled out anemia, hypothyroidism, sleep apnea, and other frequent somatic causes.

Recently, those patients with primary complaints of tiredness have been most commonly diagnosed as having *chronic fatigue syndrome* (previously and incorrectly labeled Epstein-Barr viral syndrome), a disorder characterized by fatigue lasting months to years, typically beginning soon after a viral syndrome. In addition to the fatigue, chronic fatigue syndrome is characterized by myalgias and cognitive changes such as forgetfulness and poor concentration. Although controversy still exists over the extent to which cases of chronic fatigue syndrome represent discrete postviral diagnostic syndromes, mislabeled cases of depression, or modern versions of psychasthenia, evidence continues to mount to suggest that these syndromes are discrete postinfectious entities and are not simply variants of or disguised mood or anxiety disorders.

A highly accomplished, energetic 40-year-old woman was referred for psychiatric consultation after her physicians were unable to offer a definitive physiological diagnosis despite extensive medical workup after the acute onset of profound fatigue occurring in the wake of a mild viral illness. This fatigue caused her to be totally incapacitated and bedridden for many months and left her feeling quite helpless and distraught. It was exacerbated by even small amounts of alcohol. Two independent psychiatric evaluations concluded that the patient had no psychiatric disorder. The patient developed this syndrome after jogging near Lake Tahoe. Epidemiological studies were found that reported a series of other cases of profound fatigue originating in this particular area after vigorous exercise. Various antidepressants seemed to provide partial relief, but tolerance to their positive effects developed. The fatigue slowly improved over many years; 7 years after the original symptoms, the patient continued to experience waxing and waning fatigue but at a lesser level than originally.

Disturbances in Sexual Drive

As with energy, the normal range of sexual drives is great. Some individuals are naturally lusty, whereas others have limited sexual desire. Diminished sexual drive with impotence or decreased libido is seen in a wide variety of neurological, metabolic, and other somatic syndromes. Among neurological disorders, complex partial seizures are commonly associated with hyposexuality, occurring in 50 percent of patients. Psychiatric disorders known for diminished sexual drive include depressive disorders, schizophrenia, substance abuse disorders, and marital conflict. Diminished libido, erectile dysfunction, and anorgasmia are also common sequelae of many psychotropic agents, especially strongly serotonergic antidepressants.

A depressed 36-year-old man had an excellent antidepressant response to an SSRI but developed decreased sexual interest and anorgasmia with relative preservation of erectile function. When the sexual side effects did not diminish after 4 weeks, his psychiatrist tried a number of potential antidotes. Although sildenafil (Viagra) improved his erections somewhat, his libido and orgasmic function continued to be markedly impaired. Reluctantly, he and his psychiatrist agreed to switch to a different antidepressant class that was not associated with sexual side effects.

Increased sexual activity may be seen in some neurological, drug-induced, and psychiatric disorders. Manic patients frequently exhibit hypersexual interests and behaviors to an unusual degree, compared with their euthymic interests and behaviors. Hypersexuality is occasionally seen in conjunction with epileptic syndromes or in patients who have had diencephalic injuries.

Altered sexuality, including fetishes, sadomasochism, pedophilia, and other paraphilias, may be seen as isolated psychiatric syndromes. In individuals whose previous sexual behaviors were within the bounds of social propriety for their groups, inappropriate sexual behaviors may signal early brain disease or psychosis. Cross-dressing may occur in transvestites, transgenderists, transsexuals, or, occasionally, in other psychiatric conditions.

A 54-year-old married engineer became preoccupied with viewing pornographic sites on the Internet. He had always been excited by the visual stimulation of early adolescent girls. He had never acted on these feelings, had never had an affair since being married, and, even when younger, had always had consensual sex with girls his own age. With the advent of the computer, he had become increasingly preoccupied by finding and spending significant amounts of time on Web sites devoted to photos of young girls. Eventually, he was spending 3 hours daily at these Web sites. At that point, he sought treatment for a pattern of behavior that he believed he could not control at all.

Appearance Studies show that clinicians often formulate an initial psychiatric diagnosis within 30 seconds of seeing a patient. Although approximately one-half of such initial impressions prove to be incorrect, the remainder are validated by psychiatric history and mental status examination, revealing just how much information is communicated by appearance and body language.

Among the physical disorders whose appearances suggest coexistent psychiatric conditions are acromegaly, Cushing's syndrome, Down syndrome, systemic lupus erythematosus, fetal alcohol syndrome, Klinefelter's syndrome, and Wilson's disease, to name a few. The general appearance of the skin may suggest the presence of occult psychiatric problems. The general condition and flush of the skin may reveal hypervascularity and ruddiness, suggestive of alcoholism, abscesses indicative of hypodermic needle abuse, tattoos indicative of certain group affiliations, or weathering and wasting indicative of self-neglect and malnutrition. Healed scars on the wrists and arms suggest a pattern of self-mutilation from depression, personality disturbance, or both. Patchy baldness, especially in conjunction with torn or infected cuticles, indicates trichotillomania, a syndrome of compulsive hair pulling. Psychophysiological symptoms reflecting psychiatric disturbance include urticarial reactions and neurodermatitis, the latter resulting, in part, from self-excoriation, destructive scratching secondary to compulsions, and unrelenting sensations of discomfort.

A 23-year-old woman who had recovered from a severe episode of anorexia nervosa as an adolescent had recurrent depressions and persistent personality disturbances characterized by odd and eccentric ideas, shyness, and avoidance. She became enchanted with gothic themes, spent hours on the Internet in chat rooms featuring dark and morbid poetry, and started to have herself tattooed. Within 1 year, she had tattooed every inch of her upper extremities, scalp, and torso with complex, intricate, gothic designs. She acknowledged that tattooing her skin in such an extreme manner served to mark her as deviant and to warn people away from her.

Examination of the head and neck may reveal exophthalmos or puffy eyelids, suggesting thyroid disease, marked pupillary dilation with anxiety or stimulant abuse, miosis with narcotic abuse, abnormal pupillary pigments in Wilson's disease, salivary gland enlargement in bulimia nervosa, or necrosis of the nasal septum in cocaine abuse, among other signs. Frequent sighing is a common respiratory sign in depression. Simple sighing must be distinguished from respiratory dyskinesia in psychotic patients who have been treated with neuroleptics. The latter may occur as an acute dyskinesia due to antipsychotic medication, or it may be a late manifestation and component of tardive dyskinesia.

Deviant appearance is quickly perceived by laypeople and professionals and may contribute to the frightened and stigmatizing social withdrawal by strangers, as well as acquaintances, so often experienced by psychiatric patients. Akathisia and dystonic movements and parkinsonian shuffling gait in patients taking neuroleptics (especially the older, conventional antipsychotics), as well as the dilapidated and unkempt appearance of some psychiatric patients, can immediately signal psychiatric patient status to observers. The term *Diogenes syndrome* has been used to describe old people who have filthy personal appearance and demonstrate severe self-neglect about which they have no shame.

DISTURBANCES IN THINKING

Normal Thinking *Thinking* refers to the ideational components of mental activity, processes used to imagine, appraise, evaluate, forecast, plan, create, and will. Most thought involves complex rules that are probably best currently approximated (albeit inexactly) by fuzzy-logic decision-making algorithms that use neural net technology, increasingly applied by scientists and engineers in vague situations in which all-or-none, black-or-white thinking does not apply but in which multifaceted, contradictory, and competing possibilities and biases are the rule. Most of what is known about thinking derives from the study of language as the product (and reflection) of thought, yet a great deal of thinking takes place preverbally and nonverbally. Thinking occurs in images, music, and kinesthetic sensations and in symbols other than linguistic ones. Attempts to transmit preverbal and nonverbal thought using only words are frustrating and unsatisfactory. Creative artists have considerable difficulty describing the inner states of tension and inchoate awareness from which ideas are distilled.

Ordinary thought is far from logical. Streams of conscious thought are intruded on by competing thoughts and associations and by outside stimuli, and attention is easily distracted. Ordinary conversation is marked by recurring asides, interruptions, delays, and the loss of ideas. Decisions are often made on the basis of very few cues and inadequate evidence: People jump to conclusions. Beliefs are zealously held that are not supported by evidence. Thinking in stereotypes is more common than thinking in logical categories; from an evolutionary perspective, thinking in stereotypes and by approximation has probably been more adaptive than thinking in strictly defined categories. This tendency helps account for clinicians' tendencies to make diagnoses by approximation and intuition based on prototypes and to feel less comfortable using formal lists of criteria found in statistical manuals such as DSM-IV-TR. Consistent with this notion, a recent study found that more than 60 percent of patients being treated for personality disorders by clinicians had diagnosable personality disorders when strict DSM-IV-TR criteria were applied.

Considerable variation exists among individuals regarding predominant cognitive styles, and an individual's style of thinking also shifts considerably from time to time. *Cognitive style* refers to one's predominant manner of information processing and decision making; the particular biases and distortions thinking processes make by means of augmenting, elaborating, or minimizing incoming information; and the extent to which people use careful and deliberate logic versus intuition versus thoughtless, anxiety-induced impulsivity to guide decision making. In some individuals, a particular cognitive style may come to dominate that person's repertoire so completely as to interfere with the flexible, adaptive responses required to deal with the usual variety of daily needs. An *obsessional* style of thinking is marked by attention to detail and hypervigilance concerning the possible implications of a particular thought or event. This may take the form of preoccupation with strict adherence to established rules, values, or beliefs. An obsessional style may be highly adaptive in certain situations, as in professions requiring meticulous detail such as librarians, computer programmers, and surgeons. However, excessively rigid obsessionality may be maladaptive, as when someone scrupulously sticks to the rules even when such adherence is self-destructive and short sighted. A *hysterical* style of thinking is characterized by global, diffuse, impressionistic, emotionally laden evaluations of situations in which lack of attention is given to details and nuances. This style is poorly adaptive to detail-oriented work but may be useful in the arts, certain aspects of marketing and sales, and in some social situations.

A 36-year-old attorney reported difficulty at work because he sometimes got bogged down in trivial details about cases that he could not seem to drop. His mind required him to follow small, usually irrelevant leads that offended his legalistic sensibilities even though his clients and partners had no interest in these aspects of the cases and faulted him for wasting their time and money.

Types of Thinking Because of the different ways in which both normal and abnormal thinking expresses itself, differences that are apparent to even a casual observer, attempts have been made to subtype thinking by the extent to which logical versus nonlogical thought is used. Although less commonly used than before, Sigmund Freud's division of thought into primary and secondary process thinking provides a useful description classification.

PRIMARY PROCESS Primary process thinking, the more primitive type, is typically seen in dreams but is also prominent in young children and in psychotic states. This type of thinking disregards logic, permits contradictions to exist simultaneously, disregards the linear notion of time, and is dominated by wish and fantasy. It uses symbol, metaphor, imagery, condensation, displacement, and concretism in its organization, creating the jumbled and incoherent style of thinking characteristic of dreams. Primary process thinking represents what has been loosely and metaphorically called *right brain thinking*, associated with visual images and creative thought.

SECONDARY PROCESS Secondary process thinking is characterized by logic. In contrast to primary process thinking, the secondary process uses linear notions of time, clearly delineated abstract categories, and deductive rules of logic. The abilities to think abstractly and to think in detail about future plans are characteristic of secondary process thinking. Normal secondary process thinking is also characterized by predictability, coherence, and redundancy. Words, vocal inflections, and gestures provide important contextual cues and create a sense of overall coherence to the communication. Ideas follow one another in a sequence that is understandable to the listener.

A non-Freudian typology of thought divides thinking into three types: fantasy thinking, imaginative thinking, and rational or conceptual thinking. Fantasy thinking allows the person to escape from, or deny, reality and can be seen in normal as well as pathological thinking. Everyone occasionally uses fantasy thinking when daydreaming. Some dissociative and psychotic phenomena illustrate the most pathological manifestations of fantasy thinking. Imaginative thinking merges fantasy and memory to generate plans for the future. Rational or conceptual thinking uses logic to solve problems.

Regardless of how one categorizes thought, people can fluidly shift from linear/secondary, process/rational thought to fantasy/primary, process/nonlogical thought, as in the free associative method used in psychoanalysis. During this process, individuals willfully surrender the controls that maintain secondary process thinking and switch to the less controlled modes of primary process thinking in which thoughts are loosely associated by emotional associations or based on peripheral, concrete, coincidental, loosely similar, or trivial aspects of a thought. Additionally, the fact that increases in primary process thinking can be induced in normal people under experimental conditions or with fatigue suggests that more primitive thought processes, such as those seen in psychosis, are usually inhibited by higher-order processes and that their appearance may be release phenomena—that is, nonlinear or psychotic thinking may indicate the functional absence of those overriding control systems that ordinarily sift, evaluate, and regulate the form and flow of thought before it reaches consciousness.

THOUGHT DISTURBANCES

Flow and Form Disturbances Because the underlying processes that govern thought are not understood, current systems for classifying thought abnormalities are primarily descriptive. Conventional classification separates form and flow from the content of thought, yet many types of abnormal thinking include both form and content abnormalities. Thus, although delusions are usually classified as thought content disturbances, they are also marked by formal abnormalities, such as rigidity and imperviousness of thought to external influence or to information that clearly contradicts the delusional idea.

Although *formal thought disorder* typically refers to marked abnormalities in the form and flow or connectivity of thought, some clinicians use the term broadly to include any psychotic cognitive sign or symptom.

As with energy and sexuality, normal variations in the flow and form of thought are considerable. For some people, thinking appears to be effortless—rapid and productive, exhibiting linear, goal-directed thoughts and creativity, with digressions and occasional leaps but always controlled and comprehensible. For others, thinking is a difficult exercise—a slow, painstaking process with low output, compared with other people, or "scattered," with difficulty staying with a topic or finishing a single thought. Most people experience admixtures of these extremes. Disturbances in the flow and form of thought occur with regard to rate, continuity, control, and complexity.

Thinking can be unusually slow or accelerated. Slowed (or retarded) thought, such as noted in depression, is typically goal directed but characterized by little initiative or planning. Patients experiencing retarded thought often describe feeling that even simple thought requires monumental effort, as if molasses were cluttering their thinking. These difficulties are expressed as slowness in decision making and as long latency of response, increased pause times when speech is initiated and during speech. *Thought blocking*, seen in schizophrenia, is experienced as the snapping off or as a sudden break in a train of thought, as if a wall suddenly comes down, interrupting thinking (and speaking) in mid-sentence. To an outside observer, without further explanation from the patient, thought blocking may appear identical to *thought withdrawal*, a disturbance in the control of thought in which the patient feels as if some alien force has intentionally withdrawn the thoughts from consciousness. The patient's further description and explanation of the inner experience is necessary to distinguish these two symptoms.

A 35-year-old woman with schizophrenia had a core delusion that a group of beings/spirits/forces watched over her, directing her behavior with variable intensity. At times, she began to describe a part of her thinking process to her psychiatrist, only to stop midway through, refusing to go on with the discussion. At another time, she acknowledged that she was being told by the forces that the answers to the psychiatrist's questions were too personal to divulge and that she had been instructed to stop talking.

Accelerated rates of thinking, typically accompanied by fast talking, can be seen as a normal variant. Rapid rates of speech, influenced heavily by cultural and situational factors, only sometimes reflect truly rapid thought. (For example, it is not at all clear that New Yorkers, who characteristically speak more quickly than people from some other cities, actually think at a faster rate. Similarly, auctioneers and some radio and television announcers can speak with astonishing rapidity, likely reflecting both innate capacities as well as learned psychomotor skills.) *Pressure of speech*—speech that is rapid, excessive, and typically loud—is characteristic of mania (or hypomania), stimulant intoxication, and, occasionally, anxiety. *Flight of ideas* occurs when the flow of thought increases to the point at which the train of thought switches direction frequently and rapidly. The associative links between conceptual topics during flight of ideas are comprehensible to the listener, although not without considerable effort at times. Listening to a flight of ideas that is not overwhelmingly fast can be both a dizzying and enjoyable experience for the listener, as exemplified by the successful performance style of certain contemporary comedians, notably Robin Williams.

Continuity Disturbances in the continuity of thought may take several forms. In *circumstantiality,* the flow of thought includes many digressive turns and associations, often including a great deal of unnecessary detail. Transcripts of circumstantial thought or speech are marked by multiple commas, subclauses, and parenthetic asides. Nonetheless, in circumstantial thought or speech, the speaker eventually returns to the point that was initially intended without having to be prompted by the listener.

In contrast, in *tangentiality*, the person's thought wanders further and further away from the intended point, without ever returning, so that the person may not even remember what the original point was supposed to be. Tangentiality is a mild form of *derailment* in which there is a breakdown in associations. Loose associations exemplify more severe derailment, in which the flows of ideas are no longer comprehensible to the listener because the individual thoughts seem to have no logical relation to one another. *Loose associations* are classically a hallmark feature of schizophrenia. In extreme cases, the associations of phrases and even individual words are incomprehensible, and syntax—the rules of grammar by which phrases are organized into sentences and words into phrases—may be disrupted. *Word salad* describes the stringing together of words that seem to have no logical association, and *verbigeration* describes the disappearance of understandable speech, replaced by strings of incoherent utterances.

Clang association refers to a sequence of thoughts stimulated by the sound of a preceding word. For example, a manic patient said, "I'll kill with a drill or a pill—God, I'm ill—what swill." In *echolalia,* the patient repeats a sentence just uttered by the examiner. Repetition of only the last uttered word or phrase is called *palilalia*, a symptom found most often in chronic schizophrenia.

Perseveration and stereotypy are two other associative abnormalities in which the flow of thought or speech appears to get stuck. In *perseveration*, a sentence or phrase is repeated, sometimes several times over, after it is no longer relevant. Perseveration is commonly seen in delirium and other organic mental disorders. *Stereotypy* refers to the constant repetition of a phrase or a behavior in many different settings, irrespective of context.

Disturbances in the control of thought include delusional passivity experiences and obsessional thinking. In *delusional thought passivity*, patients experience their own thoughts as being under the control of other forces. Thought passivity may take several forms: In *thought insertion,* thoughts are experienced as having been placed within the patient's mind from the outside; in *thought withdrawal,* thoughts are whisked out of the mind; in *thought broadcasting,* patients experience their thoughts as escaping their minds to be heard by others. These experiences are often combined with specific delusions of control, seemingly to explain the passivity experiences. Several of these phenomena were included by Schneider among the so-called first-rank symptoms of schizophrenia. Today, these symptoms are viewed more broadly as nonspecific psychotic symptoms, more likely to be seen in schizophrenia but not pathognomonic of the disorder.

A 42-year-old man with schizophrenia rarely went out of his house and typically believed that others were toying with him during the few conversations he had. When asked about these feelings and behaviors, he described the complete conviction that everyone could hear what he was thinking. He found this very embarrassing when in public and therefore liked to stay in his house. Additionally, when he did converse with others, he attributed their asking him questions as a form of mocking him because he was sure they knew what he was thinking anyway.

Obsessional thinking is stereotyped, repetitive, persistent thinking that is recognized as one's own thoughts. In contrast to patients with delusional thought passivity, obsessional patients do not experience their thoughts as being controlled by outside forces. Nonetheless, they experience only partial control over the obsessional thoughts. They can, with great effort, stop thinking the obsessional thoughts but cannot prevent them from recurring. Thus, characteristic of obsessions are the subjective experience of compulsion and the resistance to it. In classic obsessional thinking, insight is retained, and, as bizarre as some obsessions are, patients know that these thoughts are irrational and their own. However, more recent studies have revealed that insight into obsessional thinking is more variable than had been previously believed, at times becoming delusional. At times, obsessions may be pervasive enough to dominate the patient's consciousness. Obsessions may be simple, a sequence of words, or elaborate, such as enumerating the possible consequences of a past behavior and elaborating a cascading sequence of typically catastrophic events. Typical obsessional themes in OCD involve preoccupations with dirt and contamination, fear of harming others, symmetry, and those related to health and appearance.

Whenever she drove her car over a bump in the road, a 42-year-old woman with OCD worried that she had hit a pedestrian. Because she could not see the body, she drove around the block to look for it. After seeing no body in the road, she was transiently reassured but, within moments, became concerned that the body may have rolled under a parked car. She drove around the block for at least 30 minutes searching for the body when this obsessional thought possessed her.

Obsessional thoughts are usually seen in conjunction with compulsive behaviors, which are rituals linked to the obsessions typically constructed to undo the effects of the thought. Thus, contamination obsessions are linked to cleaning rituals, fears of harming others lead to checking rituals, and so forth.

The most prominent disturbance of thinking complexity is an impaired capacity to think abstractly. *Abstract thinking* is the ability to assume a mental set, to keep simultaneously in mind all of the aspects of a complex situation, to move from feature to feature as indicated by the situation, and to abstract common properties. Complex thinking also concerns the ability to simultaneously consider many different, vague, and subtle aspects of situations; to appreciate differing and contradictory points of view; and to integrate these multiple dimensions to form opinions that are marked by differentiatedness and nuance. Normal individuals vary greatly in their abilities to engage in abstract thinking—geniuses in mathematics and theoretical physics leave most mortals far behind. *Concrete thinking* is a disturbance in the ability to form abstract concepts, generally illustrated by literal mindedness and the inability to abstract the commonality of members of a group, for example, the fact that a flea and a tree are similar in that they are both living things. Concrete thinkers seem unable to free themselves from the literal or superficial meanings of words. Concrete thinkers may be more prone to prejudice and stereotypical thinking and more likely to manifest unidimensional or "all-or-none" reactions to complex situations. Concrete thinking can be seen in individuals with lower intelligence, organic mental disorders, and schizophrenia. Schizophrenic patients may also exhibit highly selective disturbances of abstraction.

THOUGHT CONTENT

The normal content of thought, the buzzing, booming stream of consciousness that constitutes the stuff of everyday life, comprises awareness, concerns, beliefs, preoccupations, wishes, and fantasies occurring with various degrees of clarity, vividness, differentiation, imagination, and strength. Normal thought is often illogical, containing many beliefs and prejudices that may be clearly contradictory but are nevertheless held with passion and conviction.

Belief systems are the scaffolding of thought, chains of impressions, and expectations around which plans and behaviors are organized. Belief systems may be attitudinal, setting general expectations and biases about the world that inform how incoming information is processed; examples are optimism, pessimism, and paranoia. Some beliefs are effervescent and fleeting, whereas others are pervasive, tenacious, enduring, and influential. The enduring belief systems are associated with behaviors consistent with the belief, at times dominating interpersonal relationships and lifestyles. Some beliefs are unique and private, whereas many are shared by others.

A 48-year-old man had been deeply pessimistic since childhood. Although he had no vegetative features of depression, he believed and behaved as if the world was an awful place dominated by dishonest and selfish individuals. Having any goals seemed foolish to him, given the nature of the world. He expressed these beliefs regularly to his children, to the dismay of his wife, who did not share his belief system.

Imaginative fantasy is an important component of normal thought. The vivid, eidetic imaginations of young children can produce vivid fantasies in which children become fully immersed, almost as if in hypnotic states. During latency, many children develop imaginary companions as playmates. In later years, imaginative thinking in which previously separate streams of thought playfully interact with one another to produce new ideas may be the essence of the creative reverie. Artists, writers, and creative scientists may retain access to these forms of thinking more readily than others. Meditative states of mind may facilitate the emergence of imaginative insights. Such thinking may also occur in dreams. Intrusive reveries are normal and common components of the usual adult stream of consciousness. During periods of specific deprivation, such as starvation or sexual deprivation, elaborate wish-fulfilling daydreams frequently occur.

Ideas are the contents of the stream of thought. Those that are consistent with one's sense of self, compatible with the individual's self-image, are called *ego-syntonic*. Other thoughts that conflict with one's central values are called *ego-alien* or *ego-dystonic*. An ego-dystonic impulse to kill someone, inconsistent with one's predominant value systems, may generate a counteractive ego-syntonic thought such as "you really don't mean it."

Disturbances in Thought Contents Abnormal beliefs and convictions form the core of thought content disturbances. Considerations of abnormality regarding beliefs and convictions must take the person's culture into account. Beliefs that may seem abnormal in one culture or subculture may be commonly accepted in another. For example, religious hallucinations, attributed to psychological or biological factors by contemporary Western societies, are routinely attributed to religious and spiritual causes by many other cultures. With regard to intensity of conviction, distorted beliefs range on a continuum from overvalued ideas to the determined, unshakable belief that is characteristic of fixed delusions. Abnormal beliefs and delusions are, in most circumstances, diagnostically nonspecific. Delusions are commonly seen in mania, depression, schizoaffective disorder, delirium, dementia, and substance abuse–related syndromes, as well as in schizophrenia and delusional disorders.

Overvalued ideas are unreasonable and sustained abnormal beliefs that are held beyond the bounds of reason. Patients with overvalued ideas have little or no insight into the fact that their ideas are very unlikely to be valid; however, the ideas themselves are not as patently unbelievable as most delusions. The distorted body images of body dysmorphic disorder exemplify overvalued ideas. Morbid jealousy and preoccupation with a spouse's possible infidelity may constitute an overvalued idea if no real evidence has ever existed to warrant suspicion.

> A 42-year-old man who had a brief relationship with a woman was unable to accept the fact that she no longer wanted to see him. He ruminated about every encounter they had and interpreted small gestures in the past as indicating her undying love for him. His infatuation led him to follow her repeatedly to work and school, and he pursued her relentlessly, to the point that she brought charges against him for stalking.

Ideas of reference are false personalized interpretations of actual events in which individuals believe that occurrences or remarks refer specifically to them when in fact they do not. Ideas of reference may be less firmly held than delusional beliefs.

> A 24-year-old psychotic woman from a religious background was completely distracted when anyone in the room cleared his or her throat. She explained that she interpreted throat clearing as a distinct message to her, reminding her that she was a sinner who needed to be cleaner and purer in her behaviors and thoughts.

Delusions *Delusions* are fixed, false beliefs, strongly held and immutable in the face of refuting evidence, that are not consonant with the person's educational, social, and cultural background. Thus, delusional thoughts can only be understood or evaluated with at least some knowledge of patients' interpersonal worlds, such as their involvements with religious or political groups. One of the mind's primary functions is to generate beliefs, including myths and meaning systems. These beliefs provide the individual with a sense of personal and group identity and with ways of understanding reality. They are most noticeable when shared untestable beliefs form the basis for group cohesion, as in religions and cults. Some groups adhere to their cherished beliefs despite the abundance of plausible contrary evidence—for example, the fundamentalist sects that take the biblical creation story literally. In the face of contrary evidence or grave personal threat, individuals often cling to their primary beliefs as matters of faith (i.e., alternative, nonrefutable bases for understanding). The strong faith with which religious, political, and nationalistic convictions are held, even at the cost of death, shows the power that untestable beliefs can have on behavior. Potential mental health advantages of religious beliefs have been demonstrated in epidemiological studies showing that those with a sense of personal devotion report fewer depressive symptoms.

Subjectively, delusions are indistinguishable from everyday beliefs. Therefore, the subjective experience of a delusion is no different from the subjective experience of believing that the earth is round or that one's spouse is the same person one married on his or her wedding day. Because of the identical experience of delusions and other strongly held beliefs, it is generally impossible to argue a patient out of a delusional belief. The content of delusions is highly influenced by culture. As an example, in a study comparing delusions among Austrian and Pakistani schizophrenic patients, persecutory delusions were predominant in both cultures, but differences were seen in the sources of the persecutory beliefs. Similarly, whereas centuries ago, delusions of persecution often concerned persecution by the devil and had religious connotations, persecutory delusions today often take on contemporary technological, political, and social perspectives.

> A 38-year-old schizophrenic woman was certain that the profusion of television satellite dishes in her neighborhood were all meant to beam radio signals from alien civilizations far off into the stars into her head, and that, in turn, these satellite dishes could pick up her thoughts and beam them all over the universe. She was particularly embarrassed by the fact that the sexual fantasies she frequently imagined would be publicly broadcast and that her sinfulness would become known.

Although delusions are diagnostically nonspecific, some types of delusions are more prevalent in one disorder than another. For example, although delusions of control and delusional percepts are often seen in schizophrenia, they also occur, albeit less frequently, in psychotic mood disorders. Similarly, classic mood-congruent delusions, with grandiose themes seen in mania or delusions of poverty characteristic of depression, may also be seen in schizophrenia.

Table 8–3 lists some characteristics by which delusions have been classified. *Simple delusions* contain relatively few elements, whereas *complex delusions* may contain extensive elaborations of people, spirits, motives, and situations.

Systematized delusions are usually restricted or circumscribed to well-delineated areas and are ordinarily associated with a clear sensorium and absence of hallucinations. They are often isolated

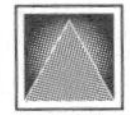

Table 8–3
Characteristics of Delusions

Simple vs. complex
Complete vs. partial
Systematized vs. nonsystematized
Primary (autochthonous) vs. secondary
Persecutory vs. nonpersecutory
How they affect behavior

from other aspects of behavior. In contrast, *nonsystematized delusions* usually extend into many areas of life, and new data—new people and situations—are constantly incorporated to further support the presence of the delusion. The patient usually has concurrent mental confusion, hallucinations, and some affective lability. Whereas the patient with a closed systematized delusional system may go about life relatively unperturbed, the patient with a nonsystematized delusion frequently has poor social functioning and often behaves in response to the delusional beliefs.

Complete delusions are those held utterly without doubt. In contrast, *partial delusions* are those in which the patient entertains doubts about the delusional beliefs. Such doubts may be seen during the slow development of a delusion, as the delusion is gradually given up, or intermittently throughout its course.

During an acute schizophrenic episode, a 23-year-old man was completely convinced that the subtle pattern of superficial veins on his legs was evidence of "astral domination" by extraterrestrial beings. After 1 week of antipsychotic medication, he believed the veins were caused by others with special powers but was less sure. Two weeks later, he denied believing that the patterns on his legs were other than superficial veins and dismissed his previous belief with a shrug.

An *autochthonous delusion* is one that takes form in an instant, without identifiable preceding events, as if full awareness suddenly bursts forth in an unexpected flash of insight like a bolt from the blue. These delusions may be quite elaborate.

After a 2-year period of gradual academic and interpersonal decline, a 21-year-old man had the sudden conviction that certain songs played on the radio used his voice in the role of lead singer. He could not explain why this would be so nor why this belief emerged suddenly when it did.

Aside from the autochthonous types, three other types of delusions have been described as primary. *Delusional percept* refers to the experience of interpreting a normal perception with a delusional meaning, one that has enormous personal significance to the patient. *Delusional atmosphere* or *delusional mood* is a state of perplexity, a sense that something uncanny or odd is going on that involves the patient but in unspecified ways. Ordinary events may take on heightened significance, but the delusional interpretations are fleeting, although the uncanny feeling stays. Typically, after a period, full-blown delusions develop, replacing the delusional mood. *Delusional memory* is the memory of an event that is clearly delusional. As an example, a patient "remembered" that his fourth-grade teacher slipped lysergic acid diethylamide (LSD) into his apple juice; this memory served to explain his psychotic disorder. The elaboration of false memories and their subsequent fixed belief may assume delusional proportions.

A young schizophrenic woman attended a "trauma group" with her roommate and gradually came to believe that she had been repeatedly sexually assaulted by her father from the time she was in the crib. What started out as vague dream-like images gradually coalesced into a series of "sensed" memories that then took on specific visual images of her father's fingers penetrating her and of his looking down at her in the crib leering. Her parents were horrified by these accusations, and there was not a shred of evidence to corroborate her increasingly venomous accusations.

Patients vary considerably in the extent to which they take action in response to delusional thoughts. Just as patients can experience delusions of their thoughts being controlled (thought passivity), they may similarly experience their feelings, behaviors, and will as controlled by outside forces. These *delusions of control* (or passivity experiences) occasionally, albeit uncommonly, result in dramatic self-destructive or aggressive behaviors, as illustrated by the murderer who called himself Son of Sam. This psychotic killer murdered a series of people in New York and claimed that he was the powerless agent of a force that required him to commit the acts. To defend themselves and others against delusional anticipated events, some patients may take bold and occasionally destructive actions.

A 38-year-old man with untreated schizophrenia was transferred from jail to hospital for evaluation and treatment after shooting (but not killing) his neighbor. He explained that the neighbor had been "hassling" him for 6 months by making noise in the middle of the night, laughing at him, and listening to his conversations through the wall. The patient explained that he shot the neighbor as a warning to back off.

Table 8–4 lists some classic types of delusions. Although less common than those involving paranoia, grandiosity, and influence, delusions of misidentification are prominently reported because of their inherently intriguing nature. In *Capgras' syndrome,* the patient believes that someone close to him or her has been replaced by an exact double. In *Frégoli's phenomenon,* strangers are identified as familiar people in the patient's life. In the *delusion of doubles*, patients believe that another person has been physically transformed into themselves.

Olfactory delusions that one emanates a foul odor are common in social anxiety syndromes, in which individuals are particularly concerned about potentially embarrassing themselves and others.

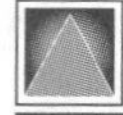

Table 8–4
Some Classic Types of Delusions

Delusions of persecution
Delusions of grandeur
Delusions of influence
Delusion of having sinned
Nihilistic delusions
Somatic delusions
Delusion of doubles (doppelganger)
Delusional jealousy (Othello syndrome)
Delusional mood
Delusional perception
Delusional memory
Delusions of erotic attachment (Clérambault's syndrome)
Delusions of replacement of significant others (Capgras' syndrome)
Delusions of disguise (Frégoli's phenomenon)
Shared delusions (*folie à deux, folie à trois, folie à famille*)

Delusions are not only seen in isolated individuals. Shared delusions may occur in couples (*folie à deux*) and in families (*folie à famille*). Many psychiatrists consider group delusions to be present in some cults as well, but exactly where the cutoff points occur between delusions and other zealous beliefs held by larger, more traditional and well-organized religious, political, and other groups is arguable.

A husband and wife appearing at a psychiatric emergency department both wore skullcaps made of sheets of aluminum foil. The reason for the caps, they concurred, was to ward off radio signals being beamed to their brains from outer space. The husband was a dominant personality who had originated this fixed delusion. His wife, a mild-mannered, passive person, seemed to have accepted her husband's interpretation of events without challenging them at all.

Disturbances of Judgment Judgment involves a complex and diverse group of mental functions that includes analytical thinking, social and ethical action tendencies, and depth of understanding or insight. Analytical thinking includes the capacity to discriminate and to weigh the pros and cons of potential alternative actions. Social and ethical action tendencies are closely related to culture and upbringing. The evidence for genetic factors in antisocial personality disorder (defined primarily by judgments that lead to criminal behaviors) points to the additional role of constitutional factors. Insight may reflect intelligence, learning, cognitive style, and the capacity to integrate intellectual knowledge with emotional awareness.

Impairments of judgment occur in many psychiatric disturbances. Anxiety states, intoxications, fatigue, and even group pressures may cause temporary impairments of judgment in otherwise normal individuals. In mood disorders, judgment may be impaired by either an exaggerated evaluation of risk or failure in depression or, conversely, of inadequate appreciation of risk or danger in mania. Organic brain damage and psychotic disorders may chronically impair any aspect of judgment in any person, regardless of premorbid character. Poor role models and deviant social backgrounds may lead to social and ethical action tendencies quite different from those of the examiner. Thus, someone raised in a criminal environment may have superb analytical judgment and self-awareness, which are, however, put to illegal use.

A 48-year-old man with bipolar disorder became severely depressed. As part of his guilt symptoms, he believed that he could no longer be a good enough husband and divorced his wife, despite her protests. When his depression remitted, he realized the depth of his poor judgment and remarried his wife.

Judgment may be impaired in one dimension and spared in others. Individuals may retain sound ethical judgment when their analytical capacities fail or may retain excellent analytical abilities for nonpersonal matters, although lacking insight into personal situations or behaviors. Thus, some people who can provide socially appropriate responses to traditional mental status examination questions, such as what one would do in a movie theater if fire broke out or what one would do with a stamped and sealed addressed envelope found in the street, might at the same time be incapable of accurately assessing crucial clinical or more personal matters specifically related to one's capacity to provide informed consent, such as the pros and cons of receiving a medication or electroconvulsive therapy (ECT); regarding judgments necessary to provide oneself with food, clothing, and shelter; or insight into one's state of health or illness. The apocryphal story about the delusional patient able to accurately evaluate and fix a broken-down car that had stymied the mechanics, ending with the patient's declaring, "I may be crazy, but I'm not stupid," indicates the selective nature of poor judgment within psychiatric disorders.

The term *insight*, usually in the context of self-awareness, has been used in a variety of ways. *Basic insight* refers to a superficial awareness of one's situation. In evaluating insight into one's psychiatric condition, basic insight allows an individual to acknowledge the presence of an illness. A deeper level of insight is operating when the patient has an intellectual appreciation of what is going on (e.g., "I have hallucinations and delusions, and my doctors have told me that I have schizophrenia and must take medication"). Still deeper levels of insight reflect more complete cognitive and emotional appreciation of a situation (e.g., "I realize that I have schizophrenia, that it impairs my judgment and social function at times, and that I will have to take medications if I am to minimize my symptoms and try to make the most of my life. I feel profoundly disappointed about this affliction because it prevents me from achieving some of the goals I've always wished for. Nevertheless, I have do my best to get over my disappointment and hurt feelings so that I can get whatever I can out of life.").

Of course, different depths of insight as self-awareness can be evaluated in many other situations, such as physical illness, quality and nature of relationships, an appreciation of strengths and weaknesses in professional situations, and so forth. In formal studies of insight using standardized instruments, lack of insight correlates with poor outcome in schizophrenia and bipolar disorder, medication noncompliance, and suicidality. Improvement of psychosis does not necessarily correlate with improved insight. Impaired insight may be associated with frontal lobe abnormalities. Insight may be as seriously impaired in mania as in schizophrenia and, contrary to earlier beliefs, may be lacking in OCD.

Judgment may be impaired by several factors, including cognitive clouding (as in disturbances of consciousness, e.g., intoxication, so that one's usual analytical abilities are impaired), self-deception, and impulsivity.

Self-deception refers to the almost universal tendency to hide certain issues about the external world or about oneself from various levels of awareness. Self-deception functions as a coping strategy, fostering or maintaining comfortable perspectives about the world and avoiding confrontation with issues and realities that inevitably stir up painful conflicts or the need for difficult actions, thereby preserving emotional calm. In addition, studies suggest that self-deception enables us to act and to be perceived as more convincing in the service of particular goals, as in romantic relationships or business dealings. Therefore, although "kidding ourselves" may sometimes reflect impaired judgment, it may at times also yield certain important strategic advantages.

Impulsive judgment describes a tendency to avoid taking the time and thought to fully understand and integrate all of the facts and levels of awareness required for optimal decision making. Impulsive judgment may occur only with certain issues or situations (such as how one picks investments), signal an impaired state (such as intoxication), or reflect a pervasive character trait.

Rapidly made judgments, and even so-called snap judgments, may not be maladaptively impulsive, even when they involve very important areas of life. Rapid decisions can be very accurate, highly adaptive, and even life-saving, especially if made against a background of great experience, wisdom, and forethought concerning the area requiring the decision.

Because, in clinical practice, the terms *insight* and *judgment* are often applied to individuals' awareness and decision making about their psychiatric status, complex motivational states that incorporate insight and judgment related to how one is dealing with one's problems, the so-called stages of readiness for change, bear mention at this point. Initially described in relation to substance abuse, including alcoholism and smoking, these stages have received considerable attention and form an important aspect of clinical assessment across other diagnostic categories such as eating disorders. Several stages have been described: (1) precontemplation: the person expresses no intention to change (may be in denial); (2) contemplation: the person acknowledges a problem and states an intention to change within several months but not right away; (3) preparation: the person intends to do something about changing in the near future and may have already made some false starts; (4) action: the individual has engaged in making sustained behavior changes; (5) maintenance: the individual has been engaged in changed behavior for more than 6 months; and (6) termination: the individual has succeeded in the change and is unlikely to ever return to the original behavior.

Disturbances of Consciousness

Consciousness can be defined as subjective awareness of the self and environment. Biologists increasingly believe that a continuum of consciousness exists, extending from lower animals through *Homo sapiens*. However, consciousness is subject to conflicting definitions and conceptualizations, and exactly where consciousness begins in evolution remains unclear. Philosophers agree that it is the subjectivity of experience, the so-called qualia of consciousness, that clearly distinguishes living consciousness from at least this generation's best versions of self-regulating automata, elegant computers, or robots. All current attempts to even approach an understanding of consciousness are very unsatisfying, and consciousness remains unexplained and as yet unexplainable from a scientific point of view. Consciousness has been viewed as an emergent property of complex biological nervous systems, as a poorly understood general property of an even more mysterious and complex universe, or as a phenomenon to be understood only in religious and spiritual terms. One of the best analyses to date of possible relationships between the construction of a brain and the possibility of consciousness has been set forth by Gerald Edelman, who believes that reflective consciousness cannot occur until complex higher-order brain systems evolve whose major functions are to monitor the experiences, activities, and results of activities of those lower-order brain systems that deal directly with appraising and responding to the external and internal environments. Such higher-order metasystems require the presence of memory so that current and immediate impressions can be checked and compared against past experiences. These metasystems may use a variety of sensor mechanisms to detect and signal their sensations or perceptions of various events. Some of these sensors may correspond to feeling states, and some may correspond initially to preverbal thought-like mechanisms that contain the capacity to develop and recognize abstract categories and, ultimately, conceptual language-based thought.

Clinically, consciousness can be considered from both qualitative as well as quantitative viewpoints. Qualitatively, consciousness does not seem to be an all-or-none phenomenon. Rather, conscious experiences may gradually and phasically shift in focus, intensity, and clarity; altered states of consciousness may occur in which some aspects of consciousness, such as sensation, perception, memory, orientation, and judgment, are enhanced or impaired relative to other aspects. Quantitatively, crude divisions can be made between states depending on the relative presence, or impairment, or total absence of consciousness. Even within the single individual, consciousness is not a unitary phenomenon. Multiple streams of thought, operating at multiple levels of preconsciousnesses appear to exist in all people almost all of the time, with various elements in these coexisting streams constantly shifting into higher or lower levels of conscious awareness. In pathological states, even more remarkable properties of consciousness are seen, for example, the existence of coconsciousness in humans who have had commissurotomies and of seemingly multiple discrete consciousnesses in patients with dissociative identity disorders.

Experiments involving patients with commissurotomies of the corpus callosum have shown the existence of two virtually separate systems of consciousness that seem to operate side by side. For example, when in the course of an experiment, the picture of a nude woman was flashed only to the right brain (the left visual field) of a commissurotomized patient, the subject verbally denied being aware of anything unusual (i.e., the left brain—the verbal brain—was unaware). But, at the same time, he started to squirm and blush, blurting out, "Oh, you have some machine!" Similarly, when a cup was presented to the right brain (left visual field) only, the patient denied seeing anything (left brain was unaware, and language output of the left brain indicated no awareness), but he was able to pick out the cup from an assortment of objects with his left hand (right brain control). That literal splitting of verbal awareness from visual–spatial awareness in the brain produces behavior that is at least superficially similar to that of patients who deny being consciously upset by an event but who react with strong visceral responses. Although this formulation is simplistic, the separate consciousness for logical–verbal and for spatial–visual awareness demonstrated in split brain experiments may be crude analogs for more highly differentiated and discrete types of awarenesses and modes of information processing. Furthermore, the very fact that there are separate and, to some extent, competing modes of consciousness may increase the likelihood of psychological distress because the various modes are capable of yielding internally conflicting views of reality.

Psychological and Physiological Factors

In ordinary states of alert consciousness, individuals are able to deploy adequate amounts of attention to their surroundings and to reflective thought. Normal people vary enormously in their ability to pay careful attention in different settings without being distracted; individual variations may reflect temperamental and cognitive style differences as well as physiological shifts within the individual. Many functions of attentive consciousness, including attention, planning, and the capacity to appropriately switch between mental tasks, so-called distractor resistant memory, have been linked to the activity of specific neurons in area 46 of the prefrontal cortex.

A sense of increased consciousness with heightened alertness, awareness, and sharper thinking may be experienced in states of highly aroused emotional states such as threat, sexual attraction, falling in love, or other high-stakes events such as hunting among primitives, sporting competitions, or performing in front of an important audience. High levels of arousal do not necessarily guarantee effective attention because optimal consciousness depends on optimal arousal. Too little arousal due to illness or fatigue may result in insufficient stimulation and mental lethargy, diminishing the sense of alertness and attentiveness, whereas too much arousal may result in hyperintense alertness but distractibility and scattered attention.

Consciousness involves, among other things, the experience of a continuous sense of self and of the environment, existing coherently in time and space. The experience of time and its passage may be altered by shifts in the level of awareness and by emotional states such as boredom, concentration, pain, and discomfort. The experience of time and space may be altered by hypnosis, marijuana, psychoactive and psychedelic drugs, and other events directly affecting brain physiology.

Disturbances in the Level of Consciousness Levels of consciousness (i.e., alertness, awareness, and attentiveness) may be pathologically increased or decreased. Such changes are diagnostically nonspecific and can occur in many different disorders. When levels of arousal and alertness are mildly elevated, as in hypomania or with the ingestion of small amounts of psychostimulants, subjective experiences are typically positive. In these situations, the person experiences intense alertness, prolonged concentrating ability, and hyperesthesias in which perceptual vividness is heightened: Colors are brighter, sounds are sharper, and touch is more intense than usual. With further increases in arousal and consciousness as seen in mania, more severe intoxications with amphetamines and cocaine, and catatonic excitement, attention fragments. Heightened alertness transforms into hypervigilance and paranoia, and hyperesthesias become unpleasant.

Diminished levels of consciousness can be described on a continuum. *Clouding of consciousness* is marked by diminished awareness of sensory cues and diminished attentiveness to the environment and to the self. Secondary process thinking is most notably compromised, and more primary process thinking emerges into consciousness. In this state, one's ability to appreciate subtleties and to think in a nuanced manner is diminished and is replaced by more dichotomous all-or-none, stereotypical thinking. The level of consciousness may fluctuate rapidly in relation to the internal physiological state or to the degree of external stimulation. In alterations of consciousness, confusion may occur with disorientation to time, place, or person. The patient is usually highly distractible and unable to pay sustained attention to a single stimulus.

Torpor is a condition in which the patient is drowsy, falls asleep easily, and shows a narrowed range of perception and slowed thinking. *Stupor* is a state of diminished consciousness in which the patient remains mute and still, although the eyes are open and may follow external objects. In the most extreme impairment of consciousness, *coma*, there is no evidence of mental activity at all. The patient essentially appears to be functioning on a decorticate or decerebrate level. In *akinetic mutism*, or *coma vigil*, patients with profound brainstem lesions appear to be awake with their eyes open, but there is in fact no evidence of consciousness. The commonly used Glasgow Coma Scale incorporates these dimensions.

Delirium, the acute confusional state, is usually characterized by a relatively abrupt onset and short duration of clouded, reduced, and fragmented attention; impaired memory and learning; perceptual and cognitive abnormalities, such as hallucinations and delusions; disrupted sleep; and other autonomic dysfunction. The level of consciousness may be consistently diminished or may fluctuate. The electroencephalogram (EEG) usually shows diffuse slowing. Typical motor abnormalities include an increase in general restlessness, fine and course tremors, and myoclonic jerks. Autonomic disturbances commonly include tachycardia, fever, elevated blood pressure, diaphoresis, and pupillary dilatation. The causes of delirium are legion, including systemic medical disorders, such as metabolic imbalances or infections, intracranial disorders due to traumatic, structural, and electrical causes, and drug intoxications and withdrawal states.

Attentional difficulties are manifest by impairments in the person's ability to deploy, focus, and sustain attention. Some attentional difficulties first appear in early childhood as developmental problems of uncertain cause and are described as attention-deficit disorders (inattentive or hyperactive types). Secondary attention-deficit difficulties may appear de novo in adulthood due to a variety of exogenous agents, psychiatric disorders, and late-life developmental and degenerative factors.

In *narcolepsy*, characterized by sudden lapses into sleep, one's usual ability to stay alert and maintain consciousness is impaired. At times, the onset of profound sleepiness is gradual, accompanied by hypnogogic phenomena, in which dream-like images invade consciousness, and at other times the shift in consciousness appears to be almost instantaneous. This syndrome, occurring in approximately 1 in 10,000 persons, is thought to be the second most frequent cause of automobile collisions after alcohol intoxication.

Altered States of Consciousness Consciousness may also be qualitatively changed, with the production of altered states. Drugs such as scopolamine (Transderm) with strong central anticholinergic properties, some seizures, and, on occasion, other conditions associated with delirium can induce *twilight states*, dream-like states of wakeful consciousness in which attention is poor, an admixture of primary and secondary process thinking appears, and patients fade in and out of alertness. Dream-like experiences intrude into the stream of conversation. Emotional outbursts or violent acts may occur during twilight states.

Mystical states of consciousness may occur in normal and pathological conditions. Intense meditation and peak or epiphanic experiences, reported by more than 10 percent of normal individuals in community surveys, may produce a sense that the self dissolves or expands, that the self fuses mystically with the cosmos, that time stops, and that universal meaning becomes clear. These perceptions may be accompanied by a sense of rejuvenation and renewed personal identity, ineffability, intense emotionality, and concurrent perceptual changes. Such experiences do not ordinarily last more than a few minutes. Many people have achieved these states through the use of psychedelic agents such as mescaline and LSD. Reports of a white light at the end of a tunnel, described by individuals using psychedelics and in near-death experiences, have been linked to specific neurophysiological pathways believed to be stimulated under these conditions.

> A 43-year-old female accountant with no prior history of spiritual or religious practice sustained a severe head injury in an automobile accident that left her comatose for approximately 6 months. When she awoke, she reported that at some point during her coma, she estimated in the third month, she experienced a profound mystical experience, which included a glorious union with God and knowing that she would not only awaken to return to life but that all was "as it should be" with the universe. After recovery, with ongoing motor impairment, she became profoundly spiritual, started attending church and teaching the Bible, and constantly evidenced a beatific glow, which she attributed to her mystical experience.

Although hypnosis lacks a consensually accepted definition, its hallmarks are selective attention, suggestibility, and dissociation. Most, but not all, people can be hypnotized to some degree. Up to 90 percent of people are capable of achieving a light trance, whereas 10 to 20 percent are capable of entering a deep trance and exhibiting remarkable hypnotic phenomena. Hypnosis occurs when the subject is in a state of heightened, not diminished, attention. EEG studies have shown hypnotized subjects to be fully awake and alert. The heightened concentration probably accounts for the unusual levels of sensory and motor performance often seen under hypnosis and self-hypnosis.

Hypnotic phenomena include hypnotically induced hallucinations (including negative hallucinations in which the subject selectively does not perceive sights, sounds, or other stimuli), anesthesia, sustained motor behaviors and acts of strength ordinarily beyond the individual's capacity, and distortions of memory (both hypermnesias and amnesia). Several phenomena that reveal the multiple nature of consciousness, for example, coconsciousness, are also demonstrable. Experiments have shown that even when a subject in deep trance has achieved profound hypnotic anesthesia and can, for example, keep a hand submerged in ice water for longer periods of time than usual, part of the hypnotized subject's consciousness continues to register exactly how painful the experience actually is and can signal the researcher about the pain, by finger movements, without the subject having any conscious awareness or disturbance. This phenomenon, called the *hidden observer*, has also been seen in postsurgical patients who, under hypnotic trance after surgery, have been able to accurately recall conversations in the operating room that occurred while they were under general anesthesia. Dissociative and psychosomatic phenomena have also been induced with hypnosis. With posthypnotic suggestion, for example, subjects may carry out complex actions without any hint that they are actually doing so because they were previously instructed to act that way under hypnosis. When asked why they are carrying out these activities, such subjects usually make up various reasons, although seemingly unaware of the real reasons for their actions. It has been suggested, not entirely facetiously, that many normal daily activities are conducted in a trance-like posthypnotic state, and although these activities are attributed to conscious intention, they may in fact be carried out due to previous suggestion. Advertisers know this well. Urticaria (hives) can be hypnotically induced and hypnotically made to disappear. Plantar warts have been successfully treated with hypnosis, and, in these conditions, diminished blood supplies to their bases have been demonstrated. It has recently been appreciated that yoga masters can exert remarkable control over basic bodily functions through self-hypnosis. As yet, little is known of the full extent to which heightened concentration may influence physiological regulation.

Suggestibility Pathological suggestibility may be seen in several clinical conditions. Automatic obedience has been described in *echolalia* (the automatic repetition of a sentence or phrase just uttered by another person), *echopraxia* (the automatic mimicking of a movement performed by another person), and *waxy flexibility* (maintaining for a prolonged period of time a posture in which one is placed), symptoms common in catatonic states. In situations of group delusions, and sometimes in cults, passive individuals adopt the delusional beliefs of stronger ones. In epidemic hysteria, as described among young women at the Salem witch trials in Arthur Miller's *The Crucible*, distorted and even delusional perceptions and beliefs may sweep over a group that has been highly aroused by a charismatic leader.

Autosuggestibility can be seen in the constructions of false memories in which an individual progressively comes to believe that something that never happened in fact occurred. Such false memories may be held with such great conviction that they are indistinguishable from the memories of real events. Because of this, memories recovered during therapy (in which there is often great pressure to "remember" certain events) cannot be taken at face value without corroboration from other sources. Various types and degrees of self-deception may be more common in individuals who are more suggestible.

DISSOCIATIVE PHENOMENA *Dissociation* refers to the splitting off from one another of what are ordinarily closely connected behaviors, thoughts, or feelings. Dissociative states are those in which there is a disturbance or alteration in the normally integrated functions of identity, memory, or consciousness and include trances, fugues, blackouts, multiple personalities (dissociative identity disorder), and dissociative frenzies. Although dissociative states are ordinarily believed to be functional in nature, arising as an adaptive defense in individuals subjected to a great deal of trauma, particularly at early ages, they occur regularly with a variety of neurological disorders, particularly those with partial complex seizures. In one series, one-third of patients with complex partial seizures had dissociative phenomena, including multiple personality. In these patients, the dissociative phenomena were not related to the seizure activity but to interictal alterations.

As in posthypnotic amnesia, elaborate activities can occur in dissociative states for which the subject has no conscious memory. This amnesia is functional in nature and may be reversed by hypnosis or drug-facilitated disinhibition, for example, with amobarbital (sodium Amytal) infusion. In many of the functional dissociative states, amnestic episodes may occur for years or decades before the patient seeks medical or psychiatric attention. *Blackouts* are periods of amnesia in alcoholism, other intoxications, or after head trauma. An alcoholic blackout period may last for hours to days, after which the person has no recollection of what transpired, although other observers attest to the fact that, during this period, the individual carried out multiple complicated behaviors. Although memory of the blackout is lost to the predominant consciousness, during subsequent reintoxication, memories of events occurring during the previous blackout may be reawakened. This phenomenon, known as *state-dependent memory*, occurs in many other conditions as well, signifying that one's ability to retrieve specific memories may be highly influenced by specific physiological alterations due to external intoxicants or other unusual physiological states.

A 43-year-old man with a 20-year history of sustained alcohol abuse was unable during a period of sobriety to recall for hospital staff the names, phone numbers, and addresses of his close friends and associates. Several weeks later, when he returned to the emergency department in an intoxicated state, he was able to recall all of those details in a reasonably straightforward manner.

Psychogenic fugue is characterized by prolonged periods in which individuals carry out very complex activities without having any recollection for their previous lives, identities, or even names. They often travel away from customary locales and assume entirely new identities. By definition, psychogenic fugue cannot be due to a neurological disorder. In comparison, the discontinuity of experience in *psychogenic amnesia* is typically more circumscribed and does not involve assuming an entirely new identity. The dissociated memories and affects often reveal themselves in disguised form such as nightmares, intrusive visual images, and conversion symptoms. Typically, in psychogenic amnesia, an individual may not be able to recollect what transpired during a specific period, for example, before the age of 9 or 10 years in the context of a traumatic childhood; during catastrophic events, such as traumatic, gruesome combat; or during less momentous events that a person prefers to forget to preserve self-esteem by denying shameful, immoral, or illegal activities.

A 28-year-old infantryman could not recollect the events of the combat situation in which he had been wounded and several of his comrades killed. Several months afterward, he participated in a series of Amytal-facilitated interviews, during which the events of combat came back to him. He recalled becoming panicky during the firefight, turning, and running away while several other soldiers in his squad, several of whom were killed, yelled to try to get him to stay in place and fight. After the interviews, he cried inconsolably and blamed himself, somewhat irrationally, for their deaths, wondering if his remaining in place and fighting might have saved their lives.

Dissociative Identity Disorder *Dissociative identity disorder*, previously known as *multiple personality disorder*, is a chronic, dissociative state in which two or more separate ongoing identities or personalities alternate in consciousness. It usually occurs in people who, as young children, were severely and repeatedly brutalized. The number of identities is variable, with some cases reporting 25 or more identities. The development of dissociated alter personalities is believed to be a last-ditch, primitive psychological defense against inescapable and unbearable traumatic situations. The personalities may be of different ages and even different sexes. Typically, the presenting identity is dysphoric, anxious, and constricted, may have headaches and periods of blackout or amnesia, and is not aware of the other personalities. A second identity is typically vivacious and uninhibited. Another identity may know all about the other personalities and has a wise perspective on the life events leading to the problems and regarding possible solutions. A classic case is described in a popular book and film *The Three Faces of Eve*.

In so-called channeling, dissociated, complex part personalities are produced in trance states in which fictitious past lives or spirit lives are created.

Ganser's Syndrome In Ganser's syndrome, the patient responds to questions by giving approximate or patently ridiculous answers, for example, in response to the question "what sound does a dog make?" the patient answers "moo." Additional features of the syndrome include alterations in consciousness, hallucinations (or pseudohallucinations), conversion phenomena, and amnesia for the episode during which these symptoms are manifest. This syndrome has most commonly been reported in prisoners and is generally believed to be a dissociative state, although organic features may contribute.

Depersonalization and Derealization *Depersonalization* refers to an alteration in one's experience and awareness of the self, leading to feelings of being unreal or detached from one's own body, of feeling like an automaton; it is often accompanied by the complaint that the individual lacks all feelings or sensory experiences. Those experiencing depersonalization frequently fear that they are going crazy. Because of this fear, patients often endure depersonalization experiences for long periods before describing them to a mental health professional. Depersonalization is also characterized by frequent internal nonaudible dialogues between the participating self and the observing self but with full awareness that both parties are the same person (a feature that distinguishes it from hallucinations). Mild sensory distortions—but not hallucinations—are commonly associated with the experience. Depersonalization is seen in a variety of neurological and psychiatric disorders and is common in complex partial seizures. It may occur in the context of depression, anxiety disorders, or certain personality disorders, or it may occur as an entity by itself. In derealization, individuals feel themselves to be real but feel that the world around them has suddenly become unreal. Derealization often, but not always, accompanies depersonalization. Transient episodes of depersonalization and derealization occur frequently in normal people, particularly during states of fatigue, sleep deprivation, or stressful situations such as bereavement, learning of a terminal diagnosis, or sudden awareness that one is about to be in an inescapable vehicle collision.

A 45-year-old mother of two underwent a breast biopsy for a suspicious lesion. Afterward, sitting in the surgeon's office, hearing him tell her that the lesion was cancerous, she recalled feeling numb and distant, saying to herself, as if from a distance, that this was all a dream. She felt as if she were living in an "alternate reality" that would disappear and return her to the real world when she left the office.

Disturbances of the Self At the most basic level, the key components of self-awareness are the reality and integrity of the self (that I am one person), the continuity of self (that I am the same person now that I was in the past and that I will be in the future), the boundaries of self (that I can distinguish between myself and the rest of the world as not-self), and activity of self (that it is *I* who is thinking, doing, feeling). Additional components of a sense of self include body image and various self-evaluations, including self-esteem and ego-ideal (ideal self). *Body image* is an individual's mental representation of his or her own body. *Self-esteem* is believed to reflect how one measures up to the desired self-image. To the extent that what one sees in oneself approximates what one would like to be, self-esteem is positive. *Ego-ideals* are fantasies of the optimum person one could ever wish to be. Any of these qualities may be disturbed in psychiatric disorders.

Within each individual is a group of social selves comprised of the roles and identities that a person assumes and that are evoked in various contexts. The presenting "self" varies depending on the people with whom one interacts, such as parents, romantic partner, child, friend, or employer, and depending on what role one assumes, such as child, parent, colleague, or lover. Accompanying each of these "selves" are various levels of objective and subjective self-awareness and self-understanding.

Disturbances in Sense of Self Disturbances of the basic elements of self-awareness may be seen in a variety of disorders. Discontinuity phenomena are characteristic of dissociative states such as psychogenic amnesias and psychogenic fugue. Depersonalization reflects a mild disturbance in the awareness of self as the agent of activity. More severe disturbance is characteristic of the psychotic passivity phenomena seen in schizophrenia. Boundary disturbances may be considered characteristic of all psychotic states regardless of diagnosis.

Disorders of self-integrity are characteristic of both dissociative identity disorders and severe borderline personality disorders in which a person's self-concept and expression of this concept to others is erratic, leading to a sense of unstable identity.

False self describes a persona or a faulty and limited superficial aspect of the personality that an individual builds up as a mechanism for adapting to a hostile world—to please, control, or negotiate with others and with himself or herself. However, the false self does not incorporate, integrate, or validate important fundamental needs, wants, values, and beliefs. Through self-deception and denial, the individual may consciously believe that this "self" constitutes his or her entire being. However, the false self is a relatively fragile construction that has usually warded off and denied fundamental strivings, which may include needs for autonomy; acting with integrity; expressing certain desires, beliefs, or talents; or other unacknowledged aspects of the self. When these warded-off needs finally break through and demand expression at various points in development, the defective false self may collapse, leading to a period of distress and identity confusion, which individuals sometimes describe as a "nervous breakdown."

Patients with pseudologia fantastica and the impostor syndrome demonstrate extreme examples of inconsistency in the sense of self. In *pseudologia fantastica*, patients compulsively spin out webs of lies, ordinarily self-aggrandizing ones, and also appear to be trying very hard to deceive themselves into believing that they are true. In the *impostor syndrome*, such fantasies are acted out by liars and impostors who seem to fervently wish that these fantasies were their reality, as if they cannot accept themselves and would be overwhelmingly ashamed to be known for who they actually are. The impostor compulsively adopts the identities of others and may, for example, show up properly attired at diplomatic functions and society galas and interact with the other guests under the assumed identity. Some famous impostors have repeatedly insinuated themselves into inner circles of high society and government.

Transsexualism is a syndrome characterized by the feeling that one was born into a body of the wrong sex and marked by the desire, starting at an early age, to be a person of the opposite sex. Male to female transsexualism is reported most often. Both psychodynamic and biological theories have been advanced to explain these unusual phenomena. Of note, studies following patients who undergo successful male to female transgender surgery have not revealed higher rates of associated psychopathology than in comparison groups.

Self-esteem is a measure of one's self-appraisal in relation to one's values and ego-ideals. Negative self-esteem is characteristic of depressive disorders, many personality disorders, and situational failures. Superficially inflated self-esteem may be seen in mania (or hypomania) or, in a fluctuating manner, with narcissistic and other personality disorders.

Although some individuals regard their ego-ideals as unattainable and are content to live as imperfect human beings, others strive to approximate their ideals. People who feel driven to achieve unattainable ideal goals or to become unrealistically perfect ideal selves are likely to be chronically dysphoric and have poor self-esteem because their attempts to become their ego-ideals are doomed to failure.

Disorders of the Will Central to the sense of self is the concept of will or volition. Psychologically, will is linked to the concepts of intentionality and of transforming awareness and knowledge into initiating action, as the bridge between desire and action. For individuals to manifest normal will, they must be aware and feel desires—and these desires must arise from within themselves. Concepts related to will that may become the focus of clinical attention when disturbed include motivation and decision making (i.e., the capacity to make choices).

Pathologically heightened will, seen primarily in manic states, is characterized by excessively intense desires and an overly facile capacity to make decisions, with complex questions being decided on in an instant. With heightened psychological energy, these individuals can start new courses of action with astonishing rapidity. Closer examination of these actions in more extreme cases, however, reveals that they share much in common with decreased will in that the intense desires and quick decisions often reflect impulsiveness, which can be considered an escape from true willing and decision making, rather than enduring desires or thoughtful decision making.

The term *abulia* has been used to describe the loss, lack, or impairment of the power to will or to execute what is in mind. Abulic individuals show a diminished sense of motive or desire and impairment in making the transition from motive and desire to execution of action. Deficiencies in will may be seen in a variety of psychiatric disorders and at the end of life, when patients have surrendered their will to live and are simply waiting to die. In schizophrenia, a diminished sense of will can be seen in passivity phenomena, already described above, as well as in other negative (or deficit) symptoms that may affect thoughts, feelings, and behaviors. These include lack of drive, impersistence at tasks, and a general inner flatness. Depressed patients also describe volitional disturbances in general apathy and anhedonia. Patients who chronically inhale solvents (e.g., glue, gasoline, toluene), smoke marijuana very heavily, and chronically use hallucinogens have a characteristic *amotivational syndrome*. The extent to which this lack of motivation results from or contributes to the chronic substance abuse is a matter of debate.

In OCD, both the obsessional thoughts and the compulsive rituals are experienced as ego dystonic and not consonant with the patient's conscious desires and will. Similarly, although patients with anorexia nervosa initially have the conscious experience of willing and controlling their intake of food, during the course of the disorder, the sense of willfulness is replaced by one of passivity, of being subjugated by obsessional thoughts and compulsive behaviors that assume control of the eating behavior.

> A 28-year-old woman with anorexia nervosa and OCD described having as mental background noise a loud audible thought that constantly tallied the caloric value not only of everything she ate but also of all the foods others in her vicinity ate or that she saw on store shelves. This other stream of thinking occurred nonstop, and, like a calculator, the thoughts constantly did sums and updated the tally for the day. These thoughts were experienced in parallel to but separate from any other thinking activities in which she happened to be engaged.

Disturbances of volition are among the more common complaints of patients with personality disturbances who request psychotherapy. Individuals with dependent personalities are characterized by difficulties in making decisions by themselves and often engage in courses of action contrary to their own desires. Similarly, individuals with passive-aggressive personalities obscure their own desires by being excessively involved in the demands made on them by others. Their courses of action do not reflect their own decisions so much as the thwarting of others' desires. People with compulsive personalities use inflexible rules, thereby precluding courses of action based on independent evaluation, individual desires, and decisions. In other situations, they are indecisive, sometimes making impulsive decisions at the last minute when forced to decide. Finally, many individuals seek treatment because of self-designated disturbances of willing: They do not know what they want, or they cannot make choices among several options, or they procrastinate excessively. Often, these problems may mask other fears—of wanting, commitment, taking initiative, hard work, success, making a mistake, being criticized, angering others, and of all the consequences related to such actions.

Disturbances of Orientation *Orientation* refers to one's awareness of time, place, and person. Accurate orientation requires the integrity of attention, perception, memory, and ideation. Impairments occur primarily in organic mental disorders (i.e., structural and toxic metabolic brain abnormalities) and occasionally in dissociative and psychotic states.

Normal individuals vary tremendously in their attention to the details of time and in the extent to which their bodies automatically keep time. Some people have reliable built-in clocks by which they can awaken themselves at precise times or accurately gauge the passage of time with uncanny accuracy, even in the absence of external cues—in a psychotherapy session, for example. Others have difficulty making judgments about time and may develop pathological lateness or habitually schedule more activities than could ever be accomplished in the available time. Poor time judgments may be seen in a variety of psychiatric disorders, such as ADHD, or as an independent problem. Benign disorientation to time is common. After a few days in a hospital bed, most people do not know exactly what the day or date is because they are not attending to or receiving their usual cues.

Pathological time disorientation can be mild or severe, with inaccuracies of estimation ranging from days to years. The dates reported by disoriented individuals may have personal significance such as those of important births, marriages, or deaths.

Because spatial cues are generally more available and obvious than temporal cues, disorientation to place often signifies a greater degree of cognitive impairment than disorientation to time and, therefore, rarely occurs in the absence of time disorientation. Disoriented people may know, more or less, the type of place they are in without knowing the specific place—patients may recognize that they are in a hospital without being able to name the hospital.

> A 79-year-old former businessman with severe dementia was able to smile responsively in appropriate circumstances and seemed to follow conversations, hiding his deficits by his well-honed social skills. When asked concretely about either time or place, he became momentarily confused and then dissembled, saying three or four half sentences that were incomprehensible and then looking plaintively toward his wife for help.

Disorientation to person, a lack of awareness of one's own identity, is typically seen only in advanced dementias such as primary degenerative dementia of the Alzheimer's type or in dissociative states. In organically induced postconcussion amnesia, transient global amnesia, and, presumably, psychogenic fugue states, knowledge of one's own identity may disappear, and a person may remain unidentified for an indefinite period until the memory for self returns.

Disturbances of Memory Memory is not a unitary phenomenon. Capacities to remember vary for the different senses and perceptions. One person may have prodigious musical memory, with the capacity to remember and reproduce whole musical pieces after one hearing, but be incapable of remembering people's names or telephone numbers. Exceptionally detailed verbal memories have been associated with obsessional cognitive styles. When individuals with extraordinary memories complain of memory loss, ordinary memory tests may be inadequate to detect their deficits, as their relative memory loss may have reduced their capacities to a point within the range of most normal people.

Memory functions have been divided into three stages: registration, retention, and recall. *Registration* (or acquisition) refers to the capacity to add new material to memory. The material may be sensory, perceptual, or conceptual and may come from the environment or from within the person. For new material to be acquired, the person must attend to the information presented, and it must then be registered through the appropriate sensory channels and then be processed or cortically organized. *Retention* is the ability to hold memories in storage. Large numbers of neurons are believed to be involved in the storage of a specific memory, and it is believed that reverberating circuits are formed in which memory traces are held by means of changes in proteins or synaptic connectivity, or both. *Recall* is the capacity to return previously stored memories to consciousness.

Newly registered material is transferred incrementally from immediate to short-term memory to long-term memory. Immediate memory lasts for 15 to 20 seconds; short-term memory (or recent memory) for several minutes up to 2 days (the time involved in new learning and its early consolidation); and long-term (or remote) memory for longer periods. Different physiological processes mediate each of these stages of memory. Because of this, processes that affect immediate or short-term memory often spare long-term memory. The processes by which memories are transferred from short-term to long-term stores are unknown.

Cognitive scientists now refer to short-term memory as *working memory*, the system that briefly stores and processes information needed for planning and reasoning. Recent studies suggest that the working memory system consists of at least two short-term memory buffers, one for verbal and another for visual memories, plus a central executive that manipulates and coordinates information stored in the two buffers for problem solving, planning, and organizing activities. Parallel processing systems involving specific areas of the prefrontal cortex and other brain areas appear to operate separately with respect to various processes concerned with working memory. For example, separate prefrontal areas appear to be involved in working memory functions concerned with object identity and spatial locations.

Other studies suggest that different types of memories are stored and retrieved by different brain systems, so that there is at least a dual memory system. The first system, sometimes called a *conditioned-emotional system*, or system for *implicit memory*, or *perceptual memory*, or *nondeclarative memory*, is present from birth, operational through life, and is addressable by situational, sensory, or affective cues. Past experiences are expressed through images, behaviors, or emotions. These memories need not involve any conscious memories of a past experience. Conditioned fear responses represent examples of memories elicited in this system. The second system, sometimes called *narrative-biographical memory*, or *explicit memory*, or *reflective memory*, or *declarative memory*, emerges during the preschool years and includes information significant to the self. Memories are addressable through intentional retrieval efforts, apart from the original learning conditions. They are identified as representing personally experienced events and compose the individual's life history, approximately equivalent to memory with consciousness or memory with awareness. Clinical studies suggest that, in at least some amnesias, implicit and explicit memory functions may be dissociated.

Disturbances in memory occur through the interruption of registration, retention, or recall.

Disturbances in Registration Registration and short-term memory retention are usually impaired in disorders that affect vigilance and attention, such as head trauma, delirium, intoxications, psychosis, spontaneous or induced seizures, anxiety, depression, and fatigue. A variety of other metabolic and structural brain disturbances can affect short-term memory as well, particularly lesions affecting the mammillary bodies, hippocampus, fornix, and closely associated areas. Patients with impaired attention and concentration who are able to demonstrate immediate recall may not be able to retain or recollect these items from short-term memory. Benzodiazepine use has been associated with working memory difficulties, especially in the elderly. Some short-acting, high-potency benzodiazepines used as sleeping pills may be particularly troublesome in this regard.

Disturbances in Retention The retention of memories is impaired in posttraumatic amnesia as well as in a number of cognitive disorders such as dementia of the Alzheimer's type and Wernicke-Korsakoff syndrome. The latter, which ordinarily results from chronic thiamine deficiency seen with alcoholism, is associated with pathological alterations in the mammillary bodies and thalamus.

Disturbances in Recall Disturbances in recall can occur even when memories have been registered and are in storage. At times, inability to recall may signify that the memory traces themselves have disappeared and are no longer retrievable. However, difficulties in recall can occur separately, as in the everyday event of forgetting the name of a person or object, only to spontaneously remember it hours or days later. In normal forgetting, more remote events are less well remembered than recent ones, and important events are most vividly retained in memory. Some demented patients may lose memories for all events occurring after a specific date or event, as if the slate has been wiped clean, but retain earlier memories. Some individuals may progressively erase memories so that they recall only earlier and earlier events. Specific types of memory functions may be subject to selectively different control mechanisms in the brain. For example, recent animal research suggests that endocannabinoids may facilitate the extinction of aversive memories, but not their acquisition or consolidation, through their selective inhibitory effects on local inhibitory networks in the amygdala.

A 27-year-old woman with PTSD symptoms related to a history of childhood physical, emotional, and sexual abuse developed a significant and persistent habit of cannabis abuse. She had tried a variety of street drugs but settled on cannabis as her drug of choice. She was certain that marijuana was far better than other drugs at enabling her to "forget" and not dwell on the past while permitting her to get about her usual day-to-day tasks and requirements.

Under usual conditions, forgotten events can be recalled with prompting, associative memories, or other forms of stimulation such as hypnosis. As described earlier, state-dependent memories are recall failures, reversed by reinstituting the context in which the memory was originally formed.

Amnesias are syndromes in which short-term and long-term memory is impaired within a state of normal consciousness. Thus, memory disturbances in delirium should, strictly speaking, not be considered amnestic syndromes. *Anterograde amnesia* is the inability to register or learn new information (and therefore to form new memories) from a specific event onward; it typically follows head trauma, states of cerebral physiological imbalance, or drug effects. Patients who receive ECT frequently have anterograde amnesias during the course of the treatments; the amnesia gradually fades over numbers of weeks. *Retrograde amnesia* is an impairment in recalling memories that were established before a traumatic event, extending backward in time for variable periods. As memory is regained, the more remote memories usually return first. A patient originally amnestic for the 3-month period before an accident may ultimately be left with amnesia for events only a day or an hour just before the accident. In organically caused retrograde amnesias, remote memories are usually intact, although amnesia may exist for more recent events. This contrasts with *psychogenic* (functional) *amnesia*, in which the periods of forgotten events may be more spotty or selective.

Hypermnesia, unusually detailed and vivid memory, may occur in gifted people, in association with obsessive-compulsive and paranoid personality traits, and in hypnotic trances. *Intrusive memories* may occur in PTSD, signaling failure of the mechanisms that usually keep unwanted memories and information out of working memory.

A 36-year-old man with mild developmental disability living on a remote and isolated ranch witnessed his brother murder a violent, drug-dealing neighbor with a shovel. The patient was implicated as an accomplice and spent several years in jail. Starting on the day of the murder and persisting on a daily basis for 5 years thereafter, the patient experienced vivid visual, olfactory, and tactile images of the murderous act—reacting with strong emotions to all of these relived sensations. The images were particularly strong when the patient lacked external stimulation and just before falling asleep.

Although many forgotten memories can be recalled in hypnotic trance, retrospective falsification and distortion may also occur under hypnosis. (Memories recalled under hypnosis usually are not accepted as evidence in court.) Retrospective falsification of memory, the development of false memories, is called *paramnesia*, also known as *fausse reconnaissance*. *Confabulation* is another common form of paramnesia in which the patient fills in memory gaps with inaccurate information. The responses given to questions by patients who confabulate may reflect past experiences or bizarre, fantastic stories. Confabulation correlates poorly with memory deficit and is believed to reflect frontal lobe dysfunction and a failure of self-monitoring. Confabulation is prominent in certain alcohol amnestic syndromes, such as Wernicke-Korsakoff syndrome, as well as other disorders of the mammillary bodies, thalamus, or frontal lobes.

Déjà vu is the sense that one has previously seen or experienced what is transpiring for the first time; it is a false impression that the current stream of consciousness has previously been recorded in memory. Related phenomena are *déjà entendu*, a sense that one has previously heard what is actually being heard for the first time, and *déjà pensé*, a feeling that one has at an earlier time known or understood what is being thought for the first time. Experiences of *jamais vu*, *jamais entendu*, and *jamais pensé* involve feelings that one has never seen, heard, or thought (respectively) things that, in fact, one has. These phenomena are all common in everyday life but may increase in states of fatigue or intoxication and in association with complex partial seizures or other psychopathological states.

Dementia is a syndrome in which the essential feature is an acquired impairment of short- and long-term memory with associated impairments of abstract thinking, judgment, personality changes, and other cortical disturbances. The symptoms always involve more than one sphere of function. In later stages, demented patients may become helpless, too confused to use a stove, and incapable of remembering the names of close relatives. They may wander into dangerous situations, oblivious of their surroundings. Dementias are caused by a variety of pathogenic processes, some of which are reversible, such as hypothyroidism and subdural hematoma, whereas others are irreversible, such as dementia of the Alzheimer's type and multiinfarct dementia. Although the characteristic cognitive disturbances seen in severe major depressive episodes are usually called *pseudodementias*, many neuropsychiatrists believe that profound cognitive dysfunction meeting criteria for dementia associated with depression should properly be labeled as a reversible dementia syndrome. The presence of pseudodementia, however, is predictive of the development of Alzheimer's disease (but not in all cases), indicating that the depression was a prodrome of the primary cognitive disorder or that the presence of pseudodementia marks those with an underlying progressive cognitive disorder.

DISTURBANCES IN PERCEPTION

Normal perception first requires that the individual be capable of receiving information as sensations. The data must then be organized to make them meaningful and comprehensible such as distinguishing figure from ground or focusing attention selectively on some part of the sensory field. The organized entities are called *percepts*. In states of sensory deficit, such as blindness, deafness, and anesthesia, perception is impaired, but perception is still possible because individuals generally perceive information about an object through several sensory modalities concurrently. The intensity of sensation and perception is affected by vigilance and attention. Highly focused attention, as in intense concentration or hypnosis, may result in unusually acute sensation and perception—hyperesthesia, hyperacusis, or extraordinary visual acuity. Focused attention may also result in the inability to sense or perceive: Deep anesthesia and negative hallucinations induced by hypnosis are simply induced failures to perceive what exists in the world.

Humans usually operate in an "average expectable environment" in which certain types and levels of sensory input are expected and for which the nervous system is primed. Excessive or inadequate stimulation in any sensory modality, levels of input that are extraordinarily intense, or the presentation of novel stimuli that are entirely different from anything previously experienced by the individual can provoke distorted perceptions in most normal people. For example, total sensory deprivation produced in carefully controlled artificial environments may elicit visual and auditory illusions and hallucinations.

Individuals generally exhibit selective perception of the world, depending on what is salient at the moment, and on his or her individual memories, emotions, fantasies, and values. Pregnant women are more likely to perceive babies around them than are people who are not as preoccupied with childbearing.

The intensity of perceptions depends on individual sensitivities as well as on mood, anxiety, and substance use. Unmedicated patients with schizophrenia have deficits in olfactory acuity. Depressed patients often describe that colors look faded, that the world looks washed out or gray, even though their capacity to recognize specific colors is unchanged. Similarly, mania is often characterized by heightened perceptions, *hyperesthesia*. When extreme, these intense perceptions are uncomfortable. Hyperesthesia can also be seen during benzodiazepine withdrawal, hallucinogen use, and, occasionally, as part of an epileptic aura.

The intensity of perception may vary with cognitive style and other psychological and neurological factors. Some individuals tend to be *augmenters* and others *minimizers* of bodily experiences. Chronic pain and some hypochondriacal syndromes may occur more commonly among somatic augmenters.

Selective deficits in the perception of emotions may occur. *Emotional aprosodies* have been described in which patients with specific neurological deficits or depression are selectively unable to recognize the expression of facial emotion. These have been linked by positron emission tomography (PET) scan to blunted activity in the right prefrontal cortex and insula.

Illusions

Perceptual distortions in estimating size, shape, and spatial relations are common even in the absence of psychiatric disorders, especially when one is fatigued or excessively aroused. *Illusions* are misinterpretations of real sensory stimuli, as when a child in a dark bedroom at night sees monsters emanating from shadows on the walls. *Pareidolia* are playful and whimsical voluntary illusions that can be seen when one looks at ambiguously defined or evanescent images such as clouds or flames in a fireplace. Both the onset and termination of these perceptions are entirely voluntary. *Trailing*, another visual illusion, is the perception that an object moving steadily in space is followed by temporally distinct, afterimages of itself. The effect is that of a series of stroboscopic photos. This phenomenon may occur with fatigue and is typically seen with marijuana and mescaline intoxication, during withdrawal from SSRIs, or, less commonly, in association with nefazodone (Serzone).

Hallucinations

Hallucinations are perceptions that occur in the absence of corresponding sensory stimuli. Phenomenologically, hallucinations are ordinarily subjectively indistinguishable from normal perceptions. Hallucinations are often experienced as being private so that others are not able to see or hear the same perceptions. The patient's explanation for this is typically delusional. Hallucinations can affect any sensory system and sometimes occur in several concurrently. When perception is altered, combinations of illusions and hallucinations, and often delusions as well, are frequently experienced together. In some studies, 90 percent of patients with hallucinations also have delusions, and approximately 35 percent of patients with delusions also have hallucinations. Children and early adolescents, however, are more likely to have hallucinations in the absence of delusions. Approximately 20 percent of patients have mixed sensory hallucinations (mostly auditory and visual) that may accompany functional, as well as organic, conditions. A given external stimulus may evoke very different perceptual distortions in different people.

> Three scientists floated in sensory deprivation tanks for long periods. One experienced a few illusions and no hallucinations; the second had many illusions and a few faint auditory and visual hallucinations; and the third had vivid, dramatic, and complex visual and auditory hallucinations.

Hallucinations are experienced by many normal people under unusual conditions. It has been estimated that between 10 and 27 percent of the general population has experienced memorable hallucinations, most commonly visual hallucinations. The large majority of self-reported hallucinations in community studies, particularly auditory hallucinations, have been associated with depressive and substance use disorders rather than frank psychotic disorders.

Hypnogogic and *hypnopompic hallucinations* are common, predominantly visual hallucinations that occur during the moments immediately preceding falling asleep and during the transition from sleep to wakefulness, respectively. Hypnagogic and hypnopompic hallucinations both occur in normal people and are also characteristic symptoms of narcolepsy. In acute bereavement, up to 50 percent of grieving spouses have reported hallucinating the voice or presence of the deceased, and after amputations, phantom limb hallucinations are common. Patients who become visually impaired often develop pseudohallucinations (i.e., visual hallucinations with preserved insight) with preserved cognitive status, the so-called Charles Bonnet syndrome. A parallel phenomenon is the emergence of hallucination, including musical hallucinations in individuals with acquired deafness. These observations suggest a "supersensitivity deprivation" hypothesis that, when deprived of important and anticipated perceptual stimuli, the mental apparatus may overinterpret any sensory stimulation as evidence of the presence of the needed objects.

A perceptual release theory suggests that hallucinations emerge from the combined presence of intense states of internal arousal and diminished sensory input (including poor attention and poor capacity to sort out relevant from irrelevant input). Thus, diminished input from the environment (as in sensory deprivation) or reduced capacity to attend to and take in the input (as in delirious states) heightens the likelihood that internal sensations, images, and thoughts are interpreted as originating in the outside environment.

Hallucinations vary according to sensory modality, degree of complexity of the hallucinated experience, the levels of conviction about their reality, the clarity of their contents, the location of their sources of origin, the degree of volitional control over them, and the degree to which the hallucination influences the person's behavior.

Auditory hallucinations range in complexity from hearing unstructured sounds, such as whirring noises or muffled whispers, to ongoing multiperson discussions about the patient. The simple auditory hallucinations are more commonly associated with organic psychoses such as delirium, complex partial seizures, and toxic and metabolic encephalopathies. Auditory hallucinations are classically associated with schizophrenia (seen in 60 to 90 percent of patients) but are also frequently seen in psychotic mood disorders. Twenty percent of manic patients and less than 10 percent of depressed patients experience auditory hallucinations.

Three types of auditory hallucinations commonly associated with schizophrenia (which, however, are also seen less commonly in patients with psychotic depressions and mania) are (1) audible thoughts described as hallucinated voices that speak aloud what the patient is thinking, (2) voices that give a running commentary on the patient's actions, and (3) hearing two or more voices arguing with each other, often about the patient, who is referred to in the third person.

A 42-year-old man with chronic schizophrenia described that he had chronic and persistent daily auditory hallucinations. Although he was not quite clear about the etiology of these voices, he surmised that they were from celestial beings. When his psychosis was relatively mild, he could hear their discussions about his behavior and heard occasional commands, which he was able to ignore. When his psychosis worsened, the voices became more critical, resulting in social withdrawal and a marked increase in depression and suicidal ideation.

While auditory hallucinations in schizophrenia are frequently mood neutral, hallucinations in patients with mood disorders are characteristically consistent with their mood. In psychotic depression, the voices may be unrelievedly critical and sadistic, whereas in mania, the voices often refer to the patient's specialness.

A 31-year-old bipolar man described a recurrent shift in the quality of auditory hallucinations associated with his changing mood states. When he was depressed, auditory hallucinations were unrelentingly critical of him, telling him that he did not deserve to live and that he should commit suicide for the good of the world. Typically, his severe depressions alternated with irritable manic states. During those periods, auditory hallucinations not only told him that he was great but also belittled and berated others in his life and sometimes instructed him to lash out and harm them when they thwarted his grandiose plans.

Command hallucinations order patients to do things. Often, the commands are benign reminders about everyday tasks: "Pick up your shoes" or "Clean off the table." However, the voices may also be frightening or dangerous, commanding acts of violence toward the self or others such as "Jump off the roof, you're not worth anything" or "Pick up the knife and kill your mother." These voices vary in insistence and persistence, and patients differ in their capacities to ignore these commands. Patients with marked passivity may be helpless in the face of command hallucinations and may feel impelled to carry out the orders. Even though one study did not find command hallucinations to be associated with a higher risk of harm to the patient or others, the presence of command hallucinations and the patient's ability to resist must be assessed carefully.

A 46-year-old woman with schizophrenia heard command hallucinations on a daily basis for the last 20 years. When her symptoms were relatively quiescent, the voices were benign, and the commands referred to daily behaviors (such as "say thank you"). Under stress, her psychosis exacerbated and the voices became louder, more insistent, and commanded more complex and dangerous behaviors, once precipitating a self-stabbing when the voices demanded it.

Visual hallucinations occur in a wide variety of neurological and psychiatric disorders, including toxic disturbances, drug withdrawal syndromes, focal CNS lesions, migraine headaches, blindness, schizophrenia, and psychotic mood disorders. Although visual hallucinations are generally assumed to characteristically reflect organic disorders, they are seen in one-fourth to one-half of schizophrenic patients, often—but not always—in conjunction with auditory hallucinations.

Visual hallucinations range from simple and elemental, in which hallucinations consist of flashes of light or geometrical figures, to elaborate visions such as a flock of angels.

Stimulation of one sensory modality sometimes evokes perceptual distortions in another. Marijuana and mescaline intoxication, for example, have been associated with *synesthesia*, an experience in which sensory modalities seem fused. This is also a normal experience for many people. Music may be experienced visually, the sound fusing with visual illusions; a tactile sensation may be experienced as a color (e.g., a hot surface may "feel red").

In certain religious subcultures, visual hallucinations may be experienced as normal. In one fundamentalist Pentecostal church, worshipers danced themselves into a frenzy, and, without using any drugs, several participants shared visions of the Virgin Mary at the altar.

A 45-year-old Hispanic farmer who lived in a rural farm area all of his life attended church regularly. He reported that he and others in his family were always aware of the presence of benevolent angels guarding over their lives. As they worked in the fields, they were often comforted by these angels, which they took to represent the souls and spirits of departed ancestors who had lived and worked in the same region for hundreds of years.

Autoscopic hallucinations are hallucinations of one's own physical self. Such hallucinations may stimulate the delusion that one has a double (*doppelganger*). Reports of near-death, out-of-body experiences in which individuals see themselves rising to the ceiling and looking down at themselves in a hospital bed may be autoscopic hallucinations. In *Lilliputian hallucinations*, the individual sees figures in very reduced size, such as midgets or dwarfs. They may be related to the perceptual distortions of *macropsia* and *micropsia*, respectively, the perceptions of objects as much bigger or smaller than they actually are.

Haptic hallucinations involve touch. Simple haptic hallucinations, such as the feeling that bugs are crawling over one's skin (formication), are common in alcohol withdrawal syndromes and in cocaine intoxication. When unkempt and physically neglectful patients complain of these sensations, they may be due to the presence of real physical stimuli, such as lice. Some tactile hallucinations—having intercourse with God, for example—are highly suggestive of schizophrenia but may also occur in tertiary syphilis and other conditions and may, in fact, be stimulated by local genital irritation. Olfactory and gustatory hallucinations, involving smell and taste, respectively, have most often been associated with organic brain disease, particularly with the uncinate fits of complex partial seizures. Olfactory hallucinations may also be seen in psychotic depression, typically as odors of decay, rotting, or death.

A 32-year-old woman with schizophrenia described that, over the 15 years of her illness, she had experienced a wide array of hallucinations. She initially noticed celestial voices, auditory hallucinations that included angelic music and comforting words. However, over the years, in conjunction with a pessimistic turn of mind, the voices became more demonic and threatening. At the same time, she began to experience somatic hallucinations, consisting of sharp, intermittent electric currents being run through her skin and genitals, which, she was convinced, were the work of evil neighbors intent on driving her out of her apartment. With medication, she was partly able to perceive these experiences as hallucinatory; however, most times, particularly when she neglected to take medications, she never doubted their authenticity.

The term *pseudohallucination* has been used in two ways. First, pseudohallucination refers to perceptions experienced as coming from within the mind (i.e., not at the boundary or outside the mind). Using this definition, loud voices that are alien, ascribed to other beings, but which the patient knows are actually within the mind rather than out in space, are pseudohallucinations. The term has also been used to describe hallucinatory experiences whose validity the patient doubts. A better term for this second phenomenon is *partial hallucination*, analogous to partial delusion. *Functional hallucinations* are rare hallucinations that occur only in connection with a specific external perception, for example, in the presence of a sound, such as running water, or a color, or a particular place. However, unlike illusions, the hallucinated sounds are not elaborations of the perception but are simply triggered only in that specific context.

Ictal hallucinations, occurring as part of seizure activity, are typically brief, lasting only seconds to minutes, and stereotyped. They may be simple images, such as flashes of light, or elaborate ones, such as visual recollections of past experiences. While the hallucinations are being experienced, the patient ordinarily experiences altered consciousness or a twilight sleep.

Migrainous hallucinations are reported by approximately 50 percent of patients with migraine. Most are simple visual hallucinations of geometrical patterns, but fully formed visual hallucinations, sometimes with micropsia and macropsia, may also occur. This complex has been called the *Alice in Wonderland syndrome* after Lewis Carroll's descriptions of the world in *Through the Looking Glass*, which mirrored some of his own migrainous experiences. In turn, these phenomena closely resemble visual hallucinations induced by psychedelic drugs such as mescaline.

A *flashback* is an intense visual reexperience of highly charged past events, which are often replays of hallucinations. They are typically associated with heavy use of hallucinogens, such as LSD and mescaline, and often occur months after the last drug ingestion. The images may be simple or complex geometrical patterns, or they may consist of previously experienced elaborate drug-induced hallucinations. Flashback phenomena may be state dependent. For example, visual hallucinations initially experienced with hallucinogens are more likely to be subsequently experienced as flashbacks when the subject is smoking marijuana. In PTSD, some complex, intrusive flashback-like images may attain a hallucinatory vividness. Images often include horrifying memories of traumatic events that may force themselves repeatedly into consciousness until they are acknowledged and worked through.

Hallucinosis is a state of active hallucination occurring in someone who is alert and well oriented. This condition is seen most often in alcoholic withdrawal, but it may also occur during acute intoxications and other drug-mediated states.

A 21-year-old man used LSD daily for 3 days, after which the visual hallucinations that first occurred while under the influence of the drug waxed and waned. He described pareidolias with distracting images of animals when he looked at traffic lights, the sky, or billboards. Trailers were common after he turned his head. Finally, he saw moving colors when he stared at any object for more than a transient time period. He assumed that these phenomena represented a lingering effect of the LSD and was not frightened by them. The hallucinations disappeared within 1 week.

Body Image Distortion Body image includes both perceptual and ideational components and may reflect primarily perceptual distortions or combinations of disturbed perception and self-appraisal, or both.

Body image disturbances can occur as normal responses to abrupt changes in the body (e.g., after amputation), in brain disease, and in psychiatric disorders. Phantom limb phenomena are classic body image problems in which an amputated limb is still felt to be present. The sensation may diminish gradually over time; the phantom feels as if it is receding into the stump.

A 53-year-old maintenance worker underwent the traumatic amputation of both legs above the knees in a motor vehicle collision. For more than a decade, after he obtained and mastered the use of bilateral prostheses, his most disturbing impairments were painful phantom limb experiences. He constantly felt as if both legs were present but raw and shattered. In spite of optimal available pain medication management, these experiences persisted, and the patient continued to search for a neurosurgeon who might alleviate the pain.

Agnosias, lack of awareness of some parts of the body, may accompany brain damage, most often of the nondominant parietal lobe. Patients with obvious motor or sensory deficits may deny that any deficit exists at all (anosognosia), or the denial may be limited to one-half of the body (hemiagnosia), usually the left side. In *hemidepersonalization syndromes*, a less common disorder (hemisomatognosia), patients feel that one of their limbs is missing, again usually on the left side. Body image distortions in which a limb feels too heavy (hyperschemazia) or weightless (hyposchemazia) can occur as a consequence of neurological conditions such as infarction of the parietal lobe. In *duplication phenomena*, patients feel as if part or all of them has doubled (e.g., they have two heads or two bodies). These rare phenomena may occur in schizophrenia, complex partial seizures, and migraine.

Dysmorphophobia refers to conditions in which patients distortedly perceive and intensely dislike the shape of a particular body part. As such, these symptoms are misnamed because there is no true phobic component such as fear or avoidant behavior. Fine lines exist between perceptual distortions and realistic but unhappy appraisals of one's body, given the high social values placed on physical appearance. Dysmorphophobia may occur in the context of some personality disorders or as an isolated disorder called *body dysmorphic disorder*. In some ways, dysmorphophobia resembles an overvalued idea. Patients may develop dysmorphophobias in relation to any body part; common concerns are hair, breasts, penis size, the shape of the nose, or the shape of the entire body. For some, changing the body part, as in rhinoplasty for those who do not like their nose, seems to effect a lasting positive change in body image, with patients becoming happier with themselves and feeling more attractive for years or lifetimes. In severe dysmorphophobia, patients may undergo multiple plastic surgeries and feel dissatisfied with every result. At times, the condition forms part of a larger and more pervasive syndrome, such as anorexia nervosa.

An attractive 19-year-old woman was preoccupied and perplexed by the fact that she perceived her eyelids as being unequal in size and shape and by the fact that the cleft in her chin was too deep. She spent hours each day in front of the mirror, trying to pose in ways that, from her perspective, did not expose these facial blemishes. She sought consultation from a plastic surgeon, who referred her for psychiatric consultation. After 2 months of treatment with an SSRI, her preoccupations with appearance diminished considerably, and she was able to turn her attention to other issues in her life.

Hypochondriacal complaints also combine perceptual and ideational distortions. Selective hypervigilance to bodily sensations may result in a higher likelihood of perceptions of unpleasant and potentially pathological body experiences among the "worried well," hypochondriacal populations, patients with somatization disorder (Briquet's syndrome), and some patients with panic disorder.

Body image distortions may, at times, be severe or bizarre. Some psychotic patients, either with schizophrenia or depression, develop somatic delusions. In depression, this often expresses itself as a delusion that part of, or the entire, body is rotting or filled with cancer. Some culture-bound syndromes in non-Western culture express themselves with body image distortions such as *koro*, in which the man fears that his penis is shrinking into his abdomen.

DISTURBANCES OF MOOD

Defining, describing, understanding, and categorizing moods have long been among the most important, and difficult, tasks in psychiatry. The language of feelings is filled with terms that seem to have mostly idiosyncratic meanings, as patients, phenomenologists, and psychiatrists all struggle both to describe inner emotions and to correlate them with external behavior. Even basic terms, such as *mood*, *affect*, *emotion*, and *feelings*, lack universal definition. The most common convention, which is used here, defines *mood* as a sustained or prevailing subjective feeling tone or range of tones. *Affect* is the moment-to-moment feeling state, sometimes rapidly shifting in response to a variety of thoughts and situations, that the clinician can observe. *Emotions* have been defined as moods and affects that are connected to specific ideas or to the physical concomitants of moods and affects. *Feelings* are the most poorly defined of all, leading Karl Jaspers to ultimately describe them as everything for which there is no other name. In common parlance, and often professionally as well, these words are sometimes used interchangeably. The term *mood disorders*, adopted for DSM-III-R and now DSM-IV-TR, replaced DSM-III-R's "affective disorders" to describe the same group of psychiatric syndromes.

Moods, affects, and emotions can be described by a number of important qualities: intensity (shallow to deep), range (broad to narrow [or flat]), stability (rigid to labile), reactivity to external events (none to much), periodicity (periodic to aperiodic), congruence with thought content (congruent [or appropriate] to incongruent), speed of resolution (rapid to slow), and viscosity (evanescent to persistent). The individual's lifelong predominant mood is one component of temperament. Thus, for example, one may be described as having a calm, buoyant, irritable, depressive, anxious, or sensitive temperament.

Moods, affects, and emotions serve as internal and external signal systems. They signal the state of the individual to others and often elicit necessary help and support from the environment. A baby's face communicates its state of need, tension, or contentment, thereby recruiting appropriate maternal interventions. As adults, much of our most important interpersonal communications is transmitted nonverbally through cues that signal the observer about our moods. Positive words communicated by a scowling or sullen face lead listeners to perceive an angry message regardless of our spoken words. Moods also have an infectious quality and serve as important ways of influencing others. Thus, when we act cheerfully toward others, they, in turn, are more likely to feel cheerful and to reciprocate that cheerfulness.

Internally, moods, affects, and emotions let individuals know how well or how poorly they are doing, allowing them, for instance, to gauge the distance between actual self-appraisal and desired self-expectations. For example, individuals who desire to master important goals and feel that they have a reasonably good chance of doing so ordinarily experience pleasant emotional states in relation to these goals. If something intervenes to prevent them from reaching these goals so that there is an insurmountable gap between their desires and the likelihood of success, they may feel hopeless. In addition to serving as signal systems, emotional states of nonspecific tension, arousal, or anger usually imply that some action is necessary to secure their discharge or release.

Emotional states and their expression are regulated by biological, psychological, and cultural influences. For example, emotional or affective lability, characterized by rapidly shifting emotions that seem unattached to the situation, typically occurs premenstrually in some women, with varying periodicity in cyclothymic individuals and in those with cluster B personality disorders, and in relation to need states such as hunger, sleep deprivation, and sexual frustration. Mood shifts have also been related to environment-related physiological influences such as seasonal changes in light. Psychological regulation of emotions may be related to specific coping mechanisms and the ability to self-soothe, which are developmentally determined. Conscious and preconscious psychological mechanisms, including varieties of self-talk, may help calm or inflame emotions. Culture factors significantly regulate emotional expression. Although the facial expressions for basic emotions are similar in all cultures studied, the range and style of emotional expression permitted in relation to specific contexts varies greatly from culture to culture and from family to family. Some cultures and families are stiff lipped and inhibit the open expression of emotion, whereas others encourage emotional display. Marked differences exist among cultures in the emotional expression of acute grief, fear, pain, and affection.

Depression The term *depression* has been used variously to describe an emotional state, a syndrome, and a group of specific disorders. When seen as part of a syndrome or disorder, depression has autonomic, visceral, emotional, perceptual, cognitive, and behavioral manifestations, as illustrated in Table 8–1. As a nonpathological, ubiquitous mood state lasting hours to days, but sometimes longer, feelings of depression are synonymous with feeling sad, blue, down in the dumps, unhappy, and miserable. Depressed mood is common and appropriate after a disappointment or loss. For most people, innate psychological resilience, alternative coping options, and supportive social networks help alleviate these brief depressive states and prevent them from becoming chronic. Some individuals have chronically depressed mood, tend to view the world as a difficult place filled with obstacles and burdens, see themselves as victimized, and lack hope for the future. The extent to which constitutional, developmental, and ongoing aversive life events contribute to this pervasive world view is unknown. People who, in early life, were deprived and traumatized may be less resilient and more prone to chronic depressive features than are others. Repeated failures and the impact of unrelenting, uncontrollable, and unpredictable negative life events may set the stage for learned helplessness in humans just as they do in animals. A subset of chronically depressed individuals may also have temperamental, biologically driven depression, often seen in conjunction with strong genetic loading for severe mood disorders.

Some depressive states are normal and common reactions to major unwelcome and undesirable life events. Normal *bereavement* best exemplifies this. In bereavement after major losses, such as the death of a parent, spouse, or child, people experience sadness, pining, and yearning but do not ordinarily have the feelings of guilt, unworthiness, and self-reproach that characterize depressive disorders. Feelings of helplessness and hopelessness may be temporarily present in bereavement, but they ordinarily pass with time. In uncomplicated cases, the process of bereavement takes 3 to 6 months in the acute phase and up to 1 year for complete resolution. Bereaved people are more likely to feel physically ill and seek general health care than at other times, and older widowers are more likely to die than age-matched nonbereaved controls. *Pathological grief reactions*, bereavements that last more than 1 year, may be seen when the surviving spouse was excessively dependent on the deceased and is unable to obtain emotional and practical (e.g., financial) support elsewhere or when the survivor is unable to grieve fully because of markedly ambivalent feelings toward the deceased. Distinguishing between pathological grief and grief triggering a depressive episode may not always be possible. The inadequate expression of grief due to incomplete bereavement is believed to be pathogenic in many subsequent psychiatric disorders. For example, impulsive acting out among adolescents who previously lost a parent is often assumed to be due to unresolved grief.

A variety of medical disorders may cause depressive syndromes. Most common among these are endocrine abnormalities, such as hypothyroidism and hyperparathyroidism, and CNS disorders such as cerebrovascular diseases and Parkinson's disease. Depressions are more common in strokes affecting left anterior lesions than other locations. Some medications, especially antihypertensive agents affecting adrenergic tone, such as reserpine (Serpasil) and possibly β-blockers, may also trigger depressions. The importance of a genetic diathesis in these iatrogenic depressions is not yet known. Depressive syndromes and disorders in general, however, are unquestionably familial and are likely to have genetic contributions, especially in depressions associated with bipolar disorder.

Cognitive features of depression are prominent. Characterizing the exact nature of the memory impairment using standardized tests has been difficult. The cognitive tasks requiring sustained effort and elaborate cognitive processing may be more disrupted in depression than are those tasks that can be accomplished more automatically. The so-called cognitive triad of depression consists of pervasive cognitive schema related to feelings of worthlessness, helplessness, and hopelessness—expectations that no one and nothing can, or is likely to, help now or in the future: "I'm not OK, the world is not OK, and it's never going to get any better."

Suicidal phenomena are of particular concern. Suicide is common in severe depressive disorders, with recent estimates of up to 9 percent of suicidal hospitalized patients ending their lives in suicide. Depressed patients compose the largest diagnostic group of all completed suicides. However, suicide occurs at high rates in many other conditions as well, notably substance abuse disorders, schizophrenia, and severe personality disorders. Suicide may occur in these conditions with or without a diagnosable comorbid depressive disorder. Depressed patients with comorbid alcohol abuse may be at particularly high risk for suicide.

Although consistent, useful, validated predictors of suicide do not exist, certain demographic features are associated with higher risk. These include being white, male, and older and living alone. In the psychiatric history, the single most important factor is that of past suicide attempts. A history of violent behavior may also predict suicide. Murderers have a very high suicide rate, especially those who murder family members during episodes of domestic violence. Among clinical signs, hopelessness, anhedonia, and severe anxiety may predict increased suicide risk. Serious physical illness in association with other risk factors, such as depression, may place a patient at higher risk. A genetic predisposition toward suicidal behavior cuts across diagnostic lines and plays a role in suicide risk. This may reflect a tendency toward impulsive behavior, correlating with low CNS levels of 5-hydroxyindoleacetic acid (5-HIAA), the major metabolite of serotonin.

Suicidal gestures and various acts of self-mutilation are also common among impulsive, dependent, and self-hating depressed people, for whom they serve as tension-releasing behaviors and as cries for help that may enlist desired social support. Because suicidal gestures have been associated with an increased risk for subsequently completed suicide, they should not be taken lightly. Such self-harm behaviors have been shown to persist in patients with borderline personality disorder well into the sixth decade of life. Contrary to earlier thinking, they do not appear to "burn out" with age. Subintentional suicide may result when suicidal gestures go awry or when reckless behavior, such as taking unnecessary risks in combat or driving while drunk, prove fatal.

Elated Moods Elated moods include euphoria, elation, exaltation, and ecstasy. They are marked by feelings of well-being and expansiveness, optimism, capability, pleasure, and grace. Such moods are normally experienced when life is going very well, when long-sought-after goals are achieved, and in states of love, religious fervor, and spiritual transcendence. Peak experiences and experiences of mystic fusion are often accompanied by feelings of exaltation and ecstasy. Sexual pleasure and some chemically mediated states of altered consciousness may also induce these feelings.

Abnormal elated moods are primarily seen as part of manic states and from the effects of certain medications and street drugs. When subtle, as in *hypomania*, the mood can be ebullient and brimming with self-confidence but with occasional irritability. Other characteristic symptoms of hypomania are increased energy, decreased need for sleep, rapidly flowing thoughts, excessive talking, inflated self-esteem with a demanding nature toward others, and diminished judgment. *Mania* is a more extreme state in which judgment and sleep are impaired to the point of marked functional disruption. As the mania exacerbates, irritability and anger increase, alternating rapidly with a brittle expansiveness. Cognitions become increasingly disorganized. Psychotic symptoms, usually involving themes of grandiosity or specialness, occur in 50 percent or more of manic patients. With increasing escalation of the manic state, thinking becomes very fragmented, psychotic symptoms are more prominent, and the syndrome may appear indistinguishable from acute schizophrenia. These three manic states—hypomania, mania, and the psychotic, fragmented manic state—have been referred to as *stage I*, *II*, and *III mania*, respectively. Manic states occur in bipolar disorder, bipolar disorder not otherwise specified, and cyclothymia and as a secondary mania caused by a variety of physical and toxic conditions. Such secondary manias may follow specific cerebral insults, accompany systemic disorders, or occur after ingestion of some drugs, including amphetamines, antidepressants, bromocriptine (Parlodel), decongestants, and corticosteroids, among others. Mania is the second most common neuropsychiatric disturbance induced by steroids, occurring in 30 to 35 percent of patients who develop steroid-induced behavioral disorders. Up to 12 percent of patients treated with levodopa (Larodopa) and bromocriptine for parkinsonism develop mania. Right hemispheric brain lesions are specifically associated with secondary mania.

Although not a DSM-IV-TR diagnosis, *hyperthymic personality* refers to personality characteristics similar to hypomania. These include unusual energy, ebullience, confidence, intensity, and so forth but without either the episodic course or the functional impairment of hypomania. Whether hyperthymic personality should be considered a bipolar spectrum disorder or refers simply to high energy individuals is still unclear.

Anxiety Like depression, the term *anxiety* refers to a number of different entities: a normal transient feeling, often with adaptive functions; a symptom seen in a wide variety of disorders; and a group of disorders in which the symptom of anxiety forms a dominant element. As a transient, disagreeable emotional state, anxiety may be adaptive, signaling anticipated or impending threat and motivating necessary action. In contrast to *fear*, the emotional state that exists when a source of threat is precise and well known, anxiety occurs when the threat is not well defined.

Patients often find it difficult to describe feelings of anxiety precisely; at its core, however, anxiety is characterized by intense negative affect, associated with an undefined threat to one's physical or psychological self. Patients use terms such as *tense*, *panicky*, *terrified*, *jittery*, *nervous*, *wound up*, *apprehensive*, and *worried*, to describe their sensations. Anxiety is additionally characterized by somatic, cognitive, behavioral, and perceptual symptoms. The somatic symptoms of anxiety are legion and often dominate; a partial list includes twitching, tremors, hot and cold flashes, sweating, palpitations, chest tightness, difficulty swallowing, nausea, diarrhea, dry mouth, and decreased libido. Cognitively, anxiety is characterized by hypervigilance, poor concentration, subjective confusion, fears of losing control or of going crazy, and catastrophic thinking. Behavioral symptoms include fearful expressions, withdrawal, irritability, immobility, and hyperventilation. Perceptual disturbances, including depersonalization, derealization, and hyperesthesia (especially hyperacusis), are also common.

Trait anxiety refers to a lifelong pattern of anxiety as a feature of temperament. Individuals with trait anxiety are skittish, are hypersensitive to stimuli, are psychophysiologically more reactive than others, and exhibit catastrophic thinking. In contrast, *state anxiety* refers to episodes of anxiety that are tightly bound to specific situations and do not persist after the provoking situation has abated. *Free-floating anxiety* is characterized by a persistently anxious mood in which the cause is unknown and in which large numbers of diverse thoughts and events all seem to trigger and compound the anxiety. In contrast, *situational anxiety* occurs only in relation to specific occasions or external stimuli, as in phobias.

Anxiety symptoms can result from numerous physical conditions as well as from other psychiatric disorders. Many endocrine, autoimmune, metabolic, and toxic disorders, as well as medication side effects, are known to generate anxiety. The psychiatrist must differentiate the response of the patient to an underlying condition (e.g., secondary anxiety) from symptoms generated by the primary disorder itself. In psychiatric populations, anxiety symptoms are prevalent among patients with psychoses, organic mental disorders, depression, and substance abuse disorders as well as in the specific anxiety disorders. In patients with schizophrenia, anxiety must be differentiated from akathisia, a common and often overlooked syndrome of subjective restlessness, anxiety, and agitation resulting from antipsychotic medication. The coexistence of anxiety symptoms and depression in major depressive disorder is substantial; anxiety symptoms, such as anxious mood and irritability, are seen in the majority of depressed patients. Additionally, one-half to two-thirds of patients with panic disorder experience a major depressive episode during their lifetime. Medication and drug effects—from acute use, side effects, or as part of withdrawal phenomena—are also common causes of anxiety. Many patients with severe anxiety become dependent on anxiolytic drugs, including benzodiazepines, other sedatives, and alcohol, for symptom relief. During attempts to discontinue these substances, or sometimes during their ongoing use, confusing admixtures of anxiety symptoms, medication effects, and withdrawal symptoms may occur.

Although all of the anxiety symptoms caused by drug use are also seen in primary anxiety disorders, perceptual disturbances, such as depersonalization and hyperesthesia, may be more common in sedative-hypnotic withdrawal syndromes than in primary anxiety disorders.

From a psychological point of view, anxiety may signal conflict between opposing desires, wishes, or beliefs on the one hand and major disequilibria generated by negative life events on the other hand. *Role strains*, conflicts among the major social roles that form a person's identity—spouse, parent, child, wage earner, professional, community member—are common sources of anxiety. The more important the conflict and the less obvious the resolution, the greater is the associated anxiety. For example, anxiety symptoms may first emerge when an individual is confronted with an unavoidable, unhappy choice, such as between sustaining a marriage or accepting a career advancement requiring a major move that is unacceptable to the spouse. At times, these conflicts may escape conscious awareness: Someone may feel anxious but not know why. Anxiety syndromes frequently result from a combination of several factors. A person in a work conflict facing an important deadline may try to alleviate initial anxiety symptoms by overwork, then ingest caffeine or amphetamines to keep alert, then become exhausted and fatigued, and ultimately use alcohol excessively to calm down, with each of these elements contributing separately to an anxiety state.

Certain developmental life situations are associated with anxiety. *Stranger anxiety* develops when infants 6 to 8 months of age begin to recognize the difference between mother and others. When children first go to school, mild anxiety symptoms are common; if the anxiety is excessive, *separation anxiety* or school phobia may result. During adult life, anxiety often centers around issues of mastery and accomplishment, both in personal and work life. *Performance anxiety*, or *stage fright*, is a specific type of pathological anxiety in which anxiety escalates to panic when public performance is required. In later life, the deterioration of one's body may engender anxiety related to feelings of helplessness and *death anxiety*.

Panic attack is a circumscribed episode of severe state anxiety lasting minutes to hours, with symptoms escalating in a crescendo pattern. The subjective experience is one of utter terror, fears that one will die, go crazy, or lose control, accompanied by many of the somatic symptoms of anxiety mentioned above, including severe chest pains, marked shortness of breath, and exhausting fatigue. Individual isolated panic attacks are common, with up to 30 percent of the general population experiencing at least one attack each year. Panic attacks occur more regularly, and typically more severely, as part of panic disorder or in association with other anxiety disorders. In classic panic disorder, the attacks are spontaneous; that is, they are not triggered by a specific, predictable environment. In contrast, panic attacks associated with other anxiety disorders are triggered by specific situations such as in social anxiety disorder by social situations or in specific phobia by confronting the feared object or situation. Patients with other psychiatric disorders may experience limited-symptom panic attacks, with episodes characterized by less intense anxiety and by fewer and milder physical symptoms such as isolated paresthesias or difficulty breathing. These limited-symptom attacks may represent aborted full-blown panic episodes that are not further exacerbated by secondary psychological reactions to the initial symptoms.

A 43-year-old man with crippling shyness and social phobia since youth started to experience increasing episodes of shortness of breath and chest pain in his late 30s. On numerous occasions, he called 911 for ambulances to take him to the local emergency room, fearing that he was having a heart attack. These episodes increased in frequency at the point in his life when his parents, who had previously supported and housed him, were becoming ill and showing signs of not being able to continue to sustain him. He gradually came to understand these episodes to be panic attacks and decreased the frequency with which he called for emergency services.

Although American psychiatry has segregated panic attacks from other forms of anxiety, assuming categorical, phenomenological, and biological differences, these distinctions are far from universally accepted. Much of European psychiatry views panic as simply an extreme form of anxiety to be understood as part of a continuum of intensity.

Phobias are irrational fears. In an effort to reduce the intense anxiety attached to phobic objects and situations, patients do their best to avoid the feared stimuli. Thus, phobias consist both of the fears and the avoidance components. The fear itself may include all the symptoms of extreme anxiety, up to and including panic. In *specific phobias*, persistent, irrational fears are provoked by specific stimuli. Table 8–5 lists some illustrative phobias. Common specific phobias include fear of dirt, excreta, snakes, spiders, heights, and blood (also termed *blood-injury phobias*).

Behavioral, psychodynamic, and biological theories have all been advanced as causes of phobias. Some well-known phobias, such as fear of animals, may result either from early traumatic events (developing

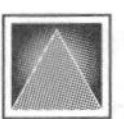

Table 8–5
Specific Phobias

Phobia	Definition
Acrophobia	Fear of heights
Agoraphobia	Fear of open spaces
Alektorophobia	Fear of chickens
Amathophobia	Fear of dust
Amaxophobia	Fear of riding in a car
Apiphobia	Fear of bees
Arachibutyrophobia	Fear of getting peanut butter stuck on the roof of the mouth
Astrapophobia	Fear of lightning
Aviophobia	Fear of flying
Blennophobia	Fear of slime
Claustrophobia	Fear of enclosed spaces
Cynophobia	Fear of dogs
Decidophobia	Fear of making decisions
Didaskaleinophobia	Fear of going to school
Electrophobia	Fear of electricity
Ephebiphobia	Fear of teenagers
Eremophobia	Fear of being alone
Gamophobia	Fear of marriage
Gatophobia	Fear of cats
Gephyrophobia	Fear of crossing bridges
Gynophobia	Fear of women
Hydrophobia	Fear of water
Kakorrhaphiophobia	Fear of failure
Katagelophobia	Fear or ridicule
Keraunophobia	Fear of thunder
Musophobia	Fear of mice
Nyctophobia	Fear of night
Ochlophobia	Fear of crowds
Odynophobia	Fear of pain
Ophidiophobia	Fear of snakes
Pnigerophobia	Fear of smothering
Pyrophobia	Fear of fire
Scholionophobia	Fear of school
Sciophobia	Fear of shadows
Spheksophobia	Fear of wasps
Technophobia	Fear of technology
Thalassophobia	Fear of the ocean
Triskaidekaphobia	Fear of the number 13
Tropophobia	Fear of moving or making changes

along the paradigm of classic Pavlovian conditioning) or from displacements of early psychodynamic conflicts. Genetic influences may also play a role in the development of phobias. For example, some individuals with blood-injury phobias, which strongly cluster among biological relatives, may be genetically predisposed by vagal responses to certain stimuli. Animal models also indicate possible biological vulnerability. Some monkeys that have never previously been exposed to snakes become panicky when placed in the presence of a snake. Because such fear responses obviously have adaptive value, it has been suggested that some human phobic responses also represent exaggerations of adaptive behaviors shaped by evolutionary biology. *Complex phobias*, more elaborate than specific phobias, involve fears related to a broader range of situations. *Agoraphobia*, the best known, means fear of the marketplace, symbolizing a fear of open spaces. Current thinking suggests that agoraphobia is a secondary reaction to panic attacks. In this view, individuals who have become terrified of having panic attacks in public retreat to the safety of their own homes, hoping to reduce the likelihood of panic attacks by avoiding places where they were once triggered and where they may feel exposed and embarrassed.

In *social anxiety disorder* (social phobia), patients become overwhelmingly anxious and fear situations in which they may be observed. In the limited type, only a few specific situations evoke the fear, such as speaking in public or using a public lavatory. In the general type, broad-based fears of social situations globally hamper the person's interpersonal life.

Aggression, Hostility, Impulsiveness, and Violence

The spectrum of aggressive emotions and behaviors is characterized by heightened vigilance in response to a sense of threat and enhanced readiness to attack. Physiological tone may be geared for a fight. Assertiveness, the adaptive aspect of these emotions, includes sensing that something needs to be done and feeling willing and competent to take constructive action. The manner and extent to which aggressive emotions can be expressed varies from society to society and from situation to situation. These emotions are among the most carefully regulated because of their potential destructiveness. Acts of aggression are on a continuum, beginning with irritability, progressing to verbal threats and intimidation, and extending to physical bullying and assault to homicide, sometimes including acts of calculated violence and sadism.

Irritability is an unpleasant feeling state characterized by inner unease. In contrast to anger, irritability does not lessen after an outburst. Often, others are more aware of an individual's irritability than is the person him- or herself. It is diagnostically nonspecific, seen in a variety of physiological states—psychotic, anxiety, and mood disorders—and as a lifelong temperamental quality. Hunger, sleepiness, sexual frustration, and pain are among the physiological triggers commonly associated with irritability.

Individual differences in the tendency toward experiencing and expressing anger and violence are biological, developmental, and cultural in origin. Some infants are irritable from birth. Subtle early birth injuries and brain anoxia may increase the susceptibility of some people to be violent. Furthermore, studies of EEG patterns in violent people show increased abnormalities, especially in those with repeated violence and violence with little or no obvious motive. Soft neurological signs are also seen in violent criminals. Biochemically, low cerebrospinal fluid (CSF) 5-HIAA has been associated with a variety of impulsive behaviors, such as violent crimes, recurrent fire setting, and violent suicide attempts.

Consistent with the hypothesis that an inverse relationship exists between central serotonergic system function and impulsive, aggressive behavior, a few double-blind, placebo-controlled studies in patients with cluster B personality disorders have demonstrated that enhancing central serotonergic function by using SSRIs reduces irritability and impulsive aggressive behavior.

A 42-year-old woman was described by those who knew her as controlling, obsessional in style, and rigid in expectations. When events in her house did not turn out as she wished or when others (husband and children) did not behave according to her demands, she became very irritable, yelling, criticizing, and berating. Eventually, she agreed to treatment with an SSRI, which markedly diminished her reactivity to events. The positive effect was far more apparent to her family members than to the patient herself.

The pathological childhood triad of bed-wetting past the age of 6 years, setting fires, and torturing animals has been associated with subsequent violent behavior in adults. Interpersonally, studies show that violence-prone individuals require more personal space around their physical person than do others. Violent individuals feel threatened when approached too closely, particularly from the rear.

Psychological and social contributions are also strong. Violence in families breeds violence, and battered children often grow up to be battering adults. Cultural norms for the expression of violence differ considerably. In some socioeconomic and ethnic groups, violent gangs organize the energies of many adolescent youth. For some, violent behavior is an adolescent socialization pattern necessary to prove one's manhood or womanhood. Like other social organizations, violent gangs have detailed rules that inhibit and govern the expression of violence. Some unpredictable and unsocialized violent people, loners, are too violent to be contained even in gangs.

Aggressive and violent behavior is diagnostically nonspecific. Violence in schizophrenia may occur as a consequence of paranoid delusions, in response to command auditory hallucinations, or secondary to passivity experiences. Manic patients and those in mixed states may be violent, often in response to minimal provocation. Violent behavior commonly occurs in patients with antisocial and borderline personalities (in the latter often self-directed as well as other directed). Violent behavior may occur in epilepsy, although rarely during true ictal periods; in frontal lobe syndromes as a "release phenomenon"; and in association with abused substances, particularly disinhibiting sedatives, such as alcohol, or stimulants such as amphetamines and cocaine, which increase irritability, aggressiveness, and paranoia.

Impulsive violence may be provoked by a number of stimuli and situations. Alcohol is perhaps the most common disinhibitor of violence. Intrafamilial violence, the most common setting for homicide, is frequently related to alcohol intoxication. In *episodic dyscontrol* and *intermittent explosive disorder*, violent behaviors typically erupt after a person has ingested alcohol, a phenomenon known as *pathological intoxication*. In these often ferocious outbursts, the individual may confront or provoke any potential target for violence, including total strangers and police, but girlfriends, wives, and parents are frequent victims. Patients with episodic dyscontrol commonly have histories of violent sexual behavior, including rape, and, often while intoxicated, speeding and reckless driving, sometimes chasing down, stopping, and attacking other motorists who they believe "get in their way."

An attractive 40-year-old woman had been highly sought after by rich and powerful men, several of whom she had married and several of whom divorced her because of her uncontrollable rages. She described herself as becoming "insanely jealous" in a flash whenever she saw her husband glancing at other attractive women, and her behavior flared out of control, particularly when she had been drinking alcohol. On one occasion, she bit off one husband's ear. She attacked another with pots and knives, nearly killing him. She recognized how serious her problems were and sought psychotherapy, medication (SSRIs were helpful), and anger management training to help her control her emotions and behaviors.

Temper Tantrums Immature individuals with persistent personality problems may not develop mechanisms to inhibit temper tantrums they displayed as children. Particularly if childhood tantrums produced the desired result, learned tantrum behaviors may persist into adult life. Although such individuals may be pleasant and sociable when life is going well, they lack the capacity to tolerate frustration and are easily provoked by threats to self-esteem and self-image and by not having their own way. When frustrated or threatened, they may act like bullies, glare, snarl, yell, shout, intimidate, pout and sulk, and sometimes be physically violent.

Displaced Rage When circumstances prevent the expression of rage directly against those people or institutions provoking frustration, other outlets for aggression are often found. Acts of violence that are either calculated or wanton may result. Cruelty to animals and fire setting may persist as adult forms of destructive behavior. Rape, an act of control, intimidation, terror, and humiliation, may also displace frustrations that are not expressed more adaptively.

Sadism may occur with or without explicit sexual gratification. Calculated cruelty conducted seemingly without anger or emotional arousal may reflect inadequate development of social morality or individual conscience, as in the conduct of torturers and some cold-blooded murderers. In some societies and under specific circumstances at certain times in history, such activity has been socially sanctioned, suggesting at least that some people lack inborn inhibitions against cruelty or violence.

A 50-year-old man with antisocial personality disorder was seen in a psychiatric emergency room for violent behavior. During the course of the assessment, he described how he had been emotionally and physically abused by a sadistic father who whipped him repeatedly until he bled and who chained him to a tree in the backyard. This man grew up feeling callous. He enjoyed intimidating and physically hurting others, as he often did in prison. With a laugh and smirk, he reflected on how he turned out to be "just like my old man."

Self-Mutilation For a variety of reasons, in many different cultures and in many different disorders, people commit acts of violence against themselves, ranging from body piercing to cutting and burning to autoamputation. Psychotic patients may perform extremely self-destructive acts short of actual suicide that often have symbolic import, such as enucleating their eyes or castrating themselves. Patients with borderline personality disorders or borderline traits may cut themselves repeatedly with broken glass or razor blades or burn themselves with cigarettes on arms, legs, breasts, or other body parts. Patients typically deny that these acts are meant to be suicidal but describe the need to feel external pain to mirror internal suffering, or to release tension, or to counteract dissociative-like numbness. Recently, self-cutting has become more common in teenagers, especially girls, as a tension-relieving mechanism.

A 20-year-old college student was taken to the emergency room by her friends, who were alarmed by the recent transverse cuts on her arms. None of the cuts were deep enough to require sutures but, even when they had healed, they left obvious small red scars on her skin. In explaining her behavior, the student described that when she was upset, such as after a fight with her boyfriend or a negative telephone call with her parents, she became agitated, and cutting herself consistently relieved the agitation and anxious feelings.

Trichotillomania is a syndrome of compulsive hair pulling, resulting in bald patches. It is often associated with other self-mutilatory behavior, such as picking the face, nails, or cuticles to the point of infection and bleeding. Trichotillomania may sometimes be related to OCD.

Children with *Lesch-Nyhan syndrome*, a developmental disability syndrome caused by a congenital metabolic abnormality, bite and pick at themselves so compulsively as to do themselves great harm and routinely require restraint. Occasionally, patients with Tourette's syndrome demonstrate compulsive self-harming behavior.

Other Disturbances of Feelings

Diminished levels of emotional intensity may be seen in anxiety disorders, mood disorders, and schizophrenia. Mild emotional flattening with blunted ability to feel joy is common in dysthymia. Some patients with narcissistic and borderline personality disorders complain of inner emptiness and pervasive boredom and ennui without demonstrating diminished affect in interviews. Similarly, patients with prominent depersonalization describe numbed emotions. Pathological levels of *blunt* or *flattened affect*, indicating markedly diminished affective expression in relation to specific thought content, may be seen in chronic schizophrenia (as part of the deficit syndrome), some organic mental syndromes, and severe depressions and as a side effect to many medications, including SSRI antidepressants, antipsychotic medications, or excessive tranquilizer use. Although the term *blunted affect* is not classically used to describe the affective flatness of severe depression, it is not always easy to distinguish between schizophrenic and depressive flatness on phenomenological grounds. *Anhedonia*, the lack of pleasurable feelings from activities that ordinarily provide pleasure, is also seen as part of severe depressions or schizophrenia. Chronically psychotic patients often exhibit emotional deterioration in which affective experience and expression are entirely unrelated to thought content. *Inappropriate affect* is incongruency of affective expression and thought content. The patient may display loud and raucous laughter or giggling in relation to bland or sad thoughts or may show grief without apparent reason. Inappropriate affect sometimes indicates that the thoughts have private meanings for the patients; the emotional expression might make better sense if the private meanings were understood. Inappropriate affect must be distinguished from affective expressions that may actually be appropriate in a given subculture or ethnic group that is unfamiliar to the observer and from defensive affect, such as the nervous laughter used to alleviate tension or ward off crying. *Affective* (or mood) *lability* is characterized by rapid emotional shifts, often within seconds to minutes. It is commonly seen during hypomanic states, late luteal phase dysphoric disorder (premenstrual syndrome), postpartum blues, other states of physiological instability, and in cluster B personality disorders.

A 51-year-old man with lifelong dysthymic disorder was treated with an SSRI. Although he had an excellent antidepressant response, 2 months after beginning treatment, he noted an affective flatness. He described not becoming as easily upset as before treatment (which both he and his wife interpreted positively), but also he believed his sense of joy, in being with his children or in nature, was markedly blunted. He enjoyed positive events but with a marked diminution of affective intensity.

Alexithymia is difficulty identifying, describing, and differentiating feelings or distinguishing between feelings and physical sensations. Alexithymic individuals often have constricted imaginations and fantasies, are preoccupied with objects and events in the outside world, and have little private, personal internal life. When distressed, the patients are simply aware of not feeling well and usually complain of somatic symptoms, leading to frustrating interactions with their physicians who cannot find physical causes for the presenting physical complaints. Some view alexithymia as a condition in which affect is communicated through somatic language.

With regard to other feeling states that may contribute to pathological conditions, recent writers have focused on the role of "shame" as a potentially important emotional mediator of specific types of narcissistic injury that may provoke states of depression, rage, PTSD, and suicide, among others.

DISTURBANCES IN MOTOR ASPECTS OF BEHAVIOR

Motor behavior is normally finely coordinated, purposeful, and adaptive, and necessary activities are usually carried out efficiently. In psychiatric disturbances, motor abnormalities can involve generalized overactivity or underactivity or manifest in a wide range of specific disorders of movement.

Overactivity

Restlessness and *agitation* are diffuse increases in body movement, usually noted as fidgeting, rapid and rhythmic leg or hand tapping, and jerky start-and-stop movements of the entire body, accompanied by inner tension. Restlessness accompanies psychiatric conditions of high emotional arousal or confusion, such as toxic states, deliria, mania, agitated depressive disorders, and anxiety disorders, as well as many medical disorders such as hyperthyroidism. In some depressive states, agitation is often accompanied by pacing and hand wringing.

Generalized overactivity, in which patients seem to have increased physical energy, is distinguished from agitation by its lack of inner tension and by more purposeful movements. It is commonly seen in mania, hypomania, and anorexia nervosa and as part of ADHD and in response to stimulating drugs and medicines.

A 25-year-old extraordinarily restless man in a psychiatric emergency room, whose glances darted incessantly around the room, paced agitatedly, picked at his skin, shifted constantly on his feet, and jiggled his arms and legs. His speech was rapid, and his mood was irritable. He had been using intravenous (IV) methamphetamine on a "run" for more than 1 week and was brought to the emergency room by relatives who were concerned that he was starting to get paranoid.

In *catatonic excitement*, much less common now than in the preneuroleptic era, patients exhibit disorganized and overactive behaviors, including frantic jumping, thrashing of limbs, and seemingly senseless menacing or attacking behaviors. Such excitement is seen in mania, periodic catatonia, catatonic forms of schizophrenia, and some culture-bound syndromes such as *amok*. *Confusional excitement* is a state of restlessness and generalized purposeless activity seen in ictal states, some acute intoxications, and deliria.

Decreased Motor Activity

Global reductions in motor activity—motor retardation—are seen in a variety of physical disorders, such as hypothyroidism, Addison's disease, some infectious and postinfectious conditions, including CFS and postpolio syndrome, and other fatiguing conditions, as well as in some organic mental disorders, intoxications, schizophrenias, and depressive disorders. Poverty of movement (akinesia, or more properly, hypokinesia) may occur in schizophrenia and as a neuroleptic side effect. Changes in the voice frequently accompany the reduced motor activity in schizophrenia and depression, with normal inflection replaced by monotonous tone and prolonged speech latency. In stuporous states, patients remain immobile, although their eyes are open, and they are apparently awake.

Conversion reactions are functional, nonphysiological, psychogenic impairments in sensory or motor functions. Common motor forms include various paralyses and pareses, including limb paralyses, ataxias, and aphonias. In *globus hystericus,* the patient is unable to swallow. Patients with *astasia-abasia* have marked unsteadiness of gait. Sensory conversion reactions include blindness, deafness, anesthesia, and analgesia. Some hyperesthesias and pain syndromes may also originate as conversion symptoms.

An 18-year-old soldier from a very rural area was brought to the emergency room at an army post during his period of basic training because his gait had become very unsteady. He was stumbling into walls and seemed unable to maintain an erect posture. He found it necessary to use crutches to ambulate. There was no history of substance use. On examination, the soldier was found to be naïve, tremulous, anxious, and homesick. He had never been away from his family before and missed them deeply. When he was reassured that he would be issued a pass to see his family, his demeanor changed, and his gait instantly improved. To the amazement of his bunkmates and drill sergeant, he was able to leave his crutches at the door. The diagnosis was astasia-abasia.

Mutism

Mutism may result from a variety of peripheral muscle and CNS conditions and from functional disorders. Mutism may occur in profound depression, catatonic states, and conversion reactions. *Elective mutism* is occasionally seen in acute adjustment disorders and some personality disturbances.

Motor Disturbances

Many motor disturbances are seen in psychiatric disorders. Some form part of the core symptoms of the disorders; some occur in disorders that, by their nature, bridge neurology and psychiatry (such as Tourette's syndrome); others are acute or chronic medication side effects.

Simple Motor Phenomena

TREMOR Tremors, involuntary oscillating movements of the limbs or head, may occur at rest or with movement. *Physiological tremors,* which are minimal at rest and increase with activity, are characterized by small amplitude and high frequency. They are characteristic of anxiety, fatigue, and toxic or metabolic disorders, such as caffeinism or hyperthyroidism, and are commonly seen in patients taking a number of different psychiatric medications, including lithium (Eskalith), valproate (Depakene), and stimulating antidepressants. *Coarse tremors,* with larger amplitude and lower frequency, are seen in Parkinson's disease and cerebellar disease. *Asterixis* is a large-amplitude flapping tremor of the hands seen in hepatic disease. *Parkinsonian* symptoms and signs may be seen in psychiatric disorders, particularly in patients taking antipsychotic medications. Symptoms include akinesias with marked decrease in normally spontaneous fidgeting, stiff gait with diminished arm swing, pill-rolling nonintention tremors (which seem to be less common in drug-induced parkinsonism, compared with the idiopathic type), expressionless soft and monotonous speech, micrographical handwriting, and cogwheel rigidity.

DYSTONIC MOVEMENTS Although dystonic movements are seen in many neurological disorders, in psychiatric patients, they are almost always secondary to the use of antipsychotic medications. Dystonic reactions consist of intermittent or sustained muscle spasms, typically of the head or neck. Common varieties include tongue spasms causing dysarthria, torticollis (neck spasm), and oculogyric crisis in which there is a forced upward gaze. Opisthotonus (spasms of paraspinal muscles leading to an arched posture) is seen less often. These reactions are most common in young males and typically occur soon after beginning or increasing the dose of a conventional antipsychotic medication.

AKATHISIA *Akathisia* is a syndrome of motor restlessness seen predominantly in the context of antipsychotic and some antidepressant medication use. It has subjective, as well as motor, components. Subjectively, patients experience muscle tension, difficulty finding a comfortable body position, and inability to stop moving; they feel as though they are "jumping out of their skin." Objectively, akathisia classically manifests by rocking from foot to foot while standing, frequently crossing and uncrossing the legs when seated, and pacing. Sleep may be disturbed because of physical discomfort. Subjective components of akathisia may be difficult to distinguish from anxiety caused by the primary disorder (typically schizophrenia). Rarely, the restlessness and inner agitation become sufficiently uncomfortable to provoke acts of violence. In pseudoakathisia, objective signs of akathisia are present, but the patient denies feeling restless.

> A 45-year-old man with OCD and Tourette's syndrome being treated with fluvoxamine (Luvox), 200 mg per day, inadvertently took 400 mg per day for 3 days. On the third day, he started to feel increasingly agitated, his legs felt restless and jittery, and he started to uncharacteristically fidget. He also noted frequent sighs in his breathing, not his usual respiratory pattern. He recalled feeling these sensations a decade earlier when a previous psychiatrist treated his Tourette's syndrome with haloperidol (Haldol) and that his psychiatrist had diagnosed akathisia. After discontinuing the fluvoxamine for 4 days, these symptoms all abated.

TARDIVE DYSKINESIA *Tardive dyskinesia* is a movement disorder that occurs only in the context of antipsychotic medication use, occasionally after many months but more commonly after years. The abnormal movements may persist with or without continued medication use or may diminish or disappear over time. The dyskinetic movements occur at rest and can usually be temporarily suppressed volitionally or by purposeful action, distraction, or sleep. The movements are varied. In the most common type, which affects the face, especially the mouth and lips, tongue thrusting, chewing movements, lip smacking, and eye blinking are seen. Another common type is characterized by choreoathetoid movements, such as writhing finger motions. In the less common but more severe truncal dyskinesias, the torso moves in thrusting motions, and respiratory dyskinesia is characterized by grunting and irregular breathing patterns. Other tardive (late) syndromes include tardive akathisia and tardive dystonia, in which the abnormal movements emerge late in treatment or on medication discontinuation.

NEUROLEPTIC MALIGNANT SYNDROME Neuroleptic malignant syndrome (NMS), a potentially fatal complication of antipsychotic medication, is characterized by muscle rigidity, fever, diaphoresis, delirium, mutism, and blood pressure abnormalities. Some view NMS as the most severe end of a spectrum that starts with antipsychotic-induced parkinsonism, progresses to extrapyramidal syndrome with fever, and then to fulminant NMS.

RABBIT SYNDROME This uncommon drug-induced extrapyramidal syndrome is often misdiagnosed as tardive dyskinesia. It most closely resembles a limited expression of a parkinsonian tremor. Patients make rapid chewing movements similar to those made by rabbits, ordinarily faster and more regular than the orofacial tic of tardive dyskinesia. The tongue is spared.

BLEPHAROSPASM *Blepharospasm* is a rapid and violent repetitive, spasmodic movement of the eyelids. These movements are often a side effect of antipsychotic or other medications but are also common in a variety of neurological disorders, including Meige's syndrome and Tourette's syndrome.

TICS *Tics* are rapid, repetitive, often spasmodic jerking involuntary movements that serve no apparent purpose. The person may try to disguise or hide the tic in a seemingly purposive movement, and the movement may ultimately be shaped into a mannerism. Tics are the central feature of tic disorders, are associated with other disorders, and may occur as a consequence of stimulant use. *Tourette's disorder* is characterized by a chronic shifting array of motor and vocal tics. The tics may include grunts, coughs, clicks, or sniffs, whereas motor symptoms may include eye blinking, tongue protrusions, facial grimacing, hopping, and twitches. Complex tics may merge into complex compulsive behaviors such as squatting, deep knee bends, and retracing steps. *Coprolalia,* characterized by sudden verbal outbursts of obscenities, occurs in less than one-third of Tourette's patients. *Mental coprolalia* is an associated feature in which obscene words or phrases suddenly intrude into consciousness in an ego-dystonic manner. Obsessive-compulsive symptoms, as well as attention-deficit symptoms, are also common in Tourette's syndrome.

SEROTONIN SYNDROME *Serotonin syndrome* is a disorder caused by excessive serotonergic input in the CNS, probably within the hypothalamus. The most common cause of serotonin syndrome is the combination of two or more medications with serotonin-enhancing properties, usually by different mechanisms. It is characterized by restlessness, myoclonus, hyperreflexia, diaphoresis, shivering, tremor, autonomic changes, including fever, and mental status changes, such as confusion.

Motor Disturbances of Schizophrenia Many of the abnormal movements ascribed to tardive dyskinesia and other antipsychotic-induced extrapyramidal syndromes have been described in chronically psychotic patients before the introduction of antipsychotic medications. In one series of 100 patients, the large majority of whom were diagnosed as schizophrenic, a review of medical records before 1955 revealed that abnormal purposive movements were found in 83 percent, mannerisms and tics in 71 percent, abnormal eye movements in 27 percent, abnormal postures or facial movements in 42 percent, and gait abnormalities in 10 percent. These findings suggest that many patients with schizophrenia have neurological symptoms not due to medications and that severe psychiatric disorders may have a neurological component as well.

CATATONIC BEHAVIORS *Catatonia* refers to a broad group of movement abnormalities usually associated with schizophrenia but also found in other disorders such as mania, depression, many neurological disorders (especially those involving the basal ganglia, limbic system, diencephalon and frontal lobes), systemic metabolic disorders, toxic drug states, and periodic catatonia. Catatonic stupor and excitement have already been noted. *Stereotypies* are repetitious, bizarre, seemingly non–goal-directed, complex organized gestures or postures that are believed to have private meanings to the patient. Examples include continuously and repeatedly crossing oneself or blessing others in a religious gesture, waving in a stylized manner, and making profane gestures. The stereotypic behaviors commonly seen in autistic children (constant spinning or rocking) may provide self-soothing, steady sensory input that helps the patients reduce the degree to which they are disturbed by the ordinarily unpredictable and uncontrollable stimulation coming from the environment. *Bizarre posturing* may also be seen in catatonia. One chronic schizophrenic patient routinely stood for hours on one leg with his arms in the air like a crane. In *echopraxia*, the patient imitates the examiner's movements and in *echolalia* imitates speech, as if in mimicry. Some catatonic patients exhibit *waxy flexibility*, maintaining unusual postures in which they have been posed for prolonged periods of time. *Negativism* may take the form of refusing to behave in a prescribed manner or resisting passive movement.

Other Movement Disturbances *Gait disturbances* in patients with psychiatric disorders include a variety of neurogenic gaits consistent with brain disease, intoxications, and medication side effects. These include the festinating gait of parkinsonism, spastic and ataxic gaits of neurological disease and psychiatric medications, waddling and reeling gaits associated with intoxications, and the nonphysiological gait disturbances seen in astasia-abasia, a form of conversion disorder. Gait mannerisms include clowning, prancing, military, and effeminate gaits.

Bruxism, chronic jaw clenching, may occur involuntarily during tension states, as an isolated occurrence during delta sleep, in which it has sometimes been associated with benzodiazepine or alcohol use, or in association with SSRI use. In severe cases, serious damage to dental enamel and temporomandibular joint pain may occur.

Myoclonus, characterized by focal muscle jerking, can be caused in psychiatric patients by certain medications, such as SSRIs or monoamine oxidase inhibitors (MAOIs). Myoclonic jerks may be difficult to distinguish from tics, but the latter often represent larger muscle groups and more highly organized motor patterns. Myoclonus may be seen at rest but is more obvious during motor activity.

Seizure-Like Behaviors In addition to the generalized, petit mal and complex partial seizures seen in some psychiatric patients, a number of nonepileptic seizure-like behaviors must be distinguished. *Breath-holding spells*, generally innocuous, impulsive, and tantrum-like phenomena, usually occur in small children who hold their breaths during moments of oppositional rage and who may faint as a result. Jerking or twitching motor movements may occur. *Temper tantrums* in young children may look like seizures, especially to the uninformed observer. The children may lie on the floor, screaming and kicking, and do not respond to the environment. *Conversion seizures* (hysterical seizures, pseudoseizures) must be differentiated from genuine epileptic seizures. Patients retain consciousness, lack abnormal reflexes, and are not incontinent. However, because so many conversion seizures occur in patients who have genuine epilepsy and who know a good deal about the condition, the differential diagnosis is sometimes difficult. *Compulsive behaviors* may occur in relation to everyday activities, such as gambling, sexual conquest, shopping, and watching TV, or in relation to substances such as alcohol, cocaine, narcotics, and food. Other compulsions involve reckless risk-taking behaviors that provide stimulation and dispel dysphoric moods. Sexual compulsive perversions, such as exhibitionism and sadomasochism, may serve similar purposes. Compulsions are seen in a variety of psychotic and nonpsychotic psychiatric disorders. The cravings that underlie compulsive behaviors are strong motivating forces, and the compulsive behaviors may regulate emotions. Unknown similarities may underlie all compulsive and addictive mechanisms. Current controversies surround the relationships of compulsive, impulsive, and addictive behaviors. Some authorities have proposed that all three should be subsumed under the rubric of a so-called reward deficiency syndrome, resulting from various combinations of gene polymorphisms governing dopamine and opioid mechanisms and including serotonin, cannabinoid, and other transmitter systems as well. From this perspective, the compulsive, impulsive, and addictive behaviors all increase the amount of dopamine and potentially other transmitters in specific brain areas. Studies in the past decade have shown that, in various subject groups, the Taq 1 a1 allele of the *DRD2* gene is associated with alcoholism, drug abuse, smoking, obesity, compulsive gambling, and several personality traits. Several other candidate genes are also under investigation. Studies have also shown that certain impulse-like behaviors may be associated with very specific genetic polymorphisms. In studies of patients with severe obesity, binge eating behavior was seen only in those individuals who had specific mutations in genes controlling the expression of melanocortin 4 receptors.

In OCD, the compulsions are ritualized, repetitive behaviors that are performed with the goal of satisfying, neutralizing, and undoing obsessional thoughts. Although intended to decrease anxiety, rituals are never more than transiently successful. The most common compulsions involve checking to make certain that gas jets and faucets have been turned off and that windows and doors are locked, hand washing, repeating certain phrases, counting objects, and placing objects in a prescribed order.

A 47-year-old woman had always been fussy about order and cleanliness but, since the birth of her child 14 years before, had become increasingly obsessed by cleanliness. She spent 3 hours daily ritualistically cleaning the apartment, using 3 to 4 rolls of paper towels daily. If a family member left even a fingerprint on a table, she became agitated and spent much time recleaning the surface and admonishing the family member.

LANGUAGE DISORDERS

Communication difficulties may be due to disorders of thinking as previously described, abnormal speech patterns in mood disturbances and schizophrenia, or primary speech fluency disorders, such as stuttering and stammering, disorders of the articulation and speech apparatus, and CNS disturbances involved in hearing and speech generation (aphasias).

Manic patients typically exhibit *pressured speech*, in which the speed of word stream is accelerated. If severe, the speech may be garbled, imprecise, and difficult to understand. Patients with psychomotor retardation depression speak slowly and monotonously and have a long speech latency in response to questions. Schizophrenic patients may exhibit a variety of speech abnormalities, including poverty of speech and poverty of content of speech (in which the amount of speaking is normal, but understanding the central message is difficult or impossible). Schizophrenic patients may also be difficult to understand because of the dysarthric effect of antipsychotic medication.

Allusory speech is vague, imprecise, and hard to comprehend because too few cues and details are provided for the listener. Such speech may be heard from some patients with schizophrenia or certain personality disorders or even normal individuals who wish to convey a sense of mystery by just being suggestive, whose suspiciousness causes them to be reluctant to spell things out clearly, or who believe that the listener is more aware of their private codes, meanings, and allusions than is the case.

Stuttering and *stammering* (ordinarily synonymous) refer to disturbances in the rhythm and fluency of speech due to blocking, convulsive repetition, or prolongation of sounds. This disorder affects males two to three times as often as females, and there is a high rate of familial transmission.

Aphasias, impairments of language produced by brain dysfunction, are ordinarily described as being fluent and nonfluent. In *fluent aphasias*, which generally reflect dysfunction in the left temporal and parietal area, patients have a normal or even elevated verbal output, sometimes with logorrhea, but they ignore the social conventions of conversation. They produce many well-articulated phrases with normal prosody, but there is little informational content. The fluent aphasias are further divided according to the extent of comprehension by the patient and the ability of the patient to repeat what the examiner says. The principal fluent aphasias are Wernicke's aphasia, conduction aphasia, anemic aphasia, and transcortical sensory aphasia.

Nonfluent aphasias are characterized by slow and poor verbal output, difficulty with spontaneous speech, omission of grammatical connecting words, and poor prosody. Patients may produce one-word replies or very short phrases. Brain lesions that cause nonfluent aphasias typically tend to occur in the anterior left hemisphere. The principal nonfluent aphasias are Broca's aphasia, transcortical motor aphasia, global aphasia, and the mixed transcortical aphasias.

In *aprosodias*, the nonverbal aspects of speech, the melody, pauses, timing, stress, accent, and intonation are impaired. Damage to the right prefrontal region has been associated with expressive aprosodias, and damage to the right temporal region and insula has been associated with receptive aprosodias.

DISTURBANCES OF INTERPERSONAL RELATIONSHIPS

Normal interpersonal relationships include relationships with parents, children, spouses, lovers, siblings, extended family members, friends, colleagues, coworkers, and members of the larger community. These relationships ordinarily help provide for the satisfaction of basic drives, for affiliative needs, and for finding purpose and meaning in life. Through stable and satisfying relationships, human needs are met for intimacy, including love, sex, and affection; to be cared for and nurtured, provide care, learn, play, relax, dominate, and be productive through mutual effort. Interpersonal relationships are carefully regulated by means of interpersonal signs and signals. The extent to which deviance from these patterns is tolerated in a given relationship varies from behavior to behavior, relationship to relationship, family to family, and culture to culture.

Disturbances in interpersonal relationships may be viewed as characteristics attributable to a single person or as characteristics of an interpersonal system. Individual disturbances are considered to be undesirable or maladaptive personality traits. When these traits are present to a significant extent and interfere with social functioning or cause distress, they may compose a personality disorder. Disturbances of interpersonal relationships have also been described at a systems level (e.g., as dyadic and family patterns of system disturbance).

Personality Traits and Disorders

Personality, variably defined, is the characteristic pattern of an individual's attitudes, behaviors, beliefs, feelings, thoughts, and values—the sum of a person's emotional, cognitive, and interpersonal attributes. Personality traits are the prominent and characteristic features of an individual's personality and do not imply psychopathology. Aspects of personality are present from early life, and personality traits are relatively stable from adolescence onward, consistent across different environments, and recognizable by friends and acquaintances. The term *personality disorder* should be reserved for those consistent patterns of thought, feeling, and behavior that are inflexible and maladaptive. Personality disturbances manifest primarily in interpersonal contexts and in this way can be viewed as interpersonal behavior disorders.

The determinants of personality are multiple and varied—innate and early biological, developmental, and environmental factors inside and outside the home. Through learning and the environment, temperamental factors (genetic or constitutional) are shaped into character.

The dimensional approach to personality and personality pathology characterizes individuals along a continuum of traits. Five dimensions of temperament have been described that appear to be somewhat independent and to have strong genetic contributions: neuroticism (highly emotional, reactive, and thin skinned, contrasting with emotional stability), extroversion (contrasting with introversion), openness (contrasting with discomfort with novel experiences), agreeableness (contrasting with contrariness), and conscientiousness (contrasting with fickleness). These temperamental attributes may have implications for the course of psychotherapies that cut across diagnostic categories.

Another dimension of personality not adequately dealt with in the DSM-IV-TR concerns moral behaviors such as honesty and integrity. The extent to which individuals behave honestly and with integrity differs considerably across individuals and in different situations. Deception and lying are common behaviors that occur in benign forms (e.g., in "white lies") and in pathological forms, psychiatrically important in antisocial and sociopathic disorders, pathological liars, and malingerers. Deception and lying may be difficult to assess clinically in the absence of additional informants. Studies of nonhuman primates indicate that, at least among chimpanzees, deception (equivalent to lying and dishonesty) is relatively common and, in some situations, adaptive.

Another personality typology characterizes personality along three dimensions related to temperamental characteristics presumed to be strongly influenced genetically: *harm avoidance*, *novelty seeking*, and *reward dependence*. High scores on the three dimensions characterize inhibition and pessimism, impulsive and exploratory behavior, and dependency and sentimentality, respectively. Different personality types can be described according to patterns of scores on the three dimensions. For example, antisocial personalities are characterized by high novelty seeking, low harm avoidance, and low reward dependence, whereas dependent characters have low novelty seeking, high harm avoidance, and high reward dependence.

DSM-IV-TR, by contrast, uses a categorical approach, yet both the large overlap among the DSM-IV-TR personality disorders and the clustering of these personality disorders into three broad groups imply a lack of clear boundaries to the currently defined categories. The three DSM-IV-TR clusters describe odd or eccentric types (cluster A); dramatic, emotional, and erratic types (cluster B); and anxious and fearful types (cluster C).

The odd or eccentric group includes paranoid, schizoid, and schizotypal personality disorders. Patients with these personality disorders have the core traits of being interpersonally distant and emotionally constricted. Paranoid personalities are quick to feel slighted and jealous, carry grudges, and expect to be exploited and harmed by others. Schizoid personalities lack friendships or close relationships with others and are indifferent to praise or criticism by others. Schizotypal personalities display odd beliefs, engage in odd and eccentric gestures and practices, and exhibit odd speech.

The dramatic, emotional, and erratic group includes borderline, histrionic, narcissistic, and antisocial personality disorders. Patients with these personality disorders characteristically have chaotic lives, emotions, and relationships. Borderline personalities are impulsive, unpredictable, angry, temperamental, unstable in relationships, compulsively interpersonal, and self-damaging with regard to sex, money, and substance use. Histrionic personalities are attention seeking, exhibitionistic, seductive, self-indulgent, exhibit exaggerated expressions of emotions, and are overconcerned with physical appearance. Narcissistic personalities tend to be hypersensitive to criticism, exploitative of others, egocentric with an inflated sense of self-importance, feel entitled to special treatment, and demand constant attention. Antisocial personalities are described almost exclusively by behavioral rather than affective or relational terms. They are truant, lie, steal, start fights, break rules, are unable to sustain work or school, and shirk everyday responsibilities.

The anxious and fearful group includes avoidant, dependent, and obsessive-compulsive personality disorders. Patients with these disorders are characterized by constricting behaviors that serve to limit risks. As examples, avoidant people avoid relationships, dependent personalities avoid being responsible for decisions, and obsessive-compulsive people use rigid rules that preclude new behaviors. Avoidant personalities are hypersensitive to rejection and are reluctant to enter close relationships in spite of strong desires for affection. Dependent personalities show excessive reliance on others to make major life decisions, stay trapped in abusive relationships for fear of being alone, have difficulty initiating projects on their own, and constantly seek reassurance and praise. Obsessive-compulsive personalities exhibit restricted expressions of warmth, tenderness, and generosity and also exhibit stubbornness with a need to be right and to control decisions; indecisive at times, they often use overly rigid application of rules and morals to the point of being inflexible.

A characteristic personality disturbance seen with frontal lobe damage is referred to as *organic personality disorder* in the tenth revision of the *International Classification of Diseases and Related Health Problems* (ICD-10) and *personality change due to a general medical condition* in DSM-IV-TR. Its features include irritability, inappropriate jocularity with euphoria, inappropriate socially disinhibited behavior, and impulsiveness. Other patients with damage to different areas of the frontal lobe, in contrast, exhibit apathy and indifference.

Interpersonal Systems Couples and families have been studied as systems in their own right, and many qualities of these systems have been identified as being clinically important. A scheme for categorizing relational disorders has been proposed for future editions of the DSM-IV-TR, but, as yet, no single generally accepted typology of family psychopathology or interactional types has been established. However, elements of marital discord and harmony have been operationalized in several standard marital inventories. Characteristics of couples and families that have received the most attention include the rules of communication, such as those governing the directness or indirectness with which disagreement and conflict are addressed; the manner (organized or chaotic) in which communications are conducted; taboo topics and secrets about which no one can openly communicate; the nature and degree of emotional expression, including affection and anger; the cohesiveness, loyalty, and compatibility of members; the nature of the members' shared identities on the one hand and their autonomous development and separateness on the other; the extent to which members treat one another respectfully or take one another for granted and use one another; the distribution of power and decision making among members; the maintenance of generational boundaries (e.g., age-appropriate performance of life roles); and the members' orientation toward and concurrence and disagreement about important values involving moral, religious, intellectual, cultural, financial, occupational, and childrearing issues, as well as aspirations, health practices, leisure activities, and other belief systems.

A characteristic family environment, called *high expressed emotion*, has been identified that defines a relapse-prone family environment in which one individual has schizophrenia, bipolar disorder, anorexia nervosa, or major depressive disorder. This interactional pattern includes demeaning, intense personal criticism ("You are rotten and lazy") and emotional overinvolvement with the identified patient. Aspects of overinvolvement can be measured by quantifying the numbers of hours of face-to-face contact and by the extent to which relatives categorically assert how the patients feel without ever bothering to ask the patients. Despite these descriptive generalizations, the specific elements of high expressed emotion families that make patients vulnerable to relapse are still obscure.

Couple and family system difficulties are most likely to erupt during predictable stressful events in the normal family life cycle, such as during the newlywed period; pregnancy and childbearing; difficult or contentious childrearing; difficulties with parents, in-laws, and other extended family; insurmountable and unanticipated financial or career problems; serious illness or death of a child or relative; the children's adolescence; departure of children from the home; infidelity; and separation.

Interpersonal *attachment styles*, based on cognitive schemas that have been linked to earlier repeated experiences with caregivers, influence how individuals perceive and act within interpersonal relationships. Specific types that have been described include insecure attachments (several subtypes include preoccupied, fearful, and anxious-ambivalent attachment), avoidant attachment (including angry-dismissive and withdrawn attachment), enmeshed attachment, unresolved attachment (in which significant losses have not been dealt with), and secure attachment styles. Specific types and subtypes have now been linked to certain types of health behaviors and clinical outcomes. For example, diabetic patients with dismissive attachment styles, a style found in approximately 25 percent of the general population and characterized by low trust of others and excessive self-reliance, show a decreased ability to collaborate with providers and have poorer glycemic control than patients with secure attachment styles. In a study at a primary care clinic, patients with insecure attachment styles reported more unaccounted for medical symptoms than others. Among these, patients with preoccupied attachment had the highest primary care costs and usefulness, whereas patients with fearful attachment had the lowest, reflecting their respective tendencies to overuse or underuse medical services.

Interpersonal Disturbances in Illness Behavior

Abnormal illness behavior (dysnosognosia) is a persistently pathological mode of experiencing, evaluating, and responding to one's own health status despite lucid and accurate appraisal and management options provided by a health professional. These behaviors can be considered as interpersonal disorders between patients and health care professionals. Central to all of these behaviors is the adoption of the sick role by the patient, who then engages in characteristic interactions with health care providers—which typically leave both the provider and the patient dissatisfied. Patients with abnormal illness behavior typically seek repeated medical evaluations from a multitude of physicians, often undergoing a series of expensive laboratory tests. At times, the level of complaints provokes unnecessary invasive laboratory examinations or surgeries, which, in turn, thereby place the patient at genuine medical risk.

Abnormal illness behaviors may be unconscious or conscious. *Unconscious abnormal illness behaviors* are those in which the patient believes the symptoms reflect some genuine illness. These behaviors may occur in somatization disorder (in which multiple symptoms and organ systems are affected), conversion disorders, somatoform pain disorder (in which no cause for the subjective level of pain can be found), and hypochondriasis (in which the primary fear is of having a serious disorder). Abnormal illness behaviors in which patients act sick when they are fully aware that they are not include malingering (in which external incentives—usually financial—are the motivating factors) and factitious disorder with physical or psychological symptoms (Munchausen's syndrome). In *Munchausen's syndrome*, patients repeatedly and compulsively present themselves for medical care with feigned or self-induced illness. These self-induced conditions may be so serious as to ultimately cause death: Some patients inject themselves with feces to cause systemic infections that then warrant hospitalization and intensive care. When the self-induced natures of the illnesses are discovered, medical staffs often become outraged at these patients. The patients rarely accept or cooperate with psychiatric care, so few have been adequately studied. Most do not appear to be psychotic, but there seems to be a disturbance in personality structure. In *Munchausen's syndrome by proxy*, a caregiver, usually a parent, induces illness in a child.

FUTURE PROSPECTS

Like psychiatric diagnostic classifications, fashions among psychiatric signs and symptoms change so that those described above must be taken in historical perspective. Characteristics once given prominence, such as the bony protuberances of the skull studied by phrenologists a century ago, are no longer accorded much importance, whereas only in the past few decades have newly described clinical phenomena, such as family, expressed emotion, and alexithymia, been appreciated. Because of the shifts in what is considered relevant and because of the current dominance of biological research, it is easy to assume that the nuances of clinical, descriptive psychopathology are mostly of historical interest. As long as the ultimate goals of clinical psychiatry are to help patients feel better and function better, attending to patients' subjective complaints with a firm knowledge of clinical descriptors will continue to be vital aspects of psychiatrists' skills.

SUGGESTED CROSS-REFERENCES

The psychiatric interview, history, and mental status examination are discussed in Section 7.1. Additional definitions of typical signs and symptoms of psychiatric illness are included in Section 7.4. Perception and cognition are discussed in Section 3.1, memory in Section 3.4, and classification of mental disorders in Section 9.1.

REFERENCES

Amador X, David A, eds. *Insight and Psychosis*. Oxford, UK: Oxford University Press; 1998.

Berrios GE, Gili M: Abulia and impulsiveness revisited: A conceptual history. *Acta Psychiatr Scand.* 1995;92:151.

Branson R, Potoczna N, Kral JG, Lentes KU, Hoehe MR, Horber FF: Binge eating as a major phenotype of melanocortin 4 receptor gene mutations. *N Engl J Med.* 2003;348:1096.

Caspi A, Sugden K, Moffitt TE, Taylor A, Craig IW, Harrington H, McClay J, Mill J, Martin J, Braithwaite A, Poulton R: Influence of life stress on depression: Moderation by a polymorphism in the 5-HTT gene. *Science*. 2003;301:291.

Ciechanowski PS, Walker EA, Katon WJ, Russo JE: Attachment theory: A model for health care utilization and somatization. *Psychosom Med.* 2002;64:660.

Cloninger RC, Svrakic DM, Przybeck TR: A psychobiological model of temperament and character. *Arch Gen Psychiatry*. 1993;50:975.

Comings DE, Blum K: Reward deficiency syndrome: Genetic aspects of behavioral disorders. *Prog Brain Res.* 2000;126:325.

Committee on the Family, Group for the Advancement of Psychiatry: A model for the classification and diagnosis of relational disorders. *Psychiatr Serv.* 1995;46:926.

Constantino JN, Cloninger CR, Clarke AR, Hashemi B, Pryzbeck T: Application of the seven-factor model of personality to early childhood. *Psychiatry Res.* 2002;109:229.

Costa PT Jr, McCrae RR: Stability and change in personality assessment: The Revised NEO Personality Inventory in the Year 2000. *J Pers Assess.* 1997;68:86.

Crichton P: First-rank symptoms or rank-and-file symptoms? *Br J Psychiatry.* 1996;169:537.

*Cummings JL. *Clinical Neuropsychiatry*. New York: Grune and Stratton; 1985.

D'Esposito M, Grossman M: The physiological basis of executive function and working memory. *Neuroscientist*. 1996;2:345.

Dhossche D, Ferdinand R, Van Der Ende J, Hofstra MB, Verhulst F: Diagnostic outcome of self-reported hallucinations in a community sample of adolescents. *Psychol Med.* 2002;32:619.

Flaum M, Arndt S, Andreasen NC: The reliability of "bizarre" delusions. *Compr Psychiatr.* 1991;32:59.

Freeman D, Garety PA, Kuipers E: Persecutory delusions: Developing the understanding of belief maintenance and emotional distress. *Psychol Med.* 2001;31:1292.

George MS, Parekh PI, Rosindky N, Ketter TA, Kimbrell TA, Heilman KM, Herscovitch P, Post RM: Understanding emotional prosody activates right hemisphere regions. *Arch Neurol.* 1996;53:665.

Goodman M, Brown JA, Deitz PM. *Managing Managed Care II: A Handbook for Mental Health Professionals*. Washington, DC: American Psychiatric Press, Inc.; 1996.

Goodwin FK, Jamison KR. *Manic-Depressive Illness*. New York: Oxford University Press; 1990.

Griffiths TD: Musical hallucinosis in acquired deafness: Phenomelonogy and brain substrate. *Brain*. 2000;123:2065.

Harvey AG: Identifying safety behaviors in insomnia. *J Nerv Ment Dis.* 2002;190:16.

Hays RD, Wells KB, Sherbourne CD, Rogers W, Spritze K: Functioning and well-being outcomes of patients with depression compared with chronic general medical illnesses. *Arch Gen Psychiatry*. 1995;52:11.

Hilgard ER. *Divided Consciousness: Multiple Controls in Human Thought and Action.* New York: John Wiley; 1977.

*Jaspers K. *General Psychopathology*. Chicago: University of Chicago Press; 1963.

Judd LL, Akiskal HS, Maser JD, Zeller PJ, Endicott J, Coryell W, Paulus MO, Kunovac JL, Leon AD, Mueller TI, Rice JA, Keller MB: A prospective 12-year study of subsyndromal and syndromal depressive symptoms in unipolar major depressive disorders. *Arch Gen Psychiatry*. 1998;55:694.

Kalechstein AD, Newton TF, Leavengood AH: Apathy syndrome in cocaine dependence. *Psychiatr Res.* 2002;109:97.

Kessler RC, McGonagle KA, Zhao S, Nelson CB, Hughes M, Eshleman S, Wittchen H-U, Kendler KS: Lifetime and 12-month prevalence of DSM-III-R psychiatric disorders in the United States: Results from the National Comorbidity Survey. *Arch Gen Psychiatry*. 1994;51:8.

Koenigsberg HW, Handley R: Expressed emotion: From predictive index to clinical construct. *Am J Psychiatry*. 1986;143:1361.

Lazare A, ed. *Outpatient Psychiatry: Diagnosis and Treatment*. 2nd ed. Baltimore: Williams & Wilkins; 1989.

Miller WR, Rollnick S. *Motivational Interviewing: Preparing People For Change*. 2nd ed. New York: Guilford; 2002.

Mintz J, Mintz LI, Arruda MJ, Hwang SS: Treatments of depression and the functional capacity to work. *Arch Gen Psychiatry*. 1992;49:761.

Montejo-Gonzalez AL, Liorca G, Izquierdo AJ, Ledesma A, Bousono M, Calcedo A, Carrasco JL, Ciudad J, Daniel E, de la Gandara J, Derecho J, Franco M, Gomez MJ, Macias JA, Martin T, Perez V, Sanchez JM, Sanchez S, Vicens E: SSRI-induced sexual dysfunction: Fluoxetine, paroxetine, sertraline, and fluvoxamine in a prospective, multicenter, and descriptive clinical study of 344 patients. *J Sex Marital Ther.* 1997;23:176.

Nayani TH, Davis AS: The auditory hallucination: A phenomenological survey. *Psychol Med.* 1996;26:177.

Nemiah J: Alexithymia: Present, past—and future? *Psychosom Med.* 1996;58: 217.

Nierenberg AA, Keefe BR, Leslie VC, Alpert JE, Pava JA, Worthington JJ, Rosenbaum JF, Fava M: Residual symptoms in depressed patients who respond acutely to fluoxetine. *J Clin Psychiatry*. 1999;60:221.

Oulis PG, Mavreas VG, Mamounas JM, Stefanis CN: Clinical characteristics of auditory hallucinations. *Acta Psychiatr Scand*. 1995;92:97.

Pilowsky I: The concept of abnormal illness behavior. *Psychosomatics*. 1990;31:207.

Prochaska JO, DiClemente CC: Transtheoretical therapy toward a more integrative model of change. *Psychother Theory Res Pract*. 1982;19:276.

Purdon SE, Flor-Henry P: Asymmetrical olfactory acuity and neuroleptic treatment in schizophrenia. *Schizophr Res*. 2000;44:221.

*Rapaport D, ed. *Organization and Pathology of Thought*. New York: Columbia University Press; 1951.

Raymond NC, Coleman E, Miner MH: Psychiatric comorbidity and compulsive/impulsive traits in compulsive sexual behavior. *Compr Psychiatry*. 2003;44:370.

Sachdev P, Loneragan C: The present status of akathisia. *J Nerv Ment Dis*. 1991;179:381.

Sansone RA, Gaither GA, Songer DA: Self-harm behaviors across the life cycle: A pilot study of inpatients with borderline personality disorder. *Compr Psychiatry*. 2002;43:215.

Schneider K. *Clinical Psychopathology*. New York: Grune and Stratton; 1959.

Schwartz CE, Wright CI, Shin LM, Kagan J, Rauch SL: Inhibited and uninhibited infants "grown up": Adult amygdalar syndrome response to novelty. *Science*. 2003;300:1952.

Shapiro D. *Neurotic Styles*. New York: Basic Books; 1965.

Sierra M, Berrios GE: The phenomenological stability of depersonalization: Comparing the old with the new. *J Nerv Ment Dis*. 2001;189:629.

*Sims A. *Symptoms in the Mind: An Introduction to Descriptive Psychopathology*. London: Bailliere Tindall; 1988.

Snaith P: Anhedonia: A neglected symptom of psychopathology. *Psychol Med*. 1993;23:957.

Sobin C, Sackeim HA: Psychomotor symptoms of depression. *Am J Psychiatry*. 1997;154:4.

*Stone MH. *Abnormalities of Personality: Within and beyond the Realm of Treatment*. New York: W.W. Norton; 1993.

Stope T, Friedman A, Ortwein G, Strobl R, Chaudry HR, Najam N, Chaudhry MR: Comparison of delusions among schizophrenics in Austria and in Pakistan. *Psychopathology*. 1999;32:225.

Tada K, Kojima T: The relationship of olfactory delusional disorder to social phobia. *J Nerv Ment Dis*. 2002;190:45.

Taylor CB, Arnow B. *The Nature and Treatment of Anxiety Disorders*. New York: Free Press; 1988.

Trumbell D: Shame: An acute stress response to interpersonal traumatization. *Psychiatry*. 2003;66:53.

Ulloa RE, Birmaher B, Axelson D, Williamson DE, Brent DA, Ryan ND, Bridge J, Baugher M: Psychosis in a pediatric mood and anxiety disorders clinic: Phenomenology and correlates. *J Am Acad Child Adoles Psychiatry*. 2002;39:337.

Westen D, Arkowitz-Westen L: Limitations of Axis II in diagnosing personality pathology in clinical practice. *Am J Psychiatry*. 1998;155:1767.

Yalom I. *Existential Psychotherapy*. New York: Basic Books; 1980.

Yudofsky SC, Hale RE, eds. *Textbook of Neuropsychiatry*. 3rd ed. Washington, DC: American Psychiatric Press; 1997.

9 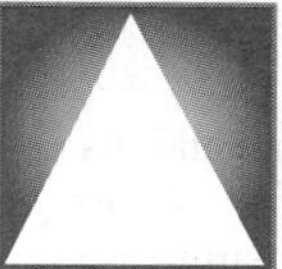

Classification in Psychiatry

▲ 9.1 Psychiatric Classification

Mark Zimmerman, M.D., and Robert L. Spitzer, M.D.

In the chapter on nosology in the first edition of the *Comprehensive Textbook of Psychiatry* (CTP), published in 1967, Henry Brill discussed the purposes and principles of classification, reviewed criticisms of the classification of mental disorders, and identified problems with applying the diagnostic manual to clinical practice. These same issues remain relevant today and are discussed in this chapter on classification as well. At the time of the first edition of the CTP, the first edition of the *Diagnostic and Statistical Manual of Mental Disorders* (DSM-I) was the official diagnostic manual, although the second edition of the *Diagnostic and Statistical Manual of Mental Disorders* (DSM-II) was published 1 year later in 1968. Brill, chairman of the American Psychiatric Association's (APA's) Committee on Nomenclature and Statistics from 1960 through 1965, delineated six advantages of the then current nomenclature: (1) widespread use, thereby facilitating communication among professionals; (2) clear definition and delineation of the disorders; (3) compatibility with the *International Classification of Diseases* (ICD) diagnostic system; (4) clear guidelines for compilation and reporting of patient diagnostic data; (5) comprehensive collection of diagnostic terms in one source; and (6) ease of use. During the 35 years after this chapter was published, the APA's diagnostic manual has been revised four times and plans are under way to revise the manual again within the next decade. Although some of the issues regarding psychiatric classification have remained the same since the first edition of the CTP, because the APA's DSM has grown in stature, political forces have increasingly voiced opinions regarding classification issues, and discussions about conceptual issues in classification have raised new questions.

The present chapter is divided into nine sections. It begins with a general description of the purposes of classification. Next, the chapter turns to the fundamental issue underlying a classification of mental disorders—the definition of mental disorder. This section includes a discussion of the impact of the operationalization of mental disorder on the epidemiology of psychiatric disorders and an examination of the core component of DSM definition of mental disorder—"a behavioral, psychological, or biological dysfunction in the individual." This section ends with a review of Jerome C. Wakefield's critique of DSM's definition of mental disorder and a review of his concept of disorder as harmful dysfunction. The subsequent three sections present an overview of the history of psychiatric classification, the history of official classifications during the past two centuries, and the recent history of classifications since the 1970s. The text revision of the fourth edition of the *Diagnostic and Statistical Manual of Mental Disorders* (DSM-IV-TR) classification is then described, highlighting and summarizing the features of disorders included in the current nomenclature. Following this is a review of issues related to the use of DSM-IV-TR, and a summary of some recent commentaries and research on the use of DSM in clinical practice. Finally, some controversies in the classification of mental disorders are described.

PURPOSES OF CLASSIFICATION

Classification is the process by which the complexity of phenomena is reduced by arranging them into categories according to some established criteria for one or more purposes. At present, the classification of mental disorders consists of specific mental disorders that are grouped into various classes on the basis of some shared phenomenological characteristics. The ultimate purpose of classification is to improve treatment and prevention efforts. Ideally, a classification of disorders is based on knowledge of etiology or pathophysiology, because this increases the likelihood of improving treatment and prevention efforts. The purposes of a classification of mental disorders involve communication, control, and comprehension.

Communication A classification enables users to communicate with each other about the disorders with which they deal. This involves using names of categories as standard shorthand ways of summarizing a great deal of information. When indicating that an individual has a particular disorder, this confers information about the cluster of clinical features that the individual is experiencing without listing all of the specific features that together constitute the disorder. For communication to be effective, there must be a high level of agreement among users of the classification.

Control *Control* of mental disorders primarily refers to the prevention of their occurrence or the modification of their course with treatment. *Control* also refers to knowledge of the course of a condition, as this too is often important in clinical management.

Comprehension Classification should provide comprehension or understanding of the causes of mental disorders and the processes involved in their development and maintenance. Disorders can, of course, be treated without knowledge of their etiology or pathophysiology. Comprehension is not an end in itself but is desired in a classification because it usually leads to more effective treatment and prevention (i.e., better control).

WHAT IS A MENTAL DISORDER?

There are many reasons why mental health professionals should care about the way in which *mental disorder* is defined. The definition of mental disorder guides distinguishing pathology from what is normal. Consequently, the definition of mental disorder can influence estimates of the prevalence of psychiatric disorders in the community, which, in turn, influences the allocation of public health expenditures. The definition of mental disorder can impact which behavioral, cognitive, and emotional perturbations are included in the classification, and the inclusion and exclusion of specific disorders from the DSM have been the source of criticism and controversy. Whether a problem is considered a disorder influences medical insurance reimbursement, and definitions of mental disorder have varied in mental health parity statutes in different states. Determination of the presence of mental disorder has potential legal implications in criminal cases and decisions regarding disability determinations. Lack of conceptual clarity regarding the definition of mental disorder can contribute to abuses of psychiatric diagnoses as a means of controlling or stigmatizing socially undesirable behavior. Finally, lack of clarity in the conceptualization of a fundamental, core issue such as the definition of mental disorder reduces confidence in the profession as an authority regarding diagnostic issues and controversies.

It should be noted that a definition of medical (nonpsychiatric) disorder is as elusive as a definition of mental disorder, although this has not been the topic of much discussion. In fact, the definition of what constitutes a medical condition may attain greater visibility during the coming years as technological advances improve the detection of pathology. For example, there has been a recent growth of facilities offering full-body imaging procedures, such as computed tomography (CT) scans, to detect occult illnesses in their early stages. The clinical significance of the early detection of abnormalities is unknown, because the natural course of the lesions detected at an early stage is unknown. Consequently, the boundary between normal variation and pathology will be challenged as the tools to detect gross abnormalities improve in the absence of understanding pathophysiological mechanisms producing clinically significant pathology.

Although it may be reassuring that difficulty in defining disorder is not limited to the mental health field, the question of what is a mental disorder should be addressed to guide the development of the classification. In contrast to most medical disorders, mental disorders are manifested by a quantitative deviation in behavior, ideation, and emotion from a normative concept. The debates over whether certain behaviors, ways of thinking, or emotional states should or should not be included in the DSM classification (i.e., should or should not be considered disorders) are grounded in ambiguities in the definition of mental disorder.

The first DSM to offer a definition of mental disorder was the third edition of the *Diagnostic and Statistical Manual of Mental Disorders* (DSM-III), and this definition has been only slightly been modified in the revised third edition of the *Diagnostic and Statistical Manual of Mental Disorders* (DSM-III-R) and the DSM-IV-TR. The history of the introduction of a definition of mental disorder into DSM-III begins in 1973, when Robert Spitzer sided with those psychiatrists and activists who wanted to remove homosexuality from DSM-II. To justify the removal of homosexuality from the DSM-II, Spitzer proposed this definition of mental disorder: "In order for a mental or psychiatric condition to be considered a psychiatric disorder, it must either regularly cause subjective distress or regularly be associated with generalized impairment in social effectiveness or functioning." With this definition, Spitzer argued that homosexuality per se does not satisfy the two requirements of his definition, because "many homosexuals are quite satisfied with their sexual orientation and demonstrate no generalized impairment in social effectiveness or functioning."

During the early years in the development of the DSM-III, Spitzer recognized that his 1973 definition of mental disorder had ignored the concept of dysfunction. With the help of many other colleagues, a new definition of mental disorder was developed, was included in DSM-III, and subsequently was modified in DSM-III-R and DSM-IV-TR. In DSM-IV-TR, mental disorder is defined as a

> clinically significant behavioral or psychological syndrome or pattern that occurs in an individual and that is associated with present distress (e.g., a painful symptom) or disability (i.e., impairment in one or more important areas of functioning) or with a significantly increased risk of suffering, death, pain, disability, or an important loss of freedom. In addition, this syndrome or pattern must not be merely an expectable and culturally sanctioned response to a particular event, for example, the death of a loved one. Whatever its original cause, it must currently be considered a manifestation of a behavioral, psychological, or biological dysfunction in the individual. Neither deviant behavior (e.g., political, religious, or sexual) nor conflicts that are primarily between the individual and society are mental disorders unless the deviance or conflict is a symptom of a dysfunction in the individual, as described above.

Definition of Mental Disorder, Psychiatric Epidemiology, and the Impairment or Distress Criterion The definition of mental disorder can potentially impact on the prevalence estimates of psychiatric and substance use disorders in epidemiological studies. Critics of the DSM have suggested that the application of the definition of mental disorder has been too broad. One possible manifestation of the expansion of the domain of mental disorder is the number of conditions identified in the DSM. Since the publication of DSM-I, the number of identified diagnoses has increased by more than 300 percent (from 106 in DSM-I to 365 in DSM-IV-TR). In fact, every revision of the DSM has been accompanied by an increase in the number of diagnoses. It has been argued that the increased number of diagnoses represents a broadening of the concept of mental disorder, and behavioral, cognitive, or emotional patterns that previously would not have been identified as pathological are reconceptualized as representing a disorder. However, a careful analysis of the increase in diagnostic labels suggests that it almost entirely represents greater specification of the forms of pathology, thereby allowing more homogeneous groups to be identified. Moreover, some of the highest epidemiological rates of mental disorders preceded the publication of DSM-III.

Since the publication of DSM-III, two large psychiatric epidemiological studies have been conducted in the United States—the Epidemiological Catchment Area (ECA) study and the National Comorbidity Study (NCS). The results of these studies were reanalyzed by applying a higher threshold to define a mental disorder—the symptoms were required to cause "a lot" of interference in the person's life or to result in treatment. On application of the clinical significance criterion, the 1-year prevalence rate of any psychiatric or substance use disorder dropped from 30.2 to 20.5 percent in the NCS and from 28.0 to 22.5 percent in the ECA study.

Impairment or Distress Criterion Considered The high prevalence rates of DSM-III and DSM-III-R psychiatric disorders in the NCS and the ECA study raised concern that the diagnostic criteria were overly inclusive, or incorrectly applied in an overly broad manner, and that they identified nondisordered individuals as disordered. Spitzer and Wakefield indicated that there were two ways in which the DSM diagnostic criteria, even when applied correctly, might nonetheless identify nondisordered individuals as having a mental disorder. One instance occurs when individuals experience normal reactions to stressful environments, and the other occurs when individuals experience mild symptoms of a disorder that are insufficiently severe to be considered a disorder. Spitzer and Wakefield labeled this the *false-positive problem* with the DSM criteria.

To reduce the problem of potential overdiagnosis, in DSM-IV-TR, the threshold to diagnose psychiatric disorders was raised by explicitly adding a clinical significance criterion to approximately one-half of the criteria sets. Precedent for this was found in the DSM-III-R criteria for social phobia, simple phobia, and obsessive-compulsive disorder (OCD). The wording of the DSM-IV-TR clinical significance criterion varies somewhat from disorder to disorder, although the most common wording is "the symptoms cause clinically significant distress or impairment in social, occupational, or other important areas of functioning." The introduction to the DSM-IV-TR manual indicates that the purpose of this criterion is to "help establish the threshold for the diagnosis of a disorder in those situations in which the symptomatic presentation by itself (particularly in its milder forms) is not inherently pathological." This criterion, however, only addresses one of the two potential causes of false positives—the labeling of mild, subthreshold conditions as disorders. The criterion does not address the issue of labeling normal reactions to stressful events as disorders.

One problem with DSM-IV-TR's clinical significance criterion is the uncertainty in how to interpret and apply it. Does *distress* refer to distress about having the symptom or distress when experiencing the symptom? In a comment on Spitzer and Wakefield's critique of the clinical significance criterion, Kenneth S. Kendler described the case of a 38-year-old woman who feared snakes since childhood. Because she lives in a metropolitan area, the only way in which this fear impacts on her life is her refusal to take her children into the snake house at the zoo. Because it is easy for her to successfully avoid snakes, her fear does not result in clinically significant impairment. Because it is unclear how the distress component of the clinical significance criterion should be interpreted, it is unclear whether this presentation warrants a diagnosis of specific phobia. The woman is highly anxious (distressed) when exposed to the fear-inducing stimuli, much more so than most people. Does this meet the distress component of the criterion? On the other hand, because exposure to snakes is successfully avoided, she denies being bothered (distressed) by having this fear. Does this mean that she does not meet the criterion? Does it mean that if she were bothered by having the fear, despite the fact that the degree of impairment is limited, then she does have a mental disorder? Spitzer and Wakefield suggest that only distress that is intrinsic to the condition should be considered when determining disorder presence or absence. If distress about having a condition is considered a defining feature of mental disorder, then false-positive diagnoses might result (e.g., Does someone who is distressed about having curly hair or being overweight have a mental disorder?).

A second problem with DSM-IV-TR's clinical significance criterion is that it is often redundant with the symptom criteria. Functional impairment is intrinsic to many disorders. For example, the symptom criterion for the disorder selective mutism is "consistent failure to speak in specific social situations (in which there is an expectation for speaking, e.g., at school) despite speaking in other situations." It is unclear how an individual can meet this criterion and not meet the additional clinical significance criterion that "the disturbance interferes with educational or occupational achievement or with social communication." Thus, the clinical significance criterion is unnecessary.

A third problem with the addition of the clinical significance criterion to the symptom criteria sets is that some individuals who have a mental disorder cannot be diagnosed as having the disorder, because the clinical significance criterion is not met. This can be considered the *false-negative problem* with the clinical significance criterion. For example, a child with frequent motor and vocal tics is not diagnosed with Tourette's syndrome unless the distress or impairment criterion is also met. This alludes to the cardinal problem of diagnosing a disorder in the absence of knowledge about underlying dysfunction. (The issue of dysfunction and its importance in defining disorder is described in greater detail in the following section.) To say that one child with tics has a disorder, because classmates, parents, or teachers are intolerant of the symptoms and are thus responsible for the child's distress or impairment, whereas another child with the same symptom expression does not have a disorder because of a different response from others, indicates that the concept of mental disorder cannot simply be based on the presence of impairment or distress. Disorders in other areas of medicine are diagnosed without explicit reference to concepts of distress and impairment, although one or the other is usually present. However, for most medical disorders, a biological abnormality or underlying dysfunction can be identified. By virtue of laboratory tests, conditions such as cancer, liver disease, and cardiac disease can be diagnosed in the absence of distress or impairment (or even the manifestation of clinical symptoms). Until underlying psychological and biological dysfunctions are identified, then the definition of mental disorder involves drawing an arbitrary line to minimize false-positive and false-negative diagnoses.

Although the nature of the underlying dysfunction may be currently unknown, the concept of disorder, as well as its differentiation from normal variation, implies the existence of an underlying disruption of normal function. Distress or impairment is not synonymous with underlying dysfunction. The same symptom presentation in two individuals may be similarly associated with comparable degrees of distress or impairment but different degrees of underlying dysfunction. Consider, for example, the evaluation of depression. The diagnosis of depressive disorder poses conceptual challenges, because multiple pathways have been well established as to their relation to the onset and maintenance of symptoms of depression. Some of the factors implicated in the cause of depression include genetic vulnerability, stressful life events, and adverse child-rearing experiences. The DSMs explicitly recognize that individuals with symptoms of depression may or may not have a disorder. Bereavement, characterized by a full depressive syndrome, is not considered a mental disorder if the symptoms last less than 2 months after a death and are not complicated by suicidal tendencies or psychosis. However, depressive symptoms after a different stressful event are considered a disorder (unless the symptoms last less than 2 weeks). Thus, two individuals can have similar symptom patterns, similar degrees of impairment, and a similar course of symptoms, yet be diagnosed differently depending on whether the stressful event precipitating the depression was or was not a loss due to death versus a different type of loss. The clinical significance criterion does not clarify how to distinguish between disorder and no disorder in this instance. Rather, there is a presumption, of unknown validity, that there is a dysfunction in mood regulation associated with a depressive syndrome after stressful life events other than a death. Consider another example in which a diagnosis of depression does not follow from application of the clinical significance criterion. Immediately after a stressful event, an individual who experiences a full depressive syndrome of brief, less than 2 weeks, duration is not diagnosed with major depressive disorder. For example, after being told unexpectedly that her husband wanted a divorce, a 35-year-old woman cried daily, developed insomnia, lost her appetite, had difficulty concentrating, felt restless and agitated, and missed some days at work. After a week, her symptoms began to improve, she returned to work, and she thought that she was coping better. A definition of disorder based on the presence of impairment and distress would classify her as having a disorder. According to DSM-IV-TR, she would not be diagnosed with major depressive disorder unless the full syndrome lasted for at least 2 weeks. A mental disorder could be diagnosed according to DSM-IV-TR—adjustment disorder—if it was concluded that the symptoms were in excess of what constitutes a normal reaction to the stressor. This indicates that the determination of disorder, then, is not simply based on symptom picture nor impairment or distress, but on the presumption of the existence of a dysfunction of an underlying regulatory mechanism that is inferred from the nature, course, and context of the symptoms.

Critique of the DSM Definition of Mental Disorder from Wakefield's Harmful Dysfunction Perspective

Explicit in the DSM-IV-TR definition of mental disorder is the requirement of underlying dysfunction, although this is sometimes not explicitly discussed, even by nosologists. For example, in discussing the issue of adding new diagnostic categories to DSM-IV-TR, the principal architects of DSM-IV-TR, when discussing the possible inclusion of minor depression and mixed-anxiety/depressive disorder noted that "there is no inherent problem in high prevalences of disorders . . . so long as it is clear that the threshold established is associated with clinically significant distress and/or disability and that the category is useful in predicting prognosis and guiding treatment." Likewise, in a recent article comparing definitions of mental disorder used in different federal and state statutes mandating parity coverage for mental health treatment, Marcia C. Peck and Richard M. Scheffler indicated that the DSM defines mental disorder as "a clinically significant behavioral or psychological syndrome or pattern that occurs in an individual . . . is associated with present distress . . . or disability . . . or with a significant increased risk of suffering." In a paper entitled "Rhinotillexomania: Psychiatric Disorder or Habit?" James W. Jefferson and Trent D. Thompson indicated that nose picking, a nearly universal practice in adults, should be considered a disorder when it becomes excessive and causes impairment or distress. No reference was made to dysfunction of underlying mechanisms. It is therefore not uncommon for discussions of the definition of mental disorder, or discussions of whether a behavioral or psychological syndrome should be characterized as a mental disorder, to focus on impairment and distress and to ignore the issue of dysfunction in underlying mechanisms. Perhaps the reason for paying less attention to this component of the definition of mental disorder is the lack of knowledge of these dysfunctions.

In a series of articles over the past 15 years, Wakefield critically examined DSM's definition of mental disorder and elaborated his own conceptualization of medical and mental disorder as *harmful dysfunction*. *Dysfunction* is defined as an inability of an internal mental mechanism to perform its intended, natural function, from an evolutionary perspective. As noted previously, the DSM's definition of *mental disorder* already includes the concept of dysfunction. However, Wakefield critiques the way that the DSM criteria operationalize the concept of dysfunction merely as statistical deviation from normative (expected) reaction. It is for that reason that DSM excludes a normative (expected) grief reaction, because it is an "expectable and culturally sanctioned response to a particular event, for example, the death of a loved one." A problem with DSM's attempt to operationalize disorder as harmful statistical deviation is the failure to consistently apply this defining principle to determine what is and what is not a disorder. Examples of conceptual inconsistency include persistent mental or behavioral states, such as gullibility, laziness, and sloppiness, that are frequently unwanted, cause distress or impairment, and are statistically deviant. Although apparently meeting DSM's conceptualization of mental disorder as harmful statistical deviation, these states are not considered disorders. Moreover, conceptual inconsistency is present even within the DSM classification. DSM's V codes are a heterogeneous collection of problems, such as phase of life problems, medication-induced movement disorders, relational problems, problems related to abuse or neglect, and malingering, that may be the focus of clinical attention, are distressing and unexpected (thereby meeting the DSM definition of mental disorder), and yet are not considered mental disorders.

Following this line of reasoning, Wakefield critiques the criteria used to diagnose adjustment disorder, which are based, in large part, on statistical deviation ("marked distress that is in excess of what would be expected from exposure to the stressor"). A possible, literal, interpretation of the adjustment disorder criteria is that individuals falling in the upper one-half of the distribution of distress after a stressful event qualify for the diagnosis.

Much of Wakefield's discussion focuses on how the definition of mental disorder must be broad enough to include conditions that are triggered by stress but not so broad that all environmentally induced perturbations in homeostasis are considered pathological. A definition that identifies the normal reactions to stresses in everyday life as disorders trivializes the concept of disorder. As Wakefield puts it,

> [T]he critical distinction that needs to be drawn is between those situations in which an environmental stress causes a breakdown of an internal mechanism such that the breakdown becomes independent of the original stress versus a natural response that is initiated and maintained directly by the ongoing stress and that would subside if the stress disappeared. The former kind of reaction is a disorder but the latter is not, according to the dysfunction conception. . . . Life naturally contains a certain amount of distress, and distress that is consistent with the natural functioning of the organism is not a disorder.

Consideration of dysfunction is also important for distinguishing between functional impairment that is indicative of disorder and impairment in functioning that instead reflects inability. Consider illiteracy and a severe reading disorder. Both are characterized by impairment in reading ability. However, illiteracy due to inadequate education is not considered a disorder, because there is no presumed underlying dysfunction. A reading disorder is diagnosed only when reading achievement is below that expected by the individual's education and intelligence (i.e., there is a presumed dysfunction in the mental process responsible for reading).

Wakefield suggests that the framers of DSM-III did not incorporate the concept of dysfunction into the criteria for individual disorders, because reliability was valued more highly than validity. Although the actual nature of the dysfunction may be unknown, Wakefield argues that it is possible for clinicians to judge whether symptoms are due to internal dysfunction. For example, Wakefield and colleagues found that clinicians could reliably agree that children growing up in violent, threatening environments who exhibit features of conduct disorder that are appropriate to the social context should not be considered to have a mental disorder. Unfortunately, Wakefield has yet to show that clinicians, for a variety of disorders, can distinguish normal reactions (e.g., depression after a loss) from harmful conditions that are the result of a dysfunction (e.g., the dysfunction of mood regulation in severe depression).

Some researchers have suggested that future psychiatric classification should focus on identifying the abnormalities of cognition, emotion, and motivation that underlie the signs and symptoms of mental disorder. Such a transition would evolve simultaneously with the development of tests to evaluate these functions and to identify abnormalities in them. This would move psychiatric classification closer to the rest of medicine, for which laboratory testing has increasingly assumed importance in identifying and classifying pathological conditions.

Harmful Dysfunction and the Definition of Mental (and Physical) Disorders The development of tests to identify underlying functional abnormalities would move psychiatric classification from a system primarily based on description closer to one based on etiology. It is sobering to realize that only 40 years ago, during the 1960s, the failure to identify underlying abnormalities was taken as evidence that the concept of mental illness was a myth. To better appreciate a harmful dysfunction definition of mental disorder, Wakefield reviewed the arguments of the critics of psychiatric classification and, in doing so, illustrated that harmful dysfunction is as relevant to defining physical disorder as mental disorder.

Thomas S. Szasz argued that a disorder requires the presence of a physical lesion, with a *lesion* being defined as an identifiable deviation in anatomical structure. The failure to identify brain lesions in individuals with medical conditions was prima facie evidence that these conditions are not disorders. Rather, the term *mental disorder* is adopted to label behavior that deviates from societal norms and to empower the medical establishment.

Wakefield identified two problems with Szasz's thesis: (1) that a lesion (i.e., a pathological anatomical structure) can be defined solely in terms of statistical deviation and (2) that *physical disorder* is defined by the presence of a lesion. The statistical deviation argument fails on two accounts. First, normal variations of anatomical structures, such as webbed toes, are not synonymous with a pathological process (i.e., dysfunction or malfunction). Second, some pathological anatomical processes, such as atherosclerosis, are not statistical deviations. Thus, the statistical deviation argument fails, because infrequent variants are not necessarily pathological, and pathological anatomical variation is not necessarily infrequent. The second component of Szasz' argument, that physical disorder is defined by the presence of a lesion, cannot account for disorders such as migraine headaches and trigeminal neuralgia, for which there are no known anatomical lesions.

Wakefield suggests that variations in structure, whether they be anatomical structures or mental mechanisms, are lesions when "the variation impairs the ability of the particular structure to accomplish the functions that it was designed to perform," and the lesion is a disorder "only if the deviation in functioning of the part affects the well-being of the overall organism in a harmful way. . . . Thus, the harmful dysfunction approach to the concept of disorder would seem to explain . . . which anatomical deviations are lesions and which lesions are disorders."

Harmful Dysfunction and Diagnostic Controversies In concluding his 1992 paper on the concept of mental disorder, Wakefield illustrated how a lack of knowledge of naturally selected mechanisms and changes in cultural mores can influence judgments about dysfunction and harm, and, consequently, determination of whether a condition is a disorder. He reviewed opinions about female orgasm during intercourse that were formed a century apart:

> According to the eminent Victorian physician and sexologist William Acton (1871), the female sexual organs do not naturally function to produce orgasm during intercourse, and the occurrence of orgasm in a woman is a form of pathology due to an excess of stimulation beyond what her body was designed to tolerate. According to Masters and Johnson (1966, 1970, 1974), orgasm during intercourse is a natural function of the female sexual organs, and lack of orgasm in a woman is a disorder due to inadequate stimulation of the sort to which her body was designed to respond. Acton and Masters and Johnson knew that there are many women who do have orgasms during intercourse and many women who do not. Acton interpreted these facts to mean that there are a lot of women who are disordered because they suffer from overstimulation, whereas Masters and Johnson interpreted these facts to mean that there are a lot of women who are disordered because they suffer from understimulation. The nonstatistical nature of function and disorder, combined with ignorance of the evolutionary history of female sexual capacities, enabled these opposite beliefs to be consistent with the same set of data and with the same concept of disorder.

Wakefield indicates that facts alone do not determine disorder status. The harm component of the disorder definition is, in part, a value judgment based on sociocultural standards. Thus, Acton and Masters and Johnson could have come to an agreement on what constitutes female orgasmic dysfunction based on evolutionary knowledge but might nevertheless have disagreed as to whether orgasm during intercourse is a desirable goal, thus disagreeing regarding the definition of female orgasmic disorder. The harmful dysfunction definition of mental disorder does not, therefore, resolve diagnostic controversies that are disputes based on values.

Problems with the Harmful Dysfunction Definition of Mental Disorder There have been conceptual critiques of the harmful dysfunction definition of mental disorder, although these have been well refuted by Wakefield. The authors agree with Wakefield's conceptual analysis of the definition of disorder, although a weakness in Wakefield's presentation is the lack of specific details in implementation. That is, it is not clear how to operationalize and incorporate the concept of dysfunction of naturally selected mechanisms into the diagnostic criteria. Wakefield simply indicates that this task needs work.

Wakefield indicates that the reason that it is important to define, in part, the DSM disorders in terms of dysfunction is to decrease the number of false-positive diagnoses. If the concept of dysfunction is incorporated into the diagnostic criteria, then some, perhaps many, persons who are currently diagnosed with a disorder will not be given such a diagnosis. Consider the following case described by Wakefield:

> The patient, a male professor in the social sciences, came to the consultation seeking antidepressant medication and medicine for insomnia. He had to present a paper in another city as part of a job interview and was afraid he could not function adequately to do so. He reported that, for the past month, he had experienced depressed mood and extreme feelings of sadness and emptiness, as well as lack of interest in his usual activities (in fact, when not with friends, he mostly stayed in bed or watched TV). His appetite had diminished, and he laid awake long into the night, unable

to fall asleep because of the pain of his sadness. He was fatigued and lacking in energy during the day and did not have the ability to concentrate on his work. There was no suicidal ideation or feelings of guilt or worthlessness. However, there was functional impairment. The patient was barely managing to meet minimal occupational obligations (e.g., he showed up at class relatively unprepared and had not attended the monthly faculty meeting or worked on his research). He also had avoided social obligations, except to be with close friends to lessen his pain.

When asked what event might have precipitated these distressing feelings, he reported, holding back tears as he spoke, that approximately a month earlier, an extremely intense and passionate 5-year love affair with a married woman (the patient was single) to whom he had been completely devoted had been ended by the woman after she made a final decision that she could not leave her husband. Both lovers had perceived this relationship as a unique, once-in-a-lifetime romance in which they had met their soul mate and had experienced an extraordinary combination of emotional and intellectual intimacy.

This individual meets the DSM-IV-TR symptom and impairment criteria for major depressive disorder. However, Wakefield argues that the loss response is "reasonably proportional" to the nature of the loss, and only on consideration of the subjective meaning of the loss can the clinician determine whether there is a dysfunction of the loss response mechanism. He further notes that such losses can trigger a "genuine" depressive disorder, and "an interesting challenge . . . is to try and formulate criteria that would distinguish truly pathological cases from normal reactions to extreme losses." It is the absence of an attempt to generate and to validate such criteria that limits the practical application of Wakefield's thesis.

HISTORY OF CLASSIFICATION

Karl Menninger and colleagues presented a compendium of classification from ancient times to the modern era. According to Menninger and colleagues, the first specific description of a mental illness appeared in approximately 3000 BC in a depiction of senile deterioration ascribed to Prince Ptah-hotep. The syndromes of melancholia and hysteria appeared in the Sumerian and Egyptian literature as far back as 2600 BC. In the Ebers papyrus (approximately 1500 BC), senile deterioration and alcoholism were described. In India, in approximately 1400 BC, a classification of psychiatric disorders was included in the medical classification system of Ayur-Veda.

Hippocrates (approximately 460 to 370 BC) is usually regarded as the one who introduced the concept of psychiatric illness into medicine. His writings described acute mental disturbances with fever (perhaps delirium), acute mental disturbances without fever (probably analogous to functional psychoses but called *mania*), chronic disturbance without fever (called *melancholia*), hysteria (broader than its later use), and Scythian disease (similar to transvestism).

Caelius Aurelianus, a fifth century physician living in the Roman Empire, described homosexuality as an affliction of a diseased mind that was found in men and women. Mental deficiency and dementia were noted by Swiss Renaissance physician Felix Platter (1536 to 1614).

Before the time of the English physician Thomas Sydenham (1624 to 1689), all illness, despite the difference in appearance between the different syndromes, was attributed to a single pathogenic process, a disturbance of the humoral balance or a disturbance in the tensions of the solid tissues. Sydenham, on the other hand, believed that each illness had a specific cause. He called for the study of morbid processes and likened the investigation of the specificity of diseases to the botanist's search for species of plants.

Philippe Pinel (1745 to 1826), a French physician, simplified the complex diagnostic systems that preceded him by recognizing four fundamental clinical types: mania (conditions with acute excitement or fury), melancholia (depressive disorders and delusions with limited topics), dementia (lack of cohesion in ideas), and idiotism (idiocy and organic dementia). Pinel thus reacted against the specific disease entity tradition of Sydenham and went back to a noncomplex hippocratic system of classification. All mental illnesses were in a category of physical illnesses called *neuroses*, which were defined as functional diseases of the nervous system—that is, illnesses that were not accompanied by fever, inflammation, hemorrhage, or anatomical lesion.

By the 19th century, mental disorder began to be regarded consistently as the manifestation of physical pathology, and scientists searched for specific lesions, parallel to the investigation of bodily diseases. Benedict-Augustin Morel (1809 to 1873) was the first to use the course of an illness as a basis for classification. His *demence precore* was not a disease entity but a particular form of the course of mental disease.

Karl Ludwig Kahlbaum (1828 to 1899), a German descriptive psychiatrist who foreshadowed Emil Kraepelin, introduced the concepts of (1) the temporary symptom complex, as opposed to the underlying disease, (2) the distinction between organic and nonorganic mental disorder, and (3) the consideration of the patient's age at the time of onset and the characteristic development of the disorder as bases for classification.

The finding made by Antoine Bayle in 1822 that progressive paresis was a specific organic disease of the brain and the discovery of Paul Broca (1824 to 1880) in 1861 that some forms of aphasia were related to definite lesions of the cortex increased attempts to base all classifications of mental disorders on demonstrated brain lesions or disturbances in vascular and nutritional physiology. Those findings led Wilhelm Griesinger (1818 to 1868) to coin the slogan "mental diseases are brain diseases." Because the knowledge of brain pathology was limited, he recognized the need for a provisional functional category for mental illnesses with as-yet-unknown somatic pathology.

In the last two decades of the 19th century, Kraepelin (1856 to 1926) synthesized three approaches: the clinical-descriptive, the somatic, and the consideration of the course of the disorder. He viewed mental illnesses as organic disease entities that could be classified on the basis of knowledge about their causes, courses, and outcomes. He brought the manic and depressive disturbances together into one illness, manic-depressive psychosis, and distinguished it, on the basis of its periods of remission, from the chronic deteriorating illness called *dementia praecox*, which Eugen Bleuler later renamed *schizophrenia*. Kraepelin also recognized paranoia as distinct from dementia praecox, distinguished delirium from dementia, and, for the first time in a classification system of mental disorders, included the concepts of psychogenic neuroses and psychopathic personalities (the "born criminal," the "unstable," "pathological liars and swindlers," and "litigious paranoiacs").

The basic approach of Kraepelin toward classification was to search for that combination of clinical features that would best predict outcome. In contrast, Bleuler (1857 to 1939) based his classification system on an inferred psychopathological process, such as a disturbance in the associative process in schizophrenia.

The personality disorders were first noted in the psychiatric literature by J. C. Prichard in 1835 with his introduction of the concepts of moral insanity and moral imbecility. In 1891, August Koch coined the phrases *psychopathic personality* and *psychopathic constitutional inferiority*.

Sigmund Freud (1856 to 1939), after studying hysteria, the prototypical neurosis, went on to divide the neuroses into the *actual neuroses*, the result of dammed-up sexual excitation, and the *psychoneuroses*, the result of unconscious conflict and compromise symptom formation. As interest in the actual neuroses diminished, the term *neurosis* came to be synonymous with *psychoneurosis*. Freud recognized only the following subtypes of neurosis: anxiety neurosis, anxiety hysteria (phobia), obsessive-compulsive neurosis, and hysteria. It was not until much later, in the American Medical Association's (AMA's) *Standard Classified Nomenclature of Disease* (1935), that reactive depression was added as an additional subtype of the neurosis, later to find its way, with other neurotic subtypes, into DSM-I and DSM-II. Freud's dynamic concepts and interest in the psychopathology of everyday life led to an expansion of the boundaries of what was considered mental illness to include mild forms of personality deviation.

As Hagop S. Akiskal and William McKinney noted, despite the advances in the understanding of mental disorders in the past 50 years, the major categories of mental disorders in the standard classification systems are based primarily on the concepts of Kraepelin and Bleuler—organic mental disorders, affective disorders, and schizophrenia—and Freud—neuroses and personality disorders.

HISTORY OF OFFICIAL CLASSIFICATIONS

The first official system for tabulating mental disorder in the United States was initially used for the decennial census of 1840. It contained only one category and lumped together the idiotic and the insane. Forty years later, in the census of 1880, the mentally ill were subdivided into separate categories for the first time (mania, melancholia, monomania, paresis, dementia, dipsomania, and epilepsy). It is sobering to realize that the conceptual issues that modern classifiers wrestle with today were well recognized by the authors of that system. In the introductory remarks to the census office report, the authors lamented about the difficulties of creating a classification system for the mentally ill:

> Much effort has been put forth to secure uniformity in the classification of the insane in every country of the world; but it seems impossible for those best qualified to form an opinion to agree upon any scheme which can be devised. Some classifications are based upon symptoms and some upon physical causes; others are a mixture of the two; and still others take into account the complications of insanity. For the purposes of the census, it seemed to us advisable to disregard all minute subdivisions and to adopt a simple analysis on the broadest possible outlines.

In 1889, the International Congress of Mental Science in Paris adopted a classification proposed by a commission headed by Morel that included 11 categories, including all those "upon which the majority (of the commission's members) was unanimous" and omitting those "upon which opinion was divided." Those early classifications are presented in Table 9.1–1.

In 1923, to conduct a special census of patients in hospitals for mental disease, the Bureau of the Census used a classification system developed in collaboration with the APA (then the American Medico-Psychological Association) and the National Committee for Mental Health. That system, consisting of 22 disorders, had been adopted by the APA in 1917 and was used until 1935, when it was revised for incorporation into the first edition of the AMA's *Standard Classified Nomenclature of Disease*. The purpose was to gather uniform statistical information in mental institutions.

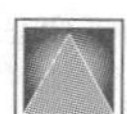

Table 9.1–1
19th Century Classifications of Mental Disorders

1840 U.S. Census	1880 U.S. Census	1889 International Congress of Mental Science
Idiocy (insanity)	Mania	Mania
	Melancholia	Melancholia
	Monomania	Periodical insanity
	Paresis	Progressive systematic insanity
	Dementia	Dementia
	Dipsomania	Organic and senile dementia
	Epilepsy	General paralysis
		Insane neuroses
		Toxic insanity
		Moral and impulsive insanity
		Idiocy, etc.

That 1935 classification was designed primarily for chronic inpatients and, therefore, proved inadequate for use with World War II psychiatric casualties, who required classifications for acute disturbances, psychosomatic disorders, and personality disorders, which were not represented in the 1935 classification. In addition, the system was considered anachronistic by the increasing number of psychodynamically oriented psychiatrists who were emerging from training programs and whose interests lay more in the treatment of private outpatients. For those reasons, shortly after World War II, the Veterans Administration and the military services developed their own systems.

In 1948, the World Health Organization (WHO) assumed the responsibility for revising what had previously been called the International List of Causes of Death and that had been revised every 10 or 20 years since its inception in 1900. The sixth revision was renamed the *Manual of the International Classification of Diseases, Injuries, and Causes of Death* (ICD-6) and contained, for the first time, a classification of mental disorders, entitled "mental, psychoneurotic, and personality disorders." It contained ten categories of psychosis, nine categories of psychoneurosis, and seven categories of disorders of character, behavior, and intelligence.

Despite the fact that American psychiatrists had participated in the development of the mental disorders section of ICD-6, the absence of such important categories as the dementias, many personality disorders, and adjustment disorders rendered it unsatisfactory for use in the United States. Other countries apparently also found the mental disorders section unsatisfactory, because only Finland, New Zealand, Peru, Thailand, and the United Kingdom made official use of it.

The lack of widespread international acceptance of that section of ICD-6 led the WHO to ask Erwin Stengel, a British psychiatrist, to investigate the situation. Stengel concluded that the lack of general acceptance of the international classification of mental disorders was due to the fact that the diagnostic terms frequently had etiological implications that were at odds with various theoretical schools of psychiatry. His suggestion was to develop a classification in which all diagnoses should be described operationally and without etiological implications in a companion glossary. (As the furor over the elimination of neuroses in DSM-III has indicated, this is not so easily done!)

In 1951, the U.S. Public Health Service commissioned a workgroup party, with representation from the APA, to develop an alternative to the mental disorders section of ICD-6 for use in this country. That document, prepared largely by George Raines and based heavily on the Veterans Administration classification system developed by William Menninger, was published in 1952 by the APA as the DSM. DSM-I included 106 diagnoses.

The significance of DSM-I was that it replaced the outdated mental disorders section of the AMA's *Standard Classified Nomenclature of Disease* and the systems devised by the military and the Veterans Administration, and, for the first time, it provided a glossary of definitions of categories. In addition, for the first time, a specialty medical association, the APA, developed what became the official American classification of mental disorders. The APA is the only medical specialty that is in charge of its official specialty classification of medical disorders.

In the definitions of the diagnostic categories, the frequent use of the term *reaction*, as in *schizophrenic reaction* and *psychoneurotic reaction*, expressed the strong environmental orientation of Adolf Meyer, and the frequent reference to defense mechanisms, particularly as an explanation of the neuroses and personality disorders, reflected the wide acceptance of psychoanalytical concepts. Despite its widespread influence and impact on American psychiatric literature, DSM-I was not universally accepted as the official nomenclature throughout the country. The New York State Department of Mental Hygiene, for example, retained the old *Standard Classified Nomenclature of Disease* until 1968.

Because most of the other countries that used the ICD also found the mental disorders section of the sixth revision unsatisfactory, the WHO sponsored an international effort to develop a classification system for mental disorders that would improve on ICD-6 and would be acceptable to all member nations. That task was coordinated in this country by the U.S. Public Health Service, which sent American representatives to the international committees preparing revisions of the mental disorders section. The eighth revision of the ICD (ICD-8) was approved by the WHO in 1966 and became effective in 1968. (The mental disorders section of the seventh revision of the ICD [ICD-7], which appeared in 1955, was identical to the mental disorders section of the sixth revision of the ICD [ICD-6].)

In 1965, the APA, which had maintained close ties with the international committees preparing ICD-8, assigned its Committee on Nomenclature and Statistics, under the chairmanship of Ernest M. Gruenberg, the task of preparing for the APA a new diagnostic manual of mental disorders based on the ICD-8 classification but defining each disorder for use in the United States. Such definitions were necessary because, when ICD-8 was first published, it did not have an accompanying glossary. It was only much later, in 1972, 4 years after DSM-II was adopted, that a glossary was published.

A draft of the second edition of the APA's DSM was circulated in 1967 to 120 psychiatrists known to have a special interest in the area of diagnosis, and it was revised on the basis of their criticisms and suggestions. After further study, the draft was adopted by the APA in 1967 and was published and officially accepted throughout the country in 1968. At approximately the same time, the General Register Office in Great Britain published its own glossary, largely written by Sir Aubrey Lewis, which interpreted the ICD-8 classification. The DSM-II classification consisted of 182 disorders in ten major categories:

1. Mental retardation. This category had been called *mental deficiency* in DSM-I and had been limited to idiopathic or familial varieties of the disorder. In DSM-II, it was subdivided according to severity and etiology.
2. Organic brain syndromes. The DSM-I distinction of acute (reversible) versus chronic (irreversible) was dropped and was replaced by the subdivision into psychoses associated with organic brain syndromes and nonpsychotic organic brain syndromes.
3. Psychoses not attributed to physical conditions listed previously. This section included the functional psychoses: schizophrenia, major affective disorders, paranoid states, and other psychoses (psychotic depressive reaction). The DSM-II category of schizophrenia included the latent type, not included in DSM-I. The DSM-I category of involutional psychotic reaction was subdivided into involutional melancholia and involutional paranoid state in DSM-II.
4. Neuroses. This category included disorders in which the chief characteristic was anxiety, whether "felt and expressed directly" or "controlled unconsciously and automatically by conversion, displacement and various other psychological mechanisms." The DSM-I subtypes were retained with the addition in DSM-II of neurasthenic neurosis, depersonalization neurosis, and hypochondriacal neurosis.
5. Personality disorders and certain other nonpsychotic mental disorders. This category included personality disorders, sexual deviation, alcoholism, and drug dependence. In DSM-I, all of those categories were subsumed under the rubric of *personality disorders*. In the personality disorders section itself, DSM-II added hysterical personality and eliminated the somewhat related DSM-I category of emotionally unstable personality.
6. Psychophysiological disorders. This group of disorders was characterized by physical symptoms caused by emotional factors and involving a single organ system, usually under autonomic nervous system innervation. The disorders were subdivided by the organ system involved.
7. Special symptoms. This category was for a small list of symptoms occurring in the absence of any other mental disorder and most likely seen in children. DSM-II added several symptoms to the DSM-I list.
8. Transient situational disturbances. This category was reserved for more or less transient disorders of any severity, including those of psychotic proportions that occurred as acute reactions to overwhelming environmental stress in persons without any apparent underlying mental disorders. Transient situational personality disorders in DSM-I did not specifically include acute reactions to stress that reached psychotic proportions, as did the category of transient situational disturbances in DSM-II.
9. Behavior disorders of childhood and adolescence. This category included six specific diagnoses. DSM-I had not provided a separate category for disorders of childhood and adolescence.
10. Conditions without manifest psychiatric disorder and nonspecific conditions. This category, not present in DSM-I, performed the function of encompassing the "conditions of individuals who are psychiatrically normal but who nevertheless have severe enough problems to warrant examination by a psychiatrist." These conditions are, therefore, not mental disorders. This category was subdivided into three groups: social maladjustment without manifest psychiatric disorder, nonspecific conditions, and no mental disorder.

Unlike DSM-I, which discouraged multiple diagnoses, DSM-II explicitly encouraged clinicians to diagnose every disorder that was present, even if one was causally related to another—for example, alcoholism secondary to a depression.

The reaction to the publication of DSM-II in 1968 was mixed. Those who were most critical of DSM-II regarded it, as one commentator stated as a "giant leap into the 19th century and a return to a kraepelinian view of mental disorders as fixed disease entities"—despite the fact that the word *disease* was limited to certain categories in the mental retardation and organic brain syndromes sections, and even though the word *illness* appeared only in the manic-depressive conditions, where it was adopted to avoid the ICD term *manic-depressive psychosis*. Karl Menninger summarized the view when he said:

> This year the APA took a great step backward when it abandoned the principle used in the simple useful nosology (DSM-I) which Dr. Will (William Menninger) worked so hard to get

installed. . . . In the interest of uniformity, in the interest of having some kind of international code of designations for different kinds of human troubles, in the interest of statistics and computers, the American medical scientists were asked to repudiate some of the advances they had made in conceptualization and in designation of mental illness.

Although child psychiatrists were pleased that DSM-II, unlike DSM-I, had a special category for children and adolescents, many were disappointed that the Group for the Advancement of Psychiatry's *Psychopathological Disorders in Childhood: Theoretical Considerations and a Proposed Classification,* which had been available for several years, was not used by the committee that developed DSM-II.

Many applauded the elimination of the term *reaction*, which had been appended to most of the DSM-I terms, as an honest retreat from the position that, by adding the term *reaction* to diagnostic labels, one thereby somehow communicates some important knowledge about the etiology of the mental disorders. As Gruenberg explained,

> The routinizing of the word "reaction" in our standard nomenclature (DSM-I) has accomplished little that is positive—it has given many psychiatrists the false notion that mental disorders are reactions of the organism to circumstances but that tuberculosis and diabetes and nephritis and measles and mumps are "things" independent of the patient's nature. For all medical diseases are also reactions of the organism to certain life circumstances and do not exist independently of the people who are sick.

Those who were most enthusiastic pointed to the potential benefits that might accrue to international research and to communication between psychiatrists of different nations because this country had adopted a system based on the ICD.

Although DSM-II was the basis for the official diagnostic manuals used in Canada, India, and several Latin American countries, other national glossaries were prepared, and they defined the ICD list of terms in their own way. The most influential glossary, other than DSM-II, was *Great Britain's Glossary of Mental Disorders,* prepared in 1968 under the direction of Aubrey Lewis.

In the absence of an internationally accepted glossary, it was inevitable that different countries would define categories somewhat differently. An important example of inconsistent definition occurred with schizophrenia. DSM-II defined *schizophrenia* broadly, consistent with the view of schizophrenia held by American psychiatrists in the 1960s, and included mild cases that most European psychiatrists would not have considered to be schizophrenia. The British glossary defined the condition more narrowly, and the differences in the reported prevalence of schizophrenia in the two countries was found to be mainly due to differences in diagnostic definition, rather than due to differences in actual rates of disorder.

In 1975, the ninth revision of the ICD (ICD-9) classification of mental disorders was published, together with a glossary, to go into effect in 1978. Although many minor changes in the ICD-8 classification and glossary were made, these were not radical changes. As with ICD-8, psychiatrists from the United States provided some limited input into the final document.

An examination of the ICD-9 classification reveals a major difficulty in developing a classification that is acceptable internationally. It is far easier to allow each country to introduce terms that are used only by that country than it is to insist that different countries use a single agreed-on terminology. Thus, as Robert E. Kendell noted, the ICD-9 classification actually includes several "alternative and quite incompatible" ways of classifying depression. For example, definitions of the categories of manic-depressive psychosis, depressed type, and depressive type of nonorganic psychosis are not mutually exclusive.

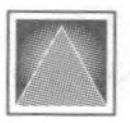

Table 9.1–2
Washington University Approach toward Establishing the Validity of a Psychiatric Diagnosis

Clinical description	Includes symptoms characteristic of the disorder, as well as demographic features, age of onset, precipitating life events, and other variables that more clearly define the clinical picture.
Delimitation from other disorders	Refers to exclusion criteria, so that individuals with other disorders who share similar clinical features are not included in the diagnostic group.
Laboratory studies	Includes biological and psychological tests.
Follow-up study	The same disorder may have variable prognosis, but, until more is known about the fundamental nature of the disorder, marked differences in outcome raise questions about the validity of the original diagnosis.
Family study	Includes family, adoption, and twin studies.

Adapted from Feighner JP, Robins E, Guze SB, et al.: Diagnostic criteria for use in psychiatric research. *Arch Gen Psychiatry.* 1972;26:57–67.

MODERN HISTORY OF CLASSIFICATION

In 1972, a group of researchers published an article in the *Archives of General Psychiatry* entitled "Diagnostic Criteria for Use in Psychiatric Research." Referred to as the *Feighner criteria* (after the lead author of the article), or the *Washington University criteria* (after the academic affiliation of the authors), for the first time, specific inclusion and exclusion criteria for different disorders were delineated. The criteria were limited to the 15 disorders that the authors considered to have been validated by empirical research. The methods of establishing diagnostic validity had been described in another paper from this group 2 years earlier and were recapitulated in the 1972 article. The Washington University five-phase approach toward establishing diagnostic validity of individual categories has dominated empirical psychiatry during the past 30 years (Table 9.1–2).

Also in 1972, Spitzer and Joseph Fleiss published a review article of studies examining the reliability of psychiatric diagnosis. They reexamined the reliability studies conducted during the 1950s and 1960s, and computed kappa coefficients of diagnostic agreement, which was then a relatively novel statistical procedure for determining the level of agreement after accounting for agreement due to chance. They concluded that the reliability of psychiatric diagnosis was poor. This established the groundwork for revising how psychiatric disorders were defined, as poor reliability limits the validity of a diagnostic system.

As part of a longitudinal study of the course of mood disorders, the Research Diagnostic Criteria (RDC) were developed along with a semi-structured diagnostic interview that evaluated these criteria. The criteria for almost every disorder originally defined by the Washington University group were modified in the RDC, and studies were subsequently conducted to compare the respective reliabilities of these criteria sets (along with the DSM-III criteria). As with the Washington University criteria, only a limited number of disorders were defined in the RDC.

DSM-III was published in 1980. Seven years later, DSM-III-R was published. Less than 1 year after the publication of DSM-III-R, plans were announced for the publication of DSM-IV. Delayed by 2 years, DSM-IV was ultimately published in 1994. Robert Spitzer was the chair of the Task Force for DSM-III and DSM-III-R, and Allen Frances the chair of the Task Force for DSM-IV.

The publication of DSM-III was received with significant comment, as it represented a marked departure from how psychiatric disorders had been previously specified and described. Although controversy surrounded some decisions, such as the removal of the term *neurosis* from the classification, the achievements of DSM-III resulted in widespread and continued adoption of its approach toward psychiatric classification.

ACHIEVEMENTS OF DSM-III

DSM-III was the first official diagnostic system to specify inclusion and exclusion diagnostic criteria. DSM-III thus followed the precedents set in the Washington University criteria and RDC for defining disorders and brought the reliable diagnostic approach used by a few research groups to the clinical community. Because an official classification system must be comprehensive and must include those disorders for which individuals seek treatment, DSM-III expanded the number of disorders defined with specified criteria from the handful in the RDC to more than 200. This required that the criteria be based on expert clinical consensus rather than systemic study. The specified diagnostic criteria of DSM-III have multiple advantages over the prototypic descriptions of DSM-II. Diagnostic reliability is better, and this is of benefit to researchers attempting to replicate another researcher's findings and to clinicians who can communicate more effectively with one another.

The specification of diagnostic criteria also enables study of the boundaries between disorders and between disorder and no disorder. Thus, the validity of the diagnostic criteria can be evaluated scientifically. In fact, it was assumed when DSM-III was published that changes would be made, and it was anticipated that these changes would follow scientific study rather than ideological debate.

DSM-III was the first official psychiatric classification to introduce a multiaxial evaluation system in which different domains of information are described on five different axes. The purpose of multiaxial evaluation is to promote a comprehensive, biopsychosocial approach toward clinical assessment. Axis I consists of all clinical disorders, except for personality disorders and mental retardation, both of which are reported on Axis II. Prominent maladaptive personality traits that do not meet criteria for a specific disorder and defense mechanisms are also noted on Axis II. Axis III is for general medical conditions that might be relevant to understanding or managing the patient's psychiatric disorder. Axis IV is for noting psychosocial and environmental problems that are relevant to the diagnosis, treatment, and prognosis of Axis I and Axis II disorders. Axis V is the global assessment of functioning (GAF) scale, a 100-point rating based on symptom severity, social functioning, and occupational functioning.

Another major achievement of DSM-III was the narrowing of the definition of schizophrenia and the requirement that, during some point in the illness, overt psychotic features must be present. The redefinition of schizophrenia brought the American system closer to the European approach toward diagnosing this disorder.

The descriptions of disorders included in DSM-III were much more detailed than the descriptions provided in DSM-II. Table 9.1–3 provides the DSM-II description of mania as an example of the brief descriptive paragraphs found in DSM-II. In contrast, the DSM-III text description of a manic episode covered six pages and included information on demographic characteristics, age of onset, familial patterns, course of illness, and differential diagnosis. (In DSM-IV-TR, this has expanded to five pages of text on a manic episode, another six pages of text to describe mixed and hypomanic episodes, and 14 more pages to describe the diagnosis of bipolar disorder.)

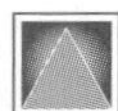

Table 9.1–3
DSM-II Description of Manic-Depressive Disorder

These disorders are marked by severe mood swings and a tendency to remission and recurrence. Patients may be given this diagnosis in the absence of a previous history of affective psychosis if there is no obvious precipitating event. This disorder is divided into three major subtypes: manic type, depressed type, and circular type.

296.1 Manic-depressive illness, manic type (manic-depressive psychosis, manic type): This disorder consists exclusively of manic episodes. These episodes are characterized by excessive elation, irritability, talkativeness, flight of ideas, and accelerated speech and motor activity. Brief periods of depression sometimes occur, but they are never true depressive episodes.

296.2 Manic-depressive illness, depressed type (manic-depressive psychosis, depressed type): This disorder consists exclusively of depressive episodes. These episodes are characterized by severely depressed mood and by mental and motor retardation progressing occasionally to stupor. Uneasiness, apprehension, perplexity, and agitation may also be present. When illusions, hallucinations, and delusions (usually of guilt or of hypochondriacal or paranoid ideas) occur, they are attributable to the dominant mood disorder. Because it is a primary mood disorder, this psychosis differs from the psychotic depressive reaction, which is more easily attributable to precipitating stress. Cases incompletely labeled as *psychotic depression* should be classified here rather than under *psychotic depressive reaction*.

296.3 Manic-depressive illness, circular type (manic-depressive psychosis, circular type): This disorder is distinguished by at least one attack of a depressive episode and a manic episode. This phenomenon makes clear why manic and depressed types are combined into a single category.

DSM-III assumed a descriptive approach to classification, because it was recognized that the etiology of psychiatric disorders was largely unknown. To facilitate the use of the diagnostic classification by clinicians with different theoretical orientations, etiological perspectives were not included in DSM-III. The basis of the disorder groupings was shared clinical features.

DSM-III, for the first time in an official classification of mental disorders, included a definition of mental disorder. As noted previously, the definition has been debated and criticized, but it at least provided a basis for discussing the relevant issues.

DSM-IV-TR CLASSIFICATION

DSM-IV was published in the midst of the criticism that it represented the third version of the DSM published within 14 years. This contrasted with the 16-year interval between DSM-I and DSM-II and the 12-year interval between DSM-II and DSM-III. Mark Zimmerman argued that the publication of three DSM editions within such a short interval could result in six problems: (1) an insufficient amount of time between DSM editions to allow the accumulation of replicated research necessary to justify a change in diagnostic criteria, thereby impeding progress in the development of a valid classification; (2) the expenditure of resources to compare the new diagnostic criteria with the old and thus divert effort toward discovering pathophysiological mechanisms; (3) difficulties in interpreting and resolving discrepant research findings based on different criteria sets; (4) an increased number of diagnostic errors because of the lack of time to learn the nuances of frequently changing diagnostic criteria; (5) impeded communication among clinicians, because three diagnostic manuals will be in widespread use; and (6) frustration from patients who have their diagnoses changed when the diagnostic manual changes. The leaders of the Task Force charged with the development of DSM-IV acknowledged concerns about the brief interval between DSM editions and indicated that DSM-IV was to be the most empirically grounded psychiatric classification system. The three components of the empirical process underpinning DSM-IV were comprehensive literature reviews, reanalyses of existing data bases, and a series of field trials comparing existing and proposed criteria sets.

Along with the proliferation of DSM versions, the 1980s and 1990s witnessed a proliferation of comment on the overall revision process, as well as specific decisions regarding behavior and cognitive patterns that were or were not included as disorders in the DSMs. Sociopolitical pressures thus assumed greater visibility (and possibly influence) in revising the classification. The ultimate political statement on classification came in the form of a referendum that was placed on the 1994 general ballot of the APA. The referendum asked the APA membership to vote on whether the tenth revision of the ICD (ICD-10) should be adopted as the official diagnostic system and the DSM-IV's publication should be postponed for 3 years. The referendum was defeated; however, the fact that a petition drive was successful in getting the issue on the ballot indicated that the level of dissatisfaction with the frequent DSM revisions was not insignificant.

DSM-IV-TR lists 365 disorders in 17 sections (Table 9.1–4), plus some diagnostic criteria proposed for further study included in the appendix. This is an increase from the 285 disorders in 17 sections in DSM-III and the 292 disorders in 18 sections in DSM-III-R. The DSM-IV-TR classification of mental disorders is provided in Table 9.1–5. In the following section, the salient features of the disorders in each section are briefly described.

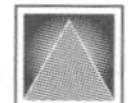

Table 9.1–4
Groups of Conditions in DSM-IV-TR

Disorders usually first diagnosed in infancy, childhood, or adolescence
Delirium, dementia, amnestic, and other cognitive disorders
Mental disorders due to a general medical condition
Substance-related disorders
Schizophrenia and other psychotic disorders
Mood disorders
Anxiety disorders
Somatoform disorders
Factitious disorders
Dissociative disorders
Sexual and gender identity disorders
Eating disorders
Sleep disorders
Impulse-control disorders not elsewhere classified
Adjustment disorders
Personality disorders
Other conditions that may be a focus of clinical attention

I: Disorders Usually First Diagnosed in Infancy, Childhood, or Adolescence

The section of disorders usually first diagnosed in infancy, childhood, or adolescence is unique in DSM-IV-TR, because the disorders grouped here are included based on the age that they are usually first diagnosed rather than shared phenomenological features. DSM-IV-TR notes that this separation is for convenience only, and it does not indicate a clear distinction between these disorders and the others in the manual.

Mental Retardation

Mental retardation is characterized by significant, below average intelligence (as demonstrated by a score below 70 on a standardized, individually administered, intelligence test) and impairment in adaptive functioning in at least two areas. *Adaptive functioning* refers to how effective individuals are in achieving age-appropriate common demands of life in areas such as communication, self-care, and interpersonal skills. Mental retardation is one of only four disorders in DSM-IV-TR in which different diagnostic code numbers are provided for different levels of severity (mild, moderate, severe, and profound).

Learning Disorders

The three specific learning disorders (reading, mathematics, and written expression) are diagnosed when performance on standardized achievement tests are substantially below expectations based on age, education, and intelligence, and these learning problems cause significant impairment in functioning. Learning disorders can be comorbid with mild mental retardation if the achievement is below that expected based on intelligence level. The context of learning difficulties is considered insofar as learning disorders are not diagnosed if low level of achievement is due to inadequate education.

Motor Skills Disorder

DSM-IV-TR lists a single motor skills disorder—developmental coordination disorder. Analogous to learning disorders, developmental coordination disorder is diagnosed when motor coordination is substantially below expectations based on age and intelligence, and when the coordination problem significantly interferes with functioning. Examples include delays in achieving developmental milestones such as crawling or walking, dropping things, and poor sports performance. The diagnosis is excluded if a specific general medical condition, such as cerebral palsy or muscular dystrophy, accounts for the symptoms.

Communication Disorders

The four specific communication disorders (expressive language disorder, mixed receptive-expressive language disorder, phonological disorder, and stuttering) are characterized by speech or language difficulties. The diagnosis of expressive and mixed receptive-expressive language disorders depends on standardized testing (similar to mental retardation and learning disorders), whereas the two articulation disorders do not. The communication disorders, similar to the learning and motor skills disorders, are only diagnosed when they cause significant impairment in functioning. The presence of subjective distress in the absence of demonstrable functional impairment would not warrant the diagnosis.

Pervasive Developmental Disorders

The four specific pervasive developmental disorders (autistic disorder, Rett's syndrome, childhood disintegrative disorder, and Asperger's syndrome) are characterized by severe difficulties in multiple developmental areas, including social relatedness, communication, and range of activity and interests. The diagnostic criteria for the social interaction deficits and repetitive and stereotypical patterns of behavior and interests are identical for autistic disorder and Asperger's syndrome. They differ in that concurrent communication deficits are required to diagnose autistic disorder and are absent in Asperger's syndrome. Also, to diagnose Asperger's syndrome, a criterion is added that the symptoms must cause clinically significant impairment in functioning; this criterion is not specified for autistic disorder.

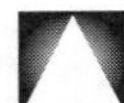

Table 9.1–5
DSM-IV-TR Classification of Mental Disorders (With *International Statistical Classification of Diseases,* Tenth Revision, Codes)

	Disorders usually first diagnosed in infancy, childhood, or adolescence (39)
	Mental retardation (41)
	Note: These are coded on Axis II.
F70.9	Mild mental retardation (43)
F71.9	Moderate mental retardation (43)
F72.9	Severe mental retardation (43)
F73.9	Profound mental retardation (44)
F79.9	Mental retardation, severity unspecified (44)
	Learning disorders (49)
F81.0	Reading disorder (51)
F81.2	Mathematics disorder (53)
F81.8	Disorder of written expression (54)
F81.9	Learning disorder NOS (56)
	Motor skills disorder (56)
F82	Developmental coordination disorder (56)
	Communication disorders (58)
F80.1	Expressive language disorder (58)
F80.2	Mixed receptive-expressive language disorder (62)
F80.0	Phonological disorder (65)
F98.5	Stuttering (67)
F80.9	Communication disorder NOS (69)
	Pervasive developmental disorders (69)
F84.0	Autistic disorder (70)
F84.2	Rett's syndrome (76)
F84.3	Childhood disintegrative disorder (77)
F84.5	Asperger's syndrome (80)
F84.9	Pervasive developmental disorder NOS (84)
	Attention-deficit and disruptive behavior disorders (85)
—.–	Attention-deficit/hyperactivity disorder (85)
F90.0	Combined type
F98.8	Predominantly inattentive type
F90.0	Predominantly hyperactive-impulsive type
F90.9	Attention-deficit/hyperactivity disorder NOS (93)
F91.8	Conduct Disorder (93)
	Specify type: childhood-onset type or adolescent-onset type
F91.3	Oppositional defiant disorder (100)
F91.9	Disruptive behavior disorder NOS (103)
	Feeding and eating disorders of infancy or early childhood (103)
F98.3	Pica (103)
F98.2	Rumination disorder (105)
F98.2	Feeding disorder of infancy or early childhood (107)
	Tic disorders (108)
F95.2	Tourette's syndrome (111)
F95.1	Chronic motor or vocal tic disorder (114)
F95.0	Transient tic disorder (115)
	Specify if: single episode or recurrent
F95.9	Tic disorder NOS (116)
	Elimination disorders (116)
—.–	Encopresis (116)
R15	With constipation and overflow incontinence *(also code K59.0 constipation on Axis III)*
F98.1	Without constipation and overflow incontinence
F98.0	Enuresis (not due to a general medical condition) (118)
	Specify type: nocturnal only, diurnal only, or nocturnal and diurnal
	Other disorders of infancy, childhood, or adolescence (121)
F93.0	Separation anxiety disorder (121)
	Specify if: early onset
F94.0	Selective mutism (125)
F94.x	Reactive attachment disorder of infancy or early childhood (127)
.1	Inhibited type
.2	Disinhibited type
F98.4	Stereotypic movement disorder (131)
	Specify if: with self-injurious behavior
F98.9	Disorder of infancy, childhood, or adolescence NOS (134)
	Delirium, dementia, and amnestic and other cognitive disorders (135)
	Delirium (136)
F05.0	Delirium due to . . . *[indicate the general medical condition] (code F05.1 if superimposed on dementia)* (141)
—.–	Substance intoxication delirium *(refer to substance-related disorders for substance-specific codes)* (143)
—.–	Substance withdrawal delirium *(refer to substance-related disorders for substance-specific codes)* (143)
—.–	Delirium due to multiple etiologies *(code each of the specific etiologies)* (146)
F05.9	Delirium NOS (147)
	Dementia (147)
F00.xx	Dementia of the Alzheimer's type, with early onset *(also code G30.0 Alzheimer's disease, with early onset, on Axis III)* (154)
.00	Uncomplicated
.01	With delusions
.03	With depressed mood
	Specify if: with behavioral disturbance
F00.xx	Dementia of the Alzheimer's type, with late onset *(also code G30.1 Alzheimer's disease, with late onset, on Axis III)* (154)
.10	Uncomplicated
.11	With delusions
.13	With depressed mood
	Specify if: with behavioral disturbance
F01.xx	Vascular dementia (158)
.80	Uncomplicated
.81	With delusions
.83	With depressed mood
	Specify if: with behavioral disturbance
F02.4	Dementia due to HIV disease *(also code B22.0 HIV disease resulting in encephalopathy on Axis III)* (163)
F02.8	Dementia due to head trauma *(also code S06.9 intracranial injury on Axis III)* (164)
F02.3	Dementia due to Parkinson's disease *(also code G20 Parkinson's disease on Axis III)* (164)
F02.2	Dementia due to Huntington's disease *(also code G10 Huntington's disease on Axis III)* (165)
F02.0	Dementia due to Pick's disease *(also code G31.0 Pick's disease on Axis III)* (165)
F02.1	Dementia due to Creutzfeldt-Jakob disease *(also code A81.0 Creutzfeldt-Jakob disease on Axis III)* (166)

(continued)

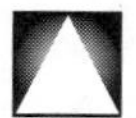

Table 9.1–5 (*continued*)

F02.8	Dementia due to . . . *[indicate the general medical condition not listed above] (also code the general medical condition on Axis III)* (167)
—.—	Substance-induced persisting dementia *(refer to substance-related disorders for substance-specific codes)* (168)
F02.8	Dementia due to multiple etiologies *(instead code F00.2 for mixed Alzheimer's and vascular dementia)* (170)
F03	Dementia NOS (171)
	Amnestic disorders (172)
F04	Amnestic disorder due to . . . *[indicate the general medical condition]* (175)
	Specify if: transient or chronic
—.—	Substance-induced persisting amnestic disorder *(refer to substance-related disorders for substance-specific codes)* (177)
R41.3	Amnestic disorder NOS (179)
	Other cognitive disorders (179)
F06.9	Cognitive disorders NOS (179)
	Mental disorders due to a general medical condition not elsewhere classified (181)
F06.1	Catatonic disorder due to . . . *[indicate the general medical condition]* (185)
F07.0	Personality change due to . . . *[indicate the general medical condition]* (187)
	Specify type: labile type, disinhibited type, aggressive type, apathetic type, paranoid type, other type, combined type, or unspecified type
F09	Mental disorder NOS due to . . . *[indicate the general medical condition]* (190)
	Substance-related disorders (191)
	[a] *The following specifiers may be applied to substance dependence:*
	Specify if: with physiological dependence or without physiological dependence
	Code course of dependence in fifth character:
	0 = Early full remission or early partial remission
	0 = Sustained full remission or sustained partial remission
	1 = In a controlled environment
	2 = On agonist therapy
	4 = Mild, moderate, or severe
	The following specifiers apply to substance-induced disorders as noted:
	[I]With onset during intoxication
	[W]With onset during withdrawal
	Alcohol-related disorders (212)
	Alcohol use disorders (213)
F10.2x	Alcohol dependence[a] (213)
F10.1	Alcohol abuse (214)
	Alcohol-induced disorders (214)
F10.00	Alcohol intoxication (214)
F10.3	Alcohol withdrawal (215)
	Specify if: with perceptual disturbances
F10.03	Alcohol intoxication delirium (143)
F10.4	Alcohol withdrawal delirium (143)
F10.73	Alcohol-induced persisting dementia (168)
F10.6	Alcohol-induced persisting amnestic disorder (177)
F10.xx	Alcohol-induced psychotic disorder (338)
.51	With delusions[I,W]
.52	With hallucinations[I,W]
F10.8	Alcohol-induced mood disorder[I,W] (405)
F10.8	Alcohol-induced anxiety disorder[I,W] (479)
F10.8	Alcohol-induced sexual dysfunction[I] (562)
F10.8	Alcohol-induced sleep disorder[I,W] (655)
F10.9	Alcohol-related disorder NOS (223)
	Amphetamine (or amphetamine-like)–related disorders (223)
	Amphetamine use disorders (224)
F15.2x	Amphetamine dependence[a] (224)
F15.1	Amphetamine abuse (225)
	Amphetamine-induced disorders (226)
F15.00	Amphetamine intoxication (226)
F15.04	Amphetamine intoxication, with perceptual disturbances (226)
F15.3	Amphetamine withdrawal (227)
F15.03	Amphetamine intoxication delirium (143)
F15.xx	Amphetamine-induced psychotic disorder (338)
.51	With delusions[I]
.52	With hallucinations[I]
F15.8	Amphetamine-induced mood disorder[I,W] (405)
F15.8	Amphetamine-induced anxiety disorder[I] (479)
F15.8	Amphetamine-induced sexual dysfunction[I] (562)
F15.8	Amphetamine-induced sleep disorder[I,W] (655)
F15.9	Amphetamine-related disorder NOS (231)
	Caffeine-related disorders (231)
	Caffeine-induced disorders (232)
F15.00	Caffeine intoxication (232)
F15.8	Caffeine-induced anxiety disorder[I] (479)
F15.8	Caffeine-induced sleep disorder[I] (655)
F15.9	Caffeine-related disorder NOS (234)
	Cannabis-related disorders (234)
	Cannabis use disorders (236)
F12.2x	Cannabis dependence[a] (236)
F12.1	Cannabis abuse (236)
	Cannabis-induced disorders (237)
F12.00	Cannabis intoxication (237)
F12.04	Cannabis intoxication, with perceptual disturbances (237)
F12.03	Cannabis intoxication delirium (143)
F12.xx	Cannabis-induced psychotic disorder (338)
.51	With delusions[I]
.52	With hallucinations[I]
F12.8	Cannabis-induced anxiety disorder[I] (479)
F12.9	Cannabis-related disorder NOS (241)
	Cocaine-related disorders (241)
	Cocaine use disorders (242)
F14.2x	Cocaine dependence[a] (242)
F14.1	Cocaine abuse (243)
	Cocaine-induced disorders (244)
F14.00	Cocaine intoxication (244)
F14.04	Cocaine intoxication, with perceptual disturbances (244)
F14.3	Cocaine withdrawal (245)
F14.03	Cocaine intoxication delirium (143)
F14.xx	Cocaine-induced psychotic disorder (338)
.51	With delusions[I]
.52	With hallucinations[I]

(*continued*)

Table 9.1–5 (*continued*)

F14.8	Cocaine-induced mood disorder[I,W] (405)
F14.8	Cocaine-induced anxiety disorder[I,W] (479)
F14.8	Cocaine-induced sexual dysfunction[I] (562)
F14.8	Cocaine-induced sleep disorder[I,W] (655)
F14.9	Cocaine-related disorder NOS (250)
	Hallucinogen-related disorders (250)
	Hallucinogen use disorders (251)
F16.2x	Hallucinogen dependence[a] (251)
F16.1	Hallucinogen abuse (252)
	Hallucinogen-induced disorders (252)
F16.00	Hallucinogen intoxication (252)
F16.70	Hallucinogen persisting perception disorder (flashbacks) (253)
F16.03	Hallucinogen intoxication delirium (143)
F16.xx	Hallucinogen-induced psychotic disorder (338)
.51	With delusions[I]
.52	With hallucinations[I]
F16.8	Hallucinogen-induced mood disorder[I] (405)
F16.8	Hallucinogen-induced anxiety disorder[I] (479)
F16.9	Hallucinogen-related disorder NOS (256)
	Inhalant-related disorders (257)
	Inhalant use disorders (258)
F18.2x	Inhalant dependence[a] (258)
F18.1	Inhalant abuse (259)
	Inhalant-induced disorders (259)
F18.00	Inhalant intoxication (259)
F18.03	Inhalant intoxication delirium (143)
F18.73	Inhalant-induced persisting dementia (168)
F18.xx	Inhalant-induced psychotic disorder (338)
.51	With delusions[I]
.52	With hallucinations[I]
F18.8	Inhalant-induced mood disorder[I] (405)
F18.8	Inhalant-induced anxiety disorder[I] (479)
F18.9	Inhalant-related disorder NOS (263)
	Nicotine-related disorders (264)
	Nicotine use disorder (264)
F17.2x	Nicotine dependence[a] (264)
	Nicotine-induced disorders (265)
F17.3	Nicotine withdrawal (265)
F17.9	Nicotine-related disorders NOS (269)
	Opioid-related disorders (269)
	Opioid use disorders (270)
F11.2x	Opioid dependence[a] (270)
F11.1	Opioid abuse (271)
	Opioid-induced disorders (271)
F11.00	Opioid intoxication (271)
F11.04	Opioid intoxication, with perceptual disturbances (272)
F11.3	Opioid withdrawal (272)
F11.03	Opioid intoxication delirium (143)
F11.xx	Opioid-induced psychotic disorder (338)
.51	With delusions[I]
.52	With hallucinations[I]
F11.8	Opioid-induced mood disorder[I] (405)
F11.8	Opioid-induced sexual dysfunction[I] (562)
F11.8	Opioid-induced sleep disorder[I,W] (655)
F11.9	Opioid-related disorder NOS (277)
	Phencyclidine (or phencyclidine-like)–related disorders (278)
	Phencyclidine use disorders (279)
F19.2x	Phencyclidine dependence[a] (279)
F19.1	Phencyclidine abuse (279)
	Phencyclidine-induced disorders (280)
F19.00	Phencyclidine intoxication (280)
F19.04	Phencyclidine intoxication, with perceptual disturbances (280)
F19.03	Phencyclidine intoxication delirium (143)
F19.xx	Phencyclidine-induced psychotic disorder (338)
.51	With delusions[I]
.52	With hallucinations[I]
F19.8	Phencyclidine-induced mood disorder[I] (405)
F19.8	Phencyclidine-induced anxiety disorder[I] (479)
F19.9	Phencyclidine-related disorder NOS (283)
	Sedative-, hypnotic-, or anxiolytic-related disorders (284)
	Sedative, hypnotic, or anxiolytic use disorders (285)
F13.2x	Sedative, hypnotic, or anxiolytic dependence[a] (285)
F13.1	Sedative, hypnotic, or anxiolytic abuse (286)
	Sedative-, hypnotic-, or anxiolytic-induced disorders (286)
F13.00	Sedative, hypnotic, or anxiolytic intoxication (286)
F13.3	Sedative, hypnotic, or anxiolytic withdrawal (287)
	Specify if: with perceptual disturbances
F13.03	Sedative, hypnotic, or anxiolytic intoxication delirium (143)
F13.4	Sedative, hypnotic, or anxiolytic withdrawal delirium (143)
F13.73	Sedative-, hypnotic-, or anxiolytic-induced persisting dementia (168)
F13.6	Sedative-, hypnotic-, or anxiolytic-induced persisting amnestic disorder (177)
F13.xx	Sedative-, hypnotic-, or anxiolytic-induced psychotic disorder (338)
.51	With delusions[I,W]
.52	With hallucinations[I,W]
F13.8	Sedative-, hypnotic-, or anxiolytic-induced mood disorder[I,W] (405)
F13.8	Sedative-, hypnotic-, or anxiolytic-induced anxiety disorder[W] (479)
F13.8	Sedative-, hypnotic-, or anxiolytic-induced sexual dysfunction[I] (562)
F13.8	Sedative-, hypnotic-, or anxiolytic-induced sleep disorder[I,W] (655)
F13.9	Sedative-, hypnotic-, or anxiolytic-related disorder NOS (293)
	Polysubstance-related disorder (293)
F19.2x	Polysubstance dependence[a] (293)
	Other (or unknown) substance-related disorders (294)
	Other (or unknown) substance use disorders (294)
F19.2x	Other (or unknown) substance dependence[a] (192)
F19.1	Other (or unknown) substance abuse (198)
	Other (or unknown) substance-induced disorders (295)
F19.00	Other (or unknown) substance intoxication (199)
F19.04	Other (or unknown) substance intoxication, with perceptual disturbances (199)
F19.3	Other (or unknown) substance withdrawal (201)
	Specify if: with perceptual disturbances

(*continued*)

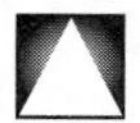

Table 9.1–5 (*continued*)

F19.03	Other (or unknown) substance-induced delirium *(code F19.4 if onset during withdrawal)* (143)
F19.73	Other (or unknown) substance-induced persisting dementia (168)
F19.6	Other (or unknown) substance-induced persisting amnestic disorder (177)
F19.xx	Other (or unknown) substance-induced psychotic disorder (338)
.51	With delusions[I,W]
.52	With hallucinations[I,W]
F19.8	Other (or unknown) substance-induced mood disorder[I,W] (405)
F19.8	Other (or unknown) substance-induced anxiety disorder[I,W] (479)
F19.8	Other (or unknown) substance-induced sexual dysfunction[I] (562)
F19.8	Other (or unknown) substance-induced sleep disorder[I,W] (655)
F19.9	Other (or unknown) substance-related disorder NOS (295)
Schizophrenia and other psychotic disorders (297)	
F20.xx	Schizophrenia (298)
.0x	Paranoid type (313)
.1x	Disorganized type (314)
.2x	Catatonic type (315)
.3x	Undifferentiated type (316)
.5x	Residual type (316)
Code course of schizophrenia in fifth character:	
	2 = Episodic with interepisode residual symptoms (*specify* if: with prominent negative symptoms)
	3 = Episodic with no interepisode residual symptoms
	0 = Continuous (*specify* if: with prominent negative symptoms)
	4 = Single episode in partial remission (*specify* if: with prominent negative symptoms)
	5 = Single episode in full remission
	8 = Other or unspecified pattern
	9 = Less than 1 year since onset of initial active-phase symptoms
F20.8	Schizophreniform disorder (317)
	Specify if: without good prognostic features/with good prognostic features
F25.x	Schizoaffective disorder (319)
.0	Bipolar type
.1	Depressive type
F22.0	Delusional disorder (323)
	Specify type: erotomanic type, grandiose type, jealous type, persecutory type, somatic type, mixed type, or unspecified type
F23.xx	Brief psychotic disorder (329)
.81	With marked stressor(s)
.80	Without marked stressor(s)
	Specify if: with postpartum onset
F24	Shared psychotic disorder (332)
F06.x	Psychotic disorder due to . . . *[indicate the general medical condition]* (334)
.2	With delusions
.0	With hallucinations
__._	Substance-induced psychotic disorder *(refer to substance-related disorders for substance-specific codes)* (338)
	Specify if: with onset during intoxication/with onset during withdrawal
F29	Psychotic disorder NOS (343)
Mood disorders (345)	
The following specifiers apply (for current or most recent episode) to mood disorders as noted:	
	[a]Severity, psychotic, and remission specifiers
	[b]Chronic
	[c]With catatonic features
	[d]With melancholic features
	[e]With atypical features
	[f]With postpartum onset
The following specifiers apply to mood disorders as noted:	
	[g]With or without full interepisode recovery
	[h]With seasonal pattern
	[i]With rapid cycling
Depressive disorders (369)	
F32.x	Major depressive disorder, single episode[a,b,c,d,e,f] (369)
F33.x	Major depressive disorder, recurrent[a,b,c,d,e,f,g,h] (369)
Code current state of major depressive episode in fourth character:	
	0 = Mild
	1 = Moderate
	2 = Severe without psychotic features
	3 = Severe with psychotic features
	Specify: mood-congruent psychotic features or mood-incongruent psychotic features
	4 = In partial remission
	5 = In full remission
	9 = Unspecified
F34.1	Dysthymic disorder (376)
	Specify if: early onset or late onset
	Specify: with atypical features
F32.9	Depressive disorder NOS (381)
Bipolar disorders (382)	
F30.x	Bipolar I disorder, single manic episode[a,c,f] (382)
	Specify if: mixed
Code current state of manic episode in fourth character:	
	1 = Mild, moderate, or severe without psychotic features
	2 = Severe with psychotic features
	8 = In partial or full remission
F31.0	Bipolar I disorder, most recent episode hypomanic[g,h,i] (382)
F31.x	Bipolar I disorder, most recent episode manic[a,c,f,g,h,i] (382)
Code current state of manic episode in fourth character:	
	1 = Mild, moderate, or severe without psychotic features
	2 = Severe with psychotic features
	7 = In partial or full remission
F31.6	Bipolar I disorder, most recent episode mixed[a,c,f,g,h,i] (382)
F31.x	Bipolar I disorder, most recent episode depressed[a,b,c,d,e,f,g,h,i] (382)

(*continued*)

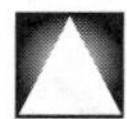

Table 9.1–5 (*continued*)

	Code current state of major depressive episode in fourth character:
	3 = Mild or moderate
	4 = Severe without psychotic features
	5 = Severe with psychotic features
	7 = In partial or full remission
F31.9	Bipolar I disorder, most recent episode unspecified[g,h,i] (382)
F31.8	Bipolar II disorder[a,b,c,d,e,f,g,h,i] (392)
	Specify (current or most recent episode): hypomanic or depressed
F34.0	Cyclothymic disorder (398)
F31.9	Bipolar disorder NOS (400)
F06.xx	Mood disorder due to . . . *[indicate the general medical condition]* (401)
.32	With depressive features
.32	With major depressive–like episode
.30	With manic features
.33	With mixed features
—.—	Substance-induced mood disorder *(refer to substance-related disorders for substance-specific codes)* (405)
	Specify type: with depressive features, with manic features, or with mixed features
	Specify if: with onset during intoxication or with onset during withdrawal
F39	Mood disorder NOS (410)
Anxiety disorders (429)	
F41.0	Panic disorder without agoraphobia (433)
F40.01	Panic disorder with agoraphobia (433)
F40.00	Agoraphobia without history of panic disorder (441)
F40.2	Specific phobia (443)
	Specify type: animal type, natural environment type, blood-injection-injury type, situational type, or other type
F40.1	Social phobia (450)
	Specify if: generalized
F42.8	Obsessive-compulsive disorder (456)
	Specify if: with poor insight
F43.1	Posttraumatic stress disorder (463)
	Specify if: acute or chronic
	Specify if: with delayed onset
F43.0	Acute stress disorder (469)
F41.1	Generalized anxiety disorder (472)
F06.4	Anxiety disorder due to . . . *[indicate the general medical condition]* (476)
	Specify if: with generalized anxiety, with panic attacks, or with obsessive-compulsive symptoms
—.—	Substance-induced anxiety disorder *(refer to substance-related disorders for substance-specific codes)* (479)
	Specify if: with generalized anxiety, with panic attacks, with obsessive-compulsive symptoms, or with phobic symptoms
	Specify if: with onset during intoxication or with onset during withdrawal
F41.9	Anxiety disorder NOS (484)
Somatoform disorders (485)	
F45.0	Somatization disorder (486)
F45.1	Undifferentiated somatoform disorder (490)
F44.x	Conversion disorder (492)
.4	With motor symptom or deficit
.5	With seizures or convulsions
.6	With sensory symptom or deficit
.7	With mixed presentation
F45.4	Pain disorder (498)
	Specify type: associated with psychological factors or associated with psychological factors and a general medical condition
	Specify if: acute or chronic
F45.2	Hypochondriasis (504)
	Specify if: with poor insight
F45.2	Body dysmorphic disorder (507)
F45.9	Somatoform disorder NOS (511)
Factitious disorders (513)	
F68.1	Factitious disorder (513)
	Specify type: with predominantly psychological signs and symptoms, with predominantly physical signs and symptoms, or with combined psychological and physical signs and symptoms
F68.1	Factitious disorder NOS (517)
Dissociative disorders (519)	
F44.0	Dissociative amnesia (520)
F44.1	Dissociative fugue (523)
F44.81	Dissociative identity disorder (526)
F48.1	Depersonalization disorder (530)
F44.9	Dissociative disorder NOS (532)
Sexual and gender identity disorders (535)	
Sexual dysfunctions (535)	
	The following specifiers apply to all primary sexual dysfunctions:
	Lifelong type, acquired type, generalized type, situational type, due to psychological factors, or due to combined factors
Sexual desire disorders (539)	
F52.0	Hypoactive sexual desire disorder (539)
F52.10	Sexual aversion disorder (541)
Sexual arousal disorders (543)	
F52.2	Female sexual arousal disorder (543)
F52.2	Male erectile disorder (545)
Orgasmic disorders (547)	
F52.3	Female orgasmic disorder (547)
F52.3	Male orgasmic disorder (550)
F52.4	Premature ejaculation (552)
Sexual pain disorders (554)	
F52.6	Dyspareunia (not due to a general medical condition) (554)
F52.5	Vaginismus (not due to a general medical condition) (556)
Sexual dysfunction due to a general medical condition (558)	
N94.8	Female hypoactive sexual desire disorder due to . . . *[indicate the general medical condition]* (558)
N50.8	Male hypoactive sexual desire disorder due to . . . *[indicate the general medical condition]* (558)
N48.4	Male erectile disorder due to . . . *[indicate the general medical condition]* (558)
N94.1	Female dyspareunia due to . . . *[indicate the general medical condition]* (558)

(*continued*)

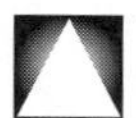

Table 9.1–5 (*continued*)

N50.8	Male dyspareunia due to . . . *[indicate the general medical condition]* (558)
N94.8	Other female sexual dysfunction due to . . . *[indicate the general medical condition]* (558)
N50.8	Other male sexual dysfunction due to . . . *[indicate the general medical condition]* (558)
__._	Substance-induced sexual dysfunction *(refer to substance-related disorders for substance-specific codes)* (562)
	Specify if: with impaired desire, with impaired arousal, with impaired orgasm, or with sexual pain
	Specify if: with onset during intoxication
F52.9	Sexual dysfunction NOS (565)
Paraphilias (566)	
F65.2	Exhibitionism (569)
F65.0	Fetishism (569)
F65.8	Frotteurism (570)
F65.4	Pedophilia (571)
	Specify if: sexually attracted to males, sexually attracted to females, or sexually attracted to both
	Specify if: limited to incest
	Specify type: exclusive type or nonexclusive type
F65.5	Sexual masochism (572)
F65.5	Sexual sadism (573)
F65.1	Transvestic fetishism (574)
	Specify if: with gender dysphoria
F65.3	Voyeurism (575)
F65.9	Paraphilia NOS (576)
Gender identity disorders (576)	
F64.x	Gender identity disorder (576)
.2	In children
.0	In adolescents or adults
	Specify if: sexually attracted to males, sexually attracted to females, sexually attracted to both, or sexually attracted to neither
F64.9	Gender identity disorder NOS (582)
F52.9	Sexual disorder NOS (582)
Eating disorders (583)	
F50.0	Anorexia nervosa (583)
	Specify type: restricting type or binge-eating and purging type
F50.2	Bulimia nervosa (589)
	Specify type: purging type or nonpurging type
F50.9	Eating disorder NOS (594)
Sleep disorders (597)	
Primary sleep disorders (598)	
Dyssomnias (598)	
F51.0	Primary insomnia (599)
F51.1	Primary hypersomnia (604)
	Specify if: recurrent
G47.4	Narcolepsy (609)
G47.3	Breathing-related sleep disorder (615)
F51.2	Circadian rhythm sleep disorder (622)
	Specify type: delayed sleep phase type, jet lag type, shift work type, or unspecified type
F51.9	Dyssomnia NOS (629)
Parasomnias (630)	
F51.5	Nightmare disorder (631)
F51.4	Sleep terror disorder (634)
F51.3	Sleepwalking disorder (639)
F51.8	Parasomnia NOS (644)
Sleep disorders related to another mental disorder (645)	
F51.0	Insomnia related to . . . *[indicate the Axis I or Axis II disorder]* (645)
F51.1	Hypersomnia related to . . . *[indicate the Axis I or Axis II disorder]* (645)
Other sleep disorders (651)	
G47.x	Sleep disorder due to . . . *[indicate the general medical condition]* (651)
.0	Insomnia type
.1	Hypersomnia type
.8	Parasomnia type
.8	Mixed type
__._	Substance-induced sleep disorder *(refer to substance-related disorders for substance-specific codes)* (655)
	Specify type: insomnia type, hypersomnia type, or parasomnia type/mixed type
	Specify if: with onset during intoxication or with onset during withdrawal
Impulse-control disorders not elsewhere classified (663)	
F63.8	Intermittent explosive disorder (663)
F63.2	Kleptomania (667)
F63.1	Pyromania (669)
F63.0	Pathological gambling (671)
F63.3	Trichotillomania (674)
F63.9	Impulse-control disorder NOS (677)
Adjustment disorders (679)	
F43.xx	Adjustment disorder (679)
.20	With depressed mood
.28	With anxiety
.22	With mixed anxiety and depressed mood
.24	With disturbance of conduct
.25	With mixed disturbance of emotions and conduct
.9	Unspecified
	Specify if: acute or chronic
Personality disorders (685)	
Note: These are coded on Axis II.	
F60.0	Paranoid personality disorder (690)
F60.1	Schizoid personality disorder (694)
F21	Schizotypal personality disorder (697)
F60.2	Antisocial personality disorder (701)
F60.31	Borderline personality disorder (706)
F60.4	Histrionic personality disorder (711)
F60.8	Narcissistic personality disorder (714)
F60.6	Avoidant personality disorder (718)
F60.7	Dependent personality disorder (721)
F60.5	Obsessive-compulsive personality disorder (725)
F60.9	Personality disorder NOS (729)

(*continued*)

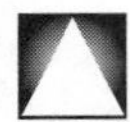

Table 9.1–5 (*continued*)

Code	Name	Code	Name
Other conditions that may be a focus of clinical attention (731)		Z63.0	Partner relational problem (737)
Psychological factors affecting medical condition (731)		F93.3	Sibling relational problem (737)
F54	. . . *[Specified psychological factor]* affecting . . . *[indicate the general medical condition]*	Z63.9	Relational problem NOS (737)
		Problems related to abuse or neglect (738)	
	Choose name based on nature of factors: (731)	T74.1	Physical abuse of child (738)
	Mental disorder affecting medical condition	T74.2	Sexual abuse of child (738)
	Psychological symptoms affecting medical condition	T74.0	Neglect of child (738)
	Personality traits or coping style affecting medical condition	T74.1	Physical abuse of adult (738)
		T74.2	Sexual abuse of adult (738)
	Maladaptive health behaviors affecting medical condition	Additional conditions that may be a focus of clinical attention (739)	
		Z91.1	Noncompliance with treatment (739)
	Stress-related physiological response affecting medical condition	Z76.5	Malingering (739)
		Z72.8	Adult antisocial behavior (740)
	Other or unspecified psychological factors affecting medical condition	Z72.8	Child or adolescent antisocial behavior (740)
		R41.8	Borderline intellectual functioning (740)
Medication-induced movement disorders (734)		R41.8	Age-related cognitive decline (740)
G21.0	Neuroleptic-induced parkinsonism (735)	Z63.4	Bereavement (740)
G21.0	Neuroleptic malignant syndrome (735)	Z55.8	Academic problem (741)
G24.0	Neuroleptic-induced acute dystonia (735)	Z56.7	Occupational problem (741)
G21.1	Neuroleptic-induced acute akathisia (735)	F93.8	Identity problem (741)
G24.0	Neuroleptic-induced tardive dyskinesia (736)	Z71.8	Religious or spiritual problem (741)
G25.1	Medication-induced postural tremor (736)	Z60.3	Acculturation problem (741)
G25.9	Medication-induced movement disorder NOS (736)	Z60.0	Phase of life problem (742)
Other medication-induced disorder (736)		**Additional codes** (743)	
T88.7	Adverse effects of medication NOS (736)	F99	Unspecified mental disorder (nonpsychotic) (743)
Relational problems (736)		Z03.2	No diagnosis or condition on Axis I (743)
Z63.7	Relational problem related to a mental disorder or general medical condition (737)	R69	Diagnosis or condition deferred on Axis I (743)
		Z03.2	No diagnosis on Axis II (743)
Z63.8	Parent–child relational problem *(code Z63.1 if focus of attention is on child)* (737)	R46.8	Diagnosis deferred on Axis II (743)

Note: An *x* appearing in a diagnostic code indicates that a specific code number is required. An ellipsis (. . .) is used in the names of certain disorders to indicate that the name of a specific mental disorder or general medical condition should be inserted when recording the name (e.g., F05.0 Delirium Due to Hypothyroidism). Numbers in parentheses are page numbers. If criteria are currently met, one of the following severity specifiers may be noted after the diagnosis: *mild, moderate,* or *severe.* If criteria are no longer met, one of the following specifiers may be noted: *in partial remission, in full remission,* or *prior history.*
HIV, human immunodeficiency virus; NOS, not otherwise specified.
From American Psychiatric Association. *Diagnostic and Statistical Manual of Mental Disorders.* 4th ed. Text rev. Washington, DC: American Psychiatric Association; 2000, with permission.

Attention-Deficit/Hyperactivity Disorder (ADHD) Since the 1990s, ADHD has been one of the most frequently discussed psychiatric disorders in the lay media because of the sometimes unclear line between age-appropriate normal and disordered behavior and because of the concern that nondisordered children are being diagnosed and treated with medication. In fact, a lawsuit was filed against the APA, charging it with being influenced by the pharmaceutical industry to include the disorder in the DSM. The central feature of the disorder is persistent inattention or hyperactivity and impulsivity, or both, that cause clinically significant impairment in functioning in two or more settings. The symptom criteria are polythetic—consisting of two lists of nine criteria (one representing the inattentive features and one representing the hyperactivity and impulsivity features) of which at least six criteria from either list are necessary for the diagnosis. Different diagnostic code numbers are provided for different subtypes (combined type, predominantly inattentive type, and predominantly hyperactive-impulsive type).

Conduct Disorder Conduct disorder, the childhood precursor of antisocial personality disorder, is characterized by a behavior pattern in which age-appropriate societal norms and rules are violated. The broad categories of the 15 diagnostic criteria are aggression toward people and animals, destruction of property, deceitfulness or theft, and serious violation of rules. Conduct disorder is the only disorder in DSM-IV-TR in which specific guidelines are provided for rating the disorder's severity, but the severity distinction is not captured by different diagnostic code numbers. The DSM-IV-TR text indicates that the context in which the features of conduct disorder are expressed should be considered when determining if the disorder is present. Thus, a child growing up in an impoverished, violent neighborhood who joins a gang and manifests features of conduct disorder for self-protection should not receive the diagnosis. On the other hand, the criteria themselves do not indicate that context should be considered.

Oppositional Defiant Disorder Oppositional defiant disorder is characterized by an ongoing pattern of negativistic, defiant, disobedient, and hostile behavior toward authority figures. Because many of the features of oppositional defiant disorder occur in nondisordered children (e.g., deliberate annoyance of others and refusal to comply with adults' requests), DSM-IV-TR includes a note in the diagnostic criteria that a criterion is met only when the behavior occurs more frequently than that of other children of the same age and developmental level. The features of oppositional defiant disorder are usually present in individuals with conduct disorder; thus, the diagnosis of oppositional defiant disorder is not also made when conduct disorder criteria are met.

Pica *Pica* refers to persistent eating of nonnutritive substances, such as dirt, paint, plaster, sand, and pebbles, that is inappropriate to developmental level and cultural practice. Pica can be diagnosed when it is secondary to another mental disorder (e.g., delusional beliefs of a chronic psychotic disorder), as long as the eating behavior is severe enough to be an independent focus of clinical attention.

Rumination Disorder The core feature of rumination disorder is the repeated regurgitation and rechewing of food after a period of normal food consumption. The diagnosis is excluded if a specific general medical condition, such as pyloric stenosis or esophageal reflux, accounts for the symptoms.

Feeding Disorder of Infancy or Early Childhood Feeding disorder of infancy or early childhood, sometimes referred to as *failure to thrive*, is characterized by weight loss or a failure to make expected weight gain in an infant or young child due to inadequate food intake. The diagnosis is excluded if a specific general medical condition accounts for the symptoms.

Tic Disorders The three specific tic disorders (Tourette's syndrome, chronic motor or vocal tic disorder, and transient tic disorder) are characterized by "sudden, rapid, recurrent, nonrhythmic, stereotyped motor movements or vocalization." The three disorders are distinguished in terms of chronicity (Tourette's syndrome and chronic tic disorder are of at least 12 months in duration; transient tic disorder is of at least 1 month in duration but less than 12 months in duration) and range of tics (Tourette's syndrome has motor and vocal tics, chronic tic disorder has motor or vocal tics, and transient tic disorder has motor or vocal tics, or both). For all three disorders, a diagnosis is only made if the symptoms cause marked distress or significant impairment in functioning.

Elimination Disorders The two specific elimination disorders (encopresis and enuresis) are characterized by repeated inappropriate passing of feces or urine, whether voluntary or involuntary. To diagnose encopresis, the child must be at least 4 years of age, and the inappropriate passage of feces must occur at least once a month for 3 months or more. For enuresis, the child must be at least 5 years of age before a diagnosis can be made, and the inappropriate voiding of urine must occur at least twice a week for 3 months or more. Subtypes are provided for each (encopresis—with or without constipation and overflow incontinence; enuresis—nocturnal only, diurnal only, and nocturnal and diurnal), although separate diagnostic codes for the subtypes are only provided for encopresis.

Separation Anxiety Disorder Separation anxiety disorder is characterized by excessive anxiety about separation from home or attachment figures beyond that expected for the child's developmental level. DSM-IV-TR notes that clinical judgment must be used to distinguish developmentally appropriate levels of separation anxiety from the excessive and impairing or distressing levels indicative of the disorder.

Selective Mutism Selective mutism is characterized by persistent refusal to speak in specific situations in which speaking is expected, despite the demonstration of speaking ability in other situations. Context is considered insofar as the diagnosis is not made if the failure to speak is attributed to lack of knowledge of the spoken language (e.g., second language of an immigrant).

Reactive Attachment Disorder of Infancy or Early Childhood Reactive attachment disorder of infancy or early childhood is characterized by one of two patterns of developmentally inappropriate social relatedness—excessively inhibited or disinhibited attachments—due to grossly pathological caregiving.

Stereotypic Movement Disorder The core feature of stereotypic movement disorder is "repetitive, seemingly driven, nonfunctional motor behavior," such as body rocking, hand waving, head banging, self-biting, and other self-mutilating behaviors. The presence of mental retardation does not exclude the diagnosis if the stereotypic behavior is sufficiently severe to be a focus of clinical attention.

II: Delirium, Dementia, and Amnestic and Other Cognitive Disorders

In a break from DSM-III-R, the disorders in this section previously were included in a section entitled "Organic Mental Syndromes and Disorders." The term *organic mental disorder* is not used in DSM-IV-TR, because it incorrectly implies that other disorders in other sections of the manual do not have an organic basis. The former DSM-III-R organic disorders section included the disorders in this section, the next section (Mental Disorders Due to a General Medical Condition Not Elsewhere Classified), and the Substance-Related Disorders section.

Delirium Delirium is characterized by a relatively rapid onset of problems in attention associated with memory impairment, disorientation, language impairment, hallucinations, or illusions. DSM-IV-TR presents separate discussions and criteria for delirium that is due to a general medical condition, substance intoxication, or substance withdrawal, although the core features of impaired attention and cognitive deficits are the same across disorders. Delirium superimposed on a preexisting vascular dementia is classified as dementia with delirium.

Dementia Dementia is characterized by memory impairment and one or more other cognitive impairments (aphasia, apraxia, agnosia, and executive functioning dysfunction). DSM-IV-TR distinguishes between five types (Alzheimer's disease, vascular, due to other general medical condition, substance-induced, and due to multiple etiologies). Alzheimer's dementia and dementia due to a general medical condition are subtyped according to the presence or absence of clinically significant behavioral disturbances (which is reflected in the fifth digit of the diagnostic code). Alzheimer's disease is also subtyped according to the patients' age of onset (which is not reflected in the diagnostic code). Vascular dementia is subtyped according to the predominant clinical characteristic (with delirium, delusions, depression, or none of the prior features) and this is reflected in the fifth digit coding.

Amnestic Disorder Amnestic disorder is characterized by clinically significant memory impairment, similar to dementia, but without the other cognitive impairments that define dementia. Two specific amnestic disorders are defined—amnestic disorder due to a general medical condition (which is subtyped as transient or chronic) and substance-induced persisting amnestic disorder.

III: Mental Disorders Due to a General Medical Condition Not Elsewhere Classified This section of mental disorders due to a general medical condition not elsewhere classified includes nine disorders due to a general medical condition (delirium, dementia, amnestic disorder, psychotic disorder, mood disorder, anxiety disorder, sexual dysfunction, sleep disorder, catatonic disorder, and personality change). Textual descriptions and diagnostic criteria are provided in this section only for catatonic disorder and personality change. The other seven disorders are described and defined in the phenomenologically relevant section to facilitate differential diagnosis, although these disorders are also listed in this section. For example, the diagnostic criteria for mood disorder due to a general medical condition are included in the mood disorders section to ensure that the clinician considers this potential cause of the presenting symptoms.

IV: Substance-Related Disorders The term *substance* in DSM-IV-TR includes what are commonly thought of as substances of abuse (alcohol, street drugs), as well as medications and toxins. Thirteen types of disorders are described (dependence, abuse, intoxication with or without delirium, withdrawal with or without delirium, dementia, amnestic disorder, psychosis, mood disorder, anxiety, sexual dysfunction, and sleep disorder). The section is organized according to the 11 specific classes of substances that may cause these disorders (alcohol, amphetamines, caffeine, cannabis, cocaine, hallucinogen, inhalant, nicotine, opioid, phencyclidine [PCP], and sedative-hypnotics). In addition, a group of *other* substances is included for substances such as anabolic steroids, nitrite inhalants, nitrous oxide, and over-the-counter and prescription drugs that are not covered by the 11 specific classes.

There is also a category for polysubstance dependence, which is diagnosed when dependence criteria are met during a 1-year period during which three or more groups of substances are used without a clear predominance of any one substance, and the dependence criteria are met for the substances as a group but not for any specific substance.

The substance-related disorders section begins with the provision of general criteria for diagnosing dependence, abuse, intoxication, and withdrawal, which can be applied to many of the substances, although substance specificity is manifest in the intoxication or withdrawal syndromes. The substance-induced disorders (psychosis, mood disorder, anxiety, sexual dysfunction, and sleep disorder) are listed with their corresponding diagnostic code numbers in this section but are described in detail in the DSM-IV-TR sections with which they share clinically similar features.

The initial section describing the general diagnostic criteria for substance dependence, abuse, intoxication, and withdrawal is followed by a discussion of the disorders associated with each of the specific substances. The section is organized by substance. Thus, all of the disorders associated with alcohol use are grouped together, followed by the disorders associated with amphetamine use, then caffeine, etc. The disorder-specific discussions of abuse and dependence refer back to the general abuse and dependence diagnostic criteria. In contrast, disorder-specific criteria for withdrawal and intoxication are presented separately for each substance.

Substance Dependence Disorders Each of the specific substances, except caffeine, can manifest a dependence syndrome. The seven criteria for substance dependence (three of which are needed to make the diagnosis) cover three major constructs: withdrawal, tolerance, and loss of control over use. Neither tolerance nor withdrawal, sometimes considered the hallmark of dependence, is necessary or sufficient to meet the diagnostic criteria for substance dependence. However, based on the presence or absence of withdrawal or tolerance, substance dependence is subtyped as with or without physiological dependence. Substance dependence is one of the few disorders in DSM-IV-TR for which remission is explicitly defined. *Complete remission* requires the absence of all criteria for at least 1 month, whereas *partial remission* refers to the presence of one or two criteria. Unique to the substance dependence disorders, the duration of the period of remission is also specified. When the period of remission is less than 12 months, then it is specified as *early remission*. This is in contrast to *sustained remission* that has persisted for at least 12 months.

Substance Abuse Disorders In contrast to DSM-III and DSM-III-R, DSM-IV-TR provides nonoverlapping criteria sets for substance dependence and abuse. Substance abuse can be diagnosed for each of the specific substances, except caffeine and nicotine. Substance abuse is characterized by a maladaptive pattern of use that results in recurrent psychosocial problems. Substance abuse is not diagnosed if the criteria for dependence have ever been met. The remission specifiers for substance dependence are not also applied to substance abuse.

Substance-Induced Disorders The symptoms of many Axis I disorders can be produced by substance use; consequently, the differential diagnosis of many psychiatric disorders includes ruling out that it is substance induced. The criteria for diagnosing substance-induced disorders are therefore placed in the phenomenologically relevant section to facilitate differential diagnosis, although these disorders are also listed in the substance-related disorders section. For example, the diagnostic criteria for substance-induced mood disorder are included in the mood disorders section to ensure that the clinician considers this potential cause of the presenting symptoms.

V: Schizophrenia and Other Psychotic Disorders The section on schizophrenia and other psychotic disorders includes eight specific disorders (schizophrenia, schizophreniform disorder, schizoaffective disorder, delusional disorder, brief psychotic disorder, shared psychotic disorder, psychotic disorder due to a general medical condition, and substance-induced psychotic disorder) in which psychotic symptoms are a prominent feature of the clinical picture. The DSM-IV-TR text notes that other disorders may also be characterized at times by psychotic features (e.g., major depressive disorder or bipolar mania with psychotic features). The grouping of disorders in this section was made to facilitate differential diagnosis and not to imply etiological links amongst the disorders in this section.

Schizophrenia Schizophrenia is generally a chronic disorder in which prominent hallucinations or delusions are usually present. The individual must be ill for at least 6 months, although he or she need not be actively psychotic during all of that time. Three phases of the disorder are defined. The *prodrome phase* refers to deterioration in function before the onset of the active psychotic phase. The active phase symptoms (delusions, hallucinations, disorganized speech, grossly disorganized behavior, or negative symptoms, such as flat affect, avolition, and alogia) must be present for at least 1 month. The residual phase follows the active phase. The features of the residual and prodromal phases include functional impairment and abnormalities of affect, cognition, and communication. If a manic or depressive syndrome occurs, its duration must be brief relative to the duration of the active phase of schizophrenia. Schizophrenia is not diagnosed if the symptoms are due to the effects of substances or a general medical condition. Schizophrenia is subtyped according to the most prominent symptoms present at the time of the evaluation (paranoid, disorganized, catatonic, undifferentiated, and residual types). The subtypes have different diagnostic code numbers. The course of the disorder can also be specified (e.g., continuous versus episodic with or without interepisode residual symptoms), although these are not reflected in diagnostic coding.

Schizophreniform Disorder Schizophreniform disorder is characterized by the same active phase symptoms of schizophrenia (delusions, hallucinations, disorganized speech, grossly disorganized behavior, or negative symptoms) but lasts between 1 and 6 months, and the prodromal or residual phase features of social or occupational impairment are absent. Similar to schizophrenia, schizophreniform disorder is ruled out if a mood episode, if present, is not brief relative to the duration of the psychotic symptoms. DSM-IV-TR does not indicate how short the mood syndrome must be to be considered *brief*, and, given that schizophreniform disorder must be less than 6 months duration, there is uncertainty in how often this exclusion criterion is relevant. Schizophreniform disorder is also excluded if the symptoms are due to the effects of substances or a general medical condition. The predicted course of the disorder can be specified (with or without good prognostic features), although this is not reflected in diagnostic coding.

Schizoaffective Disorder Schizoaffective disorder is also characterized by the same active phase symptoms of schizophrenia (delusions, hallucinations, disorganized speech, grossly disorganized behavior, or negative symptoms), as well as the presence of a manic or depressive syndrome that is *not* brief relative to the duration of the psychosis. Individuals with schizoaffective disorder, in contrast to a mood disorder with psychotic features, have delusions or hallucinations for at least 2 weeks without coexisting prominent mood symptoms. As with the other nonfunctional psychotic disorders, the symptoms are not attributable to substance use or a general medical condition. Schizoaffective disorder is subtyped as bipolar or depressive type, although this is not reflected in diagnostic coding.

Delusional Disorder Delusional disorder is characterized by nonbizarre delusions (i.e., delusions about situations that could occur in real life, such as infidelity, being followed, or having an illness). The presence of bizarre delusions or the other active phase psychotic symptoms of schizophrenia excludes the diagnosis of delusional disorder. Functional impairment is directly linked to the delusional system, and the broad-based functional decline often associated with schizophrenia is usually absent. If a manic or depressive syndrome occurs, its duration must be brief relative to the duration of the delusions. Delusional disorder is not diagnosed if the symptoms are due to the effects of substance use or a general medical condition. Delusional disorder is subtyped according to the content of the delusion, although this is not reflected in diagnostic coding.

Brief Psychotic Disorder Brief psychotic disorder requires the presence of delusions, hallucinations, disorganized speech, grossly disorganized behavior, or catatonic behavior for at least 1 day but less than 1 month. The individual returns to his or her usual level of functioning. The psychotic symptoms cannot be due to substance use or a general medical condition. Brief psychotic disorder is subtyped based on the presence or absence of markedly stressful life events or recent childbirth, although this is not reflected in diagnostic coding.

Shared Psychotic Disorder Shared psychotic disorder, also called *folie à deux*, is characterized by a delusional belief that develops in an individual involved in a close relationship with someone who has an established delusion. The content of the delusion is similar to the content in the person with the established delusion.

Psychotic Disorder Due to a General Medical Condition Psychotic disorder due to a general medical condition is diagnosed when there is evidence that hallucinations or delusions are the direct consequence of a general medical condition other than delirium or dementia. The disorder is subtyped according to whether delusions or hallucinations predominate the symptom picture, and the subtypes are coded differently.

Substance-Induced Psychotic Disorder Substance-induced psychotic disorder is analogous to psychotic disorder due to a general medical condition, except the cause of the hallucinations or delusions is substance intoxication, substance withdrawal, or a medication. The disorder is subtyped according to the predominant symptom picture and the specific substance responsible for the symptoms. The subtypes are reflected in diagnostic coding.

VI: Mood Disorders

The section on mood disorders begins with the specification of the diagnostic criteria for mood episodes (major depressive episode, manic episode, hypomanic episode, and mixed episode). The mood episode criteria are the basis for diagnosing the mood disorders; by themselves, the mood episodes are not able to be coded. The next part of the section describes the seven specific mood disorders (major depressive disorder, bipolar I disorder, bipolar II disorder, dysthymic disorder, cyclothymic disorder, mood disorder due to a general medical condition, and substance-induced mood disorder). The final part of the mood disorders section describes the many methods of subtyping, some of which are reflected in the diagnostic code.

Major Depressive Disorder The necessary feature of major depressive disorder is depressed mood or loss of interest or pleasure in usual activities. The diagnosis of major depressive disorder requires the presence of at least five of nine symptom criteria for at least 2 weeks, one of which is depressed mood or loss of interest. All symptoms must be present nearly every day, except suicidal ideation or thoughts of death, which need only be recurrent. To count toward the diagnosis, the symptom must be a change from the person's usual baseline (e.g., chronic sleep difficulty of several years duration that did not change with the onset of depressive symptoms 2 months ago does not count). To make the diagnosis, the symptoms must cause clinically significant distress or impairment and must not be due to substance use or a general medical condition. The diagnosis is excluded if the symptoms are the result of a normal bereavement and if there are psychotic symptoms in the absence of mood symptoms. The fourth digit of the five-digit diagnostic code indicates whether the individual experienced a previous episode of major depression (i.e., single episode versus recurrent episodes). The fifth digit indicates current severity, the presence of psychotic features, and, if full criteria are not met at the time of the evaluation, whether the episode is in partial or full remission. Other methods of subtyping major depression, which are not reflected in the diagnostic code, are chronicity (chronic subtype indicates an episode duration of at least 2 years); presence of catatonic, melancholic, and atypical features; association with recent childbirth (with postpartum onset, if the episode began within 4 weeks of delivery); completeness of the recovery between episodes for individuals with two or more episodes (with or without full interepisode recovery); and whether there is a seasonal pattern to the onset of recurrent episodes.

Dysthymic Disorder Dysthymic disorder is a mild, chronic form of depression that lasts at least 2 years, during which, on the majority of days, the individual experiences depressed mood for most of the day and at least two other symptoms of depression. During the 2-year period, the symptoms never get severe enough to meet criteria for a major depressive episode, although many individuals with dysthymic disorder have superimposed major depressive disorder (called *double depression*). The disorder is excluded if there is a history of mania, hypomania, or cyclothymia. The disorder is subtyped according to age of onset (early onset before 21 years of age, late onset after 21 years of age) and the presence of atypical features, although neither method of subtyping is reflected by diagnostic coding.

Bipolar I Disorder The necessary feature of bipolar I disorder is a history of a manic or mixed manic and depressive episode. Mania requires euphoric or irritable mood for at least 1 week (or any duration, if the individual is hospitalized) and at least three (if mood is euphoric) or four (if mood is irritable) of seven symptom criteria. In contrast to major depression, there is no indication that the symptoms must be present nearly every day. The diagnosis is excluded if the symptoms are the result of a general medical condition, substance use, antidepressant medication, or if there are psychotic symptoms in the absence of mood symptoms. The impairment-distress criterion for mania is different than the impairment-distress criterion for most other disorders. For most disorders, such as major depressive disorder, this criterion is worded "clinically significant distress or impairment." For a manic episode, there is no reference to distress, and the impairment must be "marked." DSM-IV-TR does not specify how "marked" differs from "clinically significant." The distress-impairment criterion for a manic episode is also met if the symptoms necessitate hospitalization or if psychotic symptoms are present. The inclusion of these other components of the impairment criterion suggests that marked impairment is more severe than clinically significant impairment. Bipolar I disorder is subtyped in many ways: type of current episode (manic, hypomanic depressed, or mixed), severity and remission status (mild, moderate, severe without psychosis, severe with psychotic features, partial remission, or full remission), the same symptom and course subtypes as major depression when the current episode is depression, and whether the recent course is characterized by rapid cycling (at least four episodes in 12 months).

Bipolar II Disorder Bipolar II disorder is characterized by a history of hypomanic and major depressive episodes. The symptom criteria for a hypomanic episode are the same as that for a manic episode, although hypomania only requires a minimum duration of 4 days. The major difference between mania and hypomania is the severity of the impairment associated with the syndrome. Hypomania is the only DSM-IV-TR disorder that is excluded if the level of impairment is too severe. The DSM-IV-TR criteria refer to observable changes in functioning but do not specify a minimum level of impairment for the diagnosis. The subtyping of bipolar II disorder is the same as bipolar I disorder, although none of the subtyping methods is reflected in diagnostic coding.

Cyclothymic Disorder The bipolar equivalent to dysthymic disorder, cyclothymic disorder, is a mild, chronic mood disorder with numerous depressive and hypomanic episodes over the course of at least 2 years. The depressive periods never meet criteria for a major depressive episode, and the hypomanic periods never meet criteria for mania, although they may meet criteria for hypomania.

Mood Disorder Due to a General Medical Condition Mood disorder due to a general medical condition is diagnosed when there is evidence that a significant mood disturbance is the direct consequence of a general medical condition other than delirium. The disorder is subtyped according to the presence of depressive symptoms not meeting criteria for a major depressive episode, depressive symptoms meeting full major depression criteria, manic features, or mixed features.

Substance-Induced Mood Disorder Substance-induced mood disorder is diagnosed when the cause of the mood disturbance is substance intoxication, withdrawal, or a medication. The disorder is subtyped according to the specific substance responsible for the symptoms, which is reflected in diagnostic coding, and the type of mood symptoms, which is not reflected in the coding.

VII: Anxiety Disorders

The section on anxiety disorders includes ten specific disorders (panic disorder, agoraphobia, specific phobia, social phobia, OCD, posttraumatic stress disorder [PTSD], acute stress disorder, generalized anxiety disorder, anxiety disorder due to a general medical condition, and substance-induced anxiety disorder) in which anxious symptoms are a prominent feature of the clinical picture. The grouping of disorders in this section was made to facilitate differential diagnosis and not to imply etiological links amongst the disorders in this section. Because separation anxiety disorder occurs in childhood, it is included in the childhood disorders section.

Panic Disorder A panic attack is characterized by feelings of intense fear or terror that come on out of the blue in situations in which there is nothing to fear and that are accompanied by at least four of a list of 13 features, the most common being heart racing or pounding, chest pain, shortness of breath or choking, dizziness, trembling or shaking, feeling faint or lightheaded, sweating, and nausea. Panic disorder is diagnosed in an individual who has experienced at least two attacks associated with 1 month or more of ongoing concern about having another panic attack, worrying about the implications of the attack, or a change in behavior because of the attacks. Panic disorder is subtyped according to the presence or absence of agoraphobia, and this is reflected in the fifth digit of the diagnostic code.

Agoraphobia Agoraphobia is a frequent consequence of panic disorder, although it can occur in the absence of panic attacks. Individuals with agoraphobia avoid (or try to avoid) situations that they think might trigger a panic attack (or panic-like symptoms) or situations from which they think escape might be difficult if they have a panic attack. Similar to the precedent of diagnosing the cooccurrence of vascular dementia and delirium as a single disorder, when panic disorder and agoraphobia are present, only a single diagnosis is made (panic disorder with agoraphobia).

Specific Phobia Specific phobia is characterized by an excessive, unreasonable fear of specific objects or situations that occurs almost always on exposure to the feared stimulus. Insight that the fear is excessive or unreasonable is required to make the diagnosis. The phobic stimulus is avoided, or, when not avoided, the individual feels severely anxious or uncomfortable. The anxiety response or avoidance causes clinically significant functional impairment or distress. The subtypes of specific phobia, based on the type of phobic stimulus (animal, environment, blood-injection-injury, or situation), are not captured by different diagnostic code numbers.

Social Phobia Social phobia is characterized by the fear of being embarrassed or humiliated in front of others. Similar to specific phobia, insight that the fear is excessive or unreasonable is required to make the diagnosis, and the phobic stimuli are avoided, or, when not avoided, the individual feels severely anxious or uncomfortable. The anxiety response or avoidance causes clinically significant functional impairment or distress. When the phobic stimuli include most social situations, then it is specified as generalized social phobia.

Obsessive-Compulsive Disorder OCD is characterized by repetitive and intrusive thoughts or images that are unwelcome (obsessions) or repetitive behaviors that the person feels compelled to do (compulsions), or both. Most often, the compulsions are done to reduce the anxiety associated with the obsessive thought. Similar to the diagnosis of specific and social phobia, at some time during the course of the disorder, the individual must exhibit some insight that the obsessions or compulsions are excessive or unreasonable. If, for most of the course of the disorder the individual does not recognize that the obsessions or compulsions are excessive, then the specifier *with poor insight* is added. The impairment-distress criterion for OCD is somewhat different than this criterion for other disorders, because it can also be met in the absence of evidence of clinically significant impairment or distress if the obsessions or compulsions are time-consuming (present for more than 1 hour per day).

Posttraumatic Stress Disorder PTSD occurs after the occurrence of traumatic events in which the individual believes that he or she is in physical danger or that his or her life is in jeopardy. PTSD can also occur after witnessing a violent or life-threatening event happening to someone else. The symptoms of PTSD usually occur soon after the occurrence of the traumatic event, although, in some cases, the symptoms develop months or even years after the trauma. The symptoms of PTSD are grouped into four categories: reaction to the event, reexperiencing symptoms, symptoms of avoidance, and symptoms of increased arousal. PTSD is diagnosed when a person reacts to the traumatic event with fear and experiences at least one reexperiencing symptom, three or more symptoms of avoidance, and two or more symptoms of hyperarousal. The symptoms must persist for at least 1 month and cause clinically significant impairment in functioning or distress. The course of the disorder (i.e., acute if less than 3 months, chronic if greater than 3 months) and timing of symptom onset in relation to the occurrence of the symptoms (i.e., with delayed onset if symptoms onset at least 6 months after the trauma) are specified, although this is not reflected in diagnostic coding.

Acute Stress Disorder Acute stress disorder occurs after the same type of stressors that precipitate PTSD, although some of the symptom inclusion criteria are different than the ones used to diagnose PTSD. Acute stress disorder is not diagnosed if the symptoms last beyond 1 month. Acute stress disorder is thus the third disorder in DSM-IV-TR that is ruled out if the symptoms persist beyond a certain amount of time (schizophreniform disorder and brief psychotic disorder are the other two). The impairment-distress criterion for acute stress disorder is somewhat different than the usual criterion, because it can be met in the absence of evidence of clinically significant impairment or distress if the symptoms "impair the individual's ability to pursue some necessary task."

Generalized Anxiety Disorder Generalized anxiety disorder is characterized by chronic excessive worry that occurs more days than not and is difficult to control. The worry is associated with symptoms, such as concentration problems, insomnia, muscle tension, irritability, and physical restlessness, and causes clinically significant distress or impairment. Generalized anxiety disorder is the only anxiety disorder that is not diagnosed if the symptoms only occur during the course of depression.

Anxiety Disorder Due to a General Medical Condition Anxiety disorder due to a general medical condition is diagnosed when there is evidence that significant anxiety is the direct consequence of a general medical condition other than delirium or dementia. The disorder is subtyped according to the presence of generalized anxiety, panic attacks, or obsessive-compulsive features, although this is not reflected in diagnostic coding.

Substance-Induced Anxiety Disorder Substance-induced anxiety disorder is diagnosed when the cause of the anxiety is substance intoxication, substance withdrawal, or a medication. The disorder is subtyped according to the specific substance responsible for the symptoms, which is reflected in diagnostic coding, and the type of anxiety symptoms, which is not reflected in the coding.

VIII: Somatoform Disorders The section on somatoform disorders includes six specific disorders (somatization disorder, undifferentiated somatoform disorder, conversion disorder, pain disorder, hypochondriasis, and body dysmorphic disorder) in which physical symptoms suggestive of a general medical condition, but not accounted for by such a condition, are a prominent feature of the clinical picture. The grouping of disorders in this section was made to facilitate differential diagnosis (i.e., the need to rule out general medical disorders) and not to imply etiological links amongst the disorders in this section.

Somatization Disorder Somatization disorder is characterized by multiple unexplained medical symptoms in diverse organ systems occurring over several years that are not explained by general medical conditions. The symptoms are grouped into four categories: pain, gastrointestinal (GI), sexual, and pseudoneurological. Symptoms from each group must be present, resulting in functional impairment or treatment, beginning before 30 years of age.

Undifferentiated Somatoform Disorder Undifferentiated somatoform disorder is a residual category for conditions characterized by unexplained medical symptoms that are not as pervasive and long-lasting as those of somatization disorder. The diagnosis is precluded by another somatoform disorder.

Conversion Disorder Conversion disorder is characterized by unexplained voluntary motor or sensory deficits that suggest the presence of a neurological or other general medical condition. Psychological conflict is determined to be responsible for the symptoms. The symptoms cause clinically significant impairment or distress or medical evaluation. The disorder is subtyped according to the type of symptom (motor, sensory, seizure, or mixed), although this is not reflected in diagnostic coding.

Pain Disorder The core feature of pain disorder is impairing or distressing pain that is the primary focus of attention. Psychological factors are determined to have an important role in the onset, severity, or maintenance of the pain. Fifth-digit coding reflects the presence or absence of a general medical condition. In addition, the course of the disorder (i.e., acute if less than 6 months, chronic if greater than 6 months) is specified, although this is not reflected in diagnostic coding.

Hypochondriasis Hypochondriasis is a distressing and impairing preoccupation with the belief of having a serious illness based on a misinterpretation of physical symptoms. After a thorough medical evaluation rules out the medical illness, the preoccupation remains. Although not a diagnostic criterion, at some time during the course of the disorder, the individual must exhibit some insight that the preoccupation is excessive or unreasonable. If there is no insight, and the belief reaches delusional intensity, then the diagnosis would be delusional disorder, somatic type rather than hypochondriasis. If, for most of the course of the disorder, the individual does not recognize that the preoccupation is excessive, then the specifier *with poor insight* is added.

Body Dysmorphic Disorder Body dysmorphic disorder is a distressing and impairing preoccupation with an imagined or slight defect in appearance. If the belief is held with delusional intensity, then delusional disorder, somatic type, might also be diagnosed. This contrasts with the decision rule for hypochondriasis that cannot be codiagnosed with delusional disorder.

IX: Factitious Disorder

Factitious disorder refers to the deliberate feigning of physical or psychological symptoms to assume the sick role. Factitious disorder is distinguished from malingering in which symptoms are also falsely reported; however, the motivation in malingering is external incentives, such as avoidance of responsibility, obtaining financial compensation, or obtaining substances. Factitious disorder is subtyped according to whether the predominant symptoms are psychological, physical, or a mixture of the two.

X: Dissociative Disorders

The section on dissociative disorders includes four specific disorders (dissociative amnesia, dissociative fugue, dissociative identity disorder, and depersonalization disorder) characterized by a "disruption in the usually integrated functions of consciousness, memory, identity, or perception." There is a hierarchical diagnostic relationship among the disorders, such that dissociative amnesia is not diagnosed when dissociative fugue or dissociative identity disorder is present, dissociative fugue is not diagnosed when the criteria for dissociative identity disorder are met, and depersonalization disorder is excluded when any of the other three dissociative disorders are present. Dissociative features, such as depersonalization, are sometimes present in other disorders and are part of the DSM-IV-TR diagnostic criteria sets for panic attacks, PTSD, acute stress disorder, and somatization disorder. DSM-IV-TR notes some controversy in the classification of conversion disorder, because it is considered to be a dissociative phenomenon in some classification schemes but is placed in the somatoform disorders section in DSM-IV-TR "to emphasize the importance of considering neurological or other general medical conditions in the differential diagnosis." This illustrates how different principles of classification might influence the organization of the classification system.

Dissociative Amnesia Dissociative amnesia is characterized by memory loss of important personal information that is usually traumatic in nature. The inability to remember is not due to normal forgetfulness, substance use, or a general medical condition; does not occur only during the course of another dissociative disorder, PTSD, or somatization disorder; and causes clinically significant impairment or distress.

Dissociative Fugue Dissociative fugue is characterized by sudden travel away from home associated with partial or complete memory loss about one's identity. At times, there is confusion about personal identity, and, at times, a new identity is assumed. The dissociation is not due to substance use or a general medical condition and causes clinically significant impairment or distress.

Dissociative Identity Disorder (Formerly, Multiple Personality Disorder) The essential feature of dissociative identity disorder is the presence of two or more distinct identities that assume control of the individual's behavior.

Depersonalization Disorder The essential feature of depersonalization disorder is persistent or recurrent episodes of depersonalization (an altered sense of one's physical being, including feeling that one is outside of one's body, physically cut off or distanced from people, floating, observing oneself from a distance, like one is in a dream, or that one's body is physically changed in shape or size). The depersonalization is not due to another psychiatric disorder, substance use, or a general medical condition, and it causes clinically significant impairment or distress.

XI: Sexual and Gender Identity Disorders

The section on sexual and gender identity disorders includes three groups of disorders—sexual dysfunctions, paraphilias, and gender identity disorder.

Sexual Dysfunctions The group of sexual dysfunction disorders is organized on the basis of the phase of sexual response that is affected. Sexual pain disorders are also included in this category. The sexual dysfunction disorders are diagnosed only when they cause marked distress or interpersonal difficulty. The two sexual desire disorders are hypoactive sexual desire disorder (lack of desire for sexual activity) and sexual aversion disorder (active avoidance of sexual contact). The two sexual arousal disorders are female sexual arousal disorder (inability to attain or maintain adequate lubrication until completion of sexual activity) and male erectile disorder (inability to attain or maintain adequate erection until completion of sexual activity). The three orgasmic disorders are female orgasmic disorder, male orgasmic disorder, and premature ejaculation. The two sexual pain disorders are dyspareunia (pain during sexual intercourse) and vaginismus (vaginal spasm interfering with sexual intercourse). Sexual dysfunction due to a general medical condition and substance-induced sexual dysfunction are also included, the subtypes of which are linked to the other sexual dysfunctions, so that these causes of sexual dysfunction are ruled out as part of the evaluation.

Paraphilias The characteristic features of paraphilias are recurrent, sexually arousing fantasies, urges, or behaviors lasting at least 6 months and involving nonhuman objects, suffering or humiliation of oneself or one's partner, or children or other nonconsenting partners. DSM-IV-TR includes eight specific paraphilias: exhibitionism (exposure of genitals to strangers), fetishism (use of nonliving objects), frotteurism (touching and rubbing against a nonconsenting person), pedophilia (attraction to children), sexual masochism (suffering pain or humiliation), sexual sadism (causing pain or humiliation to someone else), transvestic fetishism (cross-dressing), and voyeurism (observing unsuspecting individuals).

Gender Identity Disorder The characteristic feature of gender identity disorder is a persistent discomfort with one's own gender and strong cross-gender identification. Gender identity disorder is subtyped according to the individual's current age, and the subtypes are distinguished by different diagnostic codes.

XII: Eating Disorders

The section on eating disorders includes two specific disorders—anorexia nervosa and bulimia nervosa—that are characterized by abnormal eating behavior. Other disorders of eating that usually are diagnosed in infancy and childhood (i.e., pica, rumination disorder, and feeding disorder of infancy or early childhood) are included in the Disorders Usually First Diagnosed in Infancy, Childhood, or Adolescence section.

Anorexia Nervosa The core feature of anorexia nervosa is a strong fear of gaining weight or becoming fat, resulting in deliberate maintenance of low body weight. Individuals are preoccupied with their weight and body image, and their weight and perceived body shape markedly influence their self-image. An additional diagnostic criterion is required for postmenarcheal women—amenorrhea for at least three consecutive menstrual cycles. Anorexia is subtyped based on whether the individual engages in binge-eating or purging behavior (binge-eating or purging type) or maintains low weight through restricting food intake or excessive exercise (restricting type). The subtypes are not distinguished by separate diagnostic codes.

Bulimia Nervosa Individuals with bulimia nervosa engage in recurrent binge eating during which they eat an abnormally large amount of food over a short period of time. During the binge, the person feels like he or she cannot control his or her eating. To prevent weight gain from the overeating, the individual engages in compensatory behavior, such as self-induced vomiting, excessive exercise, laxative use, or going on strict diets.

XIII: Sleep Disorders

The sleep disorders are divided into four groups based on the presumed cause—primary, due to another mental disorder, due to a general medical condition, or due to substances. The sleep disorders are diagnosed only when they cause marked distress or interpersonal difficulty. The primary sleep disorders are subdivided into five dyssomnias (primary insomnia, primary hypersomnia, narcolepsy, breathing-related sleep disorder, and circadian rhythm sleep disorder) and three parasomnias (nightmare disorder, sleep terror disorder, and sleepwalking disorder).

XIV: Impulse-Control Disorders Not Elsewhere Classified

Five specific disorders of impulse control are included in this section on impulse-control disorders not elsewhere classified—intermittent explosive disorder, kleptomania, pyromania, pathological gambling, and trichotillomania. These disorders are characterized by the failure to resist urges to engage in behaviors that are harmful to the individual or others. The diagnostic criteria for three disorders, kleptomania, pyromania, and trichotillomania, are similar. The first criterion refers to repeated performance of the harmful behavior. The second criterion refers to a growing feeling of tension before performing the behavior, and the third criterion refers to tension relief or gratification after performing the behavior. For all five disorders in this section, if the behavior is attributable to another psychiatric disorder, then the impulse control disorder is not diagnosed.

Intermittent Explosive Disorder This disorder is characterized by recurrent, discrete, episodes of assaultive and violent behavior that is out of proportion to possible precipitating factors. If the behavior can be accounted for by another psychiatric disorder, such as antisocial or borderline personality disorder, bipolar disorder, or a substance use disorder, then a separate diagnosis of intermittent explosive disorder is not also made. Thus, intermittent explosive disorder is diagnosed only after other psychiatric causes of the aggressive behavior are ruled out.

Kleptomania Kleptomania is characterized by repeated stealing of items that are not needed for personal use or for their monetary value. The stealing is not done for the purpose of expressing anger or revenge. Before committing the theft, the individual experiences an increasing sense of tension that dissipates after the behavior. If the behavior is better accounted for by conduct disorder, antisocial personality disorder, or a manic episode, then a separate diagnosis of kleptomania is not also made.

Pyromania Pyromania is characterized by recurrent setting of fires because of a preoccupation or fascination with fire rather than being done for other purposes such as financial gain, political expression, revenge, or hiding of criminal behavior. Before setting the fire, the individual experiences an increasing sense of tension that dissipates after the behavior. If the behavior is better accounted for by conduct disorder, antisocial personality disorder, or a manic episode, then a separate diagnosis of pyromania is not also made.

Pathological Gambling Pathological gambling is characterized by a maladaptive pattern of gambling behavior. Although classified as an impulse control disorder, many experts draw parallels between pathological gambling and addictive disorders (i.e., substance use disorders). Of the ten criteria for pathological gambling, one refers to tolerance, one refers to an inability to control gambling behavior, and one refers to withdrawal symptoms when cutting down on or stopping gambling. The remaining criteria are a heterogeneous group of features, including psychosocial consequences of problem gambling, preoccupation with gambling, and problematic gambling behaviors (chasing after losses, gambling to escape problems, or negative emotional states).

Trichotillomania Trichotillomania is characterized by repeated hair pulling causing noticeable hair loss. The anticipatory tension criterion for trichotillomania is broader than the analogous criterion for kleptomania and pyromania. For trichotillomania, the criterion refers to an increasing sense of tension before pulling or attempts to resist pulling. Trichotillomania is the only impulse control disorder that includes an impairment-distress criterion.

XV: Adjustment Disorders

Many psychiatric disorders are precipitated or exacerbated by stressful life events. The adjustment disorder section is a residual diagnostic category that is used when the psychiatric symptoms that follow a psychosocial stressor do not meet the criteria for a specific disorder. For example, the development of depressive symptoms after a stressful event is diagnosed as a major depressive episode if the criteria for this disorder are met (i.e., at least five features of major depression for at least 2 weeks). Adjustment disorder with depressed mood, rather than depressive disorder not otherwise specified (NOS), is diagnosed only if the major depression criteria are not met. Thus, the diagnosis of a specific disorder supersedes the diagnosis of adjustment disorder, and the diagnosis of adjustment disorder supersedes the diagnosis of a not-otherwise-specified condition. Adjustment disorders are diagnosed when the person's distress in response to the event is in excess of a normative reaction to the stressor or when the symptoms cause significant impairment in functioning. Adjustment disorder is not diagnosed if the symptoms represent a bereavement reaction, although the conceptual justification for the distinction between this stressful event and other events that frequently result in psychiatric symptoms is not provided. The adjustment disorders are subtyped according to the predominant symptom picture (depressed mood, anxiety, mixed anxiety and depression, disturbance of conduct, mixed disturbance of emotions and conduct, unspecified), and this is reflected in their diagnostic code.

XVI: Personality Disorders *Personality* refers to an individual's characteristic pattern of affect, emotional regulation, behavior, motivation, cognition about self, and interactions with others that are long-standing, present since adolescence or early adulthood. Aspects of personality include the way people tend to think about themselves (e.g., self-confident or lacking confidence), how they relate to people (e.g., shy vs. friendly), how they interpret and deal with events in the environment (e.g., paranoid people believe that others are out to get them and may try to attack first before being attacked), and how an individual reacts emotionally to this situation. It is not easy to define a *healthy personality*, but, in general, it allows one to cope with the normal stress of life and to develop and to maintain satisfying friendships and intimate relationships. When long-standing patterns of thinking, behaving, and emotional response are rigid, inflexible, and cause significant distress or impairment in functioning, then a DSM-IV-TR personality disorder may be present. DSM-IV-TR includes ten specific personality disorders that are coded on Axis II.

Paranoid Personality Disorder Individuals with paranoid personality disorder are suspicious and distrustful of others. They may think that others do things just to annoy or to hurt them, and they often read hidden threats or put-downs in the comments of others. They may worry that friends or coworkers are not really loyal or trustworthy and are often reluctant to confide in others, because they believe that there is a price to pay when something personal is shared. Persons with paranoid personality disorder may have problems with anger management. They are easily slighted and hold grudges. They often find that people say things to attack their character or ruin their reputation, even though it does not seem that way to others. Individuals with paranoid personality disorder often read too much into things, take offense at things that were not meant to be critical, and often try to get back at the person they believe is attacking them. When involved in a relationship, they often worry that their partner is unfaithful.

Schizoid Personality Disorder Schizoid personality disorder is characterized by lack of emotionality and social relationships. Individuals with schizoid personality disorder are socially isolated, but this does not bother them. They usually prefer to work and do things alone. They are emotionally cold and are neither bothered by criticism from others nor joyful when complimented. Individuals with schizoid personality disorder usually do not get pleasure from many activities and often have little interest in sexual experiences with another person.

Schizotypal Personality Disorder Individuals with schizotypal personality disorder are odd and eccentric. They may dress, act, or speak in a peculiar manner. They are often suspicious and paranoid and feel anxious in social situations because of their distrust. Because of these beliefs, they have few friends. People with schizotypal personality disorder frequently feel that others are talking about them behind their back and that strangers are taking special notice of them. When walking into a room, they sometimes think that people start talking or acting differently because they are there. Individuals with schizotypal personality disorder sometimes misinterpret reality. They may mistake noises for voices and shadows or objects for people. They may believe in extrasensory perception (ESP), hexes, telepathy, and superstitions more strongly than most people, and their behavior may be influenced by these beliefs.

Antisocial Personality Disorder Antisocial personality disorder, the adult manifestation of childhood conduct disorder, is characterized by selfish, irresponsible, unlawful, and impulsive behavior that shows a lack of regard for the rights of others. Individuals with antisocial personality disorder often find it easy to lie if it serves their purpose. Physical aggression is common. Trouble at work may be the result of not arriving on time, missing too many days, not doing the work, or not following the rules. There is a general failure to conform to society's rules by engaging in illegal activities or not honoring obligations. Examples of antisocial behavior include quitting a job without other work in sight or spending money on things that one could do without, thus being unable to pay for household necessities, such as food, rent, or the utility bill. Reckless driving, speeding tickets, driving under the influence of drugs or alcohol, and ignoring recommended safety precautions are examples of a lack of regard for the safety of oneself or others. Individuals with antisocial personality disorder usually do not feel remorseful at having hurt others but instead justify or rationalize their behavior.

Borderline Personality Disorder Borderline personality disorder is characterized by emotional dysregulation, unstable interpersonal relationships, and unstable self-image. Individuals with borderline personality disorder have strong and intense emotions, often in reaction to how they perceive and believe others are treating them, and these emotions are difficult to control. Not surprisingly, individuals who have strong emotional reactions that are difficult to control often have problems in interpersonal relationships and self-image. Interpersonal relationships are affected by strong fears of being abandoned and going to extremes to keep others from leaving. At an extreme, suicide is threatened to keep someone from leaving. Relationships tend to be stormy, with many ups and downs, as the person alternates between having strong positive and negative feelings. The moods of the individual with borderline personality disorder are strong and frequently change. There are often problems with controlling anger, and anger outbursts are common. Individuals with borderline personality disorder frequently do not have a stable sense of their identity and feel empty inside much of the time. Self-destructive behavior is common. Individuals with borderline personality disorder make recurrent suicide attempts, suicide threats, or engage in self-damaging behavior, such as cutting or burning. They may also do impulsive things that can cause problems, such as gambling, spending excessive money, sexual promiscuity, excess drug and alcohol use, stealing, eating binges, or reckless driving.

Histrionic Personality Disorder In contrast to some personality disorders that are characterized by social anxiety, inhibition, and withdrawal, individuals with histrionic personality disorder are loud, overly emotionally expressive, and attention seeking. They act as if they are on stage. Individuals with histrionic personality disorder tend not to feel comfortable unless they are the center of attention. They may be flirtatious and sexually seductive and may use physical appearance to get people's attention. They often feel a close bond to someone they have just met and are quick to share personal details of their life with new acquaintances. They are often described by others as shallow.

Narcissistic Personality Disorder Individuals with narcissistic personality disorder have too high of an opinion of themselves and little regard for others, except as how others meet their needs. They see themselves as accomplishing great things that establish their superiority over others. They view themselves as special and unique and that only similarly special people could understand them. There is a sense of entitlement, and they often feel that they have earned the right to special treatment or consideration because of who they are or what they have done. Individuals with narcissistic personality disorder are often so self-absorbed that they are intolerant of others, and they lack the capacity to understand how others feel. The admiration of others is usually important, and they dream of attaining status. They may take advantage of others, if necessary, to get what is desired. Individuals with narcissistic personality disorder are often envious of others who have more than they do or believe that others are jealous of them, or both.

Avoidant Personality Disorder Avoidant personality disorder is characterized by social inhibition related to low self-esteem and sensitivity to rejection and criticism from others. Individuals with avoidant personality disorder have difficulty making friends and feel uncomfortable in social situations. It is difficult to share personal feelings and thoughts in close relationships because of the fear of being put down. Individuals with this personality disorder usually worry about making a bad impression and believe that they are not interesting or fun. Their fears of criticism and rejection can influence the type of career they choose (one that does not involve a lot of contact with people) or career advancement (turning down promotions or job opportunities that would require more contact with people).

Dependent Personality Disorder Individuals with dependent personality disorder have difficulty with self-sufficiency and have a strong need to be taken care of by others. Everyday decisions often are not made without the input of others, and others frequently make decisions about important areas of their life. Individuals with dependent personality disorder may bend over backward to the point of doing unpleasant tasks for others to get support and gratitude. It is difficult for the person with dependent personality disorder to start projects on their own, because they do not feel confident in their own abilities, and it is hard to disagree with others for fear of losing support or approval. Individuals with dependent personality disorder do not like being alone. They often believe that they cannot care for themselves, and, if a close relationship ends, they may be desperate to get into another relationship right away, even if it is not the best person for them.

Obsessive-Compulsive Personality Disorder Obsessive-compulsive personality disorder is characterized by a pattern of perfectionism, stinginess, stubbornness, orderliness, and inflexibility. Individuals with obsessive-compulsive personality disorder often spend so much time on small details that they lose sight of the main thing they were trying to do. They frequently are workaholics, who spend so much time working that they have little time for family activities, friendships, or entertainment. They are often interpersonally controlling because of their rigidity. Individuals with obsessive-compulsive personality disorder have difficulty delegating tasks or working with others unless things are done their way. Others often complain that they are too strict about moral issues and that they are cheap. Individuals with obsessive-compulsive personality disorder frequently find it difficult to throw things away, even when the object is old and worn and has no sentimental value.

XVII: Other Conditions That May Be a Focus of Clinical Attention

The conditions included in the section on other conditions that may be a focus of clinical attention are not considered mental disorders but are included because they may be the focus of clinical attention. The reasons that these conditions fail to meet the DSM-IV-TR definition for a mental disorder are not specified. Twenty-nine specific problems are listed in six groups: psychological factors affecting medical conditions, medication-induced movement disorders, other medication-induced disorders, relational problems, problems related to abuse or neglect, and others. These problems are coded on Axis I.

Psychological Problems Affecting Medical Conditions The category of psychological problems affecting medical conditions refers to those situations in which psychological factors negatively affect the course or outcome of a general medical condition or significantly increase the risk of an adverse outcome. The psychological and behavioral factors that may negatively impact on the course and outcome of a medical condition include subthreshold symptoms and personality traits that do not meet criteria for a specific mental disorder diagnosis, personality traits that undermine a therapeutic collaboration with health providers, and maladaptive behaviors, such as overeating and sedentary lifestyle.

Medication-Induced Movement Disorders The category of medication-induced movement disorders is included because of its clinical importance in treatment and differential diagnosis. Five of the six specific movement disorders described are related to the use of neuroleptics (neuroleptic-induced parkinsonism, acute dystonia, acute akathisia, tardive dyskinesia, and neuroleptic malignant syndrome). The sixth disorder is medication-induced postural tremor, which is most often associated with antidepressants and mood stabilizers. The DSM-IV-TR text includes brief descriptions of these disorders, with reference to DSM-IV-TR's appendix for a more detailed description of suggested diagnostic criteria.

Other Medication-Induced Disorders The category of other medication-induced disorders is included so that clinicians could code medication side effects that are a focus of clinical attention (e.g., severe hypotension, priapism, weight gain, and sexual dysfunction).

Relational Problems Relational problems that cause significant symptoms or functional impairment are frequently the focus of clinical attention. These problems may be associated with a mental or general medical disorder in one of the members of the relational unit. When the relationship problem is the primary focus of treatment, then the problem is coded on Axis I. If not the primary focus of treatment, the problem can be listed on Axis IV.

Problems Related to Abuse or Neglect The category of problems related to abuse or neglect includes five problems (physical abuse of child, sexual abuse of child, neglect of child, physical abuse of adult, and sexual abuse of adult) that frequently are the focus of clinical attention. Separate diagnostic codes are used when the patient is the perpetrator or victim of the abuse or neglect.

Other Conditions That May Be a Focus of Clinical Attention The last group in this class of problems includes a heterogeneous collection of 13 problems that may the focus of treatment (noncompliance with treatment, malingering, adult antisocial behavior, child or adolescent antisocial behavior, borderline intellectual functioning, age-related cognitive decline, bereavement, academic problem, occupational problem, identity problem, religious or spiritual problem, acculturation problem, and phase of life problem). Each of these problems has its own diagnostic code.

XVIII: Appendix Diagnoses

DSM-IV-TR contains proposed criteria for 20 specific disorders that were not included in the official classification but are included in an appendix, so that

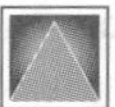

Table 9.1–6
Appendix Diagnoses in the DSM-IV-TR

Postconcussional disorder
Mild neurocognitive disorder
Caffeine withdrawal
Postpsychotic depressive disorder of schizophrenia
Simple deteriorative disorder
Minor depressive disorder
Recurrent brief depressive disorder
Premenstrual dysphoric disorder
Mixed anxiety depressive disorder
Factitious disorder by proxy
Dissociative trance disorder
Binge-eating disorder
Depressive personality disorder
Passive-aggressive personality disorder (negativistic personality disorder)

research can be conducted on their reliability, validity, and potential clinical usefulness (Table 9.1–6). Many of these disorders are currently captured by the classification under not-otherwise-specified designations (e.g., depressive disorder NOS for minor depressive disorder or premenstrual dysphoric disorder).

USING DSM-IV-TR

An 11-page introduction to DSM-IV-TR describes its history, methods of the revision process, definition of mental disorder, and issues in using a classification of mental disorders. This is followed by a cautionary statement warning against reifying the diagnostic criteria and the classification. It is noted that the specified diagnostic criteria represent guidelines for making diagnoses based on consensus opinion of current knowledge. Also, the classification may not cover all conditions for which persons seek treatment, and the inclusion of a diagnostic category in the classification does not have implications for legal decisions. After the cautionary statement, an 11-page section describes the use of the manual, and a 7-page section describes DSM-IV-TR's multiaxial diagnostic approach. The inclusion of these latter two sections is indicative of the complexity of the DSM-IV-TR classification and the potential difficulty in using it.

Multiaxial Evaluation

The DSM-IV-TR multiaxial system of evaluation, in which different domains of information are described on five different axes, was introduced in DSM-III. Proper use of DSM-IV-TR does not require the use of the multiaxial format. The purpose of multiaxial evaluation is to promote a comprehensive, biopsychosocial approach toward clinical assessment. Axis I consists of all clinical disorders, except for the personality disorders and mental retardation, both of which are reported on Axis II. Prominent maladaptive personality traits that do not meet criteria for a specific disorder and defense mechanisms are also noted on Axis II. Axis III is for general medical conditions that might be relevant to understanding or managing the patient's psychiatric disorder. In those cases in which the medical disorder causes the mental disorder, then the medical disorder is listed on Axis III, and the mental disorder is listed on Axis I as *due to a general medical condition.* Axis IV is for noting psychosocial and environmental problems that are relevant to the diagnosis, treatment, and prognosis of Axis I and Axis II disorders. When a psychosocial problem is the primary focus of treatment, then it is listed on Axis I as a *condition that may be the focus of clinical attention*, although this is not considered a mental disorder. The problem is also listed on Axis IV. Axis V is the GAF scale, a 100-point rating based on symptom severity, social functioning, and occupational functioning (see Table 7.9–2).

Multiple Disorders

Many patients have more than one psychiatric disorder. When more than one disorder is present in a patient presenting for treatment, the clinician denotes one disorder as the *principal diagnosis*. Several methods have been used by researchers in identifying principal disorders in patients with multiple psychiatric disorders. Some of the factors used to designate a principal disorder include age of onset (i.e., the principal disorder is the one that came first), relative degree of impairment (i.e., the principal disorder is the one responsible for the greatest degree of psychosocial dysfunction), and reason for seeking treatment (i.e., the principal disorder is the one that is chiefly responsible for the treatment seeking). In DSM-IV-TR, the determination of the principal diagnosis is based on the reason for the clinical service. When two disorders are nearly equally responsible for the clinical service, DSM-IV-TR acknowledges that the identification of one disorder as the principal disorder is somewhat arbitrary.

Disorder Severity

When the full criteria for a disorder are met, its severity can be specified as mild, moderate, or severe. Severity ratings are based on the number and intensity of the symptoms of the disorder and the impairment in occupational or social functioning caused by the symptoms. Although the severity specifier can be applied to all disorders, specific guidelines for making this rating are provided only for mental retardation, conduct disorder, mania, mixed manic-depressive episodes, and major depression. For each of these disorders, except conduct disorder, the disorder's severity is captured by the diagnostic code.

Remission Status

When the symptoms of a disorder are present, but the full criteria of the disorder are no longer met, then the disorder is considered in partial remission. According to DSM-IV-TR, a disorder is in full remission when no symptoms or signs of the disorder are present. Although this specifier, similar to disorder severity, can be applied to all disorders, specific guidelines for making this distinction are provided only for manic and major depressive episodes and substance dependence. For substance dependence, full remission requires that none of the diagnostic criteria has been met for at least 1 month. The definition of remission from a manic and depressive episode differs from the substance dependence remission definition in two ways. First, in contrast to a complete absence of diagnostic criteria, the DSM-IV-TR remission definition for mania and depression requires the absence of "*significant* (italics added) signs or symptoms of the disturbance." No guidelines are provided for interpreting the meaning of "significant." It is therefore unclear if the presence of one or two mild symptoms is inconsistent with the definition of remission. Second, the duration of the symptom-free interval must last at least 2 months for depression and mania, in contrast to 1 month for substance dependence. Because of the differences in defining remission for the mood and substance dependence disorders, it is unclear how to define remission for other disorders. For example, to designate anorexia as being in remission, how much residual concern, if any, about body image can remain in a patient who has regained lost weight? Or, how much discomfort, if any, can remain in a patient with a public speaking social phobia who no longer avoids public presentations? The threshold used to determine disorder remission has important implications for characterizing the longitudinal course of disorders and the effectiveness of treatment efforts and will hopefully be given more consideration in the next DSM revision.

DSM-IV-TR also differentiates between full remission and recovery. A disorder in full remission is listed as a current disorder, because it remains clinically relevant. After an unspecified period of time, based on factors such as the duration of the symptoms, the duration of the symptom-free interval, and the need for continued monitoring and prophylactic treatment, the clinician might consider the patient as having recovered from the disorder, and the disorder is no longer classified a current condition. In such cases, the clinician can list the disorder by using the specifier *prior history*.

Diagnostic Uncertainty

There are several ways of coding diagnostic uncertainty in DSM-IV-TR. The diagnosis can be deferred, or a specific diagnosis can be rendered and identified as provisional. When some information is available, not enough to diagnose a specific disorder but enough to know which class of disorder is present, then the diagnosis is *NOS*.

Clinical Conditions Not Meeting Specified Diagnostic Criteria

Clinically significant presentations sometimes do not meet the threshold for a diagnosis. This is particularly true for disorders that are defined polythetically, whereby a minimum number of features from a list are needed to make a diagnosis. To account for this, every DSM-IV-TR diagnostic class has an NOS category. For example, patients who present with fewer than five clinically significant depressive symptoms would be diagnosed with depressive disorder NOS.

Because the definition of mental disorder is based, in part, on impairment and distress, and knowledge of underlying dysfunction and etiological mechanisms is largely unknown, the DSM-IV-TR phenomenologically based classification system is unable to account for the wide diversity of clinical presentations. Similar to patients who fall below specified diagnostic thresholds, patients with atypical symptom presentations are given an NOS diagnosis in the diagnostic class that most closely resembles the clinical picture. For some NOS categories, DSM-IV-TR provides specific examples of such "atypical" presentations, and, in some instances, these symptom patterns have corresponding research diagnostic criteria that are presented in the appendix.

PSYCHIATRIC DIAGNOSIS IN CLINICAL PRACTICE

Multiple opinions about the use of the DSM system in clinical practice have been offered, two of which are described in this section. Some authors have raised concerns that clinicians have become preoccupied with eliciting signs and symptoms to make DSM psychiatric diagnoses to the exclusion of evaluating the psychosocial and psychodynamic perspectives of the patient's history. In contrast, some researchers have suggested that adherence to the DSM system is clinically important, and they have raised concerns related to clinicians' high diagnostic error rate.

In their review of DSM-III, Arnold Cooper and Robert Michels speculated that the antitheoretical approach toward classification, without superordinate principles to integrate biopsychosocial information with DSM diagnoses, would result in an overly narrow focus on determining whether diagnostic criteria are met. In their review of DSM-III-R 7 years later, they concluded that their initial concern had been realized, particularly in the clinical assessments done by the new generation of trainees. Similarly, Gary J. Tucker suggested that the improved diagnostic precision offered in the modern DSM era has resulted in narrowly focused evaluations of DSM criteria that rule in or out diagnoses but neglect the patient's life story. Signs and symptoms are accorded greater significance than coping style. These authors acknowledged that the multiaxial system of classification encourages a perspective beyond the signs and symptoms of Axis I disorders but found, in their experience, that this broader perspective is not actually taken in clinical practice. Thomas A. Widiger and Spitzer, responding to the concerns expressed in Cooper's and Michels' review of DSM-III-R, indicated that the problem lies with the teachers of the new generation of clinicians rather than the manual. They reiterated the cautionary statement in DSM-III-R that a diagnosis represents only one component of a comprehensive evaluation. Moreover, they added that their anecdotal experience in using DSM-III-R with trainees was that it stimulated a broader perspective of psychopathology, because its antitheoretical approach encouraged consideration of different models of causation and treatment.

In contrast to concerns regarding an overly narrow focus on diagnosis, in the past few years, research by several independent research groups has raised concerns about the adequacy of psychiatric diagnostic evaluations conducted in routine clinical practice, because the diagnostic assessment is not sufficiently comprehensive. For example, M. Katherine Shear and colleagues studied diagnostic accuracy in two community mental health centers, one in urban Pittsburgh and the other in rural western Pennsylvania. They found poor agreement between clinical assessments and evaluations conducted by trained raters administering the Structured Clinical Interview for DSM-IV (SCID), a semi-structured diagnostic interview commonly used by researchers to make psychiatric diagnoses. In particular, they found that, whereas clinicians frequently diagnosed adjustment disorder, the SCID interviewers made specific mood or anxiety disorder diagnoses. They also reported that more diagnostic comorbidity was identified on the SCID. In discussing their findings, Shear and colleagues questioned whether patients' outcomes were compromised by the failure to detect and to diagnose correctly treatable conditions.

In another study of community mental health patients, this one conducted in Texas, Monica R. Basco and colleagues administered the SCID to patients as a test of the usefulness of research diagnostic procedures in clinical practice. They found that supplementing information from the patients' charts with the information from the SCID resulted in more than five times as many comorbid conditions being diagnosed. A gold standard, all sources of information, diagnosis was made for all patients, and the level of agreement with this standard was higher for the SCID than the clinical diagnoses. After feedback from the SCID interview was presented to the clinicians, a change in patient care occurred in one-half of the cases.

The results of these two studies are consistent with the findings from the Rhode Island Methods to Improve Diagnostic Assessment and Services (MIDAS) project, in which diagnostic frequencies were compared in two samples—one interviewed with the SCID and the other interviewed by psychiatrists using an unstructured clinical interview. Consistent with the findings of the Texas and Pittsburgh groups, it was found that many more patients were diagnosed with two or more DSM-IV-TR Axis I disorders when research interviews were conducted than when diagnoses were based on the routine clinical evaluation. More than one-third of patients interviewed with SCID received three or more diagnoses in contrast to fewer than 10 percent of the patients assessed with an unstructured interview. Fifteen disorders were more frequently diagnosed when the SCID was used, and these differences cut across mood, anxiety, eating, somatoform, and impulse control disorder categories. Importantly, patients often desired treatment for the comorbid Axis I disorders that were not the primary reason for seeking treatment. Thus, detecting diagnostic comorbidity was important from a consumer and patient perspective. Another report from the MIDAS project examined the issue of diagnosing borderline personality disorder and found that research interviewers using the Structured Interview for DSM-IV Personality were much more likely to diagnose borderline personality disorder than clinicians. Moreover, when the information from the research interview was provided to the clinician, clinicians diagnosed borderline personality disorder more frequently; thus, it was not simply a matter of clinicians being reluctant to diagnose borderline personality disorder during the initial diagnostic evaluation.

Are these findings any cause for alarm? That is hard to say, because no research has demonstrated the clinical significance of the gap between researchers' and clinicians' diagnostic practices. Specifically, there are currently no studies that have examined the important question of whether the more accurate and comprehensive research diagnostic evaluations improve outcomes. In fact, one could argue that patients' outcomes are *not* more likely to be worse, even if diagnoses are missed.

Clinicians currently have at their disposal pharmacological agents with broad-based efficacy; consequently, diagnostic error might not be important. The new generation of medications, such as selective serotonin reuptake inhibitors (SSRIs), have been found to be effective for depression, almost all anxiety disorders, eating disorders, impulse control disorders, substance use disorders, attention deficit disorder, and some somatoform disorders. In short, most of the disorders for which individuals seek outpatient care have been found to be responsive to at least one of the new generation of antidepressant medications. Thus, it is possible that accurate and comprehensive DSM-IV-TR diagnoses are not critical after gross diagnostic class distinctions (e.g., psychotic disorder vs. mood disorder) are made. This would be consistent with the results of a survey of psychiatrists' attitudes about DSM-III and DSM-III-R conducted 10 years ago that found that only a minority of psychiatrists rated the DSMs as being important for treatment planning, determining prognosis, patient management, and understanding patients' problems.

Whether or not improved diagnostic practice would result in improved outcome, it is important to recall from the beginning of this chapter that diagnosis has more than one clinically relevant function. In addition to optimizing outcome, diagnosis is important for predicting treatment outcome. It is the opinion of the authors of this chapter that a greater percentage of the variance in outcome would be predicted by comprehensive evaluations than by clinical diagnoses. Again, this is an unstudied question.

CLASSIFICATION CONTROVERSIES

Dimensional Versus Categorical Approaches toward Classification

The introduction to DSM-IV-TR makes it clear that, although a categorical classification is described in the manual, this should not be interpreted as suggesting that the categorical approach is more reliable or valid than a dimensional approach toward classification. Put simply, a categorical system posits that there are clear boundaries between diagnostic entities or between disorder and the absence of disorder, whereas a dimensional model posits a lack of clear demarcation. Discussions of the relative merits of categorical and dimensional approaches toward the classification of mental disorders have persisted throughout the 20th century. For example, in the 1920s, Edward Mapother questioned the usefulness of classifying depressed patients as endogenous or neurotic because of the difficulty in placing many patients into one group or the other. Through the years, several statistical approaches have been used to evaluate the categorical versus dimensional approaches toward classification. These include plotting scores of symptom characteristics and determining whether the plots were consistent with a bimodal or unimodal distribution or determining linear or nonlinear relationships between symptom scores and independent variables, such as laboratory tests, family history, or treatment response. More recently, interest has grown in using Paul Meehl's taxometric methods to test for latent categories. At present, the research community is not unified in its opinion regarding the categorical-dimensional debate. Although it is apparent that there are no clearly defined boundaries distinguishing disorders from each other and from normality, much of the taxometric research is consistent with the categorical model. DSM-IV-TR's categorical approach, which is the traditional method of medical classification, seems appropriate at this time, because it is more useful in clinical practice.

Separate Disorders Versus Subtypes

Arthur C. Houts has been highly critical of the increasing number of disorders listed in each successive edition of the DSM and has suggested that this was indicative of a lack of scientific progress. Moreover, he suggested that disorders were being created that had previously not been recognized as pathology. Wakefield carefully examined the causes of diagnostic proliferation and concluded that the greater number of diagnoses listed in successive DSMs represented greater specification rather than diagnostic discoveries. In fact, he found that the increase in the number of diagnoses paralleled the increases found in the ICD classification of cardiac and GI diseases during the past 30 years.

Although the increased number of coded diagnostic entities does not generally represent the discovery of new diagnostic entities, this issue nonetheless warrants some consideration, because it has generated debate within the field between the so-called lumpers, who favor broader categories, and the splitters, who favor subclassification. Researchers are more likely to benefit from embracing the splitters' approach, as it is easier to publish findings demonstrating that a method of subclassification is associated with statistically significant differences than it is to publish null findings. Thus, there are many research articles suggesting the validity of diagnostic and (sub)classification distinctions. However, the principles guiding the incorporation of these distinctions into a classification of disorders are unwritten. Some resulting questions include the following: When is a syndrome sufficiently distinct from its near neighbors to warrant being considered a separate disorder? When is the heterogeneity amongst members of a disorder sufficient to warrant subdividing the group into more homogeneous subgroups (i.e., subtyping)? Is there a conceptual difference between distinguishing between disorders and distinguishing between subtypes of a disorder? The introduction to DSM-IV-TR does not discuss these questions.

Some examples illustrate the lack of conceptual guidelines in making these distinctions. The distinctions between bipolar and unipolar depression and psychotic and nonpsychotic depression have been demonstrated in multiple domains. Yet, unipolar and bipolar depression are considered different disorders, whereas determination of the presence of psychotic features is a method of subtyping depression. Body dysmorphic disorder is classified as a somatoform disorder. It has been conceptualized as an obsessive-compulsive spectrum disorder, and research suggests that there are many similarities and few differences between patients with body dysmorphic disorder and patients with OCD. Consider individuals with OCD who obsessively wash their hands and shower. Such individuals are not classified with body cleaning disorder. It is reasonable to suggest that body dysmorphic disorder is as representative of OCD as is body cleaning disorder.

Financial Implications of Revising the Classification Since DSM-III, the APA has made millions of dollars selling the DSMs. When plans were announced to publish DSM-IV 5 years after DSM-III-R was published, concern was raised that profit motives were responsible, at least in part, for the short interval between DSM editions. Postpublication reviews of DSM-III-R also raised such questions. It is disconcerting that financial considerations might have significantly influenced the timing of revisions of the classification. Perhaps as a result of these criticisms, the pace of DSM revisions has slowed. At the time of the writing of this chapter, it has been 8 years since the publication of DSM-IV, and DSM-V is not anticipated until the end of the decade.

However, the issue of profiting from revising the DSM manual renewed itself with the publication of the DSM-IV-TR. On the one hand, the principal architects of the DSMs have asserted that the manual is not a textbook. Despite this caveat, the detailed clinical descriptions and discussions of differential diagnosis along with up-to-date summaries of prevalence data, demographic correlates, familial patterns, and course of illness, give the DSMs the feel of a textbook, which has undoubtedly contributed to their success. Seemingly inconsistent with the assertion that the DSM should not be considered to be a textbook, the most recent version of the DSM, DSM-IV-TR, is solely an updating of the text without changes to the diagnostic criteria. This follows the typical pattern of publishing new editions of academic textbooks, such as the present one, every few years to have up-to-date summaries of scientific knowledge. Thus, despite the declaration that the DSM is not a textbook, the publication schedule suggests otherwise. The integrity of the revision process can be compromised by a conflict of interest between the scientific justification for revising and updating the manual's text and nomenclature versus fiscal gains to the APA. A potential method of reducing the tension between scientific and economic forces is to develop scientific guidelines regarding the level of significant change needed in the classification system that should trigger a revision.

SUGGESTED CROSS-REFERENCES

The psychiatric report is discussed in Section 7.3, typical signs and symptoms are discussed in Section 7.4, neuropsychological assessment is discussed in Section 7.5, clinical manifestations of psychiatric disorders are discussed in Chapter 8, and international perspectives on psychiatric diagnosis are discussed in Section 9.2.

References

Akiskal HS, McKinney W: Psychiatry and pseudopsychiatry. *Arch Gen Psychiatry.* 1973;28:367.

American Medical Association. *Standard Classified Nomenclature of Disease.* Chicago: American Medical Association; 1935.

American Psychiatric Association. *Diagnostic and Statistical Manual of Mental Disorders.* 1st ed. Washington, DC: American Psychiatric Association; 1952.

American Psychiatric Association. *Diagnostic and Statistical Manual of Mental Disorders.* 2nd ed. Washington, DC: American Psychiatric Association; 1968.

*American Psychiatric Association. *Diagnostic and Statistical Manual of Mental Disorders.* 3rd ed. Washington, DC: American Psychiatric Association; 1980.

American Psychiatric Association. *Diagnostic and Statistical Manual of Mental Disorders.* 3rd revised ed. Washington, DC: American Psychiatric Association; 1987.

American Psychiatric Association. *Diagnostic and Statistical Manual of Mental Disorders.* 4th ed, text revision. Washington, DC: American Psychiatric Association; 2000.

Basco MR, Bostic JQ, Davies D, Rush AJ, Witte B, Hendrickse W, Barnett V: Methods to improve diagnostic accuracy in a community mental health setting. *Am J Psychiatry.* 2000;157:1599–1605.

Brill H. Nosology. In: Freedman AM, Kaplan HI, Kaplan HS, eds. *Comprehensive Textbook of Psychiatry.* Baltimore: Williams & Wilkins; 1967:581–589.

Cooper A, Michels R: Book review of Diagnostic and Statistical Manual of Mental Disorders, 3rd ed, Revised (DSM-III-R). *Am J Psychiatry.* 1988;145:1300–1301.

Cooper JE, Kendell RE, Gurland BJ, Sharpe L, Copeland JRM, Simon R. *Psychiatric Diagnosis in New York and London.* London: Oxford University Press; 1972.

Endicott J, Spitzer RL: A diagnostic interview: The Schedule for Affective Disorders and Schizophrenia. *Arch Gen Psychiatry.* 1978;35:837–844.

*Feighner JP, Robins E, Guze SB, Woodruff RA, Winokur G, Munoz R: Diagnostic criteria for use in psychiatric research. *Arch Gen Psychiatry.* 1972;26:57–67.

First MB, Pincus HA: The DSM-IV text revision: Rationale and potential impact on clinical practice. *Psychiatr Serv.* 2002;53:288–292.

First MB, Spitzer RL, Williams JBW, Gibbon M. *Structured Clinical Interview for DSM-IV (SCID).* Washington, DC: American Psychiatric Association; 1997.

Follette WC, Houts AC: Models of scientific progress and the role of theory in taxonomy development: A case study of the DSM. *J Consult Clin Psychol.* 1996;64:1120–1132.

Frances AJ, Widiger TA, Pincus HA: The development of DSM-IV. *Arch Gen Psychiatry.* 1989;46:373–375.

Freud S. *Introductory Lectures on Psycho-analysis.* London: Hogarth Press; 1963.

Fulford KWM: Nine variations and a coda on the theme of an evolutionary definition of dysfunction. *J Abnorm Psychol.* 1999;108:412–420.

Gottesman II, Gould TD: The endophenotype concept in psychiatry: Etymology and strategic intentions. *Am J Psychiatry.* 2003;160:636–645.

Group for the Advancement of Psychiatry. *Psychopathological Disorders in Childhood: Theoretical Considerations and a Proposed Classification.* New York: Group for the Advancement of Psychiatry; 1966.

Gruenberg EM: How can the new diagnostic manual help? *Int J Psychiatry.* 1969;7:368.

Houts AC: The diagnostic and statistical manual's new white coat and circularity of plausible dysfunctions: Response to Wakefield, part 1. *Behav Res Ther.* 2001;39:315–345.

Jefferson JW, Thompson TD: Rhinotillexomania: Psychiatric disorder or habit? *J Clin Psychiatry.* 1995;56:56–59.

Kendell RE. *The Role of Diagnosis in Psychiatry.* Oxford: Blackwell; 1975.

Kendell R, Jablensky A: Distinguishing between the validity and utility of psychiatric diagnoses. *Am J Psychiatry.* 2003;160:4–12.

Kendler KS: Setting boundaries for psychiatric disorders. *Am J Psychiatry.* 1999;156:1845–1848.

Kihlstrom JF. To honor Kraepelin: From symptoms to pathology in the diagnosis of mental illness. In: Beutler LE, Malik ML, eds. *Rethinking the DSM.* Washington, DC: American Psychological Association; 2002:279–303.

Klerman GL, Vaillant GE, Spitzer RL, Michels R: A debate on DSM-III. *Am J Psychiatry.* 1984;141:539–542.

Kramer M. The history of the efforts to agree on an international classification of mental disorders. In: American Psychiatric Association. *Diagnostic and Statistical Manual of Mental Disorders.* 2nd ed. Washington, DC: American Psychiatric Association; 1973.

Lilienfeld SO, Marino L: Mental disorder as a Roschian concept: A critique of Wakefield's "harmful dysfunction" analysis. *J Abnorm Psychol.* 1995;104:411–420.

Lilienfeld SO, Marino L: Essentialism revisited: Evolutionary theory and the concept of mental disorder. *J Abnorm Psychol.* 1999;108:400–411.

Mapother E: Discussion on manic-depressive psychosis. *Br J Psychiatry.* 1926;2:872–876.

Meehl PE: Bootstrap taxometrics. *Am Psychol.* 1995;50:266–275.

Menninger K: Sheer verbal Mickey Mouse. *Int J Psychiatry.* 1969;7:415.

Menninger K, Mayman M, Pruyser P. *The Vital Balance: The Life Process in Mental Health and Illness.* New York: Viking Press; 1963.

Merikangas KR, Risch N: Will the genomics revolution revolutionize psychiatry? *Am J Psychiatry.* 2003;160:625–635.

Narrow WE, Rae DS, Robins LN, Regier DA: Revised prevalence estimates of mental disorders in the United States. *Arch Gen Psychiatry.* 2002;59:115–123.

Office of General Register. *A Glossary of Mental Disorders.* London: Her Majesty's Stationery Office; 1968.

Peck MC, Scheffler RM: An analysis of the definitions of mental illness used in state parity laws. *Psychiatr Serv.* 2002;53:1089–1095.

Pincus HA, Frances A, Davis WW, First MB, Widiger TA: DSM-IV and new diagnostic categories: Holding the line on proliferation. *Am J Psychiatry.* 1992;149:112–117.

Robins E, Guze SB. Establishment of diagnostic validity in psychiatric illness: Its application to schizophrenia. *Am J Psychiatry.* 1970;126:983–987.

Robins LN, Locke BZ, Regier DA. An overview of psychiatric disorders in America. In: Robins LN, Regier DA, eds. *Psychiatric Disorders in America: The Epidemiologic Catchment Study.* New York: The Free Press; 1991.

Shear MK, Greeno C, Kang J, Ludewig D, Frank E, Swartz HA, Hanekamp M: Diagnosis of nonpsychotic patients in community clinics. *Am J Psychiatry.* 2000;157:581–587.

Spitzer RL: A proposal about homosexuality and the APA nomenclature: Homosexuality as an irregular form of sexual behavior and sexual orientation disturbance as a psychiatric disorder. A symposium: Should homosexuality be in the APA nomenclature? *Am J Psychiatry.* 1973;130:1207–1216.

Spitzer RL, Endicott J, Robins E: Research diagnostic criteria: Rationale and reliability. *Arch Gen Psychiatry.* 1978;35:773–782.

Spitzer RL, Fleiss J: A re-analysis of the reliability of psychiatric diagnosis. *Br J Psychiatry.* 1974;125:341–347.

*Spitzer RL, Wakefield JC: DSM-IV diagnostic criterion for clinical significance: Does it help solve the false positives problem? *Am J Psychiatry.* 1999;156:1856–1864.

Srole L, Langner TS, Michael ST, Opler MK, Rennie TAC. *Mental Health in the Metropolis.* Vol 1. *The Midtown Manhattan Study.* New York: McGraw-Hill; 1962.

Stengel E: Classification of mental disorders. *Bull WHO.* 1959;21:601.

Szasz TS. *The Myth of Mental Illness: Foundations of a Theory of Personal Conduct.* New York: Harper & Row; 1974.

Tucker GJ: Putting DSM-IV in perspective. *Am J Psychiatry.* 1998;155:159–161.

Tuke H: French retrospective. *J Ment Sci.* 1890;36:117.

*Wakefield JC: Disorder as harmful dysfunction: A conceptual critique of DSM-III-R's definition of mental disorder. *Psychol Rev.* 1992;99:232–247.

Wakefield JC: Diagnosing DSM-IV part I: DSM-IV and the concept of disorder. *Behav Res Ther*. 1997;35:633–649.
Wakefield JC: When is development disordered? Developmental psychopathology and the harmful dysfunction analysis of mental disorder. *Dev Psychopathol*. 1997;9:269–290.
Wakefield JC. Meaning and melancholia: Why the DSM-IV cannot (entirely) ignore the patient's intentional system. In: Barren J, ed. *Making Diagnosis Meaningful: Enhancing Evaluation and Treatment of Psychological Disorders*. Washington, DC: American Psychological Association; 1998:29–72.
Wakefield JC: Evolutionary versus prototype analyses of the concept of disorder. *J Abnorm Psychol*. 1999;108:374–399.
Wakefield JC: The myth of DSM's invention of new categories of disorder: Houts' diagnostic discontinuity theses disconfirmed. *Behav Res Ther*. 2001;39:575–624.
Wakefield JC, Pottick KJ, Kirk SA: Should the DSM-IV diagnostic criteria for conduct disorder consider social context? *Am J Psychiatry*. 2002;159:380–386.
Widiger TA, Spitzer RL: Criticisms of DSM-III-R. *Am J Psychiatry*. 1989;146:566–567.
World Health Organization. *Manual of the International Classification of Diseases, Injuries, and Causes of Death*. Geneva: World Health Organization; 1948.
*Zimmerman M: Why are we rushing to publish DSM-IV? *Arch Gen Psychiatry*. 1988;45:1135–1138.
Zimmerman M, Jampala VC, Sierles FS, Taylor MA: DSM-III and DSM-IIIR: What are American psychiatrists using and why? *Compr Psychiatry*. 1993;181:360–364.
Zimmerman M, Mattia JI: Differences between clinical and research practice in diagnosing borderline personality disorder. *Am J Psychiatry*. 1999;156:1570–1574.
Zimmerman M, Mattia JI: Psychiatric diagnosis in clinical practice: Is comorbidity being missed? *Compr Psychiatry*. 1999;40:182–191.
Zimmerman M, Mattia JI: Principal and additional DSM-IV disorders for which outpatients seek treatment. *Psychiatr Serv*. 2000;51:1299–1304.

▲ 9.2 International Psychiatric Diagnosis

JUAN E. MEZZICH, M.D, PH.D., AND
CARLOS E. BERGANZA, M.D.

Diagnosis and classification in psychiatry are critical for the scientific development of this discipline across the world and for psychiatry to be able to fulfill its most important role—serving effectively the patient who presents for care. International classification and diagnosis deal with concepts central to health and health care in a global manner, an approach increasingly compelling in the interdependent world in which humans live.

A *classification of diseases* may be defined as a system of categories to which morbid entities are assigned according to some established criteria. There is not a single correct set of criteria for classifying diseases. There are many possible choices, and all of them depend on the particular purpose of a classification system and the particular interest of its various stakeholders. For the anatomist, for example, the main criteria may be the part of the body affected, whereas, for the pathologist, it may be the disease process; for the public health practitioner, it may be the etiology, and, for the clinician, it may be the particular manifestations of the illness process requiring attention. This fact points out the importance of paying attention to the needs of the multiple stakeholders of the system. However, global usability demands two sometimes conflicting requirements of the system: First, it must allow for the development of a language that is common to all those using the system, such that communication among all of them is possible to a substantial degree of intelligibility and reliability, so that fundamental aspects of the phenomena to be assessed can be understood and compared across the world. Equally important is the fact that not all users of the system have the same needs in terms of the factors that define the phenomena under study. Diagnosis in fact defines the field of medicine in general and psychiatry in particular by delineating the informational base necessary for clinical care and health promotion at the individual and public health levels. Consequently, diagnosis is also a fundamental concept for professional training and scientific research. Furthermore, it informs the conceptualization of what a case is and the methodology for its assessment in epidemiology and public health. With various degrees of systematization and explicitness, diagnostic schemas, as consensual notions and formats for describing clinical conditions, have emerged since the dawn of mankind. In every case, these notions have been embedded within their time and culture.

Building on conceptual contributions over the past two centuries in various parts of the world, and having the 100-year-old *International Classification of Diseases* (ICD) as general reference, the worldwide emphasis for advancing psychiatric diagnosis during the past several decades has been on the use of more systematic formulations of psychopathology and of explicit diagnostic criteria and rules of assignment. This has led to gains in interrater agreement (diagnostic reliability) and universal communicability of diagnostic statements. These developments, although propitious for advancements in the field, do not ensure gains in diagnostic validity or usefulness of the diagnostic enterprise. Additionally, when assessing patients in populations different from the culture in which these universalistic systems have been created, validation of such systems in the populations of interest is essential.

This has led to more recent efforts to update diagnostic validity, clinically and epidemiologically, through developments to enhance existing universalistic diagnostic systems by paying attention to local realities and the uniqueness of the individual. The first type of these developments involves adaptations of the international classification system to regional or national clinical patterns and needs. The second corresponds to idiographic or personalized formulations, such as that proposed by the World Psychiatric Association (WPA) *International Guidelines for Diagnostic Assessment* (IGDA).

KEY CONCEPTUAL AND METHODOLOGICAL DEVELOPMENTS

The classification of mental disorders improved greatly in the last two decades of the 20th century through proposals arising in different parts of the world, and it can be said that it now provides a fairly reliable operational tool. Two strategic advances emerged then as key conceptual and methodological developments for psychiatric diagnosis. One is the systematic description of psychopathological entities, and the other is a comprehensive diagnostic formulation of the clinical condition of the patient.

Systematic Description of Psychopathology

Early roots of explicit and systematized psychopathological description can be found in 19th century France, when symptoms were first used as units of analysis of abnormal behavior. Current concepts of psychiatric nosology can be traced back to the end of the 19th century, highlighted by Valentin Magnan's notion of clinical evolution in France and Emil Kraepelin's dichotomy of the major psychoses in Germany. Other significant contributions to the nosology of severe mental disorders of recent impact on psychiatric classification are the German description of cycloid psychoses, the Scandinavian concept of psychogenic psychosis, and the French delineation of *bouffée délirante*. More recently, psychopathologists from Asia, Africa, and Latin America have offered informative reports on acute transient psychoses and somatically and psychologically textured characterizations of the neuroses.

The manifestations of mental disorders constitute the focus of the so-called phenomenological description of psychopathology. That approach encouraged careful observation of clinical presentations, particularly symptom profiles, while minimizing etiological inferences. Many questions remain regarding the organization of standard nosologies, for example, the number of major classes of mental disorders, the arrangement of subclasses, and the hierarchical relationships among diagnostic categories. Furthermore, etiopathogenic perspectives—from genetics, to psychodynamics, to general systems—may, in the future, contribute enriched and more valid formulations of mental disorders.

Explicit or operational diagnostic criteria, a mainstay of modern diagnostic methodology, were persuasively proposed by the British psychiatrist Edward Stengel as a step in dealing with the widespread confusion in classification documented in his international survey, commissioned by the World Health Organization (WHO). The actual development of operational criteria was pioneered, chronologically, by José Horwitz and Juan Marconi in Latin America, Peter Berner in Austria, and John Feighner and associates in the United States. Operationalized diagnostic criteria probably represent the most conspicuous response to the need for clarity in psychiatry and are considered essential for its progress as a scientific discipline. On the other hand, the limitations of using the criteria sets include the arbitrariness often involved in setting thresholds between cases and noncases, the cumbersome nature of their use in daily practice, and the burden that they impose on meaning and usage across cultures. An approach that promises to enhance categorical definition by accommodating graded typicality and flexible boundaries involves the use of the prototypical categorization model. This is connected to the mathematical *fuzzy set theory*, and its use is being explored on particularly problematic areas of psychopathology, such as personality disorders and even schizophrenia and obsessive-compulsive disorder (OCD).

Multiaxial Diagnostic Formulation

Attempts to represent more fully the complexity of a patient's condition have emerged predominantly under the generic term *multiaxial approach.* Multiaxial diagnosis intends to portray the intricacies of the clinical condition through the systematic and separate assessment and formulation of highly informative aspects or domains. Standardized measurements, either typologies or dimensional scales, have been proposed with which to appraise each domain.

The first multiaxial schemas in psychiatry and general medicine were aimed at articulating key components of an illness. Starting in 1949, the pioneers of the field who independently proposed a methodical and almost graphical assessment of syndromes and etiology were Erik Essen-Möller and Snorre Wohlfahrt in Sweden, Maurice Lecomte and associates in France, Tadeusz Bilikiewicz in Poland, and José Leme-Lopes in Brazil.

The first multiaxial schema in general medicine was the *Systematized Nomenclature of Pathology*, which accommodated axes on topography, morphology, etiology, and symptoms. One of the latest is the *International Classification of Diseases for Oncology* (ICD-O), which focuses separately on neoplastic topography and morphology (the latter including tumor behavior and differentiation).

A more recent and far-reaching purpose of the multiaxial model is to furnish a biopsychosocial description of the patient's entire clinical condition. This encompasses not only pathologies (mental and nonmental), but also psychosocial environmental factors and the consequences of illness on the individual's functioning and quality of life. The work of John Strauss, Michael Rutter, and associates in psychiatry and of Alvin Feinstein, J. S. House, and associates in general medicine is pertinent to this objective. Among the challenges for further development of the multiaxial model are the need for greater simplicity and ease of use as well as empirical appraisal of its reliability and validity across the world.

The first national diagnostic system to incorporate a multiaxial approach was the Swedish classification of mental disorders in the late 1940s, which was based on the previously referred proposals by Essen-Möller and Wohlfahrt. More recently, the methodological developments outlined previously (phenomenological description, explicit diagnostic criteria, and multiaxial formulation) have structured the third edition and the fourth edition of the American Psychiatric Association's (APA's) *Diagnostic and Statistical Manual of Mental Disorders* (DSM-III and DSM-IV), as well as the WHO's 10th revision of the ICD (ICD-10), which has a central role for diagnosis across the world.

ICD-10

Origins of the International Classification

The origins of the ICD can be traced back to the taxonomic work of the Swedish biologist Carolus Linnaeus in the 18th century. In *Genera Plantarum*, he stated: "All the real knowledge which we possess depends on methods by which we distinguish the similar from the dissimilar. . . . We ought therefore by attentive and diligent observation to determine the limits of the genera, since they cannot be determined a priori. This is the great work, the important labor, for should the genera be confused, all would be confusion." Linnaeus stimulated scholars from all walks of life. For example, Francois Boissier de Sauvages and William Cullen developed formidable nosologies encompassing thousands of species of disease, organized into classes, orders, and genera.

Bringing these leads to fruition, the 1st International Statistical Congress held in Brussels in 1853 commissioned the Englishman William Farr and the Italian Marc d'Espine to prepare a "uniform nomenclature of causes of death applicable to all countries" as a way to obtain comparable health status information across the world. The proposals that ensued were based primarily on topographical or etiological principles. Accommodating both, Jacques Bertillón of Paris prepared the First International Classification of Causes of Death, adopted at the International Statistical Congress of 1893.

Since then, there have been revisions of the ICD approximately every 10 years. From its foundation, the WHO, created in 1948, assumed the preparation of these revisions as a constitutional responsibility. The 6th revision contained a critical expansion of the scope of the international classification by covering morbidity in addition to mortality. Correspondingly, psychiatric illness appeared for the first time in the classification with one category: mental illness and deficiency. The ninth revision of the ICD (ICD-9) had as one of its innovations the presentation of a glossary for the capsular definition of mental disorders. Although modest in informational detail, this glossary signified recognition by the WHO that the intricacy of mental problems required more than the labels used in all other chapters of the ICD.

Outline of ICD-10

Work toward the preparation of ICD-10 started in 1979, the same year in which ICD-9 was put into effect. Its developmental process involved the participation of the eight Collaborating Centers for the Classification of Diseases; specialty divisions (such as Mental Health) at the headquarters and the regional offices of the WHO; nongovernmental organizations, such as the WPA; and a miscellaneous panel of interested groups and individuals, all working under the coordination of the WHO Unit on the Development of Epidemiological and Health Statistical Services.

First to be noted in ICD-10 is its expanded scope, as indicated by its title, *International Statistical Classification of Diseases and Related Health Problems.* This expression continues the trend that, starting with an original set of causes of death, added morbidity in its fifth revision and, more recently, added problems such as disabilities and factors that influence health status, recognizing that more information is needed to deal effectively with the evolving and complex issues of health care and health promotion.

ICD-10 uses an alphanumeric code composed of a letter followed by several digits. That arrangement more than doubles the number of available categories. Splitting, rather than lumping, of categories has marked the progression of ICD revisions, which has increased the need for categorical slots. The first four characters of the code are internationally official. The 5th and 6th character fields are available for regional and special purpose adaptations. This arrangement maintains international communication while accommodating local diversity.

Another powerful and innovative concept is that ICD-10 is a family of disease and health-related classifications. At the core of the family are the 21 main chapters coded at the official three-character and four-character levels and the short tabulation lists of causes of death and morbidity. Peripherally located are the following classifications: (1) specialty-based adaptations (e.g., for oncology), in which the chief difference from the core classification lies in the further extension of the ICD codes; (2) classifications for primary care and general medical practice, characterized by the condensation of categories and emphasis on less rigorous diagnostic terminology and more immediate therapeutic usefulness; and (3) classifications of information outside the core ICD, such as that corresponding to disabilities and medical procedures. Also part of the family is the International Nomenclature of Diseases, which encompasses a list of recommended names for all diseases as well as their definitions. In contrast to the concept of nomenclature, a classification, in the words of the ICD pioneer William Farr, "groups diseases that have considerable affinity or that are liable to be confounded with each other, and therefore is likely to facilitate the deduction of general principles."

Main forms of human illness and related conditions constitute the 21 chapters as the core of ICD-10 (Table 9.2–1). New chapters structure the enlarged lists of disorders of the nervous system (Chapter VI), eye and adnexa (Chapter VII), and ear and mastoid process (Chapter VIII). The expanded chapter on neoplasms covers one full letter and shares another with blood disorders, which encompasses immunological conditions, such as acquired immune deficiency syndrome (AIDS). Also, the classification of neoplasms is multiaxial (one axis denotes topography and another morphology, i.e., histological type, and tumor invasiveness and differentiation).

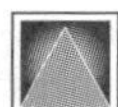

Table 9.2–1
List of Core Chapters of ICD-10

Chapter	Title
I	Certain infectious and parasitic diseases
II	Neoplasms
III	Diseases of the blood and blood-forming organs and certain disorders involving the immune mechanism
IV	Endocrine, nutritional, and metabolic diseases
V	Mental and behavioral disorders
VI	Diseases of the nervous system
VII	Diseases of the eye and adnexa
VIII	Diseases of the ear and mastoid process
IX	Diseases of the circulatory system
X	Diseases of the respiratory system
XI	Diseases of the digestive system
XII	Diseases of the skin and subcutaneous tissue
XIII	Diseases of the musculoskeletal system and connective tissue
XIV	Diseases of the genitourinary system
XV	Pregnancy, childbirth, and the puerperium
XVI	Certain conditions originating in the perinatal period
XVII	Congenital malformations, deformations, and chromosomal abnormalities
XVIII	Symptoms, signs, and abnormal clinical and laboratory findings not elsewhere classified.
XIX	Injury, poisoning, and certain other consequences of external causes
XX	External causes of morbidity and mortality
XXI	Factors influencing health status and contact with health services

From World Health Organization. *International Statistical Classification of Diseases and Related Health Problems.* 10th ed. Vol 1. Geneva: World Health Organization; 1992, with permission.

ICD-10 Classification of Mental Disorders

Mental and behavioral disorders are housed within Chapter V of ICD-10 and are coded with the letter F (Table 9.2–2). The use of the sixth letter of the Gregorian alphabet to denote chapter V is explained by the assignment of two letters to a lengthy list of conditions in chapters on infectious and parasitic diseases. After the letter F, the first digit of the Chapter V diagnostic codes denotes ten major classes of mental and behavioral disorders: F0 through F9. The second and third digits (third and fourth characters) identify progressively finer categories. For example, the code F30.2 sequentially denotes the mental chapter, mood disorders class, manic episode, and the presence of psychotic symptoms. In this manner, 1,000 four-character mental disorder categorical slots are available in ICD-10.

F0: Organic, Including Symptomatic, Mental Disorders The F0 class is etiologically based on physical disorders or conditions involving or leading to brain damage or dysfunction. The first clusters have disturbances of cognitive functions as prominent features and include the dementias (Alzheimer's, vascular, associated with other diseases, and unspecified), organic amnestic syndrome, and delirium not induced by psychoactive substances. The second cluster has as its most conspicuous manifestations alterations in perception (hallucinations), thought (delusions), mood (depressed or manic), various emotional domains (such as anxiety and dissociation), and personality.

F1: Mental and Behavioral Disorders Due to Psychoactive Substance Use In contrast to earlier classifications, the F1 class subsumes all mental disorders related to psychoactive substance use, from patterns of dependence and harmful use to various organic brain syndromes induced by substances. The diagnostic process and coding starts with identification of the substance involved (i.e., alcohol, opioids, cannabinoids, sedatives, or hypnotics, cocaine, other stimulants, hallucinogens, tobacco, volatile solvents, and other substances and combinations of them). Identified next in the code is the involved clinical condition: acute intoxication, harmful use (previously known as abuse and characterized by a pattern of use causing damage to physical or mental health), dependence syndrome, withdrawal state (with or without delirium), psychotic disorder, amnesic syndrome, residual and late-onset psychotic disorder, and other and unspecified mental disorders.

F2: Schizophrenia, Schizotypal, and Delusional Disorders The F2 class has schizophrenia as its centerpiece, a disorder characterized by fundamental and distinctive distortions of thinking and perception and by inappropriate or blunted affect. The remaining categories of nonorganic, nonaffective psychoses are considered somewhat related, phenomenologically or genetically, to schizophrenia. Particularly interesting is the cluster of acute and

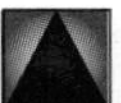

Table 9.2–2
ICD-10 Classification of Mental Disorders

F00 to F09	**Organic, including symptomatic, mental disorders**
F00	Dementia in Alzheimer's disease
F00.0	Dementia in Alzheimer's disease with early onset
F00.1	Dementia in Alzheimer's disease with late onset
F00.2	Dementia in Alzheimer's disease, atypical or mixed type
F00.9	Dementia in Alzheimer's disease, unspecified
F01	Vascular dementia
F01.0	Vascular dementia of acute onset
F01.1	Multiinfarct dementia
F01.2	Subcortical vascular dementia
F01.3	Mixed cortical and subcortical vascular dementia
F01.8	Other vascular dementia
F01.9	Vascular dementia, unspecified
F02	Dementia in other diseases classified elsewhere
F02.0	Dementia in Pick's disease
F02.1	Dementia in Creutzfeldt-Jakob disease
F02.2	Dementia in Huntington's disease
F02.3	Dementia in Parkinson's disease
F02.4	Dementia in human immunodeficiency virus (HIV) disease
F02.8	Dementia in other specified diseases classified elsewhere
F03	Unspecified dementia
A fifth character may be added to specify dementia in F00 to F03, as follows:	
.x0	Without additional symptoms
.x1	Other symptoms, predominantly delusional
.x2	Other symptoms, predominantly hallucinatory
.x3	Other symptoms, predominantly depressive
.x4	Other mixed symptoms
F04	Organic amnestic syndrome, not induced by alcohol and other psychoactive substances
F05	Delirium, not induced by alcohol and other psychoactive substances
F05.0	Delirium, not superimposed on dementia, so described
F05.1	Delirium, superimposed on dementia
F05.8	Other delirium
F05.9	Delirium, unspecified
F06	Other mental disorders due to brain damage and dysfunction and to physical disease
F06.0	Organic hallucinosis
F06.1	Organic catatonic disorder
F06.2	Organic delusional (schizophrenia-like) disorder
F06.3	Organic mood (affective) disorders
.30	Organic manic disorder
.31	Organic bipolar disorder
.32	Organic depressive disorder
.33	Organic mixed affective disorder
F06.4	Organic anxiety disorder
F06.5	Organic dissociative disorder
F06.6	Organic emotionally labile (asthenic) disorder
F06.7	Mild cognitive disorder
F06.8	Other specified mental disorders due to brain damage and dysfunction and to physical disease
F06.9	Unspecified mental disorder due to brain damage and dysfunction and to physical disease
F07	Personality and behavioral disorders due to brain disease, damage, and dysfunction
F07.0	Organic personality disorder
F07.1	Postencephalitic syndrome
F07.2	Postconcussional syndrome
F07.8	Other organic personality and behavioral disorders due to brain disease, damage, and dysfunction
F07.9	Unspecified organic personality and behavioral disorder due to brain disease, damage, and dysfunction
F09	Unspecified organic or symptomatic mental disorder
F10 to F19	**Mental and behavioral disorders due to psychoactive substance use**
F10.—	Mental and behavioral disorders due to use of alcohol
F11.—	Mental and behavioral disorders due to use of opioids
F12.—	Mental and behavioral disorders due to use of cannabinoids
F13.—	Mental and behavioral disorders due to use of sedatives or hypnotics
F14.—	Mental and behavioral disorders due to use of cocaine
F15.—	Mental and behavioral disorders due to use of other stimulants, including caffeine
F16.—	Mental and behavioral disorders due to use of hallucinogens
F17.—	Mental and behavioral disorders due to use of tobacco
F18.—	Mental and behavioral disorders due to use of volatile solvents
F19.—	Mental and behavioral disorders due to multiple drug use and use of other psychoactive substances
Four- and five-character categories may be used to specify the clinical conditions, as follows:	
F1x.0	Acute intoxication
.00	Uncomplicated
.01	With trauma or other bodily injury
.02	With other medical complications
.03	With delirium
.04	With perceptual distortions
.05	With coma
.06	With convulsions
.07	Pathological intoxication
F1x.1	Harmful use
F1x.2	Dependence syndrome
.20	Currently abstinent
.21	Currently abstinent, but in a protected environment
.22	Currently on a clinically supervised maintenance or replacement regime (controlled dependence)
.23	Currently abstinent, but receiving treatment with aversive or blocking drugs
.24	Currently using the substance (active dependence)
.25	Continuous use
.26	Episodic use (dipsomania)
F1x.3	Withdrawal state
.30	Uncomplicated
.31	Convulsions
F1x.4	Withdrawal state with delirium
.40	Without convulsions
.41	With convulsions

(*continued*)

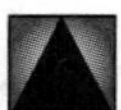

Table 9.2–2 (*continued*)

F1x.5	Psychotic disorder
.50	Schizophrenia-like
.51	Predominantly delusional
.52	Predominantly hallucinatory
.53	Predominantly polymorphic
.54	Predominantly depressive symptoms
.55	Predominantly manic symptoms
.56	Mixed
F1x.6	Amnestic syndrome
F1x.7	Residual and late-onset psychotic disorder
.70	Flashbacks
.71	Personality or behavior disorder
.72	Residual affective disorder
.73	Dementia
.74	Other persisting cognitive impairment
.75	Late-onset psychotic disorder
F1x.8	Other mental and behavioral disorders
F1x.9	Unspecified mental and behavioral disorder
F20 to F29	**Schizophrenia and schizotypal and delusional disorders**
F20	Schizophrenia
F20.0	Paranoid schizophrenia
F20.1	Hebephrenic schizophrenia
F20.2	Catatonic schizophrenia
F20.3	Undifferentiated schizophrenia
F20.4	Postschizophrenic depression
F20.5	Residual schizophrenia
F20.6	Simple schizophrenia
F20.8	Other schizophrenia
F20.9	Schizophrenia, unspecified
A fifth character may be used to classify course:	
.x0	Continuous
.x1	Episodic with progressive deficit
.x2	Episodic with stable deficit
.x3	Episodic remittent
.x4	Incomplete remission
.x5	Complete remission
.x8	Other
.x9	Period of observation less than 1 year
F21	Schizotypal disorder
F22	Persistent delusional disorders
F22.0	Delusional disorder
F22.8	Other persistent delusional disorders
F22.9	Persistent delusional disorder, unspecified
F23	Acute and transient psychotic disorders
F23.0	Acute polymorphic psychotic disorder without symptoms of schizophrenia
F23.1	Acute polymorphic psychotic disorder with symptoms of schizophrenia
F23.2	Acute schizophrenia-like psychotic disorder
F23.3	Other acute predominantly delusional psychotic disorders
F23.8	Other acute transient psychotic disorders
F23.9	Acute and transient psychotic disorders unspecified
A fifth character may be used to identify the presence or absence of associated acute stress:	
.x0	Without associated acute stress
.x1	With associated acute stress
F24	Induced delusional disorder
F25	Schizoaffective disorders
F25.0	Schizoaffective disorder, manic type
F25.1	Schizoaffective disorder, depressive type
F25.2	Schizoaffective disorder, mixed type
F25.8	Other schizoaffective disorders
F25.9	Schizoaffective disorder, unspecified
F28	Other nonorganic psychotic disorders
F29	Unspecified nonorganic psychosis
F30 to F39	**Mood (affective) disorders**
F30	Manic episode
F30.0	Hypomania
F30.1	Mania without psychotic symptoms
F30.2	Mania with psychotic symptoms
F30.8	Other manic episodes
F30.9	Manic episode, unspecified
F31	Bipolar affective disorder
F31.0	Bipolar affective disorder, current episode hypomanic
F31.1	Bipolar affective disorder, current episode manic without psychotic symptoms
F31.2	Bipolar affective disorder, current episode manic with psychotic symptoms
F31.3	Bipolar affective disorder, current episode mild or moderate depression
.30	Without somatic symptoms
.31	With somatic symptoms
F31.4	Bipolar affective disorder, current episode severe depression without psychotic symptoms
F31.5	Bipolar affective disorder, current episode severe depression with psychotic symptoms
F31.6	Bipolar affective disorder, current episode mixed
F31.7	Bipolar affective disorder, currently in remission
F31.8	Other bipolar affective disorders
F31.9	Bipolar affective disorder, unspecified
F32	Depressive episode
F32.0	Mild depressive episode
.00	Without somatic symptoms
.01	With somatic symptoms
F32.1	Moderate depressive episode
.10	Without somatic symptoms
.11	With somatic symptoms
F32.2	Severe depressive episode without psychotic symptoms
F32.3	Severe depressive episode with psychotic symptoms
F32.8	Other depressive episodes
F32.9	Depressive episode, unspecified
F33	Recurrent depressive disorder
F33.0	Recurrent depressive disorder, current episode mild
.00	Without somatic symptoms
.00	With somatic symptoms
F33.1	Recurrent depressive disorder, current episode moderate
.10	Without somatic symptoms
.11	With somatic symptoms
F33.2	Recurrent depressive disorder, current episode severe without psychotic symptoms
F33.3	Recurrent depressive disorder, current episode severe with psychotic symptoms

(*continued*)

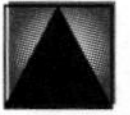

Table 9.2–2 (*continued*)

F33.4	Recurrent depressive disorder, currently in remission
F33.8	Other recurrent depressive disorders
F33.9	Recurrent depressive disorder, unspecified
F34	Persistent mood (affective) disorders
F34.0	Cyclothymia
F34.1	Dysthymia
F34.8	Other persistent mood (affective) disorders
F34.9	Persistent mood (affective) disorder, unspecified
F38	Other mood (affective) disorders
F38.0	Other single mood (affective) disorders
.00	Mixed affective episode
F38.1	Other recurrent mood (affective) disorders
.10	Recurrent brief depressive disorder
F38.8	Other specified mood (affective) disorders
F39	Unspecified mood (affective) disorder
F40 to F48	**Neurotic stress-related and somatoform disorders**
F40	Phobic anxiety disorders
F40.0	Agoraphobia
.00	Without panic disorder
.01	With panic disorder
F40.1	Social phobias
F40.2	Specific (isolated) phobias
F40.8	Other phobic anxiety disorders
F40.9	Phobic anxiety disorder, unspecified
F41	Other anxiety disorders
F41.0	Panic disorder (episodic paroxysmal anxiety)
F41.1	Generalized anxiety disorder
F41.2	Mixed anxiety and depressive disorder
F41.3	Other mixed anxiety disorders
F41.8	Other specified anxiety disorders
F41.9	Anxiety disorder, unspecified
F42	Obsessive-compulsive disorder
F42.0	Predominantly obsessional thoughts or ruminations
F42.1	Predominantly compulsive acts (obsessional rituals)
F42.2	Mixed obsessional thoughts and acts
F42.8	Other obsessive-compulsive disorders
F42.9	Obsessive-compulsive disorder, unspecified
F43	Reaction to severe stress, and adjustment disorders
F43.0	Acute stress reaction
F43.1	Posttraumatic stress disorder
F43.2	Adjustment disorders
.20	Brief depressive reaction
.21	Prolonged depressive reaction
.22	Mixed anxiety and depressive reaction
.23	With predominant disturbance of other emotions
.24	With predominant disturbance of conduct
.25	With mixed disturbance of emotions and conduct
.28	With other specified predominant symptoms
F43.8	Other reactions to severe stress
F43.9	Reaction to severe stress, unspecified
F44	Dissociative (conversion) disorders
F44.0	Dissociative amnesia
F44.1	Dissociative fugue
F44.2	Dissociative stupor
F44.3	Trance and possession disorders
F44.4	Dissociative motor disorders
F44.5	Dissociative convulsions
F44.6	Dissociative anesthesia and sensory loss
F44.7	Mixed dissociative (conversion) disorders
F44.8	Other dissociative (conversion) disorders
.80	Ganser syndrome
.81	Multiple personality disorder
.82	Transient dissociative (conversion) disorders occurring in childhood and adolescence
.88	Other specified dissociative (conversion) disorders
F44.9	Dissociative (conversion) disorder, unspecified
F45	Somatoform disorders
F45.0	Somatization disorder
F45.1	Undifferentiated somatoform disorder
F45.2	Hypochondriacal disorder
F45.3	Somatoform autonomic dysfunction
.30	Heart and cardiovascular system
.31	Upper gastrointestinal tract
.32	Lower gastrointestinal tract
.33	Respiratory system
.34	Genitourinary system
.38	Other organ or system
F45.4	Persistent somatoform pain disorder
F45.8	Other somatoform disorders
F45.9	Somatoform disorder, unspecified
F48	Other neurotic disorders
F48.0	Neurasthenia
F48.1	Depersonalization-derealization syndrome
F48.8	Other specified neurotic disorders
F48.9	Neurotic disorder, unspecified
F50 to F59	**Behavioral syndromes associated with physiological disturbances and physical factors**
F50	Eating disorders
F50.0	Anorexia nervosa
F50.1	Atypical anorexia nervosa
F50.2	Bulimia nervosa
F50.3	Atypical bulimia nervosa
F50.4	Overeating associated with other psychological disturbances
F50.5	Vomiting associated with other psychological disturbances
F50.8	Other eating disorders
F50.9	Eating disorder, unspecified
F51	Nonorganic sleep disorders
F51.0	Nonorganic insomnia
F51.1	Nonorganic hypersomnia
F51.2	Nonorganic disorder of the sleep-wake schedule
F51.3	Sleepwalking (somnambulism)
F51.4	Sleep terrors (night terrors)
F51.5	Nightmares
F51.8	Other nonorganic sleep disorders
F51.9	Nonorganic sleep disorder, unspecified
F52	Sexual dysfunction, not caused by organic disorder or disease
F52.0	Lack or loss of sexual desire
F52.1	Sexual aversion and lack of sexual enjoyment
.10	Sexual aversion
.11	Lack of sexual enjoyment
F52.2	Failure of genital response

(*continued*)

Table 9.2–2 (*continued*)

F52.3	Orgasmic dysfunction
F52.4	Premature ejaculation
F52.5	Nonorganic vaginismus
F52.6	Nonorganic dyspareunia
F52.7	Excessive sexual drive
F52.8	Other sexual dysfunction, not caused by organic disorder or disease
F52.9	Unspecified sexual dysfunction, not caused by organic disorder or disease
F53	Mental and behavioral disorders associated with the puerperium, not elsewhere classified
F53.0	Mild mental and behavioral disorders associated with the puerperium, not elsewhere classified
F53.1	Severe mental and behavioral disorders associated with the puerperium, not elsewhere classified
F53.8	Other mental and behavioral disorders associated with the puerperium, not elsewhere classified
F53.9	Puerperal mental disorder, unspecified
F54	Psychological and behavioral factors associated with disorders or diseases classified elsewhere
F55	Abuse of non–dependence-producing substances
F55.0	Antidepressants
F55.1	Laxatives
F55.2	Analgesics
F55.3	Antacids
F55.4	Vitamins
F55.5	Steroids or hormones
F55.6	Specific herbal or folk remedies
F55.8	Other substances that do not produce dependence
F55.9	Unspecified
F59	Unspecified behavioral syndromes associated with physiological disturbances and physical factors
F60 to F69	**Disorders of adult personality and behavior**
F60	Specific personality disorders
F60.0	Paranoid personality disorder
F60.1	Schizoid personality disorder
F60.2	Dissocial personality disorder
F60.3	Emotionally unstable personality disorder
.30	Impulsive type
.31	Borderline type
F60.4	Histrionic personality disorder
F60.5	Anankastic personality disorder
F60.6	Anxious (avoidant) personality disorder
F60.7	Dependent personality disorder
F60.8	Other specific personality disorders
F60.9	Personality disorder, unspecified
F61	Mixed and other personality disorders
F61.0	Mixed personality disorders
F61.1	Troublesome personality changes
F62	Enduring personality changes, not attributable to brain damage and disease
F62.0	Enduring personality change after catastrophic experience
F62.1	Enduring personality change after psychiatric illness
F62.8	Other enduring personality changes
F62.9	Enduring personality change, unspecified
F63	Habit and impulse disorders
F63.0	Pathological gambling
F63.1	Pathological fire-setting (pyromania)
F63.2	Pathological stealing (kleptomania)
F63.3	Trichotillomania
F63.8	Other habit and impulse disorders
F63.9	Habit and impulse disorder, unspecified
F64	Gender identity disorders
F64.0	Transsexualism
F64.1	Dual-role transvestism
F64.2	Gender identity disorder of childhood
F64.8	Other gender identity disorders
F64.9	Gender identity disorder, unspecified
F65	Disorders of sexual preference
F65.0	Fetishism
F65.1	Fetishistic transvestism
F65.2	Exhibitionism
F65.3	Voyeurism
F65.4	Pedophilia
F65.5	Sadomasochism
F65.6	Multiple disorders of sexual preference
F65.8	Other disorders of sexual preference
F65.9	Disorder of sexual preference, unspecified
F66	Psychological and behavioral disorders associated with sexual development and orientation
F66.0	Sexual maturation disorder
F66.1	Ego-dystonic sexual orientation
F66.2	Sexual relationship disorder
F66.8	Other psychosexual development disorders
F66.9	Psychosexual development disorder, unspecified
A fifth character may be used to indicate association with:	
.x0	Heterosexuality
.x1	Homosexuality
.x2	Bisexuality
.x8	Other, including prepubertal
F68	Other disorders of adult personality and behavior
F68.0	Elaboration of physical symptoms for psychological reasons
F68.1	Intentional production or feigning of symptoms or disabilities, physical or psychological (factitious disorder)
F68.8	Other specified disorders of adult personality and behavior
F69	Unspecified disorder of adult personality and behavior
F70 to F79	**Mental retardation**
F70	Mild mental retardation
F71	Moderate mental retardation
F72	Severe mental retardation
F73	Profound mental retardation
F78	Other mental retardation
F79	Unspecified mental retardation
A fourth character may be used to specify the extent of associated behavioral impairment:	
F7x.0	No, or minimal, impairment of behavior
F7x.1	Significant impairment of behavior requiring attention or treatment

(*continued*)

Table 9.2–2 (*continued*)

Code	Category	Code	Category
F7x.8	Other impairments of behavior	F91.2	Socialized conduct disorder
F7x.9	Without mention of impairment of behavior	F91.3	Oppositional defiant disorder
F80 to F89	**Disorders of psychological development**	F91.8	Other conduct disorders
F80	Specific development disorders of speech and language	F91.9	Conduct disorder, unspecified
F80.0	Specific speech articulation disorder	F92	Mixed disorders of conduct and emotions
F80.1	Expressive language disorder	F92.0	Depressive conduct disorder
F80.2	Receptive language disorder	F92.8	Other mixed disorders of conduct and emotions
F80.3	Acquired aphasia with epilepsy (Landau-Kleffner syndrome)	F92.9	Mixed disorder of conduct and emotions, unspecified
F80.8	Other developmental disorders of speech and language	F93	Emotional disorders with onset specific to childhood
F80.9	Developmental disorder of speech and language, unspecified	F93.0	Separation anxiety disorder of childhood
F81	Specific developmental disorders of scholastic skills	F93.1	Phobic anxiety disorder of childhood
F81.0	Specific reading disorder	F93.2	Social anxiety disorder of childhood
F81.1	Specific spelling disorder	F93.3	Sibling rivalry disorder
F81.2	Specific disorder of arithmetic skills	F93.8	Other childhood emotional disorders
F81.3	Mixed disorder of scholastic skills	F93.9	Childhood emotional disorder, unspecified
F81.8	Other developmental disorders of scholastic skills	F94	Disorders of social functioning with onset specific to childhood and adolescence
F81.9	Developmental disorder of scholastic skills, unspecified	F94.0	Elective mutism
F82	Specific developmental disorder of motor function	F94.1	Reactive attachment disorder of childhood
F83	Mixed specific developmental disorders	F94.2	Disinhibited attachment disorder of childhood
F84	Pervasive developmental disorders	F94.8	Other childhood disorders of social functioning
F84.0	Childhood autism	F94.9	Childhood disorders of social functioning, unspecified
F84.1	Atypical autism	F95	Tic disorders
F84.2	Rett's syndrome	F95.0	Transient tic disorder
F84.3	Other childhood disintegrative disorder	F95.1	Chronic motor or vocal tic disorder
F84.4	Overactive disorder associated with mental retardation and stereotyped movements	F95.2	Combined vocal and multiple motor tic disorder (Tourette's syndrome)
F84.5	Asperger's syndrome	F95.8	Other tic disorders
F84.8	Other pervasive developmental disorders	F95.9	Tic disorder, unspecified
F84.9	Pervasive developmental disorder, unspecified	F98	Other behavioral and emotional disorders with onset usually occurring in childhood and adolescence
F88	Other disorders of psychological development	F98.0	Nonorganic enuresis
F89	Unspecified disorder of psychological development	F98.1	Nonorganic encopresis
F90 to F98	**Behavioral and emotional disorders with onset usually occurring in childhood and adolescence**	F98.2	Feeding disorder of infancy and childhood
F90	Hyperkinetic disorders	F98.3	Pica of infancy and childhood
F90.0	Disturbance of activity and attention	F98.4	Stereotyped movement disorders
F90.1	Hyperkinetic conduct disorder	F98.5	Stuttering (stammering)
F90.8	Other hyperkinetic disorders	F98.6	Cluttering
F90.9	Hyperkinetic disorder, unspecified	F98.8	Other specified behavioral and emotional disorders with onset usually occurring in childhood and adolescence
F91	Conduct disorders	F98.9	Unspecified behavioral and emotional disorders with onset usually occurring in childhood and adolescence
F91.0	Conduct disorder confined to the family context		
F91.1	Unsocialized conduct disorder	F99	Unspecified mental disorder

From World Health Organization: *The ICD-10 Classification of Mental and Behavioral Disorders: Clinical Descriptions and Diagnostic Guidelines.* Geneva: World Health Organization; 1992, with permission.

transient psychotic disorders, which encompasses a heterogeneous set of acute-onset and relatively short-lived psychoses (polymorphic with or without schizophrenic symptoms, acute schizophrenia-like, and others) reportedly frequent in industrially developing countries (where most of the world population lives).

F3: Mood (Affective) Disorders The fundamental disturbance in the F3 class is a change in mood or affect, usually involving depression or elation, often accompanied by a change in level of activity. Included here are manic episode, bipolar affective disorder (characterized by recurrent episodes involving depression and elation), depressive episode, recurrent depressive disorder, persistent mood disorder (cyclothymia and dysthymia), and other and unspecified mood disorders.

F4: Neurotic, Stress-Related, and Somatoform Disorders The F4 grouping is based on a historical concept of neurosis that presumes a substantial role played by psychological causation and that mixtures of symptoms are common, particularly in less severe forms often seen in primary care. Included in this book are phobic anxiety and other anxiety disorders, OCD, reactions to severe stress and adjustment disorders, dissociative and conversion disorders, somatoform disorders, and other neurotic disorders (e.g., neurasthenia and depersonalization-derealization syndrome).

F5: Behavioral Syndromes Associated with Physiological Disturbances and Physical Factors

Included in the F5 class are eating disorders, nonorganic sleep disorders, sexual dysfunction, mental disorders associated with the puerperium and not elsewhere classified, psychological factors influencing physical disorders, and abuse of non–dependence-producing substances (e.g., antidepressants, hormones, analgesics, and many folk remedies).

F6: Disorders of Adult Personality and Behavior The F6 class includes clinical conditions and behavioral patterns that tend to persist and the expression of an individual's characteristic lifestyle and mode of relating to self and others. The main subclass involves personality disorders, which are deeply ingrained and enduring behavior patterns, manifesting as inflexible responses to a broad range of personal and social situations. An innovative category is that of enduring personality change, neither developmental nor attributable to brain damage or disease and usually emerging after catastrophic experiences or another psychiatric illness. The broad class also includes impulse, gender identity, sexual preference, and sexual development and orientation disorders.

F7: Mental Retardation Mental retardation, one of the oldest in the history of psychiatric classifications, involves arrested or incomplete mental development, characterized by impaired cognitive, language, motor, and social skills evidenced during the person's formative period and contributing to the overall level of intelligence. Its subcategories correspond to various levels of severity: mild, moderate, severe, and profound mental retardation. Extent of behavioral impairment is also coded.

F8: Disorders of Psychological Development Disorders of psychological development are characterized, as a class, by the following attributes: onset during infancy or childhood, impairment or delay of functions connected to the maturation of the central nervous system (CNS), and a steady course unlike the remissions and relapses usual in many mental disorders. The functions affected most frequently include language, visuospatial skills, and motor coordination. A major subclass encompasses a variety of specific developmental disorders, classified by the abilities involved: speech and language, scholastic skills, and motor function. The other major subclass corresponds to pervasive developmental disorders, many of which are more saliently characterized by deviance rather than delay in development but always involving some degree of delay. Most conspicuous here are childhood and atypical autistic disorder and Rett's syndrome and other childhood disintegrative disorders.

F9: Behavioral and Emotional Disorders with Onset Usually Occurring in Childhood and Adolescence The complex F9 class complements F7 and F8. Child-onset disorders included first are hyperkinetic disorders characterized by early onset, overactive and poorly modulated behavior associated with marked inattention, lack of persistent task involvement, and pervasiveness over situations and time. Conduct disorders are defined by a repetitive and persistent pattern of dissocial, aggressive, or defiant behavior. Also included in this class are emotional, social-functioning, tic, and other disorders usually starting in childhood or adolescence.

Presentations of ICD-10 by Definitional Detail

The full ICD-10 classification of mental disorders has three presentations corresponding to various degrees of definitional detail, aimed at serving different purposes and uses:

1. An abbreviated glossary containing the principal features of each disorder, for the use of statistical coders and medical librarians, published within the ICD-10 general volume
2. Clinical descriptions and diagnostic guidelines, containing widely accepted characterizations of an intermediate level of specificity, intended for regular patient care and broad clinical studies
3. Diagnostic criteria for research, characterized by more precise and rigorous definitions

Multiaxial Presentation of ICD-10 Since the late 1960s, the WHO has advanced some important initiatives on multiaxial diagnosis. One was the *Multiaxial Classification of Child Psychiatric Disorders*, first designed in 1969 and revised and expanded several times since then. Its 1975 five-axial version encompassed the following axes: psychiatric disorders, physical disorders, developmental disorders, intellectual level, and abnormal psychosocial situations. Another was the *Triaxial Classification of Health Problems for Primary Care*, which contained axes on physical, psychopathological, and social problems.

On these precedents and many others from the international literature, in the late 1980s, the WHO Mental Health Division began preparing the Multiaxial Presentation of ICD-10. The conceptual bases of this development included a critical analysis of more than 20 published multiaxial proposals originating in countries spanning three continents, which revealed important commonalties in the clinical domains covered. A second developmental principle was simplicity in the multiaxial schema, to enhance the prospects of its effective use across the world. The third principle was to base the instruments for axial assessment on components of the ICD-10 family of classifications, which had benefited from wide international consultations and field trials.

The Multiaxial Presentation of ICD-10 is composed of three axes: I, clinical diagnoses; II, disablements; and III, contextual factors. The number of axes is lower than the four or five usually included in published multiaxial schemata and constitutes a condensation of those axes most frequently included in multiaxial proposals published in the international literature, which affords a measure of content validity to the schema. The value of the simplicity of the schema is enhanced by its potential for generalization beyond psychiatric practice. Information on clinical pathology, disablement, and contextual factors appears to be relevant to all health care.

Axis I: Clinical Diagnoses Axis I accommodates mental and nonmental (general medical) disorders, underlining a fundamental commonality among all illnesses. All significant disorders identifiable in a given individual are to be listed and coded according to chapters I through XX (the disease chapters) in the core classification of ICD-10 (Table 9.2–1).

Axis II: Disablements Axis II appraises the consequences of illness in terms of impairment in the performance of basic social roles. The assessment instrument is a shortened version of the WHO Disability Assessment Scale, whose structure was condensed into four dimensions or areas: (1) personal care, (2) occupational functioning (as remunerated worker, student, or homemaker), (3) functioning with family (assessing the regularity and quality of interactions with relatives and household members), and (4) broad social behaviors (interaction with other individuals and the community at large and leisure activities).

Axis III: Contextual Factors Axis III attempts to portray the context of illness in terms of several ecological domains. These include problems related to the family or primary support group, general social environment, education, employment, housing and economic circumstances, legal issues, family history of illness, and personal life management and lifestyle. Assessment involves identifying problematic broad categories and recording specific factors. This structure is based on ICD-10 Chapter XXI (factors influencing health status and contact with health services).

Primary Health Version The ICD-10 Primary Health Version is a simple, brief classification arrangement compatible with and translatable into the ICD-10 standard classification of mental disorders (Table 9.2–3). It is linked with management aids prepared for use by primary care practitioners. The short list of categories was selected principally on the basis of importance to public health and the availability of effective and acceptable management. The centerpiece of the package is a set of pocket-sized flip-cards, one for each selected category. One side of the flip-card exhibits assessment information, such as presenting complaints, diagnostic features, and differential diagnosis. The other side displays management guidelines, such as essential information for patient and family, specific counseling for the patient and family, medication, and specialist consultation. Additional elements of the package include flow charts, symptom indexes, and a computerized version.

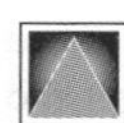

Table 9.2–3
ICD-10 Primary Health Care Categories

F00[a]	Dementia
F05	Delirium
F10	Alcohol use disorders
F11[a]	Drug use disorders
F17.1	Tobacco use
F20[a]	Chronic psychotic disorders
F23[a]	Acute psychotic disorders
F31	Bipolar disorder
F32[a]	Depression
F40[a]	Phobic disorders
F41.0	Panic disorder
F41.1	Generalized anxiety
F41.2	Mixed anxiety and depression
F43[a]	Adjustment disorder
F44[a]	Dissociative disorder (conversion hysteria)
F45	Unexplained somatic complaints
F48.0	Neurasthenia
F50[a]	Eating disorders
F51[a]	Sleep problems
F52	Sexual disorders
F70	Mental retardation
F90	Hyperkinetic (attention deficit) disorder
F91	Conduct disorder
F98.0	Enuresis

[a]More than one ICD-10 code is included.

Child and Adolescent Multiaxial Presentation of ICD-10 Chapter V Published in 1996, the version of the multiaxial presentation of ICD-10 Chapter V for use with children and adolescents is organized around six axes to serve the needs of clinicians working with this population. The taxonomic organization of the disorder categories, as well as the clinical description of each category or subcategory, follows the one presented by the clinical descriptions and diagnostic guidelines version of Chapter V for those conditions that are most relevant for children and adolescents. However, the text is reorganized to group the disorders in the particular axes this version proposes. For disorders less common in children, a mere listing of categories is included, or the text from the short version of Chapter V included in the full ICD-10 is used. The six axes that compose this system are the following: I. clinical psychiatric syndromes; II. specific disorders of psychological development; III. intellectual level; IV. medical conditions; V. associated abnormal psychosocial situations; and VI. global assessment of psychosocial disability.

Axis I describes most of the disorders included in chapter V of ICD-10, starting with the pervasive developmental disorders and the behavioral and emotional disorders with onset usually occurring in childhood or adolescence. It also includes a code (XX) for the specification of a lack of any psychiatric condition in the patient being evaluated. Axes II, III, and IV organize the corresponding disorders. Axis V, associated abnormal psychosocial situations, comprises a set of contextual factors included in Chapter XXI of ICD-10 as Z codes. Axis VI, global assessment of psychosocial disability, is an important addition in this multiaxial schema.

ADAPTATIONS OF ICD-10

The ICD-10 Classification of Mental and Behavioral Disorders is being accepted by most countries and by the WPA as the international standard in the field for statistical reporting and for clinical care and research. Emerging now is the need to harmonize international communication with recognition of cultural diversity and specific local requirements. To express this perception, several local (national and regional) adaptations, glossaries, and annotations of ICD-10 are being developed and published.

The rationale and arguments for the development of these local glossaries include the following:

- Local glossaries from across the world can serve as the fundamental bases for the preparation of bottom-up international diagnostic systems.
- Local glossaries, through their attention to various aspects of clinical reality, can facilitate the implementation of a comprehensive biopsychosocial framework, away from reductionisms of different types.
- Local glossaries can reflect the cultural integrity of different countries and human groups and can promote the value of their health-related concepts and practices.
- Local glossaries can embody and transmit the intellectual contributions of national and regional scientists and professional leaders for the benefit of the field around the world.
- Local glossaries can facilitate the effective use of international diagnostic systems by adapting the various components of these systems to national patterns and needs.

The best known of these national versions is the APA's DSM-IV-TR. In 1980, the APA published the innovative DSM-III, characterized by a phenomenological emphasis on the conceptualization and organization of mental disorders, the use of explicit diagnostic criteria, and a multiaxial formulation. It acquired wide international visibility and significantly influenced the field of psychiatric classification. After preparations for ICD-10 were started by WHO, the APA initiated the development of DSM-IV-TR, attempting this time to keep close to the international standard (which was already incorporating much of the methodological features advanced by DSM-III). Perhaps the principal attribute of DSM-IV-TR is a scholarly emphasis in its development of the basis of critical literature reviews, reanalysis of existing databases, and focused field trials.

Cuban Glossary of Psychiatry Development of the *Cuban Glossaries of Psychiatry* (GCs) started in 1975 to reflect the realities and needs of Cuba in particular, within the general framework of Latin American culture, and as an effort to contribute to the bottom-up building of international classification. The GCs have furthermore attempted to harmonize the general, represented by the existing ICD, with the local. Therefore, its authors consider the glossary to be the basic ICD-10 with only the changes and additions needed to ensure its applicability and usefulness for psychiatric care in Cuba.

As a broader conceptual framework, the GCs represent a syncretism of local historical traditions, the existing social and clinical reality of the region, and international scientific contributions. Among the many specifically Latin American contributions considered for the preparation of the GCs were the following: Honorio Delgado, a Peruvian psychiatrist, published the influential *Curso de Psiquiatría* in the middle of the 20th century, with a masterful presentation of psychopathological phenomenology and nosology. In 1954, in Rio de Janeiro, Leme Lopes published the innovative *Dimensoes do Diagnóstico Psiquiátrico,* with a pioneering multiaxial formulation of clinical conditions. The Cuban psychiatrist José Bustamante published in 1975, with anthropologist A. Santa Cruz, what can be arguably considered the first textbook of transcultural psychiatry in the world. Finally, the work of Carlos Alberto Seguín from Peru, with his volume on folkloric psychiatry, is emblematic of the rich Latin American contributions to the description of popular or culture-bound syndromes in the region.

Early Editions of the *Cuban Glossary of Psychiatry* The 1st edition of the GC (GC-1), published in 1975, constitutes an adaptation of the eighth revision of the ICD (ICD-8). Its architect was Carlos Acosta-Nodal, professor of psychiatry at Havana University, working under the auspices of Eduardo Ordaz, director of Havana Psychiatric Hospital. The GC-1 was composed of 69 adaptations of ICD-8. The 2nd edition of the GC (GC-2), published in 1983, was an adaptation of ICD-9. Its development was again chaired by Acosta-Nodal. It contained 90 modifications of ICD-9 in addition to substantive chapters devoted to historical, theoretical, and clinical aspects of psychiatry.

Third Edition of the *Cuban Glossary of Psychiatry* The current 3rd edition of the GC (GC-3) was developed under the chairmanship of Angel Otero-Ojeda from Havana University and the Havana Psychiatric Hospital (Fig. 9.2–1). It includes a number of contributions on the diagnosis of mental disorders as experienced and presented in Cuba. These encompass general psychiatry and child psychiatry. A basic objective was to maintain as much consistency as possible with ICD-10. In line with this, the coding system of ICD-10 was faithfully followed. Contributions and changes were incorporated through the employment of fifth digits in the diagnostic code or through the use of codes not used in ICD-10. The ICD-10 diagnostic guidelines for the various psychiatric disorders were also respected to the largest extent possible. In some cases, supplemental text was added. References to DSM-IV and to the ICD-10 criteria for research were often made. Of note, the GC-3 encourages diagnostic formulations based on the judicious use of all information

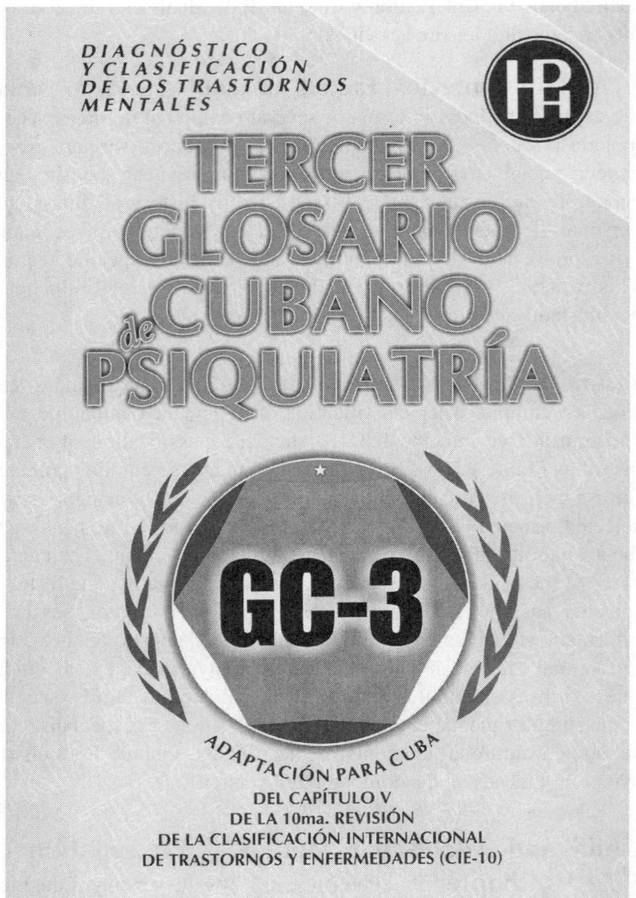

FIGURE 9.2–1 Cover of the *Third Cuban Glossary of Psychiatry,* 2000. (From Otero-Ojeda AA, ed. *Tercer Glosario Cubano de Psiquiatría.* Havana, Cuba: Hospital Psiquiátrico de La Habana; 2000, with permission.)

available and allows experienced clinicians to formulate diagnoses without strictly adhering to standard diagnostic criteria.

An interesting chapter of GC-3 is that on *syndromes of difficult placement* (sometimes referred to as *culture-based syndromes*). This includes widely known folk syndromes, such as amok, brain fag, and *susto,* as well as some syndromes and idioms of distress reported by Cuban psychiatrists. Illustrative of the latter is *abríu,* which refers to the case of certain children believed to have the power to exercise a malign supernatural influence on their relatives, particularly siblings, who, as a consequence, can experience various illnesses and even die.

Additions made in the main body of GC-3 include the following: (1) "neurotic behavior" as a qualifier in broad categories, such as mood disorders and neurotic, stress-related, and somatoform disorders; (2) diagnosis based on premorbid features for disorders of chronic or episodic source in broad categories, such as schizophrenia and related disorders and mood disorders; and (3) risky behaviors, such as suicide or substance use, which are of particular relevance to community psychiatry. An illustrative deletion was dementia in children.

Some of the most innovative contributions of GC-3 involve its multiaxial schema, which builds on the standard multiaxial presentation of ICD-10. The GC-3 multiaxial schema is as follows:

Axis I: clinical diagnosis. Mental and nonmental disorders are included as in ICD-10's multiaxial system.

Axis II: disabilities. Disablements in personal care, occupational functioning, functioning with family, and broader social functioning are included following the guidelines of ICD-10's multiaxial presentation.

Axis III: psychoenvironmental factors (adverse). Included in this axis are contextual problems listed under Axis III of the WHO's multiaxial presentation of ICD-10.

Axis IV: psychoenvironmental factors (other). Illustrative of factors considered in this axis are living alone and being particularly practical or romantic.

Axis V: maladaptive behavior and psychological needs. Included in this axis are conditions such as hypertrophic affective needs, indecisiveness, and difficulties managing hostility.

Axis VI: other significant factors. Included in this axis is miscellaneous information, such as that resulting from laboratory tests and responses to therapeutic interventions.

Latin American Guide for Psychiatric Diagnosis

Work on the GC-3 stimulated the Section on Diagnosis and Classification of the Latin American Psychiatric Association (APAL), under the leadership of Carlos Berganza (San Carlos University, Guatemala), Miguel Jorge (Escola Paulista de Medicina, Brazil), Angel Otero-Ojeda (Havana University, Cuba), and Juan E. Mezzich (Mount Sinai School of Medicine in New York and Cayetano Heredia Peruvian University in Lima) to organize the preparation of the 1st *Latin American Guide for Psychiatric Diagnosis* (GLADP) as a Latin American annotation of ICD-10. The draft was finished recently and was presented to the leadership of APAL in Guatemala City, during the XXII Latin American Congress of Psychiatry for publication and distribution.

Development of the GLADP Participants in the development of the GLADP included more than 100 psychiatrists, psychologists, and anthropologists from most countries in Latin America. They were organized into 17 work groups in charge of developing a knowledge base for issues relevant to diagnosis and classification in Latin America, such as identifying features of culture and psychiatry in the region and developing a comprehensive diagnostic formulation useful for clinicians in Latin America. Other relevant tasks included critical reviews, lexicological adjustments, annotations of ICD-10's major and specific nosological categories, and the identification and taxonomic organization of the most important cultural syndromes and idioms of distress in the region.

The project started in 1994 with a survey of 572 psychiatrists from seven Latin American countries to establish patterns of diagnostic practice in clinical work, research, and education. Overall, 91 percent of those surveyed indicated that they were using a systematic criteria-based diagnostic system in their everyday work. APA's revised third edition of the DSM (DSM-III-R) was reported as the most widely used, with ICD-9 following closely. ICD-10 was being used more frequently than DSM-IV. This was explained, in part, by the fact that DSM-IV had just been published, and the WPA was making an effort to promote the use of ICD-10 in Latin America. Training in these diagnostic systems was not satisfactory, but interest in receiving training was high among their users.

After this, the APAL Section on Diagnosis and Classification, under the leadership of Miguel Jorge, held a number of seminars at different national and regional meetings throughout Latin America to enroll a wide participation of mental health practitioners in the region. Four major conferences were carried out. The first one took place in Havana, in 1998, with the participation of more than 40 experts from Latin America, the United States, and Europe. Here, the group developed a general historical and cultural framework for the system, and the work groups were organized. The second one was on Margarita Island, Venezuela, where the first draft developed by the work groups was presented. The third major conference took place in Guadalajara, Jalisco, Mexico, in August 2000, and the latest conferences took place in Guatemala City in August, 2002, where major revisions to the text were carried out.

Main Components The GLADP is composed of four main parts: part I, historical and cultural framework; part II, comprehensive diagnostic process and formulation; part III, psychiatric nosology (includes the major classes of ICD-10 and the Latin American cultural syndromes); and part IV, appendixes (five are included: [1] lexicological glossary, [2] concepts and proposals for further study, [3] bibliography, [4] list of participants, and [5] supporters).

HISTORICAL AND CULTURAL FRAMEWORK Latin American people are heterogeneous in their ethnic, social, and cultural compositions; however, it is clear that they share a common history, language, and the way in which they view and experience their realities. Specific cultural dimensions, such as machismo, mestizaje (mixed ethnicity), and mesoginy (rejection of own origin), likely influence the way in which people adapt (successfully or otherwise) to their circumstances and give rise to behavioral manifestations reflecting pathogenic and pathoplastic influences of culture on mental disorders and other idioms of distress in the Latin American population. Of critical importance, cultural syndromes autochthonous to Latin America and receiving marginal attention in diagnostic manuals elsewhere seem clinically and epidemiologically relevant for the region. *Susto*, also known as *pasmo*, *espanto*, *jami*, and *mal de aire*, has been reported throughout the entire region. *Mal de ojo, ataque de nervios*, and others add to the list of disorders that significantly affect Latin American people living in the region or abroad and that need to be adequately described to help clinicians everywhere effectively diagnose and treat them.

COMPREHENSIVE DIAGNOSTIC ASSESSMENT AND FORMULATION The GLADP incorporates a comprehensive diagnostic model that, developed conjointly with that of the WPA IGDA, includes two components for its use: (1) a standardized diagnostic formulation and (2) an idiographic personalized formulation. A format for practical and convenient registration and codification of all relevant clinical information by the user is also included.

PSYCHIATRIC NOSOLOGY Psychiatric nosology is comprised of two components: (1) the major classes and specific categories and subcategories of ICD-10 (WHO, 1992) and (2) the organization and description of the most relevant cultural syndromes in Latin America. GLADP respects the organization and architecture of the ICD-10 nosologic system, and includes qualifying statements clearly identified as annotations to alert clinicians on the application of such categories and subcategories to Latin American people.

APPENDICES A lexicological glossary orients the users of the system on the meanings of a number of key terms for different countries in the region. Major disagreements with the architecture or the diagnostic criteria of the ICD that were expressed by participants were included in an appendix on concepts and proposals for further study, which may also inform modifications to international diagnosis systems in the future.

French Classification for Child and Adolescent Mental Disorders

After the publication of DSM-III, French child psychiatrists became concerned about its effect on their clinical practice by the emphasis that the new diagnostic system was placing on the cross sectional consideration of isolated symptoms over structural psychopathological configurations. In an effort to present French child psychiatrists with an alternative diagnostic model, a task force led by Roger Mises published, in 1988, the *French Classification for Child and Adolescent Mental Disorders* (CFTMEA). The most recent revision of this classification is now in the process of validation.

An important objective of the CFTMEA was to find definitions and diagnostic criteria of the childhood mental disorders in line with the clinical orientation of French child psychiatry. The taxonomic organization of clinical categories was based on a psychopathological approach that included an appraisal of potentials and prognosis. Because treatment in child psychiatry often offers an opportunity to change the diagnosis formulated during the first evaluation of the patient, it was considered helpful to give special consideration to clinical and psychopathological indicators of the status of a disorder as fixed or progressive and its potential consequences on the patient's mental health in the future.

CFTMEA has a wide acceptance among French child psychiatrists of diverse theoretical orientations, has been validated broadly, and is amply used in clinical, epidemiological, and outcome studies in France. It incorporates concepts of disability assessment, it proposes a biaxial approach to diagnosis, and its glossary is more inclusive than those of DSM and ICD systems without relying on symptom checklists.

CFTMEA Biaxial System The French classification is organized around two independent axes: I. basic clinical categories; and II. associated and possibly etiological factors. Axis I contains nine basic clinical categories, as follows: (1) autism and psychotic disorders; (2) neurotic disorders; (3) borderline and personality disorders; (4) reactive disorders; (5) mental retardation; (6) specific developmental disorders or disorders of instrumental functions; (7) behavior and conduct disorders, including disorders linked to the use of alcohol and other drugs; (8) psychosomatic disorders; and (9) variations from normality. Axis II divides the associated and possibly etiological factors into two headings: (1) organic factors (included here are prenatal factors, perinatal risk factors, genetic disorders, and others) and (2) environmental factors (such as mental disorders in the family; affective, educational, social, and cultural deficits; neglect and abuse; affective loses; and others).

How to Use the CFTMEA After a thorough evaluation of the patient, the clinician is asked to choose a main clinical category among the first four basic clinical categories of Axis I, which are considered to be mutually exclusive. Once this selection is considered (whether a category can be identified or not), the clinician is asked to select a complementary category among the last five basic clinical categories, which are considered not mutually exclusive. Once the clinical categories have been coded, the clinician must consider factors considered of etiological importance and others associated to the basic diagnostic categories.

Chinese Classification of Mental Disorders In China, contemporary attempts to classify mental disorders began around 1958. The first classificatory schema was published in 1979 and later was named the *Chinese Classification of Mental Disorders* (CCMD), first edition (CCMD-1) in 1981. Under the influence of the DSM and ICD systems, a number of subsequent revisions culminated in the publication of the second edition of the CCMD (CCMD-2) in 1989, the revised edition of the CCMD (CCMD-2-R) in 1995, and the third edition of the CCMD (CCMD-3) (Fig. 9.2–2) in 2001. For the first time in China, operationalized criteria for a broad range of diagnostic categories have become available. Because China has more than one-fifth of the world's population, knowledge of the CCMD is important to a broad-based psychopathology in general. Chinese people also constitute one of the fastest growing ethnic minority groups in Western societies, so understanding the CCMD may attune clinicians to certain Chinese forms of distress in an intercultural treatment context.

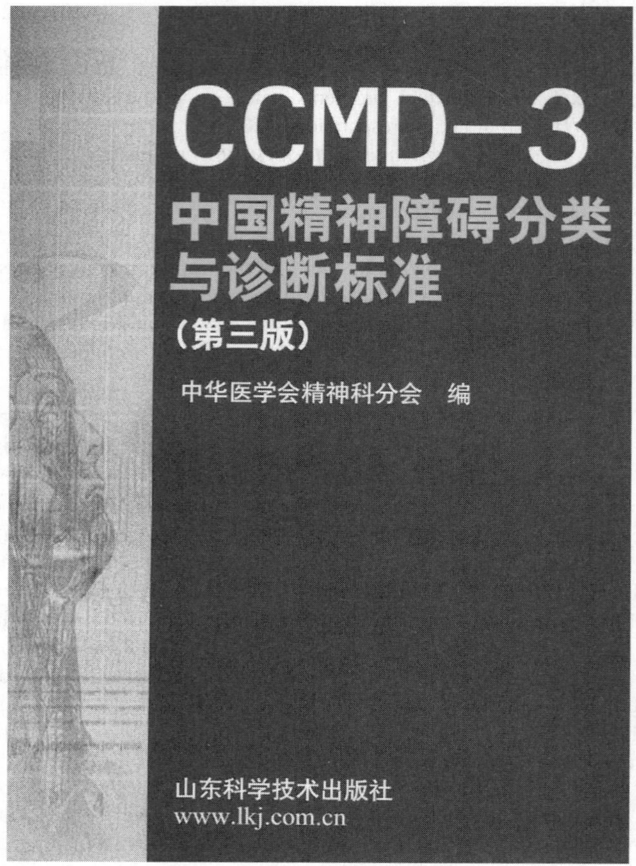

FIGURE 9.2–2 Cover of the *Chinese Classification of Mental Disorders*, 3rd ed. (From Chinese Psychiatric Association. *The Chinese Classification of Mental Disorders*. 3rd ed. Shandong, China: Shandong Publishing House of Science and Technology; 2001, with permission.)

In devising the CCMD, Chinese psychiatrists sought to harmonize with the international classification and to sustain a nosology that is useful in a vast and heterogeneous country. As a result, the CCMD and the ICD-10 share a broadly comparable architecture. However, inasmuch as symptom recognition and taxonomic strategy in psychiatry reflect the cultural norms and values of the society in which they are embedded, this blending is legitimately incomplete. The CCMD-2-R is a concise handbook of 238 pages that contains the equivalent or closest ICD-9 and ICD-10 codes (crosswalks) alongside the diagnostic headings. It contains a number of cross-culturally salient features, including particular additions (*qi-gong*–induced mental disorders and traveling psychosis), deletions (somatoform disorders, pathological gambling, and a number of personality and sexual disorders), retentions (unipolar mania and neurosis), and variations (neurasthenia, depressive neurosis, and anorexia nervosa) of standard diagnostic categories. A number of field trials have indicated adequate reliability and validity for the Chinese classification.

Third Edition of the Chinese Classification (CCMD-3) Published in April, 2001 (Fig. 9.2–2), in Chinese and English, the CCMD-3 incorporates major modifications relative to its latest predecessor, the CCMD-2-R, published 6 years earlier. It is substantially influenced by the ICD-10 and DSM-IV but contains locally salient features that are absent in the international systems. The field trials for CCMD-3 involved 114 researchers and clinicians from 41 hospitals, assessing 1,538 adult subjects and 773 child and adolescent subjects throughout the country. Reaffirming what have been the principles behind the Chinese nosological efforts, the authors propose as the main principles of the third revision the following: (1) to improve the service for patients and to meet the needs of society, (2) to fit in with Chinese cultural background and tradition, (3) to maintain the superiority of CCMD-3 to previous versions, (4) to match ICD and DSM systems as much as possible, and (5) to be concise and practical. As in its predecessor, the classification in CCMD-3 is mainly symptomatic and, to a lesser extent, etiological, respecting the taxonomic organization of ICD-10. Whenever specification of a disorder proves difficult, this is coded only as 9 (other or unspecified), instead of using the ICD-10 codes 8 (other) and 9 (unspecified).

Addition of Culture-Specific Diagnostic Categories

ICD-10 and DSM-IV lack a coded classification of culture-bound syndromes, which is often cited as a limitation of international classifications of mental disorders. By contrast, the CCMD-3 includes, illustratively, *qi-gong*–induced mental disorder as a culture-related mental disorder. *Qi-gong* is a popular trance-based exercise and healing system that consists of meditational and diverse styles of movement exercises. It is induced by using a culture-syntonic set of suggestions based on the Chinese concept of *qi* (vital energy). *Qi-gong*–induced mental disorder is believed to arise from inappropriate or excessive application of *qi-gong* or by inability to terminate the *qi-gong.* This causes the flow of *qi* to deviate from the *jing luo* conduits and to become *fire,* which may result in a variety of symptoms that do not fit into one coherent syndrome recognized in ICD-10 or DSM-IV-TR. These include *qi*-related somatic discomforts, uncontrolled motor activity, anxiety, fright, weeping, irritability, delusions, identity disturbance, hallucinations, mania, depression, and suicidal, bizarre, and violent behavior. The condition is usually brief. Treatment consists of a short course of tranquilizers and education about the proper way of practicing *qi-gong.* Relapse is uncommon.

In the Western psychiatric literature, psychosis related to traveling is uncommonly reported and is usually confined to air travel among subjects with a preexisting history of mental disorder. By contrast, the category of traveling psychosis (*lutu jinsheng bing*) arose from reports of acute psychosis developing among thousands of rural migrants who traveled in severely crammed trains over long distances in search of jobs in richer regions of China. Its principal manifestations include an acute onset, perplexity, disturbed consciousness, anxiety, persecutory delusions, horrifying illusions or hallucinations, motor excitement, impulsive and suicidal jumping off the train, and injuring others. In most cases, termination of travel, rest, and renourishment lead to recovery within a few hours to a few days. A personal or family history of mental disorder is rare. Although traveling psychosis may have an organic cause (e.g., hypercapnia, sleep deprivation, fatigue, and dehydration), its origin must be seen in the context of China's rapid market reforms, which result in marked economic regionalism and massive domestic migration. Granting traveling psychosis a special nosological status in CCMD-3 is expected to promote research into its prevention (e.g., improved conditions for traveling and regulation of migration). It also serves judicial functions, because offenders with this diagnosis may receive a better-informed verdict.

Deletion of Culturally Inappropriate Categories

Despite the common belief that Chinese people are prone to somatization, almost the whole block of somatoform disorder in ICD-10 and DSM-IV was excluded from the CCMD-2-R based on cultural reasons. However, they were again included within the group of neuroses, along with phobic disorders and neurasthenia in CCMD-3, reflecting a higher degree of compatibility with the international systems, as well as cultural changes in Chinese society. Several factors have made it difficult for Chinese psychiatrists to apply the category of somatoform disorders. Chinese patients, if given the opportunity, readily communicate dysphoria and relate somatic symptoms to psychosocial stressors. Rather than being mutually exclusive, their somatic and emotional symptoms are highly intercorrelated. Clinically, their somatization may be considered a context-dependent strategy of engaging the concern of physicians who often work at overcrowded clinics. Moreover, the hybrid (one-half Greek and one-half Latin) word *somatoform* is a terminological puzzlement to Chinese psychiatrists, who find that neuroses (including neurasthenia) are clinically more useful categories for engaging patients in treatment.

> Mrs. N. S. was a 35-year-old lower–social class housewife who presented to a psychiatric clinic with a mixture of symptoms associated with significant impairment. These included fullness in the head, weakness, worries, insomnia, cold intolerance, and difficulty in breathing for 2 years. She had previously worked as a clerk but quit to become a full-time housewife after marriage. Exploration revealed that she was burdened with caring for a teenage daughter and a 10-year-old son with childhood autistic disorder. She was also worried about the fidelity of her emotionally disengaged husband when he started to work in a nearby city for 1 to 2 days a week. Because of the absence of a persistently depressed or anxious mood, she did not meet the definitional thresholds for DSM-IV mood or anxiety disorders. Instead, she could be given the diagnosis of undifferentiated somatoform disorder according to DSM-IV or neurasthenia according to CCMD. During clinical interview, Mrs. N. S. did not think she had major depression. She was particularly puzzled by the diagnosis of undifferentiated somatoform disorder (*weifenhua quti zhangai*), which was unintelligible and experience-distancing to her. In her view, she merely had neurasthenia as a result of multiple stressors in the family. Although the Chinese psychiatrist wrote down the DSM-IV diagnosis in her case notes, he used the term *neurasthenia* to enhance clinical communication. Mrs. N. S. declined pharmacotherapy but accepted counseling readily.

From a cultural constructionist perspective, personality disorders are based on Anglo-American conceptions of personhood and codes of appropriate behavior and owe their existence to the medicalization of unvalued social behavior. Accordingly, transformations in the values of a society determine whether they are called *disease*, *sin*, or *crime*. Given the disparity between the Oriental and Occidental conceptions of personhood, queries over the contextual validity of personality disorders are to be expected. Although included as a major class in CCMD-3, personality disorders are neither common clinical diagnoses nor popular research topics in China. Published studies indicate that a high percentage of Chinese subjects fail to fall into the subtypes recognized in DSM-IV and ICD-10. Thus, anxious (avoidant) and dependent personality disorders were excluded from CCMD-2-R with the argument that many of their defining features (e.g., excessive preoccupation with being criticized or rejected in social situations and subordination of one's own needs to those of others on whom one is dependent) are normative in the Chinese culture. However, they are included in CCMD-3, along with paranoid, schizoid, dissocial, impulsive, histrionic, and anankastic personality disorders. Likewise, the category of pathological gambling, excluded in the CCMD-2-R, is returned in CCMD-3.

Retention of Diagnostic Categories Unipolar mania is no longer found in ICD-10 or DSM-IV, according to which a patient with two episodes of mania is assumed to have bipolar disorder. However, longitudinal studies indicate that recurrent mania continues to be seen in China and questions the obligatory labeling of such Chinese patients as having bipolar disorder. The possibility that they may exhibit particular biological correlates, treatment response, and outcome supported a separate nosological status in CCMD-2-R. Based on the results of its field trials, CCMD-3 also retains the concept of unipolar recurrent mania, without labeling it *bipolar disorder*, as other international systems do.

The words *neurosis* and *neurotic* have completely disappeared from the DSM-IV, whereas the ICD-10 no longer retains neurosis as a major organizing principle. Instead, neurosis is finely partitioned into a variety of anxiety and depressive disorders, resulting in a high prevalence of comorbidity being found in recent Western epidemiological studies. Among Chinese psychiatrists, *neurosis* (*shenjing zheng*) has been used as a popular descriptive and etiological concept since the 1950s. With the exception of depressive neurosis, which has disappeared as such and is now classified under the mood disorders, the class of neuroses is preserved in CCMD-3, emphasizing as its main characteristics chronicity (at least 3 months), the presence of predisposing personality and social factors, and the preservation of insight.

Variation of Diagnostic Categories By tradition, Chinese psychiatrists have confined the diagnosis of mood disorder to bipolar disorder and psychotic depression. In CCMD-2-R, chronic mild depression, such as dysthymia, was considered a form of neurosis and was subsumed under depressive neurosis. In CCMD-3, however, the classification of mood disorders has become more in line with international perspectives. The CCMD-3 adopts a relatively simple notion of depression. For the first time in China, a diagnosis of dysthymia is included in the section on mood disorders instead of the previous one on depressive neurosis. The time criterion for major depression has been changed to 2 weeks (as in ICD-10) rather than the 4 weeks demanded by CCMD-2-R, reflecting again changes in the perceptions of the depressive symptomatology by Chinese clinicians and the determination of the developers of CCMD-3 to harmonize with international practice.

Because CCMD-2-R and CCMD-3 have tightened the concept of neurasthenia according to Western epistemological assumptions (i.e., it should not be diagnosed if mood or other neurotic disorders are present), the use of this diagnosis is becoming less common among Chinese psychiatrists. However, neurasthenia remains a common clinical diagnosis among doctors in China as a whole. According to CCMD-3, it is a type of neurosis composed of any three of five nonhierarchical groups of weakness, dysphoria, excitement, nervous pain, and sleep symptoms. This flexible symptom configuration is based on ample clinical experience in China and has been supported by culturally sensitive studies of the variegated illness experience of Chinese neurasthenic patients. By contrast, DSM-IV and ICD-10 representations of neurasthenia (as an undifferentiated somatoform disorder and a chronic fatigue disorder, respectively) lack contextual validity in Chinese society.

Unlike previous versions, the CCMD-3 criteria for anorexia nervosa mostly follow the ICD-10 and the DSM-IV, reflecting the role of global influences on Chinese society, particularly in the urbanized regions of the country. However, some differences in the phenomenology of the disorder prevail, and this is reflected in diagnostic practice among Chinese clinicians. Finally, CCMD-3 retains some mental disorders relevant to Chinese psychiatry, such as homosexuality, although the tendency of clinicians seems to be to consider only those homosexuals showing distress as mentally ill.

Ms. N. F. (28 years of age, height 1.51 m [4 ft, 11 in.], ideal body weight 47 kg [103 lb]) was a single clerk who was referred to the psychiatric clinic from a gynecological unit for a 6-year history of unexplained secondary amenorrhea and weight loss from 43 kg (95 lb; body mass index, 18.9 kg/m^2) to 32 kg (70 lb; body mass index, 14.0 kg/m^2). She came from a working-class family in which the father had sexually molested her when she was 12 years of age. She experienced chronically low self-esteem and a strong sense of loss of control over her life. Since graduation from high school, she had worked continuously in a Protestant church in the hope that it would provide security for her. Ms. N. F. had always been slim and had never thought of dieting to pursue beauty. She attributed her poor food intake to loss of appetite during family dinner, when her father scolded her ruthlessly. She no longer cared how much and what she ate but sought refuge by fleeing the dining table as quickly as possible. She regarded this as a form of silent protest against him. Physical examination revealed a pubescent look and the usual signs of emaciation. Extensive investigation revealed no physical cause for the weight loss. When interviewed with the Eating Disorders module of the Structured Clinical Interview for DSM-III-R (SCID), she failed to fulfill the criteria for anorexia nervosa, and her depressive symptoms fell short of those for a major depressive episode. Ms. N. F. received individual psychotherapy for 2 years, during which family conflicts, powerlessness, and the lack of meaning in life constituted the organizing theme of her illness experience. She never mentioned the fear of fatness and sometimes challenged why the therapist, instead of understanding her lack of meaning of life, was so preoccupied with her eating behavior and body weight. She fulfilled culture-flexible diagnostic criteria for anorexia nervosa.

Regional Adaptations of ICD-10 in Other Asian Countries

The ICD-10 has been tested and is increasingly used in other Asian countries, such as India, Japan, and Korea. In Japan, for example, a recent survey revealed that more than 80 percent of educational institutions used ICD or DSM for clinical work, whereas the use of these two diagnostic systems approached 100 percent for purposes of reporting research. Available evidence indicates that it is a reasonably feasible scheme that promotes reliability and international comparisons across most diagnostic categories. Nonetheless, local modifications are required to enhance its contextual validity and to make it user friendly. For example, the Japanese Society for International Diagnostic Criteria in Psychiatry (JSIDCP) has also decided to retain a unitary concept of neurosis, which should be connected with predisposing personality traits and life events. As in CCMD-2-R, mild depression is considered a form of neurosis rather than a mood disorder, and the term *somatoform disorder* is avoided. Further examination of the discrepancies between Asian and Western nosological systems will encourage reflective self-criticism on the one hand and will contribute to an internationally valid system of psychiatric classification on the other.

TOWARD COMPREHENSIVE DIAGNOSTIC MODELS

Although the national adaptations of the ICD represent attempts at resolving the tension between universalistic and local perspectives and needs, another emerging cluster of efforts in psychiatry is aimed at integrating different informational domains and the perspectives of different evaluators in the construction of comprehensive diagnostic formulations.

Conceptual Framework The conceptual framework for these developments includes the articulation of previously divergent historical and philosophical traditions, new notions on health and health care being advanced by the WHO, and innovative developments in general health and psychiatric epidemiology. From a historical and philosophical viewpoint, the longitudinal evolution of diagnostic systems can be seen as unfolding on three parallel lines. One is represented by a synthetic, bold, and abstract platonic conceptualization of a disease entity as a sufficient descriptor of a patient's clinical condition. The second involves an analytical, textured, and experiential aristotelian viewpoint. The third is an empathetic hippocratic approach. The platonic tradition has informed the long-standing international effort to classify illnesses as reflected in the various versions of the ICD and national versions, such as DSM-IV-TR. The aristotelian perspective is reflected in the descriptions of the patient's contextualized clinical condition, using standardized typologies and scales, and has appeared under the term *multiaxial diagnostic evaluations*. The hippocratic tradition is related to recent efforts to focus on the individuality of the patient.

The WHO, through recent meetings of its executive board, is expanding its 50-year definition of *health*, proposing that it is not merely an absence of illness but a dynamic (or interactive) state of complete physical, emotional, and social well-being. Spirituality is being considered as a possible additional aspect of health. Furthermore, WHO's explorations on the description of health status is expanding its focus from disease to functioning and other positive aspects of health. One of these is quality of life, which is to be evaluated predominantly by the individual involved. Furthermore, in the formulation of its policy in *Health for All for the 21st Century,* WHO is incorporating ethics, equity, and human rights as new, important considerations.

Epidemiology, as the basic science of public health, is undergoing a substantial conceptual revision. Newer formulations go beyond the infectious disease model and the chronic disease model, calling for approaches that incorporate multiple and interactive levels of analysis, as suggested by Mervin Susser, past editor of the *American Journal of Public Health,* under the term *ecological epidemiology*.

Integrating Standardized and Idiographic Formulations Building on the traditions and developments outlined previously, the WPA is designing a more comprehensive diagnostic model as part of a project on IGDA. The model has two key components: One is a standardized multiaxial formulation that covers nosology, disabilities, contextual factors, and quality of life through typologies and scales. Such multiaxial formulation is aimed at statistically reliable measurement of key aspects of the clinical condition to facilitate sharing of diagnostic and treatment information among clinicians and across the world. The other is an idiographic or personalized formulation that focuses on the individuality of a particular patient. The idiographic formulation is aimed at providing complementary descriptive information, such as contextualized clinical problems, the positive factors of the patient, and expectations about restoration and promotion of health. It promotes engaging the patient and the family more fully in the process of clinical care, fulfilling ethical aspirations of respect to the dignity of the patient, and attending to his or her expectations in dealing with health problems and enhancing quality of life.

Development of the IGDA Project One of the roots of the WPA project on IGDA can be found in the dedicated collaboration between the WHO and WPA through its Executive Committee and its Section on Classification and Diagnostic Assessment toward the development of ICD-10, DSM-IV, recent editions of the CCMD (CCMD-2-R and CCMD-3), GC-3, and the GLADP. Also reflective of the relevant work of the WPA Classification Section on international psychiatric classification and diagnosis are three conferences held since the 1980s, during which African, Chinese, Egyptian, French, Japanese, Latin American, Russian, Scandinavian, South Asian, and U.S. perspectives were discussed, and new directions for international systems of classification and diagnosis were explored.

Another important root of the IGDA project was the International Survey on Diagnostic Assessment Procedures conducted by the WPA Section on Classification and Diagnostic Assessment in the early 1990s, which revealed a widely perceived need for more comprehensive diagnostic approaches, which should be culturally informed and generated in a truly international manner. In consideration of the previously mentioned International Survey, the Section on Classification and Diagnostic Assessment decided, in 1994, to start the development of the IGDA project. The first meeting for this purpose took place in the Bavarian town of Kaufbeuren, Germany. Since then, meetings have been held in Canada, China, France, Germany, Mexico, Turkey, and the United States. The work group for this project is composed of experts representing several theoretical approaches and fields of psychiatry. As a group, they cover all continents, consistent with the diversity of the Section membership.

Distinctive Features and Components of the IGDA Project A fundamental feature of the IGDA project involves the assessment of the psychiatric patient as a whole person, rather than just as a carrier of disease. Thus, it assumes in the clinician the exercise of scientific competence, humanistic concern, and ethical aspirations. Another essential feature is the coverage of all key areas of information (biological, psychological, and social) pertinent to describing the patient's pathology, dysfunctions, and problems, as well as his or her positive aspects or assets. A third important feature involves basing the diagnostic assessment on the interactive engagement among the clinician, the patient, and his or her family, leading to a joint understanding of the patient's clinical condition and a joint assumption and monitoring of the treatment plan. As a fourth feature, IGDA uses ICD-10 for the first three axes of its multiaxial formulation (classification of mental and general medical disorders, disabilities, and contextual factors). Alternatively, regional adaptations of ICD-10, such as DSM-IV-TR, CCMD-2-R, GC-3, or GLADP, may be used for the classification of mental disorders.

Additionally, it is important to point out the need, in the diagnostic assessment process, to use scientific objectivity and evidence-based procedures, as well as intuition and clinical wisdom to enhance the descriptive validity and therapeutic usefulness of the diagnostic formulation. Furthermore, it is critical for the effectiveness of the diagnostic enterprise to use a culturally informed framework, for the development of new diagnostic models and procedures as well as for the conduction of a competent clinical evaluation of every patient.

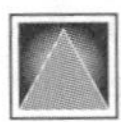

Table 9.2–4
Comprehensive Diagnostic Model Incorporated into the World Psychiatric Association International Guidelines for Diagnostic Assessment

Standardized multiaxial formulation
- I. Clinical disorders (mental and nonmental disorders)
- II. Disabilities (difficulties in fulfilling social roles in regard to personal care, occupational functioning, functioning with family, and broader social functioning)
- III. Contextual factors
- IV. Quality of life

Idiographic formulation
- I. Contextualized clinical problems
- II. Patient's positive factors
- III. Expectations about restoration and promotion of health

Table 9.2–4 presents schematically the components of the IGDA diagnostic model. The standardized multiaxial formulation of this model is basically organized according to the multiaxial presentation of ICD-10, with the addition of a fourth axis, quality of life, a multidimensional and global assessment of the patient's self-perceived well-being in areas, such as physical and emotional status; satisfaction with independent, occupational, and interpersonal functioning and with social-emotional and instrumental supports; and a sense of personal and spiritual fulfillment.

A brief description of the components of the idiographic formulation is as follows:

I. *Clinical problems and their contextualization.* These include disorders and problems, based on the Standardized Multiaxial Formulation, in language shared by the clinician, the patient, and the family, as well as key complementary information and the elucidation of pertinent mechanisms and contributory factors, from biological, psychological, social, and cultural perspectives. Important disagreements should be mentioned, and their resolution should be addressed.

II. *Patient's positive factors.* These include assets that are pertinent to the treatment of the clinical condition and to health promotion, for example, personality maturity, skills, talents, social resources and supports, and personal and spiritual aspirations.

III. *Expectations on restoration and promotion of health.* These include specific plans and hopes about what is to be achieved in treatment and about shared goals concerning health status and quality of life in the foreseeable future.

The Idiographic Formulation should be presented in natural or colloquial language to maximize flexibility and should represent the agreement reached between the clinician and the patient and the patient's family. The length of a written Idiographic Formulation could be approximately one page, and the length of an oral presentation could be approximately 5 minutes. Although this length may be advisable in general, it may vary from a short statement to a much more extensive one, depending on the time available, the purposes and format of clinical care, and other circumstances.

FUTURE DIRECTIONS

The developments of comprehensive diagnostic models and regional adaptations of ICD-10 reveal the ebullience of the diagnostic field, especially when appraised from a broad international perspective. It seems likely that the ongoing tension between universality and diversity in diagnostic systems will continue to yield innovative solutions. Emerging proposals are increasingly involving integrated assessments of health status and according pointed attention to the ethical requirements of psychiatric diagnosis. These proposals must be carefully formulated and thoughtfully and widely evaluated if they are to contribute effectively to the fulfillment of diagnosis as a conceptual and practical tool for clinical care, health promotion, and public health. It seems obvious that, in this effort, the participation of the multiple stakeholders in the health field at a global level is necessary and that those professional bodies and institutions with a global influence in the field of mental health, such as the WHO and the WPA, must fully commit themselves. Also important is the participation of national psychiatric societies active in the field, such as the APA. These considerations argue for the development of a new international classification and diagnostic system that is truly global in scope, aimed at appraising health status comprehensively and in a contextualized manner to better understand this and to better serve as the basis for effective actions toward the restoration and promotion of health in clinical and community settings. To be successful in this formidable enterprise, the enormous resources—human and otherwise—and the experience gained by the most significant experts in the field of diagnosis and classification around the globe must be enrolled, and the unique opportunities that developments in the fields of genetics, psychopharmacology, the neurosciences, and the psychosocial disciplines, as well as the enabling role of evolving informational and communication technologies linking individuals, groups, and institutions across the world, must be creatively used.

In line with the previously mentioned considerations, since 2000, the WPA, through its Section on Classification, Diagnostic Assessment, and Nomenclature, as well as a good number of its member societies, and the WHO, through its Office on Classification, Assessment, Surveys and Terminology from its Department of Evidence for Health Policy, have been actively engaged cooperatively in broadening the international base for the development of a truly integrated diagnostic system in psychiatry. As part of this effort, an international survey on the use and usage of ICD-10, DSM-IV-TR, and related diagnostic systems was conducted. It revealed that ICD-10 was the system most frequently used across the world for clinical work and training purposes, whereas DSM-IV-TR appeared to be the one most frequently used for research work. This survey also yielded a number of conceptual, methodological, and strategic recommendations for the development of future diagnostic systems.

Two major conferences have been organized with that aim in mind. The first was a 2-day symposium entitled "International Classification and Diagnosis: Critical Experience and Future Directions," hosted by the Royal College of Psychiatrists (RCP) within the framework of a WPA European Congress of Psychiatry, in London in July, 2001. This activity enrolled the participation of representatives from the WPA Executive Committee, WHO, the RCP, the APA, the Chinese Psychiatric Association, the Cuban Psychiatric Association, the APAL, the French Federation of Psychiatry, the Japanese Society of Psychiatry and Neurology, and the U. S. National Institute of Mental Health. The scientific papers originating from this symposium were published in a special double issue of *Psychopathology*, the official journal of the WPA Sections on Clinical Psychopathology and on Classification, Diagnostic Assessment, and Nomenclature.

The second major conference was a 1-day symposium entitled "International Diagnostic Systems: Interactive Integration of Perspectives and Partners" at the XII World Congress of Psychiatry in August, 2002 (Fig. 9.2–3). This event was organized with the main purpose of contributing to the integration of perspectives and partners. The first part of the symposium dealt with the integration of regional and local perspectives, focusing on the collaborative articulation of an interna-

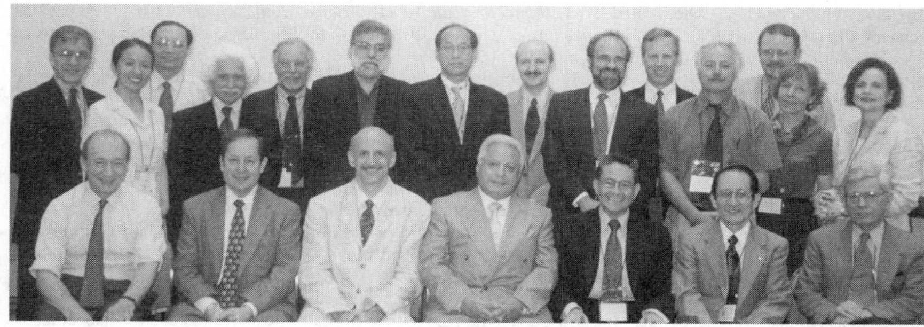

FIGURE 9.2–3 Participants at the Symposium on International Diagnostic Systems during the XII World Congress of Psychiatry in Yokohama, Japan, August, 2002. *Bottom row, left* to *right*: K. W. M. Fulford, D. A. Regier, T. B. Üstün, A. Okasha, J. E. Mezzich, Y. Nakane, A. Jablensky. *Top row, left* to *right*: C. E. Berganza, X.-H. Liu, Y. F. Chen, R. Montenegro, S. D. Kipman, L. Kirmayer, F. Lu, I. M. Salloum, M. B. First, B. Cuthbert, M. Botbol, W. Narrow, F. Quartier, M. Alegria.

tional standard with attention to local realities and needs. In addition, through the participation of the classification components of WHO, WPA, APA, and various active national and regional groups, this round table was meant to facilitate the exchange of views of current contributors to standard diagnostic systems and to encourage collaboration among these groups in prospective international diagnostic system developments. The second round table focused on integrating the perspectives of key health care stakeholders concerning the importance of diagnostic systems, an appraisal of current systems, and recommendations for future ones. The perspectives of the clinician, the biomedical and sociocultural researchers, the educator or trainer, the patient, industry, and health policy planners and the possibility of their collaborative interactions were explored.

The unfolding of these activities points out the generalized interest for improving the quality of diagnosis in psychiatry, as well as its clinical usefulness, by paying attention to what is universal about mental illness and by attending also to what is particular to the patient who presents for care in any setting across the world. The opportunities seem open for the development of a truly international diagnostic system in this field. The challenge to truly serve the person of the patient appears ready to be grasped.

SUGGESTED CROSS-REFERENCES

Section 4.1 discusses anthropology and psychiatry, whereas Section 4.4 discusses cross-cultural psychiatry. Psychiatric diagnosis is covered in Chapter 7, and the DSM-IV-TR classification is covered in Section 9.1. Neurasthenia is discussed in Chapter 15 on somatoform disorders.

References

Acosta-Nodal C, ed. *Glosario Cubano de la Clasificación Internacional de Enfermedades Psiquiátricas, (GC-1).* 1st ed. Havana, Cuba: Hosp Psiquiátr Habana; 1975.

Acosta-Nodal C, ed. *Glosario Cubano de la Clasificación Internacional de Enfermedades Psiquiátricas (GC-2).* 2nd ed. Havana, Cuba: Editorial Científico-Técnica; 1983.

Andrews G, Slade T, Peters L: Classification in psychiatry: ICD-10 versus DSM-IV. *Br J Psychiatry.* 1999;174:3.

Badley EM: An introduction to the concepts and classifications of the International Classification of Impairments, Disabilities, and Handicaps. *Disability Rehabil.* 1993;15:161.

Berganza CE: Broadening the international base for the development of an integrated diagnostic system in psychiatry. *World Psychiatry.* 2003;2:38.

*Berganza CE, Mezzich JE, Otero-Ojeda A, Jorge, MR, Villaseñor-Bayardo SJ, Rojas-Malpica C. The Latin American Guide for Psychiatric Diagnosis: A cultural overview. In: Mezzich JE, Fábrega H Jr, eds. *Cultural Psychiatry: International Perspectives.* The Psychiatric Clinics of North America; 2001;24:433.

Berlin MT, Fleck MPA: Quality of life: A brand new concept for research and practice in psychiatry. *Rev Bras Piquiatr.* 2003;25:249.

Berner P: Der Lebensabend der Paranoiker. *Wien Z Nervenheilkd.* 1969;27:115.

Berrios GE. The history of descriptive psychopathology. In: Mezzich JE, Jorge MR, Salloum JIM, eds. *Psychiatric Epidemiology: Assessment Concepts and Methods.* Baltimore: Johns Hopkins University Press; 1994.

Bramer GR: International Statistical Classification of Diseases and Related Health Problems, 10th revision. *World Health Stat Q.* 1988;41:32.

Bustamante JA, Santa Cruz A. *Psiquiatría Transcultural.* Havana, Cuba: Editorial Cientifico-Técnica; 1975.

Calles Bajo N, Valdés López G, Ceiro Valcarcel E. *Estudio Comparativo en Cuba y Africa acerca de los Conceptos Populares sobre la Enfermedad Mental.* Havana, Cuba: La Habana Empresa Bibliográfica, MINSAP; 1980.

Center for Disease Control and Prevention. International Classification of Diseases-9 (1975). Available at: http://aepo-xdv-www.epo.cdc.gov/wonder/sci_data/codes/icd9/type_txt/icd9.asp. Accessed January 12, 2003.

Chinese Medical Association. *Chinese Classification of Mental Disorders.* 2nd ed. Hunan, China: Hunan Medical University Press; 1989.

Chinese Medical Association and Nanjing Medical University. *Chinese Classification of Mental Disorders.* 2nd ed, revised. Nanjing, China: Dong Nan University Press; 1995.

*Chinese Psychiatric Association. *The Chinese Classification of Mental Disorders.* 3rd ed. Shandong, China: Shandong Publishing House of Science and Technology; 2001.

Cooper JE. The presentation of psychiatric classifications. In: Mezzich JE, von Cranach M, eds. *International Classification in Psychiatry. Unity and Diversity.* Cambridge, UK: Cambridge University Press; 1988.

Delgado H. *Curso de Psiquiatría.* Barcelona: Editorial Centífico-Médica; 1963.

Echazabal-Campos MA, Otero-Ojeda AA: Uso de sistemas taxonómicos por los psicólogos en Cuba. *Rev Hosp Psiquiátr Habana.* 1998;39:151.

Essen-Möller E, Wohlfahrt S: Suggestions for the amendment of the official Swedish classification of mental disorders. *Acta Psychiatr Scand.* 1947;47:551.

Fabrega H: International systems of diagnosis in psychiatry. *J Nerv Ment Dis.* 1994;182:256.

Fujinawa A. Overview of Japanese experiences on diagnostic classification: Past and present of the classification of mental disorders in Japan. In: Mezzich JE, Honda Y, Kastrup MC, eds. *Psychiatric Diagnosis. A World Perspective.* New York: Springer-Verlag; 1994.

Fulford KWM: Values in psychiatric diagnosis: Executive summary of a report to the chair of the ICD-12/DSM-VI Coordinating Task Force (Dateline 2010). *Psychopathology.* 2002;35:132–138.

González Menéndez R. *El Médico ante el Transtorno Psiquiátrico Menor.* 1st ed. Santiago de Cuba, Cuba: Editorial Oriente; 1989.

Horwitz J, Marconi J: El problema de las definiciones en el campo de la salud mental. Definiciones aplicables en estudios epidemiológicos. *Bol Oficinia Sanit Panam.* 1966;60:300.

House JS, Landis KR, Umberson D: Social relationships and health. *Science.* 1988;241:540.

Huttenlocher J, Hedges LV: Combining graded categories: Membership and typicality. *Psychol Rev.* 1994;101:157.

Hyman SE: Neuroscience, genetics and the future of psychiatric diagnosis. *Psychopathology.* 2002;35:139–144.

Janca A, Kastrup M, Katsching A, Lopéz-Ibor JJ, Mezzich JE, Sartorius N. *Multiaxial Presentation of ICD-10 for Use in Adult Psychiatry.* Cambridge, UK: Cambridge University Press; 1997.

Kastrup MC. Psychosocial domains in comprehensive diagnostic models. In: Costa e Silva A, Nadelson CC, eds. *International Review of Psychiatry.* Washington, DC: American Psychiatric Press; 1993.

Kendell R, Jablensky A: Distinguishing between the validity and the utility of psychiatric diagnoses. *Am J Psychiatry.* 2003;160:4.

Kessler RC: Epidemiological perspectives for the development of future diagnostic systems. *Psychopathology.* 2002;35:158–161.

Kleinman A. *Rethinking Psychiatry: From Cultural Category to Personal Experience.* New York: Free Press; 1988.

Kraepelin E. *Psychiatrie.* 5th ed. Leipzig, Germany: Barth; 1896.

Laín Entralgo P. *El Diagnóstico Médico: Historia y Teoría.* Barcelona: Salvat; 1982.

Lee S: The vicissitudes of neurasthenia in Chinese societies: Where will it go from the ICD-10? *Trancult Psychiatry.* 1994;31:153.

Lee S: Self-starvation in context: towards the culturally sensitive understanding of anorexia nervosa. *Soc Sci Med.* 1995;41:25.

Lee S: Culture in psychiatric nosology: The CCMD-2-R and international classification of mental disorders. *Cult Med Psychiatry.* 1996;20:421.

Lee S: From diversity to unity: The classification of mental disorders in 21st-century China. *Psychiatr Clin North Am.* 2001;24:421.

Lee S: Socio-cultural and global health perspectives for the development of future psychiatric diagnostic systems. *Psychopathology.* 2002;35:152–157.

Leme Lopes J. *As Dimensões do Diagnostico Psiquiátrico.* Rio de Janeiro: Agir; 1954.

Leonhard K. *Afteilung der Endogenen Psychosen.* Berlin: Akademie; 1957.

Li XJ, Li RR, Ren HX, Ren BH, Gu HX, Wu TH, Shi CW: An investigation of inducing factors associated with sudden psychiatric disorders of train passengers. *Chin J Psychiatry.* 1996;29:47.

Mezzich JE. The World Psychiatric Association and the development of ICD-10. In: Stefanis C, Rabavilas AD, Soldatos CR, eds. *Psychiatry: A World Perspective.* Amsterdam: Excerpta Medica; 1990.

Mezzich JE: An international survey on diagnostic assessment procedures. *Fortschritte Neurol Psychiatrie.* 1993;61:13.

Mezzich JE: Ethics and comprehensive diagnosis. *Psychopathology.* 1999;32:135–140.

Mezzich JE: International surveys on the use of ICD-10 and related diagnostic systems. *Psychopathology.* 2002;35:72–75.

Mezzich JE: The WPA International Guidelines for Diagnostic Assessment. *World Psychiatry.* 2002;1:36–39.

*Mezzich JE, Berganza CE, von Cranach, M, Jorge MR, Kastrup MC, Murthy RS, Okasha A, Pull CH, Sartorius N, Skodol A, Zaudig M: Essentials of WPA International Guidelines for Comprehensive Assessment. *Br J Psychiatry.* 2003;182[Suppl 45]:S37–S66.

Mezzich JE, Honda Y, Kastrup MC, eds. *Psychiatric Diagnosis: A World Perspective.* New York: Springer-Verlag; 1994.

Mezzich JE, Kleinman A, Fabrega H, Parron D. *Culture and Psychiatric Diagnosis.* Washington, DC: American Psychiatric Press; 1996.

Mezzich JE, Otero-Ojeda A, Lee S. International psychiatric diagnosis. In: Sadock BJ, Sadock VA, eds. *Kaplan & Sadock's Comprehensive Textbook of Psychiatry.* 7th ed. Vol 1. Philadelphia: Lippincott Williams & Wilkins; 2000.

Mezzich JE, Schmolke MM. Quality of life and comprehensive clinical diagnosis. In: Katsching H, Freeman H, Sartorius N, eds. *Quality of Life in Mental Disorders.* New York: John Wiley; 1997.

*Mezzich JE, Üstün TB: International classification and diagnosis: critical experience and future directions. *Psychopathology.* 2002;35:55–201.

Mezzich JE, von Cranach M. *International Classification in Psychiatry: Unity and Diversity.* Cambridge, UK: Cambridge University Press; 1988.

Misès R, Fortineau J, Jeammet P, Lang JL, Mazet P, Plantade A, Quémada N: Classification Française des troubles mentaux de l'enfant et de l'adolescent. *Psychiatrie Enfant.* 1988;31:67.

Misès R, Quemada N, Botbol M, Burzsteijn C, Garrabe J, Golse B, Jeammet P, Plantade A, Portelli C, Thevenot JP. French classification for child and adolescent mental disorders. *Psychopathology.* 2002;35:176–180.

Mundt C: Psychological perspectives for the development of future diagnostic systems. *Psychopathology.* 2002;35:145–151.

Nakane Y, Nakane H: Classification systems for psychiatric diseases currently used in Japan. *Psychopathology.* 2002;35:191–194.

Okasha A. The Egyptian diagnostic system (DMP-I). In: Mezzich JE, von Cranach M, eds. *International Classification in Psychiatry. Unity and Diversity.* Cambridge, UK: Cambridge University Press; 1988.

Orley J, Kuyken W. *International Quality of Life Assessment.* Heidelberg, Germany: Springer-Verlag; 1994.

Otero-Ojeda AA. *Adaptación Cultural del Sistema Multilaxial de la CIE-10 a través de Ejes Complementarios.* Havana, Cuba: Hospital Psiquiátrico de la Habana, Editorial Científico-Técnica; 1994.

Otero-Ojeda AA, ed. *Tercer Glosario Cubano de Psiquiatría.* Havana, Cuba: Hospital Psiquiátrico de La Habana; 2000.

Otero-Ojeda AA, Acosta Nodal C. *Características y Aportaciones Fundamentales del Tercer Glosario Cubano de Psiquiatría.* Havana, Cuba: Hospital Psiquiátrico de La Habana; 1996.

Percy C, van Holten V, Muir C. *International Classification of Diseases for Oncology* (ICD-0). Geneva: World Health Organization; 1990.

Pull C, Chaillet G. The nosological views of French-speaking psychiatry. In: Mezzich JE, Honda Y, Kastrup MC, eds. *Psychiatric Diagnosis: A World Perspective.* New York: Springer-Verlag; 1994.

Quinones C, Otero-Ojeda AA: Clarificacion psiquiatrica y psicoterapia: Uso del eje V del 3er Glosario Cubano de Psiquiatrica (mecanismos y necessidades psicopatogenicas) Psiquiatrica y Salud Integral. (*in press*).

*Regier DA, Narrow WE, First MB, Marshall T: The APA classification of mental disorders: Future perspectives. *Psychopathology.* 2002;35:166–170.

Sartorius N, Kaelber CT, Cooper JE, Roper MT: Progress towards achieving a common language in psychiatry. Results of the field trials of the clinical guidelines accompanying the WHO Classification of Mental and Behavioral Disorders in ICD-10. *Arch Gen Psychiatry.* 1993;50:115.

Seguin CA: The concept of disease. *Psychosom Med.* 1946;8:252.

Strauss JS: The person: key to understanding mental illness: Towards a new dynamic psychiatry, III. *Br J Psychiatry.* 1992;161:19.

Survey and Test Group for the CCMD-2-R: A report on the national field of the second revised edition of the Chinese classification and diagnostic criteria of mental disorders. *Chin J Psychiatry.* 1996;29:27.

United Nations Development Program (UNDP). *Human Development Report 2001: Making New Technologies Work for Human Development.* New York: Oxford University Press; 2001.

Üstün TB, Goldberg DA, Sartorius N. ICD-10. Classifying primary care mental disorders. Paper presented at: Proceedings of the 146th annual meeting of the American Psychiatric Association; May, 1993.

World Health Organization. *International Statistical Classification of Diseases and Related Health Problems.* 10th ed. Vol 1. Geneva: World Health Organization; 1992.

World Health Organization. *The ICD-10 Classification of Mental and Behavioral Disorders: Clinical Descriptions and Diagnostic Guidelines.* Geneva: World Health Organization; 1992.

World Health Organization. *The ICD-10 Classification of Mental and Behavioral Disorders: Diagnostic Criteria for Research.* Geneva: World Health Organization; 1993.

Wu CY: A clinical analysis of seventy-six cases of qigong induced psychotic disorders. *J Clin Psychol Med.* 1992;2:7.

Xu WY, Chen ZJ: An eight to ten year outcome study of unipolar mania. *Arch Psychiatry.* 1992;4:88.

10 Delirium, Dementia, and Amnestic and Other Cognitive Disorders and Mental Disorders Due to a General Medical Condition

▲ 10.1 Cognitive Disorders: Introduction and Overview

KENNETH L. DAVIS, M.D.

Cognition includes memory, language, orientation, praxis, judgment, conducting interpersonal relationships, and problem solving. Cognitive disorders not only reflect disruption in one or more of the above domains but are also frequently complicated by behavioral symptoms. Cognitive disorders exemplify the complex interface between neurology, medicine, and psychiatry in that medical or neurological conditions often lead to cognitive disorders that are, in turn, associated with behavioral symptoms. It can be argued that of all psychiatric conditions, cognitive disorders best demonstrate how biological insults result in behavioral symptomatology. The physician must carefully assess the history and context of the presentation of these disorders before arriving at a diagnosis and treatment plan. Fortunately, advances in molecular biology, diagnostic techniques, and medication management have significantly improved the ability to recognize and to treat cognitive disorders.

The aging population has resulted in a public health crisis regarding the diagnosis and management of dementia. More than 14 million Americans will develop dementia by the year 2050. With illness progression, dementia eventually disrupts all domains of cognition, thereby significantly impairing an individual's ability to function at the most basic level. Although not included in the required criteria, dementia is frequently complicated by behavioral symptoms, including agitation, delusions, and hallucinations. Not surprisingly, a tremendous amount of research has focused on the molecular biology, pathophysiology, epidemiology, phenomenology, and treatment of dementia. Judith Neugroschl and colleagues focus their review on Alzheimer's disease, the most common cause of dementia. Much progress has been made in the area of research that investigates the cognitive deficits associated with Alzheimer's disease. Many studies have elucidated the role of amyloid and neurofibrillary tangles, the pathological changes described by Alois Alzheimer more than a century ago, in the pathophysiology of Alzheimer's disease. Neuroimaging techniques have permitted visualization of the earliest structural and functional correlates of cognitive decline. Molecular biology advances have identified at least four genes that are associated with Alzheimer's disease. U.S. Food and Drug Administration (FDA) approval of cholinesterase inhibitors has transformed Alzheimer's disease from an untreatable illness less than 10 years ago to a condition for which there are effective pharmacological interventions. The ability to better identify risk factors for the subsequent development of dementia will undoubtedly provide opportunities for interventions that could delay onset and perhaps prevent the development of this devastating illness.

Although cognitive disorders may cross-sectionally present with similar symptoms, this heterogeneous group of illnesses may significantly differ in their etiologies, courses, and treatments. As a case in point, delirium and Alzheimer's disease may present with impaired recall, yet the former condition is episodic and reversible, whereas the latter illness is a neurodegenerative process for which there are only symptomatic treatments.

Steven Samuels and Neugroschl review the presentation, pathophysiology, and management of delirium. Of the cognitive disorders, delirium can be particularly difficult to diagnose because of its waxing and waning symptomatology. Given the high prevalence of delirium in the acutely ill medical patient, it behooves the clinician to anticipate the development of this condition and to search aggressively for the underlying etiology. However, there is a relative paucity of research regarding the pathophysiology and pharmacological management of delirium. In part, this fact is due to the difficulty in obtaining informed consent from delirious patients and the urgency to treat in an expedient fashion. Nonetheless, with adequate recognition of the disorder, clinicians can treat the causative factors and can appropriately manage the behavioral complications.

Martin Allan Drooker reviews cognitive disorders due to general medical condition and substances. This chapter extends previous chapters in this section through discussion of additional medical, neurological, or substance-induced causes of dementia and delirium. In contrast to other cognitive disorders, amnestic disorders are characterized by a single cognitive deficit, impaired memory. However, these syndromes are commonly associated with social and occupational functioning. Hillel Grossman reviews the range of illnesses and substances that can result in amnestic disorders. Korsakoff's syndrome provides a paradigm for recognizing how exposure to a substance (e.g., alcohol) results in focal brain injury that, in turn, causes an amnestic disorder.

Patients often develop or are evaluated for cognitive disorders in the medical setting and are not evaluated by a psychiatrist unless there are significant behavioral disturbances that interfere with day-to-day patient management. The high prevalence of psychiatric symptoms and syndromes in medically ill patients without prior psychiatric histories saliently demonstrates the physician's obligation to anticipate cognitive complications in the medical or surgical setting. Optimum treatment for cognitive disorders results from a collaborative effort between the patient's primary physician and a psychiatrist.

SUGGESTED CROSS-REFERENCES

Psychiatric clinical manifestations of specific neurological and systemic disorders are discussed in Chapter 2. Neuropsychological and intellectual assessment of adults is presented in Section 7.5, assessment of children in Section 7.7, and medical assessment and laboratory testing in Section 7.8. Discussion of substance-related disorders appears in Chapter 11, schizophrenia in Chapter 12, psychotic disorders in Section 12.16, anxiety disorders in Chapter 14, factitious disorders in Chapter 16, dissociative disorders (including dissociative amnesia) in Chapter 17, sexual dysfunctions in Section 18.1a, sleep disorders in Chapter 20, and personality disorders in Chapter 23. The psychiatric aspects of human immunodeficiency virus (HIV) infection and acquired immune deficiency syndrome (AIDS) are presented in Section 2.8. Psychological changes in normal aging (including age-related cognitive decline) are discussed in Section 51.2c, and dementia of the Alzheimer's type and other dementing disorders of late life are discussed in Section 51.3e.

REFERENCES

*Fick DM, Agostini JV, Inouye SK: Delirium superimposed on dementia: A systematic review. *J Am Geriatr Soc*. 2002;50:1723–1732.

*Hardy J, Selkoe DJ: The amyloid hypothesis of Alzheimer's disease: Progress and problems on the road to therapeutics. *Science*. 2002;297:353–356.

*Helmes E, Bowler JV, Merskey H, Munoz DG, Hachinski VC: Rates of vognitive decline in Alzheimer's disease and dementia with Lewy bodies. *Dement Geriatr Cogn Disord*. 2003;15:67–71.

*Morita T, Tei Y, Inoue S: Agitated terminal delirium and associations with partial opioid substitution and hydration. *J Palliat Med*. 2003;6:557–563.

*Wild R, Pettit T, Burns A: Cholinesterase inhibitors for dementia with Lewy bodies. *Cochrane Database Syst Rev*. 2003;3:CD003672.

▲ 10.2 Delirium

STEVEN C. SAMUELS, M.D., AND
JUDITH A. NEUGROSCHL, M.D.

Delirium is defined by the acute onset of fluctuating cognitive impairment and a disturbance of consciousness with reduced ability to attend. There are frequent associated perceptual abnormalities, sleep–wake cycle disturbances, disorganized thought process, and abnormal psychomotor activity. A significant public health problem that forebodes poor outcome, delirium is associated with cognitive and functional decline, complicates medical course, and increases resource use and mortality risk (Table 10.2–1). Unfortunately, delirium is underrecognized by health care workers. Delirium is present in 1 percent of adults in the community, in at least 10 percent of emergency department patients, in 40 percent of terminally ill patients, and in as much as one-half of hospitalized patients. Prevalence increases with patient age, complexity of medical comorbidities, and the number and frequency of medications prescribed. Delirium is most often caused by multiple etiologies, such as infection, metabolic abnormalities, endocrinopathies, substance intoxication, and withdrawal. In line with the many causes of delirium, there are several theories proposed to explain its pathophysiology. These include neurochemical abnormalities, inflammatory changes, oxidative stress, blood–brain barrier dysfunction, and interactions between these factors. An organized approach to the diagnosis and management of delirium maximizes the practitioner's effectiveness in determining and correcting the etiologies and providing safety and education to patients and caregivers. There is much research to be done on the basic and clinical aspects of delirium.

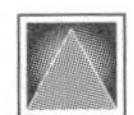

Table 10.2–1
Cost of Delirium

Cost of Delirium
Increased nursing care
Increased length of stay
Increased risk of cognitive decline
Increased risk of functional decline
Increased mortality
Delay in postoperative mobilization
Prevention of early rehabilitation
Increased rate of nursing home placement
Increased need for home care services
Increased distress to caregivers
Barrier to psychosocial closure in terminally ill patient

DEFINITION

Delirium is derived from the Latin *deliro*—to be crazy, from de- + *lira*, a furrow (i.e., to go out of the furrow), according to Stedman's 24th edition, 1982.

The revised fourth edition of the *Diagnostic and Statistical Manual of Mental Disorders* (DSM-IV-TR) defines delirium as follows:

> Foremost a disturbance of consciousness, attention, cognition, and perception. It is a common psychiatric syndrome which commonly heralds an increase in morbidity and mortality. Patients with delirium remain in the hospital longer and are more commonly discharged to long-term care facilities. Behavioral manifestations of delirium may interfere with treatment compliance and are often precipitants for psychiatric consultation. A psychiatrist should provide and/or advocate for the appropriate treatment beyond simple medical expedience.

The core symptoms of delirium include a disturbance of consciousness that is accompanied by a change in cognition that develops over a short period of time, usually hours to days, and tends to fluctuate during the course of the day (Tables 10.2–2 through 10.2–5).

HISTORY

Written descriptions of patients who would meet the current definitions of delirium date back at least 2,500 years. The examples that follow are descriptions of patients who may have been diagnosed with delirium using the current nomenclature.

In the Books of Epidemics, circa 400 BC, Hippocrates described the following case:

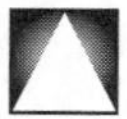

Table 10.2–2
DSM-IV-TR Diagnostic Criteria for Delirium Due to a General Medical Condition

A. Disturbance of consciousness (i.e., reduced clarity of awareness of the environment) with reduced ability to focus, to sustain, or to shift attention.

B. A change in cognition (such as memory deficit, disorientation, or language disturbance) or the development of a perceptual disturbance that is not better accounted for by a preexisting, established, or evolving dementia.

C. The disturbance develops over a short period of time (usually hours to days) and tends to fluctuate during the course of the day.

D. There is evidence from the history, physical examination, or laboratory findings that the disturbance is caused by the direct physiological consequences of a general medical condition.

Coding note: If delirium is superimposed on a preexisting vascular dementia, indicate the delirium by coding vascular dementia, with delirium.

Coding note: Include the name of the general medical condition on Axis I, for example, delirium due to hepatic encephalopathy; also code the general medical condition on Axis III.

From American Psychiatric Association. *Diagnostic and Statistical Manual of Mental Disorders.* 4th ed. Text rev. Washington, DC: American Psychiatric Association; 2000, with permission.

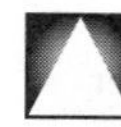

Table 10.2–4
DSM-IV-TR Diagnostic Criteria for Substance Withdrawal Delirium

A. Disturbance of consciousness (i.e., reduced clarity of awareness of the environment) with reduced ability to focus, to sustain, or to shift attention.

B. A change in cognition (such as memory deficit, disorientation, or language disturbance) or the development of a perceptual disturbance that is not better accounted for by a preexisting, established, or evolving dementia.

C. The disturbance develops over a short period of time (usually hours to days) and tends to fluctuate during the course of the day.

D. There is evidence from the history, physical examination, or laboratory findings that the symptoms in Criteria A and B developed during, or shortly after, a withdrawal syndrome.

Note: This diagnosis should be made instead of a diagnosis of substance withdrawal only when the cognitive symptoms are in excess of those usually associated with the withdrawal syndrome and when the symptoms are sufficiently severe to warrant independent clinical attention.

Code (specific substance) withdrawal delirium: alcohol; sedative, hypnotic, or anxiolytic; other (or unknown) substance.

From American Psychiatric Association. *Diagnostic and Statistical Manual of Mental Disorders.* 4th ed. Text rev. Washington, DC: American Psychiatric Association; 2000, with permission.

> Erasinus, who lived near the Canal of Bootes, was seized with fever after supper; passed the night in an agitated state. During the first day quiet, but in pain at night. On the second, symptoms all exacerbated; at night delirious. On the third, was in a painful condition; great incoherence. On the fourth, in a most uncomfortable state; had no sound sleep at night, but dreaming and talking; then all the appearances worse, of a formidable and alarming character; fear, impatience. On the morning of the fifth, was composed, and quite coherent, but long before noon was furiously mad, so that he could not constrain himself; extremities cold, and somewhat livid; urine without sediment; died about sunset.

Caelius Aurelianus, circa the fifth century AD, described another case of delirium:

> Quiet or loud laughter, singing or a state of sadness, silence, murmuring, crying or a barely audible muttering to one's self; or such a state of anger that the patient jumps up in a rage and can scarcely be held back, is wrathful at everyone, shouts,

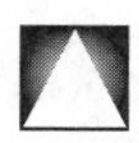

Table 10.2–3
DSM-IV-TR Diagnostic Criteria for Substance Intoxication Delirium

A. Disturbance of consciousness (i.e., reduced clarity of awareness of the environment) with reduced ability to focus, to sustain, or to shift attention.

B. A change in cognition (such as memory deficit, disorientation, or language disturbance) or the development of a perceptual disturbance that is not better accounted for by a preexisting, established, or evolving dementia.

C. The disturbance develops over a short period of time (usually hours to days) and tends to fluctuate during the course of the day.

D. There is evidence from the history, physical examination, or laboratory findings of the following:

(1) The symptoms in Criteria A and B developed during substance intoxication.

(2) Medication use is etiologically related to the disturbance.[a]

Note: This diagnosis should be made instead of a diagnosis of substance intoxication only when the cognitive symptoms are in excess of those usually associated with the intoxication syndrome and when the symptoms are sufficiently severe to warrant independent clinical attention.

Code (specific substance) intoxication delirium: alcohol, amphetamine (or amphetamine-like substance), cannabis, cocaine, hallucinogen, inhalant, opioid, phencyclidine (or phencyclidine-like substance), sedative, hypnotic or anxiolytic, other (or unknown) substance (e.g., cimetidine [Tagamet], digitalis, or benztropine [Cogentin])

[a]The diagnosis should be recorded as substance-induced delirium if related to medication use.

From American Psychiatric Association. *Diagnostic and Statistical Manual of Mental Disorders.* 4th ed. Text rev. Washington, DC: American Psychiatric Association; 2000, with permission.

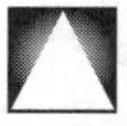

Table 10.2–5
DSM-IV-TR Diagnostic Criteria for Delirium Due to Multiple Etiologies

A. Disturbance of consciousness (i.e., reduced clarity of awareness of the environment) with reduced ability to focus, to sustain, or to shift attention.

B. A change in cognition (such as memory deficit, disorientation, or language disturbance) or the development of a perceptual disturbance that is not better accounted for by a preexisting, established, or evolving dementia.

C. The disturbance develops over a short period of time (usually hours to days) and tends to fluctuate during the course of the day.

D. There is evidence from the history, physical examination, or laboratory findings that the delirium has more than one etiology (e.g., more than one etiological general medical condition, a general medical condition plus substance intoxication, or medication side effect).

Coding note: Use multiple codes reflecting specific delirium and specific etiologies, for example, delirium due to viral encephalitis and alcohol withdrawal delirium.

From American Psychiatric Association. *Diagnostic and Statistical Manual of Mental Disorders.* 4th ed. Text rev. Washington, DC: American Psychiatric Association; 2000, with permission.

> beats himself or tears his own clothing and that of his neighbors, or seeks to hide in fear, or weeps, or fails to answer those who are not present but with the dead, as if they were in his presence; and asks for neither food nor drink, or when he does take food falls violently upon it and gulps it down unchewed, or else chews it but does not swallow it, keeping it in his mouth and after a while spitting it out. And he shuns light or darkness, experiences continuous sleeplessness or short troubled sleep; his eyes are bloodshot, the blood vessels being distended: his gaze is fixed without any blinking, or else keeps wandering about with constant blinking; sometimes he puts his hands before his eyes as if seeking to catch or remove some object which he thinks has become stuck in his eye or is flying in front of him.

Paul of Aegina, circa the seventh century AD, described yet another case:

> Attended with watchfulness, but sometimes with disturbed sleep, so that the patients' start, leap up, and cry out furiously . . . with laughter . . . and . . . with unrestrainable madness. They forget what is said and done by them, their eyes are bloodshot, and they rub them; they are sometimes squalid, sometimes filled with tears, or loaded with rheums. The tongue is rough, there is a trickling of blood from the nose, they pick at flocks of wool and gather bits of straw, and they have acute fever during the whole continuance of the disorder . . . they have the pulse small and indistinct, with a certain degree of hardness. The respiration is large and rare . . . [or] irregular, the hypochondria are retracted and have considerable heat . . . When a pituitous humour is mixed with bilious, as the cause of the disease is compound, so also is its appellation; for it is called coma vigil. When bilious humour prevails, persons so affected are troubled with watchfulness; and, when a pituitous is the cause, they lie in a state of coma. The elder writers before Galen called this disease, catochus, but since then it has been called catoche and catalepsy.

Almost 300 years ago, delirium was described by Richard Morton, circa the 18th century AD, as follows:

> Fever is caused by an increased velocity in the flow of the blood. This augmented velocity brings about delirium by interfering with the secretions of the brain glands, which were postulated to be responsible for the activation of the nerves by means of the vital fluids or the animal spirit, which circulated through them. Delirium was regarded as a waking dream, and dreams were supposed to be the result of "confounding experience by the manifold repercussions of the animal spirits which arise from the cause producing sleep and pressing the nerves so as to revert the fluctuations of their juice. In delirium, ideas are similarly excited without order or coherence by animal spirits driven into irregular fluctuation."

Almost 50 years ago, George L. Engel and John Romano postulated that delirium was a reversible cerebral insufficiency due to decreased brain metabolic activity, based on electroencephalogram (EEG) slowing in patients with delirium. In 1980, the third edition of the *Diagnostic and Statistical Manual of Mental Disorders* (DSM-III) was the first attempt to standardize delirium nomenclature. Previously, the many synonyms for delirium led to confusion among physicians within and across medical specialties. Unfortunately, the confusion persists as clinicians still use the common synonyms for delirium listed in Table 10.2–6.

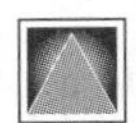

Table 10.2–6
Delirium by Other Names

Intensive care unit psychosis
Acute confusional state
Acute brain failure
Encephalitis
Encephalopathy
Toxic metabolic state
Central nervous system toxicity
Cinchonism
Paraneoplastic limbic encephalitis
Sundowning
Cerebral insufficiency
Organic brain syndrome

COMPARATIVE NOSOLOGY

Psychiatrists in the United States refer to *delirium* as the syndrome of fluctuating attention, cognitive impairment, perceptual disturbance, and sleep–wake cycle abnormalities that develop in a short time period. Neurologists may be more likely to refer to a similar syndrome as an *acute confusional state.* Others use the terms *encephalitis* or *encephalopathy.* The multiple terms used to describe delirium lead to confusion and variable thresholds to make a diagnosis. This is significant because early recognition of delirium may improve prognosis. An important consideration in creating diagnostic criteria for delirium is that, if the criteria are too stringent, mild cases of delirium may be left undiagnosed and untreated, despite being harbingers of poor outcome.

Searching for the etiology of the delirium is an essential step in the management of the delirious patient. Some nosological systems refer to the delirium solely based on cause. DSM-IV-TR subdivides delirium as to whether the causes are a general medical condition, substance withdrawal, substance intoxication, or multiple etiologies. Other classifications are more specific about cause but less specific about defining the delirium. For example, the terms *uremic* and *hepatic encephalopathy* and *limbic encephalitis* are used in the medical literature and clinical practice. *Encephalopathy* is not clearly defined, and any central nervous system (CNS) disturbance related to uremia or hepatic pathology may meet the nonspecific diagnostic criteria. *Encephalitis,* like encephalopathy, is not well defined and may represent any CNS change. For example, *limbic encephalitis* refers to paraneoplastic syndromes with CNS manifestations. *Encephalitis* and *encephalopathy* lack specificity and potentially include patients with dementia, coma, or any CNS manifestations of a disease, even if the patient does not have a delirium.

The many synonyms for delirium often confuse clinicians and researchers and create barriers to diagnosis and management (Table 10.2–6). Consistent nosology is expected to improve the ability of clinicians and researchers to refer to the same syndrome and to improve the validity and the ability to generalize research on diagnosis, factors that influence prognosis, and treatment response. The term *delirium* is emphasized in two of the preferred classification systems: the DSM-VI-TR and the *International Classification of Diseases* (ICD). Compatibility of the DSM-IV-TR and ICD is improving with collaborative efforts by the American Psychiatric Association and the World Health Organization.

DSM-IV-TR describes delirium based on signs, symptoms, time course, and etiology. If the delirium is due to a general medical condition, the history, physical examination, and laboratory studies are required to place the causative agent as a general medical condition. The conditions must be coded on Axis III, including all of the medical conditions that contribute to the delirium. Delirium due to substance intoxication or delirium due to substance withdrawal is coded if the clinical evidence, including laboratory studies, supports a toxicological syndrome (toxidrome) attributable to one or several substances or to substance withdrawal symptoms, respectively. Delirium due to multiple etiologies is the most common clinical scenario in patients with severe medical comorbidities. The delirium is coded on Axis I. The medical causes of the delirium are listed on Axis III, and the substance withdrawal or intoxication is listed on Axis I.

Coding in the ninth edition of the ICD (ICD-9) is similar to DSM-IV-TR in many respects. The specific general medical conditions and substances involved in the delirium may be coded with the ICD to a high level of specificity. The delirium itself is coded under transient organic mental disorder as acute delirium or subacute delirium. There are sections of ICD that describe accidental poisonings, with a high level of specificity for the agent. For example, if an accidental overdose of a pesticide occurred, the clinician could find this under accidental poisoning of an agricultural agent and then could choose whether the pesticide was chlorine, phosphate, or carbamate based. Delirium also can be classified as senile, presenile, or arteriosclerotic delirium. Drug withdrawal syndromes and drug-induced delirium are described with an increased specificity of coding choices when compared to the DSM-IV-TR.

EPIDEMIOLOGY

Incidence and Prevalence

Delirium is a common problem across treatment settings, and the incidence and prevalence increase with patient age and medical complexity. Higher rates of delirium are found in facilities that perform complex surgical procedures or are tertiary referral centers for severely ill patients. Physicians, nurses, and family members underrecognize delirium. This underdetection may be discerned across treatment settings as well, including primary care, emergency departments, inpatient medical, surgical, and intensive care unit (ICU) settings. There are numerous scales that are used in research to help identify delirium; these include the Confusion Assessment Method (CAM), the Delirium Rating Scale (DRS), and the Memorial Delirium Assessment Scale (MDAS). Sometimes the gold standard of an experienced clinician is also used as a benchmark. The incidence and prevalence rates for delirium across settings are shown in Table 10.2–7.

In a community aging study in Baltimore, delirium was present in 1.1 percent of those individuals older than 55 years of age. In the emergency department, delirium prevalence approaches 10 percent, with as much as 50 percent of patients presenting with altered mental state not meeting strict criteria for delirium (i.e., 40 percent have some other alteration of mental status). Some studies suggest underrecognition of delirium in the emergency department. This is concerning, as the emergency department is an important gateway into the general hospital. General medical inpatients have a delirium prevalence of 5 to 50 percent. The higher rates correspond to studies in which delirium was defined more liberally as *confusion*. The incidence of delirium in medical patients ranges from 3 to 40 percent of general medical inpatients, 15 to 25 percent of patients in the ICU, to as much as 75 percent of patients undergoing bone marrow stem cell transplant. In surgical patients, the rates may be even higher than on medical services. In general surgical units, 9 to 14 percent of patients have a delirium. Elective surgery is associated with less frequent delirium than emergent surgery, probably because of the higher level of medical acuity in patients requiring emergent interventions. The rates in cardiac surgery patients range from 7 to 35 percent, and, in surgery after hip fracture, the range is from 18 to 55 percent. Not surprisingly, terminally ill patients have a high rate of delirium (25 to 40 percent), as do elderly patients in chronic institutional settings (45 percent).

Pediatric patients, too, are at risk of delirium. The rates of delirium in children are ill defined, but the literature describes delirium in 10 to 40 percent of preschool children during emergence from anesthesia. Delirium is almost universal in severe burns and is common with high fever.

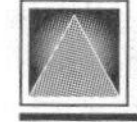

Table 10.2–7
Delirium Incidence and Prevalence in Multiple Settings

Population	Prevalence Range (%)	Incidence Range (%)
General medical inpatients	10–30	3–16
Medical *and* surgical inpatients	5–15	10–55
General surgical inpatients	N/A	9–15 postoperatively
Critical care unit patients	16	16–83
Cardiac surgery inpatients	16–34	7–34
Orthopedic surgery patients	33	18–50
Emergency department	7–10	N/A
Terminally ill cancer patients	23–28	83
Institutionalized elderly	44	33

N/A, not available.

Risk Factors and Protective Factors

Risk Factors There are numerous factors that increase a patient's risk for delirium (Table 10.2–8). These range from extremes of age to the number of medications taken. For example, pharmacokinetic and pharmacodynamic changes specific to the young and the old contribute to the increased risk as in both populations. In one study of elderly hospitalized patients, the risk of delirium was higher if the patients had vision impairment, more severe medical illness, cognitive impairment, or an elevated blood urea nitrogen (BUN) to creatinine ratio. Other studies of ICU patients suggested that hypertension, abnormal total bilirubin, smoking history, epidural use, morphine, and intravenous (IV) dopamine were associated with delirium.

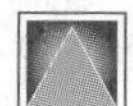

Table 10.2–8
Factors That Predispose Patients to Delirium

Vision impairment	Hypertension	Use of bladder catheter
Medical illnesses (severity and quantity)	Chronic obstructive pulmonary disease	Preoperative cognitive impairment
Cognitive impairment	Alcohol abuse	Functional limitations
Older than 70 years of age	Smoking history	History of delirium
Any iatrogenic event	Abnormal sodium level	Abnormal potassium, sodium, or glucose test
Use of physical restraints	Abnormal glucose level	Preoperative use of benzodiazepines
Malnutrition	Abnormal bilirubin level	Preoperative use of narcotic analgesics
More than three medications added	Blood urea nitrogen to creatinine ratio >18	Epidural use

Medications are another important risk factor for delirium. The risk increases with the number of medications taken and includes prescribed, illicit, herbal, and over-the-counter medications. The use of herbal and over-the-counter preparations is associated with delirium, often through interactions with other pharmaceuticals or intrinsic anticholinergic properties.

Protective Factors It is clear that good premorbid functioning before delirium predicts better outcome. Given the significant morbidity and mortality associated with delirium, interventions that prevent the occurrence of delirium or that foster early recognition have a significant impact on improving patient outcome and reduce the cost of caring for delirious patients (Table 10.2–1). A variety of interventions may improve outcome and may reduce risk. For example, educational programs that target clinicians or placement of liaison psychiatrists on orthopedic units improved coordination of care between consultants and primary care providers. Most studies demonstrated benefit in terms of decreased frequency or shorter duration of delirium and decreased length of stay compared to the usual care. Other interventions that have been studied and that demonstrate benefit include a focus on nutrition, increased rehabilitation, and attention to visual and hearing impairment.

Not all interventions have demonstrated benefit. For example, a randomized study of general medical patients older than 65 years of age compared the usual care to care by a geriatric consultant and a protocol for systematized review of patients' records. The groups, followed for as long as 8 weeks, did not differ in time to improvement from the delirium, and less than one-half of the patients in both groups demonstrated an increase in Mini-Mental State Examination (MMSE) of at least 2 points. Additionally, there were no differences between the groups in measures of delirium severity, length of stay, discharge rate to the community, living arrangements after discharge, or survival. Future interventional studies are needed to inform the debate about the content, duration, and method of educational programs that may modify the frequency, duration, and severity of delirium in various patient cohorts.

ETIOLOGY

Pathophysiology Although delirium has been described in the medical literature for at least 2,500 years, the pathophysiology of the syndrome is not understood. Several theories have been proposed. The hypotheses are speculative and are largely products from animal research (Table 10.2–9).

Although there has been research looking for a final common pathway that explains all delirium, given the heterogeneity of the etiologies and the presentations of delirium, there may not be one mechanism that encompasses the entire syndrome. To date, the proposed theories for delirium pathophysiology involve neurochemical abnormalities, alterations in metabolism, involvement of cytokines and acute phase reactants, and changes in the permeability of the blood–brain barrier. Interestingly, these systems are not mutually exclusive and may have considerable interactions.

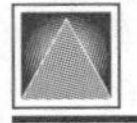

Table 10.2–9
Hypotheses about Delirium Pathophysiology

Decreased oxidative metabolism	Abnormal second messenger that uses neurotransmitter as first messenger
Reduced cholinergic function	Change in blood–brain barrier permeability
Dopamine excess	Endocrine abnormality (e.g., hypothalamic-pituitary-adrenal axis and thyroid hormone)
Norepinephrine excess	
Glutamate excess	
Serotonin imbalance	Decreased somatostatin-like reactivity
γ-Aminobutyric acid imbalance	
Decreased beta endorphin	Inflammatory hypothesis with cytokine increase
Abnormal signal transduction	

Neurochemical Neurochemical changes in acetylcholine, dopamine, glutamate, γ-aminobutyric acid (GABA), and serotonin are found in patients with delirium.

ACETYLCHOLINE The cholinergic system has been extensively studied in delirium, as it is involved with rapid eye movement (REM) sleep, attention, arousal, and memory. Anticholinergic agents have been found to cause delirium in humans and behavioral and EEG changes in animals. Assays are available to measure the anticholinergic load in the serum. The serum anticholinergic levels are increased in delirious patients and decline as delirium resolves. These assays are only used in experimental settings, as they require a great deal of expertise in interpretation and are lacking in specificity. Further support for a cholinergic component of delirium comes from the fact that cholinergic agents, such as physostigmine, have demonstrated benefit in treating anticholinergic delirium. Of interest, physostigmine has also demonstrated benefit in nonanticholinergic delirium, such as delirium from alcohol withdrawal, ketamine anesthesia, H_2 receptor antagonist delirium, and γ-hydroxybutyric acid withdrawal. This suggests the possibility of interactions between other systems and the cholinergic system in the pathophysiology of delirium.

DOPAMINE The dopaminergic system may also play a role in the pathogenesis of delirium. Dopamine is involved in maintaining and shifting attention via modulation of the frontal cortex. Antipsychotic agents that block dopamine receptors provide symptomatic relief for delirious patients and may result in a relative decrease in dopamine levels. Substances that increase dopamine, such as psychostimulants, carbidopa and levodopa (Sinemet), bupropion (Wellbutrin), or amantadine (Symmetrel), may cause delirium. As dopamine levels increase, cholinergic levels decline, possibly contributing to delirium through the interaction of the two neurotransmitter systems. Additionally, reduction in dopaminergic function is associated with alterations in oxidative metabolism.

GLUTAMATE Glutamate abnormalities are inferred in the pathophysiology of delirium. Glutamate excitatory neurotoxicity via the *N*-methyl-D-aspartate (NMDA) receptor may cause apoptosis and neuronal death and has been associated with alcohol intoxication and withdrawal, conditions that are associated with delirium. NMDA antagonists, such as phencyclidine (PCP) and ketamine, are also associated with delirium. Wernicke's encephalopathy is one example of a delirium that may involve glutamate abnormalities. Wernicke's encephalopathy is due to thiamine deficiency. Thiamine is a cofactor of several enzymes. Evidence suggests that such enzyme deficits result in focal lactic acidosis, cerebral energy impairment, and depolarization of neurons resulting from glutamate excitotoxicity.

GABA Alterations in GABA activity have been associated with delirium. In patients with hepatic encephalopathy, increased inhibitory GABA levels also are observed. An increase in ammonia levels occurs in patients with hepatic encephalopathy, which causes an increase in the amino acids glutamate and glutamine, which are precursors to GABA. In contrast, decreases in CNS GABA levels are observed in patients with delirium resulting from benzodiazepine and alcohol withdrawal.

SEROTONIN Excess and attenuated serotonin has been implicated in delirium. Support for this hypothesis comes from the classic serotonin syndrome, which is a delirium with tachycardia, tremor, diaphoresis, shivering, diarrhea, hyperreflexia, fever, ataxia, and myoclonus. Additionally, patients with hepatic pathology and delirium have elevations in serotonin. Patients who are withdrawing from serotonergic agents may also present with delirium, suggesting that the absolute levels of a single neurotransmitter may not explain delirium.

Oxidative Metabolism Alterations in oxidative metabolism may result in delirium. This may occur via a number of proposed mechanisms, including neuronal injury, reduced dopaminergic function, reduction of the synthesis and release of acetylcholine, and reduced glucose utilization. The abnormalities in oxidative metabolism may be a final common pathway for the neurotransmitter abnormalities in delirium.

Blood–Brain Barrier Alterations Delirium may be related to capillary endothelial changes that result in the disruption of the blood–brain barrier. These alterations in permeability may contribute to the pathophysiology of delirium. Cortical biopsies in patients with traumatically induced delirium from epidural and subdural hematomas demonstrate blood–brain barrier dysfunction. Other studies have proposed blood–brain barrier dysfunction in delirium tremens and primary hyperparathyroidism, a condition with many neuropsychiatric manifestations, including delirium.

Cytokines Cytokines may be implicated in the pathophysiology of delirium. Fever, infection, injury, and chemotherapy are associated with delirium and also with elevations in cytokines. Animal studies revealed clinical and EEG manifestations of delirium after administration of intraventricular interleukin-1 (IL-1), a proinflammatory cytokine. Animal studies show that IL-1 induces a reduced activity of the cholinergic system. Rodent models suggest that IL-1 administration decreases extracellular acetylcholine in the hippocampus and increases norepinephrine in the hypothalamus. Cytokines may change the endothelial permeability of the blood–brain barrier. Taken together, these findings suggest the possible central role of cytokines in the pathophysiology of delirium.

Ammonia Elevated serum ammonia levels contribute to increased glutamate and glutamine levels that are precursors to GABA. The changes in GABA activity may alter the thalamic filter of incoming stimuli to the cortex. Elevated ammonia levels have been associated with delirium due to hepatic encephalopathy, as well as delirium due to valproate, used alone or in combination with other anticonvulsant mood stabilizers. Delirium associated with hepatic encephalopathy may result from the accumulation of unmetabolized ammonia. The etiology of anticonvulsant-induced delirium is not known, but it is speculated that valproic acid (Depakene) may directly or indirectly inhibit crucial enzymes in the urea cycle.

Future Directions The basic pathophysiology of delirium may become better understood as pharmacological probes are coupled with functional neuroimaging. For example, a specific symptom cluster found in delirium may be reproduced with medication challenge, and advanced neuroimaging will allow study of the relationship between these symptoms and functional brain changes. Structural and functional neuroimaging and animal studies suggest that prefrontal cortex, anterior and right thalamus, fusiform cortex, posterior parietal cortex, and the basal ganglia may be implicated as having a role in delirium. Some authors suggest that these findings are consistent with alterations in oxidative metabolism and neurotransmitter deficits.

All told, the pathophysiology of delirium remains unclear. The effects of oxidative stress, inflammation, blood–brain barrier disturbance, endocrinopathies, and substance use and withdrawal on the neurotransmitter systems may begin to describe the complex pathophysiology of such a heterogeneous condition as delirium.

Etiologies It is clear from the previous discussion that there are many insults that may cause delirium, and, of course, most deliria are multifactorial in etiology. Examples of specific causes of delirium are listed in Table 10.2–10. The following is a discussion of some common etiologies.

Substance Intoxication Delirium The diagnosis of a substance-induced delirium is made when a medication or other chemical agent is thought to be etiologically related to the condition. The responsible substance may be determined from clinical history, physical examination, and laboratory tests, such as a toxicology screen. The goal of treatment is to remove the offending agent. A familiarity with the common toxicologic syndromes (also known as *toxidromes*) is useful, as it may guide the investigation to include screening for additional agents. Table 10.2–11 describes the common toxidromes. Additionally, an awareness of the most common drugs that are abused in a geographic region may prove to be at least as valuable in screening for substances as searching for specific signs and symptoms, especially in ingestions of multiple agents. Clinicians need to keep current with drugs of abuse, newly approved drugs, herbal preparations, and teas as potential causes of delirium.

DRUGS OF ABUSE Intoxication with a variety of drugs of abuse is known to cause a delirium. Examples include cocaine, PCP, heroin, alcohol, nitrous oxide, amphetamine and its derivatives (e.g., speed and ecstasy), and marijuana. The ever-changing choice and availability of recreational drugs obligate the clinician to keep up to date about the agents that are the newest street drugs and the cohorts that use them. Assays to determine these drugs are often not available in routine toxicology screens. Experimentation with drugs of abuse extends to synthetic compounds known as *raves*, which are often used in dance clubs. Drugs such as 3,4-methylenedioxymethamphetamine (MDMA), also known as *ecstasy*, a methamphetamine analog, have been associated with delirium and fatalities. Special K, or ketamine, an anesthetic agent often used by veterinarians, and PCP (also known as *angel dust*) are NMDA receptor antagonists and are other examples of street drugs associated with delirium. An example of the symptoms of a substance-induced delirium is described for PCP. At low to moderate doses of PCP, respirations may become rapid and shallow, with flushing, diaphoresis, numbness of the extremities, and muscular incoordination. At high doses, blood pressure, pulse rate, and respiration may drop, accompanied by nausea, vomiting, blurred vision, drooling, ataxia, dizziness, seizures, and coma. The patient may have prominent illusions, hallucinations, delusions, paranoia, disordered thinking, and catatonia, often with sparse and garbled speech.

Flunitrazepam and γ-hydroxybutyrate are other common choices of recreational drug users with the potential for delirium, as well as amnesia and sexual assault. Flunitrazepam is a benzodiazepine that causes anterograde amnesia, disinhibition, and lack of muscle control. It has been associated with violent behavior when combined with alcohol and other drugs of abuse in male juvenile delinquents who

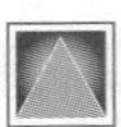

Table 10.2–10
Common Causes of Delirium

Central nervous system disorder	Seizure (postictal, nonconvulsive status, status)
	Migraine
	Head trauma, brain tumor, subarachnoid hemorrhage, subdural, epidural hematoma, abscess, intracerebral hemorrhage, cerebellar hemorrhage, nonhemorrhagic stroke, transient ischemia
Metabolic disorder	Electrolyte abnormalities
	Diabetes, hypoglycemia, hyperglycemia, or insulin resistance
Systemic illness	Infection (e.g., sepsis, malaria, erysipelas, viral, plague, Lyme disease, syphilis, or abscess)
	Trauma
	Change in fluid status (dehydration or volume overload)
	Nutritional deficiency
	Burns
	Uncontrolled pain
	Heat stroke
	High altitude (usually >5,000 m)
Medications	Pain medications (e.g., postoperative meperidine [Demerol] or morphine [Duramorph])
	Antibiotics, antivirals, and antifungals
	Steroids
	Anesthesia
	Cardiac medications
	Antihypertensives
	Antineoplastic agents
	Anticholinergic agents
	Neuroleptic malignant syndrome
	Serotonin syndrome
Over-the-counter preparations	Herbals, teas, and nutritional supplements
Botanicals	Jimsonweed, oleander, foxglove, hemlock, dieffenbachia, and *Amanita phalloides*
Cardiac	Cardiac failure, arrhythmia, myocardial infarction, cardiac assist device, cardiac surgery
Pulmonary	Chronic obstructive pulmonary disease, hypoxia, SIADH, acid base disturbance
Endocrine	Adrenal crisis or adrenal failure, thyroid abnormality, parathyroid abnormality
Hematological	Anemia, leukemia, blood dyscrasia, stem cell transplant
Renal	Renal failure, uremia, SIADH
Hepatic	Hepatitis, cirrhosis, hepatic failure
Neoplasm	Neoplasm (primary brain, metastases, paraneoplastic syndrome)
Drugs of abuse	Intoxication and withdrawal
Toxins	Intoxication and withdrawal
	Heavy metals and aluminum

SIADH, syndrome of inappropriate secretion of antidiuretic hormone.

may have been experiencing substance-induced delirium. Additionally, the agent has been found in persons who have been raped, probably used by the attacker because of its clinical effects on memory. γ-Hydroxybutyrate is a sedative hypnotic used to treat narcolepsy. It is increasingly common as a cause of stupor, and there is a risk of respiratory suppression when it is combined with other sedative agents. Additionally, withdrawal from γ-hydroxybutyrate presents in a similar manner as alcohol or benzodiazepine withdrawal.

It is important to realize that patients who abuse illicit substances are at increased risk for human immunodeficiency virus (HIV) and hepatitis B and C due to sharing needles or unprotected sexual encounters. These illnesses may increase the risk of or complicate the delirium.

Assistance in diagnosing the underlying etiology of a substance intoxication delirium is available through the local poison control center, which has a database that can identify unknown tablets and can describe likely patient responses to intoxication from most prescription and nonprescription agents, herbs, chemicals, and plants. Once the offending agent is identified, appropriate treatment may be initiated and guided through the regional poison center. Established procedures are available for the treatment of overdose of substances such as acetaminophen, aspirin, organic solvents, ethylene glycol, opioids, benzodiazepines, barbiturates, and anticholinergic agents.

Substance Withdrawal–Induced Delirium When reviewing the history and chart of a patient with delirium, the medication list should be thought of as a starting point to ask the question, "what was on this list, prescribed, over the counter, licit or illicit, last week? Yesterday?" This is especially true when a patient is admitted emergently into the hospital and is unable to give a reliable history. Any acute change in mental status can herald a substance withdrawal delirium. The diagnosis may be supported by autonomic changes or the detection of a substance or its metabolite in the urine or serum. Common substances to cause withdrawal delirium, such as alcohol, benzodiazepines, and opiates, are described in the following sections.

ALCOHOL WITHDRAWAL The classic agitated withdrawal delirium is delirium tremens. This syndrome, synonymous with severe alcohol withdrawal, presents with delirium, autonomic hyperactivity, and frequent visual and tactile hallucinations and carries a significant risk of seizures and death if untreated. Patients admitted into the hospital may present several days into admission with alcohol withdrawal and may be at risk for delirium tremens. Histories of complicated alcohol withdrawal, medical comorbidity, and elevated blood pressure are associated with an increased risk of delirium tremens.

BENZODIAZEPINE WITHDRAWAL Benzodiazepine withdrawal may appear similar to alcohol withdrawal and also may be accompanied by seizures. The onset of symptoms is dependent on the half-life of the particular benzodiazepine. For example, alprazolam (Xanax) withdrawal (short half-life) may present in 1 to 2 days, but diazepam (Diastat) withdrawal (long half-life) may present 5 to 7 days after the last dose.

OPIATE WITHDRAWAL Opiate withdrawal presents with severe flu-like syndromes, gastrointestinal (GI) cramping, diarrhea, diaphoresis, autonomic hyperactivity, and craving. Delirium may also occur with opioid withdrawal and has been reported with switching from transdermal fentanyl (Duragesic) to morphine (Duramorph). The presentation may occur because of unknown prior use of opiates in the context of abuse or prescription or methadone (Dolophine) maintenance.

Postoperative Delirium

AFTER CORONARY ARTERY BYPASS GRAFT Delirium exists in 7 to 40 percent of patients after coronary artery bypass graft (CABG). The preoperative risk factors include age, past stroke, carotid bruit, hypertension, and diabetes. The most significant intraoperative risk factor is the time on bypass pump. One outcome study of patients undergoing CABG suggested that, in patients older than 75 years of age, 37 percent had a delirium, compared to 11 percent in the 65- to 74-year-old group. Interestingly, there was no between-

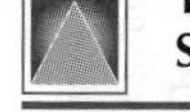

Table 10.2–11
Signs of Common Toxidromes

Substance	Pupils	Vitals	Skin	Neuromotor	Electrocardiogram	Gastrointestinal	Other	Absorption
Anticholinergic	Mydriasis	Tachycardia	Dry, flushed	Seizure, coma	QRS interval widening	Decreased bowel sounds, obstruction risk	Urinary retention	Ingestion, parenteral, ocular
Cholinergic agonist	Miosis	Bradycardia, hypotension	Flushing, sweating	Muscle cramps, tremors, seizure, paralysis	Bradycardia	Abdominal pain, vomiting, diarrhea	Bronchospasm, incontinence, lacrimation	Ingestion, ocular, inhalation
Serotonin syndrome	Mydriasis	Tachycardia, hypertension, tachypnea, fever	Flushing, diaphoresis	Lethargy, seizures, coma, hyperreflexia, myoclonus	Dysrhythmias	Diarrhea	N/A	Ingestion, parenteral
Ethanol	Eye irritation from vapors, injected conjunctiva	Hypothermia, hypotension, respiratory failure	Flushing, dermatitis	Inebriation, CNS depression, coma	Dysrhythmias	Gastritis, bleeding	Acidosis, electrolyte imbalance, hypoglycemia (children)	Ingestion, inhalation
Benzodiazepines	N/A	Hypotension, hypothermia, decreased respirations	N/A	Respiratory suppression, coma, ataxia, lethargy, slurred speech	N/A	Nausea, vomiting	Significant interaction with alcohol and opioids	Ingestion, parenteral
Cocaine	N/A	Tachycardia, hypertension, hyperthermia	N/A	Seizure, coma, CNS hemorrhage or infarct	Dysrhythmias	Bowel necrosis	Acidosis, acute respiratory distress syndrome, disseminated intravascular coagulation	Ingestion, parenteral, insufflation, topical
Sympathomimetic	N/A	Tachycardia, hypertension	Sweating	Tremulousness, seizures, intracranial hemorrhage or infarct	Dysrhythmias	Nausea, vomiting	Hypokalemia, rhabdomyolysis	Ingestion, parenteral
Opioids	Miosis	Mild hypotension, respiratory depression	Track marks indicate abuse	CNS	Dysrhythmias	Decreased bowel sounds	Hypoxia, rhabdomyolysis	Ingestion, parenteral, insufflation

CNS, central nervous system; N/A, not available.

group difference in mortality. Postoperative complications, supraventricular arrhythmia, pneumonia, and intubation duration were higher in the group of patients older than 75 years of age compared to patients 65 to 74 years of age. Other studies of CABG patients who developed a delirium suggested the possibility that biological markers of brain injury may be useful to predict which CABG patients will develop a delirium or other longer-term neuropsychiatric sequelae of CABG.

MINOR SURGICAL PROCEDURES Even minor surgical procedures have been associated with postoperative delirium. In a study of cataract surgery, 4.4 percent of patients developed postoperative delirium. Older age and premedication were associated with increased risk of developing delirium.

Delirium in Children

Common causes of delirium in children include fever, anticholinergics, anesthesia, infections, burns, endocrinopathies, head trauma, and metabolic disturbances. Less commonly, sleep apnea, sickle cell anemia, Lyme disease, HIV, neurocysticercosis, and pediatric autoimmune neuropsychiatric disorder associated with streptococcal infection have all been associated with delirium. Accidental poisonings remain a significant risk for young children, whereas substance abuse, especially with organic solvents, is a significant public health concern in older children.

DIAGNOSIS

The diagnosis of delirium is made clinically through serial observations of the patient. After a diagnosis of the syndrome is made, it is important to have a pragmatic clinical approach to identifying the underlying etiology of the delirium. This requires a systematic review to detect infections, metabolic changes, endocrine abnormalities, nutritional changes, neoplasia, medication, or substance intoxication or withdrawal. See Table 10.2–12 for one possible approach to determine the causes of delirium.

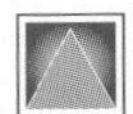

Table 10.2–12
Determining the Causes of Delirium

Gather history from patient, health care providers, friends, and family
Establish extent and acuity of the medical comorbidities with labs and diagnostic studies as appropriate
Review the medication list
Consider the medications that were recently stopped, as withdrawal may be a factor
Review for substances of abuse and dependence
Urine or serum toxicology
Consider the substances that were recently stopped, as withdrawal may be a factor (e.g., alcohol, benzodiazepines, and opiates)
Consider over-the-counter medications, herbal preparations, and teas
Establish whether there was recent exposure to anesthesia or surgery
Evaluate vital signs for autonomic changes
Check all indwelling catheters for signs of infection
Check skin for evidence of breakdown or infection
Evaluate for pain severity, duration, and intensity
Evaluate for constipation or diarrhea
Evaluate for urinary tract infection
Evaluate for acid–base disturbance
Consider deep venous thrombosis or pulmonary embolus
Consider seizure or postictal state; consider electroencephalogram
Evaluate for toxidromes (see the text for more detail)
Review laboratory studies for evidence of renal, cardiac, hepatic, pulmonary, or hematological dysfunction
Check nutritional status
Consider whether there is sensory overload or deprivation (e.g., too close to the nursing station or agitated roommate vs. glasses or hearing aide misplaced or absent)
Consider structural neuroimaging
Consider cerebrospinal evaluation
Consider additional body fluid analyses
Consider medication–medication interactions
Consider medication–over-the-counter medication interactions

Diagnosing the Delirium

Detection of a fluctuation in the ability to sustain and focus attention and impairment in cognitive functioning requires evaluation over a sufficient time period. Lucid intervals during a delirium may give a false impression to an examiner that no delirium is present. Therefore, reliance on multiple examinations over time, ideally given by the same examiner, is preferable. Questioning nursing staff, family, and friends about cognitive fluctuation, psychotic symptoms, and level of alertness may be extremely useful. Sleep–wake cycle disturbance is a significant clinical feature that may take the form of fragmented sleep, reversal of day and night, sedation during the day, and arousal during the night.

Orientation, memory, and concentration are key areas for the clinician to assess when evaluating a patient for possible delirium. Many diagnostic instruments have been developed for use in delirium patients but are limited by problems with reliability and validity. Most focus on cognition at the expense of behavioral changes. Examples of two instruments that have been validated and that are consistent with the current DSM-IV-TR definition of delirium are described in the following discussion.

The CAM is a reliable, valid, rapid, and easy-to-administer instrument to detect delirium. The diagnosis of delirium with the CAM requires an acute onset of changes or fluctuations in the course of the mental status and inattention and an altered level of consciousness or disorganized thinking. The CAM has been validated in a number of settings, including the ICU. In elderly, mechanically ventilated patients, the instrument retained high levels of validity when compared to expert clinicians using DSM-IV-TR criteria with 95 percent sensitivity and 88 percent specificity. The administration time is approximately 2 minutes. The instrument detected delirium in 83.3 percent of patients in the ICU, the highest published rate in the ICU setting. Interestingly, more than 10 percent of patients remained delirious at hospital discharge.

Another validated assessment scale for delirium is the MDAS. It is a ten-item, 30-point scale that rates disturbances in arousal, level of consciousness, psychomotor activity, and areas of cognition such as memory, attention, orientation, and thought disturbance. The MDAS can be used to follow delirium severity over time and has demonstrated reliability and validity as a measure of delirium severity in hospitalized patients with acquired immune deficiency syndrome (AIDS) and cancer. Using a cutoff score of 13 or higher for the presence of delirium, the sensitivity was 71 percent, and specificity was 91 percent.

Diagnosing Delirium in Special Populations

Delirium in Persons with Dementia

Persons with dementia may be unable to directly communicate complaints related to the development or change in a medical condition. They may be unable to report recent trauma and to describe pain, constipation, shortness of breath, nausea, changes in vision, weakness, or sensory changes. Adverse effects from the recent addition of or change in medication or over-the-counter compound may not be evident from interviewing the patient. The history of the present illness should be obtained from the patient, as well as a reliable informant, if possible. Caregiver information, physical examination, mental state examination, neurological examination, serum and urine studies, chest X-ray, electrocardiogram (ECG), and other targeted investigations should be considered, as the onset of the delirium may reflect a serious intercurrent medical illness in a patient with dementia. The medication list may reveal contributors to delirium. Moreover, recently discontinued medications may contribute to delirium. Examples include too rapid discontinuation of benzodiazepines or opiate analgesics. When serotonergic agents are discontinued too rapidly, a serotonin withdrawal syndrome may present with delirium. Patients with dementia who develop a delirium are at increased risk of long-term functional and cognitive decline, rehospitalization, long-term care placement, and mortality.

Delirium in Persons with Schizophrenia Although the literature is sparse in actual prevalence rates of delirium in schizophrenia, persons with schizophrenia carry many of the risk factors and predisposing factors for delirium, such as medical comorbidities, substance abuse, smoking history, and multiple medications. Patients with schizophrenia are also at increased risk of sexually or IV transmitted disease, including HIV and other infections, such as hepatitis B and C. Substance-induced delirium is common in schizophrenia, reflecting the high rates of substance use in this population. Additionally, medications used to treat schizophrenia may be associated with cardiovascular disease, diabetes, and weight gain. The atypical antipsychotic agents may have interactions with medications used to treat comorbid conditions and result in delirium due to drug–drug interactions. Patients with schizophrenia have developed delirium by using an herbal compound containing ephedra to combat weight gain or by combining erythromycin (E-Mycin) with clozapine (Clozaril), which results in increased clozapine levels. Additionally, clozapine withdrawal has been reported as a possible cause of delirium.

The antipsychotic agents used to treat schizophrenia may themselves cause delirium. For example, a rare medical emergency associated with antipsychotic medications is neuroleptic malignant syndrome (NMS). Signs and symptoms of NMS may include delirium, fever, rigidity, autonomic hyperactivity, leukocytosis, and increased creatine phosphokinase (CPK). Antipsychotic agents may also be associated with akathisia, a subjective feeling of restlessness that may present as severe psychomotor agitation and thus mimics a symptom of delirium. Patients taking antipsychotic agents may also develop delirium from the anticholinergic effects of typical or atypical antipsychotic agents or the associated medications used to treat the parkinsonian side effects of antipsychotic agents.

Delirium in the Terminally Ill It is important to note that terminally ill patients have high rates of delirium. The terminally ill patient may have delirium related to pain, opiates, the primary disorder, or the process of dying as the major organ systems fail.

Delirium in Children Diagnosis of delirium in children may have behavioral change as the sole manifestation. Any change of behavior or a sleep–wake problem in a young child who is not responsive to soothing from familiar figures may be an indication that an underlying medical condition or substance is at the root cause of the behavioral change. Children may be more apt to have a temporary regression of their development early in the delirium recovery.

Fever is commonly associated with delirium in children. Controversy exists regarding the degree to which one should pursue fever workup for a fever of unknown origin in a young child. Practice guidelines published in 1993 attempted to clarify the need for cultures, hospitalization, and antibiotic use. The most pressing risk is from meningitis, although other infectious sources may lead to behavioral changes and delirium in young children. Children younger than 3 years of age are given extra scrutiny for high fever but do not commonly get a lumbar puncture, even in the face of a febrile delirium. The extent of the workup is partially determined by the age of the child, as well as by the clinical presentation. Children younger than 1 month of age, independent of clinical presentation, are at an increased risk of sepsis due to neonatal risk factors. They usually receive an extensive workup that includes complete blood count (CBC); blood, urine, and cerebrospinal fluid (CSF) cultures; and chest X-ray, and they should be hospitalized for parenteral antibiotics. In general, the workup becomes less invasive with age, especially in a child 3 to 36 months of age, in whom occult bacteremia is more common than overwhelming sepsis.

CLINICAL FEATURES

Patients with delirium fluctuate in their ability to focus, to shift, and to sustain attention; are easily distractible; and demonstrate impaired memory. Associated symptoms include affective lability, psychomotor abnormalities, and misinterpretations and hallucinations. Affective symptoms often fluctuate and may include anxiety, fear, apathy, anger, euphoria, dysphoria, and irritability, all within short time periods. The perceptual disturbances are mostly visual, but they also occur in the other sensory realms. These perceptual disturbances are often disturbing to the patient and have been described as poorly organized, fragmented dreams or nightmares. Confusion and reactivity to hallucinations and disorientation may dominate the behavioral manifestations of delirium. Patients may attempt to remove IV lines, catheters, ECG leads, and other tubes or may attempt to ambulate under unsafe conditions (e.g., postoperatively).

Delirious patients are categorized on the basis of alertness and psychomotor activity. The hyperactive subtype is psychomotorically active, hypervigilant, restless, and excitable and speaks with loud or pressured speech. The hypoactive subtype is psychomotorically slowed, quiet, and withdrawn and has reduced alertness and decreased speech production. The loud patient gains the attention of others and is more likely to be diagnosed with delirium than the quiet patient who is not disturbing other patients or staff. Because delirium carries an increased risk of morbidity and mortality, the quietly delirious patient needs to be identified and appropriately evaluated and treated. A concern with the loud, hyperactive, delirious patient is the increased use of chemical or mechanical restraints that may carry the risk of neglecting the appropriate diagnostic evaluation and possibly worsening the delirium through polypharmacy.

Although increased motor activity is described as a feature in some accounts of delirium due to hyperthyroidism, anticholinergic toxicity, and alcohol withdrawal, the reliability of motor activity as an aid in differential diagnosis of delirium is not consistent. Motor activity in delirium is not consistently associated with etiology, EEG findings, cerebral blood flow, or ratings of fluctuation.

PATHOLOGY AND LABORATORY EXAMINATION

Laboratory Workup Information gained from the history, physical, and neurological examinations suggest laboratory studies to aid in determining the causes of the delirium. There is no single panel of laboratory tests that is recommended for all cases of delirium. CBC, electrolytes, liver function, renal function, thyroid function, adrenal function, glucose, calcium, magnesium, vitamin B_{12}, folate, erythrocyte sedimentation rate (ESR), rapid plasma reagin (RPR), arterial blood gas (ABG), and ECG may all be indicated. Depending on the clinical situation, HIV and hepatitis profiling may be appropriate. Urine drug and serum toxicology screens are frequently helpful. Computed tomography (CT) or magnetic resonance imaging (MRI) of the brain and EEG may be considered. Body fluid cultures and lumbar puncture may also be required.

EEG Engel and Romano (1959) postulated that delirium, "reversible cerebral insufficiency," was due to decreased brain metabolic activity based on EEG slowing. They found a correlation between decreased arousal and the disorganized background activity on EEG. In their earlier work, patients with delirium due to hypoxia demonstrated a reversal in EEG changes when they were treated with oxygen. Additionally, delirious anemic patients treated with transfusions and delirious hypoglycemic patients treated with glucose demonstrated EEG reversal back toward normal. If a patient is suspected of having a delirium, an EEG may give useful information to confirm the diagnosis. The EEG in delirium frequently demonstrates generalized slowing. If the cause of the delirium is alcohol withdrawal, fast activity may be present. In most cases, serial EEGs are most useful to establish a clinical correlation between the EEG findings and the clinical progression. The range of normal frequency on EEG may vary from 8 to 13 Hz. Therefore, a slowing may still be read as within the normal range if the baseline, healthy EEG is not known to be at a higher frequency.

Neuroimaging Structural brain imaging may detect acute or subacute conditions, such as subarachnoid hemorrhage, subdural hematomas, intracranial tumors, and vascular changes, including stroke, which may cause or contribute to a delirium. Limited evidence suggests that neuroimaging may assist in the prediction of patients who will develop a delirium. For example, the degree of white matter lesions was related to the development of delirium during an electroconvulsive therapy (ECT) course in an elderly population. Results of functional imaging have been described in case reports of patients with delirium related to hypoxia, alcohol withdrawal, and cardiac surgery. The results are too varied to be clinically useful. Functional imaging is logistically difficult in a delirious patient and, at this point, is not recommended because of lack of clinical use.

DIFFERENTIAL DIAGNOSIS

The possible DSM-IV-TR Axis I differential diagnoses for delirium include dementia with psychosis, schizophrenia or schizophreniform psychosis, posttraumatic stress disorder (PTSD), and affective disorder with psychosis.

Dementia and Delirium Delirium and dementia may be confused because of overlapping symptoms, such as disorientation and difficulty with short-term memory. The major differential points between dementia and delirium are the time to develop the condition and the fluctuation in level of attention in delirium compared to relatively consistent attention in dementia. The time to development of symptoms is usually short in delirium and, except for vascular dementia due to stroke, is usually gradual and insidious in dementia. Table 10.2–13 compares dementia and delirium to aid the clinician in the differential diagnosis between the two conditions.

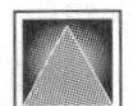

Table 10.2–13
Differentiating Dementia from Delirium

Feature	Dementia	Delirium
Onset	Slow	Rapid
Duration	Months to years	Hours to weeks
Attention	Preserved	Fluctuates
Memory	Impaired remote memory	Impaired recent and immediate memory
Speech	Word-finding difficulty	Incoherent (slow or rapid)
Sleep–wake cycle	Fragmented sleep	Frequent disruption (e.g., day–night reversal)
Thoughts	Impoverished	Disorganized
Awareness	Unchanged	Reduced
Alertness	Usually normal	Hypervigilant or reduced vigilance

Adapted from Lipowski ZJ. *Delirium: Acute Confusional States.* Oxford: Oxford University Press; 1990.

It is important to underscore that delirium and dementia are not mutually exclusive. In fact, patients with dementia are more likely than nondemented patients to develop a delirium. Any change of cognitive symptoms or behavior in a dementia patient should not be automatically attributed to the dementia without considering a general medical condition or substance as an explanation for the symptoms, especially when fluctuations in attention or sleep–wake disturbances are present. Again, a careful history should help clarify this diagnosis—that is, the dementia has a gradual, relatively stable and progressive course, whereas the superimposed delirium has caused an acute or subacute worsening in symptoms with a fluctuating course.

Schizophrenia Psychotic disorders and delirium may be confused on the basis of the active psychotic symptoms and disorganized thinking. Evaluating the rate of onset and attentional fluctuation most commonly makes the differential between schizophrenia or schizophreniform psychosis and delirium. Delirium usually has a more rapid rate of onset and fluctuation in attention. Memory problems and disorientation are more frequent in delirium than schizophrenia. The delusions in delirium are usually not as bizarre or as well systematized as in schizophrenia. Some patients with schizophrenia have concurrent dementia, further complicating the differential diagnosis. The points about differentiating dementia and delirium then become operative. Like patients with dementia, patients with schizophrenia and dementia may not have the capacity to communicate pain, acute changes in medical condition, or other basic concerns.

Affective Disorders with Psychosis Mood disorders such as depression or mania with associated psychosis may also have symptoms that overlap with delirium, such as impaired concentration, perceptual disturbances, and impaired memory. Depression may resemble a hypoactive delirium. Withdrawal, slowed speech, apathetic mood, and poor testing on cognitive scales may occur in both conditions. Depression lacks the clouding of consciousness, inattention, and variability that are present in delirium.

It is crucial to differentiate affective disorders with psychotic features from delirium because of the differences in the prognosis and treatment. It is important to consider that an untreated medical condition or substance use or withdrawal may also aggravate affective disorders. Delirium does not usually present with as significant a mood component. The psychosis seen in mood disorders with psychotic features is usually more systematized and syntonic. In contrast, the psychosis in delirium is usually more disorganized and fragmented. In psychotic mood disturbances, disorientation and fluctuation in attention are not prominent features. Impaired concentration may be present in the mood disorders, but it is the *fluctuation* in attention and concentration that provides the differential point.

If a delirium were misdiagnosed as an affective disorder with psychosis, the pharmacotherapy (usually antidepressant and antipsychotic agents) might worsen the delirium. Alternately, the medications might initially improve the symptoms, but the underlying medical condition or substance problem would remain untreated, placing the patient at further increased risk of morbidity and mortality.

Patients with a mood disorder may develop a concurrent delirium. If the presentation is unclear, an evaluation for general medical conditions or substance use or withdrawal is recommended.

COURSE AND PROGNOSIS

By the third hospital day, approximately one-half the patients who are diagnosed with delirium have been diagnosed. Symptoms of delirium usually last 3 to 5 days, but there is much variability, with slow resolution of symptoms contributing to persistent symptoms of delirium at 6 to 8 weeks for severely ill patients. Symptom resolution is frequently incomplete by hospital discharge, with as many as 15 percent of patients remaining symptomatic of delirium at 6 months. There have been numerous methodological limitations of some studies examining long-term follow-up. The presence of dementia and the level of medical comorbidity were not always controlled for, and the sample sizes were frequently small. In general, studies suggest that the increased mortality risk associated with delirium was maintained at 12, 24, and 36 months with a risk ratio of at least 2 at all time points. Additionally, at 24 months, the increased risk of cognitive and functional impairment remained.

Early recognition of delirium is hypothesized to improve prognosis by allowing clinicians to address underlying medical conditions and substances earlier in the course. Surprisingly, preventive measures to improve prognosis have demonstrated mixed results. This may be due to insufficient exposure to staff, poor retention of information presented, or other patient and clinician factors. The outcome measure used in these trials included time to delirium resolution, increase in independence in activities of daily living (ADL), decreased length of stay, and increased rate of discharge to the community rather than institutional settings. For example, one positive study demonstrated that the presence of a liaison psychiatrist on an orthopedic unit reduced the frequency of delirium and decreased the length of stay for the patients in the intervention group. Another study, which looked at whether a geriatric consultation followed by involvement of a liaison nurse with the consultant and primary team, failed to demonstrate that the intervention had any benefit. Educational intervention to physicians and nurses by means of distribution of guidelines for recognizing delirium and formal educational in-services about the guidelines failed to improve outcomes in acute care hospitals in England. Similarly, in an academic medical center in the United States, a multicomponent interventional strategy failed to reduce the rate of delirium, placement into nursing homes, need for homecare visitation, readmission rates into the hospital, and self-rated health measures, and failed to improve functional status. Adherence to nonpharmacological interventions for delirium was directly related to patient outcome in this multicomponent intervention in the United States.

TREATMENT

There are three major goals of delirium treatment. One is to find and to reverse the contributors to the delirium. The second is to ensure the patient's safety while educating patients, family, and staff. The third is the symptomatic treatment of behavioral disturbances associated with delirium. The first goal is more related to diagnosis and etiology of the causative medical conditions. The treatment of the myriad of underlying medical disorders that cause or contribute to delirium is outside the purview of this chapter. This section focuses on the second and third goals and addresses the pharmacological and nonpharmacological principles in treating delirium symptoms, as well as family and staff education. The end of this section comments on considerations specific to certain common etiologies of delirium.

Pharmacological Management of the Symptoms of Dementia

In general, it is wise not to add additional medications to the patient's regimen, unless there is a significant reason to do so. Clinical situations that might require additional medications include agitation or psychosis.

Psychosis, Agitation, or Both

Antipsychotics may be considered if psychosis, severely disorganized thought process, or extreme physical or verbal agitation places the patient or others at risk of harm.

TYPICAL ANTIPSYCHOTICS Low-dose, high-potency antipsychotic agents have been the most frequently studied agents in the treatment of delirium. They may benefit an agitated patient by allowing completion of diagnostic tests and protecting the patient and others from harm. Agents such as haloperidol (Haldol) have the longest track record in delirium management and may be given orally, intramuscularly (IM), or IV. Haloperidol is associated with less anticholinergic load than the lower-potency agents such as chlorpromazine (Thorazine) or thioridazine (Mellaril), which are not recommended in the management of delirium.

Side effects of typical antipsychotic agents that may complicate the delirium include parkinsonism and akathisia. If antipsychotics are given IV, the patient should be monitored for cardiac dysrhythmias and prolonged QTc intervals on ECG. NMS is a risk from typical and atypical antipsychotic medications.

ATYPICAL ANTIPSYCHOTICS Use of second-generation antipsychotics, such as risperidone (Risperdal), clozapine, olanzapine (Zyprexa), quetiapine (Seroquel), ziprasidone (Geodon), and aripiprazole (Abilify), may be considered on a theoretical basis for delirium management, but clinical trial experience with these agents for delirium is lacking. Ziprasidone appears to have an activating effect and may not be appropriate in delirium management. Olanzapine is available IM and as a rapidly disintegrating oral preparation. These routes of administration may be preferable for some patients with delirium who are poorly compliant with medications or who are too sedated to safely swallow medications. For patients with Parkinson's disease and delirium who require antipsychotic medications, clozapine or quetiapine have some support in the literature and are less likely to exacerbate parkinsonian symptoms.

Parkinsonism may also occur with second-generation agents. For example, risperidone is found to cause parkinsonism that may occur after several weeks to months. This delayed adverse effect is a reminder that patients with delirium who require antipsychotic agents should be tapered off these agents as soon as is clinically possible after resolution of the delirium. Outpatient follow-up for patients who remain on antipsychotics at discharge should flag the outpatient provider to attempt to reduce or discontinue the antipsychotic as soon as is clinically possible.

OTHER PHARMACOLOGIC AGENTS If an agitated patient cannot receive antipsychotics (e.g., if the patient has NMS), a benzodiazepine without active metabolites (such as lorazepam [Ativan] or oxazepam [Serax]) may be appropriate. Another delirium-related syndrome that may require short-term benzodiazepine therapy is the acute stress disorder symptoms that may occur in the wake of a delirium. Patients may develop symptoms similar to those of an acute stress disorder, such as reexperiencing the perceptual disturbances, continued disturbance in the sleep–wake cycle, hypervigilance, or notable startle response. Disorientation, psychosis, and sleep deprivation place patients at risk of perceiving delirium as a significant traumatic event. Education and support during and after symptom resolution may improve integration of the experience. Short-term use of benzodiazepines may have a role if the patient remains anxious after the delirium is resolved. It is important to rule out an acute change in medical condition or recurrence of delirium as the cause of the increased anxiety, before starting treatment.

Electroconvulsive Therapy ECT is also a treatment for delirium when other approaches have failed. It has been used as a last resort for delirious patients with severe agitation who are not responsive to pharmacotherapy, such as high doses of IV haloperidol. The ECT is usually given en bloc or daily for several days, sometimes with multiple treatments per day.

Sleep–Wake Cycle Delirium is frequently complicated by changes in the sleep–wake cycle. Attempts to restore sleep integrity may include moving the schedule of existing sedating medications to the hour of sleep or reducing or moving activating medications and stimulants such as caffeine to the morning. Brief, judicious use of sedating agents, such as zolpidem (Ambien) or trazodone (Desyrel), to reset the sleep–wake cycle may be appropriate. Care should be taken to avoid excess sedation because of risk of falls, aspiration, and inability to perform or assist with ADLs. Sedating medications may also worsen delirium because of anticholinergic side effects and indirect effects on delaying mobilization and participation in functional recovery.

Nonpharmacological Aspects of Care

Nursing Care and the Medical Team Nursing interventions are a significant portion of delirium treatment. The focus is on safety and orientation with provision of the appropriate level of stimulation and education toward the patient and family. Nursing care should follow vital sign measurements and fluid intake and output. Care should be given when feeding to reduce or to prevent aspiration. If possible, feeding should be done in the lucid intervals, with several small feedings being desirable in some cases compared to few large feedings. Explanations and reassurance that the medical team is working together to find the cause of the delirium may also be helpful. Providing sufficient and consistent staffing for the delirious patient also assists in orienting, educating, and protecting the patient. Education about delirium management empowers staff with an approach to take with patients who have delirium and their families. The psychosocial interventions deepen rapport with the patient and family and move the treatment goals forward by improving adherence and satisfaction.

Environment Attention should be paid to providing the appropriate level of stimulation and orienting cues. Orienting cues include a large clock, calendar, well-lit room, and provision of eyeglasses and hearing aides if they are required. Darkening the room at night to help with the sleep–wake cycle is also important. Objects from a patient's residence may also assist with orienting and soothing the patient. If friends and family are available to assist with orienting the patient, every effort should be made to involve them in the treatment.

Family or Companions A cooperative family member may stay with the patient to provide orientation cues, reassurance to the patient, and observational data to the nurses and physicians. The companion may offer support in the form of simple explanations that the patient is safe and education that the behavioral symptoms may be attributable to delirium. Patients with delirium who present with severe lability in mood may respond better to a companion than to mood stabilizers.

Restraints Physical restraints are overused to manage delirious, agitated patients. Several studies point toward restraint use as an aggravating factor in the escalation of agitation. Moreover, restraint use has been determined as a causal factor in death by asphyxiation in delirious elderly patients, often in combination with bed rails, and in substance intoxicated persons restrained by police in a prone position. Another study of death in restrained delirious patients in the community found a relationship between death and obesity, stimulant use, and chronic disease. Policies and training on restraint use vary by locality but are an essential component to protect the safety and welfare of patients and caregivers alike.

Patient and Family Education During the delirious episode, families can be educated as to appropriate ways to be supportive to the patient, as well as to what information is important to convey to the medical team. As the delirium symptoms resolve, the patient and family should be educated about the long-term prognosis. The knowledge about delirium's risk of increased mortality and functional and cognitive decline may be shared with the patient and family as clinically appropriate. Discussions may include information about the possibility of an acute stress-like reaction that may occur in the aftermath of a delirium. Delirium may be a profoundly upsetting experience to some patients, and they may require assistance to integrate the experience. For those patients, follow-up discussions and even brief psychotherapy should be encouraged and available.

Treatment of Specific Etiologies of Delirium

It is beyond the scope of this chapter to give specific recommendations for treating the gamut of underlying conditions that may contribute to delirium. Coordination of care with emergency physicians or internal medicine specialists may be necessary. Some common causes of delirium are discussed in the following sections.

Anticholinergic Intoxication Anticholinergic medications are associated with delirium. There may be a cumulative effect of the anticholinergic load from multiple medications. Anticholinergic poisoning almost always results in delirium and is often accompanied by physical agitation and visual hallucinations. Physical signs resulting from antimuscarinic action include widely dilated, poorly reactive pupils; warm, dry skin; dry mouth; fever; tachycardia; elevated blood pressure; constipation; and urinary retention. Use of cholinesterase inhibitors, such as physostigmine, has been shown to reduce the severity of the delirium but requires repeated dosing because of a short half-life. In a comparison study of physostigmine and benzodiazepines for anticholinergic poisoning, the physostigmine was effective, whereas the benzodiazepine was ineffective and was associated with a higher complication rate. Anticholinergic intoxication also requires cardiac monitoring. The cholinesterase inhibitors that are U.S. Food and Drug Administration (FDA)–approved for Alzheimer's disease (donepezil [Aricept], rivastigmine [Exelon], and galantamine [Reminyl]) have not been well studied as a therapeutic modality in delirium.

Wernicke's Encephalopathy Wernicke's encephalopathy is a clinical syndrome of global amnesia; ophthalmoplegia, including nystagmus; ataxia; and confusion. It is caused by thiamine deficiency as seen in alcoholism and other nutritionally deficient states, such as terminal cancer, extended hospitalization with IV fluids being the sole nutritional source, and intractable vomiting after gastric reduction. It has also been reported in hemodialysis patients. If Wernicke's encephalopathy is suspected, thiamine is administered, followed by administration of dextrose and careful monitoring for the signs and symptoms of alcohol withdrawal. Thiamine must always be given before glucose, because thiamine is a cofactor in glucose metabolism, and, if the glucose is administered first, then the brain metabolism increases, and thiamine deficiency is exacerbated. If thiamine is not immediately available, glucose should still be administered.

Substance Intoxication Substance intoxication with alcohol, benzodiazepines, opiates, or mixed compounds requires attention to the acute management of the airway and vital organ functioning. Falls and unsafe sex practices may occur in intoxicated patients and should be considered in their management. For example, an intoxicated patient with traumatic head injury and a resulting subdural hematoma might have his or her clinical presentation attributed to intoxication alone, when a diagnostic neuroimaging study of the brain would be essential. Hence, intoxicated patients should receive a thorough physical, neurological, and mental state examination, even though the details of the clinical history often await the patient's sobering up or reliance on alternate informants. Mixed substance intoxications are common. Urine and serum toxicology and knowledge of common substances of abuse aid in patient management. Another important factor to consider is whether the intoxication was a result of a suicide attempt.

The primary concern in managing a patient with substance intoxication is supportive—that is, ensuring that the patient does not have significant respiratory depression and that there are no cardiovascular abnormalities. For benzodiazepine ingestions, the benzodiazepine receptor antagonist flumazenil may be helpful; however, repeated administrations might be required. In mixed ingestions that include benzodiazepines and tricyclic antidepressants or carbamazepine (Tegretol), flumazenil may precipitate cardiac dysrhythmias or seizures. The usefulness of flumazenil in patients with hepatic encephalopathy and alcohol overdose is questionable. Opiate intoxication may cause respiratory suppression in addition to delirium. Reversal with naloxone (Narcan) or naltrexone (ReVia) may be considered with adequate support and monitoring of the cardiovascular and respiratory status. Naloxone acts through competitive binding at opioid receptors, can reverse all the receptor-mediated actions of opioids, and is indicated for patients who have significant CNS or respiratory depression. Naloxone must be administered IM or IV, has a short half-life, and may require repeated administration as the effects wear off. Naloxone administration can precipitate acute withdrawal in chronic opioid users. There are many other agents that are used in the context of emergency care as antidotes to substances ingested.

Precautions must be taken to guard against withdrawal in the case of benzodiazepines, alcohol, or opioid overdose, because withdrawal itself may cause delirium. Treatment for substance intoxication entails controlled detoxification to prevent a worsening of the delirium or even death from withdrawal. Moreover, intoxication may suggest substance abuse or dependence for which further treatment is required when the delirium resolves.

Substance Withdrawal Alcohol and benzodiazepine withdrawal are treated by replacing the offending agent with a benzodiazepine and gradually reducing the dosage of the medication. The dose of benzodiazepine should be titrated to prevent autonomic hyperactivity. In addition, thiamine, folate, and multiple vitamins are administered to patients in alcohol withdrawal because of the frequency of malnutrition and the potential for Wernicke's encephalopathy. Benzodiazepine detoxification is often performed at a slower rate than alcohol detoxification owing to the longer half-life of most benzodiazepines compared to alcohol. In addition to delirium, opioid withdrawal has a significant risk of physical discomfort to patients. Symptomatic treatment with medications such as clonidine (Catapres) is aimed at targeting GI distress, autonomic changes, and craving. Care should be taken in automatically renewing an opiate user's methadone maintenance, even if the dose was confirmed, because excess opiates may result in respiratory arrest. Time since the last use of illicit opiates or methadone, as well as use of other substances that may cause respiratory depression, should be considered. It is always possible to begin treatment at a lower dose if the clinical situation warrants it.

Treatment in Special Populations

Parkinson's Disease Parkinson's disease patients are predisposed to delirium. In Parkinson's disease, the antiparkinsonian agents are frequently implicated in causing a delirium. If there is a coexistent dementia present, delirium is twice as likely to develop in Parkinson's disease patients with dementia receiving antiparkinsonian agents than those without dementia. In delirious Parkinson's disease patients, an intensive evaluation of causes of the delirium, other than antiparkinsonian medications, is necessary. Decreasing the dosage of the antiparkinsonian agent has to be weighed against a worsening of motor symptoms. If the antiparkinsonian agents cannot be further reduced, or if the delirium persists after attenuation of the antiparkinsonian agents, clozapine is recommended as it is the best studied of the second generation antipsychotic medications. If a patient is not able to tolerate clozapine or the required blood monitoring, alternative antipsychotic agents should be considered. Quetiapine has not been as rigorously studied as clozapine and may have parkinsonian side effects, but it is used in clinical practice to treat psychosis in Parkinson's disease.

Terminally Ill Patients Not all causes of delirium are reversible, and realistic treatment expectations should be set after a discussion with the patient and caregivers. When delirium occurs in the context of a terminal illness, issues about advanced directives and the existence of a health care proxy become more significant. This scenario emphasizes the importance of early development of advance directives for health care decision making while a person has the capacity to communicate the wishes regarding the extent of aggressive diagnostic tests at life's end. The focus may change from an aggressive search for the etiology of the delirium to one of palliation, comfort, and assistance with dying.

SUGGESTED CROSS-REFERENCES

Dementia is discussed in Section 10.3, psychiatric problems in the medically ill are discussed in Chapter 24, other cognitive disorders and mental disorders due to a general medical condition are discussed in Section 10.5, amnestic disorders are discussed in Section 10.4, antipsychotics are discussed in Section 31.16, benzodiazepines are discussed in Section 31.11, alcohol-related disorders are discussed in Section 11.2, psychotic disorders are discussed in Section 12.15, consultation-liaison psychiatry is discussed in Section 24.11, and palliative care is discussed in Section 28.4.

REFERENCES

American College of Emergency Physicians: Clinical policy for the initial approach to patients presenting with altered mental status. *Ann Emerg Med.* 1999;33:251–280.

*American Psychiatric Association: Practice guideline for the treatment of patients with delirium. *Am J Psychiatry.* 1999;156[Suppl 5]:1–20.

Baraff LJ, Bass JW, Fleisher GR, Klein JO, McCracken GH Jr, Powell KR, Schriger DL: Practice guideline for the management of infants and children 0 to 36 months of age with fever without source. Agency for Health Care Policy and Research. *Ann Emerg Med.* 1993;22:1198–1210.

Bogardus ST Jr, Desai MM, Williams CS, Leo-Summers L, Acampora D, Inouye SK: The effects of a targeted multicomponent delirium intervention on postdischarge outcomes for hospitalized older adults. *Am J Med.* 2003;114:383–390.

Breitbart W, Gibson C, Tremblay A: The delirium experience: Delirium recall and delirium-related distress in hospitalized patients with cancer, their spouses/caregivers, and their nurses. *Psychosomatics.* 2002;43:183–194.

Breitbart W, Rosenfeld B, Roth A, Smith MJ, Cohen K, Passik S: The Memorial Delirium Assessment Scale. *J Pain Symptom Manage.* 1997;13:128–137.

Bucht G, Gustafson Y, Sandberg O: Epidemiology of delirium. *Dement Geriatr Cogn Disord.* 1999;10:315–318.

Cole MG, McCusker J, Bellavance F, Primeau FJ, Bailey RF, Bonnycastle MJ, Laplante J: Systematic detection and multidisciplinary care of delirium in older medical inpatients: A randomized trial. *CMAJ.* 2002;167:753–759.

Curyto KJ, Johnson J, TenHave T, Mossey J, Knott K, Katz IR: Survival of hospitalized elderly patients with delirium: A prospective study. *Am J Geriatr Psychiatry.* 2001;9:141–147.

Elie M, Rousseau F, Cole M, Primeau F, McCusker J, Bellavance F: Prevalence and detection of delirium in elderly emergency department patients. *CMAJ.* 2000;163:977–981.

Ely EW, Gautam S, Margolin R, Francis J, May L, Speroff T, Truman B, Dittus R, Bernard R, Inouye SK. The impact of delirium in the intensive care unit on hospital length of stay. *Intensive Care Med.* 2001;27:1892–1900.

Ely EW, Inouye SK, Bernard GR, Gordon S, Francis J, May L, Truman B, Speroff T, Gautam S, Margolin R, Hart RP, Dittus R: Delirium in mechanically ventilated patients: Validity and reliability of the confusion assessment method for the intensive care unit (CAM-ICU). *JAMA.* 2001;286:2703–2710.

Engel GL, Romano J: Delirium, a syndrome of cerebral insufficiency. *J Chronic Dis.* 1959;9:260–277.

*Fick DM, Agostini JV, Inouye SK: Delirium superimposed on dementia: A systematic review. *J Am Geriatr Soc.* 2002;50:1723–1732.

Folstein MF, Bassett SS, Romanoski AJ, Nestadt G: The epidemiology of delirium in the community: The Eastern Baltimore Mental Health Survey. *Int Psychogeriatr.* 1991;3:169–176.

*Goldfrank LR, Flomenbaum NE, Lewin NA, Weisman RS, Howland MA, Hoffman RS, eds. *Goldfrank's Toxicologic Emergencies.* 6th ed. Stamford, CT: Appleton & Lange; 1998.

Inouye SK: Prevention of delirium in hospitalized older patients: Risk factors and targeted intervention strategies. *Ann Med.* 2000;32:257–263.

Inouye SK, Bogardus ST Jr, Williams CS, Leo-Summers L, Agostini JV: The role of adherence on the effectiveness of nonpharmacologic interventions: Evidence from the delirium prevention trial. *Arch Intern Med.* 2003;163:958–964.

*Inouye SK, van Dyck CH, Alessi CA, Balkin S, Siegal AP, Horwitz RI: Clarifying confusion: The confusion assessment method. A new method for detection of delirium. *Ann Intern Med.* 1990;113:941–948.

Kales HC, Kamholz BA, Visnic SG, Blow FC: Recorded delirium in a national sample of elderly inpatients: Potential implications for recognition. *J Geriatr Psychiatry Neurol.* 2003;16:32–38.

Kelly KG, Zisselman M, Cutillo-Schmitter T, Reichard R, Payne D, Denman SJ: Severity and course of delirium in medically hospitalized nursing facility residents. *Am J Geriatr Psychiatry.* 2001;9:72–77.

Lerner DM, Rosenstein DL: Neuroimaging in delirium and related conditions. *Semin Clin Neuropsychiatry.* 2000;5:98–112.

Levkoff SE, Evans DA, Liptzin B, Cleary PD, Lipsitz LA, Wetle TT, Reilly CH, Pilgrim DM, Schor J, Rowe J: Delirium. The occurrence and persistence of symptoms among elderly hospitalized patients. *Arch Intern Med.* 1992;152:334–340.

*Lipowski ZJ. *Delirium: Acute Confusional States.* Oxford: Oxford University Press; 1990.

Lipowski ZJ: Delirium: How its concept has developed. *Int Psychogeriatr.* 1991;3:115–120.

Lundstrom M, Edlund A, Lundstrom G, Gustafson Y. Reorganization of nursing and medical care to reduce the incidence of postoperative delirium and improve rehabilitation outcome in elderly patients treated for femoral neck fractures. *Scand J Caring Sci.* 1999;13:193–200.

Marcantonio ER, Goldman L, Mangione CM, Ludwig LE, Muraca B, Haslauer CM, Donaldson MC, Whittemore AD, Sugarbaker DJ, Poss R: A clinical prediction rule for delirium after elective noncardiac surgery. *JAMA.* 1994;271:134–139.

McCusker J, Cole M, Abrahamowicz M, Primeau F, Belzile E: Delirium predicts 12-month mortality. *Arch Intern Med.* 2002;162:457–463.

McKhann GM, Grega MA, Borowicz LM Jr, Bechamps M, Selnes OA, Baumgartner WA, Royall RM: Encephalopathy and stroke after coronary artery bypass grafting: Incidence, consequences, and prediction. *Arch Neurol.* 2002;59:1422–1428.

Smith KM, Larive LL, Romanelli F: Club drugs: Methylenedioxymethamphetamine, flunitrazepam, ketamine hydrochloride, and gamma-hydroxybutyrate. *Am J Health Syst Pharm.* 2002;59:1067–1076.

Sternbach H: The serotonin syndrome. *Am J Psychiatry.* 1991;1486:705–713.

Tancredi DN, Shannon MW: Case records of the Massachusetts General Hospital. Weekly clinicopathological exercises. Case 30-2003. A 21-year-old man with sudden alteration of mental status. *N Engl J Med.* 2003;349:1267–1275.

Trepacz PT: Is there a final common pathway in delirium? Focus on acetylcholine and dopamine. *Semin Clin Neuropsychiatry.* 2000;5:132–148.

Van der Mast RC: Pathophysiology of delirium. *J Geriatr Psychiatry Neurol.* 1998;11:138–145; discussion, 157–158.

Young LJ, George J: Do guidelines improve the process and outcomes of care in delirium? *Age Aging.* 2003;32:525–528.

▲ 10.3 Dementia

JUDITH A. NEUGROSCHL, M.D., ALEXANDER KOLEVZON, M.D., STEVEN C. SAMUELS, M.D., AND DEBORAH B. MARIN, M.D.

This chapter first reviews the clinical diagnosis of dementia and discusses the common elements to all dementias. After this, each subtype of dementia with its own unique pathophysiology is discussed.

DEFINITION

Dementia is defined as a progressive impairment of cognitive functions occurring in clear consciousness (that is, in the absence of delirium). Dementia consists of a variety of symptoms that suggest chronic and widespread dysfunction. Global impairment of intellect is the essential feature, manifested as difficulty with memory, attention, thinking, and comprehension. Other mental functions may often be affected, including mood, personality, and social behavior. Nevertheless, the diagnosis of dementia should not be made without evidence of memory deficits and at least one other cognitive deficit. Dementia must be distinguished from mental retardation and other cognitive disorders, such as amnestic disorder, that involve impairment of only one intellectual function, memory. Although there are specific diagnostic criteria for various dementias, such as Alzheimer's disease or vascular dementia, all dementias have certain common elements, as defined by the revised fourth edition of the *Diagnostic and Statistical Manual of Mental Disorders* (DSM-IV-TR): The symptoms result in significant impairment in social or occupational functioning, and they represent a significant decline from a previous level of functioning.

HISTORY

The word *dementia* derives from the Latin word *dementatus*, meaning out of one's mind, and, as such, was potentially applicable to any state of psychopathology. Celsus probably first used the term *dementia* in the first century AD, although one of the first attempts to describe an etiology beyond old age was in the fourth century AD by Oribasius, physician to the Emperor Julian. Oribasius wrote of a disease of cerebral atrophy that caused loss of intellectual capacity and weakness of movement. It was not until the 19th century that the distinction between cognitive impairment due to dementia was separated from that caused by mental illness by Jean Etienne Dominique Esquirol, as described in his classic work, *Mental Maladies: A Treatise on Insanity*. Esquirol identified three varieties of dementia: acute, chronic, and senile. *Senile dementia* was defined as a "cerebral affection . . . characterized by a weakening of the sensibility, understanding and will" and also by marked impairments in memory, reasoning, and attention. Esquirol also described hallucinations, delusions, aggressive behavior, and motor impairments in patients with dementia.

In 1845, Wilhelm Griesinger was the first to describe senile dementia as a disease of the cerebral arteries. However, it was one of Griesinger's students, Emil Kraeplin, who later narrowed the scope of dementia by differentiating senile dementia from psychoses with cerebral arteriosclerosis, which later came to be known as *dementia praecox* and, finally, as schizophrenia. Also in the late 19th century, reports of plaques and atrophy in the brains of patients with memory deficits and mental confusion began to emerge. In 1907, Alois Alzheimer was the first to identify specific histopathological changes associated with progressive degenerative dementia. He described two cases of dementia (in 1907 and 1911) characterized by symptoms of aphasia, apraxia, agnosia, and the histopathological finding of neurofibrillary tangles and *milar foci* (plaques) that distinguished it from dementia associated with cerebral arteriosclerosis. Today, efforts continue to focus on elucidating the etiology of dementia and to further delineate the associated pathological and physiological abnormalities observed across the range of clinical presentations with specific emphasis on genetics, prevention, and treatment.

COMPARATIVE NOSOLOGY

Before the fourth edition of the *Diagnostic and Statistical Manual of Mental Disorders* (DSM-IV), dementia was categorized as a syndrome and a disorder. The third edition of the *Diagnostic and Statistical Manual of Mental Disorders* (DSM-III) described organic brain syndromes that included dementia and distinguished it from similar presentations related to substances and general medical conditions. Dementia was also listed as a group of specific disorders, including primary degenerative dementia of the Alzheimer's type, multiinfarct dementia, dementia associated with alcoholism, and dementia not otherwise specified. DSM-IV eliminated the distinction between dementia as a syndrome and dementia as a disorder and developed specific criteria to distinguish between dementia related to general medical and cerebral conditions. A recent text revision of the DSM-IV (DSM-IV-TR) has been developed with six categories of dementia: Alzheimer's type, vascular, due to other general medical conditions, due to multiple etiologies, substance-induced, and dementia not otherwise specified. The DSM-IV-TR emphasizes the necessity of resultant decline from a previously attained level of functioning to meet diagnostic criteria. In another conceptual advance from previous nosology, the DSM-IV-TR contains specific criteria to delineate etiological subcategories relying on the presence of focal neurological signs, laboratory evidence of neurological damage, or a history of significant substance abuse or contributing general medical condition.

In addition to the DSM-IV-TR, there are concurrent and overlapping methods for diagnosing dementia. The tenth edition of the *International Classification of Diseases* (ICD-10) maintains a syndromic approach applied to specific criteria and includes four dementia categories: dementia in Alzheimer's disease, vascular dementia, dementia in other diseases classified elsewhere, and unspecified dementia. The ICD-10 also has general dementia criteria that divide severity into mild, moderate, and severe. Unlike the DSM-IV-TR, the ICD-10 does not include functional impairment criteria. Instead, the ICD-10 states that cognitive decline must be sufficient to interfere with activities of daily living. The ICD-10 contains all of the dementias included in the DSM-IV-TR, with the exception of dementia due to head trauma.

The National Institute of Neurological Communicative Disease and Stroke (NINCDS) and the Alzheimer's Disease and Related Disorders Association (ADRDA) also developed another set of research criteria known as the *NINCDS-ADRDA criteria*, which combine the features of the DSM-IV-TR and the ICD-10. The NINCDS-ADRDA criteria were developed specifically for Alzheimer's disease with the intent to serve as a clinical basis for diagnosis and for use in research studies. The NINCDS-ADRDA describe specific criteria for possible, probable, and definite Alzheimer's disease. The criteria for a diagnosis of definite Alzheimer's disease require the clinical criteria for probable disease in addition to histopathological evidence from biopsy. The DSM-IV-TR criteria share features of the NINCDS-ADRDA diagnosis of probable Alzheimer's disease but add subtypes such as *with behavioral disturbance* that are a useful refinement for treatment intervention. Nevertheless, the NINCDS-ADRDA criteria for probable Alzheimer's disease make specific mention of associated psychiatric symptoms and laboratory results, such as evidence of cerebral atrophy on neuroimaging that cannot be found in the DSM-IV-TR.

Despite recent advances in molecular genetics, the linkage of dementia to specific gene expression is complicated by genetic heterogeneity, variable expression, and unclear modes of transmission. Environmental influence (e.g., education and diet) may play a significant role as well, and, combined, these elements produce a wide variety of factors that can contribute to the development of dementia. It has also become increasingly apparent that many non-Alzheimer dementias frequently coexist with Alzheimer's disease. Future nosological endeavors are likely to take all these issues into consideration. It remains necessary for now, however, to continue using phenomenological criteria to categorize the dementias.

EPIDEMIOLOGY

With the aging population, the prevalence of dementia is rising. The prevalence of moderate to severe dementia in different population groups is approximately 5 percent in the general population older than 65 years of age, 20 to 40 percent in the general population older than 85 years of age, 15 to 20 percent in outpatient general medical practices, and 50 percent in chronic care facilities. By 2050, current predictions suggest that there will be 14 million Americans with Alzheimer's disease and, therefore, more than 18 million people with dementia.

ETIOLOGY

The most common causes of dementia in individuals older than 65 years of age are: Alzheimer's disease (which accounts for approximately 60 percent), vascular dementia (15 percent), and mixed vascular and Alzheimer's dementia (15 percent). Other illnesses that account for approximately 10 percent include Lewy body dementia; Pick's disease; frontotemporal dementias; normal pressure hydrocephalus (NPH); alcoholic dementia; infectious dementia, such as human immunodeficiency virus (HIV) or syphilis; and Parkinson's disease. Some sources suggest that as much as 5 percent of dementias evaluated in clinical settings may be attributable to reversible causes, such as metabolic abnormalities (e.g., hypothyroidism), nutritional deficiencies (e.g., vitamin B_{12} or folate deficiencies), or

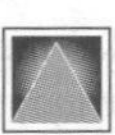

Table 10.3–1
Possible Etiologies of Dementia

Degenerative dementias
Alzheimer's disease
Frontotemporal dementias (e.g., Pick's disease)
Parkinson's disease
Lewy body dementia
Idiopathic cerebral ferrocalcinosis (Fahr's disease)
Progressive supranuclear palsy
Miscellaneous
Huntington's disease
Wilson's disease
Metachromatic leukodystrophy
Neuroacanthocytosis
Psychiatric
Pseudodementia of depression
Cognitive decline in late-life schizophrenia
Physiologic
Normal pressure hydrocephalus
Metabolic
Vitamin deficiencies (e.g., vitamin B_{12}, folate)
Endocrinopathies (e.g., hypothyroidism)
Chronic metabolic disturbances (e.g., uremia)
Tumor
Primary or metastatic (e.g., meningioma or metastatic breast or lung cancer)
Traumatic
Dementia pugilistica, posttraumatic dementia
Subdural hematoma
Infection
Prion diseases (e.g., Creutzfeldt-Jakob disease, bovine spongiform encephalitis, Gerstmann-Sträussler syndrome)
Acquired immune deficiency syndrome
Syphilis
Cardiac, vascular, and anoxia
Infarction (single or multiple or strategic lacunar)
Binswanger's disease (subcortical arteriosclerotic encephalopathy)
Hemodynamic insufficiency (e.g., hypoperfusion or hypoxia)
Demyelinating diseases
Multiple sclerosis
Drugs and toxins
Alcohol
Heavy metals
Irradiation
Pseudodementia due to medications (e.g., anticholinergics)
Carbon monoxide

dementia syndrome due to depression. See Table 10.3–1 for a review of possible etiologies of dementia.

DIAGNOSIS

The diagnosis of dementia is made by careful history, clinical examination, and selected diagnostic tests. The clinical history is most valid if corroborated with a family member or other knowledgeable informant, as patients with memory disorders are often poor historians. A social history, including occupational exposures to toxins or heavy metals, substance use, and HIV risk factors, is important in the evaluation. The medical history should include current medical conditions and their treatments, history of head trauma, cardiovascular illness, vascular risk factors, and history of transient ischemic attacks or cerebrovascular accidents (CVAs). A family history of dementia is particularly important in early-onset Alzheimer's disease or other known genetically transmitted diseases, such as Huntington's chorea. A physical and neurological examination should be performed to look for active medical problems, evidence of focal neurological signs, or movement disorders.

Another important aspect to the evaluation of a patient for a dementia is a complete mental status examination. In addition to the usual components of a mental status examination (appearance, mood, thought form and content, etc.), the clinician should evaluate of level of alertness and should conduct a screening cognitive assessment that addresses language (comprehension, fluency, etc.) and cognition. To assess cognition, the clinician must evaluate memory (as observed on interview as well as tested, such as remembering a list of words), orientation, reading, writing, speech production, calculation, abstraction, executive functioning, and constructional ability. Depending on the history, other areas may be evaluated, such as fine sensory function (e.g., two-point discrimination or graphesthesia) and visuospatial skills. There are a variety of standardized assessments used to evaluate cognition. The most common is Marshall Folstein's Mini-Mental State Examination (MMSE), a 30-point scale that covers orientation (10 points), immediate and delayed recall (6 points), naming and repeating (3 points), concentration (or concentration and calculation—spelling a word backwards or doing serial subtraction) (5 points), following a three-step command (3 points), and following a written command, copying a figure, and writing a sentence (3 points). The MMSE and other scales used for routine evaluation are subject to false-positive and -negative results, with education as a particularly confounding variable. Someone who is bright or has a high degree of education may decline markedly before their MMSE declines, whereas another person with a sixth grade education may have a score of 24 in the absence of significant impairment. These tests are useful in the context of an individual patient and must be interpreted in light of the patient's educational attainment and clinical picture. Another often-used bedside test is having the patient draw a clock set to a particular time. This is a useful tool to evaluate a number of cognitive domains, including constructional praxis and executive functioning. Nonetheless, cognitive screens are not sufficient to make or to rule out a diagnosis of dementia. More in-depth neuropsychological testing may be helpful in examining more subtle cognitive changes or in quantifying the range and pattern of abnormalities in a particular patient.

The laboratory workup should include routine blood work to evaluate hepatic and renal function, electrolyte imbalances, nutritional abnormalities, and common endocrine abnormalities (Table 10.3–2). An elevation in homocysteine is a risk factor for cardiovascular and cerebrovascular disease and may be an independent risk factor for Alzheimer's disease as well. Further tests may be suggested by the clinical history, such as serum levels of any medications, urine toxicology, urine or blood cultures, erythrocyte sedimentation rate, antinuclear antibody, HIV testing, Lyme disease antibody titers, serum levels of heavy metals, and ceruloplasmin. A spinal tap, electroencephalography (EEG), or sleep studies (polysomnography) are not considered routine but may be indicated in certain circumstances. Structural neuroimaging is very important to evaluate vascular changes, subdural hematomas, and primary or secondary central nervous system (CNS) neoplasms.

The clinical history should include the onset of symptoms, the quality of symptom progression (i.e., in a gradual and progressive manner, stepwise), a review of the cognitive domains defined in the DSM-IV-TR (Table 10.3–3), and an assessment of how the cognitive changes have affected various areas of functioning. An evaluation for other psychiatric disorders is also crucial, as severe depression may

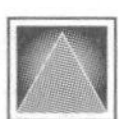

Table 10.3–2
Screening Laboratory Tests

Assessments	Rationale
Labs: complete blood count, serum electrolytes, renal and hepatic function, glucose, albumin and protein, vitamin B_{12} and folate, rapid plasma reagin (syphilis), thyroid-stimulating hormone, urinalysis	Rule out correctable or contributory causes of dementia
Imaging: computed tomography without contrast or magnetic resonance imaging	Rule out infarcts, mass lesions, tumors, and hydrocephalus
Neurological examination	Correlate imaging findings with clinical examination
Neuropsychological testing	Mini-Mental State Examination: screening test of cognitive function
	Formal description of cognitive impairments

present as dementia. In addition, schizophrenia is associated with a decrease in cognitive abilities, especially after 60 years of age.

CLINICAL FEATURES

Although the core features are the same for all dementias, the onset and course may vary. For example, a stroke followed by a dementia is, by definition, rapid in onset. Alzheimer's disease is usually insidious in onset.

The time from the onset of clinical features to presentation for evaluation varies considerably and depends on the etiology of the dementia, as well as personal and social factors, including individual and cultural attitudes and beliefs about aging, premorbid personality, and intelligence. Studies show that, although physicians are aware of the prevalence and diagnostic criteria for dementia, they often do not screen for cognitive impairment.

Cognitive Impairment

The core symptoms of cognitive dysfunction in dementia, as defined in the DSM-IV-TR, are described in the following sections.

Memory

Loss of short-term memory is often the first clinical feature that comes to the notice of patients and their relatives. Typically, memory impairment is manifested by difficulty in learning new information. As dementia progresses, retrieval of highly learned information (long-term memory) also becomes impaired. Memory deficits may be reflected in repetitiveness, missing appointments, misplacing objects, and burning meals. Topographical memory is also commonly affected, and patients may get lost. In mild-stage dementia, disorientation is usually confined to unfamiliar places. As the disease progresses, this impairment can occur in familiar environments as well. Confabulation may also occur and may manifest itself as insertion of false memories.

Mrs. Z. is a 65-year-old, college-educated, married, white woman who was brought in by her daughter for a memory evaluation because "she keeps describing events that didn't happen." For example, she meticulously described a conversation that her daughter and husband stated had never happened. She also became confused the day after Thanksgiving, being unclear whether they had already celebrated the holiday, and asked her daughter why she had bought a turkey with no legs or wings. Other examples of her memory loss included repeating questions, forgetting conversations, and losing things. Her MMSE was 25/30 (losing three points on delayed recall and two points on orientation to time).

Language

Aphasia (impaired or absent comprehension or production of speech, writing, or signs) may present as impoverished speech and can eventually progress to mutism in the severe stage. Nominal aphasia, the difficulty in naming objects, is common in the mild stage. Typically, this presents as word-finding difficulty, initially for low-frequency words (such as harmonica) but later for higher-frequency words (such as telephone). Later, fluent and nonfluent aphasias and jargon aphasia (meaningless phrases) may occur. Receptive aphasia, the inability to understand, is also common and is

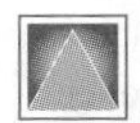

Table 10.3–3
Questions to Ask Patient and Informant Separately

Memory	Does he or she have difficulty remembering recent conversations?
	Is he or she frequently repetitive?
	Is he or she aware of current events?
	Does he or she misplace or lose things?
	Does he or she forget to turn off the stove?
Language and aphasia	Does he or she have difficulty finding the correct word?
	Is it sometimes difficult for others to understand him or her?
Orientation	Does he or she know where he or she is?
	Is he or she oriented to time (date, month, and year)?
	Does he or she forget upcoming holidays, birthdays, when to attend church, tax day, etc.?
Agnosia	Does he or she have difficulty recognizing people or places?
Activities of daily living	Does he or she have difficulty handling small sums of money?
	Does he or she have difficulty remembering short lists for shopping?
	Does he or she need assistance with eating, bathing, transfer in and out of bed, walking, toileting, grooming, or dressing?
Apraxia	Does he or she have difficulty using familiar objects (e.g., toaster)?
	Does he or she have difficulty performing simple tasks at home (e.g., making coffee, setting table, operating the television, vacuum, etc.)?
Problem solving abilities	Does he or she have difficulty relating to newspapers or television?
Executive functioning	Is he or she still able to manage finances, the checkbook, or taxes?
Social, community, and intellectual function	Has he or she lost special skills, interests, or hobbies (e.g., reading, sewing, cards, or gardening) for reasons other than physical?
	Does he or she engage in socially inappropriate behavior?
Judgment	Does he or she show problems in judgment (e.g., letting a stranger into the house)?

Adapted from Morris JC, Heyman A, Mohs RC, et al.: The Consortium to Establish a Registry for Alzheimer's Disease (CERAD). Part I. Clinical and neuropsychological assessment of Alzheimer's disease. *Neurology.* 1989;39:1159–1165.

severely disabling. An important clinical point to note is that, even when language has disintegrated completely, patients may understand nonverbal communication, such as gestures and pictures.

Mrs. R., a 74-year-old, high school–educated, married, white woman, was brought in by her family for an evaluation of her memory and word-finding difficulty. For example, she called *salad dressing* "jam," and could not think of the word *cucumber* when making a salad. On initial presentation, she was somewhat repetitive, and her MMSE was 26/30, missing three points on delayed recall and one on orientation. She was diagnosed with Alzheimer's disease, based on her difficulties in short-term memory and aphasia, normal laboratory results, no evidence of cerebral infarction, and nonfocal neurological evaluation. Three years later, her language difficulty had progressed. She sometimes gave nonsensical answers to questions and had more difficulty with comprehension. For example, when her husband asked her to go to the freezer and to get frankfurters, she brought him ice cream. She could no longer follow a three-step command. When asked to name "watch," she said, "I don't know . . . it tells time." Her short-term memory was severely impaired, yet she continued to be able to do calculations, worked at a flea market, and gave correct change. Her subsequent MMSE was 20/30, missing three points on delayed recall, two points on orientation to time, three points on naming and repeating, and two points on the three-step command.

Praxis Apraxia is the loss or diminished ability to perform coordinated motor tasks, assuming that there is no neurological or other damage to the peripheral motor apparatus. It reflects dominant parietal involvement in the dementia process. Apraxia is a major cause of loss of independence in patients, as it is reflected in the inability to cook, to dress, to wash, to go to the toilet, and to eat. Occasionally, and unwittingly, relatives add to the patient's distress by misinterpreting the inability to carry out these acts as laziness or as a lowering of standards. This is an area in which the education of relatives is important.

Mr. S. is an 81-year-old, married, white man with a master's degree who had been diagnosed with Alzheimer's disease 6 years ago. Recently, when his wife asked him to brush his teeth, he went to the bathroom and stood with the toothbrush in his hand, unable to proceed. Until 6 months ago, he was able to independently shave but then began to cut himself multiple times. His wife must now shave him with an electric razor. His other symptoms included significant difficulty with memory, language, and orientation. His MMSE was 9/30.

Gnosis Agnosia, derived from the Greek word *gnosis*, which means knowledge, is the failure to accurately recognize sensory stimuli in the absence of sensory (e.g., visual or olfactory) deficits. Visual agnosia may be reflected in the functional misuse of everyday objects (e.g., urinating in the sink). Prosopagnosia is the inability to recognize faces, even of friends and relatives. Agnosias can occur in all sensory modalities. Some demented patients may, for example, be unable to recognize familiar smells.

Mr. L. is a 78-year-old, married, Hispanic man with a college degree who was brought in by his wife because of behavioral disturbance, which was associated with not recognizing her. He would come up to her in their home, ask where his wife was, and would then become angry, insisting that she bring his wife to him. He had an approximately 6-year history of a progressive dementia and was experiencing difficulty with memory, word finding, orientation, and judgment. He was still able to play the piano at his dementia day program. His MMSE was 11/30. He initially became less agitated on a low dose of an atypical antipsychotic medication. However, his behavior progressed, and he was hospitalized after trying to strike his wife.

Executive Functioning Executive functioning is defined as the ability to plan, to sequence, to abstract, and to carry through complex tasks. Deficits in executive functioning are seen particularly in disorders affecting the frontal lobes. Executive functioning can be assessed by reviewing the patient's ability to perform at work, to pay bills, and to plan activities. Neuropsychological tests directly address executive functioning by asking the person to have flexibility in how they approach an organizational task (i.e., the ability to shift sets) or to copy complex figures, drawing a clock. These latter tests are not specific to executive functioning but can demonstrate how the patient addresses a task that involves planning and organization.

Ms. B. is a 74-year-old, retired, African-American woman with a law degree who came in for evaluation because of increased difficulty with short-term memory. She says that until approximately 8 to 10 months ago, she was always extremely organized, kept ledgers of all of her financial transactions, and had all of her papers and correspondence neatly filed. More recently, she has noted more difficulty managing the flow of papers that comes across her desk. She found that she had not paid her telephone bill but had paid her electric bill twice last month. She has no appreciable difficulty with language, and, otherwise, she and her husband deny other symptoms. Her husband states that he has started to pay the bills with her and has taken over planning of more complex social events, such as their upcoming holiday party. On testing, her MMSE was 28/30, missing only two points on delayed recall. Her neuropsychological testing showed her estimated premorbid intelligence to be in the superior range, but her memory and executive functioning were found to be in the low-normal to impaired range.

Personality and Behavioral Changes

Notwithstanding the devastating effects of the cognitive deficits described previously, it is, not infrequently, the changes in personality and behavior that families find most distressing. In assessing personality changes, the clinician must rely on close family members or friends, because the patient often does not have insight into these symptoms. Relatives may vary in their description of personality and behavioral change. Some overemphasize unpleasant behaviors, whereas others deny any changes at all.

Individuals with dementia may lose drive and initiative and become indecisive and introverted. The spectrum of emotions displayed may be narrowed, with the loss of warmth and humor. As the illness progresses, patients may sit all day in the same place, apparently doing little. This constellation of symptoms, often called *negative symptoms*, is usually characterized by prominent apathy. It is important to differentiate these latter symptoms from depression, which characteristically has prominent sadness, tearfulness, neurovegetative changes, suicidal tendency, and inappropriate guilt, among other characteristics. The negative symptoms do not respond to antidepressant medication. Abnormalities of mood are well described in the early stages of dementia. In addition, severe depression may mimic or exacerbate dementia. Mania is also occasionally seen.

In other patients, changes in behavior are reflected in agitation or disinhibition. Social skills may be lost, and there may be sexual disinhibition, use of inappropriate language, or both. Agitation may include irritability, angry outbursts, and threatening or aggressive behavior, as well as pacing and purposeless behaviors (e.g., packing and unpacking). Patients may wander, including leaving their homes in the middle of the night.

COURSE AND PROGNOSIS

Depending on etiology and severity at the time of presentation, the course and prognosis of dementia vary. Correcting potentially reversible causes is crucial, such as profound hypothyroidism, vitamin B_{12} deficiency, chronic subdural hematoma, or severe major depression. However, treatment of these reversible causes of dementia may not completely restore cognitive function. Most dementias are progressive and therefore inevitably have a poor prognosis. Modifying identifiable risk factors, such as poorly controlled hypertension in a vascular dementia, can alter progression of the illness. The time from diagnosis to death in Alzheimer's disease is usually estimated to be 8 to 10 years, and the morbidity and mortality of vascular dementia may be worse than Alzheimer's disease, presumably because of risk of further cerebrovascular events, as well as other atherosclerotic disease. The 5-year survival rate is 40 percent for patients with vascular dementia compared to 75 percent for age-matched controls.

The progression of a dementia may be complicated by other intercurrent medical illnesses, such as a stroke complicating the course of Alzheimer's disease. In general, degenerative dementias have an insidious onset and are gradually progressive. The pattern may initially include periods of more gradual decline, followed by a more rapid progression. Vascular dementia tends to have an abrupt onset and a more stepwise pattern, associated with further vascular insults, but may have a gradual and progressive course. Radiation-induced dementia may present months after radiation exposure and may have a progressive course.

Numerous scales have been developed to grade dementia severity. The simplest staging descriptors are mild, moderate, severe, and profound. The following descriptions of the stages of dementia describe typical symptoms in a variety of areas of functioning. Of course, individual patients may have patterns that do not precisely fit these descriptions, and, depending on the etiology of the dementia, the pattern may vary.

Mild stage dementia describes a state with consistent forgetfulness that is more marked for recent events, inability to function effectively in interests and more complex activities (work, community, home, or social activities), and maintained social judgment. The person may well appear intact on casual inspection. Although the patient may require prompting to perform activities of daily living (e.g., bathing and grooming), he or she is able to complete independently these tasks. Moderate stage dementia patients' long-term memory may be only slightly affected, but their short-term memory is poor. They exhibit impaired social judgment and cannot perform independently outside of the home. Activities in the home are usually limited to simple chores, and interests are severely curtailed. Severe dementia corresponds to severe memory loss, with severe deficits in long-term and short-term memory, disorientation usually to time and place, inability to independently function inside or outside of the home, requirement of help with activities of daily living (toileting, bathing, and eating), and possible incontinence. Profound dementia corresponds to a patient being unintelligible, unable to follow simple commands, incontinent, and unable to ambulate or to accomplish purposeful tasks. This latter stage may also be used to describe persons who are bedbound, are unresponsive, have swallowing difficulties, and have contractures.

TREATMENT OF DEMENTIA

In general, there are three broad types of treatment for dementia: (1) treatments to modify risk that slow the course or correct reversible causes of dementia, (2) treatments of the cognitive symptoms of dementia, and (3) treatment of associated symptoms and behaviors that may complicate the course of dementia (e.g., agitation). Accurate diagnosis of dementia allows treatment of any modifiable factors (e.g., lipid levels, hypertension, glycemic control in diabetes, vitamin deficiencies, and endocrine abnormalities) that may exacerbate the presentation or course of the dementia. The treatments for the specific dementia etiologies are discussed in the following sections on each etiology. The only dementia with a specific cognitive treatment is Alzheimer's disease.

Behavioral Disturbance Behavioral disturbance or agitation is a common reason for patients with dementia to receive psychiatric treatment. Behavioral disturbances are common in all etiologies of dementia, occurring in as much as 50 percent of community-dwelling patients and 70 to 90 percent of nursing home patients with dementia.

The domains of behavioral disturbances range from purposeless behaviors (wandering, pacing, and packing) to aggression (irritability, hitting, biting, yelling, and self injurious behaviors), sleep–wake cycle disturbances, psychotic symptoms (paranoia and visual or auditory hallucinations, or both), and resisting care (e.g., bathing and dressing). Agitation on caregiving causes great distress for patients and their caregivers.

The pathophysiology of behavioral disturbance in dementia is poorly understood. Restlessness has been hypothesized to be associated with abnormalities in the striatum, cortex, and thalamus, which may be partially mediated by γ-aminobutyric acid (GABA). Patients with dementia and agitation may have decreased serotonin, with increased postsynaptic receptor sensitivity. Studies of functional neuroimaging suggest that frontal and temporal lobe pathology is associated with agitation and psychosis. In addition, psychosis has been associated with significantly increased amyloid plaques in the presubiculum and increased neurofibrillary tangles in the middle frontal cortex.

There are a number of important issues to consider in the diagnosis of behavioral disturbance in dementia. Delirium, pain syndromes, infections, and constipation may all present as increased agitation. Because patients with more severe dementia often cannot express what is wrong, common medical conditions or pain may go undiagnosed. For instance, a postsurgical patient with a moderate dementia may have as-needed (PRN) pain medication ordered, for which he cannot verbalize a need. Another patient may be having an exacerbation of congestive heart failure and may be uncomfortable or hypoxic and thus confused and agitated. Agitation may also be precipitated by medication or substance intoxication or withdrawal. For instance, one patient with dementia may exhibit behavioral disinhibition in the context of alcohol. Another may be prescribed diphenhydramine (Benadryl) for sleep and may display increased confusion.

In the context of acute agitation, it is crucial to elicit a careful history from an informant; to assess for signs and symptoms of medical illness, substance use, or falls, or a combination of these; and to perform a complete physical examination. Laboratory work should measure electrolytes, hepatic and renal function, and complete blood count to assess for infection or anemia. An elevated blood urea nitrogen (BUN) to creatinine ratio suggests the possibility of poor hydration, which can also increase confusion and agitation. Patients with dementia may not ask for fluids and may become quite dehydrated. Changes in renal or hepatic function can also change metabolism of medications, and can cause toxicity. All medications should be reviewed. If a new medication has been added, it is important to consider drug interactions as well. In assessing agitation, it is crucial to determine the duration, frequency, and severity of symptoms, as well as the pattern of the disturbance, including which activities and caregivers are usually associated with increases in agitated behaviors.

Psychotic Symptoms Delusions and hallucinations may occur in any stage of dementia but are likely to present in the moderate stage. The most common delusions are paranoid in nature (approximately 40 percent) (e.g., suspiciousness about one's spouse, caregiver or others stealing or hiding things). Approximately 25 percent of patients with delusions are suspicious about the nature of their domicile (e.g., that they are not really in their home) or of people around them (e.g., that the person is not really a spouse, daughter, etc.). The prevalence of delusions in dementia is approximately 19 percent, and hallucinations occur in approximately 14 percent of cases. These symptoms must be differentiated from misremembering (e.g., thinking that a conversation with a relative happened 5 minutes ago instead of 50 years ago) and misperceptions (e.g., hearing a banging in the steam pipes and thinking that someone is knocking).

Disturbance of Activity Purposeless movements (pacing, packing, wandering, taking things out of drawers, and folding and unfolding items) are examples of disturbance of activity. These symptoms usually worsen with dementia severity.

Aggression Resistance to care, verbal outbursts, and physical aggression are examples of the behavioral disturbance of aggression. These symptoms may present in response to frustration at no longer being able to do certain activities or no longer being able to understand the purpose of an activity. Thus, a patient may become upset when asked to bathe or to change clothes. The patient may also respond to caregiver frustration. Aggressive behavior is quite common and is seen in approximately 25 percent of patients with moderate- and severe-stage Alzheimer's disease.

Sleep Disturbance Fragmented sleep and frequent awakenings are common. Daytime napping may also occur. Nighttime sleep disturbance, especially if associated with wandering or agitation, may be extremely disturbing and disruptive for caregivers and may precipitate nursing home placement.

Affective and Anxiety Disturbances The syndrome of diagnosable major depression is most often associated with the mild stage of dementia. Clinically, depression must be differentiated from apathy. Patients with dementia frequently have diminished interest or motivation to be involved in activities, which may be misinterpreted as depression. Sadness, tearfulness, suicidal tendency, feelings of worthlessness, and melancholia are differentiating signs of depression. Anxiety symptoms are common and may manifest as preoccupation with real or imagined upcoming appointments. This symptom is common in mild dementia (approximately 40 percent) but can be seen in moderate-stage dementia as well. Fear of being alone and increased dependence on the caregiver also increase as the disease progresses.

TREATMENT OF BEHAVIORAL DISTURBANCE

The treatment of behavioral disturbance in dementia usually involves a combination of medication and nonpharmacological and behavioral interventions. Being able to view the patient in the context of his or her environment, as well as comorbid medical conditions and dementia severity, makes the evaluation and management of behavioral disturbances the most comprehensive. Given the potential for physical concerns, substance use, and medications to manifest as agitation (e.g., pain, delirium, intoxication, and drug interactions), the first step in treating agitation is the evaluation for these possible causative etiologies. Once these concerns have been ruled out or treated, the agitation can be addressed using pharmacological and nonpharmacological mechanisms. The first step in managing a behavioral disturbance is to evaluate whether the symptom is causing difficulty in functioning or distress. If not, there is no need to intervene.

> Mrs. R., an 85-year-old woman with moderate-stage dementia, believed that a preacher would come into her home every morning at 6 AM. She would dress in her best dress, her home attendant would turn on the television, and she would watch the early morning religious program. At its conclusion, she would return to her room and change into her house dress. She was fixed in the idea that he came into her home and visited her personally and would never walk into the living room in her nightclothes or robe for fear that she would offend him. She was not agitated or disruptive, and there was no negative effect on her behavior.

Behavioral disturbance may fluctuate or may be persistent. One 5-year longitudinal study of 235 patients suggested that agitation was more persistent, whereas psychotic symptoms were only moderately so, and depressive symptoms rarely persisted.

Pharmacological Interventions

Most of the currently published literature has focused on antipsychotic medications. There is currently a large multicenter study funded by the National Institute of Mental Health (NIMH) under way to evaluate a number of different medications versus placebo in treating behavioral disturbance in Alzheimer's disease.

Antipsychotic Medications There have been large placebo-controlled trials of haloperidol (Haldol), risperidone (Risperdal), and olanzapine (Zyprexa), all of which have shown superiority of active medication versus placebo. Some studies have particularly looked at aggression and psychosis, which improved with treatment. It is important to start at a low dose and to titrate PRN, observing for side effects. Usual doses are listed in Table 10.3–4. Higher doses are associated with increased side effects. In general, the typical antipsychotics are associated with more side effects, such as tardive dyskinesia, extrapyramidal symptoms in high-potency medications, and anticholinergic effects or orthostasis in low-potency medications, than the atypical antipsychotics.

Mr. D. is a 78-year-old man with vascular dementia and an MMSE of 11/30. He is usually cooperative with care but becomes agitated and confused in the evenings. At times, he is convinced that he is not home or that someone is trying to hurt him. He occasionally becomes angry and frightened and has threatened his wife with his cane. His family has become increasingly distraught over his behavior. He was treated with a low dose of an atypical antipsychotic medication at 4 PM, which he tolerated well and which controlled his symptoms.

Trazodone Trazodone (Desyrel) is a heterocyclic antidepressant with preferential serotonin reuptake inhibition. Two small placebo-controlled studies support the use of trazodone for behavioral management. One double-blind study (N = 28) suggested that, for agitation associated with mild depressive and anxious symptoms, trazodone was superior to haloperidol. Trazodone is moderately sedating and can be used for sleep disturbance.

Mood Stabilizers Carbamazepine (Tegretol), valproic acid (Depakene), and gabapentin (Neurontin) have all been evaluated for the treatment of agitation. Most of the literature consists of open-label trials, retrospective chart reviews, and case reports. There is one placebo-controlled trial of carbamazepine with 51 patients, who showed decreased aggression and significant global improvement, and another study of valproate (N = 56) showing a trend toward improvement in agitation.

Cholinesterase Inhibitors Cholinesterase inhibitors have been described as improving behavioral symptoms in Alzheimer's disease and Lewy body dementia. Most frequently, patients with Alzheimer's disease are already taking cholinesterase inhibitors when they become agitated. Controlled studies looking at behavior as a secondary outcome measure suggest that cholinesterase inhibitors used in moderate dementia may improve anxiety, apathy, and, possibly, aggression, irritability, and disinhibition (Table 10.3–5).

Antidepressants Patients with depression complicating their dementia may be treated with antidepressants. Antidepressants all have similar efficacy, but the newer agents (e.g., selective serotonin reuptake inhibitors [SSRIs]) may be better tolerated. There is some evidence that SSRIs may improve agitation in nondepressed patients with dementia.

It is important to stress that, in pharmacologically treating a patient for agitation, one must continue to evaluate how the intervention is affecting cognition or other functioning. Although these medications are usually well tolerated and efficacious, they can cause side effects, and flexibility in changing treatment strategies is important.

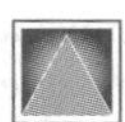

Table 10.3–5
Comparison of Acetylcholinesterase Inhibitors

Medication	Mechanism of Action	Target Dose	Comments
Tacrine (Cognex)	Inhibits AChE	120–160 mg, divided four times daily	30% elevated transaminases and severe GI intolerance.
Donepezil (Aricept)	Inhibits AChE	5–10 mg every day	May be associated with insomnia. Fewer GI symptoms.
Rivastigmine (Exelon)	Inhibits butyryl cholinesterase and AChE	6–12 mg, divided b.i.d.	Gradual titration may decrease GI side effects.
Galantamine (Reminyl)	Allosteric modulation of nicotinic receptors, weaker AChE inhibition	24–32 mg, divided b.i.d.	Gradual titration may decrease GI side effects. Least induction of AChE.

AChE, acetylcholinesterase; GI, gastrointestinal.

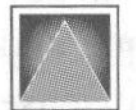

Table 10.3–4
Medication for Behavioral Disturbance in Dementia

Medication	Starting Dose	Usual Effective Dose
Haloperidol (Haldol)	0.5 mg q.d.	1–3 mg, divided
Risperidone (Risperdal)	0.25 mg q.d. or b.i.d.	1–2 mg, divided
Olanzapine (Zyprexa)	2.5 mg q.h.s. or b.i.d.	5–10 mg
Trazodone (Desyrel)	25–50 mg q.h.s. or b.i.d.	50–250 mg, divided
Carbamazepine (Tegretol)	200 mg q.h.s.	300 mg
Valproic acid (Depakote)	125 mg q.h.s.	250–1,000 mg, divided
Gabapentin (Neurontin)	100 mg q.d. or b.i.d.	300–2,400 mg, divided

b.i.d., twice a day; q.d., every day; q.h.s., every night.

Mr. P., an 86-year-old man with a 5-year history of Alzheimer's disease, was brought in by his wife because of an increase in purposeless pacing, wandering, and packing. He was prescribed an anticonvulsant and, over the course of gradual titration over 2 weeks, became more confused, would stand for long periods staring at a wall, needed to be fed, and became incontinent of urine. His MMSE declined from 18/30 to 10/30. The blood level of the medication was in a subtherapeutic range. The medication was stopped, and, over the course of 2 weeks, he returned to his previous baseline. He was referred to a day program with structured activities and was given a low dose of trazodone (25 mg) before going to the program and on returning home. This was quite effective for treating his restlessness.

Nonpharmacological Management

Behavioral interventions may reduce caregiver burden and may delay patient institutionalization. They usually aim at addressing the psychosocial or environmental reasons for the behavior. There are a number of behavioral interventions that may help address some of the agitated behaviors in dementia.

Activity Planning Activities such as exercise, socialization, predictable routines, and recreation should be maintained, if possible. Day care centers often provide safe outlets for patients and respite for caregivers. The Alzheimer's Association is an excellent resource for these programs.

ABCs The *ABCs* refers to the *a*ntecedents to disturbing behavior, the nature of the *b*ehavior, and the *c*onsequences. Interventions are based on the idea that delineating these domains can circumvent the behavior. For instance, if a patient is frustrated by not being able to do a complex task (e.g., brushing teeth), the caregiver can reduce the task into more manageable pieces (e.g., take toothbrush, wet toothbrush, squeeze toothpaste, etc.). In so doing, the patient may be able to perform each task and may regain a sense of mastery. The frustration at being unable to accomplish the overall task, which could lead to aggression, could thus be circumvented.

Environment An unfamiliar and unstructured environment can increase confusion. Adequate illumination, restoration of vision and hearing aides, reorientation to time and place, and providing familiar objects (e.g., photographs) may lessen agitation and anxiety. The use of physical restraints can increase agitation, confusion, and distress in patients. Supervision and allowance for wandering in a safe environment may be used instead of restraints.

Education Family and caregiver education, support groups, and reassurance can be extremely effective in addressing caregiver stress and can help caregivers work more effectively with demented patients.

Treatment Strategy When the pathophysiology of behavioral disturbances in dementia becomes better understood, or when there are medication trials that look at specific behavioral symptoms and their treatment as a primary outcome, it may be possible to target specific pharmacological treatment to a specific type of agitation. Currently, the literature remains equivocal.

In general, clearly defining target symptoms (e.g., hitting, paranoia, and yelling) and quantifying the frequency and severity allows for close monitoring of the efficacy of the intervention. After ruling out underlying medical conditions, pharmacological and behavioral interventions can be devised.

At this juncture, choosing an agent that, in the general psychiatric literature, has been shown to address a similar symptom (e.g., antipsychotics for aggression or psychosis) allows the clinician to create an algorithm to choose a medication class. If the first medication fails, or the side effects are intolerable, switching to another agent from the same class but with a different side effect profile or to a different class of medication may be prudent. Depending on the care-giving situation (e.g., the reliability and involvement by the caregivers), the use of various behavioral interventions or PRN medication regimens may help minimize the amount of medication needed. Hospital admission should be considered if the behavioral disturbance is so severe that the safety of the patient or the caregiver is compromised, if there is no reliable informant to observe and to report on the patient's progress, or if side effects preclude medication titration on an outpatient basis. Given the fluctuating nature of these symptoms, it is usually prudent to try to minimize medication and to attempt to discontinue medications after a period of time with good behavioral control. There is no clinical trial literature to support the continuation or discontinuation of medication, although regulations for nursing homes usually stipulate the need to attempt to decrease medications at least semiannually.

Other Treatment Issues: Caregiving for a Patient with Dementia

The burden of caring for an individual with dementia has been conceptualized as including two overall categories: subjective burden and objective burden. *Subjective burden* refers to the psychological stress experienced by the caregiver. Caregivers often experience social isolation during the course of care giving. This experience results from the fact that caring for a demented patient averages 11 hours per day. The stigma of dementia leads to the patient's and the caregiver's withholding this diagnosis from friends and family. Furthermore, healthy adults may experience discomfort in the presence of a demented individual, because the patient may have an impaired ability to communicate or may display inappropriate behaviors. Caregivers are also at increased risk of depression, sleep disturbance, and substance abuse. Caregiver stress may result in patient neglect. Lastly, the patient's agitation, sexual disinhibition, or psychotic behaviors, or a combination of these, may result in abuse of the caregiver.

Objective burden usually reflects the monetary costs associated with the caregiving process. These costs can include lost workdays, payment for medical services (e.g., medications, outpatient and emergency room visits, and hospitalizations), use of professional caregivers (e.g., social workers and paid home attendants), and institutionalization. Approximately 80 percent of dementia patients are cared for in the community by their families.

The cost of caring for individuals with Alzheimer's disease poses a significant public health burden, with annual expenses approaching 100 billion dollars in the United States. The average yearly cost of caring for a patient can be as high as $56,000. The total economic burden of caregiving for Alzheimer's patients reflects the sum of direct costs (e.g., money payments for medical care and all other goods and services related to the illness) and indirect costs (e.g., estimated monetary value associated with unpaid care and resources that are lost due to the illness). Unpaid caregiving can account for more than 60 percent of all costs. Time spent caregiving, paid and unpaid, is significantly correlated with cognitive and functional impairment.

The magnitude of caregiver burden informs the clinician about the need to address these issues during the evaluation and follow-up of dementia patients. Typically, the adult daughter takes on the responsibility of being the primary caregiver. Adult women who are their parents' caregivers have been conceptualized as the *sandwich generation*, because they care for their parents and their own children and are in the workforce as well. Optimizing the caregiver's psychological health includes education about dementia management and referral to appropriate services (e.g., counseling, support groups, and educational seminars sponsored by the Alzheimer's Association). This will undoubtedly optimize patient health as well.

ALZHEIMER'S DISEASE

Alzheimer's disease is the most common cause of dementia in the elderly. Alzheimer first described the illness in 1907 when he reported the case of a 51-year-old woman with memory loss, topographical disorientation, persecutory delusions, misidentifications, and behavioral disturbances. At her death, he examined her brain and documented the neuropathological hallmarks of amyloid plaque and neurofibrillary tangles. A definitive diagnosis of Alzheimer's disease can only be made at autopsy, using specific histopathological criteria that have been laid out by the Consortium to Establish a Registry for Alzheimer's Disease (CERAD). Clinical diagnoses are made by evaluating the course and history and by ruling out other causes of dementia, as discussed previously (Table 10.3–6). With an appropriate history and laboratory workup, Alzheimer's disease has become a diagnosis of inclusion, and the clinical accuracy in specialized centers is more than 85 percent.

Epidemiology Alzheimer's disease currently affects more than four million Americans, and the prevalence increases significantly with age. Prevalence rates from the East Boston Studies are approximately 3 percent in individuals who are 65 to 74 years of age, 18.7

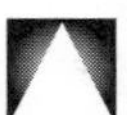

Table 10.3–6
DSM-IV-TR Diagnostic Criteria for Dementia of the Alzheimer's Type

A. The development of multiple cognitive deficits manifested by both:
  (1) Memory impairment (impaired ability to learn new information or to recall previously learned information)
  (2) One (or more) of the following cognitive disturbances:
    (a) Aphasia (language disturbance)
    (b) Apraxia (impaired ability to carry out motor activities, despite intact motor function)
    (c) Agnosia (failure to recognize or to identify objects, despite intact sensory function)
    (d) Disturbance in executive functioning (i.e., planning, organizing, sequencing, or abstracting).

B. The cognitive deficits in Criteria A1 and A2 each cause significant impairment in social or occupational functioning and represent a significant decline from a previous level of functioning.

C. The course is characterized by gradual onset and continuing cognitive decline.

D. The cognitive deficits in Criteria A1 and A2 are not due to any of the following:
  (1) Other central nervous system conditions that cause progressive deficits in memory and cognition (e.g., cerebrovascular disease, Parkinson's disease, Huntington's disease, subdural hematoma, normal-pressure hydrocephalus, and brain tumor)
  (2) Systemic conditions that are known to cause dementia (e.g., hypothyroidism, vitamin B_{12} or folic acid deficiency, niacin deficiency, hypercalcemia, neurosyphilis, or human immunodeficiency virus infection)
  (3) Substance-induced conditions.

E. The deficits do not occur exclusively during the course of a delirium.

F. The disturbance is not better accounted for by another Axis I disorder (e.g., major depressive disorder or schizophrenia).

Code based on presence or absence of a clinically significant behavioral disturbance:
  Without behavioral disturbance: if the cognitive disturbance is not accompanied by any clinically significant behavioral disturbance
  With behavioral disturbance: if the cognitive disturbance is accompanied by a clinically significant behavioral disturbance (e.g., wandering or agitation)

Specify subtype:
  With early onset: if onset is at 65 years of age or younger
  With late onset: if onset is after 65 years of age

Coding note: Also code Alzheimer's disease on Axis III. Indicate other prominent clinical features related to the Alzheimer's disease on Axis I (e.g., mood disorder due to Alzheimer's disease, with depressive features, and personality change to Alzheimer's disease, aggressive type).

From American Psychiatric Association. *Diagnostic and Statistical Manual of Mental Disorders.* 4th ed. Text rev. Washington, DC: American Psychiatric Association; 2000, with permission.

percent for individuals who are 75 to 84 years of age, and 47.2 percent for individuals older than 84 years of age. The numbers in other studies vary; for instance, another study suggested prevalence rates are approximately 0.3 percent in the age group of 60 to 69 years, 3.2 percent in the age group of 70 to 79 years, and 10.8 percent in the age group of 80 to 89 years. Overall, the prevalence of Alzheimer's disease is 3 to 5 percent of people older than 65 years of age and as much as 50 percent of people older than 85 years of age. Alzheimer's disease can also present in younger individuals (40 to 60 years of age), and this accounts for as much as 10 percent of the disease. These individuals are much more likely to have a strong family history and may have a known genetic mutation. The female to male ratio is approximately 2 to 1. Alzheimer's disease is the most common cause of dementia in the elderly, accounting for 50 to 60 percent of all dementias. Alzheimer's disease will become a greater public health problem as the society continues to gray and as the postwar baby boomers age. According to the U. S. Bureau of the Census, the percentage of the U.S. population that is older than 65 years of age will accelerate rapidly beginning in 2011, when the first baby boomers reach 65 years of age. By 2050, the number of Americans who are 65 years of age and older will have doubled, reaching 70 million people. It is estimated that, if the incidence rate does not change, by 2040, there could be 14 million affected individuals in the United States.

Etiology

The etiology of Alzheimer's disease is most likely multifactorial and may be due to an interaction of genetic susceptibilities and environmental factors. Factors that repeatedly have been implicated as risk factors for developing Alzheimer's disease include increasing age, family history, female gender, low educational status, and a history of head injury. Potential protective factors include exposure to antioxidants, nonsteroidal antiinflammatory drugs (NSAIDs), and postmenopausal estrogen replacement. To understand the possible etiologies of Alzheimer's disease, it is important to understand the known biological aberrations that have been documented.

Biology

Overproduction or decreased clearance of Aβ is implicated as a central process in the pathophysiology of Alzheimer's disease. All of the known familial mutations (Table 10.3–7) are associated with an increase in Aβ production. Aβ is a cleavage product of amyloid precursor protein (APP), which is processed in a number of ways (Fig. 10.3–1). The nonamyloidogenic α secretase cleaves APP near the plasma membrane, releasing soluble APP into circulation. In contrast, β and γ secretase cleave APP to yield amyloidogenic fragments that are usually 40 to 43 amino acids long. These fragments aggregate to form insoluble β pleated sheet fibrils and amyloid plaque.

Although its function is not known, APP may help regulate cell membrane stability or act as a receptor. Aβ has been implicated in Alzheimer's disease for several reasons: Senile plaque density correlates with cognitive impairment, Aβ deposition occurs early in the course of the illness, Aβ is known to be neurotoxic, and mutations in APP have been linked to early-onset familial Alzheimer's disease. The precise etiology of the overproduction of Aβ is not known.

The other neuropathological hallmark of Alzheimer's disease is paired helical filaments of hyperphosphorylated tau (τ) seen in the neurofibrillary tangles. τ Is a CNS protein that is involved in microtubular assembly. Microtubules are vital to normal neurotransport, and the abnormally phosphorylated τ interferes with that process. Elevations of τ are associated with neuronal injury and are seen in acute stroke, postencephalitic parkinsonism, dementia pugilistica, progressive supranuclear palsy, and subacute sclerosing panencephalitis. Hyperphosphorylated τ is the major component of neurofibrillary tangles.

NEUROCHEMISTRY Numerous neurochemical abnormalities have been demonstrated on autopsy and with functional neuroimaging in Alzheimer's disease, especially as the disease progresses. Late in the disease, these include deficits in acetylcholine (ACh), norepinephrine, serotonin, dopamine, GABA, glutamate, corticotrophin-releasing hormone, and somatostatin. These findings are significant particularly as they relate to development of potential pharmacological interventions for Alzheimer's disease.

The most robustly described neurochemical deficits are in the cholinergic system. The activity of choline acetyltransferase, the

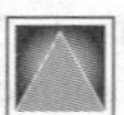

Table 10.3–7
Known Early-Onset Familial Alzheimer's Disease–Causing Mutations

Gene	Chromosome	Heritability	Age of Onset (Yrs)	Percent of Early-Onset Familial Alzheimer's Disease Cases	Comments
Presenilin-2	1	Autosomal dominant	50–90	<5	Missense mutations, ↑ $A\beta_{42}$ production
Presenilin-1	14	Autosomal dominant	33–60	50	Missense mutations, ↑ $A\beta_{42}$ production
Amyloid precursor protein	21	Autosomal dominant	43–59	<10	Missense mutations often near β or γ splice site of APP, ↑ $A\beta_{42}$ production

enzyme responsible for the final step of ACh synthesis, is substantially reduced in patients with Alzheimer's disease. This has been confirmed on autopsy of patients with at least a moderate stage of the illness but not in patients with mild illness. This is particularly evident in the nucleus basalis of Meynert and several neocortical regions. This finding has led to the development of therapies directed at the enhancement of cholinergic function.

Norepinephrine deficits have also been demonstrated in moderate-stage illness and have been the target for research on possible replacement strategies. GABA is a widely distributed inhibitory neurotransmitter. The activity of GABAergic neurons is reflected by glutamic acid decarboxylase (GAD). In Alzheimer's disease, abnormalities of GAD have been described, as have deficits in GABA, particularly in the temporal cortex. There may be changes in the number of GABA type B receptors in the hippocampus (HC) and possibly subtle changes in subunits of GABA type A receptors. The significance of this is unclear. Glutamate, an excitatory amino acid, also has been implicated in Alzheimer's disease. Changes in *N*-methyl-D-aspartate (NMDA), a glutamate receptor, have been described. Gene expression of NMDA receptors in the HC and entorhinal cortex (EC) may be altered. NMDA receptor activation plays a crucial role in learning and memory, and, thus, it seems counterintuitive that an NMDA antagonist would improve the symptomatology of Alzheimer's disease. Despite this, there have been some positive results in clinical trials using NMDA antagonists in moderate to severe Alzheimer's disease patients. Memantine, a low-affinity NMDA antagonist, is completing final trials in the United States and is currently approved for use in Europe.

GENETICS Familial aggregation and twin studies document a genetic contribution to developing Alzheimer's disease. As much as 50 percent of first-degree relatives who live to be 90 years of age develop the disease. To date, genes on chromosomes 1, 14, 19, and 21 have been implicated in Alzheimer's disease. Known genetic mutations account for approximately 2 percent of all Alzheimer's disease cases. These mutations are primarily seen in early-onset patients with strong family histories of Alzheimer's disease, and they tend to be transmitted in an autosomal dominant pattern (Table 10.3–7). Presenilin-1 (PS-1) mutations account for the majority of patients with early-onset familial Alzheimer's disease. The presenilin genes on chromosomes 1 and 14 may code for part of a proteosome that is involved in APP processing. The gene for APP is coded on chromosome 21, and it has long been noted that people with Down syndrome (trisomy 21) universally exhibit the microscopic pathology of Alzheimer's disease as they age.

Genetic studies of late-onset Alzheimer's disease (with illness onset after 65 years of age) suggest multiple possible loci that may be associated with Alzheimer's disease. Numerous candidate genes, chosen for their potential biological relevance, have been screened for the presence of polymorphisms and have been studied in Alzheimer's disease patients, and genome scans of families or sibling pairs have been evaluated for associations. The findings of these analyses are equivocal, and the number of negative studies outweighs positive ones.

The most consistent autopsy-confirmed findings are related to the *APOE* locus on chromosome 19. In addition to being a chaperone for cholesterol transport, apolipoprotein E (apoE) plays a role in redistribution of lipids associated with neurodegeneration and promotes Aβ deposition. The gene has three major alleles, *ε2*, *ε3*, and *ε4*, which code for the apoE2, apoE3, and apoE4 isoforms, respectively. The *ε3* allele is the most prevalent, with approximately 60 percent of Caucasians carrying *ε3/ε3*. Strikingly, the *e4* allele has been found in as much as 40 to 50 percent of Alzheimer's disease patients versus 16 percent of controls. The rare *ε2* allele may be protective against illness development. A gene dosage effect exists, strengthening the association between the *APOE* gene and Alzheimer's disease. Homozygosity for *ε4* confers an eightfold increased risk in developing Alzheimer's disease over *ε3/ε3*, and a 16-fold increased risk over *ε2/ε3*. Although *APOE-ε4* may be a contributing factor in the development of Alzheimer's disease, at least 50 percent of the illness is not associated with *ε4*, and, thus, the negative predictive value in finding this allele is low. Hence, *APOE* testing is not recommended for evaluating patients at risk of Alzheimer's disease.

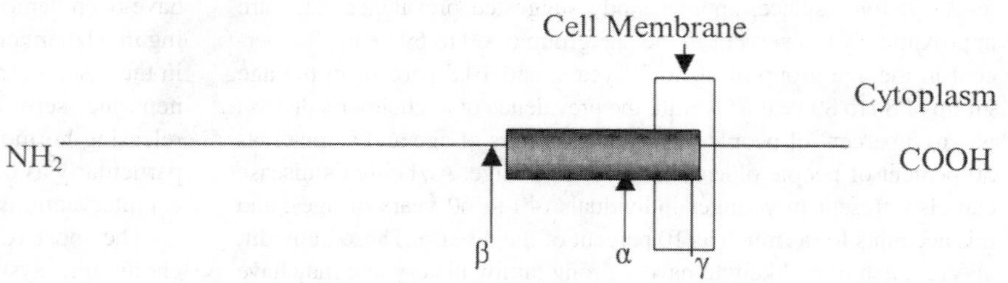

FIGURE 10.3–1 Amyloid precursor protein is cleaved by α secretase to form a soluble end product or by β and γ secretase to form 40– to 42–amino acid, amyloidogenic Aβ.

Other Possible Etiological Factors

AGE Age is the greatest risk factor for developing Alzheimer's disease. Whereas approximately 3 percent of people older than 65 years of age have Alzheimer's disease, at least 20 to 30 percent of people older than 85 years of age have Alzheimer's disease.

OXIDATIVE STRESS Oxidative stress may play a role in Alzheimer's disease. β Amyloid itself damages and kills neurons by inducing oxidative stress, as do microglia surrounding plaques. In addition, advanced glycation end products, which are also associated with Alzheimer's disease, can increase reactive oxygen production. There is also some evidence that suggests that abnormalities in mitochondrial function also may be involved in increasing oxidative stress. Thus, antioxidants may be neuroprotective. Epidemiological studies suggest that exposure to antioxidants reduces the risk of developing Alzheimer's disease, and an experimental study of patients with Alzheimer's disease who were exposed to antioxidants such as vitamin E or selegiline suggested that these agents may be able to slow the course of the illness.

INFLAMMATORY FACTORS Several lines of evidence suggest a role of the immune system in Alzheimer's disease. Population studies show that NSAID or corticosteroid use decreases the risk of developing Alzheimer's disease. Neuropathological studies demonstrate that the brains of Alzheimer's disease patients have increased concentrations of acute phase reactants, cytokines, and complement protein, when compared to aged-matched controls. Current data suggest that antiinflammatory drugs may decrease the risk of developing Alzheimer's disease but may not alter the course once the disease is manifest. There may be a differential effect among various NSAIDS, which may confound the results of current prospective studies.

ESTROGEN Basic research suggests that estrogen may play a role in Alzheimer's disease. Estrogen enhances neuronal growth and connectivity and has been shown to promote neuronal survival. It also may interact with APP processing, by increasing α secretase activity or by facilitating the function of the cholinergic system. Estrogen inhibits oxidation of lipids, lipoproteins, and nucleic acids in vitro and is protective of cells in culture against a number of insults, including β amyloid. There have been a number of population and case-control studies looking at estrogen usage and Alzheimer's disease. There is a great deal of heterogeneity in these studies, with different methods of sampling, data collection protocols, and statistical evaluations. Some studies suggest that estrogen may decrease the relative risk or delay the onset of Alzheimer's disease. Prospective studies of treatment of patients with Alzheimer's disease have been disappointing.

HEAD TRAUMA Repeated head trauma can cause a dementia syndrome (as in dementia pugilistica), and case reports have suggested that serious head injury may increase the risk of developing Alzheimer's disease. However, large prospective studies have produced mixed findings. This relationship is biologically plausible, as there is evidence that head trauma can lead to overexpression of APP, and it may increase β amyloid and neurotoxicity, possibly as a consequence of increased inflammatory activity.

NICOTINE The literature on nicotine is unclear. Prevalence data suggest an inverse relationship between smoking and Alzheimer's disease. Because people who smoke have increased mortality, they may die before the onset of illness. Incidence data have not shown a relationship. Nicotine might exert positive effects through stimulation of nicotinic receptors, and nicotine may decrease aggregation of β amyloid fragments. Nonetheless, smoking increases the risk of hypertension and cardiovascular disease and, hence, vascular dementia.

EDUCATION Epidemiological studies have suggested that people with less education are at increased risk of developing Alzheimer's disease. Functional neuroimaging findings of patients with Alzheimer's disease indicate that people with higher educational attainment or higher premorbid intellectual functioning but similar levels of dementia severity have more severe findings on neuroimaging. This suggests a protective effect of education, in that greater neuropathology is needed to produce the same clinical changes. Studies have reported that there is a relationship between cognitive decline and neocortical synaptic density in Alzheimer's disease. There is also some evidence that education can increase synaptic density.

Diagnosis and Clinical Features

The diagnostic process is as described previously in the overview of dementia. In Alzheimer's disease, the first symptom is usually a deficit in short-term memory followed by difficulty in executive functioning. Subtle difficulty with language, or visuospatial functioning may also be seen early in the disease. The clinical features are similar to those described previously in any dementia syndrome that affects cortical areas.

Pathology

Macroscopically, the brains of early Alzheimer's disease patients may appear grossly normal. As the disease progresses, widened sulci and increased ventricular size are seen. Atrophy in the temporal, parietal and frontal lobes is often most prominent.

Microscopically, the characteristic lesions of Alzheimer's disease are amyloid plaques and neurofibrillary tangles (Fig. 10.3–2). The early stages begin with relatively selective involvement of the EC and HC. Later stages involve other areas of the limbic lobes and, finally, the neocortex. Plaques contain an amyloid core that is composed of β pleated sheets of the peptide Aβ. The central core is surrounded by dystrophic neuritis, microglial cells, and reactive astrocytes. Autopsy studies have shown that Aβ deposition occurs early in Alzheimer's disease, and the amount of plaque is correlated with disease severity. Plaque cannot be well visualized with hematoxylin and eosin. Rather, amyloid stains with Congo red and exhibits birefringence or stains with silver.

The second major histopathological feature is the neurofibrillary tangle. Tangles are intracellular inclusion bodies, which contain paired helical filaments composed of abnormally phosphorylated τ proteins. Tangles also stain with silver and are difficult to visualize with hematoxylin and eosin.

Aβ deposits are not unique to Alzheimer's disease and are observed in other illnesses, such as Parkinson's disease, and normal aging. Tangles can also be seen in other conditions, but the presence of the two together in abnormally high density is pathognomonic for Alzheimer's disease.

Neuronal loss also occurs, causing atrophy with as much as 10-percent loss of the large neocortical neurons, primarily in the frontal and temporal lobes. Cholinergic neurons are affected, particularly in the basal nuclei, including the nucleus basalis of Meynert. Noradrenergic and serotonergic neurons are also affected. Other neuropathological abnormalities described in this disease include Hirano bodies. These are filamentous structures found in, or close to, pyramidal nerve cells, principally in the HC. They are invariably accompanied by gran-

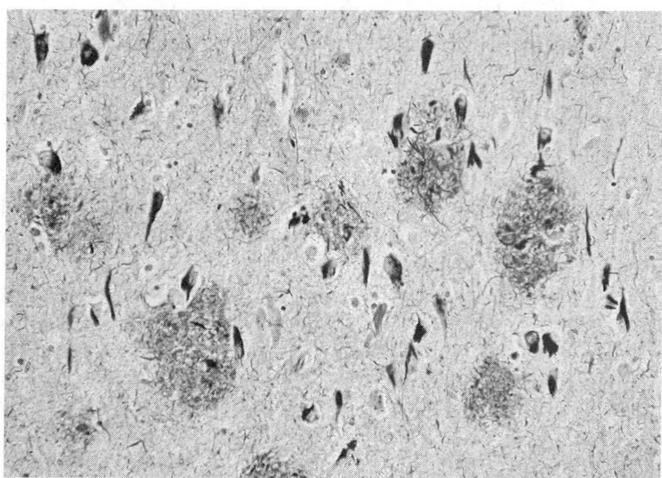

FIGURE 10.3–2 Silver staining of the hippocampus. Typical amyloid plaques and neurofibrillary tangles seen in Alzheimer's disease. (Courtesy of Dushyant Purohit, M.D., Neuropathology Division, Mount Sinai School of Medicine, New York, NY.)

ulovacuolar degeneration; these vacuoles contain dense granules. Cortical Lewy bodies have also been observed in as much as 30 percent of Alzheimer's disease cases. Lewy bodies are neuronal inclusion bodies, which are composed primarily of α-synuclein, and were first described in the substantia nigra in Parkinson's disease.

Laboratory Evaluation There are no laboratory tests that are sensitive and specific enough to use in diagnosing Alzheimer's disease. Rather, the usual battery of tests (Table 10.3–2) to exclude other diagnoses should be used. Many biological markers have been investigated, including elevated levels of cerebrospinal fluid (CSF) Aβ and τ, the presence of an *APOE-ε4* allele, and elevated homocysteine. Aβ and τ levels have too great an overlap with other dementias and normal values to be used diagnostically. *APOE* testing is not predictive of Alzheimer's disease, with particularly low negative predictive value, and thus should not be used as a diagnostic tool. Homocysteine has been shown to be a risk factor for Alzheimer's disease and cardiovascular and cerebral vascular disease, and, thus, in a clinical setting, elevated homocysteine should be tested and treated, although the effect of lowering homocysteine has not been evaluated in altering Alzheimer's disease risk. Homocysteine cannot serve as a diagnostic marker, because it is not specific for Alzheimer's disease.

Structural imaging of patients with mild cognitive impairment (MCI) and even cognitively intact elderly patients has demonstrated decreased EC or HC size, or both, in those who decline to Alzheimer's disease. This shrinkage is also seen in patients with clinically diagnosed Alzheimer's disease. This finding is not surprising, as the earliest neuropathological changes are seen in these areas. Unfortunately, accurately performing and interpreting these studies require significant expertise and, at this point, are limited to research centers. Functional imaging studies have also been used to predict decline to Alzheimer's disease in patients with MCI. The most consistent findings are of decreased parietal and temporal activation and increased metabolic recruitment (Fig. 10.3–3). There are similar concerns about the expertise needed in the use of functional imaging as an early diagnostic tool. Structural and functional imaging may be useful in the diagnostic evaluation of patients with dementia to rule out vascular or neoplastic etiologies.

Course and Prognosis At this time, researchers conceptualize Alzheimer's disease as having a long preclinical phase, followed by MCI in which the person has an isolated memory impairment, and, finally, dementia. MCI is defined as the presence of consistent memory impairment without decrements in other areas of cognition or function. Stringent definitions of MCI, such as performance on memory tests that is more than one standard deviation below age- and education-adjusted norms, discriminate MCI from normal aging. Using this definition, the conversion rate of those with MCI to frank Alzheimer's disease is as much as 15 percent per year or 50 to 70 percent over 4 to 5 years, as opposed to an approximately 1 percent per-year conversion rate in age-matched controls.

Alzheimer's disease is a progressive neurodegenerative disease. The length of time from diagnosis to death averages between 6 and 9 years. However, predicting survival time for individual patients can be difficult. There have been several possible factors identified that may predict reduced survival time. These include younger age of onset, aphasia, the presence of psychotic symptoms, male gender, and poorer cognitive performance at initial evaluation. It is well documented that mortality rates for patients with dementia are three to five times greater than those for age-matched controls.

The stages of the illness are as described previously in the section on the course of dementia. In general, patients with Alzheimer's disease lose approximately three points on the MMSE per year. Frequently, the decline is more gradual in the mild stage and then takes a more dramatic turn in the moderate stage.

Changes in the physical state may add to the morbidity of dementia. A large number of physical changes have been described as Alzheimer's disease progresses. These include weight loss, gait abnormalities, tremor, dysphagia, and urinary and fecal incontinence. Although Alzheimer's disease does not directly cause death, severely demented patients have difficulty eating and swallowing and are bedbound. Nutritional compromise, risk for aspiration, and decubitus ulcers contribute to further morbidity. Severe-stage Alzheimer's disease patients are more prone to infections (e.g., pneumonia and sepsis), which are usually the proximal cause of death. The reasons for these physical changes are poorly understood, but they are, in part, due to direct neuronal degeneration in the brain.

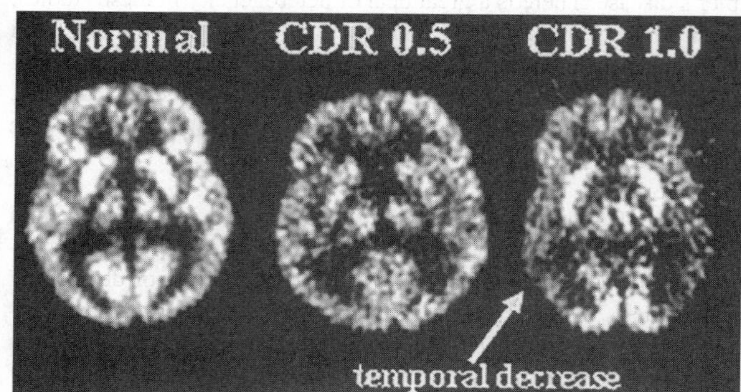

FIGURE 10.3–3 Positron emission tomography (PET) scan demonstrating decrements seen in Alzheimer's disease. The figure on the left is an [^{18}F]-2-fluoro-D-deoxyglucose PET scan from a healthy volunteer, the figure in the center is a patient with questionable Alzheimer's disease (a clinical dementia rating [CDR] scale of 0.5, loosely correlating with mild cognitive impairment), and the figure on the right is a patient with probable Alzheimer's disease (a CDR scale of 1, mild dementia). Note the frontal and temporal lobe decrease in relative glucose metabolism with probable Alzheimer's disease. (Courtesy of Monte Buchsbaum, M.D., Professor, Department of Psychiatry, Mount Sinai School of Medicine, New York, NY.)

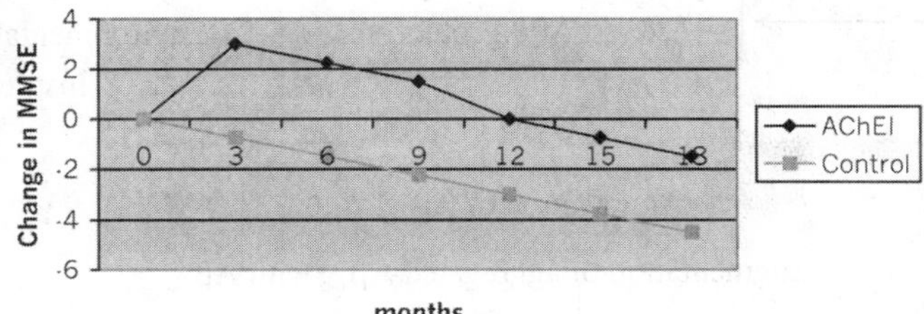

FIGURE 10.3–4 The clinical data for all of the cholinesterase inhibitors are similar. In general, over the first 3 months, there is an improvement of 1.5 to 3.0 points on Mini-Mental State Examination (MMSE). After that, there is a subsequent decline at a rate that is similar to (although possibly slower than) untreated controls. AChEI, acetylcholinesterase inhibitor.

Treatment The two strategies that are currently used in the management of the cognitive decline in Alzheimer's disease are replacement and neuroprotection. Replacement strategies focus on the neurochemical deficits in Alzheimer's disease (such as ACh or norepinephrine), whereas neuroprotective strategies aim to retard the progression of the illness by slowing further neuronal injury or loss.

The only class of drugs currently U.S. Food and Drug Administration (FDA)–approved for the treatment of Alzheimer's disease are the acetylcholinesterase inhibitors (AChEIs). These agents exemplify the replacement strategy, because they decrease the breakdown of ACh in the synapse, increasing the effective amount of ACh available. These medications are generally associated with a clinical improvement of approximately 6 to 12 months in duration (Fig. 10.3–4). After this, the patient continues to decline at a similar rate as untreated patients. When cholinesterase inhibitors were stopped, the patients most frequently fell to the level of the untreated cohort. This efficacy has been borne out in numerous longitudinal, randomized placebo-controlled trials. The agents currently available are tacrine (Cognex), donepezil (Aricept), rivastigmine (Exelon), and galantamine (Reminyl) (Table 10.3–5). Tacrine, the first medication approved by the FDA, is rarely used today because of its side effect profile (marked gastrointestinal [GI] disturbance and frequent liver function abnormalities).

Clinically, there are a number of points that should be considered in the use of AChEIs. First, a consistent finding in the clinical trials that offered open-label active medication at the end of the blind phase was that the individuals who started medication at the end of the trial never caught up with those who had started earlier. Thus, this may be suggestive of a neuroprotective effect in starting cholinesterase inhibitors early in the course of the illness. In addition, clinical trials also suggest that cholinesterase inhibitors may slow functional decline, for example, decreasing the risk of nursing home placement. In addition, in the clinical trials, stopping these medications was usually associated with marked cognitive and functional decline, and the current treatment recommendations include continuing medication as the disease progresses.

Agents have been evaluated for their neuroprotective effect to attempt to decrease the rate of progression of the illness. These include antioxidants, NSAIDS, estrogen replacement, and hydroxymethylglutaryl coenzyme A (HMG-CoA) reductase inhibitors (collectively known as *statins*). The classic antioxidant used in clinical trials is vitamin E. In doses of 1,000 IU twice a day, it was shown in one double-blind, randomized clinical trial to increase the time for moderate-stage patients to reach a poor outcome (i.e., loss of two or more activities of daily living, nursing home placement, or death), suggesting a slowing of illness progression. NSAIDS have also been evaluated, but, to date, the data from randomized clinical trials suggest that these agents may have a greater effect in protecting against the development of the disease than in slowing down its course. Interestingly, different NSAIDS have differential effects on Aβ levels on cells in culture, and previous clinical trials have focused on drugs (such as the cyclooxygenase 2 inhibitors) that may have less effect. Agents such as ibuprofen, which appear to have a greater effect in decreasing Aβ_{42} levels, will have to be assessed. Given the preponderance of women with Alzheimer's disease, estrogen has been evaluated in Alzheimer's disease. Epidemiological studies suggest that postmenopausal estrogen replacement may decrease the relative risk of developing Alzheimer's disease. A few small experimental studies showed cognitive improvement in women with Alzheimer's disease on estrogen. The most recent large multicenter trials in patients with Alzheimer's disease showed no benefit. Again, estrogen may be protective against developing Alzheimer's disease but may not significantly alter its course once the disease is manifest. Epidemiological studies suggest that increased cholesterol levels in midlife are a risk factor for subsequent development of Alzheimer's disease, and statins may decrease the risk of Alzheimer's disease. Furthermore, statin administration in cell culture and animal models decreases Aβ. Clinical trials are under way to see if these agents affect the course of Alzheimer's disease.

Pharmacotherapy is also directed at the behavioral disturbances associated with Alzheimer's disease. The most studied medications are low-dose, high-potency neuroleptics (haloperidol and risperidone). Other potentially useful agents are mood stabilizers (e.g., valproic acid and gabapentin) and antidepressants (e.g., trazodone) (Table 10.3–4).

Most patients with Alzheimer's disease inevitably require care from a multidisciplinary team that provides social, behavioral, functional, and pharmacological management. Nonpharmacological approaches to the management of Alzheimer's disease include various supportive measures, such as reality orientation and reminiscence therapy. Reality orientation depends on those in contact with the demented patient providing orienting cues. These cues may include clocks, calendars, signposts, memory boards, and verbal stimulation. In reminiscence therapy, patients are exposed to aids, including music, film, and photographs, to enhance reminiscence of past experiences. This seems to afford comfort and stimulation for patients.

A crucial part of the management of Alzheimer's dementia (and other dementias) is the provision of support to the families and other caregivers. Psychological problems in caregivers are common, including depressive and substance use disorders. Patients' behavioral problems seem to correlate highly with stress in caregivers, as well as a poor premorbid relationship between the patient and the caregiver. Caregiver education and behavior modification techniques are quite useful in managing certain behavioral disturbances in Alzheimer's disease. Self-help organizations, such as the Alzheimer's Association, can provide an invaluable means of support and education for caregivers.

New Directions in the Pharmacological Management of Alzheimer's Disease There are a number of new strategies that are being evaluated for the future management of Alzheimer's disease. Researchers have proposed the amyloid cascade, which begins with abnormal amyloid production and ends with neuronal dysfunction and death (Fig. 10.3–5). Researchers and the pharmaceutical community are evaluating different sites in this cascade to intervene to alter the progression of Alzheimer's disease.

One of the first steps in the formation of plaque is the production of Aβ. Pharmaceutical companies are actively pursuing inhibitors of

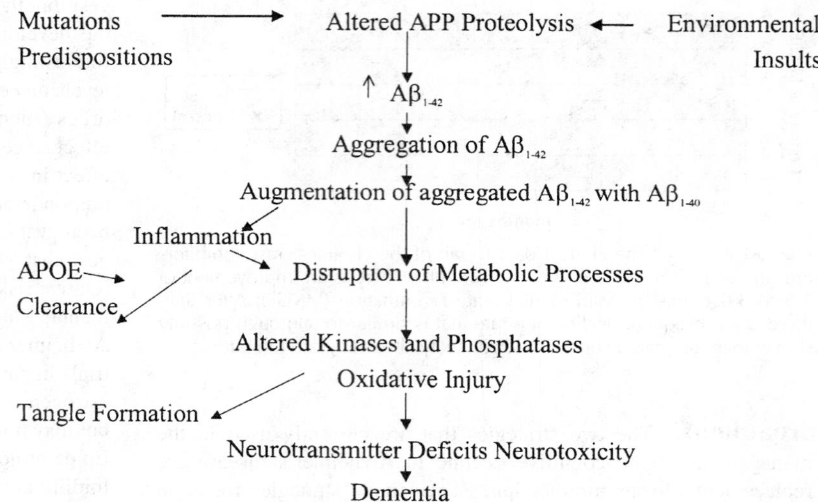

FIGURE 10.3–5 A hypothetical route to cell death and dementia, involving abnormal amyloid precursor protein (APP) proteolysis and increased Aβ, aggregation into plaque, inflammatory processes and disruption of metabolic processes, alteration of enzymes, oxidative injury and tangle formation, neurotransmitter deficits and toxicity, and, finally, cell death and dementia. (Courtesy of Kenneth L. Davis, M.D.)

β or γ secretase, and some are beginning clinical testing. The next step in the development of plaque is the aggregation of Aβ into fibrils and amyloid. Before aggregation, the Aβ is soluble and can be degraded by substances such as insulin-degrading enzyme. Agents are being studied that interfere with aggregation. Another possible strategy involves immunotherapy aimed at Aβ. Initially, active immunization vaccines were developed and found to be effective in transgenic mice at decreasing plaque. Human studies have been stalled in phase II because of serious CNS inflammatory reactions and encephalopathies. Recently, monoclonal antibodies have been tested in transgenic mice as a diagnostic measure or, potentially, as a treatment to bring CSF Aβ into the periphery.

VASCULAR DEMENTIA

Vascular dementia is the second most common cause of dementia after Alzheimer's disease. There are several important conceptual changes that have occurred over the past decade with regard to vascular dementia, and specific criteria have been developed to aid in clinical and pathological diagnosis.

History

Vascular dementia was historically referred to as *arteriosclerotic dementia*, until it became clear that cognitive impairment resulted from cerebral infarction and not vascular insufficiency alone. In the late 19th century, Otto Binswanger and Alzheimer separated dementia due to arteriosclerosis from dementia with paralysis due to neurosyphilis, a common cause of dementia at that time. In the early 20th century, Kraeplin described *arteriosclerotic insanity* as the most common cause of senile dementia, and it was thought that occluded cerebral arteries decreased blood flow to cause neuronal death, brain atrophy, and dementia. It was not until the 1970s that Alzheimer's disease was recognized as the primary cause of dementia in individuals older than 65 years of age. At that time, vascular dementia was called *multiinfarct dementia*, because it was thought that multiple vascular insults and demonstrable loss of brain tissue were necessary to manifest symptoms. Vascular dementia may be characterized by its stepwise decline, with each infarct producing acute changes and functional deterioration, but that description was omitted from the DSM-IV-TR when it became evident that a vast array of presentations and clinical courses were possible. For example, dementia may also be the result of a single, strategically located infarct found in functionally critical areas of the brain, such as the angular gyrus, thalamus, and anterior or posterior cerebral artery territories.

Comparative Nosology

According to the DSM-IV-TR, vascular dementia is diagnosed based on cognitive deficits, significant decline in social or occupational functioning, and evidence of cerebrovascular disease judged to be etiologically related to the symptoms. Cognitive deficit is defined by memory impairment and at least one other cognitive disturbance (e.g., aphasia, apraxia, agnosia, or executive functioning). Cerebrovascular disease must be apparent using neuroimaging techniques or by the presence of focal neurological signs such as weakness, hyperreflexia, and gait disturbance. In an effort to refine further the diagnosis and to aid in treatment intervention, DSM-IV-TR identifies four vascular dementia subtypes: with delirium, with delusions, with depressed mood, and uncomplicated. There is also a specifier *with behavioral disturbance* that is not coded but may apply to any of the four subtypes. The cerebrovascular condition (e.g., stroke) contributing to the dementia is listed separately on Axis III.

There are two commonly used research criteria for vascular dementia: the National Institute of Neurologic Disorders and Stroke–Association Internationale pour la Recherche et l'Enseignement en Neurosciences (AIREN), and the State of California's Alzheimer's Disease Diagnostic and Treatment Centers (ADDTC). The AIREN criteria were developed in 1993 and require three basic elements for diagnosis: cognitive loss, evidence of cerebrovascular lesions on neuroimaging, and the exclusion of other causes of dementia, such as Alzheimer's disease. The DSM-IV-TR (Table 10.3–8), on the other hand, does not require the exclusion of other causes of dementia but instead indicates that the disturbance must not be occurring in the context of a delirium. The ADDTC criteria were developed in 1992 and emphasize neuropathological confirmation of diagnosis. The ADDTC criteria delineate three categories of ischemic vascular dementia: possible, probable, and definite. Probable ischemic vascular dementia is diagnosed based on evidence of at least two strokes. Unlike the DSM-IV-TR, evidence of one stroke is sufficient for diagnosis only when there is a clear temporal relationship to symptom onset. According to the ADDTC criteria, histopathological findings plus evidence of probable disease are required to meet criteria for definite ischemic vascular dementia.

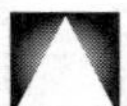

Table 10.3–8
DSM-IV-TR Diagnostic Criteria for Vascular Dementia

A. The development of multiple cognitive deficits manifested by both:
 (1) Memory impairment (impaired ability to learn new information or to recall previously learned information)
 (2) One (or more) of the following cognitive disturbances:
  (a) Aphasia (language disturbance)
  (b) Apraxia (impaired ability to carry out motor activities, despite intact motor function)
  (c) Agnosia (failure to recognize or to identify objects, despite intact sensory function)
  (d) Disturbance in executive functioning (i.e., planning, organizing, sequencing, or abstracting).
B. The cognitive deficits in Criteria A1 and A2 each cause significant impairment in social or occupational functioning and represent a significant decline from a previous level of functioning.
C. Focal neurological signs and symptoms (e.g., exaggeration of deep tendon reflexes, extensor plantar response, pseudobulbar palsy, gait abnormalities, and weakness of an extremity) or laboratory evidence indicative of cerebrovascular disease (e.g., multiple infarctions involving cortex and underlying white matter) that are judged to be etiologically related to the disturbance.
D. The deficits do not occur exclusively during the course of a delirium.

Code based on predominant features:
 With delirium: if delirium is superimposed on the dementia
 With delusions: if delusions are the predominant feature
 With depressed mood: if depressed mood (including presentations that meet full symptom criteria for a major depressive episode) is the predominant feature. A separate diagnosis of mood disorder due to a general medical condition is not given.
 Uncomplicated: if none of the previous conditions predominates in the current clinical presentation

Specify if:
 With behavioral disturbance

Coding note: Also code cerebrovascular condition on Axis III.

From American Psychiatric Association. *Diagnostic and Statistical Manual of Mental Disorders.* 4th ed. Text rev. Washington, DC: American Psychiatric Association; 2000, with permission.

Epidemiology Cerebrovascular disease is the second most common cause of dementia and may be partially responsible for as much as 30 percent of cases. Prevalence rates range from approximately 1.5 percent in people aged 70 to 75 years of age to approximately 15 percent in people older than 80 years of age. Not surprisingly, the incidence of vascular dementia increases exponentially with age, and prevalence rates are estimated to double every 5 years. In contrast to Alzheimer's disease, vascular dementia is more common in men. Vascular lesions may frequently coexist with other causes of dementia, and estimates of vascular and Alzheimer's dementias being diagnosed concurrently on autopsy are approximately 10 to 23 percent.

Etiology Cognitive impairment may result from cerebral infarction, anoxia, or hemorrhage. Infarction is typically due to arteriosclerotic plaques or thromboembolism occluding cerebral vessels. Associated risk factors include hypertension, diabetes, a history of transient ischemic attacks, and cardiac disease. Current research has focused on the role of vascular factors in Alzheimer's disease, and it has recently been observed that approximately one-third of patients with poststroke vascular dementia had preexisting memory loss and probable Alzheimer's disease. Furthermore, a reciprocal relationship may exist, whereby people with one or two lacunar strokes have been shown to require less plaque and tangle formation to manifest symptoms of dementia.

Diagnosis and Clinical Features The wide variation in symptomatology of vascular dementia in part depends on the areas of infarction. Patients may recover initially from the neurological and cognitive deficits associated with each infarct, although functional and intellectual decline eventually occur beyond a certain threshold of insult, depending on the location and extent of damage. Vascular dementia may nevertheless be distinguished from Alzheimer's dementia by its relatively sudden onset, focal neurological signs, history of stroke, and the likely presence of multiple risk factors for cerebrovascular disease. One cannot rely on the neuropsychological profile to differentiate between vascular dementia and Alzheimer's disease.

Significant small vessel disease can result in dementia. Binswanger's disease is an example of a small vessel disease. Small vessel disease typically has a subacute onset with subcortical ischemic lesions. These lesions may disrupt the frontal circuits that support executive function, motivation, and social behavior and thereby create the cognitive and behavioral manifestations of dementia. Patients may experience memory deficits, inattention, depressed mood, motor dysfunction, parkinsonism, urinary incontinence, and pseudobulbar palsy. Diagnostic criteria for subcortical vascular dementia have recently been proposed.

Laboratory Examination In addition to the frank infarction (Fig. 10.3–6) that typically results from the occlusion of major arteries, other potential neuroimaging findings are significant periventricular ischemia and deep white matter changes. Of note, white matter changes are primarily associated with hypertension and age and, although they may have some cognitive sequelae, are not usually considered the causative etiology of dementia unless they are extensive and confluent. Histopathology may reveal nonspecific demyelination and gliosis. Because of the wide range of potential etiological agents, complete laboratory evaluation is imperative and is performed according to clinical suspicion based on results of the history, physical, and neurological examinations and the MMSE, as described previously. Table 10.3–2 lists possible screening tests to consider in the initial evaluation of patients presenting with dementia to rule out a general medical condition that is potentially reversible.

Treatment The treatment of vascular dementia revolves around reducing risk factors such as hypertension and hyperlipidemia to pre-

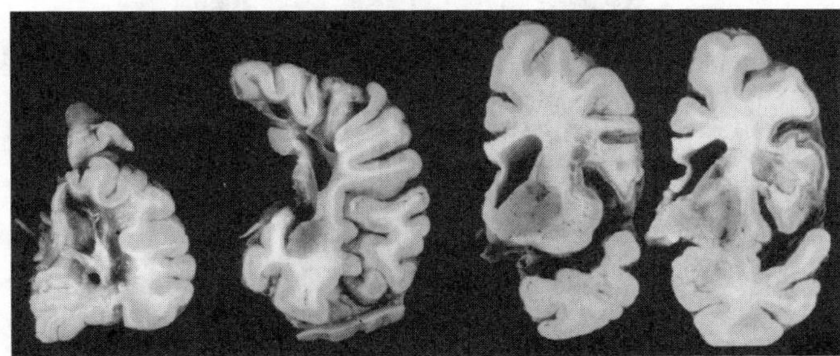

FIGURE 10.3–6 Multiinfarct dementia. This is a gross pathological specimen demonstrating multiple infarcts in the cortical and subcortical white matter, caudate nucleus, and putamen. (Courtesy of Dushyant Purohit, M.D., Neuropathology Division, Mount Sinai School of Medicine, New York, NY.)

vent additional insult. Antiplatelet medications and anticoagulation with warfarin (Coumadin) also provide protection from recurrent stroke. Likewise, in patients with significant carotid artery stenosis, surgery reduces the risk of recurrent stroke. There has been one randomized controlled trial that suggests that AChEIs may also be useful in vascular dementia. Associated psychiatric symptoms and behavioral disturbance respond to antidepressant and neuroleptic regimens, respectively, although caution must be exercised to avoid using medications with anticholinergic side effects, which may increase confusion. Examples include tricyclic antidepressants or low-potency typical antipsychotics.

BINSWANGER'S DISEASE

Binswanger's disease, a vascular dementia, is characterized by microinfarctions of white matter with sparing of the cortex (Fig. 10.3–7). It is also known as *subcortical arteriosclerotic encephalopathy*, and the hallmark is the presence of an ischemic periventricular leukoencephalopathy. Binswanger's disease produces a subcortical dementia with executive dysfunction, inattention, memory loss, slowed motor function, ataxia, incontinence, and loss of verbal fluency. Apathy, depression, behavioral disturbance, and extrapyramidal symptoms, such as parkinsonism, are also common findings. A familial form of Binswanger's disease was thought to exist, although recent developments have instead identified it as a cerebral autosomal dominant arteriopathy with subcortical infarcts and leukoencephalopathy (CADASIL). CADASIL is an autosomal dominant disorder of the small cerebral vessels that has been mapped to chromosome 19 and is characterized by transient ischemic attacks and strokes, cognitive deficits, vascular dementia, and, less frequently, migraines, mood disorders, and seizures.

DEMENTIA WITH LEWY BODIES

Dementia with Lewy bodies is the preferred term that encompasses several conditions, including senile dementia of Lewy body type, Lewy body variant of Alzheimer's disease, Lewy body dementia, diffuse Lewy body disease, and cortical Lewy body disease. The use of the term *dementia with Lewy bodies* enables clinicians and researchers to refer to the same disease state.

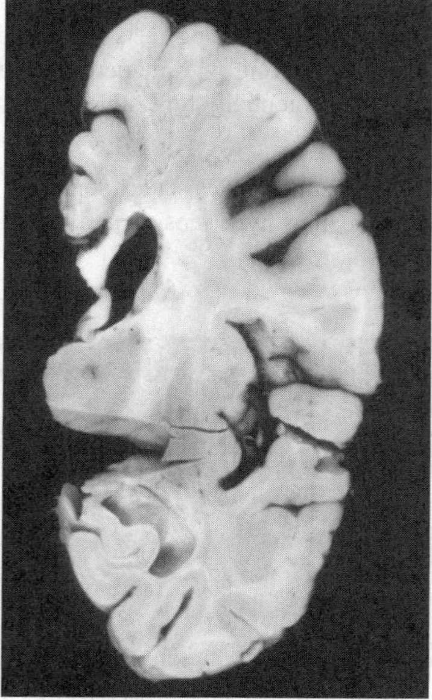

FIGURE 10.3–7 Binswanger's disease. Cross section demonstrating extensive subcortical white matter infarction, with sparing of the overlying gray matter. (Courtesy of Dushyant Purohit, M.D., Neuropathology Division, Mount Sinai School of Medicine, New York, NY.)

Dementia with Lewy bodies is a clinical diagnosis, based on a progressive dementia with parkinsonism and a fluctuation in the level of attention and the severity of the cognitive deficits. Gait and balance are often abnormal, and visual hallucinations may be a common feature. Delusions are often an associated feature. There is evidence that persons with dementia with Lewy bodies may be more susceptible to the parkinsonian side effects of antipsychotic medications. Clinical consensus criteria for dementia with Lewy bodies were published in 1996 (Table 10.3–9) but have been fraught with limitations in sensitivity and positive predictive value, although their specificity is high. When the clinical criteria were evaluated with neuropathological confirmation, one study showed 83 percent sensitivity and 95 percent specificity. Other studies have shown poorer correlations, with the sensitivity less than 50 percent. It has been suggested that adding the presence of visual hallucinations as a core criteria for the diagnosis improves the sensitivity. Of course, the use of dopaminergic drugs to address parkinsonian symptoms may confound this, as they may produce visual hallucinations.

Depending on the criteria used, dementia with Lewy bodies may be the second most prevalent dementia subtype. The clinical or neuropathological criteria often place dementia with Lewy bodies after Alzheimer's disease or vascular dementia in terms of prevalence, with the neuropathological criteria often finding dementia with Lewy bodies in as much as 25 percent of neuropathological specimens from persons with dementia. Unlike Alzheimer's disease, dementia with Lewy bodies is more likely to be seen in men than women. Prevalence rates for dementia with Lewy bodies range between 10 and 25 percent of neuropathological specimens referred for evaluation of dementia etiology in the United States or the United Kingdom but may be much lower in other countries, for example, southern India (6 to 12 percent), China (Hong Kong) (2.9 percent), and Japan (0.1 percent). This discrepancy may reflect the clinical criteria used. For example, in one clinical prevalence study in North London, the prevalence rate in patients with dementia for probable and possible dementia with Lewy bodies was 34 percent but was 10.9 percent if only cases with probable dementia with Lewy bodies were included.

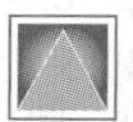

Table 10.3–9
Clinical Criteria for Dementia with Lewy Bodies (DLB)

The patient must have sufficient cognitive decline to interfere with social or occupational functioning. Of note early in the illness, memory symptoms may not be as prominent as attention, frontosubcortical skills, and visuospatial ability. Probable DLB requires two or more core symptoms, whereas possible DLB only requires one core symptom.

Core features

Fluctuating levels of attention and alertness

Recurrent visual hallucinations

Parkinsonian features (cogwheeling, bradykinesia, and resting tremor)

Supporting features

Repeated falls

Syncope

Sensitivity to neuroleptics

Systematized delusions

Hallucinations in other modalities (e.g. auditory, tactile)

Adapted from McKeith LG, Galasko D, Kosaka K: Consensus guidelines for the clinical and pathologic diagnosis of dementia with Lewy bodies (DLB): Report of the consortium on DLB international workshop. *Neurology.* 1996;47:1113–1124.

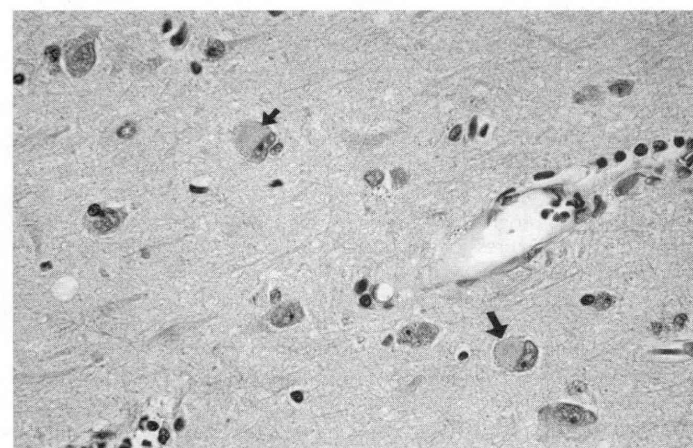

FIGURE 10.3–8 Cortical Lewy bodies (*arrows*), seen with hematoxylin and eosin staining. Lewy bodies are weakly eosinophilic, spherical, cytoplasmic inclusions. (Courtesy of Dushyant Purohit, M.D., Neuropathology Division, Mount Sinai School of Medicine, New York, NY.)

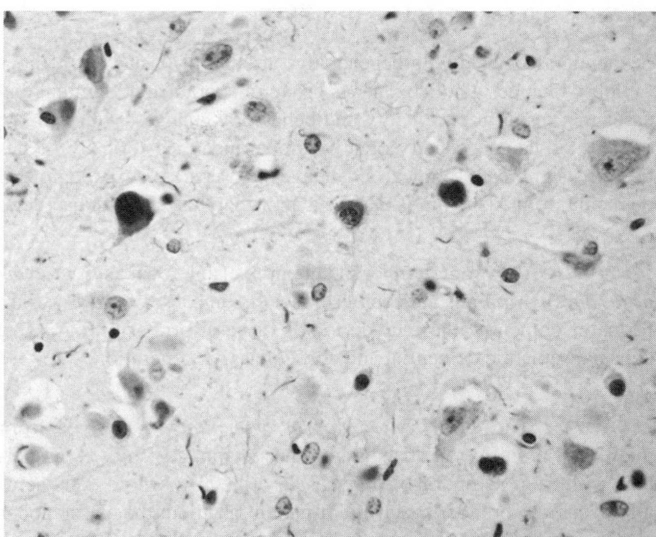

FIGURE 10.3–9 Lewy bodies—immunohistochemical staining for α-synulcein. These inclusions also stain with antibodies against ubiquitin. (Courtesy of Dushyant Purohit, M.D., Neuropathology Division, Mount Sinai School of Medicine, New York, NY.)

The pathogenesis of dementia with Lewy bodies is not clear, although the assumption is that the cortical and subcortical Lewy bodies are somehow associated with the cognitive decline and psychotic symptoms. There is some neuropathological evidence that suggests that visual hallucinations are associated with the quantity of Lewy bodies in the temporal lobes. There is also limited evidence that the pathogenesis of dementia with Lewy bodies may involve interaction between APP, Aβ, and α-synuclein.

There is no definitive laboratory test to make a diagnosis of dementia with Lewy bodies, thus, the diagnosis is made clinically. *APOE-ε4* is more common in dementia with Lewy bodies than the general population, but the *APOE-ε2* allele is not reduced. Homozygotes for *APOE-ε4* are less common in dementia with Lewy bodies when compared to Alzheimer's disease.

Neuropathological criteria for dementia with Lewy bodies require the presence of Lewy bodies in the cortical and subcortical structures. This is a distinguishing feature compared with Parkinson's disease, in which Lewy bodies are found in the substantia nigra. Lewy bodies, first identified in 1912 by Friederich Lewy, are eosinophilic, round or elongated, intracytoplasmic structures (Figs. 10.3–8 and 10.3–9). When found in the brainstem, they usually have a halo around a dense core and are stainable with hematoxylin and eosin. Cortical Lewy bodies are devoid of the halo. Lewy bodies are composed of ubiquitin or α-synuclein, which can be detected using immunohistochemical techniques.

Fifteen to 25 percent of Alzheimer's disease patients may have Lewy bodies on autopsy. They are found in the HC, EC, cingulate, and frontal and parietal cortex. Alzheimer's disease pathology does not preclude the diagnosis of dementia with Lewy bodies. Alzheimer's disease patients with dementia with Lewy bodies pathology appear to have more severe cognitive deficits as the burden of Lewy bodies in the cortical structures increases. In addition to the neuropathological overlap of dementia with Lewy bodies with Alzheimer's disease and Parkinson's disease, as much as 31 percent of dementia with Lewy bodies cases have additional vascular pathology at autopsy. Neurochemical studies suggest a cholinergic deficit earlier in the course and a decrease of choline acetyltransferase activity in dementia with Lewy bodies compared with Alzheimer's disease.

Dementia with Lewy bodies must be differentiated from Alzheimer's disease with psychotic symptoms and Parkinson's disease with dementia. As these are all clinical diagnoses, and there may be overlap between syndromes, it is important to obtain a careful clinical history, focusing on the course of the symptoms, as well as performing a careful neurological examination. Dementia with Lewy bodies patients have more pronounced visuospatial deficits and psychomotor impairments compared to Alzheimer's disease patients, but Alzheimer's disease patients have more severe memory deficits. Computerized testing reveals worsened attention with increased variability across trials in dementia with Lewy bodies patients compared to those with Alzheimer's disease. Although neuropsychological testing has shown differences between dementia with Lewy bodies, Alzheimer's disease, and vascular dementia, the tests are not able to reliably discriminate between the dementia subtypes. Functional neuroimaging studies without neuropathological confirmation have suggested the use of single photon emission computed tomography (SPECT) as an aid in the differential diagnosis of dementia with Lewy bodies, but further studies are needed. At this time, neuroimaging, like neuropsychological testing, is unable to reliably differentiate dementia with Lewy bodies from Alzheimer's disease or Parkinson's disease.

The presence of Lewy bodies in Alzheimer's disease portends a more malignant course. For example, in Alzheimer's disease patients, the number of Lewy bodies is related to a more rapid cognitive decline. Alzheimer's disease patients with parkinsonism and Lewy bodies have a more rapid rate of decline than those without Lewy bodies.

There is no specific treatment for dementia with Lewy bodies. Studies have been done with cholinesterase inhibitors, and, although there is a concern that they may worsen the parkinsonian symptoms, trials to date have not borne that out. For example, rivastigmine, a cholinesterase inhibitor, improved the dementia with Lewy bodies patients' performance on a behavioral measure and a computerized test of cognitive functioning compared to placebo in a trial of 120 dementia with Lewy bodies patients. Patients with dementia with Lewy bodies may be extremely sensitive to the extrapyramidal side effects of antipsychotic medications, and, therefore, low doses of atypical antipsychotics are usually used to treat the psychotic symptoms associated with dementia with Lewy bodies.

FRONTOTEMPORAL DEMENTIA

Dementia associated with degenerative atrophy of frontal and temporal lobes includes a heterogeneous group of sporadic and familial diseases that result in personality and behavioral changes, with variable degrees of language and cognitive impairment. Historically, it has been a significant clinical challenge to separate frontotemporal dementia from Alzheimer's disease and primary psychiatric disorders.

Definition Frontotemporal dementia, also known as *frontotemporal degeneration*, is a recent term that encompasses several variant forms of dementia that include Pick's disease, primary progressive aphasia, semantic dementia, and corticobasal degeneration.

History The term *frontotemporal dementia* was derived from the observation that the behavioral and personality changes associated with frontotemporal atrophy, as described by Arnold Pick, actually occur in a broader spectrum of patients without the classic lobar atrophy or histopathological finding of Pick bodies. *Pick's disease* used to be an overreaching term that referred to dementia associated with behavioral symptoms, aphasia, and frontotemporal atrophy on gross postmortem examination. With the advent of the term *frontotemporal dementia*, however, *Pick's disease* defines only the pathologic variant with cytoplasmic neuronal inclusions called *Pick bodies*, now recognized to be found in only a minority of cases of dementia associated with frontotemporal degeneration.

Comparative Nosology The DSM-IV-TR lists dementia due to Pick's disease within the category of dementia due to other general medical conditions, and there are no separate diagnostic criteria for Pick's disease or other frontotemporal dementias. In 1994, the Lund and Manchester Groups wrote a consensus statement proposing clinical and neuropathological criteria for frontotemporal dementia. They described it as a behavioral disorder arising from frontal and temporal cerebral atrophy and identified three patterns of histological changes: frontal lobe degeneration type, Pick type, and motor neuron disease type. Pick type was distinguished from frontal lobe degeneration type by the presence of classic Pick bodies and more "intense and circumscribed" atrophy and gliosis. The motor neuron disease type was considered to have the same gross histological changes as the frontal lobe degeneration type but was less severe in nature.

In 1998, an international workshop that included members from the Lund and Manchester Groups refined their previous consensus and developed clinical diagnostic criteria for frontotemporal lobar degeneration, now called *frontotemporal dementia*. The consensus specified features of three syndromes included within the category of frontotemporal lobar degeneration, called *frontotemporal dementia*, *progressive nonfluent aphasia*, and *semantic dementia*.

Later, in 2000, another international conference, the Work Group on Frontotemporal Dementia and Pick's Disease, reassessed the clinical and neuropathological criteria. It was the recommendation of this group to use the term *frontotemporal dementia* to categorize the many variants of clinical and pathological presentations that include Pick's disease, primary progressive aphasia (formerly *progressive nonfluent aphasia*), and semantic dementia. In another conceptual change, frontotemporal lobar degeneration came to represent a diagnosis of exclusion, used only after immunohistochemical methods fail to identify other distinctive pathological conditions. Frontotemporal lobar degeneration is now also known as *dementia lacking distinct histopathological features*.

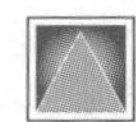

Table 10.3–10
Clinical Criteria for Frontotemporal Dementia

(1) The development of behavioral or cognitive deficits manifested by either
  (a) Early and progressive change in personality, characterized by difficulty in modulating behavior, often resulting in inappropriate responses or activities or
  (b) Early and progressive change in language, characterized by problems with expression of language or severe naming difficulty and problems with word meaning.
(2) The deficits outlined in 1a or 1b cause significant impairment in social or occupational functioning and represent a significant decline from a previous level of functioning.
(3) The course is characterized by a gradual onset and continuing decline in function.
(4) The deficits in 1a or 1b are not due to other nervous system conditions (e.g., cerebrovascular disease), systemic conditions (e.g., hypothyroidism), or substance-induced conditions.
(5) The deficits do not occur exclusively during a delirium.
(6) The disturbance is not better accounted for by a psychiatric diagnosis (e.g., depression).

From McKhann GM, Albert MS, Grossman M, Miller B, Dickson D, Trojanowski JQ: Clinical and pathological diagnosis of frontotemporal dementia. Report of the Work Group on Frontotemporal Dementia and Pick's Disease. *Arch Neurol.* 2001;58:1803–1809, with permission.

The Work Group on Frontotemporal Dementia and Pick's Disease proposed clinical criteria for frontotemporal dementia that require the presence of personality changes that result in behavioral disturbance or cognitive deficits manifested by language dysfunction. In addition, the criteria require a gradual onset of symptoms with progressive functional decline. Similar to the DSM-IV-TR dementia, these criteria also specify that deficits must cause significant impairment in social and occupational functioning, must not be due to other conditions, and must not occur solely in the context of delirium (Table 10.3–10). The Work Group also proposed neuropathological criteria to delineate five categories using τ-positive inclusion bodies, the number of microtubule-binding repeats in the insoluble τ, or the presence of ubiquitin-positive inclusion bodies as distinguishing characteristics.

Epidemiology Frontotemporal dementias have been estimated to account for between 5 and 20 percent of degenerative dementias. Clearly accepted prevalence rates are not available, but recent epidemiological studies have reported estimated rates to range between 10 and 80 per 100,000, depending on the study and the age of the sample. In younger populations (younger than 65 years of age), for example, frontotemporal dementia probably accounts for a larger percentage of total dementia cases, but overall prevalence rates remain relatively low. In older populations, Alzheimer's and vascular dementia are responsible for the vast majority of cases. It is well recognized that frontotemporal dementia is more likely to affect younger populations, and the age of onset ranges between 35 and 75 years of age. Several recent studies have found the mean age of onset to be in the sixth decade of life. Men and women are probably equally affected, and studies have documented that between 20 and 40 percent of patients have a family history of frontotemporal dementia.

Etiology The etiology remains unclear, but, in some cases, genetic linkage to chromosome 17 has been found, in addition to various τ protein mutations. On pathological examination, there may be evidence of gliosis, neuronal loss, and atrophy of the frontal and temporal cortices.

Clinical Features The Work Group on Frontotemporal Dementia and Pick's Disease identified two core clinical patterns of dementia: (1) gradual changes in personality and behavior and (2) progressive language dysfunction. The hallmark of the behavioral presentation is typically a combination of disinhibition, apathy, and limited insight. Patients may be irritable, inappropriate, impulsive, and potentially aggressive. They may exhibit perseveration of words or actions, with stereotyped behavior, mental rigidity, and inflexibility. Other disinhibition phenomena are sometimes categorized as the Klüver-Bucy syndrome of hypersexuality, hyperorality, and the need to touch and examine all objects within reach (utilization behavior).

The other presentation of frontotemporal dementia is characterized by gradual and progressive changes in language function. Depending on the nature of the dysfunction, the terms *primary progressive aphasia* and *semantic dementia* have been used to describe these patients. Patients have expressive deficits, with difficulty in word finding and naming. Early in the course of the disease, speech may be impoverished or may lack spontaneity, but there may be relative preservation of other cognitive functions, such as memory. As concentration and attention worsen, memory problems become increasingly evident. Eventually, impairments in word meaning, reading, and writing develop. With disease progression, speech may become perseverative and echolalic, with eventual mutism. Behavioral changes may also develop.

Differential Diagnosis Because the initial presentation of frontotemporal dementia may be behavioral, it is easily confused with other primary psychiatric disorders. Apathy and social withdrawal may be mistakenly treated as depression. Alternatively, disinhibition or inappropriate, bizarre, or aggressive behavior can appear manic or psychotic or can even mimic substance intoxication. In addition, frontotemporal dementia can only be considered after ruling out other potential medical causes of dementia (Tables 10.3–1 and 10.3–2).

Pathology and Laboratory Examination Frontotemporal dementia is typically characterized by asymmetrical focal atrophy of the frontotemporal regions (Fig. 10.3–10). There is underlying neu-

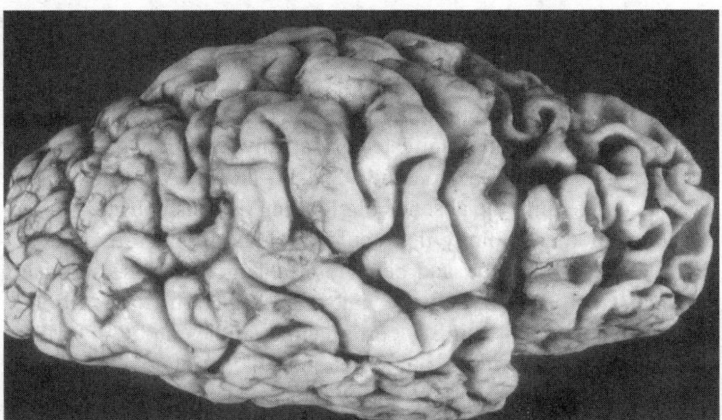

FIGURE 10.3–10 Pick's disease gross pathology. This demonstrates the marked frontal and temporal atrophy seen in frontotemporal dementias, such as Pick's disease. (Courtesy of Dushyant Purohit, M.D., Associate Professor, Department of Neuropathology, Mount Sinai School of Medicine, New York, NY.)

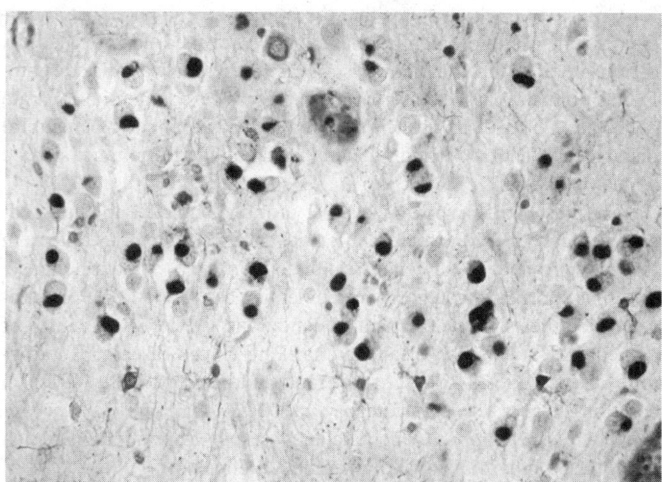

FIGURE 10.3–11 Pick bodies, demonstrated with silver staining of the hippocampus. Pick bodies are intraneuronal spherical argyrophilic inclusions. (Courtesy of Dushyant Purohit, M.D., Associate Professor, Department of Neuropathology, Mount Sinai School of Medicine, New York, NY.)

ronal loss, gliosis, and subsequent spongiform changes in the affected cortices. Pick's cells are pathognomonic in Pick's disease, and they appear swollen and stain pink on hematoxylin and eosin staining (Fig. 10.3–11). Frontotemporal dementias may also have τ-positive inclusion bodies in oligodendroglial cells and astrocytic processes. Ubiquitin-positive inclusion bodies have been described in a variant called *frontotemporal dementia with progressive motor neuron disease*, and, recently, a possible genetic marker has linked these cases to chromosome 9. Structural imaging studies with computed tomography (CT) or magnetic resonance imaging (MRI) may reveal frontotemporal atrophy. Functional imaging with SPECT and positron emission tomography (PET) have demonstrated decreased perfusion of the frontal and temporal lobes.

Treatment Frontotemporal dementia is treated symptomatically, and, to date, there is a dearth of randomized placebo-controlled trials investigating treatment for the cognitive or behavioral disturbances of these illnesses. Trazodone, antipsychotics, and anticonvulsants may help agitation and aggressive behavior. SSRIs are used for associated symptoms of depression, irritability, and apathy (see Table 10.3–4). Although decreased cholinergic activity may contribute to cognitive impairment in frontotemporal dementia, controlled trials with AChEIs are needed to support the use of these medications. Current efforts are focused on improving methods for early and accurate diagnosis.

DEMENTIA DUE TO OTHER GENERAL MEDICAL CONDITIONS

In determining whether dementia is due to a general medical condition, according to the DSM-IV-TR, there must be a temporal association between the onset or exacerbation of the underlying medical condition and the cognitive impairment. The cognitive deficits must also not be solely accounted for by Alzheimer's disease, vascular dementia, substance-induced persisting dementia, or another psychiatric illness, such as major depression (e.g., pseudodementia). The DSM-IV-TR diagnostic criteria for dementia due to other general medical conditions are identical to those for other dementias except for Criterion C, which states that there must be evidence that cognitive deficits are etiologically related to a confirmed general medical condition other than Alzheimer's disease or cerebrovascular disease. In addition, similar to the criteria for Alzheimer's dementia, separate codes are available to specify the presence or absence of behavioral disturbance. The underlying general medical condition must also be coded on Axis III.

The presence of a separate category for dementia due to other general medical conditions represents an advance from previous criteria in that they provide the clinician with the opportunity to better delineate different etiological categories of dementia. The DSM-IV-TR specifically identifies six general medical conditions as etiological causes of dementia: HIV disease, head trauma, Parkinson's disease, Huntington's disease, Pick's disease, and Creutzfeldt-Jakob disease (CJD). In addition, there is a seventh category, called *dementia due to other general medical conditions*, which includes various other etiologies, such as NPH, hypothyroidism, and vitamin B_{12} deficiency.

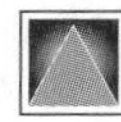

Table 10.3–11
Criteria for Clinical Diagnosis of Human Immunodeficiency Virus Type 1–Associated Dementia Complex

Laboratory evidence for systemic human immunodeficiency virus type 1 infection with confirmation by Western blot, polymerase chain reaction, or culture.

Acquired abnormality in at least *two* of cognitive abilities for a period of at least 1 mo: attention and concentration, speed of processing information, abstraction and reasoning, visuospatial skills, memory and learning, and speech and language. The decline should be verified by reliable history and mental status examination. History should be obtained from an informant, and examination should be supplemented by neuropsychological testing.

Cognitive dysfunction causes impairment in social or occupational functioning. Impairment should not be attributable solely to severe systemic illness.

At least *one* of the following:

- Acquired abnormality in motor function verified by clinical examination (e.g., slowed rapid movements, abnormal gait, incoordination, hyperreflexia, hypertonia, or weakness), neuropsychological tests (e.g., fine motor speed, manual dexterity, or perceptual motor skills), or both.
- Decline in motivation or emotional control or a change in social behavior. This may be characterized by a change in personality with apathy, inertia, irritability, emotional lability, or a new onset of impaired judgment or disinhibition.

This does not exclusively occur in the context of a delirium.

Evidence of another etiology, including active central nervous system opportunistic infection, malignancy, psychiatric disorders (e.g., major depression), or substance abuse, if present, is *not* the cause of the previously mentioned symptoms and signs.

Adapted from Working Group of the American Academy of Neurology AIDS Task Force: Nomenclature and research case definitions for neurologic manifestations of human immunodeficiency virus–type 1 (HIV-1) infection. *Neurology.* 1991;41:778–785.

Dementia Due to HIV Disease

HIV was first identified in 1983, although associated complications had been described 2 years before that time. HIV is a devastating disease that affects more than 36 million people worldwide. It has several neurological complications that are a result of the virus itself and multiple opportunistic infections. Encephalopathy in HIV infection is associated with dementia and is termed *acquired immune deficiency syndrome* (AIDS) *dementia complex*, or *HIV dementia*.

Epidemiology

AIDS dementia complex is primarily seen in patients with advanced immunodeficiency. Increased viral load predisposes patients to developing dementia. The introduction of highly active antiretroviral therapies (HAART) has reduced the incidence of dementia to less than 10 percent of patients with AIDS. Before effective antiretroviral treatments were developed, AIDS dementia complex developed in approximately 60 percent of patients. HIV is also associated with many opportunistic infections that cause neurological complications, the most common of which are cryptococcal meningitis, toxoplasmosis, cytomegalovirus (CMV) encephalitis, progressive multifocal leukoencephalopathy, neurosyphilis, and CNS lymphoma. The primary neurological conditions seen with HIV infection are peripheral neuropathy, myelopathy, and encephalopathy.

Etiology

AIDS dementia complex is probably related to neuronal loss and changes in synaptic architecture. Infected astrocytes and multinucleated macrophages may be partially responsible for the neuronal damage. Recent evidence supports the roles of envelope glycoprotein gp120, Tat, and cytokines such as tumor necrosis factor in causing neurotoxicity and resultant cellular and cognitive dysfunction. There remains a debate, however, as to whether AIDS dementia complex is a result of migration of infected peripheral cells into the CNS or whether it represents a primary CNS infection site.

Clinical Features and Diagnosis

Cognitive decline and motor slowing are the predominant characteristics of AIDS dementia complex. Cognitive changes tend to occur gradually over approximately a 6-month period, and patients often maintain insight into the nature of the decline. Concentration problems and memory impairment are frequent complaints and typically interfere with daily activities. Motor deficits are usually symmetrical, affecting the extremities, and may include ataxia, weakness, tremor, and loss of fine motor coordination. Behavioral changes and depressed mood may also occur, although with less certainty. Psychotic symptoms are rare and typically are transient if present. In late stages of the disease, AIDS dementia complex may progress to mutism, incontinence, and paraplegia. Many patients with HIV also develop a mild cognitive disorder that does not meet criteria for frank dementia but may be a precursor to AIDS dementia complex.

The diagnosis of AIDS dementia complex is made by confirmation of HIV infection and exclusion of alternative pathology to explain cognitive impairment. The American Academy of Neurology AIDS Task Force developed research criteria for the clinical diagnosis of CNS disorders in adults and adolescents (Table 10.3–11). The AIDS Task Force criteria for AIDS dementia complex require laboratory evidence for systemic HIV, at least two cognitive deficits, and the presence of motor abnormalities or personality changes. Personality changes may be manifested by apathy, emotional lability, or behavioral disinhibition. Like the DSM-IV-TR, the AIDS Task Force criteria also require the absence of clouding of consciousness or evidence of another etiology that could produce the cognitive impairment. Cognitive, motor, and behavioral changes are assessed using physical, neurological, and psychiatric examinations, in addition to neuropsychological testing. Neuroimaging studies and CSF evaluation are useful in ruling out other possible etiologies, including opportunistic infections and CNS neoplasms.

Pathology and Laboratory Examination

Neuropathological findings associated with HIV are termed *HIV leukoencephalopathy*. These are diffuse inflammatory changes with microscopic foamy macrophages and multinucleated giant cells that invade subcortical white matter. In addition to routine laboratory examinations, CSF evaluation may reveal mononuclear cells, oligoclonal bands, and elevated protein. However, these latter findings are nonspecific and are not limited to patients with AIDS dementia complex. Specific correlates of AIDS dementia complex in the CSF include elevated levels of β_2-microglobulin, neopterin, quinolinic acid, and Fas, all of which were shown to decline with antiviral treatment and decreasing viral loads. CSF is also useful to rule out the presence of cryptococcal antigen, neurosyphilis, and CMV. Neuroimaging is not diagnostic but instead may reveal pathological changes consistent with other primary diseases, such as CNS lymphoma, toxoplasma encephalitis, or progressive multifocal leukoencephalopathy. Research is focused on improving techniques such as magnetic resonance diffusion tensor imaging to better detect subtle white matter changes in HIV. In the future, magnetic resonance spectroscopy (MRS) may reliably monitor HIV brain involvement by measuring metabolites that reflect loss of neurons and glia.

Treatment Because it is clear that AIDS dementia complex is caused by HIV in the CNS and that increased viral load is associated with a greater risk of developing AIDS dementia complex, the primary goal of treatment in HIV and AIDS dementia is to control the viral load. There is a current trend to delay treatment of HIV because of concern about the inevitable evolution of the virus to become resistant over the long term and the risk of potential toxicity. The initiation of treatment is usually recommended for symptomatic infection, high viral loads (>55,000 copies per mm), or when the CD4 count falls below 350 cells per mm^3. Today, most patients are expected to reach undetectable levels of plasma virus with HAART. Current research is focused on testing resistance to improve drug selection. Scientists are also focusing on monitoring therapeutic drug levels to aid in dose selection and prevent toxicity. There are a total of 15 approved antiretroviral medications that fall within three main classes: nucleoside reverse transcriptase inhibitors, nonnucleoside reverse transcriptase inhibitors, and protease inhibitors. Special attention may be paid to choosing regimens that maximize the potential to cross the blood–brain barrier.

Dementia Due to Traumatic Brain Injury

Traumatic brain injury is defined as brain damage after external head trauma. The annual incidence is approximately two million cases, and traumatic brain injury is the leading cause of mortality in people younger than 45 years of age. Survival rates have recently improved owing to advances in trauma medicine, and this casts greater light on their morbidity, with specific focus on psychiatric complications. Head injury increases the risk of subsequently developing dementia. This is true as an immediate consequence of the injury, as a consequence of multiple head traumas (as in dementia pugilistica), or even as an independent risk factor for the development of Alzheimer's disease.

Deficits result from cortical brain damage, with the anterior temporal and orbitofrontal regions most susceptible. Cognitive impairment is common after head trauma, although the severity and duration of the deficits are related to the extent and location of damage. Other variables that significantly affect the course and nature of cognitive impairment are duration of posttraumatic amnesia, brainstem dysfunction, and degree of axonal injury.

In the acute postconcussion state, amnesia and confusion are the most common symptoms. If brain damage is extensive, memory impairment frequently persists, and disturbances of attention, language, and executive function may also develop. Patients typically complain of short-term memory deficits, such as misplacing things and difficulty recalling recent events. Episodic memory has been found to be impaired, with relative preservation of procedural memory. Disturbances in attention include concentration difficulty, impaired focus, and easy distractibility. Language disturbances vary greatly according to extent and location of damage. Deficits may range from lack of spontaneous speech to severe forms of expressive and receptive aphasia. Language impairment is typically characterized by word-finding problems, difficulty with expression, dysarthria, and dysprosody. Patients with a history of traumatic brain injury may be impulsive, with decreased motivation, poor judgment, and lack of insight. They may also exhibit concrete thinking with poor concept formation and difficulty shifting cognitive tasks.

Dementia pugilistica, or boxer's dementia, affects approximately 17 percent of retired professional boxers and is characterized by motor, cognitive, and behavioral changes. The motor abnormalities may begin with dysarthria and balance difficulties and may progress to incoordination, ataxia, and parkinsonism. Cognitive changes usually affect memory, attention, and executive functioning. The behavioral changes, which are more poorly documented, include disinhibition, irritability, paranoia, and violent outbursts. The etiology is thought to be related to multiple petechial hemorrhages in the cerebrum and cerebellum, which progress over time to gliosis or progressive cell loss. Microscopically, diffuse plaques and tangles may be seen, as are depigmentation and gliosis in the substantia nigra.

The treatment of cognitive impairment secondary to traumatic brain injury has been attempted with dopamine agonists, psychostimulants, and cholinesterase inhibitors. Some cognitive deficits have been hypothesized to occur as a result of ACh deficiency and randomized controlled trials with physostigmine have demonstrated moderate efficacy. Additional studies are needed to fully evaluate the potential role of cholinesterase inhibitors. Controlled trials with dopamine agonists have shown benefit for executive dysfunction associated with traumatic brain injury, and psychostimulants are effective for symptoms of inattention and distractibility.

Dementia Due to Parkinson's Disease

Parkinson's disease, first described by James Parkinson in 1817, is caused by an idiopathic degeneration of subcortical structures, primarily the substantia nigra. Structural damage and subsequent dopaminergic dysfunction result in significant motor abnormalities, mood disturbance, and dementia in some patients. Although the biological basis of dementia in Parkinson's disease remains unclear, the degeneration of the nucleus basalis of Meynert may contribute to cognitive impairment. The typical age of onset of Parkinson's disease is between 50 and 60 years of age, although variants may occur between one and two decades earlier. Dementia in Parkinson's disease occurs in approximately 20 to 30 percent of patients and typically affects frontal lobe executive functioning and memory. Nondemented patients also demonstrate milder cognitive deficits in visuospatial and attention shifting tasks. Neuropathology confirms the diagnosis of Parkinson's disease and is characterized by intracytoplasmic inclusions, Lewy bodies, in the substantia nigra.

The hallmark of Parkinson's disease is a movement disorder characterized by tremor, bradykinesia, and rigidity. The tremor occurs at rest bilaterally or unilaterally and may appear pill-rolling in nature. Bradykinesia is manifested by a slow and shuffling gait, blunted affect, monotonous speech, and difficulty in the initiation and execution of movement. Rigidity may also be bilateral or unilateral and is described as cogwheel rigidity, with stiffness and a superimposed jerkiness throughout flexion and extension. Depressive symptoms are a common feature of Parkinson's disease, occurring in as much as 50 percent of patients. Depressive symptoms may be related to the on–off phenomena associated with dopamine agonist treatment, in which mood symptoms worsen during the off period, coincident to changes in motoric function, and abate in the on period. The depressive syndrome associated with Parkinson's disease is typically characterized by dysphoria, irritability, hopelessness, and suicidal ideation. Psychomotor retardation is a common finding that may be associated with the major depression and the cognitive and motor impairments of the primary disease. Psychotic symptoms have also been reported in the context of depressive episodes or as the consequence of dopamine agonist treatment.

The treatment of Parkinson's disease typically includes dopamine precursors, such as levodopa (Larodopa) or the combination of carbidopa and levodopa (Sinemet). The symptoms of bradykinesia and rigidity tend to be more responsive than tremor to dopaminergic agents. Second-line agents for motor dysfunction include dopamine agonists, such as pergolide (Permax) or bromocriptine (Parlodel), and anticholinergic medications, such as benztropine (Cogentin). Selegiline (Carbex), a monoamine oxidase type B (MAO_B) inhibitor, has been shown to slow the progression of motor impairment. Randomized controlled trials with donepezil also support its use for the treatment of cognitive symptoms. Future directions of research include newer dopamine agonists, coenzyme Q, surgical treatment, and fetal neural tissue transplantation. Comorbid major depressive disorder should be treated with standard antidepressant medications and electroconvulsive therapy (ECT). ECT may temporarily improve the motor symptoms of Parkinson's disease as well.

Dementia Due to Huntington's Disease

Huntington's disease was first described by George Huntington in 1872 and has since been understood to result from an unstable trinucleotide repeat sequence (CAG) on chromosome 4. Huntington's disease is transmitted in an autosomal dominant pattern with complete penetrance. Damage occurs through neuronal loss in the caudate nucleus and putamen by a mechanism that remains unknown. Recent theories include mitochondrial dysfunction that results in neurotoxicity by the neurotransmitter glutamate. Other leading theories involve proposed abnormalities of protein metabolism and transcriptional dysregulation. The onset of Huntington's disease typically occurs between 25 and 50 years of age. A greater number of trinucleotide repeats is correlated with more severe neuronal loss, earlier age of onset, and lower cognitive performance. A juvenile form of Huntington's disease also exists, with a greater degree of motor impairment early in the course of the illness and a more rapid rate of disease progression.

Huntington's disease is characterized by psychiatric symptoms and cognitive impairment followed by pronounced motor abnormalities, including the classic choreoathetoid movements. Psychopathology may include affective disturbance, psychotic phenomena, anxiety, and personality changes. Psychiatric symptoms do not necessarily occur but, when present, are typically evident early in the disease course. Depression is a common feature of Huntington's disease, and patients are at an increased risk of suicide. As the disease progresses, patients may become apathetic or may minimize symptoms. Cognitive impairment is consistent across patients with Huntington's disease and follows a gradual, deteriorating course. Initial symptoms may include mild memory deficits with subtle difficulty in executive functioning (e.g., organizing, planning, and sequencing). Complex task performance worsens as the disease progresses, as do learning, verbal, and visuospatial abilities. Eventually, the cognitive symptoms of dementia in Huntington's may be indistinguishable from Alzheimer's disease. As the disease evolves, the choreoathetoid movements develop into more dystonic motor abnormalities and bradykinesia. Patients eventually become severely dystonic and bedridden.

As progress is made in understanding the pathophysiology of Huntington's disease, investigators have begun to develop new therapies, such as glutamate receptor antagonists, for potential use in future clinical trials aimed at slowing disease progression. Associated psychiatric features are treated symptomatically, although controlled trials are needed to assess the efficacy of antidepressants and neuroleptics. Psychotherapy may also play an important supportive role for the patient and the family.

Dementia Due to Creutzfeldt-Jakob Disease

Transmissible spongiform encephalopathy is a group of rare, but fatal, neurodegenerative diseases, which includes CJD, Gerstmann-Sträussler syndrome, fatal familial insomnia, and kuru. CJD is caused by a *proteinaceous infectious particle*, or prion. The infection produces a diffuse neurodegenerative process characterized by dementia, hypertonicity, and EEG changes.

CJD is extremely rare, and, although the onset may occur at any age, it typically begins in the 50s. Prions may incubate for decades before symptoms emerge. There may also be a genetic susceptibility to infection, as familial patterns of inheritance exist, although they represent only a minority of cases. The proposed route of transmission is through invasive body contact, such as corneal transplants or contaminated surgical instruments. Recent concern has revolved around the possibility that prion disease is more infectious than previously thought and that bovine spongiform encephalopathy in cattle may be passed to humans by ingestion and may produce a variant of CJD. The first case of the variant form of CJD was reported in 1986 and then was confirmed by histopathology in 1996. The incubation period may be 10 years. Since then, approximately 100 confirmed cases have been reported, most of which occurred in the United Kingdom.

Clinical features of CJD depend on the area of the brain affected, but initial presentations may be nonspecific and include simply lethargy and depression. The symptoms progress rapidly, over weeks, to the characteristic dementia, myoclonus, muscle rigidity, and ataxia. Death typically ensues within 1 year. Blood work and neuroimaging are unremarkable, but EEG, although nonspecific, reveals diffuse, symmetrical, rhythmic slow waves or periodic sharp and slow wave complexes, or both. Histopathology is diagnostic and shows neuronal loss, astrocyte proliferation, and a resultant spongiform appearance to the gray matter of the cortex, striatum, and thalamus. More recently, a laboratory marker has been made available that measures a protein in the CSF called 14-3-3. The role of 14-3-3 in CJD is unknown, but its presence in CSF is thought to indicate severe neuronal disruption, and it has significant diagnostic validity. Future challenges include the development of an early diagnostic test to avoid transmission through blood or organ donation. Treatment and prevention remain priorities for scientists, and efforts to elucidate the molecular mechanisms of prion disease are under way.

Dementia Due to Pick's Disease

Pick's disease is currently classified as a frontotemporal dementia by the Work Group on Frontotemporal Dementia and Pick's Disease, although the DSM-IV-TR lists it under dementia due to other general medical conditions. It is defined by the presence of Pick bodies, is characterized by personality changes and behavioral disinhibition, and typically begins before 75 years of age. Familial cases may have an earlier onset, and some studies have shown that approximately one-half of the cases of Pick's disease are familial (Figs. 10.3–10 and 10.3–11).

Dementia Due to Normal Pressure Hydrocephalus

NPH is characterized by the clinical triad of gait disturbance, cognitive impairment, and urinary incontinence. It is a fairly rare cause of dementia, with prevalence rates that vary according to the study, the clinical setting, and the diagnostic methods used. The incidence has been estimated at 2.2 per million per year, and the prevalence has been estimated at 5,000 to 10,000 patients in the United States. NPH typically occurs during the sixth or seventh decade of life, although it has been reported in children and young adults. Intraventricular CSF pressure increases due to impaired CSF flow, yet lumbar puncture does not reveal increased pressure. The etiology of the clinical deterioration is thought to be due to compression of small vessels by the dilated ventricles with resultant impairment in ventricular blood flow and perfusion deficits. This may be related to a reversal of CSF flow through the ependymal lining of the ventricle into the extracellular space of the white matter, as a compensatory mechanism for an often idiopathic obstruction to normal CSF flow. Patients with NPH have also been shown to have an increased prevalence of arterial hypertension and cerebral arteriosclerosis.

Cognitive impairments are usually characterized by memory problems, difficulty with information processing and manipulation, and generally slowed thinking. Patients tend not to demonstrate aphasia, apraxia, or agnosia, and, if present, Alzheimer's disease should be suspected. Unfortunately, the presentation of NPH is easily confused with other dementia syndromes, because ataxia and urinary incontinence can also be found in vascular dementia, Alzheimer's disease, and Parkinson's disease. Chronic alcohol abuse with subsequent frontal and cerebellar atrophy may also present with mental status changes (alcohol-related dementia) and ataxia. The urinary incontinence is a late sign and may be due to damage to the periventricular pathways extending to the bladder control center.

Enlarged cerebral ventricles on CT or MRI that are out of proportion to cerebral atrophy and lumbar puncture are diagnostic. The treatment of NPH is accomplished with shunt placement to reduce intraventricular pressure. Serial taps may also result in transient, but significant, clinical improvement. However, dementia is less likely to improve with treatment than are the other associated symptoms. A retrospective review of patients with NPH found that 30 percent of patients who underwent shunting procedures showed significant improvement. Approximately 35 percent of patients with shunts had surgical complications, and approximately 10 percent of these resulted in death or severe residual morbidity.

Dementia Due to Vitamin B_{12} Deficiency The prevalence of vitamin B_{12} deficiency has been estimated to be 15 to 44 percent in the elderly. Particularly in the population older than 70 years of age, hypochlorhydria or achlorhydria is frequently present (in 25 to 50 percent) and leads to inadequate release of protein-bound vitamin B_{12}. The prevalence of vitamin B_{12} deficiency in patients with dementia varies significantly, but the incidence of reversible vitamin B_{12} deficiency as the primary etiology is probably less than 1 percent. As a comorbid illness with dementia, however, vitamin B_{12} deficiency is a frequent finding, and several studies have documented a correlation between serum vitamin B_{12} levels and cognitive functioning in elderly patients. Some evidence also suggests that vitamin B_{12} deficiency may be more common in Alzheimer's disease. Despite this finding, other studies have contradicted the correlation between dementia and serum vitamin B_{12} levels and have also questioned the potential reversibility of dementia with vitamin B_{12} replacement. One of the proposed mechanisms by which low levels of vitamin B_{12} may influence cognition is through the disruption of methylation reactions in the CNS that could increase homocysteine levels and that may result in direct neurotoxic effects. Elevated homocysteine is also an independent risk factor for cerebrovascular disease and Alzheimer's disease.

In addition to the megaloblastic hematological changes that may be associated with vitamin B_{12} deficiency, there are several well-characterized neurological complications. The most consistently observed neurological complications are peripheral neuropathy, myelopathy, paresthesia, impaired vibratory and position sense, and symmetrical weakness. Cognitive deficits may include poor spatial copying skills, diminished episodic memory, and impaired abstract thinking. Some studies have demonstrated a worsening of cognitive functioning in dementia accompanied by vitamin B_{12} deficiency, and others have also shown impaired global cognition in subjects with vitamin B_{12} deficiency in the absence of frank dementia.

Vitamin B_{12} deficiency is traditionally diagnosed by using serum cobalamin levels, although the additional measurement of methylmalonic acid and homocysteine is more reliable and sensitive than vitamin B_{12} alone. Methylmalonic acid and homocysteine are metabolites whose levels are elevated in vitamin B_{12} deficiency and have been shown to fall with replacement therapy. Although pernicious anemia is not a common cause of vitamin B_{12} deficiency in the elderly, the Schilling test may be used to evaluate the presence of intrinsic factor. The most effective treatment is parenteral substitution with cobalamin. The initial recommended dosage is 1,000 μg daily for 1 week, then weekly for 1 month, and then monthly.

Dementia Due to Hypothyroidism Thyroid gland dysfunction is a well-recognized cause of cognitive impairment. Hypothyroidism can lead to memory problems, psychomotor slowing, and visuoperceptual and construction deficits. Cognitive deficits in hypothyroidism may be mistaken for Parkinson's dementia, Alzheimer's disease, or depression (pseudodementia), because patients may be lethargic, with flattened affect, psychomotor retardation, and decreased appetite. Studies have demonstrated clinically significant impairments on the MMSE that persist even after patients return to euthyroid states with replacement therapy. Recent evidence has led researchers to question the classic categorization of hypothyroidism as a potentially reversible cause of dementia. Given the risk of potentially irreversible dementia, and because the prevalence of hypothyroidism increases with age, routine screening in the elderly is of particular importance. The relative contributions of comorbid neurodegenerative diseases in influencing cognitive decline must also be considered. Nevertheless, it seems clear that, although the cognitive changes may be only partially reversible, proper treatment of hypothyroid states with replacement therapy provides likely benefit and possibly slows or stops progressive decline.

SUBSTANCE-INDUCED PERSISTING DEMENTIA

The DSM-IV-TR criteria for substance-induced persisting dementia are identical to those for other dementias. However, as represented by the term *persisting*, symptoms must exist "beyond the usual duration of substance intoxication or withdrawal." In addition, there must be evidence that cognitive impairments are etiologically related to the persisting effects of the substance used. Current abstinence does not preclude the presence of a substance-induced dementia, because most patients have a history of prolonged and heavy substance use. The characteristics and course of the disease depend mostly on the causative substance. Substances known to evoke a persisting dementia are alcohol, inhalants, sedatives, hypnotics, and anxiolytics. Medications such as anticonvulsants and intrathecal methotrexate have also been cited in the DSM-IV-TR to produce dementia. Toxins are a well-known cause of dementia, and frequent offenders include lead, mercury, carbon monoxide, organophosphate insecticides, and industrial solvents. Alcohol-induced persisting dementia probably has the most data to support its description, although considerable debate exists as to whether it is a distinct etiological entity or secondary to various metabolic and nutritional deficiencies associated with alcoholism. Nevertheless, alcohol related dementia is used as a paradigm of substance-induced persisting dementia for the remainder of this discussion.

Alcohol-Induced Persisting Dementia Also known as *alcohol-related dementia*, alcohol-induced persisting dementia falls within the categories of alcohol-related disorders and substance-induced persisting dementias. Prevalence rates differ considerably according to the population studied and the diagnostic criteria used, although alcohol related dementia has been estimated to account for approximately 4 percent of dementias. Milder forms of cognitive impairment are also frequently associated with chronic alcohol abuse but typically do not result in prolonged, irreversible cognitive deficit on cessation.

The causal relationship between alcohol use and dementia is complicated, and controversy exists in the literature. Alcohol, or its metabolite acetaldehyde, may have direct CNS neurotoxic effects. Dementia may also result from thiamine deficiency and subsequent cortical neuronal loss. In 1881, Karl Wernicke described a syndrome in alcoholics that consisted of abrupt onset confusion, accompanied by ataxia and abnormal eye movements, which began with nystagmus and lateral rectus or horizontal gaze paresis and progressed to complete ophthalmoplegia, usually with pupillary sparing. This syndrome became known as *Wernicke's encephalopathy*. Several years later, Sergei Sergeevich Korsakoff reported on an amnestic state with confabulation that appeared to frequently follow the encephalopathy. It has since become clear that chronic alcohol abuse impairs GI absorption of thiamine, and the resultant thiamine deficiency is the major factor in producing Wernicke's encephalopathy and Korsakoff's psychosis. In addition, alcoholism frequently results in liver disease, which, in turn, affects thiamine homeostasis, and may also directly cause neurotoxicity and cognitive impairment. Questions remain, however, as to whether dementia represents a distinct pathophysiological entity or rather is part of the constellation of symptoms seen in chronic alcohol abuse associated with liver disease and thiamine deficiency. Recent evidence suggests that alcoholic brain damage and subsequent cognitive dysfunction may be the result of a combination of direct neurotoxic insult and the metabolic effects of thiamine deficiency and liver disease.

To make the diagnosis of alcohol-induced persisting dementia, the criteria for dementia must be met. Because amnesia may also occur in the context Korsakoff's psychosis, it is important to distinguish between memory impairment accompanied by other cognitive deficits (i.e., dementia) and amnesia due to thiamine deficiency. To complicate matters, however, there is also evidence that other cognitive functions, such as attention and concentration, may also be impaired in Wernicke-Korsakoff syndrome. In addition, alcohol abuse is frequently associated with mood changes, so poor concentration and other cognitive symptoms often observed in the context of a major depression must also be ruled out.

MCIs may also exist in patients with alcohol dependence without fully meeting criteria for dementia. Recent theories have suggested that dementia may actually result from the combined effects of Korsakoff-like amnesia and the milder cognitive impairments characteristic of chronic alcohol use. These patients tend to have problem-solving and planning difficulties and perceptual-motor dysfunction, but verbal and overall IQs generally remain within the normal range. Patients with milder alcohol-related cognitive impairment may also improve significantly with sustained abstinence. Alcohol-induced persisting dementia, on the other hand, has more global and prolonged deficits.

Descriptions of alcohol-related dementia in the literature have reported many features that include memory impairment, slow mentation, disorganized thought, poor attention, impaired judgment, and disorientation. Other psychiatric symptoms may include mood lability, impulsivity, behavioral disinhibition, irritability, aggression, apathy, and paranoid ideation. In 1941, Wechsler noted that alcoholics had difficulty with abstraction, learning new material, and organizing complex perceptions. Since then, others have replicated these findings and have shown deficits to be accompanied by a relative preservation of verbal abilities. Symptoms tend to develop gradually, and this may be one way, albeit unreliably, to distinguish dementia from Wernicke-Korsakoff syndrome.

The diagnosis of alcohol-induced persisting dementia is made based on clinical evaluation. There are no pathognomonic findings, and neuroimaging studies show only nonspecific neuroanatomical changes. The most common findings on CT or MRI are cerebral atrophy and ventricular enlargement with widening of the cerebral sulci, although the relationship between radiological abnormalities and dementia is unclear. Furthermore, enlarged ventricles and widened sulci have also been found in alcohol dependence without cognitive impairment. The treatment of alcohol-induced dementia consists mainly of abstinence, although cognitive deficits persist despite cessation of drinking. Adequate nutrition and the treatment of underlying or comorbid psychiatric and medical illness are crucial.

SUGGESTED CROSS-REFERENCES

The topics in this chapter are significantly related to a number of other areas within the *Comprehensive Textbook of Psychiatry*. The reader is encouraged to review the other areas in this chapter, (Section 10.2 on delirium, Section 10.4 on amnestic disorders, and Section 10.5 on cognitive disorders due to a general medical condition), as well as Chapter 11 on substance use disorders and Section 13.7 on major depression. Section 28.4 on palliative care in dementia further explores end-of-life issues and treatment decisions in end-stage dementia.

REFERENCES

Chiu HFK: Editorial review: Vitamin B_{12} deficiency and dementia. *Int J Geriatr Psychiatry.* 1996;11:851–858.

Chui H, Gonthier R: Natural history of vascular dementia. *Alzheimer Dis Assoc Disord.* 1999;13[Suppl 3]:S124–S130.

Chui HC, Victoroff JI, Margolin D, Jagust W, Shankle R, Katzman R: Criteria for the diagnosis of ischemic vascular dementia proposed by the State of California Alzheimer's Disease Diagnostic and Treatment Centers. *Neurology.* 1992;42:473–480.

*Clifford DB: AIDS dementia. *Med Clin North Am.* 2002;86:537–550.

Cohen-Mansfield J: Nonpharmacologic interventions for inappropriate behaviors in dementia: A review, summary, and critique. *Am J Geriatr Psychiatry.* 2001;9:361–381.

Devanand DP, Jacobs DM, Tang MX, Del Castillo-Castaneda C, Sano M, Marder K, Bell K, Bylsma FW, Brandt J, Albert M, Stern Y: The course of psychopathologic features in mild to moderate Alzheimer's disease. *Arch Gen Psychiatry.* 1997;54:257–263.

Dugbartey AT: Neurocognitive aspects of hypothyroidism. *Arch Intern Med.* 1998;158:1413–1418.

Gwyther LP: Family issues in dementia: Finding a new normal. *Neurol Clin.* 2000;18:993–1010.

Hardy J, Selkoe DJ: The amyloid hypothesis of Alzheimer's disease: Progress and problems on the road to therapeutics. *Science.* 2002;297:353–356.

Helmes E, Bowler JV, Merskey H, Munoz DG, Hachinski VC: Rates of cognitive decline in Alzheimer's disease and dementia with Lewy bodies. *Dement Geriatr Cogn Disord.* 2003;15:67–71.

Kertesz A, Munoz DG: Frontotemporal dementia. *Med Clin North Am.* 2002;86:501–518.

Kindermann SS, Dolder CR, Bailey A, Katz IR, Jeste DV: Pharmacological treatment of psychosis and agitation in elderly patients with dementia: four decades of experience. *Drugs Aging.* 2002;19:257–276.

*Korczyn AD: Dementia in Parkinson's disease. *J Neurol.* 2001;248[Suppl 2]:1–4.

The Lund and Manchester Groups: Consensus statement. Clinical and neuropathological criteria for frontotemporal dementia. *J Neurol Neurosurg Psychiatry.* 1994;4:416–418.

Mahendra B. *Dementia: A Survey of the Syndrome of Dementia.* 2nd ed. Norwell, MA: MTP Press; 1987.

McKeith LG, Galasko D, Kosaka K: Consensus guidelines for the clinical and pathologic diagnosis of dementia with Lewy bodies (DLB): Report of the consortium on DLB international workshop. *Neurology.* 1996;47:1113–1124.

McKhann GM, Albert MS, Grossman M, Miller B, Dickson D, Trojanowski JQ: Clinical and pathological diagnosis of frontotemporal dementia. Report of the Work Group on Frontotemporal Dementia and Pick's Disease. *Arch Neurol.* 2001;58:1803–1809.

Morris JC: The nosology of dementia. *Neurol Clin.* 2000;18:773–785.

Naarding P, Kremer HPH, Zitman FG: Huntington's disease: A review of the literature on prevalence and treatment of neuropsychiatric phenomena. *Eur Psychiatry.* 2001;16:439–445.

Neary D, Snowden JS, Gustafson L, Passant U, Stuss D, Black S, Freedman M, Kertesz A, Robert PH, Albert M, Boone K, Miller BL, Cummings J, Benson DF: Frontotemporal lobar degeneration: A consensus on clinical diagnostic criteria. *Neurology.* 1998;51:1546–1554.

*Neugroschl J, Davis KL: Biological markers in Alzheimer'a disease. *Am J Geriatr Psychiatry.* 2002;10:660–677.

Perl DP: Neuropathology of Alzheimer's disease and related disorders. *Neurol Clin.* 2000;18:847–864.

Rao V, Lykestos CG: Psychiatric aspects of traumatic brain injury. *Psychol Clin North Am.* 2002;25:43–69.

Rapoport MJ, Feinstein A: Outcome following traumatic brain injury in the elderly: A critical review. *Brain Injury.* 2000;14:749–761.

Reisberg B, Doody R, Stoffler A, Schmitt F, Ferris S, Mobius HJ; Memantine Study Group: Memantine in moderate-to-severe Alzheimer's disease. *N Engl J Med.* 2003;348:1333–1341.

*Roman GC: Vascular dementia revisited: Diagnosis, pathogenesis, treatment, and prevention. *Med Clin North Am.* 2002;86:477–499.

Roman GC, Tatemichi TK, Erkinjuntti T, Cummings JL, Masdeu JC, Garcia JH, Amaducci L, Orgogozo JM, Brun A, Hofman A, Moody DM, O'Brien MD, Yamaguchi T, Grafman J, Drayer BP, Bennett DA, Fisher M, Ogata J, Kokmen E, Bermejo F, Wolf PA, Gorelick PB, Bick KL, Pajeau AK, Bell MA, DeCarli C, Culebras A, Korczyn AD, Bogousslavsky J, Hartmann A, Scheinberg P: Vascular dementia: Diagnostic criteria for research studies. Report of the NINDS-AIREN International Workshop. *Neurology.* 1993;43:250–260.

Sano M, Wilcock GK, van Baelen B, Kavanagh S: The effects of galantamine treatment on caregiver time in Alzheimer's disease. *Int J Geriatr Psychiatry.* 2003;18:942–950.

*Serby M, Samuels SC: Diagnostic criteria for dementia with Lewy bodies reconsidered. *Am J Geriatr Psychiatry.* 2001;9:212–216.

Shumaker SA, Legault C, Rapp SR, Thal L, Wallace RB, Ockene JK, Hendrix SL, Jones BN 3rd, Assaf AR, Jackson RD, Kotchen JM, Wassertheil-Smoller S, Wactawski-Wende J; WHIMS Investigators: Estrogen plus progestin and the incidence of dementia and mild cognitive impairment in postmenopausal women: The Women's Health Initiative Memory Study: A randomized controlled trial. *JAMA.* 2003;289:2651–2662.

Sy MS, Gambetti P, Wong BS: Human prion diseases. *Med Clin North Am.* 2002;86:551–571.

Vanneste JAL: Diagnosis and management of normal pressure hydrocephalus. *J Neurol.* 2000;247:5–114.

Wancata J, Musalek M, Alexandrowicz R, Krautgartner M: Number of dementia sufferers in Europe between the years 2000 and 2050. *Eur Psychiatry.* 2003;18:306–313.

Whyte EM, Mulsant BH, Butters MA, Qayyum M, Towers A, Sweet RA, Klunk W, Wisniewski S, DeKosky ST: Cognitive and behavioral correlates of low vitamin B_{12} levels in elderly patients with progressive dementia. *Am J Geriatr Psychiatry.* 2002;10:321–327.

Willenbring ML: Organic mental disorder associated with heavy drinking and alcohol dependence. *Clin Geriatr Med.* 1998;4:869–887.

Working Group of the American Academy of Neurology AIDS Task Force: Nomenclature and research case definitions for neurologic manifestations of human immunodeficiency virus–type 1 (HIV-1) infection. *Neurology.* 1991;41:778–785.

▲ 10.4 Amnestic Disorders

HILLEL GROSSMAN, M.D.

Perhaps no other psychiatric disorder has so captured the imagination of the public as the amnestic disorder. The notion of losing the ability to identify one's self, to recognize friends and family or even one's own life has been incorporated into countless novels, plays, and movies. The amnestic is a central literary device that allows the author to then detail the search for self and the ramifications and repercussions of such a search. Often, the rediscovery of self depends on unearthing an unspeakable trauma, the liberating force of a powerful kiss or other such manifestation of love, or simply a second head injury that mysteriously corrects the impact of the original.

Unfortunately, these fanciful dramatizations bear little resemblance to the clinical picture of amnestic disorders, neither in their clinical presentations nor in the natural course or response to treatment. Amnesia for person is rare if not unheard of. The picture of a highly intelligent, fully functional, introspective and articulate subject experiencing amnesia is also rare; more often, the amnestic has associated impairments in personality and function. The amnestic nonetheless experiences an existential predicament, the loss of a personal history and one's place in that history. Every day, if not every moment, is isolated and independent of its predecessor. The only comfort for such an existential limbo is that the subject often cannot retain awareness of his or her condition beyond fleeting and evanescent insights.

The amnestic disorders are a broad category that includes a variety of diseases and conditions that present with an amnestic syndrome. The syndrome is defined primarily by impairment in the ability to create new memories. More details regarding the syndrome and its signs, symptoms, course, and treatment are presented in the following sections.

DEFINITION (DSM-IV-TR)

The revised fourth edition of the *Diagnostic and Statistical Manual of Mental Disorders* (DSM-IV-TR) criteria are found in Tables 10.4–1 and 10.4–2. The primary criterion, Criterion A, is an impairment in memory manifested as "impairment to learn new information or inability to recall previously learned information or past events." Criterion B is the standard DSM-IV-TR requirement of functional decline in social or occupational realms, in this case deemed due to the memory disturbance. Criterion C provides the delirium and dementia rule-out: Amnestic disorders cannot be diagnosed if the patient meets criteria for delirium or a dementia. Criterion D stipulates that the memory disturbance must come about as a result of "the direct physiological effects of a general medical condition or due to the persisting effects of a substance." This distinguishes the *amnestic disorders* from *dissociative amnesia* in which the amnesia is thought to derive from psychological distress related to a life event.

Three variations of the amnestic disorder diagnosis, differing in etiology, are offered: amnestic disorder due to a general medical condition (such as head trauma), substance-induced persisting amnestic disorder (such as that due to carbon monoxide poisoning or chronic alcohol consumption), and amnestic disorder not otherwise specified for cases in which the etiology is unclear. There are two modifiers: transient, for duration less than 1 month, and chronic, for conditions extending beyond 1 month.

The DSM-IV-TR expands on these criteria with associated features and a more nuanced description. It is noted that disorientation to place and time is common, although this rarely impacts on orientation to self. Insight into the deficits is often impaired, and patients can display a striking indifference to their impairment. There may be additional deficits in realms of cognition other than memory, although these are subtle and, by definition, do not impact on functioning (otherwise the patient would be classified as having a dementia).

This definition includes several features that are open to interpretation: Although it is recognized that "pure" memory disorders do exist (patient H. M., discussed in a following section, represents the gold standard), most patients with such amnesia also show some degree of defect in other realms. *How much* impairment in other realms (e.g., personality and judgment) is allowed while still considering this a memory disorder? Are there differences in the presenting memory symptoms, course, acuity, and treatment response that influence the diagnosis? Are there subsyndromes of amnestic disorder reflecting impairments in the differing memory systems?

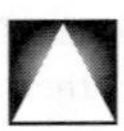

Table 10.4–1
DSM-IV-TR Diagnostic Criteria for Amnestic Disorder Due to a General Medical Condition

A. The development of memory impairment as manifested by impairment in the ability to learn new information or the inability to recall previously learned information.
B. The memory disturbance causes significant impairment in social or occupational functioning and represents a significant decline from a previous level of functioning.
C. The memory disturbance does not occur exclusively during the course of a delirium or a dementia.
D. There is evidence from the history, physical examination, or laboratory findings that the disturbance is the direct physiological consequence of a general medical condition (including physical trauma).

Specify if:
Transient: if memory impairment lasts for 1 month or less
Chronic: if memory lasts for more than 1 month

Coding note: Include the name of the general medical condition on Axis I, for example, amnestic disorder due to head trauma; also code the general medical condition on Axis III.

From American Psychiatric Association. *Diagnostic and Statistical Manual of Mental Disorders.* 4th ed. Text rev. Washington, DC: American Psychiatric Association; 2000, with permission.

Another issue relates to establishing causality or to identifying etiology for psychiatric disorders. Throughout the DSM-IV-TR, there appear variations of the previously mentioned criterion "judged to be physiologically related" to a particular medical condition or laboratory or neuroimaging finding in the context of ascribing etiology. The DSM-IV-TR gives little guidance as to how one makes this judgment of causality or relatedness of disorder to putative etiology. How low must the patient's glucose or sodium be to assume an etiological relationship? How severe must a head trauma be and what are the parameters for assessing severity before ascribing causal etiology? The answer to questions such as these can determine diagnosis, treatment, and prognosis, yet they are not questions that the DSM-IV-TR addresses.

Although disturbances in memory are fairly common, they are more often associated with global cognitive disturbances, as seen in delirium and dementia. The *pure* (or, better, *primary*) memory disturbance of amnestic disorders is rare. It is usually due to processes that produce *focal* injuries to diencephalic or mesial temporal lobe structures.

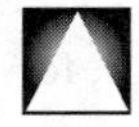

Table 10.4–2
DSM-IV-TR Diagnostic Criteria for Substance-Induced Persisting Amnestic Disorder

A. The development of memory impairment as manifested by impairment in the ability to learn new information or the inability to recall previously learned information.
B. The memory disturbance causes significant impairment in social or occupational functioning and represents a significant decline from a previous level of functioning.
C. The memory disturbance does not occur exclusively during the course of a delirium or a dementia and persists beyond the usual duration of substance intoxication or withdrawal.
D. There is evidence from the history, physical examination, or laboratory findings that the memory disturbance is etiologically related to the persisting effects of substance use (e.g., a drug of abuse or a medication).

Code [specific substance]-induced persisting amnestic disorder: alcohol; sedative, hypnotic, or anxiolytic; or other (or unknown) substance

From American Psychiatric Association. *Diagnostic and Statistical Manual of Mental Disorders.* 4th ed. Text rev. Washington, DC: American Psychiatric Association; 2000, with permission.

HISTORY

Modern studies of memory began with Herman Ebbinghaus (1850 to 1909), the German psychologist and student of Gustav Fechner, who was the first to study memory using experimental techniques. Ebbinghaus delineated learning and forgetting curves in normal adults in a variety of experimental conditions, demonstrating that memory and other higher order cognitive functions were indeed accessible to experimental study. He distinguished between long-term and short-term memory. Theodore Ribot published, in 1882, in *Les Maladies de la Memoire*, his observations of memory impairment in a variety of brain injuries. He noted that amnesia seemed to affect memories in reverse order of their development—memories of recent events were most vulnerable to loss. *Ribot's law* is now a clinical verity of retrograde amnesia.

Although the concept of a general mental deterioration, including memory loss, has been known since antiquity, the description of a discrete impairment in memory is recent. Sergei Sergeievich Korsakoff (1853 to 1900), the Russian neuropsychiatrist, began studying the long-term complications of chronic alcoholism soon after his graduation from the University of Moscow in 1875. He provided the first comprehensive descriptions of patients whose primary problems were devastation of memory. In a series of articles published between 1887 and 1891, Korsakoff described patients who developed a polyneuritis, as well as a distinct mental disorder that varied somewhat in presentation but featured memory loss prominently: "This mental disorder appears at times in the form of sharply delineated irritable weakness in the mental sphere, at times in the form of confusion with characteristic mistakes in orientation for place, time and situation and at times with an almost pure form of acute amnesia where the recent memory is well preserved though the remote past is remembered quite well."

Korsakoff called the disorder *psychosis polyneurotica*, emphasizing that the peripheral neuritis and the mental symptoms were part of the same disease. He suggested an as-yet-unknown toxic etiology for the disease: "a noxious substance disturbing the nutrition of all tissues but chiefly the nervous system." The disorder has been known for many decades as *Korsakoff's psychosis*, despite its primary manifestation being the memory deficit, and *psychosis* per se being absent or comprising confabulations only. For this reason, the terms *Korsakoff's syndrome* and *Korsakoff's dementia* are in common use and are interchangeable with the term *Korsakoff's psychosis*.

Korsakoff did not, of course, realize the connection between the disease findings and nutritional deficiency nor did he appreciate the relationship between the disorder he had described and that described by Carl Wernicke in 1881.Wernicke observed a number of patients in his Berlin clinic who presented with the now famous triad of ophthalmoplegia, gait disturbance, and confusion. Wernicke thought that this condition represented an inflammatory disease that produces punctate hemorrhages in the brainstem, particularly the occulomotor nuclei. At the turn of the century, however, some realization of the connection between Korsakoff's syndrome and Wernicke's encephalopathy emerged. Karl Bonhoeffer, in the first decade of the 20th century, described several cases of patients with Wernicke's encephalopathy who later developed a chronic amnestic disorder. In addition, descriptions of patients with a Korsakoff-like amnesia but without polyneuropathy and alcoholism came to light. Gradually, it became apparent that Wernicke's and Korsakoff's syndromes were manifestations of the same process. In the 1930s, vitamin deficiency was identified as the common etiology underlying both disorders when cases of acute Wernicke's encephalopathy were described in patients with malabsorption due to gastric carcinoma or hyperemesis of pregnancy. However, it was not until the latter half of the 20th century that neuropathological studies confirmed the singularity of pathology in Wernicke's and Korsakoff's syndromes. Maurice Victor and colleagues showed that damage to the diencephalon was the common neuropathological finding whether the clinical presentation was a Wernicke's encephalopathy or a Korsakoff's syndrome.

Victor and Raymond D. Adams advocated the term *Wernicke-Korsakoff syndrome* to emphasize the unitary nature of the disorder. Contemporary practice finds that *Wernicke's encephalopathy* is often used as the term for the acute presentation of the thiamine deficiency syndrome characterized by the famous triad. *Korsakoff's psychosis* (although not a psychosis per se) is used to refer to patients with chronic amnesic states that persist after an acute Wernicke's encephalopathy resolves or that develop insidiously on their own. The Korsakovian patient has become the paradigm for an amnestic disorder.

The association of the amnestic disorder with Korsakoff's syndrome and diencephalic degeneration was so well established that the subsequent identification in the 1950s of severely amnestic patients with pathology quite distant from the dienencephalon was astoundingly newsworthy. William Beecher Scoville and Brenda Milner described patient H. M., who, experiencing intractable seizures, underwent bilateral surgical extirpation of the medial aspect of his temporal lobes, including the hippocampi. He then demonstrated a profound loss of ability for new learning. Scoville and Milner's descriptions of H. M. were landmarks in demonstrating the essential role for the hippocampi in learning or creating new memories.

The scientific study of memory disorders bloomed in the later half of the 20th century, with the descriptions of surgical patients prompting a vast range of pathological studies, animal investigations, and the application of the nascent fields of cognitive neuroscience and neuropsychology to disorders of memory.

COMPARATIVE NOSOLOGY

DSM-I and DSM-II Earlier *Diagnostic and Statistical Manual of Mental Disorders* (DSM) versions provided skeletal definitions of the amnestic disorders. The first and second editions of the DSM subsumed them under the rubric of chronic brain syndromes associated with intoxication, reflecting the dominance of Korsakoff's syndrome as the model amnestic disorder. There was little description of the disorder or discussion of alternate conditions in which it might be seen.

DSM-III Subsequent versions of the DSM provide more detailed descriptions of the amnestic syndrome. The third edition of the DSM (DSM-III) and its revision include *amnestic syndrome* among the organic mental syndromes and disorders. The essential definition is "impairment in short- and long-term memory that is attributed to a specific organic factor." The text elaborates on the nature of the memory deficit with a variation of Ribot's law, noting that, although there is impairment in long-and short-term memory, "very remote events are remembered better than more recent events." Immediate memory, as represented by digit span or repetition, is noted to remain intact. Associated features of the amnestic syndrome are noted and include disorientation; *confabulation* (defined as "recitation of imaginary events to fill in gaps in memory"—a controversial definition); lack of insight into the deficits; and apathy, lack of initiative, and emotional blandness—"although the person is superficially friendly and agreeable, his or her affect is shallow." Although the definition stipulates that the deficits are "attributable to a specific organic factor," no guidance is offered as a basis for making such an attribution.

The DSM-III further notes that amnestic syndrome cannot be diagnosed in the course of a delirium and is to be distinguished from dementia by a lack of impairment in abstract thinking, judgment, and higher cortical function, as well as no change in personality. Amnestic syndrome is also to be distinguished from memory disturbances related to a psychological event, which is covered by psychogenic amnesia, one of the dissociative disorders.

Psychogenic amnesia is distinguished from the amnestic syndrome by its presentation and course. Psychogenic amnesia follows a traumatic event, often involving a threat of death or harm, or comes after a psychologically unacceptable event, such as a regretted one-night stand. It is not related to an *organic factor*, as stipulated for the amnestic syndrome. Psychogenic amnesia does not follow Ribot's law for typical amnesia, in which new memory recall is more impaired than recall of remote memories. It tends to present with inability to recall information relating to the traumatic event and its time frame. It can present dramatically with a global amnesia that includes the inability to recall personal history, in contrast to the amnestic syndrome in which such loss of identity is not seen. Psychogenic amnesia is noted to begin suddenly but also to terminate just as abruptly, with no residual impairment.

ICD-9 and ICD-10 The *International Classification of Diseases* (ICD) divides amnesia into two categories: amnestic (retrograde) (780.9) and amnestic (confabulatory) (294.0). The amnestic (retrograde) category encompasses a broad array of etiologies, including developmental, secondary to organic lesion, hysterical, psychogenic, and transient global. The amnestic (confabulatory) syndrome is divided into alcohol-induced (Korsakoff's syndrome), drug-induced, and posttraumatic.

DSM-IV-TR DSM-IV-TR reworked the amnestic syndrome into a group of amnestic disorders distinguished by etiology. The defining features are more succinct: "The development of memory impairment as manifested by impairment to learn new information or the inability to recall previously learned information." In contrast to earlier definitions, impairment in long- *and* short-term memory is not required. Impairment in either domain suffices. The terms *long-term memory* and *short-term memory* have been dispensed with in favor of the more specific terms referring to new learning and retention of learned material. Criterion B adds a requirement for social and occupational dysfunction, presumably to allow distinction from milder memory deficits, such as those associated with usual aging. DSM-IV-TR tries to address the issue of deficits in other cognitive domains by stipulating that, in amnestic disorders, the severity of memory impairment impinges on function, but the deficits in any other realm need be mild enough such that they do not affect function. DSM-IV-TR retains the provision that delirium and dementia must be excluded before diagnosing an amnestic disorder. DSM-IV-TR continues to require evidence that the memory disturbance is a "direct physiological consequence of a general medical condition," although the language of "organic factors" is eliminated. This reflects the conceptual shift in the nosology as a whole to allow the consideration of all potential etiologies for any diagnostic category.

In DSM-IV-TR, the cognitive disorders are branched into separate categories of delirium, dementias, and amnesic disorders, similar to the broad categories of affective disorders, anxiety disorders, etc. Although some favored the use of the term *amnesic* rather than *amnestic* to achieve consistency with the tenth edition of the ICD, this change was not made. There are four entities within the amnestic disorders category:

- Amnestic disorder due to cerebral or systemic medical conditions
- Substance-induced amnestic disorder
- Amnestic disorder due to unknown etiology
- Amnestic disorder not otherwise specified

There are no syndromic differences to the entities. The diagnoses are applied in accordance with the presumption of etiology.

EPIDEMIOLOGY

There have been no large-scale epidemiological investigations of the amnestic disorders. There are some epidemiological data related to specific disorders. Wernicke-Korsakoff syndrome is found relatively rarely at autopsy (0.4 to 2.8 percent), although microscopic evaluation of the tissue can increase the yield by 25 percent. Of note, in one series, only 20 percent of pathologically proven cases of Wernicke-Korsakoff syndrome had received the diagnosis in life, pointing to a marked underdiagnosis of this condition.

The devastating effect of amnesia on ability to live alone is demonstrated by the high prevalence of such patients in chronic care settings. In one study of long-term mental health hospitals, patients with Korsakoff's syndrome were reported to account for 5 percent of the chronic residents. A more recent survey of Scottish hospitals found Korsakoff's syndrome patients to account for 9 percent of the total hospital population.

A study of the incidence of transient global amnesia (discussed in the section Transient Global Amnesia) in Rochester, Minnesota reported 5.2 cases per 100,000 people per year.

ETIOLOGY

Amnestic disorders are, by definition, focal disorders: They involve a relatively circumscribed domain of cognition, new learning, and are the product of focal or localizing injuries. This distinguishes them from most other neuropsychiatric conditions, such as schizophrenia or Alzheimer's disease, that involve more diffuse processes. Table 10.4–3 lists several of the more common etiologies for the amnestic disorders. What is common to each of these etiologic conditions is that they cause fairly focal damage to the limbic structures vital to new learning, the hippocampus and diencephalon. They do not result in widespread cortical or subcortical damage, hence the relatively restricted deficits in memory that distinguish the amnestic disorders from the dementias. The discrete nature of these clinical symptoms and the focal nature of the etiologic lesions have made it easier to elucidate the mechanisms of normal memory formation and the pathophysiology of amnesia. The following discussion of anatomic substrates for memory derives from what has been learned from the study of amnestic patients and outlines how these specific etiologies result in the amnestic syndrome.

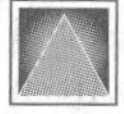

Table 10.4–3
Acute- and Insidious-Onset Etiologies for Amnestic Disorders

Acute Onset	Insidious Onset
Traumatic brain injury	Vitamin deficiencies (thiamine)
Vitamin deficiencies (thiamine)	Korsakoff's psychosis
Wernicke's encephalopathy	Malabsorption syndromes
Anoxia or hypoxia	Persistent vomiting
Postcardiac or respiratory arrest	Severe malnutrition
Postsurgical	Intracranial tumor
Thrombotic or embolic	Herpes encephalitis
Carbon monoxide poisoning	
Electroconvulsive therapy	
Transient global amnesia	
Alcohol intoxication	
Sedative-hypnotics	

Anatomic Substrates for Memory

Memory in the human brain is distributed and localized. No one memory lives in any specific brain cell or region—aspects of the memory are distributed across several regions. Yet, particular aspects of memory are localized in specific brain regions. In addition, the regions that are involved in processing memories are not the same regions that hold them in long-term storage. The localization and distribution of memory process is complex yet vital to understanding the variety of signs and symptoms in memory disorders.

Amnesia results from damage to the medial temporal lobe (*hippocampal amnesia*) or to the midline diencephalic structures (*diencephalic amnesia*). These structures, contained within the limbic memory system, are involved in the encoding of certain types of memory (explicit memories that involve conscious recollection). The limbic structures make a temporary input to the memory process but are not the final repository for long-term memories, hence, the sparing of already stored long-term memories when limbic structures are compromised. Damage to other components of the limbic system also impinge on memory formation, although the diencephalon and hippocampus are most prone to damage in the conditions that cause amnesia. It is debated whether separate hippocampal and diencephalic syndromes can be distinguished clinically. Some have postulated that diencephalic amnesia is associated with greater impairment in metamemory or awareness of memory dysfunction and a heightened tendency to confabulate. This latter aspect, however, might be related to concomitant frontal lobe involvement, as is discussed later in this chapter.

Hippocampal Amnesia

The hippocampi have primary roles in new learning and anterograde memory but not in retrograde memory. Hippocampi are involved in explicit or *declarative* memory but not in implicit memory, such as the nonconscious, automatic performance of previously learned skills (e.g., putting a golf ball or driving a car). The distinctions between explicit and implicit memory are discussed in further detail in the Associated Signs and Symptoms section.

Diencephalic Amnesia

The diencephalic structures involved in memory include the mammillary bodies, the medial dorsal thalamic nuclei, the internal medullary lamina, and the mamillothalamic tracts. The precise role of the diencephalon in memory has not yet been clarified. It is thought that these structures support the role of the hippocampi in explicit memory. Like the hippocampus, diencephalic structures are involved in explicit, but not implicit, memory functions. Degeneration of the mammillary bodies is the neuropathological hallmark of a Korsakoff's psychosis. The mammillary bodies might functionally be of importance as repositories of neurotransmitters vital to memory. Korsakoff's syndrome is the classic example of diencephalic amnesia.

Laterality

The hippocampi have hemispherical specialization similar to that of the language cortices: The left hippocampus is relatively specialized for verbal memory; the right hippocampus is specialized for nonverbal memories, such as faces, geospatial orientation, and musical memories. Unilateral damage to either hippocampus produces deficits in memory related to its function. However, profound amnestic syndromes are not seen unless there is bilateral damage.

Relevance of the Neuroanatomy of Memory to the Signs and Symptoms of Amnestic Disorders The pattern of deficits characteristic of the amnestic disorders can be understood in terms of their neuroanatomy. The conditions that cause amnesia impinge on the hippocampi or diencephalon bilaterally. Registration or attention spell is intact, as this draws primarily on frontal lobe functions that are spared. New learning, as manifested by anterograde memory, is devastated, as this depends on hippocampal and diencephalic function. Long-term memory is affected according to Ribot's law—recently formed memories that were in early stages of consolidation, still residing in the hippocampus, are vulnerable; memories of a more distant nature are protected as they are already consolidated in their host cortical regions. What can be seen from the previous discussion is that, although amnestic disorders can derive from a variety of etiologies, a common anatomical substrate is involved, the diencephalic or hippocampal structures.

Specific Conditions That Cause Amnestic Disorders

Traumatic Brain Injury (TBI) The frequency of motor vehicle accidents makes traumatic brain injury (TBI) the fastest growing etiology for amnestic disorders. The temporal lobes are at particular risk for high-speed impact-related trauma, as they abut the bony prominences of the temporal bone. Head trauma, particularly closed head injury (also known as *concussion*), produces a well-circumscribed amnestic disorder. The amnesia is anterograde and retrograde and is only obvious after the initial delirium or coma has cleared. *Anterograde* or *posttraumatic amnesia* is defined as the period between the moment of head trauma and the resumption of normal memory function. During the anterograde amnesia, the patient is unable to lay down new memories. Posttraumatic amnesia is regarded as a good measure of the severity of a head trauma and a predictor of prognosis. A posttraumatic amnesia of less than 1 hour generally predicts return to work within 1 month, whereas a posttraumatic amnesia of greater than 1 week often translates into more long-standing residual deficits and disability. The true extent of the posttraumatic amnesia can be determined after the patient has fully recovered by assessing then what his or her first reliable memories are subsequent to the head injury. *Retrograde amnesia* refers to the period *before* the head injury for which the patient is unable to recall events. Retrograde amnesia is generally shorter than posttraumatic amnesia and is not as accurate a predictor of severity or recovery.

Surgery For patients with intractable seizure disorders, the mesial temporal lobes are often the site for surgical extirpation, as mesial sclerosis is frequently the underlying pathology. Removal of hippocampal tissue can result in amnesia, as demonstrated most famously by patient H. M. H. M. was 27 years of age and of normal intelligence when he underwent bilateral surgical removal of the anterior temporal lobes. Two-thirds of each anterior hippocampus was removed. H. M. was left with an amnestic syndrome, with profound deficits in new learning but intact intelligence and no disruption of personality (although, over subsequent years of study, it became clear that he had a marked appetitive loss—he displayed no interest in sex and ate only when others suggested to eat). H. M.'s well-documented history and oft-tested capacities are paradigms of a pure amnestic disorder.

Infarctions Most of the blood supply for the hippocampi derives from branches of the posterior cerebral artery. The posterior cerebral artery territory includes the hippocampi, the limbic nuclei of thalamus, and the mesial temporal lobe. Any disease involving these arteries can result in an amnestic disorder. Thalamic strokes can present with dense anterograde amnesia without apparent motor deficits.

Intracranial Tumors Intracranial tumors, especially those involving the hypothalamus and the third ventricle can cause amnestic disorders. In his essay "The Last Hippie," Oliver Sacks eloquently describes a patient with a meningioma, left untreated for years, that ultimately invaded the diencephalon and destroyed the mesial temporal lobes. The patient was left with profound anterograde amnesia, such that he was unable to recall new information beyond minutes. Hence, he tragically relived the revelation of his father's sudden death each time this reference was made to him, and he was reinformed of his father's demise. He also had a retrograde amnesia extending back to the early 1970s, such that he persisted in a hippie world view, decades after the end of that era.

Infections Herpes simplex encephalitis is the paradigmatic infectious etiology for an amnestic disorder. Herpetic infection of the central nervous system (CNS) preferentially involves the temporal lobes and produces a hemorrhagic necrosis that can be fatal. Survivors often display a profound amnestic disorder due to destruction of medial temporal lobe structures, whereas other cognitive functions are largely intact.

Alcohol and Illicit Drugs A hallmark of the classic alcoholic *blackout* is the lack of memory for the actual blackout and for events leading up to it. This represents acute anterograde amnesia with inability to encode new memories during the period of intoxication and inability to retrieve memories encoded proximate to the blackout. Anterograde memory returns once the intoxication has dissipated, unless a second process, such as alcohol withdrawal or a Wernicke's encephalopathy, supervenes. The period of retrograde amnesia might shrink, although usually the patient does not ever regain full recall of details for events immediately preceding and during the period of intoxication. Intoxication with other common drugs of abuse, such as cocaine and heroin, is not associated with amnesia per se.

Medications Sedative-hypnotics, such as benzodiazepines and barbiturates, particularly when administered intravenously (IV), cause a *twilight* period of semiconsciousness or unconsciousness during which the patient is amnestic. There can be retrograde amnesia in addition to the anterograde amnesia, persisting until the full effects of the medication have worn off. This twilight state is often a desired goal of anesthesia or a narcotherapy. Other anesthetic agents or preanesthetic agents, such as propofol (Diprivan), can cause a similar circumscribed and transient amnesia. Sildenafil (Viagra) use has been associated, in isolated cases, with transient global amnesia, perhaps by inducing vasomotor instability.

Vitamin Deficiencies Chronic alcoholism, persistent vomiting, malabsorption syndromes, and severe malnutrition can lead to vitamin deficiencies that may lead to an amnestic syndrome. Deficiency of thiamine or vitamin B_1 has been identified as the cause of Wernicke's encephalopathy and Korsakoff's syndrome.

Neurotoxins Exposure to neurotoxins such as trimethyltin or carbon monoxide leads to a hypoxic state, as described in the following section.

ANOXIA AND HYPOXIA Anoxia and hypoxia are caused by inadequate oxygenation through respiratory, circulatory, hematological, or metabolic compromise. The hippocampi, particularly the memory-essential CA1 regions, are exquisitely sensitive to hypoxic deprivation. Hypoxia resulting from circulatory failure, such as in cardiac arrest, congestive heart failure, and shock, can produce discrete bilateral lesions in the hippocampi. Accidental or intentional carbon monoxide poisoning interferes with the oxygen transport capacity of the red blood cells and produces an anemic hypoxia that also can differentially impact the hippocampi and temporal lobe memory structures. There is necrosis of the hippocampi and, at times, the globus pallidus. The clinical picture usually involves an immediate period of coma or agitated delirium and then a chronic amnestic syndrome with typical disproportionate devastation of memory relative to other cognitive and behavioral functions.

Cardiac surgery can result in anoxic brain damage through intraoperative hypoperfusion or via release of emboli. Large emboli produce large vessel strokes, but microemboli of air, platelets, or fat can result in more circumscribed deficits. Here again, the mesial temporal lobes, including the hippocampi, demonstrate the greatest sensitivity to the hypoxia. Self-limited and chronic amnestic syndromes have been described subsequent to major cardiac surgery.

A 28-year-old man with Marfan syndrome was admitted for valve replacement surgery. He had no history of psychiatric disorder and was thought to be of normal premorbid character. He recovered consciousness soon after surgery and was alert and conversant. However, he was surprised to find himself in the hospital and had no recollection of surgery or his medical needs over the recent months. Psychiatric evaluation revealed a man in no acute distress with dense anterograde amnesia and a retrograde amnesia of approximately 3 months. He was perplexed regarding his condition but not perceptibly upset. The psychiatric consultant suggested that the stress of a major surgery had taken a toll, and the patient was retreating from the threat of mortality with his forgetting. A neurological consultant declared that this amnesia was a result of shower emboli sustained intraoperatively and suggested a recovery over days would ensue. The patient did indeed recover full memory function over the ensuing week, with a retrograde amnesia only for the days preceding the surgery. He subsequently displayed no adaptive difficulties or preoccupying existential concerns.

Electroconvulsive Therapy Immediately following an *electroconvulsive therapy* (ECT) *treatment*, patients display a postictal delirium. The duration and severity of this delirium relate to factors in the ECT administration, including the nature and dose of anesthetic agents, bilateral or unilateral electrode placement, and the stimulus parameters. Beyond this acute and self-limited delirium however, ECT produces a transient amnesia, manifested by a diminished ability to form new memories during the period of treatment. The amnesia remits within days or, at most, a few weeks after completion of treatment. The patient is left with a retrograde amnesia for many events during the days or weeks of treatment. There are rare reports of an amnesia that persists beyond the proximity of the treatment period. Some have questioned whether they represent cases of amnesia related to anesthesia related hypoxia or even subtle intratreatment stroke. It is clear that patients with preexisting dementias or other brain disorders are at higher risk for ECT-related amnesia.

Transient Global Amnesia C. Miller Fisher and Adams, in 1964, coined the term *transient global amnesia*, referring to a syndrome characterized by the sudden onset of a profound anterograde amnesia and a graded retrograde amnesia for the past weeks or months. The patient generally recalls his own identity and that of relatives or close associates but is not able to retain his immediate context even when explained to him repeatedly. Transient global amnesia typically occurs after 50 years of age and in men more commonly than women. There is no impairment of consciousness, no associated motor abnormalities, and no deficits in other cognitive domains. The patient might appear anxiously aware that something is awry or might be seemingly indifferent to his or her state.

The course is self-limiting—patients recover memory function gradually over hours to a few days and return to baseline with no residual deficits other than amnesia for the hours of the episode. The etiology is unknown. Transient global amnesia is not epilepsy. There is no disturbance of consciousness, as is typical of a partial complex seizure, or any detectable seizure activity on electroencephalogram (EEG) obtained during the event. Brain imaging is typically normal. The amnestic episode is usually not repeated. There is an association with migraine in approximately 15 percent of cases, leading to etiologic speculation of vascular instability.

Limbic Encephalitis *Limbic encephalitis* is a paraneoplastic effect of some cancers, such as small cell carcinoma of the lung. A focal inflammation of the temporal lobes is produced. The hippocampi are particularly prone to this inflammation, with a resultant amnestic disorder.

Predisposing Factors

The question of why only some alcoholics develop Wernicke-Korsakoff syndrome has led to theories regarding additional vulnerabilities. Some researchers have looked at the variety of enzymes dependent on thiamine phosphorylation and noted that particular isoforms seem predominant in those who develop Wernicke-Korsakoff syndrome. These enzymes include several that are vital for CNS metabolism, such as transketolases, pyruvate dehydrogenase, and α-ketoglutarate dehydrogenase. Moreover, enzymatic activity has been demonstrated to be decreased in autopsy specimens from patients dying from Wernicke-Korsakoff syndrome.

The issue of premorbid vulnerability is central to the development of dissociative amnesia. This type of hysterical reaction depends on the individual's character vulnerabilities rather than any biological risks. Subjects who are suggestible and prone to disproportionate investments of emotion are more likely to manifest hysterical symptoms such as a dissociative amnesia.

DIAGNOSIS AND CLINICAL FEATURES

Symptoms and Signs

Amnestic disorders of a nonhysterical nature always involve *anterograde amnesia*, meaning impaired ability to learn and to retain new information, and a lesser degree of *retrograde amnesia*, meaning impaired ability to recall previously learned information. The retrograde amnesia typically follows Ribot's law, as it is most prominent for recently learned information, with older memories being the best protected.

The following, then, are the core features of all amnestic disorders:

- There are severe deficits in new learning (anterograde amnesia).
- Attention span (roughly the same as working memory, short-term memory, immediate memory, and registration) is intact.
- General intelligence is intact.
- Retrograde amnesia is present but temporally graded, with more remote memories preserved.
- Procedural memory or the ability to learn new *tasks* as opposed to new ideas, events, or words is intact.

Amnestic subjects can also learn with priming and conditioning in laboratory circumstances. The practical usefulness of such preserved learning skills appears limited however; without the ability to consciously recall the new information, the learning accomplished is not pragmatically useful.

Korsakoff's syndrome was the first amnestic syndrome described, and it is a good clinical model for the amnestic syndrome. As noted by Korsakoff, the memory deficit involves new learning but not older established memories and knowledge. Korsakovian patients typically demonstrate a change in personality as well, such that they display a lack of initiative, diminished spontaneity, and a lack of interest or concern. These changes appear frontal lobe–like, similar to the personality change ascribed to patients with frontal lobe lesions or degeneration. Indeed, Korsakovian patients often demonstrate *executive function* deficits on neuropsychological tasks involving attention, planning, set shifting, and inferential reasoning consistent with frontal pattern injuries. For this reason, Korsakoff's syndrome is not a pure memory disorder, although it certainly is a good paradigm of the more common clinical presentations for the amnestic syndrome.

Much of what is known about memory derives from the study of patients with pure lesions of memory and discretely localized brain damage. The patient H. M., studied over several decades by a series of distinguished neuropsychologists, developed amnesia after surgical extirpation of significant portions of the medial temporal lobe bilaterally to alleviate intractable epilepsy. These well-defined lesions allowed the delineation of differential aspects of memory through descriptions of what memory capacities H. M. had lost and which were retained. H. M., although providing an invaluable lesion model for memory function, is not a typical example of a patient with an amnestic disorder. The more common etiologies of nutritional deficiency, cerebrovascular disease, tumor, and cerebral infection tend to have more widespread cerebral involvement and, therefore, at least subtle deficits in domains other than memory.

The DSM-IV-TR offers subtypes of amnestic disorders: amnestic disorder due to general medical condition, substance-induced (specifying alcohol, sedative-hypnotic, anxiolytic, or unknown substances) persisting amnestic disorder, and amnestic disorder not otherwise specified. These subtypes do not differ in clinical signs and symptoms but only in the putative etiology.

Neuropsychological and Neuroanatomical Explanations of the Signs and Symptoms of Amnestic Disorders The pattern of clinical signs described previously is understandable in terms of what is known about the neurobiology of memory. Memories are formed through a three-stage process:

1. *Acquisition* or *encoding* involves the initial reception of new knowledge by the sensory organs and its relay to the primary sensory cortex specific to that sensory modality.
2. *Consolidation* involves rehearsing this new knowledge such that a representation of it is created.
3. *Storage* involves the creation of a stable record of this knowledge with all its associated features.

A functional memory system also requires a retrieval mechanism. Retrieval is a poorly understood process. It is not clear to what extent the clinical deficits in amnestic disorders represent impairments in the acquisition, consolidation, and storage operations or the retrieval process, or a combination of processes.

Memories can be described by their temporal characteristics, that is, whether they are memories of very recent, recent, or remote events; by their content, namely, whether they are memories of events, faces, places, names rules, etc.; or by the process in which they are learned (explicitly or implicitly).

Temporal Description of Memory Temporal description of memory is the most familiar description, with clinicians routinely referring to long- and short-term memory, although the definitions of *short term* or *long term* can vary considerably. Three types or, more accurately, aspects of memory can be identified from a temporal perspective:

1. *Registration* (also known as *primary memory, working memory, immediate memory*, or *attention span*) refers to an initial retention of information that may not leave any enduring trace once full attention is diverted from it. For example, a telephone caller, lacking a paper and pencil, who receives a number from the operator can keep that number in working memory by repeating it aloud until it is dialed. The phone number is likely forgotten as soon as it is dialed and the caller stops actively trying to remember it. Information of this nature is retained in its original sensory format, such as the sound of the operator's voice reciting the phone number or a visual image of the number if it was seen in a phonebook. The information has not yet been transformed into a semantic construct, such as a word or numeric symbol. The telephone number in the previous example is retained as phonological or visual data. It is vulnerable to rapid loss, hence the caller's need to repeat the number over and over until the number is dialed. Portions of the parietal and prefrontal cortex are involved in registration or working memory, but the limbic lobe is not involved. On a clinical examination, the immediate recall of three items and the repetition of a digit span are tests of registration or working memory.
2. *New learning* is a term that is preferable to *short-term memory*, as the latter term has been used to refer to memories of varying duration, ranging from immediate recall to anything short of permanently consolidated memories. New learning involves initial encoding but also some interim consolidation of memory. New learning relies on limbic structures.
3. *Long-term* or stored memories are the permanent memories reflecting the completed process of consolidation. The neural process of consolidation is probably akin to what has been observed in simpler organisms, namely, the potentiation of specific neural circuits, such that they fire when a sensory stimulus approximating the one attached to the memory is encountered. Consolidated memories are distributed throughout the cortex, with contributions coming from the relevant areas (e.g., the emotional content of a memory from the amygdala and visual representation from the visual association cortex).

Descriptions of Memory Based on the Process of Learning or Retrieval: Implicit and Explicit Memory In addition to the temporally defined long- and short-term memory, memory can be described by whether it is consciously explicit or implicit. There is, unfortunately, a rather extensive and, at times, confusing vocabulary for describing these different aspects of memory. Figure 10.4–1 presents the more common terms in schematic outline. The primary distinction of explicit versus implicit memory is also dichotomized as *declarative* and *nondeclarative*. *Declarative (explicit) memory* refers to the ability to consciously recall facts and past events. *Nondeclarative (implicit) memory* refers to nonconscious learning, such as that used to acquire new skills (procedural memory) or that used in associative learning (conditioning).

Edouard Claperede (1873 to 1940), the French neurologist and psychologist, demonstrated this distinction memorably in his 1911 paper. Here he described a woman with a classic Korsakovian amnesia. The patient had been residing in a chronic hospital for some 5 years. She was unable to learn the name or type of facility in which

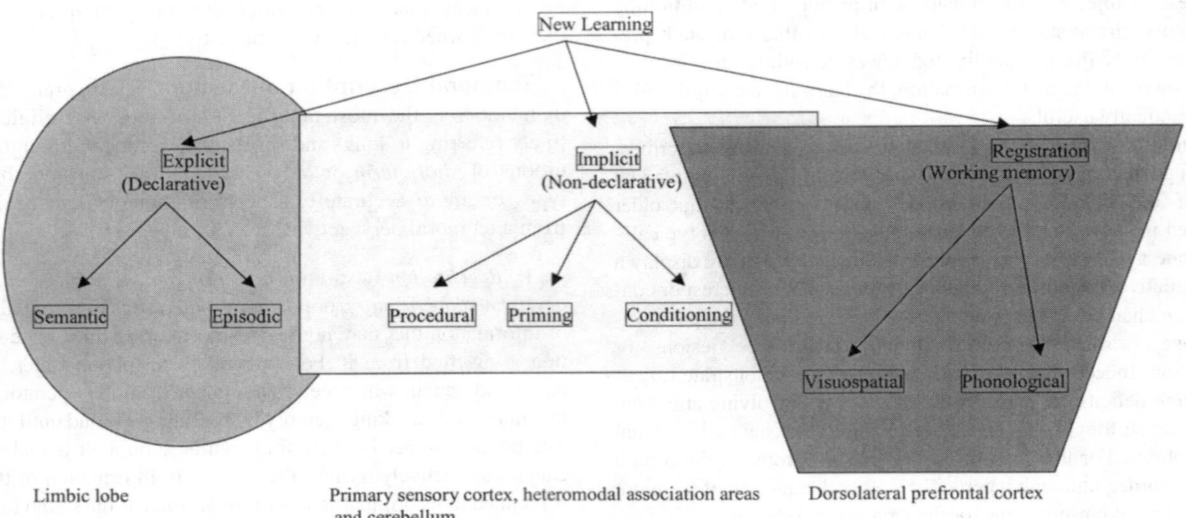

FIGURE 10.4–1 Types of learning. Note that limbic dependence is only present before consolidation. Consolidated memories are retrieved from networks distributed across the cortex and subcortical structures.

she lived but did learn her way around the facility and could independently find the route to her room. She could not state her age but could calculate it accurately if given the current date. Claperede introduced himself to this patient by shaking hands with a sharp pin hidden in his palm. When reintroduced to the patient after a sufficient lapse, the patient had no recollection of having met the doctor but refused to shake his hand, noting famously, "some people hide pins in their hands." This interaction demonstrates the severe deficits in explicit recall, as well as intact abilities to learn implicitly: The patient was unable to learn where she was and under what context she had arrived there but was able to implicitly develop geographic orientation and learn how to get to her room and what the routines were of her new residence. Moreover, although she could not learn the name or function of Professor Claperede or even recall that she had met him previously, she did develop the implicit association of pain with shaking his hand.

Implicit memory also includes conditioning, priming, and emotional learning. Conditioning entails the learning of associations through connected experiences (e.g., salivation at the sound of the bell that has become associated with dinner). The associations become connected *reflexively* and do not require conscious recall.

Deeply amnestic patients can still demonstrate learning through classical conditioning and priming. A typical priming task begins with the subject being asked to circle a letter on a list of words. The subject is not told to remember these words nor that they will be shown again. The subject is then asked to complete a list of three-letter word stems by guessing the rest of the word. One-half of the word stems derive from the original word list, and one-half of the word stems are new words. Words that were seen on the original list are completed more rapidly than the new words, even when the patient is unable to recall having seen the words earlier. Although the amnestic remains unable to recall explicitly having seen any of the original words, he or she clearly retains an implicit recognition that is evident with the enhanced rapidity with which he or she can complete the stems of those words already seen.

Aspects of Explicit and Implicit Memory Explicit or declarative memory involves *conscious* recollection of facts and events. *Semantic* memory is a term used to characterize the conscious recollection of facts and rules. *Episodic* memory is the conscious recollection of past circumstances, remote or recent. Nondeclarative or implicit memory refers to *nonconscious* recollection. Implicit memory is reflected in changes in thinking or behavior that can be attributed to a past experience without a conscious act of recall or recognition (e.g., Claperede's amnestic woman with the new handshake avoidance). *Procedural* memory refers to nonconscious recollection of motor sequences or tasks.

These distinctions are illustrated well by a naturalistic experiment conducted by the neuropsychologist, Daniel Schacter. Schacter carefully observed a memory-impaired patient with Alzheimer's disease in the natural environment of a golf course. Schacter played a round of golf with this former recreational player of fair skill on two separate occasions on two different courses. This now classic article highlights the distinction between conscious and nonconscious memory in a real-life setting. The patient had great difficulty with tasks that relied on episodic memory but did well with aspects of the game that relied on procedural or semantic memory. The patient was able to drive the ball off the tee for straight and respectable distances and could putt well enough such that, once he landed on the green, only two or three strokes were needed to hole. This suggests intact procedural memory or recollection of perceptual-motor procedures. Semantic memory was likewise intact, as the patient demonstrated good recollection of the rules and etiquette of play. He consistently hit his shots in the direction of the green, checked the label of the golf ball if he was not sure if it belonged to him, and replaced lost balls according to accepted game rules. He chose clubs appropriately to the nature of the shot ahead of him. All of these procedural tasks used *nonconscious,* implicit recollection. Indeed, when asked to explicitly recall details about what he done on a previous hole he was unable. He could not recall where he had hit the ball off the tee if there was a delay of minutes. On the second golf outing with Dr. Schacter, he could not recall at all that he had been out on a similar outing the week before. Here emerges a dissociation between explicit memory functions, such as remembering whether one golfed, and implicit or nonconscious memory functions, such as how to swing the club and the rules of play. His ability to recall rules of the game (semantic information) probably relates, in part, to this information being habitual or reflexive (e.g., one *reflexively* checks one's golf ball to see if it is indeed one's own), as well as to the fact that this information is likely well consolidated into long-term recall and hence is impervious to defects in new learning.

The amnestic patient would likely have difficulty remembering that he had golfed at any particular time (failure of episodic memory) but would likely retain the know-how for swinging a golf club or putting (procedural memory) or for how to play a hole. This dissociation of impairment relates directly to the anatomic distribution of memory functions, as described previously in the Etiology section. The amnestic patient has a predominant impairment of episodic memory ("Did I golf? When?"). This is due to the reliance of episodic memory on limbic structures such as the hippocampus and diencephalon. Episodic memory requires active, conscious recall of events or facts. This makes demands on the limbic structures that are damaged in the amnestic disorders. Basic factual knowledge (semantic memory) and procedural memory (knowledge of tasks or motor skills) are overlearned forms of knowledge that reside in the association cortices. This knowledge is fairly impervious to the local lesions and the diseases that cause amnestic syndromes. Moreover, the amnestic patient not only has the ability to access memories or knowledge in this nonconscious fashion, but also can *acquire* new knowledge implicitly, as illustrated originally by Claperede.

Implicit memory involves primary motor and sensory cortex, as well as structures other than temporal lobe or diencephalon; registration or working memory uses the dorsolateral prefrontal cortex; emotional learning (e.g., fear conditioning) involves the amygdala; priming involves the primary sensory cortex; and conditioning involves the cerebellum. Procedural memory likely involves the cerebellum and basal ganglia for the learning and retention of motor programs.

Associated Signs and Symptoms

Confabulation *Confabulation* refers to the fabrication of information spontaneously or in response to questions. Confabulation can be distinguished from conscious dissimulation or lying, as the patient believes his or her utterances and has no intent to mislead. Confabulations are not delusions per se either: They lack the systematic and fixed quality of a delusion. Two types of confabulation are noted: the more common momentary confabulations and the more rare, fantastic confabulations. Typically, confabulations arise in response to a question and have a fill-in-the-gap quality: "Did you have your breakfast?" is met with the confabulatory response of "I certainly did, let's see . . . a good breakfast at that: orange juice, eggs, bacon, and a blueberry muffin." The confabulations may not be noted until the patient is asked open-ended questions that challenge his or her recall of details. The content is mundane and related to the question at hand. *Fantastic confabulations*, on the other hand, are often offered spontaneously and are striking for their dramatic content.

A patient with a long-standing history of severe alcohol dependence was transferred to the psychiatric unit after a turbulent month on the medical service with his course complicated by alcohol withdrawal and delirium tremens. Subsequent to resolution of the delirium, the patient demonstrated a severe amnestic disorder with no ability to retain his context. He routinely identified his surroundings as a shoe factory at which he seemed to have worked in prior decades. He was generally calm and congenial and would sit in the hallway keenly watching the passers-by. He could be heard making a continual patter of comments regarding passing activities. When he heard clattering coming from a hallway closet, he immediately offered "that's them . . . little Indians . . . Nazis . . . waiting their chance . . . they pounce, one, two, three, that's it." When a female medical student hurried past he offered immediately, "her hubby is waiting, and he wants his dinner."

The fill-in-the-gaps quality of the confabulation has led many to associate confabulations with memory disorders. However, confabulations may relate more to a failure of executive function than memory dysfunction. This is clearly the case with fantastic confabulations as presented in the previous case. The notion of "little Indians" or Nazis populating the closets is striking more for its patent absurdity than for how it solves the riddle of what the noises are that are emanating from the closet. There is obviously a failure of the frontal lobe executive function responsible for inhibiting absurd interpretations and responses. This executive function has the role of censoring the hypotheses that other regions of the brain develop as explanations for sensory stimuli. Confabulation and personality change are more common in diencephalic amnesia (e.g., Korsakoff's syndrome) than in pure hippocampal amnesia, perhaps reflecting a concomitant involvement of frontal lobe structures or connections.

Personality Change The personality change seen in amnestic disorders may involve apathy or irritability, or a combination of the two. The following case illustrates the inactivity and constriction of interests that can be seen, as well as the persistent irritability and agitation that can accompany the amnesia.

A 73-year-old survivor of the Holocaust was admitted to the psychiatric unit from a local nursing home. She was born in Germany to a middle-class family. Her education was truncated due to internment in a concentration camp. She immigrated to Israel after liberation from the concentration camp and later to the United States, where she married and raised a family. Premorbidly, she was described as a quiet, intelligent, and loving woman who spoke several languages. At 55 years of age, she had a significant carbon monoxide exposure when a gas line leaked while she and her husband slept. Her husband died of carbon monoxide poisoning, but the patient survived after a period of coma. Once stabilized, she displayed significant cognitive and behavioral problems. She had difficulty with learning new information and making appropriate plans. She retained the abilities to perform activities of daily living but could not be relied on to pay bills, to buy food, to cook, or to clean, despite appearing to have retained the intellectual ability to do these tasks. She was admitted to a nursing home after several difficult years at home or in the homes of relatives. In the nursing home, she was able to learn her way about the facility. She displayed little interest in scheduled group activities, hobbies, reading, or television. She had frequent behavioral problems. She repeatedly pressed staff to get her sweets and snacks and cursed them vociferously with racial epithets and disparaging comments on their weight and dress. On one occasion, she scratched the cars of several staff with a key. Neuropsychological testing demonstrated severe deficits in delayed recall, intact performance on language and general knowledge measures, and moderate deficits on domains of executive function, such as concept formation and cognitive flexibility. She was noted to respond immediately to firmly set limits and rewards, but deficits in memory prevented long-term incorporation of these boundaries. Management involved development of a behavioral plan that could be implemented at the nursing home and empirical trials of medications aimed at amelioration of irritability.

Motor and Sensory Symptoms Motor and sensory symptoms may variably accompany an amnestic disorder, depending on the etiology. Some amnestic syndromes, such as transient global amnesia, are striking for the preservation of motor and sensory function. In contrast, the vitamin deficiencies are often accompanied by motor and sensory symptoms that persist beyond the initial recovery from acute Wernicke's encephalopathy. Patients with amnestic disorders deriving from Wernicke-Korsakoff syndrome may have gait abnormalities due to peripheral neuropathies, muscle weakness, or gait instability related to the comorbid cerebellar degeneration of chronic alcoholism. The latter may also account for the frequently seen fine motor dyscoordination. Although the more striking ocular abnormalities related to an acute Wernicke's encephalopathy often resolve with vitamin replenishment, patients might still manifest residual restriction in gaze, as well as subtle lateral nystagmus. Anosmia can accompany some amnestic disorders, such as that due to herpes simplex encephalitis and certain strokes.

As described previously, the signs and symptoms of the amnestic disorder are not restricted to the domain of memory. The following case exemplifies the more common real-life presentation of a patient with amnestic disorder. Although the primary and most obvious deficit is in memory, this patient also has obvious impairments in comportment and judgment. The latter appear as an exaggeration of premorbid traits. This case illustrates the devastating impact of memory impairment on daily functioning and the capacity to live independently.

Mrs. C. M. was an 83-year-old, twice-widowed woman who was referred for hospitalization from the office of a psychiatrist. The patient had sought assistance from the psychiatrist for the first time earlier in the week with complaints of insomnia. The day after her evaluation, she called him 12 times, seemingly unaware of each prior conversation. Information obtained from a long-standing friend filled in background and recent history. She was educated through college with some advanced training as a nurse. She was as an affluent woman accustomed to an elegant lifestyle among genteel society. She was described as having been quite demanding and critical but always refined and highly attentive to rules of etiquette and social propriety. Although the patient reported drinking "a glass of wine with my dinner," friends noted that she drank as much as 1.5 fifths of sherry per day. She had been living alone for the past 4 years subsequent to the death of her second husband. Six months before presentation, her friends noted that her personal hygiene was declining. Two months before presentation, they began receiving frequent telephone calls in which the patient seemed not to recollect previous calls. On admission, she was dressed in an elegant, although rumpled, suit, a formal hat, high-heeled shoes, and no shirt. She was malodorous. Makeup was applied unevenly, and her hair was matted beneath her hat. Speech was fluent with a sophisticated vocabulary and complex syntax. She denied pervasive mood symptoms. Affect varied from charming to irate. There were no hallucination or delusions. She scored 22/30 on the Mini-Mental State Examination (MMSE), missing points for orientation, recall, and calculation. Physical examination was remarkable for bilateral cataracts, brisk symmetrical reflexes, and a positive snout reflex. Laboratory examination, including complete blood count, serum chemistries, liver function tests, thyroid functions, rapid plasma reagin (RPR) serology, electrocardiogram (ECG), chest X-ray, and EEG, was unremarkable. A head computed tomography (CT) demonstrated mild, symmetrical sulcal and central atrophy. In the hospital, the patient's memory deficits were quite obvious. She would often approach staff with the same question or statement without any remembrance of earlier conversations. She had no recollection of the circumstances leading to hospitalization and concocted a story of having made a wrong turn at the eye clinic and then being hustled off to the psychiatric ward. Although often charming and gracious, her social interactions could be abrasive and antagonistic: She beat a hole through the office door of the ward physician with her high heel when he did not answer her knock with sufficient alacrity. She was cooperative with neuropsychological testing, although she was noted to be "rude and hostile" to the examiner. Testing estimated an average premorbid IQ and a current verbal IQ of 108. She performed well on tasks of attention, with a forward digit span of 8 and backward span of 5. Verbal fluency was intact, and grammar was fully intact. Her immediate recall of verbal text passages was within average range. After a 20-minute delay, however, she recalled none of the verbal test material nor any of visually presented information. She could perform within average range on the Trails A test, a measure of sustained attention, visual scanning, numeric sequencing, and psychomotor speed. However, she had much difficulty with the Trails B test and the Wisconsin Card Sorting Test, both of which assess executive function control and the ability to maintain and switch set readily. The testing pattern demonstrated the deficits and strengths consistent with an amnestic disorder: severe memory deficits with intact attention and other basic intellectual functions, such as language. Although immediate recall was intact, she displayed no ability to learn or to retain new information. Memory was devastated. Executive skills were impaired as well, consistent with the clinical observations of a coarsened and impulsive change in personality. In an evaluation of occupational skills in a testing kitchen, the patient repeatedly forgot that a stove surface was hot, forgot to turn off the light after removing a pot, and forgot to remove a casserole from the oven, despite reminders to do so at the appointed time. She could not recall the 911 emergency numbers. The patient's adult children and her own family lawyer met and agreed that she would require a nursing home placement. The patient contested this and argued her case convincingly in court, such that a guardian of person was appointed, and the patient was returned to her apartment with a 24-hour aide in attendance.

Assessment The assessment of a memory disorder begins even before the patient is seen. Is it the patient calling with subjective worries regarding his or her memory function or is it a friend or relative calling with concerns that the patient seems unaware of? How the patient arrives for evaluation is pertinent. Did he or she travel alone and maneuver public transportation or was he or she driven? Many patients with severe amnestic disorders are evaluated on inpatient medical or psychiatric services, where they are held out of concern for their ability to manage on their own. The typical office or bedside examination can provide many clues. The Folstein MMSE is the most widely used cognitive screen and is available in a multitude of languages. Poor performance on the ten orientation items provides a general estimate of overall cognitive function. Although the overall score may not be reflective of severe impairment, specific answers can be informative. For example, responding "1968" to the year is far more suggestive of memory impairment, perhaps a retrograde amnesia of decades, than missing the year by 1 or 2 years. Asking the patient to repeat three items assesses registration or immediate recall. Patients with amnestic disorders ought to be able to repeat these items accurately. Delirious patients, however, or patients with frontal lobe injury and impaired attention might have trouble with this elemental task. Similarly, amnestic patients ought to be able to perform the attention tasks, such as spelling *world* backwards or serial seven subtractions (provided the patient has had adequate education for these tasks), as these cognitive functions do not require use of the limbic memory system. Recall of three items after a delay is significantly impaired in amnestic disorders. Not only can the patient not recall the three items, but also category cues ("It was a coin of some sort") or even recognition cues ("Tell me if it was a penny, dime, or nickel") do not help the amnestic patient's recall. This is a classic failure of new learning, the hallmark of an amnestic disorder. The language functions of naming, repetition, reading, and writing are intact in amnestic patients, as they rely on intact temporoparietal cortical networks. The performance of a three-step command is often intact, as this task, if performed quickly enough (and with the patient repeating the instructions to himself or herself as he or she performs) is a test of working memory and the spared dorsolateral prefrontal cortex. Visuospatial function, as assessed by the copying of an interlocking pentagon, is intact. Confabulation can often be elicited by allowing for open-ended responses and some leading on (e.g., asking "haven't we met before" and then observing the patient concoct an elaborate story confirming such—"sure, you're the butcher's boy, I remember when you used to run around in your knickers, trying to stir up some trouble"). As can be seen, in amnestic disorders, even the basic bedside cognitive examination can demonstrate the striking dissociation between areas of relatively preserved cognitive functioning and the devastated memory function.

Neuropsychological testing of a more extensive nature can highlight this dissociation or can demonstrate that a seemingly focal amnesia is really accompanied by additional cognitive deficits, more consistent with a dementia. Such assessments usually include the Wechsler Memory Scale, Revised, an extensive battery that includes evaluation of immediate recall, delayed recall, verbal memory, and visual memory. Some neuropsychologists advocate a quantitative cut-off for the definition of amnestic disorder, such as a 20-point discrepancy between the intelligence quotient and memory quotients obtained on the Wechsler Intelligence Scale and the Wechsler Memory Scale, respectively.

Malingering or faked amnesia is usually suspected on clinical grounds, such as an atypical presentation (e.g., retrograde amnesia without anterograde impairment, *any* presentation with amnesia for person, or a transparently obvious circumstance of secondary gain, such as a prisoner summoned to court). There are available neuropsychological tests of symptom validity for complaints of memory deficits. These tests use forced-choice format on which malingering subjects often score below chance, indicating a deliberate attempt to answer incorrectly.

PATHOLOGY AND LABORATORY EXAMINATION

More is known about the pathological correlates of amnestic disorders than other syndromes in psychiatry, perhaps because memory can be more objectively observed and quantified than other psychiatric symptoms, such as mood or delusions.

The neuropathology of amnestic disorders has been determined from autopsy series of patients with acute Wernicke's encephalopathy or chronic Korsakoff's syndrome. Victor and Adams described the classic degeneration of the medial dorsal thalamic nuclei, the mammillary bodies, the terminuses of the fornix, and the anterior lobe and superior cerebellar vermis. All compartments of the tissue are involved, including neuronal cells, support cells, and local vasculature. The brains of Korsakoff's syndrome patients often demonstrate a generalized atrophy with some frontal predominance consistent with the clinical picture of an apathetic personality change and degraded social graces. There is necrosis of tissue surrounding the third and fourth ventricles, as well as the sylvian aqueduct. Mammillary body atrophy is the defining feature.

The cholinergic system has been studied in animals fed diets high in ethanol. They show loss of cholinergic neurons in the basal forebrain and a reduction of presynaptic cholinergic markers in the neocortex and hippocampus. Similar neurochemical pathology in humans might account for the disturbances in memory and comportment that are observed clinically.

Neuroimaging

Neuroimaging may often be unremarkable in patients with amnestic disorders, despite severe clinical deficits. This is because the structures that subserve the memory functions involved in amnesia, such as the hippocampus or the thalamic nuclei, are small, and lesions that are quite diminutive and imperceptible to CT or magnetic resonance imaging (MRI) can still affect the function of these structures significantly. Hippocampus is hard to visualize on standard CT scans, although it is seen quite clearly on MRI, particularly in the coronal view. The amnesia-causing lesion (or atrophy) in these structures can be quite small and, at times, is invisible to the untrained eye. Enlargement of the space surrounding the thalamus and hippocampus, the third ventricles, or the temporal horn of the lateral ventricles, respectively, is suggestive of disease involving these structures. Sometimes, a tiny lesion stands out within an otherwise healthy-appearing brain. This is the case with young patients who experience anoxic injury after a near drowning or carbon monoxide poisoning, in which discrete bilateral hippocampal or basal ganglia lesions may appear on MRI, with no other abnormalities detected. More often, the risk factors for amnestic disorders also predict that other brain abnormalities, such as generalized atrophy in a long-standing alcoholic who then develops a Korsakoff's syndrome, will be seen on imaging. On MRI, the mammillary atrophy is often visible. One report of a patient with acute Wernicke's encephalopathy noted visible contrast enhancement of the mammillary bodies. This contrast enhancement was no longer visible after thiamine replenishment.

DIFFERENTIAL DIAGNOSIS

Distinguishing from Delirium

Delirium can impact on any aspect of cognitive function and is therefore the most common syndrome involving memory disturbance. Delirious patients have impairment in consciousness, ranging from inattention at the subtle end of the spectrum to coma at the far end. Deliria are often manifest with global disturbances in cognition albeit with a range of severity. Amnestic disorders can be distinguished from delirium, as they occur in the absence of a disturbance of consciousness and are striking for the relative preservation of other cognitive domains.

Distinguishing from Dementias

Table 10.4–4 outlines the key distinctions between Alzheimer's dementia and the amnes-

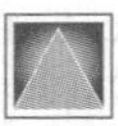

Table 10.4–4
Comparison of Syndrome Characteristics in Alzheimer's Disease and Amnestic Disorder

Characteristic	Alzheimer's Dementia	Amnestic Disorder
Onset	Insidious	Can be abrupt
Course	Progressive deterioration	Static or improvement
Anterograde memory	Impaired	Impaired
Retrograde memory	Impaired	Temporal gradient
Episodic memory	Impaired	Impaired
Semantic memory	Impaired	Intact
Language	Impaired	Intact
Praxis or function	Impaired	Intact

tic disorders. Both disorders can have an insidious onset with slow progression, as in a Korsakoff's psychosis in a chronic drinker. Amnestic disorders, however, can also develop precipitously, as in Wernicke's encephalopathy, transient global amnesia, or anoxic insults. Although Alzheimer's progresses relentlessly, amnestic disorders tend to remain static or even improve once the offending etiology has been removed. In terms of the actual memory deficits, the amnestic disorder and Alzheimer's disease still differ. Alzheimer's disease impacts on retrieval, in addition to encoding and consolidation. The deficits in Alzheimer's disease extend beyond memory to general knowledge (semantic memory), language, praxis, and general function. These are spared in amnestic disorders. The dementias associated with Parkinson's disease, acquired immune deficiency syndrome (AIDS), and other subcortical disorders demonstrate disproportionate impairment of retrieval but relatively intact encoding and consolidation and can thus be distinguished from amnestic disorders. The subcortical pattern dementias are also likely to display motor symptoms, such as bradykinesia, chorea, or tremor, that are not components of the amnestic disorders.

Distinguishing from Hysterical Phenomena Amnesia as an emotional response to a disturbing event has long been the subject of novels, plays, and films. In DSM-IV-TR, the phenomenon is called *dissociative amnesia*, a departure from the *psychogenic amnesia* nomenclature of DSM-III. The presentation for dissociative or psychogenic amnesia differs from that which has been described previously for the amnestic disorders in several fundamental ways. Dissociative amnesia involves an inability to recall circumstances related to particular events, usually of a psychologically traumatic nature. The patient may have no recollection of a specific time frame, or the amnesia might be restricted to selected events within that time frame. The period of amnesia might cover days, weeks, or even years. In contrast to the amnestic disorders, new learning or the laying down of new memories is intact. Deficits in other realms of cognition are not detectable, and there is no deterioration of personality. The course of a dissociative amnesia differs, as well. In contrast to the *gradual* shrinking of retrograde deficits seen in amnestic disorders, there can be a dramatic *sudden* return of memory in dissociative disorders once the patient is removed from the stressful environment (such as when a soldier is removed from the combat zone). The risks for developing dissociative amnesia are the risks for developing any hysterical response: an emotional personality style, heightened suggestibility, and a previous history of hysterical response (e.g., a somatic conversion reaction) to stressful circumstances. Sexual trauma is a frequently correlated experience in those with hysterical vulnerabilities. The suggestibility of these patients puts them at risk for loss of memory, as in dissociative amnesia, but also for distortions of memory, as in the false memory syndrome. The amobarbital (Amytal) interview can be useful in helping to verify diagnosis. Amobarbital (sodium pentothal) is a short-acting barbiturate, administered as a slow-push IV injection that allows the patient to fall into a partially narcotized state. Psychological defenses are dropped in this state, and the patient may be able to speak about recent stresses and concerns, as well as to demonstrate to the examiner restoration of memory for the amnestic events. Patients with brain injury–related amnesia are prone to develop a transient delirium with amobarbital rather than this restoration of cognition.

Ms. D. K. was a 19-year-old single woman referred to an outpatient psychiatric consult-liaison service with complaints of "I have trouble remembering." Three weeks before evaluation, she had an argument with her fiancé, ran out of their home, and then was assaulted and possibly raped in a downtown location. She telephoned her fiancé and informed him of the assault and her location. He retrieved her and brought her to the emergency department, where she was able to relate the course of events. Within 48 hours, however, she was no longer able to recall the details of the assault. She became amnestic to other life events, as well, including the sexual abuse she was subjected to by a stepfather and by an earlier boyfriend. She saw a neurologist 1 week later and was unable to recall her own address, workplace, or number of siblings. Neurological examination was normal, except for some difficulty with fine motor movements with her right hand. Head CT was unremarkable. Cognitive function studies demonstrated the previously mentioned amnesia for long-term events and for some overlearned information, such as her address, but no deficits in new learning, executive function, or any other cognitive domains. At the psychiatric evaluation, she scored 29/30 on the MMSE, missing one of the recall items. She could recall details of the assault and birth dates of her siblings when questioned obliquely. She related a history of sadistic sexual abuse at 9 years of age by a stepfather who raped and burnt her and of having been raped by a boyfriend as an adolescent. She reported that, since her teens, she would burn herself on her palms or arms with a cigarette lighter when feeling particularly stressed. She had never sought medical or psychiatric attention. She also had a few prior incidents of sudden-onset paralysis occurring during episodes of stress and lasting for several hours. The patient was referred for individual psychotherapy.

This case illustrates well the characteristics of a patient presenting with a dissociative amnesia. The patient's amnesia occurred subsequent to an assault and was limited primarily to events and circumstances related to this assault and prior sexual assaults. There was no impairment in new learning. The amnesia was not present until 2 days after the assault and worsened initially over the subsequent days before the memories began to return. This amnestic presentation is quite distinct from that which follows a biological insult: The selectivity of amnesia for the sexual trauma–related events, the preservation of new learning, and the progression to loss of retrograde personal memories are all highly inconsistent with amnestic disorders but quite typical of a dissociative amnesia. This patient was at heightened risk for developing a hysterical response, such as the dissociative amnesia, in this context in light of her premorbid personality vulnerabilities, such as limited frustration tolerance and a maladaptive coping repertoire that included burning herself when stressed. She also had prior episodes of hysterical paralysis.

Distinguishing from Factitious Phenomena

On rare occasions, amnesia may represent a malingered or factitious presentation. The patient may feign amnesia to avoid an undesired outcome, such as discharge from the hospital. Malingering is sometimes suspected solely because of the timing of its appearance, for example, a prisoner who develops amnesia on the eve of a scheduled appearance before an arraigning or sentencing judge. The diagnosis of factitious amnesia should be made cautiously, as some amnestic disorders (e.g., transient global amnesia) present without other indication of disease. The diagnosis is suggested when there is no evidence of an accompanying disease, and elements of the presentation and history are atypical for an amnestic disorder. A premorbid history of dissimulation and deceit, as well as a context in which the patient has obvious benefit from the assumed sick role, would raise suspicions. The clinical examination can provide clues. The examination should look for any deviations from the typical amnestic pattern of dense anterograde deficit with temporally graded retrograde amnesia. Basic knowledge, such as identification of colors, calculation skills, and orientation to self, should be intact in an amnestic disorder. On neuropsychological testing, a pattern of performance that is worse than chance or guessing suggests a manipulation of the results for deliberate failure. Typically, patients are asked to pick out words from a list that includes some words that have been shown previously. Densely amnestic patients score at least at a chance level of 50 percent accuracy simply by guessing. Malingering patients may purposely avoid the correct response, and score below chance. On tests of progressive difficulty, the malingering patient might perform poorly even on the easier tasks and may not demonstrate the graduated decrements in performance of an amnestic patient. Perseveration is more suggestive of true rather than feigned deficits.

Ganser syndrome refers to the condition described by Sigbert Ganser in the late 1890s. Ganser observed three prisoners who presented with unusual deficits comprising approximate or overshooting answers to direct questions. Some of the questions and responses he reported included: "How many fingers do you have? Eleven. Do you have a nose? I don't know. How many legs does a horse have? Three."

In Ganser syndrome, answers are provided quickly and demonstrate that the patient clearly understands the questions posed. The answers are just off the mark, although at times preposterously so. Patients might respond "I don't know" when asked their own name, might misidentify primary colors, or might make elementary mathematical errors (e.g., 2 + 2 = 5).

In current nosology, it is unclear where Ganser syndrome fits. Is it a factitious amnesia, a willful malingering by subjects seeking to avoid an undesirable circumstance by presenting themselves as ill, injured, and incapacitated? Is it more of a hysterical phenomenon, occurring in stressful circumstances to characterologically vulnerable patients? Is it a psychotic symptom, a manifestation of thought disorder? William Alywn Lishman distinguishes between the Ganser *symptom*, meaning approximate answers, and the Ganser *syndrome*, which would include a disturbance of consciousness and amnesia for the event once the symptoms have resolved. The former is fairly common and is associated with a variety of conditions, whereas the latter is quite rare and might represent a hysterical amnesia.

COURSE AND PROGNOSIS

The course of an amnestic disorder depends on its etiology and treatment, particularly acute treatment. With most of the etiologies discussed previously, the presence of a pure amnestic disorder is only identified after a more fulminant acute presentation has resolved. For example, amnesia associated with Wernicke's encephalopathy can remit entirely with rapid replacement of thiamine in adequate doses. The challenge is to recognize the acute presentation and then to provide the emergent treatment. If treatment in Wernicke's encephalopathy is not timely or effective, then the patient will likely have an enduring amnestic disorder, that is, Korsakoff's psychosis. Generally, the amnestic disorder has a static course. There is little improvement over time but also no progression. The exceptions are the acute amnesias, such as transient global amnesia, which resolves entirely over hours to days, and the amnestic disorder associated with head trauma, which improves steadily in the months subsequent to the trauma. Amnesia secondary to processes that destroy brain tissue, such as stroke, tumor, and infection, are irreversible, although, again, static, once the acute infection or ischemia has been staunched.

TREATMENT

Etiology-Specific Treatments

As true for any medical syndrome, the treatment and subsequent course of an amnestic disorder depend on its etiology. An acute-onset amnestic disorder can be a medical emergency that may respond dramatically to rapidly initiated treatment. Wernicke's encephalopathy, if treated aggressively within hours of onset, can remit with minimal residual deficits. Treatment is parenteral replacement of thiamine, usually via the IV and IM routes. Other vitamins should be replenished simultaneously. Transient global amnesia is treated expectantly with the anticipation of a gradual but full recovery of memory function over hours to days. Careful examination is necessary to exclude other potential etiologies, particularly stroke and epilepsy.

The treatment of dissociative amnesia takes advantage of the hysterical patient's suggestibility, offering strong encouragement to the patient that memory will return. The amobarbital interview or controlled narcosis can be helpful here, as a diagnostic aid, as well as a means of offering the posthypnotic suggestion of recovery.

Nonspecific Treatments

Cholinesterase inhibitors, which are approved for the symptomatic treatment of the cognitive impairment in Alzheimer's disease, have been used in isolated case reports or in small, uncontrolled series of amnestic patients (primarily Korsakovian). Reports of benefit are spotty. There have been striking reports in animal studies of reversal of alcohol-induced memory deficits with transplantation of cholinergic-rich tissue. There is no such human therapy.

Piracetam and physostigmine have been used in patients receiving ECT in an effort to diminish the anterograde amnesia associated with that procedure. No benefit has been detected.

There is a rich industry offering cognitive rehabilitation or memory enhancement. The content of these approaches differs widely. An essential premise of these programs is that memory can be encoded or recalled, or both, through means other than standard limbic loop processes. As the previous discussion indicated, this is certainly true. The amnestic can still can learn through implicit processes, such as priming and conditioning, and can use procedural and remote semantic memories. How relevant these skills are in the absence of conscious recall is debatable: Knowing or learning how to swing a golf club is of little help if one does not know how or why one is on the golf course. It has yet to be determined whether the function, independence, or even quality of life of amnestic patients is enhanced by these rehabilitative efforts.

Technology holds some promise for replacing functions lost to amnesia. Personal organizers with reminder features can be programmed to offer reminders for meals, medication taking, and appointments. However, the technological implements often fail to impact significantly on the patient's level of functioning. Again, the lack of *conscious* awareness of deficits and the inability to consciously call up memories prove critical to day-to-day functioning.

On the societal level, efforts have been made to decrease the incidence of Wernicke's encephalopathy and Korsakoff's psychosis by mandating vitamin enhancement of common foods. A survey of inpatient discharge records of 17 hospitals in greater Sydney, Australia, noted a 40-percent reduction in the incidence of Wernicke's encephalopathy and Korsakoff's psychosis in the 5 years subsequent to introduction of thiamine-enriched bread. This raises the potential protective effects for enrichment of other foodstuffs, particularly beer and wine.

SUGGESTED CROSS-REFERENCES

See Section 10.3 on dementia, Section 3.4 on memory, and Chapter 17 on dissociative disorders.

REFERENCES

*Baddeley AD, Wilson BA, Watts FN, eds. *Handbook of Memory Disorders*. Chichester, New York: John Wiley and Sons; 1995.

Benson DF, Djenderedjian A, Miller BL, Pachana NA, Chang L, Itti L, Mena I: Neural basis of confabulation. *Neurology*. 1996;46:1239–1243.

*Berrios GE, Hodges JR, eds. *Memory Disorders in Psychiatric Practice*. Cambridge, UK: Cambridge University Press; 2000.

Byrum CE, Thompson JE, Heinz ER, Krishnan KR, Tien RD: Limbic circuits and neuropsychiatric disorders. Functional anatomy and neuroimaging findings. *Neuroimaging Clin North Am*. 1997;7:79–99.

Candel I, Jelicic M, Merckelbach H, Wester A: Korsakoff patients' memories of September 11, 2001. *J Nerv Ment Dis*. 2003;191:262–265.

Carlesimo GA, Bonanni R, Caltagirone C: Memory for the perceptual and semantic attributes of information in pure amnestic and severe closed-head injured patients. *J Clin Exp Neuropsychol*. 2003;25:391–406.

Claperede E: Recognition et Moiité. *Arch Psychol*. 1911;11:79–90. In: Rapaport D, trans. *Organization and Pathology of Thought: Selected Sources*. New York: Columbia University Press; 1951.

Corkin S: What's new with the amnesic patient H.M.? *Nat Rev Neurosci*. 2002;3:153–160.

Fisher CM, Adams RD: Transient global amnesia. *Acta Neurol Scand*. 1964;40[Suppl 9]:1–82.

Kensinger EA, Clarke RJ, Corkin S: What neural correlates underlie successful encoding and retrieval? A functional magnetic resonance imaging study using a divided attention paradigm. *J Neurosci*. 2003;23:2407–2415.

Kihlstrom JF: Memory and consciousness: an appreciation of Claparède and recognition et Moiité. *Conscious Cogn*. 1995;4:379–386.

Lethem J. *Vintage Book of Amnesia: An Anthology*. New York: Vintage Books; 2000.

*Lishman WA. *Organic Psychiatry: The Psychological Consequences of Cerebral Disorder*. 3rd ed. Malden, MA: Blackwell Science; 1998.

Manns JR, Hopkins RO, Reed JM, Kitchener EG, Squire LR: Recognition memory and the human hippocampus. *Neuron*. 2003;37:171–180.

Manns JR, Hopkins RO, Squire LR: Semantic memory and the human hippocampus. *Neuron*. 2003;38:127–133.

Meulemans T, Van der Linden M: Implicit learning of complex information in amnesia. *Brain Cogn*. 2003;52:250–257.

Quinette P, Guillery B, Desgranges B, de la Sayette V, Viader F, Eustache F: Working memory and executive functions in transient global amnesia. *Brain*. 2003;126:1917–1934.

Ribot T. *Diseases of Memory: An Essay in the Positive Psychology*. New York: D Appleton and Co; 1882.

Sacks OW. The last hippie. In: *The Man Who Mistook His Wife for a Hat*. New York: Summit Books; 1985.

Schachter DL: Amnesia observed: remembering and forgetting in a natural environment. *J Abnorm Psychol*. 1983;92:236–242.

Schmolck H, Kensinger EA, Corkin S, Squire LR. Semantic knowledge in patient H.M. and other patients with bilateral medial and lateral temporal lobe lesions. *Hippocampus*. 2002;12:520–533.

Scoville WB, Milner B: Loss of recent memory after bilateral hippocampal lesions. 1957. *J Neuropsychiatry Clin Neurosci*. 2000;12:103–113.

*Squire LR, Schacter D, eds. *Neuropsychology of Memory*. 3rd ed. New York: Guilford Press; 2002.

Stuss DT, Alexander MP, Lieberman A, Levine H. An extraordinary form of confabulation. *Neurology*. 1978;28:1166–1172.

*Victor M, Adams RD, Collins GH: *The Wernicke-Korsakoff Syndrome and Related Neurologic Disorders Due to Alcoholism and Malnutrition*. 2nd ed. Philadelphia: FA Davis Co; 1989.

Victor M, Yakovlev PI: Sergei Sergeievich Korsakoff's psychic disorder in conjunction with neuritis: A translation of Korsakoff's original article with brief comments on the author and his contribution to clinical medicine. *Neurology*. 1955;5:394–406.

▲ 10.5 Other Cognitive Disorders and Mental Disorders Due to a General Medical Condition

MARTIN ALLAN DROOKER, M.D.

Increasingly, scientific views of mental illness recognize that, whether due to an identifiable anomaly (e.g., brain tumor), a neurotransmitter disturbance of unclear origin (e.g., schizophrenia), or a consequence of deranged upbringing or environment (e.g., personality disorder), all mental disorders ultimately share one common underlying theme: aberration in brain function. Treatments for those conditions, whether psychological or biological, attempt to restore normal brain chemistry. Viewed in this manner, the traditional separation of mental illness from physical illness increasingly has appeared illogical and unscientific. Before the advent of the fourth edition of the *Diagnostic and Statistical Manual of Mental Disorders* (DSM-IV) and its text revision (DSM-IV-TR), the separation of psychiatric illness into *organic* (i.e., due to an identifiable medical or neurological anomaly or psychoactive substance) and *functional* (i.e., due to unidentified factors) represented a necessary capitulation to limited understanding of the roots of mental illness, as opposed to measurable physiological differences between illnesses judged to be phenomenologically similar. Thus, the nosological shift embodied in DSM-IV and DSM-IV-TR from organic mental illness to mental illness due to a general medical condition underscores a shift in thinking about etiology. This shift is modest, not seismic, and is almost definitely transitional, based on continued limitations in the understanding of brain biochemistry.

The distinction between what are now called *primary disorders* (formerly *functional*) and *mental disorders due to a general medical condition or substance* (formerly *organic*) almost certainly will yield, over future decades, to a more unified nosology, the contour of which will depend on the nature of further scientific advance as to etiology of mental illness. The DSM-IV-TR dichotomy likely represents an improvement over the previous classification, but it should be regarded as tentative, a place to pause as further data are gleaned in the laboratory and clinical setting.

DEFINITION

DSM-IV-TR defines a *mental disorder due to a general medical condition* as a syndrome "characterized by the presence of mental symptoms that are judged to be the direct physiological consequence of a general medical condition." Similarly, a *substance-induced mental disorder* is judged to be the physiological consequence of a substance, whether a drug of abuse or prescribed medication. DSM-IV-TR emphasizes that "maintaining the distinction between mental disorders and general medical conditions does not imply that there are fundamental differences in their conceptualization, that mental disorders are unrelated to physical or biologic factors or processes, or that general medical conditions are unrelated to behavioral or psychosocial factors or processes."

The term *organic*, as used to define these mental disorders before DSM-IV, often suggested structural lesion identifiable as such. The terms *due to* and *induced* imply a shift in focus to physiological and molecular etiology.

In contrast to the general nature of the term *organic*, as used in the third edition of the DSM (DSM-III) and its revised version (DSM-III-R), DSM-IV-TR requires that the diagnosis allude to the specific medical or substance-related cause of the mental disorder (e.g., anxiety disorder due to hyperthyroidism, with generalized anxiety, and cocaine-induced psychotic disorder, with delusions). In DSM-IV-TR's multiaxial classification of mental disorders due to a general medical condition, the mental disorder is coded on Axis I, and the physical disorder is coded on Axis III.

HISTORY

For nearly two centuries, physicians and scientists interested in mental illness have struggled with issues of origin and classification. Nineteenth century physicians interested in the classification of mental illness had few tools for understanding the cellular and chemical basis of mental illness and typically worked in asylums separate from other physicians. Psychiatric units began to appear in general hospitals in growing numbers in the 1920s. This, along with the development of a variety of somatic interventions, including electroconvulsive therapy (ECT) and psychosurgery, led to increased focus on the biological basis of mental disease. In the 1930s and 1940s, individuals including George Henry and Morris Kaufman lent impetus to an evolving interest in the interface of medical and mental disorders. Psychosomatic medicine and its practitioners, consultation-liaison psychiatrists, evolved to assist nonpsychiatrists in the evaluation and management of individuals in whom psychological factors were perceived to be relevant to the development or maintenance of a host of physical disorders. These psychiatrists also were enlisted to treat the psychiatric manifestations of a variety of medical conditions. In the 1960s and 1970s, liaison activity, involving formal and informal didactic training of nonpsychiatrists by their psychiatric colleagues, was aimed at increasing awareness of the interplay between mental and medical conditions.

The middle of the 20th century witnessed several competing trends in psychiatry. Psychological theories and therapies, including psychoanalysis, grew to explain and manage even the most serious psychotic illnesses, including schizophrenia. Concurrently, psychopharmacological developments, especially the introduction of antipsychotic agents (e.g., chlorpromazine [Thorazine]), served as harbingers of sustained efforts to understand and to manage the biochemical basis of disturbed behavior. Indeed, with the close of the 20th century, leadership in psychiatry shifted from the psychological and psychodynamic theories to neuropsychiatric approaches, which have been viewed as embracing the most rigorously scientific methodologies, not unlike those used in other areas of medicine. The neuropsychiatric era has coincided with renewed emphasis on incorporation of psychiatric care into the medical mainstream, with the general hospital usually serving as the favored setting for delivery of such care.

COMPARATIVE NOSOLOGY

Historical developments were mirrored by nosological efforts. The first edition of the DSM (DSM-I) was introduced in 1952, dividing mental illness into two categories: those without clear physical or structural cause and those with identifiable acute or chronic brain impairment. The second edition of the DSM (DSM-II), introduced in 1968, maintained this dichotomy, with the latter group of disorders believed to be associated with cognitive disturbance, including memory and judgment impairment. Introduced in 1980, DSM-III defined *organic* disorders as those "associated with transient or permanent dysfunction of the brain." DSM-III and DSM-III-R recognized that *organic* could include the role of substances, that is, medications or drugs of abuse. Compared to their predecessors, DSM-III and DSM-III-R expanded the array of subtypes of organic illness, adding categories for hallucinosis, delusions, mood symptoms, anxiety symptoms, and personality disturbances, in addition to cognitive disturbances such as dementia and delirium.

DSM-IV and DSM-IV-TR, with the introduction of the concept of *due to*, abandoned the term *organic* to avoid the misconception that nonorganic, *functional* disorders were perhaps not due to biological or chemical brain aberrations. At present, functional disorders are described as primary mental disorders, and organic disorders have been divided into those induced by identifiable medical conditions (*due to a general medical condition*) and those induced by identifiable substances, prescribed or abused (*substance-induced*).

Thus, DSM-IV-TR creates a diagnostic distinction between mental disorders due to general medical conditions and those due to substances, a departure from the more unified approach adopted by DSM-III, which generally allowed for a single *organic* diagnosis defined by symptom constellation, whether due to a medical condition or substance. The dichotomy introduced by DSM-IV represents an effort at diagnostic refinement, although the distinction between substance- and medical-induced mental disorders is not meant to exclude the likelihood that evolving knowledge eventually will point to common biochemical pathways explaining mental disorders with similar phenomenological presentations.

DSM-IV-TR's diagnostic category, mental disorders due to a general medical condition, includes a broad array of psychiatric states attributable to the physiological manifestations of specific medical conditions (Table 10.5–1). In contrast to psychiatric states resulting from the emotional distress or psychological reaction to a general medical condition, this category of illness includes only those disorders in which a medical condition, through physiological means, has directly impacted on the functioning of the brain as man-

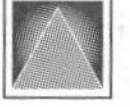

Table 10.5–1
DSM-IV-TR Classification of Mental Disorders Due to a General Medical Condition

Delirium
Dementia
Dementia due to human immunodeficiency virus disease
Dementia due to head trauma
Dementia due to Parkinson's disease
Dementia due to Huntington's disease
Dementia due to Pick's disease
Dementia due to Creutzfeldt-Jakob disease
Dementia due to other general medical conditions
Amnestic disorder
Psychotic disorder
Mood disorder
Anxiety disorder
Sleep disorder
Sexual dysfunction
Catatonic disorder
Personality change
Mental disorder not otherwise specified

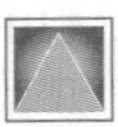

Table 10.5–2
DSM-IV-TR Classification of Substance-Induced Mental Disorders

Intoxication withdrawal
Delirium
Persisting dementia
Persisting amnestic disorder
Psychotic disorder
Mood disorder
Anxiety disorder
Sleep disorder
Sexual dysfunction
Medication-induced movement disorder
Substance-related disorder not otherwise specified

ifested by the appearance of psychiatric symptoms. These same considerations apply to substance-induced mental disorders (Table 10.5–2).

Interestingly, the tenth edition of the *International Statistical Classification of Diseases and Related Health Problems* (ICD-10) has not abandoned the *organic* nomenclature and continues a classification scheme similar to that of DSM-III and DSM-III-R. ICD-10 describes organic disorders as having a "demonstrable etiology in cerebral disease, brain injury, or other insult leading to cerebral dysfunction. The dysfunction may be primary, as in diseases, injuries and insults that affect the brain directly and selectively; or secondary, as in systemic diseases and disorders that attack the brain only as one of the multiple organs or systems of the body that are involved." Diagnoses fall within one of two categories: *organic mental disorders*, which include nonpsychoactive drug effects, and *mental and behavioral disorders due to psychoactive substance use* (Table 10.5–3).

ETIOLOGY

Mental disorders with medical, neurological, and substance-related or pharmacological roots may be divided according to a variety of classification schemes. A simple scheme divides origin into four categories: neurological, infectious and inflammatory, metabolic and endocrine, and substance-induced (Table 10.5–4).

DIAGNOSIS AND CLINICAL FEATURES

Central to diagnosis is a rigorous assessment of the course, timing, and acuity of mental symptoms; details of the individual's history, mental and physical; family history, mental and physical; review of substance exposure, including prescribed medications, over-the-counter remedies, drugs of abuse, and environmental toxins; mental status examination, including cognitive assessment (Table 10.5–5); results of physical examination, including vital signs, with emphasis on neurological findings (Table 10.5–6) and attention to specific organ systems most likely to be relevant in supporting or refuting salient diagnostic considerations; and review of pertinent laboratory and imaging studies (Table 10.5–7).

DSM-IV-TR describes three criteria that must be met for diagnosis of mental disorder due to a general medical condition:

1. There is evidence from the history, physical examination, or laboratory findings that the disturbance is the direct physiological consequence of a general medical condition.

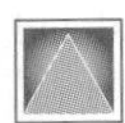

Table 10.5–3
ICD-10 Classification of Organic Mental Disorders

Organic, including symptomatic and mental disorders
Delirium
Dementia
Alzheimer's disease
Vascular
Pick's disease
Creutzfeldt-Jakob disease
Huntington's disease
Parkinson's disease
Human immunodeficiency virus disease
Dementia in other specified diseases (e.g., neurosyphilis and vitamin B_{12} deficiency)
Unspecified dementia
Organic amnestic syndrome
Other mental disorders due to brain damage and dysfunction and to physical disease
Organic hallucinosis
Organic catatonic disorder
Organic delusional (schizophrenia-like) disorder
Organic mood (affective) disorders
Organic anxiety disorder
Organic dissociative disorder
Organic emotionally labile disorder
Mild cognitive disorder
Other specified mental disorders due to brain damage and dysfunction and to physical disease
Unspecified mental disorder due to brain damage and dysfunction and to physical disease
Personality and behavioral disorders due to brain disease, damage, and dysfunction
Organic personality disorder
Postencephalitic syndrome
Postconcussional syndrome
Other organic personality and behavioral disorders due to brain disease, damage, or dysfunction
Unspecified organic personality and behavioral disorder due to brain disease, damage, and dysfunction
Organic sleep disorder
Organic sexual dysfunction
Unspecified organic or symptomatic mental disorder
Mental and behavioral disorders due to psychoactive substance use
Acute intoxication
Withdrawal state
Harmful use
Psychotic disorder
Amnestic syndrome
Residual and late-onset psychotic disorder
Other mental and behavioral disorders due to psychoactive substance use
Unspecified mental and behavioral disorder due to psychoactive substance use

2. The disturbance is not better accounted for by another mental disorder.
3. The disturbance does not occur exclusively during the course of a delirium.

Evidence of Physiological Cause

Several factors support a physiological link between a general medical condition (or substance) and a mental disorder:

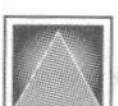

Table 10.5–4
General Medical and Substance-Induced Causes of Mental Disorders

- Neurological
  - Head trauma
  - Degenerative brain disease
    - Alzheimer's disease
    - Frontotemporal dementia
      - Pick's disease
    - Dementia with Lewy bodies
      - Parkinson's disease
    - Huntington's disease
    - Wilson's disease
  - Cerebrovascular disease
  - Demyelinating disease
    - Multiple sclerosis
  - Normal pressure hydrocephalus
  - Brain mass
    - Tumor
      - Primary
      - Metastatic
    - Other space-occupying lesion
      - Abscess
      - Subdural hematoma
- Infectious and inflammatory
  - Brain involvement alone
    - Encephalitis
    - Slow virus
  - Systemic infection or inflammation with identifiable brain involvement
    - Human immunodeficiency virus
    - Systemic lupus erythematous
  - Systemic infection or inflammation without identifiable brain involvement
    - Sepsis
    - Localized infection
    - Pneumonia
    - Urinary tract infection
- Metabolic and endocrine
  - Metabolic
    - Anemia
    - Hypoxia
    - Hypercarbia
    - Hypercalcemia and hypocalcemia
    - Renal dysfunction
    - Hepatic dysfunction
    - Acute intermittent porphyria
  - Endocrine
    - Thyroid
    - Parathyroid
    - Adrenal
    - Pheochromocytoma
  - Vitamin deficiency
    - Vitamin B_{12}
    - Thiamine
    - Niacin
    - Folate
- Substance-induced
  - Medications
    - Anticholinergic
    - Opioid
    - Sedative-hypnotic
    - Anxiolytic
    - Antidepressant
    - Corticosteroid
    - Immunosuppressant
    - Anticonvulsant
    - Antiarrhythmic
    - Antihypertensive
    - Sympathomimetic
  - Drugs of abuse
    - Alcohol
    - Cocaine
    - Phencyclidine
    - Cannabis
    - Inhalants
    - Hallucinogens
  - Other
    - Heavy metals
    - Environmental toxins

A. Presence of the general medical condition (or use of a substance), based on history, laboratory findings, imaging studies, or physical examination.

B. Temporal association between the onset, exacerbation, or remission of the general medical condition (or use of a substance) and the mental disorder. DSM-IV-TR notes that the search for a temporal link is not infallible, in that mental symptoms may occur long after the onset of a causative medical illness (e.g., psychosis due to epilepsy), or mental symptoms may occur in advance of detection of the medical problem (e.g., depression in a patient who later is diagnosed with Huntington's disease). Furthermore, treatment of the medical problem may not correct the resultant psychiatric disorder (e.g., depression that persists after hypothyroidism is corrected). Most persuasive diagnostically is treatment targeted to the general medical condition that also alleviates the mental disorder.

C. Presence of atypical features. Unusual presenting features may suggest a nonprimary mental disorder. As examples of such features, DSM-IV-TR cites atypical age of onset (e.g., first appearance of schizophrenia-like symptoms in a 75-year-old individual), unusual associated features (e.g., visual or tactile hallucinations accompanying a major depressive–like episode), diagnostic features that are more severe than would be expected based on the overall presentation (e.g., large weight loss in a patient with mild depressive symptoms), lack of family history of mental disorder, and cognitive loss out of proportion to that typically encountered in the primary mental disorder.

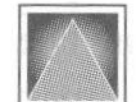

Table 10.5–5
Common Tools for Cognitive Assessment

Mini-Mental State Examination
Clock drawing
Trail-Making test
Neuropsychological testing

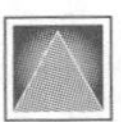

Table 10.5–6
Neurological Findings Relevant to Mental Disorder Due to General Medical Conditions or Substances

Change in consciousness
Headache
Tremor
Gait disturbance
Meningeal signs
Involuntary movements
Pathologic reflexes
Motor defect
Sensory defect
Visual defect
Auditory defect
Cranial nerve defect
Language disturbance

D. Evidence from the scientific literature of an established or frequent link between the medical condition or substance and the mental disorder (e.g., Huntington's disease and depression, Parkinson's disease and dementia, and cocaine and depression). Such evidence alone is useful but not sufficient for making a diagnostic determination in an individual case.

Disturbance Is Not Better Accounted for by Another Mental Disorder DSM-IV-TR underscores the importance of excluding primary mental disorders in diagnosing a medical or substance-induced mental disorder. At times, this is problematic, for individuals may have coexisting physical and mental disorders, the former of which do not necessarily physiologically induce the latter. For example, an individual with recurrent major depressive disorder may, in later life, develop undiagnosed hypothyroidism. Is a subsequent depressive episode primary or due to hypothyroidism? One factor supportive of a diagnosis of thyroid-induced depression would be presentation with mental symptoms not typical of the individual's earlier depressive episodes (e.g., severe fatigue). Another would be the remission of depressive symptoms in response solely to thyroid supplementation.

Another diagnostically confounding consideration is that medical conditions may impact on mental state in a nonphysiological manner, as when the medical condition acts as a psychosocial stressor. The resulting mental disorder is not diagnosed as being *due to* according to the DSM-IV-TR classification scheme. Patients with mental disorders exacerbated or induced in this fashion by medical illness generally should receive diagnosis of a primary mental disorder (e.g., adjustment disorder with depressed mood), with the medical condition listed as a stressor on Axis IV. Finally, co-occurrence of the medical and mental disorders may be purely coincidental.

Further complicating diagnosis in the medically ill is the role of substances, prescribed or abused. If evidence exists of recent or prolonged substance intoxication or withdrawal, the diagnosis of substance-induced mental disorder must be entertained, particularly if less than 4 weeks have elapsed since substance discontinuation. The exception would be substance-induced persisting disorders (i.e., primarily dementia and amnestic syndromes). Substance-induced mental disorder should be diagnosed only when symptoms are in excess of those characteristically associated with substance intoxication or withdrawal or are severe enough to warrant independent clinical attention. For example, mild depression in the context of cocaine withdrawal would not warrant independent diagnosis. Yet, depressed mood associated with active suicidal ideation, a symptom in excess of those usually related to cocaine withdrawal, would warrant a diagnosis of cocaine-induced mood disorder, with depressive features, with onset during withdrawal.

Blood and urine toxicology studies may assist in distinguishing medically induced from substance-induced mental disorders. In individuals in whom medical and substance considerations together are etiological (e.g., an individual with chronic obstructive pulmonary disease whose anxiety disorder is attributed to hypoxia but who experiences accentuated anxiety when albuterol [Proventil] is prescribed), diagnoses of mental disorder due to a general medical condition and substance-induced mental disorder are appropriate. If mental symptoms cannot adequately be separated into *primary*, *substance-induced*, or *due to a general medical condition* categories, diagnosis of *mental disorder not otherwise specified* is appropriate.

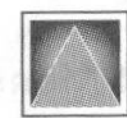

Table 10.5–7
Laboratory Examination Relevant to Mental Disorders Due to General Medical Conditions or Substances

- Blood
  - Complete blood count
  - Electrolytes
  - Glucose
  - Blood urea nitrogen and creatinine
  - Calcium, magnesium, and phosphorus
  - Liver function tests
  - Thyroid function tests
  - Serology
    - Rapid plasma reagin or Venereal Disease Research Laboratory
  - Vitamin B_{12} and folate
  - Erythrocyte sedimentation rate
  - Arterial blood gases
  - Toxicology
- Urine
  - Urinalysis
  - Toxicology
- Cerebrospinal fluid
  - Protein
  - Cells
  - Culture for infectious organisms
- Chest radiograph
- Electrocardiogram
- Brain imaging
  - Structural
    - Computed tomography
    - Magnetic resonance imaging
  - Functional
    - Positron emission tomography
    - Single photon emission computed tomography
- Electroencephalography
- Special laboratory studies
  - Blood
    - Human immunodeficiency virus
    - Ceruloplasmin
    - Drug level
  - Urine
    - Catecholamines
    - Porphobilinogens

Disturbance Does Not Occur Exclusively during the Course of a Delirium Delirium is a great pretender, the symptom constellation of which mimics many other mental disorders. In general hospital inpatient settings, at least 20 percent of patients experience delirium, the presentation of which may be subtle. When alterations in consciousness are modest, and when cognitive loss is minimal or incorrectly attributed to dementia or other nonacute cognitive states, a diagnosis of delirium easily may be missed. Instead, other accompaniments of delirium (hallucinations, paranoia, depressed mood, and anxiety) incorrectly may be perceived as the salient symptoms dictating diagnosis. In the context of acute medical illness or drug intoxication or withdrawal, clinicians must look searchingly for clues supporting delirium (fluctuating symptoms, acuity of presentation, and inattentiveness on interview) before diagnosing mental disorder (apart from delirium) due to a general medical condition or substance.

RECORDING PROCEDURES

For a mental disorder due to a general medical condition, the clinician should list on Axis I the mental disorder and the etiology (e.g., mood disorder due to hypothyroidism, with depressive features) and on Axis III the code for the general medical condition as indicated in the ninth edition, clinical modification, of the *International Classification of Diseases* (ICD-9-CM).

For substance-induced mental disorders, the relevant substance should be listed on Axis I (e.g., cannabis-induced psychotic disorder, with delusions). The diagnostician should indicate whether the mental disorder began *with onset during intoxication* or *with onset during withdrawal.*

DIAGNOSTIC CATEGORIES

DSM-IV-TR lists categories of mental disorders due to general medical conditions (Table 10.5–1) and substances (Table 10.5–2). The classification scheme is such that mental disorders due to general medical illnesses or substances, with few exceptions, are placed in categories with primary psychiatric disorders with similar phenomenology. In the shift away from the *organic* versus *functional* dichotomy, this approach implicitly recognizes current limitations in identifying physiological origin of primary and secondary (i.e., *due to* or *induced*) mental disorders. DSM-III-R placed all organic disorders in a section apart from other mental disorders. DSM-IV-TR's equivalent section is truncated, serving only as a residual category containing three diagnoses: *catatonic disorder due to a general medical condition, personality change due to a general medical condition,* and *mental disorder not otherwise specified due to a general medical condition.*

DSM-IV-TR includes decision trees for the differential diagnosis of mental disorders due to a general medical condition (Fig. 10.5–1) and for substance-induced mental disorders.

COURSE AND PROGNOSIS

Due to the vast array of general medical conditions and substances capable of inducing mental disorders, no single statement can be applied to the course and prognosis of these disorders. In general, when medical or substance factors readily correctible are identified (e.g., hyperthyroid-induced anxiety and propranolol [Inderal]–induced depression), mental symptoms may respond promptly once treatment of the causative condition is initiated. This is especially true if the mental disorder has been of brief duration. Prognosis is more guarded in progressive or long-standing disease (e.g., neurosyphilis) or substance-induced states that cannot readily be altered (e.g., use of immunosuppressant medication in post–organ transplant patients and recurrent relapses to cocaine use).

TREATMENT

Treatment is geared to correction of the underlying medical condition or removal of the offending substance. Psychopharmacological interventions also may be required, in that correction of the underlying medical or substance-induced cause alone may not result in immediate or complete remission of associated mental symptoms. In elderly and medically ill individuals, low doses of psychotropic medication initially should be used. In the absence of intolerable side effects, the clinician gradually should increase dosing until psychiatric symptoms are relieved. A common therapeutic error is the assumption that medically ill patients never require doses of psychotropic medications as high as those required by medically healthy individuals for symptom resolution.

In addition to achieving adequate dosing, the clinician must consider potential interactions between proposed psychotropic agents and nonpsychotropic medications prescribed concurrently. In many cases, these interactions are based on hepatic enzyme induction or inhibition.

Finally, as medically ill patients are more susceptible to side effects than are individuals without medical illness, medications with high incidence of cardiac, anticholinergic, sedating, or extrapyramidal side effects generally should be avoided.

Psychotherapeutic interventions in mental disorders attributable to general medical conditions often are designed to assist individuals place present medical illness within a broader framework of life coping strategies, to identify narcissistic injury inflicted by illness and debility, to correct misconceptions about illness course or suffering, and to bolster supportive relationships with family and other critical supports. Psychotherapeutic approaches may be cognitive, insight-oriented, or supportive and, depending on the medical prognosis and underlying character structure, may be short- or long-term. For mental disorders due to substance use, detoxification and continuing substance treatment may be indicated.

COGNITIVE DISORDERS DUE TO A GENERAL MEDICAL CONDITION

Cognitive disorders due to general medical conditions include delirium, dementia, and amnestic syndromes.

DELIRIUM DUE TO A GENERAL MEDICAL CONDITION

A common psychiatric diagnosis in inpatient medical and surgical settings, the presentation of *delirium* often is clouded by an array of associated, cognitive, mood, and behavioral symptoms.

Definition Delirium is characterized by disturbance of alertness and attentivenesss; cognitive or perceptual changes; and symptoms that evolve over hours or days, typically in a fluctuating manner. Not uncommonly, delirium is accompanied by mood, anxiety, or psychotic symptoms. Delirium always has one or more medical or substance-related causes.

Comparative Nosology In DSM-III-R, delirium was described as an organic mental syndrome. Qualities of inattentiveness, disorganized thinking, reduced level of consciousness, perceptual distur-

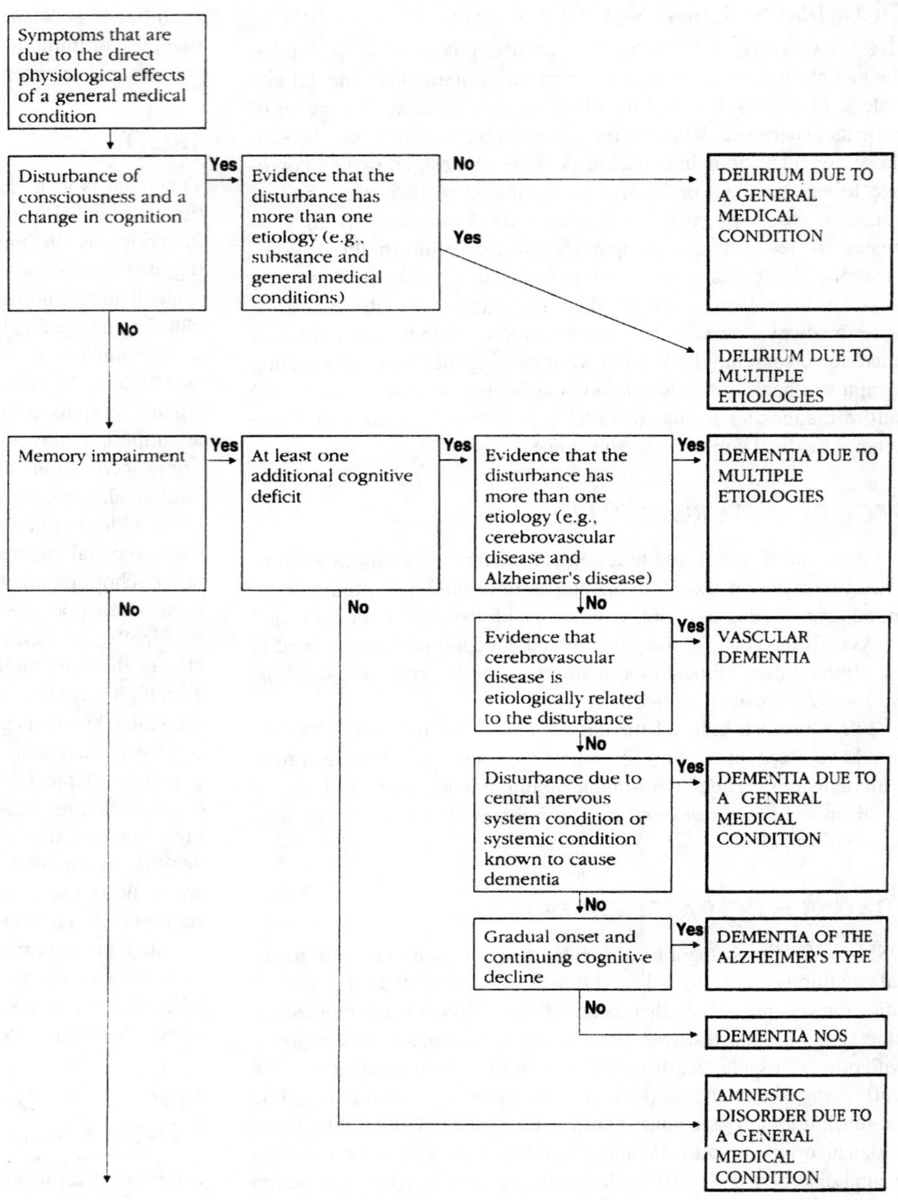

FIGURE 10.5–1 Differential diagnosis of mental disorders due to a general medical condition. NOS, not otherwise specified. (From American Psychiatric Association. *Diagnostic and Statistical Manual of Mental Disorders.* 4th ed. Text rev. Washington, DC: American Psychiatric Association; 2000, with permission.) (*continued*)

bances, sleep–wake disturbances, disorientation, memory disturbance, and acute, fluctuating course were emphasized in the description. DSM-IV and DSM-IV-TR diagnostic criteria focus on reduced consciousness and cognitive and perceptual disturbances as the most salient aspects of the presentation; disorganized thinking has been dropped as a criterion. The DSM-III-R version of delirium was attributed to *organic* factors; the DSM-IV and DSM-IV-TR versions are split into those due to a general medical condition and those that are substance-induced (including categories for delirium stemming from substance intoxication or withdrawal).

ICD-10 describes delirium as a "nonspecific organic cerebral syndrome characterized by concurrent disturbances of consciousness and attention, perception, thinking, memory, psychomotor behavior, emotion, and the sleep–wake cycle."

Epidemiology

Delirium has a point prevalence of approximately 1 percent in those older than 55 years of age but affects approximately 20 to 30 percent of individuals hospitalized for medical and surgical reasons and as much as 80 percent of patients with terminal illness near death. The elderly and individuals with preexisting cognitive impairment are at particularly high risk for development of delirium.

Etiology

The list of medical and pharmacological causes of delirium is similar to the list of general medical and substance-related causes of mental disorders cited earlier (Table 10.5–4). In addition to those causes should be added central nervous system (CNS) depressant (i.e., alcohol, benzodiazepine, and barbiturate) withdrawal.

The pathophysiology of delirium is poorly understood. Hypofunction of cholinergic systems is postulated to underlie the cognitive defects seen in delirium and probably explains the high risk of delirium associated with anticholinergic agents, particularly in individuals with preexisting cognitive dysfunction (e.g., dementia). Deficiencies

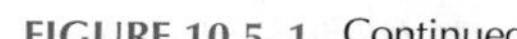

FIGURE 10.5–1 Continued

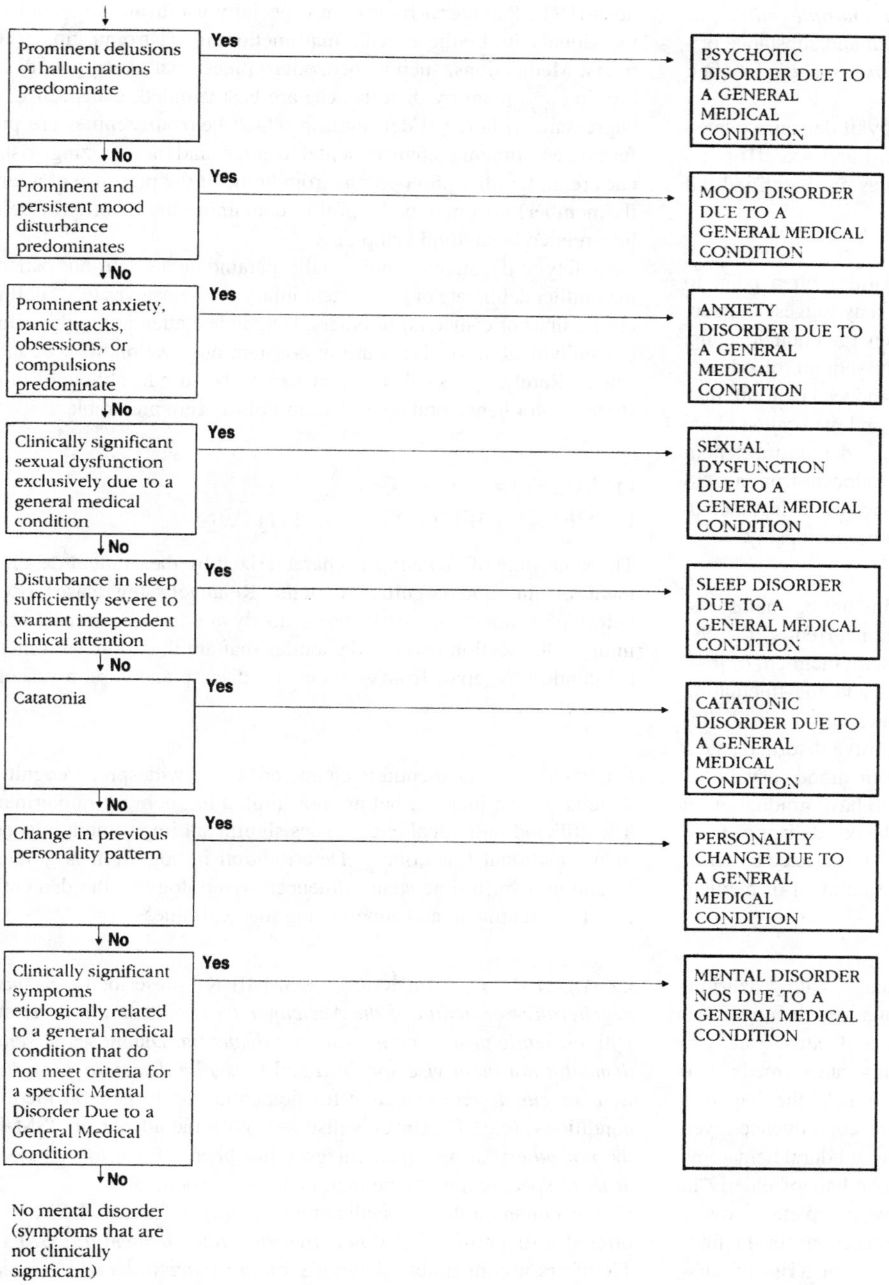

- Prominent delusions or hallucinations predominate — **Yes** → PSYCHOTIC DISORDER DUE TO A GENERAL MEDICAL CONDITION
  - **No** ↓
- Prominent and persistent mood disturbance predominates — **Yes** → MOOD DISORDER DUE TO A GENERAL MEDICAL CONDITION
  - **No** ↓
- Prominent anxiety, panic attacks, obsessions, or compulsions predominate — **Yes** → ANXIETY DISORDER DUE TO A GENERAL MEDICAL CONDITION
  - **No** ↓
- Clinically significant sexual dysfunction exclusively due to a general medical condition — **Yes** → SEXUAL DYSFUNCTION DUE TO A GENERAL MEDICAL CONDITION
  - **No** ↓
- Disturbance in sleep sufficiently severe to warrant independent clinical attention — **Yes** → SLEEP DISORDER DUE TO A GENERAL MEDICAL CONDITION
  - **No** ↓
- Catatonia — **Yes** → CATATONIC DISORDER DUE TO A GENERAL MEDICAL CONDITION
  - **No** ↓
- Change in previous personality pattern — **Yes** → PERSONALITY CHANGE DUE TO A GENERAL MEDICAL CONDITION
  - **No** ↓
- Clinically significant symptoms etiologically related to a general medical condition that do not meet criteria for a specific Mental Disorder Due to a General Medical Condition — **Yes** → MENTAL DISORDER NOS DUE TO A GENERAL MEDICAL CONDITION
  - **No** ↓
- No mental disorder (symptoms that are not clinically significant)

in arousal seen in delirium may stem from dysfunction of the reticular activating system. Hyperfunction in mesocorticolimbic dopaminergic pathways, leading to excess dopamine release, may contribute to delusions and hallucinations observed in delirium and may explain the salutary role of antipsychotic medication in management.

Diagnosis and Clinical Features

See Table 10.2–2, which lists DSM-IV-TR criteria for delirium, the cardinal symptoms of which have been described earlier. The clinician must establish the presence of a general medical condition or substance capable of causing delirium. A temporal association between the initiation of the medical condition or substance and the development of a delirium is highly suggestive of an etiological basis. Occasionally, delirium may be a harbinger of a soon-to-be-diagnosed medical problem. As a result, its diagnosis should always herald a vigorous search for cause.

Associated physical findings may assist with diagnosis of delirium. Hepatic encephalopathy may be associated with a flapping movement of the hands called *asterixis*. Autonomic hyperactivity may be observed in withdrawal from CNS depressants. Wernicke's encephalopathy related to thiamine deficiency may be associated with paralysis of gaze. Anticholinergic toxicity may be indicated by dry mucous membranes, tachycardia, and warm, flushed skin.

Time course may be diagnostically helpful: Alcohol withdrawal delirium usually commences within 24 to 72 hours of the cessation of alcohol use.

Five DSM-IV-TR diagnostic categories exist: *delirium due to a general medical condition, substance intoxication delirium, sub-*

stance withdrawal delirium, delirium due to multiple etiologies (when more that one medical origin, or a medical and substance origin, are identified), and *delirium not otherwise specified* (when insufficient etiologic evidence is present).

Recording procedures dictate that the etiology of delirium related to a general medical condition is listed on Axis I and Axis III (e.g., delirium due to pneumonia). If several etiologies are identified, all should be listed.

Laboratory Findings

Laboratory irregularities often point to the cause of delirium. Elevated white blood count may suggest an infectious origin. Hemorrhagic stroke usually is seen on brain imaging. Dehydration may be indicated by elevated serum sodium, blood urea nitrogen, and hematocrit. Diagnosis of substance-induced delirium may be facilitated by examination of urine toxicology and medication blood levels. In most deliria, electroencephalogram (EEG) demonstrates nonfocal background slowing. In delirium due to withdrawal from a CNS depressant, excess fast beta waves are observed. Severe slowing, including triphasic delta waves, may be seen in hepatic encephalopathy.

Differential Diagnosis

Due to the fluctuating nature of delirium, symptoms may not all be present concurrently, thereby confounding diagnosis, particularly in patients with incipient or low-grade deliria. Acuity of onset, inattentiveness, and the fluctuating course of symptoms, all within a medical context, assist in distinguishing delirium from slowly progressive cognitive disorders, such as dementia and amnestic syndromes, and from mood, psychotic, anxiety, and sleep disorders, all of which tend to have gradual onset and resolution. Distinguishing substance-induced delirium from delirium due to a general medical condition may be assisted by chronology of delirium symptoms and response to treatment of medical illness and removal of suspect substances.

Course and Prognosis

Most individuals with delirium recover fully, despite the often dramatic fluctuations in cognition, alertness, and mood encountered in this syndrome. Course usually is dictated by the rapidity with which the offending cause (medical or substance) is removed. Yet, if the clinician fails to make the diagnosis or to orchestrate the appropriate workup, severe consequence, even death, may ensue (e.g., delirium due to expanding subdural hematoma and alcohol withdrawal delirium). More than one-half of elderly in medical and surgical hospitals may not achieve complete recovery from delirium at the time of discharge. This may account for the finding that elderly hospitalized patients with delirium have a risk of nursing home placement that is three times that of those without delirium.

Treatment

Management of delirium is threefold: identification and correction of the underlying medical or substance cause, management of associated behavioral symptoms, and implementation of strategies designed to ensure safety of the affected individual. An aggressive search for offending medical conditions or substances should be undertaken with an aim of rapid correction. Behavioral and mental symptoms (e.g., psychosis, aggression, and psychomotor agitation) are best managed with antipsychotic medications. Increasingly, oral atypical antipsychotic agents (e.g., risperidone [Risperdal], olanzapine [Zyprexa], and quetiapine [Seroquel]) are used for this purpose. Another atypical agent, ziprasidone (Geodon), may be administered by oral and intramuscular (IM) routes. One typical antipsychotic agent, haloperidol (Haldol), has the unique advantage of three acceptable routes of administration (oral, IM, and intravenous [IV]). Parenteral routes are especially useful in noncompliant individuals or in those with malfunctioning gastrointestinal (GI) tracts. Medications, such as benzodiazepines, that exacerbate disinhibition and memory disturbances are best avoided, except in CNS depressant withdrawal delirium, in which benzodiazepines are preferred. Minimizing environmental change and maximizing visual cues (e.g., familiar photographs from home or the presence of a family member) also may be helpful in containing the severity of delirium-related behavioral symptoms.

Safety of the affected individual is paramount, as delirious patients may inflict deliberate or inadvertent injury on themselves (e.g., pulling out IV lines or catheters) or others. Heightened attention to the delirious individual, through the use of constant observation, may be indicated. Rarely, physical restraints may be used, although other strategies for behavioral control almost always are preferable.

DEMENTIA DUE TO A GENERAL MEDICAL CONDITION

The syndrome of *dementia* is characterized by the gradual development of multiple cognitive deficits. Relatively few cases occur before 65 years of age; early cases mostly are due to traumatic brain injury. This section reviews dementias that are due to general medical conditions (apart from Alzheimer's disease and cerebrovascular disease) and substances.

Definition

Dementia is characterized by widespread cognitive deficits, which include, but are not limited to, memory impairment. The afflicted individual experiences significant impairment in social or occupational functioning. Deterioration in cognition is gradual, extending over a time span influenced by etiology of the dementia, efforts at treatment, and supervening medical illness.

Comparative Nosology

DSM-III-R described *primary degenerative dementia of the Alzheimer type*, with *senile onset* and with *presenile onset*, and *multiinfarct dementia*. Diagnoses of *senile dementia not otherwise specified* and *presenile dementia not otherwise specified* were available for dementia due to general medical conditions (e.g., Parkinson's disease). With the advent of DSM-IV, the *not otherwise specified* category has been refined to include an array of specific non-Alzheimer, nonvascular dementias.

For dementia due to medications or drugs of abuse, DSM-III-R offered a diagnosis of *psychoactive substance dementia*. DSM-IV-TR offers a comparable diagnosis of *substance-induced persisting dementia*.

ICD-10 offers diagnoses for dementia in Pick's disease, Creutzfeldt-Jakob disease, Huntington's disease, Parkinson's disease, human immunodeficiency virus (HIV) disease, as well as a category for *dementia in other specified diseases* (e.g., hypercalcemia, vitamin B_{12} deficiency, epilepsy, neurosyphilis, multiple sclerosis [MS], and intoxications with nonpsychoactive substances). Also offered are categories for *unspecified dementia*, divided into *senile* and *presenile* subcategories, and *residual and late-onset psychotic disorder*, which includes dementia due to psychoactive substance use.

Epidemiology

Although Alzheimer's disease and cerebrovascular disease, individually and in combination, account for 70 to 90 percent of all dementia cases, large numbers of patients with HIV infection, Parkinson's disease, head trauma, and alcohol use disorders develop cognitive loss often culminating in dementia.

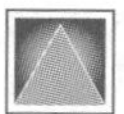

Table 10.5–8
Causes of Dementia

Neurological	Metabolic and endocrine
Degenerative	Anemia
Alzheimer's disease	Organ failure
Pick's disease	Heart
Parkinson's disease	Lungs
Huntington's disease	Kidney
Wilson's disease	Liver
Cerebrovascular disease	Thyroid
Demyelinating disease	Parathyroid
Multiple sclerosis	Adrenal
Head trauma	Vitamin deficiency
Posttraumatic dementia	Substance-induced
Dementia pugilistica	Medications
Brain mass	Sedative-hypnotic
Tumor	Anxiolytic
Subdural hematoma	Anticholinergic
Normal pressure hydrocephalus	Anticonvulsant
Infectious and inflammatory	Cardiovascular
Human immunodeficiency virus	Other
Slow viruses (e.g., Creutzfeldt-Jakob disease)	Alcohol
	Toxins
Neurosyphilis	Lead
System lupus erythematosus	Mercury
Temporal arteritis	Carbon monoxide

Etiology

Scientists postulate cholinergic deficit and inflammatory change as potential explanations for changes in neurotransmission that eventually lead to dementia. General medical conditions capable of causing dementia presumably exert their effects through one or more of these mechanisms. Medical conditions and substances that may cause dementia are listed in Table 10.5–8.

Degenerative dementias may be categorized as cortical or subcortical. Individual presentations often are mixed, particularly as dementia advances, with clinical and neuroanatomical features of both categories. Cortical dementias, including Alzheimer's disease and Pick's disease, are associated with defects in memory and executive functioning, along with aphasia, agnosia, or apraxia, or a combination of these. Subcortical dementias, including those due to HIV disease, Huntington's disease, and Parkinson's disease, involve white and deep gray matter structures and their frontal lobe projections. Early in their course, subcortical dementias present with psychomotor slowing and personality change, occasionally in advance of overt cognitive impairment.

Diagnosis and Clinical Features

The essential feature in dementia, regardless of etiology, is the presence of multiple cognitive deficits manifested by memory impairment and one or more of the following: (1) aphasia, (2) apraxia, (3) agnosia, and (4) disturbance in executive functioning (Table 10.5–9). These deficits compromise overall functioning and may be associated with change in personality and withdrawal from usual activities. Depression, delusions, or aggressive behavior may emerge as complications of dementia. Unless due to a single discrete (e.g., head injury) or reversible event, dementia tends to follow an inexorable, progressive course, usually over the course of several years, until death ensues.

In DSM-IV-TR's *dementias due to other general medical conditions*, there is evidence from the history, physical examination, or laboratory findings of a cause distinct from Alzheimer's disease or

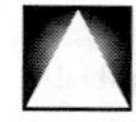

Table 10.5–9
DSM-IV-TR Criteria for Dementias Due to Other General Medical Conditions

A. The development of multiple cognitive deficits manifested by
   (1) Memory impairment (impaired ability to learn new information or to recall previously learned information)
   (2) One (or more) of the following cognitive disturbances:
      (a) Aphasia (language disturbance)
      (b) Apraxia (impaired ability to carry out motor activities, despite intact motor function)
      (c) Agnosia (failure to recognize or to identify objects, despite intact sensory function)
      (d) Disturbance in executive functioning (i.e., planning, organizing, sequencing, and abstracting)

B. The cognitive deficits in Criteria A1 and A2 each cause significant impairment in social or occupational functioning and represent a significant decline from a previous level of functioning.

C. There is evidence from the history, physical examination, or laboratory findings that the disturbance is the direct physiological consequence of a general medical condition other than Alzheimer's disease or cerebrovascular disease (i.e., human immunodeficiency virus infection, traumatic brain injury, Parkinson's disease, Huntington's disease, Pick's disease, Creutzfeldt-Jakob disease, normal pressure hydrocephalus, hypothyroidism, brain tumor, or vitamin B_{12} deficiency).

D. The deficits do not occur exclusively during the course of a delirium.

Specify:

Without behavioral disturbance

With behavioral disturbance

From American Psychiatric Association. *Diagnostic and Statistical Manual of Mental Disorders.* 4th ed. Text rev. Washington, DC; American Psychiatric Association; 2000, with permission.

cerebrovascular disease. Factors supporting the diagnosis of dementia due to a general medical condition include a temporal link between the onset of the medical condition and the development of the dementia and a known link in the scientific literature between the medical condition and dementia. Similar considerations apply to substance-induced persisting dementia.

Two subtypes of dementia due to other general medical conditions exist: *with behavioral disturbance* and *without behavioral disturbance*, based on whether the dementia is accompanied by a clinically significant behavioral problem (e.g., aggression). In both cases, the causative general medical condition is coded on Axes I and III (e.g., dementia due to Pick's disease, with behavioral disturbance).

In substance-induced persisting dementia, the offending agent is listed on Axis I (e.g., alcohol-induced persisting dementia). In addition, DSM-IV-TR provides a category for *dementia due to multiple etiologies* (e.g., the combination of Alzheimer's disease, head trauma, and alcohol); each etiology should be listed on Axis I and, when indicated, on Axis III. If specific etiology cannot be identified, *dementia not otherwise specified* is diagnosed.

When psychiatric syndromes in addition to dementia are attributable to a specific general medical condition, these should be coded on Axis I as well. For example, an individual with dementia due to hypothyroidism may also meet criteria for mood disorder due to hypothyroidism, with depressive features.

Martha Jones is a 72-year-old woman without prior psychiatric history who, over the course of 8 months, experienced a 20-lb weight gain and psychomotor slowing. She stopped marketing for groceries, halted her participation in activities at the local senior center, and failed to make rent payments for 2 months consecutively. She was admitted to the hospital with lethargy of several weeks' duration. Psychiatry was consulted to rule out depression.

Interview revealed a heavyset woman with bland and indifferent demeanor and sleepiness. Physical examination revealed edematous facial features and thinning hair, with delayed deep tendon reflexes. Ms. Jones denied that she was depressed. She was oriented to place and year but not to month. Short-term recall was one of three objects.

Laboratory studies were unremarkable, except for a thyroid-stimulating hormone level of 112 (elevated).

The psychiatry consultant diagnosed dementia due to hypothyroidism. Thyroid replacement therapy was initiated. Ms. Jones was discharged to a nursing home, where qualities of withdrawal and inactivity were noted, despite gradual cognitive improvement. A trial of methylphenidate (Ritalin) 5 mg twice daily was commenced. Gradual improvement in cognition, alertness, and energy over the course of several months allowed Ms. Jones to return home with the assistance of an aide.

In this case, factors suggesting a medical contribution to dementia include the presence of lethargy, a well-established link between hypothyroidism and dementia, and the improvement in dementia with the treatment of hypothyroidism. Psychotropic medication was required to maximize clinical response.

Dementia Due to HIV Disease One-third of asymptomatic individuals with HIV and one-half of individuals with acquired immunodeficiency syndrome (AIDS) show evidence of cognitive impairment. Those individuals with HIV-associated dementia complex appear apathetic and slowed. Gait ataxia, tremor, and a decline in handwriting skills may be present. In some cases, the dementia is not due to the effects of HIV on the CNS but rather to the effects of accompanying opportunistic lesions of the brain (e.g., toxoplasmosis and lymphoma), in which case dementia should be attributed to those lesions.

In HIV-associated dementia complex, brain magnetic resonance imaging (MRI) may show demyelination of subcortical white matter. Functional brain imaging (e.g., positron emission tomography [PET]) may demonstrate hyperactivity in the thalamus and basal ganglia in early stage HIV-associated dementia complex and hypoactivity of the temporal lobes in late stage HIV-associated dementia complex. Histopathologically, white matter and subcortical destruction are described. Spinal fluid may show lymphocytosis or elevated protein, or both; presence of white blood cells should prompt a search for a brain opportunistic infection.

Dementia Due to Head Trauma Occurring most commonly in young men, often with concurrent substance disorders, *dementia due to head trauma* usually occurs as a consequence of a single injury to the head. Head trauma is associated with abrupt acceleration or deceleration of the brain, an event that deforms neurons. This leads to temporary or sustained neuronal dysfunction, the extent of which influences the degree of recovery. If head trauma is associated with intracerebral hemorrhage, neuronal function may be further compromised. Dementia resulting from head trauma may be associated with labile affect, aggression, and irritability. This dementia rarely is progressive, except in individuals with repeated blows to the head (e.g., boxers with *dementia pugilistica*).

Dementia Due to Parkinson's Disease More than one-half of patients with Parkinson's disease experience dementia. Onset of Parkinson's disease is usually between 50 and 60 years of age. Depletion of dopaminergic and serotonergic neurons in the substantia nigra and other subcortical structures appears to underlie the movement disorder, which is characterized by bradykinesia, resting tremor, and rigidity, all of which are progressive. Dysfunction of these same neurons likely contributes to the cognitive, mood, and behavioral disturbances seen in Parkinson's disease. At autopsy, Lewy bodies are found in the substantia nigra. Treatment of the movement disorder with dopaminergic agents occasionally provokes or exacerbates psychiatric symptoms; antipsychotic medications used to treat mental symptoms may exacerbate the movement disorder. Dementia detected in elderly individuals with Parkinson's disease may be due to that disorder or to other dementing disorders, including Alzheimer's disease and cerebrovascular disease.

Dementia Due to Huntington's Disease Huntington's disease is transmitted by a single autosomal dominant gene found on the short arm of chromosome 4. Usually diagnosed in the late 30s or early 40s, Huntington's disease affects men and women equally. Offspring of affected individuals have a 50 percent chance of developing the disease. Interruption of corticostriatal connections leads to characteristic motoric, emotional, and cognitive consequences. Emotional symptoms often appear early and include irritability, depression, or psychosis. Later, cognitive disturbance appears; this is marked by psychomotor slowing, loss of spontaneity, and memory defect. Motoric abnormalities, which may present prior or subsequent to mental symptoms, include the development of choreoathetotic movements, which eventually yield to profound bradykinesia. In the striatum, reduction in levels of γ-aminobutyric acid (GABA) and acetylcholine, both of which exert an inhibitory effect on movement, leads to the characteristic movement disorder.

In late Huntington's disease, structural brain imaging, including computed tomography (CT) and MRI, may show caudate atrophy and characteristic "boxcar" ventricles. Functional imaging, such as PET, may show striatal hypometabolism.

Dementia Due to Pick's Disease Pick's disease usually appears in the sixth decade of life and has a course of 2 to 5 years. The disorder affects the frontal and temporal lobes of the brain, making this one of several forms of frontotemporal dementia. Pick's disease is characterized by personality change, including disinhibited behavior and language abnormalities, later followed by deterioration in memory. Structural brain imaging often reveals frontal atrophy. Even in the absence of structural findings, functional imaging may demonstrate frontal hypometabolism. At autopsy, intraneuronal argentophilic Pick inclusion bodies are identified.

Dementia Due to Creutzfeldt-Jakob Disease Due to a transmissible prion, that is, a slow virus, Creutzfeldt-Jakob disease is characterized by dementia; periodic bursts of EEG activity; involuntary movements, often myoclonic or choreoathetotic in nature; and ataxia. Brain imaging may show nonspecific atrophy. Postmortem microscopic examination of the brain demonstrates neuronal degeneration in cortical and subcortical gray matter. Usually, the disease develops after 40 years of age and progresses rapidly over the course of several months.

Dementia Due to Other General Medical Conditions The DSM-IV-TR residual category of *dementia due to other general medical conditions* is used for dementias that may be reversible or irreversible and that do not fall into one of the previous diagnostic categories. These dementias may present with features similar to those seen in common dementing illnesses such as Alzheimer's disease and vascular dementia, a fact that underscores the importance of performing an exhaustive laboratory and pharmacological search for reversible causes of cognitive decline in all individuals presenting with such complaints (Tables 10.5–7 and 10.5–8).

This residual category includes degenerative brain diseases such as progressive supranuclear palsy and Lewy body disease (apart from Parkinson's disease). The former is characterized by gaze paresis and axial rigidity; the latter is characterized by fluctuating cognitive symptoms, psychosis, and extreme sensitivity to the extrapyramidal side effects of antipsychotic medications.

Also included in this category is Wilson's disease. Transmitted by autosomal recessive inheritance, this disorder manifests in late adolescence or early adulthood with personality change, tremor, rigidity, and, eventually, dementia.

Dementia also may result from structural lesions and deformities of the brain (e.g., tumor, abscess, subdural hematoma, and normal pressure hydrocephalus [NPH]). Cognitive loss due to subdural hematoma may occur days, weeks, or months after a causative head injury. NPH may present with a triad of symptoms: dementia, sphincteric incontinence, and gait disorder.

Other medical disorders capable of causing dementia include: metabolic and endocrine abnormalities (e.g., hypothyroidism, hypercalcemia, liver failure, renal failure, and cardiopulmonary failure), nutritional deficiencies (e.g., thiamine and vitamin B_{12}), and inflammatory and infectious states (e.g., neurosyphilis, chronic meningitis, and systemic lupus erythematosus). Neurosyphilis, caused by *Treponema pallidum*, evolves over the course of decades; one variant, general paresis, is characterized by pupillary abnormalities, action tremor, dysarthria, seizures, and dementia that is occasionally associated with grandiose or depressive features. Substances that may cause dementia include alcohol, anticonvulsants, anticholinergic agents, sedative-hypnotic agents, mercury, and lead.

Pathophysiological mechanisms underlying the effect of general medical conditions and substances on cognition are variable and often obscure. Slowly evolving cholinergic hypofunction appears to be associated with neuronal dysfunction in a broad range of dementing illnesses. This, too, likely explains the adverse impact on cognition of drugs with anticholinergic potential.

Brain tumor and trauma directly distort neuronal structure and impede cerebral blood flow. In NPH, neuronal dysfunction may be a consequence of insufficient blood flow resulting from disruption of the pressure gradient between ventricular and subdural spaces.

In Wilson's disease, an enzymatic defect in the incorporation into ceruloplasmin of copper leads to its toxic buildup in brain, liver, kidneys and cornea. In cardiopulmonary failure and anemia, hypoperfusion or hypoxia presumably underlies impaired neuronal activity. Alcohol causes neuronal loss and glial proliferation in several regions of the brain, including the frontal lobes and temporal association areas.

Laboratory Examination Patients presenting with evidence of progressive cognitive loss should have routine blood work, including complete blood count, electrolytes, glucose, blood urea nitrogen, creatinine, liver function tests, thyroid function tests, calcium, magnesium, phosphorus, vitamin B_{12} and folate levels, and reactive plasma reagin (RPR) or Venereal Disease Research Laboratory (VDRL) tests. The last two assist in identifying neurosyphilis. Erythrocyte sedimentation rate (ESR) should be requested if inflammatory, infectious, or oncological disease is suspected. Urinalysis should be examined. Urine and serum toxicology are indicated if substance use disorders are suspected. Electrocardiogram (ECG) and arterial blood gases (ABG) may be diagnostically useful in individuals with known or suspected cardiopulmonary disease. Structural brain imaging and, occasionally, lumbar puncture and EEG should be obtained. In selected cases, special examinations are indicated (e.g., if Wilson's disease is suspected based on family history, serum ceruloplasmin will be low; ophthalmological examination will reveal the pathognomonic Kayser-Fleischer ring of the cornea). Neuropsychological testing may assist in distinguishing among different forms of dementia.

Differential Diagnosis Differential diagnosis includes Alzheimer's disease and vascular dementia, which may present similarly to, or may overlap with, dementia due to a general medical condition. When patients present with multiple possible factors contributing to dementia, the relative importance of each factor may be difficult to discern.

Also within the differential diagnosis are pseudodementia of depression, amnestic syndromes, delirium, and age-related cognitive decline. Depression and dementia both may be associated with loss of interest, appetite, and spontaneity. Clues suggestive of depression are the presence of a prior history of mood disorder, multiple unsubstantiated somatic complaints, feelings of worthlessness, and suicidal ideation. In contrast to dementia, delirium has a fluctuating, acute quality. Amnestic syndromes do not encompass the global cognitive decline typical of dementia. Age-related cognitive decline does not cause the impairment in functioning characteristic of dementia.

When attempting to discern the relative contributions of various medical or neurological illnesses or substances in the evolution of dementia in an individual case, diagnosis may be assisted by examination of chronology of dementia symptoms and response to correction of medical illness or removal of suspect substances.

Course and Prognosis The course of dementia due to a general medical condition is highly variable, depending on etiology. If dementia is attributable to a reversible cause (e.g., hypothyroidism), gradual improvement may be possible; however, if the insult has been of long duration (e.g., neurosyphilis), recovery may be incomplete or imperceptible. If dementia is attributable to an irreversible cause (e.g., Pick's disease), progressive worsening is inevitable. Substance-induced persisting dementia often improves after cessation of substance use, although some forms (e.g., alcohol-induced) may endure indefinitely.

Treatment Management techniques are most successful when a reversible dementia of short duration is identified. If dementia is due to correctable intracranial pathology, improvement may follow neurosurgical intervention (e.g., ventriculoperitoneal shunting in NPH and evacuation of subdural hematoma). Nutritional, infectious, endocrine, and cardiopulmonary conditions should be optimized. In rare cases, special pharmacotherapy may be required (e.g., symptoms of Wilson's disease respond to management with copper-chelating agents, such as penicillamine [Cuprimine]).

Regardless of etiology of dementia, psychotropic medications often are indicated in the presence of prominent behavioral or mood symptoms. Antipsychotic agents, usually atypical, commonly are used for symptoms of aggression or psychosis. Antidepressant medications and mood stabilizers (e.g., divalproex [Depakote]) may assist with labile affect, disinhibition, and tearfulness. Rarely, hormonal interventions (e.g., medroxyprogesterone [Depo-Provera]) may be considered in men with dementia who demonstrate sexually disinhibited or aggressive behavior patterns. Medications with high anticholinergic potential (e.g., thioridazine [Mellaril] and amitriptyline [Elavil]) tend to worsen cognitive loss and are best avoided. Drugs with prominent amnestic properties (e.g., benzodiazepines), too, should be avoided. The use of cholinesterase inhibitors (e.g., donepezil [Aricept] and galantamine [Reminyl]) and N-methyl-D-aspartate (NMDA)-receptor antagonists (e.g., memantine [Namenda]) is controversial. Complications of psychotropic agents include gait disturbance, drug-induced parkinsonism, and oversedation. These are best minimized by using the lowest effective dosages of selected agents and avoiding polypharmacy.

AMNESTIC DISORDER DUE TO A GENERAL MEDICAL CONDITION

In contrast to the multiple cognitive deficiencies demonstrated in dementia, individuals with *amnestic disorders* demonstrate impairment only in their ability to learn new information or to recall old information. Aphasia, agnosia, apraxia, and disturbance in executive functioning are not pronounced or, if present, do not substantially intrude on functioning. Amnestic disorders may be transient or chronic.

Comparative Nosology

In DSM-III-R, *amnestic syndrome* was categorized as an organic mental disorder. It required a finding of long- and short-term memory deficits and was attributable to the effects of a general medical condition or substance. DSM-IV and DSM-IV-TR diagnoses include: *amnestic disorder due to a general medical condition*, *substance-induced persisting amnestic disorder*, and *amnestic disorder not otherwise specified.*

ICD-10 offers the diagnoses of *organic amnestic syndrome* for states due to medical conditions and nonpsychoactive substance use and *amnestic syndrome, psychoactive substance-induced.*

Epidemiology

Amnestic disorders due to general medical conditions and substances apparently are uncommon.

Etiology

Injuries to brain regions involved with memory (e.g., middle temporal lobe structures, including hippocampus and mammillary bodies), regardless of etiology, may cause amnestic disorder. Such injuries may be due to head trauma, cerebrovascular event, hypoxia, and infections such as herpes simplex encephalitis. Transient amnestic disorder may result from disease in the vertebrobasilar system. Limbic encephalopathy, a nonmetastatic complication of carcinoma (usually small cell lung cancer), which may precede its diagnosis, is characterized by amnestic disorder and occasionally by mood and psychotic symptoms. Of substance-induced persisting amnestic disorders, the most common is due to alcohol (Korsakoff's psychosis). This syndrome results from thiamine deficiency associated with prolonged consumption of alcohol. The preceding acute state, Wernicke's encephalopathy, is characterized by confusion, ataxia, and gaze palsies. Unless thiamine is administered in the acute state, alcohol-induced persisting amnestic disorder results. Other substances that may induce amnestic disorder include anticonvulsants, lead, mercury, and carbon monoxide.

Diagnosis and Clinical Features

The critical feature in amnestic disorder, whether the result of a general medical condition or substance, is impairment in the ability to learn new information or to recall previously learned information (Table 10.5–10). The afflicted individual may confabulate, that is, create imagined experiences to fill in gaps in memory. Unlike delusions, which are fixed, confabulated stories tend to be variable. Apathy, altered personality, lack of initiative, and impairment in functioning also are aspects of amnestic disorder. As with other mental disorders due to general medical conditions and substances, a temporal association and a known link in the literature enhance the likelihood that the general medical condition or substance has caused the amnestic disorder.

The general medical condition or substance is indicated on Axis I. Etiological general medical conditions also are indicated on Axis III.

If amnestic disorder is due to a general medical condition and a substance (e.g., head injury and alcohol in an individual with alcohol dependence), amnestic disorder due to a general medical condition and substance-induced persisting amnestic disorder are diagnosed. When evidence of specific etiology is lacking, the diagnosis is amnestic disorder not otherwise specified.

Laboratory Evaluation

Structural brain imaging may reveal atrophy or enlargement of third ventricle or lateral horns related to damage to mediotemporal lobe structures. Neuropsychological testing may assist in defining the specific degree and type of memory impairment.

Differential Diagnosis

Dementia, in contrast to amnestic disorder, by definition, requires more global cognitive deficits, although both disorders impair functioning. Delirium is a more acute

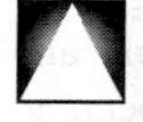

Table 10.5–10
DSM-IV-TR Diagnostic Criteria for Amnestic Disorder Due to a General Medical Condition

A. The development of memory impairment as manifested by impairment in the ability to learn new information or the inability to recall previously learned information.
B. The memory disturbance causes significant impairment in social or occupational functioning and represents a significant decline from a previous level of functioning.
C. The memory disturbance does not occur exclusively during the course of a delirium or a dementia.
D. There is evidence from the history, physical examination, or laboratory findings that the disturbance is the direct physiological consequence of a general medical condition (including physical trauma).

Specify:

Transient: if memory impairment lasts for 1 month or less

Chronic: if memory impairment lasts for more than 1 month

Coding note: Include the name of the general medical condition on Axis I, e.g., Amnestic disorder due to head trauma; also code the general medical condition on Axis III.

From American Psychiatric Association. *Diagnostic and Statistical Manual of Mental Disorders.* 4th ed. Text rev. Washington, DC: American Psychiatric Association; copyright 2000, with permission.

phenomenon and is associated with deficits in consciousness not characteristic of amnestic disorders. Predictable amnesia occurring during the course of acute substance (e.g., alcohol) intoxication or withdrawal should not be diagnosed as amnestic disorder. Dissociative amnesia usually involves inability to recall previous memories, with no deficits in recalling new information, and usually is related to emotional trauma, not a general medical condition or substance.

When medical illness and substances capable of inducing amnestic disorder coexist, differential diagnosis may be assisted by careful examination of the chronology of amnestic symptoms and the response to correction of medical disorders or removal of potentially offending substances.

Course and Prognosis

Course and prognosis of amnestic disorder due to a general medical condition are highly variable. Onset may be sudden if due to head injury or cerebrovascular event, with recovery limited by the extent of brain injury. Alcohol-induced persisting amnestic disorder improves little or not at all. In contrast, amnestic syndromes resulting from sustained heavy sedative-hypnotic use often slowly subside with cessation of substance use. Transient amnesia due to cerebrovascular insufficiency is by definition short lived but may be recurrent.

Treatment

Treatment is similar to that for dementia. Pharmacotherapy may be indicated for psychosis or mood disturbance. Psychotherapy may be limited by the core memory defect. Guidance in matters of personal hygiene, nutrition, and finance may be indicated. The affected individual should be encouraged to avoid substances that may have contributed to amnestic disorder; in some cases, formal substance treatment is indicated.

COGNITIVE DISORDERS NOT OTHERWISE SPECIFIED

Not all cognitive disorders due to general medical conditions meet criteria for dementia, delirium, or amnestic disorders. DSM-III-R placed these remaining disorders within the category *organic mental syndrome not otherwise specified.* DSM-IV-TR uses the somewhat more precise diagnosis *cognitive disorder not otherwise specified* for cognitive disorders not meeting criteria for any of the dementia, delirium, or amnestic disorders. DSM-IV-TR specifically describes two syndromes that meet research criteria for cognitive disorder not otherwise specified: *postconcussional disorder* (Table 10.5–11) and *mild neurocognitive disorder* (Table 10.5–12). ICD-10 offers comparable diagnoses of *postconcussional syndrome* and *mild cognitive disorder.*

Postconcussional Disorder

In postconcussional disorder, head injury leads to an impairment in cognitive functioning after cerebral concussion. The latter is characterized by loss of consciousness and posttraumatic amnesia and, occasionally, posttraumatic seizures, according to DSM-IV-TR research criteria. Cognitive deficiencies may exist in attention or memory. In addition, the individual may experience a series of behavioral and mood changes. Impairment in the individual's usual level of functioning is significant, yet affected individuals do not meet cognitive criteria for dementia. In addition, they demonstrate somatic and behavioral complaints not present in amnestic disorder due to head trauma.

Table 10.5–11
DSM-IV-TR Research Criteria for Postconcussional Disorder

A. A history of head trauma that has caused significant cerebral concussion.

Note: The manifestations of concussion include loss of consciousness, posttraumatic amnesia, and, less commonly, posttraumatic onset of seizures. The specific method of defining this criterion needs to be established by further research.

B. Evidence from neuropsychological testing or quantified cognitive assessment of difficulty in attention (concentrating, shifting focus of attention, or performing simultaneous cognitive tasks) or memory (learning or recalling information).

C. Three (or more) of the following occur shortly after the trauma and last at least 3 months:
(1) Becoming easily fatigued
(2) Disordered sleep
(3) Headache
(4) Vertigo or dizziness
(5) Irritability or aggression on little or no provocation
(6) Anxiety, depression, or affective lability
(7) Changes in personality (e.g., social or sexual inappropriateness)
(8) Apathy or lack of spontaneity.

D. The symptoms in Criteria B and C have their onset after head trauma or else represent a substantial worsening of preexisting symptoms.

E. The disturbance causes significant impairment in social or occupational functioning and represents a significant decline from a previous level of functioning. In school-age children, the impairment may be manifested by a significant worsening in school or academic performance dating from the trauma.

F. The symptoms do not meet criteria for dementia due to head trauma and are not better accounted for by another mental disorder (e.g., amnestic disorder due to head trauma or personality change due to head trauma).

From American Psychiatric Association. *Diagnostic and Statistical Manual of Mental Disorders.* 4th ed. Text rev. Washington, DC; American Psychiatric Association; 2000, with permission.

Differential Diagnosis

Postconcussional disorder must be distinguished from malingering, especially in circumstances in which legal action is contemplated (e.g., subsequent to an automobile accident). Individuals who, after head injury, complain of fatigue, sleep impairment, or concentration impairment may meet the criteria for major depressive disorder or, occasionally, posttraumatic stress disorder (PTSD) and should be so diagnosed. Not uncommonly, head injury occurs in young men with concurrent substance disorders, which may require independent attention.

Treatment

In individuals with postconcussional disorder, mood and anxiety symptoms may be managed psychotherapeutically and psychopharmacologically. Medications with high anticholinergic side effects (e.g., amitriptyline and diphenhydramine [Benadryl]) or amnestic potential (e.g., benzodiazepines) should be used with caution. Cognitive remediation techniques occasionally may be useful. Individuals should be encouraged to conclude litigation as rapidly as is feasible.

Mild Neurocognitive Disorder

In mild neurocognitive disorder, a general medical condition results in cognitive deficits, which, by definition, are mild, but which nonetheless intrude on prior levels of functioning. The affected individual may be able to compensate for such deficits. Yet, if the causative medical condition is progressive, an individual with this disorder eventually may meet

Table 10.5–12
DSM-IV-TR Research Criteria for Mild Neurocognitive Disorder

A. The presence of two (or more) of the following impairments in cognitive functioning, lasting most of the time for a period of at least 2 weeks (as reported by the individual or a reliable informant):
 (1) Memory impairment as identified by a reduced ability to learn or to recall information
 (2) Disturbance in executive functioning (i.e., planning, organizing, sequencing, and abstracting)
 (3) Disturbance in attention or speed of information processing
 (4) Impairment in perceptual-motor abilities
 (5) Impairment in language (e.g., comprehension and word finding).
B. There is objective evidence from physical examination or laboratory findings (including neuroimaging techniques) of a neurological or general medical condition that is judged to be etiologically related to the cognitive disturbance.
C. There is evidence from neuropsychological testing or quantified cognitive assessment of an abnormality or decline in performance.
D. The cognitive deficits cause marked distress or impairment in social, occupational, or other important areas of functioning and represent a decline from a previous level of functioning.
E. The cognitive disturbance does not meet criteria for a delirium, a dementia, or an amnestic disorder and is not better accounted for by another mental disorder (e.g., substance-related disorder or major depressive disorder).

From American Psychiatric Association. *Diagnostic and Statistical Manual of Mental Disorders.* 4th ed. Text rev. Washington, DC; American Psychiatric Association; 2000, with permission.

criteria for dementia or amnestic disorder. Examples of general medical conditions capable of causing mild cognitive loss include chronic hypoxia due to cardiopulmonary disease; hypothyroidism; early stage Alzheimer's disease; early stage HIV infection of the CNS, causing HIV-associated minor cognitive-motor disorder; and Parkinson's disease. Structural brain imaging may be completely normal, although functional brain imaging (e.g., PET) occasionally may demonstrate abnormalities suggestive of one of the more advanced cognitive disorders into which mild neurocognitive disorder may evolve.

Differential Diagnosis Early delirium may resemble mild neurocognitive loss but progresses in a more rapid and fluctuating manner. Individuals with age-related cognitive decline, with cognitive complaints due to substance use, or with cognitive complaints occurring in the absence of demonstrated findings on neuropsychological testing should not be diagnosed with mild neurocognitive disorder. Individuals in the last group occasionally meet criteria for a mood disorder.

Treatment Correction of the underlying medical disorder, when possible, may not always result in complete eradication of cognitive loss but may slow or halt further deterioration.

MOOD DISORDER DUE TO A GENERAL MEDICAL CONDITION

Mood disorders, particularly depression, accompany a range of medical problems. Often in question is the link between a medical illness and associated mood symptoms: Is the mood disturbance a physiological or psychological reaction to the medical condition? Are the two conditions (medical and psychiatric) concurrent sequelae of another factor? Is the mood syndrome responsible for exacerbation of the limitations associated with the medical condition, as might be seen in depressed individuals with fatigue and somatic complaints?

Definition To meet criteria for *mood disorder due to a general medical condition*, the diagnostician must identify mood symptoms that are a direct physiological product of a general medical condition. The mood syndrome may be depressive, manic, or mixed in presentation. The mood disturbance need not meet precise criteria for a major depressive, manic, mixed, or hypomanic episode. Mental symptoms must not be better accounted for by a primary mental disorder, for example, adjustment disorder with depressed mood, occurring as psychological response to the medical condition. The diagnosis is not made if mood symptoms occur during the course of delirium, a clinical syndrome commonly accompanied by transitory shifts in mood.

A diagnosis of *substance-induced mood disorder* relies on the appearance of mood symptoms during intoxication or withdrawal. These mood symptoms must be in excess of those usually associated with intoxication with, or withdrawal from, the substance or must be severe enough to warrant independent clinical attention.

History and Comparative Nosology DSM-III-R offered a diagnosis of *organic mood syndrome* in its section on organic mental syndromes and disorders. Seemingly more restrictive in terms of mood symptoms than the DSM-IV-TR corresponding diagnoses, organic mood syndrome was defined by symptoms similar to either a manic or major depressive episode. Mild cognitive impairment often was said to be present. Diagnosis was not made in the presence of delirium.

Commencing with DSM-IV, organic mood syndrome was bifurcated into *mood disorder due to a general medical condition* and *substance-induced mood disorder*. Apart from the etiological difference, the diagnostic criteria for the disorders are nearly identical.

ICD-10 offers the diagnosis *organic mood (affective) disorder* for "depressive, hypomanic, manic, or bipolar" symptoms due to a medical condition or nonpsychoactive substance. Mood symptoms with onset during psychoactive substance use and persisting "beyond the period during which a direct psychoactive substance-related effect might reasonably be assumed to be operating" may be diagnosed as *residual or late-onset psychotic disorder*, a term rooted in a more historical view of psychosis as a state of severe psychiatric impairment, not simply one in which delusions or hallucinations are present. Alternatively, the clinician may code ICD-10's *harmful use* diagnosis, which applies to a "pattern of psychoactive substance use that is causing damage to health," whether physical or mental.

Epidemiology Mood disorder due to a general medical condition, with depressive features, appears to affect men and women equally, in contrast to major depressive disorder, which predominates in women. As much as 50 percent of all poststroke patients experience depressive illness. A similar prevalence pertains to individuals with pancreatic cancer. Forty percent of patients with Parkinson's disease are depressed. Depressive disorders associated with terminal or painful conditions carry the greatest risk of suicide.

Etiology The array of medical illnesses that physiologically are capable of inducing a mood syndrome includes neurological disorders (e.g., Parkinson's disease, Huntington's disease, Wilson's disease, MS, cerebrovascular disease, brain tumor, temporal lobe epilepsy, and neurosyphilis); metabolic and endocrine conditions (e.g., hypo- and hyperthyroidism, hypercalcemia, hypo- and hyperadrenocorticism, hypo- and hyperparathyroidism, and vitamin B_{12} deficiency); hematological and oncological disorders (anemia and pancreatic cancer); and infectious and inflammatory states (e.g., systemic lupus erythematosus and HIV).

Prescribed substances capable of inducing mood syndromes include agents from the following categories: stimulant and sympathomimetic (e.g., methylphenidate and theophylline [Asmalix]); corticosteroid; antiparkinsonian (e.g., L-dopa [Larodopa] and bromocriptine [Parlodel]); antidepressant (inducing manic symptoms); immunosuppressant (e.g., cyclosporine [Neoral] and tacrolimus [Prograf]); antihypertensive (e.g., β-blockers and methyldopa [Aldomet]); cancer chemotherapy (e.g., vincristine [Oncovin], vinblastine [Velban], interferon, and procarbazine [Matulane]); oral contraceptives; CNS depressant (e.g., benzodiazepines and barbiturates); heavy metals; and toxins (e.g., paint and carbon monoxide).

Substances of abuse that may produce mood symptoms in intoxication include stimulants (e.g., cocaine), opioids, hallucinogens, phencyclidine (PCP), and CNS depressants (e.g., alcohol).

Substances of abuse that may produce mood symptoms in withdrawal include stimulants (e.g., cocaine) and CNS depressants (e.g., alcohol).

As in primary mood disorders, pathophysiological mechanisms by which general medical conditions and substances induce mood syndromes likely involve impact on noradrenergic, dopaminergic, serotonergic, and cholinergic neurotransmission. Substances (e.g., reserpine [Serpalan]) and medical conditions (e.g., hypoxia) capable of depleting noradrenergic function may induce depression; agents (e.g., amphetamine) that stimulate noradrenergic activity may cause mania. Many metabolic and endocrine disorders appear to induce mood syndromes by impact on the hypothalamic-pituitary-adrenal axis. Demyelinating disorders, such as MS, may cause mania associated with lesions to the hypothalamus and temporal lobes of the brain. Patchy demyelination of the CNS associated with depression is observed in vitamin B_{12} deficiency. Cerebrovascular injury may induce depression through physiological means, although precise neuroanatomical correlates require further study.

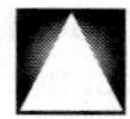

Table 10.5–13
DSM-IV-TR Criteria for Mood Disorder Due to a General Medical Condition

A. A prominent and persistent disturbance in mood predominates in the clinical picture and is characterized by either (or both) of the following:
  (1) Depressed mood or markedly diminished pleasure in all, or almost all, activities
  (2) Elevated, expansive, or irritable mood.

B. There is evidence from the history, physical examination, or laboratory findings that the disturbance is the direct physiological consequence of a general medical condition.

C. The disturbance is not better accounted for by another mental disorder (e.g., adjustment disorder with depressed mood in response to the stress of having a general medical condition).

D. The disturbance does not occur exclusively during the course of a delirium.

E. The symptoms cause clinically significant distress or impairment in social, occupational, or other important areas of functioning.

Specify:

With depressive features: if the predominant mood is depressed, but the full criteria are not met for a major depressive disorder

With major depressive–like episode: if all criteria for major depressive episode are met, except, clearly, for the criterion that the symptoms are not due to the physiological effects of a substance or a general medical condition

With manic features: if the predominant mood is elevated, euphoric, or irritable

With mixed features: if the symptoms of mania and depression are present, but neither predominates

From American Psychiatric Association. *Diagnostic and Statistical Manual of Mental Disorders.* 4th ed. Text rev. Washington, DC; American Psychiatric Association; 2000, with permission.

Diagnosis and Clinical Features

Patients with depression may experience psychological symptoms (e.g., sad mood, lack of pleasure or interest in usual activities, tearfulness, concentration disturbance, and suicidal ideation) or somatic symptoms (e.g., fatigue, sleep disturbance, and appetite disturbance), or both. Diagnosis in the medically ill may be confounded by the presence of somatic symptoms related purely to medical illness, not to depression. In an effort to overcome the underdiagnosis of depression in the medically ill, most practitioners favor including somatic symptoms in identifying mood syndromes.

In contrast to depressed individuals, those with mania present with irritable or euphoric mood, heightened energy, reduced need for sleep, and accelerated rate of thoughts. Occasionally, manic patients may engage in reckless activities with little consideration of the consequences of such behavior, such as excessive spending or risky sexual adventures.

The likelihood that a mood disorder is due to a general medical condition is increased if a temporal relationship exists between the onset, exacerbation, or remission of the medical condition and the mood disorder. Atypical features (e.g., unusual age of onset, lack of family history, and lack of prior episodes of mood disorder) also raise the likelihood of a medical basis to mood symptoms. A further supporting factor is evidence from the literature of a link between the medical condition and the development of specific mood symptoms.

Similar diagnostic considerations apply to substance-induced mood disorder. A primary mood disorder, or a mood disorder stemming from a general medical condition, is more likely if the mood symptoms develop in advance of the use of the suspect substance, persist for more than 4 weeks after cessation of use of the substance, are substantially in excess of what one would expect from the substance, or occur in an individual who previously experienced episodes of similar mood symptoms not attributable to the substance.

DSM-IV-TR provides diagnostic criteria for mood disorder due to a general medical condition *with depressive features*, *with major depressive–like episode*, *with manic features*, or *with mixed features*. In general, these criteria are less strict than for corresponding primary mood disorders. The subtype *with major depressive–like episode* is not available for substance-induced mood disorder (Table 10.5–13).

The name of the general medical condition is coded on Axis I (e.g., mood disorder due to hypothyroidism, with depressive features) and on Axis III.

If the mood disorder is substance-induced, the diagnostician may select *with onset during intoxication* or *with onset during withdrawal*, if the criteria for intoxication or withdrawal syndromes are met and if mood symptoms appear during one of those syndromes. The name of the causative substance is indicated on Axis I (e.g., cocaine-induced mood disorder, with depressive features, and with onset during withdrawal).

If mood symptoms are due to a general medical condition and a substance, both diagnoses are indicated. If mood symptoms cannot readily be attributed to a general medical condition, substance, or primary mood disorder, the clinician should diagnose mood disorder not otherwise specified.

A 45-year-old toy designer was admitted to the hospital after a series of suicidal gestures culminating in an attempt to strangle himself with a piece of wire. Four months before admission, his family had observed that he was becoming depressed: when at home, he spent long periods sitting in a chair, he slept more than usual, and he had given up his habits of reading the evening paper and puttering around the house. Within 1 month, he was unable to get out of bed in the morning to go to work. He expressed considerable guilt but could not make up his mind to seek help until forced to do so by his family. He had not responded to 2 months of outpatient antidepressant drug therapy and had made several half-hearted attempts to cut his wrists before the serious attempt that precipitated the admission.

Physical examination revealed signs of increased intracranial pressure, and a CT scan showed a large frontal-lobe tumor. (Reprinted with permission from *DSM-IV-TR Casebook*.)

In this case, provisional diagnosis recorded on Axis I is mood disorder due to brain tumor, with major depressive–like episode. Frontal lobe tumor is recorded on Axis III. This diagnosis would be supported if mood disturbance resolves after tumor resection. If it fails to do so, major depressive episode unrelated to brain tumor would also merit diagnostic consideration, especially if the individual had experienced previous such episodes earlier in life or had a family history of depression. In either case, antidepressant treatment would be appropriate for mood symptoms that fail to resolve after tumor resection.

Laboratory Evaluation Complete blood count and chemistries, thyroid function tests, serum vitamin B_{12} level, and urinalysis should be examined in all individuals with new-onset or atypical mood symptoms. Urine toxicology often is appropriate, particularly if abuse of substances is suspected. In selected cases, added laboratory studies, such as ESR, RPR, urinalysis, or lumbar puncture may be indicated. EEG or structural brain imaging, or both, should be considered in the absence of an overt medical or substance cause, the presence of cognitive impairment, or the report or presence of neurological symptoms (e.g., headache, motor or sensory loss, visual disturbance, or lethargy).

Differential Diagnosis Mood changes occurring during the course of delirium are acute and fluctuating and should be attributed to that disorder, not to mood disorder due to a general medical condition or to substance-induced mood disorder. Pain syndromes may depress mood but do so through psychological, not physiological means, and may appropriately lead to a diagnosis of primary mood disorder. In the medically ill, somatic complaints, such as sleep disturbance, anorexia, and fatigue, may be counted toward a diagnosis of major depressive episode or mood disorder due to a general medical condition, unless those complaints are purely attributable to the medical illness.

Mood disorder due to a general medical condition may be distinguished from substance-induced mood disorder by examination of time course of symptoms, response to correction of suspect medical conditions or discontinuation of substances, and, occasionally, by urine or blood toxicology results.

Course and Prognosis The course of mood disorder due to a general medical condition largely depends on the course of the underlying medical state, as well as the extent of concurrent psychiatric intervention. Similar considerations apply to substance-induced mood disorder. Prognosis for mood symptoms is best when etiological medical illnesses or medications are most susceptible to correction (e.g., treatment of hypothyroidism and cessation of alcohol use).

When such intervention is not possible (e.g., halting immunosuppressant use in an individual after kidney transplant) or fails to lead to prompt remission of mood symptoms, formal psychiatric treatment is indicated.

Treatment Pharmacotherapies should be designed to address mood symptoms while minimizing adverse interactions of prescribed antidepressant or mood-stabilizing medications with other concurrently prescribed medications. Selective serotonin reuptake inhibitors (SSRIs) used in depressive syndromes variably impact the cytochrome P450 enzyme system, thereby affecting the metabolism of other medications. Sertraline (Zoloft), citalopram (Celexa), and escitalopram (Lexapro) have a more limited impact on metabolism of other medications than do paroxetine (Paxil) and fluoxetine (Prozac). Bupropion (Wellbutrin) has stimulant properties that may be useful in the depressed, debilitated, medically ill individual. This drug must not be used in individuals with history of seizure. Mirtazapine (Remeron) may be especially useful in stimulating appetite in the anorectic or debilitated individual with depression. Similar benefit may be derived from psychostimulants, such as methylphenidate.

The clinician must recognize that medically ill individuals often are exquisitely sensitive to medication side effects and toxicities. For this reason, tricyclic antidepressants, which typically have a higher incidence of orthostatic hypotensive, anticholinergic, and cardiac conduction effects, rarely are preferred to SSRIs in the management of depression in the medically ill.

In manic or mixed mood states, divalproex is preferred to lithium (Eskalith); the latter has a low therapeutic index, with major toxicity considerations in medically ill patients at risk for dehydration or electrolyte imbalance. Other anticonvulsant agents potentially useful in mood stabilization include lamotrigine (Lamictal), carbamazepine (Tegretol), oxcarbazepine (Trileptal), and topiramate (Topamax). Drug interactions may complicate the use of anticonvulsants, particularly divalproex and carbamazepine.

In the anxious, depressed individual, caution must be exercised in the use of benzodiazepines, as these agents possess amnestic qualities that may exacerbate cognitive loss commonly present in the medically ill and elderly. When the use of benzodiazepines seems essential, agents with short half-lives (e.g., lorazepam [Ativan] and alprazolam [Xanax]) are preferred over agents with long half-lives (e.g., clonazepam [Klonopin] and diazepam [Valium]), particularly in individuals with impaired hepatic function.

In the elderly and in individuals with hepatic or renal impairment, psychotropic medications should be initiated at low dosages. Yet, if mood symptoms persist in the absence of serious toxicity or side effects, the clinician should titrate dosing upward until symptom relief is achieved, lest a premature diagnosis of treatment refractoriness be entertained. Interestingly, medically ill individuals often require psychopharmacological doses similar to those used in medically healthy individuals.

ECT, useful in severe depression (especially if associated with intense suicidal ideation), mania, and catatonia, has the advantage of being safe, highly effective, and arguably more rapid in onset than pharmacological modalities, a point of considerable importance in the debilitated, bedridden, anorectic patient for whom a feeding tube otherwise may be indicated. ECT may also be useful in patients whose GI tract is nonfunctional, thereby preventing the administration of antidepressant medications. Relative contraindications to ECT include conditions associated with increased intracranial pressure (e.g., brain tumor) or cardiac conditions associated with high risk of hemodynamic compromise (e.g., malignant arrhythmia).

Psychotherapies in the medically ill with depressed mood are geared to assisting with transition and fears regarding loss of autonomy. When pain is a factor depressing mood, this should be aggressively treated.

PSYCHOTIC DISORDER DUE TO A GENERAL MEDICAL CONDITION

Psychosis implies a departure from reality testing. Individuals with psychosis experience one or both of the following: delusions (i.e., fixed, false beliefs) and hallucinations (i.e., perception of stimuli not actually present). Psychotic symptoms may be seen in schizophrenia, *psychotic disorder due to a general medical condition*, and *substance-induced psychotic disorder*. They also may be seen in primary and secondary mood disorders, delusional disorders, cognitive disorders, and, occasionally, severe personality disorders.

Definition

DSM-IV-TR states that, in psychotic disorder due to a general medical condition, hallucinations, delusions, or both may be present and must be judged to be due to the physiological effects of a general medical condition. Importantly, delusions and hallucinations are regarded as psychotic only if the individual lacks insight into the unreality of these perceptual disturbances. The disturbance may not occur exclusively within the context of delirium and must not be better accounted for by a primary mental disorder.

Hallucinations may occur in any modality: visual, olfactory, gustatory, tactile, or auditory, or a combination of these. Delusions may involve simple or elaborate themes. They may be somatic, paranoid, religious, or grandiose.

History

Historically, the term *psychotic* was used broadly, often reserved for the most severe psychiatric conditions with the greatest impact on functioning. Thus, chronically disabling depressive illness and cognitive disorders (e.g., Korsakoff's psychosis) at one time were considered psychotic illnesses. ICD-10 continues to label severe substance-induced cognitive and mood syndromes as *residual and late onset psychotic disorders*. In focusing on hallucinations and delusions, DSM-IV-TR adheres to a narrower definition of psychosis.

Multiple theories, including those with religious, cultural, psychological, and biological aspects, have been advanced to explain the origin of psychosis. Over the course of centuries, demonic possession, moral decay, environmental stress, poor mothering, and, more recently, derangements of dopamine and serotonin metabolism have been offered.

Comparative Nosology

DSM-III-R offered two diagnoses: *organic delusional syndrome* and *organic hallucinosis*. Each diagnosis encompassed medically induced and substance-induced psychoses. Comparable DSM-IV and DSM-IV-TR psychoses are described as due to a general medical condition or substance-induced.

For psychoses stemming from general medical conditions and nonpsychoactive substances, ICD-10 provides coding for *organic delusional (schizophrenia-like) disorder* and *organic hallucinosis*. Also available is the diagnosis *psychotic disorder, psychoactive substance-induced.*

Epidemiology

Prevalence rates for these disorders are largely unknown. As much as 40 percent of individuals with temporal lobe epilepsy experience psychosis.

Etiology

Psychotic disorder due to a general medical condition is observed in diseases in these categories: neurological (e.g., Parkinson's disease, Huntington's disease, MS, visual and auditory defects, epilepsy, cerebrovascular accident, and head trauma); metabolic and endocrine (e.g., hypo- and hyperthyroidism, hypo- and hyperadrenocorticism, hypo- and hyperglycemia, hypoxia, hypercarbia, renal failure, hepatic failure, and Wilson's disease); infectious and inflammatory (e.g., systemic lupus erythematosus and HIV); and nutritional deficiency (e.g., vitamin B_{12} and thiamine).

Medications capable of inducing psychosis include agents in these categories: opioid (especially meperidine [Demerol]); anticholinergic (e.g., benztropine [Cogentin] and diphenhydramine); cardiovascular (e.g., digoxin [Lanoxin], procainamide [Promine], methyldopa); cancer chemotherapy (e.g., procarbazine); corticosteroid (e.g., prednisone [Cordrol] and dexamethasone [Decadron]); immunosuppressant (e.g., cyclosporine and tacrolimus); antiparkinsonian (e.g., L-dopa and bromocriptine); antitubercular (e.g., isoniazid [Laniazid]); sympathomimetic (e.g., theophylline and phenylephrine [Rhinall]); sedative-hypnotic, anxiolytic, and disulfiram (Antabuse).

Substances of abuse capable of inducing psychosis in intoxication include stimulants (e.g., amphetamine and cocaine), hallucinogens, PCP, inhalants, cannabis, opioids, and alcohol.

The major substance of abuse capable of inducing psychosis in withdrawal is alcohol.

Toxins capable of inducing psychosis include heavy metals, nerve gases, organophosphate insecticides, carbon monoxide, and volatile substances such as gasoline and paint.

As in primary psychoses, pathophysiological mechanisms are believed to involve alterations in metabolism of dopamine and other neurotransmitters. The importance of dopamine derangement likely accounts for the frequent association between psychosis and medical conditions (e.g., Parkinson's disease) and substances (e.g., amphetamine and L-dopa) affecting this neurotransmitter.

Diagnosis and Clinical Features

Two DSM-IV-TR subtypes exist for psychotic disorder due to a general medical condition: *with delusions*, to be used if the predominant psychotic symptoms are delusional, and *with hallucinations*, to be used if hallucinations of any form comprise the primary psychotic symptoms (Table 10.5–14).

The likelihood that psychotic symptoms are due to a general medical condition (or substance) is increased if a temporal relationship exists between the onset, exacerbation, or remission of the medical condition (or substance) and the psychotic disorder. A further supporting factor would be evidence from the literature supporting a link between the medical condition or substance and the development of psychotic symptoms. The presence of atypical features (e.g., onset after 45 years of age, lack of prior episodes of psychosis, and lack of family history of psychosis) also supports a diagnosis of psychotic disorder due to a general medical condition or substance-induced psychotic disorder.

In substance-induced psychotic disorder, symptoms must be substantially in excess of those ordinarily observed during intoxication or withdrawal or must merit independent clinical attention. Diagnosis is assisted further by the recognition that a primary psychotic disorder, or psychosis stemming from a medical illness, is more likely if the psychotic symptoms develop in advance of the use of the suspected substance, or persist for more than 4 weeks after cessation of

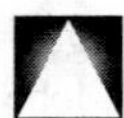

Table 10.5–14
DSM-IV-TR Criteria for Psychotic Disorder Due to a General Medical Condition

A. Prominent hallucinations or delusions.
B. There is evidence from the history, physical examination, or laboratory findings that the disturbance is the direct physiological consequence of a general medical condition.
C. The disturbance is not better accounted for by another mental disorder.
D. The disturbance does not occur exclusively during the course of a delirium.

Specify:
With delusions, if delusions are the predominant symptom
With hallucinations, if hallucinations are the predominant symptom

From American Psychiatric Association. *Diagnostic and Statistical Manual of Mental Disorders.* 4th ed. Text rev. Washington, DC; American Psychiatric Association; 2000, with permission.

use of the substance, or if prior episodes of similar psychotic symptoms could not be attributed to a substance.

For psychotic disorder due to a general medical condition, the etiological disorder is coded on Axis I (e.g., psychotic disorder due to Parkinson's disease, with delusions) and on Axis III (Parkinson's disease).

For substance-induced psychotic disorder, the responsible substance is indicated on Axis I. The diagnostician also may specify *with onset during intoxication* and *with onset during withdrawal.*

If the clinician suspects general medical and substance-induced roots to the psychosis, both diagnoses should be made. If the clinician is uncertain as to whether the psychosis is primary or induced by a medical condition or substance, the correct diagnosis is psychotic disorder not otherwise specified.

Laboratory Examination

When psychotic disorder due to a general medical condition or substance-induced psychotic disorder is suspected, complete blood count and chemistries, thyroid function tests, vitamin B_{12} level, RPR, and urinalysis should be examined. Urine toxicology usually is indicated. Structural brain imaging, EEG, and lumbar puncture should be considered for new-onset psychotic symptoms, lack of an overt etiological medical condition or substance, the presence of cognitive impairment, or the report or presence of neurological symptoms (e.g., headache, motor or sensory loss, visual disturbance, or lethargy).

Differential Diagnosis

Primary psychotic disorders, such as schizophrenia, and primary mood disorders with psychotic features may present with symptoms identical or similar to psychotic disorder due to a general medical condition; however, in primary disorders, no medical or substance cause is identifiable, despite laboratory workup. Delirium may present with psychotic symptoms, but, in contrast to psychotic disorder due to a general medical condition, delirium-related psychosis is acute and fluctuating, commonly associated with disturbance in consciousness and cognitive defects. Psychosis resulting from dementia may be diagnosed as psychotic disorder due to a general medical condition, except in the case of vascular dementia, which, according to ICD coding requirements, should be diagnosed as vascular dementia with delusions.

Unique characteristics may assist in differentiating primary from induced psychoses. Most cases of nonauditory hallucinosis are due to medical conditions, substances, or both. The converse is not true: Auditory hallucinations may occur in primary and induced psychoses. Stimulant (e.g., amphetamine and cocaine) intoxication psychosis may involve a perception of bugs crawling under the skin (formication). Temporal lobe epilepsy often is associated with olfactory hallucinations and religious delusions. Right parietal lobe lesions may induce a contralateral neglect state of delusional nature in which individuals disown parts of their bodies. Occipital lesions, whether due to tumor or cerebrovascular accident, may produce visual hallucinations.

First-rank symptoms of psychosis (i.e., thought broadcasting, thought withdrawal, and hallucinations of voices commenting or arguing) have been associated not only with schizophrenia, but also with disease of the dominant temporal lobe, including epilepsy.

When the clinician is considering the relative roles of medical conditions and substances in a patient with psychosis, diagnosis may be assisted by chronology of symptoms, response to removal of suspect substances or alleviation of medical illnesses, and toxicology results.

Course and Prognosis

The course of the underlying medical illness or substance use commonly dictates the course of psychosis due to a general medical conditions or substance, with several notable exceptions. Psychosis due to certain medications (e.g., immunosuppressants) gradually may subside even when use of those medications is continued. Minimizing dosages of such medications consistent with therapeutic efficacy often facilitates resolution of psychosis. Certain degenerative brain disorders (e.g., Parkinson's disease) may be characterized by episodic lapses into psychosis, even as the underlying medical condition advances. If abuse of substances persists over a lengthy period, psychosis (e.g., hallucinations from alcohol) may fail to remit even during extended intervals of abstinence.

Treatment

Aggressive efforts should be made to eradicate psychosis at the earliest stages, as symptoms tend to become more elaborate and ingrained over time if untreated. Apart from minimizing offending substances or treating causative medical illness, psychopharmacological and psychotherapeutic options may be considered.

Pharmacological interventions typically rely on antipsychotic agents. Atypical agents have a more favorable side effect profile than do typical agents and so are preferred. Medically ill individuals are especially susceptible to antipsychotic medication side effects (e.g., extrapyramidal signs [EPS], sedation, gait disturbance, and tardive dyskinesia). In patients with Parkinson's disease, first-line antipsychotic medication choices should include atypical agents with low incidence of EPS, such as quetiapine, olanzapine, or ziprasidone. Aripiprazole (Abilify) may represent another option. The atypical agent clozapine (Clozaril) has low incidence of EPS but is rarely selected owing to risk of agranulocytosis, which requires biweekly monitoring. For individuals who cannot or will not take oral antipsychotics, haloperidol and ziprasidone are available by IM route. Long-acting IM depot formulations of haloperidol (Haldol Decanoate), fluphenazine (Prolixin Decanoate), and risperidone (Risperdal Consta) may be useful for chronically medication-noncompliant individuals. Haloperidol may be administered IV, although this should be avoided in patients with prolonged QTc interval on ECG owing to risk of the malignant arrhythmia *torsades de points*. QTc prolongation also must be considered in using the atypical agents, especially ziprasidone, particularly when used in combination with other medications (e.g., quinidine [Cardioquin], dofetilide [Tikosyn], sotalol [Betapace], and moxifloxacin [Avelox]) that may prolong the QTc interval or in medical states associated with prolongation of the QTc interval (e.g., hypomagnesemia, hypokalemia, and congenital QT interval prolongation).

Antipsychotic agents should be dosed low when initiated, with gradual upward titration until symptoms are relieved. Anticholinergic agents (e.g., benztropine) as prophylaxis against EPS must be used with caution, or avoided entirely, as medically ill individuals often are sensitive to the cognition-impairing aspects of such agents. If EPS do occur, antipsychotic dose reduction or shift to an agent with a more favorable EPS profile (e.g., risperidone to quetiapine) may be considered before initiating an anticholinergic agent.

Psychotherapies should be geared to assisting the individual in identifying prodromal symptoms of psychosis (e.g., isolative behavior, suspiciousness, and sleep disorder) while coping with the social and occupational limitations imposed by psychosis. Most psychotherapeutic techniques are supportive and psychoeducational in nature. Psychotropic medication compliance may be impaired by limitations in the individual's insight into illness; this should be addressed in psychotherapy as well.

ANXIETY DISORDER DUE TO A GENERAL MEDICAL CONDITION

Anxiety is a ubiquitous symptom. It may be a product of an underlying anxiety disorder, primary or secondary, but often serves as a sentinel of other psychiatric disorders. It may manifest with symptoms of tension, unease, or nervousness or as full-scale panic attacks with subsequent avoidant or phobic sequelae. New-onset anxiety complaints always demand a search for underlying physiological factors.

Definition

In *anxiety disorder due to a general medical condition*, the individual experiences anxiety that causes clinically significant distress or impairment in functioning. This anxiety must represent a direct physiological, not emotional, consequence of a general medical condition. In *substance-induced anxiety disorder*, the anxiety symptoms are the product of a prescribed medication or stem from intoxication or withdrawal from a nonprescribed substance, typically a drug of abuse.

Comparative Nosology

DSM-III-R offered the diagnosis of *organic anxiety syndrome* to describe panic attacks or generalized anxiety stemming physiologically from specific organic factors. This single diagnosis covered medically induced and substance-induced anxiety syndromes. DSM-IV and DSM-IV-TR broadened the diagnosis to include obsessive-compulsive symptoms and, in the case of substance-induced anxiety, phobic symptoms.

ICD-10 offers the diagnosis of *organic anxiety disorder*, with generalized anxiety or panic aspects, for anxiety syndromes due to medical illnesses and nonpsychoactive substances. Pervasive personality and behavioral consequences due to a psychoactive substance may be diagnosed as *residual and late-onset psychotic disorder*. Alternatively, the clinician may diagnose *harmful use* of the psychoactive substance.

Epidemiology

Little data exist by which to estimate the prevalence of anxiety disorder due to a general medical condition. It is believed that medically ill individuals in general have higher rates of anxiety disorder than do the general population. Rates of panic and generalized anxiety are especially high in neurological, endocrine, and cardiology patients, although this finding does not necessarily prove a physiological link. Approximately one-third of patients with hypothyroidism and two-thirds of patients with hyperthyroidism may experience anxiety symptoms. As much as 40 percent of patients with Parkinson's disease have anxiety disorders. Prevalence of most anxiety disorders is higher in women than in men.

Etiology

Medical disorders that may induce anxiety include diseases in these categories: cardiopulmonary (e.g., arrhythmias, mitral valve prolapse, pulmonary embolism, chronic obstructive pulmonary disease, asthma, and congestive heart failure); neurological (e.g., seizure disorder, head injury, and vestibular disease); metabolic and endocrine (e.g., hyper- or hypothyroidism, hyperparathyroidism, hypoglycemia, adrenal dysfunction, pheochromocytoma, and vitamin B_{12} deficiency); and inflammatory and infectious (e.g., systemic lupus erythematosus and HIV).

Medications capable of inducing anxiety include agents in these categories: stimulant and sympathomimetic (e.g., theophylline, pseudoephedrine [Sudafed], and albuterol); antiparkinsonian, cardiovascular, antidepressant (especially SSRIs); anxiolytic (primarily when taken in as-needed fashion); corticosteroid; insulin; thyroid preparations; and caffeine preparations.

Substances of abuse that may induce anxiety symptoms in intoxication include stimulants (e.g., amphetamines, cocaine, caffeine), cannabis, PCP, inhalants, and hallucinogens.

Substances of abuse that may induce anxiety symptoms in withdrawal include alcohol, barbiturates, benzodiazepines, opioids, and nicotine.

Toxins such as carbon monoxide, paint, and gasoline fumes may induce anxiety.

Pathophysiologically, medical conditions and substances capable of inducing anxiety likely do so by derangements in noradrenergic, serotonergic, or GABA neurotransmission, or a combination of these. The locus ceruleus and limbic system appear to play key roles in modulating anxiety-related neurotransmitters. Medical conditions (e.g., hyperthyroidism, hypoxia, and pheochromocytoma) and agents (e.g., sympathomimetic agents and stimulants) that stimulate noradrenergic function increase anxiety. Postconcussive anxiety has been hypothesized to stem from injury to limbic structures.

Diagnosis and Clinical Features

Anxiety stemming from a general medical condition or substance may present with physical complaints (e.g., chest pain, palpitation, abdominal distress, diaphoresis, dizziness, tremulousness, and urinary frequency), generalized symptoms of fear and excessive worry, outright panic attacks associated with fear of dying or losing control, recurrent obsessive thoughts or ritualistic compulsive behaviors, or phobia with associated avoidant behavior (Table 10.5–15).

In anxiety disorder due to a general medical condition and substance-induced anxiety disorder, the symptoms may not be better accounted for by a primary mental disorder and must not occur exclusively during the course of a delirium. Anxiety symptoms must cause clinically significant distress or impairment in functioning.

Factors that assist in establishing the diagnosis of anxiety disorder due to a general medical condition include a temporal relationship between the onset, exacerbation, or relief of the general medical condition and anxiety symptoms; presentation that is atypical for a primary anxiety disorder (e.g., atypical age of onset and lack of family history); or an established link in the scientific literature between the general medical condition and anxiety symptoms.

Factors supportive of a diagnosis of substance-induced anxiety disorder include symptoms that, for substances of abuse, arise in the context of intoxication or withdrawal; these symptoms must be in excess of those usually associated with intoxication with, or withdrawal from, the substance and must warrant independent clinical

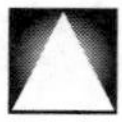

Table 10.5–15
DSM-IV-TR Criteria for Anxiety Disorder Due to a General Medical Condition

A. Prominent anxiety, panic attacks, or obsessions or compulsions predominate in the clinical picture.
B. There is evidence from the history, physical examination, or laboratory findings that the disturbance is the direct physiological consequence of a general medical condition.
C. The disturbance is not better accounted for by another mental disorder (e.g., adjustment disorder with anxiety in which the stressor is a serious general medical condition).
D. The disturbance does not occur exclusively during the course of a delirium.
E. The disturbance causes clinical significant distress or impairment in social, occupational, or other important areas of functioning.

Specify:

With generalized anxiety: if excessive anxiety or worry about a number of events or activities predominates in the clinical presentation

With panic attacks: if panic attacks predominate in the clinical presentation

With obsessive-compulsive symptoms: if obsessions or compulsions predominate in the clinical presentation

From American Psychiatric Association. *Diagnostic and Statistical Manual of Mental Disorders.* 4th ed. Text rev. Washington, DC; American Psychiatric Association; 2000, with permission.

attention. If symptoms arise in advance of substance use, persist for more than 4 weeks after substance use cessation, occur in an individual who has experienced prior similar episodes not related to substances, or are substantially more pronounced than what would be expected given the amount or duration of substance use, then another diagnosis (e.g., primary anxiety disorder or anxiety disorder due to a general medical condition) should be considered.

For anxiety disorder due to a general medical condition, three DSM-IV-TR specifiers exist: *with generalized anxiety, with panic attacks*, and *with obsessive-compulsive symptoms.* The etiological medical condition is indicated on Axis I (e.g., anxiety disorder due to pheochromocytoma, with generalized anxiety) and on Axis III.

For substance-induced anxiety disorder, the three previous specifiers, and a fourth, *with phobic symptoms*, are available. For substances of abuse, the clinician should indicate whether anxiety symptoms occurred *with onset during intoxication* or *with onset during withdrawal.* The substance is indicated on Axis I (e.g., caffeine-induced anxiety disorder, with panic attacks, and with onset during intoxication).

If the clinician believes that medical and substance factors contribute to the anxiety presentation, both diagnoses should be made. If the clinician is uncertain as to whether the anxiety disorder is primary or due to a general medical condition or substance, a diagnosis of anxiety disorder not otherwise specified is appropriate.

A 78-year-old retired lumber-company president sought help for the onset of a series of attacks in which he experienced marked apprehension, restlessness, and the need to be outdoors to relieve his sense of discomfort. He described the most recent event as having occurred at 3:00 AM a week earlier: He awoke from sleep and felt "the walls were caving in" on him. He denied that this was related to dreaming and said that he was fully awake at the time. He arose, dressed, and went outside in subzero weather; once outside, he noted gradual improvement (but not full resolution) of his symptoms. Complete resolution took a full day.

In response to pointed questioning, the patient denied dyspnea, palpitations, choking sensations, paresthesias, or nausea. He reported trembling and some sweating, together with intermittent dizziness. He imagined that he would die (or lose consciousness) if he could not "escape" from his house. He spoke of a need "to be active."

On questioning, the patient recalled a similar series of attacks almost 30 years earlier after eye surgery for an injury. He described bilateral patching of his eyes and being confined to bed for days, with his head sandbagged to preclude movement. Once ambulatory, he had experienced these attacks for more than 1 year.

The patient denied recent sleep dysfunction, change in appetite or weight, crying spells, or decreased energy. He had been taking diazepam for approximately 2 months for feelings of increased nervousness and tension. He had noted mild memory problems of late.

Further inquiry established a problem with balance and intermittent pain in the right arm and a complaint of indigestion and intermittent diarrhea. The patient had stopped gardening the past summer because of his balance problem. On examination, he was found to have a "beefy" red tongue (which he said was painful), difficulty with tandem gait and rapid alternating motion, and a mild intention tremor. He denied urinary incontinence.

Laboratory studies revealed a macrocytic anemia and vitamin B_{12} deficiency. The patient was given vitamin B_{12} replacement, and his attacks did not recur. (Reprinted with permission from *DSM-IV-TR Casebook.*)

The most important point illustrated by this case is that recurrence of mental symptoms after many years of relative quiescence of a seemingly primary mental disorder should prompt a search for a medical cause, especially in the absence of obvious precipitating factors.

Laboratory Examination

Routine laboratory studies appropriate in the evaluation of anxiety symptoms include complete blood count, electrolytes, glucose, blood urea nitrogen, creatinine, liver function tests, calcium, magnesium, phosphorus, thyroid function tests, and urine toxicology. Occasionally, additional studies may be indicated (e.g., urinary catecholamines to rule out pheochromocytoma, EEG to rule out seizure disorder, Holter monitoring to rule out cardiac arrhythmia, and ABG to rule out acute pulmonary processes). Brain imaging may be useful in ruling out demyelinating disorder, tumor, or hydrocephalus and is especially important if the anxious individual reports neurological symptoms (e.g., headache, motor or sensory changes, and dizziness), although such complaints may represent somatic manifestations of primary anxiety disorders. Lumbar puncture may be appropriate if an inflammatory or infectious cause is suspected.

Differential Diagnosis

Anxiety disorder due to a general medical condition symptomatically may resemble corresponding primary anxiety disorders. Acute onset, lack of family history, and occurrence within the context of acute medical illness or introduction of new medications or substances suggest a nonprimary cause.

Individuals with delirium commonly experience anxiety and panic symptoms, but these fluctuate and are accompanied by other delirium symptoms such as cognitive loss and inattentiveness; furthermore, anxiety symptoms diminish as delirium subsides. Patients with psychosis of any origin may experience anxiety commonly related to delusions or hallucinations. Depressive disorders often present with anxiety symptoms, mandating that the clinician inquire broadly about depressive symptoms in any patient whose primary complaint is anxiety. Dementia often is associated with agitation or anxiety, especially at night (called *sundowning*), but an independent anxiety diagnosis is warranted only if it becomes a source of prominent clinical attention. Adjustment disorders with anxiety arising within the context of reaction to medical or other life stressors should not be diagnosed as anxiety disorder due to a general medical condition.

In distinguishing anxiety due to medical illness from that due to substances, differential diagnosis may be assisted by examination of anxiety symptom chronology, response to correction or removal of suspect medical conditions and substances, and, occasionally, examination of toxicology results.

Course and Prognosis Anxiety disorder due to a general medical condition usually fluctuates in direct relation to the course of the provoking factor. Medical conditions responsive to treatment or cure (e.g., correction of hypothyroidism and reduction in caffeine consumption) often provide concomitant relief of anxiety symptoms, although such relief may lag the rate or extent of improvement in the underlying medical condition. Chronic, incurable medical conditions associated with persistent physiological insult (e.g., chronic obstructive pulmonary disease) or recurrent relapse to substance use may contribute to seeming refractoriness of associated anxiety symptoms. In medication-induced anxiety, if complete cessation of the offending factor (e.g., immunosuppressant therapy) is not possible, dose reduction, when clinically feasible, often brings substantial relief.

Treatment Pharmacologically, generalized anxiety symptoms may respond to buspirone (BuSpar), SSRIs, and benzodiazepines; the last should be used with caution in substance-abusing individuals, in patients with advanced pulmonary disease (due to risk of respiratory depression), and in those with pronounced cognitive defects. Panic symptoms may respond to SSRIs, tricyclic antidepressants (e.g., nortriptyline [Pamelor]), or benzodiazepines. High potency benzodiazepines, such as alprazolam and clonazepam, are most efficacious. Obsessive-compulsive symptoms may respond to SSRIs or clomipramine (Anafranil). When using SSRIs in anxiety disorders, starting doses should be low, so as to minimize transitory anxiogenic side effects. Tricyclic agents may be especially useful in anxiety states associated with chronic pain, but otherwise must be used with caution due to anticholinergic, orthostatic, and cardiac side effects.

Antipsychotic medications occasionally are used for time-limited management of severe anxiety, often in the context of fleeting cognitive or psychotic symptoms, as may be seen in patients treated with corticosteroids. With brief use, the risk of tardive dyskinesia is negligible. Atypical agents, owing to lower risk of EPS compared to typical agents, are preferred.

As for nonbiological therapies, if substance abuse is suspected, inpatient or outpatient treatment may be indicated. Cognitive and relaxation therapies may be useful in diminishing phobic, panic, and avoidant symptoms. Insight-oriented exploration of stressful life circumstances may be helpful once severe anxiety symptoms are contained pharmacologically.

SLEEP DISORDER DUE TO A GENERAL MEDICAL CONDITION

Several categories of sleep disturbances exist: sleep difficulties arising within the context of other mental disorders (e.g., depression, anxiety, psychosis, and dementia); sleep difficulties stemming from the direct physiological effects of a general medical condition or substance; and primary sleep disorders, which are a product of disturbances in sleep–wake cycle timing or generation. DSM-IV-TR divides primary sleep disorders into the dyssomnias (disturbance in sleep timing or quality or duration) and the parasomnias (abnormal behaviors associated with specific sleep stages, such as sleepwalking).

Definition In *sleep disorder due to a general medical condition*, the patient presents with dyssomnia or parasomnia, or a combination of the two. There must be direct evidence from history, physical, examination, or laboratory findings that a general medical condition is physiologically responsible for the sleep disturbance. In *substance-induced sleep disorder*, a medication or substance intoxication or withdrawal state is physiologically responsible. The sleep disturbance may not be better accounted for by another mental disorder, such as adjustment disorder associated with insomnia related to the stress of medical illness. Similarly, the diagnosis is not made in the context of delirium, which commonly causes sleep disturbance. Finally, the sleep disturbance must cause clinically significant distress or impairment in functioning.

Sleep-related breathing disorder (i.e., sleep apnea) and narcolepsy have unique diagnoses and therefore are specifically excluded from the diagnosis of sleep disorder due to a general medical condition.

Comparative Nosology DSM-III-R provided for *insomnia related to a known organic factor* (i.e., medical illness or substance), a category that included conditions that disturb sleep through pain and physical discomfort (e.g., arthritis and nocturnal myoclonus). This diagnosis also included physiological disturbances unique to sleep, such as sleep apnea, which have been excluded from the corresponding DSM-IV and DMS-IV-TR diagnoses. DSM-III-R also provided for *hypersomnia related to a known organic factor* (i.e., medical illness or substance), a category that included physiological disturbances unique to sleep, such as sleep apnea and narcolepsy, again excluded from the corresponding DSM-IV and DSM IV-TR diagnoses. For parasomnias related to general medical conditions or substances, DSM-III-R offered the diagnosis *parasomnia not otherwise specified.* All organic sleep diagnoses were included in the sleep disorders section of DSM-III-R, not in the organic mental disorders section reserved for cognitive, mood, psychotic, anxiety, and personality disorders with medical or substance underpinnings. This foreshadowed DSM-IV's grouping together of disorders, whether primary or induced, presenting with similar phenomenology.

ICD-10 provides for diagnosis of *organic sleep disorder*, a category that includes organic insomnia, organic hypersomnia, and narcolepsy.

Epidemiology The prevalence of sleep disorder due to a general medical condition and substance-induced sleep disorder is unknown. Elderly individuals with health issues impairing sleep (e.g., pain syndromes and cardiopulmonary disorders) and younger individuals with substance use disorders are likely at heightened risk for development of these disorders.

Etiology A variety of medical conditions and substances may contribute to sleep disturbance. Total sleep time, circadian sleep–wake cycles, and sleep architecture (i.e., characteristic patterns of nonrapid eye movement [NREM] sleep alternating with rapid eye movement [REM] sleep) may be disrupted by intrinsic brain diseases, by conditions that cause nocturnal physical distress, and by other medical conditions and substances acting through physiological mechanisms not always well understood.

Medical conditions capable of disrupting sleep include neurological disorders (e.g., dementia [especially when associated with nocturnal agitation]); movement disorders [including Parkinson's disease and Huntington's disease], stroke, and epilepsy); cardiopulmonary disorders (e.g., congestive heart failure with nocturnal dyspnea, chronic obstructive pulmonary disease, asthma, and arrhythmia); GI disorders (e.g., hepatic failure and gastroesophageal reflux); metabolic and endocrine disorders (e.g., hyper- or hypothyroidism and hyper- or hypoadrenocorticism); and pain or physical discomfort syndromes (e.g., arthritis, fibromyalgia, and diabetic neuropathy). Also included in the last category is *restless legs syndrome*, a condition characterized by aching and involuntary movement of the legs, often associated with renal failure, anemia, and diabetes mellitus.

Rare conditions associated with hypersomnia include Kleine-Levin syndrome (characterized also by hypersexuality and increased eating) and Prader-Willi syndrome (characterized also by mental retardation and obesity).

Medications that may induce sleep disorder include agents in these categories: sympathomimetic (e.g., theophylline); dopaminergic (e.g., L-dopa, methylphenidate, and bupropion); corticosteroid; psychotropic (e.g., SSRIs and sedative-hypnotic or anxiolytic agents if used sporadically); and thyroid preparations.

Substances that may induce sleep disorder during intoxication or withdrawal include alcohol, marijuana, opioids, amphetamine, cocaine, and caffeine.

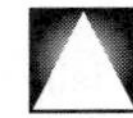

Table 10.5–16
DSM-IV-TR Criteria for Sleep Disorder Due to a General Medical Condition

A. A prominent disturbance in sleep that is sufficiently severe to warrant independent clinical attention.

B. There is evidence from the history, physical examination, or laboratory findings that the sleep disturbance is the direct physiological consequence of a general medical condition.

C. The disturbance is not better accounted for by another mental disorder (e.g., an adjustment disorder in which the stressor is a serious medical illness).

D. The disturbance does not occur exclusively during the course of a delirium.

E. The disturbance does not meet the criteria for breathing-related sleep disorder or narcolepsy.

F. The sleep disturbance causes clinically significant distress or impairment in social, occupational, or other important areas of functioning.

Specify type:

Insomnia type: if the predominant sleep disturbance is insomnia

Hypersomnia type: if the predominant sleep disturbance is hypersomnia

Parasomnia type: if the predominant sleep disturbance is a parasomnia

Mixed type: if more than one sleep disturbance is present and none predominate of comparable sexual dysfunction that was not substance-induced

From American Psychiatric Association. *Diagnostic and Statistical Manual of Mental Disorders.* 4th ed. Text rev. Washington, DC; American Psychiatric Association; 2000, with permission.

Diagnosis and Clinical Features

As with other mental illnesses due to general medical conditions, the likelihood that a sleep disorder is physiologically based is increased if the clinician can establish a temporal link between onset, cessation, or exacerbation of the general medical condition and the sleep disturbance. Other factors favoring this diagnosis include presentation atypical for corresponding primary sleep disorders and a known etiological association between the general medical condition and the sleep symptoms. Similar considerations apply with regard to substance-induced sleep disorder.

In addition, the sleep disorder must be severe enough to warrant clinical attention, must not be better accounted for by another mental disorder, does not occur exclusively during the course of a delirium, and does not meet criteria for breathing-related sleep disorder (i.e., sleep apnea) or narcolepsy. The sleep disturbance must cause clinically significant distress or impairment in functioning.

For a diagnosis of substance-induced sleep disorder, the individual must experience symptoms of sleep disturbance that are in excess of those that would normally be due to the specific substance. For drugs of abuse, the clinician must find clinical or laboratory evidence of abuse, dependence, withdrawal, or intoxication. For drugs with long half-lives (e.g., diazepam), the onset of sleep disturbance may occur as long as several weeks after abstinence, although, in general, onset of sleep disturbance more than 4 weeks after cessation of substance use suggests that the disturbance is more likely accounted for by a primary sleep disorder or a general medical condition.

DSM-IV-TR describes diagnostic criteria for sleep disorder due to a general medical condition (Table 10.5–16). Specifiers include *insomnia type*, *hypersomnia type*, *parasomnia type*, and *mixed type*. DSM-IV-TR recording procedures dictate that the medical condition be indicated on Axis I (e.g., sleep disorder due to chronic obstructive pulmonary disease, insomnia type) and on Axis III.

Substance-induced sleep disorder allows for the use of the same specifiers available for sleep disorder due to a general medical condition; also available are the specifiers *with onset during intoxication* and *with onset during withdrawal*. The responsible substance is indicated on Axis I.

If both a general medical condition and substance appear etiological, both diagnoses should be made. If evidence adequate to support neither is present, a diagnosis of dyssomnia or parasomnia not otherwise specified should be considered.

Laboratory Examination

Most general medical conditions decrease total sleep duration and increase awakenings. In addition to checking complete blood count and serum chemistries, the clinician may wish to obtain, in selected cases, thyroid function tests, urine toxicology, ECG, or arterial blood gas measurements. Sleep-related seizures produce EEG abnormalities characteristic of the underlying seizure disorder. Distinct patterns of alpha EEG activity may be observed during NREM sleep in individuals with fibromyalgia.

Differential Diagnosis

Patients with mood disorder may have sleep disturbance, but, unless this warrants independent clinical attention, efforts should be made to correcting the underlying mood syndrome, whether primary or secondary, and a diagnosis of sleep disorder should not be made. Individuals with dementia commonly experience fragmentation of sleep–wake cycles; diagnosis of sleep disorder due to a general medical condition should be made only if sleep disturbance is prominent. As sleep disturbance is a common accompaniment of delirium, an independent diagnosis of sleep disorder due to a general medical condition is not warranted.

Often, the distinction between sleep disorder due to a general medical condition and substance-related sleep disorder is complicated. For example, an individual with chronic obstructive pulmonary disease taking sympathomimetic agents may experience sleep disturbance due to these agents or to the underlying medical condition. Examination of chronology of sleep symptoms, especially as they relate to correction of associated medical conditions or removal of suspect substances, frequently proves diagnostically useful.

Course and Treatment

Sleep disorder due to a general medical condition may improve with correction of the underlying medical condition. Individuals with cardiopulmonary conditions may require adjustment in pharmacological regimens designed to facilitate comfort while recumbent. Pain syndromes may warrant heightened use of analgesics, particularly in proximity to bedtime. Restless legs syndrome may be managed with benzodiazepines, opioids, or dopaminergic agents.

Many individuals with sleep disorder benefit from provision of advice on sleep hygiene, with emphasis on avoidance of daytime napping. The individual should be encouraged to adopt regular bedtime hours. Relaxation strategies may be indicated, especially for the individual who, as bedtime approaches, experiences anxiety conditioned by an awareness of prior sleep difficulties.

Judicious use of sedative-hypnotics may be warranted to break a cycle of sleep disorder and the resultant anxiety that some patients experience. Short courses of treatment are advised. Tolerance and dependence tend to develop with extended use, compounding sleep disturbance and often inciting resistance at sedative-hypnotic taper by individuals reluctant to experience temporary withdrawal phenomena. Caution also must be used in patients with pulmonary disease due to risk of respiratory depression.

Short-acting agents, such as zolpidem (Ambien) or zaleplon (Sonata), are preferred in the elderly and in those experiencing initial insomnia. Longer-acting agents, such as flurazepam (Dalmane), risk inducing daytime hangover effect, cognitive impairment, and increased fall risk, especially in the elderly, including those with dementia. Trazodone (Desyrel) and gabapentin (Neurontin) do not cause physiological dependence; both have been successfully used in dementia-related and other sleep disturbances, including those related to the use of SSRIs. Occasionally, brief courses of atypical antipsychotic agents, such as olanzapine and risperidone, are useful in regularizing sleep in the elderly and in hospitalized patients; these agents pose little risk of inducing delirium or exacerbating cognitive impairment, to which these populations are highly susceptible. If depression is contributing to sleep disturbance, antidepressant pharmacotherapy should be considered. Tricyclic agents (e.g., nortriptyline) may be especially useful if pain contributes to sleep difficulties. Older sleep-inducing agents, such as chloral hydrate or meprobamate (Miltown), are rarely used.

James Thompson, a 62-year-old married man, has diabetic neuropathy, which contributes to bilateral leg pain and resultant middle-of-the-night awakening. Recently, after undergoing surgical resection of pancreatic cancer, Mr. Thompson began to experience difficulty falling asleep as well.

At the time of interview, Mr. Thompson reported that he was depressed and worried about his cancer diagnosis. He had concentration difficulties and loss of pleasure in usual activities. Furthermore, as bedtime approached, he acknowledged becoming extremely anxious in anticipation of sleep difficulties. Mr. Thompson slept into the late morning hours and took daytime naps to compensate for nocturnal sleep difficulties. To promote sleep, his general practitioner had prescribed diazepam, and then temazepam (Restoril), with limited success.

A trial of nortriptyline, 25 mg at bedtime, was initiated to foster pain relief and to promote sleep. When this proved only partially efficacious, trazodone, 50 mg at bedtime, was added. Mr. Thompson was instructed to establish a standard time for lying down at night and arising in the morning. Evening relaxation strategies also were identified. Nortriptyline dosing was gradually raised until an antidepressant therapeutic blood level was achieved. Psychotherapy was used to assist Mr. Thompson in coping with his medical problems and his fears of death related to his cancer diagnosis. With this regimen, pain, mood, and sleep symptoms gradually subsided.

This vignette illustrates the multifactorial nature of many medically induced and substance-induced sleep disorders: (1) the role of a medical condition (i.e., pain) in initiating sleep disturbance; (2) the interposition of another psychiatric condition (i.e., depression) in compounding the sleep disturbance; (3) the limited value of sedative-hypnotic agents, when not combined with other corrective measures; and (4) the efforts made to compensate for lost sleep by change in sleep and nap patterns, behavior that tends to exacerbate sleep disturbance.

SEXUAL DYSFUNCTION DUE TO A GENERAL MEDICAL CONDITION

Sexual dysfunction due to a general medical condition subsumes multiple forms of medically induced sexual disturbance, including erectile dysfunction, pain during sexual intercourse, low sexual desire, and orgasmic disorders. Sexual dysfunction often has psychological and physical underpinnings. The former often relate to social and cultural views of appropriate sexual functioning. The medically ill are at risk for sexual dysfunction, particularly because related psychiatric illness, including depression, sleep disturbance, and anxiety syndromes, may impair interest in, or adequacy of, sexual functioning. Chronic depression, relationship disturbances commonly found in personality-disordered individuals, and concurrent substance abuse may confound the search for etiology.

Definition

To qualify for the diagnosis of sexual dysfunction due to a general medical condition, sexual symptoms must be physiologically induced by a general medical condition and must cause interpersonal difficulty or marked distress. Furthermore, the dysfunction must not be better accounted for by another mental disorder (e.g., major depressive disorder). Similar considerations apply to *substance-induced sexual dysfunction.*

Comparative Nosology

DSM-III-R provided no allowance for sexual dysfunction attributable "exclusively to organic factors." A formal DSM-III-R diagnosis was provided if psychological factors were at least partially contributing to the sexual dysfunction. Specifiers included dysfunction that was psychogenic only, or both psychogenic and biogenic (i.e., organic). Conditions believed to be purely organic were recorded exclusively on Axis III, not on Axis I. Furthermore, sexual dysfunction diagnoses were not to be made if the dysfunction occurred exclusively within the context of another Axis I mental disorder.

DSM-III-R diagnoses included sexual desire disorders (i.e., hypoactive sexual desire disorder, sexual aversion disorder, female sexual arousal disorder, and male erectile disorder), orgasm disorders (i.e., inhibited female orgasm, inhibited male orgasm, and premature ejaculation), and sexual pain disorders (i.e., dyspareunia and vaginismus).

In contrast to DSM-III-R, DSM-IV and DSM-IV-TR incorporate into the psychiatric diagnostic nomenclature sexual dysfunction due exclusively to physiological factors. The clinician need not identify a psychological component to select a diagnosis.

ICD-10 classifies organic sexual dysfunction under *diseases of the genitourinary system.* Included are disorders such as impotence of organic origin and organic vaginismus. ICD-10 also contains diagnoses for *sexual dysfunction not caused by organic disorder or disease.* Conditions classified therein include lack of sexual desire, sexual aversion, failure of genital response (e.g., erectile dysfunction), orgasmic dysfunction, premature ejaculation, nonorgasmic vaginismus, nonorganic dyspareunia, excessive sexual drive, and other and unspecified sexual dysfunction. Less obvious is the manner in which disorders with both organic and nonorganic underpinnings are to be classified by ICD-10.

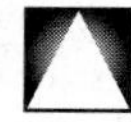

Table 10.5–17
DSM-IV-TR Criteria for Sexual Dysfunction Due to a General Medical Condition

A. Clinically significant sexual dysfunction that results in marked distress or interpersonal difficulty predominates in the clinical picture.

B. There is evidence from the history, physical examination, or laboratory findings that the sexual dysfunction is fully explained by the direct physiological effects of a general medical condition.

C. The disturbance is not better accounted for by another mental disorder (e.g., major depressive disorder).

Select code and term based on the predominant sexual dysfunction:

Female hypoactive sexual desire disorder due to . . . [insert general medical condition here]: if deficient or absent sexual desire is the predominant feature.

Male hypoactive sexual desire disorder due to . . . [insert general medical condition here]: if deficient or absent sexual desire is the predominant feature.

Male erectile disorder due to . . . [insert general medical condition here]: if male erectile dysfunction is the predominant feature.

Female dyspareunia due to . . . [insert general medical condition here]: if pain associated with intercourse is the predominant feature.

Male dyspareunia due to . . . [insert general medical condition here]: if pain associated with intercourse is the predominant feature.

Other female sexual dysfunction due to . . . [insert general medical condition here]: if some other feature is predominant (e.g., orgasmic disorder) or if no feature predominates.

Other male sexual dysfunction due to . . . [insert general medical condition here]: if some other feature is predominant (e.g., orgasmic disorder) or if no feature predominates.

From American Psychiatric Association. *Diagnostic and Statistical Manual of Mental Disorders.* 4th ed. Text rev. Washington, DC; American Psychiatric Association; 2000, with permission.

Epidemiology

Sexual behavior and functioning often have been shrouded in fear, embarrassment, or secrecy, confounding epidemiological inquiries. Little is known regarding the prevalence of sexual dysfunction due to general medical illness. In general, prevalence rates for sexual complaints are highest for female hypoactive sexual desire and orgasm problems and for premature ejaculation in men. High rates of sexual dysfunction are described in cardiac, cancer, diabetes, and HIV patients. Forty to 50 percent of individuals with MS describe sexual dysfunction. Cerebrovascular accident impairs sexual functioning, with the possibility that, in men, greater impairment follows right-hemispheric cerebrovascular injury than left-hemispheric injury. Delayed orgasm may affect as much as 50 percent of individuals taking SSRIs.

Etiology

An array of medical conditions and substances may contribute, alone or in combination with psychological factors, to sexual dysfunction. These include genitourinary conditions (e.g., prostate disease and surgery, atrophic vaginitis, uterine prolapse, pelvic infections, endometriosis, and Peyronie's disease); endocrine conditions (e.g., diabetes mellitus, hypothyroidism, hyperprolactinemia, and pituitary dysfunction); and neurological disease (e.g., spinal cord injuries, neuropathy, and MS).

Medications that may cause diminished sexual interest and orgasmic dysfunction include antihypertensive agents, antidepressant agents (particular SSRIs), anticonvulsants, and antipsychotics. Additionally, antipsychotic agents, such as haloperidol and fluphenazine, may contribute to painful orgasm. Trazodone occasionally causes priapism.

Other substances that contribute to sexual dysfunction in intoxication include amphetamine, cocaine, and other stimulants; opioids; alcohol; and sedative-hypnotics.

Diagnosis and Clinical Features

For sexual dysfunction due to a general medical condition, clinical history, physical examination, or laboratory studies must demonstrate the presence of a general medical condition that physiologically causes the sexual dysfunction. As with other mental disorders due to general medical conditions, factors that support an association between the medical illness and the sexual dysfunction include the presence of a temporal connection between the onset, exacerbation, or remission of the two conditions; atypical aspects to the presentation (e.g., unusual age or lack of family history); and a link in the scientific literature between the general medical condition and the sexual dysfunction. Diagnosis is not made if a primary mental disorder or primary sexual dysfunction better accounts for presenting symptoms.

Similar considerations apply to substance-induced sexual dysfunction. That diagnosis is not made unless sexual dysfunction is in excess of that which ordinarily would be encountered in substance intoxication and if the symptoms are severe enough to warrant independent clinical attention (Table 10.5–17).

Factors supporting a non–substance-induced (i.e., primary or general medical) origin to sexual dysfunction include symptoms beginning in advance of initiation of the substance, symptoms persisting beyond 4 weeks after use of the substance is halted, symptoms substantially in excess of what would be expected based on the type or amount or duration of substance use, or a history of prior episodes of sexual dysfunction not attributable to the substance.

For sexual dysfunction due to a general medical condition, multiple diagnostic subtypes exist, including *female hypoactive sexual desire disorder, male hypoactive sexual desire disorder, male erectile disorder, female dyspareunia, male dyspareunia, other female sexual dysfunction,* and *other male sexual dysfunction.*

The etiological medical condition is indicated on Axis I (e.g., male erectile disorder due to diabetes mellitus). The medical condition also is indicated on Axis III

For substance-induced sexual dysfunction, four diagnostic specifiers are available: *with impaired desire, with impaired arousal, with impaired orgasm,* and *with sexual pain.* In addition, the specifier *with onset during intoxication* should be used if symptoms develop during an intoxication syndrome. The etiological substance is recorded on Axis I (e.g., alcohol-induced sexual dysfunction, with impaired desire).

If a general medical condition and a substance contribute to sexual dysfunction, both diagnoses are indicated on Axis I.

Laboratory Examination

A variety of studies may be useful in identifying medical or hormonal causes of sexual dysfunction; these include serum testosterone and prolactin levels. In men, vascular studies and nocturnal penile tumescence measurements may prove helpful. Urine toxicology may be relevant if substance abuse is suspected.

Differential Diagnosis

The diagnosis of sexual dysfunction due to a general medical condition is made if the dysfunction is fully explained by the medical condition. Similarly, the diagnosis of substance-induced sexual dysfunction is made if a substance is fully explanatory. When the clinician encounters difficulty in distinguishing sexual dysfunction that may be substance-induced from that which may be due to a concurrent medical condition, differential diagnosis may be facilitated by observation after discontinuation of the suspect substance.

When psychological factors and medical (or substance) factors are judged to be contributory, the appropriate diagnosis is the primary sexual dysfunction, with the subtype *due to combined factors*. If the clinician is unable to discern origin after assessing for primary, general medical, and substance-related factors, the diagnosis of sexual dysfunction not otherwise specified is appropriate.

Sexual interest and arousal may be diminished in a variety of mood disorders (e.g., major depressive disorder), personality disorders (e.g., avoidant personality disorder), and interpersonal relationship disturbances. Sexual dysfunction under these circumstances is not traceable to specific medical conditions or substances and is not diagnosed unless it causes marked distress or interpersonal difficulty. In addition, diminished sexual interest or functioning accompanying aging is not diagnosed as sexual dysfunction due to a general medical condition.

Course and Prognosis

The course of sexual dysfunction due to a general medical condition or substance is highly variable, typically depending on etiology. Optimization of management of general medical conditions (e.g., diabetes) may ameliorate the extent or progression of sexual dysfunction. When contributory substances can be halted, or, in the case of medications, alternative agents can be used, relief of sexual dysfunction commonly ensues.

Treatment

Apart from addressing contributory medical factors and substances, treatment usually consists of psychotherapeutic and psychopharmacological interventions. Interpersonal or character issues exacerbating sexual dysfunction, including depression, anger, and relationship problems, may be dealt with in individual psychotherapy or couple's counseling. Substance counseling may be indicated.

Pharmacologically, contributory mood and anxiety disturbances must be addressed, although the clinician must consider the potentially aggravating effects on sexual function of SSRIs, which often are prescribed for these conditions. Bupropion may overcome effects of sexual dysfunction related to the use of SSRIs and may be added to the pharmacological regimen of patients who have achieved considerable psychiatric benefit from these agents.

Sildenafil (Viagra) and vardenafil (Levitra) have been used successfully to treat erectile dysfunction stemming from primary and medically induced or substance-induced sexual dysfunction. Anecdotal evidence suggests that these agents also may be useful in women with sexual arousal difficulties. Due to potentiation of hypotensive side effects, sildenafil and vardenafil must be used with caution in patients taking nitrates for coronary artery disease. With the advent of these agents, the use of penile prosthetic devices for management of erectile dysfunction has waned.

CATATONIC DISORDER DUE TO A GENERAL MEDICAL CONDITION

Before the introduction of antipsychotic medications, catatonia episodically was encountered in patients with severe mental illness. An occasional aspect of psychotic and severe mood disorders, catatonia also may be due to a general medical condition or substance.

Definition

Catatonia is a clinical syndrome characterized by striking behavioral abnormalities, often including motoric immobility or excitement, profound negativism, or echolalia (mimicry of speech) or echopraxia (mimicry of movement). To meet criteria for *catatonic disorder due to a general medical condition*, evidence must exist in the history, physical examination, or laboratory studies that the condition is due to the physiological effects of a general medical condition and is not better explained by a primary mental disorder, such as schizophrenia or psychotic depression. As with other mental disorders due to general medical conditions, the diagnosis is not made if catatonic symptoms occur exclusively within the course of delirium.

Comparative Nosology

DSM-III-R did not provide a diagnosis comparable to DSM-IV-TR's catatonia due to a general medical condition. Most mental disorders due to medical conditions are listed in the sections in DSM-IV-TR with which they share phenomenology. As no section within DSM-IV-TR exists for catatonia, the diagnosis catatonic disorder due to a general medical condition is listed in the residual section *mental disorders due to a general medical condition*.

Like DSM-III-R, DSM-IV-TR provides no specific diagnostic criteria for drug-induced catatonia. The DSM-IV-TR category of *medication-induced movement disorders* offers several diagnoses for catatonia due to antipsychotic and other medications.

ICD-10 provides a diagnosis of *organic catatonic disorder*.

Epidemiology

Catatonia is an uncommon condition. Mostly seen in advanced primary mood or psychotic illnesses, it diminished in prevalence in the second half of the 20th century with the widespread use of antipsychotic medication. Among inpatients with catatonia, 25 to 50 percent are related to mood disorders (e.g., major depressive episode, recurrent, with catatonic features), and approximately 10 percent are associated with schizophrenia. Data are scant as to catatonia's rate of occurrence due to medical conditions or substances.

Etiology

Various medical conditions may cause catatonia, among them neurological disorders (e.g., brain neoplasms and head trauma), infections (e.g., encephalitis), and metabolic disturbances (e.g., hepatic encephalopathy and hypercalcemia).

Medications capable of causing catatonia include corticosteroids, immunosuppressants, and antipsychotic (i.e., neuroleptic) agents. Catatonic qualities may be seen in extreme forms of *neuroleptic-induced parkinsonism* or may represent a manifestation of *neuroleptic malignant syndrome*, a rare, potentially life-threatening disorder associated with fever, autonomic instability, impaired consciousness, and rigidity.

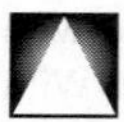

Table 10.5–18
DSM-IV-TR Criteria for Catatonic Disorder Due to a General Medical Condition

A. The presence of catatonia as manifested by motoric immobility, excessive motor activity (that is apparently purposeless and not influenced by external stimuli), extreme negativism or mutism, peculiarities of voluntary movement, or echolalia or echopraxia.
B. There is evidence from the history, physical examination, or laboratory findings that the disturbance is the direct physiological consequence of a general medical condition.
C. The disturbance is not better accounted for by another mental disorder (e.g., a manic episode).
D. The disturbance does not occur exclusively during the course of a delirium.

From American Psychiatric Association. *Diagnostic and Statistical Manual of Mental Disorders.* 4th ed. Text rev. Washington, DC; American Psychiatric Association; 2000, with permission.

Diagnosis and Clinical Features DSM-IV-TR criteria for the diagnosis of catatonic disorder due to a general medical condition include behavioral changes characteristic of catatonia; evidence from history, examination, or laboratory of a physical basis to the symptoms; and the exclusion of primary mental disorders and delirium. Behavioral changes may include motoric immobility or excessive activity, extreme negativism or mutism, peculiarities of voluntary movement, and echolalia or echopraxia. Waxy flexibility, a form of artificial posturing often evident on physical examination, is a striking and memorable finding. In lethal catatonia, a rare advanced stage of the disorder, fever and autonomic instability may conclude in death (Table 10.5–18).

The name of the general medical condition is indicated on Axis I (e.g., catatonic disorder due to hepatic encephalopathy) and on Axis III.

For catatonia related to the use of antipsychotic agents, DSM-IV-TR offers two possible Axis I diagnoses: neuroleptic-induced parkinsonism and neuroleptic malignant syndrome. For catatonia due to nonneuroleptic substances, the diagnosis of *medication-induced movement disorder not otherwise specified* is available.

Duncan Chu, a 25-year-old Asian man without prior psychiatric, substance, or medical history was brought to the hospital for evaluation of withdrawn behavior in the context of a recent break-up with his girlfriend. For the prior week, Mr. Chu's oral intake had diminished, and he had failed to go to his daily job as a computer programmer.

Psychiatry was consulted in the hospital emergency room. Mr. Chu stared ahead and demonstrated delayed reaction time in monosyllabic responses to questions. When he did speak, he acknowledged sadness due to recent break-up with his girlfriend. No evidence of psychosis was elicited. Cognitive examination demonstrated minimal defect in short-term memory. Laboratory studies and brain imaging were unremarkable. Mr. Chu had a low-grade fever of 99.5°F, which was attributed to resolving upper respiratory infection.

Mr. Chu was admitted to inpatient psychiatry to rule out depression. Low-grade fever and withdrawal, punctuated by episodic angry outbursts, persisted over the course of the subsequent two days. Mr. Chu developed a belief that staff wished to poison him; as a result, he began to refuse to eat hospital food. Haloperidol, 2 mg twice a day, was prescribed, but Mr. Chu refused to comply.

Fever rose to 101.4°F, at which point Mr. Chu was transferred to the hospital's inpatient medical service. At that time, Mr. Chu was mute, although alert. Lumbar puncture revealed lymphocytosis. Mr. Chu was diagnosed with viral encephalitis, and antiviral pharmacotherapy was initiated. On the following day, he was observed to have tonic-clonic seizure activity and was intubated for airway protection.

After extubation and defervescence, Mr. Chu remained mute. He was transferred to the hospital's rehabilitation service, where he was noted to repeat the comments and questions of various examiners. Occasionally, Mr. Chu's posture was noted to mimic the gestures of examiners or others in his environment.

Psychiatry diagnosed catatonic disorder due to viral encephalitis. Lorazepam, 0.5 mg three times daily, was initiated and then increased to 1 mg three times daily, after which spontaneous speech developed. Mr. Chu was able to cooperate with cognitive testing but demonstrated mild defects in short-term memory and orientation. Cognition slowly improved and, after 3 weeks, still on lorazepam, Mr. Chu was discharged to his parents' home. Within 2 months, lorazepam had been tapered to discontinuation, cognition had returned to normal, and Mr. Chu returned to his former employment.

This case of catatonia due to encephalitis initially was mistakenly regarded as a case of primary depression. Lack of prior psychiatric history, evolving physical findings (notably fever), and known association between encephalitis and catatonia assisted in the diagnosis. The absence of impairment in consciousness made delirium an unlikely diagnosis. Prompt improvement on lorazepam, a known treatment for catatonia, further supported the diagnosis.

Laboratory Examination No specific imaging or laboratory assessment is pathognomonic for catatonia due to a general medical condition. Neuroleptic malignant syndrome usually is associated with elevated serum creatine phosphokinase (CPK), white blood cell count, and serum transaminases.

Differential Diagnosis The diagnostician should carefully review laboratory and imaging studies and urine toxicology to rule out reversible causes of withdrawn behavior that may mimic catatonia. Patients with severe psychomotor slowing, as may be seen in advanced stages of dementia and in hypoactive delirium, may be misdiagnosed as having catatonic disorder due to a general medical condition. In medical settings, the number of patients with catatonic-like withdrawal syndromes who meet criteria for these other diagnoses vastly exceeds the number who meet criteria for catatonic disorder due to a general medical condition or substance or catatonia due to a primary psychiatric illness (e.g., major depressive disorder, with catatonic features, and schizophrenia, catatonic type).

Catatonia in severe neuroleptic-induced parkinsonism differs from that observed in neuroleptic malignant syndrome; in the latter, autonomic instability and delirium are common accompaniments, along with characteristic laboratory abnormalities.

Course and Treatment Catatonia has lethal potential, as afflicted individuals cannot care for themselves and require intensive supervision in an inpatient setting. Fluid and nutrient intake must be maintained, often with IV lines or feeding tubes. The catatonic individual must be assisted with hygiene.

Central to outcome is identification and correction of the underlying medical or pharmacological cause. Offending medications must be removed or minimized. When catatonia is due to a neurological condition (e.g., encephalitis), clinical improvement is based on the degree of reversible brain injury or impairment.

If correction of the factor judged to be etiological does not yield prompt or adequate benefit, somatic treatment options should be considered. These include administration of benzodiazepines or ECT, or both. Benzodiazepines are effective in promoting spontaneity and speech. Some theorize that these medications work by palliating fear and tension stemming from psychosis contributing to catatonia. The mechanism behind the efficacy of ECT is unknown. For neuroleptic-malignant syndrome, apart from discontinuation of the offending agent and provision of supportive care, the dopaminergic agent, bromocriptine, or the muscle relaxant, dantrolene (Dantrium), occasionally is indicated.

Antipsychotic medications should not be used in the initial management of catatonia. These medications may exacerbate the profound withdrawal and psychomotor slowing that characterize this disorder. They are best reserved for use after catatonia subsides, if psychotic thought content is evident.

PERSONALITY CHANGE DUE TO A GENERAL MEDICAL CONDITION

In *personality change due to a general medical condition*, the affected individual has sustained a personality alteration that is believed to be due to the direct physiological effects of a general medical condition. Personality traits tend to be quite durable, influencing relationships and functioning in social and occupational settings.

Definition

In personality change due to a general medical condition, the individual's pattern of behavior represents a marked alteration from previous personality. This change is judged to be the direct physiological consequence of a medical condition (e.g., head injury).

History and Comparative Nosology

For centuries, head injury has been recognized as a prime cause of personality change, and affected individuals have been described as labile, aggressive, or apathetic. In the past, when the frontal lobes of the brain were involved, the term *frontal lobe syndrome* was used.

DSM-III-R offered a diagnosis of *organic personality syndrome.* This was described as a "persistent personality disturbance, either lifelong or representing a change or accentuation of a previously characteristic trait, that is due to a specific organic factor. Affective instability, recurrent outbursts of aggression or rage, markedly impaired social judgment, marked apathy and indifference, or suspiciousness or paranoid ideation are common." Three patterns of behavior were identified: In one, lability of affect and social judgment were described as impaired. In a second pattern, apathy and indifference were the salient features. A third pattern, seen in patients with temporal lobe epilepsy, involved a tendency toward "humorless verbosity" and religiosity or paranoia. The specifier *explosive type* was applied to the syndrome if outbursts of aggression or rage were the predominant feature.

DSM-IV-TR provides for a much broader range of personality change subtypes resulting from general medical conditions. For personality change related to a substance that forms the basis for independent clinical attention, *substance-related disorder not otherwise specified* may be diagnosed.

ICD-10 provides for a diagnosis of *organic personality disorder*, described as a "significant alteration of the habitual patterns of behavior by the subject premorbidly," sometimes with "impairment of cognitive and thought functions, and altered sexuality." Another diagnosis, *postencephalitic syndrome*, is available for reversible personality changes stemming from encephalitis.

Epidemiology

Little data exist on the prevalence of personality change due to a general medical condition. It is believed that male gender, youth, and the use of substances are factors that predispose to head injury, one of the primary causes of this disorder.

Etiology

Neurological conditions, especially those affecting the frontal or temporal lobes, or subcortical structures, may lead to personality change. The frontal lobes are involved in planning and modulation of behavior; when injury occurs, lapses in social judgment and initiative may result. Orbitofrontal lesions tend to induce disinhibited behaviors and volatility of affect. Frontopolar lesions induce apathy and disengagement. Lesions in the temporal lobe affect memory, emotional response, and interpretation of events, thus contributing to the excessive seriousness and religiosity often observed in the temporal lobe epileptic. Apart from seizure activity, lesions of the frontal and temporal regions of the brain capable of inducing personality change include trauma, neoplasm, encephalitis, and cerebrovascular injury. Subcortical degenerative states associated with personality change include Huntington's disease and Wilson's disease. Frontal lobe lesions in MS may lead to personality change. Endocrine conditions, such as hypo- or hyperthyroidism or hypo- or hyperadrenocorticism, also may alter personality. Chronic alcohol use appears to have marked adverse impact on frontal lobe function, with associated personality change.

Diagnosis and Clinical Features

To qualify for the diagnosis of personality change due to a general medical condition, the personality disturbance must be persistent and must represent a change from the individual's previous characteristic personality pattern. In addition, there must be evidence from the history, physical examination, or laboratory findings that the personality change is physiologically due to a general medical condition. The diagnosis is not given if symptoms are better accounted for by another mental disorder or if they occur in the context of delirium. Personality change must cause significant distress or impairment in functioning.

Salient personality changes, influenced by region of brain injury, include affective instability, apathy, suspiciousness, or outbursts of rage vastly out of proportion to the provoking factor. In DSM-IV-TR, eight subtypes of personality change due to a general medical condition exist according to the predominant feature of the personality change (Table 10.5–19). These include *labile type*, *disinhibited type*, *aggressive type*, *apathetic type*, and *paranoid type*. *Other type* is used if the predominant feature is not captured by the previous subtypes. *Combined type* is used if the presentation has features of more than one defined subtype. *Unspecified type* serves as a residual specifier.

The name of the general medical condition is coded on Axis I (e.g., personality change due to temporal lobe epilepsy, paranoid type) and on Axis III. Similarly, substance-induced personality change that forms the basis of clinical attention is coded on Axis I (e.g., alcohol-related disorder not otherwise specified).

Elliott Davis is a 49-year-old married man without past psychiatric history who was admitted to the hospital with sudden onset of severe headache. Workup revealed subarachnoid hemorrhage due to the rupture of an intracranial aneurysm. Cerebral vasospasm, obstructive hydrocephalus, and coma ensued. Neurosurgical intervention was undertaken to clip the aneurysm and to install a ventriculoperitoneal shunt.

After a lengthy course of inpatient rehabilitation, Mr. Davis experienced outbursts of anger, episodic depressed mood, off-color remarks that verged on offensive, and impairment in his appreciation for subtlety in humor and conversation. No evidence of psychosis was observed. Family members reported that Mr. Davis always had been one to "speak his mind" and to react defensively when he felt criticized.

Brain imaging demonstrated encephalomalacia in the right frontal lobe. Mild cognitive dysfunction not rising to the level of dementia was diagnosed on neuropsychological testing.

This case illustrates personality change stemming from a direct insult to the brain. Mr. Davis meets criteria for personality change due to subarachnoid hemorrhage, labile type.

Laboratory Examination For individuals with suspected brain injury, structural imaging studies, such as MRI or CT, are indicated. EEG may yield evidence of seizure disorder. Blood work may reveal thyroid or electrolyte abnormalities or evidence of infection.

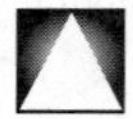

Table 10.5–19
DSM-IV-TR Criteria for Personality Change Due to a General Medical Condition

A. A persistent personality disturbance that represents a change from the individual's previous characteristic personality pattern. (In children, the disturbance involves a marked deviation from normal development or a significant change in the child's usual behavior patterns lasting at least 1 year).

B. There is evidence from the history, physical examination, or laboratory findings that the disturbance is the direct physiological consequence of a general medical condition.

C. The disturbance is not better accounted for by another mental disorder (including other mental disorders due to a general medical condition).

D. The disturbance does not occur exclusively during the course of a delirium.

E. The disturbance causes clinically significant distress or impairment in social, occupational, or other important areas of functioning.

Specify type:

Labile type: if the predominant feature is affective lability

Disinhibited type: if the predominant feature is poor impulse control, as evidenced by sexual indiscretions, etc.

Aggressive type: if the predominant feature is aggressive behavior

Apathetic type: if the predominant feature is marked apathy and indifference

Paranoid type: if the predominant feature is suspiciousness or paranoid ideation

Other type: if the presentation is not characterized by any of the previously mentioned subtypes

Combined type: if more than one feature predominates in the clinical picture

Unspecified type

From American Psychiatric Association. *Diagnostic and Statistical Manual of Mental Disorders.* 4th ed. Text rev. Washington, DC; American Psychiatric Association; 2000, with permission.

Special studies occasionally may be sought (e.g., serum ceruloplasmin in suspected Wilson's disease).

Differential Diagnosis Chronic severe illness, particularly if impacting on an individual's social or occupational functioning, mobility, and level of independence, may induce personality change, but these changes are not due to the physiological effects of the medical condition. Rather, they are due to the qualities of character and experience that the individual uses in coping with illness and physical limitation. Chronic pain syndromes may exert similar impact on personality, but such change is not attributed to direct physiological mechanisms. If the change in personality is better accounted for by cognitive, mood, anxiety, or psychotic disorder attributable to a general medical condition or to delirium, in which transient personality change is common, those disorders are diagnosed in preference to personality change due to a general medical condition. DSM-IV-TR allows for the use of this diagnosis in dementia; however, as personality change is intrinsic to dementia, the diagnosis of personality change due to dementia should be confined to individuals in whom such change is an especially prominent aspect of the clinical picture.

Personality change found in primary mental disorders should be subsumed by those diagnoses. Personality change due to a general medical condition is not to be confused with personality disorders, which are primary mental illnesses, stable and enduring, and are not due to the physiological effects of a general medical condition. Finally, personality change is an intrinsic aspect of substance dependence and should not receive specific diagnosis, unless such personality change forms the basis for clinical attention independent of the substance disorder.

Course and Prognosis Course depends on the nature of the medical or neurological insult. Personality changes resulting from medical conditions likely to yield to intervention (e.g., correction of hypothyroidism) are more amenable to improvement than are personality changes due to medical conditions that are static (e.g., brain injury after head trauma) or progressive in nature (e.g., Huntington's disease).

Treatment Psychopharmacological and psychotherapeutic interventions are designed to address behavioral and mood disturbances (e.g., aggression and irritability). For patients who experience lability of affect, anger, or impatience, anticonvulsants (e.g., valproic acid, lamotrigine, topiramate, or carbamazepine) or, occasionally, antidepressants may prove useful. Due to the impulsive character qualities seen in this disorder, caution should be taken in using medications that may be lethal in overdose (e.g., tricyclic antidepressants) or that may exacerbate disinhibition or cognitive deficits (e.g., benzodiazepines). Antipsychotic medications lower seizure threshold, a matter of concern in patients with brain injury, but may be useful in cases of severe aggression, especially if accompanied by episodic paranoid tendencies.

Psychotherapy may be supportive in nature, assisting the individual in dealing with frustrations stemming from the effects of medical illness, including social and occupational limitations. Psychoeducational and insight-oriented strategies designed to enhance awareness of the adverse effects of personality change may also have value. Family members may benefit from participation in therapies designed to enhance understanding of personality changes and to devise strategies for circumventing problematic behaviors and associated frustrations on the part of patient and family.

MENTAL DISORDER NOT OTHERWISE SPECIFIED DUE TO A GENERAL MEDICAL CONDITION

A variety of mental disorders physiologically due to general medical conditions may present with symptoms that do not meet criteria for dementing, amnestic, mood, psychotic, anxiety, sleep, sexual, catatonic, or personality syndromes secondary to medical conditions. Yet, the mental symptoms in question may impact adversely on psychological well-being or recovery from physical illness and merit psychiatric diagnosis and management.

Definition *Mental disorder not otherwise specified due to a general medical condition* is described in DSM-IV-TR as a "residual category" in which the mental disturbance is due to the physiological effects of a general medical condition but that does not meet criteria for a more specific mental disorder due to a general medical condition.

Comparative Nosology DSM-III-R provided the diagnosis of *organic mental disorder not otherwise specified.* Disturbances of consciousness due to seizure activity were offered as an example of a disturbance that might meet criteria for this diagnosis. Similarly, DSM-IV-TR cites dissociative symptoms due to complex partial seizures as suitable for diagnosis as mental disorder not otherwise specified due to a general medical condition.

ICD-10 offers the diagnosis of *organic dissociative disorder*, as well as several residual categories, including *other and unspecified mental disorder due to brain damage and dysfunction and to physical disease*.

Epidemiology Symptoms of mental disorder not otherwise specified due to a general medical condition most likely are found primarily in populations (e.g., the elderly and individuals with HIV) and settings (e.g., nursing homes and general hospital medical, surgical, and rehabilitation units) in which physical illness and debility are common.

Diagnosis and Clinical Features In many cases, symptoms are a low-grade or prodromal version of symptoms that, in a more pronounced state, would meet criteria for another mental disorder due to a general medical condition.

Jack Maxwell is an 87-year-old man who, 6 weeks after coronary artery bypass graft, complicated by pneumonia and renal insufficiency, was admitted to an inpatient rehabilitation service for management of physical deconditioning. Psychiatry was consulted to rule out depression in the context of persistent low appetite and energy associated with suboptimal participation in rehabilitation.

Mr. Maxwell reported no prior psychiatric history. He had worked as a chemist until retirement nearly two decades earlier. Laboratory examination revealed a low hematocrit of 21 and a moderately elevated blood urea nitrogen of 65.

On interview, Mr. Maxwell demonstrated psychomotor slowing and bland affect. He denied depression, hopelessness, worthlessness, or suicidal ideation. He expressed a desire to recover from his debilitated state but acknowledged uncertainty that he was capable of doing so. Mr. Maxwell complained of extreme weakness. He stated, "I just don't seem to have an appetite anymore." Cognition largely was intact, with mild short-term memory deficit.

Psychiatry diagnosed "demoralization with debilitation." A trial of methylphenidate, 5 mg twice daily, was initiated. Within 1 week, Mr. Maxwell was more energetic and reported improved appetite. Physical therapy department described Mr. Maxwell as showing improved effort and endurance.

After an extended hospital course, many patients, like Mr. Maxwell, demonstrate withdrawn behavior, anorexia, and fatigue, occasionally associated with mild cognitive loss, which do not meet criteria for cognitive or mood disorder, but which are a direct product of resolving medical illness and associated debilitation. In the absence of cardiac contraindication, management with psychostimulants may prove useful.

Treatment Apart from remedying or palliating the causative medical condition, psychopharmacological and psychotherapeutic interventions may be considered. Medication should be targeted to addressing the most salient mood or behavioral aspects of the presentation. Psychotherapy may be geared to assisting the individual in coping with the limitations imposed by medical illness. The low-grade and sporadic nature of mental symptoms accompanying mental disorder not otherwise specified due to a general medical condition occasionally limits the value or efficacy of pharmacological and psychotherapeutic interventions.

SUGGESTED CROSS-REFERENCES

Chapter 2 discusses neuropsychiatric aspects of cerebrovascular disease, head injury, HIV, and a series of other disorders affecting the CNS. Section 7.8 addresses medical assessment and laboratory testing relevant to identifying medical causes of mental disorders. Dementia and delirium are discussed in Chapter 10. Substance-related disorders, including substance-induced disorders, are categorized in Chapter 11. Other relevant discussions include schizophrenia in Chapter 12; other psychotic disorders in Section 12.16; mood disorders in Chapter 13; anxiety disorders in Chapter 14; sexual dysfunction in Chapter 18; sleep disorders in Chapter 20; and personality disorders in Chapter 23. The interface between medicine and psychiatry is discussed in Chapter 24 on psychological factors affecting medical conditions. Assessment of the older adult, including the roles of neuroimaging and neuropsychological testing, is described in Section 51.2.

REFERENCES

Abramowicz M: Drugs that cause sexual dysfunction: An update. *Med Lett Drugs Ther.* 1992;34:73.

Barry PP, Moskowitz MA: The diagnosis of reversible dementia in the elderly: A critical review. *Arch Intern Med.* 1988;148:1914.

Cassem NG: Depression and anxiety secondary to medical illness. *Psychiatr Clin North Am.* 1990;13:597.

Coslett H, Heilman K: Male sexual function: Impairment after right hemisphere stroke. *Arch Neurol.* 1986;43:1036.

DeGroen P, Craven J. Organic brain syndromes in transplant patients. In: Craven J, Rodin G, eds. *Psychiatric Aspects of Organ Transplantation.* Oxford, England: Oxford University Press; 1992.

Gibb WRG: Dementia and Parkinson's disease. *Br J Psychiatry.* 1989;154:596.

Goldberg RJ. Anxiety in the medically ill. In: Stoudemire A, Fogel BS, eds. *Principles of Medical Psychiatry.* Orlando, FL: Grune & Stratton; 1987.

Gordon WA, Hibbard MR: Poststroke depression: an examination of the literature. *Arch Phys Med Rehabil.* 1997;78:659.

*Greenloe BA, Ferrell RB, Kauffman CI, McAllister TW: Complex partial seizures and depression. *Curr Psychiatry Rep.* 2003;5:410.

Hall RC: Psychiatric effects of thyroid hormone disturbance. *Psychosomatics.* 1983;24:7.

Hall RC, Beresford TP, Blow FC. Depression and medical illness: An overview. In: Cameron OG, ed. *Presentations of Depression: Depressive Symptoms in Medical and Other Psychiatric Disorders.* New York: Wiley; 1987.

Henry GW: Some modern aspects of psychiatry in general hospital practice. *Am J Psychiatry.* 1930;86:481.

Joffe RT: A perspective on the thyroid and depression. *Can J Psychiatry.* 1990;35:754.

Kaufman MR: The role of the psychiatrist in a general hospital. *Psychiatr Q.* 1953;27:367.

Levin HS: Memory deficit after closed head injury. *J Clin Exp Neuropsychol.* 1989;12:129.

Lipowski ZJ. *Delirium: Acute Confusional States.* New York: Oxford University Press; 1990.

Lishman WA. *Organic Psychiatry*. London: Blackwell Scientific; 1998.

Navia BA. The AIDS dementia complex. In: Cummings JL, ed. *Subcortical Dementia.* New York: Oxford University Press; 1990.

Nicholas LM, Lindsey BA: Delirium presenting with symptoms of depression. *Psychosomatics.* 1995;36:471.

Pataki J, Zervas I, Jandorf L: Catatonia in a university inpatient service (1985-1990). *Convuls Ther.* 1992;8:167.

Perry TL, Hansen S, Kloster M: Huntington's chorea: deficiency of gamma-aminobutyric acid in the brain. *N Engl J Med.* 1973;288:337.

Popkin MK, Tucker G: Secondary and drug-induced mood, anxiety, psychotic, catatonic, and personality disorders: A review of the literature. *J Neuropsychiatry Clin Neurosci.* 1992;4:369.

Price RW, Brew BJ: The AIDS dementia complex. *J Infect Dis.* 1992;158:1079.

Rabins PV: Reversible dementia and the misdiagnosis of dementia: a review. *Hosp Community Psychiatry.* 1983;34:830.

Richard IH, Schiffer RB, Kurlan R: Anxiety and Parkinson's disease. *J Neuropsychiatry Clin Neurosci.* 1996;8:383.

Robinson RG, Lipsey JR, Price TR: Diagnosis and clinical management of post-stroke depression. *Psychosomatics.* 1985;26:769.

Rundell JR, Wise MG: Causes of organic mood disorder. *J Neuropsychiatry Clin Neurosci.* 1989;1:398.

*Soares CN, Poitras JR, Prouty J: Effect of reproductive hormones and selective estrogen receptor modulators on mood during menopause. *Drugs Aging.* 2003;20:85.

*Taylor WD, Steffens DC, MacFall JR, McQuoid DR, Payne ME, Provenzale JM, Krishnan KR: White matter hyperdensity progression and late-life depression outcomes. *Arch Gen Psychiatry.* 2003;60:1090.

Williams RL. Sleep disturbances in various medical and surgical conditions. In: Williams RL, Karacan I, Moore CA, eds. *Sleep Disorders: Diagnosis and Treatment.* New York: Wiley; 1988.

Winokur G: The concept of a secondary depression and its relationship to comorbidity. *Psychiatr Clin North Am.* 1990;123:567.

*Wise MG, Rundell JR, eds. *Textbook of Consultation-Liaison Psychiatry.* Washington, DC: American Psychiatric Publishing; 2002.

*World Health Organization. *Multiaxial Presentation of the ICD-10 for use in Adult Psychiatry.* Cambridge, UK: Cambridge University Press; 1997.

Zelnik T. Depressive effects of drugs. In: Cameron OG, ed. *Presentations of Depression: Depressive Symptoms in Medical and Other Psychiatric Disorders.* New York: Wiley; 1987.

11 Substance-Related Disorders

▲ 11.1 Substance-Related Disorders: Introduction and Overview

JEROME H. JAFFE, M.D., AND JAMES C. ANTHONY, PH.D., SC.M.

This chapter on the substance-related disorders is made up of separate sections organized around the syndromes associated with the use of each of the major groups of pharmacological agents that are commonly misused (abused). This section deals with issues that are common across categories of drugs: the nomenclature and diagnostic schemes of the revised fourth edition of the *Diagnostic and Statistical Manual of Mental Disorders* (DSM-IV-TR) and the tenth edition of the *International Classification of Diseases and Related Health Problems* (ICD-10), the history of substance use and dependence, epidemiology, and the etiological factors and treatment principles that appear to be common to these syndromes.

SUBSTANCE-RELATED DISORDERS IN DSM-IV, DSM-IV-TR, AND ICD-10

DSM-IV-TR does not differ from DSM-IV in the substance use disorders sections. DSM-IV-TR includes two broad categories of substance-related disorders: substance use disorders (substance dependence and substance abuse) and a diverse grouping of substance-induced disorders (such as intoxication, withdrawal, psychotic disorder, and mood disorders). Thus, in DSM-IV-TR, the topic of substance-related disorders goes beyond substance dependence and abuse and closely related problems to include a wide variety of adverse reactions not only to substances of abuse but also to medications and toxins. The medications associated with substance-induced disorders range from anesthetics to over-the-counter medications and include such diverse drug categories as anticholinergics, antidepressants, anticonvulsants, antimicrobial drugs, antihypertensive agents, corticosteroids, antiparkinsonian agents, chemotherapeutic agents, nonsteroidal antiinflammatory drugs (NSAIDs), and disulfiram (Antabuse). In addition, several categories of substance-induced disorders can be associated with a wide range of nonmedicinal toxic materials, ranging from heavy metals and industrial solvents to insecticides and household cleaning agents. DSM-IV-TR groups the diagnostic criteria for substance dependence, abuse, intoxication, hallucinogen persisting perception disorder, and withdrawal syndromes in a section titled *substance-related disorders*, whereas the other substance-related disorders (e.g., substance-induced mood disorders and substance-induced delusional disorders) are described in the sections covering delirium and other psychiatric syndromes that they most closely resemble phenomenologically (Table 11.1–1).

The section dealing with substance dependence and substance abuse presents descriptions of the clinical phenomena associated with the use of 11 designated classes of pharmacological agents: alcohol; amphetamines or similarly acting agents; caffeine; cannabis; cocaine; hallucinogens; inhalants; nicotine; opioids; phencyclidine (PCP) or similar agents; and a group that includes sedatives, hypnotics, and anxiolytics. A residual 12th category includes a variety of agents not in the 11 designated classes, such as anabolic steroids and nitrous oxide.

ICD-10 considers the disorders due to psychoactive substance use within the confines of an alphanumeric system that allows only nine categories of pharmacological agents, with one residual category to cover both multiple drug use and use of psychoactive substances not included in the nine designated categories. DSM-IV-TR and ICD-10 categorize substances comparably with the following exceptions. Caffeine and PCP are considered distinct categories in DSM-IV-TR, whereas ICD-10 includes problems related to caffeine in the category of other stimulants, such as amphetamine, and PCP must be included with hallucinogens or in the residual category. Also, ICD-10 has a special category for abuse of non–dependence-producing substances (Table 11.1–2). Specifically mentioned are antidepressants, analgesics, antacids, vitamins, and steroids or hormones.

DEFINITIONS AND DIAGNOSIS

Substance Dependence DSM-IV, DSM-IV-TR, and ICD-10 formulations for substance abuse and dependence closely follow the concepts and terminology developed in 1980 by an International Working Group sponsored by the World Health Organization (WHO) and the Alcohol, Drug Abuse, and Mental Health Administration (ADAMHA) of the United States, which defined substance dependence as follows:

> A syndrome manifested by a behavioral pattern in which the use of a given psychoactive drug, or class of drugs, is given a much higher priority than other behaviors that once had higher value. The term "syndrome" is taken to mean no more than a clustering of phenomena so that not all the components need always be present or not always present with the same intensity . . . . The dependence syndrome is not absolute, but is a quantitative phenomenon that exists in different degrees. The intensity of the syndrome is measured by the behaviors that are elicited in relation to using the drug and by the other behaviors that are secondary to drug use . . . . No sharp cut-off point can be identified for distinguishing drug dependence

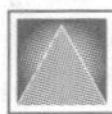

Table 11.1–1
Substance-Induced Mental Disorders Included Elsewhere in the Textbook

Substance-induced disorders cause a variety of symptoms that are characteristic of other mental disorders. To facilitate differential diagnosis, the text and criteria for these other substance-induced disorders are included in the sections of DSM-IV-TR and this textbook with disorders with which they share phenomenology.

Substance-induced delirium (Chapter 10) is included in the "Delirium, Dementia, and Amnestic and Other Cognitive Disorders" section of DSM-IV-TR.

Substance-induced persisting dementia (Chapter 10) is included in the "Delirium, Dementia, and Amnestic and Other Cognitive Disorders" section.

Substance-induced persisting amnestic disorder (Chapter 10) is included in the "Delirium, Dementia, and Amnestic and Other Cognitive Disorders" section.

Substance-induced psychotic disorder is included in the "Other Psychotic Disorders" section (Section 12.16). (In DSM-III-R, these disorders were classified as organic hallucinosis and organic delusional disorder.)

Substance-induced mood disorder is included in the "Mood Disorders" chapter (Chapter 13).

Substance-induced anxiety disorder is included in the "Anxiety Disorders" chapter (Chapter 14).

Substance-induced sexual dysfunction is included in the "Normal Sexuality and Sexual and Gender Identity Disorders" chapter (Chapter 18).

Substance-induced sleep disorder (Chapter 20) is included in the "Sleep Disorders" section.

In addition, hallucinogen persisting perception disorder (flashbacks) (Section 11.7) is included under hallucinogen-related disorder.

Adapted from *Diagnostic and Statistical Manual of Mental Disorders*. 4th ed. Text rev. Washington, DC: American Psychiatric Association; 2000.

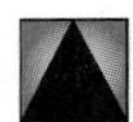

Table 11.1–2
ICD-10 Diagnostic Criteria for Abuse of Non–Dependence-Producing Substances

A wide variety of medicaments and folk remedies may be involved, but the particularly important groups are: psychotropic drugs that do not produce dependence, such as antidepressants, and laxatives and analgesics that may be purchased without medical prescription such as aspirin and paracetamol. Although the medication may have been medically prescribed or recommended in the first instance, prolonged, unnecessary, and often excessive dosage develops, which is facilitated by the availability of the substances without medical prescription.

Persistent and unjustified use of these substances is usually associated with unnecessary expense, often involves unnecessary contacts with medical professionals or supporting staff, and is sometimes marked by the harmful physical effects of the substances. Attempts to discourage or forbid the use of the substance are often met with resistance; for laxatives and analgesics, this may be in spite of warnings about (or even the development of) physical harm such as renal dysfunction or electrolyte disturbances. Although it is usually clear that the patient has a strong motivation to take the substance, no dependence or withdrawal symptoms develop, as in the case of the psychoactive substances specified in mental and behavioral disorders due to psychoactive substance use.

Identify the type of substance involved:

- Antidepressants (such as tricyclic and tetracyclic antidepressants and monoamine oxidase inhibitors)
- Laxatives
- Analgesics (such as aspirin, paracetamol, phenacetin, not specified as psychoactive mental and behavioral disorders due to psychoactive substance use)
- Antacids
- Vitamins
- Steroids or hormones
- Specific herbal or folk remedies
- Other substances that do not produce dependence (such as diuretics)
- Unspecified

From World Health Organization. *The ICD-10 Classification of Mental and Behavioural Disorders: Diagnostic Criteria for Research*. Geneva: World Health Organization; 1993, with permission.

from non-dependent but recurrent drug use. At the extreme, the dependence syndrome is associated with "compulsive drug-using behavior."

That central notion is continued in DSM-IV and DSM-IV-TR, which state:

> The essential feature of dependence is a cluster of cognitive, behavioral, and physiological symptoms indicating that the individual continues substance use despite significant substance-related problems.

The central notion in ICD-10 is virtually the same:

> . . . a cluster of behavioural, cognitive, and physiological phenomena that develop after repeated substance use and typically include a strong desire to take the drug, difficulties in controlling its use, persisting in its use despite harmful consequences, a higher priority given to drug use than to other activities and obligations, increased tolerance, and sometimes a physical withdrawal state.

Diagnostic criteria for substance dependence are shown in Table 11.1–3 (for DSM-IV-TR) and Table 11.1–4 (for ICD-10). DSM-IV-TR uses seven criteria to describe a generic concept of dependence that applies across 11 classes of pharmacological agents and requires three of seven criteria to be met if dependence is to be diagnosed. ICD-10 is based on a more dimensional concept of the dependence syndrome, but it states that a definite diagnosis of dependence should usually be made only if three or more of six criteria have been met within the previous year. Both systems use a polythetic syndrome definition in which no one specific criterion is required so long as three or more are present. However, DSM-IV-TR asks the clinician to specify whether physiological dependence—evidence of Criterion 1 (tolerance) or Criterion 2 (withdrawal)—is present or absent. Evidence indicates that physiological dependence is associated with a more severe form of the disorder.

In addition to requiring the clustering of three criteria in a 12-month period, DSM-IV-TR includes a few other qualifications. It states specifically that the diagnosis of dependence can be applied to every class of substances except caffeine. This point is admittedly controversial, and some researchers (including those who authored the section in this chapter) believe, on the basis of the same DSM-IV-TR generic criteria, that caffeine produces a distinct form of dependence, although it is usually relatively benign.

Some people consume several categories of drugs concurrently and are clearly drug dependent according to the generic criteria, but it may not be possible to ascertain whether they are dependent on any one specific class of drugs. When at least three groups of drugs are involved, DSM-IV-TR calls the condition *polysubstance dependence* (Table 11.1–5). DSM-IV-TR also makes provision for classifying substance-related disorders that cannot be classified in any of the previous categories (e.g., nitrous oxide, anticholinergics, ana-

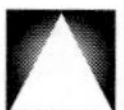

Table 11.1–3
DSM-IV-TR Diagnostic Criteria for Substance Dependence

A maladaptive pattern of substance use, leading to clinically significant impairment or distress, as manifested by three (or more) of the following, occurring at any time in the same 12-month period:
(1) Tolerance, as defined by either of the following:
(a) A need for markedly increased amounts of the substance to achieve intoxication or desired effect
(b) Markedly diminished effect with continued use of the same amount of the substance
(2) Withdrawal, as manifested by either of the following:
(a) The characteristic withdrawal syndrome for the substance (refer to Criteria A and B of the criteria sets for withdrawal from the specific substances)
(b) The same (or closely related) substance is taken to relieve or avoid withdrawal symptoms
(3) The substance is often taken in larger amounts or over a longer period than was intended.
(4) There is a persistent desire or unsuccessful effort to cut down or control substance use.
(5) A great deal of time is spent in activities necessary to obtain the substance (e.g., visiting multiple doctors or driving long distances), use the substance (e.g., chain smoking), or recover from its effects.
(6) Important social, occupational, or recreational activities are given up or reduced because of substance use.
(7) The substance use is continued despite knowledge of having a persistent or recurrent physical or psychological problem that is likely to have been caused or exacerbated by the substance (e.g., current cocaine use despite recognition of cocaine-induced depression or continued drinking despite recognition that an ulcer was made worse by alcohol consumption).

Specify if:
With physiological dependence: evidence of tolerance or withdrawal (i.e., either item 1 or 2 is present)
Without physiological dependence: no evidence of tolerance or withdrawal (i.e., neither item 1 nor 2 is present)

Course specifiers:
Early full remission
Early partial remission
Sustained full remission
Sustained partial remission
On agonist therapy
In a controlled environment

From American Psychiatric Association. *Diagnostic and Statistical Manual of Mental Disorders.* 4th ed. Text rev. Washington, DC: American Psychiatric Association; 2000, with permission.

bolic-androgenic steroids) or for an initial diagnosis of dependence or abuse when the specific drug is not known. A similar residual category is included in ICD-10, but steroids are given a distinct code. The DSM-IV-TR diagnostic criteria for other (or unknown) substance-related disorders are listed in Table 11.1–6.

Patterns of Remission and Course Specifiers Both systems deal with remission by providing distinct modifying terms that can be appended to a diagnosis of substance dependence. DSM-IV-TR terms are more varied than those of ICD-10 (Table 11.1–7). The DSM-IV-TR specifiers for remission require a period of at least 1 month, after a period of active dependence, during which no criteria of dependence are present. If a patient has not met any criteria for dependence for at least 1 month but fewer than 12 months, the course specifier is *early full* remission. If the period during which no criteria of dependence are met exceeds 12 months, the specifier of *sustained full* remission can be used. If the full criteria for dependence or abuse have not been met for less than 1 year, but one or more criteria have been present, *early partial* remission may be designated. If the period exceeds 12 months, *sustained partial* remission may be used. Two additional remission specifiers should be used when appropriate: *on agonist therapy* (includes partial agonists) and *in a controlled environment.* Thus, a heroin-dependent patient or client successfully enrolled in a methadone maintenance program for 12 months is described as in remission on agonist therapy, as are those maintained successfully on buprenorphine, a partial agonist.

Several factors, such as duration of remission and duration of a period of dependence, must be considered when deciding that a person has fully recovered and no longer warrants a diagnosis of dependence. The modifiers that describe the course of dependence in ICD-10 are similar, but specific criteria for selecting them are not provided (Table 11.1–4).

The DSM-IV-TR does not use the term "in recovery" to describe any part of the course of remission from substance use disorders. It is a term commonly used among patients who are currently abstinent while participating in 12-step programs. Many professionals who are interacting with such patients also use it. Individuals who were formerly dependent on drugs or alcohol and have been stably abstinent for many years may also refer to themselves as being "in recovery," typically to convey the idea that they are vulnerable to relapse.

Substance Abuse DSM-IV-TR defines the essential features of substance abuse as follows:

> A maladaptive pattern of substance use manifested by recurrent and significant adverse consequences related to the repeated use of substances . . . . These problems must occur recurrently during the same 12-month period . . . . [T]he criteria for Substance Abuse do not include tolerance, withdrawal, or a pattern of compulsive use and instead include only the harmful consequences of repeated use. A diagnosis of Substance Abuse is preempted by the diagnosis of Substance Dependence if the individual's pattern of substance use has ever met the criteria for Dependence for that class of substances.

Expert committees of the WHO have rejected the term "abuse" when applied to drug problems. However, DSM-IV-TR task panels have chosen to retain the concept of "substance abuse" to describe socially maladaptive behavior in connection with drug use in the absence of a history of drug dependence. That is, the progression toward drug dependence is defined by DSM-IV-TR to include the possibility of drug abuse, but once a person meets criteria for drug dependence, the possibility of drug abuse is absent with respect to each drug class recognized by the DSM-IV-TR. The DSM-IV-TR criteria for substance abuse are shown in Table 11.1–8.

Although rejecting the concept of drug "abuse," the ICD-10 includes a category of harmful use, which substantially differs from the DSM-IV-TR concept of "abuse." The concept of "harmful use" is limited to mental and physical health (e.g., hepatitis and overdose or episodes of depressive disorder resulting from heavy alcohol use). The concept specifically excludes social impairment, stating: "The fact that a pattern of use of a particular substance is disapproved of . . . or may have led to socially negative consequences such as arrest or marital arguments is not in itself evidence of harmful use." Four diagnostic criteria must be met to make the ICD-10 diagnosis of harmful use.

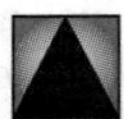

Table 11.1–4
ICD-10 Diagnostic Criteria for Mental and Behavioral Disorders Due to Psychoactive Substance Use

Mental and behavioral disorders due to use of alcohol
Mental and behavioral disorders due to use of opioids
Mental and behavioral disorders due to use of cannabinoids
Mental and behavioral disorders due to use of sedatives or hypnotics
Mental and behavioral disorders due to use of cocaine
Mental and behavioral disorders due to use of other stimulants, including caffeine
Mental and behavioral disorders due to use of hallucinogens
Mental and behavioral disorders due to use of tobacco
Mental and behavioral disorders due to use of volatile solvents
Mental and behavioral disorders due to multiple drug use and use of other psychoactive substances

Acute intoxication

G1. There must be clear evidence of recent use of a psychoactive substance (or substances) at sufficiently high dose levels to be consistent with intoxication.

G2. There must be symptoms or signs of intoxication compatible with the known actions of the particular substance (or substances), as specified below, and of sufficient severity to produce disturbances in the level of consciousness cognition, perception, affect, or behavior that are of clinical importance.

G3. The symptoms or signs present cannot be accounted for by a medical disorder unrelated to substance use, and are not better accounted for by another mental or behavioral disorder.

Acute intoxication frequently occurs in persons who have more persistent alcohol- or drug-related problems in addition. Where there are such problems, e.g., harmful use, dependence syndrome, or psychotic disorder, they should also be recorded.
The following may be used to indicate whether the acute intoxication was associated with any complications:

Uncomplicated
 Symptoms are of varying severity, usually dose dependent
With trauma or other bodily injury
With other medical complications
 Examples are hematemesis, inhalation of vomit
With delirium
With perceptual distortions
With coma
With convulsions
Pathological intoxication
 Applies only to alcohol

Acute intoxication due to use of alcohol

A. The general criteria for acute intoxication must be met.
B. There must be dysfunctional behavior, as evidenced by at least one of the following:
 (1) disinhibition
 (2) argumentativeness
 (3) aggression
 (4) lability of mood
 (5) impaired attention
 (6) impaired judgment
 (7) interference with personal functioning
C. At least one of the following signs must be present:
 (1) unsteady gait
 (2) difficulty in standing
 (3) slurred speech
 (4) nystagmus
 (5) decreased level of consciousness (e.g., stupor, coma)
 (6) flushed face
 (7) conjunctival injection

Comment

When severe, acute alcohol intoxication may be accompanied by hypotension, hypothermia, and depression of the gag reflex. If desired, the blood alcohol level may be specified.

Pathological alcohol intoxication

Note. The status of this condition is being examined. These research criteria must be regarded as tentative.

A. The general criteria for acute intoxication must be met, with the exception that pathological intoxication occurs after drinking amounts of alcohol insufficient to cause intoxication in most people.
B. There is verbally aggressive or physically violent behavior that is not typical of the person when sober.
C. The intoxication occurs very soon (usually a few minutes) after consumption of alcohol.
D. There is no evidence of organic cerebral disorder or other mental disorders.

Comment

This is an uncommon condition. The blood alcohol levels found in this disorder are lower than those that would cause acute intoxication in most people (i.e., below 40 mg/100 mL).

Acute intoxication due to use of opioids

A. The general criteria for acute intoxication must be met.
B. There must be dysfunctional behavior, as evidenced by at least one of the following:
 (1) apathy and sedation
 (2) disinhibition
 (3) psychomotor retardation
 (4) impaired attention
 (5) impaired judgment
 (6) interference with personal functioning
C. At least one of the following signs must be present:
 (1) drowsiness
 (2) slurred speech
 (3) pupillary constriction (except in anoxia from severe overdose, when pupillary dilatation occurs)
 (4) decreased level of consciousness (e.g., stupor, coma)

Comment

When severe, acute opioid intoxication may be accompanied by respiratory depression (and hypoxia), hypotension, and hypothermia.

Acute intoxication due to use of cannabinoids

A. The general criteria for acute intoxication must be met.
B. There must be dysfunctional behavior or perceptual abnormalities, including at least one of the following:
 (1) euphoria and disinhibition
 (2) anxiety or agitation
 (3) suspiciousness or paranoid ideation
 (4) temporal slowing (a sense that time is passing very slowly, and/or the person is experiencing a rapid flow of ideas)
 (5) impaired judgment
 (6) impaired attention
 (7) impaired reaction time
 (8) auditory, visual, or tactile illusions
 (9) hallucinations with preserved orientation
 (10) depersonalization
 (11) derealization
 (12) interference with personal functioning
C. At least one of the following signs must be present:
 (1) increased appetite
 (2) dry mouth

(continued)

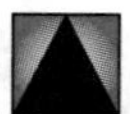

Table 11.1–4 (*continued*)

(3) conjunctival injection
(4) tachycardia

Acute intoxication due to use of sedatives or hypnotics

A. The general criteria for acute intoxication must be met.
B. There is dysfunctional behavior, as evidenced by at least one of the following:
(1) euphoria and disinhibition
(2) apathy and sedation
(3) abusiveness or aggression
(4) lability of mood
(5) impaired attention
(6) anterograde amnesia
(7) impaired psychomotor performance
(8) interference with personal functioning
C. At least one of the following signs must be present:
(1) unsteady gait
(2) difficulty in standing
(3) slurred speech
(4) nystagmus
(5) decreased level of consciousness (e.g., stupor, coma)
(6) erythematous skin lesions or blisters

Comment

When severe, acute intoxication from sedative or hypnotic drugs may be accompanied by hypotension, hypothermia, and depression of the gag reflex.

Acute intoxication due to use of cocaine

A. The general criteria for acute intoxication must be met.
B. There must be dysfunctional behavior or perceptual abnormalities, as evidenced by at least one of the following:
(1) euphoria and sensation of increased energy
(2) hypervigilance
(3) grandiose beliefs or actions
(4) abusiveness or aggression
(5) argumentativeness
(6) lability of mood
(7) repetitive stereotyped behaviors
(8) auditory, visual, or tactile illusions
(9) hallucinations, usually with intact orientation
(10) paranoid ideation
(11) interference with personal functioning
C. At least two of the following signs must be present:
(1) tachycardia (sometimes bradycardia)
(2) cardiac arrhythmias
(3) hypertension (sometimes hypotension)
(4) sweating and chills
(5) nausea or vomiting
(6) evidence of weight loss
(7) pupillary dilatation
(8) psychomotor agitation (sometimes retardation)
(9) muscular weakness
(10) chest pain
(11) convulsions

Comment

Interference with personal functioning is most readily apparent from the social interactions of cocaine users, which range from extreme gregariousness to social withdrawal.

Acute intoxication due to use of other stimulants, including caffeine

A. The general criteria for acute intoxication must be met.
B. There must be dysfunctional behavior or perceptual abnormalities, as evidenced by at least one of the following:
(1) euphoria and sensation of increased energy
(2) hypervigilance
(3) grandiose beliefs or actions
(4) abusiveness or aggression
(5) argumentativeness
(6) lability of mood
(7) repetitive stereotyped behaviors
(8) auditory, visual, or tactile illusions
(9) hallucinations, usually with intact orientation
(10) paranoid ideation
(11) interference with personal functioning
C. At least two of the following signs must be present:
(1) tachycardia (sometimes bradycardia)
(2) cardiac arrhythmias
(3) hypertension (sometimes hypotension)
(4) sweating and chills
(5) nausea or vomiting
(6) evidence of weight loss
(7) pupillary dilatation
(8) psychomotor agitation (sometimes retardation)
(9) muscular weakness
(10) chest pain
(11) convulsions

Comment

Interference with personal functioning is most readily apparent from the social interactions of the substance users, which range from extreme gregariousness to social withdrawal.

Acute intoxication due to use of hallucinogens

A. The general criteria for acute intoxication must be met.
B. There must be dysfunctional behavior or perceptual abnormalities, as evidenced by at least one of the following:
(1) anxiety and fearfulness
(2) auditory, visual, or tactile illusions or hallucinations occurring in a state of full wakefulness and alertness
(3) depersonalization
(4) derealization
(5) paranoid ideation
(6) ideas of reference
(7) lability of mood
(8) hyperactivity
(9) impulsive acts
(10) impaired attention
(11) interference with personal functioning
C. At least two of the following signs must be present:
(1) tachycardia
(2) palpitations
(3) sweating and chills
(4) tremor
(5) blurring of vision
(6) pupillary dilatation
(7) incoordination

Acute intoxication due to use of tobacco [acute nicotine intoxication]

A. The general criteria for acute intoxication must be met.
B. There must be dysfunctional behavior or perceptual abnormalities, as evidenced by at least one of the following:
(1) insomnia

(*continued*)

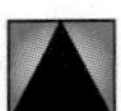

Table 11.1–4 (*continued*)

(2) bizarre dreams
(3) lability of mood
(4) derealization
(5) interference with personal functioning

C. At least one of the following signs must be present:
(1) nausea or vomiting
(2) sweating
(3) tachycardia
(4) cardiac arrhythmias

Acute intoxication due to use of volatile solvents

A. The general criteria for acute intoxication must be met.

B. There must be dysfunctional behavior, evidenced by at least one of the following:
(1) apathy and lethargy
(2) argumentativeness
(3) abusiveness or aggression
(4) lability of mood
(5) impaired judgment
(6) impaired attention and memory
(7) psychomotor retardation
(8) interference with personal functioning

C. At least one of the following signs must be present:
(1) unsteady gait
(2) difficulty in standing
(3) slurred speech
(4) nystagmus
(5) decreased level of consciousness (e.g., stupor, coma)
(6) muscle weakness
(7) blurred vision or diplopia

Comment

Acute intoxication from inhalation of substances other than solvents should also be coded here.

When severe, acute intoxication from volatile solvents may be accompanied by hypotension, hypothermia, and depression of the gag reflex.

Acute intoxication due to multiple drug use and use of other psychoactive substances

This category should be used when there is evidence of intoxication caused by recent use of other psychoactive substances (e.g., phencyclidine) or of multiple psychoactive substances where it is uncertain which substance has predominated.

Harmful use

A. There must be clear evidence that the substance use was responsible for (or substantially contributed to) physical or psychological harm, including impaired judgment or dysfunctional behavior, which may lead to disability or have adverse consequences for interpersonal relationships.

B. The nature of the harm should be clearly identifiable (and specified).

C. The pattern of use has persisted for at least 1 month or has occurred repeatedly within a 12-month period.

D. The disorder does not meet the criteria for any other mental or behavioral disorder related to the same drug in the same time period (except for acute intoxication).

Dependence syndrome

A. Three or more of the following manifestations should have occurred together for at least 1 month or, if persisting for periods of less than 1 month, should have occurred together repeatedly within a 12-month period:

(1) a strong desire or sense of compulsion to take the substance

(2) impaired capacity to control substance-taking behavior in terms of its onset, termination, or levels of use, as evidenced by: the substance being often taken in larger amounts or over a longer period than intended; or by a persistent desire or unsuccessful efforts to reduce or control substance use

(3) a physiological withdrawal state when substance use is reduced or ceased, as evidenced by the characteristic withdrawal syndrome for the substance, or by use of the same (or closely related) substance with the intention of relieving or avoiding withdrawal symptoms

(4) evidence of tolerance to the effects of the substance, such that there is a need for significantly increased amounts of the substance to achieve intoxication or the desired effect, or a marked diminished effect with continued use of the same amount of the substance

(5) preoccupation with substance use, as manifested by important alternative pleasures or interests being given up or reduced because of substance use; or a great deal of time being spent in activities necessary to obtain, take, or recover from the effects of the substance

(6) persistent substance use despite clear evidence of harmful consequences, as evidenced by continued use when the individual is actually aware, or may be expected to be aware, of the nature and extent of harm

Diagnosis of the dependence syndrome may be further specified by the following:

Currently abstinent
Early remission
Partial remission
Full remission

Currently abstinent but in a protected environment (e.g., in a hospital, in a therapeutic community, in prison, etc.)

Currently on a clinically supervised maintenance or replacement regime (controlled dependence) (e.g., with methadone; nicotine gum or nicotine patch)

Currently abstinent, but receiving treatment with aversive or blocking drugs (e.g., naltrexone or disulfiram)

Currently using the substance (active dependence)
Without physical features
With physical features

The course of the dependence may be further specified, if desired, as follows:

Continuous use
Episodic use (dipsomania)

Withdrawal state

G1. There must be clear evidence of recent cessation or reduction of substance use after repeated, and usually prolonged and/or high-dose, use of that substance.

G2. Symptoms and signs are compatible with the known features of a withdrawal state from the particular substance or substances (see below).

G3. Symptoms and signs are not accounted for by a medical disorder unrelated to substance use, and not better accounted for by another mental or behavioral disorder.

The diagnosis of withdrawal state may be further specified by using the following:

Uncomplicated
With convulsions

Alcohol withdrawal state

A. The general criteria for withdrawal state must be met.

B. Any three of the following signs must be present:

(*continued*)

Table 11.1–4 (*continued*)

(1) tremor of the tongue, eyelids, or outstretched hands
(2) sweating
(3) nausea, retching, or vomiting
(4) tachycardia or hypertension
(5) psychomotor agitation
(6) headache
(7) insomnia
(8) malaise or weakness
(9) transient visual, tactile, or auditory hallucinations or illusions
(10) grand mal convulsions

Comment

If delirium is present, the diagnosis should be alcohol withdrawal state with delirium (delirium tremens).

A. The general criteria for withdrawal state must be met. (Note that an opioid withdrawal state may also be induced by administration of an opioid antagonist after a brief period of opioid use.)

B. Any three of the following signs must be present:
(1) craving for an opioid drug
(2) rhinorrhea or sneezing
(3) lacrimation
(4) muscle aches or cramps
(5) abdominal cramps
(6) nausea or vomiting
(7) diarrhea
(8) pupillary dilatation
(9) piloerection, or recurrent chills
(10) tachycardia or hypertension
(11) yawning
(12) restless sleep

Cannabinoid withdrawal state

Note. This is an ill-defined syndrome for which definitive diagnostic criteria cannot be established at the present time. It occurs following cessation of prolonged high-dose use of cannabis. It has been reported variously as lasting from several hours to up to 7 days.

Symptoms and signs include anxiety, irritability, tremor of the outstretched hands, sweating, and muscle aches.

Sedative or hypnotic withdrawal state

A. The general criteria for withdrawal state must be met.

B. Any three of the following signs must be present:
(1) tremor of the tongue, eyelids, or outstretched hands
(2) nausea or vomiting
(3) tachycardia
(4) postural hypotension
(5) psychomotor agitation
(6) headache
(7) insomnia
(8) malaise or weakness
(9) transient visual, tactile, or auditory hallucinations or illusions
(10) paranoid ideation
(11) grand mal convulsions

Comment

If delirium is present, the diagnosis should be sedative or hypnotic withdrawal state with delirium.

Cocaine withdrawal state

A. The general criteria for withdrawal state must be met.

B. There is dysphoric mood (e.g., sadness or anhedonia).

C. Any two of the following signs must be present:
(1) lethargy and fatigue
(2) psychomotor retardation or agitation
(3) craving for cocaine
(4) increased appetite
(5) insomnia or hypersomnia
(6) bizarre or unpleasant dreams

Withdrawal state from other stimulants, including caffeine

A. The general criteria for withdrawal state must be met.

B. There is dysphoric mood (e.g., sadness or anhedonia).

C. Any two of the following signs must be present:
(1) lethargy and fatigue
(2) psychomotor retardation or agitation
(3) craving for stimulant drugs
(4) increased appetite
(5) insomnia or hypersomnia
(6) bizarre or unpleasant dreams

Hallucinogen withdrawal state

Note: There is no recognized hallucinogen withdrawal state.

Tobacco withdrawal state

A. The general criteria for withdrawal state must be met.

B. Any two of the following signs must be present:
(1) craving for tobacco (or other nicotine-containing products)
(2) malaise or weakness
(3) anxiety
(4) dysphoric mood
(5) irritability or restlessness
(6) insomnia
(7) increased appetite
(8) increased cough
(9) mouth ulceration
(10) difficulty in concentrating

Volatile solvents withdrawal state

Note: There is inadequate information on withdrawal states from volatile solvents for research to be formulated.

Multiple drug withdrawal state

Withdrawal state with delirium

A. The general criteria for withdrawal state must be met.

B. The criteria for delirium must be met.

The diagnosis of withdrawal state with delirium may be further specified by using the following:

Without convulsions
With convulsions

Psychotic disorder

A. Onset of psychotic symptoms must occur during or within 2 weeks of substance use.

B. The psychotic symptoms must persist for more than 48 hours.

C. Duration of the disorder must not exceed 6 months.

The diagnosis of psychotic disorder may be further specified by using the following:

Schizophrenia-like
Predominantly delusional
Predominantly hallucinatory
Predominantly polymorphic
Predominantly depressive symptoms
Predominantly manic symptoms
Mixed

For research purposes it is recommended that change of the disorder from a nonpsychotic to a clearly psychotic state be further specified as either abrupt (onset within 48 hours) or acute (onset in more than 48 hours but less than 2 weeks).

(*continued*)

Table 11.1–4 (*continued*)

Amnesic syndrome	***Comments***
A. Memory impairment is manifest in both: (1) a defect of recent memory (impaired learning of new material) to a degree sufficient to interfere with daily living (2) a reduced ability to recall past experiences B. All of the following are absent (or relatively absent): (1) defect in immediate recall (as tested, for example, by the digit span) (2) clouding of consciousness and disturbance of attention, as defined in delirium, not induced by alcohol and other psychoactive substances, Criterion A (3) global intellectual decline (dementia) C. There is no objective evidence from physical and neurological examination, laboratory tests, or history of a disorder or disease of the brain (especially involving bilaterally the diencephalic and medial temporal structures), other than that related to substance use, that can reasonably be presumed to be responsible for the clinical manifestations described under Criterion A. **Residual and late-onset psychotic disorder** A. Conditions and disorders meeting the criteria for the individual syndromes listed below should be clearly related to substance use. Where onset of the condition or disorder occurs subsequent to use of psychoactive substances, strong evidence should be provided to demonstrate a link.	In view of the considerable variation in this category, the characteristics of such residual states or conditions should be clearly documented in terms of their type, severity, and duration. For research purposes full descriptive details should be specified. If required, use as follows: Flashbacks Personality or behavior disorder B. The general criteria for personality and behavioral disorder due to brain disease, damage and dysfunction must be met. Residual affective disorder B. The criteria for organic mood (affective) disorder must be met. Dementia B. The general criteria for dementia must be met. Other persisting cognitive impairment B. The criteria for mild cognitive disorder must be met, except for the exclusion of psychoactive substance use in Criterion D. Late-onset psychotic disorder B. The general criteria for psychotic disorder must be met, except with regard to the onset of the disorder, which is more than 2 weeks but not more than 6 weeks after substance use. **Other mental and behavioral disorders** **Unspecified mental and behavioral disorder**

From World Health Organization. *The ICD-10 Classification of Mental and Behavioural Disorders: Diagnostic Criteria for Research.* Copyright, World Health Organization, Geneva; 1993, with permission.

Substance Withdrawal Substance withdrawal, as used in DSM-IV-TR, is a diagnostic term rather than a technical one. Thus, minor symptoms that technically are due to cessation of the use of a drug (e.g., the coffee drinker's early morning precoffee lethargy or minor headache) do not by themselves fulfill the criteria for substance withdrawal unless they are accompanied by a maladaptive behavior change and cause some clinically significant distress or impairment in social, occupational, or other important areas of functioning. DSM-IV-TR does not recognize withdrawal from caffeine, cannabis, or PCP, although some observers believe that specific signs and symptoms can be observed when those agents are abruptly discontinued after a period of heavy use. ICD-10 does describe a cannabinoid withdrawal state; accumulating evidence suggests that a cannabis withdrawal syndrome will be recognized in future revisions of the DSM-IV-TR.

Withdrawal is commonly, but not invariably, associated with the dependence syndrome. The signs and symptoms of withdrawal vary with the specific class of drug. In general, the severity of withdrawal is related to the amount of the substance used and the duration and patterns of use. Withdrawal is seen not only when the use of the substance is stopped but also when reduced use, a change in metabolism, or the administration of an antagonist results in lower levels of the drug at the relevant sites of action. Table 11.1–9 shows the DSM-IV-TR generic criteria for substance withdrawal; the ICD-10 general criteria are shown in Table 11.1–4. Specific diagnostic criteria for withdrawal from each category of drugs, to be used when the general criteria have been met, are also shown.

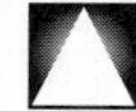

Table 11.1–5
DSM-IV-TR Diagnostic Criteria for Polysubstance Dependence

This diagnosis is reserved for behavior during the same 12-month period in which the person was repeatedly using at least three groups of substances (not including caffeine and nicotine), but no single substance predominated. Further, during this period, the dependence criteria were met for substances as a group but not for any specific substance.

From *Diagnostic and Statistical Manual of Mental Disorders.* 4th ed. Text rev. Washington, DC: American Psychiatric Association; 2000, with permission.

Substance Intoxication Intoxication is defined more narrowly in DSM-IV-TR than it might be in a pharmacology text. A variety of drugs may produce unwanted physiological or psychological effects that could be construed as intoxication (e.g., excessive sleepiness after the use of an antihistamine), but unless they are associated with maladaptive behavior, those effects do not constitute substance-induced intoxication as DSM-IV-TR defines it. Furthermore, whether a behavioral effect is maladaptive depends on the social and environmental context in which it occurs. When alcohol makes a person unusually sociable, a bit garrulous, and a little uncoordinated at a family celebration, it may not be maladaptive drinking behavior; the same behavior at a formal business meeting probably is. Similarly, ICD-10 specifies that intoxication must produce disturbances in the level of consciousness, cognition, perception, affect, or behavior that are of clinical importance. However, clinicians are to further specify which of several common complications of intoxication (e.g., trauma, delirium, convulsions) are also present. In addition, ICD-10 provides specific sets of diagnostic criteria for each of the drug categories and for multiple drugs to be used once the generic criteria for intoxication have been met. The DSM-IV-TR general criteria for substance intoxication are shown in Table 11.1–10. Also see Table 11.1–4 for the ICD-10 additional specifiers for complications of intoxication.

Substance-Induced Disorders In addition to dependence, abuse, intoxication, and withdrawal, certain psychoactive

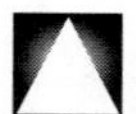

Table 11.1–6
DSM-IV-TR Diagnostic Criteria for Other (or Unknown) Substance-Related Disorders

The other (or unknown) substance-related disorders category is for classifying substance-related disorders associated with substances not shown in Table 11.1–4. Examples of these substances, which are described in more detail below, include anabolic steroids, nitrite inhalants ("poppers"), nitrous oxide, over-the-counter and prescription medications not otherwise covered by the 11 categories (e.g., cortisol, antihistamines, benztropine), and other substances that have psychoactive effects. In addition, this category may be used when the specific substance is unknown (e.g., an intoxication after taking a bottle of unlabeled pills).

Anabolic steroids sometimes produce an initial sense of enhanced well-being (or even euphoria), which is replaced after repeated use by lack of energy, irritability, and other forms of dysphoria. Continued use of these substances may lead to more severe symptoms (e.g., depressive symptomatology) and general medical conditions (liver disease).

Nitrite inhalants ("poppers"—forms of amyl, butyl, and isobutyl nitrite) produce an intoxication that is characterized by a feeling of fullness in the head, mild euphoria, a change in the perception of time, relaxation of smooth muscles, and a possible increase in sexual feelings. In addition to possible compulsive use, these substances carry dangers of potential impairment of immune functioning, irritation of the respiratory system, a decrease in the oxygen-carrying capacity of the blood, and a toxic reaction that can include vomiting, severe headache, hypotension, and dizziness.

Nitrous oxide ("laughing gas") causes rapid onset of an intoxication that is characterized by lightheadedness and a floating sensation that clears in a matter of minutes after administration is stopped. There are reports of temporary but clinically relevant confusion and reversible paranoid states when nitrous oxide is used regularly.

Other substances that are capable of producing mild intoxication include catnip, which can produce states similar to those observed with marijuana and which in high doses is reported to result in lysergic acid diethylamide–type perceptions; betel nut, which is chewed in many cultures to produce a mild euphoria and floating sensation; and kava (a substance derived from the South Pacific pepper plant), which produces sedation, incoordination, weight loss, mild forms of hepatitis, and lung abnormalities. In addition, individuals can develop dependence and impairment through repeated self-administration of over-the-counter and prescription drugs, including cortisol, antiparkinsonian agents that have anticholinergic properties, and antihistamines.

Texts and criteria sets have already been provided to define the generic aspects of substance dependence, substance abuse, substance intoxication, and substance withdrawal that are applicable across classes of substances. The other (or unknown) substance-induced disorders are described in the sections of the manual with disorders with which they share phenomenology (e.g., other [or unknown] substance-induced mood disorder is included in the mood disorders section). Listed below are the other (or unknown) substance use disorders and the other (or unknown) substance-induced disorders.

Other (or unknown) substance use disorders
Other (or unknown) substance dependence
Other (or unknown) substance abuse
Other (or unknown) substance-induced disorders
Other (or unknown) substance intoxication
Specify if:
With perceptual disturbances
Other (or unknown) substance withdrawal
Specify if:
With perceptual disturbances
Other (or unknown) substance-induced delirium
Other (or unknown) substance-induced persisting dementia
Other (or unknown) substance-induced persisting amnestic disorder
Other (or unknown) substance psychotic disorder with delusions
Specify if:
With onset during intoxication
With onset during withdrawal
Other (or unknown) substance-induced psychotic disorder with hallucinations
Specify if:
With onset during intoxication
With onset during withdrawal
Other (or unknown) substance-induced mood disorder
Specify if:
With onset during intoxication
With onset during withdrawal
Other (or unknown) substance-induced anxiety disorder
Specify if:
With onset during intoxication
With onset during withdrawal
Other (or unknown) substance-induced sexual dysfunction
Specify if:
With onset during intoxication
Other (or unknown) substance-induced sleep disorder
Specify if:
With onset during intoxication
Other (or unknown) substance-related disorder not otherwise specified

From American Psychiatric Association. *Diagnostic and Statistical Manual of Mental Disorders.* 4th ed. Text rev. Washington, DC: American Psychiatric Association; 2000, with permission.

drugs can induce syndromes that used to be called *organic mental disorders.* To avoid implying that other psychiatric disorders do not have an organic basis, DSM-IV-TR designates these syndromes as *substance-induced disorders* and recognizes the following categories: substance intoxication, substance withdrawal, substance-induced withdrawal delirium, substance-induced intoxication delirium, substance-induced persisting dementia, substance-induced persisting amnestic disorder, substance-induced mood disorder, substance-induced anxiety disorder, substance-induced psychotic disorder, substance-induced sexual dysfunction, and substance-induced sleep disorder.

When recording a diagnosis of substance-related disorder, the clinician should indicate the specific agent causing the disorder, if known, rather than the broad drug category. For example, the diagnosis should be substance-induced intoxication, pentobarbital (Nembutal), rather than substance-induced intoxication, sedative-hypnotics. However, the diagnostic code should be selected from the list of classes of substances provided in sets of criteria for the substance-induced disorder being recorded. For each of the substance-induced disorders (other than intoxication and withdrawal), the clinician should specify whether the onset occurred during intoxication or withdrawal. Thus, a specific substance-induced disorder has a three-part name delineating (1) the specific substance, (2) the context (whether the disorder occurred during intoxication or during withdrawal or occurs or persists beyond those stages), and (3) the phenomenological presentation (e.g., diazepam [Valium]–induced anxiety disorder with onset during withdrawal).

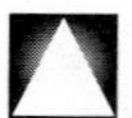

Table 11.1–7
DSM-IV-TR Course Modifiers for Substance Dependence

Six course specifiers are available for substance dependence. The four remission specifiers can be applied only after none of the criteria for substance dependence of substance abuse have been present for at least 1 month. The definition of these four types of remission is based on the interval of time that has elapsed since the cessation of dependence (early vs. sustained remission) and whether there is continued presence of one or more of the items included in the criteria sets for dependence or abuse (partial vs. full remission). Because the first 12 months after dependence are a time of particularly high risk for relapse, this period is designated *early remission.* After 12 months of early remission have passed without relapse to dependence, the person enters into sustained remission. For both early remission and sustained remission, a further designation of full is given if no criteria for dependence or abuse have been met during the period of remission; a designation of partial is given if at least one of the criteria for dependence or abuse has been met, intermittently or continuously, during the period of remission. The differentiation of sustained full remission from recovered (no current substance use disorder) requires consideration of the length of time since the last period of disturbance, the total duration of the disturbance, and the need for continued evaluation. If, after a period of remission or recovery, the individual again becomes dependent, the application of the early remission specifier requires that there again be at least 1 month in which no criteria for dependence or abuse are met. Two additional specifiers have been provided: on agonist therapy and in a controlled environment. For an individual to qualify for early remission after cessation of agonist therapy or release from a controlled environment, there must be a 1-month period in which none of the criteria for dependence or abuse are met.

The following remission specifiers can be applied only after no criteria for dependence or abuse have been met for at least 1 month. Note that these specifiers do not apply if the individual is on agonist therapy or in a controlled environment (see below).

Early full remission. This specifier is used if, for at least 1 month but for less than 12 months, no criteria for dependence or abuse have been met.

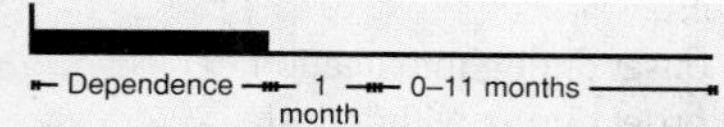

Early partial remission. This specifier is used if, for at least 1 month but less than 12 months, one or more criteria for dependence or abuse have been met (but the full criteria for dependence have not been met).

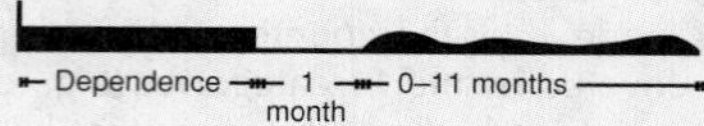

Sustained full remission. This specifier is used if none of the criteria for dependence or abuse have been met at any time during a period of 12 months or more.

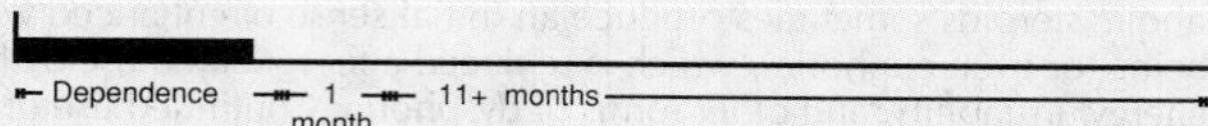

Sustained partial remission. This specifier is used if full criteria for dependence have not been met for a period of 12 months or more; however, one or more criteria for dependence or abuse have been met.

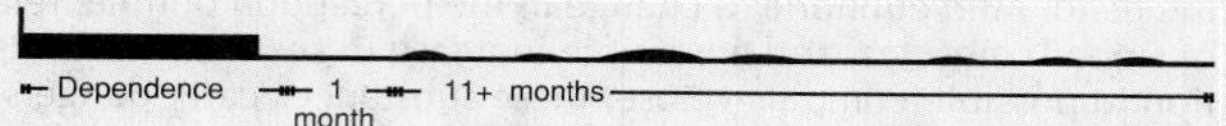

The following specifiers apply if the individual is on agonist therapy or in a controlled environment:

On agonist therapy. This specifier is used if the individual is on a prescribed agonist medication, and no criteria for dependence or abuse have been met for the class of medication for at least the past month (except tolerance to, or withdrawal from, the agonist). This category also applies to those being treated for dependence using a partial agonist or an agonist/antagonist.

In a controlled environment. This specifier is used if the individual is in an environment in which access to alcohol and controlled substances is restricted, and no criteria for dependence or abuse have been met for at least the past month. Examples of these environments are closely supervised and substance-free jails, therapeutic communities, or locked hospital units.

From American Psychiatric Association. *Diagnostic and Statistical Manual of Mental Disorders.* 4th ed. Text rev. Washington, DC: American Psychiatric Association; 2000, with permission.

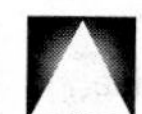

Table 11.1–8
DSM-IV-TR Diagnostic Criteria for Substance Abuse

A. A maladaptive pattern of substance use leading to clinically significant impairment or distress, as manifested by one (or more) of the following, occurring within a 12-month period:
  (1) Recurrent substance use resulting in an inability to fulfill major role obligations at work, school, or home (e.g., repeated absences or poor work performance related to substance use; substance-related absences, suspensions, or expulsions from school; neglect of children or household)
  (2) Recurrent substance use in situations in which it is physically hazardous (e.g., driving an automobile or operating a machine when impaired by substance use)
  (3) Recurrent substance-related legal problems (e.g., arrests for substance-related disorderly conduct)
  (4) Continued substance use despite having persistent or recurrent social or interpersonal problems caused or exacerbated by the effects of the substance (e.g., arguments with spouse about consequences of intoxication, physical fights)

B. The symptoms above never met the criteria for substance dependence for this class of substance.

From American Psychiatric Association. *Diagnostic and Statistical Manual of Mental Disorders.* 4th ed. Text rev. Washington, DC: American Psychiatric Association; 2000, with permission.

Table 11.1–11 shows the various disorders induced by the major categories of drugs recognized by DSM-IV-TR and indicates which disorders are seen during intoxication and which during withdrawal. Although they are not included specifically in the table, anabolic-adrenergic steroids can also induce psychotic mood, anxiety, and sleep and sexual disorders, and their withdrawal can also be associated with mood and sleep disorders. Although the current version of the table in DSM-IV (DSM-IV-TR) does not show a cannabis withdrawal syndrome, future revisions may do so.

ICD-10 takes a distinctly different approach to recording these drug-related disorders. With the first and second digits after the letter committed to designating the drug category, additional psychiatric syndromes are indicated by the use of the third and fourth digits. For example, persistent mood (affective) disorder associated with hallucinogens is designated F16.72. For the diagnosis to be made, the mood disorder needs to meet the criteria listed for mood disorders.

Evolving Terminology

The terminology used to describe the substance-related disorders has been repeatedly revised as concepts about the nature of drug-using behavior have evolved. In the 1980 third edition of the DSM (DSM-III), drug use disorders were divided into two major categories, drug abuse and drug dependence, and specific criteria for diagnosis were provided. In DSM-III-TR, adopted in 1987, the two categories were retained,

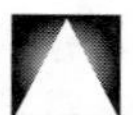

Table 11.1–9
DSM-IV-TR Diagnostic Criteria for Substance Withdrawal

A. The development of a substance-specific syndrome due to the cessation of (or reduction in) substance use that has been heavy and prolonged.
B. The substance-specific syndrome causes clinically significant distress or impairment in social, occupational, or other important areas of functioning.
C. The symptoms are not due to a general medical condition and are not better accounted for by another mental disorder.

From American Psychiatric Association. *Diagnostic and Statistical Manual of Mental Disorders.* 4th ed. Text rev. Washington, DC: American Psychiatric Association; 2000, with permission.

but the diagnostic criteria were modified. Further revisions were made for DSM-IV-TR, which adopted the terms "substance abuse" and "substance dependence," probably to eliminate the use of the more cumbersome term "alcohol and drug dependence including tobacco." For similar reasons, ICD-10 adopted the term "psychoactive substance dependence."

In much of the world literature on drug dependence, the term "dependence" is used to convey two distinct ideas: (1) a behavioral syndrome, and (2) physical or physiological dependence. *Physiological dependence* can be defined as an alteration in neural systems that is manifested by tolerance and the appearance of withdrawal phenomena when a chronically administered drug is discontinued or displaced from its receptor. Because the dual use of the word causes confusion, a 1980 ADAMHA-WHO working group recommended using "dependence" only to describe the behavioral syndrome and substituting the term "neuroadaptation" for physical dependence. Such a substitution would have emphasized several points. First, the continued use of many drugs, including some tricyclic antidepressants, some selective serotonin uptake inhibitors (SSRIs), and β-adrenergic receptor antagonists, causes neuroadaptive changes followed by withdrawal phenomena but not by drug-seeking behavior when they are discontinued. Second, neuroadaptive changes begin with the first dose of an opioid or sedative drug, and, therefore, such changes in and of themselves are not a sufficient cause (or definition) of drug dependence as a behavioral syndrome.

Why Use "Addiction"? The words "addict" and "addiction" often have pejorative connotations. Often, they are trivialized and are used to refer to frequently engaging in ordinary activities such as exercising or solving crossword puzzles. However, "addiction" continues to have the core connotation of decreased control, and some chapters in this book have retained such terms as "opioid addict" simply because they are less awkward than "severely opioid-dependent person." Here, the word "dependent," unmodified, is used to mean behaviorally dependent. The term *physiological dependence* or *physical dependence* is used to refer to the physiological changes that result in withdrawal symptoms when drugs are discontinued.

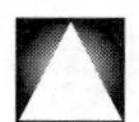

Table 11.1–10
DSM-IV-TR Diagnostic Criteria for Substance Intoxication

A. The development of a reversible substance-specific syndrome due to recent ingestion of (or exposure to) a substance. Note: Different substances may produce similar or identical syndromes.
B. Clinically significant maladaptive behavioral or psychological changes that are due to the effect of the substance on the central nervous system (e.g., belligerence, mood lability, cognitive impairment, impaired judgment, impaired social or occupational functioning) and develop during or shortly after use of the substance.
C. The symptoms are not due to a general medical condition and are not better accounted for by another mental disorder.

From American Psychiatric Association. *Diagnostic and Statistical Manual of Mental Disorders.* 4th ed. Text rev. Washington, DC: American Psychiatric Association; 2000, with permission.

COMPARATIVE NOSOLOGY

DSM-IV-TR and ICD-10 The generic concept of dependence is virtually identical in DSM-IV-TR and ICD-10. By requiring the clinician to specify whether tolerance and withdrawal are present, DSM-IV-TR appears to recognize a special significance for tolerance and physiological dependence. Some data indicate that, among alcoholics, the presence of physical dependence and, to a lesser degree, tolerance, is associated with a more severe variety of the syndrome. In practice, however, requiring evidence of these criteria does not substantially reduce the number of cases meeting the criteria for dependence in most drug categories, with the exception of hallucinogens, a class of drugs for which DSM-IV-TR does not list physiological dependence as a criterion. There is generally a high level of agreement between DSM-IV-TR and ICD-10 for making a diagnosis of dependence, although the descriptions of the criteria for determining the presence and severity of the syndrome differ. They both require that three elements of the syndrome have been present in a 12-month period. The DSM-IV-TR categorization of drug classes differs somewhat from the one used by ICD-10, which, constrained by a new alphanumeric system, uses only nine drug categories by including caffeine with amphetamine-like stimulants and PCP with other psychoactive agents.

The word *abuse* is also commonly used in ways that differ significantly from the definitions developed for use in DSM-IV-TR. In popular and legislative contexts, *drug abuse* means any use of an illegal substance or any nonprescribed use of a drug intended as a medicine as well as the harmful or excessive use of legally available substances such as alcohol and tobacco. In this chapter, the authors have chosen to use the term *illegal* in lieu of *illicit* wherever possible because illicit carries with it a moral connotation that is not carried by the term illegal. Some exceptions appear in figures taken from published works.

Despite the reliability of DSM-IV-TR and ICD-10 criteria for dependence in many European and Anglo-American cultures, several criteria (e.g., narrowing of drinking repertoire, time spent obtaining the drug, and even tolerance for the drug) have posed difficulties in other cultures, especially when dealing with alcohol. Tolerance is often misunderstood when applied to alcohol; in some cultures, holding one's liquor is a sign of manhood. Clinicians are more likely to make a diagnosis of drug dependence than alcohol dependence even when behavioral signs are comparable. In several cultures, little or no distinction is recognized among use, abuse, and harmful use of illegal drugs.

Other Perspectives The criteria for diagnosis in DSM-IV-TR and ICD-10 were developed from what is essentially a biopsychosocial model of drug dependence. In such a model, multiple factors—genetic, psychological, sociological, and pharmacological—contribute to the observed clinical syndromes. Such apparent unanimity about drug dependence should not obscure the existence of dissenting perspectives, which take several forms. In one, the biopsychosocial model is criticized as giving too much weight to biological factors and too little recognition to the notion of human will and responsibility, of medicalizing deviant behavior for the benefit of treatment professionals, and of creating universal exculpation for all those who do not live up to reasonable societal expectations. But some professionals have implicitly criticized the

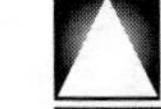

Table 11.1–11
DSM-IV-TR Diagnoses Associated with Class of Substances

	Dependence	Abuse	Intoxication	Withdrawal	Intoxication Delirium	Withdrawal Delirium	Dementia	Amnestic Disorder	Psychotic Disorders	Mood Disorders	Anxiety Disorders	Sexual Dysfunctions	Sleep Disorders
Alcohol	X	X	X	X	I	W	P	P	I/W	I/W	I/W	I	I/W
Amphetamines	X	X	X	X	I				I	I/W	I	I	I/W
Caffeine			X								I		I
Cannabis	X	X	X		I				I		I		
Cocaine	X	X	X	X	I				I	I/W	I/W	I	I/W
Hallucinogens	X	X	X		I				I[a]	I	I		
Inhalants	X	X	X		I		P		I	I	I		
Nicotine	X			X									
Opioids	X	X	X	X	I				I	I		I	I/W
Phencyclidine	X	X	X		I				I	I	I		
Sedatives, hypnotics, or anxiolytics	X	X	X	X	I	W	P	P	I/W	I/W	W	I	I/W
Polysubstance	X												
Other	X	X	X	X	I	W	P	P	I/W	I/W	I/W	I	I/W

Note: X, I, W, I/W, or P indicates that the category is recognized in DSM-IV. In addition, *I* indicates that the specifier With Onset During Intoxication may be noted for the category (except for Intoxication Delirium); *W* indicates that the specifier With Onset During Withdrawal may be noted for the category (except for Withdrawal Delirium); and *I/W* indicates that either With Onset During Intoxication or With Onset During Withdrawal may be noted for the category. *P* indicates that the disorder is Persisting.

[a]Also hallucinogen persisting perception disorder (flashbacks).

From American Psychiatric Association. *Diagnostic and Statistical Manual of Mental Disorders.* 4th ed. Text rev. Washington, DC: American Psychiatric Association; 2000, with permission.

same biopsychosocial model for not giving sufficient weight to the ideas that substance dependence is a specific primary disease (i.e., not a symptom of other psychiatric difficulties), that those who develop the disease have no control over their intake of certain substances, and that denial of the presence of a problem can be a major characteristic of the disease.

Concepts about substance dependence can be arrayed along several dimensions that are not entirely independent or orthogonal: broad versus narrow, disease versus learned behavior, and social versus medical. The narrow concept of substance dependence accepts as disorders those maladaptive behaviors associated primarily, if not exclusively, with the ingestion of substances generally accepted as pharmacological agents. Compulsive eating, gambling, running, hair pulling, and repetitive excessive sexual activities are not included among the dependence disorders, although those problems may share certain features that resemble a decreased ability to choose and are sometimes ameliorated by participation in support groups founded on principles similar to those of Alcoholics Anonymous (AA). A broad approach creates a superclass of disorders that include a number of such behaviors not involving pharmacological agents.

At the disease end of the disease-versus-behavioral syndrome dimension is a belief that dependence is not a learned behavior that can be modified or ameliorated with relearning but is a primary disorder caused by an interaction between a drug and a person with some genetic vulnerability and that only total abstinence can arrest the progression of the disease. The medical-versus-social dimension typically describes a range of views on how best to respond to problems with substances, rather than differences about the essential nature of the problems. The medical model stresses issues of assessment—treatment, planning, and record keeping—and sometimes treatment that can be rendered only by those with professional training (not necessarily physicians). The social model emphasizes the importance of social supports and integrating the person with a drug problem into a network of recovering people who can offer continuing support. The assessment and recording of progress and outcome as generally practiced by credentialed professionals are minimized.

HISTORY

The most commonly used drugs have been part of human existence for thousands of years. For example, opium has been used for medicinal purposes for at least 3,500 years, references to cannabis (marijuana) as a medicinal can be found in ancient Chinese herbals, wine is mentioned frequently in the Bible, and the indigenous people of the Western Hemisphere were smoking tobacco and chewing coca leaves generations before the arrival of the Spaniards. Some of the problems caused by alcohol and other drugs, such as drunkenness, are described in the Bible and in the writings of the ancient Greeks and Romans. As new and more concentrated forms of drugs were discovered or invented or new routes of administering them were developed, new problems related to their use emerged. In 18th-century England, for example, the alcohol-related problems seen after the introduction of cheap gin were considered more serious than those associated with beer and wine. Although, in Asia, opium smoking was a major problem in the 18th and 19th centuries, new problems related to opium were seen there and in other parts of the world after morphine, its most active alkaloid, was isolated in 1806. With the introduction of the hypodermic needle in the mid-19th century, morphine could be injected and became subject to misuse by that route. Intravenous (IV) morphine and heroin use began to spread in the early part of the 20th century. Technology also influenced the use of tobacco and the problems related to it. Although tobacco use was common by the 19th century, the serious adverse medical consequences associated with it did not emerge until the 20th century, when new methods of curing the leaves produced a mild smoking tobacco, and cigarettes were introduced. Cigarettes made common the practice of inhaling tobacco smoke deeply into the lungs. By the mid-20th century, cigarette smoking was a popular practice, and lung cancer was recognized as a consequence of cigarette use. It took an additional 20 years for it to become generally accepted that tobacco has the potential to induce dependence.

Medicalizing Excessive Drug Use

In 1810, Benjamin Rush, who is often credited as the first American physician to suggest that excessive use of alcohol was a disease rather than exclusively a moral defect, proposed the establishment of a sober house; in 1835, Samuel Woodward, a pioneer in the establishment of asylums for the insane, advocated similar asylums for inebriates. Contemporaneous with those early moves to involve medicine in dealing with excessive alcohol use was the emergence of the temperance movement and the Washingtonians—groups of reformed drunkards concerned with helping others to adopt and maintain sobriety. In the process, the Washingtonians developed many of the principles of self-help that were rediscovered by AA almost a century later. When the ideas of voluntarism and self-help, as exemplified by Washingtonian societies, failed to eliminate the problem of drunkenness, physicians began to debate more seriously the idea of coerced treatment in inebriate asylums supported by public funds. In 1870, advocates of the approach established the American Association for the Cure of Inebriates (AACI), dedicated to setting up hospitals for such people, conducting research, and teaching medical students and physicians how to treat inebriety. At first, those physicians who believed in a more spiritual, voluntary approach to the problem (neo-Washingtonians) were part of the AACI, but, gradually, the more somatically oriented factions, which advocated medically supervised asylums (and compulsory treatment when needed), gained ascendancy. Furthermore, the focus of concern was no longer limited to those who abused alcohol. Thomas Crothers, the secretary of AACI, saw inebriate asylums as places to treat all those who used any variety of intoxicant or narcotic to excess. However, very few publicly supported inebriate asylums ever opened.

Early Attitudes

The closing years of the 19th century saw growing concern about the excessive and inappropriate use of drugs, including alcohol and tobacco, as well as opiates and cocaine. First isolated from the coca leaf in 1860, cocaine came into widespread use in 1885 when pharmaceutical companies began selling it in the United States and Europe. In 1884, Sigmund Freud published a review of the potential therapeutic uses of cocaine. Some medical authorities in the United States shared his enthusiasm, and cocaine was recommended by the Hay Fever Association as a remedy for that malady. Within a few years, however, it was recognized that cocaine had the capacity to induce toxic psychosis as well as "habitual" or compulsive use and other features of a dependence syndrome. It was also recognized that long-term opiate use had dependence-inducing effects. Nevertheless, in the United States, until the beginning of the 20th century, the opium alkaloids and cocaine were still found in patent medicines that were sold over the counter without prescription for a wide variety of indications, and their labeling often did not reveal their contents.

Although achieving long-term cure of morphinism was reported to be exceedingly difficult, neither the public nor the medical profession viewed the habitual user of opium or morphine as invariably having a moral deficit. Those who had developed the morphine habit represented the entire socioeconomic spectrum, with women outnumbering men by approximately two to one. Various political and literary figures were known to use opiates but to lead otherwise productive and exemplary lives. People with emotional problems and those who had formerly used alcohol to excess were probably also overrepresented among opium users because it was not unusual at the time for physicians to prescribe opiates to control emotional problems and alcoholism. However, cocaine use and the morphine habit were also common among gamblers, petty thieves, prostitutes, and other disreputable members of society.

The problem of using the same institution for the treatment of drug users who had antisocial tendencies and those who led more conventional lives was just as vexing to early advocates of medical treatment as it is to present-day practitioners. Many proponents of inebriate asylums did not want to take responsibility for people who had frequent or serious encounters with the police because it was believed that such people made it impossible to create an atmosphere conducive to recovery. Partly to cope with the problem, even some of the proponents of a disease model of inebriety maintained the distinction between "inebriety the disease" and "intemperance the vice."

Early Control Efforts: Evolution of the Criminal Model By the late 1890s, the public and the medical community were no longer indifferent to drug use and habituation. In 1893, the Anti-Saloon League was founded, reinvigorating a temperance movement that advocated the total prohibition of alcohol. Medical texts in England, Europe, and the United States contained descriptions of morphinism, theories of its causation, and recommendations for withdrawal and postwithdrawal treatment. Some texts also described problems of cocainism. Medical authorities in the United States cautioned against overly liberal prescribing of cocaine and opiates by physicians and expressed great concern about the presence of those drugs in unlabeled proprietary over-the-counter medicines. State laws were passed that aimed at controlling the sale of opiates and cocaine, especially in patent medicines. In 1903, the cocaine in Coca-Cola was replaced by caffeine.

Partly to support the efforts of the Chinese government to control opium use in China, representatives of the United States government led the movement to negotiate an international treaty to control traffic in opium, cocaine, and related drugs. The first such treaty was signed in The Hague in 1912. Negotiators from the United States were also interested in the international control of cannabis but could not get other nations to view the substance as sufficiently problematic to warrant it. (Such control was achieved in 1925 at the Second Geneva Convention.) The Hague Convention required the signatories to pass domestic legislation controlling opiates and cocaine. The Harrison Act of 1914, the first federal legislation to regulate opiates and cocaine in the United States, was designed to restrict access to opiates and cocaine to doctors, dentists, pharmacists, and legitimate importers and manufacturers; it brought the United States into compliance with the convention.

Within the United States, state regulations concerning the sale of opiates and cocaine, the introduction of aspirin and the barbiturates, and the Pure Food and Drug Act of 1906, which required labeling of patent medicines, were already having an impact on the use of opiates in medicine when the Harrison Act was passed in 1914. Although many medical and political leaders in the United States believed that much of the problem of drug dependence resulted from careless prescribing by physicians, the Harrison Act was not originally intended to interfere with the legitimate practice of medicine or to cause special hardship for those already dependent on opiates. For several years after the Harrison Act was passed, a few cities operated clinics that prescribed morphine to people with established morphine habits. Most of those dependent on opiates before the Harrison Act became abstinent within a few years after it was passed, although generally not as a result of treatment at the clinics.

Fluctuating Attitudes Major changes had taken place in American attitudes and practices by the 1920s. The 18th Amendment to the U.S. Constitution, which prohibited the sale of alcohol, became law in 1920 and radically changed drinking behavior in the United States. Within a year after alcohol prohibition was enacted, 14 states also passed cigarette prohibition laws. Even less popular than alcohol prohibition, those anti-tobacco laws were all repealed by 1927, and by the mid-1920s, Americans were smoking 80 billion cigarettes a year. However, cocaine use, so prevalent at the turn of the century, was no longer widespread.

Disillusioned by the reluctance of morphine addicts at clinics to detoxify and by repeated relapses among those who did, doctors began to recommend (not for the first time) compulsory treatment with confinement until cure. As the new laws curtailed legitimate supplies of opiates, an illegal traffic developed to provide them to morphine addicts who could not or would not use the clinics. Increasingly, the drug sold was heroin, which had been introduced for medical use in 1898 but was quickly found by drug users to have effects quite similar to those of morphine. Many who patronized the illegal traffickers and used the clinics had histories of delinquency and criminal activity, and, eventually, that subgroup came to predominate. Reformers, moralists, and the popular press found in the opiate habit, and in the reputation of those who continued to use morphine, proof of the evils inherent in those drugs.

Negative publicity, lurid stories, medical disillusionment, and pressure from law enforcement agents combined to label the morphine clinics as medical folly and brought about their closing, the last in 1923. At the same time, a series of U.S. Supreme Court decisions implied that prescribing even small amounts of opiates or cocaine to an addict for treatment of addiction was not proper medical practice and was thus an illegal sale of narcotic drugs. Several physicians were imprisoned, and numerous others were tried, reprimanded, or otherwise harassed. By the early 1920s, people addicted to opiates were not welcome in doctor's offices, and they were often refused treatment at hospitals. *Dope addict* and *dope fiend* had become common terms, and the average layperson, as well as some otherwise well-informed members of the medical profession, appeared to believe that the opiate molecule was inherently evil. In the late 1930s, cannabis acquired a similar reputation, and in 1937, the U.S. Congress passed tax legislation prescribing criminal penalties for its use, sale, or possession. Alcohol prohibition had been repealed in 1933.

New Drug Problems The first of the barbiturate sedatives, barbital, was introduced into clinical medicine in 1903, followed over the next 30 years by scores of congeners that differed primarily in their duration of action. Within a few years after the introduction of each new compound, the first case reports of misuse, dependence, and withdrawal appeared in the medical journals, a pattern that was repeated with the nonbarbiturate sedatives, such as glutethimide (Doriden), ethchlorvynol (Placidyl), and meprobamate (Miltown), in the 1950s.

Amphetamine, first synthesized in 1887, was put into clinical use in 1932 as a drug to shrink mucous membranes. By 1935, its central stimulant effects had been recognized and found useful for treating narcolepsy, and dozens of other suggested uses soon followed. Reports that amphetamine was being used as a euphoriant began to appear in the late 1930s, but the full significance of its potential to cause harm was not appreciated until the post–World War II epidemic of IV methamphetamine addiction in Japan. That epidemic, precipitated by the sale of surplus methamphetamine tablets intended for combat troops, involved millions of people. Other amphetamine-like drugs, which have also been subject to misuse, were introduced during the 1950s and early 1960s.

The psychological effects of mescaline were already known and written about at the end of the 19th century. However, public concern about hallucinogens did not reach a high level until the 1960s, when the use of a newly discovered and exceedingly potent compound, lysergic acid diethylamide (LSD), evolved from experimentation by the intellectual elite and a few college students to more widespread use by even younger people. PCP, a general anesthetic developed in the 1950s, also became a drug of abuse in the 1960s and 1970s.

Despite repeated reports of abuse and dependence associated with barbiturates, barbiturate-like sedatives, and amphetamines and related stimulants and in spite of concerns about experimentation with LSD and related hallucinogens, there were no federal criminal sanctions related to these drugs until 1964, when authority for their control was assigned to the Food and Drug Administration (FDA). In contrast, in the 1950s, concern about heroin addiction had led to ever harsher criminal penalties for its sale or possession. Although law enforcement efforts aimed at controlling heroin use were increased, both the number of new heroin users and the crime rates continued to increase throughout the late 1960s. At about that time, there was also a sharp increase in the nonmedical use of other substances, such as cannabis and LSD, and a major epidemic of amphetamine misuse and dependence. In addition to amphetamines diverted from medical channels, supplies came from clandestine laboratories. Drug use, especially cannabis, became linked to antiestablishment attitudes, politics, and lifestyles.

Through the mid-1970s in the United States, there was a substantial increase in experimentation with cocaine followed by increases in heavy cocaine use. Starting in the late 1980s, there was an upsurge in methamphetamine use that was driven by a proliferation of illegal laboratories. Subsequently, there has been an increase in the popularity of drugs such as 3,4-methylenedioxymethamphetamine (MDMA) and γ-hydroxybutyrate (GHB), now often referred to as *club drugs* because they are typically used at marathon-like dance parties ("raves").

Evolving Treatment Approaches

Treatment for drug- and alcohol-related problems underwent several dramatic changes during the 20th century. The large specialized asylums that were advocated in the 19th century never materialized. Toward the end of the 19th century, physicians were primarily concerned with how to manage withdrawal syndromes and whether longer compulsory treatment was needed. With the advent of prohibition, the impetus to develop treatments for alcoholism declined sharply. Interest in treating opioid-dependent patients also declined as physicians became discouraged by their patients' tendency to relapse after being detoxified and as opioid use and dependence came to be seen more as criminal behaviors than as medical disorders. A few private sanatoriums continued to provide treatment for opioid dependence. By 1930, after a change in federal policy as drug-addicted prisoners began to fill the penitentiaries, the federal government established two hospitals, at Lexington, Kentucky, and Fort Worth, Texas, to provide treatment for that population and also to conduct research on opiates and opiate addiction. Treatment for barbiturate and amphetamine dependence took place largely in the mainstream of medical practice and in state hospitals, but there was no consensus on what constituted effective posthospital care.

In the mid-1930s, two recovering alcoholics rediscovered the principles of the Washingtonians, added some new principles, and initiated the self-help movement now known as *AA*. By the 1950s, this movement had begun to inspire analogous self-help efforts among other types of drug users.

The situation changed again in the early 1960s. With new outbreaks of heroin use by young people and increasing crime, the federal government and individual states attempted to respond to the problem. California initiated a civil commitment program for addicts under the administrative control of the Department of Corrections; New York City reopened Riverside Hospital to treat juvenile heroin addicts. The first follow-up studies of patients treated at the federal hospital at Lexington, Kentucky, revealed exceedingly high rates of relapse after treatment. Both the medical community and the general public demanded new ideas and solutions, including a reconsideration of providing opiate addicts with legitimate opioids through medical channels.

From 1958 to 1967, several major new approaches to treating opioid dependence were developed. Synanon, the prototype therapeutic community for treatment of chronic drug dependence, was started in California in 1958 and was soon replicated in New York with the establishment of Daytop Village and Phoenix House. Vincent Dole and Marie Nyswander showed that maintaining selected long-term heroin addicts on large daily doses of methadone (Dolophine) was effective in reducing crime and heroin use. Several research groups demonstrated that heroin addicts voluntarily tried treatment with narcotic antagonists. In the mid-1960s, New York State and the federal government legislated civil commitment programs modeled after the program in California, with an initial period of prolonged institutional care as a key element. Although many treatment programs initiated in the early 1960s continued to focus on the treatment of opioid dependence, others, especially the therapeutic communities, viewed all nonmedical drug use as stemming from similar defects in character structure and offered a generic approach to treating drug dependence.

Each of these general approaches has evolved and has incorporated findings from an unprecedented outpouring of government-funded research on treatment methods and outcome. Among the methods that found their way into both publicly supported programs and individual practices was the use of cognitive-behavioral and relapse prevention techniques.

Alcohol and Nicotine

In the 1950s, clinicians at Wilmar State Hospital in Minnesota developed a treatment program for alcoholism built on a synthesis of the medical model and the experiences of individuals recovering from alcohol dependence using the 12-step principles of AA. That treatment approach was refined and expanded at the Johnson Institute and Hazelden Foundation, also in Minnesota. The modified programs, widely adopted by others, are often referred to as *28-day programs*, *12-step programs*, or the *Minnesota model*. In the early 1970s, the effort to recognize alcoholism as a disease gained momentum, and the decision of medical insurance carriers to provide coverage for detoxification and inpatient treatment fueled an unprecedented growth of private-sector facilities offering treatment for alcoholism. Almost without exception, they were residential programs using the Minnesota model. The decriminalization of public intoxication spurred a parallel increase in alcohol treatment programs supported by the public sector.

The Surgeon General's Report of 1964 linked cigarette smoking to lung cancer and concluded that tobacco smoking was a form of dependence, although not an addiction. By the 1970s, tobacco dependence was more widely accepted as a valid clinical entity, and various treatments for it were developed. By the late 1980s, as smoking was becoming socially unacceptable, many buildings were declared smoke free, smoking was banned on most airplane flights and in many hospitals, and pharmaceutical companies began to market new products for delivering nicotine (e.g., nicotine chewing gum and transdermal patches) as aids for smoking cessation. By the late 1990s, the tobacco companies were negotiating settlements in multiple civil lawsuits by states and by individuals who had been injured by their tobacco use, and Congress had debated major tax increases on tobacco and regulation by the FDA.

Two-Tiered System

As the cocaine epidemic of the 1970s and 1980s struck the middle class, much of the large, private-sector system for treating alcoholism evolved into chemical dependency units offering similar treatments to people with alcohol problems and those with other varieties of substance dependence. By 1990, it was estimated that more than 8,000 recognized programs existed that dealt with alcoholism and other substance dependence. (The estimate at the turn of the 21st century was 12,000.) The treatment methods used varied widely in terms of settings, costs, philosophical underpinnings, and populations served. New categories of drug treatment professionals had emerged, and psychiatrists who once had considered the problems to be a low-status area successfully lobbied for the creation of a recognized subspecialty in addiction psychiatry. Treatment capacity was described as a two-tiered system with private and public sectors in which the private sector served 40 percent of the population but received 60 percent of the total expenditures for treatment. One response to the escalating cost of drug treatment services among those with private medical insurance was the rise of a managed care industry created to control costs on behalf of employers who pay for health insurance, generally by severely limiting the length of stay in hospital settings. Managed care, by refusing to recognize (and pay for) the medical necessity of inpatient treatment for most cases of drug or alcohol dependence, largely dismantled the "28-day" inpatient alcohol and drug treatment programs that had serviced patients with insurance. By the mid-1990s, managed care principles were routine in the public sector as well, and little remained of the residential component of the two-tiered system.

There are still two tiers of treatment in that some individuals with private resources or insurance have access to a wider variety of treatment opportunities. Those who do have insurance or their own funds must rely on the availability of publicly supported programs. These programs are often unable to accept new patients in a timely way. The 1990s saw increased effort to provide treatment to incarcerated individuals with drug dependence problems. Also, there was substantial expansion of "drug courts" in which judges with special interest used their authority to motivate (or coerce) drug-using offenders to accept treatment. In some cases, the treatment was largely coerced abstinence in which the court mandated frequent drug testing (usually urine tests) and specified escalating periods of incarceration for continued drug use.

Legislation and National Strategies

In 1969, Congress recognized the need to give greater attention to the problem of alcoholism and established the National Institute on Alcohol Abuse and Alcoholism (NIAAA) in the National Institute of Mental Health (NIMH). In 1970, new federal controlled substances legislation was passed, reorganizing the jumble of drug regulatory statutes that had evolved since the passage of the Harrison Act, increasing the resources for controlling the availability of illegal drugs. Shortly thereafter, the task of enforcement was given to a new agency, the Drug Enforcement Agency (DEA), which incorporated elements of the FDA and the Bureau of Narcotic and Dangerous Drugs. All drugs subject to special controls were included in one of several categories of the Controlled Substances Act (CSA).

In 1971, when U.S. troops in Vietnam were reported to be using heroin heavily, the Special Action Office for Drug Abuse Prevention (SAODAP) was established in the executive office of the president to coordinate government activities and policies relating to drug abuse and to develop and publish an overall national drug strategy. The creation of that office and the associated legislation marked a turning point in U.S. drug policy. The notion that opioid dependence was an incurable disorder, which justified the harshest of penalties in the name of prevention, was superseded by a policy that recognized that a substantial proportion of drug-dependent individuals could eventually reenter the mainstream of society. New commitments were made to basic research, epidemiology, development of new treatment methods, and evaluation of existing treatment approaches. Methadone maintenance was moved, by executive fiat, from the legal limbo of experimental status to a category that recognized its legitimacy. Regulations intended to prevent inappropriate prescribing of opioids were developed. Federal support for the expansion of community treatment programs was also greatly increased. The legislation that established SAODAP also provided the legislative framework for the National Institute on Drug Abuse (NIDA) in the Department of Health, Education, and Welfare (HEW). When it was established in 1974, NIDA became the lead agency for implementing federal policy on treatment, research, and prevention. SAODAP was ended in 1974 but was succeeded by several similar drug policy coordinating offices (currently the Office of National Drug Control Policy [ONDCP]) located within the executive office of the president.

By the early 1980s, treatment for opioid dependence was generally accepted to have demonstrable impact. However, for most patients in treatment programs, the primary drugs of choice were no longer opioids but, more typically, cannabis, stimulants, or sedatives. In the early and mid-1970s, some groups had argued for the decriminalization or legalization of cannabis. The arguments lost much of their force when it was found that in 1979 almost 10 percent of high school students were using cannabis on a daily basis. In response to what they perceived as tolerance toward cannabis use, a number of parents' organizations were formed that were committed to making all drug use unacceptable. Those groups forced NIDA to review and remove from all its publications any statements that could be interpreted as tolerating drug use. This decreased tolerance for drug use grew in parallel with a more general conservative shift in public attitudes. For example, in the 1970s, the public and the courts had rejected the use of urine testing as a means of detecting drug use in an effort to interrupt the heroin epidemic; but, starting in 1986, federal employees were required by presidential order to undergo such tests. Similar drug testing was encouraged in private industry, giving rise to new industries for detecting the presence of drugs, interpreting test results, and placing drug users in treatment.

By the 1970s, it was obvious that the major drug problems in the United States in terms of social and economic impact and health costs were alcoholism and tobacco dependence. Although the Surgeon General's Report of 1964 linking cigarettes to cancer had not produced any dramatic immediate decrease in smoking, the rate of increase in cigarette consumption among men had begun to level out. In 1988, the *Surgeon General's Report on the Health Consequences of Smoking* officially defined tobacco dependence as analogous to other varieties of drug dependence. In 1994, the FDA held hearings on the appropriateness of regulating the nicotine in tobacco as an addictive drug. Shortly thereafter, with backing from the president, the FDA assumed authority to regulate advertising of tobacco products; the White House lobbied Congress to pass legislation that would limit advertising and increase federal taxes on tobacco. Legislation was not passed. The U.S. Supreme Court rejected the FDA's assertion of authority, stating that specific congressional authority to regulate tobacco would be required. In 1998, the major tobacco manufacturers negotiated a settlement with 46 of the 50 states (the Master Settlement Agreement), which awarded the states more than $200 billion over 20 years, provided that they pass legislation that prevents any tobacco manufacturers that did not sign the agreement from selling cigarettes without paying a special tariff. This allowed the major tobacco companies to increase their prices to pay the states the agreed-on sums.

By the mid-1980s, increasing demand for the treatment of cocaine dependence, the sudden cocaine-induced deaths of several prominent athletes, and concern about the spread of human immunodeficiency virus (HIV) and acquired immune deficiency syndrome (AIDS) among IV drug users led to additional legislation that authorized the government to spend nearly $4 billion to intensify efforts against drugs and drug problems. Although most of that money was allocated to law enforcement activities, federal resources for the treatment of drug dependence and research were also substantially increased. Thereafter, the federal government created a series of offices that evolved into the Substance Abuse and Mental Health Services Administration (SAMHSA) with several constituent centers, including the Center for Substance Abuse Treatment (CSAT) and the Center for Substance Abuse Prevention (CSAP). Critics of the emphasis on supply control gained public attention when they were supported by several prominent conservative writers and economists and garnered the financial support of several well-endowed foundations. Although the more thoughtful of these critics have stopped calling for outright legalization of drugs, they have called for greater emphasis on reducing the harm related to drug use by medically prescribing heroin and other psychoactive drugs and more support for needle-exchange programs. Despite some evidence suggesting that availability of sterile needles can reduce HIV transmission, the federal government continues to ban the use of federal money for such programs.

Although largely rejected at the federal level, the general thrust toward harm reduction has gained some momentum in some states in which penalties for possession of cannabis have been reduced, and its use for medical purposes has been approved.

In 2000, Congress passed legislation that allows clinicians with special training to provide office-based treatment and to prescribe an opioid for opioid-dependent patients. Currently, the only opioid that meets the legislatively specified criteria is buprenorphine, a partial opioid agonist.

EPIDEMIOLOGY

Most of epidemiology's contributions to the understanding of the drug dependence syndromes can be sorted in relation to five main substantive rubrics plus a separate rubric for theoretical and methodological research on core concepts, measurements, and other details of research approach. The five main substantive rubrics and examples of the associated research questions are shown in Table 11.1–12.

In the field of drug dependence research, epidemiology may be known best for contributions under the rubric of "quantity." Epidemiological field surveys to quantify the burden of inebriety and habitual use of opiate drugs were added to community surveys of mental illness in the last quarter of the 19th century during the era of

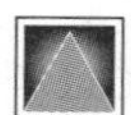

Table 11.1–12
Epidemiology's Rubrics

Five main subject matter rubrics and examples of research questions

- Quantity: How many in the population are becoming drug dependent for the first time each year?
- Location: Where, within the population, are we more and less likely to find people becoming drug dependent?
- Causes: What accounts for some people becoming drug dependent, whereas others remain unaffected?
- Mechanisms: What is the pathogenesis, natural history, and clinical course of drug dependence as observed in drug-dependent people identified in the community, compared with those identified when they are incarcerated for drug-related crimes or when they otherwise come to official attention?
- Prevention and control: What can be done to prevent or delay the onset of drug dependence and to shorten or ameliorate the burden of drug dependence when it occurs?

Adapted from Anthony JH, Van Etten ML. Epidemiology and its rubrics. In: Bellack A, Hersen M, eds. *Comprehensive Clinical Psychology*. Oxford, UK: Elsevier; 1998.

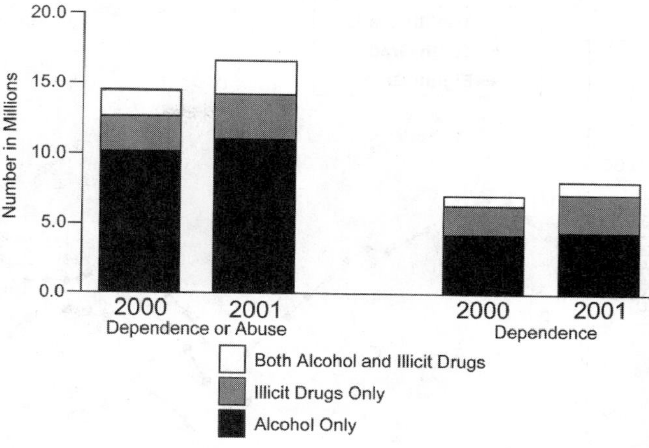

FIGURE 11.1–1 Estimates of past-year substance dependence or abuse among people 12 years of age or older in the United States, 2000 and 2001. (From National Household Survey of Drug Abuse; 2001, with permission.)

increasing concern about drunken behavior and the misuse of over-the-counter patent medicines containing opiates and cocaine.

Beginning in the 1960s, a number of distinct methods designed to gauge the extent and consequences of substance use, abuse, and dependence have been developed and have been progressively improved. Currently, the major recurring surveillance instruments in the United States are the National Household Survey on Drug Abuse (NHSDA), the Drug Abuse Warning Network (DAWN), Arrestee Drug Abuse Monitoring System (ADAM, formerly known as the *Drug Use Forecasting [DUF] program*), and the Monitoring the Future Study (MTF), also known as the *High School Survey*. In addition, data on street availability and purity of illegal drugs, drug seizures, and arrests for drug offenses are collected nationally from the DEA and the Federal Bureau of Investigation (FBI) and locally from municipal police departments. Each of these data sources has strengths and limitations. The NHSDA (recently renamed the *National Household Survey on Drug Use and Health*) annually interviews a representative sample of individuals aged 12 years and older living in households, college dormitories, homeless shelters, and rooming houses. It oversamples minority populations and certain large urban areas and focuses in detail on drug-using behaviors. It does not interview military personnel or individuals who are living on the street or in institutions (jails or hospitals). Since 2000, it has also included questions designed to measure substance dependence and abuse based on DSM-IV criteria and to determine whether respondents believe they need treatment, and it asks what type of treatment, if any, they have received in the past year. Other developments have included an increase in sample size, from less than 8,000 in the earliest survey in the 1970s to more than 50,000 in more recent years, and the deliberate probabilistic oversampling of certain metropolitan areas and disadvantaged minority groups. Because of the new sample sizes and methods, the NHSDA can now produce remarkably precise estimates. In some years, there has been assessment of suspected determinants or consequences of drug taking, such as major depression.

Analysis of the 2001 NHSDA indicates that 16.6 million people in the United States aged 12 years or older (7.3 percent of the population) could be considered to be abusing or dependent on alcohol (but not illegal drugs); 2.4 million, abusing or dependent on both alcohol and illegal drugs; and 3.2 million, abusing or dependent on an illegal drug (but not alcohol). These estimates are illustrated in Figure 11.1–1. Approximately one-half of the 16.6 million people (8.2 million) were considered substance dependent. Of those, 4.5 million were dependent on alcohol only, 2.7 million were dependent on illegal drugs but not alcohol, and 0.9 million were dependent on both alcohol and illegal drugs. When the analysis is limited to those who have used a given drug in the past year, the proportion with dependence or abuse increases. For example, 9.3 percent of past-year users of alcohol, approximately 50 percent of past-year heroin users, and 25 percent of past-year cocaine users are classified with dependence or abuse of those drugs. For past-year users of marijuana, dependence or abuse is considered present in only 16.5 percent, but because of the total number of marijuana users, the number of those with cannabis dependence or abuse (3.5 million) exceeds the number dependent on heroin and cocaine combined.

Correlates of Gender, Education, Employment, and Age of First Use

Men are twice as likely as women to be considered dependent on or abusers of alcohol or illegal drugs, (men, 10 percent; women, 4.9 percent). There is little gender difference with respect to tobacco dependence. Adults who did not complete high school are more likely than college graduates to have become dependent on illegal drugs (3.7 percent for those with less than a high school education, 0.9 percent for college graduates), although alcohol dependence or abuse is not particularly correlated with educational level. The unemployed are almost twice as likely as those employed full time to be categorized as dependent on illegal drugs or alcohol (15.4 percent, compared with 7.9 percent). Adults who first used drugs at a younger age are more likely to have developed dependence or abuse than those who started later. For example, 12 percent of those who tried marijuana by 14 years of age are classified as dependent on or abusers of an illegal drug, compared with 2 percent of those who first used at 18 years of age or older.

The Monitoring the Future survey has obtained information each year since 1975 from self-administered forms returned anonymously by high school seniors. It includes former seniors now in college and students in the eighth and tenth grades. In addition to drug use, the survey taps suspected causes and consequences of use such as perceived availability of drugs and perceived harmfulness. Although the survey depends on self-report, the trend information it provides is useful. Figure 11.1–2 shows the changes in annual use of illegal drugs by eighth-, tenth-, and 12th-grade students through 2002.

The ADAM system interviews and obtains anonymous urine specimens from a sample of arrestees in moderate-sized cities in the United States. By design, people charged with sale or possession of drugs cannot make up

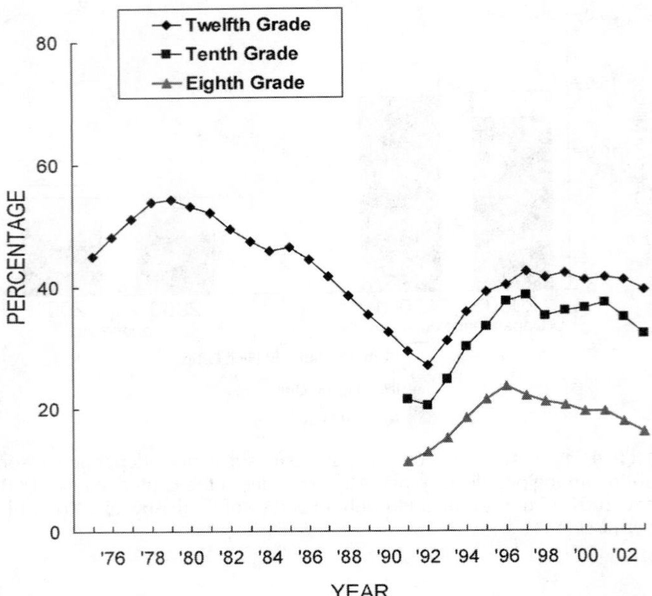

FIGURE 11.1–2 Trends in annual prevalence of an illegal drug use index for eighth, tenth, and 12th graders: percentage of students who reported use. (Courtesy of Johnston LD, O'Malley PM, Bachman JG. *Monitoring the Future National Results on Drug Use: Overview of Key Findings, 2002.* [NIH Publ. No. 03-5374]. Bethesda, MD: National Institute on Drug Abuse; 2003.)

more than 25 percent of the sample. Although it does not depend on self-reports to measure use, the ADAM results cannot be easily extrapolated to a national population, and the information that can be derived from a single urine test is limited. Nevertheless, the system obtains data from a population in which illegal drug use is high and thus provides trend data not readily available from other sources. In general, current drug use among arrestees is several times higher than among those sampled and assessed in self-reports for the national surveys.

Field survey approaches of nationally representative samples tend to be more useful and informative than incident or event reporting approaches such as DAWN. The DAWN system involves abstracting and reporting drug-related emergency room and medical examiner death event data each month of the calendar year. The DAWN system is now designed so that the reporting emergency rooms constitute a representative sample of such facilities in the continental United States. The DAWN data provide useful information on trends in the morbidity associated with various illegal drugs; but these data need to be interpreted with caution because the DAWN system reports only episodes in which a drug is part of the presenting clinical picture. For example, an increasing number of emergency room episodes associated with heroin could mean that more heroin users with AIDS-related problems are seeking primary medical care in emergency department facilities rather than that more individuals are using heroin. Similarly, reports by medical examiners of more violent deaths associated with cocaine may signal an escalation of competition among drug dealers rather than more people using cocaine. The analytical methods do not reveal the nature of the linkage between drug use and the presenting problem, which drugs (if any) played a causal role in the episode, or whether the user was a novice or a chronic user.

Comorbidity Surveys In addition to the recurring data-gathering efforts, important epidemiological information is available from two national studies that systematically interviewed representative samples of the population and used DSM-III or DSM-III-R criteria to develop estimates of current and lifetime prevalence of psychiatric disorders, including substance abuse and substance dependence. These studies are the NIMH Epidemiological Catchment Area (ECA) Study, conducted in the early 1980s, and the National Comorbidity Survey (NCS), conducted between 1990 and 1992. The ECA interviews in five areas of the United States included individuals in institutions (mental hospitals, jails, nursing homes, and so forth) and used DSM-III criteria to develop estimates of prevalence. The NCS interviews of a nationally representative sample of people not residing in institutions used DSM-III-R criteria. Although the ECA was conducted before the cocaine epidemic of the 1980s crested, and criteria for diagnosis used were altered somewhat in DSM-III-R, it nevertheless remains a landmark study of the extent of drug abuse and dependence and cooccurring psychiatric disorders.

The ECA study found that 16.7 percent of the U.S. population aged 18 years and older met the DSM-III criteria for a lifetime diagnosis of either abuse or dependence on some substance, with 13.8 percent meeting the criteria for an alcohol-related disorder, and 6.2 percent meeting the criteria for abuse or dependence of a drug other than alcohol or tobacco. The NCS found a 26.6 percent lifetime prevalence of substance abuse and dependence, substantially higher than the 16.7 percent found in the ECA. Some of this is probably due to questions in the NCS about prescription drugs that were posed when a patient reported symptoms of dependence and on differences in criteria (DSM-III vs. DSM-III-R). However, there may also have been real increases in prevalence. For illegal drugs and the nonmedical use of prescription drugs, the lifetime history of dependence in the NCS was 7.9 percent, a figure much closer to the 6.2 percent found for such drugs in the ECA study. The NCS found a 12-month prevalence estimate for any drug use disorder (including dependence and abuse) of 8.2 percent, 4.5 percent alcohol dependence, and 1.8 percent drug dependence. Except for tobacco, men are far more likely than women to use drugs and alcohol and are correspondingly more likely to have developed dependence. For example, lifetime and 12-month prevalence of alcohol dependence is 20.1 and 6.6 percent for men but only 8.2 and 2.2 percent for women, respectively.

Among the major achievements of the NCS analyses were the findings on the proportions of people who had used drugs at any time in their lives (lifetime users) who became dependent (overall and for each drug category); the demographic factors associated with use, dependence, and persistence of dependence; and the prevalence and significance of multiple psychiatric diagnoses. Dependence cannot develop if a drug is never used; thus, presenting data on the prevalence of dependence in the population as whole, including those who never used, can obscure the likelihood of dependence developing among those who do use a particular drug. In the NCS, prevalence of lifetime dependence on the broad range of illegal and nonprescribed medications was 14.7 percent, with male users only slightly more likely (16.4 percent) than female users (12.6 percent) to develop dependence. In a similar analysis of the 12-month prevalence of dependence on these drugs, the rate for the population as a whole was 1.8 percent. However, the 12-month prevalence was 3.5 percent for those who had used any of these drugs at any time in their lives, 10.3 percent for those who had used them in the past 12 months, and 23.8 percent among those who had a lifetime history of dependence. The likelihood of being drug dependent within the past 12 months, given a lifetime history of dependence, was similar for men (24.9 percent) and women (22.2 percent). Lower educational and income levels predicted a lifetime history of dependence (odds ratios greater than 2), but race, ethnicity, or living in an urban environment did not. There were also differences in the likelihood that users of a particular drug would become dependent on it. For example, for heroin, the estimated probability of having developed opioid dependence was 23 percent; for tobacco, 32 percent; for cocaine, 16.7 percent; for alcohol,

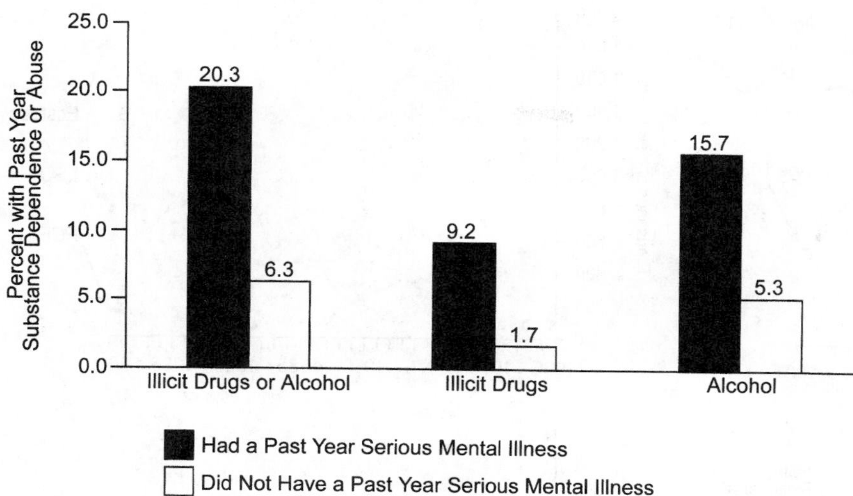

FIGURE 11.1–3 Substance dependence or abuse among adults by serious mental illness, 2001. (From National Household Survey of Drug Abuse; 2001, with permission.)

15.4 percent; but only 4.9 percent for psychedelics. Men who used alcohol were more likely to have become dependent (21.4 percent) than women (9.2 percent), possibly because they drink more than women, but genetics may also play a role.

A comparable comorbidity study conducted in England and Wales in the 1990s found, like studies in the United States, that substance-related disorders are among the most common psychiatric disorders. Alcohol dependence was found in 5 percent of the household sample (8 percent of men, 2 percent of women), in 7 percent of an institutional sample, and in 21 percent of the homeless sample. Substance use was significantly associated with higher rates of psychological morbidity. Among those not dependent on any substance, 12 percent were assessed as having a psychiatric disorder. Among those dependent on nicotine, 22 percent were assessed as having another psychiatric disorder. The rates for psychiatric comorbidity were 30 percent and 45 percent for those dependent on alcohol and other drugs, respectively.

The newest versions of NHSDA now provide some data on comorbidity and confirm the findings of the NCS that serious mental illness is strongly correlated with illegal drug use and cigarette use. Individuals with a serious mental illness are more than twice as likely to have used an illegal drug and to have been cigarette smokers. Serious mental illness is even more strongly correlated with the presence of drug abuse or dependence. This relationship is illustrated in Figure 11.1–3. In 2001, it was estimated that 3 million adults had both a serious mental illness and substance dependence or abuse in the past year. Of the 3 million, 1.6 million met criteria for abuse of or dependence on alcohol alone; 0.7 million for abuse of or dependence on both drugs and alcohol; and 0.7 million for abuse of or dependence on an illegal drug.

Comorbidity is also considered below as an etiological factor in the development of substance abuse and dependence.

Epidemics Several major overlapping drug epidemics have occurred over the past 30 years, affecting somewhat different populations. Cannabis use, which had been endemic among certain minority groups and jazz musicians, began to increase in the 1960s, especially among young people, and then spread to other segments of the population. At its peak in the mid- to late 1970s, 10 percent of high school seniors were using marijuana on a daily basis. Daily use declined to 5 percent by 1984, to 2 percent by 1991, and then reversed direction and again increased, according to the Monitoring the Future survey. Similar changes in use rates were reflected in the NHSDA.

An epidemic of heroin use also began in the early 1960s, and incidence peaked between 1969 and 1971. The population of active heroin users reached its highest levels in the early 1970s, but periodic upsurges have occurred as supplies became more available, law enforcement activity waxed and waned, and relapse rates increased among former users. In 1977, the U.S. government estimated that there were 500,000 opioid abusers and dependent users, and more recently, it revised the estimate to 320,000 occasional users and 810,000 chronic users. In general, the heroin-using population is an aging one, with a high and still growing prevalence of HIV in some areas. In 1996, the NHSDA estimated that approximately 2.3 million people had tried heroin at least once and that 245,000 had used it in the past year. However, it was believed that a large percentage of heroin users were outside the population interviewed by the survey. Data from the more recent NHSDA indicate that heroin use increased during the 1990s to levels nearly as high as those of the 1970s. The annual number of new users was estimated to range from 55,000 to 69,000 between 1989 and 1992. By 2000, the number of new heroin users per year appeared to have increased to 146,000.

The cocaine epidemic that began in the late 1960s seems to have reached its peak by 1980. In the early 1980s, according to the NHSDA, an estimated 5.8 million people in the United States (2.9 percent of the population) had used cocaine in the month before the survey. There were an estimated 1.5 million new users in 1983. The epidemic passed its peak in most segments of society by the mid-1980s, with the number of new users declining steadily until 1992. Among the heaviest users (weekly or almost weekly), use did not decline significantly, although rates among arrestees decreased in 1995. For the population as a whole, the number of new users has been increasing modestly since 1992. There were approximately 0.9 million new users in 2000.

In the early 1990s, fueled by abundant supplies of cheap methamphetamine produced illegally in many small laboratories, methamphetamine use began to increase in a number of cities in the west, southwest, and northwest of the United States. For the country as a whole, the number of new users increased from 164,000 per year at that time to 344,000 in 2000.

Changes in the annual rate of new users of various drugs over the past 30 years as deduced from the NHSDA database are shown in Figure 11.1–4.

ETIOLOGY

The model of drug dependence from which the DSM-IV-TR and ICD-10 criteria were derived conceptualizes dependence as a result of a process in which multiple interacting factors influence drug-using behavior and the loss of flexibility with respect to decisions about using a given drug. Although the actions of a given drug are critical in the process, it is not assumed that all people who become dependent on the same drug

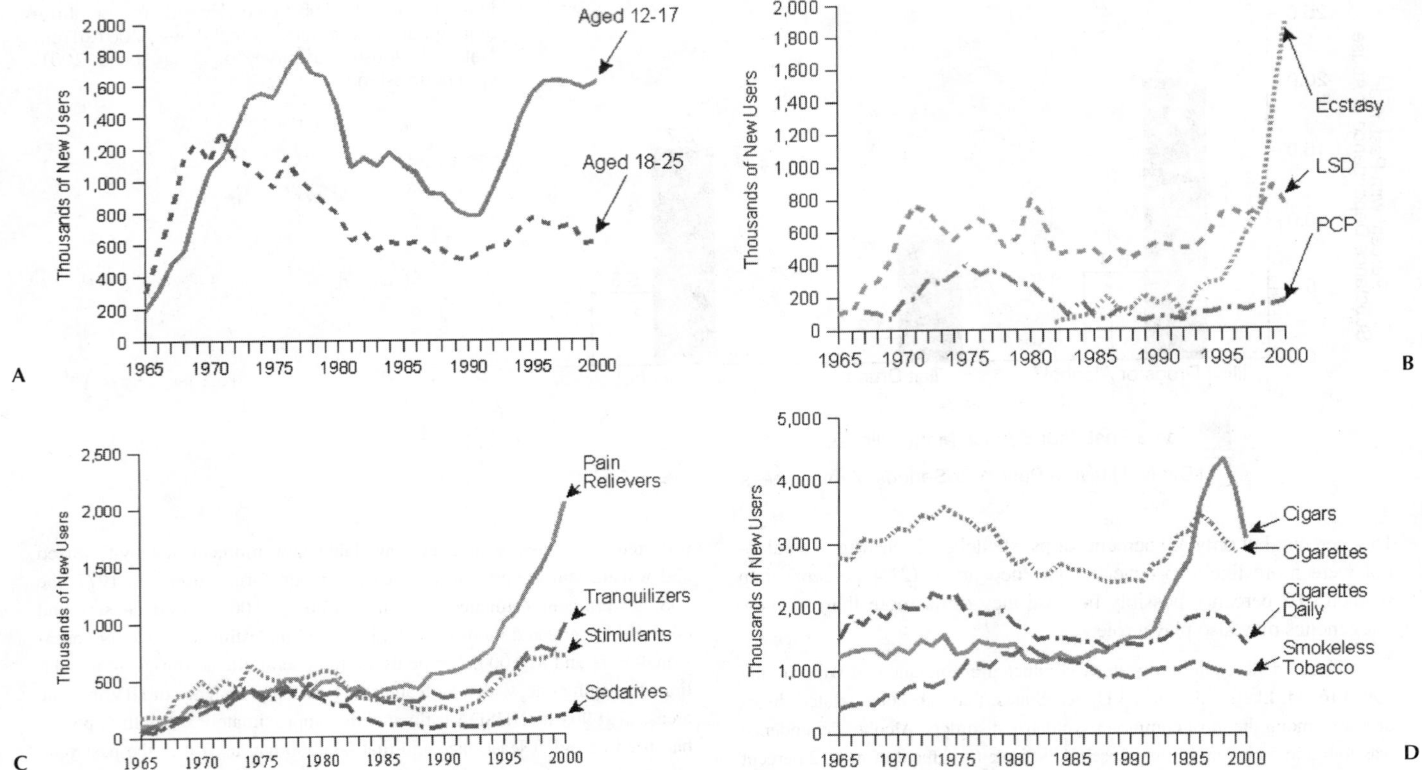

FIGURE 11.1–4 Annual number of new users (in thousands) of various drugs, 1965 to 2000. **A:** Marijuana. **B:** Ecstasy, lysergic acid diethylamide (LSD), and phencyclidine (PCP). **C:** Nonmedical users of psychotherapeutics. **D:** Tobacco. (Adapted from National Household Survey of Drug Abuse; 2001.)

experience its effects in the same way or are motivated by the same set of factors. Furthermore, it is postulated that different factors may be more or less important at different stages of the process. Thus, drug availability, social acceptability, and peer pressures may be the major determinants of initial experimentation with a drug, but other factors, such as personality and individual biology, probably are more important in how the effects of a given drug are perceived and the degree to which repeated drug use produces changes in the central nervous system (CNS). Still other factors, including the particular actions of the drug, may be primary determinants of whether drug use progresses to drug dependence, whereas still others may be important influences on the likelihood that drug use leads to adverse effects or the likelihood of successful recovery from dependence.

It has been asserted that addiction is a "brain disease," that the critical processes that transform voluntary drug-using behavior to compulsive drug use are changes in the structure and neurochemistry of the brain of the drug user. There is now more than enough evidence that such changes in relevant parts of the brain do occur. The perplexing and unanswered question is whether these changes are both necessary and sufficient to account for the drug-using behavior. Many argue that they are not, that the capacity of drug-dependent individuals to modify their drug-using behavior in response to positive reinforcers or aversive contingencies indicates that the nature of addiction is more complex and requires the interaction of multiple factors.

Figure 11.1–5 illustrates how various factors might interact in the development of drug dependence. The central element is the drug-using behavior itself. The decision to use a drug is influenced by immediate social and psychological situations as well as by the person's more remote history. Use of the drug initiates a sequence of consequences that can be rewarding or aversive and which, through a process of learning, can result in a greater or lesser likelihood that the drug-using behavior will be repeated. For some drugs, use also initiates the biological processes associated with tolerance, physical dependence, and (not shown in the figure) sensitization. In turn, tolerance can reduce some of the adverse effects of the drug, permitting or requiring the use of larger doses, which then can accelerate or intensify the development of physical dependence. Above a certain threshold, the aversive qualities of a withdrawal syndrome provide a distinct recurrent motive for further drug use. Sensitization of motivational systems may increase the salience of drug-related stimuli.

For simplicity, Figure 11.1–5 shows drug use alone as initiating that chain of consequences, but the choices a person makes over and over again are more complex. The decision is whether to use one drug or another or to engage in some behavior that does not involve drug use. Each of those decisions can initiate positive and negative consequences. Changes in the availability, costs, and consequences of alternative behaviors can also influence what appears to be compulsive use of a pharmacological agent. For example, patients in a methadone maintenance program who were using cocaine despite negative consequences (no take-home methadone) reduced their cocaine use when vouchers for goods and services were awarded for clean (negative for cocaine) urine specimens.

Social and Environmental Factors

Cultural factors, social attitudes, peer behaviors, laws, and drug cost and availability all influence initial experimentation with substances, including alcohol and tobacco. These factors also influence initial use of more socially disapproved drugs, such as cocaine and opioids, but personality factors assume a more important role. Social and environmental factors also influence continued use, although individual vulnerability and psychopathology are probably more important determinants of the

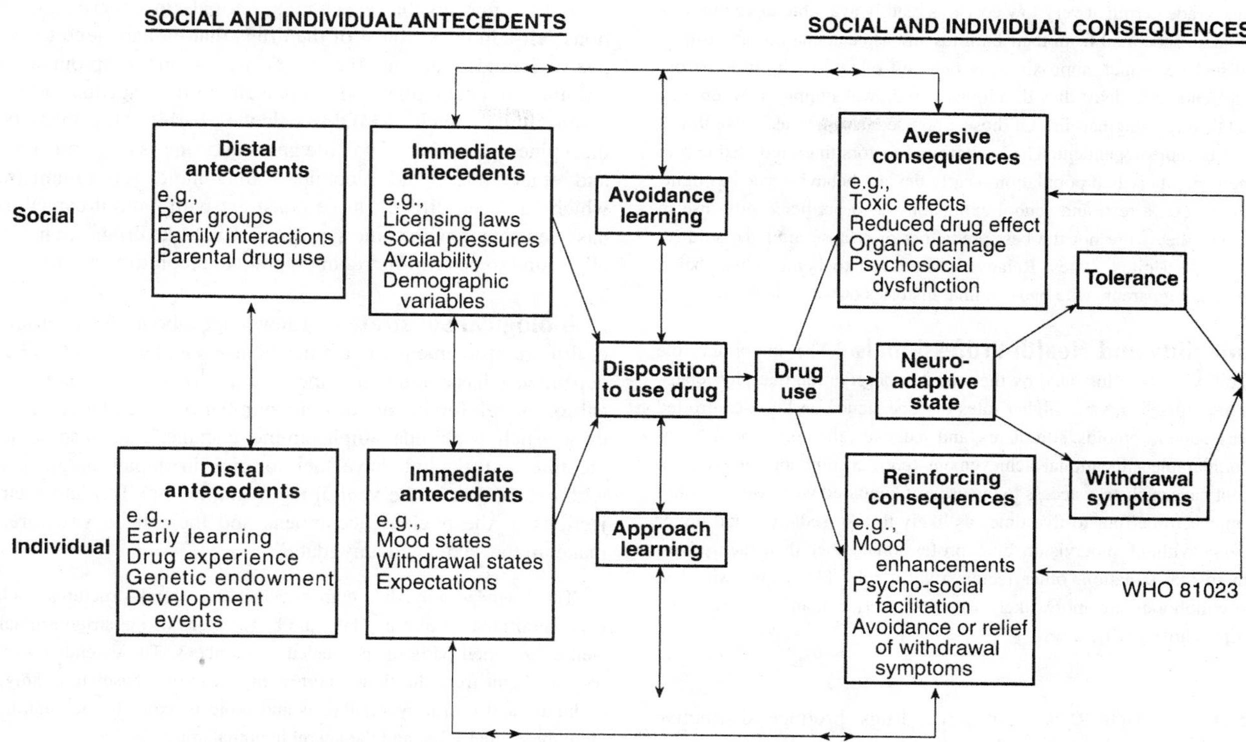

FIGURE 11.1–5 World Health Organization schematic model of drug use and dependence. (From Edwards G, Arif A, Hodgson R: Nomenclature and classification of drug- and alcohol-related problems. A WHO memorandum. *Bull WHO.* 1981;99:225, with permission.)

development of dependence. In general, the use of the less socially disapproved substances (alcohol, tobacco, and cannabis) precedes the use of opioids and cocaine, and those antecedent substances are sometimes referred to as *gateway drugs*.

Alcohol and Tobacco Substantial evidence indicates that changes in price and availability can alter the consumption of alcohol and tobacco. When an increase in sales outlets or an extension of sales hours increases the availability of alcohol, consumption tends to increase. When the cost of either alcohol or tobacco is increased in relation to disposable income (e.g., by increased taxes), consumption decreases. These factors even influence the behavior of dependent people, although perhaps not to the same degree as for those who are not dependent. Availability can be altered independently of cost, and alterations can be limited to selected populations (e.g., prohibiting sale of alcohol and tobacco to those younger than a specific age).

Social, cultural, and economic factors do not always operate synergistically but may sometimes influence consumption in opposite directions. For example, in the late 1980s, increased public awareness of how alcohol use adversely affects health resulted in a decline in its consumption. That decline occurred even though alcohol was more freely available, its cost relative to income remained constant or actually decreased, and social pressures against women drinking (unless pregnant) also decreased.

Illegal Drugs Social and cultural factors, including beliefs about the effects of a drug, frequently exert more influence on drug-use patterns than the laws that supposedly reflect such factors. For example, cannabis use increased among high school students from the early 1970s to 1979 and then decreased steadily over the next decade, although use and possession were illegal throughout the entire 18-year period, and nothing indicates that it became more expensive or less available during the 1980s (Fig. 11.1–4). An upward trend in use was noted from 1993 to 1997, although perhaps the values never reached the peak levels of 1979. Some experts believe the decline in use seen during the 1980s was linked to changing perceptions about the toxic effects of cannabis on health. The increase beginning in the 1990s was correlated with a decline in the perception of the risk of harm from regular use. Similarly, cocaine use increased in the 1970s despite high prices for the drug and high risk of criminal penalties; but after several well-publicized deaths from cocaine in the mid-1980s, prevalence of active cocaine use declined among high school seniors and in the general population even as the price of the drug declined.

Social and cultural factors profoundly influence the availability of illegal drugs; availability, in turn, influences which groups within a society are most likely to become users. Currently, illegal opioids and cocaine are more available in the inner cities of large urban areas than in other parts of the country. Such availability influences not only initial and continued drug use but also affects the relapse rates after treatment of those who live in high-availability areas. When a significant number of users of illegal drugs live in one area, a subculture evolves that supports experimentation and continued use. Many of the areas in which illegal drugs are readily available are also characterized by a high crime rate, high unemployment, and demoralized school systems—all of which serve to reduce the sense of hope and sense of self-esteem associated with resistance to use. Social and educational factors also affect the likelihood for successful recovery from drug dependence; those who find satisfying alternatives are more likely to abstain from drug use.

VIETNAM The experience of U.S. service personnel who used heroin in Vietnam provided a unique natural experiment in which the influences of availability, vulnerability, and social norms could be observed. From 1970 to

1972, high-grade heroin at very low cost was readily available to young people in Vietnam separated from their families and usual social norms. Among army enlisted personnel, approximately one-half of those who tried heroin became dependent (at least they developed withdrawal symptoms when they attempted to stop using heroin). Of those who used heroin at least five times, 73 percent became dependent. The background factors that predicted heroin use in the general civilian population—early deviant behavior, such as fighting, drunkenness, arrest, and school expulsion—also predicted drug use in Vietnam, but they were not the best predictors of relapse after the soldiers returned to the United States. Relapse was related to being white, being older, and having parents who had criminal histories or were alcoholic.

Availability and Health Professionals The important role of availability is also illustrated by the repeated observation that physicians, dentists, and nurses have far higher rates of dependence on DEA-controlled substances, such as opioids, stimulants, and sedatives, than other professionals of comparable educational achievement (e.g., accountants or lawyers) who do not have such easy access to the drugs. Compared with controls, physicians appear to be four to five times as likely to take sedatives and minor tranquilizers without supervision by a professional other than themselves. Yet even in that situation, other factors play a role. Physicians who had unhappy childhoods are more likely to self-prescribe than those who are healthier psychologically.

Drugs as Reinforcers Different drugs produce distinctive subjective states, and extensive laboratory evidence shows that people with experience can distinguish one drug class from another and can even rank different classes and doses on the basis of how much they like the effects. Yet, the hold that drugs can eventually exert on a user's behavior is not entirely a function of its initial likable or euphorigenic actions. For example, the effects of cocaine are typically described by most users as powerfully euphorigenic, producing increased self-esteem, alertness, energy, and well-being. The effects of nicotine, as described by many tobacco users, are more subtle, producing some mixture of alerting and relaxing. The subjective effects of alcohol are more likely to be described as relaxing, but are more variable, and appear to be more dependent on personality and underlying genetic variability traits and genetically influenced ethanol metabolism. Despite those differences, dependence (or addiction) can occur with each, and they appear to have shared or overlapping neural substrates for their reinforcing properties.

Almost all of the drugs that are used for their subjective effects and are associated with the development of dependence induce some degree of tolerance. In some cases, the tolerance to the toxic and aversive effects is more pronounced than the tolerance to the reinforcing and mood-elevating effects. For example, most opioid users quickly develop tolerance to opioid-induced nausea and vomiting. This may allow users to increase the dose and thus experience greater euphoric effects. Conversely, those who continue to experience aversive drug effects (such as severe flushing with alcohol) may be less likely to persist in using the drug and are at lower risk for developing dependence. Tolerant opioid users do not continue to self-administer opioids solely to prevent the highly aversive withdrawal phenomena. Interviews with heroin users have indicated that, despite some tolerance to many of the drug's effects, they continue to experience a brief euphoric effect immediately after an IV injection. Among nonalcoholic sons of alcoholic fathers, intrinsic tolerance may be a marker of biological vulnerability to developing alcohol dependence. Sons of alcoholic fathers who were more tolerant to a test dose of alcohol were far more likely to have developed alcohol dependence at 8 years' follow-up than those who were less tolerant.

With a few notable exceptions, animals in experimental situations self-administer most of the drugs that humans tend to use and abuse. Included among the drugs are μ- and δ-opioid agonists, cocaine, amphetamine and amphetamine-like agents, substituted amphetamines, such as MDMA, alcohol, barbiturates, many benzodiazepines, a number of volatile gases and vapors (e.g., nitrous oxide and ether), PCP, and nicotine. Cannabinoid self-administration, which has been difficult to demonstrate with natural cannabinoids, has been shown with some synthetics. LSD-like drugs are not generally found to be reinforcing in preclinical laboratory studies.

Biological Substrates Knowledge about the neurobiology of drug reinforcement and the mechanisms underlying tolerance and dependence has continued to increase. Pathways and structures critical for the reinforcing actions of a number of dependence-producing drugs, such as opioids, amphetamine, cocaine, and, to some degree, nicotine and alcohol, have their origins in dopaminergic neurons with cell bodies in the ventral tegmental area (VTA) and their projections to the nucleus accumbens and the related structures that make up the "extended amygdala."

The extended amygdala comprises several neural structures, including the central nucleus of amygdala, the bed nucleus of the stria terminalis, as well as the shell parts of the nucleus accumbens. The extended amygdala receives input from the limbic cortex, hippocampus, basolateral amygdala, midbrain, and lateral hypothalamus and projects axons to the ventral pallidum, the medial VTA, and the lateral hypothalamus.

The medial part of the nucleus accumbens (shell) is a particularly important site; dopamine release here is critical for the reinforcing effects of cocaine and amphetamines. It is also important for the reinforcing effects of opioids, but there are opioid receptors on neurons in the nucleus accumbens, and opioids can exert reinforcing effects at that site even when the dopaminergic terminals are destroyed. Some researchers have proposed that all positive reinforcement, including the reinforcement associated with food reward and sex, critically depends on this dopaminergic circuit.

Dopamine release from mesolimbic dopaminergic neurons may play more than one role in the genesis of drug seeking and drug dependence. Dopamine release has been postulated to facilitate learning what events and behaviors lead to important consequences for the organism and to alert the organism to pay greater attention to such events. In this way, drug-induced dopamine release leads to a greater salience of drug-using opportunities and is linked to wanting and craving.

However, the diverse categories of drugs that activate the mesolimbic dopaminergic system do so by distinct mechanisms, and most have actions on many other neural systems. Reinforcing mechanisms are also briefly described in the chapters devoted to specific drugs. Only a few examples are given here. The VTA dopaminergic neurons have both nicotinic and γ-aminobutyric acid (GABA) receptors. These neurons normally are inhibited by GABAergic activity. The GABAergic neurons acting on the VTA express μ- and δ-opioid receptors. When these receptors are activated by μ opioids, GABAergic transmission is inhibited, and the dopaminergic VTA neurons become more active and release dopamine in the nucleus accumbens. However, opioids can also act directly on neurons in the nucleus accumbens, independent of dopamine action.

As a reinforcing drug, cocaine acts primarily at the nerve endings of the serotonergic, dopaminergic, and noradrenergic neurons. When transmitters are released from those neurons into the synapse, they are transported back into the nerve endings by transporter proteins. By occupying these transporter sites, cocaine prevents the reuptake of the transmitters, thus increasing their concentration in the synapse. Cocaine's binding to the dopamine transporter is primarily responsible for its reinforcing effects, but the actions on other neurotransmitters also influence its subjective effects. Cocaine administration also produces glutamate release within the mesolimbic accumbens system, an action that is probably relevant to its capacity to change behavior because glutamate antagonists interfere with learning to associate cocaine effects to environmental stimuli.

Amphetamine also increases dopamine levels at the synapse and binds to the dopamine transporter to some degree. But amphetamine actions at the dopamine transporter are not as important as its major action, which is to displace dopamine and norepinephrine from their storage sites in the neuron and thereby lead to their release.

Alcohol, at clinically relevant concentrations, exerts its actions relatively selectively on specific receptors and neurotransmitter systems. These actions include enhancing the inhibitory action of GABAergic neurotransmitters (by increasing the sensitivity of the GABA receptor) and reducing the excitatory actions of glutamatergic neurotransmitters (by altering the response of the *N*-methyl-D-aspartate [NMDA] receptors). By its blocking actions at the NMDA receptor, ethanol can indirectly alter the release of other neurotransmitters (e.g., serotonin, dopamine, norepinephrine, glutamate, aspartate, and GABA). Low doses of alcohol increase dopamine levels in the nucleus accumbens and elevate brain serotonin concentration. Various regions of the brain differ in their sensitivity to these actions of ethanol. The endogenous opioid system may be involved in some aspects of the mood-elevating effects of alcohol because the opioid antagonist naloxone reduces alcohol self-administration in animals, and the antagonist naltrexone (ReVia) reduces relapse rates in treated alcoholics.

Mesolimbic dopaminergic neurons have multiple nicotinic cholinergic receptors on their cell bodies and terminals in the nucleus accumbens. When activated, these receptors increase dopamine release. Nicotine also increases glutamatergic activity, thereby tending to increase the activity of VTA dopaminergic neurons. This action lasts longer than nicotine's GABAergic effects, which dampen mesolimbic dopaminergic activity. Interestingly, regular exposure to nicotine-containing tobacco smoke may be more reinforcing than nicotine itself because other chemical entities in tobacco inhibit brain monoamine oxidase type A (MAO_A) and MAO_B, which are involved in the regulation of intraneuronal stores of dopamine. Presumably, this inhibition increases the amount of dopamine available for release when the dopaminergic neurons are activated.

Drugs can also act as reinforcers by terminating aversive states. Some of these actions involve dopaminergic systems, but others do not. Some researchers argue that compulsive drug use can be explained on the basis of the positive reinforcing effects of drugs without any need to invoke alleviation of withdrawal distress or any obvious source of antecedent pain or dysphoria. Furthermore, they argue, craving is primarily associated not with cues that evoke withdrawal but with those that evoke memories of positive reinforcement (euphoria). However, evidence now indicates that even when there are no obvious and dramatic withdrawal symptoms (e.g., cocaine, nicotine) adaptive changes in the reward system result in a relative dopaminergic deficiency state (measurable as decreased dopamine levels in the nucleus accumbens) when drug use is stopped or its action ceases. This deficiency state is experienced as dysphoria or anhedonia. Quite often, the same drug-using behavior that terminates this dysphoria moves the system to a hyperdopaminergic state associated with positive reinforcement (euphoria). In short, the behaviors associated with chronic drug use are typically driven by both the avoidance of dysphoria (negative reinforcement) and the pursuit of euphoria (positive reinforcement).

In animal models, such as the rat, the sensitivity of neural systems to reinforcing drugs, such as cocaine and opioids, is enhanced by corticosteroids. In animal models, a variety of stresses acting through release of corticotropin-releasing factor (CRF) and the hypothalamic-pituitary-adrenal axis can sensitize neural systems and trigger reinitiation of drug taking. There is ample clinical evidence that such stresses can act similarly in drug-dependent individuals immediately after withdrawal and for long periods thereafter. In addition, some drugs may sensitize neural systems to the reinforcing effects of the drug.

Learning and Conditioning Drug use, whether occasional or compulsive, can be viewed as behavior maintained by its consequences. Any event that strengthens an antecedent behavior pattern can be considered a reinforcer of that behavior. In that sense, certain drugs reinforce drug-taking behavior. Drugs can also reinforce antecedent behaviors by terminating some noxious or aversive state such as pain, anxiety, or depression. In some social situations, the use of the drug, quite apart from its pharmacological effects, can be reinforcing if it results in special status or the approval of friends. Social reinforcement can maintain drug use until the effects of primary reinforcement or reinforcement by alleviation of withdrawal symptoms come into play. Each use of the drug evokes rapid positive reinforcement, either as a result of the rush (the drug-induced euphoria), alleviation of disturbed affects, alleviation of withdrawal symptoms, or any combination of these effects. In addition, some drugs may sensitize neural systems to the reinforcing effects of the drug. With short-acting substances, such as heroin, cocaine, nicotine, and alcohol, such reinforcement occurs several times a day, day in and day out, creating powerfully reinforced habit patterns. Eventually, the paraphernalia (needles, bottles, cigarette packs) and behaviors associated with substance use can become secondary reinforcers, as well as cues signaling availability of the substance, and in their presence, craving or a desire to experience the effects increases. With socially acceptable substances, such as tobacco, use becomes so woven into the matrix of daily functioning that some users are reminded of the substances when performing ordinary tasks. Stresses can also act as cues that induce drug taking, particularly in the postwithdrawal period.

Researchers have used positron emission tomography (PET) and functional magnetic resonance imaging (fMRI) to study brain activity in both drug users and controls presented with drug-related stimuli (paraphernalia or video tapes). Drug users respond to the drug-related stimuli with increased activity in limbic regions, including the amygdala and the anterior cingulate, but do not respond this way to neutral stimuli. Control subjects respond minimally to both types of stimuli. Such drug-related activation of limbic areas has been demonstrated with a variety of drugs, including cocaine, opioids, and cigarettes (nicotine). Interestingly, the same regions activated by cocaine-related stimuli in cocaine users are activated by sexual stimuli in both normal controls and cocaine users.

Classical Conditioning In addition to the operant reinforcement of drug-using and drug-seeking behaviors, other learning mechanisms probably play a role in dependence and relapse. Opioid and alcohol withdrawal phenomena can be conditioned (in the Pavlovian or classical sense) to environmental or interoceptive stimuli. Such conditioning has been demonstrated in both laboratory animals and abstinent and methadone-dependent human volunteers. For a long time after withdrawal (from opioids, nicotine, or alcohol), the addict exposed to environmental stimuli previously linked with substance use or withdrawal may experience conditioned withdrawal, conditioned craving, or both. The increased feelings of craving are not necessarily accompanied by symptoms of withdrawal. The most intense craving is elicited by conditions associated with the availability or use of the substance, such as watching someone else use heroin or light a cigarette or being offered some drug by a friend. Some workers now believe that the cues that induce memories of drug-induced euphoria are more important for stimulating craving and in predisposing to relapse than either protracted or conditioned withdrawal. Those learning and conditioning phenomena can be superimposed on any preexisting psychopathology, but preexisting difficulties are not required for the development of powerfully reinforced substance-seeking behavior.

Withdrawal Syndromes and Negative Reinforcement

Although positive reinforcement is a powerful etiological factor in the genesis of cocaine, amphetamine, and (in some cases) opioid dependence, for a number of other drugs, aversive withdrawal phenomena and negative reinforcement may be equally important, or even dominant, factors. For example, in people who become dependent on benzodiazepines in the course of treatment for anxiety syndromes, when drug use is interrupted, some seem to experience a reappearance of the original symptoms, whereas others have new distressing symptoms indicating withdrawal. The use of benzodiazepines alleviates both kinds of aversive states. In either case, the drug is acting as a negative reinforcer in perpetuating drug use. Benzodiazepines can induce euphoria in alcoholic patients or in people with histories of sedative abuse, but they are not reliably euphorigenic in normal, nonalcoholic people. Benzodiazepine anxiolytic agents may induce euphoria in people who are not dependent and not anxious, but such instances are rare relative to the number who experience only relief of anxiety.

In most clinical situations, even among users of highly euphorigenic illegal drugs, the distinction between positive and negative reinforcing effects does not exist. The alcoholic, the heavy smoker, and the heroin user may experience, simultaneously or sequentially, relief of withdrawal, a sense of ease, and perhaps alleviation of dysphoria and depression. Some of the dysphoria may be a result of long-lasting dysfunction in systems subserving hedonic tone. With IV drugs, there may also be a sudden rush of intense pleasure.

Long-Lasting Changes Associated with Chronic Drug Use

After long-term use, most drugs of abuse produce adaptive changes in the brain that are manifested as acute and chronic withdrawal syndromes when drug use ceases. Other drug-induced changes in the brain appear to be related to the processes by which the memories of drug action are stored and by which drug-related stimuli acquire and retain salience. How these changes are produced, how long they persist after cessation of drug use, and how they contribute to relapse are still being explored. But much progress has occurred, as is illustrated by the example of recent changes found with chronic opioids.

OPIOIDS Tolerance and dependence on opioids involve several mechanisms. Opioid agonist binding to the opioid receptors results in an inhibition of adenylyl cyclase and lower intracellular cyclic adenosine monophosphate (cAMP) concentrations. Long-term exposure elicits compensatory upregulation of the cAMP pathway, internalization of μ and δ receptors, and a decrease in the number of G proteins, which couple the receptors to the second messengers and ion channels. Upregulation of adenylyl cyclase is mediated by the transcription factor CREB (cAMP response element–binding protein), which also plays a role in the generation of distinct and persistent Fos-like proteins. These are believed to be involved in both tolerance and sensitization. The sensitization may involve Fos-like proteins that alter the sensitivity of an α-amino-3-hydroxy-5-methyl-4-isoxazolepropionic acid (AMPA) glutamate receptor subunit. As a result of upregulation of cAMP, GABAergic neurons innervating the VTA become hyperactive when opioids are withdrawn, thus inhibiting dopaminergic neurons. Such a mechanism may account, in part, for the dysphoria and anhedonia of opioid withdrawal. In addition, chronic opioid use reduces the size of dopamine neurons in the VTA; increased production of dynorphin may also serve to inhibit dopaminergic activity at the VTA and nucleus accumbens. The glutamatergic system is also involved in opioid adaptation because NMDA receptor sensitivity is altered by opioids, and NMDA antagonists can alter the development of opioid tolerance and physical dependence. The opioid-induced changes described are believed to be only a subset of a wide range of cellular and molecular changes induced by chronic drug use.

Conditioned Withdrawal and Stress Sensitivity

In addition to the direct contribution of withdrawal phenomena to the perpetuation of drug use are the indirect effects exerted through learning mechanisms. The regular recurrence of withdrawal-induced aversive states provides ample opportunity for those states to become linked through learning to environmental cues and other mood states, and the rapid relief of withdrawal by drug use results in repeated reinforcement of drug-taking behavior. Long after there are measurable manifestations of acute withdrawal, certain moods or environmental cues can evoke components of the original withdrawal state along with urges to use the drug again. Considerable evidence shows that in former opioid addicts, stress can trigger both craving and relapse, and dysregulation of the hypothalamic-pituitary-adrenal axis persists for long periods after drug cessation.

How long withdrawal phenomena, stress sensitivity, or both continue to contribute to risk of relapse is not clear. Substantial evidence supports a withdrawal syndrome period for alcohol, opioids, and certain sedatives with subtle disturbances of mood, sleep, and cognition that persists for many weeks or months after the acute syndrome subsides. Whether the dysregulation of the hypothalamic-pituitary-adrenal axis is causally related to protracted withdrawal or has a similar time course is still uncertain.

Integrating Neurobiology and Learning

Several research groups have attempted to integrate the most recent findings from neurobiology and the role of learning to better explain how drugs gain control of behavior to produce compulsive drug use and the tendency to relapse after withdrawal.

George Koob and Michel LeMoal describe the addictive process as a "cycle of spiraling dysregulation of brain reward systems." They describe in detail the organization of the hedonic regulatory system of the brain and its interaction with systems regulating response to stress—the pituitary-adrenal axis and extrahypothalamic CRF system. The adaptive changes to chronic drug use are believed to lead to deviations in hedonic homeostasis of such magnitude that the system cannot be maintained within the normal range. Continued apparent reward function requires the mobilization of different systems, and in this sense, the system functions at a new set-point, which these researchers describe as an allostatic state. Central to this perspective is the dysregulation of hedonic tone that results from a counter-adaptive response to drug-induced excessive activation of the reward system. When drug action is withdrawn, prolonged hypoactivity follows. Failed efforts to cope with this dysregulation lead to emotional distress, which brings further negative affect and (mediated by increased levels of glucocorticoids) increased sensitivity to the rewarding effects of the drugs. At the same time, drug use alleviates the dysphoric effects of the hypofunction of the reward system. A strength of this description of the addictive process is the emphasis on the interaction of various neural systems subserving acute reinforcement, motivation effects of withdrawal, learned associations with drug effects, those systems (such as the cortico-striatal-thalamic circuits) involved in reinforcer evaluation, cognitive functioning and active inhibitory mechanisms, and the hypothalamic-pituitary-adrenal axis.

Another important contribution is the role assigned to the extrahypothalamic CRF system as well as other neuropeptide transmitters such as neuropeptide Y (NPY). During opiate, cocaine, or alcohol withdrawal, CRF increases in the central nucleus of the amygdala; microinjection of a CRF antagonist reverses the aversive effects of opioid or alcohol withdrawal. Koob and LeMoal point out that, although adrenocorticotropic hormone (ACTH)–stimulated high levels of glucocorticoids decrease the synthesis of CRF at the paraventricular nucleus, they can actually increase CRF activity at the level of the central nucleus of the amygdala.

Terry Robinson and Kent Berridge have elaborated on the role of drug-induced sensitization and alteration of brain structure in the development of addiction. The major points that form this general thesis are that addictive drugs share the ability to alter brain organization, particularly the organization of systems that subserve incentive motivation and reward. The alteration critical for the development of addiction is the sensitization of brain reward systems to drugs and drug-related stimuli. This hypersensitivity develops in those subcomponents of the brain reward system involved with assigning salience (drug wanting) to drugs to related stimuli rather than those more directly mediating drug reward or euphoria. Within this incentive-sensitization perspective, compulsive drug-seeking behavior does not require the presence of substantial or even subtle withdrawal dysphoria or the desire to obtain drug-induced euphoria. Rather, with repeated exposure, drug-related stimuli become more attractive, acquiring greater incentive value, and "grab the attention" of the drug user. In animals, drug-induced neural sensitization can be long lasting and has parallels to the long-lasting drug-seeking behavior that outlasts observable withdrawal phenomena. Sensitization (like the development of drug-dependent behavior) is not a simple consequence of drug administration but is powerfully influenced by learning and environmental context. This view helps to explain the waxing and waning long persistence of drug craving or wanting among drug-dependent individuals attempting to function in their home environments. It does not explain why the wanting so often leads to behavior even in the face of highly probably adverse consequences. The case for decreased inhibitory control is better put by Rita Goldstein and Nora Volkow.

Goldstein and Volkow elaborate a perspective that makes considerable use of data from studies of neuroimaging. This effort goes beyond the now generally accepted role of the mesolimbic dopaminergic system in accounting for the hedonic effects of addicting drugs, the role of the hippocampus and amygdala in the organization and storage of the drug experience, the hedonic deficiency (dysthymia) states that ensue after drug cessation, the biochemical and morphological dendritic changes shown to result from repeated drug administration, and the resulting salience of drug-related stimuli. What they add to these elements of addictive neurobiology are the importance of the activation of the thalamo-orbitofrontal circuit and the anterior cingulate in the experience of craving and the decreased inhibitory control over drug salient stimuli (impulsivity) due to inherent or drug-induced impairment of function of the frontal cortex, particularly the anterior cingulate.

Biological Factors—Vulnerability The children of alcoholic parents are at higher risk for developing alcoholism and drug dependence than are children of nonalcoholic parents. The higher risk for alcoholism manifests itself even when children are adopted by nonalcoholic families soon after birth. Dependence on other drugs also shows a familial pattern. The increased risk is partly due to early environmental factors (parental modeling, neglect, early child abuse) and later exposure to drugs, but genetic factors also play an important role. Numerous studies of laboratory animals have revealed genetically transmitted differences in the reinforcing effects of alcohol and various drugs, such as cocaine and opioids, and show that genetic factors powerfully influence sensitivity to toxic effects. The evidence for genetic factors in human vulnerability to alcoholism and other drug dependence is derived most convincingly from twin and adoption studies, but family studies are also revealing. Several studies of twins have found a higher concordance rate for alcoholism among identical twins than among fraternal twins. Although identical twins are generally believed to have more social contact than fraternal twins, when the effects of environmental factors are adjusted statistically, genetic factors are still found to have a major influence on the likelihood of becoming dependent. In one population-based twin study, 48 to 58 percent of the variation in liability to dependence was attributable to genetic factors; the remainder was due to general environmental influences not shared by family members.

All of the twin studies have found that genetically based vulnerability contributes substantially to the likelihood of using drugs and to becoming drug or alcohol dependent, including dependence on nicotine and caffeine. One issue that has not been entirely settled is whether the genetic vulnerability is a general, nonspecific vulnerability or is substance specific. A study of male twins in Virginia found only a nonspecific genetic vulnerability. However, a study of Vietnam–era veteran twin pairs using a somewhat different analytical approach identified both common and drug-specific genetic vulnerability factors. In that study, the importance of the nonspecific factors versus the drug-specific factors varied considerably for different drug categories. For most drugs, the variance was mostly due to a nonspecific vulnerability factor. But in the case of heroin, 54 percent of total variance was due to genetic factors, and 70 percent of this genetic variance was due to drug-specific factors. The differences concerning drug specificity between these twin studies may be due to differences in method or to the unusual experiences with heroin in Vietnam of that study population. The Collaborative Study on the Genetics of Alcoholism also found some specificity in transmission of cocaine and marijuana dependence. It seems that the existence of nonspecific genetic vulnerability factors is well established, but the role, if any, of drug-specific genetic vulnerability requires further study.

Studies of boys adopted soon after birth have shown higher rates of alcoholism among those whose biological fathers were alcoholics than among those whose biological fathers were not. Some adoption studies point toward subtypes of alcoholism among men: One is a later-onset disorder that is less severe and far more sensitive to environmental factors (type I), and the other is associated with early-onset, antisocial behavior and criminality in the biological fathers and a stronger genetic basis for the increased vulnerability (type II). The hypothesis that two genetically distinct types of alcoholism (type I and type II) exist has been criticized on the grounds that it is essentially a relabeling of the older primary-secondary categorization. In the latter, alcohol-dependent people who do not have antisocial personality disorder are designated as having *primary alcoholism*; those who first exhibit antisocial personality disorder and later develop alcoholism are designated *antisocial personality disorder with secondary alcoholism*. More recent studies of adoptees have shown that, compared with adoptees who have no biological risk or a parent with only alcoholism or only antisocial personality disorder, risk for both drug abuse or dependence is increased when substance abuse and antisocial personality disorder are present in the same biological parent. Although several research groups have been unable to use the type I and type II criteria to categorize patients with alcohol dependence accurately in clinical studies, arguments about the validity of the type I/type II categorization do not diminish the importance of genetic factors in vulnerability to developing alcohol dependence.

As many as one-third of people with alcohol dependence have no family history of the disorder. Men are more likely than women to develop alcoholism (four- to fivefold in the United States). This is true across every culture studied, probably reflecting in part stronger social sanctions on drug use and deviant behavior by women. But it is also postulated that women are less likely to drink heavily because they are less tolerant to alcohol. Women who do drink heavily run the same risk as men of developing alcoholism, and women who use illegal drugs are about as likely as men to become dependent.

Some studies have found that alcohol-dependent people are at far greater risk for developing other varieties of drug dependence. A more consistent finding is that drug-dependent people are at high risk for alcoholism and often have a family history of alcoholism. Such findings are consistent with data from the twin studies that have found general vulnerability factors.

Most researchers believe that no single gene will be found to account for the complexities of inherited risk for drug and alcohol dependence. Some genetic factors may not increase vulnerability to alcoholism but decrease it. A genetically determined variation in the activity of enzymes that metabolize alcohol (alcohol dehydrogenase and aldehyde dehydrogenase [ALDH]), common among some Asian groups, results in high levels of acetaldehyde in response to alcohol ingestion. The effect is to cause alcohol flush reaction and to exert some deterrent effect on alcohol ingestion. Alcoholism is lower among many Asian groups than among whites. Further, Asians with alcoholism are much less likely to have the inactive form of the ALDH enzyme. Also, genetically determined differences in nicotine metabolism can influence the likelihood of becoming a smoker.

Biological and Behavioral Differences Studies exploring how people with and without family histories of alcoholism might differ have involved measures of personality, drug and alcohol use patterns, psychomotor and cognitive performance, electrical activity of the brain, and endocrine responses to challenges with alcohol and other substances as well as measures of receptor numbers and affinities and enzyme activities (e.g., MAO) in peripheral tissues (e.g., blood platelets and lymphocytes). Similar studies have been conducted with offspring of men with histories of other substance use disorders. One finding that has been replicated is that, under some conditions, the electrical response of the brain that occurs approximately 300 milliseconds after a sensory stimulus (the P300 wave) has a smaller amplitude in nondrinking sons and daughters of alcoholic fathers than in control subjects without family histories of alcoholism. The decreased amplitude is believed to reflect a decreased capacity to recognize and interpret complex environmental stimuli. It has also been considered an indicator of low physiological inhibition and reflective of a maturational lag. Most studies have found no differences in intelligence among subjects with and without family histories of alcoholism. However, the results of personality studies are conflicting; some find no differences, and others find greater impulsivity, adventurousness, and sensation seeking among those with a positive family history. Studies of offspring of fathers with substance dependence have found, in addition, irritability, negative affect, and a difficult temperament. Studies of the drinking patterns of adolescent and young adult sons of alcoholic people also have not yielded consistent results; some (but not all) studies show that sons of alcoholic parents are heavier drinkers. Other studies have compared the subjective, motoric, and endocrine responses of young men with and without family histories of alcoholism after challenge exposures to alcohol and other potentially euphoriant drugs (such as benzodiazepines). Sons of alcoholic fathers seem to be more tolerant to the intoxicating effects of modest doses of alcohol, and in some (but not all) studies, higher doses of alcohol produced smaller changes in their prolactin and cortisol concentrations. Furthermore, one study found that sons who had smaller responses to test doses of alcohol at 20 years of age (i.e., were more tolerant) were fourfold more likely to have developed alcoholism 8 years later. Another study of sons of alcoholic parents found that those who had exhibited smaller electroencephalographic (EEG) alpha frequency responses to alcohol were more likely to be alcohol dependent at 10 years' follow-up.

The results of studies using benzodiazepine challenges are also not consistent; one showed a greater euphoric response to alprazolam (Xanax) in sons of alcoholic parents, and another showed no difference between positive and negative family history groups after a dose of diazepam.

A number of studies have shown that conduct disorder and early childhood aggression are associated with a substantial increase in the likelihood of early involvement with illegal drug use and development of dependence on alcohol and illegal drugs. Considerable evidence supports a role for both genetics and environmental factors in the development of conduct disorder. Antisocial personality disorder represents an independent additional risk factor for addictive disorders. The effects of antisocial personality disorder and family history of a substance-related disorder appear to be additive rather than synergistic. It seems possible that, in some of the studies of children and young people at high risk for later drug dependence, the electrophysiological differences, cognitive deficits, and personality differences reflect the presence of conduct disorder or antisocial personality disorder rather than a family history of alcoholism per se.

In a study of offspring of fathers with substance use disorders, a high composite score of neurobehavioral disinhibition (derived from measures of affect, behavior, and cognition) when measured at 10 to 12 years of age was a predictor of substance use disorder at 19 years of age. A high score at 16 years of age was a better predictor of substance use disorder than frequency of substance consumption. Interestingly, it was the presence of indicators of neurobehavioral disinhibition that was predictive and not socioeconomic status or being the son of a father with a substance use disorder.

Psychodynamic Factors and Psychopathology

Early psychoanalytical formulations postulated that drug users, in general, had either a special form of affective dysregulation (tense depression) that was alleviated by drug use or a disorder of impulse control in which the search for pleasure was dominant. More recent formulations postulate ego defects, which are evinced by the addict's inability to manage painful affects (guilt, anger, anxiety) and to avoid preventable medical, legal, and financial problems. The newer formulations postulating ego defects are to some degree the older formulations with a modest change in terminology that gives greater weight to the inability to cope with painful affects than to the intensity or abnormality of the affects per se. It is postulated that some substances pharmacologically and symbolically aid the ego in controlling those affects and that their use can be viewed as a form of self-medication. For example, it has been suggested that opioids help users control painful anger, that alcohol helps alcoholics control panic, and that nicotine may help some cigarette smokers control symptoms of depression. Although it is conceded that some of those observations may reflect problems produced by long-term use, the psychodynamic perspective is that the psychopathology is the underlying motivation for initial use, dependent use, and relapse after a period of abstinence. However, traditions of passivity and uncovering techniques derived from the psychoanalysis of neurosis are poorly suited to the treatment of most drug addicts. Further, some addicts have great difficulty differentiating and describing what they feel, a difficulty that has been called *alexithymia* (i.e., no words for feelings).

Family Dynamics One family member's substance abuse is often influenced by substance-using behaviors of others in the family, and these complex interrelationships can profoundly affect their lives. An understanding of the relationships among substance-using patients and their families is relevant for understanding the etiology of substance dependence and its treatment and for helping other family members to cope with problems associated with the substance-using behavior.

More has been written about the families of alcohol-dependent people and heroin users than about families affected by users of other drugs. Similarities between the family dynamics in these two prototypical dependencies have led researchers and clinicians to assume that certain general principles apply to all varieties of substance dependence. The observation that alcoholism is commonly found in the families of those seeking treatment for other types of dependence, that alcohol-dependent people are often dependent on other substances as well, and that those addicted to illegal drugs are often alcoholic suggests that there are common features among families with an addicted member. However, there are few data to suggest that the families of those dependent on tobacco or benzodiazepines are as dysfunctional as those affected by alcohol, opioids, or cocaine.

It is not always clear to what degree one family member's behavior is the cause of the substance-using behavior of another or is primarily a response to that behavior. Some writers emphasize that the addiction is a symptom that provides a displaced focus for conflict among other family members and that the user (the designated patient) may be playing a role in maintaining the homeostasis of a dysfunctional family. At the same time, addiction often arises in families in which one or both parents (and sometimes grandparents) have drug or alcohol problems and other psychopathology. Some characteristics commonly observed both in families of people who are alcohol dependent and of those addicted to illegal drugs are multigenerational drug dependence; a high incidence of parental loss through divorce, death, abandonment, or incarceration; overprotection or overcontrol by one parent (usually the mother) whose life is inordinately dependent on the behavior of the addicted offspring (symbiotic relationships); distant, cold, disengaged, or absent father (when the father is alive); and defiant drug-using child who appears to be engaged with peers but remains unusually dependent on the family well into adult life (pseudoindependence). The actual family dynamics are difficult to characterize because the family members' self-reports about their relationships do not reliably correspond to what outsiders observe. Such families typically do not describe themselves in the way that family therapists see them. Some workers have proposed that unresolved family grief plays a role in the genesis of drug addiction in a family member and that such families cannot deal effectively with separation because of previous losses. Despite the pathological interdependence between the addict and other family members, the addict is often described as passive, dependent, withdrawn, and unable to form close relationships.

Despite all the apparent pathology found in families, in many instances, the family brings the substance user into treatment, and the patient often believes that it is the family that is most likely to be helpful in recovery. Furthermore, clinicians now generally believe that involving families in treatment is important, if not essential, to effective intervention. One aspect of treating families is dealing with the tendency of some members to shield the patients from the consequences of their substance use, a behavior usually labeled by clinicians as *enabling* but usually experienced by the family member as loving, supporting, accepting, and protecting. A variation on family therapy, sometimes called *network therapy*, involves enlisting family members and close friends as allies of the therapist to provide social support and reinforcement of drug-abstaining behaviors. The people selected to fulfill this role function as part of a treatment team rather than as patients.

CODEPENDENCE The term *codependence* came into vogue to describe the behavioral patterns of family members who have been significantly affected by another family member's substance use or addiction. The term has been used in various ways, and there are no established criteria for codependence, a concept that some writers have expanded far beyond its origins to encompass any personality trait that involves difficulty in expressing emotions. However, many have criticized the expanded concept of codependence as a largely invalid notion based solely on anecdote. The following summary of some characteristics frequently described as aspects of codependence is not meant to imply the validity of a unitary syndrome.

One of the more agreed-on characteristics of codependence is enabling behavior. Family members sometimes feel that they have little or no control over enabling acts. Either because of social pressure to protect and support family members or because of pathological interdependencies, or both, enabling behavior often resists modification. Other characteristics of codependence include an unwillingness to accept the notion of addiction as a disease. Family members continue to behave as if the substance-using behavior were voluntary and willful (if not actually spiteful), and the user cares more for alcohol and drugs than for the members of the family. This results in feelings of anger, rejection, and failure. In addition to those feelings, the family members may feel guilty and depressed because the addict, in an effort to deny loss of control over drugs and to shift the focus of concern away from their use, often tries to place the responsibility for such use on the other family members who often seem willing to accept some or all of it.

Like the substance users themselves, family members often behave as if the substance use that is causing obvious problems is not really a problem—that is, they engage in denial. The reasons for the unwillingness to accept the obvious vary. Sometimes denial is self-protecting in that the family members believe that, if there is a drug or alcohol problem, then they are responsible.

Like the addicts themselves, codependent family members seem unwilling to accept the notion that outside intervention is needed and, despite repeated failures, continue to believe that greater willpower and greater efforts at control can restore tranquility. When additional efforts at control fail, they often attribute the failure to themselves rather than to the addict or the disease process, and along with failure come feelings of anger, lowered self-esteem, and depression.

Other Factors There are other factors that influence the pattern of use and cessation of any given substance. For example, the decision not to use a substance also has consequences that can be aversive or reinforcing, and evidence indicates that when the rewards of not using the substance are high, the likelihood of use is reduced. In addition, many of the substances associated with dependence act directly on systems that subserve both motivation and decision making, raising questions about whether use is always influenced solely by its consequences (learning processes). The cognitive processes and skills that ordinarily subserve decision making appear to be impaired by alcohol, barbiturates, cannabis, and several other categories of self-administered agents. Thus, whereas substance use is influenced by learning, the substances also alter the brain itself. This suggests additional problems and possibilities for intervention. Evidence is accumulating that limited cognitive skills reduce the likelihood of successful recovery from substance use and that coping skills can help a person avoid or deal with aversive affective states, environmental stresses, and situations that are associated with a high risk for substance use. The presence of other psychiatric disorders has a powerful influence on both the development and course of substance use disorders and is discussed separately below.

Other factors that influence the course of substance use and dependence are difficult to operationalize or teach or prescribe, but they deserve mention. Studies of the natural history of substance use indicate that recovery is powerfully influenced by the support of family and friends. Many people report that hope, faith, formal religious affiliation, or the sustaining love of some significant person are more important to their recovery than any specific treatment.

Comorbidity *Comorbidity* is the cooccurrence of two or more psychiatric disorders in a single patient. As noted earlier, a high prevalence of additional psychiatric disorders is found among people seeking treatment for alcohol, cocaine, or opioid dependence. Although opioid, cocaine, and alcohol abusers with current psychiatric problems are more likely to seek treatment, it should not be assumed that those who do not seek treatment are free of comorbid psychiatric problems; such people may have social supports that enable them to deny the impact that drug use is having on their lives. Two large epidemiological studies have shown that even among representative samples of the population, those who meet the criteria for alcohol or drug abuse and dependence (excluding tobacco dependence) are far more likely to meet the criteria for other psychiatric disorders also. In the NCS, 51 percent of those who met the criteria for a lifetime addictive disorder received at least one additional mental disorder diagnosis; in the earlier ECA study, the comparable figure was 38 percent. In the ECA study, among those diagnosed with drug dependence, the most common additional diagnosis was alcohol abuse/dependence, followed in frequency by antisocial personality disorder, phobic disorders, and major depression for men and phobic disorders, major depression, and dysthymia for women. Almost every psychiatric diagnosis was more common among those who met the criteria for drug dependence, with notable increases in odds ratios for alcoholism, antisocial personality disorder, and mania among women and for mania, antisocial personality disorder, and dysthymia among men. Both men and women with drug abuse dependence are at a substantially higher risk for schizophrenia.

In general, the probability of comorbidity is higher for those with a lifetime diagnosis of an opioid or cocaine disorder than for those with a diagnosis of cannabis abuse. Among people in prison, the comorbidity rates were even higher than in the general population; addictive disorders were found in 92 percent of prisoners with schizophrenia, 90 percent of those with antisocial personality disorder, and 89 percent of those with bipolar disorders. Among people with mental disorders seeking treatment in psychiatric specialty settings, 20 percent have a current substance abuse disorder diagnosis. More recently, it has become apparent that cigarette smoking is associated with higher probability of additional psychiatric disorders, especially mood disorders.

The findings from the NCS largely confirm the observations of the ECA study that those with substance use disorders are substantially more likely to experience other mental disorders and that those with other mental disorders are far more likely to develop substance use disorders. The NCS also underscored the finding that, although 52 percent of respondents had never experienced any DSM-III-R disorder and 21 percent had one such disorder, 13 percent had two disorders, and 14 percent had three or more disorders. Furthermore, the 12-month prevalence of a disorder was more likely among those with more than one disorder: 59 percent of all of 12-month disorders occurred in the 14 percent with a lifetime history of three or more disorders, and 89 percent of severe 12-month disorders occurred in the same group.

These findings describe rather than explain comorbidity. They do not shed much light on the question of whether, or in which cases, drug use is at least initially an adaptive effort at self-medication or whether those with a variety of psychiatric disorders are less able to cope with the effects of substance use and so are more likely to become dependent. It is also not clear whether psychiatric disorders increase the vulnerability to drug abuse and drug dependence or whether some common factor contributes to both. In some cases, however, there does appear to be a causal link between drug use and some psychiatric disorders. For example, evidence indicates that substance abuse (especially alcohol) can cause or increase the risk for depressive disorder; cocaine can increase the frequency of panic disorder; and cannabis, cocaine, and amphetamine use can aggravate or precipitate schizophrenic symptomatology. Some of these are drug-induced disorders (particularly some of the depressive symptoms seen in alcoholics) and clear with cessation of alcohol use. However, some psychiatric disorders (e.g., mood disorder and antisocial personality disorder) often antedate substance use and can be viewed as risk factors or predictors for substance abuse and dependence. This is particularly true of conduct disorder and adult antisocial behavior, in which the symptoms often begin before the onset of problematic drug use. The NCS found that the odds of developing alcohol or drug dependence increased fivefold in the presence of conduct disorder without adult antisocial behavior and 10- to 14-fold if only adult antisocial behavior or both conduct disorder and antisocial behavior were present. Of the Axis I disorders, bipolar I disorder is more strongly related to dependence on alcohol or drugs than any other mood or anxiety disorder. In general, approximately 24.5 percent of those with a 12-month addictive disorder had a mood disorder as well, and 35.6 percent had an anxiety disorder. Overall, 42.7 percent of those with a 12-month addictive disorder had at least one 12-month Axis I mental disorder. In terms of lifetime disorders, 41.0 to 65.5 percent of those with a lifetime addictive disorder have a lifetime history of at least one Axis I mental disorder, whereas 51 percent of those with one or more lifetime mental disorders (Axis I or II) have a history of one or more addictive disorders. For lifetime conduct disorder or adult antisocial behavior, the rate of lifetime substance use disorder increases to 82 percent.

Although the possibility of recall bias exists, those with both an affective and an addictive disorder usually report that depression began earlier than substance use. However, temporal relationship between two disorders does not prove causality, even when the development of the first disorder is a predictor of both the likelihood and course of the subsequent disorder. There is the possibility, as has been suggested for smoking and depression, that both disorders are linked to some third common factor. In the NCS, a more chronic course of an addictive disorder was found for those who reported earlier development of primary anxiety disorder, conduct disorder, or adult antisocial behavior but was not found with earlier onset of other mental disorders. As noted above, several current views of the etiology of drug dependence place emphasis on preexisting (genetically determined) or substance-induced deficits in the function of the prefrontal cortex not only in inhibiting responses to drug-related stimuli but in impulsivity in general.

In the NCS, cooccurring mental disorders also influence the likelihood of seeking treatment and the treatment sector from which service is sought. As mentioned, those who had a substance dependence problem were far more likely to seek and receive treatment if they also had a cooccurring mental disorder. Approximately one-third of people with a 12-month history of affective disorder received some treatment; but those who also had an addictive disorder were more likely to have received it in a specialty addiction treatment program.

A collaborative study of the genetics of alcoholism used extensive structured interviews to separate independent mood and anxiety disorders from those that occurred only within the context of active drinking or withdrawal. This study found that over a lifetime, independent mood disorder was less common in alcoholics (14 percent) than in controls (17.1 percent), although more than twice as many alcoholics (2.3 percent) as controls (1 percent) met criteria for bipolar disorder. Panic disorder and social phobia were also substantially more common as independent disorders among alcoholics. In general, in this study, the large majority of alcohol-dependent men and women did not have independent mood or anxiety disorders. This suggests that the higher rates of cooccurrence of most anxiety and affective disorders found in epidemiological studies or clinical populations probably reflect substance (alcohol)–induced anxiety and mood disorders that resolve without special intervention once drug use ceases.

Multiple Factors The biopsychosocial general model of substance dependence presented here does not attempt to assign a weight or special significance to any one factor or interaction. The implication is that for different categories of drugs, different factors may play more or less powerful causal roles in perpetuating substance use or facilitating relapse. For example, positive reinforcing effects may be more important for the development of cocaine dependence, whereas acute and protracted withdrawal phenomena may be more important in the return to opioid use after withdrawal. Even with the same substance, different factors may be more or less important for different people. Thus, the emergence of depressive symptoms may make it difficult for some cigarette smokers to quit, particularly those with a history of major depressive disorder, and those people may be helped by antidepressants. Such a multifactorial model implies that certain treatments or interventions may be more effective for one substance category than another and that, even among people using the same substances, different treatments may be indicated.

Figure 11.1–5 implies that the notion of dependence is not a property of any one element but, rather, an abstraction inferred from the relations among the elements of the system. Although it is convenient (and required by DSM-IV-TR) to see dependence as a disorder located within a person, any interpretation that overemphasizes one part of the system, whether the biology of the person, changes in the brain, social influences, or behavior, is missing part of the nature of dependence.

TREATMENT

Many people who develop substance-related problems recover without formal treatment. For those who do seek help or advice, particularly those patients with less severe disorders, relatively brief interventions are often as effective as more intensive treatments. Because these brief interventions do not change the environment, alter drug-induced brain changes, or provide new skills, a change in the patient's motivation (cognitive change) probably best explains their impact on the drug-using behavior. For those individuals who do not respond or whose dependence is more severe, a variety of interventions appear to be effective. Although each section in this chapter discusses treatment relevant to the particular substance use disorder, the clinician sees few drug-dependent people who use only one drug. (Nicotine dependence may be an exception.) For example, among patients using an illegal drug, the most common additional diagnosis is alcohol dependence.

It is useful to distinguish among specific procedures or techniques (e.g., individual cognitive-behavioral therapy, family therapy, group therapy, relapse prevention, and pharmacotherapy) and treatment programs. Most programs use a number of specific procedures and involve several professional disciplines as well as nonprofessionals who have special skills or personal experience with the substance problem being treated. The best treatment programs combine specific procedures and disciplines to meet the needs of the individual patient after a careful assessment. However, there is no generally accepted classification either for the specific procedures used in treatment or for programs making use of various combinations of procedures. This lack of standardized terminology for categorizing procedures and programs presents a problem, even when the field of interest is narrowed from substance problems in general to treatment for a single substance such as alcohol, tobacco, or cocaine. Except in carefully monitored research projects, even the definitions of specific procedures (e.g., individual counseling, group therapy, and methadone maintenance) tend to be so imprecise that one usually cannot infer just what transactions are supposed to occur. Nevertheless, for descriptive purposes, programs are often broadly grouped on the basis of one or more of their salient characteristics: whether the program is aimed at merely controlling acute withdrawal and consequences of recent drug use (detoxification) or is focused on longer-term behavioral change; whether the program makes extensive use of pharmacological interventions; and the degree to which the program is based on individual psychotherapy, AA, or other 12-step principles or therapeutic community principles. Broad program descriptions mask as much as they reveal, tend to confuse the setting with the procedures, and obscure differences in the etiological models underlying the treatments used in different programs. Further, services actually provided by the same types of programs can vary greatly in intensity and in the specific problems (legal, medical, vocational) they are intended to ameliorate.

Based on the NHSDA, approximately 3.1 million people 12 years of age or older reported receiving some form of treatment for a drug- or alcohol-related problem in 2000. Some reported treatment at more than one location. The most common treatment reported was participation in a self-help group (1.6 million). The next most frequent setting was treatment at an outpatient rehabilitation facility (1.2 million). Then, in descending order, were inpatient rehabilitation (0.87 million), mental health center (0.73 million), hospital inpatient (0.71 million), private doctor's office (0.44 million), an emergency room (0.38 million), and prison or jail (0.18 million). Figure 11.1–6 shows the drug for which people reported receiving treatment. Some of the treatments received were for drug-induced conditions other than dependence.

Not all interventions are applicable to all varieties of substance use or dependence, and some of the more coercive interventions used for illegal drugs are not applicable to substances that are legally available, such as tobacco. Changes in addictive behaviors do not occur abruptly but rather through a series of stages. Five stages in this gradual process have been proposed: precontemplation, contemplation, preparation, action, and maintenance. For some types of addiction, the therapeutic alliance is enhanced when the treatment approach is tailored to the patient's stage or readiness to change. For some drug use disorders, a specific pharmacological agent may be an important component of an intervention—for example, disulfiram, naltrexone, or acamprosate (Campral) for alcoholism; methadone, levomethadyl acetate (Orlaam) (also called L-α-acetylmethadol [LAAM]), or buprenorphine (Buprenex, Subutex) for heroin addiction; nicotine delivery devices or bupropion (Zyban) for tobacco dependence. Not all interventions are likely to be useful as resources for health care professionals. For example, young offenders with histories of drug use or dependence may be remanded to special facilities under the jurisdiction of the criminal justice system. Some

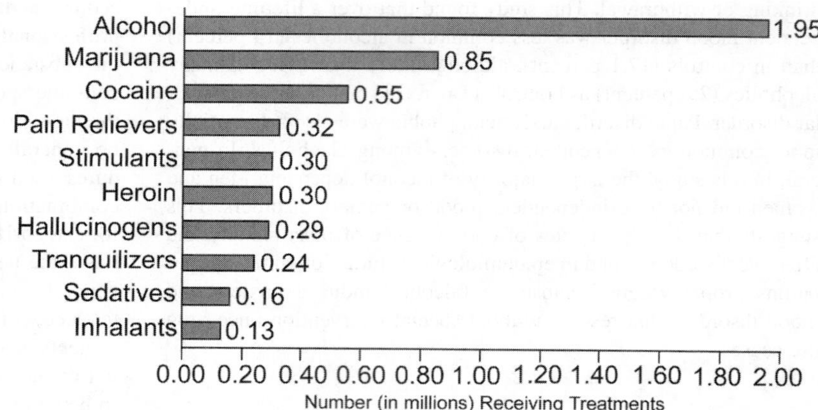

FIGURE 11.1–6 Number of U.S. community residents who received services for treatment of alcohol and other drug problems in the year before assessment, as estimated for each drug category under study. (Data from U.S. National Household Survey of Drug Abuse, 2001, with permission.)

programs for offenders (and sometimes for employees) rely almost exclusively on the deterrent effect of frequent urine testing. In contrast to the numerous studies suggesting some value for brief interventions for smoking and for problem drinking, there are few controlled studies of brief interventions for those seeking treatment for dependence on illegal drugs.

In general, for people who are severely dependent on illegal opioids, brief interventions (such as a few weeks of detoxification, whether in or out of a hospital) have limited effect on outcome measured a few months later. For those dependent on cocaine or heroin, treatment lasting as least 3 months is much more likely to result in substantial reductions in illegal drug use, antisocial behaviors, and psychiatric distress. Such a time-in-treatment effect is seen across very different modalities, from residential therapeutic communities to ambulatory methadone maintenance programs. Although some patients appear to benefit from a few days or weeks of treatment, a substantial percentage of users of illegal drugs drop out (or are dropped) from treatment before they have achieved significant benefits. Some of the variance in outcome of treatment can be attributed to differences in the characteristics of patients entering treatment and by events and conditions after treatment. However, programs based on similar philosophical principles and using what seem to be similar therapeutic procedures vary greatly in effectiveness. Some of the differences among programs that seem to be similar reflect the range and intensity of services offered. Programs with professionally trained staffs that provide more comprehensive services to patients with more severe psychiatric difficulties are more likely to be able to retain those patients in treatment and to help them to make positive changes. Differences in the skills of individual counselors and professionals can powerfully affect outcomes. Patients who have low levels of psychiatric problems tend to do well in most programs, and for these patients, the impact of specialized skills and services is more difficult to demonstrate. Such generalizations concerning programs serving illegal drug users may not hold for programs dealing with those seeking treatment for alcohol or tobacco or even cannabis problems uncomplicated by heavy use of illegal drugs. In such cases, relatively brief periods of individual or group counseling can produce long-lasting reductions in drug use. The outcomes usually considered in programs dealing with illegal drugs have typically included measures of social functioning, employment, and criminal activity as well as decreases in drug-using behavior. Treatment for alcoholism and other mental health problems generally has more limited expectations (e.g., reduction in alcohol use and symptoms of psychiatric disorders), although reduced use of health care resources subsequent to treatment is sometimes an additional measure of treatment effectiveness.

Measuring Treatment Outcome In a large multisite study of treatment, the Drug Abuse Treatment Outcome Study (DATOS; carried out from 1991 to 1993) patients were interviewed at intake and 1, 3, and 12 months after treatment. (For some types of drug use, data are now available for outcomes 5 years after original treatment entry.) As in previous multisite studies, sites selected were stable representatives of four major program types: drug-free outpatient, methadone maintenance, short-term residential (chemical dependency), and long-term residential (therapeutic community). Except at the methadone programs, which used group and individual counseling approximately equally, group counseling was the common element of the other treatments. Some antidepressant and antipsychotic agents were used in the nonmethadone programs, but they were incidental.

This study found a lower level of services available to patients seeking treatment than a decade earlier. Also, patients were older and more likely to have a variety of special medical problems (HIV, psychiatric disorders) and social needs (homelessness). Treatment outcomes were generally consistent with those of previous studies of drug treatment in the public sector. One year after treatment, there were substantial decreases in drug use. Levels of weekly or daily cocaine use at 1 year were, on average, approximately 50 percent of pretreatment levels, with greater reduction for those who participated in treatment for 3 months or more. Daily heroin use was lower among patients who remained in methadone maintenance treatment than among those who left. Although cocaine use among patients treated with methadone was somewhat lower, the reduction could not be attributed to treatment. Alcohol and marijuana use did not decline significantly. There was also no apparent decrease in suicidal thoughts or increase in employment, and, in contrast to a number of previous multisite studies, multivariate analysis in this study did not confirm the widely reported reduction in predatory or high-risk sexual behaviors, or both, for those in methadone programs. Those who stayed in long-term residential treatment for 6 months or more showed a major decrease in drug use from preadmission levels for all categories of drugs—66.4 to 22.0 percent for cocaine; 17.2 to 5.8 percent for heroin; alcohol and marijuana use reduced by more than one-half. These individuals also reported a 50 percent decrease in illegal activities and approximately a 10 percent increase in full-time employment.

The outpatient drug-free and short-term inpatient programs surveyed by DATOS had very few admissions for which heroin was the major drug problem; the most common presenting drug problem for both was cocaine, followed by alcohol and marijuana. Participation in the outpatient drug-free programs for 3 months or more was associated with a greater decrease in cocaine use at 1 year (approximately 50 percent, compared with those who stayed 3 months or less). But even 58 percent of those who stayed less than 3 months reported some decrease in cocaine use over preadmission levels. Patients who entered short-term inpatient programs also reported major decreases in drug use at 1 year, but there was no difference between those who stayed more than 2 weeks and those who stayed less than 2 weeks. Generally, the level of drug use at 1 year was predictive of drug use at the 5-year follow-up. This sustained improvement at 4 to 5 years was also noted in a follow-up of treatment programs in the United Kingdom. Although adolescents are generally reluctant to seek treatment without some external or family pressure, follow-up studies of programs specializing in adolescent treatment have found substantial and sustained decreases in drug use.

Because the decision to enter any of the programs studied in DATOS is made by the patient, the study does not give much guidance to a clinician weighing a recommendation for a specific patient. More guidance comes from a large-scale, random-assignment study of the treatment of alcoholics, which found that three distinct methods of delivering individual therapy over a 12-week period—12-step facilitation, cognitive-behavioral coping skills, and motivational enhancement (four sessions only)—produced comparable and generally quite favorable outcomes. Patient characteristics interacted significantly with the treatment in only one area, alcoholics with low-level psychiatric problems had better outcomes in terms of days of abstinence if assigned to 12-step facilitation rather than cognitive-behavioral therapy. Patients who received individual therapy after a brief period of inpatient and intensive day care treatment (aftercare) had better 1-year outcomes than those who began individual treatment as outpatients, even though their problem level at baseline was more severe.

Currently, entry into treatment rarely reflects a truly informed choice aimed at matching the characteristics and needs of the patient with the capacities and skills of a provider. Findings from studies of public sector programs serving drug users with relatively few social supports show that more intensive services, such as vocational, health, and mental health services, increase retention and produce better outcomes at follow-up. Patients who express more satisfaction with the treatment received tend to remain in treatment longer. In general, across drug categories, participation in self-help groups such as AA correlates with better short-term and long-term outcome.

Influence of Philosophical Orientation The kinds of therapeutic procedures that treatment professionals deem valuable or essential are profoundly affected by philosophical orientation. For example, one study found that many professionals who adhere to a "disease model" of substance dependence view reduction of denial, acceptance of disease, need for lifelong abstinence, commitment to recovery, and affiliation with AA as the most important elements of intervention. In contrast, dealing with responsibility, instilling motivation and confidence, teaching relapse prevention, and avoiding high-risk situations were rated highest by psychologists espousing a behavioral model of dependence. Until quite recently, even physicians were unlikely to view pharmacological interventions as having significant value in treating alcoholism or most other forms of drug dependence, although some physicians did prescribe various forms of nicotine for tobacco dependence.

Many controlled studies over many years have shown that the use of illegal opioids (heroin) can be markedly reduced by supervised administration of oral opioid agonists (methadone or LAAM) or partial agonists (buprenorphine). Because of government regulations, the use of full agonists is limited to practitioners and programs that have obtained special licenses. Data also show that naltrexone can reduce relapse rates for alcoholics after withdrawal. Controlled studies conducted in Europe show that acamprosate, a drug believed to act via actions on the glutamatergic system, can also reduce alcoholism relapse rates. At present, however, there seems to be only a modest correlation between the evidence showing that a given intervention or procedure is effective and the likelihood that it will be widely used.

Treatment of Comorbidity—Integrated versus Concurrent The treatment of the severely mentally ill (primarily those with schizophrenia and schizoaffective disorders) who are also drug dependent continues to pose problems for clinicians. Although some special facilities have been developed that use both antipsychotic drugs and therapeutic community principles, for the most part, specialized addiction agencies have difficulty treating these patients. Generally, integrated treatment in which the same staff can treat both the psychiatric disorder and the addiction is more effective than either parallel treatment (a mental health and a specialty addiction program providing care concurrently) or sequential treatment (treating either the addiction or the psychiatric disorder first and then dealing with the comorbid condition).

Services and Outcome The extension of managed care into the public sector has produced a major reduction in the use of hospital-based detoxification and virtual disappearance of longer-term residential rehabilitation programs for alcoholics. However, some managed care organizations tend to assume that the relatively brief courses of outpatient counseling that are effective with private sector alcoholic patients are also effective with patients who are dependent on illegal drugs and who have minimal social supports. For the present, the trend is to provide the care that costs least over the short term and to ignore studies showing that, for some patients, more services can produce better long-term outcomes.

Treatment is often a worthwhile social expenditure. For example, treatment of antisocial illegal drug users in outpatient settings can produce decreases in antisocial behavior and reductions in rates of HIV seroconversion that more than offset the treatment cost. Treatment in a prison setting can produce favorable decreases in postrelease costs associated with drug use and rearrests. Despite such evidence, there are problems maintaining public support for treatment of substance dependence, both in the public and private sectors. This lack of support suggests that these problems continue to be viewed, at least in part, as moral failings rather than as medical disorders.

SUGGESTED CROSS-REFERENCES

Individual sections discuss in detail the relevant substances and treatment for their related disorders: alcohol-related disorders in Section 11.2; amphetamine-related disorders, Section 11.3; caffeine-related disorders, Section 11.4; cannabis-related disorders, Section 11.5; cocaine-related disorders, Section 11.6; hallucinogen-related disorders, Section 11.7; inhalant-related disorders, Section 11.8; nicotine-related disorders, Section 11.9; opioid-related disorders, Section 11.10; PCP-related disorders, Section 11.11; sedative-hypnotic–related disorders, Section 11.12; and anabolic-androgenic steroid abuse, Section 11.13. Brief psychotherapy is covered in Section 30.9; alternative therapies, in Section 30.10; and methadone (and other maintenance therapies) in Section 31.22. Drug and alcohol abuse among elderly people is discussed in Section 51.3i.

REFERENCES

Anthony JC. Epidemiology of drug dependence. In: Galanter M, Kleber HD, eds. *Textbook of Substance Abuse Treatment*. 3rd ed. Washington, DC: The American Psychiatric Press, Inc.; 2003.

Anthony JC, Warner LA, Kessler RC: Comparative epidemiology of dependence on tobacco, alcohol, controlled substances, and inhalants: Basic findings from the National Comorbidity Survey. *Clin Exp Psychopharmacol.* 1994;2:244.

Anthony JH, Van Etten ML. Epidemiology and its rubrics. In: Bellack A, Hersen M, eds. *Comprehensive Clinical Psychology.* Oxford, UK: Elsevier; 1998.

Beirut LJ, Dinwiddie SH, Begleiter H, Crowe RR, Hesselbrock V, Nurnberger JI Jr, Porjesz B, Schuckit MA, Reich T: Familial transmission of substance dependence: Alcohol, marijuana, cocaine, and habitual smoking. *Arch Gen Psychiatry.* 1998;55:982.

Boys A, Farrell M, Taylor C, Marsden J, Goodman R, Brugha T, Bebbington P, Jenkins R, Meltzer H: Psychiatric morbidity and substance use in young people aged 13–15 years: Results from the Child and Adolescent Survey of Mental Health. *Br J Psychiatry.* 2003;182:509.

Edwards G, Arif A, Hodgson R: Nomenclature and classification of drug- and alcohol-related problems. A WHO Memorandum. *Bull WHO.* 1981;99:225.

Farrell M, Howes S, Bebbington P, Brugha T, Jenkins R, Lewis G, Marsden J, Taylor C, Meltzer H: Nicotine, alcohol and drug dependence, and psychiatric comorbidity—results of a national household survey. *Int Rev Psychiatry.* 2003;15:50.

Farrell M, Howes S, Taylor C, Lewis G, Jenkins R, Bebbington P, Jarvis M, Brugha T, Gill B, Meltzer H: Substance misuse and psychiatric comorbidity: An overview of the OPCS National Psychiatric Morbidity Survey. *Int Rev Psychiatry.* 2003;15:43.

*Gerstein DR, Harwood HJ, eds. *Treating Drug Problems.* Vol 1. Committee for the Substance Abuse Coverage Study, Division of Health Care Services, Institute of Medicine. Washington, DC: National Academy Press; 1990.

Goldstein RZ, Volkow ND: Drug addiction and its underlying neurobiological basis: Neuroimaging evidence for the involvement of the frontal cortex. *Am J Psychiatry.* 2002;159:1642.

Gossop M, Marsden J, Stewart D, Kidd T: The National Treatment Outcome Research Study (NTORS): 4–5 year follow-up results. *Addiction.* 2003;98:291.

Hser Y-I, Grella CE, Hubbard RL, Hsieh S-C, Fletcher BW, Brown BS, Anglin MD: An evaluation of drug treatments for adolescents in 4 US cities. *Arch Gen Psychiatry.* 2001;58:689.

Hubbard RL, Craddock SG, Anderson J: Overview of 5-year follow-up outcomes in the Drug Abuse Treatment Outcome Studies (DATOS). *J Subst Abuse Treatment.* 2003;25:125.

Hubbard RL, Craddock SG, Flynn PM, Anderson J, Etheridge RM: Overview of 1-year follow-up outcomes in the Drug Abuse Treatment Outcome Study (DATOS). *Psychol Addict Behav.* 1997;11:261.

Humphreys K. *Circles of Recovery: Self-Help Organizations for Addictions.* Cambridge, UK: Cambridge University Press; 2004.

*Institute of Medicine. *Broadening the Base of Treatment for Alcohol Problems.* Washington, DC: National Academy Press; 1990.

Institute of Medicine. *Pathways of Addiction.* Washington, DC: National Academy Press; 1996.

Jaffe JH. Current concepts of addiction. In: O'Brien CP, Jaffe JH, eds. *Addictive States.* Vol 70. Research Publications: Association for Research in Nervous and Mental Disease. New York: Raven; 1992.

Johnston LD, O'Malley PM, Bachman JG. *Monitoring the Future National Survey Results on Drug Use 1975–2001.* Vol I: Secondary School Students (NIH Publ. No. 01-5106). Bethesda, MD: National Institute on Drug Abuse; 2002.

Johnston LD, O'Malley PM, Bachman JG. *Monitoring the Future National Results on Drug Use: Overview of Key Findings, 2002.* (NIH Publ. No. 03-5374). Bethesda, MD: National Institute on Drug Abuse; 2003.

Kendler KS, Jacobson KC, Prescott CA, Neale MC: Specificity of genetic and environmental risk factors for use and abuse/dependence of cannabis, cocaine, hallucinogens, sedatives, stimulants, and opiates in male twins. *Am J Psychiatry.* 2003;160:687.

*Kessler RC, Crum RM, Warner LA, Nelson CB, Schulenberg J, Anthony JC: Lifetime co-occurrence of DSM-III-R alcohol abuse and dependence with other psychiatric disorders in the national comorbidity survey. *Arch Gen Psychiatry.* 1997;54:313.

Kessler RC, McGonagle KA, Zhao S, Nelson CB, Hughes M, Eshleman S, Wittchen H-U, Kendler KS: Lifetime and 12-month prevalence of DSM-III-R psychiatric disorders in the United States. *Arch Gen Psychiatry.* 1994;51:8.

Koob GF, LeMoal M: Drug addiction, dysregulation of reward, and allostasis. *Neuropsychopharmacology.* 2001;24:97.

Kreek MH, Koob GF: Drug dependence: Stress and dysregulation of brain reward pathways. *Drug Alcohol Depend.* 1998;51:23.

McLellan AT, Grissom GR, Zanis D, Randall M, Brill P, O'Brien CP: Problem-service "matching" in addiction treatment. *Arch Gen Psychiatry.* 1997;54:730.

Miller WR: Why do people change addictive behavior? The 1996 H. David Archibald lecture. *Addiction.* 1998;93:163.

Musto DF. *The American Disease. Origins of Narcotic Control.* New York: Oxford University Press; 1987.

Musto DF, ed. *One Hundred Years of Heroin.* Westport, CT: Auburn House; 2002.

*Nestler EJ: Molecular neurobiology of addiction. *Am J Addictions.* 2001;10:201.

Office of Applied Studies. *Results from the 2001 National Household Survey on Drug Abuse.* Vol I: Summary of National Findings (DHHS Publ. No. SMA 01-3758, NHSDA Series H-17). Rockville, MD: Substance Abuse and Mental Health Services Administration; 2002.

Parran TV Jr, Liepman MR, Farkas K. The family in addiction. In: Graham AW, Schultz TK, Mayo-Smith MF, Ries RK, Wilford BB, eds. *Principles of Addiction Medicine.* 3rd ed. Chevy Chase, MD: American Society of Addiction Medicine; 2003.

Prochaska JO, DiClemente CC, Norcross JC: In search of how people change. Applications to addictive behaviours. *Am Psychol.* 1992;47:1102.

Project MATCH Research Group: Matching alcoholism treatment to client heterogeneity: Project MATCH posttreatment drinking outcomes. *J Stud Alcohol.* 1997;58:2.

Regier DA, Farmer ME, Rae DS, Locke BZ, Keith SJ, Judd LL, Goodwin FK: Comorbidity of mental disorders with alcohol and other drug abuse. *JAMA.* 1990;264:2511.

Robinson TW, Berridge KC: Incentive-sensitization and addiction. *Addiction.* 2001;96:103.

Rounsaville BJ, Bryant K, Babor R, Kranzler H, Kadden R: Cross system agreement for substance use disorders: DSM-III-R, DSM-IV and ICD-10. *Addiction.* 1993;88:337.

Schuckit MA, Smith TL: An 8-year follow-up of 450 sons of alcoholic and control subjects. *Arch Gen Psychiatry.* 1996;53:202.

Schuckit MA, Tipp JE, Bucholz KK, Nurnberger JI Jr, Hesselbrock VM, Crowe RR, Kramer J: The life-time rates of three major mood disorders and four major anxiety disorders in alcoholics and controls. *Addiction.* 1997;92:1289.

*Simpson DD, Joe GW, Broome KM: A national 5-year follow-up of treatment outcomes for cocaine dependence. *Arch Gen Psychiatry.* 2002;59:538.

Simpson DD, Joe GW, Brown BS: Treatment retention and follow-up outcomes in the Drug Abuse Treatment Outcome Study (DATOS). *Psychol Addict Behav.* 1997;11:294.

Tarter RE, Kirisci L, Mezzich A, Cornelius JR, Pajer K, Vanyukov M, Gardner W, Blackson T, Clark D: Neurobehavioral disinhibition in childhood predicts early age at onset of substance use disorder. *Am J Psychiatry.* 2003;160:1078.

Tsai GE, Ragan P, Chang R, Chen S, Linnoila MI, Coyle JT: Increased glutamatergic neurotransmission and oxidative stress after alcohol withdrawal. *Am J Psychiatry.* 1998;155:726.

Tsuang MT, Lyons MJ, Meyer JM, Doyle T, Eisen SA, Goldberg J, True W, Lin N, Toomey R, Eaves L: Co-occurrence of abuse of different drugs in men. *Arch Gen Psychiatry.* 1998;55:967.

Weisner C, Matzger H, Kaskutas LA: How important is treatment? One-year outcomes of treated and untreated alcohol-dependent individuals. *Addiction.* 2003;98:901.

▲ 11.2 Alcohol-Related Disorders

MARC A. SCHUCKIT, M.D.

Alcohol use disorders are common, lethal conditions that often masquerade as other psychiatric syndromes. The average alcohol-dependent person decreases his or her life span by 10 to 15 years, and alcohol contributes to 22,000 deaths and two million nonfatal injuries each year. Fortunately, recent years have witnessed a blossoming of clinically relevant research regarding alcohol abuse and dependence, including information on specific genetic influences, the clinical course of these conditions, and the development of new and helpful treatments. This chapter attempts to bring the reader up to date on many of these new developments.

The alcohol-related disorders impact on all aspects of health care delivery systems, especially psychiatric practice. At least 20 percent of the patients in mental health settings have alcohol abuse or dependence, including individuals from all socioeconomic strata and both genders. The problems can begin early—a recent national evaluation of students on college campuses reported a 12-month prevalence for alcohol dependence of 6 percent and for abuse more than 20 percent—and alcohol has been estimated to have contributed to at least 15,000 deaths in students per year. Of particular importance to the psychiatrist are the estimated 40 to 50 percent of alcoholics who develop alcohol-induced, but temporary, clinical syndromes that resemble major depressive disorder, panic disorder, generalized anxiety disorder, and additional mood or anxiety conditions. In addition, men and women with several independent psychiatric disorders have elevated risks for the future development of alcohol-related disorders, including those with manic-depressive disease, schizophrenia, antisocial personality disorder, panic disorder, and, possibly, generalized anxiety disorder. Because the optimal short- and long-term treatments of substance-induced and independent psychiatric conditions are often different, the clinician must learn to recognize and differentiate between these conditions.

These data underscore the need for all health care providers, especially psychiatrists, to develop and maintain skills for diagnosing and treating alcohol-related disorders. At the same time, few medical practitioners have received appropriate training in dealing with these syndromes, and relatively few medical school faculty teach about substance-related conditions. The sections in this chapter help the psychiatric resident, psychiatrist, and other interested health professionals review recent developments regarding alcohol use disorders. Although these pages present data on diagnosis, the usual clinical course, new developments in genetic influences, and treatment approaches, an emphasis is placed on ways of diagnosing and treating comorbid psychiatric conditions observed in the course of alcohol abuse and dependence.

DEFINITION AND COMPARATIVE NOSOLOGY

Alcohol Use Disorder

In all diagnostic systems, the definition of alcoholism (i.e., alcohol abuse and dependence) relates to evidence of repeated impairments from alcohol in multiple areas of life functioning, despite which the person returns to drinking. The basic elements of this definition are present in the American Psychiatric Association's (APA) third edition (1980) and revised third edition (1987) of the *Diagnostic and Statistical Manual of Mental Disorders* (DSM-III, DSM-III-R, respectively) and have continued into the revised fourth edition of the DSM (DSM-IV-TR) in 1994. In this most recent manual, dependence is diagnosed as the repeated presence of at least three of seven major areas of life impairment related to alcohol that cluster together in the same 12-month period. These difficulties include tolerance, evidence of a withdrawal syndrome when the drug is discontinued or intake is decreased, potential interference with life functioning associated with spending a great deal of time using the substance, and returning to use despite evidence of physical or psychological problems. It is the syndrome of dependence for which the best data are available regarding the usual clinical course of problems, appropriateness of treatment, and potential importance of genetic factors. Although DSM-IV-TR does not require tolerance or withdrawal for dependence, recent studies have shown that a history of these phenomena, especially withdrawal, is associated with a more severe clinical course. Thus, clinicians are encouraged to subtype dependence into those syndromes with and without evidence of a physiological component (i.e., tolerance or withdrawal).

Thus, all patients with a possible alcohol use disorder should first be evaluated for the presence of alcohol dependence. For those who do not meet the criteria for this disorder, however, there is a second potential syndrome to consider, *abuse.* Here, an individual who is not dependent on alcohol demonstrates repeated problems within any 12-month period in any one or more of four potential areas of difficulties. These include repeated legal, interpersonal, social, or occupational impairments related to alcohol as well as use of alcohol in physically hazardous situations. DSM-IV-TR reformulated the concept of abuse to identify criteria that were not just a subset of those noted for dependence. Although abuse and dependence both correlate with similar background characteristics, including a family history of alcoholism, dependence has been reported to be tied to future problems for as many as 80 percent. Approximately 50 percent of those with difficulties with alcohol abuse continue to have alcohol problems, but fewer than 10 percent go on to dependence.

A similar definition of dependence is offered in the tenth revision of the *International Statistical Classification of Diseases and Related Health Problems* (ICD-10). Here, however, the threshold for diagnosis is any three of six (rather than seven) items. The criteria for ICD-10 dependence include all the concepts in DSM-IV-TR, although they are expressed and numbered differently, and some concepts are combined in a single criterion. ICD-10 also lists a second and less intense alcohol use disorder known as *harmful use.* The definition of this second syndrome is quite different from DSM-IV-TR abuse because the ICD-10 approach is based on evidence of repeated interference with psychological and physical health functioning and does not include social impairment, legal problems, or use in physically hazardous situations.

Attempts have been made to further divide alcohol dependence into additional clinically meaningful subgroups. Some authors have called for the recognition of a more severe early-onset alcohol dependence syndrome, often accompanied by criminality and dependence on other drugs, which has been labeled as *type II* or *type B alcoholism.* These approaches are consistent with the recognition that an earlier-onset alcohol dependence syndrome, like most medical and psychiatric disorders, is likely to have a more severe course, but it appears as if some of the prognostic significance of type II or B alcoholism rests with an elevated risk for a concomitant antisocial personality disorder in the early-onset group.

Severity and Remission

The DSM-IV-TR definition of dependence also attempts to better clarify the concepts of severity and remission. Regarding the former, no reliable criteria could be developed, and the manual offers the clinician the possibility of incorporating the relatively imprecise divisions of *mild* (with few symptoms), *moderate* (with functional impairment intermediate between mild and severe), and *severe* (with many symptoms); ICD-10 has no formal notation of severity.

Remission is a more complex phenomenon, and the diagnostic criteria distinguish between the high-risk period in the first 12 months of recovery and at later time points, asking the clinician to specify whether the patient is totally free of substance-related problems. The criteria also consider whether the individual is living in a controlled environment such as prison or a hospital; ICD-10 makes similar but not identical distinctions.

EPIDEMIOLOGY

Psychiatrists need to be concerned about alcoholism because this condition is common, intoxication and withdrawal mimic many major psychiatric disorders, and the usual alcoholic person does not fit the common stereotype.

Prevalence of Drinking

At some time during life, 90 percent of the population in the United States drinks, with most people beginning their alcohol intake in the early to middle teens (Table 11.2–1). By the end of high school, 80 percent of students have consumed alcohol, and more than 60 percent have been intoxicated. At any time, two out of three men are drinkers, with a ratio of persisting alcohol intake of approximately 1.3 men to 1.0 woman, and the highest prevalence of drinking is from the middle or late teens to the mid-20s.

Different groups in the United States have different rates of drinkers. Generally, groups with high education and high socioeconomic status have the highest proportion of people who currently imbibe. Among religious groups, Jews have the highest proportion who consume alcohol but the lowest number of people with alcohol dependence. Conservative Protestants and Catholics are less likely to use alcohol than liberal Protestants and Catholics. Other groups,

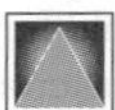

Table 11.2–1
Alcohol Epidemiology

Condition	Population (%)
Ever had a drink	90
Current drinker	60–70
Temporary problems	40+
Abuse[a]	Male: 10+ Female: 5+
Dependence[a]	Male: 10 Female: 3–5

[a]Twenty to 30 percent of psychiatric patients.

such as the Irish, have higher rates of severe alcohol problems, but they also have significantly higher rates of abstention. Very high rates of alcohol problems are found among most, but not all, American Indian and Inuit tribes.

In the United States in the mid-1990s, the average person older than 14 years of age consumed 2.2 gallons of absolute alcohol a year. This amount sounds substantial, but it is considerably less than the more than 5 gallons of absolute ethanol consumed each year at the time of the American Revolution. The current figure also represents a significant decrease from the amounts consumed during the mid-1970s and the 2.7 gallons per capita in 1981.

Alcohol Problems

Because a high proportion of people are drinkers, especially in their middle teens to mid-20s, and because the per capita consumption of alcohol is high, it is not surprising that a large proportion of people have alcohol-related problems sometime in their lives. A recent 10-year follow-up study of almost 500 men evaluated at 33 years of age found that, during the preceding decade, between one-fourth and one-third had alcohol-related blackouts, approximately one-third admitted to driving after consuming enough alcohol to be impaired, and 20 percent reported missing school or work because of either a hangover or a desire to party with alcohol rather than work.

As common and costly as these problems are, most people mature out of less severe alcohol problems with the passage of time. Thus, the average person is likely to experience fewer alcohol-related difficulties during their 30s than during their 20s, and even fewer difficulties in their 40s and 50s.

Alcohol Abuse or Dependence

The lifetime risk for alcohol dependence is approximately 10 to 15 percent for men and 3 to 5 percent for women. The rate of alcohol abuse and dependence combined may be as high as 20 percent for men and more than 10 percent for women, and the 1-year prevalence of abuse and dependence that are clinically significant is estimated at 6 percent or more. These high rates have been reported for all socioeconomic and educational levels.

The age of peak onset of alcohol problems severe enough to lead to a diagnosis of alcohol dependence is probably in the middle 20s to approximately 40 years of age. Despite multiple difficulties, most alcohol-dependent people have jobs, families, and relatively high levels of functioning. Thus, the stereotypical alcoholic person who is a homeless street person is very much the exception rather than the rule, representing only 5 percent of all people with severe, recurring alcohol-related difficulties.

Age-related differences are found in the pattern of alcohol-related problems. As is true with almost all psychiatric and many medical disorders, the earlier the onset of alcoholism, the greater likely severity and the higher the probability of a preexisting independent psychiatric condition. Therefore, when alcohol dependence is noted in a teenager, the person usually also has conduct disorder (e.g., early antisocial personality disorder). In that instance, the alcohol-related problems are likely to be associated with severe drug difficulties and antisocial problems in school and with family or peers that occurred before the onset of alcohol dependence. At the other extreme, although most alcoholic people have their problems early in life, perhaps 10 percent or so have an onset of recurring difficulties after the age of 55 years. The late onset of the disorder tends to be associated with less severe social difficulties and more subtle signs and symptoms, but a greater likelihood of associated medical problems than among younger alcoholic people.

Comorbid Conditions

The alcohol-related disorders are highly prevalent conditions, and psychiatric symptoms are common during intoxication and withdrawal. Therefore, if diagnoses are to be used to indicate prognosis and optimal treatment, an algorithm has to be developed to help the clinician disentangle temporary substance-related psychopathology from independent psychiatric syndromes. This topic is only briefly referred to in this section on epidemiology and is discussed in greater depth later in the chapter.

Up to 80 percent of alcoholic people report symptoms of sadness or anxiety during the course of their disorder. These syndromes become intense and persistent enough to meet criteria for major psychiatric conditions, such as major depressive episodes or panic disorder, in at least 40 percent. However, for even full-blown conditions, when the syndrome is only observed in the context of intoxication or withdrawal from a brain depressant, such as alcohol, the psychiatric symptoms are likely to diminish and disappear within weeks to 1 month of abstinence. These alcohol-induced mood or anxiety disorders do not have the same long-term prognoses nor require the same pharmacological treatments as independent major depressive episodes or anxiety disorders. Therefore, all the diagnostic manuals since DSM-III have warned the clinician that psychiatric syndromes developing only during intoxication or withdrawal from substances do not necessarily indicate an independent psychiatric disorder.

PHARMACOLOGY AND EFFECTS ON THE BODY

Clinicians cannot understand alcohol-related disorders without knowing something about alcohol itself.

Properties and Metabolism of Alcohol

Ethanol (beverage alcohol) is a simple molecule that is well absorbed through the mucosal lining of the digestive tract in the mouth, esophagus, and stomach. The most prominent area of uptake, however, is in the proximal small intestine, which is also the site of absorption of many of the B vitamins. Ethanol rapidly enters the bloodstream and, as a result of its high solubility in water, is distributed to almost every body system. As a consequence of its modest fat solubility, alcohol is likely to have effects on body membranes rich in fat, including neurons.

Wine, beer, and such distilled spirits as whiskey, gin, and vodka differ in their content of components other than alcohol. These *congeners* are responsible for much of the characteristic taste of the beverage and consist of combinations of methanol, butanol, aldehydes, phenols, tannins, lead, cobalt, iron, and other substances. Under certain circumstances, congeners can have physiological effects, but their potency pales in comparison with the effects of alcohol.

A standard drink of an alcoholic beverage is usually defined as containing 10 to 12 g of ethanol. In round figures, this is the amount of alcohol contained in approximately 12 oz of beer (which, in the United States, has approximately 3.6 percent ethanol), 4 oz of table wine (containing approximately 12 percent ethanol), and between 1.0 and 1.5 oz of 80-proof spirits (containing 40 percent ethanol). For an average 70-kg (155 lb) person who has an average amount of body fat, one drink is likely to raise the blood alcohol level by approximately 15 to 20 mg/dL (the same as 0.015 to 0.020 g/dL). The body subsequently metabolizes and excretes approximately one drink per hour. The rate of absorption of alcohol from the digestive tract is likely to be faster on an empty stomach than after a full meal, especially one rich in fats and carbohydrates.

After absorption into the bloodstream from the small intestine, between 2 and 10 percent of the alcohol is then excreted unchanged from the lungs or the kidneys or through sweat, but the majority is broken down in the liver. Metabolism in that organ occurs mostly through four pathways, with each resulting in the production of acetaldehyde. Most of the process occurs through the actions of alcohol dehydrogenase (ADH) in the cytosol of hepatic cells. Especially at high blood alcohol levels, some of the alcohol is also broken down in the microsomes of the smooth endoplasmic reticulum (the microsomal ethanol oxidizing system [MEOS]). The ADH process is the usual rate-limiting metabolic step, occurring relatively slowly because of the liver's need to handle the produced hydrogen ions through use of a cofactor that is in relatively short supply, nicotinamide adenine dinucleotide (NAD).

The acetaldehyde produced primarily by ADH and MEOS is then destroyed by the enzyme aldehyde dehydrogenase (ALDH) in both the liver cell cytosol and mitochondria. This step occurs rapidly, with the result that the average person does not have substantial levels of this substance. This is fortunate because, at high levels, acetaldehyde can produce histamine release and other effects that, through a variety of mechanisms, contribute to an increase and subsequent decrease in blood pressure along with nausea and vomiting.

As described later in the section on genetics of alcohol use disorders, the ALDH and ADH isoenzyme patterns of an individual are related to the risk for developing alcoholism. This is especially relevant to Asian (e.g., Japanese, Chinese, Korean) men and women, although the impact of genes that control ADH also extends to some other groups.

Alcohol as a Depressant Drug Acutely, all substances of abuse share the ability to produce changes in feeling states and subsequently increase the likelihood that a person will have a psychological drive to continue to take the substance despite potentially severe adverse consequences (psychological dependence). That effect is distinct from the physical dependence that produces the withdrawal, or abstinence syndrome, that characterizes drugs such as alcohol. However, the 300 or so diverse psychoactive drugs differ in many important ways. For example, only a few produce physiological tolerance and clinically relevant levels of withdrawal symptoms when the substance is discontinued. Some drugs (e.g., stimulants or depressants) markedly increase the chances that a person will have temporary psychoses or depressions; other drugs (e.g., opioids) do not. Some are likely to be lethal in overdose (e.g., depressants); others (e.g., cannabinols) appear to be relatively physically safe at high levels. Clinicians, therefore, are presented with a daunting challenge if they attempt to memorize all the attributes for each of the hundreds of psychoactive substances.

A useful shortcut is to place drugs of abuse into categories based on their most prominent effects at the usual doses at which they are taken. In this scheme, substances that have as their most prominent usual effects the production of somnolence and decreased neuronal activity but that are not powerful in attenuating pain are labeled as depressants or sedative-hypnotics. They include alcohol, all the benzodiazepines, and the barbiturates. These substances produce similar intoxications, are potentially lethal in overdose (especially when multiple depressant drugs are taken at the same time), produce cross-tolerance with other depressants, and are physically addicting, with similar withdrawal syndromes.

The behavioral and physiological changes observed with any substance differ with the dose, the patient's history of exposure to the drug, and clinical conditions, including physiological disorders and the patient's state of fatigue. With a drug like alcohol, the effects also change over time after intake, with more pronounced symptoms observed while the blood alcohol levels are rising than when the blood alcohol levels are falling, a phenomenon called *acute tolerance* or the *Mallenby effect.*

Neurochemical Effects of Ethanol Alcohol has major effects on most neurochemical systems, depending on the dose, with opposite actions during intoxication and withdrawal. One series of theories on the mechanisms underlying intoxication and subsequent craving focuses on changes in dopamine, tying in the effects of alcohol to the pleasure centers in the limbic system. Alcohol acutely increases dopamine and its metabolites, brain imaging reveals enhanced activity in relevant areas of the brain, and chronic drinking changes dopamine receptor numbers and sensitivity. Another key neurochemical is serotonin, with alcohol causing changes in key aspects of this transmitter and associated receptors, and levels of serotonin impact on the amount of alcohol consumed. Additional studies point out the indirect actions that alcohol has on the benzodiazepine receptor–sensitive γ-aminobutyric acid (GABA) complexes in the brain. These effects, especially actions on the GABA type A receptor ($GABA_A$), enhance the acute sedating, sleep-inducing, anticonvulsant, and muscle-relaxing effects of alcohol. Next in this abbreviated review, alcohol has potent effects on glutamate-gated ionophoric receptors, especially those that bind *N*-methyl-D-aspartate (NMDA), which are muted during intoxication and overactive during alcohol withdrawal. Finally, alcohol also acutely enhances the functioning of the opioid-related brain systems and impacts on adenosine, neurosteroids, and acetylcholine.

Tolerance With repeated administration of alcohol, larger and larger doses of the drug are required to produce the desired effect. This phenomenon, called *tolerance,* is also the ability to tolerate higher and higher doses of the substance and is the result of at least three processes. *Behavioral tolerance* reflects the ability of a person to learn how to perform tasks effectively despite the effects of alcohol. *Pharmacokinetic tolerance* is an adaptation of the metabolizing systems, including ADH and MEOS, to rid the body of alcohol rapidly. Finally, and most important, *pharmacodynamic* or *cellular tolerance* is an adaptation of the nervous system so that it can function, despite very high blood alcohol concentrations (e.g., as much as 600 mg/dL), by resisting the actions of alcohol on the cell.

Once tolerance has developed for one of the brain depressants, an individual is likely to demonstrate a similar reaction to a second drug of that class (*cross-tolerance*). Therefore, a person who has been drinking heavily, has tolerance for alcohol, and then stops drinking can be expected to require a higher dose of benzodiazepines for sleep induction. If the individual took two depressant drugs at the same time, tolerance is not likely to be observed, and the mixing of the two substances can have lethal effects.

Aspects of tolerance decrease and even disappear with consecutive weeks of abstinence. In addition, some clinicians and researchers have described a phenomenon of *reverse tolerance*, increased sensitivity, or sensitization. This is a complex situation that might relate to neurochemical adaptations or other mechanisms. For example, whether alcoholic or not, as people grow older, they have increasing levels of reaction to most brain depressants, including alcohol. Even more dramatic examples of increased reaction to alcohol are seen after severe brain damage (e.g., the consequence of an auto accident or alcohol-related brain deterioration) and after impairment in any of the major alcohol-metabolizing systems, as occurs in cirrhosis.

Craving

The state of motivation to seek out alcohol is an important component of drinking behavior. This phenomenon of craving, however, fluctuates with time and can be difficult to measure. Aspects of the drive to drink are believed to relate to classical conditioning and to also reflect neurochemical changes. On neuroimaging, presenting substance-dependent subjects with images of their drug or autobiographical stories about their substance use results in activation in the limbic system and the orbitofrontal, insular cortex, and cerebellum. These data, although mostly generated regarding cocaine, may offer useful directions for future research into ways to better understand the causes of substance dependencies and to develop more effective approaches to decrease craving and enhance treatment outcome.

Blackout

Blackout indicates a memory impairment (*anterograde amnesia*) for the period when the person was drinking heavily but remained awake. This common phenomenon is related to the ability of any brain depressant at high enough doses to interfere with the acquisition of memory. Perhaps 40 percent of teenaged and young adult males have had a blackout, and memory loss does not by itself indicate a high likelihood of alcohol abuse or dependence. The blackout, which is temporary and limited to memory problems involving a short period, is not part of the DSM-IV-TR diagnosis and is distinct from *alcohol-induced persisting amnestic disorder*, formerly known as *Wernicke-Korsakoff syndrome*.

Sleep Impairment

Alcohol intoxication can help a person fall asleep more quickly, but if the intake in an evening is more than one or two drinks, the sleep pattern can be significantly impaired. Most heavy drinkers awaken after several hours and can have problems falling back asleep. Alcohol also tends to depress rapid eye movements (REMs) and inhibit stage 4 sleep and, thus, is likely to be associated with frequent alternations between sleep stages (*sleep fragmentation*) and with more dreams late in the night as the blood alcohol level falls. Exaggerated forms of similar problems are seen in alcoholics in whom sleep stages might not return to normal for 3 or more months of abstinence.

Cerebellar Degeneration

Characterized by unsteadiness of gait, problems with standing, and mild nystagmus, cerebellar degeneration is probably caused by a combination of the effects of ethanol and acetaldehyde along with vitamin deficiencies. Treatment usually consists of total abstinence and vitamin supplementation, although complete recovery is not usual.

Other Effects on the Central Nervous System

Several rare but serious neurological and cognitive syndromes can also be observed in alcohol-dependent men and women. A thiamine deficiency, especially in the context of a preexisting vulnerability, such as a transketolase deficiency, can present as any of several neurological syndromes, including a sixth cranial nerve palsy (Wernicke's) and a severe anterograde amnesia that is out of proportion to the alcohol level of confusion (Korsakoff's). This is discussed in greater depth in the section Diagnosis and Clinical Features. Two additional central nervous system (CNS) syndromes are often fatal, including a loss of myelin in the central pons that can present as quadriplegia, lethargy, and cognitive impairment (central pontine myelinolysis) and a thinning of the corpus callosum along with a change in consciousness, ataxia, and possible dementia (Marchiafava-Bignami syndrome).

Effects on the Rest of the Body

Under certain circumstances, one to two drinks per day can have some beneficial effects. Low doses of ethanol appear to decrease the risk for myocardial infarction and thrombotic stroke, probably through decreasing platelet aggregation and enhancing the beneficial impact of high-density lipoprotein cholesterol. Additional cardioprotective action may occur through antioxidant flavinoids or the inhibition of the vasoconstrictor, endothelin-1, in the components of red wine. Low doses of alcohol have also been reported to decrease the risks for some old-age dementias, peripheral arterial disease, and gallstones.

However, any amount of alcohol is considered harmful to the developing fetus, recovering alcoholics, people taking medications that may adversely interact with alcohol, and individuals with certain medical disorders or psychiatric syndromes (such as major depressive disorder or schizophrenia) that might be intensified by alcohol. Also, the intake of more than two drinks a day is likely to increase low-density lipoprotein (LDL) cholesterol and triglycerides and to increase blood pressure, with the overall result of increasing the risk of cardiac disorders, and even low levels of alcohol may increase the risk for breast cancer. The following sections review the impact that heavy drinking can have on different body systems to help clinicians better identify alcoholic patients and educate them about the risks posed by continued drinking.

Peripheral Neuropathy

Approximately 10 percent of alcoholic people develop a deterioration of nerve functioning to the hands and feet called *peripheral neuropathy*. The symptoms include numbness of the hands and feet, often bilateral, frequently accompanied by tingling and paresthesias. Although the condition is usually relatively mild and often improves with abstinence, the pain and the numbness can result in a permanent impairment.

Gastrointestinal Problems

The gastrointestinal (GI) system can be severely affected by heavy drinking, with a relatively common problem of an acute and at times severe inflammation of the esophagus or the stomach, often accompanied by vomiting and bleeding. If gastritis occurs in the presence of dilated esophageal veins, as seen with cirrhosis, it can induce potentially lethal bleeding.

The liver and the pancreas are especially vulnerable to alcohol. In the liver, increasing alcohol doses result in the accumulation of fats and proteins in the cells, producing a reversible swelling often described as a *fatty liver*. Inflammation of the liver cells accompanied by a subsequent intense increase in some liver function tests and other signs of alcohol-induced inflammation, or hepatitis, can lead to the deposition of excessive amounts of hyalin and collagen near blood vessels, an early stage of cirrhosis, a condition only seen in approximately 15 percent of alcoholics. As damage progresses, the normal flow of blood through the liver is impaired, dilated veins or varices develop from the increased abdominal venous pressure, and fluid seeps from the liver capsule, accumulating in the abdomen as ascites. As liver failure progresses, secondary cognitive impairment can develop as various levels of hepatic encephalopathy.

Perhaps 10 percent of alcoholic people develop an inflammation of the pancreas that can present as the abdominal emergency of acute pancreatitis, which can lead to a chronic irreversible condition with associated signs of insufficiency of both sugar metabolism (a form of diabetes) and digestive enzymes. One corollary of even early-stage effects of alcohol on the liver and pancreas is an abnormality in blood sugar levels that often reverts to normal glucose tolerance with maintained abstinence.

Cerebrovascular and Cardiovascular Problems

Heavy intake of alcohol increases the blood pressure and elevates both LDL cholesterol and triglycerides, thus enhancing the risk for myocardial infarction and thrombosis. At high doses, alcohol is also a striated-muscle toxin with a resulting deterioration in the heart muscle that manifests itself as beating irregularities and signs of heart failure (*alcoholic cardiomyopathy*). Thus, it is not surprising that the leading cause of early deaths in alcoholics is cardiovascular disease. Similar levels of swelling of muscle cells and subsequent muscle pain can be observed in the skeletal muscles.

Blood-Producing Systems Alcohol intake of four to eight drinks or more per day decreases the production of white blood cells and impairs the ability of those cells to migrate to sites of infection. Such drinking can also affect the stem cells that produce the red blood components, significantly increasing the average size of the red cell (the mean corpuscular volume [MCV]), and can impair the production and the efficiency of blood platelets.

Cancer High rates of most cancers are seen in alcoholic people, especially those of the head, neck, esophagus, stomach, liver, colon, lungs, and breast tissue. An enhanced risk for breast malignancies might be seen with as few as two drinks per day, especially in women with family histories of this disease. The association with cancer probably reflects alcohol-related immune system suppression and the direct effects of ethanol on mucosal membranes. The heightened rates of malignant tumors in alcoholic people remain significant even when the possible effects of smoking and poor nutrition are considered, and this is the second leading cause of premature death in alcohol-dependent men and women.

Fetal Alcohol Effect Alcohol and acetaldehyde can have deleterious effects on the developing fetus. Both substances cross the placenta with ease and, in high enough doses, can produce fetal death and spontaneous abortion. Surviving infants of heavy-drinking mothers can evidence any mixture of the components of a syndrome that, in its full-blown form, can include severe mental retardation, a small head, a diminished physical size, facial abnormalities (including a flat bridge of the nose, an absent philtrum, and an epicanthal eye fold), an atrial septal heart defect, and syndactyly. None of these problems is reversible, and the cognitive defects and physical irregularities remain throughout life. A clinically obvious fetal alcohol syndrome has been estimated to occur in approximately 5 percent of children born to relatively heavier-drinking mothers. Because the exact amount of alcohol required and the most vulnerable periods of pregnancy have not been definitively established, all pregnant women are advised to abstain from any use of alcohol.

Other Problems In effect, high doses of alcohol adversely affect almost all body systems, cutting a decade or more off the life span even for people with higher socioeconomic and educational status. Additional body effects seen at higher rates in alcoholics include testicular atrophy; bone fractures; a host of eye effects, including cataracts; dental difficulties; skeletal muscle wasting; and, of course, the consequences of accidents.

ETIOLOGY

Many factors affect the decision to drink, the development of temporary alcohol-related difficulties in the teenage years and the 20s, and the development of alcohol dependence. The initiation of alcohol intake probably depends largely on social, religious, and psychological factors, although genetic characteristics might also contribute. However, the factors that influence the decision to drink or those that contribute to temporary problems might be different from those that add to the risk for the severe, recurring problems of alcohol dependence.

A similar interplay between genetic and environmental influences contributes to many medical and psychiatric conditions, and, thus, a review of these factors in alcoholism offers information about complex genetic disorders overall. Dominant or recessive genes, although important, only explain relatively rare conditions. Most disorders have some level of genetic predisposition that usually relates to a series of different genetically influenced characteristics, each of which increase or decrease the risk for the disorder.

It is likely that a series of genetic influences combine to explain approximately 60 percent of the proportion of risk for alcoholism, with environment responsible for the remaining proportion of the variance. Therefore, the divisions offered in this section are more heuristic than real, as it is the combination of a series of psychological, sociocultural, biological, and other factors that are responsible for the development of severe, repetitive alcohol-related life problems.

Psychological Theories A variety of theories relate to the use of alcohol to reduce tension, increase feelings of power, and decrease the effects of psychological pain. Perhaps the greatest interest has been paid to the observation that people with alcohol-related problems often report that alcohol decreases their feelings of nervousness and helps them cope with the day-to-day stresses of life. The psychological theories are built in part on the observation among nonalcoholic people that the intake of low doses of alcohol in a tense social setting or after a difficult day can be associated with an enhanced feeling of well-being and an improved ease of interactions. However, in high doses, especially at falling blood alcohol levels, most measures of muscle tension and psychological feelings of nervousness and tension are increased. Thus, tension-reducing effects of this drug might impact most on light to moderate drinkers or add to the relief of withdrawal symptoms but play a minor role in causing alcoholism. The theories that focus on alcohol's potential to enhance feelings of being powerful and sexually attractive and to decrease the effects of psychological pain are difficult to definitively evaluate.

Psychodynamic Theories Perhaps related to the disinhibiting or anxiety-lowering effects of lower doses of alcohol is the hypothesis that some people may use this drug to help them deal with self-punitive harsh superegos and to decrease unconscious stress levels. Also, classic psychoanalytical theory hypothesizes that at least some alcoholic people may have become fixated at the oral stage of development and use alcohol to relieve their frustrations by taking the substance by mouth. However, hypotheses regarding arrested phases of psychosexual development, although heuristically useful, have had little effect on the usual treatment approaches and are not the focus of extensive ongoing research. Similarly, most studies have not been able to document an "addictive personality" present in the majority of alcoholics and associated with a propensity to lack control of intake of a wide range of substances and foods. Although pathological scores on personality tests are often seen during intoxication, withdrawal, and early recovery, many of these characteristics are not found to predate alcoholism, and most disappear with abstinence. Similarly, prospective studies of children of alcoholics who themselves have no cooccurring disorders usually document high risks mostly for alcoholism. As described below, one partial exception to these comments occurs with the extreme levels of impulsivity seen in the 15 to 20 percent of alcoholic men with antisocial personality disorder, as these people have high risks for criminality, violence, and multiple substance dependencies.

Behavioral Theories Expectations about the rewarding effects of drinking, cognitive attitudes toward responsibility for one's behavior, and subsequent reinforcement after alcohol intake all contribute to the decision to drink again after the first experience with alcohol and to continue to imbibe despite problems. These issues are important in efforts to modify drinking behaviors in the general population, and they contribute to some important aspects of alcoholic rehabilitation.

Sociocultural Theories Sociocultural theories are often based on extrapolations from social groups that have high and low rates of alcoholism. Theorists hypothesize that ethnic groups, such as Jews, who introduce children to modest levels of drinking in a family atmosphere and eschew drunkenness have low rates of alcoholism. Some other groups, such as Irish men or some American Indian tribes with high rates of abstention but a tradition of drinking to the point of drunkenness among drinkers, are believed to have high rates of alcoholism. However, these theories often depend on stereotypes that tend to be erroneous, and there are prominent exceptions to these rules. For example, some theories based on observations of the Irish and the French have incorrectly predicted high rates of alcoholism among the Italians.

Yet, environmental events, presumably including cultural factors, account for as much as 40 percent of the alcoholism risk. Thus, although these are difficult to study, it is likely that cultural attitudes toward drinking, drunkenness, and personal responsibility for consequences are important contributors to the rates of alcohol-related problems in a society. In the final analysis, social and psychological theories are probably highly relevant, as they outline factors that contribute to the onset of drinking, the development of temporary alcohol-related life difficulties, and even alcoholism. The problem is how to gather relatively definitive data to support or refute the theories.

Background on Biological Contributors Although more than one-half of the proportion of risk for alcohol use disorders is explained by genes, it is likely that these represent a number of characteristics that, independently, increase or decrease the alcoholism risk. Furthermore, as is true of most genetically influenced traits, it appears as if multiple genes contribute to most of these characteristics. To give a parallel from medicine, it is likely that early-onset myocardial infarctions are genetically influenced, but some families might carry their risk through genes that relate to high blood pressure; in other families, the heightened risk might be mediated through genes causing high triglycerides; and yet others might develop early-onset heart disease related to inherited forms of cardiomyopathy. Therefore, it is not likely that any one gene causes early-onset heart attacks, and it is probable that early cardiac death reflects different biological causes in different families. Furthermore, the enhanced risk through any of these mechanisms is likely to be moderated by the type of diet, the amount of exercise, and additional influences such as smoking history. The following sections highlight data that support the importance of genetic influences in alcoholism overall and describe the possible biological mediators of the risk (Table 11.2–2).

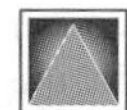

Table 11.2–2
Data Supporting Genetic Influences in Alcoholism

Close family members have a fourfold increased risk.
The identical twin of an alcoholic person is at higher risk than is a fraternal twin.
Adopted-away children of alcoholic people have a fourfold increased risk.

Importance of Genetic Influences Four lines of evidence support the conclusion that alcoholism is genetically influenced. First, there is a three- to fourfold increased risk for severe alcohol problems in close relatives of alcoholic people. The rate of alcohol problems increases with the number of alcoholic relatives, the severity of their illness, and the closeness of their genetic relationship to the person under study. The family investigations do little to separate the importance of genetics and environment, and the second approach, twin studies, takes the data a step further. The rate of similarity, or concordance, for severe alcohol-related problems is significantly higher in identical twins of alcoholic individuals than in fraternal twins in most investigations, which estimate that genes explain 60 percent of the variance, with the remainder relating to nonshared, probably adult environmental influences. Third, the adoption-type studies have all revealed a significantly enhanced risk for alcoholism in the offspring of alcoholic parents, even when the children had been separated from their biological parents close to birth and raised without any knowledge of the problems within the biological family. The risk for severe alcohol-related difficulties is not further enhanced by being raised by an alcoholic adoptive family. Finally, studies in animals support the importance of a variety of yet-to-be-identified genes in the free-choice use of alcohol, subsequent levels of intoxication, and in some consequences.

Possible Biological Mediators of the Alcoholism Risk There appears to be a series of independent characteristics that impact the alcoholism risk. First, as discussed earlier, genes on chromosome 12 that control ALDH and those on chromosome 4 that relate to ADH can decrease the alcoholism risk. The most relevant isoenzyme is the low Km ALDH2 located in the mitochondria of cells, and the gene responsible for the ALDH2*2 polymorphism is seen in approximately 50 percent of Japanese, Chinese, and Korean individuals. If a person carrying this gene is an ALDH2*2, 2*2 homozygote, they have inherited a disulfiram (or Antabuse)–like aversive reaction to alcohol because they cannot metabolize low to moderate levels of acetaldehyde and have almost no alcoholism risk. Heterozygotes (e.g., with ALDH2*2, 2*1 alleles) have a mild to modest facial flush, enhanced heart rate, and a moderately more intense (although not more aversive) response to alcohol. It has been hypothesized that the higher response may contribute to a significant decreased risk for alcohol use disorders, although the level of protection is much less for that seen for homozygotes. However, if a person with this heterozygous genotype does develop alcohol dependence, he or she may carry higher risks for damage to the brain, liver, pancreas, and testes, perhaps as a consequence of higher acetaldehyde levels when they drink. In addition, genes that impact on ADH2 and ADH3, which are more prevalent among Asian, black, and Jewish individuals, might be responsible for a slight increase in the rapidity of breakdown of alcohol, with a possible modest increase in acetaldehyde. This has been hypothesized to have a relatively small protective effect against alcohol use disorders, perhaps through enhancing the level of response to alcohol.

A second potentially important genetically influenced mechanism appears to relate to genes that impact on impulsivity, sensation seeking, and disinhibition. Studies using personality profiles and investigations incorporating electrophysiological measures of disinhibition both report that these characteristics are seen at a higher-than-expected prevalence among alcoholics, are observed in a substantial minority of children of alcohol-dependent individuals, and are strongly related to yet-to-be-identified genes. These findings might reflect the fact that more impulsive or disinhibited individuals, who, at the extreme, have the antisocial personality disorder, are both more likely to drink and less likely to demonstrate self-control when under the influence of alcohol. Consistent with this hypothesis is the fact that this type of predisposition toward substance-related disorders extends to all substances of abuse. An alternative hypothesis is that alcohol or other drugs have specific brain effects that ameliorate some of the consequences of the biological aspects of the disinhibition.

A third genetically influenced mechanism that appears to contribute to the alcoholism risk might operate through genes that enhance the vulnerability to several additional psychiatric disorders. In addition to antisocial personality disorder, two genetically influenced psychiatric disorders most closely tied to a subsequent vulnerability toward substance use disorders in general, including alcoholism, are schizophrenia and manic-depressive disease. Some investigators hypothesize that the enhanced risk for substance-related problems in these individuals is a consequence of the poor judgment that can be seen in both of these major psychiatric disorders and the hyperimpulsive state in mania. Others believe that the link between substance use disorders and these serious psychiatric conditions might reflect an overlap of genes responsible for the predisposition toward substance-related problems and those that impact on schizophrenia and bipolar disorder. Of course, it is possible that some of the relationship might occur as an individual attempts to moderate his or her psychiatric symptoms or the side effects of medications.

An additional genetically influenced characteristic impacting on the alcoholism risk involves the intensity of a person's reaction to alcohol. An ongoing study of 453 sons of alcoholics and controls, as well as their spouses and offspring, offers some relevant information. When the original subjects were evaluated at approximately 20 years of age, despite matching the two family history groups on drug use and drinking histories, at identical blood alcohol concentrations, 40 percent of the sons of alcoholics but fewer than 10 percent of the controls showed remarkably low levels of response to alcohol (i.e., they required relatively high alcohol levels for effects). The intensity of the reaction was measured by a combination of subjective feelings of intoxication, changes in motor performance while under the influence of alcohol, and alcohol-induced changes in blood hormones and electrophysiological functioning of the brain. An average of approximately 10 years later, all 453 subjects were located, and information about functioning during the follow-up period was obtained from the subject and an additional informant for 450 individuals (99.3 percent). A subsequent evaluation was carried out with 98 percent of the subjects approximately 5 years after that. At each time point, the low level of response to alcohol at approximately 20 years of age was a potent predictor of future alcoholism, with 60 percent of the sons of alcoholics who had a low response developing alcoholism by approximately 30 years of age, whereas the same was true for only 15 percent of the sons of alcoholics who showed high levels of response to the alcohol challenge.

Investigations are now under way to find specific genes that contribute to the low response to alcohol as a risk factor for alcohol use disorders, with promising findings from both candidate gene and genome scan investigations. At the same time, data are being gathered on both the original subjects and their more than 400 offspring aimed at identifying environmental factors that might operate to either enhance the alcoholism risk in the presence of a low response to alcohol or, even more important, confer resilience. Members of both generations are being followed over time.

DIAGNOSIS AND CLINICAL FEATURES

Alcohol use disorders are among the most common of the serious life-threatening behavioral or psychiatric syndromes, and the diagnosis of alcohol dependence or abuse requires a high index of suspicion for the disorder in any patient. The average man or woman presenting with severe and repetitive alcohol problems is likely to be neatly dressed, to show no signs of severe alcohol withdrawal, to have a job and a family, and to complain of a variety of physical conditions or temporary but potentially severe psychiatric complaints. Thus, the clinician must gather a history of alcohol-related life problems from the patient and, whenever possible, a resource person and must try to determine whether alcohol has caused or contributed to the psychiatric or physiological syndrome. Table 11.2–3 lists the alcohol-related disorders in DSM-IV-TR and also presents a comparable listing from ICD-10.

This section offers an overview of clinical characteristics and diagnostic criteria for a wide range of phenomena relevant to alcohol use disorders, beginning with a brief overview of comorbid psychiatric symptoms and clinically relevant thoughts on how to approach them. The section then progresses to a discussion of more general relevant diagnostic criteria, including alcohol dependence, abuse, and so on.

Diagnosing Substance-Induced Conditions

For men and women presenting with psychiatric symptoms (e.g., anxiety, depression, or psychoses) as well as evidence of alcohol-related problems, the first step is to obtain a careful history from both the patient and a resource person. Second, the clinician must emphasize syndromes that meet diagnostic criteria for major depressive disorder or full anxiety syndromes or other disorders, not just symptoms such as sadness or nervousness. Third, a timeline of relevant events from childhood to the present should be established noting (1) the approximate age of onset of alcohol problems severe and repetitive enough to justify a diagnosis of alcohol dependence (note: this is not the age of first drink or first sign of difficulty), (2) periods of abstinence of several months or more, and (3) the ages at which the patient met the criteria for any major psychiatric disorders, taking care to emphasize full-blown psychiatric clinical conditions, not isolated symptoms. If a review of the timeline reveals no evidence that the additional psychiatric syndromes either clearly antedated the severe alcohol problems or persisted for 4 or more weeks during a period of abstinence, alcoholism is the major disorder. The other psychiatric syndromes are likely to be important but temporary conditions that occurred during alcohol intoxication or withdrawal (i.e., are alcohol induced).

Depressive, anxiety, and psychotic symptoms are often seen in people with alcohol-related disorders. However, even if the psychiat-

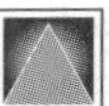

Table 11.2–3
DSM-IV-TR Alcohol-Related Disorders and Corresponding ICD-10 Disorders

DSM-IV-TR	ICD-10 Corollary
Alcohol use disorders	
Alcohol dependence	**Alcohol dependence syndrome**
Alcohol abuse	**Alcohol harmful use**
Alcohol-induced disorders	
Alcohol intoxication	**Acute intoxication due to use of alcohol**
	Uncomplicated
	With trauma or other bodily injury
	With other medical complications
Alcohol intoxication delirium	With delirium
	With perceptual distortions
	With coma
	With convulsions
No DSM-IV-TR equivalent	Pathological intoxication
Alcohol withdrawal	**Alcohol withdrawal state**
Specify if: with perceptual disturbances	Uncomplicated
	With convulsions
Alcohol withdrawal delirium	**Alcohol withdrawal state with delirium**
	Without convulsions
	With convulsions
Alcohol-induced persisting dementia	**Residual and late-onset psychotic disorder**
	Dementia
Alcohol-induced persisting amnestic disorder	**Amnesic syndrome**
Alcohol-induced psychotic disorder, with delusions	**Psychotic disorder**
Specify if: with onset during intoxication/with onset during withdrawal	Schizophrenia-like
	Predominantly delusional
	Predominantly hallucinatory
	Predominantly polymorphic
	Predominantly depressive symptoms[a]
	Predominantly manic symptoms[a]
	Mixed
	or
Alcohol-induced psychotic disorder, with hallucinations	**Residual and late-onset psychotic disorder**
	Late-onset psychotic disorder[a]
Specify if: with onset during intoxication/with onset during withdrawal	or
	Organic delusional (schizophrenia-like) disorder[b]
	or
	Organic hallucinosis[b]
Alcohol-induced mood disorder	**Organic mood (affective) disorder**[a]
Specify if: with onset during intoxication/with onset during withdrawal	or
	Residual and late-onset psychotic disorder
	Residual affective disorder
Alcohol-induced anxiety disorder	**Organic anxiety disorder**[b]
Specify if: with onset during intoxication/with onset during withdrawal	
Alcohol-induced sexual dysfunction	—
Specify if: with onset during intoxication	
Alcohol-induced sleep disorder	—
Specify if: with onset during intoxication/with onset during withdrawal	
Alcohol-related disorder not otherwise specified	**Other mental or behavioral disorder induced by alcohol**[c]
	Unspecified mental or behavioral disorder induced by alcohol

[a]These syndromes are only roughly similar in the two systems.
[b]These ICD-10 diagnoses are found in the section on organic mental disorders.
[c]Includes alcohol sexual dysfunction and alcohol sleep disorder.

ric symptoms are intense, they do not indicate a separate psychiatric syndrome when seen only during intoxication or withdrawal. In an effort to encourage clinicians and researchers to consider the entire span of clinical conditions that might be relevant to any syndrome being observed, in DSM-IV-TR, all important diagnostic entities related to a specific phenomenon (e.g., depressive disorders, anxiety disorders, psychotic disorders) are now listed within the clinically relevant sections (e.g., the mood disorder section). For the sake of clarity, conditions associated with substances are now labeled as *substance-induced disorders.*

To be termed as *substance induced*, the syndrome must be clinically meaningful and should resemble the type of disorder described within that DSM-IV-TR section (e.g., a mood disorder). There must be evidence that the clinical condition developed during, or soon after, intoxication or withdrawal from a substance (such as alcohol) that is capable of producing a relevant temporary clinical condition (such as a severe mood disturbance). The clinician and researcher are warned that the substance-induced syndrome should only be diagnosed when the psychiatric symptoms (e.g., depression) are in excess of those usually associated with intoxication or withdrawal. The diagnostic criteria further list the specific substances involved and ask that, if possible, the clinician specify whether the condition had an onset during intoxication or withdrawal. These latter modifiers are important to indicate to the clinician when additional medical and psychiatric treatment might be required. For alcohol-induced mood disorders, diagnoses can also be subtyped regarding the presence or absence of depressive, manic, or mixed features. Anxiety conditions can be further subdivided regarding the relevance of generalized anxiety symptoms, repetitive panic attacks, obsessive-compulsive symptoms, or phobic symptoms.

Hallucinations and delusions associated with intoxication or withdrawal from relevant substances are covered in the DSM-IV-TR section on psychotic disorders. When the condition is clinically relevant and when evidence exists that a substance (such as alcohol) capable of causing the psychotic symptoms is involved, a diagnosis of a substance-induced psychotic disorder (in this instance, alcohol-induced psychotic disorder) can be made. Additional criteria have been developed for alcohol-induced sexual dysfunction (Table 18.1a–20) and alcohol-induced sleep disorders.

Alcohol Dependence DSM-IV-TR provides general criteria for all substance use disorders (Table 11.1–3). These are stated in broad terms to be applied to all substances of abuse and to be flexible enough to guide the clinician's diagnoses of people from diverse cultures, both genders, and different age groups. Dependence concerns a history of an array of problems, including compulsive intake of alcohol, an increasingly important place in life occupied by the substance, and possibly evidence of physical withdrawal symptoms. Dependence criteria also concern life impairment related to the substance.

Physical dependence is a phenomenon that overlaps greatly with tolerance. As the body changes to resist the effects of alcohol, it is likely to reach a condition in which it cannot function optimally unless the brain depressant is present and in which rebound or withdrawal symptoms develop if the depressant drug is stopped quickly.

DSM-IV-TR substance dependence criteria include seven items that are subsets of the nine originally listed in DSM-III-R. These seven items are similar to the ICD-10 dependence syndrome criteria, although ICD-10 deals more directly with evidence of a compulsion to use (Table 11.1–4). In addition, although maintaining the broad concept of dependence that appeared in DSM-III-R, DSM-IV-TR asks the clinician to use the two items that deal with tolerance or withdrawal to further classify dependent people into those with and those without evidence of physiological symptoms. Recent data support the conclusion that a history of tolerance or withdrawal, especially the latter, is associated with a more severe course of alcoholism both by history and in the future.

A 39-year-old prominent businessman, Mr. G., was referred for evaluation by a clinician who was concerned that he was making little progress with the patient's mood swings and somatic complaints. Therapy, primarily using a cognitive and behavioral approach, had been instituted 6 months previously for a condition that involved depressive symptoms and irritability present most, but not all, days for the prior several years. Mr. G. had recently undergone a routine physical examination at work and was noted to have mild hypertension (blood pressure of 145/95) along with a blood test that revealed an MCV of 92.5 μm^3 and a γ-glutamyltransferase level of 43 U/L.

On interview, the patient admitted that his wife had been complaining for several years about his drinking pattern of one to two bottles of wine (i.e., 6 to 12 standard drinks) per day. She noted that the mornings after drinking he was more irritable than usual, and she complained about his restless sleep. Mr. G. had recognized potential problems and tried on several occasions to cut back on his drinking. These efforts usually resulted in periods of abstinence of between 2 and 4 weeks, followed by several months of establishing clear rules that set limits on his intake that always gave way to increased drinking as part of a celebration, business trip, vacation, or in the context of daily stresses. Mr. G. noted that once ad-lib drinking began, he slowly increased the amount consumed per day to maintain the desired effects. He denied ever experiencing full-blown alcohol withdrawal, although he did report "hangovers" lasting 6 to 12 hours but rarely going into the second day.

Alcohol Abuse The DSM-IV-TR diagnostic criteria for abuse focus on the impairment of social, legal, interpersonal, and occupational functioning in a person who is not alcohol dependent (Table 11.1–8). ICD-10 presents a diagnosis of *harmful use* that is only approximately similar to DSM-IV-TR, as the international system is limited to physical or psychological problems.

A categorical approach (e.g., abuse or dependence) has many benefits in clinical settings, including the relative ease of use while evaluating patients. However, almost by definition, there are some patients who report one or more of the dependence problems but who do not meet criteria for abuse. These men and women, sometimes referred to as *diagnostic orphans*, appear to have a clinical course that is distinct from both individuals with no alcohol-related problems and those with alcohol dependence. The patterns of problems both in the past and as established in 1- to 5-year follow-ups more closely resemble individuals with abuse, although only 10 percent of these "orphans" go on to meet criteria for abuse, and less than 5 percent go on to dependence. Future studies preparing for DSM-V-TR need to more carefully evaluate these individuals to determine whether their level of problems is significant enough to warrant altering the diagnostic system.

Alcohol Intoxication The DSM-IV-TR diagnostic criteria for alcohol intoxication are based on evidence of recent ingestion of ethanol, maladaptive behavior, and at least one of six possible physiological correlates of intoxication (Table 11.2–4). The ICD-10 criteria for acute alcohol intoxication are generally similar to DSM-IV-TR, listing seven physiological signs of intoxication, some of which, such as conjunctival injection, are not seen in DSM-IV-TR.

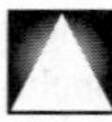

Table 11.2–4
DSM-IV-TR Diagnostic Criteria for Alcohol Intoxication

A. Recent ingestion of alcohol.
B. Clinically significant maladaptive behavior or psychological changes (e.g., inappropriate sexual or aggressive behavior, mood lability, impaired judgment, impaired social or occupational functioning) that developed during, or shortly after, alcohol ingestion.
C. One (or more) of the following signs, developing during, or shortly after, alcohol use:
 (1) Slurred speech
 (2) Incoordination
 (3) Unsteady gait
 (4) Nystagmus
 (5) Impairment in attention or memory
 (6) Stupor or coma
D. The symptoms are not due to a general medical condition and are not better accounted for by another mental disorder.

As a conservative approach to identifying blood levels that are likely to have major effects on driving abilities, the legal definition of intoxication in most states in the United States requires a blood concentration of 80 or 100 mg ethanol per dL of blood (mg/dL), which is the same as 0.08 to 0.10 g/dL. For most people, a rough estimate of the levels of impairment likely to be seen at various blood alcohol concentrations can be outlined. Evidence of behavioral changes, a slowing in motor performance, and a decrease in the ability to think clearly occurs at doses as low as 20 to 30 mg/dL, as shown in Table 11.2–5. Blood concentrations between 100 and 200 mg/dL are likely to produce a progression of the impairment in coordination and judgment to severe problems with coordination (ataxia), increasing lability of mood, and progressively greater levels of cognitive deterioration. Anyone who does not show significant levels of impairment in motor and mental performance at approximately 150 mg/dL probably has significant pharmacodynamic tolerance. In that range, most people without significant tolerance also experience relatively severe nausea and vomiting. With blood alcohol concentrations in the 200 to 300 mg/dL range, the slurring of speech is likely to become more intense, and memory impairment (*anterograde amnesia* or *alcoholic blackouts*) becomes pronounced. Further increases in blood alcohol concentration result in the first level of anesthesia, and the nontolerant person who reaches 400 mg/dL or more risks respiratory failure, coma, and death.

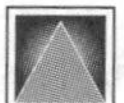

Table 11.2–5
Impairment Likely to be Seen at Different Blood Alcohol Concentrations

Level	Likely Impairment
20–30 mg/dL	Slowed motor performance and decreased thinking ability
30–80 mg/dL	Increases in motor and cognitive problems
80–200 mg/dL	Increases in incoordination and judgment errors
	Mood lability
	Deterioration in cognition
200–300 mg/dL	Nystagmus, marked slurring of speech, and alcoholic blackouts
>300 mg/dL	Impaired vital signs and possible death

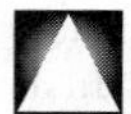

Table 11.2–6
DSM-IV-TR Diagnostic Criteria for Alcohol Withdrawal

A. Cessation of (or reduction in) alcohol use that has been heavy and prolonged.
B. Two (or more) of the following, developing within several hours to a few days after Criterion A:
 (1) Autonomic hyperactivity (e.g., sweating or pulse rate greater than 100)
 (2) Increased hand tremor
 (3) Insomnia
 (4) Nausea or vomiting
 (5) Transient visual, tactile, or auditory hallucinations or illusions
 (6) Psychomotor agitation
 (7) Anxiety
 (8) Grand mal seizures
C. The symptoms in Criterion B cause clinically significant distress or impairment in social, occupational, or other important areas of functioning.
D. The symptoms are not due to a general medical condition and are not better accounted for by another mental disorder.

Specify if:
 With perceptual disturbances

Alcohol Withdrawal

In people who have been drinking heavily over a prolonged period, a rapid decrease in blood alcohol levels might produce a variety of physical symptoms. Typical of brain depressants, including barbiturates and benzodiazepines, this *withdrawal* or *abstinence syndrome* is characterized by a group of symptoms that are the opposite of what was initially experienced with intoxication. These include a coarse tremor of the hands, insomnia, anxiety, and increased blood pressure, heart rate, body temperature, and respiratory rate—a condition labeled in DSM-IV-TR as *alcohol withdrawal* and described in Table 11.2–6. In ICD-10, the criteria for alcohol withdrawal are similar to those listed in DSM-IV-TR, with some differences in the specific items listed and the number of signs required (i.e., three) to make a diagnosis. The DSM-IV-TR criteria for alcohol withdrawal also require that the symptoms must cause clinically significant distress or impairment. Although 95 percent or more of withdrawals are limited to these mild or moderate symptoms, for 3 to 5 percent, the symptoms include convulsions or delirium.

Withdrawal phenomena are likely to begin within approximately 8 hours of abstinence, reach a peak intensity on the second or third day, and markedly diminish by the fourth or fifth day. The symptoms persist in a more mild form for as many as 3 to 6 months or more as part of a protracted withdrawal syndrome, which might contribute to relapse.

Mr. T. is a 64-year-old lawyer with a 35-year history of alcohol dependence. Alcohol-related problems have included tolerance, spending a great deal of time using alcohol (despite a relatively successful career), repeatedly giving up important business and family events because he was too intoxicated or hung over, and significant interference with his relationship with his wife. She complained about his sarcastic wit and lack of care about her areas of interest while drinking heavily.

Mr. T. had been able to stop drinking on multiple occasions in the past, at which times he experienced a tremor, anxiety, and problems sleeping. He typically self-medicated these symptoms with five or more 10-mg capsules of chlordiazepoxide per day, using pills that had been prescribed for him by his general practitioner in response to his complaints of anxiety and insomnia. Recently, Mr. T. was diagnosed with moderate hypertension and adult-onset diabetes, with the result that his family practitioner urged him to stop drinking. In recognition of his age and his associated medical problems, it was believed that withdrawal would be best treated in a medical setting.

An examination confirmed the medical diagnoses along with a mildly decreased hematocrit (38 percent). The evaluation, carried out approximately 12 hours after his most recent drink, also revealed the smell of alcohol remaining on his breath, with a blood alcohol level of 50 mg/dL. The patient demonstrated a prominent tremor of both hands along with a pulse of 110 beats per minute, a respiratory rate of 25 breaths per minute, and a blood pressure of 150/96. Mr. T. complained of feeling agitated, noted that he felt very tired but was unable to sleep, but was otherwise alert and oriented.

Alcohol Withdrawal Delirium For the small proportion of intoxications and withdrawals that are accompanied by severe cognitive symptoms, both DSM-IV-TR and ICD-10 list criteria for *alcohol intoxication delirium* and *alcohol withdrawal delirium* (Tables 10.2–2 and 10.2–3). When this agitated confusion is associated with tactile or visual hallucinations, the diagnosis of alcohol withdrawal delirium (also called *delirium tremens*) can be made. During withdrawal, some alcoholic people show one or several grand mal convulsions, sometimes called *rum fits.*

A 73-year-old professor emeritus at a university was believed to be in good health when he entered the hospital for an elective hernia repair. Perhaps reflecting his status in the community, the relatively brief history contained no detailed notes of his drinking pattern and made no mention of his γ-glutamyltransferase value of 55 U/L along with the MCV of 93.5 μm^3. Eight hours postsurgery, the nursing staff noted a sharp increase in the pulse rate to 110, an increase in blood pressure to 150/100, prominent diaphoresis, and a tremor to both hands, after which the patient demonstrated a brief but intense grand mal convulsion. He awoke extremely agitated and disoriented to time, place, and person. A reevaluation of the history and an interview with the wife documented alcohol dependence with a consumption of approximately six standard drinks per night. Over the following 4 days, the patient's autonomic nervous system dysfunction decreased as his cognitive impairment disappeared. His condition is classified as alcohol withdrawal delirium in DSM-IV-TR.

Alcohol-Induced Persisting Amnestic Disorder One of the most intensely studied alcohol-related CNS syndromes is the rare DSM-IV-TR diagnosis of *alcohol-induced persisting amnestic disorder* (Table 10.4–2), which is the result of a relatively severe deficiency in the B vitamin thiamine. Similar criteria are offered in ICD-10 as an amnesic syndrome. As mentioned briefly earlier in the section on effects of alcohol on the body, some people are at higher risk for this syndrome than are others because of a genetically influenced transketolase deficiency. The condition has been historically subdivided into (1) Wernicke's encephalopathy, with prominent ataxia and palsy of the sixth cranial nerve, a condition that tends to reverse fairly rapidly with vitamin supplementation; and (2) Korsakoff's syndrome, which is permanent in at least a partial form in perhaps 50 to 70 percent of the people affected. Korsakoff's syndrome is characterized by a pronounced anterograde and retrograde amnesia and potential impairment in visuospatial, abstract, and other types of learning. In most cases, the level of recent memory is out of proportion to the global level of cognitive impairment. The 25 percent or so of patients with Korsakoff's syndrome who are likely to recover fully and the 50 percent or so who recover partially appear to respond to 50 to 100 mg of oral thiamine a day, usually administered for many months.

Alcohol-Induced Persisting Dementia A poorly studied, heterogeneous long-term cognitive problem that can develop in the course of alcoholism is *alcohol-induced persisting dementia.* Similar syndromes are described in ICD-10 as *residual and late-onset psychotic disorder* or as *other persisting cognitive impairment.* Global decreases in intellectual functioning, cognitive abilities, and memory are observed, but recent memory difficulties are consistent with the global cognitive impairment, an observation that helps to distinguish the syndrome from alcohol-induced persisting amnestic disorder. Brain functioning tends to improve with abstinence, but perhaps one-half of all affected patients have long-term and even permanent memory and thinking disabilities. Perhaps 50 to 70 percent of these patients evidence increased size of the brain ventricles and shrinkage of the cerebral sulci, although these changes appear to be partially or completely reversible during the first year of complete abstinence.

Alcohol-Induced Conditions Reflecting the emphasis on understanding alcohol use disorders in psychiatric practice, this is an appropriate place to return to specific comorbid psychiatric conditions. Of course, individuals with alcohol use disorders have at least the same rate of most psychiatric conditions as do others in the general population and have an elevated risk for associated independent schizophrenia, manic-depressive disease, and, possibly, several of the anxiety disorders. Even more prevalent are the temporary, but potentially severe, substance-induced disorders that are distinguished from independent psychiatric conditions using the timeline method described previously. This section presents the criteria and clinical examples of some of the more common alcohol-induced conditions.

Alcohol-Induced Mood Disorder In the context of heavy and repetitive intake of any brain depressant, symptoms of severe depression are common and may be labeled as an *alcohol-induced mood disorder* (Table 13.6–18). Like DSM-III-R, ICD-10 retains this and most related substance-induced syndromes in the section on organic mental disorders labeled as an *organic mood [affective] disorder.* For long-lasting mood disturbances, ICD-10 also has the labels of *other persistent mood [affective] disorders* and *persistent mood [affective] disorder.* The diagnosis in DSM-IV-TR or ICD-10 focuses on either sadness or mania-like symptoms severe enough to impair functioning that occur only in the context of repeated heavy drinking and continue for several days to 4 weeks after abstinence.

Heavy intake of alcohol over several days results in many of the symptoms observed in major depressive disorder, but the intense sadness markedly improves within days to 1 month of abstinence. Eighty percent of alcoholic people report histories of intense depression, including 30 to 40 percent who were depressed for 2 or more weeks at a time. However, when information from patients and resource people was carefully evaluated, only 5 percent of alcoholic men and 10 percent of alcoholic women ever had depressions that met the criteria for major depressive disorder when they had not been drinking heavily.

Clinical data reveal that when even severe depression develops in alcoholic people, they are likely to improve fairly rapidly without medications or intensive psychotherapy aimed at the depressive symptoms. A recent study of almost 200 alcoholic men found that, although 40 percent had severe levels of depression after 1 week of abstinence, these symptoms markedly improved in all but 5 percent after 3 additional weeks of sobriety. At the end of several weeks to 1 month, most alcoholic patients are left with mood swings or intermittent symptoms of sadness that can resemble cyclothymic disorder or dysthymic disorder.

A consultation was requested on a 42-year-old woman with alcohol dependence who complained of persisting severe depressive symptoms despite 5 days of abstinence. In the initial stage of the interview, she noted that she had "always been depressed" and believed that she "drank to cope with the depressive symptoms." Her current complaint included a prominent sadness that had persisted for several weeks, difficulties concentrating, initial and terminal insomnia, and a feeling of hopelessness and guilt. In an effort to distinguish between an alcohol-induced mood disorder and an independent major depressive episode, a timeline-based history was obtained. This focused on the age of onset of DSM-IV-TR alcohol dependence, periods of abstinence that extended for several months or more since the onset of dependence, and the ages of occurrence of clear major depressive episodes lasting several weeks or more at a time. Despite this patient's original complaints, it became clear that there had been no major depressive episodes before her mid-20s when alcohol dependence began and that during a 1-year period of abstinence related to the gestation and neonatal period of the birth of her son, her mood had significantly improved. A provisional diagnosis of an alcohol-induced mood disorder was made. The patient was offered education, reassurance, and cognitive therapy to help her to deal with the depressive symptoms, but no antidepressant medications were prescribed. The depressive symptoms remained at their original intensity for several additional days and then began to improve. By approximately 3 weeks' abstinence, the patient no longer met criteria for a major depressive episode, although she demonstrated mood swings similar to dysphemia for several additional weeks. This case is a fairly typical example of an alcohol-induced mood disorder in an individual with alcohol dependence.

Alcohol-Induced Anxiety Disorder Anxiety symptoms fulfilling the diagnostic criteria for *alcohol-induced anxiety disorder* are also common in the context of acute and protracted alcohol withdrawal. In ICD-10, these are listed as organic anxiety disorders resembling generalized anxiety or panic disorders. Almost 80 percent of alcoholic people report panic attacks during acute withdrawal; their complaints can be intense enough for the clinician to consider diagnosing a panic disorder. Similarly, during the first 4 to 6 weeks of abstinence, people with severe alcohol problems are likely to avoid some social situations for fear of being overwhelmed by anxiety (i.e., they have symptoms resembling social phobia); their problems can at times be severe enough to resemble agoraphobia. However, when psychological or physiological symptoms of anxiety are observed in alcoholic people only in the context of heavy drinking or within the first several weeks or months of abstinence, the symptoms are likely to diminish and subsequently disappear with time alone. Only two anxiety disorders may be more closely tied to alcoholism: panic disorder and social phobia.

A 48-year-old woman was referred for evaluation and treatment of her recent onset of panic attacks. These episodes occurred two to three times per week over the past 6 months, with each lasting typically between 10 and 20 minutes. Panic symptoms occurred regardless of levels of life stress and could not be explained by current medications or medical conditions. The workup included an evaluation of her laboratory test values, which revealed a carbohydrate-deficient transferrin (CDT) level of 28 U/L, a uric acid level of 7.1 mg, and a γ-glutamyltransferase value of 47. All other blood tests were within normal limits.

The atypical age of onset of the panic attacks, along with the blood results, encouraged the clinician to probe further regarding the pattern of alcohol-related life problems with both the patient and, separately, her spouse. This step documented a history of alcohol dependence with an onset at approximately 35 years of age, with no evidence of panic disorder before that date. Nor did the patient have repetitive panic attacks beyond 2 weeks of abstinence during her frequent periods of nondrinking, which often lasted for 3 or 4 months. A working diagnosis of alcohol dependence with an alcohol-induced anxiety disorder characterized by panic attacks was made, and the patient was encouraged to abstain and was appropriately treated for possible withdrawal symptoms. Over the subsequent 3 weeks after a taper of benzodiazepines used for the treatment of withdrawal, the panic symptoms diminished in intensity and subsequently disappeared.

Alcohol-Induced Psychotic Disorder Approximately 3 percent of alcoholic people have auditory hallucinations or paranoid delusions in the context of heavy drinking and withdrawal. In DSM-III-R those problems are labeled *organic hallucinosis* or *delusional disorders.* In ICD-10, they are presented as organic delusional disorders in the organic section and as a psychotic disorder in the substance use disorders section. Many of the symptoms resemble those seen in schizophrenia, but when the psychotic features develop only in the context of alcohol problems, they are likely to clear spontaneously. The syndromes are likely to recur only if heavy alcohol intake resumes.

Alcohol-Related Disorder Not Otherwise Specified DSM-IV-TR allows for the diagnosis of *alcohol-related disorder not otherwise specified* for alcohol-related disorders that do not meet the diagnostic criteria for any of the other diagnoses (Table 11.2–7). ICD-10 offers the listings of *other* or *unspecified mental and behavioral disorders induced by alcohol.*

IDENTIFICATION IN CLINICAL SETTINGS

Establishing the diagnosis for alcohol abuse or dependence centers on obtaining from the patient and a resource person a history of the patient's life problems and the possible role played by alcohol. Up to one-third of all psychiatric patients are likely to have an alcohol problem that either caused or exacerbated the presenting clinical condition.

Prior sections of this chapter have given data about the high prevalence of alcohol use disorders and the appropriate diagnos-

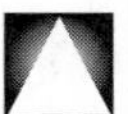

Table 11.2–7
DSM-IV-TR Diagnostic Criteria for Alcohol-Related Disorder Not Otherwise Specified

The alcohol-related disorder not otherwise specified category is for disorders associated with the use of alcohol that are not classifiable as alcohol dependence, alcohol abuse, alcohol intoxication, alcohol withdrawal, alcohol intoxication delirium, alcohol withdrawal delirium, alcohol-induced persisting dementia, alcohol-induced persisting amnestic disorder, alcohol-induced psychotic disorder, alcohol-induced mood disorder, alcohol-induced anxiety disorder, alcohol-induced sexual dysfunction, or alcohol-induced sleep disorder.

From American Psychiatric Association. *Diagnostic and Statistical Manual of Mental Disorders.* 4th ed. Text rev. Washington, DC: American Psychiatric Association; 2000, with permission.

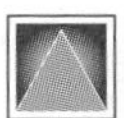

Table 11.2–8
State Markers of Heavy Drinking Useful in Screening for Alcoholism

Test	Relevant Range of Results
γ-Glutamyltransferase	>30.0 U/L
Carbohydrate-deficient transferrin	>20.0 mg/L
Mean corpuscular volume	>91.0 μm³
Uric acid	>6.4 mg/dL for men >5.0 mg/dL for women
Serum glutamic oxaloacetic transaminase (aspartate aminotransferase)	>45.0 IU/L
Serum glutamic pyruvic transaminase (alanine aminotransferase)	>45.0 IU/L
Triglycerides	>160.0 mg/dL

tic criteria. Using the information on the high prevalence, recognizing the importance of avoiding inappropriate stereotypes, and understanding the importance of substance-induced disorders combine to help the clinician identify the individual with alcohol abuse or dependence. In light of the emphasis on repetitive life problems in the relevant criteria, it is appropriate to screen all patients for life difficulties and to determine whether alcohol might have contributed to the picture. The absence of a focus on the quantity and frequency of alcohol intake in DSM-IV-TR reflects the variability in the amount of alcohol a person needs to cause repetitive problems at different ages, genders, percent body fat, associated medical conditions, and with additional medications or drugs.

Patients should be asked about patterns of problems related to accidents, interpersonal difficulties, problems at work, encounters with the law, and so on. When a problem is apparent, one can then determine the time of day, the situation, and the complaints voiced by others. If an alcohol use disorder appears probable, the diagnostic criteria can be reviewed along with a history of the quantity and frequency of alcohol intake.

Several relatively simple questionnaires can be used to preliminarily survey relevant problem areas. Two useful examples are the Alcohol Use Disorders Identification Test (AUDIT) and the Michigan Alcohol Screening Test (MAST), each of which offer a ten-item form that reviews the pattern of life problems related to alcohol. More simple instruments, such as the CAGE ([need to] *c*ut down [on drinking], *a*nnoyance, *g*uilt [about drinking], [need for] *e*ye-opener), are limited to four questions and might not be either sensitive or specific enough for many clinical settings. While the clinician may find the AUDIT or MAST useful, he or she must remember that the questionnaires do not diagnose alcohol dependence but only highlight individuals who might be especially appropriate for a more intensive clinical interview.

The process of identification can also be facilitated by the series of blood tests outlined in Table 11.2–8. These state markers of heavy drinking reflect physiological alterations likely to be observed if the patient regularly ingests four or more drinks a day over many days or weeks. One marker with a sensitivity and specificity of 60 to 80 percent is a level of 30 to 35 or more U/L of γ-glutamyltransferase, an enzyme that aids in the transport of amino acids. Because this enzyme is likely to return to normal levels after 2 to 4 weeks of abstinence, even 20 percent increases in values above those observed after 4 weeks of abstinence can be useful in identifying patients who have returned to drinking after treatment. Equally impressive results have been reported for the measure of a deglycosylated form of the protein transferrin, known as *CDT*. Using a commercially available assay, CDTect, and using a cutoff of 20 U/L, this test has a sensitivity and a specificity of 65 to 80 percent for the identification of the heavy consumption of alcohol (e.g., four to eight drinks per day for 1 week or more), although such figures might be slightly lower for women. With a biological half-life of approximately 16 days, this test can also be useful in monitoring abstinence in alcoholics. It appears that patients not identified by higher γ-glutamyltransferase values might still have elevations in CDT, so that both tests may be used for identification and abstinence-monitoring functions in alcoholics.

The MCV blood test, with perhaps 70 percent sensitivity and specificity, is useful when the size of the red blood cell is 91 μm³ or more. The 120-day life span of the red cell does not allow the test to be useful as an indicator of a return to drinking. Other tests that can be helpful in identifying patients who are regularly consuming heavy doses of alcohol include high normal values of uric acid (e.g., greater than 6.4 mg/dL), even mild elevations in the usual liver function tests, including aspartate aminotransferase and alanine aminotransferase, and elevated levels of triglycerides or LDL cholesterol.

A number of physical findings can also be useful. These include modest elevations in blood pressure; frequent bruising; cancer of the head, neck, and upper digestive tract; an enlarged liver; evidence of cirrhosis; and symptoms consistent with pancreatitis.

DIFFERENTIAL DIAGNOSIS

Once the pattern of alcohol-related life problems has been established, the diagnosis of alcohol abuse or dependence may be fairly obvious. A substantial proportion of the information presented in this chapter also helps the clinician to take the next logical step: determining whether an independent major psychiatric disorder exists. Briefly, individuals who present with clinically significant levels of depression, anxiety, or psychotic symptoms in addition to their alcoholism should be evaluated using the timeline approach to determine whether the psychiatric symptoms are likely to have been substance induced (and are thus temporary) or represent independent and longer-term psychiatric disorders. In addition, the clinical course of the psychiatric symptoms should be closely observed during the subsequent several weeks to 1 month or so of abstinence to determine whether the depression, anxiety, and other symptoms decrease in intensity over time. Although some symptoms might remain as part of a protracted withdrawal syndrome, if the disorder is substance induced, the individual should no longer fulfill criteria for the full diagnostic syndrome after 1 month or so of abstaining from alcohol.

Antisocial Personality Disorder

When the emphasis on the chronological development of symptoms is used, at least three diagnoses—*antisocial personality disorder*, *schizophrenia*, and *bipolar I disorder*—are likely to run a course independent of alcohol abuse or dependence and be true comorbid conditions. Antisocial personality disorder, listed on Axis II, begins early in life and has major effects on many aspects of life functioning. The diagnosis is based on evidence of severe antisocial behaviors in many areas beginning before the age of 15 years and continuing into adulthood. People with antisocial personality disorder are described as impulsive, frequently violent, highly likely to take risks, and unable to learn from their mistakes or to benefit from punishment. A person who carries these characteristics into adolescence, typically the time for experimentation with alcohol and drugs, can be expected to have difficulty controlling substance use. Thus, perhaps 80 percent or more of people with antisocial personality disorder are likely to develop severe alcohol problems in the course of their lives. A diagnosis of preexisting antisocial personality disorder with subsequent alcohol abuse or dependence indicates someone who is more likely than the average alcohol-dependent person to have severe coexisting drug problems, to be violent, to discontinue treatment prematurely, and to have a less-than-optimistic prognosis.

Debate continues on the optimal manner of viewing the cooccurrence of antisocial personality disorder and alcoholism, but most researchers agree that the personality disorder is a separate entity worthy of diagnosis. The genetic factors that increase the risk for antisocial personality disorder are likely to be separate from those that affect the development of alcoholism. In most treatment programs, perhaps 5 percent of alcoholic women and between 10 and 20 percent of alcoholic men have preexisting antisocial personality disorder. Other Axis II–type symptoms are often observed during intoxication and as part of the acute and protracted abstinence syndromes, but few have not been documented to predate the alcohol-related disorders. It is probably best to defer a diagnosis of most additional Axis II disorders until several months of abstinence have been observed unless the syndrome clearly antedated the alcohol use disorder.

Schizophrenia

A second disorder in which alcohol problems are more common than in the general population is schizophrenia. Characterized by what is usually a slow onset of paranoid delusions and auditory hallucinations in a clear sensorium and typically beginning in the mid-teens to the 20s, schizophrenia is likely to be severe, long lasting, and debilitating. Possibly because of a lack of long-term treatment facilities, people with schizophrenia are likely to live in inner-city areas and to spend a great deal of time on the streets. Perhaps because they use alcohol to decrease feelings of isolation or to self-medicate their symptoms, people with schizophrenia are more likely than those in the general population to go on to have severe alcohol-related life problems. Their alcohol intake is likely to undercut the effectiveness of antipsychotic medications, to increase mood swings and signs of psychoses, and to contribute to a downward course of schizophrenia that entails repeatedly revolving into and out of inpatient care. Because most alcohol treatment programs exclude actively psychotic patients, people with schizophrenia rarely appear in inpatient alcohol settings, but alcohol-related disorders are observed in 30 percent or so of schizophrenic people being treated in public mental health facilities.

> A 34-year-old unemployed, divorced white man entered treatment for alcohol dependence. His history revealed seven prior hospitalizations since the age of 23 years, with most discharge diagnoses including schizophrenia and some noting alcohol dependence. The patient was a poor historian, and no additional informants were available. However, the information from prior hospitalizations revealed that at the time of the initial inpatient stay the patient had experienced approximately 1 year of auditory hallucinations and paranoid delusions. During that time, he had not yet demonstrated severe enough problems related to alcohol or other drugs to fulfill criteria for dependence. Subsequently, a hospitalization at 28 years of age was followed by a 6-month stay in a recovery home during which the records indicated that there had been no alcohol or illicit drug use, despite which the patient continued to demonstrate auditory hallucinations and paranoid delusions without insight. The current hospitalization involved initiation of treatment of alcohol withdrawal while reevaluating and stabilizing the antipsychotic medications for this individual who demonstrated both alcohol dependence and an independent schizophrenia disorder.

Bipolar I Disorder

The third disorder in which severe alcohol problems are overrepresented is bipolar I disorder. In a manic episode, the patient is hyperexcited and impulsive, carries out most activities to excess, has poor judgment, and is likely to develop temporary alcohol problems. Although the severity of the manic symptoms usually precludes inpatient alcohol rehabilitation, alcohol-related difficulties must be evaluated in histories taken from people with manic features entering mental health facilities. However, bipolar II is difficult to evaluate in substance-dependent patients, as intoxication, withdrawal, and adjustment to frequent changes in living situations can easily mimic hypomania. This label should be reserved only for those with clear hypomanic episodes antedating the alcoholism.

Major Anxiety Disorders

Finally, there are data from recent studies that support a small but statistically significant association between independent (i.e., not alcohol induced) panic disorder and perhaps independent social phobia and alcohol dependence. One large investigation involved more than 3,000 personal interviews carried out across six centers in different parts of the United States. Although approximately 90 percent of alcohol-dependent men and women did not have an independent major anxiety disorder, and there was no evidence for a significant increased risk for most major anxiety disorders, the rates of independent panic disorder and independent social phobia were significantly higher than in controls.

Other Disorders

Debate in the literature continues about whether major depressive disorder, agoraphobia, obsessive-compulsive disorder (OCD), posttraumatic stress disorder (PTSD), and other major psychiatric diagnoses are overrepresented in the histories of alcoholic people. Several studies indicate that, when the timeline method is used and a history is obtained from multiple informants, little evidence is found for very high rates of most independent psychiatric disorders among alcoholic people other than the disorders noted above. Therefore, although the majority of alcoholic people have temporary psychiatric symptoms, they are not more likely than are people

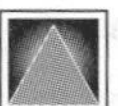

Table 11.2–9
Clinical Course of Alcohol Dependence

Age at first drink[a]	13–15 yrs
Age at first intoxication[a]	15–17 yrs
Age at first problem[a]	16–22 yrs
Age at onset of dependence	25–40 yrs
Age at death	60 yrs
Fluctuating course of abstention, temporary control, alcohol problems	—
Spontaneous remission in 20%	—

[a]Same as general population.

in the general population to carry an independent psychiatric syndrome other than the three exceptions discussed above.

Another condition worthy of comment is attention-deficit/hyperactivity disorder (ADHD). This disorder, usually diagnosed during childhood, involves learning problems, difficulties focusing attention, and, in many, problems sitting still and following through on tasks. Because these children can be disruptive in the home and school environments and reflecting the fact that many are treated with stimulant medications, such as methylphenidate (Ritalin), the question has been raised regarding the possibility that they might carry a heightened future risk for substance use disorders. Although this important issue is still the focus of active study, the data to date do not support a close tie between ADHD and alcohol use disorders or other substance-related problems in late adolescence or adulthood unless the child carries an additional risk factor, especially the precursor of antisocial personality disorder, conduct disorder.

Finally, there are interesting and complex relations between alcoholism and dependence on other drugs. Men and women with antisocial personality disorder demonstrate a marked increased risk for dependence on multiple substances, including alcohol. It is also probable that individuals with dependence on opioids and stimulants (such as cocaine and amphetamines) exhibit an increased risk for alcohol dependence, even in the absence of antisocial personality disorder. However, although, as is true for the general population, many have used other substances, most alcohol-dependent people do not meet the criteria for dependence on illicit drugs. Several recent investigations of children of alcohol-dependent men and women, as well as the large Collaborative Study on the Genetics of Alcoholism (COGA), indicated that, once the effects of antisocial personality disorder were controlled, alcohol dependence appeared to run relatively true within families, without evidence of a marked crossover between alcoholism and most other dependencies. An exception to this general rule is nicotine dependence, which has long been noted to be elevated among alcohol-dependent individuals, a finding that has been hypothesized to relate to either attempts to use nicotine to try to moderate some of the effects of high doses of alcohol or withdrawal or a possible genetic relationship between nicotine and alcohol dependence syndromes.

COURSE AND PROGNOSIS

Several recent large-scale evaluations suggest that most subgroups of alcoholics are more similar than different on the time course and prevalence of alcohol-related life difficulties. Thus, a recent comparison of alcoholic college graduates and those with only high school educations reported similar characteristics regarding most aspects of drinking patterns and many of the alcohol-related problems. The differences that do exist reflect characteristics of individuals in society in general and do not appear to indicate any unique aspects of their alcoholism. For example, as might be expected for women in the general population, compared with male alcoholics, female alcoholics have higher rates of independent depressive episodes, and slightly lower proportions of women have engaged in alcohol-related violence or have had severe alcohol-related driving problems. However, in general, the clinical courses of alcohol-dependent men and women are relatively similar. Older alcohol-dependent individuals are more likely to have medical problems, to take multiple medications, to experience more severe withdrawal syndromes, and have a less extensive social support system. Again, these characteristics reflect differences between older and younger individuals in general more than they indicate unique aspects of alcoholism in the geriatric population. Thus, although the reader is advised to take the following information as general guidelines that must be applied with common sense to subgroups of individuals, it is possible to present generalities regarding the usual clinical course of alcoholism and its treatment.

Early Course Patients with antisocial personality disorder who go on to develop alcoholism have an early onset of drinking, intoxication, and alcohol-related problems, but that scenario is not applicable to the other 80 to 90 percent of alcoholic men and 95 percent of alcoholic women. Usually, alcoholic people have their first drink (other than taking a sip from a parent's glass) between the ages of 13 and 15 years, the first intoxication is likely to occur at 15 or 16 years of age, and the first evidence of a minor alcohol-related problem is usually observed in the late teenage years. These milestones do not differ significantly from what is expected for people in the general population who do not later go on to develop alcohol abuse or dependence.

For the average person, the pattern of severe difficulties becomes apparent in the middle 20s to the middle 30s when a constellation of symptoms of relatively great severity is likely to be observed: an alcohol-related breakup of a significant relationship, a repeat alcohol-related driving or public intoxication arrest, evidence of alcohol withdrawal, being told by a physician that alcohol has harmed the person's health, or significant interference with functioning at school or work. This pattern probably does not vary much with the type of beverage used—beer, wine, or spirits.

The landmarks in Table 11.2–9 are only rough estimates and can differ greatly among people and various groups. Women, for example, are likely to begin drinking a bit later than men, but their subsequent escalation of symptoms is likely to be slightly more rapid.

Later Course Once alcohol's interference with life functioning has become apparent, unless the person permanently abstains, the future is likely to include periods of drinking problems that repeatedly alternate with periods of nondrinking and subsequent alcohol intake unassociated with problems (*temporary controlled drinking*). Abstinence often develops in response to some interpersonal, social, or legal crisis and is likely to produce only mild withdrawal symptoms. The usual alcoholic person is then likely to use the temporary cessation of drinking problems to convince themselves that alcohol is not really a cause for concern after all. Those periods of abstinence, lasting days to months, are usually followed by times during which drinking rules are established and are temporarily followed. The person is likely to consume only beer or wine (ignoring that a glass of beer, a glass of wine, and a shot of whiskey have similar amounts of alcohol) and tries to drink only at certain times of the day and under certain conditions. This period of temporary control soon leads to an escalation of alcohol intake, the accumulation of a new set of problems, and a subsequent crisis. These events, in turn, are likely to precipitate a new period of temporary abstinence, and the cycle begins again.

Thus, controlled drinking is a common but temporary condition for most alcoholic people. Those who have less severe alcohol problems, such as abuse, are probably more likely to have long-term and even permanent periods of control. However, several research projects have indicated that long-term continued control is not likely to be seen once a person meets the diagnostic criteria for alcohol dependence.

Recent follow-ups support the chronicity of the alcohol use disorders. An evaluation of approximately 1,500 subjects from primarily blue-collar families, as well as a similar follow-up of almost 450 higher functioning subjects, revealed that almost 70 percent of those with alcohol dependence continued to experience one or more of the 11 abuse or dependence criterion items during the subsequent 5 years, with highest risks for individuals who are not married, those with more severe problems at baseline, and subjects with concomitant histories of use of illicit drugs. More than one-half of the subjects with diagnoses of alcohol abuse continued their alcohol-related problems, although only 5 to 10 percent went on to dependence, as compared with approximately 3 percent of those with no alcohol use disorder at baseline.

An additional aspect of the clinical course of alcohol use disorders is worthy of mention. The lifetime risk for death by suicide may be as high as 8 to 10 percent among alcoholics, and a recent series of evaluations of more than 3,000 alcohol-dependent individuals reported that 16 percent had attempted suicide. A subsequent 5-year follow-up of a subset of this group revealed that 15 percent of those with prior attempts repeated their behavior during the interval, compared with a less than 3 percent suicide rate among those with no prior attempts. The risk for suicidal behavior among these alcohol-dependent men and women was higher for those who were younger, unmarried, had experience with illicit substances, reported a more severe course of their alcoholism, and had histories of substance-induced mood disorders.

Any discussion of the clinical course of alcoholism must include the phenomenon of spontaneous remission. Here, perhaps in response to nonspecific events or to a crisis, the alcoholic person promises to abstain and keeps the promise forever. Whatever the cause of the abstinence, approximately 20 percent or more of alcoholic people, if followed long enough, achieve permanent abstinence without formal treatment or participation in such self-help groups as Alcoholics Anonymous (AA). This outcome may be most likely for alcoholics with fewer alcohol-related problems, greater levels of life stability, and a more supportive environment.

However, if drinking continues, the alcoholic is likely to decrease his or her life span by 10 to 15 years as a result of many causes, including the marked increased risks for heart disease, cancer, accidents, and suicide among alcoholic individuals. The reasons for these enhanced mortality rates are likely to reflect the effects of alcohol described in this chapter.

Prognosis Between 10 and 40 percent of alcoholic people enter some form of treatment during the course of their alcohol problems. Although anyone might do well, there are a number of favorable prognostic signs. First is the absence of preexisting antisocial personality disorder or a diagnosis of other substance abuse or dependence. Second, evidence of general life stability with a job, continuing close family contacts, and the absence of severe legal problems also bodes well. Third, if the person stays for the full course of the initial rehabilitation (perhaps 2 to 4 weeks), the chances of maintaining abstinence are good. The combination of these three attributes predicts at least a 60 percent chance for 1 or more years of abstinence. Few studies have documented the long-term course, but researchers agree that 1-year rates are associated with a good chance for continued abstinence over an extended period.

In general, alcoholic people with preexisting independent major psychiatric disorders, such as antisocial personality disorder, schizophrenia, and bipolar I disorder, are likely to run the course of their independent psychiatric illness. Therefore, for example, clinicians must treat the patient with bipolar I disorder who has associated alcoholism with appropriate psychotherapy and lithium (Eskalith) or valproic acid (Depakene), use relevant psychological and behavioral techniques for the patient with antisocial personality disorder, and offer antipsychotic medications on a long-term basis to the patient with schizophrenia. The goal is to keep the symptoms of the independent psychiatric disorder as minimal as possible in the hope that a greater level of life stability is associated with a better prognosis for the patient's alcohol problems.

TREATMENT

The elements of treatment appropriate for patients with severe alcohol problems are fairly straightforward. The core of these efforts involves steps to maximize motivation for abstinence, helping alcoholics to restructure their lives without alcohol, and taking steps to minimize a return, or relapse, to substance-using behaviors. This cognitive and behavioral approach is similar to efforts appropriate for any long-term disorder that requires changes in lifestyles such as diabetes or hypertension. Much of the clinical challenge comes in recognizing how prevalent the alcohol-related disorders are, how often those conditions present with temporary symptoms of other psychiatric syndromes, and how to use clinical clues, physical findings, and laboratory tests to identify alcoholism.

Three general steps are involved in treating the alcoholic person once the disorder has been diagnosed: intervention, detoxification, and rehabilitation. Those approaches assume that all possible efforts have been made to optimize medical functioning and to address psychiatric emergencies. Thus, for example, the alcoholic person with symptoms of depression severe enough to be suicidal requires inpatient hospitalization for at least several days until the suicidal ideation disappears, even if it is a temporary alcohol-induced mood disorder. Similarly, the person presenting with cardiomyopathy, liver difficulties, or GI bleeding first needs adequate attention paid to the medical emergency.

The patient with alcohol abuse or dependence must then be brought face to face with the reality of the disorder (*intervention*), be detoxified if needed, and begin rehabilitation. The essentials of these three steps for alcoholic people with and without independent psychiatric syndromes are quite similar. However, in the former case, the treatments are often applied after the psychiatric disorder has been stabilized to the maximum degree possible.

Intervention The goal in this step is to break through feelings of denial and to help the patient recognize the adverse consequences likely to occur if the disorder is not treated. Intervention is a process aimed at increasing to as high a level as possible the levels of motivation for treatment and for continued abstinence.

This procedure often involves convincing patients that they are responsible for their own actions while reminding them how alcohol has created significant life impairments. The psychiatrist often finds it useful to take advantage of the person's chief presenting complaint, whether it is insomnia, difficulties with sexual performance, an inability to cope with life stresses, depression, anxiety, or psychotic symptoms. The emphasis is then placed in teaching the patient how alcohol has either created or contributed to these problems and reassuring the patient that abstinence can be achieved with a minimum of discomfort.

A physician was consulted by a 43-year-old businessman who was concerned about his wife. He had recently been confronted by their 21-year-old daughter who believed that her mother was an alcoholic. The daughter noted her mother's slurred speech on several recent occasions when the daughter called home and times during the day when the mother was apparently home but did not answer the telephone, and she observed high levels of alcohol consumption. A more detailed history revealed that, for at least the last 5 years, the husband had noted his spouse's practice of staying up after he went to bed, retiring later with alcohol on her breath. He also observed her consumption of up to 10 to 12 drinks at parties, with the resulting tendency to isolate herself from the remaining guests, her panic-like behavior regarding the need to pack liquor when they go on trips where alcohol might not be readily available, and a tremor of her hands some mornings during breakfast. The husband was given several potential courses of action, including the possibility of referring the spouse for treatment with the physician. He was advised to share his concern with his wife at a time when she was not actively intoxicated, emphasizing specific times and events when her impairment with alcohol was noted. He was also asked to consider whether a close friend of many years and the adult daughter might be included in this intervention, and it was suggested that a tentative appointment might be made with the clinician (or with an alcohol and drug treatment program) so that a next step could be established if the intervention was successful.

A physician intervening with a patient can use the same nonjudgmental but persistent approach each time an alcohol-related impairment is identified. It is the level of persistence rather than exceptional interpersonal skills that usually gets results. Most alcoholic people need a series of reminders of how alcohol contributes to each developing crisis before they seriously consider abstinence as a long-term option.

A more systematic approach to this process has been described as various forms of intervention that might fall under the heading of a brief intervention using motivational interviewing. Here, the clinician gains an alliance with the patient by demonstrating an understanding of his or her viewpoint while encouraging the individual to think through consequences associated with alcohol and the way that changing behaviors might produce benefits. During this process, it is important to recognize the patient's ambivalence toward abstinence and to show sensitivity in monitoring the person's readiness to change. Resistance on the part of the patient is best handled through discussion and problem solving rather than direct confrontation.

A recent report describes two 15-minute discussions between the clinician and patient along with a workbook that is used to review drinking problems and help the patient to understand how life cues contribute to the drinking pattern. Between the two visits, separated by approximately 1 month, the patient keeps notes of his or her usual drinking patterns. The second session is then followed by several short telephone interviews, and the process appears to have fairly promising levels of results, especially for individuals with lighter to moderate levels of alcohol problems.

Reaching out to the Family The family can be of great help in the intervention. Members must learn not to protect the patient from the problems caused by alcohol, or else the patient may not be able to generate the energy and the motivation necessary to stop drinking.

During the intervention stage, the family can suggest that the patient meet with people who are themselves recovering from alcoholism, perhaps through AA, and they themselves can attend groups, such as Al-Anon, that reach out to family members. Those support groups help family members and friends see that they are not alone in their fears, worry, and feelings of guilt. Members share coping strategies and help each other find community resources. The groups can be most useful in helping family members rebuild their lives, even if the alcoholic person refuses to seek help.

Detoxification

Most people with alcohol dependence have relatively mild symptoms when they stop drinking. If the patient is in relatively good health, adequately nourished, and has a good social support system, the depressant withdrawal syndrome usually resembles a mild case of the flu. Even intense withdrawal syndromes rarely approach the severity of symptoms described by some early textbooks.

The essential first step in detoxification is a thorough physical examination. In the absence of a serious medical disorder or combined drug dependence, severe alcohol withdrawal is unlikely. The second step is to offer rest, adequate nutrition, and multiple vitamins, especially those containing thiamine.

Mild or Moderate Withdrawal Withdrawal develops because the brain has physically adapted to the presence of a brain depressant and cannot function adequately in the absence of the drug. Giving enough of a brain depressant on the first day to diminish symptoms and then weaning the patient off the drug over the next 5 days offers most patients optimal relief and minimizes the possibility that a severe withdrawal will develop. Any depressant, including alcohol, barbiturates, or a benzodiazepine, can work, but most clinicians choose a benzodiazepine for its relative safety. Adequate treatment can be given with either short-acting drugs, such as lorazepam (Ativan), or long-acting substances such as chlordiazepoxide (Librium) and diazepam (Valium).

An example is the administration of 25 mg of chlordiazepoxide by mouth three or four times a day on the first day, with a notation to skip a dose if the patient is asleep or feeling sleepy. An additional one or two 25-mg doses during the first 24 hours can be used if the patient is jittery or shows signs of increasing tremor or autonomic dysfunction. Whatever the dosage required on the first day, the benzodiazepine can be decreased by 20 percent each subsequent day, with a resulting need for no further medication after 4 or 5 days. When using a long-acting agent, such as chlordiazepoxide, the clinician must avoid producing excessive sedation through overmedication; if the patient is sleepy, the next scheduled dose should be omitted. When taking a short-acting drug, such as lorazepam, the patient must not miss any dose because rapid changes in blood benzodiazepine concentrations may precipitate a severe withdrawal. Other depressants, including the newer anticonvulsants, such as gabapentin (Neurontin), are also effective in detoxification but have added dangers and costs.

A social model program of detoxification saves money by avoiding medications while using social supports. This less expensive regimen can be helpful for mild or moderate withdrawal syndromes. Some clinicians have also recommended β-adrenergic receptor antagonists, such as propranolol (Inderal), or α-adrenergic receptor agonists, such as clonidine (Catapres), although these medications do not appear to be superior to the benzodiazepines. Unlike the brain depressants, these other agents do little to decrease the risk of seizures or delirium.

Severe Withdrawal For less than 1 percent of alcoholic patients with extreme autonomic dysfunction, agitation, and confusion—that is, those with alcoholic withdrawal delirium, also called delirium tremens—no perfect treatment has been found. The first key step is to ask why such a severe and relatively uncommon withdrawal syndrome has occurred; the answer often relates to a concomitant medical problem that needs immediate treatment. The withdrawal symptoms can then be minimized either through the use of benzodiazepines (in which case high doses are sometimes required), or through antipsychotic agents such as haloperidol (Haldol). Once again, doses are used on the first or second day to control behavior, and the patient can be weaned off the medication by approximately the fifth day.

Another 1 percent or so of patients may have a single grand mal convulsion; the rare person has multiple fits, and the peak incidence is on the second day of withdrawal. Such patients require a neurological evaluation, but in the absence of evidence of a seizure disorder, they do not benefit from anticonvulsant drugs.

Protracted Withdrawal Finally regarding withdrawal, symptoms of anxiety, insomnia, and mild autonomic overactivity are likely to continue for 2 to 6 months after the acute withdrawal has disappeared. Although no pharmacological treatment for this syndrome appears appropriate, it is possible that some of the medications discussed below, especially acamprosate (Campral), may work, at least in part, by diminishing some of these symptoms. In any event, it is important that the clinician warn the patient that some levels of sleep problems or feelings of nervousness might remain after acute withdrawal and discuss cognitive and behavioral approaches that might be appropriate to helping the patient feel more comfortable. At least theoretically, these protracted withdrawal symptoms may enhance the probability of relapse.

Rehabilitation For most patients, rehabilitation includes three major components: (1) continued efforts to increase and maintain high levels of motivation for abstinence, (2) work to help the patient readjust to a lifestyle free of alcohol, and (3) relapse prevention. Because these steps are carried out in the context of distractions inherent in acute and protracted withdrawal syndromes and life crises, treatment requires repeated presentations of similar materials that remind the patient how important abstinence is and that help the patient develop new day-to-day support systems and coping styles.

No single major life event, traumatic life period, or identifiable psychiatric disorder is known to be a unique cause of alcoholism. In addition, the effects of any causes of alcoholism are likely to have been diluted by the effects of alcohol on the brain and the years of an altered lifestyle so that the alcoholism has developed a life of its own. This is true even though many alcoholic people believe that the cause was depression, anxiety, life stress, or pain syndromes. Research, data from records, and resource people usually reveal that the alcohol contributed to the mood disorder, accident, or life stress, not vice versa.

The same general treatment approach is used in inpatient, as well as outpatient, settings. The selection of the more expensive and intensive and perhaps a bit more effective inpatient mode often depends on evidence of additional severe medical or psychiatric syndromes, the absence of appropriate nearby outpatient groups and facilities, and the patient's history of having tried but failed in outpatient care. The treatment process in either setting involves intervention, optimizing physical and psychological functioning, enhancing motivation, reaching out to family, and using the first 2 to 4 weeks of care as an intensive period of help. Those efforts must be followed by at least 3 to 6 months of less frequent outpatient care. The latter uses a combination of individual and group counseling, the judicious avoidance of psychotropic medications unless needed for independent disorders, and involvement in such self-help groups as AA.

There are few data that indicate that it is necessary to carefully match specific aspects of the patient's history with a particular type of treatment program. In general, most investigations demonstrate relatively high rates of abstinence and improvement in life functioning regardless of the type of therapeutic approach involved.

Counseling Counseling efforts in the first several weeks to months should focus on day-to-day life issues to help patients maintain a high level of motivation for abstinence and to enhance their levels of functioning. Psychotherapy techniques that provoke anxiety or that require deep insights have not been shown to be of benefit during the early phases of recovery and, at least theoretically, may impair efforts at maintaining abstinence.

Counseling or therapy can be carried out in an individual or group setting; few data indicate that either approach is superior. The technique used is not likely to matter greatly and usually boils down to simple day-to-day counseling or behavioral or psychotherapeutic approach focusing on the here and now. To optimize motivation, treatment sessions should explore the consequences of drinking, the likely future course of alcohol-related life problems, and the marked improvement that can be expected with abstinence. Whether in an inpatient or an outpatient setting, individual or group counseling is usually offered for a minimum of three times a week for the first 2 to 4 weeks, followed by less intense efforts, perhaps once a week, for the subsequent 3 to 6 months.

Much time in counseling deals with how to build a lifestyle free of alcohol. Discussions cover the need for a sober peer group, a plan for social and recreational events without drinking, and approaches for reestablishing communication with family members and friends.

Many clinicians believe that cognitive and behavioral approaches can form a solid base to these counseling sessions. The goal of these efforts is to help the patient learn ways of coping while focusing on approaches for identifying life stresses. The clinician can use role rehearsal, modeling, and role playing while encouraging patients to practice these skills between sessions. At the same time, individuals are encouraged to identify areas of problems in day-to-day functioning, paying special attention to how they react to these challenges and the impact that substance use might have on the outcomes.

Relapse Prevention The third major component of rehabilitation efforts, relapse prevention, begins with identifying situations in which the risk for relapse is high. The counselor must help the patient to develop modes of coping to be used when the craving for alcohol increases or when any event or emotional state makes a return to drinking more likely. An important part of relapse prevention is reminding the patient about the appropriate attitude toward slips in which short-term experiences with alcohol can never be used as an excuse for returning to regular drinking. Rather, recovery is a process of trial and error; patients use slips when they occur to identify high-risk situations and to develop more appropriate coping techniques.

Importance of the Family Most treatment efforts recognize the effects that alcoholism has on the significant people in the patient's life, and an important aspect of recovery involves helping family members and close friends to understand alcoholism and how rehabilitation is an ongoing process that lasts for 6 to 12 months or more. Couples and family counseling and support groups for relatives and friends help the people involved to rebuild relationships, to learn how to avoid protecting the patient from the consequences of any drinking in the future, and to be as supportive as possible of the alcoholic patient's recovery program.

Medications If detoxification has been completed, and the patient is not one of the 10 to 15 percent of alcoholic people who have an independent mood disorder, schizophrenia, or anxiety disorder, there is little evidence in favor of prescribing psychotropic medications for the treatment of alcoholism. Levels of anxiety and insomnia that can linger for 6 months or more as part of a reaction to life stresses and protracted abstinence should be treated with behavior modification approaches and reassurance. Medications, including benzodiazepines, for these symptoms are likely to lose their effectiveness much faster than the insomnia disappears; as a result, the patient may increase the dose and have subsequent problems related to the prescribed drug. Similarly, although low levels of sadness and mood swings can linger several months, controlled clinical trials indicate no benefit in prescribing antidepressant medications or lithium to treat the average alcoholic person who has no independent or long-lasting psychiatric disorder. The mood disorder clears before the medications can take effect, and patients who resume drinking while on the medications face significant potential dangers. With little or no evidence that the medications are effective, the dangers significantly outweigh any potential benefits from their routine use.

Data from recent years support the probable modest effect of two medications in addition to the usual cognitive-behavioral approaches for treating alcohol dependence. These have been hypothesized to possibly decrease the rewarding effects of alcohol if an individual returns to drinking, diminish the symptoms of the protracted withdrawal syndrome, or, perhaps, diminish feelings of craving.

The first drug is acamprosate (Campral), which is an analog of the amino acid neurotransmitter taurine and structurally resembles GABA. Although the mechanism of action in alcoholics is unknown, acamprosate does antagonize neuronal overactivity related to the actions of the excitatory neurotransmitter glutamate, at least in part by acting as an antagonist to NMDA receptors. Thus, one possibly important mechanism for this drug may be in diminishing anxiety, mood swings, and other sleep difficulties associated with the subacute and protracted withdrawal syndrome observed after the first 4 to 5 days of alcohol abstinence.

A minimum of 15 double-blind, placebo-controlled studies that have administered the drugs for between 3 and 12 months have been published since 1985, using the usual dose of approximately 2,000 mg per day. With two exceptions, the remaining studies, including all four published investigations involving 12 months of active drug treatment, report modest but statistically significantly better outcomes with active drug during the follow-up period. The level of improvement is often in the range of 15 to 20 percent over results seen with placebo, and in most studies, rates of side effects are similar for active drug and placebo except for GI problems such as diarrhea. At least one cost-effectiveness study has indicated that the levels of improvement result in significant cost savings above and beyond the financial obligations of prescribing the drug.

The second promising medication is the long-acting, oral, opioid antagonist naltrexone (ReVia or Trexan). This agent has been marketed for many years for the treatment of acute opioid overdose as well as to help more highly motivated opioid-dependent individuals maintain abstinence through knowledge that because of the use of this blocking drug they could not achieve intoxication. Naltrexone works by blocking opioid receptors in the brain and, thus, at least indirectly changing the levels of brain activity regarding dopamine and serotonin. In alcohol-dependent individuals, naltrexone and its cousin nalmefene (Revex) have been hypothesized to decrease the rewarding effects of a drink or to diminish craving. Six double-blind, placebo-controlled studies have been published regarding the use of naltrexone in individuals with alcohol dependence along with several unpublished reports. These generally demonstrate the superiority of naltrexone to placebo on areas of drinking-related behavior similar to those evaluated for acamprosate, although the naltrexone studies have involved relatively small numbers of subjects who are evaluated over 3 months of active drug, usually as part of highly structured university-based drug trials. There are two negative studies, including a large multicenter trial that administered the drug for 6 months and found no significant differences from placebo on any of the major outcome measures, despite a nonsignificant trend for better levels of functioning associated with the active drug for several of the measures. The side effect profile of the 50 to 150 mg per day usually used in these trials is relatively benign, with the most frequent complaints involving GI upset, with possible additional problems related to a modest increase in lethargy and, perhaps, the subjective report of a dampened level of interest in activities and life events.

A third drug of possible interest in the treatment of alcoholism is the alcohol-sensitizing agent disulfiram (Antabuse), which is usually given in doses of 250 mg per day. The goal is to place the patient in a condition in which drinking alcohol precipitates an uncomfortable physical reaction, including nausea, vomiting, and changes in blood pressure. However, few data convincingly prove that disulfiram is more effective than a placebo, probably because most people stop taking the disulfiram when they resume drinking. Many clinicians have stopped routinely prescribing the agent, partly in recognition of the dangers associated with the drug itself, including mood swings, rare instances of psychosis, the possibility of an increase in peripheral neuropathies, the relatively rare occurrence of other significant neuropathies, and a rare but potentially fatal hepatitis. Moreover, patients with preexisting heart disease, cerebral thrombosis, diabetes, and a number of other conditions cannot be given disulfiram because an alcohol reaction to the disulfiram could be fatal.

Several additional medications are worth brief mention. First, a recent study evaluated the possibility that an antagonist of the serotonin 3 receptor, ondansetron (Zofran), might be better than placebo in treating alcoholics who have an early-onset severe form of their disorder associated with multiple drug dependencies and criminality. However, this drug showed no superiority to placebo for the treatment of the usual alcoholic. A second medication with some potential promise in the treatment of alcoholism is the nonbenzodiazepine antianxiety drug buspirone (BuSpar), although the effect of this drug on alcohol rehabilitation is inconsistent between studies. However, at the same time, there is no evidence that antidepressant medications, such as the selective serotonin reuptake inhibitors (SSRIs), lithium, or antipsychotic medications, are significantly effective in the treatment of alcoholism. Another physical treatment, acupuncture, has been evaluated, although the results are not promising.

Self-Help Groups Clinicians must recognize the potential importance of self-help groups such as AA. Members of AA have help available 24 hours a day, associate with a sober peer group, learn that it is possible to participate in social functions without drinking, and are given a model of recovery by observing the accomplishments of sober members of the group.

Learning about AA usually begins during inpatient or outpatient rehabilitation. The clinician can play a major role in helping patients understand the differences between specific groups. Some are comprised only of men or women, and others are mixed; some meetings are comprised mostly of blue collar men and women, whereas others are mostly for professionals; some groups place great emphasis on religion, and others are eclectic. Patients with coexisting psychiatric disorders may need some additional education about AA. The clinician should remind them that some members of AA may not understand their special need for medications and should arm the patients with ways of coping when group members inappropriately suggest that the required medications be stopped. Although difficult to evaluate using double-blind controls, most studies indicate that participation in AA is associated with improved outcomes, and incorporation into treatment programs saves money.

SUGGESTED CROSS-REFERENCES

Classification of mental disorders is discussed in Chapter 9, epidemiology in Section 5.1, and the sociocultural sciences in Chapter 4. Delirium and amnestic disorders are discussed in Chapter 10. Other substance-related disorders are discussed in Chapter 11, mood disorders are discussed in Chapter 13, anxiety disorders are discussed in Chapter 14, personality disorders are discussed in Chapter 23, and schizophrenia is presented in Chapter 12. Psychotherapies are discussed in Chapter 30.

References

Bierut LJ, Dinwiddie SH, Begleiter H, Crowe RR, Hesselbrock V, Nurnberger JI Jr, Porjesz B, Schuckit MA, Reich T: Familial transmission of substance dependence: Alcohol, marijuana, cocaine, and habitual smoking. A report from the Collaborative Study on the Genetics of Alcoholism. *Arch Gen Psychiatry.* 1998;55:982.

Connors GJ, Tonigan JS, Miller WR: A longitudinal model of intake symptomatology, AA participation and outcome: Retrospective study of the Project MATCH outpatient and aftercare samples. *J Stud Alcohol.* 2001;62:817.

Dawson DA: Alcohol and mortality from external causes. *J Stud Alcohol.* 2001;62:790.

*Fleming MF, Mundt MP, French MT, Baier Manwell L, Stauffacher EA, Lawton Barry K: Brief physician advice for problem drinkers: Long-term efficacy and benefit-cost analysis. *Alcohol Clin Exp Res.* 2002;26:36.

Hasin DS, Schuckit MA, Martin CS, Grant BF, Buchalz KK, Helzer JE: The validity of DSM IV alcohol dependence. *Alcohol Clin Exp Res.* 2003;27:244.

Heath AC, Madden PAF, Bucholz KK, Dinwiddie SH, Slutske WS, Bierut LJ, Rohrbaugh JW, Statham DJ, Dunne MP, Whitfield JB, Martin NG: Genetic differences in alcohol sensitivity and the inheritance of alcoholism risk. *Psychol Med.* 1999;29:1069.

Johnson BA, Ait-Daoud N, Prihoda TJ: Combining ondansetron and naltrexone effectively treats biologically predisposed alcoholics: From hypotheses to preliminary clinical evidence. *Alcohol Clin Exp Res.* 2000;24:737.

Johnston LD, O'Malley PM, Backman JG. *Monitoring the Future: National Survey Results on Drug Use, 1975–2002.* Vols I and II. Washington, DC: National Institute on Drug Abuse (NIH Publication #03-5375); 2003.

Kadden RM, Litt MD, Cooney NL, Kabela E, Getter H: Prospective matching of alcoholic clients to cognitive-behavioral or interactional group therapy. *J Stud Alcohol.* 2001;62:359.

Kiefer F, Holger J, Tarnaske T, Helwig H, Briken P, Holzbach R, Kempf P, Stracke R, Baehr M, Naber D, Wiedemann K: Comparing and combining naltrexone and acamprosate in relapse prevention of alcoholism. *Arch Gen Psychiatry.* 2003;60:92.

Knight JR, Wechsler H, Kuo M, Seibring M, Weitzman ER, Schuckit MA: Alcohol abuse and dependence among U.S. college students. *J Stud Alcohol.* 2002;63:263.

*Kranzler HR, Van Kirk J: Efficacy of naltrexone and acamprosate for alcoholism treatment: A meta-analysis. *Alcohol Clin Exp Res.* 2001;25:1335.

Krystal JH, Cramer JA, Krol WF, Kirk GF, Rosenheck RA: Naltrexone in the treatment of alcohol dependence. *N Engl J Med.* 2001;345:1734.

Longabaugh R, Woolard RF, Nirenberg TD, Minugh AP, Becker B, Clifford PR, Carty K, Sparadeo F, Gogineni A: Evaluating the effects of a brief motivational intervention for injured drinkers in the emergency department. *J Stud Alcohol.* 2001;62:806.

Lynskey MT, Hall W: Attention deficit hyperactivity disorder and substance use disorders: Is there a causal link? *Addiction.* 2001;96:815.

*McLellan AT, Lewis DC, O'Brien CP, Kleber HD: Drug dependence, a chronic medical illness: Implications for treatment, insurance, and outcomes evaluation. *JAMA.* 2000;284:1689.

Mundle G, Munkes J, Ackermann K, Mann K: Sex differences of carbohydrate-deficient transferrin, γ-glutamyltransferase, and mean corpuscular volume in alcohol-dependent patients. *Alcohol Clin Exp Res.* 2000;24:1400.

Narrow WE, Rae DS, Robins LN, Regier DA: Revised prevalence estimates of mental disorders in the United States: Using a clinical significance criterion to reconcile 2 surveys' estimates. *Arch Gen Psychiatry.* 2002;59:115.

Preuss UW, Schuckit MA, Smith TL, Danko GP, Bucholz KK, Hesselbrock MN, Hesselbrock V, Kramer JR: Predictors and correlates of suicide attempts over five years in 1237 alcohol dependent men and women. *Am J Psychiatry.* 2003;160:56.

Reinert DF, Allen JP: The Alcohol Use Disorders Identification Test (AUDIT): A review of recent research. *Alcohol Clin Exp Res.* 2002;26:272.

Schonfeld AM, Mattson SN, Lang AR, Delis DC, Riley EP: Verbal and nonverbal fluency in children with heavy prenatal alcohol exposure. *J Stud Alcohol.* 2001;62:239.

*Schuckit MA. *Drug and Alcohol Abuse.* 5th ed. Massachusetts: Kluwer Academic/Plenum Publishers; 2000.

*Schuckit MA: Vulnerability factors for alcoholism. In: Davis KL, Charney D, Coyle JT, Nemeroff C, eds. *Neuropsychopharmacology: The Fifth Generation of Progress.* New York: Lippincott Williams & Wilkins; 2002.

Schuckit MA, Danko GP, Smith TL, Hesselbrock V, Kramer J, Bucholz K: A five-year prospective evaluation of DSM-IV alcohol dependence with and without a physiological component. *Alcohol Clin Exp Res.* 2003;27:818.

Schuckit MA, Edenberg HJ, Kalmijn J, Flury L, Smith TL, Reich T, Bierut L, Goate A, Foroud T: A genome-wide search for genes that relate to a low level of response to alcohol. *Alcohol Clin Exp Res.* 2001;25:323.

Schuckit MA, Smith TL: The relationships of a family history of alcohol dependence, a low level of response to alcohol and six domains of life functioning to the development of alcohol use disorders. *J Stud Alcohol.* 2000;61:827.

Schuckit MA, Smith TL, Danko GP, Bucholz KK, Reich T, Bierut L: Five-year clinical course associated with DSM-IV alcohol abuse or dependence in a large group of men and women. *Am J Psychiatry.* 2001;158:1084.

Schuckit MA, Tipp JE, Bergman M, Reich W, Hesselbrock VM, Smith TL: Comparison of induced and independent major depressive disorders in 2,945 alcoholics. *Am J Psychiatry.* 1997;154:948.

Smothers B, Bertolucci D: Alcohol consumption and health-promoting behavior in a U.S. household sample: Leisure-time physical activity. *J Stud Alcohol.* 2001;62:467.

Theobald H, Johansson S-E, Bygren L-O, Engfeldt P: The effects of alcohol consumption on mortality and morbidity: A 26-year follow-up study. *J Stud Alcohol.* 2001;62:783.

Vliegenthart R, Geleijnse JM, Hofman A, Meijer WT, van Rooij FJA, Grobbee DE, Witteman JCM: Alcohol consumption and risk of peripheral arterial disease. The Rotterdam Study. *Am J Epidemiol.* 2002;155:332.

Whitfield JB, Zhu G, Duffy DL, Birley AJ, Madden PAF, Heath AC, Martin NG: Variation in alcohol pharmacokinetics as a risk factor for alcohol dependence. *Alcohol Clin Exp Res.* 2001;25:1257.

▲ 11.3 Amphetamine (or Amphetamine-like)–Related Disorders

Jerome H. Jaffe, M.D., Walter Ling, M.D., and Richard A. Rawson, Ph.D.

Amphetamine and amphetamine-like drugs are among the most widely used illicit drugs in Asia Pacific, Australia, United Kingdom, and several other Western European countries. In the United States, after a significant increase in the 1990s, methamphetamine use exceeded cocaine use in some parts of the country and brought the problem to wider attention as a matter for serious concern.

Despite important pharmacological and neurochemical differences between the amphetamine-type drugs and cocaine, the patterns of use, criteria for dependence, and toxicity associated with them are similar. In addition to amphetamine and methamphetamine, several drugs that produce similar subjective effects are considered in this section. Also briefly discussed is 3,4-methylenedioxymethamphetamine (MDMA; "ecstasy"), one of five drugs often grouped together as "club drugs."

DEFINITIONS

Amphetamine use may be associated with a number of distinct disorders of which dependence and abuse are but two. In the case of amphetamine and amphetamine-like agents, at least ten other substance-related disorders have been described.

Amphetamine dependence is defined in the revised fourth edition of the *Diagnostic and Statistical Manual of Mental Disorders* (DSM-IV-TR) as a cluster of physiological, behavioral, and cognitive symptoms that, taken together, indicate that the person continues to use amphetamine-like drugs despite significant problems related to such use (Table 11.1–3). This brief definition emphasizes the drug-using behavior itself, its maladaptive nature, and how the choice to engage in that behavior shifts and becomes constrained as a result of interaction with the drug over time. *Amphetamine abuse* is a term used to categorize a pattern of maladaptive use of amphetamine or an amphetamine-like drug, leading to clinically significant impairment or distress and occurring within a 12-month period in which the symptoms have never met the criteria for amphetamine dependence (Table 11.1–8).

The amphetamine-induced disorders include amphetamine intoxication, amphetamine withdrawal, amphetamine-induced psychotic disorder with delusions, amphetamine-induced psychotic disorder with hallucinations, amphetamine intoxication delirium, amphetamine-induced mood disorder, amphetamine-induced anxiety disorder, amphetamine-induced sleep disorder, amphetamine-induced sexual dysfunction, and amphetamine-related disorder not otherwise specified. The coding scheme of DSM-IV-TR provides distinct numbers for amphetamine dependence and amphetamine abuse, but the codes for the other amphetamine-induced disorders are common to several other substance-related disorders.

Amphetamine-type drugs with abuse potential also include methylphenidate (Ritalin) and phendimetrazine (Preludin), which are included in schedule (control level) II of the Controlled Substance Act (CSA), and diethylpropion (Tenuate), benzphetamine (Didrex), and phentermine (Ionamin), which are included in schedules III or IV of the CSA. It is presumed that all of these drugs are capable of producing all of the listed amphetamine-induced disorders. Modafinil (Provigil) also has euphorigenic effects in humans and is reinforcing in animal models. It is included in schedule IV of the CSA, but its toxicity in supratherapeutic doses and its likelihood of producing amphetamine-induced disorders are unknown.

HISTORY

Amphetamines were introduced into clinical use in the early 1930s. By late in the decade, there was some concern about amphetamine dependence, and in 1938, the first reports of amphetamine psychosis appeared. Nevertheless, between 1932 and 1946, almost three dozen medical uses of amphetamine were proposed and tried. As late as 1971, some amphetamines were available in over-the-counter nasal inhalers.

An epidemic of intravenous (IV) methamphetamine abuse and dependence occurred in Japan immediately after World War II, but until the 1960s, there was reluctance in the United States to believe that amphetamine and related drugs could cause addiction. In the mid-1960s, because of growing concern over their misuse and overuse, the Food and Drug Administration (FDA) placed these drugs under regulatory control. Nevertheless, there were enough of these drugs still on the street (believed to have been supplied primarily by diversion of legitimately produced drugs) to fuel a major epidemic of amphetamine and methamphetamine abuse in the late 1960s. This epidemic made clear the potential toxicity of amphetamines, especially when used intravenously, and such terms as "speed freaks" and "speed kills" left an enduring legacy in the popular vocabulary.

The quantity of amphetamine and amphetamine-like drugs smuggled into the country or produced illegally in clandestine laboratories continued to increase over the next decade. Although regulatory control of legitimately produced amphetamines was progressively tightened, misuse of these drugs persisted in the United States, with much of the supply coming from illicit laboratories. When it became illegal to obtain the commonly used precursor phenyl-2-propanone (P2P), illicit manufacturers found ways to produce methamphetamine from ephedrine or pseudoephedrine, or both, which was widely available in over-the-counter medications for colds and asthma. This method of synthesis, which actually yields a higher percentage of the active D-isomer of methamphetamine, was adopted by criminal organizations using large-scale laboratories and by independent producers whose small laboratories, usually located in remote rural areas, were more difficult to detect and eliminate.

In the late 1980s, it was reported that the practice of smoking crystalline methamphetamine ("ice") was on the increase, especially in Hawaii. Until the mid-1990s, however, the use of amphetamine-like stimulants continued to be overshadowed by cocaine abuse in most parts of the United States, whereas over this same period, the reverse was true in the United Kingdom, Australia, Western Europe, and Asia Pacific. In the mid-1990s, it became evident from surveys, drug testing of arrestees, and emergency room visits due to drug toxicity that methamphetamine use was increasing sharply in several areas of the United States, especially in California and some parts of the Southwest and Northwest.

At the present time, amphetamines are used legitimately almost exclusively for the treatment of narcolepsy and attention-deficit/hyperactivity disorder (ADHD), although methylphenidate is more widely prescribed for the latter indication (Chapter 39). Some amphetamine-like agents are still prescribed as appetite suppressants, but the use of amphetamine itself for that purpose has been discouraged and is illegal in some states. Amphetamines may be useful in the treatment of atypical depression, but concern about abuse potential has discouraged the controlled clinical studies that are necessary to define the specific benefits of amphetamine-like agents over traditional tricyclic antidepressants or selective serotonin reuptake inhibitors (SSRIs).

COMPARATIVE NOSOLOGY

The DSM-IV-TR diagnostic criteria for amphetamine dependence are the same generic criteria applied to other substances ranging from opioids and cocaine to alcohol. The notion of a generic concept of dependence is shared with the tenth revision of the *International Statistical Classification of Diseases and Related Health Problems* (ICD-10), published in 1999. In making a diagnosis of dependence, there is generally a high level of agreement between DSM-IV-TR and ICD-10: They use similar concepts (the dependence syndrome varying in severity), although the wording of the criteria for determining the presence and severity of the syndrome differ. Both require that three elements of the syndrome occur within a 12-month period. Although DSM-IV-TR appears to put greater stress on tolerance and physiological dependence by asking clinicians to specify if these elements are present, it is not certain whether patients who exhibit these phenomena have a distinct form of the disorder. A clearer diagnosis can be determined for patients dependent on other substances who exhibit tolerance or withdrawal—for example, those with alcohol dependence—because they can have a more severe withdrawal syndrome. One study of cocaine users found that, even if tolerance and physical dependence had not been required to make the diagnosis, there would have been approximately the same number of patients meeting the criteria for dependence.

There is a major difference between ICD-10 and DSM-IV-TR in the classification of what is called *substance abuse* in DSM-IV-TR. ICD-10 does not use the term "abuse"; instead, it includes a category of "harmful use," which is substantially different from the concept of abuse used in DSM-IV-TR. The concept of "harm" is limited to physical and mental ailments (e.g., hepatitis, cardiac damage, episodes of depression, or toxic psychosis) and specifically excludes social impairments as follows:

> Harmful patterns of use are often criticized by others and frequently associated with adverse social consequences of various kinds. The fact that a pattern of use of a particular substance is disapproved of by another person or by the culture, or may have led to socially negative consequences such as arrest or marital arguments, is not in itself evidence of harmful use.

The ICD-10 and DSM-IV-TR coding systems, which limit the number of distinct drug categories that can be recorded, also differ. ICD-10 separates cocaine-related disorders from those caused by other stimulants. Because of the limits of the coding system, the ICD-10 stimulant category includes caffeine with the amphetamines and amphetamine-like stimulants. It is not clear whether MDMA-related disorders would be included under stimulants or other drugs in the ICD-10 system.

EPIDEMIOLOGY

The National Household Survey on Drug Abuse (NHSDA) conducted in 2001 found that 7.1 percent of adults (12 years of age and older) reported lifetime nonmedical use of stimulants, a significant increase since the 4.5 percent found in the 1997 survey. Past 30-day use was reported by 1.1 percent of adults in 2001, compared with 0.3 percent in 1997. The highest rates of use in the past year (1.5 percent) were among 18- to 25-year-olds, followed by 12- to 17-year-olds. In 1993, the treatment admission rate for primary amphetamine abuse in the United States was 14 admissions per 100,000 people 12 years of age or older. By 1999, the treatment admission rate for primary amphetamine abuse in the United States as a whole had increased to 32 per 100,000 people 12 years of age or older. Thirteen states had amphetamine admission rates of at least 55 per 100,000, and eight of these had rates of 100 per 100,000 or more.

The Monitoring the Future study, a survey of students conducted since 1975, previously considered amphetamines and similar drugs together as "stimulants." Over the years, the category definition and questions pertaining to amphetamines have expanded. In 1989, "crystal meth" (or "ice") was added as a stimulant answer category. Likewise, in 1999—in response to growing concern regarding methamphetamine use in general—a full set of three questions about the methamphetamine subclass was added to the survey for all three grade levels surveyed (eighth, tenth, and 12th). The investigators now believe that, although the absolute prevalence level of methamphetamine use was probably underestimated before 1999, the shape of the overall trend curve was not distorted in their study. Among high school seniors, self-reported use of stimulants has been consistently higher than use of cocaine and crack cocaine. This study has also found that rates of amphetamine-type substance use are much higher in students and young adults than in the general U.S. population.

Baseline statistics on prevalence of use, abuse/dependence, and comorbidity are mostly drawn from two general population surveys that use accepted diagnostic criteria to measure the extent of drug abuse and dependence. These were the Epidemiologic Catchment Area (ECA) study, carried out in the early 1980s using criteria from the third edition of DSM (DSM-III), and the National Comorbidity Survey (NCS), carried out from 1990 to 1992 using criteria from the revised third edition of DSM (DSM-III-TR). The ECA report combined categories of dependence and abuse for amphetamine and amphetamine-like drugs. The 1-month, 6-month, and lifetime prevalence rates of amphetamine abuse or dependence for adults were 0.1, 0.2, and 1.7 percent, respectively. The NCS lifetime dependence rate for 15- to 54-year-olds was 1.7 percent; approximately 15 percent of respondents gave a history of some nonmedical use of stimulants; and approximately 11 percent of those respondents met criteria for dependence. New surveys are needed to provide a more current picture of the prevalence of the psychiatric disorders that are likely to have been engendered by the worldwide amphetamine epidemic.

ETIOLOGY

Drug dependence, including amphetamine and amphetamine-like substance dependence, is viewed as resulting from a process in which multiple interacting factors (social, psychological, cultural, and biological) influence drug-using behavior. This process, in some cases, leads to the loss of flexibility with respect to drug use that is the hallmark of drug dependence. According to this biopsychosocial perspective, the actions of the drug are seen as critical. However, not everyone who becomes dependent experiences the effects of a given drug in the same way or is influenced by the same set of factors. Even within the same class of pharmacological agents, different social, biological, or cultural factors may be more or less important at different stages of the process.

As with most substances, social and cultural factors influence availability and initial use of amphetamines and amphetamine-like drugs; however, strong psychological and pharmacological factors motivate continued use and the progression to dependence. Amphetamines have potent mood-elevating and euphorigenic actions in humans and are powerful reinforcers in animal models, particularly when the drug effects have rapid onset, as when they are injected or inhaled. Although there are other elements in amphetamine physical dependence syndrome, continuous use is motivated primarily by the contrast between the euphoria and sense of competence and well-being induced by the drug and the dysphoria and anhedonia associated with cessation. The contrast increases with more prolonged use of higher doses.

Comorbidity

Additional psychiatric diagnoses are quite common among those dependent on amphetamines and amphetamine-like drugs. How this comorbidity is linked etiologically to amphetamine dependence is not always clear, but epidemiological evidence shows that the presence of psychiatric disorders not necessarily induced by substance abuse (e.g., mood disorders, schizophrenia, and antisocial personality disorder) substantially increases the odds of developing substance abuse or dependence. Those with conduct disorder or antisocial personality disorder are more likely to take risks and to disregard social prohibitions against using illicit drugs. Amphetamines and amphetamine-like drugs may alleviate various psychiatric disorders or dysfunctional states in some people. For example, some users (relatively few) may find relief from adult attention-deficit disorders. The drugs may alleviate a persistent dysthymic disorder in others, and for such users, the anhedonic state after amphetamine cessation may be experienced as more intense. Still, others may have found that the drug facilitated sexual activity, increased performance, or promoted weight loss. Eventually with continued and increased use, these seemingly positive effects usually decrease or cease completely. Thus, although such factors may explain initiation or drug use on more than one occasion, they do not account for progression to dependence or abuse.

In the United States, less is known about the characteristics of young people who use amphetamines than about those who use and become dependent on cocaine and "crack." High school juniors and seniors who use illicit drugs in general perform less well in school, have poorer family relationships, report more psychological symptoms and health problems, and exhibit more delinquent behavior. Those who use cocaine and crack are the most delinquent, but reported anxiety and depression are no greater among this group than among those who do not use cocaine and crack.

Research on the temporal appearance of the syndromes indicates that, in some instances and for some syndromes, drug use predates the psychiatric disorders. In one component of the ECA study, subjects were reinterviewed 1 year later. Those who reported using amphetamines, amphetamine-like drugs, or cocaine in the time between interviews were almost eight times more likely than nonusers to have developed a depressive disorder and 14 times more likely to have experienced a panic attack. Amphetamine users report a wide range of psychiatric symptoms, most of which are correlated with high levels of drug use. These are discussed more fully below.

Genetic Factors A study of Vietnam-era twins found higher concordance rates for stimulant dependence among monozygotic twins than dizygotic twins. The analyses indicated that genetic factors and unique (unshared) environmental factors contributed approximately equally to the development of dependence. In this study, "stimulants" included cocaine, amphetamines, and amphetamine-like drugs. A substantial role for genetic factors in vulnerability to dependence in general, including stimulant dependence, was also found in studies of twins in Virginia. These studies also found a very similar underlying structure of genetic and environmental risk factors for drug abuse disorders in men and women.

Other Factors Social, cultural, and economic factors are powerful determinants of initial use, continued use, and relapse. Excessive use is far more likely to occur when amphetamines are readily available; this is amply demonstrated by the epidemics of amphetamine use in Japan and the United States and by more recent sharp increases in use that have followed the emergence of illicit large-scale and "kitchen" laboratories synthesizing cheap, relatively pure methamphetamine.

Because, in both human and animal studies, alternative positive reinforcers compete with drugs as reinforcers, the absence of such nondrug alternatives can be seen as a factor contributing to their use, especially in communities in which drugs are available, and the social pressures against their use are weak. Alternative positive reinforcers are not limited to material rewards but also include the kinds of psychological rewards associated with satisfactory interpersonal relationships and the self-esteem derived from achievements in socially acceptable endeavors.

Learning and Conditioning Learning and conditioning are also important in perpetuating amphetamine use. Environmental cues associated with amphetamine use become associated with the euphoric state so that long after cessation such cues (e.g., paraphernalia, friends who use drugs) can elicit memories that reawaken a craving for the drug. The effects of other drugs may also trigger craving for stimulants. For example, among patients seeking treatment, the continued use of alcohol, which is often consumed with stimulants, decreases the likelihood of successful cessation, probably because the alcohol acts as a trigger for craving and may also decrease the capacity to deal with craving.

Pharmacological Factors The reinforcing and toxic effects of amphetamines and amphetamine-like drugs play an important role in the genesis of amphetamine dependence and other amphetamine-related disorders. Amphetamines produce stronger and longer-lasting subjective effects than those produced by cocaine. Both categories of drugs can produce a sense of alertness, euphoria, and well-being. Performance impaired by fatigue is usually improved. There may be decreased hunger and decreased need for sleep. Patterns of toxicity are also similar, although not identical. Both amphetamines and cocaine can induce paranoia, suspiciousness, and overt psychosis that can be difficult to distinguish from paranoid-type schizophrenia; both can produce major cardiovascular toxicities. However, amphetamines and cocaine differ distinctly in their mechanisms of action at the cellular level, their duration of action, and their metabolic pathways.

Amphetamines enhance talkativeness, self-confidence, and sociability. Some people's beliefs about the capacity of these drugs to increase sexual drive and performance also play an important, if indirect, role in their reinforcing effects. Evidence for the enhancement of sexual performance by amphetamines is still largely anecdotal but seems convincing to some well-trained observers. Amphetamine users, both heterosexual and homosexual, report more frequent sexual activity with more partners than heroin users.

Mechanisms of Action Although amphetamines inhibit reuptake of monoamines to a small degree, their major action is the release of monoamines from storage sites in axon terminals, which in turn increases monoamine concentrations in the synaptic cleft. Although dopamine, norepinephrine, and serotonin are all released, most work indicates that the release of dopamine in the nucleus accumbens and related structures accounts for the reinforcing and mood-elevating effects of amphetamine; the release of norepinephrine is probably responsible for the cardiovascular effects. Unlike cocaine, which acts primarily extracellularly by binding to neurotransporters and thus inhibiting the reuptake of the neurotransmitters released into the synapse, amphetamines are taken into the neurons where they enter into the neurotransmitter storage vesicles and block the transport of dopamine into these vesicles, resulting in the extravesicular, intracellular accumulation of dopamine. This intracellular transmitter may in turn undergo oxidation with production of several highly toxic and reactive chemicals such as oxygen radicals, peroxides, and hydroxyquinones. Some of the neuronal toxicity of methamphetamine is due, therefore, not to the drug per se but to the intracellular accumulation of dopamine. Amphetamines also cause docking of the neurotransmitter vesicles at the cellular membrane and cause further leakage of the neurotransmitters into the synaptic cleft. Methamphetamine-induced increases in glutamate efflux also appear to play a role in dopaminergic neuron neurotoxicity.

Methylphenidate, widely used for the treatment of ADHD, has a mechanism of action quite distinct from that of the other amphetamine-like drugs but is generally grouped with them. Like cocaine, methylphenidate produces actions in the central nervous system (CNS) largely by blocking the dopamine transporters responsible for the reuptake of dopamine from synapses after its release. Studies suggest that the somewhat lower abuse potential of orally administered methylphenidate is due to slow occupation of dopamine transporters in the brain: It takes approximately 60 minutes for an oral dose to produce peak concentrations in the brain. In clinical studies, only one of seven normal adults reported a "high" after doses that produced blockade of 50 percent of the dopamine transporters (a degree of blockade comparable to that achieved with IV doses of cocaine). These studies and similar studies on other drugs show that reinforcing effects depend critically on the rate of change in dopamine concentrations in relevant brain circuits. Furthermore, unlike cocaine, which leaves the brain relatively rapidly, methylphenidate occupies the transporter sites for a much longer time.

Common Routes of Administration Amphetamines and amphetamine-like drugs can be taken orally, by injection, by absorption through nasal and buccal membranes, or by heating, inhalation of the vapors, and absorption through the pulmonary alveoli. As with nicotine, opioids, and freebase cocaine, inhaled amphetamine or methamphetamine is almost immediately absorbed with a rapid onset of effects. Unlike cocaine, amphetamine and methamphetamine salts can be vaporized without much destruction of the molecule, thus obviating the need for preparing a freebase form for smoking.

As with the opioids, the rapid onset of amphetamine effects from IV injection or inhalation produces an intensely pleasurable sensation referred to as a *rush*. The onset of acute effects depends on the route of administration, from seconds after smoking and injection to a few minutes after oral ingestion. The duration of the amphetamine rush has not been studied in the laboratory, but it is presumed to be shorter than the duration of elevated mood. Maximum mood effect is reached after approximately 15 minutes and lasts for 10 to 12 hours, followed by aftereffects lasting approximately 48 hours. Despite the rapid onset of action after smoked amphetamines, some users, particularly young users in Australia, United Kingdom, and Asia Pacific, make a transition from oral to IV use. Amphetamine injectors seem to be more likely than injectors of other drugs, such as heroin, to share injection equipment.

Metabolism Although amphetamine and methamphetamine are extensively metabolized in the liver, much of the ingested drug is excreted unchanged in the urine. The half-life of therapeutic doses of amphetamine ranges from 7 to 19 hours, whereas that of methamphetamine appears to be slightly longer. Both are weak bases, and half-life is considerably shorter when the urine is acidic. After toxic dosage, symptoms may take far longer (up to several days) to resolve with amphetamines than with cocaine, depending on the pH of the urine.

Tolerance and Sensitization Most amphetamine users who seek treatment report needing progressively more amphetamine to get the same euphoric effect; they have developed *tolerance*. Some tolerance also develops to the cardiovascular effects of amphetamine.

In animal models, repeated administration of amphetamine or amphetamine-like drugs (as well as cocaine) also produces a form of *sensitization* in which the response to a given dose is actually enhanced. The sensitization can be long-lasting. The paranoid states and toxic psychoses that chronic amphetamine users commonly develop are believed to be phenomena to which sensitization develops. Those who have experienced amphetamine psychosis may do so more rapidly with subsequent exposures and may even experience brief psychotic episodes as a result of stress.

Withdrawal States Amphetamine withdrawal effects are almost opposite those of intoxication—a finding not always recognized by the abuser. These effects may include fatigue, insomnia or restless hypersomnia, unpleasant dreams, hyperphagia, psychomotor agitation or retardation, dysphoria, anhedonia, and fragmented attention span. These symptoms can be intense and may be protracted.

The amphetamine withdrawal syndrome has aversive psychological qualities but is generally not deemed as physically painful as opioid withdrawal. Nevertheless, withdrawal anhedonia and fatigue may contribute to an urge to use after recent cessation. Anhedonia and dysphoria may be more important factors for those users who have come to depend on the drugs for high energy or for helping to project a confident persona, and they may be temporarily unable to function without them. For others, withdrawal dysphoria may exaggerate the intensity of an antecedent mood disorder. Studies to date have not documented a protracted amphetamine withdrawal syndrome comparable to that reported for opioids.

Mechanisms of CNS Changes The chronic administration of amphetamines results in several adaptive changes in the brain. For example, release of dopamine and resulting stimulation of dopamine receptors activates cyclic adenosine monophosphate (cAMP) within neurons in the nucleus accumbens and striatum. This activation initiates a chain of intracellular events that results in altered expression of a number of genes, some of which are mediated by phosphorylation of transcription factors such as CREB (cAMP response element–binding protein). Induction of CREB, in turn, increases expression of adenylyl cyclase. Another of the actions of CREB is to increase transcription of dynorphin in ribonucleic acid (RNA). This action is significant because dynorphin is a selective κ-opioid agonist. κ-Receptor agonists inhibit release of dopamine. Recurrent collateral axons from neurons in the nucleus accumbens are believed to release dynorphin on κ receptors at dopaminergic terminals, thus dampening excessive dopaminergic activity (Fig. 11.10–1). However, when amphetamine use is stopped, and the excessive dopamine release ceases, the compensatory high levels of dynorphin persist and further diminish dopaminergic activity, thus exaggerating the anhedonia and dysphoria of amphetamine withdrawal.

Additionally, neurons of the nucleus accumbens exhibit decreases in the concentration of G_i protein (which inhibits adenylyl cyclase) and increases in levels of cAMP-dependent protein kinase. Both of these changes may persist for weeks and are expected to upregulate the cAMP pathway. In animal models, manipulations that upregulate the cAMP pathway produce increased self-administration of cocaine (and probably of amphetamine). The persistent changes in the cAMP pathway appear to represent one mechanism of tolerance to the reinforcing effects of stimulants. Other neural mechanisms that appear to play a role in adaptation to administration of amphetamines and cocaine are cocaine- and amphetamine-regulated transcript (CART) peptides. These neurotransmitter peptides are concentrated throughout the ventral tegmental area and are also found in the nucleus accumbens. Their actions appear to be homeostatic, reversing or limiting the effects of high levels of dopamine.

The sensitization that is caused by repeated administration of amphetamine probably results from the induction and accumulation of Fos-like proteins, chronic *fos*-related antigens (FRAs) (mediated by phosphorylation of CREB). These chronic FRAs are long-lived and are distinct from Fos-like proteins seen after a single drug exposure. The accumulation of these long-lived FRAs increases locomotor and rewarding responses to cocaine and morphine and presumably to the amphetamines. The mechanism may involve changes in the makeup of glutamate (α-amino-3-hydroxy-5-methyl-4-isoxazolepropionic acid [AMPA]) receptor subunits. It has been hypothesized that these FRAs are a necessary and sufficient mechanism to account for sensitization. In addition to persistent changes in gene transcription, repeated amphetamine administration produces persistent morphological changes in neurons of the nucleus accumbens.

Glutamate and glutamate receptors play a critical role in the development of sensitization to amphetamine (and cocaine). In animals, sensitization leads to long-lasting enhancement of cocaine self-administration. Amphetamine sensitization is prevented by pretreatment with dopamine type 1 (D_1)-receptor antagonists but not D_2-receptor antagonists. Activation of D_1, but not D_2, receptors in the ventral tegmental area (VTA) increases extracellular levels of glutamate. Further, sensitization requires activation of *N*-methyl-D-aspartate (NMDA), AMPA/kainate receptors, and metabotropic glutamate receptors (mGlu).

A number of efforts have been made recently to integrate what is known about the biological changes induced by drug use and the behavioral responses to drug-related environmental stimuli and, thereby, to better understand the phenomena of addiction, particularly the tendency to relapse after a period of abstinence. One such effort emphasizes the interactions between persistent drug-induced decreases in the functional capacity of the neural systems that subserve hedonic tone and the protracted instability and increased sensitivity of the hypothalamic-pituitary-adrenal (HPA)–stress axis. Addiction is viewed as a "cycle of spiraling dysregulation of brain reward systems" and a condition in which there is a shift from the normal homeostatic range to an abnormal one—an allostatic state. Increased sensitivity to environmental stressors and release of corticotropin-releasing factor (CRF) produce responses in the dopaminergic system that are functionally equivalent to priming doses of a drug. Another perspective emphasizes the importance of drug-induced neuronal sensitization. It postulates that there is a parallel sensitization in the neural systems subserving the assignment of salience to environmental stimuli. The effect of this sensitization is that drug-related stimuli become more salient in terms of directing behavior, and that this salience is perceived as drug "wanting" or "craving." Still another effort at integration incorporates data from brain imaging studies that reveal decreased volumes in frontal cortex in many addicted subjects. The prefrontal cortex normally inhibits activity in the amygdala, which is a key area involved in emotionally charged memories, including memories of the rewarding effects of drugs that are elicited by drug-related stimuli. In this perspective, it is hypothesized that, in the addicted state, not only do drug-related stimuli evoke craving but also that there is a reduced capacity of the frontal cortex to inhibit the behavioral responses to drug "craving." Each of these efforts at synthesis is well grounded in biological and behavioral data. They are discussed more fully in Section 11.1.

Other Actions The actions of amphetamine and amphetamine-like drugs are not selective for dopamine. Amphetamine-like drugs also release norepinephrine and serotonin. Release of these transmitters may be relevant to the toxic actions of amphetamine, especially its cardiovascular toxicity.

DIAGNOSIS AND CLINICAL FEATURES

DSM-IV-TR lists a number of amphetamine (or amphetamine-like)–related disorders (Table 11.3–1) but specifies diagnostic criteria only for amphetamine intoxication (Table 11.3–2), amphetamine withdrawal (Table 11.3–3), and amphetamine-related disorder not otherwise specified (Table 11.3–4). The diagnostic criteria for the other amphetamine (or amphetamine-like)–related disorders are contained in the DSM-IV-TR sections dealing with the primary phenomenological symptom (e.g., psychosis).

Amphetamine Use Disorders The DSM-IV-TR generic criteria for dependence and abuse are applied to amphetamine and related substances (Tables 11.1–3 and 11.1–8). Depending on the dose, the route of administration, and the pattern of use, amphetamine dependence has quite variable effects on behavior, the capacity to work, and toxic consequences. With relatively low doses taken orally, behavior may be within normal limits, and dependence is manifested only by the fatigue and depressive symptoms that ensue when drug use is interrupted and by the effort devoted to ensuring a supply. With higher doses, in addition to preoccupation with getting the drug, there is often hyperactivity, restlessness, bruxism, hypertalkativeness, irritability and short-tempered behavior, decreased sleep, and decreased appetite often accompanied by weight loss. Generally, mood is elevated; the amphetamine user is gregarious and may express confidence, even some grandiosity. With very high doses and IV or pulmonary routes, behavior and judgment can be severely disrupted, dependence can develop quickly, and the likelihood of developing toxic paranoid states is high. There may also be repetitive behaviors that appear to have no rational basis, such as taking objects apart or rearranging objects. Such behaviors are believed to be analogous to the stereotypy seen when animals are repeatedly dosed with amphetamine. Severe aggressive behavior is uncommon, but it may occur during episodes of intoxication or during amphetamine-induced psychosis.

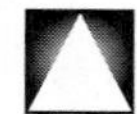

Table 11.3–1
DSM-IV-TR Amphetamine (or Amphetamine-like)–Related Disorders

Amphetamine use disorders
Amphetamine dependence
Amphetamine abuse
Amphetamine-induced disorders
Amphetamine intoxication
Specify if:
With perceptual disturbances
Amphetamine withdrawal
Amphetamine intoxication delirium
Amphetamine-induced psychotic disorder with delusions
Specify if:
With onset during intoxication
Amphetamine-induced psychotic disorder with hallucinations
Specify if:
With onset during intoxication
Amphetamine-induced mood disorder
Specify if:
With onset during intoxication
With onset during withdrawal
Amphetamine-induced anxiety disorder
Specify if:
With onset during intoxication
Amphetamine-induced sexual dysfunction
Specify if:
With onset during intoxication
Amphetamine-induced sleep disorder
Specify if:
With onset during intoxication
With onset during withdrawal
Amphetamine-related disorder not otherwise specified

From American Psychiatric Association. *Diagnostic and Statistical Manual of Mental Disorders.* 4th ed. Text rev. Washington, DC: American Psychiatric Association; 2000, with permission.

Likelihood of Progression Patients with narcolepsy and children with ADHD can take amphetamine-like drugs or methylphenidate daily for many years without developing significant tolerance to their therapeutic effects and with little escalation of dose or toxicity. When amphetamine and amphetamine-like drugs were more widely used in the treatment of obesity, relatively few patients

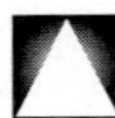

Table 11.3–2
DSM-IV-TR Diagnostic Criteria for Amphetamine Intoxication

A. Recent use of amphetamine or a related substance (e.g., methylphenidate).
B. Clinically significant maladaptive behavioral or psychological changes (e.g., euphoria or affective blunting; changes in sociability; hypervigilance; interpersonal sensitivity; anxiety, tension, or anger; stereotyped behaviors; impaired judgment; or impaired social or occupational functioning) that developed during, or shortly after, use of amphetamine or a related substance.
C. Two (or more) of the following, developing during, or shortly after, use of amphetamine or a related substance:
(1) Tachycardia or bradycardia
(2) Pupillary dilation
(3) Elevated or lowered blood pressure
(4) Perspiration or chills
(5) Nausea or vomiting
(6) Evidence of weight loss
(7) Psychomotor agitation or retardation
(8) Muscular weakness, respiratory depression, chest pain, or cardiac arrhythmias
(9) Confusion, seizures, dyskinesias, dystonias, or coma
D. The symptoms are not due to a general medical condition and are not better accounted for by another mental disorder.

Specify if:
With perceptual disturbances

From American Psychiatric Association. *Diagnostic and Statistical Manual of Mental Disorders.* 4th ed. Text rev. Washington, DC: American Psychiatric Association; 2000, with permission.

who took them daily developed dependence. Even when amphetamine-like drugs are taken for nonmedical reasons (e.g., to reduce fatigue or for euphorigenic effects), not all users progress to abuse or dependence. Although the absolute risk of such progression is not precisely known, all estimates suggest that it is high enough to justify a policy that discourages experimentation. One estimate of risk comes from a classic study, carried out in 1974 and published in 1976, of drug use among a representative sample of young men. Seventy-three percent reported having had no experience with amphetamines. Of the remaining 27 percent, almost 10 percent (or 3 percent of the total sample), reported that they used amphetamines daily. Findings from the NCS conducted in the early 1990s were remarkably similar. Approximately 15 percent of interviewees had used a stimulant other than cocaine for extramedical reasons. Of these users, 11.2 percent had become dependent on them (DSM-III-R criteria) by the time of the interview. A more recent analysis found that, among those who use cocaine, approximately 15 percent develop dependence within 10 years of first use.

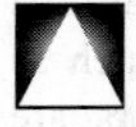

Table 11.3–4
DSM-IV-TR Diagnostic Criteria for Amphetamine-Related Disorder Not Otherwise Specified

The amphetamine-related disorder not otherwise specified category is for disorders associated with the use of amphetamine (or a related substance) that are not classifiable as amphetamine dependence, amphetamine abuse, amphetamine intoxication, amphetamine withdrawal, amphetamine intoxication delirium, amphetamine-induced psychotic disorder, amphetamine-induced mood disorder, amphetamine-induced anxiety disorder, amphetamine-induced sexual dysfunction, or amphetamine-induced sleep disorder.

From American Psychiatric Association. *Diagnostic and Statistical Manual of Mental Disorders.* 4th ed. Text rev. Washington, DC: American Psychiatric Association; 2000, with permission.

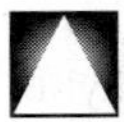

Table 11.3–3
DSM-IV-TR Diagnostic Criteria for Amphetamine Withdrawal

A. Cessation of (or reduction in) amphetamine (or a related substance) use that has been heavy and prolonged.
B. Dysphoric mood and two (or more) of the following physiological changes, developing within a few hours to several days after Criterion A:
(1) Fatigue
(2) Vivid, unpleasant dreams
(3) Insomnia or hypersomnia
(4) Increased appetite
(5) Psychomotor retardation or agitation
C. The symptoms in Criterion B cause clinically significant distress or impairment in social, occupational, or other important areas of functioning.
D. The symptoms are not due to a general medical condition and are not better accounted for by another mental disorder.

From American Psychiatric Association. *Diagnostic and Statistical Manual of Mental Disorders.* 4th ed. Text rev. Washington, DC: American Psychiatric Association; 2000, with permission.

Varied Patterns of Use There are several patterns of abuse of amphetamines and similar agents. Some people may use the drugs intermittently in relatively low doses; for example, truck drivers or students may use them to overcome fatigue or the need for sleep or to derive some positive mood effects. Some intermittent users become dependent and find it difficult to stop; some may eventually escalate the dosage. Because the drugs are no longer available legitimately for these purposes, people with that pattern of use are likely to obtain them from illicit sources.

Some people use amphetamines primarily to induce euphoria. Such users often progress to high dosages, especially if they use the drugs intravenously or by inhalation. These are obviously the most dangerous patterns of use, and they commonly lead to compulsive use or toxic effects. Although IV use initially may be intermittent, with days or weeks elapsing between episodes, such high-dose use often progresses to "sprees" or "speed runs," during which several grams of amphetamine might be smoked or injected. The runs can last for days or weeks and are commonly punctuated by episodes of toxicity (amphetamine-induced psychotic disorder with delusions or amphetamine intoxication delirium) or by brief periods of abstinence ("crashing"), generally precipitated by an interruption in the supply of the drug or exhaustion. Some clinicians have observed that in contrast to cocaine users, who prefer to smoke cocaine and use in binges interrupted by periods of cocaine abstinence, methamphetamine users are more likely to use on a daily basis and tend to change routes of administration because the drug is irritating to the nasal mucosa and lungs and for economic reasons (because smoking requires twice the amount of methamphetamine powder as injection to obtain the same effect).

High-dose amphetamine users often combine amphetamine with sedatives, benzodiazepines, or opioids to modulate the stimulant effects. Alcohol use and alcohol abuse are common concomitants of high-dose amphetamine abuse and dependence. Methamphetamine is sometimes used to reduce the sedating effects of alcohol and to facilitate and prolong socializing and sexual activity. Some observers believe that methamphetamine use increases the likelihood of multiple sex partners and the transmission of human immunodeficiency virus (HIV). In a study of gay and bisexual men who were methamphetamine injectors (and were not seeking treatment), 54 percent reported sharing needles within the preceding 30 days, and 74 percent reported exchanging sex for money or drugs. The recent increase in the use of methamphetamine in California and several western states has been predominantly among white men 25 to 34 years of age.

Comorbidity The frequent cooccurrence of other psychiatric disorders and amphetamine dependence was first noted in the 1950s. The presence of other psychiatric disorders sharply increases the odds of drug dependence in general, and drug-dependent people are more likely than the general population to meet the criteria for additional psychiatric disorders.

Patients with schizophrenia commonly use amphetamine or cocaine and develop both dependence and toxic syndromes. Some schizophrenia patients report they use stimulants to alleviate negative symptoms or adverse effects of antipsychotic agents. In fact, stimulant use generally exacerbates the negative side effects of antipsychotic drugs. Special programs involving peer-based support groups seem to be effective in linking drug-using schizophrenia patients with outpatient treatment programs.

Amphetamine-Induced Disorders

All of the disorders listed in DSM-IV-TR for cocaine (intoxication, psychotic disorder, intoxication delirium, mood disorder, anxiety disorder, sleep disorder, and sexual dysfunction) may occur in association with the use of amphetamine or amphetamine-like drugs. The clinical pictures are similar and the DSM-IV-TR diagnostic criteria and codes are identical except for substitution of the word "amphetamine" for the word "cocaine."

Amphetamine Intoxication Amphetamine intoxication can occur as a result of single doses in nontolerant individuals, but it is most commonly seen in those who are amphetamine abusers or are dependent. Some of the manifestations are exaggerated effects of the drug, including euphoria, grandiosity, restlessness, hypervigilance, talkativeness, and stereotyped repetitive behaviors. The patient is generally oriented to time, place, and situation. However, intoxication may be accompanied by visual, auditory, and tactile hallucinations or illusions. Generally, patients recognize that the symptoms are drug induced. When they do not, a diagnosis of amphetamine-induced psychotic disorder should be considered. Symptoms of amphetamine intoxication usually resolve as the drug is excreted over a period of 24 to 48 hours.

The DSM-IV-TR diagnostic criteria for amphetamine intoxication (Table 11.3–2) and cocaine intoxication (Table 11.6–2) are nearly identical. DSM-IV-TR allows for noting the presence of perceptual disturbances as a symptom of amphetamine intoxication.

Amphetamine Withdrawal The severity of the amphetamine withdrawal syndrome is presumably related to the intensity and duration of the antecedent drug use. Some elements of the syndrome (dysphoria and fatigue) can be seen after relatively brief binges or "runs" of only a few days, with some less severe aspects of "crashing" reported to occur even after 24 hours of use. During phases of the amphetamine withdrawal syndrome, users may experience severe depression that tends to resolve without special treatment when sleep normalizes.

Amphetamine users stabilized on amphetamine before withdrawal have been studied. Among the findings noted as early as 1963 were a marked shortening of time to first rapid eye movement (REM) sleep and a marked rebound in total REM sleep. A return to normal levels in some cases required several weeks.

The criteria for amphetamine withdrawal are virtually identical in DSM-IV-TR and ICD-10. Less is known about the later stages of amphetamine withdrawal, but it is likely that there are periods of increased vulnerability when stimuli previously associated with use elicit memories of drug effects and craving.

Amphetamine-Induced Psychotic Disorder and Intoxication Delirium Although amphetamine-induced psychotic disorder or intoxication delirium are usually seen only when high doses are used for a long time, such syndromes have been reported in apparently vulnerable people even after therapeutic doses given for a short time. Haloperidol (Haldol) and phenothiazines have been used to treat the psychotic syndrome. The cocaine-induced delusional syndrome is typically of short duration; however, with the amphetamine-like drugs, it may not resolve for many days after drug cessation. After recovery from either a psychotic or delirium syndrome, there may be amnesia for the entire episode or some part of it.

Psychiatrists in Japan have reported that amphetamine-induced psychosis may persist for several years and that, in the acute stage, there may be disturbance of consciousness (confusion, disorientation) in addition to the more typical mood and delusional symptoms. After recovery, people who have experienced an amphetamine-induced psychosis seem to be sensitized and experience acute paranoid psychosis on reexposure to small doses of amphetamines, and some have exacerbations in response to stress.

In animal studies, rhesus monkeys show hallucinatory-like behaviors and stereotypies in response to a low-dose amphetamine challenge as long as 28 months after a 12-week course of low-dose amphetamine exposure.

Amphetamine-Induced Mood Disorder According to DSM-IV-TR, the onset of amphetamine-induced mood disorder can occur during intoxication or withdrawal (Table 13.6–18). In general, intoxication is associated with manic or mixed mood features, whereas withdrawal is associated with depressive mood features. The manic and hypomanic symptoms often seen during amphetamine use rarely (if ever) persist beyond the period of drug use, but it is not uncommon for hypophoria, anhedonia, and depressive symptoms to persist well beyond the period of withdrawal. Patients may seek treatment for such persisting symptoms. When this occurs, the clinician should consider a diagnosis of amphetamine-induced mood disorder. However, it is often difficult to distinguish a substance-induced mood disorder from a primary mood disorder, especially in patients who have a history of depressive symptoms antedating the onset of amphetamine use. Given the pharmacology of amphetamine, it is possible that drug-induced changes could aggravate and intensify a primary depressive disorder.

Amphetamine-Induced Anxiety Disorder According to DSM-IV-TR, the onset of amphetamine-induced anxiety disorder can also occur during intoxication or withdrawal. Amphetamine, like cocaine, can induce symptoms similar to those seen in obsessive-compulsive disorder (OCD), with repetitive, stereotyped behaviors. However, these symptoms ordinarily do not persist beyond the period of drug intoxication and rarely merit a distinct diagnosis. Amphetamine-like drugs can also induce panic attacks in individuals with no previous history of panic attacks. When such episodes persist well beyond the period of drug use and require clinical attention, a distinct diagnosis should be considered.

Amphetamine-Induced Sexual Dysfunction Although amphetamine is often used to enhance sexual experiences, high doses and long-term use are associated with impotence and other sexual dysfunctions. These dysfunctions are classified in DSM-IV-TR as amphetamine-induced sexual dysfunction with onset during intoxication (Table 18.1a–20).

Amphetamine-Induced Sleep Disorder Amphetamine use can produce insomnia and sleep deprivation; people undergoing amphetamine withdrawal can experience hypersomnolence and nightmares. However, unless these disturbances persist beyond the period of drug use or well beyond withdrawal and are severe enough to merit clinical attention, they do not require a separate diagnosis.

Amphetamine-Related Disorder Not Otherwise Specified If an amphetamine (or amphetamine-like)–related disorder does not meet the criteria of one or more of the previously discussed categories, it can be diagnosed as an amphetamine-related disorder not otherwise specified (Table 11.3–4). With the increasing illicit use of designer amphetamines, syndromes may arise that do not meet the criteria outlined in DSM-IV-TR and that necessitate the frequent use of the "not otherwise specified" category. If these distinct syndromes do appear, it is hoped that future updates to the DSM will accommodate these changes to assist in their clear categorization.

Toxicity and Complications In a survey of amphetamine users in Australia, subjects reported various physical and psychological problems that they attributed to amphetamine use. Commonly reported physical symptoms were tiredness (89 percent), loss of appetite (85 percent), dehydration (73 percent), and jaw clenching (73 percent). Also reported were headaches, muscle pains, shortness of breath, and tremors. The most frequently reported psychological symptoms were mood swings (80 percent), sleep problems (78 percent); anxiety, difficulty concentrating, depression, and paranoia (each approximately 70 percent); and hallucinations and episodes of aggression and violence (each approximately 45 percent). Daily use, heavier use, and being male and unemployed were correlated with reporting more symptoms.

Amphetamines produce their most dramatic toxic effects on the CNS and the cardiovascular system. In animal models (rodents and primates), chronically administered high doses of amphetamines produce long-lasting depletion of brain norepinephrine and more selective but even longer-lasting depletion of dopamine, reductions in dopamine transporter sites (Fig. 11.3–1), and reduction in serotonergic activity.

Because these effects involve damage to both axons and axon terminals, largely sparing the cell bodies, the permanence of the damages is not known. Methamphetamine, in particular, seems capable of inducing damage to serotonergic fibers, but the noradrenergic system is largely unaffected. These effects may be due to toxic biotransformation products of excessive dopamine within the neuron. The long-lasting dopaminergic changes probably account for the altered, elevated threshold for self-stimulation in animals and the anhedonia reported by chronic amphetamine users for prolonged periods after cessation. It is not known to what degree methamphetamine use causes permanent damage in humans, but data from patients with Parkinson's disease suggest that there must be considerable damage to the dopaminergic pathways before it becomes evident in function and behavior. In monkeys, the toxic effects of chronic amphetamine use include damage to cerebral blood vessels, neuronal loss, and microhemorrhages. In humans, high doses of amphetamine have also been associated with lethal hyperpyrexia and with destructive deterioration of arterioles. High doses can also produce convulsions and ultimately coma and death.

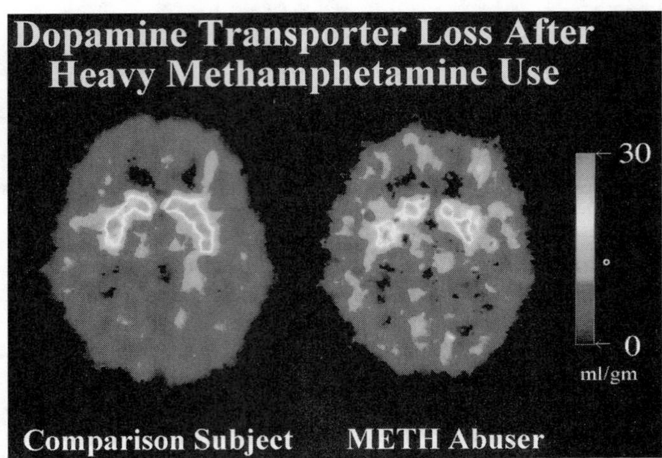

FIGURE 11.3–1 Positron emission tomography scan showing striatal dopamine transporter density in a 33-year-old male methamphetamine (METH) abuser 80 days after detoxification, compared to a 33-year-old male control subject. (See Color Plate.) (From Volkow ND, Chang L, Wang G-J, et al.: Association of dopamine transporter reduction with psychomotor impairment in methamphetamine abusers. *Am J Psychiatry.* 2001;158:377, with permission.)

Amphetamine-like drugs can cause severe cardiovascular toxicity (e.g., intracranial hemorrhage, arrhythmias, and acute cardiac failure) because of their capacity to release norepinephrine, dopamine, and serotonin and to increase blood pressure. With amphetamines, considerable tolerance develops to the effect on blood pressure. The likelihood of such cardiovascular effects is related to dose and the rapidity with which the drug is absorbed. The use of methamphetamine by smoking or IV injection is likely to result in greater cardiovascular toxicity. Amphetamine-induced hyperthermia and free radical formation are believed to be involved in causing rhabdomyolysis and the consequent renal tubular obstruction that is occasionally reported. Because amphetamine use can be associated with increased sexual activity, often accompanied by poor judgment, amphetamine users are at increased risk for venereal diseases, including HIV infection. Methamphetamine users who received highly active antiretroviral therapy but are still using have significantly higher virus loads as compared to those receiving comparable antiviral treatment whose urines are negative for methamphetamine. It is not yet clear if this is due to a direct effect of amphetamine or is a reflection of reduced compliance with treatment.

PATHOLOGY AND LABORATORY EXAMINATIONS

Amphetamine and amphetamine-like drugs can be detected for varying lengths of time in urine—usually several days, depending on frequency of use, amount of dose, and sensitivity of the testing method. Metabolites can also be detected in blood, saliva, and hair. Blood and saliva furnish a better index of current levels, whereas urine provides a longer window of opportunity for detecting use over the previous few days. Hair analysis can reveal drug use over a period of weeks to months but has little applicability in clinical situations.

Positron emission tomography (PET), magnetic resonance spectroscopy, and functional magnetic resonance imaging (MRI) studies of the brains of methamphetamine users have shown that methamphetamine users have regional brain dysfunction, which accompanies deficits in mood and cognitive function. Compared with control subjects, abstinent methamphetamine users exhibit regional neurochemical abnormalities, with relationships between relative metabolism in limbic/paralimbic regions and self-reports of depression and anxiety. Decreased dopamine transporter density has been observed in abstinent amphetamine users, but this is typically not as severe as in patients with Parkinson's disease. In one such study, dopamine transporter reduction was correlated with cognitive deficits and with years of methamphetamine use but not with dose. Another study found some recovery of dopamine transporter in some patients after several months of abstinence; but in another, striatal dopamine transporter reduction was still low in methamphetamine users who had been abstinent for several years. Motor skills and memory may remain impaired even when there is some recovery of dopamine transporter density.

DIFFERENTIAL DIAGNOSIS

The disorders associated with the use of amphetamine and amphetamine-like drugs need to be distinguished from both primary mental disorders and disorders induced by other classes of drugs. A history of the drug ingestion is important for making these distinctions. However, given the unreliability of self-reports about drug use and the likelihood that many users deny any drug use at all, laboratory testing for drugs in body fluids and histories from collaterals are very important. Disorders associated with amphetamine use cannot be easily distinguished from those associated with cocaine except by a reliable history or laboratory tests. Users of amphetamine or cocaine and related drugs may exhibit inappropriate optimism, euphoria, and expansiveness, excessive talkativeness, and a decreased need for sleep sometimes associated with irritability in the context of a clear sensorium—a pattern that is also observed in manic and hypomanic episodes of bipolar I disorder and bipolar II disorder, respectively. Those symptoms, however, may not be obvious enough to suggest their relation to drug use, and the first indication of drug dependence may be financial difficulties, an arrest for selling drugs or possessing them, or some drug-induced toxicity.

Intoxication

Amphetamine intoxication is diagnosed when the effects of the drug exceed the mood-elevating effects that users typically seek when they use amphetamines. The diagnosis of intoxication is appropriate when the drug effects are problematic enough to require differentiation from hypomanic or manic behavior.

Amphetamine and amphetamine-like drug intoxication can also be confused with phencyclidine (PCP) intoxication, although the latter is usually associated with nystagmus, motor incoordination, and some cognitive impairment. Endocrine disorders (such as Cushing's disease) and the excessive use of steroids should also be considered. Dangerously elevated body temperature and convulsions occur with methamphetamine overdoses and, if untreated, can result in death.

Psychotic Disorders

Amphetamine-induced toxic psychosis can be exceedingly difficult to differentiate from schizophrenia and other psychotic disorders characterized by hallucinations or delusions. Paranoid delusions occur in approximately 80 percent of patients and hallucinations in 60 to 70 percent. Consciousness is clear, and disorientation is uncommon. However, mood changes are common, with the user rapidly changing from friendly to hostile. The presence of repetitive and stereotypical acts associated with irritability, excitement, and vivid visual, auditory, or tactile hallucinations should raise suspicion of a drug-induced disorder. In areas and populations in which amphetamine use is common, it may be necessary to provide only a provisional diagnosis until the patient can be observed and drug test results are obtained. Even then, there may be difficulties because, in some urban areas, a high percentage of people with established diagnoses of schizophrenia also use amphetamines or cocaine. Typically, symptoms of amphetamine psychosis remit within 1 week, but, in a small proportion of patients, psychosis may last for more than 1 month.

Anxiety Disorders

Amphetamine-induced anxiety disorder must also be distinguished from panic disorder and generalized anxiety disorder.

Other Symptoms

The symptoms that may emerge during withdrawal (depression, dysphoria, anhedonia, disturbed sleep) need to be distinguished from those of primary mood disorders and primary sleep disorders. Unless the symptoms are more intense or more prolonged than is typical of amphetamine withdrawal and require independent treatment, the diagnosis should be limited to withdrawal rather than amphetamine-induced mood disorder. When a diagnosis of amphetamine-induced mood disorder is made, one must specify whether its onset was during intoxication or in withdrawal. It is also possible to specify the subtype of mood disorder (with depressive, manic, or mixed features). In differentiating amphetamine-induced mood disorder from the primary mood disorder, the critical factor is the clinician's judgment that the mood disorder was caused by the drug. An amphetamine-induced mood disorder, or mood disorder with onset during intoxication or withdrawal, usually remits within a week or two. It is appropriate, therefore, to withhold judgment about the diagnosis during the early phase of withdrawal. If depressed mood and related symptoms persist beyond a few weeks, the possibility of alternative causes should be entertained. In considering diagnostic possibilities, the clinician should consider the age of the patient at the onset of symptoms and a history of episodes of mood disorder that developed before the onset of drug use or during any long intervals when there was no significant drug abuse.

COURSE AND PROGNOSIS

The natural history of amphetamine dependence in the United States is less well documented than that of opioids or cocaine. Some researchers believe that some IV amphetamine users in the 1960s moved on to heroin use in the 1970s. However, it seems likely that many whose use was less severe simply stopped or recovered, whereas others intensified their use of alcohol.

Findings from treatment programs in California suggest that the course and prognosis for amphetamine dependence are probably similar to those for cocaine dependence. Follow-up studies of methamphetamine users treated in California in the mid-1990s also showed that a substantial percentage were no longer using methamphetamine 2 to 3 years after treatment. Among patients treated in publicly funded programs, 36 percent resumed use within 6 months, and an additional 15 percent did so within 7 to 19 months. Shorter length of treatment and involvement in selling methamphetamine predicted more rapid relapse. In a follow-up of participants in another California program that included fewer indigent patients, 80 percent reported no methamphetamine use in the 30 days before the interview; these reports were confirmed by urine tests. However, this was not a random sample. Those contacted were more likely to have completed treatment. It is also of interest that, among this group, 63 percent reported symptoms of depression during the 30 days before interview, approximately the same percentage that reported depression at treatment entry.

Japanese clinicians believe that some amphetamine users may develop persistent psychosis and that those who recover remain at high risk of reexperiencing psychosis if they use amphetamines again (sensitization). A 3- to 8-year follow-up study of 110 methamphetamine users hospitalized for drug-related problems in Japan in the 1980s found that 12 former patients had died, a mortality rate 11 times that of age- and sex-matched general population controls. However, 56 percent of those still alive had not used amphetamine-like drugs in the year before interview, and most of them also showed improvements in work and family relationships. Twenty-five percent were believed to have highly or moderately unfavorable outcomes in terms of drug use, work, and family relationships. The prognosis for Japanese convicted and imprisoned for crimes related to stimulant drug use seems as bleak as that for convicted and imprisoned drug users in the United States; 58 percent committed crimes within 1 year after release, and 98 percent committed crimes within 5 years.

TREATMENT

There are no specific, well-established treatments for dependence on amphetamine or amphetamine-like drugs and few controlled studies on the treatment of amphetamine dependence. Most casual users do not need or seek treatment. Those with moderately severe dependence obtain treatment in a variety of settings (mostly outpatient, drug free) that were not designed specifically to treat amphetamine dependence. The most severe cases, those within the criminal justice system and the homeless, generally drop out of outpatient treatment because of their complex needs or are unable to access treatment at all. Some data on treatment seeking and outcome are available for the state of California where amphetamine abuse began to increase in the early 1990s. In general, methamphetamine users in the state gave reasons for entering treatment similar to those of other substance users: personal motivation (69 percent), pressure from the criminal justice system (31 percent), and insistence from family or other significant people (22 percent). Treatment received ranged from residential and ambulatory detoxification to day treatment, 12-step activities, and case management. Although those leaving 12-step programs were more likely to have been considered treatment completers, at follow-up, patients reported similar reductions in drug use (unverified by urine tests) regardless of the treatment received and were neither more nor less successful in this respect than those receiving treatment for heroin, cocaine, or marijuana use. One psychosocial treatment strategy used a combination of group and individual counseling initially developed for crack cocaine users and was found to produce equal patient participation levels and equally good outcomes for those dependent on methamphetamine. This approach, the Matrix Neurobehavioral Model, uses a highly structured and manualized cognitive-behavioral treatment and contingency management program. A recently completed seven-site evaluation of this model suggested that such an approach can be effective across a varied group of treatment settings in a wide range of amphetamine users.

Because there are a number of similarities between amphetamine dependence and cocaine dependence, it is reasonable to assume that a number of the behavioral methods used in the treatment of cocaine dependence and described in Section 11.6 are also useful with patients who are dependent on amphetamines.

A wide variety of pharmacological agents have been explored as adjuncts to, or major elements in, the treatment of amphetamine dependence. Some have been studied in controlled trials. Virtually all of these agents had been previously tried in the treatment of cocaine dependence and produced comparably disappointing results. For example, although imipramine (Tofranil), 150 mg a day, improved treatment retention, it had no significant effect on methamphetamine use. Although an open-label trial of fluoxetine (Prozac), 20 mg a day, was reported to be useful in amphetamine dependence, success in dozens of open-label trials with cocaine-dependent patients has rarely been confirmed when the same agents were studied in double-blind, controlled trials.

In Europe and Australia, the ethics and efficacy of prescribing oral amphetamines for amphetamine users are hotly debated. This practice is allowed in the United Kingdom, although it varies from region to region, and virtually no safeguards exist against diversion of prescribed amphetamines to the illicit market. No outcome studies exist that evaluate the values and risks of this practice.

Selection of Treatment Setting

The general principles of treatment for amphetamine dependence are not very different from those for cocaine and opioid dependence, but there are fewer replicated studies on the efficacy of any particular treatment approach. As with cocaine and opioid dependence, amphetamine dependence severe enough to require formal treatment is often associated with other psychiatric diagnoses.

Patient heterogeneity requires thoughtful selection among available alternatives. Not all amphetamine users require extensive treatment; some users who are not dependent respond to external pressures, as when employers insist on careful monitoring of drug use. The executive with little history of psychopathology, a supportive social network, financial assets, and personal skills has a different prognosis and a wider range of options than does a patient who is unemployed, alienated from the family, and perhaps also using opioids. Severe depression, psychotic manifestations beyond the initial withdrawal period, and drug use that is completely out of control (i.e., repeated inability to respond to outpatient efforts) seem to be the major accepted criteria for hospitalization.

OTHER AGENTS

Substituted Amphetamines

MDMA (ecstasy) is one of a series of substituted amphetamines that also includes 3,4-methylenedioxyethylamphetamine (MDEA; "Eve"), 3,4-methylenedioxyamphetamine (MDA), 2,5-dimethoxy-4-bromoamphetamine (DOB), *para*-methoxyamphetamine (PMA), and others. These drugs produce mood-improving, stimulant, and hallucinogenic subjective effects resembling a combination of amphetamine and lysergic acid diethylamide (LSD), and in that sense, MDMA and similar analogs may represent a distinct category of drugs.

A methamphetamine derivative that came into use in the 1980s, MDMA was not technically subject to legal regulation at the time. Although it has been labeled a "designer drug" in the belief that it was deliberately synthesized to evade legal regulation, it was actually synthesized and patented in 1914. Several psychiatrists used it as an adjunct to psychotherapy and concluded that it was of value. At one time, it was advertised as legal and was used in psychotherapy for its subjective effects; however, the FDA never approved it. MDMA use in therapy raised questions of both safety and legality because the related amphetamine derivatives MDA, DOB, and PMA had caused a number of overdose deaths, and MDA was known to cause extensive destruction of serotonergic nerve terminals in the CNS. Using emergency scheduling authority, the Drug Enforcement

Agency made MDMA a schedule I drug under the CSA along with LSD, heroin, and marijuana. Despite its illegal status, MDMA continues to be manufactured, distributed, and used in the United States, Europe, Australia, and Asia Pacific. Its use is common at extended dances ("raves") popular with adolescents and young adults.

Mechanisms of Action The unusual properties of the drugs may be a consequence of the different actions of the optical isomers: the *R*(–) isomers produce LSD-like effects, and the amphetamine-like properties are linked to *S*(+) isomers. The LSD-like actions, in turn, may be linked to the capacity to release serotonin. The various derivatives may exhibit significant differences in subjective effects and toxicity. Animals in laboratory experiments self-administer the drugs, suggesting prominent amphetamine-like effects.

Subjective Effects After taking usual doses (100 to 150 mg), MDMA users experience elevated mood and, according to various reports, increased self-confidence and sensory sensitivity; peaceful feelings coupled with insight, empathy, and closeness to people; and decreased appetite. Difficulty in concentrating and an increased capacity to focus have both been reported. Dysphoric reactions, psychotomimetic effects, and psychosis have also been reported. Higher doses seem more likely to produce psychotomimetic effects. Sympathomimetic effects of tachycardia, palpitation, increased blood pressure, sweating, and bruxism are common. The subjective effects are reported to be prominent for approximately 4 to 8 hours, but they may not last as long or may last longer, depending on the dose and route of administration. The drug is usually taken orally, but it has been snorted and injected. Users have reported both tachyphylaxis and some tolerance.

The acute adverse effects reported include precipitation of episodes of panic and anxiety. Brief psychiatric disturbances that are more severe can also occur, and preexisting pathology does not appear to be a requisite for severe reactions. A healthy drug-free male subject, known to be without personal and family psychiatric illness, was given a 140-mg dose of the drug and developed a psychosis lasting 2.5 hours that included vivid auditory and visual hallucinations and a belief that people were making noise to annoy him intentionally.

After the acute effects of MDMA, there may be a combination of some diminishing residual effects gradually superseded by feelings of drowsiness, fatigue, depression, and difficulty concentrating—somewhat comparable to the crash after cessation of amphetamine use. When young adults who were Saturday-night MDMA users were compared with alcohol-only users who frequented the same club, the MDMA users reported elevated mood on the following day but feelings of depression (Beck Depression Inventory scores of approximately 12) by the fifth day. In contrast, alcohol-only users showed relatively little mood change over the 5-day period; their highest Beck depression scores (approximately 8) occurred on the second day. In a double-blind, placebo-controlled study of normal volunteers given 1.7 mg/kg of body weight of MDMA, some subjects continued to report symptoms typical of MDMA actions (suppressed appetite, jaw clenching, restlessness, heaviness in the legs, difficulty concentrating) 24 hours later. More persistent neuropsychiatric adverse effects associated with MDMA use include anxiety, depression, flashbacks, irritability, panic disorder, psychosis, and memory disturbance.

Toxicity Although it is not as toxic as MDA, various somatic toxicities attributable to MDMA use have been reported as well as fatal overdoses. It does not appear to be neurotoxic when injected into the brain of animals, but it is metabolized to MDA in both animals and humans. In animals, MDMA produces selective, long-lasting damage to serotonergic nerve terminals. It is not certain if the levels of the MDA metabolite reached in humans after the usual doses of MDMA suffice to produce lasting damage. Nonhuman primates are more sensitive than are rodents to MDMA's toxic effects and show more prolonged or permanent neurotoxicity at doses not much higher than those used by humans. Users of MDMA show differences in neuroendocrine responses to serotonergic probes, and studies of former MDMA users show global and regional decreases in serotonin transporter binding, as measured by PET. Although psychological assessment of small samples of users do not routinely find evidence of current anxiety or a mood disorder, users studied in several different countries have shown some impairment on at least one test of neuropsychological function.

Other reported toxicities include arrhythmias, cardiovascular collapse, hyperthermia, rhabdomyolysis, disseminated intravascular coagulation, acute renal failure, and hepatotoxicity. The role that contaminants in illicit MDMA play in the toxic reactions is uncertain, but significant elevations of blood pressure and temperature have been observed after administration of pure MDMA.

MDMA dependence does not appear to be a significant problem in the United States, but cases of dependence have been reported in England. Among a sample of MDMA users in Australia, 28 percent reported that problems related to the use of the drug were mostly acute reactions such as panic, paranoia, loss of reality, and hallucinations. Only 2 percent reported feeling dependent (needing to use it every day to cope), but 22 percent claimed that they knew someone who had been dependent, and 47 percent believed it was possible to become addicted. MDA, MDMA, PMA, and MDEA have all been linked to psychosis and overdose deaths. The toxic manifestations of overdose include restlessness, agitation, sweating, rigidity, high blood pressure, tachycardia, hyperpyrexia, and convulsions. Chlorpromazine (Thorazine) prevented lethality in dogs, but there are no clinical reports of its use for this purpose in humans.

There are currently no established clinical uses for MDMA, although, before its regulation, there were several reports of its beneficial effects as an adjunct to psychotherapy.

"Club Drugs" The use of a certain group of substances popularly called *club drugs* is often associated with dance clubs, bars, and all-night dance parties (raves). The group includes LSD, γ-hydroxybutyrate (GHB), ketamine, methamphetamine, MDMA (ecstasy), and Rohypnol or "roofies" (flunitrazepam). These substances are not all in the same drug class, nor do they produce the same physical or subjective effects. GHB, ketamine, and Rohypnol have been called *date rape drugs* because they produce disorienting and sedating effects, and often users cannot recall what occurred during all or part of an episode under the influence of the drug. Hence, it is alleged that these drugs might be surreptitiously placed in a beverage, or a person might be convinced to take the drug and then not recall clearly what occurred after ingestion.

Emergency department mentions of GHB, ketamine, and Rohypnol are relatively few. Of the club drugs, methamphetamine is the substance that accounts for the largest share of Drug Abuse Warning Network (DAWN) emergency department mentions and the highest number of deaths (approximately 2,600) in the 5 years from 1994 to 1998. MDMA use generated more national concern and media coverage during 1994 to 1998 because young people were disproportionately represented in emergency department visits involving club drugs. The number of emergency department visits related to MDMA, GHB, and ketamine increased significantly during this period.

Khat The fresh leaves of *Catha edulis,* a bush native to East Africa, have been used as a stimulant in the Middle East, Africa, and the Arabian peninsula for at least 1,000 years. Khat is still widely used in Ethiopia, Kenya, Somalia, and Yemen. The amphetamine-like effects of khat have long been recognized, and although efforts to isolate the active ingredient were first undertaken in the 19th century, only since the 1970s has cathinone (*S*[–]α-aminopropiophenone or *S*-2-amino-1-phenyl-1-propanone) been identified as the substance responsible for those effects. Cathinone is a precursor moiety that is normally enzymatically converted in the plant to the less active entities norephedrine and cathine (norpseudoephedrine), which explains why only the fresh leaves of the plant are valued for their stimulant effects. Cathinone has most of the CNS and peripheral actions of amphetamine and appears to have the same mechanism of action. In humans, it elevates mood, decreases hunger, and alleviates fatigue. Like amphetamine, it is self-administered by laboratory animals and produces increased locomotor activity and stereotypy. At high doses, it can induce an amphetamine-like psychosis in humans. Because it is typically absorbed buccally after chewing the leaf and because the alkaloid is metabolized relatively rapidly, high toxic blood levels are not frequently reached. Concern about khat use is linked to its dependence-producing properties rather than to its acute toxicity. It is estimated that five million doses are consumed each day despite prohibition of its use in a number of African and Arab countries.

In the 1990s, several clandestine laboratories began synthesizing methcathinone, a drug with actions quite similar to those of cathinone. Known by a number of street names (e.g., CAT, goob, and crank), its popularity is due primarily to its ease of synthesis from ephedrine or pseudoephedrine, which were readily available until placed under special controls. Methcathinone has been moved to schedule I of the CSA. The patterns of use, adverse effects, and complications are quite similar to those reported for amphetamine.

SUGGESTED CROSS-REFERENCES

The neural sciences are presented in Chapter 1 and neuropsychiatry and behavioral neurology in Chapter 2. A classification of mental disorders appears in Chapter 9. An introduction to and overview of substance-related disorders are presented in Section 11.1, cocaine-related disorders in Section 11.6, and various drugs in Chapter 31 on biological therapies, particularly sympathomimetics in Section 31.26. Schizophrenia is discussed in Chapter 12, other psychotic disorders in Section 12.16, and attention-deficit disorders in Section 39.1.

REFERENCES

Anthony JC, Warner LA, Kessler RC: Comparative epidemiology of dependence on tobacco, alcohol, controlled substances, and inhalants: Basic findings from the National Comorbidity Survey. *Exp Clin Psychopharmacol.* 1994;2:244.

Castner SA, Goldman-Rakic PS: Long-lasting psychotomimetic consequences of repeated low-dose amphetamine exposure in rhesus monkeys. *Neuropsychopharmacology.* 1999;20:10.

Ellis RJ, Childers ME, Cherner M, Lazzaretto D, Letendre S, Grant I: The HIV Neurobehavioral Research Center Group. Increased human immunodeficiency virus loads in active methamphetamine users are explained by reduced effectiveness of antiretroviral therapy. *J Infect Dis.* 2003;188:1820.

Farrell M, Marsden J, Ali R, Ling W: Methamphetamine: Drug use and psychoses becomes a major public health issue in the Asia Pacific region. *Addiction.* 2002;97:771.

Goldstein RZ, Volkow ND: Drug addiction and its underlying neurobiological basis: Neuroimaging evidence for the involvement of the frontal cortex. *Am J Psychiatry.* 2002;159:1642.

*Gorelick DA. Pharmacologic interventions for cocaine, crack, and other stimulant addiction. In: Graham AW, Schultz TK, Mayo-Smith FM, Ries RK, Wilford BB, eds. *Principles of Addiction Medicine.* 3rd ed. Chevy Chase, MD: American Society of Addiction Medication, Inc.; 2003.

*Gorelick DA, Cornish JL. The pharmacology of cocaine, amphetamines, and other stimulants. In: Graham AW, Schultz TK, Mayo-Smith FM, Ries RK, Wilford BB, eds. *Principles of Addiction Medicine.* 3rd ed. Chevy Chase, MD: American Society of Addiction Medication, Inc.; 2003.

*Green AR, Mechan AO, Elliott JM, O'Shea E, Colado MI: The pharmacology and clinical pharmacology of 3,4-methylenedioxymethamphetamine (MDMA, "Ecstasy"). *Pharmacol Rev.* 2003;55:463.

*Hall W, Hando J. Patterns of amphetamine use in Australia. In: Klee H, ed. *Amphetamine Misuse. International Perspectives on Current Trends.* Reading, Australia: Harwood Academic Publishers; 1997.

Hall W, Hando J, Darke S, Ross J: Psychological morbidity and route of administration among amphetamine users in Sydney, Australia. *Addiction.* 1996;91:81.

Jansen KLR: Ecstasy (MDMA) dependence. *Drug Alcohol Depend.* 1999;53:121.

Jaworski JN, Kozel MA, Philpot KB, Kuhar MJ: Intra-accumbal injection of CART (cocaine-amphetamine regulated transcript) peptide reduces cocaine-induced locomotor activity. *J Pharmacol Exp Ther.* 2003;307:1038.

Johnston LD, O'Malley PM, Bachman JG. *Monitoring the Future National Results on Adolescent Drug Use: Overview of Key Findings, 2001.* (NIH Publication No. 02-5105.) Bethesda, MD: National Institute on Drug Abuse; 2002.

Kalant OJ. *The Amphetamines.* Springfield, IL: Charles C. Thomas; 1973.

Kalix P: Pharmacological properties of the stimulant khat. *Pharmacol Ther.* 1990;48:397.

Kandel DB, Davies M: High school students who use crack and other drugs. *Arch Gen Psychiatry.* 1996;53:71.

Kendler KS, Prescott CA, Myers J, Neale MC: The structure of genetic and environmental risk factors for common psychiatric and substance use disorders in men and women. *Arch Gen Psychiatry.* 2003;60:929.

Kessler RC, McGonagle KA, Zhao S, Nelson CB, Hughes M, Eshelman S, Wittchen H-U, Kendler KS: Lifetime and 12-month prevalence of DSM-III-R psychiatric disorders in the United States. *Arch Gen Psychiatry.* 1994;51:8.

*Koob GF, LeMoal M: Drug addiction, dysregulation of reward, and allostasis. *Neuropsychopharmacology* 2000;24:97.

London ED, Simon SL, Berman SM, Mandelkern MA, Lichtman AM, Bramen J, Shinn AK, Miotto K, Learn J, Dong Y, Matochik JA, Kurian V, Newton T, Woods R, Rawson R, Ling R: Regional cerebral dysfunction associated with mood disturbances in abstinent methamphetamine abusers. *Arch Gen Psychiatry.* 2004;61:73.

McCann UD, Wong DF, Yokoi F, Villemagne V, Dannals RF, Ricaurte GA: Reduced striatal dopamine transporter density in abstinent methamphetamine and methcathinone users: Evidence from positron emission tomography studies with [^{11}C]Win-35,428. *J Neurosci.* 1998;18:8417.

Meng Y, Dukat M, Bridgen DT, Martin BR, Lichtman AH: Pharmacological effects of methamphetamine and other stimulants via inhalation exposure. *Drug Alcohol Depend.* 1999;53:111.

*Nestler EJ: Molecular neurobiology of addiction. *Am J Addict.* 2001;10:201.

Office of Applied Studies. *Results from the 2001 National Household Survey on Drug Abuse: Volume 1. Summary of National Findings.* National Household Survey on Drug Abuse Series H-17, DHHS publ. No. SMA 02-3758. Rockville, MD: Substance Abuse and Mental Health Services Administration; 2002.

Rawson RA, Huber A, Brethen P, Obert J, Gulati V, Shoptaw S, Ling W: Status of methamphetamine users 2-5 years after outpatient treatment. *J Addict Dis.* 2002;21:107.

Robinson TE, Berridge KC: The psychology and neurobiology of addiction: An incentive sensitization view. *Addiction.* 2000;95[Suppl 2]:S91.

Seiden LS, Sabol KE, Ricaurte GA: Amphetamine: Effects on catecholamine systems and behavior. *Ann Rev Pharmacol Toxicol.* 1993;33:639.

Solowij N, Hall W, Lee N: Recreational MDMA use in Sydney: A profile of "ecstasy" users and their experiences with the drug. *Br J Addict.* 1992;87;1161.

Stephans SE, Yamamoto BK: Methamphetamine-induced neurotoxicity: Roles for glutamate and dopamine efflux. *Synapse.* 1994;17:203.

Strang J, Sheridan J: Prescribing amphetamines to drug misusers: Data from the 1995 national survey of community pharmacies in England and Wales. *Addiction.* 1997;92:833.

Suto N, Tanabe LM, Austin JD, Creekmore E, Vezina P: Previous exposure to VTA amphetamine enhances cocaine self-administration under a progressive ratio schedule in an NMDA, AMPA/Kainate, and metabotropic glutamate receptor-dependent manner. *Neuropsychopharmacology.* 2003;28:629.

Tsuang MT, Lyons MJ, Meyer JM, Doyle T, Eisen SA, Goldberg J, True W, Lin N, Toomey R, Eaves L: Co-occurrence of abuse of different drugs in men. *Arch Gen Psychiatry.* 1998;55:967.

Vanderschuren LJ, Kalivas PW: Alterations in dopaminergic and glutamatergic transmission in the induction and expression of behavioral sensitization: A critical review of preclinical studies. *Psychopharmacology (Berlin).* 2000;151:99.

Volkow ND, Chang L, Wang G-J, Fowler JS, Leonido-Yee M, Franceschi D, Sedler M, Gatley SJ, Hitzemann R, Ding Y-S, Logan J, Wong C, Miller EN: Association of dopamine transporter reduction with psychomotor impairment in methamphetamine abusers. *Am J Psychiatry.* 2001;158:377.

Volkow ND, Wang G-J, Fowler JS, Gatley SJ, Logan J, Ding Y-S, Hitzemann R, Pappas N: Dopamine transporter occupancies in the human brain induced by therapeutic doses of oral methylphenidate. *Am J Psychiatry.* 1998;155:10.

Vollenweider FZ, Gamma A, Liechti M, Huber T: Psychological and cardiovascular effects and short-term sequelae of MDMA ("ecstasy") in MDMA-naive healthy volunteers. *Neuropsychopharmacology.* 1998;19:241.

*White FJ, Kalivas PW: Neuroadaptations involved in amphetamine and cocaine addiction. *Drug Alcohol Depend.* 1998;51:141.

Yui K, Goto K, Ikemoto S, Ishiguro T: Stress induced spontaneous recurrence of methamphetamine psychosis: The relation between stressful experiences and sensitivity to stress. *Drug Alcohol Depend.* 2000;58:67.

▲ 11.4 Caffeine-Related Disorders

ERIC C. STRAIN, M.D., AND ROLAND R. GRIFFITHS, PH.D.

Caffeine is the most widely consumed psychoactive substance in the world. Although numerous studies have documented the safety of caffeine when used in typical daily doses, there are psychiatric symptoms and disorders that can be associated with its use. Although rates for these disorders are not well established, even a low prevalence could still result in a considerable number of people with these disorders due to the widespread use of caffeine. Hence, it is important for the clinician to be familiar with caffeine, its effects, and problems that can be associated with its use.

HISTORY

Caffeine-containing foods and beverages have been consumed for hundreds, if not thousands, of years. Tea has been cultivated and consumed in China since at least 350 AD, and coffee cultivation spread from Ethiopia to Arabia in the 15th century and subsequently became a popular beverage in Arabic cultures during the 16th century. Initially, most caffeine consumption occurred in restricted geographical regions where caffeine-containing plants were indigenous. It was not until the 17th century that caffeine use began to spread, eventually achieving its current, virtually universal availability. The Dutch imported caffeine in the form of coffee from Arabic countries to Europe, where it first became popular around the middle to end of the 17th century (along with tea, tobacco, and chocolate). Medical literature during this time period described coffee as a useful beverage for a wide variety of conditions, although it is notable that coffee's use to induce sobriety was a particularly attractive feature. However, considerable controversy about whether the use of coffee was beneficial or detrimental to health was associated with its expansion into Western cultures—controversy that is mirrored in contemporary concerns over the use of caffeine.

The expansion of coffee consumption during the 17th and 18th centuries can be demonstrated by the estimate that there were between 2,000 and 3,000 coffeehouses in London by the early part of the 17th century (approximately one coffeehouse for every 200 to 300 people). The spread and popularity of coffeehouses in Europe highlight how coffee was initially a beverage consumed in public; it was only later that coffee became a beverage consumed in the home. Perhaps the most famous of the coffeehouses in London was operated by Edward Lloyd. Like most coffeehouses, Lloyd's was a center of business, especially for insurance agents, and by the end of the 18th century, Lloyd's became the well-known Lloyd's of London insurance company. However, in England, coffee use was eventually supplanted by tea consumption, with the shift in beverage preference occurring in the first half of the 18th century.

In the United States, a shift from tea to coffee use occurred in 1773 when colonists protesting British taxes threw cargoes of tea overboard in the Boston harbor—the Boston tea party. The repercussions of this event continue to the present day; the United States is now the major consumer of coffee in the world.

In the late 19th century, caffeine began appearing in various soft drink beverages. Although some caffeine contained in soft drink beverages is derived from the cola nut, most caffeine in soft drinks is added—reportedly as a flavoring agent; however, the flavoring role of caffeine in soft drinks has been challenged. In the United States, caffeine is also added to noncola soft drinks and to some bottled waters, and consumption of soft drinks has increased markedly over the past 30 years.

In the contemporary world, caffeine is integral to the economic activity of several countries. For example, only crude oil produces more foreign exchange earnings than coffee for developing countries. In the United States, coffee is the major agricultural import and in value is second only to oil among all imports. This economic and trade activity underscores the extent to which caffeine use has spread over the past four centuries so that caffeine is now available and accepted virtually everywhere in the world.

COMPARATIVE NOSOLOGY

There is no mention made of caffeine-related disorders in the first edition of the *Diagnostic and Statistical Manual of Mental Disorders* (DSM-I), which was published in 1952. In the second edition of DSM (DSM-II), published in 1968, caffeine (and, interestingly, tobacco) are explicitly excluded from consideration for a diagnosis of drug dependence, and no other mention of caffeine use disorders is included in this edition. The American Psychiatric Association first included caffeine (and tobacco) use disorders in the third edition of DSM (DSM-III) in 1980. At that time, *caffeine intoxication*—the only caffeine-related disorder in DSM-III—was included as a discrete syndrome with specific criteria for its diagnosis. Over successive editions of the DSM, caffeine intoxication has remained, and the fourth edition of DSM (DSM-IV) has included criteria for caffeine withdrawal in its appendix as a proposed category requiring further study. Currently, the revised fourth edition of DSM (DSM-IV-TR) suggests that further research is needed to establish caffeine withdrawal as a discrete syndrome. The DSM-IV-TR has also included diagnoses of caffeine-induced anxiety and caffeine-induced sleep disorders—that is, conditions in which specific caffeine-induced symptoms (anxiety, sleep disturbance) require clinical attention. Caffeine abuse and caffeine dependence are not included in DSM-IV-TR, although there is evidence that some patients can exhibit a caffeine dependence syndrome.

The tenth revision of the *International Statistical Classification of Diseases and Related Health Problems* (ICD-10) contains criteria for caffeine intoxication ("acute intoxication due to the use of other stimulants, including caffeine") and also includes several other diagnostic categories that can be applied to caffeine such as "harmful use," "dependence syndrome," and "withdrawal states from other stimulants, including caffeine." Thus, whereas DSM has tended to restrict the clinical syndromes associated with caffeine use, it is important to note that ICD-10, another prominent diagnostic system for psychiatric disorders, has a more inclusive set of conditions associated with caffeine use.

EPIDEMIOLOGY

Caffeine is found in beverages (coffees, teas, soft drinks), foods (chocolate), and medications (both prescription and over-the-counter drugs), although most caffeine consumed is derived from coffee, tea, and soft drinks. Some sources of caffeine, such as coffees and colas, are readily identifiable; others are less easily recognized. Thus, for example, noncola soft drinks can contain caffeine, and certain over-the-counter analgesics also contain caffeine. Approximately 70 percent of the soft drinks consumed in the United States contain caffeine.

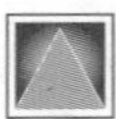

Table 11.4–1
Typical Caffeine Content of Foods and Medications

Substance	Caffeine Content
Brewed coffee	100 mg/6 oz
Instant coffee	70 mg/6 oz
Espresso	40 mg/1 oz
Decaffeinated coffee	4 mg/6 oz
Brewed tea	40 mg/6 oz
Instant tea	30 mg/6 oz
Canned or bottled tea	20 mg/12 oz
Caffeinated soda	40 mg/12 oz
Cocoa/hot chocolate beverage	7 mg/6 oz
Chocolate milk	4 mg/6 oz
Dark chocolate	30 mg/1.5 oz
Milk chocolate	20 mg/1.5 oz
Caffeinated water	100 mg/16.9 oz
Coffee ice cream or yogurt	50 mg/1 cup
Caffeinated gum	50 mg/stick
Caffeine-containing analgesics	32–65 mg/tablet
Stimulants	100–200 mg/tablet
Weight-loss aids	40–100 mg/tablet
Sports nutrition products	100 mg/tablet
Energy drinks	80 mg/8.5 oz

Adapted from Griffiths RR, Juliano LM, Chausmer AL. Caffeine pharmacology and clinical effects. In: Graham AW, Schultz TK, Mayo-Smith M, Ries RK, Wilford BB, eds. *Principles of Addiction Medicine.* 3rd ed. Chevy Chase, MD: American Society of Addiction Medicine; 2003.

Estimates of caffeine consumption require knowledge of the caffeine content of these different sources of caffeine. Also, there can be variability within categories. For example, a 6-oz cup of weak instant coffee may contain as little as 20 mg of caffeine, whereas a cup of strong drip coffee may contain as much as 150 mg. Likewise, different cola soft drinks may range in caffeine content from 23 to 71 mg per 12 oz. Table 11.4–1 provides a list of the typical caffeine content of selected caffeine-containing products.

Caffeine consumption varies by age. Figure 11.4–1 shows estimates of per capita caffeine consumption, by those who consume caffeine, for different age groups in the United States. These estimates demonstrate the wide variability in caffeine consumption for different ages. As shown in Figure 11.4–1, the average daily caffeine consumption for all ages of caffeine consumers is 2.79 mg/kg in the United States. It is worth noting that there is substantial caffeine consumption even by young children (i.e., over 1 mg/kg for children between the ages of 1 and 5 years). Worldwide, it is estimated that the average daily per capita caffeine consumption is approximately 70 mg.

In adults in the United States, the prevalence of weekly use of coffee is approximately 60 percent; of soft drinks, 50 percent; and of tea, 25 percent. More than one-half of adults consume coffee every day, with drinkers consuming an average of 3.3 cups per day. A national survey showed that 64 percent of school-age children (6 to 12 years of age) and 83 percent of adolescents (13 to 18 years of age) consume soft drinks within a 2-day period.

In the United States, it is not uncommon for the first exposure to caffeine to occur during childhood, with coffee and soft drinks each being reported as the first caffeinated beverage by approximately 40 percent of caffeine users. Onset of regular use of soft drinks occurs at an earlier age than regular use of coffee or tea. Approximately 50 percent of caffeine users consume multiple types of caffeine-containing beverages (e.g., coffee drinkers who also consume soft drinks). The average daily caffeine consumption for adult consumers of caffeine in the United States is estimated to be approximately 280 mg per day (the equivalent of approximately three cups of brewed coffee), which is less than that consumed in the United Kingdom and Sweden. Approximately 14 percent of former users of caffeine report stopping caffeine completely in response to health concerns or unpleasant side effects.

Figure 11.4–2 shows trends over 30 years in consumption of the major caffeine-containing beverages in the United States. As shown, coffee consumption has decreased modestly over the last 30 years, whereas soft drink consumption has more than doubled.

ETIOLOGY

After exposure to caffeine, continued caffeine consumption may be influenced by several different factors such as the pharmacological effects of caffeine, caffeine's reinforcing effects, genetic predispositions to caffeine use, and personal attributes of the consumer (e.g., age).

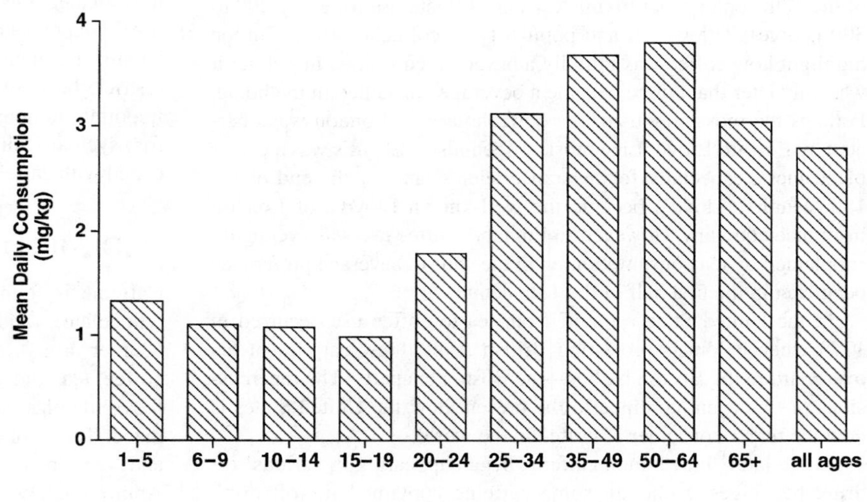

FIGURE 11.4–1 Mean daily caffeine consumption (mg/kg) for different age groups and all ages of caffeine consumers in the United States. (Adapted from Barone JJ, Roberts HR: Caffeine consumption. *Food Chem Toxicol.* 1996;34:119.)

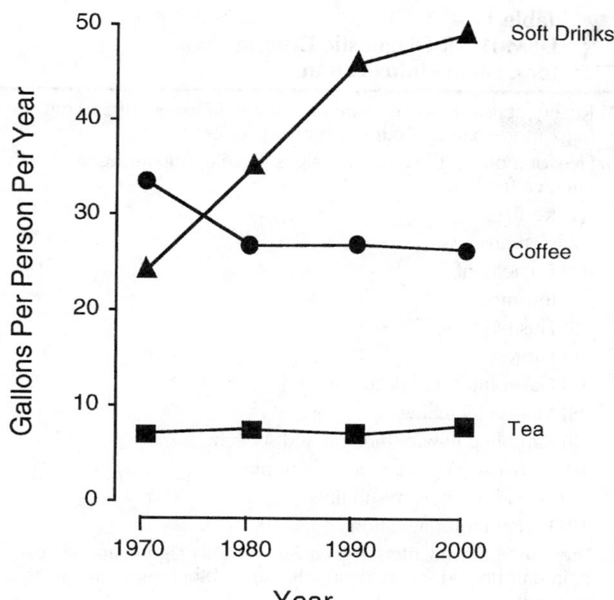

FIGURE 11.4–2 Annual per person per year consumption of caffeine in the United States from 1970 to 2000. Shown are major dietary sources of caffeine: coffee, tea, and soft drinks (i.e., flavored carbonated beverages). (Adapted from the USDA. *Food Consumption, Prices, and Expenditures, 1970–2000*; 2001.)

Pharmacology and Effects in the Central Nervous System Caffeine is a methylxanthine, as are theobromine (found in chocolate) and theophylline (typically used in the treatment of asthma). Caffeine is well absorbed from the gastrointestinal (GI) tract, with peak plasma concentrations typically occurring within 1 hour after ingestion. Caffeine is readily distributed throughout the body and is metabolized by the liver. Although there are several metabolic pathways for caffeine, it is primarily metabolized by the P450 1A2 system, and it is frequently used as a metabolic probe to assess this system's activity. The half-life of caffeine is approximately 5 hours, with large individual differences. The rate of caffeine elimination is increased by smoking, oral contraceptive steroids, cimetidine, and fluvoxamine (Luvox). Caffeine inhibits the metabolism of the antipsychotic clozapine (Clozaril) and the bronchodilator theophylline (Theo-Dur) to an extent that might be clinically significant. Caffeine metabolism is markedly slowed at the end of pregnancy.

Caffeine exerts effects throughout the body, including bronchodilation (hence the therapeutic application of caffeine and theophylline in the treatment of asthma); modest increases in blood pressure (which are reduced in caffeine-tolerant individuals); increased production of urine; increases in gastric acid secretion; and increases in plasma epinephrine, norepinephrine, renin, and free fatty acids. Centrally, caffeine affects turnover or levels of various neurotransmitters, and it functions as a central nervous system (CNS) stimulant.

Numerous investigations have examined the effects of caffeine in the CNS to understand the molecular basis for caffeine's effects. Mechanisms proposed as mediating caffeine's effects have included the inhibition of phosphodiesterases and effects on intracellular calcium (although these effects may only occur with higher doses of caffeine) and antagonism at the adenosine receptor. This latter action—adenosine receptor antagonism—appears to be the primary site of action for caffeine's effects at doses typically ingested by humans. Considerable evidence indicates an important role of dopamine in mediating the stimulant behavioral effects of caffeine.

Subjective Effects and Reinforcement Single low to moderate doses of caffeine (i.e., 20 to 200 mg) can produce a profile of subjective effects in humans that is generally identified as pleasurable. Thus, studies have shown that such doses of caffeine result in increased ratings on measures such as well-being, energy and concentration, and motivation to work. In addition, these doses of caffeine produce decreases in ratings of feeling sleepy or tired. Doses of caffeine in the range of 300 to 800 mg (the equivalent of several cups of brewed coffee ingested at once) produce effects that are often rated as being unpleasant, such as anxiety and nervousness. Although animal studies have generally found it difficult to demonstrate that caffeine functions as a reinforcer, well-controlled studies in humans have shown that people choose caffeine over placebo when given the choice under controlled experimental conditions. In habitual users, the reinforcing effects of caffeine are potentiated by the ability to suppress low-grade withdrawal symptoms after overnight abstinence. Thus, the profile of caffeine's subjective effects and its ability to function as a reinforcer contribute to the regular use of caffeine.

Genetics and Caffeine Use There may be some genetic predisposition to continued coffee use after exposure to coffee. Investigations comparing coffee or caffeine use in monozygotic and dizygotic twins have shown higher concordance rates for monozygotic twins for total caffeine consumption, heavy use, caffeine tolerance, caffeine withdrawal, and caffeine intoxication, with heritabilities ranging between 35 and 77 percent. Multivariate structural equation modeling of caffeine use, cigarette smoking, and alcohol use suggests that a common genetic factor—polysubstance use—underlines use of these three substances.

Age, Sex, and Race The relationship between long-term chronic caffeine use and demographical features, such as age, sex, and race, has not been widely studied. There is some evidence suggesting middle-aged people may use more caffeine, although caffeine use in adolescents is not uncommon. There is no known evidence that caffeine use differs between men and women, and there are no data that specifically address caffeine use for different races. There is some evidence suggesting that, for both children and adults in the United States, whites consume more caffeine than blacks.

Special Populations Cigarette smokers consume more caffeine than nonsmokers. This observation may reflect a common genetic vulnerability to caffeine use and cigarette smoking. It may also be related to increased rates of caffeine elimination in cigarette smokers. Preclinical and clinical studies indicate that regular caffeine use can potentiate the reinforcing effects of nicotine.

Heavy use and clinical dependence on alcohol is associated with heavy use and clinical dependence on caffeine. Individuals with anxiety disorders tend to report lower levels of caffeine use, although one study showed that a greater proportion of heavy caffeine consumers also use benzodiazepines. There have also been several studies showing high daily amounts of caffeine use in psychiatric patients. For example, several studies have found that such patients consume the equivalent of an average of five or more cups of brewed coffee each day. Finally, high daily caffeine consumption has also been noted in prisoners.

Personality Although attempts have been made to link preferential use of caffeine to particular personality types, results from these studies do not suggest that any particular personality type is especially linked to caffeine use.

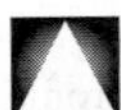

Table 11.4–2
DSM-IV-TR Caffeine-Related Disorders

Caffeine intoxication
Caffeine-induced anxiety disorder
Specify if:
With onset during intoxication
Caffeine-induced sleep disorder
Specify if:
With onset during intoxication
Caffeine-related disorder not otherwise specified

From American Psychiatric Association. *Diagnostic and Statistical Manual of Mental Disorders.* 4th ed. Text rev. Washington, DC: American Psychiatric Association; 2000, with permission.

DSM-IV-TR DISORDERS

Caffeine use can be associated with five discrete syndromes. Three of these conditions—caffeine intoxication, caffeine-induced anxiety disorder, and caffeine-induced sleep disorder—are described in DSM-IV-TR (Table 11.4–2). A fourth syndrome—caffeine withdrawal—is included in the appendix of DSM-IV-TR, and a final condition—caffeine dependence—is not included in DSM-IV-TR but is discussed here. These latter two conditions can be diagnosed using the category "caffeine-related disorders not otherwise specified," which is included in DSM-IV-TR as a substance-related disorder.

Caffeine Intoxication

Caffeine intoxication has long been recognized as a discrete syndrome associated with the use of a significant amount of caffeine (Table 11.4–3). Intoxication can be the result of an ingestion of a large amount of caffeine in a person who has not regularly consumed caffeine (a nontolerant individual) and, thus, may represent an overdose of caffeine. Alternatively, caffeine intoxication can occur in a person who chronically consumes large amounts of caffeine, which produces a more complicated clinical picture. Interestingly, although intoxication of some psychoactive substances, such as alcohol, is sought out by some people, it appears that most individuals do not actively seek repeated episodes of caffeine intoxication.

Epidemiology There have been few studies examining the prevalence of caffeine intoxication, and most of these studies have looked at selected populations (e.g., psychiatric inpatients, college students) and used ambiguous criteria. Notably, one random-digit telephone survey of caffeine use in the general community found that 7 percent of respondents had met the revised third edition of DSM (DSM-III-R) criteria for caffeine intoxication in the past year.

Comorbidity Given the limited number of studies of caffeine intoxication, it is not surprising that there is even less known about comorbid disorders associated with this condition. However, it is notable that there appears to be some association between the amount of caffeine typically consumed by individuals and certain psychiatric conditions (although it should be stressed that these are associations between the amount of caffeine consumed, not a specific diagnosis of caffeine intoxication). Thus, for example, high caffeine consumption has been noted in patients with psychiatric disorders such as bipolar I disorder, schizophrenia, and personality disorders. Excessive caffeine consumption has also been noted in people who smoke tobacco as well as heavy users of alcohol. Finally, although rare, it may be possible for a patient to develop delirium from ingesting an acute, extremely high dose of caffeine, and rare cases of suicide have been noted with excessive caffeine consumption.

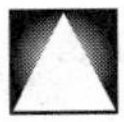

Table 11.4–3
DSM-IV-TR Diagnostic Criteria for Caffeine Intoxication

A. Recent consumption of caffeine, usually in excess of 250 mg (e.g., more than 2–3 cups of brewed coffee).
B. Five (or more) of the following signs, developing during, or shortly after, caffeine use:
(1) Restlessness
(2) Nervousness
(3) Excitement
(4) Insomnia
(5) Flushed face
(6) Diuresis
(7) Gastrointestinal disturbance
(8) Muscle twitching
(9) Rambling flow of thought and speech
(10) Tachycardia or cardiac arrhythmia
(11) Periods of inexhaustibility
(12) Psychomotor agitation
C. The symptoms in Criterion B cause clinically significant distress or impairment in social, occupational, or other important areas of functioning.
D. The symptoms are not due to a general medical condition and are not better accounted for by another mental disorder (e.g., an anxiety disorder).

From American Psychiatric Association. *Diagnostic and Statistical Manual of Mental Disorders.* 4th ed. Text rev. Washington, DC: American Psychiatric Association; 2000, with permission.

There are some patient populations that tend not to consume caffeine—patients with anxiety disorders. It has been shown that patients with generalized anxiety disorder and patients with panic disorder can be more sensitive to the effects of caffeine and that patients with panic disorder tend to have lower caffeine consumption. Thus, these may be patient populations in which there is less likelihood that caffeine intoxication is observed.

Diagnosis and Clinical Features Caffeine intoxication can present with a variety of clinical features, as shown in the criteria from DSM-IV-TR (Table 11.4–3). In addition to these signs and symptoms, reports have found patients with caffeine intoxication can have fever, irritability, tremors, sensory disturbances, tachypnea, and headaches. A general community survey indicated that the most frequent features of caffeine intoxication were diuresis, restlessness, insomnia, nervousness, excitement, and GI disturbance.

Differential Diagnosis Caffeine intoxication severe enough to come to clinical attention is probably a relatively rare condition, and several other disorders should first be considered for patients who present with features suggesting caffeine intoxication. These include other substance-related disorders, such as intoxication with other stimulants (e.g., cocaine or amphetamines), and withdrawal from drugs such as sedative-hypnotics (e.g., benzodiazepines), alcohol, or nicotine. In addition, medication adverse effects, such as akathisia, can present with features suggestive of caffeine intoxication. The final diagnosis of caffeine intoxication depends on demonstrating the ingestion of a significant quantity of caffeine before the onset of symptoms.

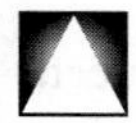

Table 11.4–4
DSM-IV-TR Diagnostic Criteria for Substance-Induced Anxiety Disorder

A. Prominent anxiety, panic attacks, or obsessions or compulsions predominate in the clinical picture.

B. There is evidence from the history, physical examination, or laboratory findings of either (1) or (2):
  (1) The symptoms in Criterion A developed during, or within 1 month of, substance intoxication or withdrawal.
  (2) Medication use is etiologically related to the disturbance.

C. The disturbance is not better accounted for by an anxiety disorder that is not substance induced. Evidence that the symptoms are better accounted for by an anxiety disorder that is not substance induced might include the following: The symptoms precede the onset of the substance use (or medication use); the symptoms persist for a substantial period of time (e.g., about a month) after the cessation of acute withdrawal or severe intoxication or are substantially in excess of what is expected given the type or amount of the substance used or the duration of use; or there is other evidence suggesting the existence of an independent non–substance-induced anxiety disorder (e.g., a history of recurrent non–substance-related episodes).

D. The disturbance does not occur exclusively during the course of a delirium.

E. The disturbance causes clinically significant distress or impairment in social, occupational, or other important areas of functioning.

Note: This diagnosis should be made instead of a diagnosis of substance intoxication or substance withdrawal only when the anxiety symptoms are in excess of those usually associated with the intoxication or withdrawal syndrome and when the anxiety symptoms are sufficiently severe to warrant independent clinical attention.

Code [specific substance]-induced anxiety disorder:

Alcohol; amphetamine (or amphetamine-like substance); caffeine; cannabis; cocaine; hallucinogen; inhalant; phencyclidine (or phencyclidine-like substance); sedative, hypnotic, or anxiolytic; other (or unknown) substance

Specify if:

With generalized anxiety: if excessive anxiety or worry about a number of events or activities predominates in the clinical presentation

With panic attacks: if panic attacks predominate in the clinical presentation

With obsessive-compulsive symptoms: if obsessions or compulsions predominate in the clinical presentation

With phobic symptoms: if phobic symptoms predominate in the clinical presentation

Specify if:

With onset during intoxication: if the criteria are met for intoxication with the substance and the symptoms develop during the intoxication syndrome

With onset during withdrawal: if criteria are met for withdrawal from the substance and the symptoms develop during, or shortly after, a withdrawal syndrome

From American Psychiatric Association. *Diagnostic and Statistical Manual of Mental Disorders.* 4th ed. Text rev. Washington, DC: American Psychiatric Association; 2000, with permission.

Course and Prognosis Caffeine has a relatively short half-life (3 to 6 hours), so caffeine intoxication typically resolves quickly and with no significant sequelae. Patients with caffeine intoxication generally have a good prognosis, although there have been isolated reports of people who have completed suicide by ingesting a massive amount of caffeine.

Treatment The first step in treating a patient presenting with evidence suggesting caffeine intoxication is to confirm the diagnosis. It is important to consider all possible sources of caffeine when considering a diagnosis of caffeine intoxication, including medications and beverages that may not be initially recognized as containing caffeine (e.g., some noncola soft drinks). Because caffeine has a relatively short half-life, short-term management of the patient can be supportive while the syndrome resolves spontaneously. For the patient who habitually consumes large amounts of caffeine and repeatedly experiences episodes of caffeine intoxication, it may be helpful to aid the patient to recognize his or her total daily caffeine consumption through the use of daily diaries and then to teach the patient about the adverse effects associated with caffeine use.

Caffeine-Induced Anxiety Disorder A caffeine-induced anxiety disorder can be panic disorder, generalized anxiety disorder, social phobia, or obsessive-compulsive disorder (OCD), although the patient does not need to fulfill all the criteria for one of these disorders to quality for a diagnosis of caffeine-induced anxiety disorder (Table 11.4–4).

There has been no work examining this caffeine-related disorder, although there have been investigations examining the relationship between caffeine use and anxiety. Patients with anxiety disorders generally consume less caffeine than control patients and experience greater self-reports of anxiety after consuming caffeine. In addition, caffeine has been used as a pharmacological probe in subjects without an anxiety disorder, and a sufficiently high dose can produce panic attacks in normal volunteer subjects.

The diagnosis of caffeine-induced anxiety disorder depends on linking the use of caffeine to the anxiety symptoms of concern. For a patient with a suspected caffeine-induced anxiety disorder, a trial of caffeine abstinence may aid in clarifying the diagnosis.

Mr. B. was a 28-year-old, single, black male graduate student who was in good health and had no history of previous psychiatric evaluation or treatment. He took no medications, did not smoke or consume alcohol, and had no current or past history of illicit drug use.

His chief complaint was that he had begun feeling mounting "anxiety" when working in the laboratory in which he was pursuing his graduate studies. His work had been progressing well, he believed his relationship with his adviser was good and supportive, and he could not identify any problems with staff or peers that might explain his anxiety. He had been working long hours but found the work interesting and had recently had his first paper accepted for publication.

Despite these successes, he reported feeling a "crescendoing anxiety" as his day progressed. He noted that by the afternoon he experienced palpitations, bursts of his heart racing, tremors in his hands, and an overall feeling of "being on the edge." He also noted a nervous energy in the afternoons. These experiences were occurring daily and seemed confined to the laboratory (although he admitted he was in the laboratory every day of the week).

When reviewing Mr. B.'s caffeine intake, it was found he was consuming excessive amounts of coffee. Staff made a large urn of caffeinated coffee each morning, and Mr. B. routinely started with a large mug of coffee. Over the course of the morning, he consumed three to four mugs of coffee (the equivalent of approximately six to eight 6-oz cups of coffee) and continued this level of use throughout the afternoon. He occasionally had a single can of caffeinated soft drink and used no other forms of caffeine on a regular basis. Mr. B. estimated he drank a total of six to eight or more mugs of coffee per day (which was estimated to be at least 1,200 mg of caffeine per day). Once pointed out to him, he realized this level of caffeine consumption was considerably higher than at any other time in his life. He admitted he liked the taste of coffee and felt a burst of energy in the morning when he drank coffee that helped him start his day.

Mr. B. and his physician developed a plan to decrease his caffeine use by tapering off caffeine. (Details of such a tapering schedule can be found in the section on Caffeine Dependence: Treatment.) Mr. B. was successful in decreasing his caffeine use and had good resolution of his anxiety symptoms once his daily caffeine use had been markedly decreased.

Caffeine-Induced Sleep Disorder Forms of a caffeine-induced sleep disorder can be insomnia, hypersomnia, parasomnia, or mixed. However, caffeine use is most frequently associated with insomnia (although there are case reports of patients who have hypersomnia in response to caffeine). Caffeine-induced sleep disorder should be diagnosed in patients with caffeine intoxication only if the sleep disturbance is in excess to that which is expected from intoxication (Table 11.4–5).

Although there are essentially no studies directly examining caffeine-induced sleep disorder, there has been work on the relationship between caffeine use and sleep. In general, ingestion of caffeine before bedtime results in a delay in sleep onset and poorer sleep quality. For some people, it has been shown that consuming 200 mg of caffeine before bedtime (the equivalent of approximately two cups of brewed coffee) can delay the onset of sleep for up to 4 hours.

Sleep disturbances secondary to caffeine use are more likely in people who are not regular consumers of caffeine. For people who consume caffeine on a daily basis, there is evidence to suggest that some tolerance occurs to the sleep-inhibiting effects of caffeine.

Caffeine can have beneficial effects when a person is sleep deprived. Studies have shown that sleep deprivation is associated with decrements in performance on a variety of tasks, and caffeine can reduce these performance decrements (although it does not completely reverse them).

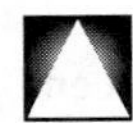

Table 11.4–5
DSM-IV-TR Diagnostic Criteria for Substance-Induced Sleep Disorder

A. A prominent disturbance in sleep that is sufficiently severe to warrant independent clinical attention.

B. There is evidence from the history, physical examination, or laboratory findings of either (1) or (2):
   (1) The symptoms in Criterion A developed during, or within 1 mo of, substance intoxication or withdrawal.
   (2) Medication use is etiologically related to the sleep disturbance.

C. The disturbance is not better accounted for by a sleep disorder that is not substance induced. Evidence that the symptoms are better accounted for by a sleep disorder that is not substance induced might include the following: The symptoms precede the onset of the substance use (or medication use); the symptoms persist for a substantial period of time (e.g., about a month) after the cessation of acute withdrawal or severe intoxication or are substantially in excess of what is expected given the type or amount of the substance used or the duration of use; or there is other evidence that suggests the existence of an independent non–substance-induced sleep disorder (e.g., a history of recurrent non–substance-related episodes).

D. The disturbance does not occur exclusively during the course of a delirium.

E. The sleep disturbance causes clinically significant distress or impairment in social, occupational, or other important areas of functioning.

Note: This diagnosis should be made instead of a diagnosis of substance intoxication or substance withdrawal only when the sleep symptoms are in excess of those usually associated with the intoxication or withdrawal syndrome and when the symptoms are sufficiently severe to warrant independent clinical attention.

Code [specific substance]-induced sleep disorder:
   Alcohol; amphetamine; caffeine; cocaine; opioid; sedative, hypnotic, or anxiolytic; other (or unknown) substance

Specify type:
   Insomnia type: if the predominant sleep disturbance is insomnia
   Hypersomnia type: if the predominant sleep disturbance is hypersomnia
   Parasomnia type: if the predominant sleep disturbance is a parasomnia
   Mixed type: if more than one sleep disturbance is present and none predominates

Specify if:
   With onset during intoxication: if the criteria are met for intoxication with the substance and the symptoms develop during the intoxication syndrome
   With onset during withdrawal: if criteria are met for withdrawal from the substance and the symptoms develop during, or shortly after, a withdrawal syndrome

From American Psychiatric Association. *Diagnostic and Statistical Manual of Mental Disorders.* 4th ed. Text rev. Washington, DC: American Psychiatric Association; 2000, with permission.

Caffeine-Related Disorder Not Otherwise Specified This category is included in DSM-IV-TR as a substance-related disorder and is to be used when the patient has a condition that is caffeine related but not diagnosable as caffeine intoxication, caffeine-induced anxiety disorder, or caffeine-induced sleep disorder (Table 11.4–6). Thus, for example, caffeine withdrawal or caffeine dependence could be coded as a caffeine-related disorder not otherwise specified.

Caffeine Withdrawal Caffeine withdrawal is included in the appendix of DSM-IV-TR with a set of diagnostic criteria to be used for further evaluation of the disorder (Table 11.4–7). Despite evidence for a discrete caffeine withdrawal syndrome, this diagnosis was not included in the body of DSM-IV-TR. The reasons provided for why it was not placed in DSM-IV-TR include concerns that there were only a limited number of symptoms (three), some symptoms were similar to each other, and the symptoms had a high prevalence in the general population and could be frequently associated with other circumstances besides caffeine withdrawal.

The research literature on caffeine withdrawal has almost doubled since DSM-IV-TR was written, and approximately 85 published reports and studies now provide an empirical basis for understanding caffeine withdrawal as a discrete diagnostic category.

Epidemiology Studies have examined caffeine withdrawal under conditions in which it is experimentally induced in a population of subjects. In a study of normal community volunteers whose average daily caffeine consumption was similar to that of the general population, 52 percent of the subjects had moderate or severe headache when caffeine withdrawal was experimentally induced under double-blind conditions; 8 to 11 percent of subjects in that study also experienced anxiety, fatigue, and depression while in withdrawal. Other similar

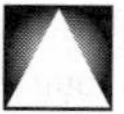

Table 11.4–6
DSM-IV-TR Diagnostic Criteria for Caffeine-Related Disorder Not Otherwise Specified

The caffeine-related disorder not otherwise specified category is for disorders associated with the use of caffeine that are not classifiable as caffeine intoxication, caffeine-induced anxiety disorder, or caffeine-induced sleep disorder. An example is caffeine withdrawal.

From American Psychiatric Association. *Diagnostic and Statistical Manual of Mental Disorders.* 4th ed. Text rev. Washington, DC: American Psychiatric Association; 2000, with permission.

studies have found that approximately one-half of subjects experience symptoms of caffeine withdrawal when it is experimentally induced (i.e., subjects undergo a double-blind discontinuation of their daily caffeine use).

There have been relatively few attempts to conduct population-based assessments of caffeine withdrawal. Such studies have usually been surveys and have found a wide range of rates of reports of caffeine withdrawal (i.e., from 8 to 41 percent). In one population-based survey, 71 percent of individuals who ended their caffeine use in an attempt to stop permanently reported experiencing DSM-IV-TR–defined withdrawal symptoms, and 24 percent reported having headache plus other symptoms that interfered with performance. In the United States, it is estimated that more than 80 percent of the adult population are regular consumers of caffeine, and even if the incidence of caffeine withdrawal is low, this still suggests that there are large numbers of people who could experience caffeine withdrawal.

Comorbidity There have been no studies that have specifically sought to determine conditions that are comorbid with caffeine withdrawal. However, patients with higher daily consumption of caffeine may be at increased risk for developing caffeine withdrawal if they miss consuming their typical dose of caffeine.

Diagnosis and Clinical Features A withdrawal condition associated with the cessation of caffeine use has been long recognized, and the most common feature noted with caffeine withdrawal has been headache. DSM-IV-TR also includes marked fatigue or drowsiness, marked anxiety or depression, and nausea or vomiting in the diagnostic criteria. However, several other signs and symptoms of caffeine withdrawal have been noted: dysphoric mood (e.g., miserable, decreased well-being/contentedness), difficulty concentrating, work difficulty, anxiety, depression, irritability, and influenza-like symptoms (e.g., nausea/vomiting, muscle aches/stiffness, hot and cold spells, heavy feelings in arms or legs; Table 11.4–8). Other effects of caffeine withdrawal include impairment in psychomotor, vigilance, and cognitive performances; increases in cerebral blood flow; and changes in quantitative electroencephalography (EEG) activity.

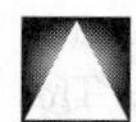

Table 11.4–7
DSM-IV-TR Research Criteria for Caffeine Withdrawal

A. Prolonged daily use of caffeine.
B. Abrupt cessation of caffeine use, or reduction in the amount of caffeine used, closely followed by headache and one (or more) of the following symptoms:
   (1) Marked fatigue or drowsiness
   (2) Marked anxiety or depression
   (3) Nausea or vomiting
C. The symptoms in Criterion B cause clinically significant distress or impairment in social, occupational, or other important areas of functioning.
D. The symptoms are not due to the direct physiological effects of a general medical condition (e.g., migraine, viral illness) and are not better accounted for by another mental disorder.

From American Psychiatric Association. *Diagnostic and Statistical Manual of Mental Disorders.* 4th ed. Text rev. Washington, DC: American Psychiatric Association; 2000, with permission.

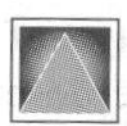

Table 11.4–8
Clinical Features of Caffeine Withdrawal

Headache
Fatigue, lethargy
Sleepiness, drowsiness
Dysphoric mood
Difficulty concentrating
Work difficulty, unmotivated
Depression
Anxiety
Irritability
Nausea or vomiting
Muscle aches or stiffness
Impaired psychomotor/cognitive performance

CAFFEINE WITHDRAWAL HEADACHE Headache is the most common feature associated with caffeine withdrawal. It is usually described as a generalized, throbbing headache that is worsened by exercise and Valsalva's maneuver and responds best to caffeine consumption. It typically begins 12 to 24 hours after the last ingestion of caffeine, although the onset can occur as long as 40 hours after the last dose. It usually resolves in 2 to 4 days, although sporadic headaches can continue for up to 11 days.

OTHER SIGNS AND SYMPTOMS OF CAFFEINE WITHDRAWAL There are several other signs and symptoms associated with caffeine withdrawal (Table 11.4–8). Patients can experience these signs and symptoms even without the concurrent presence of headache, suggesting that the other features of caffeine withdrawal are not simply secondary to the headache.

CAFFEINE WITHDRAWAL AND POSTOPERATIVE HEADACHE Headache is a frequent postoperative symptom. Patients undergoing operative procedures are required to abstain from all oral intake before the procedure, including daily dietary caffeine they typically consume. Several studies have examined whether postoperative headache could reflect caffeine withdrawal. Patients with higher daily caffeine consumption are at increased risk for developing postoperative headache. The consumption of a caffeinated beverage on the day of an operative procedure has been shown to decrease the rate of postoperative headache.

Caffeine Withdrawal and Dosage of Caffeine The risk of developing caffeine withdrawal increases as a function of increases in the daily dose of caffeine consumed. However, it should be noted that caffeine withdrawal can occur with relatively low dosages of caffeine, such as 100 mg per day (the equivalent of approximately one cup of brewed coffee). Caffeine withdrawal can also develop after as few as 3 days' exposure to moderate dosages of caffeine (e.g., 300 mg per day). Low doses of caffeine (e.g., 25 mg) are capable of suppressing the symptoms of caffeine withdrawal in individuals who stop consuming moderate doses of caffeine.

Severity of Caffeine Withdrawal Although severity of withdrawal tends to increase with increases in daily caffeine dose consumed, there are marked differences within and among individuals with regard to the incidence and severity of caffeine withdrawal. When caffeine withdrawal does occur, its severity can vary from mild to severe. In extreme cases, caffeine withdrawal has been shown to produce clinically significant distress, including impairment in daily functioning.

Caffeine Withdrawal and Age Most studies of caffeine withdrawal have determined the presence and features of caffeine withdrawal in adults. However, caffeine withdrawal has also been shown to occur in children. Like caffeine withdrawal in adults, headache and other caffeine withdrawal symptoms can occur in children.

Differential Diagnosis Several disorders should be considered in the differential diagnosis of caffeine withdrawal. Caffeine withdrawal can mimic migraine and other headache disorders, viral illnesses, sinus conditions, other drug withdrawal states (e.g., from amphetamines, cocaine), and medication reactions. The final determination of caffeine withdrawal should rest on a determination of the pattern and amount of caffeine consumption, the time interval between the last ingestion of caffeine and the onset of symptoms, and the particular clinical features presented by the patient. Resolution of symptoms by a dose of caffeine may also be useful in clarifying the diagnosis.

Course and Prognosis Caffeine withdrawal typically begins 12 to 24 hours after the last dose of caffeine and usually resolves in 2 to 7 days. Most symptoms reach their maximal intensity within the first 48 hours after cessation of caffeine use, with subsequent decreasing intensity over the following days. However, it should be noted that there can be considerable variability among people in the manifestations, severity, and time course of caffeine withdrawal. Furthermore, it has been shown that the same person can experience different symptoms and different degrees of severity of symptoms across different episodes of caffeine withdrawal.

Treatment There has been little work systematically investigating the optimal treatment for caffeine withdrawal. The symptoms of caffeine withdrawal typically resolve with the ingestion of a dose of caffeine, and a person with a provisional diagnosis of caffeine withdrawal who continues to be symptomatic after caffeine consumption has been terminated for more than 2 weeks should be carefully reevaluated and considered for other possible diagnoses. Caffeine withdrawal headaches may also respond to aspirin.

If caffeine withdrawal occurs because a person is attempting to abruptly stop all caffeine use, it may be better to attempt a tapering caffeine dosage schedule.

Ms. E. was a 32-year-old single, white woman employed full time at a local factory. She occasionally used nonsteroidal antiinflammatory drugs (NSAIDs) but was taking no regular prescription medications. She had a history of alcohol dependence, in remission for 9 years, and was otherwise in good health.

She first began consuming caffeine when she started college, and her current beverage of choice was coffee. She typically drank four to five mugs of coffee each day and preferred to drink it without cream, milk, or sugar. She estimated that 5 minutes elapsed between the time she got up in the morning and the time she had her first cup of coffee; her roommate made a pot before Ms. E. got up, and Ms. E. immediately poured a mug when she got out of bed. She spaced her mugs over the course of the day, with her last mug either after lunch or with dinner.

Physicians had recommended she cut down or stop her coffee use because of complaints of mild indigestion, but she had been unable to do so. Her roommate had also complained about her coffee use at times. Ms. E. routinely drank hot coffee in her car and had spilled it and burned herself on one occasion.

When she had stopped caffeine abruptly, Ms. E. experienced marked irritability, poor concentration, and a severe, generalized headache. When asked to rate the severity of the headache, she replied that "On a scale of one to ten, it's a 12." She also had muscle aches, low energy, lethargy, and a craving to drink a mug of coffee. On the day that she had stopped coffee use abruptly, she left work 2 hours early because of problems with concentrating on the job and went to bed several hours earlier than usual. She then returned to her usual pattern of coffee use.

Caffeine Dependence Caffeine dependence is not included in DSM-IV-TR, and DSM-IV-TR explicitly states, "A diagnosis of Substance Dependence can be applied to every class of substance except caffeine." Despite the absence of caffeine dependence in DSM-IV-TR, there is evidence supporting a diagnosis of caffeine dependence in some people with problematic caffeine consumption.

Before reviewing the features of caffeine dependence, it is important to clarify the use of the word "dependence." *Dependence* is sometimes used to indicate the presence of physical dependence—a condition characterized by physiological adaptation to the effects of a drug and usually indicated by the presence of a withdrawal syndrome when drug ingestion is discontinued. There is considerable evidence that caffeine can produce physical dependence, as indicated by the presence of caffeine withdrawal.

The term *dependence* is also used in a second way—to indicate a clinical diagnosis of dependence. Clinical diagnoses of dependence typically have included a constellation of diagnostic criteria that are loosely linked by the theme of problematic use of the drug. Included in these criteria can be evidence of physical dependence, although physical dependence is neither necessary nor sufficient to make a diagnosis of a clinical syndrome of dependence. The DSM-IV-TR criteria are used to make a clinical diagnosis of dependence.

Although there are numerous studies and reports on caffeine's ability to produce physical dependence, as evidenced by caffeine withdrawal, there is little research on whether some people who consume caffeine can develop a clinical syndrome of dependence. This is a question that only a few studies have addressed.

Epidemiology Caffeine use is common throughout the world. More than 80 percent of adults in the United States consume caffeine regularly, and their average daily caffeine consumption has been estimated to be 280 mg (the equivalent of approximately three cups of brewed coffee). Given the substantial number of people who consume caffeine regularly and their use of daily dosages that produce psychoactive effects, even a low prevalence rate of caffeine dependence could represent substantial numbers of people.

However, there has only been one study that has examined the prevalence of caffeine dependence in the general population—a random-digit telephone survey that used the generic criteria from DSM-III-R. In that study, 30 percent of caffeine consumers fulfilled diagnostic criteria for caffeine dependence, with 56 percent endorsing desire or unsuccessful efforts to cut down or control use, 28 percent reporting using more than intended, 18 percent endorsing withdrawal, 14 percent endorsing use despite knowledge of a physical or psychological problem caused by caffeine, and 8 percent reporting tolerance.

Comorbidity One study in adults (N = 16) and two in adolescents (N = 12) describe a series of case reports on caffeine dependence and report on comorbid conditions. In the study of 16 caffeine-dependent adults, approximately two-thirds of patients had a psychiatric disorder in remission, most commonly another substance abuse disorder. However, nearly one-half had a mood disorder in remission, one-fourth had an anxiety disorder in remission, and one-fifth had an eating disorder in remission. Notably, there was a clustering of nicotine dependence, caffeine dependence, and a history of an alcohol use disorder in several subjects, and this clustering of these three disorders has been noted in other studies.

Studies comparing caffeine-dependent and caffeine-nondependent adolescents have not demonstrated significant associations between caffeine dependence and psychiatric comorbidities. However, one study of high school students showed that those who reported themselves to be "addicted" to caffeine also described themselves to be more severely stressed and chronically depressed.

CAFFEINE USE AND NONPSYCHIATRIC ILLNESSES Despite numerous studies examining the relationship between caffeine use and physical illness, significant health risk from nonreversible pathological consequences of caffeine use, such as cancer, heart disease, and human reproduction, has not been conclusively demonstrated. Nonetheless, caffeine use is often considered to be contraindicated for various conditions, including generalized anxiety disorder, panic disorder, primary insomnia, gastroesophageal reflux, and pregnancy. In addition, the modest ability of caffeine to increase blood pressure and the documented cholesterol-elevating compounds of unfiltered coffee have raised the issue of the relationship of caffeine and coffee use to cardiovascular disease. Finally, there may be a mild association between higher daily caffeine use in women and delayed conception and slightly lower birth weight. However, there are studies that have not found such associations, and effects, when found, are usually with relatively high daily dosages of caffeine (e.g., the equivalent of five cups of brewed coffee per day). For a woman who is considering pregnancy, especially if there is some difficulty in conceiving, it may be useful to counsel eliminating caffeine use. Similarly, for a woman who becomes pregnant and has moderate to high daily caffeine consumption, a discussion about decreasing her daily caffeine use may be warranted.

Diagnosis and Clinical Features DSM-IV-TR provides a generic set of diagnostic criteria that are to be used for determining the presence of a substance dependence syndrome (Table 11.4–9). In addition to the results of the survey study described previously, three studies have described a series of case reports of caffeine dependence in adults (N = 16) and adolescents (N = 12). Rates of endorsement of specific dependence criteria by caffeine-dependent adults and adolescents, respectively, were 81 percent and 83 percent endorsing desire or unsuccessful efforts to cut down or control use, 94 percent and 100 percent reporting withdrawal, 94 percent and 58 percent endorsing use despite knowledge of a physical or psychological problem caused by caffeine, and 75 percent and 92 percent reporting tolerance. The validity of the diagnosis of caffeine dependence is suggested in experimental studies showing that a diagnosis of caffeine dependence prospectively predicts more severe withdrawal and a greater incidence of caffeine reinforcement.

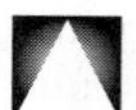

Table 11.4–9
DSM-IV-TR Criteria for Substance Dependence

A maladaptive pattern of substance use, leading to clinically significant impairment or distress, as manifested by three (or more) of the following, occurring at any time in the same 12-month period:

(1) Tolerance, as defined by either of the following:
 (a) A need for markedly increased amounts of the substance to achieve intoxication or desired effect
 (b) Markedly diminished effect with continued use of the same amount of the substance
(2) Withdrawal, as manifested by either of the following:
 (a) The characteristic withdrawal syndrome for the substance (refer to Criteria A and B of the criteria sets for withdrawal from the specific substances).
 (b) The same (or a closely related) substance is taken to relieve or avoid withdrawal symptoms.
(3) The substance is often taken in larger amounts or over a longer period than was intended.
(4) There is a persistent desire or unsuccessful efforts to cut down or control substance use.
(5) A great deal of time is spent in activities necessary to obtain the substance (e.g., visiting multiple doctors or driving long distances), use the substance (e.g., chain smoking), or recover from its effects.
(6) Important social, occupational, or recreational activities are given up or reduced because of substance use.
(7) The substance use is continued despite knowledge of having a persistent or recurrent physical or psychological problem that is likely to have been caused or exacerbated by the substance (e.g., current cocaine use despite recognition of cocaine-induced depression or continued drinking despite recognition that an ulcer was made worse by alcohol consumption).

From American Psychiatric Association. *Diagnostic and Statistical Manual of Mental Disorders.* 4th ed. Text rev. Washington, DC: American Psychiatric Association; 2000, with permission.

Differential Diagnosis When considering a possible diagnosis of caffeine dependence, it is useful to include other substance dependence syndromes in the differential diagnosis. A clinical syndrome of dependence on caffeine probably is overlooked by most clinicians because it is not included in DSM-IV-TR, and it is not widely recognized and acknowledged as a substance-related abuse disorder. Most people have no problems associated with being dependent on caffeine so long as their supply is available on a daily basis. Even if they are unable to obtain caffeine for some reason, the withdrawal syndrome is relatively short-lived and is not life-threatening.

Course and Prognosis No studies have examined the course and prognosis for patients with a diagnosis of caffeine dependence. Subjects with caffeine dependence have reported continued use of caffeine despite repeated efforts to discontinue their caffeine use.

Treatment There have been case reports describing the treatment of patients with problematic caffeine use, although there have been no systematic studies of treating patients with a confirmed diagnosis of caffeine dependence. In general, approaches have used a combination of three techniques to aid patients in decreasing or eliminating their caffeine use: gradual tapering of the daily dose, self-monitoring of daily use, and reinforcement for decreased use.

The first step in reducing or eliminating caffeine use is to have patients determine their daily consumption of caffeine. This can best be accomplished by having the patient keep a daily food diary. It is important for the patient to recognize all sources of caffeine in the diet, including different forms of caffeine (e.g., beverages, medications), and to accurately record the amount consumed. After several days of keeping such a diary, the clinician can meet with the patient, review the diary, and determine the average daily caffeine dose in milligrams.

The patient and clinician should then decide on a fading schedule for caffeine consumption. Such a schedule could involve decreases in increments of 10 percent every few days. Because caffeine is typically consumed in beverage form, the patient can use a substitution procedure in which decaffeinated beverage is gradually used in place of caffeinated beverage. A diary should continue to be maintained during this time so that the patient's progress can be monitored. The fading schedule should be individualized for the patient so that the rate of decrease in caffeine consumption minimizes withdrawal symptoms. Abruptly stopping all caffeine use should probably be avoided because withdrawal symptoms are likely to develop with sudden discontinuation of all caffeine use.

Ms. G. was a 35-year-old married, white homemaker with three children, aged 8, 6, and 2. She took no prescription medications, took a multivitamin and vitamins C and E on a daily basis, did not smoke, and had no history of psychiatric problems. She drank moderate amounts of alcohol on the weekends, had smoked marijuana in college but had not used it since, and had no other history of illicit drug use.

She had started consuming caffeinated beverages while in college, and her current beverage of choice was caffeinated diet cola. Ms. G. had her first soft drink early in the morning, shortly after getting out of bed, and she jokingly called it her "morning hit." She spaced out her bottles of soft drinks over the course of the day, with her last bottle at dinnertime. She typically drank four to five 20-oz bottles of caffeinated diet cola each day.

She and her husband had argued about her caffeinated soft drink use in the past, and her husband had believed she should not drink caffeinated soft drinks while pregnant. However, she had continued to do so during each of her pregnancies. Despite a desire to stop drinking caffeinated soft drinks, she was unable to do so. She described having a strong desire to drink caffeinated soft drinks, and if she resisted this desire, she found that she could not think of anything else. She drank caffeinated soft drinks in her car, which had a manual transmission, and noted that she fumbled while shifting and holding the soft drink and spilled it in the car. She also noted that her teeth had become yellowed, and she suspected this was related to her tendency to swish soft drink in her mouth before swallowing it. When asked to describe a time when she stopped using soft drinks, she reported that she had run out of it on the day one of her children was to have a birthday party, and she did not have time to leave her home to buy more. In the early afternoon of that day, a few hours before the scheduled start of the party, she felt extreme lethargy, a severe headache, irritability, and craving for a soft drink. She called her husband and told him she planned to cancel the party. She then went to the grocery store to buy soft drinks, and after drinking two bottles, she felt well enough to host the party.

Although initially expressing interest in decreasing or stopping her caffeinated soft drink use, Ms. G. did not attend scheduled follow-up appointments after her first evaluation. When finally contacted at home, she reported she had only sought help initially at her husband's request, and she had decided to try to cut down on her caffeine use on her own.

SUGGESTED CROSS-REFERENCES

Chapter 11 discusses substance-related disorders, anxiety disorders are discussed in Chapter 14, and sleep disorders are discussed in Chapter 20.

REFERENCES

*Barone JJ, Roberts HR: Caffeine consumption. *Food Chem Toxicol.* 1996;34:119.

Bernstein GA, Carroll ME, Dean NW, Crosby RD, Perwien AR, Benowitz NL: Caffeine withdrawal in normal school-age children. *J Am Acad Child Adolesc Psychiatry.* 1998;37:858.

Bernstein GA, Carroll ME, Thuras PD, Cosgrove KP, Roth ME: Caffeine dependence in teenagers. *Drug Alcohol Depend.* 2002;66:1.

Bruce M, Scott N, Shine P, Lader M: Anxiogenic effects of caffeine in patients with anxiety disorders. *Arch Gen Psychiatry.* 1992;49:867.

Carrillo JA, Benitez J: Clinically significant pharmacokinetic interactions between dietary caffeine and medications. *Clin Pharmacokinet.* 2000;39:127.

Cauli O, Pinna A, Valentini V, Morelli M: Subchronic caffeine exposure induces sensitization to caffeine and cross-sensitization to amphetamine ipsilateral turning behavior independent from dopamine release. *Neuropsychopharmacology.* 2003;28:1752–1759.

Dews PB, Curtis GL, Hanford KJ, O'Brien CP: The frequency of caffeine withdrawal in a population-based survey and in a controlled, blinded pilot experiment. *J Clin Pharmacol.* 1999;39:1221.

Dreisbach RH, Pfeiffer C: Caffeine-withdrawal headache. *J Lab Clin Med.* 1943;28:1212.

Durrant KL: Known and hidden sources of caffeine in drug, food, and natural products. *J Am Pharm Assoc (Wash).* 2002;42:625.

Eskenazi B: Caffeine—filtering the facts. *N Engl J Med.* 1999;341:1688.

*Fredholm BB, Battig K, Holmen J, Nehlig A, Zvartau EE: Actions of caffeine in the brain with special reference to factors that contribute to its widespread use. *Pharmacol Rev.* 1999;51:83.

Garrett BE, Griffiths RR: The role of dopamine in the behavioral effects of caffeine in animals and humans. *Pharmacol Biochem Behav.* 1997;57:533.

Gilbert RM. Caffeine consumption. In: Spiller GA, ed. *The Methylxanthine Beverages and Foods: Chemistry, Consumption, and Health Effects.* New York: Alan R. Liss; 1984.

Griffiths RR, Bigelow GE, Liebson IA: Human coffee drinking: reinforcing and physical dependence producing effects of caffeine. *J Pharmacol Exp Ther.* 1986;239:416.

*Griffiths RR, Juliano LM, Chausmer AL. Caffeine pharmacology and clinical effects. In: Graham AW, Schultz TK, Mayo-Smith M, Ries RK, Wilford BB, eds. *Principles of Addiction Medicine.* 3rd ed. Chevy Chase, MD: American Society of Addiction Medicine; 2003.

Griffiths RR, Vernotica EM: Is caffeine a flavoring agent in cola soft drinks? *Arch Fam Med.* 2000;9:727.

Griffiths RR, Woodson PP: Caffeine physical dependence: a review of human and laboratory animal studies. *Psychopharmacology.* 1988;94:437.

Harnack L, Stang J, Story M: Soft drink consumption among US children and adolescents: nutritional consequences. *J Am Diet Assoc.* 1999;99:436.

Hettema JM, Corey LA, Kendler KS: A multivariate genetic analysis of the use of tobacco, alcohol, and caffeine in a population based sample of male and female twins. *Drug Alcohol Depend.* 1999;57:69.

Hughes JR, Higgins ST, Bickel WK, Hunt WK, Fenwick JW, Gulliver SB, Mireault GC: Caffeine self-administration, withdrawal, and adverse effects among coffee drinkers. *Arch Gen Psychiatry.* 1991;48:611.

Hughes JR, Oliveto AH: A systematic survey of caffeine intake in Vermont. *Exp Clin Psychopharmacol.* 1997;5:393.

*Hughes JR, Oliveto AH, Liguori A, Carpenter J, Howard T: Endorsement of DSM-IV dependence criteria among caffeine users. *Drug Alcohol Depend.* 1998;52:99.

*James JE. *Understanding Caffeine: A Biobehavioral Analysis.* Thousand Oaks, CA: Sage; 1997.

James JE, Stirling KP, Hampton BAM: Caffeine fading: behavioral treatment of caffeine abuse. *Behav Ther.* 1985;16:15.

Kendler KS, Prescott CA: Caffeine intake, tolerance, and withdrawal in women: a population-based twin study. *Am J Psychiatry.* 1999;156:223.

Lindskog M, Svenningsson P, Pozzi L, Kim Y, Fienberg AA, Bibb JA, Fredholm BB, Nairn AC, Greengard P, Fisone G: Involvement of DARPP-32 phosphorylation in the stimulant action of caffeine. *Nature.* 2002;418:774.

McCusker RR, Goldberger BA, Cone EJ: Caffeine content of specialty coffees. *J Anal Toxicol.* 2003;27:520–522.

Nawrot P, Jordan S, Eastwood J, Rotstein J, Hugenholtz A, Feeley M: Effects of caffeine on human health. *Food Addit Contam.* 2003;20:1–30.

Oberstar JV, Bernstein GA, Thuras PD: Caffeine use and dependence in adolescents: one-year follow-up. *J Child Adolesc Psychopharmacol.* 2002;12:127.

Rogers PJ, Martin J, Smith C, Heatherley SV, Smit HJ: Absence of reinforcing, mood and psychomotor performance effects of caffeine in habitual non-consumers of caffeine. *Psychopharmacology (Berl).* 2003;167:54–62.

Silverman K, Evans SM, Strain EC, Griffiths RR: Withdrawal syndrome after the double-blind cessation of caffeine consumption. *N Engl J Med.* 1992;327:1109.

Strain EC, Mumford GK, Silverman K, Griffiths RR: Caffeine dependence syndrome: evidence from case histories and experimental evaluations. *JAMA.* 1994;272:1043.

Tinley Em, Yeomans MR, Durlach PJ: Caffeine reinforces flavour preference in caffeine-dependent, but not long-term withdrawn, caffeine consumers. *Psychopharmacology (Berl).* 2003;166:416–423.

van de Stelt O, Snel J. Caffeine and human performance. In: Snel J, Lorist MM, eds. *Nicotine, Caffeine, and Social Drinking*. Amsterdam, The Netherlands: Harwood Academic Publishers; 1998.

Weber JG, Ereth MH, Danielson DR: Perioperative ingestion of caffeine and postoperative headache. *Mayo Clin Proc*. 1993;68:842.

▲ 11.5 Cannabis-Related Disorders

WAYNE HALL, PH.D., AND LOUISA DEGENHARDT, PH.D.

HISTORY

Cannabis preparations are obtained from the plant *Cannabis sativa.* The cannabis plant has been used by humans in China, India, and the Middle East for approximately 8,000 years for its fiber and as a medicinal agent. Cannabis was introduced to Europeans in the 19th century via Napoleon's troops returning from Egypt and to Britain for medical use by a surgeon who had served in India. Cannabis was mostly used in Europe for fiber and to a lesser extent for therapeutic purposes. There was some recreational use in the Parisian bohemian demimonde in the late 19th century.

Recreational cannabis use was introduced to the United States in the 1930s from Mexico and spread via jazz musicians to cities in the northeastern United States. Its use was banned in the United States in 1938 and in most other countries by international drug control treaties in 1961. It was used in bohemian circles in the United States in the 1940s and 1950s before gradually being disseminated to the wider U.S. youth population in the late 1960s and through the 1970s and 1980s. Its use was disseminated via movies, media, and popular culture to many other developed countries in the 1970s and 1980s.

Cannabis use is still illegal in most developed societies, but it has become a common feature of youth culture, with a declining age of first use among more recent birth cohorts. Cannabis is the most widely used illicit drug worldwide (with approximately 150 million users or 3.7 percent of the world's population 15 years of age and older). It is the fourth most commonly used psychoactive drug in the United States after caffeine, alcohol, and nicotine.

CANNABIS PREPARATIONS

The cannabis plant occurs in male and female forms. The female plant contains the highest concentrations of more than 60 cannabinoids, substances that are unique to the plant. The one that is primarily responsible for the psychoactive effects that are sought by cannabis users is Δ_9-tetrahydrocannabinol (THC). THC is found in a resin that covers the flowering tops and upper leaves of the female plant. Most of the other cannabinoids are either inactive or only weakly active, although they may interact with THC.

The most common cannabis preparations are marijuana, hashish, and hash oil. Marijuana is prepared from the dried flowering tops and leaves of the plant. Its potency depends on the growing conditions, the genetic characteristics of the plant, the ratio of THC to other cannabinoids, and the part of the plant that is used. The flowering tops have the highest THC concentration, with much lower concentrations in the leaves, stems, and seeds. Varieties of cannabis cultivated for hemp fiber usually contain very low levels of THC. Cannabis plants may be grown to maximize their THC production by the "sinsemilla" method, in which only female plants are grown together.

The concentration of THC in marijuana may range from 0.5 to 5.0 percent, whereas the sinsemilla variety may contain 7 to 14 percent THC. The potency of marijuana preparations being sold in the United States has probably increased during the past several decades, although it has not increased 30-fold, as has been claimed in the popular media. Hashish, or hash, consists of dried cannabis resin. It may be light brown to almost black and may contain between 2 and 8 percent THC. Hash oil is obtained by extracting THC from hashish (or marijuana) in oil. Its color may range from clear to pale yellow–green through brown to black. The concentration of the THC in hash oil is between 15 and 20 percent.

METHODS OF USE

Cannabis is typically smoked as marijuana in a hand-rolled cigarette or "joint," which may include tobacco to assist burning. A water pipe, or "bong," is an increasingly popular way of using all cannabis preparations. Hashish may be mixed with tobacco and smoked as a joint or smoked in a pipe with or without tobacco. Because hash oil is extremely potent, a few drops may be applied to a cigarette or a joint or to the mixture in a pipe or the oil can be heated and the vapors inhaled. Whatever preparation or method of smoking is used, smokers typically inhale deeply and hold their breath to ensure maximum absorption of THC by the lungs.

The oral route of administration may also be used. Hashish may be cooked in foods and eaten. In experimental research, THC dissolved in sesame oil is swallowed in gelatin capsules. In India, cannabis may be consumed in the form of "bhang," a tea brewed from the leaves and stems of the plant. Cannabis does not lend itself to injection because THC does not dissolve in water. All but a handful of cannabis users in developed societies smoke cannabis. The chemistry and pharmacology of cannabis dictate that it be smoked. Given the preponderance of smoking as the route of administration, the reader should assume that, unless otherwise stated, cannabis is smoked.

Comparative Nosology

There is a distinction between the use and problematic use of cannabis. The existence of a dependence syndrome, and the nature of problematic cannabis use, has been an area of relatively recent research and a matter of some debate. The most recent editions of the two major diagnostic classification systems, tenth revision of the *International Statistical Classification of Diseases and Related Health Problems* (ICD-10) and the revised fourth edition of the *Diagnostic and Statistical Manual of Mental Disorders* (DSM-IV-TR), have both included categories (*harmful use* and *abuse*, respectively) that attempt to encapsulate problematic use that does not satisfy criteria for dependence but which is causing the user harm. Both classification systems have a definition of cannabis *dependence,* which is characterized by marked distress resulting by a recurring cluster of problems related to cannabis use that reflect impaired control over cannabis use despite the harms such use may be causing.

Research has suggested that ICD-10 and DSM-IV-TR classification systems agree extremely well in their identification of cases of cannabis dependence. However, each of the diagnostic systems differs slightly in their criteria for harmful use/abuse, and this is reflected in poorer agreement between the two systems on the classification of cases with respect to this diagnosis.

Epidemiology of Cannabis Use

In the United States, two major surveys of illicit drug use have been undertaken since the early 1970s. The Monitoring The Future project has surveyed

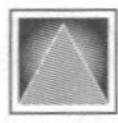

Table 11.5–1
Prevalence of Cannabis Use per 100 per Year According to the U.S. National Household Survey on Drug Abuse (2000)

Age (Yrs)	Lifetime Use	Past 12 Mos Use	Past Mo Use
12–17	18.3	13.4	7.2
18–25	45.7	23.7	13.6
26+	34.4	5.0	3.0
Total	34.2	8.3	4.8

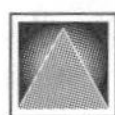

Table 11.5–3
Prevalence of Cannabis Use per 100 per Year in the 2001 U.S. Monitoring the Future Survey

Age	Lifetime Use	Past 12 Mos Use	Past Mo Use	Past Mo Daily Use
8th grade (12 yrs)	20.4	15.4	9.2	1.3
10th grade (14 yrs)	40.1	32.7	19.8	4.5
12th grade (18 yrs)	49.0	37.0	22.4	5.8
College	51.2	34.0	20.0	4.6
19–28 yrs	55.1	27.9	16.1	4.2

nationwide samples of high school seniors, college students, and young adults annually since 1975. The National Household Survey on Drug Abuse (sponsored by the National Institute on Drug Abuse [NIDA]) has surveyed household samples of adults throughout the United States since 1972.

NIDA has surveyed approximately 9,000 people 12 years of age and older in randomly selected households throughout the United States every 2 to 3 years since 1972. The survey has been conducted annually since 1991 with a sample of more than 30,000 participants.

In 2000, 34 percent of the U.S. national sample reported that they had used cannabis, 8 percent had used in the past year, and 5 percent were current users (Table 11.5–1). Lifetime use increased from 18 percent among those aged 12 to 17 years to 46 percent among those aged 26 to 34 years before declining to 34 percent among those older than the age of 35 years. Rates of discontinuation of use were high: More than two-thirds of men and three-fourths of women who had used cannabis at some time in their lives had not used it in the last year. Monthly cannabis use was more common among men (19 percent) than women (13 percent) and most common among those aged 18 to 25 years (14 percent) (Table 11.5–1).

The NIDA household survey series from 1974 to 2000 (Table 11.5–2) shows that rates of past-month cannabis use increased throughout the 1970s, peaked in 1979, and declined steadily throughout the 1980s to reach their lowest level in 1992 before increasing again in 1995.

In the Monitoring the Future project, the prevalence of cannabis use has been estimated among secondary school students, college students, and young adults (Table 11.5–3). Since 1975, approximately 15,000 high school seniors have been surveyed. The samples of college students and young adults who are surveyed each year represent a sample of those who were originally surveyed as high school seniors (approximately 14 percent) and have been followed up every 2 years. Since 1991, national samples of eighth- and tenth-grade students have also been annually surveyed.

In the 2000 survey, lifetime cannabis use increased with each older age group, but use in the past year reached a plateau in the 18- (last year of high school) to 28-year age group. Daily use peaked at 18 years of age, with 6 percent of high school seniors and 4.2 percent of 19- to 28-year-olds reporting daily cannabis use. This is much lower than the 11 percent of high school seniors in the peak year of 1978 who reported such use.

In 1982, 21 percent of the 12th graders reported that they had smoked cannabis daily for 1 month or more. This decreased to 8 percent by 1992. Daily use has been consistently higher among males than females and among those not planning to attend college. More than one-half of those who were daily users by 18 years of age began this pattern of heavy use by 16 years of age.

There have been long waves of consumption in cannabis use among American adolescents since 1975. Among 18-year-olds, lifetime prevalence peaked at 65 percent in 1980, then fell by nearly one-half by the early 1990s. Use in the past year peaked at 51 percent in 1979 and fell to 22 percent by 1992. The rate of discontinuing use also decreased (Table 11.5–4), with few of those who had used cannabis ten or more times ceasing use by 18 years of age. Most of those who ceased cannabis use had not had a great deal of experience with cannabis. The time trends in cannabis use were different from those of other drugs, suggesting that the changes in cannabis use reflected factors specific to that drug. Whereas most users of other illicit drugs also had used cannabis, trends in the use of other illicit drugs were independent of the cannabis-use trends.

After more than a decade of decreasing rates of cannabis use among American secondary students, the 1992 and 1993 surveys showed that cannabis use began to increase sharply among eighth, tenth, and 12th graders and, to a lesser extent, among college students and young adults. There was an increasing initiation rate and a higher rate of continued use. Lloyd Johnston and colleagues have argued that changes in beliefs about the risks of cannabis use were responsible for the reduction in use between 1979 and 1991 and for

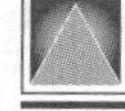

Table 11.5–2
Trends in Past Month Cannabis Use (U.S. National Household Survey on Drug Abuse 1974 to 2000)

Age (Yrs)	1974	1976	1977	1979	1985	1988	1990	1992	1995	1996	1999	2000
12–17	12.0	12.3	16.6	16.3	13.2	8.1	7.1	5.3	10.9	9.0	7.2	7.2
18–25	25.2	25.0	27.4	38.0	25.3	17.9	15.0	13.1	14.2	15.6	14.2	13.6
26+	2.0	3.5	3.3	—	—	—	—	—	—	—	2.8	3.0
26–34	—	—	—	20.8	23.1	14.7	10.9	11.4	8.3	8.4	—	—
35+	—	—	—	2.8	3.9	2.3	3.1	2.5	2.8	2.9	—	—

Note: Numbers are per 100 per year.

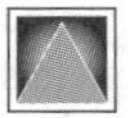

Table 11.5–4
Trends in Cannabis Use among Those in Year 12 (U.S. Monitoring the Future Study 1999)

Year	Lifetime Use	Past 12 Mos Use	Discontinuation Rate among Those Who Had Used Cannabis	
			Ever	10+ Times
1975	47	40	15	4
1980	60	49	19	5
1985	54	41	25	8
1990	41	27	34	12
1992	33	22	33	11
1993	45	36	20	8

Note: Numbers are per 100 per year.

the increase in use since 1992. They reported a strong negative correlation over time between the rates of cannabis use and the perceived risk of using cannabis and peer disapproval of use. Between 1979 and 1992, a marked increase in perceived risk and a smaller increase in personal disapproval of use preceded a large decrease in rates of use. Johnston et al. attributed the sharp upturn in cannabis use after 1992 to a preceding decline in perceived risk.

Only a small proportion of cannabis users use the drug for several years or more. The daily or near-daily use pattern over a period of years is the pattern with the greatest risk of experiencing adverse health and psychological consequences. Daily cannabis users are more likely to be male and less well educated; they are also more likely to regularly use alcohol and to have experimented with a variety of other illicit drugs, including amphetamine and other psychostimulants, hallucinogens, sedatives, and opioids.

Correlates of Cannabis Use

Age First use of cannabis typically begins in the teens, and the heaviest rates of use occur in the early 20s. Rates of cannabis use remain relatively high during the early 20s but decline thereafter. The majority of young adults who experiment with cannabis have done so by 18 years of age and rates of use decline steadily from the mid 20s into the early 30s.

Gender Rates of cannabis use in the lifetime, the past year, and the past week are consistently higher among men than women. Daily use and long-term daily use are much more common among men.

Income A positive relationship has been found between income in adolescence and early adult life and cannabis use, with those earning more money more likely to report cannabis use. In the United States, daily cannabis use is positively correlated with income and hours worked on a paid job.

Socioeconomic Status The relationship between cannabis use and socioeconomic status (SES) is weak. Higher rates of cannabis use are sometimes found among lower SES individuals, but in the past two decades, there has been no relationship between parents' education and cannabis use among 12th-grade students in the United States, with the exception that the group with lowest parental education had slightly lower cannabis use than the others. That difference may be better explained by differences in income during adolescence rather than by social class.

Ethnicity Information on the relationship between ethnicity and cannabis use is limited. Ethnic differences in one country may not generalize to others, and small sample sizes often make ethnic comparisons unreliable. Even in the very large Monitoring the Future survey, samples from several years have to be combined to make reliable comparisons between the three largest ethnic groups. These show that black students have lower rates of use in all grades than white or Hispanic students. Hispanics, on the other hand, tend to have the highest rates of use in the early grades, before the rates of school drop-out increase.

Availability In general, the more freely available a drug is, the higher its use in the population. This hypothesis has been broadly supported in the case of alcohol consumption, in which the larger the number of licensed outlets and the longer the hours of trading, the higher the levels of community alcohol consumption and alcohol-related problems. There is very little evidence to rigorously test this hypothesis in the case of cannabis use. Self-reports from surveys on how easy it is to obtain cannabis have shown very little change over long periods during which rates of cannabis use have increased and decreased in the United States.

Pharmacology of Cannabinoids

Laboratory research on animals and humans has demonstrated that the primary psychoactive constituent in cannabis is THC and its metabolites. THC acts on specific receptors or molecules in the brain and immune system. These receptors are found in areas of the brain that underlie the psychoactive and other effects of cannabis use. Two "endogenous," or naturally occurring, molecules have been discovered in the brain and body that bind to the cannabinoid receptor and mimic the action of THC.

A typical joint of between 0.5 and 1.0 g of cannabis plant contains between 5 and 150 mg of THC. Twenty to 70 percent of the THC is found in the smoke that reaches the lungs; the rest is burnt and lost in side-stream smoke. Only 5 to 24 percent of THC in the joint reaches the bloodstream when cannabis is smoked. Two to 3 mg of THC produces a brief high in an occasional user, and a single joint may provide enough THC for two or three such individuals. A heavy cannabis smoker may use five or more joints per day, whereas heavy users in Jamaica, for example, may consume up to 420 mg of THC per day.

Different methods of using cannabis lead to differing absorption, metabolism, and excretion of THC. When smoked, THC is absorbed from the lungs into the bloodstream within minutes. It is first metabolized in the lungs and then in the liver. The metabolite 9-carboxy-THC is detected in blood within minutes of smoking. Peak blood levels of THC are usually reached within 10 minutes of smoking and decrease to approximately 5 to 10 percent of their initial level within 1 hour. This rapid decline reflects the rapid conversion of THC to its metabolites and the distribution of THC to fatty tissues, including the brain.

When swallowed, THC takes 1 to 3 hours to enter the bloodstream, delaying the onset of psychoactive effects. Another metabolite, 11-hydroxy-THC, which is 20 percent more potent than THC, is found in high concentrations after being swallowed.

THC and its metabolites are highly fat soluble, so they may remain in the fatty tissues of the body for long periods. THC and its metabolites accumulate in the body because of their slow rate of clearance. They may be detected in the blood for several days and traces may persist for several weeks. THC may be stored in body fat for more than 28 days.

It has been claimed that the medical literature underestimates the adverse health effects of cannabis because it is based on research conducted on less potent forms of cannabis than have become available in the past decade. The evidence suggests that the average potency of cannabis has increased but not to the extent often claimed. Changes in patterns of cannabis use, with earlier age of first use and more regular use of more potent forms of cannabis, have probably been more important in increasing average dose of THC than any increase in the THC content of cannabis plants.

DIAGNOSTIC AND CLINICAL FEATURES

Cannabis Dependence For much of the 1960s and 1970s, cannabis was not regarded as a drug of dependence because it did not seem to produce tolerance or a withdrawal syndrome such as that seen in alcohol and opioid dependence. Views changed in the late 1970s and early 1980s with the adoption of a broader conception of drug dependence. This new conception reduced the emphasis on tolerance and withdrawal and placed more emphasis on the compulsion to use, a narrowing of the drug-using repertoire, rapid reinstatement of dependence after abstinence, and the high salience of drug use in the user's life.

Drug Dependence in DSM-IV-TR "The essential feature of Substance Dependence is a cluster of cognitive, behavioral and physiologic symptoms indicating that the individual continues use of the substance despite significant substance-related problems." A diagnosis of substance dependence is made if *three or more* of the following criteria occur at any time in the same 12-month period:

Tolerance, as defined by either of the following:
- Need for markedly increased amounts of the substance to achieve intoxication or desired effect
- Markedly diminished effect with continued use or the same amount of the substance

Withdrawal, as manifested by either of the following:
- The characteristic withdrawal syndrome for the substance
- The same (or closely related) substance is taken to relieve or avoid withdrawal symptoms

The substance is often taken in larger amounts or over a longer period than was intended.

There is a persistent desire or unsuccessful efforts to cut down or control substance use.

A great deal of time is spent in activities necessary to obtain the substance (e.g., visiting multiple doctors, driving long distances), use the substance (e.g., chain smoking), or recover from its effects.

Important social, occupational, or recreational activities are given up or reduced because of substance use.

The substance use is continued despite knowledge of having a persistent or recurrent physical or psychological problem that is likely to have been caused or exacerbated by the substance.

DSM-IV-TR *substance abuse* is defined as:

A. A maladaptive pattern of substance use leading to clinically significant impairment or distress, as manifested by one (or more) of the following, occurring within a 12-month period:
- Recurrent substance use resulting in failure to fulfill major role obligations at work, school, or home
- Recurrent substance use in situations in which it is physically hazardous (e.g., driving while intoxicated)
- Recurrent substance-related legal problems
- Continued substance use despite having persistent or recurrent social or interpersonal problems caused or exacerbated by the effects of the substance

B. The symptoms have not met criteria for substance dependence.

The Epidemiological Catchment Area (ECA) study estimated that 4.4 percent of the U.S. population had a diagnosis of cannabis abuse or dependence according to DSM-III criteria. One-third of those with lifetime cannabis abuse or dependence (38 percent) reported problems with cannabis use in the last year. Men had a higher risk of cannabis dependence than women, with the highest risk among 18- to 29-year-olds.

The most common symptoms reported by those who were cannabis dependent were requiring larger amounts (21 percent), having psychological (21 percent) or social (17 percent) problems attributed to cannabis, and inability to reduce use (8 percent). Few reported health problems (5 percent) or withdrawal sickness (3 percent). Surveys using similar methods to the ECA have produced similar estimates of the rate of cannabis dependence in Canada and New Zealand.

The National Comorbidity Survey (NCS) conducted in the United States between 1990 and 1992 found that 4.2 percent of adults met DSM-III-R criteria for cannabis dependence at some time in their lives. The proportion of people who had ever used cannabis who met criteria for cannabis dependence was 9 percent.

Risk of Cannabis Dependence People who use cannabis daily over weeks to months are most likely to become dependent. Approximately one in three daily cannabis users meet DSM-III criteria for dependence. The risk of dependence among less frequent users of cannabis is lower. In the ECA study, 17 percent of those who used cannabis more than five times met DSM-III criteria for dependence at some time in their lives. In the National Comorbidity Study, the proportion of people who had ever used alcohol, amphetamines, cannabis, cocaine, heroin, nicotine, and sedatives who met DSM-III-R criteria for dependence on each drug at some time in their lives was 32 percent for nicotine, 23 percent for heroin, 15 percent for alcohol and cocaine, and 9 percent for cannabis.

These estimates suggest the following rules of thumb about the risks of cannabis dependence. For those who have ever used cannabis, the risks of developing dependence are probably of the order of one chance in ten. Among those who use the drug more than a few times, the risk of developing dependence is from one in five to one in three. As a rule, the more often cannabis has been used and the longer it has been used, the higher the risk of dependence.

The following factors also predict a higher risk of regular involvement with cannabis: poor academic achievement, deviant behavior in childhood and adolescence, nonconformity and rebelliousness, personal distress and maladjustment, poor parental relationships, earlier use, and a parental history of drug and alcohol problems.

Clinical Populations Cannabis-dependent people seek help with cannabis-related problems in Australia, the United States, and Europe. In Australia, the proportion of cases in which cannabis was the *main* drug problem increased from 4 percent in 1990 to 7 percent in 1995. Between 1994 and 1998, cannabis was the primary drug of abuse for between 11 and 26 percent of clients of treatment agencies in the United States. Cannabis was the primary drug problem for between 2 and 16 percent of clients attending treatment agencies in the European Union in 1998.

A Swedish treatment program reported that its clients typically complained of unsuccessful attempts to stop or moderate use and frequent (often daily) intoxication despite having adverse effects connected with their cannabis use. These included sleeplessness, depression, impaired concentration and memory, and blunting of emotions.

Common symptoms among people seeking help to cease cannabis use include an inability to stop using (93 percent), feeling bad about using cannabis (87 percent), procrastinating (86 percent), loss of self-confidence (76 percent), memory loss (67 percent), and withdrawal symptoms (51 percent). Similar experiences have been reported among users in recent U.S. and Australian studies of interventions for problem cannabis use. In the Australian study, among 180 long-term cannabis users seeking help, the most common symptoms were withdrawal and use to relieve withdrawal.

Cannabis Intoxication The main reason why most young people use cannabis is to experience a "high": mild euphoria; relaxation and perceptual alterations, including time distortion; and the intensification of ordinary experiences such as eating, watching films, listening to music, and engaging in sex. When used in a social setting, the "high" may be accompanied by infectious laughter, talkativeness, and increased sociability. Cognitive changes include impaired short-term memory and attention. These make it easy for the user to become lost in pleasant reverie and difficult to sustain goal-directed mental activity. Motor skills, reaction time, motor coordination, and many forms of skilled psychomotor activity are impaired while the user is intoxicated.

Cannabis Intoxication Delirium Psychotic symptoms, such as delusions and hallucinations, are very rare experiences that may occur at very high doses of THC and perhaps in susceptible individuals at lower doses.

High doses of THC have been reported to produce visual and auditory hallucinations, delusional ideas, and thought disorder in normal volunteers. In traditional cannabis-using cultures, such as India, a "cannabis psychosis" has been reported in which the symptoms are preceded by heavy cannabis use and remit after abstinence.

The existence of a cannabis psychosis in Western cultures is still a matter of debate. In its favor are case series of cannabis psychoses and a small number of controlled studies that report characteristic differences between the symptoms of cannabis psychoses and those of psychoses in individuals who were not using cannabis at the time of hospital admission. Critics of the hypothesis emphasize the fallibility of clinical judgments about etiology, the poorly specified criteria used in diagnosing these psychoses, the dearth of controlled studies, and the striking variations in the clinical features assigned to cannabis psychoses.

Cannabis and Schizophrenia There is clinical and epidemiological evidence of an association between schizophrenia and cannabis use that suggests that cannabis use can precipitate schizophrenia or exacerbate its symptoms. But this is not the only explanation of the association: People with schizophrenia may use cannabis as a form of self-medication, or there may be other variables that explain both, such as cannabis use being a marker of other psychotogenic drug use or of vulnerability to schizophrenia.

There is good clinical and epidemiological evidence that cannabis use exacerbates the symptoms of schizophrenia in affected individuals. This includes the findings of a number of prospective studies that have controlled for confounding variables. It is also a biologically plausible relationship. Psychotic disorders involve disturbances in the dopamine neurotransmitter systems because drugs that increase dopamine release produce psychotic symptoms when given in large doses, and neuroleptic drugs that reduce psychotic symptoms also reduce dopamine levels. Cannabinoids, such as THC, increase dopamine release.

There is good prospective evidence from a Swedish conscript study that cannabis use precipitates schizophrenia in people who are vulnerable because of a personal or family history of schizophrenia. This hypothesis is consistent with the stress-diathesis model of schizophrenia in which the likelihood of developing schizophrenia is the product of stress acting on a genetic "diathesis" to develop schizophrenia. The Swedish findings have recently been confirmed in a further follow-up of the original cohort and in four other prospective studies in Israel, The Netherlands, and New Zealand. All of these studies have been able to better control for the most plausible alternative explanations of the relationship between cannabis use and schizophrenia than the original Swedish study. These studies provide strong support for the hypothesis that cannabis use, especially early-onset use, can precipitate schizophrenia in susceptible individuals.

Although it is likely, there is very little direct evidence that genetic vulnerability increases the risk that cannabis users develop psychosis. In one British study, people with a history of heavy cannabis use who developed a psychosis were ten times more likely to have a family history of schizophrenia than people with a psychosis who had not used cannabis. It is difficult to identify a genetic diathesis in the majority of cases of schizophrenia because 81 percent of people with schizophrenia do not have a first-degree relative with the disorder, and 63 percent do not have an affected first- or second-degree relative.

It seems likely that cannabis use can precipitate schizophrenia in vulnerable cases, but it is more contentious whether cannabis use can cause schizophrenia that would not otherwise have occurred. One cannot rule this possibility out, but it is unlikely to account for more than a minority of cases. Most of the 274 Swedish conscripts who developed schizophrenia had not used cannabis, and, at most, 7 percent of cases of schizophrenia could be attributed to cannabis use. Moreover, the *treated* incidence of schizophrenia, and particularly of early-onset acute cases, has declined (or remained stable) during the 1970s and 1980s when cannabis use increased among young adults in Australia and North America. Although there are complications in interpreting such trends, a large reduction in treated incidence has been observed in a number of countries, although cannabis use has increased.

Cannabis-Induced Anxiety Disorder Some users report unpleasant experiences after using cannabis. These include anxiety, panic, a fear of going mad, and depression. These are often reported by users who are unfamiliar with the effects of cannabis and by some patients given THC for therapeutic reasons. More experienced users may report these effects after swallowing cannabis because its effects may be more pronounced and of longer duration than they usually experience after smoking.

The most immediate effect of smoking cannabis is an increasing heart rate by 20 to 50 percent within a few minutes to one-quarter of an hour of smoking cannabis. Changes in blood pressure also occur. These depend on posture: Blood pressure is increased while the person is sitting and decreases while they are standing. A sudden change from lying down to standing up may produce postural hypotension and a feeling of "light-headedness" and faintness that is often the earliest indication of intoxication in naïve users. In healthy young users, these cardiovascular effects are unlikely to be of any clinical significance. They may amplify anxiety if the cannabis-induced palpitations and feeling faint are misinterpreted as symptoms of serious misadventure.

Withdrawal and Tolerance Tolerance to many of the behavioral and physiological effects of THC has been demonstrated in humans and animals. The precise mechanisms are unknown, but they probably involve changes in cannabinoid receptor function.

Early case reports of cannabis withdrawal symptoms in humans have been supported by abstinence symptoms in laboratory studies. Studies in clinical and nonclinical samples of long-term cannabis users have reported withdrawal symptoms such as anxiety, insomnia, appetite disturbance, and depression.

Regular cannabis users who are abruptly withdrawn from cannabis after 2 weeks on high doses of oral THC have complained within 6 hours of "inner unrest," and after 12 hours, they reported "irritability, insomnia, and restlessness," which were also observed by staff. These symptoms were correlated with THC dose and frequency of use and were reduced after using cannabis. Similar symptoms have been reported during the first week of abstinence in subjects who had received 210 mg of smoked cannabis a day for 4 weeks. Recent laboratory studies have reported withdrawal symptoms at much lower doses of THC given orally and by smoking. The most common symptoms were anxiety, depression, and irritability.

A controlled prospective study has been done on withdrawal symptoms among chronic cannabis users who were assessed daily on various withdrawal symptoms while in a hospital ward for 28 days. Their ratings of mood, anxiety, depression, and irritability were compared with those of two control groups of abstinent former heavy cannabis users and nonusers of cannabis. During the course of the 28 days, the chronic cannabis users showed decreases in mood and appetite; increases in irritability, anxiety, physical tension, and physical symptoms; and increased scores on the Hamilton Depression and Anxiety scales. These appeared within 24 hours and were most marked in the first 10 days, although the increase in irritability and physical tension persisted throughout the 28-day observation period.

Research using the cannabinoid antagonist SR 141716A (which immediately reverses the effects of THC) has shown that a withdrawal syndrome can be produced in rats, mice, and dogs that have been maintained on THC. The antagonist produces compressed and accentuated symptoms that are much more dramatic than the milder and more prolonged symptoms that occur under usual conditions of human use. The relatively long half-life and complex metabolism of cannabis may also result in a less intense withdrawal syndrome than drugs such as opiates.

Cannabis Disorders Not Otherwise Specified

Amotivational Syndrome The evidence that chronic heavy cannabis use produces an amotivational syndrome consists largely of case studies. Controlled field and laboratory studies have not found evidence for such a syndrome, although their value is limited by the small sample sizes and limited sociodemographical characteristics of participants of the field studies, the short periods of drug use, and the youth, good health, and minimal demands made of the volunteers in the laboratory studies. If there is such a syndrome, it is a relatively rare occurrence even among heavy, chronic cannabis users. The phenomenon may be better explained as the result of chronic intoxication in dependent cannabis users.

Cognitive Impairment The fact that cannabis use acutely impairs cognitive functioning has raised the reasonable concern that chronic use may produce cognitive impairment. The available evidence, however, suggests that the long-term heavy use of cannabis does not produce any severe or grossly debilitating impairment of cognitive function. There is no evidence, for example, that it produces anything comparable to the cognitive impairments found in chronic heavy alcohol drinkers; if it did, research to date should have detected it.

There is more recent clinical and experimental evidence, however, that the long-term use of cannabis may produce more subtle forms of cognitive impairment in the higher cognitive functions of memory, attention, and organization and in the integration of complex information. This evidence suggests that the longer the period of heavy cannabis use, the more pronounced the cognitive impairment. Nonetheless, because the impairments in performance are subtle, it remains to be determined how significant they are for everyday functioning. It also remains to be investigated whether these impairments can be reversed after an extended period of abstinence from cannabis.

A suspicion that chronic heavy cannabis use may cause gross structural brain damage was raised by a single poorly controlled study using an outmoded method of investigation, which reported that cannabis users had enlarged cerebral ventricles. Since then, a number of better-controlled studies using more sophisticated methods of investigation have consistently failed to demonstrate evidence of structural change in the brains of heavy, long-term cannabis users. These negative results are consistent with the evidence that any cognitive effects of chronic cannabis use are subtle and unlikely to manifest as gross structural changes in the brain.

Effects on Adolescent Development Cross-sectional and longitudinal studies of adolescents in the 1970s and 1980s indicate that chronic heavy cannabis use may adversely affect adolescent development in a number of ways. Interpretation of this evidence is complicated by the fact that many of the indicators of adverse development that have been attributed to cannabis use precede its use and make it more likely that a young person will use cannabis. These include minor delinquency, poor educational performance, nonconformity, and poor adjustment.

Among American adolescents in the 1970s and 1980s, the typical sequence of initiation into drug use was that the use of alcohol and tobacco preceded the use of cannabis, which, in turn, preceded the use of hallucinogens, amphetamines, and the later use of heroin and cocaine. Generally, the earlier the age of first use and the greater the involvement with any drug in the sequence, the more likely a young person was to use the next drug in the sequence.

The explanation of cannabis' role in this sequence remains contested. The evidence for the hypothesis that cannabis use has a pharmacological effect that increases the risk of using later drugs in the sequence is, at present, not compelling. More plausible hypotheses are that the sequence of drug involvement reflects a combination of the early recruitment into cannabis use of nonconforming and deviant adolescents who are likely to use alcohol, tobacco, and illicit drugs; a genetic vulnerability to become dependent on a range of substances; and socialization of cannabis users within an illicit drug–using subculture that increases the exposure, opportunity, and encouragement to use other illicit drugs. Recent prospective studies that have controlled for many of these factors have failed to eliminate the apparent "gateway effect" of cannabis.

In cross-sectional surveys of young people, cannabis use is associated with the inability to complete a high school education and with job instability in young adulthood. The complication is that those who are most likely to use cannabis have lower academic aspirations and poorer school performance *before* using cannabis than those who do not. When these differences are taken into account, the relationship between cannabis use and educational and occupational performance is much more modest. Even so, the adverse effects of cannabis and other drug use on educational performance are important because they further impair poor performance, and level of education affects choice of occupation, level of income, choice of mate, and quality of life.

There is also suggestive evidence that heavy cannabis use has adverse effects on family formation, mental health, and involvement in drug-related (but not other types of) crime. In the case of each of these outcomes, the apparently strong associations revealed in cross-sectional data are much more modest in longitudinal studies that control for associations between cannabis use and other variables that predict these adverse outcomes.

Flashbacks There are a small number of case reports of cannabis "flashbacks"—that is, experiencing symptoms of cannabis intoxication days or weeks after the individual last used cannabis. Because of their rarity and the fact that many affected individuals have also used other drugs, it is difficult to draw any conclusions about the relationship between these symptoms and cannabis use. It is often difficult to decide whether these are rare events that are coincidental with cannabis use; the effects of other drugs that are often taken together with cannabis; rare consequences of cannabis use that only occur at doses that are much higher than those used recreationally or that require unusual forms of personal vulnerability; or the results of interactions between the cannabis and other drugs.

ADVERSE EFFECTS OF CANNABIS USE

Psychomotor Effects and Driving

Cannabis intoxication impairs a wide range of cognitive and behavioral functions that are involved in driving an automobile or operating machinery. The effects are generally larger, more consistent, and more persistent in tasks that require sustained attention. Recreational doses of THC produce similar performance impairments in laboratory tests and standardized driving courses to blood alcohol concentrations of between 0.07 and 0.10 percent.

It has been difficult to estimate how these impairments affect the risk of being involved in motor vehicle accidents. Studies of the effect of cannabis on driving performance on the road have found only modest impairments because cannabis-intoxicated drivers drive more slowly and take fewer risks than alcohol-intoxicated drinkers. Cannabis users seem to be more aware of their psychomotor impairment than alcohol users.

Cannabinoids are found in between 4 and 37 percent of blood samples of accident victims, but these findings are difficult to evaluate for the following reasons. First, it has been difficult to decide whether people with cannabinoids are overrepresented among accident victims because it is not known how often cannabinoids are found in the blood of people who are *not* involved in accidents. Second, cannabinoids in blood indicate recent use, but they do not necessarily mean that the driver was intoxicated at the time of the accident. Third, many drivers with cannabinoids in their blood also have high blood alcohol levels, making it difficult to separate the effects of cannabis on accident risk from those of alcohol. Laboratory studies have suggested, however, that the separate effects of alcohol and cannabis on psychomotor impairment and driving performance are approximately additive.

There is recent evidence from controlled epidemiological studies that cannabis users are two times more likely to be involved in motor vehicle or other accidents than nonusers. This evidence is not yet as strong as comparable evidence for alcohol use, for which there are more case-controlled studies showing that people intoxicated by alcohol are overrepresented among accident victims. Cannabis users who also use alcohol are even more highly overrepresented among the victims of motor vehicle accidents.

Cardiovascular System

A few minutes to one-quarter of an hour after cannabis is smoked or swallowed, THC increases heart rate by 20 to 50 percent. This may last for up to 3 hours. Blood pressure is increased while the person is sitting and decreases on standing. In healthy young users, these cardiovascular effects are unlikely to be of any clinical significance because tolerance develops to the effects of THC, and young, healthy hearts are only mildly stressed. These effects may pose more of a risk to patients with heart disease.

The acute toxicity of cannabis, and cannabinoids generally, is very low. There are no cases of fatal cannabis poisoning in the human medical literature. Animal studies indicate that the dose of THC required to produce 50 percent mortality in rodents is extremely high in comparison with other pharmaceutical and recreational drugs. The lethal dose also increases as one moves up the phylogenetic tree, suggesting that the lethal dose in humans could not be achieved by smoking or swallowing cannabis.

The changes that cannabis causes in heart rate and blood pressure are unlikely to harm healthy young adults, but they may be less benign in patients with hypertension, cerebrovascular disease, and coronary atherosclerosis in whom cannabis smoking may pose a threat because it increases the work of the heart. The seriousness of these effects will be determined as the cohort of chronic cannabis users of the late 1960s enters the age of maximum risk for atherosclerosis in the heart, brain, and peripheral blood vessels. A recent study of the relationship between cannabis use and myocardial infarction suggests that the acute cardiovascular effects of cannabis may be life-threatening in middle-aged adults with heart disease.

Respiratory System

Regular cannabis smoking impairs the functioning of the large airways and causes symptoms of chronic bronchitis such as coughing, sputum, and wheezing. Given that tobacco and cannabis smoke contain similar carcinogenic substances and that tobacco smoke has adverse effects on the respiratory system, it is likely that chronic cannabis use also increases the risks of respiratory cancer. There is evidence that chronic cannabis smoking produces histopathological changes in lung tissues of the type that precede the development of lung cancer. Concern about the possibility of cancers caused by chronic cannabis smoking has been raised by case reports of cancers of the aerodigestive tract in young adults with a history of heavy cannabis use. A recent case-controlled study has provided the first suggestion of an increased risk of aerodigestive tract cancers among cannabis smokers.

Cellular Effects and Cancers

There is weak evidence that THC can alter cell metabolism and deoxyribonucleic acid (DNA) synthesis in the test tube. There is stronger evidence that cannabis *smoke* produces mutations in cells in the test tube and in live animals and, hence, is a potential cause of cancer. Cannabis smoke contains many of the same carcinogenic substances as cigarette smoke. If cannabis smoking causes cancer, it is most likely to be cancers of the lung and upper aerodigestive tract, which are maximally exposed to cannabis smoke.

Aerodigestive tract cancers have been reported among young adults who have been daily cannabis users, and a case-controlled study has found an association between cannabis smoking and head and neck cancer. A prospective cohort study of 64,000 adults did not find an increased incidence of head and neck or respiratory cancers, but it found increased rates of prostate cancer. The relative youth of the participants and their low rates of regular cannabis use may have reduced the ability of this research to detect an increase in respiratory cancers. Further studies are needed to clarify the issue.

There is much weaker evidence for an increased risk of cancers among children born to women who smoked cannabis during pregnancy. Three studies of very different types of cancer have reported an association with maternal cannabis use. None of these was a planned study of the role of cannabis use in these cancers, so replication of their results is required. There have not been any increases in the rates of these cancers that parallel increased rates of cannabis use over the past three decades.

Immunological Effects

Cannabinoids impair cell-mediated and humoral immunity in rodents and reduce resistance to infection by bacteria and viruses in animals. Cannabinoid receptors are expressed in cells of the immune system in animals and humans, although the significance of this for immune function is unclear. Cannabis smoke also impairs the functioning of alveolar macrophages, the first line of the body's immune defense system in the lungs. The clinical relevance of these findings is uncertain because the doses required to produce these effects have been very high, and extrapolation to the doses used by humans is complicated by the fact that tolerance may develop to these effects.

The limited experimental and clinical evidence in humans suggests that the adverse effects seen in animals are not replicated in humans. There is no conclusive evidence that cannabinoids impair immune system function in humans, as measured by T lymphocytes, B lymphocytes or macrophages, or immunoglobulin levels. There is suggestive evidence that THC impairs T-lymphocyte responses to mitogens and allogenic lymphocytes.

The clinical and biological significance of these possible effects in chronic cannabis users is uncertain. There is no epidemiological evidence of increased rates of disease among chronic heavy cannabis users, and several large prospective studies of human immunodeficiency virus (HIV)–positive homosexual men have found that cannabis use does *not* increase the risk of progression to acquired immune deficiency syndrome (AIDS).

Reproductive Effects

Chronic administration of THC disrupts male and female reproductive systems in animals, reducing testosterone secretion and sperm production, motility, and viability in males and disrupting the ovulatory cycle in females. It is uncertain whether cannabis use has these effects in humans because of the inconsistency in the limited literature on human males and the lack of research in the case of human females. There is uncertainty about the clinical significance of these effects in normal healthy young adults.

It is likely that cannabis use during pregnancy impairs fetal development, leading to smaller birth weight, perhaps as a consequence of shorter gestation and probably by the same mechanism as cigarette smoking. There is no clear evidence that cannabis use during pregnancy increases the risk of birth defects as a result of exposure of the fetus to cannabis in the uterus.

There is some evidence that infants exposed to cannabis in the uterus may show transient behavioral and developmental effects during the first few months after birth. These effects are small in comparison to those caused by tobacco use during pregnancy and have not been observed in all studies. The evidence for this consequence of cannabis use is still weak.

LABORATORY EXAMINATION

It is possible to detect cannabinoids in head hair, pubic hair, urine, sweat, saliva, and blood. Given the nature of cannabinoids and the fact that they are stored in the fat cells of the body, cannabis remains in the body for an extended period, compared with other drugs. In some cases, it may remain in urine for up to 11 weeks after use. Detection of cannabinoids is possible in hair, and some research has suggested that higher concentrations of cannabinoids may be found in pubic hair, compared with head hair. Cannabinoids may be detected in saliva and sweat, but the concentrations of cannabinoids in these fluids tend to be lower compared with urine, and in some cases, cannabinoids may not be detected using these fluids.

Cannabinoid levels in the blood vary among individuals and depend on the dose received and the individual's history of cannabis use. Blood levels of THC may range between 0 and 500 ng/mL depending on the potency of the cannabis and the time since smoking. The detection of THC in blood more than 10 to 15 ng/mL is evidence of recent use, although it is difficult to be precise about how recent. A more precise estimate of time since last use is provided by the ratio of THC to 9-carboxy-THC. Similar blood concentrations of THC and this metabolite indicate that cannabis has been used in the past 20 to 40 minutes and so suggest a high probability of intoxication, although this is less clear in regular users.

Cannabis intoxication impairs skills required to drive a motor vehicle, so it is desirable to have a measure of cannabis intoxication similar to the breath test for alcohol intoxication. The major obstacle is the lack of a simple relationship between blood levels of THC (and its metabolites) and degree of psychomotor impairment.

With repeated frequent dosing of cannabis, THC accumulates in fatty tissues in the human body, where it may remain for considerable periods. The health significance of this storage is unclear. The storage of cannabinoids *would* be serious cause for concern if THC were a highly toxic substance that remained physiologically active while stored in body fat. THC is not a highly toxic substance, and it is inactive while stored in fat. Stored cannabinoids could conceivably be released into blood, producing a "flashback," although this is likely to occur very rarely, if at all.

TREATMENT

Cannabis Dependence

Until recently, little research had been done on the type of assistance that should be given to cannabis users who seek help to stop using cannabis. Although many users may succeed in quitting without professional help, those who are unable to stop on their own need to be assisted. It is not clear what type of treatment should be provided for dependent cannabis users who have repeatedly failed to stop using cannabis and seek help.

There have been a small number of randomized controlled trials comparing group-based relapse prevention and social support in subjects who answered advertisements for help to stop using cannabis. The earliest study reported that, at 1 month after treatment, only 30 percent of their patients were still abstinent, and by the end of 1 year, only 17 percent remained abstinent.

Later studies have compared group relapse prevention intervention, individualized advice, and motivational interviewing adapted from Miller's Drinker's Check-Up with a delayed treatment condition in which participants did not receive any treatment for 4 months. At the 4-month follow-up, all three groups had reduced their cannabis use, but the two treatment groups showed the largest reduction and did not differ from each another. In the treatment groups, 37 percent were abstinent, compared with only 9 percent in the delayed treatment group. The amount of cannabis use also declined by 70 percent in the treatment groups and by 30 percent in the delayed treatment groups. Abstinence rates decreased over time, but the two treatments did not differ at 7, 13, and 16 months after treatment. Twenty-two percent of participants were abstinent throughout the 16-month study, and their abstinence was corroborated by partners and family members.

A more recent study has compared motivational enhancement to quit, motivational enhancement plus behavioral coping skills, and motivational enhancement and behavioral treatment plus incentives (vouchers for retail items) to remain abstinent. The last group had a longer period of continuous abstinence than the other two groups, which did not differ from each other. By 14 weeks' posttreatment, however, fewer than 10 percent of participants had been continuously abstinent from cannabis.

A recent Australian study has reported a comparison of a six-session cognitive-behavioral intervention with a single-session cognitive-behavioral treatment and a delayed treatment control group that was offered treatment for 4 months. Only 6.5 percent of all subjects (N = 11) were continuously abstinent during the 8-month follow-up period, and all of these were in the treatment groups. There were greater reductions in cannabis-related problems and in dependence symptoms in the two treatment groups.

To date, rates of continuous abstinence from cannabis have been low in the behavioral and cognitive treatments tested, although there have been substantial reductions in rates of cannabis use and self-reported problems related to use. Nonetheless, much more research is needed before sensible advice can be given about the best ways to achieve abstinence from cannabis. In the absence of better evidence of treatment effectiveness, people offering treatment for cannabis dependence should avoid replicating experience in the treatment of alcohol dependence in which inpatient treatment has been widely adopted in the absence of any evidence that it is more effective than outpatient forms of treatment.

There is increasing interest in the use of antidepressants to treat dependent cannabis use because of the high rates of depression reported on presentation for treatment and after cessation. Small studies have been conducted to examine the effectiveness of such a treatment, but no large randomized controlled studies have been conducted to date. This is likely to be an area of increasing research interest in the future.

Cannabis Intoxication

The adverse acute effects of cannabis (such as anxiety symptoms) can be prevented by preparing users about the cardiovascular effects they may experience. If these symptoms develop, they can usually be managed by reassurance and support.

Therapeutic Effects of Cannabinoids

When cannabinoids and cannabis are advocated for medical uses, it is primarily to relieve symptoms rather than to cure underlying diseases. The conditions for which cannabis is most commonly advocated are for symptomatic relief of nausea and vomiting caused by cancer chemotherapy, appetite loss in AIDS, and muscle spasticity and chronic pain in neurological disorders.

Analgesia

Animal studies and the biology of cannabinoid receptors suggest that cannabinoids may be useful analgesics with mild to moderate efficacy. The few controlled studies in humans have suggested that THC and other cannabinoids have modest analgesic effects on acute postoperative and chronic pain (compared with placebo) that are equivalent to 60 mg of codeine. Because patients often report adverse psychotropic effects, their use for these purposes is likely to be limited. The development of synthetic cannabinoids with fewer psychotropic effects seems a more promising way ahead than the use of THC or cannabis products.

Nausea and Vomiting

Most research on the antiemetic effects of cannabis or cannabinoids in patients receiving cancer chemotherapy was done in the 1980s using THC, nabilone, and levonantradol. Many of these studies were small in size and not well controlled. These studies showed *some* antiemetic efficacy in comparison with the antiemetic agents then available (namely, prochlorperazine [Compazine]). Clinical interest in cannabinoids decreased with the use of selective serotonin type 3 receptor agonists, such as ondansetron (Zofran), which have dramatically reduced nausea and vomiting. These provide complete control over nausea induced by cisplatin in 75 percent of cases and up to 90 percent for less emetogenic chemotherapy, whereas THC provides control in only one-third of patients. The difference in efficacy is apparent in an experimental comparison of the effects of smoked marijuana and ondansetron on nausea induced by syrup of ipecac. Marijuana had a self-reported antiemetic effect and very slightly reduced the frequency of vomiting, whereas ondansetron prevented all vomiting. Cannabinoids have a modest antiemetic effect that is offset by a high rate of adverse effects such as hypotension, dizziness, and dysphoric effects.

Wasting Syndrome and Appetite Stimulation in HIV/AIDS

THC has been shown to stimulate appetite and assist weight gain in AIDS patients in short-term trials. It has been registered for medical use for this purpose in the United States. Some patients do not like dronabinol (Marinol) because of its psychoactive side effects, the difficulty of titrating the dose, the delayed onset of effects, and the prolonged duration of the effects. There are anecdotal reports that smoked cannabis is also effective in the treatment of HIV/AIDS-associated anorexia and weight loss, but there have not been any controlled studies. A clinical trial is under way in California that examines the use of smoked cannabis in HIV-infected patients to see if they are vulnerable to immunosuppressive effects of cannabis and to infectious organisms found in cannabis.

Muscle Spasticity

Muscle spasticity is the increased resistance to passive stretch of muscles and increased deep tendon muscles. Involuntary contractions may occur that can be painful and debilitating. Approximately 90 percent of multiple sclerosis (MS) patients eventually develop muscle spasticity, as do a substantial proportion of patients with spinal cord injuries. A survey of MS patients suggested that cannabis reduced muscle spasticity, but a recent clinical trial has failed to find evidence of benefit.

Movement Disorders

Movement disorders are caused by abnormalities in areas of the brain that are connected to areas of the cortex that control motor functions. They result in abnormal skeletal muscle movements in the face, limbs, and trunk. The disorders most often mentioned as candidates for medical cannabis use are dystonia, Huntington's disease, Parkinson's disease, and Tourette's syndrome. There is limited evidence that cannabis is useful for treating any of these movement disorders. The health risks of the regular cannabis smoking that is required in people already with these health conditions provide a major limitation on its use in these disorders.

Epilepsy

There are case reports suggesting that cannabis can control epileptic seizures and one observational study that suggests that cannabis use was protective against seizures, but it has major limitations. Most of the anticonvulsant properties of cannabinoids appear to be attributable to cannabidiol (CBD) rather than to THC. Because CBD, which has no psychoactive effects, is not a controlled substance, there are no obstacles to its clinical use if its safety and efficacy are demonstrated in controlled trials.

Glaucoma

Elevated intraocular pressure is a chronic condition that produces blindness if untreated. Intraocular pressure must be controlled continuously to reduce the risk of blindness. Cannabis and THC taken orally or intravenously (IV) reduce intraocular pressure by 25 percent, but the effect lasts only 3 to 4 hours. The high doses of THC that are required to produce these effects produce side effects that preclude the lifelong use of cannabis or cannabinoids to treat glaucoma. Water-soluble cannabinoids that may be topically applied and that have no psychoactive effects may be a better prospect.

THC and other cannabinoids have not been widely used therapeutically or investigated in clinical trials. This is because, in the United States, clinical research on cannabinoids has been discouraged by regulation and the fact that THC, the most therapeutically effective cannabinoid, is the one that produces the psychoactive effects sought by recreational users. THC is also a naturally occurring substance that cannot be patented, which means that companies are unlikely to conduct research into its medical uses. The discovery of a cannabinoid receptor and the cannabinoid-like substance anandamide may encourage more basic research into the therapeutic uses of natural and synthetic cannabinoids.

SUGGESTED CROSS-REFERENCES

An overview of substance-related disorders, including substance abuse and dependence, appears in Section 11.1. Schizophrenia is discussed in Sections 12.1 and 12.2, drug-induced psychotic disorders are discussed in Section 12.16g, and substance-induced anxiety disorders are discussed in Section 14.8.

REFERENCES

Adams IB, Martin BR: Cannabis: Pharmacology and toxicology in animals and humans. *Addiction.* 1996;91:1585–1614.

Andreasson S, Allebeck P, Engstrom A, Rydberg U: Cannabis and schizophrenia: a longitudinal study of Swedish conscripts. *Lancet.* 1987;2:1483–1486.

Anthony JC, Helzer JE. Syndromes of drug abuse and dependence. In: Robins LN, Regier DA, eds. *Psychiatric Disorders in America.* New York: Free Press, MacMillan; 1991.

Anthony JC, Warner LA, Kessler RC: Comparative epidemiology of dependence on tobacco, alcohol, controlled substances and inhalants: basic findings from the National Comorbidity Study. *Clin Exp Psychopharmacology.* 1994;2:244–268.

Arseneault L, Cannon M, Poulton R, Murray R, Caspi A, Moffitt TE: Cannabis use in adolescence and risk for adult psychosis: longitudinal prospective study. *BMJ.* 2002:325:1212–1213.

Bachman JG, Wadsworth KN, O'Malley PM, Johnston L, Schulenburg J. *Smoking, Drinking and Drug Use in Young Adulthood.* Mahwah, New Jersey: Lawrence Erlbaum Associates; 1997.

Chesher G, Hall W. Effects of cannabis on the cardiovascular and gastrointestinal systems. In: Kalant H, Corrigall W, Hall W, Smart R, eds. *The Health Effects of Cannabis.* Toronto: Centre for Addiction and Mental Health; 1999:435–458.

Degenhardt L, Hall W: The association between psychosis and problematical drug use among Australian adults: findings from the National Survey of Mental Health and Well-being. *Psychol Med.* 2001;31:659–668.

Degenhardt L, Hall W, Lynskey M: The relationship between cannabis use, depression and anxiety among Australian adults: findings from the National Survey of Mental Health and Well-being. *Soc Psychiatry Psychiatr Epidemiol.* 2001;36:219–227.

Fergusson DM, Horwood JL, Swain-Campbell NR: Cannabis dependence and psychotic symptoms in young people. *Psychol Med.* 2003;33:15–21.

Fergusson DM, Horwood LJ: Does cannabis use encourage other forms of illicit drug use? *Addiction.* 2000;95:505–520.

Gerberich SG, Sidney S, Braun BL, Tekawa IS, Tolan KK, Quesenberry CP: Marijuana use and injury events resulting in hospitalization. *Ann Epidemiol.* 2003;13:230–237.

Hall W: The public health implications of cannabis use. *Aust N Z J Pub Health.* 1995;19:235–242.

Hall W, Babor T: Cannabis and public health: assessing the burden. *Addiction.* 2000;95:485–490.

Hall W, Degenhardt L: Cannabis and psychosis. *Aust N Z J Psychiatry.* 2000;34:26–34.

*Hall W, Degenhardt L, Lynskey M. *The Health and Psychological Effects of Cannabis.* National Drug Strategy Monograph No 44. Commonwealth Department of Health and Aged Care; 2001.

Hall W, Johnston L, Donnelly N. The epidemiology of cannabis use and its consequences. In: Kalant H, Corrigal W, Hall W, Smart R, eds. *The Health Effects of Cannabis.* Toronto: Addiction Research Foundation; 1999.

Hall W, MacPhee D: Cannabis use and cancer. *Addiction.* 2002;97:243–247.

Hall W, Pacula R. *Cannabis Use and Dependence: Public Health and Public Policy.* Cambridge University Press; 2003.

*Hall W, Solowij N. The adverse effects of cannabis use. *Lancet.* 1998;352:1611–1616.

Hall W, Swift W: The THC content of cannabis in Australia: evidence and policy implications. *Aust N Z J Pub Health.* 2000;24:503–508.

*Institute of Medicine. *Marijuana and Medicine; Assessing the Science Base.* National Academy Press; 1999.

*Kalant H, Corrigal W, Hall W, Smart R, eds. *The Health Effects of Cannabis.* Toronto: Addiction Research Foundation; 1999.

Lekitsos CG, Garrett E, Liang KY, Anthony JC: Cannabis use and cognitive decline in persons under 65 years of age. *Am J Epidemiol.* 1999;149:794–800.

Linszen DH, Dingemans PM, Lenior ME: Cannabis abuse and the course of recent-onset schizophrenic disorders. *Arch Gen Psychiatry.* 1994;51:273–279.

Lynskey M, Hall W: The effects of adolescent cannabis use on educational attainment: a review. *Addiction.* 2000;95:1621–1630.

Lynskey MT, Heath AC, Bucholz KK, Slutske WS: Escalation of drug use in early-onset cannabis users versus co-twin controls. *JAMA.* 2003;289:427–433.

Mittleman MA, Lewis RA, Maclure M, Sherwood JB, Muller JE: Triggering myocardial infarction by marijuana. *Circulation.* 2001;103:2805–2809.

Morral AR, McCaffrey DF, Paddock SM: Reassessing the marijuana gateway effect. *Addiction.* 2002;97:1493–1504.

Mura P, Kintz P, Ludes B, Gaulier JM, Marquet P, Martin-Dupont S, Vincent F, Kaddour A, Goulle JP, Nouveau J, Moulsma M, Tilhet-Coartet S, Pourrat O: Comparison of the prevalence of alcohol, cannabis, and other drugs between 900 injured drivers and 900 control subjects: results of a French collaborative study. *Forensic Sci Int.* 2003;133:79–85.

Programme on Substance Abuse, World Health Organization. *Cannabis: A Health Perspective and Research Agenda.* Geneva: Division of Mental Health and Prevention of Substance Abuse, World Health Organization; 1997.

Roffman RA, Stephens RS, Simpson EE, Whitaker DL: Treatment of marijuana dependence: preliminary results. *J Psychoactive Drugs.* 1988;20:129–137.

Smiley A. Marijuana: On road and driving simulator studies. In: Kalant H, Corrigal W, Hall W, Smart R, eds. *The Health Effects of Cannabis.* Toronto: Addiction Research Foundation; 1999.

*Solowij N. *Cannabis and Cognitive Functioning.* Cambridge, UK: Cambridge University Press; 1998.

Swift W, Hall W. Tolerance, withdrawal and dependence. In: Grotenhermen F, Russo E, eds. *Cannabis and Cannabinoids: Pharmacology, Toxicology and Therapeutic Potential.* New York: Haworth Press; 2002.

Tashkin D. Effects of cannabis on the respiratory system. In: Kalant H, Corrigall W, Hall W, Smart R, eds. *The Health Effects of Cannabis.* Toronto: Addiction Research Foundation; 1999.

Van Os J, Bak M, Hanssen M, Bijl RV, de Graaf R, Vedoux H: Cannabis use and psychosis: a longitudinal population-based study. *Am J Epidemiol.* 2002;156:319–327.

Verdoux H, Gindre C, Sorbara F, Tournier M, Swendsen J: Cannabis use and the expression of psychosis vulnerability in daily life. *Eur Psychiatry.* 2002;17:180S.

Zajicek J, Fox P, Sanders H, Wright D, Vickery J, Nunn AQ, Thompson A: Cannabinoids for treatment of spasticity and other symptoms related to multiple sclerosis (CAMS) study: multicenter randomised placebo-controlled trial. *Lancet.* 2003;362:1517–1526.

Zammit S, Alleback P, Andreasson S, Lundberg I, Lewis G: Self reported cannabis use as a risk factor for schizophrenia in Swedish conscripts of 1969: historical cohort study. *BMJ.* 2002;325:1199–1201.

▲ 11.6 Cocaine-Related Disorders

JEROME H. JAFFE, M.D., RICHARD A. RAWSON, PH.D., AND WALTER LING, M.D.

Few public health issues attracted as much media attention in the United States during the 1980s and early 1990s as the problems resulting from the use of cocaine and "crack." Although the intranasal use of cocaine hydrochloride in the early 1980s was associated with high-income, "jet-set" users, smokable "crack" cocaine has become an endemic drug problem in the inner cities across the United States. Epidemiological evidence has documented that the peak of this epidemic has passed in the United States, but available data indicate that rates of cocaine use are increasing in a number of European countries.

There is a wealth of new information on the neurobiology of cocaine and cocaine dependence, treatment research efforts have been extensive, and progress has been made in identifying behavioral-psychosocial treatments. However, in spite of well-funded research, there are still no clinically useful pharmacotherapies for the treatment of cocaine-related disorders.

DEFINITIONS

Substance use may be associated with a number of distinct disorders, of which dependence and abuse are but two. In the case of cocaine, the revised fourth edition of the *Diagnostic and Statistical Manual of Mental Disorders* (DSM-IV-TR) describes ten other substance-related disorders. *Cocaine dependence* is defined in DSM-IV-TR as a cluster of physiological, behavioral, and cognitive symptoms that, taken together, indicate that the person continues to use cocaine despite significant problems related to such use. With cocaine dependence, individuals find it increasingly difficult to resist using cocaine whenever it is available. It is defined in the tenth revision of the *International Statistical Classification of Diseases and Related Health Problems* (ICD-10) as a cluster of physiological, behavioral, and cognitive phenomena in which the use of cocaine takes on a much higher priority for a given individual than do other behaviors that once had a greater value. Central to these definitions is the emphasis placed on the drug-using behavior, its maladaptive nature, and how, over time, the voluntary choice to engage in that behavior shifts and becomes constrained as a result of interactions with the drug.

Cocaine abuse is a term used in DSM-IV-TR to categorize a pattern of maladaptive cocaine use leading to clinically significant impairment or distress within a 12-month period but one in which the symptoms have not met criteria for cocaine dependence. Specifically, when there is evidence of tolerance, withdrawal, or compulsive behavior associated with obtaining or administering cocaine, a diagnosis of dependence rather than abuse should be used. ICD-10 does not use the term.

Other cocaine-related disorders include cocaine intoxication, cocaine withdrawal, cocaine-induced psychotic disorder with delusions or with hallucinations, cocaine intoxication delirium, cocaine-induced mood disorder, cocaine-induced anxiety disorder, cocaine-induced sleep disorder, cocaine-induced sexual dysfunction, and cocaine-related disorder not otherwise specified (Table 11.6–1). The DSM-IV-TR coding scheme provides distinct code numbers for cocaine dependence and cocaine abuse.

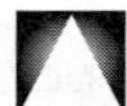

Table 11.6–1
DSM-IV-TR Cocaine-Related Disorders

Cocaine use disorders
Cocaine dependence
Cocaine abuse
Cocaine-induced disorders
Cocaine intoxication
Specify if:
With perceptual disturbances
Cocaine withdrawal
Cocaine intoxication delirium
Cocaine-induced psychotic disorder with delusions
Specify if:
With onset during intoxication
Cocaine-induced psychotic disorder with hallucinations
Specify if:
With onset during intoxication
Cocaine-induced mood disorder
Specify if:
With onset during intoxication
With onset during withdrawal
Cocaine-induced anxiety disorder
Specify if:
With onset during intoxication
With onset during withdrawal
Cocaine-induced sexual dysfunction
Specify if:
With onset during intoxication
Cocaine-induced sleep disorder
Specify if:
With onset during intoxication
With onset during withdrawal
Cocaine-related disorder not otherwise specified

From American Psychiatric Association. *Diagnostic and Statistical Manual of Mental Disorders.* 4th ed. Text rev. Washington, DC: American Psychiatric Association; 2000, with permission.

HISTORY

Purified cocaine first became commercially available in 1884. Reports of compulsive cocaine use and cocaine psychosis appeared in the European medical literature within the decade. By the beginning of the 20th century, cocaine use and dependence were not uncommon in the United States. Cocaine was an ingredient of Coca-Cola until 1900; nonprescription proprietary nostrums containing cocaine were widely promoted until the Harrison Act was passed in 1914; and 100 mg of illicit cocaine could still be bought for a quarter in the 1920s. With growing public awareness in the United States of the physical and legal risks of drug use, cocaine use and dependence declined gradually. It remained fairly common in Europe, however. Hans Maier's classic *Der Kokainismus*, published in 1926, included descriptions of relatively contemporaneous clinical cases.

There appears to have been little cocaine use and dependence from the late 1930s to the early 1970s. Although some heroin users also used cocaine, virtually no cocaine-dependent patients entered the U.S. Public Health Service Hospital at Lexington, Kentucky, in the 1960s. Starting in the 1970s and continuing throughout the 1980s, the availability of cocaine increased noticeably. For the first few years of its renewed popularity, there were few reports of cocaine toxicity and few people were reported to be seeking treatment. Some observers, apparently unaware of previous epidemics in which the compulsive nature of cocaine use and its serious toxicity had been repeatedly documented, declared cocaine to be a relatively benign drug.

In the early 1980s, "sniffing" or "snorting" (intranasal administration) of cocaine hydrochloride became a popular practice among affluent young adults. As the availability of cocaine increased and its use became increasingly destigmatized by its association with movie stars, sports heroes, and other public figures, social acceptance of cocaine use became normative in many middle- and upper-middle-class social groups. A great deal of attention was given by the media to the money and status associated with cocaine use and to the quasiromantic drama associated with cocaine trafficking.

However, as the decade progressed, cocaine use had rapidly spread throughout all economic and age levels of society, with large urban areas experiencing particularly high rates of use with the practice of inhaling vapor ("smoking") freebase forms rapidly becoming common. Whereas earlier in the decade, this way of using cocaine was usually engaged in only by individuals who could afford to buy large quantities of cocaine hydrochloride and process it into freebase form by using a home-processing procedure, major drug traffickers and the street gangs distributing cocaine now discovered that by preprocessing cocaine into smokable form ("crack"), they could easily retail it on the street and dramatically expand the market. In many large and medium-sized cities in the United States, sales of crack in $5- and $10-dosage units brought high-potency, low-cost cocaine into geographical areas already experiencing extensive poverty and unemployment. The emergence of this crack epidemic in the mid-1980s signaled an unprecedented increase of cocaine use and of the medical, legal, and social sequelae of cocaine abuse and dependence. In many U.S. cities, the crack epidemic was associated with an escalation of crime and social deterioration.

By 1985, as a result of its increasing availability and declining price, 20 million people had tried cocaine. Its toxicity became quite apparent as the number of emergency room visits for cardiovascular, neurological, and psychiatric complications increased sharply, and its capacity to induce dependence was apparent from the escalating number of requests for treatment. Increasing numbers of drug users, overdose deaths, crime, and the images of "crack babies" damaged in utero by cocaine-using pregnant women gave national visibility to the drug problem, particularly to cocaine use. Federal expenditures for law enforcement also increased sharply. Penalties for drug selling and possession were increased, and national prevention campaigns were initiated. Drug (urine) testing in the workplace became more common. Toward the end of the 1980s, casual use declined, as did the number of cocaine-related medical emergency cases seen in hospital emergency rooms. The number of heavy users did not decline as sharply, however, and urine tests of people who were arrested showed that a substantial number of criminals were still using cocaine. The drug continued to be relatively available, less costly than in the 1970s, and by the early 1990s, emergency room visits began to increase slightly. However, by the mid-1990s, drug testing of arrestees in some large cities indicated that fewer of them were using cocaine.

Problems with cocaine developed somewhat later in other parts of the world. For example, in England, Scotland, and Wales, the emergence of "crack" as a major public health problem received extensive media and political attention in 2002. In Mexico, long a transit country for cocaine on its way to the U.S. market, the late 1990s and early 21st century appear to be a period of increasing powder cocaine use among middle- and upper-class youth, whereas "crack" use is simultaneously increasing among poor street youth in Mexico City and other large central and southern Mexican cities.

COMPARATIVE NOSOLOGY

The DSM-IV-TR criteria for cocaine dependence are the same generic criteria as are applied to other psychoactive drugs. The notion of a generic concept of dependence is shared with the DSM-III-R, the fourth edition (DSM-IV), and ICD-10. Despite some changes in wording, the syndromes and criteria for making the diagnosis of dependence are similar in the two previous DSM editions and DSM-IV-TR. A generally high level of agreement also exists between DSM-IV-TR and ICD-10: They use similar concepts (the dependence syndrome varying in severity), although the wording of the criteria for determining the presence and severity of the syndrome differs. Both require that three elements of the syndrome be noted within a 12-month period. Although DSM-IV-TR appears to place greater stress than ICD-10 on tolerance and physiological dependence (because it asks clinicians to specify if these criteria are present), in practice, this has little impact on the proportion of patients seeking treatment who meet diagnostic criteria for dependence. Most patients who meet current DSM-IV-TR criteria for dependence report some tolerance, withdrawal, or both.

The ICD-10 and DSM-IV-TR differ in the classification of what is called *substance abuse* in DSM-IV-TR. ICD-10 does not use the term "abuse" but includes instead the category of harmful use, which differs substantially from the concept of abuse used in DSM-IV-TR. The concept of harm is limited to physical and mental health (e.g., hepatitis, cardiac damage, episodes of depression, or toxic psychosis). It specifically excludes social impairments, as follows:

> The fact that a pattern of use or a particular substance is disapproved of by another person or by the culture, or may have led to socially negative consequences such as arrest or marital arguments is not in itself evidence of harmful use.

EPIDEMIOLOGY

Cocaine use has fluctuated dramatically over the past four decades, not just in the United States but also in South America and in Western Europe. In the United States, the various activities aimed at estimating the extent and consequences of psychoactive drug use include, but are not limited to, the annual Monitoring the Future (MTF) study; the National Household Survey on Drug Abuse (NHSDA); the Drug and Alcohol Services Information System (DASIS), which provides national- and state-level information on the substance abuse treatment system; the Drug Abuse Warning Network (DAWN), which obtains reports form a selected group of hospital emergency department (ED) rooms and medical examiners' offices on drug-related adverse effects and deaths; and the Arrestee Drug Abuse Monitoring (ADAM) program, which obtains its data from urine tests of arrestees at selected jails. All of those estimating techniques have sampling limitations, and most do not apply standardized diagnostic criteria to substance use patterns or adverse effects. Consequently, although they provide a picture of use over time, these methods do not reveal changes in the incidence and prevalence of specific substance-related disorders such as dependence and abuse.

In the annual MTF study, substantial declines in all indicators of self-reported cocaine use among high school seniors (lifetime, past year, and past month use) between 1985 and 1992 were followed by gradual increases between 1992 and 1999. In 1999, a second peak in annual prevalence of 6.2 percent was reached. Since 1999, the annual prevalence rate has declined slightly to 5 percent in 2002. According to the NHSDA, between 1993 and 2001, annual use of cocaine fluctuated between 1.5 and 1.9 percent. During this 9-year period, the lowest annual rate—1.5 percent—was reported in 2000. In 2001, the rate cycled back to 1.9 percent. The number of current cocaine users decreased from 5.7 million in 1985 to 1.4 million in 1992. Since 1992, there have been no significant changes in the number of current cocaine users. And in 2001, an estimated 1.7 million Americans were current cocaine users (0.7 percent of the population aged 12 years and older), and 406,000 Americans were current crack users (0.2 percent).

Since 2000, NHSDA has included a set of questions on substance dependence and abuse. The questions were designed to measure dependence and abuse based on the criteria specified in DSM-IV. In 2000, 0.3 percent reported past year cocaine dependence or abuse. And in 2001, the percent rose to 0.5 percent. The difference between the 2000 and 2001 estimates was statistically significant (at the 0.05 level).

The Treatment Episode Data Set (TEDS), one of three components of DASIS, provides information on the numbers and characteristics of individuals admitted to alcohol and drug treatment. Four substances—alcohol, opiates (primarily heroin), cocaine, and marijuana/hashish—have dominated national-level treatment admissions for several years. The proportion of admissions reporting primary cocaine abuse has decreased slightly, from 17.9 percent of all admissions in 1994 to 14.4 percent in 1999.

According to the ED component of DAWN, ED cocaine mentions increased significantly over the years, from 143,337 mentions in 1994 to 193,034 mentions in 2001. The proportion of cocaine mentions in ED episodes and in all mentions, however, remained relatively stable over the same period.

ETIOLOGY

Substance dependence is currently viewed as the result of a process in which social, psychological, cultural, and biological factors influence substance-using behavior. The actions of the drug are seen as critical, but it is recognized that not everyone who becomes dependent experiences the effects of a given drug in the same way. Further, depending on the individual, different factors may be more or less important at different stages of the process, even with the same class of pharmacological agents.

Social and cultural factors largely influence the availability and initial use of cocaine and other substances. In the case of cocaine, pharmacological factors are believed important in perpetuating use and progression to dependence. Cocaine has potent mood-elevating and euphorigenic actions, especially when its effects have rapid onset, as when cocaine is injected or inhaled. Although some physical dependence develops, a physically uncomfortable, aversive withdrawal syndrome probably is less prominent in perpetuating cocaine use than that of opioids and sedatives.

Comorbidity

Additional psychiatric diagnoses are quite common among cocaine-dependent patients. It is not always evident how this comorbidity is linked etiologically to cocaine, but the epidemiological evidence clearly shows that the presence of a psychiatric disorder not related to substance abuse (e.g., mood disorders, schizophrenia, and antisocial personality disorder) substantially increases the odds of developing substance abuse and dependence. For some people, cocaine may serve to alleviate various psychiatric disorders or dysfunctional states. Some users, for example, may find relief from dysthymic disorder. Others may find that cocaine facilitates sexual activity, permits extended socializing, or counteracts the sedative effects of alcohol. However, although such factors may explain substance use on more than one occasion, they do not account for progression to dependence or abuse.

Genetic Factors

The most convincing evidence to date of a genetic influence on cocaine dependence comes from studies of twins. A study of male twins who served in the U.S. military between 1965 and 1975 found higher concordance rates for stimulant dependence (cocaine, amphetamines, and amphetamine-like drugs) among monozygotic than dizygotic twins. The analyses indicated that genetic factors and unique (unshared) environmental factors contributed approximately equally to the development of stimulant dependence. A study of male twins in Virginia found a common genetic factor exerted a strong influence on risk for illicit use and abuse/dependence for six distinct classes of drugs. Environmental factors were the major determinant of whether a particular class of drugs are used by predisposed individuals. Other studies have shown genetic contributions to attention-deficit/hyperactivity disorder (ADHD), conduct disorder, and antisocial personality disorder. Because these disorders are important risk factors for drug use and dependence, these findings also support genetic involvement in the etiology of drug dependence in general.

In animal models, it is interesting to note that laboratory animal strains differ greatly in their willingness to self-administer psychoactive drugs, including cocaine, and that strains that differ even more markedly can be developed.

Other Factors

Social, cultural, and economic factors are powerful determinants of initial use, continuing use, and relapse. Excessive use is far more likely in countries in which cocaine is readily available. Different economic opportunities may influence certain groups more than others to engage in selling illicit drugs, and selling is more likely to be carried out in familiar communities than in those in which the seller runs a high risk of arrest.

Because in both human and animal studies alternative positive reinforcers compete with drugs as reinforcers, the absence of such nondrug alternatives can be seen as a causal factor for use, especially when drugs are available and the social pressures against using them are not strong. Alternative positive reinforcers are not limited to material rewards but include psychological rewards associated with satisfying interpersonal relationships and the self-esteem that derives from achievements in socially acceptable roles. In animal models, chronic stress mediated by high levels of cortisol increases sensitivity to the reinforcing effects of cocaine and induces relapse to drug self-administration in withdrawn animals.

Learning and Conditioning

Learning and conditioning are important in perpetuation of cocaine use. Each inhalation or injection of cocaine yields a rush and a euphoric experience that reinforce the antecedent drug-taking behavior. In addition, the environmental cues associated with substance use become associated with the euphoric state so that long after a period of cessation, such cues (e.g., white powder and paraphernalia) can elicit memories of the euphoric state and reawaken craving for cocaine.

In cocaine abusers (but not in normal controls), cocaine-related stimuli activate brain regions subserving episodic and working memory and produce electroencephalographic (EEG) arousal (desynchronization). Increased metabolic activity in the limbic-related regions, such as amygdala, parahippocampal gyrus, and dorsolateral prefrontal cortex, correlate with reports of craving for cocaine, but the degree of EEG arousal does not.

Pharmacological Factors

As a result of actions in the central nervous system (CNS), cocaine can produce a sense of alertness, euphoria, and well-being. There may be decreased hunger and less need for sleep. Performance impaired by fatigue is usually improved. Like amphetamine and methylphenidate, cocaine appears to facilitate focus and disregard of distraction, an action that may have value to individuals with attention-deficit disorder. Some users believe that cocaine enhances sexual performance.

Mechanisms of Action

Cocaine inhibits the normal reuptake of monoamines from the synaptic cleft by binding to transporter proteins. Its reinforcing effects are primarily due to its actions at the dopamine transporter, producing high levels of dopamine in the synapse. Evidence suggests that stimulation of both dopamine type 1 (D_1) and D_2 receptors plays some role in dopamine's reinforcing and salience-enhancing actions. Cocaine also inhibits reuptake of norepinephrine and serotonin. The increase in norepinephrine concentration is important for some of cocaine's toxic effects.

In doses typically used by cocaine users, the drug produces increases in adrenocorticotropic hormone (ACTH) and cortisol by stimulating release of hypothalamic corticotropin-releasing hormone (CRH). Peak levels of ACTH coincide with peak plasma levels of cocaine. Dopamine and serotonin are important mediators of this effect because antagonists of these transmitters can blunt this effect of cocaine. The effect on CRH and cortisol release is similar to that observed with stress and may be linked to the increased sensitivity to stress observed in the addicted state. Acutely, cocaine also stimulates release of luteinizing hormone and follicle-stimulating hormone (FSH) and suppresses release of prolactin.

In animal models, cocaine is considered the most powerful pharmacological reinforcer of drug-taking behavior. Given free access, animals choose to self-administer cocaine rather than have food, water, or access to other animals. Death from starvation or drug toxicity is the typical consequence of unlimited cocaine access. With limited access (2 to 6 hours a day), cocaine does not gain such control over behavior, and animals may select food in preference to cocaine, depending on the dose, the amount of work they must do to get the dose, and the type and amount of food offered as alternative reinforcers.

Common Routes of Administration Cocaine can be taken by mouth, injected, absorbed through nasal and buccal membranes, or inhaled and absorbed through the pulmonary alveoli. Cocaine hydrochloride, the water-soluble form typically used for snorting or injection, is largely destroyed by the heat of burning and so is not well suited for smoking. Cocaine as freebase sublimates before it is destroyed by heat. The hydrochloride salt can be converted to the freebase form by treatment with alkali and extraction with organic solvents. Inhalation of freebase cocaine produces almost immediate absorption and a rapid onset of effects. In the 1980s, users learned to avoid the fire hazard of extracting organic solvents and still produce a crude form of freebase cocaine by heating the cocaine with sodium bicarbonate to yield *crack*, a hard, white mass that is freebase plus impurities. When smoked, this material gives off a crackling sound. In cocaine-producing countries, some users may smoke a crude intermediate product, cocaine sulfate (coca paste, pasta basica, basuca), which is usually contaminated with solvents.

As with the opioids, the rapid onset of cocaine's effects after intravenous (IV) injection or freebase inhalation produces an intensely pleasurable sensation, or rush. The cocaine rush lasts only a few minutes, whereas other psychological and physiological effects tend to decrease more slowly in parallel with decreasing concentrations in plasma.

Metabolism The half-life of a single dose of cocaine in the blood is only approximately 30 to 90 minutes. It is typically hydrolyzed by butyrylcholinesterase (plasma pseudocholinesterase) and liver esterase into inactive metabolites, most significantly benzoylecgonine and ecgonine methyl ester. The metabolite is generally detectable in urine for 24 to 72 hours after brief periods of use. With repeated high dosages (e.g., 1 to 2 g daily), cocaine or its metabolites may accumulate in body compartments (e.g., fat and the CNS), from which it is then slowly released. Consequently, using sensitive measures, cocaine may be detectable in the urine of heavy users for 2 weeks. In a study of cocaine-dependent patients admitted to an inpatient treatment unit, the average time from last reported cocaine use to first negative urine test (using a cutoff of 300 ng/mL) was 105 hours, and 20 percent had positive tests for 120 hours or longer.

The concurrent use of cocaine and alcohol may result in the accumulation of a distinct metabolite, cocaethylene. This metabolite is active and longer lasting than cocaine itself and may account for the enhancement of subjective effects and toxicity when cocaine and alcohol are used simultaneously.

Tolerance and Sensitization Patients seeking treatment often report needing progressively more cocaine to get the same effect. In laboratory studies, occasional users of cocaine have more marked cardiovascular, subjective, and endocrine responses to IV challenge doses of cocaine than subjects who are cocaine dependent. Despite the evidence for some tolerance to blood pressure elevating effects, even experienced users may sustain significant cardiovascular toxicity.

Chronic use of cocaine also produces a form of sensitization in which the response to a given dose is actually enhanced. In animals, repeated doses of CNS stimulants, such as cocaine or amphetamine, eventually elicit seizures or stereotyped behaviors not seen with initial doses. Sensitization is produced more reliably by intermittent dosing than by continuous dosing. The sensitization can be long-lasting.

The paranoid states and toxic psychoses that commonly develop in chronic cocaine users are believed to be among the phenomena to which sensitization develops. Cocaine psychosis appears more rapidly in those who have been chronic users or who previously developed psychoses.

In the laboratory, animals that develop sensitization exhibit enhanced self-administration of amphetamines and cocaine. According to several groups of researchers, sensitization phenomena play a critical role in the development of addictive behavior.

The mechanisms underlying the development of sensitization to stimulants, such as cocaine and amphetamine, have been extensively studied. Glutamate and glutamate receptors play a critical role in this phenomenon. Sensitization is prevented by pretreatment with D_1 but not D_2 receptor antagonists, and activation of D_1 but not D_2 receptors in the ventral tegmental area increases extracellular levels of glutamate. Several types of glutamate receptors appear to be involved: *N*-methyl-D-aspartate (NMDA), AMPA/Kainate, and metabotropic (mGlu). Sensitization is blocked by administration of NMDA receptor antagonists. Some data suggest that drug-induced sensitization involves alterations in a subunit of a glutamate (AMPA) receptor that is in turn caused by the accumulation of long-lasting Fos-related proteins, which in turn are mediated by CREB.

Withdrawal States The cocaine withdrawal syndrome has aversive qualities (e.g., dysphoria and anhedonia). Although withdrawal anhedonia and fatigue are not generally reported to be the most important reasons for relapse after brief withdrawal, some users who have come to depend on cocaine for high energy or to project a confident persona may be temporarily unable to function without it. For others, withdrawal dysphoria may exaggerate the intensity of an antecedent mood disorder. If a protracted cocaine withdrawal syndrome exists, it is more subtle than the syndrome associated with opioid withdrawal. It is in some ways puzzling that patients do not usually attribute craving for cocaine and relapse to withdrawal because there is considerable evidence that chronic cocaine use produces significant long-lasting changes in many parts of the brain.

COCAINE-INDUCED BRAIN CHANGES It has been found repeatedly that there are perfusion deficits in brains of cocaine-dependent subjects recently withdrawn from cocaine. This deficit is probably not related to tolerance or withdrawal, but several other findings probably are. Many (but not all) studies using positron emission tomography (PET) and single photon emission computed tomography (SPECT) to examine the brains of cocaine-dependent subjects have found a decreased number of dopamine transporters in the striatum, a finding consistent with postmortem studies. Within a few days of withdrawal, cocaine abusers show higher than normal cerebral metabolic rates in orbitofrontal cortex and basal ganglia that correlate with craving. At 1 to 4 weeks and at 3 to 4 months postwithdrawal, cocaine abusers have lower metabolic rates in the frontal cortex that correlate with symptoms of depression and decreased availability of D_2 receptors that correlates with decreased cerebral metabolic rates and years of cocaine use (Fig. 11.6–1). An increase in μ-opioid receptor binding after 4 weeks of cocaine abstinence also correlated with severity of cocaine craving.

Chronic cocaine use induces a wide range of changes in the brains of animal models; many of these changes appear to be adaptive responses, whereas others may be linked to sensitization. After a period of chronic, binge-like cocaine administration, the threshold for reinforcement increases, and dopaminergic and serotonergic transmission in the nucleus accumbens

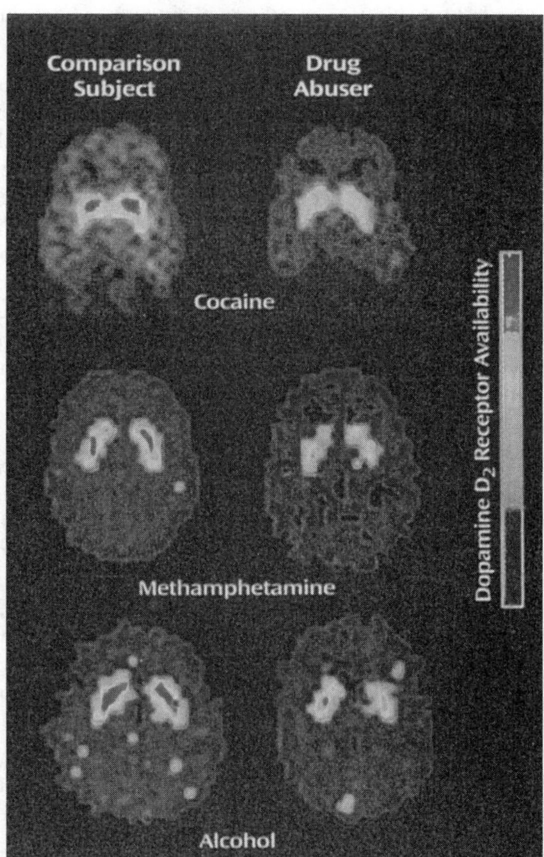

FIGURE 11.6–1 Compared with normal control subjects, dopamine type 2 (D_2) receptor binding in striatum is lower in drug users during withdrawal from cocaine, methamphetamine, and alcohol. (See Color Plate.) (From Goldstein RZ, Volkow ND: Drug addiction and its underlying neurobiological basis: Neuroimaging evidence for the involvement of the frontal cortex. *Am J Psychiatry.* 2002;159:1642, with permission.)

decreases. In addition, the density of D_1 receptors increases. Messenger ribonucleic acid (mRNA) for corticotropin-releasing factor (CRF) increases, μ- and κ-opioid receptors are upregulated, and the concentration of mRNA encoding for prodynorphin in the striatum and nucleus accumbens increases. Dynorphin, acting on κ receptors in ventral tegmental area neurons, probably serves as a negative feedback mechanism, dampening excessive dopaminergic activity. An increase in cocaine- and amphetamine-regulated transcript (CART) peptides may be another mechanism that plays a role in dampening dopaminergic activity. These distinct neurotransmitter peptides are found in the ventral tegmental area and nucleus accumbens in close proximity to γ-aminobutyric acid (GABA)ergic neurons. They appear to reverse or limit the effects of high levels of dopamine. When cocaine use ceases, enhanced dynorphin activity could contribute to reduced dopaminergic activity manifested in dysphoria and anhedonia. Neurons bearing dopamine receptors in these same brain areas show upregulation of cyclic adenosine monophosphate (cAMP)–dependent kinase and decreased concentrations of G_i protein. Both of these changes contribute to upregulation of the cAMP pathway and activation of various transcription factors, such as CREB (cAMP response element–binding protein), which results in the production of long-lasting Fos-like proteins that are distinct from those seen after acute cocaine administration. The persistent changes in the cAMP pathway probably represent one mechanism underlying tolerance. As noted above, the accumulation of Fos-like proteins, by altering a subunit of the AMPA glutamate receptor, appears to account for the development of sensitization.

With the aim of gaining a better understanding of the phenomena of addiction and postabstinence relapse, several efforts, each well grounded in both behavioral and biological data, have been made to integrate what is already known about the changes induced by drug use and the responses to drug-related stimuli in the environment. One of these efforts emphasizes the interactions between the persisting decreases in the functional capacity of neural systems subserving hedonic tone and increased sensitivity and protracted instability of the hypothalamic-pituitary-adrenocortical (HPA) stress axis. This view sees addiction as a "cycle of spiraling dysregulation of brain reward systems" in which there is a shift from a normal homeostatic state to an abnormal—allostatic—state. Increased sensitivity to environmental stressors combines with release of CRF to produce responses in the dopaminergic systems that are functionally equivalent to priming doses of a drug. Another view places emphasis on the importance of drug-induced neuronal sensitization, postulating that there is a parallel sensitization in the neural systems that subserve the assignment of salience to environmental stimuli. This sensitization causes drug-related stimuli to acquire more salience for directing behavior, and that salience is perceived as "wanting" or "craving" drugs. Still another view takes into consideration data from brain imaging studies showing that there is decreased volume of frontal cortex in many of the addicted subjects. Because the prefrontal cortex normally inhibits activity in the amygdala, which is a key area involved in emotionally charged memories, including memories of rewarding effects of drugs that can be elicited by drug-related stimuli, this perspective hypothesizes that not only do drug-related stimuli evoke craving but also that the capacity of the frontal cortex to inhibit the behavioral responses to drug craving is reduced.

DIAGNOSIS AND CLINICAL FEATURES

Table 11.6–1 lists the DSM-IV-TR cocaine-related disorders.

Patterns of Use and Abuse There are several patterns of cocaine use and abuse. For example, the indigenous people of the Andes chew coca leaves daily, but apparently very few progress to excessive use or toxicity. Although some people can use cocaine intermittently without becoming dependent, it is not clear how long such intermittent, nondependent use can continue and for what proportion of users. Cocaine use that does not cause problems for the user does not meet the DSM-IV-TR criteria for either dependence or abuse.

Among people seeking treatment for cocaine dependence (unlike opioid dependence), daily use of the drug is not the most common pattern. Instead, use may be intermittent. Intermittent use consists of episodes or binges of use, often starting on weekends and paydays and lasting until the drug supply is exhausted or toxicity develops. The runs, or binges, during which the drug may be used every 15 to 30 minutes, can last 7 or more consecutive days but typically are shorter. Although there appears to be little tolerance between binges, changes in the response to the drug occur during the binge. Euphoric effects seem less prominent, and anxiety, fatigue, irritability, and depression increase. Any pause in the drug use causes blood concentrations to drop; typically, there is dysphoria rather than a return to normal mood. If cocaine is still available, it is used to dispel the dysphoria. When the binge is interrupted or supplies have been depleted, a cocaine "crash" quickly follows. Patients report the sense of needing more cocaine to get the same effect (tolerance) more commonly than the experience of pronounced withdrawal. Some users distinguish between a brief crash and withdrawal. A substantial proportion of cocaine users seeking treatment report daily or almost daily use, often associated with daily heroin use. A small percentage of patients report using high doses for a few days a month over a long period; such people may still meet the criteria for dependence.

In the early stages, cocaine use may cause little interference with normal activities. Some people may even find that the sense of energy and heightened sense of self-confidence facilitate productive activity. Others may find that the cocaine facilitates social interaction, particularly enhancing sexual arousal and enjoyment, at least initially. The development of sexual dysfunction later in the course of use is better documented than is the enhancement.

In addition to feelings of euphoria, cocaine use may also induce concurrent feelings of anxiety, irritability, and suspiciousness. Users may commit crimes to obtain money to buy cocaine, and such crimes may involve violence. In addition, cocaine can induce paranoid ideation, and there are reports of homicide and attempted homicide during such cocaine-induced toxic states.

Cocaine is an especially powerful reinforcer when it is taken in ways that produce a rapid onset of effects. Not only do IV and intrapulmonary routes of administration produce a rapid increase in blood and brain drug concentrations and an intense rush, but especially with the smoking of freebase cocaine, an almost equally rapid decrease in blood and brain drug concentration occurs as the cocaine is redistributed and metabolized. Compared with those who use it intranasally, users who inhale freebase cocaine or inject the salt intravenously seem more likely to move from experimentation to regular, compulsive use, limited only by the availability of the drug or the money to buy it. Even in the laboratory setting, it can be shown that craving for cocaine is briefly intensified a few minutes after IV use when brain and blood concentrations are decreasing. However, although IV and pulmonary cocaine use are far more likely to result in compulsive use and dependence, the intranasal route can also lead to dependence and to the full range of cocaine toxicity (including fatalities).

Cocaine abusers frequently use sedatives or opioids to modulate the stimulant and toxic effects of the cocaine, a practice that can lead to concurrent dependence on sedatives or opioids. Sometimes an opiate, such as heroin, and cocaine are injected intravenously simultaneously; the mixture (speedball) is reportedly especially euphorigenic. Similar synergistic effects are seen when cocaine and buprenorphine (Buprenex, Subutex) are taken simultaneously. Alcohol is probably the substance most commonly used in conjunction with cocaine, and its use may become associated with cocaine use and can trigger cocaine craving in former users trying to abstain from cocaine.

Cocaine Dependence

As drug use progresses, greater priority is often given to obtaining and using cocaine than to meeting other social obligations or avoiding toxicity or arrest. The user may engage in illegal activities to raise money for cocaine or trade sex for it. At this stage, the use of cocaine is considered maladaptive and probably meets the DSM-IV-TR criteria for cocaine abuse or dependence. The DSM-IV-TR criteria for cocaine dependence are the same generic criteria applied to other substances (Table 11.1–3). A diagnosis of dependence requires a maladaptive drug use pattern that leads to clinically significant impairment or distress, as indicated by at least three of seven criteria presented in the table. DSM-IV-TR instructs the clinician to specify whether physiological dependence is present (i.e., evidence of either tolerance or withdrawal as defined in the diagnostic criteria).

Drug use to prevent withdrawal is not as dominant with cocaine dependence as with opioid dependence. However, the other criteria for dependence are common among heavy users of cocaine. Tolerance to some drug actions (e.g., euphorigenic effects) can coexist with increased sensitization to other actions (e.g., anxiogenic and psychotogenic effects).

Cocaine Abuse

Some cocaine users develop problems or adverse effects related to their drug use (i.e., their use is maladaptive) even though such use does not meet the three-criteria requirement for the diagnosis of dependence. Examples of such recurrent maladaptive patterns include use that leads to multiple legal problems; inability to meet major social, school, or work-related obligations; and continued use despite social or vocational difficulties caused by, or aggravated by, cocaine use. When one or more such substance-related problems occur in a 12-month period, but the pattern has never met the criteria for dependence, the diagnosis of cocaine abuse (Table 11.1–8) should be made.

Cocaine Intoxication

Among those who meet the criteria for cocaine abuse or dependence, certain psychiatric toxicities are common. Just as alcohol-dependent people are frequently intoxicated, cocaine users commonly develop the symptoms of cocaine intoxication during the course of a single binge. The euphoria may be accompanied by increasing suspiciousness, hypervigilance, anxiety, hyperactivity, talkativeness, and grandiosity. Users may engage in stereotyped and repetitive behaviors (e.g., disassembling and reassembling the same object). Typically, other signs and symptoms of central stimulation occur, such as tachycardia, cardiac arrhythmias, blood pressure changes, pupillary dilation, perspiration, or chills. Hallucinations may occur, including tactile hallucinations. Judgment is impaired, and confusion may occur, but insight into the drug-induced nature of the hallucinations is retained.

Any of these symptoms after the recent use of cocaine should invoke consideration of cocaine intoxication, provided they are not better accounted for by some other medical or mental disorder, and there are at least two of a number of physiological signs commonly seen with cocaine use (e.g., tachycardia and elevated blood pressure). The DSM-IV-TR diagnostic criteria for cocaine intoxication (Table 11.6–2) are identical to the criteria for amphetamine intoxication except for the substitution of the word "cocaine" for the words "amphetamine or a related substance." Any perceptual disturbances should be specified. In one study of cocaine abusers in the community, just more than one-half reported experiencing paranoia or hallucinations at some time; among those who sought treatment, 63 percent reported those symptoms. Cocaine intoxication may occur in occasional users who do not meet the criteria for abuse or dependence.

The development of paranoia does not seem to be closely related to cocaine dose. Some cocaine users develop the syndrome at far lower doses than are used by others who do not develop it. Furthermore, a person who has experienced cocaine-induced paranoia is more likely to have it recur with subsequent cocaine use. It is postulated that a change in threshold represents a form of sensitization. Cocaine use has also been linked to development of a panic disorder that outlasts the cocaine use; here too, sensitization has been postulated.

Cocaine Intoxication Delirium and Cocaine-Induced Psychotic Disorder

Whereas some paranoia or hypervigilance is typical of cocaine intoxication, and tactile and other hallucinations may also occur, cocaine use can also induce a toxic delirium and a more persistent toxic psychotic disorder characterized by suspiciousness, paranoia, visual and tactile hallucinations, and loss of insight. The hallucination of bugs (cocaine bugs) or vermin crawling under the skin (formication) is sometimes reported and is often

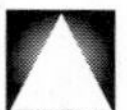

Table 11.6–2
DSM-IV-TR Diagnostic Criteria for Cocaine Intoxication

A. Recent use of cocaine.
B. Clinically significant maladaptive behavioral or psychological changes (e.g., euphoria or affective blunting; changes in sociability; hypervigilance; interpersonal sensitivity; anxiety, tension, or anger; stereotyped behaviors; impaired judgment; or impaired social or occupational functioning) that developed during, or shortly after, use of cocaine.
C. Two (or more) of the following, developing during, or shortly after, cocaine use:
 (1) Tachycardia or bradycardia
 (2) Pupillary dilation
 (3) Elevated or lowered blood pressure
 (4) Perspiration or chills
 (5) Nausea or vomiting
 (6) Evidence of weight loss
 (7) Psychomotor agitation or retardation
 (8) Muscular weakness, respiratory depression, chest pain, or cardiac arrhythmias
 (9) Confusion, seizures, dyskinesias, dystonias, or coma
D. The symptoms are not due to a general medical condition and are not better accounted for by another mental disorder.

Specify if:
 With perceptual disturbances

From American Psychiatric Association. *Diagnostic and Statistical Manual of Mental Disorders.* 4th ed. Text rev. Washington, DC: American Psychiatric Association; 2000, with permission.

associated with excoriation of the skin. A paranoid syndrome can develop within 24 hours after the beginning of a cocaine binge. When the syndrome develops in the presence of a clear sensorium, and the person retains insight into the drug-induced nature of the symptoms, it is called *cocaine intoxication*, even when there are hallucinations. When insight is lost, but the sensorium is clear, the syndrome is called *cocaine-induced psychotic disorder with delusions* or *with hallucinations*. If consciousness is disturbed (i.e., the ability to focus, sustain, or shift attention is reduced), and deficits in memory and orientation exist, the diagnosis is *cocaine intoxication delirium*.

Cocaine Withdrawal

Cocaine withdrawal phenomena have not been as thoroughly studied as those associated with opioids or alcohol. No experimental studies have been conducted in which patients with known baseline characteristics have been stabilized solely on large doses of cocaine and then abruptly withdrawn. Consequently, most data have been derived from interviews and patients' recollections or from observations of hospitalized patients whose level of drug ingestion and prior baseline characteristics can only be estimated. During the cocaine epidemic of the 1980s, approximately 50 percent of cocaine users reported experiencing some type of withdrawal when drug use was interrupted.

An early description of withdrawal based on interviews of outpatients described a three-phase syndrome in which the first phase, the crash, was characterized by agitation, depression, anorexia, and high cocaine craving. This cluster of symptoms was followed by a decrease in cocaine craving, fatigue, depression, and a desire for sleep, followed in turn by exhaustion and hypersomnia, with intermittent awakening, and hyperphagia. The second phase was reported to be heralded by normalized sleep, improved mood, and low levels of craving, but that relatively benign phase was succeeded by a return of anergia, anhedonia, anxiety, and increased cocaine craving, especially in response to stimuli previously associated with cocaine use. A third phase, extinction (which appears to represent a period of extended vulnerability to relapse rather than a phase of an extended withdrawal syndrome) was also described.

Others who have observed cocaine-dependent patients admitted to clinical and research units have not reported seeing such a complex phasic withdrawal. Instead, symptoms of depression and craving for cocaine declined steadily over several weeks. After 3 weeks, sleep, weight, and appetite were mostly comparable to those of normal controls on the same unit. Hypersomnia, disturbed sleep, hyperphagia, and excessive weight gain were not seen, nor was a severe crash observed. The phases and fluctuations in craving previously reported might have been related to environmental stimuli.

Some of the inconsistencies in the findings and symptoms associated with cocaine cessation are probably attributable to differences in the dose and duration of use and to vulnerability factors. In interviews with almost 400 cocaine abusers, including approximately 100 who were not seeking treatment, some 83 percent reported tolerance to cocaine effects (needing more to get the same effect), and 52 percent reported having undergone some type of withdrawal. Those seeking treatment were more likely to report experiencing withdrawal. Available data show no convincing evidence that a protracted cocaine withdrawal syndrome follows resolution of the signs and symptoms associated with abrupt cessation. However, abnormalities of brain function appear to persist for at least 12 weeks, and, possibly, subtle withdrawal phenomena increase vulnerability to relapse.

Although not commonly observed during recent clinical studies, severe depression, sometimes associated with suicidal ideation, is reported in the older literature on cocaine withdrawal and in occasional contemporary clinical reports. Emil Erlenmeyer reported in 1886 that depression was likely to be seen when cocaine was stopped. Maier (*Der Kokainismus*, 1926) noted that depression and apathy appeared on cessation of cocaine. To what degree the more severe depressive features are a part of withdrawal or represent the emergence of primary mood disorder is unclear.

The DSM-IV-TR diagnostic criteria for cocaine withdrawal (Table 11.6–3) specify that the syndrome follows the cessation (or reduction) of heavy, prolonged cocaine use. Further, the dysphoric mood and other symptoms (e.g., fatigue and sleep disturbances) must be intense enough to cause significant distress or impairment. Thus, the criteria are structured so that the brief dysphoria and fatigue (crash) that follow a single short binge by an occasional user do not lead to a diagnosis of withdrawal. Drug craving, often a part of cocaine withdrawal, is not included among DSM-IV-TR diagnostic criteria.

Animal Models of Withdrawal

Although there is no easily observable animal model of cocaine withdrawal comparable to that for the syndromes seen with alcohol or opioid withdrawal, animal analogs of the postuse dysphoria and anhedonia often seen in humans have been proposed. In rats, cocaine typically lowers the threshold for intracranial electrical self-stimulation. After 24 hours of cocaine self-administration, the thresholds for such self-stimulation are elevated above baseline for several days, which suggests a relative dopaminergic deficiency or insensitivity. Rats administered cocaine in a binge pattern had elevated dopamine concentrations in the nucleus accumbens during cocaine administration and below-normal concentrations during withdrawal; after 14 days of drug administration, recovery to pretreatment levels was prolonged.

Other Cocaine-Induced Disorders

Other psychiatric syndromes that may develop in the course of cocaine use include

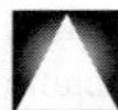

Table 11.6–3
DSM-IV-TR Diagnostic Criteria for Cocaine Withdrawal

A. Cessation of (or reduction in) cocaine use that has been heavy and prolonged.

B. Dysphoric mood and two (or more) of the following physiological changes, developing within a few hours to several days after Criterion A:
  (1) Fatigue
  (2) Vivid, unpleasant dreams
  (3) Insomnia or hypersomnia
  (4) Increased appetite
  (5) Psychomotor retardation or agitation

C. The symptoms in Criterion B cause clinically significant distress or impairment in social, occupational, or other important areas of functioning.

D. The symptoms are not due to a general medical condition and are not better accounted for by another mental disorder.

From American Psychiatric Association. *Diagnostic and Statistical Manual of Mental Disorders.* 4th ed. Text rev. Washington, DC: American Psychiatric Association; 2000, with permission.

cocaine-induced mood disorder, cocaine-induced anxiety disorder, and cocaine-induced sleep disorder. With each of those disorders, the clinician should specify whether the onset occurred during intoxication or during withdrawal. DSM-IV-TR also describes cocaine-induced sexual dysfunction and a category of cocaine-related disorder not otherwise specified (Table 11.6–4).

Cocaine-induced mood disorder can occur during use, intoxication, or withdrawal. During use and intoxication, the disorder is more likely to simulate a manic, hypomanic, or mixed episode; during withdrawal, it is more likely to involve a depressed mood. Such diagnoses are difficult to make during periods of active drug use or during the first week or two of withdrawal. Because sexual dysfunction, anxiety, and disturbed sleep are seen so commonly during cocaine use and withdrawal, the diagnoses should be made only when the disturbances or dysfunctions are judged to be in excess of that usually associated with intoxication and withdrawal and only when severe enough to require independent treatment or attention. Panic episodes that develop during cocaine use may persist for many months after cessation. Lasting vulnerability to panic attacks may be linked to sensitization phenomena.

Comorbidity The frequent cooccurrence of other psychiatric disorders and cocaine dependence was noted during the cocaine epidemic in the early part of the 20th century. The presence of other psychiatric disorders sharply increases the odds of substance dependence, and substance-dependent people are more likely than the general population to meet the diagnostic criteria for additional psychiatric disorders.

Table 11.6–4
DSM-IV-TR Diagnostic Criteria for Cocaine-Related Disorder Not Otherwise Specified

The cocaine-related disorder not otherwise specified category is for disorders associated with the use of cocaine that are not classifiable as cocaine dependence, cocaine abuse, cocaine intoxication, cocaine withdrawal, cocaine intoxication delirium, cocaine-induced psychotic disorder, cocaine-induced mood disorder, cocaine-induced anxiety disorder, cocaine-induced sexual dysfunction, or cocaine-induced sleep disorder.

From American Psychiatric Association. *Diagnostic and Statistical Manual of Mental Disorders.* 4th ed. Text rev. Washington, DC: American Psychiatric Association; 2000, with permission.

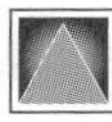

Table 11.6–5
Additional Psychiatric Diagnoses among Cocaine Users Seeking Treatment (New Haven Cocaine Diagnostic Study Results)

Psychiatric Diagnosis	Current Disorder (%)	Lifetime Disorder (%)
Major depression	4.7	30.5
Cyclothymia/hyperthymia	19.9	19.9
Mania	0.0	3.7
Hypomania	2.0	7.4
Panic disorder	0.3	1.7
Generalized anxiety disorder	3.7	7.0
Phobia	11.7	13.4
Schizophrenia	0.0	0.3
Schizoaffective disorder	0.3	1.0
Alcoholism	28.9	61.7
Antisocial personality disorder—RDC	7.7	7.7
Antisocial personality disorder—DSM-III	32.9	32.9
Attention-deficit disorder	—	34.9

RDC, Research Diagnostic Criteria.
Adapted from Rounsaville BJ, Anton SI, Caroll K, Budde D, Prusoff BA, Gawin F: Psychiatric diagnoses of treatment-seeking cocaine abusers. *Arch Gen Psychiatry.* 1991;48:43.

Among cocaine users seeking treatment, the rates of additional current and lifetime diagnoses are regularly found to be elevated. In one study, approximately 300 patients (69 percent men, average age of 28 years, and mostly lower socioeconomic class) were interviewed using the Schedule for Affective Disorders and Schizophrenia (SADS). Symptoms occurring within 10 days after the last drug use were not used in making any diagnoses. The additional psychiatric diagnoses are shown in Table 11.6–5. The most common additional lifetime diagnoses were alcoholism (62 percent), antisocial personality (33 percent), and major depression (30 percent). In this sample, depression preceded the onset of drug abuse in approximately one-third of the patients, whereas alcoholism preceded the onset of drug abuse in 21 percent.

Some studies have found that cocaine users who seek treatment have higher rates of depression and adverse consequences of drug use than those who do not. Another study found that those not seeking treatment had comparably severe cocaine use and lifetime and current psychiatric disorders and higher rates of polysubstance use and involvement with the law, but they also tended to minimize the adverse consequence of substance use and lacked pressure to seek treatment.

The prevalence of schizophrenia has generally been reported to be low among patients admitted to cocaine treatment programs, probably largely because people with schizophrenia are excluded from such programs. In fact, people with schizophrenia commonly use cocaine or amphetamine and develop both dependence and toxic syndromes, although the diagnosis is not routinely made. Depending on the geographical area, an estimated 12 to 30 percent of people with schizophrenia also abuse cocaine. It has been suggested that they use cocaine and stimulants to alleviate negative symptoms, postpsychotic depressive disorder of schizophrenia, and the side effects of antipsychotics. One nonblinded study did find fewer negative signs and more anxiety and depression among cocaine users with acute schizophrenia who had used cocaine before admission. A substantial proportion of schizophrenic patients admit having used cocaine during the months before hospitalization, but many are less candid about recent drug use, and urine tests frequently reveal recent cocaine use unsuspected by clinicians. Patients with schizophrenia who use cocaine tend to be younger and are more likely to be homeless and unemployed than psychotic patients who are not abusing drugs. Special programs involving peer-based support groups seem to be effective in linking substance-using schizophrenic patients to outpatient treatment programs.

Cocaine use may induce psychiatric syndromes (e.g., panic disorders) that may persist even after drug use is stopped. People with certain types of psychiatric disorders may be prone to experiment with cocaine or other substances, and factors that predispose to psychiatric disorders may also predispose cocaine users to become cocaine dependent.

Research on the temporal appearance of the syndromes indicates that in some instances and for some syndromes substance use antedates the psychiatric disorder. In one component of the Epidemiological Catchment Area (ECA) study, subjects were reinterviewed 1 year later. Those who reported cocaine or stimulant use in the interval were almost eight times more likely than nonusers to experience depression and 14 times more likely to have had a panic attack. Cocaine users were almost 12 times more likely to experience a manic episode.

The ECA data also show a relation between the extent of cocaine use and other psychiatric disorders. Among men 18 to 44 years of age, those who had never used cocaine or had used it less than five times had a lifetime prevalence of major depression of 7.6 percent; it was 11 percent for users who were never daily users and almost 26 percent for those who met the DSM-III criteria for cocaine abuse. Similarly, the lifetime prevalence of panic disorder was related to the extent of cocaine use.

Toxicity and Complications

High doses of cocaine can cause a wide variety of toxic effects, including cardiac arrhythmias, coronary artery spasms, myocardial infarction, and myocarditis. Other reported cardiovascular toxicities include headache, ischemic cerebral or spinal infarction, and subarachnoid or cranial hemorrhage. Toxic effects on the CNS may include seizures, hyperpyrexia, respiratory depression, and death. Cocaine-related seizures and loss of consciousness are often reported on questionnaires given to heavy users (up to 27 percent); most episodes do not lead to emergency room visits. Rhabdomyolysis, not uncommon after large doses of cocaine, may contribute to renal complications, although vasoconstriction alone may suffice to account for renal damage. Sniffing cocaine can cause ulcers of the mucosa in the nose and perforation of the nasal septum from persistent vasoconstriction. Inhaled cocaine freebase is believed to induce lung damage. Gastrointestinal (GI) necrosis, caused by vasoconstriction, has been associated with the rupture of swallowed condoms containing large amounts of cocaine. By producing placental vasoconstriction, cocaine may contribute to fetal anoxia. A list of medical complications associated with cocaine intoxication and abuse is shown in Table 11.6–6.

Seizures and respiratory depression may be related to cocaine's actions as a local anesthetic, and although the cardiovascular complications are primarily due to its effects on the reuptake of catecholamines in the peripheral nervous system, local anesthetic effects may contribute to myocardial depression. Animal studies reveal significant genetic vulnerability to various kinds of cocaine toxicities, suggesting that some of the observed toxicity in humans may not be predominantly dose dependent and predictable. Gender can influ-

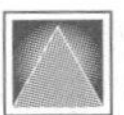

Table 11.6–6
Medical Complications of Cocaine Intoxication and Abuse

- Cardiovascular
  - Hypertension
    - Intracranial hemorrhage
    - Aortic dissection, rupture
  - Arrhythmias
    - Sinus tachycardia
    - Supraventricular tachycardia
    - Ventricular tachyarrhythmias
  - Organ ischemia
    - Myocardial ischemia and infarction
    - Renal infarction
    - Intestinal infarction
    - Limb ischemia
  - Myocarditis
  - Shock
  - Sudden death
- Central nervous system
  - Headache
  - Seizures
  - Transient focal neurological deficits
  - Cerebrovascular disorder
    - Subarachnoid hemorrhage
    - Intracranial hemorrhage
    - Cerebral infarction
    - Embolic (endocarditis)
  - Toxic encephalopathy, coma
  - Neurological complications
- Respiratory
  - Pneumomediastinum
  - Pneumothorax
  - Pulmonary edema
  - Respiratory arrest
- Metabolic and other
  - Hyperthermia
  - Rhabdomyolysis (muscle breakdown)
- Reproductive
  - Obstetrical
    - Spontaneous abortion
    - Placental abruption
    - Placenta previa
  - Premature rupture of the membranes
  - Fetal
    - Intrauterine growth retardation
    - Congenital malformations
  - Neonatal
    - Crack baby syndrome
    - Cerebral infarction
    - Delayed neurobehavioral development
- Infectious[a]
  - Acquired immune deficiency syndrome
  - Infectious endocarditis
  - Hepatitis B
  - Wound botulism
  - Tetanus

[a]Transmitted by contaminated needles or syringes.
Adapted from Benowitz NL. How toxic is cocaine? In: Bock GR, Whelan J, eds. *Cocaine: Scientific and Social Dimensions.* Ciba Foundation Symposium 166. New York: Wiley; 1992.

ence toxicity. Estrogen seems to attenuate the cerebral vasoconstrictive effects of cocaine. In volunteers given known doses of cocaine, the decrease in cerebral flow was greatest during the luteal phase of the menstrual cycle when progesterone levels are highest. Probably as a consequence of altered sensitivity of dopaminergic systems in the brain, chronic cocaine users may exhibit abnormal movements such as tics, choreoathetoid movements, and dystonic reactions. They may be particularly sensitive to neuroleptic-induced dystonias.

Cocaine use is frequently associated with increased sexual activity and sometimes the exchange of sex for cocaine. Such behaviors put cocaine users at elevated risk for venereal diseases, including infection with human immunodeficiency virus (HIV).

Treatment of Toxicity The treatment of acute cardiac emergencies is aimed at blocking the sympathomimetic effects of the drug and correcting arrhythmias. Some clinicians have recommended using combined α- and β-adrenergic receptor antagonists; however, others have advised against using adrenergic or dopaminergic blockers. Also suggested for myocardial ischemia are calcium channel blockers and nitroglycerine. Grand mal seizures may respond to diazepam (Valium). Some researchers advise using ambient cooling. In animal models, μ-agonist opioids have been found to reduce cocaine lethality.

Pathology and Laboratory Examinations

Cocaine metabolites can be detected for varying lengths of time in urine, depending on the dose of cocaine and sensitivity of the assay. They can also be detected in blood, saliva, sweat, and hair. Blood and saliva provide a better index of current concentrations, whereas urine provides a longer window of opportunity for detecting use over the previous few days. Hair analysis can reveal drug use over weeks to months but has little applicability in clinical situations.

Postmortem studies comparing tissues from cocaine users with controls found lower levels of striatal vesicular monoamine transporter protein, suggesting damage to striatal dopaminergic fibers.

Some of the insults to the CNS (e.g., cerebral infarction) are detectable by computed tomography (CT) scans or magnetic resonance imaging (MRI), but most chronic cocaine abusers who do not also abuse alcohol show no evidence of CNS structural damage when examined by these methods. However, studies using PET or SPECT have revealed a variety of functional abnormalities in the brains of recently abstinent cocaine users. Compared with controls, heavy cocaine users show perfusion defects in the cortex. Considerable improvement in cortical perfusion occurs after several weeks of abstinence, although blood flow in many instances still does not match that of normal controls. Carefully controlled studies have found that brain volumes of cocaine users are slightly smaller (show atrophy) than those of controls who do not use drugs but do not differ from those of other drug abusers. During early abstinence from cocaine (up to 1 month since last use), D_2 receptor availability is significantly reduced, compared with controls. This is also the case for heroin addicts, alcoholics, and methamphetamine abusers (Fig. 11.6–1).

Compared with normal controls and patients withdrawn from alcohol, patients withdrawn from cocaine exhibit persistent resting tremor (4 to 6 Hz, similar to that of Parkinson's disease) lasting at least 12 weeks. The tremor is subtle and is not ordinarily detected by clinical testing; no other cerebellar signs are present. They also exhibit slower reaction times in divided attention tasks that also persisted. Compared with age-matched and education-matched controls, chronic cocaine users are more likely to score in the impaired range on a neuropsychological screening battery. Impairment seems most obvious in concentration and memory, with less impairment in users who had been abstinent longer. To what extent the abnormalities in brain function are causally related to the signs and symptoms associated with cocaine cessation is uncertain.

A few early studies of cocaine addicts reported that almost all patients exhibited hyperprolactinemia lasting several weeks, which seemed consistent with a dopaminergic deficiency. However, several subsequent studies found either no evidence of hyperprolactinemia or a much lower incidence of that effect and no apparent correlation between high prolactin levels and either cocaine craving or the extent of cocaine use. Most data suggest that heavy cocaine use can, in some cases, result in prolonged periods of hyperprolactinemia. Why this occurs in some users and not others remains to be clarified.

DIFFERENTIAL DIAGNOSIS

The disorders associated with the use of cocaine need to be distinguished from both primary mental disorders and disorders induced by other classes of substances. A history of substance ingestion is important in making those distinctions. However, given the unreliability of self-reports about substance use and the likelihood that many users deny any substance use at all, laboratory testing for drugs in body fluids and histories from collaterals are important. Disorders associated with cocaine use cannot be distinguished from those associated with amphetamines and related substances except by reliable history or laboratory tests. Users of cocaine (and amphetamine and related substances) may exhibit inappropriate optimism, euphoria, expansiveness, excessive talkativeness, and a decreased need for sleep sometimes associated with irritability in the context of a clear sensorium, a pattern that is also observed in manic and hypomanic episodes of bipolar disorder. However, these symptoms may not be obvious enough to suggest their relation to substance use, and the first indication of substance dependence may be financial difficulties, an arrest for drug sale or possession, or substance-induced toxicity.

Intoxication

Cocaine intoxication is diagnosed when the effects of cocaine exceed the mood-elevating effects its users typically seek. The diagnosis of intoxication is appropriate when the effects are problematic enough to require differentiation from hypomanic or manic behavior. Cocaine intoxication can also be confused with amphetamine intoxication and phencyclidine (PCP) intoxication, although the last is usually associated with nystagmus, motor incoordination, and some cognitive impairment. Endocrine disorders (such as Cushing's disease) and excessive use of steroids should also be considered.

Toxic Psychosis

Cocaine-induced toxic psychosis can be exceedingly difficult to differentiate from schizophrenia or other psychotic disorders characterized by hallucinations or delusions. The presence of vivid visual or tactile hallucinations should raise suspicion of substance-induced disorder. In areas and populations in which cocaine use is common, it may be necessary to provide only a provisional diagnosis until the patient can be observed and substance test results are obtained. Even then there may be difficulties because, in some urban areas, a high percentage of people with established diagnoses of schizophrenia also use cocaine.

Cocaine-Induced Anxiety Disorder

Cocaine-induced anxiety disorder must also be distinguished from generalized anxiety disorder and panic disorder. Panic disorder that has its onset associated with the use of cocaine may persist well beyond the period of cocaine use.

Other Symptoms The symptoms that may emerge during withdrawal, such as depression, dysphoria, anhedonia, and disturbed sleep, need to be distinguished from those of primary mood disorders and primary sleep disorders. Unless the symptoms are more intense or more prolonged than is typical of cocaine withdrawal and so require independent treatment, the diagnosis should be limited to withdrawal rather than cocaine-induced mood disorder. When a diagnosis of cocaine-induced mood disorder is made, it is important to specify whether the onset was during intoxication or withdrawal. One can also specify the subtype of mood disorder (i.e., with depressive, manic, or mixed features). In differentiating cocaine-induced mood disorder from the primary mood disorders, the critical factor is the clinician's judgment that the mood disorder was caused by the cocaine. Generally, a cocaine-induced mood disorder, with onset during intoxication or withdrawal, remits in a week or two. It is appropriate, therefore, to withhold judgment about the diagnosis during the early phase of withdrawal. If depressed mood and related symptoms persist beyond a few weeks, alternative causes should be entertained. In reviewing diagnostic possibilities, the clinician should consider the age at which symptoms began and a history of mood episodes that developed before the onset of cocaine use or during any long intervals without significant drug abuse.

COURSE AND PROGNOSIS

Not all cocaine users develop cocaine-related disorders. However, even occasional users can experience cocaine toxicity. Among those who do develop dependence, the time from first use to problematic use ranges from a few months to 6 or more years. An analysis of data from the National Comorbidity Study found that, compared with alcohol and marijuana, cocaine dependence emerged more rapidly once use began, with 5 to 6 percent of users becoming dependent in the first year, and most dependent users having met dependence criteria within 3 years. Overall, approximately 15 to 16 percent of those who use cocaine become dependent within 10 years of first use.

The course of cocaine use is often marked by shifts from intranasal to IV use and inhalation of freebase forms. In the United States, because most people who tried cocaine did not become dependent, the decreased cocaine use in the general population in the early 1990s, which followed peak rates of self-reported use in the 1980s, does not shed much light on the natural history of cocaine dependence.

At this time, little information exists on untreated cocaine dependence, but there are findings on the course of cocaine use among those seeking treatment. A number of short-term (6-month to 2-year) follow-up studies seem to indicate that the course of dependence is more favorable for cocaine users who seek treatment than for heroin addicts who seek treatment.

In a cohort of 229 treated crack users followed for 18 months after treatment, three profiles emerged: those who continued to use throughout the period, those who cycled between use and abstinence, and those who abstained throughout the period. Those who abstained reported the greatest improvement in other areas of functioning (employment, legal, family and psychiatric), and stable abstinence was associated with longer participation in aftercare activities and 12-step program involvement.

A study of veterans living on the east coast of the United States who were randomly assigned to either an inpatient program or a day hospital program lasting 28 days found that 60 percent reported abstinence at 4 months, with approximately 56 percent of urine specimens negative for each group even at 7 months.

In a 1-year follow-up of almost 300 cocaine users, one-half treated as outpatients and one-half treated initially as inpatients, both groups showed reductions in self-reported cocaine use during the 30 days before the follow-up interview: from an average of 10 days per month at intake to 5 days for outpatients and 17 days per month at admission to 1.1 days for the group that had been inpatients. Although the data do not give the percentage of those who were entirely abstinent, the improvement levels were substantial and differed from those typically found among heroin-dependent patients seeking treatment. The prognosis appears to be even better for people with social support.

Drug Abuse Treatment Outcome Study (DATOS)

DATOS is the largest recent study of drug users seeking treatment. Approximately 3,000 patients from 81 programs were interviewed at entry and 1 year after completion of index treatment. Cocaine dependence was the most frequent primary drug problem, but some patients whose major drug problem involved heroin or alcohol also used cocaine. Among the entire sample of clients, 39 percent met criteria for antisocial personality disorder, and 14 percent met criteria for some other DSM-III-R Axis I disorder. At follow-up, 35 percent of clients who stayed in long-term residential treatment for less than 3 months and 14 percent of those who stayed longer reported weekly or more frequent cocaine use. For outpatient drug-free programs, the rates were 25 percent for those who stayed less than 3 months and 13.6 percent for those who stayed longer. Weekly or more frequent cocaine use decreased to approximately 20 percent for short-term inpatient treatment, but the drop was similar for those who stayed more than 2 weeks and those who stayed for a shorter time.

Since baseline levels of cocaine use differed, the results across program types were easier to compare when expressed as percentage reduction from pretreatment levels. Reduction in weekly or more frequent cocaine use for the long-term residential clients was 54 percent for those who stayed less than 3 months and 82 percent for who stayed more than 3 months; for outpatient drug-free clients, it was 57 percent (less than 3 months) and 87 percent (more than 3 months); for short-term inpatient clients, 79 percent (less than 2 weeks) and 74 percent (more than 2 weeks). A substantial proportion of patients were referred for additional social support and treatment after discharge, and many participated in self-help programs. The investigators concluded that there was little difference among program types but that very different types of patients self-select different treatments.

In a subsequent 5-year follow-up of a cohort of 708 subjects, weekly cocaine use was reported by 25 percent of the sample (a slight increase from the 21 percent at 1-year follow-up), and 18 percent had been arrested during the 5-year period. Poorer 5-year follow-up status was associated with more severe problems, including cocaine use frequency, at admission and lower levels of treatment exposure during their index treatment episode and during the 5-year subsequent period. The treatment benefits that were identified at 1-year follow-up did, for the most part, persist at the 5-year follow-up period. Reentry into treatment was associated with more frequent cocaine use and greater need for services at admission. Patients with highly favorable outcomes attributed improvement to motivation for change, positive influences of family, and strength from religion and spirituality.

Varieties of Remissions Treatment of cocaine dependence may have various outcomes, including, at the extremes, complete relapse to cocaine dependence or total abstinence from cocaine and related drugs for a prolonged period, more than 12 months (sustained full remission). However, sustained partial remissions occur in which, after at least 1 month when no criteria of dependence have been present, one or more criteria of abuse or dependence are again met, but over the course of 12 months, less cocaine dependence criteria have been met than the three required for full relapse. There are also situations in which these patterns are observed, but the period of observation is not a full year (early full remission and early partial remission). Any pattern of remission may be observed while the person is in a controlled environment, and that fact should be specified.

DSM-IV-TR criteria for both abuse and dependence require maladaptive use associated with distress or impairment. Technically, a person can be in sustained full remission from cocaine dependence despite occasional use, provided the drug use causes no problems or distress and does not escalate. How often such a return to occasional nonproblematic use takes place is unknown.

Cocaine and Crime

The typical interactive relation between the use of opioid drugs and crime generally holds true for cocaine users, but some significant differences exist. As with opioid users, considerable heterogeneity exists among cocaine users. Although a history of delinquency or antisocial behavior is often an antecedent to cocaine use, not everyone who uses cocaine or develops cocaine dependence engages in crime, even though the cost of using the drug may create serious financial problems. Sometimes, however, a person with no previous criminal behavior engages in a variety of illegal activities ranging from fraud and white-collar crime to drug selling, prostitution, and predatory crime just to get enough money to buy cocaine. Among people seeking treatment for any variety of substance abuse, use of cocaine is most highly correlated with income-generating crime.

In a nationwide sample of adolescents, 40 percent of serious crimes committed by the entire sample were committed by the 1.3 percent who reported using cocaine. In the late 1980s, when cocaine use decreased in the general population in the United States, it increased or merely stabilized among those arrested for a variety of serious offenses. In the late 1990s, however, cocaine use began to decline, especially among younger arrestees.

Cocaine, Aggression, and Violence

One conceptual framework for thinking about the links between violence and substance (cocaine) use involves three major causal categories: psychopharmacological effects (effects of the substances), economic compulsion (violent crimes committed to obtain money for drugs), and systemic violence (associated with the business methods and lifestyle of drug dealers). Cocaine can induce states of paranoia and aggressive behavior, a common reason why cocaine users are brought to emergency rooms. However, pharmacologically induced aggression is not the major reason why cocaine and crime, and more specifically, cocaine and violence, are linked. Among those arrested for violent crime, the primary predictors of such crime are past arrests for violent crime, poor education, and poor intellectual ability. Past arrest for violence is also associated with antisocial personality disorder. Studies of violent predatory offenders indicate that most had histories of heavy involvement with multiple substance use and with serious crime as juveniles. Among predatory offenders, high-frequency substance users are likely to use many substances, particularly heroin and cocaine, and to engage in a variety of crimes, including violent crimes, at high rates. Furthermore, many drug dealers who may not use cocaine routinely themselves resort to violence to protect or expand their customer base.

TREATMENT

Selection of Treatment Setting

The general principles of treatment for cocaine dependence do not differ much from those for other varieties of drug dependence. Patient heterogeneity requires careful assessment of the patient and thoughtful selection among alternative treatment approaches. Cocaine dependence severe enough to require formal treatment is often associated with other psychiatric diagnoses. Not all cocaine users require extensive treatment; some who are not severely dependent respond to external pressures, as when employers insist on carefully monitoring substance use. Among the factors influencing selection are the severity of dependence, other drugs being used concurrently, comorbid medical and psychiatric disorders, and the preferences of the patient and the alternatives available. Availability, in turn, is often influenced by the policies of managed care companies, the patient's resources, and the types of therapy provided locally.

Among the few reliable predictors of treatment response are the number of cocaine use days within the past 30 at the time of treatment admission and route of cocaine administration. There is considerable evidence that individuals who use cocaine on a daily or near-daily frequency or use cocaine by the injection route, or both, are more difficult to engage in outpatient treatments, are retained in treatment for shorter durations, and have poorer outcomes. These data suggest that the use of more intensive treatment (e.g., residential or inpatient settings) is preferable for individuals with these pretreatment use profiles.

In general, treatment can be initiated in intensive outpatient settings, although often third-party payers do not authorize and public sector programs cannot provide the duration of treatment or the intensity shown to be most effective. Research on treatment outcome has consistently demonstrated that individuals who are retained in outpatient treatments for longer durations (typically 90 days or more) have better outcome than those who are retained for shorter durations. In addition, in a prospective study in which cocaine-dependent individuals were randomly assigned to receive 30 days or 120 days of thrice-weekly, manualized outpatient treatment, there was a significantly superior outcome associated with the longer treatment episode. A study using random assignment found that at 4 months, working-class veterans treated in a day hospital program were about as successful in reducing their cocaine use and improving social functioning as those treated in a 28-day inpatient program. However, a somewhat higher proportion of those assigned to the inpatient setting completed the 28-day program. Currently, severe depression with suicidal ideation, psychosis, or substance use that has repeatedly failed to respond to outpatient efforts are the indications for hospitalization. A retrospective study of individuals treated for cocaine dependence in various settings found no advantage in outcome for inpatient treatment lasting more than 2 weeks.

In many instances, neither the patient nor the clinician makes the selection of the setting and type of treatment. Patients are often referred (mandated) to treatment by the criminal justice system, which often prefers long-term residential programs (therapeutic communities). The intensity and specificity of services for particular problems (i.e., medical, psychiatric, and vocational) are now considered important determinants of outcome in the specific problem areas.

Detoxification

The cocaine withdrawal syndrome is distinct from the opioid, alcohol, or sedative-hypnotic withdrawal syndrome in that there are no physiological disturbances that necessitate inpatient or residential drug withdrawal. Thus, it is generally possible to engage in a therapeutic trial of outpatient withdrawal before deciding whether a more intensive or controlled setting is required for patients unable to stop without help in limiting their access to cocaine. Patients withdrawing from cocaine typically experience fatigue, dysphoria, disturbed sleep, and some craving; some may experience depression. No pharmacological agents reliably reduce the intensity of withdrawal, but recovery over a week or two is generally uneventful. It may take longer, however, for sleep, mood, and cognitive function to recover fully.

Severity of withdrawal symptoms as measured by an instrument called the *Cocaine Symptom Severity Assessment* (CSSA) has been shown to predict treatment outcome in outpatient treatment settings. Similarly, urine toxicology results on admission are related to ability to achieve a 3-week period of abstinence during treatment. Those whose cocaine withdrawal severity is greater and those with urine tests positive for benzoylecgonine at treatment admission were less likely to achieve the study abstinence criterion.

Treatment Methods

A number of psychological and pharmacological approaches to the treatment of cocaine dependence have been explored. More than 20 different pharmacological agents have been tested in the search for drugs to facilitate withdrawal, reduce postwithdrawal craving, or prevent relapse. In general, no drug with robust therapeutic efficacy has emerged. Psychosocial approaches have included various forms of individual and group psychotherapies, drug counseling, and self-help groups.

It is generally held that total abstinence from cocaine must be the goal of treatment for those who have developed symptoms of dependence; any use at all is seen as a prodrome to relapse. However, this perspective may underestimate the benefits that accrue from treatment that results in a substantial and prolonged reduction in drug use but falls short of total abstinence. In most studies of treatment effectiveness, a significant proportion of patients report substantial reductions in use, even though they are not completely abstinent.

Psychotherapy and Behavior Modification

Psychological treatment approaches have used behavioral, cognitive-behavioral, 12-step facilitation, psychodynamic, drug counseling, and combination strategies. Two approaches, contingency management and cognitive-behavioral therapy, have received far more attention and empirical support than the others.

BEHAVIORAL APPROACHES: CONTINGENCY MANAGEMENT

Contingency management increases the frequency of a target behavior (in this case, abstinence from drugs) by reinforcing (i.e., rewarding) that behavior. In the context of drug treatment, decreased drug use or total drug abstinence (as measured by urinalysis) is the target behavior and is reinforced using cash or vouchers that may be exchanged for goods or services. In some cases, behaviors that are inconsistent with drug use, such as regular job attendance, are reinforced rather than just abstinence from drugs.

A recent review concluded that contingency management is effective in reducing the use of cocaine and other drugs as a result of both direct reinforcement (e.g., vouchers for substance-free urines) and indirect reinforcement (increased treatment retention and compliance). In some studies when the reward for drug-free urine samples is discontinued, cocaine use increases to pretreatment levels. However, in other studies, the in-treatment reductions in cocaine use persist to some degree long after the contingencies have been removed.

In one such demonstration of more lasting contingency management effects, 70 cocaine-dependent outpatients were randomly assigned to one of two experimental groups. One group earned vouchers exchangeable for retail items contingent on cocaine-free urinalysis results, whereas the second group earned vouchers independent of their urinalysis results. Patients remained in outpatient treatment for 24 weeks and were assessed at several follow-up points, up to 15 months after discontinuation of the vouchers. Results showed positive effects (i.e., increased cocaine abstinence) of the contingently delivered vouchers even 15 months after termination of the vouchers and up to 12 months after the end of treatment. Durable effects of contingency management were also seen in two studies comparing contingency management to a cognitive-behavioral approach. Both of these studies used cocaine-dependent subjects; in one of the studies, the patients were maintained on methadone for the concurrent treatment of opiate dependence. Both studies found positive effects—decreased stimulant use—of contingently delivered vouchers as long as 52 weeks after treatment entry and 36 weeks after voucher termination. Several other studies have demonstrated that the use of contingency management contributed to a significant reduction in cocaine use when used as part of a behavioral treatment package, with sustained positive effects of contingency management at 6 and 12 months. Reluctance of staff to pay addicts not to use cocaine, as well as current treatment reimbursement practices and policies, makes it unlikely that this approach will be widely used despite its potential therapeutic benefits. However, several studies have used the contingency management procedure to provide access to housing and employment opportunities. The latter "social engineering" projects have shown that the principles of positive reinforcement can be used within "world contingencies" to support abstinence from cocaine. The extent to which even these experiments are generalized to larger social service systems is unclear.

The contingency management model described above is based entirely on the use of positive reinforcement. A far older approach to stimulant use, and to drug use in general, uses a form of contingency management based on punishment of drug use rather than reward for abstinence. This approach is still in widespread use and is seen most notably in the supervision of drug-impaired professionals (such as doctors, pharmacists, nurses), athletes, employees, and a variety of offenders referred from the criminal justice system. In this framework, the individual is required to provide evidence of abstinence, usually in the form of a drug-free urine specimen. Urine tests positive for drugs generally result in adverse consequences. For a physician, this can mean loss or suspension of license to practice; for an offender, a period of incarceration. The general arrangement is often described as a contingency contract. During the period of the contract, the effect on drug-using behavior can be dramatic. However, in most cases, unless there has been additional intervention, such as participation in a 12-step program, the drug use recurs when the contract ends.

COGNITIVE-BEHAVIORAL THERAPY

Cognitive-behavioral therapy is focused on the delivery of information and development of skills that, in theory, enable a patient to discontinue drug use and avoid relapse. The techniques used within the designation of the cognitive-behavioral therapy include psychoeducation, identification of high-risk situations and warning signs for relapse, development of coping skills, development of new lifestyle behaviors, increased self-efficacy, and dealing with relapse.

Cognitive-behavioral therapy has been applied successfully across many different substances of abuse. A review of almost 25 randomized controlled trials using this approach across substances of abuse found evidence for its effectiveness in relapse prevention, as compared with no treatment. Cognitive-behavioral therapy seems to be particularly effective among patients at higher levels of addiction severity.

In one study of 128 cocaine-abusing outpatients, patients were randomly assigned to either a cognitive-behavioral therapy group or a "12-step facilitation" group for a total of 12 weeks of treatment. Participants in the 12-step facilitation group were introduced to the principles of Alcoholics Anonymous (AA) and Cocaine Anonymous (CA) and were encouraged to proceed through the first four steps and to attend outside 12-step meetings in the community. Results showed that participants who received cognitive-behavioral therapy were significantly more likely to be abstinent from cocaine both while in treatment and at a follow-up that occurred 14 weeks after treatment's end.

In addition to promoting reductions in drug use during the application of cognitive-behavioral therapy, results have sometimes shown a "delayed benefit" such that the beneficial treatment effects actually increase gradually over time, well after implementation of the techniques has ended. Three studies have reported evidence for such a delayed effect in the treatment of cocaine abuse. In two studies, nearly identical methodologies were used on two different cocaine-dependent, outpatient samples (one methadone maintained, the other not). Participants in both studies received 16 weeks of treatment and were then followed up at 26 and 52 weeks postadmission. In both studies, the beneficial effects of cognitive-behavioral therapy present during treatment were sustained or increased at follow-up points.

MOTIVATIONAL ENHANCEMENT THERAPY Motivational enhancement therapy (MET) is an approach that was initially developed for the treatment of individuals with alcohol-related disorders, but it is under considerable study for the treatment of other drug use disorders, including cocaine use. It was one of the manualized approaches evaluated in the National Institute on Alcohol Abuse and Alcoholism (NIAAA)–sponsored Project MATCH and found to produce a comparable reduction of alcohol use to the other approaches tested in that study. MET conceptualizes the human behavior change process as involving a sequential series of definable behavioral and cognitive behavioral stages. These stages, defined as *precontemplation, contemplation, action, maintenance*, and *relapse*, have been posed as a general model of habit change but specifically applied to addiction disorders within the framework of MET. The approach is designed to enhance the engagement of drug and alcohol users into treatment and to address their ambivalence toward abstinence in a constructive manner. The primary contribution of MET is that it provides an explicit set of positive reinforcement techniques and strategies that provide an alternative to confrontational approaches designed to break through patient resistance and denial. As treatment for cocaine users has become primarily delivered on an outpatient basis, and methods that promote engagement and retention in treatment have become a priority, MET has gained popularity. Although well-controlled studies have not as yet been conducted evaluating MET for the treatment of cocaine users, it is a technique that appears to be receiving a great deal of interest from practitioners.

PSYCHODYNAMIC AND INTERPERSONAL APPROACHES Psychodynamically oriented clinicians emphasize the patient's unconscious motives for using cocaine (e.g., to relieve an inner sense of emptiness or depression). Experienced clinicians with a wide range of skills believe that a combination of psychological approaches is more effective than treatments that emphasize the principles of only one approach.

GROUP PSYCHOTHERAPY TECHNIQUES Several distinct approaches to group psychotherapy with cocaine users have been described. Interpersonal group therapy focuses on relationships and uses the group interactions to illustrate the interpersonal causes of individual distress and to offer alternative behaviors. Modified dynamic group therapy is described as emphasizing character, as it manifests itself individually and intrapsychically, and in the context of interpersonal relationships with a focus on affect, self-esteem, and self-care. Both approaches share the view that the group should serve as an interpersonal anchor that leads first to more stable emotional status and enables members to face unresolved life issues. Both approaches recognize the vulnerability of the patients to narcissistic injury and the need for a supportive, empathetic environment.

Some psychotherapists emphasize that the focus in the early months of treatment must be exclusively on the disease and on achieving sobriety and recovery, but modified dynamic group therapy asserts that even early in the process, those goals are not incompatible with attention to characterological problems. Dynamic group psychotherapy assumes that substances are used as self-medication and that the people most likely to use cocaine include those whose depression, anergia, or boredom is alleviated by it. However, those who place exaggerated value on assertiveness and self-sufficiency may also find cocaine alluring. Because patients must sometimes be abstinent for at least 2 weeks before participating in this type of group therapy, the technique may be more accurately described as relapse prevention rather than treatment to induce initial cessation. Few studies bear on the effectiveness of such group therapy.

Various forms of group-based drug counseling have also been studied.

COMBINATION APPROACHES Several models have been developed that use combinations of behavioral or psychological approaches. The rationale for these approaches is that cocaine-dependent individuals have a variety of psychological-behavioral deficits that can best be addressed with a multielement treatment package. These combination approaches can be used in treatment settings that treat large numbers of substance users, such as publicly funded treatment programs, or within practice settings of individual practitioners. All of these approaches have been operationalized into treatment manuals and have been empirically evaluated to different degrees. The strength of these models is that they allow practitioners to use an integrated model to address the multiple aspects of psychological-behavioral impairment and family disruption commonly found in the lives of cocaine users. A weakness of these approaches is that it is not clear which of the specific treatment elements are critical to successful behavior change.

COMMUNITY REINFORCEMENT APPROACH The community reinforcement approach (CRA) was initially developed in the early 1980s for application in the treatment of alcoholism. In the early 1990s, it became one of the first treatment approaches with clear empirical evidence of treatment efficacy. All treatment techniques used in the model are based on principles of operant conditioning. The approach assumes that cocaine use and associated behaviors have at some time resulted in positive reinforcement and have thereby become established behaviors via this history of positive reinforcement. An initial step in this treatment approach is to conduct a functional analysis of the cocaine users' behavioral repertoire and identify the reinforcement contingencies that are maintaining the behaviors associated with cocaine use. The goal of the strategies consequently used is to find ways to reinforce behaviors that are incompatible with cocaine use. Among the specific techniques that are included in the CRA model are conjoint therapy techniques designed to promote an increase in positive couples/family interactions and improve couples/family functioning; a behavioral package of employment skills designed to improve the patient's ability to obtain and sustain fulfilling and rewarding employment; education of the patient in principles of reinforcement and principles of classic conditioning (e.g., recognize high-risk situations, understand "triggers" to use and craving) to help them understand and modify behaviors that increase their exposure to cocaine; and a program of vouchers to reinforce urine samples free of cocaine. The final element, the voucher program, is a contingency management strategy that appears to be one of the most powerful behavior change elements in the CRA package. In fact, the voucher program used in the CRA approach gave rise to the use of contingency management as an efficacious tool for reducing cocaine use as described previously.

In a study comparing the CRA approach with a 12-step–based outpatient approach, the CRA approach demonstrated significant superiority in producing a reduction in cocaine use as measured by self-report and urinalysis data. The CRA approach not only produced less cocaine use than the comparison approach but longer periods of sustained abstinence from cocaine. Further, in a subsequent report, the efficacy of this approach was sustained at 1-year follow-up assessment. Due to the extensive training required and the somewhat academic presentation of this treatment approach and rationale, there has been limited adoption of CRA in the mainstream treatment system.

NETWORK THERAPY Network therapy was developed as a specialized type of combined individual and group therapy to ensure greater success in the office-based treatment of addicted patients. Network therapy uses both psychodynamic and cognitive-behavioral approaches to individual therapy while engaging the patient in a group support network. The group, comprising the patient's family and peers, is used as a therapeutic network joining the patient and therapist at intervals in therapy sessions. The approach promotes group cohesiveness as a vehicle for engaging patients in this treatment. This network is managed by the therapist to provide cohesiveness and support and to promote compliance with treatment. Although network therapy has not received systematic controlled evaluation, it has received considerable application in the psychiatric practice because it is one of the few manualized approaches that has been designed for use by individual practitioners in an office setting.

MATRIX MODEL The matrix neurobehavioral model uses a highly structured and manualized cognitive-behavioral treatment and contingency management program. Preliminary data suggest that this approach can be effective with a wide range of cocaine users, but results from the comparison of contingency management and cognitive-behavioral therapy described below suggest that the matrix model can be made more efficient.

Comparison of Psychotherapy Methods and Programs Contingency management and cognitive-behavioral therapy approaches have been directly compared in a study of individuals with a primary diagnosis of cocaine dependence and in a study of methadone-maintained individuals who were also dependent on cocaine. The contingency management condition consisted of a 16-week voucher program in which participants could earn up to $1,200 for cocaine-negative urine samples collected thrice weekly. The cognitive-behavioral therapy condition consisted of a 16-week, thrice-weekly series of 90-minute group sessions with content based on the manual developed in the matrix model. The contingency management plus cognitive-behavioral therapy condition consisted of both sets of procedures delivered at the time of the thrice-weekly clinic visits. Study data were collected at admission, during the 16-week intervention period, at discharge, and at 26- and 52-week intervals after study admission. All study elements and parameters were identical in both studies with the exception that in the study of the methadone-maintained sample, a no cocaine treatment condition was included as a fourth group.

In these two studies, results for contingency management and contingency management plus cognitive-behavioral therapy conditions were significantly superior to the results of the cognitive-behavioral therapy and no treatment conditions during the 16-week intervention period. At the time of the 26- and 52-week follow-up interviews, the contingency management, cognitive-behavioral therapy, and contingency management plus cognitive-behavioral therapy interventions appeared to produce comparable outcomes, with all three groups demonstrating significantly superior outcomes to the no treatment condition. Interestingly, the cognitive-behavioral therapy condition appeared to produce a more substantial treatment effect at follow-up than during the 16-week study period. There was no apparent benefit of combining the two interventions, as at no point did the contingency management plus cognitive-behavioral therapy condition demonstrate superior performance to the two single intervention conditions. However, contingency management produced a rapid and substantial reduction in cocaine use and a powerful positive effect on retention in treatment, whereas the benefits of cognitive-behavioral therapy appear to emerge most robustly at points after discontinuation of the interventions.

NIDA Multisite Study A large-scale collaborative multisite cocaine treatment study sponsored by the National Institute on Drug Abuse (NIDA) compared different psychosocial treatments. After a brief period of stabilization, 487 cocaine-dependent patients were randomly assigned to one of four groups: weekly group drug counseling, group counseling plus individual drug counseling based on 12-step principles, group counseling plus individual cognitive therapy, or group counseling plus individual supportive expressive therapy. Group drug counseling was provided for 6 months; individual therapies were provided twice weekly for 3 months, then once weekly for 3 months. Therapy was manual guided, and cognitive therapy and supportive expressive therapists were fully trained professionals. Drug counselors had extensive experience with drug dependence treatment; approximately one-third were in recovery from drug dependence. All patients reported substantial reduced cocaine use, whether measured by Addiction Severity Index composite, days of cocaine use in the past month, or number of months abstinent. Follow-up occurred 1 year after treatment entry (which, for some patients, was only 6 months after completion). Patients assigned to group drug counseling plus individual drug counseling reported significantly better outcomes; patients assigned to either cognitive therapy or supportive expressive therapy stayed in treatment longer, but outcomes in terms of cocaine use or dependence were not significantly better than those for group drug counseling alone. Among patients assigned to individual counseling, 73 percent achieved 1 month of complete abstinence, and 36 percent achieved 3 consecutive months of abstinence. In the other groups, 17 to 25 percent achieved 3 months of abstinence. By 6 months posttreatment, no delayed benefits of psychotherapy had emerged. Psychiatric severity and the presence of antisocial personality disorder did not significantly affect treatment outcome.

All patients in this study participated in a stabilization phase lasting 1 to 2 weeks during which they were required to attend one group session and two case-management visits before being assigned to a specific treatment. During that time, there was attrition of less motivated patients. The therapists were highly qualified, carefully trained, used a manual to guide therapy, and were supervised. The study population was 77 percent male, 58 percent white, and 60 percent employed, with a mean age of 34 and generally low psychiatric severity. Patients taking psychotropic medication and those with schizophrenia, bipolar disorder, polysubstance dependence, or opioid dependence were excluded. However, 33 percent met criteria for alcohol dependence, 28 percent met criteria for cocaine-induced mood disorder, 14 percent met full criteria for antisocial personality disorder, and 32 percent for adult antisocial personality disorder with history of conduct disorder.

Pharmacological Agents A variety of pharmacological agents, most of which are approved for other uses, have been tested clinically for the treatment of cocaine dependence and relapse. Some of these medications are being used routinely, although little solid evidence for their efficacy has emerged. None of the pharmacological treatments that have been tried thus far are as effective in producing decreases in cocaine use as methadone, levomethadyl acetate (ORLAAM), or buprenorphine are for heroin use.

Pharmacological interventions are based on several premises, the most common of which are the following: (1) Chronic cocaine use alters dopaminergic systems so that giving up the drug is associated with a hypodopaminergic state characterized by dysphoria or anhedonia; (2) some people who use cocaine are trying to ameliorate a preexisting psychiatric disorder (such as major depressive disorder, dysthymic disorder, attention-deficit disorder, or cyclothymic disorder); (3) cocaine produces a sensitization that somehow predisposes to continued use; (4) relapse is related to memories of the reinforcing and euphoric effects of cocaine, and craving can be elicited by stress, other drugs, or environmental stimuli; and (5) interest in using cocaine can be attenuated or extinguished if its reinforcing effects can be prevented (blocked).

Methylphenidate (Ritalin) and lithium (Eskalith), respectively, have been used to treat cocaine users presumed to have preexisting ADHD or mood disorders. Those drugs are of little or no benefit for patients without the disorders, and clinicians should adhere strictly to maximal diagnostic criteria before using either of them in the treatment of cocaine dependence. In patients with ADHD, slow-release forms of methylphenidate may be less likely to trigger cocaine craving, but the impact of such pharmacotherapy of cocaine use remains to be demonstrated.

Many medications have been explored on the premise that chronic cocaine use alters the function of multiple neurotransmitter systems, especially the dopaminergic and serotonergic transmitters regulating hedonic tone, and that cocaine induces a state of relative dopaminergic deficiency. Although the evidence for such alterations in dopaminergic function has been growing, it has been difficult to demonstrate that agents theoretically capable of modifying dopamine function can alter the course of treatment, even though studies in animal models, as well as open label studies, suggested that they would be successful. Well-designed, controlled trials that obtained objective evidence of drug use have not found any of the following agents (among others) effective in reducing cocaine use: neurotransmitter precursors (e.g., dopa; tyrosine); dopaminergic agonists (bromocriptine [Parlodel]; lisuride; pergolide [Permax]); and antiparkinsonian drugs that may also affect the dopaminergic system (amantadine [Symmetrel]). Tricyclic antidepressant drugs such as desipramine (Norpramin) and imipramine (Tofranil) have also been tried. Although some double-blind studies that relied heavily on self-reports of drug use yielded some positive results, other studies have not found them significantly beneficial in inducing abstinence or preventing relapse. There is no consensus that the effects of desipramine are robust or reliable enough to justify routine use, but if it is used early in treatment, it may have some transient benefit for patients who are less severely dependent. Also tried in pilot or open studies but not confirmed as effective in controlled studies were other antidepressants such as bupropion (Wellbutrin); monoamine oxidase (MAO) inhibitors (selegiline [Eldepryl]); selective serotonin reuptake inhibitors (SSRIs; e.g., fluoxetine [Prozac]); mazindol (Sanorex); pemoline (Cylert); antipsychotics (e.g., flupenthixol); lithium; several different calcium channel inhibitors; and anticonvulsants (e.g., carbamazepine [Tegretol] and valproic acid [Depakene]). In a randomized double-blind study in Australia, cocaine users given dextroamphetamine showed some reduction in cocaine use as compared to those receiving placebo. However, given the toxicity of amphetamine and the risks of diversion and misuse, it is unlikely that this will emerge as a useful treatment in the United States.

Several agents are being developed that have not yet been tried in human studies. These include agents that selectively block or stimulate dopamine receptor subtypes (e.g., selective D_1 agonists) and drugs that can selectively block the access of cocaine to the dopamine transporters but still permit the transporters to remove cocaine from the synapse. Another approach is aimed at preventing cocaine from reaching the brain by using antibodies to bind it in the bloodstream (a so-called cocaine vaccine). Such cocaine-binding antibodies do reduce the reinforcing effects of cocaine in animal models. Also under study are catalytic antibodies that accelerate the hydrolysis of cocaine and butyrylcholinesterase (pseudocholinesterase), which appears to hydrolyze cocaine selectively and is normally present in the body.

Acupuncture Auricular acupuncture has become popular among some groups, including some drug courts and prison-based programs, as a treatment for cocaine dependence (and for other varieties of dependence behavior). Controlled studies of its efficacy for treating cocaine dependence (using sham acupuncture and attention control groups) have been conducted, but no significant differences in cocaine use (as measured by urine tests) have been shown.

Special Considerations and Special Populations

Mixed Addictions

PATIENTS MAINTAINED ON METHADONE Pharmacological agents and behavioral techniques have been used to help motivate methadone maintenance patients to reduce their cocaine use (as measured by urine tests). Some methadone programs use progressive sanctions such as decreasing take-home privileges, decreasing methadone dosage, and finally, in some cases, discharge from the program. However, one comparison study found decreasing the methadone dosage far less effective than giving 5-mg increments (up to 120 mg a day in some cases) for each cocaine-positive urine test. However, another study did not show less cocaine use among patients maintained on higher doses of methadone. Contingency management—providing small rewards, such as vouchers for goods and services, contingent on submitting a urine specimen negative for cocaine—does reduce the frequency of cocaine use, as does cognitive-behavioral therapy.

COCAINE AND ALCOHOL Although alcohol use at entry into treatment does not predict poorer outcome, continued use by the fourth week of treatment does predict reduced likelihood of achieving abstinence from cocaine. In patients dependent on both cocaine and alcohol, the opioid antagonist naltrexone (ReVia) had no effect on cocaine use. In several trials, disulfiram (Antabuse) was useful for reducing cocaine use, perhaps because it discouraged the use of alcohol, which is often associated with cocaine use.

Women, Pregnant Women, and Their Children Data suggest that, although women who seek treatment tend to be more severely drug dependent, they respond as well to treatment as do men. Women dependent on cocaine have a number of special needs, especially with respect to their physical health.

Cocaine use by pregnant women represents a hazard to the fetus. At the peak of the cocaine epidemic, 10 to 45 percent of women who received obstetrical care in some urban hospitals reported using cocaine at some time during pregnancy. The frequency and permanence of any damage sustained by the fetus continues to be a subject of controversy, but there is little question that maternal cocaine use can be associated with perinatal morbidity and mortality. Separating cocaine effects from the effects of other substances and other maternal behaviors is exceedingly difficult, but some toxicity may be due to cocaine-induced hypertension, tachycardia, and vasoconstriction, which lead to impaired placental blood flow and decreased transfer of nutrients and oxygen to the fetus. Some toxicity can occur as a result of direct effects of cocaine on the fetus. Depending on the severity of the placental and fetal effects and when they occur during gestation, the result may be teratogenic, with destruction of developing tissues or overall retardation of fetal growth. Commonly reported abnormalities in fetuses exposed to cocaine are microcephaly and structural abnormalities in brain and urinary tract development. Ischemic and hemorrhagic lesions in the newborn brain have also been reported. Spontaneous abortion, premature birth, placenta previa, and abruptio placentae are complications of pregnancy that are more common among women who use cocaine than among nonusers; low-birth-weight babies are also common.

Despite the risks, only a small percentage of the infants exhibit what might be called a *neonatal cocaine exposure syndrome*, which consists of poor feeding, irritability, tremor, and abnormal sleep patterns. Those abnormalities are most evident on the second day after birth and last for less than a week or two. Sudden infant death syndrome (SIDS) is reported to be more common among infants exposed to cocaine in utero, but because there are no controls, the evidence for this is not conclusive. The long-term neurological, cognitive, and developmental consequences of intrauterine cocaine exposure are still not clear, but after the first few months, most of these children appear to be developmentally within normal limits. Heavier cocaine use was not an independent risk factor for impairment once scores have been controlled for exposure to other drugs and relevant variables of the natal environmental. Follow-up studies have tested children 6 to 9 years of age who were exposed prenatally to cocaine and compared them with unexposed controls matched for gender, birth weight, ethnicity, and socioeconomic status. Intelligence quotient (IQ) scores did not differ and were unchanged when adjusted for caregiver IQ and home environment. In one study, however, prenatal cocaine exposure was associated significantly with lower height and weight.

There appears to be no contraindication to discontinuing cocaine abruptly during pregnancy (unlike opioids), and prompt abstinence from cocaine should be the goal of treatment.

Patients with Other Psychiatric Disorders

It is common for people with cocaine dependence who also have mood or anxiety disorders to be managed in programs that focus on the substance use problem. Several clinical reports indicate that cocaine users with bipolar disorders generally are not compliant with prescribed lithium.

Up to 10 percent of people meeting criteria for cocaine abuse also meet criteria for adult ADHD. Patients with a history of ADHD are also likely to have antisocial personality disorder. Although some studies have found that patients with antisocial personality disorder and cocaine abuse respond relatively poorly to treatment, others found improvement (reduction) in cocaine use comparable to that of patients without antisocial personality disorder. A slow-release form of methylphenidate may be less likely than other dosage forms to elicit cocaine craving, but it has not been demonstrated to reduce cocaine use.

Patients with Depression

Symptoms of depression are commonly seen in patients seeking treatment for cocaine dependence. The relation of such symptoms and of concurrent major depression to treatment outcome needs further work. The most sensible course is to treat significant depression with antidepressants only if it persists after cessation of drug use.

Patients with Schizophrenia

People with schizophrenia and other psychotic disorders who use cocaine have been managed in either primary drug treatment or psychiatric facilities. In all settings, concurrent use of alcohol and cocaine further complicates treatment. There is a growing consensus that parallel treatment in separate programs for substance dependence/abuse and schizophrenia is less effective than treatment in a comprehensive integrated program that deals with both disorders concurrently.

Intensive case management that gives patients access to social services makes it possible to treat patients with schizophrenia who abuse cocaine in the same day hospital setting as other patients. However, it may be unrealistic to require such patients to be abstinent to gain admission or to be retained in treatment, and some of the traditional rules concerning substance abuse and poor attendance may need to be relaxed. Most patients are not initially motivated to participate in abstinence-oriented programs, but when attention is paid to their individual levels of motivation, most can be engaged and moved toward active treatment.

The use of cocaine, amphetamines, and cannabis exacerbates schizophreniform disorder, and such use is not an uncommon problem. Among patients receiving public assistance or disability payments, drug use seems to increase substantially after they receive monthly checks. Patients with schizophrenia who are dependent on cocaine exhibit marked deficits in ability to learn and recall verbal information. They are also more likely to have had a history of inpatient drug treatment. Some cocaine or stimulant use may represent an attempt to alleviate negative symptoms, depression, or the side effects of antipsychotic agents, a problem that might be dealt with by using newer antipsychotic agents that have fewer extrapyramidal adverse effects, although some of these agents appear to increase plasma levels of cocaine.

SUGGESTED CROSS-REFERENCES

See Chapter 1 for a discussion of the neural sciences and Chapter 2 for a presentation of neuropsychiatry and behavioral neurology. A classification of mental disorders appears in Chapter 9. An introduction and overview of substance-related disorders is presented in Section 11.1 and amphetamine-related disorders in Section 11.3. Various drugs are discussed in the chapter on biological therapies (Chapter 31), particularly sympathomimetics in Section 31.26. Schizophrenia and other psychotic disorders are discussed in Chapter 12. Animal research and its relevance to psychiatry are discussed in Section 5.4. Cognitive-behavioral therapy is discussed in Section 48.3.

REFERENCES

Alterman AI, McLellan AT: Inpatient and day hospital treatment services for cocaine and alcohol dependence. *J Subst Abuse Treatment*. 1993;10:269.

Anthony JC, Warner LA, Kessler RC: Comparative epidemiology of dependence on tobacco, alcohol, controlled substances, and inhalants. Basic findings from the National Comorbidity Survey. *Exp Clin Psychopharmacol*. 1994;2:244.

Benowitz NL. How toxic is cocaine? In: Bock GR, Whelan J, eds. *Cocaine: Scientific and Social Dimensions*. Ciba Foundation Symposium 166. New York: Wiley; 1992.

Brown RA, Monti PM, Myers MG, Martin RA, Rivinus T, Dubreuil ME, Rohsenow DJ: Depression among cocaine abusers in treatment: relation to cocaine and alcohol use and treatment outcome. *Am J Psychiatry*. 1998;155:220.

Carroll KM, Nich C, Ball SA, McCance E, Frankforter TL, Rounsaville BJ: One-year follow-up of disulfiram and psychotherapy for cocaine-alcohol users: sustained effects of treatment. *Addiction*. 2000;95:1335.

Carroll KM, Rounsaville BJ: Contrast of treatment-seeking and untreated cocaine abusers. *Arch Gen Psychiatry*. 1992;49:464.

Carroll KM, Rounsaville BJ, Nich C, Gordon LT, Wirtz PW, Gawin FH: One year follow-up of psychotherapy and pharmacotherapy for cocaine dependence: delayed emergence of psychotherapy effects. *Arch Gen Psychiatry*. 1994;51:12.

Childress AR, Mozley PD, McElgin W, Fitzgerald J, Reivich M, O'Brien CP: Limbic activation during cue-induced cocaine craving. *Am J Psychiatry*. 1999;156:1.

Covington CY, Nordstrom-Klee B, Ager J, Sokol R, Delaney-Black V: Birth to age 7 growth of children prenatally exposed to drugs: a prospective cohort study. *Neurotoxicol Teratol*. 2002;24:489.

*Crits-Christoph P, Siqueland L, Blaine J, Frank A, Luborsky L, Onken LS, Muenz LR, Thase ME, Weiss RD, Gastfriend DR, Woody GE, Barber JP, Butler SF, Daley D, Salloum I, Bishop S, Najavits LM, Lis J, Mercer D, Griffin ML, Moras K, Beck AT: Psychosocial treatment for cocaine dependence: National Institute on Drug Abuse Collaborative Cocaine Treatment Study. *Arch Gen Psychiatry*. 1999;56:493.

Dermatis H, Galanter M, Egelko S, Westreich L: Schizophrenic patients and cocaine use: antecedents to hospitalization and course of treatment. *Subst Abus*. 1998;19:169.

Fletcher BW, Tims FM, Brown BS: Drug Abuse Treatment Outcome Study (DATOS): treatment evaluation research in the United States. *Psychol Addict Behav*. 1997;11:216.

Flynn PM, Joe GW, Broome KM, Simpson DD, Brown BS: Looking back on cocaine dependence: reasons for recovery. *Am J Addict*. 2003;12:398.

Foltin RW, Fischman MW: Effects of "binge" use of intravenous cocaine in methadone-maintained individuals. *Addiction*. 1998;93:825.

Frank DA, Jacobs RR, Beeghly M, Augustyn M, Bellinger D, Cabral H, Heeren T: Level of prenatal cocaine exposure and scores on the Bayley Scales of Infant Development: modifying effects of caregiver, early intervention, and birth weight. *Pediatrics*. 2002;110:1143.

Galanter M. Network therapy. In: Lowinson JH, Ruiz P, Millman RB, Langrod JG, eds. *Substance Abuse: A Comprehensive Textbook*. 3rd ed. Baltimore: Williams & Wilkins; 1997.

Goldstein RZ, Volkow ND: Drug addiction and its underlying neurobiological basis: neuroimaging evidence for the involvement of the frontal cortex. *Am J Psychiatry*. 2002;159:1642.

*Gorelick DA. Pharmacologic interventions for cocaine, crack, and other stimulant addiction. In: Graham AW, Schultz TK, Mayo-Smith FM, Ries RK, Wilford BB, eds. *Principles of Addiction Medicine*. 3rd ed. Chevy Chase, MD: American Society of Addiction Medication, Inc.; 2003.

*Gorelick DA, Cornish JL. The pharmacology of cocaine, amphetamines, and other stimulants. In: Graham AW, Schultz TK, Mayo-Smith FM, Ries RK, Wilford BB, eds. *Principles of Addiction Medicine*. 3rd ed. Chevy Chase, MD: American Society of Addiction Medication, Inc.; 2003.

Grella CE, Joshi V, Hser Y-I: Predictors of drug treatment re-entry following relapse to cocaine use in DATOS. *J Subst Abuse Treat.* 2003;25:145.

Higgins ST, Simon SC, Wong CJ, Heil SH, Badger GJ, Donham R, Dantona RL, Anthony S: Community reinforcement therapy for cocaine-dependent outpatients. *Arch Gen Psychiatry.* 2003;60:1043.

Hubbard RL, Craddock SG, Glynn PM, Anderson J, Etheridge RM: Overview of 1-year follow-up outcomes in the Drug Abuse Treatment Outcome Study (DATOS). *Psychol Addict Behav.* 1997;11:261.

Jaffe JH, Cascella NG, Kumor KM, Sherer MA: Cocaine-induced cocaine craving. *Psychopharmacology.* 1989;97:59.

Jaworski JN, Kozel MA, Philpot KB, Kuhar MJ: Intra-accumbal injection of CART (cocaine-amphetamine regulated transcript) peptide reduces cocaine-induced locomotor activity. *J Pharmacol Exp Ther.* 2003;307:1038.

Kampman KM, Volpicelli JR, Mulvaney F, Rukstalis M, Alterman AI, Pettinati H, Weinrieb RM, O'Brien CP: Cocaine withdrawal severity and urine toxicology results from treatment entry predict outcome in medication trials for cocaine dependence. *Addict Behav.* 2002;27:2.

Kendler KS, Jacobson KC, Prescott CA, Neale MC: Specificity of genetic and environmental risk factors for use and abuse/dependence of cannabis, cocaine, hallucinogens, sedatives, stimulants, and opiates in male twins. *Am J Psychiatry.* 2003;160:687.

Kreek MJ, Koob GF: Drug dependence: stress and dysregulation of brain reward pathways. *Drug Alcohol Depend.* 1998;51:23.

Levin FR, Evans SM, Kleber HD: Prevalence of adult attention-deficit hyperactivity disorder among cocaine abusers seeking treatment. *Drug Alcohol Depend.* 1998;52:15.

Little KY, Krolewski DM, Zhang L, Cassin BJ: Loss of striatal vesicular monoamine transporter protein (VMAT2) in human cocaine users. *Am J Psychiatry.* 2003;160:47.

Margolin A, Kleber HD, Avants SK, Konefal J, Gawin F, Stark E, Sorensen J, Midkiff E, Wells E, Jackson TR, Bullock M, Culliton PD, Boles S, Vaughan R: Acupuncture for the treatment of cocaine addiction: a randomized controlled trial. *JAMA.* 2002;287:55.

Mello NK, Mendelson JH. Cocaine, hormones, and behavior: clinical and preclinical studies. In: Pfaff, DW, Arnold A, Etgen A, Fahrback S, Rubin R, eds. *Hormones, Brain and Behavior.* St. Louis: Elsevier Science; 2002.

Mengis MM, Maude-Griffin PM, Delucchi K, Hall SM: Alcohol use affects the outcome of treatment for cocaine abuse. *Am J Addict.* 2002;11:219.

Musto D: Opium, cocaine and marijuana in American history. *Sci Am.* 1991;265:40.

Ness RB, Grisso JA, Hirschinger N, Markovic N, Shaw LM, Day NL, Kline J: Cocaine and tobacco use and the risk of spontaneous abortion. *N Engl J Med.* 1999;340:333.

*Rawson RA, McCann MJ, Huber A, Shoptaw S, Farabee D, Reiber C, Ling W. A comparison of contingency management and cognitive-behavioral approaches for cocaine dependent methadone-maintained individuals. *Arch Gen Psychiatry.* 2002;59:9.

Regier DA, Farmer ME, Rae DS, Locke BZ, Keith SJ, Judd LJ, Goodwin FK: Comorbidity of mental disorders with alcohol and other drug abuse. *JAMA.* 1990;264:2511.

Reiber C, Ramirez A, Parent D, Rawson RA: Predicting treatment success at multiple timepoints in diverse patient populations of cocaine dependent individuals. *Drug Alcohol Depend.* 2002;68:1.

Rounsaville BJ, Anton SI, Carroll K, Budde D, Prusoff BA, Gawin F: Psychiatric diagnoses of treatment-seeking cocaine abusers. *Arch Gen Psychiatry.* 1991;48:43.

Rounsaville BJ, Bryant K: Tolerance and withdrawal in the DSM-III-R diagnosis of substance dependence. *Am J Addict.* 1992;1:50.

Rounsaville BJ, Bryant K, Babor T, Kranzler H, Kadden R: Cross system agreement for substance use disorders: DSM-III-R, DSM-IV, and ICD-10. *Addiction.* 1993;88:337.

Serper MR, Bergman A, Copersine ML, Chou JC, Richarme D, Cancro R: Learning and memory impairment in cocaine-dependent and comorbid schizophrenic patients. *Psychiatry Res.* 2000;93:21.

Shearer J, Wodak A, van Beek I, Mattick RP, Lewis J: Pilot randomized double blind placebo-controlled study of dexamphetamine for cocaine dependence. *Addiction.* 2003;98:1137.

Silva de Lima M, Garcia de Oliveira Soares B, Reisser AAP, Farrell M: Pharmacological treatment of cocaine dependence: a systematic review. *Addiction.* 2002;97:931.

*Simpson DD, Joe GW, Broome KM: A national 5-year follow-up of treatment outcomes for cocaine dependence. *Arch Gen Psychiatry.* 2002;59:6.

Suto N, Tanabe LM, Austin JD, Creekmore E, Vezina P: Previous exposure to VTA amphetamine enhances cocaine self-administration under a progressive ratio schedule in an NMDA, AMPA/Kainate, and metabotropic glutamate receptor-dependent manner. *Neuropsychopharmacology.* 2003;28:629.

Tsuang MT, Lyons MJ, Meyer JM, Doyle T, Eisen SA, Goldberg J, True W, Lin N, Toomey R, Eaves L: Co-occurrence of abuse of different drugs in men. *Arch Gen Psychiatry.* 1998;55:967.

van Gorp WG, Wilkins JN, Hinkin CH, Moore LH, Hull J, Horner MD, Plotkin D: Declarative and procedural memory functioning in abstinent cocaine abusers. *Arch Gen Psychiatry.* 1999;56:85.

Wagner FA, Anthony JC: From first drug use to drug dependence: Developmental periods of risk for dependence upon marijuana, cocaine, and alcohol. *Neuropsychopharmacology.* 2002;26:479.

Wasserman GA, Kline JK, Bateman DA, Chinboga C, Lumey LH, Friedlander H, Melton L, Heagarty MC: Prenatal cocaine exposure and school-age intelligence. *Drug Alcohol Depend.* 1998;50:203.

Weddington WW, Brown BS, Haertzen CA, Cone EJ, Dax EM, Herning RI, Michaelson MA: Changes in mood, craving and sleep during short-term abstinence reported by male cocaine addicts. *Arch Gen Psychiatry.* 1990;47:861.

▲ 11.7 Hallucinogen-Related Disorders

REESE T. JONES, M.D.

Hallucinogenic drugs have been used for thousands of years. Historically, drug-induced hallucinogenic states were usually part of social and religious rituals. Recognition of profound effects of lysergic acid diethylamide (LSD) on mental functioning in 1943 markedly changed things. Unlike plant-based hallucinogens, such as psilocybin mushrooms and peyote cacti, more potent chemically synthesized hallucinogenic compounds, such as LSD, could be more readily researched, distributed, and used, leading to continued fascination with this heterogeneous group of drugs and to many thousands of scientific reports of hallucinogenic drug effects, speculations about mechanisms of action, and discussions of medical and societal problems resulting from hallucinogen distribution, use, and consequences.

DEFINITION

What drugs are properly considered hallucinogens? Classifications vary based on the classifier's specific purposes, beliefs, or prejudices. A hallucinogenic drug primarily alters perception, cognition, and mood with relatively minimal effects on memory and orientation at usually taken doses. Most commonly, definitions of hallucinogens include ergot alkaloid derivatives, such as LSD; indolealkylamines, such as psilocybin; dimethyltryptamine (DMT); and phenethylamines, such as mescaline and 3,4-methylenedioxymethamphetamine (MDMA or ecstasy), and exclude dissociative anesthetics, such as phencyclidine (PCP) and ketamine; cannabis; and stimulants, such as cocaine and most amphetamines, even though, under some circumstances, these latter drugs can produce hallucinogenic effects. Many medications can produce hallucinations, particularly at high doses; cortisone and other steroids, antidepressants, anticholinergics, and others cause a delirious, psychotic state, which sometimes includes auditory, visual, and other sensory disturbances, including hallucinations. However, these sensory symptoms are typically only one aspect of a delirium with disturbed judgment, orientation, memory, emotion, mood, and level of consciousness. Table 11.7–1 contains representative hallucinogens.

Having offered a definition for a hallucinogen, a problem remains. With uncommon exceptions, the drugs generally considered hallucinogens do not typically produce hallucinations when taken at usual doses under usual conditions. A simple definition of a *hallucination* is an experience of seeing, feeling, hearing, or smelling something not actually present in the environment, sometimes with a compelling sense of reality, but occurring without stimulation of sensory organs by ordinary sensory inputs. To call a drug a hallucinogen suggests it produces true hallucinations, that the drug user hears, sees, feels, smells, or perceives things not actually in his or her environment and is unaware that what he or she is experiencing is, in fact, not real. More typical, however, are hallucinogen-induced perceptual distortions, better termed *illusions*, resulting from drug-induced distortion of actual environmental or physical stimuli.

Alternative terms appear in the hallucinogen literature: phantastica, psychotoraxic, psycholeptic, and many others. *Psychedelic*, from the

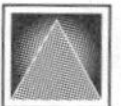

Table 11.7–1
Some Characteristic Hallucinogens

Agent	Locale	Chemical Classification	Biological Sources	Common Route	Typical Dose	Duration of Effects
Lysergic acid diethylamide	Global	Indolealkylamine	Lysergic acid, semisynthetic	Oral	75 μg	6–12 hrs
Mescaline	Southwestern United States	Phenethylamine	Peyote cactus, *Lophophora williamsii, Lophophora diffusa*	Oral	200–400 mg or 4–6 cactus buttons	10–12 hrs
Methylenedioxymethamphetamine	Global	Phenethylamine	Synthetic	Oral	50–150 mg	4–6 hrs
Psilocybin	Southern United States, Mexico, South America	Phosphorylated hydroxylated DMT	Psilocybin mushrooms	Oral	5 mg or 8 g of dried mushroom	4–6 hrs
DMT	South America, synthetic	Substituted tryptamine	Leaves of *Virola calophylla*	As a snuff, IV, smoked	0.2 mg/kg IV	30 mins
Ibogaine	West Central Africa	Indolealkylamine	*Tabernanthe iboga* powdered root	Oral	200–400 mg	8–48 hrs
Ayahuasca	South American East Amazon	Harmine, other β carbolines	Bark or leaves of liana vine	As a tea	300–400 mg	4–8 hrs
Morning glory seeds	American temperate zones	D-Lysergic acid alkaloids	Seeds of *Ipomoea violacea, Turbina corymbosa*	Orally as a tea	7–13 seeds	3 hrs

DMT, dimethyltryptamine.

Greek meaning *mind manifesting*, has successfully entered public consciousness and emphasizes valued and, for some, therapeutic effects. Psychotomimetic, meaning an imitation of psychoses, is no more accurate than alternative terms. Although sensory and other cognitive effects associated with hallucinogenic drugs have similarities to those occurring in naturally occurring psychoses, a drug-induced state does not completely mimic naturally occurring psychotic states. Newer terms such as *entheogens*, *empathogens*, or *entactogens* have supporters and justifications but often appear to be attempts to avoid using other older and value-laden terms. With unresolved imprecision acknowledged, this book uses the term *hallucinogen*.

HISTORY

Before the early 1960s, ingestion of hallucinogens in the United States was mostly limited to American Indians belonging to the Native American Church, an occasional ethnobotanist, and small groups of intellectuals, artists, and researchers. R. Gordon Wasson described Mexican Indian use of psilocybin mushrooms in 1955. LSD was discovered by Swiss chemist Albert Hofmann in 1943 and became generally available to researchers in the United States in 1949 as a drug possibly useful in psychiatric treatment and useful for studies of the pathogenesis of mental illness by producing models of psychosis. LSD was popularized in the 1960s as the mind-expanding psychedelic drug for the masses by a former Harvard professor, Timothy Leary. That latter event, as much as any single factor, accounts for location of this chapter on hallucinogens in the substance abuse section rather than somewhere else in this textbook.

Enormous scientific and popular literature describes LSD and other hallucinogen drug effects. LSD effects are prototypic of other hallucinogens. For a brief summary, it is impossible to surpass the accurate and informative personal accounts of Hofmann's discovery of LSD; Hofmann was at that time a pharmaceutical chemist in the Basel laboratories of Sandoz Pharmaceuticals.

What was unusual about LSD's hallucinogenic properties? Its extreme potency for producing profound psychic changes was remarkable. Before the potency of LSD was recognized, mescaline and other hallucinogens had been well characterized but were pharmacologically active only at milligram- or gram-per-kilogram doses. LSD is 5,000 times more potent than mescaline.

Hofmann synthesized LSD-25 in 1938 as one of a series of synthetic ergot alkaloids. LSD was number 25 in the series. When given to animals to screen for analeptic properties, LSD produced excess restlessness and no other therapeutically promising effects, so it was put aside, although Hofmann remained interested in it.

On the afternoon of April 16, 1943, shortly after synthesizing a new batch of LSD, Hofmann wrote that, while working in his laboratory, he entered a "kind of dream world." Surroundings changed in a "strange" way and became "luminous, more expressive."

> I felt uneasy and went home, where I wanted to rest. Lying on the couch with closed eyes, because I experienced daylight as unpleasantly glaring, I perceived an uninterrupted stream of fantastic pictures, with an intense kaleidoscopic play of colors. After some hours, this strange but not unpleasant condition faded away.

Hofmann assumed that he had somehow become intoxicated while working in the laboratory, perhaps from a solvent used in purifying the LSD. To test this assumption, 3 days later on Monday morning April 19, in his laboratory, he experimented by sniffing dichloroethylene vapors. Nothing special happened. He decided to test whether LSD had caused the strange sensory and psychological experience. Reasoning that he might have been exposed to a very small dose through contact with fingertips and skin absorption, he drank at 4:20 PM what he considered the smallest quantity that could be expected to produce psychological effects—0.25 mg of LSD tartrate in water. It was tasteless. At approximately 5 PM, he began to experience "dizziness, feeling of anxiety, visual distortions, symptoms of paralysis, desire to laugh."

At 5 PM, Hofmann's laboratory journal notes ended. He later wrote that it was clear at that point that LSD had caused the previous Friday's extraordinary experience because the altered perceptions were so similar but much more intense. He asked his laboratory assistant to accompany him home—by bicycle. Hofmann wrote:

On the way home my condition began to assume threatening forms. Everything in my field of vision wavered, and was distorted as if seen in a curved mirror. I had lost the feeling of time which resulted in the sensation of being unable to move from the spot, although my assistant told me later that we had traveled very rapidly. At home, I asked my companion to summon our family doctor and request milk from our neighbor. In spite of my delirious condition, I was still capable of clear and effective thinking—milk is a nonspecific antidote for poisoning. The dizziness and sensation of fainting became so strong that I could no longer hold myself erect and I had to lie down on the sofa. My surroundings had now transformed themselves in more terrifying ways. Everything in the room spun around and familiar objects and furniture assumed grotesque, threatening forms. They were in continuous motion, animated, as if driven by an inner restlessness. When the neighbor brought the milk, she was no longer Mrs. Ruch, but rather a malevolent witch with a colored mask.

Even worse than these demonic transformations of the outer world were the alterations that I perceived in myself, in my inner being. Every exertion of my will to put an end to the disintegration of the outer world, and the dissolution of my ego, seemed to be a wasted effort. The substance with which I had wanted to experiment had become a demon who had vanquished me and who scornfully triumphed over my will. I was seized by the dreadful fear of having become insane. I was taken to another world, another place, another time. My body seemed to be without sensation, lifeless, strange. Was I dying? Was this the transition? At times I believed I was outside my body, but then perceived clearly, as an outside observer, the complete tragedy of my situation. I had not even taken leave of my family (my wife, with our three children, had traveled that day to visit her parents in Lucerne). Would they ever understand that I have not experimented thoughtlessly or irresponsibly, but rather with the utmost caution?

By the time his doctor arrived, the peak intensity had passed. The doctor was puzzled by Hofmann's attempts to describe "the mortal danger which threatened my body." Hofmann's vital signs were normal. The doctor saw no reason to prescribe any medication and put Hofmann to bed.

Gradually, the intense weird feelings disappeared, and Hofmann began to enjoy the colors and shape transformations that persisted behind his closed eyes. He remarked on how remarkably each sound became transformed into optical perceptions (synesthesia). Every sound generated a changing image with its own consistent form and color. When his wife returned home, he was able to tell her what happened. He slept well and awoke the next morning refreshed with a clear head. When he walked into the garden after a spring rain, "everything glistened and sparkled . . . . The world seemed as if newly created."

Hofmann's first and unplanned serendipitous exposure was to probably a much smaller dose than the second exposure 3 days later when he took a measured 250-μg dose. Hofmann accurately characterized the self-experiment as one in which "I had not been prepared for such an overwhelming experience and because the chosen dosage had been too high." Subsequent experience with LSD has repeatedly demonstrated that lack of preparation and excessive dose more likely leads to what are now termed *bad trips*.

Although the thousands of descriptions of hallucinogen-induced states written in the subsequent 60 years vary depending on the subject, dose, setting, and expectations of the recipients and the experimenters, they all are variations on that first experience of Hofmann.

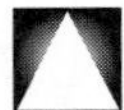

Table 11.7–2
DSM-IV-TR Hallucinogen-Related Disorders

Hallucinogen use disorders
Hallucinogen dependence
Hallucinogen abuse
Hallucinogen-induced disorders
Hallucinogen intoxication
Hallucinogen persisting perception disorder (flashbacks)
Hallucinogen intoxication delirium
Hallucinogen-induced psychotic disorder with delusions
Specify if:
With onset during intoxication
Hallucinogen-induced psychotic disorder with hallucinations
Specify if:
With onset during intoxication
Hallucinogen-induced mood disorder
Specify if:
With onset during intoxication
Hallucinogen-induced anxiety disorder
Specify if:
With onset during intoxication
Hallucinogen-related disorder not otherwise specified

From American Psychiatric Association. *Diagnostic and Statistical Manual of Mental Disorders.* 4th ed. Text rev. Washington, DC: American Psychiatric Association; 2000, with permission.

COMPARATIVE NOSOLOGY

For hallucinogen-related disorders, the revised fourth edition of the *Diagnostic and Statistical Manual of Mental Disorders* (DSM-IV-TR) lists specific diagnostic criteria only for hallucinogen intoxication and hallucinogen persisting perception disorder. Criteria for other hallucinogen-related disorders in Table 11.7–2 are in the DSM-IV-TR sections addressing the more general disorders. Although DSM-IV-TR permits specifying drug dependence as occurring with or without physiological dependence, that option does not apply to hallucinogens. Hallucinogens produce no recognized withdrawal states.

The tenth edition of the *International Statistical Classification of Diseases and Related Health Problems* (ICD-10), used throughout much of the world, makes fewer distinctions among hallucinogen-related disorders (Table 11.7–3). ICD-10 includes "harmful use" instead of abuse and omits mention of a hallucinogen-induced mood disorder and hallucinogen-induced anxiety disorder. Hallucinogen persisting perceptual disorder is not offered as a diagnostic choice, and flashbacks are considered part of a hallucinogen residual psychotic disorder. The ninth revision, clinical modification of ICD (ICD-9-CM) diagnostic terms required for Medicare and Medicaid billing do not offer the term intoxication, and ICD-9-CM does not offer a special diagnosis for one of the more common adverse events, anxiety disorder, and omits diagnosis of flashbacks and persisting perceptual disorder. To some extent, these minor inconsistencies reflect the relative rarity of adverse consequences from hallucinogen use, hence less clinical experience and data than with other drugs of abuse.

EPIDEMIOLOGY

Illicit use of hallucinogenic drugs remains popular in the United States and in Western Europe countries. In recent years, surveys in

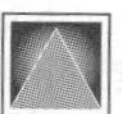

Table 11.7–3
Hallucinogen Diagnoses, DSM-IV-TR and ICD

DSM-IV-TR	ICD-9-CM	ICD-10
Hallucinogen abuse	Hallucinogen abuse	Hallucinogen harmful use
Hallucinogen dependence	Hallucinogen dependence	Hallucinogen dependence syndrome
Hallucinogen intoxication	Hallucinogen abuse	Hallucinogen acute intoxication
Hallucinogen intoxication delirium	Drug-induced delirium	Hallucinogen acute intoxication
Hallucinogen-induced mood disorder	Drug-induced organic affective syndrome	—
Hallucinogen-induced anxiety disorder	Hallucinogen abuse	—
Hallucinogen-induced psychotic disorder	Drug-induced organic delusional syndrome	Hallucinogen psychotic disorder
Hallucinogen persisting perceptual disorder	—	Hallucinogen residual psychotic disorder (flashbacks)
Hallucinogen-related disorder not otherwise specified	Unspecified drug-induced mental disorder	Other or unspecified mental or behavioral disorder induced by hallucinogen

the United States and Western Europe reported young people using hallucinogenic drugs at levels exceeding cocaine and heroin use. The National Household Survey on Drug Abuse (NHSDA) estimated that between 1965 and 1971, the number of new hallucinogen users increased tenfold from 90,000 to 900,000. Use decreased beginning in the mid-1970s. Decreased use persisted throughout the 1980s, with the drug-taking population of the United States choosing alcohol, methamphetamine, or cocaine over hallucinogens. Early in the 1990s, there was a gradual increase in hallucinogenic drug use, particularly among high school and college students and other young adults. Surveys in 1990 suggested approximately 600,000 new users; in 1996, almost one million. By 2000, the estimated number of new users increased to 1.5 million. Lifetime prevalence of hallucinogen use was 9.7 percent in 1996. More than 20 million people have used hallucinogens at least once. Lifetime prevalence is higher in whites than for Hispanics and blacks. The male to female ratio of hallucinogen use was constant across races at approximately 2:1 to 3:1.

The NHSDA survey conducted in 2001 found that 12.5 percent of people (12 years of age and older) reported lifetime use of hallucinogens, a significant increase from the 11.7 percent found in the 2000 survey. Past 30-day use, as reported by 0.6 percent of people in 2001, compared with the 0.5 percent in 2000, was a small but statistically significant increase. The highest rates of use during the past year (9.3 percent) were among 18- to 25-year-olds, followed by 12- to 17-year-olds.

Since 1975, the extent of drug use by high school students has been surveyed each year, a useful indicator of future young adult patterns. The annual prevalence of LSD use has remained less than 10 percent since 1975 but with fluctuations over the years. As was the pattern in adults, the proportion of high school seniors trying a hallucinogenic drug at least once in the prior 12 months increased from 4.4 to 8.4 percent between 1985 and 1995. However, recent trends may have leveled off. Reported LSD use by 12th graders significantly decreased from 2001 to 2002, continuing a decline that began in 1996 resulting in the lowest use rates of LSD in the history of the survey. Use of hallucinogens other than LSD, most commonly psilocybin mushrooms, showed modest but not significant declines as well. The 2002 survey also found that MDMA use decreased after significant increases during the previous few years.

ETIOLOGY

Hallucinogens are often taken by most present-day users for what might be broadly defined as recreational reasons at concerts, movies, or dances or during outdoor activities to enhance enjoyment from those or similar activities. Hallucinogen-altered consciousness includes loss of boundaries between the user and environment, changes in perception with colors and sounds distorted and intensified, and ordinary objects appearing novel or awe inspiring. Such effects serve in a way as activity enhancers. Users are usually aware the experiences are drug induced. Euphoria is usually experienced but sometimes alternates with experiences like that of dying or being born.

Use of hallucinogenic drugs, like other drug use, is the result of a process in which multiple interacting factors—social, cultural, psychological, and biological—interact to determine drug-taking behavior. With most other drugs of abuse, for some regular users, there is at some point a loss of control of drug use that is as much neurochemically determined as a result of the other factors. However, with hallucinogenic drugs, the loss of personal choice as a consequence of brain neurochemical changes appears to be less of a factor for determining future drug use, particularly progression to dependence. People continue to take hallucinogenic drugs because they find they like the effects of hallucinogenic drugs. Users report finding the experience interesting, entertaining, useful, and, for some, therapeutic or spiritual. Although ready availability of synthetic hallucinogens and relatively low cost are important determinants of use, as was the case with the older hallucinogens of plant origins, social, cultural, and psychological factors also continue to be important determinants of hallucinogen-using behavior.

To merely consider hallucinogens as mood elevators, as is sometimes the case with psychostimulants, or to view hallucinogens as drugs that produce euphoria in the simple sense of that term is inaccurate characterization of the effects on humans. Hallucinogens are not powerful reinforcers in animal models. In fact, in animal models of drug taking, hallucinogens generally appear aversive rather than reinforcing. The absence of a withdrawal syndrome (with the possible exception of MDMA) does not explain continued hallucinogen use to avoid the unpleasantness of withdrawal. Feelings of dysphoria and anhedonia are not generally associated with the cessation of hallucinogen drug use, although some users describe missing the experiences. Craving is only rarely mentioned in association with hallucinogen drug use.

PHARMACOLOGY

Hofmann's first accidental LSD exposure and his planned experiment 3 days later remain landmarks of serendipity and careful, objective reporting. His description in the section on history illustrates three characteristic hallucinogen symptom clusters: somatic, sensory, and psychological:

> Somatic symptoms include dizziness, weakness, tremors, nausea, drowsiness, paresthesias, and blurred vision.

Sensory symptoms include perceiving altered shapes and colors, difficulty in focusing on objects, a sense of sharpened hearing, and, occasionally, synesthesias.

Psychological symptoms include mood alterations ranging from happy to sad to irritable, increased feelings of tension, distorted time sense, difficulty in expressing thoughts verbally, dream-like feelings, depersonalization, and very occasionally visual hallucinations.

Structures of selected hallucinogens representative of three major groups of hallucinogens are shown in Figure 11.7–1 together with three neurotransmitters that have interesting structural similarities.

Lysergic Acid Diethylamide A large class of hallucinogenic compounds with well-studied structure–activity relationships is represented by the prototype LSD. *LSD* is a synthetic base derived from the lysergic acid nucleus from the ergot alkaloids. That family of compounds was discovered in rye fungus and was responsible for lethal outbreaks of St. Anthony's fire in the Middle Ages. The compounds are also present in morning glory seeds in low concentrations. A large number of homologs and analogs of LSD have been studied. None of them has potency exceeding that of LSD.

Physiological symptoms from LSD are typically few and relatively mild. Dilated pupils, increased deep tendon motor reflexes and muscle tension, and mild motor incoordination and ataxia are common. Increased heart rate, respiration, and blood pressure are modest in degree and variable, as are nausea, decreased appetite, and salivation.

The usual sequence of changes follows a pattern of somatic symptoms appearing first, then mood and perceptual changes, and, finally, psychological changes, although effects overlap and, depending on the particular hallucinogen, the time of onset and offset varies. The intensity of LSD effects in a nontolerant user generally is proportional to dose, with 25 μg as an approximate threshold dose.

The syndrome produced by LSD resembles that produced by mescaline, psilocybin, and some of the amphetamine analogs. The major difference among LSD, psilocybin, and mescaline is potency. A 1.5 μg/kg dose of LSD is roughly equivalent to 225 μg/kg of psilocybin, which is equivalent to 5 mg/kg of mescaline. With mescaline, there is a slower onset of symptoms and more nausea and vomiting, but in general, the perceptual effects are more similar than different.

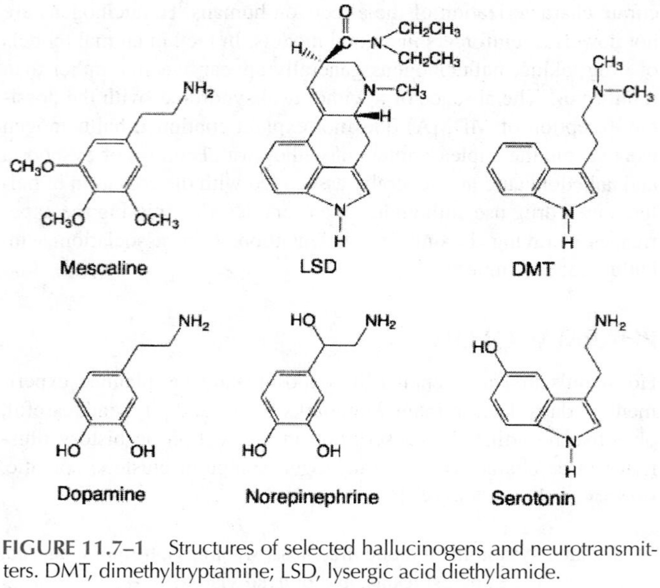

Tolerance, particularly to the sensory and other psychological effects, is evident as soon as the second or third day of successive LSD use. Four to 6 days free of LSD is necessary to lose significant tolerance. Tolerance is associated with frequent use of any of the hallucinogens. Cross-tolerance among mescaline, psilocybin, and LSD occurs, but not between amphetamine and LSD, despite the chemical similarity of amphetamine and mescaline.

LSD has been distributed as tablets, liquid, powder, and gelatin squares; but, in recent years, LSD has been commonly distributed as "blotter acid." Sheets of paper are soaked with LSD, dried, and perforated into small squares. Popular designs are stamped on the paper. Each sheet contains as many as a few hundred squares; one square containing 30 to 75 μg of LSD is one chewed dose, more or less. Planned massive ingestion is uncommon but happens by accident.

FIGURE 11.7–1 Structures of selected hallucinogens and neurotransmitters. DMT, dimethyltryptamine; LSD, lysergic acid diethylamide.

Phenethylamines *Phenethylamines* are compounds with simple chemical structures and structural similarity to the neurotransmitters dopamine and norepinephrine. Mescaline (3,4,5-trimethoxyphenethylamine), a classic hallucinogen in every sense of the term, was the first hallucinogen isolated from the peyote cactus that grows in the southwest United States and northern Mexico. Mescaline human pharmacology was characterized in 1896 and its structure verified by synthesis 23 years later. Although many psychoactive plants have been recognized dating to before recorded history, mescaline was the only structurally identified hallucinogen until LSD was described in 1943.

Mescaline Mescaline is usually consumed as peyote "buttons," picked from the small blue-green cacti *Lophophora williamsii* and *Lophophora diffusa*. The buttons are the dried, round, fleshy cacti tops. Mescaline is the active hallucinogenic alkaloid in the buttons. Use of peyote is legal for the Native American Church members in some states. Adverse reactions to peyote are rare during structured religious use. Peyote usually is not consumed casually because of its bitter taste and sometimes severe nausea and vomiting preceding the hallucinogenic effects.

Many structural variations of mescaline have been investigated and structural activity relationships fairly well characterized. One analog, 2,5-dimethoxy-4-methylamphetamine (DOM), also known as *STP*, an unusually potent amphetamine with hallucinogen properties, had a relatively brief period of illicit popularity and notoriety in the 1960s.

Another series of phenethylamine analogs with hallucinogenic properties is the 3,4-methylenedioxyamphetamine (MDA)–related amphetamines. The currently most popular and, to society, most troublesome member of this large family of drugs is MDMA, or ecstasy, more a relatively mild stimulant than hallucinogen. MDMA produces an altered state of consciousness with sensory changes and, most important for some users, a feeling of enhanced personal interactions. MDMA is discussed in more detail in Section 11.3 on amphetamine-related disorders.

Tryptamines Indolealkylamine hallucinogens contain a two-ring structure known as an *indole* and thus structurally resemble the neurotransmitter serotonin. Indoleethylamine is better known as *tryptamine*, a serotonin precursor. If the neuropharmacology of hallucinogens was simpler than it really is, phenethylamine hallucinogens would mainly interact with dopamine receptors, and tryptamines would mainly involve serotonin receptors in their brain effects. Instead, all hallucinogens bind to one or more of the serotonin receptor subtypes with agonist or partial agonist properties, and the dopamine system interacts as well.

DMT (*N,N*-dimethyltryptamine) is in many plants. DMT is also found normally in human biofluids at very low concentrations. When DMT is taken parenterally or by sniffing, a brief, intense hallucinogenic episode can result. Like mescaline in the phenethylamine group, DMT is one of the oldest, best documented, but least potent of the tryptamine hallucinogens. Synthesized homologs of DMT have been evaluated in humans and structure activity relationships reasonably well described.

Psilocybin Analogs An unusual collection of tryptamines has its origin in the world of fungi. The natural prototype is psilocybin itself. That and related homologs have been found in as many as 100 species of mushroom, largely of the *Psilocybe* genus.

Psilocybin is usually ingested as mushrooms. Many species of psilocybin-containing mushrooms are found worldwide. In the United States, large *Psilocybe cubensis* (gold caps) grow in Florida and Texas and are easily grown with cultivation kits advertised in drug-oriented magazines and on the Internet. The tiny *Psilocybe semilanceata* (liberty cap) grows in lawns and pastures in the Pacific Northwest. Psilocybin remains active when the mushrooms are dried or cooked into omelets or other foods.

Psilocybin mushrooms are used in religious activities by Mexican Indians. They are valued in Western society by users who prefer to ingest a mushroom instead of a synthetic chemical. Of course, one danger of eating wild mushrooms is misidentification and ingestion of a poisonous variety. At a large American university, 24 percent of students reported using psychedelic mushrooms or mescaline, compared with 17 percent who reported LSD use. Psilocybin sold as pills or capsules usually contains PCP or LSD instead.

Additional Hallucinogens

Ibogaine *Ibogaine* is a complex alkaloid found in the African shrub *Tabernanthe iboga*. Ibogaine is a hallucinogen at the 400-mg dose range. It has in recent years been much discussed, studied, and patented as a pharmacotherapy for heroin and other addictions using doses that range as high as 1,500 mg orally. The plant originates in Africa and traditionally is used in sacramental initiation ceremonies. The material is taken from scrapings of the plant root. Although it has not been a popular hallucinogen because of its unpleasant somatic effects when taken at hallucinogenic doses, patients exposed to ibogaine may be encountered by a psychiatrist because of the therapeutic claims.

Ayahuasca *Ayahuasca*, much discussed on Internet hallucinogen Web sites, originally referred to a decoction from one or more South American plants. The drink was made by boiling parts of a western Amazon vine (liana) that contains the alkaloids harmaline and harmine. Both of those β-carboline alkaloids have hallucinogenic properties, but the resulting visual sensory alterations are accompanied by considerable nausea. Amazon native tribes discovered that adding leaves from plants containing substantial amounts of DMT markedly enhances the visual and sacramental impact of ayahuasca. DMT itself is not active orally because it normally is destroyed by deamination enzymes in the gut, but when the two plants are ingested together, the β-carboline alkaloids inhibit the deamination enzymes that ordinarily destroy DMT. Thus, neither component in the ayahuasca plant mixture works well alone, but, when taken in combination, an extremely effective hallucinogenic agent results.

In recent years, the term *ayahuasca* has gradually evolved to refer to any mixture of two things that are hallucinogenic when taken in combination. For example, harmine and harmaline are available as fine chemicals and, when taken along with many botanicals containing DMT, result in a mixture with hallucinogenic properties.

Salvia Divinorum American Indians in northern Oaxaca, Mexico, have long cultivated and used a mint plant as a medicine and as a sacred sacrament. A relatively mild hallucinogen and little known as a hallucinogen in the United States until a few years ago, *Salvia divinorum* is now widely discussed, advertised, and sold on the Internet and is becoming generally available everywhere. It is easy to grow at home. The pure isolated active compound, salvinorin-A, is not well absorbed when taken orally, but when the plant is chewed or dried leaves smoked, it produces hallucinogen effects. Salvinorin-A, an active component in the plant, is parenterally potent, active at 250-μg doses when smoked, and of scientific and potential medical interest because it binds to the opioid κ receptor. *Salvia's* complete spectrum of effects and metabolic fate in humans has not been adequately researched.

PSYCHIATRIC DISORDERS

Hallucinogen Abuse and Dependence

Diagnosis and Clinical Features The general criteria for other substance dependence and abuse apply to hallucinogen dependence and abuse but with a less precise fit. There are no unique criteria sets for hallucinogen dependence or hallucinogen use. Tolerance develops with closely spaced repeated use to most, but not all, hallucinogen effects developing after a few successive daily doses to the perceptual and mood effects of hallucinogens but less so to autonomic and cardiovascular effects. With typical hallucinogen use patterns in which days typically pass between drug use, tolerance is not usually clinically evident. Cross-tolerance between LSD and some other hallucinogens, particularly psilocybin and mescaline, is marked but does not extend to all hallucinogens. A withdrawal syndrome after repeated use ceases is not evident. Thus, there is no DSM-IV-TR diagnosis for hallucinogen withdrawal. Hallucinogen use, even for individuals who meet the criteria for a diagnosis of dependence, is rarely more than one dose a week and usually much less frequent. Evidence of craving for hallucinogens is equivocal, with the possible exception of MDMA.

A pattern of gradually increasing drug consumption and unsuccessful efforts to decrease use is rarely reported by users nor is evidence of compulsive drug-seeking behaviors. Hallucinogen use is typically more episodic, irregular, and time limited when compared with other abused and addicting drugs.

Differential Diagnosis Sudden onset of visual hallucinations or illusions, inappropriate affect, arousal, and paranoid thinking suggest hallucinogen toxicity. However, a multitude of illicitly used drugs, prescribed medications, and non–drug-related mental illness may also account for such a clinical picture. Laboratory tests for the presence of amphetamines, cannabinoids, opiates, cocaine, benzodiazepines, and barbiturates in urine or blood are useful, as is physical examination, including careful neurological evaluation, clinical observation, and the passage of time.

Course, Prognosis, and Treatment Few people seek treatment for primary hallucinogen abuse or dependence. Hallucinogen use comes up more often as a diagnostic or treatment issue in patients experiencing anxiety, complaining of mood disorders, worried about thoughts of suicide, or experiencing symptoms of a psychosis. The role of the hallucinogen use as a precipitant remains uncertain; however, prudent advice is for an individual to stop using hallucinogens under such circumstances. With such advice and explanations why it is wise to do so, most patients give up hallucinogens, at least until the presenting symptoms are under control. Taking hallucinogens is more common in the young. No matter what the intervention, as a person grows older, hallucinogen use is likely to decrease. Pharmacotherapy for hallucinogen use or dependence is not indicated.

Hallucinogen Intoxication

Diagnosis and Clinical Features Users come to medical attention when an unexpected and unpleasant reaction follows hallucinogen drug ingestion. They present stimulated, frightened, anxious, and often fearful of losing their mind. Adverse effects of any specific hallucinogen are variable among individuals and even in the same person at different times but are more likely in people with limited hallucinogen experience. Most common, severe anxiety and panic attacks or occasionally sudden onset of intense feelings of depression and suicidal thoughts characterizes the onset as what has been termed a *bad trip*. LSD overdoses are never directly fatal, but an excessive dose or unusual sensitivity when a hallucinogen is taken in an inappropriate setting has led to fatal accidents or suicides either during or relatively soon after intoxication.

Physiological and psychological manifestations include moderately increased heart rate, elevated blood pressure, dilated pupils, mild hyperthermia, sweating, anxiety, loss of contact with reality, depersonalization, paranoia, and confusion. The DSM-IV-TR diagnostic criteria for hallucinogen intoxication are listed in Table 11.7–4.

Differential Diagnosis It is important to thoughtfully consider history of other drug ingestion or exposure and psychiatric illness and perform an adequate neurological evaluation. A urine toxicological screen for other drugs of abuse is useful, particularly because more than one drug may be involved. Information from friends or others with the patient during the previous few hours is useful. Serum, urine, or gastric content samples can be sent to analytical laboratories for specific mass spectrographic analysis, but test results are usually delayed so that initial diagnosis and treatment must be from clinical assessment. Users are not always knowledgeable about actual hallucinogen dose ingested. LSD is often sold as postage stamp–sized papers containing doses of LSD from 25 to 75 μg but, on occasion, can deliver much more. Doses of 25 μg produce mild psychological effects; doses of 200 μg are usually associated with more intense symptoms.

A diagnosis of plant hallucinogen intoxications, such as from psilocybin mushrooms, peyote, and mescaline or morning glory seeds, must usually be made by obtaining a careful history or drug samples from the patient or friends. Doses delivered from plant material are always uncertain.

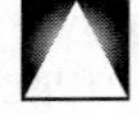

Table 11.7–4
DSM-IV-TR Diagnostic Criteria for Hallucinogen Intoxication

A. Recent use of a hallucinogen.
B. Clinically significant maladaptive behavioral or psychological changes (e.g., marked anxiety or depression, ideas of reference, fear of losing one's mind, paranoid ideation, impaired judgment, or impaired social or occupational functioning) that developed during, or shortly after, hallucinogen use.
C. Perceptual changes occurring in a state of full wakefulness and alertness (e.g., subjective intensification of perceptions, depersonalization, derealization, illusions, hallucinations, synesthesias) that developed during, or shortly after, hallucinogen use.
D. Two (or more) of the following signs, developing during, or shortly after, hallucinogen use:
 (1) Pupillary dilation
 (2) Tachycardia
 (3) Sweating
 (4) Palpitations
 (5) Blurring of vision
 (6) Tremors
 (7) Incoordination
E. The symptoms are not due to a general medical condition and are not better accounted for by another mental disorder.

From American Psychiatric Association. *Diagnostic and Statistical Manual of Mental Disorders*. 4th ed. Text rev. Washington, DC: American Psychiatric Association; 2000, with permission.

Course and Prognosis Typically, a bad trip is self-limited and, depending on the specific hallucinogen used, resolves for the most part within 6 to 12 hours or less after ingestion with no lasting sequelae. Optimal management can make things more pleasant for all concerned.

Treatment A basic principle is reassurance and supportive care. Patients experiencing intense and unpleasant hallucination intoxication can be helped by providing a quiet environment, verbal reassurance, and simply allowing the passage of time. More rapid relief is likely after oral administration of 20 mg of diazepam or, if oral administration presents problems, an equivalent parental dose of a benzodiazepine. Anxiety and other symptoms generally diminish within 20 minutes of medication administration instead of hours with only psychological and environmental support. Patients may need gentle restraint if a danger to themselves or to others, but restraint should be avoided if possible. Neuroleptic medications, particularly if given at excessive doses, may worsen symptoms and are best avoided unless the diagnosis is unclear and behavior cannot otherwise be managed.

For reasons not entirely clear, the occurrence of intense hallucinogen-induced states seeking or requiring treatment in emergency facilities has decreased markedly in recent years. Possibly a typical dose of illicit LSD taken today (25 to 50 μg) is smaller than the 100- to 200-μg doses more commonly used in the 1970s. Whether a consequence of the more modest illicit dose units sold and ingested or simply greater awareness on the part of the users and their friends about the usual time-limited course of unpleasant experiences, such cases appear less often in emergency rooms and other psychiatric treatment venues than in the 1970s.

Hallucinogen-Induced Mood Disorder

A prominent and persistent mood disturbance directly resulting from the effects of taking a hallucinogen is an essential feature. In the case of hallucinogens, this is sometimes more difficult to determine with certainty than with most other drugs of abuse. Hallucinogen effects on mood are common but usually transient for minutes or a few hours and rarely persist longer. Variability is a consistent attribute of the mood changes. Symptoms resembling those of major depression, mania, or hypomania may appear during the period of peak drug effects but do not persist much beyond the period of intoxication.

Persistent symptoms of a mood disorder sometimes were present before the use of a hallucinogen, with the drug use representing more a failed therapeutic attempt to achieve relief of symptoms rather than being causative. Hallucinogen exposure may worsen the preexisting condition. Thus, a careful history is required before making this diagnosis. Reports of suicidal feeling should be taken seriously and appropriate support and evaluation offered and not ignored as simply a drug effect that will disappear. Treatment of the persisting mood disorder should be as if the hallucinogen was not considered the major precipitant. The patient should be cautioned to avoid future hallucinogen use.

Hallucinogen-Induced Anxiety Disorder

Acute anxiety reactions during hallucinogen intoxication are one of the most common adverse consequences. The anxiety is usually related to experience of unexpected intensity of sensory distortion and feelings of loss of control. A full-blown panic state is possible. The management is oral benzodiazepines, reassurance, and explanation as described for hallucinogen intoxication.

Hallucinogen Persisting Perception Disorder

Prolonged or recurrent visual disturbances after LSD and other hallucinogen use have been recognized for a long time. For example, more than 100 years ago, Havelock Ellis, in one of the earliest accounts of a mescaline intoxication, described experiencing prolonged sensitivity to the phenomenon of light, shade, and color after ingesting mescaline. Visual sensations may recur days, weeks, or months after even a single episode of hallucinogen use. Brief symptoms lasting only a few seconds are commonly termed *flashbacks*. Sensations that present continuously, albeit with minor fluctuations, are considered hallucinogen persisting perception disorders (Table 11.7–5). That diagnosis first appeared in 1986 in the revised third edition of the DSM (DSM-III-R) as a "posthallucinogen perception disorder" and with slightly modified criteria than is in DSM-IV-TR. Hallucinogens are unique among other drug-induced disorders in DSM-IV-TR by the hallucinogen persistent perceptual disorder diagnosis.

Hallucinogen use must precede the symptom appearance and must last more than a few days after hallucinogen exposure. The intensity of the perceptual phenomenon must be sufficient to produce distress or impairment. Alternative explanations for unusual perceptual experiences must be considered before diagnosing hallucinogen persisting perception disorders, for example, visual epilepsy, migraine, delirium, dementia, schizophrenia, hypnopompic hallucinations, posttraumatic stress disorders (PTSDs), and other hallucinogen-induced disorders recognized in DSM-IV-TR.

A recent literature review covering the past 50 years concluded that the term "flashbacks" has been defined and used in so many ways as to render it valueless as a descriptor. Published studies on hallucinogen persisting perception disorders were judged methodologically inadequate. How many of the many case reports meet DSM-IV-TR criteria is impossible to determine.

Hallucinogen persisting perception disorder appears to be an occasional disorder but one that can be associated with substantial morbidity. It comes to medical attention most commonly after illicit exposure to LSD and much less often after LSD given in a treatment or research setting. Hallucinogen persisting perception disorder is less commonly reported after exposure to other hallucinogens.

Published reports do not permit even a crude estimate of hallucinogen persisting perception disorder prevalence. Considering the millions of hallucinogen doses taken by millions of people since the late 1950s, relatively few and mostly small case series have been reported.

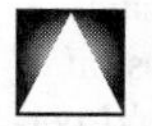

Table 11.7–5
DSM-IV-TR Diagnostic Criteria for Hallucinogen Persisting Perception Disorder (Flashbacks)

A. The reexperiencing, after cessation of use of a hallucinogen, of one or more of the perceptual symptoms that were experienced while intoxicated with the hallucinogen (e.g., geometric hallucinations, false perceptions of movement in the peripheral visual fields, flashes of color, intensified colors, trails of images of moving objects, positive afterimages, halos around objects, macropsia, and micropsia).

B. The symptoms in Criterion A cause clinically significant distress or impairment in social, occupational, or other important areas of functioning.

C. The symptoms are not due to a general medical condition (e.g., anatomical lesions and infections of the brain, visual epilepsies) and are not better accounted for by another mental disorder (e.g., delirium, dementia, schizophrenia) or hypnopompic hallucinations.

From American Psychiatric Association. *Diagnostic and Statistical Manual of Mental Disorders.* 4th ed. Text rev. Washington, DC: American Psychiatric Association; 2000, with permission.

Course and Prognosis

With nothing more than reassurance, explanation of the phenomena, and the passage of time, approximately one-half the patients with hallucinogen persisting perception disorder stop having symptoms within 5 years. Symptoms can be worsened by a variety of stimulant drugs, marijuana use, fatigue, exercise, and infections.

Etiology

Etiology remains unclear. Heightened awareness of normal visual phenomenon is one possibility. Neurochemical explanations, for example, visual processing disinhibition because of serotonin receptor dysfunction on inhibitory interneurons, are inconsistent with the absence of a relationship between the number of hallucinogen exposures and the presence of flashbacks.

Treatment

Hallucinogen persisting perception disorder causes substantial morbidity for some people seeking treatment. Treatments reported as useful include simple reassurance, supportive psychotherapy, sunglasses, neuroleptics, selective serotonin reuptake inhibitors (SSRIs), and other medications. At best, the treatment literature for hallucinogen persisting perception disorder is anecdotal, and no definitive guidance is available.

Hallucinogen-Induced Psychotic Disorders

Diagnosis and Clinical Features

What is sometimes indistinguishable from acute schizophrenic episodes can be precipitated in vulnerable individuals. Prominent hallucinations, sensory distortions, or delusions without insight that they are drug induced and persist for approximately 1 month or more after taking the hallucinogen suggest that a diagnosis of hallucinogen-induced psychotic disorder may be justified (Table 13.3–4). Because hallucinogens produce a state with many similarities to naturally occurring psychoses, the history is important in making this diagnosis. Operationally, psychotic-like symptoms and behaviors continuing more than 48 hours after hallucinogen ingestion are minimal criteria. Reported occurrence after hallucinogen exposure varies greatly, with estimates from less than 1 percent to as much as 5 percent. Highest rates are reported in patients with known psychiatric conditions who take hallucinogens and the lowest from carefully screened, healthy volunteers after experimental administration in research or treatment settings. Repeated use of hallucinogens, particularly at high doses, may be associated with the development of subsequent persistent psychotic disorders. Whether prolonged psychotic episodes occur only in predisposed individuals with underlying psychiatric disease or genetic vulnerability is unknown.

Differential Diagnosis French psychiatrist and early psychopharmacologist J. J. Moreau wrote in 1845 that some natural substances "by their brain effects produce a well defined mental illness, usually transitory but sometimes lengthy or even permanent." His statement about sums up the state of knowledge today. Hallucinogen-induced psychotic disorders with phenomenology and a clinical course indistinguishable from non–drug-induced psychotic disorders are relatively uncommon but do occasionally occur. Hallucinogens seemingly trigger a prolonged psychotic reaction in some individuals persisting weeks after the drug is used and in rare instances indefinitely. Over the past 50 years, there has been a shift in thinking whereby hallucinogens initially believed to mimic or model psychotic disorders (psychotomimetics) are now considered capable of producing psychotic disorders or at least promoting a recurrence in individuals who have had previous psychotic episodes (psychotogenic). Hallucinogens administered to psychiatric patients under controlled conditions clearly intensify or rekindle psychotic states.

When hallucinogen use became widespread in the late 1960s, they (usually LSD or cannabis) sometimes seemed to trigger long-lasting psychotic states often difficult to distinguish clinically from non–drug-related psychoses other than by the history of recent hallucinogen exposure. Such patients were often considered to be "latent schizophrenics." In fact, the most experienced LSD researchers in those early days cautioned against the experimental or therapeutic administration of LSD to individuals with a strong family history of schizophrenia because of concerns over inducing persistent psychotic states.

Patients with persistent psychoses after hallucinogen use tend to be younger with more positive and fewer negative symptoms. The relative contribution genetic vulnerability in determining hallucinogen-related psychoses remains uncertain. Epidemiological data from psychiatric hospital admission records strongly suggest that hallucinogen exposure created new cases of schizophreniform psychoses and related disorders when hallucinogen use became widespread. However, mechanisms remain uncertain. Hallucinogen use may be causing a psychosis that would in any case develop later to become evident at a younger age. Or a psychotic disorder previously unrecognized becomes evident after hallucinogens are used.

Clearly, hallucinogenic drug use is a significant risk factor for relapse in a person who has previously had a psychotic disorder. However, when administered under medical supervision, the risks of LSD and other hallucinogens appear to be relatively small. Psychotic reactions lasting more than 48 hours occurred in only 1.8 per 1,000 subjects given LSD for therapeutic reasons. When carefully screened individuals, whether healthy volunteers or patients seeking treatment, are medically screened, informed, and supervised while given reasonable doses of pure drug, adverse events both during intoxication and after are uncommon. However, when hallucinogens are used under less controlled conditions, there appears potential for serious and persistent problems.

Treatment Most important is consideration of preexisting disorders such as schizophrenia and bipolar disorders. Treatment of a persistent psychoses after hallucinogen exposure is the same as treatment for other non–drug-related psychoses with a similar clinical picture. Because many patients who present with hallucinogen-induced psychotic disorders exhibit more positive symptoms, they benefit from supportive, educational, and family therapies along with pharmacotherapy.

Hallucinogen Intoxication Delirium Although listed as an option in DSM-IV-TR, this is an uncommon disorder beginning during the acute intoxication after ingestion of hallucinogens. Because, by definition, hallucinogens are drugs that do not commonly produce a delirium, the concomitant use of other drugs or extremely high doses of hallucinogens usually is necessary to account for this condition.

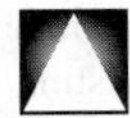

Table 11.7–6
DSM-IV-TR Diagnostic Criteria for Hallucinogen-Related Disorder Not Otherwise Specified

The hallucinogen-related disorder not otherwise specified category is for disorders associated with the use of hallucinogens that are not classifiable as hallucinogen dependence, hallucinogen abuse, hallucinogen intoxication, hallucinogen persisting perception disorder, hallucinogen intoxication delirium, hallucinogen-induced psychotic disorder, hallucinogen-induced mood disorder, or hallucinogen-induced anxiety disorder.

From American Psychiatric Association. *Diagnostic and Statistical Manual of Mental Disorders.* 4th ed. Text rev. Washington, DC: American Psychiatric Association; 2000, with permission.

Hallucinogen-Related Disorder Not Otherwise Specified Long-term lasting changes in personality appear to be a consequence of repeated and, possibly, of single exposures, although the relationships between drug effects and preexisting personality are not clear (Table 11.7–6).

Concerns first arose over adverse persistent neuropsychological toxicity from hallucinogen use in the late 1960s. Neuropsychological test performance by hallucinogen users with a history of repeated exposure on measures of memory function, problem solving, and abstract thinking reveals modest impairment at best. However, all published research has enough methodological problems so that questions of whether hallucinogens cause lasting neuropsychological change remain unanswered until larger samples of well-characterized chronic hallucinogen users are properly studied. Organic brain damage, as well as permanent changes in personality, attitude, or creativity, in people who have repeatedly used hallucinogenic drugs points to small and generally behaviorally nonsignificant changes. However, because of the typically small samples assessed in neuropsychological studies, the possibility of missing a true residual, lingering hallucinogen effect, be it adverse or beneficial, cannot be excluded.

SUGGESTED CROSS-REFERENCES

Reference to Section 11.3 on amphetamine-related disorders and to the neural sciences in Chapter 1 and neuropsychiatry and behavioral neurology in Chapter 2 may be useful. A more general discussion of substance abuse disorders (intoxication, abuse, dependence, and persisting disorders) is in Section 11.1. Section 12.8 discusses differences in presentation and course between schizophrenia and hallucinogen-related behaviors, and the phenomenology of other psychotic disorders is considered in Section 12.16. Sections 11.5 and 11.11 discuss cannabinoid- and PCP-related hallucinogenic states, respectively. MDMA psychopharmacology is discussed in Section 11.3.

REFERENCES

Abraham HD, Aldridge AM, Gogia P: The psychopharmacology of hallucinogens. *Neuropsychopharmacology.* 1996;14:285.

*Abraham HD, McCann UD, Ricaurte GA. Psychedelic drugs. In: Davis K, Charney D, Coyle J, Nemeroff C, eds. *Neuropsychopharmacology, the Fifth Generation of Progress.* New York: Lippincott Williams & Wilkins; 2002.

Aghajanian GK, Marek GJ: Serotonin and hallucinogens. *Neuropsychopharmacology.* 1999;21:16S.

Alper KR: Ibogaine: A review. *Alkaloids Chem Biol.* 2001;56:1.

Anthony JC, Warner LA, Kessler RC: Comparative epidemiology of dependence on tobacco, alcohol, controlled substances, and inhalants: Basic findings from the National Comorbidity Survey. *Exp Clin Psychopharmacology.* 1994;2:244.

Blaho K, Merigian K, Winbery S, Geraci SA, Smartt C: Clinical pharmacology of lysergic acid diethylamide: case reports and review of the treatment of intoxication. *Am J Ther.* 1997;4:211.

Boutros NN, Bowers MB Jr: Chronic substance-induced psychotic disorders: State of the literature. *J Neuropsychiatry Clin Neurosci.* 1996;8:262.

Bowers MB Jr: Psychoses precipitated by psychotomimetic drugs. A follow-up study. *Arch Gen Psychiatry.* 1977;34:832.

Bowers MB Jr, Imirowicz R, Druss B, Mazure CM: Autonomous psychosis following psychotogenic substance abuse. *Biol Psychiatry.* 1995;37:136.

*Freedman DX: The psychopharmacology of hallucinogenic agents. *Annu Rev Med.* 1969;20:409.

Glennon RA: Do classical hallucinogens act as 5-HT2 agonists or antagonists? *Neuropsychopharmacology.* 1990;3:509.

Halpern JH, Pope HG Jr: Do hallucinogens cause residual neuropsychological toxicity? *Drug Alcohol Depend.* 1999;53:247.

Halpern JH, Pope HG Jr: Hallucinogens on the Internet: A vast new source of underground drug information. *Am J Psychiatry.* 2001;158:481.

*Halpern JH, Pope HG Jr: Hallucinogen persisting perception disorder: what do we know after 50 years? *Drug Alcohol Depend.* 2003;69:109.

Hofmann A. *LSD: My problem child.* New York: McGraw Hill; 1980.

*Hofmann A. History of the discovery of LSD. In: Pletscher A, Ladewig D, eds. *Fifty Years of LSD: Current Status and Perspectives of Hallucinogens.* Pearl River, NY: Parthenon Publishing Group; 1994.

Hollister LE. *Chemical Psychoses: LSD and Related Drugs.* Springfield, IL: Thomas; 1968.

Hurlbut KM: Drug-induced psychoses. *Emerg Med Clin North Am.* 1991;9:31.

Johnston LD, O'Malley PM, Bachman JG. *Monitoring the Future National Results on Adolescent Drug Use: Overview of Key Findings, 2001.* Bethesda, MD: National Institute on Drug Abuse; 2002.

Kulig K: LSD. *Emerg Med Clin North Am.* 1990;8:551.

Lerner AG, Gelkopf M, Skladman I, Oyffe I, Finkel B, Sigal M, Weizman A: Flashback and hallucinogen persisting perception disorder: Clinical aspects and pharmacological treatment approach. *Isr J Psychiatry Relat Sci.* 2002;39:92.

Lewin L. *Phantastica: A Classic Survey on the Use and Abuse of Mind-Altering Plants.* Reprint of 1924 original ed. Rochester, VT: Park Street Press; 1998.

McKenna DJ: Plant hallucinogens: Springboards for psychotherapeutic drug discovery. *Behav Brain Res.* 1996;73:109.

McLellan AT, Woody GE, O'Brien CP: Development of psychiatric illness in drug abusers. Possible role of drug preference. *N Engl J Med.* 1979;301:1310.

Office of Applied Studies. *Results from the 2001 National Household Survey on Drug Abuse: Volume 1. Summary of National Findings.* National Household Survey on Drug Abuse Series H-17, DHHS publ. No. SMA 02-3758. Rockville, MD: Substance Abuse and Mental Health Services Administration; 2002.

Schwartz RH: LSD. Its rise, fall, and renewed popularity among high school students. *Pediatr Clin North Am.* 1995;42:403.

Sheffler DJ, Roth BL, Salvinorin A: The "magic mint" hallucinogen finds a molecular target in the kappa opioid receptor. *Trends Pharmacol Sci.* 2003;24:107.

Shulgin A. Basic pharmacology and effects. In: Laing R, ed. *Hallucinogens: A Forensic Handbook.* London: Academic Press; 2003.

Shulgin A, Shulgin A. *Pihkal, A Chemical Love Story.* Berkeley, CA: Transform Press; 1991.

Shulgin A, Shulgin A. *Tihkal: The Continuation.* Berkeley, CA: Transform Press; 1997.

Spoerke DG, Hall AH: Plants and mushrooms of abuse. *Emerg Med Clin North Am.* 1990;8:579.

Strassman RJ: Adverse reactions to psychedelic drugs. A review of the literature. *J Nerv Ment Dis.* 1984;172:577.

Strassman RJ: Hallucinogenic drugs in psychiatric research and treatment. Perspectives and prospects. *J Nerv Ment Dis.* 1995;183:127.

*Ungerleider JP, Pechnick RM. Hallucinogens. In: Galanter M, Kleber HD, eds. *The American Psychiatric Press, Textbook of Substance Abuse Treatment.* Washington, DC: American Psychiatric Press; 1994.

Vollenweider FX, Geyer MA: A systems model of altered consciousness: Integrating natural and drug-induced psychoses. *Brain Res Bull.* 2001;56:495.

▲ 11.8 Inhalant-Related Disorders

THOMAS J. CROWLEY, M.D., AND JOSEPH SAKAI, M.D.

Inhalant drugs (also called *inhalants* or *volatile substances*) are volatile hydrocarbons such as toluene, *n*-hexane, methyl butyl ketone, trichloroethylene, trichloroethane, dichloromethane, gasoline, and butane. These chemicals are sold in four commercial classes: (1) solvents for glues and adhesives; (2) propellants for aerosol paint sprays, hair sprays, frying pan sprays, and shaving cream; (3) thinners (e.g., for paint products and typing correction fluids); and (4) fuels. At room temperature, these compounds volatilize to gaseous fumes that can be inhaled through the nose or mouth, entering the bloodstream by the transpulmonary route. Despite their chemical differences, it is generally believed, although not proved, that these compounds share certain pharmacological properties.

Inhalant drugs are widely available and frequently misused, especially by adolescents. Approximately 18 percent of U.S. eighth-grade students report that they have used these substances for psychoactive effects, more than the number who have tried marijuana at that age. Most adolescents who try inhalants apparently discontinue them after one or a few times. However, for a smaller group of adolescents, especially those with comorbid conduct disorder, inhalant use may foreshadow many years of polysubstance abuse or dependence, including drug injections. Most of those people eventually shift to other drugs, although some continue daily use of inhalants themselves for many years, with major behavioral and organ pathology from the drugs' chronic toxicity. A still smaller number of adolescents die from acute inhalant toxicity, often during their first use of the drugs. Indeed, in the United Kingdom, where detailed records are available, inhalants have been a leading cause of adolescent death because, although such deaths are infrequent, adolescent deaths generally are uncommon.

DEFINITION

The section on inhalant-related disorders in the revised fourth edition of the *Diagnostic and Statistical Manual of Mental Disorders* (DSM-IV-TR) "includes disorders induced by inhaling the aliphatic and aromatic hydrocarbons . . . less commonly used are halogenated hydrocarbons . . . and other volatile compounds containing esters, ketones, and glycols." DSM-IV-TR provides two broad categories of inhalant-related disorders (Table 11.8–1). The first category is inhal-

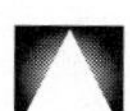

Table 11.8–1
DSM-IV-TR Inhalant-Related Disorders

Inhalant use disorders
Inhalant dependence
Inhalant abuse
Inhalant-induced disorders
Inhalant intoxication
Inhalant intoxication delirium
Inhalant-induced persisting dementia
Inhalant-induced psychotic disorder with delusions
  Specify if:
    With onset during intoxication
Inhalant-induced psychotic disorder with hallucinations
  Specify if:
    With onset during intoxication
Inhalant-induced mood disorder
  Specify if:
    With onset during intoxication
Inhalant-induced anxiety disorder
  Specify if:
    With onset during intoxication
Inhalant-related disorder not otherwise specified

From American Psychiatric Association. *Diagnostic and Statistical Manual of Mental Disorders.* 4th ed. Text rev. Washington, DC: American Psychiatric Association; 2000, with permission.

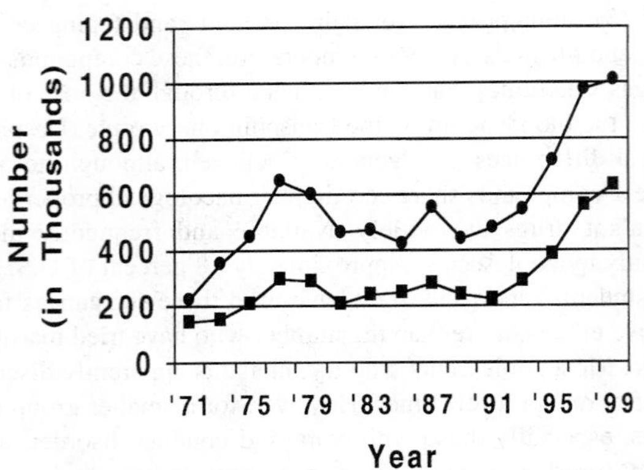

FIGURE 11.8–1 Estimated annual number of Americans beginning use of inhalants by year (odd-numbered years, 1971 to 1999). Upper line, all ages combined. Lower line, 12 to 17 years of age. (Drawn by the authors from data in Summary of Findings from the 2000 National Household Survey on Drug Abuse, NHSDA Series H-13, DHHS Publication No. [SMA] 01-3549. Substance Abuse and Mental Health Services Administration, Office of Applied Studies. Rockville, MD; 2001.)

ant use disorders (inhalant abuse and inhalant dependence), which are characterized by maladaptive patterns of inhalant use (e.g., frequency, dose, danger). The second category, inhalant-induced disorders (such as inhalant intoxication), results from the toxic effects of inhaled substances. Because of epidemiological and pharmacological differences, DSM-IV-TR excludes from the inhalant-related disorders conditions related either to anesthetic gases or to amyl and butyl nitrites, classifying these as other (or unknown) substance-related disorders; some disorders associated with those compounds are briefly discussed at the end of this chapter. Although fumes of such combustible drugs as crack cocaine and tobacco also are inhaled, DSM-IV-TR similarly places disorders related to those drugs in separate categories.

COMPARATIVE NOSOLOGY

The section on inhalant-related disorders in DSM-IV-TR lists three major categories: inhalant abuse, inhalant dependence, and inhalant intoxication. The other inhalant-related disorders have their diagnostic criteria specified in the DSM-IV-TR sections that specifically address the major symptoms. For example, inhalant-induced psychotic disorder is included with other psychotic disorders.

The tenth revision of the *International Statistical Classification of Diseases and Related Health Problems* (ICD-10) refers to inhalants as "volatile substances." ICD-10 does not use the term "abuse," which is in DSM-IV-TR, offering instead the term "harmful use." DSM-IV-TR provides no diagnosis of inhalant withdrawal (which clinicians describe but which probably is rare), whereas ICD-10 includes that diagnosis but gives no diagnostic criteria. In a study of inhalant users, the prevalence of inhalant dependence was approximately equal whether diagnoses were made by DSM-IV-TR or ICD-10 criteria, but many more users received ICD-10 harmful-use diagnoses than DSM-IV-TR abuse diagnoses.

EPIDEMIOLOGY

The impact on public health from a class of abused drugs may be indicated by the prevalence of each of these: use of the drugs, DSM-IV-TR abuse or dependence on the drugs, visits to hospital emergency departments or admissions to drug treatment programs for problems from the drugs, and deaths associated with the drugs.

Prevalence of Inhalant Use The U.S. government conducts or supports two large annual surveys of drug use. One addresses people living in American households, and the other assesses school students in the eighth, tenth, and 12th grades. Because of differences in samples and interview methods, the school survey often shows higher prevalence rates among adolescents than does the household survey, although the two usually agree well on trends over time and in their rankings of different drugs' prevalence of use.

In the latter 1990s, the household survey showed a large increase in first-time users of inhalants, and children 12 to 17 years of age contributed heavily to that increase (Fig. 11.8–1). Adolescents were most likely to start using inhalants between 14 and 16 years of age, with boys and girls being at approximately equal risk. Among American adolescents, non-Hispanic whites were most likely to try these drugs.

Figure 11.8–2, comparing year 2000 data on inhalants and marijuana from the household survey, shows "lifetime" prevalence (the proportion of respondents reporting even one episode of use) and "past month" prevalence (proportion reporting use of the drug in the previous month). Figure 11.8–2 shows that among 12- and 13-year-olds, 6.8 percent reported at least some use of inhalants, a rate higher

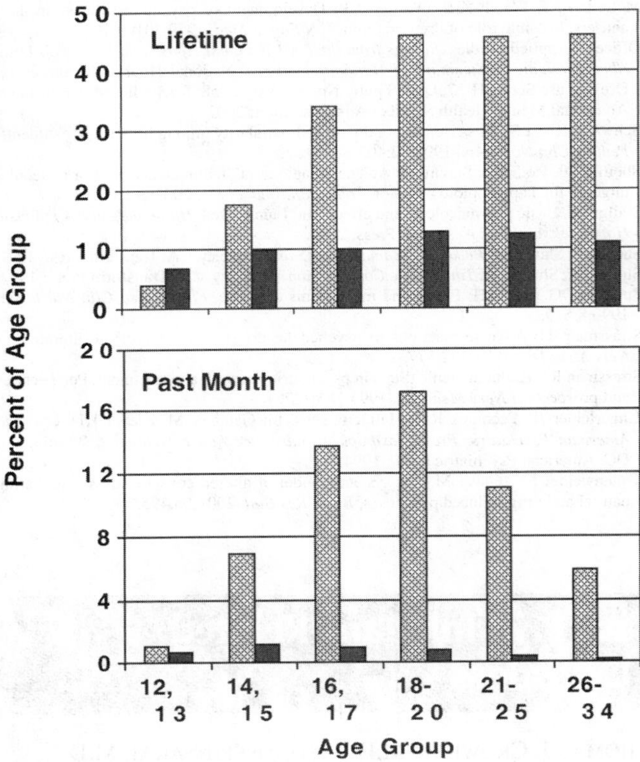

FIGURE 11.8–2 Reported use of inhalants (*solid bars*) or marijuana (*cross-hatched bars*). *Upper panel*: lifetime prevalence of any use ever reported by various age groups for the year 2000 in the National Household Survey on Drug Abuse. *Lower panel*: prevalence of reported use in the month preceding the survey. (Drawn by the authors from data in Summary of Findings from the 2000 National Household Survey on Drug Abuse, NHSDA Series H-13, DHHS Publication No. [SMA] 01-3549. Substance Abuse and Mental Health Services Administration, Office of Applied Studies. Rockville, MD; 2001.)

(at that age) than that for marijuana or any other drug addressed in the household survey. (Indeed, another American survey showed that approximately 6 percent of *fourth-grade* students had tried inhalants at least once.) The lifetime exposure rate increased to 13 percent among those 18 to 20 years of age. However, *past month* prevalence for inhalants peaked at just 1.2 percent in the 14- and 15-year-old group and declined among older groups.

Obviously, if most people who try a drug continue using it frequently, the past month prevalence rate should approach the lifetime rate, and that does not happen with inhalants. Indeed, of American adolescents who reported using inhalants once, only approximately one-half reported using more than twice, and only approximately one-third reported using more than five times. By comparison, both lifetime and past month rates for marijuana (Fig. 11.8–2) increased steadily to much higher levels than inhalants, peaking in the 18- to 20-year-old group. The government's student survey generally replicates these patterns, although prevalence rates tend to be higher in the student survey.

Prevalence of Inhalant Abuse and Dependence

Some hold that any use of substances by youngsters is "substance abuse." However, prevalence of *use* (Figs. 11.8–1 and 11.8–2) should not be confused with prevalence of DSM-IV-TR–defined *abuse.* For example, each DSM-IV-TR abuse criterion requires "recurrent" or "continued" substance use, so one-time users cannot receive that diagnosis. On the other hand, recurrent substance use in situations in which it is physically hazardous does qualify as abuse in DSM-IV-TR. Because inhalant intoxication is unpredictably and sometimes fatally toxic, any recurrent use may qualify as abuse by that criterion.

One survey of approximately 8,000 randomly sampled Americans (15 to 54 years of age) found that approximately 7 percent reported some use of inhalants but that only 0.3 percent had become dependent on the substances. Thus, only approximately 4 percent of those who had tried inhalants developed dependence on them. By comparison, almost one-third of those who had tried tobacco developed dependence on it.

Data from the authors' Center indicates that, of some 3,500 adolescents drawn from the general population of Colorado, less than 1 percent reported using inhalants more than five times. In a structured interview, only four of the subjects met DSM-IV-TR criteria for inhalant abuse, and none for inhalant dependence.

Prevalence of Inhalant-Related Emergency Department Visits

Each year, the U.S. government monitors drug-related visits to emergency departments in numerous hospitals around the country. Of some 625,000 drug-related visits to those departments in the year 2000, only approximately 1,500 (0.24 percent) were considered to involve inhalants.

Prevalence of Inhalant-Related Treatment Admissions

The U.S. government collected data on approximately 130,000 adolescent admissions to U.S. substance treatment programs during 1999. Less than 2 percent were associated with inhalant problems, and inhalants were the substances primarily contributing to the admission in only 0.4 percent of cases. More than one-half of the inhalant cases also involved alcohol and marijuana.

The authors' program has completed detailed diagnostic assessments on almost 800 adolescent patients referred for serious substance problems, usually by juvenile justice and social service agencies. Most of these patients also have comorbid conduct problems, a risk factor for inhalant involvement. Nevertheless, only 8 percent of these patients reported trying inhalants more than five times. Only 2 percent of them qualified (in structured research interviews) for DSM-IV-TR diagnoses of inhalant abuse, and another 1 percent had diagnoses of inhalant dependence. Most inhalant-dependent patients in this program also were dependent on alcohol and marijuana.

Prevalence of Inhalant Deaths

Inhalants apparently make only a small contribution to America's drug mortality. The U.S. government monitors drug death data from medical examiners' or coroners' offices in many cities. Of almost 12,000 deaths annually certified as drug induced or drug related in those areas, inhalants were involved in 1.1 percent (129 cases) in 1999, and in 0.34 percent (just 40 cases) in 2000. In 1999, approximately two-thirds of inhalant cases also involved other substances. Approximately three-fourths of inhalant deaths were among males. Racial and ethnic distributions were approximately 60 percent white, 23 percent black, 10 percent Hispanic, and 8 percent other. Seven percent of the deaths were of children 6 to 17 years of age, 12 percent were 18 to 25 years of age, and deaths were approximately equally distributed across all older age groups. By contrast, in a series collected between 1971 and 1987 in the United Kingdom, youths 15 to 19 years of age comprised more than one-half of inhalant deaths.

In summary, it appears that trying inhalants at least once is fairly common (approximately 15 percent of people by late adolescence). Many children or early adolescents (approximately 7 percent of 12- to 13-year-olds) do try inhalants, and the incidence is increasing. However, continued frequent inhalant use is rather uncommon, and the prevalence of at least monthly use decreases as youths age. Accordingly, the very limited available data suggest that inhalant abuse and dependence are rather rare in the general population. This appears to be true even among adolescents, who are more likely to use these substances. Reflecting that low prevalence in the general population, inhalant problems are the primary contributors to less than 1 in 200 adolescent admissions to substance treatment programs. Furthermore, among people of all ages visiting hospital emergency departments for drug-related problems, only approximately one-fourth of 1 percent have inhalant problems. Finally, inhalants contribute to only approximately 1 percent (or less) of American drug deaths, and other substances also are involved in most of those inhalant-related deaths.

American data show widespread experimentation with inhalants, relatively few current users, and very few inhalant emergencies or deaths, suggesting that most users try the drugs a few times and stop without mishap. Most of these users probably will not develop further drug problems, but nevertheless, the odds of such problems are much greater for them than for those who never used inhalants. For example, in a general population survey, people reporting any use of inhalants were 45 times more likely and those who had used both inhalants and cannabis were 89 times more likely than others to have injected drugs; injection, in turn, is a risk factor for infection with human immunodeficiency virus (HIV) and hepatitis C. Similarly, a prospective study of inner-city youths found that those who had used inhalants in adolescence were nine times more likely to use heroin later.

The available data suggest that most adolescents who survive a brief experimentation with inhalants and who do not have conduct disorder soon abstain from inhalants and avoid pathological outcomes. However, among adolescents with conduct disorder, perhaps one-half develop adult antisocial personality disorder. Inhalant problems in these youths often herald serious alcohol and polysubstance use in adulthood, and a few of these youths become chronic, deteriorated, inhalant-dependent adults.

The prevalence of inhalant problems in small, isolated groups or communities may deviate from larger national trends. For example, certain American Indian communities experience a high prevalence of these problems, with reported lifetime rates as high as 34 percent by eighth grade. However, a recent report on more than 1,000 adolescents from *multiple* American Indian communities found a lifetime prevalence of use (16 percent) comparable to that of the general population. Another recent study, reporting on 11,698 American Indian participants sampled from 1988 to 1997, has found a decline in lifetime inhalant use and a steady decline in the prevalence of monthly inhalant users. The authors suggest that strong prevention and educational efforts undertaken in many American Indian communities may be responsible for this change.

In some countries, many children live on the street in loose-knit juvenile gangs with little or no attachment to relatives. Among such children, inhalant use is very common, with prevalence rates reportedly exceeding 70 percent in some cities.

PHARMACOLOGY AND TOXICOLOGY

According to the household survey, the inhalants most used by American adolescents are (in descending order) gasoline, glue (which usually contains toluene), spray paint, solvents, cleaning fluids, and assorted other aerosols. Sniffing vapor through the nose or huffing (taking deep breaths) through the mouth leads to transpulmonary absorption with very rapid drug access to the brain. Breathing through a solvent-soaked cloth, inhaling fumes from a glue-containing bag, huffing vapor sprayed into a plastic bag, or breathing vapor from a gasoline can are common. Approximately 15 to 20 breaths of 1 percent gasoline vapor produce several hours of intoxication. Inhaled toluene concentrations from a glue-containing bag may reach 10,000 ppm, and vapors from several tubes of glue may be inhaled each day. By comparison, one study of just 100 ppm of toluene showed that a 6-hour exposure produced a temporary neuropsychological performance decrement of approximately 10 percent.

Toluene concentrations in blood in hospitalized intoxicated people reportedly range from 0.8 to 8.0 μg/g. Exposure at the industrial maximum of 100 ppm produces blood levels of approximately 0.5 μg/g, although moderate exercise may triple these levels through increased respiration. Brain and fat achieve higher concentrations than blood because lipophilic compounds preferentially distribute there. One positron emission tomography (PET) study in nonhuman primates has shown rapid uptake and clearance of radiolabeled toluene in specific brain regions, such as the striatum and frontal cortex. The coadministration of alcohol dramatically raises toluene concentration in blood, increasing toxicity probably through competition for hepatic metabolizing enzymes.

Approximately 20 percent of a toluene dose is excreted unchanged in the breath, but most is metabolized in the liver to hippuric acid before urinary excretion. Breath concentrations of toluene decrease by one-half within a few minutes after the end of a prolonged exposure. Blood concentrations fall more slowly, becoming undetectable 4 to 10 hours after exposure. Urinary hippuric acid remains measurable somewhat longer; hippurate to creatinine ratios greater than 1 g/g suggest toluene use, but benzoic acid food preservatives may generate false-positive hippuric acid concentrations. Hippuric acid may be formed more slowly, and thus be more persistently detectable in urine, in some Asians who have a genetically determined variant of aldehyde dehydrogenase, an enzyme involved in toluene's metabolism. Methylene chloride, which is found in products such as degreasers and paint strippers, is metabolized to carbon monoxide; use can result in carbon monoxide poisoning.

In Australia, where gasoline has contained tetraethyl lead, there is a strong correlation between length of time sniffing gasoline and blood lead levels. Some evidence suggests that lead makes an important and long-persisting contribution to the neurocognitive impairment of Australian gasoline inhalers. In remote Australian aboriginal communities, replacing leaded with unleaded gasoline reportedly did not stop users from sniffing, but it did eliminate psychotic emergencies among those sniffers. Conversely, other such communities replaced standard leaded gasoline with aviation gasoline, high in tetraethyl lead. By rapidly producing severe headaches and abdominal cramps in sniffers, this step effectively eliminated gasoline sniffing in those communities.

The cellular mechanisms of inhalant action are unclear. Hypotheses include cell membrane fluidization, interactions at γ-aminobutyric acid (GABA)–gated chloride channels, and agonism of 5-hydroxytryptamine type 3A (5-HT_{3A}) receptors, but data are very sparse. In animal studies, toluene exposure activates mesolimbic dopamine neurons. Behavioral actions in animals suggest that inhalants act like alcohol, barbiturates, and other depressants of the central nervous system (CNS). Like depressants, they produce motor stimulation at lower doses and motor suppression at higher doses as well as ataxia and loss of righting reflex. Inhalant-induced motor stimulation is attenuated by lesions of the nucleus accumbens. Inhalants also have anticonvulsant actions and show depressant-like effects in certain behavioral paradigms. Animals work to self-administer inhalants, and animals trained to press one lever when injected with alcohol or pentobarbital and another when injected with saline press the depressant-appropriate lever after exposure to toluene vapor, suggesting that the subjective experience after toluene or a depressant is similar. Moreover, test animals prefer to be in places in which they previously had been exposed to solvents. Finally, alcohol and benzodiazepines are known to potentiate inhalant effects.

Rodents develop withdrawal seizures after several days' exposure to trichloroethane, a frequently abused inhalant. The seizures are blocked by toluene, ethanol, pentobarbital, and midazolam (Versed), a benzodiazepine. Thus, inhalants can produce physical dependence, and they show cross-dependence with familiar CNS depressants.

In human subjects, low-dose (0, 75, or 150 ppm) toluene exposures for several hours produce dose-related decrements in tests of perception, memory, and manual dexterity, with increased headaches, mucosal irritation, thirst, and sleepiness.

Organ Pathology

Inhalants are associated with many potentially serious adverse effects. The most serious of these is death, which can result from respiratory depression, cardiac arrhythmias, asphyxiation, aspiration of vomitus, or accident or injury (e.g., driving while intoxicated with inhalants). Placing an inhalant-soaked rag and one's head into a plastic bag, a common procedure, may cause coma and suffocation.

Chronic inhalant users may have numerous neurological problems. Computed tomography (CT) and magnetic resonance imaging (MRI) reveal diffuse cerebral, cerebellar, and brainstem atrophy with white matter disease, a leukoencephalopathy. Single photon CT of former solvent-abusing adolescents showed both increases and decreases of blood flow in different cerebral areas. Several studies of house painters and factory workers who have been exposed to solvents for long periods also have found evidence of brain atrophy on CT scans, with decreased cerebral blood flow.

Neurological and behavioral signs and symptoms may include hearing loss, peripheral neuropathy, headache, paresthesias, cerebellar signs, persisting motor impairment, parkinsonism, apathy, poor concentration, memory loss, visual-spatial dysfunction, impaired processing of linguistic material, and lead encephalopathy. White matter changes, or pontine atrophy on MRI, have been associated with worse intelligence quotient (IQ) test results. The combination of organic solvents with high concentrations of copper, zinc, and heavy metals has been associated with the development of brain atrophy, temporal lobe epilepsy, decreased IQ, and a variety of electroencephalographic (EEG) changes.

Other serious adverse effects associated with long-term inhalant use include irreversible hepatic disease or renal damage (tubular acidosis) and permanent muscle damage associated with rhabdomyolysis. Additional adverse effects include cardiovascular and pulmonary symptoms (e.g., chest pain and bronchospasm) as well as gastrointestinal (GI) symptoms (e.g., pain, nausea, vomiting, and hematemesis). There are several clinical reports of toluene embryopathy, with signs like those of fetal alcohol syndrome. These include low birth weight, microcephaly, shortened palpebral fissures, small face, low-set ears, and other dysmorphic signs. These babies reportedly develop slowly, show hyperactivity, and have cerebellar dysfunction. Fortunately, there is no convincing evidence that toluene, the best-studied inhalant, produces genetic damage in somatic cells.

ETIOLOGY

Multiple factors contribute to the etiology of inhalant-related disorders. First, availability is important in determining the prevalence of abuse or dependence on a drug. Inhalants are cheap, available in several forms in most households, easily concealed, legal to possess, and simple to take. Second, inhalant use apparently is rewarding, both through direct pharmacological action and through the drugs' social effects. As mentioned, under certain circumstances, animals repeatedly self-administer inhalants, showing that these substances have innate reinforcing properties. In addition, adolescents usually gather in small groups to use inhalants, and being a user gains entry to the group, socially reinforcing the use. Third, inhalant users often can evade detection or punishment by parents or school authorities because the drugs quickly produce a high that passes within a few hours. Fourth, inexpensive inhalants may be one of the few exciting and novel experiences available to youths in impoverished communities providing few other reinforcers. This may help to explain the high prevalence of inhalant use on some American Indian reservations.

In addition to those extrinsic factors, at least one intrinsic factor contributes to inhalant problems. A risk-taking propensity may lead some people to the at-the-brink excitement and danger of inhalant intoxication. People with adolescent conduct disorder or adult antisocial personality disorder are prone to taking extreme risks, and many inhalant users have those disorders. Several studies suggest an association of inhalant use and conduct problems. Among youths in grades 7 through 12, inhalant users (compared with others who used no drugs or who used only cannabis or alcohol) had many characteristics suggesting conduct disorder. They accepted cheating more readily, admitted to more stealing, perceived less objection to drug use from their families, liked school less, and reported more sadness, tension, anger, and a feeling of being blamed by others. In addition, school surveys showed that solvent users were more likely to be involved with other drugs. Similarly, among youths referred to court-mandated education for minor alcohol offenses, those who also had used inhalants reported fewer school honors and more expulsions, truancy, academic failures, criminal offenses, running away, and associations with troubled peers as well as many more drug and alcohol problems. More of them also had mothers or siblings with alcohol- or drug-related problems. Some families are burdened by antisocial personality disorder and substance dependence in the adults and by conduct disorder and substance use disorders (often including inhalant abuse or dependence) in the adolescent children, and there is growing evidence that genetics play a role in these familial disorders.

Finally, two studies suggest that, even more than other drug users, inhalant users report childhood abuse or neglect.

A 14-year-old white boy was referred for inhalant problems to the authors' adolescent day-treatment substance program. The patient's mother said his biological father had abused alcohol, and the patient said that his mother had been a "speed addict." The parents divorced when the patient was 5 years of age. The patient was jailed for fighting at 12 years of age but said his mother "didn't really care." He began smoking marijuana and "huffing" spray paint two to five times per week at 13 years of age "because I was depressed"; again, he said his mother did not much care because she also was smoking marijuana then. When his mother was arrested for distributing controlled substances, he was placed in long-term residential treatment because he was considering shooting her. In that program, he briefly was treated with sertraline (Zoloft), but he "cheeked" and hoarded the pills, which were discontinued; he was said to appear less depressed without the medication. Then he was referred to the authors' program. He reported that, from 3 years of age, his biological father and a series of mother's boyfriends demeaned and ridiculed him, and his mother ignored him because of her continuing intoxications and depressions. From 4 years of age, his mother and her boyfriends, often intoxicated, struck him with belts, extension cords, paddles, fists, and sticks, and they threw shoes, spatulas, and boards at him, causing welts, bleeding, and even unconsciousness. From 5 years of age, they did not encourage school attendance, enforce household rules, or keep him clean. Between 8 and 12 years of age, he often was left alone and hungry. At 9 years of age, he first received child protective services because of abuse. He reported that when he was 11 years of age his mother purposely burned him once, leaving a scar. On structured interviews at admission, he qualified for DSM-IV-TR diagnoses of dependence on inhalants and tobacco as well as abuse of alcohol and cannabis. He also met diagnostic criteria for conduct disorder, generalized anxiety disorder, and major depression (with a very high depression rating score and several past suicide attempts). A formal aggression rating was quite high and included his report of having started more than 100 fires, often producing minor property damage. The patient received group and individual therapy and attended the program's on-site school. A psychiatrist evaluated his depression but could not obtain parental consent to use antidepressants. Family therapy continued with a previous therapist, but considerable conflict persisted between the mother and a current boyfriend. The patient reported during treatment that his mother smoked marijuana in front of him, teasing him because if he smoked it, the staff would know through urine testing. During treatment, the youth reported one episode of alcohol drinking, and frequent urine monitoring revealed amphetamines once and marijuana once. Frequent inhalant monitoring (breath samples or urinary hippuric acid) was too expensive for this publicly funded treatment program. Day treatment continued for approximately 9 months, with only modest progress. It appeared that the patient did not want treatment to end. At a follow-up attempt 4 weeks after discharge, the home phone had been disconnected.

This case highlights several important points about inhalant dependence: an association with conduct disorder and child abuse and neglect; adolescent onset; an association with abuse or dependence on other substances; family problems complicating treatment; and the impracticality of frequent biological monitoring for inhalant relapse.

INHALANT DEPENDENCE AND INHALANT ABUSE

Diagnosis and Clinical Features A diagnosis of inhalant abuse or inhalant dependence should be considered in people showing intermittent changes compatible with substance intoxication, together with an odor of organic solvents, inhalation paraphernalia, or the occasionally present perioral or perinasal papular glue-sniffers' rash. The cardinal feature of inhalant abuse is repeated use of inhalants in ways that produce a physical hazard or adverse social consequences for the user. Inhalant dependence is characterized by repeated use resulting in some combination of adverse consequences, loss of control of the drug use, and tolerance or withdrawal. Although DSM-IV-TR provides no diagnosis for inhalant withdrawal, 17 percent of inhalant users in DSM-IV's substance field trial complained of withdrawal symptoms after inhalant use. Thus, despite the absence of a separate inhalant withdrawal diagnosis, patients' complaints of withdrawal symptoms probably should be counted toward a diagnosis of inhalant dependence. ICD-10 uses the category of volatile substance dependence syndrome for inhalant dependence. ICD-10 does not include the diagnostic category of inhalant abuse, offering instead the category of harmful use of volatile substances, which is defined as a pattern of use causing damage to health.

Differential Diagnosis Three conditions should be considered. First, most adolescents who experiment with inhalants stop spontaneously after one or a few episodes of use, never meeting criteria for diagnoses of inhalant abuse or inhalant dependence. Although such use is dangerous and occasionally fatal (most often on the first try), the many spontaneous resolutions support recommendations of minimalist, nonalarmist interventions for adolescent users who do not meet criteria for diagnoses of inhalant use disorders; parents also should be involved. Firm advice to remain abstinent, coupled with education of parents on recognizing future problems, may be sufficient.

Second, polysubstance use is common in adolescent patients, and abuse or dependence on drugs other than inhalants is established through history, physical findings, and toxicological screens. Such disorders may exist in addition to, or instead of, inhalant abuse or dependence.

Third, uncontrolled and impulsive behavior during repeated inhalant intoxications may mimic aspects of, or be comorbid with, conduct disorder or antisocial personality disorder. Antisocial behavior before the onset of inhalant abuse or dependence, or in periods of abstinence, suggests the presence of these disorders.

Course and Prognosis The relatively high prevalence of inhalant use in high school surveys, and its relatively low prevalence in adulthood, led one expert to state that inhalant use "should be regarded as a passing phase or fad." However, although most inhalant users probably do not progress to serious adult disorders, the risk of such progression is much greater for those who have used inhalants than for those who have not. Studies indicate that inhalant use is associated with increased risk for future diagnoses of antisocial personality disorder and other substance use disorders. Among adult substance-dependent patients, a history of inhalant use indicated a significantly enhanced risk for antisocial personality disorder, social phobia, polysubstance use, and injection drug use. Among a group of adult heroin addicts, those who had been inhalant users appeared to be a "marginal group with particularly unfavorable developmental conditions and a specific course of addiction."

Most adolescents who progress from inhalant use to inhalant abuse or dependence eventually shift to other drugs, but some continue active inhalant dependence into adulthood. Such chronic patients may use the drugs for extended periods each day for many years; they demonstrate moderate criminal activity, weight loss, medical disease, slow and slurred speech, impaired attention and memory, and often are both dirty and louse ridden.

Tolerance occurs and, less commonly, mild withdrawal involving sleep disturbance, irritability, shakiness, sweating, fleeting illusions, and nausea. One observer reported tachycardia, delusions, and hallucinations during withdrawal.

Medical problems in chronic users may include (1) muscle weakness, sometimes with myoglobinuria and rhabdomyolysis; (2) GI problems, such as pain, nausea, vomiting, or hematemesis; (3) renal dysfunction, often with severe electrolyte imbalance; (4) cardiomyopathy; (5) hepatotoxicity; (6) pulmonary disorders (pulmonary hypertension, increased airway resistance, and acute respiratory distress); and (7) hematopoietic disorders (including elevated carboxyhemoglobin levels, methemoglobinemia, hemolytic anemia, aplastic anemia, and even acute myelocytic leukemia). Neurological problems include (1) headache, (2) paresthesias with peripheral neuropathy, (3) cerebellar degeneration or reversible cerebellar signs, (4) radiological abnormalities of widened sulci and basal cisterns, and (5) dementia (e.g., lead encephalopathy from leaded gasoline or white matter dementia from toluene).

Researchers have examined individual patients or small series of mothers who regularly used toluene during pregnancy. The studies, although they need large-scale replication, strongly suggest that such inhalant use, often with accompanying distal renal tubular acidosis in the mother, has devastating effects. Mothers may experience nausea, vomiting, abdominal pain, elevated blood pressure, and early contractions. Preterm delivery is common, and even after correction for gestational age, the infants show intrauterine growth retardation. Growth retardation continues postnatally. Dysmorphic facies, similar to those of the fetal alcohol syndrome, may occur. Perinatal infant deaths are not infrequent. The management of pregnancy in women with inhalant abuse or inhalant dependence should aim at abstinence with attention to the early detection of renal tubular acidosis, preterm labor, and fetal growth retardation.

Treatment No controlled studies guide the treatment of adults or adolescents who meet criteria for inhalant abuse or inhalant dependence. Obviously, appropriate medical care is required for the disorders' medical sequelae. In addition, vigorous treatment is needed for adolescent patients who progress from experimentation to inhalant abuse or dependence. Most of these youths have comorbid conduct disorder and are at serious risk for adverse outcomes.

Some experts assert that inhalant-dependent patients should be treated in specialized clinics, although there are no data supporting this assertion. One authority recommends that a comprehensive treatment plan include eight aspects: detoxification; a peer advocate system; assessment of physical, cognitive, and neurological deficits; building on existing strengths; developing new strengths; therapists trained in solvent abuse; attention to personal and family issues; and assistance in returning back to the community.

The author and his colleagues provide day treatment and nonhospital residential programs for adolescents 13 to 19 years of age with combined substance dependence and conduct disorder. However, treatment for these polysubstance-dependent delinquent youths is not specific by drug category (e.g., inhalants) but instead targets substance use and conduct problems generally. Most referrals are from social service and juvenile justice agencies, which pay for the treatment. Currently suicidal youths and those with recent fire setting are excluded, although many patients have past histories of these problems, together with considerable violence and gang involvement.

Treatment in these programs begins with detailed interviews addressing use and establishing diagnoses of abuse or dependence for each drug category in DSM-IV-TR. Most patients meet criteria for dependence on several substances. Interviews also address diagnoses of disorders commonly comorbid in this group: conduct disorder, attention-deficit/hyperactivity disorder (ADHD), major depressive disorder, dysthymic disorder, and posttraumatic stress disorder (PTSD). Interviews also address experiences of abuse or neglect, which are very common in these patients. Group and individual therapy is behaviorally oriented, with immediate rewards for progress toward objectively defined goals in treatment and punishments for lapses to previous behaviors. Patients attend on-site schools with special education teachers, together with planned recreational activities. The programs provide birth control consultations with Planned Parenthood. The patients' families, often very chaotic, are engaged in modifications of structural family therapy or multisystemic therapy, both of which have good empirical support. Participation in 12-step programs is required. Treatment interventions are coordinated closely with interventions by community social workers and probation officers. No medications are prescribed for inhalant abuse or dependence per se, but a child and adolescent psychiatrist often prescribes antidepressants for depression, disulfiram (Antabuse) for comorbid alcohol dependence, or bupropion (Wellbutrin) or atomoxetine (Strattera) for ADHD (stimulant medications are avoided in substance-dependent youths). Progress is monitored with urine and breath samples analyzed for alcohol and other drugs at intake and frequently during treatment. However, frequent monitoring of breath for inhalants, or of urine for hippuric acid, is too expensive for most public treatment programs. Patients who do not abstain in day treatment may transfer to residential care. Treatment usually lasts 3 to 12 months. Termination is considered successful if the youth has practiced a plan to stay abstinent; is showing fewer antisocial behaviors; has a plan to continue any needed psychiatric treatment (such as treatment for comorbid depression); has a plan to live in a supportive, drug-free environment; is interacting with the family in a more productive way; is working or attending school; and is associating with drug-free, nondelinquent peers. In many cases, of course, these goals are only partially accomplished. As with all other recommended treatments for inhalant abuse or dependence, controlled studies of long-term outcomes are lacking.

Laboratory Examinations Therapy for substance use disorders often uses repeated tests of biological samples to validate patients' reports of abstinence or use. However, with inhalants, such tests may be difficult to interpret. First, these volatile compounds have a relatively brief sojourn in the body and may be detected in urine for only a few hours after use. Second, even if the compounds occur in urine, they may volatilize out of samples during transfer or storage. Third, although hippuric acid, a toluene metabolite, can be detected longer than toluene, hippuric acid also may be produced from foods, raising a question of false-positive findings. Fourth, inhalants may bind to, or pass through, the plastic of urine cups or breath collection bags, reducing concentrations and making the compounds undetectable. Thus, the most careful monitoring for inhalants involves frequent urine samples (e.g., two or three per week) at random times, collected in tightly sealed glass containers with little or no air space, and carefully refrigerated until analysis. Analyses for inhalants usually require gas chromatography, followed by flame ionization, electron capture, or mass spectroscopic procedures. Simultaneous analyses of the ratio of the more persistent hippuric acid to creatinine may reveal recent toluene use. However, even under ideal conditions, the short half-life of inhalants makes inhalant monitoring much less valuable clinically than monitoring for many other substances. Similarly, breath samples may be collected in specially designed glass traps or in Tedlar (not Mylar) bags. However, the half-life of inhalants in alveolar air apparently is a matter of minutes, and so breath samples may be useless for monitoring treatment progress in patients who show no current signs of intoxication. Moreover, the authors have examined costs in their region for monitoring tests as a proportion of the per patient per day reimbursement rates, which must cover *all* costs of intensive day treatment. Each urine test for hippuric acid uses more than one-half and each inhalant breath test approximately 20 percent of a day's reimbursement. Each also requires approximately 1 week to complete. Thus, frequent biological monitoring for inhalants is not very practical in public treatment programs.

INHALANT INTOXICATION

Diagnosis and Clinical Features Inhalant intoxication should be considered in people showing an acute onset of behavioral disturbance, coupled with the characteristic odor of organic solvents or the presence of inhalation paraphernalia. Inhalant intoxication is an inhalant-related, clinically significant maladaptive behavioral disorder that develops during or immediately after inhalant use and (assuming survival) clears a few hours later. Intoxication signs initially may include vomiting and motor stimulation, followed by slowing, ataxia, depressed reflexes, slurred speech, disorientation, impaired judgment, lethargy, or coma. Bronchospasm, chest pain, cardiac arrhythmias or arrest, trauma, accidental burns, seizures, aspiration of vomitus, or suffocation in a plastic bag may result. Users often show slowed speech, elated mood, fearfulness, illusions, auditory and visual hallucinations, delusions, and perceptions of altered body size. The DSM-IV-TR diagnostic criteria are listed in Table 11.8–2. ICD-10 provides a comparable diagnostic category of acute intoxication due to use of volatile substances.

Laboratory Examinations As noted above, random, intermittent monitoring of biological samples has modest value for confirming self-reported abstinence in currently nonintoxicated patients with inhalant abuse or dependence because inhalants are so briefly detectable in the body. However, patients showing behavioral signs of inhalant intoxication do, in most cases, have detectable concentrations of inhalants in urine and breath. Confirming their presence may have later clinical or forensic value. Urine samples should be collected in glass vessels with little or no air space, sealed tightly, and refrigerated until analysis for inhalants themselves and for the ratio of hippuric acid (a toluene metabolite) to creatinine. Alternatively, breath samples may be collected in specially designed glass traps or in Tedlar (not Mylar) bags, and they should be analyzed for inhalants within a few hours.

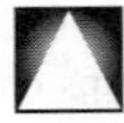

Table 11.8–2
DSM-IV-TR Diagnostic Criteria for Inhalant Intoxication

A. Recent intentional use or short-term, high-dose exposure to volatile inhalants (excluding anesthetic gases and short-acting vasodilators).
B. Clinically significant maladaptive behavioral or psychological changes (e.g., belligerence, assaultiveness, apathy, impaired judgment, impaired social or occupational functioning) that developed during, or shortly after, use of or exposure to volatile inhalants.
C. Two (or more) of the following signs, developing during, or shortly after, inhalant use or exposure:
  (1) Dizziness
  (2) Nystagmus
  (3) Incoordination
  (4) Slurred speech
  (5) Unsteady gait
  (6) Lethargy
  (7) Depressed reflexes
  (8) Psychomotor retardation
  (9) Tremor
  (10) Generalized muscle weakness
  (11) Blurred vision or diplopia
  (12) Stupor or coma
  (13) Euphoria
D. The symptoms are not due to a general medical condition and are not better accounted for by another mental disorder.

From American Psychiatric Association. *Diagnostic and Statistical Manual of Mental Disorders.* 4th ed. Text rev. Washington, DC: American Psychiatric Association; 2000, with permission.

Differential Diagnosis Differentiation from other intoxications is aided by a history of inhalant use, the presence of inhalant odor and residues on the skin or clothing, a characteristic perioral rash from contact with organic solvents, and toxicological examination of body fluids. Polysubstance use is common among solvent users, and concurrent intoxications with other drugs may be assessed by history and toxicological examinations. Despite evidence of inhalant intoxication, in comatose patients, other explanations (e.g., closed head injury) must be sought. Dextrose 50 percent for injection (50 g) and naloxone (Narcan), 2 mg intravenously (IV), help rule out coma of diabetic or narcotic origin. If delirium develops in the course of an intoxication with inhalants, the diagnosis is inhalant intoxication delirium rather than inhalant intoxication. If a mood disturbance, anxiety, or psychosis appears very prominently during an intoxication and if those symptoms are severe enough to warrant independent clinical attention, the diagnosis should be inhalant-induced mood disorder, inhalant-induced psychotic disorder, or inhalant-induced anxiety disorder, respectively.

Course and Prognosis The onset of intoxication is almost instantaneous after the inhalation of volatile hydrocarbons, given the rapid absorption of those inhalants across pulmonary membranes and their quick distribution into the brain and other lipids. Inhalant drugs are rapidly metabolized and excreted, and inhalant intoxication usually lasts a few hours or less. Unless trauma, hypoxia, cardiac arrest, burns, or other problems ensue, there probably are no lasting effects from one or a few intoxications except that each use of these reinforcing drugs may increase the probability of further use. Prolonged, repeated use causes persisting effects.

Treatment Inhalant intoxication, like alcohol intoxication, usually receives no medical attention and resolves spontaneously. However, effects of the intoxication, such as coma, bronchospasm, laryngospasm, cardiac arrhythmias, trauma, or burns, need treatment. Otherwise, care primarily involves reassurance, quiet support, and attention to vital signs and level of consciousness. Some evidence suggests that physical agitation during inhalant intoxication may precipitate cardiac arrhythmias or cardiac arrest, so the environment should be calming and reassuring. However, sedative drugs, including benzodiazepines, are contraindicated because they may potentiate inhalant effects. Because of the short half-life of inhalants, inhalant intoxication usually improves considerably after approximately 30 minutes of abstinence unless other drugs were also consumed. After resolution of the intoxication, a careful evaluation is needed, with appropriate intervention or referral for inhalant abuse or dependence, other substance use disorders, conduct disorder, or antisocial personality disorder.

INHALANT INTOXICATION DELIRIUM

DSM-IV-TR provides a diagnostic category for inhalant intoxication delirium, which is a disturbance of consciousness and a change in cognition that results from intoxication with inhalants and is not better explained by dementia. The course and treatment are like those of inhalant intoxication, but the additional confusion requires special attention to patient safety. If the delirium results in severe behavioral disturbances, short-term treatment with a dopamine receptor antagonist (for example, haloperidol [Haldol]) may be necessary. Benzodiazepines should be avoided because of the possibility of adding to the patient's respiratory depression. ICD-10 provides a comparable diagnostic category, "acute intoxication due to use of volatile substances, with delirium."

INHALANT-INDUCED PERSISTING DEMENTIA

Diagnosis and Clinical Features Studies of inhalant-caused cognitive impairment have been equivocal and have been beset by numerous methodological problems, including a focus on adolescent users with briefer lifetime exposures. But clinical and some research evidence suggests that some inhalant-using adults develop inhalant-induced persisting dementia. For example, among toluene users (average age, 29 years) studied with MRI, the neuropsychological deficits correlated strongly with the severity of cerebral white matter abnormalities, and those abnormalities appear to be caused by inhalants.

The cardinal feature of the disorder is dementia resulting from the use of inhalants. Nearly all of these people also meet the criteria for inhalant dependence. Patients with inhalant-induced persisting dementia have memory impairment and at least one of the following: aphasia (language disturbance), apraxia (impaired ability to carry out motor activities despite intact motor function), agnosia (inability to recognize or identify objects despite intact sensory function), and disturbed executive functioning (planning, organizing, sequencing, abstracting). The symptoms must significantly impair social or occupational functioning, represent a decrement from earlier functioning, not occur exclusively in the course of a delirium, and persist beyond the usual duration of inhalant intoxication. The ICD-10 category of dementia in other specified diseases classified elsewhere includes inhalant-induced persisting dementia.

Differential Diagnosis Nearly all of these patients have inhalant dependence and many are dependent on alcohol, which also produces dementia. Moreover, histories of head injury are very common among such patients. Thus, despite clear evidence of prolonged inhalant use, this disorder requires a full evaluation for the multiple causes of dementia.

Course and Prognosis

Few of these patients have been studied prospectively. Despite some reports of improvement when patients abstained from inhalants, it seems likely that most neuropsychological deficits that persist for days or weeks after intoxication continue or worsen. Moreover, as dementia progresses, patients may have less cognitive capacity to avoid relapses, complicating treatment, and each relapse may add to the accumulating cerebral toxicity.

Treatment

There is no established treatment for the cognitive and memory problems of inhalant-induced persisting dementia. Low-key street outreach and extensive social service support have been offered to severely deteriorated inhalant-dependent homeless adults. Patients may require extensive support within their families or in foster or domiciliary care.

INHALANT-INDUCED PSYCHOTIC DISORDER

The essential features of inhalant-induced psychotic disorder are prominent hallucinations or delusions judged to be due to the direct physiological effect of inhalant substances. Such psychotic symptoms sometimes develop during intoxication with inhalants, so this diagnosis applies to patients who meet criteria for inhalant intoxication but who also have psychotic symptoms in excess of those usually associated with inhalant intoxication. The psychotic symptoms must be severe enough to warrant independent clinical attention. This diagnosis is not made in the presence of inhalant intoxication delirium. The clinician can specify whether hallucinations or delusions predominate.

The course and treatment of inhalant-induced psychotic disorder are like those of inhalant intoxication. The disorder is brief, lasting a few hours to (at most) a very few weeks beyond the intoxication. Clinical evidence suggests that tetraethyl lead is a potent contributor to psychotic symptoms in countries still using leaded gasoline. Vigorous treatment of such life-threatening complications as respiratory or cardiac arrest, together with conservative management of the intoxication itself, is appropriate. Confusion, panic, and psychosis mandate special attention to patient safety. Severe agitation may require cautious control with haloperidol (5 mg/70 kg intramuscularly [IM], repeated once in 20 minutes if needed). Sedative drugs, including benzodiazepines, may potentiate and worsen inhalant intoxications.

In a randomized clinical trial, 40 hospitalized psychotic patients with revised third edition DSM (DSM-III-R) diagnoses of inhalant dependence and inhalant-induced organic mental disorder volunteered for treatment with either haloperidol (up to 40 mg per day orally) or carbamazepine (up to 1,600 mg per day orally) for up to 5 weeks. Both groups could have received intramuscular haloperidol for acute agitation. The antipsychotic response of the two groups was similar, but there were significantly fewer extrapyramidal reactions in the carbamazepine group. However, without a placebo control group, these data cannot establish that either medication was better (or worse) than no medication.

Despite similarities in name, DSM-IV-TR's inhalant-induced psychotic disorder differs from ICD-10's residual and late-onset psychotic disorder due to volatile substance use. The former is a variant of inhalant intoxication, whereas the latter is conceptualized as persisting long after direct psychoactive substance effects abate. Controversy continues as to whether inhalants produce persisting psychotic states in the absence of delirium or dementia. In ICD-10, acute intoxication due to use of volatile substances includes patients with marked psychotic symptoms arising in the course of the intoxication.

INHALANT-INDUCED MOOD DISORDER

The essential feature of inhalant-induced mood disorder is a prominent disturbance of mood judged to be due to the direct physiological effect of inhalant substances. Such mood symptoms sometimes develop during intoxication with inhalants, so this diagnosis applies to patients who meet criteria for inhalant intoxication but who also have mood symptoms in excess of those usually associated with inhalant intoxication. The mood symptoms must be severe enough to warrant independent clinical attention. The clinician can specify one of the following subtypes: with depressive features (probably the more common subtype), with manic features, or with mixed features. This diagnosis is not made in the presence of inhalant intoxication delirium. In ICD-10, acute intoxication due to use of volatile substances includes patients with marked affective symptoms arising in the course of the intoxication.

The course and treatment of inhalant-induced mood disorder are like those of inhalant intoxication. Inhalant-induced mood disorder is brief, lasting a few hours to (at most) a very few weeks beyond the intoxication. Although antidepressant or antimanic drugs are seldom appropriate for these relatively brief disorders, the risk of suicide requires a careful history and may require psychosocial treatment. Suicide has been implicated in approximately 40 percent of both inhalant-related medical examiners' death reports and inhalant-related visits to hospital emergency departments.

INHALANT-INDUCED ANXIETY DISORDER

The essential features of inhalant-induced anxiety disorder are prominent anxiety symptoms judged to be due to the direct physiological effect of inhalant substances. Such anxiety symptoms sometimes develop during intoxication with inhalants, so this diagnosis applies to patients who meet criteria for inhalant intoxication but who also have anxiety symptoms in excess of those usually associated with inhalant intoxication. The anxiety symptoms must be severe enough to warrant independent clinical attention. This diagnosis is not made in the presence of inhalant intoxication delirium. The clinician can specify one of the following subtypes: with generalized anxiety, with panic attacks, with obsessive-compulsive symptoms, or with phobic symptoms; generalized anxiety and panic attacks are probably most common. In ICD-10, acute intoxication due to use of volatile substances includes patients with marked anxiety symptoms arising in the course of the intoxication.

The course and treatment of inhalant-induced anxiety disorder are like those of inhalant intoxication. Sedative drugs, including benzodiazepines, are contraindicated because they worsen inhalant intoxication, which precipitates inhalant-induced anxiety disorder.

INHALANT-RELATED DISORDER NOT OTHERWISE SPECIFIED

The diagnosis of inhalant-related disorder not otherwise specified is reserved for inhalant-related disorders that do not fit into one of the above diagnostic categories (Table 11.8–3).

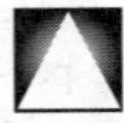

Table 11.8–3
DSM-IV-TR Diagnostic Criteria for Inhalant-Related Disorder Not Otherwise Specified

The inhalant-related disorder not otherwise specified category is for disorders associated with the use of inhalants that are not classifiable as inhalant dependence, inhalant abuse, inhalant intoxication, inhalant intoxication delirium, inhalant-induced persisting dementia, inhalant-induced psychotic disorder, inhalant-induced mood disorder, or inhalant-induced anxiety disorder.

From American Psychiatric Association. *Diagnostic and Statistical Manual of Mental Disorders.* 4th ed. Text rev. Washington, DC: American Psychiatric Association; 2000, with permission.

NITROUS OXIDE–RELATED DISORDERS

DSM-IV-TR includes nitrous oxide–related disorders among other substance-related disorders because of differences between nitrous oxide and other inhalants in modes of action and associated problems. Nitrous oxide was introduced for clinical practice in 1844 and is still a widely used inorganic gas anesthetic. It also is sold as a propellant in whipped-cream dispensers and in "whippets" for whipping cream. Not surprisingly, nitrous oxide misuse seems to appear most commonly among the health care and food service workers who use these preparations. The U.S. National Household survey estimated that, in the year 2000, two percent of 12- to 17-year-old Americans had inhaled "nitrous oxide or 'whippets'" at least once.

Nitrous oxide has a rapid onset and offset of action. It is mostly excreted in the breath with little or no biotransformation. Nitrous oxide reinforces self-administration behavior in animals. Although there is some evidence that nitrous oxide influences opioid systems, the subjective effects of the drug are not reduced by the opioid antagonist naloxone.

In studies of normal subjects without substance use disorders, some preferred inhaling nitrous oxide more than placebo, but others did not. In such studies, the drug produced feelings described as "drunk," "dreamy," "coasting or spaced out," and "pleasant bodily sensations," and those reporting more of these feelings were more likely to choose nitrous oxide over placebo.

Chronic use may produce diffuse polyneuropathy and myelinopathy with extensive, although sometimes reversible, neurological symptoms mimicking those of vitamin B_{12}–related pernicious anemia. Active vitamin B_{12} requires reduced cobalt, but nitrous oxide irreversibly oxidizes cobalt, suppressing the activity of an important enzyme, methionine synthase.

A 35-year-old male dentist with no history of other substance problems complained of problems with nitrous abuse for 10 years. This began as experimentation with what he had considered a harmless substance. However, his rate of use increased over several years, eventually becoming almost daily for months at a time. He felt a craving before sessions of use. Then, using the gas while alone in his office, he immediately felt numbness, a change in his temperature and heart rate, and an alleviation of depressed feelings. "Things would go through my mind. Time was erased." He sometimes fell asleep. Sessions might last a few minutes or up to 8 hours; they ended when the craving and euphoria ended. He had often tried to stop or cut down, sometimes consulting professionals about the problem.

Cases in the literature strongly suggest that nitrous oxide intoxication, dependence, and abuse do occur. Considering the drug's brief duration of action and users' intermittent inhalation patterns, nitrous oxide appears unlikely to produce clinically significant withdrawal. It is not clear, however, whether nitrous oxide produces other substance-related disorders. There are no clinically practical urine or breath tests for the presence of nitrous oxide. Misusers of the drug who develop neurological symptoms may have low serum concentrations of vitamin B_{12}, and remission of neurological symptoms has followed combined administration of B_{12} and folate, together with abstinence from nitrous oxide. In the absence of controlled studies of treatment for nitrous oxide use disorders, general principles for treating other substance use disorders should guide the treatment of these patients.

AMYL AND BUTYL NITRITE–RELATED DISORDERS

DSM-IV-TR includes amyl and butyl nitrite–related disorders among other substance-related disorders. The vapors of amyl nitrite, a volatile liquid, produce vasodilation and smooth muscle relaxation. Once supplied in easily "popped" glass vials, amyl nitrite found wide use as acute inhalation therapy for angina pectoris between 1867 and approximately 1980. Sublingual nitroglycerin tablets now have superseded that use. Amyl nitrite and its close relative, butyl nitrite, enjoyed a flurry of use as recreational drugs during the 1970s and 1980s. Reports from that time suggest that the use mainly was among adolescents, users of other drugs, and homosexual men. The latter group especially reported using the drugs to enhance orgasm, and these nitrites also were considered to produce a high, a feeling of wild abandon, or an altered state of consciousness. Nonmedical users called amyl nitrite vials *poppers*. Those vials' availability decreased with their declining medical use. Butyl nitrite and related compounds were then increasingly sold as "room odorizers" (but really for inhalation) under suggestive names such as Rush or Locker Room.

In one study of patients who had misused these drugs, most experienced dizziness, lightheadedness, cardiac palpitations, blurred vision, and a feeling of warmth immediately after the inhalation. Others complained of immediate headache, nasal burning, nausea, cough, dyspnea, or syncope. Nearly one-half found the experience not at all pleasant, and the others rated it only as "fair to good." Some experts believe that the drug does not have primary reinforcing effects mediated in the CNS but that certain pleasurable sensations associated with peripheral vasodilation lead to its continued use.

A few case reports document severe but nonfatal methemoglobinemia after nitrite inhalation by people genetically deficient in methemoglobin reductase. There also are reports of rapidly fatal methemoglobinemia after oral ingestion (not inhalation) of these compounds by genetically normal people. Some epidemiological studies further suggested that, among homosexual men, nitrite use might increase the risk of HIV infection or of developing Kaposi's sarcoma after HIV infection. However, those observations were heavily confounded because nitrite users tended to have more partners and to pursue unsafe sexual practices more frequently.

Considered together, the lack of a compelling instantaneous high, the immediate unpleasant feelings, and the longer-term risks from amyl and butyl nitrite seem to contribute to a rather low prevalence of use. Among Americans 12 to 17 years of age living in households, 1.7 percent said in the year 2000 that they ever had used "amyl nitrite, 'poppers', locker room odorizers, or 'Rush.'"

No studies have examined users of amyl or butyl nitrite with modern diagnostic procedures, and it is unknown how many (if any) meet criteria for intoxication, abuse, or dependence. Some people with sustained industrial exposures to nitrites experience withdrawal headaches on weekends or vacations, but it seems unlikely that intermittent, brief exposures to these short-acting drugs produce clinically significant withdrawal in recreational misusers of nitrites. There are no studies of the treatment of amyl or butyl nitrite–related disorders, and so such treatment should follow general principles for the treatment of other substance-related disorders.

SUGGESTED CROSS-REFERENCES

An overview of substance-related disorders is given in Section 11.1, hallucinogen-related disorders are discussed in Section 11.7, and phencyclidine (PCP)–related disorders are discussed in Section 11.11. Mood disorders are discussed in Chapter 13. Chapter 14 reviews anxiety disorders, and Section 12.16 covers psychotic disorders.

REFERENCES

Anthony JC, Warner LA, Kessler RC: Comparative epidemiology of dependence on tobacco, alcohol, controlled substances, and inhalants: Basic findings from the national comorbidity survey. *Exp Clin Psychopharmacol*. 1994;2:244.

*Balster RL: Neural basis of inhalant abuse. *Drug Alcohol Depend.* 1998;51:207.

Beauvais F, Wayman JC, Jumper-Thurman P, Plested B, Helm H: Inhalant abuse among American Indian, Mexican American, and non-Latino White adolescents. *Am J Drug Alcohol Abuse*. 2002;28:171.

Brouette T, Anton R: Clinical review of inhalants. *Am J Addict*. 2001;10:79.

*Cairney S, Maruff P, Burns C, Currie B: The neurobehavioral consequences of petrol (gasoline) sniffing. *Neurosci Biobehav Rev*. 2002;26:81.

*Fendrich M, Mackesy-Amiti ME, Wislar JS, Goldstein PJ: Childhood abuse and the use of inhalants: Differences by degree of use. *Am J Public Health*. 1997;87:765.

Gerasimov MR, Ferrieri RA, Schiffer WK, Logan J, Gatley SJ, Gifford AN, Alexoff DA, Marstellar DA, Shea C, Garza V, Carter P, King P, Ashby CR, Vitkun S, Dewey SL: Study of brain uptake and biodistribution of [^{11}C]toluene in non-human primates and mice. *Life Sci*. 2002;70:2811.

*Henggeler SW, Clingempeel WG, Brondino MJ, Pickrel SG: Four-year follow-up of multisystemic therapy with substance-abusing and substance-dependent juvenile offenders. *J Am Acad Child Adolesc Psychiatry*. 2002;41:868.

Hernandez-Avila CA, Orega-Soto HA, Jasso A, Hasfura-Buenaga CA, Kranzler HR: Treatment of inhalant-induced psychotic disorder with carbamazepine versus haloperidol. *Psychiatr Serv*. 1998;49:812.

Howard MO, Cottler LB, Compton WM, Ben-Abdallah A: Diagnostic concordance of DSM-III-R, DSM-IV, and ICD-10 inhalant use disorders. *Drug Alcohol Depend*. 2001;61:223.

Johnson EO, Schultz CG, Anthony JC, Ensminger ME: Inhalants to heroin: A prospective analysis from adolescence to adulthood. *Drug Alcohol Depend*. 1995;40:159.

Johnston LD, O'Malley PM, Bachman, JG. *Monitoring the Future, National Results on Adolescent Drug Abuse, Overview of Key Findings, 2000.* (NIH Publication No. 01-4923). Bethesda, MD: National Institute on Drug Abuse; 2001.

Johnston LD, O'Malley PM, Bachman, JG. *Monitoring the Future, National Survey Results on Drug Use, 1975–2000, Volume II College Students and Young Adults Ages 19–40.* (NIH Publication No. 01–4925). Bethesda, MD: National Institute on Drug Abuse; 2001.

Jones HE, Balster RL: Neurobehavioral consequences of intermittent prenatal exposure to high concentrations of toluene. *Neurotoxicol Teratol*. 1997;19:305.

Jumper-Thurman P, Beauvais F: Treatment of volatile solvent abusers. *Subst Use Misuse*. 1997;32:1883.

Kawamoto T, Koga M, Murata K, Matsuda S, Kodama Y: Effects of ALDH2, CYP1A1, and CYP2E1 genetic polymorphisms and smoking and drinking habits on toluene metabolism in humans. *Toxicol Appl Pharmacol*. 1995;133:295.

Kozel N, Sloboda Z, De La Rosa M: *Epidemiology of Inhalant Abuse: An International Perspective.* NIDA Research Monograph 148 (NIH Publication No. 95–3831). Rockville, MD: National Institute on Drug Abuse; 1995.

Lopreato GF, Phelan R, Borghese CM, Beckstead MJ, Mihic SJ: Inhaled drugs of abuse enhance serotonin-3 receptor function. *Drug Alcohol Depend*. 2003;70:11.

Lorenc JD: Inhalant abuse in the pediatric population: a persistent challenge. *Curr Opin Pediatr*. 2003;15:204.

Mackesy-Amity ME, Fendrich M: Inhalant use and delinquent behavior among adolescents: A comparison of inhalant users and other drug users. *Addiction*. 1999;94:555.

Maruff P, Burns CB, Tyler P, Currie BJ, Currie J: Neurological and cognitive abnormalities associated with chronic petrol sniffing. *Brain*. 1998;121:1903.

Neumark YD, Delva J, Anthony JC: The epidemiology of adolescent inhalant drug involvement. *Arch Pediatr Adolesc Med*. 1998;152:781.

Nicholas K, Zili S, De La Rosa M. *Research Monograph Series, Epidemiology of Inhalant Abuse: An International Perspective.* (NIH Publication No. 95–3831). Bethesda, MD: National Institute on Drug Abuse; 1995.

Novins DK, Beals J, Mitchell CM: Sequences of substance use among American Indian adolescents. *J Am Acad Child Adolesc Psychiatry*. 2001;40:1168.

Riegel AC, Ali SF, French ED: Toluene-induced locomotor activity is blocked by 6-hydroxydopamine lesions of the nucleus accumbens and the mGluR2/3 agonist LY379268. *Neuropsychopharmacology*. 2003;28:1440.

Riegel AC, French ED: Electrophysiological and behavioral studies in the rat. *Ann N Y Acad Sci*. 2002;965:281.

Rosenberg NL, Grigsby J, Dreisbach J, Busenbark D, Grigsby P: Neuropsychologic impairment and MRI abnormalities associated with chronic solvent abuse. *J Toxicol Clin Toxicol*. 2002;40:21.

*Sharp CW, Rosenberg NL. Inhalants. In: Lowinson JH, Ruiz P, Millman RB, Langrod JG, eds. *Substance Abuse: A Comprehensive Textbook.* 3rd ed. Baltimore: Williams and Wilkins; 1997.

Substance Abuse and Mental Health Services Administration, Office of Applied Studies. *Drug Abuse Warning Network Annual Medical Examiner Data 1999.* Rockville, MD; 2000.

Substance Abuse and Mental Health Services Administration, Office of Applied Studies. *Year-End 1999 Emergency Department Data from the Drug Abuse Warning Network.* DAWN Series D-20, DHHS Publication No. (SMA) 02–3634. Rockville, MD; 2000.

Substance Abuse and Mental Health Services Administration, Office of Applied Studies. Adolescent admissions involving inhalants. In: *The DASIS Report.* Rockville, MD; 2002.

Substance Abuse and Mental Health Services Administration, Office of Applied Studies. *Emergency Department Trends From the Drug Abuse Warning Network Preliminary Estimates January–June 2001 with Revised Estimates 1994–2000.* Rockville, MD; 2002.

Substance Abuse and Mental Health Services Administration, Office of Applied Studies. Inhalant use among youths. In: *The NHSDA Report.* Rockville, MD; 2002.

Substance Abuse and Mental Health Services Administration, Office of Applied Studies. *Mortality Data From the Drug Warning Network 2000.* DHHS Publication No. (SMA) 02–3633. Rockville, MD; 2002.

Walker DJ, Zacny JP: Within- and between-subject variability in the reinforcing and subjective effects of nitrous oxide in healthy volunteers. *Drug Alcohol Depend*. 2001;64:85.

Yamanouchi N, Okada S, Kodama K, Sakamoto T, Sekine H, Hirai S, Murakami A, Komatsu N, Sato T: Effects of MRI abnormalities on WAIS-R performance in solvent abusers. *Acta Neurol Scand*. 1997;96:34.

▲ 11.9 Nicotine-Related Disorders

JOHN R. HUGHES, M.D.

Although recent research and reviews have emphasized the commonalities between nicotine and other drug dependencies, nicotine dependence differs from other drug dependencies in several ways that have allowed nicotine dependence to become the most prevalent, most deadly, and most costly of the substance dependencies, and yet the most ignored. First, nicotine does not cause behavioral intoxication. As a result, nicotine-dependent persons rarely seek or are referred to psychiatrists.

Second, much of society's response to drug problems is based on how much damage drug-dependent users inflict on others. For most of its history, nicotine dependence was thought not to cause harm to others. Recently, society has recognized that nicotine dependence harms society via second-hand smoke deaths, financial costs of medical treatment, lost productivity, etc.; however, these costs are not dramatic, are quite distant, and thus are easily ignored.

Third, nicotine via tobacco is a legal drug openly promoted by several large transnational corporations. Thus, nicotine use appears legitimate, and deviant behaviors are not needed to acquire the drug. As a result, tobacco use is prevalent in persons with no psychiatric or psychological problems.

Fourth, because most of those who have stopped nicotine use have done so without treatment, a common view is that, unlike alcohol or illicit drug abusers, most smokers do not need treatment. In reality, currently, 75 percent of those who stop nicotine, alcohol, or illicit drugs do so without treatment. However, the population of smokers is changing. Today, in the developed countries, those who continue to smoke despite the large social sanctions appear to be those who are severely nicotine dependent or who have significant psychiatric problems that interfere with cessation; thus, the need for treatment will likely increase over time. Fifth, owing to the factors outlined previously, unlike alcohol and illicit drugs, few health care plans and government programs have been willing to adequately reimburse for treatment of smoking cessation.

All of these factors have discouraged psychiatrists from playing a larger role in treating nicotine dependence. Several recent events may reverse this reluctance: the growing recognition that most psychiatric patients smoke and many die from nicotine dependence; the apparently increasing dependence of remaining smokers, suggesting that many need more intensive treatments; the development of many pharmacological agents to aid smokers in stopping; and the increase in reimbursement for smoking cessation by health care plans and state health departments.

DEFINITION

Nicotine dependence and withdrawal are the two defined nicotine-related disorders in the revised fourth edition of the *Diagnostic and Statistical Manual of Mental Disorders* (DSM-IV-TR). The essential feature of any substance dependence disorder in DSM-IV-TR is that "the individual continues use of the substance despite significant substance-related problems." Because 50 percent of smokers die of a smoking-related illness, this definition clearly is applicable to nicotine use. The essential feature of withdrawal is "a substance-specific maladaptive behavioral change . . . that is due to the cessation of, or reduction in, heavy and prolonged substance use." Because nicotine withdrawal produces an observable, well-defined, time-limited syndrome in more than one-half of smokers, this definition also appears appropriate.

Nicotine abuse is not included in DSM-IV-TR, because abuse is confined to significant psychosocial problems but not physical problems, and the former is rare with nicotine use. The tenth edition of the *International Statistical Classification of Diseases and Related Health Problems* (ICD-10) includes *harmful use*, a category that is similar to abuse but that includes continued use that causes physical problems; thus, harmful use from the nicotine-containing products often occurs. Nicotine intoxication is rare. Nicotine-induced mood and other disorders are not included in DSM-IV-TR, because, although some smokers appear to have an increased incidence of depression and other psychiatric disorders after cessation, these are not thought to be nicotine-induced organic disorders but rather are thought to be due to loss of a therapeutic effect of nicotine.

HISTORY AND COMPARATIVE NOSOLOGY

Tobacco use in the New World dates back to at least 600 AD and was introduced into European culture in the 16th century. Early on, most tobacco use was via pipes, smokeless tobacco, or cigars. The cigarette became popular beginning in the early 1900s with the invention of the cigarette-making machine and the match and the use of acidifying agents to permit nicotine to enter the lower respiratory tract, where it could be rapidly absorbed into the arterial circulation. Cigarette use grew dramatically in the first half of the 20th century. The first reports of the association of smoking and disease began in the 1950s and culminated with the 1964 *Surgeon General's Report on Smoking and Health.* Use in the United States did not decline significantly until the 1970s and 1980s owing to tobacco control activities and taxation. In the 1990s and 2000s, tobacco use in the United States stabilized.

Although tobacco use in many Western nations has declined, use in developing countries is substantially increasing, in part due to relaxed marketing practices. Recent attempts by the U.S. Food and Drug Administration (FDA) and the World Health Organization to regulate and to discourage tobacco use have been only partially successful.

Nicotine dependence was widely accepted but not codified until the 1980 third edition of the DSM (DSM-III) and the ninth edition of the ICD (ICD-9) included tobacco dependence and withdrawal as disorders. The 1988 U.S. Surgeon General's *The Health Consequences of Smoking—Nicotine Addiction* comprehensively reviewed the evidence and concluded that smoking was a form of substance dependence.

EPIDEMIOLOGY

In 2002, 21 percent of Americans smoked, 24 percent were former smokers, and 55 percent never smoked cigarettes. The prevalence of pipe, cigar, smokeless tobacco, and nicotine medication use is less than 2 percent. The prevalence of smoking in the United States decreased approximately 1 percent per year between the early 1960s and the late 1980s, but it has not declined since the 1990s because of no change in initiation and cessation.

Worldwide, in the early 1990s, the prevalence of smoking in men was 47 percent, and, in women, the prevalence was 11 percent. This gender difference is large in less developed countries and small in developed countries. The prevalence of smoking has remained stable in developed countries but has significantly increased in the less developed countries since then.

The mean age of onset of smoking in the United States is 16 years of age, and few persons start after 20 years of age. How quickly dependence features appear is debatable.

In the United States, more than 75 percent of smokers have tried to quit, and approximately 50 percent try to quit each year. On a given quit attempt, only 30 percent remain abstinent for even 2 days, and only 5 to 10 percent stop permanently. However, most smokers make five to ten attempts, such that, eventually, one-half of smokers quit. In the past, 90 percent of quit attempts among U.S. smokers involved no treatment. However, with the advent of over-the-counter (OTC) nicotine medications and prescription nonnicotine medications, approximately one-third of all quits are now accompanied by medication use. The use of telephone counseling and psychotherapy is minimal.

In terms of the diagnosis of nicotine dependence per se, approximately 20 percent of people in the United States develop nicotine dependence at some point in their life, making it the most prevalent psychiatric disorder. Approximately 85 percent of current adult daily smokers are nicotine dependent. Nicotine withdrawal occurs in approximately 50 percent of smokers who try to quit.

Smoking is now as common in American women as it is in men. Smoking is more prevalent in those with lower education and income and in many, but not all, ethnic groups and is especially high in psychiatric patients (50 percent), including those with other substance use disorders (80 percent).

ETIOLOGY

Nicotine and acetylcholine bind to nicotinic-cholinergic receptors. Originally, these receptors were thought to be confined to the ganglia and neuromuscular junction but have now been found in several areas of the central nervous system (CNS). The two types of these ion-gated receptors that appear to be involved in nicotine dependence are the $\alpha 4/\beta 2$ and $\alpha 7$ subtypes. These receptors are unusual in that they quickly desensitize. This phenomenon, plus the fact that repeated use of nicotine increases, not decreases, the number of receptors, suggests that nicotine may actually act as much as an antagonist as an agonist at this receptor.

The dependence-producing effects of nicotine appear to be modulated by dopamine and glutamate release due to nicotinic receptors on dopamine cells in the ventral tegmental area and the shell of the nucleus accumbens. Nicotine also increases norepinephrine, epinephrine, and serotonin, and these increases may modulate some of the reinforcing effects from cigarettes.

Nicotine via cigarettes is rapidly absorbed directly into the arterial circulation and reaches the CNS in less than 15 seconds. Peak behavioral and cardiovascular effects occur within a few minutes. Nicotine is metabolized via the liver and has a half-life of 2 hours. Nicotine levels from smoking typically rise in the morning, plateau in the evening, and fall to near zero in the night. This pattern causes an acute tolerance, such that the first cigarettes of the day are more potent than later cigarettes.

Nicotine use, like most substance use, begins because of social reinforcement. However, with repeated exposure, many young users find the pharmacological effects of nicotine well suited to help them with the demands of adolescence. In addition, a physical dependence on nicotine usually begins within a few years, so that periods of nonuse become uncomfortable.

Nicotine dependence is due to nicotine's multiple pharmacological effects and the cigarette delivery device. Unlike many drugs of dependence, nicotine can produce several effects. For example, it can improve performance on long, fatiguing, boring tasks, decrease anger, stabilize mood, and decrease hunger. When a smoker experiences these effects, it is typically not clear how much of the effect is from nicotine combating withdrawal and bringing the smoker back to normal and how much is actual improvement above the norm. Some of nicotine's effects (e.g., performance enhancement) may occur independently of withdrawal relief. Whatever the source, these effects would appear especially helpful in adolescence, when coping skills are less than optimal.

Ironically, nicotine's lack of a typical effect of drugs of abuse—that is, intoxication—may also contribute to nicotine dependence. Lack of intoxication allows the smoker to imbibe large amounts of nicotine on a daily basis without producing a behavioral interference in daily activities, which, in turn, increases the chance of physical or psychological dependence.

The ideal reinforcer is one that occurs rapidly, frequently, and consistently, with minimal effort, and is unlikely to be punished. Nicotine via cigarettes has all these attributes. Smoking is the most rapid method to deliver a drug to the brain. It is also one of the most, if not the most, frequently reinforced behaviors. Taking 10 puffs per cigarette × 20 cigarettes per day × 365 days per year × 20 years results in millions of drug self-administrations. Because cigarettes are manufactured, they deliver precise doses of drug. Because cigarettes are legal, widely available, and inexpensive, they can be obtained with few social skills or resources. Being legal, punishment for smoking only occurs from social approbation. This combination of multiple drug effects, lack of intoxication, and method of delivery makes nicotine use often highly dependence producing.

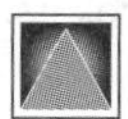

Table 11.9–1
Percent of Variation Attributable to Genetic Sources in Cigarette Smoking and Alcohol Consumption

	Genetic Variance (%)		
Substance	**Common to Both Substances**	**Substance-Specific**	**Total**
Tobacco	36	20	56
Alcohol	17	32	49

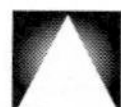

Table 11.9–2
DSM-IV-TR Nicotine-Related Disorders

Nicotine use disorder
Nicotine dependence
Nicotine-induced disorder
Nicotine withdrawal
Nicotine-related disorder not otherwise specified

From American Psychiatric Association. *Diagnostic and Statistical Manual of Mental Disorders.* 4th ed. Text rev. Washington, DC: American Psychiatric Association; 2000, with permission.

Children who are more likely to start smoking are those who have a high need to conform, low academic performance, rebelliousness, depressive symptoms, and poor self-esteem. Peer and family influences are paramount. Attention-deficit, conduct, and alcohol or drug use disorders increase the risk of initiation and maintenance of smoking.

Although not widely known, initiation and cessation of tobacco use are as heritable as alcohol dependence or abuse. Some of the genetic effects are shared with alcohol, and some are specific to tobacco (Table 11.9–1). The biological and behavioral mechanisms for genetic effects on tobacco use are not known.

DIAGNOSIS AND CLINICAL FEATURES

Table 11.9–2 lists the DSM-IV-TR nicotine-related disorders. Most of the generic criteria for substance dependence readily apply to nicotine; for example, tolerance, a withdrawal syndrome, use to avoid withdrawal, inability to stop despite repeated attempts, and continued use despite knowing that use is harmful (Table 11.9–3). Because nicotine is legal and easily available, other criteria—for example, spending a great deal of time to procure the drug and giving up activities to use the drug—are rare.

Nicotine withdrawal (Table 11.9–4) is manifested by changes in mood, insomnia, difficulty concentrating, restlessness, decreased

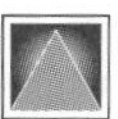

Table 11.9–3
Examples of DSM-IV-TR Nicotine Dependence Criteria

Criteria	Examples
Tolerance.	Absence of nausea, dizziness.
Withdrawal.	See Table 11.9–4.
The substance is often taken in larger amounts or over a longer period than was intended.	Most smokers do not intend to smoke 5 years later, but more than 70% continue to use.
Persistent desire or unsuccessful effort to stop.	5–10% of self-quitters are successful on each attempt; 50% of smokers have not been able to stop despite repeated attempts.
A great deal of time is spent to obtain, to use, or to recover from the drug.	Leaving work site to smoke.
Important activities are given up or reduced because of substance use.	Not taking a job because of smoking restrictions.
Use continues despite knowledge of problem caused by substance.	Many smokers have heart disease, chronic obstructive pulmonary disease, or cancer and continue to smoke.

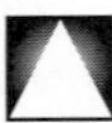

Table 11.9–4
DSM-IV-TR Diagnostic Criteria for Nicotine Withdrawal

A. Daily use of nicotine for at least several weeks.
B. Abrupt cessation of nicotine use, or reduction in the amount of nicotine used, followed within 24 hours by at least four of the following signs:
 (1) Dysphoric or depressed mood
 (2) Insomnia
 (3) Irritability, frustration, or anger
 (4) Anxiety
 (5) Difficulty concentrating
 (6) Restlessness
 (7) Decreased heart rate
 (8) Increased appetite or weight gain
C. The symptoms in Criterion B cause clinically significant distress or impairment in social, occupational, or other important areas of functioning.
D. The symptoms are not due to a general medical condition and are not better accounted for by another mental disorder.

From American Psychiatric Association. *Diagnostic and Statistical Manual of Mental Disorders.* 4th ed. Text rev. Washington, DC: American Psychiatric Association; 2000, with permission.

heart rate (average decline is eight beats per minute), and weight gain (average is 2 to 3 kg). The insomnia appears to be specific to increased awakenings and intense dreaming. Postcessation weight gain is due to increased eating and the loss of nicotine stimulation of metabolism. Craving is common, and increased coughing and decreased performance on vigilance tasks can occur. The syndrome is typically most severe with abstinence from cigarettes, intermediate with abstinence from smokeless tobacco, and least severe with abstinence from nicotine replacement products. Most withdrawal symptoms peak at 1 to 3 days and last 3 to 4 weeks; however, 40 percent of smokers have withdrawal that lasts for more than 4 weeks. In addition, craving and weight gain often persist for 6 months or more.

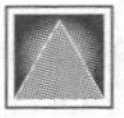

Table 11.9–5
Effect of Abstinence from Smoking on Blood Concentrations of Psychiatric Medicines

Abstinence increases blood concentrations
Clomipramine (Anafranil)
Clozapine (Clozaril)
Desipramine (Norpramin)
Doxepin (Sinequan)
Fluvoxamine (Luvox)
Haloperidol (Haldol)
Imipramine (Surmontil)
Nortriptyline (Aventyl)
Oxazepam (Serax)
Propranolol (Inderal)
Abstinence does not increase blood concentrations
Amitriptyline (Elavil)
Chlordiazepoxide (Librium)
Ethanol
Lorazepam (Ativan)
Midazolam (Versed)
Triazolam (Halcion)
Effects of abstinence are unclear
Alprazolam (Xanax)
Chlorpromazine (Thorazine)
Diazepam (Diastat)

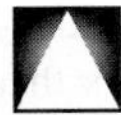

Table 11.9–6
DSM-IV-TR Diagnostic Criteria for Nicotine-Related Disorder Not Otherwise Specified

The nicotine-related disorder not otherwise specified category is for disorders associated with the use of nicotine that are not classifiable as nicotine dependence or nicotine withdrawal.

From American Psychiatric Association. *Diagnostic and Statistical Manual of Mental Disorders.* 4th ed. Text rev. Washington, DC: American Psychiatric Association; 2000, with permission.

Abstinence can also have pharmacokinetic effects. Nonnicotine chemicals in tobacco smoke activate cytochrome P450 enzymes, thereby decreasing the levels of several medications (Table 11.9–5). As a result, smoking cessation increases the concentrations of these medications. Many of these medications are psychiatric medications, and often the increase can be clinically significant; for example, haloperidol (Haldol), clozapine (Clozaril), and fluvoxamine (Luvox) concentrations increase 30 to 40 percent with abstinence.

Smoking (particularly nicotine dependence) is two to three times more prevalent among patients with mood, substance use, and other psychiatric disorders. Conversely, these psychiatric disorders are two to three times more common among current smokers than among people who have never smoked or ex-smokers. There are several possible reasons for this association; for example, shared genetic influences on smoking and psychiatric disorders, improvement by nicotine of a psychiatric disorder, modeling other psychiatric patients, and boredom. Depressive symptoms predict the likelihood of starting to smoke, the probability of becoming dependent, and the inability to stop smoking. Tobacco smoke and smokeless tobacco contain substances other than nicotine that inhibit monoamine oxidase type A (MAO_A) and monoamine oxidase type B (MAO_B), which suggests that a nonnicotine substance in tobacco may be acting as a monoamine oxidase inhibitor (MAOI) to combat depression.

Psychiatric patients may have a special need for the anxiolytic, anorexic, antiaggression, antidepressant, and cognitive-enhancing effects of nicotine. Smokers with a current or past history of most psychiatric disorders have more withdrawal on cessation and a lower rate of smoking cessation.

DSM-IV-TR also includes a residual category of nicotine-related disorders not otherwise specified; for example, abstinence-induced remission of depression (Table 11.9–6).

DIFFERENTIAL DIAGNOSIS

Many of the symptoms of nicotine withdrawal can mimic, exacerbate, or mask the symptoms of psychiatric disorders or the adverse effects of psychiatric medications; for example, akathisia, anxiety, depression, irritability, insomnia, and weight gain. Cessation of smoking appears to be able to reinitiate depression, alcoholism, and, perhaps, other psychiatric disorders in a small subgroup of smokers.

COURSE AND PROGNOSIS

Currently, one-half of ever-smokers stop smoking; however, many of those who stop unfortunately do so having already developed a smoking-related disease. Twenty percent of all mortality in the United States is due to smoking. Approximately 45 percent of smokers die of a smoking-related disease, resulting in more than 410,000 deaths per year in the United States. Smoking is a huge risk for lung cancer and chronic obstructive pulmonary disease, accounting for more than 75 percent of all deaths from these disorders. Smoking doubles the risk for cardiovascular disease deaths, but, because this disease is more prevalent, it accounts for as many smoking deaths as cancer and lung disease. The third major cause of tobacco-related mortality is chronic obstructive lung disease. Other common smoking-related diseases include low-birth-weight offspring, perinatal complications, other cancers (e.g., throat, bladder, and pancreas), and ulcers. Second-hand smoke increases the risk of cancer and heart disease in spouses and the incidence of respiratory and ear problems in children.

The tar in cigarette smoke is responsible for the cancers. Irritants and ciliotoxins appear to be responsible for lung diseases. Carbon monoxide and clotting factors appear to be the most likely causes of cardiovascular disease. The role of nicotine in cardiovascular disease appears to be much smaller than previously thought, and how many perinatal problems (including sudden infant death syndrome) are caused by carbon monoxide or by nicotine is debatable. Smokeless tobacco, pipes, and cigars cause oral cancers, especially when accompanied by heavy alcohol use.

Cessation of smoking almost eliminates the risk of heart disease in 5 years and of lung cancer in 20 years; however, the benefits of cessation are highly dependent on duration of smoking. For example, cessation of smoking before 35 years of age reverses most of the risk of smoking. Recent reviews have concluded that switching to low-tar and low-nicotine cigarettes does not improve health, in part owing to compensatory increased smoking. Also, whether newer, so-called safer cigarettes or a reduction of the number of cigarettes per day improves health is unclear.

Nicotine intoxication causes abdominal pain, dizziness, headaches, nausea, pallor, palpitations, sweating, vomiting, and weakness. Intoxication is rare, and treatment is supportive.

Although not conclusive, epidemiological, biochemical, and clinical trial data suggest that nicotine may be beneficial for dementia of the Alzheimer's type, Parkinson's disease, Tourette's syndrome, and ulcerative colitis.

TREATMENT

Several Web sites and organizations offer information on smoking treatment, including free booklets (Table 11.9–7). The guidelines for the treatment of smoking published in 2000 by the U.S. Public Health Service (USPHS) and in 1996 by the American Psychiatric Association (APA) are excellent primers. Also, most state health departments have telephone lines to assist practitioners and smokers.

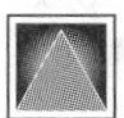

Table 11.9–7
Selected Databases of Information on Smoking Cessation Treatment and Stop Smoking Booklets

http://www.surgeongeneral.gov/tobacco	U.S. Public Health Service guidelines
http://www.treatobacco.net	World Health Organization guidelines
http://www.cancer.org	American Cancer Society
http://www.cdc.gov/tobacco	Centers for Disease Control
http://www.lungusa.org	American Lung Association
http://www.nci.nih.gov	National Cancer Institute
http://www.psych.org	American Psychiatric Association
http://www.srnt.org	Society for Research on Nicotine and Tobacco

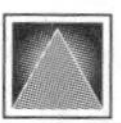

Table 11.9–8
Algorithm for the Five Rs and Five As in Treating Smoking in Psychiatric Patients

*A*sk about tobacco use.
If smoker, *a*dvise to quit.

If not ready to quit (90%):	If ready to quit (10%):
Elicit personally *r*elevant risks Discuss known *r*isks Elicit *r*ewards for quitting Elicit *r*oadblocks to quitting *R*epeat at future visit	*A*ssess prior quits and problem solve anticipated challenges. Set quit date. Decide on abrupt versus gradual cessation. *A*ssist by recommending and implementing medication and behavior therapy session on day before quit date. *A*rrange brief visit or phone call 2 to 3 days after quit date. Follow weekly. Monitor smoking, psychiatric status, and side effects. If patient lapses, discuss changing therapy. If patient relapses, state willingness to help again in near future.

Adapted from Fiore MC, Bailey WC, Cohen SJ, et al. *Treating Tobacco Use and Dependence. Clinical Practice Guideline.* Rockville, MD: Public Health Service; 2000.

All patients should be assessed for (1) smoking status, (2) motivation to quit, and (3) motivators for and barriers to quitting (Table 11.9–8). Smoking status includes current smoker, ex-smoker, or never-smoker; type of tobacco used; and frequency of use. In terms of motivation to quit, smokers can be classified as *immotives* (no plans to quit), *precontemplators* (plan to quit but not in the next 6 months), *contemplators* (plan to quit in the next 6 months), and *preparers* (plan to quit in the next month). Common motivators to quit are health concerns, effects of smoking on others, and social pressure. Common barriers to cessation are withdrawal, fear of failure, and fear of weight gain.

Psychiatrists should advise all patients who are not in crisis to quit smoking. Probably more than 90 percent of psychiatric patients are immotives or precontemplators; that is, they are not interested in quitting in the near future. The psychiatrist's role with these patients is to use the patient's concerns as motivators for cessation and to suggest ways to decrease barriers to cessation. The psychiatrist should also reintroduce cessation at later visits.

The psychiatrist should also clearly advise smoking cessation. The advice can be done in a diplomatic manner; for example, "Now that you are doing well, I want to encourage you to stop smoking." The psychiatrist should reinforce the patient's unique concerns about smoking (e.g., do not want to influence their kids to start smoking) and to suggest ways to decrease barriers to cessation (e.g., fear of weight gain). With psychiatric patients, it is often important to state one's belief that the patient has the ability to stop. Typically, the above advice has no immediate effect. However, the cumulative effect of repeating the advice at later visits and the receipt of advice from others can often motivate a quit attempt.

Among patients who are ready to stop smoking, it is best to set a quit date. Most clinicians and smokers prefer abrupt cessation, but, because there are no good data that abrupt cessation is better than gradual cessation, patient preference for gradual cessation should be respected. Brief advice should focus on the need for medication or telephone or in-person therapy, weight gain concerns, high-risk situations, making cigarettes unavailable, discussions with significant others (especially if they are smokers), and so forth. Because relapse is often rapid, the first follow-up phone call or visit should be 2 to 3 days after the quit date. These strategies have been shown to double

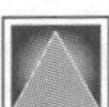

Table 11.9–9
Typical Long-Term Abstinence Rates

	Psychosocial Therapy (%)		
	None[a]	Minimal[b]	Intensive[c]
No medication	4	6	12
Medication[d]	8	12	25

[a]Includes written material.
[b]Brief advice, telephone counseling.
[c]Individual or group therapy.
[d]Proven medication as listed in Table 11.9–10.

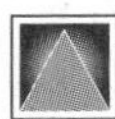

Table 11.9–10
Scientifically Proven Treatments for Smoking

Psychosocial therapy
- Behavior therapy
- Social support

Pharmacological therapies
- Bupropion (Zyban)
- Nicotine gum
- Nicotine inhaler
- Nicotine lozenge
- Nicotine nasal spray
- Nicotine patch
- Nicotine gum and patch[a]
- Bupropion and nicotine patch

Second-line pharmacological therapies
- Clonidine (Catapres)[a]
- Nortriptyline (Aventyl)[a]

[a]Not a Food and Drug Administration–approved use.

self-initiated quit rates (Table 11.9–9). The psychiatrist should also inform the patient about existing therapies (Table 11.9–10), which can often be done by referral to a state help-line.

Ms. H. was a 45-year-old patient with schizophrenia who smoked 35 cigarettes per day. She began her cigarette use at approximately 20 years of age during the prodromal stages of her first psychotic break. During the first 20 years of treatment, no psychiatrist or physician advised her to stop smoking, largely because they believed that she could not stop.

At 43 years of age, her primary care physician recommended smoking cessation. The patient attempted to stop on her own but lasted only 48 hours, partly because her housemates and friends smoked. During a routine medication check, her psychiatrist recommended that she stop smoking, and the patient described her prior attempts. The psychiatrist and the patient discussed ways to avoid smokers and had the patient announce her intent to quit and request her friends to try not to smoke around her and to offer encouragement for her attempt to quit. The psychiatrist also noted that she became irritable, slightly depressed, and restless and had insomnia during prior cessation attempts and thus recommended medications. The patient chose a nicotine patch.

The psychiatrist had the patient call 2 days after her quit attempt. At this point, the patient stated that the patch and gum were helping. One week later, the patient returned after having relapsed back to smoking. The psychiatrist praised the patient for not smoking for 4 days. He suggested that the patient contact him again if she wished to try to stop again. Seven months later, during another medication check, the psychiatrist again asked the patient to consider cessation, but she was reluctant.

Two months later, the patient called and said she wished to try again. This time, the psychiatrist and patient listed several activities that the patient could do to avoid being around friends who smoked, phoned the patient's boyfriend to ask him to assist the patient in stopping, asked the nurses on the inpatient ward to call the patient to encourage her, plus enrolled the patient in a support group for the next 4 weeks. The nicotine patch was used again, but this time the nonnicotine medication bupropion (Zyban) was added. The patient was followed with 15-minute visits for each of the first 3 weeks. She had two "slips" but did not go back to smoking and remained an ex-smoker.

DISCUSSION

Ms. H.'s psychiatrist was correct in using pragmatic plans to help the patient overcome specific problems, in following the patient with short visits or phone calls, and in recommending medication. The total amount of time spent with the patient on smoking was approximately 3 hours. Although this was not reimbursed, the psychiatrist knew that his intervention was an important contribution to the patient's health and was unlikely to be given by other care providers.

Psychosocial Therapies Behavior therapy is the most widely accepted and well-proven psychological therapy for smoking. Behavior therapy consists of several techniques, three of which are supported by good evidence. *Skills training* and *relapse prevention* identify high-risk situations and plan and practice behavioral or cognitive coping skills for these situations. *Stimulus control* refers to eliminating cues for smoking in the environment. *Rapid smoking* has smokers repeatedly smoke to the point of nausea in sessions to associate smoking with unpleasant rather than pleasant sensations. This last therapy appears effective but requires a good therapeutic alliance and patient compliance.

Intratreatment and extratreatment social support also increases abstinence. Often, behavior therapy is conducted in group settings to promote social support and to save on costs. Typically, several sessions are conducted before the quit date, and several are scheduled soon after the quit date. Less than 5 percent of smokers enroll in individual or group behavior therapies, because most smokers believe that they should be able to quit without help, treatments are generally not reimbursable, and treatment is typically offered only a few times a year. However, when behavior therapy or social support is made available via telephone, more smokers avail themselves of treatment.

Although written materials are the most common self-help format, their efficacy is small. Live-person telephone systems that tailor treatment to patient concerns are more effective, more acceptable, and available free of charge from many state health departments, pharmaceutical firms, and voluntary organizations. Other therapies, such as acupuncture, hospitalization, hypnosis, and Nicotine Anonymous (NA), have yet to be proven effective.

Pharmacological Therapies The USPHS and the APA guidelines recommend that all smokers be offered medication to aid in smoking cessation. All the medications approved by the FDA for smoking cessation double the quit rate (similar to results obtained with behavior therapy) and appear equally effective (Table 11.9–10). They produce few side-effects; less than 5 percent of patients stop medication due to adverse effects (except for nicotine nasal spray). There are no empirically verified methods to match smokers to specific medication, and, typically, smokers choose the medication they believe will be most helpful. In other substance use disorders, psychosocial therapy is thought to be essential, and pharmacotherapy is used as an aid to psychosocial therapy. In nicotine dependence, the opposite is true: Pharmacotherapy is the treatment to be offered to all, and psychosocial therapy should be added when feasible.

Nicotine Replacement Therapies Because nicotine undergoes first-pass metabolism by the liver, nongastrointestinal (non-GI) routes have had to be used to deliver nicotine. Nicotine replacement therapies are effective, presumably because they reduce nicotine withdrawal. These therapies can also be used to reduce withdrawal in patients on smoke-free wards. Replacement therapies use a short period of maintenance (6 to 12 weeks), often followed by a gradual reduction period (6 to 12 weeks). However, longer-term use may be necessary for some. Early anecdotal reports suggested that smoking and using nicotine replacement concurrently cause heart attacks; however, several studies have indicated this is not the case.

Nicotine gum is an OTC product that releases nicotine via chewing and buccal absorption. A 2-mg (for people who smoke less than 25 cigarettes per day) and a 4-mg gum variety (for people who smoke greater than or equal to 25 cigarettes per day) are available. Smokers are to use 1 to 2 pieces of gum per hour after abrupt cessation. Venous blood concentrations from the gum are one-third to one-half that of between-cigarette levels. Acidic beverages (coffee, tea, soda, and juice) should not be used before, during, or soon after gum use because these decrease absorption. Compliance with the gum has often been a problem but may be better with newer flavored gums. Adverse effects are minor and include bad taste and sore jaws. Approximately 2 percent use gum for longer than 1 year, but long-term use does not appear to be harmful. The major advantage of nicotine gum is its ability to provide relief in high-risk situations.

Nicotine patches, also sold OTC, are available in a 16-hour no-taper preparation and a 24- or 16-hour tapering preparation. Patches are administered each morning and produce blood concentrations of approximately one-half those of smoking. Compliance is high. The only major adverse effects are rashes and, with 24-hour wear, insomnia. Long-term use does not occur. Combining the nicotine patch plus the use of nicotine gum, lozenge, or inhaler in high-risk situations increases quit rates by another 5 to 10 percent. There is no substantial evidence that 24-hour versus 16-hour or taper versus no-taper patches are better.

Nicotine nasal spray, available only by prescription, produces blood concentrations more similar to a cigarette and may be especially helpful for heavily dependent smokers. However, the spray causes rhinitis, watering eyes, and coughing in more than 70 percent of patients. This product is rarely used.

Nicotine inhaler, a prescription product, was designed to deliver nicotine to the lungs, but the nicotine is actually absorbed in the upper throat. Resultant nicotine levels are similar to those for nicotine gum. The major asset of the inhaler is that it provides a behavioral substitute for smoking. These devices require frequent puffing and lose bioavailability at greater than 50°F.

The nicotine lozenge, an OTC product, is available in 4 mg (for those who smoke within 30 minutes of arising) and 2 mg (for those who do not smoke until more than 30 minutes after arising). The lozenge is held under the tongue and delivers levels of nicotine similar to gum. Because it does not require chewing, it may be more acceptable than gum for some smokers.

Nonnicotine Medications Bupropion is a prescription antidepressant medication that is approved for smoking cessation. Although its antismoking efficacy was originally believed to be due to its dopaminergic effects, it may be due to its ability to block nicotinic-cholinergic receptors. Dosages of 300 mg per day reliably double quit rates in smokers with and without a history of depression. In one study, combined bupropion and nicotine patch had higher quit rates than either alone. Adverse effects include insomnia and nausea, but these are rarely significant. The risk of seizures in those appropriately screened is less than 1 in 1,000.

Nortriptyline (Aventyl) appears to be effective for smoking cessation; however, owing to its more significant side effects than nicotine replacement or bupropion, it is typically used only when other medications have failed. Selective serotonin reuptake inhibitors (SSRIs) do not appear to be effective.

Whether other antidepressants (e.g., SSRIs or MAOIs) are effective is unclear. Importantly, the efficacy of bupropion and nortriptyline is not related to their antidepressant effects.

Clonidine (Catapres) decreases sympathetic activity from the locus ceruleus and is thereby thought to abate withdrawal symptoms. Whether given as a patch or orally, 0.2 to 0.4 mg per day of clonidine appears to double quit rates. The scientific database for the efficacy of clonidine is not as extensive or as reliable as that for nicotine replacement or bupropion, and clonidine can cause drowsiness and hypotension. Thus, clonidine is typically a second-line treatment.

Combined Psychosocial and Pharmacological Therapy

Combining medication and behavior therapy increases quit rates over either therapy alone (Table 11.9–9). Patients should be encouraged to use both. However, medications are effective in the absence of psychosocial therapy; thus, the latter should not be a requirement for the former.

Smoking Cessation Treatment in Special Populations

Behavior therapy is effective for some pregnant smokers. Use of nicotine replacement during pregnancy is debatable. The concentrations of nicotine from these medications are much lower than those from smoking, plus no carbon monoxide and tar exposure occurs. Animal studies suggest nicotine itself could be causal in sudden infant death syndrome; this is still unclear. Often, medications are reserved for pregnant smokers who have failed at cessation without medication. Nicotine replacement is effective in the elderly without excess complications; it has not been tested in smokers younger than 18 years of age. There are no known effective psychosocial or pharmacological treatments for smoking cessation in adolescents.

Smokers who have been recently diagnosed with cancer or heart disease often quit on their own; however, many do not. Despite initial anecdotal reports, nicotine replacement appears safe in those with heart disease.

Psychiatric patients who are trying to stop smoking should be encouraged to undertake psychosocial and pharmacological therapies, because these patients experience greater withdrawal symptoms and have a poorer ability to stop. In addition, these patients should be followed weekly to detect any possible exacerbation of their psychiatric problem.

Whether alcoholics should stop smoking along with or soon after stopping drinking is debatable. Current evidence suggests that, for the large majority of patients, stopping smoking does not threaten sobriety. Whether smokers with a history of alcoholism or other substance abuse need more intense therapy or different content therapy for smoking cessation is unclear.

Patients on smoke-free psychiatric wards can have withdrawal symptoms that require treatment. Because wards often lack cues for smoking, withdrawal is usually not as problematic as anticipated; thus, treatment should usually be reserved until the emergence of symptoms. If the smoker is taking passes and smoking, nicotine gum, lozenge, or inhaler is preferred, because it can be used intermittently. If the smoker is confined to the ward or is using the hospitalization to stop smoking, nicotine patches should be used because they are associated with improved compliance. All smokers should be told that the rationale for the smoke-free ward is not moral but rather is to protect nonsmokers from second-hand smoke and to prevent tempting exsmokers under stress from returning to smoking.

Non-Abstinence Goals One-half of smokers (and more than 80 percent of psychiatric patients who smoke) never stop smoking. Logically, reducing the number of cigarettes per day or switching to low-tar cigarettes should reduce the risk of harm in these smokers; however, compensatory smoking (i.e., smoking each cigarette more intensely to obtain the necessary nicotine) appears to minimize any potential benefit of these strategies. Whether using the above-described medications to reduce smoking would prevent compensatory smoking and thus would allow reduction to produce health benefits is unclear. Although some have feared that offering reduction would undermine motivation to quit, reduction appears to increase the chance of later quitting.

PREVENTION AND POLICY INITIATIVES

School-based programs to prevent the initiation of smoking have focused on methods such as education (e.g., about risks of smoking), denormalizing smoking (e.g., correcting overestimates of prevalence of smoking), skills training (e.g., refusal training), and advocacy (e.g., students demonstrate against tobacco industry). Among these, only denormalizing and skills training have good empirical support; however, even with these interventions, the long-term effect of school-based programs is not large.

Policy initiatives to reduce smoking prevalence have focused on tobacco taxation, smoking restrictions, restriction of tobacco advertising, counteradvertising via mass media, attacks on the tobacco industry as immoral, restriction of sales to minors, and warnings on cigarette packages. Among these, only taxation and mass media appear effective. Although the effects of mass media have been small, the effect of taxes is large and replicable. Taxation especially influences initiation among youth. Many of the previously mentioned initiatives have been combined into community programs under the assumption that a synergistic effect occurs. However, whether this is true is unclear.

SUGGESTED CROSS-REFERENCES

Section 11.1 provides an overview of substance abuse and substance-related disorders. Bupropion is discussed in Section 31.12. Nortriptyline is discussed in Section 31.29. Clonidine is discussed in Section 31.5.

REFERENCES

*Abrams DB, Niaura R, Brown RA, Emmons KM, Goldstein MG, Monti PM. *The Tobacco Dependence Treatment Handbook. A Guide to Best Practices.* Barlow DH, ed. New York: The Guilford Press; 2003.

Achievements in public health, 1900–1999: Tobacco use—United States, 1900–1999. *MMWR Morb Mortal Wkly Rep.* 1999;48:986–993.

Benowitz N: Nicotine addiction. *Primary Care.* 1999;26:611–631.

Benowitz NL, Peng MW: Non-nicotine pharmacotherapy for smoking cessation. Mechanisms and prospects. *CNS Drugs.* 2000;13:265–285.

Covey LS, Sullivan MA, Johnston JA, Glassman AH, Robinson MD, Adams DP: Advances in non-nicotine pharmacotherapy for smoking cessation. *Drugs.* 2000;59:17–31.

Dalack GW, Healy DJ, Meador-Woodruff JH. Nicotine dependence in schizophrenia: Clinical phenomena and laboratory findings. *Am J Psychiatry.* 1998;155:1490.

Dani JA, Heinemann S: Molecular and cellular aspects of nicotine abuse. *Neuron.* 1996;16:905.

Fiore MC, Bailey WC, Cohen SJ, Dorfman SF, Goldstein MG, Gritz ER, Heyman RB, Jaan CR, Kottke T, Lando HS, Mecklenburg RE, Mullen PD, Nett LM, Robinson L, Stitzer ML, Tommasello AC, Villejo L, Wewers ME. *Treating Tobacco Use and Dependence. Clinical Practice Guideline.* Rockville, MD: Public Health Service; 2000.

Giovino GA: Epidemiology of tobacco use in the United States. *Oncogene.* 2002;21:7326–7340.

Heath AC, Madden PAF. Genetic influences on smoking behavior. In: Turner JR, Cardon LR, Hewitt JK, eds. *Behavior Genetic Approaches in Behavioral Medicine.* New York: Plenum Press; 1995.

*Hughes JR: Possible effects of smoke-free inpatient units on psychiatric diagnosis and treatment. *J Clin Psychiatry.* 1993;54:109.

Hughes JR: Four beliefs that may impede progress in the treatment of smoking. *Tob Control.* 1999;8:323–326.

Hughes JR: Why does smoking so often produce dependence? A somewhat different view. *Tob Control.* 2001;10:62–64.

Hughes JR, Fiester S, Goldstein MG, Resnick MP, Rock N, Ziedonis D: American Psychiatric Association practice guidelines for the treatment of nicotine dependence. *Am J Psychiatry.* 1996;153:S1.

Hughes JR, Zarin DA, Pincus HA: Treating nicotine dependence in mental health settings. *J Pract Psychiatry Behav Health.* 1997;24:250.

Institute of Medicine. *Clearing the Smoke. Assessing the Science Base for Tobacco Harm Reduction.* Washington, DC: National Academy Press; 2001.

Kalman D. Smoking cessation treatment for substance misusers in early recovery: A review of the literature and recommendation for practice. *Subst Use Misuse.* 1998;33:2021–2027.

Lasser K, Boyd JW, Woolhandler S, Himmelstein DU, McCormick D, Bor DH. Smoking and mental illness: A population-based prevalence study. *JAMA.* 2000;284:2606.

*National Cancer Institute. Population Based Smoking Cessation: Proceedings of a Conference on What Works to Influence Cessation in the General Population. *Smoking and Tobacco Control Monograph No. 12.* Bethesda, MD: USDHHS, National Institutes of Health, National Cancer Institute; 2000.

National Cancer Institute. *Changing Adolescent Smoking Prevalence. Where It Is and Why. Smoking and Tobacco Control Monograph No. 14.* Bethesda, MD: USDHHS, National Institutes of Health, National Cancer Institute; 2001.

National Cancer Institute. *Those Who Continue to Smoke: Is Achieving Abstinence Harder and Do We Need to Change Our Interventions? Smoking and Tobacco Control Monograph No. 15.* Bethesda, MD: USDHHS, National Institutes of Health, National Cancer Institute; 2003.

Niaura R, Abrams DB: Smoking cessation: Progress, priorities, and prospects. *J Consult Clin Psychol.* 2002;70:494–509.

Piasecki M, Newhouse PA. *Nicotine in Psychiatry. Psychopathology and Emerging Therapeutics.* Washington, DC: American Psychiatric Press; 2002

Rabin RL, Sugarman SD. *Regulating Tobacco.* New York: Oxford University Press; 2001.

*Rigotti NA. Clinical practice: Treatment of tobacco use and dependence. *N Engl J Med.* 2002;346:506.

Shiffman S, Dresler CA, Hajek P, Gilburt SJA, Targett DA, Strahs KR: Efficacy of a nicotine lozenge for smoking cessation. *Arch Intern Med.* 2002;162:1267–1276.

Sweeney CT, Fant RV, Fagerstrom K-O, McGovern JF, Henningfield JE: Combination nicotine replacement therapy for smoking cessation. Rationale, efficacy and tolerability. *CNS Drugs.* 2001;15:453–467.

United States Department of Health and Human Services. *The Health Consequences of Smoking: Nicotine Addiction: A Report of the U.S. Surgeon General.* Washington, DC: U. S. Government Printing Office; 1988.

United States Department of Health and Human Services. *Preventing Tobacco Use Among Young People: A Report of the Surgeon General.* Washington, DC: U. S. Government Printing Office; 1994.

*United States Department of Health and Human Services. *Reducing Tobacco Use: A Report of the Surgeon General.* Atlanta, GA; U.S. Office on Smoking and Health; 2000.

Watkins SS, Koob GF, Markou A: Neural mechanisms underlying nicotine addiction; acute positive reinforcement and withdrawal. *Nicotine Tob Res.* 2000;2:19–37.

World Health Organization. *Tobacco or Health; A Global Status Report.* Geneva, Switzerland: World Health Organization; 1997.

▲ 11.10 Opioid-Related Disorders

JEROME H. JAFFE, M.D., AND ERIC C. STRAIN, M.D.

More than 20 chemically distinct opioid drugs are in clinical use throughout the world. In the developed countries, the opioid drug most frequently associated with abuse and dependence is heroin—a drug that is not used for therapeutic purposes in the United States. Dependence on opioids other than heroin is seen mostly in persons who have become dependent in the course of medical treatment, among health care professionals who have easy access to such drugs, and in those who use drugs that are diverted from medical providers and treatment programs. Virtually all of the opioid dependence and abuse seen clinically is associated with prototypical μ-agonist opioids, and all μ-agonists produce similar subjective effects. However, the patterns of use and some aspects of opioid toxicity are powerfully influenced by the route of administration and the metabolism of the specific opioid, as well as by the social conditions that determine its price and purity and the sanctions attached to nonmedical use.

DEFINITIONS

The revised fourth edition of the *Diagnostic and Statistical Manual of Mental Disorders* (DSM-IV-TR) divides *opioid-related disorders* into *opioid use disorders* (opioid abuse and opioid dependence) and nine other *opioid-induced disorders* (e.g., intoxication and withdrawal).

Opioid dependence is a cluster of physiological, behavioral, and cognitive symptoms, which, taken together, indicate repeated and continuing use of opioid drugs despite significant problems related to such use. *Drug dependence* in general has also been defined by the World Health Organization (WHO) as a syndrome in which the use of a drug or class of drugs takes on a much higher priority for a given person than other behaviors that once had a higher value. These brief definitions each have as their central features an emphasis on the drug-using behavior itself, its maladaptive nature, and on how the choice to engage in that behavior has shifted and becomes constrained as a result of interaction with the drug over time.

Opioid abuse is a term used to designate a pattern of maladaptive use of an opioid drug leading to clinically significant impairment or distress and occurring within a 12-month period, but one in which the symptoms have never met the criteria for opioid dependence.

The *opioid-induced disorders* as defined by DSM-IV-TR include such common phenomena as opioid intoxication, opioid withdrawal, opioid-induced sleep disorder, and opioid-induced sexual dysfunction. Opioid intoxication delirium is occasionally seen in hospitalized patients. Opioid-induced psychotic disorder, opioid-induced mood disorder, and opioid-induced anxiety disorder, by contrast, are quite uncommon with μ-agonist opioids but have been seen with certain mixed agonist-antagonist opioids acting at other receptors. DSM-IV-TR also includes *opioid-related disorder not otherwise specified* for situations that do not meet the criteria for any of the other opioid-related disorders.

HISTORY

Opiates have been used for at least 3,500 years, mostly in the form of crude opium or in alcoholic solutions of opium. Morphine was first isolated in 1806, and codeine was first isolated in 1832. Over the next century, pure morphine and codeine gradually replaced crude opium for medicinal purposes, although nonmedical use of opium (as for smoking) still persists in some parts of the world. The first semisynthetic opium derivative—diacetylmorphine or heroin—was introduced into medicine in 1898. The first purely synthetic drugs with morphine-like opioids, meperidine (Demerol) and methadone (Dolophine), were introduced into medical practice in the 1940s. The term *opioid* was coined to include the naturally occurring drugs derived from opium (morphine and codeine), the semisynthetic drugs produced from opium derivatives, and a wider range of totally synthetic agents bearing little chemical resemblance to morphine.

Opioid dependence, or at least opioid withdrawal, was first recognized in 1700. Opioid dependence was common by the middle of the 19th century, but it was not until later in the century that it came to be seen as an important medical problem. There was public concern about opium smoking by Chinese immigrants and the severe forms of dependence associated with the newly introduced hypodermic needle and syringe. Growing awareness of the problems created by opioid-containing patent medicines sold over the counter or casually dispensed by practitioners with minimal training generated media attention and public debate. In the United States, this debate, combined with international political considerations, led to legislation at the state and federal levels restricting opioid use to medically recognized purposes and requiring legitimate prescriptions for most use. The Harrison Act of 1914 had a profound impact on persons who were already addicted, because it was interpreted to exclude the provision of opioids to addicts as a legitimate use. Clinics that had been established specifically to provide morphine to addicts were closed, the last in 1923. Doctors were encouraged to avoid opioid addicts entirely. Detoxification efforts were a disappointment to physicians and patients because relapse was typical. An illicit traffic in opioids arose, providing drugs (mostly morphine and heroin) to persons who could no longer get them through medical channels. Addicts were arrested for possession and sale of opioids. In the early 1930s, the U.S. Public Health Service established two federal hospitals—at Lexington, Kentucky, and Fort Worth, Texas—to deal with the growing number of federal prisoners who were addicted. These hospitals provided long-term residential treatment for prisoners and for some voluntary patients. Later follow-up studies found that relapse rates were high, despite long periods of treatment. Although increasingly harsh penalties for the sale or possession of opioids were enacted, heroin addiction persisted, and its prevalence rose after World War II. By the early 1960s, some thoughtful observers recommended remedicalizing heroin distribution as a way to reduce crime associated with heroin addiction.

However, several new developments in treatment techniques sharply altered the general perception of opioid dependence as an essentially untreatable disorder. They included the development of therapeutic communities based on the Synanon model (an organization that began in California in 1958), the creation of large-scale civil commitment programs in California (1961) and New York (1965), the demonstration of the effectiveness of maintenance on oral methadone in decreasing crime and heroin use, and the development of long-acting opioid antagonists, along with the finding that some addicts were willing to take them.

Starting in the late 1960s, federal and state sources increased support for research and treatment. In response to the outbreak of heroin addiction among U.S. military personnel in Vietnam, federal support for treatment was greatly expanded and accelerated in the early 1970s. This support was not merely monetary but included legislation providing for the legitimate use of methadone and for protection of the confidentiality of patient records. The use of methadone for treating opioid addicts was restricted to specially licensed programs that were regulated by detailed federal and state regulations.

In the mid-1970s, the four dominant treatment modalities were brief detoxification, methadone maintenance, therapeutic communities, and a heterogeneous category generally designated as drug-free outpatient care. Civil commitment declined in influence and support. In the early 1980s, with the expansion of private insurance to cover treatment for alcohol abuse and drug dependence, in-hospital treatment programs based on the 12-step model pioneered in Minnesota proliferated. Although these programs were initially developed as treatments for alcohol abuse, they were gradually broadened to deal with a wider range of dependence, including opioid dependence. For a brief period, *chemical dependence* programs became an additional significant option in the array of treatments available to persons who were dependent on opioids. By the late 1980s, however, the rising cost of treatment and growing government deficits stimulated the emergence of managed care. The impact of managed care on the support for the treatment of opioid dependence has not yet been fully felt, but the availability even of short-term hospital-based treatment has virtually disappeared. In 2000, the oversight of methadone programs was changed to a system that relied more on accreditation and less on compliance with detailed government regulations. In 2001, federal legislation was passed allowing office-based physicians to prescribe an opioid (buprenorphine [Buprenex, Subutex]) for addicted patients.

COMPARATIVE NOSOLOGY

The DSM-IV-TR criteria for opioid dependence are the same generic criteria as are applied to other psychoactive drugs. The notion of a generic concept of dependence is shared with the tenth revision of the *International Statistical Classification of Diseases and Related Health Problems* (ICD-10). In the diagnosis of opioid dependence, there generally is a high level of agreement between DSM-IV-TR and ICD-10: They use similar concepts (the dependence syndrome varying in degree of severity), although the wording of the criteria for determining the presence and severity of the syndrome differs. Both require that three elements of the syndrome occur within a 12-month period.

A major difference between DSM-IV-TR and ICD-10 lies in how each defines substance abuse. ICD-10 does not use the term *abuse*. Instead, it includes a category of harmful use that is substantially different from the concept of abuse in DSM-IV-TR. However, the concept of harmful use is limited to physical and mental health (e.g., hepatitis, overdose, and skin abscess) and specifically excludes social impairments. ICD-10 states: "Harmful patterns of use are often criticized by others and frequently associated with adverse social consequences of various kinds. The fact that a pattern of use or a particular substance is disapproved of by another person or by the culture, or may have led to socially negative consequences such as arrest or marital arguments is not in itself evidence of harmful use."

DSM-IV-TR and ICD-10 also have distinctly different coding systems. ICD-10 separates for record-keeping purposes mental and behavioral disorders due to use of opioids from those caused by other categories of drugs. DSM-IV-TR limits the number of distinct drug-induced syndromes that can be recorded (except under the categories *other* and *unspecified*) as disorders induced by opioids.

EPIDEMIOLOGY

Opioid use in the United States experienced a resurgence in the 1990s, with emergency department visits related to heroin abuse doubling between 1990 and 1995. This increase in heroin use was associated with an increase in heroin purity and a decrease in its street price. In the late 1990s, there was an increase in heroin use among people who were 18 to 25 years of age and a brief upsurge in the use of oxycodone (OxyContin) from pharmaceutical sources. Methods of administration other than injecting, such as smoking and snorting, increased in popularity. The number of current heroin users has been questionably estimated to be between 600,000 and 800,000. The number of people estimated to have used heroin at any time in their lives (*lifetime users*) is estimated at approximately three million.

There are a number of activities aimed at estimating the extent and consequences of psychoactive drug use in the United States. All of the regularly recurring estimating techniques have sampling limitations, and standardized diagnostic criteria have only recently been incorporated into some of these studies. In general, these surveys may be best viewed as providing information that is useful in detecting trends over time rather than cross-sectional estimates of prevalence.

The Monitoring the Future project ("High School Senior Survey") is an annually conducted national survey of drug use that assesses a range of school-age children and young adults. Over the course of the 1990s, lifetime rates of heroin use increased for eighth, tenth, and 12th graders from 0.9 to 1.2 percent in 1991 to a peak of 2.3 to 2.4 percent in the years 1998, 1999, and 2000 and then started to decline in 2000, with the decline continuing into 2001 (rates of use between 1.7 and 1.8 percent in 2001). Rates of heroin use in the past 30 days for eighth, tenth, and 12th graders show less variability over the decade ending in 2001, with rates generally between 0.5 and 0.7 percent for most years between 1995 and 1999. However, these rates have also shown declines in 2001 for tenth and 12th graders (0.3 and 0.4 percent, respectively), although they remain elevated for eighth graders (0.6 percent).

A second national survey is the National Household Survey on Drug Abuse (NHSDA), which provides annual assessments of drug use in children and adults in the United States. In 2001, the NHSDA found that slightly more than three million persons aged 12 years or older reported using heroin at some point in their lives (an increase from 2.8 million found in 2000). However, there were considerably fewer persons who had used heroin in the past year (456,000), and an even lower number of persons who had used heroin in the past month (123,000).

Although the rates of heroin use in the past year and past month found by the NHSDA may seem quite low, it is important to note that rates of nonmedical use of pain relievers (typically opioids) are considerably higher. For example, in 2001, there were 22,133,000 persons who reported lifetime nonmedical use of a pain reliever, 8,353,000 who had such use in the past year, and 3,497,000 who had nonmedical use of a pain reliever in the past month (all increases from the number of persons who had such use in 2000). These absolute numbers are quite high, and it is also interesting to note that the ratio of past 30-day use to lifetime nonmedical use of a pain reliever (0.158) is considerably higher than the corresponding ratio of past 30-day use to lifetime use of heroin (0.040). One interpretation of these ratios is that lifetime exposure to nonmedical use of opioids is more likely to lead to past 30-day use, compared to heroin.

An alternate approach to assessing the extent of drug use is to examine the number of persons entering treatment who report use of opioids. Results from a national assessment (the Treatment Episode Data Set) for 2000 showed that there were 243,071 persons admitted for the treatment of heroin use and another 25,723 persons admitted for other opioid use. The total number of persons admitted for heroin and other opioid use was exceeded only by the number admitted for alcohol use. Heroin admissions in 2000 had increased from 168,321 persons in 1992. The states with the highest numbers of heroin admissions in the year 2000 were (in descending order) California, New York, Massachusetts, New Jersey, and Connecticut.

Two population surveys have been conducted using accepted criteria to measure the extent of drug abuse and dependence: the Epidemiological Catchment Area (ECA) Study carried out in the early 1980s using criteria from the third edition of the DSM (DSM-III) and the National Comorbidity Survey (NCS) carried out from 1990 to 1992 using the revised third edition of the DSM (DSM-III-R) criteria. The NCS found the lifetime prevalence of heroin use to be 1.5 percent overall, but with a prevalence of 2.7 percent among people who were 35 to 44 years of age, probably reflecting the peak of the heroin epidemic among adolescents and young adults in the late 1960s and early 1970s. Heroin dependence (lifetime) was 0.4 percent overall but 0.8 percent among those who were 35 to 44 years of age. Those findings indicate that approximately 32 percent of those who used heroin at the peak of the epidemic became dependent at some time in their lives.

Lifetime history of extramedical use of opioid analgesics (other than heroin) was 9.7 percent, with the highest prevalence among people who were 15 to 34 years of age, suggesting a different pattern from that of heroin. Overall, only 7.5 percent of those who used opioid analgesics outside of a medical context developed dependence as defined by DSM-III-R. Obviously, the 6-month and current prevalence rates of dependence would be lower than these lifetime rates.

The use and dependence rates derived from national surveys do not accurately reflect fluctuations in drug use among opioid-dependent and previously opioid-dependent populations. When the supply of illicit heroin increases in purity or decreases in price, use among that vulnerable population tends to increase, with subsequent increases in adverse consequences (emergency room visits) and requests for treatment.

Increases in the purity of street heroin and users' concern about the risks of human immunodeficiency virus (HIV) transmission have led to a resurgence of heroin inhalation as well as smoking (known as *chasing the dragon*). Casual users may persist in such routes of administration; however, with long-term use and increasing pharmacological tolerance, economic imperatives often lead users to switch to more efficient parenteral routes. Injecting drug users are also more likely to experience a "rush" than those using other routes of administration.

ETIOLOGY

Opioid dependence is currently seen as a biopsychosocial disorder in which multiple factors interact to influence initiation of use, continued use, and relapse after periods of abstinence. Those factors—pharmacological, social, environmental, personality, psychopathology, genetic, and familial—are the same ones that must be considered when looking at abuse and dependence on other categories of drugs. What changes in the case of the opioids is the balance of the various factors. For opioids, as for most substances, it is largely social and cultural factors that influence availability and initial use. In the case of opioid drugs, however, pharmacological factors—the initial effects and their consequences—are believed to play important roles in the perpetuation of use and of progression to dependence. Opioids have potent mood-elevating and euphorigenic actions in humans and are powerful reinforcers in animal models. This is particularly true when the effects are rapid in onset, such as when the opioids are injected or inhaled. Perhaps more than any other category of drugs, the opioids can induce long-lasting alterations in the nervous system. Some of these changes are responsible for the physical dependence that causes an aversive withdrawal syndrome when central nervous system (CNS) opioid levels decline. Other drug-induced changes that may persist for some time after withdrawal include a hyperresponsiveness to stress and a reduced responsivity for ordinary pleasurable events (hypophoria). It is not clear whether these changes should be considered part of a *protracted withdrawal* syndrome or whether they represent distinct phenomena.

Pharmacological Factors

Opioids and Opioid Receptors An opioid *agonist* is now defined as any exogenous substance that binds specifically to any of several subtypes of opioid receptor and that produces some action. Although many opioids produce actions similar to that of morphine (a prototypical μ-agonist), others may bind to various receptor subtypes in a pattern that is distinct from that of morphine, producing a dissimilar profile of actions, and may not suppress the morphine abstinence syndrome. Drugs that bind to any of the subtypes of receptors but initiate no actions are opioid *antagonists* at those receptors. Some opioids bind to receptors but cannot produce maximum effects. These are considered *partial agonists* at that receptor type.

Several opioid receptor types have been described and characterized. Three of these, μ, κ, and δ, have been recognized for some time. More recently, a fourth receptor type, OFQ/N (ORL-1), has been accepted as part of an extended family of opioid receptors. All of the opioid receptor types, including OFQ/N, are typical G-protein–coupled receptors. Receptors can be linked to second messenger systems or directly to ion channels. μ Receptors, for example, can act via G_i or G_o to directly increase potassium flux or to inhibit the action of adenylyl cyclase. Subsequent decreases in the activity of cyclic adenosine monophosphate (cAMP)–dependent protein kinases can have immediate effects on phosphorylation-dependent cellular proteins as well as long-term effects on gene expression via decreased phosphorylation of cAMP-dependent transcription factors, such as cAMP response element binding protein (CREB).

OFQ/N was identified by its high degree of homology to traditional opioid receptors. Because it did not bind any of the ligands that were bound by the classic μ, κ, or δ receptors, it was initially called an *orphan receptor*. An endogenous ligand to this orphan receptor was identified and termed *orphanin FQ* by one research group and *nociceptin* by another. It is now commonly designated OFQ/N. The peptide has been demonstrated to have analgesic and pronociceptive effects in vivo, depending on site of administration. The receptor, initially called *ORL-1*, is now more commonly designated the *OFQ/N receptor*.

Studies using specific agonists and antagonists, antisense techniques, and knock-out mice suggest the existence of subtypes of the major receptor types. Some work in mice, for example, suggests that heroin and certain other opioids exert their actions at a μ receptor subtype distinct from that at which morphine acts. However, studies in monkeys using selective opioid antagonists do not support the hypothesis that heroin acts at a distinct receptor. Subtypes of the μ receptor could explain why there is less than complete cross-tolerance between μ analgesics. Interactions among different opioid receptor types—complexes or dimerizations—may account for what appear to be receptor subtypes.

Most of the opioid drugs associated with opioid abuse and dependence are typical μ-agonists, having pharmacological profiles that are quite similar to morphine and differing primarily in terms of metabolism and pharmacokinetics. The actions of μ-agonist opioids are exerted primarily at receptors on neural tissues in the CNS, the autonomic nervous system, and, to some degree, on opioid receptors on white blood cells. These actions include analgesia, respiratory depression, changes in mood (euphoria in some persons), indifference to anticipated distress, drowsiness, decreased ability to concentrate, changes in endocrine and other functions regulated by the hypothalamus, and increased tone of smooth muscle in the gastrointestinal (GI) tract. Former heroin addicts who are given opioids report reduced anxiety, increased self-esteem, a better ability to cope with everyday problems, and a decreased sense of boredom. Given intravenously (IV), opioids produce a *rush* or *flash*, a sudden, brief sensation that is reported to be exceedingly pleasurable. Although the rush was customarily described as being much like an orgasmic sensation felt in the abdomen, in more recent interviews, addicts have described it in much more varied terms, although still as a much desired experience.

The rush, a far shorter phenomenon than a general sense of euphoria, lasts only 1 to 2 minutes and is experienced only with rapid drug intake, as with IV or intrapulmonary routes.

μ-Agonists also induce tolerance and neuroadaptive changes in the CNS that result in distressing withdrawal phenomena when the agonist is stopped after days or weeks of continuous use. In contrast, drugs that act at κ receptors, such as U-50, 488, produce some dysphoria and no significant pupillary change but still induce analgesia. Also in contrast to μ-agonists, which produce dopamine release from neurons originating in the ventral tegmental area (VTA), κ-agonists inhibit dopamine release in this pathway.

Heroin (diacetylmorphine) is more potent and more lipid soluble than morphine, thereby crossing the blood–brain barrier more rapidly and producing a more rapid onset of subjective effects and less general pruritus, an adverse effect of morphine. However, heroin is hydrolyzed quite rapidly (half-life of approximately 3 minutes) to 6-monoacetylmorphine and morphine. Its actions are probably exerted primarily through those metabolites binding to μ receptors, although 6-monoacetylmorphine may bind to δ receptors as well. Experienced addicts appear to be able to discriminate heroin from hydromorphone (Dilaudid).

In the United States, most of the μ-agonist drugs are included in schedule (control level) I (prohibited for clinical use) or schedule II (clinical use under the most restrictive prescribing controls) of the Controlled Substances Act (CSA), although some mixtures (e.g., codeine and aspirin) are in the less restrictive schedules III and IV. Buprenorphine, a partial μ-agonist now included in schedule III, was misused by opioid addicts in Europe when it was introduced there without restrictions. It is now approved for use in the United States and Europe for use in treating opioid dependence. Abuse or dependence is occasionally seen with opioids that are not prototypical μ-agonists but also have actions at other opioid receptors, such as the mixed agonist-antagonist pentazocine (Talwin). Such agents, if they are included in the CSA, may be in schedules III, IV, or V.

Several analgesics now available have actions at more than one receptor type. Some have antagonist actions at one type and agonist actions at another. For example, pentazocine has reinforcing properties and is self-administered by animals and some addicted persons, but it does not appear to exhibit a significant degree of cross-tolerance with μ-agonists and does not suppress μ-agonist withdrawal to any significant degree. It may be a weak μ-agonist and κ-agonist.

Endogenous Opioid Peptides Five distinct neurobiological opioid peptide systems or families have thus far been described. Each of these systems has a distinct genetic basis, separate biosynthetic pathways, and distinct precursor molecules. The anatomical distributions of the cells that produce and release the respective endogenous peptides are also distinct, but there is sometimes considerable overlap. These families are usually referred to as (1) the *proopiomelanocortin* (POMC), (2) the *proenkephalin*, (3) the *prodynorphin*, (4) the *proorphanin* or *pro-OFQ/N*, and (5) the *endomorphin systems*. Each precursor protein produces more than one active peptide that can be detected in body tissues.

The POMC precursor molecule contains the 91–amino acid peptide β-lipotropin, as well as adrenocorticotropic hormone (ACTH) and melanocyte-stimulating hormone (MSH). Peptides 61 to 91 in β-lipotropin make up beta-endorphin, one of the active opioid fragments produced by the POMC family. The enkephalin system consists primarily of the pentapeptides met-enkephalin (tyrosine [Tyr]–glycine [Gly]–Gly–phenylalanine [Phe]–methionine [Met]) and leu-enkephalin (Tyr-Gly-Gly-Phe-Leu). From the parent prodynorphin, the dynorphin system produces the 17–amino acid peptide dynorphin and several other active dynorphin peptides, all of which are C-terminal extensions of leu-enkephalin. They include dynorphin A (1 to 17), dynorphin A (1 to 8), dynorphin B (1 to 13), α-neoendorphin, β-neoendorphin, and others.

The proorphanin precursor molecule contains not only the 17–amino acid OFQ/N, but also another 17–amino acid peptide that is distinct from OFQ/N (Orphanin 2) and a longer peptide nocistatin. OFQ/N may have a role in stress responsiveness, learning, and memory. The endomorphins consist of two tetrapeptides that bind preferentially to the μ receptor. The roles played by OFQ/N and endomorphin peptides in the initiation and perpetuation of opioid dependence are not yet clear.

The various endogenous peptides tend to bind preferentially to one or more of the opioid receptor subtypes. For example, met-enkephalin appears to prefer δ receptors, most members of the dynorphin family of peptides display their highest affinity for κ receptors, and the endomorphins bind preferentially to μ receptors. However, beta-endorphin binds to μ receptors and δ receptors and does not appear to be as receptor selective as the other endogenous ligands. Preferential binding is not the same as exclusive binding. Peptides that bind preferentially to one set of receptors can, in high enough concentrations, exert actions at receptors for which they have lower affinities. Furthermore, posttranslational processing of some of these peptides substantially changes their receptor affinities. For example, dynorphin 1-17 binds preferentially to κ receptors, but dynorphin 1-6 also shows equivalent binding at μ and δ. Some processing produces peptides that still have receptor affinity but act functionally as antagonists. Thus, although beta-endorphin 1-31 is a potent agonist at μ and δ receptors, beta-endorphin 1-27 has one-tenth the activity and can antagonize the actions of beta-endorphin 1-31. Nocistatin, a peptide that is contained in the proorphanin molecule, produces effects that are opposite to those of OFQ/N.

Opioid Actions on Hedonic Regulation The brain regions believed to be critical in mediating the euphorigenic and positive reinforcing effects of drugs include the dopaminergic pathways originating in the VTA and projecting to the nucleus accumbens (NAc). In animals, stimulation of these areas or microinjections into this pathway are reinforcing. The dopaminergic mesocorticolimbic system also includes the amygdala, which is important for emotionally laden memories. The prefrontal, anterior, and cingulate cortices are also part of this system and are involved with drug expectation, stimulus salience, and craving. Dopaminergic input from the VTA to the NAc is thought to be the critical step in the reinforcing or euphorigenic effects of most drugs. Dopamine also appears to play a role in giving salience or importance to environmental stimuli and focuses the organism's attention and directs its behavior toward those stimuli.

μ-Agonist opioids increase the activity of VTA dopaminergic neurons by inhibiting γ-aminobutyric acid (GABA)ergic neurons, which normally inhibit VTA activity. Activation of κ receptors on the VTA dopaminergic neurons is inhibitory, causing decreased dopamine release. There are at least three types of opioid receptors on the neurons of the NAc; μ opioids have reinforcing effects at these sites that are not dependent on dopamine. Some neurons of the NAc have recurrent fibers expressing dynorphin. These recurrent fibers synapse on κ-receptor–bearing dopamine neurons in the VTA, thus creating a feedback inhibition of VTA activity (Fig. 11.10–1).

In animal models, stress and stress-related hormones can alter the sensitivity of brain structures to reinforcing effects of opioid drugs. Stress and corticotropin-releasing factor (CRF) may act by release of ACTH and glucocorticoids, but CRF may also act at other sites in the CNS. Blocking the glucocorticoid response to stress eliminates the enhanced sensitivity to morphine. There is clinical evidence that the hypothalamic-pituitary-adrenal (HPA) stress axis is unstable and hypersensitive in opioid-dependent and recently detoxified heroin

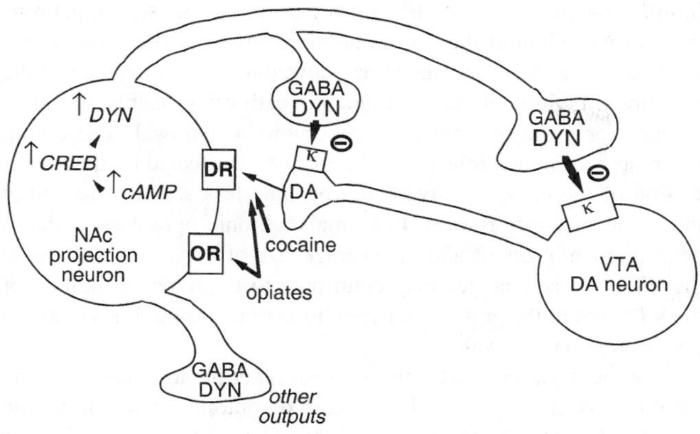

FIGURE 11.10–1 Regulation of cyclic adenosine monophosphate (cAMP) response element binding protein (CREB) by drugs of abuse. The figure shows a ventral tegmental area (VTA) dopamine (DA) neuron innervating a class of nucleus accumbens (NAc) γ-aminobutyric acid (GABA)ergic projection neuron that expresses dynorphin (DYN). DYN serves a negative feedback mechanism in this circuit: DYN, released from terminals of the NAc neurons, acts on κ opioid receptors located on nerve terminals and cell bodies of the DA neurons to inhibit their functioning. Chronic exposure to cocaine or opiates upregulates the activity of this negative feedback loop via upregulation of the cAMP pathway, activation of CREB, and induction of dynorphin. DR, dopamine receptor; OR, opioid receptor. (From Nestler EJ: Molecular neurobiology of addiction. *Am J Addict.* 2001;10:201, with permission.)

users. It is hypothesized that this hyperresponsiveness to stress may be related to relapse.

Opioids are synergistic with amphetamine or cocaine in lowering self-stimulation thresholds in animals and in inducing euphoria in humans. The neurobiological mechanisms of reinforcement of these drugs also appear to overlap .

Studies of brain glucose metabolism and cerebral blood flow in human volunteers have found striking similarities in the way in which different drugs that induce euphoria alter brain function. When subjects experienced euphoria induced by opioids or cocaine, euphoria was correlated with decreased brain glucose metabolism, especially in orbitofrontal cortex and thalamus.

Opioid Neuroadaptation, Tolerance, and Physical Dependence With μ-agonist opioids, there can be remarkable tolerance to their analgesic, respiratory-depressant, and sedative actions. Patients in Swiss heroin clinics have injected as much as 300 mg IV as a single dose. Markedly less tolerance develops to the miotic and constipating actions of opioids on the bowel. Intermediate degrees of tolerance to endocrine actions develop, and there appears to be less tolerance to the capacity of opioids to lower the threshold for electrical self-stimulation of the brain.

Heroin addicts who self-administered heroin in a research setting seemed to develop tolerance to the anxiety-relieving and mood-elevating effects of opioids and, over a period of several weeks, developed various somatic complaints and reported feeling increasingly anxious and dysphoric. Nevertheless, they were able to experience brief periods of mood elevation for 30 to 60 minutes each time that they received single injections. Interviews with heroin users indicated that they continued to experience a brief euphoric effect immediately after an injection, despite some tolerance to many of the drug effects. These data led to the conclusion that tolerant opioid users do not continue to self-administer the drugs solely to prevent the highly aversive withdrawal phenomena. Although the loss of mood-elevating effects and the appearance of hypophoria and hypochondriasis have also been observed with the long-term administration of methadone in an inpatient research setting, when heroin users with depressed mood enter methadone treatment programs, mood improves.

When tolerance to a given action develops to a μ-agonist, such as morphine, some cross-tolerance is seen with other μ-agonists. The lack of complete cross-tolerance to the analgesic actions among the μ-agonists may be a result of their binding to subtypes of μ receptors. However, when tolerance develops to a selective κ-agonist, such as the investigational drug U-50, 488, there is no cross-tolerance to μ-agonists. Similarly, opioid withdrawal phenomena can be suppressed by any opioid that acts at the same receptor but not by one that acts at another receptor; κ-agonists do not suppress withdrawal from μ-agonist–induced physical dependence. Furthermore, physical dependence induced by κ-agonists has distinct characteristics and a different pattern of withdrawal signs and symptoms.

Physical (Physiological) Dependence Physical dependence is a substance-induced change in a biological system that becomes manifest by a characteristic response pattern, the withdrawal syndrome, when the drug is removed from the body or is displaced from its receptor. In general, responses are opposite in direction to the acute agonistic effects of the drugs, that is, they are rebound hyperexcitabilities. The neuroadaptive changes induced by the repeated administration of opioids occur in cells bearing opioid receptors and in neural systems that are widespread throughout the organism. In humans, the changes begin with the first few doses. For example, if single, intramuscular (IM) doses of 15 to 18 mg of morphine are given to opioid-naïve subjects or abstinent former opioid users, large doses of naloxone (Narcan, Suboxone) (10 to 30 mg) given within 24 hours precipitate a mild μ-agonist withdrawal syndrome. However, some period of continuous receptor occupation is required before the syndrome produced by abrupt cessation reaches an intensity level high enough to be obvious to the clinical observer. Withdrawal phenomena are more intense and more readily detectable when the opioid is rapidly removed from its receptor, as happens with opioid antagonist administration.

Opioids are distinct from other classes of pharmacological agents in that not only does opioid physical dependence develop rapidly, but there also appears to be a protracted period of physiological abnormality that follows the acute opioid withdrawal syndrome. This long-lasting *protracted abstinence* syndrome, characterized by hypophoria, irritability, mood instability, and recurrent urges to use opioids, is postulated to result from opioid-induced alterations in endogenous opioid peptide systems, opioid receptors, or other intracellular proteins that are produced in neurons exposed to opioids over long periods. However, long-lasting neuronal changes can also result from indirect actions of opioids. A reduction in the size of dopaminergic neurons in the VTA has been observed in animals administered morphine over long periods. The postwithdrawal state is also characterized by HPA stress axis instability. It is postulated that the protracted abstinence syndrome and sensitivity to stress are responsible for the high rate of relapse after withdrawal.

Mechanisms of Tolerance and Physical Dependence Chronic administration of opioids induces changes in neuronal systems, several of which probably play important roles in tolerance, physical dependence, or both. Acute administration of μ or δ opioids results in G-protein–mediated inhibition of adenylyl cyclase and a decrease in cAMP concentra-

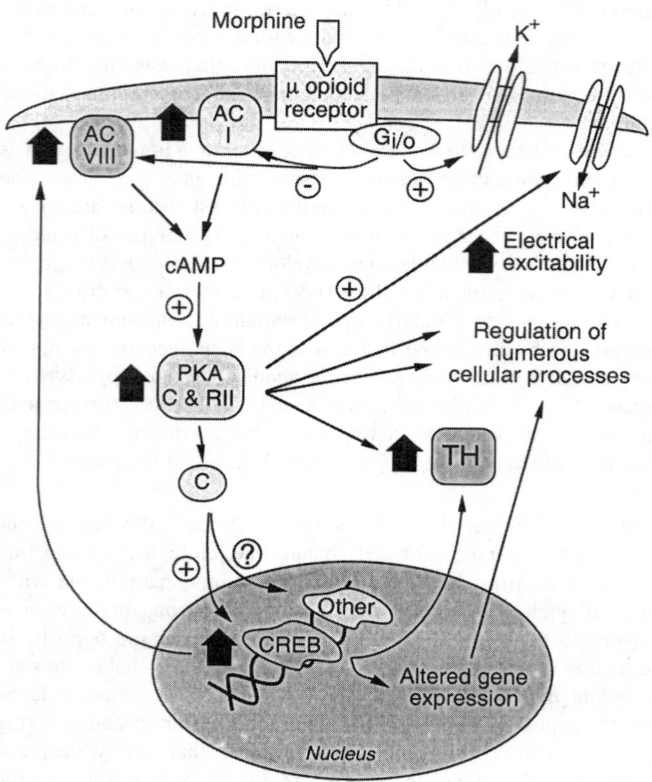

FIGURE 11.10–2 Scheme illustrating opiate actions in the locus ceruleus (LC). Opiates acutely inhibit LC neurons by increasing the conductance of an inwardly rectifying K^+ channel via coupling with subtypes of $G_{i/o}$ and by decreasing a Na^+-dependent inward current via coupling with $G_{i/o}$ and the consequent inhibition of adenylyl cyclase (AC). Reduced levels of cyclic adenosine monophosphate (cAMP) decrease protein kinase A (PKA) activity and the phosphorylation of the responsible channel or pump. Inhibition of the cAMP pathway also decreases phosphorylation of numerous other proteins and thereby affects many additional processes in the neuron. For example, it reduces the phosphorylation state of cAMP response element binding protein (CREB), which may initiate some of the longer-term changes in LC function. Upward bold arrows summarize effects of chronic morphine in the LC. Chronic morphine increases levels of AC type I (AC I) and type VIII (AC VIII), PKA catalytic (C) and regulatory type II (RII) subunits, and several phosphoproteins, including CREB and tyrosine hydroxylase (TH), the rate-limiting enzyme in norepinephrine biosynthesis. These changes contribute to the altered phenotype for the drug-addicted state. For example, the intrinsic excitability of LC neurons is increased via enhanced activity of the cAMP pathway and Na^+-dependent inward current, which contributes to the tolerance, dependence, and withdrawal exhibited by these neurons. Upregulation of AC VIII and TH is mediated via CREB, whereas upregulation of AC I and the PKA subunits appears to occur via a CREB-independent mechanism not yet identified. (From Nestler EJ: Molecular neurobiology of addiction. *Am J Addict.* 2001;10:201, with permission.)

tions. With chronic administration, there is a compensatory increase in the expression of adenylyl cyclase and the cAMP-dependent protein kinase probably mediated by effects on transcription factors such as CREB (Fig. 11.10–2). When the opioid is removed, these changes result in transiently higher cAMP concentrations and increased cellular activity.

Some aspects of withdrawal, such as excess sympathetic nervous system activation, have been attributed to the hyperexcitability that results from such an upregulation of the cAMP system in the noradrenergic neurons of the locus ceruleus. These neurons express opioid receptors, and their activity is inhibited by opioid administration. Similar changes in the cAMP pathway occur in GABAergic neurons that normally inhibit the dopaminergic neurons of the VTA. These GABAergic neurons become hyperactive during withdrawal, and the resulting inhibition of the dopaminergic pathway probably accounts, in part, for the dysphoria of acute opioid withdrawal. The opioid receptor–bearing neurons of the NAc are also affected by the upregulation of the cAMP pathway and become less sensitive to neural input that mediates reward. In animals, chronic opioid use reduces neurofilament proteins and the average size of dopamine neurons in the VTA. These changes may contribute to the hypofunctioning of the VTA and to the protracted hypophoria that is sometimes reported after opioid withdrawal.

The observation that certain α_2-adrenergic agonists such as clonidine (Catapres) or lofexidine, like opioids, can inhibit the activity of neurons in the locus ceruleus formed the background for the clinical use of α-adrenergic agonists in opioid withdrawal. These agents can suppress some of the symptoms of opioid withdrawal but are not effective in reducing dysphoria, craving, or muscle cramps.

Some aspects of tolerance may be attributable to an internalization of the μ and δ opioid receptors or to the functional decoupling of opioid receptors from their mediating G proteins. Long-term administration of opioids can upregulate G-protein receptor kinases, which, in turn, can produce a desensitization of opioid receptors (Fig. 11.10–2).

Another consequence of repeated opioid use is the intracellular accumulation of long-lasting fos-related antigens that appear to account for the development of sensitization. The mechanism may involve fos-induced changes in the makeup of a glutamate (α-amino-3-hydroxy-5-methyl-4-isoxazole propionic acid [AMPA]) receptor subunit. Glutamate receptors are involved in the neural plasticity underlying some forms of opioid tolerance, physical dependence, and sensitization. Antagonists of the ionotropic *N*-methyl-D-aspartate (NMDA) receptor inhibit the development of opioid tolerance and dependence. NMDA antagonists also inhibit conditioned opioid reward. However, the clinical usefulness of most NMDA antagonists is limited by their phencyclidine (PCP)-like side effects. Recent work has found that blockade of metabotropic glutamate receptors also inhibits the development of morphine tolerance and dependence.

Learning and Conditioning

Opioids are positive reinforcers of drug self-administration. They can also reinforce drug-seeking behavior by terminating noxious or aversive states, such as pain, anxiety, or depression (negative reinforcement). In some social situations, the use of the drug can also be reinforcing if it results in gaining special status among friends, and such social reinforcement can serve to maintain drug use until the effects of primary reinforcement or reinforcement by alleviation of withdrawal symptoms come into play. Typically, each time the drug is used, reinforcement occurs. It may be the rush, drug-induced euphoria, or alleviation of disturbed affect or of withdrawal symptoms, or a combination of those effects. Use of a short-acting opioid, such as heroin, causes such reinforcement to occur several times a day, day after day, creating a powerfully reinforced habit pattern. Eventually, the paraphernalia and hustling associated with drug use can become secondary reinforcers, as well as cues that signal drug availability, and, in their presence, craving or desire to experience drug effects increases.

In addition to this operant reinforcement of drug-using and drug-seeking behaviors, classical or pavlovian conditioning probably plays a role in relapse. In laboratory animals and human volunteers, opioid withdrawal phenomena can be conditioned to environmental or interoceptive stimuli. Animals that exhibit marked tolerance to the effects of opioids given repeatedly in one situation may exhibit toxicity when the same dose is administered in a novel environment. For long periods after withdrawal, former opioid addicts may experience conditioned withdrawal or conditioned craving when exposed to environmental stimuli previously linked to drug use or withdrawal. Conditions associated with drug use, such as watching someone else use heroin or being offered a drug by a friend, rather than conditions associated with withdrawal, elicit the most intense craving.

Integrating Neurobiology and Learning Several efforts aimed at integrating neurobiology and learning to better explain compulsive drug use and the tendency to relapse after withdrawal are described in Section 11.1 (overview). Each of these efforts at synthesis is well grounded in biological and behavioral data. They are briefly summarized here. One perspective views addiction as "a cycle of spiraling dysregulation of brain reward systems," a condition in which there is a shift from homeostasis to a new, abnormal, homeostatic set point—an allostatic state. This view places emphasis on the interactions between persistent hypofunction of the neural systems subserving hedonic tone and protracted instability and increased sensitivity of the HPA stress axis. Increased sensitivity to environmental stressors and release of CRF produce responses in the dopaminergic system that are functionally equivalent to priming doses of a drug. Another perspective emphasizes the importance of drug-induced neuronal sensitization, postulating that there is a parallel sensitization in the neural systems that subserve the assignment of salience to environmental stimuli previously associated with drug use and drug effects. As a result of this sensitization, drug-related stimuli become more salient in terms of directing behavior and are perceived as *wanting* or *craving*. Still another effort at integration incorporates data from brain imaging studies of addict volunteers that have shown decreased volume in prefrontal cortex. This brain region normally inhibits activity in the amygdala, a key area involved in emotionally charged memories, including those of the rewarding effects of drugs elicited by drug related stimuli. This view hypothesizes that, in the addicted state, not only do drug-related stimuli evoke craving, but also the capacity of frontal cortex to inhibit the usual behavioral responses elicited by craving has been diminished.

Psychological and Social Factors Social attitudes, peer pressure, and drug availability are the major determinants of experimentation with the less socially disapproved drugs. Generally, the use of tobacco, alcohol, and cannabis precedes the use of cocaine and opioids. Because, in most cases, the earlier substance use continues, most opioid or cocaine users are really multiple drug users. The presence of a significant number of opioid users in a neighborhood, town, or city creates a subculture supportive of experimentation, and continuing use of the drug usually follows. In the United States, areas in which availability of illicit opioids is high also have high crime rates, high unemployment rates, and demoralized school systems. These factors all contribute to the sense of hopelessness and the low self-esteem that reduce resistance to drug use and militate against a good prognosis once dependence develops. Along with family factors, these factors may contribute to disproportionately high rates of heroin addiction currently seen among African-American and Hispanic minorities.

A unique natural experiment in which the influence of vulnerability, social norms, and, particularly, availability could be observed was provided by the experience of U.S. service personnel who used heroin in Vietnam. During the period between 1970 and 1972, high-grade, low-cost heroin was readily available to young men separated from their families and usual social norms. Among U.S. Army enlisted men, approximately 42 percent tried heroin, and approximately one-half of those who did became physically dependent. Very few of these men, however, continued to use heroin after their return to civilian life. The importance of availability in the genesis of addiction to opioids is also illustrated by the high rates of opioid addiction among physicians, dentists, and nurses compared to other professionals with comparable educational achievement but less easy access to opioids.

Psychodynamic Factors and Psychopathology The psychodynamic perspective is that psychopathology is the underlying motivation for initial drug use, drug dependence, and relapse after a period of abstinence. More recent psychoanalytic formulations postulate ego defects, which are manifest in the addict's inability to manage painful affects (guilt, anger, and anxiety) and to avoid preventable medical, legal, and financial problems. Some addicts also appear to have great difficulty in differentiating and describing what they feel, a difficulty that has been aptly called *alexithymia* (i.e., no words for feelings). It is postulated that, pharmacologically and symbolically, opioid use helps the ego control those affects and that drug use can be viewed as a form of self-medication.

Epidemiological studies find that persons who use illicit drugs, especially those who use opioids, tend to place more value on independence and less value on academic achievement. They are also more tolerant of deviance, and a substantial number showed significant signs of delinquency before their first experimentation with opioids. A significant proportion of opioid users meet the criteria for antisocial personality disorder, even when those items that are related to illicit drug use are not applied. In Vietnam, where heroin was readily available, the use of heroin by American service personnel was powerfully predicted by the same factors that predicted use in the United States: the frequency and severity of preservice fighting, truancy, drunkenness, arrest, and school expulsion. The ECA Study and the NCS found that persons with a diagnosis of drug dependence or alcohol abuse were much more likely than were those without such a diagnosis to also have at least one other mental disorder that was present in the absence of drugs or alcohol. The rates of coexistent psychiatric disorders and substance abuse and findings of high rates of coexistent psychiatric disorders among opioid users seeking treatment do not prove causality; drug use could and does increase the risk of psychopathology. However, these data strongly support the argument that many persons are left at higher risk for initial treatment failure or relapse if treatment efforts are aimed solely at the drug-using behavior itself.

Family Factors More than 50 percent of urban heroin addicts come from single-parent families, and poor parental functioning has been consistently reported as a risk factor for opioid addiction. A retrospective study of urban men in an East Coast city compared heroin addicts, never-addicted peer controls who were associates of the addicts at 11 years of age, and never-addicted members of the community who were not associates of the addicts. Family risk factors involving deviant behaviors among family members and disruption of family structure (biological parents who had never lived together or were divorced, separated, or died before the subject reached 11 years of age) were 50 percent higher among the heroin addicts.

Typically, even in two-parent families, there are disturbed family relationships, with one parent, usually of the opposite sex, intensely involved with the addict and the other parent distant, absent, or punitive. Cross-generational alliances between the drug user and one parent against another parental figure are common. The disability of the drug-using member of the family often serves as a focus for communication among other members and sometimes may be the main motive for their remaining together; thus, the family equilibrium may be threatened by the addict's recovery.

Despite their seeming rebelliousness and precocious efforts to be independent, opioid users often remain dependent on and in close communication with families of origin well into adulthood. Interestingly, both male and female heroin addicts believe that members of their families of origin or their in-laws would be the most helpful to them in their efforts to give up drugs. Rates of alcohol and drug abuse, mental illness, and antisocial personality disorder are higher in the families of heroin users. Relatives of depressed opioid addicts tend to have higher rates of depression and anxiety but not of other disorders.

Vulnerability and Genetic Factors

Not everyone who uses an opioid becomes dependent. There is now evidence for common, drug-specific, and genetically transmitted vulnerability factors that increase the likelihood of developing drug dependence. Individuals who abuse a substance from any category are more likely to abuse substances from other categories. The common vulnerability factor is influenced by family and nonfamily environmental factors. In a study of Vietnam-era veterans, monozygotic twins were more likely than dizygotic twins to be concordant for opioid dependence. Multivariate modeling techniques indicated that not only was the genetic contribution high for heroin abuse in this group, but also a higher proportion of the variance due to genetic factors was not shared with the common vulnerability factor—that is, it was specific for opioids. A study of twins in Virginia found evidence for a common genetic vulnerability factor that influenced the likelihood that drug use would progress to dependence, but did not find a genetic vulnerability that was drug specific.

DIAGNOSIS AND CLINICAL FEATURES

Table 11.10–1 lists the DSM-IV-TR opioid-related disorders.

Opioid Intoxication

DSM-IV-TR criteria for opioid intoxication are shown in Table 11.10–2.

Opioid intoxication can vary in severity. In severe cases of opioid overdose, there is usually coma, severely depressed respiration, and pinpoint pupils. There may be gross pulmonary edema with frothing at the mouth, but X-ray evidence of pulmonary changes is seen even in less severe cases. Pulmonary edema is an opioid effect and is sometimes seen with overdoses of oral opioids that have been medically prescribed. Depending on when the patient is seen, there may also be cyanosis, cold clammy skin, and decreased body temperature. Blood pressure is decreased but only falls dramatically with severe anoxia, at which point the pupils may dilate. Cardiac arrhythmias have been reported and may be related to anoxia or to the presence of quinine as an adulterant in the opioid.

Opioid Withdrawal

The opioid withdrawal syndrome can vary greatly in intensity, depending primarily on the level of physical dependence (i.e., the chronic dose of the opioid used), the degree to which the opioid effects on the CNS were continuously exerted, the duration of use, and the rate at which the opioid is removed from the receptors. These generalizations appear to apply as well to other categories of drugs, such as barbiturates and benzodiazepines. The DSM-IV-TR diagnostic criteria for opioid withdrawal are shown in Table 11.10–3.

Although there are numerous signs and symptoms associated with opioid withdrawal, not all are uniformly present across withdrawal episodes—there can be considerable variability between persons in the particular cluster of symptoms exhibited during opioid withdrawal.

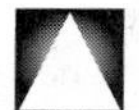

Table 11.10–1
DSM-IV-TR Opioid-Related Disorders

Opioid use disorders
Opioid dependence
Opioid abuse
Opioid-induced disorders
Opioid intoxication
Specify if:
With perceptual disturbances
Opioid withdrawal
Opioid intoxication delirium
Opioid-induced psychotic disorder, with delusions
Specify if:
With onset during intoxication
Opioid-induced psychotic disorder, with hallucinations
Specify if:
With onset during intoxication
Opioid-induced mood disorder
Specify if:
With onset during intoxication
Opioid-induced sexual dysfunction
Specify if:
With onset during intoxication
Opioid-induced sleep disorder
Specify if:
With onset during intoxication
With onset during withdrawal
Opioid-related disorder not otherwise specified

From American Psychiatric Association. *Diagnostic and Statistical Manual of Mental Disorders.* 4th ed. Text rev. Washington, DC: American Psychiatric Association; 2000, with permission.

The opioid withdrawal syndrome consists of purposive behavior, which is dependent on the observer and environment (e.g., complaints, pleas, and manipulations directed at getting more drug), and nonpurposive behavior (e.g., piloerection and dilated pupils), which is not goal oriented and is relatively independent of the observer and

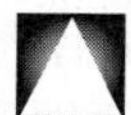

Table 11.10–2
DSM-IV-TR Diagnostic Criteria for Opioid Intoxication

A. Recent use of an opioid.
B. Clinically significant maladaptive behavioral or psychological changes (e.g., initial euphoria followed by apathy, dysphoria, psychomotor agitation or retardation, impaired judgment, or impaired social or occupational functioning) that developed during, or shortly after, opioid use.
C. Pupillary constriction (or pupillary dilation due to anoxia from severe overdose) and one (or more) of the following signs, developing during, or shortly after, opioid use:
(1) Drowsiness or coma
(2) Slurred speech
(3) Impairment in attention or memory
D. The symptoms are not due to a general medical condition and are not better accounted for by another mental disorder.

Specify if:
With perceptual disturbances.

From American Psychiatric Association. *Diagnostic and Statistical Manual of Mental Disorders.* 4th ed. Text rev. Washington, DC: American Psychiatric Association; 2000, with permission.

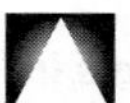

Table 11.10–3
DSM-IV-TR Diagnostic Criteria for Opioid Withdrawal

A. Either of the following:
  (1) Cessation of (or reduction in) opioid use that has been heavy and prolonged (several weeks or longer)
  (2) Administration of an opioid antagonist after a period of opioid use.

B. Three (or more) of the following, developing within minutes to several days after Criterion A:
  (1) Dysphoric mood
  (2) Nausea or vomiting
  (3) Muscle aches
  (4) Lacrimation or rhinorrhea
  (5) Pupillary dilation, piloerection, or sweating
  (6) Diarrhea
  (7) Yawning
  (8) Fever
  (9) Insomnia

C. The symptoms in Criterion B cause clinically significant distress or impairment in social, occupational, or other important areas of functioning.

D. The symptoms are not due to a general medical condition and are not better accounted for by another mental disorder.

From American Psychiatric Association. *Diagnostic and Statistical Manual of Mental Disorders.* 4th ed. Text rev. Washington, DC: American Psychiatric Association; 2000, with permission.

environment. The opioid withdrawal syndrome, although often exquisitely uncomfortable and distressing, is not, in contrast to withdrawal from alcohol or barbiturates, life threatening in healthy adults. Deaths have occurred during abrupt opioid withdrawal in debilitated patients with other medical disorders.

In the case of short-acting μ-agonist opioids, such as morphine or heroin, the first symptoms may be seen within 8 to 12 hours after the last dose of drug. In the least severe cases or early in withdrawal, symptoms may consist only of dysphoria, irritability, restlessness, and general achiness, with few objective signs. In mild syndromes, the signs and symptoms may be limited to craving, anxiety, dysphoria, yawning, perspiration, lacrimation, rhinorrhea, and restless and broken sleep. In more severe cases, as the syndrome progresses, additional signs and symptoms that may be seen include increasingly dilated pupils, piloerection (waves of gooseflesh, from which comes the term *cold turkey* to describe withdrawal), and hot and cold flashes. In severe syndromes, which, in the case of heroin and morphine, generally reach peak severity approximately 48 hours after the last dose, the patient may also experience nausea, vomiting, diarrhea, weight loss, fever (usually low grade), and increased blood pressure, pulse, and respiratory rate. Also often observed are twitching of muscles and kicking movements of the lower extremities (from which comes the phrase *kicking the habit*). It is important to remember that substantial subjective distress can develop before the more obvious physical signs. Also, when so motivated, opioid-dependent patients in early withdrawal may exaggerate the severity of distress in the hope that it will elicit higher doses of drugs for relief.

With short-acting drugs, the acute phase of the syndrome, if untreated, runs its course in 7 to 10 days. In research subjects, the acute phase was followed by a more subtle but longer-lasting phase, the protracted abstinence syndrome, that persisted for many weeks. During this phase, many physiological variables reached subnormal values, such as hyposensitivity to the respiratory stimulant effects of carbon dioxide. There was also disturbed sleep, overconcern about bodily discomfort, poor self-image, and a decreased capacity to tolerate stress. It is frequently assumed that the protracted abstinence syndrome plays a role in relapse to opioid use.

With longer-acting μ-agonist opioids such as methadone or levomethadyl acetate (ORLAAM), also known as *l*-alpha acetylmethadol (LAAM), the onset of withdrawal may be delayed for 1 to 3 days after the last dose. Although the syndrome is qualitatively similar, peak symptoms may not occur until the third to eighth day, and the symptoms may persist for several weeks.

Withdrawal from methadone, and presumably from levomethadyl acetate, is also followed by a protracted abstinence syndrome that may last for more than 6 months. If naloxone is given to a patient dependent on methadone, thereby displacing the drug abruptly from the receptors, the withdrawal is immediate in onset, can be quite severe, and persists until the naloxone is metabolized, and the residual methadone reoccupies the receptors. This phenomenon is called *precipitated withdrawal* (in contrast to spontaneous withdrawal, which occurs on abrupt cessation or a marked reduction in chronic opioid use).

Opioid withdrawal symptoms can occur after several weeks of 8 mg daily of parenteral or sublingual buprenorphine, a partial μ-agonist opioid, but such symptoms are generally not severe, although some patients are uncomfortable enough to request medications for relief of discomfort and for insomnia. After sublingual administration of 8 mg daily of buprenorphine, withdrawal symptoms are experienced within a few days after drug use is stopped, and symptoms of the acute phase reach baseline levels by 7 to 10 days. Symptoms are usually mild and consist primarily of subjective effects, such as muscle aches, dysphoria, and insomnia, rather than more dramatic autonomic signs, such as piloerection or diarrhea. If larger doses of buprenorphine have been taken (16 to 32 mg or more sublingually), drug effects can persist for several days, with onset of withdrawal symptoms delayed for 96 hours or more. This feature of buprenorphine has led to its use on an intermittent basis in some patients (e.g., at intervals of 48 to 96 hours).

Opioid Abuse and Opioid Dependence

Opioid abuse is a pattern of maladaptive use of an opioid drug leading to clinically significant impairment or distress and occurring within a 12-month period, but one in which the symptoms have never met the criteria for opioid dependence.

Opioid dependence is inferred from behaviors that indicate some decrease in volitional control over the use of an opioid drug. DSM-IV-TR specifies the criteria to be used by the clinician to decide whether the patient exhibits such a decrease in volitional control. These criteria are not specific for opioids but are believed to apply for all psychoactive agents. DSM-IV-TR does not require that any single criterion be met, and none is given special weight. Thus, the presence of tolerance and physical dependence (withdrawal) is not required. However, according to DSM-IV-TR, if tolerance and physical dependence are present, they should be noted specifically.

Because tolerance develops to many of the actions of opioid drugs after long-term use, opioid effects are not readily detected by even the careful observer. Patients maintained on large oral doses of methadone function quite normally. Physicians, nurses, and other medical personnel who use opioids, even by injection, may go undetected by their colleagues for months or years. Thus, a candid history obtained from the patient or a reliable informant is needed to make a diagnosis of dependence, although evidence of recent and long-term use can be developed by testing urine or hair for the presence of opioids.

Opioid Intoxication Delirium

Opioid intoxication delirium is most likely to happen when opioids are used in high doses, are mixed with other psychoactive compounds, or are used by a person with preexisting brain damage. Certain opioids, such as meperidine, have toxic metabolites that can accumulate, causing delirium and sometimes causing seizures. Impaired renal function increases the likelihood of accumulation.

Opioid-Induced Psychotic Disorder Opioid-induced psychotic disorder can begin during opioid intoxication. The DSM-IV-TR diagnostic criteria are contained in the section on schizophrenia and other psychotic disorders. Clinicians can specify whether hallucinations or delusions are the predominant symptoms and whether the onset occurs during intoxication or withdrawal.

Opioid-Induced Mood Disorder Opioid-induced mood disorder can begin during opioid intoxication or withdrawal and can result from chronic use (Table 11.10–3). Opioid-induced mood disorder symptoms may be of a manic, depressed, or mixed nature. A person coming to psychiatric attention with opioid-induced mood disorder usually has mixed symptoms, combining irritability, expansiveness, and depression.

Some degree of depressed mood (hypophoria) typically occurs during and for several weeks after opioid withdrawal. Opioid-induced mood disorder should not be diagnosed after opioid withdrawal unless the severity of mood disturbance exceeds what is normally encountered or persists for more than a few weeks and is of sufficient intensity to warrant independent clinical attention.

Opioid-Induced Sleep Disorder and Opioid-Induced Sexual Dysfunction Opioid-induced sleep disorder and opioid-induced sexual dysfunction are diagnostic categories in DSM-IV-TR. Hypersomnia is likely to be a more common sleep disorder among those given opioids therapeutically, but disturbed sleep (insomnia) is a common complaint of patients maintained on opioid agonists such as methadone. The most common sexual dysfunction is likely to be impotence, but patients maintained on methadone may complain of inability to achieve orgasm, rather than impotence.

Opioid-Related Disorder Not Otherwise Specified DSM-IV-TR includes diagnoses for opioid-related disorders with symptoms of delirium, abnormal mood, psychosis, abnormal sleep, and sexual dysfunction. Clinical situations that do not fit into these categories are examples of appropriate cases for the use of the DSM-IV-TR diagnosis of opioid-related disorder not otherwise specified (Table 11.10–4).

Psychiatric Comorbidity The high prevalence of additional psychiatric disorders among treated opioid-dependent patients has now been repeatedly confirmed. Currently, no subtypology of opioid-dependent patients based on psychopathology has been proposed. However, the type and severity of those additional diagnoses can influence the course of the disorder and the kind of treatment that is most likely to be effective.

Among opioid addicts seeking treatment at a program in New Haven in the 1980s, 87 percent met the Research Diagnostic Criteria (RDC) for a psychiatric disorder, in addition to opioid dependence, at some point in their lives. Other substance-related diagnoses, such as alcohol dependence, were considered additional disorders. A study of addicts seeking methadone treatment in Baltimore in the early 1990s found (using DSM-III-R criteria) a 24 percent lifetime prevalence of non–substance-related Axis I disorders, a 35 percent lifetime prevalence of Axis II disorders, and a total prevalence of additional non–substance-related diagnoses of 47 percent. In both studies, the most common diagnoses were mood disorders, alcoholism, antisocial personality disorder, and anxiety disorders (Tables 11.10–5, 11.10–6, and 11.10–7).

In the Baltimore study, cocaine dependence (65 percent) was actually higher than alcohol dependence (50 percent). Multiple psychiatric diagnoses for a given patient were common. Researchers in Europe and Australia report similar overall distributions of psychiatric disorders among opioid users seeking treatment.

Among women, depression, anxiety disorders, and borderline personality disorder were significantly more common than among male patients, and alcoholism, cannabis misuse, and antisocial personality disorder were significantly less common. The rates of current psychiatric illnesses are obviously lower than lifetime rates and vary with the treatment setting. Among the methadone patients in the Baltimore study, 5.0 percent of men and 11.2 percent of women met criteria for a current diagnosis of a non–substance-related Axis I disorder, most commonly a mood or anxiety disorder. Forty percent of the sample had a current diagnosis of cocaine dependence, and 25

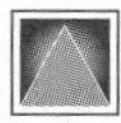

Table 11.10–5
Non–Substance-Related Axis I Psychiatric Disorders in Opioid Users

Diagnostic Category[a]	Lifetime Rate (%) (Current Rate, %) Men (N = 378)	Women (N = 338)	Total
Any Axis I disorder	15.6 (5.0)	33.4 (11.2)	24 (8.0)
Mood disorder	11.4 (2.1)	27.5 (5.3)	19.0 (3.6)
Major depressive disorder	8.7 (1.3)	23.7 (5.3)	15.8 (3.2)
Dysthymic disorder	2.4 (2.4)	4.4 (4.4)	3.4 (3.4)
Bipolar I disorder	0.8 (0.8)	0 (0)	0.4 (0.4)
Anxiety disorder	6.1 (3.4)	10.7 (6.8)	8.2 (5.0)
Simple phobia	1.9 (1.9)	5.3 (3.6)	3.5 (2.7)
Social phobia	1.9 (0.8)	3.6 (2.7)	2.7 (1.7)
Panic disorder	2.1 (0.3)	1.8 (0.9)	2 (0.6)
Agoraphobia	0 (0)	0.6 (0.3)	0.3 (0.1)
Obsessive-compulsive disorder	0.5 (0.5)	0 (0)	0.3 (0.3)
General anxiety disorder	0.8 (0.8)	0 (0)	0.1 (0.1)
Eating disorders	0 (0)	1.5 (0)	0.7 (0)
Bulimia nervosa	0 (0)	0.9 (0)	0.4 (0)
Anorexia nervosa	0 (0)	0.6 (0)	0.3 (0)
Schizophrenia	0 (0)	0.3 (0.3)	0.1 (0.1)

[a]Multiple disorders possible.
Adapted from Brooner RK, King VL, Kidorf M, et al: Psychiatric and substance use comorbidity among treatment-seeking opioid abusers. *Arch Gen Psychiatry.* 1997;54:71.

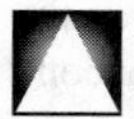

Table 11.10–4
DSM-IV-TR Diagnostic Criteria for Opioid-Related Disorder Not Otherwise Specified

The opioid-related disorder not otherwise specified category is for disorders associated with the use of opioids that are not classifiable as opioid dependence, opioid abuse, opioid intoxication, opioid withdrawal, opioid intoxication delirium, opioid-induced psychotic disorder, opioid-induced mood disorder, opioid-induced sexual dysfunction, or opioid-induced sleep disorder.

From American Psychiatric Association. *Diagnostic and Statistical Manual of Mental Disorders.* 4th ed. Text rev. Washington, DC: American Psychiatric Association; 2000, with permission.

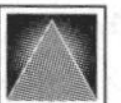

Table 11.10–6
Substance Use Disorders in Opioid Users

Diagnostic Category[a]	Lifetime Rate (%) (Current Rate, (%) Men (N = 378)	Women (N = 338)	Total
Opioid dependence	100 (100)	100 (100)	100 (100)
Cocaine			
Dependence	66.1 (39.4)	63.0 (41.1)	64.7 (40.2)
Abuse	13.0 (3.7)	11.8 (3)	12.4 (3.4)
Cannabis			
Dependence	58.7 (19.8)	42.0 (12.1)	50.8 (16.2)
Abuse	17.7 (2.6)	12.1 (2.1)	14.9 (2.4)
Alcohol			
Dependence	56.6 (29.4)	43.2 (19.5)	50.3 (24.7)
Abuse	16.1 (2.6)	9.5 (0.9)	13.0 (1.8)
Sedative			
Dependence	47.9 (17.2)	40.8 (16.6)	46.6 (16.9)
Abuse	15.3 (1.3)	10.4 (1.8)	13.0 (1.5)
Stimulant			
Dependence	19.0 (0)	19.2 (0.6)	19.1 (0.3)
Abuse	15.6 (0)	7.1 (0)	11.6 (0)
Hallucinogen			
Dependence	21.2 (1.1)	14.2 (0.3)	17.9 (0.7)
Abuse	12.7 (0)	5.6 (0)	9.4 (0)
Other substance[b]			
Dependence	15.1 (2.6)	12.7 (2.7)	14.0 (2.6)
Abuse	7.9 (0.5)	4.7 (0.6)	6.4 (0.6)

[a]Multiple diagnoses possible.
[b]Primarily inhalants, clonidine, and promethazine.
Adapted from Brooner RK, King VL, Kidorf M, et al: Psychiatric and substance use comorbidity among treatment-seeking opioid abusers. *Arch Gen Psychiatry.* 1997;54:71.

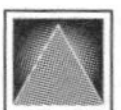

Table 11.10–7
Personality Disorders in Opioid Users

Diagnostic Category[a]	Lifetime Rate (%) Men (N = 378)	Women (N = 338)	Total
Any personality disorder	40.5	28.4	34.8
Antisocial	33.9	15.4	25.1
Avoidant	3.4	7.1	5.2
Borderline	1.3	9.5	5.2
Passive-aggressive	3.7	4.4	4.1
Paranoid	4.5	1.8	3.2
Dependent	0.5	3.0	1.7
Histrionic	0.8	2.1	1.4
Narcissistic	1.6	0.0	0.8
Obsessive-compulsive	1.1	0.3	0.7
Schizotypal	0.3	0.3	0.3
Schizoid	0.3	0.3	0.3

[a]Multiple disorders possible.
Adapted from Brooner RK, King VL, Kidorf M, et al: Psychiatric and substance use comorbidity among treatment-seeking opioid abusers. *Arch Gen Psychiatry.* 1997;54:71.

percent concurrently experienced alcoholism. Other studies have confirmed rates of current major depressive disorder in the range of 17 to 20 percent and concurrent rates of alcoholism (alcohol abuse or dependence) of 20 to 30 percent. Although stimulant dependence (other than cocaine dependence) was not seen among the patients in Baltimore, it occurs frequently in the western United States, where methamphetamine use is more prevalent.

The presence of a comorbid psychiatric condition has been shown to be associated with more severe substance abuse in some studies. In the Baltimore study, patients with comorbid psychiatric conditions were more likely to experience polysubstance abuse and to have begun abusing drugs at an earlier age. This was particularly true of patients with antisocial personality disorder.

The high rates of psychiatric comorbidity in the methadone maintenance population are by no means unique to this modality of treatment. Similar patterns of additional psychiatric disorders have been found by workers at other public clinics and by clinicians in private practice. Among patients in therapeutic communities, 60 percent reported depressive symptoms during the year before entry, 28 percent had contemplated suicide, and 13 percent had made at least one suicide attempt. Furthermore, although opioid abusers who have current psychiatric problems are more likely to seek treatment, it should not be assumed that those who do not seek treatment are free of comorbid psychiatric problems. Among the respondents in the community-based ECA study, approximately one-half of those with a substance (other than alcohol) use disorder had one or more additional psychiatric disorders (odds ratio of 4 to 5): anxiety disorder, 28.3 percent (odds ratio of 2 to 5); mood disorder, 26.4 (odds ratio of 4 to 7); antisocial personality, 17.8 percent (odds ratio of 13 to 4); and schizophrenia, 6.8 percent (odds ratio of 6 to 2). The probability of comorbidity is higher for those with a lifetime diagnosis of an opioid or cocaine disorder than for those who abuse cannabis. Widespread comorbidity was again found in the similar NCS study: 59 percent of those with a lifetime history of illicit drug abuse or dependence also met DSM-IV-TR criteria for another mental disorder, and 71 percent met the criteria for a lifetime alcohol use disorder.

PATHOLOGY AND LABORATORY EXAMINATION

In opioid abuse and opioid dependence, there may be no abnormal laboratory findings at all. Standard urine tests for heroin actually test for its main metabolite, morphine, and can usually detect morphine (heroin) for 12 to 36 hours after use. A urine test that is positive for morphine can also be caused by therapeutic doses of codeine or by the ingestion of modest amounts of poppy seeds (of the type and amount used to flavor bagels and other breads and pastries). Potent opioids, such as fentanyl (Actiq), may not be detected by standard opioid urine screens. If it is suspected that a specific opioid is being abused, it can be useful to check with a laboratory to ensure that the proper urine test is obtained, as not all opioids react with the test for morphine (e.g., methadone). Opioids with longer half-lives, such as methadone, may be detected for longer periods (4 or more days in the case of methadone) on a urine screen that tests specifically for such medications. Analysis of hair samples can provide information on drug use over the preceding 2 to 3 months. Samples of oral fluids can detect recent opioid use with approximately the same sensitivity as urine testing.

Persons who have shared injection implements often test positive for hepatitis (B and C) and for HIV. Liver enzyme tests may be elevated if there is active hepatitis. There may be positive and false-positive tests for syphilis. Chest X-rays may show evidence of pulmonary fibrosis if the person has been using injection materials contaminated with microcrystalline talc or cotton particulates. During withdrawal, white blood cell counts and cortisol levels may be elevated.

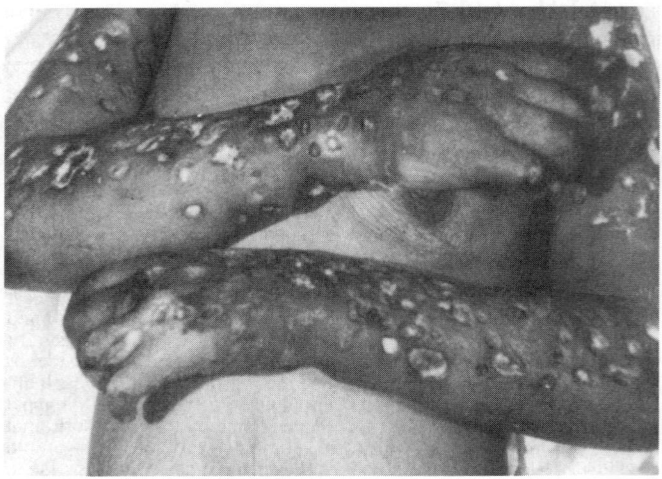

FIGURE 11.10–3 Skin popper. Circular depressed scars, often with underlying chronic abscesses, can result from skin popping. (Courtesy of Michael Baden, M.D.)

Physical findings may be unremarkable if opioids are ingested orally; snorting (insufflation) of heroin may irritate nasal membranes. Drug injectors, however, may show widespread evidence of having used unsterile injection equipment. There may be needle tracks over veins on the arms, legs, and, in some cases, the backs of the hands and the femoral and jugular veins. Infections and venous scleroses and lymph obstruction may lead to severe edema of the hands and feet. There may be skin abscesses or scars on accessible skin surfaces as a result of unsterile subcutaneous injections (Fig. 11.10–3). There may be rock-like hardening of subcutaneous and muscle tissue as a result of repeated IM injections of meperidine (often seen among health professionals). Endocarditis may produce fever and heart murmurs. In addition, a variety of neurological sequelae of IV heroin use may be detected.

DIFFERENTIAL DIAGNOSIS

The diagnosis of opioid dependence can be relatively straightforward when the patient is willing to be candid. Conversely, it can be quite taxing when the patient is motivated to conceal past patterns of opioid use, as is frequently the case among health care professionals or persons who obtain opioids from medical sources by simulating disease or greatly exaggerating the painful nature of disease actually present.

The diagnosis of opioid withdrawal is easier when the opioid is short acting and when the symptoms are accompanied by obvious physiological signs (e.g., lacrimation, rhinorrhea, and piloerection). This is not the typical case, and the clinician is often confronted by a patient complaining of various aches, pains, anxiety, and insomnia in the absence of obvious signs of withdrawal. Patients who are dependent on opioids may withhold information on the use of other classes of drugs. Because opioid withdrawal does not generally cause tremulousness, confusion, delirium, or seizures, the presence of those signs or the failure of insomnia and anxiety to respond to reasonable doses of an opioid should raise the possibility of dependence on alcohol, sedatives, or benzodiazepines.

Opioid intoxication must be differentiated from mixed intoxications in which opioids play only a minor role. In general, a failure to respond to modest doses of naloxone suggests that intoxication is caused by a nonopioid. Some patients, more typically the elderly, may respond to therapeutic doses of an μ-agonist with dysphoria and confusion; such reactions are generally short lived. They are seen more commonly with mixed agonist-antagonists. They should be considered atypical opioid intoxications rather than opioid-induced intoxication delirium or opioid-induced psychotic disorders, which, although listed in DSM-IV-TR, are quite rare. One possible exception is the state associated with the accumulation of toxic meperidine metabolites. However, even in that case, the syndrome does not usually outlast the metabolites and should probably be considered intoxication.

COURSE AND PROGNOSIS

It was once commonly believed that experimentation with illicit opioids invariably led to dependence, but it is now apparent that only a fraction of those who briefly experiment with illicit opioids develop serious problems. It is still true that those who use opioid drugs heavily—at least once a week—usually go on to use daily, at least for a brief period. Data from national surveys suggest that approximately one-third of those who experimented with heroin during the epidemic of the 1960s and 1970s became dependent on it at some point. It is likely, however, that many who go on to develop some degree of dependence recover without ever seeking formal treatment. In the St. Louis ECA study, only 20 percent of those with a lifetime history of opioid abuse had any symptom during the year before the interview.

Some persons apparently can use opioids occasionally (e.g., several times a month) over periods of months or years without becoming drug dependent. It may be that self-imposed limits on the time and place that they use drugs may help prevent progression to addiction, but drug injectors are still at risk for death from overdose, as well as for infections and other medical complications. When addiction does develop, the subsequent course of the syndrome depends on environmental factors, the characteristics of the user, the route of administration, and the specific opioid being used.

Heterogeneity of Lifestyle

Opioid addicts seeking or entering treatment in the United States and the United Kingdom exhibit a surprising heterogeneity of lifestyles, attitudes toward conventional values, and criminality. Some addicts, except for their drug use, are quite conventional, avoid criminality, work at legitimate occupations, and do not identify with the addict subculture. At the other extreme, some addicts live exclusively by illicit activities and are highly involved with other addicts. A third group appears to identify with both cultures, engaging in some criminal activities and interacting with other addicts, but living primarily on legitimate earnings. A fourth group of addicts seems not to be involved in the conventional culture or the addict subculture. They tend to be unemployed and to live on welfare, rather than on criminal earnings, and often have high levels of psychopathology. Health professionals and those who become addicted to opioids in the course of medical treatment probably constitute additional distinct subgroups.

Slips and Relapses

In the early stages of opioid use, the most typical course for the user of illicit opioids is one of periods of abstinence, voluntary or forced (by imprisonment or hospitalization), and lasting from a few weeks to many months, followed by relapse to opioid use and readdiction. Among the addicts who enter abstinence-oriented treatments, relapse occurs most often in the first 3 months; a number of studies show that at least two out of three patients relapse within 6 months. Depression and life crises (especially arguments and interpersonal losses) are associated with relapse to illicit drug use; those factors are additive. The impact of those risk factors is reduced by treatment in drug abuse programs.

The theme running through the many specific reasons given for periods of voluntary abstinence is a desire to change life patterns and weariness with the constant difficulty of trying to obtain illicit opioids. At the time of reentry into treatment, addicts are often less seriously impaired than when first treated, suggesting some residual benefit from intermittent treatment. With successful treatment episodes and with age, the duration of each drug using episode tends to shorten.

Repeated relapse is not an inevitable consequence of opioid dependence. A follow-up study of U.S. Army–enlisted personnel who became addicted during a tour of duty in Vietnam found that 88 percent of them did not become readdicted at any time during the 3 years after their return to the United States, and 56 percent had not used opioids at all. Of the soldiers who did become readdicted within the first year, 70 percent were no longer addicted when followed up in the next 2 years. Only 2 percent of the soldiers who used opioids in Vietnam (6 percent of those who tested positive for opioids at time of departure) entered treatment after their return to the United States. However, their relapse rates were as high as for civilians, with two-thirds relapsing within less than 1 year. It is possible that, among those drug users who become opioid dependent, the ones who cannot stop without formal help have a more severe form of the disorder.

In considering the natural history of opioid addiction, a distinction must be made between the course of all those who report a period of dependence (e.g., among respondents to a household survey) and the course of those who enter treatment. Those who enter treatment may have additional problems or a more severe addiction. Furthermore, opioids are rarely the sole class of drugs used. During the 1980s, a high proportion of opioid-dependent patients also abused or became dependent on cocaine. Depression was found to be a risk factor for continued cocaine use among patients in opioid treatment programs (OTPs), and cocaine use itself predicted continued heroin use and earlier discontinuation of methadone treatment. Abstinence from opioids or recovery from opioid dependence does not mean that the person has no drug problems. Standard methadone maintenance treatment programs do not appear to have any major effect in preventing cocaine use, and abuse of alcohol and other nonopioid drugs is common among patients in these programs who are no longer using other opioids.

Long-Term Prognosis

Studies from the United States and the United Kingdom support the view that opioid addiction is a disorder that eventually ends for many of those addicts who survive. This seems to be so even for those who seek treatment, a group that may have a more severe variety of the disorder. For a substantial number of these persons, it is prolonged incarceration that ends their opioid use; others stop using opioids but continue to abuse other drugs. Although there are some old opioid addicts in the United States, their numbers are few. Opinion remains divided as to just how many opioid addicts eventually achieve abstinence outside of an institution. One review of long-term follow-up studies found abstinence rates between 10 and 19 percent for drug-free treatment and between 9 and 21 percent after treatment with methadone. A 33-year follow-up of narcotic addicts remanded to the California Civil Commitment Program in the early 1960s interviewed 242 survivors. Of the original 581 heroin addicts, 49 percent were dead, a death rate more than 50 times greater than age-matched controls. Approximately 20 percent of the 242 who were followed up were currently using heroin, 14 percent were incarcerated, and 56 percent were currently abstinent, but 40 percent had used heroin within the past year. Most of the deaths involved drug-related causes or violence. Among the survivors, many had serious health problems and varying degrees of disability.

The usual measures of treatment outcome—legitimate work, crime, drug use, family relationships, and psychological adjustment—are best predicted by different pretreatment variables. Thus, pretreatment history of high levels of criminal activity most accurately predicts posttreatment criminal activity, and previous stable work history is more predictive of posttreatment gainful employment. Severity of psychological problems at the beginning of treatment, however, is a predictor of outcome on all dimensions. Opioid addicts with the least severe psychological problems appear to respond better to all treatments on all outcome measures.

In long-term follow-ups, no important differences in outcome have been found among patients treated initially by different modalities, although, over shorter follow-up periods, methadone maintenance, therapeutic communities, and drug-free programs were significantly superior to detoxification programs. Differences—or the lack thereof—among different forms of treatment may be affected by pretreatment characteristics of the patient population. For example, studies from the United States and Australia suggest that addicts electing detoxification are younger and have less psychopathology than those entering more lengthy forms of treatment.

Although a period of prolonged abstinence is a good predictor of long-term outcome, a study of heroin users in Texas found that 33 percent of those who reported 3 years of abstinence eventually relapsed. The long-term outcome for opioid dependence among persons with additional major psychiatric disorders, such as schizophrenia or bipolar I disorder, is not generally known. However, one study that specifically examined the efficacy of additional psychiatric care for dual diagnosis subjects in an outpatient drug-dependence clinic found that, although they initially had significantly greater percentages of positive urine toxicologies than patients without comorbid psychiatric conditions, they had higher retention rates in treatment and, after 6 months of treatment, had comparable success rates as the single-diagnosis group. The course of opioid dependence among medical personnel supervised by state-level organizations is far less bleak than that of heroin users who enter public sector treatment programs.

Opioids and Crime

The statistical relation between the use of illicit opioids and crime in the United States is unquestionable. Persons who use illicit opioids commit crimes more frequently than do nonusers. There are, however, questions about the degree to which one behavior causes the other. The direct tranquilizing actions of opioids ought to reduce criminal activity rather than increase it.

Historically, in countries in which crude opioids (e.g., opium and tincture of opium) were inexpensive and socially acceptable and in which it was the custom to smoke them or to take them by mouth, there was little relation between opioid use and criminal behavior. The association between opioid use and crime emerges primarily in countries such as the United States that have tried to restrict the use of opioids to legitimate medical indications but have been unable to eliminate illicit opioid traffic.

Most crimes committed by addicts are directed at getting money for drugs through shoplifting, petty theft, and drug selling; however, drug-related crimes that have the potential for violence, such as robbery, have increased. However, the relationship between drug use and crime is not one of simple cause and effect. In the United States and the United Kingdom, more than 50 percent of heroin addicts interviewed in prisons and jails or treatment programs had been arrested before their first opioid use.

In a study in Baltimore, Maryland, adolescent boys (11 to 14 years of age) who later became opioid addicts exhibited substantially more criminal behavior than did peers or age-matched nonpeers from the same community. As noted previously, there is a high incidence of antisocial personality disorder among drug users, even when the diagnostic criteria for this disorder are limited to exclude antisocial behavior engaged in solely because of the need for drugs. Although it might be argued from these data that the criminal behavior seen after the onset of addiction is merely a continuation of a criminal lifestyle, criminal activity does increase sharply after the onset of opioid addiction. Arrest rates for nondrug offenses increase from 1.5-fold to threefold after the onset of addiction, and self-reported property crimes increase to a comparable degree. However, it has also been suggested that crime is a better predictor of opioid use than opioid use is of crime and that, rather than heavy use causing crime, day-to-day success in crime enables the escalation to heavier opioid use.

Further evidence pointing to a causal relationship between opioid use and crime is the sharp reduction in self-reported criminal activity and arrests during periods of less-than-daily illicit opioid use. The decrease in crime is seen whether the decrease in opioid use is a result of effective treatment, probation, parole, or spontaneous cessation. When criminal behavior antedates opioid use, however, it is unrealistic to expect the successful treatment of opioid dependence to eliminate criminal behavior entirely. Addicts who were criminally active before opioid dependence are more likely to persist in criminal acts when they are abstinent. It is postulated that only more comprehensive treatment directed at social, psychological, and vocational factors, rather than just at illicit drug use, is likely to alter antisocial lifestyles.

Toxicity, Morbidity, Medical Complications, and Life Expectancy Opioids used orally are relatively nontoxic. Whereas long-term use, as in methadone maintenance, is associated with minor endocrine abnormalities, constipation, and some sleep disturbance, no major damage to internal organs has been noted, and no significant impact on longevity would be expected. The cognitive impairment seen with long-term alcohol and sedative use is not generally found with long-term use of oral opioids. Despite the relative safety of opioids, the life expectancy of opioid addicts, especially heroin addicts, is markedly reduced, and there may be some persistent adverse consequences related to periods of anoxia caused by drug overdoses.

Before the emergence of HIV infection among opioid injectors, estimates ranged from a twofold to a threefold increase in the expected mortality rate for older addicts to a 20-fold increase in the expected rate among young addicts. Follow-ups of treated opioid addicts in the United States indicate an overall death rate of 1.0 to 1.5 percent per year. A substantial proportion of those deaths were due to drug overdose, drug-related infections, and suicide. Homicide is also a common cause of death among urban opioid addicts in the United States. The death rate at British clinics providing clean injectable drugs to young addicts was estimated at 2 to 3 percent per year, at least 20-fold higher than the death rate of comparably aged contemporaries. Mortality rates far higher than for age-adjusted controls were also observed in Italy during a period when heroin use was not a criminal offense. The suicide rate among opioid addicts is estimated to be three times higher than in the general population. This is probably an underestimation, because it is difficult to determine how many overdose deaths are, to some degree, intentional. Risk of fatal overdose is significantly increased when tolerance is lost during abstinence, such as occurs during periods of incarceration. Risk may also be increased after discontinuation of treatment with opioid antagonists.

The advent of HIV has changed the patterns of mortality among drug users. In some areas of the United States and Europe, acquired immune deficiency syndrome (AIDS) is now an important factor in mortality among injecting drug users. HIV seroprevalence among users has a wide geographic variability and is lower in those who have been continuously in treatment. Although the death rate of heroin addicts in treatment remains higher than that of age-adjusted controls, it is substantially lower than the rate for untreated addicts.

Medical Complications Opioid drugs, properly administered, are associated with few serious medical complications. Most complications associated with opioid abuse are those associated with the route of administration. Because opioid addicts—even physicians who have access to drugs and sterile materials—tend to neglect the hygienic aspects of injecting, infections of skin and systemic organs are quite common. Filtering illicit opioids through cigarette filters or wads of cotton and injecting materials intended for oral use allows starch, talc, and other particulate contaminants to enter into the bloodstream. These particulates can cause pulmonary emboli, which can eventually result in angiothrombotic pulmonary hypertension and right ventricular failure. Staphylococcal pneumonitis may also be related to septic emboli. Endocarditis and septicemia involving lesions of the tricuspid or the aortic and mitral valves are frequent complications. Less frequent, but equally serious, complications are meningitis and brain abscess. Other frequently seen infections that can be related to injecting the substance or sharing of needles include viral hepatitis (particularly B and C), malaria, tetanus, osteomyelitis, and HIV. Syphilis transmission has also been associated with sharing of needles, although most cases are probably acquired in the usual fashion. False-positive tests for syphilis are also not uncommon among injecting drug abusers. Many opioid addicts who inject have a low-level chronic hepatitis without jaundice and may have abnormal liver function tests. In seroprevalence surveys conducted by the Centers for Disease Control and Prevention (CDC), markers of hepatitis B and C infection have been found in sera from 60 to 80 percent of drug injectors. Abnormal liver function tests, which are found in approximately two out of three heroin addicts, may persist for long periods after the cessation of injection. Comorbid alcoholism may, in some cases, contribute to the liver disease.

Other complications associated with poor IV injecting technique include chronic edema of extremities (e.g., puffy hands), probably due to lymphatic obstruction caused by contaminants and sclerosis of veins caused by the drugs or their dilutants. Chronic lymphadenopathy was common among addicts even before the advent of HIV and was also thought to be related to particulate contaminants. Subcutaneous or intracutaneous injection (known as *skin popping*) may cause widespread ulceration and disfigurement as a result of chemical necrosis or infection (Fig. 11.10–3). These injecting techniques may be used by addicts who have sclerosed their major veins. Some drug users, determined to experience the effects of the drug used IV, switch to the use of femoral and jugular veins when the surface veins of the arms and legs have become unusable. Complications associated with injection of particulate contaminated material include pulmonary hypertension (sometimes leading to cor pulmonale), occasionally seen in heroin smokers.

Additional medical complications are likely to be due to contamination of illicit opioids with other chemical substances. A number of changes found at autopsy, such as degeneration of the globus pallidus and necrosis of spinal gray matter, may fall into this category. Occasionally there are clinical manifestations in those users surviving overdose experiences. Examples are transverse myelitis, amblyopia, plexitis, peripheral neuropathy, parkinsonian syndromes, intellectual impairment, and personality changes. Pathological changes in muscles and degeneration of peripheral nerves have also been seen. Illicit laboratories sometimes produce opioid-like agents that are extremely toxic or that are so potent that even small doses are lethal. For example, 1-methyl-4-phenyl-1,2,3,6-tetrahydropyridine (MPTP), a contaminant of illegally produced meperidine, produces a severe form of parkinsonism by selective destruction of dopaminergic neurons. Although not technically a contaminant, the illicit fentanyl analog, 3-methylfentanyl (known as *China White*), is 1,000 times more potent than morphine and may have been responsible for several hundred overdose deaths.

Opioids can affect heart rhythm by lengthening the QT interval. This effect is caused by inhibition of a specific K^+ ion channel. Large increases in

QT intervals can cause serious arrhythmias, such as torsade des points. Although all opioids may be capable of exerting such effects, LAAM and methadone appear to have the lowest margin of safety, producing QT lengthening at plasma levels that are not far above those achieved in some individuals. Torsades de pointes has been reported with both LAAM and methadone.

HUMAN IMMUNODEFICIENCY VIRUS The finding that not all drug users who shared needles were infected with HIV stimulated vigorous prevention efforts aimed at recruiting patients into treatment and teaching them how to avoid infection by cleaning injection equipment properly, not sharing equipment, and not participating in high-risk sex. Outreach by community workers, coupled with specific instruction, reduces self-reported equipment sharing but has far less effect on high-risk sexual behavior. The question of whether providing injecting drug users with sterile equipment at little or no cost would substantially slow the spread of HIV infection is still controversial, but the available evidence indicates that those who inject drugs will use sterile equipment to avoid disease if the equipment is available at reasonable cost.

TUBERCULOSIS Even before the HIV epidemic, the incidence of tuberculosis was higher among heroin addicts than in the general population. Patients with compromised immune systems are far more vulnerable to developing active tuberculosis once infected, and poor compliance with antitubercular medication has led to the emergence of drug-resistant strains of the tubercle bacillus. Studies indicate that 4 to 21 percent of AIDS patients are infected with tuberculosis.

OPIOIDS AND THE IMMUNE SYSTEM μ-Opioid actions at CNS receptors can produce immunosuppressive effects (e.g., decreased natural killer–cell activity). Opioid receptors are also found on lymphocytes, and naloxone-reversible opioid effects can be demonstrated on white cells in vitro. However, the concentrations required are quite high; it seems unlikely that direct actions on white cells mediate effects on the immune system. In heroin addicts, there are changes in the ratio of helper to suppressor T cells and a suppression of cell-mediated immunity. The relation to opioid use is still unclear; the effects are probably more related to unhygienic injection practices. Natural killer–cell activity and immunoglobulins G and M are within normal limits in former heroin users maintained for several years on methadone, although abnormalities are typically observed among heroin addicts.

TREATMENT

Treatment of Opioid Intoxication (Overdose)

Overdose with an opioid agonist can produce respiratory depression and is therefore a medical emergency. The first task is to ensure an adequate airway. Tracheopharyngeal secretions should be aspirated; an airway may be inserted. The patient should be ventilated mechanically until an opioid antagonist can be administered. There are two approved opioid antagonists (naloxone, nalmefene [Revex]) that can be administered parenterally for reversal of an opioid overdose. Naloxone has a relatively short half-life (60 to 90 minutes) and must be repeatedly administered in patients who have overdosed on an opioid with a longer half-life (e.g., methadone). Initial IV naloxone dosing is approximately 0.8 mg per 70 kg of body weight. Signs of improvement—increase in respiratory rate and pupillary dilation—should occur promptly. If there is no response to the initial dosage, naloxone may be repeated after intervals of a few minutes. Nalmefene has a longer duration of action (its half-life is approximately 10 hours), and a single dose of nalmefene may be sufficient to produce sustained reversal for the duration of the effects of the opioid agonist overdose. Nalmefene's onset of effects typically occurs within minutes after IV administration, and the usual initial dose is 0.5 to 1.0 mg.

In opioid-dependent patients, too much naloxone or nalmefene may produce signs of withdrawal (precipitated opioid withdrawal), as well as reversal of overdosage. In some instances, patients may become agitated owing to precipitated withdrawal symptoms. A relative advantage of naloxone is that precipitated withdrawal effects—if they occur—are of relatively short duration. In contrast, nalmefene-precipitated withdrawal can last for hours.

In the past, it was thought that, if no response was observed after administering naloxone or nalmefene, then CNS depression was probably not solely due to opioids. However, buprenorphine is difficult to reverse with opioid antagonists, and higher doses of naloxone and nalmefene may be required for an overdose of buprenorphine. (However, the risk of respiratory depression from an overdose of buprenorphine is uncommon, as reviewed later in this chapter.)

Medically Supervised Withdrawal (Detoxification)

Opioid Agents for Treating Opioid Withdrawal

Although any opioid μ-agonist medication can be administered and then gradually reduced to alleviate opioid withdrawal symptoms, the need to use nonapproved opioids to treat withdrawal should decline as a greater number of approved medications for treatment of opioid withdrawal become available. There are now three medications approved in the United States for use in the treatment of opioid withdrawal: methadone, LAAM, and buprenorphine. Each of these is discussed here.

METHADONE There is considerable clinical experience in the use of methadone for the treatment of opioid withdrawal. Methadone can be effective in suppressing signs and symptoms of opioid withdrawal and is a safe medication when used under clinical supervision during withdrawal. Methadone can be used on an outpatient or inpatient basis.

The primary goal of inpatient treatment is to provide doses of methadone adequate to suppress withdrawal. For patients who have been using street opioids, the initial dosage of methadone is usually 10 to 20 mg orally. If signs of withdrawal persist after the first dose of methadone, the dose can be repeated after approximately 2 hours. As a general rule, initial stabilization does not require more than 40 mg of methadone during the first 24 hours. Physician addicts and others who have access to pure drugs are exceptions to that general rule and may require higher doses. If the usual daily dose of opioid (heroin, meperidine, and hydromorphone) is known, the equivalent withdrawal-suppressing dose of methadone can be calculated. For example, methadone is approximately three times as potent as morphine in suppressing withdrawal. The current tendency is to base dosage on clinical history rather than to wait for evidence of spontaneous withdrawal or to precipitate withdrawal with naloxone. After 24 to 48 hours of dose stabilization, the patient's methadone dose can be gradually reduced (for example, by reducing the dose by 10 to 20 percent per day). With close supervision and supportive resources, inpatient withdrawal with methadone can be accomplished in 7 to 10 days.

When methadone withdrawal occurs on an outpatient basis, a different set of goals and procedures can be used not only to alleviate withdrawal, but also initially to provide a dose sufficient to block the effects of illicit opioids (i.e., achieve an initial period of abstinence). Initial dosing in the first day should begin with 20 to 30 mg and should not exceed 40 mg. Over the first several days or even weeks of treatment, the dose may be raised (generally by no more than 10-mg increments per day) until cessation of illicit opioid use occurs. As the dose is being raised, patients should be monitored for evidence of sedation or other symptoms suggesting that too high a dose or rapid a dose escalation is being used. Once a period of stabilization has occurred—that is, no withdrawal symptoms and no illicit opioid use—then dose reductions can occur. Studies of outpatient methadone withdrawal show that gradual dose reductions (e.g., 3 percent per week) have a greater likelihood of success versus more rapid dose reductions (e.g., 10 percent per week). Outpatients also appear to have better outcomes when they are informed of the rate of methadone withdrawal, but there are not better outcomes when patients are allowed to self-regulate the speed at which their methadone dose is reduced. Within this paradigm, outpatient methadone dose reductions may take several months.

Outcomes from methadone withdrawal are generally quite poor. Relapse is common, and clinical experience suggests that patients are particularly vulnerable to start using illicit opioids when methadone dose drops to less than 20 to 25 mg per day. A study comparing outcomes from a 6-month methadone withdrawal that included an enriched set of psychosocial services versus continued methadone maintenance found that maintenance patients did considerably better despite efforts to optimize nonpharmacological treatments for the withdrawal group.

LAAM Although there is considerable clinical experience with methadone for the treatment of opioid withdrawal, there is little research on LAAM for this indication. Given the complexities with LAAM dosing, this medication should not be considered a typical agent for opioid withdrawal treatment, unless a patient is maintained on LAAM and wishes to withdraw.

BUPRENORPHINE Buprenorphine is a safe and effective medication for the treatment of opioid withdrawal. The parenteral form is only approved for the treatment of pain. If there is reason to use parenteral buprenorphine for treatment of withdrawal, then it is most likely that this would occur at an inpatient setting in which this form of buprenorphine is available. A typical initial dose is 0.3 to 0.6 mg IM, followed by repeated dosing two to three times per day for 1 to 2 days (i.e., a brief dose-stabilization phase). This can then be followed by dose reductions of 25 to 33 percent each day over 3 to 5 days. Buprenorphine has a relatively long duration of action, and patients typically tolerate a 3- to 5-day withdrawal with minimal evidence of withdrawal and no significant complaints of distress. Finally, it is important to note that concurrent treatment with sedating drugs—and, most especially, benzodiazepines—is contraindicated in patients being treated on an outpatient basis with buprenorphine. Case reports from France, where buprenorphine has been used extensively in the outpatient treatment of opioid dependence since 1996, indicate that there have been fatalities in patients combining parenteral buprenorphine with parenteral benzodiazepines.

The sublingual form of buprenorphine is approved for the treatment of opioid dependence and withdrawal and is marketed in two formulations: a monotherapy product (trade name: Subutex), and a combination therapy product that includes naloxone. Each form is available in two dosage strengths; a small tablet (2 mg) and large tablet (8 mg). The combination form contains a ratio of 4 to 1 for buprenorphine to naloxone (i.e., 2.0- and 0.5-mg tablets and 8- and 2-mg tablets).

Sublingual buprenorphine tablets can be used for opioid withdrawal. There is limited research on the optimal dosing withdrawal procedures for the use of sublingual buprenorphine, although some guidelines and recommendations are possible. The following recommendations assume that withdrawal is being managed on an outpatient basis. First, dosing can be once daily (unlike the usual practice of repeated daily dosing for the parenteral form). As buprenorphine is a partial opioid agonist, the first dose can precipitate mild opioid withdrawal symptoms under certain circumstances. To minimize the risk of precipitated withdrawal, it is recommended that the first dose be given when the patient is in mild spontaneous withdrawal. Patients may be started directly on the combination product—the risk of precipitating withdrawal from sublingual naloxone is extremely low, as there is poor bioavailability of naloxone by this route of administration. The first day's dose can be at least 4 mg of buprenorphine, and patients may need to be stabilized on daily doses between 8 and 32 mg to achieve adequate withdrawal suppression and abstinence from illicit opioids. Like methadone withdrawal, it is probably the case that long-duration buprenorphine withdrawals have better outcomes than shorter ones. As the smallest incremental dose of buprenorphine is 2 mg, and tablets are not scored and do not break easily, dose reductions should occur in 2-mg increments over a period of several weeks.

Conclusions Regarding Use of Opioids for Withdrawal Despite the best efforts of clinicians and the use of slow detoxification schedules, all studies to date indicate that many patients drop out before completing outpatient detoxification and that relapse rates after outpatient or inpatient detoxification are high. Relapse rates are particularly high for users of street heroin who attempt to detoxify on an outpatient basis. For such patients, extending the period of withdrawal or using a longer-acting drug, such as levomethadyl acetate, does not appear to alter the high likelihood of a rapid return to illicit opioid use. Finally, although this section focuses on the use of pharmacological aids for managing withdrawal, it is important to note the value of nonpharmacological treatments during the withdrawal period and into the postwithdrawal period as mechanisms to optimize the chance for long-term successful outcomes.

Nonopioid Medications and Nontraditional Approaches for Detoxification

α_2 Agonists Opioid withdrawal produces hyperactivity in the locus ceruleus, and this finding led to testing of α_2-agonist medications for the treatment of opioid withdrawal. Clonidine and lofexidine are the two α_2-adrenergic agonist medications commonly used for opioid withdrawal treatment.

CLONIDINE Clonidine is marketed as an antihypertensive agent. Patients stabilized on relatively low doses of opioids—for example, 30 to 40 mg of oral methadone a day—can abruptly discontinue opioid use, and clonidine can be used to attenuate withdrawal. Clonidine is given orally, starting at doses of 0.1 to 0.3 mg three to four times a day. In outpatient settings, a total dosage of greater than 1 mg per day is not recommended, although higher dosages (1.5 to 2.5 mg) have been used with hospitalized patients. The major adverse effects seen with clonidine use are hypotension, which can be quite extreme, and sedation, and the dosage must be carefully individualized. Patients in outpatient clinics who have been stabilized on methadone and who have developed a relationship with their therapists were found to be more successful in achieving abstinence when treated with clonidine than patients who were taking illicit heroin when clonidine treatment was begun. Some studies have found that outpatient detoxification with clonidine is almost as successful as detoxification using decreasing doses of methadone.

Clonidine appears to be least effective in suppressing postwithdrawal muscle aches, lethargy, insomnia, restlessness, and craving. There is no evidence that it is useful in preventing relapse after the completion of detoxification. Clonidine does appear to facilitate the detoxification of patients maintained on methadone and their subsequent stabilization on naltrexone (ReVia). Properly used, the combination of clonidine and naltrexone can shorten the period of hospitalization required for detoxification to less than 5 days. The clonidine to naltrexone technique has also been used in a day-hospital outpatient setting. Heroin addicts were given oral clonidine three times on the first day, with doses ranging from 0.1 to 0.3 mg, adjusted on the basis of dependence severity and blood pressure response; naltrexone was started on the second day. The initial naltrexone dose of 1 mg (orally) was gradually increased so that patients were receiving 40, 50, and 150 mg by days 3 to 5, respectively.

LOFEXIDINE Lofexidine is not approved for use in the United States (for opioid withdrawal or for hypertension), but it is approved and marketed in the United Kingdom for the treatment of opioid withdrawal. There has been a steady increase in sales of lofexidine in the United Kingdom since its approval, and it is more widely used than clonidine in the United Kingdom because it is believed to produce less hypotension. However, outcomes for clonidine versus lofexidine appear to be generally equivalent. Studies of lofexidine for the treatment of opioid withdrawal are currently being conducted in the United States.

Ultrarapid Detoxification

The duration of the acute phase of opioid withdrawal can be markedly shortened by using opioid antagonists to remove opioid agonists from opioid receptors. Such a procedure results in a precipitated withdrawal syndrome that is far more intense than that which occurs with mere abrupt discontinuation (spontaneous withdrawal, or going cold turkey). Building on the work of researchers who used small doses of naloxone along with benzodiazepine sedation to precipitate withdrawal and to initiate naltrexone treatment, several groups of investigators developed methods to make tolerable and to shorten further the duration of acute withdrawal. Researchers at Yale used clonidine to reduce withdrawal symptoms associated with starting naltrexone. Others added sedatives to the clonidine-naltrexone regimen. It was reported that the acute withdrawal syndrome could be shortened to less than 2 days if the procedure was initiated under full anesthesia lasting 3 to 4 hours (sometimes called *ultrarapid opioid detoxification* [UROD]).

There are little follow-up data on people who have undergone this detoxification procedure, and there is little reason to believe that ultrarapid detoxification would, by itself, be more efficacious than detoxification over 4 to 10 days. Furthermore, the costs can be considerable, given the medical intensity of the procedure (use of general anesthesia). Many clinicians have expressed the view that, because opioid detoxification using conventional methods is almost never fatal, ultrarapid detoxification subjects patients to unnecessary risks. Although this technique experienced a period of interest and use in the 1990s (including commercialization of the procedure), subsequent reviews have concluded that further research is needed to determine its relative long-term efficacy and whether it is a safe and cost-effective approach to the treatment of opioid dependence. At this point in time, it is probably best viewed as an experimental technique rather than as a mainstream procedure in medicine.

Other Techniques

Opioid withdrawal is rarely life threatening in healthy adults, and symptomatic treatments can be used to aid the motivated person during spontaneous withdrawal. These can include ibuprofen (Advil) for muscle and joint aches, promethazine (Phenergan) for nausea and vomiting, and diphenhydramine (Benadryl) for sleep.

A variety of nonpharmacological approaches to drug abstinence have been and continue to be used. Abrupt withdrawal (cold turkey) is used in some countries (e.g., Singapore) as a matter of policy, because it is believed that experiencing severe withdrawal is a deterrent to relapse. Abrupt withdrawal, coupled with considerable emotional support, is still used in some therapeutic communities. Because withdrawal stress fatalities can occur in debilitated persons (e.g., those with advanced AIDS, tuberculosis, or heart disease), some caution is indicated when using abrupt withdrawal procedures.

Acupuncture has also been used to alleviate opioid withdrawal. The acupuncture-stimulated release of endogenous opioids provides some rational basis for this approach. Although there have been numerous studies and reports of acupuncture treatment for various substance abuse disorders, there remains considerable ambiguity regarding the efficacy of this technique when used for the treatment of addictions.

Herbal medicines aimed at ridding the body of toxic substances are sometimes used in a religious or semireligious context. There is no evidence to indicate that, when those traditional approaches are used in their own cultural settings, the outcome is any better or worse than with the more medically sophisticated approaches typically used in the United States.

Treatment of Opioid Dependence

General Principles

Despite a tendency toward a greater diversity of options for the treatment of addiction in general, most opioid users treated in the United States are seen in one of four types of programs: detoxification or medically supervised withdrawal (ambulatory or residential and inpatient), usually followed by outpatient counseling; opioid maintenance (methadone, levomethadyl acetate, or buprenorphine); residential or therapeutic communities; and outpatient drug-free programs (which may be based largely on 12-step principles and which typically follow an episode of detoxification). Medically supervised withdrawal has been addressed previously in this chapter. However, it is worth reiterating that detoxification for opioid dependence with no subsequent follow-up treatment has a poor prognosis for most patients and, in some studies, produces outcomes comparable to patients on a waiting list for treatment.

A person's willingness to accept treatment may change over time as life circumstances, family relationships, and the severity and complications of the dependence change. Consideration should be given not only to the characteristics, wishes, and previous experiences of patients, but also to how they are likely to react to the particular treatments that are economically and geographically feasible.

The clinician should make it clear that treatment requires a commitment to a long-term change in lifestyle, attitude, family dynamics, and, sometimes, even geographic location and that the responsibility for making the changes belongs to the patient. If resources permit, the clinician should not rest content with making a diagnosis of opioid dependence but should make a complete psychiatric assessment and take a thorough drug use history. Most opioid users have additional psychiatric disorders and other substance-related disorders (Tables 11.10–5, 11.10–6, and 11.10–7). The severity of psychological difficulties (e.g., mood disorders, anxiety disorders, and paranoid ideation) and patterns of using drugs other than opioids are predictors of outcome in treatment. Patients should also understand, however, that, although antecedent stress, environmental conditions, and underlying psychological difficulties may have played important roles in the genesis of their drug dependence, once it is established, opioid dependence does not resolve spontaneously even if those conditions are improved. Clinicians must communicate the necessity for treating the pathological drug use as a disorder in its own right.

Goals of Treatment

The goals of treatment for opioid dependence can vary across settings and even within a particular modality of treatment, such as methadone maintenance. Although the target of opioid dependence treatment in general is to stop illicit opioid use, some therapists or programs accept a decrease in use as a sufficient goal (seeing this as having value to the user, for example, through decreasing risk for acquiring infections). Other programs may accept only complete abstinence from illicit opioid use as an acceptable clinical outcome. Other goals may relate to nonopioid drug use and non–drug use objectives (e.g., employment). Achieving sustained abstinence is a process that can take time, and decreases in illicit drug use can be a step in the direction of eventual abstinence.

HARM REDUCTION AND TREATMENT OF OPIOID DEPENDENCE The topics of harm reduction and legalization of illicit drugs are beyond the scope of this chapter. However, this chapter comments briefly on needle exchange programs that aim at providing active opioid abusers with clean needles as a way to minimize sharing of needles and syringes and thus to minimize the risk of infectious disease exposure. Evidence suggests that needle exchange programs can be effective and that they can serve as a mechanism for engaging patients in treatment that can subsequently lead to involvement in more traditional modalities, such as methadone clinics.

ROLE OF COUNSELING IN TREATMENT OF OPIOID DEPENDENCE A key feature for all modalities of opioid dependence treatment is nonpharmacological services, including counseling. Counseling services occur in outpatient, inpatient, residential, day-care, and prison settings. The program may emphasize group, individual, or family interactions, or may be designed specifically to target populations selected by age, gender, culture, race, or special status (e.g., pregnant women). Therapeutic approaches can vary widely, although, in recent years, manually driven forms of counseling have been developed (for example, for cognitive-behavioral and motivational enhancement forms of treatment), and these provide a means for better standardization of services within a treatment program, as well as guidance to counseling staff in treatment approaches.

In the context of methadone maintenance treatment programs, scheduled counseling has been shown to reduce illicit drug use substantially and to increase prosocial behaviors. The efficacy of counseling is further supported by studies showing that the quality of counseling and rapport between patient and counselor have a significant impact on outcome measures. When the dosage of methadone was held constant (e.g., at 60 mg), the addition of drug counseling on a regular basis was distinctly more effective than was emergency counseling in reducing opioid and cocaine use. When patients were provided with on-site medical, psychiatric, employment, and family counseling, the outcome was improved still further. It is reasonable to assume that the quality of counseling, psychiatric, and social services can have an impact on how opioid users not being maintained on methadone respond to treatment. In one study, detoxified heroin addicts who participated in a support group in which they learned how to avoid or to cope with situations that provoked drug cravings or feelings of withdrawal (relapse prevention) had lower relapse rates than those assigned to control groups.

ROLE OF OTHER NONPHARMACOLOGICAL TREATMENTS FOR OPIOID DEPENDENCE In addition to counseling services, other nonpharmacological treatments can serve a useful and important function in the treatment of opioid dependence. For example, monitored urine collection and testing (or other biological assessments of body fluids for drug use) provides an objective index of treatment progress. Besides this outcome function, drug testing can also serve a treatment purpose, as the patient may be further motivated to maintain abstinence because a drug test can occur as a part of the treatment process. Behaviorally based treatments, such as contingent take-home doses of methadone or voucher incentives used in cocaine treatment programs, are other forms of treatment that can be effective and powerful tools.

ROLE OF SELF-HELP GROUPS IN TREATMENT OF OPIOID DEPENDENCE Narcotics Anonymous (NA) is a self-help group of abstinent drug abusers modeled on the 12-step principles of Alcoholics Anonymous (AA). Such groups now exist in most large cities and can provide useful group support. The outcome for physicians treated in 12-step programs is generally good, but the anonymity that is at the core of the 12-step model has made detailed evaluation of its efficacy in treating opioid dependence difficult. Some methadone maintenance patients feel that 12-step self-help programs react negatively to the use of methadone, and a variant on the NA program is Methadone Anonymous (MA)—a 12-step program specifically for patients receiving methadone medication. Self-help programs can function as an important and highly useful aspect of treatment, providing a group element of support and real world experience that is not always available in the professional treatment setting.

ROLE OF MEDICATIONS IN TREATMENT OF OPIOID DEPENDENCE Specific pharmacotherapies used for maintenance treatment of opioid dependence are discussed in later sections in more detail, and medications used for detoxification have been discussed previously. Although there are several pharmacotherapies that are useful in the treatment of opioid dependence, it is not uncommon for medications to be used for relatively short periods (e.g., for medically supervised withdrawal), followed by counseling services that seek to maintain abstinence. Maintenance treatment for opioid dependence has been available for more than 30 years and can be remarkably effective.

REGULATORY CONTROL OF OPIOID DEPENDENCE TREATMENT IN THE UNITED STATES The use of opioid agonist medications (i.e., methadone and LAAM) to treat opioid dependence has historically been under significant regulatory control in the United States. For many years, *OTPs* (the term used to encompass methadone and LAAM maintenance treatment programs) were regulated by the Food and Drug Administration (FDA). In 1995, an Institute of Medicine (IOM) report recommended shifting the oversight of OTPs from the FDA regulatory system to an accreditation process under the supervision of the Substance Abuse and Mental Health Services Administration (SAMHSA). In 2001, this change was made. With this change, the federal government also explicitly and implicitly altered the practice of OTPs. These changes included the lifting of an artificial limit on maximal doses of methadone (implied to be 100 mg per day in the earlier regulations), allowed LAAM to be used on a take-home basis, and provided for more take-home doses of medications to be permitted (up to 1 month's worth after 2 years of stable treatment). In addition, the requirement that programs be accredited by an outside agency—such as the Commission on Accreditation of Rehabilitation Facilities (CARF) or the Joint Commission of Accreditation of Healthcare Organizations (JCAHO)—was a significant and substantial alteration in the operation of the OTP system.

The other major change in federal regulation of opioid dependence treatment occurred in December of 2000, when the Drug Addiction Treatment Act (DATA) was signed into law. This law allowed office-based treatment of opioid dependence with approved medications that were schedule III, IV, or V. Previously, the pharmacological treatment for opioid dependence with opioid agonist medications had been limited to the OTP system (with occasional, rare exceptions). Although there were no schedule III, IV, or V medications approved for the treatment of opioid dependence at the time that the law was passed, a review of the content of the law shows that it was designed in anticipation of buprenorphine's eventual approval. There are several implications to DATA, including the potential mainstreaming of addiction treatment into routine medical care, the opportunity to increase treatment capacity with opioid agonist medication, the expansion of treatment into areas in which OTPs are unavailable, and the opportunity to provide treatment to a population often underserved and marginalized. However, office-based buprenorphine also runs the risk of diversion and abuse, given that regulatory supervision is less stringent than that applied to OTPs. Hopefully, this treatment modality will prove to have the favorable cost to benefit ratio envisioned by its advocates.

PLACEMENT CRITERIA AND TREATMENT OF OPIOID DEPENDENCE The American Society of Addiction Medicine (ASAM) has developed patient placement criteria for use in determining the appropriate level of treatment for a patient with a substance abuse disorder. ASAM's levels of care include methadone maintenance treatment, as well as other service levels that may be used in the treatment of a patient with opioid dependence (e.g., inpatient and outpatient detoxification). Familiarity with the criteria can help guide the clinician in determining the initial treatment plan for a patient, and use of the criteria may be required by various funding agencies.

Maintenance Medications for Opioid Dependence

In the United States, there are four medications approved by the FDA for maintenance treatment of opioid dependence: methadone (available since the late 1960s), naltrexone (available since 1984), LAAM (approved by the FDA in 1993), and buprenorphine (approved by the FDA in 2002). Although there are similarities between different medications, each has unique features and certain advantages under particular clinical circumstances.

Naltrexone

The use of opioid antagonists to treat opioid dependence was originally based on the assumption that classically conditioned withdrawal symptoms and operantly reinforced drug-seeking behavior contribute to the high relapse rate typically seen after withdrawal from opioids. Theoretically, by blocking the euphoric effects of opioids, treatment with antagonists would lead to the extinction of operantly reinforced drug seeking; by preventing the reestablishment of physical dependence, treatment with antagonists also leads to the eventual extinction of conditioned withdrawal phenomena. Naltrexone is orally effective, and, when given three times a week (100 mg on weekdays and 150 mg on weekends), it completely blocks the effects of substantial doses of heroin. Its toxicity is low. However, the use of naltrexone requires the clinician to be confident that there is no longer evidence of opioid physical dependence in the patient, as a single dose of naltrexone can precipitate a withdrawal syndrome that can last several hours (given naltrexone's long duration of action). Recent treatment with antagonists has been based on empirical and laboratory observations that patients taking naltrexone experience less craving in the presence of opioid-related cues, presumably because, on a cognitive basis, they are aware that they are unable to experience the opioid effects. Naltrexone has been used in a number of clinical trials, but, in each of them, the dropout rate has been high. Curiously, these low compliance rates have not been characteristic of alcohol abusers treated with naltrexone. When naltrexone was tested in a multiclinic, double-blind study, however, few of those patients who initially expressed an interest in the drug actually took a single dose. At the 6-month follow-up, few differences were noted between the naltrexone group and the placebo control group, although the naltrexone group had fewer urine specimens positive for opioids while they were in treatment. Former opioid users sometimes report dysphoria, an adverse effect not reported when the drug is given to alcohol abusers. The only consistent side effect reported is a somewhat higher incidence of nausea.

Experienced clinicians do not think that double-blind placebo-controlled trials are the most appropriate way to assess the usefulness of long-acting antagonists. They believe that a period of 30 to 60 days of treatment with naltrexone immediately after detoxification reduces the probability of relapse to opioid use. In open studies of opioid users on probation who volunteered to take naltrexone, those on the active drug were far less likely than those randomly assigned to the placebo to violate probation and to be reincarcerated. In studies conducted in Israel and Portugal, special efforts were made to involve family members in supporting patients' compliance with naltrexone treatment, resulting in 30- to 40 percent continued abstinence rates at 1-year follow-up. In a randomized controlled study in which outpatients were given voucher incentives for taking naltrexone, compliance was significantly improved compared to control conditions of no vouchers and noncontingent vouchers. Techniques for facilitating the transfer from heroin or methadone to naltrexone (clonidine, or buprenorphine and clonidine) may increase the ease of initiating naltrexone treatment, but low compliance and high dropout rates remain unsolved problems. Another area of interest is depot preparations of naltrexone, which are under study. In a small number of volunteers, a single injection of naltrexone encased in microcapsules has been found to produce blood concentrations adequate to block the effects of street-quality heroin for approximately 30 days. It may be possible to combine depot naltrexone with a behavioral incentive, such as vouchers for treatment compliance, and to produce better outcomes than those seen in the clinical trials of oral naltrexone treatment.

Methadone

In the United States, approximately 800 outpatient maintenance programs now provide treatment with methadone or levomethadyl acetate to approximately 180,000 patients at any given time. Methadone maintenance is also used in the United Kingdom, Australia, Hong Kong, and a number of European countries. Thus, opioid maintenance is a major modality for treating opioid dependence throughout much of the world.

GENERAL PHARMACOLOGY Given acutely, methadone is a typical μ receptor agonist producing euphoria, analgesia, and other typical morphine-like effects. Given long-term by the oral route, however, methadone has several interesting properties that make it unusually useful in maintenance programs. These qualities include its reliable absorption and bioavailability after oral administration, the delay of peak plasma levels until 2 to 6 hours after ingestion, and the apparent nonspecific binding to tissues that creates a large reservoir of methadone in the body. This large reservoir, combined with slow time-to-peak effects, buffers patients against sharp peaks in subjective effects after ingestion, which, in any event, are highly attenuated as a result of tolerance. The reservoir of methadone also tends to minimize any sharp declines that would induce withdrawal. Thus, not only is the administration of methadone on a once-a-day schedule possible, but also minor variations in dosage over short periods do not induce major changes in biological effects. Although the mean plasma half-life in the naïve subject is approximately 15 hours, it ranges from approximately 22 to 56 hours in methadone-maintained patients depending on the measurement technique used. A number of commonly used therapeutic agents can induce liver enzymes and thereby can result in more rapid metabolism of methadone and in half-lives that are significantly shorter than 22 hours; some agents can inhibit metabolism.

METHADONE DOSE AND PHILOSOPHICAL DIFFERENCES AMONG PROGRAMS Methadone maintenance programs vary with respect to dosage, attitudes toward continued contrasocial behavior, medical and social services provided, and long-term goals. The original programs pioneered by Vincent Dole and Marie Nyswander emphasized methadone dosage sufficient to suppress opioid drug hunger and to induce a cross-tolerance blockade of the effects of illicit opioids, usually 80 to 120 mg per day. Patients were encouraged to remain on methadone indefinitely on the assumption that the return of opioid drug hunger after detoxification would lead to relapse and the loss of any gains achieved during treatment.

Other programs used lower doses of methadone (<50 mg per day), which were often adequate for retaining patients in treatment and partially suppressing drug-seeking behavior but not for producing adequate cross-tolerance to large doses of heroin. Such programs generally viewed maintenance as a transitional stage to eventual detoxification. Although patients may remain in treatment in these programs indefinitely, the ambiance is often more supportive of efforts at gradual withdrawal. Empirically, patients maintained on lower doses of methadone are far more likely to discontinue treatment, and those who do so are unlikely to achieve sustained abstinence from opioids. In a six-program study in the United States, the number of patients using IV heroin steadily increased after treatment was discontinued. By 12 months, 80 percent reported heroin use in the month before the interview. Because only a small percentage of these persons were actually discharged as having completed treatment, the figure is perhaps a better illustration of what happens to those who drop out.

Since publications of findings on the importance of dose in reducing opioid use and increasing retention in treatment, more programs are prescribing daily doses of methadone of 60 mg or higher. However, the proper dose is not a matter of reaching some arbitrary number. There are wide variations in rates of methadone metabolism, and some experts believe that more attention should be given to using laboratory measures of methadone plasma levels to adjust daily dosage. Data suggest that an average methadone serum level of 400 ng/mL seems adequate and that trough levels of less than 150 ng/mL are likely to be associated with some degree of withdrawal or drug hunger. Clinicians should be aware that a variety of therapeutic agents can cause a decrease in plasma levels of methadone by inducing hepatic enzymes that metabolize methadone (CYP3A4). Among those are rifampin (Rifadin), phenytoin (Dilantin), barbiturates, carbamazepine (Tegretol), and ethyl alcohol. Valproic acid (Depakene) does not accelerate metabolism. Agents that can inhibit methadone metabolism include erythromycin (E-Mycin), cimetidine (Tagamet), and ketoconazole (Nizoral). Zidovudine (Retrovir) does not alter methadone metabolism, but patients on methadone tend to have higher zidovudine levels than do controls. More methadone is excreted when urinary pH is low than when it is high; stress and other factors that lower urinary pH can result in lower plasma levels of methadone.

Patients who do not respond to methadone treatment generally continue to use illicit opioids and other illicit drugs, use alcohol to excess, attend programs irregularly, and may exhibit problematic behavior at the clinic. Such patients pose a dilemma for methadone maintenance programs, because they would probably fare worse if discharged. However, permitting them to remain demoralizes the staff and the other patients, can encourage drug use among the latter, and can lead to problems with the local community.

Long-Term Effects The relative safety of methadone maintenance in terms of organ toxicity has been firmly established. Tolerance to many of the opioid agonist actions of methadone is incomplete, however, and continuing pharmacological effects are observed. Many of these effects, such as euphoria, drowsiness, and somnolence, are more prominent in the first weeks of treatment; if the dosage level is increased too rapidly, the effects even become manifested at later points in treatment. Some effects, however, persist even after many months of treatment. Among the most common long-lasting effects are constipation, which can sometimes result in fecal impaction and intestinal obstruction; excessive sweating; complaints of decreased libido; and sexual dysfunction, for example, an inability to sustain an erection. Opioids reduce plasma levels of testosterone and follicle-stimulating hormone (FSH) for which tolerance is often incomplete, but the correlation between abnormally low plasma levels of hormones and sexual dysfunction is not high.

In general, however, indexes of HPA axis function are normal in patients maintained on long-term methadone, in contrast to the deranged function typical of active and recently detoxified heroin users. Sleep abnormalities (insomnia and nightmares) and altered electroencephalogram (EEG) sleep patterns are frequently found during the first months of methadone treatment; the EEG sleep patterns appear to return to baseline, but complaints of sleep abnormalities may persist. For a substantial percentage of patients, even those participating in programs in which dosage is adjusted, the major adverse effect is mild to moderate withdrawal symptoms before the next dose.

Tolerance to the mood-elevating effects of methadone does not develop in all patients. In double-blind studies, some patients regularly report a greater sense of well-being a few hours after ingesting their daily dose; for some patients, this effect may be an important factor in retention in treatment.

In-Treatment Outcome The majority of patients treated in methadone programs show significantly decreased opioid and nonopioid drug use, criminal behavior, and symptoms of depression and increased gainful employment. Significant differences in effectiveness across programs are owing, in some measure, to the characteristics of patients treated, but certain program features tend to make some programs more effective than others. In 1980, the average retention rate for a group of methadone clinics participating in a national prospective study was 81 percent at 1 month, 67 percent at 3 months, and 52 percent at 6 months. Higher retention rates are associated with the provision of high-quality social services (especially within the first months), higher doses of methadone (60 mg or more), allowing patients to know their dosage, the ease of accessibility, no fees or low fees, and the use of supportive, rather than confrontational, techniques.

The effectiveness of opioid maintenance treatment is powerfully influenced by the quality of the additional services provided. Effective individual drug counseling (e.g., one session per week) can result in significantly better outcome in terms of illicit opioid and cocaine use, needle sharing, crime, employment, and psychological well-being. Treatment outcome can be further improved by the provision of psychiatric services, employment counseling, and family therapy. Just as higher doses of methadone are generally more effective than lower doses, so has it been shown that higher doses of psychosocial services are more effective than lower doses. However, such additional services increase the overall cost of treatment, and, in terms of overall improved outcomes, it is more cost effective to ensure that all patients have competent standard drug counseling.

Positive behavioral change, including decreases in illicit drug use and other criminal behavior, does not typically occur immediately on entry into treatment but takes place over a period of many months. Treatments lasting less than 90 days usually have little or no impact; consequently, retention in treatment is critical. Several studies have shown a direct relation between methadone dose and the probability of treatment retention.

In Australia, patients taking doses of 80 mg or higher were twice as likely to remain in treatment than those receiving 60 to 79 mg, who were twice as likely to remain as those receiving less than 60 mg. Dosage has also been shown to have a profound effect on whether patients continue to use illicit heroin. In a study of six clinics in the United States, there was an inverse relation between methadone dosage (over the range from 20 to 80 mg daily) and the percentage of patients using heroin. Although some programs persist in using low doses that have been shown to correlate with high dropout rates and continued heroin use, their number has decreased as data on the importance of adequate dosage have become more generally accepted.

Other program factors that influence outcome and retention are the perceived range and quality of the social services provided to the patient early in the course of treatment, whether the program is flexible or confrontational and punitive about occasional illicit drug use, and the competence and quality of the program leadership and the counselors. Outcome correlates with the services actually delivered and the degree to which patients perceive that the services are those they believe are important to them. Some of the better-funded programs with better staff to patient ratios did not deliver as many services as did less well-endowed programs. The retention of drug users in treatment programs and the successful reduction of injecting drug use are particularly important in an era when such drug use often results in transmitting or acquiring HIV and other infectious illnesses. Older, black, married, and employed patients tend to remain in methadone programs longer; patients with extensive criminal backgrounds tend to drop out sooner and to perform more poorly while in treatment. The severity or duration of opioid use does not correlate with retention or performance in treatment, and patients who enter treatment under what they perceive as legal coercion show improvement comparable to that of patients who report no such external pressure.

Detoxification and Long-Term Outcome The percentage of patients remaining abstinent from opioids at 12 to 36 months after successful detoxification from opioid maintenance has ranged from 12 to 28 percent for unselected samples of patients, some of whom were discharged for violation of clinic rules. When analysis is restricted to those patients who elected to be withdrawn (with staff and patient consensus that treatment was completed), abstinence rates were substantially higher, at least over the first 6 to 12 months. Predictors of retention and positive outcome in treatment do not necessarily predict success in achieving abstinence or long-term positive outcome once withdrawal has been completed.

In general, patients with shorter drug histories and longer time in maintenance treatment but with lower dosages seem to have more success detoxifying. In one national, multiclinic follow-up study, 40 percent of former methadone patients interviewed were not using any illicit opioids and did not have any other significant drug problems 6 years after the completion of initial treatment. Other follow-up studies have found a smaller proportion of former maintenance patients who were opioid abstinent.

Although the percentage of heroin addicts maintained on methadone who eventually achieve long-term stable abstinence off methadone is not high, there is no convincing evidence that the likelihood of abstinence is higher among those treated in other modalities, once adjustment is made for various pretreatment predictors of outcome. In one study in which methadone treatment appeared to impair eventual abstinence, that disadvantage was offset by substantially lower rates of incarceration among methadone-treated patients.

LAAM Like methadone, LAAM is a μ-receptor agonist that is orally active, suppresses opioid withdrawal, and provides blockade to the effects of illicit opioids. Although levomethadyl acetate is similar to methadone in its pharmacological actions, it is converted into the active metabolites nor-acetylmethadol and di-nor-acetylmethadol that have long biological half-lives (e.g., 48 to 96 hours for di-nor-acetylmethadol). Consequently, levomethadyl acetate can be given as infrequently as three times a week, thereby reducing the inconvenience of attending a clinic daily to ingest the drug and simultaneously reducing concerns about illicit diversion. LAAM can only be provided through a clinic system (like methadone), and a relatively small number of patients are treated with LAAM. This is probably due to the restriction on its use (i.e., the clinic system), along with concerns about LAAM's safety (as described in the following discussion).

When levomethadyl acetate is abruptly discontinued, the withdrawal syndrome is slow in onset and relatively mild in intensity, but it is at least as protracted as that of methadone. Levomethadyl acetate has been shown to be equivalent to methadone in suppressing illicit opioid use and encouraging productive activity. Before its approval by the FDA, a consistent finding was that retention in treatment was lower with levomethadyl acetate than with methadone; more recently, clinicians are reporting that some patients prefer levomethadyl acetate.

Like methadone, LAAM's efficacy is dose related. A random-assignment double-blind outpatient clinical trial comparing three dose levels of levomethadyl acetate given three times a week demonstrated that higher doses were more effective in suppressing heroin use. Patients receiving the highest dose were more likely to drop out of treatment during the dose induction phase (compared to the medium and low doses), which suggests that beginning patients on LAAM requires care during the early dosing period. However, no significant difference in treatment retention was found between the three groups for the overall study period. In most cases, it is unnecessary to stabilize heroin users first on methadone, and levomethadyl acetate can be used as the initial treatment agent.

After LAAM was approved in the Unites States and Europe, cases of arrhythmias associated with LAAM use were reported to the FDA and European authorities. It was found that some patients developed prolonged QT intervals when treated with LAAM and that a potentially fatal arrhythmia (torsades de pointes) could occur. These case reports resulted in the decision to withdraw LAAM from the European market altogether. In the United States, the FDA revised LAAM's label to include a black-box warning about its potential to cause prolongation of the QT interval and the recommendation that LAAM be reserved for use as a second-line agent for the treatment of opioid dependence. Monitoring with baseline and in-treatment electrocardiograms (ECGs) should be a part of the treatment plan for patients receiving LAAM.

Despite these safety concerns, LAAM can be a useful agent for some patients. Anecdotal reports from patients treated with LAAM indicate that they feel a more level pharmacological effect, when asked to compare LAAM to previous experience with methadone. However, levomethadyl acetate has a complex pharmacology, and its use demands the clinician to exert a greater repertoire of skills than those required when prescribing methadone.

Buprenorphine Like methadone and LAAM, buprenorphine exerts its primary therapeutic effect via the μ opioid receptor. However, although methadone and LAAM are full μ-agonist opioids, buprenorphine is a partial μ-agonist. Buprenorphine was approved for opioid dependence treatment in the United States in 2002 but has been available in France for many years (where there are approximately 74,000 patients maintained on buprenorphine).

General Pharmacology Buprenorphine produces morphine-like effects at low doses, but, even when the dose is increased, the intensity of the drug's actions does not seem to exceed that produced by 30 to 60 mg of morphine. Buprenorphine has poor oral bioavailability. The product approved for opioid dependence treatment is a sublingual tablet. Early clinical studies in addicts used a sublingual, alcohol-based solution of buprenorphine, which exhibits better bioavailability than the approved tablets. Reviews of buprenorphine dosing need to be clear about which formulation (solution versus tablet) was studied.

Buprenorphine's subjective effects appear to reach a ceiling at approximately 8 to 12 mg of solution, with only modest increases in effects at 16 and 32 mg. Over this dose range, significant respiratory depression is not observed. Because of this apparent ceiling, the risk of overdose may be limited. After repeated administration, buprenorphine attenuates or blocks the subjective effects of parenterally administered μ-agonist opioids (e.g., morphine, heroin). It has been reported that, when chronically administered buprenorphine is abruptly discontinued, a generally mild opioid withdrawal syndrome develops that is delayed in onset for several days. However, well-controlled studies comparing the withdrawal syndromes of different opioid agonists have not been conducted.

Sublingual buprenorphine tablets must be water soluble to dissolve in the mouth. It is possible that persons could dissolve them for injection to experience a more pronounced acute opioid effect. To decrease this abuse potential, buprenorphine tablets containing naloxone are available in a 4 to 1 dose ratio of buprenorphine to naloxone. Because naloxone has poor sublingual bioavailability, when a combination buprenorphine-naloxone tablet is taken by the therapeutic route (sublingually), the effect is predominantly due to buprenorphine. Naloxone has good parenteral bioavailability. If a buprenorphine-naloxone tablet is dissolved and injected by a person physically dependent on opioids such as heroin, precipitated withdrawal from the naloxone occurs. Although combining buprenorphine with naloxone decreases the risk of diversion and abuse by some populations—such as persons physically dependent on full agonist opioids, such as heroin or methadone—it does not decrease potential abuse by persons who abuse but are not dependent on opioids or, possibly, by persons who are maintained on buprenorphine.

Efficacy and Safety Buprenorphine has been compared to placebo and methadone in several double-blind outpatient studies. In general, these studies have shown that buprenorphine is more effective than placebo in the treatment of opioid dependence and that 8 mg of daily sublingual buprenorphine solution is equally effective as 50 to 60 mg of daily oral methadone on measures of retaining patients in treatment and suppression of heroin use. This sublingual solution dose is probably equivalent to 8 to 16 mg of daily sublingual buprenorphine tablet. With higher doses (e.g., 16 to 32 mg sublingually), some patients experience no withdrawal for 48 to 72 hours, permitting a reduction in dosing frequency. In this respect, buprenorphine is similar to LAAM. However, although LAAM must be dosed on a less-than-daily basis, buprenorphine has the option of daily or less-than-daily dosing. When buprenorphine is provided under supervised administration, this flexibility in intermittent dosing schedules may be a clinical advantage. Although buprenorphine has attractive features in its clinical pharmacological profile, the ceiling to its effects may limit its use—especially for patients who have higher levels of physical dependence. These patients may require full agonist opioids, such as methadone or LAAM. Initial outpatient clinical trials testing buprenorphine for the treatment of opioid dependence found this medication was safe and produced a profile of adverse effects similar to other opioids, such as methadone. However, clinical experience has drawn attention to two areas of concern. A few cases of buprenorphine-related fatalities have been reported from France; virtually all of these cases were associated with parenteral abuse of a benzodiazepine (most commonly flunitrazepam [Rohypnol], a benzodiazepine not available for use in the United States). These cases suggest that patients being treated with buprenorphine should be cautioned regarding this possible medication interaction with benzodiazepines. The second area of concern with buprenorphine use has been possible hepatic toxicity. There has been some evidence that patients with underlying hepatic damage may have an exacerbation of their liver disease, as evidenced by an increase in blood liver function tests, when treated with buprenorphine. Such an effect may be more likely if the person dissolves and injects buprenorphine tablets, so that there is a sudden spike in the buprenorphine blood level. However, further clinical experience with buprenorphine maintenance will help clarify the rate at which abnormal liver function tests may occur in some buprenorphine-maintained patients with underlying liver disease.

Heroin Treatment for Opioid Dependence There have been two large studies testing heroin for the treatment of opioid dependence. Both have been conducted in Europe (Switzerland and the Netherlands), and both studies have various weaknesses and strengths. Both studies have served as focal points for what have been, at times, intense discussions of the relative merits of heroin maintenance. Despite these two efforts, it is unfortunate that there is a relative dearth of data to help inform this topic. The Swiss government initiated a research program to test the feasibility of prescribing heroin to confirmed heroin addicts who had a history of poor outcome in traditional treatments, such as methadone. Initially, the plan was to compare, through random assignment, heroin, morphine, and methadone (each administered IV). However, owing to a strong preference for IV heroin and side effects from IV morphine and methadone, the design was revised as a feasibility test and a test of concept study, with the overwhelming majority of patients receiving IV heroin. A total of more than 1,100 persons were enrolled, although reports focused on a smaller subset of 385 patients. Patients were admitted to 18 treatment centers in several Swiss cities, came to specialized clinics several times a day, and injected as much heroin as they wished. For most patients, heroin dosage first escalated rapidly but, after several weeks or months, seemed to stabilize (for the 385 patients, at 490 mg per day), albeit, in some cases, at as much as 900 mg per day IV. Most patients came to the clinic several times a day. A rich array of psychosocial services were available to patients (including medical and psychiatric care, subsidized jobs, and welfare assistance). Investigators reported that patients' overall physical and mental health improved. Earnings improved somewhat, and criminal activity declined from 69 to 10 percent, as indicated by police records. Because urine was tested for drugs only every 8 weeks, it is not certain that illicit drug use actually decreased, but patients reported a sharp decrease in illicit heroin and cocaine use. Reported use of benzodiazepines declined slowly, and alcohol and cannabis use declined little. The dropout rate was relatively low, with 69 percent retention at 18 months. Eleven new cases of HIV or hepatitis were recorded, probably due to illicit cocaine use. The annual death rate of 1 percent was far lower than that for untreated addicts and lower than that for many other treatment programs. Because of the extensive support services and the long clinic hours, the overall cost of operating these clinics (approximately $23 per patient per day) was several times higher than the cost of comparable oral methadone maintenance programs.

The second study was conducted in the Netherlands and tested heroin as a supplement to daily oral methadone maintenance (compared to continued methadone dose alone). This was a nonblind clinical trial, and the intent of the study was not to stop drug use, but to maintain persons in treatment in an effort to reduce harm exposure and to maximize the chance that enrollees would receive other services. Outcome was assessed on a variety of measures, and significant improvement was based on one of six areas of functioning (a 40 percent improvement on any one of the six was defined as success). Methadone doses were relatively low in this study, and the cost of the heroin treatment was relatively high (between approximately $40 and $70 per day). The report on the study concluded that supplemental heroin was effective, based on the primary outcome measures. Interestingly, patients in the methadone-only group also improved, although their improvement was not across as broad an array of outcome measures. One particularly perplexing feature of the study was that illicit heroin use was neither a primary outcome measure nor a reported assessment. Although this reflects the design of the study, which was not to test the efficacy of providing heroin on attenuation of illicit opioid use, the absence of some measure of illicit opioid use is surprising.

Other, Nonpharmacological Treatments for Opioid Dependence

THERAPEUTIC COMMUNITIES Although it is difficult to clearly note the onset of the *therapeutic community* (TC) mode of treatment, as precursors can be found in other forms of related treatments, in general, TCs had their start in the late 1950s and early 1960s in the United States. Since then, TCs have evolved and matured, with a body of research and writing about clinical experiences that provides evidence for their role in substance abuse treatment and information about how different TCs operate. Synanon, a TC-like program, started in California in the late 1950s, and the essential feature of TCs is that the social environment can provide a valuable and unique setting for helping the person to acquire necessary prosocial skills. The TC seeks to aid the person to grow through personal responsibility, the acquisition of social skills, and the modeling of behavior. TCs do not see treatment of substance abuse as a unidirectional process from trained staff to patients, but rather as a process that occurs through the total immersion of the person in a community with rules, structure, and therapeutic interventions that derive from member–member interactions. The goal is to effect a complete change of lifestyle, including abstinence from drugs, the development of personal honesty and useful social skills, and the elimination of antisocial attitudes and criminal behavior.

To achieve these objectives, the addict was expected to live in the TC for approximately 12 to 18 months and to participate in frequent group sessions devoted to mutual criticisms of the attitudes and behavior of the participants. The community also acts, in many respects, as a substitute family. Assumption of responsibility within the community is rewarded with increased personal freedom, material comfort, and the respect of peers. Deviation from community expectations, in terms of behavior or attitude, frequently results in harsh criticisms by staff or sometimes by the entire community. Violence and any form of drug use are totally prohibited and may result in expulsion from the community—the ultimate punishment. Although most therapeutic communities avoid the use of drugs even to ease initial withdrawal, some are more flexible regarding treatment with drugs for heavily dependent new entrants. More recently, some therapeutic communities have recognized that a high percentage of addicts have psychopathology in addition to drug dependence and thus may permit the use of prescribed antipsychotic or antidepressant medication.

Present-day therapeutic communities vary considerably in their attitudes toward professionals and in actual staffing patterns. In every community, however, at least a few ex-addicts are employed as key personnel on the staff; the ex-addicts serve as role models and as visible evidence that recovery and acceptance are possible and expected. Some therapeutic communities, such as Phoenix House, Odyssey, and Second Genesis, are or were directed by psychiatrists and employ a number of health professionals in key positions. Federally supported programs have begun to develop individualized treatment plans and to use health care professionals, such as physicians, psychologists, or master's degree–level counselors or social workers, to make initial assessments.

Although many therapeutic communities still expect residents to return to the general community after 12 to 18 months, some are experimenting with shorter periods of residence, sometimes because of pressure from funding sources. Because they require so long a period of residence, therapeutic communities obviously have little appeal to those opioid addicts who have stable and gainful employment and satisfactory personal relationships. Currently, a substantial proportion of entrants into therapeutic communities are referred by the criminal justice system. Criteria for entry have thus been modified, and external pressure to remain in treatment has been increased. Despite the external pressure, dropout rates are still high: 30 to 40 percent in the first 90 days and 50 percent within 6 months. Furthermore, the percentage of new entrants with severe psychopathology has been gradually increasing. There is substantial variation in dropout rates among ostensibly similar therapeutic communities, even after adjusting for patient characteristics.

Residence in the TC results in major reductions in drug use problems; indicators of depression also decrease significantly. Follow-up studies of graduates and dropouts indicate that patients remaining 90 days or longer exhibit significant decreases in self-reported antisocial behavior, illicit drug use, and recorded arrests, as well as substantial increases in legitimate employment. Improvement was seen in patients who met DSM-III-R criteria for antisocial personality, to approximately the same extent as those who do not. In general, for those without severe psychopathology, there is a consistent time-in-program effect that lasts as long as approximately 12 months; patients who stay longer exhibit better outcomes along all dimensions at 12-month and 5-year follow-up intervals. In some cases, patients found to be doing well have had additional treatment in other programs since leaving the TC.

OUTPATIENT DRUG-FREE PROGRAMS Such treatment programs often provide services to patients who have completed opioid withdrawal, and there are three broad levels of service contained within such programs. The first, and most intensive level of service, is a partial hospitalization program (PHP) model of treatment. Patients are typically seen at least 5 days each week and, in some PHPs, are seen 7 days per week. Days are structured, with didactic sessions mixed with psychotherapy-style groups and individual counseling sessions. PHPs often offer 5 or more hours of therapeutic interaction each day, with the amount of service provided often defined by local regulatory agencies. A step down from PHPs are *intensive outpatient programs* (IOPs). These programs typically provide services 3 days per week, and the total amount of time in treatment on each day is approximately 3 hours. Patients may graduate from a PHP to an IOP level of services. The third, and least intensive level of care, is routine outpatient counseling. This may occur once or twice per week and can consist of an individual session or group treatment, or both. A patient might be discharged from an inpatient detoxification program, attend a PHP for several weeks, and then transition to an IOP for several more weeks or even months. As treatment success becomes established, the patient may then move to meeting with a therapist once a week and perhaps may join a group of patients.

Outpatient programs often subscribe to the same goals as residential or therapeutic communities, and they can vary widely in staffing patterns, philosophy, and program content. Long-term follow-up studies suggest that these programs have an impact beyond what is seen with detoxification alone, but differences in patient characteristics make valid comparisons difficult.

PSYCHOTHERAPIES As measured by use of illicit drugs, need for ancillary psychiatric medicines, scores on scales of psychological distress, and amount of legitimate money earned, patients in methadone maintenance programs appear to benefit more when individual, analytically oriented, supportive-expressive, or cognitive-behavioral psychotherapy is added to standard drug counseling (compared to counseling alone). With such therapy, the bleak prognosis for patients with the most severe psychopathology can be improved. To best engage patients in individual therapy, the therapy should be started early and should be an integral part of the program.

Among patients maintained on methadone, one controlled study suggests that skillful family therapy in conjunction with urine monitoring is superior to standard drug counseling in fostering decreased illicit drug use. However, from a public health perspective, such additional psychotherapy for patients treated with adequate doses of methadone does not appear to be as cost effective as providing standard therapy (weekly drug counseling) to more patients. There are no controlled studies on the efficacy of individual psychotherapy in treating opioid-using patients not stabilized on methadone.

BEHAVIORAL INTERVENTIONS Methadone treatment has provided a setting in which behavioral treatments have been studied and used. For example, contingent take-home doses of methadone have been shown to be a useful mechanism for achieving therapeutic goals, such as cessation of illicit drug use. Such interventions define a mutually agreed on target that can be objectively measured (e.g., providing three consecutive urine samples that are free from illicit benzodiazepine use), which then results in a desired outcome for the patient (e.g., a take-home dose of methadone).

A second behavioral intervention that has received considerable attention and research is the use of voucher incentives. Again, a target goal is defined (e.g., a cocaine-negative urine sample), and achievement of the goal results in the earning of a monetary voucher. Typically, vouchers escalate in value as a longer duration of the target is achieved (e.g., more consecutive cocaine-negative urine samples). Patients do not receive cash payments but can use vouchers to purchase goods and services consistent with their treatment goals. Although contingent take-home doses of methadone are relatively low-cost interventions, voucher incentives have direct costs (associated with purchase of goods and services) and indirect costs (associated with staff time and effort, for example). However, novel variants of voucher incentive programs have been developed by treatment programs—for example, capitalizing on goods donated by local merchants. Interestingly, a study testing the efficacy of voucher incentives in the treatment of patients recently discharged from a detoxification program, in which opioid and cocaine use were targeted, did not find a significant difference in outcomes compared to a control, no voucher, condition.

Treatment of Special Populations

CRIMINAL JUSTICE PATIENTS There is a complex relationship between the criminal justice system, patients with substance abuse disorders, and drug-dependence treatment systems. Many patients now enter or remain in treatment because of direct coercion by the courts or correctional system, and many persons incarcerated have a concurrent substance abuse problem. Treatment of criminal justice patients includes efforts directed at persons who are incarcerated and interventions designed for persons under legal restraints but still residing in the community. The former include prison-based opioid detoxification programs, therapeutic communities, and methadone maintenance programs. Although these treatment modalities have been piloted at various sites (and, in some locations, substantial numbers of patients have been in treatment—for example, in prison-based methadone treatment), their use is the exception, rather than the rule, in most correctional settings.

Specialized interventions for opioid-dependent criminal justice patients in the community have also been developed. Probation and parole can be viewed in their own right as techniques that modify drug-using behavior. Close supervision and drug testing of parolees result in a substantial reduction in daily drug use. The efficacy of such testing and supervision depends, in part, on the way in which sanctions against use are arranged and the consistency with which such sanctions are exercised. There is evidence that probation programs that involve the use of naltrexone combined with drug counseling reduce relapse to opioid use and reincarceration rates.

PREGNANT WOMEN In general, illicit opioid use during pregnancy is associated with decreased fetal growth but not with teratological effects. Most pregnant women who continue to use heroin and other illicit drugs do not get prenatal care and deliver low-weight babies with an elevated risk for morbidity and mortality. Babies who survive may be infected with HIV and other diseases as a result of maternal high-risk behavior. Most of these risks can be substantially reduced if the mother can be retained in treatment and provided with prenatal care. Sometimes this can be accomplished in drug-free outpatient or residential programs. Using such programs usually requires initial detoxification, which must be undertaken with considerable caution, because severe opioid withdrawal early in pregnancy (before 14 weeks) can induce abortion and late in pregnancy (after 32 weeks) can induce fetal distress.

If a woman is already maintained on methadone, it is generally recommended that she remain on this medication throughout the pregnancy (given the risk of fetal distress associated with the withdrawal of methadone and the potential for relapse once withdrawal is completed). If methadone withdrawal is elected for the pregnant woman, it should be done in collaboration with clinicians experienced in perinatal addiction. Dose increases may be needed for the pregnant woman maintained on methadone because of changes in blood volume and metabolism as the pregnancy progresses, and split methadone dosing may be useful in the third trimester (when methadone metabolism and clearance increases). Babies born to mothers who have been maintained on methadone usually have evidence of neonatal opioid withdrawal, and various treatment interventions have been advocated for the neonate (although there are few controlled comparisons of these different treatments). If the use of illicit drugs can be eliminated during pregnancy, and if adequate prenatal care can be provided, infant mortality and morbidity are reduced, and, in the long run, the development and cognitive functioning of the baby are not likely to be impaired. More recent studies indicate that buprenorphine can also be used successfully in treating opioid-dependent pregnant women.

HEALTH PROFESSIONALS Health professionals often come to treatment when their drug use is discovered by colleagues or by drug enforcement agencies. Treatment generally consists of a contingency contract under which they agree to frequent drug testing and the certain revocation of their license to practice if they continue to use drugs. This contract is typically supplemented by encouragement to participate in a 12-step program or other therapy. Supervised naltrexone may occasionally be part of the regimen. Under supervision, most (as much as 85 percent) of these patients recover and are able to return to practice. Returning to specialties with easy access to opioids can pose a serious hazard to continued abstinence. For example, in one study, only 34 percent of anesthesiology residents who were abusing opioids were able to return to their specialty. For a significant percentage of the residents, the first sign of relapse was a fatal overdose.

OTHER SPECIAL POPULATIONS Certain groups of drug users are more likely to enter treatments that seem designed to deal with particular demographic groups or types of patients with a particular substance abuse problem. For example, some women may feel that only a women's treatment program will deal adequately with issues of childhood sexual abuse, spousal physical abuse, or fears of losing custody of children. Native Americans, Hispanic Americans, or Americans of African or Asian descent may feel more comfortable in programs designed to be sensitive to their cultural values. To what degree such programs are more effective than less specialized programs in retaining patients in treatment or in producing long-term behavioral change remains undetermined.

Treatment of Patients with Opioid Dependence and Additional Psychopathology

The severity of psychological disturbances—depression, anxiety, and paranoid ideation—tends to predict the overall outcome of treatment for opioid dependence. Other predictors of outcome include alcohol abuse and the use of illicit nonopioid drugs, such as cocaine. Furthermore, patients in methadone programs who meet criteria for additional nonsubstance abuse Axis I diagnoses consistently exhibit substantially higher rates of lifetime and current diagnoses of dependence on drugs other than opioids. However, the literature is not entirely consistent on the prognostic significance of additional psychopathology. In a number of studies, patients with additional psychopathology, including antisocial personality disorder, appear to do approximately as well in methadone programs or therapeutic communities as those without such diagnoses, at least in terms of reduced drug use.

Mood Disorders Some form of affective dysregulation is the most common Axis I psychiatric disorder not related to substance abuse found among opioid addicts in treatment (Table 11.10–5). Clinicians agree that those addicts with bipolar I or bipolar II disorders can benefit from treatment with mood stabilizing medications (e.g., lithium [Eskalith] and divalproex [Depakote]). Caution should be exercised when combining methadone with certain psychotropic medications—for example, carbamazepine (which may be used to treat bipolar disorder) induces methadone metabolism, which, in turn, may lead to relapse in illicit opioid use.

Although clinicians in private practice often prescribe antidepressant medications for opioid-dependent patients with major depressive disorder and minor depression, publicly supported programs often do not. The reasons for this vary. In the past, therapeutic communities were biased against the use of psychoactive agents; they seem to be less so now, and some therapeutic communities have psychiatric consultants and permit psychoactive medication when indicated. Methadone programs do not have a bias against pharmacotherapy, but many still do not commonly assess depressive symptoms, responding only when these symptoms become clinically obvious. Studies of the efficacy of antidepressant agents in the treatment of depressed opioid-dependent patients have yielded inconsistent results. It is possible that adequate antidepressant plasma concentrations may not have been achieved or that patients were not carefully selected.

In methadone-maintained patients whose depression antedated substance use or persisted for more than 1 month after admission to treatment, a double-blind study found that imipramine (Tofranil) produced significant improvements in mood, as well as self-reported decreases in the use of illicit drugs. However, as measured by urine tests, few patients achieved abstinence. In this study, the imipramine dosage was gradually increased, depending on adverse effects and response, to a maximum of 300 mg per day.

Opioid addicts tend to experience a decrease in depressive symptoms after entering treatment, regardless of whether the treatment is an opioid maintenance program or a TC. Not every patient shows spontaneous improvement, however. Because the severity of psychological impairment is a predictor of overall treatment success, the conscientious clinician will pay particular attention to persistent depression.

Anxiety Disorders Anxiety disorders rarely receive specific treatment in programs devoted to opioid dependence. A high percentage of addicts with an anxiety disorder also have dysphoria. When pharmacological treatment seems indicated, antidepressant medications would appear to be the drugs of choice, because several of these have antianxiety, antipanic, and antidepressant effects. Use of benzodiazepine medications should generally be avoided, given their abuse potential and the vulnerability of opioid-dependent persons to abuse such medications.

Schizophrenia and Other Psychotic Disorders A high percentage of patients treated in urban hospitals for psychotic disorders, including schizophrenia, also meet the criteria for a substance use disorder. In most instances, patients are abusing or are dependent on alcohol, cocaine, cannabis, or some combination of those drugs. Even in East Coast urban areas in which opioid abuse is common, opioid dependence is relatively uncommon among patients hospitalized for schizophrenia. In studies of methadone-maintained patients, prevalence rates of schizophrenia are generally less than 1 percent.

Endogenous opioids interact with dopaminergic systems, and it has been postulated that methadone can have antimanic and antipsychotic actions. There are case reports but no controlled studies of opioid users who responded poorly to traditional antipsychotic agents but whose psychotic or paranoid states responded to opioids. For patients with schizophrenia and opioid dependence, dopamine receptor antagonists are probably useful and can be combined with methadone. Methadone added to antipsychotic medication produces improvement in antipsychotic-resistant patients with paranoid schizophrenia.

Alcohol Abuse Alcoholism (alcohol abuse or dependence) is common among opioid addicts in treatment, with lifetime diagnosis rates as high as 50 percent. Several studies suggest that there is an inverse relation between alcohol use and heroin use, with alcohol use increasing as heroin use decreases as a result of treatment—a situation that reverses with relapse. In one methadone program, neither twice-weekly sessions with special AA counselors nor behavioral modification sessions with psychologists were more helpful than a control condition of standard maintenance. However, most alcohol abusers decreased their alcohol consumption, as well as their heroin use, after entering treatment, and patients and counselors who participated in treatment were enthusiastic about group sessions and expressed the belief that they were beneficial.

Disulfiram (Antabuse) can be combined with methadone without adverse effects. Large studies testing the efficacy of disulfiram in methadone-maintained, alcohol-dependent patients have not been conducted. In one moderate-sized, randomized, controlled study, disulfiram was not superior to placebo in modifying alcohol abuse or dependence among methadone-maintained patients. However, in that study, patients in both groups (disulfiram and placebo) had reductions in alcohol use. Optimal use of disulfiram in methadone-maintained patients appears to occur when there is some behavioral intervention tied to regular ingestion of the disulfiram (e.g., take-home doses of methadone).

The opioid antagonist naltrexone is approved for the treatment of opioid and alcohol abuse. In methadone-maintained patients, it is contraindicated (as it precipitates withdrawal). Theoretically, naltrexone should be an ideal medication for use in a patient with opioid and alcohol dependence, once the person has been successfully withdrawn off both, although there is no research documenting the relative success of such use.

In programs that do not use methadone, continued participation in a residential program sharply reduces alcohol use, but data on long-term outcome are lacking. Outpatient drug-free and residential programs may use AA and 12-step approaches to controlling alcohol abuse or dependence along with procedures aimed at opioid use and behavioral change.

Nicotine Dependence A study of methadone-maintained patients found that more than 90 percent had a current diagnosis of nicotine dependence. Despite the high rates of concurrent smoking found in opioid dependent patients, treatment providers often focus interventions on other drug use disorders. However, surveys suggest that many patients in treatment for opioid dependence are interested in stopping smoking. Given the health benefits associated with smoking cessation and the high rate of smoking found among opioid-dependent persons, improvement in screening and treating nicotine dependence in this population is needed.

Opioid Dependence with Other Substance Abuse Many opioid users regularly self-administer some other drug or drugs (e.g., amphetamines, cocaine, alcohol, barbiturates, benzodiazepines, or cannabinoids). In general, multidrug users have a greater range and severity of psychiatric problems. In therapeutic communities, they create more behavior problems, drop out of treatment sooner, and have poorer posttreatment outcomes. Many polysubstance users are sufficiently dependent on heroin or other opioids to qualify for treatment in methadone programs. Competent counseling has been shown to decrease cocaine use, as has the provision of positive rewards, such as vouchers or lottery tickets, contingent on urine tests that are negative for cocaine.

A retrospective study of treatment outcome for polysubstance abuse as a function of the category of drugs abused and the treatment received compared male veterans enrolled in TC treatment to those in methadone maintenance. All subjects had greater-than-average psychopathology in addition to polysubstance abuse. The groups were further categorized into opioid-stimulant, opioid-depressant, and opioid-only users. At 6-month follow-up, the opioid-only group had better outcomes on all measures than either of the other groups, with no clear superiority of either treatment approach. The opioid-stimulant group did significantly better in methadone maintenance, and the opioid-depressant group did significantly better after treatment in a TC. The researchers inferred that recovery from the depression and cognitive impairment that typically accompany the abuse of sedatives was facilitated by the prolonged abstinence afforded by treatment in a TC. Specialized facilities using TC approaches have evolved to provide treatment to drug abusers with serious psychiatric disorders, especially those who are also homeless. Their results suggest that major reductions in drug use and rehospitalization can be achieved.

SUGGESTED CROSS-REFERENCES

An overview of substance-related disorders is given in Section 11.1. Alcohol-related disorders are discussed in Section 11.2, amphetamine-related disorders are discussed in Section 11.3, and cocaine-related disorders are discussed in Section 11.6. Drug and alcohol abuse among the elderly is discussed in Section 51.3i. Posttraumatic stress disorder (PTSD) is discussed in Chapter 15, and sexual dysfunction is discussed in Section 18.1a.

REFERENCES

*American Psychiatric Association: Practice guideline for the treatment of patients with substance use disorders: Alcohol, cocaine, opioids. *Am J Psychiatry.* 1995;152[Suppl]:5.

Ball J, Ross A. *The Effectiveness of Methadone Maintenance Treatment.* New York: Springer-Verlag; 1991.

Bird SM, Hutchinson SJ: Male drugs-related deaths in the fortnight after release from prison: Scotland, 1996–99. *Addiction.* 2003;98:185.

Brooner RK, King VL, Kidorf M, Schmidt CW, Bigelow GE: Psychiatric and substance use comorbidity among treatment-seeking opioid abusers. *Arch Gen Psychiatry.* 1997;54:71.

Daglish MR, Weinstein A, Malizia A: Changes in regional cerebral blood flow elicited by craving memories in abstinent opiate-dependent subjects. *Am J Psychiatry.* 2001;158:1680.

Daws LC, White JM: Regulation of opioid receptors by opioid antagonists: Implications for rapid opioid detoxification. *Addict Biol.* 1999;4:391.

De Leon G. *The Therapeutic Community.* New York: Springer Publishing Company; 2000.

des Jarlais DC, Hagan H, Friedman SR, Friedmann P, Goldberg D, Frischer M, Green S, Tunving K, Ljungberg B, Wodak A, Ross M, Purchase D, Millson ME, Myers T: Maintaining low HIV seroprevalence in populations of injecting drug users. *JAMA.* 1995;274:1226.

Dyer KR, White JM: Patterns of symptom complaints in methadone maintenance patients. *Addiction.* 1997;92:1445.

Ernst M, London ED: Brain imaging studies of drug abuse: Therapeutic implications. *Semin Neurosci.* 1997;9:120.

Fiellin DA, O'Connor PG: Office-based treatment of opioid-dependent patients. *N Engl J Med.* 2002;347:817.

Fudala PJ, Jaffe JH, Dax EM, Johnson RE: Use of buprenorphine in the treatment of opioid addiction, II. Effects of daily and alternate-day administration and abrupt withdrawal. *Clin Pharmacol Ther.* 1990;47:525.

Goldstein RZ, Volkow ND: Drug addiction and its underlying neurobiological basis: Neuroimaging evidence for the involvement of the frontal cortex. *Am J Psychiatry.* 2002;159:1642.

Gowing LR, Farrell M, Ali RL, White JM: α2-Adrenergic agonists in opioid withdrawal. *Addiction.* 2002;97:49.

*Gutstein HB, Akil H. Opioid analgesics and antagonists. In: Harman JG, Limbird LE, eds. *Goodman & Gilman's The Pharmacological Basis of Therapeutics.* 10th ed. New York: McGraw-Hill; 2001.

Hser Y-I, Hoffman V, Grella CE, Anglin MD: A 33-year follow-up of narcotics addicts. *Arch Gen Psychiatry.* 2001;58:503.

Institute of Medicine. *Federal Regulation of Methadone Treatment.* Washington, DC: National Academy Press; 1995.

Jaffe JH, Knapp CM, Ciraulo DA. Opiates: Clinical aspects. In: Lowinson JH, Ruiz P, Millman RB, Langrod JG, eds. *Substance Abuse: A Comprehensive Textbook.* 3rd ed. Baltimore: Williams & Wilkins; 1997.

*Johnson RE, Chutuape MA, Strain EC, Walsh SL, Stitzer ML, Bigelow GE: A comparison of levomethadyl acetate, buprenorphine, and methadone for opioid dependence. *N Engl J Med.* 2000;343:1290.

Johnson RE, Jones HE, Fischer G: Use of buprenorphine in pregnancy: Patient management and effects on the neonate. *Drug Alcohol Depend.* 2003;70[Suppl 1]:S87.

Kakko J, Svanborg KD, Kreek MJ, Heilig M: 1-Year retention and social function after buprenorphine-assisted relapse prevention treatment for heroin dependence in Sweden: A randomized, placebo-controlled trial. *Lancet.* 2003;361:662.

Kendler KS, Jacobson KC, Prescott CA, Neale MC: Specificity of genetic and environmental risk factors for use and abuse/dependence of cannabis, cocaine, hallucinogens, sedatives, stimulants, and opiates in male twins. *Am J Psychiatry.* 2003;160:687.

Khantzian E, Halliday KS, McAuliffe WI. *Addiction and the Vulnerable Self.* New York: Guilford; 1990.

Kirchmayer U, Davoli M, Verster AD, Amato L, Ferri M, Perucci CA: A systematic review of the efficacy of naltrexone maintenance treatment in opioid dependence. *Addiction.* 2002;97:1241.

Kraft MK, Rothbard AB, Hadley TR, McLellan AT, Asch DA: Are supplementary services provided during methadone maintenance really cost-effective? *Am J Psychiatry.* 1997;154:1214.

Krantz MJ, Jutinsky IB, Robertson AD, Mehler PS: Dose-related effects of methadone on QT prolongation in a series of patients with torsade de pointes. *Pharmacotherapy.* 2003;23:802.

*Kreek MJ. Rationale for maintenance pharmacotherapy of opiate dependence. In: O'Brien CP, Jaffe JH, eds. *Addictive States.* Vol 30. New York: Raven Press; 1992.

Kreek MJ, Koob GF: Drug dependence: Stress and dysregulation of brain reward pathways. *Drug Alcohol Depend.* 1998;51:23.

Ling W, Charuvastra C, Collins JF, Batki S, Brown LS Jr, Kintaudi P, Wesson DR, McNicholas L, Tusel DJ, Malkerneker U, Renner JA Jr, Santos E, Casadonte P, Fye C, Stine S, Wang RIH, Segal D: Buprenorphine maintenance treatment of opiate dependence: A multicenter, randomized clinical trial. *Addiction.* 1998;93:475.

Maddox JF, Desmond DP: Ten-year follow-up after admission to methadone maintenance. *Am J Drug Alcohol Abuse.* 1992;18:289.

*McLellan AT, Arndt IO, Metzger DS, Woody GE, O'Brien CP: The effects of psychosocial services in substance abuse treatment. *JAMA.* 1993;269:1953.

Mogil JS, Pasternak GW: The molecular and behavioral pharmacology of the orphanin FQ/nociceptin peptide and receptor family. *Pharmacol Rev.* 2001;53:381.

Musto DF, ed. *One Hundred Years of Heroin.* Westport, CT: Auburn House; 2002.

Najavits LM, Weiss RD: The role of psychotherapy in the treatment of substance-use disorders. *Harvard Rev Psychiatry.* 1994;2:84.

*Nestler EJ: Molecular neurobiology of addiction. *Am J Addict.* 2001;10:201.

Neto D, Xavier M, Aguiar P, David M, Sardinha L, de Almeida C: Sequential combined treatment of heroin addicted patients in Portugal with naltrexone and family therapy. *Eur Addict Res.* 1997;3:138.

Nurco DN, Kinlock T, Balter MB: The severity of pre-addiction criminal behavior among urban, male narcotic addicts and two non-addicted control groups. *J Res Crime Delinquency.* 1993;30:293.

O'Brien CP, Childress AR, McLellan AT, Ehrman R. A learning model of addiction. In: O'Brien CP, Jaffe JH, eds. *Addictive States.* New York: Raven Press; 1992.

Popik P, Kozela E, Wrobel M, Wozniak KM, Slusher BS: Morphine tolerance and reward but not expression of morphine dependence are inhibited by the selective glutamate carboxypeptidase II (GCP II, NAALADasa) inhibitor, 2-PMPA. *Neuropsychopharmacology.* 2003;28:457.

Ritter AJ, Lintzeris N, Clark N, Kutin JJ, Bammer G, Manjari M: A randomized trial comparing levo-alpha acetylmethadol with methadone maintenance for patients in primary care settings in Australia. *Addiction.* 2003;98:1605.

Robins LN: Vietnam veterans' rapid recovery from heroin addiction: A fluke or normal expectation? *Addiction.* 1993;88:1041.

Robinson TE, Berridge KC : The psychology and neurobiology of addiction: An incentive sensitization view. *Addiction.* 2000;95[Suppl 2]:S91.

Sees KL, Delucchi KL, Masson C, Rosen A, Clark HW, Robillard H, Manys P, Hall SM: Methadone maintenance vs 180 day psychosocially enriched detoxification for treatment of opioid dependence: A randomized controlled trial. *JAMA.* 2000;283:1303.

Strain EC, Bigelow GE, Liebson IA, Stitzer ML: Moderate- versus high-dose methadone in the treatment of opioid dependence. A randomized trial. *JAMA.* 1999;281:1000.

Strang J, Griffiths P, Gossop M: Heroin smoking by "chasing the dragon": Origins and history. *Addiction.* 1997;92:673.

Tornay CB, Favrat B, Monnat M, Daeppen JB, Schnyder C, Bertschy G, Besson J: Ultra-rapid opiate detoxification using deep sedation and prior oral buprenorphine preparation: Long-term results. *Drug Alcohol Depend.* 2003;69:283.

Trujillo KA: Are NMDA receptors involved in opiate-induced neural and behavioral plasticity? A review of preclinical studies. *Psychopharmacology (Berl).* 2000;151:121.

Tsuang MT, Lyons MJ, Lyons MJ, Meyer JM, Doyle T, Eisen SA, Goldberg J, True W, Lin N, Toomey R, Eaves L: Co-occurrence of abuse of different drugs in men. *Arch Gen Psychiatry.* 1998;55:967.

▲ 11.11 Phencyclidine (or Phencyclidine-like)–Related Disorders

DANIEL JAVITT, M.D., PH.D., AND
STEPHEN R. ZUKIN, M.D.

Phencyclidine (PCP; 1-1 [phenylcyclohexyl]piperidine), also known as *angel dust*, was first developed as a novel anesthetic in the late 1950s. This drug and the closely related compound ketamine were termed *dissociative anesthetics*, because they produced a condition in which subjects were awake but apparently insensitive to, or dissociated from, the environment. The symptoms induced by PCP and ketamine closely resemble those observed in schizophrenia. As early as 1959, therefore, it was proposed that PCP psychosis might serve as a heuristically valuable model for schizophrenia. PCP entered the illicit street market in 1965. In the late 1970s, it was one of the leading drugs of abuse in the United States. Although its popularity has subsequently declined, the popularity of ketamine has been steadily increasing.

PCP and ketamine exert their unique behavioral effects by blocking *N*-methyl-D-aspartate (NMDA)–type receptors for the excitatory neurotransmitter glutamate. PCP and ketamine intoxication can present with a variety of symptoms, from anxiety to psychosis. Treatment remains largely symptomatic and supportive. Few studies have assessed medication effects on PCP or ketamine intoxication effects directly. PCP and ketamine induce psychotic symptoms that closely resemble those of schizophrenia. As such, these drugs have been frequently used in challenge studies to investigate brain mechanisms in schizophrenia. Although PCP is no longer used in controlled human studies, ketamine challenge studies are ongoing and continue to provide critical insights into schizophrenia.

HISTORY

PCP was developed in the late 1950s as a potential general anesthetic by Parke-Davis under the trade name Sernyl. Clinical trials in anesthesia were promising in that PCP did not depress vital cardiovascular and respiratory functions. In contrast to conventional general anesthetics, which induce a state of relaxed sleep, PCP induced a state of apparent catatonia, including flat facies, open mouth, fixed staring, rigid posturing, and (sometimes) waxy flexibility. Patients seemed dissociated from the environment without classic unconsciousness. For this reason, PCP was termed a *dissociative anesthetic*.

As many as one-half of patients given PCP anesthesia showed severe adverse reactions during emergence, such as agitation and hallucinations. Psychotic reactions persisting for as long as 10 days then ensued in many of these patients. PCP was used as an experimental probe of psychotomimetic mechanisms in normal and schizophrenic subjects during the late 1950s and early 1960s.

The first reported cases of PCP abuse occurred in 1965. Use escalated throughout the 1960s and 1970s. In the late 1970s, PCP was one of the most prevalent abused drugs in the United States; relatively infrequent but flamboyant and destructive episodes of PCP-induced aggressive and violent behaviors captured the public imagination and the attention of the press. The manifold and severe medical complications of PCP abuse led to an explosion of medical literature on this topic during the late 1970s and the 1980s. Over recent years, PCP abuse has declined substantially. However, it continues to be a serious public health problem.

Like PCP, ketamine was also developed in the late 1950s as a potential general anesthetic. Ketamine, like PCP, caused emergence reactions in exposed patients. Because of ketamine's shorter half-life, however, the emergence reactions are more easily managed by benzodiazepines or simple emotional support. Because it does not cause respiratory depression at anesthetic doses, ketamine remains a widely used anesthetic agent for children (who are less susceptible to its psychotomimetic effects) and medically compromised patients. Ketamine is marketed as a general anesthetic under the trade name Ketalar and as a veterinary anesthetic.

Ketamine entered the club drug scene in the 1980s, possibly as an adulterant to the more widely used drug *ecstasy* (3,4-methylenedioxymethamphetamine [MDMA]). However, ketamine rapidly became a drug of abuse in its own right, with particular popularity in the club drug or rave culture. Until recently, ketamine was not scheduled under the Controlled Substances Act and could be found in hospital pharmacies, from which diversion has frequently occurred. In 1999, ketamine was reclassified as a schedule III controlled substance by the Food and Drug Administration (FDA) and included in many states in their controlled substance legislation. Whether this will affect rates of ketamine abuse, however, remains to be seen.

EPIDEMIOLOGY

PCP, a phenylcyclohexylamine, is easily synthesized from piperazine, cyclohexanone, and potassium cyanide. The synthesis proceeds through the intermediate 1-piperidinocyclohexanecarbonitrile (PC), which is reacted with phenyl magnesium bromide to form PCP. The simplicity of this reaction, which requires almost no training or equipment, gave PCP production an economic advantage over agents that were more difficult to synthesize. The advantage did not disappear until precursors for PCP, notably piperazine, were regulated themselves. A major use for PCP has always been as an adulterant to other illicit substances, such as cocaine, methamphetamine, or lysergic acid diethylamine (LSD). Marijuana is frequently adulterated with PCP by dealers. Thus, PCP intoxication may be seen in patients who are not aware that they have taken PCP.

PCP has had many street names, including *angel dust*, *devil's dust*, *dust*, *crystal*, *cyclones*, *embalming fluid*, *wet*, *killer weed*, *mint weed*, *peace pill*, *goon*, *jet fuel*, *surfer*, *black whack*, *Illy*, *crazy Eddie*, *purple rain*, and *milk*. In combination with other drugs, it has been called *beam me up Scottie* or *tragic magic* (crack dipped in PCP); *love boat* (marijuana dipped in PCP), and *blunt* (marijuana and PCP in a cigar wrapper). Its abuse was first reported in 1965, when it had limited popularity. In the early 1970s, PCP was usually mixed with other drugs; by the late 1970s, most street samples analyzed were pure PCP. The most common routes of administration are smoking and snorting; every conceivable route of administration has been reported, including injection. Regional differences in typical routes of administration were often reported, with snorting predominating in Philadelphia and Chicago, smoking and snorting predominating in Miami, and smoking predominating in Seattle.

PCP abuse peaked between 1973 and 1979, with a smaller peak between 1981 and 1984. It is estimated that, in 1976, 9.5 percent of persons between 18 and 25 years of age had ever used PCP, increasing to 13.9 percent in 1977 and 14.5 percent in 1979. For 12- to 17-year-olds, the corresponding figures were 3 percent, 5.8 percent, and 3.9 percent, respectively. By 1988, these figures had declined to 1.2 percent for those 12 to 17 years of age and 4.4 percent for those 18 to 25 years of age. Since 1985, the highest rates of use have been in those between 26 and 34 years of age. Some 12.8 percent of high school seniors reported PCP use in 1979; this declined to approximately 3 percent from 1987 through 1995. The 1994 survey data indicate that 4.3 percent of household residents aged 12 years and older, or approximately nine million people, had used PCP at least once in their lives, up from 2.9 percent in 1985. In 1994, 478,000 people (0.02 percent) were estimated to have used PCP at least once in the prior year. Although this number is dwarfed by annual rates of marijuana (8.5 percent), cocaine (1.7 percent), inhalant (1.1 percent), and crack (0.6 percent) use, it is still significant. Rates of PCP abuse have been low but stable since that time.

PCP-related emergency department mentions increased more than fivefold between 1974 and 1979 and then declined; by 1991, PCP ranked 27th among drugs mentioned. In order, the leading cities for PCP emergency room mentions were Los Angeles, Chicago, Washington, New York City, San Francisco, Baltimore, and Philadelphia. Legal and policy changes contributed to the decline in PCP use during the 1980s. PCP was reclassified from schedule III to schedule II under the Controlled Substances Act. Reporting of production of piperidine, a major PCP precursor, was mandated. Penalties for PCP possession with intent to sell were significantly increased.

As PCP abuse has declined, ketamine abuse has increased dramatically, especially as a club drug in the rave scene. Ketamine is frequently known as *K*, *special K*, *vitamin K*, *super K*, *Kit-Kat*, or *jet*; ketamine intoxication is frequently referred to as the *K-hole* because of the dissociative and amnestic effects of the drug. Because it can be so readily combined with other drugs of abuse, it is frequently used in combination with cocaine, MDMA (ecstasy), heroin, or other party drugs—the combination sometimes being referred to as *trail mix*. Ketamine continues to be marketed as a veterinary and pediatric anesthetic. Moreover, when appropriately modified with anesthetics such as propofol (Diprivan), ketamine produces highly effective, short-acting analgesia and is being used increasingly even for adult anesthesia and postoperative pain care.

Ketamine is primarily available as an injectable prescription formulation diverted from official medical channels, although illicitly manufactured powder and tablet formulations may also be available. A typical dose is 100 to 200 mg. The street cost of ketamine in 2001 was approximately $80 per gram. Preferred routes of administration include intravenous (IV) or intramuscular (IM) injection, ingestion, smoking, or snorting.

ETIOLOGY AND PSYCHOPHARMACOLOGY

Phencyclidine, Ketamine, and *N*-Methyl-D-Aspartate (NMDA) Receptors

The unique primary central nervous system (CNS) actions of PCP and other dissociative anesthetics result from binding to high-affinity PCP receptors that are highly selective for drugs (from a variety of chemical classes) that elicit PCP-like behavioral effects. The relative potencies of such drugs in eliciting PCP-like behaviors are proportional to their potencies in competing for radioligand binding to the PCP receptor. The fundamental mechanism of action of PCP, interaction with a unique high-affinity brain binding site, was discovered in 1979. Subsequent studies demonstrated that the PCP receptor constitutes a binding site located within the ion channel of the NMDA-type glutamate receptor. Drugs that bind to PCP receptors also block NMDA-activated channels in electrophysiological and receptor binding assays. The rank order of potency of such drugs as channel blockers closely parallels their behavioral potencies and their potencies in binding to the PCP receptor. The highest densities of PCP receptors are found in the dentate gyrus, the first and second regions of the cornu ammonis (CA1 and CA2) of the hippocampus, and anterior forebrain areas, including neocortex, consistent with the ability of PCP to disrupt learning, memory, and higher cortical functions.

Unlike the other types of glutamate receptor channels, NMDA channels are permeable to Ca^{2+} as well as Na^{+}. After NMDA receptor activation, NMDA-mediated Ca^{2+} flux may lead to stimulation of calmodulin-dependent kinases with activation of postsynaptic second-messenger pathways. A unique functional property of the NMDA channel is that it is blocked in a voltage-dependent manner by the endogenous Mg^{2+} ion. The dual voltage and ligand dependence of NMDA receptors permits them to function in a hebbian manner to integrate information from multiple input streams. One stream is represented as a modulation of presynaptic glutamate release, whereas additional streams are reflected in modulation of resting membrane potential on the postsynaptic NMDA receptor-bearing dendrites. Ca^{2+} flow through open, unblocked NMDA channels may trigger long-term potentiation, which, in turn, may represent the neurophysiological substrate underlying learning and memory formation. In rodents, PCP and other NMDA antagonists induce profound memory disturbances linked to inhibition of hippocampal long-term potentiation. In humans, amnesia can be seen in PCP intoxication and ketamine anesthesia.

NMDA receptors possess two distinct agonist binding sites, one for glutamate and other excitatory amino acids (e.g., aspartate) and another for glycine and other structurally similar amino acids, such as D-serine. In vivo, glutamate and glycine–D-serine have distinct roles in receptor activation. Like most classic neurotransmitters, glutamate is released from presynaptic nerve endings in pulsatile fashion and then rapidly reabsorbed. By contrast, glycine in forebrain is neither concentrated in presynaptic nerve endings nor released in response to electrical stimulation. Furthermore, endogenous glycine concentrations are typically at or above the affinity constant of the NMDA-associated glycine site for these agents, indicating that activity-stimulated release of glycine is not required for neurotransmission. Rather, the local glycine concentration appears to set the tonic level of NMDA excitability, thus determining the degree to which presynaptic glutamate release leads to postsynaptic excitation. Glycine thus functions more as a neuromodulator than as a classic neurotransmitter. D-Serine is the only D–amino acid present in high concentration in brain. Thus, D-serine, like glycine, may help regulate the tonic excitability level of NMDA excitability. The NMDA receptor–associated glycine site is anatomically, pharmacologically, and functionally distinct from the classic strychnine-sensitive glycine receptor found primarily in hindbrain, which binds D-serine with low affinity. Glycine levels in brain are regulated by the actions of glycine transporters, which maintain subsaturating glycine levels surrounding at least some NMDA receptors. In addition to the glutamate and glycine–D-serine binding sites, the NMDA receptor complex also contains sites that are sensitive to polyamines, such as spermine and spermidine, and to redox state. Theses sites are all targets for development of anti-PCP drugs, which might also be expected to be beneficial in schizophrenia.

Opening the NMDA channel facilitates access of PCP to its receptor, accelerating the rate at which PCP-induced blockade of NMDA receptor–mediated neurotransmission takes place relative to the rate in the absence of NMDA receptor activation. In the former case, PCP gains access to its binding site rapidly via the open channel pore; in the latter case, the highly lipophilic PCP molecule gains access to its binding site via slow diffusion through the lipid bilayer.

Molecular Characterization of the Phencyclidine Receptor

The NMDA receptor complex is heteroligemeric, consisting primarily of combinations of NMDAR1 and NMDAR2 subunits. NMDAR1 is the key subunit in the formation of the receptor complex.

The large majority of NMDA receptor complexes contain an NR1 subunit; complexes may also contain variable numbers of modulatory subunits (NR2A-D). NR2B and NR2A receptors are particularly abundant in forebrain. The PCP binding site is primarily located on the NR1 subunit and overlaps the Mg^{2+} binding site. Thus, channel blockers such as PCP and ketamine have similar affinity for NR1/NR2A- and NR1/NR2B-containing receptors. However, behavioral effects of these agents may be dominated by their effects at NR1/NR2A complexes.

The glycine binding site is also contained within the NR1 subunit; thus, all NMDA receptors show glycine sensitivity. However, glycine affinity is modulated by NR2 subunits; thus, receptors containing NR2D subunits appear more sensitive to glycine than those containing NR2B subunits, which, in turn, are more sensitive than those containing NR2A subunits. Eight variants of NMDAR1 (NMDAR1a–h) have been identified, which reflect alternative messenger ribonucleic acid (mRNA) splicing. Receptors containing such variants may also have distinct sensitivities to agonists, antagonists, Zn^{2+}, and polyamines. A third NMDA subunit family, termed *NR3*, has recently been identified but is expressed primarily in brainstem and spinal cord.

NMDA receptors are primarily found postsynaptically and occur on projection neurons and interneurons. However, NMDA subunit composition varies among brain regions and cell types within a region. In some brain regions, especially in target areas of the mesolimbic-mesocortical system, NMDA receptors may also be localized presynaptically and thus may regulate release of dopamine from presynaptic terminals. It has been suggested that such receptors consist solely of NR1 subunits and thus may have a different pharmacological profile from postsynaptic receptors.

Additional CNS Actions of Phencyclidine and Ketamine At doses at least ten times those at which it exerts its unique behavioral effects by blocking NMDA receptor–mediated neurotransmission, PCP also blocks presynaptic monoamine reuptake, thus directly increasing synaptic levels of dopamine and norepinephrine. Concentrations sufficient to block monoamine reuptake may be achieved during high-dose intoxication and may contribute to the stimulatory behavioral and physiological effects of PCP seen at those doses. Ketamine, even at high doses, fails to block monoamine transporters. This observation may explain the lower incidence of episodes of extreme agitation and violence during ketamine intoxication than during PCP intoxication. At doses associated with extremely high-dose intoxication, PCP blocks neuronal Na^+ and K^+ channels, as well as muscarinic cholinergic receptors. Such effects may be relevant to the seizures observed after PCP overdose. PCP also interacts with a variety of other CNS receptors, including opiate and γ-aminobutyric acid (GABA) benzodiazepine receptors. However, most such effects take place at concentrations unlikely to be encountered in clinical situations.

Recently, in an attempt to incorporate PCP- and ketamine-induced psychosis into dopamine models of schizophrenia, it has been suggested that PCP and ketamine act as partial dopamine type 2 (D_2) receptor agonists. However, these interactions occur at PCP concentrations dramatically greater than the concentrations at which these agents interact with the PCP receptor under properly controlled experimental conditions. Similarly, in in vivo imaging studies, no direct interaction of ketamine on D_2 receptor binding has been observed. The lack of direct effect of PCP and ketamine at D_2 receptors also explains the relative insensitivity of ketamine or PCP psychosis to treatment with typical antipsychotics.

Neurotoxicity of Phencyclidine and Ketamine In animals, neurotoxic effects of PCP, ketamine, or other NMDA antagonists are observed at doses significantly greater than those required for behavioral activity. At those doses in the rat, NMDA antagonists induce neuronal vacuolization, particularly in neurons in rat posterior cingulate retrosplenial cortex (PCRS). Similar vacuolization is observed after administration of dizocilpine (MK-801), indicating that the effect is probably mediated at NMDA receptors. The effect is initially observed in layers III and IV of cortex. At lower doses (e.g., 5 mg/kg), the effect is transient, reaching a peak approximately 12 hours after PCP or dizocilpine administration and then resolving over 12 to 18 hours. Much higher doses of PCP may lead to neuronal necrosis, which is apparent even 48 hours after drug administration and is seen in hippocampus and other limbic areas as well as in the PCRS. Administration of high-dose PCP also leads to increased glucose uptake and expression of heat shock and glial fibrillary acidic protein (GFAP). Vacuolization can be inhibited by prior administration of anticholinergic, GABAergic, or antipsychotic agents and is potentiated by administration of pilocarpine (Salagen). Direct evidence of similar neurotoxic effects in humans is lacking, despite the large number of patients who have undergone ketamine anesthesia for surgery. Neurotoxicity induced by PCP, ketamine, or other NMDA antagonists may be particularly relevant to the persistent cognitive deficits observed after heavy or repeated intoxication.

Behavioral Pharmacology of Phencyclidine and Ketamine

Rodent Models Considerable species variation exists in the behavioral effects of NMDA antagonists. In rodents, these agents induce a characteristic syndrome of hyperactivity and stereotypical movements, which is only partially reversible by neuroleptics but can be more robustly antagonized by agents such as glycine or D-serine that augment NMDA receptor–mediated neurotransmission. Because the serum half-lives of PCP and ketamine are shorter, and their volume of distribution is larger in rodents than in primates, rodents typically require higher weight-adjusted doses of PCP than primates to elicit behavioral effects. Sensitization to the behavioral effects of PCP and ketamine has been detected after daily administration in rodents. Both agents also inhibit rodents' social behavior, an effect that is not reversed by typical or atypical antipsychotic agents.

The behavioral effects of PCP and ketamine are accompanied by increased release of dopamine and serotonin in multiple brain regions, including prefrontal cortex, nucleus accumbens, and striatum. Hyperactivity in rodents has traditionally been considered to reflect increased dopaminergic neurotransmission within nucleus accumbens, but more recent studies point to a critical role of prefrontal cortex as well. In contrast, PCP-induced stereotypies have traditionally been attributed to increased dopamine release within striatum.

NMDA receptors are also present in substantia nigra (A9) and ventral tegmental area (A10). Glutamatergic innervation of substantia nigra from prefrontal cortex strongly influences dopaminergic activity levels; NMDA receptors appear to be the primary mediators of glutamate-induced stimulation of midbrain dopaminergic neurons. To the extent that NMDA receptors stimulate A9 and A10 neurons, PCP would, paradoxically, be expected to diminish dopaminergic outflow from striatum and accumbens. However, direct application of PCP to A10 does not inhibit dopamine cell firing or alter dopamine release in accumbens, although it does prevent NMDA-induced neuronal activation. Thus, the behavioral effects of PCP in rodents appear to stem predominantly from its interactions within dopamine terminal fields rather than within dopaminergic midbrain nuclei.

In all regions, NMDA receptors are present on intrinsic GABAergic neurons and on glutamatergic or GABAergic outflow neurons, so that circuit level effects of NMDA blockade may be difficult to predict. For example, NMDA agonists and antagonists induce hyperactivity after acute administration into nucleus accumbens. NMDA blockade may also produce a secondary increase in glutamate release, which of itself mediates aspects of the PCP behavioral syndrome. In rodents, NMDA antagonists also produce neurophysiological deficits (e.g., disruption of prepulse inhibition) and disturbances of working memory and long-term memory formation that resemble cognitive disturbances observed in schizophrenia.

Some effects of PCP and ketamine in rodents respond preferentially to treatment with serotonin type 2A (5-HT_{2A}) receptor antagonists, such as M100,907, supporting the usefulness of atypical antagonists in the treatment of psychosis. However, despite the plethora of PCP and ketamine effects in rodents, it remains unclear which effects are most relevant to the clinical situation. The fact that rodents show hyperactivity in response to NMDA antagonists, whereas humans and nonhuman primates show predominant withdrawal symptoms, makes rodent behavioral models, in general, difficult to interpret.

Primate Models Gross behavioral effects of PCP in nonhuman primates more closely resemble the effects of the drug in humans. In monkeys, a PCP dose of approximately 0.5 mg/kg produces tranquilization in which animals appear awake but unresponsive to the environment. At 1 mg/kg, PCP induces a cataleptoid state in which animals show waxy flexibility and rigidity resembling catatonic schizophrenia. Doses of 2.5 mg/kg lead to stupor, 5 mg/kg leads to surgical anesthesia, and 15 mg/kg leads to convulsive seizures. Ketamine is approximately tenfold less potent than PCP, with doses of 5 to 10 mg/kg producing tranquilization and immobility.

Cognitive effects of PCP and ketamine have been extensively characterized in primates. Both drugs, along with other NMDA antagonists, inhibit serial response chain learning and produce delayed match to sample, which are considered animal models of working memory. Furthermore, both impair prepulse inhibition of the acoustic startle response, a putative neurophysiological marker of schizophrenia. Effective doses of PCP against prepulse inhibition, 0.25 mg/kg, are less than the level needed to produce tranquilization. During chronic treatment, PCP induces a syndrome consisting of decreased spontaneous movement and increased scanning behavior, along with inappropriate threat behavior directed toward nonexistent objects. This syndrome persists for the duration of PCP treatment and resolves thereafter. PCP effects on spontaneous activity appear to be reversible during treatment with NMDA agonists, such as glycine. In contrast, scanning behavior, which may be an animal analog of hallucinations, was affected to a lesser degree.

Ketamine produces behavioral effects in monkeys at doses of 0.5 to 2.0 mg/kg, which are likewise subanesthetic. Effects of ketamine are highly similar to those of PCP. Ketamine administration induces disturbances in long-term and working memory, prolongation of reaction time, and impairments in visual search that are strikingly similar to those observed in schizophrenia.

Pharmacokinetics of Phencyclidine PCP is highly lipid soluble and has a volume of distribution of 6.2 L/kg in humans. Significant brain concentrations are rapidly attained after inhaled, smoked, or topical administration (PCP intoxication has been documented after inadvertent wearing of clothing on which a PCP solution had been spilled). A typical street dose is approximately 5 mg (one pill, joint, or line), which results in a serum PCP concentration between 0.01 and 0.1 μM. Psychotic reactions have been observed in association with undetectable low serum concentrations (<0.02 μmol), whereas concentrations greater than 0.4 μmol induce gross impairment of consciousness. Serum concentrations greater than 1 μM are strongly associated with coma, seizures, respiratory arrest, and death. The highest recorded serum and cerebrospinal fluid (CSF) concentrations are in the range of 1 to 2 μM. Users typically titrate dosage in an effort to maximize the high while avoiding unconsciousness. Failures of judgment or variations in purity of supplies often result in inadvertent overdose, which may lead to severe medical complications. The serum half-life of PCP varies considerably among individuals, averaging approximately 20 hours. The half-life of ketamine in humans is approximately 2 hours. The lipophilicity of PCP facilitates accumulation in fatty body tissues, including the brain. PCP concentrations in brain and in adipose tissues may be more than ten times those in plasma. Mobilization of adipose stores (e.g., during exercise) may release sequestered PCP, leading to flashbacks.

Metabolism of PCP is predominantly hepatic; hydroxylase metabolites are secreted renally. PCP (negative logarithm of acid ionization constant [pK_a] = 8.5) is largely ionized in the stomach or the urinary tract. Passing through the pyloric valve, PCP enters a nonacidic environment in the small intestine in which it becomes largely nonionized and readily absorbed across the mucosal membrane, whereupon enterohepatic recalculation can account for the fluctuating clinical course so often observed in PCP intoxication.

Pharmacokinetics of Ketamine Ketamine has a briefer duration of effect than PCP. Peak ketamine levels occur approximately 20 minutes after IM injection. After intranasal administration, the duration of effect is approximately 1 hour. Ketamine is *N*-demethylated by liver microsomal cytochrome P450, especially CYP3A, into norketamine. Ketamine, norketamine, and dehydronorketamine can be detected in urine, with half-lives of 3, 4, and 7 hours, respectively. Urinary ketamine and norketamine levels vary widely from individual to individual and may range from 10 to 7,000 ng/mL after intoxication. As of yet, the relationship between serum ketamine levels and clinical symptoms has not been formally studied. Ketamine is often used in combination with other drugs of abuse, especially cocaine. Ketamine does not appear to interfere with and may enhance cocaine metabolism.

REINFORCING EFFECTS OF NMDA ANTAGONISTS

Experimental monkeys avidly self-administer large doses of PCP IV or orally. Monkeys given unlimited access to PCP maintain nearly continuous intoxication. This pattern resembles that seen with opiates and CNS depressants but differs from that seen with classical stimulants. Furthermore, in contrast to findings on opiate self-administration, monkeys self-administer doses of PCP high enough to cause marked behavioral effects. Given the similarities between behavioral effects of PCP in monkeys and humans, this research validates the clinical impression of avid human self-administration of PCP. PCP-like drugs stimulate brain reward areas, lowering the threshold for intracranial self-stimulation. Such effects, which define a classic profile for drugs abused by humans, are shared by other abused compounds, such as opiates, stimulants, and benzodiazepines, despite their differing mechanisms of action.

TOLERANCE TO NMDA ANTAGONISTS

In rats and monkeys, repeated administration of PCP daily or more frequently leads to two- to fourfold rightward shifts in dose-response curves. The major determinant of this moderate tolerance appears to be biodispositional. Much greater tolerance is induced by continuous self-administration than by intermittent dosing. Limited human data exist on PCP tolerance, but tolerance has been reported in burn patients given repeated doses of ketamine for analgesia. Tolerance has also been reported after repeated use of ketamine, with daily dosages increasing to more than 1,000 mg per day.

PHYSICAL DEPENDENCE ON NMDA ANTAGONISTS

After unlimited-access self-administration of PCP for a month or longer, severe withdrawal reactions were observed in monkeys when the drug was discontinued, including vocalizations, bruxism, oculomotor hyperactivity, diarrhea, piloerection, somnolence, tremor, and seizures. Similarly, severe reactions might be expected after PCP binges by human abusers. Despite a paucity of controlled studies of tolerance and dependence in humans, the animal literature suggests that PCP must be considered comparable to classic drugs of abuse in this respect.

LONG-TERM CONSEQUENCES OF NMDA ANTAGONISTS

Single high doses or repeated lower doses of NMDA antagonists induce structural damage in susceptible regions of rodent or primate brain. Regions that appear most sensitive to these effects are posterior cingulate and retrosplenial cortices, although effects are not confined to these regions. Neurotoxic effects of NMDA antagonists can effectively be blocked by several classes of agent, including muscarinic antagonists, GABA type A receptor ($GABA_A$) agonists or positive modulators (e.g., benzodiazepines and barbiturates), α_2-adrenergic agonists, and some, but not all, typical and atypical antipsychotics. The fact that most of these agents do not reverse PCP- or ketamine-induced psychosis or psychosis associated with schizophrenia suggests that the NMDA antagonist–induced neurotoxicity is not responsible for the psychotomimetic effects of these agents per se. However, many of the delayed neurocognitive effects of repeated PCP or ketamine abuse may be a consequence of drug-induced neurotoxicity.

During acute administration, PCP and ketamine have been shown to induce a variety of neurocognitive deficits that closely resemble those of schizophrenia. A prominent feature is difficulty in learning new information but preserved ability to retain information once learned. This pattern is similar to the pattern seen in schizophrenia but is dissimilar to the pattern seen in dementing illness, such as Alzheimer's disease. Acute administration also leads to failures of executive functioning and the ability to perform working memory tasks. As in schizophrenia, the deficit is related to inability to use new information, rather than the inability to retain information over time. PCP- and ketamine-induced cognitive deficits, however, are not limited to prefrontal processes. Thus, deficits may be observed even in such processes as mismatch negativity (MMN) generation. MMN reflects the ability of auditory cortex to respond to changes in auditory stimulation patterns.

After single, low doses, cognitive deficits resolve once the drug is cleared. The acute onset and rapid offset of cognitive dysfunction argue against the neurotoxic effects of these agents as being primarily responsible. After recreational use, however, cognitive deficits may persist even after several days of recovery. Semantic memory and attentional deficits appear most likely to persist, similar to postulated models involving prefrontal and hippocampal structural pathology. Research into persistent effects of NMDA antagonists is difficult because of lack of information regarding premorbid levels of functioning. However, if confirmed, the finding of persistent dysfunction would support the use of more aggressive intervention during acute episodes with drugs such as benzodiazepines that might prevent NMDA antagonist–induced neurotoxicity.

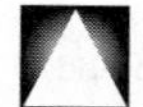

Table 11.11–1
DSM-IV-TR Phencyclidine-Related Disorders

Phencyclidine use disorders
Phencyclidine dependence
Phencyclidine abuse
Phencyclidine-induced disorders
Phencyclidine intoxication
Specify if:
With perceptual disturbances
Phencyclidine intoxication delirium
Phencyclidine-induced psychotic disorder, with delusions
Specify if:
With onset during intoxication
Phencyclidine-induced psychotic disorder, with hallucination
Specify if:
With onset during intoxication
Phencyclidine-induced mood disorder
Specify if:
With onset during intoxication
Phencyclidine-induced anxiety disorder
Specify if:
With onset during intoxication
Phencyclidine-related disorder not otherwise specified

From American Psychiatric Association. *Diagnostic and Statistical Manual of Mental Disorders.* 4th ed. Text rev. Washington, DC: American Psychiatric Association; 2000, with permission.

DSM-IV-TR DISORDERS

Table 11.11–1 lists the revised fourth edition of the *Diagnostic and Statistical Manual of Mental Disorders* (DSM-IV-TR) PCP-related disorders. Clinical presentations of PCP-induced disorders frequently fail to fit within any established diagnostic category. Mixtures of features of several categories are quite common. Frequently, the presentation varies over time as serum PCP levels fluctuate. Therefore, even the most careful single examination cannot be definitive. The absence of serious medical complications at a single time does not preclude development of such complications hours later. Delirium and psychotic features often come and go several times during intoxication. Unless serious medical complications cause irreversible cardiovascular, renal, or neurological damage, complete recovery from PCP intoxication is usually seen within 24 to 72 hours. Even in prolonged PCP-induced psychotic disorder, complete recovery is usually seen within 6 weeks.

A 17-year-old male patient was brought to the emergency room by the police, having been found disoriented on the street. As the police attempted to question him, he became increasingly agitated; when they attempted to restrain him, he became assaultive. Attempts to question or to examine him in the emergency department evoked increased agitation.

Initially, it was impossible to determine vital signs or to draw blood. Based on the observation of horizontal, vertical, and rotatory nystagmus, a diagnosis of PCP intoxication was entertained. Within a few minutes of being placed in a darkened examination room, his agitation markedly decreased. Blood pressure was 170/100; other vital signs were within normal limits. Blood was drawn for toxicological examination. The patient agreed to take 20 mg of diazepam (Valium) orally. Thirty minutes later, he was less agitated and could be interviewed, although he responded to questions in a fragmented fashion and was slightly dysarthric. He stated that he must have inadvertently taken a larger-than-usual dose of "dust," which he reported having used once or twice a week for several years. He denied use of any other substance and any history of mental disorder. He was disoriented to time and place. The qualitative toxicology screen revealed PCP and no other drugs. Results of neurological examination were within normal limits, but brisk deep tendon reflexes were noted. Some 90 minutes after arrival, his temperature, initially normal, was elevated to 38°C, his blood pressure had increased to 182/110, and he was poorly responsive to stimulation. He was admitted to a medical bed. His blood pressure and level of consciousness continued to fluctuate over the ensuing 18 hours. Results of hematological and biochemical analyses of blood, as well as urinalyses, remained within normal limits. A history obtained from his family revealed that the patient had had multiple emergency room visits for complications from PCP use during the previous several years. He had completed a 30-day residential treatment program and had participated in several outpatient programs but had consistently relapsed. The patient was discharged after vital signs and level of consciousness had been within normal limits for 8 hours. At discharge, nystagmus and dysarthria were no longer present. A referral to an outpatient treatment program was made.

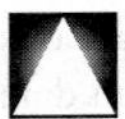

Table 11.11–2
DSM-IV-TR Diagnostic Criteria for Phencyclidine Intoxication

A. Recent use of phencyclidine (or a related substance).
B. Clinically significant maladaptive behavioral changes (e.g., belligerence, assaultiveness, impulsiveness, unpredictability, psychomotor agitation, impaired judgment, or impaired social or occupational functioning) that developed during, or shortly after, phencyclidine use.
C. Within an hour (less when smoked, snorted, or used intravenously), two (or more) of the following signs:
 (1) Vertical or horizontal nystagmus
 (2) Hypertension or tachycardia
 (3) Numbness or diminished responsiveness to pain
 (4) Ataxia
 (5) Dysarthria
 (6) Muscle rigidity
 (7) Seizures or coma
 (8) Hyperacusis
D. The symptoms are not due to a general medical condition and are not better accounted for by another mental disorder.

Specify if:
 With perceptual disturbances

From American Psychiatric Association. *Diagnostic and Statistical Manual of Mental Disorders.* 4th ed. Text rev. Washington, DC: American Psychiatric Association; 2000, with permission.

Phencyclidine and Ketamine Abuse and Dependence There have been no systematic studies of PCP abuse, dependence, or withdrawal states in humans, but primate research gives every reason to expect that they are clinically significant. Patterns of PCP and ketamine use have been documented in specific populations in which users self-administer multiple, high, daily doses continuously for weeks, months, or years. Chronic use does not cause physical dependence. Nevertheless, significant tolerance to effects of PCP or ketamine and the need for escalating doses have been documented. The avidity with which many users return to PCP or ketamine use immediately after treatment for severe intoxication or psychosis suggests that intense craving is experienced after medically supervised withdrawal. No specific treatments have been developed for PCP or ketamine abuse or dependence. Relapse can reportedly be averted with antidepressant treatment in selected patients, suggesting that some users are attracted to PCP by its antidepressant properties.

Phencyclidine Intoxication and Phencyclidine Intoxication Delirium

Diagnosis and Clinical Features The cornerstone of diagnosis of PCP intoxication (Table 11.11–2) is a history of PCP use, detection of PCP in body fluids, or both. A number of assays for PCP are available; however, for several reasons, it can be dangerous to rely on them. First, the combination of PCP's lipophilicity, long duration of action, and pK_a predicts that prominent clinical effects may be present in the absence of measurable concentrations of PCP in blood or CSF. This is particularly true for acute psychotic reactions, which have been observed at serum PCP concentrations undetectable by most assay systems. A positive assay for PCP should generally be used only qualitatively; it is particularly important not to assume that a low measured concentration predicts an uneventful recovery. pK_a considerations in relation to varying urinary and intestinal pH and enterohepatic recirculation indicate that concentrations can be expected to fluctuate. Clinical indications of significant neuronal hyperexcitability, hypertension, hyperthermia, or other physiological dysregulation should be interpreted as indicating a possible impending medical emergency. Reliance on history may also yield many false negatives, because PCP may have been misrepresented as another drug or used as an adulterant by the dealer. As PCP levels fluctuate, various mixtures of symptoms of intoxication, delirium, and psychosis are seen.

Diagnosis of ketamine abuse must be made, for the most part, without recourse to urine testing. Rapid screening assays are not generally available. Furthermore, ketamine cross-reacts unreliably with immunoassays for PCP. As with PCP, a history of ingestion is critical to making the diagnosis. Typical street doses are in the range of 100 to 200 mg. The most common complaints of ketamine abusers who present themselves to the emergency department are anxiety, chest pain, and palpitations. The most common physical manifestation of ketamine intoxication is tachycardia. Nystagmus is seen in only a minority of cases but is rotary in character when it does occur.

Physiological Bases of Intoxication, Delirium, and Medical Complications The range of clinical effects of PCP can be correlated with dose, serum PCP concentration, and interaction with several molecular target sites (Fig. 11.11–1). The CNS NMDA receptor complex would be the only system affected significantly at low PCP doses. Serum PCP concentrations as large as approximately 0.1 μmol correspond to a clinical state manifesting

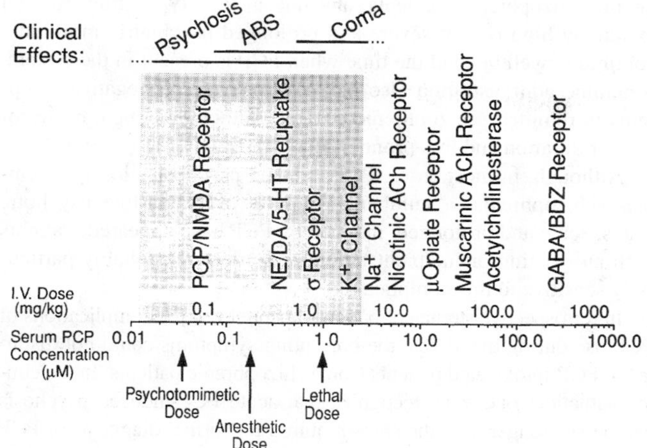

FIGURE 11.11–1 Dose range of phencyclidine (PCP) effects. The relation of dose, serum concentration, molecular target sites, and clinical effects is shown. The shaded area represents clinically relevant interactions. ABS, acute brain syndrome; ACh, acetylcholine; BDZ, benzodiazepine; DA, dopamine; GABA, γ-aminobutyric acid; 5-HT, serotonin; I.V., intravenous; NE, norepinephrine; NMDA, *N*-methyl-D-aspartate. (From Javitt DC, Zukin SR: Recent advances in the phencyclidine model of schizophrenia. *Am J Psychiatry.* 1991;148:1301, with permission.)

psychotomimetic symptoms and impaired cognition without physiological disturbances of vital functions other than nystagmus, hypertension, tachycardia, dysarthria, or hyperacusis. Serum concentrations just greater than approximately 0.1 μmol correspond to a state of delirium and, at approximately 0.3 μmol, to incipient dissociative anesthesia, with prominent numbness or diminished responsiveness to pain. At still higher doses, as additional types of receptors are occupied, acute brain syndrome accompanied by prominent neurological and cardiovascular complications is seen. Deaths from hyperthermia, status epilepticus, and hypertensive crisis have been reported. At high doses, PCP exerts direct excitatory effects on skeletal muscle endplates. These effects may underlie the many reports of superhuman strength from the late 1970s. Together with the behavioral effects of high-dose PCP, these effects probably account for muscle trauma, which, in a number of patients, has resulted in rhabdomyolysis, myoglobinuria, and renal failure. Serum concentrations of 1.0 μmol and greater are associated with coma and death. PCP-induced delirium and coma result from the combination of noncompetitive inhibition of the PCP-NMDA receptor, blockade of the reuptake sites for catecholamines and indolamines, and blockade of sodium and potassium channels and nicotinic and muscarinic cholinergic receptors.

Ketamine, because of its lower potency, shorter half-life, and decreased propensity to interact with non-NMDA binding sites, has much lower associated morbidity and mortality. Death due to uncomplicated ketamine intoxication is rare. For example, in a review of all ketamine-associated deaths in New York City between 1997 and 1999, there were no instances of fatal intoxication due to ketamine alone. In virtually all cases of fatality, ketamine was combined with other drugs, particularly opiates, with cause of death being multidrug intoxication.

NEUROLOGICAL MANIFESTATIONS The vast majority of PCP-intoxicated patients manifest horizontal, vertical, or rotatory nystagmus, which can help distinguish PCP intoxication from a naturally occurring psychotic state. Neuronal hyperexcitability is dose dependent, ranging from increased deep tendon reflexes, to opisthotonos, to focal or generalized seizures, or to status epilepticus. Focal neurological findings may arise from cerebral vasoconstriction. Coma can occur at any point during intoxication. Rotary nystagmus may also be seen during ketamine intoxication but is less common. The absence of nystagmus therefore cannot be used to exclude a diagnosis of ketamine intoxication.

BEHAVIORAL MANIFESTATIONS Clinically urgent short-term behavioral complications of PCP abuse stem from behavioral disinhibition, which can be coupled with severe agitation, panic, rage, and aggression. The disruption of sensory input by PCP can cause unpredictable, exaggerated, distorted, or violent reactions to environmental stimuli. Such reactions are more common with somewhat higher doses, at which some delirium, as well as neurological symptoms and other medical complications, is observed. The behavioral manifestations can severely compromise the clinician's ability to treat the medical complications.

CARDIOVASCULAR MANIFESTATIONS PCP-induced hypertension is dose dependent. Mild hypertension is seen in all patients with PCP intoxication. With increasing PCP dose, the panoply of sympathomimetic responses is seen; hypertensive crisis is common in association with high doses and may lead to cerebral hemorrhage. Tachycardia and mild hypertension are also seen with ketamine but are substantially less severe and unlikely to be life threatening.

AUTONOMIC MANIFESTATIONS Severe hyperthermia has been observed and can be delayed, fatal, or both. The anticholinergic properties of PCP can evoke the full spectrum of atropine-like toxicity in a dose-dependent manner and can be managed accordingly.

Differential Diagnosis Even when PCP is detected in body fluids, remember that PCP is frequently taken in combination with another drug or drugs. Depending on the analytical method used, an assay for PCP may fail to detect an intoxicating concentration of PCP. Although not conclusive or totally specific for PCP intoxication, the constellation of nystagmus, ataxia, and mild hypertension is typically observed even in mild, low-dose PCP intoxication.

Treatment Treatment of PCP intoxication aims to reduce systemic PCP levels and to address significant medical, behavioral, and psychiatric issues. For intoxication and PCP-induced psychotic disorder, although resolution of current symptoms and signs is paramount, the long-term goal of treatment is prevention of relapse to PCP use. PCP levels may fluctuate over many hours or even days, especially after oral administration. Therefore, a prolonged period of clinical observation is mandatory before concluding that no serious or life-threatening complications will ensue.

Trapping of ionized PCP in the stomach has led to the suggestion of continuous nasogastric suction as a treatment for PCP intoxication. However, this strategy can be needlessly intrusive and can induce electrolyte imbalances. Administration of activated charcoal is safer, and it binds PCP and diminishes toxic effects of PCP in animals.

Trapping of ionized PCP in urine has led to the suggestion of urinary acidification as an aid to drug elimination. However, this strategy may be ineffective and is potentially dangerous. Only a small portion of PCP is excreted in urine, metabolic acidosis itself carries significant risks, and acidic urine can increase the risk of renal failure secondary to rhabdomyolysis. Because of the extremely large volume of distribution of PCP, neither hemodialysis nor hemoperfusion can significantly promote drug clearance.

No drug is known to function as a direct PCP antagonist. Any compound binding to the PCP receptor, which is located within the ion channel of the NMDA receptor, would block NMDA receptor–mediated ion fluxes as does PCP itself. NMDA receptor mechanisms predict that pharmacological strategies promoting NMDA receptor activation (e.g., administration of a glycine site agonist drug) would promote rapid dissociation of PCP from its binding sites. However, no clinical trials of NMDA agonists for PCP or ketamine intoxication in humans have been carried out to date. Therefore, treatment must be supportive and directed at specific symptoms and signs of toxicity. Classical measures should be used for medical crises, including seizures, hypothermia, and hypertensive crisis.

Because PCP disrupts sensory input, environmental stimuli can cause unpredictable, exaggerated, distorted, or violent reactions. A cornerstone of treatment is therefore minimization of sensory inputs to PCP-intoxicated patients. Patients should be evaluated and treated in as quiet and isolated an environment as possible. Precautionary physical restraint is recommended by some authorities, with the risk of rhabdomyolysis from struggle against the restraints balanced by the avoidance of violent or disruptive behavior. Pharmacological sedation can be accomplished with oral or IM antipsychotics or benzodiazepines; there is no convincing evidence that either class of compounds is clinically superior. Because of the anticholinergic actions of PCP at high doses, neuroleptics with potent intrinsic anticholinergic properties should be avoided.

Course and Prognosis Complete recovery from PCP intoxication is the rule in the absence of major medical complications. However, many patients relapse to PCP use immediately after discharge from treatment, even for severe PCP-related complications. Intoxication usually occurs in the context of abuse, dependence, or both. Unfortunately, no specific behavioral treatments for PCP abuse and dependence have been described. Case reports indicate successful responses to residential and intensive outpatient treatment regimens with long-term follow-up, including urine monitoring with or without contingency contracting.

Phencyclidine- and Ketamine-Induced Psychotic Disorder

Diagnosis and Clinical Features Single, low IV doses (0.05 to 0.1 mg/kg) of PCP administered to normal volunteers can rapidly induce a psychotic state, lasting 4 to 6 hours, characterized by withdrawal, autism, negativism, inability to maintain a cognitive set, and concrete, impoverished, idiosyncratic, and bizarre responses to proverbs and projective testing. Some subjects show catatonic posturing. Similar effects are seen after low-dose ketamine administration (e.g., 0.2 to 0.5 mg/kg). With both drugs, negative symptoms are especially prominent and may progress to the point of mutism or catatonia. The pattern of neuropsychological impairment closely resembles that in schizophrenia, including disturbances in executive processing, working memory, and perceptual processing. An important clinical correlate of these data is that any person under the influence of even a small dose of PCP or a similar drug may have profound alterations of higher emotional functions affecting judgment and cognition, even in the absence of gross neurological findings. Well-formed hallucinations and delusions are relatively uncommon.

Challenge experiments involving recompensated schizophrenic subjects found that a single low dose of PCP can rekindle the presenting symptomatology for as long as 6 weeks, without evoking any symptoms or signs not typical of schizophrenia. Thus, schizophrenia or preschizophrenia patients abusing a PCP-type drug run an extremely high risk of severe and prolonged psychiatric morbidity, continuing well beyond the time when PCP is present in the system. Ketamine administration also induces positive and negative symptoms in remitted schizophrenic subjects, although symptoms are of shorter duration and less pronounced.

Although, in most cases, PCP-induced psychosis closely resembles schizophrenia, a number of reports of mania-like psychotic states, acute and prolonged, induced by PCP have appeared. Patients with an existing or incipient bipolar disorder are probably particularly sensitive to this complication.

In retrospective studies of patients hospitalized for complications of PCP use during the 1970s, the presenting symptoms could not distinguish PCP-intoxicated patients from schizophrenic patients. In the clinical situation, one must recognize that acute PCP-induced psychosis can persist longer than the signs required for formal diagnosis of PCP intoxication in DSM-IV-TR, particularly after low drug doses. By the time a patient comes to medical attention, psychosis may be the only notable finding. PCP-induced psychosis may remit after 4 to 6 hours or can persist for as long as 6 weeks after signs of acute physiological reactions have cleared. For acute and prolonged psychotic disorders induced by PCP, DSM-IV-TR criteria for PCP-induced psychotic disorder may fail to be met because of the absence of delusions or hallucinations, despite the presence of severe thought disorder.

In addition to its use in anesthesia, ketamine is increasingly being used for analgesia. Although it seems relatively safe during acute use, ketamine appears to be tolerated poorly during chronic administration due to cognitive and psychotomimetic side effects. Hallucinatory side effects have been observed in children as well as in adults. Nevertheless, this remains an area of active investigation. As analgesia use increases, the incidence of ketamine-induced psychotic episodes may increase as well.

Differential Diagnosis For several reasons, the differential diagnosis of PCP-induced psychotic disorder may prove challenging. First, the patient, as well as other informants, may be unaware that PCP has been used, because it may have been misrepresented as another drug or used as an adulterant. Second, PCP-induced psychosis can persist long beyond the time when PCP is detectable in blood and beyond the time when neurological and cardiovascular symptoms and signs of PCP intoxication are present. Third, careful retrospective analyses have demonstrated that frequently PCP-induced psychosis cannot be distinguished from naturally occurring schizophrenia on the basis of presenting symptoms and signs. Detection of PCP still leaves open the possibility that the patient has a preexisting psychotic disorder that has been exacerbated by PCP, a possibility that can be ruled out only by following the patient's future course.

Course and Prognosis In most cases, once any acute medical complications are successfully treated, peripheral and CNS complications, including psychosis, resolve completely within 24 to 72 hours. In the case of prolonged PCP-induced psychotic disorder, the rule is complete recovery within 4 to 6 weeks, regardless of whether antipsychotics have been administered. However, the rate of subsequent relapse to PCP use is high. Persistence of a psychotic disorder beyond 8 weeks indicates the possible presence of an underlying psychotic disorder exacerbated, but not caused, by PCP.

Treatment For acute or prolonged psychotic reactions, neuroleptics are commonly prescribed. The literature suggests that they are ineffective for most patients, but no systematic studies of this issue have been performed. Neuroleptics and benzodiazepines have been reported to be moderately effective against the agitation and behavioral disinhibition that may be present. However, the psychotic symptoms themselves often fail to respond to pharmacological treatment. As a consequence, inpatient treatment may be required throughout the course of the psychotic reaction. In animal models, atypical antipsychotics, especially clozapine (Clozaril), have proven more effective than typical antipsychotics in reversing behavioral effects of PCP. However, potential hypotensive effects of clozapine would have to be taken into account before its clinical use could be considered. To date, no clinical trials have been conducted comparing typical and atypical antipsychotics in the treatment of PCP- or ketamine-induced psychosis.

The antiepileptic drug lamotrigine (Lamictal) has been shown to prevent ketamine-induced psychotic effects, suggesting that it might have clinical efficacy in the treatment of prolonged psychosis. Several glycine site agonists, including glycine, D-serine, and D-cycloserine, have been shown to ameliorate persistent negative and cognitive symptoms of schizophrenia and so might also be considered for treatment of persistent PCP- or ketamine-induced symptoms. Effective doses of these agents are glycine, 800 mg/kg per day (approximately 60 g per day); D-serine, 30 mg/kg per day (approximately 2 g per day); and D-cycloserine, 50 mg per day.

In animals, effects of PCP are reversed by group II metabotropic agonists. In early clinical trials, prototype group II agonists, such as the compound LY354470, have shown safety and efficacy in a human anxiety model. These compounds may prove to be particularly effective in treating stress and anxiety associated with PCP or ketamine intoxication.

Phencyclidine-Induced Mood Disorder

PCP-induced mood disorder is a somewhat elusive category. A relatively small percentage of patients display a prominently elevated mood verging on hypomania after exposure to PCP. Symptoms and signs may clear as PCP concentrations decline or may progress to a PCP-induced manic state with psychotic features. In patients with a bipolar disorder, the intrinsic antidepressant properties of PCP may provoke a hypomanic or manic reaction.

Phencyclidine-Induced Anxiety Disorder

The literature provides little or no support for PCP-induced anxiety disorder as a distinct clinical entity. Preclinically, PCP and related drugs fit an anxiolytic and antidepressant profile. Distinguishing anxiety from the agitation and behavioral disinhibition observed in many patients with PCP intoxication would be difficult.

Phencyclidine-Related Disorder Not Otherwise Specified

The diagnosis of PCP-related disorder not otherwise specified is the appropriate diagnosis for a patient who does not fit into any of the previously described diagnoses (Table 11.11–3).

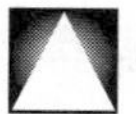

Table 11.11–3
DSM-IV-TR Diagnostic Criteria for Phencyclidine-Related Disorder Not Otherwise Specified

The phencyclidine-related disorder not otherwise specified category is for disorders associated with the use of phencyclidine that are not classifiable as phencyclidine dependence, phencyclidine abuse, phencyclidine intoxication, phencyclidine intoxication delirium, phencyclidine-induced psychotic disorder, phencyclidine-induced mood disorder, or phencyclidine-induced anxiety disorder.

From American Psychiatric Association. *Diagnostic and Statistical Manual of Mental Disorders.* 4th ed. Text rev. Washington, DC: American Psychiatric Association; 2000, with permission.

SUGGESTED CROSS-REFERENCES

Other substance-related disorders are treated in Chapter 11. Schizophrenia, a disorder related symptomatically and pathophysiologically to PCP- or ketamine-induced psychotic disorder, is discussed in Chapter 12. Delirium and its differential diagnosis are covered in Chapter 10. Amino acid neurotransmitters are covered in Section 1.5.

REFERENCES

*Anand A, Charney DS, Oren DA, Berman RM, Hu XS, Cappiello A, Krystal JH: Attenuation of the neuropsychiatric effects of ketamine with lamotrigine: Support for hyperglutamatergic effects of *N*-methyl-D-aspartate receptor antagonists. *Arch Gen Psychiatry.* 2000;57:270.

Aronow R, Miceli JN, Done AK: A therapeutic approach to the acutely overdosed PCP patient. *J Psychedel Drugs.* 1980;12:259.

Baldridge EB, Bessen HA: Phencyclidine. *Emerg Med Clin North Am.* 1990;8:541.

Balla A, Koneru R, Smiley J, Sershen H, Javitt DC: Continuous phencyclidine treatment induces schizophrenia-like hyperreactivity of striatal dopamine release. *Neuropsychopharmacology.* 2001;25:157.

*Balla A, Sershen H, Serra M, Koneru R, Javitt DC: Subchronic continuous phencyclidine administration potentiates amphetamine-induced frontal cortex dopamine release. *Neuropsychopharmacology.* 2003;28:34.

Balster RL: Clinical implications of behavioral pharmacology research on phencyclidine. *NIDA Res Monogr.* 1986;64:148.

Balster RL, Johanson CE, Harris RT, Schuster CR: Phencyclidine self-administration in the rhesus monkey. *Pharmacol Biochem Behav.* 1973;1:167.

Brust JC: Acute neurologic complications of drug and alcohol abuse. *Neurol Clin.* 1998;16:503.

Burns RS, Lerner SE: Perspectives: Acute phencyclidine intoxication. *Clin Toxicol.* 1976;9:477.

Chen G, Ensor CR, Russell D, Bohner B: The pharmacology of 1-(1-phenylcychohexyl) piperidine-HCl. *J Pharmacol Exp Ther.* 1959;127:240.

Cohen BD, Rosenbaum G, Luby ED, Gottlieb JS: Comparison of phencyclidine hydrochloride (Sernyl) with other drugs. *Arch Gen Psychiatry.* 1961;6:79.

Crowley TJ. Phencyclidine (or phencyclidinelike)-related disorders. In: Kaplan HI, Sadock BJ, eds. *Comprehensive Textbook of Psychiatry.* 6th ed. Baltimore: Williams & Wilkins; 1995.

Curran HV, Monaghan L: In and out of the K-hole: A comparison of the acute and residual effects of ketamine in frequent and infrequent ketamine abusers. *Addiction.* 2001;96:749.

Davis BL: The PCP epidemic: A critical review. *Int J Addict.* 1982;17:1137.

Deutsch SI, Mastropaolo J, Rosse RB: Neurodevelopmental consequences of early exposure to phencyclidine and related drugs. *Clin Neuropharmacol.* 1999;21:320.

Dix P, Martindale S, Stoddart PA: Double-blind randomized placebo-controlled trial of the effect of ketamine on postoperative morphine consumption in children following appendicectomy. *Paediatr Anaesth.* 2003;13:422.

Domino EF, Luby E. Abnormal mental states induced by phencyclidine as a model of schizophrenia. In: Domino EF, ed. *PCP (Phencyclidine): Historical and Current Perspectives.* Ann Arbor, MI: NPP Books; 1981.

Ellison G: The *N*-methyl-D-aspartate antagonists phencyclidine, ketamine, and dizocilpine as both behavioral and anatomical models of the dementias. *Brain Res Rev.* 1995;20:250.

Erard R, Luisada PV, Peele R: The PCP psychosis: Prolonged intoxication or drug-precipitated functional illness? *J Psychedel Drugs.* 1980;12:235.

Freeman AS, Martin BR, Balster RL: Relationship between the development of behavioral tolerance and the biodisposition of phencyclidine in mice. *Pharmacol Biochem Behav.* 1984;20:373.

Hocking G, Cousins MJ: Ketamine in chronic pain management: An evidence-based review. *Anesth Analg.* 2003;97:1730.

Itil T, Keskiner A, Kiremitci N, Holden JMC: Effect of phencyclidine in chronic schizophrenics. *Can Psychiatr Assoc J.* 1967;12:209.

Javitt DC: Management of negative symptoms of schizophrenia. *Curr Psychiatry Rep.* 2001;3:413.

*Javitt DC, Zukin SR: Recent advances in the phencyclidine model of schizophrenia. *Am J Psychiatry.* 1991;148:1301.

Krystal JH, Karper LP, Seibyl JP, Freeman GK, Delaney R, Bremner JD, Heninger GR, Bowers MB Jr, Charney DS: Subanesthetic effects of the noncompetitive NMDA antagonist, ketamine, in humans. Psychotomimetic, perceptual, cognitive, and neuroendocrine responses. *Arch Gen Psychiatry.* 1994;51:199.

Linn GS, O'Keeffe RT, Schroeder CE, Lifshitz K, Javitt DC: Behavioral effects of chronic phencyclidine in monkeys. *Neuroreport.* 1999;10:2789.

Luby ED, Cohen BD, Rosenbaum F, Gottlieb J, Kelley R: Study of a new schizophrenomimetic drug Sernyl. *AMA Arch Neurol Psychiatry.* 1959;81:363.

McCarron MM, Schulze BW, Thompson GA, Conder MC, Goetz WA: Acute phencyclidine intoxication: Clinical patterns, complications, and treatment. *Ann Emerg Med.* 1981;10:290.

McCarron MM, Schulze BW, Thompson GA, Conder MC, Goetz WA: Acute phencyclidine intoxication: Incidence of clinical findings in 1000 cases. *Ann Emerg Med.* 1981;10:237.

Misra AL, Pontani RB, Bartolemeo J: Persistence of phencyclidine (PCP) and metabolites in brain and adipose tissue and implications for long-lasting behavioural effects. *Res Commun Chem Pathol Pharmacol.* 1979;24:431.

*Moghaddam B, Adams BW: Reversal of phencyclidine effects by a group II metabotropic glutamate receptor agonist in rats. *Science.* 1998;281:1349.

*Moore KA, Sklerov J, Levine B, Jacobs AJ: Urine concentrations of ketamine and norketamine following illegal consumption. *J Anal Toxicol.* 2001;25:583.

Newmeyer JA: The epidemiology of PCP use in the late 1970s. *J Psychedel Drugs.* 1980;12:211.

Petersen RC, Stillman RC: Phencyclidine (PCP) abuse: An appraisal. *NIDA Res Monogr.* 1978;21:1.

Smith KM, Larive LL, Romanelli F: Club drugs: Methlenedioxymethamphetamine, flunitrazepam, ketamine hydrochloride and gamma-hydroxybutyrate. *Am J Health Syst Pharmacol.* 2000;59:1067.

Taffe M, Davis S, Gutierrez T, Gold L: Ketamine impairs multiple cognitive domains in rhesus monkeys. *Drug Alcohol Depend.* 2002;68:175.

Tsai G, van Kammen DP, Chen S, Kelley ME, Grier A, Coyle JT: Glutamatergic neurotransmission involves structural and clinical deficits of schizophrenia. *Biol Psychiatry.* 1998;44:667.

Umbricht D, Schmid L, Koller R, Vollenweider FX, Hell D, Javitt DC: Ketamine-induced deficits in auditory and visual context-dependent processing in healthy volunteers: Implications for models of cognitive deficits in schizophrenia. *Arch Gen Psychiatry.* 2000;57:1139.

Yanagihara Y, Ohtani M, Kariya S, Uchino K, Hiraishi T, Ashizawa N, Aoyama T, Yamamura Y, Yamada Y, Iga T: Plasma concentration profiles of ketamine and norketamine after administration of various ketamine preparations to healthy Japanese volunteers. *Biopharm Drug Dispos.* 2003;24:37.

Yesavage JA, Freeman AM III: Acute phencyclidine (PCP) intoxication: Psychopathology and prognosis. *J Clin Psychiatry.* 1978;44:664.

Zukin SR, Sloboda Z, Javitt DC: Phencyclidine (PCP). In: Lowinson JH, Ruíz P, Millman RB, Langrod JG, eds. *Substance Abuse: A Comprehensive Textbook.* 3rd ed. Baltimore: Williams & Wilkins; 1997.

▲ 11.12 Sedative-, Hypnotic-, or Anxiolytic-Related Disorders

DOMENIC A. CIRAULO, M.D., AND
OFRA SARID-SEGAL, M.D.

Abuse and dependence of therapeutic agents are influenced by several factors. Perhaps the most important determinant of sedative, hypnotic, or anxiolytic dependence is the pharmacology of the specific agents, but prescribing habits of clinicians, patient characteristics, social beliefs, and government regulations also impact the extent and patterns of anxiolytic and sedative abuse.

DEFINITION

Determining Abuse Liability

Studies of sedative, hypnotic, or anxiolytic dependence are limited by the operational definitions of abuse and dependence. Drug abuse is a sociobehavioral phenomenon, albeit with significant pharmacological origins and medical consequences.

Abuse liability can be assessed by asking a series of questions about a drug or class of drugs. By asking questions that reflect societal norms, investigators are able to obtain data concerning abuse liability through studies of illicit trafficking; population surveys of nonprescription use; audits of prescribing practices; monitoring of diversion from physician's offices, pharmacies, or manufacturing sites; emergency room treatment; and overdose deaths. Questions regarding pharmacological characteristics also predict abuse liability: Drug-induced euphoria and the development of tolerance, an abstinence syndrome, or cross-tolerance with known abusable substances may all predict risk of abuse. Finally, a number of ingenious methods for determining drug preferences in human and animal models have been developed to determine abuse liability.

The terms *abuse* and *misuse* refer to the use of a drug in a manner that is not consistent with generally accepted medical practice or social and legal custom (e.g., use without a valid prescription or use to deliberately produce intoxication, pleasure, or high). The revised fourth edition of the *Diagnostic and Statistical Manual of Mental Disorders* (DSM-IV-TR) defines abuse as a "maladaptive pattern of substance use manifested by recurrent and significant adverse consequences related to repeated use." Some authorities limit misuse to situations in which a drug is taken for a legitimate medical or psychiatric disorder but is used in a way that is not consistent with medical practice. The distinction between *abuse* and *misuse* is not widely accepted, and the terms are used interchangeably here. *Recreational use* refers to the use of drugs solely for their hedonic value. According to DSM-IV-TR, substance dependence is a "cluster of cognitive, behavioral, and physiological symptoms indicating that the individual continues use of the substance despite significant substance-related problems. There is a pattern of repeated self-administration that usually results in tolerance, withdrawal, and compulsive drug-taking behavior." The term *physiological dependence* is, according to the definition of the World Health Organization (WHO), "a pathological state brought about by a repeated administration of a drug that leads to the appearance of a characteristic and specific group of symptoms," including abstinence syndrome or discontinuance syndrome when the drug is discontinued or, in the case of certain drugs, significantly reduced. The abstinence syndrome has specific characteristics referable to the autonomic nervous system (e.g., tremor, sweating, tachycardia, and startle response) and must be clearly distinguished from recurrence of the features of the underlying disease for which the drug was originally prescribed. It can be reversed or attenuated by readministering the discontinued drug or administering a drug with cross-tolerance. Some authorities reserve the term *discontinuance syndrome* for withdrawal syndromes that develop with therapeutic agents to distinguish physiological dependence that develops throughout the course of treatment from dependence that develops from misuse of the drug. The terms are used interchangeably here.

Substances

The drugs discussed in this section are referred to as *anxiolytic* or *sedative-hypnotic drugs*. The terminology for this group of drugs is not clearly established. Their sedative or calming effects are on a continuum with their hypnotic or sleep-inducing effects. Anxiolytic drugs cover a wide spectrum of pharmacological agents, and the terminology implies more specificity than actually exists. For most of these drugs, the differentiation of their sedative, hypnotic, and anxiolytic activities has more to do with marketing than with pharmacology. The broad group of drugs that historically has been included in that class exhibits considerable variation in clinical use, toxicity, risk for abuse, and potential for diversion or recreational use. The abuse liability of those agents is classified in this section as follows: (1) benzodiazepines and functionally related drugs, (2) barbiturates, (3) and miscellaneous sedative-hypnotic drugs. In the practice of psychiatry and addiction medicine, the drugs that are most important clinically are the benzodiazepines.

ETIOLOGY AND NEUROPHARMACOLOGY

The benzodiazepines, barbiturates, and barbiturate-like substances all have their primary effects on the γ-aminobutyric acid (GABA) type A ($GABA_A$) receptor complex, which contains a chloride ion channel, a binding site for GABA, and a well-defined binding site for benzodiazepines. The barbiturates and barbiturate-like substances are also believed to bind somewhere on the $GABA_A$ receptor complex. When a benzodiazepine, barbiturate, or barbiturate-like substance does bind to the complex, it increases the affinity of the receptor for its endogenous neurotransmitter, GABA, and increases the flow of chloride ions through the channel into the neuron. Benzodiazepines have little or no effect in the absence of GABA. At high doses, barbiturates directly activate chloride channels. The influx of negatively charged chloride ions into the neuron is inhibitory, because it hyperpolarizes the neuron relative to the extracellular space.

Although all the substances in this class induce tolerance and physical dependence, the underlying mechanisms are best understood for the benzodiazepines. Long-term benzodiazepine use attenuates the receptor effects caused by the agonist. Specifically, after long-term benzodiazepine use, GABA stimulation of the $GABA_A$ receptors results in less influx of chloride than it did before benzodiazepine administration. Benzodiazepine agonists lead to several processes that result in downregulation of the $GABA_A$ receptor. Benzodiazepine agonists produce acute desensitization of the receptor (tachyphylaxis) and promote $GABA_A$ receptor sequestration in cortical neurons. Chronic administration uncouples the GABA and benzodiazepine binding sites. Receptor mechanisms underlying uncoupling are unknown, although changes in phosphorylation, altered subunit composition, and conformational changes in the receptor have been suggested. Contradictory findings have been reported with respect to alterations in receptor density. Binding affinity is not altered by chronic administration, although receptor alterations leading to uncoupling are almost certainly important in tolerance development. The changes in $GABA_A$ function do not completely explain the clinical phenomenon. For example, although patients develop tolerance to the sedative effects of benzodiazepines, the antianxiety and amnestic effects of these drugs are relatively persistent. Some investigators have suggested that alterations in receptor subunit composition account for this phenomenon.

ABUSE LIABILITY

Surveys of prescribing practices, patient-initiated dosage changes, and recreational or nonmedical benzodiazepine use along with reports from emergency rooms, medical examiners, and law enforcement agencies all suggest that benzodiazepine abuse is not a major public health problem. They are rarely used for recreational purposes, and most studies suggest that when abuse of benzodiazepines is reported, concurrent abuse of other substances is also found. The vast majority of medical and psychiatric patients use benzodiazepines appropriately, although they may be abused by patients dependent on alcohol or other drugs.

Abuse liability is evaluated, in part, by measuring the reinforcing properties of the drug. If its pharmacological effects increase behavior (i.e., self-administration of a dose or the work required to permit self-administration), then the drug is a positive reinforcer and has abuse liability. Animal and human studies have assessed the reinforcing properties of benzodiazepines.

Animal Studies Animal studies have consistently demonstrated that benzodiazepines have minimal reinforcing effects. Although a small number of studies show that animals self-administer benzodiazepines more frequently than other drugs, they are significantly less potent than other drugs of abuse (e.g., cocaine and other central nervous system [CNS] stimulants) or even many other sedative-hypnotic drugs, including most barbiturates. Studies that use the conditioned place preference paradigm have also demonstrated that benzodiazepines have minimal reinforcing effects. In some studies, diazepam (Valium) has produced place preference among laboratory rats, but to a lesser extent than classic drugs of abuse, such as morphine or amphetamine.

Animal studies using schedule-induced polydipsia (the use of intermittent food administration to the experimental animal, which promotes ingestion of fluids, including drug solutions) indicate that midazolam (Versed) is ingested more often than water, but self-administration of chlordiazepoxide (Librium) and flurazepam (Dalmane) does not differ significantly from that of water.

Another animal model predicting abuse liability consists of drug infusion in response to activity by the animal, such as lever pressing (Fig. 11.12–1). Drug infusion may allow continuous or intermittent drug availability, and rates of the administration of the drug are compared to those of the vehicle, other sedative-hypnotic drugs, and standard drugs of abuse, such as cocaine. Studies with continuous drug access suggest that triazolam (Halcion), diazepam, midazolam, clobazam (Frisium), and chlordiazepoxide have reinforcing effects; studies with intermittent drug availability show that diazepam, midazolam, triazolam, alprazolam (Xanax), lorazepam (Ativan), chlordiazepoxide, and bromazepam (Lectopam) maintain responses at a higher level than vehicle, indicating abuse liability. With the possible exception of triazolam and midazolam, in studies using this model, the benzodiazepines consistently demonstrate lower abuse liability than barbiturates other than phenobarbital, which also has relatively low abuse liability. Partial benzodiazepine receptor agonists, such as abecarnil and bretazenil, have low abuse liability in those models. Prior exposure to ethanol or sedative-hypnotic drugs may increase the reinforcing effects of benzodiazepines.

Animal studies have demonstrated that a withdrawal syndrome occurs on abrupt discontinuation of benzodiazepines. The animal models using the social interaction test and social conflict paradigms, along with isolation-induced ultrasonic vocalizations recordings, indicate that abrupt discontinuation of benzodiazepine tranquilizers may induce numerous anxiogenic responses, including decreased social interaction and increased aggressive behaviors.

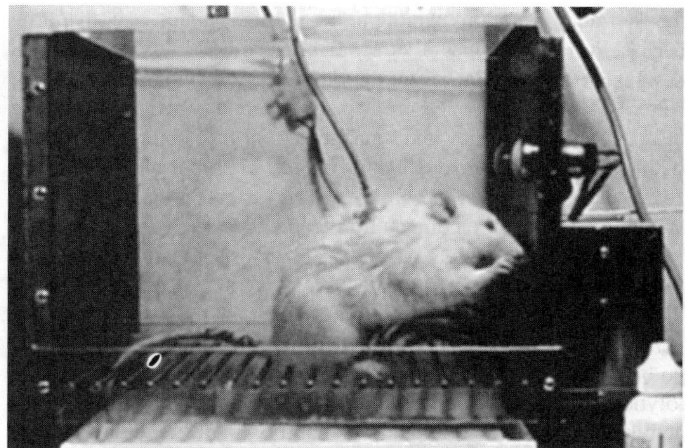

FIGURE 11.12–1 Animal in operant chamber self-administers a drug by pressing a bar to receive an infusion of a predetermined dose that is delivered from a syringe pump via a cannula implanted in its jugular vein. (Courtesy of Conan Kornetsky, Boston University School of Medicine.)

Studies that use a competitive benzodiazepine receptor antagonist, such as flumazenil (Romazicon), to precipitate withdrawal have also demonstrated the development of a withdrawal syndrome using electrophysiological measures.

Human Studies The assessment of abuse liability in humans relies on two predictive models: self-administration of benzodiazepines by experimental subjects who have a history of drug abuse and subjective responses that correlate with high abuse potential. In the first paradigm, one type of study allows subjects with a history of sedative-hypnotic dependence to self-administer orally (i.e., sample) different color-coded drugs and placebo under double-blind conditions in a simulated social environment. During subsequent sessions, they are permitted to self-administer the drug that they like the best. Some studies require that the subjects perform a task (e.g., riding a stationary bicycle) to earn doses. The abuse liability of different drugs is assessed by how often they are chosen for self-administration or by how much work a subject does to earn a dose. Scales measuring drug effect are also administered. The paradigm has the advantage of directly observing the behavior involved with ingesting the drug, albeit under somewhat artificial circumstances. It works best for former sedative-hypnotic abusers without psychiatric illness. It is probably safe to infer that those subjects are administering the drug for its hedonic value. The reason for self-administration by other subjects may not be clear. Do patients with anxiety disorder self-administer the drugs because they are effective anxiolytics or because they induce euphoria? Similarly, if subjects are in withdrawal from sedative-hypnotic drugs or ethanol, do they choose the agent that alleviates their withdrawal symptoms most effectively or the drug that produces the greatest euphoria? An additional problem with this design is that it exposes subjects to multiple doses of potentially addictive drugs.

An alternative strategy is to administer only a single dose of the test drugs and then to compare subjective responses associated with abuse liability. A set of scales, which differs slightly among laboratories, usually consists of the Morphine Benzedrine Group subscale of the Addiction Research Center Inventory (ARCI-MBG); self-reports of sedation, liking, and intensity of drug effect; monetary street value of the drug; and similarity to reference drugs of abuse. Studies demonstrate that estimates of abuse liability using this paradigm are consistent with assessments based on the self-administration model. One disadvantage of the single-dose paradigm is that it measures only subjective effects, not behavior. It also has some of the same limitations as the self-administration paradigm. Does the subject like the drug because it has a therapeutic effect or because it is intoxicating? Both designs attempt to circumvent the problem by including an adequate battery of scales that measure several different dimensions of drug effect. Dose equivalency and homogeneity of the subjects (especially with respect to a personal or family history of psychoactive substance abuse and psychiatric illness) are critical factors in the study design and in the interpretation of data from both models.

The predictive models in humans clearly establish that benzodiazepines occupy an intermediate position on the spectrum of abuse liability of sedative-hypnotic drugs. Methaqualone and barbiturates generally produce higher ARCI-MBG and drug-liking scores than do benzodiazepines. Buspirone (BuSpar), a nonbenzodiazepine anxiolytic agent (i.e., it is essentially devoid of benzodiazepine agonist activities), has little or no abuse liability in those models. With respect to differences among the benzodiazepines, the weight of the evidence suggests that diazepam has greater abuse liability than halazepam (Paxipam), oxazepam (Serax), chlordiazepoxide, or clorazepate (Tranxene). Diazepam, lorazepam, alprazolam, and triazolam exhibit similar profiles of abuse potential using those paradigms. The clinical relevance of the findings has not been adequately studied.

Flunitrazepam (Rohypnol), a benzodiazepine agonist, is not marketed in the United States but has entered the country through illegal sources in Central and South America. Reports of abuse have appeared in the clinical literature and public media. The drug has been implicated in date rape, in which flunitrazepam is added to a woman's alcoholic beverage to reduce her judgment, inhibition, and physical ability to resist sexual activity. Memory for the event may also be impaired by the combination of alcohol and flunitrazepam. A comprehensive review of the abuse liability of flunitrazepam published in 1997 concluded that little evidence suggested that the drug had higher abuse liability than other benzodiazepines, except for its preference among opioid abusers. Despite efforts by manufacturers to reformulate the drug, making it more difficult to disguise in ethanol, many countries have considered reclassifying flunitrazepam as a dangerous drug.

A review of flunitrazepam toxicity published in 2001 reported that flunitrazepam has been linked to numerous fatal intoxications in Sweden. The majority of these intoxications were suicides, but some were attributed to accidental overconsumption in combination with ethanol or other drugs. Although flunitrazepam comprised nearly one-half of all of the benzodiazepine detections in Swedish drug abuse investigations in 1997 and 1998, it made up only 30 percent of the legal sales of benzodiazepines during these years.

The weight of the evidence supports the safety and efficacy of flunitrazepam in clinical populations; however, people with alcohol or drug dependence commonly abuse it in combination with alcohol, illicit drugs, or both. Flunitrazepam is reported to be the most popular benzodiazepine among heroin addicts, and some individuals administer the drug to enhance the effects of alcohol, marijuana, or both.

Pharmacological characteristics, especially pharmacokinetics, of benzodiazepines and related compounds influence abuse liability. Some drugs (e.g., diazepam) may appear to have high abuse liability because of rapid absorption from the gastrointestinal (GI) tract after oral doses. On the other hand, pharmacodynamic differences among the drugs are not well studied. For example, little is known about differences in abuse liability between full and partial agonists or among drugs that have preferential effects on specific subtypes of the benzodiazepine receptor. Zolpidem (Ambien), for example, is an imidazopyridine hypnotic agent with a rapid onset of action and a short elimination half-life. When the drug was first marketed in the 1980s, the manufacturer presented data indicating a low abuse liability for zolpidem, but current investigations may show otherwise. Although in vitro evidence indicates that zolpidem binds preferentially to the benzodiazepine receptor with a high affinity ratio of the $\alpha 1$ and $\alpha 5$ subunits, it is unlikely that this characteristic would provide lower potential for abuse; rather, selective binding more likely explains the lack of anticonvulsant and muscle relaxant effects of the drug. Also supporting the similarity between zolpidem and classic benzodiazepines is the fact that zolpidem and triazolam depress energy metabolism in the same areas of the brain. With respect to subjective, psychomotor, and memory effects, there are no significant differences between a single 10-mg dose of zolpidem and a single 0.25-mg dose of triazolam. High doses of triazolam (0.75 mg) are identified more often as similar in effect to barbiturates, benzodiazepine, or alcohol than are high doses of zolpidem (45 mg). In the United States, New Zealand, and some European countries, zolpidem and zopiclone (Imovane) (another nonbenzodiazepine hypnotic) have been shown to have reduced efficacy after a few weeks of treatment, requiring increases in doses, which may contribute to a higher risk for abuse and dependence. In some cases, zopiclone dosages have reached levels as high as 82.5 mg per day, after an initial prescribed dosage of 3.75 to 15.0 mg per day. Dosages of zolpidem have reached 800 mg per day after an initial prescribed dose of 5 to 20 mg per day. Abrupt discontinuation of zolpidem or zopiclone after months of use has resulted in severe abstinence syndromes, which may include seizures. By 1999, the WHO Pharmacovigilance Collaborating Center in Uppsala was notified of 100 cases of zolpidem or zopiclone dependence, 45 cases of withdrawal syndromes, and 19 cases of drug misuse.

Clinical experience and research findings have identified patient characteristics that influence abuse liability. For example, when alcoholic persons and their adult children are given a single dose of alprazolam or diazepam, they have greater increases on abuse potential scales than do nonalcoholic controls without a family history of alcoholism. The differences in reinforcing effects are not attributable to pharmacokinetic differences as measured by peripheral plasma concentrations; however, pharmacodynamic differences have been noted using functional magnetic resonance imaging (MRI) and electroencephalogram (EEG) measures. When alcoholics are compared to healthy volunteers, lower prefrontal cortical GABA levels, as measured by magnetic resonance spectroscopy, are found. Studies have found that patients with prior alcohol dependence or substance abuse exhibit a clear preference for benzodiazepines in self-report models. Enhanced mood states after benzodiazepine challenges have also been found in moderate drinkers, although the confound of a family history of substance abuse has not been adequately controlled in all studies. Other findings indicate that moderate drinkers self-administer higher doses of diazepam than do light drinkers. Whether these results are drug specific or apply to the class of benzodiazepines as a whole is not known. Patients with a family history of substance abuse have reported a benzodiazepine preference in some studies. A survey of 5,000 male college students found that 23 percent of those with a positive family history of alcohol abuse reported using benzodiazepines (versus 0.9 percent of those without such a family history).

Anxiety disorder patients with a history of alcohol and substance abuse have been commonly thought to be at a higher risk for misusing benzodiazepines. A study conducted by the Harvard/Brown Anxiety Disorders Research Program (HARP) examined total daily dose, as needed (PRN) use, and continued use of benzodiazepine in patients with and without a history of alcohol dependence. That study found that prior alcohol dependence was not a strong predictor for benzodiazepine abuse.

Experimental paradigms do not provide evidence that individuals with anxiety disorders are at greater risk for benzodiazepine abuse when compared to nonanxious subjects. The fact that some anxious subjects choose diazepam over placebo in self-administration experiments underscores the limitations of the study design rather than indicating abuse potential. In such studies, it is impossible to determine if subjects choose the drug to relieve psychic distress or to experience its pleasurable effects. In clinical experience, the risk of benzodiazepine abuse in patients with anxiety disorders is low.

EPIDEMIOLOGY

Several studies have been conducted to determine the extent of benzodiazepine use by prescription and illicit means. These can be divided into the following categories: (1) number of prescriptions written and retail pharmacy sales, (2) surveys of medical use in clinical populations, (3) surveys of special clinical populations, (4) patterns of illicit use, and (5) expert opinion.

Number of Prescriptions Written and Retail Pharmacy Sales

Drug sales, as monitored by IMS Global Services, Ltd., to retail pharmacies provide one measure of benzodiazepine use. The data indicate that benzodiazepine tranquilizer sales in the United States peaked in 1973 to 1975, when annual sales were approximately 87 million prescriptions. Between 1980 and 1983, sales of benzodiazepines to retail pharmacies in the United States declined from 17.5 to 15.8 (average maintenance dose for the major indication per 1,000 inhabitants per day), but by 1985, they were back up to 17.1. Sales of drugs with long half-lives, such as diazepam and flurazepam, decreased, whereas sales of drugs with shorter half-lives, such as alprazolam, triazolam, and temazepam (Restoril), increased. From 1986 to 1989, benzodiazepine tranquilizer sales declined to approximately 56 million prescriptions.

Data indicate that the total prescription sales of benzodiazepines have undergone reductions during the last decade, with a pattern of higher sales among shorter-acting agents compared to longer-acting agents. The recent sales of anxiolytic benzodiazepines are presented in Figures 11.12–2 and 11.12–3. In addition to the trend for greater sales of shorter half-life agents, there have been changes in market share for individual agents. In 1989, alprazolam accounted for 33 percent of the U.S. market share. In 2002, alprazolam accounted for 17.1 percent of total U.S. benzodiazepine sales, an increase of 3.2 percent from 2001. Lorazepam accounted for 19 percent of the U.S. market share in 1989, and, by 2002, the drug held 12.2 percent of the market share, an increase of 0.9 percent from 2001. Diazepam held 25 percent of the U.S. market share in 1989, but only 10.9 percent in 2002, an increase of 2.5 percent from 2001. Oxazepam accounted for 0.5 percent of the U.S. market share in 2002, an increase of 0.2 percent from 2001, and clorazepate decreased from 4.8 percent of the market share in 2001 to 3 percent in 2002.

In summary, sales data support declining clinical use of benzodiazepines for treatment of anxiety disorders, which is probably attributable to the availability of alternative antianxiety agents, such as medications originally marketed as antidepressants, including selective serotonin reuptake inhibitors (SSRIs) and mixed action antidepressants. Prescription sales do not provide evidence that benzodiazepines are overprescribed.

Surveys of Medical Use in Clinical Populations

Despite problems with validity and reliability, survey data offer insight into the appropriateness of benzodiazepine use. In surveys of the U.S. population, self-reports of past-year medical use of tranquilizers or hypnotics demonstrated a 10-year downward trend of 10.9 to

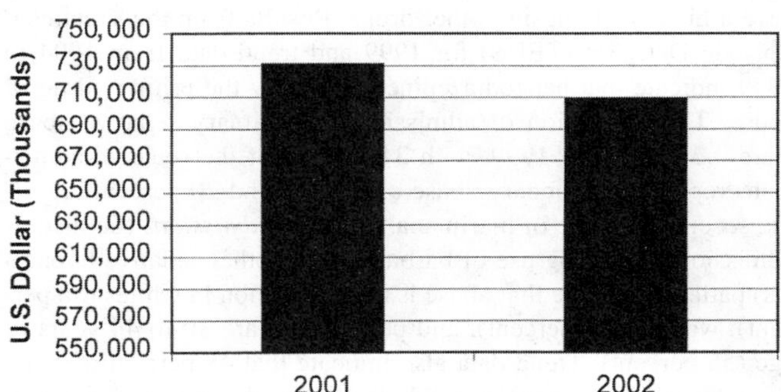

FIGURE 11.12–2 Total U.S. dollar sales of benzodiazepines, as monitored by IMS Global Services, Ltd. (From IMS Health, IMS Therapy Area Sales Report; IMS Retail Perspective & IMS Provider Perspective, 2002, with permission.)

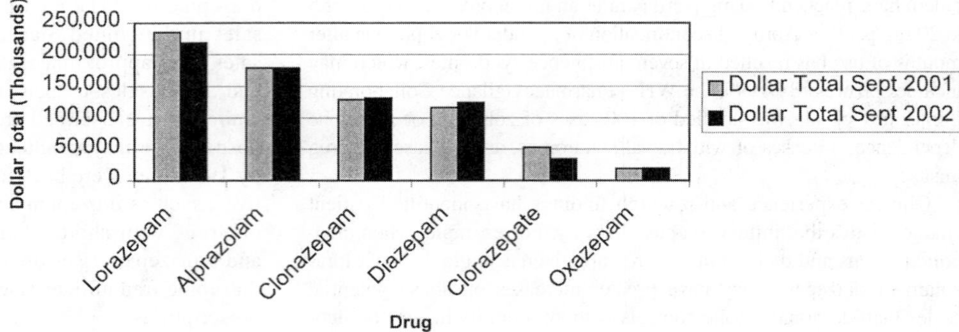

FIGURE 11.12–3 Total U.S. dollar sales of lorazepam (Ativan), alprazolam (Xanax), clonazepam (Klonopin), diazepam (Valium), clorazepate (Tranxene), and oxazepam (Serax). (From IMS Health, IMS Therapy Area Sales Report; IMS Retail Perspective & IMS Provider Perspective, 2002, with permission.)

8.3 percent and 3.5 to 2.6 percent, respectively. Most patients took benzodiazepines for less than 1 month. Long-term users were more likely to be older and to be women, and they had high levels of emotional distress and chronic health problems.

A survey of unsupervised changes in dosage indicated that 12 percent of patients had decreased their anxiolytic dosage, and 6 percent had increased it; 9 percent of patients taking hypnotics decreased their dosage, and 8 percent increased it. To put these unauthorized increases in perspective, the same survey indicated that 13 percent of patients had unauthorized increases in antidepressant dosages, and those drugs have low abuse liability. A prospective study found that patients were more likely to use antidepressants than benzodiazepines on a long-term basis, suggesting that long-term use should not, in itself, be used to measure abuse liability.

Surveys of psychiatric patients (except those diagnosed as substance abusers) have demonstrated high rates of benzodiazepine prescription but almost uniformly low abuse. In one study of 2,719 outpatients, none of the 178 patients who had received benzodiazepines was diagnosed with abuse or dependence. Studies of inpatient psychiatric patients suggest that the rate of benzodiazepine abuse or dependence ranges from 0.4 to 13.0 percent of admissions. A study from the University of Munich found that 6.7 percent of 9,408 admissions had a diagnosis of benzodiazepine abuse or dependence, approximately one-half of whom were dependent on benzodiazepines alone. Lorazepam was the most commonly abused benzodiazepine, and oxazepam was the least commonly abused benzodiazepine, even though the latter drug was the most commonly prescribed benzodiazepine in the country.

Surveys of Special Clinical Populations Substantial evidence indicates that patients who abuse benzodiazepines frequently have a history of abusing other drugs. Results from the Treatment Episode Data Set (TEDS) for 1999 and trend data from 1994 to 1999 indicate that benzodiazepines are rarely the primary drug of abuse. The proportion of admissions for primary sedative abuse were 0.2 percent in 1999, with 34 percent of the sedative admissions reporting secondary abuse of alcohol and 20 percent reporting secondary abuse of marijuana. *Sedative admissions* (defined as admissions involving use of barbiturates or other sedative-hypnotics) patterns indicate that abuse is more common in whites (86 percent), women (59 percent), and people who are 30 to 44 years of age (55 percent). Trend data also indicate that 48 percent of sedative admissions reported daily administration that was initiated after the age of 30 years.

Similar to sedatives, *tranquilizers* (defined as benzodiazepines or other tranquilizers) were reported as a primary substance of abuse by 0.3 percent of admissions. Of the admissions, alcohol was cited as secondary substance of abuse by 38 percent, marijuana was cited by 21 percent, and opiates other than heroin were cited by 15 percent. Admissions tended to involve whites (89 percent), women (58 percent), and people who were 30 to 44 years of age (53 percent). Sixty percent of admissions reported daily use of tranquilizers and reported first use after 30 years of age.

A survey of drug abuse treatment centers across the United States found that 22.6 percent of patients used minor tranquilizers (primarily benzodiazepines) weekly or more frequently. In a survey of opioid abusers in Sheffield, England, 90 percent reported benzodiazepine use daily or almost daily. Use began with a prescription in one-third of the sample. The most commonly used benzodiazepine was diazepam, and the primary goal was relief from symptoms such as insomnia, withdrawal, and anxiety rather than euphoric effect. Lower rates of benzodiazepine use were reported in French (50 percent) and German (30 percent) studies. In the last two studies, heroin addicts underreported benzodiazepine use, requiring the use of toxicological studies to detect use.

Several studies have examined rates of benzodiazepine use among patients at methadone (Dolophine) clinics. Three different U.S. clinics reported that 22, 40, and 44 percent of their patients had benzodiazepines in their urine, with European clinics reporting comparable rates. Flunitrazepam, administered orally or snorted (when available), appears to be the preferred benzodiazepine. In other countries, diazepam, alprazolam, and lorazepam are most commonly abused. In a study from Austria, patients in a methadone clinic who were asked to rate their preference for the effects of a variety of drugs reported a preference for benzodiazepines behind heroin, cocaine, all opiates, cannabis, barbiturates, and stimulants. Flunitrazepam and diazepam were the highest-rated benzodiazepines, but alprazolam was not available in Austria when the survey began. In a study in three U.S. cities, methadone-maintenance patients rated diazepam as producing the best high, with lorazepam and alprazolam also valued for their effects, and considered all three as significantly different from clorazepate, oxazepam, and chlordiazepoxide. Concern has been raised about abuse of alprazolam in methadone clinics, and at least one clinic reported that alprazolam use surpassed the use of diazepam. Patients taking methadone presumably use benzodiazepines to boost the effects of methadone, but some studies have suggested that self-medication is also an important motivating factor. Opioid abusers who use benzodiazepines are more likely to engage in other high-risk behaviors, such as needle sharing.

Cocaine abusers appear less likely to use benzodiazepines than patients in methadone clinics, with alcohol and opioids being the preferred secondary drugs of abuse. Benzodiazepines are used to attenuate the cocaine crash or to alleviate the anxiety associated with cocaine use. The patients generally use therapeutic doses of benzodiazepines on an intermittent basis.

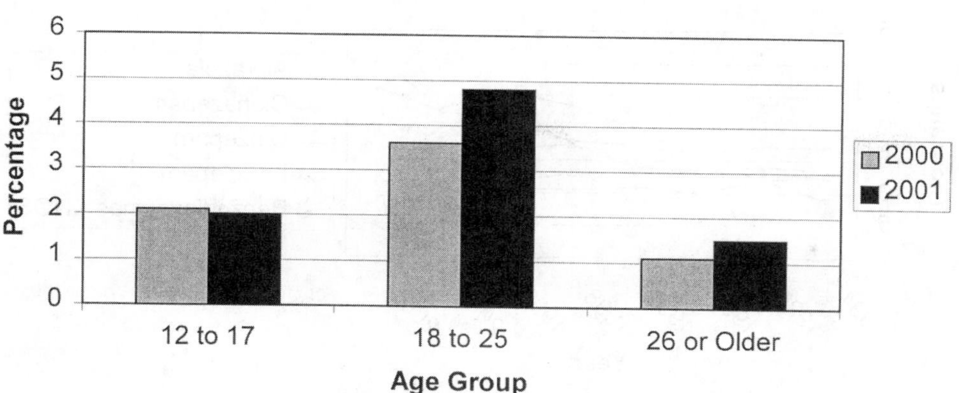

FIGURE 11.12–4 Percentages reporting illicit use of sedatives or tranquilizers within the past surveyed year.

Although the previously cited HARP study found that long-term therapeutic use of benzodiazepines did not lead to dose escalation, caution should be exercised when prescribing benzodiazepines to persons with a history of alcoholism. The majority of alcohol-dependent patients often present for such treatment without revealing the extent of their alcohol abuse to the prescribing physician. Although the American Psychiatric Association Task Force on benzodiazepine dependency recommends that "special caution" be taken when prescribing benzodiazepines to patients with history of alcohol abuse, they also acknowledge that there is a possibility that "the benefits of ongoing benzodiazepine treatment clearly outweigh the hazards" for some individuals. The benzodiazepines do, however, offer added risks because of the development of tolerance to the psychomotor and sedative effects, dependence after an intermediate term of use, a withdrawal syndrome, and the potential for cognitive changes, especially among the elderly. When patients with a history of alcohol abuse or anxiety disorders present for treatment, medical professionals must exercise clinical wisdom without unnecessarily withholding potentially effective and relatively safe medication. Because benzodiazepines appear to be more rapidly effective than antidepressants for the treatment of anxiety disorders, they are often the preferred initial pharmacological treatment. There is substantial evidence that patients with panic symptoms, especially those with a lifetime history of substance abuse, have suicide potential. With these patients, rapid symptom reduction is an important goal.

Between 16 and 25 percent of patients presenting for anxiety disorder concurrently abuse alcohol. Alcoholic women may have higher rates of concurrent use than alcoholic men. How many alcoholic patients misuse benzodiazepines is not entirely clear, but one study found that 15 percent of alcoholic outpatients who also used sedatives (mostly benzodiazepines) used them as prescribed, 24 percent used them appropriately and abused them, and 61 percent abused them. Another study reported that a little more than one-half of alcoholic outpatients with positive urine drug screens for benzodiazepines were abusing them. These data should be regarded cautiously, because treatment population surveys are biased to select only patients for whom previous therapy has failed.

It has been estimated that approximately 15 to 20 percent of all alcoholic persons presenting for treatment may be abusing benzodiazepines. Benzodiazepines are used to self-medicate withdrawal symptoms or anxiety disorders, to produce euphoria, and to enhance the effects of ethanol. Other groups may also be at high risk for benzodiazepine abuse. In England and Wales, a 1995 pilot study in prisons showed an increase in the number of urine samples that tested positive for opioids or benzodiazepines, from 4.1 percent in 1993 and 1994 to 7.4 percent in 1995. People with disabilities appear to abuse tranquilizers at as much as twice the rate of people without disabilities.

Another group that may be at higher risk for benzodiazepine toxicity are elderly patients. Recent data indicate that the overall prevalence of substance abuse disorders among geriatric psychiatry outpatients is approximately 20 percent. In the same study, 11 percent of patients were found to be dependent on benzodiazepines; a significantly higher number than the numbers that other studies have previously reported, which may be attributed to methodological differences among the different studies. Although it is unknown whether long-term administration of benzodiazepines accelerates cognitive decline, results of some studies suggest that long-term use of benzodiazepines is a risk factor for increased cognitive decline and increased risk of falls among the elderly.

Patterns of Illicit Use The National Institute on Drug Abuse's National Household Survey in 2001 found that an estimated 15.9 million Americans 12 years of age or older used an illicit drug in the month preceding the interview, which represents 7.1 percent of the population in this age group. Compared to the 2000 survey, there was a statistically significant increase of tranquilizer use from 0.4 to 0.6 percent of individuals who were 12 years of age or older. In 2001, the total percentage of the general population reporting nonmedical use of tranquilizers in their lifetime was 6.2 percent, an increase of 0.4 percent from the year before, whereas the total percentage of the general population reporting nonmedical use of sedatives in their lifetime was 3.3 percent, an increase of 0.1 percent from the year before. Figure 11.12–4 indicates the percentage of illicit use of sedatives or tranquilizers among various age groups, with the 18- to 25-year-old group reporting the greatest use.

The number of individuals reporting new nonmedical use of tranquilizers has increased steadily since 1986, with an increase from 734,000 in 1999 to 973,000 in 2000. In contrast to the data on past-year use, there were significantly more *new* users in the group of 12- to 17-year-olds than among the group of 18- to 25-year-olds.

The Drug Abuse Warning Network (DAWN) is another means of monitoring trends in drug use, although illicit and medical usage cannot be clearly differentiated. The most frequent psychotherapeutic agents mentioned in drug-related emergency department (ED) visits in 2001 were anxiolytics, sedatives, and hypnotics, which accounted for 12 percent (135,949) of total ED visits. There were also at least 100 ED mentions of γ-hydroxybutyrate (GHB) (Xyrem) in metropolitan areas. Total ED mentions of benzodiazepines have risen 14 percent from 2000 to 2001 and 39 percent between 1994 and 2001. The most frequently mentioned benzodiazepines were benzodiazepines not otherwise specified (NOS), with 30,302 mentions; alprazolam, with

FIGURE 11.12–5 Emergency department mentions of benzodiazepines. NOS, not otherwise specified.

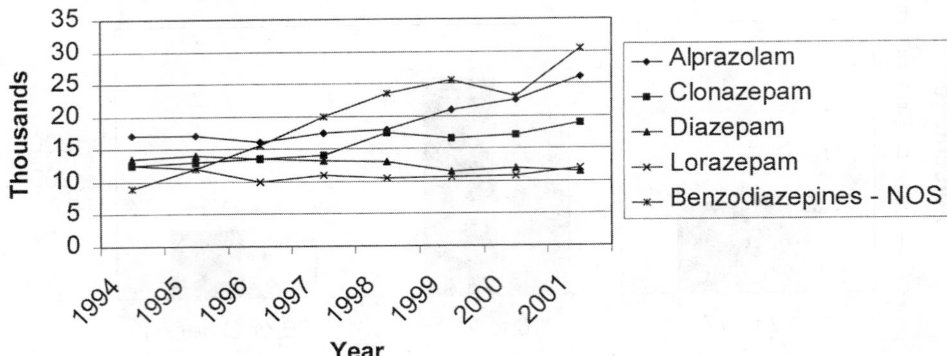

25,644 mentions; clonazepam (Klonopin), with 19,117 mentions; diazepam, with 11,447 mentions; lorazepam, with 11,902 mentions; and temazepam, with 2,637 mentions. As indicated in Figure 11.12–5, between 1994 and 2001, mentions of alprazolam rose 49 percent, mentions of clonazepam rose 57 percent, and mentions of benzodiazepines NOS rose 232 percent, whereas mentions of diazepam, lorazepam, and temazepam remained stable. Although temazepam ED mentions increased in 2001, other hypnotic benzodiazepines decreased significantly. Flurazepam decreased by 60 percent, whereas triazolam decreased 76 percent. Most presenting patients reported that their use of benzodiazepines began with nonmedical use. Only one-third of patients presenting for benzodiazepine abuse or withdrawal report that their first use occurred with a prescription while under the care of a monitoring physician.

A series of large annual surveys, designated *Monitoring the Future*, examined trends in the licit and illicit use of benzodiazepines of nationally representative samples of 12th graders throughout the United States and has been conducted since 1975. In 1991, the survey was expanded to include eighth and tenth grade students as well. The trends in the level of perceived risk and personal disapproval, as well as trends in perceived availability, are also measured by this survey

From 1977 through 1992, illicit use of tranquilizers among 12th graders declined by nearly 75 percent. During the early 1990s, tranquilizer use by 12th graders began to gradually increase, and, by 2001, 6.5 percent of 12th graders reported tranquilizer use within the past year. Past-year use among tenth graders has also been rising steadily since 1992, and past-year use among eighth graders peaked in 1996 and has since remained stable. Trends in lifetime use of tranquilizers among eighth, tenth, and 12th graders have also demonstrated gradual increases since 1992, as shown in Figure 11.12–6.

Similar to the trends found in tranquilizers, past-year use of barbiturates decreased steadily from the mid-1970s, when the usage rate was 10.7 percent, through the early 1990s, when past-year use was 2.8 percent. Since 1991, reports of past-year barbiturate use continued to gradually increase, and, by 2000, rates had risen to 6.2 percent. Since then, past-year use of barbiturates among 12th graders has leveled off at 5.9 percent. Trends in lifetime use of barbiturates have also demonstrated a gradual increase from 1991 to 2000. As indicated in Figure 11.12–7, reported lifetime usage of barbiturates among 12th graders peaked in 2000 at 9.2 percent and has since dropped to 8.7 percent. Data of lifetime use of barbiturates among eighth and tenth graders are unavailable.

The use of manufactured drugs such as GHB and flunitrazepam has recently been added to the Monitoring the Future survey. According to the same survey, in 2001, the annual prevalence of GHB was 1.1 percent in grade eight, 1.0 percent in grade ten, and 1.6 percent in grade 12. These numbers remained stable from 2000, the first year that GHB was measured. Another club drug added to the survey in 1996, flunitrazepam, also showed annual usage among eighth, tenth, and 12th graders to be approximately 1 percent. As indicated in Figure 11.12–8, the use of flunitrazepam rose minimally for 2 years and then returned to 1 percent in 1999, where it has remained.

From 1992 through 2000, *perceived availability* of tranquilizers among eighth graders declined steadily from 22.9 percent reporting “fairly easy” or “very easy” to obtain to 16.2 percent. This number

FIGURE 11.12–6 Trends in lifetime prevalence of use of tranquilizers for eighth, tenth, and 12th graders.

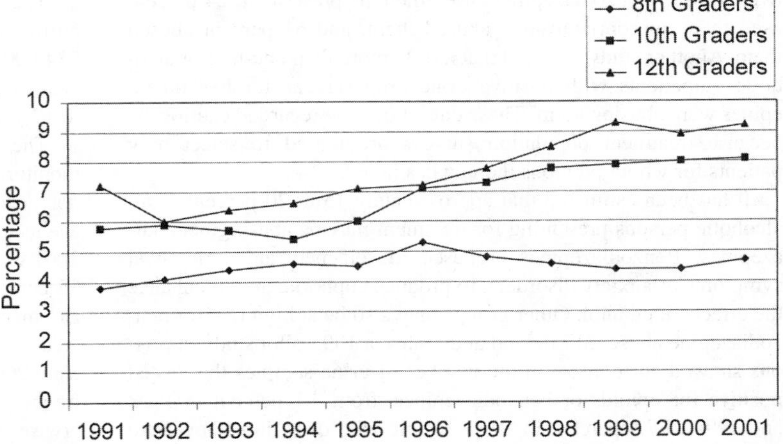

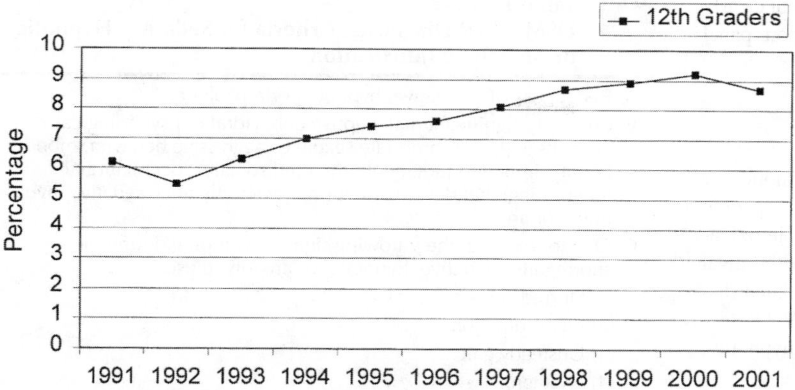

FIGURE 11.12–7 Trends in lifetime prevalence of use of barbiturates in 12th graders.

increased to 17.8 percent in 2001. The number of tenth graders reporting tranquilizers as "fairly easy" or "very easy" to obtain declined from 31.6 percent in 1992 to 27.6 percent in 2000. In 2001, perceived availability of tranquilizers among tenth graders increased to 28.5 percent. Long-term trends in perceived availability by 12th graders fell from 71.8 percent in 1975 to 33 percent in 2001. The perceived availability of barbiturates has been declining since 1975. In 1992, 27.4 percent of eighth graders reported obtaining barbiturates was "fairly easy" or "very easy." Since 1992, this percentage declined to 19.7 percent in 2001 but increased to 20.7 percent in 2001. In 1992, 38 percent of tenth graders reported obtaining barbiturates was "fairly easy" or "very easy." In 2001, the perceived availability had declined to 32.8 percent. Similarly, long-term trends of perceived availability among 12th graders has also declined from 60 percent in 1975 to 35.7 percent in 2001.

The *perceived risk* of sedative hypnotics has also been assessed by *Monitoring the Future.* When the long-term trends in harmfulness as perceived by 12th graders are examined, 34.8 percent of students reported that trying barbiturates once or twice in 1975 was perceived as harmful. A gradual decline of perceived harmfulness occurred until 1999, when it peaked at 35.1 percent. Since 1999, perception of harm has since decreased to 25.7 percent in 2001. Regular administration of barbiturates was perceived as harmful by 69.1 percent of 12th graders in 1975 and remained stable until 1994, when perception of harm decreased to 63.3 percent. Since 1994, perception of harm of regular usage of barbiturates has continued to decline to 50.3 percent in 2001.

Long-term *trends in disapproval* by 12th graders of barbiturate use have also been examined. Administration of barbiturates once or twice was disapproved of by 77.7 percent of 12th graders in 1975. Disapproval gradually increased to 90.6 percent in 1991. After 1991, disapproval began to decline to 85.9 percent in 2001. Disapproval among 12th graders of regular administration of barbiturates has fluctuated between 93 percent and 96.4 percent between 1975 and 2001.

Expert Opinion The International Study of Expert Judgment on Therapeutic Use of Benzodiazepines and Other Psychotherapeutic Medications was designed to gather systematic data on the opinions of leading clinicians concerning the benefits and risks of benzodiazepines and alternative treatments of anxiety. This survey study addressed the relative risks of benzodiazepines compared to other agents and comparative risks within the class. The expert panel assessed risk based on a drug's potential to produce tolerance, rebound symptoms, a withdrawal syndrome, and ease of discontinuation.

Two-thirds of the expert panel reported that long-term use of benzodiazepines for the treatment of anxiety disorders does not pose a high risk of dependence and abuse. Although there was agreement that the pharmacological properties of the medication may be the most important contributor to development of withdrawal symptoms, there was no consensus on whether benzodiazepines with shorter and longer half-lives have similar dependence potential. There was, however, a clear consensus that the differences in withdrawal symptoms are clinically negligible with gradual dose tapering. Because differences in abuse liability among the various benzodiazepines have not been demonstrated

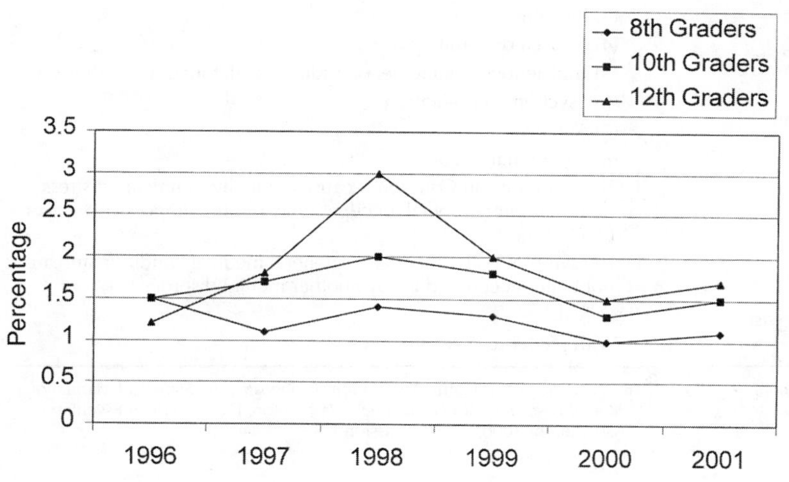

FIGURE 11.12–8 Trend in lifetime prevalence of use of flunitrazepam (Rohypnol) for eighth, tenth, and 12th graders.

in humans, and because the benefits of benzodiazepine treatment clearly outweigh the risks, the majority of physicians on the expert panel opposed increased restrictions on benzodiazepine prescribing.

DIAGNOSIS AND CLINICAL FEATURES

Diagnosis DSM-IV-TR lists a number of sedative-, hypnotic-, or anxiolytic-related disorders (Table 11.12–1) but contains specific diagnostic criteria only for sedative, hypnotic, or anxiolytic intoxication (Table 11.12–2) and sedative, hypnotic, or anxiolytic withdrawal (Table 11.12–3). Other sedative-, hypnotic-, or anxiolytic-related disorders have their diagnostic criteria outlined in the DSM-IV-TR sections that are specific for the major symptom (e.g., sedative-, hypnotic-, or anxiolytic-induced psychotic disorder).

Dependence and Abuse Sedative, hypnotic, or anxiolytic dependence and sedative, hypnotic, or anxiolytic abuse are diagnosed according to the general criteria in DSM-IV-TR for substance dependence and substance abuse.

Intoxication DSM-IV-TR contains a single set of diagnostic criteria for intoxication by any sedative, hypnotic, or anxiolytic substance (Table 11.12–2). Although the intoxication syndromes induced by all those drugs are similar, subtle clinical differences are observable, especially with intoxications that involve low doses. The diagnosis of intoxication by one of that class of substances is best confirmed by obtaining a blood sample for substance screening.

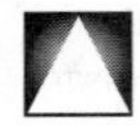

Table 11.12–1
DSM-IV-TR Sedative-, Hypnotic-, or Anxiolytic-Related Disorders

Sedative, hypnotic, or anxiolytic use disorders
Sedative, hypnotic, or anxiolytic dependence
Sedative, hypnotic, or anxiolytic abuse
Sedative-, hypnotic-, or anxiolytic-induced disorders
Sedative, hypnotic, or anxiolytic intoxication
Sedative, hypnotic, or anxiolytic withdrawal
Specify if:
With perceptual disturbances
Sedative, hypnotic, or anxiolytic intoxication delirium
Sedative, hypnotic, or anxiolytic withdrawal delirium
Sedative-, hypnotic-, or anxiolytic-induced persisting dementia
Sedative-, hypnotic-, or anxiolytic-induced psychotic disorder, with delusions
Specify if:
With onset during intoxication
With onset during withdrawal
Sedative-, hypnotic-, or anxiolytic-induced psychotic disorder, with hallucinations
Specify if:
With onset during intoxication
With onset during withdrawal
Sedative-, hypnotic-, or anxiolytic-induced mood disorder
Specify if:
With onset during intoxication
With onset during withdrawal
Sedative-, hypnotic-, or anxiolytic-induced anxiety disorder
Specify if:
With onset during withdrawal
Sedative-, hypnotic-, or anxiolytic-induced sexual dysfunction
Specify if:
With onset during intoxication
Sedative-, hypnotic-, or anxiolytic-induced sleep disorder
Specify if:
With onset during intoxication
With onset during withdrawal
Sedative-, hypnotic-, or anxiolytic-related disorder not otherwise specified

From American Psychiatric Association. *Diagnostic and Statistical Manual of Mental Disorders.* 4th ed. Text rev. Washington, DC: American Psychiatric Association; 2000, with permission.

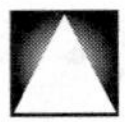

Table 11.12–2
DSM-IV-TR Diagnostic Criteria for Sedative, Hypnotic, or Anxiolytic Intoxication

A. Recent use of a sedative, hypnotic, or anxiolytic.
B. Clinically significant maladaptive behavioral or psychological changes (e.g., inappropriate sexual or aggressive behavior, mood lability, impaired judgment, impaired social or occupational functioning) that developed during, or shortly after, sedative, hypnotic, or anxiolytic use.
C. One (or more) of the following signs, developing during, or shortly after, sedative, hypnotic, or anxiolytic use:
(1) Slurred speech
(2) Incoordination
(3) Unsteady gait
(4) Nystagmus
(5) Impairment in attention or memory
(6) Stupor or coma
D. The symptoms are not due to a general medical condition and are not better accounted for by another mental disorder.

From American Psychiatric Association. *Diagnostic and Statistical Manual of Mental Disorders.* 4th ed. Text rev. Washington, DC: American Psychiatric Association; 2000, with permission.

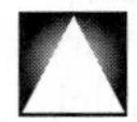

Table 11.12–3
DSM-IV-TR Diagnostic Criteria for Sedative, Hypnotic, or Anxiolytic Withdrawal

A. Cessation of (or reduction in) sedative, hypnotic, or anxiolytic use that has been heavy and prolonged.
B. Two (or more) of the following, developing within several hours to a few days after Criterion A:
(1) Autonomic hyperactivity (e.g., sweating or a pulse rate greater than 100 beats per minute)
(2) Increased hand tremor
(3) Insomnia
(4) Nausea or vomiting
(5) Transient visual, tactile, or auditory hallucinations or illusions
(6) Psychomotor agitation
(7) Anxiety
(8) Grand mal seizures
C. The symptoms in Criterion B cause clinically significant distress or impairment in social, occupational, or other important areas of functioning.
D. The symptoms are not due to a general medical condition and are not better accounted for by another mental disorder.
Specify if:
With perceptual disturbances.

From American Psychiatric Association. *Diagnostic and Statistical Manual of Mental Disorders.* 4th ed. Text rev. Washington, DC: American Psychiatric Association; 2000, with permission.

Withdrawal DSM-IV-TR contains a single set of diagnostic criteria for withdrawal from any sedative, hypnotic, or anxiolytic substance (Table 11.12–3). The clinician can specify *with perceptual disturbances* if illusions, altered perceptions, or hallucinations are present but are accompanied by intact reality testing. Benzodiazepines are associated with a withdrawal syndrome, and withdrawal from barbiturates can be life threatening. Withdrawal from benzodiazepines can also result in serious medical complications, such as seizures.

Delirium DSM-IV-TR allows diagnosis of sedative, hypnotic, or anxiolytic intoxication delirium and sedative, hypnotic, or anxiolytic withdrawal delirium (see Tables 10.2–3 and 10.2–4). Delirium that is indistinguishable from delirium tremens associated with alcohol withdrawal is more commonly seen with barbiturate withdrawal than with benzodiazepine withdrawal. Delirium associated with intoxication can be seen with barbiturates or benzodiazepines if the dosages are high enough.

Persisting Dementia DSM-IV-TR allows diagnosis of sedative-, hypnotic-, or anxiolytic-induced persisting dementia. The existence of the disorder is controversial, because whether a persisting dementia is due to the substance use itself or to associated features of the substance use is uncertain. The diagnosis needs further validation by DSM-IV-TR criteria.

Persisting Amnestic Disorder DSM-IV-TR allows diagnosis of sedative-, hypnotic-, or anxiolytic-induced persisting amnestic disorder (Table 10.4–2). Amnestic disorders associated with sedatives, hypnotics, and anxiolytics may have been underdiagnosed. One exception is the increased number of reports of amnestic episodes associated with short-term use of benzodiazepines with short half-lives (e.g., triazolam).

Psychotic Disorders The psychotic symptoms of barbiturate withdrawal can be indistinguishable from those of alcohol-associated delirium tremens. Agitation, delusions, and hallucinations are usually visual, but sometimes tactile or auditory features develop after approximately 1 week of abstinence. Psychotic symptoms associated with intoxication or withdrawal are much more common with barbiturates than with benzodiazepines and are diagnosed as sedative-, hypnotic-, or anxiolytic-induced psychotic disorders.The clinician can further specify whether delusions or hallucinations are the predominant symptoms.

Other Disorders Sedative, hypnotic, and anxiolytic use has also been associated with mood disorders (Table 13.6–18), anxiety disorders, sleep disorders, and sexual dysfunctions (Table 18.1a–20). When none of those diagnostic categories is appropriate for a person with a sedative, hypnotic, or anxiolytic use disorder, the appropriate diagnosis is sedative-, hypnotic-, or anxiolytic-related disorder NOS (Table 11.12–4).

Clinical Features and Patterns of Abuse

Oral Use Sedative, hypnotic, and anxiolytic drugs can all be taken orally, occasionally to achieve a time-limited specific effect or regularly to obtain a constant, usually mild, intoxication. The occasional use pattern is associated with young persons who take the substance to achieve specific effects: relaxation for an evening, intensification of sexual activities, and a short-lived mild euphoria. The user's personality and expectations about the substance's effects and the setting in which the substance is taken also affect the substance-induced experience. The regular-use pattern is associated with middle-aged, middle-class people who usually obtain the substance from the family physician as a prescription for insomnia or anxiety. Abusers of this type may have prescriptions from several physicians, and the pattern of abuse may go undetected until obvious signs of abuse or dependence are noticed by the person's family, coworkers, or physicians.

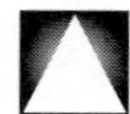

Table 11.12–4
DSM-IV-TR Diagnostic Criteria for Sedative-, Hypnotic-, or Anxiolytic-Related Disorder Not Otherwise Specified

The sedative-, hypnotic-, or anxiolytic-related disorder not otherwise specified category is for disorders associated with the use of sedatives, hypnotics, or anxiolytics that are not classifiable as sedative, hypnotic, or anxiolytic dependence; sedative, hypnotic, or anxiolytic abuse; sedative, hypnotic, or anxiolytic intoxication; sedative, hypnotic, or anxiolytic withdrawal; sedative, hypnotic, or anxiolytic intoxication delirium; sedative, hypnotic, or anxiolytic withdrawal delirium; sedative-, hypnotic-, or anxiolytic-induced persisting dementia; sedative-, hypnotic-, or anxiolytic-induced persisting amnestic disorder; sedative-, hypnotic-, or anxiolytic-induced psychotic disorder; sedative-, hypnotic-, or anxiolytic-induced mood disorder; sedative-, hypnotic-, or anxiolytic-induced anxiety disorder; sedative-, hypnotic-, or anxiolytic-induced sexual dysfunction; or sedative-, hypnotic-, or anxiolytic-induced sleep disorder.

From American Psychiatric Association. *Diagnostic and Statistical Manual of Mental Disorders.* 4th ed. Text rev. Washington, DC: American Psychiatric Association; 2000, with permission.

Intravenous Use A severe form of abuse involves the intravenous (IV) use of these substances. The users are mainly young adults intimately involved with illegal substances. IV barbiturate use is associated with a pleasant, warm, drowsy feeling, and users may be inclined to use barbiturates more than opioids because of the low cost of barbiturates. The physical dangers of injection include transmission of the human immunodeficiency virus (HIV), cellulitis, vascular complications from accidental injection into an artery, infections, and allergic reactions to contaminants. IV use is associated with rapid and profound tolerance, dependence, and a severe withdrawal syndrome. One survey reported that 28 percent of heroin addicts injected benzodiazepines, and these patients had higher rates of polydrug use, HIV risk-taking behavior, criminal activity, psychological distress, health problems, and overdose than addicts who did not inject benzodiazepines.

Benzodiazepines

Since the introduction of chlordiazepoxide in 1960, benzodiazepines have become the primary drugs used to treat anxiety and insomnia, largely replacing barbiturates and other sedative-hypnotic agents. Zolpidem, an imidazopyridine hypnotic drug, is chemically distinct from the benzodiazepines but has similar clinical effects and acts at the $GABA_A$-benzodiazepine receptor complex. The benzodiazepines have lower abuse liability than most barbiturates, pose a much lower risk when taken in overdose, and have fewer interactions with other drugs. The advantages of the benzodiazepines must be weighed against the risk for abuse and physiological dependence.

Intoxication Benzodiazepine intoxication can be associated with behavioral disinhibition, potentially resulting in hostile or aggressive behavior. The effect is perhaps most common when benzodiazepines are taken in combination with alcohol. Benzodiazepine intoxication is associated with less respiratory depression than barbiturate intoxication.

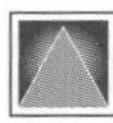

Table 11.12–5
Signs and Symptoms of the Benzodiazepine Discontinuation Syndrome

The following signs and symptoms may be seen when benzodiazepine therapy is discontinued; they reflect the return of the original anxiety symptoms (recurrence), worsening of the original anxiety symptoms (rebound), or emergence of new symptoms (true withdrawal):

- Disturbances of mood and cognition
  - Anxiety, apprehension, dysphoria, pessimism, irritability, obsessive rumination, and paranoid ideation
- Disturbances of sleep
  - Insomnia, altered sleep–wake cycle, and daytime drowsiness
- Physical signs and symptoms
  - Tachycardia, elevated blood pressure, hyperreflexia, muscle tension, agitation/motor restlessness, tremor, myoclonus, muscle and joint pain, nausea, coryza, diaphoresis, ataxia, tinnitus, and grand mal seizures
- Perceptual disturbances
  - Hyperacusis, depersonalization, blurred vision, illusions, and hallucinations

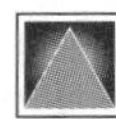

Table 11.12–6
Factors Influencing the Development of the Benzodiazepine Discontinuation Syndrome

Dosage of benzodiazepine
Duration of benzodiazepine treatment
Rate of drug taper
Psychopathology

Withdrawal Syndrome

SIGNS AND SYMPTOMS Studies in the early 1960s by Leo Hollister established that abrupt discontinuation of high doses of chlordiazepoxide or diazepam could lead to a withdrawal syndrome. More recent studies show that therapeutic doses given for weeks to months may also be associated with withdrawal syndrome.

The American Psychiatric Association's "Task Force Report on Benzodiazepine Dependence, Toxicity, and Abuse" defined *withdrawal* as a true abstinence syndrome consisting of "new signs and symptoms and worsening of preexisting symptoms following drug discontinuance that were not part of the disorder for which the drugs were originally prescribed." Many authorities have taken issue with that definition of withdrawal and prefer to distinguish withdrawal only from recurrence, not from rebound symptoms, viewing the true abstinence syndrome as consisting of rebound symptoms plus new signs and symptoms.

The signs and symptoms of the benzodiazepine discontinuation syndrome (Table 11.12–5) have been classified as major or minor, like those of the alcohol withdrawal syndrome. According to that classification, minor symptoms include anxiety, insomnia, and nightmares. Major symptoms (which are extremely rare) include grand mal seizures, psychosis, hyperpyrexia, and death.

The discontinuance syndrome may also be divided into symptoms of rebound, recurrence, and withdrawal. *Rebound symptoms* are symptoms for which the benzodiazepine was originally prescribed that return in a more severe form than they had before treatment. They have a rapid onset after termination of therapy and a brief duration. *Recurrence* refers to return of the original symptoms at or below their original intensity. The pattern and course of these symptoms reflect the anxiety disorder for which treatment was originally instituted.

Withdrawal symptoms (Table 11.12–5) are loosely categorized into four types: (1) disturbances of mood and cognition, (2) disturbances of sleep, (3) physical signs and symptoms, and (4) perceptual disturbances. Mood and cognitive symptoms are anxiety, apprehension, dysphoria, irritability, obsessive ruminations, and paranoia. Sleep disturbances include insomnia, altered sleep–wake cycle, and daytime drowsiness. Somatic symptoms are agitation, tachycardia, palpitations, motor restlessness, muscle tension, tremor myoclonus, nausea, coryza, diaphoresis, lethargy, muscle and joint pain, hyperreflexia, ataxia, tinnitus, and seizures. Perceptual disturbances include hyperacusis, depersonalization, blurred vision, illusions, and hallucinations.

The temporal sequence of symptom development is not well established, but, on the abrupt cessation of benzodiazepines with short elimination half-lives, symptoms may appear within 24 hours and peak at 48 hours. Symptoms arising from abrupt discontinuance of benzodiazepines with long half-lives may not peak until 2 weeks later. Although some investigators suggest that a subgroup of patients have withdrawal syndromes that last for many months, no medical or scientific evidence validates the existence of such a syndrome. Prolonged symptoms are almost certainly attributable to recurrence of the original anxiety or progression of the anxiety disorder itself.

RISK FACTORS Factors influencing the development of the discontinuance or withdrawal syndrome are listed in Table 11.12–6. Studies on humans and animals have attempted to identify risk factors for the development of physiological dependence. Animal studies demonstrate that the severity of withdrawal is greater with higher doses and longer periods of drug administration, but that has not been as consistently demonstrated in clinical populations. When patients are stratified into high- and low-dose groups, the withdrawal syndrome is seen to be more severe in the high-dose group. However, two recent studies, one using a daily 21-mg dose of diazepam equivalent as the cutoff separating high- and low-dose groups and the other using three groups based on diazepam daily dose (less than 6 mg, between 6 and 10 mg, and more than 10 mg), indicate no significant differences in withdrawal symptoms between groups. One possible explanation for the failure to demonstrate a consistent relation between dose and withdrawal symptoms is that subjects in clinical studies are being treated for an anxiety disorder, and, when the benzodiazepine is discontinued, the reemergence of the original anxiety symptoms may be confused with withdrawal symptoms. Furthermore, the drug dosage is probably higher in patients with the most severe disease, complicating any relation between dosage and the intensity of the discontinuance syndrome.

According to one study, withdrawal symptoms are related to treatment duration when the length of the treatment is less than 8 months but not when it is 1 year or longer. The findings of another group indicate that patients taking benzodiazepines for more than 5 years have more withdrawal symptoms than those taking them for less than 5 years.

Mild withdrawal symptoms may occur with abrupt discontinuation of therapeutic doses after 4 weeks of benzodiazepine treatment. There is a risk of rebound insomnia after a few days to 1 week of treatment with benzodiazepine hypnotic drugs with short elimination half-lives. Benzodiazepine hypnotics with longer elimination half-lives are less likely to induce rebound insomnia on abrupt discontinuation. The likelihood of a serious withdrawal syndrome increases as treatment continues, and many authorities see 4 months of treatment at therapeutic doses as a critical point in the development of clinically significant physiological dependence. That does not imply, however, that 4 months is an upper limit for treatment duration.

The risk of withdrawal is also influenced by the rate at which the drugs are discontinued. Gradual tapering of the benzodiazepines with short elimination half-lives is associated with fewer withdrawal symptoms than their abrupt discontinuation. Clinical research shows less distinct differences between gradual and abrupt discontinuation of benzodiazepines with long half-lives, because these drugs have a self-tapering action or because the period of tapering and observation in many studies is insufficient.

If benzodiazepines are abruptly discontinued, the withdrawal syndrome related to short half-life agents appears earlier and may be more intense than that with long half-life drugs. Differences in intensity have not been proved, because most studies do not monitor withdrawal symptoms for 2 weeks, which may be the time of peak symptoms with some drugs with long half-lives. Furthermore, any difference in withdrawal severity between short– and long–half-life agents is not entirely supported by animal studies. There is no difference in symptom severity of the withdrawal syndrome after animals are treated with midazolam or chlordiazepoxide, for example, because essentially all benzodiazepines, regardless of their pharmacokinetic properties in humans, are eliminated rapidly in small animal species.

The development of physiological dependence differs depending on whether it results from benzodiazepine partial agonists or full agonists. In animal models, the partial agonists bretazenil and abecarnil are associated with fewer withdrawal symptoms than are classic agonists such as diazepam or clorazepate (the prodrug for desmethyldiazepam). Clinical studies in anxious patients, however, indicate that abrupt termination of abecarnil is associated with withdrawal symptoms in some patients.

Some studies in animals indicate that periodic administration of the benzodiazepine antagonist flumazenil during the chronic administration of lorazepam, diazepam, triazolam, or clobazam may attenuate the withdrawal syndrome.

Personality traits may be a risk factor for development of the benzodiazepine withdrawal syndrome. Withdrawal severity is greater in patients with higher scores on the dependence scale of the Minnesota Multiphasic Personality Inventory 2 (MMPI-2), high prewithdrawal levels of anxiety and depression, lower educational level, and passive-dependent personality disorder.

Overdose The benzodiazepines, in contrast to the barbiturates and the barbiturate-like substances, have a large margin of safety when taken in overdoses, a feature that contributed significantly to their rapid acceptance. The ratio of lethal to effective dose is approximately 200 to 1 or higher because of the minimal respiratory depression associated with the benzodiazepines. Even when grossly excessive amounts (more than 2 g) are taken in suicide attempts, the symptoms include only drowsiness, lethargy, ataxia, some confusion, and mild depression of the user's vital signs. A much more serious condition prevails when benzodiazepines are taken in overdose in combination with other sedative-hypnotic substances, such as alcohol. In such cases, small doses of benzodiazepines can cause death. The availability of flumazenil, a specific benzodiazepine antagonist, has reduced the lethality of the benzodiazepines, because flumazenil can be used in emergency rooms to reverse the effects of the benzodiazepines.

Barbiturates

Since the advent of the benzodiazepines, barbiturate use has been limited in modern medicine. Phenobarbital is still prescribed as an anticonvulsant and as a sedative, especially for children. It is also a common component of many combination products and reduces the stimulating effects of sympathomimetic agents. Butalbital is an intermediate-acting barbiturate found in a widely used combination product that also contains acetaminophen and caffeine (Fioricet) and is approved for the treatment of muscle contraction headaches. Given the limited availability of barbiturates, it is uncommon, at least in the United States, for addiction units to treat patients dependent on barbiturates other than butalbital and phenobarbital. The barbiturates marketed currently in the United States are listed in Table 11.12–7.

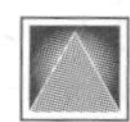

Table 11.12–7
Barbiturates and Other Sedative-Hypnotic Agents

Generic Name	Trade Name	Dose (mg)
Amobarbital	Amytal	100
Aprobarbital	Alurate	40
Butabarbital	Butisol	100
Butalbital	Many combination products (e.g., Fioricet)	100
Pentobarbital	Nembutal	100
Secobarbital	Seconal	100
Chloral hydrate	Aquachloral Supprettes, Generic	500
Ethchlorvynol	Placidyl	500
Glutethimide	Generic	250
Meprobamate	Miltown	400

Note: The substitution technique for sedative-hypnotic withdrawal requires calculation of equivalent doses of phenobarbital to replace the sedative-hypnotic agent that the patient is taking. The above are doses of various sedative-hypnotic agents for which a 30-mg dose of phenobarbital should provide adequate coverage of a withdrawal syndrome. Daily doses of phenobarbital should rarely exceed 600 mg using this protocol.

A major disadvantage of the use of the barbiturates is the development of pharmacokinetic and pharmacodynamic tolerance. *Tolerance* is defined as reduced drug response as a result of decreased drug concentration at the site of action, usually the result of increased drug metabolism (pharmacokinetic) or of cellular adaptive changes with unchanged or higher drug concentrations at the site of action (pharmacodynamic). Pharmacodynamic tolerance begins after acute doses and continues to develop over weeks to months. Tolerance to the mood-altering and sedative effects develops to a greater extent than does tolerance to the lethal effects, increasing the risk of accidental overdose.

Intoxication When barbiturates and barbiturate-like substances are taken in relatively low doses, the clinical syndrome of intoxication is indistinguishable from that associated with alcohol intoxication. The symptoms include sluggishness, incoordination, difficulty in thinking, poor memory, slowness of speech and comprehension, faulty judgment, disinhibition of sexual and aggressive impulses, a narrowed range of attention, emotional lability, and exaggeration of basic personality traits. The sluggishness usually resolves after a few hours, but the impaired judgment, distorted mood, and impaired motor skills may remain for 12 to 24 hours, depending primarily on the half-life of the abused substance. Other potential symptoms are hostility, argumentativeness, moroseness, and (occasionally) paranoid and suicidal ideation. The neurological effects include nystagmus, diplopia, strabismus, ataxic gait, positive Romberg's sign, hypotonia, and decreased superficial reflexes.

Dependence and Withdrawal Physiological dependence may develop after a daily dose of 400 mg of pentobarbital (Nembutal) for 3 months; abrupt discontinuation results in paroxysmal abnormalities on the EEG in approximately 30 percent of patients. At a daily dose of 600 mg of pentobarbital for 1 to 2 months, a withdrawal syndrome characterized by anxiety, insomnia, anorexia, tremor, and EEG changes occurs in approximately one-half of patients, and 10 percent may have a single seizure. At higher dosages of 800 to 2,200 mg per day for several weeks to months, abrupt discontinuation leads to minor symptoms, which include apprehension and uneasiness, insomnia, muscular weakness, twitches, coarse tremors, myoclonic jerks, postural faintness and orthostatic hypotension, anorexia, vomiting, and EEG changes, within 24 hours of the last dose. Minor symptoms may persist as long as 2 weeks. At high doses, major symptoms develop. As many as 75 percent of patients may have grand mal seizures on the second or third day after withdrawal, and two-thirds have more than one seizure. The interictal EEG shows four spike-wave discharges per second. Two-thirds of these patients develop delirium between the third and eighth day of withdrawal, which is sometimes accompanied by hypothermia, which may be fatal. Disorientation, visual hallucinations, and frightening dreams may precede the onset of full delirium. Delirium may be exceedingly difficult to reverse, even with large doses of a barbiturate; thus, clinicians should never wait for the appearance of withdrawal symptoms before instituting therapy. The duration of the withdrawal syndrome is between 3 and 14 days; most end by the eighth day.

Overdose Barbiturates are lethal when taken in overdose, because they induce respiratory depression. In addition to intentional suicide attempts, accidental or unintentional overdoses are common. Barbiturates in home medicine cabinets are a common cause of fatal drug overdoses in children. As with benzodiazepines, the lethal effects of barbiturates are additive to those of other sedative-hypnotic drugs, including alcohol and benzodiazepines. Barbiturate overdose is characterized by induction of coma, respiratory arrest, cardiovascular failure, and death.

The lethal dose varies with the route of administration and the degree of tolerance for the substance after a history of long-term abuse. For the most commonly abused barbiturates, the ratio of lethal to effective dose ranges between 3 to 1 and 30 to 1. Dependent users often take an average daily dose of 1.5 g of a short-acting barbiturate, and some have been reported to take as much as 2.5 g per day for months. The lethal dose is not much greater for the long-term abuser than it is for the neophyte. Tolerance develops quickly to the point at which withdrawal in a hospital becomes necessary to prevent accidental death from overdose.

Miscellaneous Sedative-Hypnotic Drugs

The drugs discussed in the following sections have little or no role in modern therapeutics. However, prescriptions for some have been increasing, especially in New York, where a 1989 triplicate prescription program has led to a 44 percent decline in benzodiazepine prescribing in retail pharmacies, a 60 percent decline in the Medicaid program, and a 30 percent decline in Blue Cross Blue Shield programs. Corresponding prescription increases of 125 percent for meprobamate (Miltown), 29 percent for ethchlorvynol (Placidyl), and 136 percent for chloral hydrate (Aquachloral Supprettes) have been reported.

The older sedative-hypnotics drugs are similar in effect to the barbiturates, and they lead to tolerance and physiological dependence. The withdrawal syndrome is similar to the barbiturate withdrawal syndrome, and the protocols described for barbiturates should be used for safe withdrawal of patients dependent on those drugs.

Meprobamate Meprobamate, a carbamate derivative, has weak efficacy as an antianxiety agent. At clinical doses in humans, it has minimal muscle-relaxant effects, but it may have a mild analgesic effect in musculoskeletal pain and may potentiate analgesics. Typical daily doses are between 1,200 and 1,600 mg, with a maximum of 2,400 mg, in three or four divided daily doses. A discontinuance syndrome occurs after several weeks of treatment with a daily dose of 2,400 mg, and mild symptoms may be seen with long-term therapy at doses of 1,600 mg daily. Onset of the discontinuance syndrome occurs within 12 to 48 hours after abrupt discontinuation and lasts for an additional 12 to 48 hours. Seizures may be common in withdrawal from meprobamate, and reports published in the 1970s suggest that serious withdrawal symptoms are more common with meprobamate than with barbiturates. Fatalities from overdose have been reported after doses as low as 12 g. The manufacturer offers the following guidelines for blood concentration: 5 to 20 μg/mL is the normal range with recommended doses; 30 to 100 μg/mL is associated with mild to moderate overdose, with patients in stupor or light coma; 100 to 200 μg/mL is associated with serious overdose, deeper coma, and fatalities; concentrations greater than 200 μg/mL are associated with more fatalities than survivals. Meprobamate induces microsomal enzymes and may exacerbate intermittent porphyria.

Chloral Hydrate Chloral hydrate is used as a hypnotic in doses of 0.5 to 2.0 g. After oral administration, it is rapidly transformed to trichloroethanol, the metabolite responsible for its pharmacological activity. It is also effective in blocking experimentally induced seizures; however, anticonvulsive and hypnotic doses are similar in humans, making the benzodiazepines and barbiturates better choices for anticonvulsive medications.

At high doses, chloral hydrate may produce respiratory depression, hypotension, gastric necrosis, depressed cardiac contractility, and a shortened refractory period. Even at therapeutic doses, it is associated with gastric distress and flatulence. Somnambulism, disorientation, and paranoid ideation may occur. Tolerance and physiological dependence develop with long-term use, and the withdrawal syndrome is similar to the barbiturate abstinence syndrome. Several drug interactions occur with chloral hydrate, including displacement of oral anticoagulants and acidic drugs from protein binding sites by the metabolite trichloroacetic acid. When combined with furosemide (Lasix), flushing, tachycardia, hypotension or hypertension, and diaphoresis have been reported. It potentiates the effects of ethanol, and it should not be used in patients with intermittent porphyria. Fatalities from overdose may occur with as little as 4 g, although patients have survived after taking 30 g.

Ethchlorvynol Ethchlorvynol is a rapidly acting sedative-hypnotic agent with anticonvulsant and muscle-relaxant properties. Recommended doses are 500 to 1,000 mg. Initial effects (which may include euphoria) occur 15 to 30 minutes after an oral dose, and plasma levels peak at 1 to 1.5 hours. The elimination half-life of the parent compound is 10 to 20 hours. The duration of the hypnotic effect is approximately 5 hours. Long-term use of ethchlorvynol has been associated with toxic amblyopia, scotoma, nystagmus, and peripheral neuropathy, which are usually reversible on drug discontinuation. IV self-administration may cause pulmonary edema.

Idiosyncratic reactions of excitement and stimulation have been described. Hypersensitivity reactions with urticaria and rare fatal thrombocytopenia may also arise. It should not be used in patients with intermittent porphyria. Tolerance, physiological dependence, and a withdrawal syndrome are seen with long-term administration. Lethal doses are typically between 10 and 25 g; one person was reported to have died after taking 2.5 g with ethanol, and one patient survived but was in a coma for 7 days after taking 50 g.

Glutethimide and Methyprylon Glutethimide and methyprylon (no longer marketed in the United States) are piperidinedione sedative-hypnotic drugs that have high liability for abuse. Glutethimide resembles the barbiturates in most respects but differs from them in having significant anticholinergic activity. An overdose can cause ileus, bladder atony, mydriasis, hyperpyrexia, myoclonic jerks, and convulsions. A lethal dose is between 10 and 20 g; intoxication may be seen at a dose of 5 g. An unusual characteristic of glutethimide is that a withdrawal syndrome can occur in patients taking therapeutic doses (0.5 to 3.0 g daily), even when they have not stopped taking the drug. The abstinence syndrome includes tremulousness, nausea, tachycardia, fever, tonic muscle spasms, and grand mal seizures. Withdrawal from a combination of glutethimide and antihistamine has caused catatonia and dyskinesia. When glutethimide is taken with codeine (the street name is a *load*), a euphoria similar to that with heroin results. In these patients, detoxification may require opioid withdrawal and sedative withdrawal.

Methaqualone Methaqualone is no longer available in the United States, and much of what is sold on the street as methaqualone is actually diazepam. Methaqualone is a quinazoline with sedative, anticonvulsive, local anesthetic, and antispasmodic activity. It has antitussive effects comparable to those of codeine and weak antihistaminic activity. During the 1960s and 1970s, those in the drug culture considered it to provide the ultimate high of all sedative-hypnotic agents, producing euphoria comparable to that from heroin. Chronic users may take daily doses between 75 mg and 2 g, with an average daily dose of 775 mg. Adverse effects include peripheral neuropathy, nightmares, somnambulism, gastric discomfort, and urticaria. Death has been reported after 8 g, but one report attributed most deaths under the influence of methaqualone to accidents due to impairment produced by the drug. Tolerance and physiological dependence are seen with chronic dosing.

An overdose of methaqualone may result in restlessness, delirium, hypertonia, muscle spasms, convulsions, and (in high doses) death. Unlike barbiturates, methaqualone rarely causes severe cardiovascular or respiratory depression, and most fatalities result from combining methaqualone with alcohol.

γ-Hydroxybutyrate The abuse potential of GHB is becoming an area of concern among physicians in the United States. GHB was used for decades in Europe with a limited number of reported adverse effects and abuse. However, beginning in the late 1980s, when clinical use of GHB as a dietary supplement, growth promoter, and mild sedative became more prevalent, public health officials began inquiring about its safety and efficacy. By the early 1990s, concern that GHB was developing into a popular drug of abuse and evidence that GHB was being used as a recreational club drug led to U.S. Food and Drug Administration (FDA) removal of GHB from the market. The FDA has recently approved GHB as a treatment for narcolepsy, marketed under the trade name Xyrem. Also, it is still possible to obtain products containing GHB and its precursors through the Internet and various health food stores.

GHB is a naturally occurring short-chained fatty acid naturally distributed throughout the CNS. It is synthesized in the brain from GABA via deamination to succinic semialdehyde (SSA) by GABA aminotransferase. Other precursors of GHB such as 1,4-butanediol and γ-butyrolactone may have important roles as well. GHB activity is terminated by synaptic reuptake and subsequent metabolism of SSA to succinate, which is further degraded to carbon dioxide and water. Although the half-life of GHB is reported as 30 to 50 minutes, its pharmacokinetics are nonlinear, so that high doses may take considerably longer to clear from the body.

The pharmacologic actions of GHB are mediated through specific GHB receptors that are G-protein coupled. GHB may also bind to GABA type B ($GABA_B$) receptors, although some investigators believe that the affinity is so low that this may not be of physiological importance. Other data suggest that weak $GABA_B$ agonist activity has been demonstrated in studies that have shown that $GABA_B$ antagonists block GHB effects and that the $GABA_B$ agonist baclofen (Lioresal) produces effects similar to GHB. Euphoric effects of GHB may be mediated by enhanced dopamine release in the striatum and mesolimbic system.

Early testing of GHB found that dose-dependent sedation and anesthetic properties could be produced in both humans and laboratory animals. Recent testing has shown that, when administered at high doses, GHB produces EEG changes associated with epileptiform patterns, supporting initial thoughts that GHB induced cataleptic states rather than true sedation in some animals. However, further investigations of GHB's influence on EEG patterns have shown that lower doses of GHB produce patterns consistent with physiological sleep. Unlike other hypnotics, GHB has been shown to increase slow wave sleep, stages III and IV, and to increase rapid eye movement (REM) episodes. These developments have supported the use of GHB in the treatment of narcolepsy.

Animal models assessing the abuse potential of GHB have not provided strong evidence of abuse potential. Studies of rhesus monkeys using a substitution procedure have shown that rates of self-administration of GHB were relatively low when compared to those of positive controls, indicating that GHB has minimal reinforcing effects and low abuse potential. Some conditioned place preference and self-administration models in rodent populations have been more suggestive of reinforcing properties of GHB; however, further investigations must be conducted.

Abuse liability testing in humans is limited. In drug discrimination studies, consistent cross substitution of GHB with benzodiazepines and barbiturates has not been shown. There have been reports that cross substitution does occur between GHB and $GABA_A$ agonists and ethanol, but this occurs only within a narrow dose range and appears inconsistently.

Despite limited data, the development of tolerance and dependence has been shown in animals. Data from rodent studies indicate that tolerance to motor impairment and sedative effects caused by GHB administration does occur. Physical dependence to GHB has not been directly examined in controlled animal studies; however, tolerance studies using repeated administration of GHB have not reported the occurrence of withdrawal symptoms after discontinuation.

There have been no formal studies monitoring the potential of GHB to produce tolerance and dependence in humans, and evidence gathered from case reports has been contradictory and inconclusive. Quantitative data on the prevalence of licit and illicit use of GHB are currently unavailable, but monitoring systems have recently added it to annual surveys.

Determining the risk of GHB administration in humans is difficult owing to insufficient laboratory testing of GHB intoxication, limited availability of data reporting blood and tissue levels of hospitalized patients, coingestion of alcohol, or other drugs in clinical cases. GHB in combination with other CNS depressants, especially ethanol, creates amplified CNS depression and has been found to result in acute intoxication, often requiring medical attention. Similar to benzodiazepines and barbiturates, when GHB and alcohol are combined, memory impairment, confusion, increased sleep, and unconsciousness are likely to occur. This has led to concern about its potential to increase the risk of sexual assaults on unsuspecting women (i.e., date rape). Other adverse effects include mild hypothermia, dizziness, nausea, vomiting, weakness, loss of peripheral vision, agitation, hallucinations, decreased respiratory effort, and coma. GHB alone has not been found to precipitate seizures in humans, and reported incidences could be the result of concurrent sympathomimetic drug ingestion or a misinterpretation of clonic movements produced by the high doses of GHB. Reports have indicated that GHB has been linked to deaths in humans; however, the majority of these cases involve GHB in combination with ethanol or methamphetamines. Clinical guidelines for management of overdose and withdrawal are not based on systematic investigations. Patients who overdose on GHB are treated with supportive care, and most patients regain consciousness within several hours, although there have been reports that complete recovery may require several days. Treatment of the abstinence syndrome is usually managed with benzodiazepines, although clinical reports suggest these are inconsistently effective.

TREATMENT

Withdrawal

Benzodiazepines Guidelines for the treatment of benzodiazepine discontinuance syndrome and the clinical management of withdrawal are presented in Table 11.12–8. The most common clinical situations that require medically supervised withdrawal from the benzodiazepines involve patients with anxiety disorders or chronic insomnia who have been maintained on therapeutic doses of benzodiazepines for several months or years, patients taking supratherapeutic doses of benzodiazepines for treatment-resistant types of anxiety or because of inappropriate dosage escalation, and patients who abuse benzodiazepines as part of a mixed abuse pattern (e.g., those who use benzodiazepines to self-medicate alcohol withdrawal or to end a cocaine run).

In planning a rational withdrawal, clinicians should remember the factors that influence the development of physiological dependence. The risk of withdrawal is greatest in patients taking high doses over long periods. The onset of withdrawal and its peak severity are earlier with agents with short half-lives, and, if they are not tapered, withdrawal from them may be more severe than that from agents with long elimination half-lives, although the last point has not been definitively established. Concurrent use of other sedative-hypnotic agents (e.g., barbiturates or ethanol) may alter the time course and severity of the benzodiazepine withdrawal syndrome.

TAPERING The basic principle underlying safe withdrawal is gradual tapering of the benzodiazepine dosage. In cases of detoxification from therapeutic doses, the daily dose is known, and the tapering protocol is easily calculated. Anyone taking a benzodiazepine for 2 weeks or longer should be tapered from the drug. Initially, the dose is reduced by approximately 10 to 25 percent, and the patient is observed for any signs and symptoms of withdrawal. Withdrawal signs appear earlier for drugs with short half-lives than for drugs with long half-lives. Subsequent reductions depend on how the patient responds to initial changes and require individualization based on careful observation of the patient's condition after each dose change.

In some cases, patients taking high therapeutic doses of a benzodiazepine for a year or more may require several months or longer to stop the medication completely, not primarily for pharmacological reasons, but so they can learn alternative strategies for coping with anxiety. Most patients taking midrange therapeutic doses for a shorter time tolerate weekly reductions ranging from 10 to 25 percent. Most authorities agree that the last phases of drug discontinuation are the most difficult for the patient, and it may be necessary to slow the taper rate or to stop the taper entirely. The adjunctive use of nonbenzodiazepine medications may be useful in these circumstances.

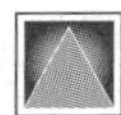

Table 11.12–8
Guidelines for Treatment of Benzodiazepine Discontinuance Syndrome

Evaluate and treat concomitant medical and psychiatric conditions.

Obtain drug history and urine and blood samples for drug and ethanol assay.

Determine required dose of benzodiazepine or barbiturate for stabilization, guided by history, clinical presentation, drug-ethanol assay, and (in some cases) challenge dose.

Detoxification from supratherapeutic dosages:

- Hospitalize if there are medical or psychiatric indications, poor social supports, or polysubstance dependence or if the patient is unreliable.
- Some clinicians recommend switching to a longer-acting benzodiazepine for withdrawal (e.g., diazepam [Valium], clonazepam [Klonopin]); others recommend stabilizing on the drug that the patient was taking or on phenobarbital.
- After stabilization, reduce dosage by 30% on the second or third day and evaluate the response, keeping in mind that symptoms that occur after decreases in benzodiazepines with short elimination half-lives (e.g., lorazepam [Ativan]) appear sooner than with those with longer elimination half-lives (e.g., diazepam).
- Reduce dosage further by 10–25% percent every few days, if tolerated.
- Use adjunctive medications if necessary—carbamazepine (Tegretol), gabapentin, β-adrenergic receptor antagonists, divalproex (Depakote), clonidine (Catapres), and sedative antidepressants have been used, but their efficacy in the treatment of the benzodiazepine abstinence syndrome has not been established.

Detoxification from therapeutic dosages:

- Initiate 10–25% percent dose reduction and evaluate response.
- Dose, duration of therapy, and severity of anxiety influence the rate of taper and the need for adjunctive medications.
- Most patients taking therapeutic doses have uncomplicated discontinuation.

Psychological interventions may assist patients in detoxification from benzodiazepines and in the long-term management of anxiety.

Detoxification from supratherapeutic dosages of benzodiazepines may require a slightly different approach. Most clinicians hospitalize such patients because of the greater medical risks associated with supratherapeutic dosage withdrawal. Patients may be tapered using the benzodiazepine that they have been taking or switched to a drug with a long elimination half-life, such as diazepam or clonazepam, using the dose equivalencies listed in Table 11.12–9 to determine the initial daily dose. The estimated equivalent dose is then administered in divided doses on day 1 to ensure that an accurate history and appropriate equivalency are established. Some clinicians stabilize patients on that dose for 2 to 3 days; others prefer to reduce the dose by 30 percent on the second day, followed by 5 to 10 percent daily reductions. The use of carbamazepine (Tegretol) or divalproex (Depakote) in high-dosage withdrawal often permits even larger daily reductions in the benzodiazepine dose. Most high-dose detoxification can be completed in 2 weeks or less using this protocol. For some patients, the dose cannot be reduced that rapidly, however, and slower, longer tapers are sometimes necessary. The efficacy of anticonvulsants for the treatment of the benzodiazepine discontinuance syndrome has not been established, although clinical experience to date is encouraging.

When the physician knows that the patient has been taking supratherapeutic doses but cannot determine the exact dose, 20 mg of diazepam may be given to estimate tolerance. The dose should be repeated every 2 hours until mild sedation occurs. The total dose

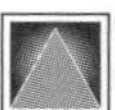

Table 11.12–9
Approximate Therapeutic Equivalent Doses of Benzodiazepines

Generic Name	Trade Name	Dose (mg)
Alprazolam	Xanax	1
Chlordiazepoxide	Librium	25
Clonazepam	Klonopin	0.5–1.0
Clorazepate	Tranxene	15
Diazepam	Valium	10
Estazolam	ProSom	1
Flurazepam	Dalmane	30
Lorazepam	Ativan	2
Oxazepam	Serax	30
Temazepam	Restoril	20
Triazolam	Halcion	0.25
Quazepam	Doral	15
Zolpidem	Ambien	10
Zaleplon	Sonata	10

required to induce mild sedation is then considered the initial dose, and the detoxification proceeds as described previously.

Some concerns have been raised regarding a lack of cross-tolerance between triazolobenzodiazepines and other benzodiazepines. Those concerns are based entirely on anecdotal reports and are not supported by controlled trials or experimental data. Case reports suggest that diazepam does not adequately treat the withdrawal syndrome from alprazolam and that the combination of chlordiazepoxide and diazepam fails to attenuate withdrawal symptoms from triazolam, although questions have been raised concerning the adequacy of the diazepam doses in those cases. Others report that lorazepam can successfully treat triazolam withdrawal and that clonazepam can be substituted for alprazolam in patients with panic disorder. If the primary drug that the patient is taking is not going to be used in the withdrawal protocol, clonazepam or lorazepam may be the best drug to use when detoxifying patients who have been taking supratherapeutic dosages of triazolobenzodiazepines. It is not clear whether higher doses of diazepam would have alleviated the alprazolam withdrawal syndrome in the published case reports. Some authorities recommend the use of phenobarbital in such cases.

DETOXIFICATION FROM MULTIPLE DRUGS OF ABUSE Polysubstance abuse may present special problems for safe withdrawal. The most common polysubstance abuse pattern influencing medical management of detoxification from benzodiazepines is the concurrent use of alcohol, opioids, and cocaine. Combination with alcohol alters the time course and increases the severity of the sedative withdrawal syndrome. Adequate dosages of a benzodiazepine usually suffice for safe withdrawal; however, in rare instances, even large dosages of diazepam can be ineffective, and switching to a barbiturate becomes necessary.

When supratherapeutic doses of benzodiazepines are abused with large amounts of opioids, it is best to discontinue the former drug first and then stabilize the patient on methadone or some oral opioid. When the period of risk for major symptoms of sedative-hypnotic withdrawal passes, opioid withdrawal may begin. Addiction to low or moderate dosages of benzodiazepines or opioids often permits simultaneous withdrawal from both classes of drugs.

Benzodiazepines are often used to terminate a cocaine or other psychostimulant run or to decrease anxiety induced by cocaine. Benzodiazepines used intermittently in that manner usually do not require detoxification. The chronic use of high doses of benzodiazepines with cocaine is less common but does require medically supervised benzodiazepine tapering. The cocaine abstinence syndrome is characterized by depression, irritability, lethargy, lack of motivation, hypersomnolence, confusion, and drug craving. The clinical presentation of the sedative-hypnotic withdrawal syndrome may be altered by recent cocaine use and is best monitored by carefully measuring vital signs (e.g., increases in pulse, temperature, and blood pressure).

Some clinicians prefer to use phenobarbital for detoxification of patients with mixed-drug abuse. A dose of phenobarbital equivalent to the benzodiazepine and other sedatives the patient is taking is calculated (Tables 11.12–7 and 11.12–9) or, preferably, the dose is determined from a challenge test, and the patient is stabilized on that amount in divided daily doses for the period of peak risk of withdrawal. The maximum daily dose of phenobarbital is 600 mg. After stabilization, phenobarbital dose is reduced by 30 to 60 mg every 2 or 3 days.

ADJUNCTIVE MEDICATIONS Several adjunctive medications are used to treat the benzodiazepine withdrawal syndrome, but in no case has their efficacy been consistently supported in controlled trials nor is there evidence that any specific adjunctive medication is superior to another.

Carbamazepine, given in doses that achieve the therapeutic concentrations for treatment of seizures, may partially attenuate the withdrawal syndrome from benzodiazepines. Initial dosages are 200 mg twice a day, although some clinicians recommend a single dose of 400 mg at bedtime to take advantage of the sedative effect. If initial doses are well tolerated, carbamazepine is increased to 600 mg on the second or third day. Typical total daily doses range from 400 to 800 mg. After several days of treatment, benzodiazepine dosage is tapered. Despite reports that tapering can be completed within a week, even from supratherapeutic dosages, some patients require a slow taper that lasts several weeks. Carbamazepine can be tapered quickly 2 to 4 weeks after the last benzodiazepine dose. Carbamazepine may not be successful in withdrawing patients with panic disorder, because it is ineffective in blocking panic attacks, but it has shown some success even in these patients, as long as a slow benzodiazepine taper is used. The efficacy of other anticonvulsants is undetermined, but clinical experience suggests that valproate may reduce withdrawal symptoms as well. Enteric-coated tablets of divalproex (Depakene) are used in starting dosages of 500 to 1,000 mg divided in two or three daily doses. Dosages are increased to achieve serum concentrations of 50 to 120 μg/mL. Some clinicians prefer to use daily loading doses of 20 mg/kg. For patients who abuse alcohol and benzodiazepines, valproate should be avoided when liver enzyme activities are three times their normal values. Gabapentin (Neurontin) may also reduce benzodiazepine withdrawal symptoms, but experience is limited.

The α-adrenergic receptor antagonists may also attenuate withdrawal symptoms. Propranolol (Inderal) in doses of 60 to 120 mg may reduce the symptoms of benzodiazepine withdrawal, although tachycardia and elevated blood pressure are the primary symptoms affected, whereas the subjective sense of discomfort and dysphoria persists. The α-adrenergic receptor antagonists do not have prophylactic effects against seizures and should not be used in monotherapy for withdrawal. Nevertheless, in some cases, propranolol or atenolol (Tenormin), 50 to 100 mg, may be helpful adjuncts to withdrawal treatment.

Clonidine (Catapres), 0.1 mg twice a day to 0.2 mg three times a day or as a patch, has been used in the treatment of low-dose benzodiazepine withdrawal with variable results. Clonidine does not provide protection against withdrawal seizures. It may be effective only when used before withdrawal symptoms develop.

Although antidepressants have not been rigorously studied in the treatment of benzodiazepine withdrawal, many experienced clinicians prescribe them. Agents with well-established antipanic and sedative effects may be useful adjunctive medications for patients whose anxiety recurs during taper or after drug discontinuation. Imipramine (Tofranil), amitriptyline (Elavil), doxepin (Adapin, Sinequan), nefazodone (Serzone), trazodone (Desyrel), SSRIs, and monoamine oxidase inhibitors (MAOIs) may all be useful in that role. Melatonin is a useful treatment for insomnia during withdrawal.

PSYCHOLOGICAL TREATMENTS Specific psychological treatments for withdrawal have not been widely studied. Cognitive behavioral strategies for anxiety management have been applied to patients withdrawing from benzodiazepines with mixed results. Patients who meet the criteria for generalized anxiety disorder are poor candidates for relaxation training.

Many practitioners believe that successful withdrawal requires transmitting to the patient a sense of control over the withdrawal symptoms. In support of this belief, placebo substitution is associated with fewer withdrawal symptoms after drug discontinuation than is withdrawal without placebo. Apparently, the belief that one is taking an effective medication is enough to reduce symptoms.

One way to foster a sense of control over withdrawal symptoms is to link the symptoms of anxiety to environmental intrapsychic stressors. Cognitive restructuring teaches patients about the withdrawal syndrome and helps them identify and relabel withdrawal symptoms as anxiety, thus permitting the implementation of adaptive coping strategies, which include systematic desensitization, in vivo graded exposure, and group problem solving. Using a diary to record mood states and their precipitants sometimes helps cognitive restructuring. A diary may also alert the clinician to maladaptive responses to benzodiazepine withdrawal, such as increased alcohol consumption.

The concept of *cognitive coping* should be introduced to patients, and examples of self-statements (talking to oneself) that are applicable to withdrawal and anxiety management should be discussed and provided as flash cards. They include such statements as "I feel nervous now, but it won't last," "I feel bad, but it's not worse than when I had the flu," or "I feel uncomfortable, but nothing bad is going to happen to me." Self-statements should be short, simple, and relevant to the patient.

Patients are encouraged to be active participants in developing their withdrawal schedule. Clinicians should be flexible about the rate of taper and should encourage the patient to join in the withdrawal process, especially those who are withdrawing from therapeutic doses. It is often useful to request that patients choose which doses should be decreased or eliminated according to their perceived need. For some patients, setting a maximum permissible daily dose may be necessary.

LONG-TERM OUTCOME Few adequately designed follow-up studies have been carried out on patients who terminated benzodiazepine treatment. Many studies suffer from sample selection bias, diagnostic heterogeneity of the sample, and failure to assess environmental factors or to control for concurrent psychotherapy or psychoactive medication; however, despite those shortcomings, several interacting findings have emerged.

In one study of patients who had discontinued benzodiazepines from 10 months to 3.5 years earlier, 70 percent were no longer taking benzodiazepines and had few or no symptoms, 22 percent were not taking benzodiazepines but required other psychotropic medications, and 8 percent had returned to benzodiazepine use. Another study assessed patients who were evaluated for a discontinuation program 3 to 6 years earlier and found that 45 percent were not using benzodiazepines, although some were using other psychoactive medication. Of those who successfully completed the tapering program, 73 percent were benzodiazepine free at follow-up, compared to 39 percent of patients who entered but did not complete the program, and 14 percent of patients who did not participate in the program. Another study of patients treated for benzodiazepine dependence found that 56 percent of benzodiazepine-free (no use during the preceding month) patients had moderate to severe anxiety, and 38 percent had moderate to severe depression at 1- to 5-year follow-up. A different study found that, even though 66 percent of patients were not taking benzodiazepines at follow-up, 75 percent had taken them at some time during the 5 years after entering a discontinuation program.

The follow-up studies suggest that most patients can successfully discontinue taking benzodiazepines. They also indicate that some patients experience recurrent anxiety that requires alternative psychoactive medication or reinstitution of benzodiazepine therapy. However, a subgroup of patients who discontinue benzodiazepines actually shows improvement in anxiety over pretapering levels, which suggests that those who continue to have significant symptoms of anxiety or depression while taking a benzodiazepine should probably undergo a drug-free trial period. The value of a structured program for discontinuation and the substitution of medications with low abuse liability are supported in several studies. There appears to be no relation between long-term outcome (i.e., not using benzodiazepines at follow-up) and the duration of treatment or the specific benzodiazepine that was discontinued. Some evidence suggests that low doses of benzodiazepines predict successful discontinuation, although other studies have found weak or no correlation between dose and return to benzodiazepine use.

Barbiturates There are three common methods of establishing the barbiturate dosage required for safe withdrawal: (1) administration of a test dose of pentobarbital to determine tolerance, (2) calculation of required doses based on estimated equivalencies, and (3) administration of phenobarbital loading doses.

In the first method, the initial step is to determine tolerance. Once intoxication has subsided but before withdrawal symptoms have developed, an oral dose of 200 mg of pentobarbital is administered on an empty stomach, and the effects are observed after 1 hour to determine the stabilization dose (Table 11.12–10). If no changes are observed, the test is repeated 3 hours later using 300 mg. If there is still no response, the total requirement may exceed 1,600 mg per day. The calculated daily dose is divided and given every 4 to 6 hours for a 2- to 3-day stabilization period. Daily dose reductions are usually 10 percent of the stabilization dose, but withdrawal regimens must be individualized. Phenobarbital may be substituted for pentobarbital for stabilization and withdrawal at one-third of the dose.

The second method of barbiturate detoxification requires calculating the equivalent hypnotic dose of phenobarbital on the basis of the dosage of barbiturate or other sedatives the patient reports taking, also taking into consideration any alcohol consumed. A dose of 30 mg of phenobarbital is substituted for an equivalent hypnotic dose of the sedative. The patient is stabilized for the period of peak vulnerability to withdrawal, 2 to 3 days for sedative-hypnotic agents with short half-lives, and reductions of 30 to 60 mg of phenobarbital are made every 2 or 3 days. Clinicians using this method report that only rarely are doses of phenobarbital greater than 600 mg required. The procedure is not recommended, however, because published equivalencies are only approximations, and patients vary greatly in their metabolism and pharmacodynamic response to the same dose

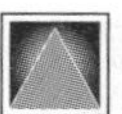

Table 11.12–10
Pentobarbital (Nembutal) Test Dose Procedure for Barbiturate Withdrawal

Symptoms after Test Dose of 200 mg of Oral Pentobarbital	Estimated 24-Hr Oral Pentobarbital Dose (mg)	Estimated 24-Hr Oral Phenobarbital Dose (mg)
Level I: Asleep, but arousal is possible; withdrawal symptoms not likely	0	0
Level II: Mild sedation; patient may have slurred speech, ataxia, and nystagmus	500–600	150–200
Level III: Patient is comfortable; no evidence of sedation; may have nystagmus	800	250
Level IV: No drug effect	1,000–1,200	300–600

Adapted from Ciraulo DA, Shader RI, eds. *Clinical Manual of Chemical Dependence.* Washington, DC: American Psychiatric Press; 1991. Data from Ewing JA, Bakewell WE: Diagnosis and management of depressant drug dependence. *Am J Psychiatry.* 1967;123:909.

of the sedative. Furthermore, animal studies indicate that cross-tolerance among the various anxiolytic and sedative-hypnotic agents is not complete. Furthermore, the method relies on the patient's history of drug use, which is often unreliable. Plasma concentrations can establish which sedatives have been ingested and may indicate the degree of tolerance when clinical correlations are made. Estimation of tolerance (and thus determination of dosage requirements) is best made after a test dose or a loading dose is administered. Tables 11.12–7 and 11.12–9 list approximate equivalencies of selected barbiturates, benzodiazepines, and sedatives.

The final method for medical withdrawal from barbiturates involves using loading doses of phenobarbital. According to the original protocol, 120-mg doses are administered every 1 to 2 hours until three of five signs are present—nystagmus, drowsiness, ataxia, dysarthria, or emotional lability—or, if patients are in withdrawal, until abstinence symptoms abate. No additional drug is administered, and, because of its long half-life, the drug self-tapers. Patients are assessed before each dose. Some clinicians have modified the protocol to use doses of 60 mg every 1 to 2 hours and to use a gradual taper rather than abrupt discontinuation. The originators of the protocol reported a mean loading dose of 1,440 mg, with hourly doses sometimes required for 15 to 20 hours. They have also administered phenobarbital IV at 0.3 mg/kg per minute, with close medical supervision, for medically ill patients.

Overdose The treatment of overdose of the general class of substances involves gastric lavage, activated charcoal, and careful monitoring of vital signs and CNS activity. Overdose patients who come to attention while awake should be kept from slipping into unconsciousness. Activated charcoal should be administered to delay gastric absorption. If the patient is comatose, the clinician must establish an IV fluid line, monitor the patient's vital signs, insert an endotracheal tube to maintain a patent airway, and provide mechanical ventilation, if necessary. Hospitalization of a comatose patient in an intensive care unit is usually required during the early stages of recovery from such overdoses.

SUGGESTED CROSS-REFERENCES

Substance-related disorders are discussed throughout Chapter 11, with an introduction, overview, and relevant general tables in Section 11.1. Biological therapies are the focus of Chapter 31; benzodiazepines are covered in Section 31.11, MAOIs are covered in Section 31.19, and serotonin-specific reuptake inhibitors are covered in Section 31.24.

REFERENCES

Allison C, Pratt JA: Neuroadaptive processes in GABAergic and glutamatergic systems in benzodiazepine dependence. *Psychopharmacol Ther.* 2003;98:171.

Barnes EM: Use-dependent regulation of $GABA_A$ receptors. *Int Rev Neurobiol.* 1996;39:53.

Bruce SE, Vasile RG, Goisman RM, Salzman C, Spencer M, Machan JT, Keller MB: Are benzodiazepines still the medication of choice for patients with panic disorder with or without agoraphobia? *Am J Psychiatry.* 2003;160:1432.

Busto UE, Romach MK, Sellers EM: Multiple drug use and psychiatric comorbidity in patients admitted to the hospital with severe benzodiazepine dependence. *J Clin Psychopharmacol.* 1996;16:51.

Ciraulo DA, Barnhill JG, Ciraulo AM, Sarid-Segal O, Knapp C, Greenblatt DJ, Shader RI: Alterations in pharmacodynamics of anxiolytic in abstinent alcoholic men: Subjective responses, abuse liability, and encephalographic effects of alprazolam, diazepam, and buspirone. *J Clin Psychopharmacol.* 1997;37:64.

Ciraulo DA, Nace EP: Benzodiazepine treatment of anxiety or insomnia in substance abuse patients. *Am J Addict.* 2000;9:276–284.

Ciraulo DA, Sands BF, Shader RI: Critical review of liability for benzodiazepine abuse among alcoholics. *Am J Psychiatry.* 1988;145:1501.

*Ciraulo DA, Sarid-Segal O, Knapp C, Ciraulo AM, Greenblatt DJ, Shader RI: Liability to alprazolam abuse in daughters of alcoholics. *Am J Psychiatry.* 1996;153:956.

Costa E, Guidotti A: Benzodiazepines on trial: A research strategy for their rehabilitation. *Trends Pharmacol Sci.* 1996;17:192.

Darke S: Benzodiazepine use among injecting drug users: Problems and implications. *Addiction.* 1994;89:379.

de las Cuevas C, Sanz E, de la Fuente J: Benzodiazepines: More "behavioural" addiction than dependence. *Psychopharmacology.* 2003;167:297.

De Wit H, Griffiths RR: Testing the abuse liability of anxiolytic and hypnotic drugs in humans. *Drug Alcohol Depend.* 1991;28:83.

Druid H, Holmgren P, Ahlner J: Flunitrazepam and evaluation of use, abuse, and toxicity. *Forensic Sci Int.* 2001;122:136–141.

*Dunne DL: Long term use of sedative and hypnotic medication. *Arch Gen Psychiatry.* 1999;56:355.

DuPont RL: Abuse of benzodiazepines: The problems and the solutions. *Am J Drug Alcohol Abuse.* 1988;14[Suppl]:1.

Elsesser K, Sartory G, Maurer J: The efficacy of complaints management training in facilitating benzodiazepine withdrawal. *Behav Res Ther.* 1996;34:149.

Evans SM, Critchfield TS, Griffiths RR: Abuse liability assessment of anxiolytics/hypnotics: Rationale and laboratory lore. *Br J Addict.* 1991;86:1625.

Evans SM, Funderburk FR, Griffiths RR: Zolpidem and triazolam in humans: Behavioral and subjective effects and abuse liability. *J Pharmacol Exp Ther.* 1990;255:1246.

Evans SM, Griffiths RR, de Wit H: Preference for diazepam, but not buspirone, in moderate drinkers. *Psychopharmacology.* 1996;123:154.

Farre M, Teran MT, Cami J: A comparison of the acute behavioral effects of flunitrazepam and triazolam in healthy volunteers. *Psychopharmacology.* 1996;125:1.

Gilson SF, Chilcoat HD, Stapleton JM: Illicit drug use by persons with disabilities: Insights from the National Household Survey on Drug Abuse. *Am J Public Health.* 1996;86:1613.

Greenblatt DJ, Harmatz JS, Zinny MA, Shader RI: Effect of gradual withdrawal on the rebound sleep disorder after discontinuation of triazolam. *N Engl J Med.* 1987;317:722.

Griffiths RR, Bigelow G, Liebson I: Human drug self-administration. Double-blind comparison of pentobarbital, diazepam, chlorpromazine, and placebo. *J Pharmacol Exp Ther.* 1979;210:301.

Griffiths AN, Jones DM, Richens A: Zopiclone produces effects on human performance similar to flurazepam, lormetazepam and triazolam. *Br J Clin Pharmacol.* 1986;21:647.

Griffiths RR, Lamb RJ, Ator NA, Roache JD, Brady JV: Relative abuse liability of triazolam: Experimental assessment in animals and humans. *Neurosci Biobehav Rev.* 1985;9:133.

Griffiths RR, Lamb RJ, Sannerud CA, Ator NA, Brady JV: Self-injection of barbiturates, benzodiazepines and other sedative-anxiolytics in baboons. *Psychopharmacology.* 1991;103:154.

Hayward P, Wardle J, Higgitt A, Gray J: Changes in "withdrawal symptoms" following discontinuation of low-dose diazepam. *Psychopharmacology.* 1996;125:392.

Hobbs WR, Rall TW, Verdoorn TA. Hypnotics and sedatives: Ethanol. In: Gilman AG, Rall TW, eds. *Goodman and Gilman's The Pharmacological Basis of Therapeutics.* 9th ed. New York: Pergamon; 1996.

Hutchinson MA, Smith PF, Darlington CL: The behavioral and neuronal aspects of the chronic administration of benzodiazepine anxiolytic and hypnotic drugs. *Prog Neurobiol.* 1996;49:73.

Ito T, Suzuki T, Wellman SE, Ho IK: Pharmacology of barbiturate tolerance/dependence: $GABA_A$ receptors and molecular aspects. *Life Sci.* 1996;59:169.
Kales A, Manfredi RL, Vgontzas AM, Bixler EO, Vela BA, Fee EC: Rebound insomnia after only brief and intermittent use of rapidly eliminated benzodiazepines. *Clin Pharmacol Ther.* 1991;49:468.
Lejoyeux M, Solomon J, Ades J: Benzodiazepine treatment for alcohol-dependent patients. *Alcohol Alcoholism.* 1998;33:6.
Lillsunde P, Korte T, Michelson L, Portman M, Pikkarainen J, Seppala T: Drugs usage of drivers suspected of driving under the influence of alcohol and/or drugs. A study of one week's samples in 1979 and 1993 in Finland. *Forensic Sci Int.* 1996;77:119.
Malcom R, Brady KT, Johnston AL, Cunningham M: Types of benzodiazepines abused by chemically dependent inpatients. *J Psychoactive Drugs.* 1993;25:315.
Mueller TI, Goldenberg IM, Gordon AL, Keller MB, Warshaw MG: Benzodiazepine use in anxiety disorder patients with and without a history of alcoholism. *J Clin Psychiatry.* 1996;57:2.
Mumford GK, Evans SM, Fleishaker JC, Griffiths RR: Alprazolam absorption kinetics affects abuse liability. *Clin Pharmacol Ther.* 1995;57:356.
Nicholson KL, Balster RL: GHB: New and novel drug of abuse. *Drug Alcohol Depend.* 2001;63:1–22.
Nutt DJ, Costello MJ: Rapid induction of lorazepam dependence and reversal with flumazenil. *Life Sci.* 1988;43:1045.
Paterniti S, Dufouil C, Alperovitch A: Long-term benzodiazepine use and cognitive decline in the elderly: The epidemiology of vascular aging study. *J Clin Psychopharmacol.* 2002;22:285–293.
Piercey MF, Hoffmann WE, Cooper M: The hypnotics triazolam and zolpidem have identical metabolic effects through the brain: Implications for benzodiazepine receptor subtypes. *Brain Res.* 1991;554:244.
Podhorna J: The experimental pharmacotherapy of benzodiazepine withdrawal. *Curr Pharm Design.* 2002;8:23–43.
Posternak MA, Mueller TI: Assessing the risks and benefits of benzodiazepines for anxiety disorders in patients with a history of substance abuse or dependence. *Am J Addict.* 2001;10:48–68.
Rickels K, Case WG, Schweizer E, Garcia-Espana F, Fridman R: Benzodiazepine dependence: Management of discontinuation. *Psychopharmacol Bull.* 1990;26:63.
Rickels K, Case W, Schweizer E, Garcia-Espana F, Fridman R: Long-term benzodiazepine users 3 years after participation in a discontinuation program. *Am J Psychiatry.* 1991;148:757.
Rickels K, Case WG, Schweizer EE, Swenson C, Fridman RB: Low-dose dependence in chronic benzodiazepine users: A preliminary report of 119 patients. *Psychopharmacol Bull.* 1986;22:407.
Rickels K, Fox IL, Greenblatt DJ, Sandler KR, Schless A: Clorazepate and lorazepam: Clinical improvement and rebound anxiety. *Am J Psychiatry.* 1988;145:312.
Roache JD, Henningfield JE, Jaffe JH, Klein S, Sampson A: Reinforcing effects of triazolam in sedative abusers: Correlation of drug liking and self administration measures. *Pharmacol Biochem Behav.* 1995;50:171.
Roy-Byrne PP, Dager SR, Cowley DS, Vitaliano P, Dunner DL: Relapse and rebound following discontinuation of benzodiazepine treatment of panic attacks: Alprazolam versus diazepam. *Am J Psychiatry.* 1989;146:860.
Rush CR, Griffiths RR: Zolpidem, triazolam, and temazepam: Behavioral and subject-rated effects in normal volunteers. *J Clin Psychopharmacol.* 1996;16:146.
*Salzman C: Addiction to benzodiazepines. *Psychiatr Q.* 1998;69:251.
Sellers EM, Ciraulo DA, Dupont RL, Griffiths RL, Kosten TR, Romach MK, Woody GE: Alprazolam and benzodiazepine dependence. *J Clin Psychiatry.* 1994;54:64.
*Simmons MM, Cupp MJ: Use and abuse of flunitrazepam. *Ann Pharmacother.* 1998;32:117.
Spiegel DA, Bruce TJ, Gregg SF, Nuzzarello A: Does cognitive behavior therapy assist slow-taper alprazolam discontinuation in panic disorder? *Am J Psychiatry.* 1994;151:876.
Steentoft A, Worm K, Pedersen CB, Sprehn M, Mogensen T, Sorensen MB, Nielsen E: Drugs in blood samples from unconscious drug addicts after the intake of an overdose. *Int J Legal Med.* 1996;108:248.
Tehrani MH, Barnes EM: Sequestration of gamma-aminobutyric acid α receptors on clathrin-coated vesicles during chronic benzodiazepine administration in vivo. *J Pharmacol Exp Ther.* 1997;283:384–390.
Uhlenhuth EH, Balter MB, Ban TA, Yang K: International study of expert judgment on therapeutic use of benzodiazepines and other psychotherapeutic medications: IV. Therapeutic dose dependence and abuse liability of benzodiazepines in the long-term treatment of anxiety disorders. *J Clin Psychopharmacol.* 1999;19[Suppl]:2.
Uhlenhuth EH, De Wit H, Balter MB, Johanson CE, Mellinger GD: Risks and benefits of long-term benzodiazepine use. *J Clin Psychopharmacol.* 1988;8:161.
*Vorma H, Naukkarinen H, Sarna S, Kuoppsalami K: Long-term outcome after benzodiazepine withdrawal treatment in subjects with complicated dependence. *Drug Alcohol Abuse.* 2003;70:309.
Woods JH, Katz JL, Winger G: Benzodiazepines: Use, abuse, and consequences. *Pharmacol Rev.* 1992;44:151.
Woods JH, Wigner G: Current benzodiazepine issues. *Psychopharmacology.* 1995;118:107.
Woods JH, Winger G: Liability of flunitrazepam. *J Clin Psychopharmacol.* 1997;17[Suppl]:1S.
Zawertailo LA, Busto UE, Kaplan HL, Greenblatt DJ, Sellers EM: Comparative abuse liability and pharmacological effects of meprobamate, triazolam, and butabarbital. *J Clin Psychopharmacol.* 2003;23:269.
Zawertailo LA, Busto U, Kaplan HL, Sellers EM: Comparative abuse liability of sertraline, alprazolam, and dextroamphetamine in humans. *J Clin Psychopharmacol.* 1995;15:117.

▲ 11.13 Anabolic-Androgenic Steroid Abuse

HARRISON G. POPE, JR., M.D., AND KIRK J. BROWER, M.D.

The *anabolic steroids* are a family of drugs comprising the natural male hormone testosterone and a group of more than 50 synthetic analogs of testosterone, synthesized over the last 60 years (Table 11.13–1). These drugs all exhibit various degrees of *anabolic* (muscle building) and *androgenic* (masculinizing) effects. Thus, they should more correctly be called *anabolic-androgenic steroids* (AAS). Note that it is important not to confuse the *AAS* (testosterone-like hormones) with *corticosteroids* (cortisol-like hormones such as hydrocortisone and prednisone). Corticosteroids have no muscle-building properties and, hence, little abuse potential; they are widely prescribed to treat numerous inflammatory conditions such as poison ivy or asthma. AAS, by contrast, have only limited legitimate medical applications, such as in the treatment of hypogonadal men, the wasting syndrome associated with human immunodeficiency virus (HIV) infection, and a few specific diseases such as hereditary angioedema and Fanconi's anemia. However, AAS are widely used illicitly, especially by boys and young men seeking to gain increased muscle mass and strength either for athletic purposes or simply to improve personal appearance.

HISTORY

Testosterone was first synthesized in 1935, and, by the 1940s, various synthetic derivatives of testosterone had appeared. Both the ana-

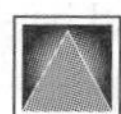

Table 11.13–1
Examples of Commonly Used Anabolic Steroids

Compounds usually administered orally
Fluoxymesterone (Halotestin, Android-F, Ultandren)
Methandienone (formerly called methandrostenolone; Dianabol)
Methyltestosterone (Android, Testred, Virilon)
Mibolerone (Cheque Drops[a])
Oxandrolone (Anavar)
Oxymetholone (Anadrol, Hemogenin)
Mesterolone (Mestoranum, Proviron)
Stanozolol (Winstrol)
Compounds usually administered intramuscularly
Nandrolone decanoate (Deca-Durabolin)
Nandrolone phenpropionate (Durabolin)
Methenolone enanthate (Primobolan Depot)
Boldenone undecylenate (Equipoise[a])
Stanozolol (Winstrol-V[a])
Testosterone esters blends (Sustanon, Sten)
Testosterone cypionate
Testosterone enanthate (Delatestryl)
Testosterone propionate (Testoviron, Androlan)
Testosterone undecanoate (Andriol, Restandol)
Trenbolone acetate (Finajet, Finaplix[a])
Trenbolone hexahydrobencylcarbonate (Parabolan)

Note: Many of the brand names listed above are foreign but are included because of the widespread illicit use of foreign steroid preparations in the United States.
[a]Veterinary compound.

bolic and androgenic actions of these drugs were quickly recognized; they were reportedly first used by Adolf Hitler's troops in World War II to increase aggressiveness, although this claim has never been verified. In the late 1930s and early 1940s, a number of psychiatric investigations suggested that testosterone possessed antidepressant properties. The hormone was believed to be especially effective for the "male climacteric" and was frequently prescribed in Europe and in the United States for depressed middle-aged men. With the advent of electroconvulsive therapy (ECT) and standard antidepressant medications, however, the use of AAS for psychiatric purposes rapidly waned. The last several years, however, have seen renewed interest in the therapeutic effects of AAS: Controlled investigations have suggested that testosterone supplementation produces antidepressant effects in men with HIV infection and in men refractory to conventional antidepressants.

By the 1950s, athletes had recognized the value of AAS. The first reported use of these drugs in athletics was apparently by the Russians in 1954, followed within a few years by elite athletes from many other countries. Over the next three decades, the use of AAS rapidly expanded among athletes at all levels, especially in sports requiring muscle mass and strength such as bodybuilding, powerlifting, football, and field events such as the shot put. During the 1960s and 1970s, many placebo-controlled studies tested whether AAS were truly effective for gaining muscle mass. The results of these studies were frequently equivocal, usually because the studies used dosages and durations of AAS administration far below those used by actual athletes in the field. On the basis of these studies, many reputable textbooks and reviews in pharmacology and endocrinology concluded that steroids were ineffective for athletic purposes. Athletes who had actually used these drugs and who were aware of the enormous muscle gains that they could produce tended to hold the medical profession in great contempt for its ignorance; consequently, these athletes often discounted medical warnings about the possible physical and psychiatric dangers of these agents.

By the late 1980s and early 1990s, medical professionals increasingly acknowledged that AAS were indeed highly effective for achieving muscle gains and that use of these agents had approached epidemic proportions in the United States. Preliminary reports also began to document adverse psychiatric and medical consequences associated with using high-dose AAS for nonmedical purposes. These trends led to increasing concern about the public health consequences of using AAS, and, in 1991, the U.S. Congress passed the Steroid Trafficking Act, adding AAS to the list of Schedule III controlled substances and placing jurisdiction over these substances in the hands of the Drug Enforcement Administration (DEA). Based on widespread anecdotal experience with users of AAS, it seems as if this legislative change has had a marked effect in that it has led to a diminished supply of genuine steroids on the black market and a greatly increased number of counterfeit steroids with no pharmacological effects. However, unlike many of the other drugs of abuse, AAS may be purchased legally without a prescription in many countries and can be sent illicitly by mail to the United States (e.g., to post office boxes). This pattern makes interdiction difficult and ensures that a substantial supply of genuine steroids will be available to illicit users in the United States for the foreseeable future.

Although the general public is quite familiar with many forms of illicit substance abuse, most laypersons and, arguably, even most physicians are surprisingly unfamiliar with the effects of AAS or the extent of their use. In particular, most people are unaware that, without massive doses of AAS, it is virtually impossible to achieve the combination of low body fat and high muscularity exhibited by many competition bodybuilders and professional athletes. Because athletes and their promoters have large personal and financial motivations to deny such drug use, the public has been hoodwinked for decades about the magnitude of the AAS problem. However, recent years have seen mounting scandals and revelations about AAS use by elite athletes in the Olympics and other competitions as well as by prominent members of professional sports teams. Public awareness has also increased in response to reports of premature deaths in athletes known or suspected to have taken AAS.

COMPARATIVE NOSOLOGY

Psychiatric syndromes associated with use of AAS are cited in the fourth revised edition of *Diagnostic and Statistical Manual of Mental Disorders* (DSM-IV-TR) under the general category of other substance-related disorders. The tenth revision of *International Statistical Classification of Diseases and Related Health Problems* (ICD-10) classifies steroid-related disorders under abuse of non–dependence-producing substances along with agents such as antacids and laxatives. A rapidly growing body of literature, however, now supports a syndrome of AAS dependence and withdrawal together with several AAS-induced psychiatric disorders. The best established among the latter are a syndrome of hypomanic or manic symptoms associated with steroid use and a depressive syndrome associated with steroid withdrawal. This chapter parallels the standard terminology of DSM-IV-TR for other drugs of abuse, discussing anabolic steroid dependence and abuse, anabolic steroid–induced mood disorder, anabolic steroid–induced psychotic disorder, and anabolic steroid–induced disorder not otherwise specified.

EPIDEMIOLOGY

Use of AAS is widespread among men in the United States but is much less frequent in women. Among the most reliable data regarding the prevalence of steroid use are those from the National Household Survey on Drug Abuse (NHSDA). This survey, which has been conducted regularly since 1971, included questions about AAS in 1991 and 1994. Findings from this survey in 1994 indicated that approximately 890,000 American men and approximately 190,000 American women reported having used AAS at some time during their lives. Approximately 286,000 men and 26,000 women were estimated to have used steroids within the past year. Among the number of individuals estimated to have used these drugs during the past year, nearly one-third, or 98,000, were between 12 and 17 years of age. Various studies of high school students in the United States have produced even higher estimates of the prevalence of anabolic steroid use among adolescents. For example, one study of 3,403 12th-grade boys in 46 public and private hospitals in the United States found that 6.6 percent reported current or past use of AAS, with two-thirds of the users reporting that they had first tried these drugs when they were 16 years of age or younger. Across studies of high school students, it is estimated that 3 to 12 percent of males and 0.5 to 2.0 percent of females have used AAS during their lifetimes. One possible criticism of these results, however, is that some students may have misunderstood the survey questions and claimed that they had used AAS when, in fact, they had used only corticosteroids prescribed to them for conditions such as asthma or dermatological problems. Even allowing for this possible source of error, however, it is evident that rates of anabolic steroid use among American adolescents are high.

The current high rates of steroid use among younger individuals appear to represent an important shift in the epidemiology of steroid use. As recently as the mid-1970s, use of these drugs was largely confined to competition bodybuilders, other elite weight-training athletes, and elite athletes in other sports. Currently, however, it appears that an increasing number of young men, and occasionally even young women, may be using these drugs purely to enhance personal appearance rather than for any athletic purpose.

Individuals with one form of substance abuse are often found to abuse other substances as well, especially alcohol, and some studies document polysubstance use among those who take illicit AAS. However, other anabolic steroid users report that they carefully abstain from using drugs such as alcohol and cocaine because they are concerned with maximizing their muscularity or athletic ability. Anabolic steroid users, especially those involved in competition bodybuilding, may use a wide variety of other *ergogenic* (performance-enhancing) drugs to gain muscle, lose fat, or lose water for bodybuilding competitions. Other drugs commonly used by competitive bodybuilders are thyroid hormones, such as liothyronine (Cytomel) and levothyroxine (Synthroid); human growth hormone and its daughter compound, somatomedin-C (insulin-like growth factor-1 [IGF-1]); insulin; dehydroepiandrosterone (DHEA); androstenedione; sympathomimetic agents, such as amphetamines, ephedrine, and pseudoephedrine (Sudafed); β-adrenergic receptor agonists, such as clenbuterol; the amino acid derivative γ-hydroxybutyrate (GHB); various laxatives and diuretics; the opioid agonist-antagonist nalbuphine (Nubain); and others. Drug combinations in humans are poorly studied, although animal studies reveal that AAS may sensitize the brain to the rewarding properties of amphetamine, enhance voluntary alcohol intake, and increase cocaine-related seizures. In humans, drug combinations may also lead to adverse interactions. One postmortem study, for example, found that 11 of 34 deaths among users of AAS were related to polysubstance use.

PHARMACOLOGY

Chemistry All steroid drugs—including AAS, estrogens, and corticosteroids—are synthesized in vivo from cholesterol and resemble cholesterol in their chemical structure. Testosterone has a four-ring chemical structure containing 19 carbon atoms (Fig. 11.13–1). Most synthetic derivatives of testosterone are produced by one or more of the following modifications: (1) forming an ester at the C-17-β-hydroxyl group, (2) adding an alkyl group to the C-17-α position, or (3) altering the structure at a different carbon site.

Aqueous testosterone suspension is essentially inactive when ingested by the oral route because of first-pass metabolism in the liver and is only briefly active when injected because it is rapidly absorbed and metabolized. Synthetic AAS overcome these problems. Testosterone esters (such as testosterone cypionate [Depo-Testosterone] and testosterone enanthate [Delatestryl]) confer the advantage of slower absorption than testosterone when injected, and their effects last from 2 to 4 weeks. Testosterone esters are hydrolyzed to testosterone after they are absorbed, so these agents can be monitored by blood concentrations. Testosterone is metabolized in part to dihydrotestosterone, which is up to ten times more potent than testosterone as an androgen, and in part to the estrogen estradiol, which accounts for some of the adverse effects seen in men, such as gynecomastia. Testosterone is also metabolized to so-called neurosteroids in the brain. The effects of testosterone depend both on the balance of metabolic enzymes and on the concentration of androgen receptors in a particular tissue. The C-17-alkylated synthetic AAS make oral administration possible, but once-daily use is generally required.

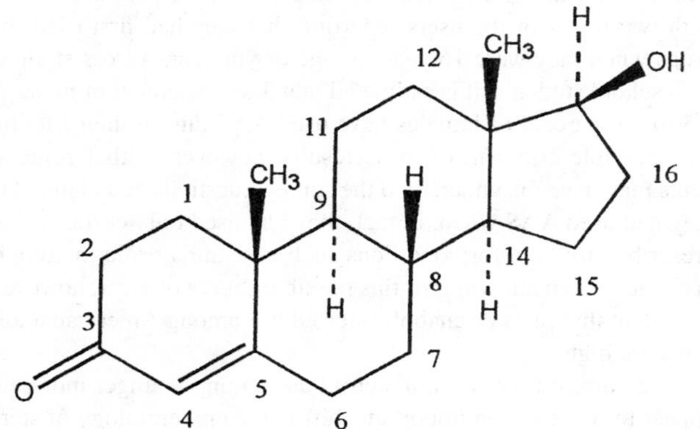

FIGURE 11.13–1 Molecular structure of testosterone.

Pharmacodynamics AAS bind androgen receptors in the cytoplasm of cells. The androgen-receptor complex is then translocated to the cell nucleus, where it augments gene transcription and, ultimately, new protein synthesis. The anabolic steroid effects desired by illicit users result especially from new protein synthesis in muscle tissue. The mechanism of action for psychoactive effects is poorly understood, but a recent experimental study reported significantly higher levels of 5-hydroxyindoleacetic acid (5-HIAA) in the cerebrospinal fluid (CSF) of methyltestosterone- versus placebo-treated men. Moreover, 5-HIAA levels correlated significantly with certain AAS-associated effects, including increased energy, diminished sleep, and sexual arousal. Animal studies suggest that AAS-induced increases in vasopressin and substance P may be associated with aggressive behavior. In addition, testosterone can be enzymatically converted in the brain to neurosteroids that have psychoactive effects. Finally, AAS may have reinforcing effects through their actions on opioid and dopamine systems, as is discussed below.

Normal testosterone plasma concentrations for men range from 300 to 1,000 ng/dL. Generally, 200 mg of testosterone cypionate taken every 2 weeks restores physiological testosterone concentrations in a hypogonadal male. A eugonadal male who initiates physiological dosages of testosterone has no net gain in testosterone concentrations because exogenously administered AAS shut down endogenous testosterone production via feedback inhibition of the hypothalamic-pituitary-gonadal axis. Consequently, illicit users take higher-than-therapeutic dosages to achieve supraphysiological effects. The dose–response curve for anabolic effects may be logarithmic, which could explain why illicit users generally take 10 to 100 times the therapeutic dosages. Doses in this range are most easily achieved by taking combinations of oral and injected AAS, which illicit AAS users often do. Transdermal testosterone, available by prescription for testosterone replacement therapy, may also be used.

Effects on Specific Organs and Systems The first effects of endogenous androgens are to induce male sexual differentiation in the fetus. Accumulating evidence suggests that fetal and perinatal androgens cause sexual dimorphism of the brain (at least in nonhuman mammals) as well as differentiation of the sexual organs. During puberty, testosterone levels increase in boys to produce male secondary sex characteristics. The phallus, prostate, and seminal vesicles all grow and develop, and testosterone and gonadotropins are involved in sperm production. Androgens cause the larynx to enlarge, the vocal cords to lengthen and thicken, and the voice to deepen. A male pattern of body hair develops, including hair on the face and chest. Sebaceous glands grow and increase their secretions, predisposing the adolescent to acne. Bones and muscles also grow during puberty as a result of androgen stimulation. Exogenous administration of AAS to a prepubertal male also induces all these effects.

In adults, physiological levels of testosterone continue to be important for spermatogenesis, although abnormally high levels suppress spermatogenesis by inhibiting release of luteinizing hormone (LH), which is also required for spermatogenesis. Exogenous AAS increase muscle growth, promote mineralization of bones, and stimulate erythropoiesis by increasing erythropoietin levels and by direct action on the bone marrow.

Therapeutic Indications AAS are primarily indicated for testosterone deficiency (male hypogonadism), hereditary angioedema (a congenital skin disorder), and some uncommon forms of anemia caused by bone marrow or renal failure. In women, they are given, although not as first-choice agents, for metastatic breast cancer, osteoporosis, endometriosis, and adjunctive treatment of menopausal symptoms. In men, they have been used experimentally as a male contraceptive and for treating major depressive disorder and sexual disorders in eugonadal men. Recently, they have been used to treat wasting syndromes associated with acquired immune deficiency syndrome (AIDS). As mentioned earlier, controlled studies have also suggested that testosterone has antidepressant effects in some HIV-infected men with major depressive disorder, and is also a supplementary (augmentation) treatment in some depressed men with low endogenous testosterone levels who are refractory to conventional antidepressants.

Adverse Reactions The most common adverse medical effects of AAS involve the cardiovascular, hepatic, reproductive, and dermatological systems. In general, the more common adverse effects tend to be cosmetic and are reversible on cessation of AAS. Serious, life-threatening effects occur rarely, but the long-term consequences of nonmedical AAS use have been little studied. It is established that the orally active C-17-alkylated AAS are generally more toxic to the liver and more likely to adversely affect cholesterol levels than the injectable testosterone esters. A recent report revealed a shortened life span in mice exposed to high-dose AAS, but the generalizability to humans is unknown. Nevertheless, a recent 12-year follow-up of 62 powerlifters in Finland, suspected to have used AAS, found that eight (13 percent) had died, a rate 4.6 times higher than in a matched population sample of 1,094 men. The causes of death were suicide (three cases), acute myocardial infarction (three), hepatic coma (one), and non-Hodgkin's lymphoma (one).

AAS produce an adverse cholesterol profile by increasing levels of low-density lipoprotein cholesterol and decreasing levels of high-density lipoprotein cholesterol. High-dose use of AAS may also activate hemostasis. AAS are widely reported to increase blood pressure, although most controlled studies do not confirm this. Nevertheless, the adverse effects on cholesterol and hemostasis have led to concerns of increased coronary artery disease and atherosclerosis among users of AAS. Isolated case reports of myocardial infarction, cardiomyopathy, left ventricular hypertrophy, and stroke among users of AAS, including fatalities, have appeared, but there are no epidemiological studies that assess the risk to the cardiovascular and cerebrovascular systems from using high-dose, illicit AAS. Fortunately, changes in cholesterol levels are reversible when AAS are discontinued.

Liver effects include cholestatic jaundice, benign and malignant liver tumors, and peliosis hepatis (blood-filled cysts that may rupture and cause death), although all these effects are rare. At least one fatality from prostatic cancer has been reported in association with AAS. The case was a 40-year-old bodybuilder, and the early onset of his cancer strongly implicated his use of AAS in its etiology. AAS use may also induce benign prostatic hypertrophy.

AAS-induced endocrine effects in men include testicular atrophy and sterility, both usually reversible after discontinuing AAS, and gynecomastia, which may persist until surgical removal. In women, shrinkage of breast tissue, irregular menses (diminution or cessation), and masculinization (clitoral hypertrophy, hirsutism, and deepened voice) can occur. Masculinizing effects in women may be irreversible, although this issue has not been well studied. Androgens taken during pregnancy could cause masculinization of a female fetus. Dermatological effects include acne and male pattern baldness. Abuse of AAS by children has led to concerns that AAS-induced premature closure of bony epiphyses could cause shortened stature. Other uncommon adverse effects include edema of the extremities due to water retention, exacerbation of tic disorders, sleep apnea, and polycythemia.

Laboratory Findings The use of AAS can be associated with elevations in liver function tests such as bilirubin, lactate dehydrogenase (LDH), alkaline phosphatase, aspartate aminotransferase (AST, or SGOT), and alanine aminotransferase (ALT). However, elevations in LDH, ALT, and AST, as well as the muscle enzyme creatine phosphokinase (CPK), are common in weight-training athletes, even in the absence of AAS use, as a result of muscle trauma from intensive weightlifting. The enzyme γ-glutamyl transaminase (GGT), which is present exclusively in liver and not in muscle, may be more useful to distinguish frank liver toxicity from mere muscle trauma in users of AAS.

An altered cholesterol profile (decreased levels of high-density lipoprotein cholesterol and increased levels of low-density lipoprotein cholesterol) is seen especially with oral administration of the C-17-alkylated AAS. Total cholesterol and triglyceride concentrations may also be elevated. Increases in the hematocrit and hemoglobin levels may occur relative to a patient's baseline values, although the hematocrit is rarely abnormally elevated unless AAS are combined with erythropoietin, as some endurance athletes have done.

Endocrine Tests AAS inhibit the release of LH and follicle-stimulating hormone (FSH), resulting in lower serum levels. Serum testosterone and estradiol levels vary with the particular agent and timing of the sample. For example, the use of supraphysiological doses of testosterone esters increases both testosterone and estradiol levels, whereas the exclusive use of most other AAS decreases these hormonal levels. Similarly, testosterone and estradiol levels are decreased during AAS withdrawal because of the lingering inhibition of the hypothalamic-pituitary-gonadal axis.

Other Tests Semen analysis may reveal decreased sperm count and motility as well as abnormal sperm morphology. Left ventricular hypertrophy can be found on the electrocardiogram (ECG), although nonusers can have left ventricular hypertrophy on the basis on intensive strength training alone. An echocardiogram can rule out impaired diastolic function, which has been reported in some AAS users with left ventricular hypertrophy.

ETIOLOGY

The major reason for taking illicit AAS is to enhance either athletic performance or physical appearance. Taking AAS is reinforced because they can produce the athletic and physical effects that users desire, especially when combined with proper diet and training. Further reinforcement derives from winning competitions and from social admiration for physical appearance. AAS users also perceive that they can train more intensively for longer durations with less fatigue and with decreased recovery times between workouts.

The dramatic effects of AAS on muscle growth are illustrated in Figure 11.13–2, which compares a "natural" bodybuilder who has never used these drugs with a bodybuilder of identical height and body fat who has used AAS extensively.

Although the anabolic or muscle-building properties of AAS are clearly important to those seeking to enhance athletic performance and physical appearance, psychoactive effects may also be important in the persistent and dependent use of AAS. Anecdotally, some AAS users report feelings of power, aggressiveness, and euphoria, which become associated with and can reinforce AAS taking.

Cross-sectional studies have delineated a number of demographic and psychosocial differences between users and nonusers of AAS. In general, males are more likely to take AAS than females, and athletes are more likely to take AAS than nonathletes. Some studies have suggested that adolescent AAS use is associated with higher levels of childhood antisocial traits and lower levels of parental supervision. Among weight lifters, one study found that both AAS users and individuals thinking about using AAS (high-risk group) were more likely than those not thinking about using AAS (low-risk group) to spend increased time each week lifting weights, to be training specifically for a bodybuilding competition, to use nonsteroidal substances for training enhancement (such as vitamins, amino acids, protein supplements, stimulants, and so-called natural testosterone releasers), and to know other AAS users. Interestingly, the high-risk nonuser group was more likely than either the low-risk group or the AAS users to "feel not big enough." Indeed, recent investigations have suggested that some male and female weight lifters may have muscle dysmorphia, a form of body dysmorphic disorder in which the individual feels that he or she is not sufficiently muscular and lean. Individuals with muscle dysmorphia may perceive themselves to be much smaller and weaker than they actually are, causing this disorder to formerly be called *reverse anorexia nervosa*. By extension, the risk factors for dependent use may overlap with those for initial use. One study found higher doses of AAS and more dissatisfaction with body image among dependent users than nondependent users, suggesting that both pharmacological factors and self-perceptions were risk factors for dependence on AAS.

Another recent cross-sectional study compared 48 AAS users with a very similar group of experienced weight lifters who reported no use of AAS. In comparison to the nonusers, AAS users reported higher levels of conduct disorder and other antisocial traits, including much greater use of other illicit drugs, during the time before their first use of AAS. Although both groups described similar family background and childhood experiences, AAS users reported poorer relationships with their fathers. At the time that they first started lifting weights, the AAS users reported significantly lower confidence about their body appearance than nonusers. Collectively, the findings of available studies suggest that the combination of body-image concerns and antisocial traits may create a particularly high risk for AAS use.

ANABOLIC STEROID DEPENDENCE AND ABUSE

The possibility of anabolic steroid dependence was mentioned in the scientific literature as early as 1980. Three case reports appeared in the medical literature between 1988 and 1990, which described young men who initially took AAS to enhance their weight lifting and bodybuilding activity and later used the drugs to combat depression when they tried to stop using them. The men reported feeling addicted and sought professional help to stop using illicitly obtained AAS because they were unable to accomplish discontinuation on their own.

At least 162 other cases of AAS dependence were documented in the medical literature between 1990 and 2000. Several research groups used the revised third edition of DSM (DSM-III-R) criteria for substance dependence to diagnose steroid dependence in samples of weight lifters taking illicit AAS. One group made presumptive DSM-III-R diagnoses using an anonymous, self-administered questionnaire and found responses suggestive of dependence on AAS in 57 percent of 49 men. Self-reported diagnostic symptoms and their frequencies included taking more AAS than intended (51 percent), difficulty cutting down or controlling use (16 percent), continuing to use despite adverse consequences (37 percent), tolerance (18 percent), and withdrawal (84 percent). In addition to a desire to take more AAS (52 percent) and headaches (20 percent), the most frequently reported withdrawal symptoms were depressive in nature and included fatigue (43 percent), depressed mood (41 percent), restlessness (29 percent), anorexia (24 percent), insomnia (20 percent), and decreased libido (20 percent). Another research group, using the same methods and questionnaire, also found a 57 percent rate of dependence among 21 AAS users.

Three other research groups, all of which diagnosed dependence with a face-to-face interview and the Structured Clinical Interview for DSM-III-R (SCID), reported somewhat lower rates of AAS dependence (25 percent of 88 AAS users, 14.3 percent of 77 users, and 26 percent of 50 users). Similarly, 23 percent of 100 users met DSM-IV criteria for AAS dependence in an Australian sample. Finally, a study of 91 inpatient substance abuse treatment programs identified 68 AAS users, of whom 69 percent were judged to meet DSM-III-R criteria for AAS dependence. The wide range of prevalence rates across the seven studies (14 to 69 percent) probably reflects differences in sampling and differences in diagnostic methods, so the true prevalence of dependence among AAS users and in the general population is unknown.

Published observations suggest that women may also manifest dependence on AAS, but female dependence on male hormones appears to be relatively rare when compared with men. To the authors' knowledge, only two cases of AAS dependence in women had been reported in the medical literature through the first half of 2002, with the first case published in 1998. Importantly, there appear to be no reported cases of anabolic steroid dependence in patients who were prescribed AAS for legitimate medical indications such as hypogonadism or anemia. Thus, physicians probably need not be concerned about dependence when legitimately prescribing AAS at therapeutic doses.

Etiology

The mechanism of dependence on AAS is not firmly established. For example, some authors have argued that AAS dependence represents a compulsive attachment to athletic activities, such as weight lifting—accompanied by feeling high when actively participating in those activities—rather than to any psychoactive properties of the AAS themselves. According to this view, AAS are taken more for their "muscle-active" than for their psychoactive properties, and any feelings of euphoria result from satisfying workouts or from the social rewards for having a big and muscular body.

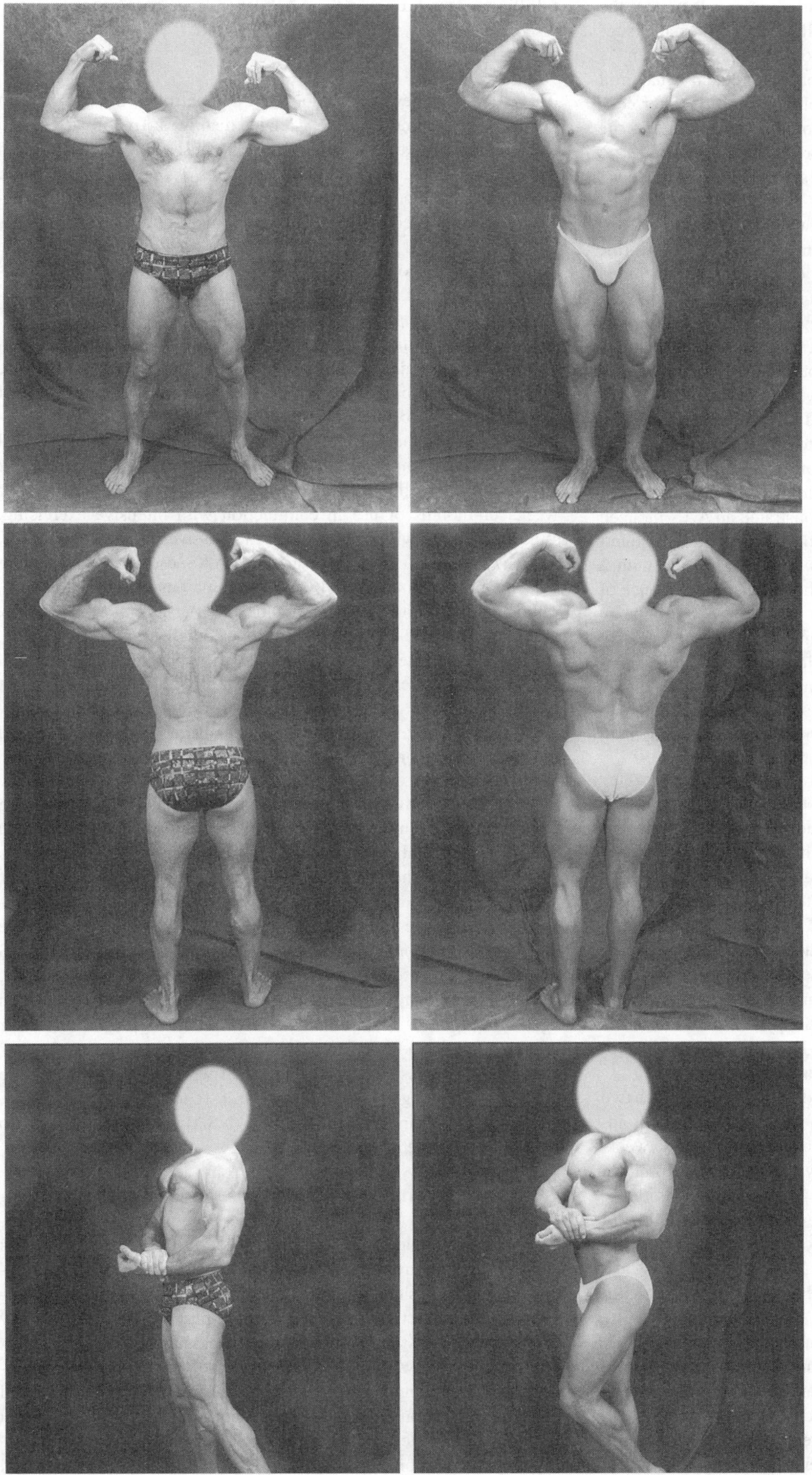

FIGURE 11.13–2 Physical effects of anabolic steroid use. These photographs compare a "natural" bodybuilder who has never used anabolic steroids (*left*) with a man who has used large doses of anabolic steroids over several years (*right*). Both men are 67 in. tall and have 7 percent body fat. The man on the left weighs 170 lbs and represents approximately the maximum degree of muscularity obtainable without drugs. His fat-free mass index is 25.4 kg/m^2 by the formula of Elena Kouri et al. The man on the right weighs 213 lbs and has a fat-free mass index of 31.7 kg/m^2. Note that the muscle hypertrophy from steroid use is particularly marked in the upper body in the pectoralis, deltoid, trapezius, and biceps muscles. Any man significantly more muscular than the man on the left has almost certainly abused anabolic steroids.

Nevertheless, several controlled studies in humans document the mood-altering properties of AAS, and preliminary studies also suggest that AAS are effective in treating major depressive disorder. As mentioned above, one recent study in humans correlated behavioral changes with levels of a serotonin metabolite in the CSF after controlled administration of an anabolic steroid. AAS also mimic the electroencephalographic (EEG) patterns produced by dopaminergic stimulants in humans. In animal studies, several lines of evidence suggest that AAS have reinforcing effects. Hamsters, for example, have been shown to self-administer testosterone, suggesting a primary reinforcing effect despite an apparent lack of social rewards. Similarly, mice and rats in some studies developed a conditioned place preference to settings in which they received testosterone but not placebo injections. Some evidence suggests that the conditioned place preference is mediated by a neurosteroid metabolite of testosterone. Finally, AAS bind to specific receptors in the brain and alter neurotransmitter functioning, albeit in ways that are not fully elucidated. A recent study of male rats revealed that treatment with nandrolone decanoate altered dopamine receptor densities in the ventral tegmental area and nucleus accumbens, portions of the brain postulated to be involved in the reinforcing action of other abused drugs such as cocaine. Another study in rats demonstrated an AAS-induced increase in endogenous opioid concentrations in the ventral tegmental area. However, a study of three rhesus monkeys, treated with 2 weeks of high-dose AAS, found that they did not display evidence of increased opioid tolerance or dependence.

In addition to positive reinforcement mechanisms, the negative reinforcement mechanisms of avoiding withdrawal symptoms, particularly depression, and avoiding the feeling of being too small may contribute to AAS dependence. In summary, it is likely that both "myoactive" and psychoactive effects contribute to the development of dependence on AAS.

Course and Prognosis No longitudinal studies of dependent AAS users have been published to date. Based on two case reports, it appears that AAS dependence can develop within 9 to 12 months after initiating use. In these cases, users took supratherapeutic doses and combined multiple anabolic steroid drugs, including both oral and injectable forms. However, dependence has also been described in a male weight lifter who used a single oral agent at three times the therapeutic dose for nearly 9 years. Severity of dependence is also variable. In one study, 8.2 percent of 49 anabolic steroid users reported six or more DSM-III-R dependency symptoms, which is consistent with severe dependence.

Some authors have speculated that withdrawal from AAS has two phases, with phase 1 lasting 1 week or less and consisting of opioid-like withdrawal symptoms. Phase 2 begins within the first week, consists of depressive symptoms, and may last for several months. Other than one case report, however, there is no published evidence of opioid-like withdrawal symptoms after the discontinuation of AAS. One study in rhesus monkeys did not demonstrate naloxone-induced opioid withdrawal symptoms after 2 weeks of high-dose testosterone injections. Conversely, the evidence for depressive withdrawal symptoms is more compelling.

Few users of AAS seek substance abuse treatment. One study estimated that anabolic steroid users accounted for less than 0.1 percent of patients entering treatment programs for substance abuse. The low number of documented treatment cases stands in contrast to the large number of Americans estimated to use AAS illicitly (400,000 per year) and to be at risk for developing dependence (14 to 69 percent of users). However, it is not clear that most individuals fulfilling research criteria for AAS dependence require treatment to discontinue use.

Treatment Few descriptions and no controlled trials have been published of treatment for AAS-related disorders. Treatment is based on a comprehensive assessment, including history, mental status and physical examinations, and laboratory tests. As in the case of other psychiatric disorders, treatment should address both the primary disorder and associated biological, psychological, and social factors. As in the case of other substance use disorders, treatment must motivate AAS users to discontinue use, ameliorate withdrawal-related symptoms, target associated psychiatric disorders, and address psychosocial triggers to relapse.

Abstinence is the treatment goal of choice for patients manifesting AAS abuse or dependence. To the extent that users of AAS abuse other addictive substances (including alcohol), traditional treatment approaches for substance-related disorders may be used. Nevertheless, AAS users may differ from other addicted patients in several ways that have implications for treatment. First, the euphorigenic and reinforcing effects of AAS may only become apparent after weeks or months of use in conjunction with intensive exercising. When compared with immediately and passively reinforcing drugs, such as cocaine, heroin, and alcohol, AAS use may entail more delayed gratification. Second, AAS users may manifest greater commitment to culturally endorsed values of physical fitness, success, victory, and goal directness than users of other illicit drugs. Finally, AAS users are often preoccupied with their physical attributes and may rely excessively on these attributes for self-esteem. Treatment therefore depends on a therapeutic alliance that is based on a thorough and nonjudgmental understanding of the patient's values and motivations for using AAS.

AAS Withdrawal Supportive therapy and monitoring are essential for treating AAS withdrawal because suicidal depressions can occur. Hospitalization may be required when suicidal ideation is severe. Patients should be educated about the possible course of withdrawal and reassured that symptoms are time limited and manageable. Antidepressant agents are best reserved for patients whose depressive symptomatology persists for several weeks after AAS discontinuation and who meet criteria for major depressive disorder. Selective serotonin reuptake inhibitors (SSRIs) are the preferred agents because of their favorable adverse effect profile and their effectiveness in the only reported case series of treated AAS users with major depressive disorder. Physical withdrawal symptoms are not life threatening and do not ordinarily require pharmacotherapy. Nonsteroidal antiinflammatory drugs (NSAIDs) may be useful to treat musculoskeletal pain and headaches.

Endocrine Pharmacotherapies Various endocrine pharmacotherapies for AAS withdrawal have been proposed on theoretical grounds, including testosterone substitution and taper, human chorionic gonadotropin, and estrogen blockers. Endocrine pharmacotherapies have as their goal the restoration of hypothalamic-pituitary-gonadal axis functioning. Hypothalamic-pituitary-gonadal activity can remain depressed for 12 or more weeks after cessation of prolonged, high-dose AAS use and resembles hypogonadotropic hypogonadism. Although most AAS users eventually recover normal endocrine function, anecdotal evidence suggests that occasional heavy AAS users experience prolonged and possibly even irreversible suppression of hypothalamic-pituitary-testicular axis function after discontinuing AAS. However, there are no studies demonstrat-

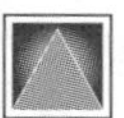

Table 11.13–2
Relationship of Weekly Steroid Dosage to Prevalence of Mood Disorders

	No. (%) of Subjects Displaying Mood Disorders[b]			
Weekly Steroid Dose[a] (No. of Users)	**Manic Episode**	**Hypomanic Episode**	**Major Depressive Disorder**	**Total[c]**
Low (N = 12)	0	1 (8)	0	1 (8)
Medium (N = 51)	0	5 (10)	3 (6)	7 (14)
High (N = 25)	4 (16)	3 (12)	7 (28)	11 (44)

[a]Low represents less than 300 mg per week of testosterone or equivalent; medium, 300 to 1,000 mg per week; and high, more than 1,000 mg per week.
[b]Significance of relationship between increasing doses of steroids and prevalence of mood disorders by two-sided trend test: manic episode, $P = .01$; major depressive disorder, $P = .003$; total, $P = .004$.
[c]Total is less than sum of individual categories because some individuals displayed both a manic or hypomanic episode and a major depressive episode in association with steroids.
From Pope HG Jr, Katz DL: Psychiatric and medical effects of anabolic-androgenic steroid use: A controlled study of 160 athletes. *Arch Gen Psychiatry.* 1994;51:375, with permission.

ing the efficacy of endocrine pharmacotherapies for treating illicit AAS users during withdrawal, so their use remains experimental and cannot be routinely recommended. Consultation with an endocrinologist is highly recommended.

ANABOLIC STEROID–INDUCED MOOD DISORDERS

Irritability, aggressiveness, hypomania, and frank mania associated with anabolic steroid use probably represent one of the most important public health issues associated with these drugs. Although athletes using these drugs have long recognized that syndromes of anger and irritability (sometimes called *roid rage*) could be associated with AAS use, these syndromes were little recognized in the scientific literature until the late 1980s and 1990s. Since then, a series of observational field studies of athletes has suggested that some AAS users develop prominent hypomanic or even manic symptoms during AAS use. In a recent review of 12 such studies, 11 reported at least some such effects in association with anabolic steroid use, with an apparent association between the dosage of AAS used and the frequency of psychiatric effects. Specifically, in individuals using the equivalent of 300 mg of testosterone a week or less, psychiatric effects appear rare; in individuals taking intermediate dosages, between 300 and 1,000 mg of testosterone equivalent per week, mood syndromes appear more common; and in individuals taking the equivalent of more than 1,000 mg a week, mood syndromes become quite common and are occasionally severe.

The association of AAS dosage with psychiatric effects is illustrated by examining individual studies. At the low end of the dosage range, for example, one study of 53 men examined individuals who were using a mean dose of only 318 mg of testosterone or equivalent a week. The men in this study exhibited essentially no psychiatric changes during use of AAS. By comparison, another study examined 71 men and six women who were using a mean dose estimated as somewhat more than 500 mg a week. The authors of this study noted that one (1.3 percent) of the subjects developed mania and six (7.8 percent) developed hypomania. One subject (1.3 percent) described major depressive disorder during AAS use, and five (6.5 percent) subjects reported major depressive disorder in association with AAS withdrawal. Five (6.5 percent) of the 77 users in this study reported a suicide attempt during a period of withdrawal from AAS use. At the high end of the dosage range, a third study examined 39 men and two women who had used a mean of 750 mg per week. In this study, five (12 percent) of the subjects reported a manic syndrome, and five (12 percent) reported psychotic symptoms at some time in association with AAS use. Interestingly, among the eight subjects reporting manic or psychotic symptoms or both in this study, the average weekly dose was approximately 900 mg. A further illustration of the relationship between AAS dosage and the prevalence of psychiatric syndromes is provided in Table 11.13–2, which provides the frequency of hypomanic, manic, and major depressive syndromes reported among 88 users of AAS in one study in which the users are grouped on the basis of the maximum dosage of AAS used. Psychiatric syndromes are almost absent at the lowest dosages but affected nearly one-half of the individuals using dosages equivalent to 1,000 mg or more of testosterone a week.

Observational field studies, however, are subject to a number of methodological limitations common to retrospective studies of this nature. First, subjects are being asked to describe psychiatric symptoms that may have occurred well in the past and that therefore may be colored by recall bias. Second, these subjects were generally taking drugs obtained on the black market that were of unknown potency or authenticity. Thus, assumptions regarding the nature and dosage of the drugs are necessarily crude at best. Third, selection bias may influence which subjects present for interviews in observational studies: Subjects who have experienced prominent psychopathology in association with AAS use might be either more likely or less likely to participate. Fourth, expectational effects and influences from the subculture of the gymnasium may greatly influence subjects' reactions to AAS. For example, an individual lifting weights regularly in a "hard-core" gymnasium might be primed to expect increases in his or her irritability and aggression with AAS use, even if such changes do not actually occur.

Laboratory studies using AAS in normal volunteers avoid most of these limitations but are subject to problems of their own. Specifically, most laboratory studies, including endocrinological investigations, physiological studies, and studies using AAS to treat various medical conditions, have used very modest doses of testosterone or other AAS, rarely exceeding the equivalent of 300 mg of testosterone a week. Furthermore, such studies have rarely attempted to measure psychiatric effects systematically. Not surprisingly, these studies have generally failed to note prominent psychiatric changes in their subjects. As a result, some such studies have erroneously concluded that AAS lack psychiatric effects. This error is similar to that of many earlier negative studies of the effects of AAS on muscle growth, again because the studies typically used doses far less than those actually used by athletes in the field.

Recently, four newer laboratory studies have appeared in which normal male volunteers were given dosages of 500 mg per week or

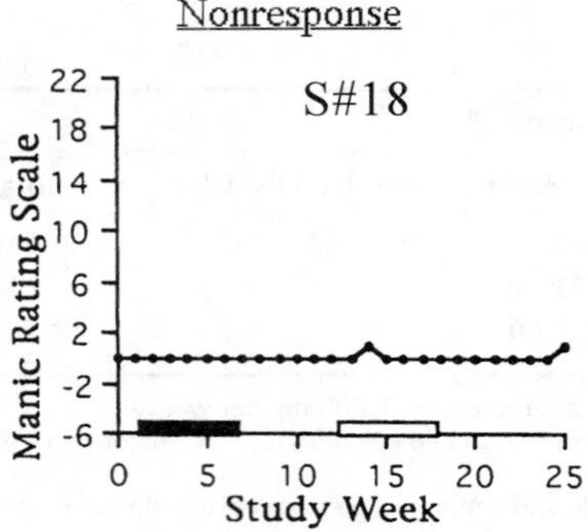

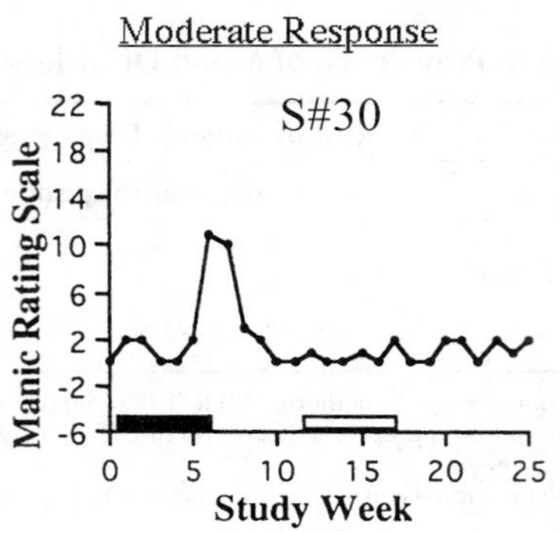

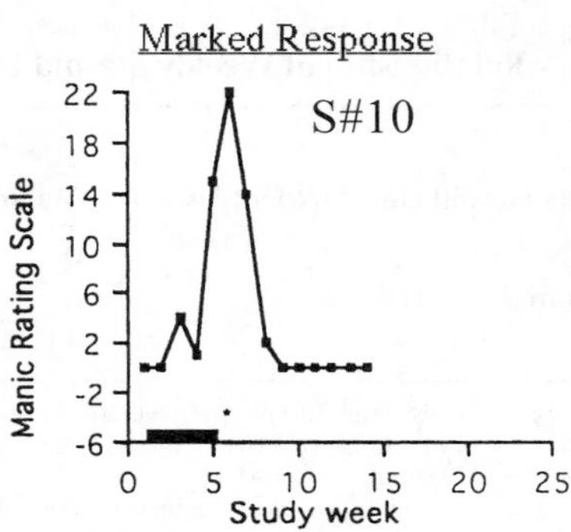

FIGURE 11.13–3 Examples of nonresponse, moderate response, and marked response to testosterone versus placebo on the Young Manic Rating Scale. The black bar represents the period of testosterone cypionate administration in each subject. Testosterone was administered in gradually increasing doses (150 mg per week for the first 2 weeks, 300 mg per week for the next 2 weeks, and 600 mg per week for the final 2 weeks of the period). The white bar represents the period of placebo administration. A 6-week washout period was interposed between the two treatment periods to minimize carryover effects.

more of testosterone or equivalent under placebo-controlled, double-blind conditions. These studies represent the first available controlled investigations that have used doses of AAS more closely approximating those used by actual AAS abusers. Of 109 men receiving such dosages in these four studies combined, five exhibited prominent hypomanic or manic syndromes during AAS exposure. These subjects displayed levels of symptomatology that might be expected to seriously impair normal social or occupational functioning; one subject studied even requested that he be placed in seclusion on the ward in which the study was conducted. By contrast, however, the great majority of the men in these four studies exhibited very few behavioral changes with high dosages of AAS. Thus, it appears that most individuals taking AAS, even at fairly high dosages, experience few psychiatric effects, although an occasional individual may develop a severe manic or hypomanic reaction. At present, the mechanism of these reactions is unknown; they may represent an idiosyncratic phenomenon unrelated to premorbid psychiatric function.

Figure 11.13–3 shows changes in ratings of manic symptoms in three subjects who received testosterone cypionate in dosages up to 600 mg a week versus inert placebo, each for periods of 6 weeks in a double-blind, crossover design. Subjects varied widely in their response to testosterone. The subject on the left side of the figure exhibited virtually no change in manic ratings during either the testosterone or placebo periods; the subject in the middle displayed a modest increase in manic symptoms in association with testosterone but not sufficient to significantly affect his social or occupational functioning. By contrast, the subject on the right displayed a marked manic reaction, approaching the range of patients hospitalized for treatment of manic episodes, requiring the investigators to discontinue testosterone administration 1 week earlier than planned. The symptoms of mania resolved promptly within 2 weeks after discontinuation of testosterone.

It is difficult to extrapolate from these findings to estimate the frequency of prominent hypomanic or manic reactions among AAS users in the field. Illicit users may use higher dosages than could ethically be administered in the laboratory; such users may take several different AAS together ("stacking"); they may use alcohol or other drugs while taking AAS; and of course they do not screen themselves with the same care as is the case in a laboratory study. Finally, some users may become more sensitized to the psychiatric effects of AAS after using them for multiple courses over time; because most of the subjects in available laboratory studies were steroid naïve before treatment, they may not be representative of actual AAS users in the field. For all these reasons, the crude rate of approximately 5 percent previously estimated may represent a lower bound for the true prevalence of AAS-induced hypomanic and manic syndromes in the overall population of users.

A possible serious consequence of AAS-induced mood disorders may be violent or even homicidal behavior. Several published reports have anecdotally described individuals with no apparent history of psychiatric disorder, no criminal record, and no history of violence, who committed violent crimes, including murder, while under the influence of AAS. In a number of cases, AAS use has been cited in criminal trials as a possible mitigating factor in the defense of such individuals. Although a causal link is difficult to establish in these cases, evidence of AAS use has frequently been presented in forensic settings as a possible mitigating factor in criminal behavior. One recent study of 133 sequential, newly incarcerated male felons found that three (2.3 percent) reported committing violent crimes while under the influence of AAS.

At least one published study, together with anecdotal experience, suggests that violence associated with AAS is frequently directed at women. In one study that specifically examined this issue, 23 male AAS users were compared with 14 male nonusers, using the Conflict Tactics Scales to assess users' relationships with their girlfriends or spouses. Significant differences emerged on several of these scales between users on drugs and nonusers and between users on drugs and the same users when off drugs.

AAS-induced depressive syndromes have generally not been reported in laboratory studies but have been documented in field studies. Case reports of completed suicides associated with AAS withdrawal have also appeared. In some instances, it appears that a brief and self-limited syndrome of depression occurs on AAS withdrawal, probably as a result of the depression of the hypothalamic-pituitary-gonadal axis after exogenous AAS administration. Such syndromes might be expected to occur more often in the field than in laboratory settings because athletes typically take AAS for longer intervals than occurs in the laboratory, resulting in more pronounced neuroendocrine depression and shrinkage of the testes.

Not all depressive syndromes of this nature, however, are self-limited. Some reports have described episodes of depression that continued for months after discontinuing AAS and which required treatment with fluoxetine (Prozac), tricyclic antidepressant agents, or ECT. Again, however, given the uncontrolled and retrospective nature of these observations, it is difficult to judge the true frequency of such syndromes in the field.

ANABOLIC STEROID–INDUCED PSYCHOTIC DISORDER

Psychotic symptoms are rare in association with anabolic steroid use but have been described in a few cases, primarily in individuals who were using the equivalent of more than 1,000 mg of testosterone a week. Usually, these symptoms have consisted of grandiose or paranoid delusions, generally occurring in the context of a manic episode, although occasionally occurring in the absence of a frank manic syndrome. In most cases reported, psychotic symptoms have disappeared promptly (within a few weeks) after the discontinuation of the offending agent, although temporary treatment with antipsychotic agents was sometimes required. As with manic reactions to AAS, the mechanism for these seemingly idiosyncratic psychotic reactions is unknown. It is interesting to note, however, that the chemically related family of hormones, corticosteroids, also produces idiosyncratic manic and psychotic symptoms in occasional individuals, although creating few psychiatric effects in the great majority of patients. The mechanism of action of these idiosyncratic effects with corticosteroids is also unknown.

ANABOLIC STEROID–RELATED DISORDER NOT OTHERWISE SPECIFIED

Occasional anecdotal reports have described decreases in symptoms of anxiety disorders, such as panic disorder and social phobia, during AAS use and exacerbations of these disorders during AAS withdrawal. Conversely, some individuals report increases in anxiety symptoms while taking AAS. However, no systematic data are available on these entities.

Anabolic steroid use may frequently be associated with use of other licit and illicit ergogenic drugs. Thus, athletes may exhibit both physical and psychiatric morbidity associated with the use of these other drugs and also may develop apparent abuse and dependence of multiple ergogenic drugs, although this syndrome has been poorly characterized in the literature to date. For example, use of ephedrine and other central nervous system (CNS) stimulants to promote fat loss may lead to insomnia, anxiety, and other features of stimulant abuse and dependence syndromes. Use of large doses of adrenal hormones, such as DHEA and androstenedione, may lead to masculinizing effects in female athletes. DHEA may also possess antidepressant properties, although data in this area remain limited. Use of excessive dosages of thyroid hormones may produce psychiatric effects similar to those seen in thyrotoxicosis. In a recent anonymous questionnaire study of 334 men attending Boston-area gyms, 18 (5.4 percent) reported use of AAS. Of these, 14 (78 percent) reported use of ephedrine-containing substances, 15 (83 percent) reported use of adrenal hormones, such as androstenedione, and four (22 percent) reported illicit use of thyroid hormones.

Recent data also suggest that AAS use may serve as a "gateway to the use of opioid agonist/antagonists, such as nalbuphine, or to use of frank opioid agonists such as heroin." One study in New Jersey found that 21 (9 percent) of 227 sequential men, admitted for treatment of opioid dependence, had apparently been introduced to opioids through AAS; they reported that they had first learned about opioids from fellow AAS users and had subsequently first purchased opioids from the same individual who had sold them AAS. A subsequent study of men admitted for substance dependence treatment in Massachusetts produced similar findings.

Mr. A. is a 26-year-old, single white man. He is 69 in. tall and presently weighs 204 lbs with a body fat of 11 percent. He reports that he began lifting weights at 17 years of age, at which time he weighed 155 lbs. Within 1 year of beginning his weight lifting, he began taking AAS after obtaining them through a friend at his gymnasium. His first cycle of AAS, lasting for 9 weeks, involved methandienone (Dianabol), 30 mg orally a day, and testosterone cypionate, 600 mg intramuscularly (IM) a week. During these 9 weeks, he gained 20 lbs of muscle mass. He was so pleased with these results that he took five further cycles of AAS over the course of the next 6 years. During his most ambitious cycle, approximately 1 year ago, he used testosterone cypionate, 600 mg per week; nandrolone decanoate (Deca-Durabolin), 400 mg per week; stanozolol (Winstrol), 12 mg per day; and oxandrolone (Anavar), 10 mg per day.

During each of the cycles, Mr. A. noted euphoria, irritability, and grandiose feelings. These symptoms were most prominent during his most recent cycle, when he felt invincible. During this cycle, he also noted a decreased need for sleep, racing thoughts, and a tendency to spend excessive amounts of money. For example, he impulsively purchased a $2,700 stereo system when he realistically could not afford to spend more than $500. He also became uncharacteristically irritable with his girlfriend and on one occasion put his fist through the side window of her car during an argument—an act inconsistent with his normally mild-mannered personality. After this cycle of AAS ended, he became moderately depressed for approximately 2 months, with hypersomnia, anorexia, markedly decreased libido, and occasional suicidal ideation.

Mr. A. smoked marijuana almost daily during his last 2 years of high school and continues to smoke at least twice a week. He has experimented briefly with hallucinogens, cocaine, opiates, and stimulants but has rarely used them in the last 5 years. However, he has used a number of drugs to lose weight in preparation for bodybuilding contests. These include ephedrine, amphetamine, triiodothyronine, and thyroxin. Recently, he has also begun to use the opioid agonist-antagonist nalbuphine (Nubain) intravenously (IV) to treat muscle aches from weight lifting. He reports that IV nalbuphine use is widespread among other anabolic steroid users of his acquaintance.

Mr. A. exhibits characteristic features of muscle dysmorphia. He checks his appearance dozens of times a day in mirrors or when he sees his reflection in a store window or even in the back of a spoon. He becomes anxious if he misses even one day of working out at the gym and acknowledges that his preoccupation with weight lifting has cost him both social and occupational opportunities. Although he has a 48-in. chest and 19-in. biceps, he has frequently declined invitations to go to the beach or a swimming pool for fear that he looks too small when seen in a bathing suit. He is anxious because he has lost some weight since the end of his previous cycle of AAS and is eager to resume another cycle of AAS in the near future.

SUGGESTED CROSS-REFERENCES

An overview of substance-related disorders is given in Section 11.1; mood disorders are discussed in Chapter 13 and psychotic disorders in Chapter 12. Body dysmorphic disorder is covered in Chapter 15.

REFERENCES

Bahrke MS, Wright JE, Strauss RH, Catlin DH: Psychological moods and subjectively perceived behavioral and somatic changes accompanying anabolic-androgenic steroid use. *Am J Sport Med.* 1992;20:717.

Bahrke MS, Yesalis CE, Kopstein AN, Stephens JA: Risk factors associated with anabolic-androgenic steroid use among adolescents. *Sports Med.* 2000;29:397–405.

*Bhasin S, Storer TW, Berman N, Callegari C, Clevenger B, Phillips J, Bunnell TJ, Tricker R, Shirazi A, Casaburi R: The effect of supraphysiologic doses of testosterone on muscle size and strength in normal men. *N Engl J Med.* 1996;335:1.

Bidwill MJ, Katz DL: Injecting new life into an old defense: Anabolic steroid-induced psychosis as a paradigm of involuntary intoxication. *Univ Miami Entertainment Sport Law Rev.* 1989;7:1.

Bronson FH, Matherne CM: Exposure to anabolic-androgenic steroids shortens life span of male mice. *Med Sci Sport Exerc.* 1997;29:615.

Brower KJ: Withdrawal from anabolic steroids. *Curr Ther Endocrinol Metab.* 1997;6:338.

*Brower KJ: Anabolic steroid abuse and dependence. *Curr Psychiatry Rep.* 2002;4:377.

Brower KJ, Blow FC, Hill EM: Risk factors for anabolic androgenic steroid use in men. *J Psychiatr Res.* 1994;28:369.

Buckley WA, Yesalis CE, Friedl KE, Anderson W, Streit A, Wright J: Estimated prevalence of anabolic steroid use among male high school seniors. *JAMA.* 1988;260:3441.

Catlin DH. Effects and complications of anabolic androgenic steroids. In: Karch SB, ed. *Handbook on Drug Abuse.* Boca Raton, FL: CRC Press; 1998.

Clancy GP, Yates WR: Anabolic steroid use among substance abusers in treatment. *J Clin Psychiatry.* 1992;53:97.

*Daly RC, Su TP, Schmidt PJ, Pickar D, Murphy DL, Rubinow DR: Cerebrospinal fluid and behavioral changes after methyltestosterone administration: Preliminary findings. *Arch Gen Psychiatry.* 2001;58:172.

Forbes GB, Porta CR, Herr BE, Griggs RC: Sequence of changes in body composition induced by testosterone and reversal of changes after drug is stopped. *JAMA.* 1992;267:397.

Gruber AJ, Pope HG Jr: Psychiatric and medical effects of anabolic-androgenic steroid use in women. *Psychother Psychosom.* 2000;69:19.

Isacsson G, Garle M, Ljung EB, Asgard U, Bergman U: Anabolic steroids and violent crime—an epidemiological study at a jail in Stockholm, Sweden. *Compr Psychiatry.* 1998;39:203.

Johansson P, Lindqvist A, Nyberg F, Fahlke C: Anabolic androgenic steroids affects alcohol intake, defensive behaviors and brain opioid peptides in the rat. *Pharmacol Biochem Behav.* 2000;67:271.

Kanayama G, Cohane G, Weiss RD, Pope HG Jr: Past anabolic-androgenic steroid use among men admitted for substance abuse treatment—an underrecognized problem? *J Clin Psychiatry.* 2003;64:156.

Kanayama G, Pope HG Jr, Cochane G, Hudson JI: Risk factors for anabolic-androgenic steroid use among weightlifters: a case-control study. *Drug Alcohol Depend.* 2003;71:77–86.

Kanayama G, Pope HG Jr, Hudson JI: "Body image" drugs: A growing psychosomatic problem. *Psychother Psychosom.* 2001;70:61.

Kashkin KB, Kleber HD: Hooked on hormones: An anabolic steroid addiction hypothesis. *JAMA.* 1989;262:3166.

Kindlundh AM, Lindblom J, Bergstrom L, Wikberg JE, Nyberg F: The anabolic-androgenic steroid nandrolone decanoate affects the density of dopamine receptors in the male rat brain. *Eur J Neurosci.* 2001;13:291.

Kouri EM, Pope HG Jr, Katz DL, Oliva PS: Fat-free mass index in users and non-users of anabolic-androgenic steroids. *Clin J Sport Med.* 1995;5:223.

Lin GC, Erinoff L, eds. *Anabolic Steroid Abuse.* (DHHS Publication No. ADM 91-1720). Washington, DC: U.S. Government Printing Office; 1990.

Madea B, Grellner W: Long-term cardiovascular effects of anabolic steroids. *Lancet.* 1998;352:33.

Malone DA Jr. Pharmacological therapies of anabolic androgenic steroid addiction. In: NS Miller, MS Gold, eds. *Pharmacological Therapies for Drug and Alcohol Addictions.* New York: Marcel Dekker; 1995.

Malone DA Jr, Dimeff RJ: The use of fluoxetine in depression associated with anabolic steroid withdrawal: A case series. *J Clin Psychiatry.* 1992;53:130.

Malone DA Jr, Dimeff R, Lombardo JA, Sample BRH: Psychiatric effects and psychoactive substance use in anabolic-androgenic steroid users. *Clin J Sport Med.* 1995;5:25.

Olivardia R, Pope HG Jr, Hudson JI: "Muscle dysmorphia" in male weightlifters: A case-control study. *Am J Psychiatry.* 2000;157:1291.

Parssinen M, Seppala T: Steroid use and long-term health risks in former athletes. *Sport Med.* 2002;32:83.

Pope HG Jr, Katz DL: Homicide and near-homicide by anabolic steroid users. *J Clin Psychiatry.* 1990;51:28.

Pope HG Jr, Katz DL: Psychiatric and medical effects of anabolic-androgenic steroid use. *Arch Gen Psychiatry.* 1994;51:375.

Pope HG Jr, Katz DL: Psychiatric effects of exogenous anabolic-androgenic steroids. In: Wolkowitz OM, Rothschild AJ, eds. *Psychoneuroendocrinology for the Clinician.* Washington, DC: American Psychiatric Press; 2003:331–358.

*Pope HG Jr, Kouri EM, Hudson JI: The effects of supraphysiologic doses of testosterone on mood and aggression in normal men: A randomized controlled trial. *Arch Gen Psychiatry.* 2000;57:133.

Pope HG Jr, Kouri EM, Powell KF, Campbell C, Katz DL: Anabolic-androgenic steroid use among 133 prisoners. *Compr Psychiatry.* 1996;37:322.

Rosellini RA, Svare BB, Rhodes ME, Frye CA: The testosterone metabolite and neurosteroid 3alpha-androstanediol may mediate the effects of testosterone on conditioned place preference. *Brain Res Rev.* 2001;37:162.

Schumacher J, Muller G, Klotz KF: Large hepatic hematoma and intraabdominal hemorrhage associated with abuse of anabolic steroids. *N Engl J Med.* 1999;340: 1123.

Su TT, Pagliaro M, Schmidt PJ, Pickar D, Wolkowitz OM, Rubinow DR: Neuropsychiatric effects of anabolic steroids in male normal volunteers. *JAMA.* 1993;269:2760.

Thiblin I, Lindquist O, Rajs J: Cause and manner of death among users of anabolic androgenic steroids. *J Forensic Sci.* 2000;45:16.

Yates WR, Perry P, MacIndoe J, Holman T, Ellingrad V: Psychosexual effects of three doses of testosterone in cycling and normal men. *Biol Psychiatry.* 1999;45:254.

*Yesalis CE, ed. *Anabolic Steroids in Sport and Exercise.* 2nd ed. Champaign, IL: Human Kinetics; 2000.

Yesalis CE, Kennedy NJ, Kopstein AN, Bahrke MS: Anabolic-androgenic steroid use in the United States. *JAMA.* 1993;270:1217.

12 Schizophrenia and Other Psychotic Disorders

▲ 12.1 Concept of Schizophrenia

Robert W. Buchanan, M.D., and
William T. Carpenter, Jr., M.D.

Schizophrenia is a clinical syndrome of variable, but profoundly disruptive, psychopathology that involves cognition, emotion, perception, and other aspects of behavior. The expression of these manifestations varies across patients and over time, but the effect of the illness is always severe and is usually long-lasting.

HISTORY

Written descriptions of symptoms commonly observed today in patients with schizophrenia are found throughout recorded history. Early Greek physicians described delusions of grandeur and paranoia and deterioration in cognitive functions and personality. Because these symptoms are not unique to schizophrenia, it is uncertain whether these behaviors were associated with what is currently called schizophrenia. Indeed, several scholars have argued that schizophrenia is of relatively recent origin.

Schizophrenia emerged as a medical condition worthy of study and treatment in the 18th century. By the 19th century, the various psychotic disorders were generally viewed as insanity or madness, and the movement to conceptualize these disorders as regrettable afflictions replaced the view of insanity as a reprehensible behavior. Many clinical categories were described during the middle to late 19th century, but a general approach capable of integrating the diverse manifestations of mental illness into distinguishable clinical syndromes was lacking.

A major impediment to distinguishing schizophrenia from other forms of psychoses was the existence of another common illness, general paresis of the insane. The mental manifestations of general paresis were quite diverse and overlapped extensively with schizophrenic symptomatology. The cause of syphilitic insanity was subsequently traced to a spirochetal infestation, and malaria-induced fever therapy proved partially effective. Antibiotics were eventually found to provide effective treatment and prevention. The identification and treatment of general paresis is one of the great stories of medical science. The identification of syphilitic insanity reduced the heterogeneity of madness and enabled Emil Kraepelin to delineate the two other major patterns of insanity—manic-depressive psychosis and dementia praecox (or dementia of the young)—and to group together under the diagnostic category of dementia praecox the previously disparate categories of insanity, such as hebephrenia, paranoia, and catatonia. In differentiating dementia praecox from manic-depressive disorder, Kraepelin emphasized what he believed to be the characteristic poor long-term prognosis of dementia praecox, as compared to the relatively nondeteriorating course of manic-depressive illness. Kraepelin went on to describe the two principal pathophysiological or disease processes occurring in dementia praecox (*Dementia Praecox and Paraphrenia*, 1919):

> On the one hand we observe a weakening of those emotional activities which permanently form the mainsprings of volition. In connection with this, mental activity and instinct for occupation become mute. The result of this part of the process is emotional dullness, failure of mental activities, loss of mastery over volition, of endeavor, and of ability for independent action. The essence of personality is thereby destroyed, the best and most precious part of its being, as Griesinger once expressed it, torn from her. . . .
>
> The second group of disorders, which gives dementia praecox its peculiar stamp . . . consists in the loss of the inner unity of the activities of intellect, emotion, and volition in themselves and among one another. Stransky speaks of an annihilation of the "intrapsychic co-ordination". . . this annihilation presents itself to us in the disorders of association described by Bleuler, in incoherence of the train of thought, in the sharp change of moods as well as in desultoriness and derailments in practical work. But further, the near connections between thinking and feeling, between deliberation and emotional activity on the one hand, and practical work on the other is more or less lost. Emotions do not correspond to ideas.

The description of the destruction of the personality provides a conceptual framework for the avolitional or negative symptom component of the illness, and the description of "the loss of the inner unity of activities" process provides a conceptual framework for the positive symptoms of schizophrenia.

In 1911, Eugen Bleuler, recognizing that dementia was not a usual characteristic of dementia praecox, suggested the term *schizophrenia* (splitting of the mind) for the disorder. Bleuler introduced the concept of primary and secondary schizophrenic symptoms; his four primary symptoms (the four As) were abnormal associations, autistic behavior and thinking, abnormal affect, and ambivalence. Of these four symptoms, Bleuler viewed as central to the illness the loss of association between thought processes and among thought, emotion, and behavior. Examples of these losses of associations are a patient laughing on receiving news of the death of a loved one, the introduction of magical thinking and peculiar concepts into an ordinary discussion, and the sudden display of angry behavior without experiencing anger (or an understandable provocation).

Bleuler's view that a dissociative process is fundamental to schizophrenia and that this process underlies a wide variety of the symptom manifestations of schizophrenia has provided a major paradigm for conceptualizing the illness, that is, that in spite of its various manifestations, schizophrenia is a single disease entity in which there is extensive similarity in etiology (cause) and pathophysiology (mechanism) across all patients with the disorder. In this view, a neurophysiological disturbance of indeterminate origin and nature occurs that is manifested as dissociative processes adversely influencing the development of mental capacities in the areas of thought, emotion, and behavior. Depending on the individual's adaptive capacity and environmental circumstances, this fundamental process could lead to secondary disease manifestations, such as hallucinations, delusions, social withdrawal, and diminished drive.

There are many parallels in medicine for the previously mentioned single-disease model. Patients with type I diabetes mellitus share an impairment in insulin metabolism, but the secondary manifestations may vary considerably, depending on which organ systems are involved. Similarly, patients with temporal lobe epilepsy share a common pathophysiological mechanism but present with a myriad of different signs and symptoms. The diverse manifestations of syphilitic insanity perhaps best illustrate the usefulness of this disease entity approach for schizophrenia.

The major alternative etiopathophysiological model conceptualizes schizophrenia as a clinical syndrome rather than as a single disease entity. This view holds that, although patients with schizophrenia share a sufficient commonality of signs and symptoms to validly differentiate them from patients with other forms of psychosis (e.g., affective disorders and toxic psychoses), more than one disease entity is eventually found within this syndrome. This view is supported by the existence of numerous risk factors, the implication of multiple genes, and the heterogeneity in clinical presentation, treatment response, and clinical course. The demonstration over the past 50 years that mental retardation is a clinical syndrome comprised of multiple disease entities rather than a single disease entity best illustrates this construct. Schizophrenia currently maintains the status of a clinical syndrome in the absence of evidence for the existence of a single disease entity.

There are other competing models for conceptualizing schizophrenia, that, although seriously debated in the past, are presently dismissed as demonstrably invalid or so seriously reductionistic as to not account for major observations associated with the illness. Nondisease models, such as the societal reaction theory (a sane reaction to an insane world) or Thomas Szasz's theory that schizophrenia is a myth enabling society to manage deviant behavior, cannot adequately account for the distribution of schizophrenia among biological relatives, the range of early developmental risk factors, the associated functional and structural brain abnormalities, the normalizing effects of drug treatment, or the extensive similarity and lifetime prevalence and clinical manifestations of schizophrenia across widely divergent cultures. Narrow framework disease models that attempt to account for the illness solely at the level of psychological mechanisms are also demonstrably inadequate in accommodating the known facts of the illness. Genetic or immunovirological causal factors cannot be addressed by reductionistic theories operating at the psychological or social levels. The many biological, psychological, and social factors relevant to the understanding and treatment of the person with schizophrenia requires a broad medical model and eschews reduction to any single level of the functioning organism.

Recent scientific advances have confirmed current concepts of schizophrenia and suggested that the nosology of psychotic illness will continue to evolve. Family studies have provided an important validation of Kraepelin's original formulation of dementia praecox and manic-depressive psychosis as separate disorders. These studies have repeatedly shown that biological relatives of patients with schizophrenia have an increased risk of schizophrenia and schizophrenia spectrum disorders, whereas biological relatives of patients with a major affective disorder have an increased risk for affective disorders. The separation is not complete, but it is supportive of the two disorders as independent disease entities. Twin studies indicate that the genetic distinction between schizophrenia and major affective disorders is even more robust when considering concordance rates among monozygotic twins. There is also evidence that the presence of the deficit form of schizophrenia (i.e., schizophrenia with primary negative symptoms) increases the relative risk of schizophrenia and decreases the relative risk for other mental illness in biological relatives. These results suggest that some subtypes of schizophrenia may breed true. In contrast, there are emerging data from linkage analyses conducted in families selected for the presence of bipolar disorder, other major affective disorders, or schizophrenia that suggest that there is remarkable overlap of chromosomal areas suspected to be the location of genes contributing to disease liability. It now appears likely that a number of genes confer liability for major psychiatric disorders and that these genes may overlap across current diagnostic boundaries. Initial gene expression findings from postmortem tissue also suggest this overlap, and nosologists will soon be challenged to reconceptualize classification of these illness syndromes.

In summary, schizophrenia is appropriately and accurately conceptualized as a disease process. Although it is possible that a unifying etiology and pathophysiology will eventually be uncovered that will account for all, or almost all, cases, it seems more likely that more than one disease entity exists within the clinical syndrome of schizophrenia, with each having a distinguishable etiology and pathophysiology. Any reductionistic approach to the description or explanation of the disorder cannot adequately account for the range of relevant information and facts. A broad medical model that integrates factors ranging from the molecular to the psychosocial level of organization is necessary to describe schizophrenia, to account for the range of pathogenic influences, and to provide for treatment and rehabilitation. With suggestions of extensive overlap in genetic vulnerability across current schizophrenia and affective disorder disease classes, a remarkable reconceptualization of nosology may be required in the near future.

EPIDEMIOLOGY

Schizophrenia is a leading worldwide public health problem that exacts enormous personal and economic costs. Schizophrenia affects just less than 1 percent of the world's population. If schizophrenia spectrum disorders are included in the prevalence estimates, then the number of affected individuals increases to approximately 5 percent. The concept of schizophrenia spectrum disorders is derived from observations of psychopathological manifestations in the biological relatives of patients with schizophrenia. Diagnoses (and approximate lifetime prevalence rates [percent of population]) for these disorders are schizoid personality disorder (fractional percentage), schizotypal personality disorder (1 to 4 percent), schizoaffective psychosis (<1 percent), and delusional disorder (fractional percentage). The relationship of these disorders to schizophrenia in the general population is unclear, but in family pedigree studies, the presence of a proband with schizophrenia significantly increases the prevalence of these disorders among biological relatives.

Schizophrenia is found in all societies and geographical areas. Although comparable data are difficult to obtain, incidence and lifetime prevalence rates are roughly equal worldwide. There is a slightly greater incidence of schizophrenia in men than women. There is a greater incidence of schizophrenia in urban versus rural areas. This difference had previously been attributed to the *social drift* phenomenon, in which afflicted or vulnerable individuals tend to lose their occupation and social niche and drift toward pockets of poverty and inner city areas. However, recent studies have confirmed the increased incidence in urban areas, with the relative risk for schizophrenia related to the degree of urbanization. Schizophrenia also tends to be more severe in developed versus developing countries. Occasional geographic areas of increased prevalence of schizophrenia are interesting in terms of illness etiology. For example, a northern Scandinavian, isolated population appears to have a gene pool enriched for schizophrenia vulnerability, probably brought to the region generations ago by two immigrating families.

Patients with schizophrenia are at increased risk for substance abuse, especially nicotine dependence. As much as 90 percent of patients may be dependent on nicotine. Patients with schizophrenia are also at increased risk for suicidal and assaulting behavior. Suicide is a major cause of death of patients with schizophrenia, and approximately 10 percent of patients commit suicide.

Because schizophrenia begins early in life, causes significant and long-lasting impairments, makes heavy demands for hospital care, and requires ongoing clinical care, rehabilitation, and support services, the financial cost of the illness in the United States is estimated to exceed that of all cancers combined. In 1990, the direct and indirect costs of schizophrenia were estimated at $33 billion. The locus of care has shifted dramatically over the last 50 years from long-term hospital-based care to acute hospital care and community-based services. In 1955, approximately 500,000 hospital beds in the United States were occupied by the mentally ill—the majority of these with a diagnosis of schizophrenia. The figure is now less than 250,000 hospital beds.

Deinstitutionalization has dramatically reduced the number of beds in custodial facilities, but an overall evaluation of its consequences is disheartening. Many patients have simply been transferred to alternative forms of custodial care (in contrast to treatment or rehabilitative services), including nursing home care and poorly supervised shelter arrangements. Others have been released to communities often unable or unwilling to provide the minimal requirements for clinical care or humane support. For more fortunate patients, the burden of care has shifted to the family, creating an extremely difficult hardship for large numbers of families in this country. The estimate of the overall financial burden to these families is in the billions of dollars. The less fortunate patient may have no place to live, may be forced to live in circumstances of isolation and hopelessness, or may end up in jail. Patients with a diagnosis of schizophrenia are reported to account for 15 to 45 percent of homeless Americans. Modern-day managed care and other economic factors place further pressure to reduce bed use, with still marginally prepared communities and a relative dearth of alternative care systems. Continuity-of-care systems that include assertive outreach programs and supervised housing and emergency care provide an effective alternative to hospital-based care for many patients, but costs are substantial, and it has not proven feasible to simply shift cost from impoverished public hospital sectors.

ETIOLOGY

The etiological process or processes by which a causal agent creates the pathophysiology of schizophrenia are not yet known. However, there is considerable evidence from family, twin, and adoptive studies that genetic factors make a robust contribution to the etiology of schizophrenia, with genetic factors established as relevant to some, perhaps all, cases. Linkage and association genetic studies have been used to delineate these factors and have provided strong evidence for eight linkage sites: 1q21-22, 6p22-24, 6p21-22, 8p21-22, 10p11-15, 13q14-32, 15q13-15, and 22q11-13. Further analyses of these chromosomal sites have led to the identification of specific candidate genes, and the best current candidates are alpha-7 nicotinic receptor, *DISC 1*, *GRM 3*, dysbindin, *COMT*, *NRG 1*, *RGS 4*, and *G 72*. Each of these genes appears to make a small contribution to schizophrenia vulnerability. What other genes are involved and what combinations are necessary for disease are not known. It is also not yet determined how the proteins they produce contribute to the pathophysiology of schizophrenia.

Risk factor studies have also identified a number of potential environmental factors that may contribute to the development of schizophrenia. These include gestational and birth complications, exposure to influenza epidemics or maternal starvation during pregnancy, Rhesus (Rh) factor incompatibility, and an excess of winter births. The nature of these factors further suggests a neurodevelopmental pathological process in schizophrenia, but the exact pathophysiological mechanisms associated with these risk factors is not known. There are interesting reports that a subgroup of patients with the avolitional component of the illness, defined by criteria for the deficit syndrome, do not share in the winter birth excess but rather show a summer birth excess, suggesting the possibility of a separate disease entity within the schizophrenia syndrome. A number of speculations regarding viral and immune mechanisms, sometimes posited as an explanation of the season of birth risk factor, are plausible, but no virus or immune mechanism has yet been established as an etiological factor in schizophrenia. Finally, substance abuse has been identified as a risk factor for developing schizophrenia.

A central conceptual issue in the investigation of the etiology of schizophrenia is whether schizophrenia is a neurodevelopmental or a neurodegenerative disorder. Is the cause of schizophrenia to be found in the failure of the normal development of the brain, or is it to be found in a disease process that alters a normally developed brain? Both, of course, may be true, because the schizophrenia syndrome probably represents more than one disease process, or a developmental abnormality may increase the risk for the subsequent occurrence of a neurodegenerative disorder. Although Kraepelin believed that schizophrenia had an early onset and was a chronic deteriorating disorder, the examination of the clinical course of the illness has not been helpful in clarifying this issue. Kraepelin eventually came to believe that there were multiple possible outcome types. This has been verified in European and North American long-term follow-up studies, in which as many as eight course types are typically described. Furthermore, subtle neurological manifestations, cognitive dysfunction, and disturbances in affect are often present early in the course of illness, usually before the onset of hallucinations and delusions, and perhaps from birth. However, it is not clear whether these abnormalities reflect abnormal brain development or are the consequences of an early lesion to a normal brain, nor is it clear whether the early morbid picture progresses into the full manifestation of psychosis or whether early morbidity represents a vulnerability state susceptible to expressing psychosis in the context of a later lesion or stressful new demands on cognition and interpersonal skills later in adolescence and early adulthood, or both. In any case, it is clear that the illness process usually plateaus within the first 5 to 10 years of psychosis and does not manifest progressive deterioration throughout the course. Late life improvement, perhaps based on lessened intensity of the psychotic component of the illness, is more typical than continued progression.

The neuropathological investigation of schizophrenia has produced somewhat less ambiguous results. Although there are sporadic reports of gliosis in schizophrenic brains, which may indicate the presence of a neurodegenerative disease process and subsequent neuropathological response, the majority of studies have failed to document the presence of gliosis. The absence of gliosis does not necessarily preclude a neurodegenerative process, because an apoptotic pathology in early development might not be associated with gliosis. However, in combination with reports of abnormal cell migration and other markers of abnormal development, the preponderance of postmortem evidence is consistent with the neurodevelopmental hypothesis of schizophrenia. Further support for a neurodevelopmental pathophysiology comes from neuropsychological, cognitive psychological, and neuroimaging findings in first-episode cases, which tend to be similar to findings in more chronic cases, although longitudinal imaging studies have suggested that patients with schizophrenia may exhibit accelerated cortical or subcortical tissue loss. Perhaps even more decisive are abnormalities in morphological features, which are believed to be developmental in nature and are associated with at least some forms of schizophrenia. Such findings range from abnormalities in peripheral development, such as finger ridge formation, to abnormal cell migration to landmarks of abnormal brain development, such as asymmetry of the planum temporale. The consistency with which the known data point to early deviations in the development of the central nervous system (CNS) has been useful in focusing theory and investigative work.

The explosion of information on the neurobiology of brain development has led to considerable new knowledge on the potential mechanisms of pathogenic influences. It is now clear that subtle deviations in the development of the brain could create dysfunctions associated with specific behaviors. Postmortem findings of abnormalities in neural plate formation, which suggest a deviation in programmed cell migration or reduced cell density, provide intriguing support for the proposition that the developmental process that establishes normal brain cytoarchitecture may have gone awry in schizophrenia. Another view is that the brain has established extensive redundancy during the developing years and that the fine-tuning that is necessary for efficient functioning involves eliminating certain nerve cells and many of the synapses connecting cells. A failure to adequately prune nerve cells and synapses or to err in selection for pruning could, in theory, underlie dysfunctions that later lead to schizophrenia symptoms. Altered nerve cell migration or pruning is speculative but illustrates plausible mechanisms by which risk factors could alter normal brain development in schizophrenia.

Principal hypotheses regarding causation include altered genes, neuroimmunovirology factors, and hypoxic or neurotoxic damage during gestation and birth.

Altered Expression of Genes Schizophrenia and schizophrenia-related disorders (i.e., schizotypal, schizoid, and paranoid personality disorders; schizophreniform disorder; and other nonaffective psychotic disorders) occur at an increased rate among the biological relatives of patients with schizophrenia. This increased rate is most dramatically illustrated in the case of monozygotic twins, who have identical genetic endowment and an approximately 50-percent concordance rate for schizophrenia. This rate is four to five times the concordance rate in dizygotic twins or the rate of occurrence found in other first-degree relatives (i.e., siblings, parents, or offspring). The role of genetic factors is further reflected in the drop-off in the occurrence of schizophrenia among second- and third-degree relatives, in whom one would hypothesize a decreased genetic loading. The finding of a higher rate of schizophrenia among the biological relatives of an adopted-away person who develops schizophrenia, as compared to the adoptive, nonbiological relatives who rear the patient, has provided further support to the overwhelming pedigree and twin study evidence suggesting a significant genetic contribution to the etiology of schizophrenia. However, the monozygotic twin data clearly demonstrate the fact that individuals who are genetically vulnerable to schizophrenia do not inevitably develop schizophrenia; environmental factors must be involved in determining a schizophrenia outcome. If a vulnerability-liability model of schizophrenia is correct in its postulation of an environmental influence, then other biological or psychosocial environmental factors may prevent or cause schizophrenia in the genetically vulnerable individual.

A major obstacle to delineating which genes are involved in schizophrenia is the fact that the modes of genetic transmission in schizophrenia are unknown. No current model (e.g., single-gene dominant or recessive, polygenetic, multifactorial, or latent trait) satisfactorily accounts for the data. Determining the mode of transmission in a putative genetic disorder requires a known phenotype and genetic homogeneity across the pedigrees. Neither of these conditions is met in schizophrenia. Nonetheless, to understand the etiology of schizophrenia, it will eventually be necessary to identify the actual genes and their products and to determine the molecular and neurobiological consequences that lead to schizophrenia pathophysiology.

Postgenomic era technologies provide an opportunity to accelerate discovery of molecular mechanisms. The application of gene expression methods, gene discovery techniques, and proteomic technology to postmortem brain tissue has the potential to identify specific cell types, genes, and proteins involved in the molecular cascade. Still early in development, these approaches offer solid potential for discovery of molecular targets as candidates for etiology and for drug development. Substantial technological and data analytical problems remain to be resolved. The delineation of the different phenotypic manifestations of the schizophrenic genes or markers of the phenotypes is critically important, for case ascertainment and in moving genetic inquiry closer to the neuronal effects of schizophrenia-related genes. Measures of oculomotor physiology (e.g., smooth pursuit eye movements), information processing (e.g., the continuous performance task and forced span-of-apprehension test), and sensory gating (e.g., P50) are prominent candidate markers. These measures have been found to distinguish patients with schizophrenia and their biological relatives from control groups. The P50 sensory gating phenomena marker is of particular interest, because it captures a basic neuronal property, whose dysfunction could be explanatory of schizophrenia pathophysiology. In linkage studies, the P50 measure has been used to define the schizophrenia phenotype, and positive linkage has been found on an area of chromosome 15 near the site of the gene for the $\alpha7$ nicotinic receptor. This receptor is thought to mediate the normal P50 sensory gating mechanism.

It has proven exceedingly difficult to progress from evidence confirming a genetic contribution to the etiology of schizophrenia to evidence implicating specific genes in the disease. Nonetheless, the area of genetic investigation is highly promising, because there is unequivocal evidence for a genetic contribution to some, perhaps all, forms of the illness, and there is presently an explosion of knowledge and techniques relevant to discovering the genetic basis for human disease. Linkage analysis has quickly moved from a few marker probes to banks of hundreds, which enables the entire genome to be examined with probes spaced along all chromosomes. Analytical techniques have been developed to evaluate polygenetic disorders, and gene substructure techniques now enable investigators to focus on candidate genes found to distinguish schizophrenia and normal control brains.

Neuroimmunovirology

Immune and viral hypotheses of schizophrenia are as old as scientific knowledge in these areas. Louis Pasteur confirmed that a virus could cause a neuropsychiatric disease when he isolated the rabies virus in 1881. However, schizophrenia is not an acute encephalitis or a fulminating infection. More subtle pathophysiological mechanisms are involved that make it more difficult to establish etiology. Furthermore, the epidemiological data supporting an infectious theory, although interesting, are weak. Schizophrenia may have a north to south prevalence gradient (south to north in the Southern hemisphere), may be endemic to a few areas (e.g., northern Sweden), has a winter birth excess, and, similar to multiple sclerosis (MS), has monozygotic twin discordance. However, it has been difficult to conduct definitive studies of immunovirological hypotheses because any potential marker of an immune or viral process associated with schizophrenia is applicable to only some cases of schizophrenia and is subject to interpretation as being secondary to conditions associated with the disease (e.g., crowding of chronically hospitalized patients, exposure of chronic patients living in low socioeconomic circumstances, and poor health habits).

Viral theories remain popular, despite the difficulty in validating any particular version. Their popularity stems from the fact that several specific viral theories have the power to explain the particular localization of pathology necessary to account for a range of manifestations in schizophrenia without overt febrile encephalitis. There are six general pathogenic models of viral and immune pathophysiology relevant to schizophrenia. These are retroviral infection, current or active viral infection, past viral infection, virally activated immunopathology, autoimmune pathology, and secondary influences (i.e., in utero exposure to maternal infection).

Retroviral Infection

A retrovirus can insert itself into the genome and thereby alter the expression of the host's own genes and the genes of the host's offspring toward the development of schizophrenia (the virogene hypothesis). There is conflicting evidence for the hypothesis. Retroviral sequences have been identified in postmortem brain tissue from patients with schizophrenia. In contrast, retrovirus-associated enzymes that would be present in an active infection but not in a virogene scenario have not been successfully identified.

Current or Active Viral Infection

Viruses with an affinity for the CNS have been postulated to be involved in the etiology of schizophrenia. It is envisioned that a neurotropic virus infects nerve cells in discrete parts of the brain and causes sustained alterations in the functioning of the involved neural systems or that byproducts of a viral infection have direct toxic effects on nerve cell functioning. An alternative formulation of this hypothesis is based on the observation that viruses can infect the brain, with substantive disease manifestations only showing up many years later. In theory, this could account for the subtle early manifestations frequently observed in schizophrenic patients that are followed by more intense symptom manifestations 10 to 30 years later.

A substantial challenge to either formulation of the current or active viral infection hypothesis is the absence of direct evidence substantiating a viral etiology, including the lack of physical signs of encephalitis (e.g., lymphocytic infiltrate) in postmortem tissue and the failure to recover or to isolate a putative agent.

Past Viral Infection

The past viral infection hypothesis posits a virus infecting certain brain tissues early in life to create a vulnerability to schizophrenia or as a causal mechanism for the initial illness processes that later lead to the picture of classical schizophrenia. The resulting tissue damage produces long-lasting alterations in neural systems, leading to schizophrenia manifestations without persistent viral infection.

Virally Activated Immunopathology

One of two general mechanisms is proposed in the category of virally activated immunopathology. The first is based on the observation that viruses are normally endogenous to the human brain and have a discontinuous or focal distribution in the brain. Periodic viral reactivation of these foci normally does not result in psychotic symptoms. However, in an individual with a genetically or environmentally determined abnormal immune response to viruses, it is hypothesized that viral reactivation would result in an induction of schizophrenic psychopathology. This theory regards the products of immunoreactivity as the mediators of the pathogenic influence. The second mechanism in this category is that the virus may induce the host to fail to recognize its own tissues as "self" and, as a consequence, to mount a destructive immune response. The virus may do this by altering some cellular component, such as normally cryptic neural cell surface proteins, causing it to stimulate a host response. A cytotoxic or antibody response would cause direct interference of nerve cell function by destruction of the cells or, in the case of receptor proteins, altered neurotransmission.

Autoimmune Pathology

Schizophrenia has been hypothesized to be an idiopathic autoimmune disease, such as rheumatoid arthritis or systemic lupus erythematosus, wherein, for reasons not entirely clear but probably involving genetics, some tissues are not recognized as self and become the target of immune response.

Secondary Influences: In Utero Exposure to Maternal Infection

A number of epidemiological studies have reported that women who are exposed to influenza epidemics during the second trimester of pregnancy are more likely to give birth to offspring at increased risk for schizophrenia. This observation raises the possibility that some attribute of maternal infection, such as fever or cytokine activation, perturbs normal brain development during the period of active neural cell migration. This interesting etiological lead has been challenged by studies that have attempted to assess whether the mother was actually infected, rather than simply being exposed to an epidemic. There is also evidence that prenatal rubella infection may increase the risk for development of schizophrenia and other nonaffective psychotic disorders.

Birth and Pregnancy Complications

Studies, across a broad range of methodological approaches, have repeatedly demonstrated an association between obstetrical complications and an increased risk of schizophrenia. Prospective, population-based studies suggest three major classes of complications that are associated with schizophrenia: (1) pregnancy complications (i.e., bleeding, diabetes, preeclampsia, and Rh incompatibility), (2) abnormal fetal growth and development (i.e., low birth weight, congenital malformations, and reduced head circumference), and (3) delivery complications (i.e., asphyxia, emergency cesarean section, and uterine atony). However, the mechanisms underlying these associations have not been established. The following plausible explanations, which are not mutually exclusive, guide present-day research.

- The genes that create vulnerability for schizophrenia may also alter early embryonic development in a manner that leads to increased likelihood of birth and pregnancy complications.

- Early gestational adverse events influence the developing brain and create an increased risk for birth complications and schizophrenia. The potential role of Rh incompatibility as a risk factor for schizophrenia is an interesting example of this proposition.
- Gestational or birth complications may cause hypoxic damage. Brain regions most frequently implicated as deviant in schizophrenia (e.g., hippocampus) are among the most sensitive areas in the developing brain to hypoxia.

PATHOPHYSIOLOGY

Because schizophrenia represents a disturbance in some, but not all, brain functions, it is reasonable to suppose that specific brain regions or neural circuits are involved and that the manifestations of schizophrenia must necessarily involve altered processing of physiological information; this altered processing would be, in turn, dependent on disturbances of cytoarchitectural, biochemical, or electrophysiological properties of the neural systems, or a combination of these.

Throughout most of this century, examination of postmortem brain tissue has been the principal source of data bearing on the neuroanatomy of schizophrenia. Early reference to schizophrenia as "the graveyard of neuropathology" was not because of a lack of neuropathological findings but rather because of the lack of a discernible pattern in the frequently observed pathological findings and the possibility that deviations were artifactual in nature or were a consequence, rather than a cause, of the disease. For example, head trauma and viral infections affecting the brain would be more common in crowded custodial hospitals than in typical comparison groups. Moreover, the widespread use of antipsychotic drugs in the treatment of schizophrenia introduced additional artifacts in the investigation of brain pathophysiology. Finally, knowledge of brain and behavioral relationships was not sufficiently detailed to guide neuropathological inquiry during much of this century.

Scientists have long been keenly aware of the necessity for the development of noninvasive techniques to study brain structure and function in living patients. This is particularly important in the absence of valid animal models. During the middle one-third of the 20th century, pneumoencephalography (PEG) provided substantial evidence for enlarged brain ventricles, suggesting diminished tissue in schizophrenia compared to controls. Electroencephalography (EEG) provided information on cortical surface electrical activity, but neither PEG nor EEG techniques could provide a comprehensive evaluation of human brain structure or function.

The development of structural (e.g., computerized axial tomography [CAT] and magnetic resonance imaging [MRI]) and functional (e.g., positron emission tomography [PET], single photon emission computed tomography [SPECT], functional MRI, magnetoencephalography, and magnetic resonance spectroscopy) in vivo imaging techniques have made possible a more detailed view of brain structure and physiology. These techniques have become available at a time when a better understanding of the interconnections between cortical and subcortical structures and their implications for brain and behavior relations is emerging from preclinical studies of the brain. CAT studies have replicated the PEG observation of enlarged ventricles and have further shown that a substantial proportion of patients with schizophrenia, in comparison to normal controls, exhibits increased sulcal widening. These results suggest that patients with schizophrenia may have relatively less brain tissue, a condition that could represent a failure to develop or a subsequent loss of tissue. MRI, with its enhanced gray and white matter resolution, is able to provide a far more detailed assessment of specific brain structures. Studies using MRI have found evidence in patients with schizophrenia for decreased cortical gray matter in the prefrontal and temporal cortex; cerebral white matter fiber tract alterations; decreased volume of limbic system structures, for example, the amygdala, hippocampus, and entorhinal cortex and the thalamus; and increased volume of basal ganglia nuclei. These findings are consistent with the findings of neuropathological examinations of postmortem tissue, including ultrastructural examination, which, in some cases, indicate cell loss, misalignment of cells, altered membrane and intracellular structure and protein expression, or a combination of these.

Structural findings may help clarify the meaning of altered patterns of function. Functional imaging studies have documented abnormal patterns of glucose metabolism or blood flow during performance of specific cognitive tasks. These techniques are also able to provide insights into the functional neuroanatomy of the various symptom complexes that characterize patients with schizophrenia. Functional imaging studies of actively hallucinating patients have implicated components of the language and anterior cingulate basal ganglia thalamocortical neural circuits (Fig. 12.1–1). In contrast, several studies have demonstrated an association of primary, enduring negative symptoms and decreased glucose metabolism or blood flow of the dorsolateral prefrontal and the inferior parietal cortices (Fig. 12.1–2).

Present-day knowledge of the pathophysiology of schizophrenia is acquired from the study of living subjects by using structural and functional imaging and anatomically relevant symptom and neurocognitive assessment techniques. These technologies are supplemented by advances in postmortem biochemical, molecular, and

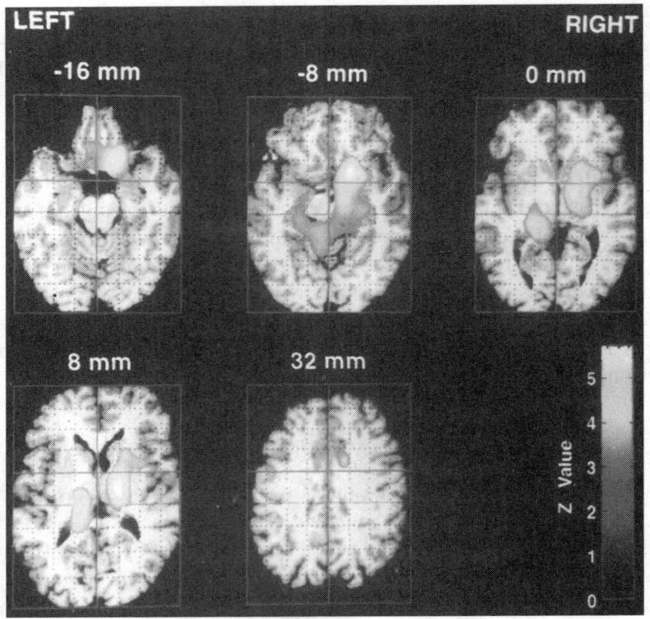

FIGURE 12.1–1 Axial sections demonstrating brain areas with significantly increased activity during auditory verbal hallucinations in the group study. Functional positron emission tomography results (threshold at $Z > 3.09$, $P < .001$, by reference to the unit normal distribution) are displayed, superimposed on a single structural T1-weighted magnetic resonance imaging scan that has been transformed into the Talairach space for anatomical reference. Section numbers refer to the distance from the anterior commissure–posterior commissure line, with positive numbers being superior to the line. The areas of activation extend into the amygdala bilaterally and into the right orbitofrontal cortex. Although these regions of extension are consistent with the limbic paralimbic component of activity during hallucinations and may contribute to drive and affect in this context, definitive statements cannot be made in the absence of discrete maxima. (See Color Plate.) (From Silbersweig DA, Stern E, Frith C, et al.: A functional neuroanatomy of hallucinations in schizophrenia. *Nature.* 1995;378:1769, with permission.)

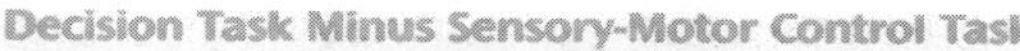

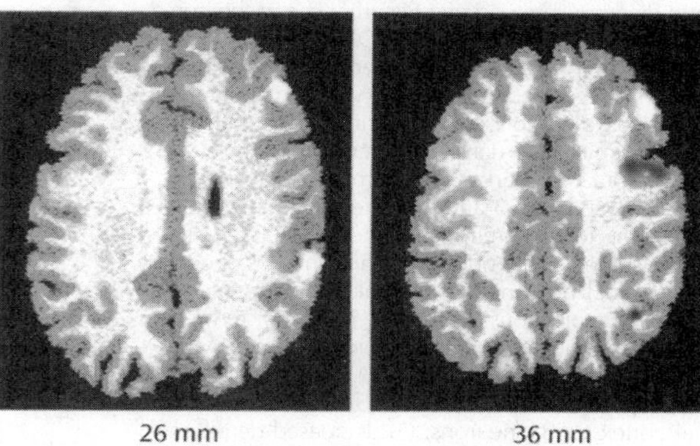

FIGURE 12.1–2 Brain regions activated more in ten schizophrenic patients without primary negative symptoms than in eight patients with primary negative symptoms deficit schizophrenia during a sensory-motor control task and a decision task. As shown in the **left panel**, the regions significantly more activated in nondeficit than deficit patients during the control task were the right and left middle frontal cortex. Right cluster size: 104 voxels with a maximum Z score of 2.61. Left cluster size: 316 voxels with a maximum Z score of 3.98. As shown in the **right panel**, the regions significantly more activated in the nondeficit patients during the decision task were the right middle frontal two clusters and inferior parietal cortices. Right frontal cluster sizes: 299 voxels with a maximum Z score of 4.81 and 138 voxels with a maximum Z score of 3.28. Right inferior parietal cluster size: 185 voxels with a maximum Z score of 3.32. (From Lahti AC, Holcomb HH, Medoff DR: Abnormal patterns of regional cerebral blood flow in schizophrenia with primary negative symptoms during an effortful auditory recognition task. *Am J Psychiatry.* 2001;158:1797–1808, with permission.)

structural evaluations to test increasingly sophisticated neuroanatomical and biochemical theories of schizophrenia.

Major Neuroanatomical Theories

Over the last 25 years, there has been a gradual evolution from conceptualizing schizophrenia as a disorder that involves discrete areas of the brain to a perspective that views schizophrenia as a disorder of brain neural circuits. These neural circuit models of the pathophysiology of schizophrenia posit that a structural or functional lesion disrupts the functional integrity of the entire circuit. There are several factors that have contributed to this change in perspective. First, the delineation of the neuroanatomy of the different neurotransmitter pathways has led to an increased appreciation of how different brain regions are connected with each other and how cortical and subcortical structures are able to reciprocally regulate the function of each other. For example, the identification of the mesolimbic and mesocortical dopaminergic pathways contributed to the development of neuroanatomical hypotheses implicating the prefrontal cortex or limbic system, or both, in the pathophysiology of schizophrenia. The further delineation of the reciprocal regulatory pathways between the prefrontal cortex and the limbic system, particularly the hippocampus, led to more recent formulations of these hypotheses, in which limbic and prefrontal neuroanatomical models of schizophrenia have been integrated into a single unifying neurodevelopmental theory of schizophrenia. These hypotheses propose that an early developmental lesion of the dopaminergic tracts to the prefrontal cortex results in the disturbance of prefrontal and limbic system function and leads to the positive and negative symptoms and cognitive impairments observed in patients with schizophrenia.

Prefrontal cortex and limbic system hypotheses are the predominant neuroanatomical hypotheses of schizophrenia. The demonstration of decreased prefrontal gray or white matter volumes, or both; prefrontal cortical interneuron abnormalities; disturbed prefrontal metabolism and blood flow; decreased hippocampal and entorhinal cortex volume; disarray or abnormal migration of hippocampal and entorhinal neurons, or both, provides strong support for the involvement of these brain regions in the pathophysiology of schizophrenia. Of particular interest in the context of neural circuit hypotheses linking the prefrontal cortex and limbic system are studies demonstrating a relationship between hippocampal morphological abnormalities and disturbances in prefrontal cortex metabolism or function, or both.

A second contributing factor to the adoption of a neural circuit conceptual framework has been the increased understanding of how the brain is organized into local microcircuits, consisting of the connections among afferent and efferent neurons and interneurons (Fig. 12.1–3), and macrocircuits. An example of the latter are the segregated parallel basal ganglia thalamocortical neural circuits, which connect the cerebral cortex, through the basal ganglia, with the thalamus (Fig. 12.1–4). Each of these circuits is hypothesized to subserve a discrete range of functions. A number of investigators have used these circuits as a starting point for their hypotheses of schizophrenic pathophysiology. These hypotheses primarily differ from each other on their point of emphasis. For example, integrating data from animal studies and neurobehavioral and functional and structural imaging studies in humans, it has been hypothesized that dysfunction of the anterior cingulate basal ganglia thalamocortical circuit underlies the production of positive psychotic symptoms, whereas dysfunction of the dorsolateral prefrontal circuit underlies the production of primary, enduring, negative or deficit symptoms.

A third factor has been the elucidation of the neural basis of cognitive functions observed to be impaired in patients with schizophrenia. The observation of the relationship among impaired working memory performance; disrupted prefrontal neuronal integrity; altered prefrontal, cingulate, and inferior parietal cortex; and hippocampal blood flow provides strong support for disruption of the normal working memory neural circuit in patients with schizophrenia. Similarly, the delineation of the neural circuits for language and attention and information processing has influenced the conceptualization of schizophrenia pathophysiology. The classical language circuit, which includes Broca's and Wernicke's areas and associated cortical and subcortical structures, has been hypothesized to be involved in the production of hallucinations, delusions, and positive formal thought disorder. This hypothesis is the most important alternative to the anterior cingulate hypothesis for positive psychotic symptoms. The involvement of this circuit, at least for auditory hallucinations, has been documented in a number of functional imaging studies contrasting hallucinating versus nonhallucinating patients.

Sensory processing abnormalities are routinely observed in patients with schizophrenia. The type of abnormalities range from disturbances in sensory gating to disturbances in visual information processing. The latter impairments have been argued to be selec-

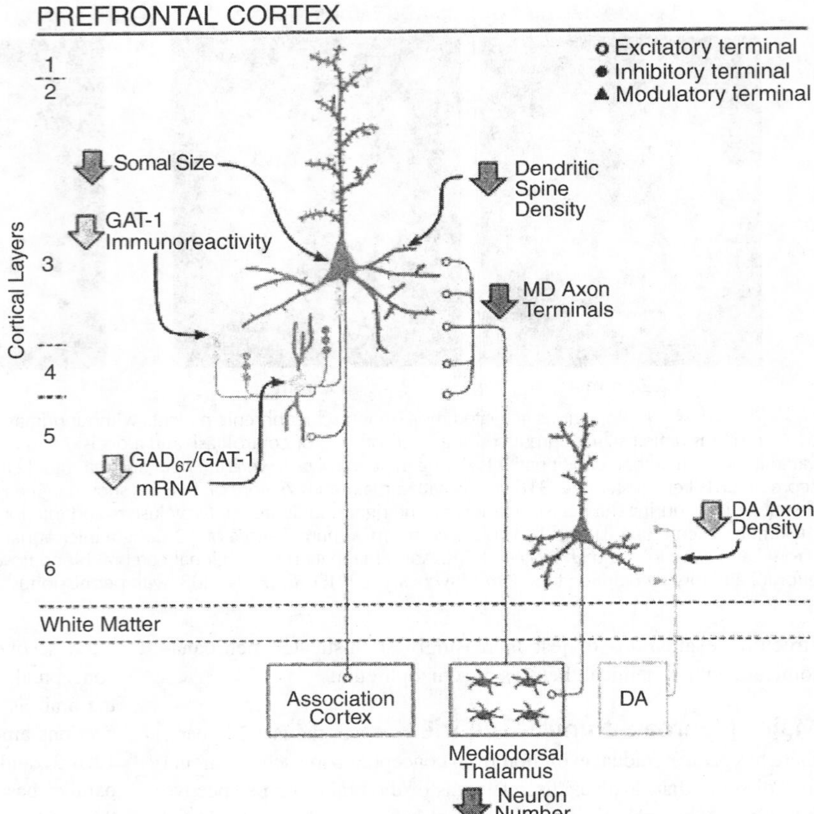

FIGURE 12.1–3 Cortical circuitry in schizophrenia. Schematic diagram summarizing disturbances in the connectivity between the mediodorsal (MD) thalamic nucleus and the dorsal prefrontal cortex in schizophrenia. Postmortem studies have reported that subjects with schizophrenia have (1) decreased number of neurons in the MD thalamic nucleus; (2) diminished density of parvalbumin-positive varicosities, a putative marker of thalamic axon terminals, selectively in deep layers 3 and 4, the termination zone of MD projections to the prefrontal cortex; (3) preferential reduction in spine density on the basilar dendrites of deep layer 3 pyramidal neurons, a principal synaptic target of the excitatory projections from the MD; (4) reduced expression of the messenger ribonucleic acid (mRNA) for glutamic acid decarboxylase (GAD_{67}), the synthesizing enzyme for γ-aminobutyric acid (GABA), in a subset of prefrontal cortex GABA neurons; (5) decreased density of GABA transporter (GAT-1)–immunoreactive axon cartridges, the distinctive, vertically arrayed axon terminals of GABAergic chandelier neurons, which synapse exclusively on the axon initial segment of pyramidal neurons; and (6) decreased dopamine (DA) innervation of layer 6, the principal location of pyramidal neurons that provide corticothalamic feedback projections. (From Lewis DA, Lieberman JA: Catching up on schizophrenia: Natural history and neurobiology. *Neuron.* 2000;28:325, with permission. See this article for additional details and references.)

tively related to negative symptoms. The overlap between brain regions that have been implicated in the production of negative symptoms and the visual information processing neural circuit, which includes inferior and superior parietal and prefrontal cortices, caudate and thalamic nuclei, and the reticular activating system, provides a neuroanatomical rationale for the relationship between these two dimensions of schizophrenia and a conceptual framework for future studies of the neuroanatomy of negative symptoms.

The development of neural circuit hypotheses offers tremendous advantages to the investigation of the neuroanatomy of schizophrenia. First, these hypotheses more accurately reflect the actual organization of the brain. Second, computational models of neural circuit hypotheses can be developed to investigate how perturbations of circuit function can lead to signs and symptoms of schizophrenia. Neural circuit models have been created for the cognitive and symptom manifestations of schizophrenia. Third, neural circuit hypotheses provide a conceptual framework for hypothesis-testing studies and optimize the interpretation of information derived from current brain imaging and postmortem studies. Finally, the use of neural circuit models implicates brain regions not typically conceptualized as being central to the neuroanatomy of schizophrenia. The thalamus and cerebellum are but two examples of this issue.

Major Biochemical Theories Information is processed in neural circuits through the transmission of an electrical signal through a nerve cell axon and across synapses to postsynaptic receptors on other nerve cell components. Nerve cells generally receive, process, and send signals to and from thousands of other cells. The transmission of the signal across the synapse and the processing of the signal within a cell require a complex series of biochemical events. The entire operation involves a number of steps requiring large amounts of energy and involving gene expression and the synthesis and degradation of proteins. It is evident that physiological function in any brain system involves the chemistry of that system and that dysfunction can emanate from these biochemical processes. It is, therefore, natural to presume that the biochemistry of the brain plays a fundamental role in the disruptions of brain function involved in schizophrenia. The move from a general concept of the biochemistry of schizophrenia to specific theories is based on three principal sources of knowledge. The first source is an ever-increasing understanding of intracellular communication from the cell membrane to the genetic material of the nucleus and of intercellular communication through the various neurotransmitter systems of the brain. The second is increased knowledge of the basic pharmacology of behavior and cognitive functions. The third is knowledge of the mechanism of action of drugs that can induce schizophrenia-like behaviors or that alter symptom expression in patients with schizophrenia. These three sources of knowledge have led to biochemical hypotheses involving dopamine, noradrenaline, serotonin, acetylcholine, glutamate, and several neuromodulatory peptides or their receptors. Because there are many possibilities, it is important to understand the general development of a biochemical hypothesis of schizophrenia. The dopamine hypothesis is the most prominent and enduring hypothesis.

Dopamine and Schizophrenia The hyperdopaminergic hypothesis of schizophrenia arose from two sets of observations of drug action on the dopaminergic system. Drugs that increase dopamine system activity, such as amphetamine, cocaine, L-dopa, and methylphenidate (Ritalin), can induce a paranoid psychosis that is

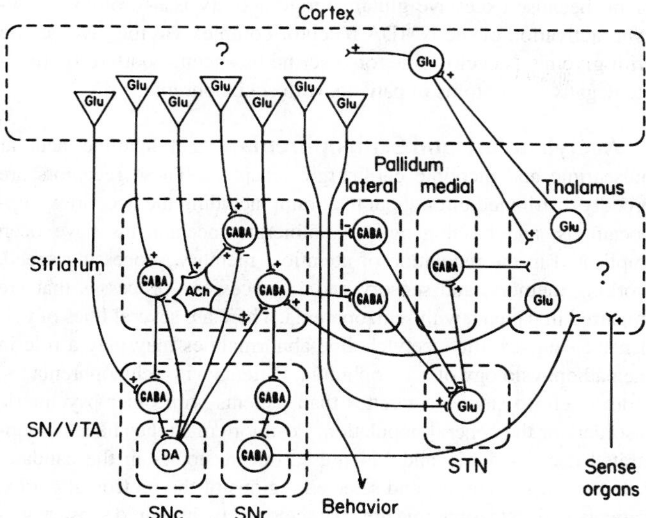

FIGURE 12.1–4 A tentative scheme of interactions between glutamate (Glu) and dopamine (DA) in the basal ganglia. The cholinergic interneuron in the striatum is a large, spiny cell with a rich collateral network that can be assumed to make synaptic contacts with a large number of other striatal cells. The cholinergic interneuron receives a cortical glutamatergic input on its soma, while its axon terminals are in synaptic contact with medium-sized, spiny γ-aminobutyric acid (GABA)ergic output neurons. Only two such GABA neurons are shown, but, in reality, it is reasonable to assume that one cholinergic neuron innervates many GABAergic neurons. The cholinergic interneuron also makes contact (although perhaps not forming a real synapse) with dopaminergic nerve terminals. From the way in which the synapses are drawn here, the cortex would be able to control the activity in the GABAergic output neurons projecting to the thalamus via the medial segment of the globus pallidus (partly via the subthalamic nucleus [STN] and substantia nigra pars reticulata [SNr]). In this manner, the cortex can selectively suppress impulse flow in one subpopulation of GABAergic projection neurons while facilitating impulse flow in another subpopulation, thus presumably enabling a meaningful behavior by suppressing irrelevant locomotor programs. The importance of glutamatergic pathways for maintaining a purposeful behavior is revealed by the primitive locomotor pattern that results from treatment with the *N*-methyl-D-aspartate antagonist MK-801.

For the sake of simplification, the different thalamic nuclei are not shown. Conceivably, striatopallidothalamic neurons can influence the entire thalamus via, for example, the reticular nucleus, which communicates with all other thalamic nuclei. Apart from the corticostriatal glutamatergic pathway, there are at least three other corticifugal systems that the cortex can use to protect itself from overstimulation: (1) the corticonigral projection; (2) the corticothalamic projection, which terminates in the thalamic intralaminar nuclei, from which a thalamostriatal projection originates; and (3) the corticosubthalamic projection. ACh, acetylcholine; SN, substantia nigra; SNc, substantia nigra pars compacta; VTA, ventral tegmental area. (From Carlsson M, Carlsson A: Interactions between glutamatergic and monoaminergic systems within the basal ganglia-implications for schizophrenia and Parkinson's disease. *Trends Neurosci.* 1990;13:896, with permission.)

similar to some aspects of schizophrenia. When administered to patients with schizophrenia, these compounds may produce a transitory worsening of hallucinations, delusions, and thought disturbance. In contrast, drugs that have the capacity to block postsynaptic dopamine receptors reduce the symptoms of schizophrenia. Substantial evidence supports the role of postsynaptic dopamine blockade as an initiating factor in a cascade of events responsible for the therapeutic action of antipsychotic drugs. Other mechanisms, such as depolarization blockade, have been implicated as plausible explanations for long-term antipsychotic effects. That these actions are actually corrective for the pathophysiological disturbance in schizophrenia is suggested by the capacity of dopamine-stimulating drugs to worsen symptoms of schizophrenia or to induce psychosis. This rationale for the role of dopamine excess, particularly for the positive symptom aspect of schizophrenia, is compelling.

However, despite the compelling rationale for the role of dopamine in schizophrenia, testing the hypothesis has proven problematic. In general, clinical studies, across a broad range of indices of dopamine metabolism, have been characterized by marked variability in results. Studies aimed at measuring abnormal concentrations of dopamine or its metabolites in blood, urine, and spinal fluid are confronted by problems that are almost insurmountable. In large fluid compartments, alterations in dopamine metabolism associated with schizophrenia represent only a minor contribution to the particular index of dopamine metabolism; spinal fluid necessarily provides a summation of total brain activity, most of which is not considered germane to schizophrenia, and blood and urine provide even more indirect indices.

Imaging studies have produced more compelling evidence for dopamine involvement. Several studies have used the following paradigm to investigate abnormal dopamine metabolism: Patients with schizophrenia are infused with an indirect dopamine agonist (e.g., amphetamine), and then the extent to which radioligand occupancy of postsynaptic dopamine receptors is reduced by competition with endogenous dopamine is determined. The comparison of pre- and postinfusion radioligand occupancy provides an index of dopamine release and reuptake rates. These studies have demonstrated excessive dopamine release in patients with schizophrenia, which may be related to the severity of their positive psychotic symptoms. PET studies of dopamine receptor distribution and the density of receptor expression offer an alternative approach for examining the dopamine hypothesis. This approach has been used to document an increase in dopamine type 2 (D_2) receptors in the caudate nucleus of drug-free patients with schizophrenia and has been applied to other dopamine receptors (i.e., D_1 receptor) and brain regions, including the prefrontal and anterior cingulate cortices. There is evidence of altered D_1 and D_2 receptor distribution in these areas, but replication of these preliminary results is required.

Finally, there is the potential for the relatively precise biochemical study of dopamine in postmortem tissue, but here, as with the use of body fluids, sources of artifact and imprecision have been difficult to manage. The concentration of a neurotransmitter in any tissue is altered as cellular components break down after death and as small differences in dissection from brain to brain take place. The administration of antipsychotic drugs during life almost always confounds the biochemistry of postmortem tissue, and one can rarely be sure of the extent to which any biochemical finding is directly related to the schizophrenic disease process. In addition, there are a large number of candidate areas for brain dysfunction, so that one may easily examine the wrong location. It is also quite possible that brain areas may exhibit biochemical dysfunction during discrete periods of development but that these abnormalities are no longer present at the time of death or that the biochemistry of death may obscure the biochemistry of life. Despite these methodological limitations, postmortem studies have confirmed the elevation of striatal D_2 postsynaptic receptors observed in PET studies. There have also been reports of increased dopamine concentrations in the amygdala, decreased density of the dopamine transporter, and increased numbers of dopamine type 4 (D_4) receptors in entorhinal cortex.

Although conclusive evidence for the hyperdopaminergic hypothesis has been elusive, the hypothesis remains a viable explanation for the positive symptoms of schizophrenia. It is a particularly robust proposition for explaining the effect of antipsychotic drugs. Interestingly, in the context of the investigation of the hypothesis, recent studies have suggested the possibility that a dopamine deficiency may also occur in patients with schizophrenia. For example, several studies have observed that patients with negative symptoms have lower plasma or cerebrospinal fluid (CSF) homovanillic acid (HVA) concentrations. Also, patients with influenza encephalitis, who were mistaken for having schizophrenia, tended to have emotional dullness and low drive. Similarities in these cases with aspects of Parkinson's disease (which is known to involve loss of dopamine neurons) and the fact that some of these postencephalitic patients developed Parkinson's disease lend support to a dopamine deficiency hypothesis for the negative symptom aspect of schizophrenia. In addition, antipsychotic drugs, which are dopamine antagonists, produce behaviors suggestive of negative symptoms of schizophrenia in animals and humans free of mental illness. These observations have led to a reformulation of the dopamine hypothesis, which incorporates the possibility of concomitant dopamine excess and deficiency. Dopamine excess would be restricted to the dopaminergic pathways projecting to the basal ganglia and limbic system and would account for the positive psychotic symptoms, whereas dopamine deficiency would be restricted to the mesocortical pathways and would account for the negative symptoms of schizophrenia.

Glutamate and Schizophrenia Glutamate is the major excitatory neurotransmitter in the brain and mediates cortical–cortical, cortical–subcortical, and thalamic–cortical transmission. Glutamate binds to ionotropic and metabotropic receptors. The ionotropic receptors include the *N*-methyl-D-aspartate (NMDA) receptor complex, kainate, and α-amino-3-hydroxy-5-methyl-4-isoxazolepropionic acid (AMPA). Interest in the possible role of glutamate in the pathophysiology of schizophrenia has emerged from an increased understanding of the role of NMDA in the regulation of behavior and cognition; an increased understanding of the interactions between glutamatergic and dopaminergic, cholinergic, and γ-aminobutyric acid (GABA)ergic systems; observations of abnormal NMDA receptor binding in the prefrontal cortex and abnormal NMDA messenger ribonucleic acid (mRNA) expression in the hippocampus in patients with schizophrenia; and observations of the acute and chronic effects of phencyclidine (PCP) and related compounds. Acute administration of PCP produces symptoms that have been argued to mimic the positive and negative symptoms of schizophrenia. Chronic PCP administration produces a hypodopaminergic state in the prefrontal cortex; a state that has been argued to result in negative symptoms. PCP occupies receptors within the open calcium channels of the NMDA receptor complex, thereby blocking ion flow. PCP and its analog, ketamine, interfere with glutamatergic transmission. In addition to the observation of schizophrenia-like symptomatology in humans abusing PCP, ketamine has been used in the experimental laboratory and has been observed to produce transitory mild manifestations of positive and negative symptoms in normal volunteers and a transitory and mild worsening of positive symptoms in patients with schizophrenia. Activation of dopamine receptors inhibiting glutamatergic neurons or decreased NMDA-mediated inhibition of dopamine neurons, directly or through the actions of GABAergic interneurons, could be associated with a dopamine-excess psychosis. There is also emerging evidence to support the involvement of the other two ionotropic receptors. Postmortem studies have documented abnormal kainate and AMPA receptor binding in the cerebral cortex and abnormal AMPA mRNA expression in the hippocampus of patients with schizophrenia. These considerations support a hypoglutamatergic hypothesis for schizophrenia pathophysiology and predict a therapeutic effect for compounds activating the NMDA receptor complex. This is a difficult strategy to implement, because excessive glutamatergic activity is neurotoxic; however, activation of the NMDA receptor complex via the glycine site with glycine, D-cycloserine, or D-serine has been reported to alleviate negative symptoms in patients with schizophrenia.

Acetylcholine and Schizophrenia Acetylcholine acts at muscarinic and nicotinic cholinergic receptors. These receptors are broadly distributed throughout the brain, including the neocortex, hippocampus, and basal ganglia. Cholinergic mechanisms have been implicated in the regulation of attention, memory, processing speed, working memory, and sensory gating processes—processes that are impaired in patients with schizophrenia. There are several lines of evidence to suggest that acetylcholine abnormalities may play a role in the pathophysiology of schizophrenia. Patients with schizophrenia are more likely to smoke cigarettes than patients with other psychiatric disorders or the general population. Postmortem studies have demonstrated decreased M1 and M4 muscarinic receptors in the caudate-putamen, hippocampus, and selected regions of the prefrontal cortex. Patients with schizophrenia are characterized by impaired sensory gating, including impaired performance on the P50 sensory gating paradigm. The α7 nicotinic receptor plays an important role in normal sensory gating function, smoking reverses P50 impairments in patients with schizophrenia, and, in families with patients with schizophrenia, impaired P50 performance is linked with the chromosome 15 region that contains the gene for the α7 nicotinic receptor. Patients with schizophrenia have been shown to have decreased α7 nicotinic receptors in the hippocampus. The α4β2 nicotinic receptor has been shown to regulate dopamine, serotonin, GABA, and glutamate release, which suggests that this receptor may play a pivotal role in the regulation of neurotransmitter systems that are involved in cognition. Postmortem studies have demonstrated abnormal regulation of these receptors in patients with schizophrenia.

The glutamatergic and cholinergic hypotheses exemplify a major transition that has occurred recently in the biochemistry of schizophrenia. Before this transition, observations of drug actions in schizophrenia first led to clinical treatment and then to the advancement of the pathophysiological theory of schizophrenia. With the ever-increasing knowledge of the neural organization of the brain and of the various properties and receptor sites of neurotransmitters, it is now possible to postulate pathophysiological theory first and then attempt to derive new clinical treatment from theory. There is now reason for substantial optimism that new treatment approaches will be developed more rapidly in the future, based on a broader range of pathophysiological hypotheses and the availability of animal models for aspects of the illness not therapeutically responsive to dopamine blockade–based medications.

Other Neurotransmitters and Neuromodulators Any neurotransmitter involved in neural systems subserving behaviors whose disruption could result in symptoms of schizophrenia is naturally of interest in schizophrenia theory and research. The rich innervation of the frontal cortex and limbic system with serotonergic neurons, the modulatory effect of these neurons on dopaminergic neurons, and the involvement of these pathways in the regulation of a broad range of complex functions have led several investigators to posit a pathophysiological role for serotonin in schizophrenia. These hypotheses have taken various forms over the course of the last five decades. In the early 1950s, a serotonergic deficiency hypothesis was proposed for schizophrenia. Observations of hallucinations in subjects who had ingested lysergic acid diethylamide (LSD), a compound that is chemically similar to serotonin and blocks serotonin receptor sites, furthered the hyposerotonin hypothesis. However, drugs that decrease serotonin activity tend to reduce schizophrenic symptoms (e.g., reserpine [Serpalan] and clozapine [Clozaril]) and have diminished interest in the deficiency hypothesis. Of greater current interest are hypotheses positing a serotonin excess as causative of positive and negative symptomatology. The robust serotonergic antagonist activity of clozapine and other new or second-generation antipsychotics, coupled with the demonstrated effectiveness of clozapine for positive symptoms in chronic, treatment-resistant patients, has contributed to the current emphasis on this proposition. However, several studies have raised questions about the efficacy of serotonin antagonists for negative symptoms broadly defined or persistent, primary negative symptoms. Moreover, pharmacological modification of serotonin systems with specific serotonergic agents has not produced impressive clinical results.

A similar rationale can be applied to construct hypotheses implicating norepinephrine in the psychopathology of schizophrenia. Anhedonia, that is, the impaired capacity for emotional gratification and the decreased ability to experience pleasure, has long been noted to be a prominent feature of schizophrenia. A selective neuronal degeneration within the norepinephrine reward neural system could account for this aspect of schizophrenic symptomatology. However, biochemical and pharmacological data bearing on this proposal are inconclusive. As with dopamine and serotonin, there have been noradrenergic excess and deficiency pathophysiological hypotheses.

GABA is the major inhibitory neurotransmitter. There have been several studies that have documented GABAergic interneuron abnormalities in the prefrontal cortex of patients with schizophrenia. GABAergic interneurons regulate glutamatergic activity and are also involved in hippocampal sensory gating neural circuits. Benzodiazepines have been shown to have a modest antipsychotic effect. These considerations provide a strong rationale for a GABAergic role in the pathophysiology of schizophrenia.

Neuromodulatory hypotheses focus on the fact that neuropeptides, such as substance P and neurotensin, are colocalized with the catecholamine and indolamine neurotransmitters and influence the action of these neurotransmitters. Alterations in neuromodulatory mechanisms could facilitate, inhibit, or otherwise alter the pattern of firing in these neuronal systems. Explorations of neuromodulator hypotheses are preliminary and inconclusive.

Integrative Hypotheses The natural evolution of pathophysiological hypotheses of schizophrenia is the development of comprehensive models that integrate neuroanatomical and biochemical hypotheses. The superimposition of the neurotransmitters involved in the connections among cortical, basal ganglia, and thalamic structures that comprise the basal ganglia thalamocortical neural circuits is a prime example of this approach (Fig. 12.1–3). The cerebral cortex, through glutamate projections from the cortex to the basal ganglia, facilitates the performance of selected behaviors while inhibiting others. The excitatory glutamatergic neurons terminate on GABAergic and cholinergic neurons that, in turn, provide a feedback mechanism for glutamatergic excitation and suppress or excite dopaminergic neurons and other neurons. This regulatory activity can enable the cortex to protect itself from overstimulation from thalamocortical neurons. The elucidation of the neuroanatomy and biochemistry of cortical microcircuits has also served as a starting point for the articulation of pathophysiological hypotheses of schizophrenia. These integrative models provide a framework for identifying potential neurotransmitter targets for drug development, as well as providing explanatory models for the observed effects of pharmacological agents in patients with schizophrenia, for example, PCP-induced psychotic symptoms mediated through the interactions of glutamate and other neurotransmitter systems in the neocortex, basal ganglia, or limbic system structures, or a combination of these.

DIAGNOSIS

Issues relating to the validity and reliability of schizophrenia diagnoses are a distant echo in discussions of classification. Current attention is conceptual and theoretical. Is schizophrenia one disease or many? What are the endophenotypes? Where will future boundaries between schizophrenia and affective psychoses be drawn? Will the various functional psychoses of the last century turn out to be one psychotic illness on a severity continuum? What are the implications of multigenetic and multifactorial etiological constructs?

Although 20th century views of schizophrenia varied substantially across time and diagnostic schools, there has been substantial agreement among diagnosticians throughout the world and between seemingly divergent diagnostic approaches in the recognition of typical cases of schizophrenia, at least where the presence of positive psychotic symptoms was required. Although many pathological manifestations can be viewed on a continuum with normal behavior, there is little difficulty in distinguishing schizophrenia from normality and validating the presence of a disease. In the past, major areas of disagreement between diagnostic approaches involved broad versus narrow concepts, whether positive psychotic symptoms were required, whether dissociative thought disorder was required in all cases, and which symptoms could be considered of first rank in differential diagnosis. In general, systems with broad criteria and emphasis on psychosocial pathology included more subtle cases with greater likelihood of diagnostic disagreement but also increased validity for genetic studies using family pedigree data. The concept of schizophrenia spectrum pathology was introduced in this regard and led to the development of schizoid and schizotypal personality disorder constructs.

The importance of operationalized diagnostic criteria and differential diagnosis increased with the development of specific pharmacological interventions. The variability in diagnostic criteria was underscored in the 1960s, when it was convincingly demonstrated that U.S. diagnosticians used a much broader and less defined construct of schizophrenia than their U.K. counterparts. Application of reliable research diagnostic criteria suggested greater validity for the U.K. clinical diagnoses, prompting the concern that a broad construct of schizophrenia inadvertently included two categories of patients ill-suited for antipsychotic drug therapy. The first category was patients with bipolar or major depressive disorders with psychotic features, who, if erroneously considered to have schizophrenia, were administered antipsychotic medication rather than the more specific and effective treatments available for patients with these disorders (i.e., antidepressant drugs, lithium [Eskalith], and electroconvulsive therapy [ECT]). The second category included patients with schizophrenia spectrum personality disorders. These patients were sometimes misdiagnosed as having schizophrenia and, as a consequence, were likely to be administered drug treatments designed for the positive symptoms of schizophrenia that provided little benefit and subjected them to substantial risk.

A considerable body of research during the 1960s and 1970s clarified many diagnostic issues and set the stage for the development of a diagnostic system implemented in the American Psychiatric Association's third edition of the *Diagnostic and Statistical Manual of Mental Disorders* (DSM-III). The DSM-III approach, with specified symptom-based diagnostic criteria and demonstrated reliability, is now the accepted diagnostic system in North America and throughout the international research community. The use of this approach has led to the reliable and consistent differential diagnosis of schizophrenia, which has enhanced scientific and clinical communication and has substantially increased the likelihood of the effective use of diagnostically specific treatments. The current revised fourth edition of the *Diagnostic and Statistical Manual of Mental Disorders* (DSM-IV-TR) and the tenth edition of the *International Classification of Diseases* (ICD-10) diagnostic approaches are extensions of this approach.

The close connection of diagnosis and drug treatment has been the dominant paradigm in drug development and is regarded as essential in registration studies seeking U. S. Food and Drug Administration (FDA) approval of new drugs and new indications. Schizophrenia and bipolar patients are studied separately to determine antipsychotic efficacy, and an approved drug indication is specifically related to the diagnostic class in which it is tested. This paradigm is about to shift. An early indication of the limitation of this paradigm was a little-noted observation of the influential 1960s U.S.–U.K. study. In the United States, the broad application of a schizophrenia diagnosis was associated with an increased rate of antidepressant drug therapy in patients with schizophrenia. A depressed patient with schizophrenia and a patient with psychotic depression are both potential candidates for antipsychotic and antidepressant therapy. Beginning with observations in the 1970s, which suggested that schizophrenia is best conceptualized as a syndrome comprised of three semi-independent domains of psychopathology, an alternative paradigm has been introduced requiring understanding of treatment effects on specific psychopathological domains. Drug and psychosocial therapies have turned out not to be antischizophrenic but antipsychotic. For this reason, and data relating to endophenotypes and neuroanatomy, the field is moving beyond diagnosis in characterizing and grouping patients.

Beyond Diagnosis A valid diagnostic system is essential for clinical and epidemiological purposes and is an important initial consideration in treatment, especially in longer-term relapse prevention and maintenance therapy. However, diagnosis at the syndrome level is not adequate for the scientific study of the multiple etiopathophysiologies of schizophrenia. The disease class paradigm has led to the development of treatment for psychosis but has limited treatment discovery for other key features of the illness.

The traditional approach to reducing the heterogeneity of the schizophrenia syndrome has been to delineate subtypes and to attempt to confirm or to disprove their validity. The classical subtypes, disorganized (DSM-IV-TR) or hebephrenia (ICD-10), paranoid, catatonic, and simple schizophrenia, represent the most frequently used subtype approach for reducing heterogeneity. Although important differences, such as age of onset and pattern of symptom development, validate these subtypes, the classical subtypes have not provided a strong heuristic for the study of etiology and pathophysiology.

An alternative approach to syndromic heterogeneity is the domains of psychopathology construct. In this approach, important clinical features of the syndrome are defined, and those that are relatively independent from other features are selected as domains forming the basic unit of study. Symptoms of schizophrenia usually segregate into three semi-independent symptom complexes: (1) hallucinations and delusions; (2) disorganized behavior, including positive formal thought disorder, bizarre behavior, and inappropriate affect; and (3) negative symptoms, including restricted affective experience and expression, diminished drive, and poverty of speech. Longitudinal studies provide support for the independence and stability of these domains, at least when negative symptoms are primary to the disease process. These results support a paradigm shift. The neuroanatomy of schizophrenia becomes the neuroanatomy of each domain, for example, and treatment efficacy has to be evaluated domain by domain.

The domains of psychopathology approach has been extensively applied to the investigation of primary negative symptoms. These symptoms differ from other domains with respect to their familial heritability; neuroanatomy, as evidenced in structural and functional neuroimaging studies; and response to antipsychotic treatment. Long-term outcome, season of birth, and age of onset are also distinctive. These results provide strong support for the heuristic value of this approach and raise the hope that this approach to heterogeneity reduction will provide more decisive data in studies of etiopathophysiology and neuroanatomy and explicit information regarding the efficacy profile of pharmacological treatments. In this approach, an interesting challenge relates to the question of why these domains, semi-independent within individuals with schizophrenia, cooccur in the syndrome. One interesting outcome is the possibility that some domains may help define specific disease entities within the syndrome. Substantial evidence exists that this is the case when patients with the deficit form of schizophrenia, which is defined by the presence of enduring, primary, negative symptoms, are distinguished from those with the nondeficit form of schizophrenia.

Cognitive Impairment For diagnosis, the three symptom domains constitute the principal diagnostic considerations. However, schizophrenia is associated with a broad array of cognitive impairments, including impaired attention/information processing, reasoning and problem-solving, social cognition, processing speed, verbal and visual learning and memory, and working memory functions. Attention, language, memory, and processing speed impairments are critically important and account for much of the variance in poor social and occupational functional outcomes. On a theoretical level, attention, working memory, and, possibly, verbal memory impairments may be liability and vulnerability markers and may be used to define schizophrenia phenotypes. Cognitive impairments may be useful in the early detection of individuals at high risk for the future development of schizophrenia. They may provide a basis for creating new models for treatment development. Moreover, the neuropsychological assessment of cognitive impairments permits probabilistic anatomical inferences, and the use of cognitive tasks that assess these impairments have become increasingly important in guiding functional neuroimaging studies.

The relationship among cognitive impairments and the symptoms of schizophrenia is unclear. For many years, cognitive impairments were conceptualized as the psychological foundations of symptom manifestations. However, there is a large body of evidence that has documented the relative independence of cognitive impairments and positive psychotic symptoms. For example, clinical trials have repeatedly demonstrated that large changes in positive symptom status can occur without a corresponding improvement in cognitive function reflected in cognitive or neuropsychological test performance. The use of the three symptom complex model and less complicated cognitive paradigms may lead to the elucidation of possible relationships between the various cognitive impairments and the symptom complexes.

In summary, the clinical manifestations of schizophrenia are well known. The conceptualization of schizophrenia as a clinical syndrome, which is importantly distinguished from bipolar affective and other psychotic disorders, has been validated. Diagnostic research has produced some modification in classification and has demonstrated the adequacy of the reliability and validity of current approaches. It has also produced a reasonable degree of uniformity in international usage that serves clinical and scientific purposes. Because the clinical syndrome of schizophrenia probably represents more than one pathological process, specifically addressing the etiology, pathophysiology, and treatment of specific symptom domains offers important new power to research designs. The future may bring a more dramatic evolution of the concept, as the basis for genetic and psychopathological overlap between major classes is understood.

COURSE, PROGNOSIS, AND OUTCOME

In his pioneering description of schizophrenia, Kraepelin argued that schizophrenia was characterized by an early onset followed by a chronic and deteriorating course with a defect end state. Bleuler suggested that a chronic deteriorating course was a frequent, but not a necessary, outcome. He rejected dementia as the defect end state. However, neither of these early workers took into account the extent to which these observations were based on chronic, institutionalized patient populations. There are now extensive longitudinal outcome data on patients who were treated before and after the introduction of antipsychotic medication, which support a more optimistic prognostic picture. Although schizophrenia is always a serious disease, it is now clear that patients with the disorder may follow a variety of courses over the long term, including some that are relatively benign. However, it remains true that, although the disease does not always progress to a deteriorated end state, there are substantial and enduring adverse consequences for most patients.

The course of illness is sometimes more benign in female patients with schizophrenia. Possible reasons include the following: (1) Estrogen may modify dopamine pathophysiology; (2) female patients may have a better response to antipsychotic drugs; (3) the deficit form of schizophrenia is a predominantly male disease; and (4) egocentric cultures are traditionally more stressful for men.

The course of illness can be divided into four major epochs: premorbid, onset of illness, middle course, and late course.

Premorbid Epoch

The *premorbid epoch* refers to symptom manifestations before the onset of overt, positive psychotic symptoms. Twenty-five to 50 percent of patients with schizophrenia exhibit impaired behavior or subtle symptom manifestations. These abnormalities may present as diminished social drive; decreased emotional responsivity; withdrawn, introverted, suspicious, or impulsive behavior; idiosyncratic responses to ordinary events or circumstances; and short attention span, delayed developmental milestones, or poor motor and sensorimotor coordination, or a combination of these. The presence of social behavior disturbances have been picked up as early as infancy by workers who have noticed a lack of responsiveness and emotional expression in infants who later developed schizophrenia. *Childhood asociality*, a trait that has previously been referred to as a poor prognostic indicator, is probably more appropriately conceptualized as the early morbid manifestations of negative or deficit symptomatology. Cognitive difficulties are observed during preteen and teenage years in children at high risk for developing schizophrenia. Patients may also exhibit impaired premorbid scholastic and occupational development or poor premorbid adjustment in these domains. These functional impairments may reflect early morbid features related to negative symptom and cognitive impairments, the effect of subtle disorganization or reality distortion pathology, or developmental strength or weakness that interacts with disease pathology to determine course. Their presence is associated with poorer prognosis.

Onset of Illness

The *second epoch*, onset of illness, typically refers to the onset of positive psychotic symptoms (i.e., hallucinations and delusions, formal thought disorder, and disorganization). The onset of positive psychotic symptoms is insidious in approximately one-half of the patients, with the earliest signs of psychotic illness occurring years before the florid or overt manifestation of psychosis. In other cases, onset is relatively acute, with onset of positive psychotic symptoms marking a sharp deviation in life trajectory. Patients with the insidious type of onset are likely to have a poor intermediate course and poor long-term course. In contrast, patients with normal development and ordinary personality attributes, who experience a relatively sudden appearance of hallucinations, delusions, and disorganized thought, vary widely in terms of intermediate and long-term outcome of the disorder, some having good long-term outcomes and others having poor long-term outcomes. Duration of untreated psychosis (DUP) is now a focus of early intervention research. The hypothesis that longer DUP causes a worse outcome (i.e., positive psychotic symptoms are toxic hypothesis) is difficult to evaluate, because insidious onset is a robust poor prognostic factor, and insidious onset cases routinely come to diagnosis and treatment later in the psychotic course than acute onset cases.

There is a gender difference in age of onset. In men, there is a unimodal onset of positive symptoms, with peak incidence from 18 to 25 years of age. In contrast, women exhibit a bimodal distribution in the onset of positive symptoms. The first peak occurs between 20 and 35 years of age, and the second peak occurs after 40 years of age.

Middle Course

The *middle course-of-illness epoch* may be subdivided into two subepochs. The first 5 to 10 years of illness is frequently characterized by multiple exacerbations of positive psychotic symptoms, during which a patient may return to an asymptomatic baseline between episodes or may remain actively psychotic without achieving full recovery. This subepoch is followed by a plateau phase, in which patients experience a stabilization of their symptoms, and the number of exacerbations decreases.

Recent studies have made it evident that the underlying deterioration associated with schizophrenia principally occurs during the onset of illness and the first half of the middle phase, rather than over the remaining course of illness. However, complications caused by the illness lead to ever-increasing impediments to normal existence, so that secondary effects may be progressive, even though the primary psychopathology has reached a plateau. For example, patients who live in understimulating environments lose social skills and work capabilities, even if their symptom levels improve. Effective treatment late in the course of a chronic disease diminishes illness, but it does not restore lost experience and opportunity—nor does it overcome stigma. A history of disabling schizophrenia is a serious social and occupational burden, regardless of the degree of recovery.

Late Course

In the *late course-of-illness epoch*, there is a tendency for the intensity of positive psychotic symptoms to diminish with age, and many patients with long-term impairments regain some degree of social and occupational competence. Although the illness becomes less disruptive and easier to manage, the effects of years of dysfunction are rarely overcome. It would be highly unusual for an individual with a chronic form of the illness to gain the niche in society and the quality of personal life that would have been possible had the illness not been present. More typically, patients continue to manifest direct signs of the illness process throughout their life. Twenty- to 40-year follow-up studies provide a basis for estimating that approximately 55 percent of patients with schizophrenia have moderately good outcomes, and 45 percent have more severe outcomes. These figures are more optimistic than earlier views for at least two reasons. First, sample selection was broader and more representative. Second, effective treatments, which make a considerable difference in the short-term course, also have a modest impact on the long-term course.

Although no present treatment approach can prevent or cure schizophrenia, some approaches have had remarkable remedial effects on course. Although not subject to scientific verification, there is considerable evidence from a large body of clinical experience that a form of schizophrenia referred to as *devastating schizophrenia*, which represented approximately 15 percent of the cases before the introduction of antipsychotic medication, now represents less than 5 percent of the cases. This form of the illness had an acute, rather than insidious, onset but paradoxically led to an unrelenting course. There is another line of evidence, also difficult to substantiate empirically, which suggests that the earlier the antipsychotic medication is initially administered in the course of schizophrenia, the more benign the course. In patients with established diagnoses of schizophrenia, clinicians consider it prudent to detect and to initiate treatment as early as possible during an acute symptom exacerbation. Using the same rationale, the initial treatment should also be undertaken as early as the initial detection of the disease process permits. Studies of first-episode patients suggest that the onset of psychosis may, on the average, precede diagnosis and treatment by almost 2 years, and the onset of negative symptoms can be traced back even further. These studies also suggest that earlier initiation of pharmacological treatment improves outcome in first-episode patients. However, as noted previously, the association of insidious onset with poor prognosis confounds the interpretation of the benefits of decreased length of DUP on future course of illness.

There is now increasing interest in establishing reliable methodology for the detection and treatment of individuals who are at immediate risk for having an initial episode of schizophrenia but who have not yet manifested overt positive psychotic symptoms, to ascertain whether future course is thereby substantially affected. The earliest manifestations of illness are usually nonspecific, and it would be difficult to initiate antipsychotic drug treatment in the large population of young people manifesting suspiciousness, eccentric behavior, social withdrawal, low motivation, magical ideation, and the like. Second-generation antipsychotic medications have a reduced extrapyramidal and dysphoric adverse effect profile, lending impetus to the early intervention approach based on presumptions of increased safety and tolerability. Preliminary studies suggest that early intervention approaches can have a beneficial impact on the early course of illness. The long-term impact of these interventions is not known. Moreover, early intervention often initiates long-term treatment, and some second-generation antipsychotics may increase cardiovascular and diabetic risk factors—an important consideration when treating young patients.

There is considerable evidence suggesting that the prophylactic use of antipsychotic medication reduces the relapse rate by more than one-half. This fact is largely responsible for the substantial reduction in inpatient care and the transition to community-based treatment. The level of success associated with this major shift in the setting in which schizophrenia is treated and the serious shortcomings associated with shifting care to unprepared communities are noted in the discussion on treatment and rehabilitation.

There are social determinants of outcome that are best understood in a cultural context. The course of schizophrenia tends to be more benign in developing countries than in developed countries. This difference in course is generally understood as representing a psychosocial influence on course rather than cultural differences in the causes of schizophrenia. The incidence and lifetime prevalence of the disease appear to be relatively comparable across cultures and societies. One compelling construct is that the sociocentric structures of developing countries place less demand on individual performance and provide a more broadly supportive interpersonal environment than do the egocentric cultures of the more developed nations. The latter nations, with their marked emphasis on individual accomplishment and productivity, are more demanding and stressful for those with impaired drive or impaired mental functioning. Rather than finding an appropriate, usually reduced level of functioning, the patient with schizophrenia in Western industrialized societies tends to be isolated, with greatly reduced opportunities for work and meaningful social contacts. Indicative of this lack of involvement, unemployment rates for patients with schizophrenia are upward of 80 percent in the United States.

TREATMENT AND REHABILITATION

The history of the care and treatment of patients with schizophrenia is replete with instances of humane and inhumane approaches. From a practical and moral standpoint, the value of humane care is intrinsic and does not rest on scientific evaluation of efficacy. There is a large body of literature and scientific data regarding the pharmacological and psychosocial treatment and rehabilitation of patients with schizophrenia. The general conclusions of this accumulated information are presented in the following discussion.

Pharmacological Interventions Before 1952, there were no generally applicable treatments of demonstrated effectiveness. Reserpine had been used with some limited success, and electroconvulsive treatment was important in reducing symptoms in the most acutely disturbed cases. However, it was not until the introduction of chlorpromazine (Thorazine) in France in 1952 and in North America in 1954 that the modern era of effective pharmacological therapeutics for schizophrenia began.

The antipsychotic drugs used to treat schizophrenia have a wide variety of pharmacological properties, but all share the capacity to antagonize postsynaptic dopamine receptors in the brain. Conventional antipsychotics are often referred to as *neuroleptics* because of their neurological side effects. New or second-generation antipsychotics are less likely to exhibit these effects, and they have been referred to as *atypical antipsychotics*. The generally recognized clinical effect of antipsychotics is to diminish positive psychotic symptom expression and to reduce relapse rates. Although sedation may be a side effect, and diminished anxiety may be a clinical effect, the primary value of these drugs is for their remedial effect on positive psychotic symptoms and not for their sedating or tranquilizing properties. In fact, their antipsychotic efficacy extends beyond schizophrenia to include positive psychotic symptoms associated with illnesses other than schizophrenia. In contrast to positive psychotic symptoms, conventional antipsychotics have not been shown to be effective for primary, enduring, negative or deficit symptoms or the cognitive impairments observed in patients with schizophrenia.

Antipsychotic drugs are used throughout the world for four primary clinical purposes: (1) to manage acute positive psychotic symptom disturbances, (2) to induce remission from positive psychotic symptom exacerbations, (3) to maintain the achieved clinical effect over prolonged periods of time (maintenance therapy), and (4) to prevent relapses or new episodes of positive psychotic symptom expression (prophylactic therapy). The clinical intent is to administer the drugs in a manner that increases patient compliance and avoids illness exacerbations due to patients discontinuing their medication. It is now recognized that optimal treatment involves the integration of antipsychotic drug treatment with psychosocial treatment approaches and rehabilitation techniques.

The first second-generation antipsychotic to be available for clinical use was clozapine. Clozapine has a unique mechanism of action and was shown during the 1970s to have a differential effect on patients resistant to the therapeutic effects of conventional antipsychotics. However, there is an approximately 1 percent risk of agranulocytosis associated with the use of clozapine. This potentially lethal cessation in the production of white blood cells was associated with a series of deaths in Finland during the mid-1970s and led to a decreased use of clozapine in Europe and failure to market the drug in the United States. Interest in clozapine was rekindled by the results of a large-scale multicenter study in chronic, treatment-resistant inpatients with schizophrenia. The study yielded convincing evidence of the superior efficacy of clozapine for ameliorating positive psychotic symptoms in treatment-resistant patients. Consistent with the worldwide experience in the late 1970s and early 1980s, the study also showed that clozapine can be used with relative safety within the context of careful monitoring for agranulocytosis. The development of clozapine represented the first incremental gain in the effectiveness of the pharmacological agents used to treat schizophrenia since the original introduction of chlorpromazine.

The demonstration that clozapine can be effective in some patients for whom conventional antipsychotics are not has spawned considerable interest in the development of new antipsychotics for the treatment of schizophrenia. Over the last decade, five new antipsychotics have been introduced: risperidone (Risperdal), olanzapine (Zyprexa), quetiapine (Seroquel), ziprasidone (Geodon), and aripiprazole (Abilify). These new drugs were introduced in the hope that they would share the superior efficacy of clozapine, but without the risk of agranulocytosis and the other side effects that have limited the use of clozapine. However, although these new medications appear to be as effective for positive psychotic symptoms as the conventional antipsychotics, none of them has been proven to have superior efficacy for this aspect of the illness. Their main advantage over the conventional antipsychotics is their substantially decreased extrapyramidal side effect burden. This decreased side effect burden may result in their apparently greater effectiveness and appears to have reduced the incidence of long-lasting motoric side effects (i.e., persistent dystonia and tardive dyskinesia). Several of the second-generation antipsychotics also appear to have greater benefit than the conventional antipsychotics for the treatment of depressive symptoms and the prevention of relapse and rehospitalization. These considerations have led to the second-generation antipsychotics replacing conventional antipsychotics as the first line of pharmacological treatment for first-episode and chronic patients with schizophrenia.

The second-generation antipsychotics are not without their limitations. Several of these agents have been associated with the development of clinically significant metabolic disturbances, including weight gain, hyperlipidemias, and new-onset type II diabetes mellitus. Patients with schizophrenia are already at increased risk for cardiovascular disease because of their lifestyle, and the occurrence of these side effects only places these patients at greater risk for adverse cardiovascular events. Long-term studies will eventually clarify whether the decreased risk of extrapyramidal side effects, including tardive dyskinesia, warrants the increased risk of these metabolic side effects.

There is considerable interest in whether the novel pharmacological properties of the second-generation antipsychotics will lead to increased efficacy for the negative symptom and cognitive impairment illness components. A number of studies have indicated that second-generation antipsychotics are more effective than conventional antipsychotics for negative symptoms, but differences are usually related to concurrent changes in extrapyramidal or depressive symptoms or excessive dosages of the conventional antipsychotic comparator drug. In studies that have controlled for these potential sources of artifact, the apparently superior efficacy of the second-generation antipsychotics disappears. A similar story is emerging for the comparative efficacy of second-generation and conventional antipsychotics for cognitive impairments. Conventional antipsychotics have been observed to have little impact on cognitive function, even when their use has resulted in significant improvement in the positive psychotic symptom component of the illness. This lack of benefit suggests that these agents may have inherent toxic effects on cognition, especially when used in higher dosages. Second-generation antipsychotics improve performance on neuropsychological measures of cognitive functions, but the effect is relatively modest, and patients continue to exhibit considerable cognitive impairments in comparison to normal controls. The differential cognitive effect between second-generation and conventional antipsychotics is less pronounced when second-generation antipsychotics are compared to lower doses of conventional antipsychotics.

The limitations of conventional and second-generation antipsychotics for the negative symptoms and cognitive impairment components of schizophrenia have led to the investigation of the usefulness of pharmacological augmentation strategies for these components. A series of studies have supported the potential usefulness of glutamatergic agents that bind to the glycine site of the NMDA glutamatergic receptor for the treatment of primary, enduring, negative or deficit symptoms. Glycine, D-cycloserine, and D-serine have produced encouraging results in preliminary controlled clinical trials. Other augmentation strategies for these symptoms include the use of dopamine and serotonergic and noradrenergic agents.

The delineation of the pharmacology of normal cognition has also led to the investigation of augmentation strategies in the treatment of cognitive impairments. The potential usefulness of cholinergic and dopaminergic and other pharmacological agents is currently being investigated.

Augmentation strategies have also been used to treat positive psychotic symptoms that fail to respond to antipsychotic treatment, including clozapine. However, lithium, antiepileptics, antidepressants, and antianxiety agents have not been shown to substantially reduce these symptoms. Some small patient subgroups may be differentially responsive to a class of drugs other than antipsychotics, but, in the absence of the capacity to identify in advance which patients respond favorably, it is difficult to prove or to disprove this proposition. In contrast, these drugs may be effective for cooccurring anxiety, depressive, manic, and aggressive symptoms. The emerging trend for patients with persistent positive psychotic symptoms is to treat these patients with multiple antipsychotic drugs. There is currently no empirical basis for this treatment strategy.

ECT was frequently used in the treatment of patients with schizophrenia before the introduction of antipsychotic drugs. ECT is particularly effective in the treatment of catatonic stupor and excitement but generally produces results similar to those obtained with antipsychotics, that is, a reduction of positive symptoms rather than a reversal of long-term functional impairments. Although ECT is safe and painless, its use is restricted, in part by litigation and societal attitudes, but also because any therapeutic advantage gained in an initial series of treatments is not easily maintained. Also, there is currently no compelling evidence that ECT is effective in antipsychotic-resistant patients. For all of these reasons, drug treatment approaches are generally preferred.

Psychosocial Interventions The debate over whether patients should be treated with pharmacological or psychosocial treatments has given way to the search for how these treatments should be optimally integrated. Controlled clinical trials have conclusively demonstrated that intensive psychotherapy is less effective than pharmacological treatment, that it is not superior to less expensive, less ambitious psychosocial forms of psychotherapy, and that it should no longer be considered as an alternative to the use of antipsychotic drugs. In addition, studies have repeatedly demonstrated that supportive forms of psychosocial treatment are entirely compatible with drug treatment and can increase the effectiveness of overall treatment, reduce the amount of medication necessary, enhance patient participation in the full range of treatment, and optimize social and occupational functioning. Especially impressive are studies documenting the considerable additional benefit achieved in reducing relapse and hospitalization rates when family therapy and education programs are added to maintenance pharmacological treatment. These studies make clear that psychosocial and rehabilitative interventions have become essential components of the comprehensive treatment of patients with schizophrenia.

Psychosocial and rehabilitation interventions include cognitive behavior therapy for treatment-resistant positive psychotic symptoms; supportive, problem-solving, educationally oriented psychotherapy; family therapy and education programs aimed at helping patients and their families understand the patient's illness, reduce stress, and enhance coping capabilities; social and living skills training; supported employment programs; and the provision of supervised residential living arrangements. The development and increased use of psychosocial services have been complemented by the evolution of services designed to decrease the use of inpatient hospital services and to maintain the patient in the community. Assertive community treatment teams are designed to provide intensive outreach services to patients who are unable to be maintained in the community with traditional outpatient clinical treatment. Crisis management services, including 24-hour crisis beds and partial hospitalization programs, represent alternatives to hospitalization during periods of symptom exacerbation.

The development of these services reflects the ongoing shift in the treatment of the patient with schizophrenia from a hospital-based to a community-based system of care. When optimal treatment with these services is provided, the rewards of therapeutic accomplishment, reduction in morbidity, and economic cost benefits are profound and rival therapeutic accomplishments found anywhere in medicine. The demonstrated benefits of these services challenge the field to establish an adequate community-based treatment approach prepared to meet the challenges and demands of broad-based integrated treatment. Society has failed to meet the challenge of providing evidence-based treatment to most people who have schizophrenia.

A new and future challenge is the organization of intervention in the prepsychotic and early psychotic phases of illness. Clinical prudence requires early identification and treatment, but the earliest indicators are usually not psychotic features. Psychosocial treatment for nonpsychotic illness manifestations needs to be developed, just as pharmacological treatments for cognitive impairments and negative psychopathology are required if prepsychotic treatment is to address early morbid features in patients at high risk for psychosis.

FUTURE DIRECTIONS

The field is at the beginning of a new century of opportunity for major breakthroughs in the treatment and prevention of schizophrenia. The 20th century closed with substantial progress in defining brain anatomy and function associated with this illness syndrome. Candidate diseases within the syndrome were hypothesized, and postmortem findings ranged from the microanatomical to gene expression candidates for pathophysiology. Chromosome locations and candidate genes were identified, and new methodologies based in postgenomic technology were put into place. Progress with physiological and cellular phenotypes has positioned the field for more sure-footed and rapid advance on genotype discovery in schizophrenia. Although the multifactorial and multigenetic etiology of the syndrome is certain, new paradigms providing heuristic advantage in the classification of psychopathological phenomena provide a means of addressing the problem of syndromic heterogeneity. Multidisciplinary work has become critical, and the schizophrenia investigator of today is likely to be engaged in translational research using postgenomic technology and bioinformatics.

Although opportunities are great, so are the remaining challenges. Cognitive impairments and primary negative symptoms are largely responsible for the poor functional outcome and low quality of life of most persons with schizophrenia. Will new molecular targets result in the first efficacious treatments for these illness components? What knowledge of etiopathophysiology is required to discover primary and secondary prevention interventions? Will the multiple genes involved in risk so overlap with affective and other disorders that current classification of diseases will be invalidated? Will the many common and small contributors to risk and the many and varied pathophysiological results require a new disease paradigm? The sections in Chapter 12 show the substantial clinical progress and future scientific promise relating to schizophrenia. The complexity of this most distinctively human disease syndrome, however, assures that the conquest of schizophrenia will be one of medicine's most difficult challenges.

SUGGESTED CROSS-REFERENCES

A more detailed discussion of etiology, brain structure and function, clinical features, and somatic and psychosocial treatments are presented in other sections of Chapter 12. A detailed introduction to areas of neuroscience and cognitive science relevant to schizophrenia is provided in Section 1.2 on functional neuroanatomy, Section 1.3 on neuronal development and plasticity, Sections 1.15 and 1.16 on brain imaging, Section 1.17 on basic molecular genetic neuroscience, and Section 3.1 on perception and cognition.

REFERENCES

Blyler CR, Gold JM. Cognitive effects of typical antipsychotic treatment: Another look. In: Sharma T, Harvey P, eds. *Cognition in Schizophrenia*. New York: Oxford University Press; 2000.

Breier A, Su T-P, Saunders R, Carson RE, Kolachana BS, De Bartolomeis A, Weinberger DR, Weisenfeld N, Malhotra AK, Eckelman WD, Pickar D: Schizophrenia is associated with elevated amphetamine-induced synaptic dopamine concentrations: Evidence from a novel positron emission tomography method. *Proc Natl Acad Sci U S A*. 1997;94:2569.

*Buchanan RW, Breier A, Kirkpatrick B, Ball P, Carpenter WT Jr: Positive and negative symptom response to clozapine in schizophrenic patients with and without the deficit syndrome. *Am J Psychiatry*. 1998;155:751.

Cahn W, Pol HE, Lems EB, van Haren NE, Schnack HG, van der Linden JA, Schothorst PF, van Engeland H, Kahn RS: Brain volume changes in first-episode schizophrenia: A 1-year follow-up study. *Arch Gen Psychiatry*. 2002;59:1002.

Cannon M, Jones PB, Murray RM: Obstetric complications and schizophrenia: Historical and meta-analytic review. *Am J Psychiatry*. 2002;159:1080.

Carlsson A: Neurocircuitries and neurotransmitter interactions in schizophrenia. *Int Clin Psychopharmacol*. 1995;3:21.

*Carpenter WT, Buchanan RW, Kirkpatrick B, Tamminga C, Wood F: Strong inference, theory testing, and the neuroanatomy of schizophrenia. *Arch Gen Psychiatry*. 1993;50:825.

Csernansky JG, Mahmoud R, Brenner R: The Risperidone-USA-79 Study Group: A comparison of risperidone and haloperidol for the prevention of relapse in patients with schizophrenia. *N Engl J Med*. 2002;346:16.

Davis JM, Chen N, Glick ID: A meta-analysis of the efficacy of second-generation antipsychotics. *Arch Gen Psychiatry*. 2003;60:553.

*Egan MF, Goldberg TE, Kolachana BS, Callicott JH, Mazzanti CM, Straub RE, Goldman D, Weinberger DR: Effect of COMT Val108/158 Met genotype on frontal lobe function and risk for schizophrenia. *Proc Natl Acad Sci U S A*. 2001;98:6917.

Freedman R: Schizophrenia. *N Engl J Med*. 2003;349:1739.

Freedman R, Coon H, Myles-Worsley M, Orr-Urtreger A, Olincy A, Davis A, Polymeropoulos M, Holik J, Hopkins J, Hoff M, Rosenthal J, Waldo MC, Reimherr F, Wender P, Yaw J, Young DA, Breese CR, Adams C, Patterson D, Adler LE, Kruglyak L, Leonard S, Byerley W: Linkage of a neurophysiological deficit in schizophrenia to a chromosome 15 locus. *Proc Natl Acad Sci U S A.* 1997;94:587.

Gao WJ, Goldman-Rakic PS: Selective modulation of excitatory and inhibitory microcircuits by dopamine. *Proc Natl Acad Sci U S A.* 2003;100:2836.

Goff DC, Tsai G, Levitt J, Amico E, Manoach D, Schoenfeld DA, Hayden DL, McCarley R, Coyle JT: A placebo-controlled trial of D-cycloserine added to conventional neuroleptics in patients with schizophrenia. *Arch Gen Psychiatry.* 1999;56:21.

Goldberg TE, Egan MF, Gscheidle T, Coppola R, Weickert T, Kolachana BS, Goldman D, Weinberger DR: Executive subprocesses in working memory: Relationship to catechol-*O*-methyltransferase Val158Met genotype and schizophrenia. *Arch Gen Psychiatry.* 2003;60:889.

Green MF, Marder SR, Glynn SM, McGurk SR, Wirshing WC, Wirshing DA, Liberman RP, Mintz J: The neurocognitive effects of low-dose haloperidol: A two-year comparison with risperidone. *Biol Psychiatry.* 2002;51:972.

Heresco-Levy U, Javitt DC, Ermilov M, Mordel C, Silipo G, Lichenstein M: Efficacy of high-dose glycine in the treatment of enduring negative symptoms of schizophrenia. *Arch Gen Psychiatry.* 1999;56:29.

*Kirkpatrick B, Buchanan RW, Ross DE, Carpenter WT Jr: A separate disease within the syndrome of schizophrenia. *Arch Gen Psychiatry.* 2001;58:165.

Lahti AC, Holcomb HH, Medoff DR, Weiler MA, Tamminga CA, Carpenter WT Jr: Abnormal patterns of regional cerebral blood flow in schizophrenia with primary negative symptoms during an effortful auditory recognition task. *Am J Psychiatry.* 2001;158:1797.

*Leonard S, Gault J, Hopkins J, Logel J, Vianzon R, Short M, Drebing C, Berger R, Venn D, Sirota P, Zerbe G, Olincy A, Ross RG, Adler LE, Freedman R: Association of promoter variants in the α7 nicotinic acetylcholine receptor subunit gene with an inhibitory deficit found in schizophrenia. *Arch Gen Psychiatry.* 2002;59:1085.

Lewis DA, Lieberman JA: Catching up on schizophrenia: Natural history and neurobiology. *Neuron.* 2000;28:325.

Lieberman JA, Fenton WS: Delayed detection of psychosis: Causes, consequences, and effect on public health. *Am J Psychiatry.* 2000;157:1727.

Mirnics K, Middleton FA, Stanwood GD, Lewis DA, Levitt P: Disease-specific changes in regulator of G-protein signaling 4 (RGS4) expression in schizophrenia. *Mol Psychiatry.* 2001;6:293.

Mortensen PB, Pedersen CB, Westergaard T, Wohlfahrt J, Ewald H, Mors O, Andersen PK, Melbye M: Effects of family history and place and season of birth on the risk of schizophrenia. *N Engl J Med.* 1999;340:603.

Schooler NR, Keith SJ, Severe JB, Matthews SM, Bellack AS, Glick ID, Hargreaves WA, Kane JM, Ninan PT, Frances A, Jacobs M, Lieberman JA, Mance R, Simpson GM, Woerner MG: Relapse and rehospitalization during maintenance treatment of schizophrenia. *Arch Gen Psychiatry.* 1997;54:453.

Shergill SS, Brammer MJ, Fukuda R, Williams SC, Murray RM, McGuire PK: Engagement of brain areas implicated in processing inner speech in people with auditory hallucinations. *Br J Psychiatry.* 2003;182:525.

Stefansson H, Sigurdsson E, Steinthorsdottir V, Bjornsdottir S, Sigmundsson T, Ghosh S, Brynjolfsson J, Gunnarsdottir S, Ivarsson O, Chou TT, Hjaltason O, Birgisdottir B, Jonsson H, Gudnadottir VG, Gudmundsdottir E, Bjornsson A, Ingvarsson B, Ingason A, Sigfusson S, Hardardottir H, Harvey RP, Lai D, Zhou M, Brunner D, Mutel V, Gonzalo A, Lemke G, Sainz J, Johannesson G, Andresson T, Gudbjartsson D, Manolescu A, Frigge ML, Gurney ME, Kong A, Gulcher JR, Petursson H, Stefansson K: Neuregulin 1 and susceptibility to schizophrenia. *Am J Hum Genet.* 2002;71:877.

Straub RE, Jiang Y, MacLean CJ, Ma Y, Webb BT, Myakishev MV, Harris-Kerr C, Wormley B, Sadek H, Kadambi B, Cesare AJ, Gibberman A, Wang X, O'Neill A, Walsh D, Kendler KS: Genetic variation in the 6p22.3 gene DTNBP1, the human ortholog of the mouse dysbindin gene, is associated with schizophrenia. *Am J Hum Genet.* 2002;71:337.

▲ 12.2 Schizophrenia: Scope of the Problem

JOHN LAURIELLO, M.D., JUAN R. BUSTILLO, M.D., AND SAMUEL J. KEITH, M.D.

Schizophrenia is a chronic, pervasive, disabling, and potentially terminal illness that affects a significant proportion of the world population. Given its severity, the illness affects the patient, his or her family, and society. The following section endeavors to explore the wide scope of such a devastating illness. Schizophrenia has been a long misunderstood condition to patients, their families, society, and, remarkably, too many in the medical and psychological fields. There have been a number of books and movies, produced for the general public, that have attempted to explain the illness with a varied degree of success; notable examples are *I Never Promised You a Rose Garden* and *A Beautiful Mind.* In many cases, the stories revolve around one person's struggle with schizophrenia. In *A Beautiful Mind,* the experiences of John Nash, a brilliant mathematician and the recipient of the Nobel Prize in Economics, are described in a way that has improved the public's understanding of the illness. However, the particular experience of John Nash's eventual development of *reality testing* and his return to better functioning is unusual and does not fully describe the experiences of many with schizophrenia. For these other patients, symptoms remain, and reality testing is not fully realized. Moreover, they are unable to function at an adequate level to be self-sufficient. They pose an unfortunate burden to their families, who, with the patient, are the everyday heroes of their own stories. To their community, they incur a cost in direct and indirect value that is borne by all, with varying degrees of willingness.

This section first details the overall costs of the illness and how this cost is broken down and borne. Schizophrenia is truly an "illness without borders," and individuals from remote rural areas to highly industrialized countries share a relatively stable prevalence of the disorder. How the illness is regarded, treated, and paid for may differ, however. There have been national estimations of the cost of schizophrenia from developed and underdeveloped countries. Finally, the section considers how the treatment of schizophrenia compares to other medical illnesses and how, to general surprise, it fares well.

The lifetime prevalence of schizophrenia worldwide can be approximated at 1 percent of any given adult population. One percent of adult Americans with schizophrenia would be approximately two million people according to the 2000 U.S. Census. That is the equivalent to the population of the state of New Mexico! Worldwide, that population could be in the tens of millions. Because it is a chronic but not immediately fatal illness, this is a population that is ill over a long period of time. One estimate of the life expectancy for a person with schizophrenia is 20 percent shorter than the general population. In 2000, the overall life expectancy in the United States was 76 years, so, following the estimate above, the life expectancy of a person with schizophrenia would be 60 years. If the average age of onset for schizophrenia is 25 years of age, that means, on average, that an individual with schizophrenia must contend with the illness for 35 years. With the improvements in treatment, it is not unusual for patients with schizophrenia to reach an even older age, and there is now an expertise in the geriatric treatment of schizophrenia. Thirty-five years of an illness means a long period of burden on family that is often transferred from parent to sibling or even child. Thirty-five years of an illness means 35 years of possible exposure to effective but strong medications with inherent side effects. Thirty-five years means that these patients must be assured adequate living conditions, at least a subsistence allowance, and repeated hospitalizations, if and when necessary.

UNMET NEEDS

In many ways, schizophrenia is a bellwether condition for psychiatric illnesses as a whole, and general conclusions about mental illness are applicable to schizophrenia, if not worse for that condition. A recent interim 2002 report from the U.S. President's New Freedom Commission on Mental Health paints a grim portrait of mental illness treatment in the United States. The report describes five main barriers to access of care. These include

Fragmentation and gaps in care for children
Fragmentation and gaps in care for adults

High unemployment and disability for people with serious mental illness

Older adults not receiving care for mental illness

Mental health and suicide prevention not being a national priority.

Fragmented care is especially problematic with an illness like schizophrenia that necessitates a multisystemic interdisciplinary approach. Psychiatrists, nurses, case managers, and vocational rehabilitation experts, to name just a few, are integral members of a treatment team. However, large gaps exist in many communities for such a team. First, finding psychiatrists with the requisite skills and experience in treating patients with schizophrenia may be lacking, especially in rural areas of the country. Vocational and case management must also be available, and, if available, referrals to housing and job placement must also be found. High unemployment and the need to find meaning and vocation while experiencing schizophrenia are paramount and are discussed further in the section. Older individuals with schizophrenia require specialty care, as medical illnesses and behavioral problems may appear or worsen with older age. Likewise, preventing schizophrenia is an area of intense interest, especially identifying early premorbid symptoms and intervening before the illness reaches full manifestation. Finally, the issue of suicide is underappreciated but is a real, potential outcome for people with schizophrenia, so it must be recognized and dealt with whenever it appears.

PHARMACOECONOMICS OF SCHIZOPHRENIA

Direct and Indirect Cost of Schizophrenia There have been several estimates of the cost of schizophrenia over the last 50 years, beginning with Rashi Fein's 1958 landmark study for the Commission on Mental Illness. Fein's critical contribution to the field was the inclusion of direct and indirect costs of the illness. Direct costs, usually the more obvious of the two, include the upfront treatment expenditures for the patient. Dorothy Rice broke down the direct costs in her 1999 paper on the economic impact of schizophrenia in the United States. This was an update of her previous work with Leonard Miller on 1985 estimates inputting 1990 economic data and indicators. Direct costs included mental health organizations (i.e., community mental health centers, treatment centers, etc.), short-stay (acute) hospitals, physician and other professionals, nursing homes, medications, and support costs. Her estimation of the direct costs equaled $17.3 billion, a little more than one-half of the total costs of $32.5 billion. The indirect costs included the morbidity and mortality associated with such a pervasive, chronic illness. The indirect costs assumed estimates of loss of productivity and governmental support needed to maintain the patient. In addition, the cost of pain and suffering of the patient and their family and the heavy burden that families have to take on to support their ill relative were approximated. Rice estimated that the loss of productivity due to the illness and the inherent 20 percent shortened life expectancy accounted for $12 billion (36.9 percent of the $32.5 billion total), whereas the remaining costs accounted for the remaining $3.5 billion. This cost was much higher than earlier estimates. John G. Gunderson and Loren R. Mosher had estimated a high-end cost in 1975 of schizophrenia in the United States to be $15 billion, one-half of the 1990 estimate! Rice and Miller's 1985 estimates totaled $22.7 billion and had grown $10 billion in just 5 years.

The cost of schizophrenia is not an isolated problem to the United States, and all countries contend with the illness as well as their resources can accommodate. In other Western industrialized countries, the cost is similar to that in the United States, although the particulars of the delivery and support may differ. In the United Kingdom, the National Health Service accounts for 38 percent of the total cost, and local county authorities account for 12 percent, with one-half of the costs estimated from indirect expenditures. An estimate of the 1992 and 1993 costs of schizophrenia in the United Kingdom by Martin Knapp was 2.6 billion pounds. In an analysis by Julian F. Guest and Ron F. Cookson, the cost for the first 5 years of all patients diagnosed with schizophrenia was 862 million pounds. A 1988 estimate for the cost of treating schizophrenia in Australia was 1 billion, up from 310 million Australian dollars in 1976. Moreover, an Australian study by Gavin Andrews and colleagues put the total cost (direct and indirect) of treating schizophrenia at six times the cost of treating myocardial infarction. In non-Western countries, the cost is more difficult to determine, and many of the needs of these patients are not met because of other drastic national priorities for the general population. A study by Toyin G. Suleiman and colleagues in Nigeria highlights difficulties in the poorer countries. In Nigeria, the authors describe a dire lack of social welfare programs and nursing homes that reduces governmental support, leaving nearly all costs to families. Most sensitive to the problems of devaluation and poverty is the access to newer medications that are clearly more expensive and hence unavailable in countries like Nigeria.

Examples of Schizophrenia Costs

Family Burden Families often bear a substantial amount of the burden of any illness in a relative, and this is especially true in schizophrenia. The notion that schizophrenia could be traced to maladaptive parenting (e.g., schizophrenogenic mother) was damning and grossly incorrect. Families no longer consider themselves a cause but still are obligated to care for their children, spouse, or parent. The concept of *expressed emotion* (EE) tries to acknowledge that families with relatives with any illness may consciously or unconsciously criticize or unfairly blame the patient. Likewise, infantilizing or enabling the patient may be similarly nonproductive. A great deal of study and work with families has improved the relationships and prognoses of many patients with schizophrenia.

> Mrs. B. had cared for her son with schizophrenia for more than 20 years. They generally had a good and loving relationship. However, often, when her son became psychotic, he would scream at the voices, and she would need to stay with him and calm him, because she feared being evicted from her apartment. After numerous trials of failed medications, her son began to receive clozapine (Clozaril) for treatment-resistant psychosis. Although not cured, he was able to attend a day program for the first time in 20 years and to return to watercolor painting, something he had excelled in before his illness. For his mother, it was the first time she could remember that she could leave him and spend some time alone or with her friends. The medication had had a profound effect on the patient and his mother.

Despite all this effort, families must still contend with the mismatch between what the patient was or could have been and the possibility of relapses, violence, and suicide. One of the authors of this section (J.L.) has called schizophrenia the *illness of lost opportunities*, and this applies to the patient and his or her loved ones. The National Alliance for the Mentally Ill (NAMI) grew out of the need for families to support and advocate better research and care for their relative. NAMI has been an unqualified success but still does not have the national recognition of other family groups, such as Mothers Against Drunk Driving (MADD). A survey of state mental health programs examined the number and type of services offered to families with severe mental illness such as schizophrenia. Of 44 states queried, 73 percent did not have a clear policy for delivering services to families, although 80 percent reported that they supported family programs, most often *family-to-family* programs, such as NAMI, with only 61 percent reimbursing providers for family services. This is despite an extensive literature supporting the efficacy of such supportive interventions.

Vocational Loss Competitive employment (these are jobs acquired through the same avenues as the general population and are not supported by government programs or transfer payments) has been estimated at less than 20 percent for severely mentally ill persons and probably less for patients with chronic schizophrenia. One important goal of any medical treatment is to maintain patients as functional and independent in the community as possible. Disincentives to work, such as governmental cuts or pay backs for employment while on assistance, have been steadily reduced or eliminated. Supported employment programs are attempts to go beyond traditional vocational rehabilitation (e.g., transitional or sheltered employment), aiming to improve success in competitive employment. Individual placement programs (IPPs) that immerse and support patients at the job site have shown promise. The goal is permanent, competitive employment, substituting individualized on-the-job training and ongoing support (in lieu of preoccupational training) and enlisting the client's interests and preferences. A recent study by Anthony F. Lehman and colleagues studied the effects of an IPP compared to a more traditional psychosocial program without an emphasis on job placement. The results showed that the IPP was statistically better than the more general psychosocial program. Twenty-seven percent versus 7 percent were competitively employed. However, the authors also pointed out the low level of job retention by any patient who had gotten a competitive job. Employment retention in other studies has also been disappointing, with dropout rates greater than 40 percent. Although vocational programs may help patients attain entry-level positions, there is no evidence that the programs confer longer-term employment benefits for patients (i.e., transitioning to higher-level jobs and educational and training opportunities) or satisfying careers. However, paid employment may have beneficial effects on nonvocational outcomes and is not associated with increased rates of relapse or other negative outcomes.

Ms. J. B. had never worked in her life, having been diagnosed with schizophrenia at 20 years of age while still in college. For many years, she attempted to find a job on her own but could keep them for only a short time. Through the suggestion of her psychiatrist and case manager, she enrolled in a state-supported vocational program. She received basic employment information and was then placed in a job with a job coach. The first two jobs did not go well; she had difficulty with office work and large groups. Her job coach noted that she liked gardening, so her third job placement was on a small grounds keeping crew for an apartment complex. She did quite well in this position and was praised by her boss as being dependable and hard working.

Stigma One of the most widespread and insidious costs of mental illness and schizophrenia in particular is the stigma associated with the illness. Stigma includes negative attitudes and stereotypes directed at patients with schizophrenia, as well as their families. Stigma can manifest itself internally by the patient as a belief that they are defective and undeserving; by the family, who may marginalize the relative; and by society, which may discriminate and place barriers to the person's full integration into their community. A survey of patients with schizophrenia supports the belief that patients internalize many of these negative beliefs. Study participants were interviewed using the Consumer Experiences of Stigma Questionnaire (CESQ). Seventy-three of 74 participants reported at least one stigma experience. Seventy percent of patients worried about being viewed unfavorably because of their illness, and 58 percent avoided telling others about having schizophrenia. One-half of the patients had personally witnessed offensive comments about mental illness, and 43 percent had seen or heard such negative comments in the media.

Mr. R. W. had been treated successfully for his paranoid thoughts and had been symptom free for more than 1 year. In the last few sessions with his psychiatrist, he had mentioned a desire to start dating again. He had met a woman, and she seemed to be interested in him. Their first date had gone well, and, on the second date, they went to a movie that had a character with schizophrenia. Mr. R. W. told his date that he had been diagnosed with schizophrenia. The woman seemed to take the information in stride, but, when Mr. R. W. called for a third date, she did not answer or call back. Later, he told his psychiatrist that he had been wrong in telling her so soon, and he would be reluctant to do so in the future.

In a community survey for the World Psychiatric Association's Global Campaign to Fight Stigma and Discrimination Because of Schizophrenia, respondents were queried on attitudes about people with schizophrenia. Twenty percent of respondents felt they would be unable to maintain a friendship with a person with schizophrenia, 50 percent would not be able to room with a person with schizophrenia, and 75 percent could not see themselves marrying someone with the illness. In this survey, greater contact did not appear to improve acceptance, but greater knowledge of the illness favored more accepting attitudes. Moreover, the conceptualization that schizophrenia is a dangerous and violent disorder was perpetuated by individual anecdotes but was never compared to the general level of violence among the general population, in which schizophrenia fares the same or even better.

Stigma is carried not only by the patients, but also by their families. Often, families feel ostracized by their extended family and friends when a relative is identified as having schizophrenia. The circumstances of the first admission or subsequent readmissions can involve the police or similar actions at the family home, creating a lasting negative impression by landlords and neighbors. The fear that schizophrenia is a violent illness isolates the family even more. Finally, the lack of societal acceptance that this is an illness that requires emotional and financial support is extremely hurtful to families. Insurance coverage for all mental illnesses often lags behind the coverage for other chronic illnesses, and the widespread support to finance treatment and research for schizophrenia is nearly absent. Would there be any enthusiasm for a telethon or march on Washington, DC for support of people with schizophrenia?

One solution to reducing stigma is the creation of public awareness of the illness as a treatable biological illness similar to other more accepted medical conditions (e.g., diabetes and heart disease). In one study of attitudes about patients with schizophrenia, the more personal historical contact with friends, acquaintances, and family members with schizophrenia, the less dangerous they were perceived. In the same study, providing data about violence and schizophrenia also reduced the perception that the patients were inherently violent. The change in attitude through first person contact and accurate information presents an avenue to the reduction of stigma for those with schizophrenia and a hope for better integration.

WORLDWIDE IMPACT OF SCHIZOPHRENIA

The fundamental concept of schizophrenia was developed during the late 19th and early 20th century in central Europe by physicians who carved out a psychotic syndrome separate from senile dementias and manic-depressive illness. This concept assumed the presence of a disease of the brain usually manifested in early adulthood with a constellation of psychotic symptoms (culturally dissonant behaviors that suggested a major break in reality testing, such as delusions and hallucinations), a propensity for chronicity, and a serious impact on the subject's ability to function interpersonally and occupationally.

The emphasis given to the various components of the definition (early onset, characteristic psychotic symptoms, chronicity, and severity of impact) has been modified by different theoreticians, but the core concept has proven itself to be heuristically and clinically useful and remains. However, despite much research, no validating factor external to the definition of the clinical syndrome, with enough sensitivity and specificity, has been identified. Hence, issues of cross-cultural comparability had to be considered. That is, if *schizophrenia* is defined by a cluster of behaviors considered deviant in a specific cultural context, and no test can yet prove the presence of the disease entity in a specific individual, is the syndrome present in different cultures to the same extent and is it recognized as deviant by the community? Is it manifested in a similar way? Does it have a serious functional impact?

Emil Kraepelin recognized the importance of these issues and made a trip to the Far East specifically to document whether schizophrenia was present in non-Western cultures. Subsequently, several psychiatrists documented in a more or less systematic way the presence of the syndrome in various Asian and African communities. These studies generally supported the universality of schizophrenia but suffered from various methodological limitations, such as cross-sectional or retrospective observations, nonoperationalized definitions, lack of standardized instruments, and biases in the selection of cases. Fortunately, in the 1960s, 1970s, and 1980s, the World Health Organization (WHO) implemented large, sophisticated, multinational studies specifically designed to address cross-cultural issues. The two main studies are the International Pilot Study of Schizophrenia (IPSS) and the Determinants of Outcome Study (DOS).

International Pilot Study of Schizophrenia

This first major effort in cross-cultural psychiatric research began in 1968 and was implemented in the early 1970s. A primary goal was to establish the feasibility of large-scale international psychiatric studies and to lay the groundwork for future epidemiological studies of schizophrenia. Other aims were to explore whether schizophrenia existed in different parts of the world, to identify common and differing clinical presentations of the disorder, and to investigate the course and outcome among different cultures.

Young patients (age range of 18 to 44 years of age) admitted for psychotic symptoms to a psychiatric facility in nine centers were included. The centers were: Aahrus (Denmark), Agra (India), Cali (Colombia), Ibadan (Nigeria), London (Britain), Moscow (Union of Soviet Socialist Republics), Prague (Czechoslovakia), Taipei (Taiwan), and Washington, DC (United States). Explicit inclusion and exclusion criteria were used to select patients without known *organic* or chronic deteriorated psychoses. Field workers were trained to apply standardized psychiatric interviews in eight different languages, and satisfactory interrater reliability was achieved.

Among the 1,202 patients included, 811 received diagnoses of schizophrenic disorders, the rest having mainly affective and other psychoses. As expected, in all centers, subjects with schizophrenia were identified. Despite the important cultural, political, and economic differences among the nine participating countries, the symptomatology expressed was remarkably similar: Patients and their relatives complained of changes in behavior resulting in occupational or interpersonal problems. Subjects were preoccupied with unsupported beliefs of persecution or invasion of mind and body by alien forces and persistent, distressing perceptual experiences of bodiless voices or complex visual imagery.

Two years later, 75 percent of the initial patients were reinterviewed with the same instruments. Detailed data on the presence of multiple psychotic and nonpsychotic symptoms, the pattern of course, and social function were collected. Also, a composite measure of overall outcome (based on the level of remission, the total percentage of follow-up time in a psychotic episode, and the severity of social dysfunction) was assessed. An important finding was that, although the majority of patients (56 percent) had intermediate outcomes (more than one psychotic episode), a substantial proportion (26 percent) had good outcomes (only one episode), and only a minority (18 percent) experienced poor outcomes with unremitting psychosis, multiple episodes, or severe social impairment.

A more striking finding related to outcome in *developed* versus *developing* countries. This dichotomy was defined based on standard socioeconomic measures such as infant mortality, causes of death, literacy, etc. In the three developing countries, India, Nigeria, and Colombia, better outcomes were found than in the subjects from the developed countries. For example, 48 and 57 percent of the subjects from India and Nigeria, respectively, were rated as having best outcomes, compared to the developed countries' low percentages of such outcomes (6 to 23 percent). Conversely, between 11 and 31 percent of patients in developed countries had the worst outcomes, compared to a smaller percentage (5 and 15 percent) from Nigeria and India, respectively.

Seventy-six percent of the initial cohort was reevaluated after 5 years. Again, patients from developing countries had better outcomes than subjects from the developed centers. Other clinical and demographic factors were significantly related to a better outcome: female gender, acuteness of onset, diagnosis of schizoaffective disorder, and shorter duration of symptoms before assessment. Furthermore, psychosocial characteristics at initial examination such as not being married, social isolation, premorbid personality dysfunction, and poor sexual adjustment all predicted poor social functioning at 5 years' follow-up. Nevertheless, regardless of the inclusion of these other factors in a statistical model, the dichotomy of developing versus developed centers and acuteness of onset remained the most significant predictors of outcome.

Despite the strengths of this landmark study, important limitations must be considered when interpreting the significance of the findings. First, attrition was different across sites and was especially high in the Nigerian site (50 percent at 2 years and 41 percent at 5 years). This raises the issue of potential self-selection for follow-up among the subjects living in rural areas in countries with worse transportation infrastructure. Hence, it is possible that researchers were less able to recontact some of the sickest patients living in the more remote villages. However, attrition in the other developing centers was not particularly high.

Another limitation relates to the comparability of the patients recruited across sites. That is, perhaps a larger proportion of subjects in the developing sites were initially misclassified as having schizophrenia when they really had a more benign, short-lived type of psychotic disorder. In support of this contention, a high proportion of patients who experienced relapses at the Indian site were rediagnosed with affective or reactive psychoses (28 percent at 2 years). Also, a more acute pattern of onset, which robustly predicted outcome, was more common among the developing countries. However, the effect of center type remained after controlling statistically for acuteness of onset.

Finally, because the IPSS sample was not an epidemiological cohort, and because obstetric complications are a well-described risk factor for schizophrenia, it is possible that, in the poorer countries with higher infant mortality, a significant proportion of children at risk for the more severe forms of schizophrenia died before reaching adulthood and manifesting the disorder. To address this and other limitations and to better understand the important finding of better outcome in developing countries, the DOS was implemented.

Determinants of Outcome Study

The centers participating in the DOS were Aarhus (Denmark), Agra and Chandigarh (India), Cali (Colombia), Dublin (Ireland), Honolulu and Rochester (United States), Ibadan (Nigeria), Moscow (Union of Soviet Socialist Republics), Nagasaki (Japan), Nottingham (Britain), and Prague (Czechoslovakia). The Chandigarh center included two sites, a rural one and an urban one. Six of the 12 centers had participated in the IPSS.

Incidence

Data acquisition began in 1978, which involved a case-finding strategy of prospective surveillance of psychiatric, other medical, and social services during a 2-year period. Through this methodology, subjects seeking help for possible psychotic disorders for the first time in their lives were identified. The case-finding network also included other community agencies, such as religious institutions and traditional healers, providing a better coverage of incident cases than the IPSS, although not as comprehensive as a door-to-door epidemiological survey of the community. Hence, estimates of incidence of schizophrenia were possible in seven of the centers able to fully implement the case-finding strategy. Patients were selected early in the illness by restricting inclusion only to younger individuals (15 to 54 years of age) and to those who had made a first contact with any helping agency in the preceding 3 months. Standardized, reliable diagnostic and rating instruments were used in native languages and subjects.

The annual incidence of new cases of broadly defined schizophrenia (including the ninth edition of the *International Classification of Diseases* [ICD-9] categories of schizophrenia, paranoid state, and various reactive and unspecified psychoses) varied between 1.5 and 4.2 per 100,000 population at risk among the centers. A narrower definition that included the presence of Schneiderian first-rank symptoms (the more bizarre delusions and hallucinations consistent with the experience of invasion of the self by alien agencies) resulted in similar incidences (0.7 to 1.4 per 100,000 population) across sites. These values closely resemble those reported in several sophisticated epidemiological studies performed in Western countries and again support the universality of schizophrenia.

Demographic and Clinical Characteristics

A total study population of 1,379 was selected. The group was clearly identified early in the course of illness, and the majority (86 percent) had experienced symptoms for less than 1 year. As expected, the study population was young, with 78 percent of subjects being younger than 35 years of age and evenly divided between men and women. However, men predominated (58 percent) among the subjects younger than 35 years of age, whereas women were older at the time of entry: 62 percent of the patients in the range from 35 to 54 years of age were women. This pattern of earlier age of onset for men was not different between the developing and developed countries and replicated findings from the IPSS.

The reasons for seeking help given by relatives were remarkably similar: in more than 90 percent of cases, these involved behavior or speech perceived as bizarre and a deterioration of performance of the daily routine. A smaller percentage of cases (10 to 25 percent) involved the risk of suicide or violence to others as an important reason for initiating contact. The symptom profiles across developing and developed countries were more striking for their similarities than their differences. Negative symptoms of neglect of usual activities and social withdrawal were most often identified as the earliest manifestations, before the more florid psychotic (or positive) symptoms such as delusions and hallucinations became apparent. More than one-half of the patients experienced first-rank (Schneiderian) symptoms, and these subjects were more likely to have various other psychotic symptoms at the same time. Although similarly present across developing and developed countries, the Schneiderian symptoms were not specific to schizophrenia and failed to predict outcome. However, in developing countries, visual hallucinations were somewhat more frequent, whereas depressive symptoms tended to occur more often in the developed centers. On the whole, the pattern or mixture of possible psychotic and nonpsychotic symptoms was quite similar among the various centers. The great majority (96 percent) of patients were considered ill enough to warrant prescription of antipsychotic medications.

Content of Symptoms and Cultural Themes

To further assess similarities and differences in the content of the psychotic symptomatology and whether content reflects certain salient themes specific to a culture, two sites, Agra (India) and Ibadan (Nigeria), were further evaluated. The perceptions of the patient's behavioral disturbance from a close relative were more systematically assessed. An instrument developed for this purpose, with comparable psychometric properties, was used in both centers. In India, the patients projected a more self-centered, emotional, and agitated quality. It can be speculated that these expressions of self-centeredness reflect central Indian societal values of mystical life and the strong emphasis on family, severely distorted by the illness.

In Nigeria, the relatives described the schizophrenia patients as highly suspicious, with many persecutory delusional and hallucinatory experiences. These themes can be interpreted as consistent with a Nigerian world view of distrust of those around and that disease is somehow the product of negative forces purposely unleashed against the sick individual. Although the clinical presentation of the disease is remarkable mostly by the similarities across different cultures, and this is consistent with the universality of schizophrenia, these additional findings support the common-sense view that the content of even bizarre symptoms is, to some extent, drawn from important local cultural themes. Hence, some of the major global sociopolitical changes of the last two decades are probably linked to less frequent delusional preoccupations of communist takeover and perhaps more common themes of control through computer microtechnology and being infected with acquired immune deficiency syndrome (AIDS).

TWO-YEAR OUTCOME Seventy-eight percent of patients were reassessed at 1 and 2 years. The majority of subjects (50 percent) only had one episode, and a minority (15 percent) experienced an unremitting, continuous psychotic process. Approximately 33 percent had two or more episodes followed by remissions. The most benign remitting course was clearly more common among patients in developing countries (58 percent) than in developed centers (45 percent). Conversely, the most severe unremitting course was more frequent among developed (20 percent) than developing (12 percent) countries. Likewise, severely impaired social functioning was more common (43 percent) in developed than developing (32 percent) centers. These differences were apparent, although patients in developed countries were more likely to take antipsychotic medications for longer periods. Hence, in this independent and more representative sample of previously untreated, early schizophrenia, the important and surprising cross-cultural findings from the IPSS were replicated.

The most important predictors of a good outcome were, as in the IPSS, origin from a developing center and acuteness of onset. Fifty-four percent of patients had an acute onset (symptoms developed in a week or less), with a higher proportion of such cases in developing countries. However, after statistically controlling for type of onset, the significant effect of the center remained. Outcomes were not related to presence of the narrower, Schneiderian diagnosis but were worse for diagnoses of paranoid and hebephrenic schizophrenia. Other predictors of good outcome were being married, female gender, better adjustment in adolescence, more frequent contacts with friends, and no use of street drugs. Again, statistical modeling of these variables failed to eliminate the most robust effects of the category of developing versus developed countries and the acuteness of onset.

Family Environment, Expressed Emotion, and Outcome George W. Brown and James L. Birley, in 1968, demonstrated, and several others in Western countries have replicated that schizophrenia patients returning to families originally rated as high in EE are more likely to relapse during the following year. EE is an empirically derived index of the frequency of specific negative comments (criticism, overinvolvement, and hostility) made by live-in relatives about the person with schizophrenia during a structured interview. It was also determined that the impact of high EE was only apparent if the patient experienced significant face-to-face contact with the critical, hostile, or overinvolved family members and that this effect was not mediated through medication compliance. Furthermore, this literature supported the development of various psychotherapeutic and behavioral strategies proven effective to reduce the risk of psychotic relapse in schizophrenia.

The DOS provided the opportunity to examine family characteristics and their impact on outcome in a subgroup of the sample. EE was assessed among live-in relatives of patients with schizophrenia in the Chandigarh (India) center (the rural and urban sites) and the Aarhus (Denmark) center. The same EE standardized instruments were used in both countries. Fifty-four percent of households were classed as high in EE in Aarhus, compared to only 23 percent in Chandigarh. Within the Chandigarh sample, urban families were more often classified as high in EE (30 percent) than the rural households (8 percent).

After 1 year of follow-up, families in Chandigarh were reassessed (this follow-up was not completed at the Danish site). Despite the low frequency of relapse (14 percent), the schizophrenia patients residing in families rated as high in EE at baseline were more likely (31 percent) to relapse than those from low-EE households (9 percent). After 1 year, the majority (79 percent) of high-EE families had changed to low EE. These findings replicated several other longitudinal Western studies and suggested that some emotional characteristics in the family of residence may, in part, be related to the better outcome evident in developing countries.

However, there are caveats to this interpretation. The number of subjects and families reassessed was small, and there were no reports of a clear correlation between reductions in EE and relapse. It is possible that a high EE status may be a consequence of the relapse itself (or of patients being more severely ill). Proving a causal role of EE for psychotic relapse requires a controlled family therapy study with the aim of reducing relapse through an effect on EE and that includes interim EE assessments. One such study from England did find reductions on patient relapse and on families' EE with the experimental family therapy. However, similar changes from high to low EE were reported in the relatives in the control group. This would not be expected if EE was a stable dimension with a simple causal role in relapse.

Interpretation and Summary of WHO Studies

What is the meaning of the better prognoses of persons with schizophrenia in developing or non-Western countries? It has been speculated that developing countries are more *sociocentric*, with an emphasis on social relations and a range of rules, roles, and conventions consistent with living in a village. This may sustain long-term relationships and may make isolation less likely even for the disabled. Western, industrialized societies can be labeled as more *egocentric*, with relationships more likely to be bilateral and subject to constant reevaluation and revocation. Also, the fierce competition in the job market with frequent moves to new locations for employment in developed countries may be less likely to foster a stable, structured environment that allows persons with schizophrenia to recuperate at their own pace.

As mentioned previously, family milieu (EE) has been found to be related to psychotic relapse in the West and in one developing site (Chandigarh, India) of the DOS. Persons with schizophrenia, like several other groups with chronic relapsing psychiatric and nonpsychiatric illnesses, appear to be more vulnerable to excessive emotional demands within and outside of the family. Perhaps, in the developing countries, the more traditional family with extended kinship ties provides more consistent support. Conversely, the more common nuclear family in Western industrialized communities may end up placing heavier demands on fewer relatives, usually parents and siblings who may become overwhelmed by the responsibility and may relate to the patient more critically.

Finally, the possibility of differential survival, with more children at risk for schizophrenia growing up and developing the most severe forms of the illness in industrialized countries with better health care systems, remains. However, the DOS finding of similar incidence of schizophrenia among developed and developing countries argues against this explanation.

In summary, these two landmark WHO studies have produced consistent evidence that the disorder defined in the Western medical literature as schizophrenia exists in different communities and cultures. This condition is, indeed, perceived by the community as a disorder, that is, a change in the individual that is inconsistent with the local behavioral norms and that requires help. Although the clinical presentation is heterogeneous, and there are no pathognomonic signs or symptoms, the pattern of symptomatology is more remarkable by its similarities than by its differences among the various study sites. The rate of occurrence of new cases is also similar across countries, as is the gender and age patterns of presentation (younger onset in males). These characteristics support the concept that the same nonaffective psychotic disease occurs worldwide.

Outcome, in terms of remission of psychosis and functional reintegration to society, is heterogeneous within schizophrenia and is by no means uniformly malignant, as originally conceptualized by Kraepelin. Approximately one-half of total cases have a single episode with good functional recovery. Predictors of good outcome include acute onset, better premorbid function, and female gender. Better outcomes are clearly more common in developing countries for still unknown reasons. These studies do not support the original kraepelinian concept that the majority of patients with schizophrenia deteriorate and fail to recover.

However, using a definition of schizophrenia that emphasizes chronicity and includes a minimum length of psychosis (at least 1 month) and functional deterioration (at least 6 months), like the current revised fourth edition of the *Diagnostic and Statistical Manual of Mental Disorders* (DSM-IV-TR), most likely identifies a subgroup with worse prognosis. For example, recent follow-up data from the Hillside, New York first-episode schizophrenia study suggest that *recovery*, defined as full symptom remission, fulfillment of age-appropriate expectations, performance of daily living skills without supervision, and engagement in social interaction, is rare, despite high rates of symptom response and compliance with pharmacological treatment: Only 17 percent of the subjects met cumulative criteria for recovery by 5 years. Although generally young, patients in the Hillside cohort had a mean length of illness of approximately 16 months when identified and were referred to a specialized tertiary level care psychiatric center. Hence, these patients were not *acute* when compared to the IPSS and DOS samples. This is consistent with the WHO studies' findings of the importance of acuteness of onset and premorbid function in terms of outcome. Data acquired with a more sophisticated assessment of psychosocial outcome, less dependent on the level of symptomatology, will become available in the future for a subgroup of the DOS sample. This will permit a more precise look at the extent of return to full premorbid level of social function across different cultures.

COMPARABILITY OF SCHIZOPHRENIA TO OTHER CONDITIONS

A considerable knowledge about the illness of schizophrenia has been accumulated over the past 50 years since antipsychotic medication was introduced. The position of leading clinicians changed from not using medication, because it might interfere with psychodynamic interventions, to the development of highly technical interpersonal interventions to be used in coordinated treatment plans. There are many questions that remain to be answered. Included among them are

- Does the addition of a highly intensive psychosocial intervention contribute to better outcomes?
- Does a psychosocial program rely on "more is better" or are there specific gains made from specific treatments?
- Are continuity and constancy of treatment more important than intensity?
- With limited resources, should community treatment programs orient toward enhanced pharmacology or enhanced psychosocial treatment?

Although the answers to these questions remain elusive for the most part, the field currently has sufficient knowledge to assist in the development of a sophisticated treatment program to reliably treat people with schizophrenia. Throughout a treatment program, efficacy and effectiveness must be matched with dignity and informed choice. It is not an issue of what is done to or for patients, but rather it is what to do with patients that will ultimately make the difference. The advent of advocacy groups has empowered a formerly disenfranchised population. In addition, their families are no longer seen as pariahs but as valued members of the overall therapeutic environment.

Psychiatric treatment of schizophrenia, as well as most treatment of mental illness, has changed but is not always considered a science. For reasons that remain elusive, psychiatry, and the patients it serves, has not received the recognition that its science deserves. Whether it is a part of the stigma that attends a psychiatric diagnosis is unclear. It is interesting to note that these prevailing negative views are completely independent of the actual data about the field. For more than 40 years, psychiatry has developed and actually led science in the art of clinical trials—the testing of treatments. Although accepted medical practices in other branches of medicine have come under question as to their efficacy (e.g., low-fat diets and arthroscopy for the knee), psychiatry has built a credible database that examines proposed treatments thoroughly and fairly. When hemodialysis was proposed as a treatment for schizophrenia in the mid-1970s, the scientific community tempered its therapeutic excitement until clinical trials were able to demonstrate that this was not an effective treatment for this illness. However, the science of psychiatry goes much further. A careful evaluation of the base of clinical trials found the following:

> In a comparative evaluation of 6-month trial data for schizophrenia and two treatment approaches to stenosed arteries, psychiatric treatment outcomes in schizophrenia were superior to angioplasty and atherectomy. That failure to achieve remission in schizophrenia may approach 40 percent at the 6-month interval is generally accepted and looked at as a disappointment; that angioplasty and atherectomy have 50 percent or more restenosis at 6 months is less well acknowledged. If the reader doubts this, just look at how these two domains of medicine—psychiatry and procedural cardiology—are treated by insurers! Some may argue that in psychiatry more than just a single medicine is applied, here a single procedure of atherectomy or angioplasty is compared to a broader arsenal of treatments. One can compare a single medicine in a drug trial to another area of internal medicine.

Comparing the results of a 1-year outcome with an atypical medication, risperidone (Risperdal), to the results of six leading antihypertensive medications, there is a sizable advantage in favor of maintenance of remission for the psychiatric treatment. *Relapse* was defined in the psychiatric treatment as

- Psychiatric hospitalization
- Physician judgment that increased care is necessary *and* a Positive and Negative Syndrome Scale (PANSS) score increase of 25 percent relative to baseline or increase by ten points, if baseline less than or equal to 40
- Deliberate self-injury
- Emergence of clinically significant suicidal or homicidal ideation
- Violent behavior resulting in significant injury to another person or property damage
- Significant clinical deterioration defined by a Clinical Global Impression of Change (CGIC) score of 6.

Relapse for the antihypertensive medication was defined as, once the diastolic pressure was brought below 95, it could it be kept there at the end of 1 year. The results for the antipsychotic medication showed a 23 percent relapse rate at 1 year; the average for the six antihypertensive medications was 48 percent.

It is obvious that the field of psychiatry has done well in the conduct of clinical trials. Psychiatrists should not apologize for the results. Psychiatrists are in an era of ever-increasing budget demands in health care. Achieving parity in insurance coverage has reached the national stage. All that is necessary is for psychiatric treatments and the patients they help to be given a level playing field. Effective treatments are theoretically available; they need to have delivery assured in the real world.

Significance of Treatment Delivery The specifics of pharmacological and psychosocial treatments have been thoroughly covered in other chapters. It is clear that the treatments for schizophrenia have improved in both domains. Pharmacologically, the advent of antipsychotic medications that provide superior efficacy, while reducing extrapyramidal side effects, has been a welcome advance. That patients were persuaded to take the conventional antipsychotic medications of an earlier period is a testament to how powerful the therapeutic relationship with patients is. The older treatments added increasing stigma to an illness that was already stigmatizing. The fixed facial expression, the lack of arm swing, the distinctive tremor, and the facial movements and tics all served to point out how different a patient with schizophrenia was. In any situation, it was no challenge to identify a patient on conventional antipsychotic medications. Furthermore, such side effects as akathisia or restless leg were not only stigmatizing, but also highly intolerable to the patient.

Psychosocial treatments have also advanced. The basic principles of consistent, continuous contact with a patient with schizophrenia are critical to apply. The past 40 years have seen many of the high-intensity, high-technology psychosocial treatments fall victim to carefully done research. Psychoanalysis with schizophrenia is rarely used, after the major study of intensive psychotherapy at McLean Hospital and Boston University showed that the more ill a patient with schizophrenia was, the less likely he or she was to tolerate intensive psychotherapy. Despite this differential attrition—the more ill patients dropping out of the intensive (three times a week) psychotherapy, and yet remaining in the good clinical management group (30 minutes a week), the only measures that showed any advantages favored the good clinical management group. Intensive family management programs have followed a similar pattern. When compared to consistent low-intensity family programs, advantages for the intensive programs in schizophrenia have been hard to find. That working with families, considering them as important treatment allies, is a critical ingredient in the success of any treatment program for schizophrenia is undeniable. Just how intensive or specific the technology needs to be is unknown. Furthermore, despite their widespread success in clinical trials, the family psychosocial technologies have not gained the critical acceptance and use in most treatment programs. Newer approaches, for example, cognitive behavior treatments, hold considerable promise and, given their widespread acceptance in depression, may find better uptake in the treatment community than some of the other therapies.

Nothing said previously should be taken as a disparagement of psychosocial interventions for schizophrenia. On the contrary, successful treatment, including pharmacotherapies, must be imbedded in the context of a relationship model. As noted previously, psychiatrists have asked patients to take medications with severe and stigmatizing side effects. These patients only take such medications in the context of a meaningful, trusting, and supportive relationship. Unless the clinician fully understands the patient and the impact of this illness on him or her, the likelihood of medication adherence is low. Even with this relationship, optimal medication management and adherence may be difficult.

Adherence Adherence to medication regimens is a universally difficult task. When the terms *partial adherence or compliance* or *nonadherence or compliance* are used, they are not used as an accusation; they are used to comment on human nature. There are compelling data that demonstrate that only approximately 40 percent of patients with asthma or rheumatoid arthritis are fully compliant with their medication. With schizophrenia, the data are even more sobering. A recent large database study showed that less than 10 percent of patients with schizophrenia refilled their prescriptions appropriately through the course of 1 year. The mean number of days patients were without medication was 4 months. A second finding from this study comparing an atypical medication to conventional medication prescription refills was that, although the patients on the atypical antipsychotic were more likely to refill their prescription than those on conventional antipsychotic medication, the difference was only 15 days, and, given that the average length of time without medication was almost 4 months, this difference would not be clinically significant. Psychiatrists are aware of this difficulty with compliance, yet seem to have done little to offset it. A recent survey of community psychiatrists on the degree of difficulty to produce compliance sufficient to produce therapeutic efficacy found that only weight reduction and exercise programs were as difficult as schizophrenia (Fig. 12.2–1).

In many ways, the partially compliant patient presents a more difficult problem for the clinician than does the fully noncompliant one. Patients who refuse medication, never fill prescriptions, and fail to keep follow-up appointments are easily identified and clearly require a different approach to treatment. The partially compliant patient, on the other hand, is difficult to identify. Most patients believe they are taking their medication as prescribed, when, in reality, 60 to 70 percent are not. Further, the current treatment philosophy of maintaining patients on the lowest therapeutic dose, although helpful for side effects, may increase the impact of missed doses to the point that they fall below the therapeutic threshold. In the past, when large doses of medication were the rule, missing occasional doses had less potential to be damaging.

The impact of not meeting the lowest therapeutic dose threshold can be seen in either incomplete recovery, lack of full functioning, or return of symptoms and relapse. The reversal of symptoms, secondary to medication absence, once they have started is also difficult. There have now been five studies evaluating the difference between continuous medication and medication given only at the onset of prodrome or early symptoms. The results of these studies are universally negative for the intervention at symptom exacerbation. Relapse is twice as likely using such a strategy, and yet, many patients themselves adopt such an as-needed medication strategy (Fig. 12.2–2).

For many patients, the onset of schizophrenia is their first contact with a chronic and persistent illness. Approximately 50 percent of people who develop schizophrenia have it before 25 years of age. Before 25 years of age, most people's experience with illness has been with time-limited illnesses, such as bacterial infection or a broken bone, in which they take or apply the treatment for a period of time, stop the treatment, and everything returns pretty much to normal, until their next episode. That is not the case with schizophrenia; yet patients often apply this model to it. In addition, people with schizophrenia have neurocognitive issues that affect attention, persistence, and attitude, all of which make medication taking more difficult. The results of the model of illness and the neurocognitive deficits lead to problems with medication compliance and cycles of repeated relapses.

There are also some interesting studies under way pointing to the role of medication in preventing or delaying the onset of schizophrenia. At the present time, these results must be seen as preliminary, but they do shed light on the importance of medication compliance. In a study from Australia, patients with subthreshold symptoms of schizophrenia were treated for 6 months and then followed up for 6 additional months. Those who were assigned a pharmacological intervention had significantly fewer progressions to the first episode

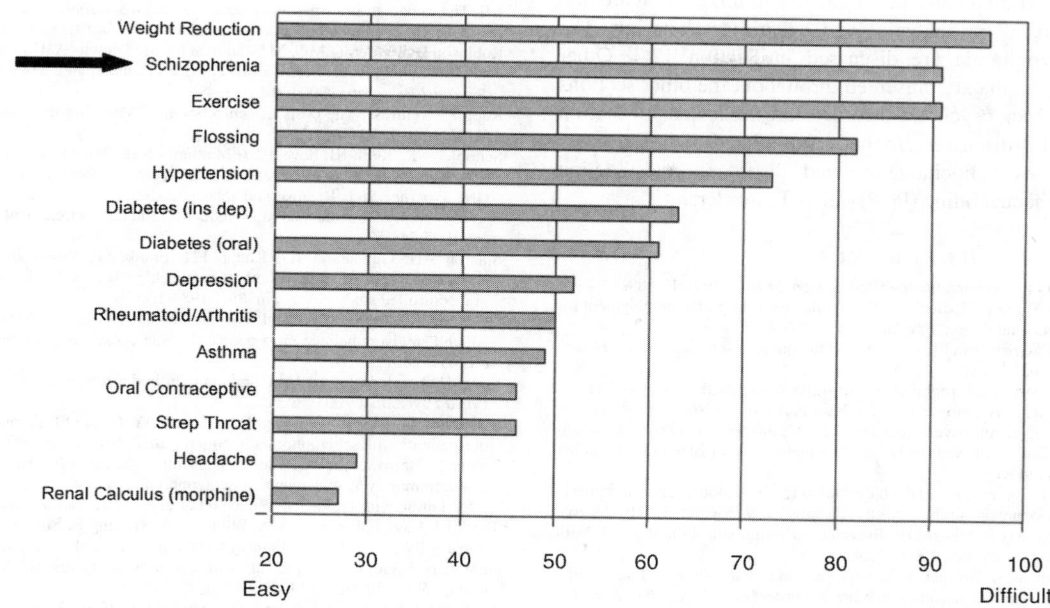

FIGURE 12.2–1 Degree of difficulty to produce adherence sufficient for therapeutic effect. ins dep, insulin dependent.

of psychosis at the 6-month treatment end than those who were not assigned a pharmacological intervention. By the 12-month evaluation, the differences between the two groups were no longer significant. A further analysis, however, found that those patients who had been assigned to the pharmacological intervention *and were adherent to it* maintained the protection of the medication for the full 12 months.

Psychiatrists have generally considered psychotic episodes and relapse to be negative outcomes in schizophrenia, and, indeed, they are. What is becoming clearer, however, is that, with each episode, patients seem to lose something that they do not recapture. In one study of first episode patients, the time to remission after a first episode was 47 days; after a second episode, the time to remission was 76.5 days; and, after a third episode, the time to remission was 130 days. Each successive episode required longer to return to a remitted state. The cause for this deterioration has recently received attention from neuroimaging studies that suggest that a neurodegenerative process may be occurring. Although controversial, these findings of medication adherence offering protection against the development of an initial psychotic episode and the neurodegeneration imaging studies certainly give potential added support to medication compliance being a critical ingredient in treatment paradigms. In reality, it may not matter whether there is a biological component or whether it is a matter of demoralization, the simple fact remains that multiple relapses are detrimental to overall outcome in schizophrenia. It is incumbent on the clinician to emphasize that schizophrenia is not like other illnesses that the patient may have experienced. Furthermore, initially, families frequently use a similar model, because they so want their developing adolescent or young adult to realize the potential that was once so clearly on their path. It is hard for a clinician to consider removing this expectation and hope. On the other hand, the greatest hope for the patient may result from an acceptance that this is a persistent illness that turns out most positively only if treatment is accepted. The clinician needs to be in a position of preventing further deterioration, encouraging full remission, and returning the patient, over time, to productivity. Currently, only 20 percent of patients with schizophrenia will be competitively employed—and employment and independent living are important milestones of success. If psychiatrists are able to increase treatment compliance—pharmacologically and psychosocially—from the start of subthreshold or early psychosis, psychiatrists can contribute to far greater success in an illness that has known all too little.

In conclusion, the issue of schizophrenia encompasses a wide scope. The illness casts a long shadow and spares no particular culture or society, although outcome may differ depending on geography. The problem poses significant costs on society, and this cost appears to be escalating each year. On a positive note, although the diagnosis of schizophrenia has often been stigmatizing, successful interventions, psychosocial and pharmacological, have been developed. These interventions have not been uniformly recognized but are comparable or better than treatments of other medical illnesses.

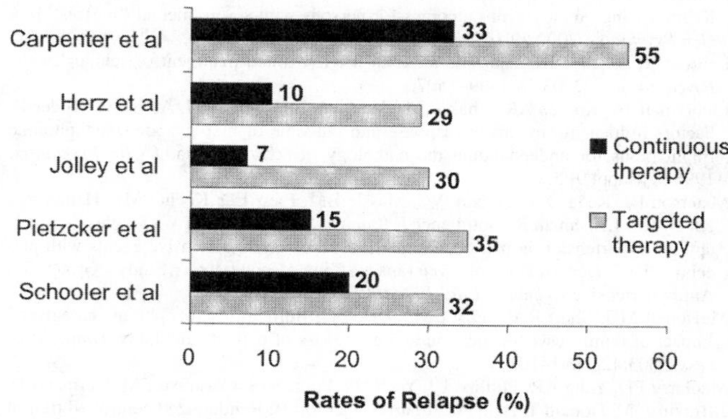

FIGURE 12.2–2 Continuous versus target maintenance. Rates of relapse after 1 year. (From Kane JM: Schizophrenia. *N Engl J Med.* 1996;334:34–41, with permission.)

SUGGESTED CROSS-REFERENCES

Some of the methods and concepts applicable to this section are discussed in Section 5.2 on statistics and experimental design. The genetics of schizophrenia are discussed in Section 12.3. Other aspects of schizophrenia are presented throughout the other sections of Chapter 12. Other psychotic disorders are reviewed in Section 12.15. Section 11.3 discusses amphetamine-related disorders, Section 11.7 discusses hallucinogen-related disorders, and Section 11.11 discusses phencyclidine (PCP)–related disorders.

REFERENCES

Andrews G: The cost of schizophrenia revisited. *Schizophr Bull.* 1991;17:389.

Bond GR, Drake RE, Mueser KT, Becker DR: An update on supported employment for people with severe mental illness. *Psychiatr Serv.* 1997;48:335.

Brown GW, Birley JL: Crises and life changes and the onset of schizophrenia. *J Health Soc Behav.* 1968;9:203.

Burke DT: Monetary cost of schizophrenia to Australia. *Med J Aust.* 1986;144:723.

Byerly M, Fisher R, Rush AJ, Holland R, Varghese F. A Comparison of Clinician vs. Electronic Monitoring of Antipsychotic Adherence in Schizophrenia. Poster presentation at: American College of Neurology and Psychiatry Annual Meeting; December 2002; San Juan, Puerto Rico.

Conley RR, Mahmoud R: A randomized double blind study of risperidone and olanzapine in the treatment of schizophrenia or schizoaffective disorder. *Am J Psychiatry.* 2001;158:765.

*Crisp AH, Gelder MG, Rix S, Meltzer HI, Rowlands OJ: Stigmatisation of people with mental illnesses. *Br J Psychiatry.* 2000;177:4.

Csernansky JG, Mahmoud R, Brenner R: The comparison of risperidone and haloperidol for the prevention of relapse in patients with schizophrenia. *N Engl J Med.* 2002;346:16.

Dickerson FB, Sommerville J, Origoni AE, Ringel NB, Parente F: Experiences of stigma among outpatients with schizophrenia. *Schizophr Bull.* 2002;28:143.

Dixon L, Goldman H, Hirad A: State policy and funding of services to families of adults with serious and persistent mental illness. *Psychiatr Serv.* 1999;50:551.

Ferriman A: The stigma of schizophrenia. *BMJ.* 2000;320:522.

Guest JF, Cookson RF: Cost of schizophrenia to UK society: An incidence-based cost-of-illness model for the first 5 years following diagnosis. *Pharmacoeconomics.* 1999;15:597.

Gunderson JG, Mosher LR: The cost of schizophrenia. *Am J Psychiatry.* 1975;132:9.

*Jablensky A, Sartorius N, Ernberg G, Anker M, Korten A, Cooper JE, Day R, Bertelsen A: Schizophrenia: Manifestations, incidence, and course in different cultures. A World Health Organization ten-country study. *Psychol Med Monogr Suppl.* 1992;20:1–97.

Katz M, Marsella A, Dube KC, Olatawura M, Takhashi R, Nakane Y, Wynne L, Gift T, Brennan J, Sartotius N, Jablensky A: On the expression of psychosis in different cultures: Schizophrenia in an Indian and a Nigerian community. *Cult Med Psychiatry.* 1988;12:331.

Keith SJ, Kane JM: Partial compliance and patient consequences in schizophrenia: Our patients can do better. *J Clin Psychiatry*. 2003;64(11):1308–1315.

*Keith SJ, Matthews SM: The value of psychiatric treatment: Its efficacy in severe mental disorders. *Psychopharmacol Bull.* 1993;29:427.

Kemp R, Hayward P, Applewhaite G, Everitt B, David A: Compliance therapy in psychotic patients: Randomised controlled trial. *BMJ.* 1996;312:345.

Knapp M: Costs of schizophrenia. *Br J Psychiatry.* 1997;171:509.

Kommana S, Mansfield M, Penn DL: Dispelling the stigma of schizophrenia. *Psychiatr Serv.* 1997;48:1393.

Kyngas HA. Compliance of adolescents with asthma. *Nurs Health Sci.* 1999;1:195.

*Leff J, Sartorius N, Jablensky A, Korten A, Ernberg G. The International Pilot Study of Schizophrenia: Five year follow-up findings. *Psychol Med.* 1992;22:131.

Leff J, Wig N, Ghosh A, Bedi H, Menon D, Kuipers L, Korten A, Ernberg G, Day R, Sartorius N, Jablensky A: Influence of relatives' expressed emotion on the course of schizophrenia in Chandigarh. *Br J Psychiatry.* 1987;151:166.

Lehman A: Vocational rehabilitation in schizophrenia. *Schizophr Bull.* 1995;21:645.

Lehman AF, Goldberg R, Dixon LB, McNary S, Postrado L, Hackman A, McDonnell K: Improving employment outcomes for persons with severe mental illnesses. *Arch Gen Psychiatry.* 2002;59:165.

Lenroot R, Bustillo JR, Lauriello J, Keith SJ: Integrated treatment of schizophrenia. *Psychiatr Serv*. 2003;54:1499–1507.

Lieberman JA, Koreen AR, Chakos M, Sheitman B, Woerner M, Alvir JM, Bilder R: Factors influencing treatment response and outcome of first-episode schizophrenia: Implications for understanding the pathology of schizophrenia. *J Clin Psychiatry.* 1996;57[Suppl 9]:5.

Materson BJ, Reda D, Cushman WC, Massie BM, Freis ED, Kochar MS, Hamburger RJ, Fye C, Lakshman R, Gottdiener J, Ramirez EA, Henderson W: Single-drug therapy for hypertension in men: A comparison of six antihypertensive agents with placebo. The Department of Veterans Affairs Cooperative Study Group on Antihypertensive Agents. *N Engl J Med.* 1993;328:914.

McDonell MG, Short RA, Berry CM, Dyck DG: Burden in schizophrenia caregivers: Impact of family psychoeducation and awareness of patient suicidality. *Family Process.* 2003;42(1):91–103.

McGorry PD, Yung AR, Phillips LJ, Yuen HP, Francey S, Cosgrave EM, Germano D, Bravin J, McDonald T, Blair A, Adlard S, Jackson H: Randomized controlled trial of interventions designed to reduce the risk of progression to first episode psychosis in a clinical sample with subthreshold symptoms. *Arch Gen Psych.* 2002;59:921.

McGuire TG: Measuring the economic costs of schizophrenia. *Schizophr Bull.* 1991;17:375.

Newman SC, Bland RC: Mortality in a cohort of patients with schizophrenia: A record linkage study. *Can J Psychiatry.* 1991;36:239.

Penn DL, Kommana S, Mansfield M, Link BG: Dispelling the stigma of schizophrenia: II. The impact of information on dangerousness. *Schizophr Bull.* 1999;25:437.

*Rice DP: The economic impact of schizophrenia. *J Clin Psychiatry.* 1999;60[Suppl 1]:4.

Robinson DG, Woerner MG, McMeniman M, Medelowitz A, Bilder RM: Symptomatic and functional recovery from a first episode of schizophrenia or schizoaffective disorder. *Am J Psychiatry*. 2004;161:473–479.

Rupp A, Keith SJ: The costs of schizophrenia: Assessing the burden. *Psychiatr Clin North Am.* 1993;16:413.

Schooler NR, Keith SJ, Severe JB, Matthews SM, Bellack AS, Glick ID, Hargreaves WA, Kane JM, Ninan PT, Frances A, Jacobs M, Lieberman JA, Mance R, Simpson GM, Woerner MG: Relapse and rehospitalization during maintenance treatment of schizophrenia. The effects of dose reduction and family treatment. *Arch Gen Psychiatry.* 1997;54:453.

Stanton AH, Gunderson JG, Knapp PH, Frank AF, Vannicelli ML, Schnitzer R, Rosenthal R: Effects of psychotherapy in schizophrenia: Design and implementation of a controlled study. *Schizophr Bull.* 1984;10:520.

Struening EL, Perlick DA, Link BG, Hellman F, Herman D, Sirey JA: The extent to which caregivers believe most people devalue consumers and their families. *Psychiatr Serv.* 2001;52:1633.

Stuart H, Arboleda-Flórez JA: Community attitudes toward people with schizophrenia. *Can J Psychiatry.* 2001;46:245.

Suleiman TG, Ohaeri JU, Lawal RA, Haruna AY, Orija OB: Financial cost of treating out-patients with schizophrenia in Nigeria. *Br J Psychiatry.* 1997;171:364.

Tarrier N, Barrowclough C, Vaughn C, Bamrah JS, Porceddu K, Watts S, Freeman H. The community management of schizophrenia: A controlled trial of a behavioural intervention with families to reduce relapse. *Br J Psychiatry.* 1988;153:532.

Topol EJ, Laya F, Pinkerton CA, Whitlow PL, Hofling B, Simonton CA, Masden RR, Serruys PW, Leon MB, Williams DO: A comparison of directional atherectomy with coronary angioplasty in patients with coronary artery disease. The CAVEAT Study Group. *N Engl J Med.* 1993;329:221.

Velligan DI, Newcomer J, Pultz J, Csernansky J, Hoff AL, Mahurin R, Miller AL: Does cognitive function improve with quetiapine in comparison to haloperidol? *Schizophr Res.* 2002;53:239.

Viller F, Guillemin F, Briancon S, Moum T, Suurmeijer T, van den Heuvel W: Compliance to drug treatment of patients with rheumatoid arthritis: A 3-year longitudinal study. *J Rheumatol.* 1999;26:2114.

Wig N, Menon D, Bedi H, Kuipers L, Ghosh A, Day R, Korten A, Ernberg G, Sartorius N, Jablensky A: Expressed emotion and schizophrenia in north India. II. Distribution of expressed emotion components among relatives of schizophrenic patients in Aarhus and Chandigarh. *Br J Psychiatry.* 1987;151:160.

World Health Organization. *Schizophrenia: An International Follow-up Study*. Chichester, UK: John Wiley and Sons; 1979.

▲ 12.3 Schizophrenia: Genetics

BRIEN P. RILEY, PH.D., AND KENNETH S. KENDLER, M.D.

The goal of this section is to provide an overview of the current state of knowledge of the genetic epidemiology and molecular genetics of schizophrenia. The discussion of genetic epidemiology focuses on the following key questions: Is schizophrenia a familial disorder? To what extent is any familial aggregation of schizophrenia due to genetic versus environmental factors? What is the nature of the psychiatric disorders that are transmitted within families? As the section argues that genetic factors play an important role in the familial transmission of schizophrenia, the discussion of molecular genetics of schizophrenia focuses on two additional questions: What kinds of genetic transmission mechanisms appear most likely? What are the current status and future prospects for identifying specific genes that predispose to schizophrenia?

IS SCHIZOPHRENIA FAMILIAL?

The most basic question in the genetics of schizophrenia is whether the disorder aggregates (or "runs") in families. Technically, familial aggre-

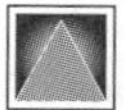

Table 12.3–1
Summary Results of Major Recent Family Studies of Schizophrenia That Included a Normal Control Group, Personal Interviews with Relatives, and Blind Diagnosis of Relatives

			First-Degree Relatives of Schizophrenic Probands			First-Degree Relatives of Control Probands				
Author, Yr	Diagnostic Criteria	Controls	BZ	N	Schizophrenia MR (%)	BZ	N	Schizophrenia MR (%)	P	Correlation in Liability (r) ± Standard Error
Tsuang, 1980[a]	Consensus senior Iowa clinicians	Screened surgical patients	362	20	5.5	475	3	0.6	.00002	0.36 ± 0.04
Baron, 1985	RDC, DSM-III	Screened acquaintances	329	19	5.8	337	2	0.6	.0001	0.37 ± 0.04
Kendler, 1985[a]	DSM-III	Screened surgical patients	703	26	3.7	931	2	0.2	8×10^{-8}	0.38 ± 0.03
Frangos, 1985	DSM-III	Controls	478	26	5.4	536	6	1.1	.0001	0.28 ± 0.04
Coryell, 1988	RDC	Screened volunteers	72	1	1.4	160	0[b]	0	Nonsignificant	0.23 ± 0.12
Gershon, 1988	RDC chronic schizophrenia	Volunteers	97	3	3.1	349	2	0.6	.038	0.25 ± 0.09
Kendler, 1992	DSM-III-R	Unscreened general population controls	276	18	6.5	428	2	0.5	.000004	0.41 ± 0.04
Maier, 1993[c]	RDC	Unscreened general population controls	435	17	3.9	320	1	0.3	.001	0.36 ± 0.04
Taylor, 1993	DSM-III	Screened medical patients	335	9	2.7	264	0[b]	0	.000003	0.33 ± 0.04
Parnas, 1993[c,d]	DSM-III-R	Screened controls	192	31	16.2	101	2	1.9	.0001	0.41 ± 0.04
Erlenmeyer-Kimling, 1995[c,d]	DSM-III-R	Screened controls	54	6	11.1	93	0[b]	0	.002	0.53 ± 0.08

BZ, *bezugsziffer* (total lifetime equivalents of risk); MR, morbid risk; RDC, Research Diagnostic Criteria.
[a]Studies on partially overlapping data sets; results include relatives with only hospital records.
[b]For the purpose of calculating a correlation in liability, one-half a case of illness in controls is assumed.
[c]Prevalence rather than MR reported.
[d]Offspring only.

gation means that a close relative of an individual with a disorder is at increased risk for that disorder, compared with a matched individual chosen at random from the general population. The section reviews family studies of schizophrenia examining primarily first-degree relatives (parents, full siblings, and offspring), as little systematic information on more distant relationships has been gathered in recent years.

Early Family Studies In a 1967 review paper, Edith Zerbin-Rudin listed 17 major family studies of schizophrenia involving first-degree relatives. By 1980, at least nine other major studies had been reported. All of these studies consistently showed a substantially greater risk for schizophrenia in the close relatives of schizophrenics than was expected in the general population.

However, nearly all of these studies had three important methodological limitations. First, no control groups were used so that the rates of schizophrenia in the general population required for comparison had to be derived from the literature. Second, diagnoses were made nonblind, with the research team always knowing that the individual being evaluated was a relative of a schizophrenic individual. Third, neither structured personal interviews nor operationalized diagnostic criteria were used. In fact, in many of the early studies, it is unclear how many individuals were personally examined and how many were evaluated from indirect information such as reports of relatives or doctors or from hospital notes.

Modern Family Studies In the early 1980s, several research groups questioned the validity of earlier family studies of schizophrenia. Perhaps, they suggested, the evidence for the familial aggregation of schizophrenia results from consistent biases in the previous studies. In addition, they were concerned that the diagnostic approach to schizophrenia in these earlier studies might have been overly broad. When "narrowly" diagnosed, they argued that the familial aggregation of schizophrenia might be weak or absent. Since 1980, 11 major family studies of schizophrenia have been reported that used blind diagnoses, control groups, personal interviews, and operationalized diagnostic criteria. These studies permit a more rigorous evaluation than has hitherto been possible of the degree to which schizophrenia aggregates in families.

The key results from these studies are summarized in Table 12.3–1. This table contains the diagnostic criteria used in the study, the nature of the control proband group, and the probability value (i.e., the probability of observing such a difference in the rates of schizophrenia in the two groups by chance if the true rates were identical). The term *proband* refers to the individual through whom the family was identified for study. A typical family study of schizophrenia begins with two types of probands: those with schizophrenia and a matched group of control probands. Relatives of these probands are systematically assessed. Table 12.3–1 also presents the lifetimes at risk in the assessed relatives of schizophrenia and control probands and the morbid risk for schizophrenia in the two groups. The term *lifetimes at risk* is the sum for all assessed relatives of the proportion of their lifetime risk for schizophrenia they have completed. The term *morbid risk,* or MR, is a statistic commonly used in genetics and equals the total proportion of individuals who are expected to be affected with a disorder in a given population if all members of that population have completed their age at risk. Finally, the table includes the *correlation of liability*. If schizophrenia is due to several genetic and environmental factors that act approximately additively in influencing an individual's liability or predisposition to schizophrenia, then this figure represents the degree of correlation between first-degree relatives in overall risk of the disease. This is a useful figure because it combines into a single statistic the risk figures for schizophrenia in relatives of schizophrenic and control probands. The *higher* the correlation of liability, the *stronger* is the degree of familial aggregation of schizophrenia.

Before addressing the major results summarized in this table, two preliminary comments are in order. First, the sample of relatives studied varies very widely in the different investigations. For example, the lifetimes at risk in relatives of schizophrenics range more than tenfold, from more than 700 to 54. On average, the larger studies provide more stable statistical estimates for the true risk of schizophrenia in relatives of schizophrenic and control probands. Second, various diagnostic criteria were used in the different studies. However, eight studies used either the third edition of the *Diagnostic and Statistical Manual of Mental Disorders* (DSM-III), Research Diagnostic Criteria (for chronic schizophrenia), or the revised DSM-III (DSM-III-R) criteria, all of which require, in addition to specified psychotic symptoms, at least 6 months of illness, usually with functional impairment. Third, whereas nine of the studies examined all available first-degree relatives (parents, full siblings, and offspring), two studies examined only offspring.

There are five major conclusions that can be drawn from the large body of work summarized in the table. First, the risk for schizophrenia in relatives of schizophrenic probands varies widely across studies, from a low of 1.4 percent to a high of 16.2 percent. Much of this fluctuation can probably be explained by differences in diagnostic criteria or statistical fluctuations in small samples (the lowest risk is found in the smallest study). However, it remains possible that there are true population differences in the risk for schizophrenia in relatives of schizophrenic probands.

Second, the risk for schizophrenia in the relatives of nonpsychiatric control probands is relatively similar across studies, ranging—with the exception of the study of Josef Parnas et al.—from only 0.2 to 1.1 percent, corresponding closely to the range of risks for schizophrenia found in general population studies.

Third, in every study, the risk for schizophrenia was higher in the relatives of schizophrenic probands than in relatives of control probands. Across these studies, the risk of schizophrenia was, on average, 11 times greater in relatives of schizophrenic probands than in relatives of matched control probands. Fourth, in all but one study, the difference in risk for schizophrenia in the relatives of schizophrenic and control probands was quite unlikely to occur by chance (i.e., $P < .05$). In a number of studies, the probability values were very low (i.e., <.001), indicating that such differences in risk were *extremely* unlikely to occur by chance.

Finally, although there was some variation, the correlation in liability for all studies fell in the range from +0.23 to +0.53, with a weighted mean across the 11 studies of +0.35. Most of the largest studies that used relatively narrow diagnostic criteria for schizophrenia obtained correlations of liability in the narrow range of +0.32 to +0.41, as the highest and lowest correlations in the table come from, respectively, the smallest and next to smallest studies. These results suggest that most of these studies can be seen as replications of one another because they are providing us with similar results regarding the degree of familial aggregation of schizophrenia. The correlation of liability between first-degree relatives in the range of +0.30 to +0.40 indicates a relatively strong degree of familial aggregation.

Family Studies: Summary In conclusion, the questions raised in the early 1980s about the degree of familial aggregation of typical adult-onset schizophrenia can now be addressed satisfactorily. The results of a large number of recent, carefully performed family studies support the conclusions of earlier and less methodologically rigorous investigations in finding that schizophrenia strongly aggregates in families. The familial aggregation of schizophrenia appears to be quite substantial when schizophrenia is defined using modern, relatively narrow diagnostic criteria such as those found in DSM-III and DSM-III-R. On average, the risk for schizophrenia in the relatives of controls is between 0.5 and 1.0 percent, compared with between 3 and 7 percent in relatives of schizophrenic probands in most studies. The best estimate of the correlation in liability to schizophrenia in first-degree relatives is probably between +0.3 and +0.4.

Recently, results of the first methodologically rigorous family study of childhood-onset schizophrenia have been reported. Compared with parents of both matched normal controls and children with attention-deficit/hyperactivity disorder (ADHD), parents of childhood-onset schizophrenia had a more than tenfold increased risk for schizophrenia, supporting the hypothesis of etiological continuity between childhood-onset and adult-onset schizophrenia.

TO WHAT EXTENT IS THE FAMILIAL AGGREGATION OF SCHIZOPHRENIA DUE TO GENETIC VERSUS ENVIRONMENTAL FACTORS?

Resemblance among relatives can be due either to shared environment (nurture) or shared genes (nature), or both. A major goal in psychiatric genetics is to determine the degree to which familial aggregation for a disorder like schizophrenia results from environmental versus genetic mechanisms. Although sophisticated analysis of family data can begin to make this discrimination, nearly all of the knowledge about this problem in schizophrenia comes from twin and adoption studies.

Twin Studies Twin studies are based on the assumption that monozygotic (MZ) and dizygotic (DZ) twins share a common environment to approximately the same degree. However, MZ twins are genetically identical, whereas DZ twins (like full siblings) share, on average, only one-half of their genes in common. Whereas the validity of the second assumption is beyond question, the first, or "equal environment" assumption, has been a focus of considerable controversy.

Several studies have shown that measures of the social environment (e.g., sharing friends, attitudes of parents and teachers) are more highly correlated among young MZ than among young same-sex DZ twins. These results at first appear to suggest that the equal environment assumption is false. However, there is another possible interpretation. Although similarity in environment might make MZ twins more similar, it is also plausible that, by behaving alike, MZ twins seek out or create more similar environments for themselves. These two alternative hypotheses have been subject to empirical evaluation in a number of studies, nearly all of which suggest that the environmental similarity of MZ twins is the *result* and not the cause of their behavioral similarity. Although probably not exactly true, current evidence from an increasingly wide range of studies supports the general validity of the equal environment assumption of twin studies.

Results are available from 13 major twin studies of schizophrenia (Table 12.3–2). None of these, however, meets all of the methodological criteria outlined above for family studies and an additional criterion that zygosity assignment be made blind with respect to

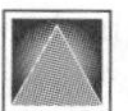

Table 12.3–2
Concordance with Respect to Probands and the Heritability of Liability to Schizophrenia in the Major Twin Studies Reported to Date

			Probandwise Concordance[a]				
			Monozygotic		Same-Sex Dizygotic		
Author	**Country**	**Year**	**N**	**%**	**N**	**%**	**Heritability of Liability (± Standard Deviation)**
Luxenburger	Germany	1928	14/22	64	0/13	0	[b]
Rosanoff et al.	United States	1934	24/41 to 50/66	61	7/53 to 14/60	13	0.84 ± 0.26 to 0.63 ± 0.26
				76		23	
Essen-Möller	Sweden	1941	7/11	64	4/27	15	0.87 ± 0.36
Kallmann	United States	1946	191/245	78	59/318	19	0.90 ± 0.13
Slater	England	1953	28/41	68	11/61	18	0.73 ± 0.21
Inouye	Japan	1963	33/55	60	2/11	18	0.66 ± 0.35
Kringlen	Norway	1967	31/69	45	14/96	15	0.61 ± 0.20
Fischer	Denmark	1973	14/23	61	12/43	28	0.41 ± 0.29
Gottesman and Shields	England	1972	15/26	58	4/34	12	0.86 ± 0.32
Tienari	Finland	1975	7/21	33	6/42	14	0.53 ± 0.33
Kendler and Robinette	United States	1983	60/194	31	18/277	6	0.71 ± 0.04[c]
Onstad et al.	Norway	1991	15/31	48	1/28	4	0.87 ± 0.08[c]
Cannon et al.	Finland	1998	40/87	46	18/195	9	0.83 ± 0.09

[a]Concordance rates are not age-corrected. Estimates of the heritability of liability are based on population risks for schizophrenia either provided in the study or estimated by the reviewer. For further details regarding figures in this table, see the Kendler et al. (1983) studies with multiple reports; the latest or most complete report was chosen for analysis.
[b]Cannot be calculated because none of the dizygotic pairs was concordant.
[c]Correlation in liability in monozygotic twins is reported rather than the standard heritability of liability, so standard error is substantially lower.

psychiatric diagnosis. Some studies come closer than others. For example, a variety of different clinicians made diagnoses from blind case abstracts in the original report from the Maudsley twin series of Irving Gottesman and James Shields. These same case records have more recently been examined using modern operationalized criteria with similar overall results. In the study by Kenneth Kendler and Dennis Robinette from the National Academy of Science-National Research Council (NAS-NRC) Registry, psychiatric diagnoses were collected from a wide variety of clinical settings in which clinicians could not possibly have been aware of any research hypotheses. Furthermore, it could be shown that zygosity assignment was not biased with respect to psychiatric diagnosis. The new Norwegian and Finnish studies used the high-quality twin and psychiatric registries in Norway and Finland and, thus, should be representative of all treated cases of illness. Whereas the Norwegian study was based on personal psychiatric assessments and performed with structured instruments and DSM-III-R operationalized criteria, the Finnish study used previously recorded hospital and disability diagnoses. The sample size of the Finnish study was relatively large (253 pairs), whereas the Norwegian sample was of much more modest size (52 pairs). However, both studies relied on self-report zygosity measures, and the interviews and diagnoses in the Norwegian study were performed nonblind.

Although all these studies agree that probandwise concordance for schizophrenia (the risk for schizophrenia in the co-twins of a schizophrenic proband twin) is much higher in MZ than in DZ twins, the absolute rates of concordance vary widely. Two factors are probably responsible for most of this variation. First, some studies used a broader definition of schizophrenia than others. Second, some studies obtained most of their proband twins from chronically hospitalized populations, whereas others used population-based registries in which milder cases commonly occur. Twin studies have often, but not always, found a positive relationship between concordance and severity of illness.

Both the diagnostic approach to schizophrenia and the method of ascertaining probands should equally affect concordance rates in MZ and DZ twins. Therefore, a better method of comparing results across studies is a summary statistic based on concordance in both MZ and DZ twins. One of the best of these is the heritability of liability as calculated from the correlations in liability in MZ and DZ twins. This statistic ranges from 0.0 if genetic factors play no role in susceptibility to a disorder to a maximum of 1.0 if genes entirely determine disease risk. Because this statistic is based on the polygenic multifactorial threshold model, which may or may not be appropriate for schizophrenia, these results should be regarded as only one plausible way of approximating reality. Nonetheless, the major twin studies of schizophrenia agree in estimating the heritability of liability of schizophrenia at between 0.6 and 0.9 (Table 12.3–2). These results suggest that genetic factors play a major role in the familial transmission of schizophrenia.

Genetic theory predicts that if all the familial aggregation of schizophrenia was due to genetic factors, then the heritability of liability should be approximately double the correlation in liability found in first-degree relatives (because, on average, first-degree relatives share one-half of their genes in common). Comparing the results of Tables 12.3–1 and 12.3–2 indicates that, at least as a rough approximation, this hypothesis is supported. The range of the heritability of liability to schizophrenia calculated from twin studies is approximately twice the range of the correlation in liability to schizophrenia found in first-degree relatives in most family studies.

Twin studies also provide two tests for the role of nongenetic familial transmission in the liability to schizophrenia. First, one can ask whether the correlation in liability in DZ twins is more than one-half that which is predicted in MZ twins if only additive genetic factors are operating. A review of all major twin studies to date suggests that nongenetic factors may play at most a modest role in the transmission of schizophrenia. Second, the risk for schizophrenia in DZ co-twins can be compared with that in siblings of schizophrenic probands. Although having the same degree of genetic relationship to the affected proband, DZ co-twins certainly share more of the familial environment than do ordinary siblings. Several twin studies have suggested that a difference in risk does exist between these two groups. However, such a difference has not been consistently found across all studies and was *not* found in the recent Norwegian small-sample twin family study of schizophrenia.

Adoption Studies Adoption studies can clarify the role of genetic and environmental factors in the transmission of schizophrenia by studying two kinds of rare but informative relationships: (1) individuals who are genetically related but do not share familial–environmental factors, and (2) individuals who share familial–environmental factors but are not genetically related. Table 12.3–3 summarizes, in the order discussed, the major adoption studies of schizophrenia, reporting raw data and statistical tests. The summary here is organized by the kind of adoption design used.

Three studies have compared the adopted-away offspring of schizophrenic parents with the adopted-away offspring of matched controls. In the first of these, Leonard Heston found a significant excess of schizophrenia in adopted-away offspring of schizophrenic versus control mothers. The second such study was performed in Denmark under the direction of David Rosenthal and found results in a similar direction, which, however, fell short of statistical significance, particularly when only parents with a consensus diagnosis of schizophrenia or schizophrenia spectrum were included. This study has been the subject of a blind reanalysis using DSM-III criteria, which, when including only biological parents with a consensus diagnosis of schizophrenia from the original investigators, found a significant excess of schizophrenia spectrum in adopted-away offspring of schizophrenic versus control parents. The third, and by far the largest, such study was performed in Finland under the direction of Pekka Tienari. This study also found a highly statistically significant excess of schizophrenia and schizophrenia spectrum disorders in the adopted-away offspring of schizophrenic mothers, compared with the adopted-away offspring of matched control mothers.

Another major adoption strategy used for studying schizophrenia begins with ill adoptees rather than with ill parents. The full implementation of this design permits two separate experiments: (1) a test for the etiological role of shared environmental factors by comparing the nonbiological adoptive relatives of the schizophrenic and the control adoptees, and (2) a test for the etiological role of genetic factors by comparing the biological relatives of the schizophrenic and control adoptees who were raised in households away from their ill relatives. This strategy has been used by Seymour Kety and colleagues in a series of adoption studies carried out in Denmark. The first, or Copenhagen, sample began with 34 adoptees located in Copenhagen who received a consensus diagnosis of chronic, borderline, or acute schizophrenia. These adoptees and their matched controls had been separated from their biological parents at an early age and raised by individuals with whom they had no biological relationship. The first report on this series was based on hospital abstracts of all relatives located by the population and psychiatric registries available in Denmark. Schizophrenia and related disorders were significantly concentrated only in the biological relatives of the schizophrenic adoptees. The next phase of this project involved personal interviews of all available and cooperative relatives. After these interviews had been dictated into English and blinded, a diagnostic review of these also indicated a substantial concentration of schizophrenia spectrum disorders only in the biological relatives of the schizophrenic adoptees.

A second sample beginning with 41 schizophrenia spectrum adoptees from outside of Copenhagen (termed the *Provincial sample*) has also been collected. On the basis of personal interviews with biological and adoptive relatives, the results basically replicated the parallel findings from the Copenhagen sample. Schizophrenia and the spectrum disorders were significantly more common in the biological relatives of schizophrenic versus control adoptees, whereas these disorders were equally uncommon in the two groups of the adoptive relatives. In an independent review of the interviews from both the Copenhagen and Provincial samples using DSM-III criteria, Kendler and Alan Gruenberg replicated and extended all the major earlier findings of Kety and coworkers.

Because twin studies contain no parent–offspring pairs, they are not helpful in clarifying whether parents influence their children's risk for schizophrenia in ways other than passing on their genes. However, several adoption strategies have been used to clarify the role of parent–offspring environmental transmission (termed *vertical cultural transmission* [VCT]) in schizophrenia. First, if offspring of schizophrenics in part "learn" schizophrenia from their parents, then decreasing the amount of contact between schizophrenic parents and their children should decrease their risk for illness. Two studies have produced results inconsistent with this hypothesis. Jerry Higgins et al. compared the adopted-away offspring of schizophrenic parents with naturally reared offspring of schizophrenics. Although the sample size was small (23 offspring in each group), follow-up personal interviews indicated a nonsignificant excess of schizophrenia in the adopted-away offspring, compared with those children reared by a schizophrenic parent. In a variation of a full adoption study, a similar design was used in Israel to compare 25 offspring of schizophrenics reared in a kibbutz (in which children are raised together in children's houses, although still having considerable contact with their parents) with 25 offspring of schizophrenics raised in conventional nuclear family settings in towns elsewhere in Israel. A follow-up interview in adulthood with these offspring revealed that the risk for DSM-III schizophrenia was actually higher (nonsignificantly) in the kibbutz-reared (13 percent) than in the town-reared offspring (8.7 percent). Including the schizophrenia spectrum disorders, this difference was even greater (26.1 vs. 13.0 percent), although still short of statistical significance. Both of these results are inconsistent with the VCT hypothesis.

A second way to address the VCT hypothesis is to look at the risk for schizophrenia in the adopted-away offspring of normal individuals reared by schizophrenic parents. Although limited by a small sample size and a small number of parents with typical schizophrenia, Paul Wender et al. found no evidence for increased rates of illness in such adoptees.

Third, VCT of schizophrenia predict that among adopted individuals who become schizophrenic, schizophrenia should be overrepresented in their adoptive parents, who culturally "transmit" schizophrenia. In Kety's Copenhagen and Provincial samples, no excess cases of schizophrenia or related spectrum conditions were seen in the adoptive parents of the schizophrenic adoptees. In separate samples, Wender et al. twice studied psychopathology in the adoptive parents of schizophrenics. The first of these studies found evidence for an excess of severe psychopathology in the adoptive parents of schizophrenics. In the second study, which the authors believed was better controlled, no such increase was found.

Fourth, because step-siblings of schizophrenics are exposed to the same schizophrenogenic rearing environment as the schizophrenic person but lack the biological relationship to the parents, VCT also predicts an excess of schizophrenia in step-siblings of schizophrenics. Two studies have been unable to find an excess risk for schizophrenia in relatively small samples of step-siblings of schizophrenic probands.

In summary, twin and adoption studies provide strong and consistent evidence that genetic factors play a major role in the familial aggregation of schizophrenia. Evidence for a role for nongenetic familial factors is less clear; some studies suggest that they may con-

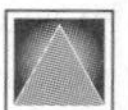

Table 12.3–3
Summary Results of Major Adoption Studies of Schizophrenia

Author, Yr	Location	Diagnosis in Relatives	Relationship of Index Group to Schizophrenic Proband	Affected N	Affected %	Control Group	Affected N	Affected %	P	Comments
Heston, 1966	Oregon	Schiz	AAO	5/47	10.6	AAO of normals	0/50	0	.01[a]	—
Rosenthal et al., 1971	Denmark	Schiz spect	AAO	14/52	26.9	AAO of controls	12/67	17.9	.12[a]	Including only parents in whom judges agreed on a schiz spect diagnosis.
Lowing et al., 1983[b]	Denmark	Schiz spect	AAO	11/39	28.2	AAO of controls	4/39	10.3	.02[a]	Independent analysis of the study by Rosenthal et al.; biological parents restricted to DSM-II schiz; spect in offspring defined by DSM-III as schiz and as schizotypal and schizoid personality disorders.
Tienari, 2000	Finland	Schiz spect	AAO	17/164	10.4	AAO of controls	4/197	2.0	.0007	Schiz spect defined using DSM-III-R criteria as schiz, schizoaffective, and schizophreniform disorder and schizotypal personality disorder.
Kety et al., 1975	Denmark	Schiz spect	BRAS ARAS	24/173 2/74	13.9 2.7	BRAC ARAC	6/174 5/91	3.4 5.5	.0003[a] NS[c]	Greater Copenhagen sample using both hospital abstracts and personal interviews; biological rels of schiz adoptees include both first- and second-degree rels; results reported excluding schizoid personality from spectrum.
Kety, 1994	Denmark	Schiz spect	BRAS ARAS	22/171 0/71	12.9 0	BRAC ARAC	3/121 0/55	2.5 0	<.005 NS[c]	The Provincial Danish Adoption Study based on personal interviews.
Kendler and Gruenberg, 1994	Denmark	Schiz spect	BRAS ARAS	9/38 0/30	23.7 0	BRAC ARAC	5/107 1/102	4.7 1.0	.001[b] NS[c]	Independent analysis of personal interviews from Kety's Copenhagen and Provincial studies using DSM-III criteria: results from index adoptees with DSM-III schiz; only first-degree biological rels considered. In rels, schiz spect is defined as schiz, schizoaffective disorder, mainly schizophrenic, and schizotypal and paranoid personality disorders.

AAO, adopted-away offspring; ARAS, adoptive relatives of adopted schizophrenics; ARC, adoptive relatives of adopted controls; BRAC, biological relatives of adopted controls; BRAS, biological relatives of adopted schizophrenics; NS, nonsignificant; rels, relatives; schiz, schizophrenia or schizophrenics; spect, spectrum.
[a]Represents statistical test for genetic transmission of liability to schiz. Values of *P* are one-tailed.
[b]Represents independent analyses of previous studies, not new investigations.
[c]Represents statistical test for cultural transmission of liability to schizophrenia. Values of *P* are two-tailed.

tribute modestly to the familial aggregation of schizophrenia, but the majority of studies find no evidence for significant nongenetic familial factors for schizophrenia.

HOW NARROW OR BROAD ARE THE PSYCHIATRIC DISORDERS THAT ARE TRANSMITTED WITHIN FAMILIES?

The first systematic family study of schizophrenia, performed by Ernst Rüdin in Emil Kraepelin's newly established Psychiatric Institute in Munich in 1916, found that siblings of schizophrenic patients had increased rates not only of schizophrenia but of other potentially related psychotic disorders as well. Since that time, a major focus of family, twin, and adoption studies of schizophrenia has been to clarify more precisely the nature of the psychiatric syndromes that occur in excess frequency in relatives of schizophrenic patients. This effort has been greatly aided by the emergence of operationalized diagnostic criteria in psychiatry that permit more precise and reliable diagnoses.

On the level of psychopathological syndromes, four heuristic hypotheses can be articulated about the nature of the liability to schizophrenia that is transmitted in families: (1) a general liability to all psychiatric illnesses; (2) a liability to poor psychosocial functioning, oddness, suspiciousness, and so forth; (3) a liability to many forms of psychosis; and (4) a specific liability to typical schizophrenia. These hypotheses are useful because each generates a different prediction about the kinds of psychiatric disorders that should be seen in excess in families of schizophrenics.

A General Liability to All Psychiatric Illnesses?

The first hypothesis predicts that the risk for all major forms of psychiatric illness should be increased in relatives of schizophrenics. The hypothesis is consistent with the unitary hypothesis of mental disorders, which postulates that all psychiatric illness is on a single continuum with schizophrenia at the most deviant end. This hypothesis can be best evaluated in modern family studies and in reanalyses of major adoption studies that have used similar diagnostic criteria and normal control groups. In the modern family studies that have examined this question, there is nearly uniform agreement that the rates of anxiety disorders and substance dependence disorders are not increased in relatives of schizophrenic versus matched control probands. Somewhat more controversy surrounds the question of the familial relationship between schizophrenia and affective illness. The majority of family and adoption studies that have examined this question report similar rates for unipolar and bipolar illness in relatives of schizophrenic and control probands. However, several recent studies have found a significantly greater risk for unipolar illness in the relatives of schizophrenic probands. The reason for these discrepant findings remains a subject of debate.

A Liability to Schizophrenia or to Schizophrenia Spectrum Disorders?

Both of the two chief architects of the concept of schizophrenia, Kraepelin and Eugen Bleuler, noted that some close relatives of patients with schizophrenia, although never psychotic, had odd or eccentric personalities that were clinically reminiscent of schizophrenia. Since that time, similar observations have been made by a number of clinicians and researchers. The first, and probably the most influential, rigorous study of what may be termed these *schizophrenia-related personality disorders* was made by Kety and colleagues in the Danish adoption studies referred to above. Based on a blind diagnostic review with their own diagnostic criteria, Kety and colleagues found a statistically significant excess rate of borderline and uncertain schizophrenia in the biological relatives of schizophrenic versus control adoptees.

More recent applications of operationalized criteria have replicated and extended these earlier findings in support of the second hypothesis. Since 1983, 11 family studies have examined the risk for *schizophrenia spectrum*, defined as schizotypal or paranoid personality disorder using DSM-III or DSM-III-R criteria, in relatives of schizophrenic and matched normal control probands (Table 12.3–4). These studies included two reanalyses of different Danish adoption samples, a Finnish adoption sample, four family studies conducted in the United States, and one family study each conducted in Greece, Ireland, and Germany. The absolute rates of schizotypal and paranoid personality disorder in both relatives of schizophrenic and control probands differ widely across studies. This might be expected because of the quite different approaches used for the assessment of these personality disorder syndromes. However, every study found that schizotypal or paranoid personality was more common in relatives of schizophrenic versus control probands, and this difference was statistically significant in 9 of the 11 studies. In aggregate, these results provide strong support for the second hypothesis articulated above—that the familial liability to schizophrenia is in part reflected by a set of personality traits related to social isolation, oddness, and suspiciousness.

Recent family and adoption studies of schizophrenia have also provided substantial data in favor of the third hypothesis articulated above—that what is transmitted in families of individuals with schizophrenia is a liability to many forms of psychosis. In most, but not all, studies that have examined this question, the risk for nonschizophrenic psychotic disorders (such as schizophreniform disorder, schizoaffective disorder, delusional disorder, and psychosis not otherwise specified [NOS]) is increased in relatives of schizophrenic probands, compared with that seen in relatives of controls. Furthermore, although examined in fewer studies, the risk for schizophrenia appears to be usually increased in the relatives of probands with nonschizophrenic psychotic disorders.

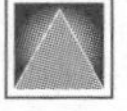

Table 12.3–4
Summary Results of Major Family and Adoption Studies Using Personal Interviews to Examine Risk for DSM-III and DSM-III-R Schizotypal or Paranoid Personality Disorder in First-Degree Relatives of Schizophrenic and Normal Control Probands

		Relatives of Schizophrenic Probands			Relatives of Control Probands			
			SPD or PPD			SPD or PPD		
Author, Yr	**Study Group**	**BZ**	**N**	**MR ± SE**	**BZ**	**N**	**MR ± SE**	***P***
Lowing, 1983	Adopted-away offspring	39	6	15.4 ± 5.8	39	3	7.7 ± 4.3	.29
Kendler, 1994[a]	Biological relatives of adoptees	35	6	17.1 ± 6.4	106	4	3.8 ± 1.9	.01
Tienari, 1997[a]	Adopted-away offspring	184	8	4.3 ± 1.2	203	1	0.5 ± 0.5	.01
Baron, 1985	Nuclear family study	329	72	21.9 ± 2.3	337	16	4.7 ± 1.2	$<10 \times 10^{-9}$
Frangos, 1985	Nuclear family study	478	13	2.7 ± 0.7	536	3	0.6 ± 0.3	.006
Coryell, 1988	Nuclear family study	72	3	4.2 ± 2.3	160	4	2.5 ± 1.2	.49
Gershon, 1988	Nuclear family study	108	3	2.8 ± 1.6	380	0	0	.01
Kendler, 1993	Nuclear family study	319	26	8.2 ± 1.5	580	10	1.7 ± 0.5	.000003
Parnas, 1993	Nuclear family offspring only	192	41	21.3 ± 3.0	101	5	5.0 ± 2.2	<.0001
Maier, 1994	Nuclear family study	289	6	2.1 ± 0.8	320	1	0.3 ± 0.3	.04
Erlenmeyer-Kimling, 1995[a]	Nuclear family offspring only	44	4	9.1 ± 4.3	90	1	1.1 ± 1.1	.02

BZ, *bezugsziffer* (lifetimes at risk); MR, morbid risk; PPD, paranoid personality disorder; SE, standard error; SPD, schizotypal personality disorder.
[a]Prevalence reported rather than MR.

Another specific test of the third hypothesis is to examine the frequency of psychotic affective illness in relatives of schizophrenics. In large-scale family studies both in Iowa and in Ireland, Kendler and colleagues found that, although relatives of schizophrenics were not at increased risk for affective illness, if affectively ill, they were more than twice as likely to become psychotic as affectively ill relatives of controls. Furthermore, in both studies, compared with controls, relatives of probands with psychotic affective illness were at increased risk for schizophrenia.

In summary, results to date provide strong evidence against the validity of hypotheses 1 and 4. The familial predisposition to schizophrenia is neither completely nonspecific nor highly specific. Results are available to strongly support the second hypothesis and also to provide some evidence in favor of the third hypothesis. Current evidence suggests that the familial liability to schizophrenia increases not only the risk for narrowly defined schizophrenia but also for schizotypal and paranoid personality disorder and probably several nonschizophrenic psychotic illnesses. These findings provide an increasingly complex but informative picture of the nature of the transmitted liability to schizophrenia.

Liability to Symptomatic Aspects of Schizophrenia

The contributions of familial and genetic factors to the overall liability to schizophrenia are reviewed above. However, the influence of familial–genetic factors could also impact on the *specific* liability to individual schizophrenic symptoms, symptom dimensions, or syndromes. This possibility can be evaluated by examining the clinical features of pairs of relatives affected with schizophrenia.

The earliest attempts to address this question examined whether the classic Kraepelinian subtypes "ran true" in families. Results of earlier studies were conflicting, but most recent studies using modern operationalized criteria have been generally negative. Efforts at examining whether specific clinical features of schizophrenia are correlated in pairs of affected relatives have been fewer but more successful. Every study to date has found significant correlations of certain clinical features in pairs of affected relatives, but the specific features (e.g., course, thought disorder, intensity of delusions) have not been consistent across studies, perhaps because of modest sample sizes. The largest such study to date found that global course and outcome, as well as all major symptoms except hallucinations, were significantly correlated in 256 Irish sibling pairs concordant for schizophrenia. Three symptom factors—*negative symptoms*, *positive symptoms*, and *affective symptoms*—were also all significantly but modestly correlated in these pairs. Sibling resemblance for five statistically defined schizophrenic syndromes also substantially exceeded chance expectation.

A recent analysis of the Maudsley twin series examined symptom dimensions in identical and fraternal twin pairs concordant for schizophrenia. Patterns consistent with a genetic effect (i.e., correlations stronger in identical than in fraternal pairs) were found for disorganized, negative, manic, and general psychotic symptom dimensions. To date, these studies suggest that the clinical manifestations of the schizophrenic syndrome are significantly influenced by familial factors that are probably at least in part genetic. If genetic factors are largely responsible, at least two different mechanisms could be at work. First, there might be *modifier* genes that do not directly contribute to disease risk but influence the manifestations of the illness in affected individuals. Second, *genetic heterogeneity* for schizophrenia could exist in which distinct genetic loci predispose to different subforms of illness. Symptom resemblance then arises because affected relatives tend to have the same subform. Further research is needed to discriminate between these two possibilities.

WHAT KINDS OF GENETIC TRANSMISSION MECHANISMS APPEAR MOST LIKELY?

The conclusion that genes account for a substantial proportion of the risk for schizophrenia and related psychiatric disorders naturally leads to an interest in understanding the mechanisms underlying such genetic transmission. Is the risk for schizophrenia the result of many genes of small individual effect, or can a single gene, acting alone, transmit a major risk of developing schizophrenia? For many years, genetic epidemiological studies have been carried out with the goal of answering these questions. However, for reasons discussed below, most of these questions have not yet been definitively answered.

The major genetic–epidemiological approach to this question before the advent of linkage studies was statistical modeling either of risk figures for the various classes of relatives of schizophrenia or of the observed pattern of schizophrenia within systematically collected samples of nuclear families or extended pedigrees. This latter technique is called *complex segregation analysis*. In contrast to linkage analysis, complex segregation analysis examines phenotypes only and *not* genetic marker information. Both these strategies compare the observed patterns of co-occurrence of schizophrenia among family members of close versus more distant genetic relationship with the degree of sharing expected under alternative genetic models.

Studies of the patterns of risk for schizophrenia in major classes of relatives (e.g., MZ and DZ co-twins, parents, siblings, offspring, nieces and nephews) have usually concluded that the familial transmission of schizophrenia *cannot* be explained solely by a single major locus (SML). In particular, the concordance rate in MZ twins (approximately 50 percent) is too high relative to the risk in siblings and DZ twins (5 to 10 percent). Such a pattern is more consistent with multiple interacting (or epistatic) loci.

With regard to complex segregation analysis, the results to date have been frustratingly inconclusive, although more frequently inconsistent than consistent with an SML etiology for schizophrenia. Given the genetic complexity of schizophrenia, it is likely that even the most mathematically sophisticated methods of complex segregation analyses are, as analytical tools, too blunt to provide definitive answers.

WHAT IS THE CURRENT STATUS AND WHAT ARE THE FUTURE PROSPECTS FOR IDENTIFYING SPECIFIC GENES THAT PREDISPOSE TO SCHIZOPHRENIA?

For background, the reader is referred to general reviews of molecular genetic mechanisms, basic strategies and statistical methods used for gene mapping, and a general review of linkage studies in psychiatry based on deoxyribonucleic acid (DNA) polymorphisms.

Approaches: Linkage and Association Two fundamentally distinct strategies have been used in attempts to find specific genes that confer susceptibility to schizophrenia: tests of *linkage* and *association*. The chapter briefly reviews current progress using both of these methods. The major difference between these two approaches is that association studies are generally focused on candidate genes, whereas linkage makes no assumption about specific genes involved in etiology. Because of their fundamental differences, the two approaches have generally been considered separately. As shall be seen, more recent association studies have tended to follow linkage evidence and have produced the most exciting current results. The authors, therefore, treat these topics as related rather

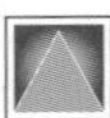

Table 12.3–5
Characteristics of Classic Mendelian Disorders versus Schizophrenia

Characteristics	Mendelian Disorders	Schizophrenia
Penetrance[a]	Usually complete—MZ concordance ~100%	Incomplete—MZ concordance 30–70%
Phenocopies	Usually absent	Present
Diagnostic boundaries	Clear	Uncertain
Locus heterogeneity within families	Never	Uncertain, but likely
Locus heterogeneity across families	Variable, but often absent	Uncertain, but likely

MZ, monozygotic.
[a]The probability of illness given the disease-predisposing genotype.

than separate and focus on association studies that have been led by the evidence for linkage.

Linkage Studies of Schizophrenia—Preface

Linkage has proved to be a method of immense power for simple or Mendelian disorders in which a small number of families can usually unambiguously produce strong evidence for linkage to a small chromosomal region. As discussed below, despite much effort, such a result has not emerged for schizophrenia. Why? As outlined in Table 12.3–5, schizophrenia differs from Mendelian disorders in at least five critical ways, all of which make successful linkage studies much more difficult.

First, most Mendelian disorders are *fully penetrant*—that is, if you inherit a disease mutation and live through the period of risk, you always have the disorder. As outlined above, the pattern of illness in families—in which first-degree relatives of schizophrenic probands have a risk of schizophrenia of approximately 5 to 8 percent—and the concordance rate in MZ twins (40 to 55 percent) are inconsistent with the action of a highly penetrant SML. Unlike in Alzheimer's disease—in which a well-recognized series of pedigrees exist in which the disorder segregates as a Mendelian dominant—no one has ascertained pedigrees in which schizophrenia is transmitted as a classic Mendelian disorder. Finally, the offspring of unaffected MZ co-twins have an elevated risk of illness, suggesting that cases of schizophrenia cannot be simply divided into "genetic" and "sporadic" forms. These results all suggest that, in aggregate, genes involved in the etiology of schizophrenia have *reduced penetrance*—that is, one can carry a susceptibility allele(s) for schizophrenia and not manifest the illness. For this reason, the terms *liability* or *predisposing alleles* or *variants* are used in the subsequent discussion.

Second, for most Mendelian conditions, in all individuals who manifest typical symptoms of the disease, the symptoms are due to the disease mutation. For schizophrenia, this is not true, as schizophrenia-like symptoms can be produced by drugs of abuse and more rarely by metabolic or neurological conditions. These are called *phenocopies*.

Third, in nearly all Mendelian disorders, disease development is independent of the environment. This is not the case in schizophrenia, however, in which several environmental risk factors, including season of birth, obstetric complications, and intrauterine influenza infections, have been shown to increase risk of illness.

Fourth, in most Mendelian disorders, there is an obvious discontinuity between affected and unaffected individuals. Diagnostic boundaries are less clearly delineated for psychiatric illness and are the subject of continued debate in linkage studies. As noted above, it is uncertain what the correct phenotypic boundaries are for schizophrenia to use in linkage and association studies.

Fifth, the mutations that cause Mendelian disorders are sufficiently rare that, for all practical purposes, the same disease locus is responsible for all the cases of illness in a pedigree. Schizophrenia is much more common, and it is plausible, although unproven, that in many high-density families, two or more loci are contributing to disease susceptibility. Across families, the pattern with Mendelian disorders is variable. In most disorders, mutations at a single locus are responsible for all known cases of illness (e.g., Huntington's disease, cystic fibrosis). However, for some Mendelian syndromes (e.g., limb-girdle muscular dystrophy and retinitis pigmentosa), a number of distinct loci, usually on different chromosomes, have been found in different subsets of families. Critically, within an individual family, the same locus and mutation are responsible for all cases of disease. Given that schizophrenia is not a disease but rather a broad behavioral syndrome and given the great complexity of the human brain, it is plausible that mutations in many different genes might result in this condition. This particular issue has a number of ramifications, which merit some discussion.

Epidemiological data from schizophrenia suggest that the population frequencies of liability variants are likely to be orders of magnitude greater than the frequency of even the most common single-gene mutations (such as cystic fibrosis, which has a carrier frequency of 2.5 percent). The implication is that, even within families, variants in distinct genes may predispose different affected family members to illness. Current models hypothesize that variants in many genes can increase liability to schizophrenia (a *polygenic* model of total population risk) and that a few of these loci predispose an individual to schizophrenia (an *oligogenic* model of individual risk). One immediately apparent problem is that the current approaches treat loci individually, but the risk associated with an individual locus is likely to be small and may be dependent on the genotypes at other loci (an *epistatic* model of risk). The evidence supporting both polygenic and epistatic models of risk suggests that an additional problem is *stochastic sampling variation,* the random variation of predisposing loci represented in family or case-controlled samples. Stochastic sampling variation (along with concerns about the power of small samples) is widely believed to be responsible for much of the difficulty in replicating linkage results.

In summary, the tight 1 to 1 relationship that exists between disease mutation and phenotype that is characteristic of Mendelian genetic disorders does not apply to schizophrenia. Locus heterogeneity both within and between families is likely to further complicate this picture. These problems all mean that the signal to noise ratio for linkage studies is much greater for schizophrenia. As is true in any experimental design, the lower the signal to noise ratio, the larger the sample size that is required to reliably detect an effect. This principle is particularly applicable to linkage studies of complex diseases such as schizophrenia. As has been demonstrated by a range of formal power analyses, much larger sample sizes are likely to be required to detect linkage reliably for schizophrenia than are needed for the genetically simple Mendelian disorders. All of these issues should be borne in mind when assessing the evidence for specific chromosomal locations that follows.

Linkage Analysis Methods and Early Studies

Linkage results are most commonly a statistic called a *LOD score*—for *l*ogarithm of the *od*ds. A LOD score is the logarithm, to the base 10, of the likelihood of the observed data given linkage divided by the likelihood of that same data given no linkage. So, LOD scores of +3 and –2 mean that the likelihood that the observed families are linked is 10^3 or 1,000:1 and 10^{-2} or 0.01:1.00, respectively. LOD scores require the specification of a genetic model and are thus termed *parametric*. Because linkage analysis is likelihood based and likelihood-based tests can be maximized over one or more parameters, a common technique is to vary parameters and use likelihood maximization to choose the best parameter value. Thus, the focus of linkage analysis is often comparison of the relative likelihood of the data under one parameter value compared with another. Variations of the LOD score that allow for heterogeneity or that assess only the affected individuals in a sample have been applied to address some of the problems outlined above, but this chapter does not distinguish between these in the discussion that follows. An alternative approach, widely used in complex traits, is *nonparametric* linkage analysis. All classes of relatives have predefined probabilities of sharing zero, one, or two marker alleles at a random locus. These nonparametric statistics are based on testing for deviations from expected allele sharing distributions and avoid the problem of specifying a model, which, as seen above, is very difficult for schizophrenia.

Early linkage studies of schizophrenia before the current era of highly informative genetic markers were performed using a limited range of traditional polymorphisms (e.g., blood groups, proteins, and red cell enzymes). The genome coverage provided by these studies was meager.

Association Studies of Schizophrenia—Preface

Association studies examine whether individuals affected by a disease more frequently have a particular allele at some "candidate" genetic locus than individuals not affected by the disease. This association can occur for two reasons. Either the allele being studied *directly* influences risk for the disorder or, more commonly, the allele is in *linkage disequilibrium* (LD) with the disease-predisposing mutation. LD means that specific alleles at two nearby loci tend to be inherited together and is a reflection of the evolutionary history of variation in a region. LD occurs because a new variant (i.e., marker or mutation) always arises on a *specific* background chromosome and initially only exists in conjunction with the other alleles present on that background. It is seen when one variant is close enough to another that the original association created when the newer variant arose, or entered into a population through a population bottleneck, has not had time to be broken apart by genetic recombination. High degrees of LD between loci therefore generally imply spatial proximity, which is why association studies cover much smaller regions of the genome than do linkage studies. In addition, association can occur for spurious reasons unrelated to disease etiology, such as *population stratification*, in which the cases and controls come from different population groups or subgroups, and observed genotypic differences are due to this population difference rather than to true association between marker and phenotype. Although linkage—the cosegregation of a marker and a disease—is a family-based phenomenon, LD is a population phenomenon and relies on the specific population history of the marker and disease mutation.

Association Analysis Methods and Early Studies

Association studies have two important advantages when compared with linkage studies. First, individual patients can be studied. Second, under many circumstances, association studies are considerably more powerful than linkage studies at detecting genes of modest effect. However, they have two disadvantages. First, they "scan" much smaller regions of the genome than do linkage studies. Practically, this means that association studies must be used for candidate genes only. Currently, a genome scan using the association method is technically, but not fiscally, feasible. Second, obtaining proper controls for association studies can be difficult and can lead to false positives, especially in the presence of population stratification.

Recently, a new approach to association studies that solves this problem has been adopted. Transmission disequilibrium testing assesses whether certain alleles, or *haplotypes*, the combination of alleles on one of the pair of chromosomes, are transmitted to affected individuals more often than expected by chance. By studying individual patients and their parents, researchers can use as a "virtual control group"—the parental genes that did not get transmitted to the patient.

Certainly, the longest history of LD studies in schizophrenia has involved the HLA region on chromosome 6p. The earlier literature suggested the possibility of replicated positive associations with HLA A9 and B5 and negative associations with BW35. Furthermore, the positive association with the A9 allele was particularly noted in cases of paranoid schizophrenia. More recent reports, using molecular genetic genotyping methods, have focused on possible associations of schizophrenia with DQB1 and DRB1 HLA loci.

Association studies in schizophrenia (and other psychiatric disorders) have tended in the past to focus on a limited set of "usual suspect" genes, generally those coding for receptors, transporters, and synthetic or degradatory enzymes in neurotransmitter pathways. Results from these studies have generally not been particularly exciting. As polymorphic markers became available near or within neurotransmitter receptors, many reports have examined association between schizophrenia and serotonin and especially dopamine receptors. Sometimes, these studies used polymorphisms within the gene, such as the Ser311Cys structural polymorphism within the dopamine type 2 (D_2) receptor gene, a glycine to serine missense polymorphism at position 9 in the N-terminal extracellular domain of the D_3 receptor and the 48 base-pair sequence repeat in the D_4 receptor. Few replicated findings have emerged to date—although there is a suggestion in some, but not all, studies of excess homozygosity at the D_3 receptor gene in patients with schizophrenia. A European multicenter collaborative group recently reported evidence for a modest association (odds ratio [OR], approximately 1.2) between schizophrenia and the T102C polymorphism in the 5-hydroxytryptamine type 2A (5-HT_{2A}) receptor. Although association studies remain a major interest in attempting to clarify the nature of the genetic liability to schizophrenia, it is probably fair to conclude that a powerful, widely replicated finding has yet to emerge from this technique alone.

Molecular Genetic Studies of Schizophrenia—Current State of the Field

Space limitations preclude an exhaustive review of linkage studies of schizophrenia here. Instead, the authors review selective current developments. Twenty-five complete or nearly complete genome scans for schizophrenia (in which markers are placed at 10- to 20-centimorgan [cM] intervals over the entire human genome) have now been published on small to moderate-sized high-density family sets. None of these scans has revealed evidence for a large SML for schizophrenia. Consistent with the evidence reviewed above, these results suggest that the existence of a single susceptibility locus that accounts for a large majority of the genetic variance for schizophrenia either in individual families or in populations is unlikely. A smaller number of genome scans examining specific clinical features of the illness (such as neuropsychological deficits; age at onset; and positive, negative, and disorganized symptoms) have been published. Finally, two metaanalyses of genome scan data using different statistical approaches and six metaanalyses of specific chromosomal regions have been published.

Although reviewed elsewhere in this volume, a very brief review of genetic marker types and their designations should assist the reader in understanding the material that follows. Most of the results discussed below come from studies of a particular kind of DNA polymorphism, the *tandem repeat* polymorphism. *Tandem repeats* are variable numbers of a repeating unit of nucleotides. Tandem repeat units exist in all sizes, from mononucleotides (rarely used due to the difficulty of accurate genotyping) through di- (the most common and most commonly used), tri-, tetra-, and pentanucleotides. The frequency of polymorphisms of various unit sizes in the genome is generally inversely correlated with the length of the tandem repeat unit. They are referred to variously as *microsatellites*, *short tandem repeats* (STRs), *simple sequence repeats* (SSRs), or *AC repeats* (after the most common dinucleotide repeat sequence). The alleles of these markers are different segment lengths due to different numbers of the tandemly repeated unit. This marker type is very common and tends to be extremely polymorphic (i.e., to have many alleles) and therefore to have high *heterozygosity* (the proportion of individuals who have two different alleles at the marker locus). As a result of the high heterozygosity, they also tend to be extremely *informative*, in which information content is defined as the probability that the allele transmitted to a given offspring from a given parent can be unambiguously determined. Most linkage studies are performed using microsatellite markers. Nomenclature for markers of this type are "D numbers," which identify the chromosome on which the marker locus maps and the historical order in which the marker was identified. Thus, the 278th microsatellite identified on chromosome 22 (one discussed shortly) has D number D22S278.

In contrast, single-nucleotide polymorphisms (SNPs) are genetic variations at a single base and have only two alleles, lower heterozygosity, and lower information content. Association and LD studies tend, in general, to use SNPs as the marker of choice; whereas large numbers of alleles (and therefore high information content) are useful for linkage, lower allele numbers and lower information content are more appropriate for association studies. Nomenclature for these markers varies, but in discussions presented here, the authors tend to use the "common allele-position-rare allele" convention. A variant with A as the more frequent allele and G as the rarer allele at base 18 of a hypothetical gene is named A18G. Numbering of the position can vary depending on whether it was identified in the context of complementary DNA (cDNA) studies (in which the position refers to the transcript and thus does not include intronic sequences) or genomic studies (in which position includes intronic sequence). The first base of the methionine start codon is always given the number 1, regardless of the two distinctions above. Bases in the upstream region before the start codon are given negative numbers. When SNPs occur in coding sequence and alter amino acid sequence, they often are based on the amino acid change and position rather than the nucleotide change and position. Examples of both can be seen in the discussion of candidate gene studies above (Ser311Cys polymorphism in the D_2 receptor gene and the T102C polymorphism in the 5-HT_{2A} receptor gene).

Over the course of the last decade, tentative evidence for replicated linkages for schizophrenia susceptibility loci has begun to be seen. To date, eight regions appear most promising on the basis of individual reports of genome-wide linkage studies; in historical order, these are 22q12-q13, 8p22-p21, 6p24-p22, 13q14-q32, 5q22-q31, 10p15-p11, 6q21-q22, and 15q13-q14. These are reviewed in some detail. Several caveats should be noted, however. First, the interpretation of these results is quite controversial, particularly as the definition of "replication" for linkage to a complex trait remains uncertain. Second, in the interest of brevity, discussion of studies that do not find evidence for linkage in these selected regions has been omitted, but it is important to bear this selective bias in mind when considering the data that follow. Many samples do not provide supportive evidence for these regions. Third, discussion of a number of other less well-supported regions has been omitted; more detailed information about other issues in linkage analysis of schizophrenia and putative linkage regions can be found elsewhere.

Chromosome 22q12-q13.1 Linkage Studies

Initial evidence for linkage to chromosome 22q came from three markers spanning approximately 23 cM in the 22q13.1 region in the Maryland family sample. A collaborative replication study in a total of 217 multiplex pedigrees with groups from Virginia, Great Britain, and France followed but did not confirm the linkage in the new samples.

From a number of attempted replications, two samples were positive: pedigrees from Utah and high-density English and Welsh pedigrees. After increasing the size of the Maryland family sample, the most significant marker in their genome scan was the same dinucleotide repeat polymorphism, D22S278, as that showing maximum evidence for linkage in the English and Welsh families. Eleven groups contributed data for this marker to the first collaborative schizophrenia linkage study. There was excess sharing of alleles in these 620 affected sibling pairs ($P = .006$), particularly in 296 pairs with data available from both parents ($P = .001$). It is important to note, however, that the authors calculated that this locus is likely to account for *no more* than 2 percent of total variance in liability. Two further samples of families from Germany and from England and the United States also supported this putative linkage. The role of this region in liability to schizophrenia remains unclear, although the number of positive findings seem unlikely to have occurred by chance. Results are summarized in Figure 12.3–1.

Additional interest in this region of 22q came from a known chromosomal rearrangement. The cosegregation of chromosomal anomalies or rearrangements with phenotypes resembling a particular disease has provided useful clues to the locations of the gene(s) involved, most notably in the positional cloning of the dystrophin (or *DMD*) gene. Velocardiofacial syndrome is caused by deletions at 22q11 near these linkage results for schizophrenia. Historically, approximately 10 percent of patients with velocardiofacial syndrome were believed to present with a psychotic phenotype, but more recent studies suggest much higher rates of 25 to 29 percent. Conversely, preliminary results suggest that approximately 2 percent of adult-onset and 6 percent of childhood-onset schizophrenic patients have microdeletions in this region, in excess of the estimated general population frequency of such deletions of 0.025 percent. Although statistically significant, this excess of deletions is probably not enough to explain significant population attributable risk. The authors must thus conclude that variation in genes in this region in individuals *without* a deletion may contribute to liability.

Chromosome 22q12-q13.1 Candidate Genes

COMT The velocardiofacial syndrome critical region contains the gene for catechol-*O*-methyltransferase (COMT) located at 22q11, which is involved in the synthesis and degradation of catecholamines and is genetically and functionally polymorphic, with a

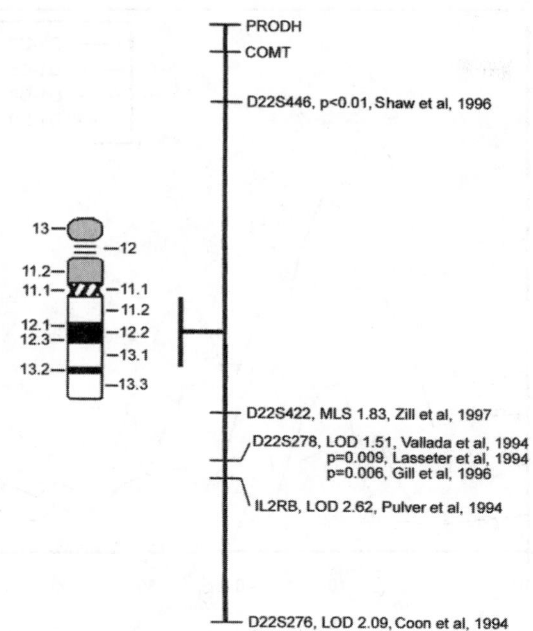

FIGURE 12.3–1 Locations of positive results on chromosome 22. LOD, logarithm of the odds.

variable amino acid, Val158Met. Val and Met alleles are of almost identical frequency. Most studies of the *COMT* gene have tested for association with the low activity (Met) allele (with mixed results). One recent report suggests that the high activity (Val) allele, through increased catabolism of dopamine in the prefrontal cortex, may slightly increase the risk of schizophrenia and may explain some of the observed differences in cognitive performance and prefrontal cortical functioning between cases and controls.

Another study examined *COMT* in a homogeneous population of Ashkenazi Jewish individuals from Israel and used the largest case-control sample for schizophrenia yet reported. Three of these SNPs genotyped in the *COMT* gene showed significant association with schizophrenia in 720 cases and 2,000 to 4,000 controls. In agreement with the study above, an association was found with the homozygous high activity genotype (Val/Val) and with the two other SNPs tested. Interestingly, differences between men and women for allele and genotype frequencies, strength of association, and population attributable risk were seen at all three loci individually and in haplotype analyses. Overall, the study found that the population attributable risk for COMT in females was 32.2 percent, whereas that in males was 13.5 percent. Although the population attributable risk estimates need to be interpreted with caution due to the evidence for an epistatic model of risk discussed above, they suggest that 32.2 percent of female patients and 13.5 percent of male patients *would not have been affected* if liability variants in this gene were not present in the population. No such observation of a differential effect of a gene in males and females has previously been reported.

PRODH2 Work in samples of adult-onset and childhood-onset cases gave evidence for association with the *PRODH2* gene, which codes for proline dehydrogenase, a widely expressed mitochondrial enzyme. This locus is also within the deletion region. In this study, the evidence for association of markers in *PRODH2* was significant in both adult-onset and childhood-onset samples and somewhat stronger in the childhood-onset sample. Marker data from a third independent sample of cases and controls trended toward the results seen for the adult-onset sample but did not reach conventional significance. However, analysis of the childhood-onset subset of this case-control sample was significant for association of the same marker alleles with disease.

Chromosome 8p22-p21 Linkage Studies

The Maryland family sample also gave the first evidence of linkage to chromosome 8p22-p21. A multicenter collaborative linkage study supported this putative locus with excess allele sharing at D8S261. Data from Canadian, Irish, mixed U.K./Icelandic, and Icelandic pedigrees all support a locus on 8p. These replication results are spread across approximately 15 megabases (Mb) of sequence. Further analyses of the Maryland sample subdivided by diagnosis positioned the peak result 5 Mb centromeric of the original finding. One of the key points to note is that, although numerous samples support a locus on this chromosome, comparison between individual studies is consistent with the possibility of multiple genes in the region. For example, if only the Irish and Icelandic samples are considered, both support a locus on 8p, but both are negative at the other's peak position. Results are summarized in Figure 12.3–2.

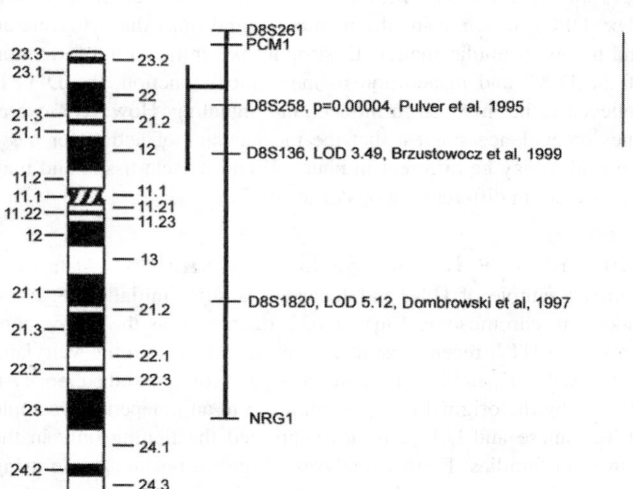

FIGURE 12.3–2 Locations of positive results on chromosome 8. LOD, logarithm of the odds.

Chromosome 8p22-p21 Candidate Genes

NRG1 After obtaining linkage evidence to chromosome 8p in their Icelandic families, Kari Stefansson et al. performed fine mapping with 50 markers across a 30-cM interval. Analysis of these markers identified two risk haplotypes spanning a region of approximately 1 Mb within the gene for neuregulin (*NRG1*). Case-control samples from Ireland and Scotland have provided additional support for this locus and for the specific haplotypes identified in the Icelandic cases. Neuregulin is expressed in central nervous system (CNS) synapses and appears to have a role in the expression and activation of neurotransmitter (including glutamate) receptors.

PCM1 Follow-up work in the case and control samples from the United Kingdom has identified association in the pericentriolar material (*PCM1*) gene. The product of this gene is a protein associated with microtubules and involved in neuronal transport. Along with evidence for association, magnetic resonance imaging (MRI) studies of brain morphology comparing cases with and without associated *PCM1* alleles and two sets of controls showed significant reductions of gray matter volume in the left orbitofrontal cortex of the cases with the associated *PCM1* alleles, compared with the other cases and both control groups.

PPP3CC Parallel strands of evidence for the involvement of the calcineurin A gamma (CNAγ) subunit gene (*PPP3CC*) in schizophrenia were also reported recently. Calcineurin is a dimeric calcium-dependent serine/threonine phosphatase composed of a regulatory (CNB) subunit and one of three catalytic (CNA) subunits and is highly expressed in the CNS. First, conditional knock-out mice lacking CNB expression in forebrain display certain behaviors similar to those observed in schizophrenic patients, including decreased social interaction, impaired prepulse and latent inhibition, and severe working memory deficits. Second, case/control association testing of calcineurin-related genes, which focused on those mapping to regions with previous linkage evidence, identified association with both individual markers and marker haplotypes in *PPP3CC* (chromosome 8p21.3). Neither of the genes encoding the CNB (chromosome 2p14) or CNAα (chromosome 4q24) subunits gave evidence for association. Results from *PCM1* and *PPP3CC* both await replication in other samples.

Chromosome 6p24-p22 Linkage Studies The first evidence for linkage of schizophrenia to the 6p region came from studies of Irish families with a high density of disease. In data from 16 markers, evidence for linkage was modest under a narrow diagnostic model but increased substantially as the diagnostic definition broadened to include spectrum disorders. Evidence for linkage decreased when the definition was broadened further to include nonspectrum disorders. The relationship between diagnostic breadth and evidence for linkage in this sample is illustrated in Figure 12.3–3.

To date, eight independent reports of analyses of this region of 6p have been published. Studies of the Maryland, German, and mixed German and Israeli pedigrees supported linkage to 6p24-p22. A family sample from Quebec found supportive evidence for a schizophrenia susceptibility locus in some, but not all, families. A large, multigenerational family from Sweden supported this linkage in a single branch of the family; a haplotype of markers within the putative linked segment was found to segregate with schizophrenia. A large, multicenter collaboration detected significant excess allele sharing in this region. Results are summarized in Figure 12.3–4.

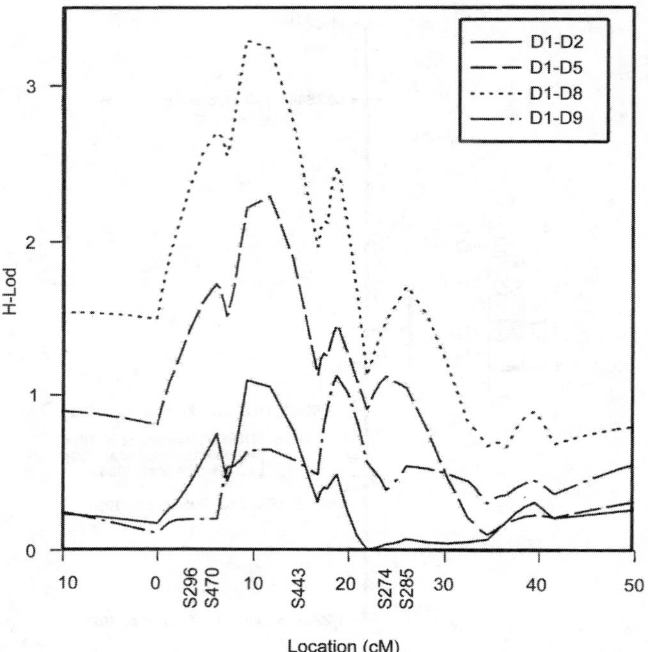

FIGURE 12.3–3 The relationship between diagnostic breadth and evidence for linkage on chromosome 6p in the Irish high-density family sample. LOD, logarithm of the odds.

Chromosome 6p24-p22 Candidate Genes: *DTNBP1* Follow-up work in the Irish family set demonstrated a positive association in the dystrobrevin binding protein 1 (*DTNBP1*) gene. Subsequent reanalysis of the association data revealed a risk haplotype of SNP markers in this gene. Replication studies have been generally supportive: Five studies of seven independent samples gave positive support for the association, and two studies of two independent samples did not.

The function of *DTNBP1* is unknown and must currently be considered in relation to the proteins it is known to interact with. It was first identified as a binding partner of both α- and β-dystrobrevins, which are binding partners of dystrophin, a large, membrane-associated protein expressed at highest levels in muscle and brain and mutated in Duchenne's and Becker's muscular dystrophy. In muscle, dystrophin is associated with the dystrophin-associated protein complex (DPC), which spans the membrane and links the cytoskeleton and the extracellular matrix. Dystrophin is central to the formation of the DPC, and in addition to mechanical function, the DPC is believed to be involved in intracellular signaling. However, several lines of evidence suggest that the mechanisms of action for these molecules may be different in neuronal and muscle tissue and may be different in different regions of the brain.

Chromosome 13q14-q32 Linkage Studies Data from a mixed sample of U.K. and Japanese families initially suggested linkage to chromosome 13q14.1-q32, of interest as the region contains the 5-HT_{2A} receptor gene. Preliminary data from the Maryland and mixed U.K. and Icelandic samples gave some initial support. An attempt by the original group to replicate in an independent sample of Taiwanese and U.K. families supported the finding only in the European families. Further analyses of the European sample using slightly different methods yielded positive data at two markers

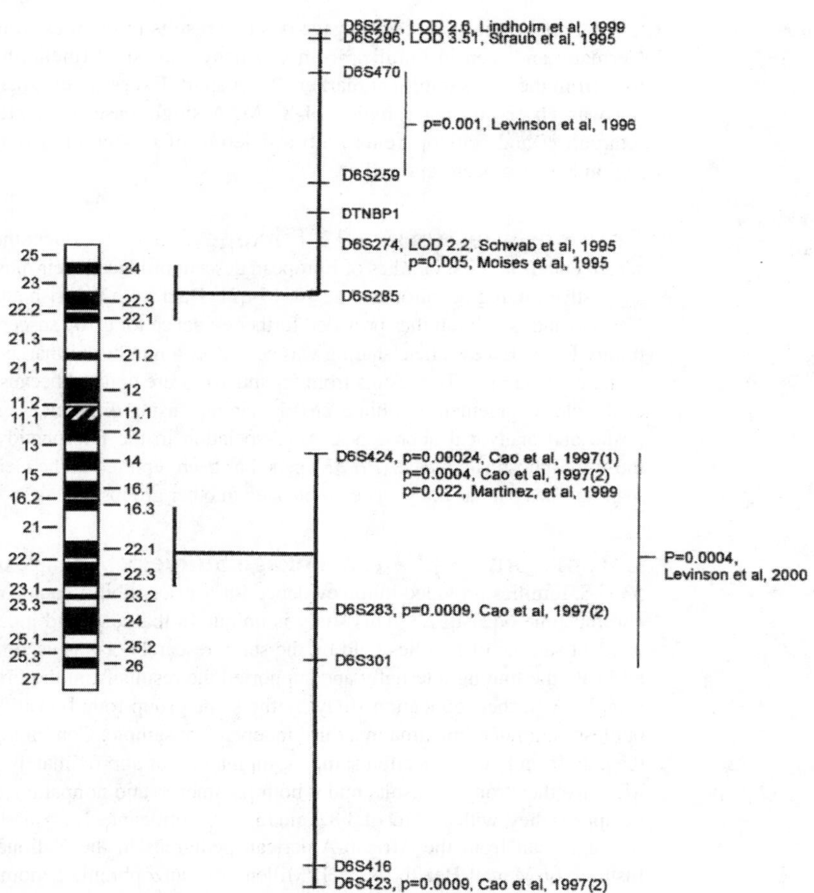

FIGURE 12.3–4 Locations of positive results on chromosome 6. LOD, logarithm of the odds.

located at 13q32, but they were separated by a region in which the values of the statistics dropped almost to zero.

Genome scan data from a mixed U.K. and U.S. sample gave positive evidence but was extremely distant from other findings in the region. The Maryland family sample gave modest evidence for linkage under a recessive model; nonparametric analysis of the same data was highly significant. Marker data in narrowly defined Canadian pedigrees gave fairly strong evidence for linkage. The results from chromosome 13 are particularly difficult to interpret because of the very large distances between positive markers. Unlike chromosome 6, in which two distinct regions have been detected in different samples, there has been little agreement about the site of greatest evidence on 13q. Overall, the combined linkage reports are spread over a region of approximately 60 Mb, containing approximately 120 known or putative genes. On the other hand, although locations are much less certain on chromosome 13q than in other linkage regions, this chromosome has produced some of the most significant linkage evidence seen in the studies of schizophrenia. Results are summarized in Figure 12.3–5.

Chromosome 13q14-q32 Candidate Genes: *G72* and *DAAO*

An elegant recent study examined markers in the distal 5 Mb of this broad linkage region, site of one of the most significant findings on chromosome 13. Nearly 200 SNPs were tested across the region and identified two regions of association. In one of these regions, two genes called *G72* and *G30* were investigated. Of note, the exons of these genes could not be predicted by any computational method tested, suggesting that they are highly novel in their sequence and organization. Both genes show alternative transcripts in brain and other tissues. Association studies of SNPs within *G72* have not yet provided a clear pattern. One of these is nonsynonymous and is significant alone. The nature of the amino acid change (lysine to arginine) is conservative but has major consequences in some proteins. However, the overall pattern of results is probably most consistent with the existence of further unidentified predisposing variants in this gene.

D-Amino acid oxidase (encoded by the gene *DAAO*) was identified as a binding partner of, and appears to be activated by, the product of *G72*. *DAAO* was screened for association evidence, and four SNPs tested were significantly associated. Results of this kind (showing association in two interacting genes in the same sample) are rare, so this study had a unique opportunity to test for an epistatic genetic interaction. Evidence for epistasis (the combined risk when both loci are considered is greater than the sum of the risks for the two individual loci) was observed for one pair of *DAAO* and *G72* genotypes, supporting a potential interaction between them in risk for schizophrenia.

Chromosome 5q22-q31 Linkage Studies

The first widely noted positive evidence for linkage in schizophrenia, and the first study to use DNA polymorphisms, was reported by Robin Sherrington et al. in 1988. Following up on the report of an association of schizophrenia with a partial trisomy of chromosome 5q, they examined the proximal region of the trisomy, including the 5q11.2 breakpoint, with two RFLP polymorphisms in seven U.K. and Icelandic families. The strong evidence they reported for linkage in this region could not be replicated by many other groups nor by the original investigators themselves.

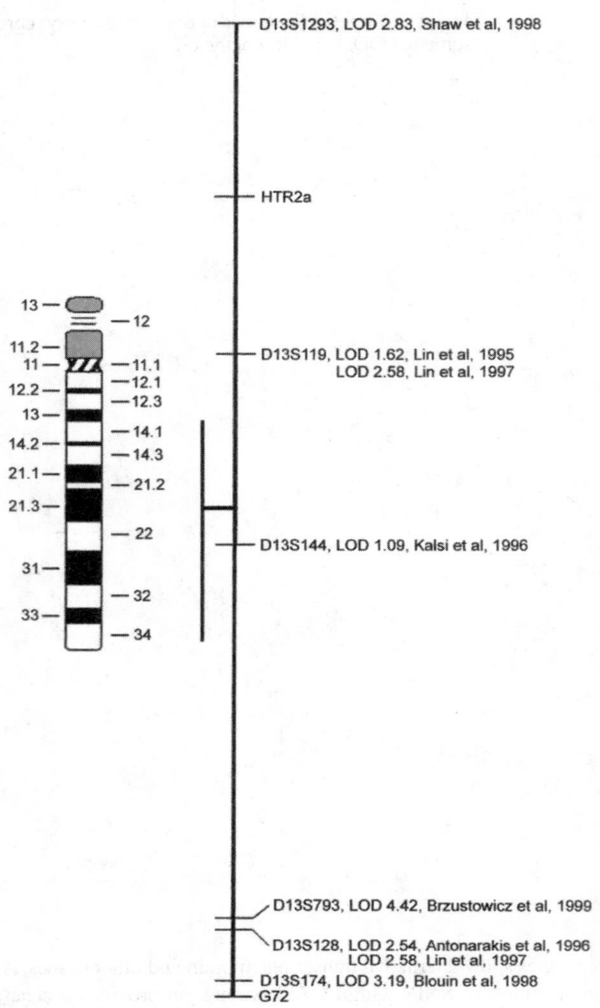

FIGURE 12.3–5 Locations of positive results on chromosome 13. LOD, logarithm of the odds.

Two groups have found suggestive evidence of linkage on chromosome 5q22-q31 in a region distinct from that in earlier studies. Data from the Irish sample was positive under a narrow diagnostic model. Analyses with a broader disease definition resulted in substantial reduction in the statistics. Results were positive (although of variable magnitude) across the entire set of 14 markers spanning 45 cM of this region.

Markers in the same region gave positive results in families from Germany and then in families from Germany and Israel (including four from the first sample) at markers 2 cM apart. Excess allele sharing was observed over a region of 8 cM. A single case of mental retardation and schizophrenia with a deletion of this chromosome region has also been reported.

Chromosome 10p15-p11 Linkage Studies Genome screen data from U.S. families of European descent produced their most suggestive finding on chromosome 10p15-q21. Data from the Irish and German and Israeli families provided further evidence for a 10p susceptibility locus. Excess allele sharing was seen over a number of markers in the latter sample. The results from 5q and 10p were unusual because of the close agreement (within 5 cM) in samples using different diagnostic and analytical approaches. An association in the phosphatidyl inositol 5-phosphate kinase (*PIP5K*) gene has been reported in the German families but has not yet been replicated in other groups.

Chromosome 6q21-q22 Linkage Studies A sample of 53 U.S. families provided initial evidence for a susceptibility locus on chromosome 6q21-q22.3. This study is unique in that a second independent sample of families held by the same researchers was used to replicate the finding internally and supported the results from the first sample. A further replication study by the same group found positive but less significant maxima in a third independent sample. Combining the data from both replication samples, an interval of approximately 8 Mb gave the strongest results under both parametric and nonparametric approaches, with a LOD of 3.82 and highly significant excess allele sharing. Data from the African-American pedigrees in the National Institute of Mental Health (NIMH)/Millenium schizophrenia genome screen provided support for these findings. The markers positive in this latter sample flank the 8-Mb region of interest above. Results are summarized in Figure 12.3–4. A collaborative study of these last four regions gave highly significant evidence for a schizophrenia susceptibility locus on 6q21-q22 and modest support across a much larger region of chromosome 10p but did not support a locus on 5q or 13q.

Chromosome 15q13-q14 The first evidence for a possible chromosome 15 schizophrenia susceptibility locus was the report of linkage of an evoked potential abnormality common in schizophrenics and relatively rare in controls to chromosome 15q13-q14. The abnormality is believed to reflect a sensory-gating deficit, a decreased capacity to filter out repetitive stimuli, and it segregates as a single gene trait in families. Linkage evidence was strongest for a

FIGURE 12.3–6 Locations of positive results on chromosome 15. LOD, logarithm of the odds.

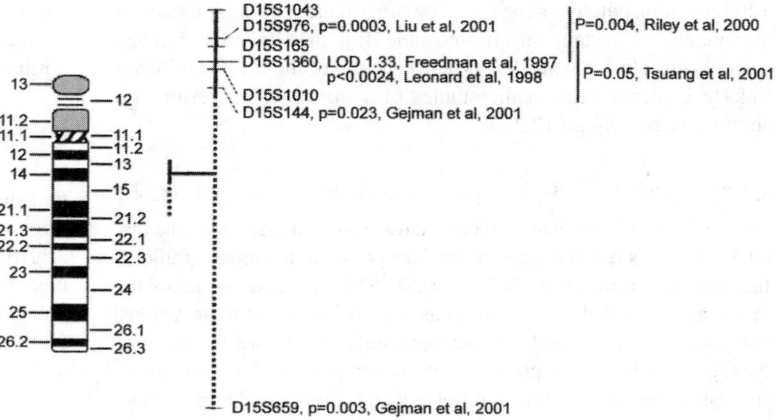

marker in intron 2 of the α7 nicotinic cholinergic receptor subunit gene (*CHRNA7*), which gave a highly significant LOD score when tested against the sensory-gating phenotype and a positive but nonsignificant LOD when tested against schizophrenia. In addition to the positional evidence, this gene is an attractive candidate because of the high incidence of smoking in schizophrenics and because both nicotine and clozapine (Clozaril) ameliorate the sensory-gating deficit.

Data from South African Bantu families in a dense marker set around *CHRNA7* gave positive nonparametric evidence across the entire map. Analysis of marker haplotypes in the Bantu families gave significant evidence for overtransmission of one marker haplotype to affected individuals, consistent with a susceptibility allele existing on this haplotype. Analyses by the original group in an independent sample detected highly significant excess allele sharing at D15S1360.

Four recent studies found additional supportive evidence for a susceptibility locus in this region: in Taiwanese families, a Veterans Affairs Cooperative sample, Azorean families, and another sample of U.S. families. The last result is some distance away from the others, which are tightly clustered around the *CHRNA7* gene. Results are summarized in Figure 12.3–6. Screening of the *CHRNA7* promoter region for polymorphisms has shown that the identified variants all reduce expression of *CHRNA7* and that the variants are significantly more common in cases than in controls. Sensory gating was significantly poorer in those controls with a promoter variant than in those without.

Current Linkage Regions: Summary

Results in these areas share at least two of the following three features: (1) They have been replicated in at least two other samples in addition to the one in which they were first reported, (2) they have not been replicated in all studies, and (3) a collaborative effort has pooled results across many groups and produced suggestive results. These regions represent a wide range of results: narrow (5q, 10p, 15q) to very broad (8p, 13q) regions of chromosomes, those supported (6p, 6q, 8p) or not (5q, 13q) by replication in collaborative studies, and those with positive evidence in candidate genes (22q, 6p, 8p, 10p, 13q, 15q) and those without (5q, 6q). Currently, all of the regions and candidate genes discussed in the sections above are promising, but further assessment of each is still needed, both to clarify patterns of linkage or association and to elucidate their contribution to the neurobiology of schizophrenia.

Metaanalyses of Genome Screen Data

Metaanalysis of whole genome screen data offers a different kind of insight into the mechanisms of complex trait genetics: Because many samples, and therefore more data, are included, they represent a first approximation of a very large, multisample genome screen. Two different statistical approaches for such metaanalyses have been published. One combines the significance levels reported in the original genome screens after correcting each value for the size of the suggested region. Four different statistics are calculated using this approach, the most important of which (the replication multiple scan probability) excludes the most significant study (to assess the overall evidence without being biased by the most extreme single result). Results from the first approach were significant for chromosomes 8p, 13q, and 22q. One limitation of the statistical approach used is that no new information about potential regions of interest can be detected with it.

The second method ranks 30-cM bins of the genome from most positive to least positive for each study and then sums the ranks for each bin. Significance levels are calculated by simulation. Because this method uses not significance levels but the actual marker LOD scores, it is possible to identify regions of the genome that are of potential interest on the basis of modest positive results occurring in the same region across many studies but which may have been overlooked due to the issues of signal to noise ratio and stochastic sampling variation discussed earlier. Results of the second approach supported linkage to chromosomes 6p, 8p, and 10p of the previously identified regions discussed above.

However, the strongest evidence for a potential locus was on chromosome 2q, a region suggested by only a few studies and not widely followed up, and on 3p, the site of an early linkage finding in the Maryland sample that could never be replicated by subsequent studies. Finally, significant evidence of linkage was also detected for two regions never previously implicated by an individual study, on chromosomes 11q and 14p. These results are being followed up currently.

Chromosomes 9q34.3, 4q24-q32, 18, and 1q32-q41

Four additional chromosome regions deserve brief mention, although the evidence for their involvement in schizophrenia is less well replicated and less certain. Two studies have found positive evidence on chromosome 9q34.3, very close to the q telomere. This region contains two genes of potential interest, dopamine β-hydroxylase (*DBH*) and the central subunit of the *N*-methyl-D-aspartate (NMDA) receptor (*NR1*). The first of these has been tested directly in one sample and did not produce positive evidence. However, both neurochemical and transgenic mouse studies support a possible role for NR1 in liability to schizophrenia.

In one sample, a cluster of three markers on 4q24-q32 gave some evidence for involvement in liability to schizophrenia. This region has been a focus of attention in studies of bipolar disorder. Some evidence in support of this region was observed in Irish, U.S. and Australian, and Finnish family samples.

Interest in chromosome 18 began with several reports of the cooccurrence of psychiatric disorders and chromosomal anomalies, and linkage evidence between this chromosome and bipolar disorder has also been reported. Two replication attempts in schizophrenia samples after the putative bipolar linkage were negative, but several positive results have been reported in markers and candidate genes in the mixed German and Israeli sample with and without the inclusion of affective disorder families and in data from Welsh families.

Interest in chromosome 1 in schizophrenia began with reports of a balanced 1:11 translocation segregating with serious mental illness in a large pedigree from Scotland. The chromosome 1 breakpoint lies at 1q42.1, and two groups reported suggestive linkage findings in this region in a population isolate from Finland and in the Maryland sample. Ongoing work in the Scottish pedigree has now identified three genes disrupted by the breakpoint and, of potential interest in psychotic illness more generally, in this region. Genome scans of families from Finland and Canada have also provided evidence for a chromosome 1 locus, although the chromosomal position varies between these studies, making interpretation difficult. A recent study of pedigrees from the United States and India detected association in the regulator of G-protein signaling 4 (*RGS4*) gene. In this study, the same markers in the same 10-kilobase region were associated in both samples, although different specific marker haplotypes gave this evidence in the U.S., compared to the Indian, families.

Linkage Studies of Schizophrenia: Summary

The field of linkage studies of schizophrenia continues to change rapidly and may have altered considerably by the time this chapter is read. Certainly, the most important development in the last several years has been the emergence of a number of replicated findings and the identification of associations within genes in these target regions. Given the vast number of statistical tests that are now performed in most linkage studies (many markers, several diagnostic models, several genetic models, often several different linkage programs), the true type I (or false-positive) error rate emerging from any individual study is nearly impossible to quantify. It remains a major concern that results of quite high apparent statistical significance could occur by chance alone because so many tests are performed.

Therefore, replication is critical. However, there are many reasons why a "true" finding might not be replicated, including genetic variation between populations and differences in statistical power, diagnostic methods, and statistical approaches. Given the evidence of replication across several groups for regions on 22q, 8p, 6p, 13q, 5q, 10p, 6q, and 15q, it seems increasingly unlikely that all of these regions represent false positives. It is difficult to conceive of an inherent bias that produces spuriously positive results across multiple groups (especially given the wide differences between studies described above) in the same chromosomal region.

A further important development in the field has been the recent emergence of results from total genome scans for other complex disorders, including type 1 and type 2 diabetes mellitus, multiple sclerosis (MS), inflammatory bowel disease, and asthma. These studies may hold important lessons for the attempts to understand schizophrenia. For insulin-dependent diabetes and MS, a "major" gene appears to exist in the HLA region that has been detected in nearly all studies. However, in other regions, nonreplication across groups is as frequent as replication. This is also the pattern seen in initial studies of asthma. In one study of asthma, a genome scan in sibling pairs from three different U.S. ethnic groups showed almost no replication for putative regions of linkage across the three samples. These results suggest that the difficulties in detecting replicable linkages for schizophrenia may not be unique to the psychiatric disorders but rather may reflect a general pattern of problems associated with linkage studies of complex disorders. When the simple and powerful 1:1 relationship between gene and phenotype that is seen in Mendelian disorders breaks down, linkage studies change from a relatively straightforward, although arduous, task to an uncertain and murky endeavor. Detecting genes of modest effect size for complex, moderately heritable diseases is likely to prove a difficult task.

Schizophrenia Candidate Genes: Summary

The collected evidence for the current best set of candidate genes for schizophrenia susceptibility displays both similarities and contrasts to the summary of linkage evidence presented above. The reported associations for two of these candidates, *DTNBP1* and *NRG1*, have been replicated in other samples. Critically, positive replications outnumber negative ones by two or three to one for both genes. *RGS4*, although showing some evidence of replication, has provided weaker support in follow-up studies. Other candidates, such as *G72/DAAO*, *PRODH2*, and *COMT* await the collection of sufficient data to interpret the validity of the original studies.

One particularly exciting shared feature of most of the candidates discussed above is that they can be related to potential pathophysiology through dysfunction in glutamatergic neurotransmission, which may be an important systemic element in the etiology of schizophrenia. Although a detailed discussion of this theory is outside the scope of this chapter, recent reviews by Paul Harrison and Michael Owen of the genetic evidence and by Bita Moghaddam of the neuroscience evidence discuss the positions of the gene products of *NRG1*, *COMT*, *PRODH2*, *DAAO*, *G72*, and *RGS4* in the biochemical and functional pathways influencing the glutamatergic system. Of the current best candidates, only the gene product of *DTNBP1* does not yet fit easily into this framework.

FUTURE DIRECTIONS

The evidence is strong that schizophrenia is a familial disorder and that the familial aggregation of schizophrenia is due largely, although probably not entirely, to genetic factors. Whatever the familial predisposition that operates for schizophrenia, it not only "codes" for the classic, deteriorating psychotic disorder but also increases liability to "schizophrenia-like" personality disorders and probably for some other nonschizophrenic nonaffective psychoses. Two decades of research using statistical methods have not clearly delineated the mode of transmission of schizophrenia, a result that is understandable given its likely complexity.

Advances in molecular and statistical genetics have opened up realistic opportunities to localize on the human genome the specific genes that influence the liability to schizophrenia. Association studies have yet to provide convincing evidence for the role of a range of candidate genes in the etiology of schizophrenia. Genome scan strategies have, however, provided several regions, including chromosomes 5q, 6p, 6q, 8p, 10p, 15q, and 22q, in which a number of groups have found evidence for linkage. Although false-positive findings cannot be ruled out, it is likely that one or more of these regions do contain one or more susceptibility genes for schizophrenia. This belief is supported by an emerging number of identified positional candidate genes that, in some cases, are now being replicated in independent samples. Given the major focus on this area of multiple research groups throughout the world, it is likely that, within several years, these or other loci might emerge as widely replicated susceptibility genes for schizophrenia. If this occurs, it will represent a true watershed event in the history of schizophrenia research.

Although the step of gene identification will itself represent a major advance, it will also represent the beginning of several new lines of research, including (1) rational drug design based on knowledge of basic pathophysiology, (2) characterization of genotype–phenotype relationships based on knowledge of specific pathogenic mutations, (3) identification of environmental risk factors that interact with specific genes, and (4) realistic prevention research given the ability to identify high-risk individuals.

SUGGESTED CROSS-REFERENCES

Population genetics in psychiatry is discussed in Section 1.17, and genetic linkage analysis of the psychiatric disorder is discussed in Section 1.18.

REFERENCES

Asarnow RF, Nuechterlein KH, Fogelson D, Subotnik KL, Payne DA, Russell AT, Asamen J, Kuppinger H, Kendler KS: Schizophrenia and schizophrenia-spectrum personality disorders in the first-degree relatives of children with schizophrenia: The UCLA family study. *Arch Gen Psychiatry*. 2001;58:581–588.

Blouin JL, Dombroski BA, Nath SK, Lasseter VK, Wolyniec PS, Nestadt G, Thornquist M, Ullrich G, McGrath J, Kasch L, Lamaca M, Thomas MG, Gehrig C, Radhakrishna U, Snyder SE, Balk KG, Neufeld K, Swartz KL, DeMarchi N, Papadimitriou GN, Dikeos DG, Stefanis CN, Chakravarti A, Childs B, Housman DE, Kazazian HH, Antonarakis SE, Pulver AE: Schizophrenia susceptibility loci on chromosomes 13q32 and 8p21. *Nat Genet*. 1998;20:70–73.

Brzustowicz LM, Hodgkinson KA, Chow EWC, Honer WG, Bassett AS: Location of a major susceptibility locus for familial schizophrenia on chromosome 1q21-q22. *Science*. 2000;288;678–682.

Brzustowicz LM, Honer WG, Chow EWC, Little D, Hodgkinson K, Bassett A: Linkage of familial schizophrenia to chromosome 13q32. *Am J Hum Genet*. 1999;65;1096–1103.

Cannon TD, Kaprio J, Lonnqvist J, Huttunen M, Koskenvuo M: The genetic epidemiology of schizophrenia in a Finnish twin cohort: A population-based modeling study. *Arch Gen Psychiatry*. 1998;55;67–74.

Cao Q, Martinez M, Zhang J, Sanders AR, Badner JA, Cravchik A, Markey CJ, Beshah E, Guroff JJ, Maxwell ME, Kazuba DM, Whiten R, Goldin LR, Gershon ES, Gejman PV: Suggestive evidence for a schizophrenia susceptibility locus on chromosome 6q and a confirmation in an independent series of pedigrees. *Genomics*. 1997;43:1–8.

Cardno AG, Holmans PA, Rees MI, Jones LA, McCarthy GM, Hamshere ML, Williams NM, Norton N, Williams HJ, Fenton I, Murphy KC, Sanders RD, Gray MY, O'Donovan MC, McGuffin P, Owen MJ: A genomewide linkage study of age at onset in schizophrenia. *Am J Med Genet*. 2001;105:439–445.

Chowdari KV, Mirnics K, Semwal P, Wood J, Lawrence E, Bhatia T, Deshpande SN, Thelma BK, Ferrell RE, Middleton FA, Devlin B, Levitt P, Lewis DA, Nimgaonkar VL: Association and linkage analyses of RGS4 polymorphisms in schizophrenia. *Hum Mol Genet.* 2002;11:1373–1380.

*Chumakov I, Blumenfeld M, Guerassimenko O, Cavarec L, Palicio M, Abderrahim H, Bougueleret L, Barry C, Tanaka H, La Rosa P, Puech A, Tahri N, Cohen-Akenine A, Delabrosse S, Lissarrague S. Picard FP, Maurice K, Essioux L, Millasseau P, Grel P, Debailleul V, Simon AM, Caterina D, Dufaure I, Malekzadeh K, Belova M, Luan JJ, Bouillot M, Sambucy JL, Primas G, Saumier M, Boubkiri N, Martin-Saumier S, Nasroune M, Peixoto H, Delaye A, Pinchot V, Bastucci M, Guillou S, Chevillon M, Sainz-Fuertes R, Meguenni S, Aurich-Costa J, Cherif D, Gimalac A, Van Duijn C, Gauvreau D, Ouelette G, Fortier I, Realson J, Sherbatich T, Riazanskaia N, Rogaev E, Raeymaekers P, Aerssens J, Konings F, Luyten W, Macciardi F, Sham PC, Straub RE, Weinberger DR, Cohen N, Cohen D: Genetic and physiological data implicating the new human gene G72 and the gene for D-amino acid oxidase in schizophrenia. *Proc Natl Acad Sci U S A.* 2002;99:13675–13680.

DeLisi LE, Shaw SH, Crow TJ, Shields G, Smith AB, Larach VW, Wellman N. Loftus J, Nanthakumar B, Razi K, Stewart J, Comazzi M, Vita A, Heffner T, Sherrington R: A genome-wide scan for linkage to chromosomal regions in 382 sibling pairs with schizophrenia or schizoaffective disorder. *Am J Psychiatry.* 2002;159:803–812.

Egan MF, Goldberg TE, Kolachana BS, Callicott JH, Mazzanti CM, Straub RE, Goldman D, Weinberger DR: Effect of COMT Val108/158 Met genotype on frontal lobe function and risk for schizophrenia. *Proc Natl Acad Sci U S A.* 2001;98:6917–6922.

Gerber DJ, Hall D, Miyakawa T, Demars S, Gogos JA, Karayiorgou M, Tonegawa S: Evidence for association of schizophrenia with genetic variation in the 8p21.3 gene, PPP3CC, encoding the calcineurin gamma subunit. *Proc Natl Acad Sci U S A.* 2003;100:8993–8998.

Gill M, Vallada H, Collier D, Sham P, Holmans P, Murray R, McGuffin P, Nanko S, Owen M, Antonarakis S, Housman D, Kazazian H, Nestadt G, Pulver AE, Straub RE, MacLean CJ, Walsh D, Kendler KS, DeLisi L, Polymeropoulos M, Coon H, Byerley W, Lofthouse R, Gershon E, Golden L, Crow T, Freedman R, Laurent C, Bodeau-Pean S, d'Amato T, Jay M, Campion D, Mallet J, Wildenauer DB, Lerer B, Albus M, Ackenheil M, Ebstein RP, Hallmayer J, Maier W, Gurling H, Curtis D, Kalsi G, Brynjolfsson J, Sigmundson T, Petursson H, Blackwood D, Muir W, St. Clair D, He L, Maguire S, Moises HW, Hwu H-G, Yang L, Wiese C, Tao L, Liu X, Kristbjarnason H, Levinson DF, Mowry BJ, Donis-Keller H, Hayward NK, Crowe RR, Silverman JM, Nancarrow DJ, Read CM: A combined analysis of D22S278 marker alleles in affected sib-pairs: Support for a susceptibility locus for schizophrenia at chromosome 22q12. *Am J Med Genet Neuropsychiatr Genet.* 1996;67:40–45.

Gottesman II. *Schizophrenia Genesis: The Origins of Madness.* New York: W. H. Freeman; 1991.

Gurling HM, Kalsi G, Brynjolfson J, Sigmundsson T, Sherrington R, Mankoo BS, Read T, Murphy P, Blaveri E, McQuillin A, Petursson H, Curtis D: Genomewide genetic linkage analysis confirms the presence of susceptibility loci for schizophrenia, on chromosomes 1q32.2, 5q33.2, and 8p21-22 and provides support for linkage to schizophrenia, on chromosomes 11q23.3-24 and 20q12.1-11.23. *Am J Hum Genet.* 2001;68:661–673.

*Harrison PJ, Owen MJ: Genes for schizophrenia? Recent findings and their pathophysiological implications. *Lancet.* 2003;361:417–419.

Kendler KS, Gruenberg AM, Kinney DK: Independent diagnoses of adoptees and relatives as defined by DSM-III in the Provincial and National samples of the Danish Adoption Study of Schizophrenia. *Arch Gen Psychiatry.* 1994;51:456–468.

Kendler KS, McGuire M, Gruenberg AM, O'Hare A, Spellman M, Walsh D: The Roscommon Family Study: I. Methods, diagnosis of probands and risk of schizophrenia in relatives. *Arch Gen Psychiatry.* 1993;50:527–540.

Kety SS, Wender P, Jacobsen B, Ingraham LJ, Jansson L, Faber B, Kinney DK: Mental illness in the biological and adoptive relatives of schizophrenic adoptees: Replication of the Copenhagen study in the rest of Denmark. *Arch Gen Psychiatry.* 1994;51:442–455.

Levinson DF, Holmans P, Straub RE, Owen MJ, Wildenauer DB, Gejman PV, Pulver AE, Laurent C, Kendler KS, Walsh D, Norton N, Williams NM, Schwab SG, Lerer B, Mowry BJ, Sanders AR, Antonarakis SE, Blouin JL, Deleuze JF, Mallet J: Multicenter linkage study of schizophrenia candidate regions on chromosomes 5q, 6q, 10p, and 13q: Schizophrenia linkage collaborative group III. *Am J Hum Genet.* 2000;67:652–663.

*Levinson DF, Lewis CM, Wise LH, Schizophrenia Collaborative Linkage Group: Genome scan meta-analysis of schizophrenia and bipolar disorder, part II: Schizophrenia. *Am J Hum Genet.* 2003;73:17–33.

Levinson DF, Mahtani MM, Nancarrow DJ, Brown DM, Kruglyak L, Kirby A, Hayward NK, Crowe RR, Andreasen NC, Black DW, Silverman JM, Endicott J, Sharpe L, Mohs RC, Siever LJ, Walters MK, Lennon DP, Jones HL, Nertney DA, Daly MJ, Gladis M, Mowry BJ: Genome scan of schizophrenia. *Am J Psychiatry.* 1998;155:741–750.

Levinson DF, Wildenauer DB, Schwab SG, Albus M, Hallmayer J, Lerer B, Maier W, Blackwood D, Muir W, Clair DS, Morris S, Moises HW, Yang L, Kristbjarnarson H, Helgason T, Wiese C, Collier DA, Holmans P, Daniels J, Rees M, Asherson P, Roberts Q, Cardno A, Arranz MJ, Vallada H, Ball D, Kunugi H, Murray RM, Powell JF, Nanko S, Sham P, Gill M, McGuffin P, Owen MJ, Pulver AE, Antonarakis SE, Babb R, Blouin J-L, DeMarchi N, Dombroski B, Housman D, Karayiorgou M, Ott J, Kasch L, Kazazian H, Lasseter VK, Loetscher E, Luebbert H, Nestadt G, Ton C, Wolyniec PS, Laurent C, de Chaldee M, Thibaut F, Jay M, Samolyk S, Petit M, Campion D, Mallet J, Straub RE, MacLean CJ, Easter SM, O'Neill FA, Walsh D, Kendler KS, Gejman PV, Cao Q, Gershon E, Badner J, Beshah E, Zhang J, Riley BP, Rajagopalan S, Mogudi-Carter M, Jenkins T, Williamson R, DeLisi LE, Garner C, Kelly M, LeDuc C, Cardon L, Lichter J, Harris T, Loftus J, Shields G, Comasi M, Vita A, Smith A, Dann J, Joslyn G, Gurling H, Kalsi G, Brynjolfsson J, Curtis D, Sigmundsson T, Butler R, Read T, Murphy P, Chen AC-H, Petursson H, Byerley W, Hoff M, Holik J, Coon H, Nancarrow DJ, Crowe RR, Andreasen A, Silverman JM, Mohs RC, Siever LJ, Endicott J, Sharpe L, Walters MK, Lennon DP, Hayward NK, Sandkuijl LA, Mowry BJ, Aschauer HN, Meszaros K, Lenzinger E, Fuchs K, Heiden AM, Moises HW, Kruglyak L, Daly NJ, Tara C: Additional support for schizophrenia linkage on chromosomes 6 and 8: A multicenter study. *Am J Med Genet Neuropsychiatr Genet.* 1996;67:580–594.

Millar JK, Christie S, Semple CAM, Porteous DJ: Chromosomal location and genomic structure of the human translin-associated factor X gene (TRAX; TSNAX) revealed by intergenic splicing to DISC1, a gene disrupted by a translocation segregating with schizophrenia. *Genomics.* 2000;67:69–77.

Millar JK, Wilson-Annan JC, Anderson S, Christie S, Taylor MS, Semple CAM, Devon RS, St. Clair DM, Muir WJ, Blackwood DHR, Porteous DJ: Disruption of two novel genes by a translocation co-segregating with schizophrenia. *Hum Mol Genet.* 2000;9:1415–1423.

*Moghaddam B: Bringing order to the glutamate chaos in schizophrenia. *Neuron.* 2003;40:881–884.

Paunio T, Ekelund J, Varilo T, Parker A, Hovatta I, Turunen JA, Rinard K, Foti A, Terwilliger JD, Juvonen H, Suvisaari J, Arajarvi R, Suokas J, Partonen T, Lonnqvist J, Meyer J, Peltonen L: Genome-wide scan in a nationwide study sample of schizophrenia families in Finland reveals susceptibility loci on chromosomes 2q and 5q. *Hum Mol Genet.* 2001;10:3037–3048.

Riley BP, McGuffin P: Linkage and associated studies of schizophrenia. *Am J Med Genet Semin Med Genet.* 2000;97:23–44.

Schwab SG, Knapp M, Mondabon S, Hallmayer J, Borrmann-Hassenbach M, Albus M, Lerer B, Rietschel M, Trixler M, Maier W, Wildenauer DB: Support for association of schizophrenia with genetic variation in the 6p22.3 gene, dysbindin, in sib-pair families with linkage and in an additional sample of triad families. *Am J Hum Genet.* 2003;72:185–190.

Shifman S, Bronstein M, Sternfeld M, Pisante-Shalom A, Lev-Lehman E, Weizman A, Reznik I, Spivak B, Grisaru N, Karp L, Schiffer R, Kotler M, Strous RD, Swartz-Vanetik M, Knobler HY, Shinar E, Beckmann JS, Yakir B, Risch N, Zak NB, Darvasi A: A highly significant association between a COMT haplotype and schizophrenia. *Am J Hum Genet.* 2002;71:1296–1302.

Stefansson H, Sarginson J, Kong A, Yates P, Steinthorsdottir V, Gudfinnsson E, Gunnarsdottir S, Walker N, Petursson H, Crombie C, Ingason A, Gulcher JR, Stefansson K, St. Clair D: Association of neuregulin 1 with schizophrenia confirmed in a Scottish population. *Am J Hum Genet.* 2003;72:83–87.

*Stefansson H, Sigurdsson E, Steinthorsdottir V, Bjornsdottir S, Sigmundsson T, Ghosh S, Brynjolfsson J, Gunnarsdottir S, Ivarsson O, Chou TT, Hjaltason O, Birgisdottir B, Jonsson H, Gudnadottir VG, Gudmundsdottir E, Bjornsson A, Ingvarsson B, Ingason A, Sigfusson S, Hardardottir H, Harvey RP, Lai D, Zhou M, Brunner D, Mutel V, Gonzalo A, Lemke G, Sainz J, Johannesson G, Andresson T, Gudbjartsson D, Manolescu A, Frigge ML, Gurney ME, Kong A, Gulcher JR, Petursson H, Stefansson K: Neuregulin 1 and susceptibility to schizophrenia. *Am J Hum Genet.* 2002;71:877–892.

*Straub RE, Jiang Y, MacLean CJ, Ma Y, Webb BT, Myakishev MV, Harris-Kerr C, Wormley B, Sadek H, Kadambi B, Cesare AT, Gibberman A, O'Neill FA, Walsh D, Kendler KS: Genetic variation in the 6p22.3 gene DTNBP1, the human ortholog of mouse dysbindin, is associated with schizophrenia. *Am J Hum Genet.* 2002;71:337–348.

Straub RE, MacLean CJ, Ma Y, Webb BT, Myakishev MV, Harris-Kerr C, Wormley B, Sadek H, Kadambi B, O'Neill FA, Walsh D, Kendler KS: Genome-wide scans of three independent sets of 90 Irish multiplex families and follow-up of selected regions in all families provides evidence for multiple susceptibility genes. *Mol Psychiatry.* 2002;7:542–559.

Tang JX, Zhou J, Fan JB, Li XW, Shi YY, Gu NF, Feng GY, Xing YL, Shi JG, He L: Family-based association study of DTNBP1 in 6p22.3 and schizophrenia. *Mol Psychiatry.* 2003;8:717–718.

Van Den Bogaert A, Schumacher J, Schulze TG, Otte AC, Ohlraun S, Kovalenko S, Becker T, Freudenberg J, Jonsson EG, Mattila-Evenden M, Sedvall GC, Czerski PM, Kapelski P, Hauser J, Maier W, Rietschel M, Propping P, Nothen MM, Cichon S: The DTNBP1 (Dysbindin) gene contributes to schizophrenia, depending on family history of the disease. *Am J Hum Genet.* 2003;73:1438–1443.

van den Oord EJ, Sullivan PF, Jiang Y, Walsh D, O'Neill FA, Kendler KS, Riley BP: Identification of a high-risk haplotype for the dystrobrevin binding protein 1 (DTNBP1) gene in the Irish study of high-density schizophrenia families. *Mol Psychiatry.* 2003;8:499–510.

Wilcox MA, Faraone SV, Su J, Van Eerdewegh P, Tsuang MT: Genome scan of three quantitative traits in schizophrenia pedigrees. *Biol Psychiatry.* 2002;52:847–854.

▲ 12.4 Schizophrenia: Environmental Epidemiology

ALAN S. BROWN, M.D., MICHAELINE BRESNAHAN, PH.D., M.P.H., AND EZRA S. SUSSER, M.D., DR.P.H.

In the search for the causes of schizophrenia, there is a resurgence of interest in the role of epidemiological studies. Earlier work on the epidemiology of schizophrenia focused largely on determining basic parameters, such as incidence and prevalence. More recently, however, investigators have placed additional focus on identifying environmental risk factors for this disorder. The strongest evidence that schizophrenia has environmental etiologies derives from studies of monozygotic (MZ) twins. It has been known for many years that the rate of discordance for schizophrenia among MZ twins is approximately 50 percent. Since it can be presumed that these twin pairs share all of their genes, it is likely that environmental factors account for the discordance. This has inspired epidemiological researchers to embark on investigations aimed at examining the effect of environmental factors on schizophrenia risk.

This section provides a selective review of the epidemiology of schizophrenia focusing on worldwide distribution and changes over time. Next, it reviews the major environmental etiologies of schizophrenia from a life course perspective. Particular attention will be paid to factors operating early in development. Finally, this section elaborates on future directions necessary to refine and expand current understanding of the role of environmental factors in schizophrenia.

EPIDEMIOLOGY

The search for environmental causes of schizophrenia begins, as with most diseases, in the examination of the descriptive epidemiology of the disorder. The goal is to establish the overall incidence rate of disease, differences in the rates of disease in a society over time, and differences in the rates of disease between societies, with the expectation that distribution of disease will contribute to an understanding of the nature and determinants of the disorder.

Overall Incidence Rate

In a recent review of 27 schizophrenia-incidence studies published between 1985 and 1997, William Eaton reported that the mean annual incidence across studies was 0.2 per 1,000, and the range was 0.04 to 0.58 per 1,000. This review restricted focus to studies in which cases were identified from both inpatient and outpatient services in a defined geographic area and were diagnosed by a psychiatrist. Even with these limitations, the fourteenfold variation in rates observed across these studies is likely due, in part, to differences in methods of individual studies. It is noteworthy that, across these studies, ten different diagnostic definitions were used. The majority of rates reported in the review adopted "broad" criteria for case definition (International Classification of Diseases, eighth edition [ICD-8], ICD-9, traditional diagnosis, Present State Examination [PSE] SPO). Similar recent studies not included in the review reporting incidence based on ICD-10 or the revised third edition of the *Diagnostic and Statistical Manual of Mental Disorders* (DSM-III-R) criteria report rates at or below the mean in this review article.

Differences over Time

In the exploration of environmental etiologies, secular trends over years and decades may provide the first evidence of changes in environmental factors influencing disease. Time trends have played a central role in the historical epidemiology of schizophrenia. In the 19th century, perceived increases in "madness" were a matter of great public concern and debate. Contemporary analysts have speculated that these increases were related to the occurrence of schizophrenia, giving rise to the notion that schizophrenia is a modern disease. For most of the 20th century, it was assumed that the incidence of schizophrenia was relatively unchanging. This assumption was challenged beginning in the 1980s, and the subject has been the topic of ongoing research interest.

More than a dozen reports of declining incidence, first observed in the late 1960s and 1970s in several developed countries (e.g., Scotland, England, Wales, New Zealand, Denmark), have been published. The decline was usually reported as a *period trend*—that is, a trend in rates reported over calendar years rather than over birth years. If the period trend is attributable to a decline in the underlying incidence of disease, rather than to other sources of artifact, it would signal a change in the processes operating around the time of disease onset.

The validity of the observed trend as reflecting changes in underlying incidence of schizophrenia has been questioned on several grounds. Changes in the underlying structure of the population in a given region—age, gender, ethnic, and socioeconomic composition—could also account for declines in dynamic populations. An "aging" of the population over time could account for declining rates as the proportion at highest risk of new disease declines. Studies failing to stratify on age or perform age standardization are vulnerable to this influence.

Changes in treatment systems over time could also account for the decline. The period of declining incidence coincided with a period of great service change in developed countries, marking a shift from inpatient to community care. Studies relying on first admissions, as opposed to studies relying on first treatment contact, are vulnerable to the influence of these treatment-system changes. Changes in diagnostic practices could also account for the period decline. The shift could be triggered by the introduction of effective treatments for other disorders, changes in diagnostic fashion, or a movement toward the application of narrower criteria.

Among the potential alternative explanations for the period trend, the movement toward a narrower diagnosis of schizophrenia has not been ruled out as an explanation for the decline. Judith Allardyce and colleagues demonstrated the impact of diagnosis on trends in first-contact patients in Scotland. Whereas the incidence of clinically diagnosed schizophrenia based on administrative record declined over the period of 1979 to 1999, the incidence of computer-generated Operational Criteria (OPCRIT) Checklist for Psychotic Illness ICD-10– and DSM-IV–diagnosed schizophrenia based on case notes showed no such decline. The authors of this study suggested that the decline in clinical diagnosis reflected a movement to apply more restrictive criteria in clinical practice.

The evidence is not entirely consistent. There have also been other reports of approximately stable rates and reports of increasing rates of first admissions and first treatment contacts. A study examining incidence in southeast London reported a near doubling in rates of OPCRIT-diagnosed Research Diagnostic Criteria schizophrenia and DSM-III-R schizophrenia over a 30-year period (1965 to 1997). Although changes in age and gender composition of the population were adjusted for, other potentially significant changes in the underlying population (e.g., change in ethnic composition) could explain these findings.

Time trends in the incidence of schizophrenia have also been assessed over birth cohorts (mapping incidence rates by birth years), although fewer studies have adopted this strategy. A decline in incidence rates observed over birth cohorts would suggest that at least part of an observed secular decline is determined by processes occurring early in life: nutritional and infectious factors during pregnancy and early childhood and obstetric factors influenced by prevailing treatment practices are all plausible (see Early Development Environmental Factors, below). Again, several studies showed a decline in incidence. Two studies have used age-period-cohort analysis to disentangle the period and cohort effects and examine their relative contribution to the decline. Noriyoshi Takei and colleagues found that most of the decrease in clinical diagnosis of schizophrenia in Scotland between 1966 and 1990 was accounted for by period effects (88 percent), but there was still a small cohort effect.

Difference across Societies

Most, if not all, complex diseases exhibit variations in distribution across societies. Nonetheless, the prevailing belief with respect to schizophrenia is one of uniform incidence.

In searching for evidence of environmental influences in the etiology of disease, a contrast between low- and high-income societies can be informative. The transition from low- to high-income countries implies not only an economic transition, but also a social transition and an epidemiological transition. The overall health profiles of low- and high-income countries are vastly different. One would expect the mental health profiles to be different as well. Although there are observable differences across high- and low-income countries in some psychiatric disorders (e.g., anorexia nervosa), in others, the difference is less than would be expected.

To begin to evaluate systematic differences in incidence across societies requires simultaneous observation in multiple sites using uniform methodology. To date, the most comprehensive such effort to be undertaken is the landmark World Health Organization (WHO) Ten Country Study. Beginning in 1978, the Ten Country Study examined incidence, course, and outcome of schizophrenia in developed and developing countries. First-contact patients with nonaffective psychosis were identified over a 2-year period within each of 13 catchment areas. Methods of assessment and diagnosis were equivalent across sites. Eight sites had sufficiently complete case ascertainment to yield incidence rates. Of the eight sites reporting incidence, two were in India—urban Chandigarh and rural Chandigarh—and the remaining six were largely urban catchment areas in Denmark, Ireland, the United Kingdom, Russia, Japan, and the United States.

The most widely reported finding was that the incidence of schizophrenia *narrowly defined* did not vary significantly across sites. This finding is often cited as evidence for a uniform distribution of schizophrenia worldwide. Whether this evidence actually supports such a claim is a matter of debate. The narrow definition of schizophrenia was based on CATEGO S+ criteria, derived from cross-sectional assessment of first-rank symptoms. This diagnosis demonstrates poor agreement with the diagnosis of schizophrenia under contemporary criteria. Furthermore, the representativeness of the sites in terms of "worldwide" sampling has been questioned. Specifically, among the sites reporting incidence, only two were in a developing country, one of which is in a modern urban area.

The second finding was that the incidence of schizophrenia *broadly defined* varied significantly across sites, with the highest incidence rates reported by the two developing country sites. Comparing the sites reporting the highest and lowest incidence rates indicates that the magnitude of variation is 2.5–fold. The importance of variation in broadly defined schizophrenia—a diagnostic category that is overinclusive relative to current conceptions of schizophrenia—is also unclear. The incidence of nonaffective acute remitting psychosis was approximately tenfold higher in developing country sites, compared to developed country sites in this study. The inclusion of transient psychotic disorders under the diagnosis of broad schizophrenia, however, does not explain the reported difference in rates. Rediagnosing cases meeting broad criteria under modern criteria may shed light on these findings with respect to schizophrenia per se.

The Ten Country Study also found a significantly higher occurrence of catatonic schizophrenia in developing country settings. Catatonic schizophrenia was diagnosed in 10 percent of cases in developing countries (including sites not providing incidence reports), whereas it was extremely rare in developed country settings.

Thus, the evidence can be interpreted as suggesting relatively uniform distribution (a narrow interpretation) or as suggesting systematic variation across developed and developing societies (a broad interpretation). At present, it is not clear which is the more appropriate interpretation. Subsequent studies from the Caribbean tend to support the latter. In each of three intermediate-income countries (Jamaica, Trinidad, and Barbados), rates reported for CATEGO SPO schizophrenia were higher than those reported by WHO for developed country sites, except Moscow, and were more similar to those reported by developing country sites.

Urban–Rural Differences In the 19th century, perceived increases in rates of insanity coincided with rapid urbanization in Europe and the United States. Historical analysis of data from the U.S. 1880 census enumerating "defective, dependent, and delinquent classes" showed that living in an urban setting was associated with an increased risk of being classified as insane. A difference in rates of schizophrenia across the urban–rural continuum persists to the present day in developed country settings. The discrepancy in rates between urban and rural environments has usually been attributed to selective migration or social drift of individuals as a consequence of illness or its prodrome. Current research, however, suggests that an urban setting may, indeed, represent an environmental risk for schizophrenia.

The urban risk factor has been recently addressed in several large population cohort studies investigating place of birth, upbringing, and residence at onset. The developing line of evidence confirms an association between urbanicity and risk of schizophrenia and suggests that the urban risk factor operates early in life. The association between place of upbringing and risk of schizophrenia was evaluated by Glyn Lewis and colleagues in a study examining 49,191 male Swedish conscripts. Survey data obtained at conscription were linked to data from the national psychiatric care registry, encompassing 15 years of follow-up. Lewis and colleagues found that the risk of schizophrenia was 1.65 times higher among men brought up in cities, compared to those brought up in rural areas. In a large Danish population-based cohort of 1.75 million people, Preben Bo Mortensen and colleagues found a dose–response relationship between urbanicity at birth and schizophrenia; the relative risk associated with birth in the capital in comparison to birth in a rural area was 2.4. The salience of early exposure was reinforced in a study by Machteld Marcelis and colleagues that reported urban residence at onset was not associated with risk of schizophrenia, after controlling for place of birth. The timing of the risk during early life is, however, uncertain. Intriguing findings examining residence from birth to age 15 suggest that urban risk may be cumulative over childhood.

This line of evidence supports a meaningful urban–rural difference in risk of schizophrenia based on early exposure. These findings are not likely to be fully explained by selective migration or urban–rural differences in diagnostic practices or access to care. The cause or causes of the urban–rural difference are, however, unknown. A range of individual and contextual factors have been put forward to explain the difference, including infection, obstetric complications, diet, toxins, household crowding, and sociocultural challenges. There may also be protective factors in rural areas that are as yet uninvestigated.

Neighborhood Effects In a landmark 1936 study, Robert E. L. Faris and H. Warren Dunham reported that the highest first admission rates of schizophrenia were concentrated in central areas of Chicago and declined moving out toward the periphery. It was hypothesized that in areas with the highest rates, neighborhood characteristics—social disorganization and consequent social isolation—contributed to the occurrence of the disease. Edward Hare, building on the concept of social isolation, found a higher incidence of schizophrenia in areas of Bristol that had a higher proportion of single-person households. Whether these neighborhoods acted to foster the development of schizophrenia could not be determined, however, because the findings could also be explained by individuals at risk of schizophrenia selectively migrating into these communities.

The importance of neighborhood context as an influence on individual risk has been more clearly shown in two recent studies. Jim van Os found a higher risk for schizophrenia among single individuals living in neighborhoods with fewer single people. This suggests that personal characteristics that place one at risk for schizophrenia can be enhanced by certain contexts. Similarly, elevated rates among ethnic minorities living in largely nonminority communities have been reported.

Immigration A classic finding in the history of schizophrenia research is Ornulv Odegaard's observation in 1932 of higher rates of psychosis among Norwegian immigrants in the United States. Since then, numerous studies have found higher incidence rates of schizophrenia in some immigrant populations; the majority of recent findings emanate from Europe. Elevated rates have been reported in immigrant groups from low- and high-income regions, for example, Surinamese immigrants in the Netherlands, Afro-Caribbean immigrants in the United Kingdom, and Scandinavian immigrants in Denmark.

This line of research has been elaborated in the United Kingdom with respect to Afro-Caribbean immigrants and their children. The elevated risk of schizophrenia in this group is striking; some have estimated the risk at four to eight times that of white residents in the United Kingdom. Furthermore, the risk appears to be greater for second-generation than for first-generation immigrants, implicating environment in the host country. The principal threats to the validity of these results include inaccuracy of rates due to under-enumeration of the resident immigrant population, pathways to care that result in greater identification of cases among immigrants, and misdiagnosis based on cultural misunderstanding or bias. To a greater or lesser extent, each of these issues has been addressed, and the weight of evidence continues to support meaningful differences.

The factors that underlie this particular immigrant effect have yet to be identified. Selective migration, obstetric complications, premorbid neurological illness, infections, and cannabis use have been hypothesized, but no convincing evidence has emerged to explain the differential. This has led some to search for sociocultural explanations, such as discrimination against immigrants. Recent findings in a Danish population-based cohort of increased risk of schizophrenia among native-born Danes with a history of foreign residence in childhood, as well as foreign-born residents and residents with a foreign-born mother, suggest that investigating migration per se may lead to new insights in this area.

ETIOLOGY

Early Development Environmental Factors As implied in the introduction to this chapter, a key question with regard to etiological factors is not whether environmental exposures play a role in schizophrenia but, rather, what are the precise factors and what is the period of development during which they operate. Increasing evidence suggests that a considerable proportion of environmentally caused cases occur after an exposure that impairs the development of the brain and that increases the liability to schizophrenia in adulthood. This hypothesis is supported by clinical and epidemiological studies, indicating a tendency for neurocognitive, behavioral, and neuromotor impairments in preschizophrenic children, a higher rate of minor physical anomalies, and brain abnormalities—including ventriculomegaly, diminished hippocampal volume, and an increased rate of cavum septum pellucidum—at the first episode of illness. This latter neuroimaging finding is of particular interest because cavum septum pellucidum ordinarily dissipates by the time of birth, providing further evidence that schizophrenia has its origins in early development. Taken together, much of this work forms the theoretical backbone for a neurodevelopmental hypothesis of schizophrenia. Because these studies are elaborated in detail in Section 12.5, the reader is referred to that section for more information.

A second critical line of investigation supporting an early developmental insult is the consistent demonstration that births of schizophrenia cases appear to cluster with regard to the date and the place of birth. A consistent excess of schizophrenia, approximately 5 to 15 percent, has been demonstrated among individuals who were born during the late winter and early spring. An interesting series of subsequent studies has demonstrated that patients with the deficit syndrome of schizophrenia are more likely to have been born during the summer months. With regard to place of birth, several prior studies have shown that the relative risk of schizophrenia is increased for persons born in urban, as compared to nonurban, settings.

Obstetric Complications The studies reviewed above have inspired a growing number of investigations aimed at identifying associations between specific early developmental factors and risk of schizophrenia. The vast majority of studies in this area have relied on data collected at the time of birth, and, thus, the most reliable data in such studies relate to the perinatal and neonatal periods of development. These factors, generally referred to as obstetric complications, have been examined in relation to schizophrenia, using both case-control and population-based designs. Given the large number of such studies and heterogeneity between studies, this section will focus on three published metaanalyses that cover nearly all of the major investigations in this area.

The first, and most recent, is that of Mary Cannon and colleagues. Given potential methodological limitations of case-control studies, the study limited the analysis to only those studies that used population-based registers or cohorts; standardized, prospectively collected obstetric information; and comparison subjects from the general population. The authors found significant estimates for three main categories of obstetric complications: complications of pregnancy (bleeding, preeclampsia, diabetes, and rhesus [Rh] incompatibility), abnormal fetal growth and development (low birth weight, congenital malformations, and small head circumference), and complications of delivery (asphyxia, uterine atony, and emergency cesarean section).

In the second metaanalysis, J. R. Geddes and S. M. Lawrie included all published studies with nonschizophrenic control groups and those that stated the method of diagnosis of schizophrenia and the measurement of obstetric complications. Although specific obstetric complications were not examined, the authors reported a pooled-odds ratio of 2.0 (95 percent confidence interval [CI], 1.6–2.4) for the development of schizophrenia.

In a third metaanalysis, Geddes and colleagues investigated individual patient data from 12 case-control studies, all of which used the Lewis-Murray Scale to quantify the presence of obstetric complications. This design was chosen to improve the comparability between the results. The authors found significant associations between schizophrenia and premature rupture of membranes, prematurity (gestational age less than 37 weeks), and use of resuscitation or incubator and borderline significant associations between schizophrenia and low birth weight (<2,500 g) and forceps delivery.

Twin studies have shed further light on the role of obstetric complications in schizophrenia. Pairs that contained one or more twins with schizophrenia (both discordant and concordant) had increased obstetric complications compared to healthy twin pairs. In the discordant twin pairs, however, complications of labor and delivery, especially prolonged labor, were found at increased rates. The rate of prolonged labor was also high in discordant twin pairs in which the second-born twin developed schizophrenia.

As discussed by the authors of these papers, there are a number of potential limitations that affect the interpretability of these results. First, the possibility of ascertainment bias and confounding may have affected the results of a number of studies, particularly the case-control studies. Second, a number of "exposures," such as low birth weight, are likely to be caused by a number of specific prenatal influences or by prematurity, each of which may be a more proximate etiological factor. Third, an insufficient number of studies examined interactive or subgroup effects, such as family history, sex, or age of onset. One metaanalysis worth noting in this regard found that the relationship between obstetric complications and schizophrenia was confined to patients younger than age 25 years. Fourth, the findings of Geddes and Lawrie suggested the possibility of publication bias against small negative studies. Fifth, there appeared to be evidence of significant heterogeneity between the case-control and cohort studies included in the Geddes and Lawrie study and discordance between studies that used birth records as compared to maternal recall in the Geddes and colleagues study.

Understandably, then, the results of this body of literature, including the results of the metaanalyses described above, are somewhat conflicting. The most commonly proposed pathogenic mechanism is fetal or perinatal hypoxia, as it appears to be common to many of the complications with positive associations. Although hypoxia may represent a "final common pathway" to the development of schizophrenia after these obstetric insults, it is unclear whether the individual obstetric complications examined in these studies are a primary cause of hypoxia or whether they result from other noxious insults earlier in development. In addition, the effects of hypoxic insults may differ markedly from one another, depending on the type and the timing of the obstetric complication.

Abnormal fetal growth has been proposed as a second general mechanism that leads to schizophrenia. As reviewed above, findings such as low birth weight and diminished head circumference are consistent with such a mechanism. If environmental insults are involved, they would be expected to retard growth during the prenatal period. It is, however, unclear which types of prenatal environmental factors are responsible for these findings in schizophrenia. Certainly, several prenatal factors have been well established as causes of low birth weight. Prenatal exposures are reviewed in the following section.

Studies of Specific Prenatal Factors The studies reviewed above have helped considerably in advancing our understanding of the etiologies of schizophrenia and have provided further data to support the neurodevelopmental hypothesis of schizophrenia. More recently, however, substantial attention has shifted to investigations that focus on the prenatal period of development. These studies have examined a variety of prenatal risk factors, including viral infection, immunological dysfunction, nutritional deficiency, and toxic exposures.

One of the chief reasons for the acceleration on research in this area is that, in order to rigorously investigate the role of prenatal factors, the collection of the data should optimally begin during pregnancy, rather than during birth. Fortunately, several birth cohorts with prospectively collected data during pregnancy have recently passed through the age of risk for schizophrenia. A second reason for an increased focus on the prenatal period is that some of these cohorts contain more refined data on the prenatal experience and maternal serum specimens drawn during pregnancy, which permit the examination of more specific in utero insults. This section discusses both ecological studies that gave rise to hypotheses on specific prenatal insults as risk factors for schizophrenia and then elaborates on the birth cohort studies that are more definitively testing these factors in the etiology of schizophrenia.

INFLUENZA Prompted by studies that demonstrated a clustering of schizophrenia births in the winter and spring months, investigators began to examine whether subjects who were in utero during influenza epidemics evidenced an increased risk of schizophrenia. In the first study of this type, Sarnoff Mednick and colleagues showed that Finnish subjects who were in the second trimester of fetal development during the 1957 type A2–influenza epidemic had a significantly increased occurrence of schizophrenia than subjects who were not in utero during the second trimester. Since then, many studies in Europe, the United States, Japan, and Australia, using similar research designs, have attempted to replicate the finding. Positive associations between second-trimester exposure to influenza and schizophrenia have been shown in Great Britain, Japan, and, to some degree, in Australia. Other studies that attempted to relate the annual prevalence of influenza epidemics over many decades have largely confirmed these results. There have, however, been several studies that failed to replicate this association, including studies with some notable methodological strengths, such as complete case ascertainment and relatively large numbers of cases.

In the only two cohort studies of this relation, no associations were found; however, these studies were limited by small sample sizes, and the first used maternal recall after the pregnancy to define the infection.

Therefore, when considered as a group, the results are equivocal. One likely reason for the discrepant findings is misclassification of exposure, especially through the use of ecological data (i.e., influenza epidemics in a population) or maternal reports of infection. To attempt to surmount this limitation, a recent study used serologic measures of influenza infection obtained during pregnancies enrolled in a population-based birth cohort. The serum samples were prospectively obtained in all pregnancies giving rise to birth cohort members, and schizophrenia in the offspring was diagnosed mostly by direct research-based interviews. Serologically documented influenza exposure in the first trimester was associated with a sevenfold increase in risk of schizophrenia (and related spectrum disorders), and influenza during early to midgestation, a period of pregnancy that overlapped the second trimester, was associated with a threefold increased schizophrenia risk. The results were unchanged after adjustment for several confounders. The population-attributable risk of schizophrenia after early gestational influenza exposure was as high as 21 percent, suggesting that approximately one-fifth of schizophrenia cases might not have occurred if influenza exposure had been prevented. These results provide the first serologic evidence of a relation between prenatal influenza and schizophrenia.

OTHER VIRAL INFECTIONS If prenatal exposure to influenza is a risk factor for schizophrenia, then it is reasonable to consider other infectious agents in the etiology of this disorder. Previous ecological studies have demonstrated associations between schizophrenia and prenatal exposure to measles, varicella-zoster, polio, and mumps. As in the influenza work described above, investigators have more recently used birth cohort designs with more refined measures of infectious exposures. Alan S. Brown and colleagues examined the risk of schizophrenia in a birth cohort with prospectively documented prenatal exposure to a group of several respiratory infections. In contrast to ecological studies, the exposure was documented from obstetric records in individual pregnancies. The authors found a significant, greater than twofold increased risk of schizophrenia in subjects exposed to these infections during the second trimester. Upper respiratory tract infections were especially increased among subjects who later developed schizophrenia.

In a second study, Brown and colleagues examined the risk of schizophrenia (and spectrum disorders) in a birth cohort with known exposure to rubella. In the Rubella Birth Defects Evaluation Project (RBDEP), pregnant women who were clinically documented with prenatal exposure to rubella were recruited for a follow-up of the sequelae of rubella infection in the offspring. Rubella infection was serologically confirmed in the majority of mothers and offspring. In a follow-up study in midadulthood, Brown and colleagues demonstrated that more than 20 percent of the offspring of rubella-exposed pregnancies were diagnosed with schizophrenia spectrum disorders. Although the numbers were small, the effect appeared to be strongest for rubella exposure during the first 2 months of gestation, similar to studies of other sequelae of rubella that established that the greatest vulnerability to teratogenic events occurs in early gestation. A further finding that lends credence to the association is that nearly 90 percent of rubella-exposed schizophrenia spectrum cases, compared to only 33 percent of rubella-exposed controls, had a decline in intelligence quotient (IQ) between childhood and adolescence. Increases in neuromotor and behavioral abnormalities were also demonstrated in the rubella-exposed schizophrenia cases, compared to rubella-exposed controls. These findings suggest that prenatal rubella exposure may have led to a deviant neurodevelopmental trajectory—an ultimate outcome of which was schizophrenia spectrum disorders.

In a study on the National Collaborative Perinatal Project, serologic specimens were collected during pregnancy to investigate the relation between late pregnancy antibody to several infectious agents and schizophrenia. Among the seven agents examined, a significant association was demonstrated between maternal immunoglobulin G (IgG) antibody to herpes simplex virus type 2 (HSV-2) and schizophrenia. One caveat of this study is that IgG antibodies can stay elevated for many years after infection, and, thus, it is unclear whether active HSV-2 infection occurred during pregnancy in these cases.

CYTOKINES The demonstration of relationships between in utero exposure to several infectious agents and risk of schizophrenia suggest that they share a common pathogenic mechanism. Proinflammatory cytokines are robustly elevated after exposure to most infectious pathogens and are known to orchestrate the immune response to these agents. Investigators have therefore begun to examine whether maternal cytokine levels are increased during pregnancies that gave rise to offspring with schizophrenia, as compared to pregnancies resulting in control offspring. In one recent study, maternal second-trimester levels of interleukin-8 (IL-8) were significantly elevated in pregnancies of schizophrenia offspring. No differences were found for three other cytokines in that study, including interleukin-1β (IL-1β), interleukin-6 (IL-6), and tumor necrosis factor alpha (TNF-α). In a smaller study using prenatal serum specimens, increased late gestational maternal TNF-α was found in pregnancies giving rise to cases of psychosis (which included, but was not limited to, schizophrenia). Although in utero exposure to infectious agents is the most likely explanation, it is also possible that other inflammatory processes may be involved. For instance, elevated cytokine levels have been associated with both preeclampsia and increased maternal body mass index, and each of these prenatal factors has been associated with schizophrenia.

Nutritional Factors

DUTCH HUNGER WINTER The first evidence that prenatal malnutrition may play a role in schizophrenia was derived from the studies of the Dutch Hunger Winter of 1944 to 1945. This famine, which occurred toward the end of World War II, precipitated by a Nazi blockade of the Netherlands, was accompanied by other unfortunate circumstances. This led to severe caloric restriction by a substantial proportion of the Dutch population; the famine was most severe in the western Netherlands. Nearly 22,000 people died as a result of the famine, and there was substantially decreased fertility, increased mortality, and diminished birth weight. Unlike most other famines, it was time limited, and the extent and timing of caloric restriction and psychiatric outcomes were well documented. Thus, this tragic event also prevented a unique opportunity to investigate the role of prenatal malnutrition during specific periods of development to psychiatric disorders.

In a psychiatric follow-up of this cohort, Ezra S. Susser and colleagues investigated the relation between prenatal exposure to the Dutch famine and risk of schizophrenia and related disorders. The authors found that exposure to the peak of the famine during the periconceptional period was associated with a significant, twofold increased risk of schizophrenia. In a subsequent study, this cohort exposed to famine in early gestation also showed an increase in risk of schizoid personality disorders.

These findings appear to be specific to major psychiatric disorders, as Brown and colleagues did not demonstrate an association between prenatal famine during this period of gestation and risk of schizophrenia. The authors did demonstrate, however, that famine exposure later in gestation was related to an increased risk of major affective disorders. This finding indicates that the timing of the gestational insult may play an important role in the type of psychiatric disorder that arises, with a more severe disorder resulting from a prenatal insult that occurs earlier in development.

These effects may be explained by a number of nutritional and nonnutritional factors. Nutritional factors include general malnutrition or a micronutrient deficiency. One additional finding from the Dutch famine study that lends credence to a micronutrient deficiency is that the risk of congenital neural defects (mostly neural-tube defects) was also increased in the birth cohort exposed periconceptionally to severe famine. Prenatal folate deficiency has been established as a risk factor for neural-tube defects. Interestingly, folate deficiency occurs commonly during pregnancy, and neural-tube defects show no clear gradient across rich and poor societies. This suggests that prenatal folate deficiency may be a candidate risk factor for schizophrenia, even in societies in which famine is rare or nonexistent. Nonetheless, protein-calorie malnutrition or deficiencies of other micronutrients, such as essential fatty acids or retinoids, should also be considered, as each adversely affects brain development. Furthermore, ingestion of toxic substances, such as tulip bulbs, or of animals, such as cats, that may have harbored infectious organisms could have played an etiological role. Finally, the excessive stress may have increased activation of the hypothalamic-pituitary-adrenal axis, leading to secretion of cortisol, which has been shown to damage development of the hippocampus and other brain structures implicated in schizophrenia. Other prenatal stressors are suspected to increase risk of schizophrenia.

MATERNAL BODY MASS INDEX A second factor that relates to maternal nutrition is body mass index (BMI, defined as kg/m^2). High maternal BMI is associated with poor pregnancy outcomes, including neural-tube defects. To further examine this question in the Prenatal Determinants of Schizophrenia Study, Catherine Schaefer and colleagues examined the relationship between maternal BMI to the development of schizophrenia spectrum disorders in the offspring. A graded increase was shown in risk of schizophrenia as BMI increased; the risk was nearly threefold for offspring of mothers in the highest BMI category (greater than 30). Although these results seem counterintuitive, in a high-income society, obesity is a common indicator of suboptimal nutritional status. In addition, it was known that during the period of the study (1959 to 1966), overweight pregnant women were advised to markedly limit food intake, and amphetamines were commonly prescribed for this purpose. Each of these interventions, in addition to increased hemostatic factors associated with obesity, may have adversely influenced the development of the fetal brain. Given that more than 20 percent of reproductive-age women are considered to be obese, the attributable risk for schizophrenia resulting from elevated BMI might be substantial. A recent study suggests that maternal hypertension, which frequently cooccurs with obesity, increases the risk of schizophrenia in the offspring.

Rhesus Incompatibility Rh incompatibility has been investigated as a risk factor for schizophrenia. Rh incompatibility occurs when an Rh-negative mother gives birth to an Rh-positive child. The maternal antibodies elicited by the fetal Rh antigen cross the placenta and damage the developing fetal brain, causing a variety of neurodevelopmental problems; the risk is highest for second- and later-born offspring, because Rh sensitization has already occurred in such offspring from a first Rh-positive pregnancy. Motivated in part by this literature, J. Megginson Hollister and colleagues examined whether Rh-incompatible second- and later-born male offspring had an increased risk of schizophrenia; a significant, twofold increase in risk was observed. Two other studies support this association.

Prenatal Stress Some, although not all, studies of schizophrenia support an etiological role for prenatal stress. In 1978, in the first of these studies, Matti O. Huttenen and Pekka Niskanen found an increased risk of schizophrenia among offspring who were in utero when their fathers were killed during wartime. Van Os and John Paul Selten reported a twofold increase in risk of schizophrenia among individuals who were in utero during the Nazi occupation of the Netherlands; the effect was strongest for the first trimester.

Environmental Factors throughout the Lifespan

Demographic Factors Some of the earliest studies have demonstrated consistent relationships between several demographic factors and risk of schizophrenia. Although some of these associations may be explained by factors occurring early in life, the period or periods during which they have their impact have not been precisely localized.

SOCIOECONOMIC STATUS The most frequent demographic factor examined in relation to risk of schizophrenia is socioeconomic status. For many years, investigators have shown that subjects who lived in poorer neighborhoods tended to have higher rates of schizophrenia. This association has spawned a lively debate with regard to the direction of causality. In the first hypothesis, known as the *social selection* (or *drift*) *hypothesis*, it has been argued that the psychopathology and impaired functioning in schizophrenia lead to a decline in social status. In the second, known as the *social causation hypothesis*, it is argued that factors associated with poverty, such as malnutrition, stress, and poor medical care, result in schizophrenia. Considerable evidence supports the social drift hypothesis, although some studies, including a recent population-based case-control study, indicate that low paternal social class and residence in a deprived area at birth are associated with an increased risk of schizophrenia. On the other hand, two other studies reported that high paternal socioeconomic status at birth was linked to an increased risk of schizophrenia, although a small sample size (in one study) and lack of follow-up through the age of risk in these latter studies may have explained these latter results.

PATERNAL AGE A second demographic factor that has been strongly associated with risk of schizophrenia is paternal age. To date, seven studies have demonstrated that advanced paternal age of the father at the time of the offspring's birth is associated with a higher occurrence of schizophrenia in the offspring. Studies that have investigated schizophrenia risks stratified by paternal age groups have demonstrated a monotonic relationship. The risk appears to increase substantially at age 35 to 40 years. De novo mutations in the male sperm cell line have been suggested as a potential explanation, because such mutations increase exponentially with advancing paternal age. Other evidence supporting the de novo mutation hypothesis includes the observation that the schizophrenic offspring of older, compared to younger, fathers are less likely to have a family history of schizophrenia. However, other factors, including genetic predisposition of fathers who have children at later ages and a different rearing environment by older fathers, have not yet been ruled out as causal explanations.

SUBSTANCE ABUSE Several, although not all, studies have reported increased rates of substance abuse in patients with schizophrenia. Among psychoactive substances, studies have suggested that rates of amphetamine, hallucinogen, and cannabis abuse are increased in schizophrenic patients. One key question raised, however, is what is the nature of the cause–effect relationship—that is, do patients with schizophrenia use substances to alleviate the symptoms of the illness, or do these substances increase the risk of schizophrenia? Although studies have shown that substance abuse begins before illness onset in the majority of schizophrenic patients, the insidious nature of the onset of schizophrenia does not rule out the possibility of "self-medication" of symptoms. There is also the possibility of a common antecedent (e.g., social adjustment) that is a risk factor for both substance use and for schizophrenia.

There has been particular interest in the association between cannabis and schizophrenia, based on both biological plausibility and public health ramifications. Sven Andreasson and colleagues examined this association in a cohort of 45,570 Swedish conscripts. Data on drug use were obtained from questionnaires completed at the time of conscription and linked to the national psychiatric care registry. Cannabis use predicted risk of schizophrenia during 15 years of follow-up. Those reporting high levels of use (more than 50 occasions) were at sixfold increased risk of schizophrenia compared to nonusers. The Swedish cohort was revisited in a subsequent study capturing 27 years of follow-up. The risk profile was found to be the same. In the later follow-up study, more comprehensive measures were taken by Stan Zammit and colleagues to identify and control for factors potentially confounding the association, including diagnosis at conscription, IQ score, poor social integration, disturbed behavior, cigarette smoking, and place of upbringing. Adjusting for these factors reduced the odds for heavy cannabis users by approximately half to a threefold elevation in risk.

Research in this area is rapidly developing. There is some evidence indicating that cannabis use increases the risk of any level of psychotic symptoms and the risk of a severe level of psychotic symptoms in a dose–response fashion among individuals known to be free of psychotic symptoms at baseline. There is also a suggestion that initiating cannabis use earlier as opposed to later in adolescence may be more damaging. If the association between cannabis use and schizophrenia is shown to be causal, this would provide a clear target for prevention efforts and a significant source of preventable cases.

Traumatic Brain Injury Previous studies have suggested increased rates of traumatic brain injury (TBI) in schizophrenia. In these studies, the occurrence of TBI schizophrenia usually precedes the onset of schizophrenia by several to many years, suggesting that the disorder is not an organic psychosis (i.e., a DSM-IV-TR psychosis due to a general medical condition). Compared to healthy controls, the risk of schizophrenia was increased by threefold to tenfold after TBI. Due to the relative lack of studies in this area, further work is needed to establish TBI as a risk factor for schizophrenia.

Viral Infection in Adulthood As reviewed above, many studies have examined whether prenatal exposure to influenza and other viral infections is associated with risk of schizophrenia. There have, however, also been studies that have examined whether adult subjects with schizophrenia have an increase in viral antibodies or nucleotide sequences. One of the most commonly studied is Borna disease virus (BDV). Some previous studies have detected increased seroprevalence to BDV in patients with schizophrenia, as well as other neuropsychiatric disorders, although other investigations have failed to detect the association. Differences in assay methods and potential contamination with cross-reactive antigens have been raised as potential explanations for the discrepancies. Other investigators have examined viral nucleic acid sequences in postmortem brains of patients with schizophrenia. Alla M. Taller and colleagues found no amplified sequences for 12 different viruses, including cytomegalovirus, Epstein-Barr virus, herpes simplex, measles, rubella, and influenza. A recent study has demonstrated a greater than fivefold increase in the proportion of schizophrenia subjects with retroviral sequences in the cerebrospinal fluid (CSF), as compared to controls. Strong homology was found to the endogenous retroviral species HERV-W. Infection with exogenous retroviruses is one potential cause, although it is also possible that it resulted from increased transcription of endogenous retroviruses, which may be caused by a variety of nonviral factors. One key limitation of all of these studies is their cross-sectional design, which does not allow for the delineation of cause–effect relationships.

FUTURE DIRECTIONS

Population-Based Birth Cohort Studies

A *population-based birth cohort* is a sample of subjects who are born within a specified geographic region or time or both and who are drawn from the general population of that region. Subjects in the cohort are then followed up for the outcome of interest, in this case, for schizophrenia. As exemplified by some of the studies discussed above, research designs that focus on these cohorts have several intrinsic merits. First, they feature data collected prospectively and at or near the time of their occurrence. This results in improved reliability and validity and diminishes the potential for recall bias, in which the parents of subjects are more likely to remember a particular exposure if an adverse outcome occurs. Second, they are less likely to be affected by selection bias, especially if the population sampled is representative of the population at risk and the control subjects are representative of the source population. Third, if the follow-up is frequent, they permit the minimization of bias by allowing the application of methods for adjustment of loss to follow-up.

Several population-based birth cohorts throughout the world are presently "coming of age" for risk of schizophrenia. Several of the findings reviewed above were made possible by studies of these cohorts. Perhaps the most valuable of these cohorts are those that collected prospective, detailed, and medically documented data during pregnancy and the early perinatal/neonatal period and that obtained serum and other biological samples during these periods. As illustrated above, these birth cohorts are leading to the examination of potential risk factors for schizophrenia that could not be investigated in previous studies. Work aimed at extending the findings on early to midgestational infections and measures of the maternal and fetal immune response are under way. With regard to nutritional factors, exposures including homocysteine, vitamin B_{12}, retinoids, and essential fatty acids are being investigated. Studies of prenatal toxic exposures such as lead are under way, and polychlorobiphenyls (PCBs) and methylmercury may be targeted in future investigations. Studies of prenatal hormonal exposures, including thyroid, sex steroids, and stress-related hormones, are also being considered in future work.

By harnessing the power of advanced methods of serologic analyses, many of these risk factors may soon be analyzed simultaneously for a fraction of the current cost and provide a substantial saving in the quantity of sera used. Because the serologic data are largely being collected in birth cohorts with a comprehensive database that includes early developmental events, parental background, and demographic factors, investigators are able to investigate factors that may confound or mediate observed associations between these variables. As novel hypotheses unfold from research on neurodevelopmental and other biological pathways, new candidate risk factors will be tested in these population-based birth cohorts.

Gene–Environment Interaction

As briefly reviewed above, it is unlikely that, in most cases, environmental factors act alone in increasing the vulnerability for schizophrenia. Rather, many experts believe that they act in concert with mutated genes. Consequently, several models of gene–environment interaction have been developed, including additive, multiplicative, and synergistic effects. Under an additive model, the effect of one factor (gene) is not dependent on the other factor (environmental exposure). To calculate the risk of disease, one merely adds the individual effects. Under a synergistic effects model, the combined effect of the two factors is greater than the sum of their individual effects.

There is some evidence of interaction between genetic and environment factors in studies of schizophrenia. Family history studies suggest that birth during the winter and spring months interacts with genetic vulnerability for schizophrenia. Patients born during these months had higher risk of schizophrenia than did their relatives. With regard to the Afro-Caribbean finding discussed earlier, one study demonstrated that the risk of schizophrenia was higher in the British-born siblings of the schizophrenia probands than among their Afro-Caribbean–born parents. The authors suggested that prenatal rubella infection may have interacted with genetic vulnerability in this ethnic group, because only the second generation would have been exposed in utero to infectious illnesses such as rubella.

Twin studies of schizophrenia have provided additional evidence in support of a gene–environment interaction hypothesis. In a landmark study, the offspring of affected and unaffected MZ twins had similar rates of schizophrenia. One interpretation of these findings is that an environmental exposure was necessary for the expression of the genotype. In a second twin study, the concordance rates of schizophrenia in MZ twin pairs likely to be monochorionic (i.e., sharing a chorion) was substantially higher than MZ twin pairs that were dichorionic (i.e., having separate chorions). Because it is more likely that a prenatal environmental exposure was shared between both members of monochorionic twin pairs than both members of dichorionic pairs, this suggests an interaction between shared genes and in utero exposures in schizophrenia. Finally, high-risk studies have provided some evidence for gene–environment interaction. It was demonstrated that individuals at high genetic risk for schizophrenia, compared to low-risk offspring, evidenced a greater effect of obstetric complications on ventricular enlargement.

Although these different study paradigms provide an indication of an interaction between genetic and environmental factors in schizophrenia, they are relatively few in number, often involve small sample sizes, and the genetic and environmental "factors" included in them are only proxy measures. Thus, they must be interpreted with caution until more rigorously designed studies are conducted.

Studies of Brain Structure and Function

This section has heretofore presented evidence for associations between environmental factors and schizophrenia. Yet, to prove that these factors are etiological in nature, several additional steps are necessary. One of the most critical steps is to substantiate the biological plausibility of these associations. The fundamental question relevant to plausibility concerns the mechanisms by which these risk factors lead to structural and functional alterations in the brain that contribute to the pathophysiology of schizophrenia. Two strategies for addressing this issue are discussed below.

Clinical Studies of Brain Structure and Function

A wealth of evidence indicates that patients with schizophrenia have a number of brain anomalies that likely play a role in the disorder. With regard to brain structure, investigations have demonstrated, among other findings, ventriculomegaly, diminished cortical volume and thickness, decreased hippocampal volume, and elevated rates of cavum septum pellucidum in patients with schizophrenia as compared to healthy controls. Many investigations have attempted to link obstetric complications with these brain anomalies. Several, although not all, of these studies have suggested that patients with increased structural brain anomalies, especially ventriculomegaly, were more likely to have been affected by obstetric complications. Still, these studies are limited by several factors, including relatively crude measures of obstetric complications and the use of computed tomography (CT) scans rather than magnetic resonance imaging (MRI) (in most cases). In a recent study that used MRI, perinatal hypoxia was associated with diminished volume of the hippocampus. A recent study of discordant MZ twins using MRI demonstrated associations between labor-delivery complications and decreased hippocampal volume in the ill twin, and obstetric complications in general were related to increased ventricular size in the ill twin.

Studies of obstetric complications in schizophrenia that use functional brain measures are less common and, thus far, consist exclusively of neuropsychological measures. In one study, obstetric complications were correlated with perseveration on the Wisconsin Card Sorting Test, although this finding was not replicated in a subsequent investigation. A second study showed that errors in the Trail Making Test, which requires mental set-shifting (an executive function), were associated with obstetric complications.

This work argues that at least some of the brain abnormalities in schizophrenia may have their origin in obstetric insults. Because of the importance of the prenatal period in neuronal generation, migration, and differentiation, studies in population-based birth cohorts using more sophisticated neuroimaging techniques are currently under way to examine the relation to prenatal risk factors and structural and functional brain abnormalities.

Animal Models A promising direction in investigating the mechanisms by which environmental factors lead to brain anomalies found in schizophrenia is the use of models that attempt to replicate these anomalies. Several animal models have focused on the effects of early development insults. One of the most commonly cited is that of Barbara Lipska, Daniel Weinberger, and colleagues. In this animal model, a rodent is given a hippocampal lesion during the neonatal period, and behavioral, physiological, and morphometric studies are conducted throughout the animal's life span. These investigators have demonstrated excessive dopamine-mediated behaviors and neurochemical abnormalities that emerge during adulthood, but not during early life, similar to the period of onset of schizophrenia.

S. Hossein Fatemi and colleagues have examined the effect of prenatal influenza infection on proteins demonstrated to be abnormal in postmortem brains of patients with schizophrenia. In this study, rats exposed to influenza at gestational day 9 had a marked decrease in the number of reelin-producing Cajal-Retzius cells in the cortex and hippocampus. This finding is of particular interest because reelin plays an important role in neuronal migration, and the timing of this migration coincides well with the epidemiological studies of prenatal influenza described in the previous section. Some studies have demonstrated diminished reelin in postmortem brains of patients with schizophrenia. Additional work has shown that prenatal immune activation is associated with endophenotypic markers of schizophrenia, including disrupted latent inhibition, increased sensitivity to amphetamine, and morphological alterations in the hippocampus and entorhinal cortex.

IMPLICATIONS OF THIS WORK

One primary implication of work on environmental risk factors for schizophrenia is that it may promote strategies for prevention. If associations between environmental risk factors and schizophrenia are confirmed, it is conceivable that they may lead to new public health measures. With regard to the neurodevelopmental area of research, such measures could become routinely incorporated into obstetric practice. Considerable experience already exists with regard to mass public health programs that have virtually eliminated viral central nervous system (CNS) teratogens such as rubella and vitamin deficiencies such as folic acid—both of which are associated with neural-tube defects. Such programs may serve as a model for initiatives aimed at preventing schizophrenia. For example, if the influenza findings reviewed above are confirmed, the use of vaccinations to nonpregnant women of reproductive age may prevent up to one-fifth of schizophrenia cases. On a more general level, improved prenatal and perinatal care, a problem largely found in impoverished areas of the United States and the Third World, may have an even more pronounced effect on lowering the risk of schizophrenia, as these interventions may simultaneously eliminate a number of potential risk factors for schizophrenia. With regard to later development, if head trauma is confirmed as a risk factor for schizophrenia, such simple measures as seatbelts or cycling helmets may conceivably prevent cases of schizophrenia.

A second implication of this work relates to studies on early intervention. Such work aims to identify children and adolescents who are at greatest risk for developing schizophrenia, for the purpose of medical and psychosocial treatments that may prevent or ameliorate the course of schizophrenia. Such factors include behavioral problems, subthreshold psychotic symptoms, and social dysfunction. The incorporation of data on early developmental risk factors may help to supplement these predictors, especially if those risk factors with the largest effect sizes and population-attributable risk are used.

A third implication of these studies is the elucidation of pathogenic mechanisms. As reviewed above, the use of animal models has already served to identify the process by which a prenatal insult can lead to outcomes that resemble those found in schizophrenia. One potential result of this work is to identify novel brain disturbances that would never before have been considered from clinical studies that examine large groups of patients who are likely to manifest significant etiological heterogeneity. The identification of new, etiologically linked brain disturbances may have potential for the discovery of new drug targets for schizophrenia.

A fourth implication is the identification of vulnerability genes. If schizophrenia results from an interaction between environmental risk factors and vulnerability genes, the use of samples with homogeneous environmental etiologies may facilitate the identification of causal genes.

The role of epidemiology in the identification of etiologies of schizophrenia is assuming increasing importance. Thus far, the most robust findings are for early life influences. A large body of literature indicates that complications of labor and delivery may be risk factors for the disorder, although a number of findings are conflicting. This work does suggest, however, that factors associated with fetal and perinatal hypoxia and abnormal fetal growth may play an especially important etiological role.

More recent work has focused on specific prenatal environmental etiologies, inspired, in part, by highly informative birth cohorts that have recently matured into the age of risk for schizophrenia. These cohorts have provided serum and other biological specimens that have permitted more rigorous testing of the neurodevelopmental hypothesis of schizophrenia than previous studies that relied on ecological data. This work is yielding more definitive findings that certain prenatal environmental insults are especially involved in the etiology of schizophrenia. These include the following: viral exposures (influenza, rubella), immunological dysfunction (cytokine elevations), nutritional deficiency, Rh incompatibility, and prenatal stress. Despite these advances, considerable work remains. The data from population-based birth cohort studies that prospectively evaluate prenatal exposures in schizophrenia have only begun to be mined. Studies on the potential influence of genetic mutations that likely interact with many of these environmental exposures are under way and will certainly benefit from the findings of the Human Genome Project and new molecular genetic approaches. Investigations aimed at linking our knowledge of environmental risk factors for schizophrenia with disturbances in structure and function of the brain promise to yield valuable information on the pathogenesis of this condition. New, high-risk studies with high-quality data on environmental exposures—and state-of-the-art methodologies for probing neuroanatomy and neurophysiology—should help to reveal the trajectory of the early illness manifestations. The coupling of epidemiologic investigations and animal models in translational research paradigms should further expand current knowledge of etiopathogenesis.

Environmental epidemiology has potentially profound implications not only for understanding the causes of schizophrenia, but also for improving our efforts at prevention. Epidemiological studies have played a very important role in eradicating or reducing the incidence of many of humankind's scourges, including illnesses induced by infection (rubella, smallpox), nutritional deficits (folic acid, vitamin A), and toxins (lead). Additional benefits of this field of work include measures aimed at early intervention, the elaboration of pathogenic mechanisms, and the identification of vulnerability genes. Aided by advances in epidemiological methods, neurobiological techniques, and unique samples of subjects, one can anticipate that the next decade of research on environmental epidemiology holds great promise for the ultimate eradication of schizophrenia.

SUGGESTED CROSS-REFERENCES

Information about genetics relevant to this section can be found in Section 1.17 on population genetics and Section 1.18 on genetic linkage analysis of psychiatric disorders. The treatment of schizophrenia, including psychosocial and psychoeducational approaches, is covered in Section 12.16.

References

Allardyce J, Morrison G, Van Os J, Kelly J, Murray RM, McCreadie RG: Schizophrenia is not disappearing in south-west Scotland. *Br J Psychiatry.* 2000;177:38–41.

Andreasson S, Allebeck P, Engstrom A, Rydberg U: Cannabis and schizophrenia. A longitudinal study of Swedish conscripts. *Lancet.* 1987;2(8574):1483–1486.

Arseneault L, Cannon M, Poulton R, Murray R, Caspi A, Moffitt TE: Cannabis use in adolescence and risk for adult psychosis: Longitudinal prospective study. *BMJ.* 2002;325(7374):1212–1213.

Bhugra D, Hilwig M, Hossein B, Marceau H, Neehall J, Leff J, Mallett R, Der G: First-contact incidence rates of schizophrenia in Trinidad and one-year follow-up. *Br J Psychiatry.* 1996;169(5):587–592.

Boydell J, Murray RM. Urbanization, migration and risk of schizophrenia. In: Murray RM, Jones PB, Susser E, van Os J, Cannon M, eds. *The Epidemiology of Schizophrenia.* Cambridge University Press; 2003.

Boydell J, Van Os J, Lambri M, Castle D, Allardyce J, McCreadie RG, Murray RM: Incidence of schizophrenia in south-east London between 1965 and 1997. *Br J Psychiatry.* 2003;182:45–49.

Bresnahan M, Menezes P, Varma V, Susser E. Geographical variation: Developing and developed countries. In: Murray RM, Jones PB, Susser E, van Os J, Cannon M, eds. *The Epidemiology of Schizophrenia.* Cambridge University Press; 2003.

Brewin J, Cantwell R, Dalkin T, Fox R, Medley I, Glazebrook C, Kwiecinski R, Harrison G: Incidence of schizophrenia in Nottingham. A comparison of two cohorts, 1978–80 and 1992–94. *Br J Psychiatry.* 1997;171:140–144.

*Brown AS: Prenatal infection and adult schizophrenia: A review and synthesis. *Int J Ment Health.* 2001;29:22–37.

Brown AS, Begg MD, Gravenstein S, Wyatt RJ, Bresnahan M, Babulas VP, Susser ES: Serologic evidence for prenatal influenza in the etiology of schizophrenia. *Arch Gen Psychiatry.* 2004.

Brown AS, Cohen P, Harkavy-Friedman J, Babulas V, Malaspina D, Gorman JM, Susser ES: Prenatal rubella, premorbid abnormalities, and adult schizophrenia. *Biol Psychiatry.* 2001;49(6):473–486.

Brown AS, Hooton J, Schaefer CA, Zhang H, Petkova E, Babulas V, Perrin M, Gorman JM, Susser ES: Elevated maternal interleukin-8 levels and risk of schizophrenia in adult offspring. *Am J Psychiatry.* 2004.

Brown AS, Schaefer CA, Wyatt RJ, Goetz R, Begg MD, Gorman JM, Susser ES: Maternal exposure to respiratory infections and adult schizophrenia spectrum disorders: A prospective birth cohort study. *Schizophr Bull.* 2000;26(2):287–295.

Brown AS, Susser ES, Lin SP, Neugebauer R, Gorman JM: Increased risk of affective disorders in males after second trimester prenatal exposure to the Dutch hunger winter of 1944–45. *Br J Psychiatry.* 1995;166(5):601–606.

*Cannon M, Jones PB, Murray RM: Obstetric complications and schizophrenia: Historical and meta-analytic review. *Am J Psychiatry.* 2002;159(7):1080–1092.

Cannon TD, Van Erp TG, Rosso IM, Huttunen M, Lonnqvist J, Pirkola T, Salonen O, Valanne L, Poutanen VP, Standertskjold-Nordenstam CG: Fetal hypoxia and structural brain abnormalities in schizophrenic patients, their siblings, and controls. *Arch Gen Psychiatry.* 2002;59(1):35–41.

Cantor-Graae E, Pedersen CB, McNeil TF, Mortensen PB: Migration as a risk factor for schizophrenia: A Danish population-based cohort study. *Br J Psychiatry.* 2003;182:117–122.

Dohrenwend BP, Dohrenwend BS. *Social Status and Psychological Disorder: A Causal Inquiry.* New York: Wiley-Interscience; 1969.

Eaton WW. Evidence for universality and uniformity of schizophrenia around the world: Assessment and implications. In: Gattaz WF, Hafner H, eds. *Search for the Causes of Schizophrenia*, 4th ed. Berlin: Springer-Verlag; 1999.

Faris DE, Dunham W. *Mental Disorders in Urban Areas.* Chicago: University of Chicago Press; 1939.

Fatemi SH, Emamian ES, Kist D, Sidwell RW, Nakajima K, Akhter P, Shier A, Sheikh S, Bailey K: Defective corticogenesis and reduction in reelin immunoreactivity in cortex and hippocampus of prenatally infected neonatal mice. *Mol Psychiatry.* 1999;4(2):145–154.

Fukuda K, Takahashi K, Iwata Y, Mori N, Gonda K, Ogawa T, Osonoe K, Sato M, Ogata S, Horimoto T, Sawada T, Tashiro M, Yamaguchi K, Niwa S, Shigeta S: Immunological and PCR analyses for Borna disease virus in psychiatric patients and blood donors in Japan. *J Clin Microbiol.* 2001;39(2):419–429.

Geddes JR, Lawrie SM: Obstetric complications and schizophrenia: A metaanalysis. *Br J Psychiatry.* 1995;167(6):786–793.

Geddes JR, Verdoux H, Takei N, Lawrie SM, Bovet P, Eagles JM, Heun R, McCreadie RG, McNeil TF, O'Callaghan E, Stober G, Willinger U, Murray RM: Schizophrenia and complications of pregnancy and labor: An individual patient data metaanalysis. *Schizophr Bull.* 1999;25(3):413–423.

Hare E: Mental illness and social conditions in Bristol. *J Ment Sci.* 1956;102:349–357.

Harrison G, Fouskakis D, Rasmussen F, Tynelius P, Sipos A, Gunnell D: Association between psychotic disorder and urban place of birth is not mediated by obstetric complications or childhood socio-economic position: A cohort study. *Psychol Med.* 2003;33:723–731.

Harrison G, Gunnell D, Glazebrook C, Page K, Kwiecinski R: Association between schizophrenia and social inequality at birth: Case-control study. *Br J Psychiatry.* 2001;179:346–350.

Hickling FW, Rodgers-Johnson P: The incidence of first contact schizophrenia in Jamaica. *Br J Psychiatry.* 1995;167(2):193–196.

Hoek HW, Brown AS, Susser E: The Dutch famine and schizophrenia spectrum disorders. *Soc Psychiatry Psychiatr Epidemiol.* 1998;33(8):373–379.

Hollister JM, Brown AS. Rhesus incompatibility and schizophrenia. In: Susser E, Brown AS, Gorman JM, eds. *Prenatal Exposures in Schizophrenia.* Washington, D.C.: American Psychiatric Press, Inc.; 1999.

Jablensky A, Sartorius N, Ernberg G, Anker M, Korten A, Cooper JE, Day R, Bertelsen A: Schizophrenia: Manifestations, incidence and course in different cultures. A World Health Organization ten-country study. *Psychol Med Monogr Suppl.* 1992;20:1–97.

Karlsson H, Bachmann S, Schroder J, McArthur J, Torrey EF, Yolken RH: Retroviral RNA identified in the cerebrospinal fluids and brains of individuals with schizophrenia. *Proc Natl Acad Sci U S A.* 2001;98(8):4634–4639.

Lewis G, David A, Andreasson S, Allebeck P: Schizophrenia and city life. *Lancet.* 1992;340(8812):137–140.

Likpin I, Schneemann A, Solbrig MV: Borna disease virus: Implications for human neuropsychiatric illness. *Trends Microbiol.* 1995;3(2):64–69.

Marcelis M, Takei N, Van Os J: Urbanization and risk for schizophrenia: Does the effect operate before or around the time of illness onset? *Psychol Med.* 1999;29(5):1197–1203.

McGuffin P, Owen MJ, Farmer AE: Genetic basis of schizophrenia. *Lancet.* 1995;346(8976):678–682.

*Mednick SA, Machon RA, Huttunen MO, Bonett D: Adult schizophrenia following prenatal exposure to an influenza epidemic. *Arch Gen Psychiatry.* 1988;45(2):189–192.

*Mortensen PB, Pedersen CB, Westergaard T, Wohlfahrt J, Ewald H, Mors O, Andersen PK, Melbye M: Effects of family history and place and season of birth on the risk of schizophrenia. *N Engl J Med.* 1999;340(8):603–608.

Murray RM, Jones PB, Susser E, van Os J, Cannon M, eds. *The Epidemiology of Schizophrenia.* Cambridge University Press; 2003.

Odegaard O: Emigration and insanity. *Acta Psychiatr Neurol Scan Suppl.* 1932;4:1–206.

Pedersen CB, Mortensen PB: Evidence of a dose-response relationship between urbanicity during upbringing and schizophrenia risk. *Arch Gen Psychiatry.* 2001;58(11):1039–1046.

Phillips P, Johnson S: How does drug and alcohol misuse develop among people with psychotic illness? A literature review. *Soc Psychiatry Psychiatr Epidemiol.* 2001;36(6):269–276.

Schaefer CA, Brown AS, Wyatt RJ, Kline J, Begg MD, Bresnahan MA, Susser ES: Maternal prepregnant body mass and risk of schizophrenia in adult offspring. *Schizophr Bull.* 2000;26(2):275–286.

Selten JP, Cantor-Graae E, Nahon D, Levav I, Aleman A, Kahn RS: No relationship between risk of schizophrenia and prenatal exposure to stress during the Six-Day War or Yom Kippur War in Israel. *Schizophr Res.* 2003;63:131–135.

Sorensen HJ, Mortensen EL, Reinisch JM, Mednick SA: Do hypertension and diuretic treatment in pregnancy increase the risk of schizophrenia in offspring? *Am J Psychiatry.* 2003;160:425–429.

South MA, Sever JL: Teratogen update: The congenital rubella syndrome. *Teratology.* 1985;31(2):297–307.

Susser E, Mojtabai R. Epidemiology of schizophrenia research: The untapped potential. In: Gattaz WF, Hafner H, eds. *Search for the Causes of Schizophrenia,* 4th ed. Berlin: Springer-Verlag; 1999.

Susser E, Wanderling J: Epidemiology of nonaffective acute remitting psychosis vs. schizophrenia. Sex and sociocultural setting. *Arch Gen Psychiatry.* 1994;51(4):294–301.

Susser ES, Schaefer CA, Brown AS, Begg MD, Wyatt RJ: The design of the prenatal determinants of schizophrenia study. *Schizophr Bull.* 2000;26(2):257–273.

Takei N, Lewis G, Sham PC, Murray RM: Age-period-cohort analysis of the incidence of schizophrenia in Scotland. *Psychol Med.* 1996;26(5):963–973.

Taller AM, Asher DM, Pomeroy KL, Eldadah BA, Godec MS, Falkai PG, Bogert B, Kleinman JE, Stevens JR, Torrey EF: Search for viral nucleic acid sequences in brain tissues of patients with schizophrenia using nested polymerase chain reaction. *Arch Gen Psychiatry.* 1996;53(1):32–40.

Torrey EF, Bowler AE, Clark K: Urban birth and residence as risk factors for psychoses: An analysis of 1880 data. *Schizophr Res.* 1997;25(3):169–176.

Van Os J, Driessen G, Gunther N, Delespaul P: Neighbourhood variation in incidence of schizophrenia. Evidence for person-environment interaction. *Br J Psychiatry.* 2000;176:243–248.

Van Os J, Selten JP: Prenatal exposure to maternal stress and subsequent schizophrenia. The May 1940 invasion of The Netherlands. *Br J Psychiatry.* 1998;172:324–326.

Zammit S, Allebeck P, Andreasson S, Lundberg I, Lewis G: Self reported cannabis use as a risk factor for schizophrenia in Swedish conscripts of 1969: Historical cohort study. *BMJ.* 2002;325(7374):1199.

Zuckerman L, Rehavi M, Nachman R, Weiner I: Immune activation during pregnancy leads to a postpubertal emergence of disrupted latent inhibition, dopaminergic hyperfunction, and altered limbic morphology in the offspring: A novel neurodevelopmental model of schizophrenia. *Neuropsychopharmacology.* 2003;10:1778–1789.

▲ 12.5 Developmental Model of Schizophrenia

Robin M. Murray, M.D., D.Sc., F.R.C.P., and
Elvira Bramon, M.D.

HISTORICAL PERSPECTIVE

The idea that early-onset psychosis has a neurodevelopmental origin was common in the later part of the 19th century. Thomas Clouston, a lecturer in psychiatry at the University of Edinburgh, used the term *developmental insanity* to describe a highly familial psychosis with a poor outcome that occurred predominantly in young men. In Clouston's words in 1891, "Adolescent insanity has also this peculiarity; it occurs just before maturity. It is the last cortical developmental disease." However, Emil Kraepelin's concept of dementia praecox as a progressively deteriorating illness displaced the developmental ideas for almost a century. Then, in the mid-1980s, Robin Murray and Shôn Lewis in Europe and Daniel Weinberger in North America revived the debate with new evidence supporting the neurodevelopmental theory.

Nearly 20 years after its reformulation, the neurodevelopmental theory has become widely accepted, and few doubt that schizophrenia has a developmental component. However, the simple model postulated initially failed to explain the full complexity of schizophrenia. The precise mechanisms by which early developmental risk factors impact brain development and then, only much later, lead to full-blown psychosis and why the age of onset of psychotic symptoms could vary so dramatically all remained unexplained by the early neurodevelopmental hypothesis. There has been much recent discussion over what causes the onset of psychosis, and there appear to be three main possibilities. First, there may be late developmental changes; these may interact with earlier pathology or act "ab initio." Second, there may be dopaminergic sensitization. Third, there may be neurodegeneration, either ab initio or secondary to the psychosis or other psychiatric symptoms. Furthermore, the neuropathology studies by Joyce Kovelman and Arnold Scheibel and by Hans Jacob and Helmut Beckman—which suggested aberrant neural migration and formed a major pillar for the neurodevelopmental hypothesis—proved remarkably difficult to replicate.

The neurodevelopmental–neurodegenerative discussion is under constant review as new data become available. In recent years, growing evidence indicates that the mesolimbic–dopaminergic pathways play a crucial role in the neurodevelopmental model. Dopamine sensitization might be the link between deviant brain development and the vulnerability to develop psychosis later on in life under certain environmental influences. The current neurodevelopmental theory has thus evolved to successfully integrate both biological data and psychosocial evidence.

RISK FACTORS OPERATING VERY EARLY IN LIFE

Prenatal and Perinatal Events

The association between pregnancy or delivery complications and schizophrenia has been a crucial element in the developmental theory of schizophrenia. Aaron Rosanoff and colleagues first described this association in 1934 in a series of schizophrenic twins and suggested that schizophrenia could "at least in part result from birth trauma." However, little further research was carried out for 40 years. Then, a number of case-control studies reported an excess of pregnancy and perinatal problems among patients with schizophrenia. These early data were summarized in two metaanalyses, which confirmed a modest association between the global term *obstetric complications* and the later development of schizophrenia. However, the metaanalyses were criticized on the basis that the individual studies that contributed to them were small and heterogeneous in their methodology. Most relied on maternal interviews rather than medical records and were therefore subject to potential recall bias. The metaanalyses also raised concerns about selection and publication biases. More vigorous methods were needed.

Table 12.5–1 summarizes a number of large, well-designed longitudinal studies that have been published in the last decade. Most of this work has been conducted using population and hospital registers in Northern Europe and has allowed for an optimal selection of controls from the same populations. What makes this research so valuable is its use of prospective obstetric data from birth records or registers, as it has become possible to measure exposure to specific obstetric complications much more accurately. Despite occasional inconsistencies, these large studies support the notion that exposure to obstetric complications is a risk factor for schizophrenia.

A recent metaanalysis of population-based studies has pooled together very large samples and has made it possible to reliably iden-

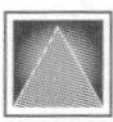

Table 12.5–1
Register-Based Studies of Obstetric Complications (OCs) and Schizophrenia

Study	Sample and Method	Main Findings
Jones et al. (1998)	1966-born cohort with 11,017 Finnish subjects. Linked psychiatric and obstetric case registers. Follow-up at age 28 yrs.	76 Subjects had developed schizophrenia at age 28 yrs. Schizophrenic patients were significantly more likely than controls to have had perinatal brain damage or to be premature.
Hultman et al. (1999)	Swedish population-based cohort study. Comparison of obstetric records for 167 patient–control pairs linked to psychiatric register.	Schizophrenic patients were more likely than controls to have OCs, especially if male. Schizophrenia was associated with multiparity and maternal bleeding in pregnancy.
Dalman et al. (1999)	Same cohort as Hultman et al. Follow-up of 507,516 children born in the late 1970s.	238 Subjects developed schizophrenia during follow-up period. Schizophrenia was associated with OCs. Preeclampsia was the strongest individual risk factor.
Kendell et al. (1996)	115 case-control pairs from the Scottish population born 1971–1974. Linked obstetric and psychiatric records.	Schizophrenia was associated with a significant excess of OCs, especially preeclampsia and infants requiring hospital neonatal care.
Kendell et al. (2000)	Reanalysis of same Scottish sample.	Selection bias was detected in the control group of the 1996 study. Reanalysis showed no significant association between OCs and schizophrenia.
Byrne et al. (2000)	Compared obstetric records of 431 patient–control pairs. Linked with psychiatric case register.	Global rate of OCs did not differ between patients and controls. Male patients with a young onset had significantly more OCs than controls.
Cannon et al. (2000)	Prospective cohort study (NCPP). Comparison of 72 patients, 63 unaffected siblings, and 7,941 controls.	The odds of schizophrenia increase linearly with increasing number of hypoxia-associated OCs.
Rosso et al. (2000)	1955 Finnish birth cohort. 80 patients, 61 unaffected siblings, and 56 matched controls.	Hypoxia-associated OCs significantly increase the odds of early-onset schizophrenia (but not of later-onset schizophrenia).
Zornberg et al. (2000)	Prospective cohort study (NCPP). 603 individuals born between 1959 and 1966 were followed for 23 yrs after early childhood assessments.	Hypoxic-ischaemia–related fetal or neonatal OCs were associated with striking increase in risk for schizophrenia and other nonaffective psychoses (5.7% vs. 0.4% for nonexposed).
Brown et al. (2001)	Comparison of 70 young adults from the rubella-exposed 1964 birth cohort against 1,510 unexposed controls from the ECA and the Albany and Saratoga studies.	The subjects prenatally exposed to rubella demonstrated a substantially higher risk for nonaffective psychosis compared to the unexposed controls (RR, 5.2).
Wahlbeck et al. (2001)	Cohort study of 7,086 Finnish subjects. Linked obstetric and school health records with psychiatric register.	Intrauterine and childhood malnutrition was associated with increased lifetime risk to develop schizophrenia.
Dalman et al. (2001) Thomas et al. (2001)	Case-control studies recruiting from the Stockholm psychiatric register. Included 524 patients with schizophrenia and 1,043 controls matched by age, gender, and hospital and parish of birth. OC data were obtained from birth records.	There was a strong association between signs of asphyxia at birth and schizophrenia, with an odds ratio of 4.4. The increased risk of schizophrenia associated with OCs (asphyxia in particular) was not significantly modified by gender, maternal history of psychosis, or age of onset. Limited statistical power.
Sorensen et al. (2003)	Data from the Copenhagen Perinatal Cohort of 7,866 individuals born between 1959 and 1961 linked to the Danish National Psychiatric Register.	84 Cases of schizophrenia were found (1.1% prevalence). Children of mothers with hypertension in pregnancy plus diuretic treatment were at significantly greater risk of developing schizophrenia (odds ratio, 4.0). In pregnancies complicated by hypertension, diuretics may interfere with aspects of fetal neurodevelopment.

CI, confidence interval; ECA, Epidemiologic Catchment Area; NCPP, National Collaborative Perinatal Project; RR, relative risk.

tify a number of specific obstetric complications as risk factors for schizophrenia. These complications are listed in Table 12.5–2, in descending order of the risk they convey. Diabetes during pregnancy, low birth weight, emergency cesarean section, congenital malformations, uterine atony, asphyxia, and a few other obstetric complications emerged as some of the most clear risk factors for later development of schizophrenia. Although the overall effect of obstetric complications is modest, some researchers believe that the association may be stronger for certain subgroups, for example, those cases with early onset of symptoms.

The biological mechanism underlying the link between obstetric complications and schizophrenia remains elusive. However, from the early data to the recent, higher-quality studies, findings point toward fetal or neonatal hypoxia as a potential mechanism. The National Collaborative Perinatal Project suggested a dose–effect relationship for hypoxia, and those subjects who experienced three or more hypoxia-related obstetric complications were at least five times more likely to develop schizophrenia than controls without obstetric complications. A plausible explanatory model is that of gene–environment interactions; thus, those with a genetic liability to schizophrenia may be especially vulnerable to the toxic effects of hypoxia on the developing brain.

Other Early Environmental Hazards Individuals born in late winter or early spring have a slightly increased risk (7 to 10 percent) of developing schizophrenia later. This points toward an etiological agent acting during gestation, birth, or early childhood rather than around the time of onset. A number of studies suggest that this seasonal effect could be secondary to exposure to maternal influenza during winter, but other research fails to find such a link. Intrauterine rubella infection has also been suggested as a potential candidate. Stephen Buka and colleagues were fortunate to be able to retrieve blood samples taken during pregnancy in the early 1960s from mothers of 27 subjects who, several decades later, developed psychosis. The maternal samples—and those taken from mothers of controls—were searched for evidence of perinatal pathogens capable of affecting brain development. The offspring of women with elevated levels of immunoglobin G (IgG) and IgM and antibodies to herpes simplex during pregnancy were

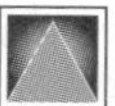

Table 12.5–2
Main Findings from Metaanalysis of Registered-Based Studies of Obstetric Complications (OCs) in Schizophrenia

OC	Schizophrenia Sample Exposed to OC/Total	Comparison Sample Exposed to OC/Total	Pooled Odds Ratio	95% CI	*P* Value
Diabetes in pregnancy	3/237	3/1,909	7.76	1.37–43.90	<.03
Placental abruption	3/308	1,643/508,352	4.02	0.89–18.12	.07
Birth weight <2 kg	6/504	78/10,926	3.89	1.40–10.84	.009
Emergency cesarean section	20/818	1,595/507,863	3.24	1.40–7.50	.006
Congenital malformations	10/737	6,144/508,781	2.35	1.21–4.57	<.02
Uterine atony	27/659	16,913/507,703	2.29	1.51–3.50	<.001
Rhesus-related risk factors	18/759	2,911/17,537	2.00	1.01–3.96	<.05
Asphyxia	60/1,109	119/2,297	1.74	1.15–2.62	.008
Bleeding in pregnancy	34/1,223	9,367/524,972	1.69	1.14–2.52	.009
Birth weight <2.5 kg	60/1,294	19,343/536,045	1.67	1.22–2.29	.002
Preeclampsia	75/1,712	18,286/510,275	1.36	0.99–1.85	.05

Note: Main results from a metaanalysis gathering all population-based studies of OCs in schizophrenia. These OCs, listed in descending order of the risk they convey, significantly increase the risk of developing schizophrenia.
CI, confidence interval.
From Cannon M, Jones PB, Murray RM: Obstetric complications and schizophrenia: Historical and meta-analytic review. *Am J Psychiatry.* 2002;159:1080, with permission.

at increased risk of developing schizophrenia and other psychotic illnesses in adulthood.

Additional early hazards that have an impact on the mother can compromise fetal development. Thus, gestational diabetes mellitus and maternal malnutrition have been associated with an increased risk for the offspring of developing schizophrenia. Indeed, a number of investigators have produced evidence suggesting that maternal stress (e.g., during war or floods) also increases risk. However, these findings require replication and a plausible mechanism to explain how such diverse hazards to the fetus could increase the risk of schizophrenia. One unifying hypothesis proposes a dysregulation of the hypothalamic-pituitary-adrenal (HPA) axis. Although typically associated with mood disorders, the contribution of glucocorticoid-related neurotoxicity to schizophrenia is receiving growing support. In vitro investigations show how high levels of glucocorticoids reduce neuronal size and dendritic arborization, which has been observed in schizophrenia. High plasmatic glucocorticoid levels are also associated with reductions in hippocampal volume, such as those described in first episodes of psychosis. Thus, patients with schizophrenia show heightened levels of cortisol in response to a number of diverse biological challenges, including physical and psychological stresses, and such elevated cortisol levels could impair neurodevelopment.

Finally, recent research demonstrates that the window of opportunity for risk-increasing insults is wider than was previously thought and that events in early childhood can compromise brain development and maturational changes. For example, infants exposed to viral infections affecting the central nervous system (CNS) were five times more likely to develop schizophrenia than those unexposed. Similarly, there is some evidence that brain injury in early childhood may also increase the risk of developing schizophrenia later.

Markers of Prenatal Deviant Development

It is well established that the morphogenesis of the brain, the craniofacial region, and epidermal ridges are intimately related. Ectodermal development is known to occur during the first and second trimesters of life, and disturbances of development at this time can cause defects in cranial and facial features, as well as in hands and feet. An increase in the prevalence of these minor physical anomalies is a consistent finding among patients with schizophrenia, as compared to controls. Similarly, epidermal ridges (also known as *dermatoglyphicals*) appear on the hand between weeks 12 and 15 of life, and, after this period, they remain unchanged. People with schizophrenia display an excess of apparently innocent changes in the patterns and counts of their dermatoglyphicals.

Although epidermal ridges on the fingers and palm may not reveal the future, they certainly provide useful information about a patient's early life. Minor physical anomalies and dermatoglyphical alterations have been interpreted as markers of disrupted prenatal development. They show that an insult (whether genetic, environmental, or both) occurred during early to mid-gestation. This insult leaves an obvious trace in the skin or other physical features, and it does so precisely at a time when the brain, another ectodermal derivate, is undergoing its genesis.

Minor physical anomalies and dermatoglyphical changes are, of course, no proof of abnormal brain development, but they certainly raise suspicions. There is preliminary support for the idea that dermatoglyphical changes may be indirect indicators of aberrant brain development. One study has reported an association between abnormal dermatoglyphical ridge counts and cerebral structural abnormalities measured by magnetic resonance imaging (MRI) in patients with schizophrenia. Furthermore, compared to controls, patients with schizophrenia present an excessive asymmetry of ridge counts between left and right hands, which correlates with their more prevalent mixed-handedness. The above findings have been interpreted as two related markers pointing toward a greater developmental instability in schizophrenia, probably affecting the brain.

ARE CHILDREN WHO EVENTUALLY DEVELOP SCHIZOPHRENIA DIFFERENT FROM PEERS WHO REMAIN WELL?

If the brain of the schizophrenic individual has been subject to deviant development very early in life, one might expect that his or her development in childhood would not be entirely normal. Consequently, there has been much recent interest in the childhood antecedents of schizophrenia. In one of the earliest studies, Barbara Fish and colleagues followed a small group of newborn babies for 10 years, and those who developed schizophrenia, as well as the offspring of schizophrenic mothers, showed delays in physical, motor, and cognitive development. What Fish termed *pandevelopmental retardation* was not so much a fixed neurological defect as a disorganized timing and integration of neurological maturation and, in some cases, could be identified in as early as the first month. She interpreted these developmental delays affecting multiple sensorimotor systems as consistent with an "inherited, congenital neurointegrative defect" that was associated with schizophrenia.

Elaine Walker and colleagues examined home movies of children who would become schizophrenia patients years later and noted more postural and upper limb movement abnormalities than in their well siblings. These abnormalities were most noticeable in the first 2 years of life and ameliorated thereafter, raising the possibility of ongoing recovery from an early lesion. Walker's study had a relatively small sample; however, the use of videos provided strong evidence, which was assessed by several raters who were blind for outcome. Although these early retrospective studies were original and interesting, they were potentially subject to bias. To fully understand the childhood antecedents of schizophrenia, stronger, more representative studies were needed.

Evidence from Large Population-Based Cohorts

A series of large cohort studies, summarized in Table 12.5–3, were published through the 1990s. The 1946 British Birth Cohort Study followed up more than 5,000 children for over 40 years. Compared to controls, the 30 children who went on to develop schizophrenia had delayed motor milestones, particularly walking. During their childhoods, the 30 children had three times the number of speech problems as controls, and low educational-test scores also emerged as a significant risk factor for schizophrenia. A preference for solitary play, as well as behaviors indicating poor social competence, were predictors of schizophrenia. An independent cohort from the British National Child Development Study, with a similar design, provided further evidence that gender and the development of social abilities during childhood are important influences on the risk for psychosis and other psychiatric disorders.

Another prospective cohort study from Philadelphia compared premorbid measures of children who later developed schizophrenia with measures of their relatives who remained healthy, as well as with measures of controls. Both patients and relatives performed significantly worse than the controls—but did not differ from each other—on verbal and nonverbal cognitive tests taken in childhood. Early social maladjustment, motor coordination deficits, and behavioral and language dysfunction (e.g., echolalia, inappropriate laughter, or unintelligible speech) were significantly increased in both those who later developed schizophrenia and their siblings. Hence, premorbid social, cognitive, and motor dysfunctions were significant indicators of vulnerability to schizophrenia—such vulnerability being the result of familial (genetic and shared environmental) factors.

Mary Cannon and colleagues compared elementary school records of 400 preschizophrenic children and the same number of healthy controls born in Helsinki, Finland. Poor performance in sports and handicrafts, which may indicate motor coordination deficits, were risk factors for schizophrenia. This finding is consistent with the high-risk and other birth-cohort studies and, also, with the poor motor coordination seen on childhood videotapes described earlier.

Further evidence of impaired development in schizophrenia came with the Northern Finland 1966 cohort, which documented the ages at which participants learned to stand, walk, and control bladder and bowel functions and considered how they related to adult risk of mental illness. Delayed milestones increased the risk for later psychosis in a linear fashion. Thus, being precocious implied a certain degree of protection from psychosis. There was no such association between milestones and nonpsychotic disorders.

A multidisciplinary study of human development enrolled more than 1,000 children born in Dunedin, New Zealand, and monitored them as they grew up. When participants became 26 years of age, they were given psychiatric assessments with the aim of linking adult mental illness with premorbid risk factors in childhood and adolescence. Of the cohort, 3.7 percent were diagnosed with a schizophreniform disorder, 2.0 percent were diagnosed with mania, and 28.5 percent had a nonpsychotic anxiety or mood disorder. Compared to controls, those who fulfilled diagnostic criteria for any adult psychiatric disorder had had more emotional and interpersonal problems when they were children. Furthermore, significant impairments in neuromotor, language, and cognitive development were present only in those children who were later diagnosed with schizophreniform disorder. Thus, neuromotor, language, and other cognitive developmental impairments in early childhood are risk factors specifically associated with schizophreniform disorder in adult life.

A child psychiatrist had interviewed the Dunedin children at age 11 years, searching for any evidence of early psychopathology. Interestingly, those children who reported unusual quasipsychotic experiences had a 16-fold increased risk of schizophreniform disorder as adults. This study demonstrates a certain continuity of psychotic symptoms from childhood to adulthood and indicates that delusions have their origins often more than a decade before clinical psychosis is formally diagnosed. It is also interesting that this and several of the other cohort studies all point to receptive language deficits as being particularly noticeable in preschizophrenic individuals. Much research indicates that auditory hallucinations are disorders of inner language. Therefore, it is not surprising that children who have impaired language perception are more prone to misperceive their own inner speech as an external voice in adult life.

COULD INTELLECTUAL ABILITY PREDICT SCHIZOPHRENIA? COHORTS OF YOUNG SOLDIERS

The Swedish Army Study examined nearly 50,000 eighteen-year-old male conscripts. By the age of 30 years, 195 had been hospitalized with schizophrenia and a similar number with nonschizophrenic psychosis. There was a highly significant association between low intelligence quotient (IQ) scores at age 18 and the subsequent development of schizophrenia. Indeed, the relationship between schizophrenia and IQ was linear at all levels of intellectual ability, with risk gradually increasing as IQ decreased. The risk for nonschizophrenic psychoses was also higher in those with lower IQ, but the effect was less marked and nonlinear. The effect size of the low-IQ risk factor exceeded that of any other known environmental risk factors. The association between low IQ and schizophrenia could be directly causal, with cognitive impairment leading to false beliefs and perceptions. Alternatively, the association could be indirect, with factors such as abnormal brain development increasing the risk for schizophrenia and, incidentally, causing the lower IQ.

A similar study conducted on the Israeli Army assessed nearly 10,000 new conscripts who were 16 to 17 years of age. Deficits in social functioning, organizational ability, and intellectual functioning predicted later hospitalization for schizophrenia. There was a linear relationship between IQ and risk of schizophrenia, and the

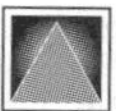

Table 12.5–3
Childhood Antecedents of Schizophrenia: Summary of Population Cohort Studies

Study	Sample and Follow-Up Period	Main Findings
The 1946 British Birth Cohort Jones et al. (1994)	>5,000 Children followed over 40 yrs.	30 Children developed schizophrenia. They showed delayed motor milestones and had more speech problems, lower educational test results, and poorer social competence during childhood.
British National Child Development Study Done et al. (1994)	All births in Britain during 1 wk in March, 1958, were followed for 28 yrs. 2,000 randomly selected controls were compared to cases requiring psychiatric admission.	Cases: 40 schizophrenia, 35 affective psychoses, and 79 neurotic disorders. Teachers provided measurements of social skills and performance in childhood. Those who developed schizophrenia had significantly more social maladjustment than controls, especially if male. Children who went on to develop affective psychoses did not differ much from controls. Preneurotic children, especially if female, manifested poorer social adjustment than controls.
Swedish Army Study David et al. (1997)	<50,000 18-yr-old men conscripted into Swedish army 1969–1970. Psychiatric outcomes by age 30 examined.	195 Soldiers of the cohort had been admitted to hospital with schizophrenia, and another 192 had been admitted with nonschizophrenic psychosis. There was a highly significant association between low IQ scores at age 18 yrs and the subsequent development of schizophrenia.
Israeli Army Study Davidson et al. (1999)	<10,000 16- and 17-yr-old men conscripted into Israeli army.	Deficits in social functioning, organizational ability, and intellectual functioning predicted later hospitalization for schizophrenia. There was a linear inverse relationship between IQ and risk of schizophrenia.
Finnish school records study Cannon et al. (1999 and 2002)	400 Preschizophrenic children and 400 control children born in Helsinki, 1951–1960.	Comparison of elementary school records between cases and controls. Poor performance in sports and handicrafts, which may indicate motor coordination deficits, were risk factors for schizophrenia. In this sample of schizophrenia cases, poor educational attainment and poor grades for attention at school were significantly associated with the risk of criminal offending in adulthood.
Philadelphia Study Bearden et al. (2000)	72 Patients with schizophrenia, 62 of their unaffected relatives, and 7,941 controls.	Both patients and relatives performed significantly worse than controls on verbal and nonverbal cognitive tests at the ages of 4 and 7 yrs. Early social maladjustment, motor coordination deficits, and behavioral and language dysfunction (e.g., echolalia, inappropriate laughter, or unintelligible speech) were significantly increased in those who later developed schizophrenia and their siblings. Therefore, premorbid social, cognitive, and motor dysfunctions are significant indicators of vulnerability to schizophrenia.
Northern Finland 1966 cohort Isohanni et al. (2001 and 2003)	>12,000 Babies followed until 31 yrs of age. Psychiatric outcomes by age 30 examined.	Cases: 100 schizophrenia, 55 other psychoses, and 315 miscellaneous nonpsychotic mental disorders. The ages when participants learned to stand, to walk, and to control bladder and bowel functions were compared across groups. Delayed milestones increased the risk for later psychosis in a linear fashion. This association was specific for psychotic disorders. Development at age 1 did not relate to clinical course of schizophrenia as measured by number and duration of hospital admissions. Early developmental deviation in motor function could be a phenotypic marker of vulnerability to schizophrenia.
Dunedin Study Cannon et al. (2002)	>1,000 Babies born in Dunedin, New Zealand, 1972–1973. Psychiatric assessment at age 26 yrs provides adult diagnoses.	At age 26 yrs, 3.7% had a schizophreniform disorder, 2.0% were diagnosed with mania, and 28.5% had a nonpsychotic anxiety or mood disorder. Compared to controls, those with any adult psychiatric diagnosis had more emotional and interpersonal problems when they were children. Neuromotor, language, and other cognitive developmental impairments in childhood emerged as risk factors specifically associated with schizophreniform disorder in adult life. Children reporting unusual quasipsychotic experiences at age 11 yrs had a 16-fold increased risk of schizophreniform disorder at age 26 yrs.

IQ, intelligence quotient.

authors suggest that low IQ is itself a causal factor that increases the risk of schizophrenia. Lower intellectual ability could act independently, or it could be one of the means by which other genetic or environmental influences exert their effect—or both. The authors suggest that low IQ could compromise information processing, eventually leading to the psychopathology of schizophrenia, or, alternatively, that high IQ may be protective.

Support has also come from genetic studies for the idea that subtle intellectual deficits may be causally linked to schizophrenia. First, studies of the relatives of schizophrenic individuals have indicated that they show similar but milder cognitive deficits. Second, and very recently, Richard Straub and colleagues have produced evidence that certain variants of the dysbindin gene on chromosome 6 are linked to schizophrenia and, furthermore, that these alleles are associated with lower IQ. In a similar vein, a genetic variant at the catechol-*O*-methyltransferase locus, which influences the breakdown of frontal dopamine, appears to slightly impair executive function and has been weakly associated with schizophrenia. Such genetically determined impairments of cognition should, of course, be apparent long before the onset of frank psychosis. The wealth of data from population-based prospective studies has provided sound evidence that people who develop schizophrenia often experience developmental deviances that are manifest in early childhood or adolescence. There also seems to be a continuum between early, mild psychotic-like experiences and a clinical diagnosis of psychosis later in life. However, these general-population cohorts require a huge effort over very long periods to gather a relatively small number of cases. Furthermore, they provide restricted information about potential risk factors, and such risk factors tend to be demographic and nonspecific variables. This has led to the search for more targeted samples in the so-called high-risk studies.

Development of Young People at Increased Risk for Psychosis: Evidence from High-Risk Projects Family studies have reported numerous deficits in neural, cognitive, and behavioral domains that are promising markers of liability to schizophrenia spectrum disorders. Such research on families aims to identify unaffected gene carriers to ultimately increase the power of molecular studies searching for genetic risk factors. These valuable subclinical samples of relatives are also being used in a longitudinal way to obtain phenotypic indicators that may successfully predict future cases of psychoses. Reliable predictors of outcome would lead to earlier and more targeted therapeutic interventions. Thus, during the 1960s and 1970s, a number of centers set out to collect and follow high-risk samples, that is, children and young individuals with an increased chance of developing psychosis based on their family history. This design is free from the biases of retrospective research and has also allowed assessments of exposure to more specific putative risk factors for schizophrenia and other psychoses, as such risk factors are largely environmental and developmental.

The New York High-Risk Project recruited offspring of patients with schizophrenia, of patients with affective disorders, and of unaffected parents. The three groups of children were examined with extensive tests measuring their early cognitive abilities, social behavior and development, and their psychiatric morbidity when they became adults. The majority of neurobehavioral measures studied—for example, general and social intelligence, executive function (as measured by the Wisconsin Card Sorting Test), and early behavior—were significantly impaired in the offspring of schizophrenia patients, as compared to the other two groups of children. However, on follow-up, only some specific measures showed potential to predict which of the at-risk children would develop schizophrenia in adulthood. For example, if substance abuse was accounted for, adult outcomes could be differentiated successfully on the basis of behavioral disturbances in childhood (including discipline problems, tantrums, and family fights). Children who would later develop adult schizophrenia displayed significantly more behavioral problems than children who would develop either affective disorders or addictions or those who were to remain well as adults. Furthermore, attention, verbal memory, and gross motor skill deficits were substantially more prevalent among children destined to develop schizophrenia, and demonstrated a remarkable sensitivity to predict schizophrenia, ranging from 50 to 83 percent. Interestingly, they were also relatively specific indexes of risk for schizophrenia, as opposed to risk for affective disorder outcomes.

The Edinburgh High-Risk Project started in 1994 and is now producing its initial results. High-risk subjects were 16 to 25 years old and, although they were well at entry, they had two close relatives with schizophrenia. These high-risk young people are being followed up and compared against a demographically similar sample of first-episode patients and healthy individuals free from family history of psychosis. Initial findings revealed an association between schizotypal traits and psychotic symptoms and suggest that those at-risk subjects who have higher schizotypy scores are at increased risk to develop schizophrenia. Assessments of childhood behavior were obtained via maternal interviews at entry and follow-up. Withdrawn, delinquent, and aggressive behaviors in adolescents at risk emerged as significant early predictors of developing schizophrenia. Compared to people who remained well, those subjects who went on to develop schizophrenia showed impaired memory function. Although this seems consistent with the literature, the Edinburgh High-Risk Project is still ongoing, and a longer follow-up period is required to confirm these preliminary findings.

In summary, high-risk studies concur in showing that 25 to 50 percent of children born to parents with schizophrenia have developmental abnormalities, especially poor motor coordination in early childhood and attention and information-processing deficits later. The large population cohorts are also consistent with the presence of deviances and changes in children who develop schizophrenia as adults. The measures of premorbid deviance described to date have substantial sensitivity and specificity to predict clinical outcomes in groups at genetic risk, but the childhood indicators are a very long way from being extrapolated to the general population in any early detection campaign (Fig. 12.5–1).

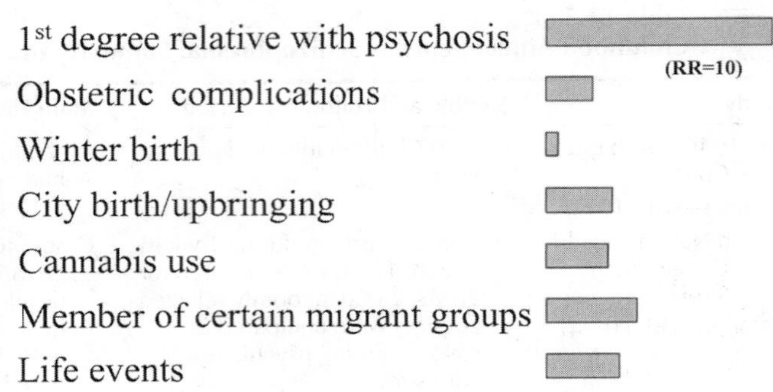

FIGURE 12.5–1 Individual risk factors and their effect sizes. RR, relative risk. (From Bramon E, Kelly J, Van Os J, Murray M: The cascade of increasingly deviant development that culminates in the onset of schizophrenia. *Neurosci News*. 2004;4:5–19, with permission.)

Research into the Prodromal Phase of Psychosis

Although many questions remain unanswered regarding the etiology and pathophysiology of schizophrenia, its natural course has been well described. In many cases, the symptoms on which the diagnosis is based are preceded by a period of nonspecific psychopathology that lasts 1 to 2 years on average: the *prodromal phase*.

Prodromal symptoms involve attenuated psychotic experiences (such as ideas of reference, magical thinking, and illusions) or, alternatively, full-blown positive symptoms of very brief duration. They also include nonspecific mood, anxiety, or cognitive symptoms, as well as social withdrawal and a nonspecific decline in function. Obviously, these prodromal phenomena overlap with disorders other than schizophrenia, and they can even be seen as part of a continuum between psychiatric illness and mental distress in the healthy subject. Only certain thresholds of intensity and duration make the prodromal experience pathological, and, in any case, it always remains largely unspecific. Thus, the term *prodromal* can be somewhat misleading in that it can be perceived as inevitably leading to the onset of schizophrenia, when, in fact, it is better described as substantial risk of imminent psychosis onset. But how substantial? How imminent?

Prodromal cases are understood as vulnerable individuals at ultra-high risk for developing a psychotic disorder imminently. They include subjects with classic prodromal experiences as described above and also, given the relevance of genetic risk factors, individuals with schizotypal traits or a family history of psychosis showing functional decline.

Patrick McGorry and colleagues in Melbourne, Australia, started a study with the aims of early detection and intervention in the prodromal phase of psychosis. After following prodromal cases for 1 year, it was found that more than 40 percent of the cases became clinically psychotic. Some variables emerged as highly significant predictors of conversion to psychosis (for example, long duration of prodrome, poor functioning at intake, low-grade psychotic features, and disorganization), and combining several of those predictors pro-

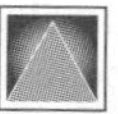

Table 12.5–4
Cohorts of Prodromal Samples and Their Chances of Transition to Psychosis

Study	Sample	Follow-Up	Rate of Transition (%)	Main Findings
Germany				
Klosterkötter et al. (2001)	160 Prodromals from 695 referrals for a second opinion	9.6 yrs, on average	49.4	BSABS predicted conversion to schizophrenia with sensitivity, 98%; specificity, 59%; PPV, 70%; and NPV, 96%. Thought, language, perception, and motor disturbances showed the highest predictive accuracy.
Norway				
Larsen et al. (2001)	10 Prodromals	1 yr	40	Clinical trial of supportive psychotherapy (no antipsychotic drugs used) in prodromal states. Ongoing study, results are preliminary.
United Kingdom				
Morrison et al. (2002)	23 Prodromals from general practice referrals	6–12 mos	22	Randomised Controlled Trial of Cognitive Therapy (versus monitoring) in prodromal states. Prodromals showed significantly higher scores of schizotypy, metacognitive beliefs, and dysfunctional self-schemas than healthy controls.
United States				
Lencz et al. (2003)	32 Young at-risk persons	2 yrs' mean follow-up	25	Help-seeking adolescent and young adults with increased risk for schizophrenia based on their family history and/or their clinical symptoms. The severity of positive symptoms could predict the development of psychosis with sensitivity, 0.88; specificity, 0.75; and PPV, 0.54.
Woods et al. (2003)	59 Prodromals	1 yr treatment and 1 yr follow-up	33 (preliminary result)	Randomized double-blind, placebo-controlled trial of olanzapine. After an 8-wk treatment, the olanzapine group had significant symptomatic improvement and weight gain, compared to cases on placebo. Authors developed a structured interview to predict which prodromal cases will transition to psychosis.
Australia				
Yung et al. (2003)	49 Prodromals from 162 referrals	1 yr	40.8	Combining several clinical predictors gave sensitivity, 86%; specificity, 91%; PPV, 80%; and NPV, 94%. Long duration of prodrome, poor functioning at intake, low-grade psychotic symptoms, depression, and disorganization were highly significant predictors of psychosis.

Note: Cohort studies that follow patients with prodromal symptoms allow estimation of the probability for the transition from prodromal case to schizophrenia or other psychoses.
BSABS, Bonn Scale for the Assessment of Basic Symptoms; NPV, negative predictive value; PPV, positive predictive value.

duced good levels of sensitivity and specificity. The study illustrates that, with relatively short follow-up periods, there is scope for predicting which at-risk subjects will develop full-blown psychosis.

With some variations in the definition of *prodrome*, Joachim Klosterkötter and colleagues from the Bonn Early Recognition Study conducted the longest follow-up of a large prodromal sample and had similar findings. After an average of approximately 9 years, and without any specific intervention, half of their prodromal subjects developed schizophrenia. They examined the Bonn Scale for the Assessment of Basic Symptoms (BSABS) as a tool to predict transition to schizophrenia. The scale revealed an excellent ability to exclude transition to psychosis accurately, as false negatives are rare. However, this was in a sample that was very likely to develop psychosis, and there is little evidence that instruments such as the BSABS could be useful to identify prodromal cases in the general population.

Additional ongoing studies of the prodrome are summarized in Table 12.5–4. A number of them are clinical trials assessing whether early intervention during the prodromal phase, including treatment with low doses of antipsychotics, can help. This field is not free from controversy or ethical dilemmas. For example: Can early treatment during the prodrome prevent psychosis or improve its outcome? Given that the majority of prodromals do not develop psychosis, will the potential benefits of treating them outweigh the risks of side effects and stigma? Whatever the answers to these questions prove to be as more research unfolds, it is clear that the prodrome of psychosis holds important clues for etiological research into the disease in general and the developmental model in particular.

At present, there are a number of ongoing studies of prodromal samples. Their findings are summarized in Table 12.5–4 and coincide with the above to indicate conversion rates from one-third to one-half. These differences are clearly explained by variations in the manner in which prodromal subjects are recruited and selected and the degree of therapeutic interventions applied in each project. Although prodromal symptoms seem to be strong risk factors and, therefore, promising predictors of psychosis, all studies to date are conducted on highly selected samples. These symptoms will surely be much weaker predictors if applied to the general population. Furthermore, from the stage of prodrome, it is possible to transition to schizophrenia but certainly also to affective and other psychoses. In any case, this research shows how preexisting nonspecific psychopathology can help to predict the subsequent development of psychosis. The prodromal period has been reported to last 1 to 2 years on average, although it can be much longer. Certainly, identifying at-risk subjects sooner and more reliably would produce a better understanding of the way symptoms develop during the early stages of psychosis and of what constitutes early-risk factors. Efforts are being made to use neuroimaging, neuropsychology, electrophysiology, and other techniques, as well as clinical data, to obtain more accurate and reliable predictors of later psychosis. The study of developmental markers among prodromal subjects will undoubtedly contribute new insights to the developmental model of schizophrenia.

THE BRAIN IN SCHIZOPHRENIA: FINDINGS FROM IMAGING RESEARCH

It is well established that, compared to controls, people with schizophrenia display volumetric changes in certain brain structures. The most consistent deviances described are an increase in ventricular size and subtle global and regional gray matter volume reductions. In a recent metaanalysis, Ian Wright and colleagues reviewed MRI brain scans of more than 1,500 patients and a similar number of healthy volunteers. They reported a 26 percent enlargement in ventricular volume and a clear reduction in mean cerebral volume among schizophrenic subjects. Subtle yet significant volume reductions associated with schizophrenia have been found for specific areas, including superior temporal gyrus and medial temporal lobe regions (amygdala, hippocampus, and parahippocampal gyrus).

Recently, voxel-based methods of analyzing structural MRI images have enabled the whole brain to be examined and have implicated, in particular, the medial temporal region, insula, and anterior cingulate. These brain regions identified by MRI largely coincide with the postmortem anatomical findings.

Could Subtle Brain Deviances in Schizophrenia be Developmental in Origin?

MRI studies in first-onset psychosis or in relatives of patients, as well as other evidence, suggest that at least some of the subtle brain deviances described in schizophrenia may be due to abnormal brain development.

MRI Findings Present at the Onset of Psychosis

There have been numerous reports of enlargement of lateral and third ventricles in first-onset and early-onset cases of schizophrenia. Reduced volumes of several structures, such as cortical gray matter, thalamus, left hippocampus–amygdala, and left posterior–superior temporal gyrus, have also been demonstrated consistently during the earliest stages of the disease. Abnormalities that are present at the onset of psychosis cannot be explained adequately by disease progression or medication effects.

Brain Asymmetry Reductions One additional piece of evidence points toward fetal life. The normal brain is typically asymmetrical, and the development of brain asymmetry is usually complete by the middle of the third trimester of gestation. A number of studies revealed a reduced asymmetry in several brain areas in schizophrenia, including the planum temporale and fronto-occipital areas. A recent metaanalysis, reviewing handedness, language, and anatomical studies, confirms the decreased anatomical and functional cerebral lateralization in schizophrenia. The reduced asymmetry found in several brain structures in schizophrenia is, therefore, likely to originate during fetal life and may be indicative of a disruption in brain lateralization during neurodevelopment.

Developmental Brain Lesions Furthermore, there is an excess of rare congenital cerebral lesions in patients with schizophrenia, such as aqueduct stenosis, arachnoid and septal cysts, agenesis of the corpus callosum, and cavum septum pellucidum. However, such abnormalities are distinctly unusual, and, generally, the deviant findings associated with schizophrenia are much more subtle. Indeed, it is an open question whether these differences in brain structure found between people with schizophrenia and normal subjects are brain abnormalities that are an intrinsic part of the disease process itself. Alternatively, they might be regarded as risk factors, deviations within the normal range, which increase the chances that an individual will develop schizophrenia.

MRI Findings in the Unaffected Relatives of Patients

The environmental factors discussed earlier have only a modest effect in increasing risk and generally operate in the context of genetic predisposition. The genetic component to schizophrenia has been well established, and, recently, two large twin studies have confirmed that a high proportion of the variance in liability to schizophrenia is due to additive genetic effects.

A number of investigators have asked whether the first-degree relatives of people with schizophrenia show any of the same brain structural deviations as their schizophrenic kin. The Maudsley Family Study examined MRI scans of patients and well relatives from families with a single case of schizophrenia, as well as multiply affected families. Based on patterns of affected cases observed within pedigrees, healthy relatives that appeared most likely to carry genes of risk for schizophrenia showed substantial enlargements of lateral and third ventricles. On the other hand, those relatives with lower chances of transmitting susceptibility genes did not differ significantly from controls. Other studies of unaffected relatives have also reported enlarged ventricles, as well as reduced volumes of cortical gray matter, thalamus, and amygdala–hippocampal complex. The brain structure deviations described among unaffected relatives cannot be explained by the pathological process of psychosis. These morphological changes are more likely to be a manifestation of familial risk factors, possibly genes influencing brain development. Indeed, in the Maudsley Family Study, the greater the genetic loading, the smaller the total gray matter volume.

Is Brain Deviance Associated with Early Environmental Hazards? An interesting relationship between early environmental risk factors and brain structural deviance has emerged. In particular, a history of fetal hypoxia is associated with increased structural brain abnormalities among schizophrenia patients. Although there is no full agreement, several studies have also suggested a link between obstetric complications and increased ventricular volume and reduced hippocampal volumes. The Maudsley Family Study samples showed that those patients with schizophrenia who experienced obstetric complications had reduced hippocampal volumes compared to patients with a family history of psychosis but who were free from obstetric complications. Thus, decreased hippocampal volume in schizophrenia could be, in part, a consequence of early environmental hazards, and, again, this finding points toward fetal hypoxia as one likely causal link between severe obstetric complications and cerebral damage in schizophrenia. However, other studies show that the unaffected relatives of people with schizophrenia have decreased hippocampal volumes. It is likely that both genetic and early environmental factors impinge on hippocampal development in schizophrenic individuals; indeed, those carrying susceptibility genes may be especially sensitive to early environmental insults.

DO NEUROPATHOLOGY AND HISTOPATHOLOGY STUDIES IMPLICATE EARLY DEVELOPMENTAL DEVIANCE?

Neuropathological studies have largely confirmed the neuroimaging data concerning gross anatomy, but there has been much less consistency in the histopathological findings. It is well established that, during the second trimester of fetal life, there is an enormous neuronal migration from the periventricular germinal matrix to the cortex. Three very influential papers published during the mid-1980s and early 1990s suggest that this migration was disturbed in schizophrenia, leading to entorhinal cortex heterotopias and hippocampal neuronal disarray. Unfortunately, the studies could not be replicated. Questions have been raised about the design of histopathology studies of schizophrenia. The samples tend to be small and the procedures and areas of interest are often heterogeneous. Given the subtlety of the alterations sought in so-called functional psychoses, these methodological issues might have resulted in false initial reports or hampered the chances of replication.

The reductions in cortical volume described by in vivo imaging studies have a close correlate in postmortem examinations. Rather than loss of neurons, histopathological studies in schizophrenia consistently report what has been termed *loss of neuropil*, that is, reductions in neuronal size, dendritic spine density, and length. Such changes affect cortical areas, especially frontal cortex, hippocampus, and cingulate gyrus. They also show reductions of synaptic proteins and synaptic gene expression. In other words, patients have smaller neurons with fewer dendritic arborization, and this leads to increased neuronal density. How this loss of neuropil affects subcortical areas is less clear, but the dorsomedial thalamus is probably affected. The cytoarchitectural deviances described, such as decreased neuronal size and aberrant synaptic and dendritic organization, could certainly be due to early maldevelopment. However, later-life environmental influences and even the process of aging cannot be ruled out as a cause of the neuropil reduction in schizophrenia.

There is no evidence of the classic signs of neurodegeneration in the brains of people with schizophrenia, and the general absence of gliosis in schizophrenia strongly argues against an adult-onset degenerative process. However, a wealth of evidence shows that a substantial reorganization of cortical connections, involving a programmed synaptic pruning process, takes place during adolescence in humans. This elimination of redundant synaptic connections is thought to lead to a more efficient use of neural networks that allows the adolescent to develop increasingly complex and mature cognitive abilities. Irwin Feinberg introduced the importance of pruning of cortical neurons during adolescence in schizophrenia. He proposed that there might be a flaw in this peri-pubertal progressive synapse elimination. Matcheri Keshavan and colleagues further developed Feinberg's pruning hypothesis by integrating new data from diverse in vivo neurobiological measures that are well characterized in schizophrenia. Thus, neuropathological studies report reductions in frontal gray matter volumes, an increase in neuronal density, and loss of synaptic markers. Phosphorus magnetic resonance spectroscopy indicates failure of new synapse production and excessive synapse reduction. Functional imaging studies report findings of "hypofrontality" and are compatible with neuropsychological assessments revealing prefrontal-type cognitive deficits. All of these observations coincide in supporting the idea that schizophrenia may be associated with an excess of the normal pruning of the prefrontal cortex that occurs during adolescence. These ideas of aberrant pruning of synapses during adolescence have become known as the *late neurodevelopmental model*.

These ideas are not, of course, new. More than a century ago, Clouston related the onset of developmental insanity to maturational changes in the adolescent brain. He stated:

> Then what a change in the mental activity of the brain does the period of puberty cause. Looking at the matter from the combined point of view of physiologists and psychologists, we must connect the new development of the affective faculties, the new ideas, the new interests in life, the new desires and organic cravings, the new delight in certain sorts of poetry and romance, with a new evolution of function in certain parts of the brain that had lain dormant before.

A 23-year-old woman was referred for psychiatric assessment after she became verbally aggressive in a public place. She had an extensive family history of mental illness: The patient's paternal uncle had schizophrenia successfully treated with depot antipsychotics, and, although no reliable details were available, two siblings of her paternal grandfather had several breakdowns—one had undergone a frontal lobotomy, and the other had a child with mental retardation. As for early environmental hazards, her mother suffered German measles about the time of conception. There were no additional problems during pregnancy, but at birth, the patient was small for her age and required forceps delivery. Thereafter, she did not thrive and, in fact, lost weight, at which point she was admitted to a children's hospital and received a diagnosis of celiac disease. Her parents said she had been slow in passing her milestones. They were told that she had a learning disability, but she managed to stay in normal schooling, struggling until the age of 16. After leaving school, she tried to take several training courses and jobs as a beauty therapist and as a nursery assistant, but they did not last and she became increasingly isolated. By the age of 19, she became frightened and suspicious and started to develop paranoid delusions. She reported hearing voices of people swearing at her and giving her orders and ultimately "trying to wind [me] up." She laughed inappropriately, her behavior became disorganized, and her self-care declined dramatically. She was admitted to the hospital, diagnosed with a psychotic illness, and antipsychotic treatment was started. She responded to the drugs rapidly and was discharged without psychotic symptoms; however, her compliance with treatment was irregular and she needed five subsequent short admissions over a period of 5 years. When not in the hospital, she lived relatively independently in a supervised residential home. She did not work but kept herself busy with numerous activities, from aerobics to horse riding. This is a case in which genetic risk factors interacted with very early environmental hazards to jeopardize brain development—hence the low IQ—and finally resulted in the onset of symptoms of schizophrenia during late adolescence.

WHAT THE SIMPLE NEURODEVELOPMENTAL MODEL FAILS TO EXPLAIN

Why Does Damage Occurring in Early Life Cause Symptoms Decades Later? One of the main challenges to the initial developmental theory was to explain how hazards occurring in fetal or prenatal life could cause psychotic symptoms so many years later. Brain maturation is a prolonged process that continues well after adolescence. The early developmental model proposed one possible explanation in which lesions lie silent until maturational processes expose neuronal circuits that are deviant but not functional during childhood. Although the damage takes place very early in life, maturational changes are also required to reveal any malfunction and symptoms. Animal models have given some support to this view. Hippocampal lesions made to rat pups remain relatively silent until puberty, and aberrant behaviors only appear in their adult life. Thus, it is possible that an early developmental insult to a critical brain area, such as the hippocampus, may have delayed manifestations.

Could damage compromising brain maturation rather than organogenesis be sufficient to lead to schizophrenia? The *late* as opposed to the *early* developmental model postulates that at least some of the crucial developmental abnormalities occur during adolescence. As described in the neuropathology section above, the human brain undergoes a maturational process involving programmed synaptic elimination throughout adolescence. Keshavan

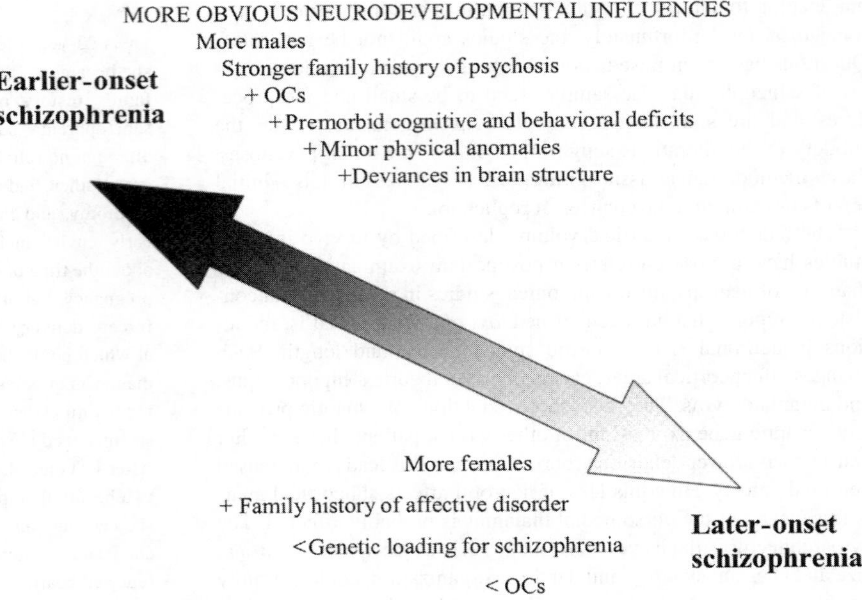

FIGURE 12.5–2 Factors that influence the age of onset of schizophrenia. OCs, obstetric complications.

postulated that schizophrenia might result from an excessive synaptic pruning. Perhaps the best evidence in support of this comes from the study of children who developed schizophrenia before age 13 years. These individuals show a pattern of loss of cortical volume, which appears to spread from the back to the front of the brain as they go through adolescence. There is also some evidence from studies prospectively examining individuals as they develop psychosis.

What, however, could cause such aberrant pruning? Human neurodevelopment, the pruning processes in particular, is under genetic regulation. Thus, genes of risk for schizophrenia might exert some of their effects by compromising cortical maturation. In view of the possibility that experience and learning may influence the selective survival of certain synapses, it is conceivable that the social environment may also help shape brain maturation. Thus, genetic risk factors, environmental events, or their interactions may interfere with the synaptic pruning that takes place in the maturing cortex throughout adolescence, finally leading to the schizophrenia syndrome.

Late-Onset Schizophrenia A key difficulty for the early neurodevelopmental model is the question of why the onset of frank psychosis does not occur until several years after the supposed developmental lesion or lesions. The late developmental model successfully covers the onset in the second decade of life by invoking brain maturational events in adolescence. However, people develop schizophrenia throughout adult life into old age, and late-onset patients, especially those who show relatively normal premorbid adjustment, are difficult to account for by deviant brain development and maturation alone.

What factors influence the age of onset of psychosis? Onset is generally earlier in male patients than in female. Furthermore, patients with a family history of schizophrenia tend to have an earlier age of onset compared to those cases with less genetic risk, regardless of gender. As noted earlier, obstetric complications in gestation and delivery may result in earlier onset. Other indicators of aberrant neurodevelopment, such as premorbid cognitive and behavioral deficits, minor physical anomalies, and deviances in brain structure, have also been associated with early onset of schizophrenia.

Furthermore, patients with late-onset psychosis seem to carry less genetic loading for schizophrenia, and their relatives are at higher risk for affective disorders. A potential explanation is that patients with late-onset schizophrenia may, in fact, have a different illness, possibly with etiological factors in common with affective psychosis. Alternatively, the symptoms may arise from brain degeneration (Fig. 12.5–2).

One may conclude that the role of neurodevelopmental impairment is most marked in early-onset schizophrenia, but it becomes progressively less obvious in patients with increasing age of onset. In other words, only a proportion of the variance in liability to schizophrenia can be attributed to impaired brain development.

IS THERE EVIDENCE OF DEGENERATION?

The neurodevelopmental hypothesis struggles to adequately explain the malignant course with deterioration shown by some patients over time. A number of studies claiming progression of morphological abnormalities after the onset of psychosis have reopened the question of whether a neurodegenerative process might play a part in earlier-onset schizophrenia.

Is There Progression of Brain Deviances in Schizophrenia? Conflicting Imaging Evidence Lynn DeLisi and colleagues performed a prospective follow-up of first-episode cases of schizophrenia and age-matched controls for almost 10 years and compared the rate of change over time in the size of certain brain structures. There were differences in the rate of change in the first 4 years in the overall volumes of left and right hemispheres and right cerebellum and in the area of the isthmus of the corpus callosum. The authors interpreted these changes over time as evidence for a subtle active brain process in the first few years of a schizophrenic illness. A number of other studies of first-episode patients have also found apparent progression of brain deviances affecting a number of different structures. Jeffrey Lieberman and colleagues examined more than 100 first-onset patients, half of whom were followed for up to 6 years. They confirmed the presence of ventricular enlargement and hippocampal volume reductions at the time of the first episode. They found no overall change in brain volumes but a progressive increase in ventricular volume in those patients with poor outcome. However, they found no further reductions in cortical or hippocampal volumes over time.

Another longitudinal study focusing on childhood-onset schizophrenia reported that brain abnormalities were progressing during adolescence but became stable in early adulthood. Further work from the same group using high-resolution MRI scans showed that, compared to 12 matched controls, 12 adolescent early-onset patients had accelerated gray matter loss over a 5-year follow-up period.

Christos Pantelis and colleagues examined a small group of subjects who were at very high risk for psychosis on the basis of family history, schizotypal traits, decline in functioning, or demonstration of very brief or attenuated psychotic experiences. After 1 year, half of the cohort made a transition toward a full-blown psychotic disorder. Compared to those who remained well, subjects who subsequently developed psychosis showed left-sided reductions in parahippocampal, fusiform, and orbitofrontal cortex. The authors concluded that this process started in the prodromal phase of the illness, even before clinical psychotic symptoms were expressed.

Reports of progression of structural abnormalities are more common in, but not confined to, first-episode and early-onset cases. Stephen Wood and colleagues reported a reduction of whole-brain volume in both first-episode and chronic patients after a relatively short follow-up of approximately 2 years. Daniel Mathalon and colleagues reported that patients with chronic schizophrenia had accentuated loss of frontotemporal gray matter and enlargement of ventricular and sulcal cerebrospinal fluid (CSF) spaces at an average 4-year follow-up. Tomoyuki Saijo and colleagues conducted one of the longest studies, with up to 10 years' coverage, and reported progressive lateral ventricular enlargement in a small sample of patients. Several studies agree that progression of brain deviance over time is associated with a more severe clinical course and poorer outcome.

However, not all imaging cohort studies of first-episode patients agree with these progressive morphological changes. Gustav DeGreef and colleagues found no variation in cortical or ventricular volumes over a 1- to 2-year period. Similarly, Anthony James and colleagues report no progression of ventricular enlargement found in adolescent-onset patients after an average follow-up of approximately 3 years.

Making Sense of the Controversy over Progressive Brain Deviance

The evidence from imaging cohorts indicates that pathological changes are already present at the onset of illness. Some of those changes involving frontal lobes and superior temporal gyrus may be progressive. Ventricle size in schizophrenia is probably not static, and there is substantial enlargement during the early stages of the illness, which tends to stabilize later on.

However, as Weinberger and McClure point out, there are numerous methodological difficulties associated with longitudinal quantitative neuroimaging research. Studies discussed above include imaging techniques of different resolution. The sample sizes tend to be small and the matching of controls and cases is, in some studies, far from optimal. The influence of prescribed medication and substance misuse remains largely unknown and provides room for confounding.

This putative progression of morphological changes has been interpreted as evidence in favor of neurodegenerative processes in schizophrenia. However, there is no indication from neuropathological studies that the findings of volume decrements on follow-up MRI studies reflect neurodegeneration. Finally, if there were progressive changes in the brain during the first few years after onset of psychosis, how is it that, at the same time, neuropsychological studies show cognitive function to be either static or improving? Any plausible degenerative theory based on progression requires an explanation of this curious paradox.

It is worth noting that many studies reporting progression of structural changes have been performed on younger patients in their first episode of illness or with onset in childhood or adolescence, when the brain is still at a crucial stage of development. Thus, one explanation for the confusion over whether there is progression of brain changes after onset of psychosis is that those changes noticed are, in fact, changes associated with late brain development, as suggested by Judith Rapoport and colleagues. It may be that maturation accentuates the trajectory of neurodevelopmental deviance in already compromised brains, without the need to invoke an additional neurodegenerative process. Thus, patients presenting in childhood or adolescence may show the brain structural consequences of exaggerated adolescent synaptic pruning, but those samples composed of adult patients may show little change.

IS THERE A ROLE FOR SOCIAL RISK FACTORS?

The theory that schizophrenia is simply a brain disorder remained unchallenged from the late 1970s to the late 1990s. Thus, the initial neurodevelopmental model implied that symptoms of schizophrenia were simply a consequence of the development of aberrant neural networks. However, there is convincing evidence that social risk factors play a crucial role in the development of schizophrenia (Fig. 12.5–2). Although there is a clear association between certain social risk factors and schizophrenia, the direction of causality has not always been demonstrated.

COULD AN ADVERSE UPBRINGING CONVEY HIGHER RISK FOR SCHIZOPHRENIA?

In the British 1946 cohort, 4-year-old children rated as having a poor mother–child relationship had a sixfold increase in risk for developing schizophrenia later in life. Of course, this does not indicate whether poor mothering was a causal risk factor or whether deviances inherent to the preschizophrenic children made them less able to form a close bond with their mother. Children with known genetic risk for schizophrenia were found to be more likely to develop the disorder if they lived on a kibbutz rather than in a family home. Overall, kibbutz children did not have the worst outcomes, suggesting that these genetically at-risk children inherited a vulnerability to the social environment. Another cohort study examined more than 3,000 Finns born in the 1950s who were temporarily isolated from their families because a relative had developed tuberculosis. At birth, they were placed in adequate nursing homes for an average period of 7 months. Compared to more than 6,000 suitably matched controls, the index cases had a similar incidence of schizophrenia and other psychoses after a follow-up period of 28 years. Thus, temporary family separation with adequate care is unlikely to increase the risk for schizophrenia. Adoption studies have a crucial say in this matter. Offspring from schizophrenic mothers who were adopted away at birth were more likely to develop the illness if they were reared in adverse circumstances, as compared to those raised in loving homes by stable adoptive parents.

Effect of Being Born or Brought Up in a City Several studies in the 1990s indicated that being born or brought up in a city increased the risk for schizophrenia. In one of the most impressive studies, conducted with a Danish national sample, the relative risk (RR) of schizophrenia associated with urban birth was 2.4. Furthermore, there was a dose–response relationship, and the larger the town of birth, the greater the risk, suggesting a causal effect. Because so many people are born and live in cities, a relatively small increase in risk would cause a large increase in numbers of people with the disease. Indeed, they calculated that the population attributable risk for urban birth was 34.6 percent, compared to 9.0 percent or 7.0 percent for having a mother or father with schizophrenia, respectively. A similar population attributable risk had previously been reported in data from Holland, where, in addition, it was shown that the effect of urban birth, urban upbringing, or both, is not confounded by urban residence in adult life. A further analysis of the above Danish study has shown that the association between urbanization and schizophrenia is based on continuous or repeated exposures during upbringing—not just urban birth. There is, indeed, a dose–response relationship between urban upbringing and risk for schizophrenia, again, suggesting a causal link. Finally, a recent Swedish population cohort, in which more than 690,000 individuals were followed up for almost 10 years, confirmed that urban, compared to rural, birthplace was associated with increased risk of adult onset schizophrenia and other nonaffective psychoses (hazard ratios were 1.24 and 1.63, respectively). Causal factors underlying this association appeared to operate independently of risks associated with obstetric complications or parental educational status. As pointed out by Jim Van Os and colleagues in their study of a Dutch population, it could be better explained by a gene–environment interaction: Although both urbanicity and a family history of psychosis emerged as risk factors, it was the combination of the two that dramatically increased the risk for schizophrenia.

Risk Associated with Isolation The Swedish conscript study discussed earlier also looked at the interaction of premorbid personality and social isolation. Young men who felt they were more sensitive than their peers, had fewer than two close friends. and did not have a girlfriend had an increased risk of later developing the disorder. Once again, this raises the question of whether these characteristics are an expression of a schizoid or schizotypal personality or whether they are, themselves, independent risk factors. Until proven otherwise, it is wise to consider that both may be true. In other words, individuals with a schizoid or schizotypal personality may be less able to make social relationships, and, at the same time, the social isolation itself may cause them to become increasingly deviant. Van Os and colleagues found that people who were single had a slightly higher risk of developing psychosis if they lived in a neighborhood with fewer single people, as compared to a neighborhood with many other single people. The authors suggested that single status might give rise to perceived (or actual) social isolation if most other people were living with a partner. The question of whether social isolation increases the risk of schizophrenia (or, rather, whether a close relationship may be protective) was also raised by Assen Jablensky and colleagues. They showed that marriage had a protective effect for men, and that this was not simply a consequence of better-adjusted men being more likely to marry. There is consistent evidence for an association between social isolation and schizophrenia; however, the direction of causality remains to be elucidated.

Migration Effect As far back as the 1930s, Örnulv Ödegaard noted that Norwegian migrants to the United States were at increased risk of schizophrenia. More recently, Preben Mortensen and colleagues studied a population cohort of more than 2 million Danes. Compared to subjects who were born in Denmark to Danish mothers, those born outside Denmark had a significantly higher risk of developing schizophrenia. RRs ranged between 2 and 4 for different birth origins. The increased risk also applied to second-generation migrants, particularly those who had lived abroad before the age of 15 years.

The most striking findings on the migration issue have come from the United Kingdom, where numerous studies have reported an increased incidence of schizophrenia among Afro-Caribbean people. Misdiagnosis and increased neurodevelopmental insult have been largely ruled out as explanations. A high genetic predisposition also seems unlikely, since those living in the Caribbean do not share the increased risk. Morbid risks for schizophrenia were similar for parents and siblings of whites and first-generation Afro-Caribbean patients. However, the morbid risk for siblings of second-generation Afro-Caribbean patients was approximately seven times higher than that for their white counterparts. The study suggests the presence of an environmental agent that is operating on this particular population in the United Kingdom but not in the Caribbean. Social isolation and alienation have been put forward as plausible culprits. Finally, it appears that the incidence of schizophrenia in migrants is greatest when they live in areas with few other migrants; again, one possible explanation is the relative isolation and lack of social support. Thus, migration, possibly by way of its potential isolating effect, is a risk factor for schizophrenia.

Abuse of Illegal Drugs and Risk for Schizophrenia

It is well established that dopamine-releasing drugs can precipitate psychosis. Persecutory or bizarre delusions, as well as hallucinations and thought disorder, are well documented in experimental studies using drug challenges with healthy volunteers and patients. Whereas cocaine and amphetamine are well-accepted risk factors for psychosis, the role of cannabis has been less clear and, until recently, was considered a relatively innocuous substance in terms of triggering psychosis. More recent research shows that repeated exposure to cannabis also induces alterations in dopamine transmission. Cannabis is well known to trigger brief psychotic episodes in controls and to exacerbate preexisting psychotic symptoms. However, could it actually contribute to the onset of psychosis?

A reevaluation of the Swedish Army Study discussed previously reveals that cannabis is, indeed, associated with increased risk of schizophrenia in a dose-dependent way. Heavy cannabis consumption at the age of 18 years is associated with a more than sixfold increased risk of developing schizophrenia later. This association is not explained by concurrent use of other drugs, such as cocaine or amphetamine. The confounding effects of premorbid personality traits predisposing to both cannabis use and schizophrenia have also been accounted for and ruled out in this sample. All participants were thoroughly screened for psychiatric diagnosis at the time of conscription. More than half of those who admitted to heavy cannabis use had a preexisting psychiatric diagnosis. However, even when these individuals were excluded, cannabis consumption remained a risk factor for later psychosis. Although a small number of participants with prodromal schizophrenia may have increased cannabis use as a consequence of their illness, this would not apply to the vast majority of the cohort, and, therefore, "self medication" alone is unlikely to explain the results.

Recently, the above ideas have been replicated in a cohort of children followed up in Dunedin, New Zealand. Using cannabis in adolescence increased the risk of developing schizophreniform psychosis, even after psychotic symptoms preceding the onset of cannabis use are controlled for, indicating that cannabis abuse is not secondary to preexisting psychosis. Furthermore, earlier use of cannabis confers greater risk than if the drug is used in late adolescence.

Despite the evidence that dopamine-releasing drugs are risk factors for psychosis, the vast majority of users come to no such harm, indicating that further vulnerabilities must interplay in the association between drugs and psychosis. Philip McGuire and colleagues showed that the relatives of patients with cannabis-associated psychosis had an increased risk of developing schizophrenia. Chiken Chen noted findings similar for methamphetamine use in a large Taiwanese sample. Those methamphetamine abusers who developed psychosis were distinguished from those who remained unaffected by their greater frequency of schizoid and schizotypal traits in childhood and by a more extensive family history of psychosis. Thus, it may be that some individuals abuse drugs because they already have psychiatric problems, and, among them, it is those who have a genetic predisposition to psychosis who are particularly likely to develop this illness.

Adverse Life Events and Stress

Three prospective studies have found an association between life events and onset of psychosis. Stressful life events in the 3 weeks preceding onset or relapse of symptoms seemed important—although, the effect size was greater in affective psychosis than in schizophrenia. Again, the direction of the relationship between life events and psychosis has been questioned. It is difficult to fully rule out the possibility that the actual adverse events might have been precipitated by preexisting psychopathology or personality traits of the patient.

However, there are emerging lines of evidence in support of the role of stress in causing or precipitating psychosis. Experiments in which animals are exposed to developmental insults show how they become particularly vulnerable to social stress. The same has been postulated for humans and could explain why an adverse environment could have particularly detrimental effects on a developmentally compromised individual.

There is growing interest regarding how environmental and psychosocial risk factors as described above can link with psychosis. By what mechanism could isolation, migration, city upbringing, abuse of drugs, and other environmental adversities generate psychotic symptoms?

DOPAMINE SENSITIZATION: LINKING BRAIN DEVELOPMENT, ENVIRONMENTAL STRESS, AND SYMPTOMS IN SCHIZOPHRENIA

The evidence discussed thus far helps to illuminate the development of the child at risk for schizophrenia. However, what is the mechanism that converts a socially isolated youngster with some deficits in cognition and unusual ideas into a floridly psychotic patient? Some answers can be found by exploring the effect of developmental insults on mesolimbic dopamine systems.

As is well known, the dopamine hypothesis of schizophrenia is derived from the evidence that all antipsychotic drugs block dopamine type 2 (D_2) receptors, whereas dopamine agonists can elicit positive symptoms of the illness. This long-standing theory has been bolstered by in vivo imaging evidence, which directly implicates dopamine dysregulation in the pathogenesis of the positive psychotic symptoms. For example, a series of single photon emission computed tomography (SPECT) and positron emission tomography (PET) studies has demonstrated that patients with acute schizophrenia release excessive amounts of dopamine in response to an amphetamine challenge and that there is a clear relationship between the degree of this release and severity of psychotic symptoms. Thus, there is strong evidence of heightened dopaminergic transmission, predominantly a presynaptic dysregulation, in patients with schizophrenia. However, because dopamine dysregulation is not apparent among patients with schizophrenia in remission, it is probably more of a "state" abnormality associated with active symptoms of psychosis rather than a permanent trait of the illness. Thus, abnormality of dopamine is necessary, but not sufficient, to explain psychosis. The key question is now thus: How, exactly, does a neurotransmitter such as dopamine fuel psychotic experiences?

Dopamine As a Mediator of Emotional Response to Stimuli

There is wide agreement regarding dopamine's role in reward and reinforcement, as well as in its negative counterparts—that is, aversive stimuli and behavioral extinction, respectively. Changes in dopamine firing are observed during the anticipation and the experience of either pleasurable or dreaded stimuli. Dopamine appears to be a neurochemical mediator for events with innate rewarding or aversive effects, but, more importantly, this is also the case for neutral stimuli that become associated with the rewarding effects. The mesolimbic–dopaminergic system is thought to be crucial in the attribution of emotional relevance, or salience, to stimuli and, ultimately, in influencing goal-oriented behavior.

Much research supports dopamine as a central mediator of emotional salience and motivation in the normal response to stimuli. Shitij Kapur has extended this idea to acute psychosis, which he regards as "a disorder of dopamine-induced aberrant salience." Under normal circumstances, a stimulus-bound release of dopamine mediates the attribution of emotional relevance or salience to stimuli, and such salience is accordingly reflected in appropriate thoughts and behaviors. However, in acute psychosis, there is an exaggerated dopamine transmission, out of synchrony with any stimuli. This dopamine dysregulation leads to the assignment of inappropriate emotional and motivational relevance to external and internal stimuli. This aberrant attribution of salience is perpetuated in the absence of any further stimulus, since it is generated by abnormal neurochemistry. Kapur suggests that delusions develop as an attempt to provide an explanation or interpretation for this misattributed emotional relevance. Hallucinations can be understood as resulting from increased salience being given to internal representations of perceptions or memories.

Dopamine Sensitization

On the basis of recent animal and human imaging research, it is postulated that this dopamine dysregulation arises from the development of sensitization of mesolimbic–dopaminergic systems. Long-term sensitization is a process whereby repeated exposure to a stimulus such as a substance or a stressor results in an enhanced response to subsequent exposures. The phenomenon has been well characterized in rodents. Sensitization only becomes apparent after withdrawal and reexposure to a stimulus and,

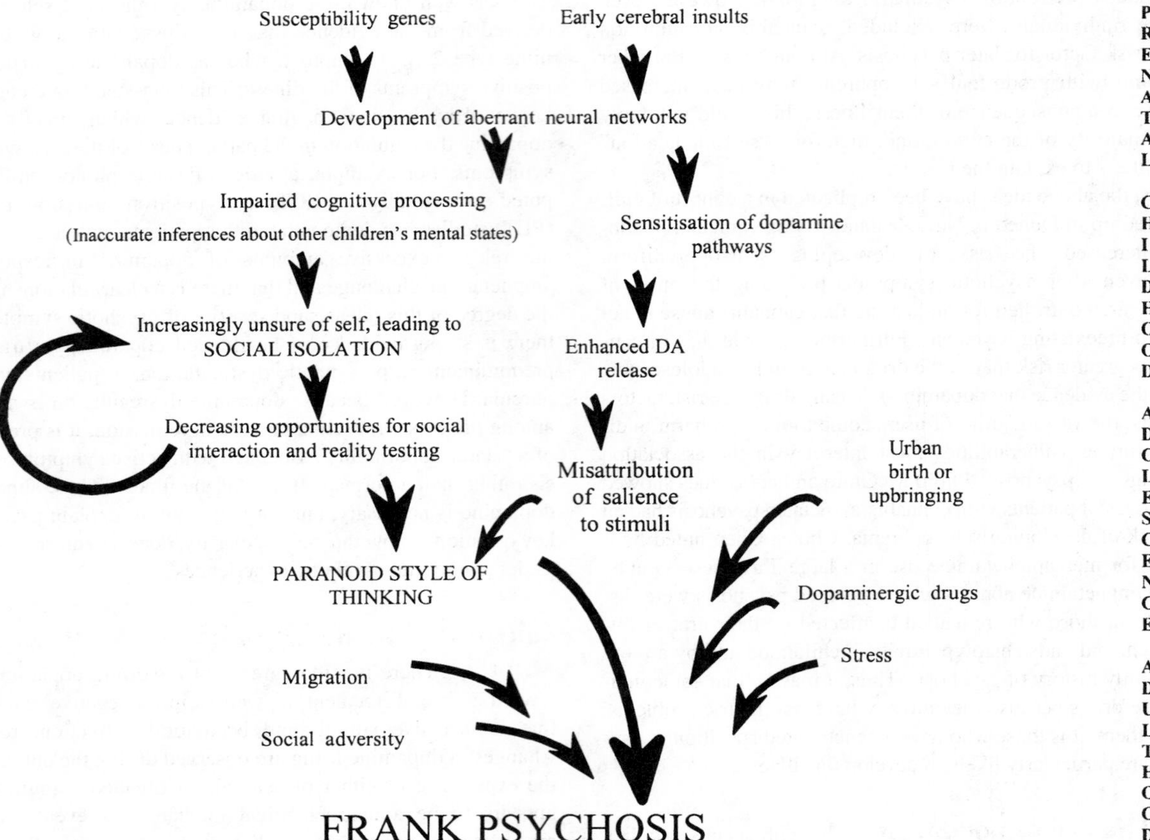

FIGURE 12.5–3 The cascade of increasingly abnormal development that culminates in the onset of full-blown psychosis. Also shown are the main risk factors for psychosis over life. DA, dopamine.

therefore, can be expressed months or even years after it was induced. Vulnerability to sensitization is dependent on stages of brain development; for example, amphetamine-induced sensitization is not produced in rats before 3 weeks of postnatal life. It is well documented that patients with schizophrenia are particularly vulnerable to the psychotogenic effects of such stimulants and, more important, even in those cases of first exposure to the drug. This has given rise to the term *endogenous sensitization* in schizophrenia. The most clear neurochemical manifestation of a sensitized state is the excessive dopamine release induced by psychostimulant drugs. Brain imaging tools have been used to measure dopamine transmission in vivo and support the hypothesis that dysfunctional dopamine systems in schizophrenia result from sensitization phenomena. However, the imaging studies also show that such sensitization may stabilize during periods of clinical remission, and antipsychotic-induced blockade of dopaminergic receptors might allow a progressive extinction of this sensitized state.

Impact of Developmental Insults on Dopamine Pathways Dopamine sensitization is a link between a biological dysfunction and symptoms of schizophrenia, but how is it caused? A plausible explanation is that abnormal neural development can lead to a vulnerability to sensitization of dopamine pathways and ultimately result in an impaired control over mesolimbic–dopaminergic transmission. The relevance of early neural insults for dopamine sensitization is demonstrated by studies showing how animals subject to perinatal brain lesions develop dopamine systems, which are particularly prone to such dysregulation when they become mature. For example, B. K. Lipska and colleagues reported that artificial lesions to the hippocampus in neonatal rats remain relatively silent until adult life. Then the animals develop hyperresponse to amphetamine and to stress that manifests with abnormalities in behavior, electrophysiology, and neuroimaging. Interestingly, analogous damage to adult rats did not produce such deleterious effects. Barbara Lipska's model mimics many of the abnormalities that are found in schizophrenia, but, of course, it results from an artificial lesion. Patricia Boksa and colleagues have shown that birth by cesarean section, a more physiological perinatal stress, also induces altered mesocorticolimbic dopamine transmission in the rat, together with increased adult behavioral responses to amphetamines and to stress. In humans, there is also evidence that perinatal injury can induce subcortical dopaminergic overactivity. Özlem Kapucu and colleagues used SPECT to examine 20 infants with hypoxic-ischemic brain damage and noted that striatal D_2 receptor density decreased as the severity of the injury increased. A similar impact on dopamine-receptor populations and transmission might arise from abnormal cortical pruning in the context of schizophrenia. There is substantial evidence from both animal and human research that alterations in cortical development might impair the capacity of dopamine pathways to respond normally to stress. This failure of homeostatic and buffering mechanisms results in a process of endogenous sensitization, which produces the positive symptoms seen in schizophrenia.

In summary, deviant neural development in early life leads to mesolimbic–dopaminergic neurons that become hyperresponsive to environmental influences, such as drugs or stress, that can manifest years later. As sensitization establishes, smaller and smaller stressors can induce an excessive release of dopamine. The enhanced and dysregulated dopaminergic transmission mediates the aberrant attribution of salience to internal and external stimuli, which ultimately manifest as psychotic symptoms (Fig. 12.5–3).

FUTURE DIRECTIONS

Genetic epidemiological and molecular studies imply that liability to develop schizophrenia is inherited, not through a single major gene, but through a number of genes of small effect. Some of those genes are probably shared with other psychotic conditions, such as bipolar disorder, and some are likely to be involved in the control of neurodevelopmental processes underlying cognitive capacities (for example, neuregulin-1, dysbindin, or catechol-*O*-methyltransferase genes). Studies of the relatives of patients with schizophrenia indicate that families transmit relatively innocent minor developmental deviations—for example, slight alterations in brain structure, neurophysiology, or neurocognition. However, when a child is unlucky enough to inherit several of these traits—and is exposed to environmental hazards such as obstetric complications—then the cumulative effect puts that individual on a trajectory of increasing deviance.

High-risk and cohort studies demonstrate that children who eventually develop schizophrenia are slow to walk and talk and show an excess of subtle emotional, neuromotor, and cognitive difficulties, particularly in coordination and receptive language. These neurocognitive problems and difficulties in interpersonal relations lead preschizophrenic children to become increasingly isolated from their peers, and, by their early teens, they are more likely to harbor odd and paranoid ideas. These quasipsychotic ideas and neuropsychological and social deviances that are present many years before the clinical illness are not simply epiphenomena of an early lesion, but are also part of the causal pathway to psychosis.

A plausible model is that this cascade of increasingly deviant development is then compounded by brain maturational changes during adolescence, which result in a process of dopamine sensitization, leading to a lability of the dopamine response to stress. This developmentally compromised individual is, therefore, more susceptible to the effects of dopamine-releasing drugs and other stress-generating risk factors, such as migration, isolation, or being brought up in a city. Excessive dopamine release in mesolimbic pathways is thought to underlie an aberrant attribution of motivational salience to stimuli that crystallizes into psychotic experiences. Developmental insults leading to sensitization of dopaminergic pathways provide a mechanism through which a cascade of increasing deviance interacts with further psychosocial risk factors to culminate in the onset of psychotic symptoms.

SUGGESTED CROSS-REFERENCES

Neurochemical hypotheses of schizophrenia are discussed in Sections 1.4, 1.5, and 1.6, and information regarding neuroimaging studies of schizophrenia can be found in Section 12.6. Chapter 38, Pervasive Developmental Disorders, discusses early psychosis and prodromal research. Information on the genetics of schizophrenia can be found in Section 12.3.

REFERENCES

Andreasson S, Engstrom A, Allebeck P, Rydberg U: Cannabis and schizophrenia—a longitudinal study of Swedish conscripts. *Lancet*. 1987;2(8574):1483–1486.

Arseneault L, Cannon M, Poulton R, Murray RM, Caspi A, Moffitt TE: Cannabis use in adolescence and risk for adult psychosis: Longitudinal prospective study. *BMJ*. 2002;325:1212–1213.

*Cannon M, Jones PB, Murray RM: Obstetric complications and schizophrenia: Historical and meta-analytic review. *Am J Psychiatry*. 2002;159(7):1080–1092.

Cannon TD, van Erp TGM, Rosso IM, Huttunen M, Lonnqvist J, Pirkola T, Salonen O, Valanne L, Poutanen VP, Standertskjold-Nordenstam CG: Fetal hypoxia and structural brain abnormalities in schizophrenic patients, their siblings, and controls. *Arch Gen Psychiatry*. 2002;59(1):35–41.

Cantor-Graae E, Pedersen C, Mortensen PB: Migration as a risk factor for schizophrenia: A Danish population-based cohort study. *Schizophr Res*. 2002;53(3):33–34.

Clouston T. *The Neuroses of Development*. Edinburgh: Oliver & Boyd, 1891.

Dazzan P, Murray RM: Neurological soft signs in first-episode psychosis: A systematic review. *Br J Psychiatry*. 2002;181:S50–S57.

*DeLisi LE: Defining the course of brain structural change and plasticity in schizophrenia. *Psychiatry Res*. 1999;92:1–9.

Feinberg I: Schizophrenia: Caused by a fault in programmed synaptic elimination during adolescence? *J Psychiatr Res*. 1982–1983;17(4):319–334.

Harrison G, Fouskakis D, Rasmussen F, Tynelius P, Sipos A, Gunnell D: Association between psychotic disorder and urban place of birth is not mediated by obstetric complications or childhood socio-economic position: A cohort study. *Psychol Med*. 2003;33:723.

Harrison PJ: The neuropathology of schizophrenia—a critical review of the data and their interpretation. *Brain*. 1999;122:593–624.

Ho BC, Andreasen NC, Nopoulos P, Arndt S, Magnotta V, Flaum M: Progressive structural brain abnormalities and their relationship to clinical outcome—a longitudinal magnetic resonance imaging study early in schizophrenia. *Arch Gen Psychiatry*. 2003;60:585.

*Kapur S: Psychosis as a state of aberrant salience: A framework linking biology, phenomenology, and pharmacology in schizophrenia. *Am J Psychiatry*. 2003;160:13.

Keshavan MS: Development, disease and degeneration in schizophrenia: A unitary pathophysiological model. *J Psychiatr Res*. 1999:33(6):513–521.

Keshavan MS, Anderson S, Pettegrew JW: Is schizophrenia due to excessive synaptic pruning in the prefrontal cortex—the Feinberg hypothesis revisited. *J Psychiatr Res*. 1994:28(3):239–265.

Klosterkotter J, Hellmich M, Steinmeyer EM, Schultze-Lutter F: Diagnosing schizophrenia in the initial prodromal phase. *Arch Gen Psychiatry*. 2001;58:158.

Lahuis B, Kemner C, Van Engeland H: Magnetic resonance imaging studies on autism and childhood-onset schizophrenia in children and adolescents—a review. *Acta Neuropsychiatrica*. 2003;15:140.

Larsen TK, Friis S, Haahr U, Joa I, Johannessen JO, Melle I, Opjordsmoen S, Simonsen E, Vaglum P: Early detection and intervention in first-episode schizophrenia: A critical review. *Acta Psychiatrica Scandinavica*. 2001;103:323.

Laurelle M: The role of endogenous sensitization in the pathophysiology of schizophrenia: Implications from recent brain imaging studies. *Brain Res Brain Res Rev*. 2000;31:371–384.

Lawrie SM, Whalley HC, Abukmeil SS, Kestelman JN, Miller P, Best JJK, Owens DGC, Johnstone EC: Temporal lobe volume changes in people at high risk of schizophrenia with psychotic symptoms. *Br J Psychiatry*. 2002;181:138–143.

Lencz T, Smith C, Auther A, Cornblatt B: Severity of baseline positive symptoms predicts psychosis in adolescents prodromal for schizophrenia. *Schizophr Res*. 2003;60:20.

Lewis DA, Levitt P: Schizophrenia as a disorder of neurodevelopment. *Annu Rev Neurosci*. 2002;25:409–432.

Lipska BK, Weinberger DR: Genetic-variation in vulnerability to the behavioral-effects of neonatal hippocampal damage in rats. *Proc Natl Acad Sci U S A*. 1995:92(19): 8906–8910.

Maki P, Veijola J, Joukamaa M, Laara E, Hakko H, Jones PB, Isohanni M: Maternal separation at birth and schizophrenia—a long-term follow-up of the Finnish Christmas Seal Home Children. *Schizophr Res*. 2003;60:13.

Marcelis M, Takei N, van Os J: Urbanization and risk for schizophrenia: Does the effect operate before or around the time of illness onset? *Psychol Med*. 1999;29(5):1197–1203.

McDonald C, Grech A, Touopoulou T, Schulze K, Chapple B, Sham P, Walshe M, Sharma T, Sigmundsson T, Chitnis X, Murray RM: Brain volumes in familial and non-familial schizophrenic probands and their unaffected relatives. *Am J Med Genet*. 2002;114(6):616–625.

Miller P, Byrne M, Hodges A, Lawrie SM, Owens DGC, Johnstone EC: Schizotypal components in people at high risk of developing schizophrenia: Early findings from the Edinburgh High-Risk Study. *Br J Psychiatry*. 2002;180:179–184.

Morrison AP, Bentall RP, French P, Walford L, Kilcommons A, Knight A, Kreutz M, Lewis SW: Randomised controlled trial of early detection and cognitive therapy for preventing transition to psychosis in high-risk individuals—study design and interim analysis of transition rate and psychological risk factors. *Br J Psychiatry*. 2002;181:S78.

Murray RM, Lewis SW: Is schizophrenia a neurodevelopmental disorder? *Br Med J (Clin Res Ed)*. 1987;295(6600):681–682.

Murray RM, Ocallaghan E, Castle DJ, Lewis SW: A neurodevelopmental approach to the classification of schizophrenia. *Schizophr Bull*. 1992;18(2):319–332.

Pedersen CB, Mortensen PB: Evidence of a dose-response relationship between urbanicity during upbringing and schizophrenia risk. *Arch Gen Psychiatry*. 2001;58(11):1039–1046.

Schulze K, McDonald C, Frangou S, Sham P, Grech A, Toulopoulou T, Walshe M, Sharma T, Sigmundsson T, Taylor M, Murray RM: Hippocampal volume in familial and nonfamilial schizophrenic probands and their unaffected relatives. *Biol Psychiatry*. 2003;53:562.

Selemon LD, Goldman-Rakic PS: The reduced neuropil hypothesis: A circuit based model of schizophrenia. *Biol Psychiatry*. 1999;45(1):17–25.

Shenton ME, Dickey CC, Frumin M, McCarley RW: A review of MRI findings in schizophrenia. *Schizophr Res.* 2001;49(1–2):1–52.

Sorensen HJ, Mortensen EL, Reinisch JM, Mednick SA: Do hypertension and diuretic treatment in pregnancy increase the risk of schizophrenia in offspring? *Am J Psychiatry.* 2003;160:464.

Sugarman PA, Craufurd D: Schizophrenia in the Afro-Caribbean community. *Br J Psychiatry.* 1994;164:474–480.

Van Os J, Driessen G, Gunther N, Delespaul P: Neighbourhood variation in incidence of schizophrenia—evidence for person-environment interaction. *Br J Psychiatry.* 2000;176:243–248.

Walker E: Risk factors and the neurodevelopmental course of schizophrenia. *Eur Psychiatry.* 2002;17:363–369.

Woods SW, Breier A, Zipursky RB, Perkins DO, Addington J, Miller TJ, Hawkins KA, Marquez E, Lindborg SR, Tohen M, McGlashan TH: Randomized trial of olanzapine versus placebo in the symptomatic acute treatment of the schizophrenic prodrome. *Biol Psychiatry.* 2003;54:453.

*Wright IC, Rabe-Hesketh S, Woodruff PWR, David AS, Murray RM, Bullmore ET: Metaanalysis of regional brain volumes in schizophrenia. *Am J Psychiatry.* 2000;157(1):16–25.

*Yung AR, Phillips LJ, Yuen HP, Francey SM, McFarlane CA, Hallgren M, McGorry PD: Psychosis prediction: 12-month follow up of a high-risk ("prodromal") group. *Schizophr Res.* 2003;60:21.

▲ 12.6 Neuroimaging in Schizophrenia: Linking Neuropsychiatric Manifestations to Neurobiology

Raquel E. Gur, M.D., Ph.D., and Ruben C. Gur, Ph.D.

NEUROIMAGING: THE SPEARHEAD OF A NEUROPSYCHIATRIC PERSPECTIVE

The severe behavioral manifestations of schizophrenia have continued to provide an impetus for efforts at understanding the neurobiology of this complex disorder. Advances in neuroimaging have reached a point at which the convergence of evidence permits several conclusions that link clinical features of schizophrenia to dysfunctional brain systems. Noteworthy advances bridge between clinical and basic neuroscience research, address mechanisms underlying schizophrenia, and have implications for treatment. The contribution of neuroimaging to this effort has been to document abnormalities in whole brain, as well as regional, morphology and physiology in a way that serves to integrate clinical, neurobehavioral, and basic research. In the 5 years since the previous edition of this textbook, the literature on neuroimaging in schizophrenia has nearly doubled compared to the literature that has been available since the inception of imaging in the late 1970s. Clearly, it is impossible to update all aspects of neuroimaging in schizophrenia. Instead, this chapter will highlight the main findings, focusing on the integration of brain and behavior.

As the field of neuroimaging has evolved, complementary progress has also been made in behavioral neurosciences. Such progress includes the development and application of more precise and efficient measures of neurobehavioral domains, the incorporation of emotion processing and olfaction as probes of limbic function, and improved transitions between human and animal paradigms. There is an increased recognition that schizophrenia is characterized by selective cognitive, emotive, and olfactory processing deficits, against a background of global impairment. The nature of the deficit and findings of impaired performance in unaffected family members have contributed to a shift from examining the genetics of diagnostic categories to a focus on endophenotypic markers, with parallel paradigms in humans and animals. Such work opens the way to the application of microarray technology in genetic analyses and the study of cellular and molecular abnormalities in diverse brain regions. Considered jointly, these advances establish firm foundations for hypothesis-driven research that systematically examines core neurobiological abnormalities underlying schizophrenia. The integration of neurobehavioral and neuroimaging paradigms, essential for functional neuroanatomical investigations, also makes it possible to address fundamental questions. Growing evidence indicates that abnormalities in brain development play formative roles in the pathophysiology of schizophrenia. Examination of neuroleptic-naïve, first-episode patients in neurobehavioral and neuroimaging studies helps evaluate the presence of abnormalities at disease onset. Repeated measures can longitudinally address questions regarding disease progression. This section will first present a summary of neurobehavioral studies that provide the probe to brain systems that underlie the disorder and then highlight neuroimaging studies across diverse methods.

The diversity of methods reflects, to some extent, the complexity of the brain and schizophrenia. It is perhaps useful to highlight the main classes of neuroimaging methods in the context of the cascade leading from brain to behavior. The cascade begins at the anatomical substrate and proceeds through the initiation of electrical pulses triggering neurotransmitter release, a process that eventuates in relaying the signal for action (Fig. 12.6–1). The process requires energy metabolism. Although far from the cellular level, neuroimaging methods can yield information on every step in this cascade. Magnetic resonance imaging (MRI) technologies can provide morphometric parameters of neuroanatomy. Event-related electrophysiological methods (electroencephalography [EEG]/event-related potential [ERP]), based on surface electrodes, as well as magnetoencephalography (MEG), yield information on activity of neuronal aggregates with high temporal and improving spatial resolution. Metabolic biochemical activity can be measured with magnetic resonance spectroscopy (MRS), and functional MRI (fMRI) yields measures of cerebral blood flow (CBF) change. Positron emission tomography (PET) provides functional measures of oxygen and glucose metabolism and of CBF, as well as measures of neurotransmitter function. Single photon emission computed tomography (SPECT) can also evaluate both CBF and receptor function. Together, they afford an impressive arsenal for assessing and studying brain structure and function. New methods are being developed, such as MRI sequences sensitive to the direction and degree of proton diffusion. Because diffusion is greatest along the axonal axis, tensor diffusion imaging (TDI) can trace neuronal fiber tracts, enabling a transition from volumetric measures to tracing connectivity.

NEUROBEHAVIORAL DEFICITS IN SCHIZOPHRENIA

The clinical presentation of schizophrenia is associated with a range of behavioral changes and aberrations that do not directly constitute a part of the clinical characterization but are, nonetheless, salient and crippling. These deficits cover a broad range of behavior, including cognition, emotion, and sensory domains. Understanding the nature and contributions of these impairments is essential for developing models of neural systems involved in schizophrenia.

Cognition Impaired cognition in schizophrenia, leading to early conceptualizations of "dementia praecox," was well supported by numerous applications of psychological measures. Earlier studies

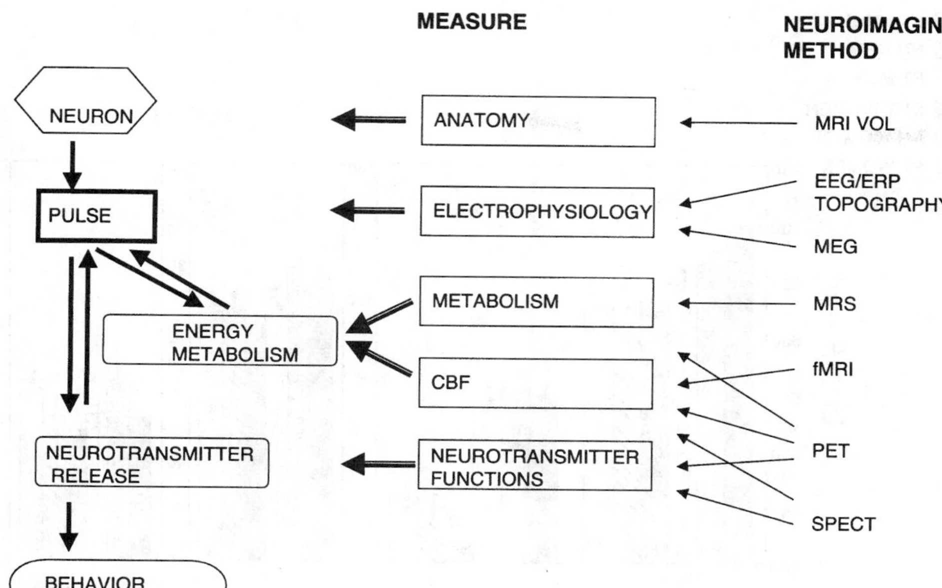

FIGURE 12.6–1 A schematic presentation of the imaging methods that yield measures pertinent to stages in the cascade from neuronal activity to behavior. CBF, cerebral blood flow; EEG, electroencephalography; ERP, event-related potential; fMRI, functional magnetic resonance imaging; MEG, magnetoencephalography; MRI, magnetic resonance imaging; MRS, magnetic resonance spectroscopy; PET, positron emission tomography; SPECT, single photon emission computed tomography; VOL, volume. (From Gur RC, Gur RE: Neuroimaging applications in the elderly. *Am J Geriatric Psychiatry*. 2002; 10:5, with permission.)

commonly focused on single domains, such as attention, and did not associate cognitive aberrations with functional brain systems. Neuropsychological batteries, which have been initially developed and applied in neurological populations, attempt to link behavioral deficits to brain function. This line of research in schizophrenia, with diverse test batteries, has consistently indicated diffuse dysfunction related to frontotemporal systems, with relatively greater impairment in executive functions and in learning and memory.

Examination of cognition in relation to clinical status has advanced understanding of the nature and scope of impairment in schizophrenia. Two lines of research have been particularly useful in the efforts: the evaluation of new-onset patients and longitudinal follow-up. Neurocognitive deficits are evident at initial clinical presentation, before treatment initiation. Therefore, studying new-onset patients avoids confounding due to the possible consequences of treatment, hospitalization, and social isolation that may contribute to compromised function. Furthermore, it has been observed in longitudinal studies that the cognitive deficits do not show appreciable amelioration with symptomatic relief associated with treatment. However, some neurocognitive domains have improved with treatment, perhaps more so with atypical neuroleptics. Yet, methodological issues limit conclusions, as most studies applied typical neuroleptics in a relatively high dose. Furthermore, neurocognitive measures have shown limited, albeit consistent, relation to clinical symptoms but appear more closely related to functional outcome. Although the literature evaluating the specificity of deficits in schizophrenia is limited, the profile and severity seem different from other disorders with psychotic features, such as bipolar disorder. Thus, early evaluation may have diagnostic and treatment implications.

Neuropsychological studies have found impairments in multiple domains, including perception, attention, visuospatial abilities, language, memory, emotion, executive function, and coordination. Within this pattern of diffuse impairment, attention, working and episodic memory, and executive functioning are more severely impaired. Several brain systems are implicated by these deficits. The attention-processing circuitry includes brainstem-thalamo-striato-accumbens-temporal-hippocampal-prefrontal-parietal regions. Deficits in working memory implicate the dorsolateral prefrontal cortex, and the ventromedial temporal lobe is implicated by deficits in episodic memory. A dorsolateral-medial-orbital-prefrontal cortical circuit mediates executive functions. These are obviously complex systems, and impairment in one may interact with dysfunction in others. Studies with large samples are needed to test models of underlying pathophysiology.

Emotion In addition to the marked cognitive impairment, emotion-processing deficits have also been noted in schizophrenia, and a growing literature indicates their contribution as neurobehavioral probes. Emotional impairment in schizophrenia is clinically well established, manifesting in flat, blunted, inappropriate affect and depression. Studies have reported emotion-processing deficits in identification, discrimination, and recognition of facial expressions. Although these deficits may represent a component of the generalized cognitive impairment, they relate to symptoms and neurobiological measures, encouraging further research. Animal and human investigations have implicated the limbic system, primarily the amygdala, hypothalamus, mesocorticolimbic dopaminergic systems, and cortical regions, including orbitofrontal, dorsolateral prefrontal, temporal, and parts of parietal cortex.

Olfaction Patients with schizophrenia are impaired in their ability to detect and identify odors. Olfactory deficits are present at the onset of illness, do not relate to disease severity or treatment, and are possibly progressive. It is unclear whether the deficits are part of the generalized neurocognitive impairment, but they are evident even when patients perform similarly to healthy participants on tasks designed as control measures. The neuroanatomical differences noted in MRI studies of patients relative to healthy controls suggest that olfactory bulb changes and medial temporal lobe abnormalities could mediate the observed behavioral aberrations.

Linking Deficits to Brain Function The link between neurobehavioral deficits and brain dysfunction can be examined both by correlating individual differences in performance with measures of brain anatomy and through the application of neurobehavioral probes in functional imaging studies. With these paradigms, the

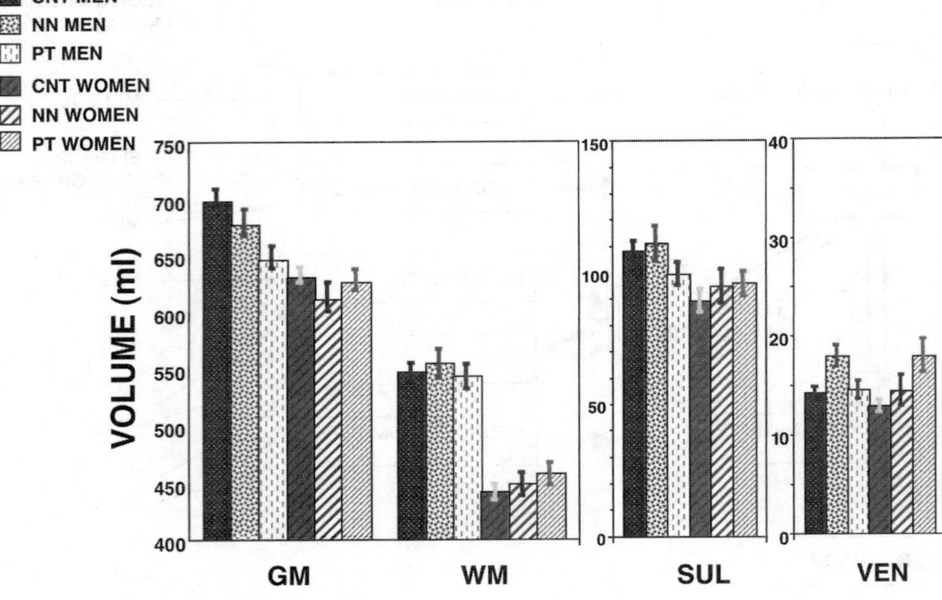

FIGURE 12.6–2 Whole-brain volumes for parenchyma (gray matter [GM] and white matter [WM]) and cerebrospinal fluid (CSF) compartments (sulci [SUL] and ventricle [VEN]) in healthy men and women (control [CNT]) and in people with schizophrenia (neuroleptic-naïve [NN] and previously treated [PT]). (Adapted from Gur RE, Turetsky BI, Bilker WB, Gur RC: Reduced gray matter volume in schizophrenia. *Arch Gen Psychiatry.* 1999;56:905.)

topography of brain activity in response to engagement in tasks in which deficits have been noted in patients can be investigated. Thus, there is "on-line" correlation between brain activity and performance that permits direct examination of brain behavior relations.

NEUROANATOMICAL STUDIES IN SCHIZOPHRENIA

Neuroanatomical correlates of impaired performance have provided the foundation for current thinking about brain regulation of behavior. As noted in the previous section, the behavioral aberrations manifested in schizophrenia implicate diffuse abnormalities likely to involve several brain systems. Defining the neuroanatomical differences and possible changes associated with schizophrenia is, arguably, a prerequisite for understanding its neural substrates and interpreting functional studies of brain physiology and neurochemistry. Structural morphometric studies have applied reliable computerized segmentation methods for obtaining volumetric measures. The improvement in precision of neuroanatomical parameters has yielded some consistency in effects and correlations with clinical and neurobehavioral measures. This section briefly highlights and illustrates these research efforts, starting with whole-brain effects, and then describes some regional effects.

Brain and Cerebral Spinal Fluid Segmentation

Multiple studies with MRI examining whole-brain and cerebrospinal fluid (CSF) volumes have indicated smaller brain volume and increased CSF in patients with schizophrenia relative to healthy people. The increase is more pronounced in ventricular than sulcal CSF. There is, however, considerable overlap between patients and healthy people, suggesting that abnormalities at the level of whole brain may characterize only subtypes of patients with schizophrenia. Brain and CSF volumes have been related to phenomenological and other clinical variables, such as premorbid functioning, symptom severity, and outcome. Abnormalities in these measures are likely to be more pronounced in patients with poorer premorbid functioning, more severe symptoms, and worse outcome. The concept of *brain reserve* that has been suggested in other disorders, such as Alzheimer's disease, may apply to schizophrenia as well. Thus, normal brain and CSF volumes are preliminary indicators of protective capacity. As understanding of how brain systems regulate behavior in health and disease has improved, it has become possible to take advantage of neuroimaging to examine specific brain regions implicated in the pathophysiology of schizophrenia.

Gray Matter and White Matter Segmentation Gray matter and white matter tissue segmentation, particularly feasible with thin-sliced, T1-weighted MRI sequences, provides anatomical information supplementing the demarcation of brain and CSF. Gray matter changes have been found during adolescence and in the course of the normal aging process. Gray–white segmentation is critical in developmental studies in which age-related decreases in gray matter may be obscured by simultaneous increases in total brain and cranial volumes. This image-processing methodology can help determine whether tissue loss and disorganization in schizophrenia are primarily gray matter deficits or whether abnormalities in white matter are also involved. Several studies using segmentation methods have indicated that gray matter volume reduction characterizes individuals with schizophrenia. This reduction is apparent in neuroleptic-naïve, first-episode patients and supports the growing body of work indicating that schizophrenia is a neurodevelopmental disorder (Fig. 12.6–2).

Regional Volumes In evaluating specific regions, the most consistent findings are of reduced volumes of temporal lobe, superior temporal gyrus, and medial temporal lobe structures. Other brain regions have also been noted to have reduced volumes, although less consistently. These include the prefrontal cortex, parietal lobe, thalamus, basal ganglia, cerebellar vermis, and olfactory bulbs. The application of diverse methods may partly explain discrepant results. For example, morphometric prefrontal studies differed in magnetic field, scanning parameters, slice thickness and contiguity, image processing, and regions examined. Consequently, findings seem inconsistent, with some noting no differences between patients and healthy participants, and others observing volume reduction in gray matter, white matter, or both tissue compartments.

Relatively few studies have related sublobar volumes to clinical or neurocognitive measures. Higher right orbitofrontal volume was

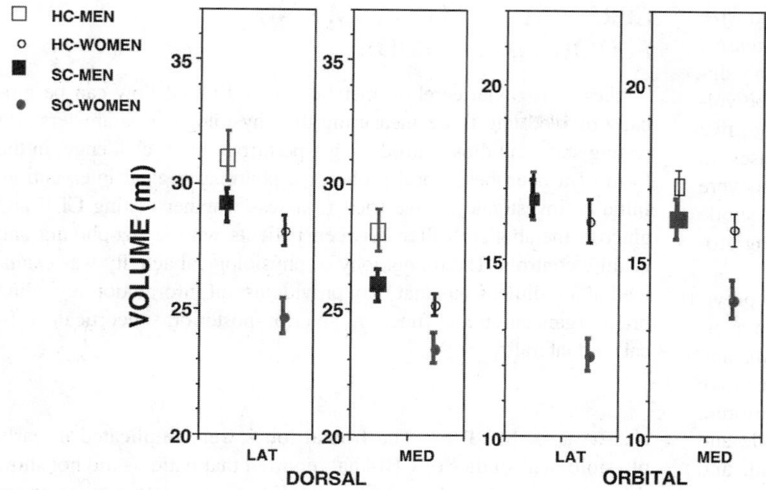

FIGURE 12.6–3 Volume of frontal subregions in healthy controls (HC) and in patients with schizophrenia (SC). LAT, lateral; MED, medial. (From Gur RE, Cowell PE, Latshaw A, et al.: Reduced dorsal and orbital prefrontal gray matter volumes in schizophrenia. *Arch Gen Psychiatry.* 2000;57:761, with permission.)

associated with positive symptom severity in men with schizophrenia in one study, and dorsolateral volume was related to performance on abstraction, attention, and memory in another study. Despite sample sizes and partial inclusion of subfrontal regions, these studies support the hypothesis that increased volume is associated with better performance. In a sample of 70 patients and 81 healthy participants, reduced gray matter volume was observed in the dorsolateral prefrontal cortex (Fig. 12.6–3). The effects were moderated by sex for dorsomedial and orbital regions: In men with schizophrenia, reduced volume was specific to the dorsolateral prefrontal sector, whereas in women, it was reduced in both the orbital and dorsal regions. Greater volume reductions were associated with higher symptom severity and poorer cognitive function.

For the temporal lobe, global lower volume was reported, as well as reduced gray matter but not reduced white matter, with lateralization to the left hemisphere. Regional analysis indicated decreased volume in temporolimbic structures, including the hippocampus (Fig. 12.6–4), parahippocampal gyrus, and amygdala. However, the results are not consistent, and some studies did not report differences in these regions. A metaanalysis examined 18 studies measuring hippocampal volumes, sometimes combined with amygdala. Bilateral hippocampal reduction had a significant effect size, and adding amygdala further increased it. Laterality effects were inconclusive. Cortical temporal regions, especially the superior temporal gyrus, have also been evaluated. Reduced volume has been observed in anterior, posterior, and total superior temporal gyrus and was related to severity of auditory hallucinations and thought disorder. However, other studies have not noted a decrease in superior temporal gyrus volume.

More recently, efforts have focused on identifying neuroanatomical substrates that may relate to clinical subtypes. For example, patients were divided by whether their memory suggested cortical or subcortical dementia. Patients with cortical deficits were more likely male with an earlier age at disease onset and had reduced temporal lobe gray matter. Patients who had memory deficits characteristic of subcortical dementia had ventricular enlargement and more negative symptoms.

Longitudinal Studies

Of note is that the observed volume reductions in schizophrenia are evident at first presentation before treatment. The question of progression of parenchymal tissue loss has been addressed in relatively few studies. Longitudinal studies applying MRI have examined first-episode patients. This is an informative population because the design enables prospective follow-up starting early in the course of illness. One group of investigators found no ventricular changes in a follow-up of 13 patients and 8 controls conducted 1 to 2 years after the initial study. Another study evaluated 16 patients and five controls 2 years after a first psychotic

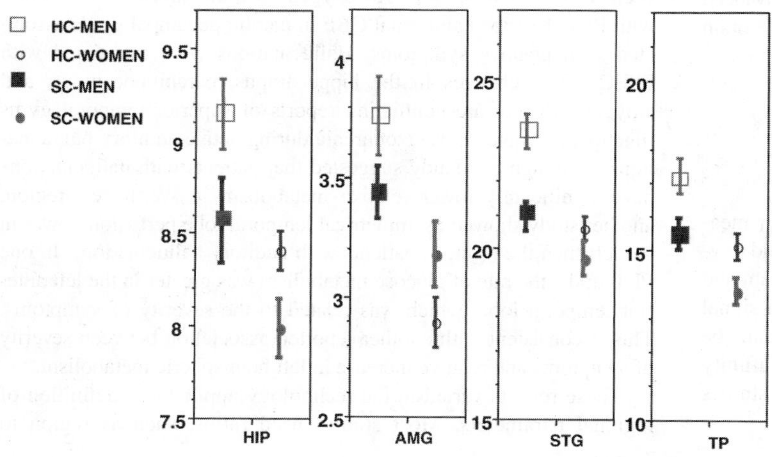

FIGURE 12.6–4 Volume of temporal subregions in healthy controls (HC) and in patients with schizophrenia (SC): controls minus patients. AMG, amygdala; HIP, hippocampus; STG, superior temporal gyrus; TP, temporal pole. (From Gur RE, Turetsky BI, Cowell PE, et al.: Temporolimbic volume reductions in schizophrenia. *Arch Gen Psychiatry.* 2000;57:769, with permission.)

episode. Patients showed no consistent change in ventricular size with time, although there were individual increases or decreases. With a slightly larger group of 24 patients and six controls, no significant changes were observed in ventricular or temporal lobe volume at follow-up. Subsequently, 20 of these patients and five controls were rescanned over 4 years, and greater decreases in whole-brain volume and enlargement in left ventricular volume were observed in patients. The authors of the study concluded that subtle cortical changes may occur after the onset of illness, suggesting progression in some cases.

In a longitudinal study, 40 patients (20 first-episode, 20 previously treated) and 17 healthy participants were rescanned an average of 2.5 years later. The volumes of whole brain, CSF, and frontal and temporal lobes were measured. The severity of negative and positive symptoms was assessed, medications were monitored, and neurobehavioral functioning was evaluated. First-episode and previously treated patients had smaller whole-brain, frontal, and temporal lobe volumes than controls at intake. Longitudinally, reduction in frontal lobe volume was found only in patients, whereas temporal lobe reduction was also seen in controls. The association between volume reduction and symptom change differed between patient groups, but in both first-episode and previously treated patients, volume reduction was associated with decline in some neurobehavioral functions.

The question of specificity of neuroanatomical findings to schizophrenia was addressed in a recent study that evaluated 13 patients with first-episode schizophrenia, 15 patients with first-episode affective psychosis (mainly manic), and 14 healthy comparison subjects longitudinally, with scans separated by 1.5 years. The investigators reported that patients with schizophrenia had progressive decreases in gray matter volume over time in the left superior temporal gyrus compared with both other groups. The existence of neuroanatomical abnormalities in first-episode patients indicates that brain dysfunction occurred before clinical presentation. However, the longitudinal studies suggest evidence of progression in which anatomical changes may impact some clinical and neurobehavioral features of the illness in some patients.

MRI findings have been most consistent for gray matter volume reduction. More recently, white matter changes have also been reported. The availability of diffusion tensor imaging will enhance the efforts to examine compartmental abnormalities. The growing understanding of brain development and MRI data obtained from children suggests that the neuroanatomical neuroimaging literature in schizophrenia is consistent with diffuse disruption of normal maturation. Thus, there is clear evidence for structural abnormalities in schizophrenia associated with reduced cognitive capacity and less clear evidence for structural abnormalities with symptoms. Future work, perhaps with more advanced computerized parcellation methods, is needed to better chart the brain pathways that are most severely affected.

FUNCTIONAL IMAGING STUDIES OF SCHIZOPHRENIA

Functional imaging methods examine brain activity through measures related to energy metabolism, such as rates of glucose and oxygen use and CBF. Methods include PET for glucose metabolism and CBF, SPECT for CBF, and fMRI for measuring changes in signal intensity attributable to CBF. Neuroreceptor function can be assessed using methods for measuring receptor density and affinity at presynaptic and postsynaptic sites. Both PET and SPECT studies have been conducted in people with schizophrenia.

CEREBRAL METABOLISM AND BLOOD FLOW STUDIES

Studies of regional cerebral metabolism and blood flow can be globally divided into those measuring the physiological parameters at a resting state and those introducing a perturbation, or challenge, in the form of a neurobehavioral probe or a pharmacological intervention. Initially, investigators have tried to assess whether resting CBF and glucose metabolism differ between patients with schizophrenia and healthy controls. The topography of physiological activity was examined along dimensions that may provide useful information regarding brain organization and function: anterior–posterior, subcortical–cortical, and laterality.

Resting Baseline The frontal lobes were implicated in early physiological studies of CBF that reported that patients did not show the normal pattern of increased anterior CBF relative to posterior CBF. This hypofrontal disturbance in the anterior–posterior gradient has been supported by some, but not all, studies of resting CBF with the xenon-133 (^{133}Xe) and SPECT and glucose metabolism with PET. The relationship between this pattern of metabolic activity and clinical variables has also been examined. Duration of illness and negative symptoms were associated with decreased frontal metabolic activity. Longer course of illness and more severe negative symptoms were associated with lower anteroposterior gradient.

Differences in resting values between patients and controls were also found in laterality indices, suggesting relatively higher left hemispheric values in more severely ill patients. Furthermore, improvement in clinical status correlated with a shift toward lower left hemispheric metabolism relative to right hemispheric metabolism. This supports hypotheses derived from behavioral data concerning lateralized abnormalities in schizophrenia.

After assessing global, anterior–posterior, and laterality dimensions, investigators have begun the study of functional changes in brain systems linked to other impaired behavior in schizophrenia. Dysfunction in temporal limbic structures, including the hippocampus and temporal cortex, is supported by neuroanatomical and neuropsychological studies. Lateralized abnormalities in these regions, with greater left than right hemispheric dysfunction, are implicated by characteristic clinical features of schizophrenia, such as thought disorder, auditory hallucinations, and language disturbances. PET studies of temporal lobe metabolism include findings of both increased and decreased glucose use. Decreased metabolism was also noted in the hippocampus and anterior cingulate cortex.

Metabolism and flow pattern in temporolimbic regions have also been related to symptoms. An oxygen-15 (^{15}O)–labeled water study with PET described abnormal CBF in parahippocampal gyrus associated with positive symptoms. Hallucinations were associated with SPECT flow changes in the hippocampus, parahippocampus, and amygdala. There are conflicting reports of superior temporal gyrus functional changes in schizophrenia during active auditory hallucinations. Although one study suggested that patients with hallucinations have significantly lower relative metabolism in Wernicke's region, another study showed asymmetrical temporal lobe perfusion, lower in the left than the right, in patients with auditory hallucinations. In one PET study, the rate of glucose metabolism was greater in the left anterior temporal lobe, which was related to the severity of symptoms. This is consistent with another reported association between severity of symptoms and relative increase in left hemispheric metabolism.

These reports varied in the technology applied and definition of regional parameters. Most studies used ratios, such as region to whole brain or anterior to posterior, rather than absolute values of activity. Inconsistencies in findings could also be related to sample size, heterogeneity, analytical approaches, and individual techniques. Most studies included relatively small samples of patients that varied in important clinical factors, such as chronicity, symptom subtypes and severity, level of functioning, and history of treatment. Furthermore, inclusion criteria varied, and some laboratories applied more stringent criteria related, for example, to history of comorbidity of substance abuse and head trauma with loss of consciousness. Another potential source of variability in results is the definition of resting state. Some studies used reduced sensory input, and others used sensory stimulation to standardize this condition. However, several studies have examined the reproducibility of resting baseline measures with relatively unstructured conditions (i.e., eyes open and ears unoccluded, with ambient noise kept to a minimum). These studies found very high reproducibility among healthy subjects and patients with schizophrenia.

Given the demonstrated reliability of the standardized resting baseline condition, it is important to include such a condition in physiological neuroimaging studies. A standardized resting baseline serves three main purposes. First, it permits comparison across studies within a center as technology evolves and patient characteristics change. Without a common resting baseline condition it would be impossible to determine the source of differences in results. Second, it enables comparability across centers. Imagine the need to explain why two centers using the same or similar tasks find evidence for different regional abnormalities in schizophrenia. If resting baseline values are available and are comparable in the two samples, different task effects could be legitimately attributed to theoretically meaningful sources, such as task condition or symptomatic variability. Third, it provides a reference point for evaluating whether a given task or condition has increased neural activity. In studies that have included such a condition, cognitive activation was consistently shown to increase cortical activity in both patients and controls relative to a resting baseline. Using a resting baseline condition enables the investigator to make much stronger statements in the interpretation of regional effects. Rather than being restricted to statements that a given region has changed in its activation relative to the remainder of the brain, resting baseline availability permits stating whether the task has induced increased neural activity.

Functional changes in the basal ganglia have been examined with PET and SPECT. Several PET studies implicate basal ganglia dysfunction in schizophrenia. The withdrawal–retardation factor (emotional withdrawal, blunted affect, and motor retardation) of the Brief Psychiatric Rating Scale (BPRS) has been negatively correlated with PET basal ganglia metabolic activity. Neuroleptic-naïve patients were reported to have relatively increased blood flow in the left globus pallidus. Other PET studies report decreased basal ganglia metabolism in schizophrenia, whereas still others found increased basal ganglia metabolic rates after administration of neuroleptic medication.

Thus, although the contribution of PET metabolic and blood flow studies so far has been to add to the growing evidence implicating basal ganglia involvement in schizophrenia, the exact nature of the dysfunction remains unclear. In particular, the relationship between basal ganglia and frontal lobe activity in schizophrenia needs further scrutiny. There is emerging evidence, revealed by structural and functional imaging, of a dynamic interrelationship between the various key regions. One study showed that patients with schizophrenia not only fail to activate dorsolateral prefrontal cortex in response to the Wisconsin Card Sorting Test, but they also fail to inhibit caudate activation. Hence, in patients with schizophrenia, basal ganglia continue to show relatively increased flow in caudate during performance of the task, as opposed to healthy controls, who seem to demonstrate a reciprocal relationship in which relative blood flow decrease in the basal ganglia is associated with increasing perfusion to the frontal region.

Activation Studies

Measures of CBF and metabolism during the performance of cognitive tasks tend to accentuate differences between patients and controls. Perhaps even more important, such measures are critical for establishing the link between behavioral deficits and the ability of brain regions to become activated in response to task demands. This expectation has been supported in studies that used neurobehavioral probes.

The general approach in the field has been to work from hypotheses derived from neurobehavioral data, which associate behavioral measures with regional brain function. Task selection can be made to include a target task, in which patients are expected to have differential deficit, and control tasks. Patients are then compared to healthy participants in the pattern of task-induced changes in regional brain activity. This has now become the established research paradigm, and significant progress has been made in elucidation of brain systems underlying healthy and pathological behavior.

Early studies obtained CBF resting and performance measures. Although no differences were noted in overall or hemispheric CBF between patients and controls at resting baseline, distinct abnormalities were seen when physiological activity was measured in response to cognitive probes. The nature of the dysfunction was related to the hypothesis examined. For example, pursuing the laterality hypothesis, tasks were administered with demonstrated links to left (verbal) and right (spatial) hemispheric functioning. Healthy controls showed the expected greater left hemispheric increase for the verbal task and greater right hemispheric increase for the spatial task. However, patients with schizophrenia had a bilaterally symmetrical activation for the verbal task and greater left hemispheric activation for the spatial task. Thus, patients did not show the normal left hemispheric dominance for the verbal task and, instead, showed left hemispheric overactivation for the spatial task. Similarly, distinct abnormalities were reported in the dorsolateral prefrontal region during activation with the Wisconsin Card Sorting Test of abstraction and mental flexibility, which is sensitive to frontal lobe damage. The application of this paradigm to the study of monozygotic twins discordant for schizophrenia revealed that all affected twins had reduced dorsolateral prefrontal cortex CBF response compared to discordant co-twins. Furthermore, negative symptoms, which have been related to frontal lobe dysfunction, showed a negative correlation with frontal CBF during performance of executive but not control tasks.

Probing brain systems with specific tasks has also been advanced in SPECT and in CBF studies with PET. These methods have also indicated abnormalities in patients with schizophrenia with a range of tasks, including memory and executive and attentional measures (Fig. 12.6–5).

In a PET study of cerebral blood flow with oxygen-15–labeled water, research participants performed word encoding and word retrieval tasks. While patients with schizophrenia has similar performance to healthy controls, they had reduced cerebral activity in left frontotemporal areas during episodic encoding. These regions were activated during subsequent retrieval, but reduced activation during encoding correlated with poorer recognition performance. This may reflect impaired strategic use of semantic information to organize encoding and facilitate retrieval in schizophrenia. Applying the same PET methodology, another study examined the effects of encoding

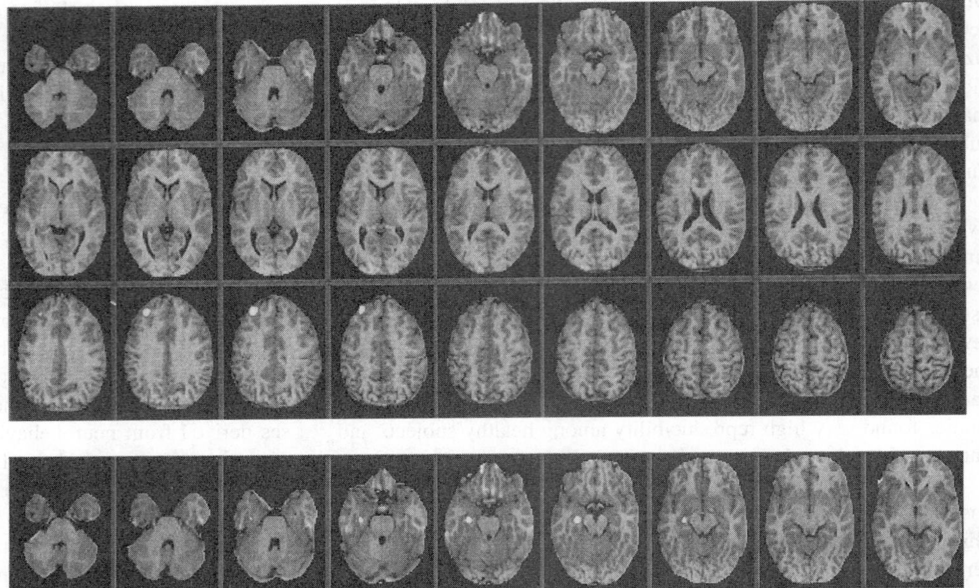

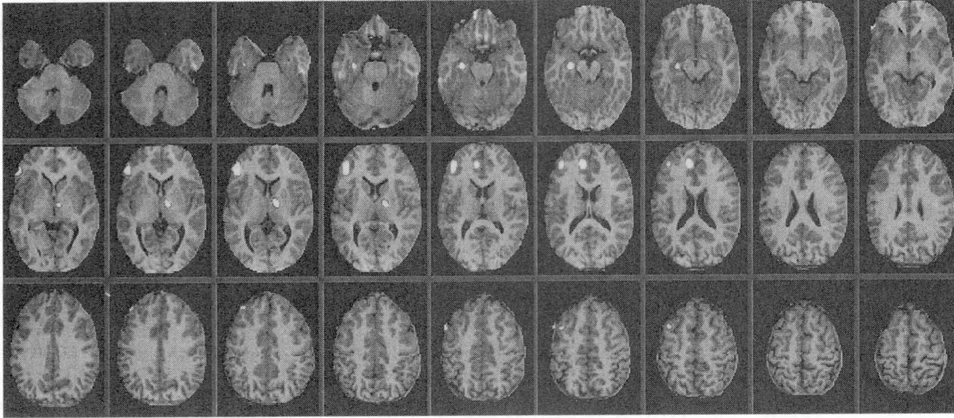

FIGURE 12.6–5 Penn Word Retrieval Test. Positron emission tomography study of memory activation in schizophrenia. **A:** During word encoding, healthy controls (N = 23) show increased activity in the left prefrontal and superior temporal regions relative to patients (N = 23). **B:** During word recognition, controls show greater activation than patients in left prefrontal, left anterior cingulate, left mesial temporal lobe, and right thalamus. (See Color Plate.) (From Ragland JD, Gur RC, Raz J, et al.: Effect of schizophrenia on frontotemporal activity during word encoding and recognition: A PET cerebral blood flow study. *Am J Psychiatry.* 2001;158:1114, with permission.)

interventions, such as item repetition and the formation of semantic associations, on hippocampal activity. Healthy controls recalled more words, but both groups improved performance after encoding intervention. However, the pattern of brain activity differed. In healthy controls, but not in participants with schizophrenia, increased hippocampal blood flow was observed. In patients, greater activation of prefrontal regions was noted during word retrieval.

The consistent finding emerging is lack of normal regional activation in response to task and activation in some regions not seen in healthy subjects. These results suggest that brain systems recruited for the performance of specific tasks in healthy people are not engaged in a similar manner in patients with schizophrenia. What might account for such aberrations? Genetic liability, neurodevelopmental abnormalities in which brain systems fail to achieve maturity, or the impact of a psychotic process that interrupts normally developed structures and processes? Does therapeutic intervention ameliorate the abnormal signature? How specific are the results to schizophrenia? These are some of the questions yet to be answered that can be addressed with neuroimaging.

Functional MRI The introduction of fMRI is an exciting, more recent development in functional imaging research. fMRI methods offer several potential advantages over PET for imaging brain function, including higher spatial resolution, higher temporal resolution, noninvasiveness and lack of ionizing radiation, direct correlation with anatomical imaging, greater repeatability, and economy. Disadvantages of fMRI techniques include the presence of loud background noise generated by the gradient shifts, difficulties in presenting stimuli and performing tasks in the magnet bore, claustrophobia, low signal-to-noise ratio for most methods, and lack of quantitation in physiological units for most methods. Many of these disadvantages can be overcome through the use of specialized equipment compatible with the MRI environment. These methods will be described briefly, because they are recent and hold potential for functional imaging in schizophrenia.

The blood oxygen level dependent (BOLD) method has been most widely applied to fMRI, with results replicating previous PET studies. The technique relies on magnetic susceptibility effects of deoxyhemoglobin, which cause regional decreases in signal in imaging sequences that are sensitive to susceptibility (e.g., echoplanar or routine gradient echo sequences). With regional brain activation studies, a net increase in signal intensity is observed in regions known to be activated by the task. The increase in image intensity corresponds to a local decrease in deoxyhemoglobin. This finding is attributed to a greater increase in regional blood flow than in regional oxygen consumption, a notion supported by PET measurements of blood flow and oxygen consumption with regional brain activation. A wide variety of pulse sequences can be used to obtain BOLD measures. Many simple activation paradigms have been tested, and activation has been observed with both fast and slow imaging. A typical response is a 1 to 25 percent change in regional image intensity that develops over 3 to 8 seconds after task initiation. Susceptibility effects of deoxyhemoglobin are field dependent. Thus, a scanner with 1.5-tesla field strength would typically record signal changes with functional activation of approximately 0.25 to 5.0 percent, whereas, at 4 tesla, changes up to 25 percent have been observed. The main advantages of ultrafast imaging are that time

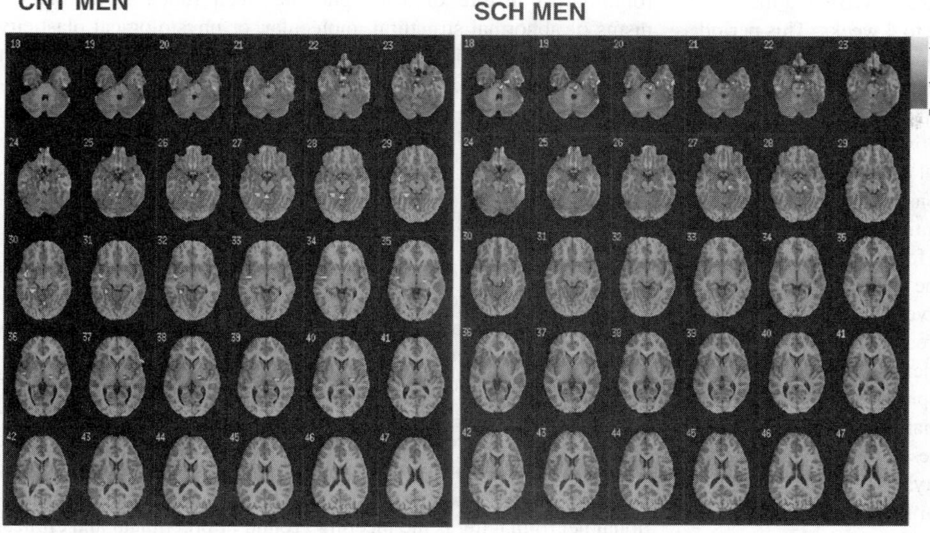

FIGURE 12.6–6 Functional magnetic resonance imaging study of emotion processing in schizophrenia, minus age discrimination. Healthy men (control [CNT]) show greater activation in the amygdala relative to men with schizophrenia (SCH). (See Color Plate.) (From Gur RE, McGrath C, Chan RM, et al.: An fMRI study of facial emotion processing in schizophrenia. *Am J Psychiatry*. 2002; 159:1992, with permission.)

course of signal change can be observed and multislice imaging can be carried out in a reasonable period.

Arterial spin tagging (quantitative perfusion imaging) uses magnetization tagging of endogenous arterial water to determine perfusion of brain parenchyma by comparing images obtained with and without labeling of the arterial supply. The method is analogous to steady-state techniques used in PET, as the regional signal intensity is dependent on the arterial blood flow that delivers labeled spins and the T1 relaxation rate, which causes the labeling to decay. This technique has the important advantage of providing quantitative CBF parameters. Furthermore, perfusion is measured in brain parenchyma directly and is, thus, better localized than measurements obtained using an intravascular tracer, which is most sensitive to venous outflow effects. There may also be less motion sensitivity than with BOLD.

The transition from isotopic methods to fMRI for measuring regional brain activation has been embraced by investigators, because of the advantages offered. Consequently, numerous experiments have applied neurocognitive paradigms in fMRI studies aimed at dissecting complex behavior. Most of these studies have involved healthy people, applying the BOLD method using blocked designs and, more recently, event-related paradigms. Relative to the wide range of neurocognitive processes examined in healthy people, there have been fewer fMRI studies in schizophrenia. Studies have reported abnormal activity in response to motor tasks, working memory, attention, word fluency, emotion processing, and medication effects in 1.5-tesla scanners. More recent investigations have been conducted in higher fields. These functional neuroimaging studies have successfully linked deficits in performance to abnormalities in activation patterns.

In one study of word memory, patients had reduced activation in anterior prefrontal, posterior cingulate, and retrosplenial areas during word encoding. The word recognition task was associated with reduced activation in the patients' dorsolateral prefrontal and limbic/paralimbic regions. Yet, higher activity was observed in bilateral anterior prefrontal cortices. Thus, it appears that patients do not recruit the same neural circuitry as healthy people.

Given the documented deficits in emotion processing associated with schizophrenia, fMRI studies have targeted emotion circuitry with neurobehavioral probes using predominately facial stimuli. Overall, studies have reported reduced limbic activation in schizophrenia both for mood induction effects and for emotion discrimination tasks. For example, in one study, participants viewed facial displays of happiness, sadness, anger, fear, and disgust, and neutral faces. Their task alternated between emotion and age discrimination with a cross-hair reference condition interleaved. Patients and healthy controls did not differ in performance on either task. However, there were voxels in the left amygdala and bilateral hippocampus in which controls had significantly greater activation than patients. Failure to activate limbic regions during emotional valence discrimination may explain emotion-processing deficits in patients with schizophrenia. Although the lack of limbic recruitment did not significantly impair simple valence discrimination performance in this clinically stable group, it may impact performance of more demanding tasks (Fig. 12.6–6).

Methodological Considerations and Treatment Effects

Task difficulty and effort must be investigated to understand the mechanisms through which disturbed behavior emanates from abnormal activation. Differences in activation patterns can be difficult to interpret in the face of differences in performance. The underlying assumption in the measurement of brain activation is that neuronal activity drives mental effort. Given comparable basal abilities, greater activation should relate to better performance. However, in schizophrenia, it is unclear how a finding of reduced or increased activation should be interpreted. One approach is to make the tasks easy so that patients and controls perform equally. However, the truncated performance range in the healthy group limits the ability to associate performance to brain activation. More difficult tasks in which individual differences can be examined are necessary to better understand abnormal brain circuitry.

A host of clinical variables requires attention in functional imaging studies. These variables include patient subtype, severity of symptoms, and treatment status. The complexity of the studies and their typically small samples result in limited conclusions. Considering treatment, the pharmacological status of patients undergoing metabolic and blood flow studies has varied. Research has ranged from investigations in which neuroleptics were considered a variable to be controlled to those in which pharmacological intervention was introduced in a standardized fashion to examine treatment effects on the regional metabolic landscape. The washout period in studies that attempted to control the effects of neuroleptics on CBF and metabolism has typically been short, ranging from 2 to 4 weeks. This period is a compromise between what is feasible and what is desirable. A large sample of unmedicated men with schizophrenia underwent a PET cerebral glucose metabolism study, and cortical-striatal-thalamic circuitry was evaluated. Low metabolic activity in medial frontal cortical regions and the basal ganglia, as well as an impaired lateralization pattern in frontal and temporal regions, was observed in the patient group. The inclusion of neuroleptic-naïve, first-episode patients is particularly informative when the focus of the study is the effects of pharmacological intervention. The study of neuroleptic-naïve patients before pharmacological intervention permits evaluation of the disease state separate from its treatment. The pattern of abnormalities is evident in first-episode patients across studies that examined differences between their first episode and episodes of previously treated patients. This suggests that disruption in normal brain processes is already apparent at the presentation of illness and cannot be attributed to treatment or chronicity.

A repeated-measures longitudinal design has been applied in a limited number of functional imaging studies. In addition to examining the symptom severity over time, this paradigm is particularly useful when pharmacological intervention is standardized. One study compared the effects of thiothixene (Navane) and haloperidol (Haldol) in chronic patients who were scanned off medication and after 4 to 6 weeks on medication. A different pattern of global and regional glucose metabolism was seen in the two groups. In another study, PET scans were obtained at weeks 5 and 10 of a double-blind, crossover trial of haloperidol and placebo in 25 patients with schizophrenia. Low relative metabolism in the striatum on placebo was associated with improved symptomatology. Responders to treatment had increased metabolism in the striatum after treatment. Nonresponders failed to show such a change and had more marked hypofrontality on medication. In a subsequent study, 12 patients were scanned before and 4 to 6 weeks after treatment with clozapine (Clozaril) or thiothixene. The drugs had a differential effect, with clozapine increasing metabolism and thiothixene decreasing metabolism in the basal ganglia (right more than left). Henry Holcomb and colleagues, in a repeated-measures design, studied glucose metabolism in 12 patients when on a fixed dose of haloperidol and 5 and 30 days after drug withdrawal. No differences were observed between metabolism on medication and after 5 days of discontinuation. However, at 30 days, decreased metabolism was noted in the caudate, putamen, and anterior thalamus, whereas there was an increase in the frontal cortex and anterior cingulate. The authors of the study concluded that the basal ganglia is the site of primary antidopaminergic action of haloperidol and that other changes observed are mediated through the striatal-thalamic-cortical pathways. The integration of pharmacological and neurobehavioral probes is a potentially powerful approach. For example, it was noted that in patients with schizophrenia, there was enhanced activation of the anterior cingulate after administration of apomorphine, suggesting a modulating role for dopamine.

Application of neurobehavioral probes during functional imaging studies is a productive avenue in the effort to define involvement of neural systems in the pathophysiology of schizophrenia. Such neurobehavioral probes document deficits in performance associated with abnormal brain activation, perhaps sparing the sensory domain and implicating the ventromedial temporal lobe, prefrontal cortices, and limbic subcortical nuclei, which mediate memory, executive functioning, and attention. These systems are characterized by dynamic plasticity, high connectivity, and vulnerability to insult, consistent with the hypothesis that abnormal plasticity is a core neurobiological feature of schizophrenia. Such fundamental mechanisms of abnormal structural, molecular, or physiological plasticity should be evident throughout the central nervous system (CNS) but most prominently expressed in neural systems mediating activity-dependent cognitive processes of attention, memory, and executive functioning.

NEURORECEPTOR STUDIES

Study of Neuroreceptors The study of neuroreceptors is another critical window for assessing brain function and can give insight on the nature of neurochemical abnormalities in schizophrenia. Because advances in elucidating the pathophysiology of schizophrenia require understanding of neurotransmitter function, the application of PET and SPECT to the study of receptors is an important domain with treatment implications. These efforts are guided both by an extensive psychopharmacological literature and by advances in basic neuroscience on neuroreceptor subtyping. Functional neuroimaging is the meeting ground of preclinical and clinical neuropharmacology. Human neuroreceptor PET studies have built on progress with in vitro binding measurements of receptor density and affinity and neuroreceptor autoradiography.

PET and SPECT Studies Earlier work with radioligands for PET studies focused on the dopamine type 2 (D_2) receptor. The psychotic symptoms noted in schizophrenia have been associated with dysfunction of dopamine, which is targeted in treatment with neuroleptics. Two major methodologies for quantitative measurement were developed and applied in the study of schizophrenia. One set of studies applied [^{11}C]*N*-methylspiperone and reported that patients relative to controls have higher D_2 maximal binding capacity (B_{max}) values. A second set of studies using [^{11}C]raclopride reported similar B_{max} and distribution coefficient (K_d) values in patients and controls. These apparent differences have been discussed and summarized extensively and are likely related to multiple factors, including patient variables, ligand properties, and PET modeling methods. Because the ligands differ in binding properties and sensitivity to endogenous dopamine, studies permitting a more direct comparison have been instructive. For example, the reproducibility of the [^{11}C]*N*-methylspiperone finding in a study of seven neuroleptic-naïve patients and seven controls before and after administration of 7.5 mg of haloperidol was examined. Consistent with a previous quantitative PET study of [^{11}C]raclopride binding, there were no differences between patients and controls pretreatment, and, after haloperidol, the specific binding of [^{11}C]*N*-methylspiperone was reduced by 80 to 90 percent. In further efforts, the initial results obtained with [^{11}C]*N*-methylspiperone were replicated in a new sample of drug-naïve patients with schizophrenia. Other data revealed that D_2 density increased in psychotic patients but not in nonpsychotic patients with bipolar disorder. The degree of increase was comparable to that reported in schizophrenia. This raises questions regarding the specificity of the dopamine hypothesis to schizophrenia versus other disorders with psychotic features.

Other ligands have also been applied. For example, D_2 striatal dopamine receptors were evaluated with [^{76}Br]bromospiperone in PET studies of untreated patients with schizophrenia compared to healthy people. There was no increase in striatum to cerebellum ratios of D_2 receptors in patients relative to controls, and no relation to symptoms or subtypes emerged. A PET study with ^{11}C-FLB 457, a radioligand for extrastriatal D_2 dopamine receptors, examined 11 drug-naïve men with schizophrenia and 18 healthy controls. Extrastriatal binding potential differences were observed in the anterior cingulate cortex, where patients had a 12.5 percent reduction relative to controls.

The D_2 receptor SPECT ligand iodide-benzamide [^{123}I]iodobenzamide (IBZM) has been applied in studying dopamine D_2 receptors in patients with schizophrenia. In earlier work, a large sample of 56 patients was evaluated and a semiquantitative analysis of D_2 receptor binding was calculated (basal ganglia to frontal cortex ratio of activity). The basal ganglia to frontal cortex ratios in patients taking typical neuroleptics were significantly lower than those of the neuroleptic-free patients but not lower than those of patients taking the atypical agents clozapine and remoxipride. No overall elevation of D_2 receptor binding was observed when comparing 20 patients off medications and 20 controls, a finding similar to PET studies that examined D_2 receptor occupancy.

D_1 dopamine receptor function in schizophrenia was also examined in PET studies. ^{11}C-labeled SCH23390 with high and low specific radioactivity was administered to ten neuroleptic-naïve patients and ten controls. There were no differences between the two groups in receptor density and affinity measured in the caudate nucleus, the putamen, and several neocortical regions. Other ligands are currently being applied to evaluate serotonergic and muscarinic function with both PET and SPECT ligands.

Receptor Function and Clinical Response

The study of neuroreceptors can also address issues related to the relationship between receptor function and clinical signs, such as akathisia, commonly seen in patients treated with conventional neuroleptics. Thus, for example, PET studies at low and high doses of [^{11}C]SCH23390, a selective D_1 dopamine receptor antagonist, were conducted in healthy people. Transient akathisia occurred only when binding in the basal ganglia was at a high level, with 45 to 59 percent occupancy. The D_2 dopamine receptor antagonist [^{11}C]raclopride was measured in 13 patients with schizophrenia and 20 healthy participants. Akathisia was associated in patients and controls with maximal ligand binding in the basal ganglia. Other clinical features have been evaluated in relation to receptor function. Treatment resistant patients did not differ from neuroleptic responders in degree of D_2 receptor occupancy by the neuroleptic agents. The regional distribution and kinetics of haloperidol binding were studied with [^{18}F]haloperidol in a PET study of five patients with schizophrenia examined while on haloperidol and after a drug washout and nine controls. Wide regional distribution of the ligand was evident in the cerebellum, basal ganglia, and thalamus, in contrast to the specific binding to the basal ganglia of [^{18}F]*N*-methylspiroperidol. Thus, small structural differences among butyrophenones are associated with changes in kinetics and distribution.

Typical and Atypical Antipsychotics

PET neuroreceptor methods have also been applied in the study of atypical antipsychotic drugs compared to typical antipsychotic drugs. The properties of clozapine binding to D_1 and D_2 dopamine receptors were examined in an open study of 5 patients relative to 22 patients treated with typical neuroleptics. Clozapine induced lower D_2 occupancy (38 to 63 percent), whereas D_2 receptor occupancy with typical neuroleptics at conventional doses was 70 to 89 percent. Neuroleptic-induced extrapyramidal syndromes were associated with higher D_2 occupancy. In a follow-up study, the relationship between D_2 receptor occupancy and antipsychotic drug effect was examined in a double-blind study using [^{11}C]raclopride. Seventeen patients with schizophrenia were randomly assigned to three groups treated with a varied dose of raclopride. A PET study was conducted at steady state on 13 patients during the third to fourth week of treatment. A curvilinear relationship between plasma concentration of raclopride and D_2 receptor occupancy was obtained. A significant relationship was noted between D_2 receptor occupancy and Brief Psychiatric Rating Scale percent change as a measure of outcome. The D_2 receptor occupancy in patients who had extrapyramidal side effects was higher than in patients with no extrapyramidal side effects. Further work examined D_1, D_2, and 5-hydroxytryptamine type 2 (5-HT_2) receptor occupancy in 17 patients treated with clozapine (125 to 600 mg per day) applying [^{11}C]SCH23390, ^{11}C-raclopride, and [^{11}C]*N*-methylspiperone. D_2 receptor occupancy (20 to 67 percent) was lower than for typical neuroleptics (70 to 90 percent), D_1 receptor occupancy (36 to 59 percent) was higher than that reported for typical neuroleptics (0 to 44 percent), and 5-HT_2 receptor occupancy was high (84 to 94 percent). Thus, clozapine shows a combination of relatively high D_1, low D_2, and very high 5-HT_2 receptor occupancy values, with serum concentrations not predictive of degree of receptor occupancy. In a PET study of [^{11}C]raclopride, another group of investigators determined D_2 receptor occupancy induced by 2 mg per day of haloperidol for 2 weeks in seven patients. High levels of D_2 occupancy (53 to 74 percent) were noted with substantial clinical improvement. A similar investigation in nine patients receiving 2 to 6 mg per day of risperidone (Risperdal) showed receptor occupancy (66 to 79 percent) similar to that of typical neuroleptics and higher than that of clozapine.

Another study that illustrates the implications of this line of research to treatment evaluated seven first-episode or drug-free patients. They were treated with risperidone, 6 mg per day for 4 weeks, and then 3 mg per day for 2 weeks. PET studies were performed after 4 and 6 weeks, with [^{11}C]raclopride to measure D_2 receptor occupancy and [^{11}C]*N*-methylspiperone to measure 5-HT_{2A} receptor occupancy. Participants were treatment responsive, and none had extrapyramidal side effects when entering the study. At the 6-mg-per-day dose, mean D_2 receptor occupancy was 82 percent (range, 79 to 85 percent), 5-HT_{2A} receptor occupancy was 95 percent (range, 86 to 109 percent), and 6 patients had developed extrapyramidal side effects. After dose reduction to 3 mg per day, D_2 receptor occupancy ranged from 53 to 78 percent, and 5-HT_{2A} receptor occupancy range was 65 to 112 percent. Three patients still had extrapyramidal side effects at the reduced dose. This suggests that treatment with 4 mg per day of risperidone can achieve a beneficial antipsychotic effect with a minimal risk of extrapyramidal side effects. A recent study examined the relationship between D_2 receptor occupancy level and subjective experience in patients with recent-onset schizophrenia. Patients were randomly assigned to 6 weeks of double-blind treatment with either olanzapine, 7.5 mg per day, or haloperidol, 2.5 mg per day. Receptor occupancy was assessed with IBZM SPECT. Receptor occupancy between 60 and 70 percent was associated with optimal subjective experience, but variability was evident. This indicates the need for individual titration of dose to reach optimal occupancy.

These research paradigms illustrate the integration of functional neuroimaging with pharmacological research. Incorporation of these strategies into psychopharmacological studies of schizophrenia with available and new therapeutic agents can advance the field and guide treatment intervention.

METABOLITE STUDIES: MR SPECTROSCOPY

MRS provides analytical qualitative and quantitative data on cellular metabolism and molecular structure. It has been used to study metabolism in vitro and in vivo in animals and humans. Spectral localization methods permit the measurement of hydrogen-1 (^{1}H) and phosphorus-31 (^{31}P) nuclear magnetic resonance (NMR) spectra from precisely localized volumes of interest, and this provides the basis for applying these techniques to study brain diseases. Because the technology is fundamentally similar to that used in MRI, several groups have developed approaches that integrate these two modalities into a single examination.

There is a growing literature using this method to investigate the underlying metabolism of neuropsychiatric disorders, including schizophrenia. Early work in the field applied ^{31}P methods to the study of schizophrenia, reporting hypofunction in the dorsolateral prefrontal cortex in neuroleptic-naïve patients. In the patients, the levels of inorganic phosphate were decreased and the levels of adenosine triphosphate (ATP) were increased. These latter results were interpreted as reflecting hypofunction of the dorsal prefrontal cortex. This interpretation is consistent with reports of decreased blood flow and decreased use of glucose in this region, as summarized above. A follow-up case report described a patient who exhibited in the ^{31}P MRS spectra similar to those reported for schizophrenia well before the onset of psychotic symptoms. This finding led the investigators to propose that MRS may be of value in examining high-risk subjects, such as family members of patients with schizophrenia, for the presence of spectral abnormalities. Another group reported ^{31}P MRS results consistent with these findings. This suggests the possibility of dysfunction in the normal process of programmed synaptic pruning, critical in brain maturation. Abnormal pruning could result in neuronal loss, as well as upregulation of the postsynaptic dopaminergic receptors. These changes observed by ^{31}P clearly suggest that there should be alterations in the levels of the compounds routinely detectable by localized proton MRS.

There has been considerable interest in obtaining solvent suppressed proton spectra in humans. Technical advances have made it possible to relate MRS measurements to the underlying biochemistry occurring in the tissue being sampled. *N*-acetylaspartate (NAA), found by NMR in glia and neurons but not on astrocytes, has been proposed as an index of neuronal integrity. The measurements of amino acids present in the brain have been promising. There is approximately 12 mM of glutamate (Glu) present in the brain, making it, by far, the most abundant amino acid. The rate of Glu synthesis and oxidation is different in astrocytes and neurons. Two important products of Glu metabolism are glutamine (Gln), which is formed from Glu by Glu synthetase located in astrocytes, and γ-aminobutyric acid (GABA), which is an inhibitory neurotransmitter. Aspects of the metabolism of these compounds and the influence of this metabolism on MRS spectral appearance have been examined. Glu is largely confined by barriers in permeability to the tissue in which it is formed. Gln can be converted to Glu at the site of neurotransmitter activity by glutaminase, which is present in neurons. The combination of two enzymes, Gln synthetase (converts Glu to Gln) and glutaminase (converts Gln to Glu), acts as a sort of cycle to maintain the concentrations of Glu and Gln. The levels of GABA and Glu were determined by MRS in cultured preparations of cortical neurons and cerebellar granule cells. Extracts of granule cells contained large amounts of Glu, whereas the neuronal cells contained large amounts of GABA.

Detection of these compounds in vivo in clinical studies showed elevated levels of Gln in patients with chronic hepatic encephalopathy, and spectral editing methods can be applied to determine the levels of Glu in the human brain. The concentrations of Glu reported were in excellent agreement with literature values. The measurement of Glu in these studies was referenced to the concentration of the total creatine present (9.6 mM) in the brain. The key feature in this methodology was the use of short echo delays (12 milliseconds) to obtain estimates of the Glu present. Thus, MRS can be used to measure the levels of these amino acids, and the levels of these compounds may provide some insights into the activity of the excitatory (Glu) and inhibitory (GABA) neurotransmitters present in the tissue being sampled. Based on these methodological advances, studies applying spectroscopy in schizophrenia have increased.

The levels of Glu, Gln, and NAA were acquired at 4.0 tesla from 21 first-episode, neuroleptic-naïve patients with schizophrenia. The Gln level was significantly higher in the left anterior cingulate cortex and thalamus of patients compared to healthy subjects, and no differences were noted for other metabolites. The findings support the role of glutamatergic activity in the pathophysiology of schizophrenia. The lack of difference between patients and controls in the levels of NAA, a finding reported in other studies of first-episode, neuroleptic-naïve patients, may relate to the brain region sampled. Regions of interest examined differ in MRS studies and have included the dorsolateral prefrontal cortex, medial temporal lobe, anterior cingulate, and thalamus. Studies that have reported lower NAA concentration in the mediodorsal region of the thalamus included chronically treated patients with schizophrenia.

With growing experience and application of MRS, metabolite measures have been related to clinical variables, including symptoms and treatment. For example, in a study of 36 patients with schizophrenia, a regionally selective negative correlation was reported between prefrontal NAA to creatine ratio and negative symptoms. In a repeated-measures design, the investigators also evaluated 23 patients when stable on antipsychotics for at least 4 weeks and when off medications for at least 2 weeks. When treated, patients had higher NAA measures in the dorsolateral prefrontal cortex, suggesting a region-specific effect. To examine whether glutamatergic activity may contribute to the therapeutic effect of olanzapine (Zyprexa), Glu concentrations were measured in serum and were estimated in cingulate cortex in a within-subject design. Ten patients with schizophrenia were initially evaluated when treated with conventional neuroleptics, and the study was repeated 8 weeks after a crossover to olanzapine. Brain Glu activity did not change significantly in the group, but concentrations increased with an improvement in negative symptoms.

MRS technology has provided estimates of brain concentrations of important cerebral metabolites, which are related to neuronal function and have been implicated in the pathophysiology of schizophrenia. Advances in magnetic field strength, data acquisition, and processing will enhance spatial and temporal resolution. Such progress, linked to other measures of cerebral function in the physiological and neurobehavioral domains, holds promise for the elucidation of pathophysiology and the understanding of therapeutics.

CHALLENGES AND FUTURE DIRECTIONS

Considerable progress with a range of neuroimaging technologies has been made in efforts to advance the understanding of the neurobiology of schizophrenia. However, the underlying mechanisms at play remain elusive. Difficulties in identifying mechanisms are endemic to disorders of complex behavior. No gene; pathological lesion; cellular, molecular, or neurochemical abnormality; or specific neural system has been recognized as being central to schizophrenia. Instead, abnormalities are evident at many levels of neurobehavioral and neurophysiological processing and in multiple neural systems—from the cerebellum to diencephalon to primary, association, and limbic cortices and the olfactory bulb. These diffuse abnormalities, which implicate neurodevelopmental aberrations, are not fully expressed as a disorder until after brain development and maturation are largely completed.

The recognition that the underlying pathological processes of schizophrenia are present throughout the CNS suggests that there may be some core defects in neurotransmission whereby the ability of neurons to respond to and process stimuli is curtailed. However, within the context of global abnormalities, some neural systems are differentially affected. Brain regions with greater vulnerability, such as the hippocampus, prefrontal cortex, and olfactory system, are dynamic and maintain a high degree of plasticity during brain maturation and thereafter.

Both structural and functional neuroimaging studies suggest that diffuse abnormalities are evident in neuroleptic-naïve, first-episode patients with schizophrenia and can be linked to neurobehavioral and neuropsychiatric manifestations. These research methods can be applied as endophenotypic measures to informative populations in genetic paradigms, such as individuals at high risk. Furthermore, evidence for progressive changes in some patients, perhaps associated with some treatments, encourages longitudinal studies.

In the context of the overall effort in neurobiological research in schizophrenia, functional neuroimaging studies have contributed to advance the understanding of brain dysfunction related to neurobehavior and neuropharmacology. The field has reached some maturity in developing appropriate paradigms, and there is now a need for adequate sample size in patient and healthy populations, with attention to clinical heterogeneity and variability in brain function in relation to gender and age.

One of the major challenges in this research is the integration of neuroimaging data, across anatomical and functional measures, with clinical and neurobehavioral variables. A potential strength of functional neuroimaging is the integration of data on neuroreceptor function, metabolites, and metabolic activity. Ultimately, dysfunctional neurotransmitter systems translate to aberrant metabolism. Because CBF and metabolism reflect neuronal activity, relating these domains is prerequisite for understanding the neurobiology of schizophrenia. As new receptor subtypes are cloned and radioligands are developed and available for human studies, it will be necessary to know which neuroreceptor measures result in increased neuronal activity and, in turn, how regional activation relates to behavior.

Thus, although new receptor ligands, improved resolution, and the development of methods for MR spectroscopy and flow measures are welcome and exciting, it is unlikely that the neural basis of schizophrenia will be found simply by applying the right method with sufficient resolution. Rather, it seems that the harder and longer route of understanding the interaction among the brain's structural integrity, regional activity, and neuroreceptors as they affect the clinical and neurobehavioral manifestations of schizophrenia must be undertaken.

These challenges are compounded by the absence of suitable animal models for the disorder as currently phenotypically defined, buttressing the need to identify endophenotypes that can be studied in both humans and animals. The identification of such endophenotypes in schizophrenia that have their counterparts in rodents enables investigation of the genetic, molecular, biochemical, anatomical, and physiological aspects of these behaviors. The technological developments in animal imaging will enhance the capabilities to conduct translational research. This top-down–bottom-up interchange holds great promise for advancing the understanding of the pathophysiology of schizophrenia.

SUGGESTED CROSS-REFERENCES

Functional neuroanatomy is covered in Section 1.2. The neural basis of schizophrenia psychopathology is further discussed in Section 12.7.

References

Andreasen NC, O'Leary DS, Watkins GL, Ponto LL, Hichwa RD: Neural mechanisms of anhedonia in schizophrenia: A PET study of response to unpleasant and pleasant odors. *JAMA*. 2001;286:427.

Bertolino A, Callicott JH, Mattay VS, Weidenhammer KM, Rakow R, Egan MF, Weinberger DR: The effect of treatment with antipsychotic drugs on brain *N*-acetylaspartate measures in patients with schizophrenia. *Biol Psychiatry*. 2001;49:39.

Crespo-Facorro B, Paradiso S, Gur RC, Ragland JD, Moberg PJ, Bilker WB, Kohler C, Siegel SJ, Gur RE: Computerized neurocognitive scanning II: The profile of schizophrenia. *Neuropsychopharmacology*. 2001;25:777.

de Haan L, van Bruggen M, Lavalaye J, Booij J, Dingemans PM, Linszen D: Subjective experience and D2 receptor occupancy in patients with recent-onset schizophrenia treated with low-dose olanzapine or haloperidol: A randomized, double-blind study. *Am J Psychiatry*. 2003;160:303.

Gur RE: Temporolimbic volume reductions in schizophrenia. *Arch Gen Psychiatry*. 2000;57:769.

*Gur RE, Chin S: Laterality in functional brain imaging studies in schizophrenia. *Schizophr Bull*. 1999;25:141.

Gur RE, Cowell PE, Latshaw A, Turetsky BI, Grossman RI, Arnold SE, Bilker WB, Gur RC: Reduced dorsal and orbital prefrontal gray matter volumes in schizophrenia. *Arch Gen Psychiatry*. 2000;57:761.

Gur RE, Cowell P, Turetsky BI, Gallacher F, Cannon T, Bilker W, Gur RC: A follow-up magnetic resonance imaging study of schizophrenia. *Arch Gen Psychiatry*. 1998;55:145.

Gur RE, McGrath C, Chan RM, Schroeder L, Turner T, Turetsky BI, Kohler C, Alsop D, Maldjian J, Ragland JD, Gur RC: An fMRI study of facial emotion processing in schizophrenia. *Am J Psychiatry*. 2002;159:1992.

Gur RE, Turetsky BI, Cowell PE, Finkelman C, Maany V, Grossman RI, Arnold SE, Bilker WB, Heinrichs RW, Zakzanis KK: Neurocognitive deficit in schizophrenia: A quantitative review of the evidence. *Neuropsychology*. 1998;12:426.

Hofer A, Weiss EM, Golaszewski SM, Siedentopf CM, Brinkhoff C, Kremser C, Felber S, Fleischhacker WW: Neural correlates of episodic encoding and recognition of words in unmedicated patients during an acute episode of schizophrenia: A functional MRI study. *Am J Psychiatry*. 2003;160:1802.

Honey GD, Bullmore ET, Soni W, Varatheesan M, Williams SCR, Sharma T: Differences in frontal cortical activation by a working memory task after substitution of risperidone for typical antipsychotic drugs in patients with schizophrenia. *Proc Natl Acad Sci U S A*. 1999;96:13432.

Honey GD, Sharma T, Suckling J, Giampetro V, Soni W, Williams SC, Bullmore ET: The functional neuroanatomy of schizophrenic subsyndromes. *Psychol Med*. 2003;33:1007.

Karlsson P, Farde L, Halldin C, Sedvall G: PET study of D(1) dopamine receptor binding in neuroleptic-naive patients with schizophrenia. *Am J Psychiatry*. 2002;159:761.

Kasai K, Shenton ME, Salisbury DF, Hirayasu Y, Lee CU, Ciszewski AA, Yurgelun-Todd D, Keshavan MS, Stanley JA, Pettegrew JW: Magnetic resonance spectroscopy in schizophrenia: Methodological issues and findings—part II. *Biol Psychiatry*. 2000;48:369.

Kikinis R, Jolesz FA, McCarley RW: Progressive decrease of left superior temporal gyrus gray matter volume in patients with first-episode schizophrenia. *Am J Psychiatry*. 2003;160:156.

Kohler CG, Gur RC, Gur RE: Emotional processes in schizophrenia: A focus on affective states. In: Borod JC, ed. *The Neuropsychology of Emotion*. Oxford: Oxford University Press, 2000.

Lim KO, Hedehus M, Moseley M, de Crespigny A, Sullivan EV, Pfefferbaum A: Compromised white matter tract integrity in schizophrenia inferred from diffusion tensor imaging. *Arch Gen Psychiatry*. 1999;56:367.

*Lyoo IK, Renshaw PF: Magnetic resonance spectroscopy: Current and future applications in psychiatric research. *Biol Psychiatry*. 2002;51:195.

Manoach DS, Gollub RL, Benson ES, Searl MM, Goff DC, Halpern E, Saper CB, Rauch SL: Schizophrenic subjects show aberrant fMRI activation of dorsolateral prefrontal cortex and basal ganglia during working memory performance. *Biol Psychiatry*. 2000;48:99.

Mitelman SA, Shihabuddin L, Brickman AM, Hazlett EA, Buchsbaum MS: MRI assessment of gray and white matter distribution in Brodmann's areas of the cortex in patients with schizophrenia with good and poor outcomes. *Am J Psychiatry*. 2003;160:2154.

Moberg PJ, Agrin, RN, Gur RE, Gur RC, Turetsky BI, Doty RL: Olfactory dysfunction in schizophrenia: A qualitative and quantitative review. *Neuropsychopharmacology*. 1999;21:325.

Nelson MD, Saykin AJ, Flashman LA, Riordan HJ: Hippocampal volume reduction in schizophrenia as assessed by magnetic resonance imaging: A meta-analytic study. *Arch Gen Psychiatry*. 1998;55:433.

Nyberg S, Eriksson B, Oxenstierna G, Halldin C, Farde L: Suggested minimal effective dose of risperidone based on PET-measured D2 and 5-HT2A receptor occupancy in schizophrenic patients. *Am J Psychiatry*. 1999;156:869.

Pearlson GD, Marsh L: Structural brain imaging in schizophrenia: A selective review. *Biol Psychiatry*. 1999;46:627.

Ragland JD, Gur RC, Raz J, Schroeder L, Smith RJ, Alavi A, Gur RE: Effect of schizophrenia on frontotemporal activity during word encoding and recognition: A PET cerebral blood flow study. *Am J Psychiatry*. 2001;158:1114.

Saykin AJ, Shtasel DL, Gur RE, Kester DB, Mozley LH, Stafiniak P, Gur RC: Neuropsychological deficits in neuroleptic-naïve, first-episode schizophrenic patients. *Arch Gen Psychiatry*. 1994;51:124.

*Sharma T, Harvey P, eds. *Cognition in Schizophrenia*. Oxford: Oxford University Press, 1999.

*Shenton ME, Dickey CC, Frumin M, McCarley RW: A review of MRI findings in schizophrenia. *Schizophr Res*. 2001;49:1.

Stanley JA, Pettegrew JW, Keshavan MS: Magnetic resonance spectroscopy in schizophrenia: Methodological issues and findings—part I. *Biol Psychiatry*. 2000;48:357.

Suhara T, Okubo Y, Yasuno F, Sudo Y, Inoue M, Ichimiya T, Nakashima Y, Nakayama K, Tanada S, Suzuki K, Halldin C, Farde L: Decreased dopamine D_2 receptor binding in the anterior cingulate cortex in schizophrenia. *Arch Gen Psychiatry*. 2002;59:31.

*Tauscher J, Kapur S: Choosing the right dose of antipsychotics in schizophrenia: Lessons from neuroimaging studies. *CNS Drugs*. 2001;15:671.

Theberge J, Bartha R, Drost DJ, Menon RS, Malla A, Takhar J, Neufeld RW, Rogers J, Pavlosky W, Schaefer B, Densmore M, Al-Semaan Y, Williamson PC: Glutamate and glutamine measured with 4.0 T proton MRS in never-treated patients with schizophrenia and healthy volunteers. *Am J Psychiatry*. 2002;159:1944.

Turetsky BI, Moberg PJ, Mozley LH, Moelter ST, Agrin RN, Gur RC, Gur RE: Memory-delineated subtypes of schizophrenia: Relationship to clinical, neuroanatomical, and neurophysiological measures. *Neuropsychology*. 2002;16:481.

Weiss AP, Schacter DL, Goff DC, Rauch SL, Alpert NM, Fischman AJ, Heckers S: Impaired hippocampal recruitment during normal modulation of memory performance in schizophrenia. *Biol Psychiatry*. 2003;53:48.

▲ 12.7 Schizophrenia: Neuropathology

ROSALINDA C. ROBERTS, PH.D., AND
CAROL A. TAMMINGA, M.D.

Schizophrenia is an active area of medical research directed toward understanding disease mechanisms, with the hope that an informed illness pathophysiology will lead to rational treatments. Several approaches are used for exploring schizophrenia mechanisms; characteristically, these involve persons with schizophrenia or family members, because knowledge of clinical aspects of illness is a strength of the field. Studies of clinical presentation (including symptoms and cognitive characteristics), clinical signs (electroencephalogram [EEG], eye tracking, and evoked potential [EP]), in vivo brain characteristics (regional cerebral blood flow [rCBF], receptor characteristics, and volume), and postmortem brain characteristics (histology, electron microscopy, and neurochemistry) have all been used to generate information. Because the answers to schizophrenia pathophysiology are still unknown, it is impossible to say which are the critical pieces of information and which data are epiphenomena or confounds. Nonetheless, the pace of discovery, both preclinical research of brain mechanisms and clinical studies of changes in schizophrenia, is impressive and can be served by timely updates of findings to allow the pathophysiology puzzle to coalesce.

One of the important databases in schizophrenia research involves analyses from postmortem brain tissue. Studies of brain tissue from deceased persons with schizophrenia involve a rare opportunity to examine the tissue of interest in the illness. Elements of pathophysiology must exist in schizophrenia tissue. However, the confounds are legion, and the study material can be affected by in-life conditions (e.g., chronic medication, trauma, and institutionalization) and postmortem handling (e.g., postmortem interval [PMI], time to freezer, perimortem anoxia, and dissection approaches). Thus, the task of discovering the schizophrenia signal among identified changes has not been easy. Moreover, the identification of relevant brain regions on which to focus is also a matter of broad discussion and, sometimes, controversy.

Pathological studies of schizophrenia were an active area of research at the turn of the 20th century, but the popularity diminished when no definitive lesions were identified by using the best techniques of the day (this was in the face of "real" lesions in other brain diseases, such as Parkinson's and Alzheimer's diseases). Still, today, no such gross visible lesions have been discovered in schizophrenia. However, with the development of important new laboratory methodologies for brain research, new kinds of abnormalities are being evaluated in postmortem tissue for disease relevance. It is the purpose of this section to draw attention to the newest elements of postmortem brain research in schizophrenia and to tie together current findings into testable hypotheses.

Of course, data are inevitably collected and organized from an implied or explicit perspective. The hypothesis that schizophrenia is localized to one particular brain area draws investigations into that region. The emerging reality that complex mental and motor performances are systems phenomena can also influence data collection. Previous research can contribute to identifying irrelevant or uninvolved mechanisms, as well as to discovering pathophysiology. For example, because gliosis appears not to exist in schizophrenia tissue, the likelihood of cerebral inflammation contributing critically to pathophysiology schizophrenia becomes relatively low. Therefore, processes associated with tissue inflammation are not likely players in illness pathophysiology like infections, ischemia, neurodegeneration, or autoimmune phenomena. Moreover, without gliosis, evidence is accumulating to support the existence of an early developmental process, which creates the opportunity for or predisposes to later schizophrenia. Pathology localized to cerebral regions (e.g., frontal, limbic, and basal ganglia) or general cerebral pathology (e.g., synaptic changes and mitochondrial changes) and pathology affecting function of a neural system remain viable possibilities.

POSTMORTEM ANALYSIS: CHALLENGES OF THE METHOD

The neuropathology of schizophrenia has been studied since the late 1800s, and reports exist of abnormalities in many brain regions. One of the challenges of postmortem neuropathological observations in schizophrenia is that the changes that are seen are widespread, often subtle, not specific to the disease, and not found in all individuals with the disease. There is no gross lesion that identifies the schizophrenic brain, such as the massive shrinkage of the caudate nucleus in Huntington's disease or the loss of dopamine neurons in the substantia nigra (SN) in Parkinson's disease. Moreover, many of the abnormalities that are detected in the brains of patients with schizophrenia are not selective and are associated with other psychiatric conditions as well. Finally, there are many nonreplication studies, due, in part, to the problems of the differing methodology, the heterogeneity of the disease, the course of the illness, and chronic medication effects. Thus, no single brain lesion may be necessary or sufficient to diagnose schizophrenia. These complications of studying the neuropathology of schizophrenia have led to the infamous quote of Fred Plum in 1972 that "schizophrenia is the graveyard of neuropathologists."

There are certain challenges in postmortem research that are not limited to the study of schizophrenia but are characteristic of human brain research in general. Postmortem tissue itself is often compromised by long PMIs, poor preservation, or harsh fixation of the tissue, which are often incompatible with the application of histochemical, neurochemical, or electron microscopic techniques. Other confounding factors include medications used to treat medical conditions and drug and alcohol abuse. In addition, postmortem samples are often skewed to a particular type of case by the technical and practical aspects of tissue procurement. Thus, adequate or representative sampling of the population can be difficult. Moreover, there is a great deal of heterogeneity within control human populations, let alone those with mental illness, and this can impact on studies of the brain.

TISSUE CHARACTERISTICS AND STRATEGIES FOR COLLECTION

There are several sources for postmortem tissue, including medical examiners' cases, willed body programs, tissue and organ donor resources, and chronically hospitalized patients. Each has its own set of advantages and disadvantages. Some of the confounds of postmortem research can be minimized by careful attention to tissue collection. There are several tissue characteristics that make a collection optimal. An important feature is to collect tissue not only from schizophrenia cases and matched normal controls, but also from other psychiatric control groups, such as bipolar, depressed, or suicide, or a combination of these. Relatively short PMIs of less than 24 hours—less than 8 hours, whenever possible—are important or crucial depending on the tissue use and lessen the confounds of postmortem artifacts. For electron microscopy, the PMIs have to be less than 7 to 8 hours. A broad age range is important to avoid confounding findings due to aging. Rarely, if at all, are postmortem brains from neuroleptic-free subjects available, and obtaining brains that have been antipsychotic free for a period of time before death is difficult but not impossible. This tissue is particularly valuable. Another troublesome confounding factor in postmortem research is the high incidence of drug and/or alcohol abuse in mentally ill patients. Eliminating such tissue from a collection is possible but not always practical, especially if there are other limiting factors (such as short PMIs). Limiting the percentage of cases with drug and/or alcohol abuse and having a similar proportion of such cases across groups helps to control for this problem. Tissue from subjects with sufficient clinical information to make revised fourth edition of the *Diagnostic and Statistical Manual of Mental Disorders* (DSM-IV-TR) subdiagnoses is desirable as well. Premortem assessments of patients are valuable, but, because people with schizophrenia are diagnosed in young adulthood and live relatively normal life spans, a donors' clinic is not nearly as practical as for some neurological disorders, in which the time interval between diagnosis and death is relatively short (a few years).

REGIONAL BRAIN EXAMINATION

Abnormalities in postmortem schizophrenic tissue have been reported in many areas of the brain. This section focuses on the regions that have received the most attention.

Prefrontal Cortex

Interest in pathology of the prefrontal cortex is based on behavioral, as well as human imaging, data. It has long been noted that several symptoms or signs of schizophrenia mimic those found in persons with prefrontal lobotomies or *frontal syndromes*. Moreover, human brain imaging studies, predominantly functional, have indicated prefrontal deficits. Regardless of whether this deficit is primary or a confound of chronic medication use or psychological deficits, it has effectively signaled the prefrontal cortex for detailed postmortem study. Not surprisingly, there is considerable evidence from postmortem brain that supports anatomical abnormalities in the prefrontal cortex in schizophrenia.

The neocortex consists of six layers that have connections to each other, as well as to different cortical and subcortical structures. The neuropil, the area between neuronal and glial cell bodies, consists mainly of a dense network of dendrites, dendritic spines, axons, and axon terminals. In the cerebral cortex from patients with schizophrenia, a decrease in the thickness of the gray matter in postmortem work has been reported. Stereological studies in the prefrontal cortex have shown that the neuronal density is increased, whereas the total number of neurons is not changed. These data suggest that the thinning of gray matter is due, in large part, to a loss of neuropil. Other studies have shown that there is a decrease in the somal size (70 to 140 percent), including the soma of pyramidal cells, which undoubtedly also contributes to the thinning of the cortical gray matter. Smaller neuronal somata have been interpreted to reflect a reduction in the dendritic arborization of these cells, as somal size is correlated with the size and extent of the dendritic tree.

A variety of anatomical and other techniques have indicated defects in presynaptic elements. Microarray studies show decreased expression of many genes involved in synaptic function. Immunocytochemical studies using markers of axon terminals (e.g., synaptophysin, γ-aminobutyric acid [GABA], GABA transporter [GAT]) find reductions in axon terminal density in several areas of the prefrontal cortex. General markers of axon terminals, such as synaptophysin (a synaptic vesicle protein) or SNAP25 (a synaptosomal protein), have been used to estimate synaptic number in various Brodmann's areas (BA) in postmortem brains in schizophrenia. A decrease in synaptophysin immunoreactivity of 15 to 30 percent has been observed in BA46 and BA9; these changes do not appear to be due to antipsychotic medication. Immunoblotting data for synaptophysin show a robust decrease of 30 to 50 percent in BA9, BA10, and BA20. Other markers of axon terminals, such as SNAP25, show a decrease of 32 to 56 percent in BA9 and BA10.

The magnitude of the synaptic loss, combined with the observation that losses of synaptic markers are in many, if not all, cortical layers, suggests that multiple sources of terminals are affected. Data from immunohistochemical studies localizing particular proteins, enzymes, or transmitters have confirmed this. GAT immunoreactivity marks GABAergic terminals, some of which are the terminals of chandelier cells that form synapses on the axon initial segments of pyramidal neurons in layer III. The configuration formed by the immunoreactive terminals around the initial segments has been termed *axon cartridges*. Approximately a 40 percent decrease in labeled cartridges has been found in subjects with schizophrenia. The number of labeled cartridges is normal in a comparison of a psychiatric control group and neuroleptic-treated animals and is more severely decreased in schizophrenic subjects off medication, suggesting that this change is not caused by neuroleptic medication. In addition to a decrease in GAT-labeled terminals, there are reports of a decrease in parvalbumin-labeled terminals, which are thought to arise from the thalamus. In addition, there is a report of a decrease in number of terminals labeled with tyrosine hydroxylase, the synthesizing enzyme for dopamine. Whether the decrease in the number of immunoreactive structures represents a decrease in the number of synapses or a loss of immunoreactivity in the terminals is unclear at this time. That noted, the data indicate abnormalities in several types of terminals arising from neurons within and extrinsic to the cortex.

Postsynaptic structures are affected as well. One method of identifying dendrites is by the immunocytochemical localization of microtubule-associated protein (MAP2). Quantitative analysis of MAP2 stained prefrontal and occipital cortex from schizophrenic subjects reveals a 31 to 42 percent decrease in the area fraction labeled by MAP2 in BA9 and BA32, with no changes noted in primary visual cortex. Studies in the prefrontal cortex using the Golgi method, a technique that impregnates the entire cell (but only approximately 1 percent of all of the cells), reveal shorter abnormally shaped dendrites consistent with the MAP2 findings. Golgi studies also show a reduction in the number of dendritic spines on pyramidal neurons in the prefrontal cortex. Dendritic spines are protrusions on dendrites that provide more surface area to the dendrite and are the targets of the majority of synapses on a neuron, especially excitatory synapses. The reduction in spine number indicates a reduced number of synapses, particularly those of the asymmetrical type. In summary, there are numerous reports that are consistent with the reduced neuropil hypothesis.

Other Cortical Areas

There is marked regional heterogeneity in cortical pathology in schizophrenia. Neuropathological abnormalities are reported in other regions of frontal cortex and in the temporal, parietal, occipital, and limbic lobes (reviewed in the next section) as well. Even though other cortical regions have not been studied as thoroughly as the prefrontal and limbic cortex, these two cortical regions do appear to be the most affected among cortical regions. Some, but not all, abnormalities that are found in the prefrontal cortex are seen elsewhere in the cortex, whereas other areas appear to be far less affected. Primary visual cortex, once thought to be a control region lacking significant pathology, has recently been shown to have structural abnormalities. For example, increased neuronal density, decreased synaptophysin protein and messenger ribonucleic acid (mRNA), and decreased GAP43 mRNA are reported in BA17. An increase in neuronal density in BA17 is present but is not as robust as in prefrontal cortex, and not all reports of synaptophysin show decreases, possibly due to methodological differences.

Other regions of cortex show varying degrees of abnormalities. BA10 in frontal cortex of schizophrenia cases shows decreases in several measures, including gray level index, the density of small neurons, the density of parvalbumin labeled neurons, the number of dendritic spines in layer III, reelin protein and mRNA, synaptophysin protein, and SNAP25 protein. There are no changes in GFAP protein or mRNA and no changes in glial cell density or neuronal somal size. Normal neuronal and glial size and no changes in packing density of neurons or glia are observed in Broca's area (BA44). In BA47, there are reports of decreased neuronal and glial cell density, whereas only neurons are reduced in size.

The temporal lobe is a functionally diverse region including medial temporal limbic structures, primary auditory cortex, and temporal association cortex. In BA22 and BA20, there are reports of decreased reelin protein, mRNA and reelin-labeled cells, decreased dendritic spine density, decreased synaptophysin mRNA in BA22 and protein in BA20, increased GAP43 protein and decreased SNAP25 protein in BA20. Some changes in the temporal lobe have to do with asymmetry and are described in the section Loss of Asymmetry, whereas medial temporal lobe pathology is described in the section Limbic System.

There is also evidence for a mismigration of neurons in the prefrontal, parietal, and temporal cortex of brain of schizophrenia patients. During embryogenesis, cortical neurons are born in the ventricular zone and migrate to the cortical subplate, where they wait before migrating into the cortical plate to form the six layers of the cortex. This neuronal migration into the cortex is thought to be complete by the end of the second trimester in primates. With the use of several markers (MAP2, MAP5, and SMI-32), a number of studies found an abnormal density of cells in the subcortical white matter of postmortem schizophrenia patients. These cells are thought to be remnants of subplate neurons and therefore may indicate an incomplete migration of neurons into the cortex. Investigators also used nicotinamide adenine dinucleotide phosphate (NADPH)–diaphorase as a marker of these subplate remnants. Normally, these neurons are found in high levels in the superficial white matter, with a smaller population found dispersed throughout the cortical layers. In the prefrontal and temporal cortices of postmortem brain of schizophrenia patients, the majority of these neurons are found in the deeper white matter, with few located in the cortical mantle. This apparent shift in the distribution of this subpopulation of neurons is interpreted as representing altered migration of neurons into the cortex or a failure of programmed cell death. These findings are consistent with a neurodevelopmental disturbance occurring at approximately the second trimester of gestation.

Limbic System

Using in vivo functional imaging findings as a putative predictor of location of cerebral pathophysiology in schizophrenia implicates the limbic cortex. Studies from multiple laboratories have implicated the anterior cingulate cortex in some aspects of schizophrenia pathophysiology. The hippocampus is not only smaller in size in schizophrenia, but is also functionally abnormal. Consequently, a postmortem focus on histology and neurochemical pathology in limbic cortex has a rational basis in clinical testing and is being pursued.

Considerable pathology has already been defined in the postmortem limbic cortex in schizophrenia. The primary limbic structures in brain (namely, hippocampus, cingulate cortex, anterior thalamus, and mammillary bodies) and their intimately associated cortical areas (entorhinal cortex) have been found to regularly display pathological abnormalities. These are abnormalities of cell size, cell number, area, neuronal organization, and gross structure. Moreover, the entorhinal cortex has been observed to show abnormalities of cellular organization in layer II neurons. It is interesting to recall that structural changes on magnetic resonance imaging (MRI) and functional changes in positron emission tomography (PET) have targeted the same areas for interest in schizophrenia pathophysiology. The consistency of this localizing pathology, despite the variety of concrete findings, is striking across technically different studies. As increasingly sophisticated and diverse neuropathological techniques are applied to this analysis, important findings will emerge. Earlier studies reported alterations in superficial cellular organization (for example, in layer II) in entorhinal cortex, with layer II cells trailing into the lower cortical layers, again consistent with a neuronal migratory failure in this area. Another study found cingulate and middle frontal cortex to have more neurons present in lower rather than in superficial layers, again consistent with a concept of migratory failure. Other kinds of developmental studies have focused on changes in structural or growth-related elements, or both, in the neurons themselves, which would disturb normal development. The early observations of hippocampal neuronal disarray in schizophrenia are consistent with the recently reported selective loss of two microtubule-associated proteins (MAP2 and MAP5) in schizophrenic postmortem hippocampal tissue. Markers of axon terminals, such as synaptophysin, synapsin, and SNAP25, are decreased in hippocampus as well.

Despite the growing consensus that there are limbic cortical abnormalities in schizophrenia, there is a lack of consistent evidence for which neuroanatomical defects exist in the hippocampi and entorhinal cortices in the postmortem brains of schizophrenics. Daniel R. Weinberger highlights several studies describing cytoarchitectural abnormalities in the entorhinal cortex (including the specific loss of NADPH-diaphoreses neurons) as providing the best evidence for neuropathological defects. However, the gross abnormalities in entorhinal cytoarchitecture, such as abnormal sulci and islands in layer II, were not observed in a large study by Bruton or in tissue from the Maryland Brain Collection. Other studies have reported significant reductions in the volumes or cross-sectional areas of the entorhinal cortex or hippocampus in schizophrenics compared to controls, but these results have not been uniformly replicated. With respect to cell counts, there are reports of decreases in the density of hippocampal neurons, especially in the fourth region of the cornu ammonis (CA4) in the left anterior hippocampus and significant reductions in the total number of hippocampal neurons in hippocampal CA1 and CA2, CA3, and CA4 regions. However, using a systematic stereological study design, Stephan Heckers and colleagues could not find any significant differences in hippocampal cell number or regional neuronal volume between the hippocampi of 13 schizophrenics and 13 gender- and age-matched controls. Francine M. Benes did not find any changes in pyramidal cell density, although she found pyramidal cell size reduction in all regions of the hippocampus (CA1 through CA4) in this study.

In the anterior cingulate cortex, there has been a series of studies suggesting pathology related to loss or deficiency of small GABA-containing interneurons. Benes first showed an alteration in neuronal clustering in the anterior cingulate of schizophrenia subjects, suggesting perhaps a change in macrocolumn processing. She noted a decrease in cell size in the anterior cingulate (and prefrontal and motor cortex) and an increase in vertical axon numbers. Then, after dividing neurons into pyramidal cells and small neurons, she reported a decrease in number of small neurons in cingulate cortex layers II through VI. Finally, she reported an increase in GABA receptor density in layers II and III of the anterior cingulate cortex.

Several alterations in neurochemical measures of glutamatergic and related transmitter function in the postmortem schizophrenic hippocampus or the related dorsoventral temporal cortex, or both, have been identified. Although there appears to be no change in the density of hippocampal *N*-methyl-D-aspartate (NMDA) glutamate receptors, kainate binding, particularly in CA2, has been found to be reduced in several studies, but not consistently. Reduced levels of non-NMDA receptor binding and lower concentrations of non-NMDA receptor mRNA have been reported in CA3. Moreover, the glutamate receptor subunit mRNAs for $GluR_2$ and kainic acid (KA_2) and $GluR_2$ have been found to be selectively reduced in schizophrenic hippocampus, and a higher flip-flop isoform ratio has been identified for α-amino-3-hydroxy-5-methyl-4-isoxazolepropionic acid (AMPA) receptors. $GluR_1$ through $GluR_7$ mRNA subunits appeared unchanged in one study of schizophrenia in all brain areas evaluated, whereas another study found $GluR_1$ message diminished in the parahippocampal gyrus and $GluR_2$ message reduced in hippocampal subfields. Binding to NMDA receptors NR1 and NR2B has been found increased in superior temporal cortex. Aspartate binding, putatively to presynaptic elements, has been reported to be reduced or unchanged in schizophrenic temporal cortex. The reduced hippocampal synaptophysin levels reported are consistent with a decrease in the density of synapses in hippocampus in schizophrenia. Within temporal cortex, but not in hippocampus, some evidence supports increased glutamate concentrations in schizophrenia; moreover, glutamate and GABA release appear to be reduced in postmortem schizophrenic tissue. Changes in the GABA type A ($GABA_A$) receptor density, in GABA release, and in glutamate-related transmitters and their enzymes in hippocampus have been reported in the illness. Often, more pronounced or significant changes have been found within the left hemisphere of the temporal cortex, when compared to the right hemisphere. Taken as a whole, these data indicate possible instability in markers of ionotropic glutamate transmission in hippocampus in this illness.

Thalamus The thalamus is connected to specific regions within the cortex as well as to basal ganglia and limbic system structures. Although some studies of the thalamus as a whole show no evidence of volume shrinkage or neuronal loss, studies that have examined particular subnuclei have reported such abnormalities. The medial dorsal nucleus of the thalamus, which has reciprocal connections with the prefrontal cortex, has been reported by several, but not by all, investigators to contain a reduced number of neurons. The total number of neurons, oligodendrocytes, and astrocytes is reduced by 30 to 45 percent in schizophrenic subjects. This putative finding does not appear to be due to the effects of antipsychotic drugs, as the volume of the nucleus is similar in size between schizophrenics treated chronically with medications and neuroleptic-naive subjects. Not only are the number of cells decreased, but the cell size is also smaller. The volume of and neuronal density and size within the pulvinar are also smaller in schizophrenic subjects as compared to controls. Moreover, there is a recent report of volume reduction and decreased neuron number in the left, but not right, ventral lateral posterior nucleus. Although thalamic cell loss may not be confined to only these three subnuclei, it does not appear to be a universal finding in all thalamic subnuclei, as the centromedian nucleus does not show similar changes.

Basal Ganglia The neostriatum is a basal ganglia structure composed of the caudate nucleus and the putamen, which play a role in motor skills, cognition, and behavior. The striatum is an important area to consider in schizophrenia for several reasons. Damage to the striatum from neurodegenerative diseases such as Huntington's disease or stroke can produce psychiatric, even psychotic, symptoms and cognitive deficits similar to those in schizophrenia. The striatum is a major site of convergence of dopaminergic and glutamatergic systems, both of which have been implicated in the disease process. Drugs used to treat hypokinetic movement disorders such as Parkinson's disease, which target the striatum (i.e., dopamine agonists), can produce hallucinations and delusions. Moreover, the striatum is one of the brain regions that has been seen to manifest several types of abnormalities in schizophrenia. Reports of metabolic abnormalities include diminished metabolism, notably in neuroleptic-naïve subjects, as well as decreased striatal metabolism associated with auditory hallucinations.

Electron microscopic studies have shown several abnormalities in the striatum in terms of spine size, synaptic organization, mitochondria, and astrocytes. In the striatum, dendritic spines receive the majority of cortical inputs. Individual spines receive converging glutamatergic cortical inputs and dopaminergic nigral inputs. Therefore, spines are a site of convergence of these two brain regions and transmitter systems, both of which have been implicated in the pathophysiology of schizophrenia. The functional implication of smaller spines may be alterations in synaptic transmission and efficacy, the conductance of the action potential through the spine or the biochemical microenvironment at the synapse. Interestingly, striatal dendritic spines in rats chronically treated with haloperidol (Haldol) show no differences in spine size but do show reductions in spine number, suggesting that the report of smaller spines in schizophrenic cases does not appear to be a neuroleptic effect.

There are changes in basal ganglia synaptic organization and ultrastructural abnormalities. In a subset of schizophrenia tissue, the density or proportion, or both, of symmetric synapses was lower in the caudate versus the putamen, implying an imbalance in inhibitory synaptic transmission. The density of perforated synaptic profiles, cortical afferents thought to be involved in synaptic turnover and cognition, was lower in the striatum of the schizophrenic group compared to the control groups. The density of axodendritic synaptic profiles, particularly the asymmetrical type, which are probably thalamic in origin, was decreased in the caudate in a subset of the schizophrenic cases that did not have tardive dyskinesia. The proportion of asymmetrical axospinous synaptic profiles was elevated in the caudate in comparison to normal controls. The variety of synapses affected in the schizophrenic group implies the involvement of several neuronal circuits. Although the average size of axon terminals appears similar in schizophrenic subjects as compared to normal subjects, and many of the terminals are normal in appearance, some are reported to be swollen or degenerated. Synaptic length in patients versus controls has been reported to be similar or longer, with thicker postsynaptic densities. The capacity for compensatory responses in the caudate nucleus of patients with schizophrenia, as suggested by changes in the size of the postsynaptic density, is unclear at this time and needs further exploration. Concentric lamellar bodies, which are unusual inclusions and indicative of pathology, are observed in axons, as well as glial cells. Fewer mitochondria also characterize the striatum of schizophrenic subjects and are described later in the Mitochondria section.

Light microscopic findings have also been reported in the striatum of cases with schizophrenia. There are fewer cholinergic interneurons. Neurochemically, deficits have been reported in uptake sites for glutamate and GABA, decreases in enkephalin, and increases in the concentration of serotonin. Dopamine receptors are characteristically upregulated, commonly thought secondary to chronic medication. Because of this direct drug action, neurochemical differences in monoamine systems within basal ganglia are often ascribed to treatment, not to illness. The caudate nucleus has been observed to display augmentation of presynaptic dopamine function and reduced levels of neurotensin receptors. There are conflicting data on whether AMPA receptor sites are increased in density in the caudate nucleus in schizophrenia. One report indicates that there is an increase that is not due to neuroleptic treatment, whereas another report confirms the increase but attributes the change to suicide.

Some abnormalities observed in the striatum of schizophrenics, such as enlarged size, are thought to be due to chronic neuroleptic effects. The size increase is not massive, usually ranging from 5 to 8 percent, and has been more recently localized to the anterior part. In some studies, this volume change is not significant, unless the ratio of striatal volume to the rest of the hemisphere is analyzed. Nevertheless, it should be taken into consideration in data interpretation in studies in which this volume change might impact on the results, such as cell counts or synaptic counts. For the most part, the decreases in cell counts or synapse counts are of a much larger magnitude than the increase in striatal size and are thus not negated by this antipsychotic-induced effect. The cellular compartment responsible for the increased size of the striatum has not been identified at this time.

There have been astonishingly few neuropathological studies of the SN in schizophrenic subjects. Neurons in the SN are pale in medial regions and appear swollen or degenerating. The cell volume of the SN pars compacta (SNc) neurons in preneuroleptic era schizophrenic cases was reported to be reduced in the medial part of the SNc, and there was a reduction in the volume of the lateral SNc by approximately 20 percent. Glial cells appeared normal in terms of absolute number, but nuclear size was observed to be 30 percent smaller than normal. More recent data show that SNc neurons have altered patterns of neurophysin labeling. At the electron microscopic level, smaller axon terminals, hyperplasia of mitochondria, and abnormal lamellar structures have been reported, although in a small sample size.

GENERAL CEREBRAL PATHOLOGY

Although some pathologic abnormalities are peculiar to specific brain regions, other changes are observed across brain regions.

Cerebral Ventricular Enlargement The cerebral ventricles, particularly the lateral and third ventricles, are enlarged in schizophrenia, a finding that is well replicated as shown by Weinberger and colleagues in a mixture analysis of more than 1,000 cases and controls. Ventricular enlargement has been identified in postmortem studies, as well as in vivo studies, and implies possible volume reduction of the surrounding cerebral tissue. The magnitude of the ventricular enlargement can be robust, with some patients showing ventricles up to 40 percent larger than those of controls. Although ventricular enlargement in patients with schizophrenia is present for the group as a whole and appears to be correlated with genetic risk factors, there is considerable overlap in the range of ventricular size between persons with schizophrenia and controls. Ventricular enlargement is not unique to schizophrenia but is pronounced in a number of other central nervous system (CNS) diseases, particularly diseases characterized by neurodegeneration of structures adjacent to the ventricles, such as Huntington's disease, in which the caudate nucleus degenerates. However, ventricular enlargement in schizophrenia does not appear to be due to a neurodegenerative process, because there are no obvious signs of neuronal loss and no increase in the number of glial cells.

The lateral ventricle is the ventricle of the cerebral hemispheres, whereas the third ventricle is found in the diencephalon. Enlargement of these structures would suggest shrinkage of the adjacent brain matter. The gray matter structure adjacent to the third ventricle is the thalamus, for which reductions in volume have been reported. It is unclear whether the magnitude in volume of thalamic shrinkage can totally account for the expanded third ventricle. The nuclei that abut the lateral ventricle are not reported to be smaller or shrink to a much smaller magnitude than can account for the enlargement of the ventricle. For example, the gray matter structure adjacent to the anterior horn and body of the lateral ventricle is the caudate nucleus, which is slightly enlarged in neuroleptic-treated people with schizophrenia. The posterior horn of the lateral ventricle extends into the occipital lobe, for which reports of shrinkage are minimal. The inferior horn of the lateral ventricle extends into the temporal lobe, and, certainly, medial temporal lobe structures, such as the hippocampus, are reported to be smaller in the brains of schizophrenic subjects. However, the enlargement of the inferior horn of the ventricle may not be totally accounted for by the magnitude of the shrinkage of the hippocampus. Therefore, the possibility of white matter shrinkage exists. Certainly, shrinkage of white matter, the volume of which is extensive, could account for a significant portion of the enlargement of the lateral ventricles. In fact, MRI studies report white matter shrinkage in the medial temporal lobe, anterior limbs of the internal capsule, and superior occipital frontal fasciculus.

Loss of Asymmetry Many brain structures are normally lateralized in the human, with area or volume being consistently larger in one hemisphere or the other. Some asymmetries are related to lateralized functions, such as language. The observation of abnormal cerebral asymmetry in schizophrenia has been studied since 1879 by Crichton-Brown. Many studies of schizophrenia have shown an absence or reversal of the normal cerebral asymmetries found in controls. These disruptions in normal asymmetry are thought to reflect abnormalities during development. The main regions in which this asymmetry has been noted in neuropathological studies are in the left superior temporal gyrus, a reversal of the normally larger left planum temporale, and a loss of the normally larger left sylvian fissure. Moreover, certain abnormalities in the brains of patients with schizophrenia are restricted to or are worse in one hemisphere (usually the left) over the other. To cite a few examples, schizophrenia subjects show thinning of the left parahippocampal gyrus, left temporal horn enlargement, reduction in size of the left medial temporal lobe, and loss of synaptic proteins from the left thalamus.

Mitochondria Functional mitochondria are critical for proper neuronal function and health. Mitochondria produce more than 95 percent of the cellular energy via the electron transport chain. In addition, mitochondria buffer intracellular calcium and are the main source of reactive oxygen species (ROS) and of proapoptotic and antiapoptotic factors. Mitochondria have the capacity to change their shape, to fuse and to divide in response to metabolic demands, and to change location within a cell by moving along microtubules and, to some extent, actin. Neurons require a great deal of energy, in the form of adenosine triphosphate (ATP), to maintain the concentration gradient across the cell membrane and to repolarize after an excitatory postsynaptic potential (EPSP). Mitochondrial dysfunction leads to impairment in repolarization, the production of ROS, and apoptosis.

Several studies have implicated mitochondria in schizophrenia. Imaging studies have shown reduced ATP production in the temporal lobe of patients with schizophrenia compared to normal controls. Mitochondrial transcripts have been found to be abnormal in frontal cortex patients, with schizophrenia encoding mitochondrial ribosomal ribonucleic acid (rRNA) or part of cytochrome oxidase subunit II. Another study using complementary deoxyribonucleic acid (cDNA) microarray analysis found decreases in transcripts linked to mitochondrial energy production, such as the malate shuttle system, and the tricarboxylic acid (TCA) cycle. Complex I and complex IV of the electron transport chain have been found to be altered in the brains or in the blood of patients with schizophrenia. Reductions in complex IV activity have been reported in the frontal cortex (43 to 53 percent) and caudate nucleus (30 to 63 percent). Interestingly, the putamen shows an increase in complex IV activity, which is negatively correlated with intellectual and emotional impairments. Complex I activity in platelets has been shown in several studies to be increased (190 percent) in schizophrenic patients who are acutely or chronically psychotic but to be reduced (53 percent) in patients with residual schizophrenia. This deficit, which implies impairment of mitochondrial function, has been observed in other diseases associated with motor disorders.

Anatomical abnormalities in mitochondria have been reported in several brain regions, including the cortex and basal ganglia. In electron microscopic studies, Natalya A. Uranova and colleagues have reported that patients with schizophrenia have fewer mitochondria in the anterior limbic cortex and caudate nucleus. Fewer mitochondria (20 percent) have been reported throughout the neuropil in the striatum. The loss of mitochondria in glial elements also appears to contribute to the overall loss of mitochondria from the neuropil. Another ultrastructural study has shown fewer mitochondria, particularly fewer ultrastructurally intact ones, in striatal astrocytes in schizophrenia cases. In addition, a decrease in mitochondrial number was also reported in oligodendrocytes in the striatum and frontal cortex. This same group has reported hypoplasia of mitochondria in axon terminals synapsing onto dopamine neurons in the SNc.

Cerebral metabolic rate is thought to reflect, in part, synaptic activity. Changes in *synaptic activity* may be due to many things, including changes in synaptic density or changes in the energy stores at the synapse within the axon terminal. Thus, abnormalities in metabolism in the schizophrenic brain may be due to abnormal number or function of mitochondria, organelles that produce energy within the cell. Fewer mitochondria may be a primary deficit of the disease, or mitochondria may die as an epiphenomenon of the disease. Alternatively, mitochondria may be sequestered in neuronal somata located extrinsically or intrinsically to the nucleus in which they appear to be lost from the neuropil (e.g., the striatum). An inability of mitochondria to move into axon terminals or dendrites could account for a decreased number of mitochondria in the neuropil in these structures. Because mitochondria move around the neuron along microtubules between the soma and processes, damage to cytoskeletal elements may lead to a failure of proper mitochondrial movement. In fact, preliminary observations in the SN of drug-treated rats and schizophrenic subjects suggest structural abnormalities in dopaminergic neurons. The loss of mitochondria from terminals and dendrites by whatever mechanism may not totally account for the decreased frequency observed in the neuropil of schizophrenic cases.

The extent to which abnormalities in mitochondrial morphology, number, enzymatic activity, and gene transcripts are the effect of antipsychotic drug treatment is an important consideration. This has been partially addressed in many of the aforementioned studies by studying drug-free patients and the reaction of mitochondria to antipsychotic drug use in experimental animals. For example, rats chronically treated with haloperidol show a decrease in the number of mitochondria and an increase in their size, a change that is more striking in the rats that developed vacuous chewing movements, a rodent model of tardive dyskinesia. Although the size, but not the number of mitochondria, partially recovered after a drug withdrawal period of 1 month, total recovery might be possible after longer periods of withdrawal. The functional implications of larger mitochondria or more of them, or both, assuming that they are healthy, are that there are increased energy demands present in the structures containing them. Alternatively, enlarged mitochondria may reflect impaired energy metabolism if they are swollen or exhibit compromised structural integrity. Identifying the particular subsets of striatal neurons that manifest these mitochondrial changes and determining whether the mitochondria are functioning properly are necessary to adequately interpret the functional implications of these changes.

Expression of Developmental Proteins The migration of neurons from the ventricular zone to their proper positioning in the cortex requires a multitude of neural events, including start signals, cell–cell recognition, cell adhesion, motility, and stop signals. Because schizophrenia may have a developmental component, researchers have focused their attention on some of the molecules thought to play a role in this process. Neurotrophin-3 (NT-3), brain-derived neurotrophic factor (BDNF), ciliary neurotrophic factor (CNTF), basic fibroblast growth factor (bFGF), glia-derived neurotrophic factor (GDNF), growth associated protein (GAP43), epidermal growth factor (EGF), and reelin are all developmentally active proteins and are among likely candidates to be abnormal in schizophrenia.

Reelin is thought to help guide newly arriving migrating neurons to their proper destination, although the precise mechanism is presently unknown. Patients with schizophrenia are reported to have a significant (50 percent) reduction in the normal levels of reelin and its transcript in all of the brain areas examined (prefrontal and temporal cortex, hippocampus, caudate nucleus, and cerebellum). Interestingly, although reelin levels are normal in patients with some psychiatric disorders such as unipolar depression, reelin levels are also decreased in patients with bipolar disorder.

Neural cell adhesion molecules (N-CAMs), which are important for the motility of neurons during migration, have also been found to be changed in the postmortem brain of schizophrenia patients. N-CAM levels are found to be increased in the brains of people with schizophrenia; however, more N-CAMs are found in their polysialylated form, rendering neurons less mobile. The 105- to 115-kDa N-CAM is increased in cerebrospinal fluid (CSF), prefrontal cortex, and hippocampus. Schizophrenia has also been associated with changes in the expression of neurotrophic factors that regulate growth and survival during early neuronal differentiation and migration. BDNF supports survival and differentiation of developing and mature neurons, including dopamine neurons. Increases in BDNF concentrations have been reported in cortical areas, whereas decreases have been observed in hippocampus of patients when compared to controls. GAP43, a protein important for axon growth, targeting, and synaptogenesis is also found to be altered in schizophrenia. EGF levels are decreased in prefrontal cortex of schizophrenic subjects, whereas EGF receptor expression is higher than normal in cortex. The change does not appear to be an effect of antipsychotic drugs, as EGF levels are low in young, drug-free patients, and there is no change in animals chronically treated with antipsychotic drugs.

In summary, the neuropathological evidence clearly supports disturbances in early neurodevelopment. However, neurodevelopment is not limited to perinatal life. In fact, there are many "developmental" changes that occur at different stages of postnatal life, including neurite pruning, neurogenesis, apoptosis, neurite proliferation, axonal myelination, and structural brain changes. Many of the neuropathological abnormalities observed in schizophrenia may therefore be the result of neurodevelopmental lesions or insults that leave the brain more vulnerable to any number of further changes that may coincide with the clinical onset of schizophrenia or acute psychotic relapses.

Synaptic Connections Normal synaptic organization and reorganization or plasticity depend on presynaptic and postsynaptic structures. Spines are plastic structures that respond to experimental or environmental manipulation, or both, quickly and in a variety of ways. For instance, changes in spine size, shape, or density occur after deafferentation, after long-term potentiation, in response to complex environments, in association with seizures, and in response to hormonal changes. Alterations in spine number may simply be a reflection of the relatively impoverished environment that persons with schizophrenia experience. Alternatively, if this defect is present at the onset of disease, it may be one of the anatomical substrates of impaired function. Synaptic density is directly related to the number of terminals and spines. Synaptic density is highest in childhood at approximately 2 years of age, with a 30 to 40 percent decline in adolescence after extensive pruning, settling in a relatively stable level in adulthood. It is noteworthy that the clinical onset of schizophrenia and the appearance of psychotic symptoms are coincident with the completion of the intense pruning that occurs in adolescence. Interestingly, computer models simulating synaptic pruning in the cortex indicate that excessive pruning leads to hallucinations. The impaired ability of dendritic spines to remodel could lead to spine loss and, consequently, pruning back of axon terminals that no longer have appropriate targets. Alternatively, many presynaptic proteins are abnormal in several regions of the schizophrenic brain, and a problem with normal synapse formation could arise at the presynaptic site. Loss of dendritic spines is thought not to be caused by neuroleptic treatment; evaluation of preneuroleptic era brain tissue would potentially support this conclusion. The question of what occurs first, loss of postsynaptic spines or loss of axon terminals, is unanswered and certainly deserves attention. Pharmacological agents that target spine and axon survival, formation, plasticity, and synaptic function may be of therapeutic use.

ANIMAL MODELS

Because the use of chronic antipsychotic treatment is virtually ubiquitous in schizophrenia, it is an inevitable confound in the study of postmortem material. Thus, animal models to control for anatomical and neurochemical change secondary to chronic drug treatment have an important place in working up putative illness differences. Chronic treatments in animals have been favored that approximate the duration of treatment in the human condition, perhaps 6 to 12 months in the rodent. Moreover, setting the dose of drug for the animal as one that produces clinical therapeutic plasma levels in the rodent is favored. It is already known that structural and anatomical changes accompany dopamine-receptor blockade, not only dopamine-system changes. Thus, knowledge of both of these from animal experiments can suggest parallel changes in human tissue as drug-induced not disease-induced.

Anatomical Changes Animal studies show a myriad of structural changes in the brains of animals treated with antipsychotic drugs, which aid in the interpretation of the data from postmortem work. Although dopamine receptors are blocked almost immediately, structural and physiological changes take weeks to develop. Interestingly, there are striking differences in anatomical changes after short (3 weeks) versus long-term (>4 months) treatment, indicating that neuroleptic-induced plasticity is a dynamic and evolving process. Moreover, most of the neuroleptic-induced changes reverse—at varying lengths of time—after drug withdrawal. Many of the drug-induced changes seen in experimental animals predict changes in the postmortem schizophrenic tissue. Antipsychotic drugs appear to normalize or to normalize partially some of the pathology seen in the postmortem tissue, resulting in the problem of undetected pathology that is normalized by treatment.

Chronic haloperidol treatment results in ultrastructural alterations in the striatum, including reduced synaptic and mitochondrial density and hypertrophied mitochondria. Short-term treatment with haloperidol produces the opposite effect in the striatum and little effect in the limbic system. Perforated synapses, which are cortical glutamatergic synapses, are reported by some, but not all, investigators to be increased in number in the striatum by haloperidol but not by clozapine (Clozaril). Olanzapine (Zyprexa), chronically given, produces no changes in synaptic organization in the striatum. Haloperidol treatment produces opposite effects on enkephalin and substance P, resulting in an increase in enkephalin mRNA and a decrease of substance P mRNA in the striatum. The number of striatal interneurons expressing somatostatin or acetylcholine is decreased by haloperidol as well. Neuroleptic-induced morphological changes are not confined to the striatum, as alterations have been reported in other regions. There are reports of an increased number of synapses or the size of axon terminals, or both, in the cortex and the SN. The SN displays fewer tyrosine hydroxylase (TH)–labeled neurons after treatment with haloperidol, owing to diminished expression of TH rather than cell death, as this measure returns to normal on drug withdrawal.

Neurochemical Changes In rats treated for 6 months with antipsychotics, a first-generation drug (haloperidol) increased dopamine type 2 (D_2) receptors in striatum, decreased glutamic acid decarboxylase (GAD) mRNA and $GABA_A$ receptors in globus pallidus (GP), decreased dopamine type 1 (D_1) in the substantia nigra pars reticularis (SNr) and increased $GABA_A$ receptors, and, finally, increased $GABA_A$ receptors in the mediodorsal (MD) thalamus. In contrast, the second-generation antipsychotics (olanzapine, sertindole [Serlect]) failed to increase D_2 receptors in striatum, failed to show GAD mRNA changes in GP or any changes in SNr, and produced no MD thalamic alteration in $GABA_A$ receptors. However, all the antipsychotics increase GAD mRNA in the reticular nucleus of the rat thalamus, suggesting this as a part of the mechanism of their antipsychotic action. These ubiquitous drug-induced changes throughout basal ganglia and thalamus suggest caution in interpreting postmortem monoamine findings in these dopamine-rich regions.

Schizophrenia is a uniquely human disease with many symptoms that are impossible to assess in animals, such as hallucinations, delusions, and thought disorder. To date, there are several animal models of schizophrenia that partially replicate certain, but not all, constellations of abnormalities. There are several strategies for producing animal models, including pharmacological manipulations, mutations for particular neurotransmitters or developmental proteins, and brain lesions during fetal, neonatal, or adult life. Animal models, not of drug action, but of disease mechanism, can serve postmortem studies by suggesting and confirming parallel mechanisms in disease tissue and in the animal model tissue. Of the existing animal models of schizophrenia, most are useful, and some are controversial. Examples include models of cognitive deficits, such as social learning, or abnormal sensory gating and problems with working memory. An experimental model of impaired working memory has been developed by Patricia S. Goldman-Rakic and colleagues. Monkeys with lesions of the dorsolateral prefrontal cortex have been shown to be a useful model of this cognitive deficit. Developmental animal models include fetal irradiation in monkeys, which produces thalamic abnormalities, and a model of prenatal influenza infection, as well as neonatal hippocampal lesions, developed in rodents. There are models of psychosis (e.g., with phencyclidine [PCP] or ketamine) and even of protein specific abnormalities (e.g., with an animal knock out or knock down). For example, the reeler heterozygote mouse displays several abnormalities that are homologous to those found in schizophrenia. Regardless of the model, a match between anatomy or chemistry in the disease versus the model would be supportive of an illness connection.

FUTURE DIRECTIONS

Although the answers to the questions of pathophysiology in schizophrenia are not yet known, it is clear that this answer is complicated. Current studies across laboratories using different techniques find a variety of tissue changes in the illness. These changes are in several different, but not all, brain regions. Some pathology is validated by more than one laboratory, often with different methods. The issue of so much nonreplication in schizophrenia pathology is troubling and often frustrating. Certainly, one issue to account for this is the inherent confounds in postmortem study that were already discussed. The observation that people with schizophrenia do not all have identical brain abnormalities may not be simply due to technical problems and must give clues to etiology. However, even given this, it is likely that many of the pathological changes will be found to be truly associated with the illness, and many of the CNS regions will be found to be pathological. There are several ways to interpret this problem and to construct subsequent experiments to test the implicit questions. One would like to assume that schizophrenia has multiple pathophysiologies and is a medical syndrome rather than a discrete disease. Experiments have looked for and have found differences in schizophrenia subgroups that are consistent with the idea that different clinical subgroups have distinct pathology. An alternative and perhaps complementary speculation is that schizophrenia is a CNS systems' illness, involving one or more functional circuits, such as the limbic system or the prefrontal cortex, or both, and that the pathology rests somewhere within a circuit, but not always in the same location. It is conceivable that an abnormality in one of several nodes in a circuit will result in the final common pathway being disrupted and the multiple manifestations of the disease resting on the specific system components affected. This scenario implies and allows for a complex and potentially highly variable pathology but that is a fixed system in which the pathology is found and whose malfunction can produce the symptoms of the illness.

It is clear that the pace of discovery in this area suggests a finite time to a definitive discovery. The level of productivity and experimentation is high. Resources exist and new technologies are being applied. The "graveyard" association has now been lost and has been replaced with great scientific opportunity.

SUGGESTED CROSS-REFERENCES

Chapter 1 covers neural sciences, including neuroanatomy (Sections 1.2 and 1.3) and imaging (Sections 1.15 and 1.16). Psychiatric aspects of child neurology are covered in Section 2.13.

REFERENCES

Arnold SE, Rioux L: Challenges, status, and opportunities for studying developmental neuropathology in adult schizophrenia. *Schizophr Bull.* 2001;27:395.

*Benes FM: Emerging principles of altered neural circuitry in schizophrenia. *Brain Res Brain Res Rev.* 2000;31:251.

Benes FM, Berrett S: GABAergic interneurons: Implications for understanding schizophrenia and bipolar disorder. *Neuropsychopharmacology.* 2001;25:1.

Ben-Shachar D: Mitochondrial dysfunction in schizophrenia: A possible linkage to dopamine. *J Neurochem.* 2002;83:1.

Bunney BG, Potkin SG, Bunney WE: Neuropathological studies of brain tissue in schizophrenia. *J Psychiatr Res.* 1997;31:159.

Cullen TJ, Walker MA, Parkinson N, Craven R, Crow TJ, Esiri MM, Harrison PJ: A postmortem study of the mediodorsal nucleus of the thalamus in schizophrenia. *Schizophr Res.* 2003;60:157.

Daniel DG, Goldberg TE, Gibbons RD, Weinberger DR: Lack of a bimodal distribution of ventricular size in schizophrenia: A Gaussian mixture analysis of 1056 cases and controls. *Biol Psychiatry.* 1991;30:887.

DeLisi LE: Defining the course of brain structural change and plasticity in schizophrenia. *Psychiatry Res.* 1999;92:1.

Gao XM, Sakai K, Dean B, Conley RR, Roberts RC, Tamminga CA: Ionotropic glutamate receptors and expression of NMDA receptor subunits in subregions of human hippocampus: Effects of schizophrenia. *Am J Psychiatry.* 2000;157:1141.

Goldman-Rakic PS: The physiological approach: Functional architecture of working memory and disordered cognition in schizophrenia. *Biol Psychiatry.* 1999;46:650.

*Harrison PJ: The neuropathology of schizophrenia: A critical review of the data and their interpretation. *Brain.* 1999;122:593.

Ingvar DH, Franzen G: Abnormalities of cerebral blood flow distribution in patients with chronic schizophrenia. *Acta Psychiatr Scand.* 1974;50:425.

Jones LB, Johnson N, Byne W: Alterations in MAP2 immunocytochemistry in areas 9 and 32 of schizophrenic prefrontal cortex. *Psychiatry Res.* 2002:114:137.

Kung L, Conley R, Chute DJ, Smialek J, Roberts RC: Synaptic changes in the striatum of schizophrenic cases: A controlled postmortem ultrastructural study. *Synapse.* 1998;28:125.

Kung L, Roberts RC: Mitochondrial pathology in human schizophrenic striatum: A postmortem ultrastructural study. *Synapse.* 1999;31:67.

Lewis DA, Cruz DA, Melchizky DS, Pierri JN: Lamina-specific deficits in parvalbumin-immunoreactive varicosities in the prefrontal cortex of subjects with schizophrenia: Evidence for fewer projections from the thalamus. *Am J Psychol.* 2001;158:1411.

*Lewis DA, Lieberman JA: Catching up on schizophrenia: Natural history and neurobiology. *Neuron.* 2000;28:325.

Lewis DA, Pierri JN, Volk DW, Melchitzky DS, Woo TW: Altered GABA neurotransmission and prefrontal cortical dysfunction in schizophrenia. *Biol Psychiatry.* 1999;46:616.

Lewis DA, Volk DW, Hashimoto T: Selective alterations in prefrontal cortical GABA neurotransmission in schizophrenia: A novel target for the treatment of working memory dysfunction. *Psychopharmacology (Berl).* 2003 (*E-pub ahead of print*).

Lieberman JA: Is schizophrenia a neurodegenerative disorder? A clinical and neurobiological perspective. *Biol Psychiatry.* 1999;46:729.

Medoff DR, Holcomb HH, Lahti AC, Tamminga CA: Probing the human hippocampus using rCBF: Contrasts in schizophrenia. *Hippocampus.* 2001;11:543.

Pierri JN, Volk CL, Auh S, Sampson A, Lewis DA: Somal size of prefrontal cortical pyramidal neurons in schizophrenia: Differential effects across neuronal subpopulations. *Biol Psychiatry.* 2003;54:111.

Roberts RC, Conley R, Kung L, Peretti FJ, Chute DJ: Reduced striatal spine size in schizophrenia: A postmortem ultrastructural study. *Neuroreport.* 1996;7:1214.

*Selemon LD: Regionally diverse cortical pathology in schizophrenia: Clues to the etiology of the disease. *Schizophr Bull.* 2001;27:349.

*Selemon LD, Goldman-Rakic PS: The reduced neuropil hypothesis: A circuit based model of schizophrenia. *Biol Psychiatry.* 1999;45:17.

Selemon LD, Mrzljak J, Kleinman JE, Herman MM, Goldman-Rakic PS: Regional specificity in the neuropathologic substrates of schizophrenia: A morphometric analysis of Broca's area 44 and area 9. *Arch Gen Psychiatry.* 2003;60:69.

Selemon LD, Rajkowska G: Cellular pathology in the dorsolateral prefrontal cortex distinguishes schizophrenia from bipolar disorder. *Curr Mol Med.* 2003;3:427.

Shirakawa O, Tamminga CA: Basal ganglia GABAA and dopamine D1 binding site correlates of haloperidol-induced oral dyskinesias in rat. *Exp Neurol.* 1994;127:62.

Tamminga CA. Neuropsychiatric aspects of schizophrenia. In: Yudofsky SC, Hales RE, eds. *American Psychiatric Press Textbook of Neuropsychiatry.* 3rd ed. Washington, DC: American Psychiatric Press; 1997.

Tamminga CA, Thaker GK, Buchanan R, Kirkpatrick B, Alphs LD, Chase TN, Carpenter WT: Limbic system abnormalities identified in schizophrenia using positron emission tomography with fluorodeoxyglucose and neocortical alterations with deficit syndrome. *Arch Gen Psychiatry.* 1992;49:522.

Tamminga CA, Vogel M, Gao X, Lahti AC, Holcomb HH: The limbic cortex in schizophrenia: Focus on the anterior cingulate. *Brain Res Brain Res Rev.* 2000;31:364.

Uranova NA, Casanova MF, DeVaughn NM, Orlovskaya DD, Denisov DV: Ultrastructural alterations of synaptic contacts and astrocytes in postmortem caudate nucleus of schizophrenic patients. *Schizophr Res.* 1996;22:81.

Uranova N, Orlovskaya D, Vikhreva O, Zimina I, Kolomeets N, Vostrikov V, Rachmanova V: Electron microscopy of oligodendroglia in severe mental illness. *Brain Res Bull.* 2001;55:597.

Weinberger DR: Cell biology of the hippocampal formation in schizophrenia. *Biol Psychiatry.* 1999;45:395.

Weinberger DR, Berman KF: Prefrontal function in schizophrenia: Confounds and controversies. *Philos Trans R Soc Lond B Biol Sci.* 1996;351:1495.

▲ 12.8 Schizophrenia: Clinical Features and Psychopathology Concepts

BRIAN KIRKPATRICK, M.D., AND CENK TEK, M.D.

SYMPTOMS IN A BROADER CONTEXT

Contemporary diagnostic criteria for *schizophrenia* define it as an idiopathic psychotic disorder in which affective syndromes are absent or play a relatively less important role clinically than do psychotic symptoms. (See Tables 12.8–1 and 12.8–2 for the diagnostic criteria from the revised fourth edition of the *Diagnostic and Statistical Manual of Mental Disorders* [DSM-IV-TR] and the tenth edition of the *International Statistical Classification of Diseases and Related Health Problems* [ICD-10], respectively. In this chapter, quotations without attribution are from the DSM-IV-TR.)

However, the concept of psychosis is vague, and there is no widely accepted definition. The DSM-IV-TR Glossary Association *Diagnostic and Statistical Manual of Mental Disorders* (DSM) cites multiple definitions: hallucinations and delusions, with or without insight; a mental impairment that "grossly interferes with the capacity to meet ordinary demands of life"; a "gross impairment in reality testing"; or the symptoms in the DSM diagnostic criteria—hallucinations, delusions, disorganized speech, grossly disorganized behavior, or catatonic behavior.

However, the view that the psychopathology of schizophrenia consists exclusively of psychotic symptoms is incomplete. Many other psychiatric problems, as well as medical conditions, are also found in schizophrenia, and some of these are quite distressing or impairing or may even be life threatening. For many patients, psychotic symptoms may not be the most important psychopathological problem that they have. For instance, in outpatients, the cognitive impairment found in schizophrenia has a stronger relationship to the level of functioning than does the severity of psychotic symptoms. In addition, people with schizophrenia have an increased mortality rate compared to the general population, and psychopathological problems such as depression, drug abuse, and polydipsia probably make a much greater contribution to this increase in mortality than do psychotic symptoms per se.

If clinicians focus exclusively on psychotic symptoms when they consider the psychopathology of schizophrenia, they miss other problems that could be treated. For instance, the neuropsychiatric syndromes other than psychosis that are found in schizophrenia, such as depression and obsessive-compulsive symptoms, often respond to specific drug treatments, and drug abuse may improve with psychosocial treatments. Impaired insight can interfere with treatment adherence, but some aspects of impaired insight may improve with psychoeducation. One can also anticipate that, within a few years, there will be effective treatments for the cognitive impairment of schizophrenia, as well as for the primary negative symptoms found in some patients. Therefore, the evaluation of schizophrenia should consist of much more than evaluation of psychotic symptoms, and a broad evaluation will only become more imperative with time.

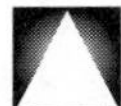

Table 12.8–1
DSM-IV-TR Criteria for Schizophrenia

A. Characteristic symptoms: Two (or more) of the following, each present for a significant portion of time during a 1-month period (or less, if successfully treated):
Delusions
Hallucinations
Disorganized speech (e.g., frequent derailment or incoherence)
Grossly disorganized or catatonic behavior
Negative symptoms (i.e., affective flattening, alogia, or avolition).
Note: Only one Criterion A symptom is required if delusions are bizarre or hallucinations consist of a voice keeping up a running commentary on the person's behavior or thoughts or two or more voices conversing with each other.

B. Social and occupational dysfunction: For a significant portion of the time since the onset of the disturbance, one or more major areas of functioning, such as work, interpersonal relations, or self-care, is markedly below the level achieved before the onset (or when the onset is in childhood or adolescence, failure to achieve expected level of interpersonal, academic, or occupational achievement).

C. Duration: Continuous signs of the disturbance persist for at least 6 months. This 6-month period must include at least 1 month of symptoms (or less, if successfully treated) that meet Criterion A (i.e., active-phase symptoms) and may include periods of prodromal or residual symptoms. During these prodromal or residual periods, the signs of the disturbance may be manifested by only negative symptoms or two or more symptoms listed in Criterion A present in an attenuated form (e.g., odd beliefs, unusual perceptual experiences).

D. Schizoaffective and mood disorder exclusion: Schizoaffective disorder and mood disorder with psychotic features have been ruled out because (1) no major depressive episode, manic episode, or mixed episode has occurred concurrently with the active-phase symptoms or (2) if mood episodes have occurred during active-phase symptoms, their total duration has been brief relative to the duration of the active and residual periods.

E. Substance and general medical condition exclusion: The disturbance is not due to the direct physiological effects of a substance (e.g., a drug of abuse or a medication) or a general medical condition.

F. Relationship to a pervasive developmental disorder: If there is a history of autistic disorder or another pervasive developmental disorder, the additional diagnosis of schizophrenia is made only if prominent delusions or hallucinations are also present for at least 1 month (or less, if successfully treated).

From American Psychiatric Association. *Diagnostic and Statistical Manual of Mental Disorders.* 4th ed. Text rev. Washington DC: American Psychiatric Association; 2000, with permission.

Psychopathology and Etiology

To understand the psychopathology of schizophrenia, it helps to put the study of symptoms in a broader context. Specifically, research on the environmental risk factors that are associated with an increased risk of schizophrenia helps put the signs and symptoms of the disorder in perspective.

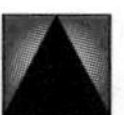

Table 12.8–2
ICD-10 Criteria for Schizophrenia

Definition

The schizophrenic disorders are characterized in general by fundamental and characteristic distortions of thinking and perception and by inappropriate or blunted affect. Clear consciousness and intellectual capacity are usually maintained, although certain cognitive deficits may evolve in the course of time. The disturbance involves the most basic functions that give the normal person a feeling of individuality, uniqueness, and self-direction. The most intimate thoughts, feelings, and acts are often felt to be known to or shared by others, and explanatory delusions may develop, to the effect that natural or supernatural forces are at work to influence the afflicted individual's thoughts and actions in ways that are often bizarre. The individual may see himself or herself as the pivot of all that happens. Hallucinations, especially auditory, are common and may comment on the individual's behavior or thoughts. Perception is frequently disturbed in other ways: Colors or sounds may seem unduly vivid or altered in quality, and irrelevant features of ordinary things may appear more important than the whole object or situation. Perplexity is also common early on and frequently leads to a belief that everyday situations possess a special, usually sinister, meaning intended uniquely for the individual. In the characteristic schizophrenic disturbance of thinking, peripheral and irrelevant features of a total concept, which are inhibited in normal directed mental activity, are brought to the fore and are used in place of those that are relevant and appropriate to the situation. Thus, thinking becomes vague, elliptical, and obscure, and its expression in speech sometimes becomes incomprehensible. Breaks and interpolations in the train of thought are frequent, and thoughts may seem to be withdrawn by some outside agency. Mood is characteristically shallow, capricious, or incongruous. Ambivalence and disturbance of volition may appear as inertia, negativism, or stupor. Catatonia may be present. The onset may be acute, with seriously disturbed behavior, or insidious, with a gradual development of odd ideas and conduct. The course of the disorder shows equally great variation and is by no means inevitably chronic or deteriorating (the course is specified by five-character categories). In a proportion of cases, which may vary in different cultures and populations, the outcome is complete, or nearly complete, recovery. The sexes are approximately equally affected, but the onset tends to be later in women.

Although no strictly pathognomonic symptoms can be identified, for practical purposes, it is useful to divide the previously mentioned symptoms into groups that have special importance for the diagnosis and that often occur together, such as:

(a) Thought echo, thought insertion or withdrawal, and thought broadcasting;

(b) Delusions of control, influence, or passivity, clearly referred to body or limb movements or specific thoughts, actions, or sensations; delusional perception;

(c) Hallucinatory voices giving a running commentary on the patient's behavior or discussing the patient among themselves or other types of hallucinatory voices coming from some part of the body;

(d) Persistent delusions of other kinds that are culturally inappropriate and completely impossible, such as religious or political identity or superhuman powers and abilities (e.g., being able to control the weather or being in communication with aliens from another world);

(e) Persistent hallucinations in any modality, when accompanied by fleeting or half-formed delusions without clear affective content or by persistent, overvalued ideas, or when occurring every day for weeks or months on end;

(f) Breaks or interpolations in the train of thought, resulting in incoherence or irrelevant speech or neologisms;

(g) Catatonic behavior, such as excitement, posturing, waxy flexibility, negativism, mutism, and stupor;

(h) Negative symptoms, such as marked apathy, paucity of speech, and blunting or incongruity of emotional responses, usually resulting in social withdrawal and lowering of social performance; it must be clear that these are not due to depression or to neuroleptic medication;

(i) A significant and consistent change in the overall quality of some aspects of personal behavior, manifested as loss of interest, aimlessness, idleness, a self-absorbed attitude, and social withdrawal.

Diagnostic guidelines

The normal requirement for a diagnosis of schizophrenia is that a minimum of one clear symptom (and usually two or more, if less clear-cut) belonging to any one of the groups listed previously as (a) through (d) or symptoms from at least two of the groups referred to as (e) through (h) should have been clearly present for most of the time during a period of 1 month or more. Conditions meeting such symptomatic requirements but of duration less than 1 month (whether treated or not) should be diagnosed in the first instance as acute schizophrenia-like psychotic disorder and are classified as schizophrenia if the symptoms persist for longer periods.

Viewed retrospectively, it may be clear that a prodromal phase in which symptoms and behavior, such as loss of interest in work, social activities, and personal appearance and hygiene, together with generalized anxiety and mild degrees of depression and preoccupation, preceded the onset of psychotic symptoms by weeks or even months. Because of the difficulty in timing onset, the 1-month duration criterion applies only to the specific symptoms listed previously and not to any prodromal nonpsychotic phase.

The diagnosis of schizophrenia should not be made in the presence of extensive depressive or manic symptoms, unless it is clear that schizophrenic symptoms antedated the affective disturbance. If schizophrenic and affective symptoms develop together and are evenly balanced, the diagnosis of schizoaffective disorder should be made, even if the schizophrenic symptoms by themselves would have justified the diagnosis of schizophrenia. Schizophrenia should not be diagnosed in the presence of overt brain disease or during states of drug intoxication or withdrawal.

From World Health Organization. *The ICD-10 Classification of Mental and Behavioural Disorders: Diagnostic Criteria for Research*. Geneva: World Health Organization; 1992, with permission.

A seminal study in the epidemiology of schizophrenia was the finding in a Finnish sample that the death of the father before a child's birth increased the child's risk of psychosis in adult life, compared to children whose fathers died during the first year of the child's life. The risk was greatest if the father's death occurred during the third, fifth, ninth, or tenth 4-week period of gestation. Subsequent studies—the first by some of the researchers involved in the paternal death study—have repeatedly found that influenza and other infectious diseases, including polio and measles, increase the risk of schizophrenia in the offspring if the mother is infected during the second or early third trimester of gestation. The common threads of the Finnish study and these studies of infectious diseases are, first, a stress response in the mother and, second, the importance of the timing of the stress. More recently, several psychological stressors have also been associated with an increased risk of schizophrenia in adult life in people whose mothers faced the stress during the second or early third trimester of gestation.

In animal models, prenatal stress causes alterations in many brain systems. Given the epidemiological evidence on schizophrenia, one would therefore expect the brain of the child exposed to a robust maternal stress response to have changes in many systems and, possibly, many behaviors as well. Such is the case with schizophrenia. Anatomical changes outside of the brain are also found in the disorder. For instance, as a group, people with schizophrenia have subtle abnormalities in the head and face, in dermatoglyphics, in the branching of peripheral nerves, and in immunological variables.

In short, the psychopathological abnormalities of schizophrenia are not restricted to psychotic symptoms but include many disturbances of thought, emotion, and behavior. That is,

- Schizophrenia is not just a psychotic disorder but a neurodevelopmental disorder in which psychosis is found.
- Schizophrenia is not just a psychotic disorder but a disorder of many brain functions.
- Schizophrenia is not just a brain disorder but a disorder with manifestations in many parts of the body.

HISTORICAL CONCEPTS

Psychotic forms of mental illness have been recognized for many centuries. For instance, at the end of the 18th century, Haslam Morel gave detailed descriptions of patients with psychotic symptoms. However, an organized effort to identify specific psychotic disorders first developed in the 19th century, when efforts to delineate specific diseases in other areas of medicine resulted in significant advances in medical science and improvements in public health. In the mid-1800s, Morel attempted to link causes, symptoms, course, and outcome to define specific psychotic syndromes.

The delineation of the disorder now recognized as schizophrenia is largely owing to the efforts of German-speaking psychiatrists in the second half of the 19th century. Ewald Hecker (1843 to 1909) provided the first strong description of hebephrenia, although the concept probably derived from the work of his supervisor, Karl Kahlbaum (1828 to 1899), who had also coined the term *catatonia*. In 1871, Hecker described *hebephrenia* as a psychosis with early onset and a poor prognosis; patients exhibited formal thought disorder and a "silly" affect (which would be called *inappropriate affect* today). Emil Kraepelin (1856 to 1926) subsequently suggested that catatonia, hebephrenia, and some other forms of psychosis represented one disease, which he termed *dementia praecox* or *premature dementia* (a term borrowed from Morel). Kraepelin distinguished this illness from affective psychosis. His conceptualization of these two disorders is essentially what is used today.

Other advances in medicine facilitated Kraepelin's observations. The discovery that a microbe caused syphilis showed that the pathophysiology of psychotic disorders could be found, especially if the course of illness were considered along with the clinical picture. An understanding of tertiary syphilis also decreased the heterogeneity of psychosis, making it possible to distinguish other groups of psychotic patients.

Kraepelin, a keen clinical observer, noticed the course of a group of mental illnesses starting in "near relation to the period of youth" with "varied initial clinical presentations" that eventually led to a mental deterioration. He clearly delineated this illness, dementia praecox, from affective psychosis and the dementias of later life. Kraepelin made his observations during the period in which other neurologists and neuropathologists were describing the histological correlates of Alzheimer's disease and other neuropsychiatric conditions. He assumed that dementia praecox had a neurological or metabolic origin, but he noted that at the time there was no evidence for such an origin. Kraepelin first suggested that dementia praecox invariably had a poor course and outcome. However, in later years, he changed his position, reporting that 24 percent of his cases showed improvement, and 13 percent recovered.

Kraepelin provided detailed case presentations, which were intended to be used as templates for reaching a diagnosis. In his view, the characteristic symptoms of dementia praecox were found in the presence of intact memory, physical perception, and consciousness. Those characteristic symptoms were impaired perceptual interpretation; impaired attention; decreased interest in the outer world; hallucinations, usually auditory and unpleasant; feeling that one's thoughts were being influenced by some outside force; impaired train of thought; incoherence of thought (inferred from incoherent speech); stereotypies; mannerisms; diminished mental efficiency; impaired insight and judgment; delusions; emotional dullness; and negativism. He stressed that symptoms could be present in various combinations, and no single symptom was found in all cases.

Another important contributor to the disease concept of schizophrenia was the Swiss psychiatrist Eugen Bleuler, who coined the term *schizophrenia*. Bleuler respected Kraepelin's disease description and classification system but attempted to apply Sigmund Freud's ideas to the phenomenology of illness. Bleuler disliked the term *dementia praecox*, as he observed that the deterioration that he observed was unlike the dementia of old age and did not have to occur in early life. Although Bleuler is credited for showing that the illness did not inevitably result in serious deterioration, he thought a full recovery was not possible. It is also notable that, although Bleuler gives credit to Kraepelin for the definition of a disease entity, he himself regarded schizophrenia as a group of illnesses.

In contrast to Kraepelin, Bleuler defined a set of *fundamental symptoms*, which he thought were present in all cases and during all stages. These were a disturbance of *associations*, or thought disorder; changes or lack of emotional reactions, or *affect*; *ambivalence* in emotions, will, and thought; *autism*, that is, detachment from reality; and impaired *attention*. In addition to these, he also defined a set of *accessory symptoms*; although these arose from the individual's psychological reaction to the environment and life events, the disease process created a predisposition to experience them. These accessory symptoms were hallucinations, delusions, illusions, catatonic symptoms, and other kinds of behavioral abnormalities. Accessory symptoms may present at any time, in different combinations, or may not be present at all.

In the United States, a less medical or physiological view of schizophrenia developed in the late 19th and early 20th centuries. According to Adolph Meyer, psychotic symptoms were reactions to life events. He did not believe that schizophrenia was a discrete disease entity, but rather he believed that psychotic symptoms represented habit patterns that were exaggerations of normal behavior. Harry Stack Sullivan and other psychiatrists and psychologists influenced by Freud emphasized disturbed interpersonal relationships in people with schizophrenia. With increasing research on the neurobiological basis of schizophrenia, the influence of Meyer and Sullivan has decreased.

EVOLUTION OF DIAGNOSTIC CRITERIA

Bleuler and Kraepelin provided detailed descriptions of the symptoms of schizophrenia. However, Bleuler's obligatory symptoms could be applied rather broadly and arbitrarily, especially as he suggested that the symptoms of schizophrenia occur in a spectrum that is on a continuum with normal behavior. This view and the influence of psychoanalysis contributed to the broad definition of schizophrenia used by American psychiatrists in the middle years of the 20th century.

However, other trends eventually led to the widespread acceptance of explicit diagnostic criteria for schizophrenia (as well as other neuropsychiatric disorders), which resulted in a narrowing of the category in American practice. First, explicit criteria were being developed and used with success in other areas of medicine. Second, several studies showed that American psychiatrists did not have good agreement on

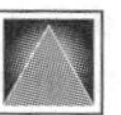

Table 12.8–3
Frequency of Some Symptoms of Schizophrenia in Different Regions of the World in the International Pilot Study of Schizophrenia, World Health Organization (Percentage of the Patients Who Have the Symptom)

	Total (811 Patients)	North America (Washington, DC)	South America (Cali)	Asia, India (Agra)	Asia (Taipei)	Western Europe (London and Aarhus)	Eastern Europe (Moscow and Prague)
Lack of insight	84	49	93	86	97	88	90
Suspiciousness	60	68	53	59	81	59	47
Delusions of persecution	52	45	40	54	68	63	35
Ideas of reference	55	43	66	66	72	60	47
Delusions of reference	50	46	60	60	58	60	43
Flat affect	52	46	50	50	55	68	37
Auditory hallucinations (any type)	42	25	56	56	51	40	35
Auditory hallucinations (voices speak to patient)	36	Not rated	55	55	48	39	26
Thought alienation	34	25	40	40	40	50	24

diagnoses; that is, two psychiatrists often did not give the same diagnoses to patients. This problem with interrater reliability existed within American psychiatry and between Americans and Europeans. An influential study of the latter problem was the United States–United Kingdom Cross National Project. In the study, a group of researchers armed with standardized interviews studied diagnostic practices in hospitals in London and in the state of New York. Roughly 60 percent of admissions in New York state hospitals were diagnosed with schizophrenia, whereas the diagnosis was approximately one-half as frequent in London. The British psychiatrists diagnosed schizophrenia in a manner similar to those of research diagnoses, but roughly one-half of the patients diagnosed with schizophrenia in New York did not have schizophrenia when standardized criteria were used. However, if these criteria were applied, the prevalence rate in both countries was similar. The discrepancy between diagnostic patterns of U.S. and U.K. psychiatrists was replicated in a videotape study that involved a large number of psychiatrists on both sides of the Atlantic.

Another groundbreaking study that contributed to the drive for explicit diagnostic criteria was the International Pilot Study of Schizophrenia (IPSS), performed under the auspices of the World Health Organization (WHO). In this study, more than 1,000 patients were interviewed in nine countries using a structured diagnostic interview, the Present State Examination (PSE). The study revealed that the disease manifested itself in a relatively similar manner in diverse cultures. It also revealed that it was possible to develop uniform diagnostic criteria with good interrater reliability and that structured diagnostic interviews could be used across different cultures around the world. A summary of the frequency of various symptoms seen in schizophrenia in the sites of the IPSS is presented in Table 12.8–3.

A third factor encouraging the development of diagnostic criteria for schizophrenia was the advent of effective medications for neuropsychiatric disorders. The efficacy for psychosis of chlorpromazine and related drugs and the relative lack of efficacy of lithium and antidepressants—a pattern that helped validate Kraepelin's diagnostic boundaries—increased support for defining discrete disorders.

The first edition of the *Diagnostic and Statistical Manual of Mental Disorders* (DSM-I) was published by the American Psychiatric Association in the 1950s. It was greatly influenced by Meyer and defined *schizophrenic reactions* rather than an illness. The work of German psychiatrist Kurt Schneider (1887 to 1967) was influential in subsequent diagnostic systems. Schneider identified symptoms that he thought were pathognomonic for schizophrenia (Table 12.8–4); he named these *first-rank symptoms*. He argued that the presence of these symptoms, in the absence of an underlying physical illness, was particularly valuable in determining the diagnosis of schizophrenia. Other symptoms, which he called *second-rank symptoms*, were not as specific but were also frequently seen in schizophrenic patients. Some of Schneider's first-rank symptoms are still part of contemporary diagnostic criteria. However, later studies have shown that first-rank symptoms are not so specific to schizophrenia as Schneider thought and can be seen in other types of psychosis. At the level of clinical symptoms, truly pathognomonic symptoms do not exist for schizophrenia.

After DSM-I, several important diagnostic criteria sets were developed. In the United States, the efforts of psychiatrists at Washington University in St. Louis were particularly important. The Feighner criteria, which defined a small number of disorders, were followed by the more extensive Research Diagnostic Criteria (RDC). The RDC included a longitudinal dimension in differential diagnosis. The RDC was the precursor for the third edition of the *Diagnostic and Statistical Manual of Mental Disorders* (DSM-III), which was the first DSM to articulate clear-cut diagnostic criteria for neuropsychiatric disorders. The WHO's *International Classification of Diseases* (ICD) also evolved over the same period.

DIAGNOSIS AND COMPARATIVE NOSOLOGY

As there are no validated diagnostic markers for schizophrenia, diagnosis is based as much on the exclusion of other psychotic disorders as the presence of specific patterns of symptoms. Current diagnostic criteria are imperfect in terms of their relationship to validating variables. For instance, some chromosomal linkages are specific to schizophrenia, and others are specific to bipolar disorder, but some linkages relate to both disorders. However, contemporary diagnostic criteria have been validated to a considerable extent by studies of course of illness and treatment response.

The current versions of the DSM and ICD diagnostic systems are DSM-IV-TR and ICD-10 (Tables 12.8–1 and 12.8–2). These diagnostic criteria sets undergo extensive field tests and, despite some differences, are largely concordant with each other in their definition of schizophrenia. Both reflect a significant narrowing of the diagnosis of schizophrenia compared to common practice in the United States in the middle 20th century. The major difference between these systems lies in the longitudinal course criteria, with DSM-IV-TR requiring 6 months as opposed to 1 month, and in deterioration

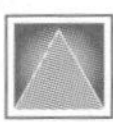

Table 12.8–4
First-Rank Symptoms of Kurt Schneider

Audible thoughts	Hearing one's own thoughts. These are actual hallucinations, but the source can be identified by the patient as his or her own thoughts.
Voices heard arguing	Hallucinations of more than one voice talking to each other; conference type auditory hallucinations. Subject can be of anything.
Voices heard commenting on one's actions	Hallucinations of a voice or voices that continuously comment on the patient's behavior simultaneously with the action; running commentary type of auditory hallucinations.
The experience of influences playing on the body (somatic passivity experiences)	A feeling that strange influences are at work in one's body. These experiences of physical interference may be attributed to devices, rays, suggestion, etc.
Thought withdrawal and other interference with thought	Thought withdrawal is a feeling that other people are taking the thoughts away. Thought insertion is a feeling that other people are intruding their thoughts on the patient.
Diffusion of thought or thought broadcasting	Thoughts are believed to be no longer private but shared (or perceived) by others.
Delusional perception	Delusional perception is different than a delusion. An abnormal, self-referenced meaning is attached to a genuine perception without any emotional or rational justification. As the meaning of it, rather than the perception itself, is altered, it is a disturbance of thought.
All feelings, impulses (drives), and volitional acts that are experienced by the patient as the work or influence of others	Influences working on the patient's will. It is experienced by the patient as some alien control.

in social and occupational function, which is required by DSM-IV-TR but not ICD-10. In addition, ICD-10 includes a simple schizophrenia subtype, which does not require the presence or a history of psychotic symptoms. This subtype is not present in DSM-IV-TR.

The DSM-IV-TR symptomatic criterion (Criterion A) requires the presence of a characteristic symptom or symptoms for at least 1 month or for less time if it is successfully treated. If this psychotic symptom is a hallucination of a running commentary or of two or more voices conversing (both Schneiderian first-rank symptoms), or if there is a bizarre delusion, then only one symptom is required to meet Criterion A. Otherwise, there must be (1) two psychotic symptoms of the following type—hallucinations, delusions, disorganized speech, or grossly disorganized or catatonic behavior—or (2) the presence of one of these psychotic symptoms and a negative symptom (affective flattening, alogia, or avolition).

The DSM-IV-TR criteria do not make a distinction between primary or idiopathic negative symptoms and those negative symptoms that are secondary to such causes as depression or drug-induced extrapyramidal symptoms. However, it is common clinical sense that secondary negative symptoms are not sufficient for Criterion A, as is noted in the text of the DSM-IV-TR.

In ICD-10, the symptom criterion is defined in more detail than in DSM-IV-TR and has a greater emphasis on Schneiderian first-rank symptoms. ICD-10 also makes a clear distinction between primary and secondary negative symptoms. Another important difference from DSM-IV-TR is the strict requirement of a 1-month duration of symptoms; duration of less than 1 month does not meet the criteria, even if the patient is treated successfully.

Diagnostic Criteria: Functioning

In addition to the cross-sectional criteria, DSM-IV-TR requires the presence of significant deterioration in one or more major areas of functioning, such as work, interpersonal relations, or self-care. When the onset is in childhood or adolescence, failure to achieve the expected level of function in these areas satisfies this criterion.

ICD-10 does not require functional deterioration for a diagnosis of schizophrenia. It also states in the text that the deterioration is not inevitable.

Diagnostic Criteria: Duration

In addition to the cross-sectional and functional deterioration criteria, DSM-IV-TR requires a total duration of at least 6 months. Within this 6-month period, 1 month of active-phase symptoms, that is, clear-cut psychosis, as described previously, must be present. DSM-IV-TR allows a shorter acute psychotic period if successful and timely treatment of symptoms has been instituted. The rest of the 6-month period may include continuing psychotic symptoms, prodromal symptoms preceding clear-cut psychosis, or residual symptoms after the resolution of psychotic symptoms. Residual symptoms may be attenuated forms of psychotic symptoms, such as odd beliefs, magical thinking, and ideas of reference that are not at the level of (not sufficiently severe to be considered) delusions; odd perceptual experiences not at the level of hallucinations; peculiar or concrete thinking; vague speech; or odd behavior that is not as severe as gross disorganization. Alternatively, residual symptoms can include negative symptoms. If the 6-month duration criteria cannot be met in the presence of other criteria, then a diagnosis of *schizophreniform disorder* should be made. The DSM-IV-TR criteria for schizophreniform disorder are presented in Table 12.8–5.

ICD-10 only requires a duration of 1 month. It acknowledges the possibility of a prodromal phase in the text, but it is clearly specified that this period should not be included in the required 1-month duration of psychotic symptoms. That is, according to ICD-10, regardless of treatment, if the psychotic phase lasts less than 1 month, then a diagnosis of acute schizophrenia-like psychotic disorder should be

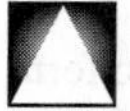

Table 12.8–5
DSM-IV-TR Criteria for Schizophreniform Disorder

A. Criteria A, D, and E of schizophrenia are met.
B. An episode of the disorder (including prodromal, active, and residual phases) lasts at least 1 month but less than 6 months. (When the diagnosis must be made without waiting for recovery, it should be qualified as *provisional.*)

Specify if:
- Without good prognostic features
- With good prognostic features: as evidenced by two (or more) of the following:
  - Onset of prominent psychotic symptoms within 4 weeks of the first noticeable change in usual behavior or functioning
  - Confusion or perplexity at the height of the psychotic episode
  - Good premorbid social and occupational functioning
  - Absence of blunted or flat affect

From American Psychiatric Association. *Diagnostic and Statistical Manual of Mental Disorders.* 4th ed. Text rev. Washington DC: American Psychiatric Association; 2000, with permission.

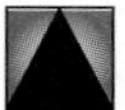

Table 12.8–6
ICD-10 Criteria for Acute Schizophrenia-Like Psychotic Disorder

An acute psychotic disorder in which the psychotic symptoms are comparatively stable and fulfill the criteria for schizophrenia but have lasted for less than 1 month. Some degree of emotional variability or instability may be present, but not to the extent described in acute polymorphic psychotic disorder.

Diagnostic guidelines

For a definite diagnosis:

(a) The onset of psychotic symptoms must be acute (2 weeks or less from a nonpsychotic to a clearly psychotic state);

(b) Symptoms that fulfill the criteria for schizophrenia must have been present for the majority of the time since the establishment of an obviously psychotic clinical picture;

(c) The criteria for acute polymorphic psychotic disorder are not fulfilled.

If the schizophrenic symptoms last for more than 1 month, the diagnosis should be changed to schizophrenia.

Includes:

Acute (undifferentiated) schizophrenia
Brief schizophreniform disorder
Brief schizophreniform psychosis
Oneirophrenia
Schizophrenic reaction

From World Health Organization. *The ICD-10 Classification of Mental and Behavioural Disorders: Diagnostic Criteria for Research.* Geneva: World Health Organization; 1992, with permission.

made. The ICD-10 criteria for acute schizophrenia-like psychotic disorder are presented in Table 12.8–6.

Diagnostic Criteria: Exclusions

DSM-IV-TR requires that mood disorders and schizoaffective disorder be ruled out. The patient should not meet the criteria for a mood episode (manic or depressive) during the psychotic phase, or, if there is a mood episode concomitant with active-phase symptoms, then its duration should be brief relative to the duration of the psychotic illness (including residual symptoms).

According to ICD-10, a patient with a depressive or manic episode can still meet the criteria for schizophrenia, if the criteria for schizophrenia have been met before the onset of the mood episode.

DSM-IV-TR excludes a diagnosis of schizophrenia if the symptoms are a direct physiological effect of a substance, a drug of abuse or a medication, as well as when the symptoms are due to another neurological or medical condition. Although worded differently, in effect, ICD-10 has the same exclusion.

DIAGNOSTIC SUBTYPES

The diagnostic subtypes of schizophrenia in DSM-IV-TR and ICD-10 are similar and reflect little change from Kraepelin's classification scheme. However, these subtypes appear to have weak relationships to biological variables, and their long-term stability is weak as well, with patients often changing their subtype over the course of their illness. (The paranoid subtype appears to have more stability than the other subtypes.) For these reasons, the standard subtypes—paranoid, disorganized, catatonic, and undifferentiated—have limited clinical usefulness.

Paranoid Schizophrenia

The hallmark feature of paranoid schizophrenia is the presence of one or more delusions and frequent auditory hallucinations. Although in other contexts, *paranoid* means

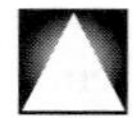

Table 12.8–7
DSM-IV-TR Diagnostic Criteria for Paranoid Schizophrenia

A type of schizophrenia in which the following criteria are met:

Preoccupation with one or more delusions or frequent auditory hallucinations.

None of the following is prominent: disorganized speech, disorganized or catatonic behavior, or flat or inappropriate affect.

From American Psychiatric Association. *Diagnostic and Statistical Manual of Mental Disorders.* 4th ed. Text rev. Washington DC: American Psychiatric Association; 2000, with permission

persecutory, in the context of the paranoid subtype, the delusions and hallucinations need not be persecutory. The contents of the auditory hallucinations are often related to the content of the delusions.

In DSM-IV-TR, the diagnosis of the paranoid subtype is largely made by exclusion. As some of the worst prognostic features (disorganized speech, disorganized behavior, and flat or inappropriate affect) are excluded, this subtype has a relatively favorable prognosis.

The diagnostic criteria for paranoid schizophrenia in DSM-IV-TR and ICD-10 are presented in Tables 12.8–7 and 12.8–8.

Disorganized (or Hebephrenic) Schizophrenia

The subtype of disorganized (or hebephrenic) schizophrenia was first described by Hecker, who used the term *hebephrenia*, a term that is retained in ICD-10. The hallmark of the subtype is thought disorder, although, in DSM-IV-TR, disorganized behavior and flat or inappropriate affect are also required. Delusions and hallucinations, if present, are often fragmentary. Poor premorbid function, an insidious onset, a continuous course, and a poor prognosis are typical of this subtype.

DSM-IV-TR and ICD-10 criteria are presented in Tables 12.8–9 and 12.8–10.

Catatonic Schizophrenia

Catatonia was first described by Kahlbaum, who described a syndrome with prominent motor and behavioral symptoms. Kraepelin and Bleuler regarded catatonia as part of schizophrenia, a position that is reflected in current diagnostic systems (Tables 12.8–11 and 12.8–12). However, catatonic symptoms can be found in affective disorder as well as schizophrenia. In developed countries, catatonia is probably much less prevalent now than in the past, perhaps owing to widespread early treatment of psychosis.

The criteria for the catatonic subtype require two of five characteristic symptoms: immobility (stupor or *catalepsy*, the latter of which is a rigid maintenance of a body position over an extended period of time); excessive purposeless motor activity; *negativism* ("apparent motiveless resistance to instructions or attempts to be moved"); peculiar movements (posturing, stereotypies, mannerisms, or grimacing); or *echolalia* or *echopraxia* (respectively, in DSM-IV-TR, "pathological, parrotlike, and apparently senseless repetition of a word or phrase just spoken by another person" and an involuntary "repetition by imitation of the movements of another").

Undifferentiated Schizophrenia

The category of *undifferentiated schizophrenia* is defined for the patients who meet the criteria for schizophrenia but cannot clearly be classified into one of the subtypes described previously. Diagnosis is by exclusion of other subtypes.

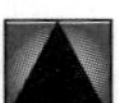

Table 12.8–8
ICD-10 Diagnostic Criteria for Paranoid Schizophrenia

Definition

This is the commonest type of schizophrenia in most parts of the world. The clinical picture is dominated by relatively stable, often paranoid, delusions, usually accompanied by hallucinations, particularly of the auditory variety, and perceptual disturbances. Disturbances of affect, volition, and speech and catatonic symptoms are not prominent.

Examples of the most common paranoid symptoms are:

(a) Delusions of persecution, reference, exalted birth, special mission, bodily change, or jealousy;

(b) Hallucinatory voices that threaten the patient or give commands or auditory hallucinations without verbal form, such as whistling, humming, or laughing;

(c) Hallucinations of smell or taste or of sexual or other bodily sensations; visual hallucinations may occur but are rarely predominant.

Thought disorder may be obvious in acute states, but, if so, it does not prevent the typical delusions or hallucinations from being described clearly. Affect is usually less blunted than in other varieties of schizophrenia, but a minor degree of incongruity is common, as are mood disturbances such as irritability, sudden anger, fearfulness, and suspicion. Negative symptoms, such as blunting of affect and impaired volition, are often present but do not dominate the clinical picture.

The course of paranoid schizophrenia may be episodic, with partial or complete remissions, or chronic. In chronic cases, the florid symptoms persist over years, and it is difficult to distinguish discrete episodes. The onset tends to be later than in the hebephrenic and catatonic forms.

Diagnostic guidelines

The general criteria for a diagnosis of schizophrenia must be satisfied. In addition, hallucinations or delusions, or both, must be prominent, and disturbances of affect, volition, and speech and catatonic symptoms must be relatively inconspicuous. The hallucinations usually are of the kind described previously in (b) and (c). Delusions can be of almost any kind of delusions of control, influence, or passivity, and persecutory beliefs of various kinds are the most characteristic.

Includes:

Paraphrenic schizophrenia.

Differential diagnosis: It is important to exclude epileptic and drug-induced psychoses and to remember that persecutory delusions might carry little diagnostic weight in people from certain countries or cultures.

Excludes:

Involutional paranoid state (F22.8)

Paranoia (F22.0)

From World Health Organization. *The ICD-10 Classification of Mental and Behavioural Disorders: Diagnostic Criteria for Research.* Geneva: World Health Organization; 1992, with permission.

Residual Schizophrenia The classification of residual schizophrenia is used for patients who have had at least one psychotic episode in the past and have met the criteria for schizophrenia, but no longer have psychotic symptoms (Tables 12.8–13 and 12.8–14). However, they exhibit continuing evidence of illness with negative symptoms, residual symptoms, or both that are attenuated forms of psychotic symptoms. The condition can be chronic or may be a transition to a complete remission of the illness.

Other Subtypes Two other subtypes that are not included in DSM-IV-TR or ICD-10 deserve mention in this context.

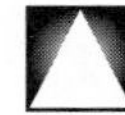

Table 12.8–9
DSM-IV-TR Diagnostic Criteria for Disorganized Schizophrenia

A type of schizophrenia in which the following criteria are met:

All of the following are prominent:

Disorganized speech

Disorganized behavior

Flat or inappropriate affect

The criteria are not met for catatonic type.

From American Psychiatric Association. *Diagnostic and Statistical Manual of Mental Disorders.* 4th ed. Text rev. Washington DC: American Psychiatric Association; 2000, with permission.

Simple Schizophrenia Defined by Bleuler as a separate subtype, *simple schizophrenia* is not included in DSM-IV-TR but is retained in ICD-10 (Table 12.8–15). Psychotic symptoms are not prominent, but there is a predominance of negative symptoms, residual symptoms of the type that would be seen in residual schizophrenia, insidious onset, odd behavior, and decrease of social function.

Deficit Schizophrenia The subtype of deficit schizophrenia appears to be stable over time but is not included in DSM or ICD-10. The hallmark is prominent idiopathic or primary negative symptoms, which are enduring. Patients with deficit schizophrenia

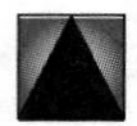

Table 12.8–10
ICD-10 Diagnostic Criteria for Hebephrenic Schizophrenia

Definition

A form of schizophrenia in which affective changes are prominent, delusions and hallucinations fleeting and fragmentary, behavior irresponsible and unpredictable, and mannerisms common. The mood is shallow and inappropriate and often is accompanied by giggling or self-satisfied, self-absorbed smiling or by a lofty manner, grimaces, mannerisms, pranks, hypochondriacal complaints, and reiterated phrases. Thought is disorganized, and speech is rambling and incoherent. There is a tendency to remain solitary, and behavior seems empty of purpose and feeling. This form of schizophrenia usually starts between 15 and 25 years of age and tends to have a poor prognosis because of the rapid development of negative symptoms, particularly flattening of affect and loss of volition.

In addition, disturbances of affect and volition and thought disorder are usually prominent. Hallucinations and delusions may be present but are not usually prominent. Drive and determination are lost, and goals are abandoned, so that the patient's behavior becomes characteristically aimless and empty of purpose. A superficial and manneristic preoccupation with religion, philosophy, and other abstract themes may add to the listener's difficulty in following the train of thought.

Diagnostic guidelines

The general criteria for a diagnosis of schizophrenia must be satisfied. Hebephrenia should normally be diagnosed for the first time only in adolescents or young adults. The premorbid personality is characteristically, but not necessarily, rather shy and solitary. For a confident diagnosis of hebephrenia, a period of 2 or 3 months of continuous observation is usually necessary to ensure that the characteristic behaviors described previously are sustained.

Includes:

Disorganized schizophrenia

Hebephrenia

From World Health Organization. *The ICD-10 Classification of Mental and Behavioural Disorders: Diagnostic Criteria for Research.* Geneva: World Health Organization; 1992, with permission.

Table 12.8–11
DSM-IV-TR Diagnostic Criteria for Catatonic Schizophrenia

A type of schizophrenia in which the clinical picture is dominated by at least two of the following:

- Motoric immobility, as evidenced by catalepsy (including waxy flexibility) or stupor
- Excessive motor activity (that is apparently purposeless and not influenced by external stimuli)
- Extreme negativism (an apparently motiveless resistance to all instructions or maintenance of a rigid posture against attempts to be moved) or mutism
- Peculiarities of voluntary movement, as evidenced by posturing (voluntary assumption of inappropriate or bizarre postures), stereotyped movements, prominent mannerisms, or prominent grimacing
- Echolalia or echopraxia

From American Psychiatric Association. *Diagnostic and Statistical Manual of Mental Disorders*. 4th ed. Text rev. Washington DC: American Psychiatric Association; 2000, with permission.

have been reported to differ from other patients with schizophrenia in terms of risk factors, course of illness, family history of schizophrenia, functional and structural imaging variables, neurocognitive measures, and response to treatment. There is less comorbidity with substance abuse and with symptoms of anxiety and depression. The condition is seen more in men than in women, and the onset is often insidious. Premorbid function and quality of life are worse than in other patients with schizophrenia. Although the usefulness of this subtype is clear in the context of research, its clinical usefulness, in terms of dictating treatment, is not well established to date, and patients with deficit schizophrenia can be classified in one of the subtypes in the DSM-IV-TR or ICD-10.

DIFFERENTIAL DIAGNOSIS

The psychotic and negative symptoms of schizophrenia can be mimicked by other psychiatric, medical, and neurological disorders. Some of the known causes for schizophrenia-like symptoms are presented in Table 12.8–16. As there are no pathognomonic signs or symptoms and no laboratory or imaging tests that would aid in the diagnosis, a careful history, a mental status examination, and an exclusion of other causes are necessary for reaching a valid diagnosis. Special attention to differential diagnosis should be paid in first episode cases, for cases with atypical features (such as a rapid onset or onset at a late age), after a medical disorder or a new medical treatment, for onset after substance use, or for a presentation with changes in sensorium.

A good history with a careful review of systems, basic laboratory tests, and a careful physical examination help differentiate many of the medical illnesses that may cause psychotic symptoms. Specific neurological disorders that may mimic some symptoms of schizophrenia may present further challenge in differential diagnosis and may necessitate the use of specific diagnostic studies, such as electroencephalogram (EEG), magnetic resonance imaging (MRI) scans, cerebrospinal fluid (CSF) analysis, and serology. Some commonly used medications (e.g., L-dopa, steroids, and anticholinergics), including some that are available over the counter (e.g., antihistamines, including histamine 2 blockers), may cause symptoms mimicking schizophrenia.

The effects of drugs of abuse present a particular challenge in the differential diagnosis of schizophrenia. Psychotic symptoms are

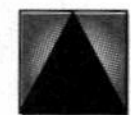

Table 12.8–12
ICD-10 Diagnostic Criteria for Catatonic Schizophrenia

Definition

Prominent psychomotor disturbances are essential and dominant features and may alternate between extremes, such as hyperkinesis and stupor, or automatic obedience and negativism. Constrained attitudes and postures may be maintained for long periods. Episodes of violent excitement may be a striking feature of the condition.

For reasons that are poorly understood, catatonic schizophrenia is now rarely seen in industrial countries, although it remains common elsewhere. These catatonic phenomena may be combined with a dream-like (oneiroid) state with vivid scenic hallucinations.

Diagnostic guidelines

The general criteria for a diagnosis of schizophrenia must be satisfied. Transitory and isolated catatonic symptoms may occur in the context of any other subtype of schizophrenia, but, for a diagnosis of catatonic schizophrenia, one or more of the following behaviors should dominate the clinical picture:

(a) Stupor (marked decrease in reactivity to the environment and in spontaneous movements and activity) or mutism;
(b) Excitement (apparently purposeless motor activity, not influenced by external stimuli);
(c) Posturing (voluntary assumption and maintenance of inappropriate or bizarre postures);
(d) Negativism (an apparently motiveless resistance to all instructions or attempts to be moved or movement in the opposite direction);
(e) Rigidity (maintenance of a rigid posture against efforts to be moved);
(f) Waxy flexibility (maintenance of limbs and body in externally imposed positions);
(g) Other symptoms, such as command automatism (automatic compliance with instructions) and perseveration of words and phrases.

In uncommunicative patients with behavioral manifestations of catatonic disorder, the diagnosis of schizophrenia may have to be provisional until adequate evidence of the presence of other symptoms is obtained. It is also vital to appreciate that catatonic symptoms are not diagnostic of schizophrenia. A catatonic symptom or symptoms may also be provoked by brain disease, metabolic disturbances, or alcohol and drugs and may also occur in mood disorders.

Includes:

- Catatonic stupor
- Schizophrenic catalepsy
- Schizophrenic catatonia
- Schizophrenic flexibilitas cerea

From World Health Organization. *The ICD-10 Classification of Mental and Behavioural Disorders: Diagnostic Criteria for Research.* Geneva: World Health Organization; 1992, with permission.

expected effects of hallucinogenic drugs such as lysergic acid diethylamide (LSD) and phencyclidine (PCP), but cocaine and amphetamines can also cause hallucinations and delusions. Hallucinogens typically cause vivid, usually nonauditory, hallucinations but may cause other problems as well. PCP can also cause a catatonic-like presentation or persecutory delusions. Amphetamines and like substances may induce a psychosis that may present with persecutory delusions and may closely mimic schizophrenia. The chronic use of substances such as organic solvents and marijuana is also reported to be associated with apathy or an amotivational syndrome that may mimic the negative symptoms of schizophrenia. Withdrawal from alcohol, as well as barbiturates and other sedative-hypnotic drugs, can present with psychotic symptoms. A complicating factor is that comorbidity with substance abuse is high in schizophrenia. The order of onset of substance abuse and the onset of psychotic or prodromal symptoms of schizophrenia is helpful but not completely

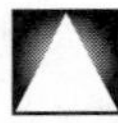

Table 12.8–13
DSM-IV-TR Diagnostic Criteria for Residual Schizophrenia

A type of schizophrenia in which the following criteria are met:

- Absence of prominent delusions, hallucinations, disorganized speech, and grossly disorganized or catatonic behavior.
- There is continuing evidence of the disturbance, as indicated by the presence of negative symptoms or two or more symptoms listed in Criterion A for schizophrenia, present in an attenuated form (e.g., odd beliefs and unusual perceptual experiences).

From American Psychiatric Association. *Diagnostic and Statistical Manual of Mental Disorders*. 4th ed. Text rev. Washington DC: American Psychiatric Association; 2000, with permission.

indicative in the differential diagnosis of schizophrenia and a substance-induced psychotic disorder.

It is not clear that schizophrenia and schizoaffective disorder are entirely separate disease entities, and the differential diagnosis between these two disorders is often difficult (see the criteria for schizoaffective disorder in Table 12.8–17). However, clinical management strategies for these two disorders are often different, so it is a clinically useful diagnostic distinction. The diagnosis of schizoaffective disorder requires a depressive, mixed, or manic mood episode and a concomitant psychosis, as well as euthymic periods of at least 2-weeks' duration when the psychotic or negative symptoms of schizophrenia are apparent. Mood episodes should be present for a substantial period of the total duration of the illness. One notable point is that a major depressive episode requires the presence of depressed mood; anhedonia alone is not sufficient.

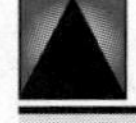

Table 12.8–14
ICD-10 Diagnostic Criteria for Residual Schizophrenia

Definition

A chronic stage in the development of a schizophrenic disorder in which there has been a clear progression from an early stage (comprising one or more episodes with psychotic symptoms meeting the general criteria for schizophrenia) to a later stage characterized by long-term, although not necessarily irreversible, negative symptoms.

Diagnostic guidelines

For a confident diagnosis, the following requirements should be met:

(a) Prominent negative schizophrenic symptoms (i.e., psychomotor slowing; underactivity, blunting of affect; passivity and lack of initiative; poverty of quantity or content of speech; poor nonverbal communication by facial expression, eye contact, voice modulation, and posture; poor self-care and social performance);

(b) Evidence in the past of at least one clear-cut psychotic episode meeting the diagnostic criteria for schizophrenia;

(c) A period of at least 1 year during which the intensity and frequency of florid symptoms, such as delusions and hallucinations, have been minimal or substantially reduced, and the negative schizophrenic syndrome has been present;

(d) Absence of dementia or other organic brain disease or disorder and of chronic depression or institutionalization sufficient to explain the negative impairments.

If adequate information about the patient's previous history cannot be obtained, and it therefore cannot be established that criteria for schizophrenia have been met at some time in the past, it may be necessary to make a provisional diagnosis of residual schizophrenia.

Includes:

- Chronic undifferentiated schizophrenia
- "Restzustand"
- Schizophrenic residual state

From World Health Organization. *The ICD-10 Classification of Mental and Behavioural Disorders: Diagnostic Criteria for Research*. Geneva: World Health Organization; 1992, with permission.

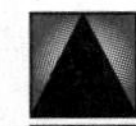

Table 12.8–15
ICD-10 Diagnostic Criteria for Simple Schizophrenia

Definition

An uncommon disorder in which there is an insidious but progressive development of oddities of conduct, inability to meet the demands of society, and decline in total performance. Delusions and hallucinations are not evident, and the disorder is less obviously psychotic than the hebephrenic, paranoid, and catatonic subtypes of schizophrenia. The characteristic negative features of residual schizophrenia (e.g., blunting of affect and loss of volition) develop without being preceded by any overt psychotic symptoms. With increasing social impoverishment, vagrancy may ensue, and the individual may then become self-absorbed, idle, and aimless.

Diagnostic guidelines

Simple schizophrenia is a difficult diagnosis to make with any confidence, because it depends on establishing the slowly progressive development of the characteristic negative symptoms of residual schizophrenia without any history of hallucinations, delusions, or other manifestations of an earlier psychotic episode and with significant changes in personal behavior, manifested as a marked loss of interest, idleness, and social withdrawal.

Includes:

- Schizophrenia simplex

From World Health Organization. *The ICD-10 Classification of Mental and Behavioural Disorders: Diagnostic Criteria for Research*. Geneva: World Health Organization; 1992, with permission.

A patient with a major depressive episode may present with delusions and hallucinations, whether the patient has a unipolar or bipolar mood disorder. Delusions seen with psychotic depression are typically mood congruent and involve themes such as guilt, self-depreciation, deserved punishment, and incurable illnesses. In mood disorders, psychotic symptoms resolve completely with the resolution of depression. A depressive episode that is this severe may also result in loss of functioning, decline in self-care, and social isolation, but these are secondary to the depressive symptoms and should not be confused with the negative symptoms of schizophrenia.

A full-blown manic episode often presents with delusions and sometimes hallucinations. Delusions in mania are most often mood congruent and typically involve grandiose themes. The flight of ideas seen in mania may, at times, be confused with the thought disorder of schizophrenia. Special attention during mental status examination of a patient with flight of ideas is required to note whether the associative links between topics are conserved, although the conversation is difficult for the observer to follow because of the patient's accelerated rate of thinking.

In delusional disorder, although the hallmark of the illness is presence of one or more delusions, these lack the bizarre quality of schizophrenic delusions and may be quite plausible. Aside from the effects of the delusions, function may remain normal (see the criteria in Table 12.8–18).

Anxiety disorders usually do not pose a problem in the differential diagnosis of schizophrenia. An exception to this may be a severe form of obsessive-compulsive disorder (OCD) in which the content of obsessions are rather odd, compulsive rituals are strange, and insight into symptoms is more limited than is usual with OCD patients. Special care should be exercised in the mental status exam-

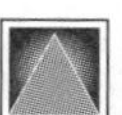

Table 12.8–16
Some of the Known Causes for Schizophrenia-Like Symptoms

- General medical
  - Wilson's disease
  - All endocrinopathies, especially of thyroid and adrenal
  - Systemic lupus erythematosus and other connective tissue diseases
  - Porphyrias
  - Vitamin B_{12} deficiency
  - Thiamine deficiency
  - Pellagra
  - Homocystinuria
  - Some chromosomal abnormalities (e.g., fragile X, XXY, and XO)
  - Fabry's disease
  - All deliriums
- Neurological
  - All brain tumors, especially frontal lobe
  - Epilepsy, especially with temporal and frontal lobe foci
  - Traumatic brain injury
  - All central nervous system infections, especially by herpesvirus, human immunodeficiency virus, and Creutzfeldt-Jakob disease, rickettsiae
  - Neurosyphilis
  - Huntington's disease
  - Parkinson's disease
  - Pick's disease
  - Multiple sclerosis
  - Normal pressure hydrocephalus
  - All dementias and delirium
  - Metachromatic leukodystrophy
- Substances, medications, and toxins
  - Substances of abuse
    - Phencyclidine
    - Lysergic acid diethylamide
    - Cocaine
    - Hallucinogenic mushrooms and other plants
    - Alcohol, acute and chronic use, and withdrawal; also Wernicke-Korsakoff syndrome and alcoholic hallucinosis
    - Barbiturate and benzodiazepine (withdrawal)
    - Amphetamine and related stimulants
    - Marijuana, chronic use
  - Medications
    - Glucocorticoids and other steroids, including over-the-counter dehydroepiandrosterone
    - Anticholinergic medications, including medications with anticholinergic side effects
    - L-Dopa
    - Histamine 2 (H_2) blockers
    - Digitalis
    - Disulfiram (Antabuse)
    - Ephedra and related herbs and medicines
    - Quinolones
    - Selegiline (Carbex)
    - Isoniazid (Laniazid)
    - Topiramate (Topamax)
  - Toxins
    - Heavy metals, arsenic, manganese, lead, mercury, thallium
    - Carbon monoxide
    - Volatile hydrocarbons (also as substance of abuse)
    - Organophosphates
- Psychiatric
  - Any mood disorder with psychotic features
  - Schizoaffective disorder
  - Schizophreniform disorder
  - Brief psychotic disorder
  - Delusional disorder
  - Postpartum psychosis
  - Shared psychotic illness (folie a deux)
  - Any type of dementia
  - Delirium with any etiology
  - Obsessive-compulsive disorder
  - Autism and related disorders
  - Schizotypal personality disorder
  - Schizoid personality disorder
  - Paranoid personality disorder
  - Some culture bound syndromes
  - Malingering
  - Borderline personality disorder

ination to inquire about the presence of obsessions and to note the patterns of rituals and their anxiety-relieving function.

Some personality disorders, especially of the paranoid, schizoid, and schizotypal varieties, may feature symptoms resembling features of schizophrenia. However, by definition, clear-cut psychotic symptoms are not present.

Disorders with dementia, such as Alzheimer's disease, may present with delusions, hallucinations, and a presentation that may resemble the thought disorder of schizophrenia as a consequence of loss of cognitive function. Even in late-onset cases, schizophrenia does not present with frank memory loss.

In settings such as emergency rooms and forensic and disability assessment situations, malingering should be included in the differential diagnosis.

With the widespread use of antipsychotic medications, early administration of these medications may change the initial presentation of schizophrenic psychosis, posing problems for diagnosis. The longitudinal course of the illness should clarify the diagnosis.

Finally, as in all psychiatric diagnoses, special care should be exercised when diagnosing patients who belong to cultures or subcultures that are different from that of the clinician.

MEASUREMENT

Any consumer of the research literature on schizophrenia needs to have some understanding of the instruments used to quantify the psychopathology of schizophrenia. Instruments intended to make a diagnosis usually are used simply to note the presence or absence and, sometimes, the duration of particular signs and symptoms. In contrast, other instruments are used to quantify the severity of symptoms, especially the change in severity over time. This second group of instruments forms the backbone of randomized clinical trials. Some of these instruments are designed to be relatively comprehensive measures of psychopathology, whereas others focus on particular symptom areas. Some instruments originally designed to make a diagnosis, such as the Schedule for Affective Disorders and Schizophrenia (SADS), have also been scaled so that they can measure

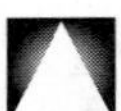

Table 12.8–17
DSM-IV-TR Criteria for Schizoaffective Disorder

Diagnostic criteria for 295.70 schizoaffective disorder

A. An uninterrupted period of illness during which, at some time, there is a major depressive episode, a manic episode, or a mixed episode concurrent with symptoms that meet Criterion A for schizophrenia.

Note: The major depressive episode must include Criterion A1: depressed mood.

B. During the same period of illness, there have been delusions or hallucinations for at least 2 weeks in the absence of prominent mood symptoms.

C. Symptoms that meet criteria for a mood episode are present for a substantial portion of the total duration of the active and residual periods of the illness.

D. The disturbance is not due to the direct physiological effects of a substance (e.g., a drug of abuse or a medication) or a general medical condition.

Specify type:

Bipolar type: if the disturbance includes a manic or a mixed episode (or a manic or a mixed episode and major depressive episodes)

Depressive type: if the disturbance only includes major depressive episodes

From American Psychiatric Association. *Diagnostic and Statistical Manual of Mental Disorders*. 4th ed. Text rev. Washington DC: American Psychiatric Association; 2000, with permission.

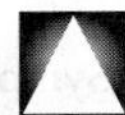

Table 12.8–18
DSM-IV-TR Criteria for Delusional Disorder

A. Nonbizarre delusions (i.e., involving situations that occur in real life, such as being followed, poisoned, infected, loved at a distance, or deceived by spouse or lover or having disease) of at least 1-month duration.

B. Criterion A for schizophrenia has never been met.

Note: Tactile and olfactory hallucinations may be present in delusional disorder if they are related to the delusional theme.

C. Apart from the impact of the delusions or its ramifications, functioning is not markedly impaired, and behavior is not obviously odd or bizarre.

D. If mood episodes have occurred concurrently with delusions, their total duration has been brief relative to the duration of the delusional periods.

E. The disturbance is not due to the direct physiological effects of a substance (e.g., a drug of abuse or a medication) or a general medical condition.

Specify type (the following types are assigned based on the predominant delusional theme):

Erotomanic type: delusions that another person, usually of higher status, is in love with the individual.

Grandiose type: delusions of inflated worth, power, knowledge, identity, or special relationship to a deity or famous person.

Jealous type: delusions that the individual's sexual partner is unfaithful.

Persecutory type: delusions that the person (or someone to whom the person is close) is being malevolently treated in some way.

Somatic type: delusions that the person has some physical defect or general medical condition.

Mixed type: delusions characteristic of more than one of the previously mentioned types, but no one theme predominates.

Unspecified type.

From American Psychiatric Association. *Diagnostic and Statistical Manual of Mental Disorders*. 4th ed. Text rev. Washington DC: American Psychiatric Association; 2000, with permission.

severity and change, but these are not as widely used as the instruments originally designed to measure severity.

Diagnostic Instruments Studies of interrater reliability have shown that a failure to ask the same questions contributes to disagreements about diagnosis. To deal with this problem, highly structured interviews that, in effect, consist of lists of questions about symptoms and their duration have been developed to eliminate this source of variance. Most of these instruments are designed to make the differential diagnosis of schizophrenia versus schizoaffective disorder and affective disorder and therefore have many items related to those diagnoses as well. The PSE was the first important instrument of this kind and was designed to generate diagnoses according to the ICD. The PSE has evolved into the Schedule for Clinical Assessment in Neuropsychiatry (SCAN). The SCAN is also intended to generate ICD diagnoses and has become important in international public health research, especially in international cooperative studies.

Another structured interview, the SADS, was developed to be used with the RDC. However, in most research settings in the United States, the Structured Clinical Interview for DSM-IV-TR (SCID) is now used instead. A number of other diagnostic instruments exist; some have special applications. For instance, the Operational Checklist for Criteria for Psychotic Illnesses (OCCPI) is often used in studies based on chart material. The OCCPI is designed to be used with diagnostic software, OPCRIT. The Schedule for the Deficit Syndrome is another instrument used to make a diagnosis within the heterogeneous syndrome of schizophrenia.

Severity Measures Among the comprehensive severity and change measures, the most important are the brief psychiatric rating scale (BPRS) and the Positive and Negative Syndrome Scale (PANSS), which is essentially an expansion of the BPRS. In schizophrenia treatment trials sponsored by the pharmaceutical industry, the PANSS is used more often than is the BPRS. Both of these instruments have several *factors*, or groups of symptoms related to a single concept, such as positive symptoms or depression. Although the total score is often reported for treatment trials, it is a relatively meaningless measure, and the factors are usually the focus of the trial.

Of the more narrowly focused severity rating scales, the most important is the Scale for the Assessment of Negative Symptoms (SANS). The SANS has 25 items, which are organized into five subscales: affective flattening, alogia, anhedonia, avolition, and attention (Table 12.8–19). The SANS played an important role in the study of negative symptoms, as it was the first widely accepted measure of this specific aspect of psychopathology. It is used often in treatment trials, as well as in other kinds of studies of schizophrenia.

The Hamilton Rating Scale for Depression (HRSD) originated in the field of depression research but is often used in schizophrenia treatment trials. However, the motor side effects of antipsychotic drugs and the idiopathic negative symptoms of schizophrenia can complicate the rating of depression in people with psychosis. The Calgary Depression Scale is less vulnerable to these problems than is the HRSD and increasingly is being used in place of other measures of depression.

HETEROGENEITY

Specific inclusion and exclusion criteria for the diagnosis of schizophrenia first became widely accepted in the United States with the

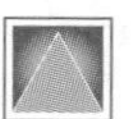

Table 12.8–19
Items in the Scale for the Assessment of Negative Symptoms (SANS)

Affective flattening or blunting
Unchanging facial expression
Decreased spontaneous movements
Paucity of expressive gestures
Poor eye contact
Affective nonresponsivity
Inappropriate affect
Lack of vocal inflections
Global rating of affective flattening
Alogia
Poverty of speech
Poverty of content of speech
Blocking
Increased latency of response
Global rating of alogia
Avolition-apathy
Grooming and hygiene
Impersistence at work or school
Physical anergia
Global rating of avolition-apathy
Anhedonia-asociality
Recreational interests and activities
Sexual interest and activity
Ability to feel intimacy and closeness
Relationships with friends and peers
Global rating of anhedonia-asociality
Attention
Social attentiveness
Inattentiveness during mental status testing
Global rating of attention

advent of DSM-III. This change in the field has had important benefits for patients, but the criteria can give the misleading impression that most patients with schizophrenia have a similar clinical presentation. In fact, patients with schizophrenia vary greatly with respect to their signs and symptoms: Some have hallucinations but no delusions, some have delusions but no hallucinations, some have both, some have marked disorganization with negative symptoms but neither hallucinations nor delusions, and so on. Other aspects of their symptoms—frequency, duration, impact on the patient's function, and the degree of distress that the symptoms cause—also vary greatly, as do other aspects of the psychopathology of schizophrenia. Nor is the pattern of comorbidity—the neuropsychiatric impairments other than psychosis that are so common in schizophrenia—consistent across patients.

Some patients function well and lead full lives, but most people with schizophrenia lead lives that are a great deal more difficult, limited, and unhappy than would be the case without the disorder. Their occupational accomplishments, relationships, general health, and satisfaction with their lives all suffer.

PHASES OF ILLNESS

The manifestations of schizophrenia appear to originate in utero, and the symptoms of the disorder continue throughout adult life for many patients. However, these manifestations change over the life span. The *typical* course of the disorder is presented here, but it is important to remember that course of illness also varies greatly among patients.

Although some children meet the criteria for schizophrenia, in most patients, flagrant psychosis does not appear until adolescence (usually late adolescence) or early adulthood. Nonetheless, as a group, people who do not meet the criteria for the disorder until they are in adult life appear to have a number of subtle problems in function in childhood and adolescence. (The individual patient may have many or none of these problems.) These include poor social relationships, mild motor problems (including mild, abnormal, involuntary movements and a lack of coordination), and cognitive problems, such as poor memory, processing speed, and attention. Therefore, although it is often said that schizophrenia has its onset in late adolescence or early adulthood, it is more accurate to say that flagrant psychosis usually has its onset at that time.

Although there is a peak in incidence in late adolescence or early adulthood, it should be noted that there is variation in first age of onset. Moreover, although there is a decline in incidence after that age, there is another incidence peak in later life, beginning at approximately 60 years of age. This late-life onset group has received relatively little study. Much more is known about the group of patients with onset in middle age, who as a group appear to have a higher percentage of women than is the case among patients with a more typical age of onset, as well as less severe negative symptoms and less cognitive impairment.

Typically, one can discern a first episode of psychosis. However, this may be preceded by a period of deteriorating function and nonspecific symptoms lasting weeks, months, or years, during which the patient often has increasing isolation and distress, often with depression and anxiety. This period of deterioration is sometimes called a *prodrome*, although, in the context of schizophrenia, there is another meaning for this word, which is described in the following discussion. When the onset of flagrant psychosis is gradual—over a period of many months or a few years, rather than within a few weeks—such an onset is said to be *insidious*.

After the first episode, there is considerable variation in the degree of recovery of function and in the persistence or nonpersistence of psychotic symptoms. Patients may be left with no psychotic symptoms, with subtle psychotic-like symptoms such as illusions and fleeting ideas of reference, or with mild psychotic symptoms. In some patients, the psychotic symptoms never improve greatly after the first or second episode. In a minority of patients, the psychotic symptoms are devastatingly severe and persistent.

The onset and course of the comorbid neuropsychiatric syndromes found in schizophrenia, such as depression, obsessive-compulsive symptoms, and polydipsia, have received little study.

In most patients, it is possible, with antipsychotic treatment, to discern clinically significant variation in the severity of psychotic symptoms; as a consequence, for most patients, it is meaningful to talk about episodes, relapses, or exacerbation. In this chapter, such an episode is called an *exacerbation of psychotic symptoms*. This can be a confusing issue, as some patients have no psychotic symptoms between these episodes, whereas others have fairly severe symptoms that worsen. In patients with an episodic course, *prodrome* has a meaning other than the period of deterioration before the first onset of psychosis, namely, the period that precedes a clear-cut increase in psychotic symptoms in a patient with a previous episode or episodes of psychosis. During this type of prodrome, which can last days or weeks, the patient may have increasing depression, anxiety, irritability, and mild psychotic-like symptoms before the appearance of clear-cut or worsening psychotic symptoms.

As explained in the following discussion, it is useful to distinguish between negative symptoms broadly defined and negative symptoms narrowly defined. Broadly defined negative symptoms can be found in many patients with the onset of flagrant psychosis or in the prodromal phase leading up to the first episode. In the patient with a subsequent episode, negative symptoms may also be part of the prodrome that precedes an exacerbation of psychosis.

From the perspective of the entire life span, the degree of recovery is highly variable across patients. Some patients have a single episode, with essentially full recovery, whereas others have severe psychotic symptoms from the time of their first episode until death. The typical course is for these symptoms to be most severe during the first 5 to 10 years after the onset of flagrant psychosis, with a degree of gradual subsequent improvement. However, recovery from psychosis is not the only kind of recovery that is, in theory, possible in schizophrenia, as people with schizophrenia may have any of several other problems as well. Recovery from these other aspects of the psychopathology of schizophrenia has received relatively little study. However, overall level of function appears to improve, on average, in later life, so there may be some recovery from some of these problems as well. Unfortunately, cognitive function, when impaired, and narrowly defined negative symptoms, if present, do not appear to improve with time.

PSYCHOTIC SYMPTOMS

An effort to place psychotic symptoms in a broader context and to include the other symptoms of schizophrenia as central parts of the illness does not mean that psychotic symptoms are not important. Psychotic symptoms can be terribly distressing for the person who has them, can create enormous barriers between people with schizophrenia and others, and can be the direct cause of severe impairments of function. Indirectly, psychotic symptoms can also lead to death, for instance, via a command hallucination to commit suicide or from accidents due to a patient's being distracted or disorganized.

Concepts of the psychopathology of psychosis in schizophrenia have changed considerably since the 1980s. An important influence on this change was the publication of the many descriptive statistical studies—usually using factor analysis—of the signs and symptoms of schizophrenia. A rather consistent pattern of four factors has emerged from these studies. The first factor consists of hallucinations and delusions. That is, in patients, the severity of hallucinations is significantly correlated with the severity of delusions. Together, these two kinds of symptoms are termed *reality distortion*. Another group of symptoms, termed *disorganization*, does not correlate with the severity of reality distortion, that is, it is possible for a patient to have one of these problems—reality distortion or disorganization—but not the other (although some patients experience both). *Negative symptoms*, as well as a cluster of *anxiety and depressive symptoms*, constitute two other symptom clusters, the severity of which varies independently of the severity of the other clusters. By definition, all patients with schizophrenia have psychotic symptoms (reality distortion or disorganization) at some point in the course of their illness, but there is no single pattern of psychotic symptoms.

The existence of this factor structure (i.e., these statistical relationships) outside of schizophrenia has been demonstrated in bipolar disorder and the schizophrenia spectrum (the nonpsychotic personality disorders that have a genetic relationship to schizophrenia), and it may exist in the general population as well. The generalized nature of these factors, that is, these statistical relationships, may reflect some underlying neurobiological independence, anatomical or otherwise, in these symptom clusters. There is some research that suggests reality distortion, disorganization, and narrowly defined negative symptoms have different neural substrates.

Hallucinations

Hallucinations consist of abnormal perceptions in any of the senses: hearing, vision, touch, olfaction, or taste. DSM-IV-TR states that a hallucination has the "compelling sense of reality of a true perception but . . . occurs without external stimulation of the relevant sensory organ."

In schizophrenia, *auditory hallucinations* receive the most attention, but hallucinations also occur in all of the other senses. Patients and clinicians often refer to *voices*, and patients with schizophrenia frequently have the experience of what seems to be speech or other recognizable sounds. Such hallucinations are *formed*. However, word fragments and unformed auditory hallucinations, which may consist of sounds that are not like speech or are inchoate, also occur. *Command hallucinations* consist of instructions spoken to the patients; some patients feel compelled to obey these commands. The commands may be trivial or even silly or may urge dangerous actions. A *running commentary* consists of hallucinated comments on the patient's actions. Some patients experience the voices of multiple people, who may talk to each other; the DSM-IV-TR refers to "two or more *voices conversing* with each other."

Visual hallucinations, like auditory hallucinations, can be formed, with recognizable objects, such as people, animals, and faces, or unformed, consisting of lights or vague shapes. The clinical rule of thumb that a visual hallucination implies the presence of a medical or neurological condition other than schizophrenia is not reliable, although such conditions should receive careful consideration in a patient with a new onset of schizophrenia or a change in long-standing psychotic symptoms.

The *olfactory hallucinations* found in schizophrenia are often unpleasant, such as the smell of burning rubber or of an offensive body odor. *Tactile hallucinations* include a sensation of being touched or struck; a feeling of pressure; distortions in body size, such as the feeling that a limb has expanded or contracted; and a sensation that a limb is moving when it is not or that something is moving under the skin. *Gustatory hallucinations* can consist of any taste.

An *illusion* consists of a misperception or misinterpretation of a real external stimulus. Illusions are not rare in schizophrenia. The distinction between a hallucination and an illusion, which seems so crisp when reading their definitions, is not always clear.

Delusions can be characterized in terms of the degree of the patient's insight into the reality of the experience; the hallucinations' frequency, intensity, and modality; the patient's emotional response; and the hallucinations' relationship to any delusions. These characteristics of delusions vary greatly across patients and, often, for the individual patient over time.

Delusions

A *delusion* is "a false belief based on incorrect inference about external reality that is firmly sustained despite what almost everyone else believes, and despite what constitutes incontrovertible and obvious proof or evidence to the contrary. The belief is not one ordinarily accepted by other members of the person's culture or subculture."

Many kinds of delusions are found in schizophrenia. Of particular importance is a *bizarre delusion*, which "involves a phenomenon that the person's culture would regard as totally implausible." That is, a bizarre delusion consists of a belief in something that cannot occur. In contrast, a nonbizarre delusion involves something that could happen but has not. For example, a delusion that one's spouse is unfaithful is not bizarre, as such things do happen (and *delusional jealousy* is common). A delusion that space monkeys have come down from their spaceship and put a radio transmitter in the patient's teeth and that they are now using it to control the patient's movements is bizarre, as this does not happen. An *erotomanic delusion* entails the belief that another person is in love with the patient; the object of the delusion is often famous or powerful. A *grandiose delusion* is a belief that the person has a special role or special powers. A *delusion of control* is the belief that one's feelings, thoughts, or actions are being controlled by someone or something other than oneself. A *delusion of reference* is the belief that events and people refer to the patient or are intended to deliver a message to the patient. The message is often critical or hostile. A patient with a *persecutory delusion* believes that he or she is being treated with malice, that is, "being attacked, harassed, cheated, persecuted, or conspired against." A *somatic delusion* concerns the patient's body and usually has the content that the patient is ill or has some other bodily abnormality. Patients with such delusions may experience pain in that area of the body and may insist on repeated examination. A *delusion of thought broadcasting* is the experience or conviction that the patient's thoughts are being "broadcast" and can therefore be heard by other people. A patient with the *delusion of thought insertion* believes that thoughts have been placed in his or her mind.

Patients with schizophrenia may also have unusual ideas that do not quite meet the definition of a delusion. For instance, an *idea of reference* has content similar to a delusion of reference, but the belief "may be transitory, not held firmly, or vague." In general, an *overvalued idea* is an "unreasonable and sustained belief that is maintained with less than delusional intensity (the person is able to acknowledge the possibility that the belief may not be true)."

As is the case for hallucinations, the characteristics of delusions can vary with clinical state for the individual state and are not uniform for all patients. Insight (conviction of the reality of the delusion), the time spent thinking about the delusional idea, and the emotional response to the delusion all vary greatly among patients and, often, for a patient over time.

Disorganization Bizarre or disorganized speech has long been recognized as part of the psychopathology of schizophrenia. The cluster of symptoms that is now termed *disorganization* and the disorganized subtype in DSM-IV-TR overlap with the older concept of hebephrenia. The hallmark of disorganization and of the disorganized subtype is *formal thought disorder*, so called because it is the form or organization of speech, rather than the content of speech, that is abnormal, as is the case with a delusion. It is, however, a common mistake to refer to *delusions* as *thought disorder*. From disorganized speech, one infers a disorganization in thinking. Disorganized speech is sometimes called *positive formal thought disorder* to distinguish it from negative thought disorder, which consists of poverty of speech (few words spoken and little information conveyed). In contrast, *poverty of content of speech* (many or a normal number of words spoken and little information conveyed) is another form of positive formal thought disorder. Other symptoms that correlate with disorganized speech and behavior and that are considered part of the disorganization syndrome or dimension include inappropriate affect and poorly sustained attention. Problems in attention can be found with formal mental status examination or can be manifested in managing activities of daily living, such as preparing a simple meal.

One can distinguish degrees of disorganization in speech. The less severe forms include vagueness, mild distractibility, and overinclusiveness (giving more details than are needed). More severe forms of thought disorder include *derailment*, which is a "pattern of speech in which a persons' ideas slip off one track onto another that is completely unrelated or only obliquely related. This disturbance occurs between clauses, in contrast to incoherence, in which the disturbance is within clauses." Incoherence is "speech or thinking that is essentially incomprehensible to others because words or phrases are joined together without a logical or meaningful connection. . . . This has sometimes been referred to as word salad to convey the degree of linguistic disorganization." *Blocking* is the phenomenon of a patient's suddenly losing the thread of his or her own thoughts or speech, that is, the patient experiences an interruption of thought processes—the mind goes blank.

Some research suggests patients with marked formal thought disorder have biological differences from other patients with schizophrenia, including differences in age of onset (earlier), gender composition (more often male), and some neuroanatomical differences.

Kraepelin provided a detailed description of aspects of disorganization:

> Patients lose in a most striking way the faculty of logical ordering of their trains of thought . . . the most unnatural combinations of heterogeneous ideas are formed, because their incongruity is not perceived. . . . The most evident truths are not recognized, the greatest contradictions are thoughtlessly accepted . . . the patients' mental association often has that peculiarly bewildering incomprehensibility, which distinguishes them from other forms of confusion. It constitutes the essential foundation of incoherence of thought.
>
> In less severe cases this is shown only in increased facility of distraction . . . in passing without any connection from one subject to another, in the interweaving of superfluous phrases and incidental thoughts. . . . A patient who was quite sensible, when asked to copy the fable of the "greedy dog," performed the exercise correctly as far as the sentence: "But when he snapped at it, his own piece of meat fell from his mouth, and sank in the water," then, however, continued:
>
> "And as now her present condition depends wholly on what Dr. J. M. plans for the future, who wishes to make himself acquainted with what is in connection with it, and of whose condition she wished to be again acquainted with, which he wished on his own desire. Now he had nothing at all but what was yours, which seems to lose what was his, but he himself tried to lose it, the fortune which for him was trying to be acquired," and so on.
>
> [M]ore striking is the departure from the given idea in the answer of a patient who was asked what year it was:
>
> "O I know nothing, what shall I say? Fire, fire! O you old beast, devil, wretch, dog, slaughtered, slaughtered! It's cold in the wood; hurrah! Damn it a million times, beast of a cat, slaughtered."
>
> In certain circumstances the incoherence may go on to complete loss of connection and to confusion. An example of this is given in the following answer of a patient to the questions: Are you ill?
>
> "You see as soon as the skull is smashed and one still has flowers (laughs) with difficulty, so it will not leak out constantly. I have a sort of silver bullet which held me by my leg, that one cannot jump in, where one wants, and that ends beautifully like the stars . . ."

NEGATIVE SYMPTOMS

The so-called negative symptoms of schizophrenia have become the focus of a great deal of attention in recent years. For instance, clinical trials often have negative symptoms as the principal, or one of the principal, outcome measures. These symptoms are not only associated with much of the impairment of function found in the disorder, but also cause much of that impairment.

The negative symptoms that are listed among the characteristic symptoms (Criterion A) in the DSM-IV-TR criteria for schizophrenia are *affective flattening*, *alogia*, and *avolition*. *Affect* is "a pattern of observable behaviors that is the expression of a subjectively expe-

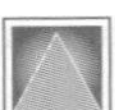

Table 12.8–20
Items in Other Negative Symptom Scales

Negative scale from the Positive and Negative Syndrome Scale (PANSS):
- Blunted affect
- Emotional withdrawal
- Poor rapport
- Passive or apathetic social withdrawal
- Difficulty in abstract thinking
- Lack of spontaneity and flow of conversation

Negative symptom (anergia) factor from the Brief Psychiatric Rating Scale (BPRS):
- Blunted affect
- Psychomotor retardation
- Emotional withdrawal
- (Some investigators include disorientation in this factor as well)

rienced feeling state." *Blunted affect* is a "significant reduction in the intensity of emotional expression." *Flat affect* is at the extreme end of affective blunting or flattening: "absence or near absence of any signs of affective expression."

There are three aspects to consider when assessing blunting of affect: facial expression, expressive gestures and other body language, and modulation of the voice. The intensity and frequency of facial expressions are important; however, an unchanging expression of anger, sadness, or depression is not what is important for the diagnosis of schizophrenia. Expressive gestures, such as hand movements and head nods, are part of body language, which can include movements such as leaning forward or back and turning the body toward or away from the interviewer. Modulation of the voice includes changes in the rate, volume, and pitch of speech, all of which vary frequently in normal speech. Blunted affect should be distinguished from *inappropriate affect*, which is a "discordance between affective expression and the content of speech or ideation" and belongs to the disorganization syndrome.

DSM-IV-TR defines *alogia* as an "impoverishment in thinking that is inferred from observing speech and language behavior. There may be brief and concrete replies to questions and restriction in the amount of spontaneous speech (poverty of speech)." In contrast, *poverty of content of speech* (a component of the disorganization syndrome) is speech that is "adequate in amount but conveys little information because it is overconcrete, overabstract, repetitive, or stereotyped."

Avolition is an "inability to initiate and persist in goal-directed activities. When severe enough to be considered pathological, avolition is pervasive and prevents the person from completing many different types of activities." There is an ambiguity in this definition, as there are many causes of avolition, such as depression, anxiety, suspiciousness, and physical illness, as well the amotivational syndrome found in some patients with schizophrenia that is not due to these other problems but is part of schizophrenia. (In other disorders, neurologists refer to this impairment as *apathy*.) The avolition in the DSM-IV-TR criteria for schizophrenia should be restricted to this amotivational syndrome.

Negative Symptoms Broadly Defined

The term *negative symptom* is associated with a great deal of confusion. Much of what is written about negative symptoms is unintentionally misleading, and this lack of clarity interferes with advances in the field of schizophrenia, from thinking about pathophysiology to the design and interpretation of clinical trials. First, as commonly used in clinical settings, the boundaries of negative symptoms—that is, which signs and symptoms are negative—are an issue on which clinicians often disagree. Most would consider blunted affect and poverty of speech to be negative symptoms but often disagree on whether depression, for instance, is as well. Negative symptom rating scales have helped enormously in this regard by defining these symptoms for research purposes. These rating scales are also important, because they are used in drug trials, which in turn influence clinicians' thinking. In research, there are three widely used measures: the negative symptom factor of the BPRS, the negative symptom subscale of the PANSS, and the SANS (Tables 12.8–19 and 12.8–20).

Use of the term *negative symptoms* suggests that these are a separate group of impairments, distinct from other aspects of psychopathology of schizophrenia, but an examination of the items in these rating scales reveals that this is not entirely the case. For instance, it is often stated that negative symptoms are better predictors of quality of life than is the severity of psychotic symptoms. However, in the SANS, the items for grooming and hygiene, impersistence at work or school, and recreational interests and activities (as well as others) *measure* quality of life and level of function directly. To some extent, the same problem can be found in the other widely used measures of negative symptoms.

To understand the problems associated with the concept of negative symptoms, it is useful to distinguish between negative symptoms broadly defined and negative symptoms narrowly defined. When referring to *negative symptoms*, clinicians often have in mind the unemotional, apathetic patient, who was described by Kraepelin:

> Now if we make a general survey of the psychic clinical picture of dementia praecox . . . there are apparently two principal groups of disorders which characterize the malady. On the one hand we observe a weakening of those emotional activities which permanently form the mainsprings of volition. In connection with this, mental activity and instinct for occupation becomes mute. The result of this part of the morbid process is emotional dullness, failure of mental activities, loss of mastery over volition, of endeavor, and of ability for independent action. The essence of personality is thereby destroyed, the best and most precious part of its being, as Griesinger once expressed it, torn from her. With the annihilation of personal will, the possibility of further development is lost, which is dependent wholly on the activity of volition. . . . It is worthy of note . . . that memory and acquired mental proficiency may occasionally be preserved in a surprising way when there is complete and final destruction of the personality itself.

In contrast to the negative symptoms that are rated with the SANS, PANSS, and BPRS, Kraepelin is clearly talking about an enduring impairment. In addition, negative symptoms due to such problems as depression or drug side effect, rather than to the disorder of schizophrenia itself, are not what Kraepelin was trying to describe. In other words, he was describing enduring, idiopathic symptoms.

There have been a number of efforts to delineate the psychopathology of the apathetic patient described by Kraepelin, in terms of a dimension and as a subtype. The concept of anhedonia overlaps with enduring, idiopathic negative symptoms (although anhedonia can be transitory and can result from other causes, such as anxiety and serious depression). Timothy Crow's type II schizophrenia, which was characterized by blunted affect and poverty, was an important step in the development of a negative symptoms subtype and was followed by Nancy Andreasen's *negative schizophrenia*, which was defined by a high score on the SANS.

Kraepelin's description represents the narrow definition of negative symptoms: the patient with an enduring amotivational syndrome that is not due to such other causes as depression or medication side effects. In contrast, the rating scales represent a broader definition. Although patients with the syndrome Kraepelin described would have high scores on the widely used negative symptom rating scales, so would many other patients, because there are many causes of negative symptoms other than schizophrenia itself. For instance, serious depression, which is common in schizophrenia, may result in blunted affect, poverty of speech, social withdrawal, poor hygiene, poor participation in social and recreational activities, poor rapport, and poor occupational function, all of which have corresponding items in these rating scales. However, antidepressants may greatly improve these symptoms in a depressed patient but do not treat the enduring, idiopathic negative symptoms of schizophrenia. Similarly, severe psychotic symptoms—regardless of the presence or absence of depression—can also result in high scores on many of these same negative symptom rating scale items, which often decrease with an improvement in psychosis.

Narrowly Defined Negative Symptoms: Deficit Schizophrenia In the 1980s, criteria were promulgated for a subtype of schizophrenia characterized by enduring, idiopathic negative symptoms. These patients were said to exhibit the *deficit syndrome*. This group of patients is now said to have *deficit schizophrenia* (see the criteria for that putative disease diagnosis in Table 12.8–21). Patients with schizophrenia who do not meet the criteria are said to have *nondeficit schizophrenia*. The symptoms used to define deficit schizophrenia are strongly intercorrelated, although various combinations of the six negative symptoms in the criteria can be found.

What is distinctive about the criteria for this subtype is that a differential diagnosis of the cause of the negative symptoms is required, and the negative symptoms must be enduring. With training, good interrater reliability is possible. The deficit-nondeficit categorization also has considerable long-term stability.

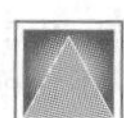

Table 12.8–21
Diagnostic Criteria for Deficit Schizophrenia

At least two of the following six features must be present, and of clinically significant severity:
- Restricted affect
- Diminished emotional range
- Poverty of speech
- Curbing of interests
- Diminished sense of purpose
- Diminished social drive

Two or more of these features have been present for the preceding 12 months, and always were present during periods of clinical stability (including chronic psychotic states). These symptoms may or may not be detectable during transient episodes of acute psychotic disorganization or decompensation.

Two or more of these enduring features are also idiopathic, that is, not secondary to factors other than the disease process. Such factors include
- Anxiety
- Drug effect
- Suspiciousness
- Formal thought disorder
- Hallucinations or delusions
- Mental retardation
- Depression

The patient meets DSM-IV-TR criteria for schizophrenia.

Compared to nondeficit patients, deficit schizophrenia patients are remarkable for (1) their poor function, which cannot be explained by severe psychotic symptoms, drug abuse, depression, anxiety, or suspiciousness, all of which are less severe in deficit than nondeficit patients, and (2) a lack of distress over this poor function, along with a near absence of awareness of impairment. Deficit patients are isolated and seriously impaired but largely uncomplaining.

This group of patients appears to have a disease that is separate from that of other patients with schizophrenia, as the two groups differ on the dimensions used throughout medicine to distinguish diseases: signs and symptoms, course of illness, risk and etiological factors, pathophysiological correlates, and treatment response. Several studies suggest that this pattern of findings is not due to the deficit patients simply having a more severe form of the same pathophysiology affecting other subjects with schizophrenia.

The psychopathological differences between deficit and nondeficit schizophrenia can be summarized as follows:

Relative to *signs and symptoms*, deficit patients have more severe negative symptoms but also less emotionality (depression, guilt, hostility, and anxiety) and a decreased prevalence of drug abuse. They also have slightly less severe delusions with a social content, including suspiciousness. The cognitive impairment of deficit patients is also greater than that found in nondeficit schizophrenia.

Deficit patients have a more severe *course of illness* than nondeficit patients, with a higher prevalence of abnormal involuntary movements before administration of antipsychotic drugs and poorer social function before the onset of psychotic symptoms. The onset of their first psychotic episode is more often insidious, and they show less long-term recovery of function than do nondeficit patients. (The deficit-nondeficit categorization is a better predictor of long-term outcome than are negative symptoms broadly defined.) Deficit patients are also less likely to marry than are other patients with schizophrenia. However, despite their poorer level of function and greater social isolation, both of which should increase a patient's stress and, therefore, the risk of serious depression, deficit patients appear to have a decreased risk of major depression and probably have a decreased risk of suicide as well.

Deficit patients' *risk factors* differ from those of nondeficit patients; deficit schizophrenia is associated with an excess of summer births, whereas nondeficit patients have an excess of winter births. Deficit schizophrenia may also be associated with a greater familial risk of schizophrenia and of mild, deficit-like features in the nonpsychotic relatives of deficit probands. Within a family with multiply affected siblings, the deficit-nondeficit categorization tends to be uniform. The deficit group also has a higher prevalence of men.

The psychopathology of deficit patients impacts on treatment; their lack of motivation, lack of distress, greater cognitive impairment, and asocial nature undermine the efficacy of psychosocial interventions, as well as their adherence to medication regimens. Their cognitive impairment, which is greater than that of nondeficit subjects, also contributes to this lack of efficacy.

OTHER NONPSYCHOTIC SYMPTOMS

People with schizophrenia have many neuropsychiatric and medical problems other than hallucinations, delusions, disorganization, and negative symptoms. Psychotic symptoms can often be controlled with appropriate medications, so these nonpsychotic symptoms are often more impairing, relative to social and occupational function, than are the patient's hallucinations, delusions, or formal thought disorder, especially in nondeficit patients. Some of these nonpsychotic symptoms also contribute to the increased mortality and physical morbidity found in schizophrenia. These abnormalities are so common and so important that they should be considered an integral part of the disorder of schizophrenia.

Estimates of the prevalence of these other problems within schizophrenia may come from population-based (epidemiological) studies or from clinical samples. Both kinds of studies have important limitations. Clinical samples are subject to a number of biases that can cause the extent of comorbidity to be overestimated, relative to the true prevalence of comorbidity within the population of all people with schizophrenia. Epidemiological studies, on the other hand, are likely to have many more false-positive and false-negative diagnoses of schizophrenia than are clinical samples. Despite these limitations, it is clear that, in schizophrenia, impairments other than psychotic symptoms are so common as to be the rule; therefore, the clinician is obligated to determine the extent to which the patient is burdened by these other problems.

Depression

It is useful to distinguish in schizophrenia, as in other disorders, between depressive symptoms and a depressive syndrome or depressive episode (major depression). Estimates of the percent of patients with schizophrenia who experience major depression at some point during their lives (lifetime prevalence) have been as high as 80 percent, but most estimates are in the range of one-fourth to one-third of patients. Point prevalence—the percentage of patients with a depressive syndrome at a single point in time—may be as high as 10 percent in inpatients, and approximately one-half of that in outpatients.

The term *postpsychotic depression* once dominated the research on depression in schizophrenia. This term has lost a great deal of its popularity, as it is problematic on several counts. First, the term implies that a serious depression is a direct response to the experience of psychosis. Patients' depressive symptoms tend to increase during a psychotic exacerbation but also usually improve as the psychosis resolves. Moreover, many patients develop depressive syndromes so long after an exacerbation of psychosis that to call them *postpsychotic* is largely meaningless. Depressive symptoms also often precede psychosis, in two senses: (1) Before the first episode of clear-cut psychosis, most patients have a period of nonpsychotic symptoms that lasts weeks to months and that frequently includes depressive symptoms, and (2) in patients with a previous history of psychotic symptoms, a subsequent psychotic exacerbation may be preceded by symptoms that include depressive mood, anxiety, irritability, and increasing psychotic-like experiences. As is the case in other disorders, anxiety is associated with depression in schizophrenia.

Psychiatry has struggled for many years with the nosology of psychosis associated with affective syndromes. One school of thought in American psychiatry considered the presence of depressive or manic episodes almost to be a negative pathognomonic sign, that is, the presence of an affective episode ruled out the diagnosis of schizophrenia. This view has been discredited by longitudinal studies, which have found that serious depression and, to a lesser extent, manic episodes are common in schizophrenia. Studies of genetics, other risk factors, pathophysiology, and treatment response have also undermined this view. It seems likely that, within a few years, research will lead to a marked revision of the nosology of psychotic and affective disorders.

Increasingly, psychiatrists prescribe antidepressants for patients with schizophrenia who meet criteria for a major depressive episode. Among patients in the midst of an exacerbation of their psychotic symptoms, improvement in psychotic symptoms is associated with an improvement in depressive symptoms, so the prescription of an antidepressant is often deferred, as improvement in the psychotic symptoms may quickly make the antidepressant unnecessary. However, antidepressants are often indicated in patients with schizophrenia and, because of the risk of suicide, may be lifesaving.

Although the symptom profile of depression that is found in schizophrenia is similar to that of nonpsychotic patients, depression appears to occur most frequently in schizophrenia patients who have particular characteristics. Patients who are aware that they are ill are more likely to have depressive symptoms, whereas those with deficit schizophrenia appear to be relatively immune to depression, despite their poorer function and social isolation. Suspiciousness may be associated with an increased risk of depression, cross sectionally and subsequently. Alcohol use is also associated with depression within schizophrenia.

Manic syndromes in the context of schizophrenia have been studied much less than depression. However, such episodes do occur in patients with narrowly defined schizophrenia, and the presence of manic symptoms, or even the presence of a full manic syndrome, does not by itself rule out the diagnosis of schizophrenia.

Suicide

Attempted and completed suicide rates are significantly increased in schizophrenia. It has been reported that suicide attempts are made by 20 to 50 percent of the patients; as many as 10 percent of patients eventually kill themselves. These numbers reflect an approximately 20-fold increase over the suicide rate in the general population.

There are several possible contributors to this extremely high rate of suicide, including command hallucinations and drug abuse. However, probably the most important factor is the presence of a major depressive episode. Demographic and clinical features that have been associated with suicide include young age (and being in the early course of illness), male gender, single marital status, depressive symptoms and hopelessness, more severe illness, frequent relapses, recent hospitalization, good insight, higher cognitive function, higher socioeconomic background, poor social functioning, and lack of social support. From these factors emerge the profile of the patient at greatest risk: a young man who once had high expectations but who has recently realized that his dreams are not likely to come true. However, suicide should never be dismissed as a possibility on the basis of demographics.

Cognitive Impairment

An important development in the understanding of the psychopathology of schizophrenia is an appreciation of the importance of cognitive impairment in the disorder. In outpatients, cognitive impairment is a better predictor of level of function than is the severity of psychotic symptoms. Patients with schizophrenia typically exhibit subtle cognitive dysfunction in the domains of attention, executive function, working memory, and episodic memory. Although a substantial percentage of patients have normal intelligence quotients, it is possible that every person who has schizophrenia has cognitive dysfunction compared to what he or she would be able to do without the disorder. Although these impairments cannot function as diagnostic tools, they are strongly related to the functional outcome of the illness and, for that reason, have clinical value as prognostic variables, as well as for treatment planning.

The cognitive impairment seems already to be present when patients have their first episode and appears largely to remain stable over the course of early illness. (There may be a small subgroup of patients who have a true dementia in late life that is not due to other cognitive disorders, such as Alzheimer's disease.) Cognitive impairments are also present in attenuated forms in nonpsychotic relatives of schizophrenia patients.

The cognitive impairments of schizophrenia have become the target of pharmacological and psychosocial treatment trials. It is likely that effective treatments will become widely available within a few years, and these are likely to lead to an improvement in the quality of life and level of functioning of people with schizophrenia.

The impairment observed in schizophrenia was noted by the early students of the disease. Kraepelin and a contemporary, Busch, conducted experiments on the retention of perceived material and observed deficits in intervals as short as 30 seconds. These experiments, which were also cited by Bleuler, are similar to some current-day neuropsychological paradigms that test working memory, in which patients with schizophrenia frequently exhibit impairments. Today, there is renewed interest in cognitive impairment, which is frequently cited as a core feature of the illness. In *Dementia Praecox*, Kraepelin noted that "It was evident that they could not make the effort to retain and to reproduce what they really saw. . . . This behavior without doubt nearly related to the disorder of attention which we frequently find conspicuously developed in our patients." Likewise, in *Dementia Praecox or the Group of Schizophrenias,* Bleuler noted a similar impairment: "The facilitating as well as the inhibiting properties of attention are equally disturbed."

Polydipsia and Other Repetitive Behaviors Some patients with schizophrenia ingest an enormous amount of fluids, sometimes exceeding 5 L per day. This polydipsia is an important but neglected aspect of the abnormal behavior found in schizophrenia, as some patients' fluid intake leads to electrolyte concentrations that are so low as to induce water intoxication—that is, an altered mental status due to low electrolyte concentrations—and even cardiac arrhythmias and death. Schizophrenia is associated with an increased mortality rate, compared to the general population, and polydipsia contributes to this.

Polydipsia is also found in some other neuropsychiatric syndromes, including autism, but it is more common in schizophrenia. As is the case for many nonpsychotic problems in schizophrenia, estimates of the prevalence of this problem vary greatly, from 3 percent to as high as 25 percent in some studies. Fewer than one-third of polydipsic patients also have a history of water intoxication. Polydipsic patients appear usually to drink normal amounts of water per bout of drinking but have these bouts much more frequently.

Chronic hyponatremia is found in a fraction of polydipsic patients. Polydipsia appears or worsens during psychotic exacerbations in some patients, but many patients exhibit polydipsia when their psychotic symptoms are relatively well controlled. Patients with a chronic hyponatremia may be at particular risk of water intoxication during an exacerbation of their psychotic symptoms.

A consideration of the biology of polydipsia is beyond the scope of this chapter, but the existence of two physiological groups deserves mention here, because of the evidence that these two groups have some behavioral differences. One group of patients with polydipsia is able to maintain its serum electrolytes, despite the consumption of large volumes of fluids, whereas the other group overwhelms its fluid system and has decreased electrolyte concentrations. There is some evidence that the second, hyponatremic group may overlap significantly with deficit, as opposed to nondeficit, schizophrenia.

Patients with schizophrenia often manifest a number of other repetitive behaviors, including pica, bulimia, and the hoarding of a variety of objects. These repetitive behaviors, other than polydipsia, are usually found in severely ill patients. Several such behaviors may be found in some patients, but they do not covary within a population of patients. The exception is the combination of smoking and polydipsia, which tend to cooccur.

Alcohol, Tobacco, and Other Drug Use Drug abuse is common in schizophrenia. In clinical populations, the lifetime prevalence of any drug abuse (other than tobacco) is often much greater than 50 percent; in epidemiological studies, the prevalence can be 40 to 50 percent. For all drugs of abuse (other than tobacco), abuse is associated with poorer function.

The issue of whether drug abuse causes schizophrenia or is a consequence of the illness is controversial and beyond the scope of this chapter. There is evidence consistent with both possibilities. Certainly, it is common for family members to attribute their relative's schizophrenia to drug abuse during adolescence.

Smoking Smoking has a high prevalence in schizophrenia; in clinical samples, the prevalence can be nearly 90 percent. This prevalence is higher than in other groups with neuropsychiatric disorders. Such estimates are probably biased, but, in a population-based study, schizophrenia patients had a prevalence that was 63 percent higher than that in the general population. Smoking probably contributes to the increased mortality found in schizophrenia and decreases the blood concentrations of some antipsychotics. Although in some instances, the patient may, as a consequence of this change in drug concentrations, be more comfortable (because of decreased side effects), other methods of helping patients be comfortable while taking antipsychotic drugs are obviously preferable.

There are suggestions that the increased prevalence in smoking is due, at least in part, to brain abnormalities in nicotinic receptors. A specific polymorphism in a nicotinic receptor has been linked to genetic risk for schizophrenia, and nicotine administration appears to improve some cognitive impairments in schizophrenia. Among patients who smoke habitually, cigarette withdrawal also appears to decrease cognitive function. Hence, patients may seek nicotine via smoking because they feel better in more than one way.

Alcohol Alcohol abuse is also a serious problem in schizophrenia. In one population-based study, the lifetime prevalence of alcohol within schizophrenia was 40 percent, whereas the prevalence in the previous year was 17 percent; for the general population, these prevalence figures were 34 percent and 10 percent. Alcohol abuse increases risk of hospitalization and, in some patients, may increase psychotic symptoms.

Cannabis and Other Drug Abuse Population-based studies suggest that people with schizophrenia also have an increased prevalence of abuse of other common street drugs. In an epidemiological study, 16 percent of subjects with schizophrenia reported a lifetime history of nonalcohol substance misuse. Cannabis is of particular note, because it is associated with schizotypal symptoms—that is, mild, psychotic-like symptoms—in nonpatient populations. Abnormalities in brain cannabinoid receptors that are not due to cannabis use may also exist in schizophrenia.

The use of amphetamine, cocaine, and similar drugs should raise particular concern, because of their marked ability to increase psychotic symptoms.

Motor Abnormalities

Involuntary Movements Because they are overt, observable behaviors, abnormal movements should also be considered part of the psychopathology of schizophrenia. Many currently available antipsychotic medications can cause abnormal involuntary movements with chronic use. This drug-induced motor syndrome is called *tardive dyskinesia*. However, studies conducted before the use of antipsychotic agents and studies of drug-free patients in the modern era have repeatedly found that patients with schizophrenia have a surprisingly high prevalence of such movements in the absence of antipsychotic treatment. (Parkinson-like movement disorders may also have an increased prevalence in schizophrenia, but the evidence is less conclusive.) As abnormal movements are also found in other conditions, one might think that this association is due to bias. However, psychiatric patients with a variety of diagnoses have been compared to schizophrenia patients from the same hospital, and schizophrenia has proven to have a higher prevalence of spontaneous movement than the other disorders. One estimate of the prevalence of spontaneous dyskinetic movements in schizophrenia by age was 4 percent in first-episode patients, 12 percent for patients ill for several years who were younger than 30 years of age, 25 percent for patients between 30 and 50 years of age, and 40 percent for those 60 years of age or older.

Other evidence also suggests that, for some patients, abnormal movements are an integral part of the disease process of schizophrenia. For instance, longitudinal studies have shown that motor dysfunction is present in children who later develop schizophrenia. In addition, subjects with schizotypal personality disorder also have an increased prevalence of abnormal movements, compared to matched controls and subjects with other personality disorders. The evidence is relatively consistent in suggesting that deficit patients have an increased prevalence of such movements before antipsychotic treatment; there is somewhat less evidence that hebephrenic patients also have an increased risk.

Kraepelin gave a vivid description of involuntary movements in patients with schizophrenia:

> The spasmodic phenomena in the musculature of the face and of speech, which often appear, are extremely peculiar disorders. Some of them resemble movements of expression, wrinkling of the forehead, distortion of the corners of the mouth, irregular movements of the tongue and lips, twisting of the eyes, opening them wide, and shutting them tight, in short, those movements which we bring together under the name of making faces or grimacing; they remind one of the corresponding disorders of choreic patients. . . . Connected with these are further, smacking and licking with the tongue, sudden sighing, sniffing, laughing, and clearing the throat. But besides, we observe specially in the lip muscles, fine lightning-like or rhythmical twitchings, which in no way bear the stamp of voluntary movements. . . . Several patients continually carried out peculiar sprawling, irregular, choreiform, outspreading movements, which I think I can best characterize by the expression "athetoid ataxia."

Other Motor Abnormalities The motor manifestations of catatonia have been described previously. Catatonia has long been considered a hallmark of schizophrenia, but it is also found in affective disorder.

Subtle abnormalities in motor behavior have been found in children who develop schizophrenia in adult life. Mild incoordination is common. Mannerisms are also found. Both of these problems persist into adult life.

Kraepelin described mannerisms, which he defined as "morbidly changed forms" of movement:

> Even simple movements can show such changes. Sometimes they are carried out with too great an expenditure of force, or unnecessary groups of muscles take part in them, or too much of the limb is employed, so that they become ungraceful and clumsy; or they are not rounded off, they begin and end jerkily and appear therefore stiff, wooden, and angular. Other patients again arrive at the aim of the movement not by the nearest way, but by round-about ways with all sorts of changes and interpolations; they add flourishes by which the movements become unnatural, affected and manneristic. . . . Grasping is done with fingers spread out; speaking is accompanied with loud hawking and grunting or with smacking movements of the lips, the face is distorted by spasmodic grinning.

Obsessive-Compulsive Symptoms In some patients, distinguishing obsessions and compulsions from psychotic symptoms can be difficult. For instance, if a patient frequently hears voices that comment on an odor coming from the patient, and that patient washes multiple times during the day, it may be difficult to distinguish whether this behavior represents a true compulsion or psychosis. The DSM-IV-TR states that schizophrenic symptoms "are not ego-dystonic and not subject to reality testing." This boundary between a compulsion and an action due to a psychotic experience can be difficult to discern. An idea or behavior can be ego-syntonic at one point but not later; in addition, the qualities of being ego-syntonic and ego-dystonic exist on a continuum.

Nonetheless, obsessions and compulsions that can be distinguished from psychotic symptoms per se are common in schizophrenia. Investigators have estimated the prevalence of obsessions and compulsions within schizophrenia—that is, the number of patients with significant obsessions or compulsion—as well as the prevalence of schizophrenia patients who meet the DSM-IV-TR criteria for OCD (aside from the exclusion criterion of schizophrenia). In clinics, estimates for the prevalence of significant obsessive-compulsive symptoms typically range from 15 to 25 percent; the estimates for a syndrome that meets DSM criteria for OCD are slightly lower. The group of patients with these symptoms probably has poorer function than the group that does not.

Panic Attacks Panic attacks have received relatively little attention in the context of schizophrenia, but some studies suggest that panic attacks essentially identical to those found in primary panic disorder are relatively common in patients with schizophrenia. Estimates of the prevalence of panic attacks in clinical samples are typically 25 to 40 percent. The results of one study suggest that panic attacks may be part of the prodrome preceding the first onset of schizophrenia. An association between panic attacks and paranoid schizophrenia, rather than other subtypes, has been replicated. Psychotic symptoms may transiently increase during a panic attack. In one family study, the prevalence of panic disorder was higher in the families of schizophrenia and panic disorder probands than in the families of control subjects; the prevalence in the schizophrenia families did not differ from that in the families of panic disorder probands.

Insight A common feature of schizophrenia is poor insight, that is, a lack of awareness that the patient has a problem. People with schizophrenia have poorer insight than patients with depression but may not have more impairment of this kind than do bipolar patients.

In recent years, sophisticated instruments for quantifying insight have been developed, in which different aspects of insight can be considered independently. For instance, a patient may acknowledge that his or her symptoms are unusual but may deny that they are caused by an illness. Alternatively, the patient may acknowledge that he or she was ill but may deny that there is any risk that the symptoms could return. One can also extend the concept of insight to aspects of function, as well as to symptoms. Thus, one can distinguish awareness of *symptoms*, of *impairment*, of the *views other people have* of the patient, of the causes of the impairment (called *attribution*), of the *need for treatment*, and of the *effects of treatment*.

Within each of these realms, insight is not an all-or-nothing phenomenon. A patient may have excellent insight into one aspect of the illness—for instance, that his or her voices are abnormal—but may lack insight into another aspect, for instance, that the medications decrease the severity of the voices. Within a realm of insight, the patient's understanding can also be partial: One patient may be convinced that voices, for instance, are not due to an illness, whereas another patient may think it is possible that his voices are due to an illness but may not be sure.

Insight can also vary over time. Educating a patient may change his or her level of insight, and clinical improvement in other aspects of the illness may be associated with improved insight. Resolution of an exacerbation of psychotic symptoms can be associated with better insight.

A number of explanations for the poor insight of schizophrenia have been proposed. Psychosis itself—that is, the inability to discern reality—has been blamed, whereas others have argued that poor insight may serve as a protective defensive mechanism, especially as depression is associated with good insight. However, many researchers in this area have come to believe that some aspects of poor insight are due to neuropsychological impairments, that is, to a large extent, impaired insight has a neurological basis.

Deficit schizophrenia patients appear to have particularly poor insight. This may be related to their poorer cognitive impairment.

Mortality

Mortality in schizophrenia is significantly higher than that of the general population. Death from unnatural causes is fourfold the expected rate and accounts for almost 40 percent of this increased risk; the leading cause of unnatural death is suicide. However, the death rate from accidents and homicide is also approximately twice the expected rate.

Violence

The association between violence and schizophrenia is controversial, and the research on violence and schizophrenia produces mixed results. There is a lack of a common definition for violence, and sampling bias is common in studies. Clearly, the proportion of violence in society attributable to schizophrenia is small. That said, patients with schizophrenia are probably slightly more likely to commit violent acts than are members of the general population but are significantly less likely than patients with many other psychiatric disorders, most notably, substance abuse and personality disorders. Comorbid substance abuse increases the risk of violence, and violent patients are more likely to be acutely psychotic. Reported incidences of violent acts are much lower after the first contact with psychiatric care compared to the period before psychiatric care is instituted. Finally, the approximate annual risk of homicidal acts among patients with schizophrenia is reported to be small: 1 in 3,000 for men and 1 in 33,000 in women.

Patients with schizophrenia also have an increased risk of being the victims of violence.

SOMATIC COMORBIDITY

People with schizophrenia have a risk of death from natural causes that is approximately 1.5 times the expected rate, and the disorder is also associated with poorer general health status than that of the general population. There are many possible causes for this association. As a group, people with schizophrenia struggle with decreased social function and a downward drift in socioeconomic status, with associated poor access to medical care; comorbid substance abuse, including the use of tobacco; the side effects of the medications that are used to treat schizophrenia; impaired cognitive function; and comorbid neuropsychiatric disorders such as polydipsia that can have a direct impact on health.

Interestingly, people with schizophrenia also have a well-established decrease in risk of rheumatoid arthritis and may have a decrease in the risk of allergies. These negative associations may be related to the mild immunological changes found in schizophrenia.

Obesity

Patients with schizophrenia appear to be more obese, with higher body mass indexes than age- and gender-matched cohorts in general population. This is due, at least in part, to the effect of many antipsychotic medications, as well as poor nutritional balance and decreased motor activity. This weight gain, in turn, contributes to an increased risk of cardiovascular morbidity and mortality, an increased risk of diabetes, and other obesity-related conditions such as hyperlipidemia and obstructive sleep apnea.

Diabetes Mellitus

Schizophrenia is associated with an increased risk of type II diabetes mellitus (DM). This is probably due, in part, to the association with obesity noted previously, but there is also evidence that some antipsychotic medications cause DM through a direct mechanism. Some studies that predate the use of antipsychotic medications also suggested that schizophrenia is associated with diabetes; hence, the widespread developmental problems found in schizophrenia may include metabolic abnormalities.

Cardiovascular Disease

Many antipsychotic medications have direct effects on cardiac electrophysiology. In addition, obesity, increased rates of smoking, diabetes, hyperlipidemia, and a sedentary lifestyle all independently increase the risk of cardiovascular morbidity and mortality.

HIV

Patients with schizophrenia appear to have a risk of human immunodeficiency virus (HIV) infection that is 1.5 to two times that of the general population. This association is thought to be due to increased risk behaviors, such as unprotected sex, multiple partners, and increased drug use.

Chronic Obstructive Pulmonary Disease

Rates of chronic obstructive pulmonary disease are reportedly increased in schizophrenia compared to the general population. The increased prevalence of smoking is an obvious contributor to this problem and may be the only cause.

Rheumatoid Arthritis

Patients with schizophrenia have approximately one-third the risk of rheumatoid arthritis that is found in the general population. This inverse association has been replicated several times.

EVALUATION AND TREATMENT IN A BROADER CONTEXT

The framework for understanding the psychopathology of schizophrenia presented in this chapter, which has emphasized the importance of the nonpsychotic, as well as the psychotic, aspects of the disorder, is part of the broader trend to view schizophrenia as a neurodevelopmental disorder. This neurodevelopmental framework has an important practical advantage for patients. If clinicians understand that, in the evaluation of a patient with schizophrenia, evaluation of the psychosis alone is not sufficient, patients are more likely to receive effective treatment for the many problems other than psychosis that confront people with schizophrenia. Psychotic symptoms, as terrible as they can be, are probably not the principal reason that people with schizophrenia have, on average, a shorter life span than does the general population. Depression, metabolic problems, and drug abuse probably make much greater contributions to this problem. In addition, for many patients, psychotic symptoms are not the reason that they experience emotional anguish or the principal reason that their level of function is significantly impaired. Clinicians need to pay attention to the broad manifestations of this disorder.

SUGGESTED CROSS-REFERENCES

For further information on the neurodevelopmental theory of schizophrenia, the reader is encouraged to read Section 12.5. Section 12.9 provides further detail on the cognitive impairments found in schizophrenia. Aspects of differential diagnosis are discussed in more depth in Section 12.15 (other psychotic disorders).

References

Amador XF, Flaum M, Andreasen NC, Strauss DH, Yale SA, Clark SC, Gorman JM: Awareness of illness in schizophrenia and schizoaffective and mood disorders. *Arch Gen Psychiatry.* 1994;51:826.

Arndt S, Andreasen NC, Flaum M, Miller D, Nopoulos P: A longitudinal study of symptom dimensions in schizophrenia. Prediction and patterns of change. *Arch Gen Psychiatry.* 1995;52:352.

American Psychiatric Association. *Diagnostic and Statistical Manual of Mental Disorders.* 4th ed., text revision. Washington, DC: American Psychiatric Association; 1994.

Berrettini WH: Are schizophrenic and bipolar disorders related? A review of family and molecular studies. *Biol Psychiatry.* 2000;48:531.

Bleuler E. *Dementia Praecox, or the Group of Schizophrenias.* New York: International Universities Press; 1952.

Buchanan RW, Carpenter WT: Domains of psychopathology: An approach to the reduction of heterogeneity in schizophrenia. *J Nerv Ment Dis.* 1994;182:193.

Carpenter WT Jr, Kirkpatrick B: The heterogeneity of the long-term course of schizophrenia. *Schizophr Bull.* 1988;14:645.

*Castle DJ, Murray RM: The epidemiology of late-onset schizophrenia. *Schizophr Bull.* 1993;19:691.

Cooper JE, Kendell RE, Gurland BJ, Sharpe L, Copeland JRM, Simon R. Institute of Psychiatry, Maudsley Monographs, Number 20. *Psychiatric Diagnosis in New York and London: A Comparative Study of Mental Hospital Admissions.* London: Oxford University Press; 1972.

Fenton WS: Prevalence of spontaneous dyskinesia in schizophrenia. *J Clin Psychiatry.* 2000;61[Suppl 4]:10.

Goldman MB: A rational approach to disorders of water balance in psychiatric patients. *Hosp Community Psychiatry.* 1991;42:488.

Green AI, Canuso CM, Brenner MJ, Wojcik JD: Detection and management of comorbidity in patients with schizophrenia. *Psychiatr Clin North Am.* 2003;26:115.

*Green MF: What are the functional consequences of neurocognitive deficits in schizophrenia? *Am J Psychiatry.* 1996;153:321.

Gross-Isseroff R, Hermesh H, Zohar J, Weizman A: Neuroimaging communality between schizophrenia and obsessive compulsive disorder: A putative basis for schizo-obsessive disorder? *World J Biol Psychiatry.* 2003;4:129.

Hafner H: Onset and course of the first schizophrenic episode. *Kaohsiung J Med Sci.* 1998;14:413.

Harris EC, Barraclough B: Excess mortality of mental disorder. *Br J Psychiatry.* 1998;173:11.

Heun R, Maier W: Relation of schizophrenia and panic disorder: Evidence from a controlled family study. *Am J Med Genet.* 1995;60:127.

Hoenig J. Schizophrenia: Clinical section. In: Berrios GE, Porter R, eds. *A History of Clinical Psychiatry: The Origin and History of Psychiatric Disorders.* New York: New York University Press; 1995.

Hoff AL, Kremen WS: Is there a cognitive phenotype for schizophrenia? The nature and course of the disturbance in cognition. *Curr Opin Psychiatry.* 2002;15:43.

*Kirkpatrick B, Buchanan RW, Ross DE, Carpenter WT. A separate disease within the syndrome of schizophrenia. *Arch Gen Psychiatry.* 2001;58:165.

Koenig JI, Kirkpatrick B, Lee P: Glucocorticoid hormones and early brain development in schizophrenia. *Neuropsychopharmacology.* 2002;27:309.

*Kraepelin E. *Dementia Praecox and Paraphrenia.* Edinburgh: E & S Livingstone; 1919.

McCreadie RG: Scottish Comorbidity Study Group. Use of drugs, alcohol and tobacco by people with schizophrenia: Case-control study. *Br J Psychiatry.* 2002;181:321.

McGlashan TH, Fenton WS: Classical subtypes for schizophrenia: Literature review for DSM-IV. *Schizophr Bull.* 1991;17:609.

McGrath JJ, Feron FP, Burne TH, Mackay-Sim A, Eyles DW: The neurodevelopmental hypothesis of schizophrenia: A review of recent developments. *Ann Med.* 2003;35:86.

Moberg PJ, Turetsky BI: Scent of a disorder: Olfactory functioning in schizophrenia. *Curr Psychiatry Rep.* 2003;5:311.

Niemi LT, Suvisaari JM, Tuulio-Henriksson A, Lonnqvist JK: Childhood developmental abnormalities in schizophrenia: Evidence from high-risk studies. *Schizophr Res.* 2003;60:239.

Palmer BW, McClure FS, Jeste DV: Schizophrenia in late life: Findings challenge traditional concepts. *Harv Rev Psychiatry.* 2001;9:51.

Ratakonda S, Gorman JM, Yale SA, Amador XF: Characterization of psychotic conditions. Use of the domains of psychopathology model. *Arch Gen Psychiatry.* 1998;55:75.

Schneider K. *Clinical Psychopathology.* New York: Grune & Stratton; 1959.

*Siris SG: Depression in schizophrenia: Perspective in the era of "atypical" antipsychotic agents. *Am J Psychiatry.* 2000;157:1379.

Siris SG: Suicide and schizophrenia. *J Psychopharmacol.* 2001;15:127.

Tibbo P, Warneke L: Obsessive-compulsive disorder in schizophrenia: Epidemiologic and biologic overlap. *J Psychiatry Neurosci.* 1999;24:15.

Walsh E, Buchanan A, Fahy T: Violence and schizophrenia: Examining the evidence. *Br J Psychiatry.* 2002;180:490.

World Health Organization. *Report of The International Pilot Study of Schizophrenia.* Vol 1. Geneva: World Health Organization; 1973.

▲ 12.9 Schizophrenia: Cognition

James M. Gold, Ph.D., and Michael F. Green, Ph.D.

NEUROCOGNITION IN SCHIZOPHRENIA

The study of the cognitive impairment has become one of the central issues in schizophrenia research over the last decade, as evidenced by a surge in publications addressing aspects of the issue. A computerized search of the Medline database using neuropsychology and schizophrenia as linked key words reveals a publication rate of 1.5 papers per year from 1970 to 1979, 10.8 papers per year during the 1980s, 49.6 papers per year during the 1990s, and 72 papers per year since 2000. This recent interest builds on a long and rich clinical and experimental tradition dating back to the original clinical descriptions of the illness. For Emil Kraepelin, abnormalities in cognitive functioning were fundamental to the illness, providing strong leads about the likely site of underlying neuropathology. He reasoned that abnormalities of the frontal and temporal lobes were implicated by the impairments observed in "higher intellectual abilities," because "these are the faculties which our patients invariably suffer profound loss in contrast to memory and acquired capabilities . . . the peculiar speech disorders resembling sensory aphasia and the auditory hallucinations which probably point to the temporal lobe being involved." Thus, on the basis of clinical observation and inference, Kraepelin identified schizophrenia as a disorder involving multiple brain areas and cognitive functions, with an emphasis on aspects of attention and cognitive control that remain the central topics of contemporary research.

This section provides an overview of many of the central issues in the study of cognitive performance in schizophrenia. The literature in this area is voluminous and defies comprehensive review. Therefore, the approach of this section is deliberately selective, as it emphasizes the most clinically relevant areas in which the literature has provided the most robust, reproducible findings and in which the study of cognitive functioning has shed important light on the nature of the illness. These areas include (1) cognitive deficits as developmental precursors, (2) the deficit pattern observed in first-episode patients, (3) the course of cognitive impairment, (4) the relationship between clinical symptoms and cognition, (5) the role of individual differences, (6) cognitive deficits as risk markers for the illness, (7) the importance of cognition for functional outcome, and (8) the impact of pharmacological treatment on cognitive functioning. In addition, this section addresses some of the basic theoretical issues raised by cognitive findings, including the issue of whether it is possible to provide an

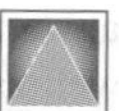

Table 12.9–1
Major Cognitive Constructs and Representative Measures

Construct	Examples of Tests	Description
Episodic memory	California Verbal Learning Test	*Episodic memory* refers to the ability to acquire and to retain new information in long-term storage. Typically, this type of memory is assessed with a list of words or brief stories.
Working or immediate memory	Digit span, letter number span, N-Back Test	*Working memory* refers to the ability to maintain a limited amount of information for a brief time (usually a few seconds), such as when one retains a telephone number long enough to make a call. The working memory system allows for the maintenance of information and the manipulation or use of this information in the service of other cognitive operations.
Vigilance or sustained attention	Versions of the continuous performance test	Vigilance involves maintaining a readiness to respond to a particular target stimulus and not to respond to nontargets over a period of time. Vigilance is typically measured by tests in which a series of briefly presented stimuli appear on a computer screen, and subjects are asked to respond only to selected targets.
Executive functioning	Wisconsin Card Sorting Test; Tower of Hanoi	*Executive functioning* refers to volition, planning, purposive action, and self-monitoring of behavior. Card-sorting tests are frequently used to assess executive functioning. These tests assess the subject's ability to attain, to maintain, and to shift cognitive set.
Verbal fluency	Controlled Oral Word Association Test	Verbal fluency tests measure one's ability to generate words that begin with a certain letter or that belong to a certain semantic category, such as animals.
Early visual processing	Span of apprehension, visual masking	Measures of early visual processing evaluate basic stages of visual processing, such as detection and identification of visual stimuli. Assessments of these processes usually involve the brief, tachistoscopic presentation of visual stimuli on a screen.
Psychomotor skills	Grooved peg board, finger tapping	Psychomotor abilities are usually assessed with tests of motor speed or dexterity. Motor speed is measured with rapid, repetitive finger movements, and dexterity is assessed with tasks that involve fine manual manipulation.
Language and verbal knowledge	Vocabulary, Boston Naming Test	Language or verbal knowledge tests require subjects to provide definitions of words or the correct name for drawings of common objects.
Speed of processing	Digit symbol	Processing speed tasks typically involve simple cognitive operations. Thus, all subjects are able to perform the task, and the critical dependent measure is how many items they are able to complete in a specific period of time.

integrative explanatory account of the accumulated literature in terms of the fundamental processes that are implicated by the deficits documented in the empirical literature. See Table 12.9–1 for brief definitions of many of the key cognitive constructs and examples of clinical measures that are commonly used in this literature.

HISTORICAL OVERVIEW

The central role of cognitive impairment in the theoretical conceptualizations of Kraepelin and Eugen Bleuler provided a strong stimulus for the use of experimental methods to provide a more specific and detailed examination of the nature of cognitive impairment in the illness. Although this older literature is well beyond the scope of this review, there are a few highlights that are worthy of particular mention. In 1945, David Rappaport and colleagues published a two-volume work, *Diagnostic Psychological Testing*, summarizing their findings on the effect of psychiatric illness on a broad battery of intellectual, memory, reasoning, and personality tests. In describing chronic schizophrenic patients, Rappaport noted that these patients have their greatest impairments in "judgment, attention, concentration, planning ability and anticipation," as well as significant difficulties in new learning, abstract reasoning, and the overall efficiency of intellectual functioning. Although Rapaport and colleagues interpreted these findings within a psychodynamic context, the basic empirical data documented in their work are consistent with contemporary research findings. These findings were not unique, as major research efforts from multiple laboratories were devoted to the study of deficits in abstract reasoning, intellectual functioning, and aspects of attention. The program of experimental research led by David Shakow is particularly notable in the breadth of topics addressed, ranging from sensory functioning, learning impairment, intellectual decline, to reaction time. In attempting to account for the overall nature of the deficit in schizophrenia, Shakow implicated an impairment of cognitive control processes, presaging contemporary notions of executive control failures. He stated that patients had difficulty maintaining an appropriate "generalized set" to guide selective processing of environmental stimuli, as well as response selection. With such a set impairment, "the rudderless nature of the controls is revealed by present behavior that is unrealistic. . . . Performance is unstable and either markedly loose or extremely rigid. The person seems to be working at a level considerably below true capacity." Shakow's conceptualization is strikingly close to current formulations suggesting that the critical deficit in schizophrenia involves the control and modulation of cognitive processing rather than any discrete localized form of computation.

The fact that these early investigators were able to identify many of the critical empirical findings and conceptual issues in the contemporary schizophrenia literature 40 to 50 years before the development of standardized diagnostic criteria is remarkable and suggests that these cognitive impairments are truly strong *signals*. However, the prevailing psychodynamic zeitgeist considered schizophrenia to be a *functional* rather than *organic* disorder. Indeed, at the same time that these observations were being published, major theoretical accounts of schizophrenia continued to emphasize the role of early childhood experience and parenting in the genesis of schizophrenia. Thus, the cognitive data were not widely considered as direct evidence of cortical compromise in schizophrenia.

Schizophrenia As a Brain Disease

The scientific zeitgeist changed dramatically at the close of the 1970s in the face of multiple lines of evidence that schizophrenia reliably involved abnormalities of brain structure, as well as function. Three influential review papers examining the diagnostic accuracy of neuropsychological tests in distinguishing between functional and organic disorders all came to similar conclusions: Neuropsychological tests reliably differentiated *functional* from *organic* patients, except in chronic schizophrenia, in which classification approached chance levels. These reviews were published nearly contemporaneously with the first computed tomography (CT) studies that documented ventricular enlargement in patients with schizophrenia. This combination of evidence led to the straightforward conclusion that the reason that patients with schizophrenia performed as if they had brain damage was because they, in fact, had structural brain abnormalities. This confluence of evidence marks a clear dividing line in schizophrenia research. The direct in vivo imaging evidence of ventricular enlargement in schizophrenia had a profound effect on the larger community of clinicians and researchers in legitimizing the idea that schizophrenia was a brain disease, supplanting psychodynamic views on the etiology of the disorder. Furthermore, the rapid growth of clinical neuropsychology as a discipline occurring in the 1980s led to a dramatic increase in the number of studies explicitly motivated by an effort to use cognitive measures as a means of interrogating the neural systems involved in schizophrenia. It is the work that grew from this intellectual soil that is reviewed in the following discussion.

COGNITIVE DEFICITS AS DEVELOPMENTAL PRECURSORS

Most contemporary discussions about the etiology of schizophrenia assume that multiple interacting factors are involved, ranging from adverse in utero events, to underlying genetic vulnerability, to environmental stresses. These early adverse environmental events and genetic liability are thought to interact with brain maturational processes, culminating with the onset of frank psychotic symptoms, most typically in the late teenage years. However, this neurodevelopmental framework suggests that the abnormalities in neural function that later lead to clinically symptomatic illness might be evident far earlier in other aspects of behavior, with cognition being a likely indicator of risk. Note that this perspective implies that the concept of *premorbid* intellectual function needs to be reconceived as *prepsychotic* intellectual function, as it is assumed that the essence of the *morbid* process has shaped the developmental process.

Retrospective studies of the childhood intellectual performance of patients who later developed schizophrenia began in the 1960s and 1970s. In general terms, the literature supports the idea that a subtle compromise of childhood intellectual function (on the order of 5 to 7 intelligence quotient [IQ] points) is characteristic of patients with schizophrenia. Such deficits were most reliably observed in studies contrasting the intellectual performance of future patients to healthy control children (drawn form the same school class, for example). Deficits have also been documented in some, but not all, studies in which sibling controls were examined. This pattern of results raises the possibility that siblings may also have a form of intellectual compromise relative to nonfamily controls. Although highly suggestive of a common, likely genetically mediated compromise of intellectual development in patients and siblings, this literature also has a number of important limitations, including the absence of operational diagnostic criteria and issues of sampling bias that are common in retrospective research designs.

Prospective Studies These methodological issues have been addressed by a number of recent independent studies that have examined epidemiological samples, studied prospectively from early in development, in which it was possible to link these data with adult psychiatric diagnostic information contained in patient registries or hospital records. In the first such study, a group of British investigators was able to examine a cohort of more than 5,000 children, all of whom were born in a single week in 1946. This birth cohort was prospectively studied on multiple occasions from early infancy into middle age. A wide range of data was collected over time, ranging from early developmental milestones, to educational achievement testing, to social-behavioral data based on maternal interview. Based on the follow-up data, as well as mental health registry information, it was possible to identify 30 members of the original cohort who met diagnostic criteria for schizophrenia as adults. These 30 cases were then compared to the rest of the cohort on the developmental variables of interest. Future cases sat, stood, walked, and talked at slightly later ages than controls, with more frequent speech problems noted by their doctors. On academic testing, future cases demonstrated deficits on verbal, nonverbal, and mathematics measures. These deficits were apparent at 8 years of age, with an amplification of the deficit by 15 years of age (with effect sizes ranging from 0.2 to 0.6 across measures and time). Importantly, there was a linear trend between intellectual performance and later risk for schizophrenia, suggesting that the overall result could not be attributed to a severely impaired subgroup. In the behavioral realm, future cases were noted to prefer solitary play at 4 and 6 years of age, with increased self-report of social anxiety by 13 years of age, something noted by teacher reports at 15 years of age. Thus, this study demonstrates that the later development of schizophrenia is preceded by subtle alterations in neurological, cognitive, and social functioning, with varying manifestations across the course of early and adolescent development. The basic findings of this landmark study have been replicated in other birth cohort studies, including an American study that documented IQ deficits on the order of 7 points observed at 4 years of age. Interestingly, in the American study, the intellectual performance of future patients did not differ from their siblings, replicating the result pattern observed in some of the earlier studies discussed previously, suggesting that intellectual compromise may be genetically mediated. As in the English study, the entire score distribution appeared to be shifted in the future patient group: Future cases were overrepresented at lower performance levels and underrepresented at the higher performance levels.

Military Inductee Studies The results from these birth cohort designs are supported by large sample studies of military inductees. These studies linked prospectively obtained data to diagnostic information contained in mental health registries. In a population-based Israeli study, subjects received an extensive intellectual and academic assessment at 16 years of age, and these data were linked to follow-up diagnostic information. Comparing more than 500 patients with individually matched controls, future patients demonstrated significant deficits on all intellectual measures, with effect sizes ranging from 0.3 to 0.6 on different measures (equivalent to approximately 4 to 9 IQ points). Importantly, future cases of nonpsychotic bipolar disorder did not demonstrate any evidence of intellectual impairment relative to controls, suggesting that the schizophrenia finding is relatively specific and does not reflect risk for psychiatric maladjustment. The results of this study are consistent with a Swedish military conscript study of 50,000 subjects using case registry information about later psychiatric diagnosis. In the Swedish study, there was again a linear relationship between IQ and schizophrenia risk. The results of these large epidemiological studies are remarkably consistent and suggest that a subtle compromise of intellectual function is a risk factor for schizophrenia. These findings are consistent with evidence from high-risk research designs in which the offspring of parents with schizophrenia have been studied. Such studies have also revealed deficits in overall IQ or in more specific cognitive functions, such as in attention and short-term memory during early childhood and adolescence (family studies are discussed more thoroughly in the section Family Studies). It should be noted that the magnitude of impairment observed on general measures of intellectual and academic ability appears to be amplified on more specific measures of attentional function, as documented in the high-risk literature, suggesting the latter may be more sensitive measures of schizophrenia liability.

Two aspects of these findings are relevant for considering the course of schizophrenia and the issue of heterogeneity among patients. First, an overall estimate of approximately a one-third to one-half standard deviation deficit in intellectual ability observed before onset of psychotic symptoms appears to be fairly consistent across studies and can serve as a baseline for evaluating the extent of deficit observed in ill adult patients. In addition, several of these studies have emphasized the linear relationship between measures of intellectual function and schizophrenia. Such a relationship suggests that schizophrenia risk is a quantitative, rather than an all-or-none, phenomenon. This would imply that efforts to subgroup patient samples along simple binary dimensions (intellectually impaired versus nonimpaired) will likely fail to represent accurately the continuous nature of the underlying distribution.

DEFICIT PATTERN OBSERVED IN FIRST-EPISODE PATIENTS

The vast majority of neuropsychological studies in the schizophrenia literature before the past decade were conducted in chronically ill patient populations, often drawn from long-term inpatient facilities. This sampling bias raises the possibility that the deficit pattern documented in many studies from the 1970s and 1980s might reflect the impact of numerous uncontrolled variables, including the effect of institutionalization itself and the possible effect of long-term pharmacological treatment, or might represent an effect of illness severity and duration, with most studies sampling the most severely afflicted patients with a long history of chronic illness. These concerns stimulated a series of independent studies of patients assessed at the time of their first psychotic episode, in some studies before the initiation of pharmacological treatment. In several instances, the study groups were generated from consecutive admissions to major treatment facilities, and the resulting patient samples are likely fairly representative of the illness in general or, at a minimum, representative of the ill population that requires intensive treatment. Thus, the results of these studies provide potentially compelling evidence concerning the role of confounding factors in estimating the severity of cognitive impairment in schizophrenia and further yield a critical baseline measure in considering the course of cognitive impairment in schizophrenia.

There is a remarkable degree of consistency in findings reported from studies based in New York City; Philadelphia; Long Island, New York; and Iowa: Patients studied at first episode present clear evidence of neuropsychological impairment, with overall performance levels at least one standard deviation below that of healthy controls (the equivalent of an IQ of 85 relative to the control mean of 100). This overall level of performance impairment is clearly more severe than the subtle deficits documented in the developmental precursor literature reviewed previously. This contrast strongly supports the inference that significant intellectual decline occurs near the time of symptom onset. The precise timing of this deterioration is not clear: It is possible that intellectual decline occurs before the onset of frank symptoms (for example, over the preceding 1 to 3 years), or it may be more proximal to the development of psychosis.

Two Forms of Impairment

Combining the evidence from the developmental precursor and first-episode literature, it appears that two distinct forms of intellectual impairment are characteristic of schizophrenia: (1) deficits that arise early in development and (2) deficits that arise in the context of clinical illness. These two types of deficits are conceptually, as well as temporally, distinct: Developmentally based deficits limit the normal acquisition of cognitive skills, as seen on measures of intelligence and academic ability. This developmental compromise is relatively subtle, requiring sensitive formal testing and comparison to well-matched control populations. In contrast, illness-onset–related deficits appear to represent an actual decline in function: They reflect a compromise in the ability to access, to deploy efficiently, and to coordinate the cognitive skills that were successfully acquired during the developmental period. Illness-onset deficits tend to be far more severe than developmentally based deficits and are obvious in the context of clinical interaction.

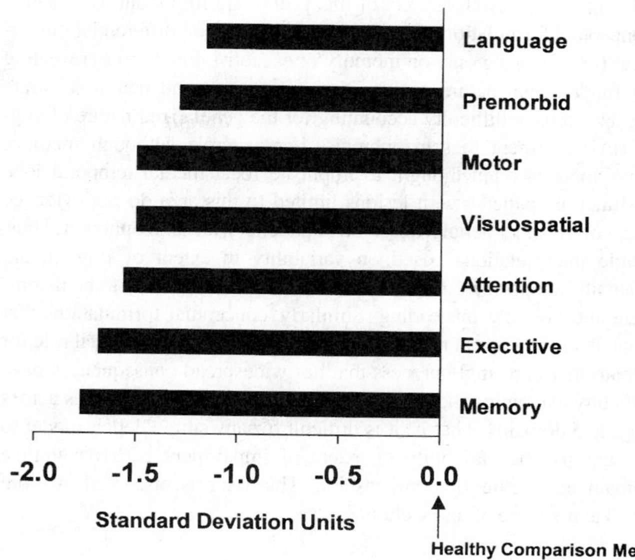

FIGURE 12.9–1 Performance of first-episode patients on seven summary cognitive scales relative to a healthy comparison group. Each summary score is a composite based on multiple individual tests of that construct. Patient performance is expressed in standard deviation units derived from the comparison group: The healthy comparison group has a mean score of 0 on each summary score. Note that patients score at least 1 standard deviation unit below the healthy comparison group on all scales. (Data adapted from Bilder RM, Goldman RS, Robinson D, et al.: Neuropsychology of first-episode schizophrenia: Initial characterization and clinical correlates. *Am J Psychiatry.* 2000;157:549.)

General and Specific Deficits

Although the breadth of general illness-onset–related intellectual decline is impressive, there is considerable variability in the extent of impairment noted across cognitive domains, with some functions (typically memory in many studies) demonstrating somewhat more severe impairment than observed in other cognitive domains. This point is illustrated in Figure 12.9–1, based on a sample of 94 first-episode patients, which shows impairment averaging approximately 1.5 standard deviation units across seven cognitive domains. Even the least impaired cognitive domain score was more than 1 standard deviation below that observed in controls, with a maximal impairment of 1.75 standard deviation units. Statistical analyses revealed that the memory and executive scales were differentially more impaired when compared to the mean of the other scales. Conversely, patients demonstrated a relative strength on the language scale that was significantly less impaired than the overall mean.

The results from this study appear to be quite representative of the first episode literature, which provides robust evidence for (1) a substantial deficit spanning all measured aspects of cognition relative to healthy controls and (2) variation in the extent of impairment across domains, with evidence from multiple studies suggesting that memory and executive function are the two domains most likely to show modest differential impairment. Both aspects of this profile are important to consider. Conceptual formulations that emphasize the areas of differential impairment (i.e., focusing only on memory or executive function) as revealing the fundamental nature of cognitive impairment and neural substrate implicated have difficulty accounting for the generalized nature of cognitive impairment in schizophrenia. For example, although memory impairment is often thought to implicate focal medial temporal lobe dysfunction, patients with lesions limited to this area do not evidence many of the other deficits observed in patients with schizophrenia. Thus, profile interpretations based on variability in extent of impairment, when all functions are impaired to some degree, are likely to be incomplete and possibly misleading. Similarly, conceptual formulations that emphasize the general nature of the deficit or that posit a critical role for impairment in a single process that has widespread consequences have difficulty explaining the fact that the extent of impairment varies across cognitive domains. That is, it is difficult for any single deficit model to account for the variability in extent of impairment across cognitive domain in a straightforward fashion. This issue is discussed in more detail at the close of this section.

COURSE OF COGNITIVE IMPAIRMENT

The question of whether schizophrenia involves a progressive form of intellectual decline or a more stable form of impairment has been the focus of considerable controversy beginning with Kraepelin's description of the syndrome. There is a great deal of evidence that the illness involves a decline of intellectual function from the highest level achieved before the onset of psychotic symptoms superimposed on more subtle developmentally based compromise. The key question is whether the process that leads to intellectual decline occurs over a limited period of time. That is, if there is some type of destructive process that leads to a loss of intellectual function, it is certainly plausible that the severity or duration of this process varies across patients, thereby producing evidence of illness progression. There are several types of evidence that can be brought to bear on this question. Repeated longitudinal assessment is the most powerful study design to document cognitive course of illness. Recent longitudinal studies of first-episode and more chronically ill samples have failed to document clear, reliable evidence of progressive intellectual deterioration in patients with schizophrenia. Earlier studies used cross-sectional designs, comparing the extent of impairment demonstrated by patient samples of varying age relative to controls, to reach the same conclusion. Thus, multiple study designs and literature reviews argue against the idea that schizophrenia is an illness that involves progressive intellectual decline.

On the other hand, evidence suggesting progressive decline has come from several studies that have contrasted the cognitive performance of first-episode patients to that observed among more chronically ill patient groups and have found somewhat more severe impairments in the latter. The interpretation of such findings, however, is not straightforward, given the potential confound of sampling bias. That is, it is likely that the best-outcome portion of first-episode samples is not represented in chronically ill samples, perhaps accounting for the evidence of worse performance over time. Another approach to this issue is to compare the level of impairment observed in first-episode patients (the sample shown in Fig. 12.9–1) to that documented in the literature overall, a literature comprised primarily of study groups with long-established illness, as shown in Figure 12.9–2.

It is striking that, nearly without exception, the deficits in first-episode patients are highly similar to those documented in the overall literature. Although the results of only one first episode are represented in the figure, roughly comparable results have been reported from multiple first-episode studies. Thus, across study designs there is a great deal of evidence to suggest that the level of impairment observed at first episode is basically stable, at least through middle age.

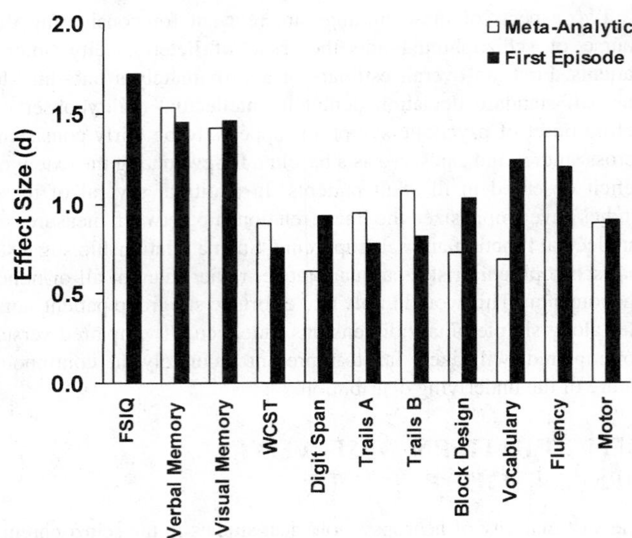

FIGURE 12.9–2 Effect size (d) comparisons between first-episode patients and metaanalytic findings in schizophrenia. The metaanalysis was based primarily on the performance observed in studies of chronically ill patients. Note that the overall profile of impairment across tests is remarkably similar across first-episode patients and the metaanalytic findings. FSIQ, Full-Scale Intelligence Quotient; WCST, Wisconsin Card Sorting Test. (Metaanalytic findings in this figure were adapted from Heinrichs RW. *In Search of Madness: Schizophrenia and Neuroscience.* New York: Oxford University Press; 2001. First-episode results were calculated as d scores and adapted based on data presented by Bilder RM, Goldman RS, Robinson D, et al.: Neuropsychology of first-episode schizophrenia: Initial characterization and clinical correlates. *Am J Psychiatry.* 2000;157:549.)

Aging

It is important to note that the vast bulk of the schizophrenia research literature has been conducted in young and middle-aged patients. Thus, the possibility that the illness may interact with processes implicated in normal aging has not been widely studied. This is an important limitation of the literature. Normal aging has a marked impact on cognitive functioning, and there is evidence of substantial individual differences in cognitive aging among healthy subjects. Importantly, there is highly suggestive evidence that high-ability subjects (better educated, higher IQ) show less marked effects of normal and abnormal aging. This effect is typically referred to as *cognitive reserve.* In essence, higher levels of education and cognitive ability are thought to provide a type of buffering effect on the negative impact of aging and disease.

Therefore, there is reason to suspect that patients with schizophrenia, insofar as they demonstrate deficits from early in development, as well as pronounced illness-onset–related deficits, may be unusually susceptible to the deleterious effects of aging on cognitive performance. There is some empirical evidence that is consistent with this suggestion. A number of groups have documented severely impaired levels of cognitive performance in elderly schizophrenia study groups, at times indistinguishable from the severity of impairment observed in frankly demented patient groups. As reviewed previously, such severe levels of impairment are not characteristic of schizophrenia through middle age. Although these findings may reflect sample bias (i.e., only the most impaired patients are found in chronic care institutions), they may also represent an interaction of sample bias with aging. That is, these highly impaired subjects, severely lacking in cognitive reserve, are most likely to show pronounced negative effects of aging. Note that this possibility does not imply that schizophrenia is a progressive disease. Instead, the findings in these unusual patient groups raise the possibility of an interaction effect involving disease severity, lack of cognitive reserve, and aging. Given the aging of the population overall, further research in this area will become increasingly important for the development of rational treatment strategies for this portion of the patient population.

RELATIONSHIP BETWEEN COGNITIVE PERFORMANCE AND SYMPTOMS

Widespread acceptance of the evidence that cognitive impairment was a direct reflection of the neuropathology of schizophrenia was slowed by the common sense clinical concern that symptoms interfere with the test performance of patients. Thus, active hallucinations might interrupt the ability to sustain task performance, delusions might lead patients to misconstrue the testing situation or task demands in a highly idiosyncratic fashion, formal thought disorder might compromise the types of verbal expression required to respond to test questions, and poverty of speech and amotivational behavior might compromise engagement in the assessment procedures.

Independence of Cognition and Symptoms Although these concerns seem clinically intuitive, there are five lines of evidence that suggest that cognitive performance is surprisingly independent of symptom severity and type. First, there is evidence that many patients demonstrate clear cognitive impairments before the onset of psychotic symptoms. Second, there is evidence that many of the first-degree relatives of patients also demonstrate cognitive impairments, despite the fact that they do not have any evidence of psychosis. Third, there is evidence that patients demonstrate similar levels of impairment during periods of clinical remission as levels of impairment experienced when these patients are more acutely symptomatic. This literature demonstrates that cognitive impairment may occur in the absence of symptoms diagnostic of schizophrenia. Fourth, there is evidence that conventional and new-generation antipsychotic treatments may have marked effects on the clinical symptoms of the illness, with only rather subtle effects on cognitive performance. This is fairly direct evidence that cognitive impairment and symptoms are largely independent, and, by inference, it suggests that these two dimensions must be mediated by different neural systems: One system is powerfully modulated by antipsychotic medications, with the other system far less responsive.

Correlational Designs The fifth, and perhaps most direct, piece of evidence concerning the relationship of symptoms and cognition comes from studies that have examined the correlation between symptom severity and type and measures of cognitive performance. Such correlational analyses have been reported in dozens of studies with widely disparate findings, ranging from studies documenting a complete lack of relationship between all types of symptoms and cognitive performance, to studies documenting specific associations between particular cognitive measures and specific types of symptoms, to studies showing rather modest relationships. These disparities suggest that methodological issues, including sample size, chronicity, severity of illness, and symptom measurement instrumentation, may be important determinants of study results.

Despite the size and complexity of this literature, some general trends can be discerned. In metaanalytic reviews examining the clinical and symptomatic correlates of memory, executive function, and attention impairments, positive symptom severity failed to correlate with performance in all three of these cognitive domains, whereas consistent, albeit modest, effect size correlations were found with negative symptom severity. These metaanalytic findings are consistent with findings from two recent studies of first-episode patients in which detailed cognition-symptom correlation data were presented, facilitating the calculation of average correlations between 30 individual cognitive tests and symptoms in one study and between 8 summary cognitive domain scores in the other. The average correlation of positive symptoms and cognitive performance was –0.06 and –0.19 in these two studies, the negative symptom average correlations were –0.14 and –0.29, and the average correlations of disorganization and cognition were 0.04 and –0.08. As is immediately apparent from a consideration of these correlations, there is little relationship between ratings of positive and disorganization symptoms and cognitive performance, whereas negative symptoms show the most consistent association with cognitive performance. At a minimum, the results of these two studies are sufficient to support a conclusion that substantial cognitive impairment may occur that cannot be attributed to symptom severity. As noted previously, such striking independence of symptoms and cognition is not always observed, particularly in more chronically ill and severely symptomatic study groups. In such study populations, more robust associations have sometimes been documented, particularly involving negative and disorganization symptoms.

Even if the association of symptoms and cognition is modest, it is still possible that it can be a guide to identifying neural systems that are implicated by the disorder. Some broad trends can be discerned from the literature that bears on this issue. Given some of the similarities between negative symptoms and the behavioral sequela of frontal lobe injuries, one might expect a selective relationship between severity of negative symptoms and measures typically thought to assess frontal lobe cognitive function. The evidence on this point is somewhat disappointing, as it appears that the negative symptoms are related to cognition more broadly, including visual and perceptual functions that likely implicate the functional integrity of posterior brain systems. Studies of patients with severe persistent negative symptoms, patients with the so-called deficit syndrome, underscore this point. These studies suggest relatively general cognitive differences with substantial evidence of impairment on functions likely mediated by the parietal cortex, such as aspects of sensory motor processing. By similar reasoning, positive symptoms might be expected to correlate with memory performance, as both are thought to result from limbic system dysfunction. As noted previously, however, the relationship between these two domains is quite weak. There is some evidence that formal thought disorder and other aspects of behavioral disorganization may show somewhat selective relationships with measures of semantic memory, context processing, and inhibitory control. Thus, there is some suggestive evidence for symptom-cognition specificity. However, the anatomy implicated is widely distributed rather than focal.

Cognitive Mechanisms It is likely that further progress in this area will require the use of cognitive measures designed to assess specific cognitive processes thought to be involved in specific symptom generation (i.e., delusions of control rather than an overall measure of delusion severity) rather than the correlation of clinical neuropsychological measures with broad symptom assessments. It is important to make a conceptual distinction between the cognitive mechanisms involved in symptom generation versus the cognitive mechanisms and systems that underlie adaptive intellectual performance when considering this question. The symptoms of schizophrenia clearly involve cognitive mechanisms, that is, auditory hallucinations must be mediated through language and perceptual mechanisms; delusions must be mediated through reasoning, inference, and judgment; and formal thought disorder must involve language processing. Thus, there is no question that symptoms involve cognitive processes, and there is a large and growing literature that addresses the specific cognitive architecture of different types of symptoms. However, the evidence suggesting relative independence of symptoms and neuropsychological performance strongly suggests that the specific cognitive mechanisms implicated by symptom formation are not the same cognitive mechanisms implicated by the intellectual deficits of patients. The fact that some significant correlations have been reported in the literature suggests that symptom formation and cognitive ability measures may involve partially overlapping elements of the far wider neural networks that mediate each of these domains. On the whole, however, it appears that the cognitive impairments of schizophrenia are relatively independent of the symptomatic features of the illness.

ROLE OF INDIVIDUAL DIFFERENCES

The fact that the group mean profile of cognitive impairment is highly reliable across numerous independent studies and appears to be highly reliable within an individual patient over time may create the erroneous impression that all patients exemplify this clinical prototype. In fact, there is substantial heterogeneity among patients in overall level of impairment and in the specific pattern of impairment that is observed. Although such variability in level and pattern of impairment may be important clinically, it is important to put such variability in the appropriate interpretive context. The range of *normal* cognitive performance is wide: That is, Full-Scale IQs ranging from 85 to 115 are considered normal by definition, yet there is little question that individuals differing by 30 IQ points are likely to demonstrate a number of important differences in educational and occupational achievement. Furthermore, there is a large factor in analytical literature demonstrating that many aspects of cognitive performance are at least partially independent from one another. Thus, substantial variability across different cognitive functions is the rule, not the exception, among healthy individuals. Therefore, substantial variability among patients in level and pattern of performance is to be expected and is fundamentally a normal phenomenon. No doubt, this type of performance variability reflects meaningful genetic and environment differences across individuals, and there is every reason to expect that patients will demonstrate similar effects.

There is, however, one clear implication of normal variability in cognitive function: It proves to be difficult to use cognitive measures as diagnostic measures for schizophrenia. Any cut score is likely to misclassify many healthy subjects drawn from the lower end of the normal distribution as ill (poor specificity) and similarly misclassifies highly performing patients as healthy (poor sensitivity). To illustrate this point, it is informative to consider the cognitive performance of monozygotic twins who are discordant for schizophrenia. In one such study, the performance of the ill twin was, almost without exception, below the level found in the well twin, suggesting nearly 100 percent sensitivity of a number of test measures to diagnostic status when variance related to genetic factors is controlled through a direct comparison to a twin. Importantly, many of the ill twins in this series demonstrated superior cognitive performance relative to the well twins from other families. That is, the signature of impairment is not absolute performance level but, instead, current performance level relative to the level that might have been expected on the basis of genetic and social and environmental factors. On most measures, a small minority of the ill twins scored beyond the bottom of the range observed among the group of healthy twins from all the families. If schizophrenia involves a modest overall downward shift in the cognitive performance distribution, only a few subjects should be expected to perform below the lower limits of the healthy range. Importantly, such a shift results in a significant portion of patients continuing to perform in the healthy range, despite the fact that they clearly have experienced an illness-related compromise of cognitive performance.

Normal Neuropsychological Performance? A number of recent studies have addressed the question of whether neuropsychological impairment can be detected in every patient with schizophrenia. Typically, such studies isolated a highly performing subgroup of patients from a larger sample and examined their cognitive profile in detail relative to healthy controls. A variety of approaches have been used to identify this subgroup, ranging from including subjects considered normal on the basis of a blind clinical rating of test performance to including subjects for whom current IQ and premorbid estimates were similar, suggesting an absence of cognitive decline, or to including subjects with a high current IQ. The subgroups (comprising approximately 20 to 25 percent of the total patient sample) identified by each of these approaches continue to demonstrate more subtle, circumscribed evidence of cognitive impairment, with deficits noted in memory, attention, and executive function from one or more of the studies taking this methodological approach. Not surprisingly, the extent of impairment described in these subgroups has been relatively mild and, at times, appears to be highly focal, limited to one or two aspects of cognitive performance, in contrast to the group mean profile of extensive impairment. In addition, it appears that there is a small number of subjects for whom no clear evidence of impairment can be discerned. Such patients raise the possibility that cognitive morbidity may not be an inevitable feature of the illness. However, in the absence of twin or family comparison subjects, the question remains whether such patients are truly unimpaired relative to their level of expected performance or whether they are simply high-ability subjects who have experienced a rather mild form of intellectual compromise that leaves them still well within the normal range. In summary, based on available evidence, it appears that some form of cognitive impairment is unquestionably characteristic of the vast majority of patients with schizophrenia and is likely characteristic of all patients when the role of normal individual differences is considered.

COGNITIVE DEFICITS AS RISK MARKERS FOR SCHIZOPHRENIA

The fact that cognitive abnormalities have been documented from the early childhood years of patients who develop the clinical syndrome in adulthood suggests that these deficits may represent risk markers for the illness. Logically, such cognitive impairments can be attributed to genetic or environmental factors (or their interaction). Two main study designs have been used to examine the role of cognitive deficits as risk markers: (1) genetic high-risk predictive designs and (2) studies of clinically unaffected adult family members of ill probands. Studies of the offspring of parents with schizophrenia, so-called high-risk study designs, have been largely motivated by the desire to find early cognitive or behavioral indicators that have a strong predictive relationship to long-term clinical outcomes. For instance, multiple studies have assessed aspects of attentional performance in preadolescent or adolescent samples and have found that attention impairment was related to later clinical outcome: Many subjects, who, as adults, developed schizophrenia or spectrum disorders, demonstrated impairments of attention many years before such clinical symptomatic abnormalities were expressed. Thus, findings from high-risk designs reveal early cognitive markers directly tied to the clinical phenotype. In light of the previous discussion of individual differences, it is not surprising that cognitive measures have somewhat modest sensitivity and specificity as risk markers for the clinical phenotype. Importantly, the findings of high-risk studies, taken by themselves, only provide suggestive, rather than unambiguous, evidence of genetic effects. That is, given the evidence that schizophrenia risk likely involves genetic and environmental factors (recall that the schizophrenia risk is only approximately 50 percent in monozygotic twin pairs), abnormalities evident in childhood that have a strong relationship to later outcome could also represent the influence of nongenetic environmental effects.

Cognition As an Endophenotype More direct evidence of genetically mediated cognitive deficits can be seen in family studies examining the performance of clinically unaffected adult relatives of ill patients. Cognitive abnormalities observed in nonpsychotic family members are often considered to be *endophenotype markers*, indicators of a genetically transmitted neurobiological abnormality that is associated with the illness but that also occurs among relatives who do not manifest the full clinical phenotype. Such cognitive markers may present a much more tractable problem for genetic analysis than the clinical phenotype: These abnormalities occur more often than the clinical phenotype, can be measured with more precision than the clinical phenotype, can sometimes be modeled in experimental animals, and likely have a much simpler genetic architecture than the clinical phenotype. Thus, cognitive markers may be useful in increasing the power of genetic linkage studies. In this type of linkage study, cognitive performance, rather than the clinical phenotype, is used to classify subjects as *affected*, thereby increasing the power to discern genetic effects due to the increased frequency of cognitive abnormalities compared to the expression of the clinical phenotype (i.e., diagnosis of schizophrenia). Cognitive performance can also be used to evaluate the significance of candidate genes that are considered relevant to schizophrenia based on their neurobiological properties. For example, recent studies have documented single gene effects from two genes (one involved with dopamine function, the other with acetylcholine) on aspects of cognitive performance (sensory gating and working memory) that are known to be impaired in schizophrenia.

Family Studies The challenges facing these approaches are considerable in light of the complexity and contradictory nature of the findings that have been documented in family studies. Three central findings have emerged from family studies: (1) Nearly every cognitive abnormality found in ill patients has also been documented among clinically unaffected family members, generally at a lesser severity than among patients. (2) However, unlike the patient literature, there is far more variability across family studies in the extent and type of abnormalities reported. (3) There is contradictory evidence about the extent to which these cognitive abnormalities are truly independent of the symptoms of the disorder. That is, there is clear evidence that impairment occurs among nonpsychotic family members. However, it is possible that subdiagnostic threshold levels of symptoms may be important correlates of cognitive performance among relatives. Each of these issues is discussed briefly in the text that follows.

The range of abnormalities detected in nonpsychotic first-degree relatives closely resembles the range of abnormalities reliably observed in patients when data are combined across studies. The abnormalities range from elementary deficits in sensory gating, in which patients and relatives fail to show a normal reduced response to the second of a pair of auditory stimuli, to the most complex aspects of reasoning and problem solving. A substantial literature documents abnormalities in smooth pursuit eye movements, in early visual processing, in working memory, and in multiple aspects of attention. The deficit profile that has emerged from family studies closely approximates the patient profile, and studies that have compared patients, relatives, and controls have generally found that the performance of relatives generally falls somewhere between that observed in patients and that found in healthy controls.

Thus, there is robust evidence that many, if not all, of the cognitive abnormalities observed in patients are likely genetically mediated to some degree. Despite this broad similarity of the patient and relative profile, it is important to note that the literature in this area is quite contradictory, with multiple studies finding a particular task impaired in samples of relatives and with other studies failing to document such a deficit. This type of discordance should be expected, given the fact that siblings share, on average, 50 percent of their genetic material with their ill family member. Thus, a substantial portion of first-degree relatives in every study is likely not to have the genes of interest. This fact likely underlies many of the inconsistencies of the literature.

This literature highlights the importance of studies showing that ill and well family members reliably share the same cognitive abnormalities. In this approach, ill probands are separated into those with and those without a specific type of cognitive impairment in comparison to unrelated healthy controls, using a variety of cut points for impairment (for example, one, two, or three standard deviations below the healthy control mean). The relatives of impaired probands are much more likely to demonstrate impairment on the same cognitive measure than the relatives of probands with intact performance on that measure. A major challenge facing the field is to determine how many independent dimensions are implicated by the array of behavioral findings, as this will help define the number of genetic factors that need to be identified. In a recent study at the National Institute of Mental Health (NIMH), it was found that the impairments observed on multiple measures appear to be largely independent of one another, suggesting the presence of multiple independent genes linked to different aspects of cognitive performance. The challenge of unraveling the genetics of cognitive impairment in schizophrenia converges at this point with the study of the genetics of normal cognition. That is, the developing basic science literature concerning the role of single and multiple genes in mediating general and specific aspects of cognition will be an important foundation for the study of cognitive endophenotypes.

There is less agreement in the field about the association of subthreshold symptomatic features and cognitive impairment. Many of the studies in the field simply segregate relatives into those who meet diagnostic criteria for schizophrenia spectrum disorders versus those who do not. Using this approach, it appears that many of the cognitive findings do not appear to be related to the presence of psychiatric illness. However, other investigators have advocated the use of an expanded clinical phenotype. In this approach, family members are considered to be clinically *affected* if they demonstrate subthreshold levels of symptom expression, that is, they demonstrate only one or two of the four or five symptoms or traits required to meet standard diagnostic criteria for schizophrenia spectrum disorders. Using this approach, it appears that smooth pursuit eye tracking abnormality may be primarily found among clinically affected relatives, whereas multiple studies using a more conventional approach to diagnosis have reported that such abnormalities are unrelated to psychiatric diagnosis. As a broad generalization, it does appear that many of the cognitive abnormalities reported among relatives are more frequent and more severe in those relatives who also demonstrate psychiatric abnormalities, even when these symptoms are not severe enough or pervasive enough to meet diagnostic criteria for a psychotic spectrum disorder.

Genetic and Environmental Contributions There is also contradictory evidence concerning whether the transition from risk to illness is best conceptualized as representing simply a matter of severity of cognitive impairment or whether there are specific

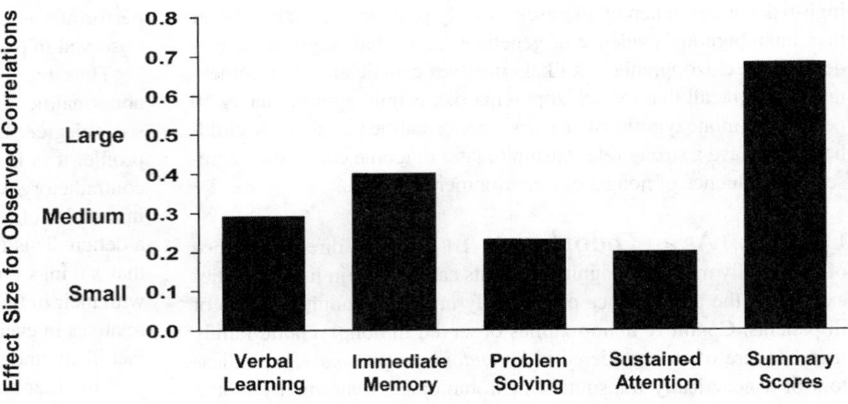

FIGURE 12.9–3 Cognition and functional outcome: strengths of relationship. These metaanalytic results demonstrate the strength of association observed between specific cognitive domains and aspects of functional outcome. Note that the cognition-outcome relationship is enhanced when summary cognitive scores are examined. (Data adapted from Green MF, Kern RS, Braff DL, et al.: Neurocognitive deficits and functional outcome in schizophrenia: Are we measuring the "right stuff"? *Schizophr Bull.* 2000;26:119.)

forms of cognitive impairment that can be attributed to nongenetic factors. As noted previously, relatives tend to perform between the level of impairment observed in ill patients and the normative level of controls across multiple measures. This would suggest a relatively straightforward, quantitative *severity* model: More severe impairment is associated with illness. Alternately, there is some evidence consistent with the idea that, although much of the cognitive impairment in schizophrenia is heritable, some impairment may not be under strong genetic control, implying the role of environmental factors. For example, one family study and another of discordant monozygotic twins came to similar conclusions in segregating attention and memory measures. In both studies, impairments of attention were shared by probands and their presumed gene-carrying relatives at similar levels of impairment. However, also in both studies, impairments of episodic memory were found specifically in ill probands and not among the relatives. This would suggest that episodic memory might be a sensitive marker of clinical illness rather than risk and that it is a form of impairment that cannot be explained on the basis of genetic factors. Arguing against this hypothesis is the fact that multiple family studies have documented episodic memory impairments in clinically unaffected relatives. Further study of this question is needed, given the importance of the issue of whether it is possible to account for the basic cognitive profile in schizophrenia solely on the basis of genetic factors or whether certain forms of impairment are under less exclusive genetic control and instead implicate a variety of environmental factors.

IMPORTANCE OF COGNITION FOR FUNCTIONAL OUTCOME

The functional consequences of the cognitive deficits of schizophrenia have only recently been appreciated. As mentioned previously, earlier studies of cognition in schizophrenia were focused on attempts to define and to characterize the cognitive deficits in this illness, not to understand their implications for adaptive and social functioning. Despite some earlier findings that higher intelligence was linked to better functioning in schizophrenia, it was not until that 1990s that studies started to explore systematically the consequences of cognitive deficits for patients' daily functioning. For example, do cognitive deficits make it difficult for patients to catch the right bus, to prepare a meal, to keep a job, or to maintain communication with their families? In essence, these studies used cognitive deficits to understand the disability of schizophrenia, as opposed to underlying neural circuits.

Although the studies in this area vary widely, they tend to have several features in common, making it possible to summarize the findings. Most of the studies involved a brief cognitive battery, often including measures of memory, attention, and executive control. Studies typically examined one category of functional outcome, including (1) community adaptation (e.g., social functioning, occupational functioning, and degree of independent living), (2) success in psychosocial rehabilitation programs, or (3) performance on simulated interpersonal tasks conducted in a laboratory. Across studies, despite some negative findings, cognitive deficits show highly consistent relationships to all three of these types of functional outcome. The magnitudes of these relationships are demonstrated in Figure 12.9–3, which shows the effect sizes between several key cognitive areas (executive functions, types of memory, and vigilance) and functional outcome. Most of these relationships are medium effect sizes, meaning that they should be clinically noticeable, in addition to being statistically significant. When summary scores of cognition are used (e.g., a composite or a global score) instead of individual cognitive constructs, the magnitude of the relationships with functional outcome is even stronger.

Cognitive deficits may account for some of the heterogeneity in the course of illness. Long-term follow-up data indicate that work and social functioning in schizophrenia remain impaired, but, on average, they do not deteriorate significantly with increasing duration of illness. Most striking is the marked heterogeneity in the level and the course of social and work functioning over time, with some patients showing stability, others showing improvement, and others showing deterioration. Recent studies have examined the long-term predictive importance of cognition for functional outcome. These studies indicate that cognitive assessments can predict functional outcome 2 to 15 years later. In addition, when patient functioning is assessed repeatedly, it appears that baseline cognition is a good predictor of the slope of change in social behavior; patients with good cognitive abilities tend to show improvement over time, whereas more cognitively impaired patients demonstrate stable forms of impairment. One explanation for these findings is that relatively stable cognitive abilities determine whether a patient is able to acquire the skills needed for an improved course of functioning in the community over time.

Differential Prediction of Outcome Domains It is possible that some cognitive measures are more strongly related to functional outcome than others. If so, remediation efforts would be wisely directed at the measures with the closest connections to outcome. In a series of metaanalyses, memory for lists of words (secondary or episodic memory) seemed to be especially related to all types of functional outcome compared to other cognitive tasks. However, the construct with the strongest relationships may depend on the specific type of outcome. For example, vocational success (which typically places a range of social and cognitive demands on the individual) may depend more on speed of processing (the rate at which subjects are able to complete rapid perceptual and motor output tasks). For success on psychosocial rehabilitation programs, verbal learning deficits may be particularly important. Several studies have found that, compared to patients with good memory, patients with poor memory start out demonstrating lower levels of knowledge for the material and have a more shallow learning slope for acquisition of new material.

These findings have a large amount of face validity. It is logical that verbal memory would be related to success on social skills training programs, because participants need to encode and to retain material presented by trainers and through videotapes. It is reasonable that encoding, retention, sequencing, and executive control are cognitive prerequisites that are needed for success with activities of daily living (such as maintaining hygiene, taking mass transportation, communicating socially, and preparing meals). These daily tasks, called *instrumental life skills*, form the building blocks for adequate functioning in the community. Likewise, speed of processing may be important for vocational success when the job places time demands on the individual.

If these cognitive abilities are basic requirements of daily functioning in general, then the relationships between cognition and outcome should be seen in disorders other than schizophrenia. Indeed, cognitive deficits appear to take a toll on functioning in disorders as diverse as multiple sclerosis (MS), acquired immune deficiency syndrome (AIDS), and head injury, even in a nonclinical elderly sample. One can conclude that cognitive abilities such as memory and vigilance help people navigate through the world, and this is as true for schizophrenic patients as it is for elderly retirees. Considering that these associations are diagnostically nonspecific, it is somewhat surprising that it took so long for them to be demonstrated.

Although the relationships between cognitive deficits and functional outcome have been demonstrated rather consistently across studies, the mechanisms for the relationships are not known. Cognitive abilities may have a direct relationship with aspects of functional outcome. Alternatively, cognitive deficits may be related to functional outcome through some intervening process that, in turn, is a more direct determinant of functional outcome. Such intervening variables may include social cognition (e.g., identifying emotions in faces or voices) or learning potential (ability to acquire new information). If there are intervening variables, identifying them becomes a critical next step to understand the nature of the relationships and also to guide new treatment targets. Along these lines, several psychosocial programs have started to target problems in identifying emotions in faces.

In contrast to cognitive deficits, psychotic symptoms (hallucinations and delusions) are relatively poor predictors and correlates of functional outcome. The successful control of positive psychotic symptoms with antipsychotic medications has not led to dramatic improvement in functional outcome and a reduction in disability for the illness. This discrepancy is explained by the relative independence of symptomatic and functional outcome. It is likely that other types of clinical symptoms, such as formal thought disorder, are more associated with functional outcome than are hallucinations and delusions. Among clinical features of schizophrenia, it appears that the deficit syndrome (i.e., persistent negative symptoms, including avolition) is a strong predictor of functional outcome.

IMPACT OF PHARMACOLOGICAL TREATMENTS ON COGNITIVE FUNCTIONING

Because cognitive deficits are core features of schizophrenia, and because they are related to functional outcome, they have become logical targets of intervention. Exploring interventions for the cognitive deficits of schizophrenia is a recent endeavor, one that has grown rapidly over the past decade. One can divide intervention approaches for cognition into two general categories: compensatory and restorative. A *compensatory* approach is one that attempts to work around the cognitive deficit to improve daily activities or to increase the benefits of rehabilitation. In this approach, there is no attempt to alter the underlying deficit; instead, there is an attempt to take the deficit into consideration in the development of a treatment plan. Examples of compensatory approaches include *errorless learning* methods in rehabilitation and the use of environmental cues for memory deficits. A *restorative* approach, in contrast, is one that is intended to improve the underlying deficit. Restorative approaches can be pharmacological or nonpharmacological (e.g., cognitive remediation). This section focuses on the pharmacological restorative approach and briefly surveys the evidence on cognitive effects of antipsychotic medications.

First-Generation Antipsychotics

In general, first-generation antipsychotic medications had minimal effects on cognition. There are a few exceptions, including some reports of beneficial effects on vigilance and some reports of detrimental effects on motor speed. Nonetheless, it is safe to conclude that the first-generation medications had minimal effects on cognition, in stark contrast to their beneficial effects on psychotic symptoms. This discrepancy in treatment success between clinical and cognitive features of the illness provides additional support for the relative independence of these areas of outcome.

Although first-generation antipsychotic medications do not appear to affect cognitive abilities directly, they may have an indirect detrimental effect through the coadministration of anticholinergic medications. The anticholinergic medications that are frequently given with first-generation antipsychotic medications for the treatment of motor side effects (e.g., benztropine [Cogentin]) are disruptive to certain cognitive abilities, particularly components of memory.

Second-Generation Antipsychotics

In contrast to the first generation of medications, the cognitive effects of second-generation antipsychotic agents appear more promising. Initial observations with clozapine (Clozaril) suggested that it improved verbal fluency, which is the ability to generate words within a certain time period. Since these initial studies with clozapine, all of the second-generation medications have been compared to conventional antipsychotic medications on batteries of cognitive tasks. In the past few years, several literature reviews and a metaanalysis have concluded that the second-generation antipsychotic medications have cognitive benefits compared to first-generation medications. The studies in this literature clearly have numerous methodological limitations (e.g., many of the early studies were open-label within-group switch studies). Nonetheless, this conclusion is bolstered by considering the consistency across open-label studies, as well as results from several double-blind, randomized studies.

The reviews of the literature have focused on three of the newer antipsychotic medications (clozapine, risperidone [Risperdal], and olanzapine [Zyprexa]), and, based on more recently published studies, the conclusions of benefits relative to first-generation medications seem equally applicable to other second-generation medications (quetiapine [Seroquel] and ziprasidone [Geodon]). At this time, there are no convincing data to support cognitive superiority of one second-generation medication over another. It is possible that newer antipsychotic medications may influence certain areas of cognition more than others (that is, certain medications may differentially impact specific cognitive functions, but the data are only suggestive at this time). There is speculation that the most recently approved antipsychotic medication, aripiprazole (Abilify), may have beneficial cognitive effects due to its unusual mechanism of action (partial agonist at the dopamine type 2 [D_2] receptor), but it has not yet been adequately tested in this regard.

Although the newer antipsychotic medications offer cognitive advantages relative to first-generation medications, they clearly do not normalize the cognitive impairment characteristic of schizophrenia. As mentioned previously, relatively subtle deficits are present in preschizophrenic individuals before the onset of any clinical symptoms of schizophrenia, so it may be unreasonable to expect a medication to bring cognition up to normal levels. However, even with reduced expectations, the total amount of cognitive benefit in second-generation versus first-generation medications is fairly modest. Considering the entire difference between patients and controls in cognition, the newer medications make up approximately one-fourth to one-third of that difference, leaving plenty of room for additional improvement.

It should be emphasized that the comparisons between second-generation and first-generation medications have almost always involved typical or higher (by U.S. standards) doses of first-generation medications. This dosing pattern leaves open the question of whether the same results would have been achieved if low doses had been used. In fact, based on a 2-year study of a low-dose first-generation medication, it seems likely that the cognitive advantages of second-generation medications can be attenuated or eliminated when low doses of a comparator are used. If the advantages of the second-generation medications depend on the dose of the first-generation medication, it raises the possibility that the second-generation medications are less cognitively detrimental than the first-generation medications, instead of being truly beneficial for cognition.

The cognitive studies of the second-generation medications have served well to focus attention on the importance of cognitive deficits in schizophrenia, and cognition is now considered to be a legitimate treatment target by clinicians and by the pharmaceutical industry. However, if larger cognitive benefits are to be expected, it may be necessary to consider pharmacological agents other than antipsychotic medications. As mentioned previously, the magnitude of the difference between first-generation and second-generation medications is modest (although significant) and not large enough to normalize the performance of patients. In addition, if the newer antipsychotic medications are better for cognition than first-generation medications, it is an accident. The second-generation medications were developed for better safety and tolerability, not with the goal of enhancing cognitive functioning. It has been argued that it is now time to select compounds dedicated to the cognitive deficits in schizophrenia, and this requires a move to other types of medications.

Adjunctive medications (used in addition to a stable dose of antipsychotic medications) specifically intended to improve cognition in schizophrenia are starting to be explored. For example, several studies have been conducted using glycinergic agents. Initial trials with D-cycloserine (a modulator of the glycine site of the glutamate *N*-methyl-D-aspartate [NMDA] receptor) have shown mixed results in terms of cognitive benefits. Other types of agents under investigation include an ampakine (a positive modulator at the glutamate α-amino-3-hydroxy-5-methyl-4-isoxazolepropionic acid (AMPA) receptor and a serotonin type 1A (5-HT_{1A}) agonist. The results from these preliminary trials are promising, and studies with adequate statistical power are under way.

ARE THERE MULTIPLE INDEPENDENT COGNITIVE DEFICITS IN SCHIZOPHRENIA?

The long list of cognitive deficits in schizophrenia is impressive, but it leaves one wondering whether the diverse array of problems can be explained in a more parsimonious manner. That is, might it be possible to account for many, if not all, of the observed deficits on the basis of a much smaller number of core impairments? This issue has notable implications; it is difficult to answer questions about the underlying pathophysiology of cognitive deficits or about the treatment of cognitive deficits until there is a clearer sense of how many separate deficits are involved. The picture is complicated by the fact that many cognitive tests are intercorrelated, in patients and in normal subjects. That is, although different tasks assess different cognitive functions (probably mediated, at least in part, by different neural systems), subjects who score well in one domain tend to score well in others as well. This pattern of positive intercorrelation is evidence that many cognitive abilities are only partially independent of one another, with most major cognitive domains reflecting general ability to a significant degree. This raises the possibility that the broad deficit pattern in schizophrenia could reflect an impairment of general cognitive ability, at a superordinate level, rather than at the level of the more discrete, independent aspects of cognition that are typically discussed in the literature (i.e., memory and attention). However, this well-replicated correlational finding does not rule out the possibility of specific core impairments, as many different cognitive functions share certain key components. For example, a prominent deficit in working memory would be expected to impact multiple cognitive domains, including language comprehension, arithmetic skills, and problem solving (among many others), given the critical role of transient information storage in these cognitive operations. Thus, the broad deficit pattern in schizophrenia does not eliminate the possibility that a much smaller number of core deficits may explain the variety of impairments that are common. Such key deficits would then become the focus for studies of pathophysiology, genetics, and treatment. The search for parsimony in this area has been conducted in two ways: empirical approaches that examine patterns in large patient databases and theoretical approaches that attempt to isolate core deficits. The following discussion gives examples of each.

Psychometric Approaches

One way to generate clues about underlying cognitive deficits in schizophrenia is to evaluate the effect sizes of the differences between patients and controls on a range of cognitive tasks. If the effect sizes are similar across tasks, it suggests the presence of a common underlying deficit. If the effect sizes noted across tasks differ, the tasks with the larger differences are likely to be closer to the underlying core deficits. As reviewed previously, the size of the patient deficit varies across cognitive constructs from medium to large effects (approximately 0.5 to 1.5 standard deviations), implicating multiple, likely independent, deficits. The magnitude of deficits in verbal learning, executive control, and speed of processing tends to be larger than others, implicating these areas as possible core deficits, and is typically attributed to frontal-temporal lobe dysfunction.

It is important to note that fully normal performance is rarely observed in any cognitive domain. Thus, the deficits in schizophrenia vary in magnitude, not in their presence or absence. This fact critically limits the ability of neuropsychological measures to point to discrete, localized forms of impairment, because all areas of the brain appear to be compromised to some extent. In addition, the pattern of uneven impairment across cognitive functions could logically result from a single underlying deficit that had differential effects on different cognitive functions. As an analogy, in Parkinson's disease, an abnormality in a single neurotransmitter system (dopamine) has dramatic motor effects coupled with more subtle cognitive effects, given the differential involvement of dopamine in motor versus many cognitive systems. Thus, the comparison of effect sizes on psychometric measures can only provide hints as to which cognitive and neural systems are maximally compromised in the illness. A more refined view of the nature of cognitive deficits requires the use of multivariate approaches (e.g., principal component analyses and structural equation modeling), but such approaches are, so far, rare in the schizophrenia literature.

Theoretical Approaches Theoretical approaches, typically based on models from cognitive science in normal subjects, have also been used to find parsimony in the range of cognitive deficits. Three examples are briefly described: (1) the use of context, (2) limited processing resources, and (3) basic perceptual deficits.

Context Processing Several different groups using different approaches have concluded that a loss of the ability to use context information can explain many of the cognitive problems in schizophrenia. As mentioned previously in the section Historical Overview, an early integrative theory of schizophrenia was Shakow's theory of *segmental set* that developed starting in the 1930s. The idea was that most tasks and daily activities need to be broken into segments. To accomplish the tasks, one needs to work on the individual segments, while at the same time retaining the mental set for the overall goal. According to Shakow, a basic problem in schizophrenia is that the big picture (the set, or the context) is easily lost. More recently, the interest in context comes from computer modeling of cognition. The goal of these studies is to take computer models of normal cognition and to modify them to develop a computer model that mimics the performance of schizophrenic patients. The intention was to try to find a core cognitive component based on computer simulation results that can explain a range of performance deficits. One promising lead occurred when a *context module*, similar to a working memory function, was included in the computer model. When damage to the context module was programmed, the results of the computer simulations were good at predicting the performance of schizophrenic patients on several different types of tests. These simulations were seen as support for a basic problem in processing of context (e.g., working memory), and this deficit was speculatively linked to a deficit in prefrontal dopaminergic function. The context processing deficit model provides a principled account for multiple areas of deficit in schizophrenia that implicate failures in the control and modulation of cognitive processing, a clear strength of the model. It is less clear that the model can account for deficits in sensory-perceptual processing or in basic aspects of memory function that do not appear to involve a major role for strategy, the use of context information, or other forms of top-down control over elementary functions. However, the context-processing model provides evidence that it may be possible to account for a wide array of apparently different types of cognitive failure on the basis of a single underlying deficit. It remains for future modeling and empirical research to delineate the impairments that can, and those that cannot, be explained on the basis of a context-processing deficit.

Processing Resources A second approach has been to explain deficits on a variety of tasks according to how much attention they demanded. In this account, attention is regarded as a limited resource, and people are thought to vary in the amount of resources they have available to support cognitive processing. It has been proposed that many of the performance deficits in schizophrenia can be explained parsimoniously as the result of a reduced availability of attentional resources. Limitations in this attentional resource could arise because schizophrenic patients have smaller than normal amounts of attentional resources or because they do not allocate their attentional resources efficiently. For example, some of their processing resources might be tied up in unimportant mental activities, and not enough is left over for important cognitive tasks. If patients have problems with the amount or allocation of attentional resources, this impairment should be most evident on tasks that require substantial attentional resources, with relatively intact performance on tasks that are not as resource intensive. This prediction works well for many tasks, but it is not as well suited for explaining deficits on certain tests of early visual perception and sensory gating. These tasks do not seem to require great mental effort, but patients show deficits nonetheless. At a theoretical level, this account is not specific about the nature of processing resources and the boundaries between attention and other cognitive systems. Thus, it has been difficult to definitively confirm or falsify the model.

Perceptual Impairments A third theoretical approach has emphasized the importance of deficits on perceptual tasks. It may be possible to explain a variety of cognitive deficits in terms of abnormalities in basic perception. The idea is that a problem in perception causes an initial disruption that leads to a cascade of events resulting in problems in other aspects of cognition, including memory and attention. One advantage of focusing on perception in this context is that the underlying neural systems are better established for perceptual processes than for other, more complex, aspects of cognition. One example is a series of recent studies in visual perception that have tried to probe two different visual pathways: magnocellular and parvocellular. The anatomy and characteristics of these pathways are well established, and tests have been devised to probe them separately. Much of the evidence suggests that the magnocellular pathway is especially affected in schizophrenia. Another example is to use visual perception tests to explore underlying neural oscillations. Tests of sensory gating and visual masking have suggested that schizophrenia patients have abnormalities in high-frequency cortical oscillations, specifically frequencies in the gamma range (30 to 70 Hz). These gamma range oscillations are involved in normal human perception and cognition. A failure to generate or to maintain activity in the gamma range may explain a wide range of phenomena in schizophrenia, including problems in perceptual organization and working memory. Hence, perceptual tasks can be used to explore underlying neural systems that may be the root cause of a variety of observed performance deficits.

FUTURE DIRECTIONS

Future studies of cognitive function in schizophrenia are likely to be shaped by developments in basic cognitive neuroscience, functional neuroimaging, and behavior genetics. The clinical neuropsychological assessment approaches that have been the mainstay of schizophrenia research have been extremely valuable in documenting the presence of cognitive impairment in schizophrenia and the importance of cognition for functional outcome but have limited ability to isolate specific cognitive deficits and neural systems, because most clinical tests involve multiple cognitive operations. To isolate specific deficits, the field will need to turn increasingly to basic cognitive neuroscience behavioral methods and functional neuroimaging techniques. The integration of cognitive neuroscience methods with genetic approaches should provide a much clearer picture of the nature of cognitive impairment in schizophrenia, the neural substrate that is implicated, and the basic neurobiology of the illness. This type of basic research, coupled with advances in understanding the relationship between aspects of cognition and functional outcome, should inform the next generation of clinical assessment approaches. Such an understanding is critical for the development of rational pharmacological approaches directed at enhancing cognitive function as a key to reducing the disability of schizophrenia.

SUGGESTED CROSS-REFERENCES

Perception and cognition are discussed in Section 3.1, and brain models are covered in Section 3.5. Cognitive assessment in children is covered in Section 7.7. Section 3.3 covers learning theory.

References

Aleman A, Hijman R, de Haan EHF, Kahn RS: Memory impairment in schizophrenia: A meta-analysis. *Am J Psychiatry.* 1999;156:1358.

Barch DM, Carter CS, MacDonald AW 3rd, Braver TS, Cohen JD: Context-processing deficits in schizophrenia: Diagnostic specificity, 4-week course, and relationships to clinical symptoms. *J Abnorm Psychol.* 2003;112:132.

*Bilder RM, Goldman RS, Robinson D, Reiter G, Bell L, Bates JA, Pappadopulos E, Wilson DF, Alvir JM, Woerner MG, Geisler S, Kane JM, Lieberman JA: Neuropsychology of first-episode schizophrenia: Initial characterization and clinical correlates. *Am J Psychiatry.* 2000;157:549.

Blyler CR, Gold JM. Cognitive effects of typical antipsychotic treatment: Another look. In: Sharma T, Harvey PD, eds. *Cognition in Schizophrenia.* New York: Oxford University Press; 2000.

Brekke JS, Long JD: Community-based psychosocial rehabilitation and prospective change in functional, clinical, and subjective experience variables in schizophrenia. *Schizophr Bull.* 2000;26:667.

Cannon TD, Huttunen MO, Lonnqvist J, Tuulio-Henriksson A, Pirkola T, Glahn D, Finkelstein J, Hietanen M, Kaprio J, Koskenvuo M: The inheritance of neuropsychological dysfunction in twins discordant for schizophrenia. *Am J Hum Genet.* 2000;67:369.

*Cohen JD, Barch DM, Carter C, Servan-Schreiber D: Context-processing deficits in schizophrenia: Converging evidence from three theoretically motivated cognitive tasks. *J Abnorm Psychol.* 1999;108:120.

Doniger GM, Foxe JJ, Murray MM, Higgins BA, Javitt DC: Impaired visual object recognition and dorsal/ventral stream interaction in schizophrenia. *Arch Gen Psychiatry.* 2002;59:1011.

Egan MF, Goldberg TE, Gscheidle T, Weirich M, Rawlings R, Hyde TM, Bigelow L, Weinberger DR: Relative risk for cognitive impairments in siblings of patients with schizophrenia. *Biol Psychiatry.* 2001;50:98.

Frith CD. *The Cognitive Neuropsychology of Schizophrenia.* Hillsdale, NJ: Lawrence Erlbaum Associates; 1992.

Goff DC, Tsai G, Manoach DS, Coyle JT: Dose-finding trial for D-cycloserine added to neuroleptics for negative symptoms in schizophrenia. *Am J Psychiatry.* 1995;152:1213.

Goldberg TE, Egan MF, Gscheidle T, Coppola R, Weickert T, Kolachana BS, Goldman D, Weinberger DR: Executive subprocesses in working memory: Relationship to catechol-*O*-methyltransferase Val158Met genotype and schizophrenia. *Arch Gen Psychiatry.* 2003;60:889.

Green MF. *Schizophrenia Revealed: From Neurons to Social Interactions.* New York: W. W. Norton & Company, Inc.; 2001.

*Green MF, Kern RS, Braff DL, Mintz J: Neurocognitive deficits and functional outcome in schizophrenia: Are we measuring the "right stuff"? *Schizophr Bull.* 2000;26:119.

Harvey PD, Silverman JM, Mohs RC, Parrella M, White L, Powchik P, Davidson M, Davis KL: Cognitive decline in late-life schizophrenia: A longitudinal study of geriatric chronically hospitalized patients. *Biol Psychiatry.* 1999;45:32.

Heinrichs RW. *In Search of Madness: Schizophrenia and Neuroscience.* New York: Oxford University Press; 2001.

Hyman SE, Fenton WS: What are the right targets for psychopharmacology? *Science.* 2003;299:350.

*Javitt DC, Liederman E, Cienfuegos A, Shelley A: Panmodal processing imprecision as a basis for dysfunction of transient memory storage systems in schizophrenia. *Schizophr Bull.* 1999;25:763.

Jones P, Rodgers B, Murray R, Marmot M: Child developmental risk factors for adult schizophrenia in the British 1946 birth cohort. *Lancet.* 1994;344:1398.

Keefe RS, Silva SG, Perkins DO, Lieberman JA: The effects of atypical antipsychotic drugs on neurocognitive impairment in schizophrenia: A review and meta-analysis. *Schizophr Bull.* 1999;25:201.

Kraepelin E. *Dementia Praecox and Paraphrenia.* Huntington, NY: Robert E. Krieger Publishing; 1971.

Kremen WS, Seidman LJ, Pepple JR, Lyons MJ, Tsuang MT, Faraone SV: Neuropsychological risk indicators for schizophrenia: A review of family studies. *Schizophr Bull.* 1994;20:103.

Leonard S, Gault J, Hopkins J, Logel J, Vianzon R, Short M, Drebing C, Berger R, Venn D, Dirota P, Zerbe G, Olincy A, Ross RG, Adler LE, Freedman R: Association of promotor variants in the alpha7 nicotinic acetylcholine receptor subunit gene with an inhibitory deficit found in schizophrenia. *Arch Gen Psychiatry.* 2002;59:1085.

Lezak MD. *Neuropsychological Assessment.* 3rd ed. New York: Oxford University Press; 1995.

Mohamed S, Paulsen JS, O'Leary D, Arndt S, Andreasen N: Generalized cognitive deficits in schizophrenia. *Arch Gen Psychiatry.* 1999;56:749.

Nuechterlein KH, Dawson ME, Green MF: Information-processing abnormalities as neuropsychological vulnerability indicators for schizophrenia. *Acta Psychiatr Scand.* 1994;90:71.

Pinkham AE, Penn DL, Perkins DO, Lieberman JA: Implications of a neural basis for social cognition for the study of schizophrenia. *Am J Psychiatry.* 2003;160:815.

Rapaport D, Gill M, Schafer R. *Diagnostic Psychological Testing.* Chicago: Year Book Publishers; 1945.

Rund BR: A review of longitudinal studies of cognitive functions in schizophrenia patients. *Schizophr Bull.* 1998;24:425.

Saykin AJ, Shtasel DL, Gur RE, Kester DB, Mozley LH, Stafiniak P, Gur RC: Neuropsychological deficits in neuroleptic naïve patients with first-episode schizophrenia. *Arch Gen Psychiatry.* 1994;51:124.

Schechter I, Butler PD, Silipo G, Zemon V, Javitt DC: Magnocellular and parvocellular contributions to backward masking dysfunction in schizophrenia. *Schizophr Res.* 2003;64:91.

Shakow D. *Adaptation in Schizophrenia: The Theory of Segmental Set.* New York: John Wiley and Sons; 1979.

Sharma T, Harvey PD. *Cognition in Schizophrenia. Impairments, Importance, and Treatment Strategies.* Oxford, UK: Oxford University Press; 2000.

Smith TE, Hull JW, Huppert JD, Silverstein SM: Recovery from psychosis in schizophrenia and schizoaffective disorder: Symptoms and neurocognitive rate-limiters for the development of social skills. *Schizophr Res.* 2002;55:229.

Spencer KM, Nestor PG, Niznikiewicz MA, Salisbury DF, Shenton ME, McCarley RW: Abnormal neural synchrony in schizophrenia. *J Neurosci.* 2003;23:7407.

*Weinberger DR, Egan MF, Bertolino A, Callicott JH, Mattay VS, Lipska BK, Berman KF, Goldberg TE: Prefrontal neurons and the genetics of schizophrenia. *Biol Psychiatry.* 2001;50:825.

▲ 12.10 Schizophrenia: Sensory Gating Deficits and Translational Research

Robert Freedman, M.D.

Persons with schizophrenia confront an existential question that has engaged philosophers and others who have considered the problem of perception. No one knows with absolute certainty whether his or her brain accurately portrays reality. In the course of normal existence, that dilemma is only rarely probed, but, for many persons with schizophrenia, it is one of the most troubling aspects of their psychosis.

For medical students who are first introduced to a person with schizophrenia, the dilemma at first may seem to be a pretense. A perfectly composed woman announces to the students that she hears commands from space ships that she can ignore only with the greatest difficulty. They counter, with polite questions that nonetheless hint at incredulity: "You hear messages from space ships?" With humor, she counters: "With my graduate degree in classics, I had hoped for Marcus Aurelius, but instead I got Star Trek." She tells them that voices from the space ships caused her to wander alone down dark streets and alleys, that she drank to intoxication to quiet their insistent and often critical tone, that for years they had threatened her with harm if she revealed them to anyone, and that no amount of reality testing ever blunted their force. The students confront her still politely, but more insistently, the questions coming slightly louder, each word enunciated for emphasis: "The . . . space . . . ships. . . . You hear them." She is equally insistent, and her insistence seems to slightly anger the students: "I was once a bright young student, just like all of you, but my life took a different turn. I hear messages from space ships." Finally, someone says aloud what everyone is thinking: "But you have a graduate degree from a major university, and you know that there is no such thing as space ships that send messages." "I realize that," she replies, "but I still cannot ignore them." Everyone is frustrated at this inconsistency between her intellect and her delusional belief, and the professor gets notes from the class: "Please don't bring actresses to class and tell us that they have schizophrenia."

There is no direct way to study the pathophysiology of hearing messages from space ships. Certainly, animal models do not seem applicable, and there is no direct way of assessing how this patient's neuronal activity generates the messages. Her disorder is obviously complex; it involves more than just hearing the voices from the space ship. She also feels compelled to react to their commands, and it is yet to be explored what they are saying that she finds so disturbing. Other patients readily point out that the voices mirror their worst thoughts about themselves. Although few people may share the space ship communication, most people occasionally experience their worst thoughts about themselves in almost voice-like form. The medical students sometimes acknowledge thoughts about their suitability for medicine or their ability to pass next week's test, thoughts that can have an insistent quality that may transcend their acknowledgment that the rigorous admission process to medical school (and the excellence of the instruction that they receive) make the fears somewhat unrealistic.

Certainly, when one considers fully the messages from the space ship, it is difficult to conceptualize their pathophysiology in any simple way. The messages command attention, comment on specific facets of the patient's life, evoke emotion, and compel a decision to act or not to act on their commands. All aspects of higher brain function—attention, perception, memory registration and retrieval, affect regulation, and executive function—are involved. Some investigators have concluded that such phenomena are inherently too complicated to analyze and that it would be better to search for simpler phenomena that might also demonstrate abnormal brain function in persons with schizophrenia. An analogy might be a computer diagnostic program. When it is obvious that a computer is misprocessing words, the diagnostic does not consist of a spelling bee. Rather, the computer is asked to process a series of 0s and 1s, to determine if one of its chips has a malfunction.

SENSORY GATING ABNORMALITIES IN SCHIZOPHRENIA

One of the simplest brain functions is habituation, the decreased response to repeated sensory stimuli. One paradigm that has been used to assess this function is the measurement of the electrophysiological response to repeated simple sounds. When two sounds are delivered approximately 0.5 seconds apart, normal subjects have a significantly decreased response to the second sound. Everyone hears both sounds, but the brain's overall activation to the second sound is reduced. The response is not restored until approximately 8 seconds later. This can be demonstrated with a tape recorder. Clap twice quickly, then wait 8 seconds, and clap twice again. When one replays the tape, as one waits 8 seconds for the second set of sounds, one may wonder if a mistake was made in the recording or if the tape was rewound to the wrong place. By 8 seconds, it seems like the sounds will not repeat themselves, even if one is certain that two sets have been recorded. The first sound of the next pair seems to come almost unexpectedly; it seems like a novel stimulus, despite the fact that one recorded it oneself. The second of the pair is a quite different experience. It seems more predictable, like a rhythm. Thus, although the two sounds of the pair are identical, they are perceived quite differently, solely as a function of the time between the stimuli. This phenomenon is a simple demonstration of an elementary form of habituation, termed *sensory gating*. Psychologists have theorized that sensory gating has a protective role. The brain's ability to process a stimulus fully, by registering all of its sensory components and comparing them against full experience, is limited, compared to the vast array of stimuli in the environment. A simplification that many organisms have found effective is to exclude repeated stimuli, of which the second click of the pair of clicks is an example, so that they can respond more vigorously to novel stimuli, like the first click. Determining that information is repeated requires minimal processing, so that the decision itself does not require much brain activity. Because the sensory gating or filtering is at such an elementary level, this mechanism is sometimes referred to as an *inhibitory sensory gating mechanism*, because it seems to regulate the flow of sensory information to higher brain centers. As is seen in a subsequent section, the gating is initially performed in the brainstem reticular formation. Furthermore, some processing occurs despite the filtering of the repeated information, so that the brain can always access the information if it needs it. If the rhythm of clapping is varied, or if the second clap in one of a series of paired claps is omitted, it is easily noticeable, but as long as everything is predictable, the response to the second sound remains diminished.

The electrophysiological response of the brain to the sounds is measured using the P50 component of the auditory evoked response, an electrically positive (P) wave that occurs 50 milliseconds after the stimulus and that is recorded from the vertex of the head. The neuronal response of the brain to the stimulus is robust enough that the electrical field associated with it can be recorded through the scalp and skull. However, signal averaging is necessary to separate the response from the other activity of all other brain areas, which together compose the electroencephalogram (EEG). In practice, the response to 80 to 120 pairs of clicks is averaged. The amplitude of the response to the second sound is significantly diminished in amplitude compared to the first for normal subjects. Patients with schizophrenia lack much of this inhibition. Normals generally diminish the second amplitude by at least 50 percent. Most schizophrenics do not (Fig. 12.10–1).

This abnormality is not unique to schizophrenia. It also occurs in the manic phase of bipolar disorder, particularly in the acute phase, or in bipolar patients who have psychosis. However, the abnormality is not seen in attention-deficit/hyperactivity disorder (ADHD), so that it seems more related to specific disturbances of the brain in

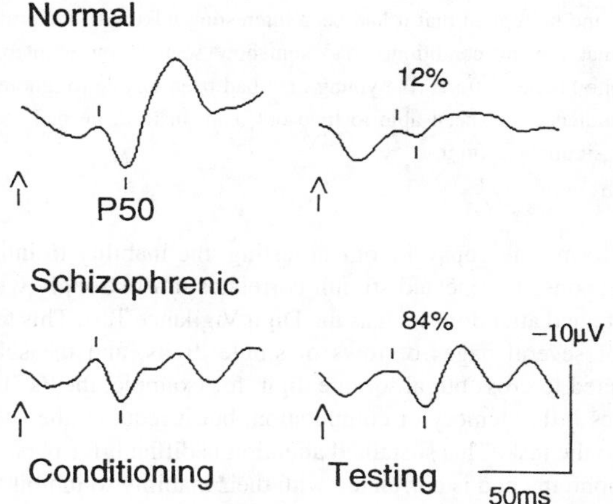

FIGURE 12.10–1 Auditory evoked potentials recorded from scalp surface in response to two identical clicks, which occurred at the arrows. For a normal subject, the response to the first click has larger amplitude waveforms than the response to the second. The first stimulus is called the *conditioning stimulus*, because it conditions or activates inhibitory mechanisms whose strength is tested by the response to the second, or test, stimulus. For a person with schizophrenia, the response to the conditioning stimulus is similar to that of the normal subject, but there is little or no inhibition of response to the second stimulus. The P50 wave, which is frequently measured in such experiments, is shown as a downward deflection between the tic marks. The amplitude of the second response relative to the first is shown expressed as percentage.

psychosis, rather than to a general problem in attention. In schizophrenia, the abnormality is relatively constant. It does not vary with clinical state, acutely psychotic or in remission, and it does not vary with the pattern of symptoms, so that patients with positive and negative symptoms or deficit symptoms have abnormalities. It thus appears to be a reflection of a rather enduring trait that is part of the underlying neurobiology of chronic schizophrenia.

The P50 inhibitory abnormality is not the only abnormality in sensory gating observed in schizophrenia. A similar abnormality is a deficiency in the inhibition of the startle response. Normally, persons startle to loud sounds by blinking their eyes or contracting their forehead and neck muscles. However, if the sound is preceded by 50 to 200 milliseconds of a low tone, then the startle response is diminished. This phenomenon, called *prepulse inhibition of startle*, is also diminished in schizophrenia. The P50 inhibitory abnormality and prepulse inhibition of startle occur over relatively brief time courses, involving stimuli that occur within a second of each other. The relatively brief time course suggests that specific neuronal circuits might be malfunctioning.

It cannot be directly determined how this elementary dysfunction is related to more complex dysfunctions, such as messages from space ships, but the abnormality also appears to be related to other observations that schizophrenics have difficulty with processing sounds and other sensory stimuli. During acute psychoses in particular, patients describe how sounds and lights seem to flood their consciousness in an uncontrollable way. They describe a state sometimes referred to as *hypervigilance*, in which stimuli in their environment seem to command their attention. Sometimes, it is obvious that these are stimuli that most persons would ignore.

A young man who had schizophrenia was being interviewed in a classroom that also contained an air conditioner. Everyone could hear the air conditioner, but the members of the audience were able to apportion most of their attention to what the professor and patient were saying to each other. As the interview concluded, the professor thanked the young man, and he replied that it had been interesting talking to the professor, but that the air conditioner had somehow seemed more interesting. Despite his best efforts, the young man had been unable to ignore what the audience had been able to tune out, and, instead, he had ascribed some significance to it.

In formal neuropsychological testing, the inability to inhibit the P50 response to repeated stimuli correlates most strongly with tests of sustained attention, such as the Digit Vigilance Test. This test consists of several pages of rows of single digits, and the subject is instructed to cross out all of one digit, for example, the 7s. The task requires little memory or computation, but it requires the subject to stick to the task. This sustained attention is difficult for persons with schizophrenia and is correlated with their inability to inhibit the P50 response. The implication is that the patients' inability to perform consistently on the task may be due, in part, to their ability to inhibit their response to competing stimuli in the environment. Diminished performance on psychological tests has been related to other difficulties in patients' lives. Diminished ability to pay attention, as measured on tasks such as the Digit Vigilance Test, is correlated with the inability to form social relationships. Thus, the simple problem in inhibition of response to repeated stimuli could reflect a defect in a simple neuronal mechanism that underlies an entire range of behaviors, from simple gating of sensitivity to noise in the environment to the ability to engage in more complex social interactions.

Patients develop various ways to handle this problem in sensory gating. Many times, they withdraw and avoid contact with others, perhaps because they cannot process the wealth of stimuli that occur in social environments. Some patients deliberately give themselves other stimuli that they can control. For example, one schizophrenia patient uses a machine that makes wave sounds and increases its intensity to overcome other sounds in his environment that he cannot control. His family knows that he is particularly ill when the wave sounds increase. In psychiatric hospitals, seclusion rooms are used in part to help acutely ill patients by diminishing the amount of sensory stimulation that they are exposed to. A subsequent section describes how medications and other substances affect the neuronal circuits involved in sensory gating.

SENSORY GATING ABNORMALITIES AS A NEURONAL DYSFUNCTION

The P50 response to repeated stimuli has an analog in several laboratory animal species. Normal rodents, cats, and monkeys respond to repeated stimuli with the diminished responses. Although animals may not be a good model for schizophrenia itself, the details of neuronal circuitry involved in sensory inhibition cannot be analyzed in human beings, because invasive electrophysiological recordings at the single neuron level are not possible. Therefore, animal models have a particular role in the investigation of which neuronal mechanisms might be involved in sensory gating. In rodents, a P20 response is recorded from the skull surface and has properties similar to the human P50. In the rodent, depth electrodes find the hippocampus to be the source of the wave, and the principal neurons of the hippocampus discharge on the rising phase of the P20 wave. The P20, as recorded at the skull surface, is likely the summed excitatory postsynaptic potential (EPSP) of the principal neurons of the hippocampus as they respond to the synaptic inputs carrying the information from the sound. The hippocampus contains two major regions, the dentate gyrus and horn of Ammon or cornu ammonis (CA). The CA is divided into four regions, CA1 through CA4. CA3 appears to be the principal source of P20. The hippocampus is not a primary sensory processing area. Rather, it is concerned with interpreting the significance of sensory stimuli, to orient the organism to its environment. Sound reaches CA3 through two quite different pathways. One is the classical lemniscal pathway. Sound is converted into neural activity by the cochlea of the ear, and it then reaches the cochlear nucleus through the auditory nerve. The cochlear nucleus projects to the superior olivary nucleus and then to the inferior colliculus through a major brainstem pathway called the *lateral lemniscus*. The colliculus, in turn, projects to the midbrain thalamic nucleus concerned with sound, the medial geniculate. The medial geniculate projects to the forebrain primary auditory cortex in the temporal lobe. The primary auditory cortex then projects to a series of secondary association cortices, which eventually project to the entorhinal cortex. This cortex then projects to the dentate gyrus, as well as directly to the CA3 principal or pyramidal neurons, through a pathway that directly penetrates the hippocampal formation, called the *perforant path*. Transmission throughout this pathway, from the auditory nerve to the perforant path, responds to both of the paired sounds in the previously mentioned paradigm. The path thus preserves the information contained in a continuous stream of auditory information, such as speech or music.

The second path to the hippocampus diverges within the lateral lemniscus. The nucleus of the lateral lemniscus projects to the

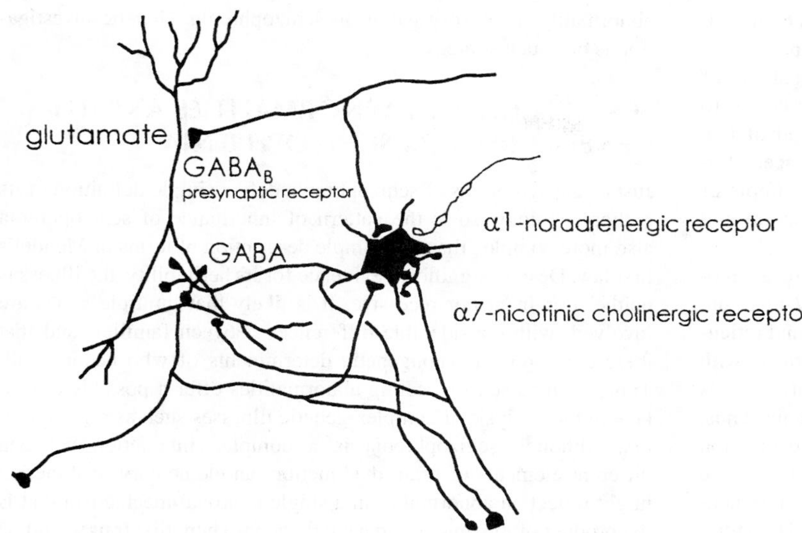

FIGURE 12.10–2 Neuronal circuitry responsible for inhibition in the hippocampus. Pyramidal neurons *(left)* respond to excitatory inputs that activate glutamate receptors on their dendrites. These same excitatory inputs also activate inhibitory interneurons (shown in *black, right*), which then decrease the release of excitatory neurotransmitter onto the pyramidal neurons. In addition, pyramidal neurons themselves excite the interneurons. In the conditioning-testing paradigm, the first stimulus would activate this inhibitory mechanism, so that the response to the second stimulus would be diminished. The response of inhibitory neurons is enhanced by further excitation from cholinergic inputs coming into the hippocampus from the septal area. These cholinergic inputs activate α7 nicotinic receptors on the interneuron, which cause the interneuron to increase its release of its inhibitory neurotransmitter γ-aminobutyric acid (GABA). When enough GABA is released, it reaches GABA type B (GABA$_B$) presynaptic receptors on the excitatory inputs to the pyramidal cells and inhibits the release of glutamate. This inhibitory mechanism is set into motion by the first, or conditioning, stimulus, and it then blocks the response to the second, or test, stimulus.

medial reticular formation, at the caudal portion of the pons. The reticular neurons here project into the spinal cord, where they mediate the startle response, and also into the ventral forebrain and midbrain, where they synapse on the cholinergic nuclei, including those of the medial septal nucleus. Medial septal neuron axons enter the hippocampus through the fornix, a fiber tract that ascends in the septum pellucidum to form the fimbria, which envelop the hippocampus with projections. Region CA3 has especially prominent cholinergic innervation. The nucleus of the lateral lemniscus responds to both sounds. The reticular formation does not, and neither does the medial septal nucleus. Although cholinergic fibers project to all hippocampal neurons, the projection is especially prominent on inhibitory interneurons, which inhibit the principal pyramidal neurons by a variety of synaptic mechanisms.

Thus, there is a convergence of two different pathways at the hippocampus. The perforant pathway carries much information as a constant stream, and the fimbria-fornix sets the inhibitory tone that determines how that information is received. A single stimulus activates an entire population of pyramidal neurons, some quite strongly and others less strongly. Inhibitory neurons generally project to a number of pyramidal neurons, so that they can control the sensitivity of many pyramidal neurons to stimuli. If the inhibitory tone is low, the population of hippocampal pyramidal neurons is responsive to all stimuli, but it has a corresponding loss of focus, because all the neurons are responding. If the inhibitory tone is high, then the population as a whole is less responsive, but it is better able to use its processing capacity for a specific task, for example, it can process the professor's words and not the air conditioner's hum. CA3 projects to CA1, the primary memory area of the hippocampus, which is responsible for short-term learning. This capacity is limited, so CA3 has the important role of determining what should be transmitted to CA1. The cholinergic regulation of the inhibitory neurons is critical to determining the range of information to which the CA3 responds.

A number of neurotransmitters are involved in this process. Glutamate is a nearly universal excitatory neurotransmitter. It is responsible for excitation of the inhibitory interneurons and the pyramidal neurons themselves. The simultaneous activation of the inhibitory interneurons and the pyramidal neurons is an example of feed-forward inhibition, which is common in the central nervous system (CNS). The inhibitory interneurons inhibit pyramidal neuron responses by several mechanisms, all involving the neurotransmitter γ-aminobutyric acid (GABA). GABA activates chloride channels through one set of receptors, located on the cell body and dendrites of the pyramidal neuron, which prevent the pyramidal neuron membrane from reaching the threshold for initiating action potentials. Activation of a second set of receptors, called GABA type B (GABA$_B$) receptors, many of which are located on the presynaptic terminals of afferents to the pyramidal neurons, prevents release of glutamate from the afferents, so that the pyramidal neurons do not respond to the incoming stimuli, because no glutamate has been released onto their dendrites. Figure 12.10–2 summarizes some of these features.

All glutamate receptor types are involved in the excitation of pyramidal neurons. Interneurons require specific activation of *N*-methyl-D-aspartate (NMDA)–type glutamate receptors, which require a more prolonged depolarization. Part of that depolarization depends on the simultaneous activation of cholinergic synapses from the medial septal nucleus. The receptor type here is the α7 nicotinic receptor. Acetylcholine activates a variety of muscarinic and nicotinic receptors. Nicotinic receptors are so named because they also respond to nicotine. NMDA receptors and α7 receptors admit calcium into the neuron when their channels are opened by glutamate or acetylcholine.

Nicotinic and muscarinic cholinergic receptors are activated by acetylcholine. Their differences occur because the different receptors are generated by different genes, and the different receptor types have different functions in the brain. They may be found on different types of neurons, and they may also have different mechanisms. α7 Nicotinic receptors, for example, are found in number of areas, but they are especially prominent on inhibitory interneurons in the hippocampus and the thalamus. Their role in admitting calcium to the cell is more prominent than other cholinergic receptors. However, the feature that most easily distinguishes different types of nicotinic receptors is their differential response to antagonists. One such antagonist is α-bungarotoxin, a snake toxin that was known to bind to receptors in the brain, as well as to the neuromuscular junction, which is also a nicotinic receptor. The nature of α-bungarotoxin binding in the brain was not clear at the time when it was initially demonstrated that α-bungarotoxin infused into the brains of rats caused them to lose their inhibition of response to the second stimulus. No other class of cholinergic antagonists caused a similar loss. Subsequently, the gene for this receptor was cloned. It is called α7, because it was the seventh nicotinic receptor to be cloned, and it resembled the α or acetylcholine-binding subunit of the neuromuscular junction receptor, the first nicotinic receptor to be cloned. The receptor itself is thought to be comprised of five identical α7 units that combine to form a channel. When acetycholine molecules contact α7 units, they twist slightly, an example of protein allosterism, to form an opening that admits calcium and other ions into the cell.

α7 Nicotinic receptors, as measured by the binding of antagonists such as α-bungarotoxin or by antibodies to the α7 nicotinic receptor, are reduced in the hippocampus, frontal cortex, and reticular thalamic nucleus of postmortem brain tissue from patients with schizophrenia. The reduction is approximately 50 percent of levels found in tissue from persons who did not have schizophrenia. Thus, there is some evidence that the ability of the receptor to function may be decreased. However, the reduction should be viewed in the larger context of a more general decrease in the number of interneurons, particularly in the hippocampus and frontal cortex. Therefore, it is not clear whether the lower expression of α7 receptors may not simply be part of a decrease in inhibitory neurons. Either possibility is consistent with the decreased inhibitory function demonstrated by the reduced inhibition of P50 evoked potentials.

Other neurotransmitters also have modulatory roles. Dopamine increases the response of cortical neurons to incoming stimuli, so that more of their activity is transmitted to the hippocampus. Serotonin, through serotonin type 2A (5-HT_{2A}) receptors, increases the release of glutamate onto the pyramidal neurons. Norepinephrine interferes with the calcium influx produced by α7 and NMDA receptors.

As complicated as this schema seems, it is a simplified version of a number of neuronal mechanisms that support the response of the brain to a simple stimulus. Any of these neuronal mechanisms can malfunction in schizophrenia, but the specific lack of inhibition in the sensory gating paradigm implicates the interneuron, with its NMDA and α7 nicotinic synapses. The animal model suggests candidate neuronal mechanisms, but other strategies must be used to determine which of these candidates is actually responsible for the abnormality in sensory gating in schizophrenia. Genetic investigation is one such strategy.

SENSORY GATING ABNORMALITIES AND THE GENETIC RISK FOR SCHIZOPHRENIA

Just as the symptoms of schizophrenia defy a simple definition of its pathophysiology, so is the pattern of inheritance of schizophrenia also more complex than any simple description of terms of Mendel's first law. Despite significant evidence for its heritability, the illness is neither dominant nor recessive. It is likely that multiple genes are involved, with considerable differences between families, and that there are significant nongenetic determinants of who becomes ill. Traits such as sensory gating abnormalities offer a possible advantage in the analysis of complex genetic illnesses such as schizophrenia. Although schizophrenia is a complex interaction between different elements of brain dysfunction, an elementary dysfunction might reflect an abnormality in a single neuronal mechanism that is the product of dysfunction in a single gene. Then, that trait would be distributed in families in accordance with Mendel's first law, and its distribution could be mapped onto the human genetic map using genetic linkage techniques. Because schizophrenia itself does not have Mendelian distribution in families, it would be expected that some persons in the families might have the abnormality in sensory gating but might not have schizophrenia.

The family in Figure 12.10–3 is an example of what was found. The sex of all individuals in the family has been disguised, the order of their birth has been changed, and some members of the family have been removed from the diagram to protect the family's identity. The two persons with schizophrenia in the family have abnormal P50 inhibition. So does one of the parents; the other parent had died before the study was undertaken. Several of their siblings have abnormal P50 inhibition as well. Polymorphisms, generally differences in the numbers of particular repeated sequences of nucleotides in the introns or non–amino acid–coding portion of genets, were mapped across all the chromosomes in these families. Some of the families showed a correspondence between the inheritance of the

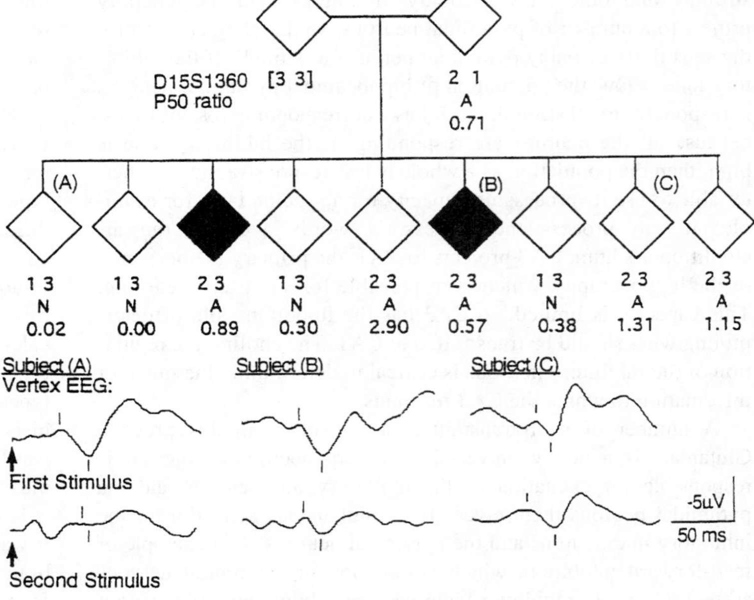

FIGURE 12.10–3 Inheritance of P50 inhibition (shown as the ratio of the test to the conditioning amplitude) and alleles of D15S1360 in a family with two individuals with schizophrenia (*darkened symbols*). The two alleles of D15S1360 are linked to the abnormality in P50 inhibition, as well as to schizophrenia itself. EEG, electroencephalogram.

P50 abnormality and the inheritance of polymorphisms at a specific location on chromosome 15. This location was subsequently shown to be the location of *Ch*olinergic *R*eceptor *N*icotinic *A*lpha-*7* gene (*CHRNA7*), that is, the gene for the α7 nicotinic receptor subunit.

A deoxyribonucleic acid (DNA) clone containing *CHRNA7* was scanned for new repeated sequences, one of which, D15S1360, is shown in Figure 12.10–3. This sequence is in intron 2 of *CHRNA7*. In this particular family, there are three lengths of the D15S1360 repeat, which are labeled 1 through 3 in Figure 12.10–3. Each individual has two copies of D15S1360, one on each chromosome. The living parent's two chromosomes can be distinguished by the two different copies. During meiosis, when the egg or sperm is formed, one copy is selected at random for inclusion. The other copy comes from the other parent's sperm or egg. The living parent transmits allele 2 or copy of D15S1360 to approximately one-half the children, and allele 1 to the other half. Although the other parent had died by the time of this study, it can be deduced that this parent has two copies of allele 3, because each of the children has received an allele 3. At other nearby markers, this deceased parent's two chromosomes are distinguishable, just as for the living parent with D15S1360. Thus, this family provides evidence for inheritance of P50 inhibition at D15S1360, by comparing the pattern of transmission of D15S1360 with the distribution of abnormal P50 inhibition. A maximum likelihood analysis is used to compare the probability that D15S1360 marks the site of a gene that is linked to the trait of abnormal P50 inhibition to the probability that the codistribution of marker and trait occurred by chance. In the initial study of nine families, of which the family in Figure 12.10–3 is part, this odds ratio was 5.3, expressed as a common or base 10 logarithm. The probability was thus greater than 100,000 to 1.

The probability that schizophrenia itself is inherited at this locus was suggestive but not as significant. The difference occurs for several reasons. First, many fewer individuals in the families have schizophrenia than have abnormal P50 inhibition, so that the number of times that D15S1360 is associated with schizophrenia is fewer than the number of times it is associated with abnormal P50 inhibition. Second, there were occasional individuals in the families who had schizophrenia, but normal P50 inhibition. These individuals did not have the same D15S1360 genotypes as other members of the family who had schizophrenia and abnormal P50 inhibition. Therefore, they diminished the association between schizophrenia and D15S1360. Such individuals are reminders that the genetics and neurobiology of schizophrenia are much more heterogeneous than the genetics and neurobiology of a simple measure like P50 inhibition. In families with multiple individuals with schizophrenia, it is sometimes assumed that schizophrenia always occurs by the same mechanism, but it is also possible that the multiple cases have occurred because there are several different causes of schizophrenia possible in the family.

Genetic linkage studies involving markers in the chromosome 15q14 region have now been pursued by a number of investigators, using schizophrenia as the phenotype. Eight studies have found evidence for linkage in this region, but others have not. The odds ratios have approached 10,000 in some studies. Genetic linkage to bipolar disorder, particularly psychotic variants, has also been observed in this region.

The DNA of the *CHRNA7* gene has been sequenced to determine if it contains abnormalities in persons with schizophrenia that could explain how inheritance at this chromosomal site causes α7 nicotinic receptors to fail. The principal part of any gene is its exons, which contain the nucleotides that code for the amino acid of the peptide product, in this case the α7 nicotinic receptor subunit. This code is normal, so that it is likely that the receptor has a normal structure. However, there are changes in the promoter of the gene, which is a region next to the first exon that controls how abundantly the gene is transcribed into messenger ribonucleic acid (mRNA). These changes, most of which are changes in a single nucleotide, cause the gene to have modestly decreased expression, so that there would be fewer α7 nicotinic receptors. In fact, studies of postmortem brain tissue from schizophrenics have demonstrated fewer α7 nicotinic receptors in several brain areas in schizophrenia, including the hippocampus, frontal cortex, and the thalamus. As was found with genetic linkage, the abnormalities in the promoter of *CHRNA7* are more closely associated with abnormal P50 inhibition than they are with schizophrenia itself.

As detailed elsewhere in this volume, that are many genetic loci that contribute to the risk for schizophrenia. The relative strength of each contribution is unknown, and the genes at each of these loci are just beginning to be identified. Some of these genes may also influence various aspects of sensory gating. For example, a gene that modifies the response of NMDA receptors has been identified as one of the putative genes involved in transmission of risk for schizophrenia.

In comparing the neurobiology and genetic inheritance of P50 inhibition with schizophrenia, it is thus obvious that P50 inhibition is one element in the pathogenesis of schizophrenia but that it is neither necessary nor sufficient to cause the illness. No other genetic locus or neurobiological trait has been found to have an obligate role in the pathogenesis of all cases of schizophrenia. Thus, P50 inhibition fulfills the requirement of Mendel's first law of genetics, in that it segregates or distributes itself in families as a discrete trait, which is now shown to be linked to a specific genetic location.

However, its significance in the pathogenesis of schizophrenia can better be considered from the perspective of Mendel's second law, which proposes that genetic or biologically different traits should segregate independent of each other in a family. In addition to abnormalities in sensory gating, there are other abnormalities in schizophrenia. Two others that are commonly described are abnormalities in dopaminergic neurotransmission and diminished volume of the hippocampus. There are many others as well, but, for the purposes of illustration, these two suffice. In addition to sensory gating abnormalities, schizophrenic persons often have higher dopaminergic neurotransmission, as measured by increased plasma levels of dopamine metabolites, and smaller hippocampal volumes, perhaps reflecting decreased numbers of neurons or smaller neurons. As predicted by Mendel's second law, these additional traits are independent of abnormal P50 inhibition in the families of schizophrenics. Family members who do not have schizophrenia but who have abnormal P50 inhibition have normal hippocampal volume and normal dopaminergic neurotransmission. Higher dopamine metabolite levels and diminished hippocampal volume are found in other members of the family who do not have schizophrenia, but, generally, they do not have elevated levels of dopamine metabolites or diminished hippocampal volume. Thus, none of the three traits causes schizophrenia, and any of them can be found in someone who does not have schizophrenia.

There are several corollaries of the proposal that schizophrenia occurs because of the convergence of several independent abnormalities. One corollary is that each abnormality has to have a high prevalence in the general population. If three traits are required, the prevalence of schizophrenia, approximately 0.01, or 1 percent, must be equal to the product of the prevalence of the three traits. If they have equal prevalence, then each of them would be present in 0.22, or 22 percent, of the population. For *CHRNA7*, the frequency of promoter polymorphisms in the general population is in this range. A second corollary is that each independent abnormality should have a phenotype, even if it occurs in a person who does not have schizophrenia. Persons with abnormalities in P50 inhibition in the families of a proband with schizophrenia themselves have some evidence for schizotypal characteristics, although few fulfill diagnostic criteria for schizotypal personality disorder.

It has long been noted that some individuals who are close relatives of a proband with schizophrenia may be unusually creative or successful. Whether or not these persons have specific abnormalities in P50 inhibition or any other neurobiological risk factor is, of course, unknown. One provocative example is the 19th century philosopher Arthur Schopenhauer. Schopenhauer made fundamental contributions to the understanding of the role of the will in mental function. His father died by suicide, and his paternal grandfather had died insane. Schopenhauer himself was cynical, aloof, and suspicious of others. He slept with a loaded gun; refused to go to barbers because he feared their razors; and kept his smoking pipes in a locked cabinet, so that they could not be contaminated. In his essay, "On Noise," he wrote about his sensory gating disturbance: "I have long held the opinion that the amount of noise which anyone can hear undisturbed stands in inverse proportion to his mental capacity, and may therefore be regarded as a pretty fair measure of it. . . . Noise is a torture to all intellectual people."

SENSORY GATING ABNORMALITIES AND THE TREATMENT OF SCHIZOPHRENIA

A somewhat simplified model of the pathophysiology of schizophrenia can be constructed from the three traits. The model proposes that the normal function of the brain is to process sensory stimuli into an accurate view of the world and that disordered thinking arises from disordered perception. Dopamine increases the sensitivity of neurons to stimuli, so that it acts as a volume or gain control, increasing the amount of response that all neurons have for stimulation. Heightened awareness is not in itself pathological; it is part of the normal fight-or-flight reaction when individuals are in novel situations or under stress or need to enhance their responses. Sensory gating mechanisms, which could be considered in the model as a second step in processing, allow the brain to decrease the amount of information that it needs to process by diminishing the response to redundant information. The elimination of redundant information, such as repeated sounds, enables the brain to save its resources, that is, the responses of neurons in its memory circuits, for novel stimuli or for stimuli whose importance is recognized by other mechanisms. If one is reading this book in a library, one may appreciate the ability to filter or to tune out redundant sounds, so that one can concentrate on this chapter, yet still be able to respond when the person next to one unexpectedly asks one for coffee. Finally, information, appropriately filtered, reaches the brain's memory systems, where new information is compared with already learned information, and, if appropriate, new memories are formed. The capacity for these last tasks is thought to be rather limited, compared to the amount of information potentially available through the senses. In schizophrenia, increased dopamine levels cause neurons to respond to many stimuli; the excess responses cannot be filtered, because sensory gating mechanisms are abnormal; and the memory capacity is diminished, because the hippocampus is smaller. As a consequence, inaccurate memories are recorded. At first, these are the basis for a suspicion that something is wrong. Patients often trace their delusions and hallucinations back to an ambiguous perception: "I was bending over to get a drink and I thought that a teacher behind me called me an alien, but I am not sure. I cannot get that thought out of my mind—she called me an alien."

Failure of any one of the three mechanisms by itself is not pathological. Heightened stress leads to hypervigilance, which could be beneficial in a new situation, such as a new job. Decreased sensory gating may prevent the premature exclusion of information, so that more features of the world remain available to higher brain areas, resulting in a more novel, creative view of the world. Diminished memory capacity would not seem to have an advantage, but diminished intelligence by itself does not result in schizophrenia.

Treatment of schizophrenia has primarily been directed toward blocking increased dopaminergic neurotransmission, which is the target of the neuroleptic antipsychotic drugs. Sensory gating mechanisms are not directly targeted by any medication. Nicotine activates $\alpha7$ nicotinic receptors at relatively high doses, compared to most of the other nicotinic receptors, and thereby causes schizophrenic subjects to be able to inhibit their P50 response to the second stimulus. Smoking two to three cigarettes in 10 minutes is generally adequate, but the effect is lost within 15 minutes, and, thereafter, the receptors remain desensitized for a prolonged period of time. Desensitized receptors cannot be activated by the patient's only acetylcholine or by additional nicotine, so that, despite the transient positive effect, the net effect of smoking is to increase receptor dysfunction.

Persons with schizophrenia are among the most likely to smoke heavily in the population. By inhaling deeper and holding the smoke longer, they extract approximately 50 percent more nicotine per cigarette than other smokers. Schizophrenic persons are not protected from the health risks of smoking, although some data suggest a relative protection from lung cancer, compared to comparably smoking nonschizophrenic persons. There is no protection from the cardiovascular risk. Therefore, despite the transient effect on sensory gating, nicotine is not a treatment of schizophrenia.

Nonetheless, the most currently effective drug for schizophrenia, clozapine (Clozaril), also normalizes P50 inhibition, a property not shared with any older or newer antipsychotic drugs currently available. Furthermore, clozapine is the only drug that decreases patients' cigarette smoking. Clozapine's effects on the inhibition of auditory responses have been studied in animal models and appear to be the result of increased acetylcholine release, which activates $\alpha7$ nicotinic receptor. The mechanism of the increased acetylcholine release is not known, but it could reflect clozapine's antagonism of a variety of serotonergic receptors that normally diminish acetylcholine release.

No treatment currently available can restore lost hippocampal neurons or those in other brain areas concerned with processes such as memory. However, head protection through seat belts, bicycle helmets, and the like has become a general social mandate, which may be helpful in preventing schizophrenia and other brain illnesses whose severity is affected by head injury. The selection of dopaminergic neurotransmission as the prime target for therapy of schizophrenia is already being questioned, because of its possible negative impact on the cognition of schizophrenias. Some day, historians of the treatment of schizophrenia may wonder why psychiatrists and pharmacologists focused on this mechanism, when it was obvious that the ability to increase neuronal sensitivity to stimuli is critical to psychosocial and cognitive functions. Early 21st century psychiatrists may acquire a reputation not dissimilar to George Washington's learned doctors.

SENSORY GATING ABNORMALITIES AND THE DEVELOPMENT OF SCHIZOPHRENIA

One of the mysteries of the brain is that it constructs itself with the same genes and gene products that it later uses for its function in information processing. The $\alpha7$ nicotinic receptor is no exception. It is expressed on neurons as soon as they are generated from primordial neuroepithelium. The receptor remains at high levels in many areas, including the hippocampus and several areas of the cerebral cortex, until other innervation is established. Recent evidence suggests that NMDA-type glutamate receptors are constructed in concert with earlier expressed $\alpha7$ nicotinic receptors. Despite these apparently helpful effects of nicotinic receptors in the early development of neuronal connections, they are potentially harmful as well. Because they admit calcium through their ion channels, α7 receptors can kill immature neurons by admitting too much calcium. The excess calcium causes apoptosis or programmed cell death when it occurs before the neurons have developed calcium-binding proteins to buffer cytoplasmic calcium levels. Thus, abnormalities in the number of α7 nicotinic receptors could have profound developmental effects, in addition to their eventual effects on signal processing in mature animals. The role of α7 nicotinic receptors or any of the other genetic and neurobiological elements associated with schizophrenia in brain development is not yet known, nor is it known to what extent abnormalities in the developmental role of α7 receptors predispose individuals to the later development of psychoses. Nevertheless, primary prevention of schizophrenia will have to take into account the likelihood of a significant developmental role of genes such as *CHRNA7*. It is possible that genetic abnormalities cause much of pathology that is later manifested as schizophrenia by the time the individual has passed the perinatal developmental period.

SENSORY GATING ABNORMALITIES AND THE STORY OF SCHIZOPHRENIA

Let this chapter now return to the patient who heard messages from space ships. If she is compared to the medical school class, who fear that they will somehow fail in their medical education, there are some commonalities and some differences. Both are self-critical and self-doubting. However, whereas the class can put aside their fears and doubts to study effectively, the patient cannot. When she is acutely psychotic, the fear overwhelms her, and she responds to its demands, in the form of commands from the space ship, against her better judgment. The most bizarre aspect, however, is the concept of the space ship. Why has she created the space ship? It would seem that the phenomenon is so overwhelming to her that she has created a story to explain it. She is a bit disappointed in the originality of the story, but it is a story that nonetheless organizes a number of features of her problem. First, it reflects the incredible degree of the disorganization of her perception, so that her own thoughts are not longer recognizable to her. Second, it reflects the chronicity of her problem. Persons under acute stress rarely come up with the idea of space ships. Psychotic patients describe how, over the course of months to years, their understanding of an external force trying to control them deepens. First, they notice that something is amiss in their perception of the external world. Then, they suspect that another person may be offending them, perhaps by whispering about them. Finally, they realize the extent of the forces allied against them. The police, the Central Intelligence Agency (CIA), or aliens are observing, communicating, and then directly influencing their brain. The *influencing machine*, the idea that a machine could influence the patient's brain, superseded the devil as a preferred paranoid delusion in the 19th century. Obviously, space ships are the 21st century variant.

The author of this section included a story of how dysfunction in an elementary neuronal mechanism could be related to the genetic risk for schizophrenia. A story implies that not all of the aspects of the problem are fully proven; a story means that at least part of the information relies on imagination. Indeed, there are no rigorous standards of scientific proof that allow movement with confidence from one level of analysis, for example, molecular or neurobiological, to another, for example, psychological or behavioral, so that there is an element of imagination that draws parallels and links between these different levels of analysis in a *translational story*. The great German microbiologist Robert Koch put forth postulates in the 19th century that describe standards of proof for how a microbe, such as the tuberculosis bacillus that he discovered, can be related to a human illness, that is, consumption. The microbe had to be isolated from an ill person, it had to be grown in pure culture, then it had to infect a new case, and then, finally, it had to be isolated from that new case. There are, as yet, no similar postulates for relating a gene to a neuronal function, to a psychological function, and, finally, to auditory hallucinations. Thus, one is left with a story, one that has not yet reached scientific postulate status. Part of the problem is that so little of how the brain develops and functions is yet understood. For example, the detailed study of the α7 receptor's role in perception may eventually be eclipsed by consideration of its earlier role in development.

It may be fitting that the space ship itself is a story, created to explain the inexplicable. Indeed, it is argued that the brain evolved to tell stories, to turn the mysterious into the predictable, by developing models of what is happening that can be used to predict the future. In some cases, the stories explain how the gods manipulate the heavenly bodies, so that the seasons become predictable, and crops can be planted and harvested. In other cases, the stories summarize fears about the unpredictable, when the gods' wrath causes devastation. Stories of people who have schizophrenia are also contained within that great human tradition, a reflection of the havoc wreaked by their brain dysfunction expressed in a uniquely human way.

SUGGESTED CROSS-REFERENCES

The genetics of schizophrenia are covered in Sections 1.17 and 1.18. Perception and cognition are discussed in Section 3.1. Brain models of the mind are covered in Section 3.5.

REFERENCES

Adler LE, Hoffer LD, Wiser A, Freedman R: Normalization of auditory physiology by cigarette smoking in schizophrenic patients. *Am J Psychiatry.* 1993;150:1856–1861.

Adler LE, Pachtman E, Franks R, Pecevich M, Waldo MC, Freedman R: Neurophysiological evidence for a defect in neuronal mechanisms involved in sensory gating in schizophrenia. *Biol Psychiatry.* 1982;17:639–654.

Benes FM, Berretta S: GABAergic interneurons: Implications for understanding schizophrenia and bipolar disorder. *Neuropsychopharmacology.* 2001;25:1–27.

Bickford PC, Luntz-Leybman V, Freedman R: Auditory sensory gating in the rat hippocampus: Modulation by brainstem activity. *Brain Res.* 1993;607:33–38.

Braff DL, Geyer MA, Swerdlow NR: Human studies of prepulse inhibition of startle: Normal subjects, patient groups, and pharmacological studies. *Psychopharmacology.* 2001;156:234–258.

Broadbent DE. *Decision and Stress.* London: Academic Press; 1971.

Cannon TD, Zorrilla LE, Shtasel D, Gur RE, Gur RC, Marco EJ, Moberg P, Price RA: Neuropsychological functioning in siblings discordant for schizophrenia and healthy volunteers. *Arch Gen Psychiatry.* 1994;51:651–661.

Chumakov I, Blumenfeld M, Guerassimenko O, Cavarec L, Palicio M, Abderrahim H, Bougueleret L, Barry C, Tanaka H, La Rosa P, Puech A, Tahri N, Cohen-Akenine A, Delabrosse S, Lissarrague S, Picard FP, Maurice K, Essioux L, Millasseau P, Grel P, Debailleul V, Simon AM, Caterina D, Dufaure I, Malekzadeh K, Belova M, Luan JJ, Bouillot M, Sambucy JL, Primas G, Saumier M, Boubkiri N, Martin-Saumier S, Nasroune M, Peixoto H, Delaye A, Pinchot V, Bastucci M, Guillou S, Chevillon M, Sainz-Fuertes R, Meguenni S, Aurich-Costa J, Cherif D, Gimalac A, Van Duijn C, Gauvreau D, Ouelette G, Fortier I, Realson J, Sherbatich T, Riazanskaia N, Rogaev E, Raeymaekers P, Aerssens J, Konings F, Luyten W, Macciardi F, Sham PC, Straub RE, Weinberger DR, Cohen N, Cohen D: Genetic and physiological data implicating the new human gene G72 and the gene for D-amino acid oxidase in schizophrenia. *Proc Natl Acad Sci U S A.* 2002;99:13675–13680.

Clementz BA, Geyer MA, Braff DL: Multiple site evaluation of P50 suppression among schizophrenia and normal comparison subjects. *Schizophr Res.* 1998;30:71–80.

Cornblatt BA, Malhotra AK: Impaired attention as an endophenotype for molecular genetic studies of schizophrenia. *Am J Med Genet.* 2001;105:11–15.

Cullum CM, Harris JG, Waldo M, Smernoff E, Madison A, Nagamoto HT, Griffith J, Adler LE, Freedman R: Neurophysiological and neuropsychological evidence for attentional dysfunction in schizophrenia. *Schizophr Res.* 1993;10:131–141.

Curtis L, Blouin JL, Radhakrishna U, Gehrig C, Lasseter VK, Wolyniec P, Nestadt G, Dombroski B, Kazazian HH, Pulver AE, Housman, Bertrand D, Antonarakis SE: No evidence for linkage between schizophrenia and markers at chromosome 15q13-14. *Am J Med Genet.* 1999;88:109–112.

Durant W. Schopenhauer. In: *The Story of Philosophy.* New York: Simon and Schuster; 1953:227–264.

Elvevag B, Kerbs KM, Malley JD: Autobiographical memory in schizophrenia: An examination of the distribution of memories. *Neuropsychology.* 2003;17:402–409.

*Freedman R: Schizophrenia. *N Engl J Med.* 2003;349:1738–1749.
Freedman R, Adams CE, Leonard S: The alpha 7-nicotinic acetylcholine receptor and the pathology of hippocampal interneurons in schizophrenia. *J Chem Neuroanatomy.* 2000;20:299–306.
*Freedman R, Coon H, Myles-Worsley M, Orr-Urtreger A, Olincy A, Davis A, Polymeropoulos M, Holik J, Hopkins J, Hoff M, Rosenthal J, Waldo MC, Yaw J, Young DA, Breese CR, Adams C, Patterson D, Adler LE, Kruglyak L, Leonard S, Byerley PW: Linkage of a neurophysiological deficit in schizophrenia to a chromosome 15 locus. *Natl Acad Sci.* 1997;94:587–592.
George TP, Vessicchio JC, Termine A, Sahady DM, Head CA, Pepper WT, Kosten TR, Wexler BE: Effects of smoking abstinence on visuospatial working memory function in schizophrenia. *Neuropsychopharmacology.* 2002;26:75–85.
Goldberg TE, Egan MF, Gscheidle T, Coppola R, Weickert T, Kolachana BS, Goldman D, Weinberger DR: Executive subprocesses in working memory: Relationship to catechol-*O*-methyltransferase Val158Met genotype and schizophrenia. *Arch Gen Psychiatry.* 2003;60:889–896.
Goldman-Rakic PS, Muly EC 3rd, Williams GV: D(1) receptors in prefrontal cells and circuits. *Brain Res Brain Res Rev.* 2000;31:295–301.
*Green MF: What are the functional consequences of neurocognitive deficits in schizophrenia. *Am J Psychiatry.* 1996;1534:321–330.
Green MF, Marder SR, Glynn SM: The neurocognitive effects of low-dose haloperidol: A two-year comparison with risperidone. *Biol Psychiatry.* 2002;51:972–978.
Greene R: Circuit analysis of NMDAR hypofunction in the hippocampus, in vitro, and psychosis of schizophrenia. *Hippocampus.* 2001;11:569–577.
Guan ZZ, Zhang X, Blennow K, Nordberg A: Decreased protein level of nicotinic receptor alpha7 subunit in the frontal cortex from schizophrenic brain. *Neuroreport.* 1999;10:1779–1782.
Heckers S, Rauch SL, Goff D, Savage CR, Schacter DL, Fischman AJ, Alpert NM: Impaired recruitment of the hippocampus during conscious recollection in schizophrenia. *Nat Neurosci.* 1998;1:318–323.
Leonard S, Gault J, Hopkins J, Logel J, Drebing C, Vianzon R, Short M, Berger R, Robinson M, Freedman R: Promoter variants in the $\alpha 7$ nicotinic acetylcholine receptor subunit gene are associated with an inhibitory deficit found in schizophrenia. *Arch Gen Psychiatry.* 2002;59:789–802.
McEvoy JP, Freudenreich O, Wilson WH: Smoking and therapeutic response to clozapine in patients with schizophrenia. *Biol Psychiatry.* 1999;46:125–129.
*Mullen R: The problem of bizarre delusions. *J Nerv Ment Dis.* 2003;191:546–548.
Pickar D, Labarca R, Doran AR: Longitudinal measurement of plasma homovanillic acid levels in schizophrenic patients. Correlation with psychosis and response to antipsychotic treatment. *Arch Gen Psychiatry.* 1986;43:669–676.
Seidman LJ, Faraone SV, Goldstein JM, Kremen WS, Horton NJ, Makris N, Toomey R, Kennedy D, Caviness VS, Tsuang MT: Left hippocampal volume as a vulnerability indication for schizophrenia: A magnetic resonance imaging morphometric study of non-psychotic first degree relatives. *Arch Gen Psychiatry.* 2002;59:839–849.
Selemon LD, Goldman-Rakic PS: The reduced neuropil hypothesis: A circuit based model of schizophrenia. *Biol Psychiatry.* 1999;45:17–25.
Suddath RL, Christianson GW, Torrey EF: Anatomical abnormalities in the brains of monozygotic twins discordant for schizophrenia. *N Engl J Med.* 1990;322:789–794.
van der Gaag M, Hageman MC, Birchwood M: Evidence for a cognitive model of auditory hallucinations. *J Nerv Ment Dis.* 2003;191:542–545.
*Venables P: Input dysfunction in schizophrenia. *Prog Exp Personality Res.* 1964;1:1–47.
Waldo MC, Cawthra E, Adler LE: Auditory sensory gating, hippocampal volume, and catecholamine metabolism in schizophrenics and their siblings. *Schizophr Res.* 1994:12:93–106.
Weinberger DR: Implications of normal brain development for the pathogenesis of schizophrenia. *Arch Gen Psychiatry.* 1987;44:660–669.

▲ 12.11 Schizophrenia: Psychosocial Treatment

FAITH B. DICKERSON, PH.D., M.P.H., LISA DIXON, M.D., M.P.H. AND ANTHONY F. LEHMAN, M.D., M.S.P.H.

Schizophrenia is a pervasive psychiatric disorder that typically has its onset in early adulthood and persists for the remainder of the lifespan. The etiology of schizophrenia is unknown but is presumed to be biological. Multiple lines of evidence suggest the presence of brain abnormalities in affected individuals. Despite its biological underpinnings, schizophrenia exerts its effects in psychological realms; perceptions, thinking, and emotion are often disrupted. As such, schizophrenia has long been the focus of psychosocial and psychotherapeutic interventions.

Adding to the impetus for psychotherapeutic treatments is the fact that the experience of schizophrenia is often baffling and frightening to the affected individual. Patient accounts attest to the feelings of horror and aloneness that may accompany psychotic symptoms. The person with schizophrenia may feel alienated from and shunned by others. Friendships and work roles may be lost. Self-devaluation and despair are not uncommon, and approximately 10 to 13 percent of individuals with schizophrenia ultimately kill themselves.

For the families of individuals with schizophrenia, the illness can likewise be perplexing and burdensome. The ill relative may present with intense behavioral and emotional disturbances. Family members often experience difficulties in understanding and dealing with such problems. An estimated 60 to 75 percent of persons with schizophrenia live with their families, who thus are frequently the primary care providers. Even for family members who are not present on a day-to-day basis, the illness can lead to considerable distress.

In the current era, psychotherapy and other psychosocial treatments are provided in combination with medication, which is highly effective at reducing psychotic symptoms and is now considered an essential component of treatment for schizophrenia. However, the benefits of medications for the illness are incomplete. Many patients with schizophrenia persist in having residual symptoms, even when adhering to medication regimens that conform to current treatment standards. Full recovery from the illness is uncommon, and only approximately one-third of patients with schizophrenia have an outcome that is considered favorable, even with the widespread availability of antipsychotic medications.

The location of treatment for schizophrenia has changed markedly in recent decades. Before the advent of neuroleptic medications in the mid-1950s, and even for the following two decades, treatment for schizophrenia was offered primarily in hospital settings. Hence, many of the earlier studies of psychotherapy for schizophrenia were performed with patients in institutional environments. With the cumulative effects of deinstitutionalization, the location of treatments, including psychotherapy and psychosocial interventions, has shifted to nonhospital settings.

INDIVIDUAL PSYCHOTHERAPY

Psychoanalysis and Psychodynamic Psychotherapy

Psychoanalysis was the dominant paradigm in American psychiatry during much of the 20th century, so it is not surprising that this approach was applied to the treatment of individuals with schizophrenia. Within a psychodynamic framework, symptoms of psychosis are understood as secondary to early intrapsychic and interpersonal experiences. In addition, symptoms are seen as having specific meaning for the person based on conflicts beyond the person's awareness. Psychotherapy within a psychodynamic approach aims to help elucidate the psychological origin of symptoms and enable the person to resolve the psychological problems on which symptoms are presumably based. In keeping with the tenets of psychoanalytic therapy, treatment is seen as offering the patient a *corrective* emotional experience in the long-term relationship with the therapist.

After the introduction of neuroleptic medication the 1950s and the availability of a clearly effective treatment for schizophrenia, the benefits of psychotherapeutic approaches for the disorder were increasingly called into question. Controlled studies performed at Camarillo State Hospital in the 1960s indicated that medication treatment was superior to psychodynamic psychotherapy and to milieu therapy when the treatments were rigorously compared. Further research performed at McLean Hospital in the 1980s also failed to support the specific benefits of psychodynamic therapy for this population.

In the McLean study, psychodynamic therapy was compared to another psychotherapy approach, reality adaptive supportive psychotherapy, which was not based on psychodynamic principles. The psychodynamic, insight-oriented therapy focused on patient–therapist transference, on significant events in the patient's past and present life, and on development of psychological insight. The supportive therapy approach aimed to provide supportive counseling, practical advice, and encouragement around medication compliance. Patients with schizophrenia were randomly assigned to a treatment group and were maintained on antipsychotic medication. Therapy was provided by experienced clinicians in both approaches. Results of the study showed that the supportive therapy was superior on most of the outcomes that were measured. There was no significant difference between groups with regard to improvement in psychiatric symptoms at the end of the study.

The McLean study was criticized on methodological grounds. For example, broad outcome measures were used rather than measures more closely linked to the therapy process. Use of broad outcomes may have biased the study against finding an effect for psychodynamic therapy. On the other hand, one could argue that if therapy does not have an effect on persons' symptoms and role functioning, the benefits of the approach for persons with schizophrenia may be limited.

Also adding to the pessimism about orthodox dynamic psychotherapy in persons with schizophrenia were follow-up studies of patients with schizophrenia treated with intense psychodynamic psychotherapy at Chestnut Lodge Hospital in Maryland and the New York State Psychiatric Institute. Many of these patients remained seriously disabled by their schizophrenia and there was a significant rate of suicide. Although the follow-up studies lacked a comparison group, the relatively poor outcomes of the patients further dimmed enthusiasm for the use of intense psychotherapy for schizophrenia.

More recent opinion holds that intensive psychodynamic psychotherapy may be toxic for patients with schizophrenia. Criticism is particularly focused on therapies that are emotionally intrusive and those that promote regression. Therapy that is too intense or stimulating may be disruptive for patients with schizophrenia and may lead to poor outcomes. Rejection of intensive psychodynamic therapies does not negate the importance of psychotherapy that encourages the persons to share their illness experiences and to discuss the meaning that they attach to these experiences. Illness-related events may affect each individual differently and may be understood in the unique context of the person's life.

Supportive Psychotherapy

Supportive therapy is a form of psychotherapy that is not clearly defined and that has not been the subject of many direct studies for the treatment of individuals with schizophrenia. Although there is little scientific evidence about the efficacy of this treatment approach, it is frequently provided to patients with the disorder. The elements of supportive therapy, as discussed in the text that follows, often overlap with elements in other therapeutic approaches. Supportive therapy may also overlap with more informal sources of support and counseling that persons with schizophrenia may receive from friends or family members and peers, as well as from staff in psychiatric rehabilitation and housing programs.

Supportive therapy is focused on the here and now of the patient's life and aims to help the patient define reality more clearly and solve practical problems. Supportive approaches foster the patient's positive feelings toward the therapist and provide a safe forum for the expression of feelings. Therapeutic issues may include the human concerns raised by having a persistent psychiatric illness, problems in managing the disorder, and normal problems of living that may take on added difficulty because of the schizophrenia illness. The specific strategies that comprise supportive counseling may include providing reassurance, offering explanations and clarification, and giving guidance and suggestions.

The potential benefits of supportive therapy for patients with schizophrenia are several. Regular and supportive interaction with a psychotherapist may help sustain a patient with schizophrenia and may reduce the patient's feelings of aloneness and despair. Given the high rate of completed suicide among individuals with schizophrenia, interventions that may reduce suicidal ideas and behaviors are of high importance.

A positive relationship with the prescribing psychiatrist may also enhance the patient's adherence to prescribed medication. There is a high rate of medication nonadherence in schizophrenia, which often leads to a recurrence of florid psychotic symptoms. Therefore, the benefits of a supportive psychotherapeutic relationship between the patient and the psychiatrist should not be underestimated. An example of a case treated with supportive therapy is described in the following case study.

A 33-year-old man from a middle-class family experienced the onset of paranoid delusions and auditory hallucinations at 17 years of age, shortly after graduating from high school. Before that, he was an introverted but good student. The first 6 years of his illness were marked by four hospitalizations totaling nearly 3 years, recurrent aggressive acts toward others, and frequent noncompliance with medications. Despite those problems, he completed 1 year of community college during that time but was unable to hold a job for more than 4 months or to live on his own.

Six years ago, after his last hospitalization, which spanned 6 months, and during which he was highly assaultive, a more intensive effort at supportive psychotherapy was implemented. The initial sessions focused on educating him about his diagnosis and the reasons for continuing the antipsychotic medication—at the time, 1 cc of fluphenazine (Prolixin Decanoate) every 2 weeks. He was reluctant to continue the medication, because he felt too sleepy and did not entirely believe that he had a mental illness. Instead, he believed that his problems arose from the social abuse that he had experienced from other students in high school several years earlier. However, he agreed to work with the psychiatrist to gradually decrease the dosage, rather than stopping the medication abruptly.

After the establishment of that medication contract, the patient spent several therapy sessions talking about his feelings of paranoia and of being out of control of his life, his rage at perceived past harassment by others, and his extreme frustration about feeling like a "wimp and a loser." He stated that his frequent aggressive outbursts and fights in the hospital had been conscious efforts to prove his manhood. To increase the patient's sense of control, the therapist switched the medication from depot to tablet form and gradually reduced the dosage until mild paranoia reemerged. Thereafter, the patient was compliant with the medication at a dosage of 5 mg of oral fluphenazine per day.

Over the past 3 years, the patient has continued to discuss his feelings of rage as an adolescent, his poor self-esteem, and his feelings of shame. He has remained nonpsychotic, and, although frequently frustrated about his general level of disability relative to his much more successful brothers, he completed a vocational rehabilitation training program, works full-time at a manual labor job, and lives in his own apartment. Supportive therapy sessions have decreased gradually from weekly to monthly, with the option of scheduling extra sessions when needed. In those sessions, he continues to seek advice about practical problems—such as dating, dealing with a boss that he does not like, and techniques for feeling relaxed with others—and about such psychological issues as his shame about his illness, his ambivalence about his parents' attempts to continue to support him, and his confusion about how to integrate his intense emotional experiences of alienation in high school with the concept of having a brain disorder, schizophrenia.

Patients highly rate supportive counseling. A survey of patients performed in Maryland in the mid-1990s sampled their opinions about what they sought and valued in their interactions with psychotherapists. The group of 212 persons was drawn from persons who attended psychosocial rehabilitation programs, almost all of whom were receiving individual psychotherapy. Among the major diagnostic groups, the largest number of persons in the sample, nearly 40 percent, had a diagnosis of schizophrenia. The vast majority of respondents noted that psychotherapy had brought positive changes to their lives. In terms of the type of psychotherapy, 81 percent of the respondents with schizophrenia expressed preference for brief, less frequent sessions of reality-oriented therapy as opposed to longer, more frequent sessions of insight-oriented therapy. Across the whole sample, the qualities in a therapist that were the most highly rated were friendliness and someone who was an expert on the patient's type of illness. Therapeutic issues that were considered to be the most important included independence, the development of self-esteem, the achievement of hope, and employment.

Cognitive Behaviorally Oriented Psychotherapy

Cognitive behavioral strategies, which have been established as efficacious for the treatment of anxiety and depression, have been extended to the treatment of schizophrenia and other psychotic disorders. Most of the research in this area has been carried out in the last 10 to 15 years. Although cognitive behavioral therapies are often presented as a distinct school of psychotherapy, it is important to point out that they share elements with other therapeutic approaches and have borrowed from these other approaches. Like the supportive therapies, the cognitive behaviorally oriented therapies place a high premium on the rapport between patient and therapist. Like the psychodynamic approaches, some forms of cognitive behaviorally oriented psychotherapy may foster the patient's search for psychological meaning to the illness. Cognitive behaviorally oriented psychotherapy may also emphasize a presumed continuity between so-called normal and psychotic experience in an effort to understand and to normalize the patient's experience.

The cognitive behaviorally oriented psychotherapies for schizophrenia have emerged largely from the United Kingdom. The psychotherapies draw on the tenets of cognitive therapy originally developed in the United States for the treatment of anxiety and depression. Within a cognitive behavioral model, a person's behavior and actions are determined by the person's thoughts and attributions. Emotional distress is assumed to be associated with faulty thinking, which, if modified, can alter emotional responses.

Proponents of cognitive behaviorally oriented psychotherapy for schizophrenia acknowledge the biological basis of the disorder and actively promote medication adherence. This psychotherapy also targets psychotic symptoms. To accomplish this goal, the psychotherapist does not directly confront the patient's psychotic symptoms. Instead, the therapist strives to develop a *collaborative empiricism* with the patient; the patient and therapist together rationally examine the patient's beliefs and symptoms.

Cognitive behaviorally oriented psychotherapy for schizophrenia generally starts with several sessions assessing the patient's specific symptoms and the distress associated with the symptoms. Coping strategies that the patient has used may also be reviewed. The patient's preferences about topics of concern in part determine the focus of the subsequent sessions. Specific therapeutic strategies are then applied to address the specific problems that have been identified. The therapy aims to address issues systematically over a fixed number of sessions. Homework exercises may be suggested, and the material from these experiences may be used as material for discussion. To illustrate cognitive behaviorally oriented psychotherapy, one such approach is described in more detail, along with studies that have assessed its efficacy.

Normalizing cognitive behavioral therapy, which was developed by psychiatrists in the United Kingdom, follows distinct stages that are described in a treatment manual and illustrated in Figure 12.11–1. In the engagement phase, the patient and therapist examine the antecedents of the patient's psychotic illness and develop a shared formulation that emphasizes the psychological processes that may be operative. The formulation places a premium on explanations that help normalize the patient's symptoms. Throughout this and other phases, the need for medication compliance is emphasized.

Next in the sequence, the therapist focuses on any coexisting anxiety and depression, using established cognitive behavioral techniques. Then, the therapist turns to specific positive psychotic symptoms that the patient experiences. Strategies to deal with hallucinations include an analysis of the patient's beliefs about the origins and nature of the voices. Useful tools to address hallucinations include the patient's completing voice diaries, reattributing the causes of the voices, and generating coping strategies, such as focusing or distraction. If the patient experiences delusions, these are addressed with successive questions that are used to find the underlying beliefs. The therapist addresses thought disorder by repeatedly asking the patient to fill in the gaps in the stream of conversation and to clarify neologisms. Negative symptoms may also be addressed, but only after work has been completed on positive symptoms.

In a clinical trial of this cognitive behaviorally oriented approach, patients who were referred by clinicians were randomly assigned to receive the cognitive behaviorally oriented therapy or *befriending*, a supportive therapy interaction. Therapy was delivered over a 9-month period, and patients received an average of 19 individual sessions from psychologists and psychiatrists experienced in this method. Results of the study indicate that befriending and cognitive behavioral interventions resulted in significant reductions in positive and negative symptoms. However, those patients in the cognitive behaviorally oriented psychotherapy group continued to improve at the time of a 9-month follow-up after the therapy had ended.

In a further study of this approach, a larger group of patients was assigned to cognitive behaviorally oriented therapy or treatment as usual. Specially trained community nurses provided the cognitive behaviorally oriented psychotherapy. The therapy also included illness education that was delivered in educational booklets that were developed especially for the study. Results of the study indicate that patients in the cognitive behaviorally oriented psychotherapy showed an improvement in overall symptomatology, insight, and depression compared to the control group. The patients who received the cognitive behaviorally oriented psychotherapy rated the intervention as "very helpful."

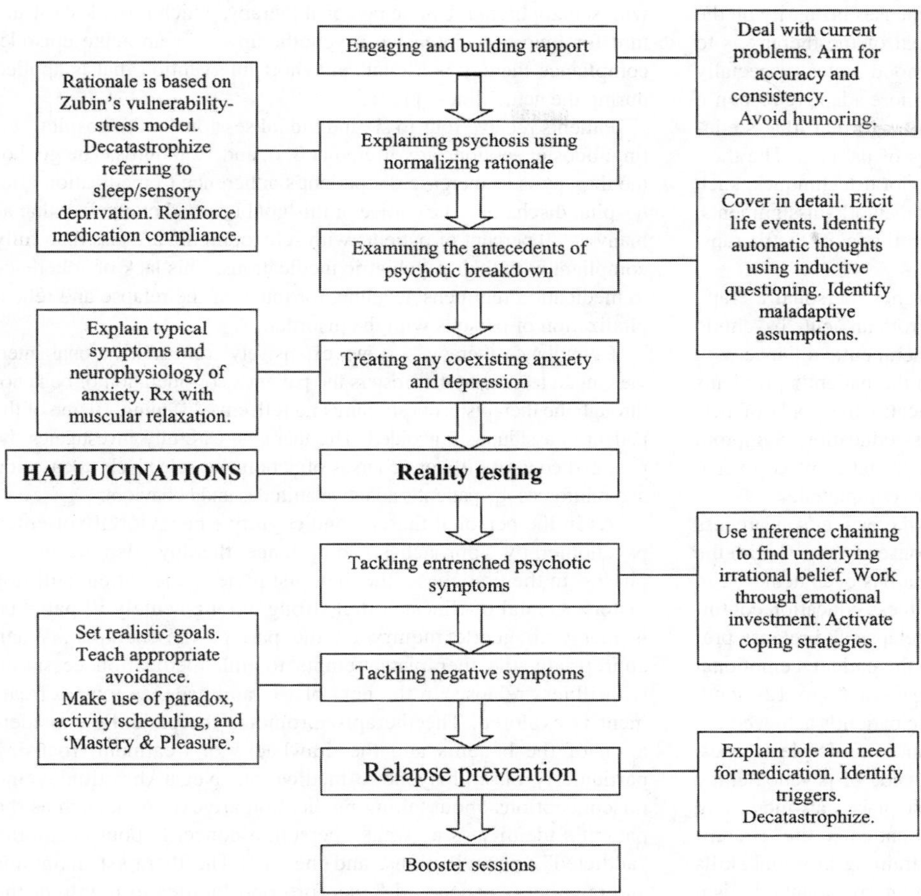

FIGURE 12.11–1 All patients have followed a flexible course of cognitive therapy with sessions of variable length. Most have progressed through these stages. Rx, treatment. (From Kingdon DG, Turkington D. *Cognitive-Behavioral Therapy of Schizophrenia.* New York: Guilford Press; 1994, with permission.)

Although the cognitive behaviorally oriented psychotherapies hold promise for the treatment of schizophrenia, limitations in these approaches and in the understanding of their active ingredients need to be emphasized. First of all, as in any psychotherapy intervention for patients with schizophrenia, some patients with the disorder may be unwilling to participate. Selectivity of patients is a major issue in the evaluation of studies of this kind. In the original study of normalizing therapy described previously, all participants had had distress about their symptoms and were specifically referred for the intervention. In the follow-up study provided by the community nurses, the patient inclusion criteria were broader.

Cognitive deficits, prevalent among patients with schizophrenia, may make it difficult for patients to engage in an approach that requires at least some conceptual abilities. Poor insight or denial of illness symptoms also make engagement in cognitive behaviorally oriented therapy difficult. Although illness insight is often a goal of the therapy, some acknowledgment of the presence of a disorder may be an important starting point. In fact, some trials of cognitive behaviorally oriented psychotherapy, including the study cited previously, may require the patient to have some distress about symptoms to participate effectively.

In addition to questions about the selectivity of patients, another question about the cognitive behaviorally oriented psychotherapy for schizophrenia concerns the extent of the treatment gains. Although reductions in illness symptoms and in the distress about these symptoms are major accomplishments, studies have not been consistent in showing a transfer of these gains to the patient's social and role functioning. An additional issue concerns the interaction between cognitive behaviorally oriented psychotherapy and other concomitant treatments. It is unclear how cognitive behaviorally oriented therapy may enhance or may duplicate other psychosocial interventions. In addition, most of the studies that have been performed have not carefully controlled psychiatric medications, nor has there been careful study of how these approaches may fare among patients treated with newer antipsychotic medications.

Implementation and dissemination of cognitive behaviorally oriented therapy pose significant challenges. Most studies of cognitive behaviorally oriented psychotherapy for schizophrenia have taken place in the United Kingdom, so the applicability to American patients and to the American health care system remains to be established. In addition, the requirement of specialty training to deliver the therapy makes implementation of the therapy difficult.

Other Individual Psychotherapy Approaches

Given the pervasive problems of persons with schizophrenia, it is not surprising that other broad-based models of psychotherapy have been developed for persons with this disorder. Again, it is important to note that these psychotherapeutic approaches may overlap with each other in terms of their treatment elements and specific psychotherapeutic strategies. Three other psychotherapy models are described in the following sections to illustrate the innovative and specialized therapies that have been developed and studied for persons with this disorder.

Personal Therapy

Developed by clinician researchers at the Western Psychiatric Institute and Clinic in Pittsburgh, Pennsylvania, personal therapy is a disorder-specific and intense psychotherapy for individuals with schizophrenia. The therapy focuses primarily on the patient's affective dysregulation. A major goal of the therapy is to develop an understanding of the patient's mood states, especially negative affects, and to promote the patient's more adaptive response to emotional stresses. Personal therapy includes formal illness educational workshops delivered to small groups of patients. The therapy also incorporates more traditional, behavioral techniques, such as modeling, practice, feedback, and homework assignments. Behavioral exercises, consistent with the overall goal of the therapy, are focused on the awareness of self and others.

Unlike some other psychotherapy approaches, personal therapy is staged to the patient's degree of recovery from an acute psychotic episode. The first phase aims to establish a therapeutic alliance with an emphasis on the therapist's empathy with the patient's problems and symptoms. A therapeutic contract explicates the goals of personal therapy. This phase also includes illness education. Symptom stabilization is the goal. This treatment usually takes place over 6 months or until the objectives of this phase are completed.

In the next phase, the therapist focuses on the patient's awareness of interpersonal stressors and individual responses to stress, with the goal of maintaining the symptom stability that has been achieved in addition to making psychological progress. Illness education continues. The therapist provides education about relapse and relapse prevention and helps the patient identify cues to the patient's emotional distress. This phase of therapy typically spans a 6- to 12-month period. The third phase of therapy includes the patient's achievement of consistent social perceptions and performance in role-play scenes. These skills are then applied in situations outside of psychotherapy sessions. In this therapy phase, the therapist places an increasing emphasis on the relationship between the patient's life circumstances and internal mood states. Advanced training in social skills may be undertaken in such areas as managing interpersonal criticism and conflict. Attention also focuses on the demands that the patient experiences in work and relationships.

This ambitious therapy approach was tested in a trial in which personal therapy was compared to family therapy and to supportive psychotherapy. The therapy was delivered to patients who were recently discharged from the hospital and was provided over a 3-year period. Despite careful attention to the development of this specialized therapy, results of the study did not show any significant difference in relapse rates among the treatment groups; the overall relapse rate was 29 percent, which is considered low by some standards. Patients receiving personal therapy did have more improvements in psychosocial functioning over the course of the study than did patients in the other treatment conditions. Furthermore, the mean score for personal therapy patients changed on the 100-point Global Assessment Scale from 47 to 64 over the 3-year treatment period. This improvement underscores the importance of attempting to replicate this study in another treatment setting.

In evaluating the effect of personal therapy for those living with family members versus those living independently, results suggest that personal therapy lowered the rate of relapse among the former group but was associated with an increased rate of relapse among the latter group. The reasons for this differential effect are unclear and await further study. However, this finding raises interesting questions regarding how social and environmental circumstances of patients may determine intervention outcomes and how various forms of psychosocial interventions may be synergistic.

Compliance Therapy Compliance therapy differs from the personal therapy described previously and highlights the range of specialized interventions that have been developed for individuals with schizophrenia. Unlike personal therapy, which provides a structure for long-term intensive psychotherapy after an acute episode, compliance therapy is a relatively short intervention that is applied during the acute illness phase.

Patients receive four to six individual sessions in the hospital setting; booster sessions are offered at 3, 6, and 12 months. The goal of the therapy is to increase the patient's adherence to medication after hospital discharge. The choice of this goal is based on the fact that as many as 80 percent of patients with schizophrenia are less than fully compliant with their psychiatric medications. This lack of adherence to medication regimens accounts for much of the relapse and rehospitalization of persons with the disorder.

Compliance therapy borrows extensively from motivational interviewing, a technique that fosters the patient's consideration of behavior through the therapist's questioning and reflective listening. Blame of the patient is assiduously avoided. The therapist carefully investigates the pros and cons of different courses of action and selectively focuses on and reinforces the patient's adaptive attitudes and behaviors.

As in the personal therapy and cognitive behaviorally oriented psychotherapy approaches, compliance therapy also occurs in phases. In the first phase, the therapist reviews the patient's illness history. Denial of illness, often strong among acutely ill patients, is met with gentle inquiry on the part of the therapist. When appropriate, the therapist attempts to link medication cessation with illness relapse. In the next phase, ambivalence toward treatment is explored. The therapist promotes the patient's consideration of the benefits and the drawbacks of treatment, focusing particularly on antipsychotic medication. Negative attitudes and misconceptions about taking medication are explored, such as the patient's identity as a "weak" person, a concern about becoming "addicted" to medications, and the like. The therapist maintains an empathetic stance and looks for opportunities to highlight the benefits of medication adherence. A sample dialogue, reprinted from Roisin Kemp's and colleagues' "Compliance Therapy: An Intervention Targeting Insight and Treatment Adherence in Psychotic Patients," between a therapist and patient in the middle phase of a compliance therapy intervention is as follows (from phase 2: exploring ambivalence to treatment):

> The patient, James, has a delusion that he was Christ and therefore did not need medication. He was intelligent, good rapport had been established, and he had shown himself to be receptive to discussion of alternative arguments. He confirms his belief by regularly using a grid of words, asking certain questions, and observing flashes of light fall on individual words, which he interpreted as communication from God.
>
> James: "I see a flash . . . then I know I'm Christ. So that means I'm not ill and don't need medication. Sometimes I can see that it's not true. . . . But what would cause it if not heavenly forces?"
>
> Therapist: "Let's consider for a minute that there could be another explanation. You've set up this grid and you're in an expectant mood. I could well imagine that you might be very focused on certain words."
>
> James: "Well, that wouldn't cause the flashes, would it?"
>
> Therapist: "I think sometimes if one is concentrating hard, images can seem to shimmer a bit. I was wondering too if you always see these flashes when you use your grid or just sometimes."
>
> James: "Not always. I think maybe the communication doesn't always work."
>
> Therapist: "Or, looking at it another way, could these instances be chance events, or the result of your own expectations?"

This kind of logical disputation can expose defective reasoning and possibly leads to a drop in self-esteem. Therefore, one needs to point out that all people are prone to errors such as jumping to conclusions (arbitrary inference), getting things out of context (selective abstraction), and taking things personally (personalization). People are prone to do this especially when they are under stress or are hypervigilant, that is, in a watchful mood.

James went on to reveal the consequences of forsaking his delusion:

> James: "I can see what you're saying. If I tell myself it is just images or my own mind . . . it makes me a bit sad to think that . . . I've been taken over with it for a year and a half."
>
> Therapist: "You've been caught up with thinking about it for some time. . . . That's pretty heavy stuff. I can image it could be a burden at times."
>
> James: "Yes, it's baffling. It tires me out mentally."
>
> Therapist: "So, can you think of any advantages in being less preoccupied with it, would you have more energy for the things you enjoy?"

During the third phase, the therapy focuses on medication as a strategy to enhance the patient's quality of life. An effort is made to destigmatize the use of medication by underscoring the high prevalence of mental disease for which medications are advised. The routine use of medications for many common nonpsychiatric medical disorders is also emphasized. Psychiatric medications are presented as a kind of insurance policy to staying well. Medication adherence is linked with the patient's personal goals, such as maintaining a job or a personal relationship.

Compliance therapy was studied in a clinical trial with acutely ill hospital patients with schizophrenia in the United Kingdom. Compared to a nonspecific counseling approach matched for one-to-one therapy time, compliance therapy was more effective in terms of patients' illness insight, attitudes about medication, medication compliance, and global functioning. Gains persisted during an 18-month follow-up period in the two-thirds of patients who were available at follow-up.

Psychotherapy for First-Episode Psychosis In addition to interventions focused on persistently ill patients, some researchers and practitioners are placing heightened emphasis on specialized interventions for patients experiencing their first episode of psychotic symptoms. These interventions are driven by advances in treatment and by concerns that many patients do not enter treatment until well after the onset of symptoms and disability. A leading example is an intervention developed by a team of clinicians in Australia that is called *cognitively oriented psychotherapy for early psychosis* (COPE).

The following observations provide the underpinning for this intervention. The illness course during the 2 to 5 years after the first psychotic episode is highly predictive of the long-term course of the disorder and the person's long-term degree of disability. Although more than 80 percent of persons achieve remission from a first acute psychotic episode, close to 50 percent relapse by 2 years after the index hospital discharge. If an intervention can be provided to improve the person's adjustment to the illness and to enhance recuperation from the first episode, the future course of the disorder may be improved. The goal is to reduce the number and severity of further illness episodes.

In the COPE intervention, psychotherapy is provided individually over a 1-year period to persons who have had a first episode of psychosis, many of whom go on to have a diagnosis of schizophrenia. In most instances, the COPE therapy is initiated after the acute psychotic symptoms have subsided. There are four foci to the intervention, not addressed in a fixed order or exclusively at any point during the therapy: assessment, engagement, adaptation, and secondary morbidity. Assessment is focused on identifying the major psychological issues, for example, the person's attribution of illness symptoms and the effect of the illness on the person's self-image. As in many of the other approaches discussed so far, the COPE therapist develops an agenda collaboratively with the patient during this phase. The next major focus of the treatment includes illness education, as well as a focus on social withdrawal, issues related to stigma, and problems of motivation. Secondary symptoms, such as anxiety and depression, also are addressed. Unlike the cognitive behavioral strategies discussed in an earlier section, the target symptoms in COPE are not positive symptoms. Positive symptoms have typically responded to psychopharmacology in first episode patients. Instead, the intervention focuses on the person's response to the disorder and on the reduction of further illness morbidity.

Results from a pilot study of the COPE approach show that patients receiving the COPE intervention had better outcomes than did a group of patients who did not have access to case management and other specialized treatment services after the index hospitalization. Patients receiving the COPE intervention showed only a slight advantage over those who also received case management and other services but who refused the specific COPE psychotherapy. At the 1-year follow-up, there was not a significant difference among the three groups in terms of rates of relapse and hospital readmission. Specialized psychotherapy for first-episode patients may be a helpful intervention, but an understanding of the benefits of a psychotherapeutic intervention for this group of patients awaits future study.

GROUP PSYCHOTHERAPY

Group psychotherapies for schizophrenia encompass several approaches: groups that are relatively unstructured and are focused on supportive interpersonal interactions within the group; groups that are primarily didactic and focused on illness education and medication adherence; and groups that deliver a cognitive behaviorally oriented intervention for symptom management. All of these interventions are variations of interventions that may be delivered in an individual format.

Also within the realm of group interventions for schizophrenia are groups that focus on rehabilitation goals, such as skills training.

Supportive Group Therapy Systematic investigation of supportive group therapy for schizophrenia has been limited. The completed studies of the last several decades have been mostly in outpatient settings. In this approach, patients are encouraged to discuss their problems and feelings in a therapy atmosphere that fosters sharing, group cohesion, and a sense of belonging and mutual support. The therapist uses open-ended questions along with empathy, warmth, and reflection to facilitate the group process. Patients are encouraged to set personal goals and to enlist the help of other group members in discussing the difficulties and strategies for obtaining these goals. Although the pursuit of personal objectives is promoted, the therapy does not provide structured training or formal homework assignments. Therapy typically occurs over an extended period of months.

Many patients with schizophrenia have deficits in social functioning and smaller social networks than do persons without major mental illness. Therefore, a group approach that promotes socialization would seem to be clinically relevant and beneficial for persons with schizophrenia, beyond therapy delivered individually. However, the few studies of supportive group therapy with this population typically have used interventions that are not clearly formulated. Studies also have not included a comparison treatment condition, adding to the difficulty of drawing conclusions. Other studies that have directly compared supportive group therapy and specific skills training groups have tended to favor the more direct and focused approaches.

Group Illness Education Education about schizophrenia and its treatment may be delivered to patients in a group format, as well as individually. Although there have been no systematic comparisons between group and individual formats, it is possible that the small group setting might have advantages in fostering patients' learning through participation with other patients in the give and take of the therapy process. Providing therapy in a group may also be more efficient for clinical settings that treat large numbers of patients with schizophrenia.

Despite the wide appeal of illness education for schizophrenia and its implementation in many clinical settings, the approach has not been widely standardized or studied. Illness education groups differ in their content and focus. Most groups aim primarily to provide information about schizophrenia, including the types of illness symptoms, the relapse signs, the stress vulnerability model of the disorder, medications, and other treatments. Other topics may include medication side effects, stressors and coping strategies, community resources, and comorbid conditions such as substance abuse. Although many of these issues may be addressed to some extent by a psychiatrist or psychotherapist providing treatment to an individual patient, the illness education format is likely to cover these topics more extensively and systematically.

On the whole, research indicates that group interventions for illness and medication education improve knowledge about the specific topics that are taught but do not substantially influence other outcomes, such as social functioning or relapse prevention. Programs that include behavioral components related to medications are more likely to affect patients' actual medication adherence.

Group Cognitive Behaviorally Oriented Psychotherapy A final group approach to be considered here is one that offers cognitive behaviorally oriented psychotherapy for positive psychotic symptoms. The particular intervention presented focuses on auditory hallucinations. However, it is conceivable that additional specialized therapy approaches, focused on other target psychotic symptoms, could also be developed.

The group hallucination-focused intervention comes from the United Kingdom, as do most of the other cognitive behaviorally oriented psychotherapies for schizophrenia. Patients selected for the group have hallucinations that are distressing and that have persisted despite medication treatment. A total of six weekly group sessions and one follow-up session is offered. Each session is focused on a particular topic and follows a semistructured format. Group topics include sharing of personal experiences about voices, models of hallucinations, and effective coping strategies for voices. In a pilot study of this approach, patients in the group experienced greater improvements in the perceived power and distress associated with the voices than did patients who did not receive the intervention. They also reported an increased number and effectiveness of coping strategies. The developers of this approach promote it as a less costly format than individual cognitive behaviorally oriented psychotherapy. The group approach may have additional benefits over an individually delivered therapy, but this question awaits further study.

FAMILY INTERVENTIONS

Family interventions for schizophrenia were first developed in the 1950s and 1960s, an era dominated by psychodynamic approaches. In the family therapy of this era, it was assumed that problems in the patient's early upbringing or in the quality of the relationships in the patient's family caused schizophrenia. Concepts that were used to describe the presumed family pathology included *double-bind interactions*, *marital schism and skew*, *communication deviance*, and *family scapegoats*. Families often were implicitly or even explicitly held accountable for the illness of their family member. Within this context, family therapy attempted to correct the presumed dysfunctions in family dynamics that were understood as contributing to the patient's illness.

The idea that family interactions play a significant role in the etiology of schizophrenia has now been discredited. Careful studies have shown that families with schizophrenia on the whole do not differ significantly from other families. In addition, family therapy interventions based on family pathology models generally did not alter the course of the illness. Unfortunately, the blaming of families went a long way to alienate family members from mental health professionals. The pathologizing of families also impeded collaboration between families and professional treaters, both of whom are often actively involved in the patient's care.

As interest in family therapy for schizophrenia declined, another model of family interaction emerged that seemed to explain the variable rates of relapse among individuals with schizophrenia. Known as *expressed emotion*, this concept was based on an observed association between specific characteristics of family–patient interactions, such as criticality and patient relapse after the initial onset of the illness. It is important to note that the label of *expressed emotion* does not well characterize the full range of observations embedded in the rating of *expressed emotion*, which subsumes such components as hostility, criticism, and emotional overinvolvement. Nonetheless, the association has been replicated by a number of clinical investigators. In this model, family attitudes are not viewed as etiologically related to the development of schizophrenia but are seen as contributing to the recurrence of psychotic episodes. It followed that interventions with families that reduce the level of *expressed emotion* might reduce the risk of relapse.

The level of families' expressed emotion is assessed by a semistructured interview that was developed in the United Kingdom, the Camberwell Family Interview. In this interview, family members are asked about their experiences surrounding the patient's admission to the hospital, with an emphasis on questions about arguments or irritability within the family. The responses of family members are rated on a number of variables, three of which make up the expressed emotion construct: criticism, hostility, and emotional overinvolvement. The Camberwell Family Interview was updated in the 1970s to include two other important variables. The amount of face-to-face contact between the patient and family members was computed, and 35 hours per week was considered to be *high contact*. Also included as an important variable was whether the patient took antipsychotic medication.

A number of clinical trials have been performed to evaluate the effectiveness of family interventions. These interventions were based on the idea that increasing the supportive interactions within the family setting may prevent, or at least reduce, the risk of relapse. These studies were initially performed in the United Kingdom and have also been carried out in the United States. In some of these studies, only patients living in families with high expressed emotion were included. In other studies, patients from families with high or low expressed emotion were included, and the outcomes of the two groups were compared. Results of these studies overall suggest that family interventions reduce the rate of relapse among patients. However, the usefulness of the expressed emotion concept in the implementation and success of family interventions is uncertain.

The reasons for this uncertainty include the fact that a clear association has not been found between the effectiveness of family interventions and reductions in families' levels of expressed emotion. Also, the cause-and-effect relationship implied by the expressed emotion model—that family attitudes trigger relapse—has not been established. It is uncertain whether emotionally charged elements in a family environment contribute to relapse or whether clinical characteristics of patients that are associated with relapse may elicit negative family responses. In addition, the idea of expressed emotion may have been overextended. In an effort to explain relapse, expressed emotion was linked to deficits in arousal and in processing complex emotions on the part of individuals with schizophrenia. Generalizing from ratings obtained from a verbal interview to the pathophysiology of schizophrenia is a big step. Also, the role of culture was overlooked, as family expectations in non–Anglo Saxon cultures were found to differ. Finally, although not attributing the onset of schizophrenia to families, the expressed emotion construct does suggest that families may be toxic and implicates family members in their relatives' relapse. As such, the expressed emotion concept has been perceived by many as another form of blaming families, although clearly the originators of this concept did not intend for this to happen. Overall, there is no doubt that the initial observation of the link between expressed emotion and relapse provides important clues regarding how to optimize the environment of persons with schizophrenia, but more research, conducted within a context that is sensitive to the concerns and perceptions of family members, is necessary.

Several types of programs have been developed and studied for the family members of persons with schizophrenia. Starting in the 1970s, clinical investigators in Britain, based on initial findings about the relationship between expressed emotion and relapse, developed a program of family treatment for individual families. An assessment of each family in their own home identified interpersonal conflicts that became the focus of resolution efforts. Also included in the intervention was a relatives' group, not including patients, that provided a forum for mutual sharing and support. An additional education component presented information about schizophrenia and its treatment. This family program was compared with routine care over a 9-month period. Results indicated significantly lower relapse rates among patients in the family intervention group.

Specific family interventions have also been developed and carried out in the United States. In one of the first such programs, investigators at University of California Los Angeles in the 1970s developed a short-term family crisis intervention for patients and their families. The intervention was provided immediately after the patient's hospital discharge. The family intervention group received six sessions delivered to individual families that were focused on family problems and coping strategies. Two different doses of antipsychotic medication, standard doses as opposed to lower doses, were also compared. Over a 6-month period, patients receiving the family intervention and the standard dose of medication experienced the lowest relapse rate.

Another group of clinical researchers in Los Angeles in the 1980s developed a more extensive family intervention program. In this program, in-home sessions with the patient and family members provided information about schizophrenia and also training in problem-solving skills. After the first 9 months of individual family sessions, multifamily group sessions were held. Patients, all from families evaluated to have high expressed emotion, were randomized to receive the family treatment or individual patient management only. Results at 9-month and 2-year follow-ups strongly favored the family intervention group in terms of reduced relapse rates and symptom severity. In this study, the behavioral family management model placed a high premium on teaching specific coping and problem-solving skills to families.

A separate group of investigators in Pittsburgh developed a more complex and multifaceted psychosocial intervention that included a family treatment component. The family intervention focused sequentially on developing an alliance with the family, providing information and suggestions about managing the illness and delivering an intensive workshop with other families. Skills learned during the workshop were then applied in individual family therapy sessions that included the patient. A study of this family intervention compared patients receiving only the family intervention to a second group receiving the family intervention and social skills training, to a third group receiving only social skills training, and to a fourth group in a control condition; all patients received regular medication. Results indicated that persons who received the family intervention in combination with the skills training had the lowest rate of relapse; persons receiving the family intervention alone and the skills training alone had the next lowest relapse rate, and the control group had the highest rate.

More recent studies of family intervention for patients with schizophrenia have been performed in other countries and cultural groups. For example, a large-scale study with more than 3,000 patients in China in the early 1990s assigned patients individually to a group family psychoeducation condition or to routine services provided by a primary care clinic. The family psychoeducation consisted of ten standardized lectures and then discussion sessions provided by a psychiatrist over a 1-year period. The patients in the family intervention condition had significantly better rates of relapse, symptom severity, ability to work, and treatment compliance.

Family interventions that have proven to be effective in reducing relapse rates and, in some cases, improving other patient and family outcomes vary in terms of their specific format, content, and duration. However, common elements from these programs can be identified. In all of these programs, schizophrenia is presented as an illness that is biologically based and that requires medication treatment. The interventions also present information about specific symptoms, illness course, signs of relapse, and specific treatments. In effective programs, the family intervention is part of an overall treatment package that provides active pharmacotherapy and other standard treatments. The most successful programs also last at least 9 months.

In contrast, family interventions that produce good outcomes do *not* include a focus on family communication or interpersonal family relationships as related to the *etiology* of schizophrenia. They also do not include a retrospective review of family history and family conflicts. Instead, the focus is on the here and now, on current symptoms and stresses, and on ways to cope with and solve problems that are related to the patient's illness.

Another set of elements common to these effective family interventions concerns the role of families in the treatment. The interventions stress the competence of families, not their pathology. The interventions aim to enable families to deal with symptoms and crises that are presented by the schizophrenia illness of their relative.

The relationship between family members and mental health professionals is ideally a collaborative one. Although family interventions have been mostly focused on patient outcomes, such as reduced relapse rates, family interventions may also target variables that are assessed on the part of family members, such as family burden and family distress. Evidence now suggests that family psychoeducational interventions reduce family burden.

Although a positive, forward-looking approach is the most helpful to families in dealing with a family member with schizophrenia, it is also important to acknowledge the negative emotions that families may feel. Multiple-family groups allow for sharing and mutual support among persons from different families.

Many family members experience guilt about their relative's schizophrenia and voice a concern about whether the illness was caused by poor parenting or some other deficit in the family member's upbringing. Although family blaming has largely disappeared from the explanation of schizophrenia that is provided to families by health professionals, the attitude lingers among some providers. Older family members may also approach current treatment with strong memories and resentments of treatment received in the 1960s and 1970s, when family-blaming views were widely promulgated. Family members also commonly experience anger, not only about the unfairness of the relative's persistent and disabling illness, but about a health care system that may often fall short of meeting their relative's needs. For some family members, these concerns may be channeled into advocacy activities that serve to promote more public awareness about mental illness and the deficiencies of the service delivery system.

Demoralization and depression also are common themes among families. There may be chronic grief about the lost potential and restricted life of the relative with schizophrenia. For many families, helping to care for the ill relative creates objective burdens in their day-to-day lives. Such burdens may take the form of draining family finances to supplement the relative's income and to pay for treatment costs, as well as the time and energy necessary to provide direct personal support. Subjective burdens experienced by families include guilt, anger, and depression. Family members also may worry about the welfare and safety of their relative with schizophrenia. Fears about suicide and violence are not uncommon. Often, there are concerns among aging family members about the provision of care for their relative after they, the family members, are no longer available to provide it. Advocacy and support organizations may offer families information about how to constructively plan for this eventuality.

Taken as a group, carefully performed clinical studies support the efficacy of family education and other services to families in meeting the psychological needs of families and in reducing the likelihood of relapse on the part of the ill relative. Results of selected studies underscore the effectiveness of this approach. However, there are several questions that have yet to be resolved.

First, what are the necessary or optimal ingredients of an effective family intervention? Providing information about schizophrenia and practical advice, promoting the development of coping strategies, and fostering emotional support are the basic core elements, but what about more intense behavioral skills and communication training delivered to individual families?

Results are informative from a large clinical trial in the 1990s, the Treatment Strategies in Schizophrenia Study. Performed at five sites, this study compared various combinations of medication strategies and specified family treatment methods. All families received basic psychoeducation and monthly support groups. Families in an applied family management program received, in addition, individualized illness education conducted in the family home and training focused on communication and problem-solving skills. More than 300 acutely ill patients with schizophrenia were randomized to one of the two family and three medication conditions. At the end of the 2-year follow-up period, results revealed no significant difference between the family conditions in the rate of patient relapse or rehospitalization. It is important to note that patients in both family conditions received basic family services; only 25 percent of patients in both family conditions who received the optimal medication strategy were rehospitalized, a rate that is lower than those found in other studies that have included a no family intervention condition. This study does not support the superiority of an intensive family intervention that involves home visits and specific training in communication and problem-solving skills.

Second, what are the most appropriate formats for family sessions? Some interventions involve work with individual families, some provide multiple-family groups, and some combine the two formats. Studies performed in New York comparing multiple-family formats with individual family formats have shown some relative benefit of the multiple-family group; however, this issue is open to further study. The one study site that was in the largely black community of Harlem, New York City, did not show superiority of the multiple-family format over the single-family format.

Multiple-family group interventions have been studied in other settings as well, including at a capitated community mental health center in the state of Washington. The intervention involves small group multifamily meetings. Three initial sessions are held with the patients present and focus on information about schizophrenia. The following sessions, which take place over 12 months, include family members and patients together and are focused on problem-solving and coping skills to address individual goals. In a study of this intervention, patients enrolled in the study all had regular contact with their families and were randomly assigned to the family intervention or to standard care that included case management. Results of the study indicate that patients in the family intervention experienced significantly reduced negative symptoms compared to those receiving standard care.

Third, which families should receive which family interventions? As previously discussed, the early family education interventions based on the expressed emotion concept were generally targeted for families with high expressed emotion. This selection criterion tends not to be used in more recent studies. Most of the clinical trials of family interventions also recruited patients while they were in the acute hospital setting. In the current era, use of hospitalization has been reduced, and more care is provided in outpatient settings. Newer studies have sometimes recruited patients who are receiving community-based services, as in the study described from Washington state.

Fourth, what is the appropriate timing of the intervention? Several studies performed in the 1990s, all from outside of the United States, provided family interventions early in the course of schizophrenia. In a series of studies performed in the Netherlands, the addition of an intensive behavioral family management program to individual outpatient therapy did not improve relapse rates among recent-onset schizophrenia patients. The limited benefits of the specialized intervention may have been due, in part, to the fact that the comparison condition did provide some family education. The study's authors raised questions about the appropriateness of the intensive family intervention for families of new-onset patients, who may believe that the illness may not recur. The authors also noted that the intervention might add to family stress, specifically if communication skills are taught to families who already possess these skills.

Dissemination and Future Directions Despite the fact that family interventions have been established as effective for families of patients with schizophrenia, they are often not available in treatment settings. A study by the Schizophrenia Patient Outcomes Research Team (PORT) found that, in the mid-1990s, only 31 percent of a sample of persons with schizophrenia who had regular family contact reported that their family received information about schizophrenia. In general, the education provided to family members tends to be from informal contact with clinicians rather than from a specific or formalized program.

The limited dissemination of family interventions for schizophrenia is likely due to several factors. Mental health professionals and administrators may underestimate the value of these services. Clinicians are rarely trained in providing family psychoeducation and are often overextended with other activities and services that have a higher priority than family work.

Other factors at the level of the clinical setting may also discourage the practice of family intervention. Concern about patient confidentiality can become an obstacle in clinicians' willingness to discuss patients with family members, although this can be overcome in most cases. Logistical problems, such as scheduling and billing, may be present. There may also be outdated attitudes toward families on the part of clinicians that include a family-blaming model of the etiology of schizophrenia.

Attitudes of patients and families may also contribute to an underuse of family interventions in schizophrenia. Family members may already feel burdened and may be reluctant to commit themselves to regular meetings. They may also feel stigmatized by having a relative with schizophrenia and may be reluctant to share their concerns with others. They may also fear criticism from mental health professionals. Patients may worry about including family members in their treatment, especially if their own alliance with care providers or with family members is fragile.

More extensive dissemination of family interventions may emerge from the demands of family advocates and also from standards of care that accompany evidence-based treatment guidelines. In the meantime, volunteer peer-led family education programs have developed to fill the need for family education. An example of such a program is the Family-to-Family Education Program (FFEP) sponsored by the National Alliance for the Mentally Ill (NAMI), the leading advocacy and support organization in the United States for persons with serious mental illness. FFEP is a mutual assistance family program that is organized and led by trained volunteers from families of persons who have mental illness.

The FFEP is a 12-week program combining education about mental illness with specific support mechanisms to help families understand and cope with their family member with mental illness. Curriculum topics from this program are shown in Table 12.11–1. The program has been implemented in 45 U.S. states with the help of 3,000 volunteer teachers. A preliminary study of the program's effectiveness has been performed with participants in six counties in the state of Maryland. Results indicate that participating family members experienced reduced subjective burden and increased empowerment over the period of the intervention compared to a waiting period, gains that were sustained at a 6-month follow-up. The impact of these benefits on patient outcomes is unknown.

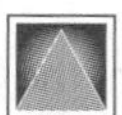

Table 12.11–1
Curriculum in Family Education

Class 1	Introduction: special features of the course; learning about the normative stages of emotional reactions to the trauma of mental illness; belief systems and principles; goals for family member with mental illness; understanding illness symptoms as a double-edged sword.
Class 2	Schizophrenia, major depression, mania, schizoaffective disorder: diagnostic criteria; characteristic features of psychotic illnesses; questions and answers about getting through the critical periods in mental illness; keeping a crisis file.
Class 3	Mood disorders, borderline personality disorder, anxiety disorders, dual diagnosis: Types and subtypes of depression and bipolar disorder; diagnostic criteria for borderline personality disorder, panic disorder and obsessive-compulsive disorder; cooccurring brain and addictive disorders; telling our stories.
Class 4	Basics about the brain: functions of key brain areas; research on functional and structural brain abnormalities in the major mental illnesses; chemical imbalances in the brain; pathophysiology of brain cells and neurogenesis; genetic research; infectious and developmental second hits, which may cause mental illness; the biology of recovery: National Alliance for the Mentally Ill Science and Treatment video.
Class 5	Problem-solving skills workshop: how to define a problem; sharing problem statements; solving the problem; setting limits.
Class 6	Medication review: how medications work; basic psychopharmacology of the mood disorders, anxiety disorders, and schizophrenia; medication side effects; key treatment issues; stages of adherence to medications; early warning signs of relapse.
Class 7	Inside mental illness: understanding the subjective experience of coping with a brain disorder; problems in maintaining self-esteem and positive identity; gaining empathy for the psychological struggle to protect one's integrity in mental illness.
Class 8	Communication skills workshop: how illness interferes with the capacity to communicate; learning to be clear; how to respond when the topic is loaded; talking to the person behind the symptoms of mental illness.
Class 9	Self-care: learning about family burden; sharing in relative groups; handling negative feelings of anger, entrapment, guilt, and grief; how to balance one's life.
Class 10	The vision and potential of recovery: learning about key principles of rehabilitation and model programs of community support; a first-person account of recovery from a consumer guest speaker.
Class 11	Advocacy: challenging the power of stigma in one's life; learning how to change the system; meet and hear from people advocating for change.
Class 12	Review, sharing, and evaluation: certification ceremony; party!

From Burland J. Family-to-Family Education Program of the National Alliance for the Mentally Ill (NAMI). Arlington, VA: NAMI; 2001, with permission.

INTEGRATING PSYCHOSOCIAL AND MEDICATION TREATMENTS

Antipsychotic medication has been established as the single most effective treatment for schizophrenia. However, for many persons, medication is a necessary, but not sufficient, treatment to achieve optimal clinical improvement. As described in this chapter, there are several psychotherapeutic and psychosocial interventions with established efficacy for schizophrenia. These interventions are now recommended for the treatment of schizophrenia and are included in the updated PORT guidelines for schizophrenia. A section of the updated guidelines that pertains to the interventions discussed in this section is presented in Table 12.11–2.

It is important to note that pharmacotherapy was not controlled or studied in most of the research supporting the specific psychosocial treatments. A few studies have investigated different combina-

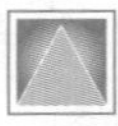

Table 12.11–2
Recommendations for Psychosocial Treatment from the Schizophrenia Patient Outcomes Research Team (PORT): Updated Treatment Recommendations, 2003

For most persons with schizophrenia, the combination of psychopharmacological and psychosocial interventions improves outcomes. A number of psychosocial treatments have demonstrated efficacy. These include family interventions and cognitive behaviorally oriented psychotherapy. In the same way that psychopharmacological management must be individually tailored to the needs and preferences of the patient, so too should the selection of psychosocial treatments. All persons with schizophrenia should be provided with education about their illness and indications for treatments. The key elements of illness education include information about schizophrenia symptoms, medications and other treatments, and strategies for relapse prevention. Medication adherence should be addressed as part of education about medication. Similarly, in the absence of compelling reasons otherwise, families should be provided with education and invited to have ongoing contact with the treatment team.

Recommendation: family intervention

Persons with schizophrenia and their families who have ongoing contact with each other should be offered a family intervention, the key elements of which include a duration of at least 9 mos, illness education, crisis intervention, emotional support, and training on how to cope with illness symptoms and related problems.

Recommendation: cognitive behaviorally oriented psychotherapy

Persons with schizophrenia who have residual psychotic symptoms while receiving adequate pharmacotherapy should be offered adjunctive cognitive behaviorally oriented psychotherapy. The key elements of this intervention include a shared understanding of the illness between the patient and therapist, identification of target symptoms, and the development of specific cognitive and behavioral strategies to cope with these symptoms.

tions of psychosocial treatments and medication-dosing strategies. In most of these studies, the combination of a specialized psychosocial intervention and a standard dose of medication achieved the best results. These studies were all carried out with patients receiving first-generation antipsychotic medications. There is some indication that use of the newer psychopharmacological agents may improve the effectiveness of psychosocial treatments. The reduced side effects of the newer medications may render patients more energetic and available to participate in psychosocial interventions. Little research has been undertaken to date on the combination of second-generation antipsychotic medications and psychosocial interventions; this topic remains an important one for future investigations.

A major problem in understanding the interaction between medication and psychosocial treatments is the fact that many of the specialized psychosocial treatments are not widely practiced by mental health practitioners or available to patients with schizophrenia in usual clinical settings. The reasons for the lack of dissemination of family interventions have been discussed earlier in this chapter. Similar factors may apply to other psychosocial therapies.

In general, psychosocial therapies are time consuming and expensive to deliver. Medication costs are usually paid from sources outside of the mental health system, from general health insurance funds. By contrast, the costs of psychosocial treatment for schizophrenia are typically borne by clinical settings, many of which have limited resources. To the extent that state-of-the-art psychosocial interventions require more time or are perceived to require more time, there may be little incentive to implement them. Generally, they are not marketed by their developers and are not mandated by regulatory agencies nor are they reimbursed at a higher rate than more generic services.

More work is needed to implement the psychosocial interventions that are known to be effective, to promote the development of innovations in psychosocial treatment, and to optimize the interaction of psychosocial and medication treatments. Similar to any chronic illness, the treatment of schizophrenia requires a multimodal approach to obtain the best outcomes.

SUGGESTED CROSS-REFERENCES

For further information related to the assessment of the patient with schizophrenia, see Section 7.1. Section 12.2 is important for a full understanding of the syndrome. For information about rehabilitation approaches, see Section 12.13. An overview of all the psychotherapies is provided in Chapter 30.

References

Buckley PF, Lys C: Psychotherapy and schizophrenia. *J Psychother Pract Res.* 1996;5:185–201.

Coursey RD: Psychotherapy with persons suffering from schizophrenia: The need for a new agenda. *Schizophr Bull.* 1989;15:349–353.

Coursey RD, Keller AB, Farrell EW: Individual psychotherapy and persons with serious mental illness: The clients' perspective. *Schizophr Bull.* 1995;21:283–301.

*Dickerson FB: Cognitive behavioral psychotherapy for schizophrenia: A review of recent empirical studies. *Schizophr Res.* 2000;16:71–90.

*Dixon L, Adams C, Lucksted A: Update on family psychoeducation for schizophrenia. *Schizophr Bull.* 2000;26:5–20.

*Dixon LB, Lehman AF: Family interventions for schizophrenia. *Schizophr Bull.* 1995;21:631–641.

Dixon L, Lyles A, Scott J, Lehman A, Postrado L, Goldman H, McGlynn E: Services to families of adults with schizophrenia: From treatment recommendations to dissemination. *Psychiatr Serv.* 1999;50:233–238.

Durham RC, Guthrie M, Morton RV, Reid DA, Treliving LR, Fowler D, Macdonald RR: Tayside-Fife clinical trial of cognitive-behavioural therapy for medication-resistant psychotic symptoms. *Br J Psychiatry.* 2003;182:303–311.

Falloon IR, Boyd JL, McGill CW, Razani J, Moss HB, Gilderman AM: Family management in the prevention of exacerbations of schizophrenia: A controlled study. *N Engl J Med.* 1982;306:1437–1440.

Fenton WS: Evolving perspective on individual psychotherapy for schizophrenia. *Schizophr Bull.* 2000;26:47–72.

Goldstein J, Rodnick EH, Evans JR, May PR, Steinberg M: Drug and family therapy in the aftercare of acute schizophrenics. *Arch Gen Psychiatry.* 1978;38:1169–1177.

Gumley A, O'Grady M, McNavy L, Reilly J, Power K, Norrie J: Early intervention for relapse in schizophrenia: Results of a 12-month randomized controlled trial of cognitive behavioural therapy. *Psychol Med.* 2003;33:419–431.

Hogarty GE, Greenwald D, Ulrich RL, Kornblith SJ, DiBarry AL, Cooley S, Carter M, Flesher S: Three-year trials of personal therapy among schizophrenic patients living with or independent of family, II: Effects on adjustment of patients. *Am J Psychiatry.* 1997;154:1514–1524.

Hogarty GE, Kornblith SJ, Greenwald D, DiBarry AL, Cooley S, Flesher S, Reiss D, Carter M, Ulrich RL: Personal therapy: A disorder-relevant psychotherapy for schizophrenia. *Schizophr Bull.* 1995;21:379–393.

Hogarty GE, Kornblith SJ, Greenwald D, DiBarry AL, Cooley S, Ulrich RL, Carter M, Flesher S: Personal therapy: Three-year trials of personal therapy among schizophrenic patients living with or independent of family, I: Description of study and effects on relapse rates. *Am J Psychiatry.* 1997;154:1504–1513.

Kemp R, David A, Hayward P: Compliance therapy: An intervention targeting insight and treatment adherence in psychotic patients. *Behav Cogn Psychother.* 1996;24:331–350.

Kemp R, Hayward P, Applewhaite G, Everitt B, David A: Compliance therapy in psychotic patients: Randomized controlled trial. *BMJ.* 1996;312:345–349.

Kemp R, Kirov G, Hayward P, Everitt B, David A: Randomized controlled trial of compliance therapy: 18 Month follow-up. *Br J Psychiatry.* 1998;172:413–419.

*Kingdon DG, Turkington D. *Cognitive-Behavioral Therapy of Schizophrenia.* New York: Guilford Press; 1994.

Lefley HP: Expressed emotion: Conceptual, clinical, and social policy issues. *Hosp Community Psychiatry.* 1992;43:591–598.

Lehman AF, Kreyenbuhl J, Buchanan RW, Dickerson FB, Dixon LB, Goldberg R, Green-Paden LD, Tenhula WN, Boerescu D, Tek C, Sandson N: The Schizophrenia Patients Outcomes Research Team (PORT): Updated treatment recommendations. *Schizophr Bull.* 2003 (*in press*).

Lenroot R, Bustillo JR, Lauriello J, Keith SJ: Integrated treatment of schizophrenia. *Psychiatr Serv.* 2003;54:1499–1507.

Marder SR: Integrating pharmacological and psychosocial treatments for schizophrenia. *Acta Psychiatr Scand.* 2000;102[Suppl 407]:87–90.

Marder SR, Wirshing WC, Mintz J, McKenzie J, Johnston K, Eckman TA, Lebell M, Zimmerman K, Liberman RP: Two-year outcome of social skills training and group psychotherapy for outpatients with schizophrenia. *Am J Psychiatry.* 1996;53:1585–1592.

McFarlane WR, Dixon L, Lukens E, Lucksted A: Family psychoeducation and schizophrenia: A review of the literature. *J Marital Fam Ther.* 2003;29:223–245.

McGlashan TH: The Chestnut Lodge follow-up study. II. Long-term outcome of schizophrenia and the affective disorders. *Arch Gen Psychiatry.* 1984;41:586–601.

Mueser KT, Berenbaum H: Psychodynamic treatment of schizophrenia: Is there a future? *Psychol Med.* 1990;20:253–262.
Mueser KT, Corrigan PW, Hilton DW, Tanzman B, Schaub A, Gingerich S, Essock SM, Tarrier N, Morey B, Vogel-Scibilia S, Herz MI: Illness management and recovery: A review of the research. *Psychiatr Serv.* 2002;53:1272–1284.
Rector NA, Seeman MV, Segal ZV: Cognitive therapy for schizophrenia: A preliminary randomized controlled trial. *Schizophr Res.* 2003;63:1–11.
Schooler NR, Keith SJ, Severe JB, Matthews SM, Bellack AS, Glick I, Hargreaves WA, Kane J, Ninan PT, Allen F, Jacobs M, Lieberman JA, Mance R, Simpson GM, Woerner MG: Relapse and rehospitalization during maintenance treatment of schizophrenia: The effects of dose reduction and family treatment. *Arch Gen Psychiatry.* 1997;54:453–463.
*Scott JE, Dixon LB: Psychological interventions for schizophrenia. *Schizophr Bull.* 1995;21:621–630.
Sensky T, Turkington D, Kingdon D, Scott JL, Scott J, Siddle R, O'Carroll M, Barnes TR: Randomized controlled trial of cognitive-behavioural therapy for persistent symptoms in schizophrenia resistant to medication. *Arch Gen Psychiatry.* 2000;57:165–172.
Turkington D, Kingdon D, Turner T: Effectiveness of a brief cognitive-behavioural therapy intervention in the treatment of schizophrenia. *Br J Psychiatry.* 2002;180:523–527.
Zygmunt A, Olfson M, Boyer CA, Mechanic D: Interventions to improve medication adherence in schizophrenia. *Am J Psychiatry.* 2002;159:1653–1664.

▲ 12.12 Schizophrenia: Somatic Treatment

JOHN M. KANE, M.D., AND STEPHEN R. MARDER, M.D.

The pharmacotherapy of schizophrenia has undergone substantial changes since the last edition of this book. The second-generation antipsychotics (referred to as *serotonin–dopamine antagonists,* or *SDAs,* in this text) have become the dominant agents for treating schizophrenia. The widespread use of these agents has revealed both their advantages and limitations. In well-managed inpatient units and outpatient clinics, extrapyramidal symptoms, including dystonias, parkinsonism, and akathisia, are uncommon events. In addition, patients are substantially more comfortable on their medications. The greatest advantages of the second-generation antipsychotics may become apparent when these agents are administered during long-term treatment. Emerging evidence suggests that second-generation agents may be associated with better outcomes during maintenance treatment and may facilitate success in psychosocial treatments and rehabilitation. On the other hand, mental health providers have become increasingly concerned about other side effects, such as weight gain, risk of diabetes, and cardiac arrhythmias.

HISTORY

The history of somatic therapies in schizophrenia can be divided into two eras, with the discovery of chlorpromazine (Thorazine)—the first clearly effective antipsychotic drug—as the dividing line. Before the introduction of antipsychotics in the early 1950s, several treatments had been administered to individuals with psychotic illness, with results that are difficult to interpret because careful research methods in psychiatry had not been developed. During the late 19th and early 20th centuries, schizophrenia was viewed as an illness associated with an inevitable deterioration into dementia. As a result, patients were frequently hospitalized for long periods of time. Somatic treatments were used to help control the most severe symptoms of the disorder and make hospitals safer. Sedating agents, such as bromides and barbiturates, were used to control agitation and physical treatments, such as hydrotherapy and wet sheet packs, were also used for their calming effects. In the early 1920s, sleep treatment with barbiturates was introduced. This treatment was based on the observation that patients tended to improve after an overdose of barbiturates. The method involved maintaining patients in a highly sedated state for days, during which they would awaken only for necessary activities, such as eating and personal hygiene.

Insulin coma treatment was introduced during the 1930s. Patients were administered gradually increasing doses of insulin until a coma was introduced. After an hour of monitoring, glucose was administered, terminating the coma. Patients were commonly administered as many as 20 comas. Insulin coma was widely used in the treatment of psychosis, suggesting that it may have been somewhat effective. Unfortunately, it was never exposed to adequate research trials, and it remains unclear if the treatment was effective. It was abandoned when antipsychotics were introduced.

In 1935, Moniz proposed prefrontal lobotomy as a treatment for serious mental illnesses. The support for this treatment came from animal studies in which frontal lobe extirpations in monkeys resulted in an animal that appeared less easily frustrated. Although there is a remarkable lack of controlled studies comparing psychosurgery to other treatments, the use of frontal lobotomy was common before the introduction of effective antipsychotics. Although reports suggest that lobotomy may have been effective in reducing severe psychotic symptoms, it also resulted in deteriorations in other areas. After lobotomies, patients frequently demonstrated personality deterioration with impulsive and psychopathic behaviors, as well as impairments in concept formation and the ability to plan. Psychosurgery was abandoned as a treatment for schizophrenia after the introduction of effective antipsychotic medications.

Convulsive therapies were developed after it was observed that some patients improved after a seizure. Drugs such as camphor and pentylenetetrazol (Metrazol) were used initially to induce seizures but were abandoned after Ugo Cerletti and Lucino Bini proposed the use of electrically-induced convulsions. In its early days, electroconvulsive therapy (ECT) was administered without anesthetics or muscle relaxants. The lack of anesthetics inspired fear in many patients, and the lack of muscle relaxants led to injuries from forceful muscle contractions. ECT continues to have a role in certain types of schizophrenia and is discussed in a later section.

The first effective antipsychotic medications were probably derived from extracts of the rauwolfia plant. Publications from the 1930s and 1940s suggested that these agents were effective for both hypertension and psychosis. Reserpine, the most potent of the rauwolfia alkaloids, was introduced in the early 1950s and was widely prescribed in the United States and elsewhere for schizophrenia and other psychotic illnesses. Studies comparing reserpine to dopamine receptor antagonists suggested that their efficacy was similar. However, reserpine's side effects, particularly depression, led most clinicians to prefer the dopamine receptor antagonists. Thus, reserpine is only rarely used for managing psychosis.

The discovery of chlorpromazine in the early 1950s may be the most important single contribution to the treatment of a psychiatric illness. Henri Laborit, a surgeon in Paris, noticed that administering chlorpromazine to patients before surgery resulted in an unusual state in which they seemed less anxious regarding the procedure. In 1952, he convinced Jean Delay and Pierre Deniker and other psychiatrists to administer chlorpromazine to psychotic and excited patients. The effects were extraordinary. Chlorpromazine was effective at reducing hallucinations and delusions, as well as excitement. It was also noted that it caused side effects that appeared similar to parkinsonism. The use of chlorpromazine spread rapidly through the psychiatric hospitals in Paris and, eventually, to the rest of the world. Because chlorpromazine was relatively easy to administer to a large number of patients, it was partially responsible for a substantial reduction in the number of patients in psychiatric hospitals.

Thioridazine (Mellaril) and fluphenazine (Permitil, Prolixin), as well as newer classes of drugs, such as the butyrophenones (e.g., haloperidol [Haldol]) and the thioxanthenes (e.g., thiothixene [Navane]), were developed after the introduction of chlorpromazine. Although these newer agents differed in their potency and side effect profiles, all were similar in their effectiveness. Clozapine (Clozaril), the first effective antipsychotic with negligible extrapyramidal side effects, was discovered in 1958 and first studied during the 1960s. However, in 1976, it was noted that clozapine was associated with a substantial risk of agranulocytosis. This property resulted in delays in the introduction of clozapine. In 1990, clozapine finally became available in the United States, but its use was restricted to patients who responded poorly to other agents. The introduction of risperidone (Risperdal) in 1994, olanzapine (Zyprexa) in 1996, quetiapine (Seroquel) in 1997, ziprasidone (Geodon) in 2001, and aripiprazole (Abilify) in 2002, have given clinicians new alternatives for treating a large number of patients with schizophrenia. These newer agents have replaced older drugs as the standard treatments for schizophrenia.

PHASES OF TREATMENT IN SCHIZOPHRENIA

Somatic treatment differs depending on the phase of a patient's illness. The acute stage is usually characterized by psychotic symptoms that require immediate clinical attention. These symptoms may represent a first psychotic episode or, more commonly, a relapse in an individual who has experienced multiple episodes. Treatment during this phase focuses on alleviating the most severe psychotic symptoms. After the acute phase, which usually lasts from 4 to 8 weeks, patients usually enter a stabilization phase in which acute symptoms have been controlled. However, patients remain at risk for relapse if treatment is interrupted or if the patient is exposed to stress. During this stabilization phase, treatment focuses on consolidating therapeutic gains, with similar treatments as those used in the acute stage. This phase may last as long as 6 months after recovery from acute symptoms. The third stage is the stable, or maintenance, phase when the illness is in a relative stage of remission. The goals during this phase are to prevent psychotic relapse and to assist patients in improving their level of functioning.

EFFECTIVENESS OF ANTIPSYCHOTIC MEDICATIONS

A large body of evidence supports the effectiveness of antipsychotics for schizophrenia. Many of these studies were carried out in the 1960s, when there was skepticism about whether these agents were truly antipsychotic or simply more effective tranquilizers. An evaluation of these studies by the 1995 Schizophrenia Patient Outcomes Research Team (PORT) found that approximately 70 percent of patients treated with an antipsychotic achieved remission. In contrast, only approximately 25 percent of patients treated with placebo were remitted. Most studies compared one or more antipsychotics with either a placebo or an agent, such as phenobarbital, that served as a control. Antipsychotics were found to be more effective than either placebo or tranquilizers.

EFFECTIVENESS OF ECT IN SCHIZOPHRENIA

ECT has been studied in both acute and chronic schizophrenia. Studies in recent-onset patients indicate that ECT is about as effective as antipsychotic medications and more effective than psychotherapy. Other studies suggest that supplementing antipsychotic medications with ECT is more effective than antipsychotic medications alone. Studies of ECT in chronic schizophrenia have been less promising. There are anecdotal reports indicating that ECT is effective in patients who are poor responders to antipsychotic medications. Overall, these results suggest that ECT probably has a limited role in schizophrenia. Patients should receive trials of antipsychotics before receiving ECT. If these medications are ineffective, acutely ill patients can be treated with ECT. Antipsychotic medications should be administered during and after ECT treatment.

TREATMENT OF ACUTE EPISODES

Indications for Somatic Treatment

Nearly all schizophrenia patients with acute psychotic symptoms will benefit from an antipsychotic medication. Aside from relieving the patient from symptoms, there is some evidence indicating that lengthy delays in initiating drug treatment may alter the long-term course of schizophrenia. This evidence is summarized in a review by Richard J. Wyatt, who found that delays in treatment, usually of 6 months or more, were associated with a greater need for hospital treatment and a worse social and vocational outcome. Some other studies, but not all, suggest that a longer time between the first onset of psychosis and the initiation of treatment is related to a worse outcome. Many of the studies reviewed by Wyatt have important limitations, such as comparison of individuals treated during different decades and lack of randomization. However, a definitive study will never be carried out to determine whether withholding treatment worsens the long-term course of schizophrenia. As a result, it is probably prudent for clinicians to consider the possibility that untreated psychosis can result in a type of permanent damage.

These data do not mean that all patients need to be treated immediately. There are circumstances in which the management of a patient may improve if drug treatment is delayed several days. A brief delay may permit clinicians to develop a more thorough diagnostic evaluation and rule out causes of abnormal behavior, such as substance abuse, extreme stress, medical illnesses, and other psychiatric illnesses.

Assessment

Whenever possible, patients should receive a physical examination with a neurological examination, a mental status examination, and a laboratory evaluation before medications are started. Blood tests for complete blood cell count (CBC); electrolytes; fasting glucose; lipid profile; and liver, renal, and thyroid function should be ordered. Other evaluations that should be considered are pregnancy tests in women and human immunodeficiency virus (HIV) and syphilis tests when relevant. Individuals with schizophrenia are at a higher risk for cardiovascular disease than the population at large. As a result, an electrocardiogram (EKG) should probably be done at the onset of treatment for many patients with cardiac risk factors. The presence of movement disorders, particularly preexisting tardive dyskinesia, should be assessed, as this may influence the selection of an antipsychotic.

Because antipsychotics are relatively safe drugs, treatment can usually begin before the results of laboratory tests are known. An exception is clozapine treatment, which should only begin after the patient is confirmed as having a normal CBC. Under emergent conditions—for example, when patients refuse to cooperate with an evaluation—antipsychotics can be administered before a medical evaluation.

Selection of an Antipsychotic Drug

Antipsychotics can be categorized into two main groups: the older conventional antipsychotics, which have also been called *first-generation antipsychotics*, or *dopamine receptor antagonists*, and the newer second drugs, which have been called *second-generation antipsychotics*, or *SDAs*. The terms dopamine receptor antagonist and SDA are based on the theory that the antipsychotic effects of dopamine receptor antagonists result from the blockade of dopamine type 2 (D_2) receptors and the SDAs differ in having effects related to their ratio of D_2 and 5-hydroxytryptamine type 2A (5-HT_{2A}) antagonism. (There is some doubt as to whether the unique properties of these agents are related to this mechanism.) The dopamine receptor antagonists are further categorized as being low-, mid-, or high-potency, with the higher-potency drugs having a greater affinity for D_2 receptors and a greater tendency to cause extrapyramidal side effects. Low-potency drugs are less likely to cause extrapyramidal side effects but are more likely to cause postural hypotension, sedation, and anticholinergic effects.

If a history of an antipsychotic response is not available, there are other factors that can influence drug selection (Table 12.12–1). These have been considered by a number of groups who have developed evidence-based guidelines, including the Texas Medication Algorithm Project (TMAP), the Schizophrenia PORT, and the Mount Sinai Consensus Conference. All of these groups recommend the preferential use of SDAs, particularly for first-episode patients. The Mount Sinai Conference recommended reserving dopamine receptor antagonists for patients who respond without demonstrating extrapyramidal side effects, for patients who have demonstrated that they respond better to dopamine receptor antagonists than SDAs, and for those who are managed with depot antipsychotics. However, the recent marketing of a long-acting injectable form of risperidone will alter that recommendation. The different guidelines agree that patients who do not respond to SDAs should have a trial of clozapine.

There is no evidence that any one SDA is more effective than any other, except for clozapine's advantage for treatment-refractory patients. (The authors of this chapter have reviewed the studies in which first- and second-generation antipsychotics were compared and have concluded that, although some of these studies found statistically significant differences, these differences were small and could be explained by the comparison of different or nonoptimum doses.) The selection of an antipsychotic should be based on other factors, including a patient's history of drug treatment, his or her preference of one drug over another, and the side effects that the patient and the clinician are most anxious to avoid.

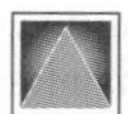

Table 12.12–1
Factors Influencing Antipsychotic Selection

Factor	Consider
Subjective response	A dysphoric subjective response to a particular drug predicts poor compliance with that drug
EPS sensitivity	Clozapine, quetiapine, and other SDAs
Tardive dyskinesia	Clozapine, quetiapine, and other SDAs
Poor medication compliance or high risk of relapse	Oral form of a long-acting antagonist (risperdone, haloperidol, or fluphenazine in the United States.)
Pregnancy	Probably haloperidol (most data supporting its safety)
Cognitive symptoms	SDA
Negative symptoms	SDA
Treatment refractory	Clozapine
Side effects	
Weight gain	Ziprasidone or aripiprazole
Diabetes	Ziprasidone or aripiprazole
Prolactin elevation	SDA other than risperidone
Sedation	Ziprasidone or aripiprazole

EPS, extrapyramidal side effects; SDA, serotonin–dopamine antagonist.

Route of Administration

The decision regarding route of administration is usually straightforward. Under most conditions, patients should be treated with an oral antipsychotic. Short-acting intramuscular drugs are useful when the patient refuses oral dosing and when a rapid onset is helpful. Intramuscular administration of most antipsychotics results in peak plasma levels in approximately 30 minutes with clinical effects emerging within 15 to 30 minutes. Most orally administered antipsychotics result in a peak plasma level in 1 to 4 hours after administration.

Long-Acting Injectable Antipsychotics

Antipsychotic medications can also be administered as long-acting injectable compounds. These drugs differ from short-acting compounds in that they are released slowly over a period of several weeks and, as a result, can take days or weeks to achieve maximum serum concentration and weeks to months to achieve steady state. Thus, the drugs are helpful for continuation and maintenance treatment, but not for rapid acute treatment. Some oral supplementation is necessary while peak plasma levels are being achieved. Fluphenazine and haloperidol have been formulated as esters formed between the alcohol group of the drug and a long-chain fatty acid. After injection, the drug is slowly released from the injection site by enzymatic hydrolysis of the ester and diffusion of the free drug.

Recently, a long-acting form of risperidone has been marketed using a microsphere formulation in which risperidone is embedded in a matrix of glycolic acid–lactate copolymer and suspended in an aqueous solution. Gradual hydrolysis of the copolymer leads to release of the active drug over a period of several weeks.

Starting Antipsychotics

Before starting an antipsychotic, clinicians should describe to patients the medication that is being prescribed, its target symptoms, and its possible side effects. It is particularly important to describe side effects such as akathisia, as this can be misinterpreted as agitation under some circumstances. Patients who are severely disturbed may be unable to participate meaningfully in this discussion. However, most will benefit from information about the goals of treatment and important risks associated with antipsychotic medication. Because patients with schizophrenia may be suspicious, it is particularly important to emphasize that patients can participate as collaborators in interpreting medication effects. Because psychotic individuals may be dependent on the help and support of their families, it is frequently helpful to involve one or more family members in decision making regarding drug treatment.

In some settings and locations, it is necessary for patients to give written or verbal consent before receiving an antipsychotic medication. This can be a dilemma for patients who are conceptually disorganized and find it difficult to understand the risks and benefits of drug treatment. Under these circumstances, clinicians should adjust the complexity of the discussion to the patient's state of mind. Thus, it may be appropriate to provide a limited amount of information that focuses on the most common acute side effects of the medication when the patient is most seriously impaired. As the patient improves, clinicians may then elaborate on the costs and benefits of medication. For example, detailed discussions about tardive dyskinesia or weight side effects associated with chronic treatment may be deferred until the patient has improved and long-term maintenance is being considered.

It is also important for psychiatrists to evaluate whether acutely disturbed patients are able to participate meaningfully in decisions about their medication. Clinicians should become familiar with local and state laws that affect a patient's right to refuse or accept drug treatment. The most difficult situation is when a patient who desperately needs medication refuses it. Under some conditions, family members who have been educated about schizophrenia may be helpful in convincing patients to accept medication. Every locality has provisions for treating patients against their will under emergency conditions. Some permit involuntary treatment when certain conditions are met. As patients improve, the great majority will eventually accept their own need for medication. Many localities now have laws allowing for compulsory outpatient treatment, particularly for patients who have a history of violent or aggressive behavior.

Dosage Selection Finding the best dose for an antipsychotic is both difficult and important. The difficulty exists because the physician is often unable to titrate dose against clinical effects, due to the delay between a clinical intervention and the patient's clinical response. In some individuals, there is a delay of days or even weeks between the time when a medication is started and when the patient eventually responds. However, antipsychotic response usually begins in the first week and accumulates over time. Preclinical findings indicate that the neurochemical response to antipsychotics is complex and includes an initial blockade of central dopamine receptors, followed by delayed decrease in dopamine turnover. Researchers have often assumed a greater delay in antipsychotic response when proposing preclinical models of drug effect than is supported by recent clinical reports.

Although high doses of a dopamine receptor antagonist can be associated with extrapyramidal side effects, some patients are able to tolerate antipsychotics at very high doses. This is particularly true for nonsedating, high-potency drugs. This observation has led clinicians to raise the prescribed doses in hope that higher doses will lead to greater improvement than moderate doses. This belief resulted in a substantial increase in the average dose of antipsychotics prescribed in the United States during the 1970s and 1980s. During this period, many psychiatrists prescribed doses above 1,000 mg of chlorpromazine equivalents (or 20 mg of haloperidol) on a routine basis, whereas others reserved high-dose treatment for patients who remained symptomatic on lower doses.

A number of dosage comparison studies have failed to support the routine use of higher doses. That is, when groups of patients are assigned to higher doses, such as more than 2,000 mg of chlorpromazine or 40 mg of haloperidol, the rate of improvement and the amount of improvement are no greater than for those assigned to more moderate doses. Moreover, many clinicians are prescribing doses of second-generation antipsychotics—particularly olanzapine and quetiapine—that are substantially higher than those that are recommended. At present, there is no evidence from controlled trials that supports these higher doses. Clinicians are sometimes impressed by individuals who require these higher doses, suggesting that there is a small group of patients who should be treated with high doses. However, most patients who are receiving these high doses are only partial responders to an antipsychotic and have endured dosage increases that were not associated with improvement.

There are only limited data from controlled trials to assist clinicians in finding the best dose of clozapine. The mean dose of clozapine prescribed differs between Europe and the United States, with Europeans commonly treating with less than 300 mg of clozapine per day and clinicians in the United States often prescribing 500 mg or more. These experiences support the practice of treating most clozapine patients with doses in the range of 300 to 500 mg per day. However, side effects, particularly sedation and orthostatic hypotension, are often limiting factors that prevent clinicians from reaching a targeted dose. Although some patients have an optimal response in doses between 600 and 900 mg, the risk of seizure increases substantially in this dose range. More recent studies suggest that patients are more likely to respond to clozapine at plasma levels of 350 ng/mL or higher, suggesting that measuring plasma levels may be useful for poor responders.

Large multicenter trials indicate that risperidone is most effective at 4 to 8 mg per day. Higher doses may lead to extrapyramidal side effects, without an advantage in increased effectiveness. In the United States, the average dosage of risperidone prescribed for schizophrenia is slightly more than 4 mg per day. This suggests that a reasonable practice would be to manage patients with schizophrenia with 4 mg of risperidone and increase the dose if they do not respond after 4 to 6 weeks. Olanzapine is usually effective in the range of 10 to 20 mg per day, although a number of case reports describe individuals who demonstrated optimal responses at doses of 25 mg and higher. Case reports also identify patients who have demonstrated substantial improvements when doses of quetiapine were raised well above 800 mg. At this time, there is no evidence that prescribing doses of ziprasidone greater than 160 mg per day increases its effectiveness.

A number of recent findings suggest a reasonable strategy for treating acute schizophrenia. The dose of an antipsychotic that is likely to be effective is the dose that occupies an appropriate number of D_2 receptors. For dopamine receptor antagonists, this is approximately 80 percent of receptors. The therapeutic response depends on processes that occur after these receptors have been occupied for a period of time. This observation is supported by findings from both positron emission tomography (PET) scanning and the measurement of plasma homovanillic acid, which suggest that clinical improvement is not associated with the immediate effects of the drug on dopamine receptors, but on processes that occur later.

Therefore, the goals of the first days of treatment are to administer a drug dose that occupies an adequate proportion of dopamine receptors and to keep the patient comfortable until the drug is effective. If a patient does not respond in the first or second week, this may predict poor response, but many would argue that an adequate trial should last at least 4 weeks. Also, the strategy of using medications on an as-needed basis as a guide to finding the optimal dose makes very little sense, as the immediate and delayed responses are very different.

Managing Agitation in Acute Psychosis Agitation in acute schizophrenia can result from disturbing psychotic symptoms, such as frightening delusions or suspiciousness, or from other causes, including stimulant abuse or extrapyramidal side effects, particularly akathisia. Patients with akathisia can appear agitated when they experience a subjective feeling of motor restlessness. Differentiating akathisia from psychotic agitation can be difficult, particularly when patients are incapable of describing their internal experience. If patients are receiving an agent associated with extrapyramidal side effects, usually a first-generation antipsychotic, a trial with an anticholinergic antiparkinson medication or propranolol (Inderal) may be helpful in making the discrimination.

Clinicians have a number of options for managing agitation that results from psychosis. Antipsychotics and benzodiazepines can result in relatively rapid calming when psychotic patients are agitated. An advantage of an antipsychotic is that a single intramuscular injection of haloperidol, fluphenazine, olanzapine, or ziprasidone will often result in calming without an excess of sedation. Low-potency antipsychotics are often associated with sedation and postural hypotension, particularly when they are administered intramuscularly. Intramuscular ziprasidone and olanzapine are similar to their oral counterparts in not causing substantial extrapyramidal side effects during acute treatment. This can be an important advantage over haloperidol or fluphenazine, which can cause frightening dystonias or akathisia in some patients. A rapidly dissolving oral formulation of olanzapine (Zydis) may also be helpful as an alternative to an intramuscular injection.

Benzodiazepines are also effective for agitation during acute psychosis. Lorazepam (Ativan) has the advantage of reliable absorption when it is administered either orally or intramuscularly. The combination of lorazepam with a high-potency antipsychotic has been found to be safer and more effective than large doses of DAs in controlling excitement and motor agitation. Moreover, the use of benzodiazepines may reduce the amount of antipsychotic that is needed to control psychotic patients.

MANAGING SIDE EFFECTS

Patients will frequently experience side effects of an antipsychotic before they experience clinical improvement. Whereas a clinical response may be delayed for days or weeks after drugs are started, side effects will often begin almost immediately. For low-potency drugs, these side effects are likely to include sedation, postural hypotension, and anticholinergic effects, whereas high-potency drugs are likely to cause extrapyramidal side effects.

This early onset of side effects is important because a patient's interpretation of a drug's effectiveness is often associated with how that drug makes the patient feel. Moreover, one of the challenges of treating acutely psychotic individuals is maintaining the trust of individuals who may misinterpret experiences and become suspicious. Warning patients about the potential side effects of medication can lead to prompt management and will often improve the trust between patient and clinician. Moreover, minimizing adverse effects can have long-lasting effects, as one of the powerful predictors of drug reluctance or drug refusal is an earlier experience of side effects.

Extrapyramidal Side Effects One of the most widely accepted benefits of the new generation antipsychotics is their reduced propensity to cause extrapyramidal side effects. Some debate has centered around the comparator drugs and dosages used in establishing these benefits, but even relatively low doses of high-potency, conventional antipsychotics (e.g., haloperidol, 4 mg per day) are associated with more extrapyramidal side effects than recommended doses of SDAs. These side effects can occur, however, and, because many patients around the world continue to receive conventional antipsychotic drugs, awareness of extrapyramidal side effects remains critical.

The most common and troubling form of extrapyramidal side effect is akathisia, a side effect consisting of a subjective feeling of restlessness along with restless movements, usually in the legs or feet. Patients who experience severe akathisia will often pace continuously or move their feet restlessly while they are sitting. Some complain that they are unable to feel comfortable, regardless of what they do. Severe akathisia can cause patients to feel anxious or irritable, and some reports suggest that severe akathisia can result in aggressive or suicidal acts.

Researchers have estimated that 25 to 75 percent of patients treated with a high-potency, conventional DA will experience akathisia. This side effect can be difficult to assess and is frequently misdiagnosed as anxiety or agitation. Akathisia is also thought to be a correlate of poor antipsychotic drug response.

Because patients may experience akathisia as irritability or agitation, asking patients whether they are restless or if they have difficulty sitting still can be helpful in early stages of treatment. At this point, a dosage adjustment, a β-blocker, or an anticholinergic antiparkinson drug may provide considerable relief. Also, patients who have a history of developing severe akathisia and respond poorly to these treatments are likely to do better if they are treated with a new-generation antipsychotic.

Dystonias are probably the most frightening type of extrapyramidal side effect. They are intermittent or sustained muscular spasms and abnormal postures affecting mainly the musculature of the head and neck but sometimes the trunk and lower extremities. Common forms of dystonia include abnormal positioning of the neck, impaired swallowing (dysphagia), hypertonic or enlarged tongue, and deviations of the eyes (oculogyric crisis). These reactions usually appear within the first few days of therapy. Dystonias are more likely to occur in younger patients, particularly young men.

Antipsychotic-induced parkinsonism consists of tremor, muscular rigidity, and a decrease in spontaneous movements. All of these features resemble the movement disorder in idiopathic parkinsonism. Examination usually reveals a positive glabella tap. This motor disturbance affects approximately 30 percent of patients who are chronically treated with traditional antipsychotics. The first evidence of drug-induced parkinsonism may be a diminished arm swing or decreased facial expressiveness. Risk factors for antipsychotic-induced parkinsonism include increasing age, dose, a history of parkinsonism, and underlying basal ganglia damage.

When patients develop extrapyramidal side effects, clinicians have a number of alternatives. These include reducing the dose of the antipsychotic (which is most commonly a dopamine receptor antagonist), adding an antiparkinson medication, and changing the patient to an SDA that is less likely to cause extrapyramidal side effects. The most effective antiparkinson medications are the anticholinergic antiparkinson drugs. Although these medications are frequently effective, they also cause their own side effects, including dry mouth, constipation, blurred vision, and, often, memory loss. Also, these medications are often only partially effective, leaving patients with substantial amounts of lingering extrapyramidal side effects. Centrally acting β-blockers, such as propranolol, are frequently effective for treating akathisia. Most patients respond to dosages between 30 and 90 mg per day.

If conventional antipsychotics are being prescribed, clinicians may consider prescribing prophylactic antiparkinson medications for patients who are likely to experience disturbing extrapyramidal side effects. These include patients who have a history of extrapyramidal side effect sensitivity and those who are being treated with relatively high doses of high-potency drugs. Prophylactic antiparkinson medications may also be indicated when high-potency drugs are prescribed for young men who tend to have an increased vulnerability for developing dystonias. Again, these patients should be candidates for newer drugs.

Some individuals are highly sensitive to extrapyramidal side effects at the dose that is necessary to control their psychosis. For many of these patients, medication side effects may seem worse than the illness itself. These patients should be treated routinely with an SDA, as these agents result in substantially fewer extrapyramidal side effects than the dopamine receptor antagonists. These highly sensitive individuals may actually experience extrapyramidal side effects on an SDA. Risperidone may cause extrapyramidal side effects at higher doses—for example, more than 6 mg—and olanzapine may cause mild akathisia at higher doses.

Tardive Dyskinesia and Other Tardive Syndromes

As with extrapyramidal side effects, tardive dyskinesia is far less common with the SDAs than with conventional drugs. Although there is a lack of very long-term data, prospective studies lasting 6 months or longer are consistent in demonstrating a significantly lower risk of tardive dyskinesia with new-generation drugs (i.e., clozapine, risperidone, olanzapine, quetiapine) than comparator drugs, such as haloperidol. Fewer data are currently available with ziprasidone and aripiprazole, but early experience certainly suggests a low risk with those drugs as well. These results were somewhat expected in that early occurring extrapyramidal side effects are a significant risk factor for tardive dyskinesia. However, the risk of tardive dyskinesia is not absent with SDAs, and it is important for clinicians to be aware of the identification and management of tardive dyskinesia even when patients are treated with SDAs. Tardive dyskinesias commonly consist of abnormal, involuntary movements of the mouth, face, tongue, trunk, and extremities. The oral–facial movements occur in approximately three-fourths of tardive dyskinesia patients and can include lip smacking, sucking, and puckering, as well as facial grimacing. Other movements might include irregular movements of the limbs, particularly choreoathetoid-like movements of the fingers and toes and slow, writhing movements of the trunk. Younger patients with tardive dyskinesia tend to develop slower athetoid movements of the trunk, extremities, and neck.

The abnormal movements of tardive dyskinesia are usually reduced by voluntary movements of the affected areas and are increased by voluntary movements of unaffected areas. The abnormal movements of tardive dyskinesia are usually increased with emotional arousal and absent when the individual is asleep. According to the diagnostic criteria in DSM-IV-TR, the abnormal movements should be present for at least 4 weeks and patients should have been exposed to an antipsychotic for at least 3 months. The onset of the abnormal movements should occur either while the patient is receiving an antipsychotic or within 4 weeks of discontinuing an oral antipsychotic or 8 weeks after the withdrawal of a depot antipsychotic.

Prevalence surveys indicate that 20 to 30 percent of patients who are chronically treated with a conventional dopamine receptor antagonist will exhibit symptoms of tardive dyskinesia. Three to five percent of young patients receiving a dopamine receptor antagonist develop tardive dyskinesia each year. The risk in elderly patients is much higher. Although seriously disabling dyskinesia is uncommon, a small proportion can affect walking, breathing, eating, and talking. Individuals who are more sensitive to acute extrapyramidal side effects appear to be more vulnerable to developing tardive dyskinesia. Patients with organic mental illness and affective disorders may also be more vulnerable to tardive dyskinesia than those with schizophrenia.

An American Psychiatric Association Task Force on Tardive Dyskinesia issued a report in which they made a number of recommendations for preventing and managing tardive dyskinesia. These include (1) establishing objective evidence that antipsychotic medications are effective for an individual; (2) using the lowest effective dose of antipsychotic; (3) prescribing cautiously with children, elderly patients, and patients with mood disorders; (4) examining patients on a regular basis for evidence of tardive dyskinesia; (5) considering alternatives to the antipsychotic being used, obtaining informed consent, and considering dosage reduction when tardive dyskinesia is diagnosed; (6) considering a number of options if the tardive dyskinesia worsens, including discontinuing the antipsychotic or switching to a different drug. Clozapine has been shown to be effective in reducing severe tardive dyskinesia or tardive dystonia.

Regular monitoring for tardive dyskinesia should be a component of management strategies with antipsychotics. The monitoring should be particularly careful for those patients with an increased risk for tardive dyskinesia, such as elderly patients, patients who are sensitive to extrapyramidal side effects, and individuals with affective illness. Routine monitoring should include examination every 3 to 6 months, and monitoring for high-risk groups should be carried out every 3 months.

Other Side Effects

Sedation and postural hypotension can be important side effects for patients who are being treated with low-potency dopamine receptor antagonists, such as chlorpromazine and thioridazine and clozapine. These effects are often most severe during the initial dosing with these medications. As a result, patients treated with these medications—particularly clozapine—may require weeks to reach a therapeutic dose. Although most patients develop tolerance to sedation and postural hypotension, sedation may continue to be a problem. In these patients, daytime drowsiness may interfere with a patient's attempts to return to community life.

All of the dopamine receptor antagonists, as well as risperidone, elevate prolactin levels, which can result in galactorrhea and irregular menses. There is also concern that long-term elevations in prolactin and the resultant suppression in gonadotropin-releasing hormone can cause clinically important suppression in gonadal hormones. These, in turn, may have effects on libido and sexual functioning. There is also concern that elevated prolactin may cause decreases in bone density and lead to osteoporosis. The concerns about hyperprolactinemia and sexual functioning and bone density are based on experiences with prolactin elevations related to tumors and other causes. It is unclear if these risks are also associated with the lower elevations that occur with prolactin-elevating drugs.

Before the introduction of SDAs, elevated prolactin was a consequence of treatment with all antipsychotics. Clozapine, olanzapine, ziprasidone, quetiapine, and aripiprazole do not appear to elevate prolactin above normal levels. As a result, when patients demonstrate side effects related to prolactin, such as galactorrhea or menstrual disturbances, changing patients to a prolactin-sparing agent may be effective.

Side Effects of Clozapine

As noted in Section 31.25, clozapine has a number of side effects that make it a difficult drug to administer. The most serious is a risk of agranulocytosis. This potentially fatal condition occurs in approximately 0.3 percent of patients treated with clozapine during the first year of exposure. Subsequently, the risk is substantially lower. As a result, patients who receive clozapine in the United States are required to be in a program of weekly blood monitoring for the first 6 months and biweekly monitoring thereafter.

Clozapine is also associated with a higher risk of seizures than other antipsychotics. The risk reaches nearly 5 percent at doses over 600 mg. Patients who develop seizures with clozapine can usually be managed by reducing the dose and adding an anticonvulsant, usually valproate (Depakene). Myocarditis has been reported to occur in approximately 5 patients per 100,000 patient years. Other side effects with clozapine include hypersalivation, sedation, tachycardia, weight gain, fever, and postural hypotension.

Health Monitoring in Patients Receiving Antipsychotics

Patients with schizophrenia are more likely than the population at large to suffer from a number of illnesses, including coronary heart disease, diabetes, and hypertension. The high prevalence of these illnesses may explain why individuals with schizophrenia have a significantly shorter life expectancy than the population at large. The risk of these illnesses is partly explained by the lifestyles of many patients, which may include smoking, poor dietary habits, and obesity. In addition, there is increasing evidence that certain antipsychotics—but not all—can cause weight gain.

A metaanalysis by David B. Allison and coworkers estimated the amount of weight gain associated with moderate doses of several antipsychotics over 10 weeks. Among the drugs studied, the mean increases were clozapine, 4.45 kg; olanzapine, 4.15 kg; sertindole, 2.92 kg; risperidone, 2.10 kg; and ziprasidone, 0.04 kg. Other large studies suggest that certain antipsychotics—particularly clozapine and olanzapine—are associated with an increase in the risk of diabetes and hyperlipidemias.

A group of mental health and medical experts met in New York in October, 2002, to discuss guidelines for monitoring the health of individuals with schizophrenia. There was a consensus that psychiatrists should monitor a number of health indicators including body mass index (BMI), fasting blood glucose, and lipid profiles. If clinicians follow the recommendation that patients should be weighed and their BMI calculated for every visit for 6 months after a medication change, it will have a major effect on psychiatric practice. On the other hand, adherence to some or all of the recommended practices may improve the health of patients with schizophrenia.

NEGATIVE, MOOD, AND COGNITIVE SYMPTOMS

Negative symptoms and cognitive impairments are associated with a substantial amount of the social and vocational disability in schizophrenia. This observation has resulted in a reappraisal of the goals of treatment, placing a greater emphasis on treatment strategies for decreasing the severity of these impairments. Most of the attention has focused on negative symptoms.

William T. Carpenter, Jr., has made an important contribution to this area by classifying negative symptoms into primary and secondary categories. Secondary negative symptoms are those symptoms that may result from other conditions, such as depression or extrapyramidal side effects. Extrapyramidal side effects are a common cause of secondary negative symptoms, particularly when patients are experiencing akinesia, a side effect that can be manifest in decreased speech, decreased motivation, and decreased spontaneous gestures. In addition, positive or psychotic symptoms can result in secondary negative symptoms. A common example is the patient who is withdrawn or uncommunicative as a result of suspiciousness.

The management of secondary negative symptoms begins with the management of the condition that caused these symptoms. For depression, this may include the addition of an antidepressant medication; for extrapyramidal side effects, this may involve the addition of an antiparkinson medication, a dose reduction, or a change to an antipsychotic—usually an SDA—that is associated with fewer extrapyramidal side effects.

If the previously mentioned causes of secondary negative symptoms have been ruled out, the patient is likely to be demonstrating a type of enduring primary negative symptom. There is some evidence to suggest that the SDAs are more effective in treating negative symptoms than conventional agents. However, it is unclear if these effects are related to a reduction in secondary negative symptoms. Until this issue is decided by adequate controlled studies, it is probably reasonable for clinicians to consider changing to an SDA for patients with substantial negative symptoms.

Patients with schizophrenia frequently experience impairments in memory, attention, and information processing. These cognitive impairments can also interfere with the social and vocational rehabilitation of patients, even when their psychotic symptoms have been well controlled. As with negative symptoms, cognitive impairments can be secondary to other causes, such as substance abuse or drug side effects. The anticholinergic effects of either an antipsychotic or an antiparkinson medication, such as biperiden (Akineton) or benztropine (Cogentin), can cause cognitive impairments that are difficult to distinguish from symptoms that are part of the schizophrenia illness. Decreasing the use of anticholinergic medication by changing to drugs that do not require antiparkinson medications—particularly SDAs—may be helpful. There is also evidence suggesting that clozapine, risperidone, and other SDAs may be more effective at treating cognitive impairments than dopamine receptor antagonists.

SUICIDAL BEHAVIOR

Patients with schizophrenia and schizoaffective disorder are at considerable risk for suicidal behavior. Approximately 20 to 40 percent of patients make suicide attempts, and 10 percent succeed. Suicidal behavior appears to be an independent domain from psychosis; however, depression and comorbid substance abuse increase the risk. Based on a large-scale study of clozapine (vs. olanzapine) in patients at risk for suicide, clozapine has recently received a new indication for the prevention of suicidal behavior.

STRATEGIES FOR POOR RESPONDERS

When patients with acute schizophrenia are administered an antipsychotic medication, approximately 60 percent will improve to the extent that they will achieve a complete remission or experience only mild symptoms; the remaining 40 percent of patients will improve but still demonstrate variable levels of positive symptoms that are resistant to the medications. Rather than categorizing patients into responders and nonresponders, it is more accurate to consider the degree to which the illness is improved by medication. Some resistant patients are so severely ill that they require chronic institutionalization. Others will respond to an antipsychotic with substantial suppression of their psychotic symptoms but demonstrate persistent symptoms, such as hallucinations or delusions.

Before considering a patient a poor responder to a particular drug, it is important to assure that they received an adequate trial of the medication. A 4- to 6-week trial on an adequate dose of an antipsychotic represents a reasonable trial for most patients. If patients demonstrate even a mild amount of improvement during this period, it may be reasonable to wait, as data from groups of patients indicate that patients may improve at a steady rate for 3 to 6 months. If the patient is receiving a drug with adequate data to define a therapeutic level, it may also be helpful to confirm that the patient is receiving an adequate amount of the drug by monitoring the plasma concentration. This information is available for a number of antipsychotics, including haloperidol, clozapine, fluphenazine, trifluoperazine (Stelazine), and perphenazine (Trilafon). A very low plasma concentration may indicate that the patient has been noncompliant or, more commonly, only partially compliant. It may also suggest that the patient is a rapid metabolizer of the antipsychotic or that the drug is not being adequately absorbed. Under these conditions, raising the dose may be helpful. If the level is relatively high, clinicians should consider whether side effects may be interfering with therapeutic response.

If the patient is responding poorly, many clinicians will consider raising the dose above the usual therapeutic level. The use of high doses in poor medication responders has been studied under a number of circumstances. Nearly all studies found that higher doses were not associated with greater improvement than conventional doses. This suggests that changing to another drug is more likely to be helpful than changing to a high dose.

If a patient has responded poorly to a conventional dopamine receptor antagonist, it is unlikely that this individual will do well on another dopamine receptor antagonist. Studies suggest that a poor response to one dopamine receptor antagonist is likely to be followed by a poor response to another. This suggests that changing to an SDA is more likely to be helpful.

There is substantial evidence indicating that clozapine is effective for patients who respond poorly to dopamine receptor antagonists. Double-blind studies comparing clozapine to other antipsychotics indicated that clozapine had the clearest advantages over conventional drugs in patients with the most severe psychotic symptoms, as well as in those who had previously responded poorly to other antipsychotics. The most definitive evidence of clozapine's advantages in this population comes from a multicenter trial reported by John Kane in which clozapine was compared with chlorpromazine. Patients in this study were a severely psychotic group of individuals who had failed in trials with at least three antipsychotics. Clozapine was significantly more effective than chlorpromazine in nearly every dimension of psychopathology, including both positive symptoms and negative symptoms. This study found that 30 percent of patients treated with clozapine met improvement criteria by the end of the 6-week trial. Studies with a longer duration indicate that as many as 60 percent of patients are likely to meet these same improvement criteria when maintained on clozapine for 6 months.

There is also evidence suggesting that risperidone and olanzapine may be helpful when a dopamine receptor antagonist is only partially effective. At least one controlled trial with each of these drugs has shown superiority to conventional antipsychotics in poor or partial responders, or "noninferiority" to clozapine. However, other studies suggest clozapine to be superior. A number of metaanalyses have been conducted supporting clozapine's superiority in treatment-resistant patients. Given clozapine's side effects profile, a case can be made for the practice of first trying patients on risperidone or olanzapine when they have responded poorly to a DA. However, if patients do not respond adequately, a trial of clozapine is clearly warranted.

MAINTENANCE THERAPY

During the stable, or maintenance, phase, patients are usually in a relative state of remission with only minimal psychotic symptoms. The goals during this stage are to prevent patients from experiencing psychotic relapse and to assist patients in improving their level of functioning. Pharmacotherapy plays an important part in both of these goals. Medications are effective in preventing or delaying psychotic relapse and may also be an important adjunct in managing functional impairments that may interfere with rehabilitation. The art of maintenance treatment results from the unfortunate problem that medication side effects can sometimes interfere with these goals. In addition, titrating dosage in maintenance treatment can be very difficult because the relapse or exacerbation that can result from too low a dose is not likely to occur for weeks to months.

Drug and Route of Administration for Maintenance Therapy

Stable patients who are maintained on an antipsychotic have a much lower relapse rate than patients who have their medications discontinued. Although studies differ, pooling large amounts of data suggests that 16 to 23 percent in a year will experience a relapse while receiving medications and 53 to 72 percent will relapse without medications. Clinicians are often tempted to discontinue medications in patients who have been well and stable for prolonged periods of time. Unfortunately, these patients also have high relapse rates when their medications are discontinued. Other evidence indicates that patients who experience relapses while they are receiving an antipsychotic have milder episodes than patients who relapse on no medication. It has also been suggested that patients who had their medications discontinued are more likely to show dangerous behavior and be admitted involuntarily.

As previously discussed, tardive dyskinesia has been a major concern in establishing the benefit-to-risk ratio of long-term treatment. Even with the conventional antipsychotics, experts agreed that the benefits of maintenance treatment outweighed the risks. As newer medications have been introduced with a substantively reduced risk of tardive dyskinesia, one of the major concerns about long-term treatment has been diminished.

The evaluation of the benefit-to-risk ratio has been particularly challenging in those patients who have experienced only one psychotic episode and have responded well to treatment. It is important to recognize that, although many such patients achieve remission, recovery (which includes sustained, relatively normal social and vocational adjustment) is far less common.

In recent years, it has been well established that even patients who have had only one episode have a 4 in 5 chance of relapsing at least once over the next 5 years and that stopping medication increases this risk fivefold.

At the same time, it is often difficult for late adolescents or young adults to accept the nature of their illness and the need for ongoing pharmacotherapy. This represents a psychotherapeutic and psychoeducational challenge to clinicians and underscores the importance of combining psychosocial treatments, family therapy, rehabilitation, and pharmacological management.

Although published guidelines do not make definitive recommendations about the duration of maintenance treatment after the first episode, recent data suggest that 1 or 2 years might not be adequate. This is a particular concern when patients have achieved good employment status or are involved in educational programs, as they have an enormous amount to lose if they experience another psychotic episode.

It is generally recommended that multi-episode patients receive maintenance treatment for at least 5 years, however, the implication that discontinuing medication at that point is not without substantial risk is a mistake, and many experts would recommend pharmacotherapy on an "indefinite" or "for the foreseeable future" basis.

The first 3 to 6 months after an acute episode or relapse is a period of particular vulnerability. With short lengths of hospital stay, adequate linkages with ambulatory programs are critical to insure continuity of care. After stabilization for 6 months, most experts recommend gradual dosage reduction. However, there are very few studies helping to define minimum maintenance dose for new-generation oral medications. Given reduced concern regarding tardive dyskinesia and the lack of a clear dose–response curve for weight gain, one could argue that there is less incentive to define lowest effective dose for maintenance treatment with these agents.

There are emerging data that the SDAs are more effective in preventing relapse than the conventional drugs. At present, our impression is that this advantage is not simply due to enhanced compliance. Although there are data suggesting some improvement in adherence with the new-generation drugs, these differences are modest at best.

Noncompliance rates with long-term antipsychotic treatment are very high. Average estimates suggest that 40 to 50 percent of patients become noncompliant within 1 or 2 years. Given the high rates of relapse after discontinuation of medication and the potentially severe consequences (loss of job, interference with school, family burden, suicide risk, homelessness, aggressive or violent behavior), attempts to enhance adherence are critical. Although psychosocial treatments focusing on compliance can be helpful, the use of long-acting injectable medication should be considered as a preventive measure and not just reserved for patients who have repeatedly experienced noncompliance and consequent relapse.

Pooling data from numerous double-blind studies show overall significant advantages for long-acting medication in comparison to oral medication, particularly when only long-term studies are included. If anything, these trials underestimate the impact of guaranteed medication, as the nature of clinical trials are such that highly selected, relatively compliant patients are included and the careful monitoring entailed is not representative of routine clinical care.

There are a number of potential advantages of long-acting injectable medication. First, clinicians know immediately when noncompliance occurs and have some time to initiate appropriate interventions before the medication effect dissipates. Second, there is less day-to-day variability in blood levels, potentially making it easier to establish minimum effective dose. Third, many patients who have had experience with such treatment often prefer it.

With the availability of second-generation, long-acting injectable medications, the benefit-to-risk ratio is also enhanced.

INTEGRATING PHARMACOTHERAPY AND PSYCHOSOCIAL TREATMENT

Most patients with schizophrenia will benefit from a combination of pharmacotherapy and psychosocial treatments. Recent improvements in both domains suggest that the overall outcome of this disorder can be improved if patients receive the optimal forms of both treatments at the appropriate stage of their illness. Both studies and clinical experience suggest that psychosocial treatments are probably most effective when patients have recovered from severe psychotic episodes. During the acute psychotic phase, clinical management should emphasize maintaining cooperativeness and trust. This is particularly important when there is overt suspiciousness or a tendency to misinterpret the intentions of the treatment team. A successful strategy is likely to include clear explanations of the rationale for treatment and possible drug side effects. Because family members may be important allies in assuring cooperativeness, family psychoeducation programs have been demonstrated to be helpful during this phase.

It is difficult to generalize about the interactions of drugs and psychosocial treatments for stable patients, because psychosocial treatments can be quite different in their content and their goals. Nevertheless, a number of important treatment principles can be drawn from the literature on combining treatments. The first is that psychosocial treatments are most likely to be effective when patients have been effectively stabilized on drugs. Early studies by Gerard Hogarty indicated that psychosocial treatments could actually lead to a worse outcome when outpatients with schizophrenia were treated with a placebo. Other studies indicate that patients are most likely to respond to psychosocial treatments when their condition is stable. For example, a recent study with social skills training found that patients who received a type of pharmacotherapy that minimized the proportion of time that they were in a psychotic state also demonstrated the greatest improvements in social adjustment.

Psychosocial treatments may also improve the response to pharmacotherapy by improving medication compliance. This was suggested in a study in which patients received a form of family treatment that also encouraged medication compliance. In addition, specific group sessions focused on compliance have been shown to be helpful. Other studies have indicated that psychosocial treatments, particularly family treatment, may decrease the amount of stress the patient experiences within the family and that this, in turn, decreases the amount of antipsychotic medication required by the patient.

The introduction of newer antipsychotics may result in much greater interest in psychosocial interventions. Patients who receive newer agents may be better candidates for psychosocial treatments when treatment with these agents is associated with improvements in negative and cognitive symptoms, as well as reduced side effects. Also, patients who are improved on clozapine, risperidone, olanzapine, or other drugs may initially appear ready to return to community life. However, these individuals then experience a series of frustrating failures at work, school, or in social relationships, which indicate that a drug alone may not be sufficient to prepare them for their new roles.

SUGGESTED CROSS-REFERENCES

For further information related to assessment of the patient with schizophrenia, see Section 7.4 on typical signs and symptoms of psychiatric illness and Section 7.9 on psychiatric rating scales. Chapter 12 on schizophrenia is important for a full understanding of the syndrome. To appreciate the antipsychotic medications, see Sections 31.16 and 31.25 on antipsychotic drugs. Because other medications are used to augment antipsychotic medications, see the other sections of Chapter 31 on biological therapies.

REFERENCES

*Agid O, Kapur S, Arenovich T, Zipursky RB: Delayed-onset hypothesis of antipsychotic action: A hypothesis tested and rejected. *Arch Gen Psychiatry*. 2003;60:1228–1235.

Allison DB, Mentore JL, Heo C, Chandler LP, Cappelleri JC, Infante MC, Weiden PJ: Antipsychotic-induced weight gain: A comprehensive research synthesis. *Am J Psychiatry*. 1999;156:1686–1696.

Bollini P, Pampallona S, Orza MJ, Adams ME, Chalmers TC: Antipsychotic drugs: Is more worse? A meta-analysis of the published randomized control trials. *Psychol Med*. 1994;24:307–316.

Carpenter WT Jr., Heinrichs DW, Wagman AMI: Deficit and nondeficit forms of schizophrenia: The concept. *Am J Psychiatry*. 1988;145:578–583.

Cramer JA, Rosenheck R: Compliance with medication regimens for mental and physical disorders. *Psychiatry Serv*. 1998;49:196–201.

*Davis JM, Chen M, Glick ID: A meta-analysis of the efficacy of second-generation antipsychotics. *Arch Gen Psychiatry*. 2003;60:553–564.

Falloon IRH, Liberman RP. Behavioral family interventions in the management of chronic schizophrenia. In: McFarlane WR, ed: *Family Therapy in Schizophrenia*. New York: Guilford Press; 1983.

Hogarty GE, Anderson CM, Reiss DJ, Kornblith SJ, Greenwald DP, Jabna CD, Medonia MJ: Family psychoeducation, social skills training, and maintenance chemotherapy in the after-care treatment of schizophrenia: I. One year effects of a controlled study on relapse and expressed emotion. *Arch Gen Psychiatry*. 1986;43:633–642.

Hogarty GE, Anderson CM, Reiss DJ, Kornblith SJ, Greenwald DP, Ulrich RF, Carter M: Family psychoeducation, social skills training, and maintenance chemotherapy in the after-care treatment of schizophrenia: II. Two-year effects of a controlled study on relapse and adjustment. *Arch Gen Psychiatry*. 1991;48:340–347.

Janicak PG, Davis JM, Preskorn SH, Ayd FJ. *Principles and Practice of Psychopharmacology*. Baltimore: Williams and Wilkins; 1993:93–184.

*Kane JM, Eerdekens M, Lindenmayer JP, Keith SJ, Lesem M, Karcher K: Long-acting injectable risperidone: Efficacy and safety of the first long-acting atypical antipsychotic. *Am J Psychiatry*. 2003;160:1209–1222.

Kane JM, Honigfeld G, Singer J, Meltzer H: Clozapine for the treatment-resistant schizophrenic: A double-blind comparison versus chlorpromazine/benztropine. *Arch Gen Psychiatry*. 1988;45:789–796.

Kane JM, Marder SR, Schooter NR, Wirshing WC, Umbricht D, Baker RW, Wirshing DA, Safferman A, Ganguli R, McMeniman M, Borenstein M: Clozapine and haloperidol in moderately refractory schizophrenia: A 6-month randomized and double-blind comparison. *Arch Gen Psychiatry*. 2001;58:965–972.

*Leucht S, Barnes TR, Kissling W, Engel RR, Correll C, Kane JM: Relapse prevention in schizophrenia with new generation anti-psychotics: A systematic review and exploratory meta-analysis of randomized, controlled trials. *Am J Psychiatry.* 2003;160:1209–1222.

*Marder SR, Hubbard JW, Van Putten T, Midha KK: The pharmacokinetics of long-acting injectable neuroleptic drugs: Clinical implications. *Psychopharmacology.* 1989;98:433–439.

Metlzer HY, Alphs L, Green AL, Altamura AC, Anand R, Bertholdi A, Bourgeois M, Chouinard G, Islam Z, Kane JM, Krishnan R, Lindenmayer J-P, Potkins A, for the InterSePT Study Group: Clozapine treatment for suicidality in schizophrenia. *Arch Gen Psychiatry.* 2003;60:82–91.

Robinson D, Woerner M, Alvir J, Bilder R, Goldman R, Geisler S, Koreen A, Sheitman B, Chakos M, Mayerhoff D, Lieberman J: Predictors of relapse following response from a first episode of schizophrenia or schizoaffective disorder. *Arch Gen Psychiatry.* 1999;56:241–247.

▲ 12.13 Psychiatric Rehabilitation

ROBERT E. DRAKE, M.D., PH.D., AND
ALAN S. BELLACK, PH.D.

Psychiatric rehabilitation denotes a wide range of interventions designed to help people with disabilities due to mental illness improve their functioning and quality of life by enabling them to acquire the skills and supports needed to be successful in usual adult roles and in the environments of their choice. Normative adult roles include living independently, attending school, working in competitive jobs, relating to family, having friends, and having intimate relationships. Psychiatric rehabilitation emphasizes independence rather than reliance on professionals, community integration rather than isolation in segregated settings for persons with disabilities, and patient preferences rather than professional goals.

Psychiatric rehabilitation has become a fundamental component of the treatment for schizophrenia. Specific approaches to rehabilitation are consistent with current knowledge regarding the etiology, pathophysiology, manifestations, treatment, and course of the disorder. Recent evidence, reviewed in other chapters, indicates that schizophrenia is a brain disease, or set of diseases, causally related to genetic factors or prenatal and perinatal insults, or both. Although the definitive neurobiological substrate of the disorder remains to be defined, many patients manifest neurodevelopmental abnormalities, such as subtle attentional, cognitive, and neuromotor signs, which are evident in childhood, long before the onset of overt psychotic illness. Research on schizophrenia shows abnormalities of neural structure, circuitry, and function. Clinically, the disorder is characterized by positive symptoms of psychosis, such as hallucinations and delusions; negative symptoms, such as lack of motivation and poverty of speech; cognitive deficits, such as problems with memory and executive functioning; and psychosocial difficulties, such as poor social role performance, unemployment, high rates of substance abuse, and increased risks for homelessness, victimization, and other problems. Long-term follow-up studies have consistently shown, over many decades, that a small percentage of schizophrenia patients recover completely, but the great majority continue to be plagued by symptoms, cognitive difficulties, and psychosocial problems for decades.

Antipsychotic medications, including the new generation of antipsychotics, are demonstrably effective in reducing positive symptoms and have a modest effect on negative symptoms, but have limited impact on cognitive impairment and psychosocial functioning. For the great majority of patients, medications help with symptom control but do not restore premorbid levels of functioning or produce normative role performance. Moreover, 20 percent or more of schizophrenia patients have psychotic symptoms that do not respond to antipsychotic medications, and many additional patients have residual symptoms. Thus, medications for schizophrenia should be considered palliative, and it seems unlikely that medications will restore normal brain function in the context of a serious neurodevelopmental brain disorder. Furthermore, medications cannot be expected to reverse the consequences of impaired learning, failure to master adult developmental tasks, and social withdrawal.

Therefore, current approaches to the treatment of schizophrenia involve multidimensional interventions to ameliorate multiple impairments and impact different domains. *Psychiatric rehabilitation* refers to interventions that aim to improve role performance. Traditionally, rehabilitation has been distinguished from treatment in that it focuses on improving functional performance rather than on controlling symptoms or illness. Further, rehabilitation specialists sometimes argue that they focus on the patient's strengths rather than their deficits. In practice, however, these distinctions rapidly blur, and many interventions could be considered treatment or rehabilitation. For example, several cognitive-behavioral and skills training interventions emphasize improving skills for managing the illness, as well as for enhancing functional status, and most interventions take strengths and deficits into account. The distinction between rehabilitation and treatment is, therefore, somewhat arbitrary. In this book, several interventions for schizophrenia could be classified as treatment or rehabilitation, and a selection of current interventions has been divided up for the sake of illustration.

HISTORY

Current approaches to psychiatric rehabilitation represent the confluence of several historical traditions. In the 19th century, the reform movement called *moral treatment* emphasized putting people with mental illness in benign environments and normal roles. Moral treatment recognized that participation in education, work, social activities, and other normal roles could have a healthful effect.

In the United States, government programs for employment of people with disabilities were started after World War I for persons with physical disabilities and were subsequently extended to those with psychiatric disabilities in 1943. These programs transferred ideas and approaches from physical rehabilitation to the practice of psychiatric rehabilitation and focused psychiatric rehabilitation on the domain of employment.

Deinstitutionalization and the development of community mental health centers in the 1950s and 1960s not only changed the locus of care for persons with schizophrenia to the community, but also promoted interest in making services accessible, comprehensive, and germane for normative environments and roles. The National Institute of Mental Health and, later, the Center for Mental Health Services of the Substance Abuse and Mental Health Services Administration helped to develop the community mental health ideology that is called the *community support system model.* Following this model, community mental health programs for persons with schizophrenia now assume concepts and services such as case management, assertive outreach, coordination, integration, continuity, advocacy, self-help, supported employment, supported education, and supported housing. The focus of community mental health rapidly transitioned from reversing the disabling effects of institutionalization to preventing disability in young adults with severe psychiatric illness who had minimal experience in hospitals.

In the early years of deinstitutionalization, patients and nonprofessionals came together to form psychosocial self-help clubs, such as Fountain House in New York and Horizon House in Philadelphia, to promote mutual aid and self-help. The early self-help clubs were rapidly transformed into a range of psychosocial rehabilitation centers around the country. Despite great diversity, psychosocial rehabilitation centers consistently emphasized mutual support; strategies for coping with real-life environments; health promotion rather than a focus on illness; normative roles, such as worker; and belief in the potential for productivity. Current ideas regarding psychiatric rehabilitation derive directly from these activities.

Developments in the fields of skills training and environmental modification have directly stimulated modern approaches to rehabilitation. Skills training methods derived from social learning principles have been applied to numerous areas of everyday functioning—for example, daily living tasks, social activities, employment, education, housing, relating to the health care system, and managing one's illnesses. Approaches to making environments more accommodating are considerably more diverse. They extend from collaborative work with families, using psychoeducational approaches, to a wide range of tactics used in the community to remove barriers faced by people with mental illness related to societal stigma, legal constraints, economic disincentives, and rigidities in the health care system.

Finally, the consumer-initiated movement called *recovery* became an influential ideology for advocates and mental health care systems during the 1990s. Although consumers resist a simple definition of recovery, the ideology includes hope, self-management of illness, and pursuit of personal goals, which typically involve normative adult roles. Because rehabilitation has always been patient-centered, recovery goals for most patients are isomorphic with their rehabilitation goals.

SPECIFIC APPROACHES TO REHABILITATION

As the field of psychiatric rehabilitation has expanded dramatically over the past two decades, numerous approaches have been developed and tested. Many incorporate a core approach to skills training, which includes a functional analysis, stepwise development, behavioral practice and role playing, social and tangible reinforcement, shaping, coaching, prompting, and generalization activities. These are illustrated later in this chapter by the description of social skills training and substance abuse rehabilitation. Others make extensive use of environmental accommodations and supports. The descriptions of supported employment and substance abuse rehabilitation illustrate these approaches. Other approaches focus more on changing society to reduce stigma and enable people with schizophrenia to perform successfully in normative adult roles. Although not discussed here, many laws and regulations, such as the Americans with Disabilities Act and the Ticket to Work legislation, are aimed at altering social restrictions that have prevented people with disabilities from succeeding in competitive employment.

This review presents four common approaches to psychiatric rehabilitation as examples of current practices. These examples are not meant to reflect the full range of available approaches, but rather to illustrate the goals, techniques, and supporting research.

Vocational Rehabilitation

Impairment of vocational role performance is a common complication related to schizophrenia. Studies across the United States show that less than 15 percent of patients with severe mental illnesses, such as schizophrenia, are employed. Nevertheless, studies also show that competitive employment is a primary goal for 50 to 75 percent of schizophrenia patients. Due to patient interests and historical factors discussed earlier, vocational rehabilitation has always been a centerpiece of psychiatric rehabilitation.

Many approaches to helping people with schizophrenia achieve employment were developed over the last half-century. Most of these involved train-and-place models in which extensive preemployment assessments and preparatory experiences, such as sheltered work trials, were used to evaluate and improve the patient's attitudes, skills, appearance, readiness, and other abilities presumed necessary to obtain and sustain competitive employment. Evaluations of these stepwise approaches to vocational rehabilitation found that they did not improve the rate of competitive employment; most patients became discouraged, disengaged, or stalled during preparatory experiences.

Supported Employment In the late 1980s, the emphasis of vocational rehabilitation began to shift to place-and-train models, termed *supported employment*, which were borrowed from the field of developmental disabilities. Supported employment emphasizes individualized placement based on a rapid job search without extensive preemployment assessment or training. After being placed in jobs of their choice, patients are helped to learn the skills and provided the supports needed to be successful. This typically involves part-time employment, and jobs often begin at just a few hours per week and expand over time. The focus is on mainstream jobs in the competitive labor market, owned by the employee rather than the rehabilitation program, with regular pay at or above minimum wage and supervision by the employer. According to the federal definition, supported employment involves

> competitive work in integrated work settings . . . consistent with the strengths, resources, priorities, concerns, abilities, capabilities, interests, and informed choices of the individuals, for individuals with the most significant disabilities for whom competitive employment has not traditionally occurred; or for whom competitive employment has been interrupted or intermittent as a result of a significant disability.

Supported employment is provided in a wide variety of service contexts, including community mental health centers, community rehabilitation programs, clubhouses, and psychiatric rehabilitation centers. Although the evidence suggests that supported employment is optimally effective only when clients concurrently receive adequate mental health treatment, supported employment is not limited to a specific service model.

Several features of supported employment have been codified into a standardized approach called *Individual Placement and Support* (IPS). The principles of IPS evolve as research demonstrates how to improve employment outcomes. IPS is thus considered to be synonymous with evidence-based supported employment for persons with psychiatric disabilities. The IPS features of supported employment are as follows:

Competitive employment. The goal of supported employment is to aid patients in securing competitive employment in work settings integrated in a community's economy. The great majority of patients who seek a vocational program want competitive employment, particularly if they are encouraged to believe that they can work. If patients want volunteer work or education instead, they can be helped to achieve these goals using the same techniques. Few patients prefer sheltered jobs, unless they have been socialized into low expectations.

Rapid job search. Searching for jobs occurs early in the process of supported employment rather than after lengthy preemployment assessment, training, or work trials. In practice, this means focusing on a job search rapidly and typically finding a first job within 3 months.

Integration of rehabilitation and mental health. Vocational rehabilitation is considered an integral component of mental health treatment rather than a separate service. Optimally, employment specialists are integrated into multidisciplinary teams. The teams can be assertive community treatment teams or any other form of multidisciplinary team. The critical process is that employment specialists meet regularly with the multidisciplinary team and collaborate on helping the patients to achieve their goals for employment.

Patient preferences. Services are based on patients' preferences and choices rather than on providers' judgments. Patients are more satisfied and stay in jobs longer when the jobs are consistent with their preferences for employment. Programs that place all patients in similar jobs because the jobs are readily available do not have as much success.

Continuous and comprehensive assessment. Assessment occurs primarily in the course of community work experiences. Many schizophrenia patients have little work experience. Thus, the best way to understand their skills, needs, and motivation is to try part-time jobs in the community. As patients experience jobs, they learn more about their own preferences.

Ongoing support. Follow-along supports are tailored to the individual patient's needs and continued indefinitely. The multidisciplinary team provides a range of supports over time, with help from different members of the team as appropriate. Greater intensity of support is provided during times of crisis.

Existing supported employment programs for people with psychiatric disabilities subscribe to some or all of these principles, and research shows that programs with greater fidelity produce better employment outcomes. By 1995, a national survey identified 36,000 people with mental illness employed in supported employment positions. Since then, nearly all state mental health and vocational rehabilitation authorities have rapidly expanded supported employment programs.

Supported employment is usually provided by college graduates with some experience in human services and with supervision by a master's-level vocational specialist. The supported employment worker focuses specifically on vocational assessment, placement, and support, but the multidisciplinary team is involved throughout. The case manager encourages patients to try employment and usually provides access to employment services. The team psychiatrist is critical in communicating optimism regarding work; in making sure that the patient's symptoms, medications, and coping strategies are considered in developing an optimal job match; and, often, in adjusting medications when the patient goes to work. The entire team may help in finding a job and providing supports. For example, the case manager may help with problem solving related to interpersonal difficulties on the job, the social worker may help by meeting with the family to understand their concerns about employment, and the psychiatrist may provide extra medications to help with initial anxiety on the job or decrease medications to reduce side effects that interfere with working.

The key to a successful job is finding an optimal match; the job should fit the patient's interests, abilities, ways of coping with illness, needs regarding benefits, and other important features. Trying different jobs is often necessary to find the right job match. The following vignette illustrates a successful job match.

Antonio is a 45-year-old man who has been a client of a mental health agency for more than 10 years. He attended the rehabilitative day treatment program until it was converted to a supported employment program. His case manager encouraged him to think about the possibility of working part-time. Antonio told his case manager that he could not work because of his schizophrenia and because he was helping to raise his two kids and needed to be home at 3 PM, when they returned from school everyday. The case manager explained to Antonio that getting a job does not necessarily mean working 40 hours a week and that lots of people in the agency's supported employment program were working in part-time jobs, even jobs that only require a few hours a week.

Antonio agreed to meet one of the employment specialists to discuss the possibility of work. Over the next couple of weeks, the employment specialist met with Antonio several times, read his clinical record, and talked with his case manager and psychiatrist. The employment specialist learned that Antonio loved to drive his car. He also learned that Antonio had attendance problems in past jobs because he felt unappreciated. The employment specialist found Antonio to be a sociable and likable person.

Antonio told the employment specialist that he was willing to do any job. He did not have one specific job in mind. After discussing options with Antonio and with the team, the employment specialist suggested a job at Meals on Wheels as a driver for the lunch delivery. Antonio was hired and loved it right from the start. Absenteeism was never a problem, because he liked driving around and knew that people were counting on him for their meals. The hours were perfect (10 AM to 2 PM), so he could be at home when his kids returned from school. He became good friends with the other workers. He told his case manager that it was wonderful to be bringing home a paycheck again. And best of all, he said, was that his kids saw him going to work just like their friends' dads.

Research on Supported Employment Several findings from the recent research on vocational rehabilitation are consistent. First, supported employment interventions that focus on direct and individualized placements with follow-along supports are more effective than traditional approaches. There is no evidence that interventions that focus on preemployment skills training improve vocational outcomes of any kind, including type, quality, amount, length, and satisfaction related to employment. The role of skills training once the patient is in a job remains unclear, but many supported employment programs provide such training as part of follow-along support.

Second, the evidence favoring supported employment over other approaches to vocational rehabilitation is relatively sound. The research includes a series of studies showing that conversion of rehabilitative day centers to supported employment programs leads to higher rates of employment without negative outcomes. A number of randomized, controlled trials also show that supported employment produces better employment outcomes, including higher rates, earnings, hours, and tenure of competitive employment. These controlled studies demonstrate the following regarding supported employment: it is more effective than sheltered workshops and traditional rehabilitation programs, it is more effective when clients are enrolled immediately after referral instead of first receiving prevocational preparation, and it is more effective when provided by a single agency that combines clinical and vocational services than when the two services are provided by separate agencies. Moreover, the magnitude of the effect is substantial. For example, typical rates of employment are three times higher in supported employment programs than in the comparison conditions. These trials are summarized in Figure 12.13–1.

Third, all types of patients appear to have greater success in supported employment than in traditional vocational programs.

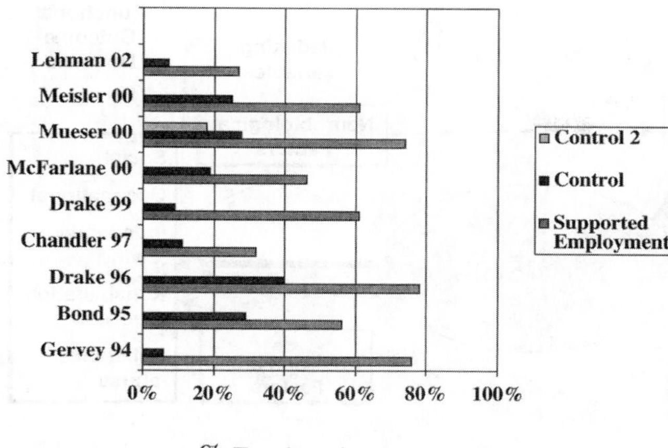

FIGURE 12.13–1 Randomized, controlled trials of supported employment.

Although survey data show that patients who enter supported employment programs are typical of other community mental health center patients, several subgroups have been studied. Patients with better vocational histories have greater success than do those with minimal work experience, but patients with poor vocational histories, nevertheless, have greater success in supported employment than in comparison programs. Controlled trials have also demonstrated that supported employment is effective with minority groups, specifically African-American and Latino patients, with dually diagnosed patients, and with inner city residents who have been recently homeless.

Fourth, although clinicians fear that high expectations will destabilize schizophrenia patients, there is no evidence that supported employment services produce clinical instability, higher rates of relapse, or other untoward outcomes. Conversely, patients who are currently in competitive employment appear to benefit in numerous ways and report higher satisfaction with services, better self-esteem, and greater quality of life. One study showed that patients who worked consistently (more than half of the months) during an 18-month project were improved in several other areas of adjustment, whereas similar patients who worked the same amount in sheltered settings showed no improvements in any of these areas.

Fifth, there is evidence that supported employment is effective for typical patients, in large programs, and in large service systems. For example, a number of mental health centers have increased their rate of competitive employment for patients with severe and persistent mental illness (mostly schizophrenia patients) from less than 10 to 40 percent or more and sustained these improvements over years, and several states have successfully shifted their state-wide system of vocational services toward supported employment.

Despite the success of supported employment, several concerns have been raised. For example, critics question whether jobs obtained through supported employment are good jobs, have reasonable job tenure, lead to careers, and really enable people to get off benefits. They also question what happens to patients who do not succeed in supported employment. Most of the research on supported employment is unfortunately limited by relatively short-term follow-ups. Nevertheless, there is evidence that patients themselves express high satisfaction with the jobs and stay in first jobs for 4 to 6 months, which is typical of the general population starting first jobs. More important, three long-term follow-up studies (4 to 12 years) indicate that initial high employment rates and satisfaction with supported employment are maintained over time. However, only a small minority of patients get off benefits completely. New regulations, such as legislation that allows patients to purchase extensions of their Medicaid insurance, may impact benefits. More longitudinal research is critical.

Social Skills Rehabilitation

Social dysfunction is a defining characteristic of schizophrenia. People with the illness have difficulty fulfilling social roles, such as worker, spouse, and friend, and have difficulty meeting their needs when social interaction is required (e.g., negotiating with merchants, requesting assistance to solve problems). Social dysfunction is semi-independent of symptomatology and plays an important role in the course and outcome of the illness. As shown in Table 12.13–1, social competence is based on three component skills: (1) social perception, or receiving skills; (2) social cognition, or processing skills; and (3) behavioral response, or expressive skills. Social perception is the ability to accurately read or decode social inputs. This includes accurate detection of affect cues, such as facial expressions and nuances of voice, gesture, and body posture, as well as verbal content and contextual information. Social cognition involves effective analysis of the social stimulus, integration of current information with historical information, and planning of an effective response. This domain is also referred to as *social problem solving*.

Behavioral response or expressive skills include the ability to generate effective verbal content, speak with appropriate paralin-

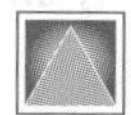

Table 12.13–1
Components of Social Skill

Expressive behaviors
- Speech content
- Paralinguistic features
  - Voice volume
  - Speech rate
  - Pitch
  - Intonation
- Nonverbal behaviors
  - Eye contact (gaze)
  - Posture
  - Facial expression
  - Proxemics
  - Kinesics

Receptive skills (social perception)
- Attention to and interpretation of relevant cues
- Emotion recognition

Processing skills
- Analysis of the demands of the situation
- Incorporation of relevant contextual information
- Social problem solving

Interactive behaviors
- Response timing
- Use of social reinforcers
- Turn taking

Situational factors
- Social "intelligence" (knowledge of social mores and the demands of the specific situation)

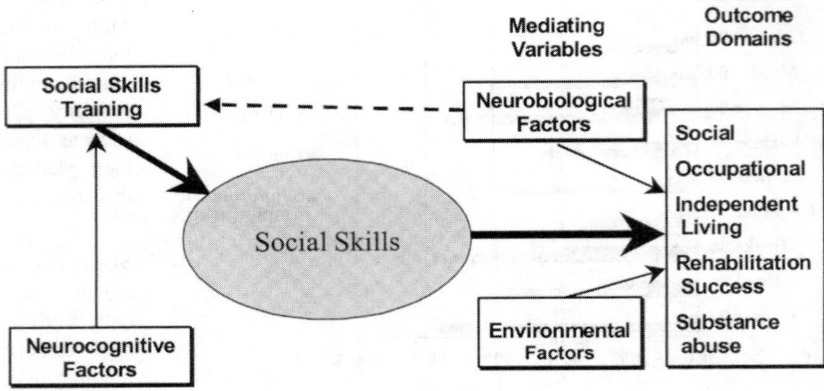

FIGURE 12.13–2 A model of the role of social skills, social skills training, and mediators on functional outcomes.

guistic characteristics, and use suitable nonverbal behaviors, such as facial expression, gestures, and posture. Effective social behavior requires the smooth integration of these three component processes so as to meet the demands of the specific social situation. Effective social behavior also involves more macrolevel response styles, including turn taking and provision of social reinforcement.

The term *skill* is used to emphasize that social competence is based on a set of learned abilities rather than traits, needs, or other intrapsychic processes. Conversely, ineffective social behavior is often the result of social skill deficits. Many elemental aspects of social skill, such as sharing and turn taking, are learned in childhood, whereas more complex behavioral repertoires, such as dating and job interview skills, are generally acquired in adolescence and young adulthood. Some elements of social competence, such as the perception of facial expressions of affect, are probably genetically hardwired at birth. Nevertheless, research suggests that virtually all social behaviors can be modified by experience or training.

Social dysfunction is hypothesized to result from three circumstances: when individuals do not know how to perform appropriately, when they do not use skills in their repertoire when they are called for, and when appropriate behavior is undermined by socially inappropriate behavior. Each of these circumstances appears to be common in schizophrenia. First, there is good reason to believe that people with schizophrenia do not learn key social skills. Children who later develop schizophrenia in adulthood have been found to have subtle attention deficits in childhood that may interfere with the development of social relationships and the acquisition of basic social skills. Second, schizophrenia often strikes first in late adolescence or young adulthood, a critical period for mastery of adult social roles and skills, such as dating and sexual behaviors, work-related skills, and the ability to form and maintain adult relationships. Third, many individuals with schizophrenia gradually develop isolated lives punctuated by periods in psychiatric hospitals or community residences. Such events remove clients from their "normal" peer group, provide few opportunities to engage in age appropriate social roles, and limit social contacts to mental health staff and other severely ill clients. Under such circumstances, people with schizophrenia do not have the opportunity to acquire and practice appropriate adult roles. Moreover, skills mastered earlier in life may be lost due to disuse or lack of reinforcement by the environment during periods of chronic illness. Fourth, cognitive impairment is a relatively universal feature of schizophrenia and is associated with deficits in social cognition, including social perception and social problem solving. One area of cognitive dysfunction that appears to be of particular relevance is difficulty with the integration of contextual information, or the ability to see the relevance of previous experience to current events and use experience to guide future behavior. This disability makes it difficult for people with the illness to adjust their behavior to situational demands and prior social experiences.

Social skill deficits are widespread, albeit not ubiquitous, in people with schizophrenia and tend to be relatively stable over time. They are also resistant to treatment with antipsychotics, including new-generation medications. This is not surprising, given that social dysfunction results, in part, from failure to acquire critical skills in childhood and early adulthood, from social isolation and withdrawal, and from environmental pressures, rather than from discrete problems in neurotransmitter systems.

Social Skills Training As illustrated in Figure 12.13–2, social skills are hypothesized to play a major role in functional outcomes domains, although other factors influence community functioning as well. The model also postulates that skill deficits can be reduced with a structured behavioral intervention called *social skills training*. The basic technology for teaching social skills was developed in the 1970s and has not changed substantially in the intervening years. Based on social learning principles, social skills training emphasizes the role of behavioral rehearsal in skill development rather than discussion. The training process is more analogous to the way motor skill would be taught, as opposed to the conversational interactions typical of psychotherapy. Complex social repertoires, such as making friends and dating, are first broken down into discrete steps or component elements, analogous to the way a music teacher would break a difficult piece of music into simpler segments. For example, initiating conversations requires first gaining the other person's attention via introductory remarks, asking general questions, following up with specific questions, and sharing information with first-person statements. Nonverbal and paralinguistic behaviors are similarly segmented. Patients are first taught to perform the elements and then gradually learn to smoothly combine them through shaping and reinforcement of successive approximations.

The primary modality of social skills training is role play of simulated conversations. The trainer first provides instructions on how to perform the skill and then models the behavior to demonstrate how it is performed. After identifying a relevant social situation in which the skill might be used, the patient engages in role play with the trainer. The trainer next provides feedback and positive reinforcement, which are followed by suggestions for how the response can be improved. The sequence of role play followed by feedback and reinforcement is repeated until the patient can perform the response adequately. Training is typically conducted in small groups (six to eight patients), in which case patients each practice role playing for three to four trials and provide feedback and reinforcement to one another. Teaching is tailored to the individual—for example, a highly impaired group member might simply practice saying no to a simple request, whereas a less cognitively impaired peer might learn to negotiate and compromise.

The content of training programs is organized into curricula, such as job interview skills, medication management skills (how to communicate with health care providers), dating skills, and assertion skills. Duration of training can range from four to eight sessions for a very circumscribed program, such as safe sex skills, to 6 months to 2 years for a comprehensive program including conversation skills, making friends, soliciting help, assertiveness, and dealing with problems in group living situations. Regardless of duration, training sessions are typically held three to five times per week. As with acquiring any skill, the less frequent or more dispersed the sessions, the greater the loss or forgetting of skill between sessions. Training is structured so as to minimize demands on neurocognitive capacity. Extensive use is made of audiovisual aides, with instructions presented in handouts and on flip charts or white boards, as well as delivered orally. Material is presented in brief units, there is frequent repetition and review, and patients are required to verbalize instructions and express plans (what the person will say) before engaging in role play. An attempt is made to produce overlearning so that responses can be elicited relatively automatically in the environment (i.e., with minimum demand on analytical and problem solving skills). Individuals delivering social skills training are generally bachelor's- or master's-level clinical staff, and two therapists are employed whenever possible (one person directs the session, and the second serves as role play partner).

Richard M. was a single, white man first diagnosed with schizophrenia at age 22, when he was a freshman at college. He was hospitalized briefly but was unable to return to school and moved back home with his parents. He attended a day treatment program intermittently over the next 6 years, before he was referred for help with getting a job and dating.

Richard had missed out on a critical period of adult development and had never learned dating skills or the social skills needed to get or maintain a job. He was appropriately groomed and did not present himself as a patient, but he seemed quite uncomfortable in social interactions. He scarcely made eye contact, staring at the floor when he spoke, and did not initiate conversation, responding to questions with brief answers.

Richard was invited to participate in a social skills training group for 3 months with six other patients. The focus of the group was employment skills. Patients were taught critical social skills for getting and maintaining a job, such as how to participate in job interviews; how to approach a supervisor to understand how to do a job or for help with work-related problems; how and when to make requests or explain problems, such as getting to work late because of traffic or needing to leave early to go to a doctor's appointment; and socializing with coworkers. Simultaneously, Richard was enrolled in a supported employment program and worked with a case manager to find a job as a computer support person. He found a 24-hours-per-week job at a small company and continued to attend the skills group, using the sessions to work on interpersonal issues at work, including engaging in casual conversation with coworkers and dealing with unreasonable requests from people.

When the vocational skills group ended, Richard was scheduled for a dating group with seven other male and female patients who had similar interests. This group focused on finding someone to date, dating etiquette, asking someone out (or being asked out), appropriate conversation for dates, sexual interactions, and safe sex practices. In addition to role play and discussion, the group shared ideas on how to meet people and what to do on dates.

Richard responded well to treatment. He had maintained the computer job at follow-up, 6 months after he concluded the dating skills group. His case manger also reported that he had a girlfriend, a woman that he had met at his church group. He had also expressed an interest in enrolling in college classes at night. He was still living at home with his parents, but, for the first time, was seriously considering what he would need to do to move out.

Research on Social Skills Training The basic social skills training strategy was refined and validated in a number of single case studies and small group designs conducted in the 1970s and 1980s. These early reports were followed by a series of randomized, controlled trials that have provided a clearer picture of areas in which social skills training is and is not effective.

The specific skills training program that has been most widely studied is the University of California, Los Angeles (UCLA), Social and Independent Living Skills Program. This program was designed for ease of dissemination and includes carefully crafted videotapes and instruction manuals for both trainers and patients. Training involves standard skills training techniques (e.g., role play, modeling) and includes modules (curricula) covering seven areas: medication management, symptom management, recreation for leisure, conversation skills, substance abuse management, workplace fundamentals, and community reentry (skills for the transition from inpatient to outpatient environments).

One carefully conducted study compared 1 year of intensive group social skills training to supportive group therapy, in the context of a low-dose pharmacotherapy trial. Social skills training consisted of two modules from the UCLA program (medication management and symptom management) administered twice a week for 6 months, followed by once-per-week skills training. There were highly significant differences favoring the social skills training group at the end of training, and these were maintained for a 1-year follow-up. Both groups manifested improvements in symptomatology. The pharmacotherapy component of the trial consisted of low-dose fluphenazine decanoate (Prolixin) supplemented by either oral fluphenazine or placebo during prodromes. Social skills training produced significantly greater improvement in social role functioning than did supportive group therapy, especially for subjects who received active drug supplementation. Social skills training also decreased the risk of relapse among subjects receiving placebo.

One of the critical questions about social skills training concerns transfer of training, or generalization of newly learned skills to the community. There is scant evidence for spontaneous generalization from office-based training to the community, consistent with the behavioral aphorism that generalization must be programmed. That is, treatment must bridge the gap between office-based training and the community by systematically prompting and reinforcing desired behavior or by engaging significant others in the community to do so, or both. One creative study examined this premise by supplementing office-based training with community-based case management to encourage patients to use their newly acquired skills. Subjects were randomly assigned to 6 months of social skills training or occupational therapy each, followed by 18 months of follow-up case management.

Over the 2-year trial, social skills training produced significantly greater improvements than occupational therapy in independent living skills in the community, although the differences tended to decrease after the 6-month active treatment phase ended.

The case management approach has been refined with an intervention called in vivo amplified skills training (IVAST), which combines standard skills training with intensive case management. The case manager helps support completion of homework assignments, identifies and reinforces opportunities to use trained skills, and establishes links with support systems (e.g., significant others) in the community to reinforce use of newly learned skills. Examples of case management activities include helping a patient to make a doctor's appointment, to use public transportation, and to attend social activities. IVAST requires careful assessment of individual skills and needs and the extent to which the living environment is concordant with the patient's capacity to succeed. The case manager/trainer helps develop skills and shape the environment as needed, rather than putting the onus for success on the patient. One study compared 60 weeks of office-based skills training to IVAST, which supplemented the office-based training with weekly sessions in the community. Subjects were randomly assigned to one of the two skills conditions, and half of each psychosocial group was randomly assigned to receive either risperidone (Risperdal) or haloperidol (Haldol). There were significant increases in social functioning for both skills training conditions, but IVAST resulted in greater and more rapid improvement. There were no medication effects or medication by skills training interactions, consistent with previous studies indicating that even effective antipsychotic treatment does not substantially affect social functioning in the community. These two studies suggest that IVAST is a promising new approach that warrants further investigation by other research groups.

Neurocognitive impairment is relatively universal among people with schizophrenia, and there is good evidence that these cognitive factors influence social functioning. A number of studies have also demonstrated that cognitive impairment influences performance in social skills training, including verbal memory, executive functioning, and vigilance. Skills training techniques are designed to minimize the demands on cognitive capacity so that most patients can benefit from training. However, patients with significant deficits in memory, executive functioning, or attention learn more slowly than patients with more moderate cognitive impairment and have difficulty acquiring more complex skills. The goals and pace of training sessions are typically adjusted to accommodate for differences in learning capacity, but an alternative approach that has sparked considerable interest is to combine skills training with cognitive remediation strategies.

Integrated psychological therapy (IPT) is a multistage intervention that provides core training in cognitive skills and social perception that are thought to be prerequisites for effective social functioning before moving on to more prototypical skills training strategies. Training is conducted in a small-group format for 6 months or longer and consists of a variety of structured exercises designed to give patients practice in reasoning, verbal memory, social problem solving, and social perception in a reinforcing social context. A series of studies has provided modest support for the IPT program, but the value of the cognitive training per se has been unclear.

There have been numerous reviews of the social skills training literature since 1990. The literature is limited by wide variability in methodology, outcome criteria, assessment instruments, and subject populations in different trials, but nearly all reviews have concluded that social skills training is substantially effective. The main areas of agreement are on the following points.

First, social skills training is not substantially effective for reducing symptoms or preventing relapse. Social skills training may affect these domains indirectly by teaching skills that help to reduce social failures that would otherwise cause sufficient stress to precipitate exacerbations of symptoms, but social skills training is basically a targeted treatment that can achieve important social outcomes when applied in conjunction with other critical interventions, including pharmacotherapy, case management, and substance abuse treatment, as well as environmental supports, such as housing.

Second, social skills training is clearly effective in increasing the use of specific social behaviors and improving functioning in the specific domains that are the primary focus of the treatment. Social skills training techniques have become a standard component of interventions for a variety of behavioral problems in which social skills are a component, such as teaching patients to start a conversation, teaching substance abusers how to refuse drugs, and teaching people at risk for human immunodeficiency virus (HIV) how to negotiate for safe sex.

Third, social skills training has a positive impact on social role functioning, although the findings for this outcome domain are not entirely consistent. The most critical question about social skills training, which has not been clearly answered, is the extent to which learning in the clinic translates into either specific behavioral changes or generally improved role functioning in the community.

Fourth, social skills training appears to have a positive effect on satisfaction and self-efficacy. Patients feel more self-confident in social situations after training.

Substance Abuse Rehabilitation

Substance use disorder (which includes abuse or dependence on alcohol or other drugs and is often termed *substance abuse*) is the most common and clinically significant comorbidity with schizophrenia. Approximately 50 percent of adults with schizophrenia have cooccurring substance abuse and are therefore considered dually diagnosed (although most have multiple diagnoses rather than just two disorders). Substance use disorders complicate their lives in myriad ways, leading to increased symptoms, relapses, hospitalizations, violence, incarceration, unstable housing, homelessness, victimization, family problems, and serious medical problems, such as HIV and hepatitis.

In the early 1980s, along with recognition of the problem of dual diagnosis in community-based systems of care, clinicians and researchers discerned that parallel treatment in which the patient was expected to go back and forth between mental health providers and substance abuse providers in separate agencies and systems was ineffective, because few patients were able to negotiate relationships in two systems and integrate treatment recommendations from separate providers. Commonly, patients were excluded from, dropped out of, or extruded from one or both treatment systems. For example, patients were often ineligible for housing in substance abuse programs because they were taking psychotropic medications for their mental illness and dismissed from mental health housing programs because they were using alcohol or street drugs.

Dual Diagnosis Programs

Efforts also began in the 1980s to combine, or integrate, mental health and substance abuse interventions for people with dual disorders. Clinical programs have evolved rapidly as more has been learned about helping people with dual, or cooccurring, disorders recover from their substance use disorders. Several features of integrated dual diagnosis treatment are associated with better outcomes and thus are considered evidence-based principles. These principles are as follows:

Integration. All of the recent studies support the basic notion of combining, or integrating, mental health and substance abuse interventions. *Integration* means that one clinician or team takes responsibility for helping the patient learn to manage and recover from both illnesses. Mental health and substance abuse interventions are not only combined, but also specifically tailored to fit persons with cooccurring disorders. The patient does not have to travel to different programs, resolve the inconsistencies of conflicting messages, or relate to independent clinicians. Integration must occur at the level of clinical interaction—the communication between practitioner and patient. It does not mean that programs or systems of care exchange memoranda of agreement. System-level or agency-level integration is not sufficient to impact patient outcomes. Most programs accomplish integration by establishing multidisciplinary teams, which include substance abuse treatment experts, mental health experts, and others with expertise in housing, vocational services, and so on.

Stage-wise interventions. Effective programs incorporate the concept of stages of treatment. In the simplest conceptualization, stages of treatment include (1) engaging the patient in a trusting relationship, (2) helping the engaged patient develop the motivation to pursue recovery, (3) helping the motivated patient to acquire skills and supports for controlling illnesses and pursuing personal goals, and (4) helping the patient in stable remission to develop and use strategies for preventing relapses.

Rather than moving linearly through stages, patients sometimes enter services at advanced levels, sometimes skip over or pass rapidly through stages, and often relapse to earlier stages. Moreover, they may be in different stages with respect to recovery from mental illness and from substance abuse. Nevertheless, the concept of stages has proven useful to program planners and clinicians, because patients at different stages respond to different stage-specific interventions. For example, patients at the engagement stage typically need attention given to basic needs and to establishing a relationship with a clinician, whereas abstinence-oriented group interventions are appropriate and central for patients in the active treatment stage.

Assertive outreach. Many dually diagnosed patients have difficulty in accessing services and participating consistently in treatment. Effective programs therefore provide assertive outreach, usually through some combination of intensive case management, meetings in the patient's residence, and social network interventions. For example, homeless persons with dual diagnosis often benefit from outreach, from help with housing and other basic needs, and from time to develop a trusting relationship before formal treatment. These approaches often enable them to engage in and maintain needed relationships with a consistent provider over months and years.

Motivational interventions. The majority of dual diagnosis patients have little readiness for abstinence-oriented treatment. Many also have given up attempts to manage their psychiatric illnesses or to pursue education, employment, or other personal goals, because they are discouraged and overwhelmed by two chronic illnesses. To counter these problems, effective programs incorporate motivational interventions that are designed to help develop readiness for more definitive interventions aimed at illness self-management. For example, patients who are so demoralized, symptomatic, or confused that they mistakenly believe that alcohol and cocaine are helping them cope better than medications do require education, support, and counseling to develop hope and a realistic understanding of illnesses, drugs, treatments, and goals. Motivational interventions involve helping individuals to identify their own goals and then to recognize, through a systematic examination of ambivalence, that not managing their illnesses interferes with attaining those goals.

Counseling. Once patients become motivated to manage their own illnesses, they need to develop skills and supports to control symptoms and to pursue an abstinent lifestyle. Effective programs provide some form of counseling that promotes cognitive and behavioral skills at this stage. The counseling takes different forms and formats (e.g., group, individual, family, or a combination). These approaches often incorporate motivational sessions at the beginning of counseling and, as needed, in subsequent sessions rather than as separate interventions.

Social support interventions. In addition to helping the patient build skills for illness self-management and pursuit of goals, effective programs also focus on strengthening the immediate social environment to help the patient modify behavior. These activities, which recognize the role of social networks in recovery from dual diagnosis, comprise peer group, social network, or family interventions. Different group interventions can be effective, provided the patient attends consistently, suggesting that the social support, rather than the specific model of treatment, may be the critical component.

Long-term perspective. Effective programs recognize that recovery tends to occur over months or years. People with severe mental illness and substance abuse do not usually develop stability and functional improvements quickly, even in intensive treatment programs, unless they enter treatment at an advanced stage. Instead, they tend to improve over months and years, in conjunction with a consistent dual diagnosis program. Effective programs therefore take a long-term, community-based perspective that includes rehabilitation activities to prevent relapses and enhance gains. For patients who do not respond to treatment in the community, long-term residential care is often used.

Comprehensiveness. Learning to lead a symptom-free, abstinent lifestyle that is satisfying and sustainable typically requires transforming many aspects of one's life (i.e., habits, ways of managing stress, friends, activities, and housing). Therefore, effective programs address substance abuse and mental illness in all aspects of the program and service system rather than as a discrete substance abuse treatment intervention. Inpatient hospitalization, assessment, crisis intervention, medication management, money management, laboratory screening, housing, and vocational rehabilitation incorporate special features that are tailored specifically for dual diagnosis. For example, housing and vocational programs can be used to support the dually diagnosed individual in acquiring skills and supports needed for recovery.

Raymond was a single, 26-year-old African-American man with schizophrenia and polydrug addiction. After becoming ill in his mid-teens, he dropped out of high school, lost contact with his family, and ended up homeless in a large eastern city. He rarely used medications and did not comply with outpatient treatment. Increasingly, his only sober time was during brief stays in jail after arrests for minor crimes. He had been assaulted on the streets many times.

Raymond was assigned to a new assertive community treatment team after a brief hospitalization and detoxification. Team members approached Raymond in shelters and on the streets. He initially refused medications and treatment, but he was glad to have the help in finding housing and getting back on Social Security benefits and Medicaid insurance. Team members gradually formed a trusting relationship with

Raymond over the course of several hospitalizations, arrests, and detoxifications. He agreed to take medications, which the team delivered each day to his apartment. When Raymond became less psychotic, he agreed to have someone else manage his money until he could learn the skills to do so, live in a residential program for people with dual disorders, and try employment. As he gradually improved, despite several relapses of substance abuse, he was helped to find a part-time job as a groundskeeper in a local cemetery, to develop sober friends through dual diagnosis and Narcotics Anonymous (NA) groups, and to reconnect with his family for weekly telephone conversations. After 3 years with the assertive community treatment team, Raymond reported that he was much happier leading an abstinent life and having friends he could trust and a job that he was proud of.

Research on Dual Diagnosis Programs Beginning in the mid-1990s, controlled research studies of comprehensive dual diagnosis programs began to appear. Although these studies demonstrate a variety of positive outcomes, they are also limited by serious methodological problems, including inconsistency of interventions, heterogeneity of patients, difficulties with measures, variable lengths of follow-up, small samples, failure to engage patients, high attrition, and treatment drift.

Table 12.13–2 shows a summary of the recent controlled studies, including design, participants, interventions, and outcomes. This table includes true experiments (randomized studies) and quasi-experiments (controlled studies with nonequivalent comparison groups). Because most of these studies take place in the context of comprehensive mental health services, this table focuses on substance abuse treatment components and on substance abuse as an outcome.

Several features of these 11 studies warrant attention. First, there are few true experiments, and the true experiments have limitations, such as those described above. Second, eight studies address comprehensive outpatient programs, and three address residential programs. Even among the outpatient and residential studies, however, there is little consistency of specific experimental interventions or of control group interventions. Thus, no two studies are strictly comparable.

Third, the participants in most of these studies are heterogeneous diagnostically with respect to mental illness diagnoses, substance abuse diagnoses, treatment history, and other important characteristics, such as motivational level. Heterogeneity can, of course, easily obscure outcomes.

Fourth, because dual diagnosis patients are difficult to engage and retain in treatment, attrition was high in many studies. Studies that included assertive outreach tended to have much better retention in treatment and research.

Fifth, studies examined various aspects of substance abuse, using a variety of measures. Compared with non–mentally ill substance abusers, patients with cooccurring disorders tend to use smaller amounts of substances, have different consequences of their use, and have less of the physiological syndrome of dependence. These distinctions render traditional instruments less useful, but few new instruments have been validated, and a consensus has not yet developed on how best to assess substance use in dually diagnosed patients. Nevertheless, the relatively consistent finding is that the experimental groups do better on at least one substance abuse outcome (and usually on other outcomes, such as hospitalization, not shown in Table 12.13–2), whereas the control or comparison groups never do better and often do worse on a variety of outcomes.

Given the complexity and noncomparability of studies, any consistent findings are remarkable. The most consistent finding is that programs with greater integration of mental health and substance abuse interventions tend to have better outcomes. However, few other specific elements are consistent across studies. In fact, because of heterogeneity and other design problems, it is impossible at this point to say that any specific intervention is effective for dual diagnosis patients. This was the conclusion of an earlier Cochrane review that considered only the most rigorous studies. Such a conclusion ignores the principle of evidence-based medicine that clinicians should use the best available evidence within a hierarchy of evidence. It also ignores the observation that several principles of care are consistent across many successful dual diagnosis programs. Thus, an alternative interpretation is that, while interventions are refined and until research on specific interventions and combinations is available, the existing evidence should be used to abstract principles of dual diagnosis programs that appear to be effective. Taking this approach, the several principles of dual diagnosis treatment that were outlined earlier can be identified.

Cognitive Rehabilitation

Increased recognition of the prevalence and importance of neurocognitive deficits over the last decade has stimulated increasing interest in remediation strategies. Much of the work in this area has focused on psychopharmacological approaches, especially on the new-generation antipsychotics. New-generation medications appear to have a positive effect on neurocognitive test performance, but the effect size for any of the medications is small to medium, and there is little evidence that these medications have a clinically meaningful impact on neurocognitive functioning in the community. As a result, there has been a parallel interest in the potential for psychosocial approaches, referred to alternately as *cognitive rehabilitation* or *cognitive remediation*. This body of work is distinguished from cognitive-behavioral therapy and cognitive therapy, which focus on reducing psychotic symptoms.

Two reports in the late 1980s rekindled interest in the possibility of cognitive rehabilitation. One study, discussed earlier, attempted to combine cognitive training with higher-level social skills training in IPT. This innovative work has had tremendous heuristic value.

A second study at the National Institutes of Health (NIH) found that patients with schizophrenia were unable to benefit from explicit instructions and practice on the Wisconsin Card Sorting Test (WCST), a widely used test of executive functioning. The study was linked to data demonstrating that patients had diminished prefrontal blood flow in dorsolateral prefrontal cortex while responding to the WCST, implying that schizophrenia was marked by an unmodifiable abnormality of the dorsolateral prefrontal cortex. The NIH work stimulated a series of mostly successful laboratory demonstrations that WCST performance deficits, albeit widespread, are neither endemic to the illness nor immutable. For example, one study demonstrated that WCST performance could be enhanced by financial reinforcement and specific instructions. Other laboratories have since produced comparable and enduring effects using similar training strategies and extended practice alone.

Cognitive remediation strategies have since been shown to improve performance on other measures of information processing as well, including so-called trait markers, such as span of apprehension, that were assumed to be stable characteristics of the illness. One study provided subjects with extensive practice on a motor dexterity task and either a visual reading task or a dot spatial memory task. Improved performance was gradually shaped over 10 weeks. A majority of subjects reached normative levels on the reading and dot tasks, and most showed improvement on the dexterity task as well. Other studies have produced modest improvements on a variety of

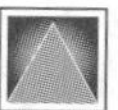

Table 12.13–2
Recent Controlled Studies of Dual Diagnosis Interventions

Study	Design	Participants	Interventions	Outcomes
Godley et al., 1994	Experiment, treatment for 2 yrs	N = 38 dual diagnosis patients	Integrated intensive case management plus substance abuse counseling vs. nonintegrated services	Intensive case management group had fewer days of drug use.
Jerrell and Ridgely, 1995	Quasi-experiment, treatment for 18 mos	N = 132 dual diagnosis patients	Behavioral skills training vs. 12-step counseling: case management vs. 12-step counseling	Behavioral skills training group had fewer substance abuse symptoms than 12-step group.
Drake et al., 1997	Quasi-experiment, treatment for 18 mos	N = 217 homeless, dual diagnosis patients	Integrated intensive case management, substance abuse counseling, and housing supports vs. nonintegrated services	Integrated treatment group had greater treatment progress and greater reductions in alcohol severity.
Carmichael et al., 1998	Experiment in 2 sites: quasi-experiment in 1 site	N = 208 dual diagnosis patients	Integrated mental health and substance abuse treatment vs. nonintegrated treatment	Integrated treatment group had greater improvement in alcohol abuse and drug abuse.
Ho et al., 1998	Quasi-experiment, 6-mo treatment intervals	N = 179 dual diagnosis patients	Integrated day treatment plus assertive community treatment and skills training vs. integrated day treatment	The group with enhanced assertive community treatment and skills training had greater rates of abstinence.
Drake et al., 1998	Experiment, treatment for 3 yrs	N = 203 dual diagnosis patients	Integrated assertive community treatment plus substance abuse counseling vs. nonintegrated services	Integrated treatment group had greater treatment progress and decreased alcohol severity.
Kasprow et al., 1999	Quasi-experiment, outcome at discharge after several yrs of residential treatment	N = 385 dually diagnosed veterans	Residential treatment facilities that specialized in integrated mental health and substance abuse treatment vs. similar residential facilities that specialized in substance abuse treatment	Patients in integrated treatment had faster return to independent community living but no differences in substance abuse outcomes.
McHugo et al., 1999	Quasi-experiment, treatment for 3 yrs	N = 87 dual diagnosis patients	Assertive community treatment teams with high fidelity for dual diagnosis treatment vs. similar teams with low fidelity	Patients in high-fidelity programs had greater reductions in alcohol and drug use and higher rates of substance abuse remission.
Brunette et al., 2001	Quasi-experiment	N = 86 dual diagnosis patients, follow-up 1 yr after residential treatment	Long-term integrated mental health and substance abuse residential treatment (average, 400 days) vs. short-term integrated residential treatment (average, 66 days)	Patients discharged from long-term programs were more likely to maintain abstinence.
Barraclough et al., 2001	Experiment, treatment for 9 mos	N = 36 patients with schizophrenia and substance abuse	Motivational counseling, family psychoeducation, and cognitive behavioral therapy vs. usual services	Experimental group had more days of abstinence.
Aguilera et al., 2001	Quasi-experiment	N = 225 dual diagnosis patients	Residential treatment with integrated mental health and substance abuse interventions vs. residential treatment with substance abuse focus	Integrated treatment group had more successful program completers and less recidivism, but substance abuse outcomes not reported.

attention tasks using practice, shaping, and errorless learning, a behavioral strategy designed to minimize failure.

These laboratory studies involve brief trials designed to demonstrate that cognitive performance could be enhanced, not to show clinically significant changes in performance. However, a recent review of the literature identified 15 studies in which the duration and intensity of training were sufficient to produce a clinical impact. Most of these clinical investigations examined the impact of training on measures that were independent of tasks used in training, whereas the laboratory trials primarily demonstrated change on the same neurocognitive tests used in training or on close parallels. Length of training ranged from 5 weeks to 5 months, with multiple training sessions per week. The targets of training have included verbal memory, problem solving and executive functions, attention, social perception, and work performance. Some studies focused narrowly on single cognitive domains, whereas others targeted a range of functions. Training strategies have similarly been quite diverse, including self-guided practice on computer tasks that mirror neurocognitive tests, self-guided practice on commercially produced educational materials, intensive individual training using paper-and-pencil neurocognitive test materials, and small group discussions and naturalistic rehearsal of social cognition. Overall, the data are promising, with most studies generating small to medium effect sizes.

Several representative studies illustrate key points and warrant comment. One study of cognitive remediation therapy, an intervention that focuses on executive functioning (i.e., cognitive flexibility, working memory, and planning), used a sophisticated training model based on principles of errorless learning, targeted reinforcement, and guided practice on cognitive tasks administered in one-on-one therapy sessions. Training media included paper-and-pencil games and neurocognitive tests. A preliminary trial yielded improvement on several neuropsychological measures and modest retention of training effects over a 6-month follow-up interval. A companion neuroimaging study demonstrated meaningful changes in cortical activation among a subgroup of patients who responded positively to the intervention, suggesting that the effects may extend beyond simple practice-related improvements on training tasks. A limitation of this program is that it uses a highly tailored individual treatment model and demands high levels of therapist skill to slowly shape patient behavior. However, the focus on executive functioning and the carefully thought out training/teaching strategy warrant further study, especially if a small group version can be developed.

An alternative approach capitalizes on the ease of standardization and flexibility provided by computer software. One study reported positive results for a program that provided self-directed practice on basic attention, memory, and reasoning tasks (e.g., visual tracking, list learning, pyramids). The emphasis was on repetitive practice of elementary neurocognitive skills (working memory, attention) that are assumed to be the basis for higher-level cognitive processes. There was minimal teaching/training; patients primarily engaged in self-guided practice at a computer. Results from this study indicate significant changes in several domains of neurocognition. However, cognitive rehabilitation was integrated into a supported work program, and patients were paid for hours spent on the computer tasks, which may limit generalizability, because patients may not be willing to participate without financial remuneration.

Another cognitive remediation approach, the neuropsychological educational approach to remediation (NEAR), uses commercially available educational software. The tasks are more like games than repetitive exercises and, therefore, are interesting to many subjects. They have built-in feedback mechanisms to guide performance, and difficulty level can be tailored to the individual. The tasks all require the use of multiple cognitive processes, with an emphasis on higher-order executive functions. The intervention is administered in an open classroom format in which patients attend on an ad lib basis, select tasks they are interested in working on each day, and move at their own pace. The approach emphasizes self-guided practice, rather than structured training, to foster intrinsic motivation for learning and allow patients to enhance their preferred problem-solving styles.

The contrast between self-guided practice and the intensive teaching approach underscores several major questions facing the field. First, can cognitive impairment best be considered a problem of reduced capacity, or is it a problem of downstream integration? That is, do patients have limited attention or working memory stores that make it impossible to perform higher-level cognitive tasks, or are there problems in neurocircuitry that prevent the smooth integration of attentional inputs and memory traces? A related question is whether the problem is primarily in basic functions, such as attention and working memory, or in higher-order processing, such as executive functioning. Of course, both problems could apply to different groups of patients and both could be present in the same patients. To the extent that the impairment involves reduced attentional or working memory capacity, repetitive practice might be sufficient to enhance functioning. To the extent that it is a failure in problem solving or reasoning, it seems likely that teaching would play a critical role.

If the problem is more in the domain of downstream integration of inputs, it is not clear how one would proceed to improve functioning. In fact, data from neuroimaging studies suggest that patients use inefficient neurocognitive operations and are unable to use appropriate (i.e., normal) neural circuits to perform cognitive tasks. For example, when faced with difficult working reasoning or working memory tasks, patients tend to show diffuse increases in cerebral blood flow in several areas of the brain, whereas healthy controls tend to have blood flow increases solely in frontal regions. It is as if patients are unable to focus their cognitive resources in brain regions that are critical for good task performance. Consequently, practice on elementary functions, with or without training, may improve performance on the specific task practiced, but it may not be sufficient to normalize functioning or lead to transferable gains. Conversely, training on higher-order functions may not increase efficiency. One study showed that cerebral activation on a control task increased among patients who did well in their remediation program, whereas it decreased among normal controls on retesting. These data could suggest that patients might have learned to compensate for their impairment by using more effort to do the task or by using different brain regions than those used by nonpatients.

A more general question concerns the potential for cognitive change. The rehearsal-only approaches assume something akin to an exercise model of neurocognitive function, which may not accurately reflect the neurodevelopmental nature of schizophrenia and the uncertain malleability of the adult brain. A compensatory approach that capitalizes on existing strengths, teaches new strategies for meeting cognitive demands, and uses environmental supports may be more appropriate. An example of a compensatory approach is cognitive adaptation training (CAT), in which case managers provide patients with home-based strategies to help structure their living environment to maximize the likelihood that they can complete requisite activities of daily living. Examples include posting reminders about appointments inside the door of the apartment, listing items of clothing to be worn on the closet door, and placing medications in a location that makes it maximally likely that the patient will see it and be reminded to take it. Prompts and other environmental aides are individually tailored to the patients' level of apathy, disinhibition, and executive dysfunction. CAT can be administered in a time-limited fashion but may be a lifelong service for severely impaired patients. One recent study found that 9 months of CAT was superior to an attention placebo and standard outpatient care on positive symptoms, negative symptoms, motivation, community functioning, global functioning, and incidence of rehospitalization.

Judging the potential for cognitive rehabilitation based on existing trials (analog or clinical) is difficult due to the risk of type II error (e.g., incorrectly concluding that it is ineffective). It may be safe to conclude that a particular strategy is not effective, but one cannot extrapolate from any single trial to the broader domain. For example, a particular technique that fails to produce an effect in ten training sessions might be effective after 50. Ten sessions of practice on computerized memory tasks may not be sufficient to produce a generalizable increase in processing capacity, but meaningful changes may become apparent after 100 sessions. Alternatively, an innovative program based on a different conceptual model of training or dysfunction could produce clinically significant results. No technique has yet demonstrated the ability to produce clinically meaningful changes in neurocognitive capacity or shown that training has a significant impact on community functioning. However, this is a young research area, and existing approaches are promising. There are also some innovative developments in pharmacological treatment for other disorders involving cognitive impairment, such as the use of supplemental cholinergic agents in Alzheimer's disease and adrenergic agents for attention-deficit disorder. Such drugs might help increase cognitive capacity and thereby enable patients to be more responsive to rehabilitation strategies that target higher-order processes. It is likely that, over the next decade, knowledge about brain function and the potential for pharmacological and psychosocial strategies, alone and in combination, will increase dramatically.

ETHICAL ISSUES

The ethics of conducting rehabilitation strategies are generally the same as for conducting other psychotherapies. However, two issues come up regularly: avoiding infantilization and maintaining confidentiality. The first concerns the risk of viewing the patient as unable to make adult choices, such as whether to participate in rehabilitation, where to live, whether or not to work, and whether or not to use drugs and alcohol. Although it may be more of a value than an ethical standard, psychiatric rehabilitation is based on the assumption that the practitioner and the patient are in a partnership to facilitate recovery and improve quality of life. The basic model involves collaboration and shared decision making and does not portray the practitioner as authority or parental figure. When patients make what appear to be bad choices, the practitioner must consider the patient's right to choose and whether the choice is dangerous versus simply not the choice the practitioner would make. If the choice is, in fact, potentially harmful, a collaborative process of considering alternatives is more likely to produce good choices than an authoritative, admonitory approach.

Failure to consider the patient as a partner also leads to violations of confidentiality. Practitioners sometimes assume that they are the primary arbiters of what information to share with parents, other clinicians, and other agencies. In fact, in most circumstances that do not involve the safety of patients or others, the patient should be the arbiter of what information is shared with whom. For example, in supported employment, the patients always determine whether to disclose information about their illnesses to employers.

SUGGESTED CROSS-REFERENCES

Section 12.14 provides outcome information on treatment programs in schizophrenia. Chapter 30 discusses psychotherapy methods, including cognitive therapy (Section 30.6) and dialectical behavior therapy (Section 30.8) that also have been used in treating schizophrenia.

References

Anthony W, Cohen M, Farkas M, Gagne C. *Psychiatric Rehabilitation*, 2nd ed. Boston: Center for Psychiatric Rehabilitation; 2002.

Barraclough C, Haddock G, Tarrier N, Lewis S, Moring J, O'Brien R, Schofield N, McGovern J: Randomized controlled trial of motivational interviewing and cognitive behavioral intervention for schizophrenia patients with associated drug or alcohol misuse. *Am J Psychiatry*. 2001;158:1706.

Becker DR, Drake RE. *A Working Life for People with Severe Mental Illness*. New York: Oxford University Press; 2003.

*Bellack AS, Gold JM, Buchanan RW: Cognitive rehabilitation for schizophrenia: Problems, prospects, and strategies. *Schizophr Bull*. 1999;25:257.

Bellack AS, Mueser KT, Gingerich S, Agresta J. *Social Skills Training for Schizophrenia: A Step-by-Step Guide*. New York: Guilford Press; 1997.

Bond GR, Becker DR, Drake RE, Rapp CA, Meisler N, Lehman AF, Bell M: Implementing supported employment as an evidence-based practice. *Psychiatric Serv*. 2001;52:313.

Bond GR, Resnick SG, Drake RE, Xie H, McHugo GJ, Bebout RR: Does competitive employment improve nonvocational outcomes for people with severe mental illness? *J Consult Clin Psychol*. 2001;69:489.

Brenner HD, Roder V, Hodel B, Kienzle N, Reed D, Lieberman RP. *Integrated Psychological Therapy for Schizophrenic Patients (IPT)*. Goettingen, Germany: Hogrefe & Huber Publishers; 1994.

Cook J, Razzanno L: Vocational rehabilitation for persons with schizophrenia. *Schizophr Bull*. 2000;26:87.

Dilk MN, Bond GR: Meta-analytic evaluation of skills training research for individuals with severe mental illness. *J Consult Clin Psychol*. 1996;64:1337.

*Drake RE, Essock S, Shaner A, Carey KB, Minkoff K, Kola L, Lynde D, Osher FC, Clark RE, Rickards L: Implementing dual diagnosis services for clients with severe mental illness. *Psych Serv*. 2001;52:469.

Drake RE, Mercer-McFadden C, Mueser KT, McHugo GJ, Bond GR: A review of integrated mental health and substance abuse treatment for patients with dual disorders. *Schizophr Bull*. 1998;24:589.

Eckman TA, Wirshing WC, Marder SR, Liberman RP, Johnston-Cronk K, Zimmerman K, Mintz J: Technology for training schizophrenics in illness self-management: A controlled trial. *Am J Psychiatry*. 1992;149:1549.

Ganju V. Implementation of evidence-based practices in state mental health systems: Implications for research and effectiveness studies. *Schizophr Bull*. 2003;29:125–131.

Glynn SM, Marder SR, Liberman RP, Blair K, Wirshing WC, Wirshing DA, Ross D, Mintz J: Supplementing clinic-based skills training with manual-based community support sessions: Effects on social adjustment of patients with schizophrenia. *Am J Psychiatry*. 2002;159:829.

*Heinssen RK, Liberman RP, Kopelowicz A: Psychosocial skills training for schizophrenia: Lessons from the laboratory. *Schizophr Bull*. 2000;26:21.

Herz MI, Marder SR. *Schizophrenia: Comprehensive Treatment and Management*. New York: Lippincott Williams & Wilkins; 2002.

Lehman AF, Goldberg R, Dixon LB, McNary S, Postrado L, Hackmann A, McDonnell K: Improving employment outcomes for persons with severe mental illness. *Arch Gen Psychiatry*. 2002;58:165.

Liberman RP. *Handbook of Psychiatric Rehabilitation*. Boston: Allyn and Bacon; 1992.

*Liberman RP. *Social and independent living skills: The community reentry program*. Los Angeles: Author; 1995

Mueser KT, Drake RE, Bond GR: Recent advances in psychiatric rehabilitation. *Harv Rev Psychiatry*. 1997;5:123.

Mueser KT, Noordsy DL, Drake RE, Fox L. *Integrated Treatment for Dual Disorders: Effective Intervention for Severe Mental Illness and Substance Abuse*. New York: Guilford Press; 2003.

Rapp CA. *The Strengths Model: Case Management with People Suffering from Severe and Persistent Mental Illness*. New York: Oxford Press; 1998.

Spaulding WD, Reed D, Sullivan M, Richardson C, Weiler M: Effects of cognitive treatment in psychiatric rehabilitation. *Schizophr Bull*. 1999;25:657.

Stein LI, Santos AB. *Assertive Community Treatment of Persons with Severe Mental Illness*. New York: W.W. Norton; 1998.

Twamley EW, Jeste DV, Bellack AS: A review of cognitive training in schizophrenia. *Schizophr Bull*. 2003;29(2):359–382.

*Velligan DI, Bow-Thomas CC, Huntzinger C, Ritch J, Ledbetter N, Prihoda TJ, et al. Randomized controlled trial of the use of compensatory strategies to enhance adaptive functioning in outpatients with schizophrenia. *Am J Psychiatry*. 2000;157:1317.

Wykes T, Reeder C, Corner J, Williams C, Everitt B: The effects of neurocognitive remediation on executive processing in patients with schizophrenia. *Schizophr Bull*. 1999;25:291.

Wykes T, van der Gaag M: Is it time to develop a new cognitive therapy for psychosis—cognitive remediation therapy (CRT)? *Clin Psychol Rev*. 2001;21:1227.

▲ 12.14 Schizophrenia: Integrative Treatment and Functional Outcomes

Wayne S. Fenton, M.D.

Providing individualized care in a least restrictive or most integrated setting is a core value of psychiatric medicine related to the treatment of schizophrenia. Patients with this disorder who would have been long-term residents of psychiatric institutions a generation ago are now treated in community settings. In later stages of this deinstitutionalization, more disturbed patients continue to be moved from downsized or closing institutions to communities often ill prepared to care for them. Although research has yielded effective treatments for many aspects of schizophrenia, surveys of routine care indicate that science-based treatment approaches are not available in many communities—a "science to service gap" that leaves many individuals little access to the best available care. As a result, the burden of schizophrenia for both patients with schizophrenia and their family members remains high.

The history of schizophrenia treatment over the 20th century is a contentious one, characterized by often acrimonious ideologically driven debates between authorities embracing biological and psychosocial models of etiology and therapeutics. As part of a broad shift in medicine from reliance on traditional authority and theory-based standard practices to reliance on systematic assessment and compilation of research evidence from clinical trials, *evidence-based practice* is rapidly becoming the basis for rationally informing treatment decisions in schizophrenia and other psychiatric disorders. This approach assumes that both individual patient care decisions and health policies should promote access to treatments based on rigorous scientific information concerning the efficacy (outcomes), costs, and cost-effectiveness of alternative treatment approaches. Although comprehensive surveys of the treatment outcome literature for particular disorders are periodically commissioned, no single scientific or governmental agency is responsible for defining "official" evidence-based treatment practice for mental illness. Rather, ongoing support for treatment research aims to maintain a dynamic and growing body of scientific evidence bearing on the usefulness of new and existing treatments. Thus, knowledge of evidence-based practice requires current and continuous familiarity with the scientific literature related to the treatment of mental disorders.

Because of the significance of schizophrenia as a public health problem, National Institutes of Mental Health (NIMH), Substance Abuse and Mental Health Services Administration (SAMHSA), and Agency for Health Care Policy and Research (AHCPR) have supported research to identify best-practice models both for treatment of individuals with mental disorders and for the organization and delivery of mental health services within a public mental health system. Important recent compilations of evidence-based treatment practice for patients with schizophrenia and other common mental illness include

U.S. Department of Health and Human Services. *Mental Health: A Report of the Surgeon General.* Rockville, MD: U.S. Department of Health and Human Services, Substance Abuse and Mental Health Services Administration, Center for Mental Health Services, National Institutes of Health, National Institutes of Mental Health; 1999.

American Psychiatric Association. *Practice Guidelines for Treatment of Patients with Schizophrenia.* Washington, DC: American Psychiatric Press; 1997.

Lehman AF, Steinwachs DM, the Co-Investigators of the PORT Project: At issue: translating research into practice: The Schizophrenia Patient Outcomes Research Team (PORT) treatment recommendations. *Schizophr Bull.* 1998;24:1–10.

Cochrane Schizophrenia Group. Abstracts of Cochrane Reviews. The Cochrane Library, Issue 4; 2003. Available at: http://www.mediscope.ch/cochrane-abstracts/g060index.htm.

In assessing levels of evidence associated with the treatment of schizophrenia, the randomized, controlled trial is the "gold standard" for evaluating treatment efficacy. In these studies, patients are randomly assigned to two or more treatment options, and outcome is assessed, often by independent raters who are unaware of what treatment the patient has received. Evidence is strongest for the efficacy of treatments tested in many randomized clinical trials. Evidence is weaker for treatments in which fewer formal trials are available, and data are supplemented or supplanted by expert opinion.

MISCONCEPTIONS AND LIMITS OF EVIDENCE-BASED PRACTICE

A major criticism of evidence-based practice is that it ignores intuition, experience, and clinical judgment; deemphasizes the importance of the physician–patient relationship; and renders the practice of medicine sterile and formulaic. Contrary to these criticisms, most proponents of evidence-based practice agree that "a cookbook is not a cook." Aspects of the "art of medicine" can only be derived from the opinions and experience of exceptional clinicians who demonstrate excellent judgment in making complex clinical management decisions and who have a gift for precise observation, careful diagnosis, and the ability to make human contact with difficult, frightened, or withdrawn patients. The history of medicine and psychiatry, however, is filled with examples of compelling clinical intuition that later has proved incorrect. Therefore, although valuing expert clinical problem-solving skills, an evidence-based practice approach ultimately strives to extract testable and teachable practices used by expert clinicians to rigorously evaluate their validity.

TREATMENT INTEGRATION

Evidence-based practice is defined by randomized clinical trials supported by expert opinion. By design, randomized trials focus on evaluating the efficacy or effectiveness of a specific treatment element or management strategy in achieving specific anticipated outcomes. Thus, although the evidence base derived from these trials is informative about the usefulness of specific interventions in defined patient groups, it provides less guidance with respect to defining an overall strategy for integrating effective elements into a comprehensive, individualized treatment plan. Evidence-based practice provides a menu of efficacious treatments from which a clinician may select. What particular combination of interventions is optimal for a particular patient with a particular type of schizophrenia at a particular phase of illness is an aspect of clinical practice that can be called *treatment integration.* Effective treatment integration strategies are more difficult to rigorously test and often must be specified in terms of principles and priorities and in terms of clinical reasoning.

No single treatment can ameliorate the myriad symptoms and disabilities associated with schizophrenia. As articulated in the American Psychiatric Association's *Practice Guidelines for the Treatment of Patients with Schizophrenia,* therapeutic efforts must be comprehensive, multimodal, and empirically titrated to the individual patient's response and progress. Although there is currently no cure for schizophrenia, the skillful application of pharmacological, psychotherapeutic, rehabilitation, and community support interventions can limit illness morbidity and mortality, improve patient outcome, and enhance quality of life.

As with individuals with other long-term medical disorders, many patients with schizophrenia need comprehensive and continuous care over prolonged periods. To the extent that both biological and psychosocial factors are critical determinants of the course and outcome of schizophrenia, a psychiatrist may be in the best position to coordinate and integrate the various treatments required and provide continuity of care over time.

Each component of a comprehensive treatment plan for a patient with schizophrenia targets specific aspects of the disorder and its common sequelae. Pharmacological interventions target positive, negative, and disorganized symptom domains, mood symptoms, and cognition. Rehabilitation efforts target deficits in self-care, social, or vocational skills and provide structure in the form of someplace to be and something productive to do. Access to appropriate entitlements, treatment services, housing, and social support is the goal of community support programs. Individual psychotherapy addresses the human aspects of adaptation to a serious psychiatric disorder and targets problems such as denial, demoralization, treatment compliance, personal relationships, and self-esteem. Psychotherapy focuses on understanding the patient's beliefs, attitudes, aspirations, and experiences. The coordination, timing, and titration of all specific treatment elements is informed by this understanding and by an ongoing assessment of individual patient needs that can often best be achieved within a long-term physician–patient relationship.

ASSUMPTIONS GUIDING INTEGRATIVE TREATMENT OF SCHIZOPHRENIA

Integrative treatment of schizophrenia is based on assumptions about the disorder that recognize the joint contributions of biological, psychological, and social/environmental factors:

A stress-diathesis or vulnerability-stress model represents the best available integration of data pertinent to the etiology, course, and outcome of schizophrenia. This model postulates that schizophrenia results from a dynamic interaction between environmental or experiential stress in a person who is "vulnerable" to react to this stress with schizophrenic symptom formation.

The vulnerabilities to schizophrenia are likely to be multiple and heterogeneous. Aspects of vulnerability are undoubtedly genetic, although some may be acquired environmentally through intrauterine, birth, and postnatal developmental complications. Some of the relatively enduring difficulties observed among subgroups of patients are (1) deficits in information processing and maintaining a steady focus of attention; (2) dysfunctions in psychophysiology suggesting deficits in sensory inhibition and autonomic responsivity; (3) impairments in working memory, executive functioning, abstract thinking, and social competence; and (4) general coping deficits, such as anhedonia, a propensity to cognitive and perceptual distortions, overvaluing threat, under-appraising abilities, and extensive use of denial.

The vulnerability to schizophrenia is seen as a relatively enduring proclivity to developing overt clinical symptoms; vulnerability is likely to be manifest as a set of stable traits present premorbidly, at onset, and during acute episodes and remissions. At the same time, vulnerability is not static but shaped epigenetically over time by environmental influences; a "stress" sufficient to precipitate relapse at one time, for example, may be less likely to do so at a later point when new coping strategies or better supports have been acquired.

The stress side of the vulnerability-stress model postulates that a variety of stressors (internal or external events requiring adaptation) can precipitate the emergence of symptoms in a vulnerable individual. Given biologically based vulnerability, the onset, course, and outcome of an individual's disorder may be shaped by interactions between the person and the environment. Among psychosocial factors, stressful life events, cultural milieu (egocentric vs. sociocentric), social class, social network size and density, and emotional quality of the living environment have been demonstrated to be associated with the onset or course of schizophrenia.

Illness course is understood as a dynamic product of the affected individual's adaptive assets and vulnerabilities interacting over time with various stresses. In a highly vulnerable individual, sufficient stress can precipitate intermediate (prodromal or relapse-prodrome) states of dysfunction that amplify preexisting cognitive, affective-autonomic, and social coping deficits. In the absence of adaptive strategies or environmental supports, these interact negatively with the existing stressors to magnify their effect in a downwardly spiraling process that ends in a full-blown clinical syndrome. Clinical experience indicates that the stresses associated with illness onset or exacerbation are highly individualized, rendering generalization about the typical nature of such stresses difficult. Stresses may be primarily biochemical (as in substance abuse), environmental (as in leaving for college, joining the armed services, breaking up with a girlfriend), or social (poverty, unemployment).

Schizophrenia is heterogeneous, as are individuals afflicted with it. The clinical diversity of schizophrenia in relation to vulnerabilities and risk factors, age and type of onset, manifest signs and symptoms, longitudinal course, and long-term outcome suggests that the disorder may be heterogeneous with regard to underlying etiology. Symptom dimensions in schizophrenia include positive symptoms (delusions, hallucinations), disorganized symptoms (thought disorder, bizarre behavior), deficit symptoms (anhedonia, avolition, affective flattening), cognitive deficits, and depressive symptoms or suicidality. Individual patients may show symptoms from one, two, or all of these domains. Illness heterogeneity is partially captured by currently available subtyping systems: Paranoid schizophrenia, for example, is associated with good premorbid functioning, late age of onset, many positive symptoms, intermittent illness over the first several years, and a comparatively high likelihood of good outcome despite a higher risk of suicide; the deficit form of schizophrenia is characterized by poor premorbid functioning, earlier onset, severe and enduring negative symptoms, a low risk of suicide, and often persistent lifelong disability. An etiology-based subtyping that allows for precise longitudinal prediction for individual patients is not, however, available. At a minimum, schizophrenic illnesses of greater and lesser severity and "virulence" can be identified and the "biological" vulnerability of individuals may differ.

As with the illness itself, individuals afflicted with schizophrenia differ substantially in adaptive capacities, intelligence, and instrumental and verbal competence. Furthermore, the degree of social support available to them varies greatly. In general, the greater the level of instrumental skills acquired before the onset of illness (work or educational experience, experience with relationships, experience living independently), the better positioned the individual is to recover or maintain functioning once the illness has become established. For some patients, the inability to acquire much in the way of adaptive skills may represent the product of the lifelong vulnerability underlying the tendency to the illness. For other patients, a particularly "virulent" form of schizophrenia may catastrophically erode adequate premorbid skills, resulting in substantial permanent disability. Other patients with good premorbid abilities may be left after an acute episode with their skills and competence largely intact.

Schizophrenia is a developmental disorder with a phasic course. Systematic investigation of longitudinal course has only recently begun, and the understanding of illness phases is preliminary. Phases may include (1) prodromal periods during which a highly individualized constellation of symptoms that represent early manifestation of clinical decompensation emerge; (2) acute or active phases, often associated with the full-blown emergence of positive symptoms superimposed onto preexisting deficits; (3) subacute, convalescent, or stabilization phases characterized by gradual restoration of some functioning, perhaps associated with postpsychotic depression; (4) moratoriums or adaptive plateaus characterized by a gradual reconstitution of identity, gathering of support, and strengthening of skills; (5) change points or shifts in functioning over a relatively brief period, initiated by the patient's own desires or pressure from others and associated with the potential for either quantum improvement or decompensation; and (6) end-state or stable plateaus, relatively enduring periods of stability characterized by greater or lesser fixed deficits or chronic levels of positive symptoms. Alternatively, schizophrenia can be divided into epochs such as the onset, middle-course, and late-course epochs.

Outcome in schizophrenia is variable. Functional outcome in schizophrenia is variable in at least two respects: (1) Among groups of patients, there is substantial interindividual differences observed in both short-term treatment response and longer-term disability or degree of recovery; and (2) for any given individual, outcome is not unitary but may vary considerably across different domains of functioning.

Current knowledge concerning the outcome of schizophrenia derives largely from follow-up studies of patients assessed at an index time period (often hospital admission or discharge) and evaluated some years later. One metaanalysis indexed 320 studies with an average follow-up duration of 6 years conducted between 1895 and 1991. Fewer studies have a follow-up duration of 15 to 30 years. Contrary to the Kraeplinian view of schizophrenia as a disease inevitably leading to deterioration, follow-up studies all find a range of outcomes among patients with schizophrenia from fully recovered to continuous and severe incapacity. Differences in the percentage of patients achieving good outcomes across studies can be attributed to differing sample characteristics and diagnostic approaches: When schizophrenia is diagnosed "broadly" to include patients with varying durations of illness, outcome tends to be more favorable. When diagnostic systems (such as the revised fourth edition of the *Diagnostic and Statistical Manual of Mental Disorders* [DSM-IV-TR]) that require evidence of established chronicity are used, the proportion of patients found to be recovered is less. Additional factors consistently associated with better long-term outcome include the absence of substance abuse, later onset of illness, better premorbid skills and functioning, more favorable initial treatment response, the absence of deficit symptoms and cognitive deficits, the preservation of affect, including depression, and female gender. As described elsewhere in this section, data concerning the early course of schizophrenia are increasingly derived from prospective studies of first episode or patients in the prodromal phase of illness.

Early studies of schizophrenia classified patient outcomes in global terms such as "deteriorated," "improved," or "recovered." Beginning with the research of John Strauss and William Carpenter in the 1960s, global ratings of schizophrenia outcome were resolved into component dimensions of functioning that were found to be semi-independent or only loosely linked. Symptom severity, social functioning, occupational functioning, and relapse frequency are major dimensions of patient outcome. These are considered semi-independent insofar as they are only moderately correlated so that, for example, symptom severity is not necessarily associated with work disability. As noted above, symptomatic outcome is now specified in terms of multiple component symptom dimensions. Among symptom dimensions, cognitive deficits and negative, or deficit, symptoms are most predictive of social, occupational, and functional outcome. Because these are symptom dimensions for which available medications are least effective, considerable research is focused on developing psychosocial or pharmacological approaches to understanding and remedying cognitive deficits and negative symptoms.

Research indicates that patients, family members, and clinicians may place differing value on various dimensions of outcome. Thus, in addition to objective measures of symptom severity and functioning, objective and subjective quality of life and achievement of self-defined goals are considered increasingly important dimensions of treatment outcome.

Recovery is a concept introduced in the lay writings of mental health consumers in the 1980s and, in part, reflects a turnabout in attitudes as a result of the consumer movement and self-help activities. Recovery has been described as a process, an outlook, a vision, and a guiding principle. The overarching message, supported by contemporary research, is that hope and restoration of a meaningful life are possible despite serious mental illness. Beyond a narrow medical view of mental illness, recovery implies restoration of identity, self-esteem, and meaningful roles in society. On a practical level, the recovery movement is evidenced by greater participation of consumers and families in the design and oversight of services and service systems, the creation and support of family and consumer-operated services to supplement traditional care, active efforts to eliminate stigma associated with mental illness, and the creation of new definitions of outcome that are expanded to emphasize self-esteem, empowerment, optimism, and self-efficacy.

INTEGRATED TREATMENT: THE CLINICAL RELATIONSHIP

In an era in which resources available for the care of patients with serious mental illness are shrinking, the clinical relationship is at risk of being devalued in the treatment of schizophrenia. As in the management of other chronic diseases, however, multiple treatment modalities must be selectively applied over time and modified in relation to changing individual circumstances. This creates the need for someone to orchestrate and coordinate treatment and maintain responsibility for the overall treatment plan. As is true in medicine generally, the quality of the doctor–patient relationship sets the stage for a therapeutic alliance and continuity of care, which is a major determinant of treatment adherence and, hence, the success of all prescribed therapies. In combination with antipsychotic medication, some form of individual therapy in which the therapist maintains responsibility for integrating treatment elements is likely the most common treatment offered to patients with schizophrenia in the United States. Surveys of patients and their families consistently rank individual psychotherapy along with medication prescribing among the most highly valued services provided by mental health practitioners.

Relative to hundreds of studies that have evaluated pharmacological agents in schizophrenia, very few clinical trials of individual psychotherapy have been conducted over the past four decades. These trials, often initiated in the context of factionalism between psychologically and biologically oriented psychiatry, have generally been of greater value in dislodging firmly held but incorrect beliefs about the effectiveness of specific types of individual psychotherapy than in pointing to what does work.

Individual psychotherapy is defined most broadly as a professional relationship in which the technical expertise of the physician is directed in an effort to promote the patient's recovery or to relieve suffering. At a minimum, this physician–patient relationship provides the context in which symptoms and disabilities are assessed, consent and collaboration for treatment obtained, and the effects of interventions are evaluated. More ambitious goals, appropriate for selected patients in settings in which time and resources allow, can include the exploration of maladaptive patterns of living through careful scrutiny of relationships with others and the therapeutic relationship itself. Most psychotherapy, as actually practiced, falls somewhere in between, requiring from the therapist a broad base of medical and psychological skills. A psychiatrist providing psychotherapy for schizophrenic patients should probably be prepared to give an intramuscular (IM) injection, interpret transference, or give a patient a ride to work.

Current approaches to the clinical relationship represent an amalgamation of practices described by the term *flexible psychotherapy.* This approach draws from perspectives and techniques derived from the historical traditions of investigative and supportive psychotherapy to accommodate the heterogeneity of schizophrenia and the individuals who have it. Because techniques drawn from these traditions continue to shape contemporary perspectives on the clinical relationship, selected elements of investigative and supportive psychotherapy are summarized below.

CLINICAL RELATIONSHIP IN INVESTIGATIVE PSYCHOTHERAPY

History Psychotherapy for schizophrenia in the United States originated as a modification of psychoanalysis. Early psychoanalysts, such as Abraham Brill, advocated an active effort to promote "rapport" and arouse the patient's interest in his or her own malady. In time, he observed that confidence in and a "passive attachment" to the physician could develop so that the latter might become a bridge between the patient and reality. Observing difficulties schizophrenia patients had in maintaining relationships led Harry Stack Sullivan to formulate the paradigm of "interpersonal psychiatry" in the 1940s. Psychopathology was viewed as difficulties in living arising largely from personal and social relations and as personality warps believed to be the lasting residue of earlier unsatisfactory interpersonal experiences. The predecessors of ego and self-psychology, "interpersonal psychiatry" and "psychodynamic psychotherapy" became dominant paradigms in American psychiatry in the 1940s, 1950s, and 1960s.

Goals The goal of intensive psychotherapy is alleviation of the patient's emotional difficulties and elimination of symptoms. This is accomplished by undertaking a thorough scrutiny of the patient's life history (especially the history of his or her interpersonal relationships), reviewing the realities of the patient's current relationships and life situation, and understanding the historical roots of maladaptive interpersonal patterns as reflected in the doctor–patient relationship and in daily life.

Technical Approach Therapist attributes cited as important in investigative psychotherapy include a basic respect for the patient that stems from a conviction that the patient's problems are not too different from one's own. Aloofness, rigidity, and critical pomposity are discouraged, and the psychotherapist should be willing to admit when he or she is wrong. Intensive psychotherapy must be conducted in a setting of mutual safety and is conversational: Free association is discouraged as aggravating disorganization.

Examining transference (patient's reactions to the therapist) is expected in investigative psychotherapy and is considered useful in allowing the patient to understand distorted perceptions and respond more realistically to people in his or her current life. Countertransference (therapist's feelings that arise in work with schizophrenic patients) can include discouragement, fear, worthlessness, hatred, contempt, guilt, rage, envy, or lust. The therapist's ability through introspection to understand, rather than act on, these reactions is a defining feature of the clinical relationship. Feelings evoked by the patient can serve as a source of information about the patient's state of mind and as a means of understanding how others typically react and respond to the patient. Successful management of countertransference allows the therapist to create a "holding" relationship with the patient that creates an environment of interpersonal safety.

The literature on intensive psychotherapy describes interventions that correspond to different phases of therapy: (1) establishing a relationship, (2) elucidating the patient's experience in the here and now, (3) tolerating the mobilized transference and countertransference, and (4) integrating the patient's experiences into an expanded perspective of the self.

Establishing a relationship with the schizophrenic patient can be challenging. Consistency, straightforwardness, and an active effort to establish rapport are advocated. Within bounds, a reasonable degree of self-disclosure on the therapist's part can help counter distortions by allowing the patient to get a fix on the therapist as a person. A relationship should be sought on the patient's terms. At times, engaging in activity (walking or playing a game) or finding a neutral topic of common interest (sports, music) further promotes establishing a relationship. If successful, a background feeling of security and predictability increasingly characterizes the therapy.

Elvin Semrad viewed the core tasks of psychotherapy as helping the patient acknowledge, bear, and put into perspective his or her feelings and painful life experiences. Acknowledging the patient's feelings and painful experiences becomes pertinent once a relationship has been established. Strategies for elucidating affects include listening, narrowing the focus, seeking concrete detail, acknowledging feelings (especially loss, anger, sadness), and naming or labeling emotions. Examining the patient's day-to-day life in detail allows the therapist to develop a picture of the patient's difficulties, frustrations, and characteristic reactions to others.

Tolerating affects correspond to Semrad's concept of "bearing" painful feelings that have been acknowledged. Simply stated, patients experience themselves being accepted, negative emotions and all, and, learning from the therapist's example, become better able to accept unwanted aspects of themselves.

Broadening patients' understanding of themselves and their situations corresponds to the third part of Semrad's triad: helping patients put into perspective their painful affects, life experiences, and maladaptive solutions. Providing insight is one way of integrating the patient's experiences into an expanded perspective of the self. Emotional insight, gained by direct experience in the doctor–patient relationship, is emphasized. This phase of therapy should leave the patient with a more accepting and complex view of himself or herself as a person capable of experiencing the full range of human emotions. Passivity is seen as an active choice, and patients recognize that continued progress depends on their willingness to attempt new solutions in their daily lives.

CLINICAL RELATIONSHIP IN SUPPORTIVE PSYCHOTHERAPY

History Supportive psychotherapy has been favored by biologically and pharmacologically oriented clinicians. In theory and technique, it is grounded in the medical model in which the patient is seen as having an organically based illness requiring treatment from a physician. As described by Talcott Parsons, the medical model implies essential elements of expected behavior for both the physician and patient. These elements define the physician's and patient's respective roles, relationship, and responsibilities.

According to Parsons, the physician's role is characterized by four key qualities: (1) universalistic, (2) functionally specific, (3) affectively neutral, and (4) collectivity oriented. The universalistic norm requires the physician to treat all patients alike, according to scientific and medical standards. The role is functionally specific in that the physician is seen as a specialist in health and disease who is expected to limit attention to circumscribed areas involving medical matters. Affective neutrality prevents the doctor from entering too sympathetically into the patient's situation, allowing for steadfastness of judgment and the exercise of emotional control. Finally, collectivity orientation, as opposed to self-orientation, demands that the doctor treat the patient according to the patient's needs and health standards of the community.

The role of the patient, as is the role of the physician, is defined by expected behavior that involves both rights and obligations. First, the person who is ill is exempt from normal social responsibilities and excused from customary obligations so that he or she may attend to the process of getting well. A second right is exemption from responsibility for illness—the illness is not considered the patient's fault, and the patient has the right to receive care. At the same time, the patient has the obligation to want to get well, obtain technically competent help, and cooperate with treatment.

Goals

In contrast to the ambitious aims of personality change associated with the intensive therapy tradition, the short- and long-term goals of supportive psychotherapy are comparatively modest. These include (1) relief from the immediate crisis or direct reduction of acute disequilibrium, (2) removal of symptoms to premorbid levels, (3) reestablishment of psychic homeostasis through a strengthening of defenses, (4) sealing over psychotic experiences and conflicts, (5) the circumscribed fostering of adaptation, and (6) mobilization and preservation of healthy aspects of the patient to enable optimal functioning and minimize the impact of persistent deficits. Supportive therapy uses the physician–patient relationship to create a background of adequate clinical care that supports the prescription of effective pharmacological interventions. Functional or social recovery, rather than personality change, is the primary aim of treatment.

Technical Approach

The overall technical approach of supportive psychotherapy is one of pragmatism in which the physician, based on medical and psychiatric expertise, helps the patient interpret and adapt to reality. As such, the therapist uses techniques that include defining reality, offering direct reassurance, giving advice on current problems of living, urging modification of expectations, and actively organizing the environment for patients who cannot do so themselves. To help stabilize the patient's environment, the therapist often maintains close contact with the patient's family or other treaters and may intervene on the patient's behalf with family, employers, and social agencies.

Eliciting and tracking symptomatology and targeting symptoms for psychopharmacological intervention are major foci for the supportive psychotherapist. Psychopathology is interpreted in a medical context as the unwanted emergence of signs of illness. The basic content of psychotherapy focuses on teaching and relearning—the patient is educated regarding the nature of the illness and taught to monitor symptoms and act promptly to suppress his or her exacerbation. The therapist fosters positive transference as a benign authority; positive feelings are treated as real. Negative transference is avoided. The therapist may become very active in helping the patient learn new ways of adapting and may use or prescribe cognitive, behavioral, or social skill training techniques.

HIERARCHY OF CLINICAL NEEDS

Contemporary scientific assumptions about schizophrenia suggest that patients' clinical needs and associated therapeutic tasks can be ordered hierarchically. To treat schizophrenia, a variety of interventions and strategies, including methods derived from traditions of supportive and investigative psychotherapy, may be required. The crucial question becomes which interventions are of potential value for a particular individual at a particular phase of illness. As outlined in Table 12.14–1, different clinical needs assume greater importance during different illness phases. In addition, although some tasks are clearly relevant for all patients receiving integrated treatment; others, particularly those relating to the goals of intensive psychotherapy, are pertinent for only a small subgroup of patients. This model, which has been termed *flexible psychotherapy*, assumes the therapist's capacity to "shift gears" flexibly and change roles with all patients based on changing circumstances, always holding in mind the goal of helping the patient accept, learn about, and self-manage what may often be a chronic and devastating illness.

Consideration of the patient's schizophrenia subtype, current and premorbid functioning, and self-defined treatment goals is relevant to the determination of appropriate treatment tasks. For patients with severe hebephrenic or deficit forms of schizophrenia, for example, the most humane and practical goal may be establishing a supportive ongoing treatment within a sheltered setting that minimizes stress and provides for basic human needs. For the majority of patients who reside in the community, some degree of psychoeducation and rehabilitative tasks should be planned with the aim of minimizing acute relapses and promoting maximal functioning and quality of life. A primary focus on investigative tasks is reserved for motivated patients who have established a good working relationship with their therapist and exhibit an interest in and ability to make constructive use of such techniques. Attunement to psychological concerns may be particularly important for patients who have a dramatic response to new medications. Here, removed from its outmoded etiological assumptions and overly ambitious aims, the substantial clinical knowledge derived from the tradition of investigative psychotherapy can be applied pragmatically in a contemporary context.

Although many of the tasks outlined in Table 12.14–1 overlap with the concerns and expertise of other service providers, all should be the concern of the individual psychotherapist and a focus for individual psychotherapy. A focus on higher-level educational and psychological tasks is generally inappropriate in the presence of overwhelming difficulties in obtaining basic human services. Thus, the necessary first goal of psychotherapy with a homeless person may be direct assistance in finding housing. Although other professionals may be relied on to accomplish specific tasks, physicians/therapists should consider themselves responsible for ensuring the results of these efforts.

The following general treatment strategies are common to all of the specific therapeutic tasks outlined:

Evaluation. A thorough evaluation of the patient initiates the treatment process. During medical assessment and stabilization, this includes ruling out identifiable physical conditions, assessing competence to consent to treatment and dangerousness, and determining the responsivity of symptoms to acute pharmacological intervention. Psychosocial assessment inventories aim to measure the degree to which the patient's adaptive capacities measure up against the stresses and demands of his or her living environment. Efforts to establish a supportive ongoing treatment test the patient's capacity to trust and rely on another human being for support and guidance. When

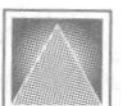

Table 12.14–1
Flexible Psychotherapy: Therapeutic Tasks, Interventions, Goals, and Evidence-Based Practice

Therapeutic Task and Level	Clinical Focus	Interventions	Goals	Illness Phase	Evidence-Based Practice
Medical assessment and stabilization	Crisis intervention Psychiatric, medical diagnosis Safety Acute symptom management	Clinical, medical, neurological assessment Hospitalization or community alternative short-term care Directive and supportive communication, limit setting Pharmacological treatment	Diagnose or rule out medical, neurological disorders Ensure safety Minimize effect of acute episode on life situation (housing, job, family) Effect rapid symptom reduction	Prodromal, acute	ACT Day hospital Crisis residencies Pharmacological algorithms and guidelines
Psychosocial assessment and case management	Stress and vulnerabilities Social supports Living arrangements, daily activities Adaptive capacities Access to economic and treatment resources	Skilled psychological and psychosocial assessment Evaluation of human service needs Linkage with social service, human service, and community support services	Mobilize social support Assess postepisode psychosocial service needs, including day treatment, supportive housing, if needed Ensure access to all required entitlements Enlist cooperation of family or other caregivers	Subacute, convalescent, stabilization	ACT Compliance therapy Family psychoeducation Acute-phase CBT
Establish supportive treatment	Treatment relationship and alliance Denial, suspiciousness, disorganization Self-esteem	Continued medication—attention to complaints and medication adverse effects Support, positive regard, reassurance, bolstering defenses Promote comfort with therapist and treatment—encourage	Encourage sufficient acceptance of illness to allow cooperation with treatment Promote trust in therapist and comfort with therapeutic routine Support strengths, adaptive defenses Monitor for relapse	Early maintenance, moratorium, or adaptive plateau	ACT Family psychoeducation Post–acute-phase CBT Integrated dual diagnosis treatment
Psychoeducation	Understanding and acceptance of illness Human concerns associated with disability Self-management of illness	Teaching and support Identification of individual-specific stresses Awareness of individual-specific prodromal and active symptoms Determine lowest effective prophylactic medication dose	Relapse prevention Learning stress management strategies Self-recognition of prodromal symptoms Establish maintenance regime Collaborative self-management of illness	Maintenance, moratorium, change points	Maintenance medication guidelines (e.g., PORT) Personal therapy Family psychoeducation CBT for treatment resistant symptoms
Rehabilitation or habilitation tasks	Social, vocational, self-care skills Learning or relearning Establishing realistic expectations Adaptation to deficits	Attention to details of daily self-care, social and occupational functioning Modeling and practice of new skills Cognitive, problem solving, social skills enhancement Environmental intervention, family education, supported employment	Promote highest adaptive functioning within limitations imposed by defeats Promote activities that enhance self-esteem through accomplishment and productivity Encourage activities that improve quality of life Promote attainment of self-defined goals Learn strategies that allow functioning despite deficits	Maintenance, end state, stable plateau	Personal therapy Social skills training Place and support vocational services Group therapy (social skills oriented) Integrated dual diagnosis treatment
Investigative/insight-oriented tasks	Conflicts, interpersonal relationships, life goals	Exploration of feelings, conflicts, ambivalence Focus on past events, life history Examination of important relationships, including relationship with therapist Interpretation	Integrating psychosis into expanded concept of self Construction of life narrative Working through conflicts Improved capacity of intimacy and productivity	Selected and motivated patients during stable periods	No evidence-based approaches

ACT, assertive community treatment; CBT, cognitive-behavioral therapy; PORI, Patient Outcomes Research Team.

applicable, psychoeducational, rehabilitative, and investigative interventions are preceded by an assessment of the patient's cognitive strengths and deficits, allowing interventions to be formulated that match the patient's talents.

Continuous reevaluation. The fluid nature of schizophrenia and an individual's adaptation to it over time demands periodic reassessment of course, prognosis, phase of illness, and target problems. As these change, so do treatment goals. Providing concrete support in the form of a ride to work may be helpful early in the effort to promote vocational rehabilitation but later may promote unwarranted dependency and prolong disability.

Timing. The phasic natural history of schizophrenia requires attention to when particular therapeutic tasks are attempted. For many patients, to minimize stress and forestall relapse, relatively little beyond assessment, stabilization with medication, and establishment of a supportive ongoing treatment should be attempted during the first 6 to 12 months after an acute episode. Once the patient is asymptomatic and shows signs of revitalization, rehabilitation and more complex psychoeducational elements may be gradually introduced.

Titration. Treatment interventions should be applied with graded increases of intensity and complexity. Higher-level therapeutic tasks should be attempted and higher levels of work or social functioning expected only after completion and consolidation of earlier gains. Substantial rehabilitation, for example, rarely is possible until progress has been made in attaining a stable supportive treatment relationship. Likewise, there is evidence that early, active, and ambitious psychologically oriented treatment may be disorganizing or toxic for certain patients. In general, treatment changes should be pursued cautiously, modifying only one element at a time.

Integration with psychopharmacology. Each of the tasks outlined above takes acute and prophylactic antipsychotic drugs as given for most patients. Control and prevention of psychotic symptoms using the lowest effective dosage of medication is the overall treatment goal. Decisions regarding pharmacological management are often linked to the relative success or failure of accomplishing various psychotherapeutic tasks. Considerable psychoeducation, for example, should be accomplished before attempting maintenance medication dose reduction or the initiation of a targeted (intermittent) medication strategy. Long-acting injectable neuroleptics may be useful for patients unable to tolerate the daily reminder of illness associated with oral medication or for patients unable to maintain a reliable treatment relationship.

Shared decision making as ideal of clinical relationship. Patients' expectations have changed considerably since Parsons' classic description of the sick role. Access to knowledge through the media, Internet, and direct patient marketing has rendered patients and families more knowledgeable than at any time in history; organizations representing patients have a stronger voice in health care and information itself; the source of professional authority is no longer the exclusive possession of the profession. Concurrently, an "acute care" conception of disease is being supplanted by recognition that much of disease burden derives from long-term or chronic conditions. In many instances, this change is associated with a shift in the goals of medical care from "cure" to "disease management." For many patients, "illness self-management" becomes a significant treatment goal. "Shared decision making" is a promising template for the physician–patient relationship that is an alternative to both the "paternalistic model," in which the physician unilaterally renders an opinion from on high, and "pure consumerism," which reduces the physician to a dispassionate technocrat dispensing information concerning statistical risks and benefits of alternate treatment approaches. The model embraces the inherent vulnerability of the patient facing serious illness who must make decisions with serious consequences: the patient who wants to know "What would you do if you were in my shoes, doctor?" At the same time, shared decision making recognizes that the relative importance placed on risks, outcomes, and side effects by the doctor and patient are not necessarily congruent, so that meaningful physician contribution to patient decision making requires understanding of the patient as an individual with unique values and priorities. The key component of a therapeutic alliance appears to be the ability of the doctor and patient to negotiate shared goals and work collaboratively together toward their accomplishment, although cognitive deficits, treatment-resistant symptoms, or a lack of insight experienced by some patients with schizophrenia can render this extremely difficult to the extent that possible identification of shared goals and shared decision making represent valuable ideals for treatment.

As outlined in Table 12.14–1 and described in detail elsewhere in this section, specific evidence-based practices have been developed that are appropriate for application at various illness phases. Research-based medication algorithms and guidelines are available to inform both acute and maintenance treatment. Evidence-based psychosocial approaches address a range of clinical issues, including enhancing medication adherence in the postacute illness phase, providing individual and family psychoeducation to enhance disease management skills and reduce relapse, and providing assertive community treatment to maintain a therapeutic relationship with mistrustful, nonadherent, or repeatedly relapsing patients. Equally essential tasks include teaching social skills during stable illness phases, managing cooccurring substance abuse and mental illness with integrated treatment approaches based on stages of change models, promoting employment through place and support models of rapid vocational training, and developing or strengthening behavioral strategies to manage medication-resistant treatment.

CLINICAL REASONING

Although the variability of schizophrenia precludes a treatment algorithm applicable to all clinical situations, principles of clinical reasoning that guide treatment planning within the framework of a hierarchy of clinical needs can be articulated. Research evidence derived from groups of patients notwithstanding, determining the efficacy of any particular intervention for an individual patient often devolves to clinically informed trial and error. Under these circumstances, the probability of success can be enhanced by an effort to be systematic and scientific in administering and evaluating interventions.

Identify Target Symptoms for Intervention Neither psychopharmacological nor psychosocial interventions remedy all aspects of schizophrenia; rather, they target narrow and specific dimensions of symptoms or disability. If a new medicine is to be tried, it is useful to specify in advance what symptoms or behaviors the trial aims to address and by what criteria it is evaluated as successful or not. Similarly, the target symptoms, behaviors, or goals of a trial of a psychosocial intervention should be narrowly identified to later assess the intervention's effectiveness. A medication change cannot be expected to obviate an intractable psychosocial problem such as unemployment or homelessness; likewise, a trial of assertive community treatment might enhance medication compliance but does not in and of itself decrease symptoms.

Try New Treatments for a Sufficient Time and at a Sufficient Dose

Pressures to try new treatments often arise in the context of either long-standing dissatisfaction with the results of prior approaches or because of the emergence of new problems or crises. Because of a sense of urgency, patients, families, and clinicians may wish to see immediate results and become impatient if they are not forthcoming. This pressure can be exacerbated by utilization review schemes that demand frequent changes as evidence of "active treatment." With respect to medication, it is important to recognize that, although generalized effects, such as sedation, increased sleep, and decreased aggression, may be seen within a few days, full antipsychotic effects may require a trial at an adequate dose that lasts up to several months. Likewise, nearly all psychosocial interventions take time to demonstrate efficacy. For these reasons, to the extent possible, the target dose and duration of a treatment trial should be specified in advance, and sufficient time should be allowed to assess intervention efficacy. Without providing a trial at an adequate dose and for an adequate duration, a potentially useful intervention may be abandoned as ineffective.

Change One Treatment Element at a Time

Urgent pressure for immediate improvements can also lead to the rapid prescription of multiple medications. Under these circumstances, if the patient's symptoms improve, it is impossible to determine which element alone or in combination with others is responsible for the improvement. As a result, the risk of exposure to an unnecessary medication is high. If the patient's condition worsens, it is difficult to determine whether the combination treatment itself is responsible for the worsening or whether one of the changes alone could have been of value. Changing one medication at a time is often the only strategy that allows clear inferences about treatment efficacy for an individual patient. This principle also extends to psychosocial treatments and combined medication/psychosocial interventions. The best time to start a new job, for example, may not be during a medication change. If symptoms reemerge, it is difficult to determine whether the medication or additional psychosocial stress is responsible.

Initiate Changes Gradually

With respect to starting medications, the axiom "start low, go slow" is often recommended. Although imaging receptor occupancy and pharmacogenomics may some day allow precise prediction of medication dose and individual side-effect vulnerability, at present, it is only observed that patients vary in sensitivity to medications in a way that cannot be predicted in advance. Rapid dose escalation runs the risk of passing through an optimal dose range and inadvertently crossing a dosage threshold for side effects. A thorough medication trial often requires a gradual dose escalation to determine optimal individual treatment response. Conversely, during maintenance-phase treatment, a gradual dosage reduction to determine the lowest dose effective in preventing the recurrence of symptoms is often warranted. Particularly for patients with a history of rapid relapse after medication discontinuation, switching antipsychotic medications should be accomplished with a gradual cross-titration that may last weeks or more. The principle of gradualism can also apply to psychosocial treatments and life changes generally. A long-inactive patient might be advised to try one or two classes or take a part-time job as a trial rather than plunge into full-time school or work.

Avoid Major Treatment Changes during Periods of Stress or When the Cost of Relapse Is High

Periods of psychosocial stress create an unstable baseline against which to evaluate the impact of changes in treatment. Although symptom exacerbations associated with stress may necessitate instituting new treatments or other supports, elective changes in treatment, such as planned medication changes, might be delayed until a stressful period abates. Moves, changes in important relationships and periods of loss, failure, or success can be potentially destabilizing stresses. As is true for all people, periods of stress are not the optimal time for making important and irreversible life decisions. Similarly, major changes in treatment are best avoided when the cost of relapse is high, such as when starting school or a new job.

Balance Expectations

Despite available treatments, schizophrenia remains associated with substantial long-term disability. At the same time, recovery is increasingly possible. An aggressive approach to treatment embraces each new treatment advance as representing the potential for further improvement and better functioning. Its guiding axiom is "Never give up hope." At the same time, patients and families have suffered as a result of unrealistic expectations, and patients who have maintained a reasonable degree of functioning have been destabilized by abandoning adequate treatment in the search for something better. Thus, at times, "Better may be the enemy of good." These competing perspectives must be skillfully balanced in relation to what is known about predictors of outcome in schizophrenia and the individual patient and family's expectations and tolerance for risk.

Treatment Integration—Organization of Services

Integrated treatment for patients with schizophrenia requires an organizational infrastructure that is adequately funded and allows patients flexible access to a full continuum of medical and psychosocial services. As described in the 1999 Report of the Surgeon General, a community support system (CSS) model forms the conceptual basis of contemporary organization of services for patients with severe and persistent mental illness. This model is predicated on the belief that individuals with serious mental illness can become citizens of their communities if provided with support and access to both specialized mental health services as well as mainstream resources such as housing and vocational opportunities. The CSS concept was designed by NIMH in the 1980s with extensive participation from the field and is defined as "an organized network of caring and responsible people committed to assisting a vulnerable population meet their needs and develop their potentials without being unnecessarily isolated or excluded from the community." Although the CSS concept was articulated before extensive development of evidence-based practices and some of its language is outdated, the general principles of care organization articulated remain valid.

The CSS concept delineates ten essential components that are needed to provide adequate opportunities and services for people with long-term mental illness (Table 12.14–2). The CSS model defines *principles* for the organization of mental health services that can be actualized in any number of specific administrative or oversight structures. Central to the model, however, is the concept of a coherent, responsible, and accountable system of care. Twenty years of experience attempting to implement the CSS model suggests factors that can differentiate a functioning system from an incoherent or uncoordinated service configuration. Specifically, effective and successful systems are characterized by

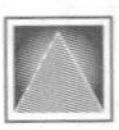

Table 12.14–2
Essential Components of Community Support System Model for Organization of Care

Location of clients/outreach: Locate clients, reach out to inform them of available services, and assure their access to needed services and community resources by arranging for transportation, if necessary, or by taking the services to the clients.

Assistance in meeting basic human needs: Help clients meet basic human needs for food, clothing, shelter, personal safety, and general medical and dental care, and assist them to apply for income, medical, housing, and other benefits that they may need and to which they are entitled.

Mental health care: Provide adequate mental health care, including diagnostic evaluation; prescription, periodic review and regulation of psychotropic drugs as needed; and community-based psychiatric, psychological and/or counseling and treatment services.

24-Hr crisis assistance: Provide 24-hr quick-response crisis assistance directed toward enabling both the client and involved family and friends to cope with emergencies while maintaining the client's status as a functioning community member to the greatest possible extent. This should include around-the-clock telephone services, on-call trained personnel, and options for either short-term or partial hospitalization or for temporary community housing arrangements for crisis stabilization.

Psychosocial and vocational services: Provide comprehensive psychosocial services, including a continuum of high to low expectation services and environments designed to improve or maintain clients' abilities to function in normal social roles. Some of these services should be available on an indefinite-duration basis and should include, but need not be limited to, services that train clients in daily and community living skills; help clients develop social skills, interests, and leisure time activities; and help clients find and make use of appropriate employment opportunities and vocational services.

Rehabilitative and supportive housing: Provide a range of rehabilitative and supportive housing options for people not in crisis who need a special living arrangement. The choices should be broad enough to allow each client an opportunity to live in an atmosphere offering the degree of support necessary while also providing incentives and encouragement for clients to assume increasing responsibility for their lives.

Assistance/consultation and education: Provide back-up support, assistance, and education to families, friends, landlords, and employers to maximize benefits and minimize problems for clients.

Natural support systems: Recognize and involve natural support systems, such as consumer and family self-help groups, consumer-run service alternatives, neighborhood networks, churches, community organizations, and commerce and industry.

Protection of client rights: Establish grievance procedures and mechanisms to protect client rights both in and outside of mental health or residential facilities.

Case management: Facilitate effective use by clients of formal and informal helping systems by designating a single person or team responsible for helping the client to make informed choices about opportunities and services, assuring timely access to needed assistance, providing opportunities and encouragement for self-help activities, and coordinating all services to meet the client's goals.

From Stroul BA: *Crisis residential services in a community support system: Report to the NIMH Crisis Residential Services Project.* Rockville, MD: National Institute of Mental Health; 1987, with permission.

Provision of a continuum of care that can flexibly provide individualized services to patients with varying levels of disability across the full spectrum, from minimal support to comprehensive inpatient or long-term highly supervised community support.

Continuity of care across service levels—in a system providing continuity of care, one or more clinicians remain involved in an individual patient's care regardless of where in the system the patient is being treated at any particular time. For example, if a patient living in the community is hospitalized, the designated clinician responsible for coordinating the overall treatment plan maintains contact with both the patient and the hospital treatment team during the acute care episode, insures that hospital staff are adequately informed regarding the patient's needs, and participates in discharge planning and aftercare.

The system incorporates and integrates *all* components of the CSS model. Providing adequate mental health services is virtually useless, for example, in the absence of meeting basic human service needs for food, clothing, and shelter.

An effective and coherent system maintains responsibility and accountability for clients who fall into "overflow" care settings such as the criminal justice and homeless systems. Clients falling into these systems remain the responsibility of the CSS, and a designated responsible clinician works to ensure continuation of service provision and coordinated return to more stable and integrated living situations.

An effective system offers a full menu of evidence-based practices to ensure that mental health services offered are science based and most likely to deliver desired patient outcomes.

An effective system ensures accountability by incorporating a meaningful data management and quality assurance capacity. In addition to satisfaction surveys, accountability is assured by measuring and reporting "hard process measures" (such as days to first appointment after hospital discharge, outreach visits to clients in jails and homeless shelters per month, percent of missed appointments followed up by outreach phone call or home visit) and measuring and reporting "hard outcome measures" (such as hospitalization rates, rates of homelessness, rates of arrest and incarceration, suicide attempts, patient deaths, competitive employment rates, and client functional status). A meaningful data management and quality assurance capacity ensures that the CSS can proactively identify and correct deficiencies and creates a culture of continuous quality improvement.

EMPIRICALLY BASED INDIVIDUAL PSYCHOTHERAPY

Illness Phase–Specific Cognitive-Behavioral Therapy

In the past decade, disease-specific cognitive-behavioral interventions that target problems experienced by patients with schizophrenia have been tested in randomized clinical trials. Developed largely in the United Kingdom and designed to be added onto "routine clinical care," including pharmacological management, these time-limited treatments focus on illness phase–specific issues.

Acute-Phase Cognitive-Behavioral Therapies *Compliance therapy* is a four- to six-session intervention for acutely ill inpatients that targets improved attitude toward medication and postdischarge adherence as treatment goals. Based on motivational interviewing, the treatment involves nonjudgmental exploration of the patient's attitudes and beliefs about medication, assessment of sources of ambivalence, and an effort to link medication adherence with the patient's self-defined goals. Studies have documented better postdischarge adherence and longer community survival at 18 months for patients receiving this brief intervention. A more intensive inpatient cognitive-behavioral therapy program (3 hours per week, with postdischarge booster sessions for 8 weeks) in combination with family education sessions has been found to reduce the duration of acute psychosis, severity of residual symptoms, and relapse over a 9-month postdischarge follow-up period. Acute-phase treatment packages for first-episode patients with and without medication-resistant positive symptoms have been described and are currently undergoing testing.

Post–Acute-Phase Cognitive-Behavioral Therapies Post–acute-phase cognitive-behavioral therapy targets delusions and hallucinations that have not fully responded to pharmacological treatment. Conceptually, these treatments are based on the observation that patients are able to discover, learn, and use coping strategies to decrease symptom severity or distress associated with medication-resistant symptoms. Techniques used derive from individualized assessment and vary based on individual patient preference. They may include belief modification, self-management techniques, and coping strategy enhancements, such as attention switching, attention narrowing, increasing or decreasing social activity, modifying sensory input, using relaxation strategies, and psychoeducation. In vivo practice and homework assignments are often prescribed and an overall attempt to build on coping methods already used by the patient. Clinical trials of post–acute-phase cognitive-behavioral therapy added to routine care have demonstrated a superior effect on residual positive symptoms, illness exacerbations, and days spent in hospital care relative to generic supportive therapy or befriending. A postacute combination cognitive-behavioral therapy integrating motivational interviewing, cognitive-behavioral therapy, and family intervention for patients with comorbid schizophrenia and substance abuse disorders has yielded a reduction in positive symptoms and exacerbations and an increase in number of days abstinent over a 12-month period from baseline to follow-up. Moving from efficacy to effectiveness, one preliminary controlled study demonstrated the usefulness of integrating techniques from cognitive-behavioral therapy into routine general psychiatric practice.

Although results from randomized controlled trials demonstrate an advantage of adding time-limited cognitive-behavioral therapy to usual care for patients with schizophrenia at both the acute and post-acute phases of illness, not all studies have been positive, and substantial refusal and drop-out rates indicate that these treatments are not appropriate for all patients. Those studies that have evaluated predictors of response have pointed to subjective distress (e.g., ego-dystonic symptoms) and some pretreatment insight as predictors of patients most likely to benefit from targeted cognitive-behavioral therapy interventions. Because of these considerations, most reviews conclude that, although results from cognitive-behavioral therapy trials are promising, further research is required to define for which patients and under what conditions these treatments are optimal. Because nearly all research on cognitive-behavioral therapy has taken place in the context of the U.K. National Health Service, generalizability to other care settings is an additional concern, particularly insofar as effective cognitive therapies for depression have been available in the United States for decades, but few clinicians are trained in these methods, and they have had a very limited impact on routine clinical care.

Personal Psychotherapy Although reflecting clinical practice, treatment integration based on the hierarchy of clinical needs described as *flexible psychotherapy* has not been formally assessed. Similar in overall outlook to flexible psychotherapy, however, *personal therapy* was developed by Gerry Hogarty and his colleagues at the University of Pittsburgh as a form of individual treatment and a strategy for treatment integration that is sufficiently operationalized to allow empirical testing. Personal therapy is designed for recently discharged outpatients with chronic or subchronic schizophrenia. Its objective is to enhance personal and social adjustment and forestall late (third-year) relapse. It is a disorder-specific treatment that accommodates neuropsychological aspects of schizophrenia and attempts to avoid the adverse effect of poorly timed interventions.

Within a stress-vulnerability model, individual-specific stress, often interpersonal, is seen as precipitating affective dysregulation. This loss of control over mood is seen as resulting in poorly reasoned dysfunctional behavior that negatively influences the reciprocal behavior of others in a cycle that may end in relapse. Based on individual patients' needs, personal psychotherapy uses a range of interventions to promote patients' self-awareness and foresight and equip patients with adaptive strategies that facilitate self-monitoring and self-control of affect.

Personal psychotherapy includes three phases, each with explicitly defined goals and corresponding interventions. The achievement of these goals is carefully assessed before the patient advances to the next level of treatment. Phases of treatment, goals, and operational criteria defining readiness to move to more advanced phases are summarized in Table 12.14–3. Within each phase, the exposure of patients to specific interventions is varied based on individual need. Although the therapy was designed to be given over a 3-year time span, patients spend as much time at each level as required to meet advancement criteria, and not all patients progress through all three phases. Personal therapy is administered against a backdrop of psychopharmacological treatment that aims to minimize side effects by using the lowest medication dose needed to prevent symptom exacerbation.

Investigators at the University of Pittsburgh completed two 3-year randomized controlled trials of personal therapy for newly discharged patients with schizophrenia and schizoaffective disorders. Patients residing with their family were assigned to supportive therapy, personal therapy, family psychoeducation/management, or a combination of the latter two treatments. Patients living alone, who were generally more disabled, were assigned to personal therapy or supportive therapy.

Results indicated that personal therapy was remarkably well accepted by patients participating in the trials. Over 3 years, only 8 percent of patients receiving personal therapy and 23 percent of patients in contrasting treatments were dropped for noncompliance or administrative reasons. The efficacy of personal therapy in relapse reduction was tied to residential status. Patients receiving personal therapy who were living with family experienced fewer relapses. The more impaired group of patients receiving personal therapy who were living alone experienced a greater rate of relapse. Consistent with the clinical dictum that psychologically oriented treatments can be futile or harmful when applied before basic human service needs are addressed, personal therapy patients who relapsed were more likely to have unstable housing and difficulty securing food and clothing.

Independent of relapse reduction, personal therapy produced substantial differential improvements in social adjustment and role performance. Although improvements in social adjustment among patients receiving supportive and family therapy reached a plateau at 12 months, the personal adjustment of personal therapy patients continued to improve in the second and third postdischarge years with no evidence of a plateau. Relative to supportive and family therapy, individual psychotherapy was superior in promoting a progressive improvement in psychosocial adjustment (Fig. 12.14–1).

Hogarty and his colleagues at the University of Pittsburgh have recently completed a trial of a *recovery phase* intervention termed *cognitive enhancement therapy* for patients who have successfully proceeded through phases of personal psychotherapy. This treatment integrates pharmacological treatment with computer-based attention training exercises and small group–based psychological treatment aimed at promoting abstract thinking, problem solving, and greater

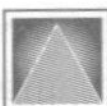

Table 12.14–3
Personal Therapy: Goals, Techniques, and Criteria for Advancement

Treatment Phase	Initiation Criteria	Goals	Techniques
Phase I (3–6 mos)	? Residential stability	Therapeutic joining Stabilization Treatment contract Basic psychoeducation (stress-vulnerability model) Establish lowest effective medication dose	Supportive techniques (acceptance, empathy, problem solving) Basic stress identification and avoidance Support gradual resumption of responsibilities Basic social skills training Basic psychoeducation workshop
Phase II (6–18 mos)	Positive symptoms stable Maintenance dose of medication achieved Can maintain attention for 30 mins Basic understanding of illness Regularly attends appointments Appropriate basic social skills	Self-awareness of affective, cognitive, behavioral states Awareness of individual stressors, internal cues of stress Learn self-protective strategies Awareness of individual dysfunctional responses to stress Improved social perception and functioning	Individualized psychoeducation Encourage self-reflection Exploration of individual vulnerabilities, stresses Teach basic relaxation techniques (if patient is interested) Exercises to improve social perception, teach basic conflict management (role play)
Phase III (18–36 mos)	Continued clinical stability Recognition of role of stress as potential precipitant of psychosis Regular participation in role-playing exercises (if social skills deficit present) Evidence of accurate social perception Identification of at least one affect and physical or cognitive cue of vulnerability Basic relaxation technique learned	Learn relationship between life circumstance and internal state Learn relationship between felt affect and expressions of affect Learn to predict significant others' reactions to expressions of affect Learn criticism management Recognize prodrome, need for prophylactic medication—avoid late relapse	Investigation of individual-specific responses to stress Exploration of individual strengths and persistent limitations Carefully timed vocational and resocialization initiatives Advanced relaxation and social skills exercises

ability to recognize the thoughts and affects of others. Preliminary data from this evaluation suggest that this targeted approach may be useful in alleviating deficits in social cognition in stable outpatients with schizophrenia who experience persistent cognitive deficits. As with cognitive-behavioral therapy, further research and replication are required to fully assess the usefulness of this approach.

SPECIAL ISSUES

Medication Compliance

Noncompliance with effective psychopharmacological treatments during both acute and maintenance therapy is a major cause of morbidity among patients with schizophrenia. When prolonged or repeated, noncompliance contributes to a downwardly spiraling cycle of relapse, recidivism, and deterioration of social and instrumental functioning. Empirical correlates of noncompliance include (1) patient-related factors (greater illness severity or grandiosity, lack of insight, substance abuse comorbidity), (2) medication-related factors (dysphoric medication side effects, ineffective or excessively high dosages), (3) environmental factors (inadequate support of supervision, practical barriers), and (4) clinician-related factors (poor therapeutic alliance). Available research underscores the multiplicity of explanations for reduced compliance and highlights the necessity of an individualized assessment. Of particular relevance to psychotherapy are patients' health beliefs and the psychological meanings attached to their illness and its treatment.

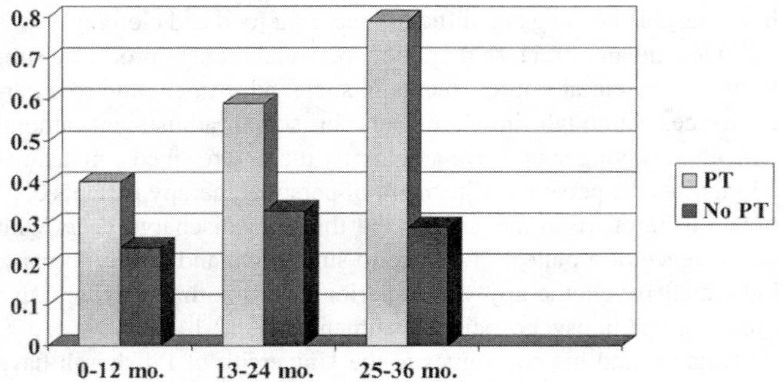

FIGURE 12.14–1 Personal therapy (PT). Social adjustment of patients receiving PT (N = 74) and other treatments (N = 77) in a 3-year trial. (Adapted from Hogarty GE, Greenwald D, Ulrich RF, et al.: Three year trials of personal therapy among schizophrenic patients living with or independent of family II: Effects on adjustment of patients. *Am J Psychiatry.* 1997;154:1514.)

Among the psychological meanings associated with medication noncompliance, the following have been described: (1) pervasive denial about having an illness and needing treatment; (2) reactive efforts to regain control of one's life and maintain a sense of self-cohesion by organizing in opposition to the will of others; (3) the concrete equation of taking medication with being ill (if I need drugs, I must be sick; the higher the dose, the sicker I am; I'll stop being ill if I stop taking drugs); (4) lack of knowledge or incorrect beliefs about medications (taking drugs is a sign of weakness); (5) paranoid views of medication as being poison, controlling, or damaging; (6) secondary gain from psychosis—grandiose delusional gratification, escape from normal expectations and responsibilities; (7) pain and anguish accompanying symptom reduction with its attendant recognition that one has been ill and that the illness is severe; (8) displacement from transference, such as discontinuing medication as an expression of anger toward therapist or family; and (9) an expression of unconscious ambivalence or fear of autonomy—as in discontinuing medication immediately before beginning a new job or rehabilitation program.

The variety of possible factors related to noncompliance points to the need for a broad and flexible approach that applies a range of interventions based on current knowledge of psychopharmacology and sound dynamic understanding of the individual patient. General recommendations for improving compliance in the context of the clinical relationship have included: (1) conveying interest and concern about medication by asking specific questions about how much medication is being taken, effects, and side effects; (2) assuming many patients at times take more or less medication and creating a therapeutic environment in which such "experiments" are legitimized and can be talked about; (3) involving patients to the greatest extent possible in their own medication treatment, such as by allowing self-regulation of dosage within bounds; (4) arranging for the taking of medication under the supervision of family, friends, or others and enlisting their support for medication; (5) offering direct praise and support for medication compliance; (6) providing education in the areas of medication side effects, relapse prevention, and the biological basis of major mental illness; (7) promoting self-monitoring through record keeping and other behavioral interventions; (8) attending to and building the therapeutic relationship as a lever to change; and (9) helping the patient experience activities that promote self-esteem and compete with psychosis as sources of gratification.

The choice of specific interventions for medication noncompliance should be based on a differential diagnosis that generates hypotheses regarding which specific factor(s) is operative in the individual patient. When lack of knowledge and cognitive deficit are major factors in noncompliance, specific cognitive and behavioral procedures have been developed to enhance cognitive mastery and skill attainment. When noncompliance represents the wish to regress, ambivalence about functioning, or an expression of anger, dynamic exploration and interpretation are required. When severe disorganization is a major factor, arrangements for supervised medication administration may be necessary.

Finally, it must be recognized that some patients who appear to be clear candidates for benefiting from medication continue to refuse despite all efforts. These circumstances can arouse reactions in the therapist that are not helpful, such as telling the patient to seek treatment elsewhere out of anger or wishing to hurt the patient through abandonment. Another unproductive countertransference is withholding advice or support that might be of use to the patient to see him or her "learn their lesson" by experiencing a full-blown relapse. Allowing the noncompliant patient who leaves treatment against medical advice to do so with dignity can set the stage for greater collaboration should the patient return in the future.

Circumstances requiring the therapist to initiate commitment or involuntary administration of medication also typically evoke powerful countertransference. After such coercive interventions, the clinician may experience considerable guilt about or fear of the patient. At such a time, the therapist is tempted to discontinue all contact and turn the patient over to another clinician, rationalizing that a therapeutic alliance is never again possible after such heavy-handed acts. Experience demonstrates that such an assessment is usually a distortion that more often serves the needs of the clinician than the patient. After resolution of such an episode, many patients may express gratitude for the therapist's action and in hindsight recognize that they were in need of treatment.

Suicide and Suicide Prevention

Suicide is probably the single leading cause of premature death among people with schizophrenia, with long-term rates of suicide in this population estimated to be 10 to 13 percent. Distressingly often, suicide in schizophrenia seems to occur "out of the blue," without prior warnings or expressions of verbal intent. Some data suggest that those patients with the best prognosis (few negative symptoms, preservation of capacity to experience affects, better abstract thinking) can paradoxically also be at highest risk for suicide. These patients frequently declined from a higher level of premorbid functioning and had an intermittent illness that, during periods of remission, allowed them to retain the capacity to reflect on their life situation and illness. This profile points to the importance of attunement to the human aspects of adapting to a severe and recurrent illness, including the potential for despair, damage to self-esteem, and hopelessness. For patients who recover from an episode with insight and recognition of what has happened, assisting the patient to acknowledge, bear, and put the illness and its disabilities into perspective can be a useful psychotherapeutic approach.

Specific recommendations for suicide prevention include recognizing actuarially defined high-risk patients (e.g., male, young, those with concurrent depression, recent loss or rejection, prior suicide attempts, limited external support), providing additional monitoring and support during high-risk periods (e.g., immediately after hospital discharge), and using specific targeted psychopharmacological and psychosocial interventions for comorbid depression and substance abuse. Several studies have shown that two-thirds or more of schizophrenic patients who commit suicide have seen an apparently unsuspecting clinician within 72 hours of death. Consequently, clinicians should be active in directly asking patients if they are experiencing suicidal ideation and documenting the resulting assessment; if not directly asked, schizophrenia patients may not reveal their intent. A large recent pharmacological study suggests that clozapine (Clozaril) may have particular efficacy in reducing suicidal ideation in schizophrenia patients with prior hospitalizations for suicidality. Epidemiological studies indicate that up to 80 percent of schizophrenia patients may have a major depressive episode at some time in their lives. After stabilization of acute psychotic symptoms with antipsychotic medications, adjunctive antidepressant medications have been shown to be effective in alleviating cooccurring major depression in schizophrenia.

Cooccurring Substance Abuse

Many studies indicate that individuals with severe mental illness, including schizophrenia, are at increased risk for cooccurring substance abuse disorders. In the Epidemiological Catchment Area Study, 17 percent of the general population, but 48 percent of persons with schizophrenia, met criteria for substance abuse disorders. Substance abuse disorder dual diagnoses are more common in patients who are young, male, single, less educated, and who have a history of conduct disorder or family history of substance abuse. The most commonly abused substance is alcohol, followed by cannabis and cocaine. Medication nonadherence, frequent emergency department visits, homelessness, and incarceration correlate with cooccurring substance abuse disorders. Although people with serious mental illness who abuse substances appear less likely to develop medical sequelae associated with continuous heavy substance abuse, they may be more sensitive to the destabilizing effect of alcohol or drug use. More than 100 studies of patients with schizophrenia indicate that dual diagnosis is associated with adverse outcomes such as frequent relapse, rehospitalization, violence, incarceration, depression, suicide, sexually transmitted diseases, increased treatment costs, and family burden.

Although it has been suggested that patients with serious mental illness may abuse substances to "self-medicate" negative symptoms or the extrapyramidal side effects of antipsychotic medications, patients' self-reported reasons for use tend to be similar to others with substance abuse disorders: to combat loneliness, social anxiety, boredom, and insomnia. Because of poverty, many people with schizophrenia may live in neighborhoods where drugs are readily available.

In the United States, mental illness and substance abuse treatment settings have been fiscally, administratively, and ideologically separated, with the federal government funding the bulk of substance abuse treatment and state governments funding mental illness treatment facilities. As a consequence, patients were often advised to seek definitive treatment in one system before being referred to the other. Alternatively, patients in one system were referred to the other for consultation. Too often, this resulted in a complete lack of access to any treatment for patients with cooccurring schizophrenia and substance abuse: These patients were judged to be appropriate for the mental health system because they were substance abusers and not inappropriate for the substance abuse system because of mental illness.

To remedy this situation, integrated mental illness–substance abuse treatment models have been developed in recent years. These models use the same clinician or team of clinicians, working in one setting to provide coordinated mental illness and substance abuse interventions. According to Drake and Mueser, effective integrated programs are characterized by a number of features:

Most are developed within existing outpatient mental health programs that have a full array of community support services in place.

Awareness of substance abuse disorders permeates all aspects of the program and services provided and are not isolated as a single discrete substance abuse intervention.

Recognizing the difficulty that dual diagnosis patients have maintaining treatment adherence, programs provide continual outreach and close monitoring techniques to build and maintain consistent therapeutic relationships.

Programs recognize that treatment must be long-term and anticipate the need for treatment participation over months and years.

Programs recognize that most dual diagnosis patients have little readiness for abstinence-oriented substance abuse disorder treatment, and rather than only treat highly motivated patients, programs incorporate motivational interventions designed for patients who do not recognize substance abuse disorders or are not yet motivated to change. Motivational interventions help patients to identify their personal goals and clarify the role of substance use in impeding achievement of those goals.

Because of the frequent cooccurrence of substance abuse disorders, all patients with schizophrenia should be screened for substance abuse history; mental health treatment programs should use formal screening tools as part of intake assessments. Denial of substance abuse on the face of clinical and psychosocial instability should trigger more detailed assessment, including obtaining information from family or case managers. Assessment also involves evaluating the patient's awareness of the consequences of substance abuse and readiness to change. Four stages of treatment—engagement, persuasion, active treatment, and relapse prevention—have been described. Case management to address human service needs such as housing, entitlements, social isolation, medical care, and rehabilitation are particularly important for this population. Furthermore, in the context of comprehensive integrated treatment, "close monitoring" techniques such as medication supervision, protective payeeships, guardianships for medications, urine drug screens, supported housing, and outpatient commitment can also be of value.

With respect to pharmacological treatment, some evidence suggests that second-generation antipsychotics, particularly clozapine (Clozaril), may facilitate the reduction of substance abuse in patients with schizophrenia. Bupropion (Wellbutrin), in combination with behaviorally oriented smoking cessation programs, may be useful in promoting tobacco cessation for schizophrenia patients.

HIV Risk Reduction The human immunodeficiency virus (HIV) epidemic is among the most serious public health problems of modern times. Since the 1990s, more than a dozen studies have reported elevated HIV infection rates in people with serious mental illness, the majority of whom have schizophrenia. A large recent study of 931 consecutively admitted patients in three states reported an HIV seroprevalence rate of 3.1 percent; eight times the reported U.S. population rate. Prevalence rates for hepatitis B (HBV) and hepatitis C (HCV) infection were 23.4 and 19.6 percent, respectively—rates 5 and 11 times that of the general population, respectively. Data from predominantly urban samples, which overrepresent ethnic minorities and people living in poverty, report higher HIV rates. Elevated HIV and sexually transmitted disease (STD) infection rates in people with severe mental illness may be a result of the fact that these people are more likely to engage in high-risk behaviors such as using injection drugs, having multiple sexual partners and high-risk partners (such as intravenous [IV] drug users), engaging in sexual exchange for money or drugs, and rarely using condoms. In one survey, anal sex appeared to be common among people with schizophrenia, although the majority of men who had sex with men did not classify themselves as gay. At the same time, HIV knowledge deficits may be more prevalent among people with schizophrenia and referrals for screening less common. This may in part be due to clinicians' erroneous beliefs that people with schizophrenia are rarely sexually active.

As is true for people generally, merely giving information about HIV and acquired immune deficiency syndrome (AIDS) does not change behavior. Interventions that are effective are based on models of behavioral change that, in addition to knowledge per se, target health beliefs and attitudes, motivation to reduce risk behavior, skills needed to accomplish behavior change (such as condom negotiation skills with partners), and barriers to behavioral change, such as lack of access to condoms. Several randomized trials have used these principles to develop targeted interventions for people with schizophrenia, with promising results. Many HIV prevention interventions described in the literature share methods used successfully to improve other skill deficits in patients with schizophrenia, including small group formats, emphasis on cognitive and behavioral skill building, and efforts to encourage skill use in real-life situations. Also similar to general skill-oriented rehabilitative approaches, HIV prevention interventions require integration with other treatment modalities, particularly substance abuse treatment and attention to basic human service issues such as housing and income supports. Long-term risk reduction has yet to be documented with any specific intervention, suggesting that ongoing attention to risk reduction is required. When specific interventions are not available, clinicians should be cognizant of the fact that patients with schizophrenia are at particularly high risk for HIV, HBV, and HCV; assess risk behavior; and endeavor to integrate risk reduction strategies into available treatments. For patients with cognitive disturbances, obtaining informed consent for screening may require greater prescreening educational efforts.

PRACTICAL CONSIDERATIONS IN OUTPATIENT ASSESSMENT

When scheduling an initial outpatient visit for a patient with schizophrenia, the clinician should set aside sufficient time (1.5 to 2.0 hours) to conduct a thorough preliminary assessment. If the referral is initiated over the phone by someone other than the patient, it is useful to use the phone contact to obtain a cursory outline of the patient's history and current mental status. Information about symptom severity, current medications, and current and past suicidality and aggression should be sought with the aim of determining whether outpatient evaluation can proceed safely. If preliminary contacts suggest the possibility of a need for hospitalization or other acute care, specific information about what acute care resources the patient is eligible to access should be obtained.

It is common for patients with schizophrenia to arrive for a first appointment accompanied by a family member, case manager, or other caregiver. After introduction to the patient and those arriving with him or her, an initial assessment interview can be conducted with the patient alone. In this interview, the clinician may need to make an active effort to promote the patient's comfort. This can be done, for example, by offering coffee, pointing out the specific place to sit, outlining what will be discussed, and, if necessary, patterning the assessment interview with a specific set of questions. With the patient's permission, it is then often useful to spend some time alone with the accompanying family member or other caregiver. This interview allows the person accompanying the patient to express specific concerns or worries in private and can provide important additional information about the patient's situation. Refusing contact with the patient's family under the banner of "confidentiality" is almost always ill advised. During an initial assessment, patients rarely object to such contacts, which can be presented in a matter-of-fact manner as a standard part of the initial consultation.

Ideally, the outcome of the initial visit is a mutually agreed on plan for further assessment or treatment. This plan should include the frequency and duration of visits, payment, medication regimen, and arrangements for the patient or caregivers to reach the physician (or other team member) in the event of a crisis between scheduled appointments. Attention should also be given to practical considerations, such as transportation to appointments, and how and where prescriptions are filled. If psychotherapy is recommended, a general statement of its methods and goals may be useful ("We will meet so that we can talk together, better understand your difficulties, and work with you on your medications to improve your situation."). In addition, defining some mutually agreed on area (problem, concern, goal, medication side effect) in which the therapist can be seen as potentially useful to the patient sets the stage for a positive therapeutic relationship.

The frequency and duration of clinical visits are individualized. If psychotherapy is used, 45- to 50-minute sessions are most common in an outpatient setting, but the frequency of visits may be increased during periods of clinical instability or if insight-oriented psychotherapy is prescribed. Less-frequent visits of shortened duration (15 to 20 minutes) may be negotiated during periods of stability for patients who have learned to self-manage their illness or for those who find contact with a clinician aversive, disorganizing, or irrelevant.

In addition to setting the stage for establishing a working relationship with the patient, the clinician's management of the initial interview should promote collaboration with the patient's family member, case manager, or other caregiver. Both the patient and the caregiver can be told that the patient's confidentiality is respected, but should the therapist at any time believe a relapse or other dangerous situation is developing, the help of family or other caregivers will be solicited. The family can be encouraged to contact the clinician should they develop concerns and the frequency of future family contacts should be agreed on. Family or caregiver support is crucial to the outcome of treatment and is most likely extended to a clinician who is believed to be empathic, responsive to concerns, and available.

SUGGESTED CROSS-REFERENCES

Section 12.13 provides information on rehabilitation. Other treatment methods are discussed in Chapter 30 (psychotherapies) and Chapter 31 (biological therapies).

REFERENCES

Alanen YO. *Schizophrenia: Its Origins and Need-Adapted Treatment.* London: H. Karnac, Ltd.; 1997.

American Psychiatric Association: Practice guidelines for the treatment of patients with schizophrenia. *Am J Psychiatry.* 1997;154[Suppl]:1–63.

Barrowclaugh C, Haddock G, Tarrier N, Lewis SW, Moring J, O'Brien R, Schofield N, McGovern J: Randomized controlled trial of motivational interviewing, cognitive behavior therapy, and family intervention for patients with comorbid schizophrenia and substance use disorders. *Am J Psychiatry.* 2001;158:1706–1713.

Book HE: Some psychodynamics of non-compliance. *Can J Psychiatry.* 1987;32:115.

*Bustillo JR, Lauriello J, Horan WP, Keith SJ: The psychosocial treatment of schizophrenia: An update. *Am J Psychiatry.* 2001;158:163–175.

Deegan PE: Recovery and empowerment for people with psychiatric disabilities. *J Soc Work Health Care.* 1997;25:11–24.

Dickerson FB: Cognitive behavioral psychotherapy for schizophrenia: A review of recent empirical studies. *Schizophr Res.* 2000;43:71–90.

Dixon L, Adams C, Luckstead A: Update on family psychoeducation for schizophrenia. *Schizophr Bull.* 2000;26:5–20.

*Drake RE, Mueser KT: Psychosocial approaches to dual diagnosis. *Schizophr Bull.* 2000;26:105–118.

Fenton WS: Community interventions. *Curr Opin Psychiatry.* 2000;13:189–194.

Fenton WS: Depression, suicide and suicide prevention in schizophrenia. *Suicide Life Threat Behav.* 2000;30:134–149.

Fenton WS: Evolving perspectives on individual psychotherapy of schizophrenia. *Schizophr Bull.* 2000;26:47–72.

*Fenton WS, Blyler CR, Heinssen RK: Determinants of medication compliance in schizophrenia: Clinical and empirical correlates. *Schizophr Bull.* 1997;23:637.

Frank AF, Gunderson JG: The role of the therapeutic alliance in the treatment of schizophrenia: Relationship to course and outcome. *Arch Gen Psychiatry.* 1990;47:228.

Haddock G, Barrowclough C, Tarrier N, Moring J, O'Brien R, Schofield N, Quinn J, Palmer S, Davies L, Lowens I, McGovern J, Lewis S: Cognitive-behavioural therapy and motivational intervention for schizophrenia and substance misuse. 18-Month outcomes of randomized controlled trial. *Br J Psychiatry.* 2003;183:418–426.

Hatfield AB, Gearson JS, Coursey RD: Family members' ratings of the use and value of mental health services: Results of a national NAMI Survey. *Psychiatr Serv.* 1996;27:825–831.

Heinssen RK, Liberman RP, Kopelowicz A: Psychosocial skills training for schizophrenia: Lessons from the laboratory. *Schizophr Bull.* 2000;26:21–46.

Hogarty GE, Greenwald D, Ulrich RF, Kornblith SJ, DiBarry AL, Cooley S, Carter M, Flesher S: Three year trials of personal therapy among schizophrenic patients living with or independent of family II: Effects on adjustment of patients. *Am J Psychiatry.* 1997;154:1514.

Hogarty GE, Kornblith SJ, Greenwald D, DiBarry AL, Cooley S, Flesher S, Reiss D, Carter M, Ulrich R: Personal therapy: A disorder-relevant psychotherapy for schizophrenia. *Schizophr Bull.* 1995;21:379–393.

Kelly JA: HIV Risk reduction interventions for persons with severe mental illness. *Clin Psychol Rev.* 1997;17:293–309.

Kemp R, Kirov G, Everitt P, Haywood P, David A: Randomized controlled trial of compliance therapy: 18 Month follow-up. *Br J Psychiatry.* 1998;172:413–419.

Lehman AF, Fischer EP, Postrado L, Delahanty J, Johnstone BM, Russo PA, Crown WH: The Schizophrenia Care and Assessment Program Health Questionnaire (SCAP-HQ): An instrument to assess outcomes of schizophrenia care. *Schizophr Bull.* 2003;29:247–256.

Lehman AF, Goldberg R, Dixon LB, McNary S, Postrado L, Hackman A, McDonnell K: Improving employment outcomes for persons with severe mental illnesses. *Arch Gen Psychiatry.* 2002;59:165–172.

*Lehman AF, Steinwachs DM, the Co-Investigators of the PORT Project: At issue: Translating research into practice: The Schizophrenia Patient Outcomes Research Team (PORT) treatment recommendations. *Schizophr Bull.* 1998;24:1–10.

Lenroot R, Bustillo JR, Lauriello J, Keith SJ: Integrated treatment of schizophrenia. *Psychiatr Serv.* 2003;54:1499–1507.

Noordsy DL, Green AI: Pharmacotherapy for schizophrenia and cooccurring substance use disorders. *Curr Psychiatry Rep.* 2003;5:340–346.

Parsons T. *The Social System.* Glencoe, IL: The Free Press; 1951.

Rako S, Mazer H, eds. *Semrad: The Heart of a Therapist.* New York: Jason Aronson; 1980.

Rosenberg SD, Goodman LA, Osher FC, Swartz MS, Essock SM, Butterfield MI, Constantine NT, Wolford GL, Salyers MP: Prevalence of HIV, hepatitis B, and hepatitis C in people with severe mental illness. *Am J Public Health.* 2001;91:31–37.

Rosenheck R, Tekell J, Peters J, Cramer J, Fontana A, Xu W: Does participation in psychosocial treatment augment the benefits of clozapine? *Arch Gen Psychiatry.* 1998;55:618–625.

Stroul BA: *Crisis residential services in a community support system: Report to the NIMH Crisis Residential Services Project.* Rockville, MD: National Institute of Mental Health; 1987.

Twamley EW, Jeste DV, Bellack AS: A review of cognitive training in schizophrenia. *Schizophr Bull.* 2003;29:247–256.

*U.S. Department of Health and Human Services. *Mental Health: A Report of the Surgeon General.* Rockville, MD: U.S. Department of Health and Human Services, Substance Abuse and Mental Health Services Administration, Center for Mental Health Services, National Institutes of Health, National Institutes of Mental Health; 1999.

Weiden P, Havens L: Psychotherapeutic management techniques in the treatment of outpatients with schizophrenia. *Psychiatr Serv.* 1994;45:549–555.

Winston A, Pinsker H, McCullough L: A review of supportive psychotherapy. *Hosp Community Psychiatry.* 1986;37:1105–1114.

Zygmunt A, Olfson M, Boyer CA, Mechanic D: Interventions to improve treatment adherence in schizophrenia. *Am J Psychiatry.* 2002;159:1653–1664.

▲ 12.15 Schizophrenia Spectrum: Pathology and Treatment

MING T. TSUANG, M.D., PH.D., WILLIAM S. STONE, PH.D., STEPHEN J. GLATT, PH.D., AND STEPHEN V. FARAONE, PH.D.

INTRODUCTION AND HISTORY

Schizophrenia is a complex disorder in both its etiology and its presentation. The illness has been studied for more than a century, but much remains unknown about its origins, development, pathology, and treatment. Progress in unraveling these mysteries has accelerated in the last 30 years. The introduction of improved study methods, such as brain imaging technologies, neuropsychological assessment, and molecular genetic techniques, has provided the impetus for such advancement. Another source of progress involves a gradually evolving reconceptualization of the disorder and the nature and extent of its spectrum.

One component of this evolving view is the idea that schizophrenia may represent a point—or end point—on a continuum of deficit rather than a discrete disease entity. The notion of a "spectrum" of schizophrenias, comprised of schizophrenia and a number of related—but generally milder—conditions, is not new. The concept was advanced by Eugen Bleuler, who foreshadowed the current state of the field in his 1911 work, *Dementia Praecox, or the Group of Schizophrenias*. The classification of specific disorders in the schizophrenia spectrum is a more recent advance due largely to diagnostic refinements in the revised fourth edition of the *Diagnostic and Statistical Manual of Mental Disorders* (DSM-IV-TR) and the tenth revision of *International Statistical Classification of Diseases and Related Health Problems* (ICD-10) and to the use of behavioral genetic and other family study paradigms. These methods have provided the strongest evidence for the inclusion of schizoaffective disorder and schizotypal personality disorder in the spectrum and moderate evidence for the inclusion of paranoid and schizoid personality disorder. Recently, the authors proposed research criteria for another syndrome, called *schizotaxia*, which extends the spectrum further. Each of these disorders shares some clinical features with schizophrenia and may also share etiological elements. If this last point is correct, the disorders may share common treatment targets as well, which is significant for at least two reasons. First, successful treatments, particularly in the more severe spectrum disorders, may be useful in the treatment of milder related disorders. Second, successful treatments for the less severe disorders may be relevant for the potential early intervention in, and even prevention of, the development of more severe disorders in the spectrum.

The remainder of this section briefly summarizes the current understanding of schizophrenia as a benchmark for evaluating the knowledge about the underlying pathology and effective management of related schizophrenia-spectrum disorders. Other sections in this section focus more on schizophrenia itself. Similarities among the schizophrenia-spectrum disorders are noted, although an emphasis is placed on identifying and explaining the differences between these conditions. The section closes with a discussion that anticipates changes that may emerge in the methods used to study, treat, and, ultimately, prevent these conditions.

THEORETICAL ISSUES

Although inclusion in the schizophrenia spectrum is not arbitrary, there are no widely accepted rules for determining whether a syndrome warrants inclusion. Rather, two traditional lines of evidence have been used to make this distinction. The first of these criteria is that a disorder should show some clinical similarity to schizophrenia. The second criterion for inclusion in the schizophrenia spectrum is that a disorder should aggregate in families that are affected by schizophrenia, as evidence of both the genetic and nongenetic etiological similarities of the disorder to schizophrenia.

Clinical Similarities to Schizophrenia Regarding this first criterion, there is a clear gradient of clinical similarity between various disorders and schizophrenia according to the criteria presented in the American Psychiatric Association's DSM-IV-TR. The diagnosis of schizophrenia is based on fulfilling the criteria in Table 12.15–1, which include clinical features of the disorder that must be met and the exclusion of other conditions that may mimic its symptoms such as mood disorders, general medical conditions, or pervasive developmental disorders. Social dysfunction appears to be a cardinal feature of the illness, whereas the specific Criterion A symptoms present may dictate which subtype of schizophrenia is diagnosed; yet the presence of at least two symptoms (or in the case of severe delusions or hallucinations, only one symptom) is essential for the diagnosis of schizophrenia. For example, the presence of disorganized speech and behavior paired with flat or inappropriate

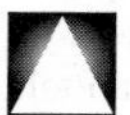

Table 12.15–1
Summary of DSM-IV-TR Diagnostic Criteria for Schizophrenia

A. Characteristic symptoms: Two (or more) of the following, each present for a significant portion of time during a 1-month period (or less if successfully treated):
   (1) Delusions
   (2) Hallucinations
   (3) Disorganized speech
   (4) Grossly disorganized or catatonic behavior
   (5) Negative symptoms, i.e., affective flattening, alogia, or avolition
   Note: Only one Criterion A symptom is required if delusions are bizarre or hallucinations consist of a voice keeping up a running commentary on the person's behavior or thoughts, or two or more voices conversing with each other.

B. Social/occupational dysfunction: One or more major areas of functioning, such as work, interpersonal relations, or self-care, are markedly below the level achieved before the onset.

C. Duration: Continuous signs of the disturbance persist for at least 6 months.

D. Schizoaffective and mood disorder exclusion: Schizoaffective disorder and mood disorder with psychotic features have been ruled out.

E. Substance/general medical condition exclusion: The disturbance is not due to the direct physiological effects of a substance or a general medical condition.

F. Relationship to a pervasive developmental disorder: If there is a history of autistic disorder or another pervasive developmental disorder, the additional diagnosis of schizophrenia is made only if prominent delusions or hallucinations are also present for at least 1 month (or less if successfully treated).

From American Psychiatric Association. *Diagnostic and Statistical Manual of Mental Disorders*. 4th ed. Text rev. Washington, DC: American Psychiatric Association; 2000, with permission.

affect may be indicative of disorganized type schizophrenia if catatonic features are not exhibited. Delusions and hallucinations are prominent markers of paranoid type schizophrenia, especially in the absence of disorganized or catatonic features and affective disturbance. In the catatonic subtype of schizophrenia, motoric dysfunction is featured prominently. However, the pattern of presentation of specific symptoms comprising Criterion A does not always conform to the patterns of any specific type of schizophrenia. In that case, a diagnosis of undifferentiated type schizophrenia may be indicated.

An important way of conceptualizing schizophrenia, and one that is repeated throughout the schizophrenia spectrum in varying proportions, involves the presence of positive and negative symptoms. Although these are not the only dimensions along which symptoms vary (e.g., disorganization may be an independent factor, at least in some spectrum disorders), they represent many of the fundamental clinical problems in schizophrenia and related disorders. *Positive symptoms* refer to symptoms that are present in schizophrenia and contribute to thought disorder and psychosis (e.g., delusions and hallucinations most prominently, but also milder forms of magical thinking, ideas of reference, odd speech or behavior, and perceptual illusions) but are not generally present in the general population. *Negative symptoms* refer to thoughts and behaviors that are generally present in the general population but occur at abnormally low levels in schizophrenia (e.g., range of affect and the capabilities to enjoy aspects of the environment, the company of others, and close interpersonal relationships).

To some extent, positive and negative symptoms occur independently of each other. Although all patients with DSM-IV-TR–defined schizophrenia show positive symptoms (e.g., delusions or hallucinations) during the course of their illness, some patients present with a particularly prominent loading of either positive (e.g., DSM-IV-TR schizophrenia, paranoid type) or negative (e.g., DSM-IV-TR schizophrenia, residual type) symptoms. Moreover, antipsychotic medications are generally more effective at reducing positive symptoms (especially the older, "typical" neuroleptics) than they are at reducing negative symptoms (or neuropsychological deficits). Different balances of positive and negative symptoms also characterize spectrum conditions. For example, individual patients with paranoid personality disorder show a preponderance of positive symptoms, patients with schizotypal personality disorder may show a preponderance of either positive ("positive schizotypy") or negative ("negative schizotypy") symptoms, and individuals with schizoid personality disorder or "schizotaxia" show a preponderance of negative symptoms.

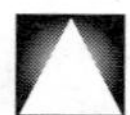

Table 12.15–2
Summary of DSM-IV-TR Diagnostic Criteria for Schizoaffective Disorder

A. An uninterrupted period of illness during which, at some time, there is either a major depressive episode, a manic episode, or a mixed episode concurrent with symptoms that meet Criterion A for schizophrenia.

B. During the same period of illness, there have been delusions or hallucinations for at least 2 weeks in the absence of prominent mood symptoms.

C. Symptoms that meet criteria for a mood episode are present for a substantial portion of the total duration of the active and residual periods of the illness.

D. The disturbance is not due to the direct physiological effects of a substance or a general medical condition.

From American Psychiatric Association. *Diagnostic and Statistical Manual of Mental Disorders.* 4th ed. Text rev. Washington, DC: American Psychiatric Association; 2000, with permission.

Schizoaffective Disorder

According to these diagnostic standards, schizoaffective disorder can be seen as having significant symptom overlap with schizophrenia in addition to its affective features (Table 12.15–2). In fact, based on the requirements of the diagnosis of schizoaffective disorder, which specify that Criterion A of schizophrenia must be satisfied and that delusions or hallucinations must be present, schizoaffective disorder shares more than any other disorder in common with schizophrenia clinically. Of the two subtypes of schizoaffective disorder, the depressive type is believed to lie nearer the schizophrenia spectrum, whereas the bipolar type is believed to have its foundation closer to that of traditional mood disorders. Nevertheless, there is evidence that both subtypes are on a disease continuum that includes schizophrenia, suggesting that the traditional boundary between schizophrenia and mood disorders may be somewhat artificial.

Schizotypal Personality Disorder

Among the several personality disorders that have clinical features in common with schizophrenia, schizotypal personality disorder is the most similar in terms of the number of shared criteria and the degree of impairment (Table 12.15–3). This is due in part to the fact that the diagnosis of schizotypal personality disorder is based on the presence of both social and cognitive deficits, which are also central to the diagnosis of schizophrenia itself. In fact, the features of schizotypal personality disorder reflect those of schizophrenia but with less severity. For example, the ideas of reference, odd beliefs, magical thinking, unusual perceptual experiences, and suspiciousness that characterize schizotypal personality disorder are reminiscent of the delusions and hallucinations of paranoid type schizophrenia (i.e., positive symptoms), whereas the odd thinking, speech, and behavior of this personality disorder resemble the analogous—but more severe—features of disorganized type schizophrenia. Furthermore, the appearance of affective disturbance, the lack of close friends, and the excessive social anxiety

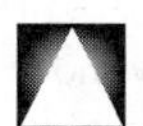

Table 12.15–3
Summary of DSM-IV-TR Diagnostic Criteria for Schizotypal Personality Disorder

A. A pervasive pattern of social and interpersonal deficits marked by acute discomfort with, and reduced capacity for, close relationships, as well as by cognitive or perceptual distortions and eccentricities of behavior, beginning by early adulthood and present in a variety of contexts, as indicated by five (or more) of the following:
   (1) Ideas of reference (excluding delusions of reference)
   (2) Odd beliefs or magical thinking that influences behavior and is inconsistent with subcultural norms
   (3) Unusual perceptual experiences, including bodily illusions
   (4) Odd thinking and speech
   (5) Suspiciousness or paranoid ideation
   (6) Inappropriate or constricted affect
   (7) Behavior or appearance that is odd, eccentric, or peculiar
   (8) Lack of close friends or confidants other than first-degree relatives
   (9) Excessive social anxiety that does not diminish with familiarity and tends to be associated with paranoid fears rather than negative judgments about self

B. Does not occur exclusively during the course of schizophrenia, a mood disorder with psychotic features, another psychotic disorder, or a pervasive developmental disorder.

From American Psychiatric Association. *Diagnostic and Statistical Manual of Mental Disorders.* 4th ed. Text rev. Washington, DC: American Psychiatric Association; 2000, with permission.

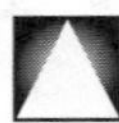

Table 12.15–4
Summary of DSM-IV-TR Diagnostic Criteria for Paranoid Personality Disorder

A. A pervasive distrust and suspiciousness of others such that their motives are interpreted as malevolent, beginning by early adulthood and present in a variety of contexts, as indicated by four (or more) of the following:
  (1) Suspects, without sufficient basis, that others are exploiting, harming, or deceiving him or her
  (2) Is preoccupied with unjustified doubts about the loyalty or trustworthiness of friends or associates
  (3) Is reluctant to confide in others because of unwarranted fear that the information will be used maliciously against him or her
  (4) Reads hidden demeaning or threatening meanings into benign remarks or events
  (5) Persistently bears grudges (i.e., is unforgiving of insults, injuries, or slights)
  (6) Perceives attacks on his or her character or reputation that are not apparent to others and is quick to react angrily or to counterattack
  (7) Has recurrent suspicions, without justification, regarding fidelity of spouse or sexual partner

B. Does not occur exclusively during the course of schizophrenia, a mood disorder with psychotic features, or another psychotic disorder and is not due to the direct physiological effects of a general medical condition.

From American Psychiatric Association. *Diagnostic and Statistical Manual of Mental Disorders*. 4th ed. Text rev. Washington, DC: American Psychiatric Association; 2000, with permission.

commonly seen in schizotypal personality disorder are easily recognizable as diluted forms of the essential social dysfunction of schizophrenia (i.e., negative symptoms).

Paranoid Personality Disorder

Paranoid personality disorder is characterized by a pervasive distrust and suspiciousness of others in which malevolent motives are ascribed to others without sufficient basis (Table 12.15–4). Although paranoid personality disorder as a whole shares only this single group of symptoms with schizophrenia, these features are central to the diagnosis of paranoid type schizophrenia; thus, the inclusion of paranoid personality disorder in the group of schizophrenia-spectrum disorders seems warranted.

Schizoid Personality Disorder

In the same vein, there is also good reason to include schizoid personality disorder in the group of schizophrenia-spectrum disorders. The principal clinical feature of schizoid personality disorder is a consistent pattern of social dysfunction, ranging from aversion of social relationships to restricted affective expression in interpersonal settings (Table 12.15–5), symptoms that are similar to (but less pronounced than) the social dysfunction that is a fundamental feature of schizophrenia.

Schizotaxia

It is important to note that, although the above-named disorders represent the major DSM-IV-TR diagnostic entities that are typically included in the discussion of schizophrenia-spectrum illnesses, other conditions (both those that are and those that are not recognized in the DSM-IV-TR) share clinical features with schizophrenia and may also belong to the family of schizophrenias. This is significant because a thorough comprehension of schizophrenia-spectrum pathology and treatment requires that the continuum of disorder be understood in its entirety. The study of related conditions could provide a twofold benefit by filling the gaps in the understanding of the schizophrenia spectrum as a whole and by enhancing the understanding of schizophrenia and other specific disorders in the spectrum.

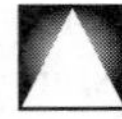

Table 12.15–5
Summary of DSM-IV-TR Diagnostic Criteria for Schizoid Personality Disorder

A. A pervasive pattern of detachment from social relationships and a restricted range of expression of emotions in interpersonal settings, beginning by early adulthood and present in a variety of contexts, as indicated by four (or more) of the following:
  (1) Neither desires nor enjoys close relationships, including being part of a family
  (2) Almost always chooses solitary activities
  (3) Has little, if any, interest in having sexual experiences with another person
  (4) Takes pleasure in few, if any, activities
  (5) Lacks close friends or confidants other than first-degree relatives
  (6) Appears indifferent to the praise or criticism of others
  (7) Shows emotional coldness, detachment, or flattened affectivity

B. Does not occur exclusively during the course of schizophrenia, a mood disorder with psychotic features, another psychotic disorder, or a pervasive developmental disorder and is not due to the direct physiological effects of a general medical condition.

From American Psychiatric Association. *Diagnostic and Statistical Manual of Mental Disorders*. 4th ed. Text rev. Washington, DC: American Psychiatric Association; 2000, with permission.

Schizotaxia is a putative syndrome not described in the DSM-IV-TR that could prove crucial to the discussion of schizophrenia-spectrum pathology and treatment. As originally formulated by Paul Meehl, schizotaxia represented the genetic predisposition to schizophrenia that led, almost invariably, to either schizotypy or schizophrenia, depending on environmental circumstances. Even with the consideration of a liability to schizophrenia receiving widespread conceptual support among researchers, the concept of schizotaxia was reformulated only recently as a meaningful clinical syndrome as well as a relatively specific reflection of the vulnerability to schizophrenia. In this view, schizotypy and schizophrenia are viewed as only two of the possible outcomes of schizotaxia. In addition, schizotaxia is viewed currently as a condition that (1) emerges as a result of the interaction between a genetic predisposition toward illness and the biological consequences of early adverse environmental experiences (e.g., pregnancy complications); (2) includes meaningful, definable clinical and neuropsychological symptoms; (3) remains a stable syndrome in many individuals; and (4) is similar conceptually and phenomenally to negative schizotypal personality disorder. Clinically, initial attempts to define schizotaxia focus on negative symptoms and neuropsychological dysfunction in nonpsychotic relatives of schizophrenic patients. In contrast, it is also likely that the syndrome will come to include additional neurobiological (e.g., structural brain abnormalities) and social deficits.

Familial Aggregation with Schizophrenia

The criterion of clinical similarity to schizophrenia clearly identifies several disorders that can be assigned to the schizophrenia spectrum with varying degrees of certainty based on the extent of their similarity to schizophrenia. Schizoaffective disorder is at the top of this list and schizoid and paranoid personality disorders at the bottom. Yet, there is no clear benchmark for how much similarity warrants inclusion among the schizophrenia-spectrum disorders. Thus, additional standards are helpful in making the distinction between conditions that merely share some symptoms with schizophrenia (e.g., substance-induced psychotic disorder or other "phenocopies") and those that may have a common origin and a shared pathology. The second criterion listed above (i.e., the disorder should show familial aggregation with schizophrenia) is useful for this purpose.

Even with this standard in mind, the level of evidence for inclusion in the schizophrenia spectrum varies widely from condition to condition. Early researchers, such as Emil Kraepelin, noted an increased frequency of schizophrenia-related phenomena among the family members of patients with the disorder. Subsequent research in genetic epidemiology has characterized and quantified the excess of schizophrenia-spectrum pathology in these relatives more precisely.

Schizoaffective Disorder The evidence from more than a dozen family studies (that compared rates of schizoaffective disorder between the relatives of schizophrenic patients and control subjects), twin studies (that compared concordance rates of schizoaffective disorder and schizophrenia in monozygotic and dizygotic twin pairs), and adoption studies (that compared rates of schizoaffective disorder between biological and adoptive relatives of patients with schizophrenia) illustrated the genetic relationship between schizophrenia and schizoaffective disorder. The rate of schizoaffective disorder among the family members of patients with schizophrenia can be as high as 9 percent, well above the rates of schizoaffective disorder among relatives of control subjects as well as the general population (less than 1 percent).

Schizophrenia-Spectrum Personality Disorders Nonpsychotic schizophrenia-spectrum conditions have also been studied in this manner to determine their familial clustering with schizophrenia. It is apparent that many relatives of patients with schizophrenia have maladaptive personality traits, including impaired interpersonal relationships, social anxiety, and constricted emotional responses. Less frequently, mild forms of thought disorder, suspiciousness, magical thinking, illusions, and perceptual aberrations have been observed. This composite set of personality characteristics points to elevated rates of schizotypal, schizoid, or paranoid personality disorders among the relatives of schizophrenic patients, but not all of these have received the same level of support for a familial relationship to schizophrenia.

Schizotypal personality disorder shows the strongest familial link with schizophrenia, with rates of the personality disorder 1.5 to 5.0 times higher among the relatives of schizophrenic patients than in the relatives of controls or in the general population. Furthermore, the results of twin and adoption studies again establish that the disorder appears not only to have a familial relationship with schizophrenia but a significant genetic link as well.

Investigations of paranoid and schizoid personality disorders have not provided a similar level of evidence for a familial association with schizophrenia. In fact, some studies found no increase in the rate of paranoid personality disorder among the first-degree relatives of schizophrenic patients when compared with the rates observed in the family members of control subjects. Schizoid personality disorder has a slightly stronger relationship with schizophrenia, but evidence for a familial aggregation with schizophrenia remains weak overall. Based on the superficial clinical similarities of these two personality disorders in relation to schizophrenia, it is indeed surprising that neither disorder shows a stronger genetic etiological relationship to schizophrenia.

Schizotaxia Finally, it is interesting that schizotaxia, which is conceptualized as the genetic liability toward schizophrenia and defined currently by negative symptoms and neuropsychological dysfunction, is relatively common among the nonpsychotic relatives of patients with schizophrenia. In contrast to schizotypal personality disorder, which occurs in less than 10 percent of the adult relatives of schizophrenic individuals, the core symptoms of schizotaxia range from 20 to 50 percent among the first-degree relatives of schizophrenic patients. Because it has not received formal acceptance as a diagnostic entity, genetic epidemiological studies of schizotaxia are far less common than for other schizophrenia-spectrum disorders. Thus, although a genetic basis for the familial aggregation of schizotaxia in families of a schizophrenic patient is presumed, twin and adoption studies have yet to verify this genetic hypothesis. Further, it is not yet known if the relatives of patients with other schizophrenia-spectrum disorders exhibit higher rates of schizotaxia.

Summary Not surprisingly, the evidence for inclusion in the schizophrenia spectrum is strongest for those disorders that share the most clinical features with schizophrenia (e.g., schizoaffective disorder and schizotypal personality disorder). It is also possible that either the observed relationships may be an artifact of the much greater level of research attention that has been devoted to the analysis of these two disorders relative to schizoid and paranoid personality disorders, or they may result from the relatively low prevalence of the latter two conditions. As paranoid and schizoid personality disorders are examined more extensively for familial links with schizophrenia and as more subjects with these conditions become available for study, these conditions may be found to cluster at a higher, lower, or comparable frequency as schizoaffective disorder and schizotypal personality disorder in families that are affected by schizophrenia.

PATHOLOGY

Brain Structure The pathology of schizophrenia is complex and elusive. The earliest investigations into the underlying biological dysfunction of the illness were limited by available technology that could analyze the gross differences in the brain. Even with current technologies available to study the brain being considerably more sophisticated, it is still useful to examine superficial configurations of the brain as well as the structure of deeper brain regions because many such anomalies in the brains of patients with schizophrenia appear related to the disorder. Structural abnormalities exist in a plethora of cortical and subcortical brain structures in schizophrenic patients, as determined by both postmortem tissue analyses and structural brain imaging techniques such as magnetic resonance imaging (MRI). Abnormalities in some structures, however, are identified more consistently than they are in other structures. These include, for example, increased volume in the lateral ventricles and decreased volumes in the dorsolateral and medial prefrontal cortices, cingulate and paracingulate cortices, hippocampus, parahippocampal and superior temporal gyri, septum pellucidum, and thalamus. The nature and extent of these structural abnormalities often differ between individual patients and their families or between research samples. Their overall reliability nonetheless adds to the view that they are core features of schizophrenia.

The integrity of brain structure in schizoaffective disorder has not received much research attention independent from schizophrenia; rather, patients with schizoaffective disorder tend to be examined jointly with patients who have schizophrenia, reflecting the close proximity of the former to the latter on the continuum of clinical features and (presumed) etiology. The limited number of studies that have investigated the state of the brain in schizoaffective disorder still provide only mixed evidence for common morphology in the two disorders. In fact, these studies have not noted as many structural deficits. For example, features sometimes seen in schizophrenic patients (such as striatal enlargement and cerebral volume reductions) were each noted in only one of three existing studies of schizoaffective patients. In contrast, ventricular enlargement, characteristic of schizophrenia, was observed in two of three studies. In view of the heterogeneous results often reported in structural studies of schizophrenia, such differences are not surprising across just three studies. Considering this, the similarities with schizophrenia (e.g., enlarged ventricles) should probably receive more weight than the differences at this point. More work is clearly needed in this area along with the recognition that schizoaffective disorder, depressed type, may differ etiologically from schizoaffective disorder, bipolar type.

Consistent with the notion of schizotypal personality disorder as a related and less severe disorder in the schizophrenia spectrum, a review of the relevant literature demonstrates that many (but not all) of the structural abnormalities present in schizophrenia are also apparent in schizotypal personality disorder. For example, individuals with schizotypal personality disorder show brain abnormalities in the superior temporal and parahippocampal gyri, lateral ventricles, thalamus, and septum pellucidum that are similar to those seen in people with schizophrenia. By contrast, medial temporal lobe abnormalities and lateral ventricular enlargement are not prominent in schizotypal personality disorder. If the structural differences observed between schizotypal personality disorder and schizophrenia relate directly to the clinical differences between the disorders, this implicates enlargement of the ventricles in addition to the deterioration of the medial temporal lobes in the emergence of psychosis that separates the two disorders phenomenologically. This hypothesis remains to be rigorously tested.

Although structural brain imaging and postmortem tissue analysis have not yet been conducted on individuals with schizoid or paranoid personality disorders, structural abnormalities in the nonpsychotic relatives of schizophrenic patients are now becoming widely recognized. Compared with controls, this subgroup of relatives has significant volume reductions bilaterally in the amygdala-hippocampal region, thalamus, and cerebellum and significantly increased volumes in the pallidum. Relatives of patients with schizophrenia may also exhibit lower volumes in other medial limbic and paralimbic structures, including the anterior cingulate and paracingulate cortex, insula, and parahippocampal gyrus.

Brain Function Functional neuroimaging studies of the brain, in which the metabolic activity of distinct brain regions is measured during activities, are less common than structural brain imaging studies. Consequently, they do not provide as much insight into the pathological neural bases of schizophrenia and schizophrenia-spectrum disorders. With this caveat in mind, it does appear that abnormal patterns of brain activation in functional neuroimaging studies of schizophrenia are generally localized to regions in which structural abnormalities also occur. The same may be true for the spectrum conditions as well, although some anomalies in structure and function do not overlap in schizophrenia and are thus unlikely to overlap in schizophrenia-spectrum conditions. It has been relatively difficult to integrate all of the reports of functional brain abnormalities in schizophrenia due to methodological differences among studies. The most important of these involves differences in patterns of brain activation resulting from the differences in cognitive demands. Thus, functional brain images acquired from patients with schizophrenia performing a wide variety of tasks in different studies (e.g., a problem-solving task, an auditory vigilance task, and a verbal memory task) are not readily combinable. Furthermore, studies seeking analogous deficits on consistently deficient processes in schizophrenia (e.g., motor task performance, verbal fluency, auditory attention) in patients with schizoaffective disorder, or schizoid or paranoid personality disorders, remain to be performed. Because of this, although functional brain imaging is a powerful tool that will undoubtedly influence the understanding of most schizophrenia-spectrum disorders and their treatment in the foreseeable future, it has yet to do so.

The exception to this generalization is schizotypal personality disorder, for which a small but important body of work exists. The limited number of reports of functional abnormalities in schizotypal personality disorder is important because the picture that emerges from these studies further justifies the personality disorder's position in the schizophrenia spectrum. For example, abnormalities in frontal activation in schizotypal personality disorder mimic those of schizophrenia, with the important difference that, in schizotypal personality disorder, additional brain regions are recruited to accomplish tasks requiring frontal lobe activation. Moreover, resting metabolic activity in dopamine-containing subcortical nuclei (particularly, the putamen) is increased among schizotypal individuals relative to controls and to patients with schizophrenia, whereas during performance of a verbal working memory task (a domain that is among the most impaired in schizophrenic patients and among their nonpsychotic relatives), individuals with schizotypal personality disorder exhibited reduced activation relative to controls.

As stated above, the functional integrity of the brain has not been investigated in individuals with schizoid personality disorder; therefore, the evidence for functional abnormalities in paranoid personality disorder is essentially anecdotal at this point. For example, frontal lobe dysfunction has been reported to mimic paranoid personality in case studies. Nonpsychotic relatives of patients with schizophrenia, however, have received more attention in this regard, and findings of functional brain abnormalities in this group (which also contains individuals with schizotaxia) appear to be robust and reliable. For example, relatives show abnormal brain activation patterns while performing working memory tasks with interference. Such tasks normally produce activation in the lateral and medial prefrontal cortex, posterior parietal and precuneal cortex, and thalamus but do so to a greater extent in relatives. This increase in activation is not due to a greater intensity of activity. It is due to more widespread brain activation. Furthermore, relatives exhibit more bilateral activation on working memory tasks, with or without interference, than do control subjects. These findings indicate at least one or both of two possibilities: (1) Relatives demonstrate a compensatory exertion of inefficient neural circuitry in attempting to perform an effortful task to produce accurate output; and (2) they have abnormal connectivity in the circuitry required to perform these tasks. These functional data complement structural MRI abnormalities and add to evidence of brain abnormalities in adult, nonpsychotic relatives of patients with schizophrenia.

Neurotransmission Although many functional imaging methods measure "brain activation" by quantifying energy consumption, the functional abnormalities in the brains of people with schizophrenia do not simply reflect a different pattern of blood flow or oxygenation or glucose use (although these may be indicated). Rather, these differences are believed to be the observable consequence of altered neurotransmission. Thus, by proxy, functional brain-imaging differences give some indication of underlying neurochemical and neurophysiological pathology.

For decades, the central dopamine systems were considered the prime neural substrates of schizophrenic symptomatology with good reason. The evidence supporting dopaminergic dysfunction in schizophrenia is voluminous, although specific mechanisms are still in need of clarification. The "dopamine hypothesis" of schizophrenia pathology was derived partly from observations that typical antipsychotic medications blocked dopamine type 2 (D_2) receptors, whereas indirect dopamine agonists, such as amphetamine, produced psychotic symptoms that resembled schizophrenia. The initial and most basic form of the dopamine hypothesis asserted that schizophrenia results from dopaminergic hyperactivity. Later reformulations focused on relationships between hyperactivity in mesolimbic dopamine neurons and dopaminergic hypoactivity in the prefrontal cortex. An exclusively dopaminergic hypothesis of schizophrenia is too simplistic to explain the development, yet with either the phenomenology or the heterogeneity of the disorder, there is considerable (although necessarily indirect) evidence for both cortical dopaminergic hypoactivity and subcortical dopaminergic hyperactivity in schizophrenia.

Schizophrenic patients often show lower levels of dopamine-β-hydroxylase (the enzyme that converts 3,4-dihydroxyphenylalanine to dopamine) and lower plasma levels of homovanillic acid (a dopamine metabolite). Conversely, elevated levels of homovanillic acid have been reported among the most severely psychotic patients. It is difficult to reconcile such findings, particularly given the coarse level of analysis such as the plasma. Still, such data may be indicative of relative imbalances between distributed dopamine systems (such as mesolimbic and mesocortical dopamine projections) rather than a global hyperactivity of all dopamine neurons.

A slightly more proximal data source for measuring dopaminergic system dysfunction in schizophrenic patients is cerebrospinal fluid (CSF). Early work suggested that the levels of homovanillic acid in CSF correlated with levels of anxiety and agitation among schizophrenic patients; later studies showed that a correlation with the severity of psychosis (especially positive symptoms) was also evident in schizophrenia. The ability of antipsychotic medications to reduce CSF levels of homovanillic acid in schizophrenic patients is consistent with the dopamine hypothesis. Yet, although elevated levels of homovanillic acid in schizophrenia are associated primarily with positive symptoms, relatively few studies reported the inverse relationship with negative symptoms (i.e., higher levels of negative symptoms associated with lower levels of homovanillic acid).

Neuroimaging techniques offer perhaps the best current methods for noninvasive examination of aspects of neurotransmission. Methods such as positron emission tomography and single photon emission computed tomography are not capable of visualizing actual neurotransmission but can provide indirect indices by selectively measuring the occupancy of particular proteins in specific neurotransmitter receptors. To date, the application of such methods has illustrated that dopamine transporter occupancy is not altered in schizophrenia, even early in the disease process or in patients experiencing their first psychotic episode. D_2 receptors have been found on a reliable basis to be occupied to a greater extent in schizophrenic patients than in controls; at least a subset of patients exhibits greater D_2 receptor density. Serotonin 2A receptors and γ-aminobutyric acid (GABA) A receptors do not appear to be altered reliably in the schizophrenic brain.

The diversity of clinical symptoms in schizophrenia, the likely multifactorial polygenic mode of inheritance in most cases, the multiple neurochemical actions of atypical antipsychotic medications, such as clozapine (Clozaril), and the demonstration of numerous neurochemical and morphological abnormalities all underlie the view that multiple biochemical deficits contribute to the etiology of schizophrenia. Thus, aside from dopaminergic dysfunction, abnormalities in glutamate neurotransmission are becoming central to the working hypotheses of the pathology of schizophrenia. Much of this attention is derived from the fact that glutamate is a ubiquitous excitatory neurotransmitter in the central nervous system (CNS), which allows it to interact with many other transmitter systems, including dopamine (thus, dopamine dysfunction is presumed to follow from glutamatergic abnormality). *N*-methyl-D-aspartate (NMDA) and α-amino-3-hydroxy-5-methyl-4-isoxasolepropionate glutamate receptors in the nucleus accumbens modulate dopaminergic neurons in the nucleus accumbens and in the frontal cortex, but the effect of glutamate differs at the two sites. The presence of presynaptic glutamate receptors on dopamine neurons in the frontal cortex generally results in facilitation of dopamine function, whereas dopamine reuptake is inhibited and its release facilitated by glutamate in the nucleus accumbens. This means that agents interfering with glutamate transmission facilitate cortical dopaminergic hypoactivity and subcortical hyperactivity, a finding consistent with the dopamine hypothesis of schizophrenia.

Further evidence for a role of glutamate in schizophrenia is derived from the fact that it is a critical neural substrate of cortical-level processing and cognition, and manipulations of glutamatergic function in schizophrenia reduce negative symptoms and improve cognition. In fact, glutamatergic antagonists, such as phencyclidine (PCP), elicit psychotic symptoms from nonschizophrenic individuals that resemble the illness, and they exacerbate symptoms in patients with schizophrenia. PCP acts by binding to a site on the NMDA receptor that blocks the influx of calcium and other cations through the ion channel, which then blocks receptor function. The effects of NMDA antagonists are not limited to positive symptoms. PCP and ketamine (another glutamatergic antagonist), for example, produce negative symptoms and cognitive deficits in verbal declarative memory and executive functions in normal subjects. Furthermore, administration of ketamine to patients with schizophrenia worsens psychotic symptoms and neuropsychological deficits. It is interesting to note that administration of certain NMDA agonists, such as cycloserine, ameliorates clinical symptoms and possibly cognitive deficits.

Although the continued endorsement of dopaminergic and glutamatergic dysfunction in schizophrenia is well grounded in the research findings, debate continues about the nature of these disruptions. One of the major questions regarding the role of these neurotransmitters (especially dopamine, which is modulated by glutamate) in schizophrenia is whether this represents the cause or the consequence of the activity. Because of the noninvasive techniques that must be used to study human subjects and the fact that patients with schizophrenia are usually not available for study until the onset of the illness, it has been difficult to establish whether these dopaminergic abnormalities precede the illness and contribute to its genesis or are a consequence of psychosis or pharmacological treatments. Generally, studies of nonmedicated, first-episode patients confirm that these abnormalities are largely in place before illness onset. Additional work currently under way in first-episode patients needs to be evaluated before this conclusion is considered definitive.

A few studies have focused on neurotransmission in schizotypal personality disorder. In one, CSF levels of homovanillic acid were increased among patients with schizotypal personality disorder relative to controls, which was associated with positive symptoms. Similar findings were obtained when plasma homovanillic acid was assessed as an estimation of central dopaminergic activity. Interestingly, lowered homovanillic acid levels were obtained in a sample of subjects with schizotypal personality disorder who were relatives of patients with schizophrenia, compared with relatives of schizophrenic patients with either other personality disorders or relatives without a diagnosis. When the influence of negative symptoms was removed statistically by treating it as a covariate, a positive correlation between homovanillic acid and positive symptoms reemerged, similar to previous findings. Taken together, these findings point to a relationship between lowered homovanillic acid levels and negative symptoms and elevated homovanillic acid levels and positive symptoms. Neurochemical data on patients with schizoid or paranoid personality disorders are notably lacking.

More significant than studies of schizotypal individuals, studies of nonpsychotic, nonschizotypal relatives of schizophrenic patients can prove useful for evaluating the timeline of neurotransmitter dysfunction in schizophrenia because these individuals, by definition, have not had psychotic symptoms or taken antipsychotic medications. Any differences between these individuals and normal controls can be viewed as a consequence of the underlying predisposition toward illness rather than as a function of the emergence of the disorder or its treatment. In this context, it is notable that first-degree relatives of schizophrenic patients do show lower circulating levels of homovanillic acid when compared with a normal control group. Remarkably, plasma homovanillic acid is also inversely correlated with negative symptom scores, whereas it is positively correlated with attenuated positive symptom scores on the Positive and Negative Syndrome Scale. The inverse correlation with negative symptom scores (i.e., higher levels of negative symptoms associated with lower levels of homovanillic acid) is particularly consistent with the diagnostic criterion of elevated negative symptoms in schizotaxia. It is also consistent with the findings described above for schizophrenia and schizotypal personality disorder. The crucial determination of whether individuals who meet diagnostic criteria for schizotaxia show more, less, or the same amount of homovanillic acid reductions as nonschizotaxic relatives of patients with schizophrenia has not yet been made. Other aspects of neurochemical function, such as glutamatergic neurotransmission, also have yet to be investigated in depth in relatives and particularly in schizotaxia.

Schizophrenia research is evolving toward molecular methods that promise to shed light on the pathology of the disease and, ultimately, its etiology. The true molecular etiology of schizophrenia is being uncovered only slowly. As is typical, research into the molecular biological basis of schizophrenia-spectrum disorders will likely evolve even more slowly. Examination of these disorders at increasingly microscopic levels of analysis, including genomic and proteomic levels, is necessary before a full picture of their foundations is revealed. The challenge for the coming years is to clarify specific pathological proteins that give rise to these disorders. In addition to the significant treatment possibilities that such discoveries will facilitate, the elucidation of the genes that code for these proteins will reveal many of the common etiological components underlying disorders in the schizophrenia spectrum. Moreover, such data will provide the basis for understanding how environmental and biological factors combine to determine one's placement along the schizophrenia spectrum and, as a consequence, also the most appropriate intervention and treatment strategies.

TREATMENT

The treatment of schizophrenia has evolved with time due to a growing awareness of the biological underpinnings of the disease accented by small doses of serendipity. Once the pharmacological treatment of choice, typical neuroleptics, such as haloperidol (Haldol), are being replaced in most patients by newer antipsychotic medications with higher efficacy and a lower propensity for undesirable side effects. Currently, atypical antipsychotics, such as risperidone (Risperdal), quetiapine (Seroquel), olanzapine (Zyprexa), and ziprasidone (Geodon), comprise the first line of treatments for schizophrenia. Due to the small but significant possibility of serious side effects, clozapine is mainly still reserved for treatment-resistant cases. Psychopharmacological treatments are by far the most effective tool for treating schizophrenia, but psychotherapeutic and psychosocial interventions remain important, especially as adjuncts to pharmacological treatment.

Schizoaffective Disorder Advances in the treatment of schizophrenia have thus far benefited patients with severe spectrum disorders, such as schizoaffective disorder, far more than they have patients with "milder" spectrum disorders, such as schizotypal, schizoid, and paranoid personality disorders, or schizotaxia. Based on its confluence of affective and psychotic features (and the fact that diagnostic inaccuracy may cause schizophrenic and bipolar-disordered patients to receive this diagnosis), schizoaffective disorder is often examined for clinical responsiveness to both mood-stabilizing and antipsychotic medications. A review of these studies dictates a relatively obvious treatment regimen for both bipolar and depressive types of schizoaffective disorder. Historically, either typical antipsychotics or lithium alone were used to manage some cases of the bipolar type of schizoaffective disorder, whereas the coadministration of these two compounds was more effective and, thus, preferable. For the treatment of the depressive type of schizoaffective disorder, combined treatment with antipsychotics and antidepressants was not superior to treatment with antipsychotics alone. However, the efficacy of these treatment strategies has not been evaluated in controlled clinical trials. This is currently of little consequence because these routines are no longer the preferred strategies for the management of the disorder. A newer generation of medications has largely supplanted lithium and typical antipsychotic treatments for many patients.

More recent data suggest that newer mood stabilizers, such as valproate (Depakene) and carbamazepine (Tegretol), and novel antipsychotics, such as clozapine and risperidone, have greater efficacy. Accordingly, their use is increasing, whereas the use of diazepam (Valium) and typical antipsychotics has diminished. For example, a 1,150-mg dose of divalproex (Depakote) can improve Clinical Global Impression Scale scores in 75 percent of bipolar-type schizoaffective-disordered patients, with very few of these patients having serious side effects that merit discontinuation. A mean dose of 643 mg per day of carbamazepine lowers adherence more than lithium administration; but for those in whom it is well tolerated, carbamazepine reduces hospitalization, recurrence, and concomitant psychotropic medication usage, especially among those with depressive-type schizoaffective disorder.

A regimen of 4.7 mg per day of the atypical antipsychotic risperidone has been shown to lower Young Mania Rating Scale scores by 18 points after 6 weeks, Positive and Negative Syndrome Scale scores by 20 points, Hamilton Rating Scale of Depression scores by 6.6 points, and Clinical Global Impressions scores by one point after 4 weeks. Also, when compared with haloperidol, risperidone is better tolerated and provides better symptom relief on at least a subset of clinical scales. For example, risperidone is 14 percent more effective than haloperidol in reducing scores on the Positive and Negative Syndrome Scale and greater than 60 percent more effective in lowering scores on the Hamilton Rating Scale of Depression but is less effective on the Clinician-Administered Rating Scale for Mania. It is important to recognize that treatment protocols involving either or both of the newer mood stabilizers or atypical antipsychotics are not effective for some patients and that their efficacy has been refuted in selected research reports. Yet, the majority of work on schizoaffective disorder suggests that these newer mood stabilizers and antipsychotics can effectively relieve symptoms alone or in combination for a satisfactory proportion of patients.

A new wave of atypical antipsychotics has also shown promise for the treatment of schizoaffective disorder. For example, olanzapine is significantly more effective than haloperidol at doses of 5 to 20 mg in treating both the depressive and bipolar types of the disorder. In relative terms, olanzapine is most effective in treating those who are currently manic or depressed. Furthermore, the drug is tolerated better than haloperidol, with fewer serious side effects, but the likelihood of weight gain is higher with olanzapine. Ziprasidone also has dose-related efficacy on total scores of the Brief Psychotic Rating Scale and Clinical Global Impression Scale, with optimum effects observed at approximate doses of 160 mg per day. As a group, the atypical antipsychotics may have better efficacy for schizoaffective disorder than even for schizophrenia itself, possibly due to their greater affinity for serotonin 1A, 1D, and 2 receptors.

Antiepileptic agents, including gabapentin (Neurontin) and lamotrigine (Lamictal), may also be useful adjunctive treatments for schizoaffective disorder and may be effective when administered alone. Gabapentin can produce symptom relief in as many as 75 percent of schizoaffective-disordered patients at a dose of 1,440 mg per day and may be especially effective in helping treatment-resistant cases, suggesting that wider usage of this compound may be indicated in the future if controlled clinical trials support this high level of effectiveness. Lamotrigine was effective in limited trials at dosages as low as 200 mg per day but showed maximal effects on mood stability and paranoid symptoms at a dosage of 400 mg per day.

Nonpharmacological, biologically oriented therapies have shown limited promise as effective treatments for schizoaffective disorder in the absence of adjunctive pharmacological management. For example, maintenance electroconvulsive therapy (ECT) was effective in a subgroup of patients with schizoaffective disorder, whereas bright light therapy and repetitive transcranial magnetic stimulation (TMS) were each reported to help one patient with schizoaffective disorder in case studies. More empirical work is needed before advocating these procedures for widespread use in the treatment of schizoaffective disorder.

Schizophrenia-Spectrum Personality Disorders

Compared with the literature on treatments of schizophrenia or schizoaffective disorder, there are considerably fewer reports on treatments for schizotypal, schizoid, and paranoid personality disorders. Literature reviewed for the Quality Assurance Project (1990) included 294 papers focusing on the treatment of personality disorders. Only 31 of these studies related to the treatment of schizophrenia-spectrum personality disorders, and a limited number of these reported treatment outcomes in a quantitative manner. Moreover, many studies of pharmacotherapeutic intervention in personality disorders have examined subjects with extensive comorbidity, thus making conclusions regarding the specific personality disorder of interest difficult to interpret. Subjects with comorbid schizotypal and borderline personality disorders are perhaps the most frequent among this mixed group of subjects.

Although such flawed methods still appear in the scientific literature, overall trends indicate that they are becoming phased out in favor of methodologically sound studies with more "pure" or "refined" diagnostic groups. Still, although the need for diagnostic accuracy and precision is well recognized, well-designed studies in this area remain scarce. General treatment recommendations are presented below, along with selected examples of outcome studies whenever they are available and informative for the selection of a particular treatment.

Schizotypal Personality Disorder

Because schizotypal personality disorder is a complex and (probably) etiologically heterogeneous disorder, it is not likely that one treatment approach is useful for all patients. Different treatments and combinations of therapies are more likely to be the most useful for different presentations of the disorder.

Patients with schizotypal personality disorder often view their worlds as odd and threatening places. As with most personality disorders, psychotherapeutic intervention is indicated, whereas the prospect of pharmacotherapy (other than for acute phases of the illness) largely remains an unrealized goal. Rapport and trust between the clinician and patient can be difficult to establish in schizotypal personality disorder, but these elements are crucial for the success of any therapy.

In light of the frequent occurrence of paranoia and suspiciousness and a limited tolerance for social interactions (among other positive symptoms, negative symptoms, and neuropsychological deficits), exploratory psychotherapeutic approaches by themselves are less likely to facilitate positive change than are approaches that emphasize supportive and cognitive-behavioral therapies. Such approaches often emphasize concrete interim goals and stipulate explicit means of attaining them. Because individuals with this disorder may decompensate during times of stress and experience transient episodes of psychosis, they also benefit from techniques to facilitate stress reduction (e.g., relaxation techniques, exercise, yoga, and meditation). Evidence does exist that at least some individuals with schizotypal features are likely to seek treatment in times of stress.

Some of the methods used successfully in other neurodevelopmental disorders that share one or more features with schizotypal personality disorder (e.g., cognitive deficits in attention-deficit/hyperactivity disorder [ADHD]) might also prove useful in the treatment of this condition. As a consequence, in addition to psychiatric symptoms, other issues should be addressed in therapy, including an understanding of the patient's cognitive strengths and weaknesses. This may help patients confront and cope with long-standing difficulties in their lives. For instance, individuals may present with deficits in attention, verbal memory, or organizational skills that have contributed to failures in a variety of educational, occupational, and social endeavors and reinforced negative self-images and the experience of performance anxiety. Knowledge of their more circumscribed cognitive capabilities might allow patients to reframe their difficulties in a more benign manner and also facilitate a more realistic selection of personal, educational, and occupational goals.

To some extent, deficits in specific cognitive domains can also be attenuated. For example, deficits in the acquisition, organization, and retrieval of information may be reduced by standard procedures for these types of difficulties (e.g., writing information down in a "memory notebook," use of appointment books, rehearsal of new information, and a focus on one activity at a time, among others). In addition, social skills training and family therapy may help relieve signs of social anxiety and overcome feelings of isolation from others, even if anxiety about being in a group likely hinders their participation in these types of interventions. Intensive case management and day hospital admission may also prove helpful (but more costly) when necessary.

Although the psychotherapeutic interventions discussed above are reasonable and appropriate for use in treating schizotypal personality disorder, more research is needed to determine which approaches are most effective. As noted above, there is a paucity of such studies at the present time. It is clear that little therapeutic change is seen after a course of insight-oriented psychotherapy. In one retrospective study, the Global Assessment Scale was measured in patients with several diagnoses on admission to a psychiatric hospital. One of these groups was diagnosed with the third edition of the DSM (DSM-III) schizotypal personality disorder. Another group consisted of patients with schizotypal personality disorder and comorbid borderline personality disorder. Patients remained hospitalized for an average of 16.6 months and were followed up an average of 13.6 years after primary treatment consisting of intensive psychoanalytical therapy. Patients admitted with schizotypal personality disorder demonstrated significant improvement at follow-up. The concern remains that, after such a long follow-up period, treatment effects are difficult to discern from the effects of other potentially intervening variables, such as life events, or simply the passage of time. In a study of former inpatients given retrospective DSM-III diagnoses of schizotypal personality disorder approximately 15 years after treatment, subjects with pure schizotypal personality disorder showed, at best, only moderate levels of function at follow-up.

Marginally beneficial effects of day hospitals on the outcome of schizotypal personality disorder have also been documented. An intensive treatment regimen consisting of psychodynamically oriented individual and group therapy, art therapy, and daily community meetings for an average of 5.5 months produced little change on either the Global Symptom Index or the Health Sickness Rating Scale. At follow-up, there was a moderate decrease in symptoms, but global functioning remained poor.

The few investigations into the usefulness of medications in treating schizotypal personality disorder used small numbers of subjects and combined samples of schizotypal and borderline personality disorders. As a result, conclusions about the effectiveness of treatment must be conservative. Typical antipsychotics, in particular, reduce positive symptoms or depressed mood in times of acute stress, but the high incidence of adverse side effects discourages their widespread use at other times, including the more chronic, stable (i.e., noncrisis) phases of the disorder. The newer antipsychotics may be more appropriate for this purpose, but clinical trials are needed to assess their efficacy. Other types of medication have shown generally nonspecific effects. For example, fluoxetine (Prozac) is commonly tested for efficacy in schizotypal personality disorder, and it was shown to reduce scores on several scales of the Hopkins Symptom Checklist in a combined group of patients with DSM-III-R schizotypal and borderline personality disorder. By contrast, in groups consisting solely of patients with schizotypal personality disorder, the reductions were not significant. The possibility of treatments to reduce negative and cognitive features of schizotypal personality disorder merits consideration and is considered further in the discussion of treatments for schizotaxia.

Schizoid Personality Disorder As with schizotypal personality disorder, the presentation and presumed causes of schizoid personality disorder are likely to be multifactorial. The heterogeneity of the disorder, its chronic nature, and its characterization by negative symptoms that do not generally foster an optimal therapeutic atmosphere, make this personality disorder difficult to treat. In addition to these limitations, the virtual absence of outcome studies of the disorder complicates the advancement of general treatment recommendations; nevertheless, some agreed-on treatment options are presented below.

The isolation, anhedonia, and restricted affect of schizoid personality disorder can only be ameliorated under optimal clinical conditions consisting of solid rapport and a stable therapeutic environment in which the patient can learn to rely on the support provided by the clinician, especially during times of crisis. Existing studies support the role of cognitive-behavioral therapies in developing social skills and increasing interpersonal sensitivity, although supportive (rather than insight-oriented) psychotherapy is generally considered useful. Psychodynamic approaches are not likely to be well tolerated. Practical, goal-oriented strategies have better chances of success. Thus, concrete and agreed-to treatment objectives with supportive, behavioral, and psychosocial treatment strategies are indicated most clearly. Group therapy may increase interpersonal skills and overall social motivation, but, in general, only relatively high-functioning patients may tolerate it. Pharmacological intervention in schizoid personality disorder has not been advocated traditionally except to attenuate anxiety or depression during crises. As with schizotypal personality disorder, the hope is that research will lead to psychopharmacological management strategies in the future. The general recommendations provided above need to be validated experimentally, as they are based more on practical guidelines than they are on clinical outcome studies.

Paranoid Personality Disorder Individuals with paranoid personality disorder rarely present themselves for treatment. Not surprisingly, there has been little outcome research to suggest which types of treatment are most effective with this disorder. Research studies that have examined the effects of various treatments on paranoid symptoms have usually done so within the context of other conditions such as anxiety disorders or posttraumatic stress disorder (PTSD). Studies of "pure" paranoid personality disorder are almost nonexistent. Family or group therapies are generally ineffective and are not recommended. Due to the patient's characteristic mistrust, a supportive, client-centered environment is the optimal setting for therapeutic change. As with the other schizophrenia-spectrum personality disorders, building rapport is difficult, also due to the fundamentally guarded nature of the disorder. Stability in the therapeutic setting is critical to increase the patient's trust. It is critical that the clinician remain objective and supportive rather than confrontational when treating the patient's paranoid ideas, just as it is for delusions of schizotypal personality disorder. An honest, practical, goal-oriented approach that does not present too much insightful observation or interpretation may work best with paranoid patients.

Pharmacological treatment and management of paranoid personality disorder is not widely supported, but certain medications can be useful during the more severe bouts of illness. For example, diazepam can reduce severe anxiety, whereas administration of a neuroleptic or atypical antipsychotic may be indicated if decompensation becomes severe. These medications should be used sparingly to prevent the emergence of countertherapeutic effects emerging from the patient's underlying mistrust and fear of being manipulated.

Schizotaxia Evidence has been presented that the social dysfunction, negative symptoms, and neuropsychological deficits observed in many of the schizotaxic, nonpsychotic relatives of schizophrenic patients can be ameliorated by various treatment strategies. The negative symptoms of this condition, along with social deficits, can be treated at least partially by some of the same psychotherapeutic and psychosocial methods that are effective in treating schizotypal and schizoid personality disorders. This point also reflects conceptual similarities between schizotaxia and negative schizotypal personality disorder. In addition to these methods, psychopharmacological interventions may become possible in the foreseeable future.

The feasibility of this view was examined in a recent pilot study with nonpsychotic first-degree relatives of patients with schizophrenia.

Subjects who met Research Diagnostic Criteria for schizotaxia, which included moderate levels of negative symptoms and moderate deficits in two or more neuropsychological domains (i.e., attention/working memory, long-term verbal memory, or executive functions), were treated with low doses of risperidone, one of the newer antipsychotic medications. Of eight subjects who met criteria for schizotaxia (out of 27 who were assessed), six subjects agreed to enter the treatment protocol. The dose of risperidone started at 0.25 mg per day and increased gradually to a maximum of 2 mg per day over a 2-week period. The course of treatment was 6 weeks. Negative symptoms decreased in five out of six subjects, and in three cases, these improvements were substantial (e.g., total scores on the Scale for Assessment of Negative Symptoms were reduced by approximately 50 percent), with effects more modest in two cases (total scores on the Scale for the Assessment of Negative Symptoms were reduced by approximately 25 percent). Five out of six cases also showed substantial improvements (of one to two standard deviations) in attention and working memory over the 6-week period. The sixth subject, who had lower overall cognitive abilities, did not demonstrate improvement in clinical or cognitive measures. The inability of that subject to improve raises the possibility that minimal levels of ability were necessary for improvement, at least in the treatment domains assessed in this study. Side effects of the medication were temporary and primarily mild. Replication of these effects in a larger double-blind research design could be significant for the treatment of schizotaxia. Early intervention and prevention efforts in schizophrenia could benefit in the future as well.

FUTURE OF SCHIZOPHRENIA-SPECTRUM DISORDER RESEARCH AND TREATMENT

The understanding of the pathology of schizophrenia and its treatment has advanced greatly over the last century. Exponential gains have been made in the last three decades. This knowledge has had tangible impacts on the disease: Inpatient admissions and their length of stay in psychiatric hospitals have decreased steadily, and more patients are managing their disease effectively, especially through the use of psychotropic medication. These advances have also benefited the understanding of other schizophrenia-spectrum disorders, particularly the more severe conditions such as schizoaffective disorder and schizotypal personality disorder. Yet, whereas schizophrenia still holds many secrets from researchers and clinicians, it is these schizophrenia-spectrum disorders that remain truly enigmatic. This is not a function of a greater complexity of these conditions relative to schizophrenia. Schizophrenia is certainly among the most complex disorders known to humans. Instead, this lack of understanding is a direct function of the amount of research that these conditions have received, due either to their lower prevalence or to lesser severity, or both, than schizophrenia. This situation is improving (e.g., there are now numerous investigations into the psychopathology and neurobiology of schizotypal and nonschizotypal nonpsychotic relatives of patients with schizophrenia), but there is a particular need to explore novel treatment options across the schizophrenia spectrum.

At present, the gaps in the knowledge of both the pathology and the treatment of various schizophrenia-spectrum disorders lead to several recommendations:

In recognition of schizoaffective disorder as a separate disease entity from schizophrenia, subsequent studies of the condition should ascertain only subjects who are diagnosed with schizoaffective disorder. These patients must be studied separately from schizophrenic patients or schizoaffective-disordered patients with comorbidity to clarify the position of schizoaffective disorder on clinical, etiological, and treatment spectrums that include schizophrenia and schizophrenia-spectrum personality disorders. Studies that present data pooled from schizophrenic subjects and those with schizoaffective disorder only serve to complicate the conclusions that can be drawn for either disorder. The clinical similarity of the two disorders should not be assumed to reflect any etiological, pathological, or treatment similarities between the conditions until their apparent proximity on the schizophrenia spectrum can be established definitively. Moreover, it is essential that in recognition of the heterogeneity of schizoaffective disorder that the depressed and bipolar subtypes be considered separately before they are combined into a single group.

Some of the same issues apply to schizotypal personality disorder. This disorder should be studied alone rather than in combination with different personality disorders (e.g., borderline personality disorder). Much of what is known now about the treatment of schizotypal personality disorder comes from studies of such heterogeneous samples. As with schizoaffective disorder, a true understanding of this condition can only be obtained when "pure" cases are examined. Also, like schizoaffective disorder, schizotypal personality disorder may be heterogeneous. Unlike schizoaffective disorder, this is not reflected in the psychiatric nomenclature. Treatment strategies for negative schizotypy can be identical to those suggested for schizotaxia.

All aspects of schizoid and paranoid personality disorders should be studied more extensively. This has been a low priority historically due to the lesser severity of these conditions relative to the other schizophrenia-spectrum disorders, their low prevalence in the population, and the low likelihood of these individuals becoming available for study. Sample pooling and multisite collaborations may be necessary to generate samples with adequate power for differentiating between these disorders and the other schizophrenia-spectrum disorders on neurobiological underpinnings and treatment outcomes.

Schizotaxia (and its clinical and pathological characteristics) needs more study, both as a clinical syndrome in its own right and as a marker for the susceptibility to schizophrenia and maybe other schizophrenia-spectrum conditions. This highly prevalent condition among the nonpsychotic relatives of individuals with schizophrenia has significant clinical impact not only at the individual level but at the societal level as well. If some of the deficits associated with schizotaxia can be remedied as effectively as initial data indicate, further research into this condition and its treatment may yield great benefits for patients and their families.

All of these conditions should be studied using rigorous diagnostic criteria, well-defined diagnostic boundaries, and, eventually, biologically based phenotypes. Because of diagnostic uncertainty, classification of these conditions is never perfect. This reality can introduce unreliability into studies of their pathology and treatment. New research is identifying biologically based phenotypes that segregate in families affected by schizophrenia and schizophrenia-spectrum conditions. If these alternate phenotypes can be measured more reliably than diagnostic categories, they may provide an effective basis for disease dissection and etiological discovery in the near future. Candidate biological phenotypes include deficient prepulse inhibition, eye tracking dysfunction, neurological signs, biochemical abnormalities, characteristic auditory evoked potentials, neuroimaging-assessed brain abnormalities, and neuropsychological impairment.

The point that stands out about the data on the pathology and treatment of schizophrenia-spectrum conditions is not what is known or what is not but rather what remains to be investigated. For example, particularly promising therapies (such as cognitive-behavioral therapies and atypical antipsychotic administration) have yet to be examined systematically for effectiveness in the schizophrenia-spectrum personality disorders. When the above recommendations are heeded, this mysterious group of disorders will come under control one by one, eventually leading to their early detection and intervention and, ultimately, to their prevention.

SUGGESTED CROSS-REFERENCES

The reader is encouraged to refer to the related schizophrenia sections on genetic epidemiology (Section 12.3), clinical features and psychopathology concepts (Section 12.8), pharmacotherapy (Section 12.12), and psychosocial treatment (Section 12.11).

References

Battaglia M, Torgersen S: Schizotypal disorder: At the crossroads of genetics and nosology. *Acta Psychiatr Scand.* 1996;94:303–310.

Bleuler E. *Dementia Praecox or the Group of Schizophrenias.* New York: International Universities Press; 1950.

Carlsson A, Waters N, Holm-Waters S, Tedroff J, Nilsson M, Carlsson ML: Interactions between monoamines, glutamate, and GABA in schizophrenia: New evidence. *Ann Rev Pharmacol Toxicol.* 2001;41:237–260.

Coryell WH, Zimmerman M: Personality disorder in the families of depressed, schizophrenic, and never-ill probands. *Am J Psychiatry.* 1989;146:496–502.

*Dickey CC, McCarley RW, Shenton ME: The brain in schizotypal personality disorder: A review of structural MRI and CT findings. *Harv Rev Psychiatry.* 2002;10:1–15.

Faraone SV, Green AI, Seidman LJ, Tsuang MT: "Schizotaxia": Clinical implications and new directions for research. *Schizophr Bull.* 2001;27:1–18.

Faraone SV, Kremen WS, Lyons MJ, Pepple JR, Seidman LJ, Tsuang MT: Diagnostic accuracy and linkage analysis: How useful are schizophrenia spectrum phenotypes? *Am J Psychiatry.* 1995;152:1286–1290.

Faraone SV, Seidman LJ, Kremen WS, Pepple JR, Lyons MJ, Tsuang MT: Neuropsychological functioning among the nonpsychotic relatives of schizophrenic patients: A diagnostic efficiency analysis. *J Abnorm Psychol.* 1995;104:286–304.

Faraone SV, Seidman LJ, Kremen WS, Toomey R, Pepple JR, Tsuang MT: Neuropsychological functioning among the nonpsychotic relatives of schizophrenic patients: A four-year follow-up study. *J Abnorm Psychol.* 1999;108:176–181.

Faraone SV, Seidman LJ, Kremen WS, Toomey R, Pepple JR, Tsuang MT: Neuropsychological functioning among the nonpsychotic relatives of schizophrenic patients: The effect of genetic loading. *Biol Psychiatry.* 2000;48:120–126.

*Getz GE, DelBello MP, Fleck DE, Zimmerman ME, Schwiers ML, Strakowski SM: Neuroanatomic characterization of schizoaffective disorder using MRI: A pilot study. *Schizophr Res.* 2002;55:55–59.

Gruen R, Asnis L, Lord S: Familial transmission of schizotypal and borderline personality disorders. *Am J Psychiatry.* 1985;142:927–934.

Harrison P: The neuropathology of schizophrenia: A critical review of the data and their interpretation. *Brain.* 1999;122:593–624.

Heckers S: Neuroimaging studies of the hippocampus in schizophrenia. *Hippocampus.* 2001;11:520–528.

Kendler KS, McGuire M, Gruenberg AM, O'Hare A, Spellman M, Walsh D: The Roscommon Family Study. III. Schizophrenia-related personality disorders in relatives. *Arch Gen Psychiatry.* 1993;50:781–788.

Kurachi M: Pathogenesis of schizophrenia: Part II. Temporo-frontal two-step hypothesis. *Psychiatry Clin Neurosci.* 2003;57:9–15.

*Meehl PE: Schizotaxia, schizotypy, schizophrenia. *Am Psychol.* 1962;17:827–838.

Rogers KL, Winokur G. The genetics of schizoaffective disorder and the schizophrenia spectrum. In: Tsuang MT, Simpson JC, eds. *Handbook of Schizophrenia Volume 3: Nosology, Epidemiology, & Genetics.* New York: Elsevier; 1988.

Seidman LJ, Faraone SV, Goldstein JM, Goodman JM, Kremen WS, Matsuda G, Hoge EA, Kennedy D, Makris N, Caviness VS, Tsuang MT: Reduced subcortical brain volumes in nonpsychotic siblings of schizophrenic patients: A pilot MRI Study. *Am J Med Genet (Neuropsychiat Genet).* 1997;74:507–514.

Seidman LJ, Faraone SV, Goldstein JM, Goodman JM, Kremen WS, Toomey R, Tourville J, Kennedy D, Makris N, Caviness VS, Tsuang MT: Thalamic and amygdala-hippocampal volume reductions in first degree relatives of schizophrenic patients: An MRI-based morphometric analysis. *Biol Psychiatry.* 1999;46:941–954.

Seidman LJ, Faraone SV, Goldstein JM, Kremen WS, Horton NJ, Makris N, Toomey R, Kennedy D, Caviness VS, Tsuang MT: Left hippocampal volume as a vulnerability indicator for schizophrenia: A magnetic resonance imaging morphometric study of nonpsychotic first-degree relatives. *Arch Gen Psychiatry.* 2002;59:839–849.

Seidman LJ, Wencel HE: Genetically mediated brain abnormalities in schizophrenia. *Curr Psychiatry Rep.* 2003;5:135–144.

Siever LJ, Koenigsberg HW, Harvey P, Mitropoulou V, Laruelle M, Abi-Dargham A, Goodman M, Buchsbaum M: Cognitive and brain function in schizotypal personality disorder. *Schizophr Res.* 2002;54:157–167.

*Soares JC, Innis RB: Neurochemical brain imaging investigations of schizophrenia. *Biol Psychiatry.* 1999;46:600–615.

Squires-Wheeler E, Skodol AE, Bassett A, Erlenmeyer-Kimling L: DSM-III-R schizotypal personality traits in offspring of schizophrenic disorder, affective disorder, and normal control parents. *J Psychiat Res.* 1989;23:229–239.

Stone WS, Glatt SJ, Faraone SV. The biology of schizotaxia. In: Stone WS, Faraone SV, Tsuang MT, eds. *Early Clinical Intervention and Prevention of Schizophrenia.* Totowa, NJ: Humana Press; 2004:339–353.

*The Quality Assurance Project: Treatment outlines for paranoid, schizotypal and schizoid personality disorders. The Quality Assurance Project. *Aust N Z J Psychiatry.* 1990;24:339–350.

Tsuang MT, Gilbertson MW, Faraone SV. Genetic transmission of negative and positive symptoms in the biological relatives of schizophrenics. In: Marneros A, Tsuang MT, Andreasen N, eds. *Positive vs. Negative Schizophrenia.* New York: Springer-Verlag; 1991:265–291.

Tsuang MT, Stone WS, Gamma F, Faraone SV: Schizotaxia: Current status and future directions. *Curr Psychiatry Rep.* 2003;5:128–134.

Weiss AP, Schacter DL, Goff DC, Rausch SL, Alpert NM, Heckers S: Impaired hippocampal recruitment during normal modulation of memory performance in schizophrenia. *Biol Psychiatry.* 2003;53:48–55.

▲ 12.16 Other Psychotic Disorders

This section describes six disorders included in the section on "other psychotic disorders" in the fourth revised edition of the *Diagnostic and Statistical Manual of Mental Disorders* (DSM-IV-TR). It also describes culture-bound syndromes and the tenth revision of *International Statistical Classification of Diseases and Related Health Problems* (ICD-10) category of acute and transient psychoses. The disorders in this section occur less frequently than schizophrenia or psychotic mood disorders but can have profound short- or long-term psychosocial consequences. As a group, these disorders are more poorly understood than schizophrenia and, in their initial stages, can be difficult to distinguish from other forms of psychosis. Table 12.16–1 provides an overview of the clinical features of the disorders described in this section and compares them to other disorders that have similar characteristics.

12.16a Acute and Transient Psychotic Disorders and Brief Psychotic Disorder

Ramin Mojtabai, M.D., Ph.D., M.P.H.

Acute psychotic disorders with a remitting course have a long history. Along with the classic syndromes of schizophrenia and affective psychoses, Emil Kraepelin (1856 to 1926) discussed amentia—a psychotic disorder with remitting course and favorable outcome, originally described by Theodor Meynert (1833 to 1898). Similar psychotic syndromes were described by other 19th- and 20th-century European psychiatrists under various terms, such as *cycloid psychosis, bouffée délirante, reactive psychosis,* and others, as briefly described in Table 12.16a–1. At the same time, investigators reported a high prevalence of acute benign psychotic episodes in Africa, the Caribbean islands, and India. The descriptions of these psychotic syndromes are rather similar—a remarkable observation because these descriptions grew out of different psychiatric traditions separated by national and linguistic boundaries. They all portray a psychotic condition with acute onset and remitting course. Nevertheless, the multiplicity of the descriptions and labels has been

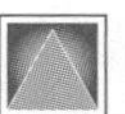

Table 12.16–1
Overview of Onset and Characteristic Features of Selected Psychotic Disorders

Disorder	Onset	Positive Symptoms	Negative Symptoms	Mood Symptoms	Duration of Symptoms	Functioning
Nonaffective psychotic disorders						
Schizophrenia	Acute or insidious	Two or more present for at least 1 mo: delusions, hallucinations, disorganized speech, disorganized or catatonic behavior	Affective flattening, avolition, anhedonia.	If present, duration is brief.	At least 6 mos with active phase of at least 1 mo	Social and occupational dysfunction for a significant portion of the time
Schizophreniform disorder	Usually acute	Same as schizophrenia	If present, consider as poor prognostic feature.	If present, duration is brief.	1–6 mos, including prodrome, active, and residual phases	Impairment during episode; full return to premorbid level within 6 mos
Brief psychotic disorder; ICD-10 acute and transient disorder (ATPD)[a]	Acute; specifiers: with or without marked stressor; postpartum	Same as schizophrenia	Absent.	May be present but do not meet criteria.	1 day–1 mo (up to 3 mos for ATPD)	Impairment during episode; full return to premorbid level after remission
Schizophrenia: paranoid type	Same as schizophrenia	Delusions or hallucinations, or both	Not prominent.	Same as schizophrenia.	Same as schizophrenia	Same as schizophrenia, except functioning tends to be somewhat better
Delusional disorder	Usually insidious	Only nonbizarre delusions; tactile or olfactory hallucinations may be present if related to delusional theme	Absent.	Usually present. If criteria for mood disorder are met, duration is brief.	At least 1 mo	Apart from the impact of the delusion, functioning is not markedly impaired
Psychosis not otherwise specified	Variable; specifiers include postpartum	Present but do not meet criteria for any other psychotic disorder	Absent.	May be present but do not meet criteria.	Variable	Not significantly impaired
Psychotic mood disorders						
Schizoaffective disorder	Acute or insidious	Same as schizophrenia	Usually less severe and less chronic than schizophrenia.	Symptoms meeting episode criteria present for significant portion of time.	Same as schizophrenia; delusions or hallucinations present for 2+ wks in the absence of prominent mood symptoms	Same as schizophrenia
Major-depressive disorder with psychosis	Variable; specifiers include postpartum	Only in presence of mood episode	Absent, but some mood symptoms (anhedonia, avolition) may be difficult to distinguish.	Depressed mood or anhedonia with other symptoms of depression.	2+ wks	Impairment during episode
Mania with psychosis	Acute; specifiers include postpartum	Only in presence of mood episode	Absent.	Abnormally elevated, expansive, or irritable mood with other symptoms of mania.	1 wk; any duration if hospitalization is required	Impairment during episode
Mixed episode with psychosis	Variable	Only in presence of mood episode	Absent.	Criteria for both mania and depression.	Same as mania with psychosis	Impairment during episode

ATPD, acute and transient psychotic disorders.
[a]Some may be classified as culture-bound syndromes.
Table by L.J. Fochtmann, M.D.; E.J. Bromet, Ph.D.; R. Mojtabai, M.D., Ph.D.; S. Fennig, M.D.; B. Naz, M.D., and G.A. Carlson, M.D.

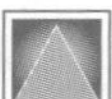

Table 12.16a–1
Partial Listing of the Classic Descriptions of Acute and Transient Psychotic Disorders

Diagnosis	Publications	Description
Amentia	Meynert T: Amentia, die Verwirrtheit. *Jahrb Psychiatr Neurol.* 1889;9:1.	A psychotic illness with acute onset characterized by confusion and perplexity; agitation; rapidly changing, vivid hallucinations and delusions; misidentification phenomena; anxiety; and apprehension, first introduced by Theodore Meynert (1833–1898). An association with physical illness and exhaustion was noted in some patients. Full recovery occurs in a few weeks or months. Although somewhat influential at its time, amentia never produced much interest in later years.
Cycloid psychosis	Kleist K: Über zykloide, paranoide und epileptoide Psychosen und über die Frage der Degenerations-psychosen. *Schweizer Arch Neurol Psychiat.* 1928;23:1. Leonhard K: Cycloid psychoses-endogenous psychoses which are neither schizophrenic nor manic depressive. *J Ment Sci.* 1961;107:632. Perris C, Brockington IF. Cycloid psychoses and their relation to the major psychoses. In: Perris C, Struwe G, Jansson B, eds. *Biological Psychiatry.* Amsterdam: Elsevier; 1981:447–450.	A psychotic disorder with acute onset and good prognosis but frequent recurrences, characterized by confusion, mood-incongruent delusions, hallucinations, overwhelming anxiety, deep feelings of happiness or ecstasy, motility disturbances of akinetic or hyperkinetic type, a particular concern with death, mood swings, and rapid change in symptoms within an episode. Two variants of the disorder were first described by Karl Kleist (1879–1960): confusional insanity characterized by contrasting phases of confused excitement and stupor and motility psychosis characterized by contrasting phases of hyperkinesis and akinesis. A third variant, anxiety-elation psychosis, was introduced by Karl Leonhard (1904–1988). The diagnosis of cycloid psychosis is still used by German, Scandinavian, and other European psychiatrists and was influential for the formulation of acute and transient psychotic disorders in ICD-10. Carlo Perris and Ian Brockington introduced a set of explicit criteria for the diagnosis of cycloid psychosis in 1981.
Bouffée délirante	Magnan V, Legrain M. *Les Dégénérés (Etat Mental et Syndromes Episodiques).* Paris: Rueff et Cie; 1895. Pull CB, Pull MC, Pichot P: Nosological position of schizoaffective psychoses in France. *Psychiatr Clin.* 1983;16:141.	A psychotic disorder with acute onset in a person without previous psychiatric history. The episode remits completely with no residual symptoms. The episodes are characterized by delusions, hallucinations, depersonalization and derealization, confusion, mood change, and changing symptoms during the course of episode. Episodes are not due to organic or substance use. The syndrome was introduced by Valentin Magnan (1835–1916) and Paul-Maurice Legrain (1860–1939) in 1895 as caused by degeneration, a 19th-century view that attributed mental illness to the spread of modern civilization and urban life. Although this etiological formulation is no longer accepted, the diagnosis is still used by French-speaking clinicians in Europe, West Africa, and the Caribbean. The concept of *bouffée délirante* was influential in formulation of the ICD-10 acute and transient psychotic disorders. Due to its common occurrence in Africa and the Caribbean, it is also categorized as a culture-bound syndrome in the DSM-IV-TR. Charles Pull and colleagues proposed a set of explicit diagnostic criteria for *bouffée délirante* in 1983.
Psychogenic or reactive psychosis	Wimmer A. *Psykogene Sindssygdomsformer.* Copenhagen, Denmark: St. Hans Hospitals Jubilæumsskrift; 1916.	A psychotic disorder with acute onset after external stress. Compared with schizophrenia, the onset is more likely to be acute and later in life. Premorbid adjustment tends to be better than in schizophrenia. There are more affective and confusional symptoms and fewer bizarre symptoms, and there is less family history of schizophrenia. Prognosis is better than schizophrenia. Diagnoses of psychogenic or reactive psychoses were popular among Scandinavian psychiatrists in the early part of the 20th century and continued to be used throughout the past century but found limited use outside of these countries.
Schizophreniform psychosis or disorder	Langfeldt G. *The Schizophreniform States.* Copenhagen, Denmark: Ejnar Munksgaard; 1939. American Psychiatric Association. *Diagnostic and Statistical Manual.* 3rd ed. Washington, DC: American Psychiatric Press; 1980.	The Norwegian psychiatrist Gabriel Langfeldt (1937–1966) introduced the concept of schizophreniform psychosis as a condition with sudden onset after an identifiable precipitating factor and good outcome in an individual with well-adjusted premorbid personality. The patients often present disturbance of mood and clouding of consciousness. The term, but not the concept, was adopted by the DSM-III as a nonaffective psychotic syndrome with schizophrenic symptoms, which is distinguished from schizophrenia by a duration of less than 6 mos. The concept of schizophreniform in the latter sense was perpetuated in the later editions of the DSM.
Oneirophrenia	Meduna LJ. *Oneirophrenia: The Confusional State.* Urbana, IL: The University of Illinois Press; 1950.	Ladislas von Meduna (1896–1964) described oneirophrenia in 1939 as a syndrome characterized by acute onset of confusion, nightmare or dream-like quality of all perceptions (hence the term "oneirophrenia"), extreme fear and anxiety, delusions, and visual hallucinations. The prognosis is generally good with full recovery. Meduna proposed an endocrinological explanation for the syndrome.
Hysterical psychosis	Hollander MH, Hirsch SJ: Hysterical psychosis. *Am J Psychiatry.* 1964;120:1066.	Although the term *hysterical psychoses* had been in use since the early 20th century, Marc Hollander and Steven Hirsch presented the first formal description of the syndrome in 1964. These authors described a psychotic episode with sudden and dramatic onset related to a profoundly upsetting event in the context of a "hysterical" personality. Symptoms include hallucinations, delusions, depersonalization, and disorganized behavior. The episode seldom lasts longer than 1–3 wks.

one of the major barriers to better understanding and classification of these psychoses. In more recent years, there have been attempts to surpass these barriers by defining a syndrome based on the common features of the traditional descriptions. The introduction of the acute and transient psychotic disorders in the tenth revision of *International Statistical Classification of Diseases and Related Health Problems* (ICD-10) is important in this context.

The historical roots of the revised fourth edition of the *Diagnostic and Statistical Manual of Mental Disorders* (DSM-IV-TR) diagnosis of brief psychotic disorder, similar to ICD-10 acute and transient psychotic disorders, are to be found in European psychiatry. The Scandinavian concept of reactive or psychogenic psychosis was especially influential in the formulation of the third edition of the DSM (DSM-III) brief reactive psychosis diagnosis, which, in DSM-IV and DSM-IV-TR, was replaced by brief psychotic disorder. The change was partly motivated by the observation that many cases of brief psychosis are not precipitated by a marked stressor and, hence, are not "reactive." Nonetheless, the DSM-IV and DSM-IV-TR distinguish between brief psychotic disorder with and without marked stressors and indicate that brief psychotic disorder with marked stressor is equivalent to the brief reactive psychosis.

DEFINITIONS

Acute and transient psychotic disorders are defined by ICD-10 as psychotic conditions with onset within 2 weeks and full remission within 1 to 3 months. A more detailed description along with criteria for specific conditions under this general rubric is presented in Table 12.16a–2. These conditions do not have a designated place in the DSM-IV-TR. Many of the cases of ICD-10 acute and transient psychotic disorder would be categorized as schizophreniform disorder, brief psychotic disorder, or psychotic disorder not otherwise specified (NOS) in DSM-IV-TR. Nevertheless, historical tradition and the available empirical evidence justify classifying these conditions under one diagnostic rubric.

Brief psychotic disorder is defined by DSM-IV-TR as a psychotic condition that involves the sudden onset of psychotic symptoms, which lasts 1 day or more but less than 1 month. Remission is full, and the individual returns to the premorbid level of functioning. Thus, most individuals diagnosed with brief psychotic disorder under DSM-IV-TR are classified as having acute and transient psychotic disorders under ICD-10. DSM-IV-TR criteria for brief psychotic disorder are presented in Table 12.16a–3.

COMPARATIVE NOSOLOGY

Acute and transient psychotic disorders have been the subject of a long nosological debate. Some authors argue that these conditions should be considered as an independent group of disorders—a "third psychosis" along with the two classic syndromes of schizophrenia and mood disorder. Others view these psychoses as variants of schizophrenia or mood disorders, pointing to their diagnostic instability as evidence. Probably, both views are correct. The group of acute and transient psychotic disorders likely includes atypical variants of schizophrenia and mood disorders as well as patients with "genuine" nonschizophrenic, nonaffective acute and transient psychotic disorders. A consensus seems to be emerging that this latter group should be categorized separately.

There have been few empirical studies of the diagnostic stability of the ICD-10 category of acute and transient psychotic disorders, and these studies have had mixed results. One study from Denmark reported that approximately one-half of the patients with an original diagnosis of acute and transient psychotic disorders met the criteria for other psychotic disorders at 1-year follow-up. Other studies from Germany and India found that only 16 to 27 percent of patients met criteria for other diagnoses at 2- to 3-year follow-ups. Most changes in diagnosis at follow-up were into the mood disorder category. Although meeting criteria for a manic or depressive episode excludes a diagnosis of acute and transient psychotic disorder, ICD-10 notes that "emotional turmoil, with intense transient feelings of happiness and ecstasy or anxieties and irritability" is frequently present. These mood features may, in fact, be atypical features of a mood disorder. Thus, further refining the diagnosis of acute transient psychotic disorders by excluding these features may improve the diagnostic stability of this disorder.

Two other refinements to the ICD-10 diagnosis have been proposed: first, extending the duration criteria to 6 months; second, forgoing subclassification into the specific conditions. Studies show that the duration of nonaffective psychoses with acute onset and remitting course is typically longer than the 1 to 3 months specified in the ICD-10 and extends up to 6 months in many individuals.

Critics have also noted that subclassification into specific disorders is not supported by current clinical or research evidence. Furthermore, these conditions are relatively rare, especially in Western countries, and it is unlikely that future studies will include enough patients from each specific disorder to be able to reliably examine the validity of these specific disorders.

There is no specific place for acute and transient psychotic disorders in the DSM-IV-TR. As a result, these patients are classified under a number of different diagnostic categories. The large majority meets criteria for schizophreniform disorder, brief psychotic disorder, or psychotic disorder NOS, although the actual proportions that receive each diagnosis vary considerably across studies. In the DSM-IV field trial for schizophrenia and other psychotic disorders, of all individuals meeting the ICD-10 criteria for acute and transient psychotic disorders, 42 percent also met the revised DSM-III (DSM-III-R) criteria for schizophreniform disorder, 21 percent for psychotic disorder NOS, and only 13 percent for brief reactive psychosis. In contrast, in a study from Germany, 62 percent of those with acute and transient psychotic disorders also met the DSM-IV criteria for brief psychotic disorder, 31 percent for schizophreniform disorder, and 5 percent for psychotic disorder NOS. Part of the difference in the results of the two studies may be due to differences in the criteria of DSM-III-R brief reactive psychosis and DSM-IV brief psychotic disorder.

Although acute onset is described in the text of the DSM-IV-TR as an essential feature of brief psychotic disorder and, in the criteria for schizophreniform disorder, as a specifier for favorable prognosis, it is not a diagnostic criterion for any of the above DSM-IV-TR diagnoses. As a result, many patients with transient psychosis with a nonacute onset are also given these diagnoses.

Brief psychotic disorder's predecessor, brief reactive psychosis, was introduced in DSM-III as a psychotic condition lasting less than 2 weeks that followed a significant psychosocial stressor and that involved emotional turmoil and one of the symptoms of loosening of associations, delusions, hallucinations, or disorganized or catatonic behavior. This diagnosis was maintained in the DSM-III-R, but the allowable duration of symptoms was extended to 1 month. In DSM-IV and DSM-IV-TR, this diagnosis was replaced by brief psychotic disorder, eliminating an identifiable psychosocial stressor as a diagnostic criterion. Furthermore, the DSM-III and DSM-III-R criterion of emotional turmoil was removed from the DSM-IV and DSM-IV-TR criteria for brief psychotic disorder. The aim of the revisions in successive editions of the DSM was to broaden the scope of the diagnosis of brief psychotic disorder. However, the impact of these revisions on the validity of the diagnosis is not known.

Few studies have examined the stability of the brief psychotic disorder diagnosis. In a prospective epidemiological study of a first-

Table 12.16a–2
ICD-10 Diagnostic Criteria for Research for Acute and Transient Psychotic Disorders

F23: Acute and transient psychotic disorders

G1: There is acute onset of delusions, hallucinations, incomprehensible or incoherent speech, or any combination of these. The time interval between the first appearance of any psychotic symptoms and the presentation of the fully developed disorder should not exceed 2 weeks.

G2: If transient states of perplexity, misidentification, or impairment of attention and concentration are present, they do not fulfill the criteria for organically caused clouding of consciousness as specified for F05.-, Criterion A.

G3: The disorder does not meet the symptomatic criteria for manic episode (F30.-), depressive episode (F32.-), or recurrent depressive disorder (F33.-).

G4: There is insufficient evidence of recent psychoactive substance use to fulfill the criteria for intoxication (F1x.0), harmful use (F1x.1), dependence (F1x.2), or withdrawal states (F1x.3 and F1x.4). The continued moderate and largely unchanged use of alcohol or drugs in amounts or with the frequency to which the individual is accustomed does not necessarily rule out the use of F23; that must be decided by clinical judgment and the requirements of the research project in question.

G5: Most commonly used exclusion clause. There must be no organic mental disorder (F00–F09) or serious metabolic disturbances affecting the central nervous system (not including childbirth). A fifth character should be used to specify whether the acute onset of the disorder is associated with acute stress (occurring 2 weeks or less before evidence of first psychotic symptoms): F23.x0 without associated acute stress, F23.x1 with associated acute stress. For research purposes, it is recommended that change of the disorder from a nonpsychotic to a clearly psychotic state is further specified as either abrupt (onset within 48 hours) or acute (onset in more than 48 hours but less than 2 weeks).

F23.0: Acute polymorphic psychotic disorder without symptoms of schizophrenia

A. The general criteria for acute and transient psychotic disorders (F23) must be met.

B. Symptoms change rapidly in both type and intensity from day to day or within the same day.

C. Any type of either hallucinations or delusions occurs, for at least several hours, at any time from the onset of the disorder.

D. Symptoms from at least two of the following categories occur at the same time:

(1) Emotional turmoil, characterized by intense feelings of happiness or ecstasy, or overwhelming anxiety or marked irritability

(2) Perplexity or misidentification of people or places

(3) Increased or decreased motility to a marked degree

E. If any of the symptoms listed for schizophrenia (F20.0–F20.3), Criteria G(1) and (2), are present, they are present only for a minority of the time from the onset (i.e., Criterion B of F23.1 is not fulfilled).

F. The total duration of the disorder does not exceed 3 months.

F23.1: Acute polymorphic psychotic disorder with symptoms of schizophrenia

A. Criteria A, B, C, and D of acute polymorphic psychotic disorder (F23.0) must be met.

B. Some of the symptoms for schizophrenia (F20.0–F20.3) must have been present for the majority of the time since the onset of the disorder, although the full criteria need not be met (i.e., at least one of the symptoms in Criteria G1[1]a to G1[2]c).

C. The symptoms of schizophrenia in Criterion B above do not persist for more than 1 month.

F23.2 Acute schizophrenia-like psychotic disorder

A. The general criteria for acute and transient psychotic disorders (F23) must be met.

B. The criteria for schizophrenia (F20.0–F20.3) are met, with the exception of the criterion for duration.

C. The disorder does not meet Criteria B, C, and D for acute polymorphic psychotic disorder (F23.0).

D. The total duration of the disorder does not exceed 1 month.

F23.3 Other acute predominantly delusional psychotic disorders

A. The general criteria for acute and transient psychotic disorders (F23) must be met.

B. Relatively stable delusions or hallucinations are present but do not fulfill the symptomatic criteria for schizophrenia (F20.0–F20.3).

C. The disorder does not meet the criteria for acute polymorphic psychotic disorder (F23.0).

D. The total duration of the disorder does not exceed 3 months.

F23.8: Other acute and transient psychotic disorders

Any other acute psychotic disorders that are not classifiable under any other category in F23 (such as acute psychotic states in which definite delusions or hallucinations occur but persist for only small proportions of the time) should be coded here. States of undifferentiated excitement should also be coded here if more detailed information about the patient's mental state is not available, provided that there is no evidence of an organic cause.

F23.9: Acute and transient psychotic disorder, unspecified

From World Health Organization. *The ICD-10 Classification of Mental and Behavioural Disorders: Diagnostic Criteria for Research.* Geneva: World Health Organization; 1992, with permission.

admission cohort from Suffolk County, New York, only 27 percent of subjects receiving a consensus research diagnosis of brief psychotic disorder at the 6-month follow-up maintained this diagnosis when reevaluated at the 24-month follow-up. Another 9 percent were rediagnosed as schizophreniform disorder and 18 percent as psychotic disorder NOS. The remainder were rediagnosed either as mood disorders (27 percent), schizophrenia (9 percent), or other conditions (9 percent). In contrast, a study of consecutive psychotic admissions from Halle, Germany, indicated that 83 percent of the patients initially diagnosed with brief psychotic disorder did not change diagnosis when reevaluated 2 years later. However, unlike the Suffolk County study, which formulated consensus diagnoses based on all available longitudinal information, the German study used cross-sectional diagnosis at the time of follow-up; hence, episodes between initial evaluation and follow-up were not taken into consideration when determining diagnostic stability. Furthermore, unlike the Suffolk County study, the German study was not a first-admission study. Changes in diagnosis are more likely in the early course of psychotic conditions.

EPIDEMIOLOGY

Acute and transient psychotic disorders are rare, especially in industrialized settings. As a result, there are little accurate data on their incidence or prevalence. An epidemiological study based on data from an

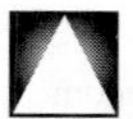

Table 12.16a–3
DSM-IV-TR Criteria for Brief Psychotic Disorder

A. Presence of one (or more) of the following symptoms:
(1) Delusions
(2) Hallucinations
(3) Disorganized speech (e.g., frequent derailment or incoherence)
(4) Grossly disorganized or catatonic behavior

Note: Do not include a symptom if it is a culturally sanctioned response pattern.

B. Duration of an episode of the disturbance is at least 1 day but less than 1 month, with eventual full return to premorbid level of functioning.

C. The disturbance is not better accounted for by a mood disorder with psychotic features, schizoaffective disorder, or schizophrenia and is not due to the direct physiological effects of a substance (e.g., a drug of abuse, a medication) or a general medical condition.

Specify if:

With marked stressor(s) (brief reactive psychosis): if symptoms occur shortly after and apparently in response to events that, singly or together, would be markedly stressful to almost anyone in similar circumstances in the person's culture

Without marked stressor(s): if psychotic symptoms do not occur shortly after or are not apparently in response to events that, singly or together, would be markedly stressful to almost anyone in similar circumstances in the person's culture

With postpartum onset: if onset within 4 weeks postpartum

From American Psychiatric Association. *Diagnostic and Statistical Manual of Mental Disorders.* 4th ed. Text rev. Washington, DC: American Psychiatric Association; 2000, with permission.

international study reported that the incidence was ten times higher in developing countries, compared with industrialized countries, and two times higher in women, compared with men. The annual incidence rates per 10,000 in this study were 0.49 in men and 0.88 in women in developing countries and 0.04 in men and 0.10 in women in industrialized countries. These psychoses comprised 35 percent of all first-contact nonaffective psychoses in developing countries, compared with only 6 percent in industrialized countries. The definition of acute and transient psychotic disorders in this study was somewhat different from the ICD-10. With regard to gender distribution, however, these results are similar to those reported from clinical studies of ICD-10 acute and transient psychotic disorders as well as cycloid psychosis, *bouffée délirante*, and other similar syndromes.

Age of onset is in the early to mid-20s in the developing countries and in the mid-20s to mid-30s in industrialized countries. The most common specific disorder in the group of ICD-10 acute and transient psychotic disorders is acute polymorphic psychotic disorder without symptoms of schizophrenia, comprising between one-third and one-half of all cases of acute and transient psychotic disorders, followed in frequency of occurrence by acute polymorphic psychotic disorder with symptoms of schizophrenia.

Brief psychotic disorder is perhaps even less common than acute and transient psychotic disorders. In a sample of more than 1,000 cases of nonorganic psychotic or major affective disorder hospitalized in a German university hospital, these conditions comprised only 2.5 percent of the cases. Similarly, in the Suffolk County first-admission cohort, a primary diagnosis of brief psychotic disorder was found in only 2 percent of individuals. A study of U.S. Air Force recruits during basic training reported a 6-week incidence rate of 1.43 cases of DSM-III-R brief reactive psychosis per 100,000 recruits. However, this number may overestimate the incidence rate in the general population because basic training is a particularly stressful period.

Similar to acute and transient psychotic disorders, brief psychotic disorder is more common among women than men. Also similar to acute and transient psychotic disorders, age of onset of brief psychotic disorder in industrialized settings might be higher than in developing countries.

ETIOLOGY

Little is known about the etiology of acute and transient psychotic disorders and even less about brief psychotic disorder. The available evidence for acute and transient psychotic disorders points to both biological and sociocultural factors. In one study from India, for example, a history of antecedent fever was reported in 47 percent of individuals with an acute and transient psychotic disorder. In all patients, the fever had resolved before the onset of psychotic symptoms, making it unlikely that the psychosis was the direct effect of a medical disorder (e.g., infection). Similar reports from other developing country settings and classic European psychiatric literature also note high rates of febrile illness before the development of acute and transient psychotic disorders, which may, in part, explain the higher incidence of these disorders in developing country settings in which infectious diseases are common. Few family studies of ICD-10 acute and transient psychotic disorders or brief psychotic disorders have been conducted. A study from India reported a higher risk of acute transient psychotic disorders and a lower risk of schizophrenia and mood disorders in the first-degree relatives of probands, compared with schizophrenia probands. Similar results were obtained in family studies of cycloid psychosis and reactive psychosis in other settings.

The high incidence rate of acute and transient psychotic disorders in developing country settings has naturally led to speculations about the role of sociocultural factors in the etiology of these syndromes. It has been suggested that rapid cultural change and modernization in the developing countries expose individuals to loss of status and stress arising from role confusion, making individuals vulnerable to psychotic reactions.

"Acute stress" (within approximately 2 weeks of onset of psychosis) has been noted by ICD-10 as a feature in some individuals with acute and transient psychotic disorders. However, the actual proportion of patients who experience acute stress in this time frame varies considerably across studies, ranging from 10 to 69 percent, highlighting the difficulty of reliably assessing such stress. Assessment of acute stress is also complicated by lack of a clear definition of such stress in ICD-10 and the possible impact of recall bias. Furthermore, the stressors likely vary according to social and cultural context. Thus, for example, among women in developing countries, departure from or return to their parental village was a major stressor in one study, whereas among men in these settings, job-related problems were the main stressor.

Similarly, with or without "marked stressor(s)" is noted by DSM-IV-TR as a specifier for brief psychotic disorder. However, there are very little reliable data on the proportion of cases that are preceded by such stressors.

Clinical lore suggests an association between preexisting personality disorders and both acute and transient psychotic disorders and brief psychotic disorder. This association has also been noted in the text of DSM-IV-TR. However, reliable assessment of premorbid personality disorders in patients with psychotic conditions is often difficult and may be affected by recall bias or residual psychotic symptoms. This point was highlighted in a Danish study of acute and transient psychotic disorders in which the majority of patients were diagnosed with a preexisting personality disorder shortly after recovery from psychosis, whereas 1 year later, only a minority received such diagnosis.

Finally, a psychodynamic formulation of brief reactive psychosis links this condition to deficient ego strength. According to this formulation, psychosis occurs in response to an intense emotionally stressful event that, in the absence of support in the environment, overwhelms the individual's ego defense mechanisms.

DIAGNOSIS AND CLINICAL FEATURES

Acute and Transient Psychotic Disorders Recognition of acute and transient psychotic disorders early in their course is difficult. In the first few weeks of the illness, there are no certain indicators that distinguish acute and transient psychotic disorders from other nonaffective psychotic disorders with acute onset. Furthermore, even in retrospect, assessing the duration of a psychotic episode and distinguishing spontaneous remission from remission due to antipsychotic medication treatment is often difficult. Therefore, a definitive diagnosis of acute and transient psychotic disorder is often only possible retrospectively and when extensive information on the patient's past history is available.

The ICD-10 provides a sequence of three "key features" to be used for diagnosing acute and transient psychotic disorders. In the order of priority, these features are: (1) an *acute onset* (within 2 weeks); (2) presence of *typical syndromes*, which are the basis for the subcategorization into specific disorders; and (3) the presence of associated *acute stress* (within approximately 2 weeks of onset). *Acute onset* is defined as "a change from a state without psychotic features to a clearly abnormal psychotic state, within a period of 2 weeks or less." Time to onset should be distinguished from time from onset to the maximum severity of illness. The maximum severity of illness may be reached weeks after onset. Similarly "prodromal periods of anxiety, depression, social withdrawal, or mildly abnormal behaviour" should not be counted in assessing time to onset. Thus, acute onset is still recorded even if the individual reports weeks or months of these prodromal symptoms before the onset of illness. ICD-10 also suggests that a distinction be made between acute onset, as described above, and abrupt onset—that is, onset within 48 hours, noting that the latter may be associated with even better outcome.

With regard to the second key feature, a *typical syndrome*, two syndromes are described in ICD-10: a polymorphic syndrome and a typical schizophrenic syndrome. The polymorphic syndrome consists of marked hallucinations, delusions, and perceptual disturbances that change from day to day or even from hour to hour. This state is frequently associated with symptoms of emotional turmoil, "with intense transient feelings of happiness and ecstasy or anxieties and irritability." Although mood symptoms might be present, the criteria for a manic or depressive disorder episode are not met. The following example from the ICD-10 casebook illustrates these features:

Mrs. C. is a 25-year-old Frenchwoman who was brought by ambulance to a hospital emergency department in the city in which she lived. Her husband reported that she had been perfectly normal until the previous evening, when she had come home from work complaining that "strange things were going on" at her office. She had noticed that her colleagues were talking about her, that they had been quite different all of a sudden, and that they had started behaving as if they were acting a part. Mrs. C. was convinced that she had been put under surveillance and that someone was listening in on her telephone conversations. All day she had been feeling as if she were in a dream. When she looked in the mirror, she had seemed unreal to herself. She had become increasingly anxious, incoherent, and agitated during the course of the day and had not been able to sleep at all during the night. She had spent most of the night looking out of the window. Several times she pointed at the crows in a nearby tree and told her husband, "The birds are coming."

In the morning, Mr. C. found his wife on her knees as if she were praying. She knocked her head repeatedly against the floor and talked in a rambling way, declaring that she had been entrusted with a special mission, that her boss was a criminal, there were spies everywhere, and something terrible would happen soon. All of a sudden, she calmed down, smiled at her husband, and told him that she had decided to convert from Catholicism to Islam. At that stage, she became quite elated, started laughing and shouting, and declared that she and her husband could pray to the same god from then on. Shortly afterward, she was terrified again and accused her husband of trying to poison her.

Mrs. C. was brought up in a town in the west of France where her parents owned a small restaurant. She did well in school, went on to college, and trained as an interpreter. During her training, she met her future husband, who had come to France from Algeria to train as an interpreter himself. Because both she and her husband were agnostics, the fact that they came from different religious backgrounds had never been a problem. She took a job with an administration related to the European Communities, and her husband found a position with an international interpreting company. The couple was doing well; they had bought a nice house on the outskirts of Mrs. C.'s hometown and were planning to have a child in the near future.

Mrs. C.'s parents were in good health. She had a brother and two sisters. At 18 years of age, her younger sister had had a nervous breakdown and in the ensuing years had been hospitalized repeatedly in a psychiatric hospital with a diagnosis of schizophrenia.

Both Mrs. C. and her husband refrained from drinking alcohol and were strongly opposed to any kind of drugs, including prescription medicines.

Mr. C. described his wife as an outgoing, sociable, and perfectly normal woman. However, he was quite worried about what was happening, all the more because she appeared to have symptoms resembling those he had observed in his sister-in-law.

On admission, Mrs. C. was frightened and bewildered but was oriented in time, place, and person. She was restless and constantly changed position, standing and sitting, moving about the room, shouting and screaming, weeping and laughing. She talked in a rambling way, shifting from one subject to another without any transition. Something criminal was going on at her office, she said, and she had discovered a secret plot. There were microphones hidden everywhere, she added, and "the birds are coming." She wondered whether the physician was a real physician or a spy in disguise. She went on to speak about "my mission," declared that Jesus had been a false prophet, that Muhammad was the real prophet, and that she would convince the world of what was right and wrong. She then began to explain that the truth was to be found in numbers. The digit "3" signifies good, she said, and the digit "8" represents evil. Suddenly she started to weep, explaining that her parents had died and that she wished to join them in heaven.

During the first days of hospitalization, Mrs. C. continued presenting a rapidly changing symptomatology. Her mood frequently shifted from sadness to elation, and the content of her delusions changed from persecution to mysticism. On several occasions she came out of her room and complained that she had heard people speaking about her, even when there was no one in the vicinity. When asked to describe what she was hearing, she spoke of voices coming from the corridor. She firmly denied that the voices might emanate from within her own body.

The physical examination did not reveal any abnormality. Results of blood tests, including thyroid function, were within normal limits, as were all other special investigations such as an electroencephalogram (EEG) and brain scan.

Mrs. C. was treated with 30 mg of haloperidol [Haldol] during the first week and with one-half this dose for the following week. After 2 weeks, all of her symptoms had disappeared, and she was discharged on medication. She was seen once a week in the outpatient department for another month, during which the medication was progressively reduced and then stopped completely. Two months after the onset of the delusional episode, the patient continued to be free of symptoms.

DISCUSSION

Mrs. C.'s symptoms began abruptly (i.e., over <48 hours) and included unsystematized polymorphous delusions, auditory hallucinations, rapidly fluctuating changes in mood, depersonalization, and derealization. She had no clouding of consciousness, suggesting that her symptoms did not result from delirium. Her symptoms had resolved within 2 weeks of illness onset and did not recur over a several-month period despite tapering of her antipsychotic, suggesting that her symptoms were not the result of schizophreniform disorder or schizophrenia. Consequently, because she had no symptoms of schizophrenia and no precipitating stressor, Mrs. C.'s diagnosis is best described as acute polymorphic psychotic disorder, without symptoms of schizophrenia and without associated acute stress.

The schizophrenic syndrome requires that the ICD-10 symptom criteria for schizophrenia be met for the majority of the time since the onset but less than 1 month. The schizophrenic syndrome might be associated with the polymorphic syndrome as in acute polymorphic psychotic disorder with symptoms of schizophrenia or stand alone as in acute schizophrenia-like psychotic disorder, as the following excerpt from the ICD-10 casebook illustrates:

Mr. T. was a 25-year-old Moroccan. He was unemployed, having given up his studies in mechanical engineering. Mr. T.'s mother had just gotten into bed one evening when she smelled smoke coming from her son's room. She rushed in and found Mr. T. fanning the flames of a smoldering heap of clothes. She attempted to stop him, but he violently pushed her away, so she ran outside for help. Several neighbors came to her aid and overpowered Mr. T., who tried to stop them from entering the house. The neighbors managed to put out the blaze, but not before it had destroyed Mr. T.'s room and much of his mother's. Mr. T. was admitted to the psychiatric clinic after this incident. Before setting fire to the house, he had become increasingly violent toward his family. The current episode of difficulties started 10 days previously, when he had begun smoking hashish and seemed to lose interest in his studies. He started neglecting his appearance and became excessively preoccupied with religious duties and mystical topics. He became particularly aggressive toward his mother and began accusing her of having behaved sinfully in the past.

Mr. T. came from a family of average socioeconomic status. He started school at the age of 6 years. He was well adjusted, and his school grades were very good. He was able to obtain a grant to continue in higher education and began to study mechanical engineering. His parents separated when he was 3 years of age. At the time of Mr. T.'s admission to the clinic, his father was 62 years of age but had had no contact with his son. His mother was 48 years of age and had remarried 10 years before. Mr. T. was brought up by an uncle and attended boarding schools. His mother was in regular contact with him and even did some household chores for the uncle because he was not married. Mr. T. was well adjusted socially. He was outgoing and had many friends, both male and female. He first smoked hashish during adolescence and was reported to smoke it occasionally. He was cheerful but temperamental. He was interested in sports and traveling abroad and was said to have good religious and moral standards. Although Mr. T. had had no serious physical illnesses, when he was 22 years of age, he had been in a traffic accident and was treated for a cut on his scalp. No fracture was noted. He had attended the university hospital's psychiatric outpatient department that same year, complaining of problems of adjustment after starting his university studies. He stopped attending the outpatient department while still being evaluated and was never given a diagnosis.

Physical examination of Mr. T. showed no abnormalities. Complete blood cell count, liver functions, erythrocyte sedimentation rate, and blood urea nitrogen were normal, as was brain mapping. On admission, the patient was overtly irritable, agitated, disheveled, and unshaven. There was no manneristic behavior, nor were there stereotypies or other catatonic behavioral features. He complained of nervous tension only. During conversation, he stopped abruptly and said he was unable to remember what he was going to say.

Three days after the incident, when he was asked about his attempt to burn down the house, Mr. T. said he was carrying out "holy justice" because his mother was a sinful woman. He explained that if he had succeeded in burning the house down, "those who have to be punished" would have gone to hell, and their past would have been reduced to ashes. He had not been successful, he said, because a neighbor had secretly reported him to the police.

Asked whether he ever heard voices, he said he sometimes heard the orders of evil spirits. However, these voices had not affected his behavior, he said, because they were not directed toward him. Rather, the reason he was able to hear the spirits was simply because he was carrying out a special holy mission. There was no evidence of cognitive impairment or of pyromania.

DISCUSSION

Mr. T. first showed signs of mental distress when he was 22 years of age. However, there is no information as to whether a disorder began developing at that time and continued insidiously. Therefore, the current illness must be regarded as a solitary episode that began 10 days before his admission to the clinic. Mr. T. has overt signs and symptoms of a thought processing disorder (blocking), delusions (e.g., carrying out holy justice), and clear hallucinatory experiences. He had a clear-cut psychotic state that fulfills the criteria for ICD-10 schizophrenia, except that the time criterion (i.e., symptoms lasting at least 1 month) is not fulfilled. The diagnosis was therefore acute schizophrenia-like psychotic disorder. According to the description of this category in ICD-10, if the schizophrenia symptoms last more than 1 month, the diagnosis should be changed to paranoid schizophrenia.

It should be noted that there is concurrent hashish smoking, and the possibility of a psychotic disorder induced by psychoactive substance use is present. The information about Mr. T.'s physical state revealed neither signs of intoxication (e.g., reddening of the conjunctiva or increased heart rate) nor any abnormality in the liver tests. Nevertheless, a provision for schizophrenia-like psychotic disorder due to use of cannabinoids should be made. This diagnosis can be made only when the patient remits with no residual symptoms of the psychotic state.

The ICD-10 section on acute and transient psychotic disorders defines *acute stress* as "events that would be regarded as stressful to most people in similar circumstances, within the culture of the person concerned." ICD-10 mentions "bereavement, unexpected loss of partner or job, marriage, or the psychological trauma of combat, terrorism and torture," as typical examples of acute stress.

A diagnosis of acute and transient psychotic disorder requires ruling out typical manic or depressive episodes, alcohol or drug intoxication, delirium, dementia, and mental disorders due to medical etiologies.

DSM-IV-TR Brief Psychotic Disorder The diagnosis of brief psychotic disorder is based on the presence of one or more psychotic symptoms, including delusions, hallucinations, disorganized speech, and disorganized or catatonic behavior. Although sudden onset is discussed as an essential feature of brief psychotic disorder in the text of DSM-IV-TR, it is not included in the diagnostic criteria. Similar to the ICD-10 diagnostic criteria for acute and transient psychotic disorders, DSM-IV-TR criteria for brief psychotic disorder allow for specifiers indicating presence or absence of *marked stressor(s)*. These are defined as events that are "markedly stressful to almost anyone in similar circumstances in the person's culture." The manual does not specify stressors that qualify as marked stressors, but examples reported in the literature include serious surgery or medical illness, stress of immigration, war and other mass violence, torture, and even intensive training programs such as military training. The following excerpt from the DSM-IV-TR casebook presents an example of a young man who experienced an episode of brief psychotic disorder during military training:

A Norwegian lumberman was admitted to the psychiatric ward of a hospital shortly after starting his required military duty at 20 years of age. During the first week after his arrival at the military base, he believed the other recruits looked at him in a strange way. He watched the people around him to see whether they were out "to get" him. He heard voices calling his name several times. He became increasingly suspicious and after another week had to be admitted to the psychiatric department at the University of Oslo. There he was guarded, scowling, skeptical, and depressed. He gave the impression of being very shy and inhibited. His psychotic symptoms disappeared rapidly when he was treated with an antipsychotic drug. However, he had difficulties in adjusting to hospital life. Transfer to a long-term mental hospital was considered; but after 3 months, a decision was made to discharge him to his home in the forest. He was subsequently judged unfit to return to military services and was struck from the military lists.

The patient, the eldest of five siblings, was the son of a farm laborer in one of the valleys of Norway. His father was an intemperate drinker who became angry and brutal when drunk. The family was very poor, and there were constant quarrels between the parents. As a child, the patient was inhibited and fearful and often ran into the woods when troubled. He had academic difficulties and barely passed elementary school.

When the patient became older, he preferred to spend most of his time in the woods, where he worked as a lumberman from 15 years of age. He had his own horse, lived in a log cabin, and disliked being with people. He sometimes took part in the youth dances in the village. Although never a heavy drinker, he often got into fights in the village when he had a drink or two. At the age of 16 years, he began to keep company with a girl 1 year his junior who sometimes kept house for him in the woods. They eventually became engaged.

DISCUSSION

The Norwegian psychiatrist who provided this case made the Scandinavian diagnosis of reactive psychosis, paranoid type. The patient displays the typical features of the disorder: reaction to extreme stress that exacerbates underlying psychological conflicts in which the prognosis for full recovery is very good. To label a psychosis reactive, the psychic trauma must be considered of such significance that the psychosis does not appear in its absence. There must be a temporal connection between the trauma and the onset of the psychosis, and the content of the psychotic symptoms must reflect the traumatic experience. In this case, for an extremely shy and isolated man, military service was a much more serious stressor than for an ordinary person of the same age.

According to DSM-IV-TR, the differential diagnosis is between delusional disorder and brief psychotic disorder. The nonbizarre delusion that he was being persecuted suggests delusional disorder, persecutory type; but delusional disorder requires a duration of at least 1 month, and this patient apparently recovered from his psychotic symptoms within a few weeks. Therefore, the diagnosis is brief psychotic disorder because this diagnosis applies to psychotic illnesses of at least 1 day but no more than 1 month, with eventual full return to premorbid functioning, as in this case. The importance of the stressor could be indicated on Axis IV.

Although the lumberman has had a tendency toward social isolation and difficulties with peers as an adolescent, there is insufficient information to justify a personality disorder diagnosis. Therefore, the presence of schizoid personality traits on Axis II shall be simply noted.

FOLLOW-UP

The patient was reinterviewed by hospital personnel at 4, 7, and 23 years after his admission. He has had no recurrences of any psychotic symptoms and has been fully employed since 6 months after he left the hospital. He married the young woman to whom he was engaged, and at the last follow-up, he had two grown children.

After leaving the hospital, the patient worked for 2 years in a factory and then as lumberman. For the last 20 years, he has managed a small business, which he has run well. He has been happy at work and in his family life. He has made an effort to overcome his tendency toward isolation and has several friends. Among other duties, he has been chairman of a sheep-rearing association in the country. He is well liked in the village.

The patient believes that his natural tendency is to be socially isolated and that his disorder was connected with the fact that in the military situation he was forced to deal with other people.

Although in this case, the temporal order of stressor and psychotic episode was clear, it is not always easy to determine whether a specific stressor was a precipitant or consequence of the illness. Other sources of information, such as information from spouse or friends, about the level of functioning before the onset of episode, as well as history of similar responses to similar stressors in the past, may be helpful in determining the order of events. The DSM-IV-TR criteria for brief psychotic disorder also allow for a "with postpartum onset" specifier for episodes starting within 4 weeks' postpartum.

Although emotional turmoil and confusion are not among the diagnostic criteria for brief psychotic disorder, they are noted as typical experiences in the text of DSM-IV-TR. The text also notes rapid shifts from one intense affect to another in some cases. A study of brief reactive psychosis from Swaziland, southern Africa, also notes that cases in that setting are characterized more by volatile affect and behavior, altered states of consciousness, and dissociative experiences than by clear-cut psychotic symptoms.

DSM-IV-TR diagnosis of brief psychotic disorder requires ruling out typical mood disorders, schizoaffective disorder, schizophrenia, substance-induced disorder, and disorders that are due to a general medical condition.

PATHOLOGY AND LABORATORY EXAMINATION

There are no laboratory tests for acute and transient psychotic disorders or brief psychotic disorder. There is also very little information on the biochemical, physiological, and anatomical correlates of these disorders. Most available data are based on work by European investigators on cycloid psychosis—many cases of which likely meet the criteria for ICD-10 acute transient psychotic disorders or DSM-IV-TR brief psychotic disorders.

Auditory evoked potential studies in patients with cycloid psychosis recorded P300 peaks over the left hemisphere, similar to normal controls. In contrast, in patients with residual schizophrenia, P300 peaks are located over the right hemisphere. Right-lateralized P300 peaks are related to structural and functional abnormalities of the left temporal lobe. Furthermore, a higher P300 amplitude, compared with normal controls, was noted in the cycloid psychosis patients, suggesting a higher level of arousal.

This finding is consistent with a regional cerebral blood flow (CBF) study of cycloid psychosis that recorded increased hemispheric blood flow during the psychotic episode with return to normal after remission. There was a direct relationship between the severity of symptoms and arousal, on the one hand, and the degree of increase in blood flow, on the other. No such increase in hemispheric blood flow has been noted during the acute episodes of mood disorders or schizophrenia.

Results of computed tomography (CT) scan studies have also distinguished cycloid psychosis from schizophrenia. Although studies of schizophrenia have consistently shown evidence of enlarged ventricles and dilated cerebral fissures, patients with cycloid psychosis show little or no evidence of such deficits.

Finally, researchers from Japan have noted hypothalamic-pituitary axis abnormalities in subsets of female patients with recurrent atypical psychoses who are more likely to experience episodes at the time of menstruation and parturition.

DIFFERENTIAL DIAGNOSIS

A definitive diagnosis of acute and transient psychotic disorders or brief psychotic disorder early in the first episode of illness is difficult if not impossible. Unless the psychosis has fully remitted, it is impossible to know the duration of an episode of illness. Therefore, during the first few days or weeks of an episode, the diagnosis is usually provisional.

A provisional ICD-10 diagnosis of acute polymorphic psychotic disorder without symptoms of schizophrenia is changed to a diagnosis of ICD-10 persistent delusional disorder or other nonorganic psychotic disorder if the illness lasts more than 3 months. Similarly, a diagnosis of acute polymorphic psychotic disorder with symptoms of schizophrenia is changed to ICD-10 schizophrenia if the episode lasts more than 1 month (note that the minimum duration criterion for schizophrenia in ICD-10 is different from DSM-IV-TR).

Good prognosis of acute and transient psychotic disorders, variability of symptoms, and the presence of mood symptoms sometimes make differentiation from mood disorders difficult. Presence of a full mood syndrome that meets the ICD-10 criteria for a manic or a depressive episode excludes diagnosis of acute and transient psychotic disorders.

Similar considerations apply to the distinctions between DSM-IV-TR brief psychotic disorders and mood disorders. The duration of an episode of brief psychotic disorder is defined as less than 1 month. If the duration of illness (from prodrome through recovery) exceeds 1 month, the diagnosis needs to be changed to schizophreniform disorder, schizophrenia, delusional disorder, or psychotic disorder NOS, depending on other symptoms and the duration of illness.

When successful treatment leads psychotic symptoms to remit within 1 month, it is also difficult to distinguish brief psychotic disorder from other longer-lasting disorders. In such instances, the presence of continued residual symptoms or impairment may be helpful in making a diagnosis. In other individuals, however, only the long-term course of illness can resolve diagnostic uncertainties.

Perhaps the most critical differential diagnostic issue for both acute and transient psychotic disorders and brief psychotic disorder is to rule out delirium, dementia, psychotic disorder due to medical illness, and drug or alcohol intoxication or withdrawal. Careful physical and laboratory examination is often indicated. Toxicological screens and imaging studies may also be indicated. A positive drug or alcohol screen does not necessarily rule out a diagnosis of acute and transient psychotic disorder or brief psychotic disorder. Some patients with these conditions may use substances in an attempt to reduce their symptoms. The temporal relationship between the onset of psychosis and the substance use may be helpful in differentiating a substance-induced psychotic episode from a non–substance-induced one. Symptoms that persist for many days after all traces of the substance are eliminated from blood and urine support diagnoses of acute and transient psychotic disorders or brief psychotic disorder.

Both acute and transient psychotic disorders and brief psychotic disorder may be associated with confusion and perplexity, making it difficult to distinguish these disorders from delirium or medical causes of psychosis. Diurnal variation of consciousness, which is a characteristic of delirium, may also be confused with variable "polymorphic" psychotic symptoms seen in the acute and transient psychotic disorders. However, compared with delirium, changes in consciousness in acute and transient psychotic disorders are generally less severe and less persistent. Furthermore, a medical cause of delirium can often be identified through history, physical examination, laboratory tests, or imaging studies.

Acute psychotic episodes have been reported in a number of medical conditions, including head trauma, cerebral anoxia, epilepsy, and endocrinological disorders such as hyper- or hypothyroidism. Many of these episodes are associated with disturbances of consciousness. Differential diagnosis is often based on a thorough medical history and physical examination as well as laboratory investigations.

COURSE AND PROGNOSIS

Acute and transient psychotic disorders, by definition, have a favorable early course—full remission within 1 to 3 months is a diagnostic criterion in ICD-10. Although there are few first-admission studies that allow for reliable assessment of course and outcome, the available evidence indicates that most of the recovered patients remain well in ensuing years, and even among those who experience further episodes, these episodes are transient, and the outcome is generally favorable. A study from India reported that 47 percent of first-admission patients with ICD-10 acute and transient psychotic disorders had further episodes during a 3-year follow-up. A second first-admission study from Germany similarly reported a 46 percent relapse rate during 3 to 7 years of follow-up. Yet another first-admission study from Suffolk County, New York, reported recurrence of psychotic episodes in 38 percent of patients in a 4-year follow-up. Although the rate of recurrence has been higher in some other studies, patients often recover fully from their episodes and only approximately 6 to 18 percent of patients have any residual symptoms at a later point of time. A 12-year follow-up study from India also reported favorable long-term outcome, at least in that setting. The long-term course and outcome of acute and transient psychotic disorders in industrialized settings have not been studied. In one study, the risk of suicidal behavior during the episodes of acute and transient psychotic disorders was as high as in schizophrenia or bipolar disorder.

Brief psychotic disorder also, by definition, has a benign early course—all cases fully remit within 1 month. Some, however, experience relapses. In a study of consecutive admissions from Halle, Germany, 70 percent experienced relapses during a 2-year follow-up. Nevertheless, the social functioning of these individuals was much better than individuals with schizophrenia—more than 90 percent were living independently, and more than one-half were employed.

FUTURE DIRECTIONS

Better understanding of the etiology, epidemiology, course, and treatment of acute remitting psychoses is hampered by the multiplicity of diagnostic labels and systems. Reaching consensus on a uniform diagnosis is the first priority for research and practice. Introduction of the diagnostic group of acute and transient psychotic disorders in ICD-10 is a useful point of departure. Further revisions of this diagnosis in ICD-11 and inclusion of a corresponding category in the DSM-V could further improve communication among researchers and practitioners.

SUGGESTED CROSS-REFERENCES

Related materials on psychoses of brief duration can be found in Sections 12.16b and 12.16f.

References

Beighley PS, Brown GR, Thompson JW: DSM-III-R brief reactive psychosis among Air Force recruits. *J Clin Psychiatry.* 1992;53:283.

Collins PE, Wig NN, Day R, Varma VK, Malhotra S, Misra AK, Schanzer B, Susser E: Psychosocial and biological aspects of acute brief psychoses in three developing country sites. *Psychiatr Q.* 1996;67:177.

Cooper J, Singh SP. Acute and transient psychoses. In: Henn F, Sartorius N, Helmchen H, Lauter H, eds. *Contemporary Psychiatry, Vol. 3, Specific Psychiatric Disorders.* Berlin: Springer-Verlag; 2001.

Das SK, Malhotra S, Basu D: Family study of acute and transient psychotic disorders: Comparison with schizophrenia. *Soc Psychiatry Psychiatr Epidemiol.* 1999;34:328.

Flaum M, Amador X, Gorman J, Bracha HS, Edell W, McGlashan T, Pandurangi A, Kendler KS, Robinson D, Lieberman J, Ontiveros A, Tohen M, McGorry P, Tyrrell G, Arndt S, Andreasen NC. DSM-IV field trial for schizophrenia and other psychotic disorders. In: Widiger TA, Frances AJ, Pincus HA, Ross R, First MB, Davis W, Kline M, eds. *DSM-IV Sourcebook.* Vol. 4. Washington, DC: American Psychiatric Association; 1998.

Guinness EA: I. Relationship between the neuroses and brief reactive psychosis: Descriptive case studies in Africa. *Br J Psychiatry.* 1992;160[Suppl 16]:12.

Hatotani N: The concept of "atypical psychoses": Special reference to its development in Japan. *Psychiatry Clin Neurosci.* 1996;50:1.

*Jablensky A: Classification of nonschizophrenic psychotic disorders: A historical perspective. *Curr Psychiatry Rep.* 2001;3:326.

Jabs BE, Pfuhlmann B, Bartsch AJ, Cetkovich-Bakmas MG, Stober G: Cycloid psychoses—from clinical concepts to biological foundations. *J Neural Transm.* 2002;109:907.

Jäger MDM, Hintermayr M, Bottlender R, Strauss A, Moller HJ: Course and outcome of first-admitted patients with acute and transient psychotic disorders (ICD-10:F23): Focus on relapses and social adjustment. *Eur Arch Psychiatry Clin Neurosci.* 2003;253:209.

Jørgensen P, Bennedsen B, Christensen J, Hyllested A: Acute and transient psychotic disorder: A 1-year follow-up study. *Acta Psychiatr Scand.* 1997;96:150.

Malhotra S, Malhotra S: Acute and transient psychotic disorders: Comparison with schizophrenia. *Curr Psychiatry Rep.* 2003;5:178.

*Menuck M, Legault S, Schmidt P, Remington G: The nosologic status of the remitting atypical psychoses. *Compr Psychiatry.* 1989;30:53.

Mojtabai R, Susser ES, Bromet EJ: Clinical characteristics, 4-year course, and DSM-IV classification of patients with nonaffective acute remitting psychosis. *Am J Psychiatry.* 2003;160:2108.

*Mojtabai R, Varma VK, Susser E: Duration of remitting psychoses with acute onset. Implications for ICD-10. *Br J Psychiatry.* 2000;176:576.

Perris C. *A Study of Cycloid Psychoses.* Copenhagen: Munksgaard; 1974.

Pillmann F, Balzuweit S, Haring A, Bloink R, Marneros A: Suicidal behavior in acute and transient psychotic disorders. *Psychiatry Res.* 2003;117:199.

*Pillmann F, Haring A, Balzuweit S, Bloink R, Marneros A: The concordance of ICD-10 acute and transient psychosis and DSM-IV brief psychotic disorder. *Psychol Med.* 2002;32:525.

Pillmann F, Haring A, Balzuweit S, Marneros A: A comparison of DSM-IV brief psychotic disorder with "positive" schizophrenia and healthy controls. *Compr Psychiatry.* 2002;43:385.

Pull CB, Chaillet G. The nosological views of French-speaking psychiatry. In: Mezzich JE, Honda Y, Kastrup MC, eds. *Psychiatric Diagnosis: A World Perspective.* Berlin: Springer-Verlag; 1994.

Sajith SG, Chandrasekaran R, Sadanandan Unni KE, Sahai A: Acute polymorphic psychotic disorder: Diagnostic stability over 3 years. *Acta Psychiatr Scand.* 2002;105:104.

Schwartz JE, Fennig S, Tanenberg-Karant M, Carlson G, Craig T, Galambos N, Lavelle J, Bromet EJ: Congruence of diagnoses 2 years after a first-admission diagnosis of psychosis. *Arch Gen Psychiatry.* 2000;57:593.

Strakowski SM: Diagnostic validity of schizophreniform disorder. *Am J Psychiatry.* 1994;151:815.

Susser E, Varma VK, Mattoo SK, Finnerty M, Mojtabai R, Tripathi BM, Misra AK, Wig NN: Long-term course of acute brief psychosis in a developing country setting. *Br J Psychiatry.* 1998;173:226.

*Susser E, Wanderling J: Epidemiology of nonaffective acute remitting psychosis vs schizophrenia: Sex and sociocultural setting. *Arch Gen Psychiatry.* 1994;51:294.

12.16b Schizophreniform Disorder

BUSHRA NAZ, M.D., LAURA J. FOCHTMANN, M.D., AND EVELYN J. BROMET, PH.D.

HISTORY

In 1939, the Norwegian psychiatrist Gabriel Langfeldt introduced the concept of schizophreniform disorder by showing that patients with initial symptom profiles consistent with schizophrenia could be divided into two groups based on their subsequent course. One group had a poor course and was referred to as *typical schizophrenia,* and the other group had a relatively better course and outcome and was referred to as *schizophreniform disorder.* Forty years later, the term *schizophreniform disorder* was officially included in the third edition of the *Diagnostic and Statistical Manual of Mental Disorders* (DSM-III) under "psychotic disorders not elsewhere classified." Nevertheless, the concept of schizophreniform disorder as envisioned by Langfeldt deviates significantly from that adopted by the DSM-III. Langfeldt described a condition with sudden onset and benign course associated with mood symptoms and clouding of consciousness, whereas DSM-III described a condition distinguishable from schizophrenia only with regard to duration—the prodromal, active, and residual phases of the illness must last more than 2 weeks but less than 6 months. Indeed, when the charts of 55 of Langfeldt's original patients diagnosed with schizophreniform psychosis were reevaluated, most patients met the revised DSM-III (DSM-III-R) criteria for mood disorder rather than schizophrenia.

The DSM-III concept of schizophreniform disorder was maintained in future editions. DSM-III-R added the requirement that the illness not meet the criteria for brief reactive psychosis (i.e., duration of symptoms of less than 1 month) and that the presence or absence of a series of good prognostic features be specified. DSM-III-R also dropped the Criterion B of schizophrenia (impairment in functioning) from the diagnostic criteria of schizophreniform disorder. This diagnosis was maintained with little change in the fourth edition of DSM (DSM-IV) and the revised DSM-IV (DSM-IV-TR).

There are conflicting data on the diagnostic stability of DSM-IV-TR schizophreniform disorder. One study found that all patients in a

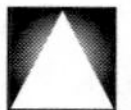

Table 12.16b–1
DSM-IV-TR Criteria for Schizophreniform Disorder

A. Criteria A, D, and E of schizophrenia are met.
B. An episode of the disorder (including prodromal, active, and residual phases) lasts at least 1 month but less than 6 months. (When the diagnosis must be made without waiting for recovery, it should be qualified as "provisional.")

Specify if:

Without good prognostic features

With good prognostic features: as evidenced by two (or more) of the following:

(1) Onset of prominent psychotic symptoms within 4 weeks of the first noticeable change in usual behavior or functioning
(2) Confusion or perplexity at the height of the psychotic episode
(3) Good premorbid social and occupational functioning
(4) Absence of blunted or flat affect

From American Psychiatric Association. *Diagnostic and Statistical Manual of Mental Disorders.* 4th ed. Text rev. Washington, DC: American Psychiatric Association; 2000, with permission.

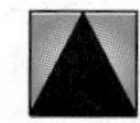

Table 12.16b–2
ICD-10 Diagnostic Guidelines for Acute Schizophrenia-Like Psychotic Disorder

A. The onset of psychotic symptoms must be acute (2 weeks or less from a nonpsychotic to a clearly psychotic state).
B. Symptoms that fulfill the criteria of schizophrenia must have been present for the majority of time.
C. The criteria for acute polymorphic psychotic disorder are not fulfilled.

If the psychotic symptoms last for more than 1 month, then the diagnosis should be changed to schizophrenia.

From World Health Organization. *The ICD-10 Classification of Mental and Behavioural Disorders: Diagnostic Criteria for Research.* Geneva: World Health Organization; 1992, with permission.

first-episode cohort who were initially diagnosed with schizophreniform disorder were subsequently diagnosed with schizophrenia or schizoaffective disorder at 2-year follow-up. Other studies have found that 30 to 50 percent of patients receiving the diagnosis schizophreniform disorder at their first hospitalization maintain this diagnosis over time. In the absence of longitudinal follow-up, these findings underscore the importance of regarding the diagnosis of schizophreniform disorder as provisional.

COMPARATIVE NOSOLOGY

The nosology of schizophreniform disorder has changed very little since it was first introduced into the DSM-III in 1980. In DSM-IV, schizophreniform disorder is conceptualized as a variant of schizophrenia. Thus, the first criterion specifically requires that a patient meet Criterion A for schizophrenia—that is, two or more of the following symptoms: delusions, hallucinations, disorganized speech, grossly disorganized or catatonic behavior, or negative symptoms. The first criterion further specifies that the patient does not have schizoaffective or mood disorder with psychotic features (schizophrenia Criterion D) or a substance or general medical condition (schizophrenia Criterion E). The second criterion differentiates the disorder from schizophrenia by requiring a 1- to 6-month duration of the prodromal, active, and residual phases. Thus, if the duration is less than 1 month, the diagnosis might be brief psychotic disorder. If the duration of illness extends beyond 6 months, the diagnosis might be changed to schizophrenia (Table 12.16b–1).

One of the difficulties in making the diagnosis of schizophreniform disorder is that its validity depends on observing a patient for more than 6 months after onset of psychosis. In the event that the diagnosis is made before 6 months have elapsed, it is considered provisional. Another difficulty is in dating the onset of the prodromal phase, particularly when it evolves insidiously. Without a distinct symptom onset, it becomes difficult to decide whether the illness is actually of 1- to 6-months' duration.

The tenth revision of *International Statistical Classification of Diseases and Related Health Problems* (ICD-10) contains a conceptually similar category to schizophreniform disorder, namely, acute schizophrenia-like psychotic disorder. For this disorder, patients fulfill the ICD-10 criteria for schizophrenia, but the duration is less than 1 month. Most important, the onset of symptoms must be acute ("2 weeks or less from a nonpsychotic to a clearly psychotic state"). Thus, in contrast to the DSM-IV, ICD-10 is more specific about the nature of the onset of psychotic symptoms (Table 12.16b–2).

EPIDEMIOLOGY

There are currently no data on the prevalence rate of schizophreniform disorder per se. In part, this is because the reliability of reports about psychotic symptoms given to lay interviewers in community surveys is very poor. Thus, the National Comorbidity Survey (NCS), in which a diagnostic interview was administered to a representative sample of the U.S. population, included a clinician reinterview to verify the psychotic symptoms endorsed during the Composite International Diagnostic Interview (CIDI) administered by the lay interviewer. Although separate rates were not given for schizophreniform disorder, the lifetime prevalence rate of five clinician-diagnosed DSM-III-R disorders (schizophrenia, schizophreniform disorder, schizoaffective disorder, delusional disorder, and atypical psychosis) was 6.9 per 1,000. The only other available data are from a similarly conducted national survey in Holland of approximately 7,000 individuals aged 18 to 64 years. The lifetime prevalence rates were 3.7 per 1,000 for DSM-III-R schizophrenia, schizoaffective disorder, and schizophreniform disorder combined.

ETIOLOGY

Although no etiology has been established for schizophreniform disorder, risk factors have been evaluated. For schizophrenia and schizophreniform disorder combined, the National Comorbidity Survey (NCS) found that unemployment; residing in a metropolitan area; low income; being separated, widowed, or divorced; young age; low education; and living with nonrelatives were associated with receiving the diagnosis. In a birth cohort from New Zealand followed up at 26 years of age, risk factors for schizophreniform disorder per se included obstetric and early neonatal complications (e.g., low American Pediatric Gross Assessment Record [APGAR] score, hypoxia, small for gestational age) and impairments in neuromotor performance, receptive language, and cognitive development. Other childhood risk factors included emotional problems, psychotic symptoms elicited at 11 years of age, and cannabis use.

Few studies to date have examined biological or neurophysiological precursors of schizophreniform disorder. However, as with schizophrenia, patients with schizophreniform disorder seem to be more likely to have enlarged ventricles. In one study, rates of ventricular enlargement were comparable in patients with chronic schizophrenia and those with first-episode schizophreniform disorder. In addition, left ventricular enlargement in patients with schizophreniform disorder was correlated with a progression of illness to schizophrenia or schizoaffective disorder. Thus, although the available evidence is sparse, it seems reasonable to hypothesize that there are shared risk factors and etiological factors for schizophreniform disorder and for schizophrenia.

DIAGNOSTIC AND CLINICAL FEATURES

Schizophreniform disorder is an acute psychotic disorder that has a rapid onset and lacks a long prodromal phase. Although many patients with schizophreniform disorder may experience functional impairment at the time of an episode, they are unlikely to report a progressive decline in social and occupational functioning. The initial symptom profile is the same as that of schizophrenia in that two or more psychotic symptoms (hallucinations, delusions, disorganized speech and behavior, or negative symptoms) must be present. Schneiderian first-rank symptoms are frequently observed. There is also an increased likelihood of emotional turmoil and confusion, the presence of which may indicate a good prognosis. Although negative symptoms may be present, they are relatively uncommon in schizophreniform disorder and are considered poor prognostic features. In a small series of first-admission schizophreniform patients, one-fourth had moderate to severe negative symptoms. Almost all were initially categorized as "schizophreniform disorder without good prognostic features," and 2 years later, 73 percent were rediagnosed with schizophrenia, compared with 38 percent of those with "good prognostic features."

By definition, patients with schizophreniform disorder return to their baseline state within 6 months. In some instances, the illness is episodic, with more than one episode occurring after long periods of full remission. However, if the combined duration of symptomatology exceeds 6 months, then schizophrenia should be considered.

Ms. V. was a 30-year-old white woman from a working-class family. She was born prematurely and as a toddler had a seizure disorder that was treated with phenobarbital (Luminal, Solfoton) for 1 year. She did well in school but dropped out in the 12th grade, obtained a General Educational Development (GED) diploma, and began working at 18 years of age. She described her adolescence as a time when she was happy, outgoing, and had several friends. She married at 21 years of age and had two children, but 9 months before her initial hospitalization, she and her husband separated. Ms. V. began working in a local factory, and she and her children moved in with her mother. About 6 weeks before her initial admission, Ms. V. started feeling that drug dealers and gangsters were out to hurt her and that people were poisoning her food. She also did not let her children eat, fearing they would die from food poisoning. She was admitted to the hospital for 2 weeks but did not receive any medications at that time. Three weeks after discharge, she was readmitted with the same symptoms and also experienced thought broadcasting, thought insertion, and olfactory hallucinations. She was treated with haloperidol (Haldol) and was discharged after 1 month. She later moved to Florida with her mother and children, worked full time, and remained free of symptoms without treatment for 9 years. At that time, she again became psychotic, but after treatment with olanzapine (Zyprexa) for 1 month, she recovered fully and resumed her usual social and occupational functioning.

DISCUSSION

Ms. V. presented with an acute psychotic disorder that had a rapid onset without a significant prodromal phase. Her symptoms lasted approximately 3 months but were otherwise typical of those seen in schizophrenia and included persecutory ideas, thought insertion, thought withdrawal, and olfactory hallucinations. She had an additional episode of illness approximately 10 years later, but her total duration of symptoms still remained less than 6 months. Between episodes, she returned to her premorbid level of social and occupational functioning. Of note, Ms. V. had been born prematurely, a possible obstetric risk factor for development of schizophreniform disorder. Although she had a history of seizure disorder as a child and olfactory hallucinations with her initial episode of illness, there was no evidence that a seizure disorder was contributing to her psychotic presentation. Thus, a diagnosis of schizophreniform disorder is most appropriate for Ms. V.

Mr. C. was 19 years of age when he was first admitted to a psychiatric inpatient unit. In the second grade, he was diagnosed with a learning disability and subsequently attended special education classes. His mother described him as a quiet boy who got along well with his peers. After graduating from high school, he lived with his mother and did clerical work. Before his first admission, Mr. C. became despondent, withdrawn, agitated, and had difficulty sleeping. He began to act bizarrely, talking to himself, laughing inappropriately, and warning his sister that the Mafia was after them. He was hospitalized and treated with antipsychotic medication but left the hospital against medical advice after 2 weeks. His symptoms worsened rapidly, and he was readmitted to the hospital. He was treated with perphenazine (Trilafon) and discharged 5 weeks later. Over the next 2 months, he required two further hospitalizations for recurrent delusions and auditory hallucinations before being stabilized on medications. By 6 months after his index admission, Mr. C. was asymptomatic, and he functioned well for the next 4 years. At that point, his doctor tried to reduce Mr. C.'s medication, and he again became floridly psychotic. His antipsychotic medication was again increased, with good control of his symptoms and a reasonable level of functioning. By 10-year follow-up, he had several friends, had gotten married, and had two children. Nevertheless, he had been unable to finish college and continued to receive disability benefits.

DISCUSSION

Mr. C. was a participant in a longitudinal, first-admission cohort study (the Suffolk County Mental Health Project). His initial episodes of psychosis, when diagnosed after the initial baseline interview, met criteria for schizophreniform disorder. However, with longitudinal follow-up, it became clear that his symptoms recurred without antipsychotic treatment, even after many years of being free of psychotic symptoms. Consequently, he was rediagnosed as having schizophrenia, emphasizing the provisional nature of the schizophreniform disorder diagnosis and the importance of longitudinal observation in confirming the diagnosis.

DIFFERENTIAL DIAGNOSIS

It is important to first differentiate schizophreniform disorder from psychoses that can arise from medical conditions. This is accomplished by taking a detailed history and physical examination and, when indicated, performing laboratory tests or imaging studies. A detailed history of medication use, including over-the-counter medications and herbal products, is essential because many therapeutic agents may also produce an acute psychosis. Although it is not always possible to distinguish substance-induced psychosis from other psychotic disorders cross-sectionally, a rapid onset of psychotic symptoms in a patient with a significant substance history should raise the suspicion of a substance-induced psychosis. A detailed substance use history and toxicological screen are also important for treatment planning in an individual with a new onset of psychosis.

The duration of psychotic symptoms is one of the factors that distinguish schizophreniform disorder from other syndromes. Schizophrenia is diagnosed if the duration of the prodromal, active, and residual phases lasts for more than 6 months, whereas symptoms that occur for less than 1 month indicate a brief psychotic disorder. In DSM-IV-TR, a diagnosis of brief psychotic disorder does not require that a major stressor be present.

To distinguish mood disorders with psychotic features from schizophreniform disorder is sometimes difficult. Furthermore, both the Epidemiologic Catchment Area (ECA) study and the NCS have found schizophreniform disorder and schizophrenia to be highly comorbid with mood and anxiety disorders. Additional confounds are that mood symptoms, such as loss of interest and pleasure, may be difficult to distinguish from negative symptoms, avolition, and anhedonia. Some mood symptoms may also be present during the early course of schizophrenia. Again, a thorough longitudinal history is important in elucidating the diagnosis because the presence of psychotic symptoms exclusively during periods of mood disturbance is an indication of a primary mood disorder.

COURSE AND PROGNOSIS

For individuals whose diagnosis remains schizophreniform disorder after longitudinal follow-up, the illness course is usually benign. In general, these patients have met criteria for "good prognostic features" on first presentation. These features include: onset of psychotic symptoms within 4 weeks of the first noticeable change in usual behavior or functioning, confusion or perplexity at the height of the psychotic episode, good premorbid social and occupational functioning, and absence of blunted or flat affect. The first patient described above (Ms. V.) illustrates the characteristics and course of an individual diagnosed with schizophreniform disorder with good prognostic features. In this patient, the onset of psychotic symptoms occurred within 1 week, her premorbid functioning was good, she did not display a flat affect, and she had a relatively benign course.

Although the DSM-IV-TR states that the presence of two or more good prognostic features provides a reasonable way to distinguish between patients with a good or poor prognosis, some patients with two or more positive prognostic features have a mixed or poor course. The second patient described earlier (Mr. C.) had an acute onset and reasonable premorbid functioning, yet his clinical course was relatively poor, and his diagnosis at the 10-year follow-up point was schizophrenia.

Mr. C.'s case also illustrates the difficulty in judging the course of the disorder and establishing a precise diagnosis when a patient's symptoms are modified by active treatment. With Mr. C., the diagnosis became clearer when his medications were decreased and his psychotic symptoms recurred. Had this event not occurred, Mr. C.'s diagnosis may have remained schizophreniform disorder.

Individuals classified as "without good prognostic features" often have a course that resembles that of patients initially diagnosed with schizophrenia. For many of these patients, their diagnosis indeed changes to schizophrenia with longitudinal observation.

SUGGESTED CROSS-REFERENCES

A more detailed review of schizophrenia is presented in Chapter 12. Acute and transient disorders are discussed in Section 12.3a.

References

*Benazzi F: Outcome of schizophreniform disorder. *Curr Psychiatry Rep.* 2003;5:192.

*Bergem AL, Dahl AA, Guldberg C, Hansen H: Langfeldt's schizophreniform psychoses fifty years later. *Br J Psychiatry.* 1990;157:351.

Cannon M, Caspi A, Moffit TE, Harrington H, Taylor A, Murray RM, Poulton R: Evidence for early-childhood, pan-developmental impairment specific to schizophreniform disorder: Results from a longitudinal birth cohort. *Arch Gen Psychiatry.* 2002;59:449.

DeLisi LE, Hoff AL, Kushner M, Calev A, Stritzke P: Left ventricular enlargement associated with diagnostic outcome of schizophreniform disorder. *Biol Psychiatry.* 1992;32:199.

*Kendler K, Gallagher TJ, Abelson JM, Kessler RC: Lifetime prevalence, demographic risk factors, and diagnostic validity of nonaffective psychosis as assessed in a US community sample: The National Comorbidity Survey. *Arch Gen Psychiatry.* 1996;53:1022.

Kim-Cohen J, Caspi A, Moffitt TE, Harrington H, Milne BJ, Poulton R: Prior juvenile diagnoses in adults with mental disorder: Developmental follow-back of a prospective-longitudinal cohort. *Arch Gen Psychiatry.* 2003;60:709.

*Langfeldt G. *The Schizophreniform States.* Copenhagen, Denmark: Ejnar Munksgaard; 1939.

*Naz B, Bromet EJ, Mojtabai R: Distinguishing between first-admission schizophreniform disorder and schizophrenia. *Schizophren Res.* 2003;62:51.

Weinberger DR, DeLisi LE, Perman GP, Targum S, Wyatt RJ: Computer tomography in schizophreniform disorder and other acute psychiatric disorders. *Arch Gen Psychiatry.* 1982;39:778.

12.16c Delusional Disorder and Shared Psychotic Disorder

Shmuel Fennig, M.D., Laura J. Fochtmann, M.D., and Evelyn J. Bromet, Ph.D.

HISTORY

Delusional disorders, which were once referred to as *paranoid disorders*, have been recognized since the time of the ancient Greeks, who defined *paranoia* as "insanity" or "madness." In the 19th century, Karl Kahlbaum offered a taxonomy that included a group of disorders labeled paranoia whose symptoms were primarily intellectual. Richard von Krafft-Ebbing presented delusions as the main symptom of paranoia. In the fourth and sixth editions of his textbook, Emil Kraepelin described paranoia as stable, nonbizarre, well-systematized delusions with a chronic course, although the course lacked the typical deterioration of dementia praecox. "One invariably observes the insidious development of a permanent unshakable delusional system from inner causes in which clarity and order of thinking, willing and action are completely preserved . . . ." Paranoia kept its position despite the further development of the dementia praecox concept and the introduction of paraphrenia in the eighth edition of Kraepelin's textbook. The distinction between paranoid disorder and paranoid schizophrenia was maintained by Eugen Bleuler. However, Kurt Kolle followed up Kraepelin's patients and showed that their pattern of deterioration was similar to that of patients with dementia praecox. This view was expressed in the second edition of the *Diagnostic and Statistical Manual of Mental Disorders* (DSM-II), in which paranoid states were regarded as possible variants of schizophrenia.

Shared delusional disorder was first described in 1860 by Jules Baillarger, who called the syndrome *folie à communiquée*, and later described by Charles Lasègue and Jules Falret, who gave the syndrome the commonly used name *folie à deux* in 1877. Over the years, many other names, including *shared psychotic disorder*, *shared delusional disorder*, and *induced psychotic disorder*, have been used to describe this syndrome in which two individuals with a close and generally long-term relationship share the same delusional belief.

COMPARATIVE NOSOLOGY AND DESCRIPTION OF DIAGNOSTIC SUBTYPES

The nosological status of delusional disorder as a separate entity has been the subject of debate since Kraepelin first described his concept of paranoia. Three viewpoints have evolved: The first is that delusional disorder is a variant of schizophrenia; the second is that it is a variant of mood disorder; finally, the third is Kraepelin's original position, namely, that paranoia is a third form of psychosis distinct from both schizophrenia and mood disorder. The revised third edition of the DSM (DSM-III-R) and the fourth edition of the DSM (DSM-IV) accepted the Kraepelinian definition of paranoia. For clarity and to encompass other types of delusions, it was called *delusional disorder*, and the word paranoid was dropped. The emphasis is on the presence of nonbizarre delusions lasting for more than 1 month without prominent hallucinations. The duration of the delusions is the only diagnostic feature that departs from Kraepelin's original description. DSM-IV also emphasized the relative preservation of functioning. In contrast to schizophrenia, impaired functioning in delusional disorder can only be as a consequence of the delusions themselves. For example, if a woman with an erotomanic delusion about her boss is fired from work after harassing him, this is a consequence of the delusion. DSM-IV acknowledged the difficulty of differentiating obsessive-compulsive disorder (OCD) with lack of insight from delusional disorder; in these instances, it allows both diagnoses to be made. Similarly, with body dysmorphic disorder with an overvalued idea, the distinction from a somatic delusion is sometimes difficult to make, and DSM-IV allows these two diagnoses to coexist (Table 12.16c–1).

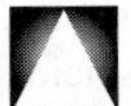

Table 12.16c–1
DSM-IV-TR Diagnostic Criteria for Delusional Disorder

A. Nonbizarre delusions (i.e., involving situations that occur in real life, such as being followed, poisoned, infected, loved at a distance, or deceived by spouse or lover, or having a disease) of at least 1 month's duration.

B. Criterion A for schizophrenia has never been met. **Note:** Tactile and olfactory hallucinations may be present in delusional disorder if they are related to the delusional theme.

C. Apart from the impact of the delusion(s), or its ramifications, functioning is not markedly impaired, and behavior is not obviously odd or bizarre.

D. If mood episodes have occurred concurrently with delusions, their total duration has been brief relative to the duration of the delusional periods.

E. The disturbance is not due to the direct physiological effects of a substance (e.g., a drug of abuse, a medication) or a general medical condition.

Specify type (the following types are assigned based on the predominant delusional theme):

Erotomanic type: delusions that another person, usually of higher status, is in love with the individual

Grandiose type: delusions of inflated worth, power, knowledge, identity, or special relationship to a deity or famous person

Jealous type: delusions that the individual's sexual partner is unfaithful

Persecutory type: delusions that the person (or someone to whom the person is close) is being malevolently treated in some way

Somatic type: delusions that the person has some physical defect or general medical condition

Mixed type: delusions characteristic of more than one of the above types, but no one theme predominates

Unspecified type

From American Psychiatric Association. *Diagnostic and Statistical Manual of Mental Disorders*. 4th ed. Text rev. Washington, DC: American Psychiatric Association; 2000, with permission.

The tenth revision of *International Statistical Classification of Diseases and Related Health Problems* (ICD-10) has a similar description of delusional disorder but avoids the definition of bizarre delusions by requiring that the delusions be "other than those listed as typically schizophrenic" (i.e., other than completely impossible or culturally inappropriate or Schneiderian first rank) (Table 12.16c–2). In ICD-10, the duration of the delusion has to be more than 3 months. Both DSM-IV and ICD-10 allow the presence of transient, nonprominent hallucinations. In the ICD-10, delusional disorders that are acute (more than 1 month and less than 3 months) are classified as acute and transient psychotic disorders. Theoretically, the DSM-IV might include individuals with less severe disorders than ICD-10, but in reality, delusional disorder is typically chronic in nature, and thus both systems most likely include similar patients.

The heart of both diagnostic classifications is the presence of nonbizarre or nonschizophrenic delusions. Delusions have traditionally been regarded as beliefs that are fixed, false, and not ordinarily accepted by other members of one's culture or subculture. Although delusional beliefs are often held with absolute conviction and are not amenable to reason (DSM-III-R), empirical studies have demonstrated that the strength of delusions may be dimensional. For example, levels of conviction may fluctuate, and delusional beliefs may be partially responsive to evidence or reason. As a result, the revised DSM-IV (DSM-IV-TR) definition acknowledges that delusions may show varying levels of conviction.

According to DSM-IV, delusions are deemed bizarre "if they are clearly implausible, not understandable, and not derived from ordinary life experience." Kraepelin proposed that the delusions of schizophrenic patients were "... extraordinary, sometimes wholly nonsensical," compared with the typical delusions of paranoid or bipolar patients. Similarly, Karl Jaspers distinguished two groups of delusions—those that were "psychologically irreducible" and those that he called "delusion like ideas" that emerged "from shattering, mortifying, guilt provoking ... experience." Kurt Schneider enumerated a list of delusions and hallucinations that he believed were pathognomonic of schizophrenia and thus classified them as first-rank symptoms. These symptoms included certain auditory hallucinations (audible thoughts, voices arguing about or discussing the person's actions), delusions of passivity (somatic passivity, thought withdrawal, thought insertion, "made feelings," "made impulses," and "made" volitional acts), delusions of thought broadcasting, and "delusional perception." These symptoms, in Jasper's terms, are not psychologically reducible—that is, understandable for the patient's affect, a determination requiring an empathic or phenomenological interview. In DSM-III-R and DSM-IV, the examples given for bizarre delusions are taken from the first-rank Schneiderian symptoms. The degree to which those symptoms and bizarre delusions define different phenomena remains unclear. In the DSM-III-R, a *bizarre delusion* is defined as "... involving phenomena that the person's culture would regard as totally implausible, e.g. ... thought broadcasting, and being controlled by a dead person." In the text accompanying the DSM-IV, *bizarre delusions*, as noted above, are defined as "... clearly implausible and not understandable and not derived from ordinary life experience." In the ICD-10, on the other hand, the distinction between bizarre delusions that are or are not Schneiderian is explicitly considered in the criteria. Research has shown that the reliability of the assessment of first-rank Schneiderian symptoms is quite good and better than that for bizarre delusions.

The DSM-IV lists five specific subtypes of delusional disorder based on their content: persecutory, jealousy, somatic-hypochondriac, grandiose, and erotomanic. It also allows for mixed and unspecified types. Indeed, it is sometimes legitimate to diagnose jealous, grandiose, and persecutory themes in one patient.

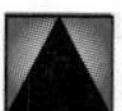

Table 12.16c–2
ICD-10 Diagnostic Criteria for Delusional Disorders

A. A delusion or a set of related delusions, other than those listed as typically schizophrenic in Criterion G1(1)b or d for paranoid, hebephrenic, or catatonic schizophrenia (i.e., other than completely impossible or culturally inappropriate), must be present. The commonest examples are persecutory, grandiose, hypochondriacal, jealous (zelotypic), or erotic delusions.
B. The delusion(s) in Criterion A must be present for at least 3 months.
C. The general criteria for schizophrenia are not fulfilled.
D. There must be no persistent hallucinations in any modality (but there may be transitory or occasional auditory hallucinations that are not in the third person or giving a running commentary).
E. Depressive symptoms (or even a depressive episode) may be present intermittently, provided that the delusions persist at times when there is no disturbance of mood.
F. There must be no evidence of primary or secondary organic mental disorder as listed under organic, including symptomatic, mental disorders or of a psychotic disorder due to psychoactive substance use.

Specification for possible subtypes

The following types may be specified if desired: persecutory, litiginous, self-referential, grandiose, hypochondriacal (somatic), jealous, erotomanic.

Other persistent delusional disorders

This is a residual category for persistent delusional disorders that do not meet the criteria for delusional disorder. Disorders in which delusions are accompanied by persistent hallucinatory voices or by schizophrenic symptoms that are insufficient to meet criteria for schizophrenia should be coded here. Delusional disorders that have lasted for less than 3 months should, however, be coded, at least temporarily, under acute and transient psychotic disorders.

Persistent delusional disorder, unspecified.

From World Health Organization. *The ICD-10 Classification of Mental and Behavioural Disorders: Diagnostic Criteria for Research.* Geneva: World Health Organization; 1993, with permission.

Persecutory Type Persecutory type is the archetype of delusional disorder. The individual who has this subtype is convinced that he or she is being persecuted or harmed. The persecutory beliefs are often associated with querulousness, irritability, and anger, and the individual who acts out his or her anger may at times be assaultive or even homicidal. At other times, such individuals may become preoccupied with formal litigation against their perceived persecutors. In contrast to persecutory delusions of schizophrenia, the delusions are systematized, coherent, and nonbizarre. Social functioning in areas not concerned with the delusion itself is not compromised. The ICD-10 recognizes this type of delusional disorder more explicitly than the DSM-IV. In some of these individuals, the demarcation between normality, pathological behavior, overvalued ideas, and delusion may not be clear. In addition, the following features are often seen: determination to succeed against all the odds; a tendency to identify barriers as conspiracies; an endless crusading spirit to right a wrong; a driven quality—getting agonizing pleasure from pursuing the cause; saturating the field with multiple complaints; unsociability and quarrelsome behavior; and the belief that defeat is unacceptable. Rather than surrender, the paranoid person appeals as often as the legal system permits. The following patient illustrates the paranoid form of delusional disorder:

Mrs. S., 62 years of age, was referred to a psychiatrist because of complaints of not being able to sleep. Before this episode, she worked full time taking care of children, played tennis almost every day, and managed her household chores. Her chief complaint was that her downstairs neighbor wanted to get her to move away and was doing a variety of things to harass her. At first, she based her belief on certain looks that he gave her and damage done to her mailbox, but later she believed he might be leaving empty bottles of cleaning solutions in the basement, so she would be overcome by fumes. As a result, the patient was fearful of falling asleep, convinced that she might be asphyxiated and not awaken in time to get help. She felt somewhat depressed and believed her appetite might be diminished from the stress of being harassed. However, she had not lost weight and still enjoyed playing tennis and going out with friends. At one point, she considered moving to another apartment but then decided to fight back. The episode had gone on for 8 months when her daughter persuaded her to have a psychiatric assessment. She was pleasant and cooperative in the interview. Except for the specific delusion and mild depressive symptoms, her mental status was normal.

Her past history revealed that she was depressed 30 years before after the death of a close friend. She saw a counselor for several months, which she found helpful, but was not treated with medication. For the current episode, she agreed to take medications, although she believed her neighbor was more in need of treatment than she was. Her symptoms improved somewhat with risperidone (Risperdal), 2 mg PO every night, and clonazepam (Klonopin), 0.5 mg PO every morning and every night.

DISCUSSION

This patient presented with a single delusion regarding her neighbor that was within the realm of possibility (i.e., not bizarre). Other areas of her functioning were normal. Although mild depressive symptoms were present, they did not meet criteria for major depressive disorder. Her prior symptoms of depression appeared to be related to a normal bereavement reaction and had not required pharmacotherapy or hospitalization. Thus, her current presentation is one of delusional disorder, persecutory type, and not major depressive disorder with psychotic features. In terms of treatment, the ability to create a working alliance with the patient, avoiding the discussion of the veracity of her delusion and focusing on her anxiety, depression, and difficulty falling asleep enabled her psychiatrist to introduce the medications with quite beneficial results.

Jealous Type As a part of the human condition, jealousy can act as a survival mechanism that enables us to defend our clan. In reality, jealousy can be transformed from normal jealousy to pathological jealousy to jealousy that qualifies as "delusional" jealousy. The decision about when jealousy becomes pathological is thus, in part, socially determined.

The most common delusion of jealousy is the belief that one's spouse is unfaithful. In some instances, some degree of infidelity may actually be occurring, yet the magnitude of the jealous response and the "evidence" accumulated to support accusations of unfaithfulness take on a delusional quality. Jealousy is dangerous, for it not only evokes anger but also arms the jealous individuals with a sense of righteous indignation to justify their acts of aggression. Jealousy focuses primarily on the partner and can sometimes lead to harm or actual homicide of the partner or others. The following patient illustrates these qualities of delusions of jealousy.

F.M. was a 51-year-old married, white man who lived with his wife in their own home and worked full time driving a sanitation truck. He was admitted to the hospital reporting that he was depressed because his wife was having an affair. He began to follow her, kept notes on his observations, and badgered her constantly about this, often waking her up in the middle of the night to make accusations. Shortly before admission, these arguments led to physical violence, and he was brought to the hospital by police. He was treated with thioridazine (Mellaril), 50 mg by mouth every night, and noted that he was less worried about his wife's behavior. He was seen by a psychiatrist monthly, but on follow-up 10 years later, he continued to believe that his wife was unfaithful. His wife noted that he sometimes became agitated about the delusion but that he generally controlled the impulse to act on it.

DISCUSSION

This patient experienced a fixed, encapsulated delusion of jealousy that did not interfere with his other activities. That he was able to exert some control over acting on the delusional belief suggested that it diminished in power over time. Although he initially reported feeling somewhat depressed over his wife's perceived infidelity, he did not have other symptoms suggestive of a major depressive episode.

Erotomanic Type In erotomania, which has also been referred to as *de Clérambault syndrome* or *psychose passionelle*, the patient has the delusional conviction that another person, usually of higher status, is in love with him or her. Such patients also tend to be solitary, withdrawn, dependent, and sexually inhibited as well as having poor levels of social or occupational functioning. The following operational criteria for the diagnosis of erotomania have been suggested: (1) a delusional conviction of amorous communication, (2) object of much higher rank, (3) object being the first to fall in love, (4) object being the first to make advances, (5) sudden onset (within a 7-day period), (6) object remains unchanged, (7) patient rationalizes paradoxical behavior of the object, (8) chronic course, and (9) absence of hallucinations.

In addition to the erotomanic subtype of delusional disorder, it is important to recognize that erotomanic symptoms may also occur in the context of other psychiatric disorders. In fact, the majority of patients with erotomania have a diagnosis other than delusional disorder.

The phenomenon of stalking is also linked, at times, to erotomania. Most definitions of stalking include the following elements: A pattern of intrusive behavior akin to harassment occurs; an implicit or explicit threat emanates from the pattern of behavior; and the target experiences considerable fear as a result. Stalkers most often persecute their targets by unwanted communications, which consist of frequent telephone calls, letters, e-mail, graffiti, notes, or packages. Typically, stalkers also follow their target and make unwelcome or intrusive and unexpected appearances in his or her public domain. In slightly more than one-half of individuals, stalking ceases within 1 year, whereas, in one-fourth, it lasts for 2 to 5 years. In some, the violence may escalate until the stalker actually murders the victim or his or her children, or both. In the United States, for example, it is estimated that approximately one-fourth of forensic stalking cases culminate in significant violence.

"Simple obsessional" stalkers make up the bulk of those who stalk and follow someone after a real relationship has terminated. Usually, they are motivated by intense resentment after perceived abuse or rejection. The "classic" erotomanic stalker often has psychosis and is usually a woman with the delusional belief that an older man of higher social class or social esteem is in love with her. A small proportion of these stalkers have the erotomanic type of delusional disorder. Psychotic stalking can also be associated with different psychotic disorders, including bipolar disorder, major depressive disorder, or schizophrenia. One well-known example of the latter is John Hinckley Jr., who engaged in stalking behavior and attempted to assassinate President Ronald Reagan in an effort to impress and win over his secret love, Jodie Foster, who had not responded to the many letters and poems he had left her.

The following patient illustrates delusional disorder, erotomanic type, with stalking:

Mrs. D. was a 32-year-old nurse, married with two children, when she was referred to the clinic by her supervisor from a local hospital. She had assaulted one of the residents, claiming he was in love with her. She had worked in the hospital for 12 years and was considered a good nurse. She had previously fallen in love with another physician on the staff of the hospital. Her current delusion began when the young physician entered a room in which she was lying in bed after cosmetic surgery and pointed at her. She had not known him before, but at that moment, she became convinced that he was in love with her. She tried to approach him several times by letter and phone, and although he did not respond, she was sure he was trying to hide his love from her. She was convinced that he was trying to transmit his love through looks he gave her and through the tone of his voice. The resident met her and denied being in love with her, but she began stalking him. At that point, the head nurse forced her to go for a consultation. She was treated for several months during which she continued to work at the same unit and was able to avoid contact with the resident. She insisted that her husband did not know about this. She refused any medications. The therapist arranged a three-way meeting with himself, the patient, and the resident. As a result of this meeting, there was a small reduction in the intensity of her belief, but she continued to maintain it nonetheless. She subsequently agreed to take antipsychotic medications and was given perphenazine, 16 mg per day, but there was no improvement. She continued to hold her belief, and the delusion subsided only after the resident moved to another hospital.

DISCUSSION

This patient's presentation demonstrates a number of the features of the erotomanic type of delusional disorder. In particular, her delusion began abruptly with what she perceived to be a specific response to her by the resident. She rationalized his lack of apparent interest in her, and her delusional conviction that he was in love with her persisted even after being confronted and despite treatment with antipsychotic medications. The presence of a previous episode speaks to the often chronic nature of the disorder, albeit with a different person being the object of her delusions. The absence of hallucinations and the preservation of her ability to function are also consistent with a delusional disorder rather than a diagnosis of schizophrenia.

Somatic Type The somatic type of delusional disorder is the only one that was not included in Kraepelin's original description of paranoia. It is diagnosed when the central themes of the delusional system are of a hypochondriacal or somatic nature. As a result, in the older literature, this type of delusional disorder is sometimes referred to as *monosymptomatic hypochondriasis*. As with other subtypes of delusional disorder, the patient must have a clear sensorium, and the symptoms may not result from an underlying physical illness or a psychiatric disorder other than delusional disorder.

The onset of symptoms with the somatic type of delusional disorder may be gradual or sudden. In most patients, the illness is unremitting, although the severity of the delusion may fluctuate. Hyperalertness and high anxiety also characterize patients with this subtype. Some themes recur, such as concerns about infestation in delusional parasitosis, preoccupation with body features with the dysmorphic delusions, and delusional concerns about body odor, which are sometimes referred to as *bromosis*. In delusional parasitosis, tactile sensory phenomena are often linked to the delusional beliefs. In Europe, delusional parasitosis is generally believed to represent a primary hallucination with an accompanying secondary delusion that explains the sensory perception, whereas in the United States, the sensory phenomena associated with delusional parasitosis are viewed as components of a systematized and encapsulated delusion.

Patients with the somatic type of delusional disorder rarely present for psychiatric evaluation, and when they do, it is usually in the context of a psychiatric consultation/liaison service. Instead, patients generally present to a specific medical specialist for evaluation. Thus, these individuals are more often encountered by dermatologists, plastic surgeons, urologists, acquired immune deficiency syndrome (AIDS) specialists, and sometimes dentists or gastroenterologists.

Ms. G. was a 56-year-old homemaker and mother of two who was hospitalized in the burn unit for wound care and skin grafting after sustaining chemical burns to her trunk and extremities. Six months before admission, Ms. G. had become increasingly convinced that minute bugs had burrowed underneath her skin. She tried to rid herself of them by washing multiple times each day with medicated soap and lindane shampoo. She also visited several dermatologists and had shown them samples of "dead bugs" for them to examine under the microscope. All told her there was nothing wrong with her and suggested that her problems were psychiatric in nature. She became increasingly distressed by the infestation and worried that the bugs might invade her other organs if not eradicated. Consequently, she decided to asphyxiate the bugs by covering her body with gasoline and holding it against her skin with plastic wrap. She noted that her skin became red and felt as though it were burning, but she viewed this as a positive sign that the bugs were being killed and writhing around as they died. Several hours after she had applied the gasoline, her daughter came to the house, saw Ms. G.'s condition, and took her to the hospital. When evaluated in the burn unit, Ms. G. spoke openly of her concerns about the bugs and was still unsure whether they were present or not. At the same time, she recognized that it had been a mistake to try to kill them with gasoline. She was oriented to person, place, and time and had no other delusional beliefs or auditory or visual hallucinations. She said her mood was "OK," although she was realistically concerned about the extensive treatment that she required and the difficult process of recovering from her injury. She reported no suicidal ideas or intent before admission and had no history of psychiatric treatment. She also did not report any use of substances except for drinking several beers socially approximately twice each month. During her stay in the hospital, she was treated with haloperidol in doses of up to 5 mg per day, with improvement in her concerns about the infestation. She continued to cooperate with treatment for her burns.

DISCUSSION

This patient demonstrates a classic presentation of delusional parasitosis, including the repeated visits to other physicians and the absolute conviction that the infestation is present. The lack of a significant history of alcohol or substance use suggests that the sensation of bugs crawling on her skin was not associated with substance intoxication or withdrawal.

Grandiose Type

Grandiose type of delusion in the absence of mania is rarely encountered in clinical practice, and it is debatable whether it should be classified as a distinct subtype of delusional disorder. The subtyping seems to be historical because this subtype was included in Kraepelin's description of paranoia. Many paranoid patients have a flare of grandiosity in their thoughts, but it is rarely elaborated into a full-blown delusion.

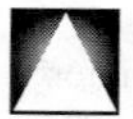

Table 12.16c–3
DSM-IV-TR Diagnostic Criteria for Shared Psychotic Disorder

A. A delusion develops in an individual in the context of a close relationship with another person(s) who has an already-established delusion.
B. The delusion is similar in content to that of a person who already has the established delusion.
C. The disturbance is not better accounted for by another psychotic disorder (e.g., schizophrenia) or a mood disorder with psychotic features and is not due to the direct physiological effects of a substance (e.g., a drug of abuse, a medication) or a general medical condition.

From American Psychiatric Association. *Diagnostic and Statistical Manual of Mental Disorders*. 4th ed. Text rev. Washington, DC: American Psychiatric Association; 2000, with permission.

Mixed Type

Mixed type includes individuals who exhibit more than one of the preceding types simultaneously.

Unspecified Type

Although the preceding themes are most commonly observed among individuals with delusional disorder, other delusions may occur as well. Examples include the misidentification syndromes such as Capgras' syndrome, in which others are viewed as having been replaced by an identical impostor, or Fregoli syndrome, in which another familiar person is believed to be disguised as someone else. In Cotard's syndrome, individuals report that they have lost all of their possessions, status, and strength as well as their entire being, including their organs.

Shared Psychotic Disorder

In shared psychotic disorder, one individual develops a delusional belief in the context of a close relationship with another person or people who already have an established delusional idea. Although shared psychotic disorder usually involves two individuals, it may involve more than two individuals, including entire family units. The key features of the disorder are the unquestioning acceptance of the other individual's delusional beliefs and the temporal sequence of development of the disorder, with one of the individuals having an earlier onset. In DSM-III, the persecutory nature of the shared delusions is emphasized, but in DSM-III-R, the nature of the shared delusion is broadened to include all types of delusional beliefs. DSM-IV maintains this broader definition of the type of delusional beliefs and includes the proviso that the symptoms are not better accounted for by another psychotic disorder, a psychotic mood disorder, a substance-induced disorder, or a general medical condition (Table 12.16c–3).

Although persecutory delusional beliefs are most commonly seen in shared psychotic disorder, comprising approximately 70 percent of patients in one study, religious, grandiose, and somatic delusions may also be observed, as the following example illustrates:

Mrs. B., a 59-year-old woman, presented to the emergency department for evaluation of upper-thigh pain of 9 months' duration. She reported that, on a prior visit to another hospital, she had received an injection of an antiemetic medication in her left thigh while experiencing intense nausea and vomiting from a viral syndrome. Several weeks after that emergency department visit, she began to experience discomfort in her thigh that was typically a sharp pain, exacerbated by movement, but which was occasionally a dull pain that occurred even while motionless. She stated that she was convinced that the needle tip had broken off in her thigh and was continuing to cause her discomfort. She demanded that an X-ray of her leg be done and that a surgeon be called to remove the remaining portion of the needle. Physical examination showed no deformity or discoloration over the site of the reported discomfort and no tenderness on palpation. Neurological examination was nonfocal, and sensation was symmetrical and intact throughout. An X-ray of the left thigh disclosed no evidence of any object and showed no other abnormality. When this information was presented to the patient and her husband, they became outraged. Mr. B. stated that he could not believe that five different hospitals had not been able to locate the retained piece of needle because he and his wife could feel it themselves. They both demanded to see a surgeon and refused to leave the emergency department until one was contacted. It was at this point that a psychiatric consultation was requested. Neither Mr. nor Mrs. B. had any history of psychiatric disorder. They had been married for 40 years and had no children. Mr. B. had worked as an accountant until his retirement 5 years previously, and Mrs. B. was a homemaker. Neither described themselves as having many friends, and they generally spent their time together at home, reading, gardening, or watching television. Mr. B. stated that at first he couldn't believe that a piece of the needle could have broken off in his wife's leg, but after the pain persisted for several months and his wife pointed out the irregular areas in her thigh, he became convinced that the needle was there and that something needed to be done about it. They both denied any plans to take legal action against the original facility and stated that their only goal was to have the problem addressed. They rejected all suggestions that psychiatric intervention might be of help, and Mrs. B. signed herself out of the emergency department.

DISCUSSION

Mr. and Mrs. B. are typical of individuals who develop a shared delusional disorder in that they are socially isolated and have a close, longstanding relationship. Shared psychotic disorders are most commonly seen in spouses, in a parent and a child, or in close siblings (often sisters) who have lived together for a long time. The development of the delusional belief in Mr. B. occurred over time and was subsequent to the onset of Mrs. B.'s delusions. Their rejection of psychiatric intervention is typical of many individuals with delusional disorders, including shared psychotic disorder.

CLINICAL ASSESSMENT

The first step in the clinical assessment is establishing whether a delusion exists. Some statements that initially seem to be delusional may, in fact, be true. In contrast, reports of circumstances that initially seem believable may only be clearly identified as delusions as the symptoms worsen, the delusion becomes less encapsulated, or more information comes to light. Several clinical examples illustrate these points:

Mr. R. was a 56-year-old member of his country's diplomatic corps who was brought to the psychiatric emergency department by police. Mr. R. had been stopped by police after he was noted to be driving erratically through a local highway tunnel. When approached by the police officers, he became agitated and combative, striking several people and demanding that he be released. He ultimately told police that a group of individuals from a rival political group in his country was trying to have him killed and that he needed to leave the United States immediately. Rather than arresting Mr. R., the police brought him to the emergency department for psychiatric evaluation.

On arrival in the emergency department, he remained quite agitated and fearful, inspecting the room for hidden cameras or microphones. He was initially suspicious of the interviewer, inquiring about the interviewer's background, but ultimately communicated the same history that he had given to police. Throughout the interview, Mr. R. remained guarded, apprehensive, and hyperalert. He repeatedly told the interviewer that, although he knew his story seemed far-fetched, it was entirely true.

Given Mr. R.'s apparent delusional beliefs and his potential for dangerousness to others on the basis of his striking the police officers and driving erratically, hospitalization was recommended. Mr. R. said he would feel safe being on a locked psychiatric unit and agreed to the admission "until other arrangements can be made." A few hours later, several other members of the diplomatic corps arrived at the hospital and, with Mr. R.'s permission, spoke with the psychiatrist. Mr. R.'s coworkers presented their identification, reiterated Mr. R.'s story, stated that Mr. R.'s life was in danger and that a private plane was waiting at the airport to take Mr. R. to safety. They asked that Mr. R. be released. Mr. R. was noticeably relieved by their appearance at the hospital and asked to be discharged to their custody. Because Mr. R.'s beliefs no longer appeared to be delusional and because there was no evidence that he posed a danger to others if being driven to the airport by his coworkers, Mr. R. was discharged from the hospital.

Mr. T. was 42 years of age when he was brought to a psychiatrist for evaluation. He lived with his parents and four brothers. His chief complaint was that his business partner was trying to force him to quit by giving him too much work. Although he appeared outwardly calm, Mr. T. complained of nervousness and restlessness. He also noted an inability to sleep at night, feeling that his neighbor was making noise on purpose. Mr. T.'s brother corroborated that the neighbor was being quite noisy at night and did not seem to respond to requests to be quieter. The psychiatrist prescribed hypnotic and anxiolytic medication.

Three days later, the psychiatrist received a phone call from the patient's brother who requested that Mr. T. be seen emergently. On arriving at the psychiatrist's office, Mr. T. appeared quite anxious and perplexed. He stated that the noises had grown louder and were now present throughout the day. He also was convinced that other people besides his neighbor and his business partner were trying to harm him. Mr. T.'s brother now reported that Mr. T.'s beliefs had no basis in reality.

The initial evaluations of Mr. R. and of Mr. T. illustrate some of the inherent difficulties in diagnosing delusional disorder. Certain behavioral features, such as hypersensitivity, guardedness, evasiveness, secretiveness, litigiousness, overly detailed descriptions, hostility, and humorlessness, are characteristic of the delusional patient yet are not pathognomonic. The patient may also be secretive, vague, and not voluntarily provide the clinician with necessary details. At other times, the patient may see no need to convey information, believing that the interviewer is part of the "conspiracy" and already knowledgeable about its specifics. For example, the patient may view the interview as a staged game in which both parties know the hidden meanings behind the overt text. As a result, certain phrases are commonly heard from individuals with persecutory ideas in the context of delusional disorder (e.g., "Don't play games with me," "You know what 'they' have been doing"). Characteristic observations or reports about the patient's behavior (e.g., checking for microphones, checking the spouse's clothes) may also lend support to the diagnosis. Even with such observations, it is sometimes difficult to distinguish between a true observation, a firm belief, an overvalued idea, and a delusion. Confabulation

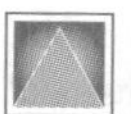

Table 12.16c–4
Potential Medical Etiologies of Delusional Syndromes

Disease or Disorder Class	Examples
Neurodegenerative disorders	Alzheimer's disease, Pick's disease, Huntington's disease, basal ganglia calcification, multiple sclerosis, metachromatic leukodystrophy
Other central nervous system disorders	Brain tumors, especially temporal lobe and deep hemispheric tumors; epilepsy, especially complex partial seizure disorder; head trauma (subdural hematoma); anoxic brain injury; fat embolism
Vascular disease	Atherosclerotic vascular disease, especially when associated with diffuse, temporoparietal, or subcortical lesions; hypertensive encephalopathy; subarachnoid hemorrhage, temporal arteritis
Infectious disease	Human immunodeficiency virus/acquired immune deficiency syndrome, encephalitis lethargica, Creutzfeldt-Jakob disease, syphilis, malaria, acute viral encephalitis
Metabolic disorder	Hypercalcemia, hyponatremia, hypoglycemia, uremia, hepatic encephalopathy, porphyria
Endocrinopathies	Addison's disease, Cushing's syndrome, hyper- or hypothyroidism, panhypopituitarism
Vitamin deficiencies	Vitamin B_{12} deficiency, folate deficiency, thiamine deficiency, niacin deficiency
Medications	Adrenocorticotropic hormones, anabolic steroids, corticosteroids, cimetidine, antibiotics (cephalosporins, penicillin), disulfiram, anticholinergic agents
Substances	Amphetamines, cocaine, alcohol, cannabis, hallucinogens
Toxins	Mercury, arsenic, manganese, thallium

may also be difficult to distinguish from delusions, although delusions are usually more systematized. Often, the extremeness and inappropriateness of the patient's behavior rather than the simple truth or falsity of the belief indicate its delusional nature. Consequently, when evaluating individuals with possible delusional disorder, the most sensible approach is to gather as much data as possible from many sources and then use clinical judgment in determining whether a threshold indicating psychopathological disturbance has been passed.

DIFFERENTIAL DIAGNOSIS

In making a diagnosis of delusional disorder, the first step is to eliminate medical disorders as a potential cause of delusions. Many medical conditions may be associated with the development of delusions (Table 12.16c–4), at times accompanying a delirious state.

Toxic-metabolic conditions and disorders affecting the limbic system and basal ganglia are most often associated with the emergence of delusional beliefs. Complex delusions occur more frequently in patients with subcortical pathology. In Huntington's disease and in individuals with idiopathic basal ganglia calcifications, for example, more than 50 percent of patients demonstrated delusions at some point in their illness. After right cerebral infarction, types of delusions that are more prevalent include anosognosia and reduplicative paramnesia (i.e., individuals believing they are in different places at the same time). Capgras' syndrome has been observed in a number of medical disorders, including central nervous system (CNS) lesions, vitamin B_{12} deficiency, hepatic encephalopathy, diabetes, and hypothyroidism. Focal syndromes have more often involved the right rather than the left hemisphere. Delusions of infestation, lycanthropy (i.e., the false belief that the patient is an animal, often a wolf or "werewolf"), heutoscopy (i.e., the false belief that one has a double), and erotomania have been reported in small numbers of patients with epilepsy, CNS lesions, or toxic-metabolic disorders.

In dementia syndromes of all types, 15 to 50 percent of individuals experience delusions. Although a minority of patients have complex, well-systematized delusions, most of these delusions are simple. Persecutory delusions are particularly common in early dementia and in some individuals may be the first manifestation of dementing illness.

Once medical conditions, delirium, and dementia have been eliminated as possible diagnoses, the use of medications and substances must be explored as possible contributors to the patient's delusions. Among the substances of abuse, amphetamines and cocaine are most likely to result in delusional beliefs, typically persecutory in nature. Prescribed substances, over-the-counter medications, and herbal products, such as ephedra, may also be associated with the development of delusions.

In differentiating delusional disorder from other psychotic disorders, a number of factors need to be taken into consideration. Individuals with schizophrenia often have hallucinations or disorganized thoughts or behavior that are not present in delusional disorder. The presence of bizarre delusions is also characteristic of schizophrenia, although difficulties in reliably judging the bizarreness of delusions may cloud this distinction. In addition, prominent negative symptoms or a deterioration in function from previous premorbid levels suggests a diagnosis of schizophrenia.

Mood disorders are also common in the differential diagnosis of delusional disorder. Mood symptoms are highly prevalent in delusional disorders. For many individuals, symptoms of depression may seem to be an understandable response to the perceived delusional experiences (e.g., feeling overwhelmed and demoralized over "harassment" by neighbors or coworkers). In addition, given the prevalence of mood disorders, many individuals who present with a delusional disorder have had a history of depression. Somatic, grandiose, or persecutory delusions that are similar to those observed in patients with delusional disorder may also be seen in individuals with psychotic mood disorders. In distinguishing mood disorders with psychotic features from delusional disorder, it is therefore important to determine whether a full mood syndrome (e.g., manic, depressed, or mixed episode) is present or whether milder mood symptoms are present that do not meet criteria for a mood disorder. It is also important to consider the temporal pattern of symptom onset and progression and recognize that, over time, the boundaries between mood disorder and delusional disorder generally become clear.

Perhaps most difficult in terms of differential diagnosis is differentiating among an overvalued idea, an obsession with lack of insight, and a delusion. For example, the somatic type of delusional disorder may be easily confused with hypochondriasis. In hypochondriasis, there is a preoccupation with fears of having, or the idea that one has, a serious disease, and this is based on the person's misinterpretation of bodily symptoms. In addition, the preoccupation persists despite appropriate medical evaluation and reassurance. Although the patient may be briefly relieved and begin to doubt this conviction of illness for a short while after each evaluation, the fear generally emerges again. Although many individuals with hypochondriasis have some realization of the excessive nature of their fears, a form of hypochondriasis "with poor insight" has been described. It can be difficult to draw the line between these "poor insight" patients and actual delusional disorder. In most individuals with hypochondriasis, however, there is a longer pattern of being preoccupied with physical symptoms, and the preoccupations generally are not limited to a single symptom or organ system.

In body dysmorphic disorder, there is a preoccupation with a slight or imagined defect in appearance. These individuals may recognize that their view of their appearance is distorted, yet a significant proportion of individuals with body dysmorphic disorder hold their beliefs with delusional intensity. Thus, when criteria for both disorders are met, both body dysmorphic disorder and delusional disorder somatic type may be diagnosed.

Similarly, reality testing may be poor in some individuals with OCD. The DSM-IV diagnosis of OCD assumes that the individual recognizes at some time that the obsessions or compulsions are excessive or unreasonable. Nonetheless, patients show varying degrees of insight into the validity of their beliefs, and some individuals do not usually recognize that their symptoms are unreasonable. In DSM-IV, these individuals are diagnosed as having OCD "with poor insight." If the obsession reaches "delusional proportions," DSM-IV suggests that delusional disorder or "psychotic disorder not otherwise specified" be diagnosed in addition to OCD. The common occurrence of such dual diagnoses is suggested by one sample of 49 OCD patients in which one-third of subjects also met DSM-IV criteria for delusional disorder.

Particularly when persecutory ideas are present and patients are guarded about sharing full details of their delusional beliefs, it may be difficult to differentiate delusional disorder from a paranoid personality disorder. Again, the longitudinal history is important in establishing a diagnosis of a personality disorder and also in determining whether delusions are now superimposed on the individual's premorbid personality. If a patient has paranoid personality disorder before the onset of psychosis and after the psychosis has subsided, then such individuals are diagnosed with both delusional disorder (Axis I) and paranoid personality disorder (Axis II).

ETIOLOGY

The etiology of delusional disorder is not known. Studies of epidemiological and genetic risk factors are difficult to conduct because the diagnosis of delusional disorder is unstable, and it occurs infrequently, comprising approximately 2 to 8 percent of admissions for nonorganic psychosis.

Psychodynamic theories about the origin of paranoid delusions suggest that paranoia is a protective psychological response to different types of stress or conflict that represent a profound threat to self-esteem or to the self (e.g., fear of the unknown, "homosexual panic," adjustment to immigration). The paranoid response to threat is an affective withdrawal from intimate ties and an intense effort to retain the appearance of normalcy. In addition, the defensive mechanism of projection is used to alleviate these intolerable feelings. In certain individuals, the paranoid defense escalates to a distinct maladaptive state that fails in its aim to reduce anxiety and further disrupts the patient's capacity to function. At its extreme, this series of psychic events is postulated to result in the development of a delusional disorder.

Another theory of the etiology of delusional disorder is based on research by cognitive and experimental psychologists and suggests that people with persecutory delusions selectively attend to threatening information, jump to conclusions on the basis of insufficient information, attribute negative events to external personal causes, and have difficulty in envisaging others' intentions and motivations. Chris Frith suggested that delusions of reference and persecution, as well as misidentification syndrome, exemplify this inability to represent and interpret the beliefs, thoughts, and intentions of other people. It has also been suggested that a person with delusional disorder has a biologically driven perceptual anomaly that involves vivid and intense sensory input. Other differences in the perceptions and thought processes of delusional patients may also shape the expression of delusional beliefs. Relative to controls, for example, people with delusional disorder may show a tendency to seek less information before reaching decisions (reasoning bias) and, hence, jump to conclusions on the basis of less evidence. The bias may be more pronounced with emotionally salient material. People with persecutory delusions may preferentially attend to threat-related stimuli (attentional bias) and preferentially recall threatening episodes, thereby reinforcing the delusional belief.

In shared psychotic disorder, etiological theories are primarily based on family and interpersonal dynamics. In general, individuals who develop a shared delusion tend to have had a submissive role in the relationship with the individual who was first to develop a delusional disorder. In other dyads, the person who develops the shared delusion may be particularly impressionable due to personality factors or intellectual limitations. Social isolation due to personality factors, poverty, language difficulties, or geographical isolation may also be a contributor.

COURSE AND PROGNOSIS

The course of the disorder has been difficult to study for a number of reasons, which include the relatively small proportion of psychotic patients with delusional disorder, the unstable nature of the diagnosis, and the tendency for delusional disorder patients to avoid treatment by medical professionals in general and by psychiatrists in particular. The age of onset of delusional disorder is generally in the mid- to late 30s and, in the Suffolk County, New York, series, the vast majority of individuals had an insidious onset regardless of the age at hospitalization. In addition, the course in patients with delusional disorder generally appears to be less chronic and to have less associated deterioration than the course of patients with schizophrenia or schizoaffective disorder. Although the specific delusions may persist and remain fixed, they are generally stable. Functioning tends to be preserved and negative outcomes from the disorder typically occur when individuals are unable to refrain from acting on their delusional beliefs. For example, in the handful of patients with a stable diagnosis of delusional disorder in the Suffolk County series noted above, almost all patients resumed their previous level of functioning after discharge from the hospital. The impact of age of onset with course is unclear, with some studies showing more favorable prognosis with earlier age of onset and some showing no effect of age of onset on course. In some studies, the presence of precipitating factors has been associated with better outcome along with female sex and being married. With respect to number of hospitalizations and degree of functional impairment, overall functioning appears somewhat more favorable for the jealousy subtype of delusional disorder; however, better clinical outcomes have also been observed in patients with persecutory delusions, compared with those with delusions of grandeur or jealousy. The presence of comorbid diagnoses, particularly depression, may be an additional complicating factor that negatively influences the course of the disorder.

Because of the relative rarity of shared delusional disorder, which has been estimated to occur in less than 1 percent of admissions for psychosis, the clinical course and prognosis are unclear, although some reports of successful treatment are present in the literature.

SUGGESTED CROSS-REFERENCES

Conditions to be differentiated from delusional disorders are discussed in Chapter 12 (schizophrenia), Chapter 13 (mood disorders), Chapter 15 (somatoform disorders), Chapter 24 (paranoid personality disorder), and Chapter 10 (mental disorders due to a general medical condition). OCD is covered in Chapter 14 (on anxiety disorders). Aging and psychiatric disorders in the elderly are covered in Chapter 51.

References

*Cameron NA. Paranoid conditions and paranoia. In: Arieti S, ed. *American Handbook of Psychiatry*. New York: Basic Books; 1959.

Copeland JR, Dewey ME, Scott A, Gilmore C, Larkin BA, Cleave N, McCracken CF, McKibbin PE: Schizophrenia and delusional disorder in older age: Community prevalence, incidence, comorbidity, and outcome. *Schizophr Bull*. 1998;24:153.

Eisen JL, Rasmussen SA: Obsessive compulsive disorder with psychotic features. *J Clin Psychiatry*. 1993;54:373.

*Fennig S, Craig TJ, Bromet EJ: The consistency of DSM-III-R delusional disorder in a first-admission sample. *Psychopathology*. 1996;29:315.

Freud S. Psychoanalytic notes upon an autobiographical account of a case of paranoia (dementia paranoides). In: *Standard Edition of the Complete Work of Sigmund Freud*. Vol. 12. London: Hogarth Press; 1966.

Fricchione GL, Carbone L, Bennett WI: Psychotic disorder caused by general medical condition, with delusions: Secondary "organic" delusional syndromes. *Psychiatr Clin North Am*. 1995;18:363.

Frith CD. *The Cognitive Neuropsychology of Schizophrenia*. New York: Psychology Press; 1992.

Garety PH, Freeman D: Cognitive approaches to delusions: A critical review of theories and evidence. *Br J Clin Psychol*. 1999;38:113.

Goldstein RL, Laskin AM: De Clerambault's syndrome (erotomania) and claims of psychiatric malpractice. *J Forensic Sci*. 2002;47:852–855.

Gralnick A: Folie a deux—the psychosis of association: A review of 103 cases and the entire English literature, with case presentations. *Psychiatr Q*. 1942;16:230.

Jaspers K. *General Psychopathology*. Vols. 1 and 2. Translated by Hoenig J and Hamilton MW. Baltimore: The Johns Hopkins University Press; 1997.

Jorgensen P: Course and outcome in delusional disorders. *Psychopathology*. 1994;27:373.

Kamphuis JH, Emmelkamp PM: Stalking—a contemporary challenge for forensic and clinical psychiatry. *Br J Psychiatry*. 2000;176:206.

*Kendler KS: Demography of paranoid psychosis (delusional disorder). *Arch Gen Psychiatry*. 1982;39:890.

Lasègue C, Falret J: La folie à deux. *Ann Med. Psychol*. 1877;18:321. (English translation by Michaud R: *Am J Psychiatry*. 1964;121:1.)

Maher BA, Spitzer M. Delusions. In: Adams HE, Sutker PB, eds. *Comprehensive Handbook of Psychopathology*. 2nd ed. New York: Plenum; 1993.

Manschreck TC: Delusional disorder: The recognition and management of paranoia. *J Clin Psychiatry*. 1996;57[Suppl 3]:32.

McAllister TW: Neuropsychiatric aspects of delusions. *Psychiatr Ann*. 1992;22:269.

Menzies RP, Fedoroff JP, Green CM, Isaacson K: Prediction of dangerous behavior in male erotomania. *Br J Psychiatry*. 1995;166:529.

Munro A. *Delusional Disorder*. New York: Cambridge University Press; 1999.

*Opjordsmoen S, Retterstol N: Delusional disorder: The predictive validity of the concept. *Acta Psychiatr Scand*. 1991;84:250.

Pearn J, Gardner-Thorpe C: Jules Cotard (1840–1889): His life and the unique syndrome which bears his name. *Neurology*. 2002;58:1400–1403.

Riecher-Rossler A, Hafner H, Hafner-Ranabauer W, Loffler W, Reinhard I: Late-onset schizophrenia versus paranoid psychoses: A valid diagnostic distinction? *Am J Geriatr Psychiatry*. 2003;11:595–604.

Rosenfeld B: Recidivism in stalking and obsessional harassment. *Law Hum Behav*. 2003;27:251–265.

*Sacks MH: Folie a deux. *Compr Psychiatry*. 1988;29:270.

Wehmeier PM, Barth N, Remschmidt H: Induced delusional disorder. A review of the concept and an unusual case of folie á famille. *Psychopathology*. 2003;36:37–45.

12.16d Schizoaffective Disorder

Shmuel Fennig, M.D., Laura J. Fochtmann, M.D., and Gabrielle A. Carlson, M.D.

HISTORY

Emil Kraepelin divided the psychoses into dementia praecox with a progressive deterioration and manic-depressive illness with a remitting course; however, his rich clinical examples included many patients with features of both disorders. Others, such as Johannes Lange, Karl Bowman, and William Dunton, also described intermittent forms of dementia praecox that included periods of excitement or depression along with gradual deterioration in functioning. Eugen Bleuler considered that the existence of mood and schizophrenic symptoms during the same episode did not alter the diagnosis of schizophrenia and pointed out the need for prolonged observation to correctly differentiate schizophrenia from manic-depressive psychosis. Jacob Kasanin was the first to coin the term *schizoaffective psychosis*. He based his observation on a distinct subgroup of nine young patients with good premorbid functioning, a sudden onset of both schizophrenic and mood symptoms, and good outcome. However, a review of his detailed case histories shows that all of these individuals would be diagnosed as having psychotic mood disorder under the revised fourth edition of the *Diagnostic and Statistical Manual of Mental Disorders* (DSM-IV-TR). Nevertheless, schizoaffective disorder has survived as a construct and constitutes a distinct category in the section on schizophrenia and other psychotic disorders in DSM-IV-TR.

COMPARATIVE NOSOLOGY

In current diagnostic systems, patients can receive the diagnosis of schizoaffective disorder if they fit into one of the following six categories: (1) patients with schizophrenia who have mood symptoms, (2) patients with mood disorder who have symptoms of schizophrenia, (3) patients with both mood disorder and schizophrenia, (4) patients with a third psychosis unrelated to schizophrenia and mood disorder, (5) patients whose disorder is on a continuum between schizophrenia and mood disorder, and (6) patients with some combination of the above.

The Research Diagnostic Criteria (RDC) were the first to define specific criteria for this disorder. Specifically, *schizoaffective disorder* was defined as the acute cooccurrence of a full mood syndrome and one of a set of "core schizophrenic" symptoms such as bizarre delusions, first-rank symptoms, or hallucinations. Distinctions were made between schizoaffective-depressed and schizoaffective-manic as well as between chronic and nonchronic subtypes. Another critical distinction was between the "mainly schizophrenic subtype," which required poor premorbid functioning and persistence of psychosis for more than 1 week and the "mainly affective subtype," in which premorbid functioning was good, and psychosis did not persist for more than 1 week. This distinction was based on clinical evidence that persistent psychosis predicted poor response to mood disorder treatments. In a number of well-designed family studies, relatives of patients with the affective subtype of schizoaffective disorder and patients with mood disorders were found to have increased rates of mood disorders in comparison with normal control families but not increased rates of schizophrenia. Such patients also exhibited a greater response to mood disorder treatment. In contrast, patients with the schizophrenic subtype of schizoaffective disorder showed an increased prevalence of schizophrenia in their relatives.

Under the third edition of DSM (DSM-III), disorders involving full affective syndromes with schizophrenia-like symptoms were classified as mood disorders with mood-incongruent symptoms. As long as the schizophrenic symptoms occurred at the same time as the mood disturbance, the patient was considered to have a mood disorder. The DSM-III grouped schizoaffective disorder under "Psychotic Disorders Not Elsewhere Classified" and relegated it to a residual category, making it a diagnosis of last resort. In the revised DSM-III (DSM-III-R), schizoaffective disorder became more clearly defined with the specification that ". . . there have been delusions or hallucinations for at least two weeks, but no prominent mood symptoms" and that "the duration of all episodes of a mood syndrome has not been brief relative to the total duration of the psychotic disturbance." DSM-IV-TR incorporated the stricter time frame of 1 month's duration of schizophrenia symptoms and required an "uninterrupted period of illness during which at some time, either there is a Major Depressive Episode, a Manic Episode, or a Mixed Episode concurrent with symptoms that meet Criterion A for Schizophrenia." DSM-IV-TR also elaborated more on the criterion of duration of the mood symptoms relative to the psychotic symptoms. In the tenth revision of *International Statistical Classification of Diseases and Related Health Problems* (ICD-10), schizoaffective disorder is a distinct entity and can be applied to patients who have cooccurring mood symptoms and schizophrenic-like mood-incongruent psychosis.

EPIDEMIOLOGY

No general population study has determined the prevalence or incidence of schizoaffective disorder. However, general population surveys do reveal a high degree of comorbidity between schizophrenia and mood disorders. In the Epidemiologic Catchment Area (ECA) study, which administered the DSM-III version of the Diagnostic Interview Schedule to samples of the general population in five locations in the United States, depression was highly comorbid with schizophrenia (odds ratio of 14). An even stronger relationship existed between schizophrenia and bipolar mood disorder (odds ratio of 46). However, in the ECA, the agreement between lay and clinician diagnoses of schizophrenia was very poor. In the National Comorbidity Study, using more rigorous diagnostic methodology to ascertain DSM-III-R disorders in a representative sample of the U.S. population, 66 people were diagnosed with schizophrenia out of more than 8,000 who were interviewed. Eighty-one percent of these individuals also received a lifetime diagnosis of a mood disorder (59 percent with major depressive disorder and 22 percent with bipolar disorder).

Also unstudied are the risk factors for schizoaffective disorder. In clinical samples, gender differences among individuals with schizoaffective disorder parallel those seen in mood disorders, with approximately equal numbers of men and women with the bipolar subtype and a more than twofold female to male predominance among the depressed subtype of schizoaffective disorder.

ETIOLOGY

Schizoaffective disorder and schizophrenia have frequently been combined in etiological research. As a result, little is known about the distinctive etiological factors associated with schizoaffective disorder per se. As with schizophrenia, however, schizoaffective disorder may be a neurodevelopmental disorder. In addition, genetic factors may play a role because research has also shown that relatives of probands with schizoaffective disorder have significantly higher rates of mood disorder than relatives of probands with schizophrenia and significantly higher rates of schizophrenia than relatives of probands with mood disorder.

DIAGNOSTIC AND CLINICAL FEATURES

The DSM-IV-TR diagnostic criteria for schizoaffective disorder are listed in Table 12.16d–1, and the ICD-10 diagnostic criteria for schizoaffective disorder are listed in Table 12.16d–2.

According to DSM-IV-TR, the first requirement in making a diagnosis of schizoaffective disorder is that the psychotic illness meet Criterion A for schizophrenia—that is, there are delusions, hallucinations, bizarre behavior, or negative symptoms. Concurrent with the psychotic symptoms, there needs to be a depressive or a manic episode that meets the full criteria for such an episode. To distinguish depressive symptoms from negative symptoms of schizophrenia, the DSM-IV-TR criteria for schizoaffective, depressed type, emphasize that Criterion A1 of a major depressive episode must be fulfilled (i.e., the presence of "depressed mood" and not simply anhedonia or loss of interest).

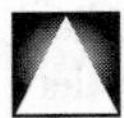

Table 12.16d–1
DSM-IV-TR Diagnostic Criteria for Schizoaffective Disorder

A. An uninterrupted period of illness during which, at some time, there is either a major depressive episode, a manic episode, or a mixed episode concurrent with symptoms that meet Criterion A for schizophrenia.

Note: The major depressive episode must include Criterion A1: depressed mood.

B. During the same period of illness, there have been delusions or hallucinations for at least 2 weeks in the absence of prominent mood symptoms.

C. Symptoms that meet criteria for a mood episode are present for a substantial portion of the total duration of the active and residual periods of the illness.

D. The disturbance is not due to the direct physiological effects of a substance (e.g., a drug of abuse, a medication) or a general medical condition.

Specify type:

Bipolar type: if the disturbance includes a manic or a mixed episode (or a manic or a mixed episode and major depressive episodes)

Depressive type: if the disturbance only includes major depressive episodes

From American Psychiatric Association. *Diagnostic and Statistical Manual of Mental Disorders.* 4th ed. Text rev. Washington, DC: American Psychiatric Association; 2000, with permission.

Determining whether an individual patient fulfills the DSM-IV-TR criteria for schizoaffective disorder also requires that the clinician take a detailed temporal history of the onset and offset of mood and psychotic symptoms. In addition, the patient must be able to clearly distinguish when mood and psychotic symptoms started and stopped. Because both types of symptoms can begin or end insidiously and because retrospective reporting is inherently unreliable, this is not always a simple task for either the clinician or the patient. Without adequate information on the length of psychosis and mood symptoms, it is difficult to know whether Criterion B (psychotic symptoms in the absence of the mood syndrome) and Criterion C (mood symptoms occurring for a substantial portion of the duration of the active and residual periods of illness) are fully met. In this context, the term "substantial portion" typically requires that mood symptoms are present during 15 to 30 percent of the total illness duration. This requirement makes the diagnosis of schizoaffective disorder unstable because it requires the exercise of clinical judgment, and any fluctuations in mood can lead to a change of diagnosis. Hence, in a series of close to 700 first-admission patients with psychotic features, 6 percent received a diagnosis of schizoaffective disorder at hospital discharge, but only one-half of these (3 percent of the total) met DSM-III-R criteria for schizoaffective disorder on review by the research psychiatrists. Two years later, only one-third of those initially diagnosed with schizoaffective disorder were again diagnosed with this disorder, with one-third diagnosed with schizophrenia and one-third diagnosed with an affective psychosis. Thus, with strict application of the DSM-IV-TR criteria, the diagnosis of schizoaffective disorder is limited to a small group of individuals. Furthermore, the requirement that mood symptoms be present for a substantial portion of the total illness, by definition, delineates a group of chronically ill and relatively treatment-resistant individuals.

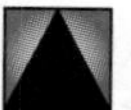

Table 12.16d–2
ICD-10 Diagnostic Criteria for Schizoaffective Disorders

G1. The disorder meets the criteria for one of the affective disorders of moderate or severe degree, as specified for each category.

G2. Symptoms from at least one of the groups listed below must be clearly present for most of the time during a period of at least 2 weeks (these groups are almost the same as for schizophrenia):

(1) Thought echo, thought insertion or withdrawal, thought broadcasting (Criterion G1[1]a for paranoid, hebephrenic, or catatonic schizophrenia)

(2) Delusions of control, influence, or passivity, clearly referred to body or limb movements or specific thoughts, actions, or sensations (Criterion G1[1]b for paranoid, hebephrenic, or catatonic schizophrenia)

(3) Hallucinatory voices giving a running commentary on the patient's behavior or discussing the patient among themselves or other types of hallucinatory voices coming from some part of the body (Criterion G1[1]c for paranoid, hebephrenic, or catatonic schizophrenia)

(4) Persistent delusions of other kinds that are culturally inappropriate and completely impossible but not merely grandiose or persecutory (Criterion G1[1]d for paranoid, hebephrenic, or catatonic schizophrenia) such as has visited other worlds, can control the clouds by breathing in and out, can communicate with plants or animals without speaking

(5) Grossly irrelevant or incoherent speech or frequent use of neologisms (a marked form of Criterion G1[2]b for paranoid, hebephrenic, or catatonic schizophrenia)

(6) Intermittent but frequent appearance of some forms of catatonic behavior such as posturing, waxy flexibility, and negativism (Criterion G1[2]c for paranoid, hebephrenic, or catatonic schizophrenia)

G3. Criteria G1 and G2 above must be met within the same episode of the disorder and concurrently for at least part of the episode. Symptoms from both G1 and G2 must be prominent in the clinical picture.

G4. The disorder is not attributable to organic mental disorder or to psychoactive substance–related intoxication, dependence, or withdrawal.

Schizoaffective disorder, manic type

A. The general criteria for schizoaffective disorder must be met.

B. Criteria for a manic disorder must be met.

Other schizoaffective disorders

Schizoaffective disorder, unspecified

Comments

If desired, further subtypes of schizoaffective disorder may be specified, according to the longitudinal development of the disorder, as follows:

Concurrent affective and schizophrenic symptoms only

Symptoms as defined in Criterion G2 for schizoaffective disorders

Concurrent affective and schizophrenic symptoms beyond the duration of affective symptoms

Note: This diagnosis depends on an approximate "balance" among the number, severity, and duration of the schizophrenic and affective symptoms.

From World Health Organization. *The ICD-10 Classification of Mental and Behavioural Disorders: Diagnostic Criteria for Research.* Geneva: World Health Organization; 1992, with permission.

DIFFERENTIAL DIAGNOSIS

The critical step in every differential diagnosis is determining whether a substance use disorder or a medical disorder could account for the patient's symptoms. A mood disorder or a psychotic disorder due to a general medical condition is diagnosed when evidence from the history, physical examination, or laboratory tests indicates that the symptoms are the direct physiological consequence of a specific general medical condition. A wide range of medical etiologies, including neurological disorders, infectious diseases, metabolic abnormalities, and endocrinopathies, may result in a combination of psychosis and mood change that may resemble schizoaffective disorder. Similarly, prescribed medications and abused substances may produce mood change and psychosis either with chronic use, acute intoxication, or withdrawal. For example, alcohol can predispose to a depressive-like state through either acute or chronic use and can also produce hallucinosis. The chronic use of cannabis may precipitate psychosis, but it can lead to an anergic state that shares many features with depression ("amotivational syndrome"). Chronic cocaine use may similarly be associated with psychosis as well as changes in mood. Thus, careful screening for medical disorders and substance use disorders is an essential aspect in the differential diagnosis of schizoaffective disorder.

In distinguishing between schizoaffective disorder and mood disorder with psychotic features, several elements should be taken into consideration. Many clinicians do not assess the relative persistence of psychotic and mood symptoms between acute episodes, and others expand schizoaffective disorder to include chronic psychosis with a few prominent mood symptoms as well as mood disorders with an acute, severely psychotic presentation. Patients often view depression as more understandable or socially acceptable than psychosis and may retrospectively emphasize the duration of depressive symptoms in their illness. It is also difficult by history alone to disentangle negative symptoms from depressive symptoms. By the same token, without a clear history of a euphoric mood, manic episodes may retrospectively be viewed as an episode of acute psychosis associated with agitation or irritability. Thus, it is important to take a thorough history using information from as many informants as possible to delineate whether criteria were met for both a mood episode and schizophrenia. Such a temporal history can also be useful in distinguishing a mood disorder, typically depression, that is superimposed on schizophrenia. In actual practice, it is also important to note that the diagnosis of schizoaffective disorder may only become clear with longitudinal follow-up, as illustrated in the following examples:

Mr. C. was a 24-year-old man with no previous psychiatric history. Pregnancy, birth, early development, and adjustment through army service as a paramedic were normal. After discharge from the army, he began to study law but then quit school and traveled around Asia, where he used cannabis. Family members who saw him during this time noticed several changes: He insisted on changing his name, he began to isolate himself, and he believed that he was the heir of the Dali Lama. When he became aggressive and argumentative, he was brought home and hospitalized. On admission, he was dressed like a Tibetan monk with his head shaved. Although oriented to time and place, he had delusions of grandeur, stating that he was the most clever man on the planet and was the ancestor of the Messiah. He was also suspicious, arrogant, and argumentative. On laboratory assessment, he was also found to have hepatitis A. He was treated with perphenazine (Trilafon), 28 mg per day, and ultimately discharged to outpatient treatment. He tried again to attend law school but could not persist for more than 1 year before quitting. When his psychiatrist agreed to stop his antipsychotic medications, he relapsed 1 month later. His second admission occurred after a manic episode during which he spent money lavishly, had angry outbursts, was excessively talkative, was hyperactive, and believed he was the Messiah. He was treated with haloperidol (Haldol), 5 mg per day, and lithium (Eskalith), 1,200 mg. After discharge and another attempt at law school, he traveled to India. He was brought home, rehospitalized with another manic episode, and discharged on depot antipsychotic medications. After being rehospitalized because of extrapyramidal side effects, he was begun on olanzapine (Zyprexa), 20 mg per day, and valproic acid, 1,000 mg per day. During that hospitalization, his mood seemed more depressed, but he did not meet criteria for an episode of major depressive disorder. During the subsequent 5 years, he remained out of the hospital and had no episodes of mood disorder. He was careful to avoid using cannabis or other substances. He does not work but functions well as a husband and father. From time to time, he has thoughts that he might be hurt by other people inflicting injury on his liver (a somatic delusion), but these thoughts never last more than a few days.

DISCUSSION

The first diagnostic issue was determining whether the psychosis was due to a general medical condition or to substance abuse/dependence. This seemed unlikely because hepatitis rarely is associated with the development of an acute manic syndrome. Although cannabis use can precipitate psychosis, the patient's psychotic symptoms and mood disturbance also occurred in the absence of substance use. In addition, the patient's longitudinal course was not consistent with either a substance-induced disorder or a psychosis due to a general medical condition. Although Mr. C.'s mood episodes were distinct, there were clear psychotic symptoms in the absence of a mood episode, making schizoaffective disorder a more appropriate diagnosis than bipolar disorder. In addition, his course reflected a lack of return to premorbid function in spite of reasonable control of his symptoms with an antipsychotic and a mood-stabilizing anticonvulsant. The duration of mood symptoms relative to the total illness duration was significant, approximately fitting the often suggested criterion of 30 percent for schizoaffective disorder.

Mrs. P. was a 47-year-old, divorced, unemployed woman who lived alone and was chronically psychotic despite treatment with olanzapine, 20 mg per day, and citalopram (Celexa), 20 mg per day. She believed that she was getting messages from God and the police department to go on a mission to fight drug dealers. She also believed that the Mafia was trying to stop her in this pursuit. The onset of her illness began at 20 years of age, when she experienced the first of several depressive episodes. She also described periods when she felt more energetic, talkative, had decreased need for sleep, and was more active, sometimes cleaning her house the whole night. Approximately 4 years after the onset of her symptoms, she began to hear "voices" that became stronger when she got depressed, but that were still present and continued to disturb her even when her mood was euthymic. Approximately 10 years after her illness began, she developed the belief that policemen were everywhere and that the neighbors were spying on her. She was hospitalized voluntarily. Two years later, she had another depressive episode, and the voices told her she could not live in her apartment. She was tried on lithium, antidepressants, and antipsychotic medications but continued to be chronically symptomatic with mood symptoms as well as psychosis.

DISCUSSION

Mrs. P. demonstrates a "classic" presentation of schizoaffective disorder in which clear depressive and hypomanic episodes are present in combination with continuous psychotic illness and first-rank symptoms. Her course is typical of many individuals with schizoaffective disorder.

COURSE AND PROGNOSIS

Although the course and prognosis of schizoaffective disorder may vary, outcome is generally poorer than for patients with mood disorder but somewhat better than for patients with schizophrenia. In the Suffolk County, New York, first-admission series, 75 percent of patients with this disorder did not remit fully over the first 2 years of follow-up, compared with 87 percent of patients with schizophrenia and 22 and 40 percent of those with psychotic bipolar disorder and psychotic depressive disorder, respectively.

SUGGESTED CROSS-REFERENCES

A more detailed review of schizophrenia is presented in Chapter 12. Mood disorders are covered in Chapter 13.

REFERENCES

*Bowman KM, Raymond AF. A statistical study of delusions in the manic-depressive psychoses. In: *Proceedings of the Association for Research in Nervous and Mental Diseases*. Vol. XI. Baltimore: Williams & Wilkins Co.; 1931.

Dunton WR: The cyclic forms of dementia praecox. *Am J Insanity*. 1910;66:465.

Jarbin H, Ott Y, von Knorring A: Adult outcome of social function in adolescent-onset schizophrenia and affective psychosis. *J Am Acad Child Adolesc Psychiatry*. 2003;42:176–183.

*Kasanin J: The acute schizoaffective psychoses. *Am J Psychiatry*. 1933;13:97.

Kelose JR: Arguments for the genetic basis of the bipolar spectrum. *J Affect Dis*. 2003;73:183–197.

*Kendler KS, McGuire M, Gruenberg AM, Walsh D: Examining the validity of DSM-III-R schizoaffective disorder and its putative subtypes in the Roscommon family study. *Am J Psychiatry*. 1995;152:755.

Kessler RC, McGonagle KA, Zhao S, Nelson CB, Hughes M, Eshleman S, Wittchen HU, Kendler KS: Lifetime and 12-month prevalence of DSM-III-R psychiatric disorders in the United States: Results from the National Comorbidity Survey. *Arch Gen Psychiatry*. 1994;51:8.

Kilzieh N, Wood AE, Erdman J, Raskind M, Tapp A: Depression in Kraepelinian schizophrenia. *Comp Psychiatry*. 2003;44:1–6.

Lange J. *Katatoiche Erscheininngen in Rahmen Manisher Erkrankungen*. Berlin: Julius Springer; 1922.

Marneros A: The schizoaffective phenomenon: The state of the art. *Acta Psychiatrica Scandinavica*. 2003;108:29–33.

Regnold WT, Thapar RK, Marano C, Gavirneri S, Kondapavuluru PV: Increased prevalence of type 2 diabetes mellitus among psychiatric inpatients with bipolar I affective and schizoaffective disorders independent of psychotropic drug use. *J Affective Disorders*. 2003;70:19–26.

Robins LN, Regier DA, eds. *Psychiatric Disorders in America: The Epidemiological Catchment Area Study*. New York: The Free Press (Macmillan); 1991.

*Schwartz JE, Fennig S, Tanenberg-Karant M, Carlson G, Craig T, Galambos N, Lavelle J, Bromet EJ: Congruence of diagnoses 2 years after a first-admission diagnosis of psychosis. *Arch Gen Psychiatry*. 2000;57:593.

*Winokur G, Tsuang MT. *The Natural History of Mania, Depression and Schizophrenia*. Washington, DC: APA Press; 1996.

12.16e Postpartum Psychosis

BUSHRA NAZ, M.D., LAURA J. FOCHTMANN, M.D., AND EVELYN J. BROMET, PH.D.

The postpartum period is a time of enormous physical, social, and emotional changes. Almost 85 percent of women experience some type of mood disturbance, such as mood lability or tearfulness, during the postpartum period. Postpartum psychosis is relatively rare and can occur as part of postpartum mood disorder or as a separate entity. In the 19th century, two French physicians, Jean Esquirol and Louis Victor Marce, carefully described the clinical profiles of more than 100 women with postpartum psychosis. Thus, its occurrence has been well documented for many years.

COMPARATIVE NOSOLOGY AND CLASSIFICATION

In the revised fourth edition of the *Diagnostic and Statistical Manual of Mental Disorders* (DSM-IV-TR), the diagnosis of "brief psychotic disorder with postpartum onset" is given when psychosis occurs within 4 weeks of delivery and mood symptoms are not present. If the psychosis lasts longer than 1 month, then other diagnoses, such as schizophreniform disorder, should be considered. More typically, postpartum psychosis occurs together with mood symptoms. In such situations, the patient is given a diagnosis of a mood disorder with the specifier of postpartum onset.

The tenth revision of *International Statistical Classification of Diseases and Related Health Problems* (ICD-10) assumes that most patients with puerperal mental illness are not distinguishable from patients with mood disorders or schizophrenia. When this is not possible, the diagnosis of "mental and behavioral disorders associated with the puerperium, not elsewhere classified" is given.

EPIDEMIOLOGY

The incidence of postpartum psychosis is approximately 1 to 2 per 1,000 births, with psychotic symptoms appearing within the first week after childbirth in most individuals. In a review of 20 studies of hospitalized patients with puerperal psychosis, approximately one-fifth of postpartum psychoses were unassociated with toxicity, mood disorder, or schizophrenia.

The most important risk factor for developing a postpartum psychosis is previous history. The risk of puerperal relapse is as high as 70 percent. Other risk factors include primigravida, being unmarried, cesarean section, having a female child, and previous personal or family history of psychiatric illness. Fetal distress and offspring abnormalities (neurological abnormalities, cyanosis, neonatal polycythemia, thrombocytopenia) have also been identified as risk factors.

ETIOLOGY

The etiology of postpartum psychosis is not known. Although the role of hormonal changes after delivery has been evaluated, there is insufficient evidence to draw firm conclusions about the effects of female reproductive hormones on the neuronal system in relation to postpartum psychosis. One hypothesis is that the sharp decline in estrogen after delivery contributes to the onset of postpartum psychosis. Another theory holds that a rapid, approximately 30-fold drop in progesterone levels may contribute to the onset of postpartum psychiatric disorder.

In the last trimester of pregnancy, cortisol levels are also increased, with total and free plasma cortisol and 24-hour urinary cortisol levels similar to those seen in mild Cushing's syndrome. After peaking during labor and delivery, cortisol levels also return to baseline gradually over approximately 1 month. One small study found that post-dexamethasone cortisol levels were significantly elevated in women with postpartum psychosis, but all of the patients had mood symptoms. Thus, the role of cortisol in postpartum nonaffective psychosis remains to be investigated.

Thyroid hormone concentrations are also high during pregnancy and decrease during postpartum period. Approximately 10 percent of women are diagnosed with hypothyroidism in the postpartum period. Thyroid dysfunction, particularly hypothyroidism, may produce psychiatric symptoms. In relation to postpartum psychosis, there is the suggestion of a disturbance in the hypothalamic-pituitary axis, with one study reporting blunted thyroid-stimulating hormone (TSH) response to thyrotropin-releasing hormone (TRH).

DIAGNOSTIC AND CLINICAL FEATURES

In the DSM-IV-TR, the diagnostic specifier of postpartum psychosis is applied in the mood disorders, brief psychotic disorder, and psychosis not otherwise specified (NOS) sections if the onset of symptoms occurs within 4 weeks of delivery.

The clinical prodrome for postpartum psychosis in general can include insomnia, fatigue, sadness, irritability, and emotional lability. The psychosis itself can develop dramatically and quickly. For postpartum patients with mood disorder, the presenting symptoms of psychosis can include auditory hallucinations, confusion, nihilistic delusions, grandiose delusions, and delusions of guilt. Among puerperal women with schizophrenia, auditory hallucinations, agitation, persecutory delusions, delusions of control, formal thought disorder, disorientation, and confusion are frequently seen. Additional transient symptoms may occur that resemble mild delirium, including inability to sustain attention, distractibility, poor recent memory, labile mood, bewilderment, and transient delirious states.

The delusions often specifically pertain to the newborn infant such as that the newborn is possessed by the devil, has special powers, or is destined to meet a terrible fate. There may also be obsessional thoughts regarding violence to the child. However, infanticide is rare. The following vignette describes a patient with postpartum psychosis:

Mrs. Z. is a 30-year-old high school teacher living in Lagos, Nigeria. She is married and has five children. The birth of her last child was complicated by hemorrhage and sepsis, and she was still hospitalized on the gynecology service for 13 days after delivery when her gynecologist requested a psychiatric consultation. Mrs. Z. was agitated and seemed to be in a daze. She said to the psychiatrist: "I am a sinner. I have to die. My time is past. I cannot be a good Christian again. I need to be reborn. Jesus Christ should help me. He is not helping me." A diagnosis of postpartum psychosis was made. An antipsychotic drug, chlorpromazine (Thorazine), was prescribed, and Mrs. Z. was soon well enough to go home. Three weeks later, she was readmitted, this time to the psychiatric ward, claiming she "had had a vision of the spirits" and was "wrestling with the spirits." Her relatives reported that at home she had been fasting and "keeping a vigil" through the nights and was not sleeping. She had complained to the neighbors that there was a witch in her house. The witch turned out to be her mother. Mrs. Z.'s husband, who was studying engineering in Europe, hurriedly returned and took over the running of the household, sending his mother-in-law away and supervising Mrs. Z.'s treatment himself. She improved rapidly on an antidepressant medication and was discharged in 2 weeks. Her improvement, however, was short-lived. She threw away her medications and began to attend mass whenever one was given, pursuing the priests to ask questions about scriptures. Within 1 week, she was readmitted. On the ward, she accused the psychiatrist of shining powerful torchlights on her and taking pictures of her, opening her chest, using her as a guinea pig, poisoning her food, and planning to bury her alive. She claimed to receive messages from Mars and Jupiter and announced that there was a riot in town. She clutched her Bible to her breast and accused all the doctors of being "idol worshippers," calling down the wrath of her god on all of them. After considerable resistance, Mrs. Z. was finally convinced to accept electroconvulsive treatment, and she became symptom free after six treatments. At this point, she attributed her illness to a difficult childbirth, the absence of her husband, and her unreasonable mother. She saw no further role for doctors, called for her priest, and began to speak of her illness as a religious experience that was similar to the experience of religious leaders throughout history. However, her symptoms did not return, and she was discharged after 6 weeks of hospitalization.

FOLLOW-UP

During the following year, Mrs. Z. had several brief relapses with vivid and frightening dreams, which she described as a loose connection between reality and dream. Her priest believed that she was going through a difficult religious experience. Her mother believed that witchcraft might be the source of her problems and proposed a traditional religious solution. However, it was her husband who prevailed, and each relapse was treated with medication.

Mrs. Z. returned to the psychiatry department 2 years later to visit with staff. Her functioning was back to normal, although she reported occasional experiences of "spirits" for which she supplied a religious explanation. She did not require further psychiatric support.

DISCUSSION

From the perspective of DSM-IV-TR, psychotic symptoms with a duration of at least 1 day and no more than 1 month that occur in the absence of full mood syndrome and are not due to the direct effects of a substance or a general medical condition are diagnosed as brief psychotic disorder. Because the onset was within 4 weeks of childbirth, the postpartum specifier is applied. This diagnosis is provisional, depending on whether recovery occurs within 1 month. The DSM-IV-TR classification does not adequately deal with recurrent and apparently brief postpartum psychotic experiences separated by periods of full remission. Therefore, the only option is to reapply the diagnosis of brief psychotic disorder. The duration of her third episode was more ambiguous; however, that she became symptom free after six electroconvulsive treatments suggests that remission may have occurred within 1 month, which again justifies the same diagnosis. If there were significant residual symptoms that necessitated the 6-week hospital stay, then the diagnosis is changed to schizophreniform disorder.

COURSE AND PROGNOSIS

Although postpartum psychosis has an excellent prognosis, it also has a high recurrence rate and can be associated with subsequent nonpuerperal episodes. The overall prognosis depends on the diagnostic entity. For brief psychotic disorder and for affective psychoses, the overall prognosis is reasonably good. Schizophrenia is associated with an increased likelihood of chronic disability.

The implications of postpartum disorder have been described in relation to the child. Postpartum psychosis itself, as an extreme form of postpartum disease, should also be seen as potentially impacting on the relationship between mother and child and the child's developmental picture. Child abuse and neglect should also be watched for. Although rare, infanticide is more likely to occur in postpartum psychosis than in other postpartum psychiatric disorders. In addition, postpartum psychosis is often missed by both physicians and family members, with potentially dire consequences.

SUGGESTED CROSS-REFERENCES

Mood disorders are covered in Chapter 13. Section 28.1 discusses psychiatry and reproductive medicine.

REFERENCES

Ahokas A, Aito M: Role of estradiol in puerperal psychosis. *Psychopharmacology.* 1999;147:108.

*Brockington IF, Winokur G, Dean C. Puerperal psychosis. In: Brockington IF, Kumar R, eds. *Motherhood and Mental Illness.* London: Academic Press; 1982.

Davidson J, Robertson E: A follow-up study of post partum illness, 1946–1978. *Acta Psychiatrica Scand.* 1985;71:451.

*Kendell RE, Chalmers JC, Platz C: Epidemiology of puerperal psychoses. *Br J Psychiatry.* 1987;150:662.

*McNeil TF, Blennow G: A prospective study of postpartum psychoses in a high-risk group. *Acta Psychiatr Scand.* 1988;78:478.

*Ndosi NK, Mtawali ML: The nature of puerperal psychosis at Muhimbili National Hospital: its physical comorbidity, associated main obstetric and social factors. *Afr J Reprod Health.* 2003;6:41.

Paykel ES, del Campo AM, White W, Horton R: Neuroendocrine challenge studies in puerperal psychoses: Dexamethasone suppression and TRH stimulation. *Br J Psychiatry.* 1991;159:262.

Rehman AU, St. Clair D, Platz C: Puerperal insanity in the 19th and 20th centuries. *Br J Psychiatry.* 1990;156:861.

Sharma V: Pharmacotherapy of postpartum psychosis. *Expert Opin Pharmacother.* 2003;4:1651.

Sharma V, Mazmanian D: Sleep loss and postpartum psychosis. *Bipolar Disord.* 2003;5:98.

12.16f Culture-Bound Syndromes with Psychotic Features

RAMIN MOJTABAI, M.D., PH.D., M.P.H.

For some Western-trained clinicians, it is difficult to imagine that a well-defined and relatively common psychiatric condition, such as anorexia nervosa, is specific to the European culture and is rarely encountered in other cultural settings. Anorexia nervosa is, in fact, a prime example of *culture-bound* or *culture-specific syndromes*—a diverse group of conditions that are specific to a cultural setting.

The revised fourth edition of the *Diagnostic and Statistical Manual of Mental Disorders* (DSM-IV-TR) defines *culture-bound syndromes* as

> Recurrent, locality-specific patterns of aberrant behavior and troubling experience that may or may not be linked to a particular DSM-IV diagnostic category. Many of these patterns are indigenously considered to be "illnesses," or at least afflictions, and most have local names. Although presentations conforming to the major DSM-IV categories can be found throughout the world, the particular symptoms, course and social response are very often influenced by local cultural factors. In contrast, culture-bound syndromes are generally limited to specific societies or culture areas and are localized, folk, diagnostic categories that frame coherent meanings for certain repetitive, patterned, and troubling sets of experiences and observations (p. 898).

This definition highlights two important characteristics of culture-bound syndromes. First, culture-bound syndromes are not culturally influenced presentations of "major" psychiatric disorders (i.e., those cataloged in the Western diagnostic and classification systems such as DSM-IV-TR and the tenth revision of *International Statistical Classification of Diseases and Related Health Problems* [ICD-10]). For example, reports from some non-Western cultural settings indicate that somatic symptoms predominate in the picture of major depression in these settings. These patients, however, should be diagnosed as cases of major depression and treated as such. Second, culture-bound syndromes are folk categories, incorporating beliefs about etiology of the condition and its treatment as well as specific symptom patterns. This characteristic has profound implications for assessment and proper management of culture-bound syndromes.

Although most conditions categorized as culture-bound syndromes in the DSM-IV-TR or ICD-10 are not associated with psychotic features, some do present with such features. Differentiation of these conditions from other universally encountered psychotic conditions, such as schizophrenia and affective psychoses, has important implications for management of these patients.

It is also important to note that clinicians working in developing countries have for many years noted higher rates of psychotic conditions with acute onset and remitting course. One epidemiological study found the incidence of such psychotic conditions to be ten times higher in developing country settings than industrialized settings. Most of these individuals, however, likely meet the ICD-10 criteria for acute and transient psychotic disorders or the DSM-IV-TR brief psychotic disorder, schizophreniform disorder, or psychotic disorder not otherwise specified (NOS) and, hence, may not be considered culture-bound syndromes.

COMPARATIVE NOSOLOGY

The culture-bound syndromes occupy an ambiguous status in both DSM-IV-TR and ICD-10, reflecting the controversies in the field. Many investigators argue that culture-bound syndromes can only be properly understood within their cultural context, hence ruling out attempts at categorizing them under DSM-IV-TR or ICD-10 diagnostic categories. Others appreciate the culture-specific characteristics of these syndromes but argue that they should be regarded as variants of already-known categories of psychopathology that are cataloged in the formal diagnostic manuals. DSM-IV-TR and ICD-10 seem to hold an intermediate position. Both manuals provide lists of the culture-bound syndromes as appendices. Both also categorize some culture-bound syndromes under specific diagnostic categories in the texts of the manuals.

The culture-bound syndromes were first introduced as a list of 25 conditions in appendix I in DSM-IV and were reintroduced with little change in DSM-IV-TR (Table 12.16f–1). In addition, a number of these same syndromes were discussed as examples of "possession trance" under the category of dissociative disorder NOS in the text of the manual. According to the DSM-IV-TR, "Possession trance involves replacement of the customary sense of personal identity by a new identity, attributed to the influence of a spirit, power, deity, or other person and associated with stereotyped 'involuntary' movements or amnesia." *Amok*, *bebainan*, *latah*, *pibloktoq*, *ataque de nervios*, and possession states reported from India were discussed as examples of possession trance.

ICD-10 similarly introduced a listing of culture-bound syndromes as an appendix. Three of these same syndromes (*dhat*, *koro*, and *latah*) were also discussed as examples of "other specified neurotic disorders." This category is described in ICD-10 as comprising "mixed disorders of behaviour, beliefs, and emotions which are of uncertain etiology and nosological status and which occur with particular frequency in certain cultures." ICD-10 also notes that, due to their strong association with cultural beliefs and behavior pattern, these syndromes are best regarded as not delusional. Some other culture-bound syndromes are likely classifiable in the category "trance and possession disorders" in the ICD-10.

EPIDEMIOLOGY

There is a dearth of epidemiological data about culture-bound syndrome. This is partly due to the lack of explicit diagnostic criteria for these syndromes. In the absence of such criteria, ascertainment is difficult because of discrepancies in the use of each diagnostic term by clinicians. Patients may report having experienced the same culture-bound disorder despite wide variations in their actual symptoms. Using a patient self-report method, for example, 16 percent of a general population sample in Puerto Rico reported having experienced *ataque de nervios*, one of the better-studied culture-bound syndromes reported in Latino populations. The prevalence was approximately 75 percent among patients in mental health clinics.

ETIOLOGY

Speculation about the etiology of culture-bound syndromes has mostly focused on sociocultural factors. Mass social stressors, such as ethnic conflict, rapid modernization, cultural transformation, and social alienation have all been implicated in epidemics of culture-bound syndromes of *koro* and in cases of *latah* and *amok*. It has also been hypothesized that the themes of culture-bound syndromes reflect the value systems and preoccupations of the respective culture. Virility and reproductive ability are major determinants of a person's worth in many non-Western cultures in which cases of *koro* syndrome are encountered. Similarly, the Japanese emphasis on the importance of social evaluations has been implicated in the etiology of *taijin kyofusho*, a culture-bound syndrome with features similar to social anxiety.

A study of the distribution of the "brain fag" syndrome—characterized by headache and visual and cognitive symptoms—in secondary school children in Swaziland, southern Africa, suggested an association with urbanization. Thirty-four percent of children in rural areas, compared with only 6 percent in elite schools in the capital, presented with symptoms.

DIAGNOSIS AND CLINICAL FEATURES

The growing waves of immigration from the developing countries to the United States and western Europe over the past few decades has meant that, for many Western-trained clinicians, culture-bound syndromes are no longer exotic curiosities of distant lands. Assessing people suspected to have culture-bound syndromes often requires a basic understanding of the formulations of health and illness in the patient's culture. Such understanding does not only help with reaching a diagnosis but also facilitates communication with the patient and the family and is conducive to a trusting relationship with them.

Differentiation of pathological behaviors from culturally normal patterns of behavior is crucial. Some behavior patterns, such as those observed in trance rituals and possession cults, may appear abnormal to an outsider. However, these behaviors are clearly recognized as normal by other members of the culture. The patients themselves and the families could serve as the primary source for cultural information necessary for distinguishing between these normal behaviors and psychopathology. It is safe to assume that the index behavior is beyond the normal range when the patient or the family seek professional help for that behavior.

Missing a culture-bound syndrome in assessing a patient from another culture may lead to inappropriate diagnosis and treatment, as illustrated by the following excerpt from the *DSM-IV-TR Casebook*.

Mrs. O., agitated and screaming, was brought to the emergency room of a city hospital by her family, complaining of severe left-sided facial pain. The previous week, after she heard that her former husband had remarried in the Dominican Republic, she had become increasingly agitated and developed insomnia and anorexia. She moved into her mother's home with her two children and that day developed the facial pain. By the time she was seen by the attending psychiatrist, Mrs. O. was alternately mute and mumbling unintelligibly in Spanish and English. She was given small doses of an antipsychotic medication with no response. Because of her behavior, she was admitted to the psychiatric ward for further evaluation.

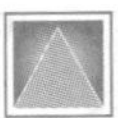

Table 12.16f–1
Culture-Bound Syndromes in DSM-IV-TR

amok A dissociative episode characterized by a period of brooding followed by an outburst of violent, aggressive, or homicidal behavior directed at people and objects. The episode tends to be precipitated by a perceived slight or insult and seems to be prevalent only among men. The episode is often accompanied by persecutory ideas, automatism, amnesia, exhaustion, and a return to premorbid state after the episode. Some instances of *amok* may occur during a brief psychotic episode or constitute the onset or an exacerbation of a chronic psychotic process. The original reports that used this term were from Malaysia. A similar behavior pattern is found in Laos, Philippines, Polynesia (*cafard* or *cathard*), Papua New Guinea, and Puerto Rico (*mal de pelea*) and among the Navajo (*iich'aa*).

ataque de nervios An idiom of distress principally reported among Latinos from the Caribbean but recognized among many Latin-American and Latin-Mediterranean groups. Commonly reported symptoms include uncontrollable shouting, attacks of crying, trembling, heat in the chest rising into the head, and verbal or physical aggression. Dissociative experiences, seizure-like or fainting episodes, and suicidal gestures are prominent in some attacks but absent in others. A general feature of an *ataque de nervios* is a sense of being out of control. *Ataques de nervios* frequently occur as a direct result of a stressful event relating to the family (e.g., news of the death of a close relative, a separation or divorce from a spouse, conflicts with a spouse or children, or witnessing an accident involving a family member). People may experience amnesia for what occurred during the *ataque de nervios*, but they otherwise return rapidly to their usual level of functioning. Although descriptions of some *ataques de nervios* most closely fit the DSM-IV description of panic attacks, the association of most *ataques* with a precipitating event and the frequent absence of the hallmark symptoms of acute fear or apprehension distinguish them from panic disorder. *Ataques* span the range from normal expressions of distress not associated with having a mental disorder to symptom presentations associated with the diagnoses of anxiety, mood, dissociative, or somatoform disorders.

bilis and colera (also referred to as *muina*) The underlying cause of these syndromes is believed to be strongly experienced anger or rage. Anger is viewed among many Latino groups as a particularly powerful emotion that can have direct effects on the body and can exacerbate existing symptoms. The major effect of anger is to disturb core body balances (which are understood as a balance between hot and cold valences in the body and between the material and spiritual aspects of the body). Symptoms can include acute nervous tension, headache, trembling, screaming, stomach disturbances, and, in more severe cases, loss of consciousness. Chronic fatigue may result from the acute episode.

boufée delirante A syndrome observed in West Africa and Haiti. This French term refers to a sudden outburst of agitated and aggressive behavior, marked confusion, and psychomotor excitement. It may sometimes be accompanied by visual and auditory hallucinations or paranoid ideation. The episodes may resemble an episode of brief psychotic disorder.

brain fag A term initially used in West Africa to refer to a condition experienced by high school or university students in response to the challenges of schooling. Symptoms include difficulties in concentrating, remembering, and thinking. Students often state that their brains are "fatigued." Additional somatic symptoms are usually centered around the head and neck and include pain, pressure or tightness, blurring of vision, heat, or burning. "Brain tiredness" or fatigue from "too much thinking" is an idiom of distress in many cultures, and resulting syndromes can resemble certain anxiety, depressive, and somatoform disorders.

dhat A folk diagnostic term used in India to refer to severe anxiety and hypochondriacal concerns associated with the discharge of semen, whitish discoloration of the urine, and feelings of weakness and exhaustion. Similar to *jiryan* (India), *sukra prameha* (Sri Lanka), and *shen-k'uei* (China).

falling out or blacking out These episodes occur primarily in the southern United States and Caribbean groups. They are characterized by a sudden collapse, which sometimes occurs without warning but is sometimes preceded by feelings of dizziness or "swimming" in the head. The individual's eyes are usually open, but the person claims an inability to see. The person usually hears and understands what is occurring around him or her but feels powerless to move. This may correspond to a diagnosis of conversion disorder or a dissociative disorder.

ghost sickness A preoccupation with death and the deceased (sometimes associated with witchcraft) frequently observed among members of many American Indian tribes. Various symptoms can be attributed to ghost sickness, including bad dreams, weakness, feelings of danger, loss of appetite, fainting, dizziness, fear, anxiety, hallucinations, loss of consciousness, confusion, feelings of futility, and a sense of suffocation.

***hwa-byung* (also known as *wool-hwa-byung*)** A Korean folk syndrome literally translated into English as "anger syndrome" and attributed to the suppression of anger. The symptoms include insomnia, fatigue, panic, fear of impending death, dysphoric affect, indigestion, anorexia, dyspnea, palpitations, generalized aches and pains, and a feeling of a mass in the epigastrium.

koro A term, probably of Malaysian origin, that refers to an episode of sudden and intense anxiety that the penis (or, in women, the vulva and nipples) will recede into the body and possibly cause death. The syndrome is reported in south and east Asia, where it is known by a variety of local terms such as *shuk yang, shook yong,* and *suo yang* (Chinese); *jinjinia bemar* (Assam); and *rok-joo* (Thailand). It is occasionally found in the West. Koro at times occurs in localized epidemic form in east Asian areas. The diagnosis is included in the Chinese Classification of Mental Disorders, Second Edition (CCMD-2).

latah Hypersensitivity to sudden fright, often with echopraxia, echolalia, command obedience, and dissociative or trance-like behavior. The term *latah* is of Malaysian or Indonesian origin, but the syndrome has been found in many parts of the world. Other terms for the condition are *amurakh, irkunii, ikota, olan, myriachit,* and *menkeiti* (Siberian groups); *bah tschi, bah-tsi, baah-ji* (Thailand); *imu* (Ainu, Sakhalin, Japan); and *mali-mali* and *silok* (Philippines). In Malaysia, it is more frequent in middle-aged women.

locura A term used by Latinos in the United States and Latin America to refer to a severe form of chronic psychosis. The condition is attributed to an inherited vulnerability, to the effect of multiple life difficulties, or to a combination of both factors. Symptoms exhibited by people with *locura* include incoherence, agitation, auditory and visual hallucinations, inability to follow rules of social interaction, unpredictability, and possible violence.

mal de ojo A concept widely found in Mediterranean cultures and elsewhere in the world. *Mal de ojo* is a Spanish phrase translated into English as "evil eye." Children are especially at risk. Symptoms include fitful sleep, crying without apparent cause, diarrhea, vomiting, and fever in a child or infant. Sometimes adults (especially women) have the condition.

nervios A common idiom of distress among Latinos in the United States and Latin America. A number of other ethnic groups have related, although often somewhat distinctive, ideas of "nerves" (such as *nevra* among Greeks in North America). *Nervios* refers both to a general state of vulnerability to stressful life experiences and to a syndrome brought on by difficult life circumstances. The term *nervios* includes a wide range of symptoms of emotional distress, somatic disturbance, and inability to function. Common symptoms include headaches and "brain aches," irritability, stomach disturbances, sleep difficulties, nervousness, easy tearfulness, inability to concentrate, trembling, tingling sensations, and *mareos* (dizziness with occasional vertigo-like exacerbations). *Nervios* tends to be an ongoing problem, although variable in the degree of disability that is manifest. *Nervios* is a very broad syndrome that spans the range from patients free of a mental disorder to presentations resembling adjustment, anxiety, depressive, dissociative, somatoform, or psychotic disorders. Differential diagnosis depends on the constellation of symptoms experienced, the kind of social events that are associated with the onset and progress of nervios, and the level of disability experienced.

pibloktoq An abrupt dissociative episode accompanied by extreme excitement of up to 30 minutes' duration and frequently followed by convulsive seizures and coma lasting up to 12 hours. It is observed primarily in arctic and subarctic Eskimo communities, although regional variations in name exist. The individual may be withdrawn or mildly irritable for a period of hours or days before the attack and typically reports complete amor her clothing, break furniture, shout obscenities, eat feces, flee from protective shelters, or perform other irrational or dangerous acts.

(*continued*)

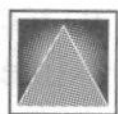

Table 12.16f–1 (*continued*)

***qi-gong* psychotic reaction** A term describing an acute, time-limited episode characterized by dissociative, paranoid, or other psychotic or nonpsychotic symptoms that may occur after participation in the Chinese folk health-enhancing practice of *qi-gong* ("exercise of vital energy"). Especially vulnerable are individuals who become overly involved in the practice. This diagnosis is included in CCMD-2.

rootwork A set of cultural interpretations that ascribe illness to hexing, witchcraft, sorcery, or the evil influence of another person. Symptoms may include generalized anxiety and gastrointestinal complaints (e.g., nausea, vomiting, diarrhea), weakness, dizziness, the fear of being poisoned, and sometimes fear of being killed ("voodoo death"). Roots, spells, or hexes can be put or placed on other people, causing a variety of emotional and psychological problems. The hexed person may even fear death until the root has been taken off (eliminated), usually through the work of a root doctor (a healer in this tradition), who can also be called on to bewitch an enemy. Rootwork is found in the southern United States among both African-American and European-American populations and in Caribbean societies. It is also known as *mal puesto* or *brujeria* in Latino societies.

***sangue dormido* ("sleeping blood")** This syndrome is found among Portuguese Cape Verde Islanders (and immigrants from there to the United States) and includes pain, numbness, tremor, paralysis, convulsions, stroke, blindness, heart attack, infection, and miscarriage.

***shenjing shuairuo* ("neurasthenia")** In China, this is a condition characterized by physical and mental fatigue, dizziness, headaches, other pains, concentration difficulties, sleep disturbance, and memory loss. Other symptoms include gastrointestinal problems, sexual dysfunction, irritability, excitability, and various signs suggesting disturbance of the autonomic nervous system. In many patients, the symptoms meet the criteria for a DSM-IV mood or anxiety disorder. This diagnosis is included in CCMD-2.

***shen-k'uei* (Taiwan); *shenkui* (China)** A Chinese folk label describing marked anxiety or panic symptoms with accompanying somatic complaints for which no physical cause can be demonstrated. Symptoms include dizziness, backache, fatigability, general weakness, insomnia, frequent dreams, and complaints of sexual dysfunction (such as premature ejaculation and impotence). Symptoms are attributed to excessive semen loss from frequent intercourse, masturbation, nocturnal emission, or passing of "white turbid urine" believed to contain semen. Excessive semen loss is feared because of the belief that it represents the loss of one's vital essence and can thereby be life threatening.

shin-byung A Korean folk label for a syndrome in which initial phases are characterized by anxiety and somatic complaints (general weakness, dizziness, fear, anorexia, insomnia, gastrointestinal problems), with subsequent dissociation and possession by ancestral spirits.

spell A trance state in which individuals "communicate" with deceased relatives or with spirits. At times, this state is associated with brief periods of personality change. This culture-specific syndrome is seen among African Americans and European Americans from the southern United States. Spells are not considered to be medical events in the folk tradition but may be misconstrued as psychotic episodes in clinical settings.

***susto* ("fright" or "soul loss")** A folk illness prevalent among some Latinos in the United States and among people in Mexico, Central America, and South America. *Susto* is also referred to as *espanto, pasmo, tripa ida, perdida del alma,* or *chibih. Susto* is an illness attributed to a frightening event that causes the soul to leave the body and results in unhappiness and sickness. Individuals with *susto* also experience significant strains in key social roles. Symptoms may appear any time from days to years after the fright is experienced. It is believed that, in extreme cases, *susto* may result in death. Typical symptoms include appetite disturbances, inadequate or excessive sleep, troubled sleep or dreams, feelings of sadness, lack of motivation to do anything, and feelings of low self-worth or dirtiness. Somatic symptoms accompanying susto include muscle aches and pains, headache, stomachache, and diarrhea. Ritual healings are focused on calling the soul back to the body and cleansing the person to restore bodily and spiritual balance. Different experiences of *susto* may be related to major depressive disorder, posttraumatic stress disorder, and somatoform disorders. Similar etiological beliefs and symptom configurations are found in many parts of the world.

taijin kyofusho A culturally distinctive phobia in Japan in some ways resembling social phobia in DSM-IV. This syndrome refers to an individual's intense fear that his or her body, its parts or its functions, displease, embarrass, or are offensive to other people in appearance, odor, facial expressions, or movements. The syndrome is included in the official Japanese diagnostic system for mental disorders.

zar A general term applied in Ethiopia, Somalia, Egypt, Sudan, Iran, and other North-African and Middle-Eastern societies to the experience of spirits possessing an individual. People possessed by a spirit may experience dissociative episodes that may include shouting, laughing, hitting the head against a wall, singing, or weeping. Individuals may show apathy and withdrawal, refusing to eat or carry out daily tasks, or may develop a long-term relationship with the possessing spirit. Such behavior is not considered pathological locally.

CCMD-2, *Chinese Classification of Mental Disorders*, 2nd edition.

On the ward, Mrs. O. was agitated and had outbursts of bizarre behavior. For example, she suddenly snatched another patient's purse or grabbed at gold chains around a male patient's neck. Once she ate plastic flowers from a vase. She appeared sad, frightened, and disheveled. She reported ideas of reference and command auditory hallucinations of her daughter's voice telling her to kill herself. She received larger doses of antipsychotic medication. Although there was some decrease in her agitation, she continued intermittently to display bizarre behavior.

On the following day, a family meeting was held with Mrs. O., her mother, daughter, and son. It now became clear that when Mrs. O. heard that her ex-husband had remarried she became terrified that he would no longer support her and their children. A meeting was scheduled with the ex-husband the next day to discuss these issues at which he indicated his intention to continue to pay child support. After this meeting, there was a pronounced change in Mrs. O. Her psychotic symptoms resolved, and her intermittent episodes of agitation stopped. Her medication was tapered and discontinued without recurrence of symptoms. Having returned to her previous level of functioning, she was discharged after 1 week of hospitalization.

DISCUSSION

This case is presented as an example of a culture-specific syndrome that is not recognized in the official classification of mental disorders. *Ataques de nervios* is a sudden, dramatic, but transient change in behavior observed in people from Spanish-speaking countries after the occurrence of major stress. It is sometimes attributed to malevolent spirits. It generally involves dissociative symptoms and frequently symptoms that suggest a panic attack, such as palpitations, chest tightness, shortness of breath, and dizziness. There may also be, as in this case, bizarre behavior and frankly psychotic symptoms such as hallucinations. The disturbance usually begins in the presence of family members, and the family often mobilizes to provide support and even removal of the stressor. Although in this case the hallucinations and incoherence, lasting only a few days, support an official diagnosis (DSM-IV-TR) of brief psychotic disorder, it is a serious mistake to ignore the fundamental difference between this seemingly psychotic disorder and other psychotic disorders in which stress and dissociation do not play a major role. In retrospect, the failure to recognize that this was not the usual psychotic disorder and that complete recovery was to be expected was undoubtedly responsible for the inappropriate administration of the antipsychotic medication.

Cases of this syndrome raise the interesting question of whether it is appropriate to give a pathological diagnosis to a condition, such as *ataques de nervios*, because it can be considered a culture-specific expression of distress, analogous to normal bereavement. One could argue that had this woman received the necessary social support from her family, she would have recovered quickly and never would have required medical care.

Mrs. O. experienced the remarriage of her ex-husband as very stressful, although it is not clear whether this would be markedly stressful to almost anyone in similar circumstances in the person's culture. However, because it is clearly the stress of her ex-husband's remarriage that has precipitated this episode, if one were to make the DSM-IV-TR diagnosis of brief psychotic disorder, one would add with marked stressor.

Uncritical labeling of a problem behavior as a culture-bound syndrome on the basis of bizarre symptoms or the statements of the patient and family can also be detrimental. Patients and their families often use cultural terms, such as *nervios* or *ataque de nervios*, loosely as generic expressions for emotional or physical pain or as "idioms of distress"—somewhat like the term "nervous breakdown" in the modern American-English culture. It is therefore important to go beyond these generic terms and ask the patients or their families to specifically describe the problem behaviors and experiences. In addition, Arthur Kleinman and his colleagues suggest asking the patients and the families a few simple questions that help elicit their cultural beliefs about the illness, including questions such as what they call the illness, what they believe to be its cause, what they believe to be the course or the outcome, and what treatments they expect or accept.

Another important caveat in assessing culture-bound syndromes is the differentiation between ethnicity and culture. Ethnic backgrounds of the patients are not necessarily indicators of their cultural affiliations. Patients from immigrant groups undergo various degrees of acculturation as a result of exposure to the culture of their adoptive country. Assessing the level of acculturation is therefore important in assessing these patients.

Infectious diseases and nutritional deficiencies are common among low-income immigrant populations in Western settings and may present with psychological complaints or behavioral manifestations. Similarly, serious psychiatric disorders, such as schizophrenia and major depression, do occur with similar rates in different cultural settings and should be diagnosed and treated as such.

In many patients with culture-bound syndromes, the criteria for various DSM-IV-TR disorders are also met, especially mood and anxiety disorders. For instance, in a study from Puerto Rico, 63 percent of the patients who reported *ataques de nervios* met the criteria for a DSM-IV-TR psychiatric disorder or a substance disorder, compared with 28 percent of the rest of the sample. Therefore, assessment of these other disorders should be an integral part of assessment of culture-bound syndromes.

DIFFERENTIAL DIAGNOSIS

The major challenge in differential diagnosis of culture-bound syndromes is distinguishing among these conditions and the major psychiatric disorders in DSM-IV-TR and ICD-10, particularly psychotic and dissociative conditions. As noted above, this differentiation has to rely on both the presenting symptoms and the patient's cultural background. Such differentiation often has important treatment implications.

Some of the uncommon psychotic symptoms present a surface resemblance to culture-bound syndromes. For instance, *koro*-like beliefs about receding genitalia have been reported among patients with psychotic disorders in Western cultural settings. Also, symptoms of echopraxia and echolalia noted in some patients with schizophrenia in Western settings are similar to behavioral and verbal manifestations of *latah*. As noted, these behaviors only bear a surface resemblance to culture-bound syndromes. The terminology used for culture-bound syndromes should not be used for describing these conditions.

COURSE AND PROGNOSIS

Course of culture-bound syndromes is generally favorable. Most of these conditions present as self-limiting episodes after stressful events. This conclusion, however, is based on anecdotal reports because no formal follow-up studies of these conditions have been published.

SUGGESTED CROSS-REFERENCES

Cultural psychiatry issues are also discussed in Sections 4.2, 4.3, 4.4, and 9.2 (international perspectives on psychiatric diagnosis). Culture-bound syndromes are discussed in Chapter 27.

REFERENCES

Baer RD, Weller SC, de Alba Garcia JG, Glazer M, Trotter R, Pachter L, Klein RE: A cross-cultural approach to the study of the folk illness *nervios*. *Cult Med Psychiatry*. 2003;27:315.

Guarnaccia PJ, Lewis-Fernandez R, Rivera Marand M: Toward a Puero Rican popular nosology: *Nervios* and *ataque de nervios*. *Cult Med Psychiatry*. 2003;27:339.

Guarnaccia PJ, Rogler LH: Research on culture-bound syndromes: New directions. *Am J Psychiatry*. 1999;156:1322.

Guinness EA: III. Profile and prevalence of the brain fag syndrome: Psychiatric morbidity in school population in Africa. *Br J Psychiatry*. 1992;160[Suppl 16]:42.

*Jilek WG, Jilek-Aall L. Culture-specific mental disorders. In: Henn F, Sartorius N, Helmchen H, Lauter H, eds. *Contemporary Psychiatry, Vol. 2, Psychiatry in Special Situations*. Berlin: Springer-Verlag; 2001.

*Kleinman A, Parron DL, Fabrega H, Good BJ, Mezzich JE. Culture in DSM-IV. In: Widiger TA, Frances A, Pincus HA, Ross R, First MB, eds. *DSM-IV Sourcebook*. Vol. 3. Washington, DC: American Psychiatric Press; 1997.

Kukoyi O, Carney CP: Curses, madness, and mefloquine. *Psychosomatics*. 2003;44:339.

Lopez-Ibor JJ Jr: Cultural adaptations of current psychiatric classifications: Are they the solution? *Psychopathology*. 2003;36:114.

Mezzich JE, Kirmayer LJ, Kleinman A, Fabrega H, Parron DL, Good BJ, Lin K-M, Manson SM: The place of culture in DSM-IV. *J Nerv Ment Dis*. 1999;187:457.

*Mezzich JE, Kleinman A, Fabrega H, Parron DL. *Culture and Psychiatric Diagnosis*. Washington, DC: American Psychiatric Press; 1995.

Parzen MD: Toward a culture-bound syndrome-based insanity defense? *Cult Med Psychiatry*. 2003;27:131.

*Simons RC, Hughes CC. *The Culture-Bound Syndromes: Folk Illnesses of Psychiatric and Anthropological Interest*. Dordrecht, The Netherlands: D. Reidel Publishing Company; 1985.

Susser E, Wanderling J: Epidemiology of nonaffective acute remitting psychosis vs schizophrenia. Sex and sociocultural setting. *Arch Gen Psychiatry*. 1994;51:294.

*Tseng W-S. *Handbook of Cultural Psychiatry*. San Diego: Academic Press; 2001.

12.16g Psychosis Not Otherwise Specified

SHMUEL FENNIG, M.D., AND LAURA J. FOCHTMANN, M.D.

Under the umbrella of psychosis not otherwise specified (NOS), there is a variety of clinical presentations that do not fit within current diagnostic rubrics. Indeed, in the revised fourth edition of the *Diagnostic and Statistical Manual of Mental Disorders* (DSM-IV-TR), there are no specific diagnostic criteria for this category. Rather, it includes "psychotic symptomatology (i.e., delusions, hallucinations, disorganized speech, grossly disorganized or catatonic behavior) about which there is inadequate information to make a specific diagnosis or about which there is contradictory information, or disorders with psychotic symptoms that do not meet the criteria for any specific Psychotic Disorder."

The DSM-IV-TR provides several examples:

Postpartum psychosis that does not meet criteria for mood disorder with psychotic features, brief psychotic disorder, psychotic disorder due to a general medical condition, or substance-induced psychotic disorder

Psychotic symptoms that have lasted for less than 1 month but that have not yet remitted so that the criteria for brief psychotic disorder are not met

Persistent auditory hallucinations in the absence of any other features

Persistent, nonbizarre delusions with periods of overlapping mood episodes that have been present for a substantial portion of the delusional disturbance

Situations in which the clinician has concluded that a psychotic disorder is present but is unable to determine whether it is primary, due to a general medical condition, or substance induced

Even in carefully executed follow-up studies of psychiatric patients, 5 to 10 percent receive a diagnosis of psychosis NOS after 2 to 3 years of follow-up. Comorbid substance use is one of the most frequent confounding variables in establishing a specific diagnosis because substance use can be found in more than one-half of all patients admitted to the hospital with psychotic symptoms.

Parallel to the diagnosis of psychosis NOS in DSM-IV-TR, the tenth revision of *International Statistical Classification of Diseases and Related Health Problems* (ICD-10) includes the category "Other Acute and Transient Psychotic Disorders." This category is used for "any other acute psychotic disorders that are not classifiable under any other category in the section of acute and transient psychotic disorder (such as acute psychotic states in which definite delusions or hallucinations occur but persist for only small proportions of the time). States of undifferentiated excitement should also be coded here if more detailed information about the patient's mental state is not available, provided that there is no evidence of an organic cause." For brief episodes, there is no qualifier of time: "Acute polymorphic psychotic disorder without symptoms of schizophrenia" states that "any type of either delusions or hallucinations occurs, for at least several hours, at any time from the onset of the disorder."

EPIDEMIOLOGY

There is minimal information about the prevalence of this diagnosis in the community. In clinical practice, psychosis NOS is often used with first-admission patients when there is inadequate information to make a diagnosis or when a more severe diagnosis, such as schizophrenia, is being avoided because of the unreliability of initial cross-sectional diagnoses. For example, in Suffolk County, New York, between 1989 and 1995, 26 percent of first admissions with a psychotic condition were given a diagnosis of psychosis NOS by the treating clinician, whereas 12 percent were given this diagnosis by the research team. Among patients diagnosed with psychosis NOS by the clinicians, the most common diagnosis by the research team was schizophrenia (23 percent) followed by psychosis NOS (19 percent). As noted above, the application of this diagnosis decreases after first admission. In the Suffolk series, by the 6-month follow-up, only 4.8 percent were diagnosed by the research team with psychosis NOS, and by 24 months' follow-up, the rate was 3.9 percent. In samples from Ireland, Italy, and Germany, a diagnosis of psychosis NOS was given to 2 to 12 percent of patients with psychosis.

CLINICAL FEATURES

The category of psychosis NOS includes psychotic episodes presenting with delusions, hallucinations, disorganized speech, and grossly disorganized or catatonic behavior about which there is inadequate information to make a specific diagnosis or about which there is contradictory information. It also includes disorders with psychotic symptoms that do not meet the criteria for any specific psychotic disorder, such as patients who present to the hospital with persistent auditory hallucinations that are not accompanied by mood disturbance and that are not pathognomonic for schizophrenia or any other DSM-IV-TR category. Another group of patients who receive a diagnosis of psychosis NOS are those with long-standing delusions accompanied by functional impairment (thus excluding a diagnosis of delusional disorder) without other symptoms of schizophrenia.

Psychosis NOS is also used when a clinician is unable to determine whether the psychosis is primary, is due to a general medical condition, or is substance induced. Medical contributors to psychosis are often chronic, and many individuals do not have a sufficient period of abstinence from substance use to be able to make such distinctions. In addition, some substances can cause prolonged psychotic symptoms, further confounding clinical diagnosis. For example, studies done in the 1970s with phencyclidine (PCP) could not distinguish patients with a PCP-induced psychosis from patients with schizophrenia. In fact, the extent to which the use of certain illicit substances contributes to the etiology of psychosis remains unknown.

The following example describes a patient with no history of substance abuse:

R. W. was 21 years of age when he was brought to a psychiatric emergency service because of strange behavior. He had no history of drug or alcohol abuse or dependence. While visiting relatives in Las Vegas, he began to think that his uncle was out to get him. This feeling grew stronger, and his father was not able to convince him that it was not true. This episode lasted for 5 hours. He was hospitalized for 1 week, and his psychotic symptoms cleared immediately with no medications. Over the next 10 years, he continued to have short episodes of psychosis, usually associated with lack of sleep. A typical episode occurred when the patient went to Canada with his girlfriend. At that time, he had not slept for 2 days. He was happy and excited because it was one of his first trips with his girlfriend. At the hotel, he reported suspicions that people were looking at him, following him, and wanting to hurt him. He became so frightened that he did not eat his dinner. He finally left the restaurant with his girlfriend and went to sleep. He reports waking up the next day and feeling fine. The whole incident lasted approximately 3 hours.

DISCUSSION

This patient had repeated brief episodes of psychosis, ranging from several hours to several days and often associated with inadequate sleep. He did not meet the criteria for any other psychotic disorder based on the duration of symptoms. His psychotic episodes did not last long enough to meet the criteria for brief psychotic disorder, which requires a duration of symptoms of at least 1 day. He also did not meet criteria for delusional disorder, which require that the symptoms last for at least 1 month.

SUGGESTED CROSS-REFERENCES

A more detailed review of schizophrenia is presented in Chapter 12. Mood disorders are covered in Chapter 13.

REFERENCES

Chabrol H: Chronic hallucinatory psychosis: Bouffe d'elirante, and the classification of psychosis in French psychiatry. *Curr Psychiatry Rep*. 2003;5:137–191.

Chaudron LH, Pies RW: The relationship between postpartum psychosis and bipolar disorder: A review. *J Clin Psychiatry*. 2003;64:1284–1292.

Degenhardt L, Hall W, Lynskey M: Testing hypotheses about the relationship between cannabis use and psychosis. *Drug Alcohol Depend*. 2003;71:37–48.

Fennig S, Bromet EJ, Craig T, Jandorf L, Schwartz JE: Psychotic patients with unclear diagnoses. *J Nerv Ment Dis*. 1995;183:207.

Kendler KS, Walsh D: Schizophreniform disorder, delusional disorder and psychotic disorder not otherwise specified: Clinical features, outcome, and familial psychopathology. *Acta Psychiatr Scand*. 1995;91:370–378.

Mojtabai R, Susser ES, Bromet EJ: Clinical characteristics, 4-year course, and DSM-IV classification of patients with nonaffective acute remitting psychosis. *Am J Psychiatry*. 2003;160:2108–2115.

Peralta V, Cuesta MJ: The nosology of psychotic disorders: A comparison among competing classification systems. *Schiz Bull*. 2003;29:413–425.

Serretti A, Rietschel M, Lattuada E, Krauss H, Schulze TG, Muller DJ, Maier W, Smeraldi E: Major psychoses symptomatology: Factor analysis of 2241 psychotic subjects. *Eur Arch Psychiatry Clin Neurosci*. 2001;251:193–198.

12.16h Treatment of Other Psychotic Disorders

LAURA J. FOCHTMANN, M.D.

As with schizophrenia or psychotic mood disorders, the treatment of patients with other psychotic disorders is complex and needs to consider both the specific features of the disorder as well as specific and unique features of the individual patient. Furthermore, the development of a treatment plan is not simply a single event that occurs with the initiation of care but, rather, is an ongoing process that continues throughout treatment. Changes in the treatment plan may be prompted by additional information from the patient, family, or other significant individuals about the patient's symptoms, response to treatment, psychiatric or medical history, psychosocial situation, or cultural context. The appropriateness of the treatment plan should also be reassessed with symptomatic worsening or with symptoms that persist for extended periods without apparent or full response to treatment. For patients whose symptoms have resolved, reassessments of the treatment plan help determine whether continuing follow-up care is indicated.

The treatment planning process begins during the initial evaluation of the patient with the formulation of a multiaxial diagnosis that guides the selection of specific interventions discussed below. In addition, the initial evaluation helps determine whether the patient's symptoms require specific treatment or whether they represent an acute and transient psychotic reaction or a culturally based syndrome that will resolve without treatment. As an additional element of the initial evaluation, it is important to understand the patient's conceptualization of his or her symptoms. In discussing symptoms, patients of differing cultural or ethnic backgrounds may have differing explanations for their symptoms or use differing vocabularies in describing their experiences. In this regard, family members and others within the patient's support network may be able to provide helpful information about the sociocultural context in which symptoms are occurring. In exploring the meaning of symptoms with the patient, it is helpful to inquire about the onset of the symptoms, the patient's understanding of what may have caused the symptoms, and the reasons the symptoms began when they did. It is also important to ask whether the patient sees a need for treatment and, if so, what therapeutic approaches seem most helpful.

Understanding the patient's view of his or her symptoms has many advantages in planning treatment and facilitating treatment adherence. By emphasizing that the clinician is interested in the unique aspects of the patient's experience, such an inquiry may help in building rapport. In addition, it conveys respect and appreciation for the patient's views and an openness by the clinician to understand different perspectives, including cultural factors. Obtaining patient feedback about treatment lays the groundwork for a collaborative approach to treatment planning in which the clinician actively seeks and incorporates patient input. An in-depth understanding of the patient's symptoms can aid in diagnosis-specific treatment planning by suggesting the presence of specific culture-bound syndromes. However, the patient's answers to such questions may also reveal the extent of a delusional system or the absence of insight into having an illness. Through understanding the meaning of the patient's symptoms, the clinician may become aware of specific related fears, anxieties, or other affective responses that may impact on treatment planning. For example, in a patient with delusional jealousy or erotomania, the clinician may learn that the patient is feeling spurned and, as a result, is angrily planning violent revenge. Alternatively, in a patient with persecutory delusions in the context of delusional disorder, the patient's overwhelming anxiety about being in danger may serve as a means for establishing a positive therapeutic relationship and offering antipsychotic medication. Thus, a thorough understanding of the patient's symptoms and the meaning of those symptoms to the patient aids in arriving at an individualized plan of treatment that is most likely to be effective.

In developing an individualized treatment plan for individuals with other psychotic disorders, several elements should be taken into consideration. For all patients who present with psychotic symptoms, the clinician needs to determine the most appropriate setting for providing treatment. Most patients respond best to a combination of therapeutic approaches, including pharmacotherapy, psychotherapy, psychosocial therapies, and other interventions, such as patient and family education, support groups, 12-step programs, or involvement of traditional healers. The indications for these therapeutic approaches and their integration into an overall plan of treatment for individuals with other psychotic disorders are described in more detail below. In addition, the treatment plan should address any comorbid diagnoses that are present. Given the relatively high rates of alcohol and other substance use disorders among individuals with psychoses, it is particularly important to identify and incorporate treatment for these disorders into the treatment plan.

DETERMINING A TREATMENT SETTING

In determining an initial setting for treatment, the clinician may choose among a continuum of options, ranging from involuntary or voluntary hospitalization to partial hospital or intensive outpatient programs to continuing day treatment to assertive community treatment to office-based outpatient treatment. The specific setting that is selected should optimize the safety of the patient while simultaneously providing care in the setting that is least restrictive and most likely to facilitate long-term stability of the patient's illness. Because the optimal setting for treatment varies for each individual over time, clinicians should regularly review whether the current setting of care is most appropriate for the patient's needs.

In determining whether a patient is best managed on an inpatient or outpatient basis, it is essential to consider the degree to which the patient may pose a risk to him- or herself or to others. Although it is impossible to predict suicidal or homicidal behavior with certainty even in an intensive treatment setting, hospitalization offers a higher level of observation and a greater ability to make rapid adjustments in treatment than other settings of care. Thus, inpatient admission is often needed for individuals who appear to be at relatively high risk of acute harm to themselves or others.

Although evidence is limited, rates of suicide attempts and suicide appear to be increased in individuals with acute and transient psychosis, postpartum psychosis, schizophreniform disorder, and schizoaffective disorder, as compared with the general population. The presence of suicidal ideas or a recent suicide attempt further increases short-term risk and requires additional inquiry to determine whether other risk factors for suicide are present, including specific suicidal plans or intent. Patients with delusional disorder may attempt suicide after becoming demoralized by the ongoing nature of their perceived persecution by others. Other patients may harm themselves in an effort to protect their family members from injury. Examples might include women with postpartum psychosis who believe that they are possessed and in danger of harming their infant or patients with delusional disorder who believe that the criminal element will target their family if they remain alive. Still, other patients may harm themselves without suicidal intent in an effort to address their delusional beliefs. An example of this is an individual with delusional parasitosis who covers his or her skin with a caustic substance in an effort to stop the infestation.

Hospitalization may also be indicated when history or mental status examination suggests that the patient is at an increased risk of harming others. In addition to specific ideation or plans of harm to others, risk is greater in individuals with a past history of aggressiveness or violent or explosive outbursts. Patients who are agitated or hostile during the interview are also likely to be at an increased risk of aggressive behavior toward others. The specific content of the patient's psychotic experience may also provide clues to an increased short-term likelihood of risk. Examples might include a mother who believes her child to be the offspring of Satan or someone with delusional disorder who believes specific individuals are planning to kill him or her. Misidentification syndromes may also lead a patient to harm others. For example, a patient who believes his or her spouse has been kidnapped and "switched" with an impostor may try to harm the "impostor" to learn where the "real" spouse is being held captive. Patients may also manifest violent or disorganized behavior with culture-bound syndromes (e.g., *amok*). The possibility of suicide/homicide should also be considered. For example, with untreated postpartum psychosis, rates of infanticide have been estimated to be as high as 4 percent. Patients with delusional jealousy or erotomania may also be at increased risk of suicide/homicide. These issues should therefore be considered in determining an appropriate setting for care.

In addition to the potential risks of dangerousness to self or others, a number of other factors may suggest a need for inpatient treatment. Patients with minimal insight into the need for treatment and those with a history of poor treatment adherence may require hospitalization for acute stabilization at lower levels of potential risk than individuals who adhere to treatment and are in a stable, ongoing therapeutic relationship. Hospitalization may also be indicated to carry out essential medical assessments or treatment, such as electroconvulsive therapy (ECT), if the patient's level of psychosis prevents these from being performed as an outpatient. The ability to observe patients in a controlled setting may also be helpful in establishing a psychiatric diagnosis and rapidly implementing treatment. This can be particularly helpful in patients with comorbid medical disorders in whom medical monitoring may be important with initiation of treatment and in individuals with comorbid substance use disorders in whom continuing substance use may confound diagnosis and treatment. If the ideal setting for treatment is not available in the community, a higher level of care may also be required. For example, a patient who may be able to be managed in a partial hospitalization program may need inpatient care instead if partial hospital or intensive outpatient follow-up is not readily obtainable. The presence of family and community supports is also important in this regard. An individual who resides with a supportive family or who is living in a supervised housing setting may be managed safely as an outpatient, whereas the same level of symptoms may necessitate hospitalization in an individual who is homeless or lives alone.

For patients who do not require inpatient treatment, partial hospital or intensive outpatient programs provide a setting for acute stabilization and more extensive monitoring of symptoms and treatment response than office-based outpatient care. Continuing day treatment programs and assertive community treatment programs are typically used to maintain stabilization and facilitate treatment adherence for individuals with a more chronic illness course. Individuals with schizoaffective disorder and some individuals with delusional disorder, for example, might receive particular benefit from the ongoing structure and multidisciplinary approach afforded by treatment in these settings.

ANTIPSYCHOTIC AGENTS

For treatment of psychotic disorders other than schizophrenia and psychotic mood disorders, the antipsychotic agents are, not surprisingly, the primary class of medications used. The challenge for the clinician is in determining whether treatment with an antipsychotic is or is not indicated and, if so, the duration of treatment that is required. For patients with an acute onset of symptoms that is consistent with an acute and transient psychosis, antipsychotic medication may or may not be required depending on the severity of the symptoms. In some individuals, the use of oral or short-acting injectable antipsychotic medications on an acute or "as needed" basis is sufficient to control psychotic symptoms without need for ongoing antipsychotic therapy. Similarly, most individuals with culture-bound syndromes do not require treatment with an antipsychotic medication.

For individuals with a provisional diagnosis of schizophreniform disorder, antipsychotic treatment is generally indicated. In fact, some evidence suggests that outcomes may be worse if long delays occur before antipsychotic treatment is initiated. Less clear is the duration of treatment that is needed with schizophreniform disorder. For individuals followed after a first episode of illness, most studies show an increased risk of relapse if antipsychotic medication is discontinued during the first 6 months of treatment. Those with the best outcomes had antipsychotic medication doses maintained at 80 to 100 percent of the dose used in treating the acute episode of illness. For individuals whose psychosis resolves entirely with a full return to baseline levels of functioning, many clinicians recommend a gradual tapering of antipsychotic medication after 6 months of treatment, with careful monitoring for recurring symptoms or functional decline.

Individuals with postpartum psychosis generally require acute treatment with an antipsychotic medication. Many episodes of postpartum psychosis occur in the context of an underlying mood disorder, and for these individuals, antipsychotic medications may be slowly tapered and discontinued 6 to 12 months after the acute illness episode has resolved. Those individuals with postpartum exacerbations of psychosis in the context of another psychotic disorder are more likely to require ongoing antipsychotic treatment.

In schizoaffective disorder, initial and maintenance antipsychotic treatment is an important element of treatment. Yet to be proved, however, is whether antipsychotic medication can control both the psychosis and the mood symptoms of schizoaffective disorder or whether adjunctive treatment is needed with antidepressants, lithium (Eskalith) or mood-stabilizing anticonvulsants, or both. In patients with treatment-resistant schizoaffective disorder, as in patients with treatment-resistant schizophrenia, clozapine (Clozaril) often produces a positive therapeutic response. In addition to treating hallucinations and delusions, case report literature suggests that clozapine may help in stabilizing mood and diminishing suicidality in individuals with schizoaffective disorder. More recent evidence from a randomized controlled trial also suggests a beneficial effect of clozapine on suicidality in schizoaffective disorder.

Patients with delusional disorder often lack insight into having an illness and are reluctant to take antipsychotic medications. Nonetheless, although response rates in patients with delusional disorder are frequently said to be lower than response rates in other psychotic disorders, patients with delusional disorder can clearly benefit from antipsychotic medications. For those whose delusions do respond to treatment, clinical observations suggest that long-term antipsychotic administration is needed to maintain remission.

In treating patients with the foregoing psychotic disorders, most recommendations on the choice of specific antipsychotic medications come from the knowledge of these agents in the treatment of schizophrenia and case series observations rather than well-designed clinical trials. Some evidence from randomized double-blind trials is available that shows the efficacy of antipsychotic medications in the short-term treatment of schizoaffective disorder. However, these findings are primarily from subgroup analyses of patients in clinical trials that included individuals with schizophrenia and schizophreniform disorder as well as schizoaffective disorder. In addition, changes in the diagnostic criteria for schizoaffective disorder over the past several decades have made it difficult to pool data from older studies to subject them to metaanalyses.

With the exception of clozapine, the second-generation antipsychotics (e.g., risperidone [Risperdal], olanzapine [Zyprexa], quetiapine [Seroquel], ziprasidone [Zeldox], aripiprazole [Abilify]) are preferred over first-generation agents because of their more favorable side-effect profile. Like the other second-generation antipsychotic agents, clozapine is less often associated with acute extrapyramidal side effects and has a much lower likelihood of inducing tardive dyskinesia or neuroleptic malignant syndrome. At the same time, because clozapine treatment can be associated with the rare but potentially fatal side effects of agranulocytosis and myocarditis, its use is generally reserved for individuals whose psychosis does not respond to other antipsychotic treatments. In addition, the need for regular monitoring of white blood cell counts leads some patients to be reluctant to consider clozapine treatment. Among the other second-generation antipsychotics, the choice of a particular medication is generally based on the side-effect profile of the medication, the patient's history of response, and the potential for interactions with other medications that the patient may be taking. In individuals who do not respond to second-generation agents, first-generation antipsychotics may be used.

In women with postpartum psychosis who are breast-feeding, choice of a specific medication should consider the possible effects on the infant. All antipsychotics are present in breast milk to some degree, and all have been noted by the American Academy of Pediatrics to have an effect on the nursing infant that is unknown but of possible concern. Nonetheless, for mothers who choose to breast-feed, it may be preferable to choose an antipsychotic medication with a shorter half-life and collect breast milk when levels are at their lowest. Use of a second-generation agent (with the exception of clozapine) may also be preferable, with less likelihood of short- and long-term adverse effects.

For patients with frequent recurrences of illness relating to poor treatment adherence, use of a long-acting injectable formulation should be considered. Of the second-generation antipsychotic medications available, only risperidone is available in a long-acting injectable formulation (Risperdal Consta). If long-acting injectable forms of first-generation antipsychotics are used, the potential for greater side effects from depot forms of these medications (e.g., haloperidol decanoate, fluphenazine decanoate) needs to be weighed against the benefits of improved medication adherence for the individual patient.

Case report literature suggests that the first-generation antipsychotic pimozide (Orap) may be of particular value in treating individuals with delusional disorder, in general, and those with delusional parasitosis, in particular. However, other case reports suggest that antipsychotics other than pimozide may also be effective in patients with delusional disorder. Thus, an initial trial of a second-generation antipsychotic agent is warranted in such patients, given the increased risk of adverse effects with pimozide, including extrapyramidal side effects, neuroleptic malignant syndrome, tardive dyskinesia, QTc prolongation, and malignant arrhythmias with reports of sudden death at doses of more than 20 mg per day.

Regardless of whether a first- or second-generation antipsychotic agent is selected for use, the selected dosage should be at the lowest possible level to minimize adverse effects as well as costs. Often, in an effort to shorten the length of the psychosis, shorten hospital stays, or minimize the likelihood of hospitalization, there is a tendency, fueled by financial or utilization reviewing pressures, to rapidly and aggressively increase medication dosages. However, full resolution of a psychotic episode may take weeks to months, and the benefits of an increment in medication dose are not immediately apparent. Thus, adjustment of medication dosages should occur gradually with frequent assessments to determine response or emergence of adverse effects. In particular, when adjusting antipsychotic dosages, it is important to assess for signs of akathisia that may be difficult to distinguish from psychotic agitation. Antipsychotic-induced akinesia may also be difficult to distinguish from negative symptoms of psychosis or from depressive symptoms, particularly in individuals with schizoaffective disorder. When extrapyramidal symptoms do emerge with antipsychotic treatment, these may need to be addressed through the use of adjunctive anticholinergic agents or amantadine. For patients with akathisia, concomitant treatment with propranolol (Inderal) or a benzodiazepine may be helpful. If significant extrapyramidal side effects persist, reductions in medication dosage or a change to a medication with fewer side effects may also be indicated.

It is also important to recognize that individuals from differing racial or ethnic backgrounds may metabolize antipsychotics differently and have differing patterns of response or sensitivity to adverse effects. For example, in East Asians, required dosages of antipsychotic medications are typically much less than those in white individuals. Such factors need to be taken into consideration when initiating and adjusting dosages of antipsychotic medication during treatment.

BENZODIAZEPINES

Treatment with benzodiazepines may be useful in several situations when treating individuals with psychotic disorders. For individuals who experience agitation or severe anxiety, benzodiazepines can be used on a short-term basis while the patient's diagnosis and need for antipsychotic treatment are being clarified. For some patients with acute and transient psychotic episodes or culture-bound syndromes, short-term use of a benzodiazepine alone may be sufficient to treat anxiety, agitation, or insomnia and permit resolution of symptoms. In addition, because agitation and severe anxiety may increase the likelihood of suicidal behaviors, short-term use of benzodiazepines can also be beneficial in this regard. As noted above, benzodiazepines may also be helpful in treating akathisia in patients receiving antipsychotic medication. Catatonic features of psychotic disorders are another indication for treatment with benzodiazepines, with most studies using moderate to high doses of lorazepam (Ativan). In treating fearfulness and anxiety associated with persecutory delusions, patients with delusional disorder may find short-term benzodiazepine treatment to be more acceptable at first than treatment with antipsychotics. Attending to the patient's feelings of anxiety and treating those effectively may contribute to a positive therapeutic relationship in which the patient is more willing to consider antipsychotic treatment.

In general, the clinician wants to choose a moderate- to long-acting benzodiazepine such as lorazepam or clonazepam (Klonopin). Although diazepam (Valium) and chlordiazepoxide (Librium) also are long-acting benzodiazepines, their metabolism to long-acting active metabolites makes them less useful in this context. Before prescribing a benzodiazepine on a short-term basis, the clinician should consider whether the patient has a history of a substance use disorder. Although a history of a substance use disorder does not preclude benzodiazepine treatment if it is otherwise indicated, for such patients, it may be preferable to choose other options for management of agitation (e.g., use of a sedating antipsychotic). When treating women with postpartum psychosis, it should be recognized that the effects of benzodiazepines in breast-fed infants are unknown but have been noted by the American Academy of Pediatrics to be of possible concern.

In patients with severe agitation, "as needed" doses of benzodiazepines may be given orally or parenterally for rapid sedation alone or in combination with antipsychotic medication. Of the benzodiazepines, the rapid intramuscular (IM) absorption and onset of action of lorazepam make it best suited for parenteral use. Often, administration of IM lorazepam in combination with an IM antipsychotic agent (e.g., ziprasidone, haloperidol) permits more rapid control of agitation with lower overall doses of medication than the use of either agent alone.

LITHIUM AND MOOD-STABILIZING ANTICONVULSANTS

The use of lithium and anticonvulsant medications, such as valproic acid (Depakene), carbamazepine (Tegretol), and oxcarbazepine (Trileptal), is common in the treatment of individuals with schizoaffective disorder. However, evidence from well-designed clinical trials is limited. In one older study that assessed the prophylactic effect of lithium in patients with schizoaffective disorder, no specific benefits of treatment were noted, with serum levels in the subtherapeutic to low therapeutic range (0.45 to 0.60 mEq/L). In another more recent study that compared lithium with carbamazepine over an average of 2.5 years of maintenance therapy, carbamazepine was associated with fewer adverse effects and, in patients with the depressive type of schizoaffective disorder, produced a superior response. In contrast, the overall drop-out rate was greater for patients treated with carbamazepine, and the response to the two medications did not differ in other subgroups of patients with schizoaffective disorder. However, because serum levels of each medication were again in the low therapeutic range, these results are also difficult to interpret and require replication. There is some evidence that maintenance treatment with lithium in patients with broadly defined schizoaffective disorder may diminish the risk of suicide attempts and suicide as is clearly seen in individuals with bipolar disorder. Again, however, most of the available studies have not included patients with well-defined diagnoses of schizoaffective disorder or separated subgroups of patients with schizoaffective disorder from those with other mood or psychotic disorders. Thus, in the absence of well-designed clinical trials, in making the decision to use lithium or mood-stabilizing anticonvulsants in treating schizoaffective disorder, the risks and benefits for the individual patient should be weighed. If such medications are prescribed, the suggested use and therapeutic levels of these medications in bipolar disorder should serve as a guide to treatment planning.

Treatment with lithium or mood-stabilizing anticonvulsants is also commonly recommended for women with postpartum psychosis. Reports in the literature primarily involve the use of lithium during the postpartum period and are uncontrolled. However, the substantial overlap between postpartum psychosis and bipolar disorder makes it likely that many women with postpartum psychosis show comparable therapeutic benefits to those observed in patients with bipolar disorder. In addition, women with postpartum psychosis may similarly benefit from maintenance treatment with these agents.

If short-term or maintenance treatment is chosen for women with postpartum psychoses, carbamazepine and valproic acid are noted to be generally compatible with breast-feeding. In contrast, lithium should be used with caution in mothers who are breast-feeding their infants because serum levels in the infant may be one-third to one-half of maternal levels. Lamotrigine (Lamictal), which has also been used in the treatment of patients with bipolar disorder, should be used cautiously as well. Although its full effects in the infant are unknown, therapeutic serum levels of lamotrigine can be observed in the breast-fed infant and may produce a risk of rash and Stevens-Johnson syndrome.

The use of lithium or anticonvulsants for management of patients with the tenth revision of *International Statistical Classification of Diseases and Related Health Problems* (ICD-10) acute and transient psychotic disorders, culture-bound syndromes, or delusional disorders has not been evaluated. However, there are case reports of effective use of lithium in treating cycloid psychosis and good prognosis schizophrenia.

ANTIDEPRESSIVE AGENTS

Use of adjunctive antidepressive agents is common in individuals with other psychotic disorders. In choosing a specific antidepressant, the clinician should review the patient's history of antidepressant treatment, including treatment responses, the adequacy of the treatment course in terms of dosage and duration of therapy, and any associated side effects of treatment. In general, antidepressant treatment is initiated with a serotonin reuptake inhibitor (e.g., citalopram [Celexa], escitalopram [Lexapro], fluoxetine [Prozac], paroxetine [Paxil], sertraline [Zoloft]), venlafaxine (Effexor), or mirtazapine (Remeron). These medications are generally well tolerated, with fewer side effects and much greater safety in overdose than either tricyclic antidepressants or monoamine oxidase inhibitors (MAOIs). Factors, such as interactions with other medications and the side-effect profile of the specific agents, should also be considered. For example, patients with prominent insomnia may respond better to a less activating antidepressant, whereas those with prominent fatigue may benefit from a more activating agent. In addition, as with antipsychotic medications, metabolism and side-effect profiles of antidepressive agents may vary across racial or ethnic groups. Bupropion (Wellbutrin) may also be used, although its dopamine-enhancing properties may make it more likely to worsen psychosis, and it is less likely to be useful in patients with prominent anxiety. With nefazodone (Serzone), the risk of hepatic failure, although small, makes it less appropriate for use as a first-line agent. Trazodone may be useful for its sedative properties but appears to be less effective as an antidepressant than other agents, at least at readily tolerated doses.

Antidepressants are frequently indicated in treating individuals with a major depressive episode in the context of schizoaffective disorder. In such patients, the choice of a specific antidepressant follows the general guidelines for antidepressant choice in treating depressive episodes in patients with bipolar disorder. In addition, in weighing the benefits and risks of antidepressant treatment, the possibility of precipitating a manic episode or increasing mood cycling should be taken into consideration.

Antidepressive agents have also been widely used in treating postpartum depression. Their use in postpartum psychosis is less clear and depends on whether prominent symptoms of depression are also present. For women who plan to breast-feed, there are no data suggesting that one antidepressant is safer than another. Although complications of neonatal exposure to antidepressants appear to be rare, the effects of longer-term exposure on the developing brain are not known.

In individuals with the somatic type of delusional disorder, particularly with body dysmorphic delusions, antidepressants with significant serotonin reuptake–blocking properties (i.e., SSRIs, clomipramine [Anafranil]) may be specifically useful, at least according to a number of case reports. Given the diagnostic overlap between such patients and those with severe obsessions or psychotic depression, a trial of an SSRI in combination with an antipsychotic may be worthwhile if antipsychotic therapy alone is ineffective.

Antidepressants have also been noted to be effective in several culture-bound syndromes. One retrospective study examined the use of fluvoxamine (Luvox) or clomipramine in 48 individuals with *taijin kyofusho*. Of the 33 individuals who continued in treatment for 6 months, 48 percent were classed as treatment responders. In a study of 93 men with *dhat* syndrome who were randomized to receive lorazepam, imipramine, vitamins, or counseling, both active pharmacological treatment conditions had a greater response rate than placebo. In addition, both had significantly greater response rates and lower rates of drop-outs at 4 weeks than did counseling. Delusions of fatal contagion, observed within Hmong refugees of Southeast Asia, have also been noted to respond to treatment with tricyclic antidepressants. Antidepressant treatment may also be considered for individuals with other culture-bound syndromes that have prominent symptoms of anxiety or depression, particularly if such symptoms persist despite culturally based interventions.

ELECTROCONVULSIVE THERAPY

No clinical trials have examined the use of ECT in psychotic disorders other than schizophrenia or depressive or manic episodes with psychotic features. Studies do show that, in psychotic mood disorders, ECT works rapidly and is highly efficacious in treating depression, mania, and psychosis. Although response rates are significantly lower in individuals with schizophrenia, some patients who have not responded to treatment with antipsychotics do show clear responses to ECT. In addition to decreasing psychosis and normalizing mood, suicidal ideation has also been shown to resolve rapidly with ECT treatment. Thus, it is not surprising that case reports suggest the usefulness of ECT in individuals with treatment-resistant schizoaffective disorder as well as in women with postpartum psychosis. The rapidity of the response to ECT is also likely to be of benefit in postpartum psychosis by diminishing the effects of prolonged illness on mother–infant attachment. Although the risks of cognitive effects with ECT need to be taken into consideration, the use of bilateral electrode placement for ECT is more likely to prove effective than unilateral electrode placement.

PSYCHOTHERAPIES

For most individuals with the psychotic disorders discussed in this chapter, some form of supportive psychotherapy is helpful. On the other hand, insight-oriented therapies are rarely indicated. The goals of supportive therapy include facilitating treatment adherence and providing education about the illness and its treatment. Other educational efforts may focus on the impact that social or physical isolation, psychosocial stressors, or sleep deprivation may have on mood and on psychosis. Often, patients may need realistic guidance and assistance surrounding issues such as insurance coverage or medical care and follow-up.

The psychotherapeutic relationship also provides an emotionally secure setting in which the patients can discuss their psychotic experiences and also think about pragmatic strategies for coping with those experiences and their aftermath. For individuals whose symptoms do not fully respond to pharmacotherapy, the clinician may help the patients learn to speak about their experiences only to those who are understanding. For example, individuals with delusional disorders often encounter problems from making repeated phone calls to police to discuss persecutory fears or having repeated contacts with objects of their erotomanic delusions. In psychotherapy, they may learn to recognize these behaviors as creating more difficulties for themselves and may learn to stop acting on their delusional ideas even when such beliefs are still present. For some individuals, cognitive therapeutic approaches may be helpful in this regard. During psychotherapy, discussion of the unrealistic nature of delusional beliefs should be done gently and only after rapport with the patient has been established. By definition, delusional beliefs are fixed, and this is particularly true in patients with delusional disorders who, if confronted, present elaborate evidence and rationales supporting their delusional ideas. At the same time, one should not simply agree with the delusional belief because this only leads the patient to be suspicious of the clinician if the delusional ideas begin to subside with treatment. Instead, the clinician can emphasize that people have differing views on many things, but that should not keep them from working together in a collaborative fashion to address other issues that help the patient to function better with less emotional distress.

Similar approaches to supportive psychotherapy can be used for individuals with psychotic symptoms in the context of schizophreniform disorder, schizoaffective disorder, or postpartum psychosis. Some patients with schizoaffective disorder or postpartum psychosis may also benefit from interpersonal psychotherapy or cognitive-behavioral therapy, particularly if depressive symptoms are prominent.

For individuals from a different cultural background than the clinician and particularly those with a culture-bound syndrome, consideration of cultural aspects is an essential ingredient of the psychotherapeutic process and is important in establishing rapport, engaging the patient in treatment, and collaborating with the patient in developing a treatment plan. For some patients, psychotherapy may worsen rather than improve symptomatology. For example, Western-based psychotherapies that value and promote individual independence may conflict with culturally important values such as family or community unity and harmony. Thus, before beginning psychotherapy with an individual with a culture-bound syndrome, it is generally helpful to speak with the patient, the patient's family, or traditional healers or others with expertise in the patient's culture. Depending on the specific culture-bound syndrome, specific forms of psychotherapy may be indicated such as Morita therapy for the treatment of *shinkeishitsu.* Consultation with culturally informed individuals helps the clinician determine whether psychotherapy is, in fact, indicated and, if so, helps delineate a culturally appropriate framework for treatment.

CULTURAL AND TRADITIONAL HEALERS

Many individuals with culture-bound syndromes initially seek treatment from cultural or traditional healers or other alternative providers of care. In other instances, either when symptoms are severe or have not responded to traditional treatments, patients may be referred to Western-trained practitioners for care. In addition to consulting with cultural or traditional healers for information about cultural beliefs and background, some have suggested the possible usefulness of collaborating with indigenous healers. Such decisions should be made on an individualized basis and depend on the patient's symptoms and the wishes of the patient and family as well as the flexibility of the available healers. When patients are simultaneously being seen by Western-trained clinicians and cultural or traditional healers, it is also important to note whether patients are simultaneously receiving psychotropic medications and teas or herbal preparations that may interact or alter serum levels of prescribed medications. Ideally, collaboration and coordination of treatment between caregivers minimize confusion for the patient and optimize treatment.

PSYCHOSOCIAL TREATMENTS

Although specific clinical trials of psychosocial treatments have not been conducted in individuals with schizoaffective disorder or delusional disorder, it is likely that the benefits from such treatments that have been shown for patients with schizophrenia are also observed for individuals with these disorders. Improvements in adaptive functioning may also occur with vocational rehabilitation, social skills training, or psychosocial clubhouse programs. Intensive case management services and programs for assertive community treatment may assist in coordination of care as well as in providing other supportive and treatment resources. Such programs should be considered for individuals with schizoaffective disorder or delusional disorder, particularly those with frequent relapses or hospitalizations.

PATIENT AND FAMILY EDUCATION, INCLUDING SUPPORT AND SELF-HELP GROUPS

As noted above, patient education is an essential element of treatment for individuals with any psychotic disorder. In addition, randomized controlled trials in schizophrenia suggest that long-term psychoeducational family programs are of benefit to individuals with schizophrenia and their families. Some of these trials have also included individuals with schizoaffective disorder, suggesting that such formal psychoeducational programs are likely to be of benefit in these patients as well.

Although controlled trials are lacking, family education is similarly important to the treatment of the other psychotic disorders discussed in this chapter. Goals of family education, like goals of patient education, generally include providing information about the illness and its treatments and learning to identify early signs of relapse of illness. Illness-specific educational efforts may be particularly difficult because less is known about the course and treatments for these disorders than for schizophrenia or psychotic mood disorders. In addition, schizophreniform disorder and postpartum psychosis commonly evolve into other diagnoses with differing prognoses. These uncertainties should be discussed openly with patients and families. Although patients and family members may be more knowledgeable about culture-bound syndromes, interactions with Western-trained practitioners of differing cultural backgrounds and uncertainties about nontraditional treatments may also be stressful and should be discussed.

Medication teaching may also be complex because patients may be taking multiple medications of differing classes with differing side-effect profiles. In addition to specific information on each medication, patients and families should also understand that medications interact, and adverse effects may result from addition of other prescribed medications, over-the-counter preparations, and herbal or natural products. Thus, they should be educated about the importance of contacting the clinician before taking any such additional preparations.

The new onset of psychosis, recurrent psychotic symptoms, or psychiatric hospitalizations is generally quite distressing to patients as well as family members. For individuals with postpartum psychosis, family members are also dealing simultaneously with the care of an infant, and the implications that the patient's illness has for her own future and that of her baby. Later in the follow-up period, women with postpartum psychosis and their partners may need education about the likelihood of recurrent episodes of illness with future pregnancies so that appropriate planning of contraception or future pregnancies can occur.

For patients with delusional disorder, family members may be incorporated into the patient's delusional system (e.g., delusional jealousy, misidentification syndromes, shared delusions). Educating these family members about the patient's illness and the nature of delusional beliefs is essential. For individuals with shared delusions, family therapy may be necessary.

Many patients or families find it helpful to become involved with a self-help group or a support group such as the local chapter of the National Alliance for the Mentally Ill. However, it is also important to consider the composition of the specific support group before suggesting that patients or families attend. Support groups in which most individuals are dealing with chronic psychiatric illness may not be immediately relevant or may actually seem threatening to individuals who are dealing with acute manifestations of psychosis in themselves or their family members. Individuals with substance use disorders or those who have family members with substance use disorders may similarly benefit from attending a 12-step program on a regular basis.

SUGGESTED CROSS-REFERENCES

The reader is encouraged to read the relevant sections on treatment in the chapters on schizophrenia (Sections 12.8, 12.9, and 12.10), mood disorders (Sections 13.7, 13.8, and 13.9), cultural psychiatry (Section 4.1), reproductive medicine (Section 28.1), and Chapters 29, 30, and 31, as well as the American Academy of Pediatrics guidelines for the use of psychotropics during pregnancy and lactation.

REFERENCES

American Academy of Pediatrics: Transfer of drugs and other chemicals into human milk. *Pediatrics.* 2001;108:776.

American Psychiatric Association. *The Practice of Electroconvulsive Therapy: Recommendations for Treatment, Training, and Privileging: A Task Force Report of the American Psychiatric Association.* 2nd ed. Washington, DC: American Psychiatric Press; 2001.

American Psychiatric Association. Practice Guideline for the Treatment of Patients with Schizophrenia. 2nd ed. *Am J Psychiatry.* 2004;161[Suppl]:1–56.

Bhatia MS, Malik SC: Dhat syndrome—a useful diagnostic entity in Indian culture. *Br J Psychiatry.* 1991;159:691.

Ciapparelli A, Dell'Osso L, Bandettini di Poggio A, Carmassi C, Cecconi D, Fenzi M, Chiavacci MC, Bottai M, Ramacciotti CE, Cassano GB: Clozapine in treatment-resis-

tant patients with schizophrenia, schizoaffective disorder, or psychotic bipolar disorder: A naturalistic 48-month follow-up study. *J Clin Psychiatry.* 2003;64:451–458.
Dolder CR, Lacro JP, Leckband S, Jeste DV: Interventions to improve antipsychotic medication adherence: Review of recent literature. *J Clin Psychopharmacol.* 2003;23:389–399.
Expert consensus panel for optimizing pharmacologic treatment of psychotic disorders. Expert consensus guideline series. Optimizing pharmacologic treatment of psychotic disorders. *J Clin Psychiatry.* 2003;64[Suppl 12]:2–97.
*Fishman BM, Bobo L, Kosub K, Womeodu RJ: Cultural issues in serving minority populations: Emphasis on Mexican Americans and African Americans. *Am J Med Sci.* 1993;306:160.
Greil W, Ludwig-Mayerhofer W, Erazo N, Engel RR, Czernik A, Giedke H, Muller-Oerlinghausen B, Osterheider M, Rudolf GA, Sauer H, Tegeler J, Wetterling T: Lithium vs carbamazepine in the maintenance treatment of schizoaffective disorder: A randomised study. *Eur Arch Psychiatry Clin Neurosci.* 1997;247:42.
*Guscott RG, Steiner M: A multidisciplinary treatment approach to postpartum psychoses. *Can J Psychiatry.* 1991;36:551.
Harrigan SM, McGorry PD, Krstev H: Does treatment delay in first-episode psychosis really matter? *Psychol Med.* 2003;33:97.
Hodes R: Cross-cultural medicine and diverse health beliefs: Ethiopians abroad. *West J Med.* 1997;166:29.
Janicak PG, Keck PE Jr, Davis JM, Kasckow JW, Tugrul K, Dowd SM, Strong J, Sharma RP, Strakowski SM: A double-blind, randomized, prospective evaluation of the efficacy and safety of risperidone versus haloperidol in the treatment of schizoaffective disorder. *J Clin Psychopharmacol.* 2001;21:360.
Kane JM, Carson WH, Saha AR, McQuade RD, Ingenito GG, Zimbroff DL, Ali MW: Efficacy and safety of aripiprazole and haloperidol versus placebo in patients with schizophrenia and schizoaffective disorder. *J Clin Psychiatry.* 2002;63:763.
Keck E Jr, Reeves KR, Harrigan EP: Ziprasidone in the short-term treatment of patients with schizoaffective disorder: Results from two double-blind, placebo-controlled, multicenter studies. *J Clin Psychopharmacol.* 2001;21:27.
*Levinson DF, Umapathy C, Musthaq M: Treatment of schizoaffective disorder and schizophrenia with mood symptoms. *Am J Psychiatry.* 1999;156:1138.
*Lin KM, Cheung F: Mental health issues for Asian Americans. *Psychiatr Serv.* 1999;50:774.
Maeda F, Nathan JH: Understanding *taijin kyofusho* through its treatment, Morita therapy. *J Psychosom Res.* 1999;46:525.
Meltzer HY, Alphs L, Green AI, Altamura AC, Anand R, Bertoldi A, Bourgeois M, Chouinard G, Islam MZ, Kane J, Krishnan R, Lindenmayer JP, Potkin S: Clozapine treatment for suicidality in schizophrenia: International Suicide Prevention Trial (InterSePT). *Arch Gen Psychiatry.* 2003;60:82.
Muller-Oerlinghausen B, Ahrens B, Grof E, Grof P, Lenz G, Schou M, Simhandl C, Thau K, Volk J, Wolf R: The effect of long-term lithium treatment on the mortality of patients with manic-depressive and schizoaffective illness. *Acta Psychiatr Scand.* 1992;86:218.
*Munro A, Mok H: An overview of treatment in paranoia/delusional disorder. *Can J Psychiatry.* 1995;40:616.
Opler LA, Klahr DM, Ramirez PM: Pharmacologic treatment of delusions. *Psychiatr Clin North Am.* 1995;18:379.
Pang KY: *Hwabyung*: The construction of a Korean popular illness among Korean elderly immigrant women in the United States. *Cult Med Psychiatry.* 1990;14:495.
Potkin SG, Alphs L, Hsu C, Krishnan KR, Anand R, Young FK, Meltzer H, Green A, InterSePT Study Group: Predicting suicidal risk in schizophrenic and schizoaffective patients in a prospective two-year trial. *Biol Psychiatry.* 2003;54:444–452.
Tran PV, Tollefson GD, Sanger TM, Lu Y, Berg PH, Beasley CM Jr: Olanzapine versus haloperidol in the treatment of schizoaffective disorder: Acute and long-term therapy. *Br J Psychiatry.* 1999;174:15.

▲ 12.17 Schizophrenia and Other Psychotic Disorders: Special Issues in Early Detection and Intervention

SCOTT W. WOODS, M.D., AND
THOMAS H. MCGLASHAN, M.D.

The treatment of schizophrenia has improved substantially since the 1950s. With the best of modern treatments, most patients are now able to live in the community instead of in the hospital and are able to engage actively in ongoing rehabilitation efforts. Full recovery, however, continues to be the exception rather than the rule, and many patients are left with a degree of chronic, if stable, disability

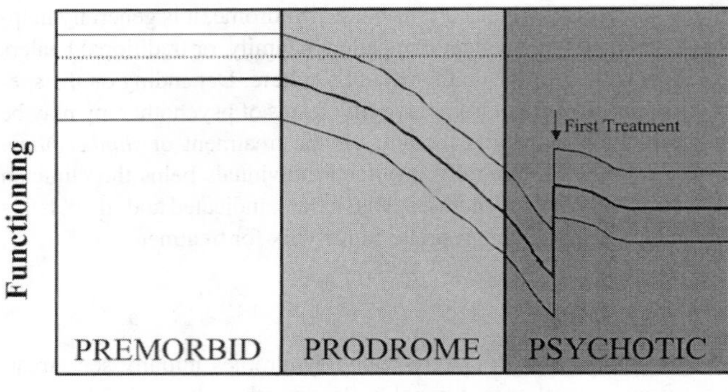

FIGURE 12.17–1 Phases of illness in schizophrenia. A schematic representation of the early course of illness in schizophrenic patients. Time is displayed on the ordinate and global functioning on the abscissa. The dotted line represents 100 percent of age-adjusted, average normal functioning. The line in bold illustrates the average course of a group of patients with schizophrenia over premorbid, prodromal, and psychotic phases. Function generally declines rapidly during prodromal phase, as well as early in the psychotic phase. The duration of time between onset of psychosis and the first antipsychotic treatment is known as the *duration of untreated psychosis.* Variability in course is expressed by the upper and lower hairline time-course curves, which illustrate the wide range that is observed across patients throughout the course of illness.

that remains refractory to current treatments. In recent years, early detection and intervention has attracted increasing interest as a potential paradigm to prevent the development of chronic disability and to augment the efficacy of medications and psychosocial therapies. This chapter will elaborate on that perspective and its rationale, promises, and limitations, with an emphasis on early detection and early intervention during the prodromal phase.

PHASES OF SCHIZOPHRENIA

The course of schizophrenia has been divided conceptually into three phases of illness (Fig. 12.17–1). The first phase is known as the *premorbid phase*, a period of asymptomatic, usually subtle, and generally stable impairments starting from birth. The next phase is the *prodromal phase*, a symptomatic period of escalating severity usually beginning after puberty and lasting 1 to 2 years. Not all schizophrenic patients remember a period of prodromal symptoms, but, according to retrospective accounts, 80 to 90 percent do. The next phase is the *psychotic phase*, beginning with the first frankly psychotic symptoms. Patients are considered to have passed the threshold of frank psychosis when they no longer retain insight into the unreality of their emerging symptoms but instead express conviction that hallucinatory experiences and delusional beliefs are really happening. Patients who have recently experienced onset of psychosis are said to be in their *first episode* of illness. Evidence indicates that, for most patients, severity of illness continues to escalate after onset for at least a few years. Diagnostic criteria have thus far been standardized, generally accepted by psychiatrists, and codified in the revised fourth edition of the *Diagnostic and Statistical Manual of Mental Disorders* (DSM-IV-TR) only after patients have entered the psychotic phase.

Premorbid Phase Information about the premorbid phase is available primarily from three sources: birth cohort studies, studies of children at genetic risk, and longitudinal studies of other groups.

Birth cohort studies indicate that children who later become schizophrenic score 0.5 to 1.0 standard deviation below the control mean on tests of intelligence quotient (IQ). Recently, a study conducted by Michael Davidson and colleagues linked the Israeli Draft Board Registry with the Israeli National Psychiatric Hospitalization Case Registry and determined which draft board tests in healthy male adolescents were associated with hospitalization for schizophrenia 1 to 10 years later. People who later developed schizophrenia had significant deficits in social functioning, organizational ability, and intellectual functioning compared to those who did not. Some of the subjects who developed schizophrenia early on within the 1 to 10–year window may have been evaluated during the prodromal phase rather than the premorbid phase.

The long-term prediction findings from six studies of young children at genetic risk for schizophrenia have suggested that in genetically at-risk individuals, several factors were associated with long-term psychosis or schizophrenia spectrum outcomes, including maternal influenza during gestation, obstetrical complications (OCs), neurointegrative deficits in infancy, separation during the first year of life, social and affective and motor coordination deficits in early childhood, attentional dysfunction in childhood, social dysfunction later in childhood, attention-deficit neurobehavioral deficits and poor motor coordination in preadolescence, teacher-rated behaviors in adolescence, and absence of protective family environments.

The predictive power of early self-experienced cognitive deficits for the subsequent development of schizophrenia has been investigated by Joachim Klosterkotter and colleagues using the Bonn Scale for the Assessment of Basic Symptoms (BSABS). A total of 160 patients were studied, all of whom had been referred for evaluation because the referring clinician perceived them to be at risk for later development of schizophrenia. At initial examination, none had shown psychotic symptoms. At reexamination on the average of 9.6 years later, a very high proportion (49 percent) had developed a schizophrenic disorder. Several of the early self-experienced cognitive deficits were reported to have particularly high sensitivity, specificity, and positive predictive power among this population whose a priori risk was extremely high. Several of the best predictive basic symptoms resemble attenuated positive symptoms studied by other groups (e.g., visual perception disturbances, acoustic perception disturbances, derealization, unstable ideas of reference, and thought interferences). The BSABS may be capturing some symptoms characteristic of the prodromal phase, as well as premorbid deficits.

Lastly, a long-term psychosis-risk study testing prospectively established criteria administered psychosis-proneness scales to psychology undergraduate students at a large U.S. university by Loren Chapman and colleagues. The high-scoring students on the Perceptual Aberration or Magical Ideation Scales were hypothesized a priori to develop psychosis at a higher rate over a 10-year period than lower-scoring controls. Ten of 182 high-scoring students (positive predictive value [PPV], 5.5 percent) had developed psychosis by the 10-year follow-up, as compared to 2 of 153 controls. Post-hoc analyses incorporating information from the Social Anhedonia Scale were able to increase the PPV for psychosis to 21 to 24 percent. This group also reported a partial prospective replication in a new sample. The Chapman Scales may also be capturing symptoms characteristic of the prodromal phase in addition to premorbid deficits.

Three patterns of functioning have been described during the premorbid phase: stable-good, stable-poor, and deteriorating. The degree of premorbid phase impairment and its time course are variable across individuals—so much so that some studies have identified superior functioning as a risk factor for schizophrenia. Variability in course continues to be characteristic of schizophrenia in its later phases as well.

Despite the promise of this line of research, development of diagnostic criteria for the premorbid phase still appears to be premature. Findings derived from exploratory methods should be tested in new samples from the vantage of prospective hypothesis testing, and the prospective findings among U.S. college students appear thus far to have a false-positive rate of case prediction that is too high to justify intervention efforts.

Prodromal Phase

The prodromal phase is the first symptomatic period. The prodromal phase almost always begins after puberty and is associated with a rapid decline in functioning (Fig. 12.17–1) and escalating symptoms.

Psychotic Phase

The course of first-episode schizophrenia is variable across patients. Predictors of relatively good outcome include prominence of affective symptoms, late onset, acute onset, and relative absence of negative symptoms. On the average, however, the authors' review indicates that first-episode schizophrenia patients appear to show a continued decline in functioning over the next few years, with stabilization afterwards.

Short DUP appears to be another predictor of good outcome. DUP is the period of time after onset of the psychotic phase and before the first antipsychotic medication treatment (Fig. 12.17–1). The mean DUP for first-episode samples is often 1 to 2 years. DUP can be very long—10 years or longer in some individuals. The distribution of DUP is heavily skewed to the right, so that the median DUP of first-episode samples is almost always much shorter than the mean. Reducing DUP may offer therapeutic advantages, as is discussed below.

EARLY DETECTION AND EARLY INTERVENTION

Detection and intervention are said to be *early* if patients are identified and treated early in the first episode of illness or during the prodromal or premorbid phases. When patients are identified and treated shortly after onset in the first episode, they are considered to have experienced a short DUP.

Relationship

If intervention to prevent schizophrenia were to be attempted in the general population, such efforts would constitute *primary prevention*, or *universal prevention*. Increasing access to and use of prenatal care would be an example of a possible primary prevention. Intervention delivered to asymptomatic individuals who are selected based on the presence of risk markers during the presumed premorbid phase would be termed *secondary prevention*, or *selective prevention*. Intervention delivered during the presumed prodromal phase to individuals who are symptomatic but have not developed the full syndrome is considered to be another type of secondary prevention, termed *indicated prevention*. Lastly, when delivered to patients who already meet full criteria for the psychotic phase of schizophrenia, intervention that aims to reduce disability or mortality would be considered *tertiary prevention*.

Rationale

The most basic rationale for early detection and intervention arises from the escalation of the patient's severity of illness during the prodromal and early active phases. Increased severity of illness is potentially associated with greater suffering and greater risk of suicide, violence, derailment from psychosocial developmental trajectories, and socially alienating, self-stigmatizing behaviors. Early intervention can potentially be delivered before

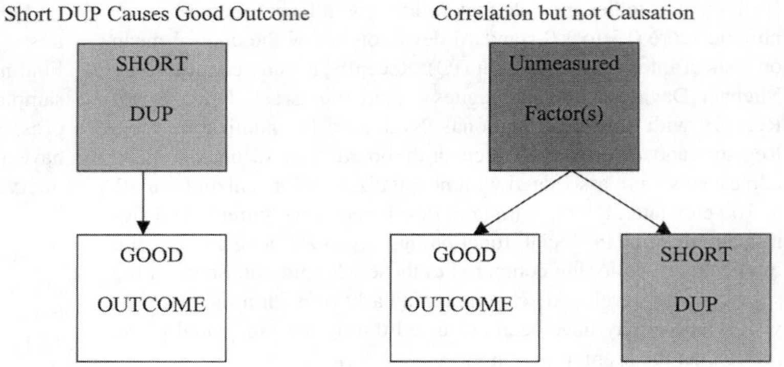

FIGURE 12.17–2 Possible relationships between duration of untreated psychosis (DUP) and outcome. The statistically significant correlation that has been observed in most observational studies between DUP and treatment outcome is consistent with either of two interpretations. One possibility is that shorter DUP directly causes better treatment outcome, perhaps because the treatment somehow interrupts a process of deterioration that is still active in patients with short DUP (*left panel*). The other possibility is that short DUP and better outcome are both consequences of some other factor or factors that have not yet been measured (*right panel*).

such suffering and risks have occurred, thus providing a type of tertiary prevention. This potential is generally recognized in the psychiatric clinical and research communities, and, as a result, early detection and intervention programs are being organized with increasing frequency.

Additionally, possible benefits of early detection and intervention are more hypothetical and have become the subjects of active current empirical investigation.

Possibility of Better Treatment Outcome One hope for early intervention is that earlier treatment may be associated with more complete long-term resolution of symptoms and diminished residual disability, a type of secondary prevention. Theoretically speaking, this question would be best addressed by randomized experiments either before or after onset. For many years now, however, it has been considered unethical after onset to assign patients at random to briefer DUP (immediate treatment) versus longer DUP (delayed treatment), except for very brief periods under careful observation. Thus, after onset, the question of whether earlier intervention is associated with better long-term outcome has been primarily addressed in naturalistic designs where DUP is not manipulated experimentally.

Many studies of this type have been conducted, and the results are mixed, although the bulk of the evidence suggests that shorter DUP is associated with better clinical outcomes. No formal metaanalysis of this body of studies has been published yet, but recent comprehensive reviews report that approximately two-thirds of 25 studies showed a significant association between shorter DUP and better outcome on one or more measures, and none showed a significant association between longer DUP and better outcome on any measure.

When formal metaanalyses are conducted, it will be important to take into account the possibility of a critical window of deterioration within the period of DUP. Specifically, studies that intervened with first-episode patients who, despite being in their first episode nevertheless had very long DUP, perhaps should not be properly considered as examples of early intervention. Conversely, samples where DUP was relatively short overall may not have a sufficient range of DUP to be sensitive to a DUP effect.

It is important to appreciate that data from these naturalistic designs are consistent with either of two interpretations, as shown in Figure 12.17–2. One possibility is that shorter DUP causes better treatment outcome directly, perhaps because the treatment somehow interrupts a process of deterioration that is still active in patients with short DUP. The other possibility is that short DUP and better outcome are both consequences of some other factor or factors that have not been measured. Factors that have been considered for this role include acuity of onset and premorbid functioning. One study has suggested that DUP was somewhat stronger than and somewhat independent from premorbid functioning as a predictor of outcome. In this study, DUP and acuity of onset were not significantly correlated, which argues against DUP being a proxy for acuity of onset. Another study similarly found that premorbid functioning and DUP were not strongly correlated, which argues against poor premorbid functioning being a cause of long DUP.

Some studies have examined the effect of DUP on outcome using a nonrandomized longer DUP control group. One study conducted by Patrick McGorry and colleagues used a pre-post design to investigate outcomes before and after the institution of a first-episode program that aimed to detect schizophrenia early and reduce DUP. DUP was reduced somewhat by the program from a mean of 227 weeks to a mean of 175 weeks, and the patients detected somewhat earlier demonstrated better functioning and had spent less time in the hospital at 1-year follow-up compared to first-episode patients treated after usual detection. Recently, a second study from one of the authors has made use of a quasiexperimental design to investigate the possible effect of DUP on outcome. This research group mounted an extensive early detection campaign in Rogaland County, Norway, and will compare outcomes of care among first-episode patients treated after usual detection at the same time in two "control" counties in Norway and Denmark. Early detection was achieved by an intensive, multilevel campaign of community education about psychosis and its treatment, including provider trainings, billboards, mailings, and radio and television advertisements. Long-term outcome data are not yet available, but preliminary pre-post data from within Rogaland County suggest that DUP had been robustly reduced from a mean of 114 weeks to a mean of 25 weeks.

Because there is, as yet, no established standard of care for patients in the presumed prodromal phase, randomized studies are possible in this population to determine whether earlier treatment is associated with more complete long-term resolution of symptoms and diminished residual disability. The few studies that have been conducted are reviewed in a later section.

Possibility of Preventing Structural Brain Degeneration and Cognitive Decline Small reductions in cerebral gray-matter volume and larger increases in cerebral ventricular volume are characteristic of patients with established schizophrenia as a group. Qualitatively similar findings have been described at the time of the first episode. Thus, structural deficits have already been present before onset of illness as it is currently defined and identified.

Correspondingly, a variety of neuropsychological weaknesses are also characteristic of patients with established schizophrenia as a group. Similar findings have been described at the time of the first episode. These observations suggest the need to investigate earlier intervention in the hope of influencing deficit processes earlier in their development. The literature on progression of the structural and neuropsychological findings after onset is mixed, however. Some recent studies have detected continued progression of structural deficits after onset among first-episode patients. Whether currently available treatments can retard or halt any structural or neuropsychological progression after onset remains unknown.

SYMPTOMATIC PRODROME FOR SCHIZOPHRENIA AND ITS HISTORY

A prodromal phase of schizophrenic disorders has been recognized since the time of Eugene Bleuler. Historically, the prodrome concept as applied to schizophrenia has been limited to a retrospective viewpoint in the same way that the prodrome as a more general concept in medicine has historically been retrospective. In this context, patients can be described as having been prodromal only after they have experienced onset of schizophrenia.

COMPARATIVE NOSOLOGY

Because the prodrome for schizophrenia has been historically limited to retrospective conceptualizations, the use of the term to describe patients prospectively can be viewed as a misnomer. The other most common terms used for these patients, employed by Patrick McGorry and colleagues, are *at-risk mental state*, or ARMS, and *patients at ultra-high risk*. The authors favor the term *prodromal* for its familiarity, brevity, and inclusion of the notion that the state is symptomatic.

EPIDEMIOLOGY

The incidence of schizophrenia is approximately 1 new patient per year per 10,000 persons in the population. A recent metaanalysis indicates that men are approximately 1.4 times more likely to develop schizophrenia than are women. The average age of onset of the psychotic phase of schizophrenia is in the early twenties, with onset being somewhat earlier in males. Careful epidemiologic studies of the schizophrenia prodrome have not been conducted, but the incidence of truly prodromal patients is likely to be approximately 1 in 10,000 as well, with an average age 1 to 2 years younger than the age of onset for schizophrenia. Because the age of onset is younger in men, any oversampling bias among clinical populations of prodromal patients toward a younger age would likely alter the gender ratio of the sample. In other respects, the epidemiology of the prodrome should mirror the epidemiology of schizophrenia itself. On the other hand, to the extent that current prodromal criteria identify false-positive cases, the epidemiology of the prodrome may be expected to differ from that of schizophrenia.

DIAGNOSIS AND CLINICAL FEATURES

Most studies, including the seminal work of Heinz Hafner and colleagues, indicate that largely nonspecific symptoms related to anxiety and mood predominate early in the prodrome. These are usually followed by or accompanied by negative symptoms, such as loss of volition and social withdrawal, and cognitive changes, such as difficulty with attention and concentration. Positive symptoms (perceptual abnormalities, ideas of reference, and suspiciousness) develop late and herald the relatively imminent onset of psychosis.

Prospective Prodromal Diagnostic Criteria

Prospective diagnostic criteria for the schizophrenic prodrome that predict onset of psychosis in the near future have been recently developed, based on review of retrospective descriptions and studies of preliminary criteria. These criteria were initially proposed by Patrick McGorry and colleagues and have been revised by the authors (Table 12.17–1). As described above, these criteria identify a symptomatic patient group that is at high risk for progression to frank first-episode psychosis within the next year. The criteria describe three prodromal subgroups, based on attenuated positive symptoms (attenuated posi-

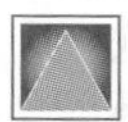

Table 12.17–1
Diagnostic Criteria for Prodromal Syndromes

Prodromal Syndromes	Diagnostic Criteria
Attenuated positive symptom syndrome (APSS)	Abnormal unusual thought content, suspiciousness, grandiosity, perceptual abnormalities, and/or organization of communication that is below the threshold of frank psychosis.
	AND
	These symptoms have begun or worsened in past year.
	AND
	These symptoms occur at least once/week for last month.
	AND
	Psychosis ruled out.
Brief intermittent psychotic syndrome (BIPS)	Frankly psychotic unusual thought content, suspiciousness, grandiosity, perceptual abnormalities, and/or organization of communication.
	BUT
	These symptoms have begun in the past 3 months.
	AND
	The symptoms occur currently at least several minutes per day at least once/month.
	AND
	Psychosis ruled out.
Genetic risk + functional deterioration (G/D)	First-degree relative with history of any psychotic disorder.
	OR
	Schizotypal personality disorder in patient.
	AND
	Substantial functional decline in the past year.
	AND
	Psychosis ruled out.
Rule out psychosis	Frankly psychotic unusual thought content, suspiciousness, grandiosity, perceptual abnormalities, and/or organization of communication.
	AND
	Symptoms are disorganizing or dangerous.
	OR
	Symptoms occur more than 1 hr/day more than 4 times/wk in the past month.

Note: Prospective diagnostic criteria for the schizophrenic prodrome that predict onset of psychosis in the near future (see text). These criteria have identified a symptomatic patient group that is at high risk for progression to frank first-episode psychosis within the next year. Four sets of criteria are shown that describe three prodromal syndromes and the threshold for frank psychosis. The three prodromal syndromes are based on APSS, BIPS, or G/D. In the research setting, the criteria are operationalized using a structured diagnostic interview and standardized rating scales.

tive symptom syndrome [APSS]), brief psychotic symptoms (brief intermittent psychotic syndrome [BIPS]), or genetic risk plus functional deterioration (G/D). In the research setting, the criteria are operationalized using a structured diagnostic interview and standardized rating scales. The authors have developed and use the Structured Interview for Prodromal Syndromes (SIPS) and the Scale of Prodromal Symptoms (SOPS). These instruments have been translated into 14 different languages. Other instruments also have been developed for similar purposes, such as the Comprehensive Assessment of At Risk Mental States and the BSABS.

In the authors' experience, most prodromal patients meet the APSS criteria, and only a few answer the G/D criteria without also meeting APSS. For example, at baseline, in a clinical trial conducted by the authors where enrollment has been completed, 53 out of 60 patients (88 percent) met APSS criteria, including six who met APSS and G/D criteria simultaneously. An additional seven enrolled patients met only G/D criteria. In the authors' experience, the BIPS subtype appears to be fairly rare. No patients meeting BIPS criteria were enrolled in the authors' clinical trial. In another sample, 35 of 49 prodromal patients (71 percent) met APSS criteria, whereas 18 of 49 (37 percent) met G/D, and 12 of 49 (24 percent) met BIPS, with moderate overlap among all three groups. The G/D criteria were designed to permit inclusion based on a family history of psychosis, rather than a family history of schizophrenia per se. This decision was made because relatives of probands with schizophrenia are not only more likely to be diagnosed with schizophrenia than relatives of controls, but are also more likely to be diagnosed with psychotic affective disorders, according to some studies.

Symptoms, Distress, and Impairment of Prodromal Patients

Prodromal diagnostic criteria require that patients be currently symptomatic, and patients so identified appear to represent a newly recognized clinical population. Prodromal patients appear to represent a clinical population for at least four reasons: (1) their symptoms can be highly distressing to them and their families, (2) the patients and their families are often treatment seeking, (3) they show evidence of functional impairment, and (4) they show evidence of cognitive impairment. Examples of the subjective distress that can be associated with prodromal symptoms are provided in the case reports below. Most patients in the authors' experience have previously sought and received psychiatric services, including medications. Global Assessment of Functioning scores (full range, 0 to 100) have been reported to average below 50 in the authors' sample. Lastly, the authors' unpublished data show that prodromal patients as a group achieved scores between those of first-episode patients and those of unaffected subjects on a wide variety of neuropsychological tasks.

PATHOLOGY AND LABORATORY EXAMINATION

At the moment, there are no findings from pathological or laboratory examinations that are pathognomonic for the schizophrenia prodrome. A recent magnetic resonance imaging (MRI) study has reported that cerebral gray-matter volume is reduced in true positive prodromal patients in a variety of cortical regions. Gray matter volume deficits increased in these patients during the interval between initial diagnosis as prodromal and conversion to psychosis. The volume deficits appear small in magnitude, however, and, as for established schizophrenia, the effect size is also likely to be small so that the prodromal distribution of volumes overlaps substantially with that of the control group. A substantial degree of overlap would mean that MRI scanning would probably not be useful as a diagnostic test in individual cases. When there is substantial overlap on a test between pathological cases and controls, either test sensitivity is likely to be low (high rate of false-negative diagnoses) or test specificity is likely to be low (high rate of false-positive diagnoses), no matter what cutoff score is chosen to define the border between normality and abnormality.

Good medical practice, however, suggests that patients suspected of being prodromal for schizophrenia should receive a physical examination and routine laboratory examinations of blood and urine to screen for known medical conditions that can be responsible for incipient psychosis.

DIFFERENTIAL DIAGNOSIS

The differential diagnosis of the schizophrenia prodrome is a broad one. In addition to early cases of known medical conditions that can be responsible for incipient psychosis, several other conditions must be considered.

Perhaps the most frequent and most difficult differential diagnostic issue occurs with regard to depression with psychotic features. Depressive symptoms are common in schizophrenic patients throughout the natural history of the illness, including during its early stages, as well as the prodromal early phase. Although depressive symptoms are common among prodromal patients, in the authors' experience, most prodromal patients do not meet criteria for a full depressive syndrome. In the authors' sample of prodromal patients, scores on a commonly used depression-rating scale were significantly lower than in samples of patients with major depression. In general, the depressive mood in prodromal patients is experienced as a loss of emotional feeling and as discouragement rather than true sadness, self-blame, or even irritability. Some patients say they must feel depressed, although they are not sure what depression feels like, because others have told them depression must be the cause of their difficulties. Prodromal patients may complain of loss of energy, interest, or concentration or experience initial insomnia, and some can experience suicidal thoughts. Few, however, complain of melancholic symptoms such as early waking, loss of appetite or weight, or feeling guilty. Depression with psychotic features, on the other hand, is typically associated with a full depressive syndrome and often with melancholia. Moreover, depression with psychotic features has been classically associated with older age groups rather than with adolescence or young adulthood.

Other diagnoses that must be considered in the differential include schizotypal personality disorder, borderline personality disorder, attention-deficit disorder (ADD), and obsessive-compulsive disorder (OCD). Schizotypal personality disorder is described as having onset during adolescence and is characterized by attenuated positive symptoms similar to those of the prodrome. The two conditions are distinguished by course—in the prodrome, the symptoms are progressive, and in schizotypal personality, they are enduring but stable. When brief psychotic episodes under stress are accompanied by a pattern of intense but unstable interpersonal relationships and impulsivity, a diagnosis of borderline personality is made rather than a BIPS prodromal state. It is also unusual for the brief psychotic episodes of borderline personality to have begun in the past 3 months (Table 12.17–1). ADD usually has onset before puberty, and new onset of attentional difficulties after puberty should occasion careful inquiry about the attenuated positive symptoms that characterize prodromal patients. Lastly, when prodromal patients experience intrusive thoughts, they are generally less stereotyped, less unambivalently ego alien, less frequently associated with classic OCD themes such as contagion or inadvertent harm to others, and less often associated with compulsive behavior.

CASE HISTORIES

Prodromal patients can meet criteria for any one prodromal syndrome by itself or any two or all three prodromal syndromes simultaneously. The following disguised case histories are revised from an earlier publication from the authors to illustrate patients meeting each type separately. Each was one of the first 100 patients evaluated in the authors' Prevention through Risk Identification, Management, and Education (PRIME) prodromal research clinic.

CASE ONE: ATTENUATED POSITIVE SYMPTOM SYNDROME

Adrienne was a 15-year-old white girl in the tenth grade who lived with her widowed mother and younger sister. For the 6 months since the start of the school year, she had become increasingly angry, down, and withdrawn from her girlfriends, whom she felt were secretly talking about her disparagingly. Her depressive symptoms prompted her mother, who herself had been treated for depression over the last decade, to seek consultation.

In her evaluation, Adrienne acknowledged worrying that her girlfriends only "pretended" friendship. These concerns occurred approximately once every 2 weeks and were, in hindsight, by her own account, usually mistaken. She also wondered at times if people could read her mind, especially when she was thinking about them, but she also said she must be "crazy" to think this way. She experienced problems understanding schoolwork, rereading texts several times to comprehend meaning. She felt unmotivated, had difficulty completing her work, procrastinated frequently, and suffered a fall in grades from As to Cs in two of her classes. She also felt confusion once or twice a month, during which time she would forget what she was talking about in midconversation.

Adrienne was judged to meet the APSS criteria. The attenuated positive symptoms included unusual thought content (people reading her mind) and suspiciousness (people talking about her negatively). She reported no grandiosity or perceptual abnormalities and displayed no thought disorganization.

Adrienne assented and her mother consented for Adrienne to participate in a placebo-controlled clinical trial. Gradually, over a 5-month period, Adrienne reported an increased severity of some of her symptoms. She withdrew further from her friends and reported perceptual abnormalities in the form of her name being called in the wind or hearing a radio playing music when not turned on. She became increasingly fearful of being attacked sexually by men and refused to shower out of fear that the scene from *Psycho* would be reenacted. This symptom was judged to have crossed into the psychotic range. Despite the symptom severity, however, her everyday life remained the same, and her psychotic symptom was not considered disorganizing or dangerous. Adrienne was judged to have converted to psychotic disorder when the symptom remained prominent more than half the time over the next few weekly assessments. Double-blind medication was stopped, and she was offered and accepted open-label–rescue antipsychotic medication.

CASE TWO: BRIEF INTERMITTENT PSYCHOTIC SYNDROME

Barry was a 17-year-old junior in high school who lived with his parents and younger brother. His parents were first-generation immigrants who met and married in the United States. There was no family history of mental illness. Barry's problems began in the ninth grade when he became depressed and withdrawn and had difficulties concentrating and sleeping for 2 months. The same problems resurfaced in his junior year.

At his initial evaluation, Barry was guarded and affectively constricted. He said there were people who held grudges against him and wanted to beat him up. The week before his evaluation, he avoided two classmates because he thought he heard them calling him queer and felt he was in danger of being attacked. When questioned in detail, he acknowledged that the other two students probably had not called him queer, but he had been sure of it at that moment. Barry had similar experiences four to five other times over the prior 3 months, never lasting more than a few minutes and never leading to confrontation. Barry had mild conceptual disorganization manifest as occasional circumstantial thinking but no other unusual thought content or grandiosity. Functionally, his grades had slipped from Bs to Ds, and he was in danger of having to repeat his junior year.

Barry was judged to meet the BIPS criteria. He had moments of paranoia that were of delusional intensity but not acutely disorganizing or dangerous and too short-lived to meet duration criteria for presence of psychosis.

CASE THREE: GENETIC RISK AND FUNCTIONAL DECLINE PRODROMAL SYNDROME

Cameron was a 16-year-old male junior in high school. He was the youngest of three children. One of his two older sisters had been treated for schizophrenia for 3 years. Cameron had felt depressed for approximately 3 months before his referral and was treated with an antidepressant with moderate success. Nevertheless, he continued to feel tired, to sleep a great deal, to have trouble concentrating, and to have fleeting thoughts about hurting himself. Once in the month before evaluation, when riding in the car with his mother, he became acutely worried that they were being followed by the car behind them. One month before referral, Cameron thought he heard the television playing when it was off. Most striking and problematic were several negative symptoms. Cameron felt unmotivated to do anything other than spend long hours on his computer. This indifference included schoolwork, and he was failing four of his five classes and attending school only approximately 60 percent of the time. He felt uncomfortable around friends and preferred to be alone. He complained of not having feelings when it was normal to have them. Cameron was brought for evaluation by his mother, who was concerned that he was showing symptoms similar to those she had seen before her daughter's psychotic break.

Cameron participated passively in the evaluation. He acknowledged depression and negative symptoms. His mother indicated he "seemed to have two minds" about these. On the one hand, he acknowledged concern and kept promising to begin engaging in activities "tomorrow." On the other hand, he never did. Cameron discounted his concern about having been followed as a product of his imagination.

Most striking were the number and strength of Cameron's negative symptoms and his concomitant deterioration in functioning both academic and socially. His Global Assessment of Functioning score was judged to have fallen 40 points in the past year. This functional decline plus the family history of schizophrenia in a first-degree relative satisfied the Genetic Risk and Functional Decline Prodromal Syndrome. His positive symptoms appeared either too mild or too infrequent to meet APSS or BIPS criteria.

COURSE AND PROGNOSIS

Diagnostic criteria for the schizophrenia prodrome based on the patient's presenting symptoms (Table 12.17–1) have been highly predictive of the development of psychosis within the next 12 months in studies published by two groups. Criteria developed by Patrick McGorry and colleagues in Melbourne, Australia, have shown a prospective risk of conversion or PPV of 40.8 percent within the first 12 months in 49 prodromal patients. Similar criteria used by the authors at the PRIME Clinic in New Haven have shown a prospective risk of conversion of 50 percent within the first 12 months in 14 prodromal patients who received no specific treatment (Fig. 12.17–3). Moreover, none of 20 patients diagnosed as nonprodromal converted. Unpublished data from the authors' clinical trial revealed that, of 29 prodromal patients randomly assigned to placebo, 13 became psychotic within 2 years (44.8 percent), six completed 2 years without converting to psychosis, and ten dropped out so that outcome at 2 years is unknown. Among patients with known 2-year outcomes, 13 of 19 became psychotic (68.4 percent). Three conversions occurred in the first month, two each in months 2, 3, and 5, and one each in months 8, 10, 14, and 24.

A conversion to psychosis rate of 40 percent or more has been considered high enough to indicate beginning preventive intervention studies in prodromal patients. These studies have targeted improvement in the patients' current symptoms, as well as the prevention of schizophrenia.

It must be emphasized that, although current prodromal diagnostic criteria have a high PPV for the development of psychosis, they do make some false-positive diagnoses. The precise extent of false-positive diagnoses will not be known until large numbers of patients are followed for substantially longer than 1 year. Expected sources of false positives include subjects with new-onset schizotypal personality disorder that then remains stable over time and Axis I conditions such as bipolar disorder, major depression, or OCD. In the Melbourne sample described above, the 12-month outcomes were described as "no diagnosis" in 24 percent and "nonpsychotic Axis I diagnosis" in 31 percent. In the authors' sample described above, most of the patients who did not progress to schizophrenia remained prodromal, and the prodromal symptoms remitted by 12 months in only a few (Fig. 12.17–3). Depending on how the diagnostic criteria are used, some of the nonpsychotic outcomes may represent *false false positives*, meaning cases of illness that would be useful to detect. However, a proportion of the prodromal patients at the time of initial diagnosis may be undergoing "transient emotional turmoil" that will remit spontaneously. These last cases would clearly be *true false positives*.

Prodromal diagnostic criteria must surely also produce some false-negative diagnoses. Thus far in the authors' experience, however, no cases initially not meeting the prodromal diagnostic criteria have progressed to psychosis within the next year (Fig. 12.17–3). Interestingly, however, several such patients have subsequently progressed to the point of meeting prodromal criteria (Fig. 12.17–3).

		OUTCOME			
		Psychotic	Prodromal	Not	
SIPS	Prodromal	7	5	2	14
	Not	0	2	18	20
		7	7	20	34

FIGURE 12.17–3 Outcome at 12 months among untreated patients meeting and not meeting prodromal diagnostic criteria as determined by the Structured Interview for Prodromal Syndromes (SIPS) used by the authors at the Prevention through Risk Identification, Management, and Education (PRIME) Clinic in New Haven. Among the patients initially diagnosed as prodromal, 50 percent (7 out of 14) progressed to schizophrenic psychosis within 12 months. Most of the initially prodromal patients who did not progress to psychosis remained prodromal (five out of seven), and the prodromal symptoms remitted by 12 months in only two. None of patients diagnosed as nonprodromal progressed to psychosis. Two (of 20) such patients have subsequently progressed to the point of newly meeting prodromal criteria. Patients who do not initially meet full criteria should be asked to return if symptoms worsen. If psychotic versus not psychotic within 12 months is considered the relevant binary categorical outcome, the sensitivity of the criteria as implemented with the SIPS is 100 percent, specificity is 74 percent, and PPV is 50 percent.

Thus, it is important to emphasize that current prodromal diagnostic criteria are not designed to identify all patients who are truly prodromal, but rather those prodromal patients who are at imminent risk for progression to psychosis. Patients who do not initially meet full criteria should be asked to return if symptoms worsen.

As mentioned earlier, recent studies that attempted to predict schizophrenia onset over a longer, 10-year period reported predictive signs and symptoms that may have been observed in some of their subjects during the prodromal phase. These signs and symptoms included social deficits and deficits in organizational ability and intellectual functioning; self-perceived cognitive deficits, including perceptual abnormalities similar to those described just above; and perceptual aberrations, magical ideation, and social anhedonia.

Prodromal patients who progress to psychosis (the true-positive cases) during careful monitoring may be said to have experienced onset of first-episode psychosis with zero DUP. Relatively little is known about the course of treated illness in such patients, but the authors' small case series suggests that hospitalization is only rarely needed and that remissions of high functional quality are the rule, at least over the short term.

TREATMENT

Only two controlled studies addressing treatment needs of prodromal patients have been completed. Both studies have evaluated treatment with newer atypical antipsychotic medications. Part of the rationale for beginning such prodromal intervention studies included the perception that the risks of using antipsychotic medications appeared to have been reduced with the advent of the new agents.

The first trial, from Melbourne, randomized prodromal patients to open-label risperidone (Risperdal) plus usual care (N = 31), versus usual care alone (N = 28). Risperidone-treated patients received cognitive therapy concomitantly, but usual-care patients did not. Six-month conversion to psychosis rates were 9.7 percent for the risperidone and cognitive therapy treatment and 35.7 percent for usual care ($P < .05$). Risperidone was discontinued after 6 months, and patients were followed for another 6 months. Some patients in whom medication had been discontinued went on to convert to psychosis during the medication-free follow-up interval. The study used an open-label design and assessed severity of illness at fixed 6-month intervals, often when patients were no longer receiving the treatment to which they were randomized. Perhaps as a consequence, although the randomized groups in the previous study differed on rates of conversion to psychosis over 6 months, no significant differences were observed on severity of illness ratings. The results of this study provide strong support for the ability of an atypical antipsychotic medication to prevent progression to psychosis among prodromal patients. The observation that patients randomized to risperidone converted to psychosis after risperidone was discontinued suggests the need for studies of longer-term medication administration. Because the medication and cognitive therapy were bundled together in this study, it is not possible to ascribe the beneficial effects observed separately to risperidone, separately to cognitive therapy, or to a combination effect of the two treatments. Because the risperidone was prescribed in open-label fashion, the contribution of placebo effects to the benefit observed also cannot be estimated.

The authors have conducted a double-blind, placebo-controlled trial of olanzapine (Zyprexa) in 60 prodromal patients. Patients were to continue under random assignment for 1 year. Individual and family psychosocial interventions with supportive and psychoeducational components were available to each patient in both arms of the trial. Analyses of the first 8 weeks of treatment focusing on symptomatic improvement were conducted. The main finding was that patients randomized to olanzapine improved to a significantly greater degree over an 8-week period than did patients randomized to placebo on the SOPS prodromal rating scale. Olanzapine-treated patients gained significantly more weight, but other safety results, including EPS ratings, were generally similar in the olanzapine and placebo groups. Longer-term analyses are under way.

FUTURE DIRECTIONS

Prodromal patients are not only at high risk of conversion to psychosis in the near term, but they are also symptomatic, functionally impaired, and treatment seeking. As many as several hundred thousand patients may become prodromal worldwide each year. Currently, relatively little is known about the overall balance between the benefits and risks that medication treatment brings to prodromal patients, and, thus, continued treatment research is critically needed to guide clinical practice for these individuals. This treatment research must proceed with careful attention to study design and risks and benefits of the design for participants, along with careful attention to informed consent and decisional capacity in these patients and their families and to stigma potentially associated with treatment or untreated symptoms. If data supportive of short-term antipsychotic treatment for prodromal patients continue to emerge, the next important studies will need to investigate optimal duration of treatment.

Simultaneously, several other research agendas related to prodromal patients should also receive attention, including research aimed at improving the predictive power of current diagnostic criteria for the prodrome. Several other domains of measurement have the potential to improve diagnostic efficiency for prodromal patients, including assessment of negative symptoms, structural and functional brain imaging, neuropsychological testing, electrophysiology studies, and genetic studies. The potential influence of diagnostic comorbidity at first identification of the prodrome should also be better studied.

It is possible that medication treatments that are only somewhat effective or even ineffective in patients who have developed chronic schizophrenia may be quite useful in the early stages of illness. Thus, future studies should look beyond antipsychotic medications to test potential treatments that target theoretical mechanisms that may underlie early progression of illness. Neurobiological processes that may account in part for early progression of schizophrenic illness could include excessive oxidative stress and hypofunction of the *N*-methyl-D-aspartate (NMDA) subtype of glutamate receptors, or both. Potential drug treatments that may be beneficial for prodromal or early first-episode patients based on these mechanisms of action include vitamins E and C, selenium, fatty acid supplementation, antioxidant medications, lamotrigine (Lamictal), GABAergic agonists, α_2-adrenergic agonists, serotonin-2A receptor agonists, and glycine agonists. Each of these strategies deserve clinical trials in prodromal or early first-episode patients.

Lastly, if, after onset, long DUP predisposes the patient with schizophrenia to follow a course of chronic disability, then long DUP in first-episode patients is a public health problem of the first magnitude. Recent work confirming that DUP can be reduced paves the way for increasing implementation of early-detection programs within routine clinical service systems. Early-detection programs aimed at reducing DUP in first-episode patients also will detect prodromal cases. Even if prodromal intervention research does not continue to support the value of early intervention in the prodromal phase, longitudinal monitoring of prodromal patients offers what may be the best route to minimizing DUP. Those prodromal patients who progress to psychosis during monitoring can then be treated with virtually zero DUP. Early-detection programs within the clinical service delivery system then offer opportunities for services research to determine whether improved long-term patient outcomes and societal cost savings from prevented hospitalizations and foregone disability pensions result.

SUGGESTED CROSS-REFERENCES

The reader is encouraged to refer to the sections on electrophysiology studies (Section 1.14), neuropsychological testing (Section 2.1), medical assessment and laboratory testing (Section 7.8), epidemiology of schizophrenia (Section 12.4), structural and functional brain imaging in schizophrenia (Section 12.6), genetics of schizophrenia (Section 12.3), clinical features of schizophrenia (Section 12.8), clinical features of mood disorders (Section 13.6), obsessive-compulsive disorder (Chapter 8), personality disorders (Chapter 23), and attention-deficit disorder (Chapter 39).

REFERENCES

Aleman A, Kahn RS, Selten JP: Sex differences in the risk of schizophrenia: Evidence from metaanalysis. *Arch Gen Psychiatry*. 2003;60:565.

Bleuler E. *Dementia Praecox or the Group of the Schizophrenias*. New York: International Universities Press; 1911.

Chapman LJ, Chapman JP, Kwapil TR, Eckblad M, Zinser MC: Putatively psychosis-prone subjects 10 years later. *J Abnorm Psychol*. 1994;103:171.

Davidson L, McGlashan TH: The varied outcomes of schizophrenia. *Can J Psychiatry*. 1997;42:34.

Davidson M, Reichenberg A, Rabinowitz J, Weiser M, Kaplan Z, Mark M: Behavioral and intellectual markers for schizophrenia in apparently healthy male adolescents. *Am J Psychiatry*. 1999;156:1328.

Hafner H, Maurer K, Loffler W, Fatkenheuer B, an der Heiden W, Riecher-Rossler A, Behrens S, Gattaz WF: The epidemiology of early schizophrenia. Influence of age and gender on onset and early course. *Br J Psychiatry Suppl*. 1994;23:29–38.

Harrison PJ: The neuropathology of schizophrenia. A critical review of the data and their interpretation. *Brain*. 1999;122:593.

Heinrichs RW. *In Search of Madness: Schizophrenia and Neuroscience*. Oxford, U.K.: Oxford University Press; 2001.

Jones P, Rodgers B, Murray TM, Marmot M: Child development risk factors for adult schizophrenia in the British 1946 birth cohort. *Lancet*. 1994;3:1398.

Kenny JT, Freedman L. Cognitive impairment in early stage schizophrenia. In: Zipursky RB, Schulz SC, eds. *The Early Stages of Schizophrenia*. Washington, DC: American Psychiatric Publishing, Inc.; 2002.

Klosterkotter J, Hellmich M, Steinmeyer EM, Schultze-Lutter F: Diagnosing schizophrenia in the initial prodromal phase. *Arch Gen Psychiatry*. 2001;58:158.

*Larsen TK, McGlashan TH, Johannessen JO, Friis S, Guldberg C, Haahr U, Horneland M, Melle I, Moe LC, Opjordsmoen S, Simonsen E, Vaglum P: Shortened duration of untreated first episode of psychosis: Changes in patient characteristics at treatment. *Am J Psychiatry*. 2001;158:1917.

Lieberman JA, Perkins D, Belger A, Chakos M, Jarskog F, Boteva K, Gilmore J: The early stages of schizophrenia: Speculations on pathogenesis, pathophysiology, and therapeutic approaches. *Biol Psychiatry*. 2001;50:884.

Mathalon DH, Sullivan EV, Lim KO, Pfefferbaum A: Progressive brain volume changes and the clinical course of schizophrenia in men: A longitudinal magnetic resonance imaging study. *Arch Gen Psychiatry*. 2001;58:148.

McGlashan TH: Duration of untreated psychosis in first-episode schizophrenia: Marker or determinant of course? *Biol Psychiatry*. 1999;46:899–907.

McGlashan TH, Miller TJ, Woods SW. A scale for the assessment of prodromal symptoms and states. In: Miller TJ, Mednick SA, McGlashan TH, Libiger J, Johannessen JO, eds. *Early Intervention in Psychotic Disorders*. The Netherlands: Kluwer Academic Publishers; 2001.

McGlashan TH, Zipursky RB, Perkins DO, Addington J, Miller TJ, Woods SW, Hawkins KA, Hoffman R, David S, Tohen M, Breier A: A randomized double blind clinical trial of olanzapine vs. placebo in patients at risk for being prodromally symptomatic for psychosis. I. Study rationale and design. *Schizophr Res*. 2003;61:7–18.

McGorry PD, Edwards J, Mihalopoulos C, Harrigan SM, Jackson HJ: EPPIC: An evolving system of early detection and optimal management. *Schizophr Bull*. 1996;22:305.

*McGorry PD, Yung AF, Phillips LJ, Yuen HP, Francey S, Cosgrave EM, Germano D, Bravin J, Adlard S, McDonald T, Blair A, Adlard S, Jackson H: Randomized controlled trial of interventions designed to reduce the risk of progression to first-episode psychosis in a clinical sample with subthreshold symptoms. *Arch Gen Psychiatry*. 2002;59:921.

Miller TJ, McGlashan TH, Rosen JL, Cadenhead K, Ventura J, Cannon TD, McFarlane W, Perkins DO, Pearlson GD, Woods SW: Prodromal assessment with the Structured Interview for Prodromal Syndromes and the Scale of Prodromal Symptoms: Predictive validity, inter-rater reliability, and training to reliability. *Schiz Bull*. 2003;29:703.

Miller TJ, McGlashan TH, Rosen JL, Somjee L, Markovitch P, Stein K, Woods SW: Prospective diagnosis of the prodrome for schizophrenia: Preliminary evidence of interrater reliability and predictive validity using operational criteria and a structured interview. *Am J Psychiatry*. 2002;159:863.

Miller TJ, Woods SW, Rosen JL, McGlashan TH: Treatment of psychosis at onset. *Am J Psychiatry*. 2002;159:153.

Miller TJ, Zipursky RB, Perkins DO, Addington J, Woods SW, Hawkins KA, Hoffman R, Preda A, Epstein I, Addington D, Lindborg S, Tohen M, Breier A, McGlashan TH: A randomized double blind clinical trial of olanzapine vs. placebo in patients at risk for being prodromally symptomatic for psychosis. II. Recruitment and baseline characteristics of the "prodromal" sample. *Schizophr Res*. 2003;61:19–30.

Mrazek PJ, Haggerty RJ, eds. *Reducing Risks for Mental Disorders: Frontiers for Preventive Intervention Research*. Washington, DC: National Academy Press; 1994.

Olin SC, Mednick SA: Risk factors of psychosis: Identifying vulnerable populations premorbidly. *Schizophr Bull*. 1996;22:223.

*Pantelis C, Velakoulis D, McGorry PD, Wood SJ, Suckling J, Phillips LJ, Yung AR, Bullmore ET, Brewer W, Soulsby B, Desmond P, McGuire PK: Neuroanatomical abnormalities before and after onset of psychosis: A cross-sectional and longitudinal MRI comparison. *Lancet*. 2003;361:281.

Preda A, Miller TJ, Rosen JL, Somjee L, McGlashan TH, Woods SW: Treatment histories of patients with a syndrome putatively prodromal for schizophrenia. *Psychiatr Serv*. 2002;53:342.

*Woods SW, Breier A, Zipursky RB, Perkins DO, Addington J, Miller TJ, Hawkins KA, Marquez E, David SR, Tohen M, McGlashan TH: Randomized trial of olanzapine vs. placebo in the symptomatic acute treatment of patients meeting criteria for the schizophrenic prodrome. *Biol Psychiatry*. 2003;54:453.

Woods SW, Miller TJ, McGlashan TH: The prodromal patient: Both symptomatic and at risk. *CNS Spectrums*. 2001;6:223.

Wright IC, Rabe-Hesketh S, Woodruff PW, David AS, Murray RM, Bullmore ET: Meta-analysis of regional brain volumes in schizophrenia. *Am J Psychiatry*. 2000;157:16.

Yung AR, McGorry PD: The prodromal phase of first-episode psychosis: Past and current conceptualizations. *Schizophr Bull*. 1996;22:353.

Yung AR, Phillips LJ, McGorry PD, McFarlane CA, Francey S, Harrigan S, Patton GC, Jackson HJ: Prediction of psychosis. A step towards indicated prevention of schizophrenia. *Br J Psychiatry*. 1998;172:14.

*Yung AR, Phillips LJ, Yuen HP, Francey SM, McFarlane CA, Hallgren M, McGorry PD: Psychosis prediction: 12-Month follow up of a high-risk ("prodromal") group. *Schizophr Res*. 2003;60:21.

13 Mood Disorders

▲ 13.1 Mood Disorders: Historical Introduction and Conceptual Overview

HAGOP S. AKISKAL, M.D.

CLINICAL AND PUBLIC HEALTH SCOPE OF MOOD DISORDERS

Prevalence For nearly 2,500 years, mood disorders have been described as one of the most common illnesses of humankind, but only recently have they commanded major public health interest. The World Health Organization (WHO) has ranked depression fourth in a list of the most urgent health problems worldwide. The U.S. Agency for Health Care Policy and Research, a federal agency concerned with medical practice from a public health perspective, devoted two volumes to depression out of the first ten it has published on such topics as pain, hypertension, diabetes mellitus, and coronary artery disease. University of California psychiatrist Kenneth Wells demonstrated that the disability induced by depression compares with and often exceeds those of such diseases. Moreover, there are now data from several sources indicating that the morbidity and mortality from many of these diseases are increased with depressive comorbidity.

Depressive disorders afflict one out of five women and one out of ten men at some time during their lives. Depressive episodes alternating with mania or hypomania represent the domain of bipolar disorders. Increasingly, the conventional figure of 1 percent for bipolar disorders in the general population is challenged, and there are now convincing data that this group of disorders may account for 5 percent of the population and up to 50 percent of all depressions. The enlargement of the boundaries for bipolar disorder is largely due to better detection of the bipolar II subtype (depression plus hypomania rather than mania). The current evidence for and the clinical, therapeutic, and public health implications of such a broadened bipolar concept have been summarized in a World Psychiatric Association monograph.

Despite the availability of effective treatments, many persons with mood disorders are disabled, and rates of suicide (which occurs in approximately 15 percent of depressive patients, especially in those with bipolar II disorder) are high in young and, particularly, elderly men. Although depressive disorders are more common in women, more men than women die of suicide. High-profile cases of infanticide recently publicized on television have brought into the public's awareness the role of the reproductive cycle in severe postpartum psychosis and, more generally, the high burden of all forms of depression in women.

The suboptimal outcome of mood disorders documented in recent research reports cannot be ascribed to underdiagnosis and undertreatment alone for several reasons. First, Gerald Klerman and colleagues have suggested that the incidence of mood disorders may be increasing in younger age groups, especially in cohorts born in the 1960s, and may be associated with rising rates of alcohol and substance abuse. Second, mood disorders, once believed to be essentially adult disorders, are increasingly diagnosed in children and adolescents. Third, clinical studies suggest higher rates of chronicity, recurrence, and refractoriness than previously believed. For instance, chronicity, reported by Emil Kraepelin to occur in no more than 5 percent in the early 20th century in Germany, is now seen in varying degrees in one out of three affectively ill patients. Nonetheless, outcome studies coming from university centers tend to overestimate the proportion of cases with less favorable prognosis, and, undeniably, many patients seen in private practice experience a favorable outcome. Also, not unexpectedly, current data indicate that depressed patients treated by psychiatrists in private settings receive much better care than those in other settings.

Concepts of Mood Disorders In the European tradition, the broader rubric of *affective disorder* (which subsumes mood and anxiety disorders) has been conceptualized along two influential schools. Aubrey Lewis and his followers from the Maudsley school have promoted a continuum model—from anxiety disorders to mild neurotic depressions to severe endogenous and psychotic depressions. The Newcastle school, led by Martin Roth, has sharply demarcated those conditions from one another. Although vestiges of both approaches are still influential in clinical and basic research, their significance is presently overshadowed by European studies in Germanophone countries that subdivide mood disorders on the basis of polarity: unipolar (depressive episodes only) and bipolar (depressive episodes plus manic, hypomanic, or mixed episodes). That subdivision, in part supported by studies in the United States, has served as the basis for much recent research into the biology, treatment, and classification of mood disorders, and is reflected in the fourth edition of the *Diagnostic and Statistical Manual of Mental Disorders* (DSM-IV-TR) and the tenth revision of the *International Statistical Classification of Diseases and Related Health Problems* (ICD-10). Despite such official sanction, many authorities today continue to see considerable continuity between recurrent depressive and bipolar disorders. This has led to widespread discussion and debate about the bipolar spectrum, which incorporates classic bipolar disorder, bipolar II, and recurrent depressions.

Emerging data also tend to favor a continuum between juvenile and adult mood disorders. This is based on the pioneering contributions by Elva Poznanski at the University of Michigan, as well as the work of Leon Cytrin and colleagues at the National Institute of Mental Health (NIMH), Gabrielle Carlson in collaboration with Dennis Cantwell at the University of California at Los Angeles, and Joachim Puig-Antich at Columbia University in New York.

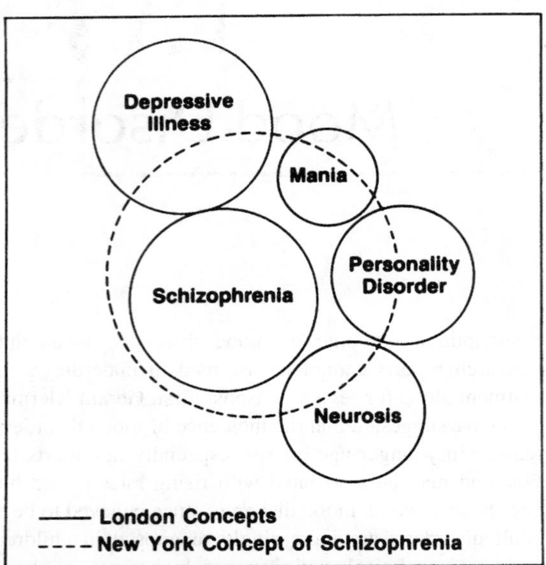

FIGURE 13.1–1 Comparison of British (London) and U.S. (New York) concepts of schizophrenia. (Adapted from Cooper JE, Kendell RE, Garland BJ, et al. *Psychiatric Diagnosis in New York and London*. London: Oxford University Press; 1972.)

Childhood bipolarity, too, is receiving increasing clinical attention, thanks to the seminal work of Elizabeth Weller and colleagues, originally conducted at Ohio State University. In addition, clinical observations at the University of Tennessee by the present author on the juvenile offspring of adult patients with bipolar disorder have led to a greater appreciation of the bipolar nature of complex clinical presentations of affective illness in the juvenile offspring and kin of adult bipolar probands. More recent work by Biederman's group at Harvard suggests intriguing links between pediatric bipolar disorder and attention-deficit/hyperactivity disorder (ADHD).

Current concepts of mood disorders in the United States embrace a wide spectrum, including many conditions previously diagnosed as schizophrenia, personality disorder, or neurosis. The diagnostic shift occurred in part as a result of the U.S.–U.K. Diagnostic Project, which demonstrated that schizophrenia was being diagnosed at the expense of mood disorders (Fig. 13.1–1). Conceptual boundaries were further broadened by the availability of new and effective treatments and by the unacceptable risk for tardive dyskinesia and suicide in persons with misdiagnosed mood disorders. More generally, present research interest in mood disorders in the United States emanated from a landmark 1969 NIMH conference on the psychobiology of affective illnesses: The NIMH Collaborative Depression Study—a long-term prospective project deriving directly from recommendations made at the conference—has legitimatized the broader perspective.

Morbidity and Mortality

Unfortunately, findings published by Martin Keller and colleagues in the 1980s documenting gross undertreatment of mood disorders continue to describe the current treatment landscape worldwide. Whatever changes have occurred in diagnostic practice do not appear to have significantly affected the morbidity and mortality of mood disorders. This is all the more scandalous because the 1990s have seen new classes of user-friendly antidepressant and mood-stabilizing agents, as well as depression-specific psychotherapies. In the author's opinion, this state of affairs results, in part, from the fact that clinical exposure to mood disorders in both specialized (psychiatric) and primary care (general medical) training is suboptimal. Mood disorders, as highly prevalent and lethal disorders, must command a greater share in the clinical curriculum of both psychiatrists and general medical practitioners. As most mood disorders are chronically relapsing conditions, long-term exposure to patients with these disorders in mood or bipolar clinics should be obligatory training for young doctors. Unfortunately, few academic centers have such clinics, and those that exist are largely devoted to research. The primary goal of these clinics is the execution of research protocols rather than gaining clinical experience in caring for such patients.

Nearly half of all cases of depression, just like those with adult-onset diabetes, remain undetected for years or inadequately controlled—both of which seem to lag behind hypertension, in which early detection and treatment have significantly reduced complications such as stroke. Efforts by patient-advocacy organizations—often in concert with national psychiatric organizations and governmental mental health agencies—appear to be increasing public and government awareness of mood disorders. Ultimately, however, the challenge is to provide all primary care physicians with the requisite hands-on experience in this prevalent group of disorders. User-friendly tools to detect suicidal patients in the general medical sector would further enhance preventive efforts. These would require significant changes in the structure of health care, including, but not limited to, the greater participation of nurses and social workers as liaisons in primary mental health and continuity of care for depressed or suicidal patients.

Because mood disorders underlie 50 to 70 percent of all suicides, effective treatment of these disorders on a national level should, in principle, drastically reduce this major complication of mood disorders. That elderly depressed patients, often with medical comorbidity, constitute the highest risk group for suicide yet escape clinical detection and treatment is particularly problematic for public health. A small-scale Swedish study undertaken by Rihmer and Rutz, although not specifically targeted to the elderly, has yielded promising results in this regard. In addition, clinical findings in recurrent mood disorders have clearly shown the value of lithium prophylaxis in the prevention of suicide and overall mortality. Emerging data suggest that such benefits may accrue from all efficacious treatments for mood disorders.

DEFINITIONS

Mood disorders encompass a large group of psychiatric disorders in which pathological moods and related vegetative and psychomotor disturbances dominate the clinical picture. Known in previous editions of DSM as *affective disorders*, the term *mood disorders* is preferred today because it refers to sustained emotional states, not merely to the external (affective) expression of the present emotional state. Mood disorders are best considered as syndromes (rather than discrete diseases) consisting of a cluster of signs and symptoms, sustained over a period of weeks to months, that represent a marked departure from a person's habitual functioning and tend to recur, often in periodic or cyclical fashion.

Major Depressive Disorder and Bipolar Disorder

Major depressive disorder (unipolar depression) is reported to be the most common mood disorder. It may manifest as a single episode or as recurrent episodes. The course may be somewhat protracted—up to 2 years or longer—in those with the single-episode form. Whereas the prognosis for recovery from an acute episode is good for most patients with major depressive disorder, three out of four patients experience recurrences throughout life, with varying degrees of residual symptoms between episodes. *Bipolar disorders* (previously called *manic-depressive psychosis*) consist of at least one hypomanic, manic, or mixed episode. *Mixed episodes* represent a simultaneous mixture of depressive and manic or hypomanic manifestations. Although a minority of patients experience only manic episodes, most bipolar disorder patients experience episodes of both polarity. Manias predominate in men, depression and mixed states in women. The bipolar disorders were classically described as psychotic mood disorders with both manic and major depressive episodes (now termed *bipolar I disorder*), but recent clinical studies have shown the existence of a spectrum of ambulatory depressive states that alternate with milder, short-lived periods of hypomania rather than full-blown mania (bipolar II disorder). Bipolar II disorder, which is not always easily discernible from recurrent major depressive disorder, illustrates the need for more research to elucidate the relation between bipolar disorder and major depressive disorder.

Dysthymia and Cyclothymia

Clinically, major depressive episodes often arise from a low-grade, intermittent, and protracted depressive substrate known as *dysthymic disorder*. Likewise, many instances of bipolar disorders, especially ambulatory forms, represent episodes of mood disorder superimposed on a cyclothymic background, which is a biphasic alternating pattern of numerous brief periods of hypomania and numerous brief periods of depression. Dysthymic and cyclothymic disorders represent the two prevalent subthreshold mood conditions roughly corresponding to the basic temperamental dysregulations described by Kraepelin and Ernst Kretschmer as predisposing to affective illness.

It is not always easy to demarcate full-blown syndromal episodes of depression and mania from their subthreshold counterparts commonly observed during the interepisodic periods. The subthreshold conditions appear to be fertile terrain for interpersonal conflicts and postaffective pathological character developments that may ravage the lives of patients and their families. In North America—and some Western European countries—many such patients end up being labeled with *borderline personality disorder*, which, unfortunately, often tends to obscure the affective origin of the presenting psychopathology.

Cyclothymic and dysthymic conditions also exist in the community without progression to full-blown mood episodes. As such, they are best considered, respectively, as trait bipolar and trait depressive conditions. Understanding the factors that mediate transition from trait to clinical state is important for preventing manic and major depressive episodes.

Other Subthreshold Mood States

Epidemiological studies in both Europe and North America have also revealed other subsyndromal conditions with depressive and hypomanic manifestations with few symptoms (oligosymptomatic mood states) and of short duration (brief episodes). Variously referred to as *minor*, *subsyndromal*, *brief*, or *intermittent*, these descriptions do not merely represent arbitrary lowering of diagnostic thresholds, but herald increasing realization of their importance in early detection of at-risk individuals—as has happened in other medical fields (e.g., diabetes mellitus and essential hypertension). If disabling mood disorders afflict 5 to 8 percent of the general population (Epidemiologic Catchment Area [ECA] study), milder but still clinically significant mood disorders would raise lifetime rates to 17 percent (National Comorbidity Study [NCS]); if subclinical mood states are added, that figure doubles to involve a third of the general population (as reported, for instance, by Kenneth Kendler and colleagues). New evidence from both Europe and the United States has shown that bipolar spectrum conditions (bipolar I, bipolar II, and bipolar disorder not otherwise specified [NOS] in formal diagnostic manuals such as DSM-IV-TR and ICD-10) may account for at least 50 percent of all mood disorders in the community and in psychiatric practice.

Comorbidity in mood disorders involves considerable overlap with anxiety disorders. As summarized in an NIMH monograph, anxiety disorders can occur during an episode of depression, may be a precursor to the depressive episode, and, less commonly, may occur during the future course of a mood disorder. Those findings suggest that at least some depressive disorders share a common diathesis with certain anxiety disorders. More recent clinical experience suggests intriguing comorbidity patterns between bipolar II disorder on one hand and panic, obsessive-compulsive, and social phobic states on the other. Furthermore, bipolar I and II disorders are particularly likely to be complicated by use of alcohol, stimulants, or both. In many cases, the alcohol or substance abuse represents attempts at "self-treatment" of the depression and associated anxiety or insomnia (or both) and, in the case of mania and hypomania, attempts to maintain or enhance the positive moods and energy. Finally, physical illness—both systemic and cerebral—occurs in association with depressive disorders with a greater frequency than expected by chance alone. Unless properly treated, such depression negatively impacts the prognosis of the physical disorder. More provocatively, there is current reawakening in the contribution of cerebral and cardiovascular factors to the origin of late-onset psychotic depressions (previously classified as *involutional melancholia*).

An integrated framework of pathogenesis is necessary for understanding psychopharmacological, somatic, and psychotherapeutic approaches in the clinical management of patients with mood disorders. A historical perspective on current developments is also a valuable lesson in the study of mood disorders.

GRECO-ROMAN DESCRIPTIONS

Much of what is known today about mood disorders was described by the ancient Greeks and Romans, who coined the terms *melancholia* and *mania* and noted their relation. The ancients also hypothesized a temperamental origin for those disorders. Much of modern thinking about mood disorders (e.g., the work of French and German schools in the middle and latter part of the 19th century, which influenced current British and American concepts) can be traced back to these ancient concepts.

Melancholia

Hippocrates (460 to 357 BC) described melancholia ("black bile") as a state of "aversion to food, despondency, sleeplessness, irritability, and restlessness." Thus, in choosing the name of the condition, Greek physicians (who may have borrowed the concept from ancient Egyptians) postulated the earliest biochemical formulation of any mental disorder. They believed that the illness often arose from the substrate of the somber melancholic temperament, which, under the influence of the planet Saturn, made the spleen secrete black bile, ultimately leading to mood darkening through its influence on the brain. Greek descriptions of the clinical manifestations of depression and of the temperament prone to melancholia are reflected in the DSM-IV-TR in the subdepressive lethargy, self-denigration, and habitual gloom of the person with dysthymic disorder.

One Hippocratic aphorism recognized the close link between anxiety and depressive states: "Patients with fear of long-standing are subject to melancholia." Hippocrates, who described the first historical case of melancholia, may have also been the first to describe a depressive mixed state, an activated form of depression:

A woman of Thasos became morose because of a justifiable grief, and although she did not take to her bed, she suffered from insomnia, loss of appetite . . . she complained of fears and *talked much*; she showed despondency and . . . *talked at random and used foul language*... many intense and continuous pains . . . *she leapt up and could not be restrained* . . . (emphases by author).

According to Galen (131 to 201 AD), melancholia manifested in "fear and depression, discontent with life, and hatred of all persons." A few hundred years later, another Roman, Aurelianus, citing the now-lost works of Soranus of Ephesus, amplified the role of aggression in melancholia (and its link to suicide) and described how the illness assumed delusional coloring: "Animosity toward members of the household, sometimes a desire to live and at other times a longing for death, suspicion on the part of the patient that a plot is being hatched against him."

In addition to natural melancholia, which, presumably, arose from an innate predisposition to overproduce the dark humor and led to a more severe form of the malady, Greco-Roman medicine recognized such environmental contributions to melancholia as immoderate consumption of wine, perturbations of the soul due to the passions (e.g., love), and disturbed sleep cycles. Autumn was considered the season most disposing to melancholy.

Mania A state of raving madness with exalted mood was noted by the ancient Greeks, although it referred to a somewhat broader group of excited psychoses than that in modern nosology. Its relation to melancholia was probably noted as early as the first century BC, but, according to Aurelianus, Soranus discounted it. Nonetheless, Soranus had observed the coexistence of manic and melancholic features during the same episode, consisting of continual wakefulness and fluctuating states of anger and merriment and, sometimes, of sadness and futility. Thus, Soranus seemed to have described what today are called *mixed episodes* in DSM-IV-TR and ICD-10. Natural melancholy was generally considered a chronic disorder, but Soranus noted the tendency for attacks to alternate with periods of remission.

Although others before him hinted at it, Aretaeus of Cappadocia (circa 150 AD) is generally credited with making the connection between the two major mood states: "It appears to me that melancholy is the commencement and a part of mania." He described the cardinal manifestations of mania as it is known today:

> There are infinite forms of mania, but the disease is one of them. If mania is associated with joy, the patient may laugh, play, dance night and day, and go to the market crowned as if a victor in some contest of skill. The ideas the patients have are infinite. They believe they are experts in astronomy, philosophy, or poetry.

Aretaeus described the extreme psychotic excitement that could complicate the foregoing clinical picture of mania:

> The patient may become excitable, suspicious, and irritable; hearing may become sharp. . .[and they might] get noises and buzzing in the ears; or may have visual hallucinations; bad dreams and his sexual desires may get uncontrollable; aroused to anger, he may become wholly mad and run unrestrainedly, roar aloud; kill his keepers, and lay violent hands upon himself.

Noting the fluctuating nature of symptoms in the affectively ill, Aretaeus commented: "They are prone to change their mind readily; to become base, mean-spirited, illiberal, and in a little time extravagant, munificent, not from any virtue of the soul, but from the changeableness of the disease." Aretaeus was thus keenly aware of the characterological distortions so commonly manifested during the different phases of cyclical mood disorders.

Finally, consolidating the knowledge of several centuries, Aretaeus described mania as a disease of adolescent and young men given intermittently to "active habits, drunkenness, lechery" and an immoderate lifestyle (what today might be called *cyclothymic disorder*). Exacerbations were most likely to occur in the spring.

Affective Temperaments The concept of health and disease in Greco-Roman medicine was based on harmony and balance of the four humors, of which sanguine humor was deemed the healthiest. But even a desirable humor such as blood, which made persons habitually active, amiable, and prone to jest, could, in excess, lead to the pathological state of mania. The melancholic temperament, dominated by black bile and predisposed to pathological melancholia, was described as lethargic, sullen, and given to brooding or contemplation; its modern counterparts are depressive personality disorder (now in a DSM-IV-TR appendix) and its clinical expression as dysthymic disorder (included in both ICD-10 and DSM-IV-TR). A long tradition dating back to Aristotle (384 to 322 BC) attributed creative qualities to the otherwise tortured melancholic temperament in such fields as philosophy, the arts, poetry, and politics. The remaining two temperaments, choleric and phlegmatic, were less desirable, as yellow bile made persons choleric (irritable, hostile, and given to rage) and phlegm made them phlegmatic (indolent, irresolute, and timid). The choleric and phlegmatic temperaments would probably be recognized today as borderline personality disorder and avoidant or schizoid personality disorder, respectively.

Many of the original Greek texts on melancholia were transmitted to posterity through medieval Arabic texts such as those of Ishaq Ibn Imran and Avicenna (and their Latin rendition by Constantinus Africanus). In describing different affective states, Avicenna developed the theory of the temperaments to its fullest. He speculated that a special form of melancholia supervened "if black bile be mixed with phlegm" when the illness was "coupled with inertia, lack of movement, and quiet." Further, mania was not necessarily linked to the sanguine (what today is termed *hyperthymic*) temperament, as many forms of excited madness were believed to represent a mixture of black and yellow bile.

Avicenna further observed that the mixture of anger and restlessness in melancholia indicated that the disease was manic in nature and that the appearance of such signs and symptoms along with violence heralded the transition from melancholia to mania. Avicenna was prescient in this respect, because these activated, irritable depressions with racing thoughts have yet to receive the DSM-IV-TR "blessing" for being classified as bipolar mixed states. Those elaborations on Galen's temperamental types might be considered the forerunners of current personality dimensions, deriving mood states from various mixtures of neuroticism and introversion-extroversion. (What both ICD-10 and DSM-IV-TR describe as *cyclothymic disorder* represents the intense mood lability of high neuroticism coupled with cyclic alternation between extroversion and introversion.) Speculation on how diverse depressive phenomena could be understood as a mix of humors anticipated modern multiple-transmitter hypotheses of depression. Ishaq Ibn Imran summarized the existing knowledge of melancholia by considering the interaction of genetic factors ("injured prenatally as the result of the father's sperm having been damaged") with a special temperament given to "mental overexertion"—although not necessarily physical overactivity—that, in turn, was associated with "disruption of the correct rhythms of sleeping and waking." Those views, too, have a very modern ring to them.

MODERN ERA

The first English text (Fig. 13.1–2) entirely devoted to affective illness was Robert Burton's *Anatomy of Melancholy,* published in 1621. A scholarly review of medical and philosophical wisdom accumulated in past centuries, it also anticipated many modern developments. The concept of affective disorder endorsed by Burton was rather broad (as it always has been in the United Kingdom), embracing mood disorders and many disorders that are today considered somatoform disorders, including hypochondriasis. Although he described "causeless" melancholias, Burton also categorized the various forms of love melancholy and grief. Particularly impressive was his catalogue of causes, culminating in a grand conceptualization:

> Such as have Saturn misaffected in their genitures such as are born of melancholy parents as offend in those six non-natural things, are of a high sanguine complexion, are solitary by nature, great students, given to much contemplation, lead a life out of action, are most subject to melancholy. Of sexes both, but men more often. Of seasons of the year, autumn is most melancholy. Jobertus excepts neither young nor old.

Burton's six nonnatural things referred to such environmental factors as diet, alcohol, biological rhythms, and perturbations induced by passions such as intense love. Burton himself did not definitively indicate age prevalences. Like nearly all of his predecessors, he favored male (rather than the currently reported female) preponderance. Finally, Burton considered both the melancholic (contemplative) and the sanguine (hot-blooded) temperaments to be substrates of melancholia. Burton's work thus linked certain forms of depression with the softer expressions of the manic disposition, or bipolar II disorder, from which he himself appears to have suffered.

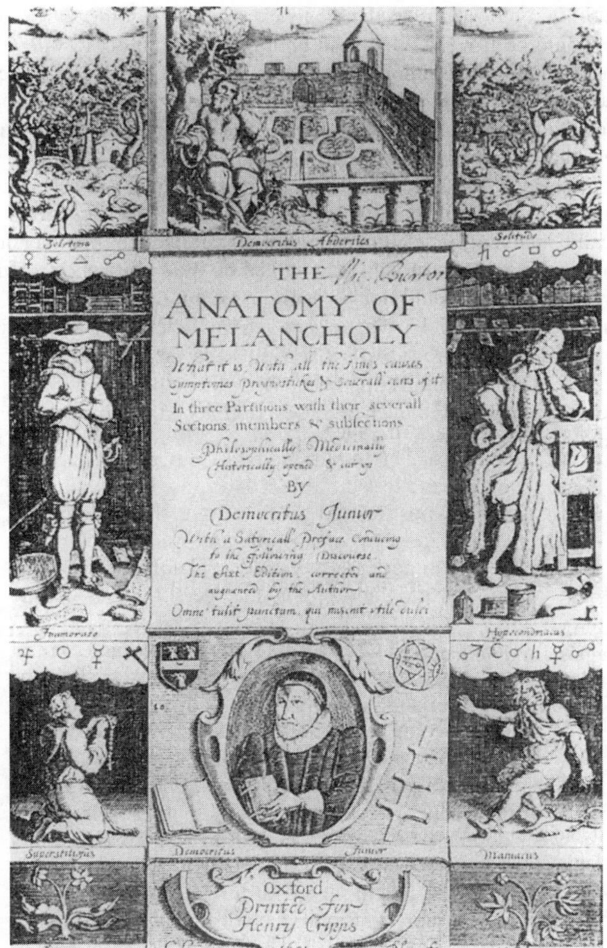

FIGURE 13.1–2 Frontispiece of Robert Burton's *Anatomy of Melancholy* (1621).

The 18th and 19th centuries introduced humane hospital care of the mentally ill, thereby permitting systematic clinical observation of the psychopathology and outcome of mood disorders.

Concept of Affective Disorder Although Celsus (circa 30 AD) had described "forms of madness that go no further than sadness," the French alienist Jean-Philippe Esquirol (1840) may have been the first psychiatrist in modern times to suggest that a primary disturbance of mood might underlie many forms of depression and related paranoid psychoses. Until Esquirol's work, melancholia had been categorized as a form of insanity (i.e., ascribed to deranged reasoning or thought disturbance). Esquirol's observations on melancholic patients led him to postulate that their insanity was partial (dominated by one delusion, a monomania) and that "the symptoms were the expression of the disorder of the affections. The source of the evil is in the passions." He coined the term *lypemania* (from the Greek, "sorrowful insanity") to give nosological status to a subgroup of melancholic disorders that were affectively based. Esquirol cited Benjamin Rush (1745 to 1813), the father of American psychiatry, who had earlier described *tristimania*, a form of melancholia in which sadness predominated.

Esquirol's influence led other European psychiatrists to propose milder states of melancholia without delusions, which were eventually categorized as simple melancholias and, ultimately, as primary depressions. Such descriptions culminated in the Anglo-Saxon psychiatric term *affective disorder*, coined by Henry Maudsley (1835 to 1918), the renowned British psychiatrist after whom the London hospital is named.

Manic-Depressive Illness and the Question of Psychogenic Depressions Although the connection between mania and depression had been rediscovered sporadically since it was first described 2,000 years ago, the clinical work that finally established *circular insanity* (Jean-Pierre Falret's term) and *folie à double forme* (Jules Baillarger's term) as discrete nosologic entities with both depressive and manic poles was undertaken by these two Esquirol disciples in the 1850s. That accomplishment built on Philippe Pinel's reforms, which championed humane treatment of the mentally ill in Paris around the turn of the 18th century and emphasized systematic clinical observations of patients, which were detailed in case records. French alienists made longitudinal observations on the same patient from one psychotic attack into another. Furthermore, Esquirol had introduced chronicling events in statistical tables. Thus, the Hippocratic approach to defining a particular case by its onset, circumstances, course, and outcome was applied by French alienists in studying the affectively ill. The humanitarian reforms introduced in the 19th century ensured that standards of general health and nutrition would improve the outlook for the mentally ill—especially those with potentially reversible disorders such as affective disorders—who could now be discharged from the asylums. The French school, by segregating the nondeteriorating mood disorders from other types of insanity, then paved the way for the Kraepelinian system.

Kraepelin's (1856 to 1926) unique contribution was not so much his grouping together of all the forms of melancholia and mania, but his methodology and painstaking longitudinal observations, which established manic-depressive illness as a nosological entity and (he hoped) a disease entity. His rationale was that (1) the various forms had a common heredity measured as a function of familial aggregation of manic and depressive cases, (2) frequent transitions from one to the other occurred during longitudinal follow-up of patients, (3) a recurrent course with illness-free intervals characterized most cases, (4) the superimposed episodes were commonly opposite to the patient's habitual temperament—that is, mania could be superimposed on a depressive temperament and depression on a hypomanic temperament—and (5) both depressive and manic features could occur during the same episode (mixed states). Kraepelin's synthesis was developed as early as the sixth (1899) edition of his *Lehrbuch der Psychiatrie* and most explicitly stated in the opening passages of the section on manic-depressive psychosis in the eighth edition (published in four volumes, 1909 to 1915):

> Manic-depressive insanity includes on the one hand the whole domain of so-called periodic and circular insanity, on the other hand simple mania, the greater part of the morbid states termed melancholia and also a not inconsiderable number of cases of confusional insanity. Lastly, we include here certain slight and slightest colorings of mood, some of them periodic, some of them continuously morbid, which on the one hand are to be regarded as the rudiment of more severe disorders, on the other hand, pass over without boundary into the domain of personal predisposition.

For Kraepelin, the core pathology of clinical depression consisted of lowered mood and slowed (retarded) physical and mental processes. In mania, by contrast, the mood was elated, and both physical and mental activity were accelerated. His earlier observations on what he termed *involutional melancholia* (referring to 40- to 65-year-old patients with extreme anxiety, irritability, agitation, and delusions) had led him to separate that entity from the broader manic-depressive rubric. But, in the eighth edition of *Lehrbuch der Psychiatrie,* he united melancholia with the manic-depressive group, with the justification that it was a special form of mixed state and that follow-up conducted by his pupil Dreyfus had demonstrated unmistakable excited phases.

The classification of mood disorders is still evolving. Karl Leonhard in 1957, Jules Angst in 1966, Carlo Perris in 1966, and George Winokur, Paula Clayton, and Theodore Reich in 1969, working independently in four different countries, proposed that depressive disorders without manic or hypomanic episodes (unipolar depressive disorder) that appear in middle age and later are distinct from depressive episodes that begin at earlier ages and alternate with manic or hypomanic episodes (bipolar disorder). The main difference between the two affective subtypes is the greater familial loading for mood disorder—especially for bipolar disorder—among bipolar disorder probands.

Kraepelin had conceded the occurrence of psychogenic states of depression occasioned by situational misfortune. However, he believed manic-depressive illness was hereditary—yet he could not document postmortem anatomopathological findings in the brains of manic-depressive patients. Therefore, manic-depression had to be considered a functional mental disorder in which brain disturbances were presumed to lie in altered physiological functions. Such biological factors were deemed absent in the psychogenic depressions. Thus, Kraepelin's classification of mood disorders is both dualistic and unitary. It is dualistic to the extent that he designated them as either psychologically occasioned or somatically caused. It is unitary with respect to disorders in the latter group, which have been termed *endogenous affective disorders* (i.e., due to internal biological causes). In other words, Kraepelin restricted the concept of clinical depression to what DSM-TR-IV terms *major depressive disorder with melancholic features*. Moreover, he postulated a continuum between that condition and what DSM-IV-TR and ICD-10 now term *bipolar disorders*.

As summarized in Table 13.1–1, until recently, endogenous depressions were contrasted with those of exogenous cause (i.e., external and, presumably, psychogenic causes). Transitions between the two groups are so frequent, however, that the two-type thesis of depression has been largely abandoned in official classifications in North American psychiatry and most parts of the world. In one study conducted by the author's mood clinic team in Memphis during the 1970s, 100 patients with neurotic depression (the prototype of exogenous depression), prospectively followed over 3 to 4 years, developed episodes with endogenous, psychotic, and even bipolar features (Table 13.1–2). Nonetheless, the endogenous–exogenous dichotomous grouping still has a few adherents in England and Australia who continue to research its potential for clinical predictions. Such research generally attempts to validate the various subtypes on the basis of their clinical characteristics rather than presumed cause. Today, most mood disorder experts would probably agree that depressive illness has endogenous and exogenous components in most patients presenting clinically. This does not necessarily imply that a continuum exists between all forms of depressive disorders, but suggests that neurotic and endogenous clinical features are not the best way to capture the heterogeneity of these disorders. Consensus would be less likely reached on how to delimit clinical depressive disorder from comorbid disorders such as the various anxiety disorders, substance use disorders, and personality disorders. Clarifying the boundaries between those disorders has emerged as a principal challenge in the classification of mood disorders.

Cartesian thinking in 17th-century France conceptually separated mind from body, thereby providing physicians autonomy over the somatic sphere, free from interference by the Church. The dichotomous paradigm ensured that the study of the two aspects of the human organism would not be confounded by the complexities of mind–body interactions. That is one reason Kraepelin's descriptive observations have proved valuable to subsequent generations of clinicians. Furthermore, his approach exemplifies the best tradition of scientific humanism in medicine: Description and diagnostic categorization of an individual patient are necessary for the physician to

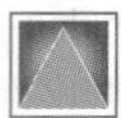

Table 13.1–1
Overlapping Dichotomies of Affective Disorders That Are Not Necessarily Synonymous

Manic-depressive	Psychogenic
S (somatic) type	J (justified) type
Autonomous	Reactive
Endogenous	Exogenous
Psychotic	Neurotic
Acute	Chronic
Major	Minor
Melancholic	Neurasthenic
Typical	Atypical
Primary	Secondary
Biological	Characterological

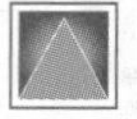

Table 13.1–2
Three- to Four-Year Prospective Follow-up in Neurotic Depressions (N = 100)

Diagnosis and Outcome	N[a]
Manic episode	4
Hypomanic episode	14
Psychotic depression	21
Endogenous depression	36
Episodic course	42
Unstable characterological features	24
Social invalidism	35
Suicide	3

[a]The total exceeds 100 because more than one outcome was possible in each patient.

Summarized from Akiskal H, Bitar A, Puzantian V, et al.: The nosological status of neurotic depression: a prospective 3- to 4-year examination in light of the primary-secondary and unipolar-bipolar dichotomies. *Arch Gen Psychiatry.* 1978;35:756, with permission.

apply the knowledge gained from past observation of similarly described and diagnosed patients. One limitation to the Kraepelinian approach is that because of its biological reductionism, it is not sufficiently articulate to account for mind–body interactions in the genesis of mental disorders.

Depressions as Psychobiological Affective Reaction Types Bridging the divide between psyche and soma was the ambition of Swiss-born Adolf Meyer (1866 to 1950), who dominated psychiatry from his chair at Johns Hopkins University during the first half of the 20th century. Meyer coined the term *psychobiology* to emphasize that both psychological and biological factors could enter into the causation of depressive and other mental disorders. Because of the nascent state of brain science during Meyer's time, he was more adept at biography than biology and, therefore, paid greater attention to psychosocial causation. He preferred the term *depression* (pressed down) to *melancholia* because of its lack of biological connotation. He conceived of depressive states in terms of unspecified constitutional or biological factors interacting with a series of life situations beginning at birth or even at conception. From that viewpoint arose the unique importance accorded personal history in depressive reactions to life events.

Meyer's terminological revision left a somewhat confusing legacy in that the term *depression* is now applied to a broad range of affective phenomena ranging from sadness and adjustment disorders to clinical depression and bipolar disorders. Repercussions can be seen in the low threshold for diagnosing major depressive disorder in DSM-IV-TR, which makes it difficult to differentiate major depressive disorder from transient life stresses that produce adjustment disorder with depressed mood. Nosological nuances to which Meyerians paid little attention, such as the difference between melancholic depression and more mundane depressions, are not just a matter of semantics. To the extent that those two forms of depression are seen in different clinical settings, hypotheses based on one population may not apply to the other. For instance, uncontrollable traumatic events may have taught study subjects to feel helpless or to view the world in a negative light, but that does not equate with clinical depression; nor does the process appear to be specific to depression. Failure to make such nosological distinctions further clouds interpretations of the results of trials comparing psychotherapy and pharmacotherapy for depressive disorders.

On the other hand, the Meyerian emphasis on biographical factors for the patient represented a more practical approach to depth psychology. Recent sociological interpretations of depression can also be traced to Meyer's work. But, in final analysis, the Meyerian concern for the uniqueness of the individual has proved heuristically sterile. It deemphasizes what is diagnostically common to different individuals, thereby obscuring the relevance of accrued clinical wisdom for the index patient. For that reason, the Meyerian approach, after enjoying clinical popularity for several decades in North America, has given way to neo-Kraepelinian rigor. However, the psychobiological vision of bridging biology and psychology, one of the major preoccupations of psychiatric thought and research today, owes much to Meyer's legacy.

CONTEMPORARY MODELS OF DEPRESSION

From classical times through the early part of the 20th century, advances in the understanding of mood disorders involved conceptual shifts from supernatural to naturalistic explanations; from reductionistic, unitarian theories of causation to pluralistic theories; and from dualism to psychobiology. Knowledge of those conceptual developments provides a useful base from which to scrutinize models and concepts of mood disorder developed later in the 20th century. The new approaches, derived from competing theoretical positions, have generated models for understanding various aspects of mood disorders, particularly depressive disorders (Table 13.1–3).

The formative influence of early experience as it is dynamically shaped by emerging mental structures during development is the common denominator for the psychoanalytic concepts of psychopathological phenomena. By contrast, behavioral approaches in their more traditional formulations focus on the pathogenetic impact of proximate contexts. The cognitive approaches, which are akin to the behavioral–pathogenetic tradition, nonetheless concede that negative styles of thinking might mediate between proximate stressors and more remote experiences. In explaining the origin of mood disorders, all three schools—psychoanalytic, behavioral, and cognitive—emphasize psychological constructs. The biological models, however, are concerned with defining the somatic mechanisms that underlie or predispose individuals to morbid affective experiences. The schism between psychological and biological conceptualizations is an instance of the mind–body dichotomy that has characterized the Western intellectual tradition since Descartes. After all, psychological and somatic approaches represent merely convenient investigational strategies that attempt to bypass the methodological gulf between mental and neural structures. The ultimate aim is to understand how mood disorders develop within the psychoneural framework of a given person.

Aggression-Turned-Inward Model Sigmund Freud was initially interested in a psychoneural project for all mental phenomena. Limitations of the brain sciences of the day led him to adopt instead a model that relied on a concept of mental function borrowed from physics. The notion that depressed affect is derived from retroflexion of aggressive impulses directed against an ambivalently loved internalized object was actually formulated by his Berlin disciple Karl Abraham and later elaborated by Freud. Abraham and Freud hypothesized that turned-in anger was intended as punishment for the love object that had thwarted the depressed patient's need for dependency and love. Because, in an attempt to prevent the traumatic loss, the object had already been internalized, the patient then became the target of his or her own thanatotic impulses. A central element in those psychic operations was the depressed patient's ambivalence toward the object, which was perceived as a frustrating parent. Aggression directed at a loved object (parent) was therefore attended by considerable guilt. In the extreme, such ambivalence, guilt, and retroflexed anger could lead to suicidal behavior.

According to this model, depression is an epiphenomenon of the transduction of thanatotic energy, a reaction that takes place in the closed hydraulic space of the mind. Freud's earlier writings had similarly portrayed anxiety as being derived from the transformation of dammed-up sexual libido. Although Freud envisioned that psychoanalytic constructs would one day be localized neuroanatomically, the hydraulic mind is a metaphor that does not refer to actual physiochemical space in the brain.

The conceptualization of emotional behavior as an arena of incompatible forces confined to a psyche that is relatively impervious to current influences outside the organism is the major liability of the aggression-turned-inward model and, perhaps, of orthodox psychoanalysis itself. Although the sexual energy transduction hypothesis of anxiety has been discarded in modern psychoanalytic thought, in modified version, the aggression-turned-inward model continues to be used in clinical conceptualization today. The lingering popularity of the model may be due, in part, to its compatibility with the clinical observation that many depressed patients

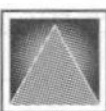

Table 13.1–3
Major Models of Depression

Proponents (Year)[a]	Model	Mechanism	Scientific and Clinical Implications
Karl Abraham (1911)	Aggression turned inward	Transduction of aggressive instinct into depressive affect	Hydraulic mind closed to external influences; nontestable
Sigmund Freud (1917) John Bowlby (1960)	Object loss	Disruption of an attachment bond	Ego-psychological; open system; testable
Edward Bibring (1953)	Self-esteem	Helplessness in attaining goals of ego ideal	Ego-psychological; open system; social and cultural ramifications
Aaron Beck (1967)	Cognitive	Negative cognitive schemata as intermediary between remote and proximate causes	Ego-psychological; open system; testable; predicts phenomenology; suggests treatment
Martin Seligman (1975)	Learned helplessness	Belief that one's responses will not bring relief from undesirable events	Testable; predicts phenomenology; predicts treatment
Peter Lewinsohn (1974)	Reinforcement	Low rate of reinforcement, or reinforcement presented noncontingently; social deficits might preclude responding to potentially rewarding events	Testable; predicts phenomenology; predicts treatment
Joseph Schildkraut (1965) William Bunney and John Davis (1965) Alec Coppen (1968) I. P. Lapin and G. F. Oxenkrug (1969) David Janowsky et al. (1972) Arthur Prange et al. (1974) Larry Siever and Kenneth Davis (1985)	Biogenic amine (neurochemical)	Impairment or dysregulation of aminergic transmission	Testable; reductionistic; explains phenomenology and opposite episodes; suggests treatment
Bernard Carroll et al. (1981)		Impaired glucocorticoid and mineralocorticoid receptors (neuroendocrine)	Testable; reductionistic; explains phenomenology; explains anxious comorbidity; suggests treatment
Alec Coppen and D. M. Shaw (1963) Peter Whybrow and Joseph Mendels (1968) Robert Post (1990)	Neurophysiological	Electrophysiological disturbances leading to neuronal hyperexcitability and/or kindling	Testable; reductionistic; explains phenomenology and recurrence; suggests treatment
Hagop Akiskal and William McKinney (1973) Frederick Goodwin and Kay Jamison (1990)	Final common pathway	Stress-diathesis interaction converging on midbrain mechanisms of reward and biological rhythms	Testable; integrative, psychobiological; pluralistic; explains phenomenology; suggests treatment

[a]Dates provided for the models refer to the original paper or work in which they first appeared. In some instances, the bibliography at the end of the section provides references reflecting more updated thinking by those authors.

Updated from Akiskal H, McKinney W: Overview of recent research in depression: integration of 10 conceptual models into a comprehensive clinical frame. *Arch Gen Psychiatry*. 1975;32:285.

suffer from lack of assertion and outwardly directed aggressiveness. However, a substantial number of hostile, depressed patients are also encountered in clinical practice (indeed "depression with anger attacks" has been recently described), and clinical improvement in most patients typically leads to decreased, not increased, hostility. Such observations shed doubt on the aggression-turned-inward mechanism as a universal explanation for depressive behavior. Finally, little evidence exists to support the contention that outward expression of anger has therapeutic value in clinical depression.

Outwardly directed hostility in depression is not a new clinical observation; in fact, Greco-Roman physicians had noted it. Hostility is best considered a manifestation rather than a cause of depressive disorder, especially when the disorder is attended by mixed bipolar features. The hostility of the depressed patient can also be understood as an exaggerated reaction to frustrating love objects, as secondary to self-referential attribution, or simply as nonspecific irritability of an ego in affective turmoil; this could, in part, be a function of a concurrent personality disorder from the erratic cluster. Such common-sense explanations that do not invoke unobservable hydraulic transmutations have greater appeal from heuristic and clinical perspectives.

Object Loss and Depression

Object loss refers to traumatic separation from significant objects of attachment. Ego-psychological reformulations of the Abraham–Freud conceptualization of depression have paid greater attention to the impact of such losses on the ego, deemphasizing the id-libidinal and related hydraulic aspects. The depressant impact of separation events often resides in their symbolic meaning for a person rather than in any arbitrary objective weight that the event may have for clinical raters. However, love loss, bereavement, and other exits from the social scene, as defined by the London psychiatrist Eugene Paykel, are presently the concepts most commonly used in practice and research.

Although love melancholy had been described since antiquity, the two affective states were systematically compared for the first time in Freud's 1917 paper on mourning and melancholia. According to current data, the transition from grief to pathological depression occurs in no more than 10 percent of adults and 20 percent of children. These figures suggest that such transition occurs largely in persons predisposed to mood disorders.

John Bowlby of the Tavistock Clinic, London, did a comprehensive clinical investigation of the attachment that the child establishes with the mother or mother substitutes during development, a bond considered the prototype for all subsequent bonds with other objects. Like many psychoanalytic explanations of adult symptom-formation, the object loss model is formulated as a two-step hypothesis, consisting of early breaks in affectional bonds, which provide the behavioral predisposition to depression, and adult losses, which are said to revive the traumatic childhood loss and so precipitate depressive episodes. However, the role of proximate separations in provoking depressive reactions rests on more solid clinical evidence than the hypothesized sensitization resulting from developmental object loss. That realization has led Bowlby to regard childhood sensitization resulting from early deprivation as a generic characterological vulnerability to a host of adult psychopathological conditions.

Compared with aggression turned inward, object loss is more directly relevant to clinical depression, yet it is still pertinent to question whether it is an etiological factor. Studies at the Wisconsin Primate Center have indicated that optimal homeostasis with the environment is most readily achieved when the individual is securely attached to significant others, and the dissolution of such ties appears relevant to the emergence of a broad range of psychopathological disturbances rather than depression per se. A related methodological question is whether object loss operates independently of other etiological factors. For instance, a history of early breaks in attachment may reflect the fact that one or both of the patient's parents had mood disorder, with resultant separation, divorce, suicide, and so forth.

On balance, the ego-psychological object loss model is conceptually superior to its id-psychological counterpart. In postulating an open system of exchange between a person and the environment, the model permits consideration of etiological factors other than separation, such as heredity, character structure, and adequacy of social support—all of which might modulate the depressant impact of adult separation events. Conceptualizing the origin of depression along those lines is in the mainstream of current ideas of adaptation, homeostasis, and disease. An important treatment implication is the value of social support in preventing relapse and mitigating chronicity of depression. That is, indeed, an ingredient in the interpersonal psychotherapy of depression, which can be conceptualized as a form of brief, focused, and practical psychodynamic therapy.

Loss of Self-Esteem and Depression Reformulation of the dynamics of depression in terms of the ego suffering a collapse of self-esteem represents a further conceptual break with the original id-psychological formulation; depression is said to originate from the ego's inability to give up unattainable goals and ideals. The model further posits that the narcissistic injury that crushes the depressed patient's self-esteem is imposed by the internalized values of the ego rather than the hydraulic pressure of retroflected thanatotic energy deriving from the id. Because the construct of the ego is rooted in social and cultural reality, loss of self-esteem may result from symbolic losses involving power, status, roles, identity, values, and purpose for existence. Thus, the existential and sociocultural implications of depression conceived as a derivative ego state provide the clinician with a far more flexible and pragmatic tool for understanding depressed persons than the archaic hydraulic metaphors related to libidinal vicissitudes. That model represents one of the first attempts to formulate depression in terms that subsequent psychological theory and research could operationalize in more testable form.

Self-esteem is part of the habitual core of the individual and, hence, is integral to the personality structure. Indeed, low self-esteem conceived as a trait is a major defining attribute of the depressive (melancholic) personality. Although it is understandable that such individuals can easily sink into melancholia in the face of environmental adversity, it is not obvious why persons with apparently high self-esteem (e.g., those with hypomanic and narcissistic personalities) also succumb to melancholy with relative ease. To explain such cases, one must invoke an underlying instability in the system of self-esteem that renders it vulnerable to depression. The opposite is also known to occur; that is, manic episodes may develop from a baseline of low self-esteem, as in the case of bipolar disorder patients with antecedent traits of shyness, insecurity, and dysthymia.

The foregoing considerations suggest that the vicissitudes of self-esteem deemed central to the model of depression as loss of self-esteem are manifestations of a more fundamental mood dysregulation. In classic psychoanalysis, such dysregulation is considered to be of constitutional origin. In general, attempts by psychoanalytic writers to account for bipolar oscillations have not progressed beyond metapsychological jargon, with the notable exception of denial of painful affects as a mechanism in the phenomenology of mania.

Cognitive Model The cognitive model, developed by Aaron Beck at the University of Pennsylvania, hypothesizes that thinking along negative lines (e.g., thinking that one is helpless, unworthy, or useless) is the hallmark of clinical depression. In effect, depression is redefined in terms of a cognitive triad, according to which patients think of themselves as helpless, interpret most events unfavorably vis-à-vis the self, and believe the future to be hopeless. In more recent formulations in academic psychology, these cognitions are said to be characterized by a negative attributional style that is global, internal, and stable and that exists in the form of latent mental schemata that generate biased interpretations of life events.

Because the cognitive model is based on retrospective observations of already depressed persons, it is virtually impossible to prove that causal attributions such as negative mental schemata precede and, therefore, predispose to clinical depression; they can just as readily be regarded as subclinical manifestations of depression. The theoretical importance of the cognitive model lies in the conceptual bridge it provides between ego-psychological and behavioral models of depression. It has also led to a new and widely accepted system of psychotherapy that attempts to alter the negative attributional style, to alleviate the depressive state, and, ultimately, to fortify the patient against future lapses into negative thinking, despair, and depression.

The cognitive model, therefore, has the cardinal virtue of focusing on key reversible clinical dimensions of depressive illness, such as helplessness, hopelessness, and suicidal ideation, while providing a testable and practical psychotherapeutic approach. That approach, however, is less likely to succeed in patients with the full-blown melancholic manifestations of a depressive disorder. It is doubtful that negative cognitions alone could account for the profound disturbances in sleep, appetite, and autonomic and psychomotor functions encountered in melancholic depressions. Furthermore, conceptualizing a multifaceted malady such as depression largely or solely as a function of distorted cognitive processes is reminiscent of pre-Esquirolian notions that emphasized impaired reasoning in the development of depression. Finally, recent extensions or modifications, or both, of cognitive therapy in association with behavioral therapy (cognitive-behavioral therapy) for all emotional disorders (and even for schizophrenia) are reminiscent of earlier global claims of the psychodynamic perspective.

Learned Helplessness Model The learned helplessness model is, in some ways, an experimental analog of the cognitive model. The model proposes that the depressive posture is learned from past situations in which the person was unable to terminate undesirable contingencies. The model is based on experiments in dogs that were prevented from taking adaptive action to avoid unpleasant electrical shock and, subsequently, showed no motivation to escape such aversive stimuli, even when escape avenues were readily available. Armed with evidence from many such experiments, University of Pennsylvania psychologist Martin Seligman postulated a trait of learned helplessness (a belief that it is futile to initiate personal action to reverse aversive circumstances) formed from the cumulation of past episodes of uncontrollable helplessness.

The learned helplessness paradigm is a general one and refers to a broader mental disposition than depression. Thus, it is potentially useful in understanding such diverse conditions as social powerlessness, defeat in sporting events, and posttraumatic stress disorder (PTSD). In addition, past events might shape a characterological cluster, consisting of passivity, lack of hostility, and self-blame, relevant to certain depressive phenomena. The low hostility observed in some patients during clinical depression could, for instance, be ascribed to the operation of such factors. Learned helplessness could thereby provide plausible links between aspects of personal biography and clinical phenomenology in depressive disorders. Therapeutic predictions for alleviating depression and related psychopathological states capitalize on new cognitive strategies geared to modifying expectations of uncontrollability and the negative attributional style. This illustrates how insights gained from experimental paradigms can be combined fruitfully to address clinical disorders.

Nonetheless, the clinician should be wary of unwarranted clinical extrapolations. For example, some therapists have argued that the depressed patient's passivity is "manipulative," serving to obtain interpersonal rewards. It has also been suggested that such factors have a formative influence on the development of the depressive character. That interpretation appears more relevant to selected aspects of depression than to the totality of the disorder. Depressive behavior and verbalizations clearly have a powerful interpersonal impact, but casting depression as merely a masochistic lifestyle developed to secure interpersonal advantages represents a mechanistic circular argument that could be viewed as disrespectful of the clinical agony of patients with mood disorders. Finally, although most formulations focusing on helplessness have emphasized acquisition through learning, recent experimental research in animals tends to implicate genetic factors in the vulnerability of learning to behave helplessly. The value of the helplessness paradigm may reside in its utility to predict a variety of subthreshold affective disturbances generic to civilian reactions to adversity and trauma.

Depression and Reinforcement

Other behavioral investigators, including, notably, Oregon psychologist Peter Lewinsohn, have developed clinical formulations of depression that hinge on certain deficits in reinforcement mechanisms. According to the reinforcement model, depressive behavior is associated with lack of appropriate rewards and, more specifically, with receipt of noncontingent rewards. The model identifies several contributory mechanisms. Some environments may consistently deprive persons of rewarding opportunities, thereby placing them in a chronic state of boredom, pleasurelessness, and, ultimately, despair. That reasoning, however, may offer more insight into social misery than clinical depression. A more plausible postulated mechanism is the provision of rewards that are not in response to the recipient's actions; in other words, the gratis provision of what a person considers undeserved rewards may lead to lowering of self-esteem. Predisposition to depression is formulated in terms of inadequate social skills, which are hypothesized to decrease a person's chances of responding to potentially rewarding contingencies in the environment. Indeed, recent research on the relationship between personality and depression suggests that such deficits might underlie certain depressive states. Therefore, psychotherapeutic approaches designed to enlarge a patient's repertoire of social skills may prove valuable in preventing some types of depression.

The concepts of depression that have been derived from behavioral methodology and developed in the past several decades are scientifically articulate and, therefore, testable approaches to clinical depression. However, the important distinction between depression on self-report inventories and clinical depression tends to be overlooked in investigations testing the reinforcement paradigm. Furthermore, the behavioral model does not address the distinct possibility that reinforcement deficits may, in part, represent the psychomotor deficits of depressive illness. Nevertheless, by focusing on reward mechanisms, the behavioral model provides a conceptual bridge between purely psychological and emerging biological conceptualizations of depression.

Biogenic Amine Imbalance

Formulation of sophisticated biological explanations of mood disorders had to await development of neurobiological techniques that could probe the parts of the brain involved in emotions. Although the complex physiology of the limbic-diencephalic centers of emotional behavior generally cannot be directly observed in humans, much has been learned from animal work. The limbic cortex is linked with both the neocortex, which subserves higher symbolic functions, and the midbrain and lower brain centers, which are involved in autonomic control, hormonal production, and sleep and wakefulness. Norepinephrine-containing neurons are involved in many functions that are profoundly disturbed in melancholia, including mood, arousal, appetite, reward, and drives. Other biogenic amine neurotransmitters that mediate such functions are the catecholamine dopamine—especially important for drive, pleasure, sex, and psychomotor activity—and the indoleamine serotonin, which is involved in the regulatory control of affects, aggression, sleep, and appetite. Cholinergic neurons, secreting acetylcholine at their dendritic terminals, are generally antagonistic in function to catecholaminergic neurons.

Although the opioid system might, on experimental and theoretical grounds, also serve as one of the neurochemical substrates for mood regulation, in the author's opinion, no cogent model of mood disorders involving that system has appeared to date. Likewise, biochemical formulations of mood disorders have paid relatively little attention to the major excitatory brain neurotransmitter glutamate and the inhibitory neurotransmitter γ-aminobutyric acid (GABA).

Biogenic Amine Hypotheses

Joseph Schildkraut at Harvard University and William Bunney and John Davis at NIMH published the first formal hypothesis connecting depletion or imbalance of biogenic amines (specifically norepinephrine) and clinical depression. The serotonin counterpart of the model was emphasized in the models proposed by Alec Coppen in England and I. P. Lapin and G. F. Oxenkrug in Russia. Both catecholamine and indoleamine hypotheses were essentially based on two sets of pharmacological observations. First, reserpine (Serpasil), which decreases blood pressure by depleting biogenic amine stores, precipitates clinical depression in some patients. Second, antidepressant medications, which alleviate clinical depression, raise the functional capacity of the biogenic amines in the brain. This style of thinking is known as the *pharmacological bridge*, extrapolating from evidence on the mechanism of drug action to the neurotransmitter pathologies presumed to underlie a given psychiatric disorder. Such pharmacological strategies have been of heuristic value in developing research methods for investigation of mood disorders and schizophrenia. Indeed, the research methodology developed by the relatively few investigators working in this area during the past half century is among the most elegant in the history of psychiatry.

Variations of the biogenic amine model assign somewhat different relative weights to the biogenic amines norepinephrine and serotonin in the development of pathological mood states. Arthur Prange and colleagues at the University of North Carolina formulated a permissive biogenic amine hypothesis in which serotonin deficits permit expression of catecholamine-mediated depressive or manic states. That hypothesis was supported by subsequent animal research showing that an intact serotonin system is necessary for optimal functioning of noradrenergic neurons. Omission of tryptophan from the diet of antidepressant-responsive depressed patients may annul the efficacy of the antidepressant; among healthy volunteers, that special diet also induces sleep electroencephalographic characteristics of clinical depression. Although such findings are provocative, the precursor-loading strategy to increase the brain stores of serotonin (e.g., with L-tryptophan) has not been unequivocally successful in reversing clinical depression. Dietary loading with catecholamine precursors has fared even worse than serotonin-precursor loading in the treatment of depression.

The cholinergic-noradrenergic imbalance hypothesis proposed by David Janowsky and colleagues represents yet another attempt to elucidate the roles of biogenic amines. This hypothesis, along with the related cholinergic supersensitivity hypothesis developed by J. Christian Gillin, has been tested extensively at the University of California at San Diego. Subsequent formulations by Larry Siever and Kenneth Davis at the Mount Sinai Hospital in New York have refocused on noradrenergic dysregulation. The model assumes oscillation from one output mode to the other at different phases of depressive illness. In a provocative extrapolation from that model, bipolar depression would have low noradrenergic output, but many instances of major depressive disorder, as with some anxiety disorders, could be biochemically conceptualized as high-output conditions.

Despite more than four decades of extensive research and indirect evidence, however, no deficiency or excess of biogenic amines in specific brain structures has been shown to be necessary or sufficient for the occurrence of mood disorders. It has not been possible to either confirm the putative role of central norepinephrine in depression or to discard it altogether. The role of dopamine as formulated, among others, by the Italian pharmacologist Gian Luigi Cessa, although studied less extensively than that of norepinephrine, deserves greater recognition, as it may have relevance to atypical and bipolar depression as well as to mania.

Preliminary data from a small brain imaging study has shown blunted serotonin responsivity in prefrontal and temporoparietal areas in unmedicated patients with major depressive disorder. Such data, considered in the context of the overall serotonin literature in depression, is provocative but not conclusive and serves to illustrate the fact that the case for serotonergic disturbance in depression continues to be based on indirect evidence. Moreover, the putative permissive role of serotonin is better documented for aggressive suicide attempts. Serotonergic dysfunction might subserve other conditions characterized by lack of inhibitory control, among them, obsessive-compulsive disorder (OCD), panic disorders, bulimia nervosa, certain forms of insomnia, alcoholism (alcohol abuse or dependence), and a host of impulse-ridden personality disorders. Such considerations have led Dutch psychiatrist Herman van Praag and colleagues to postulate a dimensional neurochemical disturbance generic to a large group of disorders within the traditional nosology. This hypothesis might be variously regarded as a challenge to psychiatric nosology or as a statement of the need to supplement clinical classification with biochemical parameters. Both interpretations are in line with clinical observations during the past two decades testifying to the high prevalence of comorbidity in depressive, other emotional disorders, and certain impulse-control disorders.

It is implied that the foregoing postulated biochemical faults are genetically determined. Although biogenic amine models of mood disorders were developed retrospectively from the pharmacological action of antidepressant and thymoleptic agents, they have stimulated development of new classes of antidepressants with more selective action on specific neurotransmitter receptors. Their introduction has virtually revolutionized the treatment of depression. Yet the fundamental biochemistry of mood disorders is still far from being understood. Curiously, although selective in action, the new compounds working on the serotonin system have broad effectiveness in a variety of mood-related conditions, such as dysthymic disorder, PTSD, OCD, panic disorder, social phobia, bulimia nervosa, and borderline personality disorder. Such data indirectly favor the hypothesis of an underlying biological commonality to several of these disorders. The foregoing considerations have, in turn, led to a provocative formulation of an increasingly prevalent "social syndrome" in populations experiencing social disruption, immigration, and abuse and characterized by anxiety, depression, violence-proneness, impulsivity, and suicidality—reflecting a perturbed serotonin system, the oldest, most basic brain structure involved in human socialization and territoriality, coping with stress, danger, and survival.

New antidepressants with dual action on both serotonergic and noradrenergic receptors and emerging data on their possible greater efficacy in melancholic depressions do suggest that the biochemistry of mood disorders involves more complex dysregulation than is implied in single-neurotransmitter hypotheses. The work of George Henninger and colleagues at Yale University further suggests that monoamines better explain how antidepressants facilitate recovery from depression than being the fundamental causes of depression. Moreover, emerging biochemical paradigms are moving away from distal biochemical lesions to focus on molecular perturbations closest to the putative genetic underpinnings of mood disorders. Originally tied to the mechanism of action of mood stabilizers in bipolar disorder, such work is exploring second messenger systems, phosphorylation G proteins, signal transduction, deoxyribonucleic acid (DNA) transcription, and messenger ribonucleic acid (RNA) translation. Again, such search for molecular mechanisms represents "backward logic" from the putative mechanism of action of selected thymoleptic agents. The same can be said about Frederick Petty's GABAergic and Shih-Jen Tsai's brain-derived neurotrophic factor (BDNF) hypothesis in the origin of bipolar disorder.

Neuroendocrine Links Functionally inadequate mobilization of neurotransmitters in the face of continued or repeated stress, as indirectly reflected in pathological modification of noradrenergic and serotonergic receptor function, could represent neurochemical final common pathways of homeostatic failure. Such mechanisms could also provide links with psychoendocrine dysfunction; the hypothesized neurotransmitter deficits may underlie the disinhibition of the hypothalamic-pituitary-adrenal axis, characterized by steroidal overproduction, the most widely studied endocrine disturbance in depressive illness. When challenged with dexamethasone (Decadron), the altered axis resists suppression, thereby offering Bernard Carroll's team (then at the University of Michigan) the possibility of developing the dexamethasone suppression "test" (DST) for melancholia. Presently, this procedure is of uncertain specificity for depressive illness, and, thus, is unsuitable to serve as a diagnostic test. However, that line of research has been useful in pathogenetic understanding. For instance, it led to the demonstration by the Emory University's Charles Nemeroff of increased concentrations of corticotropin-releasing factor (CRF) in the cerebrospinal fluid (CSF) of patients with major depressive disorder. CRF also appears relevant to the pathophysiology of anxiety disorders, such as panic disorder, and PTSD. The research of Florian Holsboer's group at Munich's Max Planck Institute has shown impaired glucocorticoid and mineralocorticoid receptor function in these disorders, with relevant pathophysiological and therapeutic implications.

Another neuroendocrine index of noradrenergic dysregulation, blunted growth hormone response to the α_2-adrenergic receptor agonist clonidine (Catapres) likewise points to limbic-diencephalic disturbance. However, studies performed in the United States suggest that it is positive in both endogenous depression and severe anxiety disorder (panic disorder). Thyroid-stimulating hormone (TSH) blunting upon thyrotropin stimulation, another common neuroendocrine disturbance in depression, also shows limited specificity.

What is remarkable, however, is that the DST, clonidine, and thyrotropin challenge data, in aggregate, identify most persons with clinical depression. Such evidence of midbrain disturbance argues for considering clinical depression to be a legitimate disease. The disease concept of depression is further buttressed by computed tomography (CT) scans showing enlarged pituitary and adrenal glands, a state marker of depressive illness.

Stress and Depression The concept of a pharmacological bridge implies two-way traffic. The hypothesized chemical aberrations may be primary or genetically based. Provision should also be made, however, for the likelihood that psychological events that precipitate clinical depression might initiate or exacerbate neurochemical imbalance in vulnerable subjects. That suggestion is supported by studies in animals in which early separation from peers and inescapable frustration effect profound alterations in the turnover of biogenic amines and in postsynaptic receptor sensitivity. Thus, in genetically predisposed persons, environmental stressors might more easily lead to perturbations of limbic-diencephalic neurotransmitter balance. Finally, in vulnerable individuals, especially during the formative years of childhood, psychological mechanisms might more easily perturb midbrain neurochemistry. Traumatic experiences appear particularly potent in this regard. The hippocampus has been the subject of intense recent research as the possible neuro-anatomical substrate linking such loss and trauma to adult depression. Ongoing ingenious experimental paradigms in primates and rodents continue to explore the role of early experience and stress in subsequent depressive-like behaviors in these animals. In humans, a new provocative finding indicates that a polymorphism of the serotonin transporter gene would identify who among traumatized children would develop adult depression. Likewise, a polymorphism of the monoamine oxidase (MAO) A gene plays a significant role in determining who among battered children will grow into an adult sociopath. Animal models of mania are sparse and problematic.

Neurophysiological Approaches

Neuronal Hyperexcitability Lithium is known to replace intracellular sodium and hyperpolarize the neuronal membrane, thereby decreasing neuronal excitability. Abnormalities in neuronal electrolyte balance (an excess of residual sodium, defined by radioisotope techniques) and hypothesized secondary neurophysiological disturbances were the focus of British investigations by Alec Coppen and colleagues in the early 1960s. The existing data appear compatible with the hypothesized movement of excess sodium into the neuron during an episode of mood disorder and redistribution toward the preillness electrolyte balance across the neuronal membrane during recovery. Intraneuronal sodium leakage is postulated in both depressive and manic disorders but deemed more extreme in the latter. Because the harmonious activity of the neuronal cell and, by implication, that of a group of neurons depends on the electrical gradient maintained across its membrane by differential distribution of sodium, abnormalities in sodium concentrations and transport are hypothetically relevant to the production of an unstable state of neurophysiological hyperexcitability. In formulating their thesis of neurophysiological arousal in melancholic states, Joseph Mendels and Peter Whybrow (both of whom have worked at the University of Pennsylvania) have capitalized on the foregoing electrolyte disturbances. The view that mania represents a more extreme electrophysiological dysfunction in the same direction as depression violates the common-sense notion of symptomatological "opposition" between the two kinds of disorder, yet, it may, in part, account for the existence of mixed states in which symptoms of depression and mania coexist. The NIMH team led by Frederick Goodwin first showed that a substantial minority of depressed patients with a bipolar substrate respond to lithium salts, which further supports the concept of a neurophysiological common denominator to mania and depression. Perturbations of calcium metabolism also appear relevant to bipolar patients. Therapeutic implications of this observation (e.g., the use of calcium channel inhibitors in bipolar I disorder) have not yielded consistent results. Finally, rubidium, another alkali metal, has been explored in the depressive phase of bipolar disorders, again with inconclusive results.

Rhythmopathy European studies have shown that depressed patients are phase advanced in many biological rhythms, including the latency to the first rapid eye movement (REM) in sleep. Shortened REM latency, which has been extensively studied by David Kupfer and colleagues at the University of Pittsburgh, has been proposed as another laboratory "test" for depressive disorder. Shortened REM latency may serve as a trait marker for depression, because it has been found in dysthymia and so-called borderline personality, as well as among the clinically "well" offspring of adults with major depression.

Formulations of circadian rhythms by Thomas Wehr and Norman Rosenthal, working at NIMH, have focused on abnormalities on brain regulation of temperature, activity, and sleep cycles. Others have investigated the role of the pineal hormone melatonin in mood disorders, without achieving consistent results. The application of circadian rhythm research concepts to women with mood disorders has also led to imaginative methods, but, again, without definitive characterization of the neurophysiologic faults.

At a basic level, instrumental REM sleep deprivation in neonates has been recently shown to lead to adult "depression-like" behaviors in rats. In human studies, sleep deprivation and exposure to bright white light has been shown to correct phase disturbances and thereby terminate depressive episodes, especially in subjects with periodic and seasonal depressions. It has even been shown that the average citizen is light deprived, and that phototherapy can benefit even those without clear-cut seasonal patterns. Unfortunately, except for their use in mild seasonal depressions and suppression of sleep deprivation to prevent hypomania in bipolar disorder, the foregoing circadian studies have not had a palpable impact on practice. Their application in the large segment of mood-disordered patients remains cumbersome, if not elusive. Their impact can be better assessed at the level of theory. Although the specificity and efficacy of these neurophysiological indices and manipulations for clinical depression and bipolar disorder require more extensive research, cumulatively, they point to midbrain dysregulation as the likely common neurophysiological substrate of affective disorders. The foregoing considerations further suggest that the ancient Greeks, who ascribed melancholia to malignant geophysical influences, did not indulge in mere poetic metaphor. The ancients had observed the disturbed circadian patterns and advocated their readjustment to restore euthymia.

Affective Dysregulation A major challenge for research in mood disorders is to characterize the basic molecular mechanisms that underlie the neurophysiological rhythmopathies, which, in turn, might account for the recurrent nature of the affective pathology as envisioned by Kraepelin. This means that in the most typical recurrent forms of the disorders, the constitutional foundations (manifested as cyclothymic and dysthymic traits and/or a broad range of emotional disequilibrium covered by the rubric of "neuroticism") are so unstable that the illness may run its entire course more or less autonomously, with the environment largely serving to turn on and off the more florid phases (episodes). Parisian psychiatrist Jean Delay, a pioneer in psychopharmacology in the 1950s, has also emphasized affective dysregulation as the fundamental pathology in the spectrum of mood disorders. Robert Post (at NIMH) hypothesized that the electrophysiological substrates could be so kindled that an oligoepisodic disorder initially triggered by environmental stressors could assume an autonomous and polyepisodic course. He hypothesizes that this phenomenon might occur because neuronal perturbations brought about by stressors in the early course of mood disorders get incorporated into the DNA. This fascinating kindling hypothesis, however, does not seem to pertain to garden-variety mood disorders, but those with extreme cyclicity. The monograph on manic-depressive illness by Fred Goodwin and Kay Jamison presents in-depth arguments for this cyclical paradigm of thymopathy.

THEORETICAL SYNTHESIS

Pathophysiological Understanding

Modern psychobiology attempts to link experience and behavior to the central nervous system (CNS). Building conceptual bridges between the psychological and biological approaches to mood disorders requires sophisticated strategies that go beyond the Cartesian notion of limited mind–body interactions through the pineal gland and the generalizations of the Meyerian school.

In collaboration with William McKinney in 1973, the author developed the conceptual framework that considers the affective syndromes as the final common pathway of various psychological and biological processes. The overarching hypothesis is that psychological and biological etiological factors converge in reversible deficits in the diencephalic substrates of pleasure and reward. Those areas of the brain subserve the functions that are disturbed in melancholia and mania. The integrative model links the central chemistry and physiology of reward mechanisms with the object loss and behavioral models of depression, both of which give singular importance to the depressant role of loss of rewarding interpersonal bonds. A key element of the model is the circadian disturbances observed since ancient times in both depressive and manic syndromes. Both syndromes are conceptualized as clinical manifestations of a disordered limbic system with its subcortical and prefrontal extensions. The brain imaging studies in melancholic patients by Wayne Drevets, originally at Washington University, have visualized limbic disturbances extending into subcortical structures and occurring primarily in those with a familial diathesis for depression; the amygdala appears to be the focal limbic structure in the latter studies. Clinical experience and research data suggest that multiple factors described below converge to produce or exacerbate dysregulation in these brain regions, leading to the final common pathway of clinical depression. The data on mania are more tentative and will be mentioned when relevant.

Heredity Current evidence indicates a significant genetic role in the causation of bipolar and recurrent major depressive disorders. Although it is not known exactly what is inherited, and biological endophenotypes have not been delineated, temperamental dysregulation might be hypothesized to fulfill the role of a behavioral endophenotype. The depressive inheritance may translate into impaired coping under stress (neuroticism), and bipolar inheritance might translate into affective dysregulation (cyclothymia), involving over- and underreactivity to life situations, circadian events, and biological stressors. Whatever the precise nature of the inherited fault or excess, current research suggests that heritability involves a broad spectrum of disorders, including milder affective states, as well as temperamental inclinations. Recent findings, both from clinical and genetic investigations, have emphasized the importance of broad affective phenotypes that incorporate panic and anxiety reactivity within both traditional unipolar and bipolar disorders. For instance, the affective dysregulation underlying bipolar disorder can manifest in euphoria, irritability, depression, panic attacks, and social anxiety. Such tendencies are observed among both patients and their first-degree relatives. Genetic heterogeneity is likely and may involve inheritance of a single dominant gene with variable penetrance in some families or specific subtypes, or oligogenic inheritance in the majority of cases. Different genetic mechanisms will, in all likelihood, involve more than one disorder (e.g., depression and generalized anxiety; bipolar I disorder, psychosis, stimulant abuse, and dipsomania; bipolar II disorder, panic disorder, and bulimia nervosa). Another distinct possibility is that some forms of schizophrenia, bipolar I and II disorders, and recurrent depressions lie on an oligogenic bipolar spectrum. A polymorphism involving the short alleles of the serotonin transporter gene appears relevant to depressive dispositions. The genetic mechanism involving mood reactivity and panic appear to be subserved by chromosome 18q. The partial overlap of manic and schizophrenic phenomenology might be related to a polymorphism in the GRK3 system.

Developmental Predisposition Parents with mood disorders are often in conflict, which may lead to separation, divorce, and suicide. It can be said that heredity often determines the type of environment into which the child predisposed to mood disorder is born. Developmental object loss, although not specifically involved in causing mood disorder, might modify the expression of the illness, possibly by leading to earlier-onset, more severe episodes, and an increased likelihood of personality disorder and suicide attempts. The serotonin transporter polymorphism mentioned above appears to mediate the relationship between early trauma and depression. Likewise, this polymorphism appears relevant to neuroticism and suicide attempts.

Temperament Since ancient times, persons prone to mania and melancholia have been described as possessing certain temperamental attributes, representing variations on the theme of what today is subsumed under cyclothymic, dysthymic, and anxious-inhibited temperaments, as well as the traits of high neuroticism describing emotionality. Many monozygotic twins discordant for full-blown mood disorders studied by Aksel Bertelsen's Danish research team exhibited affective instability with temperamental moodiness, which strongly suggests that such attributes are genetically determined. Research conducted by Kendler's team at the Medical College of Virginia further suggests that several of the temperamental attributes might be transmitted as part of the genetic liability to mood disorders. The author's research has identified such temperaments in the prepubertal offspring of parents with bipolar I disorders, suggesting that they precede by years to decades the overt onset of major mood disorder episodes. The high expressed emotion atmosphere and the negative critical remarks by relatives and affectively unstable patients documented in the recent psychological literature on mood disorders often reflect the interpersonal clashes between patients and their temperamentally intense relatives. Thus, temperaments appear intimately involved in generating much interpersonal friction, emotional arousal, and sleep loss (just to cite common perturbations), thereby eliciting many of the life stressors that precipitate affective episodes. The use of stimulant drugs either to self-treat lethargy or enhance hypomanic traits could further contribute to episode precipitation. As for the depressive disposition, the work of Maria Kovacs at the University of Pittsburgh has shown that dysthymia in children evolves into major depressive episodes postpubertally, of which a proportion switch to bipolar states. These data cohere with the work of the present author conducted at the University of Tennessee, Memphis, showing shortened REM latency in early-onset dysthymic subjects. The familial bipolar diathesis revealed in the Tennessee work, along with its tendency to switch to hypomania, suggest commonalities between depressive and bipolar II disorders.

Life Events Most individuals do not develop clinical depression when exposed to environmental adversity. Such adversity seems to play a pathogenic role primarily in those with an affective diathesis. In fact, the work of Kendler at the Medical College of Virginia indicates that genetic factors might underlie the depressive disorder patients' susceptibility to life events. Furthermore, current data suggest that social stressors in the onset of depression are more relevant to the first few episodes of the illness. The evidence linking such events to mania is less convincing. At any rate, stressful events often appear to be triggered by the temperamental instability that precedes clinical episodes. Interpersonal losses are common events in the lives of individuals with intense temperaments. The arousal and sleep loss associated with such events can precipitate both depressive and manic states.

A recent study by Peter McGuffin's team at the Institute of Psychiatry, London, raised the possibility that one mechanism by which heredity produces depression is the creation of environmental adversities in the lives of individuals predisposed to this illness. This work is now replicated by independent groups of investigators. Whatever the origin of environmental adversity, it is common clinical experience that loss represents an important, perhaps even central, theme in clinical depression. Variables that seem to modulate the impact of adult losses include concurrent life events, resultant changes in lifestyle, lack of interpersonal support, deficient social skills, and the symbolic meaning of the putative loss. The research program of George Brown and his followers in London capitalizes on the foregoing considerations, particularly the importance of early and proximate losses in socioeconomically disadvantaged women who lack supportive relationships. However, that conceptualization downplays the degree to which the social context of the depression reflects the dysthymic temperamental liabilities of those depressed women. Recent research indicates that even social support is determined to a considerable degree by the genetic mechanisms that underlie mood disorders. Indeed, the short alleles of the serotonin transporter gene are now implicated in mediating between adverse events and clinical depression.

Biological Stressors Many physical diseases and pharmacological agents are known to precede the onset of both depressive and manic episodes. Like psychosocial stressors, however, they do not generally seem to cause de novo episodes but mobilize them in persons with a personal and family history of mood disorders. Thyroid disturbances have a role in practice because they are associated with rapid cycling in bipolar patients, especially women; lithium is often contributory to such disturbances occurring in the depressions in which bipolar women are not uncommonly "stuck."

Sex Clinical and epidemiological studies concur in suggesting that women are at higher risk for mood disorders, with the risk highest for depression. This now appears to be, in part, a function of anxious-depressive traits represented by neuroticism. These traits have strong genetic determinants. Women have higher concentrations of monamine oxidase (the enzyme that breaks down monamine transmitters) in the brain and more precarious thyroid status. In addition, low estrogen and high progesterone concentrations have been postulated as possible mediating factors in postpartum depressions, premenstrual accentuation of affective instability, and women's vulnerability to the depressant effect of steroidal contraceptives. Finally, recent data point to the role of estradiol in depressions occurring during the transition to menopause. Personality factors might also be relevant to the sex differences in depression. In recent collaborative work with University of Pisa psychiatrist Giulio Perugi, the author has proposed the hypothesis that female sex might favor greater expression of dysthymic attributes, whereas hyperthymic traits appear favored by male sex. Those considerations tend to parallel, respectively, the *ruminative* and *active* cognitive response styles reported by Susan Nolen-Hoeksema, originally at Stanford University, to distinguish the sexes. What specific sex-related biographical factors might interact with sex-related biological factors to produce such trait differences is, at present, largely unknown. An intriguing possibility is that women, because of temperamental inclination to depressive cognitions, might react more intensely to childhood adversities, as well as be more specifically vulnerable to adult stressors related to bonding with men and child rearing. Research by Mark George and colleagues has raised the provocative possibility that women overrespond to sad circumstances over a lifetime, thereby permanently altering anterior limbic and prefrontal brain function in a "depressive" direction. The high prevalence of anxious-depressive conditions in women—most pronounced at the clinical level—might be linked, hypothetically, to an evolutionary adaptive advantage conferred by traits of fear, inhibition, and avoidance to women who bear the responsibility of pregnancy and child rearing. The higher prevalence of minor depressions in women, rediscovered in a recent Danish study, are in line with the foregoing hypothesis.

The integrative model presented here (Fig. 13.1–3) goes beyond the general provisions of the unified approach developed three decades ago. It is submitted that, at least in the highly recurrent forms of the malady, affective temperaments represent the intermediary stage between remote (hereditary) and proximate (stressful) factors and that limbic-diencephalic dysfunction is best characterized as the biological concomitant of the clinical manifestations of the affective syndromes. Like the temperamental dysregulations, these biological disturbances represent a putative stage in the pathogenetic chain. They emerge as temperamental instabilities that react to, provoke, or invite life events, substance use, and alterations in circadian rhythms—which, in turn, appear to usher in the behavioral, emotional, and cognitive manifestations of the illness. It is finally relevant to point out that biological stressors such as hormonal disturbances and traumatic brain injury appear to compromise limbic-diencephalic function as their depressant mechanism.

Therapeutic Perspectives The foregoing integrative model mandates the joint use of somatic-pharmacological and psychosocial

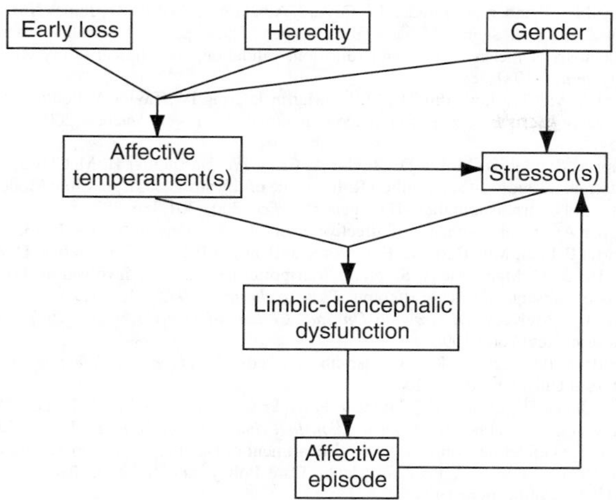

FIGURE 13.1–3 An integrative pathogenetic model of mood disorders.

interventions. Although the milder forms of mood disorders can be managed with psychotherapy, somatic treatments are usually required to reverse the biological disturbances in melancholia before the patient can respond to interpersonal feedback. Depressive disorders with psychotic features often necessitate more definitive somatic interventions, such as electroconvulsive therapy (ECT). Continued psychopharmacological treatment is also effective in decreasing rates of relapse and future recurrence in most. Today, bipolar disorder, as well as most forms of depression, are considered lifelong illnesses needing indefinite maintenance pharmacotherapy.

Psychosocial therapy by skilled clinicians can provide support, combat demoralization, change maladaptive self-attributions, and improve conjugal and vocational functioning. Recent fascinating data support the notion that psychosocial interventions such as cognitive-behavioral therapy modulate cortical-limbic function described earlier as the final common pathway of depressive illness. Whether such therapy can also modify personality traits to fortify the patient against new episodes is a future research challenge. In the author's view, it may prove more profitable to attempt to help patients explore professional and object choices that match their temperamental proclivities and assets, which, in turn, might provide them greater harmony and adaptation in life. Although much needs to be learned about the indications for medication and psychotherapy in different subtypes of mood disorders, research to date not only does not support a negative interaction between the two forms of treatment, but, on selected parameters, suggests additive and even synergistic interaction. There is a great need for patients, their families, and clinicians to understand how a biologically driven illness like depression should be approached from a pragmatic psychotherapeutic perspective.

The challenge for psychiatric research in the decade ahead is to elucidate the basic mechanisms whereby the predisposing, precipitating, and mediating variables reviewed here and others yet to be identified interact to produce the final common path of decompensation in melancholia. Because of the heterogeneity of depressive conditions presenting as a psychobiological final common clinical syndrome and because antidepressant agents, irrespective of specificity to one or another biogenic amine, are approximately equally effective in two-thirds of those with depressive disorders, the antidepressant agents may be acting not on the primary lesions of these disorders but on a neurochemical substrate distal to the underlying biological faults. Choice of antidepressants is still highly determined by the side effect profile least objectionable to a given patient's physical status, temperament, and lifestyle. That so many different classes of antidepressants—with different mechanisms of action—have been marketed since the 1990s represents indirect evidence for heterogeneity of putative biochemical lesions. The investigation of central neurotransmitter receptor function continues to occupy much current effort to delineate the mechanism of antidepressant action and side effects of classic agents, as well as the new compounds that have made the treatment of depression "clinician and patient friendly." Whether study of specific receptors will unravel the molecular mystery of depression remains to be seen. Since the 1990s, studies have begun on antidepressant and mood-stabilizing effects on molecular mechanisms believed to be closer to the "genetic underpinnings" of mood disorders. Herein is the promise of the future, a new generation of psychiatrists conversant with both clinical phenomenology and molecular biology. Data suggest that the biological specificity of genetic factors in mood disorders might be translated into distinct temperamental dysregulations, which, in turn, might predispose to different affective subtypes.

Returning to the therapeutic arena, mounting clinical evidence indicates that, in a special subgroup of depressed patients with bipolar disorder, antidepressants might provoke mixed episodes, hypomanic episodes, or both, and possibly increase later cycling. The kindling-sensitization model suggests the utility of anticonvulsant medication on episode escalation and might represent yet another example of pathophysiological intervention. Whatever the merit of this model, the 1990s have witnessed intense clinical and research interest and U.S. Food and Drug Administration (FDA) approval of clinical introduction of divalproex (Depakote) and lamotrigine (Lamictal) for bipolar disorder, and many other promising anticonvulsants are being developed for that disorder. Anticonvulsant mood stabilizers appear to possess a broad spectrum of activity on bipolar disorders, including mixed dysphoric and rapid-cycling forms. Lithium, by contrast, seems more specific to euphoric or "classic" mania. On the other hand, the introduction of olanzapine (Zyprexa), risperidone (Risperdal), and quetiapine (Seroquel), atypical antipsychotics, for mania raises intriguing questions about a common neural substrate for schizophrenic and manic disorders.

Psychoeducational interventions geared to disturbed rhythms of the disorder represent another example of rational therapeutics. Mood clinics should help patients and their significant others to dampen stimulation so that it is kept at an optimal level for depressed patients with cyclothymic traits. All offending drugs (e.g., cocaine, caffeine, and sedative-hypnotic agents) should be gradually eliminated and circadian disruptions and sleep loss minimized. The greater challenge is learning how to curb the ill-advised actions of patients with cyclical depressions. Psychoeducation and psychotherapy have the task of ameliorating the resulting social problems. Compliance with mood-stabilizer regimens that, for many, would attenuate episodes and prevent such sequelae is difficult to achieve. Further research on treatment or medication-adherence techniques is needed for promoting more efficient use of mood stabilizers.

It is tempting to suggest that biogenic amines, the "humors" of modern psychobiology, play the same heuristic role as the ancient humors did for many centuries. The black humor, appropriately evoked in the construct of melancholia in DSM-IV-TR, may not have the same claim for etiological relevance to depressive disorders as norepinephrine and serotonin, but at least has a classic heritage. Dopamine, by contrast, may represent the sanguine humor that drives hypomanic temperaments and manic behavior. When genetic factors contributing to clinical depression and mania are discovered, in all likelihood, they will be more linked to temperamental dispositions than to full-blown affective disease phenotypes. The clinician will still need to interpret the myriad of influences that impinge on such inclinations to produce disease in an individual patient—that is, fundamental scientific advances in mood disorders, rather than diminishing the role of practitioners, will actually increase it. Regretfully, despite destigmatization efforts and a rich armamentarium of therapeutic developments, the actual clinical care of affectively ill at the severe end of the spectrum continues to be grossly inadequate. More research will not improve this dismal situation unless the human and social dimensions of severe mood disorders are addressed with the requisite clinical and public health policies. Caring for the mentally ill is a dimension distinct from evidence-based treatments along psychopharmacological and psychotherapeutic lines: It requires the allocation of human resources and integrated mental health structures geared to the total patient.

In any discipline, scientific truth is a function of its technology, but understanding the phenomena under consideration is a matter of philosophical temperament that seeks integration and the hope for a unified vision. Research into the causes and treatment of mood disorders has generated abundant recent data suitable for integration into theory and practice, and conceptualizing the origin and treatment of mood disorders can no longer be justified on the grounds of ideological preference alone.

SUGGESTED CROSS-REFERENCES

Sections 13.2 through 13.9 cover the various aspects of mood disorders in great detail.

REFERENCES

Abraham K. Notes on the psychoanalytical investigation and treatment of manic-depressive insanity and allied conditions. In: *Selected Papers of Karl Abraham.* Hogarth Press: London; 1948.

Adams F, ed. *Aretaeus of Cappadocia: The Extant Works of Aretaeus, the Cappadocian.* Sydenham Society: London; 1856.

Ahrens B, Muller-Oerlinghausen M, Schou M, Wolf T, Alda E, Grof P, Grof G, Lenz C, Simhandl K, Thau P, Vestergaard R, Muller HJ: Excess cardiovascular and suicide mortality of affective disorders may be reduced by lithium prophylaxis. *J Affect Disord.* 1995;33:67.

Akiskal HS: Dysthymia and cyclothymia in psychiatric practice a century after Kraepelin. *J Affect Disord.* 2001;62:17–31.

Akiskal HS, Downs J, Jordan P, Watson S, Daugherty D, Pruitt DB: Affective disorders in referred children and younger siblings of manic-depressives: mode of onset and prospective course. *Arch Gen Psychiatry.* 1985;4:996.

*Akiskal HS, McKinney WT: Depressive disorders: toward a unified hypothesis. *Science.* 1973;182:20.

Akiskal HS, Yerevanian BI, Davis GC, King D, Lemmi H: The nosologic status of borderline personality: clinical and polysomnographic study. *Am J Psychiatry.* 1985;142:192–198.

Angst F, Stassen HH, Clayton PJ, Angst J: Mortality of patients with mood disorders: follow-up over 34–38 years. *J Affect Disord.* 2002;68:167–181.

Barrett TB, Hauger RL, Kennedy JL, Sadovnick AD, Remick RA, Keck PE, McElroy SL, Alexander M, Shaw SH, Kelsoe JR: Evidence that a single nucleotide polymorphism in the promoter of the G protein receptor kinase 3 gene is associated with bipolar disorder. *Mol Psychiatry.* 2003;8:546–557.

Beck AT. *Depression: Causes and Treatment.* University of Pennsylvania Press: Philadelphia; 1967.

Berger M, Vollmann J, Hohagen F, Konig A, Lohner H, Voderholzer U, Riemann D: Sleep deprivation combined with consecutive sleep phase advance as a fast-acting therapy in depression: an open pilot trial in medicated and unmedicated patients. *Am J Psychiatry.* 1998;155:1134–1135.

*Bertelsen A, Harvald B, Hauge M: A Danish twin study of manic-depressive disorders. *Br J Psychiatry* 1997;130:330.

Biederman J, Mick E, Faraone SV, Spencer T, Wilens TE, Wozniak J: Pediatric mania: a developmental subtype of bipolar disorder? *Biol Psychiatry.* 2000;48:458–466.

Bowlby J: Process of mourning. *Int J Psychoanal.* 1961;45:317.

Brown GW, Harris T: Social origins of depression: *A Study of Psychiatric Disorder in Women.* London: Tavistock; 1978.

Brown ES, Varghese FP, McEwan BS: Association of depression with medical illness: does cortisol play a role? *Biol Psychiatry.* 2004;55:1–9.

Bunney WE Jr, Davis JM: Norepinephrine in depressive reactions: a review. *Arch Gen Psychiatry.* 1965;13:483.

Carlson GA, Cantwell DP: Unmasking masked depression in children and adolescents. *Am J Psychiatry.* 1980;137:445–449.

Carroll BJ, Feinberg M, Greden IF, Tarika J, Albala AA, Haskett RF, James NM, Kronfol Z, Lohr N, Steiner M, de Vigne JP, Young E: A specific laboratory test for the diagnosis of melancholia: standardization, validation, and clinical utility. *Arch Gen Psychiatry.* 1981;38:15.

Caspi A, McClay J, Moffitt TE, Mill J, Martin J, Craig IW, Taylor A, Poulton R: Role of genotype in the cycle of violence in maltreated children. *Science.* 2002;297:851–854.

Caspi A, Sugden K, Moffit TE, Taylor A, Craig IW, Harrington H, McClay J, Mill J, Martin J, Braithwaite A, Poulton R: Influence of life stress on depression: Moderation by a polymorphism in the 5-HTT gene. *Science.* 2003;301:386–389.

Coppen A: The biochemistry of affective disorders. *Br J Psychiatry.* 1967;113:1237.

Courtet P, Picot MC, Bellivier F, Torres S, Jollant F, Michelon C, Castelnau D, Astruc B, Buresi C, Malafosse A: Serotonin transporter gene may be involved in short-term risk of subsequent suicide attempts. *Biol Psychiatry.* 2004;55:46–51.

Cytryn L, McKnew D. *Growing Up Sad: Childhood Depression and Its Treatment.* Norton: New York; 1996.

Davidson RJ, Scherer KR, Goldsmith HH, eds. *Handbook of Affective Sciences.* Oxford University Press; 2003.

Delay J. *Les Déglements de L'humeur.* Paris: Presses Universitaires de France; 1946.

Depression Guideline Panel. *Depression in Primary Care: Volumes 1 & 2.* Clinical Practice Guideline, Number 5. U.S. Department of Health and Human Services, Public Health Service, Agency for Health Care Policy and Research. Rockville, MD: AHCPR Publication; 1993.

Drevets WC: Neuroimaging abnormalities in the amygdala in mood disorders. *Ann N Y Acad Sci.* 2003;985:420–444.

Espiritu RC, Kripke DF, Ancoli-Israel S, Mowen MA, Mason WJ, Fell RL, Klauber MR, Kaplan OJ: Low illumination experienced by San Diego adults: association with atypical depressive symptoms. *Biol Psychiatry.* 1994;35:403–407.

Feng P, Ma Y: Instrumental REM sleep deprivation in neonates leads to adult depression-like behaviors in rats. *Sleep.* 2003;26:990–996.

Frasure-Smith N, Lesperance F: Depression—a cardiac risk factor in search of a treatment. *JAMA.* 2003;289:3171–3173.

Freeman EW, Sammel MD, Liu L, Gracia CR, Nelson DB, Hollander L: Hormones and menopausal status as predictors of depression in women in transition to menopause. *Arch Gen Psychiatry.* 2004;61:62–70.

Freud S. Mourning and melancholia. In: *Standard Edition of the Complete Psychological Works of Sigmund Freud.* Vol 4. London: Hogarth Press; 1975.

George MS, Ketter TA, Parekh PI, Horwitz B, Herscovitch P, Post RM: Brain activity during transient sadness and happiness in healthy women. *Am J Psychiatry.* 1995;152:341.

Gershon ES, Hamovit J, Guroff JJ, Dribble E, Leckman JF, Sceery W, Targum SD, Numberger JI, Goldin LR, Bunney WE: A family study of schizoaffective, bipolar I, bipolar II, unipolar, and normal control probands. *Arch Gen Psychiatry.* 1982;39:1157.

Gessa GL: Dysthymia and depressive disorders: dopamine hypothesis. *Eur Psychiatry.* 1996;11:123.

Gilbody S, Whitty P, Grimshaw J, Thomas R: Educational and organizational interventions to improve the management of depression in primary care: a systematic review. *JAMA.* 2003;289:3145–3151.

Gillin JC, Sitaram N, Duncan WC: Muscarinic supersensitivity: A possible model for the sleep disturbance of primary depression? *Psychiatry Res.* 1979;1:17.

Gilmer WS, McKinney WT: Early experience and depressive disorders: human and non-human primate studies. *J Affect Disord.* 2003;75:97–113.

Goldapple K, Segal Z, Garson C, Lau M, Bieling P, Kennedy S, Mayberg H: Modulation of cortical-limbic pathways in major depression: treatment-specific effects of cognitive behavior therapy. *Arch Gen Psychiatry.* 2004;61:34–41.

*Goodwin FK, Jamison KR. *Manic-Depressive Illness.* New York: Oxford University Press; 1990.

Heninger GR, Delgado PL, Chamey DS: The revised monoamine theory of depression: a modulatory role for monoamines, based on new findings from monoamine depletion experiments in humans. *Pharmacopsychiatry.* 1996;29:2.

Hippocrates. Epidemics III. In: Jones WHS, tr. *Hippocrates.* Vol 1. Cambridge: Harvard University Press; 1923.

Holsboer F: The role of peptides in treatment of psychiatric disorders. *J Neural Transm Suppl.* 2003;64:17–34.

Jackson SW. *Melancholia and Depression: From Hippocratic Times to Modem Times.* New Haven: Yale University Press; 1986.

Janowsky DS, El-Yousef MK, Davis JM, Sekerke HJ: A cholinergic-adrenergic hypothesis of mania and depression. *Lancet.* 1972;1:632.

Jorge RE, Robinson RG, Moser D, Tateno A, Crespo-Facorro B, Arndt S: Major depression following traumatic brain injury. *Arch Gen Psychiatry.* 2004;61:42–50.

Keller MB, Klerman GL, Lavori PW, Fawcett JA, Coryell W, Endicott J: Treatment received by depressed patients. *JAMA.* 1982;248:1848.

Kendler KS: Social support: a genetic-epidemiological analysis. Am J Psychiatry. 1997;154:1398.

Kendler KS, Gardner CO, Prescott CA: Toward a comprehensive developmental model for major depression in women. *Am J Psychiatry.* 2003;159:1133–1145.

Kendler KS, Karkowski-Shuman L: Stressful life events and generic liability to major depression: genetic control of exposure to the environment? *Psychol Med.* 1997;27:359.

Kendler KS, Neale MC, Kessler RC, Heath AC, Eaves LJ: A longitudinal twin study of personality and major depression in women. *Arch Gen Psychiatry.* 1993;50:853.

Klerman GL, Lavori PW, Rice J, Reich T, Endicott J, Andreasen NC, Keller MB, Hirschfield RM: Birth-cohort trends in rates of major depressive disorder among relatives of patients with affective disorder. *Arch Gen Psychiatry.* 1985;42:689.

Kovacs M, Akiskal HS, Gatsonis C, Parrone PL: Childhood-onset dysthymic disorder: clinical features and prospective naturalistic outcome. *Arch Gen Psychiatry.* 1994;51:365–374.

*Kraepelin E. *Manic-Depressive Insanity and Paranoia*. Edinburgh: Livingstone; 1921.
Krishman KR: Pituitary size in depression. *J Clin Endocrinol Metab*. 1991;72:256.
Kupfer DJ: REM latency: a psychobiologic marker for primary depressive disease. *Biol Psychiatry*. 1976;11:159.
Lapin IP, Oxenkrug GF: Intensification of the central serotoninergic processes as a possible determinant of the thymoleptic effect. *Lancet*. 1969;1:132.
Leonhard K, Berman R, tr. *The Classification of Endogenous Psychoses*. New York: Irvington; 1979.
Lesch KP, Bengel D, Heils A, Sabol SZ, Greenberg BD, Petri S, Benjamin J, Muller CR, Hamer DH, Murphy DL: Association of anxiety-related traits with a polymorphism in the serotonin transporter gene regulatory region. *Science*. 1996;274:1483.
Lewinsohn PM, Youngren MA, Grosscup SJ. Reinforcement and depression. In: Depue RE, ed. *The Psychobiology of Depressive Disorders; Implications for the Effects of Stress*. New York: Academic Press; 1979.
Lewis A: States of depression: their clinical and aetiological differentiation. *Br Med*. 1938;J2:875.
*Maj M, Akiskal HS, Lopez-Ibor JJ, Sartorius N, eds. *Bipolar Disorder, World Psychiatric Association Series Evidence and Experience in Psychiatry*. London: John Wiley & Sons; 2002.
Manji HK, McNamara R, Chen G, Lenox RH: Signalling pathways in the brain: cellular transduction of mood stabilization in the treatment of manic-depressive illness. *Aust N Z Psychiatry*. 1999;33[Suppl]:S65–S83.
Mann JJ, Malone KM, Diehl DJ, Perel J, Cooper TB, Mintun MA: Demonstration in vivo of reduced serotonin responsivity in the brain of untreated depressed patients. *Am J Psychiatry*. 1996;153:174.
McGuffin P, Katz R, Bebbington P: The Camberwell Collaborative Depressive Study: III. Depression and adversity in the relatives of depressed probands. *Br J Psychiatry*. 1988;152:775.
McMahon FJ, Simpson SG, McInnis MG, Badner JA, MacKinnon DF, DePaulo JR: Linkage of bipolar disorder to chromosome 18q and the validity of bipolar II disorder. *Arch Gen Psychiatry*. 2001;58:1025–1031.
Murray CJL, Lopez AD, eds. *The Global Burden of Disease*. Geneva: World Health Organization; 1996.
Nazroo JY, Edwards AC, Brown GW: Gender differences in the onset of depression following a shared life event: a study of couples. *Psychol Med*. 1997;27:9.
Nemeroff CB, Widerlov E, Bissette G: Elevated concentrations of CSF corticotropin-releasing factor-like immunoreactivity in depressed patients. *Science*. 1984;226:1342.
Nestler EJ, Barrot M, DiLeone RJ, Eisch AJ, Gold SJ, Monteggia LM: Neurobiology of depression. *Neuron*. 2002;34:13–25.
Niculescu AB, Akiskal HS: Sex hormones, Darwinism and depression. *Arch Gen Psychiatry*. 2001;58:1083–1084.
Nolen-Hoeksema S, Morrow J, Frederickson BL: Response styles and the duration of episodes of depressed mood. *J Abnorm Psychol*. 1993;102:20.
Olsen LR, Mortensen EL, Bech P: Prevalence of major depression and stress indicators in the Danish general population. *Acta Psychiatr Scand*. 2004;109:96–103.
Parry BL, Haynes P: Mood disorders and the reproductive cycle. *J Gend Specif Med*. 2000;3:53–58.
Perugi G, Akiskal HS, Pamacciotti S, Massini S, Toni C, Milanfranchi A, Musetti L: Depressive comorbidity of panic, social phobic and obsessive compulsive disorders: Is there a bipolar II connection? *J Psychiatr Res*. 1999;33:53–61.
Perugi G, Musetti L, Simonini E, Piagentini F, Cassano GB, Akiskal HS: Gender mediated clinical features of depressive illness: the importance of temperamental differences. *Br J Psychiatry*. 1990;157:835–841.
Petty F: GABA and mood disorders: a brief review and hypothesis. *J Affect Disord*. 1995;34:275–281.
Post RM: Transduction of psychosocial stress into the neurobiology of recurrent affective disorder. *Am J Psychiatry*. 1992;149:999.
Poznanski E, Zrull JP: Childhood depression: clinical characteristics of overtly depressed children. *Arch Gen Psychiatry*. 1970;23:8.
Prange AJ Jr, Wilson IC, Lynn CW, Alltop LB, Stikeleather RA: L-Tryptophan in mania: contribution to a permissive hypothesis of affective disorders. *Arch Gen Psychiatry*. 1974;30:56.
Puig-Antich J. Affective disorders in children and adolescents. In: Meltzer HY, ed. *Psychopharmacology: The Third Generation of Progress*. New York: Raven; 1987.
Rihmer Z, Rutz W, Pihlgren H: Depression and suicide on Gotland: an intensive study of all suicides before and after a depression-training programme for general practitioners. *J Affect Disord*. 1995;35:147.
Rihmer Z, Kiss K: Bipolar disorders and suicidal behaviour. *Bipolar Disord*. 2002;(Suppl 1);21–25.
Roth RM, Barnes TR: The classification of affective disorders: a synthesis of old and new concepts. *Compr Psychiatry*. 1981;22:54–77.
Rutz W: Rethinking mental health: a European WHO perspective. *World Psychiatry*. 2003;2:125–127.
Schildkraut JJ: The catecholamine hypothesis of affective disorders: a review of supporting evidence. *Am J Psychiatry*. 1995;22:509–522.
Schulberg HC: Treating major depression in primary care practice. Eight-month clinical outcomes. *Arch Gen Psychiatry*. 1996;53:913.
Seligman MD. *Helplessness: On Depression, Development and Death*. San Francisco: Freeman; 1975.
Siever LJ, Davis KL: Overview: toward a dysregulation hypothesis of depression. *Am J Psychiatry*. 1985;142:1017.
Tsai S-J: Is mania caused by overactivity of central brain-derived neurotrophic factor? *Med Hypotheses*. 2004;62:19–22.
Unutzer J: Diagnosis and treatment of older adults with depression in primary care. *Biol Psychiatry*. 2002;52:285–292.
van Praag HM, Kahn RS, Asnis GM, Wetzler S, Brown SL, Bleich A, Kom ML: Denosologization of biological psychiatry or the specificity of 5-HT disturbances in psychiatric disorders. *J Affect Disord*. 1987;13:1.
Wehr TA, Rosenthal NE: Seasonality and affective illness. *Am J Psychiatry*. 1989;146:829.
Weller EB, Weller RA: Bipolar disorder in children: misdiagnosis, underdiagnosis, and future diagnosis. *J Am Acad Child Adolesc Psychiatry*. 1995;34:709.
Whybrow P, Mendels J: Toward a biology of depression: some suggestions from neurophysiology. *Am J Psychiatry*. 1969;125:45.
Wilhelm K, Parker G, Hadzi-Pavlovic D: Fifteen years on: evolving ideas in researching sex differences in depression. *Psychol Med*. 1997;27:875.
Winokur G, Clayton PJ, Reich T. *Manic-Depressive Illness*. St. Louis: Mosby; 1969.
Yerevanian BI, Koek RJ, Mintz J: Lithium, anticonvulsants and suicidal behavior in bipolar disorder. *J Affect Disord*. 2003;73:223–228.
Zis KD, Zis A: Increased adrenal weight in victims of violent suicide. *Am J Psychiatry*. 1987;144:1214.

▲ 13.2 Mood Disorders: Epidemiology

Zoltán Rihmer, M.D., Ph.D., and Jules Angst, M.D.

Community epidemiological studies in the field of psychiatry provide several important and clinically useful pieces of information on the prevalence and other characteristics (e.g., risk factors, social correlates, use of health care) of mood disorders that cannot be extrapolated from everyday clinical practice. Inpatient and outpatient populations (the most severe and frequently comorbid cases) are not representative of all patients with mood disorders, because many subjects do not seek treatment. Until the first decades of the 20th century, when psychiatry existed only within the walls of psychiatric institutes, it was believed that schizophrenia and (manic) depressive disorders were equally frequent but relatively rare disorders. However, due to the great development in the classification and treatment of psychiatric disorders that has occurred since the second half of the 20th century, clinical studies of this period clearly suggest that depressive disorders—even in the clinical population—are much more common than schizophrenia. The two main sources of this observation are (1) the steady and marked decrease of the clinical practice of misdiagnosis of depression or mania, or both, as schizophrenia and (2) the fact that the most recent classification systems (the revised fourth edition of the *Diagnostic and Statistical Manual of Mental Disorders* [DSM-IV-TR] and the tenth revision of the *International Classification of Diseases and Related Health Problems* [ICD-10]) have made the diagnoses of depressive disorders and bipolar disorders more inclusive. The latter, however, does not suggest an irrational dilution of the diagnostic category of depression and mania, as DSM-IV-TR major depressive or dysthymic disorder, as well as bipolar disorder (by definition), has an especially strong negative impact on an individual's daily functioning and quality of life, comparable to several other major medical disorders, such as diabetes and heart disease.

The increased interest in psychiatric epidemiology in the last decades of the 20th century owes much to the international development in methodology. With the worldwide introduction of operational criteria for well-defined psychiatric diagnostic categories via DSM-III (1980), DSM-IV-TR (2000), and ICD-10 (1993), it became possible to perform large-scale, cross-sectional, longitudinal, and cross-national community surveys and studies of patients in nonpsychiatric settings. Specific new instruments for assessing different

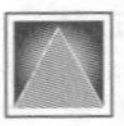

Table 13.2–1
Different Clinical Manifestations of Unipolar Depression as Defined by Severity and Duration Threshold

Severity Threshold	Duration Threshold		
Number of DSM-IV-TR Symptoms Required	<2 Wks	2 Wks–2 Yrs	>2 Yrs
2 (mild)	—	Subsyndromal symptomatic depressive disorder	—
3–4 (medium)	—	Minor depressive disorder	Dysthymic disorder
5 or more (severe)	Recurrent brief depressive disorder	Major depressive disorder	Chronic major depressive disorder

psychiatric syndromes and disorders were developed, including the following: the Diagnostic Interview Schedule (DIS) (the most widely used), the Composite International Diagnostic Interview Schedule (CIDI), the Mini International Diagnostic Interview (MINI), and the Schedule for Clinical Assessment in Neuropsychiatry (SCAN), which is capable of generating DSM-IV-TR and ICD-10 diagnoses. The modern epidemiological studies, applying the above-mentioned new instruments with refined diagnostic criteria, have found higher prevalence rates for specific mood disorders than the earlier studies based on unstructured clinical interviews. However, these studies are not free from shortcomings. Inaccurate recall of the interviewed subject can bias the lifetime prevalence rates, and the low or lacking sensitivity of these instruments to subthreshold syndromes seriously affects the prevalence of current psychopathology. Many individuals in the community may show some (a few or more) depressive symptoms that do not reach the severity or duration threshold for specific mood disorders in the DSM-IV-TR system but, nevertheless, also have substantial morbidity and dysfunction. These mood states are frequently called *subthreshold*, or *subsyndromal*, disorders, and evidence suggests that they are the less severe forms of major depressive or bipolar disorders, that they can be the precursors of further full-blown major mood syndromes, and that they can represent a residual state of major depression as a result of incomplete recovery from it. On the other hand, treatment of these subsyndromal disorders before they become severe or syndromal is important for preventing their progression and eliminating the risk of subsequent complications, primarily suicide and, secondarily, substance abuse disorders. However, the term subthreshold, or subsyndromal, can easily cause confusion, as it depends on the cutoff line of the severity and duration thresholds of the given syndrome. If syndromal level is defined as major depression, dysthymic disorder, minor depressive disorder, and recurrent brief depressive disorder can be considered subsyndromal, or subthreshold, disorders, because, in the case of dysthymic and minor depressive disorders, the required severity is below the threshold, or syndromal, level and, in the case of recurrent brief depressive disorder, the required duration is below the threshold, or syndromal, level (Table 13.2–1). Therefore, besides major depressive episode and dysthymic disorder, recurrent brief depressive disorder and minor depressive disorder (as well as recurrent brief hypomania) are well-defined and valid diagnostic categories that can also be considered in clinical practice and epidemiological research.

Despite the strict diagnostic thresholds for specific mood disorders in the DSM-IV-TR and other diagnostic systems, the distinction of milder mood disorders from the normal variation of mood is sometimes problematic. It is frequently the consequence of the fact that depression and anxiety commonly overlap with each other at the subsyndromal level of dysthymia/minor depression and any anxiety disorder. Patients suffering from this mixed anxiety-depressive disorder may exhibit the same disability as do threshold depressives and could also be classified as patients in clinical practice and as cases in further epidemiological surveys.

The two most influential epidemiological studies came from the United States: the Epidemiological Catchment Area Study (ECA) in 1981 and the National Comorbidity Survey (NCS) in 1991. The first investigation was performed in five sites throughout the United States (New Haven, Baltimore, St. Louis, Durham, and Los Angeles), included more than 18,000 community and institutionalized subjects (18 years of age or older), and used the DIS for case identification. More than 8,000 people from a nationwide sample (between the ages of 15 and 54 years) in which a modified version of CIDI was used as a diagnostic instrument participated in the NCS. During the years 2001 and 2002, the NCS was replicated (NCS-R) in the 48 contiguous states of the Unites States, including 9,090 household residents aged 18 years or older. In addition, several large-scale, cross-sectional, and national and international community studies, as well as surveys in primary care, were performed recently in many countries outside the United States, including Canada, Australia and New Zealand, Germany, France, the United Kingdom, Switzerland, Spain, Italy, the Netherlands, Lebanon, Taiwan, Korea, Greece, Norway, Finland, and Hungary. The data presented in this chapter are derived from North American and other community-based studies on the frequency, distribution, and clinical correlates of unipolar depressive disorders and bipolar illness.

PREVALENCE AND INCIDENCE OF MOOD DISORDERS IN THE COMMUNITY

Unipolar and bipolar depressive disorders, including their different clinical manifestations, are the most frequent psychiatric illnesses both in the community and in a variety of clinical settings. In addition to their frequent and serious complications (e.g., suicide, substance use disorders), they are strongly associated with limitations in well-being and daily functioning that are equal to or greater than those of several chronic medical conditions.

Unipolar Depression The ECA study reported that the lifetime and 1-year prevalence rates of major depressive disorder were 4.9 percent and 2.7 percent, respectively. Most likely due to the different methodology used in the NCS (i.e., the lower threshold for case identification with CIDI), the lifetime, 1-year, and current prevalence figures (17.1 percent, 10.3 percent, and 4.9 percent, respectively) were much higher. Most recent results of the NCS-R on the prevalence of CIDI/DSM-IV major depressive disorder showed that the major depression prevalence estimates were intermediate between the ECA and NCS estimates: the lifetime and 12-month prevalence of major depressive disorder in the NCS-R were 16.2 and 6.6 percent, respectively, and the mean episode duration was 16 weeks. The major depressive disorder usually was associated with substantial symptom severity, Axis I comorbidity, and role impairment. In the Zurich cohort study, the life-

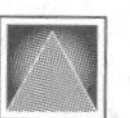

Table 13.2–2
Lifetime, 1-Year, and Current (1-Month) Prevalence Rates of Unipolar Depressive Disorders According to Eight Large-Scale Population Studies Conducted in the United States and Europe

		Lifetime Prevalence (%)	1-Yr Prevalence (%)	Current Prevalence (%)
Major depressive episode	Range	5–17	3–10	2–7
	Average	12	7	4
Dysthymic disorder	Range	3–6	3	3
	Average	5	—	—
Minor depressive disorder	Range	10	2	—
	Average	—	—	—
Recurrent brief depressive disorder	Range	16	4–8	5
	Average	—	6	—
Full unipolar spectrum		20–25	10–15	5–10

Adapted from Angst, 1998; Ayuso-Mateos et al., 2001; Kessler et al., 1994; Kessler et al., 1997; Lépine et al., 1997; Regier et al., 1988; Szádóczky et al., 1998; and Weissman et al., 1996.

time prevalence of major depression was estimated to be approximately 16 to 20 percent. The lifetime, 1-year/6-month, and current (1-month) prevalence rates of different forms of DSM-IV-TR unipolar depressive disorder, according to the eight major community surveys using specific diagnostic instruments (DIS, CDI, MINI, SCAN) performed in the United States and Europe, are shown in Table 13.2–2. It should be noted that, because of the tendency to forget over time (particularly in the case of male subjects), period prevalence rates and lifetime prevalence rates are less reliable than current (point) prevalence rates. However, when attempting to estimate the number or rate of people with any kind of unipolar depressive disorder in the population at any given time or time period, one should be cautious, as the true values are substantially lower than the sum of the prevalence rates of different depressive subgroups. This is due to the fact that one patient might have more than one diagnosis, because different forms of unipolar depression show a substantial overlap cross-sectionally and longitudinally. In addition, a patient's diagnosis may change over time—for example, from dysthymic disorder to major depressive disorder and vice versa (double depression), or from recurrent brief depressive disorder to major depressive disorder (combined depression). A cross-national comparison of studies conducted using DIS in ten different countries all over the world published lifetime and 1-year prevalence rates of major depression for people between the ages of 18 and 65, standardized to U.S. age and sex distribution. The lifetime rates varied between 1.5 percent and 19.0 percent. The lowest figures were found in Taiwan, Hong Kong, and Korea, and the highest figure was found in Beirut, Lebanon. The 1-year prevalence rates ranged from 0.8 percent in Taiwan to 5.8 percent in New Zealand.

Incidence is defined by the number of new cases of the given disorder per 100,000 of the population over 1 year. Incidence dates are difficult to obtain, because their collection relies on prospective studies. The yearly incidence of a major depressive episode in the ECA study was 1.59 percent (women, 1.89 percent; men, 1.10 percent). In the Swedish Lundby study, the annual first incidence of depression was 0.76 percent for women and 0.43 for men, and, up to the age of 70 years, the cumulative probability of first-episode depression was 45 percent in women and 27 percent in men. Similarly, in Hungary (another European country in which the suicide rate is high), up to the age of 60 years, the cumulative probability of a first-episode DIS-DSM-III-R major depression was 32 percent for women and 18 percent for men.

Based on the prevalence and incidence rates of unipolar depressive disorders, it should be concluded that depressive disorders are quite common in Western societies. The prevalence of depression in Far Eastern countries, however, is lower, probably due to cultural differences regarding such areas as psychosocial stressors and alcohol and drug consumption. Investigating the differences between ethnic groups—whites, African Americans, Hispanics, and Asian Americans—a recent study from the United States found that, after adjusting for demographic factors, Asian Americans had the lowest prevalence of both major depressive and dysthymic disorders. This suggests that the prevalence rate of major depressive episode (and bipolar I) disorder in Far Eastern countries reported by the Cross-National Collaborative Group could, in fact, be lower. In addition, differences in diagnostic instruments and in other aspects of methodology may also explain some discrepancies regarding the varying prevalence of depression in Western countries.

Bipolar Disorders

Although clinical and epidemiological research of bipolar disorder has been a relatively neglected area in the past, this illness is receiving more and more attention. Until recently, bipolar disorder was equated with classic manic-depressive (i.e., bipolar I) disorder, and the lifetime prevalence of bipolar disorder was found to be approximately 1 percent. However, if the diagnosis of bipolar II disorder (major depression with hypomania, but not with mania)—a valid, reliable, and quite stable clinical diagnosis (which has become a specific diagnostic category in DSM-IV-TR)—was considered, much higher lifetime prevalence rates of the broadly defined bipolar disorders, up to at least 5 percent, were reported. The emerging epidemiology of bipolar disorders is a result of not only this important step (i.e., recognition of the fact that hypomania is as important an indicator of bipolarity as mania), but also the use of DSM-IV-TR criterion of a minimum duration of hypomania shorter than 4 days, as hypomania lasting 2 or 3 days has been well validated. Finally, it is also evident that psychotic and mixed (dysphoric) forms of elated/excited mood states can be seen frequently in otherwise typical manic-depressive (bipolar I) disorder and that these clinical presentations do not automatically mean schizoaffective illness or agitated depression. The correct identification of bipolar II illness has important implications, and not only for epidemiological research. In the absence of mood stabilizers, antidepressants alone may worsen the course of bipolar II disorder by inducing hypomania, rapid cycling, and mixed states, but there is a lack of placebo-controlled studies in this field. As in the case of unipolar depressive disorders, clinical and research evidence strongly suggest that the milder (subthreshold or subsyndromal) forms of bipolar mood states (i.e., cyclothymic disorder and recurrent brief hypomania) represent clinically less severe forms and, frequently, the precursors of the full-blown bipolar disorders. In contrast to this, bipolar II disorder is surprisingly stable over time: In patients with at least a 5-year history of major mood disorder, bipolar II diagnosis rarely progresses to bipolar I disorder.

There are far fewer large-scale community surveys on bipolar disorder than there are on unipolar depression. Because hypomania is frequently not recognized by the probands and recall bias can also affect the results, bipolar II disorder is difficult to diagnose in clinical practice, particularly in normal populations. Therefore, the presently available figures probably underestimate the true frequency of milder forms of bipolar spectrum disorders. In spite of this, data available at present from the United States and from some European countries are sufficient to conclude that bipolar spectrum disorders are more prevalent in the community, as earlier believed, and that bipolar II disorder may be the most common clinical phenotype. The lifetime, 1-year, and current (1-month) prevalence rates of different clinical forms of bipolar disorder are shown in Table 13.2–3. The lifetime and 1-year prevalence rates of bipolar I disorder have been reported to be up to 2.4 percent and 1.3 percent, respectively, whereas the point prevalence rates are approximately 0.5 percent. As for bipolar II disorder, its lifetime prevalence has been found to be between 0.3 and 3.0 percent. If the full bipolar spectrum is considered, the lifetime prevalence rates range between 2.6 and 7.8 percent. In the ECA study, the lifetime prevalence rate of bipolar I (manic) disorder was 0.8 percent and the 6-month prevalence was 0.5 percent. Because the lifetime prevalence rate of bipolar II disorder was 0.5 percent, the figure for lifetime total bipolarity (bipolar I plus bipolar II) was 1.3 percent. However, in a 2003 paper in which ECA data were reanalyzed, the addition of subthreshold bipolarity (mostly bipolar II and beyond) to bipolar I produced a total lifetime prevalence of 6.4 percent. In the NCS, which used a different diagnostic instrument, the lifetime and 1-year prevalence rates of bipolar I disorder were 1.6 percent and 1.3 percent, respectively. The study of the Cross-National Collaborative Group on the epidemiology of major depression and bipolar disorder found relatively consistent lifetime rates for bipolar disorders across the seven countries studied. As in the case of major depression, the lowest figures for DSM-III bipolar I (manic-depressive) disorder were found again in the Far Eastern countries (0.3 percent in Taiwan and 0.4 percent in Korea), whereas the highest rates emerged in New Zealand (1.5 percent) and the United States (0.9 percent). In the remaining three countries (Canada, Puerto Rico, and Germany), the figures were 0.6 percent, 0.6 percent, and 0.5 percent, respectively.

There are a few reports on the annual incidence of bipolar illness. Some data on bipolar I (manic) disorder are available, but all reports found its annual incidence to be very low, ranging between 0.01 and 0.003 percent. Considering, however, the milder forms of the full bipolar spectrum (e.g., cyclothymic disorder, hypomania), the yearly incidence figures could be much higher. Mania rarely presents itself as a classic (euphoric) syndrome, as, in approximately 20 percent of the cases, psychotic symptoms (either mood-congruent or mood-incongruent) also color the clinical picture. Furthermore, mixed mood states occur, on the average, in 40 percent of bipolar I (manic) patients over a lifetime, whereas rapid cycling course (more than four distinct affective episodes per year), affecting approximately 20 percent of all bipolar patients, more often arises from a bipolar II than a bipolar I baseline.

In sum, recent epidemiological studies show that, in addition to unipolar major depressive disorders, the community prevalence and clinical significance of the full bipolar spectrum also represents a major public health problem.

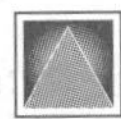

Table 13.2–3
Lifetime, 1-Year, and Current (1-Month) Prevalence Rates of Bipolar I, Bipolar II, Cyclothymic Disorder, and Hypomania

	Lifetime Prevalence (%)	1-Yr Prevalence (%)	Current Prevalence (%)
Bipolar I disorder	0–2.4	0.9–1.3	0.4–0.5
Bipolar II disorder	0.3–4.8	—	—
Cyclothymia	0.5–6.3	0.5–1.4	—
Hypomania[a]	2.6–7.8	—	—
Full bipolar spectrum	2.6–7.8	0.5–1.4	0.4–0.5

[a]Including recurrent brief hypomania (lasting only 1 to 3 days and, therefore, not reaching the diagnostic criteria of DSM-IV-TR hypomania).
Adapted from Angst, 1998; Kessler et al., 1994, 1997; Szádóczky et al., 1998; and Weissman et al., 1996.

DEMOGRAPHIC FACTORS

Sex The most consistent finding across all of the studies on the prevalence and incidence of unipolar major depression is that it is approximately twofold more common among women than men. This gender difference begins in early adulthood, is most pronounced in people between the ages of 30 and 45, and also persists in the elderly. Because there are no data (aside from biological–hormonal differences) that show that female gender per se means increased vulnerability for depression, increased stress sensitivity, maladaptive coping strategies, and multiple social roles (all of which are frequently seen in women) and substance use disorders that can mask depressive symptoms (more frequently seen in men) have been suggested for the explanation of the gender difference. In addition to these psychosocial theories, recent studies show that because prior anxiety disorders are more common in women, preceding anxiety disorder may also be a significant factor contributing to the higher depressive morbidity in women. Thus, gender difference in unipolar major depression seems to result from the complex interaction of the mentioned biological and psychosocial variables. Minor depressive disorder and recurrent brief depressive disorder are also more common among women, but the difference is not so marked as that in major depression.

In contrast to unipolar depression, the gender ratio in bipolar disorder (all subtypes combined) is approximately 1:1. However, among bipolar II patients and in special subpopulations (mixed/dysphoric mania, winter depression, bipolar depression with atypical clinical features, rapid cycling bipolar disorder), women are overrepresented. Looking at the depression–mania continuum as a whole spectrum, there is a clear trend: the higher the depressive component, the higher the proportion of women. Consequently, in the rare cases of unipolar mania (manic episode without any major or minor depression), men are markedly overrepresented. The gender differences in lifetime prevalence rates are more marked than in 1-year and current prevalence rates, which may be attributable—at least in part—to the stronger male tendency to forget previous episodes and deny emotionally negative events. Recent population-based epidemiological surveys showed that the lifetime prevalence and 1-year prevalence of major depression, dysthymia, and bipolar disorder were much higher among people with same-sex sexual behavior, particularly in the case of men.

Age Depressive disorders show much higher lifetime prevalence among people younger than 45 years, but the age of onset differs

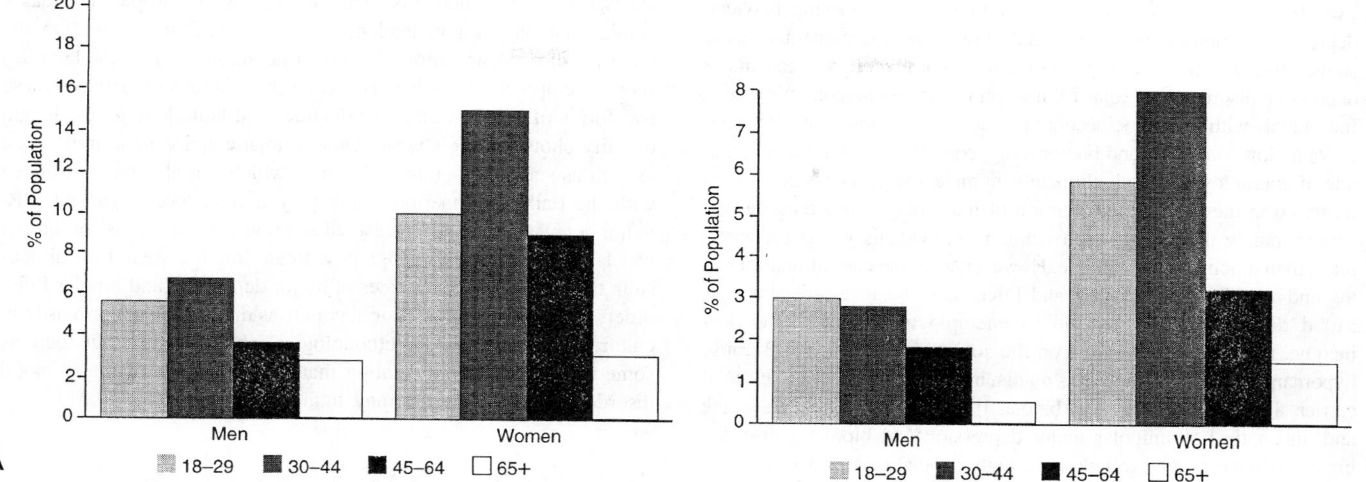

FIGURE 13.2–1 Lifetime **(A)** and current (1-month) **(B)** prevalence of major depressive disorders by age and gender. (Data derived from the Epidemiological Catchment Area Study.) (Adapted from Blazer DG: Mood disorders: epidemiology. In: Sadock BJ, Sadock VA: *Kaplan and Sadock's Comprehensive Textbook of Psychiatry*, 7th ed. Philadelphia PA: Lippincott Williams & Wilkins; 2000:1300.)

between unipolar and bipolar and familial and nonfamilial cases. The average age of onset of recurrent unipolar major depressive episode falls between the ages of 30 and 35 years, whereas single-episode major depression that often lacks family history of mood disorders usually begins some years later. The genetic predisposition for depression decreases with age. However, social stressors appear to place younger individuals at a greater risk for depression than elderly ones. On the other hand, isolation, loss of interpersonal contacts, medical disorders, and disability play a more important role in the development of depression in later life. Early-onset depression is associated with a higher female to male ratio than late-onset depression. Because major depressive disorder is a frequent and highly recurrent illness, the probability of recurrence does not decrease with age. The incidence of major depressive disorder in old age is lower in both sexes, but first incidence and prevalence of minor depressive disorder show the opposite trend. The incidence of unipolar major depressive disorder in the postpartum period is just slightly increased, but this is not the case in the postmenopausal years. The lifetime and current prevalence of major depressive episode by age and gender, based on the data from the ECA study, are shown in Figure 13.2–1. Pure (primary) dysthymic disorder typically starts in late adolescence or early adulthood, but, in the absence of appropriate treatment, almost all cases develop later into major depression. The first incidence of dysthymia is also common in old age, but this is typically the consequence of the adverse psychosocial and biological conditions frequently seen among the elderly.

The age of onset of bipolar disorder, most commonly around 20 years of age, is substantially (about 10 years) lower than that of unipolar depression. In more than half of the cases, onset is before the age of 20, frequently in late adolescence. In contrast to this, first-onset mania is very rare among elderly people. The age of onset in bipolar I and bipolar II disorders are similar, but there is a slight tendency for higher age of onset in bipolar II patients. The incidence of the depressive phase of bipolar disorder after childbirth is relatively high, and the majority of patients with "postpartum depression" have bipolar disorder. Like unipolar depression, bipolar patients with positive family history of mood disorders are significantly younger at the beginning of the illness and need less stressors to precipitate the illness than those lacking such history.

Race and Ethnicity

It is well known that cultural differences may influence the clinical presentation of depression and mania, leading to unreliable figures in prevalence studies performed by standard methodology. However, comparing the data of whites, African Americans, and Hispanics, both the ECA study and the NCS showed that if social class, education, and residency were controlled, the prevalence of unipolar major depressive episode and bipolar I disorders did not show significant variation based on race and ethnicity.

However, a recent American study found that, after adjusting for demographic factors, Asian Americans had lower lifetime prevalence of depressive disorders.

SOCIAL VARIABLES

Marital Status

The relationship between marital status and mood disorders is quite complex. For example, being single, divorced, or separated can be either a risk factor for depression or the result of the adverse life events generated by depressive or manic psychopathology, or both. Major depressive disorder and bipolar illness are most frequent among divorced, separated, or widowed individuals. Single women have lower rates of depression than married women do, but the opposite is true for men. However, being single as a result of having never married, as a result of the dissolution of a difficult marriage, and as a result of widowhood represent three very different conditions. The risk of a major depressive episode is very high among recently widowed individuals of all ages, but is particularly high in the elderly. Patients with mood disorder are overrepresented among the divorced, and the rate of family breakdown (separation, divorce) is elevated slightly in dysthymic patients, substantially in major depressive patients, and markedly in bipolar I and bipolar II patients. The presence of mania, hypomania, or major depression is a strong predictor for future separation or divorce, which can cause serious distress for the patients and for their spouses and may generate negative life events for their children. These early negative life events (e.g., parental loss before adolescence) are well known predisposing factors for adult mood disorders, particularly in the case of family loading (case of subjects with positive family history of mood disorders).

Socioeconomic Factors

Although the relationship between depressive symptoms and low social class is well documented, most studies found only a weak (but consistent) correlation between major depressive disorder or bipolar I illness and lower socioeconomic status. Individuals with lower socioeconomic status have a lower level of educational, lower income, and poorer living conditions, as well as a higher rate of unemployment and, ultimately, homelessness. As has been demonstrated in the NCS, the proportion of major depressive episode was approximately three times higher among individuals without a workplace than among those with one. However, as in the case of marital status and mood disorder, cause and effect may be reversed here, too. Mood disorder can easily lead to unemployment, divorce, or low income, resulting in regression on the social hierarchy scale. Because hypomania is not as disruptive as mania, in terms of academic and social carrier, the educational level of bipolar II patients is above the average and, in contrast to unipolar major depression and bipolar I disorder, bipolar II patients tend to belong to higher social classes and are relatively overrepresented among socially active, creative people.

Residence

As urban communities are more stressful than rural ones, it is not surprising that most studies performed in Western societies concluded that major depression was more frequent in urban residents than in their rural counterparts. In the ECA study, this rural–urban difference also persisted after controlling for marital status, race, and socioeconomic status. The results of the NCS show that respondents living in rural areas had approximately 40 percent lower odds of 1-year comorbidity of three or more mental disorders than did those living in urban areas. The urban–rural distinction tells us little about the real living and social conditions in general, but it can be a good marker for the density of the population and for other important sociological variables.

SEASONAL AND GEOGRAPHIC VARIABLES

Seasonal Factors

Despite the fact that more than two-thirds of patients with recurrent major mood disorders show irregular seasonal patterns individually, statistically, spring and fall are the peak times for depression, just as summer is for mania. Because seasonal affective disorders (fall–winter depression and spring–summer depression) occur in approximately 20 to 25 percent of the patients with recurrent major mood disorders, it is possible that the seasonal pattern observed in unipolar depression and bipolar disorders in general is the consequence—at least in part—of the characteristic annual rhythms of these specific seasonal subtypes. The seasonal profiles of committed and attempted suicides, the prescription of antidepressants and ECT, and the availability of L-tryptophan (the main precursor of serotonin) are very similar to the seasonal onset of major depression. However, acute and long-term pharmacotherapy of mood disorders (more precisely, its cessation) can change the seasonal pattern of depression and mania, which should be taken into account either in planning studies or in the interpretation of the results. On the other hand, the decreasing seasonal variation in suicides that has been observed in many countries in the last two decades may reflect, among others, the reduced rate of depression-related suicides in the given population.

Geographic Trends

There is a general, but weak, trend for lower prevalence of depression and higher rate of mania in regions located closer to the Equator. Consistently, at least in the Northern Hemisphere, winter depression (which affects between 1 and 6 percent of the community) seems to be more frequent in countries situated farther from it. A significant positive correlation was found between prevalence of winter depression and latitude in North America (where its prevalence is twice as high as in Europe), whereas a similar, but only slight, tendency was observed in Europe. On the other hand, the distribution of summer depression across the latitudes shows the opposite tendency. However, the relationship between these two forms of seasonal affective disorder and latitude (e.g., the length of daily photoperiod) is weak. Other climatic and genetic influences, as well as social and cultural factors—which can also be interrelated with the daily photoperiod—may play a role, too. In the NCS-R, major depressive disorder (seasonal and nonseasonal forms combined) was largely unrelated to geography. Regarding the West–East dimension, the lower prevalence rates of major depressive and bipolar I disorders reported from Far Eastern countries may be related primarily to cultural differences and methodological shortcomings, but there is some recent evidence indicating that the prevalence of major mood disorders in these countries may, in fact, be lower.

PSYCHOSOCIAL FACTORS

Social Stressors

Social stressors, in general, have been well recognized as risk factors for mood disorders. However, different kinds of social stressors (i.e., childhood vs. adulthood events, acute vs. chronic stressors, positive vs. negative life events) can play different roles in the predisposition and precipitation of depressive or manic disorders. In the case of major depression and bipolar disorder, the association of acute stressors and the onset of illness become progressively weaker with the increasing number of previous episodes, and patients at high genetic risk for mood disorders commonly experience depressive or manic episodes without any negative life event. In the development of major mood disorders, chronic stressors (e.g., unemployment, difficult marriage) play a more important role than specific, acute stressors. However, accumulation of stressful negative life events is the strongest predisposing factor. The higher level and, probably, the different nature of social stressors in individuals living in urban communities may be among the main sources accounting for their higher psychiatric morbidity. The fact that subjective perception of life events is more important than the event itself makes the estimation of the causative role of life events more difficult. On the other hand, it has also been demonstrated that acute, positive life events (that are quite rare in Western communities) can also precipitate either major depression or mania in vulnerable individuals. Negative life events should not be considered as only predisposing or precipitating factors, as they are frequently the result of the behavior of patients with major depressive disorder and, particularly, patients with bipolar disorder.

Social Support

Social support can improve coping and modify (e.g., reduce or eliminate) the occurrence of psychosocial stressors or the adverse consequences of them. The consistent finding in the literature that living alone, having low socioeconomic status, and being unemployed are significant risk factors for mood disorders. In other words, it means that weak or lacking social support (including social network, social interaction, and instrumental support) can also be considered a major risk factor. However, regarding social interactions, the frequency of the interactions is more important than the amount. Poor social support is related to onset, relapse, and recurrence of depression, but there is no evidence for the excess of depression among women caused by reduced social support.

COMORBIDITY

Individuals with major mood disorders are at an increased risk of having one or more additional comorbid Axis I disorders. The most frequent disorders are alcohol abuse or dependence, panic disorder, obsessive-compulsive disorder (OCD), and social anxiety disorder. Conversely, individuals with substance use disorders and anxiety disorders also have an elevated risk of lifetime or current comorbid mood disorder. In both unipolar and bipolar disorder, men more frequently present with substance use disorders, whereas women more frequently present with comorbid anxiety and eating disorders. In general, bipolar patients more frequently show comorbidity of substance use and anxiety disorders than do patients with unipolar major depression. In the ECA study, the lifetime history of substance use disorders, panic disorder, and OCD was approximately twice as high among patients with bipolar I disorder (61 percent, 21 percent, and 21 percent, respectively) than in patients with unipolar major depression (27 percent, 10 percent, and 12 percent, respectively). The figures in the latter group also highly exceeded the corresponding rates in the general population. Recent clinical and epidemiological studies show that, if bipolar II disorder is also considered, comorbidity of substance use disorders and anxiety disorders is the highest in the bipolar II subgroup. Because comorbid substance use disorders and anxiety disorders worsen the prognosis of the illness and markedly increase the risk of suicide among unipolar major depressive and bipolar patients, the data presented above are consistent with previous findings showing that bipolar patients (particularly bipolar II patients) are at the highest risk of suicide. These findings also indicate that Axis I comorbidity might be among the most important contributing factor to that risk. However, there is a substantial overlap between mood and substance use disorders. The National Alcohol Epidemiology Survey, conducted in the United States with more than 42,000 community residents, showed that, out of the population studied, 16 percent had had a lifetime history of alcohol use disorder and major depression. Among these patients, 41 percent were classified with primary depression, 17 percent were classified with concurrent depression, and 42 percent were classified with secondary depression. This finding supports and extends the results of previous studies conducted among alcoholics in treatment and has strong diagnostic and treatment implications.

USE OF HEALTH SERVICES

Despite the great progress in the diagnosis and treatment of depressions in the last two decades, they still remain underdiagnosed and undertreated. North American and European surveys show that approximately half of those who develop mood disorders seek treatment for them, but only a small fraction (about one-third) of recognized depressives receive appropriate treatment. The results of the NCS-R also showed that 52 percent of persons with 12-month prevalence of major depressive disorder received health care treatment for their depression, but the treatment was adequate in fewer than half such cases. An increasing rate of health service utilization is related to increasing severity of depression and to comorbid psychiatric and medical disorders. Despite the fact that many patients with depressive disorders seek help in primary care, general practitioners still have difficulties recognizing and treating depression. The current prevalence of major depression in primary care is approximately 10 to 15 percent and that of dysthymic disorder is approximately 6 to 8 percent. Paradoxically, because severe major depression is much more common among those with comorbid chronic medical disorders, depressions with significant somatic comorbidity, in particular, remain unrecognized in primary care. Data from the NCS show that, in individuals with two or more chronic physical illnesses, the 1-year prevalence of severe major depression is fourfold higher than that of individuals without such conditions. Women more often seek treatment for their depression and are more compliant with the treatment than are men, but, unfortunately, "male depression" is less frequently recognized. Because there is no gender difference in the response to antidepressant pharmacotherapy, these facts can help to explain the so-called suicide paradox—that is, despite the fact that major depression is much more common in women, it is men who are markedly overrepresented among suicide victims. Besides general practitioners, other professionals (i.e., internists, cardiologists, neurologists) also frequently see depressed patients. The point prevalence of major depressive disorder in acute (medical–surgical hospital) care is also higher than 10 percent, a figure well in excess of the point prevalence rate for the general population. Concomitant depression increases the morbidity and mortality from concurrent medical illness, and patients with simultaneous medical disorder and depression are less compliant with treatment and take longer to recover than nondepressed medical patients.

Depressed patients, particularly those who go unrecognized, frequently seek general health care, but depression, if correctly identified, can be effectively treated even in primary care. On the other hand, despite the fact that more than half of suicide victims contact different levels of health care 4 weeks before committing suicide, the rate of adequate antidepressive pharmacotherapy among depressed suicide victims is disturbingly low. However, epidemiological and clinical studies, as well as the steadily increasing use of antidepressants (the latter is accompanied by a constant decline in suicide rates in North America, Australia, and Europe), indicate that, in the last decade of the 20th century, the referral, recognition, and successful treatment of depression increased, suggesting that the prognosis for depressive illness, in general, is getting better and better.

HISTORICAL TRENDS

The ECA, the NCS, and some other epidemiological studies have suggested that there was a clear increase in the cumulative lifetime rates of major depressive disorder both in women and in men, (i.e., more recent birth cohorts were exposed to an increased risk of major depression). These cohort differences, however, were not limited to major depression but applied to a wide range of other diagnoses as well. Recent retrospective and prospective studies show that there has been no direct evidence for a marked increase in the incidence and prevalence of depression over the past decades. The observed changes are mainly due, in particular, to artifacts of memory and, to a lesser degree, to higher subjective awareness, better definitions and methods of case identification, redistribution by age and sex (with higher rates among younger women being of recent origin), and increase in childhood-onset mood disorders.

SUGGESTED CROSS-REFERENCES

An overview of epidemiology is given in Section 5.1. Social origins of mood disorders are discussed in Section 4.2. Classification of mental disorders is presented in Chapter 9. Specific review of the genetics of mood disorders can be found in Section 13.3. The role of stress in the etiology of psychiatric disorders is discussed in Section 24.9. Suicide is discussed in detail in Section 29.1. The epidemiology of psychiatric disorders in late life is reviewed in Section 51.1b.

REFERENCES

Akiskal HS: Bipolarity: beyond classic mania. *Psychiatr Clin North Am.* 1999;22(3).

Akiskal HS: Validating the bipolar spectrum. *J Affect Disord.* 2003;73:1–2.

Akiskal HS, Bourgeois ML, Angst J, Post R, Möller H-J, Hirschfeld R: Re-evaluating the prevalence of and diagnostic composition within the broad clinical spectrum of bipolar disorders. *J Affect Disord.* 2000;59:S5.

*Angst J. The emerging epidemiology of hypomania and bipolar II disorder. *J Affect Disord.* 1998;50:143.
Angst J: The prevalence of depression. In: Briley M, Montgomery SA. *Antidepressant Therapy at the Dawn of the Third Millennium.* London: Martin Dunitz; 1998.
Ayuso-Mateos JL, Vázquez-Barquero JL, Dowrick C, Lehtinen V, Dalgard OS, Casey P, Wilkinson C, Lasa L, Page H, Dunn G, Wilkinson G: Depressive disorders in Europe: prevalence figures from the ODIN study. *Br J Psychiatry.* 2001;179:308.
Beekman ATF, Deeg DJH, van Tilburg T, Smit JH, Hooijer C, van Tilburg W: Major and minor depression in later life: a study of prevalence and risk factors. *J Affect Disord.* 1995;36:65.
*Blazer DG: Mood disorders: epidemiology. In: Sadock BJ, Sadock VA. *Kaplan and Sadock's Comprehensive Textbook of Psychiatry.* 7th ed. Philadelphia: Lippincott Williams & Wilkins; 2000.
Chen Y-W, Dilsaver SC: Comorbidity of panic disorder in bipolar illness: evidence from the Epidemiologic Catchment Area Survey. *Am J Psychiatry.* 1995;152:280.
Freeman MP, Freeman SA, McElroy SL: The comorbidity of bipolar and anxiety disorders: prevalence, psychobiology, and treatment issues. *J Affect Disord.* 2002;68:1.
*Goodwin FK, Jamison KR. *Manic-Depressive Illness.* New York: Oxford University Press; 1990.
Grant BF, Hasin DS, Dawson DA: The relationship between DSM-IV alcohol use disorders and DSM-IV major depression: examination of the primary-secondary distinction in a general population sample. *J Affect Disord.* 1996;38:113.
Hall WD, Mant A, Mitchell PB, Rendle VA, Hickie IB, McManus P: Association between antidepressant prescribing and suicide in Australia, 1991–2000: trend analysis. *Br Med J.* 2003;326:1008.
Jackson-Triche ME, Sullivan G, Wells KB, Rogers W, Camp P, Mazel R: Depression and health-related quality of life in ethnic minorities seeking care in general medical settings. *J Affect Disord.* 2000;58:89.
Judd LL, Akiskal HS: The prevalence and disability of bipolar spectrum disorders in the U.S. population: re-analysis of the ECA database taking into account subthreshold cases. *J Affect Disord.* 2003;73:123.
Kessler RC, Berglund P, Demler O, Jin R, Koretz D, Merikangas KR, Rush JA, Walters EE, Wang PS: The epidemiology of major depressive disorder. Results from the National Comorbidity Survey Replication (NCS-R). *JAMA.* 2003;289:3095.
*Kessler RC, McGonagle KA, Zhao S, Nelson CB, Hughes M, Eshleman S, Wittchen H-U, Kendler KS: Lifetime and 12-month prevalence of DSM-III-R psychiatric disorders in the United States. Results from the National Comorbidity Survey. *Arch Gen Psychiatry.* 1994;51:8.
Kessler RC, Rubinow DR, Holmes C, Abelson JM, Zhao S: The epidemiology of DSM-III-R bipolar I disorder in a general population survey. *Psychol Med.* 1997;27:1079.
Kessler RC, Walters EE, Forthofer MS: The social consequences of psychiatric disorders, III: probability of marital stability. *Am J Psychiatry.* 1998;155:1092.
Kessler RC, Zhao S, Blazed DG, Swartz M: Prevalence, correlates, and course of minor depression and major depression in the national comorbidity survey. *J Affect Disord.* 1997;45:19.
Lecrubier Y: Is depression under-recognised and undertreated? *Int Clin Psychopharmacol.* 1998;13(Suppl 5):3.
Lépine J-P, Gastpar M, Mendlewicz J, Tylee A: The first pan-European study DEPRES (Depression Research in European Society). *Int Clin Psychopharmacol.* 1997;12:19.
Maj M, Sartorius N. *Depressive Disorders. WPA Series Evidence and Experience in Psychiatry.* Chichester: John Wiley and Sons; 1999.
Mersch PPA, Middendrop HM, Bouhuys AL, Beersma DGM, van den Hoofdakker RH: Seasonal affective disorder and latitude: a review of the literature. *J Affect Disord.* 1999;53:35.
Murphy JM, Larid NM, Monson RR, Sobol AM, Leighton AH: A 40-year perspective on the prevalence of depression. *Arch Gen Psychiatry.* 2000;57:209.
Parker G, Hadzi-Pavlovic D: Is any female preponderance in depression secondary to a primary female preponderance in anxiety disorders? *Acta Psychiatr Scand.* 2001;103:252.
Piccinelli M, Wilkinson G: Gender differences in depression. *Br J Psychiatry.* 2000;177:486.
Regier DA, Boyd JH, Bruke JD, Rae DS, Myers JK, Kramer M, Robins LN, George LK, Karno M, Locke BZ: One-month prevalence of mental disorders in the United States. *Arch Gen Psychiatry.* 1988;45:977.
Rihmer Z, Kiss K: Bipolar disorders and suicide risk. *Clin Appr Bipol Disord.* 2002;1:15.
Rorsman B, Graesbeck A, Hagnell O, Lanke J, Öhman R, Öjesjö L, Otterbeck L: A prospective study of first-incidence depression: the Lundby study, 1951–1972. *Br J Psychiatry.* 1990;156:336.
Standfort TGM, de Graaf R, Bijl RV, Schnabel P: Same-sex sexual behavior and psychiatric disorders. Findings from the Netherlands Mental Health Survey and Incidence Study (NEMESIS). *Arch Gen Psychiatry.* 2001;58:85.
Stewart WF, Ricci JA, Chee E, Hahn SR, Morgenstein D: Cost of lost productive work time among US workers with depression. *JAMA.* 2003;289:3135.
Szádóczky E, Papp Z, Vitrai J, Rihmer Z, Füredi J: The prevalence of major depressive and bipolar disorders in Hungary. Results from a national epidemiologic survey. *J Affect Disord.* 1998;50:153.
*Weissman MM, Bland RC, Canino GJ, Faravelli C, Greenwald S, Hwu H-G, Joyce PR, Karam EG, Lee C-K, Lellouch J, Lépine J-P, Newman SC, Rubio-Stipec M, Wells E, Wickramaratne PJ, Wittchen H-U, Yeh E-K: Cross-national epidemiology of major depression and bipolar disorder. *JAMA.* 1996;276:293.
Wilhelm K, Mitchell P, Slade T, Brownhill S, Andrews G: Prevalence and correlates of DSM-IV major depression in an Australian national survey. *J Affect Disord.* 2003;75:155.
Wittchen H-U, Höfler M, Meister W: Prevalence and recognition of depressive syndromes in German primary care settings: poorly recognized and treated? *Int Clin Psychopharmacol.* 2001;16:121.
Young AS, Klap R, Sherbourne CD, Wells KB: The quality of care for depressive and anxiety disorders in the United States. *Arch Gen Psychiatry.* 2001;58:55.

▲ 13.3 Mood Disorders: Genetics

JOHN R. KELSOE, M.D.

The familial nature of mood disorders is commonly observed by clinicians, patients, and families. Numerous family and twin studies have long documented the heritability of these disorders. Recently, however, the primary focus of genetic studies has been the identification of specific susceptibility genes using molecular genetic methods. Fueled by powerful tools from the Human Genome Project, this work is now poised to discover multiple disease genes in the coming years. The discovery of such disease genes will have a far-reaching and direct impact on clinical practice and requires that clinicians be familiar with this rapidly evolving area. The identification of susceptibility genes may lead to the development of deoxyribonucleic acid (DNA) tests to aid in diagnosis and in prediction of treatment response. These genes will also point to novel targets for drug discovery and the development of new medications with distinct efficacy profiles. The public is also increasingly aware of genetic issues, and the clinician is frequently called on to interpret these complex data for patients and families. In this chapter, the genetic epidemiology of mood disorders is reviewed and possible models of genetic transmission are considered. An overview of the methods of positional cloning is then presented, and the current state of such studies in mood disorders is reviewed. Lastly, the clinical and ethical issues raised by these impending genetic discoveries are discussed.

GENETIC EPIDEMIOLOGY

By determining the rates of illness in different types of relatives, genetic epidemiological studies can provide a great deal of information about the familial and genetic nature of a disorder. The following questions can be addressed: Are mood disorders familial? Are they genetic? What portion of the etiology is genetic? How are the genes for mood disorder transmitted? How do different forms of mood disorder differ in their genetic transmission? How are different forms of mood disorder related to each other?

Numerous such studies have been conducted in the 20th century and provide much information about the genetic transmission of mood disorders. However, these studies must be considered in the light of their various methodological limitations. Foremost of these is the range of diagnostic methods employed. Many of these studies were conducted before the distinction between unipolar and bipolar illnesses; thus, the statistics from these studies pool both illnesses. Similarly, many of these studies preceded the introduction of operationalized diagnostic criteria. Thus, it may not be clear exactly how the diagnoses were made, and it is difficult to compare or pool the results across studies. In the more recent studies that distinguish unipolar and bipolar disorder, bipolar disorder has received more attention because of its greater degree of familiality. Other methodological issues that are important to such studies include ascertainment bias. If the results of a study are to be meaningfully generalized to the population, it is critical that the subjects to be studied are selected in a systematic and nonbiased fashion. For example, if probands (the first ill subject identified in a family) are selected based on their strong family history, then the results of a family study may inaccurately indicate a strong familial rate of illness in the population. A similar error will be made if ill family members are preferentially selected for study. Systematic ascertainment methods attempt to avoid such biases by studying all patients who present within a certain environment, such as a mood disorders clinic. Another limitation, for reasons of feasibility in many of these studies, is the use of the family history method. In this approach, the rates of illness in family members of a proband are determined by systematically questioning the proband about his or her family. Although there are several excellent standardized instruments for the family history method, this method is inherently less accurate than the direct interview method in which each family member is interviewed to make a diagnosis.

Family Studies

Family studies address the question of whether a disorder is familial. More specifically: Is the rate of illness in the family members of someone with the disorder greater than that of the general population? Typically, all subjects with the disorder in a given environment or population will be identified and questioned regarding illness in their first-degree relatives. The rates of illness are then compared to either the rates in the general population or the rates in first-degree relatives of control subjects. Rates of illness are typically adjusted for age to indicate the morbid risk.

Table 13.3–1 illustrates several such studies of bipolar disorder. The studies indicate a morbid risk of bipolar disorder in first-degree relatives of bipolar probands that ranges between 3 and 8 percent. The ratio of risk to family members divided by the population rate of illness is a genetic parameter typically notated as λ. Compared to a rate of 1 percent in the general population, bipolar disorder has a λ value of approximately 7, indicating a strong familial risk. Similarly, studies of families of unipolar probands reveal morbid risks for unipolar disorder among first-degree relatives that are elevated two- to threefold over the general population. These data strongly support the familial nature of mood disorders. Furthermore, unipolar disorder is generally found at an elevated rate in the families of bipolar probands, and the rate of bipolar disorder is elevated in the families of unipolar probands. In fact, unipolar disorder is typically the most common form of mood disorder in families of bipolar probands. This familial overlap suggests some degree of common genetic underpinnings between these two forms of mood disorder.

Twin Studies

The family study data clearly indicate that mood disorders are familial. However, such studies are unable to distinguish whether it is genetic or environmental factors that mediate the familial transmission. Families might share a variety of different environmental factors that could transmit the illness. Such factors might be behavioral in nature, but they could also be shared exposure to infectious agents, toxins, and other brain insults. Twin studies provide the most powerful approach to separating genetic from environmental factors, or "nature" from "nurture." Many strategies for twin studies have been used, but, most commonly, both monozygotic (MZ) and same-sex dizygotic (DZ) twin pairs are identified in which one twin has a mood disorder. The other twins are then examined to determine the proportion of twin pairs in which both twins are affected. This is termed the *concordance rate*. Typically, twin pairs are selected who have been raised together so that environmental factors are shared equally. Thus, a difference in concordance rate between the MZ and DZ pairs reflects the role of heritable genetic factors. An alternative powerful strategy is to study twin pairs raised apart; however, such samples are much more difficult to obtain.

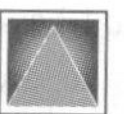

Table 13.3–1
Selected Family Studies of Bipolar Disorders

Study, Yr	Relatives at Risk	Morbid Risk (%) Bipolar	Morbid Risk (%) Unipolar
Fieve et al., 1984	2,171	6.6	9.0
Gershon et al., 1982	598	8.0	14.9
Rice et al., 1987	557	5.7	23.0[a]
Sadovnick et al., 1994	1,102	3.5	5.7

[a]Observed rates rather than morbid risk.

Table 13.3–2 summarizes several twin studies of mood disorders. Considering unipolar and bipolar disorders together, these studies find a two- to fourfold increase in concordance rate for mood disorder in the MZ twins compared to the DZ twins. This is the most compelling data for the role of genetic factors in mood disorders. It is equally noteworthy that the concordance rate for MZ twins is not 100 percent. This is clear evidence that nonheritable environmental factors also play a significant role in mood disorders. In studies that distinguish bipolar from unipolar disorders, the MZ to DZ concordance ratio for bipolar–bipolar pairs is higher than that for unipolar–unipolar pairs. This indicates a greater role for genetics in bipolar disorders than in unipolar disorders. Furthermore, the rate of unipolar disorder is elevated in the MZ co-twins of bipolar probands, and, to a lesser extent, the rate of bipolar disorder is elevated in the co-twins of unipolar probands. This is consistent with the family data and argues for a genetic overlap between bipolar and unipolar disorder.

Adoption Studies

Adoption studies provide an alternative approach to separating genetic and environmental factors in familial transmission. A variety of limitations of twin studies have been raised, including the argument that parents treat MZ twins and DZ twins differently, so environment is not equally shared. Adoption studies have been conducted using a variety of experimental designs, but the most common is the adoptee-as-proband strategy. In this approach, probands are identified who have a mood disorder and were adopted at birth. Through this event, nature is separated from nurture. The rates of psychiatric illness are then determined in both the biological and adoptive parents.

Only a limited number of such studies have been reported, and their results have been mixed. One large study found a threefold increase in the rate of bipolar disorder and a twofold increase in unipolar disorder in the biological relatives of bipolar probands. Similarly, in a Danish sample, a threefold increase in the rate of unipolar disorder and a sixfold increase in the rate of completed suicide in the biological relatives of affectively ill probands

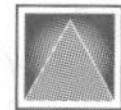

Table 13.3–2
Selected Twin Studies of Mood Disorders

Study, Yr	Monozygotic Twins No. Twin Pairs	Monozygotic Twins Concordance (%)	Dizygotic Twins No. Twin Pairs	Dizygotic Twins Concordance (%)
Rosanoff et al., 1935	23	69.6	67	16.4
Kallman, 1954	27	92.6	55	23.6
Bertelsen, 1979	55	58.3	52	17.3
Kendler et al., 1993	154	69.7	326	34.9

were reported. Other studies, however, have been less convincing and have found no difference in the rates of mood disorders. Overall, these results are supportive of the role of genetics and consistent with the twin data. However, difficulty obtaining subjects and the resulting small sample sizes may be some of the reasons these data are less strong than the twin data.

MODE OF TRANSMISSION

If mood disorders are in large part caused by genetic factors, then what is the nature of their genetic transmission? Segregation analysis of the family study data has been used to attempt to answer this question. Are mood disorders the result of one or of a few genes transmitted in a Mendelian fashion? Or, do many genes interact to predispose an individual to illness? As detailed below, different modes of transmission result in different patterns of inheritance of illness. By examining these patterns in families, one may attempt to distinguish the different possible modes of transmission. For example, in a simple dominant genetic disorder, one would expect to observe that half of the children of an affected parent are also affected. In a recessive disorder, only one-fourth of the children of two nonaffected carriers should be affected. More complex modes of inheritance involving multiple genes result in other patterns of illness that can be sought in the family data. Typically, in segregation analysis, the predicted patterns of several different models of transmission are tested to see which one best fits the observed family data.

The results of such analyses have been mixed. Several such analyses have been inconclusive and excluded all tested models of transmission. However, other, more recent analyses using large samples and more sophisticated genetic models have supported the presence of an autosomal dominant major locus. Other studies have supported a multifactorial-threshold model for mood disorders. In these models, the effects of multiple genes add together to produce a unitary predisposition common to all affective disorders. Different mood disorders result at different thresholds in this single underlying genetic liability. X-linkage has also been argued based on the observation that female relatives of bipolar probands have a twofold higher risk for unipolar disorder. This is also supported by evidence for decreased male-to-male transmission in bipolar disorder. It is difficult to draw any definitive conclusions from such complex and inconsistent data. It seems likely that the complexity results from the presence of multiple genes with multiple modes of transmission. In the face of such heterogeneity, the sample sizes and statistical methods used may have limited power to consistently demonstrate a given mode of transmission. The data do suggest that, of the many genes most likely operating in mood disorders, some have a major effect on predisposition, and these major genes are likely autosomal dominant or, perhaps, X-linked. Consistent with such heterogeneity, recent analyses have argued for more complex modes of transmission in which multiple genes interact to predispose to illness.

Several other intriguing results emerge from the family study data. Subjects with mood disorders are more likely than is expected by chance to marry spouses who also have mood disorders. This is termed *assortative mating* and leads to a higher rate of families in which the illness can be traced to both the mother's and the father's sides of the family than would be expected by chance. Such bilineal families may play an important role in the interaction of multiple genes in the population. Family studies have also indicated that the rate of mood disorders is increasing over time in the population. This is termed the *cohort effect* and is illustrated in Figure 13.3–1. Among family members of bipolar probands, those born more recently have a higher risk for bipolar disorder and an earlier age of onset. The cause of the cohort effect is unknown. It has been speculated to be a result of changing environmental stresses in society, an artifact of recollection, or, possibly, an indication of a genetic effect termed *anticipation*, which will be discussed further below.

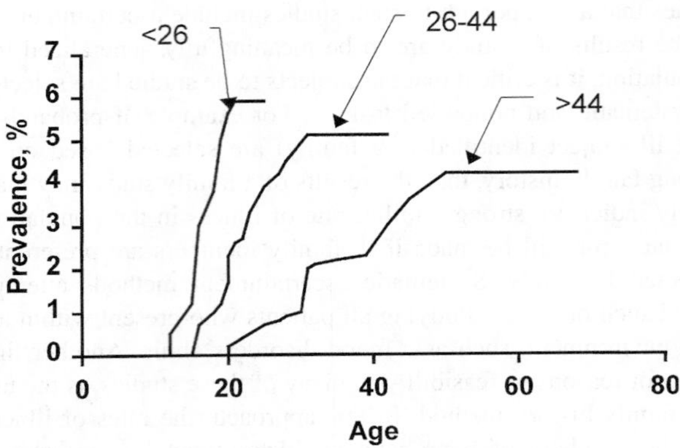

FIGURE 13.3–1 Age-related penetrance curves for bipolar disorder. The risk for bipolar disorder among relatives of bipolar probands is depicted as a function of age. The probability of having bipolar disorder, or penetrance, increases with age. The cohort effect is illustrated by the different age-dependent risk curves for relatives within three different age groups. Relatives born more recently have a higher rate of bipolar disorder and an earlier age of onset. (From Rice J, Reich T, Andreasen NC, et al.: The familial transmission of bipolar illness. *Arch Gen Psychiatry.* 1987;44:441–447, with permission.)

GENETIC RELATIONSHIPS WITHIN THE SPECTRUM OF MOOD DISORDERS

The genetic relationship between the various forms of mood disorder has been a much studied and debated topic. Bipolar and unipolar disorders are widely felt to have some sort of common genetic underpinning, although its exact nature is unclear. The twin and family data reviewed above argue for unipolar disorder occurring in the twins or other relatives of bipolar probands at a greater rate than that expected by chance. However, it is less clear that bipolar disorder occurs in the relatives of unipolar probands at an elevated rate. Twin studies indicate that "polarity" is usually consistent in MZ twins—in other words, bipolar–bipolar or unipolar–unipolar pairs are much more common than bipolar–unipolar pairs. Yet bipolar–unipolar pairs do occur. These data suggest that bipolar and unipolar disorders are genetically neither completely identical nor completely distinct. Rather, there is a partial genetic similarity. A possible model for the relationship between these genes and disorders is illustrated in Figure 13.3–2. In this model, some or all of the genes for bipolar disorder may also result in unipolar disorder. In addition, there is a larger pool of genes that predispose only to unipolar disorder. Therefore, unipolar disorder would be clearly elevated in families with bipolar disorder. However, because only a minority of cases of unipolar disorder results from bipolar genes, only a small elevation in the rate of bipolar disorder would be seen in the relatives of unipolar probands.

This model also predicts that a portion of those with unipolar disorder carry genes that may also predispose to bipolar disorder. Such patients have been said to have "bipolar III" disorder by some writers and have been the subject of much discussion and investigation. They are presumably identified by a family history of bipolar disorder or a history of developing hypomania or mania only in response to antidepressant treatment. Similarly, some authors have described a hypomanic-like personality style termed *hyperthymic tempera-*

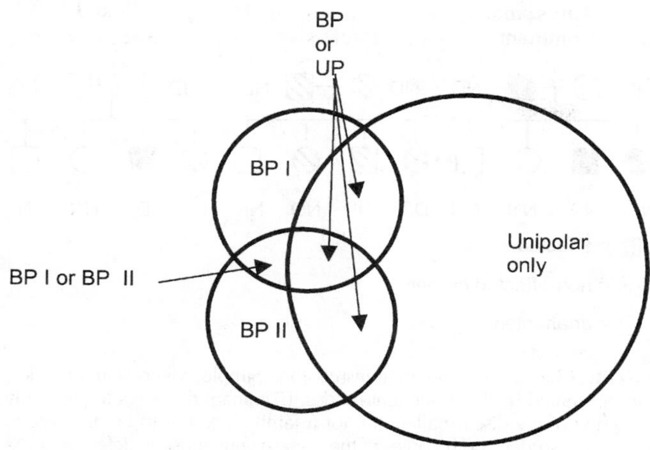

FIGURE 13.3–2 A model of genetic relationships among mood disorders. This model of the relationship between genes for bipolar and unipolar disorders (BP and UP) posits that the majority of genes for bipolar disorder can predispose to either bipolar or unipolar disorder. Among genes for bipolar disorder, some preferentially predispose to bipolar I, some to bipolar II, and others can predispose to either form of illness. A larger set of genes predisposes only to unipolar disorder. This model predicts that a subset of those with unipolar disorder carry genes that may also predispose to bipolar disorder.

ment. Unipolar patients with hyperthymic temperament likely carry some bipolar genes. Such hyperthymic unipolar patients are more likely to have a family history of bipolar disorder and to develop mania spontaneously. These unipolar patients with a bipolar genetic diathesis may also be more likely to respond to lithium augmentation of antidepressant treatment. These data suggest the possibility that bipolar disorder is one extreme of a quantitative trait that extends into normal behavior and personality variants. This is consistent with a quantitative genetic trait as described below.

Other forms of mood disorders have also been postulated to be, at least to some extent, genetically distinct. Several studies have reported that, although the risk for bipolar I is similar in the relatives of bipolar I or bipolar II probands, the risk for bipolar II is greater than that for bipolar I in the relatives of bipolar II probands. This suggests that bipolar II, to some extent, breeds true and that a subset of the genes for bipolar disorder predisposes preferentially to bipolar II. Bipolar disorder with psychotic features is more commonly found in the families of probands with psychotic symptoms, suggesting that bipolar disorder with psychotic features may be a genetically distinct form of illness. Comorbid panic disorder may also tend to cooccur in families and be associated with more rapid switching. However, studies of bipolar patients with rapid-cycling illness find that the presence of rapid cycling in the proband has no impact on the risk for mood disorders or rapid cycling in relatives. Thus, it seems that rapid cycling alone is not a distinct genetic subform of bipolar disorder.

The genetic relationship of schizoaffective disorder to mood disorders is a complex question that involves the role of psychosis in the genetics of mood disorders. The genetic nature of schizoaffective disorder also bears on the genetic relationship between schizophrenia and mood disorders. Studies examining familial risks in relatives of schizoaffective patients have led to inconsistent results, some finding an increased risk of schizophrenia and some an increased risk of bipolar disorder. A possible explanation is that schizoaffective disorder represents a mixture of patients, some with bipolar and some with schizophrenia diatheses. This is supported by data that find an increased rate of bipolar disorder among the relatives of probands with the bipolar subtype of schizoaffective disorder. Schizophrenia has also been reported to be increased among the relatives of probands with the depressive type of schizoaffective disorder. Alternatively, it has been proposed that the Kraepelinian distinction between the disorders is not valid and that both schizophrenia and mood disorders lie at the extremes of a spectrum of a common genetic liability. It is intriguing that recent linkage studies, as reviewed below, may be beginning to provide possible support for the existence of some genetic loci common to both schizophrenia and bipolar disorder. A more definitive understanding of the genetic relationships between these different forms of illness will likely require identification of the specific genes involved.

SUMMARY OF THE GENETIC FEATURES OF MOOD DISORDERS

The above data argue that mood disorders are not simple genetic traits. There is no one gene that consistently causes illness in all cases in a simple and predictable fashion. In genetic terms, there is not a 1-to-1 relationship between the genes (genotype) and the expressed trait (phenotype) that is transmitted in a simple Mendelian fashion. Therefore, mood disorders are said to be complex genetic disorders rather than simple Mendelian traits. What are the factors that contribute to this complexity?

The twin data provide compelling evidence that genes explain only 50 to 70 percent of the etiology of mood disorders. Environment or other nonheritable factors must explain the remainder. Therefore, it is a predisposition or susceptibility to disease that is inherited. The probability that someone will manifest a trait given that they have a certain genotype is termed the *penetrance* of the gene. Mood disorders are said to have reduced penetrance (less than 100 percent). Furthermore, the penetrance of mood disorder genes increases with age, from a low risk for illness in childhood to a maximum in adulthood. The cohort effect, as described above and illustrated in Figure 13.3–1, further complicates the relationship of penetrance to age, causing it to vary with the date of birth. Thus, in families of people with mood disorders, there are likely individuals who have the genes for mood disorder but do not develop the disease. These are termed *nonpenetrant carriers*. The converse of this situation is individuals who have mood disorder but do not have the genes. Such individuals with purely environmentally caused disease are termed *phenocopies*. These factors conspire to produce an indirect relationship between genes and disease.

Variable expressivity refers to the phenomenon of the same gene or group of genes resulting in a variety of different forms of illness. The twin data clearly demonstrate this for mood disorders. Identical twins with identical genomes are observed in which one twin has bipolar and the other has unipolar disorder. Nonheritable factors must play a role in the specific manifestation of the predisposition to mood disorder. Such variability in expression is not unique to psychiatric disorders. For example, in neurofibromatosis, ill individuals range in manifestations and severity from those with only pigmented retinal lesions to others with multiple large tumors. Such a range in expression results from the same disease gene.

Of the various factors complicating the genetic transmission of mood disorders, the most significant and most challenging for gene mapping efforts is genetic heterogeneity. *Heterogeneity* refers to the likely role of multiple genes in the etiology of illness. Ultimately, only the identification of multiple disease genes will convincingly demonstrate the presence of genetic heterogeneity. However, the segregation analyses described above provide strong suggestion of its likely presence. There are several critical questions regarding the nature of heterogeneity in mood disorders: How many genes are involved? How large an effect does each gene have? In what ways do the genes interact to produce illness? These questions define a variety of models of heterogeneity, which are described below. Such models can be broadly grouped into those in which disease results from a few genes of major effect (major loci) and those in which disease derives from the combined action of many genes of small effect (polygenic or oligogenic). The answers to these questions are not currently known for mood disorders. However, as described above, the segregation analyses suggest a mixture of genes of both large and small effect, which are transmitted in a variety of ways.

Evidence for several other complex forms of genetic transmission have also been reported for mood disorders. Some studies of bipolar disorder have indicated that the illness is more likely to be transmitted through mothers than through fathers. Such parent-of-origin effects imply a genetic phenomenon called *imprinting*. In imprinting, a genetic locus is processed differently in male meiosis than it is in female meiosis, such that different traits result from maternal transmission than result from paternal transmission. Angelman's and Prader-Willi syndromes are examples. These are two different mental retardation syndromes that result from different maternal or paternal imprinting of the same locus on chromosome 15. The bipolar data suggest that the penetrance of bipolar genes may be affected by imprinting rather than different phenotypes.

Another non-Mendelian genetic phenomenon reported in mood disorders is anticipation. In disorders displaying anticipation, the severity of the illness increases and the age of onset decreases with successive generations. This is generally associated with genetic mutations involving trinucleotide repeat expansions. In disorders such as Huntington's disease or fragile X mental retardation, the disease gene contains a region of DNA in which a three-nucleotide sequence is repeated a variable number of times. For reasons currently not well understood, the number of repeats increases in successive generations until the gene's function is disrupted and illness results. Anticipation involving both increasing severity of illness and decreasing age of onset has been reported for bipolar disorder. Indirect evidence for the presence of trinucleotide repeat expansions has also been reported, however, no specific gene manifesting such a mutation has been described.

COMPLEX GENETIC DISORDERS

Simple Mendelian Traits

As described above, complex genetic disorders are simply those that are not transmitted in classic Mendelian patterns. A review of Mendelian transmission thus provides a useful background for a discussion of complex genetic traits.

Simple Mendelian traits are characterized by genetic homogeneity; one gene transmits the trait with complete penetrance. Figure 13.3–3 illustrates the three primary modes of Mendelian transmission. In genetic terminology, different forms of a given gene are termed *alleles*. A disease gene may have either a normal, nonmutated allele or a mutated, disease-causing allele. In dominant genetic disorders, only one copy of the disease allele is necessary to cause illness. Dominant illnesses are typically transmitted in a vertical fashion from grandparent to parent to child. In the simplest case, half of the children of an affected parent will have the disease. In recessive disorders, both copies of the disease gene must be defective for disease to result. Heterozygotes with only one disease allele are non-affected carriers. Disease typically results from the mating of two nonaffected carriers. One-fourth of the resulting children will be homozygous for the disease allele and, hence, ill. Recessive illnesses typically appear in a horizontal pattern in families (i.e., in cousins). It is important to understand that it is the nature of the mutation in the gene that determines whether it is transmitted in a dominant or recessive fashion. Recessive mutations typically deactivate genes that are expressed in excess. Therefore, an adequate amount of gene product can be produced by only one functioning copy. In dominant disorders, the amount of gene product expressed may be critical. A reduction in gene dosage, resulting from only one functioning copy, leads to illness. Alternatively, a dominant mutation may result in overfunctioning of the gene, which results in illness. X-linked disorders are characterized by the presence of the disease gene on the X chromosome. They also may be either dominant or recessive. X-linked dominant disorders are more common in women, whereas X-linked recessive disorders are more common in men. Father-to-son transmissions are impossible in X-linked disorders, as it is the Y sex chromosome that is transmitted.

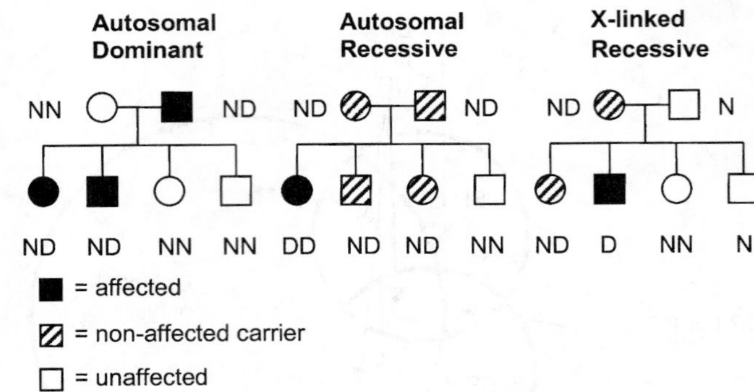

FIGURE 13.3–3 Mendelian transmission. Simple Mendelian disorders are transmitted by three different modes. Dominant disorders require only one copy of the disease allele (D) for a family member to be affected. In recessive disorders, both copies of the disease gene must be defective. In X-linked disorders, the disease gene is carried on the X chromosome. N, normal allele.

Heterogeneity Models

Of the variety of factors that distinguish complex disorders from Mendelian disorders, the most important is the presence of multiple genes or genetic heterogeneity. Multiple genes may combine to produce illness in a variety of different ways, as illustrated in Figure 13.3–4. These heterogeneity models fall into two categories based on genetic effect size. In *single major locus models*, only one disease gene is necessary to produce illness in a given individual. In an *interfamilial heterogeneity model*, one gene transmits the predisposition to illness in each family. However, there are different predisposing genes in different families. In an *intrafamilial heterogeneity model*, any one of multiple genes within the same family can transmit the illness.

In oligogenic or polygenic transmission models, multiple genes of smaller effect interact to predispose to illness. In these models, one gene by itself is unlikely to cause illness. Rather, the probability of illness increases with the number of different genes involved. The term *oligogenic* is used when a smaller number of genes are involved, as opposed to *polygenic*, which is used when a larger number of genes are involved. In an *additive polygenic model*, each gene contributes a certain probability (penetrance) of manifesting the disorder. The total genetic liability to illness is then the sum of the probabilities contributed by all of the polygenes. In Figure 13.3–4, under the additive model, the disease alleles for genes A and B alone each convey a 40 percent probability of illness. Individuals who carry the disease alleles for both A and B have an 80 percent risk for illness. The total risk is simply the sum of the risks for each individual polygene. In the epistatic

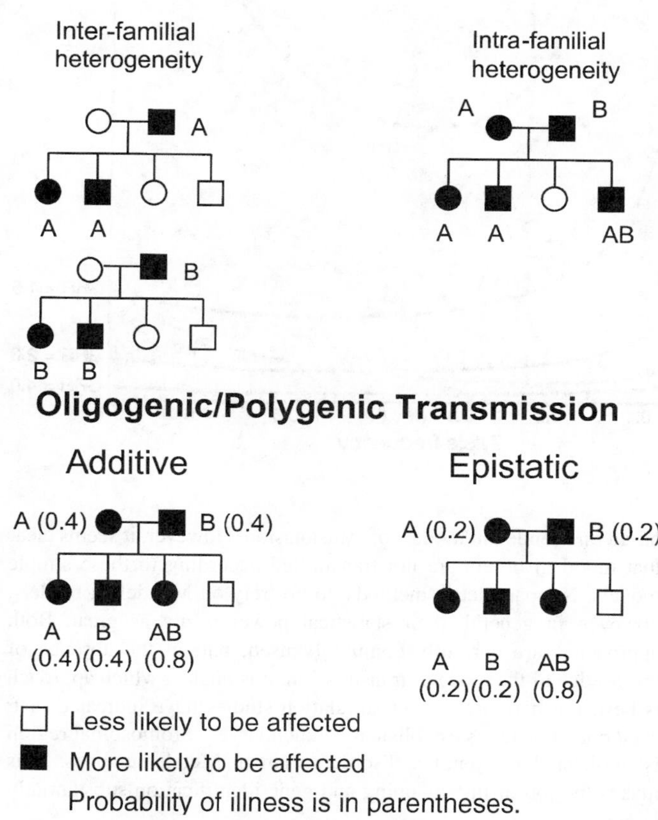

FIGURE 13.3–4 Models of heterogeneity. Several different models for the role of multiple genes in genetic disorders. In single major locus heterogeneity models, a single gene is primarily responsible for the predisposition to illness in an individual. However, different single major loci may act in different families or within the same family. In oligogenic models, multiple genes, each of smaller effect, typically interact to produce the susceptibility to illness. (Probability of illness is in parentheses.) In an additive model, the effects of these genes simply add together. In epistatic models, the overall effect is greater than the sum of each gene acting separately.

model, the disease alleles at genes A and B each convey a relatively small effect alone. However, individuals with the disease alleles for both A and B have a risk for illness that is greater than the sum of risks for A and B. In the example in Figure 13.3–4, A and B each convey a 20 percent risk alone. The affected daughter with the AB genotype, however, has an 80 percent risk for illness. Epistatic interactions have been observed in many organisms and frequently reflect a "two-hit" effect on a biological system. For example, a neurotransmitter system may be able to tolerate a defect in gene A by increasing the activity of gene B. Similarly, gene B may be able to compensate for a defect in A such that individuals with defects in A or B alone may have only a limited risk for illness. However, if both A and B are defective, the system is unable to compensate and the risk for illness goes up considerably.

Quantitative Traits One of the many difficulties in studies of psychiatric genetics is the definition of *affected.* Variable expressivity results in a variety of disorders from similar genotypes. It is frequently not clear which of these disorders should be considered affected for the purposes of genetic analyses. An alternative to such dichotomous definitions of phenotype is the use of quantitative phenotypes. Many biological variables are obvious quantitative phenotypes, such as blood pressure and height. However, it is not immediately obvious which mood disorder is "worse" or "more" than another. Nevertheless, quantitative phenotypes have been applied with some success to mood disorders. An example is the multiple-threshold model described above. Although quantitative phenotypes can be the result of single major loci, the concept has evolved historically in connection with polygenic traits. In such models, each polygene contributes in either an additive or epistatic fashion to the value of the quantitative phenotype. Quantitative models offer a useful alternative to the dichotomous approach to phenotype. However, the basic problem is that mood disorder phenotypes are more complex than either the dichotomous or quantitative genetic models.

POSITIONAL CLONING OF COMPLEX DISORDERS

Positional cloning refers to the use of molecular genetic methods to identify disease genes based on their chromosomal location. Such studies, directed at the identification of specific disease genes, are the focus of most recent research efforts in the genetics of mood disorders. The methods and strategies of positional cloning are reviewed in more detail elsewhere in this text. A brief description here will preface a review of the problems faced in such studies of mood disorders and some of their potential solutions.

DNA markers are segments of DNA of known chromosomal location, which are highly variable between individuals. They are used to track the segregation of specific chromosomal regions within families affected with a disorder. When a marker is identified whose alleles consistently cosegregate with disease in families, it is said to be *genetically linked.* This implies that a gene for the disorder is physically near the marker on a chromosome. The Human Genome Project has provided thousands of such markers and precisely mapped them to chromosomal locations. By using several hundred markers, one can systematically survey the genome in search of markers linked to a disease. In this fashion, novel disease genes can be identified based on their chromosomal location rather than their physiological function. It is this ability to identify novel genes without relying on knowledge of their function or of the pathophysiology of the disorder that makes positional cloning such a powerful approach. This approach has led to the successful identification of genes for numerous diseases such as Huntington's disease and cystic fibrosis.

The statistics of linkage analysis are either parametric or nonparametric. Parametric analyses assume a certain model of inheritance (e.g., dominant or recessive) and then test the marker data for the probability of fitting that assumed model. Nonparametric analyses do not require an assumption of model of inheritance. Instead, affected family members are tested for significantly increased sharing of marker alleles. The affected sibling pair method is an example of this approach. More recently, methods have been developed for the nonparametric analyses of all affected relative pairs in families. Parametric methods generally have greater power to detect linkage if the correct model is used. Nonparametric methods have less power but are not vulnerable to error resulting from the use of an incorrect model of inheritance. The logarithm of odds (LOD) score is a commonly used statistic in linkage studies. The LOD score is the logarithm of the odds for linkage divided by the odds against linkage. Depending on the study design, a LOD score of approximately 3.3 is the conventionally accepted threshold for statistical significance.

When a chromosomal region is identified by genetic linkage studies in families, the disease gene has typically been localized to a region of between 5 and 30 million base pairs of DNA, which might

FIGURE 13.3–5 Sample sizes required to detect linkage or association for different risk allele frequencies and effect sizes. The number of pairs of subjects necessary to detect a disease gene by linkage or a disease allele by association is depicted as a function of the frequency of that allele in the population. Dashed lines illustrate the power of linkage using a sibling pair strategy, and solid lines show the power of association using a case-control sample. Each are calculated for differing genotype relative risks (GRR), which are the frequencies of disease in those with the allele divided by the rate in the general population. Although linkage has good power for strong gene effects (GRR = 4.0), very large sample sizes are required for smaller gene effects (GRR = 2.0). Association, however, requires much smaller sample sizes even for small gene effects. (From Risch N, Merikangas K: The future of genetic studies of complex human diseases. *Science.* 1996;273: 1516–1517, with permission.)

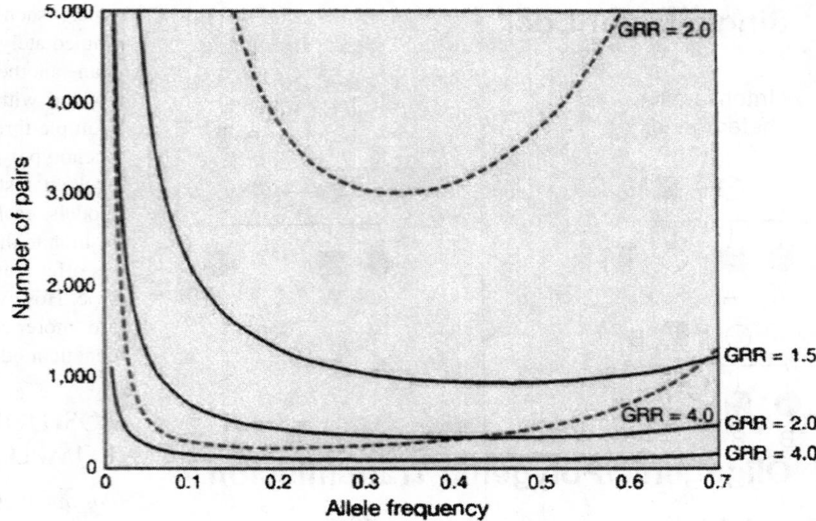

contain several hundred genes. Genetic association studies may then sometimes be useful to more finely map the disease gene within this region. In these studies, markers are tested for significant differences in the frequencies of their alleles between unrelated groups of affected subjects and control subjects. Such differences may reflect the presence of linkage disequilibrium and indicate that the marker is very near the disease gene. Until recently, physical mapping methods were used to identify the exact disease gene. Recently, this has dramatically changed, as the Human Genome Project has mapped almost all human genes, providing powerful new tools for positional cloning.

Difficulties of Mapping Complex Disorders In simple Mendelian traits, there is a 1-to-1 correspondence between genotype and phenotype. Everyone in a family who has the disorder has the gene, and everyone who has the gene has the disorder. This allows extraction of maximal information regarding the possible cosegregation of marker and disorder in linkage studies. However, both reduced penetrance and phenocopies loosen the connection between genotype and phenotype and thereby reduce the statistical power of linkage methods to identify genes. In complex disorders, it is not clear that nonaffected individuals did not receive the disease allele, nor is it certain that affected individuals did. This translates directly into the need for larger samples of families for study.

Variable expressivity and difficulty in diagnosis introduce further uncertainty in modeling genetic transmission. It is not clear which of the spectrum of mood disorders should be considered affected. If the definition of affected is too narrow, then valuable information from family members with more subtle forms of illness may be lost. However, if the definition of affected is too broad, too many phenocopies may be included as affected, which introduces error. Most linkage studies currently use a hierarchy of different definitions of illness, which range from narrow to broad. For example, a narrow model might include as affected only those with bipolar disorder. A broad model would include bipolar disorder and recurrent major depression. The difficulty in making behavioral diagnoses adds further complexities. Psychiatric diagnoses rely on the accuracy of the individual's memories and judgments about behavior that depend on the context of one's life and environment.

Other difficulties arise out of the limitations of statistical methods. The most powerful statistical methods currently available are based on Mendelian models of transmission. However, it seems clear that mood disorders are not transmitted according to these simple models. Nonparametric methods do not rely on Mendelian models, however, in general, their statistical power is not as great. Both approaches are currently commonly used, but, in the absence of knowledge of the mode of transmission, it is unclear which approach is best. Furthermore, recent simulation studies have indicated that, even once linkage is established, a much larger chromosomal region is implicated in complex disorders than in Mendelian ones. This makes the job of fine mapping and gene identification substantially larger.

The greatest problem facing positional cloning studies is clearly heterogeneity. If mood disorders result from a relatively small number of genes of large effect, then they will be identified soon. However, if a large number of genes, each of small effect, are involved, then identifying them will require large sample sizes or a different approach altogether. Current data suggest that the number of genes probably lies somewhere between these extremes. The cost of heterogeneity in terms of sample size is illustrated in Figure 13.3–5. This simulation study, using affected sibling pairs, indicates that if a gene is present in less than 25 percent of families under study, the total number of families required to detect linkage increases substantially.

Multigene models, such as epistatic or additive gene interactions, also pose significant problems for mapping complex traits. As described above, if two genes interact epistatically, each gene considered alone may show only limited evidence of association or linkage. Only by considering both genes simultaneously can the genes be readily detected, as most of the genetic effect is in the interaction between the genes. Although it is likely that epistatic effects are present, it is currently unclear how important they are in the genetic transmission of mood disorders.

Solutions for Mapping Complex Disorders Despite these challenges, powerful new tools and strategies are enabling gene identification in mood disorder. Many of these new developments involve the use of more sophisticated statistical methods. Several new methods of nonparametric analysis have been developed that do not require assumptions about mode of transmission and that use linkage information with greater efficiency. New approaches have also been developed for the analysis of multigene interactions. One of the areas of greatest growth is the development of methods for genetic mapping using association and linkage disequilibrium. These mathematical tools use information from the new, very-high-density map developed by the Human Genome Project. These approaches will be used for the fine mapping of genes within linkage peaks and for whole-genome association studies using tens or hundreds of thousands of markers.

One of the most important developments for mapping genes is the availability of large sample sizes. If mood disorders are highly heterogeneous and epistasis is present, large sample sizes are required to detect both the genes and the gene–gene interactions. Fortunately, studies have recently been completed that have collected more than 800 families with bipolar disorder. Projects to collect thousands of bipolar cases and controls are now beginning in preparation for large association studies. Samples of this size should enable the detection of small gene effects and facilitate analysis of epistasis. Family samples are also being collected from a variety of founded genetic isolates. Such populations may have lower genetic heterogeneity, facilitating gene-mapping studies. They also may have a simpler genetic population structure because of the absence of mixtures of populations that may facilitate genetic studies.

Various approaches to refining the phenotype may improve the odds of success in linkage studies. Studying subforms of an illness whose genetic distinctness is supported by epidemiological data may allow investigators to reduce the number of genes under study. For example, bipolar II disorder or lithium-responsive illness may represent distinct subsets of bipolar genes. Such subforms of illness may be easier to map. Similarly, measures of personality or affective temperament may also provide more sensitive approaches to detecting the phenotype or may also separate different subforms of illness. Intermediate phenotypes or endophenotypes may also be useful in this regard. Intermediate phenotypes are biological markers associated with illness and segregate in families. Sleep electroencephalogram (EEG) measures and sensitivity to various pharmacological challenges are examples of such possible markers. Biochemical measures in lymphoblastoid cell lines may also be useful endophenotypes. Intermediate phenotypes can be used to identify psychiatrically well family members who carry susceptibility genes. In this way, these biological markers display a higher penetrance than the psychiatric disorder itself and, thus, capture more genetic information from family members. Furthermore, they may also reflect biologically distinct subforms of illness.

New Tools from the Human Genome Project The last few years have seen dramatic advances in the Human Genome Project that now provide powerful tools for the analysis of complex traits. The most important of these is the completed sequence of the human genome. This sequence has enabled the mapping of most human genes. This mapping was also made possible by large-scale efforts to sequence all messenger ribonucleic acids (mRNAs) from numerous tissues. Short fragments of expressed genes called *expressed sequence tags* (ESTs) could then be matched to genomic sequence data to identify genes in the sequence. One of the most surprising outcomes of this work is that there were fewer human genes than had been previously believed: approximately 35,000 instead of 100,000. Now, instead of laboriously cloning the genes within a region implicated by linkage, researchers can look up the genes in a chromosomal segment, the complete sequence of those genes, and the DNA between the genes. This obviates a laborious process in fine mapping and facilitates a systematic approach to gene identification.

The identification of almost all human genes has also made possible comprehensive studies of RNA or gene expression. Thousands of genes can now be placed on microarrays that can then be hybridized to the RNA from a tissue. By detecting the amount of fluorescently labeled mRNA binding to the genes on the array, the level of expression of thousands of genes can be examined simultaneously. This technology can be used to study animal models of disease or postmortem brain to identify possible candidate genes for illness.

After the sequencing of the human genome, attention has focused on studies of variation in human sequencing. Sequencing of genomic regions in many individuals has confirmed the idea that humans differ from each other at approximately 1 base pair in 1,000. The majority of these differences are changes in single bases termed *single-nucleotide polymorphisms* (SNPs). More than 2 million of these have now been identified across the genome. To exploit these high-density markers, a variety of high-throughput methods have been developed to genotype SNPs. These developments will soon make it possible to conduct genome-wide association studies. As described above, association is the study of allele frequencies in populations, as opposed to linkage, which is the study of segregation in families. Association has greater power to detect genes of smaller effect. However, to detect association or linkage disequilibrium, the marker must be very close to the disease mutation on the order of 5 to 50 kilobases. This requires a very large number of markers and, until recently, was not considered feasible. However, these new advances may soon make it possible to screen the entire genome for association. This approach, in combination with the statistical methods mentioned above, promises greater power to unravel complex disorders.

GENETIC LINKAGE AND ASSOCIATION STUDIES: RESULTS TO DATE

The search for genes for mood disorders has, to date, focused primarily on bipolar disorder, because of the stronger evidence for its genetic basis. In its early years, this search had a series of ups and downs of reported findings and subsequent nonreplications likened to the highs and lows of the illness itself. Such high-profile nonreplications led to frustration among investigators and concern that false-positive linkage results might be common. Many investigators argued for highly conservative thresholds for the statistical significance of linkage results to adequately guard against such events. However, subsequent experience has indicated that such strongly positive results are relatively uncommon. Furthermore, simulation studies of heterogeneous or polygenic disorders have shown that nonreplications should be expected, even for real loci, until adequate data are accumulated to convincingly demonstrate linkage.

Recently, a number of positive results have emerged that are quite encouraging in terms of the ability of linkage analysis to successfully identify genes for bipolar disorder. These results meet criteria not only for statistical significance, but also for significant replication. Furthermore, as more genome scans are conducted in more and larger samples, the same loci have been repeatedly, although not consistently, identified. This provides hope that at least some loci are common enough and have a large enough effect that they may be identified using feasible family samples.

However, with the increasing number of studies done, a large portion of the genome has come to be implicated. Many of these regions may simply reflect false-positives, but it also could indicate that there are more genes for the illness than had been previously thought. This remains a fundamental question in this field. This work began with the assumption of a few genes transmitted in a largely Mendelian fashion. However, the current linkage data suggest a larger number of genes, possibly in the dozens. However, it is possible that many more genes are involved. If the number of genes is more than a few dozen, they may be very difficult to detect by linkage for two reasons: The effect size of each gene within the population may be too small; and, given the 20- to 30-Mb length of most linkage peaks, the loci may be too close together to be resolved by linkage. If this is the case, then association may be the genetic tool of choice. Fortunately, as described above, tools from the Human Genome Project will soon make possible such high-resolution association studies. Association studies of candidate genes have already begun to yield some replicable results. This field is now entering an exciting phase as strong, replicable results begin to appear as the result of many studies and larger samples. Strong evidence is also emerging for a few specific genes. The coming years will likely see the replicable identification of many novel genes for mood disorders.

Linkage Studies of Bipolar Disorder This field began with two studies that initially reported strong evidence for linkage but was soon followed by several failures to replicate these results in other family samples and, later, in additional studies of the same family samples. One of the first reports of linkage to bipolar disorder was a study of the Old Order Amish in southeastern Pennsylvania. This group is particularly useful for genetic studies, because they have remained genetically isolated from the rest of society since their immigration from Germany and Switzerland in the 1700s. Strong evidence of linkage (LOD of 4.8) was initially reported to markers on 11p15. However, in subsequent analyses of an expanded version of the same family, the evidence for linkage was much reduced. Miron Baron and colleagues obtained a similar result in their studies of the X chromosome and bipolar disorder. An initial strong linkage result later could not be replicated. These initial false starts led to some skepticism about this approach. They also suggested that these were not simple Mendelian traits, but rather complex traits involving multiple genes. These initial results also altered the expectations for such studies; many studies would be required to obtain replication and determine which results were real.

Table 13.3–3 summarizes some of the chromosomal regions that have been reported to be linked to bipolar disorder. These studies have been conducted in a wide range of family samples varying in number of families, size of families, genetic strategy (e.g., sibling pair), and geographical and ethnic origin. Many of these results meet statistical significance, and some have been replicated with statistical significance. Almost all of these regions have been implicated to some degree in more than one study.

Several regions on chromosome 18 have been reported to be linked to bipolar disorder. The first of these was a region near the centromere on 18p. Subsequent studies of chromosome 18 replicated these findings near the centromere and also identified a second region on 18q. These studies found linkage to 18q to preferentially occur in families in which affective illness was transmitted through the mother, suggesting a possible parent-of-origin effect. Other studies of a genetic isolate in Costa Rica reported evidence of linkage to two separate sites, one on each end of chromosome 18. Together, these data suggest the presence of as many as four different loci on this one chromosome. Only further studies and the identification of the actual genes will confirm whether this many genes actually exist on 18.

A locus on distal 21q has also been extensively studied and implicated in multiple studies of bipolar disorder. Xq, which was reported in 1987 and, later, not replicated, has returned as a region of interest in studies of a Finnish population. Chromosome 12q was first suspected based on the identification of a Welsh family in which bipolar disorder cosegregated with a rare skin disease, Darier's disease. The skin disease was subsequently mapped to 12q, leading investigators to examine this region in families with bipolar disorder who did not have Darier's disease. Linkage of markers in this region to bipolar disorder was reported in Welsh families and also in a large isolate in Quebec. 22q was first implicated in psychiatric illness by the observation of psychotic and mood symptoms in adolescents

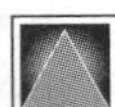

Table 13.3–3
Selected Chromosomal Regions with Evidence of Linkage to Bipolar Disorder

Chromosome	Reference	Result
4p16	Blackwood et al., 1996	LOD of 4.1
4q35	Adams et al., 1998	LOD of 3.19
6q	Dick et al., 2003	LOD of 2.2
8p	Ophoff et al., 2002	$P<10^{-4}$
10p12	Foroud et al., 2000	LOD of 2.5
10q25	Cichon et al., 2001	LOD of 2.86
12q23-24	Dawson et al., 1995; Morissette et al., 1999	LOD of 2.47
13q32	Detera-Wadleigh et al., 1999	LOD of 3.5
16p13	Ewald et al., 1995	LOD of 2.65
17q	Dick et al., 2003	LOD of 2.4
18p11	Berrettini et al., 1994	LOD of 2.6
18q21	Stine et al., 1995	LOD of 3.51, in paternal pedigrees
18q22-23	Freimer et al., 1996	LOD of 3.7
21q22.3	Straub et al., 1994	LOD of 3.4
22q11-q12	Kelsoe et al., 2001	LOD of 3.8
Xq26-q28	Baron et al., 1987; Pekkarinen et al., 1995	LOD of 2.09; LOD of 3.1

LOD, logarithm of odds.

with a 22q11 deletion syndrome called *velocardiofacial syndrome*. Subsequently, this and other regions of this chromosome have shown linkage or association to both schizophrenia and bipolar disorder.

Several linkage studies have found evidence for the involvement of specific genes in clinical subtypes. The linkage evidence on 18q, described above, has been shown to be derived largely from bipolar II–bipolar II sibling pairs and from families in which the probands had panic symptoms. Similarly, lithium-responsive bipolar disorder has been employed as a specific phenotype to identify loci linked to a putatively genetically distinct form of illness. Evidence has also been reported that families with bipolar disorder and psychotic symptoms may be preferentially linked to regions on chromosomes 13 and 22. These intriguing results suggest a high level of specificity of gene to phenotype and are in contrast with other studies described below that argue for the nonspecific nature of susceptibility genes.

It is difficult to interpret the large number of linkage results in studies of bipolar disorder and to determine which of the loci reported are most likely to represent real susceptibility genes. Fortunately, the accumulation of multiple complete scans of the genome in different family sets and the development of ways to apply metaanalysis methods to linkage data has enabled a systematic approach to this question. Metaanalysis methods examine the results of multiple studies and calculate statistics that test the strength of a finding across multiple data sets. One such study examined 11 published genome scans of bipolar disorder using a method called *multiple scan probability*. This analysis identified 13q and 22q as the two regions with strongest evidence for linkage to bipolar disorder and as those most clearly replicated. Another analyzed data from 18 family sets using the Genome Scan Meta-Analysis (GSMA) method. This analysis reported support for regions on chromosomes 9p, 10q, and 14q.

Genetic Overlap between Bipolar Disorder and Schizophrenia As linkage results have accumulated for genome scans of both bipolar disorder and schizophrenia over the last decade, it has become increasingly apparent that there is a sub-

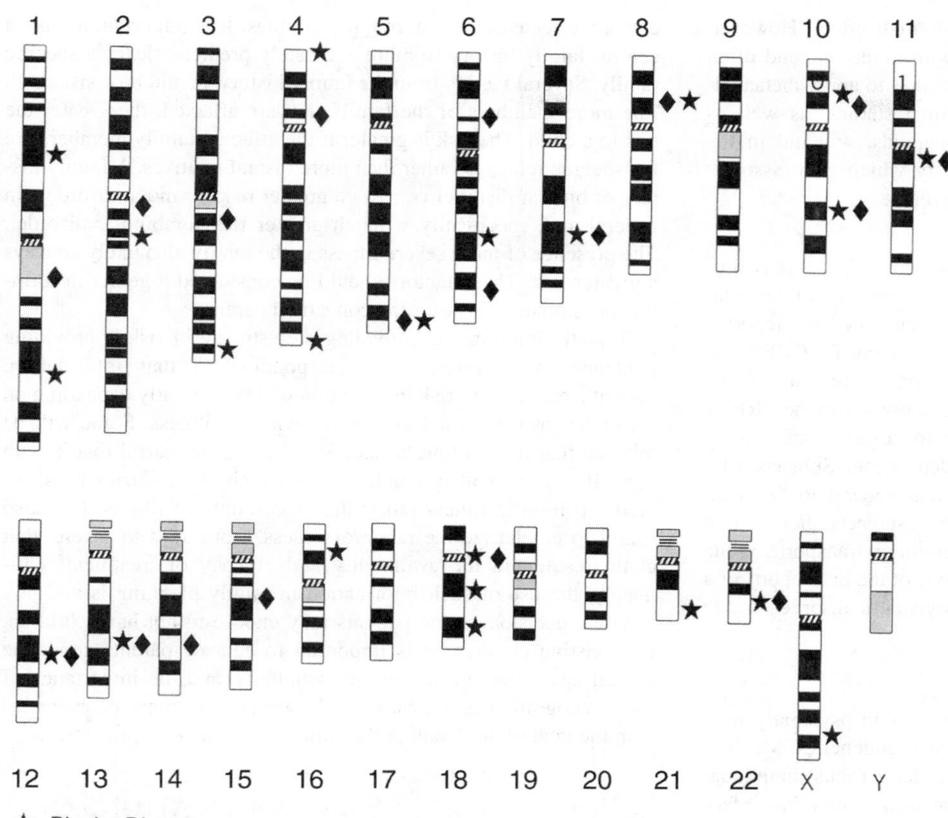

FIGURE 13.3–6 Overlap between putative genetic loci for bipolar disorder and schizophrenia.

stantial overlap between loci identified for the two disorders. This remarkable and unexpected result suggests that a substantial portion of the susceptibility genes for each disorder are the same. Figure 13.3–6 illustrates this phenomenon by summarizing some of the more prominent reports of linkage for these illnesses. At least nine regions, the majority for each disorder, have been implicated in both disorders. Because each linkage region is quite large and typically spans hundreds of genes, it is impossible to know at this point that the same genes are involved in each disorder in these regions. However, the degree of this overlap suggests that at least some genes are shared. This possibility is unexpected in light of the substantial family history literature, which, for the most part, has argued that each disorder "breeds true." These studies have examined how often schizophrenia is seen in the relatives of bipolar probands and vice versa. However, this possibility resonates with the common clinical observation of schizoaffective disorder and psychotic mood disorders. It is also consistent with the "spectrum" concept of major psychoses, which placed schizophrenia and bipolar disorder at opposite ends of a spectrum. Such a possible genetic overlap is also consistent with more recent family studies, which have shown schizoaffective disorder and other psychotic mood disorders to occur at equal frequencies in the offspring of schizophrenic and bipolar probands.

Association and Candidate Gene Studies of Bipolar Disorder

Numerous candidate genes have also been examined for their possible role in the susceptibility to mood disorders. The candidates that have been examined are largely genes involved in catecholamine or serotonin neurotransmission. Tyrosine hydroxylase regulates the biosynthesis of catecholamines. It has been shown to have a tetranucleotide repeat polymorphism in intron 1 that influences expression and is associated with bipolar disorder. Brain-derived neurotrophic growth factor (BDNF) is a gene involved in the development and maintenance of catecholaminergic neurons. It maps to 11p15 and has been reported to be associated with bipolar disorder. The serotonin transporter mediates the active reuptake of serotonin from the synapse and is the site of action of selective serotonin reuptake inhibitor (SSRI) antidepressants. It has been associated with both susceptibility to bipolar disorder and response to SSRI medications.

Several genes have recently been reported as possible successes of positional cloning—that is, the responsible genes within linkage peaks. G-protein receptor kinase 3 (GRK3) mediates the desensitization of dopamine type 1 (D_1) receptors and other receptors in response to agonist stimulation. It maps to 22q11 and has been implicated in bipolar disorder by both linkage and association. G72 is a gene on chromosome 13q that may indirectly modulate the effect of serine on *N*-methyl-D-aspartate (NMDA) receptors. This region on 13q has been reportedly linked to both bipolar disorder and schizophrenia. The G72 gene was first identified in studies of schizophrenia and later shown in several studies to also be associated with bipolar disorder. This may be the first specific gene identified that plays a role in both disorders. XBP1 is a gene involved in the endoplasmic reticulum stress response. It was first identified in microarray gene expression studies of lymphoblastoid cell lines from twins with bipolar disorder. It maps to a region on 22q linked to bipolar disorder. Variants in the gene were reported to be associated with illness.

This is only a partial summary of the numerous genes that have been tested for association with mood disorders. Studies of this nature have great power to detect genes of small effect. However, this literature is currently very complex, with numerous and often conflicting studies. There are now enough studies to apply metaanalysis methods for many of these genes. Such studies, as well as efforts to better standardize association methods, will aid in the interpretation of these data and help identify which gene associations are the strongest and most likely to be real.

Studies of Unipolar Depression

Until recently, only limited attention had been paid to gene-mapping studies of unipolar depression. However, a genome linkage scan has now been reported that found very strong evidence of linkage to the locus for CREB1 on chromosome 2. Eighteen other genomic regions were found to be linked; some of these displayed epistatic interactions with the CREB1 locus. Another study has reported evidence for a gene–environment interaction in the development of major depression. Subjects who underwent adverse life events were shown in general to be at an increased risk for depression. However, of such subjects, those with a variant in the promotor region of the serotonin transporter gene showed the greatest increase in risk. This is one of the first reports of a specific gene–environment interaction in a psychiatric disorder.

PHARMACOGENETICS

One of the first clinical applications of genetics in psychiatry may come from the newly emerging field of pharmacogenetics. Medication responses in mood disorders frequently have robust individual differences. Though response has been related to some clinical factors, genetic differences likely play a major role. The strongest result in this field to date involves a repeat variant in the promoter region of the serotonin transporter gene. This variant has been shown to influence the expression of the protein that is the site of action of SSRIs. It has also been associated in several studies with response to SSRIs and response to lithium. The risk for antidepressant-induced mania has also been shown to be associated with this gene. Although studies of this area is relatively new, it promises a powerful tool for future clinicians who one day may use a DNA test panel to optimize the selection of medications for individual patients, thereby reducing the trial and error involved in medication treatment.

GENETIC COUNSELING

Based on the observation of psychiatric illness in their own families or the increasing public awareness of psychiatric genetics, patients frequently ask clinicians three questions: Are mood disorders genetic? What is the risk to my children or grandchildren? Is there a blood test for the gene? The answer to the last question is the easiest: Currently, there is no blood test available. However, it is likely that such a test will be available at some point, possibly in the near future, and with it will come a variety of serious practical and ethical issues, which are discussed below. The answer to the first question is also easy: Yes, mood disorders are genetic, as is evidenced by the large body of epidemiological data summarized in this chapter. However, it is important that patients understand that mood disorders are only in part genetic. The twin studies argue strongly that only 50 to 70 percent of the etiology of mood disorders is genetic. Therefore, it is a predisposition to illness that is inherited and interacts with other nonheritable factors.

The risk to children and grandchildren is the more difficult question and the one that deserves the greatest consideration. The family data indicate that if one parent has a mood disorder, a child will have a risk for mood disorder of between 10 and 25 percent. If both parents are affected, this risk roughly doubles. It is important to take a careful family history to more accurately predict risk for a specific family. Several factors from the family history should be considered. The more members of the family that are affected, the greater the risk to a child. The risk is greater if the affected family members are first-degree relatives rather than more distant relatives. A family history of bipolar disorder conveys a greater risk for mood disorders in general and, specifically, a much greater risk for bipolar disorder. The presence of more severe illness in the family also likely conveys a greater risk. These factors should be considered together in forming an estimate of risk for the concerned parent.

Equally important to providing the estimate of risk is providing guidance in interpreting and responding to that information. Patient's reactions to risk information will vary greatly depending on his or her own personal experience with the illness. Some will be relieved that it is so low, whereas others will be fearful that it is so high. It is important to emphasize that their child carries a risk or predisposition to illness rather than a certainty of illness. It is also useful to emphasize the range of illness, from mild to severe, that could result and the availability and efficacy of treatment. Ultimately, the use of such information in family planning is a highly personal decision. Some patients may choose to not have children. For existing children, it is important to educate parents about the typical age of onset, presenting symptoms, and the importance of early recognition and treatment. However, this must be balanced with the goal of not labeling the child or being overly protective.

FUTURE DIRECTIONS AND IMPLICATIONS OF IDENTIFYING SUSCEPTIBILITY GENES

It is the gradual accumulation of a large body of data that has led to the successful replications described above. Thus, in the near future, gene-mapping studies will likely continue using current strategies. As still more data are accumulated, it is likely that further reported loci will be replicated, whereas others will prove to be false positives. The development and study of the large samples required will necessitate large collaborative efforts between multiple groups of investigators using common diagnostic and genetic methods. The availability of the high-density SNP map will facilitate the identification of disease genes in linkage peaks. In the near future, genome-wide association studies may enable studies to detect larger numbers of genes of smaller effect. Such data will facilitate the testing of multigene models. Ultimately, a more comprehensive understanding of the genetics of mood disorder may entail complex models of the interaction of numerous genes. As a better understanding of environmental effects becomes available, these will be incorporated into such models. Although some environmental effects may be nonspecific, it seems likely that at least some will reflect specific gene–environment interactions. Such interactions may be difficult to detect and will add substantial complexity to the overall model of mood disorder genetics. At this point, it seems promising that most genes for mood disorders can be identified through such large, though tractable, projects.

What will be the implications of this knowledge? The most immediate impact may well be on public opinion. Psychiatrically ill persons have long experienced the stigma and discrimination that portions of the public impose out of fear and ignorance. The acceptance of major mental illnesses as brain disorders has been slow. The definitive identification of genetic causes may have a highly beneficial impact on public understanding and acceptance.

This knowledge should also have a dramatic impact on understanding of pathophysiology and approaches to treatment for mood disorders. Most current theories of pathophysiology are based on the mode of action of therapeutic agents, which were, for the most part, discovered serendipitously. The site of action of therapeutic drugs is not necessarily either the site of the genetic defect or the primary site of the pathophysiology. The identification of disease genes may point to entirely new systems involved in the pathophysiology or components of currently implicated systems that were not previously known. It is hoped that such an understanding may lead to the rational drug design long sought by patients, clinicians, and pharmaceutical companies. The result may be new drugs that act via completely novel mechanisms, possibly with greater efficacy and specificity. Further down the genetic road lies the prospect of gene therapy for mood disorders. In this approach, DNA is used as a therapeutic agent delivered to the relevant tissues by engineered viruses or other vectors. Such artificially delivered DNA can be used to provide the correct version of a defective disease gene. Alternatively, a disease process might be ameliorated by changing the expression of other regulatory genes. Such an approach goes straight to the root of biology and pathology and offers the prospect of an extremely powerful and completely new treatment modality. The application of this approach to psychiatric disorders is likely in the relatively distant future and faces formidable problems.

The identification of disease genes will likely have a major impact on diagnosis and nosology. Just as the diagnosis of jaundice has given way to a classification scheme based on pathophysiology, it is likely that, in the future, the diagnosis of major mood disorders may be specific to disease mechanism. Mechanism-specific diagnoses may dictate the use of different, more specific, and more effective treatments. Lastly, such knowledge will carry with it danger and responsibility. Premorbid DNA testing that would indicate the degree of genetic vulnerability to major mood disorders could become available. Those with psychiatric disorders will then face the same issues of genetic testing currently faced by families with Huntington's disease or breast cancer: Will at-risk family members want such information? How will they use it? How will they cope with it? How can psychiatrists assist them in these decisions? Lastly, how can patients be protected from discrimination based on such information?

In summary, genetic studies promise a new era of understanding and treatment of mood disorders. Identification of genes alone will not elucidate pathophysiology but will merely point the way for the application of modern neuroscience methods in the equally large task of understanding mechanisms. Recent results suggest that such guidance may not be far away.

SUGGESTED CROSS-REFERENCES

A general review of basic molecular genetics is provided in Section 1.10. Principles of population genetics are discussed in Section 1.17. The concepts and methods of linkage analysis and their application to psychiatry are reviewed in Section 1.18. The epidemiology of mood disorders is discussed in Section 14.2.

REFERENCES

Adams LJ, Mitchell PB, Fielder SL, Rosso A, Donald JA, Schofield PR: A susceptibility locus for bipolar affective disorder on chromosome 4q35. *Am J Hum Genet.* 1998;62:1084–1091.

Akiskal HS: The prevalent clinical spectrum of bipolar disorders: beyond DSM-IV. *J Clin Psychopharmacol.* 1996;16:4S–14S.

*Badner JA, Gershon ES: Meta-analysis of whole-genome linkage scans of bipolar disorder and schizophrenia. *Mol Psychiatry.* 2002;7:405–411.

Baron M, Risch N, Hamburger R, Mandel B, Kushner S, Newman M, Drumer D, Belmaker RH: Genetic linkage between X-chromosome markers and bipolar affective illness. *Nature.* 1987;326:289–292.

Barrett TB, Hauger RL, Kennedy JL, Sadovnick AD, Remick RA, Keck PE Jr, McElroy SL, Alexander M, Shaw SH, Kelsoe JR: Evidence that a single nucleotide polymorphism in the promoter of the G protein receptor kinase 3 gene is associated with bipolar disorder. *Mol Psychiatry.* 2003;8:546–557.

Berrettini WH, Ferraro TN, Goldin LR, Weeks DE, Detera-Wadleigh S, Nurnberger JI Jr, Gershon ES: Chromosome 18 DNA markers and manic-depressive illness: evidence for a susceptibility gene. *Proc Natl Acad Sci U S A.* 1994;91:5918–5921.

*Bertelsen A. A Danish twin study of manic-depressive disorders. In: Schou M, Stromgren E, eds. *Origin, Prevention and Treatment of Affective Disorder.* London: Academic Press; 1979:227–239.

Blackwood DH, He L, Morris SW, McLean A, Whitton C, Thomson M, Walker MT, Woodburn K, Sharp CM, Wright AF, Shibasaki Y, St. Clair DM, Porteous DJ, Muir WJ: A locus for bipolar affective disorder on chromosome 4p. *Nat Genet.* 1996;12:427–430.

*Caspi A, Sugden K, Moffitt TE, Taylor A, Craig IW, Harrington H, McClay J, Mill J, Martin J, Braithwaite A, Poulton R: Influence of life stress on depression: moderation by a polymorphism in the 5-HTT gene. *Science.* 2003;301:386–389.

Cichon S, Schmidt-Wolf G, Schumacher J, Muller DJ, Hurter M, Schulze TG, Albus M, Borrmann-Hassenbach M, Franzek E, Lanczik M, Fritze J, Kreiner R, Weigelt B, Minges J, Lichtermann D, Lerer B, Kanyas K, Strauch K, Windemuth C, Baur MP, Wienker TF, Maier W, Rietschel M, Propping P, Nothen MM: A possible susceptibility locus for bipolar affective disorder in chromosomal region 10q25–q26. *Mol Psychiatry.* 2001;6:342–349.

Dawson E, Parfitt E, Roberts Q, Daniels J, Lim L, Sham P, Nothen M, Propping P, Lanczik M, Maier W, Reuner U, Weissenbach J, Gill M, Powell J, McGuffin P, Owen M, Craddock N: Linkage studies of bipolar disorder in the region of the Darier's disease gene on chromosome 12q23-24.1. *Am J Med Genet.* 1995;60:94–102.

Detera-Wadleigh SD, Badner JA, Berrettini WH, Yoshikawa T, Goldin LR, Turner G, Rollins DY, Moses T, Sanders AR, Karkera JD, Esterling LE, Zeng J, Ferraro TN, Guroff JJ, Kazuba D, Maxwell ME, Nurnberger JJ, Gershon ES: A high-density genome scan detects evidence for a bipolar-disorder susceptibility locus on 13q32 and other potential loci on 1q32 and 18p11.2. *Proc Natl Acad Sci U S A.* 1999;96:5604–5609.

Dick DM, Foroud T, Flury L, Bowman ES, Miller MJ, Rau NL, Moe PR, Samavedy N, el Mallakh R, Manji H, Glitz DA, Meyer ET, Smiley C, Hahn R, Widmark C, McKinney R, Sutton L, Ballas C, Grice D, Berrettini W, Byerley W, Coryell W, DePaulo R, MacKinnon DF, Gershon ES, Kelsoe JR, McMahon FJ, McInnis M, Murphy DL, Reich T, Scheftner W, Nurnberger JI Jr.: Genomewide linkage analyses of bipolar disorder: a new sample of 250 pedigrees from the National Institute of Mental Health Genetics Initiative. *Am J Hum Genet.* 2003;73:107–114.

Egeland JA, Gerhard DS, Pauls DL, Sussex JN, Kidd KK, Allen CR, Hostetter AM, Housman DE: Bipolar affective disorders linked to DNA markers on chromosome 11. *Nature.* 1987;325:783–787.

Erlenmeyer-Kimling L, Adamo UH, Rock D, Roberts SA, Bassett AS, Squires-Wheeler E, Cornblatt BA, Endicott J, Pape S, Gottesman II: The New York High-Risk Project. Prevalence and comorbidity of axis I disorders in offspring of schizophrenic parents at 25-year follow-up. *Arch Gen Psychiatry.* 1997;54:1096–1102.

Ewald H, Mors O, Flint T, Koed K, Eiberg H, Kruse TA: A possible locus for manic depressive illness on chromosome 16p13. *Psychiatr Genet.* 1995;5:71–81.

Fieve RR, Go R, Dunner DL, Elston R. Search for biological/genetic markers in a long-term epidemiological and morbid risk study of affective disorders. *J Psychiatr Res.* 1984;18:425–445.

Foroud T, Castelluccio PF, Koller DL, Edenberg HJ, Miller M, Bowman E, Rau NL, Smiley C, Rice JP, Goate A, Armstrong C, Bierut LJ, Reich T, Detera-Wadleigh SD, Goldin LR, Badner JA, Guroff JJ, Gershon ES, McMahon FJ, Simpson S, MacKinnon D, McInnis M, Stine OC, DePaulo JR, Blehar MC, Nurnberger JI Jr: Suggestive evidence of a locus on chromosome 10p using the NIMH genetics initiative bipolar affective disorder pedigrees. *Am J Med Genet.* 2000;96:18–23.

Freimer NB, Reus VI, Escamilla MA, McInnes LA, Spesny M, Leon P, Service SK, Smith LB, Silva S, Rojas E, Gallegos A, Meza L, Fournier E, Baharloo S, Blankenship K, Tyler DJ, Batki S, Vinogradov S, Weissenbach J, Barondes SH, Sandkuijl LA. Genetic mapping using haplotype, association and linkage methods suggests a locus for severe bipolar disorder (BPI) at 18q22-q23. *Nat Genet.* 1996;12:436–441.

Gershon ES, Hamovit J, Guroff JJ, Dibble E, Leckman JF, Sceery W, Targum SD, Nurnberger JI, Goldin LR, Bunney WE: A family study of schizoaffective, bipolar I, bipolar II, unipolar, and normal control probands. *Arch Gen Psychiatry.* 1982;39:1157–1167.

Heun R, Maier W: The distinction of bipolar II disorder from bipolar I and recurrent unipolar depression: results of a controlled family study. *Acta Psychiatr Scand.* 1993;87:279–284.

Kallman F. Genetic principles in manic-depressive psychosis. In: Hoch PH, Zubin J, eds. *Depression.* New York: Grune & Stratton; 1954:1–24.

Kelsoe JR: Arguments for the genetic basis of the bipolar spectrum. *J Affect Disord.* 2003;73:183–197.

Kelsoe JR, Ginns EI, Egeland JA, Gerhard DS, Goldstein AM, Bale SJ, Pauls DL, Long RT, Kidd KK, Conte G, Housman DE, Paul SM: Re-evaluation of the linkage relationship between chromosome 11p loci and the gene for bipolar affective disorder in the Old Order Amish. *Nature.* 1989;342:238–243.

Kelsoe JR, Spence MA, Loetscher E, Foguet M, Sadovnick AD, Remick RA, Flodman P, Khristich J, Mroczkowski-Parker Z, Brown JL, Masser D, Ungerleider S, Rapaport MH, Wishart WL, Luebbert H: A genome survey indicates a possible susceptibility locus for bipolar disorder on chromosome 22. *Proc Natl Acad Sci U S A.* 2001;98:585–590.

Kendler KS, Pedersen N, Johnson L, Neale MC, Mathe AA: A pilot Swedish twin study of affective illness, including hospital- and population-ascertained subsamples. *Arch Gen Psychiatry.* 1993;50:699–700.

MacKinnon DF, Xu J, McMahon FJ, Simpson SG, Stine OC, McInnis MG, DePaulo JR: Bipolar disorder and panic disorder in families: an analysis of chromosome 18 data. *Am J Psychiatry*. 1998;155:829–831.
MacKinnon DF, Zandi PP, Gershon ES, Nurnberger JI Jr., DePaulo JR Jr: Association of rapid mood switching with panic disorder and familial panic risk in familial bipolar disorder. *Am J Psychiatry*. 2003;160:1696–1698.
Martinez MM, Goldin LR: The detection of linkage and heterogeneity in nuclear families for complex disorders: one versus two marker loci. *Am J Hum Genet*. 1989;44:552–559.
McInnis MG, McMahon FJ, Chase GA, Simpson SG, Ross CA, DePaulo JR Jr: Anticipation in bipolar affective disorder. *Am J Hum Genet*. 1993;53:385–390.
McMahon FJ, Simpson SG, McInnis MG, Badner JA, MacKinnon DF, DePaulo JR: Linkage of bipolar disorder to chromosome 18q and the validity of bipolar II disorder. *Arch Gen Psychiatry*. 2001;58:1025–1031.
McMahon FJ, Stine OC, Meyers DA, Simpson SG, DePaulo JR: Patterns of maternal transmission in bipolar affective disorder. *Am J Hum Genet*. 1995;56:1277–1286.
Meloni R, Leboyer M, Bellivier F, Barbe B, Samolyk D, Allilaire JF, Mallet J: Association of manic-depressive illness with tyrosine hydroxylase microsatellite marker. *Lancet*. 1995;345:932.
Mendlewicz J, Rainer JD: Adoption study supporting genetic transmission in manic-depressive illness. *Nature*. 1977;268:327–329.
Morissette J, Villeneuve A, Bordeleau L, Rochette D, Laberge C, Gagne B, Laprise C, Bouchard G, Plante M, Gobeil L, Shink E, Weissenbach J, Barden N: Genome-wide search for linkage of bipolar affective disorders in a very large pedigree derived from a homogenous population in Quebec points to a locus of major effect on chromosome 12q23-q24. *Am J Med Genet*. 1999;88:567–587.
Nielsen DA, Goldman D, Virkkunen M, Tokola R, Rawlings R, Linnoila M: Suicidality and 5-hydroxyindoleacetic acid concentration associated with a tryptophan hydroxylase polymorphism. *Arch Gen Psychiatry*. 1994;51:34–38.
Ophoff RA, Escamilla MA, Service SK, Spesny M, Meshi DB, Poon W, Molina J, Fournier E, Gallegos A, Mathews C, Neylan T, Batki SL, Roche E, Ramirez M, Silva S, De Mille MC, Dong P, Leon PE, Reus VI, Sandkuijl LA, Freimer NB: Genome-wide linkage disequilibrium mapping of severe bipolar disorder in a population isolate. *Am J Hum Genet*. 2002;71:565–574.
Pekkarinen P, Terwilliger J, Bredbacka PE, Lonnqvist J, Peltonen L: Evidence of a predisposing locus to bipolar disorder on xq24-q27.1 in an extended Finnish pedigree. *Genome Res*. 1995;5:105–115.
Potash JB, Chiu YF, MacKinnon DF, Miller EB, Simpson SG, McMahon FJ, McInnis MG, DePaulo JR Jr: Familial aggregation of psychotic symptoms in a replication set of 69 bipolar disorder pedigrees. *Am J Med Genet*. 2003;116B:90–97.
Potash JB, Zandi PP, Willour VL, Lan TH, Huo Y, Avramopoulos D, Shugart YY, MacKinnon DF, Simpson SG, McMahon FJ, DePaulo JR Jr, McInnis MG: Suggestive linkage to chromosomal regions 13q31 and 22q12 in families with psychotic bipolar disorder. *Am J Psychiatry*. 2003;160:680–686.
Rice J, Reich T, Andreasen NC, Endicott J, van Eerdewegh M, Fishman R, Hirschfeld RM, Klerman GL: The familial transmission of bipolar illness. *Arch Gen Psychiatry*. 1987;44:441–447.
Rosanoff AJ, Handy L, Plesset IR: The etiology of manic-depressive syndromes with special reference to their occurrence in twins. *Am J Psychiatry*. 1935;91:725–762.
Sadovnick AD, Remick RA, Lam R, Zis AP, Yee IM, Huggins MJ, Baird PA: A mood disorder service genetic database: morbidity risks for mood disorders in 3,942 first-degree relatives of 671 index cases with single depression, recurrent depression, bipolar I or bipolar II. *Am J Med Genet*. 1994;54:132–140.
Segurado R, Detera-Wadleigh SD, Levinson DF, Lewis CM, Gill M, Nurnberger JI Jr, Craddock N, DePaulo JR, Baron M, Gershon ES, Ekholm J, Cichon S, Turecki G, Claes S, Kelsoe JR, Schofield PR, Badenhop RF, Morissette J, Coon H, Blackwood D, McInnes LA, Foroud T, Edenberg HJ, Reich T, Rice JP, Goate A, McInnis MG, McMahon FJ, Badner JA, Goldin LR, Bennett P, Willour VL, Zandi PP, Liu J, Gilliam C, Juo SH, Berrettini WH, Yoshikawa T, Peltonen L, Lonnqvist J, Nothen MM, Schumacher J, Windemuth C, Rietschel M, Propping P, Maier W, Alda M, Grof P, Rouleau GA, Del Favero J, Van Broeckhoven C, Mendlewicz J, Adolfsson R, Spence MA, Luebbert H, Adams LJ, Donald JA, Mitchell PB, Barden N, Shink E, Byerley W, Muir W, Visscher PM, Macgregor S, Gurling H, Kalsi G, McQuillin A, Escamilla MA, Reus VI, Leon P, Freimer NB, Ewald H, Kruse TA, Mors O, Radhakrishna U, Blouin JL, Antonarakis SE, Akarsu N: Genome scan meta-analysis of schizophrenia and bipolar disorder, part III: bipolar disorder. *Am J Hum Genet*. 2003;73:49–62.
Spence MA, Flodman PL, Sadovnick AD, Bailey-Wilson JE, Ameli H, Remick RA: Bipolar disorder: evidence for a major locus. *Am J Med Genet*. 1995;60:370–376.
Stine OC, Xu J, Koskela R, McMahon FJ, Gschwend M, Friddle C, Clark CD, McInnis MG, Simpson SG, Breschel TS, Vishio E, Riskin K, Feilotter H, Chen E, Shen S, Folstein S, Meyers DA, Botstein D, Marr TG, DePaulo JR: Evidence for linkage of bipolar disorder to chromosome 18 with a parent-of-origin effect. *Am J Hum Genet*. 1995;57:1384–1394.
Straub RE, Lehner T, Luo Y, Loth JE, Shao W, Sharpe L, Alexander JR, Das K, Simon R, Fieve RR, Lerer B, Endicott J, Ott J, Gilliam TC, Baron M: A possible vulnerability locus for bipolar affective disorder on chromosome 21q22.3. *Nat Genet*. 1994;8:291–296.
Tsuang MT, Faraone SV: *The Genetics of Mood Disorders*. Baltimore: Johns Hopkins University Press; 1990.
*Zubenko GS, Maher B, Hughes HB III, Zubenko WN, Stiffler JS, Kaplan BB, Marazita ML: Genome-wide linkage survey for genetic loci that influence the development of depressive disorders in families with recurrent, early-onset, major depression. *Am J Med Genet*. 2003;123B:1–18.

▲ 13.4 Mood Disorders: Neurobiology

MICHAEL E. THASE, M.D.

Biological factors have been implicated in the pathogenesis of depression since antiquity. It has only been since the 1960s, however, that the methods have been available to study these processes. Knowledge has advanced steadily as experimental methods have become progressively more sophisticated, moving from assays of monoamine metabolites in peripheral specimens to direct measurement of cerebral metabolism and gene activity. This chapter reviews the conceptual underpinnings of and updates research on the neurobiology of depressive disorders. Evidence of disturbances in brain function is examined in relation to the diverse clinical presentations, varied longitudinal courses, and differential response to a wide range of therapies that characterize the depressive disorders.

CLINICAL PHENOMENOLOGY

The signs, symptoms, and subjective experiences associated with depression have long suggested dysfunction of basic central nervous system (CNS) processes. With respect to cortical function, depression involves multiple disturbances of information processing. Most depressed people automatically interpret experiences from a negative perspective, and their access to memory is negatively biased. In more severe depressive states, cognition and problem-solving skills are further compromised by poor concentration and decreased ability to use abstract thought. A virtual monologue of negative thoughts and images seems to run on autopilot, and, unlike normal states of sadness, ventilation to a confidante has little beneficial effect. In more extreme cases, delusions or hallucinations, or both, grossly distort reality testing. These neurocognitive changes point to dysfunction involving the hippocampus, prefrontal cortex (PFC), and other limbic structures.

Another biologically based characteristic of depression involves decreased interest and a loss of mood reactivity: Spontaneous, goal-directed activities decrease, and events that *should* improve mood have little or no effect. One correlate of loss of interest is decreased reinforcer salience. Even basic appetitive functions, such as appetite and libido, are diminished in severe depression. Anhedonia and decreased consummatory behavior point to dysfunction of the neural circuits involved in the anticipation and consummation of rewards, which involve the thalamus, hypothalamus, nucleus accumbens, and PFC.

Alterations in the initiation, expression, and spontaneity of movement are common in severe depression. Decreased animation, or *psychomotor retardation*, is sometimes accompanied by a superimposed state of agitation. In addition to the pacing and frequent postural shifts, stereotypical signs or behaviors, such as a furrowed brow, hair pulling, biting at the lips or nail beds, and compulsive scratching, are observed in severe depressive states. Anhedonia and psychomotor disturbances are more pronounced with advancing age, with agitation typically limited to the most severe depressive syndromes. These observable signs point to dysfunction of subcortical circuits connecting the thalamus, basal ganglia, and striatum. Almost all depressed people report fatigue and an inability to feel refreshed by sleep, whether they have insomnia or they sleep too much. Although insomnia is more common, hypersomnolence is not uncommon before 40 years of age and is associated with other signs of vegetative reversal, such as increased appetite and weight gain. Insomnia, especially after 50 years of age, includes more specific sleep disturbances, such as difficulty maintaining sleep and early morning awakening. Such *terminal* insomnia is, in turn, linked to diurnal mood variation, in which morning is the worst time of the day. Disturbances of these normally well-entrained circadian rhythms further point to dysregulation of thalamic and brainstem regions.

The coaggregation or (albeit imperfect) clustering of these signs and symptoms forms the basis for several of the classical subtypes of depression. For example, anhedonia, loss of mood reactivity, and psychomotor disturbance are more commonly associated with weight loss, terminal insomnia, or diurnal mood disturbance, or a combination of these. This constellation forms the basis of the syndrome of *melancholia* (also known as *autonomous*, *biological*, *psychotic*, or *endogenous depression*). As these depressions often recur without the provocation of a significant stressor, they were presumed to have an *internal* (i.e., neurobiological) etiology. The fact that such depressions were slow to remit spontaneously yet were quite responsive to electroconvulsive therapy (ECT) further reinforced perceptions of underlying biological dysfunction. The stable nature of this syndrome over the centuries has been recognized explicitly by the contemporary use of the ancient Greek term *melancholia*, even though black bile was long ago ruled out as an etiological factor!

By contrast, the depressions commonly seen in young adult life more often seemed inextricably tied to interpersonal problems and other psychosocial difficulties. The terms *nonendogenous* and *reactive* were used to represent the observation that younger depressed people tended to be plagued by stressful life events. The association of an early age of onset with comorbid anxiety further solidified impressions that younger depressed patients had a *neurotic* disorder. Another hallmark of a putatively neurotic disorder, chronicity, also characterized many early-onset depressions. The presumed primacy of psychosocial factors in neurotic or nonendogenous depression was further suggested by less than gratifying responses to ECT and, subsequently, tricyclic antidepressants (TCAs). That the onset of depression in early life may, of course, distort personality development, limit one's repertoire of coping skills, and alter drug responsivity (i.e., pathoplasty) was overlooked.

Within the relatively broad grouping of nonendogenous depression was a subgroup characterized by *reverse* neurovegetative symptoms (i.e., increased appetite, weight gain, and hypersomnolence). As the patients treated by the hospital-based psychopathologists seldom had such symptoms, this presentation was considered to be atypical. However, as clinical research shifted to ambulatory settings, and contact with milder, younger depression increased, this *atypical* depression became more commonplace. Nevertheless, the notion of atypicality was reinforced by relatively poorer response to ECT and TCAs as compared to monoamine oxidase inhibitors (MAOIs).

RISK FACTORS

Genetic Influences

Mood disorders and suicide clearly run in families, yet the contributions of nature and nurture have provoked intense debates for decades. It is now well established that bipolar affective disorder is more heritable than other mood disorders, that an early age of onset is associated with greater heritability, and that heritability increases in proportion to the amount of shared genetic material. Thus, identical twins have greater heritable risk than fraternal twins, who are at approximately the same risk of other first-degree relatives (i.e., siblings and parents). First-degree relatives, in turn, have greater shared risk than half-siblings, grandparents, or cousins. Research comparing same-sex fraternal and identical twins and studies using the adopted-away paradigm further demonstrated that heritable risk transcends environmental influences. Research using modern molecular genetic methods will eventually lead to identification of the gene products that transmit this risk.

Although the significance of genetics cannot be disputed, considerable variability exists within and across groups with comparable heritable risks. For example, identical twins do not have 100-percent concordance of bipolar affective disorder. Early-onset depressions are more heritable, and, conversely, late-onset mood disorders (i.e., after 60 years of age) have the lowest rates of heritability. In some pedigrees, men are at greater risk for alcoholism and sociopathy, and women are at greater risk for depression. There is some evidence that environmental experiences may influence whether a woman develops depression or a generalized anxiety disorder. Genetics thus constitute just one pathway of vulnerability or, perhaps more accurately, a platform on which other biopsychosocial risk factors are expressed.

Predispositions to various emotional states (i.e., mood set points or temperament) appear to be partly heritable. Of particular importance is a temperament characterized by excessive emotional reactivity and behavioral inhibition. This temperament, which can be recognized in infancy, is associated with enduring vulnerability to depression and anxiety. Childhood onset of dysthymia similarly presages extremely high rates of depression and bipolar disorder in adulthood. Modern theories of temperament and personality converge around several related dimensions, including high levels of harm avoidance (neuroticism) and low levels of novelty seeking (introversion).

ETIOLOGY OF EMOTIONS

Some consider depression to be an extreme expression of sadness, a normal mood, with elation to be the healthier counterpart of the euphoria of mania. Such continuity between normal and pathological mood states is illustrated by bereavement. On the one hand, grief is a universal experience, yet, on the other hand, it can segue into a severe and disabling depressive state. Although there are less obvious parallels to mania, the intensity of new romantic love or other peak emotional experiences is associated with changes in perception, cognition, behavior, and judgment that border on manic excitement. The euphorigenic effects of cocaine and other psychostimulants amply document that the hard wiring for manic states exists in many if exposed to the right neurochemical milieu.

There is now considerable evidence that several basic emotions are observed across human cultures. Sadness and crying, for example, may be a universally recognized interpersonal distress signal. Moreover, the capacity to recognize the emotional states of others develops at such an early age that innate processes are undoubtedly implicated.

At the risk of anthropomorphizing excessively, basic emotional states are also observable across mammalian species. Behavioral predispositions toward aggressivity (or passivity) and social dominance (or subordination) appear to extend across vertebrate species. However, by virtue of a large neocortex, *Homo sapiens* is distinguished by a greater capacity to modify expression of basic emotional states via integration, abstraction, and synthesis of complex symbolic representations, communication of experiences to others in direct or elaborated forms, and development of self-concepts that guide behavior in relation to others and an anticipated future. The domains of competence are similarly broader and diverse. Whereas a highly competent primate may quickly gain a position of dominance if placed in a new troupe, only the human can intentionally misrepresent his or her competence, conceal his motivations, or be thwarted by archival documentation of past behaviors.

When compared to other mammals, the relatively greater importance and intensity of attachment bonds facilitate the protracted task of human childrearing and enhance the advantages of kinship. Indeed, for hundreds of thousands of years, the ancestors of *Homo sapiens* lived in a world in which the survival into adulthood was uncommon. It is only in the past few centuries that average life expectancy has exceeded 40 years. Young humans are arguably the most vulnerable of mammals and certainly remain dependent on their caregivers for the longest period of time. Although perhaps politically incorrect, certain divisions of labor no doubt increased the chances of viable offspring and may have slowly shaped gender differences in affectivity and affiliated behavior. By contrast, the profound changes in social systems and lifestyles that have taken place in the past several centuries have forced adaptations that are too rapid for natural selection. In relative terms, the breathtaking sociocultural and technological changes of the 20th century in the industrialized world have taken place in less than 0.00001 of hominid experience! The stressors faced in modern life thus present complexities that, despite such a large neocortex and complex social systems, sometimes overwhelm basic adaptive capacities.

EMOTIONAL PROCESSING AND THE BRAIN

Modern affective neuroscience focuses on the importance of four brain regions in the regulation of normal emotions: the PFC, the anterior cingulate, the hippocampus, and the amygdala (Fig. 13.4–1). The PFC is viewed as the structure that holds representations of goals and appropriate responses to obtain these goals. Such activities are particularly important when multiple, conflicting behavioral responses are possible or when it is necessary to override affective arousal. There is evidence of some hemispherical specialization in PFC function. For example, left-sided activation of regions of the PFC is more involved in goal-directed or appetitive behaviors, whereas regions of the right PFC are implicated in avoidance behaviors and inhibition of appetitive pursuits. Subregions in the PFC appear to localize representations of behaviors related to reward and punishment.

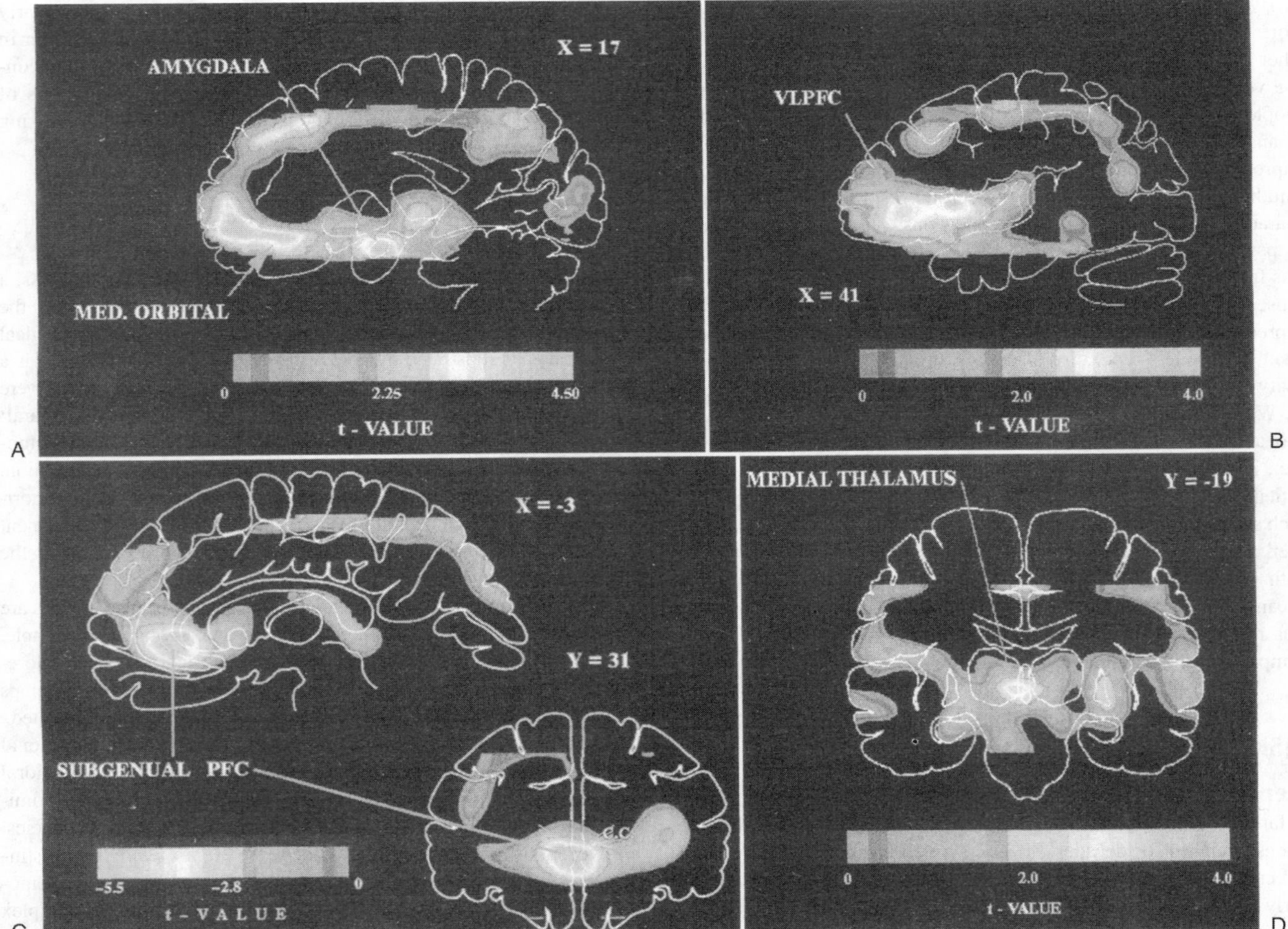

FIGURE 13.4–1 Composite coronal and sagittal sections of positron emission tomography scans show areas in which cerebral glucose metabolism is decreased in depressed patients relative to matched healthy controls. PFC, prefrontal cortex; VLPFC, ventrolateral prefrontal cortex. (See Color Plate.) (From Wayne Drevets, M.D.; and from *Annu Rev Med* 2002;49 by Annual Reviews, http://www.annualreviews.org, with permission.)

The anterior cingulate cortex (ACC) is thought to serve as the point of integration of attentional and emotional inputs. Two subdivisions have been identified: an affective subdivision in the rostral and ventral regions of the ACC and a cognitive subdivision involving the dorsal ACC. The former subdivision shares extensive connections with other limbic regions, and the latter interacts more with the PFC and other cortical regions. It is proposed that activation of the ACC facilitates effortful control of emotional arousal, particularly when goal attainment has been thwarted or when novel problems have been encountered.

The hippocampus is most clearly involved in various forms of learning and memory, including fear conditioning, as well as inhibitory regulation of the hypothalamic-pituitary-adrenal (HPA) axis activity. Emotional or contextual learning appears to involve a direct connection between the hippocampus and the amygdala.

The amygdala appears to be a crucial way station for processing novel stimuli of emotional significance and coordinating or organizing cortical responses. Located just above the hippocampi bilaterally, the amygdala has long been viewed as the heart of the limbic system. Although most research has focused on the role of the amygdala in responding to fearful or painful stimuli, it may be ambiguity or novelty, rather than the aversive nature of the stimulus per se, that brings the amygdala on line.

STRESS AND ANIMAL MODELS OF DEPRESSION

Studies of rodents, dogs, cats, and nonhuman primates have demonstrated that acute stress responses involve activation of central and peripheral components of two interactive psychoneuroendocrine systems, the cortical HPA axis and the sympathomedullary (SM) axis. Acute responses to stress are phenomenologically and neurobiologically more akin to fear and anxiety than depression. However, whereas stress initially signals threat, it is loss, the anticipation of loss, and the loss of hope that provoke sadness and despair.

Acute stress activates cell bodies of norepinephrine (NE) neurons in the locus ceruleus, whose ascending axons signal noradrenergically mediated increases in cortical arousal and whose descending axons signal increased adrenergic (predominantly epinephrine) output by the sympathetic nervous system and adrenal medulla. Behaviorally, the perception of acute stress elicits perceptual vigilance, preparedness for response, and inhibition of consummatory activities, such as foraging and pursuit of sexual activity.

Stress simultaneously triggers and releases corticotropin-releasing hormone (CRH) from neurons in the hypothalamus and cerebral cortex. CRH not only activates synthesis and release of adrenocorticotrophic hormone (ACTH) from the anterior pituitary, which, in turn, triggers release of cortisol and other glucocorticoids (from the adrenal cortex), but also synergistically increases locus ceruleus activity and, directly or indirectly, increases synthesis of other stress-reactive gene products and antiinflammatory responses. The acute response to stress is counterbalanced by homeostatic or adaptive mechanisms. These include feedback inhibition by glucocorticoid receptors in the hippocampus and pituitary, downregulation of postsynaptic noradrenergic receptors, and inhibitory auto- and heteroreceptors on presynaptic NE neurons. As is discussed subsequently, parallel input from serotoninergic, γ-aminobutyric acid (GABA), and glycinergic neurons exert dampening or inhibitory effects.

Exposure to prolonged, inescapable stress is associated with numerous adaptations in neurobehavioral responses. Although CRH levels in the brain and corticosteroid levels in the periphery may remain elevated, levels of NE, serotonin (5-HT), dopamine (DA), and GABA in the brainstem and forebrain eventually decrease. Animals trapped in such a state cease trying to resist or to escape and show decreased grooming and appetitive behavior. The behavior persists outside of the experimental situation. There are significant individual differences in the development of such learned helplessness, as well as differences across pedigrees, strains, and species. Conversely, antidepressant drugs have been shown to prevent, to attenuate, or to reverse learned helplessness across species.

Studies of the experiences of primates in the wild, of course, are more relevant to the stresses faced by people than a rat's response to inescapable, painful, electric shock. These naturalistic studies demonstrate not only that central 5-HT activity is partly under genetic control, but also that a fall from a dominant role within a primate social hierarchy results in decreased 5-HT neurotransmission and increased HPA. In the wild, animals with low levels of the serotoninergic metabolite 5-hydroxyindoleacetic acid (5-HIAA) are likely to be more aggressive, more socially subordinate, and less sexually active. When social status is manipulated by creating a new troupe from a cohort of subordinate primates, a new dominance hierarchy emerges, and the more dominant animals experience a corresponding increase in 5-HT function. Conversely, during times of adversity, such as drought or famine, it is the socially dominant primates that experience the largest increases in HPA activity.

Maltreatment and Early Adversity

Physical, verbal, and sexual abuse have an indelible effect on one's life trajectory. Although maltreatment has been well documented in the pathogenesis of posttraumatic stress disorder (PTSD) and borderline personality disorder for decades, it has only recently been shown that such a history results in a two- to threefold increase in risk of depression and is associated with important phenomenological and biological differences in depressive states.

Studies of animal models confirm that lasting alterations in neuroendocrine and behavioral responses can result from severe early stress. Animal studies further indicate that even transient periods of maternal deprivation can alter subsequent responses to stress. This vulnerability has been shown to be the result of enduring changes in gene expression. For example, activity of the gene coding for the neurokinin *brain-derived neurotrophic growth factor* (BDNF) is decreased after chronic stress, as is the process of neurogenesis. Protracted stress thus can induce changes in the functional status of neurons and, eventually, cell death. Recent studies in depressed humans indicate that a history of early trauma is associated with increased HPA activity accompanied by structural changes (i.e., atrophy or decreased volume) in the cerebral cortex.

MONOAMINE SYSTEMS: FUNCTION AND DYSFUNCTION

An area of scientific inquiry is chosen, in part, because of the knowledge base and experimental paradigms available to investigators. In the early 1960s, Nobel prize–winning research had just elucidated the importance of monoamines in neurotransmission. Moreover, it was possible to measure the metabolites of the catecholamine NE in various body fluids and 5-HIAA, the principal metabolite of 5-HT, in cerebrospinal fluid (CSF). Visualization of the functional brain, by contrast, was essentially limited by the low sensitivity of recording neuronal activity from the surface electrodes used for electroencephalograms (EEGs). Thus, although the paroxysmal spikes in electrical activity caused by epileptogenic foci or the diffuse slowing associated with delirium could be documented, the more subtle changes in brain activity or metabolism associated with affective states could not.

In addition, there were multiple lines of evidence from pharmacological studies implicating perturbations of monoamine systems in the therapeutic and iatrogenic effects of various medications. The relevant pharmacotherapies of the time, the TCAs and MAOIs, were known to increase the amount of neurotransmitter available at monoamine synapses. The amine-depleting compound reserpine (Serpalan) was known to cause depression as a side effect. Intoxication with potent noradrenergic agonists, such as amphetamine and cocaine, also was known to induce states of sleepless euphoria and activated psychosis, followed by a crashing, depression-like withdrawal.

The early monoamine hypotheses formulated by Joseph J. Schildkraut, Alexander H. Glassman, Arthur J. Prange, Jr., John Davis, Herman van Praag, Jonathan Cole, and others have undergone much revision, and it is now known that these ancient neuromodulatory systems comprise only a small fraction of the brain's neurons. Nevertheless, the critical importance of NE and 5-HT neurotransmission in the pathophysiology and treatment of mood disorders remains unquestioned. A third important monoamine, the catecholamine DA, was thought to play a greater role in the pathophysiology and treatment of schizophrenia and thus received less emphasis. Nevertheless, over time, evidence of DA dysfunction in at least some forms of depression has emerged. Knowledge about postsynaptic receptor families, presynaptic auto- and heteroreceptors, second messengers, neurokinins, and gene transcription factors has added layers of complexity to the original monoamine hypotheses. Even more so, since the mid-1960s, there has been a progressive shift away from focusing on disturbances of single neurotransmitter systems in favor of studying neurobehavioral systems, neural circuits, and more intricate neuroregulatory mechanisms. The monoaminergic systems are thus now viewed primarily as broader, neuromodulatory systems, and disturbances are as likely to be secondary or epiphenomenal effects as they are directly or causally related to etiology and pathogenesis.

Noradrenergic Systems The cell bodies of almost all noradrenergic neurons in the brain are located in the locus ceruleus of the brainstem and project rostrally to the hypothalamus, basal ganglia, limbic system, and cerebral cortex. This diffuse distribution belies NE's role in initiating and maintaining limbic and cortical arousal, as well as modulation of other neuronal systems. Noradrenergic projections to the amygdala and hippocampus are implicated in emotional memory and behavioral sensitization to stress, and prolonged activation of the locus ceruleus contributes to the state of learned helplessness. The medial forebrain bundle (MFB) is the key ascending NE pathway to anterior cortical structures. Stimulation of the MFB elicits increased levels of goal-directed and reward-seeking behavior. Sustained stress eventually results in decreased MFB neurotransmission, which may account for anergia, anhedonia, and diminished libido in depression. The locus ceruleus also is the origin of neurons that project rostrally to interact with the cell bodies of the sympathetic nervous system and, hence, the adrenal medulla. The locus ceruleus is phasically active. Increased activity is provoked by perception of novel stimuli; decreased activity accompanies eating and sleeping. As noted previously, there is an additive interaction (i.e., positive feedback loop) between noradrenergic neurons in the locus ceruleus and CRH from the hypothalamus, as well as cortical regions. Other negative feedback loops must exert inhibitory control over this alerting synergism to prevent sustained pathological activation. For example, increased noradrenergic output stimulates α_2 heteroreceptors on colocalized inhibitory 5-HT neurons, and a sustained increase in CRH drives results in decreased hypothalamic release of ACTH, which blunts HPA activity. Changes in cognitive processing of sensory input can further dampen corticolimbic and sympathoadrenal responses to sustained threatening or painful stimuli.

Serotoninergic Systems Serotoninergic neurons project from the brainstem dorsal raphe nuclei to the cerebral cortex, hypothalamus, thalamus, basal ganglia, septum, and hippocampus. 5-HT pathways have inhibitory and facilitatory functions in the brain. For example, much evidence suggests that 5-HT is an important regulator of sleep, appetite, body temperature, metabolism, and libido. Moreover, 5-HT inhibits aggressive behavior across mammalian and reptilian species. Serotoninergic neurons projecting to the suprachiasmatic nucleus (SCN) of the hypothalamus help regulate circadian rhythms (e.g., sleep–wake cycles, body temperature, and HPA axis function). 5-HT also permits or facilitates goal-directed motor and consummatory behaviors in conjunction with NE and DA.

As noted previously, there is some evidence that 5-HT neurotransmission is partly under genetic control. Nevertheless, 5-HT tone shows a seasonal fluctuation, and, whereas acute stress increases 5-HT release transiently, chronic stress eventually causes decreased 5-HT activity and depletion of 5-HT stores. Chronic stress may also increase synthesis of 5-HT type 1A (5-HT_{1A}) autoreceptors in the dorsal raphe nucleus, which further decrease 5-HT transmission. Elevated glucocorticoid levels tend to enhance 5-HT functioning and thus may have significant compensatory effects in chronic stress.

Dopaminergic Systems There are four relatively discrete DA pathways in the brain. The tuberoinfundibular system projects from cell bodies in the hypothalamus to the pituitary stalk, exerting inhibitory control over prolactin secretion. The nigrostriatal system originates from cell bodies in the substantia nigra and projects to the basal ganglia, regulating involuntary motor activity. The cell bodies of the mesolimbic pathway are located in the ventral tegmentum and project diffusely to the nucleus accumbens, amygdala, hippocampus, medial dorsal nucleus of the thalamus, and cingulate gyrus. This pathway modulates emotional expression, learning and reinforcement, and hedonic capacity. The fourth DA pathway, also originating in the ventral tegmentum, is the mesocortical pathway, which projects to the orbitofrontal and the prefrontal cortical regions. The mesocortical pathway helps regulate motivation, concentration, and initiation of goal-directed and complex executive cognitive tasks. Decreased mesocortical and mesolimbic DA activity has obvious implications in the cognitive, motor, and hedonic disturbances associated with depression. Across pathways, increased DA activity is potentiated by nicotinic inputs and glucocorticoids, and DA levels are inversely correlated with indices of brain 5-HT activity.

Summary of Research on Monoamines in Depression After nearly 30 years of research, it can be concluded that subsets of depressed people manifest one or more abnormalities of monoamine neurotransmission. Decreased central NE activity can be inferred, in part, from decreased urinary excretion of the metabolite 3-methoxy-4-hydroxyphenylglycol (MHPG). However, a partly overlapping subgroup of patients manifests elevated circulating levels of NE and its metabolites. This suggests a dissociation of NE activity in the MFB and SM systems. Functionally increased noradrenergic activity is also reflected by blunted α_1, β, and β-coupled second messenger (i.e., cyclic adenosine monophosphate [cAMP]) responses.

Chronic treatment with NE reuptake inhibitors (NRIs) (the antidepressants desipramine [Norpramin], nortriptyline [Aventyl], maprotiline [Ludiomil], bupropion [Wellbutrin], and reboxetine) causes a time-dependent decrease in firing of NE neurons and down-regulation of postsynaptic β receptors. The antidepressant effects of NRIs are reversed by transiently decreasing the availability of NE in the brain by administration of the NE synthesis inhibitor α-methyl-p-tyrosine (AMPT).

5-HT dysfunction has been documented in overlapping subgroups of patients using a variety of methods, ranging from low CSF levels of 5-HIAA to decreased regional cerebral metabolism in response to a 5-HT agonist, such as D-fenfluramine. 5-HT dysfunction also is reflected by blunted responses to specific (e.g., the specific 5-HT_{1A} compound ipsapirone) and nonselective (e.g., L-tryptophan or D-fenfluramine) agonists, decreased neuroendocrine responses, and decreased 5-HT uptake sites on blood platelets. As discussed subsequently, decreased 5-HT neurotransmission also can be inferred from the findings of HPA and EEG sleep studies. Dietary depletion of L-tryptophan induces 5-HT mediated abnormalities in a subset of vulnerable individuals. Likewise, L-tryptophan depletion reverses responses to MAOIs and selective serotonin reuptake inhibitors (SSRIs).

Low levels of the DA metabolite homovanillic acid have been implicated in psychomotor retardation. Some evidence suggests that increased DA activity, perhaps mediated by elevated glucocorticoid levels or lower levels of the enzyme DA β-hydroxylate, may contribute to development of delusions and hallucinations.

Other Neurotransmitter Disturbances

Acetylcholine (ACh) is found in neurons that are distributed diffusely throughout the cerebral cortex. Cholinergic neurons have reciprocal or interactive relationships with all three monoamine systems. Abnormal levels of choline, which is a precursor to ACh, have been found at autopsy in the brains of some depressed patients, perhaps reflecting abnormalities in cell phospholipid composition. Cholinergic agonist and antagonist drugs have differential clinical effects on depression and mania. Agonists can produce lethargy, anergia, and psychomotor retardation in normal subjects, can exacerbate symptoms in depression, and can reduce symptoms in mania. These effects generally are not sufficiently robust to have clinical applications, and adverse effects are problematic. Antidepressants, via their serotonergic or adrenergic effects, may decrease cholinergic function, although direct anticholinergic effects are unrelated to antidepressant activity.

In an animal model of depression, strains of mice that are super- or subsensitive to cholinergic agonists have been found to be prone to or more resistant to developing learned helplessness. Cholinergic agonists can induce changes in HPA activity and sleep that mimic those associated with severe depression. Indeed, some remitted patients with mood disorders, as well as their never-ill first-degree relatives, have a trait-like increase in sensitivity to cholinergic agonists. Cholinergic supersensitivity is attenuated by manipulations that increase noradrenergic activity and is intensified by interventions that reduce inhibitory 5-HT input. GABA has an inhibitory effect on ascending monoamine pathways, particularly the mesocortical and mesolimbic systems. Reductions of GABA have been observed in plasma, CSF, and brain GABA levels in depression. Animal studies have also found that chronic stress can reduce and eventually can deplete GABA levels. By contrast, GABA receptors are upregulated by antidepressants, and some GABAergic medications have weak antidepressant effects.

The amino acids glutamate and glycine are the major excitatory and inhibitory neurotransmitters in the CNS. Glutamate and glycine bind to sites associated with the *N*-methyl-D-aspartate (NMDA) receptor, and an excess of glutamatergic stimulation can cause neurotoxic effects. Importantly, there is a high concentration of NMDA receptors in the hippocampus. Glutamate may thus work in conjunction with hypercortisolemia to mediate the deleterious neurocognitive effects of severe recurrent depression. There is emerging evidence that drugs that antagonize NMDA receptors have antidepressant effects.

SECOND MESSENGERS AND INTRACELLULAR CASCADES

The binding of a neurotransmitter and a postsynaptic receptor triggers a cascade of membrane-bound and intracellular processes mediated by second messenger systems. Receptors on cell membranes interact with the intracellular environment via guanine nucleotide-binding proteins (G proteins). The G proteins, in turn, connect to various intracellular enzymes (e.g., adenylate cyclase, phospholipase C, and phosphodiesterase) that regulate utilization of energy and formation of second messengers, such as cyclic nucleotide (e.g., cAMP and cyclic guanosine monophosphate [cGMP]), as well as phosphatidylinositols (e.g., inositol triphosphate and diacylglycerol) and calcium-calmodulin.

Second messengers regulate the function of neuronal membrane ion channels, neurotransmitter synthesis and release, and protein kinase activity. Protein kinase, for example, catalyzes phosphorylation, an energy-liberating process involved in the synthesis and degradation of neuroreceptors, ion channels, G proteins, and gene transcription and translation factors. Some studies have reported abnormalities in platelet adenylate cyclase activity, phosphoinositide hydrolysis, intracellular calcium metabolism, and G-protein function in depressive disorders. Moreover, antidepressants may initiate a series of intracellular reactions that turn down synthesis of CRH and monoamine receptors and turn on peptides, such as BDNF. There is also increasing evidence that mood stabilizing drugs act on G proteins or other second messengers.

Alterations of Hormonal Regulation

HPA Activity As noted previously, elevated HPA activity is a hallmark of mammalian stress responses and one of the clearest links between depression and the biology of chronic stress. Hypercortisolemia in depression suggests one or more of the following central disturbances: decreased inhibitory 5-HT tone; increased drive from NE, ACh, or CRH; or decreased feedback inhibition from the hippocampus.

Evidence of increased HPA activity is apparent in 20 to 40 percent of depressed outpatients and 40 to 60 percent of depressed inpatients. Older patients, particularly those with highly recurrent or psychotic depressive disorders, are the most likely to manifest increased HPA activity. Although hypercortisolism is one of the best-replicated biological correlates of melancholia or endogenous depression, it is hardly a specific abnormality. For example, a short period of starvation or several weeks of partial sleep deprivation can induce hypercortisolism in otherwise healthy people.

Elevated HPA activity in depression has been documented via excretion of urinary free cortisol (UFC), 24-hour (or shorter time segments) intravenous (IV) collections of plasma cortisol levels, salivary cortisol levels, and tests of the integrity of feedback inhibition. A disturbance of feedback inhibition is tested by administration of dexamethasone (Decadron) (0.5 to 2.0 mg), a potent synthetic glucocorticoid, which normally suppresses HPA axis activity for 24 hours. Nonsuppression of cortisol secretion at 8:00 AM the following morning or subsequent escape from suppression at 4:00 PM or 11:00 PM is indicative of impaired feedback inhibition. Hypersecretion of cortisol and dexamethasone nonsuppression are imperfectly correlated (approximately 60 percent concordance). A more recent development to improve the sensitivity of the test involves infusion of a test dose of CRH after dexamethasone suppression.

Neither the sensitivity nor the specificity of these tests of feedback inhibition is sufficient for use as a diagnostic test, and adrenocortical hyperactivity (albeit usually less prevalent) is observed in mania, schizophrenia, dementia, and other psychiatric disorders. Nonsuppression may implicate a loss of inhibitory hippocampal glucocorticoid receptors more so than increased CRH drive, which also may account for the strong age dependence of cortisol nonsuppression. As noted previously, dexamethasone nonsuppression in adulthood is also associated with a history of early trauma, which may result from a permanent reduction in synthesis of glucocorticoid receptors or premature death of these developmentally vulnerable hippocampal neurons.

Elevated HPA activity in depression is typically not associated with the physical stigmata of Cushing's syndrome but is sufficient to be implicated in the genesis of neurocognitive and neuroimmunological disturbances. Patients with increased HPA activity are typically less responsive to attention placebo interventions and psychotherapy. Hypercortisolemic depressed patients thus may have a relatively greater need for active pharmacotherapy or ECT. Hypercortisolism does, however, usually resolve with effective treatment. When persistent despite effective treatment, increased HPA activity is associated with a high risk of relapse. This is presumably a consequence of incomplete resolution of the pathophysiology of the depressive episode. One implication of these relationships is that interventions that suppress HPA activity, including dexamethasone and the cortisol synthesis inhibitor ketoconazole (Nizoral), are sometimes used to treat patients with more refractory depressive disorders. Drugs that directly antagonize central CRH receptors are being developed as possible antidepressants.

Thyroid Axis Activity Approximately 5 to 10 percent of people evaluated for depression have previously undetected thyroid dysfunction, as reflected by an elevated basal thyroid-stimulating hormone (TSH) level or an increased TSH response to a 500-mg infusion of the hypothalamic neuropeptide thyroid-releasing hormone (TRH). Such abnormalities are often associated with elevated antithyroid antibody levels and, unless corrected with hormone replacement therapy, may compromise response to treatment.

An even larger subgroup of depressed patients (e.g., 20 to 30 percent) shows a blunted TSH response to TRH challenge. This type of response would usually suggest hyperthyroidism, yet few depressed patients have clinically significant elevations of thyroid hormones. A blunted TSH response in a euthyroid person thus may result from pituitary downregulation consequent to increased TRH drive. As neurons containing TRH have been identified in a variety of cortical regions, this abnormality may have a suprahypothalamic origin. Increased central TRH secretion, in turn, could result from a homeostatic response to decreased noradrenergic neurotransmission. Joffe and colleagues further speculate that the therapeutic benefit of 1-triiodothyronine (T_3) augmentation therapy is mediated by a dampening of this failed homeostatic response. To date, the major therapeutic implication of a blunted TSH response is evidence of an increased risk of relapse despite preventive antidepressant therapy. Of note, unlike the dexamethasone suppression test (DST), blunted TSH response to TRH does not usually normalize with effective treatment.

Growth Hormone Growth hormone (GH) is secreted from the anterior pituitary after stimulation by NE and DA. Secretion is inhibited by somatostatin, a hypothalamic neuropeptide, and CRH. Pulsatile GH secretion follows a 24-hour circadian rhythm, with a characteristic secretory surge during the first few hours of sleep. The most consistent finding in depression is a blunted GH response to clonidine, an α_2-receptor agonist. Secretory responses after the onset of sleep or the administration of nonselective adrenergic agonists, such as desipramine, are also blunted in depression.

Although the hypothalamus has the highest concentrations of somatostatin, significant concentrations are also found in the amygdala, hippocampus, nucleus accumbens, PFC, and locus ceruleus. In addition to inhibition of GH release, somatostatin inhibits release or antagonizes the effects of CRH, GABA, and TSH. Decreased CSF somatostatin levels have been reported in depression, and increased levels have been observed in mania.

Prolactin Prolactin is released from the pituitary by 5-HT stimulation and inhibited by DA. Most studies have not found significant abnormalities of basal or circadian prolactin secretion in depression, although a blunted prolactin response to various 5-HT agonists has been described. This response is uncommon among premenopausal women, suggesting that estrogen has a moderating effect.

Alterations of Sleep Neurophysiology Sleep is regulated by complex, temporally and environmentally cued interactions between the monoamine neuromodulatory systems, neuroendocrine secretion, and neuropeptides. At the broadest levels, there is a seasonal or circannual tendency for longer and deeper sleep in winter and a circadian propensity for the onset of sleep (i.e., after dark and after midday). Onset of sleep is promoted by a surge in secretion of the pineal hormone melatonin (after the onset of darkness). Sleep onset is followed by the nocturnal surge in GH secretion, which occurs within the first 90 minutes of sleep onset. A reduction of core body temperature and diurnally low levels of cortisol secretion further promote the maintenance of sleep. Orchestrated across each 24-hour period is an oscillating, 90-minute, infraradian cycle defined by rapid eye movement (REM) sleep. Within each cycle, there is a characteristic progression from light to deeper levels of sleep (defined by different types of EEG activity), culminating in the paradoxical central activation of REM sleep, during which most of the night's dreaming occurs. An 8-hour night of sleep thus includes four or five nonrapid eye movement (NREM)–REM cycles. The propensity for deep sleep is greatest within the first 3 hours after sleep onset. REM sleep periods, by contrast, tend to become longer and more intense across the night.

Prefrontal cortical metabolism is normally decreased during NREM sleep, a time of physical and metabolic rest. The frontal cortex is essentially off line during deep sleep, and the predominate rhythm of brain activity consists of slow (delta) desynchronized waves of thalamocortical origin. REM sleep, by contrast, is characterized by fast, low-amplitude electrical activity and increased glucose metabolism in the limbic system. REMs are under the direct control of cholinergic neurons in the pons, which are tonically inhibited by the reticular activating system (predominately by histaminergic and noradrenergic neurotransmission) during wakefulness. During sleep, inhibitory 5-HT projections from the dorsal raphe nuclei phasically suppress REM. Pharmacological manipulations that increase central cholinergic activity lighten sleep and increase phasic REM activity. Dietary depletion of 5-HT and exogenous administration of glucocorticoids similarly can increase phasic REM indices. Injections of CRH and ingestion of potent noradrenergic agonists decrease total sleep time, reduce slow wave sleep, and suppress REM sleep.

Depression is associated with a premature loss of deep (slow wave) sleep and an increase in nocturnal arousal. The latter is reflected by four types of disturbance: (1) an increase in nocturnal awakenings, (2) a reduction in total sleep time, (3) increased phasic REM sleep, and (4) increased core body temperature. The combination of increased REM drive and decreased slow wave sleep results in a significant reduction in the first period of NREM sleep, a phenomenon referred to as *reduced REM latency*. Results of family and twin studies suggest that these related abnormalities are partly heritable. Consistent with the expected behavior of a heritable trait, reduced REM latency and deficits of slow wave sleep typically persist after recovery of a depressive episode. Blunted secretion of GH after sleep onset is associated with decreased slow wave sleep and shows similar state-independent or trait-like behavior. Difficulties maintaining sleep and increased phasic REM sleep are associated with hypercortisolism and increased limbic blood flow and glucose metabolism; although some forms of pharmacotherapy can distort sleep profiles, recovery from depression usually is accompanied by at least a partial reversal of these abnormalities. The combination of reduced REM latency, increased REM density, and decreased sleep maintenance identifies approximately 40 percent of depressed outpatients and 80 percent of depressed inpatients. False-negative studies are commonly seen in younger, hypersomnolent patients, who may actually experience an increase in slow wave sleep during episodes of depression. Approximately 10 percent of otherwise healthy individuals have abnormal sleep profiles, and, like dexamethasone nonsuppression, false-positive cases are not uncommonly seen in other psychiatric disorders.

Despite clear limitations as a diagnostic test, EEG sleep recordings continue to be an important research tool. For example, patients manifesting a characteristically abnormal sleep profile have been found to be less responsive to psychotherapy and to have a greater risk of relapse or recurrence and may benefit preferentially from pharmacotherapy. Most antidepressants suppress REM sleep, probably by directly or indirectly activating postsynaptic 5-HT_{1A} receptors. The efficacy of antidepressants that do not suppress REM sleep, such as nefazodone (Serzone) and bupropion, warrants further study, especially in patients with pathologically increased REM sleep. Antidepressant effects on sleep maintenance and slow wave sleep are more variable and appear to be mediated by antihistaminic effects and antagonism of 5-HT type 2 (5-HT_2) receptors.

STRUCTURAL AND FUNCTIONAL BRAIN IMAGING

Computed axial tomography and *magnetic resonance imaging* (MRI) scans have permitted sensitive, noninvasive methods to assess the living brain, including cortical and subcortical tracts, as well as white matter lesions. The most consistent abnormality observed in the depressive disorders is increased frequency of abnormal hyperintensities in subcortical regions such as periventricular regions, the basal ganglia, and the thalamus. More common in bipolar I disorder and among the elderly, these hyperintensities appear to reflect the deleterious neurodegenerative effects of recurrent affective episodes. Ventricular enlargement, cortical atrophy, and sulcal widening also have been reported in some studies. Some depressed patients also may have reduced hippocampal or caudate nucleus volumes, or both, suggesting more focal defects in relevant neurobehavioral systems. Diffuse and focal areas of atrophy have been associated with increased illness severity, bipolarity, and increased cortisol levels.

Positron emission tomography (PET) and functional MRI scanning are currently the most powerful methods for visualizing brain activity during rest and various states of activation. Normal sadness is associated with an increase in blood flow and neuronal activity in the thalamus and medial PFC. This appears to be a nonspecific change associated with diverse emotional responses. More specific activation is seen in the left amygdala, hippocampal formation, and parahippocampal gyrus. Sadness generated by one's own thoughts (as opposed to a video scenario) and anticipatory anxiety are associated with a relative increase in blood flow to the anterior insular cortex.

The most widely replicated PET finding in depression is decreased anterior brain metabolism, which is generally more pronounced on the left side. From a different vantage point, depression may be associated with a relative increase in nondominant hemispheric activity. These abnormalities have been observed in unipolar and bipolar depressions and appear to be somewhat state dependent. Furthermore, there is a reversal of hypofrontality after shifts from depression into hypomania, such that there are greater left hemisphere reductions in depression compared to greater right hemisphere reductions in mania. Other studies have observed more specific reductions of reduced cerebral blood flow or metabolism, or both, in the dopaminergically innervated tracts of the mesocortical and mesolimbic systems in depression. Again, there is evidence that antidepressants at least partially normalize these changes.

In addition to a global reduction of anterior cerebral metabolism, increased glucose metabolism has been observed in several limbic regions, particularly among patients with relatively severe recurrent depression and a family history of mood disorder (Fig. 13.4–2). During episodes of depression, increased glucose metabolism is correlated with intrusive ruminations. Increased paralimbic metabolism appears to be reversible with effective pharmacotherapy, but, in one study, the abnormality reemerged when recently remitted patients were restudied off medication. If truly state independent, paralimbic hypermetabolism could represent an emotional amplifier that helps distort the signal of relatively minor stressors in those at high risk for recurrent depression.

IMMUNOLOGICAL DISTURBANCE

Depressive disorders are associated with several immunological abnormalities, including decreased lymphocyte proliferation in response to mitogens and other forms of impaired cellular immunity. These lymphocytes produce neuromodulators, such as corticotropin-releasing factor (CRF), and cytokines, peptides known as *interleukins*. There appears to be an association with clinical severity, hypercortisolism, and immune dysfunction, and the cytokine interleukin-1 may induce gene activity for glucocorticoid synthesis.

SUMMARY

Major depressive disorder is associated with a myriad of neurobiological disturbances, perhaps as varied as the range of clinical presentations and treatments. When broadly viewed as *traits* (inherited or acquired) or *states* (abnormalities only apparent during episodes of illness), these disturbances begin to show some degree of coherence. State-dependent abnormalities, for example, tend to coaggregate in patients with more severe syndromes, classified as *endogenous depression* or *melancholia*. These more classical syndromes are more common in older individuals, particularly those with recurrent or psychotic depressions. The changes in brain function associated with severe depression include increased phasic REM sleep, poor sleep maintenance, hypercortisolism, impaired cellular immunity, reductions of anterior cerebral blood flow and glucose metabolism, and

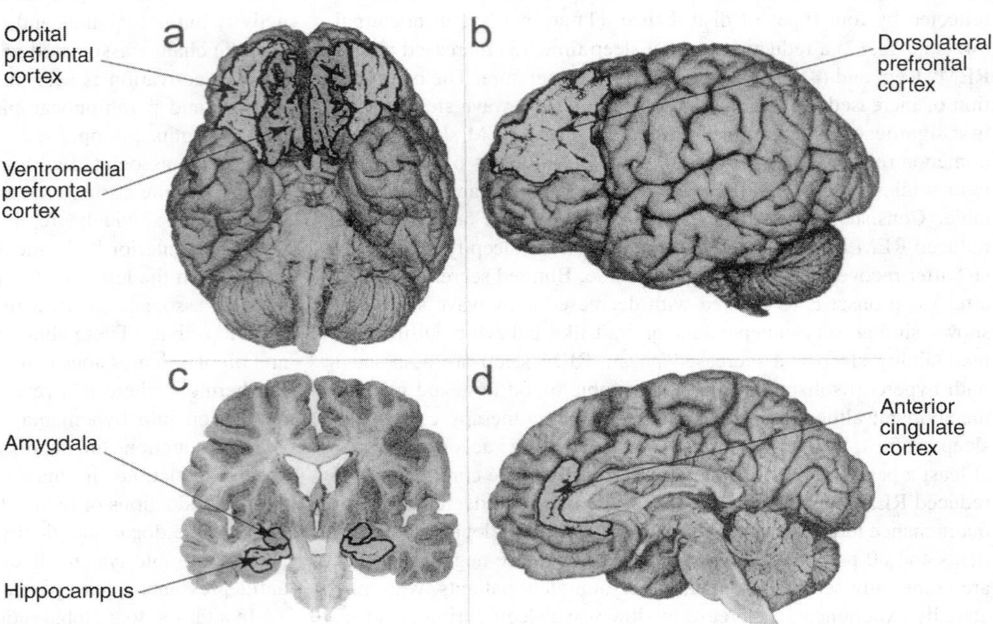

FIGURE 13.4–2 Key brain regions involved in affect and mood disorders. **a:** Orbital prefrontal cortex and the ventromedial prefrontal cortex. **b:** Dorsolateral prefrontal cortex. **c:** Hippocampus and amygdala. **d:** Anterior cingulated cortex. (See Color Plate.)

increased glucose metabolism in the amygdala. Such changes suggest, almost without exception, the consequences of an exaggerated and sustained stress response. Once manifest in this form, the depressive episode tends to be longer, more disabling, more prone to relapse, and more likely to benefit from pharmacotherapy or ECT (vis à vis non-specific or psychotherapeutic interventions).

Trait-like abnormalities include decreased slow wave sleep, reduced REM latency, and blunted nocturnal GH secretion. These abnormalities are associated with an early age of onset and increased vulnerability to recurrent illness. The heritability of these abnormalities, which at least partly reflects decreased 5-HT inhibition of exaggerated stress responses, is inferred from family studies and other at-risk paradigms.

Examples of more persistent, but acquired abnormalities may include global and focal changes, cortical atrophy, hypertrophy of the adrenal cortex, periventricular hyperintensities, and alterations in CRH synthesis. Blunted TSH response (to a TRH infusion) and dexamethasone nonsuppression may represent *hybrids*, in that these abnormalities can be slow to normalize and, when persistent after remission, convey a high risk of relapse.

Although specific genes have not yet been identified, there is no doubt that vulnerability to mood disorders is, for some, heritable. This type of heritability is most likely polygenetic and, in all likelihood, will be best understood through models that include gene–environment interactions. Nevertheless, increased heritability is associated with an earlier age of onset, greater comorbidity, increased risk of recurrent illness, and an increased likelihood of hypomanic or manic episodes. Is it ironic that two of the more heritable forms of mood disorder, early onset chronic depressions and bipolar depression, are relatively less likely to be associated with state-dependent neurobiological disturbances? Different genetic vulnerabilities, different clinical presentations, and age-dependent differences in the effects of depression on brain function depression are likely to explain this apparent paradox.

Aging and the accumulating consequences of recurrent depressive episodes are inextricably connected. However, the diseases of aging that ravage brain function definitely increase the risk of depression and decrease responsivity to conventional forms of treatment. The late-onset form of depression associated with cerebral atherosclerosis illustrates the subtle interplay between brain function and mood disorder.

Ultimately, depression remains a fundamentally human experience, partly because people can all relate to sadness, grief, and the heartbreak of lost love and partly because of the contrived nature of experiments that subject animals to prolonged, inescapable stress. Strong and sustaining affective bonds and an enduring sense of self-worth and competence are simply too important, and assaults on these fundamental aspects of well-being are too frequent for some humans to withstand without becoming depressed. That some are more vulnerable to depression than others is without question, as is the association of stress, depression, and numerous, reproducible changes in brain function. Understanding the mechanisms of successful and unsuccessful adaptation and elucidating the alterations in brain function that predispose to and maintain depressive disorders represent the best hope to prevent and to relieve the misery and suffering of tens of millions of people.

SUGGESTED CROSS-REFERENCES

Monoamine neurotransmitters are discussed in Section 1.4, and the contributions of the neural sciences in general are the focus of the other sections of Chapter 1. Biological therapies are covered in Chapter 31.

References

Barden N: Modulation of glucocorticoid receptor gene expression by antidepressant drugs. *Pharmacopsychiatry.* 1996;29:12.

Belanoff JK, Kalehzan M, Sund B, Fleming Ficek SK, Schatzberg AF: Cortisol activity and cognitive changes in psychotic major depression. *Am J Psychiatry.* 2001;158:1612.

Bremner JD, Innis RB, Salomon RM, Staib LH, Ng CK, Miller HL, Bronen RA, Krystal JH, Duncan J, Rich D, Price LH, Malison R, Dey H, Soufer R, Charney DS: Positron emission tomography measurement of cerebral metabolic correlates of tryptophan depletion-induced depressive relapse. *Arch Gen Psychiatry.* 1997;54:364.

Commons KG, Connolley KR, Valentino RJ: A neurochemically distinct dorsal raphe-limbic circuit with a potential role in affective disorders. *Neuropsychopharmacology.* 2003;28:206.

*Davidson RJ, Pizzagalli D, Nitschke JB. The representation and regulation of emotion in depression. Perspectives from affective neuroscience. In: Gotlib IH, Hammen CL, eds. *Handbook of Depression.* New York: Guilford Press; 2002.

Delgado PL, Charney DS, Price LH, Aghajanian GK, Landis H, Heninger GR: Serotonin function and the mechanism of antidepressant action reversal of antidepressant-induced remission by rapid depletion of plasma tryptophan. *Arch Gen Psychiatry.* 1990;47:411.

*Drevets WC: Functional neuroimaging studies of depression: The anatomy of melancholia. *Ann Rev Med.* 1998;49:341.

Duman RS, Heninger GR, Nestler EJ: A molecular and cellular theory of depression. *Arch Gen Psychiatry.* 1997;54:597.

Evans DL, Ten Have RT, Douglas SD, Gettes DR, Morrison M, Chiappini MS, Brinker-Spence P, Job C, Mercer DE, Wang YL, Cruess D, Dube B, Dalen EA, Brown T, Bauer R, Petitto JM: Association of depression with viral load, CD8 T lymphocytes, and natural killer cells in women with HIV infection. *Am J Psychiatry.* 2002;159:1752.

Farmer A, Mahmood A, Redman K, Harris T, Sadler S, McGuffin P: A sib-pair study of the temperament and character inventory scales in major depression. *Arch Gen Psychiatry.* 2003;60:490.

*Frodl T, Meisenzahl EM, Zetsche T, Born C, Groll C, Jäger M, Leinsinger G, Bottlender R, Hahn K, Müller H-J: Hippocampal changes in patients with a first episode of major depression. *Am J Psychiatry.* 2002;159:1113.

Frodl T, Meisenzahl EM, Zetzsche T, Born C, Jäger M, Groll C, Bottlender R, Leinsinger G, Müller H-J: Larger amygdala volumes in first depressive episode as compared to recurrent major depression and healthy control subjects. *Biol Psychiatry.* 2003;53:338.

Goetz RR, Wolk SI, Coplan JD, Ryan ND, Weissman MM: Premorbid polysomnographic signs in depressed adolescents: A reanalysis of EEG sleep after longitudinal follow-up in adulthood. *Biol Psychiatry.* 2001;49:930.

Goldapple K, Segal Z, Garson C, Lau M, Bieling P, Kennedy S, Mayberg H: Modulation of cortical-limbic pathways in major depression. *Arch Gen Psychiatry.* 2004;61:34.

Higley JD, Thompson WW, Champoux M, Goldman D, Hasert MF, Kraemer GW, Scanlan JM, Suomi S, Linnoila M: Paternal and maternal genetic and environmental contributions to cerebrospinal fluid monoamine metabolites in rhesus monkeys (*Macaca mulatta*). *Arch Gen Psychiatry.* 1993;50:615.

Holsboer F. Neuroendocrinology of mood disorders. In: Bloom FE, Kupfer DJ, eds. *Psychopharmacology: The Fourth Generation of Progress.* New York: Raven Press; 1995.

Johansson C, Willeit M, Smedh C, Ekholm J, Paunio T, Kieseppa T, Lichtermann D, Praschak-Rieder N, Neumeister A, Nilsson L-G, Kasper S, Peltonen L, Adolfsson R, Schalling M, Partonen T: Circadian clock-related polymorphisms in seasonal affective disorder in their relevance to diurnal preference. *Neuropsychopharmacology.* 2003;28:734.

Keck ME, Welt T, Müller MB, Uhr M, Ohl F, Wigger A, Toschi N, Holsboer F, Landgraf R: Reduction of hypothalamic vasopressinergic hyperdrive contributes to clinically relevant behavioral and neuroendocrine effects of chronic paroxetine treatment in a psychopathological rat model. *Neuropsychopharmacology.* 2003;28:235.

Kegeles LS, Malone KM, Slifstein M, Ellis SP, Xanthopoulos E, Keilp JG, Campbell C, Oquendo M, Van Heertum RL, Mann JJ: Response to cortical metabolic deficits to serotonergic challenge in familial mood disorders. *Am J Psychiatry.* 2003;160:76.

Kempermann G, Kronenberg G: Depressed new neurons: Adult hippocampal neurogenesis and a cellular plasticity hypothesis of major depression. *Biol Psychiatry.* 2003;54:499.

*Kendler KS, Gardner CO, Prescott CA: Toward a comprehensive development model for major depression in women. *Am J Psychiatry.* 2002;159:1133.

Künzel HE, Binder EB, Nickel T, Ising M, Fuchs B, Majer M, Pfennig A, Ernst G, Kern N, Schmid DA, Uhr M, Holsboer F, Modell S: Pharmacological and nonpharmacological factors influencing hypothalamic-pituitary-adrenocortical axis reactivity in acutely depressed psychiatric inpatients, measured by the Dex-CRH test. *Neuropsychopharmacol.* 2003;28:2169.

Lampe IK, Hulshoff HE, Janssen J, Schnack HG, Kahn RS, Heeren TJ: Association of depression duration with reduction of global cerebral gray matter volume in female patients with recurrent major depressive disorder. *Am J Psychiatry.* 2003;160:2052.

Liotti M, Mayberg HS, McGinnis S, Brannan SL, Jerabek P: Unmasking disease-specific cerebral blood flow abnormalities: Mood challenge in patients with remitted unipolar depression. *Am J Psychiatry.* 2002;159:1830.

Maes M, Meltzer HY. The serotonin hypothesis of major depression. In: Bloom FE, Kupfer DJ, eds. *Psychopharmacology: The Fourth Generation of Progress.* New York: Raven Press; 1995.

Nemeroff CB: New vistas in neuropeptide research in neuropsychiatry: Focus on corticotropin-releasing factor. *Neuropsychopharmacology.* 1992;6:69.

Newport DJ, Heim C, Owens MJ, Ritchie JC, Ramsey CH, Bonsall R, Miller AH, Nemeroff CB: Cerebrospinal fluid corticotropin-releasing factor (CRF) and vasopressin concentrations predict pituitary response in the CRF stimulation test: a multiple regression analysis. *Neuropsychopharmacology.* 2003;28:569.

Petty F: GABA and mood disorders: A brief review and hypothesis. *J Affect Disord.* 1995;34:275.

Phillips ML, Drevets WC, Rauch SL, Lane R: Neurobiology of emotion perception II: Implications for major psychiatric disorders. *Biol Psychiatry.* 2003;54:515.

Sanacora G, Mason GF, Rothman DL, Hyder F, Ciarcia JJ, Ostroff RB, Berman RM, Krystal JH: Increased cortical GABA concentrations in depressed patients receiving ECT. *Am J Psychiatry.* 2003;160:577.

Sapolsky RM: Glucocorticoids and hippocampal atrophy in neuropsychiatric disorders. *Arch Gen Psychiatry.* 1999;57:925.

Shelin YI, Gado MH, Kraemer HC: Untreated depression and hippocampal volume loss. *Am J Psychiatry.* 2003;160:1516.

Thase ME, Dubé S, Bowler K, Howland RH, Myers JE, Friedman E, Jarrett DB: Hypothalamic-pituitary-adrenocortical activity and response to cognitive behavior therapy in unmedicated, hospitalized depressed patients. *Am J Psychiatry.* 1996;153:886.

*Thase ME, Jindal R, Howland RH. Biological aspects of depression. In: Gotlib IH, Hammen CL, eds. *Handbook of Depression.* New York: Guilford Press; 2002.

Vythilingam M, Heim C, Newport J, Miller AH, Anderson E, Bronen R, Brummer M, Staib L, Vermetten E, Charney DS, Nemeroff CB, Bremner JD: Childhood trauma associated with smaller hippocampal volume in women with major depression. *Am J Psychiatry.* 2002;159:2072.

Williams RB, Marchuk DA, Gadde KM, Barefoot JC, Grichnik K, Helms MJ, Kuhn CM, Lewis JG, Schanberg SM, Stafford-Smith M, Suarez EC, Clary GL, Svenson IK, Siegler IC: Serotonin-related gene polymorphisms and central nervous system serotonin function. *Neuropsychopharmacology.* 2003;28:533.

▲ 13.5 Mood Disorders: Intrapsychic and Interpersonal Aspects

JOHN C. MARKOWITZ, M.D., AND BARBARA MILROD, M.D.

The criteria listed in the revised fourth edition of the *Diagnostic and Statistical Manual of Mental Disorders* (DSM-IV-TR) reliably define *mood disorders* but do not completely describe them or explain how patients experience them. Depressed patients suffer emotionally, cognitively, and physically. This chapter describes three key theoretical approaches that have been applied to mood disorders: psychoanalytic-psychodynamic, cognitive, and interpersonal. They vary in their frequency of use in clinical practice and in the amount of research they have received.

Theory has uses and limitations. Theory can help organize thinking about depression and can pinpoint aspects of the syndrome. A theory can provide a narrative thread or focus to anchor a clinical formulation and to give coherence to a therapy. A theoretical approach is indeed necessary for clinicians to impose order on the overwhelming amount of clinical data with which patients present for treatment. Theories may also allow the psychiatrist to make predictions about treatment mechanisms and outcomes. An organizing theoretical framework is as essential to structuring a psychotherapy as grammar is to speech. Hence, understanding the theoretical backgrounds of psychotherapies is crucial for the psychotherapeutic clinician.

Theories should be considered approximations of the truth, needful of testing and subject to disconfirmation. Dogma and ideology have done psychiatrists and other mental health professionals more harm than good, for example, in separating psychotherapy and pharmacotherapy into opposing camps—a rift from the 1950s that is only now being healed. In as much as the etiology of mood disorders is complex and remains unknown, and no theory can comprehensively explain it, rigid adherence to any theory is likely to lead to clinical problems. The best clinicians may be those who can understand and use multiple theories but can flexibly decide on the optimal theoretical perspective to apply to a given patient's illness and then persevere in using that model for an appropriate course of treatment.

Psychodynamic theory has the longest historical tradition. Cognitive theory and psychodynamic theory largely focus on intrapsychic phenomena, whereas interpersonal theory, the newest and least formally developed, focuses more on interpersonal, extrapsychic reality. Aspects of cognitive and interpersonal theories derive from psychoanalysis. Each approach provides a potentially useful explanation of the plight of the depressed patient. Although the usefulness of therapies derived from cognitive theory (cognitive-behavioral therapy [CBT]) and interpersonal theory (interpersonal psychotherapy [IPT]) have been better tested for depression than has psychodynamic therapy to date, no theory of depression has been formally empirically tested.

PSYCHODYNAMIC ASPECTS OF MOOD DISORDERS

A contemporary psychoanalytic understanding of mood disorders includes a comprehensive focus on biological underpinnings, cognitive function, and interpersonal situation and style. What is unique to psychoanalysis is its attention to intrapsychic, unconscious pressures in its consideration of psychological symptoms, including mood disorders. This chapter focuses largely on psychoanalytic theories of depression, although it should be noted that exciting, early-outcome research in psychodynamic treatment of depression is currently under way. To present a description of intrapsychic aspects to mood disorders, several basic psychoanalytic ideas about mental life must be defined:

1. From a psychodynamic view, mental life exists on two levels: within the realm of consciousness and also within a less accessible realm, described as *the unconscious*. Psychic or emotional symptoms arise from aspects of mental life that are at least in part unconscious. This is true of mood disorders.

2. Psychoanalysts have found it useful to conceptualize the mind as comprising three basic theoretical psychic structures: *the id, the ego,* and *the superego*. In brief, *the id* is the aspect of the mind that subsumes the drive derivatives and desires. *The ego* serves as an intermediary between the id and the external world. It contains many intrapsychic functions, including motor action, perception, self-esteem, the relationship to reality, and the ability to modulate the drives and anxiety. Defense mechanisms, which are unconscious mechanisms used to modulate the drives and anxiety, are ego functions. *The superego* comprises the person's value system. The superego can punish and reward the person, depending on whether or not his or her actions are consonant with his or her moral values.

3. *Moods are pervasive ego states* that color the entire ego with the same affect state. Unlike simple affective responses to events, they are not focused, but general, because the affect is too strong or because the ego is too weak to contain a focused response. Because moods are generalized states, they always involve some degree of denial of the opposite feelings. From a psychoanalytic vantage, moods always carry an unconscious significance, notwithstanding their well-documented biological and neurotransmitter underpinnings.

4. Since Sigmund Freud's discovery of the importance of the unconscious in everyday mental life and of individuals' capacity to shut off unwanted, painful, emotionally laden experiences using defense mechanisms, the understanding of moods and symptoms has been enhanced by the recognition that these psychic phenomena represent a breakthrough of *unconscious fantasy* into consciousness. Persistent unconscious fantasies often underlie people's psychological symptoms, dreams, personalities, and important life choices.

5. Freud initially described another central principle in the organization of mental life: that *people unconsciously avoid unpleasure* and that ideas that produce unpleasure are screened from consciousness by *repression* or processes that are now called *defenses*. Clinically, the degree to which *unpleasure* is avoided varies from patient to patient, and Freud later modified his original theory about people avoiding unpleasure. In *Beyond the Pleasure Principle*, he attempted to describe intrapsychic mechanisms that could account for phenomena in which the pursuit of pleasure is given up for the more fundamental need to discharge intense emotional tensions to protect the individual. Major depression is a condition in which the person is living beyond the pleasure principle.

PSYCHOANALYTIC DESCRIPTIONS OF MAJOR DEPRESSION

Psychoanalytic formulations highlight the phenomenology of aspects of major depression, helping make the emotional backdrop of the illness more understandable. Although these theories provide a clinically rich set of ideas that can be useful in the treatment of such patients, it should be emphasized that no theoretical positions are supported by systematic research. The field of psychoanalysis has been fairly resistant to research. These psychoanalytic formulations, despite their differences, are not mutually exclusive. This chapter outlines some of these formulations and provides illustrative clinical examples.

Response to Loss and Anger Turned Inward The classic psychoanalytic understandings of depression were stated by Karl Abraham, Freud, and Sandor Rado and emphasized depressives' reactions to object loss, in reality or in fantasy. In these formulations, the profound response to loss occurs in part because the current loss invokes an earlier, childhood loss, also of a fantastical or realistic nature. These authors noted depressives' ambivalent or hostile object relations, along with object attachments characterized by excessive dependency, laced with an emphasis on need gratification in emotionally charged relationships. Major depression occurs only after the tie to the object is shattered. In *Mourning and Melancholia*, Freud highlighted the way in which depressed patients irrationally attack themselves. In his formulation, this occurs because aspects of an ambivalent object become internalized or incorporated into the patient's sense of self, and hostility directed toward the object is instead directed at the self. This state of affairs serves to preserve the relationship with the other person (the object) in reality.

Solomon Asch described a variation on these dynamics in which some patients become depressed not because of object loss, but because of the maintenance of a submissive tie to the object. This tie is maintained because the patient perceives separation to be an aggressive act with destructive consequences. Rage at having to play this part is directed toward the self, as the patient feels devalued because of the submission.

Joseph Sandler and Walter G. Joffe, also focusing on the phenomenon of loss leading to depression, culled the Hampstead Index, a comprehensive clinical registry of childhood responses to abandonment and loss, for cases of childhood depression. They inferred that depression is a basic affective response to loss. They emphasized that more than just the other person is lost and that the child feels he or she has also lost a sense of self in relationship to the lost object or a previous set of feelings about the self. Thus, as Freud and Abraham also noted, they emphasize a symbiotic or narcissistic tie to the object. They saw future depressives as struggling against feelings of helplessness and injured self-esteem in childhood.

Ms. A., a 26-year-old woman, presented with severe major depression in the context of her boyfriend Mr. B.'s expressing increasing anger at her and his saying that he wanted to move out of their home. Ms. A., an anxious person at baseline, took to her bed for several weeks, closing the blinds so that no light could enter her room. She stopped eating, lost weight, and slept most of the time. She dropped out of school and took a leave of absence from work. She thought almost constantly of suicide, although she had not picked a method, and her deep commitment to her religion made this an unacceptable choice. In her first session, she spoke about how worthless she felt, and how she blamed herself for her boyfriend wanting to break up with her. She said that she thought she was too "pointless," "anxious," and "boring" for him and that her presence stifled him. She expressed no anger toward Mr. B. at the time of her presentation, saying that she "understood" why he was being like this. She also said she hoped that this was just a "bad phase" that he would get over, although he told her repeatedly that he was dating another woman. In psychotherapy, it gradually emerged, however, that, over the past month, Mr. B. had been breaking dishes and furniture at their home. He yelled at Ms. A. almost constantly. This patient's depression remitted with psychodynamic psychotherapy only as she became aware of her own murderous rage toward Mr. B., at which time she began to view herself in a less negative and denigrated manner.

Guilt Melanie Klein postulated that depressed patients fear that they cannot protect an idealized or good internalized "other" from destructive impulses that are full of rage. Although emphasizing a different facet of major depression, this view coincides with Freud's focus on the destruction of the object tie in major depression. As a result, the depressive's characteristic guilt, inhibitions, and punitive superego develop. However, not all depressions are characterized by excessive guilt, and Klein's description applies only to this subset of patients. Klein also highlighted the danger that depressives foresee in triumphing over parents or siblings via any life success: Success is experienced as aggressively humiliating to loved ones or as damaging to others. Klein noted that idealization and devaluation are manic defenses against the guilt and sense of loss experienced in the resulting depression.

Ms. C., a 23-year-old woman, became acutely depressed when she was accepted to a prestigious graduate school. Ms. C. had been working diligently toward this acceptance for the past 4 years. She reported being "briefly happy, for about 20 minutes" when she learned the good news but rapidly slipped into a hopeless state in which she recurrently thought of the pointlessness of her aspirations, cried constantly, and had to physically stop herself from taking a lethal overdose of her roommate's insulin. In treatment, she focused on her older brother, who had regularly insulted her throughout the course of her life, and how "he's not doing well." She found herself worried about him. She mentioned that she was not used to being the "successful" one of the two of them. In connection with her depression, it emerged that Ms. C.'s brother had had a severe, life-threatening, disfiguring pediatric illness, requiring much family time and attention throughout their childhood. Ms. C. had become "used to" his insulting manner toward her. In fact, it seemed that she required her brother's abuse of her not to feel overwhelmed by survivor guilt about being the "healthy, normal" child. "He might insult me, but I look up to him. I adore him. Any attention he pays to me is like a drug," she said. Ms. C.'s acceptance to graduate school had challenged her defensive and essential compensatory image of herself as being less successful, or damaged, in comparison to her brother, thereby overwhelming her with guilt. Her depression remitted in psychodynamic psychotherapy as she better understood her identification and fantasy submission to her brother.

Impairment in Self-Esteem Regulation A general trait of patients with major depression is the loss of self-regard. Yet, loss of self-regard can occur in the absence of depression. Edward Bibring disagreed with Klein's formulation that emphasized the importance of a punitive superego and argued that conflicts about aggression and object loss were secondary determinants in depression. He viewed depression instead as resulting from a sense of helplessness, impaired self-esteem, and self-directed anger triggered by failures to live up to the narcissistic aspirations of any developmental phase.

Charles Brenner also deemphasized the classic psychoanalytic focus on object loss, seeing a depressive propensity as equally likely to connect with organizing fantasies of narcissistic injury and, particularly, of castration. These fantasies are accompanied by reactive aggression against those blamed for the painful affects, with consequent guilt.

Mr. D., a 39-year-old successful and aggressive lawyer, had "never been depressed a day in [his] life" before developing a kidney stone that required a 5-day hospital stay full of medical interventions. He was well on discharge but developed major depression, with lethargy, decreased energy, hopelessness, and weight loss. He cried all the time. "I feel like a big, fat failure," he announced. Handsome but insecure, Mr. D. prided himself on his physical prowess and appearance and on his ability to attract the amorous attentions of "beautiful women." "I'm not supposed to be sick," he said, "especially down there. It makes me feel old, ugly, and unattractive. Disgusting, in fact." In describing his experiences in the hospital, he reported that the humiliation or narcissistic blow to his self-esteem resulting from the illness and hospitalization had so overwhelmed him ("I was hooked up to these disgusting tubes—even in my penis!" he wailed) that he had uncharacteristically not even complained about being placed into a four-bed hospital room with three homeless people who hadn't showered. "I figured they were in control, so I didn't even think about it," he said. His remitted in psychoanalysis with therapeutic exploration of the way in which the hospitalization had, in fantasy, felt like a castration.

Many contemporary psychoanalysts amplify on these models in their understanding of depression, while acknowledging the prominence of impaired self-esteem regulation. Edith Jacobson emphasized the development of self and object representations in depressive patients. She noted depressed patients' disappointment with parental figures, resulting in devaluation and degradation of their images and of self-representation, especially when a mature separation had not been achieved.

Inadequacy of Early Caregivers Psychoanalysts have given a personal, intrapsychic face to the well-known epidemiological observation of the connection between parental (particularly maternal) depression and subsequent depression in children. Heinz Kohut described depression as connected to experiences of profound emptiness in patients whose parents were unable to empathize with their early affective experiences. Such is the case for many depressed patients, as many parents of depressed patients are themselves depressed. These patients crave compensatory relationships (self-object relationships, mirroring experiences, and idealizing relationships), leaving them vulnerable to disappointment, as real relationships do not live up to these compensatory fantasies.

Leo Stone highlighted depressives' refusal to accept the separateness and autonomy of the object. Again, this view emphasizes the symbiotic tie to the object to compensate for an incomplete sense of self. Stone said that depressives unconsciously coerce objects; they are disappointed in them and are prone to envy and rage because of an early history of oral frustration. Aggressive fantasies about disappointing and hurting loved ones give rise to the severe guilt with which these patients struggle.

Ms. E., a 21-year-old college student, presented with major depression and panic disorder since early adolescence. She reported hating herself, crying constantly, and feeling profoundly hopeless in part because of the chronicity of her illness. Even at the time of presentation, she noted her sensitivity to her mother's moods. "My mother's just always depressed, and it makes me so miserable, I just don't know what to do," she said. "I always want something from her, I don't even know what, but I never get it. She always says the wrong thing, talks about how disturbed I am, stuff like that, makes me feel bad about myself." In one session, Ms. E. poignantly described her childhood: "I spent a lot of time with my mother, but she was always too tired, she never wanted to do anything or play with me. I remember building a house with blankets over the coffee table and peeking out, spying on her. She was always depressed and negative, like a negative sink in the room, making it empty and sad. I could never get her to do anything." This patient experienced extreme guilt in her psychotherapy when she began to talk about her mother's depression. "I feel so bad," she sobbed. "It's like I'm saying bad things about her. And I love her so much, and I know she loves me. I feel it's so disloyal of me." Her depression remitted in psychodynamic psychotherapy as she became more aware of and better able to tolerate her feelings of rage and disappointment with her mother.

Sidney Blatt, a psychoanalytic researcher, contrasts *anaclitic* depressives, anxiously attached individuals who struggle with excessive dependence on others, with *introjective* depressives, who are compulsively self-reliant. Blatt contends that anaclitic patients experience more feelings of loneliness, helplessness and weakness; introjectives experience a sense of worthlessness, self-criticism, and guilt.

PSYCHOANALYTIC FORMULATIONS OF DYSTHYMIA

Psychoanalysts have largely written about major depression, but some have also addressed dysthymia. Asch noted underlying masochistic pathology in dysthymic patients, a view that has been deemphasized by contemporary dysthymia researchers, who have underlined that chronic depression can appear phenomenologically like underlying masochistic character structure, simply because of its chronicity. Mardi Horowitz emphasizes the "pleasure of revenge" in the patient's defeating of all those around him or her through failure, hopelessness, and negativity, and he regards this as more important than the experience of personal suffering for many such patients. David Milrod describes the rewarding and punitive aspects of superego function in response to narcissistic injury in patients with chronic dysthymia and self-pity.

Ms. F., a 20-year-old college student, came to psychotherapy complaining of chronic depression. She described herself as "dull, but difficult too." Although she enjoyed school, she had trouble finding things outside of school that she enjoyed doing. She was bored, lethargic, and unhappy most of the time. Although she had friends and a boyfriend—albeit a man much less desirable than she might otherwise have been expected to find—she resented their demands on her time, often because she found herself upset when she was with them. Her relationships with her boyfriend, some of her closer friends, and her mother were characterized by intermittent "crises": events when Ms. F. felt ignored, criticized, and abused by them, and she wound up locking herself in her room to cry, sometimes for days. As psychotherapy unfolded, it became clear that her boyfriend was demanding of her time, yet rarely actually spoke to her. For example, he preferred to have her "around" while he worked on his computer for hours on end, but, when he went out "to hang out," he preferred to spend time with his friends, without her. Ms. F. handled this situation with a combination of resignation and resentment: She stayed with him while he worked, then often ignored him at parties that they both attended to "get back at him." In psychodynamic psychotherapy, her dysthymia and passive masochism resolved at the same time, enabling her to stop feeling worthless in social situations and with her boyfriend and to become more assertive in all of her relationships.

SYNTHESIS: DYNAMICS OF DEPRESSION

Features common to many psychoanalytic theories of depression include feelings of exquisite narcissistic vulnerability stemming from a variety of sources, including early loss or experiences with parents perceived as traumatically unempathetic, frustrating, or rejecting. A sense of helplessness or inadequacy in relation to these experiences, with accompanying fantasies of damage or castration, contributes to this vulnerability. The resulting impairment in self-esteem regulation is common to all depressed patients, who are prone to self-images of being unlovable, damaged, or inadequate.

Depressed patients perceive that they have failed to live up to their ambitions or to their moral values in the ego ideal, the intrapsychic mechanism that triggers guilt in depression. Many psychoanalysts hypothesize that the resulting aggression toward a frustrating parent or toward the self as damaged contributes decisively to the propensity toward depression. In depressed patients, aggression is largely self-directed. Guilt (conscious or unconscious) or shame results from the patient's perceived sense of failure, with a diminished sense of self. Difficulties in self-esteem regulation contribute to a self-representation of being bad or shamefully out of control, aggravating the original problem in a vicious cycle.

The *sine qua non* of depression is aggression directed toward the self-representation, which proves uncontainable and spreads to a mood state. This may arise from a withdrawal of positive or *libidinal* supplies to the self-representation and replacement with aggression in the following ways: (1) by not living up to personal aspirations (giving rise to shame, rather than guilt); (2) by not living up to the ego ideal (precipitating guilt); and (3) in an interpersonal depression, as described by Freud, in which a symbiotic bond to an ambivalent object tie is shattered. From a psychoanalytic perspective, this latter type of depression is associated with more primitive pathology, and these patients are more likely to be in a borderline or psychotic spectrum, because of the nature of the primitive, symbiotic interpersonal bond. These different pathways trigger a common self-assessment of being worthless, bad, inadequate, or unlovable. The resulting hostility directed toward the self is a core feature of depression.

Retroflected hostility has been pinpointed in the historical psychoanalytic literature as also contributing to borderline and obsessional pathology. Indeed, many patients with these underlying character structures also experience major depression. From a psychoanalytic perspective, the essential feature of all depressions is the self-directed aggression that becomes a mood state. Difficulty with self-esteem regulation, which is not an essential component of other syndromes, is always prominent in depression, coupled with aggression turned inward that exacerbates guilt and shame.

PSYCHOANALYTIC FORMULATIONS OF MANIA

From a psychoanalytic perspective, the clinical presentation of mania arises as a result of a global, massive regression that affects all three psychic structures: the id, the ego, and the superego. The regression leads to a primitive mental state in which there is a reinstatement of the pleasure principle. In *Group Psychology and Analysis of the Ego*, Freud described mania as a fusion of the ego with its superego. Less cryptically, psychoanalysts have highlighted a common organizing fantasy in manic patients of a fantasy incorporation or mystical union of the patient with someone of great power, often an aristocrat or God, as in the story of St. Theresa's mystical union with God. Such organizing fantasies, couched in sexual and oral terms, magically impart a sense of omnipotence and specialness to the patient, highlighting one aspect to the common phenomenology of mania. Bertram D. Lewin notes that, in mania, early relationships with both parents that had become desexualized during the process of superego formation during latency become resexualized during the manic episode and that, in fantasy, the manic patient is identified with both partners (male and female) during the sexual act. The states of mania and of hypomania involve massive use of the defense mechanism of denial, in which aspects of reality are entirely ignored. One author hypothesized that the manic episode was precipitated by the need to control the memory and the experience of intolerable pain. In this way, mania represents a defensive reaction, different from depression, in response to pain and distress.

Ms. G., a 42-year-old housewife and mother of a 4-year-old boy, developed symptoms of hypomania and, later, of frank mania without psychosis, when her only son was diagnosed with acute lymphocytic leukemia. A profoundly religious woman who had experienced 10 years of difficulty with conception, Ms. G. was a devoted mother. She reported that she was usually rather "down." Before her son's illness, she used to joke that she had become pregnant with him by divine intervention. When her son was diagnosed and subsequently hospitalized, he required painful medical tests and emergency chemotherapy, which made him ill. The doctors regularly barraged Ms. G. with bad news about his prognosis during the first few weeks of his illness.

Ms. G. was ever present with her son at the hospital, never sleeping and always caring for him, yet the pediatricians noted that, as the child became more debilitated, and the prognosis became more grim, she seemed to bubble over with renewed cheerfulness, good humor, and high spirits. She could not seem to stop herself from cracking jokes to the hospital staff during her son's painful procedures, and, as the jokes became louder and more inappropriate, the staff grew more concerned. During her subsequent psychiatric consultation (requested by the pediatric staff), Ms. G. reported that her current "happiness and optimism" were justified by her sense of "oneness" with the mother of God, Mary. "We are together now, she and I, and she has become a part of me. We have a special relationship," she winked. Despite these statements, Ms. G. was not psychotic and said that she was "speaking metaphorically, of course, only as a good Catholic would." Her mania resolved when her son achieved remission and was discharged from the hospital.

COGNITIVE THEORY OF DEPRESSION

Learning theory long has been a branch of behavioral psychology. The disgruntled psychoanalyst Aaron Beck, finding that psychoanalytic theory did not sufficiently explain dreams of depressed patients, developed a theory of depression based on educating the patient about his or her negative thinking, or cognitions. Beck and colleagues then successfully tested CBT, a treatment built on this theory, in clinical trials. The cognitive model is based on the recognition that people are not objective; rather, an individual's idiosyncratic perception of events affects his or her emotions and behaviors. Depressed individuals perceive reality in subjectively depressed ways. Elaborate discussions of cognitive theory exist, and cognitive explanations have been extended from their original depressive origins to a range of psychopathology. Brad A. Alford and Beck argue that cognitive theory provides a comprehensive and coherent paradigm for psychopathology.

Beck's initial observations about major depression have a salience and simplicity worth repeating. He noted that depressed patients tend to have characteristically skewed and negative thoughts about (1) themselves, (2) their environment, and (3) the future, a damning cluster that he termed the *cognitive triad*. Indeed, depressed individuals frequently report negative thinking about themselves: "I'm a loser," "Everything I do goes wrong," "I'm weak and defective," etc. The environment appears hostile and overwhelming: "Even if I felt capable—which I don't—there's no way I could cope with what I have to do"; "My friends will react badly if I try to speak up"; "She will reject me." Finally, not only do things look grim in the present, but there is also no prospect of relief in the future: "It's never going to get any better." These three aspects of negative perspective converge to provide a convincingly, despairingly bleak and mood-congruent view of the world. This outlook helps explain why depressed patients see no way out of their misery and contemplate suicide.

Cognitive theory has explored the form as well as the content of thinking characteristic of depressed patients. Not only are cognitions skewed to the negative and pessimistic, but particular types of distortions also occur. Depressed individuals tend to engage in all-or-nothing, dichotomous thinking: If things are not entirely one way, they must be the opposite. Depressed individuals make arbitrary (negative) inferences about events, selectively abstract negative details out of context, overgeneralize (concluding negative rules from single instances), magnify (the negative) and minimize (the positive), and take personally events that may not be directly about them. Depressed patients *catastrophize,* leaping from one imagined worst-case scenario to the next in disastrous cascade: "H. will take what I said as an insult, and will never speak to me again, and will tell all our friends. Then no one will like me, I'll be all alone, and my social life will be ruined forever." They selectively seek out negative evidence, failures, and setbacks that confirm their theories of defectiveness, while ignoring or discounting the successes they have as flukes:

Mr. J., a 19-year-old college sophomore, made two mistakes on a test. Although his overall grade was high, and the mistakes themselves appeared minor to the therapist, he took them as proof that he was defective and deficient. His perfect score on the next test, by contrast, he discounted as "luck . . . the teacher was being easy on me," but not as any evidence of his personal competence.

If, while depressed, one considers oneself to be a loser, one pays most attention to outcomes that fit that schema.

Beck made the important point that the depressed outlook is not objective but irrational. *Automatic thoughts* of characteristically self-deprecatory and hopeless nature pop involuntarily into the patient's head. Because these thoughts are mood congruent, depressed individuals find them believable. The negative thinking characteristic of depressed patients is damaging in two respects. First, it is painful and depressing: Many patients are barraged with negative ideas about themselves and their situation, in effect, a stream of insults. Second, these thoughts tend to inhibit action: If one knows that one is an incompetent person who is going to fail, one will also have thoughts such as "Why bother?" Depressive thinking patterns not only hurt, but they also paralyze individuals into inaction, which then leaves them more time to ruminate on their inactivity ("I'm not doing anything with my life") and to suffer self-criticism. The deterioration of productive behavior due to negative thinking will then lead to more things going wrong in the patient's life, providing more examples of the patient's incompetence and reinforcing the negative thinking.

The case examples above provide good examples of self-critical thinking that, in cognitive theory, would be understood as the irrational, *automatic* thoughts of a depressed patient: Ms. A. felt "pointless" and "boring"; Mr. D. felt "like a big, fat failure," "old, ugly, and unattractive . . . disgusting"; and Ms. F. felt herself to be "dull, but difficult too."

Immediate and specific negative cognitions ("He doesn't like me") fit into larger, more basic and stable patterns of self-conception called *schemas* or *core beliefs*. For depressed patients, these tend to be global, negative, all-or-nothing assumptions based on early childhood experience: "If I do something imperfectly, it's (and I'm) worthless"; "If I'm not in total control, I'm completely helpless," etc. Early cognitive theory presented such negative thinking as a cause rather than an effect of depression. Although cognitions are clearly an important aspect of depression, it seems naïve, at this point, to expect that this is the single etiology of a complex and multidetermined syndrome that has genetic and environmental components. Hence, over time, cognitive theory has tended to back away from that etiological stance.

A general cognitive explanation of a major depressive episode is that a vulnerable individual, perhaps predisposed by biology and by negative schemas based on early childhood, experiences a current life situation that evokes *automatic* thoughts. For example, a relatively minor setback at work might activate underlying schemas by eliciting the thoughts, "I've done a bad job," and, therefore, "I'm a terrible worker," and "I've let the company and my coworkers down," "My boss hates me," and, therefore, "I'll never succeed," and "I'm a failure." A disagreement in a relationship might rouse ideas such as, "K. doesn't like me," evoking and seemingly confirming the more general core beliefs: "I'm a terrible person," "I'm a lousy parent," and, furthermore, "No one could possibly love me." The onset of these thoughts and accompanying depressive symptoms further compromises functioning, reinforcing the negative outlook. As mood darkens and the negative thoughts become ever more credible and pervasive, the patient gives up activities ("Why bother?") and feels still more helpless and hopeless.

Cognitive therapy, the treatment that follows from this approach, includes a Socratic discussion and evaluation of the patient's thoughts, weighing the evidence supporting and contradicting such thoughts. The patient actively tests hypotheses based on automatic thoughts ("I'll fail at whatever I do") by attempting various selected behaviors. As the patient learns to recognize the irrational nature of depressive thinking, he or she can challenge it rather than simply believing it and can begin to extinguish such thinking, replacing automatic irrational thoughts with rational responses. Outcome research repeatedly has shown that this approach is efficacious in treating mood disorders and other psychiatric syndromes.

Dysthymic and Bipolar Disorders Cognitive theory has not been particularly altered for dysthymic disorder. Rather, chronicity of depression would simply seem to ingrain negative core beliefs more deeply. Cognitive behavioral analysis system of psychotherapy (CBASP), an eclectic treatment that James P. McCullough developed specifically to treat chronic depression, postulates that chronically depressed patients fail to behave appropriately in interpersonal encounters. CBASP combines elements of cognitive, behavioral, psychodynamic, and interpersonal therapies in focusing on the patient's behaviors and thinking in interpersonal encounters, including those with the therapist.

Cognitive-behavioral treatments have been developed not only for unipolar depression, but also as an adjunct to medication for bipolar disorder. Mania may be viewed as the mirror of depression, wherein overvalued positive ideas ("I'm special," "I'm the greatest") automatically arise, again distorting reality, but this time in the opposing direction. Thinking itself accelerates in mania. By and large, cognitive theory has had less to say about manic than depressed states, and adaptations of cognitive therapies for mania are more practical than theoretical. They focus on psychoeducation about the illness and behavioral stabilization, such as maintaining a regular sleep schedule, and emphasize the importance of adherence to pharmacotherapy (M. Basco, *personal communication*, 2002).

Aspects of cognitive theory have been tested for unipolar depression, with sometimes contradictory results. CBT, which directly addresses depressive negative cognitions and helps patients weigh their evidence rather than simply believing them, has repeatedly demonstrated efficacy as a treatment for major depression and does improve negative cognitions. Yet, other antidepressant treatments relieve depression and improve cognitions without specifically addressing cognitions, and behavioral activation—a behavioral approach without the cognitive component—has been shown to be as efficacious as CBT. Efficacious treatments for depression may spread from a particular theorized target to generalized benefits.

Comparison to Psychodynamic Theory Cognitive theory does not contradict and, to some degree, overlaps with psychoanalytic theory. The treatments emerging from these theories differ greatly, however, in large part owing to their differing definitions of the role of the therapist, their handling of the therapeutic relationship, and their approach to the meaning of that relationship—in psychoanalytic terms, the *transference*. Both theories focus on intrapsychic processes and on self-critical thinking, but cognitive theory emphasizes the distinction between rational and irrational thinking and their connection to mood rather than to unconscious fantasy.

INTERPERSONAL THEORY OF DEPRESSION

Interpersonal theory dates back to the era after World War II, when it arose as a heretical response to the more intrapsychic emphasis of psychoanalysis. Psychoanalytic theory emphasized the importance of early life experience, and many therapists at that time saw the patient's psychic structure as essentially formed by the end of adolescence. Psychiatrists such as Adolf Meyer, Harry Stack Sullivan, Erich Fromm, and Frieda Fromm-Reichmann challenged then-current theory by emphasizing the influence of the real impact of current life events on their patients' psychopathology, focusing on environmental and interpersonal encounters rather than underlying intrapsychic drives and structures.

Sullivan coined the term *interpersonal* as a rubric for considering current life experience. He scrutinized communications in the social field, a more *external* outlook than traditional psychoanalysis. The interpersonal theorists worked mainly with inpatients diagnosed with schizophrenia in a prepharmacological era. Although their work stirred great controversy at the time, and a Sullivanian school still exists distinct from the psychoanalysis of drives and ego psychology, Sullivan was trained in psychoanalysis and did not entirely disagree with his forebears. Over time, the rift between Sullivanians and other psychoanalysts has narrowed.

The consideration of current interpersonal factors gained currency over succeeding decades, and it is now mainstream clinical thinking that current life events and interpersonal functioning affect and are affected by psychopathology. A school of interpersonal psychoanalysis—not particularly focused on mood disorders—arose. Psychoanalytically trained therapists, such as Silvano Arieti and Jules Bemporad, emphasized interpersonal factors in the treatment of depressed patients. Jack C. Anchin and Donald J. Kiesler have reviewed other interpersonally based psychotherapies. None of these theories has received empirical testing.

Researchers did develop a host of related data about interpersonal issues associated with depression. For example, research showed that interpersonal supports protect an individual against depression: Having a confidant to talk to reduces the risk of developing a depressive episode. Major life stressors, including the death of a significant other, struggles in important relationships, and upheavals such as a change in marital status, housing, job status, or physical health have been shown to increase the risk of depressive episodes in vulnerable individuals. Moreover, the onset of depressive episodes leads to deterioration in relationships and social functioning.

John Bowlby postulated that people have an evolutionarily determined, instinctual drive to form emotional attachments. Animal evidence now supports this theory. This basic component of human nature ensures infant survival: Children need to have parents nearby or available for feeding and protection. As children develop, they begin to explore their environment, gradually moving out from the *secure base* of their attachment figure. Disruptions in this early caregiving connection may lead to vulnerability of attachment style. For example, loss of one's mother in the first decade of life has been shown to be a risk factor for subsequent depression. Children with insecure childhood attachments may not learn to ask for help from others. When such vulnerable individuals face stressors or feel an absence or inadequacy of interpersonal supports during times of stress, they may be helpless to respond effectively and may be prone to developing symptoms. Furthermore, individuals with insecure attachment styles may have difficulty in developing comfortable relationships on which they can rely for support in times of need.

Depressed individuals have great difficulty in interpersonal functioning. They tend, guiltily, to see other people's needs as more important than their own. Their passive, self-abnegating outlook means that the depressed person's needs likely go unmet and that they view their environment as painful and burdensome. Moreover, depressed patients expect that they feel painful and burdensome to others. They guiltily try to meet other people's needs and to act normal when they do not feel normal. Such activity is exhausting and relatively ungratifying.

Research by Zlotnick et al. and others has shown that depressed patients report more negative interactions and fewer positive interactions with other people than do other individuals. Whereas depressive symptoms may initially evoke sympathy from others, this soon turns to irritation as depressed individuals express helplessness and hopelessness and have difficulty in maintaining social functioning. Hence, they tend to withdraw from social relationships, in which they fear that they will bother other people or be unable to defend themselves from criticism or rejection. This diminishes social supports and leaves the depressed individual feeling alienated, isolated, and misunderstood.

In the 1970s, when Gerald L. Klerman, Myra M. Weissman, and their colleagues were conducting a randomized controlled trial of outpatients with major depressive episodes, they recognized that many such patients received psychotherapy in community treatment. They sought accordingly to add psychotherapy to their trial but realized that it was unclear then (as now) of what such community psychotherapy consisted. They then developed IPT as a manual, time-limited treatment for outpatients with major depressive disorder based on interpersonal and attachment theories as well as empirical evidence of the psychosocial nature of depression. IPT is thus one specific therapeutic application of more general interpersonal theory. IPT demonstrated efficacy for major depression in this and in subsequent outcome trials.

In simplest terms, interpersonal theory as applied to IPT can be understood as a link between mood and events. For all people, upsetting external events evoke a sad or demoralized mood: In lay terms, they are "depressing." For biologically or environmentally predisposed individuals, however, a sufficiently disturbing life event can trigger an episode of major depression. Examples of such life events are the death of a significant other (complicated bereavement), a problematic relationship (role dispute), or other major life change (role transition). Once a depressive episode starts, its symptoms compromise functioning, producing more negative life events in a vicious downward cycle. This formulation seems straightforward, even commonsensical, but depressed patients have a peculiar amnesia for external events and tend to blame themselves for how they feel or to see the depressed state as who they are. It can be helpful clinically to remind them that they are ill, not defective, and that outside events may have contributed to their distress.

IPT therapists do not propose this as an etiological theory of depression but as a pragmatic one: The depressive mood episode can be linked to a precipitating life event or to consequent life events that become the focus for treatment. The IPT therapist defines major depression as a medical illness—a treatable medical problem that is not the patient's fault—and links it to an interpersonal focus, such as a role dispute. The therapeutic contract for the patient is to solve the interpersonal focus within a time-limited period. Solving the interpersonal problem is at once a realistic relief (e.g., improving a marriage), relieves depressive symptoms, and builds interpersonal skills that may hopefully protect against future interpersonal triggers and depressive episodes. Typical areas of interpersonal skill building are issues such as self-assertion, confrontation, effective expression of anger, and the taking of social risks.

Clinicians armed with differing theories approach the same material in different ways. IPT seeks a life event or interpersonal situation as a plausible and pragmatic fiction on which to focus a time-limited treatment in which the patient can work on interpersonal skills. For example, the case of Ms. A. might be conceptualized as major depression arising in the context of a role dispute with her boyfriend, Mr. B. Had she been treated in IPT, the focus might have been on recognition and appropriate expression of her own anger as part of learning to renegotiate that relationship. Alternatively, or additionally, clinical judgment might have defined the break-up of that relationship as a role transition that Ms. A. needed to mourn and to accept to move on to better relationships or activities. Ms. C.'s difficulty in tolerating her acceptance to graduate school might similarly be considered a role transition, as might Mr. D.'s bout of renal stones. Medical illnesses, even if transient, frequently provoke role transitions by shifting a patient's perception of his life trajectory; Mr. D. may have interpreted his hospitalization as evidence of his fading potency, aging, and mortality. Ms. E.'s situation might conceivably be defined as a role transition—adjusting to college life away from her mother—or as a role dispute with her mother.

Dysthymic Disorder An adaptation of IPT has been developed for dysthymic disorder, but differences in the treatment are largely those of technique. Patients with chronic depression tend to be socially isolated (Ms. F. is slightly unusual in having a boyfriend, although her choice of boyfriend was in keeping with the disorder) and invariably have interpersonal difficulties. If the syndrome began early in life, as is often the case, patients may never have developed important communication skills. They tend to be passive and unassertive and to experience self-assertion as selfish, rather than as a healthy and sometimes necessary negotiation of one's own goals in life, and anger as a bad feeling rather than as a useful interpersonal signal that someone is bothering them. Even if they have had such capabilities in the past, interpersonal functioning will have eroded under the pounding discouragement of chronic depression. Chronicity breeds resignation and entrenches maladaptive interpersonal patterns.

As in the treatment of acute major depression, IPT for dysthymic disorder normalizes these feelings as inevitable human emotions and as useful signals of interpersonal encounters. The patient learns to tolerate a modicum of selfishness as a healthy motivation to achieve happiness, of anger and confrontation as necessary forms of self-defense against the demands of others, and of social risk-taking as uncomfortable but necessary to get ahead in life. Role playing in therapy helps prepare patients to achieve these goals.

Bipolar Disorder There is no real adaptation of interpersonal theory for mania. Ellen Frank and colleagues have adapted IPT for bipolar patients as an adjunctive treatment to pharmacotherapy by combining it with a behavioral strategy. Interpersonal social rhythms therapy (IPSRT) is a hybrid of IPT and social zeitgeber theory, which stresses the importance of maintaining diurnal structure through regular patterning of events or social rhythms. In particular, this involves ensuring a regular bedtime to prevent the loss of sleep that often triggers a manic episode. As with CBT for bipolar disorder, this represents more of a clinically reasonable, pragmatic extension of an already established treatment than a theoretical evolution.

SUMMARY

Psychoanalytic, cognitive, and interpersonal theories all provide insights into mood disorders. None is received truth, and all are surely incomplete. This chapter has not covered all theories of mood disorder: Biological, behavioral, feminist, and many other theories have been proposed for depression. Psychoanalytic, cognitive, and interpersonal theories each capture important aspects of complex syndromes. Each may be useful to therapists and patients in conceptualizing the patient's status and in organizing his or her treatment.

SUGGESTED CROSS-REFERENCES

The reader is encouraged to refer to related mood disorders sections: historical and conceptual overview (Section 13.1), epidemiology (Section 13.2), clinical features (Section 13.6), treatment of depression (Section 13.7), treatment of bipolar disorders (Section 13.8), and psychotherapy (Section 13.9), as well as the sections on psychotherapies (Chapter 30), psychiatric treatment in child psychiatry (Chapter 48), and the treatment of psychiatric disorders in geriatric psychiatry (Section 51.4).

REFERENCES

Abraham K. A short study of the development of the libido, viewed in the light of mental disorders (1924). In: *Selected Papers on Psychoanalysis.* London: Hogarth Press; 1927:418–501.

Abraham K. Notes on the psycho-analytical investigation and treatment of manic-depressive insanity and allied conditions (1911). In: *Selected Papers on Psychoanalysis.* London: Hogarth Press; 1927:137–156.

Alford BA, Beck AT. *The Integrative Power of Cognitive Therapy.* New York: Guilford; 1997.

American Psychiatric Association. *Diagnostic and Statistical Manual of Mental Disorders.* 4th ed. Washington, DC: American Psychiatric Association; 1994.

Anchin JC, Kiesler DJ, eds. *Handbook of Interpersonal Psychotherapy.* New York: Pergamon Press; 1982.

Arieti S, Bemporad J. *Severe and Mild Depressions.* New York: Basic Books; 1978.

Asch S: Depression: Three clinical variations. *Psychoanal Stud Child.* 1966;21:150–170.

Asch S. The analytic concepts of masochism: A re-evaluation. In: Glick R, Meyers D, eds. *Masochism: Current Analytic Perspectives.* Hillsdale, NJ: Analytic Press; 1988:93–116.

Basco M, Rush AJ. *Cognitive-Behavioral Therapy for Bipolar Disorder.* New York: Guilford Press; 1996.

*Beck AT, Rush AJ, Shaw BF, Emery G. *Cognitive Therapy of Depression.* New York: Guilford Press; 1979.

Beck JS. *Cognitive Therapy: Basics and Beyond.* New York: Guilford Press; 1995.

Bemporad J: Psychotherapy of the depressive character. *J Am Acad Psychoanal.* 1976;4:347–372.

Bibring E. The mechanics of depression. In: Greenacre P, ed. *Affective Disorders.* New York: International Universities Press; 1953:13–48.

Blatt S: Contributions of psychoanalysis to the understanding and treatment of depression. *J Am Psychoanal Assoc.* 1998;46:723–752.

Bowlby J. *Attachment and Loss.* New York: Basic Books; 1973.

Bowlby J: Developmental psychiatry comes of age. *Am J Psychiatry.* 1998;145:1–10.

Brenner C: Affects and psychic conflict. *Psychoanal Q.* 1975;44:1–28.

Brown GW, Harris T. *The Social Origins of Depression: A Study of Psychiatric Disorder in Women.* New York: Free Press; 1978.

Cohen MB, Baker G, Cohen RA, Fromm-Reichmann F, Weigert EA: An intensive study of twelve cases of manic depressive psychoses. *Psychiatry.* 1954;17:103–137.

Crits-Christoph P, Connoly MB, Gallop R: Early improvement in manual-guided cognitive and dynamic psychotherapies predicts 16-week remission status. *J Psychother Pract Res.* 2001;10:145–154.

Eells TD, ed. *Handbook of Psychotherapy Case Formulation.* New York: Guilford Press; 1997.

Ehlers CL, Frank E, Kupfer DJ: Social zeitgebers and biological rhythms: A unified approach to understanding the etiology of depression. *Arch Gen Psychiatry.* 1988;45:948–952.

Frank E, Swartz HA, Kupfer DJ: Interpersonal and social rhythm therapy: Managing the chaos of bipolar disorder. *Biol Psychiatry.* 2000;48:593–604.

Freud S. Studies on hysteria. In: Strachey J, ed. *Standard Edition of the Complete Psychological Works of Sigmund Freud.* Vol 2. 1895:1–183.

Freud S. Two principles of mental functioning. In: Strachey J, ed. *Standard Edition of the Complete Psychological Works of Sigmund Freud.* Vol 12. 1911:223.

*Freud S. Mourning and melancholia. In: Strachey J, ed. *Standard Edition of the Complete Psychological Works of Sigmund Freud.* Vol 14. 1915:237–258.

Freud S. Beyond the pleasure principle. In: Strachey J, ed. *Standard Edition of the Complete Psychological Works of Sigmund Freud.* Vol 18. 1920:3–67.

Freud S. Group psychology and analysis of the ego. In: Strachey J, ed. *Standard Edition of the Complete Psychological Works of Sigmund Freud.* Vol 18. 1921:69–143.

Freud S. The ego and the id. In: Strachey J, ed. *Standard Edition of the Complete Psychological Works of Sigmund Freud.* Vol 19. 1923:3–66.

Hofer MA. An evolutionary perspective on anxiety. In: Roose SP, Glick RA, eds. *Anxiety as Symptom and Signal.* Hillsdale, NJ: Analytic Press; 1995:17–38.

Horowitz M: On the difficulty of analyzing character. *J Clin Psychoanal.* 1999;8:212–217.

Jacobson E: Transference problems in the psychoanalytic treatment of severely depressed patients. *J Am Psychoanal Assoc.* 1954;2:595–605.

*Jacobson E. *Depression: Comparative Studies of Normal, Neurotic, and Psychotic Conditions.* Madison, CT: International Universities Press; 1971.

Jacobson NS, Dobson K, Truax PA, Addis ME, Koerner K, Gollan JK, Gortner E, Prince SE: A component analysis of cognitive-behavioral treatment for depression. *J Consult Clin Psychol.* 1996;64:295–304.

Kafka F. *The Castle.* New York: A. A. Knopf; 1930.

Klein M: Mourning and its relation to manic-depressive states. *Int J Psychoanal.* 1940;21:125–153.

Klerman GL. Ideological conflicts in integrating pharmacotherapy and psychotherapy. In: Beitman BD, Klerman GL, eds. *Integrating Pharmacotherapy and Psychotherapy.* Washington, DC: American Psychiatric Press; 1991.

*Klerman GL, Weissman MM, Rounsaville BJ, Chevron ES. *Interpersonal Psychotherapy of Depression.* New York: Basic Books; 1984.

Kohut H. *The Analysis of the Self.* New York: International Universities Press; 1971.

Levitan HL: The relationship between mania and pain. *Bull Meninger Clin.* 1977;41:145–161.

Lewin BD. *The Psychoanalysis of Elation.* New York: WW Norton; 1950.

Lewin BD. Analysis and structure of a transient hypomania (1932). In: Arlow JA, ed. *Selected Works of Bertram D. Lewin.* Richmond, VA: William Byrd Press; 1973:57–70.

Lewin BD. Comments on hypomanic and related states (1941). In: Arlow JA, ed. *Selected Works of Bertram D. Lewin*. Richmond, VA: William Byrd Press; 1973:78–84.
Markowitz JC. *Interpersonal Psychotherapy for Dysthymic Disorder*. Washington, DC: American Psychiatric Press; 1998.
Markowitz JC, Svartberg M, Swartz HA: Is IPT time-limited psychodynamic psychotherapy? *J Psychother Pract Res*. 1998;7:185–195.
McCullough JP Jr. *Treatment for Chronic Depression: Cognitive Behavioral Analysis System of Psychotherapy*. New York: Guilford Press; 2000.
Miller L, Warner V, Wickramaratne P, Weissman MM: Self-esteem and depression: Ten year follow-up of mothers and offspring. *J Affect Disord*. 1999;52:41–49.
*Milrod D: Self-pity, self-comforting, and the superego. *Psychoanal Stud Child*. 1972;27:505–528.
Milrod D: Psychoanalytic theory of depression: Identification, orality, anxiety. *Psychoanal Stud Child*. 1988;43:83–100.
Rado S: The problem of melancholia. *Intl J Psychoanal*. 1928;9:420–438.
Rudden M, Busch FN, Milrod B, Singer M, Aronson A, Roiphe J, Shapiro T: Panic disorder and depression: A psychodynamic exploration of comorbidity. *Int J Psychoanal*. 2003;84:997–1015.
Sandler J, Joffe WG: Notes on childhood depression. *Int J Psychoanal*. 1965;46:88–96.
Shapiro T: The concept of unconscious fantasy. *J Clin Psychoanal*. 1992;1:517–524.
Stone L: Psychoanalytic observations on the pathology of depressive illness: Selected spheres of ambiguity or disagreement. *J Am Psychoanal Assoc*. 1986;34:329–362.
Sullivan HS. *The Interpersonal Theory of Psychiatry*. New York: WW Norton; 1953.
Weissman MM, Markowitz JC, Klerman GL. *Comprehensive Guide to Interpersonal Psychotherapy*. New York: Basic Books; 2000.
Zlotnick C, Kohn R, Keitner G, Della Grotta SA: The relationship between quality of interpersonal relationships and major depressive disorder: Findings from the National Comorbidity Study. *J Affect Disord*. 2000;59:205–215.

▲ 13.6 Mood Disorders: Clinical Features

HAGOP S. AKISKAL, M.D.

HETEROGENEITY OF MOOD DISORDERS

Terminology Mood disorders are characterized by pervasive dysregulation of mood and psychomotor activity and by related biorhythmic and cognitive disturbances. The rubric of *affective disorder*, which, in some European classifications, also subsumes morbid anxiety states, is increasingly being replaced by the nosologically more delimited concept of *mood disorder*. Thus, *mood disorder* is now the preferred term in the World Health Organization's (WHO's) tenth edition of the *International Statistical Classification of Diseases and Related Health Problems* (ICD-10) and the American Psychiatric Association's (APA's) fourth edition of *Diagnostic and Statistical Manual of Mental Disorders* (DSM-IV). Although this chapter refers to the diagnostic criteria in the revised fourth edition of DSM (DSM-IV-TR) (2000), this text revision is essentially identical to the DSM-IV (1994). Official mood disorder categories in current use include bipolar disorders (with manic or hypomanic, depressive, or mixed episodes) and major depressive disorders, and their respective attenuated variants known as *cyclothymic* and *dysthymic disorders*. The term *unipolar* is avoided in DSM-IV-TR, because major depressive disorder, especially when early in age at onset, is an unstable diagnosis and is liable to switch to bipolar. Conditions that, in earlier editions of these manuals, were categorized as *endogenous depression*, *involutional melancholia*, and *psychotic depressive reaction* have been incorporated into major depressive disorder. Although *depressive neurosis* is parenthetically mentioned in DSM-IV-TR as a condition corresponding to dysthymic disorder, many such patients do meet criteria for major depressive disorder. Although the neurotic-endogenous distinction has been officially deleted, the term *melancholic features* is now used to qualify major depressive disorders in which biological concomitants predominate. The American and international classifications recognize the common occurrence of mixed anxiety-depressions, which underscores the value of the broader *affective disorder* rubric. It is presently uncertain whether classic neurasthenic conditions, which have recently reemerged and overlap to some extent with the so-called chronic fatigue syndrome, should be classified under this broad rubric.

Recent Diagnostic Trends The reshuffling and reclassification of various affective conditions into the mood disorders chapter of the APA classification has, on balance, considerably broadened their boundaries. This change reflects, in part, developments in pharmacotherapy that have resulted in considerable alleviation of suffering for persons whose illnesses fall short of and sometimes beyond the boundaries of classic mood disorders. As a result, a person with recurrent mood disorders who would have been disabled can now expect to lead a life relatively free of major episodes and major personal and occupational disruptions. Such gratifying results have, in turn, helped destigmatize this group of disorders. Destigmatization has been further facilitated by published self-revelations of famous persons with depressive and bipolar disorders. Unfortunately, access to competent mental health care is not available to large segments of the populations. Moreover, destigmatization, which has led to global efforts to detect and to treat mood disorders—particularly depression—in public and private sectors, may have had unintended sequelae. Despite the obvious public health advantages of such destigmatization, some authorities nonetheless now contend that a global *depression-centric* perspective has emerged in psychiatric and general medical sectors at the expense of bipolar disorders and may have led to overtreatment with antidepressants and unmasking of latent bipolar disorders. Others believe the opposite to be true—that it is bipolar disorder that is overdiagnosed and mood stabilizers that are overused. Existing data, however, indicate that, on balance, it is the continuing underdiagnosis of bipolar disorder that presents the greatest threat to public health.

Spectrum of Mood Disorders The foregoing considerations notwithstanding, the increasing clinical diagnosis of major depressive and bipolar disorders should not be dismissed as mere therapeutic fad. External validating strategies, such as familial-genetic studies and prospective follow-up, can now be used to buttress the broadened concept of mood disorders, including that of bipolar disorder. New research comparing monozygotic and dizygotic twins has demonstrated that the genetic propensity to mood disorders embraces entities that extend beyond endogenous depression (melancholia in DSM-IV-TR) to subsume a larger variety of depressions, including some encountered in persons in the community who have never received psychiatric treatment. Although such data might seem counterintuitive to those who would restrict depression to a core primary "biological" disease, they suggest that the constitutional predisposition for affective dysregulation occurs in as many as one of every three persons. That ratio is similar to the proportion of those who progress to a full depressive syndrome after bereavement, rhesus monkeys developing depressive-like behavior after a separation paradigm, and dogs that develop learned helplessness after inescapable shock. The fact that these rates are considerably higher than those observed in clinical populations suggests that many subjects possess protective factors against major depressive episodes; alternatively, the data suggest that other factors determine which person with emotional distress becomes a clinical case. A

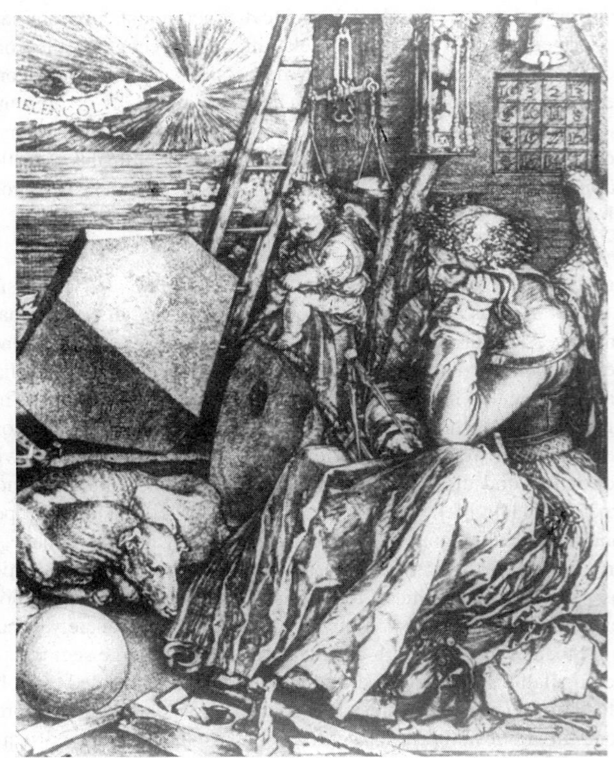

FIGURE 13.6–1 *Melancholia* (1514) by Albrecht Dürer.

great deal might therefore be revealed about the nature of pathological affective processes through study of self-limiting affective conditions on the border of mood disorders.

Current evidence from long-term prospective studies indicates that the course of mood disorders consists of various gradations of affective oscillations from the subsyndromal level to the syndromic level. Major episodes represent an operational convention to define a clinical threshold. Subchronic course, dominated by subthreshold symptoms, occurs in 50 to 60 percent. This is equally true for major depressive disorder and bipolar disorders. Detecting the illness in its subthreshold stage and treating interepisodic subthreshold phases are important clinical considerations.

The suffering and dysfunction resulting from mood disorders are among the most common reasons for consulting psychiatrists and other physicians. In fully developed cases of depression, all activity stops—including creative powers—and life is grim and in total disarray (as portrayed in Albrecht Dürer's masterpiece, Fig. 13.6–1). Interestingly, the ladder and the angel-like portrayal of the melancholic subject in this wood block promise that the illness that can bring descent into the hell of depression can also permit ascent into the heavens and creativity. Such creativity, however, is largely limited to a few talented individuals with the milder forms of bipolarity. Many with the manic extremes of the illness have poor judgment and insight, refuse treatment, and suffer a deteriorative course.

All great physicians of the past, beginning with Hippocrates, have devoted considerable space in their general medical texts to the clinical characterization of melancholic and manic states, as well as their alternations in the same patient. The relationship of anxious and melancholic states was also known. A broad spectrum of affective disturbances—ranging from the relatively mild temperamental variants (represented in the official American nosology by dysthymic and cyclothymic disorders) to their severest forms (including what, today, is considered mood disorder with mood-congruent and mood-incongruent psychotic features)—have been described in classical medical and psychiatric treatise. Finally, classical authors noted that melancholia and certain physical diseases shared seasonal exacerbation and described the common occurrence of alcohol indulgence, especially in those prone to mania. These boundary problems continue to pose challenges today, with the addition of substance use disorders.

AFFECTS, MOODS, TEMPERAMENTS, AND MORBID MOOD STATES

Ethological Considerations *Affects* and *moods* refer to different aspects of emotion. Affect is communicated through facial expression, vocal inflection, gestures, and posture and (according to current ethological research) is intended to move human beings and other primates to appraise whether a person is satisfied, distressed, disgusted, or in danger. Thus, joy, sadness, anger, and fear are basic affects that serve a communicative function in primates, as well as many other mammalian species.

Affects tend to be short-lived expressions, reflecting momentary emotional contingencies. Moods convey sustained emotions; their more enduring nature means that they are experienced long enough to be felt inwardly. Moods are also manifested in subtle ways, and their accurate assessment often requires empathic understanding by the interviewer. The words that subjects use to describe their inner emotions may coincide with the technical terms used by researchers or clinicians and often vary from one culture to another. Furthermore, the inward emotion and the prevailing affective tone may be discordant. This conflict could be due to deliberate simulation (i.e., the subject does not wish to reveal his or her inner emotion), or it could result from a pathological lesion or process that has altered the emotions and their neural substrates. Thus, evaluating moods and affective expression requires considerable clinical experience. Such evaluation is obviously of great importance in differential diagnosis. Finally, it is of great usefulness in the therapeutic process; the admonition to "go after the affect" in psychotherapy helps to find where it hurts, thereby making treatment possible.

Sadness and Joy The normal emotions of sadness and joy are part of everyday life and should be differentiated from major depressive disorder and mania. Sadness, or normal depression, is a universal human response to defeat, disappointment, or other adversities. The response may be adaptive, in an evolutionary sense, by permitting withdrawal to conserve inner resources, or it might signal the need for support from significant others. Transient depressive periods also occur as reactions to certain holidays or anniversaries, as well as during the premenstrual phase and the first week postpartum. Termed, respectively, *holiday blues*, *anniversary reactions*, premenstrual tension, and *maternity blues*, they are not psychopathological per se, but those predisposed to mood disorder may develop clinical depression during such times. As premenstrual tension is described later in the chapter under its clinically relevant extreme expression termed *premenstrual dysphoric disorder* as an example of depression not otherwise specified (where DSM-IV-TR has placed it), this section focuses on other normative mood continua.

Grief Normal bereavement or grief, considered the prototype of reactive depression, occurs in response to significant separations and losses, such as death, divorce, romantic disappointment, leaving familiar environments, forced emigration, or civilian catastrophes. DSM-IV-TR tends to limit the concept of normal grief to loss due to the death of a loved one—a condition that it considers as an exclusionary criterion for major depression. However, the work of Elie Karam and colleagues showed that bereavement and other losses associated with the civil war in Lebanon served as potent forces in depression formation. The same was true for the losses due to the earthquake in Armenia. The boundary behavior and clinical depression are blurred in reactions to such complex losses. In addition to depressed affect that is appropriate to the loss, bereavement reactions are characterized by the prominence of sympathetic arousal and restlessness believed to represent, from an evolutionary perspective, physiological and behavioral mechanisms to facilitate the search for the lost object. Like other adversities, bereavement and loss do not generally seem to cause depressive disorder, except in those predisposed to mood disorder. Reactions to major catastrophes might represent a partial exception.

Elation The positive emotion of elation is popularly linked to success and achievement. However, paradoxical depressions may also follow such positive events, possibly because of the increased responsibilities that often have to be faced alone. Elation is conceptualized psychodynamically as a defense against depression or as a denial of the pain of loss, as exemplified by *maniacal grief*, a rare form of bereavement reaction in which elated hyperactivity may replace the expected grief. The character of the "merry widow" in operatic music seems to be of similar derivation.

Other pseudomanic states include the brief energetic and unusually lucid periods encountered in dying patients or in those who need to take superhuman action in the face of unusual duress, both of which have been conceptualized as a *flight into health*. In predisposed persons, such reactions might be the prelude to a genuine manic episode. Sleep deprivation, which commonly accompanies major stressors, might represent one of the intermediary mechanisms between stressor and adverse clinical outcome.

Affective Temperaments Another mediating factor between normal and pathological moods is temperament. Most persons have a characteristic pattern of basal affective oscillations that defines their temperament. For instance, some are easily moved to tears by sad or happy circumstances, whereas others tend to remain placid. Normally, oscillations in affective tone are relatively minor, tend to resonate with day-to-day events, and do not interfere with functioning. Some exhibit greater variability of emotional responses whereby, with no obvious provocation, the person alternates between normal mood and sadness or elation. Temperament traits tend to cluster into basic types. A worrying temperament associated with generalized anxiety disorder is often complicated by depressive episodes. It may be as prevalent as 5 percent of the general population, and it overlaps, to some extent, with the depressive temperament; such inclination to melancholy makes the person more easily sink into sad moods and occurs in 3 to 6 percent of the general population. The hyperthymic temperament, in which the person is naturally inclined toward cheerful moods, has been reported in 4 to 8 percent; the cyclothymic temperament, swinging between cheerful and sad moods, characterizes 4 to 6 percent of young adults. All four types have an early insidious onset and tend to persist throughout adult life. Interestingly, these temperaments may be the prelude to episodes of depressive or hypomanic and manic polarity, which underscores the inherent instability of temperamental inclinations. Marked irritable-explosive traits occur in 2 to 3 percent of young subjects and tend to attenuate by middle age. Current data suggest that such traits often coexist with the mood-labile cyclothymic type, representing the dark "borderline" side of this temperament.

An examination of the traits associated with these temperaments can provide the rationale for the hypothesis about the social and evolutionary functions that they subserve (Table 13.6–1). Thus, the person with a depressive temperament is hard working, dependable, sensitive to the suffering and needs of others, and suitable for jobs that require long periods of devotion to meticulous detail; such persons are said to shoulder the burdens of existence without experiencing its pleasures. A person with the hyperthymic temperament, endowed with high levels of energy, extroversion, and humor, assumes leadership positions in society or excels as a performer in media or entertainment; they are also successful from a Darwinian perspective in that they are adept in amorous advances and engender a large number of offspring. In talented persons, the cyclothymic temperament, which alternates between sadness and elation, could provide the inspiration for love and for the emotional intensity needed for composing music, writing poetry, and painting. One with the irritable temperament might be best suited for a military career or even revolutionary action. The danger with persons with extreme temperaments is that they could swing too far in one or the other direction, or in both directions (i.e., major depressive, manic, or mixed episodes). Use of such substances as alcohol, caffeine, and other stimulants might further destabilize affective regulation in persons with those attributes. Some adolescent girls with irritable cyclothymia might develop the extreme emotional disequilibrium that, in contemporary psychiatry, is considered borderline personality disorder. Temperament concepts can enrich understanding of the boundary between normal moods and emotional disorders and can supplement the somewhat arid DSM-IV-TR descriptors of personality disorders with valuable information about individual vulnerability and assets.

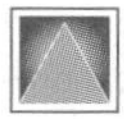

Table 13.6–1
Attributes, Assets, and Liabilities of Depressive and Hyperthymic Types Derived from Classic Concepts of Temperaments

Depressive	Hyperthymic
Gloomy, incapable of fun, complaining	Cheerful and exuberant
Humorless	Articulate and jocular
Pessimistic, and given to brooding	Overoptimistic and carefree
Guilt-prone, low self-esteem, and preoccupied with inadequacy or failure	Overconfident, self-assured, boastful megalomaniac
Introverted with restricted social life	Extroverted and people seeking
Sluggish, living a life out of action	High energy level, full of plans
Few but constant interests	Versatile with broad interests
Passive and "sensitive"	Overinvolved and meddlesome
Reliable, dependable, and devoted	Uninhibited and stimulus seeking

Morbid Mood States

Mood disorders represent abnormal or extreme variations of mood and associated manifestations and are characterized by the following features: pathological mood change, endoreactive moods, recurrence, and impairment.

Pathological Mood Change Pathological moods are distinguished from their normal counterparts by being out of proportion to any concurrent stressor or situation; being unresponsive to reassurance; being sustained for weeks, months, and, sometimes, years; and having a pervasive effect on the person, such that judgment is seriously compromised by the mood.

Endoreactive Moods Depression and mania are diagnosed, respectively, when sadness or elation is overly intense and continues beyond the expected impact of a stressful life event. Indeed, the morbid mood might arise without apparent or significant life stress. The pathological process in mood disorders is thus partly defined by the ease with which an intense emotional state is released and, especially, by its tendency to persist autonomously even when the offending stressor is no longer operative. Rather than being endogenous (i.e., occurring in the absence of precipitants), mood disorders are best conceptualized as endoreactive (i.e., once released, they tend to persist autonomously). The homeostatic dyscontrol of mood, which is part of a more pervasive mood dysregulation, resists reversal to the habitual baseline affective tone. DSM-IV-TR, which tends to disparage theory and to adhere to a descriptive level of operationalism, gives insufficient weight to this fundamental characteristic of mood disorders. Indeed, the current understanding of clinical depression is that it is due to underlying biological—putative genetic—factors that compromise coping with life stressors.

Recurrence In a more descriptive vein, what sets mood disorders apart from their normal emotional counterparts is the clustering of signs and symptoms into discrete syndromes that typically recur on an episodic basis or pursue an intermittent, subthreshold course over the span of many years, if not a lifetime. Cyclic course and, in some cases, regular periodic recurrence are other signs of mood dysregulation that are particularly relevant to bipolar disorder.

Impairment Normative reactions to adversity and stress, including biological stress, typically consist of transient admixtures of anxiety and dysphoria that are best captured under the DSM-IV-TR rubric of adjustment disorder with mixed emotional features. That is, self-limiting reactions are best qualified broadly as normal affective states that produce little, if any, impairment in the main areas of functioning.

Although anxiety, irritability, and anger do occur in various types of mood disorders, pathologically sustained mood states of depression and elation characterize those disorders. Morbid mood states (mood disorders) then consist of protracted emotional reactions that deepen or escalate, respectively, into clinical depression or mania, with a tendency to recur or to evolve into unremitting chronicity in 15 to 20 percent of cases. The contribution of temperamental peculiarities to such outcomes should be apparent. The impaired functioning characteristic of mood disorders is thus based on a combination of factors, including severity, autonomy, recurrence, and chronicity of the clinical features.

To recapitulate, dysregulation in mood disorders can take different forms. It could be expressed as a single severe episode that persists autonomously for many months and sometimes years, or it might recur with episodes of varying severity, years apart or in rapid succession, with or without interepisodic remission. In general, the earlier the age at onset, the more likely are recurrences, especially those of bipolar nature. Thus, depending on the course of the illness, impairment could be state dependent and could occur during an episode, or it could extend into the interepisodic period. According to National Institute of Mental Health (NIMH) estimates, on average, a woman with bipolar disorder spends 12 years in florid episodes (often hospitalized), loses 14 years from a productive career and motherhood, and has her life curtailed by 9 years. More recent weekly prospective observations over up to two decades in the NIMH Collaborative Study of Depression have shown that patients with bipolar disorder I are symptomatic 47 percent of the time, and bipolar disorder II patients are symptomatic 53 percent of the time, much of it spent in subthreshold depression. In this study, unipolar major depressive disorder was even more pervasive, with subacute chronicity 59 percent of the time.

Recent observations have also revealed another pattern of impairment. In dysthymic and cyclothymic disorders, which represent an intensification of temperamental instability, impairment is not due to the severity of the mood disturbance per se but to the cumulative impact of the dysregulation beginning in the juvenile or early adult years and continuing unabated or intermittently over long periods; hence, the frequent confusion with character pathology. Here, the impairment is more subtle but nonetheless is pervasive. Persons with cyclothymic disorder tend to be dilettantes, whereas those with dysthymic disorder often lead morose and colorless lives. The fundamental causes of mood disorders must be sought in the preclinical expressions in the offspring of adults with these disorders.

PSYCHOPATHOLOGY

Depressive Syndrome Like other illnesses, depressive disorder clusters into signs and symptoms that constitute what DSM-IV-TR and ICD-10 term *major depressive episode* (Table 13.6–2). These criteria attempt to set an operational threshold for depressive

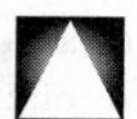

Table 13.6–2
DSM-IV-TR Criteria for Major Depressive Episode

A. Five (or more) of the following symptoms have been present during the same 2-week period and represent a change from previous functioning; at least one of the symptoms is (1) depressed mood or (2) loss of interest or pleasure.

Note: Do not include symptoms that are clearly due to a general medical condition or mood-incongruent delusions or hallucinations.

(1) Depressed mood most of the day, nearly every day, as indicated by subjective report (e.g., feels sad or empty) or observation made by others (e.g., appears tearful). *Note:* In children and adolescents, can be irritable mood.

(2) Markedly diminished interest or pleasure in all, or almost all, activities most of the day, nearly every day (as indicated by subjective account or observation made by others).

(3) Significant weight loss when not dieting or weight gain (e.g., a change of more than 5 percent of body weight in a month) or decrease or increase in appetite nearly every day. *Note:* In children, consider failure to make expected weight gains.

(4) Insomnia or hypersomnia nearly every day.

(5) Psychomotor agitation or retardation nearly every day (observable by others, not merely subjective feelings of restlessness or being slowed down).

(6) Fatigue or loss of energy nearly every day.

(7) Feelings of worthlessness or excessive or inappropriate guilt (which may be delusional) nearly every day (not merely self-reproach or guilt about being sick).

(8) Diminished ability to think or to concentrate or indecisiveness, nearly every day (by subjective account or as observed by others).

(9) Recurrent thoughts of death (not just fear of dying), recurrent suicidal ideation without a specific plan, or a suicide attempt or a specific plan for committing suicide.

B. The symptoms do not meet criteria for a mixed episode.

C. The symptoms cause clinically significant distress or impairment in social, occupational, or other important areas of functioning.

D. The symptoms are not due to the direct physiological effects of a substance (e.g., a drug of abuse, a medication) or a general medical condition (e.g., hypothyroidism).

E. The symptoms are not better accounted for by bereavement, that is, after the loss of a loved one, the symptoms persist for longer than 2 months or are characterized by marked functional impairment, morbid preoccupation with worthlessness, suicidal ideation, psychotic symptoms, or psychomotor retardation.

From American Psychiatric Association. *Diagnostic and Statistical Manual of Mental Disorders.* 4th ed. Text rev. Washington, DC: American Psychiatric Association; 2000, with permission.

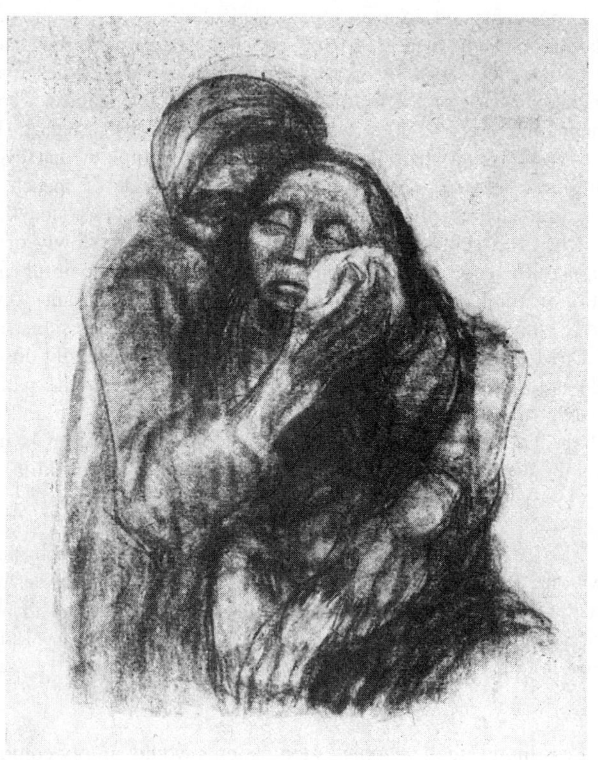

FIGURE 13.6–2 *Death Giving Comfort* by Kaethe Kollwitz (1867 to 1945).

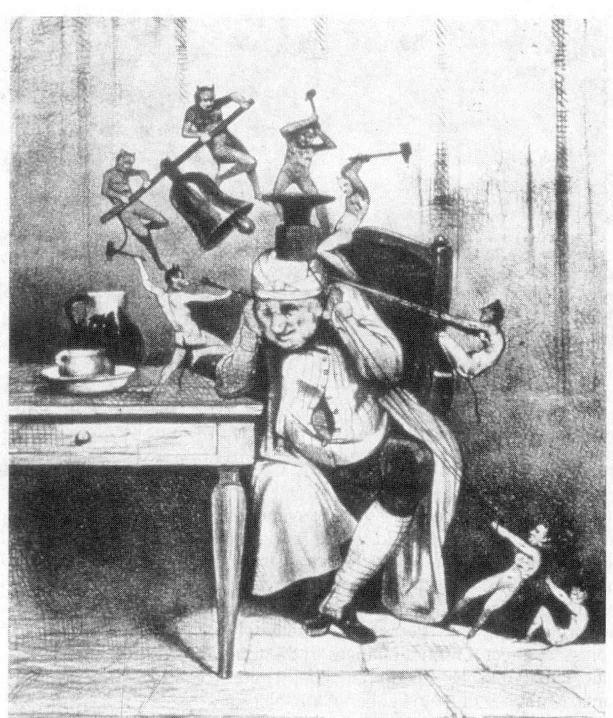

FIGURE 13.6–3 *Headache* by Honoré Daumier (1808 to 1879).

disorder based on a specified number of items and their temporal patterns. The diagnosis of clinical depression cannot be accomplished by a checklist: The DSM-IV-TR diagnostic criteria for major depressive disorder provide a general guide. Only after an in-depth phenomenological approach can a clinician ascertain diagnosis of a depressive disorder. Disturbances in all four spheres (mood, psychomotor activity, cognitive, and vegetative) should be ordinarily present for a definitive diagnosis of major depressive disorder, although that is not specified in DSM-IV-TR.

Mood Disturbances Mood change, usually considered the *sine qua non* of morbid depression, manifests in a variety of disturbances, including (1) painful arousal, (2) hypersensitivity to unpleasant events, (3) insensitivity to pleasant events, (4) insensitivity to unpleasant events, (5) reduced anticipatory pleasure, (6) anhedonia or reduced consummatory pleasure, (7) affective blunting, and (8) apathy. The phenomenology and psychometric properties of this broad range of mood disturbances are under investigation at the Salpêtrière Hospital in Paris. The focus in the description that follows is primarily on painfully aroused mood (depression) and diminished capacity for pleasure (anhedonia), two mood disturbances given selective weight in DSM-IV-TR and ICD-10.

DEPRESSED MOOD The term *depressed mood* refers to negative affective arousal, variously described as *depressed*, *anguished*, *mournful*, *irritable*, or *anxious*. These descriptions tend to trivialize a morbidly painful emotion, typically experienced as worse than the severest physical pain. Thus, depressed mood has a somatic quality that, in the extreme, is indescribably painful. Even when not so severe, depressive suffering is qualitatively distinct from its "neurotic" counterparts, taking the form of groundless apprehensions with severe inner turmoil and torment. This description is particularly apt for middle-aged and elderly persons, who were once considered to be experiencing *involutional melancholia*. The sustained nature of the mood permits no respite, although it tends to lift somewhat in the evening. Suicide may represent an attempt to find deliverance from such unrelenting psychic torment; death can be experienced as comforting (Fig. 13.6–2).

Patients with a milder form of the malady typically seen in primary care settings might deny experiencing mournful moods and instead complain of physical agony from headache (Fig. 13.6–3), epigastric pain, precordial distress, and so on, in the absence of any evidence of diagnosable physical illness. Such conditions have been described as *depressio sine depressione* or *masked depression*. In such cases, commonly observed in older patients, the physician should corroborate the presence of mood disturbance by the depressed affect in the patient's facial expression, vocal inflection, and overall appearance.

ANHEDONIA AND LOSS OF INTEREST Paradoxically, the heightened perception of pain in many persons with depressive disorder is accompanied by an inability to experience normal emotions. Patients exhibiting the disturbance may lose the capacity to cry, a deficit that is reversed as the depression is lifting.

In evaluating anhedonia, inquiring whether the patient has lost the sense of pleasure is not enough; the clinician must document that the patient has actually given up previously enjoyed pastimes. When mild, anhedonia evidences with a decreased interest in life. Later, patients complain that they have lost all interest in things. This is best illustrated by William Shakespeare in Hamlet's disgust: "How weary, stale, flat, and unprofitable seem to me all the uses of the world" (Act I, Scene II). In the extreme, patients lose their feelings for their children or spouses, who once were a source of joy. Thus, the hedonic deficit in clinical depression might represent a special instance of a more pervasive inability to experience emotions.

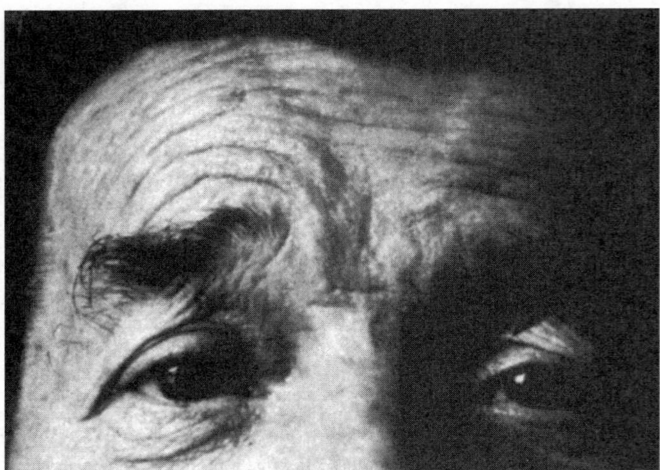

FIGURE 13.6–4 The Swiss neuropsychiatrist Otto Veraguth described a peculiar triangle-shaped fold in the nasal corner of the upper eyelid. The fold, often associated with depression, is referred to as *Veraguth's fold*. The photograph illustrates this physiognomic feature in a 50-year-old man during a major depressive episode. Veraguth's fold may also be seen in persons who are not clinically depressed, usually while they are harboring a mild depressive affect. Distinct changes in the tone of the corrugator and zygomatic facial muscles accompany depression, as shown on electromyograms. (Courtesy of Heinz E. Lehmann, M.D.)

Patients with severe depression may complain of being emotionally cut off from others and experience depersonalization and a world that seems strange to them (derealization). The impact of the loss of emotional resonance can be so pervasive that patients may denounce values and beliefs that had previously given meaning to their lives. For instance, members of the clergy might present with the complaint that they no longer believe in the Church and that they have lost God. The inability of the person with depressive disorder to experience normal emotions (commonly observed among young depressed patients) differs from the schizophrenic patient's flat affect in that the loss of emotions is itself experienced as painful; that is, the patient suffers immensely from the inability to experience emotions.

Psychomotor Disturbances In depression, psychomotor changes consist of abnormalities in the motor expression of mental and emotional activity. In severe cases, these changes manifest in specific facial features (Fig. 13.6–4).

PSYCHOMOTOR AGITATION Although agitation (pressured speech, restlessness, hand wringing, and hair pulling) is the more readily observed abnormality, it appears to be less specific to the illness than retardation (slowing of psychomotor activity). Psychophysiological studies have documented that such slowing often coexists with agitation.

PSYCHOMOTOR RETARDATION Underlying many of the deficits seen in clinical depression, some authorities believe psychomotor retardation to be the core, or primary, pathology in mood disorders. Morbid depression—what patients describe as being "down"—can be understood in terms of moderate to extreme psychomotor slowing. The patient experiences inertia, being unable to act physically and mentally. Recent brain imaging research that has revealed subcortical (extrapyramidal system) disturbances in mood disorders tends to support the centrality of psychomotor dysfunction in these disorders.

Long neglected in psychopathological research, psychomotor retardation can be measured with precision. The Salpêtrière Retardation Scale developed by Daniel Widlocher and colleagues places special emphasis on the following disturbances: (1) paucity of spontaneous movements; (2) slumped posture with downcast gaze (Fig. 13.6–5); (3) overwhelming fatigue (patients complain that everything is an effort); (4) reduced flow and amplitude of speech and increased latency of responses, often giving rise to monosyllabic speech; (5) a subjective feeling that time is passing slowly or has stopped; (6) poor concentration and forgetfulness; (7) painful rumination or thinking that dwells on a few (usually unpleasant) topics; and (8) indecisiveness or an inability to make simple decisions.

DSM-IV-TR places greater emphasis on the more easily observable objective or physical aspects of retardation. For the patient, however, the subjective sense of slowing is as pervasive and disabling. This more psychological dimension of retardation is most reliably elicited from depressed persons with good verbal skills.

Ms. A., a 34-year-old literature professor, presented to a mood clinic with the following complaint: "I am in a daze, confused, disoriented, staring. My thoughts do not flow, my mind is arrested. . . . I seem to lack any sense of direction, purpose. . . . I have such an inertia, I cannot assert myself. I cannot fight; I have no will."

Less linguistically sophisticated patients would simply complain of an inability to perform household chores or difficulty in concentrating on their studies. Such psychomotor deficits, in turn, underlie depressed patients' diminished efficiency or their inability to work.

PSEUDODEMENTIA The slowing of mental functions can be so pronounced in elderly persons that they experience memory difficulties, disorientation, and confusion.

STUPOR Psychomotor slowing in young persons is sometimes so extreme that patients might slide into a stupor, unable to participate even in basic biological functions, such as feeding themselves. Such an episode is often the precursor of bipolar disorder, which later declares itself in a manic episode. Today, depressive disorder is diagnosed in its earlier stages, and subtle stupor is much more likely to be encountered clinically.

A 20-year-old male college student seen in the emergency room spoke of "being stuck—as if I have fallen into a black hole and can't get out." Further evaluation revealed that the patient was metaphorically describing his total loss of initiative and drive and was engulfed by the disease process. A clinician without the requisite phenomenological training might consider such a patient bizarre and perhaps even psychotic. Yet, the patient responded dramatically to fluoxetine (Prozac) and, in 2 weeks, was back in school.

Cognitive Disturbances The cognitive view of depression considers negative evaluations of the self, the world, and the future (the negative triad) central to understanding depressed mood and behavior, but it is equally likely that the depressed mood colors perceptions of the self and others or that disturbed psychomotor activity leads to negative self-evaluations. Therefore, instead of being considered causal, the cognitive triad in depression is best approached empirically as a psychopathological manifestation of depression. Faulty thinking patterns are clinically expressed as (1) ideas of dep-

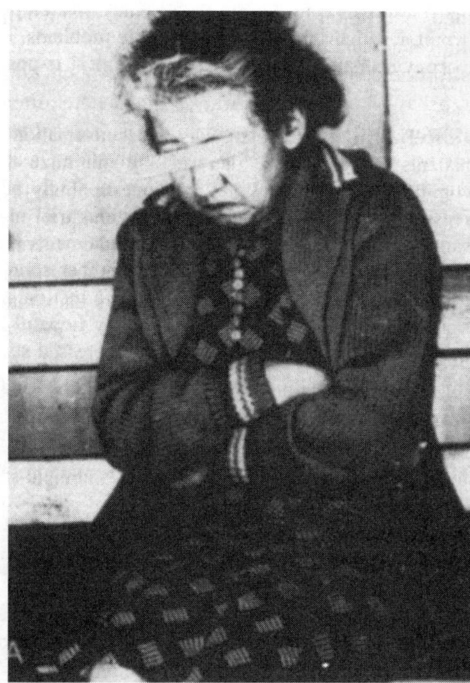

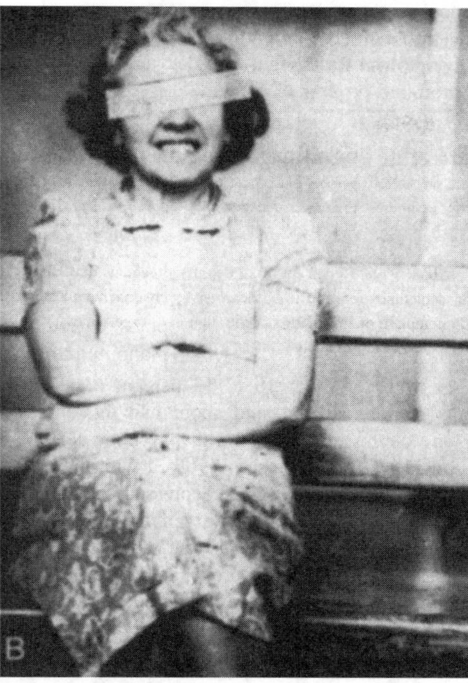

FIGURE 13.6–5 A 38-year-old woman during a state of deep retarded depression **(A)** and 2 months later, after recovery **(B)**. Note the turned-down corners of her mouth, her stooped posture, her drab clothing, and her hairdo during the depressed episode. (Courtesy of Heinz E. Lehmann, M.D.)

rivation and loss; (2) low self-esteem and self-confidence; (3) self-reproach and pathological guilt; (4) helplessness, hopelessness, and pessimism; and (5) recurrent thoughts of death and suicide.

The essential characteristic of depressive thinking is that the patient views everything in an extremely negative light. The self-accusations are typically unjustified or are blown out of proportion, as in the case of a middle-aged woman who was tormented by guilt, because, as a child, she had not repaid a nickel that she had borrowed from a classmate. Some of the thoughts may verge on the delusional. For instance, an internationally renowned scientist complained that he was "nothing." Self-evaluations that indicate an extremely low image of one's self might, nonetheless, reflect an accurate perception of one's impairment from psychomotor retardation.

MOOD-CONGRUENT PSYCHOTIC FEATURES In depressive disorder with psychotic features (Table 13.6–3), negative thinking acquires grossly delusional proportions and is maintained with such conviction that the thoughts are not amenable to change by evidence to the contrary. According to Kurt Schneider, delusional thinking in depression derives from humankind's four basic insecurities—those regarding health, financial status, moral worth, and relationship to others. Thus, severely depressed patients may have delusions of worthlessness and sinfulness, reference, and persecution: They believe that they are being singled out for their past mistakes and that everyone is aware of their incompetence. Persecutory ideation in depression is often *prosecutory* in that it derives from the belief that one deserves punishment for such transgressions. A severely depressed man may feel so incompetent in all areas of functioning, including the sexual sphere, that he may suspect his wife of having an affair (delusion of infidelity).

Other depressed persons believe that they have mismanaged their finances in such a way that their children will starve (delusions of poverty); that they are harboring an occult illness, such as cancer or the acquired immune deficiency syndrome (AIDS) (delusions of ill health); or that parts of their bodies are missing (nihilistic delusions). In more severe illness, the patient might feel that the world has changed and that calamity and destruction await everyone. In rare tragic instances, a parent with such delusions might kill his or her young children to save them from moral or physical decay and then commit suicide. In women with psychotic depression, infanticide is most likely to occur in the postpartum period, often leading to all types of inappropriate interpretations in the media. Finally, a minority of depressed persons have fleeting auditory or visual hallucinations with extremely unpleasant content along the lines of their delusions (e.g., hearing accusatory voices or seeing themselves in coffins or graveyards). All of these psychotic experiences are genuine affective delusions or hallucinations. They are mood congruent in the sense that they are phenomenologically understandable in light of the prevailing pathological mood.

MOOD-INCONGRUENT PSYCHOTIC FEATURES Sometimes so-called first-rank or schneiderian-type symptoms can arise in the setting of a major depressive episode.

A 42-year-old civil servant said that she was so paralyzed by depression that she felt that she had no personal initiative and volition left; she believed that some malignant force had taken over her actions and that it was commenting on every action that she was undertaking. The patient recovered fully with thymoleptic medication. There is no reason to believe that, in this patient, the feelings of somatic passivity and running commentary indicated a schizophrenic process.

Thus, with proper phenomenological probing, certain classes of apparently mood-incongruent psychotic experiences listed in DSM-IV-TR can be understood as arising from the pathological mood and the profound changes in psychomotor activity that accompany them. (In other instances, the clinician must seek a history of alcohol or substance use disorder or withdrawal as a putative explanation for mood incongruence in psychotic depression.) In brief, incidental schneiderian first-rank symptoms should not distract from the diag-

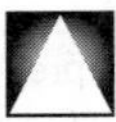

Table 13.6–3
DSM-IV-TR Criteria for Severity, Psychotic, and Remission Specifiers for Current (or Most Recent) Major Depressive Episode

Note: Code in fifth digit. Mild, moderate, severe without psychotic features, and severe with psychotic features can be applied only if the criteria are currently met for a major depressive episode. In partial remission and in full remission, they can be applied to the most recent major depressive episode in major depressive disorder and to a major depressive episode in bipolar I or II disorder only if it is the most recent type of mood episode.

Mild: Few, if any, symptoms in excess of those required to make the diagnosis. Symptoms result in only minor impairment in occupational functioning or in usual social activities or relationships with others.

Moderate: Symptoms or functional impairment between *mild* and *severe.*

Severe without psychotic features: Several symptoms in excess of those required to make the diagnosis. Symptoms markedly interfere with occupational functioning or with usual social activities or relationships with others.

Severe with psychotic features: Delusions or hallucinations. If possible, specify whether the psychotic features are mood-congruent or mood-incongruent:

Mood-congruent psychotic features: Delusions or hallucinations whose content is entirely consistent with the typical depressive themes of personal inadequacy, guilt, disease, death, nihilism, or deserved punishment.

Mood-incongruent psychotic features: Delusions or hallucinations whose content does not involve typical depressive themes of personal inadequacy, guilt, disease, death, nihilism, or deserved punishment. Included are such symptoms as persecutory delusions (not directly related to depressive themes), thought insertion, thought broadcasting, and delusions of control.

In partial remission: Symptoms of a major depressive episode are present, but full criteria are not met, or there is a period without any significant symptoms of a major depressive episode lasting less than 2 months after the end of the major depressive episode. (If the major depressive episode was superimposed on dysthymic disorder, the diagnosis of dysthymic disorder alone is given once the full criteria for a major depressive episode are no longer met.)

In full remission: During the past 2 months, no significant signs or symptoms of the disturbance were present.

Unspecified.

From American Psychiatric Association. *Diagnostic and Statistical Manual of Mental Disorders.* 4th ed. Text rev. Washington, DC: American Psychiatric Association; 2000, with permission.

nosis of an affective psychosis if otherwise typical signs and symptoms of mood disorder are present.

HOPELESSNESS AND SUICIDE Given that most, if not all, clinically depressed patients find themselves locked in the private hell of their negative thoughts, it is not surprising that many untreated or inadequately treated patients give up hope of ever recovering and kill themselves. The suicide attempt is not, however, undertaken in the depth of melancholia. When asked if she had any suicide plans, one severely depressed patient of the author replied, "Doctor, I don't exist—I am already dead."

Thus, the risk of suicide is less pronounced during acute severe depression. Emil Kraepelin observed that it is when psychomotor activity is improving, yet mood and thinking are still dark, that the patient is most likely to muster the requisite energy to commit the suicidal act. Aaron Beck's work has shown that hopelessness on mental status evaluation in a patient recovering from depression should alert the clinician to the possibility of such an outcome. The discovery of a therapeutic modality that could achieve improvement of psychomotor, mood, and cognitive components in tandem will constitute a major clinical advance.

There is no basis for the common belief that inquiring about suicide provokes such behavior. On the contrary, patients are often relieved that the physician appreciates the magnitude of their suffering. Suicidal ideation is commonly expressed indirectly (e.g., in a wish not to wake up or to die from a malignant disease). Some depressed persons are tormented with suicidal obsessions and are constantly resisting unwanted urges or impulses to destroy themselves. Others might yield to such urges passively (e.g., by careless driving or by walking into high-speed traffic). A third group harbors elaborate plans, carefully preparing a will and taking out insurance. Deliberate planning indicates a high suicidal risk. The foregoing examples are not exhaustive; they are meant to remind clinicians in charge of depressed patients to be alert always to the possibility of suicide.

Vegetative Disturbances The Greeks considered depression a somatic illness and ascribed it to black bile; hence, the term *melancholia.* The mood change in depressive disorder is accompanied by measurable alterations of biorhythms that implicate midbrain dysfunction. Once the changes occur, they tend to be independent of the environment throughout much of the episode, and, as a consequence, they do not respond to interpersonal feedback of a pleasant or upbeat nature. The biological concomitants of melancholia include profound reductions in appetite, sleep, and sexual functioning, as well as alterations in other circadian rhythms, especially matinal worsening of mood and psychomotor performance. These disturbances are central to the DSM-IV-TR concept of melancholia (Table 13.6–4), a form of depression in which such biological concomitants predominate. An equally prominent subgroup of depressed persons exhibits a reversal of the vegetative and circadian functions, with increases in appetite and sleep—and sometimes in sexual functioning—and an evening worsening of mood; in this atypical pattern (Table 13.6–5), patients characteristically exhibit mood reactivity and sensitivity to rejection. Marked retardation might herald a manic switch, whereas atypicality should raise the suspicion of bipolar II disorder.

ANOREXIA AND WEIGHT LOSS The most reliable somatic indicators of depressive disorder include anorexia and weight loss. In addition to being a hypothalamic-based disturbance in depression, anorexia might be secondary to blunted olfactory or taste sensations or a decreased enjoyment of food, or (rarely) it might result from a delusional belief that the food has been poisoned.

Inanition, especially in elderly persons, can lead to malnutrition and electrolyte disturbances that represent medical emergencies in their own right. If weight loss is severe, especially after 40 years of age, the psychiatrist should first use appropriate medical consultation to rule out the likelihood of an occult malignancy.

WEIGHT GAIN Overeating, decreased activity, or both may result in weight gain. In middle-aged patients, it may aggravate preexisting diabetes mellitus, hypertension, or coronary artery disease. In younger patients, especially women, weight problems may conform to a bulimic pattern that is often the expression of the depressive phase of a bipolar disorder with infrequent hypomanic periods (bipolar II disorder).

INSOMNIA Sleep disturbance, a cardinal sign of depression, often is characterized by multiple awakenings, especially in the early hours of the morning, rather than by difficulty falling asleep. The light sleep of a depressed person, in part a reflection of the painful arousal of the disorder, tends to prolong the depressive agony over 24 hours. Thus, deep stages of sleep (III and IV) are decreased or deficient. The attempt to overcome the problem by drinking alcohol may initially succeed but ultimately aggravates

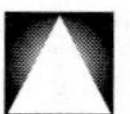

Table 13.6–4
DSM-IV-TR Criteria for Melancholic Features Specifier

Specify if:

With melancholic features (can be applied to the current or most recent major depressive episode in major depressive disorder and to a major depressive episode in bipolar I disorder or bipolar II disorder, only if it is the most recent type of mood episode)

A. Either of the following, occurring during the most severe period of the current episode:
 (1) Loss of pleasure in all, or almost all, activities
 (2) Lack of reactivity to usually pleasurable stimuli (does not feel much better, even temporarily, when something good happens)

B. Three (or more) of the following:
 (1) Distinct quality of depressed mood (i.e., the depressed mood is experienced as distinctly different from the kind of feeling experienced after the death of a loved one)
 (2) Depression regularly worse in the morning
 (3) Early morning awakening (at least 2 hours before usual time of awakening)
 (4) Marked psychomotor retardation or agitation
 (5) Significant anorexia or weight loss
 (6) Excessive or inappropriate guilt

From American Psychiatric Association. *Diagnostic and Statistical Manual of Mental Disorders.* 4th ed. Text rev. Washington, DC: American Psychiatric Association; 2000, with permission.

the sleep patterns and insomnia. This is also true for sedative-hypnotic agents, which are often prescribed by the busy general practitioner who has not spent enough time diagnosing the depressive condition. Although sedatives (including alcohol) effectively reduce the number of awakenings in the short term, they are not effective in the long run, because they further diminish stage III and stage IV sleep. They are not antidepressants, and they tend to prolong the depression.

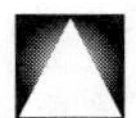

Table 13.6–5
DSM-IV-TR Criteria for Atypical Features Specifier

Specify if:

With atypical features (can be applied when these features predominate during the most recent 2 weeks of a current major depressive episode in major depressive disorder or in bipolar I disorder or bipolar II disorder when a current major depressive episode is the most recent type of mood episode, or when these features predominate during the most recent 2 years of dysthymic disorder; if the major depressive episode is not current, it applies if the feature predominates during any 2-week period).

A. Mood reactivity (i.e., mood brightens in response to actual or potential positive events).

B. Two (or more) of the following features:
 (1) Significant weight gain or increase in appetite
 (2) Hypersomnia
 (3) Leaden paralysis (i.e., heavy, leaden feelings in arms or legs)
 (4) Long-standing pattern of interpersonal rejection sensitivity (not limited to episodes of mood disturbance) that results in significant social or occupational impairment

C. Criteria are not met for with melancholic features or with catatonic features during the same episode.

From American Psychiatric Association. *Diagnostic and Statistical Manual of Mental Disorders.* 4th ed. Text rev. Washington, DC: American Psychiatric Association; 2000, with permission.

HYPERSOMNIA Young depressed patients, especially those with bipolar tendencies, often exhibit excessive sleep and have difficulty getting up in the morning.

Kevin, a 15-year-old boy, was referred to a sleep center to rule out narcolepsy. His main complaints were fatigue, boredom, and a need to sleep all the time. Although he had always started the day somewhat slowly, he now could not get out of bed to go to school. That alarmed his mother, prompting sleep consultation. Formerly a B student, he had been failing most of his courses in the 6 months before referral. Psychological counseling, predicated on the premise that his family's recent move from another city had led to Kevin's isolation, had not been beneficial. Extensive neurological and general medical workup had also proven negative. He slept 12 to 15 hours per day but denied cataplexy, sleep paralysis, and hypnagogic hallucinations. During psychiatric interview, he denied being depressed but admitted that he had lost interest in everything except his dog. He had no drive, participated in no activities, and had gained 30 pounds in 6 months. He believed that he was "brain damaged" and wondered whether it was worth living like that. The question of suicide disturbed him, as it was contrary to his religious beliefs. These findings led to the prescription of desipramine (Norpramin) in a dosage that was gradually increased to 200 mg per day over 3 weeks. Not only did desipramine reverse the presenting complaints, but it also pushed him to the brink of a manic episode.

The affective nature of the disorder in such patients is often unrecognized, and their behavior is attributed to "laziness." The vignette also illustrates the emergence of manic behavior during antidepressant treatment. Such shifts in polarity are common in major depressive disorder and necessitate revising the diagnosis to a bipolar disorder (contrary to the admonitions of DSM-IV-TR). Hypersomnia associated with lethargy should actually raise strong suspicion of bipolar disorder in young depressives. In the elderly, organic or brain pathology should be suspected.

CIRCADIAN DYSREGULATION Many circadian functions, such as temperature regulation and cortisol rhythms, are disrupted in major depressive disorder. Disturbances of sleep rhythms, however, have received the greatest research focus. These include deficits in stage IV or delta sleep, as well as more intense rapid eye movement (REM) activity in the first one-third of the night. More specific to depressive disorders—whether suffering from insomnia or hypersomnia—nearly two-thirds of patients exhibit a marked shortening of REM latency, the period from the onset of sleep to the first REM period. This abnormality is observed throughout the depressive episode and may also be seen during relatively euthymic periods in persons with recurrent depression. The occurrence of short REM latency in the younger clinically well relatives of the affectively ill suggests that neurophysiological abnormalities might precede the overt psychopathological manifestations of the illness; on closer scrutiny, these "well" relatives are often found to meet criteria for subthreshold mood conditions, such as dysthymic disorder, intermittent depression, or labile temperament.

Few data exist on the consistency of sleep electroencephalographic (EEG) abnormalities in patients from episode to episode. However, clinical experience suggests that a patient observed over time (even during the same episode) may exhibit insomnia and morning worsening of mood and activity during one period of the disorder and hypersomnia extending to late morning hours during another period. In either case, persons with depressive disorder are characteristically tired in the morning, which means that even prolonged sleep is not refreshing for them. The propensity to exhibit such divergent patterns of sleep disturbance is more likely in bipolar disorders. Patients with major depressive disorder tend to exhibit insomnia more stereotypically episode after episode; despite extreme fatigue, they rarely oversleep. Such fatigue coexisting with negative affective arousal is even more exhausting.

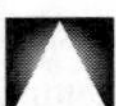

Table 13.6–6
DSM-IV-TR Criteria for Seasonal Pattern Specifier

Specify if:

With seasonal pattern (can be applied to the pattern of major depressive episodes in bipolar I disorder, bipolar II disorder, or major depressive disorder, recurrent).

A. There has been a regular temporal relationship between the onset of major depressive episodes in bipolar I disorder or bipolar II disorder or major depressive disorder, recurrent, and a particular time of the year (e.g., regular appearance of the major depressive episode in the fall or winter).

Note: Do not include cases in which there is an obvious effect of seasonal-related psychosocial stressors (e.g., regularly being unemployed every winter).

B. Full remissions (or a change from depression to mania or hypomania) also occur at a characteristic time of the year (e.g., depression disappears in the spring).

C. In the last 2 years, two major depressive episodes have occurred that demonstrate the temporal seasonal relationships defined in Criteria A and B, and no nonseasonal major depressive episodes have occurred during that same period.

D. Seasonal major depressive episodes (as described previously) substantially outnumber the nonseasonal major depressive episodes that may have occurred over the individual's lifetime.

From American Psychiatric Association. *Diagnostic and Statistical Manual of Mental Disorders.* 4th ed. Text rev. Washington, DC: American Psychiatric Association; 2000, with permission.

SEASONALITY Another classic biorhythmic disturbance in mood disorders is seasonal (especially autumn-winter) accentuation or precipitation of depression. Most of those patients experience increased energy and activation, if not frank hypomania, in the spring. In the fall and winter, they complain of fatigue, tend to crave sugars, and overeat and oversleep. The hypersomnia in some of these patients is associated with delayed (rather than short) REM latencies. These data suggest dysregulation of circadian rhythms in depressive disorders rather than mere phase advance. Given the biphasic nature of the clinical phenomenology, some autumn-winter depressions belong to the bipolar spectrum (type II). Although autumn-winter depression has received the greatest attention, there also exist summer depressions; the former appear related to reduction of daylight (photoperiods), and the latter appear related to increased temperature. The DSM-IV-TR criteria for seasonal pattern specifiers are listed in Table 13.6–6.

SEXUAL DYSFUNCTION Decreased sexual desire is seen in depressed men and women. In addition, some women experience temporary interruption of their menses. Depressed women are often unresponsive to lovemaking or are disinclined to participate in it, a situation that could lead to marital conflict. Psychotherapists might mistakenly ascribe the depression to the marital conflict and might devote unnecessarily zealous psychotherapeutic attention to conjugal issues. Decreased or lost libido in men often results in erectile failure, which may prompt endocrinological or urological consultation. Again, depression may be ascribed to the sexual dysfunction rather than the reverse, and definitive treatment may be delayed by the focus on the sexual complaint. The author is aware of some men with depressive disorder who were subjected to permanent penile implants before receiving more definitive treatment for their depression. This is less likely to occur in the sildenafil (Viagra) era, but even treatment with such agents would not necessarily resolve the impotence in clinically depressed patients without competent treatment of the mood disorder. Selective serotonin reuptake inhibitors (SSRIs) typically aggravate the sexual dysfunction, whereas bupropion (Wellbutrin) tends to improve it.

A small subgroup of persons with depressive disorder may exhibit increased sexual drive or activity of a compulsive nature. These patients tend to have other atypical features as well; hence, the increased sexual drive can be considered the *fifth reverse vegetative sign* (after evening worsening of mood, initial insomnia, hypersomnia, and weight gain). The author is aware of several patients who derive temporary reversal of their depression after intense sexual encounters. In these depressed persons, increased sexual drive, intensity, or both may indicate a mixed episode of bipolar disorder (type II). Further scrutiny in such cases often reveals a premorbid cyclothymic or hyperthymic temperament. Current data suggest that, depending on the breadth of the criteria used, 30 to 70 percent of depressions with atypical features belong to the bipolar spectrum.

Manic Syndrome

As with clinical depression, the psychopathology of mania (Table 13.6–7) can be conveniently discussed under mood, psychomotor, circadian, and cognitive disturbances. The clinical features of mania are generally the opposite of those of depression. Thus, instead of lowered mood, thinking, activity, and self-esteem, there is elevated mood, a rush of ideas, psychomotor acceleration, and grandiosity. Despite those contrasts, the two disorders share such symptoms as irritability, anger, insomnia, and agitation. Actually, an excess of the latter symptoms of escalating intensity suggests a mixed phase or mixed episode (Table 13.6–8) of mania and depression occurring simultaneously. DSM-IV-TR does not specifically mention the foregoing signs and symptoms, which recent research has identified as clinical pointers toward mixed states. Manic and mixed episodes represent the hallmark of what

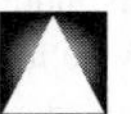

Table 13.6–7
DSM-IV-TR Criteria for Manic Episode

A. A distinct period of abnormally and persistently elevated, expansive, or irritable mood, lasting at least 1 week (or any duration if hospitalization is necessary).

B. During the period of mood disturbance, three (or more) of the following symptoms have persisted (four, if the mood is only irritable) and have been present to a significant degree:

(1) Inflated self-esteem or grandiosity
(2) Decreased need for sleep (e.g., feels rested after only 3 hours of sleep)
(3) More talkative than usual or pressure to keep talking
(4) Flight of ideas or subjective experience that thoughts are racing
(5) Distractibility (i.e., attention too easily drawn to unimportant or irrelevant external stimuli)
(6) Increase in goal-directed activity (socially, at work or school, or sexually) or psychomotor agitation
(7) Excessive involvement in pleasurable activities that have a high potential for painful consequences (e.g., engaging in unrestrained buying sprees, sexual indiscretions, or foolish business investments)

C. The symptoms do not meet criteria for a mixed episode.

D. The mood disturbance is sufficiently severe to cause marked impairment in occupational functioning or in usual social activities or relationships with others or to necessitate hospitalization to prevent harm to self or others, or there are psychotic features.

E. The symptoms are not due to the direct physiological effects of a substance (e.g., a drug of abuse, a medication, or other treatment) or a general medical condition (e.g., hyperthyroidism).

Note: Manic-like episodes that are clearly caused by somatic antidepressant treatment (e.g., medication, electroconvulsive therapy, or light therapy) should not count toward a diagnosis of bipolar I disorder.

From American Psychiatric Association. *Diagnostic and Statistical Manual of Mental Disorders.* 4th ed. Text rev. Washington, DC: American Psychiatric Association; 2000, with permission.

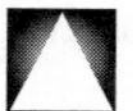

Table 13.6–8
DSM-IV-TR Criteria for Mixed Episode

A. The criteria are met for a manic episode and a major depressive episode (except for duration) nearly every day during at least a 1-week period.
B. The mood disturbance is sufficiently severe to cause marked impairment in occupational functioning or in usual social activities or relationships with others or to necessitate hospitalization to prevent harm to self or others, or there are psychotic features.
C. The symptoms are not due to the direct physiological effects of a substance (e.g., a drug of abuse, a medication, or other treatment) or a general medical condition (e.g., hyperthyroidism).
Note: Mixed-like episodes that are clearly caused by somatic antidepressant treatment (e.g., medication, electroconvulsive therapy, or light therapy) should not count toward a diagnosis of bipolar I disorder.

From American Psychiatric Association. *Diagnostic and Statistical Manual of Mental Disorders.* 4th ed. Text rev. Washington, DC: American Psychiatric Association; 2000, with permission.

was once termed *manic-depressive psychosis* and is currently termed *bipolar I disorder*.

Although milder or hypomanic features (Table 13.6–9) can contribute to success in business, leadership roles, and the arts, recurrences of even mild manic symptomatology are typically disruptive. The elated mood tends to produce overoptimism concerning one's abilities, which, coupled with the impulsivity characteristic of mania, often leads to disaster. Thus, accurate and early diagnosis is paramount.

Classic mania, as formulated in the DSM-IV-TR operationalism of manic episode (Table 13.6–7), is relatively easy to recognize. Misdiagnosis was once rampant in North American practice, as clinicians confused severe mania with schizophrenia and confused its milder variants with normality or with narcissistic and sociopathic personality disorders. Like the misdiagnosis of depressive conditions, such errors of clinical judgment are due to a lack of familiarity with the phenomenology of the classic illness. Again, DSM-IV-TR criteria provide only a guideline. The actual diagnosis requires careful history and phenomenological understanding by an empathic observer. The manic patient lifts the observer's mood and makes the examiner smile and even laugh but can also be irritating. The patient's speech is fast and may even appear to the novice psychiatry student as "loose," but it also can often be witty. Finally, the behavior is typically dramatic, expansive, and jesting. Although not specifically listed in DSM-IV-TR, current research indicates that social disinhibition and pathological overfamiliarity with strangers represent cardinal features of mania and can be contrasted with the withdrawal of most schizophrenic patients. For the experienced clinician, the overall gestalt experienced in the presence of manic patients is emotionally and qualitatively distinct from that of persons with schizophrenia or frontal lobe diseases; the latter conditions tend to leave the examiner cold. These considerations become clearer when the clinical observer systematically examines the psychopathology of mania in the areas of mood, behavior, and thinking.

Mood Disturbance

Mood disturbance in mania represents a contrast to that observed in depression, but not entirely.

MOOD ELEVATION The mood in mania is classically one of elation, euphoria, and jubilation, typically associated with laughing, punning, and gesturing.

LABILITY AND IRRITABILITY The prevailing positive mood in mania is not stable, and momentary crying or bursting into tears is common.

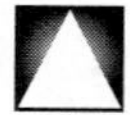

Table 13.6–9
DSM-IV-TR Criteria for Hypomanic Episode

A. A distinct period of persistently elevated, expansive, or irritable mood, lasting throughout at least 4 days, that is clearly different from the usual nondepressed mood.
B. During the period of mood disturbance, three (or more) of the following symptoms have persisted (four, if the mood is only irritable) and have been present to a significant degree:
(1) Inflated self-esteem or grandiosity
(2) Decreased need for sleep (e.g., feels rested after only 3 hours of sleep)
(3) More talkative than usual or pressure to keep talking
(4) Flight of ideas or subjective experience that thoughts are racing
(5) Distractibility (i.e., attention too easily drawn to unimportant or irrelevant external stimuli)
(6) Increase in goal-directed activity (socially, at work or school, or sexually) or psychomotor agitation
(7) Excessive involvement in pleasurable activities that have a high potential for painful consequences (e.g., the person engages in unrestrained buying sprees, sexual indiscretions, or foolish business investments)
C. The episode is associated with an unequivocal change in functioning that is uncharacteristic of the person when not symptomatic.
D. The disturbance in mood and the change in functioning are observable by others.
E. The episode is not severe enough to cause marked impairment in social or occupational functioning or to necessitate hospitalization, and there are no psychotic features.
F. The symptoms are not due to the direct physiological effects of a substance (e.g., a drug of abuse, a medication, or other treatment) or a general medical condition (e.g., hyperthyroidism).
Note: Hypomanic-like episodes that are clearly caused by somatic antidepressant treatment (e.g., medication, electroconvulsive therapy, or light therapy) should not count toward a diagnosis of bipolar II disorder.

From American Psychiatric Association. *Diagnostic and Statistical Manual of Mental Disorders.* 4th ed. Text rev. Washington, DC: American Psychiatric Association; 2000, with permission.

Also, the high is so excessive that many patients experience it as intense nervousness. When crossed, patients can become extremely irritable and hostile. Thus, lability and irritable hostility are as much features of the manic mood as is elation. In mixed manic states, they dominate the clinical picture, giving rise to what is now termed *dysphoric mania* (and what Kraepelin had characterized as *anxious-depressive mania*).

Psychomotor Acceleration

Accelerated psychomotor activity, the hallmark of mania, is characterized by overabundant energy and activity and rapid, pressured speech. Subjectively, the patient experiences an unusual sense of physical well-being (eutonia).

FLIGHT OF IDEAS Thinking processes are accelerated, subjectively experienced as flight of ideas, and thinking and perception are unusually sharp. The patient may speak with such pressure that associations are difficult to follow; such clang associations are often based on rhyming or chance perceptions and can be lightning fast. The pressure to speak may continue despite the development of hoarseness (a characteristic shared with some politicians on the campaign trail!).

IMPULSIVE BEHAVIOR Manic patients are typically impulsive, disinhibited, and meddlesome. Pathological familiarity with total strangers is also a feature not specifically listed in the DSM-IV-TR schema for mania, yet it is one of its cardinal signs. They are intrusive in their increased involvement with others, leading to friction with family members, friends, and colleagues. They

Table 13.6–10
DSM-IV-TR Criteria for Catatonic Features Specifier

Specify if:

With catatonic features (can be applied to the current or most recent major depressive episode, manic episode, or mixed episode in major depressive disorder, bipolar I disorder, or bipolar II disorder)

The clinical picture is dominated by at least two of the following:

(1) Motoric immobility as evidenced by catalepsy (including waxy flexibility) or stupor
(2) Excessive motor activity (that is apparently purposeless and not influenced by external stimuli)
(3) Extreme negativism (an apparently motiveless resistance to all instructions or maintenance of a rigid posture against attempts to be moved) or mutism
(4) Peculiarities of voluntary movement as evidenced by posturing (voluntary assumption of inappropriate or bizarre postures), stereotyped movements, prominent mannerisms, or prominent grimacing
(5) Echolalia or echopraxia

From American Psychiatric Association. *Diagnostic and Statistical Manual of Mental Disorders.* 4th ed. Text rev. Washington, DC: American Psychiatric Association; 2000, with permission.

are distractible and move quickly, not only from one thought to another, but also from one person to another, showing heightened interest in every new activity that strikes their fancy. They are indefatigable and engage in various activities in which they usually display poor social judgment. Examples include preaching or dancing in the street; abuse of long-distance calling; buying new cars, hundreds of records, expensive jewelry, or other unnecessary items; paying the bills of total strangers in bars; giving away furniture; impulsive marriages; engaging in risky business ventures; gambling; and sudden trips. Such pursuits can lead to personal and financial ruin.

DELIRIOUS MANIA An extremely severe expression of mania (once known as *Bell's mania*), delirious mania involves frenzied physical activity that continues unabated and leads to delirium and disorientation—a life-threatening medical emergency. This complication, the manic counterpart of stupor, is rare today. (There is no need to invoke here the concept of catatonic features as advocated by DSM-IV-TR [Table 13.6–10]. The DSM-IV-TR position is terminologically confusing and phenomenologically imprecise.)

Vegetative Disturbances

Vegetative disturbances are more difficult to evaluate in mania than in depression.

HYPOSOMNIA Hyposomnia is the cardinal sign of decreased need for sleep—the patient sleeps only a few hours but feels energetic on awakening. Some patients may actually go sleepless for several days. This could lead to dangerous escalation of manic activity, which might continue despite signs of physical exhaustion.

INATTENTION TO NUTRITION There does not seem to be a clinically significant level of appetite disturbance as such, but weight loss may occur because of increased activity and neglect of nutritional needs.

SEXUAL EXCESSES Although hypersexuality is a cardinal sign of mania, it is not listed separately in the DSM-IV-TR criteria. Instead, it is diluted in Criteria B6 and B7 (Table 13.6–7). The sexual appetite is typically increased and may lead to sexual indiscretion. Married women with previously unblemished sexual lives may associate with men below their social status. Men typically overindulge in alcohol, frequent bars, and may squander their savings on prostitutes. The sexual misadventures of manic patients result in marital disasters and, hence, the multiple separations or divorces that are almost pathognomonic of the disorder. The sexual excesses of bipolar patients are even more problematic today, in view of the specter of AIDS.

Cognitive Distortions

Manic thinking is overly positive, optimistic, and expansive.

GRANDIOSITY, LACK OF INSIGHT, AND POOR JUDGMENT The patient exhibits inflated self-esteem and a grandiose sense of confidence and achievements. Behind that facade, however, may be a vague and painful recognition that the positive self-concepts do not represent reality. However, such insight (if present at all) is transient, and manic patients are notoriously refractory to self-examination and insight. Denial and lack of insight, cardinal psychological derangements of mania, are not listed in the DSM-IV-TR criteria for manic episode or bipolar disorders. This is a serious omission, because it is this lack of insight—coupled with poor judgment—that leads manic patients to engage in activities that harm themselves and their loved ones. It also explains, in part, their nonadherence with medication regimens during the manic phase.

DELUSION FORMATION Manic patients often harbor delusional beliefs, including delusions of exceptional mental and physical fitness and talent; delusions of wealth, aristocratic ancestry, or other grandiose identity; delusions of assistance (i.e., well-placed persons or supernatural powers are assisting their endeavors); or delusions of reference and persecution, based on the belief that enemies are observing or following them out of jealousy at their special abilities. At the height of mania, patients may even see visions or hear voices congruent with their euphoric mood and grandiose self-image (e.g., they might see images of heaven or hear cherubs chanting songs to praise them). The denial characteristic of mania—and the frequently psychotic nature of episodes—means that clinicians must routinely obtain diagnostic information about past episodes from significant others. Lack of insight also unfortunately means that hospitalization must often be arranged on an involuntary basis.

MOOD-INCONGRUENT PSYCHOSIS Psychosis in the setting of mania and mixed manic episodes is typically mood congruent. The sense of physical well-being and mental alacrity is so extraordinary that it is understandable why manic patients believe that they possess superior powers or perhaps are great scientists or famous reformers. Moreover, their senses are so vivid that reality appears richer and more exotic and can be easily transformed into a vision.

Likewise, their thoughts are so rapid and vibrant that they feel that they can hear them. Thus, certain first-rank schneiderian-type symptoms that have been traditionally considered mood incongruent can be understood phenomenologically to arise from the powerful mental experiences of mania.

A 37-year-old engineer had experienced three manic episodes for which he had been hospitalized; all three episodes were preceded by several weeks of moderate psychomotor retardation. Although he had responded to lithium (Eskalith) each time, once outside the hospital, he had been reluctant to take it and eventually refused to do so. Now that he was "euthymic," after his third and most disruptive episode during which he had badly beaten his wife, he could more accurately explain how he felt when manic. Mania, he experienced as "God implanted in him," so he could serve as "testimony to man's communication with God." He elaborated as follows: "Ordinary mortals will never, never understand the supreme manic state which I'm privileged to experience every few years. It is so vivid, so intense, so compelling. When I feel that way, there can be no other explanation: To be manic is, ultimately, to be God. God himself must be supermanic: I can feel it when mania enters through my left brain like laser beams, transforming my sluggish thoughts, recharging them, galvanizing them. My thoughts acquire such momentum, they rush out of my head, to disseminate knowledge about the true nature of mania to psychiatrists and all other ordinary mortals. That's why I will never accept lithium again—to do so is to obstruct the divinity in me." Although he was on the brink of divorce, he would not yield to his wife's plea to go back on lithium.

The vignette illustrates the possibility that even some of the most psychotic manifestations of mania represent explanatory delusions, the patient's attempt to make sense of the experience of mania. The DSM-IV-TR criteria for severity and psychotic specifiers for manic and mixed episode (Tables 13.6–11 and 13.6–12) are more concerned with operational rigor than with the phenomenological sophistication needed to understand such core manic experiences. (Many manic patients abuse alcohol and stimulants to enhance their mental state; mood incongruence can sometimes be explained on that basis.)

HYPOMANIA VERSUS MANIA Nonpsychotic and nondisruptive variants of mania are much more common and are recognized by DSM-IV-TR as hypomanic episodes. They are the historical clinical marker for bipolar II. Diagnostically, history of hypomania is preferably obtained from significant others who have observed the patient; the experience is often pleasant, and the subject may be unaware of it or may tend to deny it. Others experience irritable or dysphoric hypomanic episodes, which may be difficult to recognize clinically because of a stereotype that emphasizes the positive aspects of hypomania. DSM-IV-TR stipulates that marked impairment in functioning does not occur, and patients often feel that they benefit from the energy and confidence of hypomania. This is true if hypomania is mild and "sunny." Certainly, many, especially those with "darker" irritable activation, do experience impairment in occupational and interpersonal functioning over time. DSM-IV-TR stipulates a minimum duration of 4 days for hypomania; however, current evidence indicates that bipolar II disorder with long (≥4 days) and short (2 to 3 days) hypomania are indistinguishable on the basis of bipolar family history. It is therefore recommended that the threshold for detecting the duration of hypomania be set at 2 days. Ultimately, the duration of hypomanic experiences might be less important than the fact that they recur. In other words, brief recurrent hypomanias, even if duration is 1 day, interspaced with major depressive episodes, can be taken as presumptive evidence for bipolar II. Finally, although DSM-IV-TR states that treatment-emergent hypomania in a depressed patient does not count toward a diagnosis of bipolarity, prospective observations show that nearly all such episodes are followed eventually by spontaneous hypomania (or mania); moreover, family history for bipolar disorder is comparable on patients with spontaneous and antidepressant-associated hypomania. In brief, antidepressant-associated hypomanias are best considered as a genetically less penetrant variant of bipolarity (which, in the literature, are often referred to as *bipolar III disorders*).

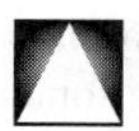

Table 13.6–11
DSM-IV-TR Criteria for Severity, Psychotic, and Remission Specifiers for Current (or Most Recent) Manic Episode

Note: Code in fifth digit. Mild, moderate, severe without psychotic features, and severe with psychotic features can be applied only if the criteria are currently met for a manic episode. In partial remission and in full remission, they can be applied to a manic episode in bipolar I disorder only if it is the most recent type of mood episode.

Mild: Minimum symptom criteria are met for a manic episode.

Moderate: Extreme increase in activity or impairment in judgment.

Severe without psychotic features: Almost continual supervision is required to prevent physical harm to self or others.

Severe with psychotic features: Delusions or hallucinations. If possible, specify whether the psychotic features are mood-congruent or mood-incongruent:

- **Mood-congruent psychotic features:** Delusions or hallucinations whose content is entirely consistent with the typical manic themes of inflated worth, power, knowledge, identity, or special relationship to a deity or famous person.
- **Mood-incongruent psychotic features:** Delusions or hallucinations whose content does not involve typical manic themes of inflated worth, power, knowledge, identity, or special relationship to a deity or famous person. Included are such symptoms as persecutory delusions (not directly related to grandiose ideas or themes), thought insertion, and delusions of being controlled.

In partial remission: Symptoms of a manic episode are present, but full criteria are not met, or there is a period without any significant symptoms of a manic episode lasting less than 2 months after the end of the manic episode.

In full remission: During the past 2 months, no significant signs or symptoms of the disturbance were present.

Unspecified.

From American Psychiatric Association. *Diagnostic and Statistical Manual of Mental Disorders*. 4th ed. Text rev. Washington, DC: American Psychiatric Association; 2000, with permission.

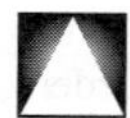

Table 13.6–12
DSM-IV-TR Criteria for Severity, Psychotic, and Remission Specifiers for Current (or Most Recent) Mixed Episode

Note: Code in fifth digit. Mild, moderate, severe without psychotic features, and severe with psychotic features can be applied only if the criteria are currently met for a mixed episode. In partial remission and in full remission, they can be applied to a mixed episode in bipolar I disorder only if it is the most recent type of mood episode.

Mild: No more than minimum symptom criteria are met for a manic episode and a major depressive episode.

Moderate: Symptoms or functional impairment between *mild* and *severe*.

Severe without psychotic features: Almost continual supervision required to prevent physical harm to self or others.

Severe with psychotic features: Delusions or hallucinations. If possible, specify whether the psychotic features are mood-congruent or mood-incongruent:

- **Mood-congruent psychotic features:** Delusions or hallucinations whose content is entirely consistent with the typical manic or depressive themes.
- **Mood-incongruent psychotic features:** Delusions or hallucinations whose content does not involve typical manic or depressive themes. Included are such symptoms as persecutory delusions (not directly related to grandiose or depressive themes), thought insertion, and delusions of being controlled.

In partial remission: Symptoms of a mixed episode are present, but full criteria are not met, or there is a period without any significant symptoms of a mixed episode lasting less than 2 months after the end of the mixed episode.

In full remission: During the past 2 months, no significant signs or symptoms of the disturbance were present.

Unspecified.

From American Psychiatric Association. *Diagnostic and Statistical Manual of Mental Disorders*. 4th ed. Text rev. Washington, DC: American Psychiatric Association; 2000, with permission.

DIAGNOSTIC CLASSIFICATION

The classification of mood disorders in DSM-IV-TR subsumes a large variety of patients seen in private, public, ambulatory, and inpatient settings. The main demarcation in that large clinical terrain is between bipolar and depressive disorders. Thus, bipolar disorders range from the classic manic and depressive episodes, often of psychotic intensity (bipolar I disorder), to recurrent major depressive episodes, alternating with hypomanic episodes (bipolar II disorder), and cyclothymic mood swings. Likewise, depressive disorders include those with psychotic severity, melancholia, atypical features, and dysthymic variants.

Major and specific attenuated subtypes are distinguished on the basis of severity and duration. In dysthymic and cyclothymic disorders, a partial mood syndrome consisting of such subthreshold features as subdepressive and hypomanic periods is maintained, intermittently or continuously, for at least 2 years. Subdepressive periods dominate in dysthymia; in cyclothymia, they alternate with brief hypomania. The onset is typically in adolescence or childhood, and most persons with these diagnoses first seen clinically in young adulthood have had low-grade mood symptoms for 5 to 10 years. Major mood disorders, which generally begin much later in life, require the presence of a full manic episode or a full depressive episode—sustained for at least 1 and 2 weeks, respectively—and an episodic course, typically permitting recovery or remission from episodes. DSM-IV-TR recognizes that as many as one-third of persons with major depressive disorders fail to achieve full symptomatic recovery and should thus be qualified as chronic or in partial remission. They are no longer considered dysthymic (the misleading convention in the third edition of the DSM [DSM-III]).

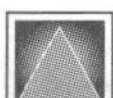

Table 13.6–13
Differentiating Characteristics of Bipolar and Unipolar Depressions

	Bipolar	Unipolar
History of mania or hypomania (definitional)	Yes	No
Temperament and personality	Cyclothymic and extroverted	Dysthymic and introverted
Sex ratio	Equal	More women than men
Age of onset	Teens, 20s, and 30s	30s, 40s, and 50s
Postpartum episodes	More common	Less common
Onset of episode	Often abrupt	More insidious
Number of episodes	Numerous	Fewer
Duration of episode	3–6 mos	3–12 mos
Psychomotor activity	Retardation > agitation	Agitation > retardation
Sleep	Hypersomnia > insomnia	Insomnia > hypersomnia
Family history		
Bipolar disorder	Yes	±
Unipolar disorder	Yes	Yes
Alcoholism	Yes	Yes
Pharmacological response		
Most antidepressants	Induce hypomania-mania	±
Lithium carbonate	Prophylaxis	±

Dichotomy or Continuum?

Although, in the extreme, bipolar and depressive disorders can be discriminated clinically and therapeutically (Table 13.6–13), clinical observations testify to a vast overlap between those extremes. Thus, the distinctions between the various affective subtypes are not as hard and fast as DSM-IV-TR attempts to portray. For instance, full-blown bipolar disorder can be superimposed on cyclothymic disorder that tends to persist after the resolution of manic or major depressive episodes. Even more common is major depressive disorder complicating cyclothymic disorder, which should be reclassified as an important course variant of bipolar II disorder. Likewise, recent evidence indicates that dysthymic disorder may precede major depressive disorder in as many as one-third of cases. Moreover, as much as 50 percent of persons with major depressive disorder during long-term prospective follow-up develop hypomanic or manic episodes and should be reclassified as having bipolar disorder. In some, if not many, instances, apparent switching of polarity might simply be due to earlier misclassification of bipolar disorder as major depressive disorder. Finally, unexpected crossing from dysthymic disorder to hypomanic or manic episodes has also been described, suggesting that some forms of dysthymic disorder are subaffective precursors of bipolar disorder. The author's work has led to the concept of *subbipolar dysthymia* (not a formal category in DSM-IV-TR) to bring clinical attention to this subgroup of patients. Such observations are in line with Kraepelin's historic attempt to bring all mood disorders under one rubric. Epidemiological studies in the community have also shown much fluidity between various subthreshold and major mood disorders.

Heterogeneity undoubtedly exists among mood disorders. But the classic unipolar-bipolar distinction might not be the best way to capture it. The foregoing observations suggest that much of the recurrent depressive terrain might be *pseudo-unipolar* (i.e., soft bipolar). The clinical significance of these considerations lies in the fact that many DSM-IV-TR subtypes of mood disorders are not pure entities, and considerable overlap and switches in polarity take place. They also provide some rationale, for instance, for why lithium or other mood stabilizer augmentation may be effective in some apparently unipolar depressions; such patients do not necessarily experience brief spontaneous hypomanic episodes but instead often exhibit a high baseline level of hyperthymic traits. Finally, several studies have shown that bipolar patients with cyclothymic premorbid adjustment and interepisodic adjustment are at considerable risk for *antidepressant-induced rapid cycling*, defined as a rapid succession of major episodes with few or no intervals of freedom.

Such considerations further testify to the wisdom of supplementing major mood diagnoses with temperamental attributes. DSM-IV-TR only makes subtle or oblique hints concerning this and instead provides the practitioner with an unwieldy, if not useless, array of episode and course specifiers. In the end, it all boils down to whether or not there is interepisodic remission (Table 13.6–14).

As Kraepelin illustrated in his monograph, course is best captured graphically. DSM-IV-TR only provides examples of this for depressive disorders (Fig. 13.6–6) and limits itself to four patterns. Kraepelin, after diagramming 18 illustrative patterns for the entire spectrum of manic-depressive illness, declared that the illness pur-

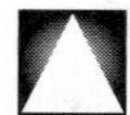

Table 13.6–14
DSM-IV-TR Criteria for Longitudinal Course Specifiers

Specify if (can be applied to recurrent major depressive disorder or bipolar I or II disorder):

With full interepisode recovery: if full remission is attained between the two most recent mood episodes

Without full interepisode recovery: if full remission is not attained between the two most recent mood episodes

From American Psychiatric Association. *Diagnostic and Statistical Manual of Mental Disorders.* 4th ed. Text rev. Washington, DC: American Psychiatric Association; 2000, with permission.

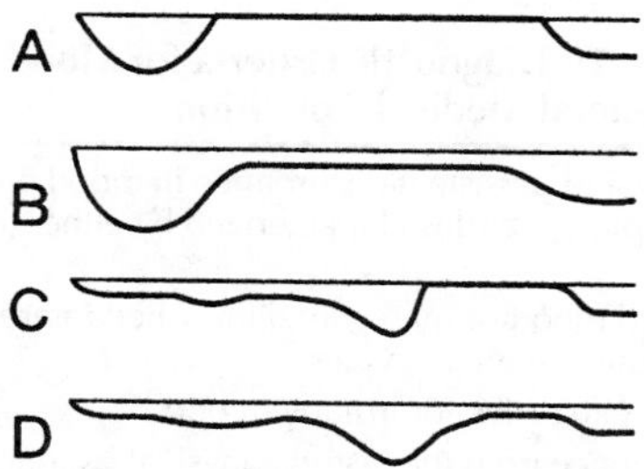

FIGURE 13.6–6 Graphs depicting prototypical courses. **A:** Course of major depressive disorder, recurrent, with no antecedent dysthymic disorder and a period of full remission between the episodes. This pattern predicts the best future prognosis. **B:** Course of major depressive disorder, recurrent, with no antecedent dysthymic disorder but with prominent symptoms persisting between the two most recent episodes (i.e., partial remission is attained). **C:** Rare pattern (present in fewer than 3 percent of persons with major depressive disorder) of major depressive disorder, recurrent with antecedent dysthymic disorder but with full interepisode recovery between the two most recent episodes. **D:** Course of major depressive disorder, recurrent, with antecedent dysthymic disorder and no period of full remission between the two most recent episodes. This pattern, commonly referred to as *double depression,* is seen in approximately 20 to 25 percent of persons with major depressive disorder. (From American Psychiatric Association: *Diagnostic and Statistical Manual of Mental Disorders.* 4th ed. Text rev. Washington, DC: American Psychiatric Association; 2000, with permission.)

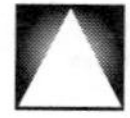

Table 13.6–15
DSM-IV-TR Diagnostic Criteria for Major Depressive Disorder, Single Episode

A. Presence of a single major depressive episode.
B. The major depressive episode is not better accounted for by schizoaffective disorder and is not superimposed on schizophrenia, schizophreniform disorder, delusional disorder, or psychotic disorder not otherwise specified.
C. There has never been a manic episode, a mixed episode, or a hypomanic episode. **Note:** This exclusion does not apply if all of the manic-like, mixed-like, or hypomanic-like episodes are substance or treatment induced or are due to the direct physiological effects of a general medical condition.

If the full criteria are currently met for a major depressive episode, *specify* its current clinical status or features, or both:

Mild, moderate, severe without psychotic features, or severe with psychotic features
Chronic
With catatonic features
With melancholic features
With atypical features
With postpartum onset

If the full criteria are not currently met for a major depressive episode, *specify* the current clinical status of the major depressive disorder or features of the most recent episode:

In partial remission, in full remission
Chronic
With catatonic features
With melancholic features
With atypical features
With postpartum onset

From American Psychiatric Association. *Diagnostic and Statistical Manual of Mental Disorders.* 4th ed. Text rev. Washington, DC: American Psychiatric Association; 2000, with permission.

sued an indefinite number of courses. Although not represented in the official U.S. and international classifications, some of these course patterns are of considerable interest today. For instance, a biphasic course (a sequence in which episodes of opposite polarity succeed each other and then are followed by a free interval) is relevant to treatment response. Thus, depression followed by mania or hypomania—compared to mania or hypomania followed by depression—appears, on the basis of replicated studies, to be less responsive to lithium.

DEPRESSIVE DISORDERS

The broad category of depressive disorders includes major depressive disorder, dysthymic disorder, and depressive disorder not otherwise specified.

Major Depressive Disorder Episodes usually begin over a prodromal period of weeks to months. The DSM-IV-TR diagnosis of major depressive disorder requires (1) dysphoric mood or decreased interest in usual activities and (2) at least four additional classic depressive signs and symptoms, (3) which must be sustained for at least 2 weeks, and (4) which cannot be explained by another process known to cause depressive symptoms, such as normal bereavement, certain physical conditions commonly associated with depression, or another mental disorder. It can be a single episode or, commonly, recurrent, or both (Tables 13.6–15 and 13.6–16).

Comorbid Physical Disease The foregoing considerations raise the question of whether major depressive disorder should be limited to depressions of unknown etiology (i.e., those without documented physical causes). The DSM-IV-TR approach has basically been that, when the cause is known, the condition should be diagnosed as mood disorder due to a general medical condition (Table 13.6–17), which must be specified, or substance-induced mood disorder (Table 13.6–18). The problem with this approach is that many common medical factors historically associated with depression do not seem to be causative in the etiological sense but rather are triggering agents in otherwise predisposed persons. This is analogous to the situation with life events, which no longer are used in making distinctions between reactive and endogenous subtypes of depression. A more troubling implication is that major depressive disorders without demonstrable physical disease are not medical or otherwise biological. More importantly, there appears to be no reliable or valid way for a clinician to decide that a depressive condition is due to a specified medical condition. For this reason, it is generally more practical to diagnose the depressive disorder on Axis I and to specify the contributing physical condition on Axis III. In brief, the designation *due to a general medical condition* is cumbersome and redundant. The author considers major depressive disorder to represent the final common pathway of multifactorial interacting factors—physical and psychological—a syndrome that should be diagnosed irrespective of presumed cause.

Diagnostic Threshold Another question concerning the DSM-IV-TR definition of major depressive disorder relates to the threshold at which a constellation of depressive features becomes a condition distinct from the ordinary blues. Within the current definition, if a person responds to a setback with lowered spirits and self-doubt, difficulty in sleeping and concentration, and decreased sexual interest for 14 days, he or she would qualify for the diagnosis of a major depressive disorder of mild intensity. Many clinicians would consider such a condition a relatively minor departure from normality, probably no more than an adjustment disorder. Obviously, crite-

Table 13.6–16
DSM-IV-TR Diagnostic Criteria for Major Depressive Disorder, Recurrent

A. Presence of two or more major depressive episodes.

Note: To be considered separate episodes, there must be an interval of at least 2 consecutive months in which criteria are not met for a major depressive episode.

B. The major depressive episodes are not better accounted for by schizoaffective disorder and are not superimposed on schizophrenia, schizophreniform disorder, delusional disorder, or psychotic disorder not otherwise specified.

C. There has never been a manic episode, a mixed episode, or a hypomanic episode. **Note:** This exclusion does not apply if all of the manic-like, mixed-like, or hypomanic-like episodes are substance or treatment induced or are due to the direct physiological effects of a general medical condition.

If the full criteria are currently met for a major depressive episode, *specify* its current clinical status and/or features:

Mild, moderate, severe without psychotic features, or severe with psychotic features
Chronic
With catatonic features
With melancholic features
With atypical features
With postpartum onset

If the full criteria are not currently met for a major depressive episode, *specify* the current clinical status of the major depressive disorder or features of the most recent episode:

In partial remission or in full remission
Chronic
With catatonic features
With melancholic features
With atypical features
With postpartum onset

Specify if:

Longitudinal course specifiers (with and without interepisode recovery)
With seasonal pattern

From American Psychiatric Association. *Diagnostic and Statistical Manual of Mental Disorders.* 4th ed. Text rev. Washington, DC: American Psychiatric Association; 2000, with permission.

ria other than signs, symptoms, and duration are necessary to differentiate a major depressive disorder from adjustment reactions to life situations. The presence of the following characteristics might assist in such a differentiation.

- By definition, a major depressive disorder should be incapacitating. Previously, much attention was paid to the interpersonal consequences of depression. Recent evidence indicates that measurable deficits in work performance are often early manifestations. Afflicted persons also do not benefit from taking leisure time, and, hence, prescribing vacations is futile.
- Major depressive disorder is usually perceived as a break from a person's usual or premorbid self, which can be so striking that patients may feel as though they are losing their minds. The important point is that the patient and significant others can usually relate the onset of the illness to a given month or quarter of a year, which is not true, for instance, for dysthymic disorder.
- Major depressive disorder is often experienced by the patient as qualitatively distinct from grief or other understandable reactions to loss or adversity. William James described it as follows:

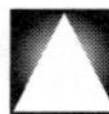

Table 13.6–17
DSM-IV-TR Diagnostic Criteria for Mood Disorder Due to a General Medical Condition

A. A prominent and persistent disturbance in mood predominates in the clinical picture and is characterized by either (or both) of the following:

(1) Depressed mood or markedly diminished interest or pleasure in all, or almost all, activities

(2) Elevated, expansive, or irritable mood.

B. There is evidence from the history, physical examination, or laboratory findings that the disturbance is the direct physiological consequence of a general medical condition.

C. The disturbance is not better accounted for by another mental disorder (e.g., adjustment disorder with depressed mood in response to the stress of having a general medical condition).

D. The disturbance does not occur exclusively during the course of a delirium.

E. The symptoms cause clinically significant distress or impairment in social, occupational, or other important areas of functioning.

Specify type:

With depressive features: if the predominant mood is depressed but the full criteria are not met for a major depressive episode

With major depressive-like episode: if the full criteria are met (except Criterion D) for a major depressive episode

With manic features: if the predominant mood is elevated, euphoric, or irritable

With mixed features: if the symptoms of mania and depression are present but neither predominate.

Coding note: Include the name of the general medical condition on Axis I, for example, mood disorder due to hypothyroidism, with depressive features; also code the general medical condition on Axis III.

Coding note: If depressive symptoms occur as part of a preexisting vascular dementia, indicate the depressive symptoms by coding the appropriate subtype, for example, vascular dementia, with depressed mood.

From American Psychiatric Association. *Diagnostic and Statistical Manual of Mental Disorders.* 4th ed. Text rev. Washington, DC: American Psychiatric Association; 2000, with permission.

> There is a pitch of unhappiness so great that the goods of nature may be entirely forgotten, and all sentiment of their existence vanish from the mental field. For this extremity of passion to be reached, something more is needed than adversity; the individual must in his own person become the prey of pathological melancholy. Such sensitiveness and susceptibility of mental pain is a rare occurrence where the nervous constitution is entirely normal: one seldom finds it in a healthy subject even where he is the victim of the most atrocious cruelties of outward fortune; it is an active anguish, a sort of psychical neuralgia wholly unknown to healthy life.

Two additional features, when present, would further validate the diagnosis of major depressive disorder.

- History of past episodes.
- Consecutive-generation family history of mood disorder—especially when a large number of family members are afflicted with depression or mood disorder—is characteristic of clinical depression. For instance, one study that prospectively followed persons with minor or neurotic depression found that such pedigrees predicted the development of future major episodes. DSM-IV-TR makes no provision for considering such familial factors in diagnostic decisions. In clinical practice, these factors would strongly weigh whether depression is taken seriously.

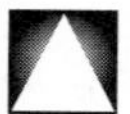

Table 13.6–18
DSM-IV-TR Diagnostic Criteria for Substance-Induced Mood Disorder

A. A prominent and persistent disturbance in mood predominates in the clinical picture and is characterized by either (or both) of the following:
  (1) Depressed mood or markedly diminished interest or pleasure in all, or almost all, activities
  (2) Elevated, expansive, or irritable mood.
B. There is evidence from the history, physical examination, or laboratory findings of (1) or (2):
  (1) The symptoms in Criterion A developed during, or within a month of, substance intoxication or withdrawal.
  (2) Medication use is etiologically related to the disturbance.
C. The disturbance is not better accounted for by a mood disorder that is not substance induced. Evidence that the symptoms are better accounted for by a mood disorder that is not substance induced might include the following: The symptoms precede the onset of the substance use (or medication use); the symptoms persist for a substantial period of time (e.g., approximately 1 month) after the cessation of acute withdrawal or severe intoxication or are substantially in excess of what would be expected, given the type or amount of the substance used or the duration of use; or there is other evidence that suggests the existence of an independent non–substance-induced mood disorder (e.g., a history of recurrent major depressive episodes).
D. The disturbance does not occur exclusively during the course of a delirium.
E. The symptoms cause clinically significant distress or impairment in social, occupational, or other important areas of functioning.

Note: This diagnosis should be made instead of a diagnosis of substance intoxication or substance withdrawal only when the mood symptoms are in excess of those usually associated with the intoxication or withdrawal syndrome and when the symptoms are sufficiently severe to warrant independent clinical attention.

Code [specific substance]-induced mood disorder:
  Alcohol; amphetamine (or amphetamine-like substance); cocaine; hallucinogen; inhalant; opioid; phencyclidine (or phencyclidine-like substance); sedative, hypnotic, or anxiolytic; other (or unknown) substance.

Specify type:
  With depressive features: if the predominant mood is depressed
  With manic features: if the predominant mood is elevated, euphoric, or irritable
  With mixed features: if symptoms of mania and depression are present and neither predominates.

Specify if:
  With onset during intoxication: if the criteria are met for intoxication with the substance, and the symptoms develop during the intoxication syndrome
  With onset during withdrawal: if criteria are met for withdrawal from the substance, and the symptoms develop during, or shortly after, a withdrawal syndrome.

From American Psychiatric Association. *Diagnostic and Statistical Manual of Mental Disorders*. 4th ed. Text rev. Washington, DC: American Psychiatric Association; 2000, with permission.

Single-Episode and Recurrent Subtypes A significant minority, perhaps one-third, of all major depressive episodes does not recur (Table 13.6–15). Such patients tend to be older and less likely to have a positive family history for mood disorders and have a more protracted (1 to 2 years) course of the disorder. Patients with single-episode major depressive disorder should be distinguished from those experiencing their first episodes of recurrent major depressive disorder (Table 13.6–16). The latter group tends to be younger, and the disorder is more likely to have been preceded by a depressive temperament or dysthymic disorder. Those who switch to bipolar disorder are more likely to have experienced recurrent depressions (≥5 episodes).

Research has established that recurrent major depressive disorders are more familial than their single-episode counterparts. The average length of episodes is 6 months, whereas the mean interval between episodes tends to vary (typically years). The mean number of major episodes over a lifetime, according to retrospective and prospective studies, is five to six, in contrast to an average of eight to nine major episodes in bipolar disorder. These figures are probably underestimates in that they are typically ascertained on the basis of clinical referral or hospitalization, or both.

Melancholic Features In DSM-III, the neurotic-endogenous distinction was deleted. Neurotic depression was largely absorbed by dysthymic disorder and the major depressive disorders that complicate it; endogenous depression became *melancholic features*, a qualifying phrase for major depressive disorders in which anhedonia, guilt, and psychomotor-vegetative disturbances dominate the clinical picture (Table 13.6–4). DSM-IV-TR retains these conventions.

Although the foregoing conventions have received much criticism, they are based on solid data from independent studies. Thus, *neurotic depression*, defined as a reactive (i.e., precipitated) nonpsychotic depression of mild to moderate intensity with predominant anxiety and characterological pathology, does not seem to constitute a distinct nosological entity. Although such a presentation is common in clinical practice, well-conducted studies in the United States and Germany have shown that the prospective follow-up course of those patients is heterogeneous, including melancholic and even psychotic depressions and, in some instances, bipolar transformation. The progression of a precipitated, relatively mild depression (reactive illness) to severe psychotic depression (or one with melancholic autonomy) during prospective observation suggests that so-called endogenous depressions may have their onset in milder depressions, that neurotic and psychotic depressions do not necessarily refer to distinct disorders but to disorders that differ in severity, and that the presence of precipitating stress carries little diagnostic weight in differentiating subtypes of depression (although the absence of such stress might be used to support a melancholic level of major depressive disorder).

At the heart of the concept of morbid depression is its autonomy from stresses that may have precipitated it and its general unresponsiveness to other environmental input. This is embodied in Donald Klein's concept of *endogenomorphic depression*, which could be precipitated and mild (endoreactive), while exhibiting disturbances of hedonic mechanisms refractory to current interpersonal contexts. Many authorities believe that such features dictate the need to use somatic approaches to reverse the maladaptive autonomy and to restore response to interpersonal feedback; that is, psychotherapeutic approaches are deemed largely ineffective until the autonomy is somatically lysed.

Given the somatic connotation of the ancient concept of *melancholia*, the APA classification has officially adopted it as the preferred nosological term for the revised concept of endogenetics; hence, the prominence of the vegetative and biorhythmic features accorded to it in DSM-IV-TR. However, the APA diagnostic schema risks confusing endogenous depression with another classic concept of mood disorder, that of *involutional melancholia*.

Atypical Features Reverse vegetative signs with rejection sensitivity, often contrasted to melancholia on phenomenological and pharmacological grounds, represent a major depressive disorder qualifier occurring in as many as one-third of all major depressive disorders. As mentioned earlier—and to be discussed in greater detail later in this chapter—atypical features are so common in bipolar disorder, especially bipolar II disorder, that some consider them to be clinical markers for soft bipolar disorders. Although there is no consensus on this question, before diagnosing major depressive disorder in such cases, it is clinically wise to exclude bipolar II disorder.

Psychotic Features Ten to 15 percent of major depressive disorders, usually from the rank of those with melancholic features, develop into delusional depressions. In young persons, they tend to be retarded, even stuporous, and are best considered initial episodes of a bipolar disorder until proven otherwise. More typically, psychotic depression that develops for the first time after 50 years of age often presents with severe agitation, delusional guilt, hypochondriacal preoccupations, early morning awakening, and weight loss. The premorbid adjustment of such patients is classically characterized as *obsessoid*. Their mournful-anxious mood and agitation are autonomous, being refractory to psychological interventions, and they endure great psychic suffering. Except for the fact that generally one to two episodes occur in late-onset (so-called involutional) depressions, they represent a severe variant of DSM-IV-TR melancholia. Kraepelin's postulation of a cerebrovascular basis for such cases makes the ventricular enlargement and white matter opacities reported in psychotic depressions of some interest. Their etiological specificity for persons with late onset psychotic depression has been controversial, however, because younger (more bipolar) persons with psychotic depression may exhibit similar findings. Brain imaging findings tend to be correlated with the neurocognitive deficits observed in psychotic depressions. Those features do not seem to define a distinct depressive subtype, but one of greater severity that some authorities now classify as *vascular depressions*. Finally, despite attempts to suggest a neurochemical uniqueness based largely on the need for antipsychotic treatment in the acute phase of many of those patients, familial and other external validations have failed to support psychotic depression as a separate entity; hence, the decision in DSM-IV-TR to use psychotic features as a specifier for major depressive episode (Table 13.6–3). Emerging data, nonetheless, might eventually force a change in this convention. For instance, William Coryell and collaborators in the NIMH collaborative study of depression have shown psychotic depression to be the most consistent unipolar subtype across episodes. Alan Schatzberg's work, originally conducted at Harvard, likewise underscores the uniqueness of psychotic depression based on neuroendocrine and putative neurochemical considerations. Finally, consideration should be given to Athanasios Koukopoulos' clinical formulation that many agitated psychotic depressions might represent mixed states (i.e., activated depressions that belong to the bipolar spectrum).

Chronic Depression The DSM-IV-TR criteria for chronic specifier appear in Table 13.6–19. The clinical situation, however, is much more complex than these conventions. For instance, the symptom profile in chronic depressions usually displays low-grade intensity rather than severe syndromic chronicity. Severe depressive disorder, in its psychotic forms, is so agonizing that the patient is at risk of committing suicide before the disorder has a chance to become chronic. More commonly, the psychotic symptoms respond to medication or to electroconvulsive therapy (ECT), but residual depressive symptoms may linger for a long time. In other persons with chronic depressions, the chronicity arises from more mundane (nonpsychotic) major depressive episodes, depressive residua following one or several clinical episodes that fail to remit fully. Instead of the customary remission within 1 year, the patients are ill for years. The level of depression varies, fluctuating between syndromic illness and milder symptoms. Recent landmark analyses from the NIMH collaborative study of depression by Lewis Judd and colleagues have actually shown that as many as 60 percent of major depressive disorder patients have a subthreshold fluctuating chronic course.

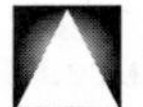

Table 13.6–19
DSM-IV-TR Criteria for Chronic Specifier

Specify if:

Chronic (can be applied to the current or most recent major depressive episode in major depressive disorder and to a major depressive episode in bipolar I or II disorder, only if it is the most recent type of mood episode).

Full criteria for a major depressive episode have been met continuously for at least the past 2 years.

From American Psychiatric Association. *Diagnostic and Statistical Manual of Mental Disorders.* 4th ed. Text rev. Washington, DC: American Psychiatric Association; 2000, with permission.

Rather than exhibiting a frankly depressive mood, many persons with chronic depression experience deficits in their ability to enjoy leisure and to display an attitude of irritable moroseness. They also show a sense of resignation, generalized fear of an inability to cope, adherence to rigid routines, and inhibited communication. Such deficits, along with the irritable humor, tend to poison their conjugal lives: Their marriages are typically in a state of chronic deadlock, leading neither to divorce nor to reconciliation. In other patients, the residual phase is dominated by somatic features, such as sleep and other vegetative or autonomic irregularities. That these interpersonal, conjugal, and autonomic manifestations represent unresolved depression is shown by persistent sleep EEG (especially REM and delta phase) abnormalities that are indistinguishable from their acute counterparts. Regrettably, self-treatment with ethanol or iatrogenic benzodiazepine dependence, rather than definitive treatment for the ongoing low-grade depression, is common.

Failure to recover from major depressive disorder is associated with increased familial loading for depression, disabled spouses, deaths of immediate family members, concurrent disabling medical disease, use of depressant pharmacological agents, and excessive use of alcohol and sedative-hypnotic agents. Social support is often eroded in persons with residual depression, through the death or illness of significant others. Therefore, a thorough medical evaluation and socially supportive interventions should be essential ingredients of the overall approach to these patients.

Interpersonal disturbances in such patients are usually secondary to the distortions produced by long-standing depression. Therefore, observed pathological characterological changes—clinging or hostile dependence, demanding tendencies, touchiness, pessimism, and low self-esteem—are best considered as *postdepressive personality* changes. A dangerous stereotypical thinking holds that, because a patient has not responded adequately to standard treatments (the illness has become chronic), the disorder must have a characterological substrate. The long duration of the disorder often leads the patient to identify with the failing functions of depression, producing the self-image of being a depressed person. This self-image itself represents a malignant cognitive manifestation of the depressive disorder and dictates vigorous treatment targeted at the mood disorder.

Dysthymic Disorder Dysthymia (Table 13.6–20) is distinguished from chronic depressive disorder by the fact that it is not a sequel to well-defined major depressive episodes. Instead, in the most typical cases, patients complain that they have always been depressed. Thus, most cases are of early onset, beginning in childhood or adolescence and certainly by the time patients reach their 20s. A late-onset subtype, much less prevalent and not well characterized clinically, has been identified among middle-aged and geriatric populations, largely through epidemiological studies in the community.

Although the dysthymic disorder category in DSM-IV-TR can occur as a secondary complication of other psychiatric disorders, the core concept of dysthymic disorder refers to a subaffective disorder with (1) low-grade chronicity for at least 2 years, (2) insidious onset with origin often in childhood or adolescence, and (3) persistent or intermittent course. Although not part of the formal definition of dysthymic disorder, the family history is typically replete with depressive and bipolar disorders, which is one of the more robust findings supporting its link to primary mood disorder.

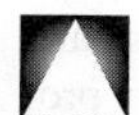

Table 13.6–20
DSM-IV-TR Diagnostic Criteria for Dysthymic Disorder

A. Depressed mood for most of the day, for more days than not, as indicated by subjective account or observation by others, for at least 2 years. **Note:** In children and adolescents, mood can be irritable, and duration must be at least 1 year.

B. Presence, while depressed, of two (or more) of the following:
   (1) Poor appetite or overeating
   (2) Insomnia or hypersomnia
   (3) Low energy or fatigue
   (4) Low self-esteem
   (5) Poor concentration or difficulty making decisions
   (6) Feelings of hopelessness

C. During the 2-year period (1 year for children or adolescents) of the disturbance, the person has never been without the symptoms in Criteria A and B for more than 2 months at a time.

D. No major depressive episode has been present during the first 2 years of the disturbance (1 year for children and adolescents); that is, the disturbance is not better accounted for by chronic major depressive disorder or major depressive disorder, in partial remission.

   Note: There may have been a previous major depressive episode, provided that there was a full remission (no significant signs or symptoms for 2 months) before development of the dysthymic disorder. In addition, after the initial 2 years (1 year in children or adolescents) of dysthymic disorder, there may be superimposed episodes of major depressive disorder, in which case both diagnoses may be given when the criteria are met for a major depressive episode.

E. There has never been a manic episode, a mixed episode, or a hypomanic episode, and criteria have never been met for cyclothymic disorder.

F. The disturbance does not occur exclusively during the course of a chronic psychotic disorder, such as schizophrenia or delusional disorder.

G. The symptoms are not due to the direct physiological effects of a substance (e.g., a drug of abuse, a medication) or a general medical condition (e.g., hypothyroidism).

H. The symptoms cause clinically significant distress or impairment in social, occupational, or other important areas of functioning.

Specify if:
   Early onset: if onset is before 21 years of age
   Late onset: if onset is at 21 years of age or older.

Specify if (for most recent 2 years of dysthymic disorder):
   With atypical features.

From American Psychiatric Association. *Diagnostic and Statistical Manual of Mental Disorders.* 4th ed. Text rev. Washington, DC: American Psychiatric Association; 2000, with permission.

Social Adjustment Dysthymic disorder is typically an ambulatory disorder compatible with relatively stable social functioning. However, the stability is precarious; recent data document that many patients invest whatever energy they have in work, leaving none for leisure and family or social activities, which results in marital friction. These empirical findings on the work orientation of persons with dysthymic disorder echo earlier formulations in the German and Japanese literature. For instance, Kraepelin described such persons as follows: "Life with its activity is a burden which they habitually bear with dutiful self-denial without being compensated by the pleasures of existence."

The dedication of persons with dysthymic disorder to work has been suggested to be an overcompensation and a defense against their battle with depressive disorganization and inertia. Nevertheless, Ernst Kretschmer suggested that such persons are the "backbone of society," dedicating their lives to jobs that require dependability and great attention to detail. Epidemiological studies have demonstrated that some persons with protracted dysthymic complaints, extending over many years, have never experienced clear-cut depressive episodes. Some of them may seek outpatient counseling and psychotherapy for what some clinicians might consider *existential depression*, with feelings of being empty and lacking any joy in life outside their work. Such persons have been described as leading "monocategorical existences." Others present clinically because their low-grade dysphoria has intensified into a major depression disorder.

Course An insidious onset of depression dating back to late childhood or the teens, preceding any superimposed major depressive episodes by years or even decades, represents the most typical developmental background of dysthymic disorder. A return to the low-grade depressive pattern is the rule after recovery from superimposed major depressive episodes, if any; hence, the designation *double depression* as a prominent course pattern illustrated in DSM-IV-TR for depressive illness (Fig. 13.6–6). This pattern, commonly seen in clinical practice, consists of the baseline dysthymic disorder fluctuating in and out of depressive episodes. The more prototypical patients with dysthymic disorder often complain of having been depressed since birth or of feeling depressed all the time. They seem, in the apt words of Kurt Schneider, to view themselves as belonging to an "aristocracy of suffering." Such descriptions of chronic gloominess in the absence of more objective signs of depression earn these patients the label of *characterological depression.* The description is further reinforced by the fluctuating depressive picture that merges imperceptibly with the patient's habitual self and thus raises uncertainty as to whether dysthymic disorder belongs in Axis I or Axis II. This conceptual uncertainty notwithstanding, given the confluence of data on the efficacy of many classes of antidepressants, dysthymic patients should not be denied the potential benefit of antidepressants.

Clinical Picture The profile of dysthymic disorder overlaps with that of major depressive disorder but differs from it in that symptoms tend to outnumber signs (more subjective than objective depression). This means that marked disturbances in appetite and libido are uncharacteristic, and psychomotor agitation or retardation is not observed. This all translates into a depression with attenuated symptomatology. However, subtle endogenous features are not uncommonly observed: inertia and anhedonia that are characteristi-

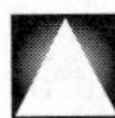

Table 13.6–21
DSM-IV-TR Alternative Research Criterion B for Dysthymic Disorder

B. Presence, while depressed, of three (or more) of the following:
(1) Low self-esteem or self-confidence, or feelings of inadequacy
(2) Feelings of pessimism, despair, or hopelessness
(3) Generalized loss of interest or pleasure
(4) Social withdrawal
(5) Chronic fatigue or tiredness
(6) Feelings of guilt, brooding about the past
(7) Subjective feelings of irritability or excessive anger
(8) Decreased activity, effectiveness, or productivity
(9) Difficulty in thinking, reflected by poor concentration, poor memory, or indecisiveness

From American Psychiatric Association. *Diagnostic and Statistical Manual of Mental Disorders.* 4th ed. Text rev. Washington, DC: American Psychiatric Association; 2000, with permission.

cally worse in the morning. Because patients presenting clinically often fluctuate in and out of a major depression, the core DSM-IV-TR criteria for dysthymic disorder tend to emphasize vegetative dysfunction, whereas the alternative Criterion B for dysthymic disorder (Table 13.6–21) in a DSM-IV-TR appendix lists cognitive symptoms.

Although dysthymic disorder represents a more restricted concept than its parent, neurotic depression, it is still quite heterogeneous. Anxiety is not a necessary part of its clinical picture, yet dysthymic disorder is often diagnosed in patients with anxiety and neurotic disorders. That clinical situation is perhaps to be regarded as a secondary or *anxious dysthymia* or, in the framework of Peter Tyrer, as part of a *general neurotic syndrome*. For greater operational clarity, it is best to restrict dysthymic disorder to a primary disorder, one that cannot be explained by a non-mood disorder. The essential features of such primary dysthymic disorder include habitual gloom, brooding, lack of joy in life, and preoccupation with inadequacy. Dysthymic disorder then is best characterized as long-standing, fluctuating, low-grade depression, experienced as part of the habitual self and representing an accentuation of traits observed in the depressive temperament. Dysthymia then can be viewed as a more symptomatic form of that temperament, introduced in a DSM-IV-TR appendix as a depressive personality disorder (Table 13.6–21). Sleep EEG data indicate that many persons with dysthymic disorder at baseline exhibit the sleep patterns of those with acute major depressive disorder, providing support for the constitutional nature of the disorder. Further evidence for that position comes from studies demonstrating high rates of familial affective disorder in dysthymic disorder or depressive temperament, or both.

The clinical picture of dysthymic disorder that emerges from the foregoing description is quite varied, with some patients proceeding to major depression, whereas others manifest the pathology largely at the personality level. The foregoing considerations suggest that a clinically satisfactory operationalism of dysthymia must include symptomatic, cognitive, and trait characteristics.

A 27-year-old, male, grade-school teacher presented with the chief complaint that life was a painful duty that had always lacked luster for him. He said that he felt "enveloped by a sense of gloom" that was nearly always with him. Although he was respected by his peers, he felt "like a grotesque failure, a self-concept I have had since childhood." He stated that he merely performed his responsibilities as a teacher and that he had never derived any pleasure from anything he had done in life. He said that he had never had any romantic feelings; sexual activity, in which he had engaged with two different women, had involved pleasureless orgasm. He said that he felt empty, going through life without any sense of direction, ambition, or passion, a realization that itself was tormenting. He had bought a pistol to put an end to what he called his "useless existence" but did not carry out suicide, believing that it would hurt his students and the small community in which he lived.

Dysthymic Variants Dysthymia is not uncommon in patients with chronically disabling physical disorders, particularly among elderly adults. Dysthymia-like clinically significant subthreshold depression lasting 6 or more months has also been described in neurological conditions, including stroke. According to a recent WHO conference that generated a book, this condition aggravates the prognosis of the underlying neurological disease and therefore deserves pharmacotherapy. Ongoing studies should provide more explicit clinical recommendations on this topic.

Prospective studies on children have revealed an *episodic course* of dysthymia with remissions, exacerbations, and eventual complications by major depressive episodes, 15 to 20 percent of which might even progress to hypomanic, manic, or mixed episodes postpuberty. Persons with dysthymic disorder presenting clinically as adults tend to pursue a chronic unipolar course that may be complicated by major depression. They rarely develop spontaneous hypomania or mania. However, when treated with antidepressants, some of them may develop brief hypomanic switches that typically disappear when the antidepressant dose is decreased. Although DSM-IV-TR would not allow the occurrence of such switches in dysthymia, systematic clinical observation has verified their occurrence in as many as one-third of dysthymic patients. In this special subgroup of persons with dysthymic disorder, the family histories are often positive for bipolar disorder. These patients represent a clinical bridge between major depressive disorder and bipolar II disorder.

Depressive Disorder Not Otherwise Specified

DSM-IV-TR criteria for the depressive disorder not otherwise specified category are presented in Table 13.6–22. The DSM-IV-TR then lists a hodgepodge of conditions that do not hang together by any coherent theme. It is unclear what is nonspecific about these conditions, when no less than six entities are specified! What follows are descriptions of several of these entities and related conditions that are commonly used in the epidemiological, clinical, or pharmacological literature, which the architects of DSM-IV-TR simply decided do not deserve recognition. The conditions described in the following discussion go beyond the DSM-IV-TR depressive disorder not otherwise specified categories. In the opinion of the present author, depressive disorder not otherwise specified might be justified when the depressive features do not coalesce into a full syndrome, failing to meet the 2-week duration threshold, especially when they occur in association with other disorders or life situations or physiological conditions, or both.

Minor Depressive Disorder In so-called minor depression (Table 13.6–23), observed in primary care settings, the depression is subthreshold, milder than major depressive disorder, and yet not protracted enough to be considered dysthymic. These varied manifestations of depression argue for a continuum model (Fig. 13.6–7) as originally envisaged by Kraepelin. Lewis Judd and collaborators at the University of California at San Diego have suggested that sub-

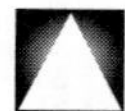

Table 13.6–22
DSM-IV-TR Diagnostic Criteria for Depressive Disorder Not Otherwise Specified

The depressive disorder not otherwise specified category includes disorders with depressive features that do not meet the criteria for major depressive disorder, dysthymic disorder, adjustment disorder with depressed mood, or adjustment disorder with mixed anxiety and depressed mood. Sometimes depressive symptoms can present as part of an anxiety disorder not otherwise specified. Examples of depressive disorder not otherwise specified include:

1. Premenstrual dysphoric disorder: In most menstrual cycles during the past year, symptoms (e.g., markedly depressed mood, marked anxiety, marked affective lability, and decreased interest in activities) regularly occurred during the last week of the luteal phase (and remitted within a few days of the onset of menses). These symptoms must be severe enough to markedly interfere with work, school, or usual activities and must be entirely absent for at least 1 week postmenses.
2. Minor depressive disorder: episodes of at least 2 weeks of depressive symptoms but with fewer than the five items required for major depressive disorder.
3. Recurrent brief depressive disorder: depressive episodes lasting from 2 days to as long as 2 weeks, occurring at least once a month for 12 months (not associated with the menstrual cycle).
4. Postpsychotic depressive disorder of schizophrenia: a major depressive episode that occurs during the residual phase of schizophrenia.
5. A major depressive episode superimposed on delusional disorder, psychotic disorder not otherwise specified, or the active phase of schizophrenia.
6. Situations in which the clinician has concluded that a depressive disorder is present but is unable to determine whether it is primary, due to a general medical condition, or substance induced.

From American Psychiatric Association. *Diagnostic and Statistical Manual of Mental Disorders.* 4th ed. Text rev. Washington, DC: American Psychiatric Association; 2000, with permission.

threshold depressive symptoms—without necessarily meeting the criterion for mood change—might actually represent the most common expressions of a depressive diathesis. From such a subsyndromal symptomatic depressive base, individuals predisposed to depressive illness are said to fluctuate in and out of the various DSM-IV-TR and subthreshold subtypes of depressive disorders. This viewpoint is presently most cogent for subsyndromal symptomatic depression that follows major depressive disorder, a strong predictor of subsequent frequent relapse or chronic course. There is an important message for the clinician here: Treat subsyndromal symptomatic depression residual to major depressive disorder.

Premenstrual Dysphoric Disorder In view of the higher prevalence of depressive disorders in women, premenstrual affective changes—dysphoria, tension, irritability, hostility, and labile mood—have received clinical and, more recently, research attention. The attempt to establish a specific premenstrual dysphoric disorder beyond this more normative premenstrual tension has neglected the occurrence of premenstrual eutonia, increased energy, and sexual drive. The not uncommon occurrence of these positive emotions, along with the labile mixed affective manifestations, tends to point toward a bipolar phenomenon. Although women with severe premenstrual complaints appear to have higher rates of lifetime major mood disorders, a recent twin study found that genetic and environmental factors contributing to premenstrual depression and major depressive disorders are largely distinct. Furthermore, events such as migraine, epileptic attacks, and panic states may, in some instances, be associated with the premenstrual phase. The foregoing considerations suggest the hypothesis that premenstrual psychobiological changes exacerbate different neuropsychiatric disorders to which women are otherwise predisposed. Whether the exaggerated premenstrual variability in emotional equilibrium constitutes a specific mood disorder or a more familiar affective disorder variant (e.g. mixed panic-depressive, bipolar) must await more definitive studies.

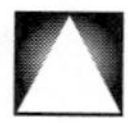

Table 13.6–23
DSM-IV-TR Research Criteria for Minor Depressive Disorder

A. A mood disturbance, defined as follows:
 (1) At least two (but less than five) of the following symptoms have been present during the same 2-week period and represent a change from previous functioning; at least one of the symptoms is (a) or (b):
  (a) Depressed mood most of the day, nearly every day, as indicated by subjective report (e.g., feels sad or empty) or observation made by others (e.g., appears tearful). **Note:** In children and adolescents, can be irritable mood.
  (b) Markedly diminished interest or pleasure in all, or almost all, activities most of the day, nearly every day (as indicated by subjective account or observation made by others).
  (c) Significant weight loss when not dieting or weight gain (e.g., a change of more than 5 percent of body weight in a month) or decrease or increase in appetite nearly every day. **Note:** In children, consider failure to make expected weight gains.
  (d) Insomnia or hypersomnia nearly every day.
  (e) Psychomotor agitation or retardation nearly every day (observable by others, not merely subjective feelings of restlessness or being slowed down).
  (f) Fatigue or loss of energy nearly every day.
  (g) Feelings of worthlessness or excessive or inappropriate guilt (which may be delusional) nearly every day (not merely self-reproach or guilt about being sick).
  (h) Diminished ability to think or to concentrate or indecisiveness, nearly every day (by subjective account or as observed by others).
  (i) Recurrent thoughts of death (not just fear of dying), recurrent suicidal ideation without a specific plan, or a suicide attempt or a specific plan for committing suicide.
 (2) The symptoms cause clinically significant distress or impairment in social, occupational, or other important areas of functioning.
 (3) The symptoms are not due to the direct physiological effects of a substance (e.g., a drug of abuse or a medication) or a general medical condition (e.g., hypothyroidism).
 (4) The symptoms are not better accounted for by bereavement (i.e., a normal reaction to the death of a loved one).

B. There has never been a major depressive episode, and criteria are not met for dysthymic disorder.

C. There has never been a manic episode, a mixed episode, or a hypomanic episode, and criteria are not met for cyclothymic disorder. **Note:** This exclusion does not apply if all of the manic-like, mixed-like, or hypomanic-like episodes are substance or treatment induced.

D. The mood disturbance does not occur exclusively during schizophrenia, schizophreniform disorder, schizoaffective disorder, delusional disorder, or psychotic disorder not otherwise specified.

From American Psychiatric Association. *Diagnostic and Statistical Manual of Mental Disorders.* 4th ed. Text rev. Washington, DC: American Psychiatric Association; 2000, with permission.

Recurrent Brief Depressive Disorder Now in a DSM-IV-TR appendix (Table 13.6–24), recurrent brief depressive disorder

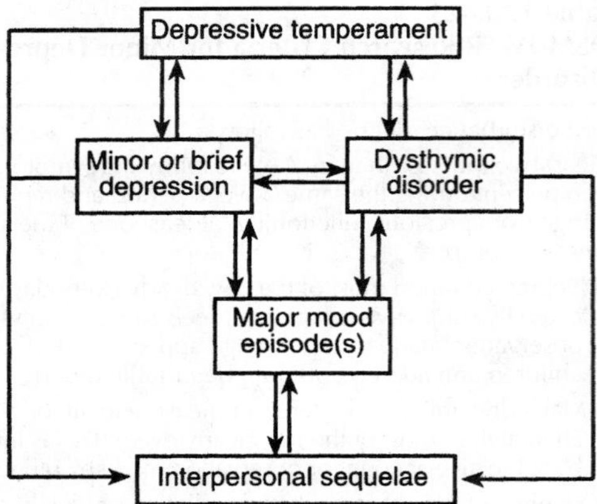

FIGURE 13.6–7 Relation of various depressive conditions supporting a spectrum concept. (From Akiskal HS: Dysthymia: Clinical and external validity. *Acta Psychiatr Scand.* 1994;89[Suppl]:19, with permission.)

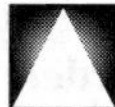

Table 13.6–24
DSM-IV-TR Research Criteria for Recurrent Brief Depressive Disorder

A. Criteria, except for duration, are met for a major depressive episode.
B. The depressive periods in Criterion A last at least 2 days but less than 2 weeks.
C. The depressive periods occur at least once a month for 12 consecutive months and are not associated with the menstrual cycle.
D. The periods of depressed mood cause clinically significant distress or impairment in social, occupational, or other important areas of functioning.
E. The symptoms are not due to the direct physiological effects of a substance (e.g., a drug of abuse or a medication) or a general medical condition (e.g., hypothyroidism).
F. There has never been a major depressive episode, and criteria are not met for dysthymic disorder.
G. There has never been a manic episode, a mixed episode, or a hypomanic episode, and criteria are not met for cyclothymic disorder. **Note:** This exclusion does not apply if all of the manic-like, mixed-like, or hypomanic-like episodes are substance or treatment induced.
H. The mood disturbance does not occur exclusively during schizophrenia, schizophreniform disorder, schizoaffective disorder, delusional disorder, or psychotic disorder not otherwise specified.

From American Psychiatric Association. *Diagnostic and Statistical Manual of Mental Disorders.* 4th ed. Text rev. Washington, DC: American Psychiatric Association; 2000, with permission.

derives from British work on young adults with frequent suicide attempts and epidemiological studies conducted in a young adult cohort in Zurich. It is described as short-lived depressions that usually recur on a monthly basis but are *not* menstrually related. They could coexist with major depressive disorder or dysthymic disorder and with hypomania. Again, the existence of hypomanic-prone recurrent brief depressive disorder argues for a bridge between depressive and bipolar II disorders. Such patients are believed to be more prevalent in primary care than in psychiatric settings. Those seen in psychiatric settings are likely to be given Axis II diagnoses, such as borderline personality disorder. The current nosological status of recurrent brief depressive disorder is uncertain, but it testifies to Kraepelin's observation that many transitional forms link the depressive temperament to affective episodes: "A permanent gloomy stress in all the experiences of life usually perceptible already in youth, and may persist without essential change throughout the whole of life (or) there is actually an uninterrupted series of transitions to periodic melancholia in which the course is quite indefinite with irregular fluctuations and remissions."

Reactive Depression Classically, *reactive depression* is defined as resulting from a specific life event. In an ideal case, the depression would not have occurred without the event (e.g., love loss) to which it is a reaction. It continues as long as the event is present, and it terminates with the reversal of the event (e.g., return of the lover). Depressions exhibiting all of those features are almost never seen in clinical practice. With interpersonal support, most people can face life's reverses, which explains why reactive depression tends to be self-limiting. Hence, adjustment disorder is the more appropriate diagnosis for many cases of reactive depression.

Chronic Demoralization Conceptually, however, one can envision chronically unsatisfactory life situations that might lead to chronic helplessness. However, such a condition, which could warrant the designation of chronic reactive depression, is a contradiction in terms. The question often raised is why a person would continue to stay in the situation. Sometimes psychodynamic authors invoke the concept of masochism to explain why certain persons cannot rid themselves of painful life situations, implying that they somehow contribute to their maintenance. Current thinking is that some of those presumed self-defeating traits are more situation specific than previously believed and might resolve with the elimination of the situation. So-called self-defeating features then are best considered psychodynamic mechanisms rather than indicators of a specific personality. At the present stage of knowledge, they do not deserve to be raised to the level of a nosological entity (hence, their disappearance from DSM-IV-TR). Chronic adjustment disorder might describe the chronic demoralization observed among some individuals stuck in chronically unsatisfactory life situations. Others might fulfill the criteria for dysthymia. Finally, if the chronically unsatisfactory life conditions involve conjugal violence and trauma, posttraumatic stress disorder (PTSD) may be the appropriate diagnosis.

Neurasthenia A century-old term developed by the American neuropsychiatrist George Beard, *neurasthenia* refers to a more chronic stage of anxious-depressive symptomatology. The anxiety generated by overstimulation is so excessive that it is replaced by a chronic disposition to irritability, fatigue (especially mental fatigue), lethargy, and exhaustion. It is as if the patient's mind refuses to take on new stresses. The clinical picture described by Beard suggests that anxious manifestations were preeminent in his time. They included headache, scalp tenderness, backache, heavy limbs, vague neuralgias, yawning, dyspepsia, palpitations, sweating hands and feet, chills, flushing, sensitivity to weather changes, insomnia, nightmares, pantaphobia, asthenopia, and tinnitus.

Although the diagnosis of neurasthenia is now used more in China than in the rest of the world, the recent worldwide popularity of the concept of chronic fatigue syndrome attests to the clinical acumen of classic physicians. Despite much energy invested in finding a viral or immunological cause, current descriptions tend to suggest an anxiety or mood disorder basis for many, but certainly not all, of those with the syndrome. Some neurasthenic patients would meet the criteria for major depressive disorder with atypical features and history of panic and phobic disorders. What circumstances would lead anxiety or depression to manifest primarily in fatigue is as elusive as it was 100 years ago. Like many other patients presenting to primary care settings with somatic complaints, those with chronic fatigue tend to denounce psychiatric diagnoses as inadequate explanations for their ills.

Postpsychotic Depressive Disorder of Schizophrenia

DSM-IV-TR describes postpsychotic depressive disorder of schizophrenia as follows:

> The essential feature is a Major Depressive Episode that is superimposed on, and occurs only during, the residual phase of Schizophrenia. The residual phase of Schizophrenia follows the active phase (i.e., symptoms meeting Criterion A) of Schizophrenia. It is characterized by the persistence of negative symptoms or of active-phase symptoms that are in an attenuated form (e.g., odd beliefs, unusual perceptual experiences). The superimposed Major Depressive Episode must include depressed mood (i.e., loss of interest or pleasure cannot serve as an alternate for sad or depressed mood). Most typically, the Major Depressive Episode follows immediately after remission of the active-phase symptoms of the psychotic episode. Sometimes it may follow after a short or extended interval during which there are no psychotic symptoms. Mood symptoms due to the direct physiological effects of a drug of abuse, a medication, or a general medical condition are not counted toward postpsychotic depressive disorder of Schizophrenia.

According to DSM-IV-TR, persons whose presentation meets those proposed criteria (Table 13.6–25) would be diagnosed as having depressive disorder not otherwise specified. As already pointed out, *not otherwise specified* represents such a hodgepodge of clinical situations that the designation *depressive disorder not otherwise specified* is at best meaningless and at worst countertherapeutic. In all postpsychotic depressions, one must first exclude a missed bipolar diagnosis. Negative symptoms due to classic antipsychotics—especially depot phenothiazines and those due to the residuum of schizophrenia once positive symptoms are brought under control—should be distinguished from the depressive episodes that complicate the course of schizophrenia in young, intelligent patients. This phenomenon is so common (at least 30 percent of patients with schizophrenia) that it can be considered as part of the natural course of schizophrenia rather than a separate nosological entity.

Primary versus Secondary Depressive Disorder Not Otherwise Specified

DSM-IV-TR finalizes its list of depressive disorder not otherwise specified categories by referring to situations in which the physician has deemed that a depressive disorder exists but is uncertain whether it is secondary to a delusional disorder, alcohol or substance abuse, or physical disease. The differentiation of mood disorders from nonaffective conditions is described later in this chapter, under differential diagnosis. Suffice it to say here that, from a therapeutic point of view, whether a depression is deemed clinically significant and in need of treatment should not be based on whether or not it is secondary to another disorder.

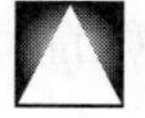

Table 13.6–25
DSM-IV-TR Research Criteria for Postpsychotic Depressive Disorder of Schizophrenia

A. Criteria are met for a major depressive episode.
   Note: The major depressive episode must include Criterion A1: depressed mood. Do not include symptoms that are better accounted for as medication side effects or negative symptoms of schizophrenia.

B. The major depressive episode is superimposed on and occurs only during the residual phase of schizophrenia.

C. The major depressive episode is not due to the direct physiological effects of a substance or a general medical condition.

From American Psychiatric Association. *Diagnostic and Statistical Manual of Mental Disorders.* 4th ed. Text rev. Washington, DC: American Psychiatric Association; 2000, with permission.

BIPOLAR DISORDERS

Four bipolar disorder categories are included in DSM-IV-TR: bipolar I disorder, bipolar II disorder, cyclothymic disorder, and bipolar disorder not otherwise specified.

Bipolar I Disorder

Typically beginning in the teenage years, the 20s, or the 30s, the first episode of bipolar I disorder could be manic, depressive, or mixed. One common mode of onset is mild retarded depression or hypersomnia for a few weeks or months, which then switches into a manic episode. Others begin with a severely psychotic manic episode with schizophreniform features; only when a more classic manic episode occurs is the affective nature of the disorder clarified. In a third group, several depressive episodes occur before the first manic episode. A careful history taken from significant others often reveals hyperthymic or cyclothymic traits that antedated the frank onset of manic episodes by several years, if not longer.

Single manic episode (Table 13.6–26) describes patients having a first episode of mania (most such patients eventually develop depressive episodes). The remaining subcategorization is used to specify

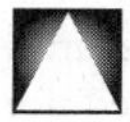

Table 13.6–26
DSM-IV-TR Diagnostic Criteria for Bipolar I Disorder, Single Manic Episode

A. Presence of only one manic episode and no past major depressive episodes.
   Note: *Recurrence* is defined as a change in polarity from depression or an interval of at least 2 months without manic symptoms.

B. The manic episode is not better accounted for by schizoaffective disorder and is not superimposed on schizophrenia, schizophreniform disorder, delusional disorder, or psychotic disorder not otherwise specified.

Specify if:
   Mixed: if symptoms meet criteria for a mixed episode.

If the full criteria are currently met for a manic, mixed, or major depressive episode, *specify* its current clinical status or features, or both:
   Mild, moderate, severe without psychotic features, or severe with psychotic features
   With catatonic features
   With postpartum onset

If the full criteria are not currently met for a manic, mixed, or major depressive episode, *specify* the current clinical status of the bipolar I disorder or features of the most recent episode:
   In partial remission or in full remission
   With catatonic features
   With postpartum onset

From American Psychiatric Association. *Diagnostic and Statistical Manual of Mental Disorders.* 4th ed. Text rev. Washington, DC: American Psychiatric Association; 2000, with permission.

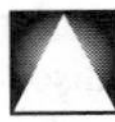

Table 13.6–27
DSM-IV-TR Diagnostic Criteria for Bipolar I Disorder, Most Recent Episode Manic

A. Currently (or most recently) in a manic episode.
B. There has previously been at least one major depressive episode, manic episode, or mixed episode.
C. The mood episodes in Criteria A and B are not better accounted for by schizoaffective disorder and are not superimposed on schizophrenia, schizophreniform disorder, delusional disorder, or psychotic disorder not otherwise specified.

If the full criteria are currently met for a manic episode, *specify* its current clinical status or features, or both:
Mild, moderate, severe without psychotic features, or severe with psychotic features
With catatonic features
With postpartum onset

If the full criteria are not currently met for a manic episode, *specify* the current clinical status of the bipolar I disorder or features of the most recent manic episode, or both:
In partial remission or in full remission
With catatonic features
With postpartum onset

Specify if:
Longitudinal course specifiers (with and without interepisode recovery)
With seasonal pattern (applies only to the pattern of major depressive episodes)
With rapid cycling

From American Psychiatric Association. *Diagnostic and Statistical Manual of Mental Disorders.* 4th ed. Text rev. Washington, DC: American Psychiatric Association; 2000, with permission.

the nature of the current or most recent episode in patients who have had recurrent mood episodes (Tables 13.6–27 through 13.6–31). For clinicians and researchers alike, it is more meaningful to chart a patient's course in color over time—for example using red for manic, blue for depressive, and violet for mixed episodes, with hypomanic, dysthymic, and cyclothymic periods drawn in the appropriate colors on a smaller scale between the major episodes. Life

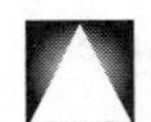

Table 13.6–28
DSM-IV-TR Diagnostic Criteria for Bipolar I Disorder, Most Recent Episode Hypomanic

A. Currently (or most recently) in a hypomanic episode.
B. There has previously been at least one manic episode or mixed episode.
C. The mood symptoms cause clinically significant distress or impairment in social, occupational, or other important areas of functioning.
D. The mood episodes in Criteria A and B are not better accounted for by schizoaffective disorder and are not superimposed on schizophrenia, schizophreniform disorder, delusional disorder, or psychotic disorder not otherwise specified.

Specify if:
Longitudinal course specifiers (with and without interepisode recovery)
With seasonal pattern (applies only to the pattern of major depressive episodes)
With rapid cycling

From American Psychiatric Association. *Diagnostic and Statistical Manual of Mental Disorders.* 4th ed. Text rev. Washington, DC: American Psychiatric Association; 2000, with permission.

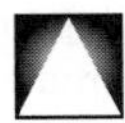

Table 13.6–29
DSM-IV-TR Diagnostic Criteria for Bipolar I Disorder, Most Recent Episode Mixed

A. Currently (or most recently) in a mixed episode.
B. There has previously been at least one major depressive episode, manic episode, or mixed episode.
C. The mood episodes in Criteria A and B are not better accounted for by schizoaffective disorder and are not superimposed on schizophrenia, schizophreniform disorder, delusional disorder, or psychotic disorder, not otherwise specified.

If the full criteria are currently met for a mixed episode, *specify* its current clinical status or features, or both:
Mild, moderate, severe without psychotic features, or severe with psychotic features
With catatonic features
With postpartum onset

If the full criteria are not currently met for a mixed episode, *specify* the current clinical status of the bipolar I disorder or features of the most recent mixed episode, or both:
In partial remission or in full remission
With catatonic features
With postpartum onset

Specify if:
Longitudinal course specifiers (with and without interepisode recovery)
With seasonal pattern (applies only to the pattern of major depressive episodes)
With rapid cycling

From American Psychiatric Association. *Diagnostic and Statistical Manual of Mental Disorders.* 4th ed. Text rev. Washington, DC: American Psychiatric Association; 2000, with permission.

events, biological stressors, and treatment can be indicated by arrows on the time axis. This approach, originally championed by Kraepelin, is routinely used in mood or bipolar clinics to chart retrospectively the past course of illness in mood disorders, especially bipolar disorders. Robert Post at the NIMH has developed this approach into systematic clinical science. Its adoption for clinical use was recommended by an international conference that took place in Barcelona. Recent data from the NIMH Collaborative study—using a prospective method of life charting—of bipolar I disorder clinical cohorts followed in five major U.S. medical centers have shown more depression, especially its subthreshold variants, during an average of 12 years of follow-up. These patients were actually symptomatic nearly 50 percent of the weeks through the entire follow-up, suggesting a more pervasive course of illness than previously appreciated. Although such data indicate some degree of tertiary care bias in favor of patients willing to be retained in a long-term study, they underscore a clinical reality faced by many clinicians in their daily practice.

On average, manic episodes predominate in youth, and depressive episodes predominate in later years. Although the overall sex ratio is approximately one to one, men, on average, undergo more manic episodes, and women experience more mixed and depressive episodes. Bipolar I disorder in children is not as rare as previously thought; however, most reported cases are in boys, and mixed-manic (dysphoric-explosive) and rapid-cycling presentations are the mode. Childhood-onset depression must also be considered a major risk for ultimate bipolar transformation. This is based on the following characteristics: (1) early age at onset; (2) even sex ratio; (3) prominence of irritability, labile moods, and explosive anger, suggesting mixed episodes; (4) questionable response to antidepressants, hypomanic switches, or both; (5) high recurrence rate after depression; and (6) familial affective loading.

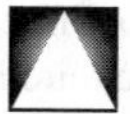

Table 13.6–30
DSM-IV-TR Diagnostic Criteria for Bipolar I Disorder, Most Recent Episode Depressed

A. Currently (or most recently) in a major depressive episode.
B. There has previously been at least one manic episode or mixed episode.
C. The mood episodes in Criteria A and B are not better accounted for by schizoaffective disorder and are not superimposed on schizophrenia, schizophreniform disorder, delusional disorder, or psychotic disorder not otherwise specified.

If the full criteria are currently met for a major depressive episode, *specify* its current clinical status or features, or both:

Mild, moderate, severe without psychotic features, or severe with psychotic features
Chronic
With catatonic features
With melancholic features
With atypical features
With postpartum onset

If the full criteria are not currently met for a major depressive episode, *specify* the current clinical status of the bipolar I disorder or features of the most recent major depressive episode, or both:

In partial remission or in full remission
Chronic
With catatonic features
With melancholic features
With atypical features
With postpartum onset

Specify if:

Longitudinal course specifiers (with and without interepisode recovery)
With seasonal pattern (applies only to the pattern of major depressive episodes)
With rapid cycling

From American Psychiatric Association. *Diagnostic and Statistical Manual of Mental Disorders*. 4th ed. Text rev. Washington, DC: American Psychiatric Association; 2000, with permission.

Mania can also first appear after 65 years of age, although a diligent search often reveals a past mild, forgotten, or untreated depressive or excited episode in earlier years.

Acute Mania Mania typically escalates over a period of 1 to 2 weeks; more sudden onsets have also been described. The DSM-IV-TR criteria (Table 13.6–7) stipulate (1) a distinct period that represents a break from premorbid functioning, (2) a duration of at least 1 week, (3) an elevated or irritable mood, (4) at least three to four classic manic signs and symptoms, and (5) the absence of any physical factors that could account for the clinical picture. The irritable mood in mania can deteriorate to cantankerous behavior, especially when the person is rebuffed. Such patients are among the most aggressive seen in the emergency room. Florid grandiose psychosis with paranoid features, a common presentation of mania, further contributes to the aggression. Alcohol use, observed in at least 50 percent of bipolar I patients (often during the manic phase), further disinhibits the patient and might lead to a dangerous frenzy. Such patients may attack loved ones and hurt them physically. So-called crimes of passion have been committed by patients harboring delusions of infidelity on the part of spouses or lovers, usually when under the influence of alcohol.

The genesis of delusional, hallucinatory, even first-rank, psychotic experiences in mania has already been described. Recent research has documented that most types of formal thought disorders are common to schizophrenic and mood psychoses; only poverty of speech content

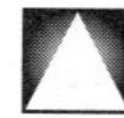

Table 13.6–31
DSM-IV-TR Diagnostic Criteria for Bipolar I Disorder, Most Recent Episode Unspecified

A. Criteria, except for duration, are currently (or most recently) met for a manic, a hypomanic, a mixed, or a major depressive episode.
B. There has previously been at least one manic episode or mixed episode.
C. The mood symptoms cause clinically significant distress or impairment in social, occupational, or other important areas of functioning.
D. The mood symptoms in Criteria A and B are not better accounted for by schizoaffective disorder and are not superimposed on schizophrenia, schizophreniform disorder, delusional disorder, or psychotic disorder not otherwise specified.
E. The mood symptoms in Criteria A and B are not due to the direct physiological effects of a substance (e.g., a drug of abuse, a medication, or other treatment) or a general medical condition (e.g., hyperthyroidism).

Specify if:

Longitudinal course specifiers (with and without interepisode recovery)
With seasonal pattern (applies only to the pattern of major depressive episodes)
With rapid cycling

From American Psychiatric Association. *Diagnostic and Statistical Manual of Mental Disorders*. 4th ed. Text rev. Washington, DC: American Psychiatric Association; 2000, with permission.

(vagueness) emerges as significantly more common in schizophrenia. Finally, posturing and negativism occur in mania (and, in the author's view, do not warrant the designation of catatonic features as advocated by DSM-IV-TR). Although not specifically mentioned in the DSM-IV-TR definition, confusion, even pseudodemented presentations, can occur in mania. Mania is most commonly expressed as a phase of bipolar I disorder, which has strong genetic determinants. Available evidence does not permit separating recurrent mania without depressive episodes from that type as a distinct nosological entity.

Secondary Mania Although there is some suggestion that postpartum mania without depression is distinct from familial bipolar I disorder (in which depressive, manic, and especially mixed manic episodes occur in the postpartum period), the evidence for a distinct puerperal mania is not compelling at this time (hence, the decision in DSM-IV-TR to include the postpartum-onset specifier, rather than a separate mood disorder diagnosis). Mania without prior bipolarity can arise in the setting of such somatic illnesses as thyrotoxicosis, systemic lupus erythematosus or its treatment with steroids, rheumatic chorea, multiple sclerosis (MS), Huntington's disease, cerebrovascular disorder, diencephalic and third ventricular tumors, head trauma, complex partial seizures, syphilis, and (most recently) AIDS. The family history is reportedly low in such cases, suggesting a relatively low genetic predisposition and, thus, a lower risk of recurrence. These patients do not easily fit into the DSM-IV-TR category of mood disorder due to a general medical condition (Table 13.6–17), because most of the conditions appear to be cerebral. Such factors must always be diligently sought in manias of late life.

Less well-defined forms of mania are the so-called reactive manias. Personal loss and bereavement are hypothesized to be triggering factors, and the reaction is conceptualized psychodynamically as a denial of loss. Although such explanations may be plausible in individual cases, no systematic data suggest that these patients differ in family history from persons with other manias. The same is generally true for depressed patients who switch to hypomania or mania after abuse of stimulant drugs, treatment with antidepressants, or sleep deprivation. In all of these situations, a bipolar diathesis is usually manifest in a family history of mania or in spontaneous excited episodes during prospective observation. First-onset manic episodes can also occur in persons who abruptly abstain from alcohol after one or more decades of chronic use and then develop classic bipolar I disorder.

Chronic Mania DSM-IV-TR does not specifically address the diagnostic questions posed by the 5 percent of bipolar I disorder patients who have a chronic manic course. These cases commonly represent deterioration of course dominated by recurrent manic episodes grafted on a hyperthymic baseline. Noncompliance with pharmacological treatment is the rule. Recurrent excitement is personally reinforcing, subjective distress is minimal, and insight is seriously impaired. Thus, the patient sees no reason to adhere to treatment. Episodic or chronic alcohol abuse, prevalent in such patients, has been suggested as a contributory cause of the chronicity. Some authorities further consider comorbid cerebral pathology responsible for nonrecovery (and increased mortality) from manic excitements occurring in late life.

Grandiose delusions (e.g., delusions of inventive genius or aristocratic birth) are not uncommon in chronic mania and may lead to the mistaken diagnosis of paranoid schizophrenia. Because of their social deterioration, Kraepelin subsumed such patients under the category *manic dementia*. Organic factors, such as head trauma and chronic alcohol abuse, may contribute to the deterioration. Nonschizoid premorbid adjustment, a family history of bipolar I disorder, and the absence of flagrant formal thought disorder can be marshaled in establishing the affective basis of these poor-prognosis manic states.

Bipolar Mixed Phase Momentary tearfulness and even depressed mood are commonly observed at the height of mania or during the transition from mania to retarded depression. These transient labile periods, which occur in most bipolar I disorder patients, must be contrasted with mixed episodes proper.

The latter, variously referred to as *mixed mania* or *dysphoric mania*, are characterized by dysphorically excited moods, irritability, anger, panic attacks, pressured speech, agitation, suicidal ideation, severe insomnia, grandiosity, and hypersexuality, as well as persecutory delusions and confusion. Severely psychotic mixed states that involve hallucinations and schneiderian symptoms risk being labeled *schizoaffective*. A correct diagnosis helps to avoid conventional antipsychotic drugs known to exacerbate the depressive component; in such patients, failure to use mood stabilizers can prolong the patient's misery.

New research data from mood centers worldwide on mixed mania suggest that dysphoric mania—mania and full-blown depression occurring simultaneously—is relatively uncommon. Two to four depressive symptoms from the list of depressed mood, helplessness, hopelessness, fatigue, anhedonia, guilt, and suicidal ideation, impulses, or both in the setting of a manic syndrome, appear to suffice for the diagnosis of mixed manic states, which occur in 50 percent of patients with bipolar disorder sometime during their lives. Mixed states occur predominantly in women in whom mania is superimposed on a depressive temperament or a dysthymic baseline. These considerations suggest that the DSM-IV-TR concept of mixed episode (Table 13.6–8) as a cross-sectional mixture of mania and depression is simplistic and phenomenologically naïve. The emerging conceptualization of mixed mania is a manic state intruding on long-term depressive traits. Other mixed manic states, especially in men, often arise from the interaction of substance or alcohol use in bipolar I disorder.

Depressive Phase Psychomotor retardation, with or without hypersomnia, marks the uncomplicated depressive phase of bipolar I disorder. Onset and offset are often abrupt, although onset can also occur gradually over several weeks. Patients may recover into a free interval or may switch directly into mania. Switching into an excited phase is particularly likely when antidepressants have been used. However, not all patients develop mania after antidepressant treatment of bipolar depression. Some develop a mixed agitated depression; indeed, patients may be stuck for many months in a severe depressive phase with some manic admixtures, such as racing thoughts and sexual arousal. DSM-IV-TR does not specifically recognize a mixed depressive phase, with few manic symptoms occurring during full-blown depression. Such recognition is necessary, because these patients do not need continued aggressive antidepressant therapy, but rather mood stabilizers, ECT, or both.

Delusional and hallucinatory experiences are less common in the depressive phase of bipolar I disorder than in the manic and mixed manic phases. Stupor is the more common psychotic presentation of bipolar depression, particularly in adolescents and young adults. Pseudodemented organic presentations appear to be the counterpart of stupor in elderly adults.

Cyclothymic Disorder An attenuated bipolar disorder that typically begins insidiously before 21 years of age, cyclothymic disorder is characterized in DSM-IV-TR by frequent short cycles of subsyndromal depression and hypomania (Table 13.6–32). The author's research has revealed alternating patterns of moods, activity, and cognition (Table 13.6–33), which are more explicit than the DSM-IV-TR criteria; they have the added advantage of having been validated. The course of cyclothymia is continuous or intermittent, with infrequent periods of euthymia. Shifts in mood often lack adequate precipitants (e.g., sudden profound dejection with social with-

Table 13.6–32
DSM-IV-TR Diagnostic Criteria for Cyclothymic Disorder

A. For at least 2 years, the presence of numerous periods with hypomanic symptoms and numerous periods with depressive symptoms that do not meet criteria for a major depressive episode. **Note:** In children and adolescents, the duration must be at least 1 year.

B. During the previously mentioned 2-year period (1 year in children and adolescents), the person has not been without the symptoms in Criterion A for more than 2 months at a time.

C. No major depressive episode, manic episode, or mixed episode has been present during the first 2 years of the disturbance.

Note: After the initial 2 years (1 year in children and adolescents) of cyclothymic disorder, there may be superimposed manic or mixed episodes (in which case bipolar I disorder and cyclothymic disorder may be diagnosed) or major depressive episodes (in which case bipolar II disorder and cyclothymic disorder may be diagnosed).

D. The symptoms in Criterion A are not better accounted for by schizoaffective disorder and are not superimposed on schizophrenia, schizophreniform disorder, delusional disorder, or psychotic disorder not otherwise specified.

E. The symptoms are not due to the direct physiological effects of a substance (e.g., a drug of abuse or a medication) or a general medical condition (e.g., hyperthyroidism).

F. The symptoms cause clinically significant distress or impairment in social, occupational, or other important areas of functioning.

From American Psychiatric Association. *Diagnostic and Statistical Manual of Mental Disorders*. 4th ed. Text rev. Washington, DC: American Psychiatric Association; 2000, with permission.

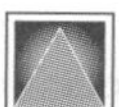

Table 13.6–33
Clinical Features of Cyclothymic Disorder

Biphasic dysregulation characterized by abrupt endoreactive shifts from one phase to the other, each phase lasting for a few days at a time, with infrequent euthymia.

Behavioral manifestations

Introverted self-absorption versus uninhibited people seeking

Taciturn versus talkative

Unexplained tearfulness versus buoyant jocularity

Psychomotor inertia versus restless pursuit of activities

Subjective manifestations

Lethargy and somatic discomfort versus eutonia

Dulling of senses versus keen perceptions

Slow-witted thinking versus sharpened thinking

Shaky self-esteem alternating between low self-confidence and overconfidence

Pessimistic brooding versus optimism and carefree attitudes

Updated from Akiskal HS, Khani M, Scott-Strauss A: Cyclothymic temperamental disorders. *Psychiatr Clin North Am.* 1979;2:527.

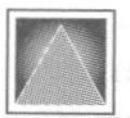

Table 13.6–34
Evolving Spectrum of Bipolar Disorders

Bipolar $^1/_2$: schizobipolar disorder

Bipolar I: core manic-depressive illness

Bipolar I$^1/_2$: depression with protracted hypomania

Bipolar II: depression with discrete spontaneous hypomanic episodes

Bipolar II$^1/_2$: depression superimposed on cyclothymic temperament

Bipolar III: depression plus *induced* hypomania (i.e., hypomania occurring solely in association with antidepressant or other somatic treatment)

Bipolar III$^1/_2$: prominent mood swings occurring in the context of substance or alcohol use or abuse

Bipolar IV: depression superimposed on a hyperthymic temperament

Adapted from Akiskal HS, Pinto O: The evolving bipolar spectrum: Prototypes I, II, III, IV. *Psychiatr Clin North Am.* 1999;22:517–534.

drawal for a few days switching into cheerful, gregarious behavior). Circadian factors may account for some of the extremes of emotional lability, such as the person's going to sleep in good spirits and waking up early with suicidal urges. The mood changes of cyclothymia are best described as *endoreactive* in the sense that endogenous overreactivity seems to determine the sudden shifts in mood and behavior (e.g., falling in love with a person one has just met and as quickly falling out of love).

Mood swings in these ambulatory patients are overshadowed by the chaos that the swings produce in their personal lives. Repeated romantic breakups or marital failures are common because of interpersonal friction and episodic promiscuous behavior. Uneven performance at school and work is also common. Persons with cyclothymic disorder are dilettantes; they show great promise in many areas but rarely bring any of their efforts to fruition. As a result, their lives are often a string of improvident activities. Geographical instability is a characteristic feature; easily attracted to a new locale, job, or love partner, they soon lose interest and leave in dissatisfaction. Polysubstance abuse, which occurs in as many as 50 percent of such persons, is often an attempt at self-treatment.

Bipolar II Disorder

Research conducted during the past three decades has shown that, between the extremes of manic-depressive illness defined by at least one acute manic episode, which could be mood-congruent or -incongruent (bipolar I disorder), and strictly defined major depressive disorder without any personal or family history of mania (pure unipolar disorder), there exists an overlapping group of intermediary forms characterized by recurrent major depressive episodes and hypomania. Table 13.6–34 summarizes the author's observations in defining the clinical subtypes within this intermediary realm best described as *soft bipolarity*. The most accepted of the subtypes is bipolar II disorder (with spontaneous hypomania), elevated to the status of a nosological entity in DSM-IV-TR (Table 13.6–35). Current data worldwide indicate that bipolar II disorder is actually more prevalent than bipolar I disorder. This certainly appears true in the outpatient setting, in which an average of 50 percent of persons with major depressive disorder have been reported to conform to the bipolar II disorder pattern.

The following self-description provided by a 34-year-old poet illustrates the pattern:

> I have known melancholy periods, lasting months at a time, when I would be literally paralyzed: All mental activity comes to a screeching halt, and I cannot even utter one word. I become so dysfunctional that I was once hospitalized. Although the paralysis creeps into me insidiously—often lasting months—it typically reverses within hours. I am suddenly alive and vibrant, I cannot turn off my brain neither during the day nor at night; I usually go on celebrating like this for many days, needing no more than few hours of slumber each day.

This vignette is nearly identical to the autobiographical description provided by the British poet William Cowper three centuries earlier: "I have known many a lifeless and unhallowed hour . . . long intervals of darkness interrupted by short returns of peace and joy. . . . For many succeeding weeks to rejoice day and night was all my employment. Too happy to sleep much, I thought it was lost time that was spent on slumber."

Although some hypomanias last for weeks, the hypomania at the end of depressive episodes in most bipolar II disorder patients does not persist long; it is usually measured in days. As discussed earlier, hypomanias with short duration (<4 days) are familially similar to those with longer duration (≥4 days). Hence, the recommendation in the clinical research literature to lower the DSM-IV-TR threshold for hypomania to 2 days rather than 4 days. Another common form of bipolar II disorder is major depressive disorder, superimposed on cyclothymic disorder, in which hypomania precedes and follows major depressive disorder, the entire interepisodic period characterized by cyclothymic mood instability. Such patients tend to have an unstable course, stormy interpersonal relationships, and more irritable and hostile hypomanic episodes—hence confused with borderline personality disorder. Current data indicate that cyclothymic and noncyclothymic bipolar II disorder have similar rates of familial bipolarity, which suggests that the borderline characterological features represent a complication of the unstable course that cyclothymia imparts to bipolar II disorder. Such individuals with unstable course have high risk of suicide—indeed, the high burden of suicide in mood disorders appears to be due to bipolar II disorder, based on research in Budapest. Descriptively, *hypomania in bipolar II disorder* can be defined as mini manic episodes occurring spontaneously. Bipolar II disorder—especially when major depressions are superimposed on cyclothymia—is thus best characterized as cyclical or *cyclothymic depression.*

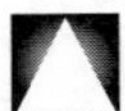

Table 13.6–35
DSM-IV-TR Diagnostic Criteria for Bipolar II Disorder

A. Presence (or history) of one or more major depressive episodes.
B. Presence (or history) of at least one hypomanic episode.
C. There has never been a manic episode or a mixed episode.
D. The mood symptoms in Criteria A and B are not better accounted for by schizoaffective disorder and are not superimposed on schizophrenia, schizophreniform disorder, delusional disorder, or psychotic disorder not otherwise specified.
E. The symptoms cause clinically significant distress or impairment in social, occupational, or other important areas of functioning.

Specify current or most recent episode:

Hypomanic: if currently (or most recently) in a hypomanic episode

Depressed: if currently (or most recently) in a major depressive episode.

If the full criteria are currently met for a major depressive episode, *specify* its current clinical status or features, or both:

Mild, moderate, severe without psychotic features, or severe with psychotic features. Note: Fifth-digit codes cannot be used here, because the code for bipolar II disorder already uses the fifth digit.

Chronic
With catatonic features
With melancholic features
With atypical features
With postpartum onset

If the full criteria are not currently met for a hypomanic or major depressive episode, *specify* the clinical status of the bipolar II disorder or features of the most recent major depressive episode (only if it is the most recent type of mood episode), or both:

In partial remission, in full remission. Note: Fifth-digit codes cannot be used here, because the code for bipolar II disorder already uses the fifth digit.

Chronic
With catatonic features
With melancholic features
With atypical features
With postpartum onset

Specify if:

Longitudinal course specifiers (with and without interepisode recovery)

With seasonal pattern (applies only to the pattern of major depressive episodes)

With rapid cycling

From American Psychiatric Association. *Diagnostic and Statistical Manual of Mental Disorders.* 4th ed. Text rev. Washington, DC: American Psychiatric Association; 2000, with permission.

The depressive episodes of patients with bipolar disorder often have admixtures (e.g., flight of ideas and increased drives and impulsivity in sexual and other domains). These are best regarded as depressive mixed states, basically ignored in the DSM-IV-TR schema. Depressive mixed states are not as severe as dysphoric mixed states but are refractory to antidepressants nonetheless. Current Italian research conducted by Franco Benazzi and the present author indicates that such depressive mixed states occurs in as much as 60 percent of cases of bipolar II disorder and as much as 30 percent of cases of "unipolar" major depressive disorder. Both groups have similar rates of familial bipolarity, suggesting that one out of three patients with "unipolar" depression belongs to the bipolar II spectrum.

Hypomania The common denominator of the soft spectrum of bipolar disorders is the occurrence of hypomania as episode or trait. *Hypomania* in DSM-IV-TR (Table 13.6–9) refers to a distinct period of at least a few days of mild elevation of mood, sharpened and positive thinking, and increased energy and activity levels, typically without the impairment characteristic of manic episodes. It is not merely a milder form of mania. Hypomania occurring as part of bipolar II disorder rarely progresses to manic psychosis, and insight is relatively preserved. Hypomania is distinguished from mere happiness in that it tends to recur (happiness does not!) and can sometimes be mobilized by antidepressants. In cyclothymic disorder, it alternates with mini depressions; in hyperthymic temperament, it constitutes the person's habitual baseline. These definitions, developed by empirical research by the author, recognize three patterns of hypomania: *episodes* heralding the termination of a retarded depressive state (bipolar II disorder), cyclic alternation with mini depressions (cyclothymic disorder), and an elevated baseline of high mood, activity, and cognition (hyperthymic or chronic hypomanic *traits*).

Because hypomania is experienced as a rebound relief from depression or as a pleasant, relatively short-lived, ego-syntonic mood state, persons with bipolar II disorder rarely report it spontaneously. Skillful questioning is thus required to make the diagnosis of soft bipolar conditions; as in mania, collateral information from family members is crucial. In interviewing the patient, it is customary to use questions along these lines: "Have you had a distinct sustained high period when your mood was so intense that you felt nervous, you were endowed with such energy that others could not keep up with you, and when your thinking and perceptions were unusually vivid or rapid?" These are based on DSM-IV-TR criteria (Table 13.6–9), which require high or irritable mood as a prerequisite (Criterion A). Many bipolar patients react to inquiries about "high moods" or "high periods" with a negative: "I am not a manic-depressive!" In collaboration with Benazzi, the authors have recently shown that it is best first to inquire about signs and symptoms referring to behavioral activation (Criterion B) and, once the requisite number of such activation criteria are met, to return to the mood items (Criterion A). Once energized periods are remembered, the patient is more likely to recall the mood change associated with these periods.

Clinical and epidemiological studies in the United States and Europe have revealed a richer range of hypomanic manifestations than those listed in the DSM-IV-TR, including an increase in cheerfulness and jocularity; gregariousness and people seeking; greater interest in sex; talkativeness, self-confidence, and optimism; and decreased inhibitions and sleep need. The clinician must ascertain that those experiences were not due to stimulant or alcohol withdrawal. Depressive and hypomanic periods are often not easily discerned, because chronic caffeine use, stimulant abuse, or both may complicate the depression. In such instances, diagnosis should be deferred for 1 month after detoxification.

When in doubt, direct clinical observation of hypomania—sometimes elicited by antidepressant pharmacotherapy—provides definitive evidence for the bipolar nature of the disorder. Unfortunately, DSM-IV-TR denies bipolar status to treatment-emergent hypomanic episodes. As discussed previously in this chapter, current evidence is strongly supportive of the bipolar nature of such hypomanias. In the research literature, these are often considered as *bipolar III disorder* (not an official term in DSM-IV-TR).

Seasonal Patterns Seasonality is observed in many cyclic depressions, often with autumn or winter anergic depression and energetic periods in the spring. This natural propensity explains why phototherapy may provoke mild hypomanic switches. Although not specifically identified by DSM-IV-TR, seasonal depressions conform, in large measure, to the bipolar II disorder or bipolar III disorder pattern. Furthermore, preliminary evidence suggests that treatment with classic antidepressants disrupts the baseline seasonality, with the depressive phase appearing in the spring and summer. The changes that antidepressants induce in seasonal depressions probably represent a special variant of the rapid-cycling phenomenon.

Temperament and Polarity of Episodes New systematic clinical observations have revealed that bipolar II disorder (characterized predominantly by depressive attacks) arises more often from a hyperthymic or cyclothymic baseline, whereas bipolar I disorder (defined by manic attacks) not uncommonly arises from the substrate of a depressive temperament. In line with these observations, a prospective 11-year NIMH study of major depressive disorder patients who switched to bipolar II disorder showed that *mood-labile* (cyclothymic) and *energetic-active* (hyperthymic) temperament traits were highly specific (86 percent) and reasonably sensitive (42 percent) predictors of such an outcome.

Bipolarity is conventionally defined by the alternation of manic (or hypomanic) and depressive episodes. The foregoing data on temperaments suggest that a more fundamental characteristic of bipolarity is the reversal of temperament into its "opposite" episode (in the case of the bipolar II disorder spectrum, from cyclothymia and hyperthymia to major depression). Such findings suggest that the intrusion of cyclothymic and hyperthymic traits into a depressive episode may underlie the instability of the bipolar II disorder subtype and could partly explain why bipolar II depression often has mixed features. These considerations may have important implications for preventing recurrence. For instance, a prospective study of the onset of bipolar disorder in the offspring or siblings of adults with the disorder found that children with depressive onsets as their first episode (which were usually treated with antidepressants) had significantly higher rates of recurrence than those with manic or mixed onsets (treated with lithium) during a 3-year prospective observation. It appears that temperamental instability in the depressive group might have predisposed them to the cycling effect of antidepressants.

Alcohol and Substance Abuse New evidence supports the high prevalence of alcohol and substance abuse in mood disorder subtypes, especially those with interepisodic cyclothymia and hyperthymia. The relation appears particularly strong in the teenage and early adult years, when the use of such substances often represents self-medication for the mood instability. It is not just self-treatment for selected symptoms associated with the down or up phases (e.g., alcohol to alleviate the insomnia and nervousness characteristic of both phases), it also augments certain desired ends (e.g., stimulants to enhance high-energy performance and sexual behavior associated with hypomania). Alcohol may be sought both for its disinhibiting effects and for sedation to calm the nervousness of the high periods. How many display alcohol and substance abuse secondary to an underlying bipolar diathesis remains to be determined. However, in view of findings suggesting a link between polysubstance abuse and suicide in adolescents with bipolar familial backgrounds, the use of mood stabilizers in these adolescents should be strongly considered. Although alcohol and stimulant use continues into adult years in a considerable number of bipolar disorder patients, such use is often unrelated to familial alcoholism and frequently tends to dwindle during long-term follow-up, which supports the self-medication hypothesis.

Rapid-Cycling Bipolar Disorder *Rapid cycling* is defined as the occurrence of at least four episodes—of retarded depression and hypomania (or mania)—per year (Table 13.6–36). Thus, rapid cyclers are rarely free of affective symptoms and experience serious vocational and interpersonal incapacitation. Lithium is only modestly helpful to those patients, as are traditional antipsychotic agents; most antidepressants readily induce excited episodes and thus aggravate the rapid-cycling pattern. A balance among mood stabilizers, atypical antipsychotic drugs, and antidepressants may be difficult to achieve. Antidepressants should be avoided, because every provoked hypomania is followed by depression, and the roller-coaster is further prolonged. Many such patients require frequent hospitalization, because they develop explosive excitement and precipitous descent into severe psychomotor inhibition. The disorder is a roller-coaster nightmare for the patient, significant others, and the treating physician. Treating these patients is an art. Lamotrigine (Lamictal), a new mood stabilizer that stabilizes "from below," has been reported efficacious in this group of patients.

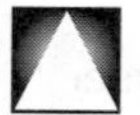

Table 13.6–36
DSM-IV-TR Diagnostic Criteria for Rapid Cycling Specifier

Specify if:

With rapid cycling (can be applied to bipolar I disorder or bipolar II disorder).

At least four episodes of a mood disturbance in the previous 12 months that meet criteria for a major depressive, manic, mixed, or hypomanic episode.

Note: Episodes are demarcated by partial or full remission for at least 2 months or a switch to an episode of opposite polarity (e.g., major depressive episode to manic episode).

From American Psychiatric Association. *Diagnostic and Statistical Manual of Mental Disorders.* 4th ed. Text rev. Washington, DC: American Psychiatric Association; 2000, with permission.

As expected, rapid cycling commonly arises from a cyclothymic substrate, which means that most rapid cyclers have bipolar II disorder. Factors favoring its occurrence include (1) female gender; (2) borderline hypothyroidism; (3) menopause; (4) temporal lobe dysrhythmias; (5) alcohol, minor tranquilizer, stimulant, or caffeine abuse; and (6) long-term, aggressive use of antidepressant medications. Most clinically identified patients are bipolar II women in middle age or upper social classes. Rapid cycling is uncommon from a bipolar I disorder base.

Leadership and Creativity Persons with hyperthymic temperament and soft bipolar conditions in general possess assets that permit them to assume leadership roles in business, the professions, civic life, and politics. Increased energy, sharp thinking, self-confidence, and eloquence represent the virtues of an otherwise stormy life.

Creative achievement is relatively uncommon among those with the manic forms of the disorder, which are too severe and disorganizing to permit the necessary concentration and application. Notable artistic achievements are found among those with soft bipolar disorders, especially cyclothymic disorders. Psychosis, including severe bipolar swings, is generally incompatible with creativity. That conclusion, based on systematic studies by the author and Kareen Akiskal, tends to refute the romantic tendency to idolize insanity as central to the creative process. As talent is the necessary ingredient of creativity, how might soft bipolarity contribute? The simplest hypothesis is that depression might provide insights into the human condition, and the activation associated with hypomania helps in producing the artistic work. A more profound interpretation suggests

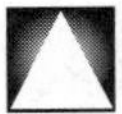

Table 13.6–37
DSM-IV-TR Diagnostic Criteria for Bipolar Disorder Not Otherwise Specified

The bipolar disorder not otherwise specified category includes disorders with bipolar features that do not meet criteria for any specific bipolar disorder. Examples include the following:

1. Rapid alternation (over days) between manic symptoms and depressive symptoms that meet symptom threshold criteria but not minimal duration criteria for manic, hypomanic, or major depressive episodes.
2. Recurrent hypomanic episodes without intercurrent depressive symptoms.
3. A manic or mixed episode superimposed on delusional disorder, residual schizophrenia, or psychotic disorder not otherwise specified.
4. Hypomanic episodes, along with chronic depressive symptoms, that are too infrequent to qualify for a diagnosis of cyclothymic disorder.
5. Situations in which the clinician has concluded that a bipolar disorder is present but is unable to determine whether it is primary, due to a general medical condition, or substance induced.

From American Psychiatric Association. *Diagnostic and Statistical Manual of Mental Disorders*. 4th ed. Text rev. Washington, DC: American Psychiatric Association; 2000, with permission.

that the repeated self-doubt that comes with recurrent depression might be an important ingredient of creativity, because original artistic or scientific expression is often initially rejected, and the self-confidence that accompanies repeated bouts of hypomania can help in rehearsing such ideas or expressions until they are perfected. Finally, the tempestuous object relations associated with bipolarity in the parent's or the patient's life often create the unique biographical landmarks that might be immortalized in an artistic medium.

Bipolar Disorder Not Otherwise Specified

The criteria for bipolar disorder not otherwise specified are listed in Table 13.6–37. In this section, certain conditions are described that are on the edge of the better-defined categories of bipolar disorders. Although they are commonly observed in clinical practice, there is a relatively sparse literature on them.

Ultrarapid Cycling In these patients, hypomanic or manic and depressive episodes alternate rapidly over a few days. In many, the alternation occurs in a regular fashion. The episodes in such cycling patients have greater amplitudes than in cyclothymia, leading to marked impairment. They can be considered as intermediary between cyclothymia and full-blown rapid cycling. Of considerable theoretical and methodological interest, they are difficult to manage clinically. Some individuals with this condition learn to change their work days such that they coincide with the hypomanic periods.

Recurrent Brief Hypomania This hypomanic counterpart of recurrent brief depressive disorder is best conceptualized as a variant of soft bipolarity described previously. It tends to coincide with cyclothymic depression, in which hypomanias are short (<4 days).

Hysteroid Dysphoria Hysteroid dysphoria combines reverse vegetative signs with the following characteristics: (1) giddy responses to romantic opportunities and an avalanche of dysphoria (angry-depressive, even suicidal, responses) to romantic disappointment; (2) impaired anticipatory pleasure, yet the capability to respond with pleasure when such is provided by others (i.e., preservation of consummatory reward); and (3) craving for chocolate and sweets, which contain phenylethylamine compounds and sugars believed to facilitate cellular and neuronal intake of the amino acid L-tryptophan, hypothetically leading to synthesis of endogenous antidepressants in the brain. The use of the epithet *hysteroid* was used to convey that the apparent character pathology was secondary to a biological disturbance in the substrates governing affect, drives, and reward. The intense, unstable life of the patient with hysteroid dysphoria suggests links to cyclothymic disorder or bipolar II disorder. This suggestion is further supported by the Columbia group's tendency to subsume those patients under atypical depressions (some of which, as indicated, have bipolar affinities). Like patients with bipolar depression, they respond preferentially to monoamine oxidase inhibitors (MAOIs). In brief, hysteroid dysphoria appears to be a variant of bipolar II disorder with cyclothymic-irritable traits. Such patients are often relegated to the realm of borderline personality. Recent formulations deriving from the Pisa–San Diego Collaboration suggest that cyclothymic traits represent the underlying diathesis of atypical depression, borderline personality, and bipolar II.

Bipolar III and IV Disorders In bipolar III disorder (which is not an official nosological term), evidence of bipolarity is softer, such as a brief episode of an antidepressant-mobilized switch. As discussed previously, family history for bipolar disorder is often positive in such patients. In those in whom the pharmacologically mobilized excursion is brief and occurs rarely, the premorbid temperament is often depressive in tone, suggesting that an exogenous *activating* factor is needed to unmask the bipolar diathesis. Such cases raise the possibility that some phenotypically unipolar depressed patients are nonetheless constitutionally bipolar.

In bipolar IV disorder (again, not a formal DSM-IV-TR entity, which likewise can be subsumed under bipolar disorder not otherwise specified), discrete hypomanic episodes do not occur. Instead the patient's habitual temperamental baseline is sunny, overenergetic, and overoptimistic (hyperthymic). Depending on the threshold of traits used in determining the presence of hyperthymia, bipolar IV disorder patients may constitute 10 to 20 percent of those with major depressive disorder. The presence of marked narcissistic traits is a helpful clinical clue that a clinically depressed patient might belong to the group of those with hyperthymic depressions.

Primary versus Secondary Bipolar Disorder Not Otherwise Specified DSM-IV-TR finally suggests that, when the clinician is uncertain whether distinct bipolar signs and symptoms are due to physical or alcohol or substance use disorders, bipolar disorder not otherwise specified is the proper diagnosis. The contribution of medical etiologies to manic states has already been described; such patients usually respond quite well to currently available antimanic and mood-stabilizing agents given for the duration of the episode. As for the comorbidity of bipolar and alcohol or substance use disorders, it is best to recognize both sets of disorders, to ensure that competent treatment is provided to both. Dual diagnosis programs are ideally suited for such a task, although, in the author's experience, the contribution of bipolar disorder to the morbidity of these dually diagnosed patients is often underestimated, if not ignored. Thereby, the opportunity to treat both conditions with mood stabilizer combinations is lost.

MOOD DISORDERS NOT OTHERWISE SPECIFIED

After all diagnostic information has been obtained, some patients with affective symptoms do not meet the specific criteria for the mood conditions described thus far, nor do they fit the examples listed in the not otherwise specified categories for depressive and bipolar disorders. DSM-IV-TR lists "acute agitation" as an example. Another example that the author has encountered in his practice are individuals with acute suicidal ideation of an ego-dystonic nature, not accompanied by other affective symptoms. Family or close follow-up, or both, often suggests a more discrete mental condition. Mood disorder not otherwise specified is a statistical concept for filing purposes and not a clinical description. In general, the author prefers to consider such cases as undiagnosed mood disorders. However, two hybrid conditions, which have not been specifically addressed elsewhere in this chapter, can be conveniently discussed here.

Mixed Anxiety-Depressive Disorder

The inclusion of anxious depressive states in a DSM-IV-TR appendix acknowledges the simultaneous occurrence of anxious (e.g., the threat that loss represents) and depressive (e.g., the despair of loss) cognition in a person confronted with a major aversive life situation. The admixture implies that the psychopathology progresses from anxiety to depression, that the patient's mental state is still in flux, and that the ongoing dynamics partly explain the subacute or chronic nature of the disorder. Anxious depression serves to point to the common presence of anxiety in depressive states, especially its greater visibility when the depression is less prominent. Patients with the latter presentation are reportedly most prevalent in general medical settings. This should not come as a surprise, because depressive symptoms that motivate medical consultation commonly complicate generalized anxiety states with a subthreshold level of symptomatology. Some authorities argue that neurotic depressions arise as maladaptive responses to anxiety and, on that basis, suggest retaining the *neurotic depression* rubric. Recent preliminary genetic data indirectly support the contention that certain (unipolar) depressive and (generalized) anxiety states are related. However, more research is needed before such an entity can be unequivocally accepted as an official nosological category. The difficulty is that, as currently defined, anxious depressions are heterogeneous. In patients refractory to anxiolytic or antidepressant treatment, practitioners must entertain the diagnosis of a complex bipolar II disorder with mixed features. Indeed, recent familial-genetic investigations suggest that bipolar II disorder with panic attacks might represent a special form of bipolar disorder.

Atypical Depression

Although a delimited version of atypical depression was incorporated into DSM-IV-TR as *atypical features* (Table 13.6–5) to qualify the cross-sectional picture of depressive disorders (and has been described earlier in this chapter in relation to major depressive disorder), this construct is much broader in the clinical research literature. Originally developed in England and currently under investigation at Columbia University in New York, *atypical depression* refers to fatigue superimposed on a history of somatic anxiety and phobias, together with reverse vegetative signs (mood worse in the evening, insomnia, tendency to oversleep and to overeat). Sleep is disturbed in the first one-half of the night in many persons with atypical depressive disorder, so irritability, hypersomnolence, and daytime fatigue would be expected. The temperaments of these patients are characterized by sensitive traits. The MAOIs and serotonergic antidepressants seem to show some specificity for such patients, which is the main reason that atypical depression is taken seriously.

Other research suggests that reverse vegetative signs can be classified as (1) the anxious type just described or (2) a subtle bipolar subtype with protracted hyperphagic-hypersomnic-retarded dysthymic disorder with occasional brief, extroverted, hypomanic-type behavior, often elicited by antidepressants. Increasing evidence indicates considerable affinity between atypical depression and bipolar II and III disorders. Furthermore, many patients with dysthymic disorder exhibit atypical features at various times. Actually, atypical depression might be an artifact of the DSM-IV-TR definition of hypomania of 4 or more days. Recent Italian research suggests that many patients with atypical depression meet criteria for brief hypomania or cyclothymic disorder. Such patients also resemble those with hysteroid dysphoria, the precursor of the construct of atypical depression.

In brief, the categories of not otherwise specified in the DSM-IV-TR mood disorders schema largely reflect inadequacies of the operational approach to capture patients whose symptomatology falls between or on the boundaries of more classic diagnoses.

DIFFERENTIAL DIAGNOSIS

A missed mood disorder diagnosis means that the disorder does not receive specific treatment, which has serious consequences. Many such persons drop out of school or college, lose their jobs, get divorced, or may commit suicide. Those with unexplained somatic symptoms are frequent users of the general health system. Others are unwell, despite interminable psychotherapy. Some, treated with conventional neuroleptics, develop tardive dyskinesia unnecessarily. As with other medical disorders for which specific treatments are available, accurate diagnosis and early treatment are within the purview of all physicians and mental health professionals. Psychiatrists, in particular, should develop the competence to detect the entire spectrum of mood disorders. Despite massive educational efforts, underdiagnosis and undertreatment of mood disorders remain serious problems worldwide. The most pernicious of these is down-playing the mood component because a personality disorder is given undue prominence.

Although much enthusiasm was generated a decade ago about the potential use of certain biological markers (e.g., REM latency, dexamethasone-suppression test [DST], and thyrotropin-releasing hormone [TRH] test) to corroborate the differentiation of mood disorder from adjacent disorders, no definitive progress justifies their routine use in clinical practice. The same is true, at least for now, for brain imaging, neuropsychological testing, and genetic screening. Faced with unusual or confusing presentations, a systematic clinical approach is still the best method in differential diagnosis (1) to detail all clinical features of the current episode, (2) to elicit a history of more typical major mood episodes in the past, (3) to assess whether the presenting complaints recur periodically or cyclically, (4) to substantiate adequate social functioning between periods of illness, (5) to obtain a positive family history for classic mood disorder and to construct a family pedigree, and (6) to document a history of unequivocal therapeutic response to thymoleptic medication or ECT in the patient or the family.

Using the foregoing validating approach, one can examine the affective links of many DSM-IV-TR disorders currently listed under mood disorders not otherwise specified, as well as controversial nosological entities currently categorized as nonmood disorders. The latter include conduct disorders, borderline personality disorder, impulse-control disorders, polysubstance abuse, psychotic disorder not otherwise specified, pain disorder, hypochondriasis, hypoactive sexual desire disorder, circadian rhythm sleep disorder and delayed sleep-phase type, bulimia nervosa, and adjustment disorder (with work inhibition). These conditions place special emphasis on selected affective features, such as disinhibited behavior, temperamental behavior, mood lability, vegetative disturbances, and psychomotor anergia. This discussion first briefly considers the differential diagnostic problem *within* affective states—such as that between grief and melancholia, anxiety versus depressive disorder, and unipolar versus bipolar disorders—before embarking on a systematic examination of the differential diagnosis of mood disorders with their more classic boundaries.

Normal Bereavement Bereaved persons exhibit many depressive symptoms during the first 1 to 2 years after their loss, so how can the 5 percent of bereaved persons who have progressed to a depressive disorder be identified?

- Grieving persons and their relatives perceive bereavement as a normal reaction, whereas those with depressive disorder often view themselves as sick and may actually believe they are losing their minds.
- Unlike the melancholic person, the grieving person reacts to the environment and tends to show a range of positive affects.
- Marked psychomotor retardation is not observed in normal grief.
- Although bereaved persons often feel guilty about not having done certain things that might have saved the life of the deceased loved one (guilt of omission), they typically do not experience guilt of commission.
- Delusions of worthlessness or sin and psychotic experiences in general point toward mood disorder.
- Active suicidal ideation is rare in grief but common in major depressive disorder.
- "Mummification" (i.e., keeping the belongings of the deceased person exactly as they were before his or her death) indicates serious psychopathology.
- Severe anniversary reactions should alert the clinician to the possibility of psychopathology.

In another form of bereavement depression, the patient simply pines away, unable to live without the departed person, usually a spouse. Although not necessarily pathological by the foregoing criteria, such persons do have a serious medical condition. Their immune function is often depressed, and their cardiovascular status is precarious. Death can ensue within a few months of that of a spouse, especially among elderly men. Such considerations (highlighted in the work of Sidney Zisook and his San Diego colleagues at the University of California) suggest that it would be clinically unwise to withhold antidepressants from many persons experiencing an intensely mournful form of grief. The case vignette from the author's private practice illustrates this point:

A 75-year-old widow was brought to treatment by her daughter because of severe insomnia and total loss of interest in daily routines after her husband's death 1 year before. She had been agitated for the first 2 to 3 months and thereafter "sank into total inactivity—not wanting to get out of bed, not wanting to do anything, not wanting to go out." According to her daughter, she was married at 21 years of age, had four children, and had been a housewife until her husband's death from a heart attack. Past psychiatric history was negative; premorbid adjustment had been characterized by compulsive traits. During the interview, she was dressed in black, appeared moderately slowed, and sobbed intermittently, saying "I search everywhere for him. . . . I don't find him." When asked about life, she said "everything I see is black." Although she expressed no interest in food, she did not seem to have lost an appreciable amount of weight. Her DST result was 18 mg/dL. The patient declined psychiatric care, stating that she "preferred to join her husband rather than get well." She was too religious to commit suicide, but, by refusing treatment, she felt that she would "pine away . . . find relief in death and reunion."

Anxiety Disorders Anxiety symptoms, including panic attacks, morbid fears, and obsessions, are common during depressive disorders, and depression is a common complication of anxiety states.

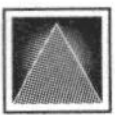

Table 13.6–38
Unique Cross-Sectional Profiles of Clinical Anxiety and Depression

Anxiety	Depression
Hypervigilance	Psychomotor retardation
Severe tension and panic	Severe sadness
Perceived danger	Perceived loss
Phobic avoidance	Loss of interest—anhedonia
Doubt and uncertainty	Hopelessness—suicidal
Insecurity	Self-deprecation
Performance anxiety	Loss of libido
	Early-morning awakening
	Weight loss

From Akiskal HS: Toward a clinical understanding of the relationship of anxiety and depressive disorders. In: Maser JP, Cloninger CR, eds. *Comorbidity of Mood and Anxiety Disorders.* Washington, DC: American Psychiatric Press; 1990, with permission.

Systematic British studies have shown that early-morning awakening, psychomotor retardation, self-reproach, hopelessness, and suicidal ideation are the strongest clinical markers of depression in that differential diagnosis. On follow-up of depressed patients, the manifestations tend to remit, whereas those with anxiety states continue to exhibit marked tension, phobias, panic attacks, vasomotor instability, feelings of unreality, and perceptual distortions, as well as hypochondriacal ideas. A predominance of such anxiety features antedating the present illness suggests the diagnosis of an anxiety disorder. Because anxiety disorders rarely first appear after 40 years of age, late appearance of marked anxiety features strongly favors the diagnosis of melancholia. The clinical picture is often one of morbid groundless anxiety with somatization, hypochondriasis, and agitation. The depressive nature of the illness is further supported by a superior response to ECT. Periodic monosymptomatic phobic and obsessional states exist that can be regarded as affective equivalents on the basis of a family history of mood disorders and their response to thymoleptic agents. Recent data from a large clinical series suggest that 15 percent of cases have hypomanic symptoms; these patients are best considered to have bipolar II disorder and are treated with lithium salts. Social phobias often usher in adolescent depression, even a bipolar II disorder; the latter is particularly likely when the phobia is paired with alcohol abuse.

The psychopathological differentiation of anxiety and depressive states has not been entirely resolved. Cognitive factors may differentiate them best (Table 13.6–38). Although recurrent (especially retarded) major depressive disorder is a distinct disorder from anxiety states, at least some forms of depression may share a common diathesis with anxiety disorders, particularly generalized anxiety disorders. Before assigning patients to such a putative mixed anxiety-depressive group (not yet an official nosological entity), the clinician must note that anxiety that arises primarily during depressive episodes is best considered as epiphenomenal to depressive disorder. The same is generally true for anxiety symptoms that occur in a person with depressive disorder who is using alcohol or sedative-hypnotic or stimulant drugs. Finally, anxiety symptoms could be prominent features of mixed bipolar states, as well as complex partial seizures.

Major Depressive Disorder versus Bipolar Disorder

This "internal" boundary question of whether a patient has major depressive disorder versus bipolar disorder has been discussed extensively throughout this chapter. It has emerged as a major challenge in clinical practice. Numerous studies have shown that bipolar disorder is not only confused with personality, substance use, and schizophrenic disorders, but also with depressive and anxiety disorders. Prospective and other systematic studies have shown that each of the following features—especially in combination—is predictive of bipolar disorder:

- Early age at onset
- Psychotic depression before 25 years of age
- Postpartum depression, especially one with psychotic features
- Rapid onset and offset of depressive episodes of short duration (<3 months)
- Recurrent depression (more than five episodes)
- Depression with marked psychomotor retardation
- Atypical features (reverse vegetative signs)
- Seasonality
- Bipolar family history
- High-density three-generation pedigrees
- Trait mood lability (cyclothymia)
- Hyperthymic temperament
- Hypomania associated with antidepressants
- Repeated (at least three times) loss of efficacy of antidepressants after initial response
- Depressive mixed state (with psychomotor excitement, irritable hostility, racing thoughts, and sexual arousal *during* major depression)

More broad indicators of bipolarity include the following conditions, none of which, by themselves, clinch a bipolar diagnosis but should raise clinical suspicion in that direction: agitated depression, cyclical depression, episodic sleep dysregulation, or a combination of these; refractory depression (failed antidepressants from three different classes); depression in someone with an extroverted profession, periodic impulsivity, such as gambling, sexual misconduct, and wanderlust, or periodic irritability, suicidal crises, or both; and depression with erratic personality disorders.

Personality Disorders

The state dependency of most personality measures is well documented. Accordingly, as appropriately exhorted by DSM-IV-TR, clinicians should refrain from using personality disorder labels in describing patients with active affective illness and should focus instead on competent treatment of the mood disorder. Unfortunately, such advice is not always heeded. Even in those with chronic or subthreshold mood disorders, personality maladjustment is best considered postaffective, arising from the distortions and conflicts that affective disturbances produce in the life of the patient. The most problematic of the personality labels used in those with mood disorders is borderline personality disorder, usually applied to teenage and young adult women. The DSM-IV-TR diagnostic criteria for the disorder indicate a liberal mélange of low-grade affective symptoms and behavior. Table 13.6–39 shows that the overlap between borderline personality and mood disorders is extensive, so that giving a *borderline* diagnosis to a person with mood disorder is redundant. Use of personality disorder diagnoses may lead to neglect of the mood disorder or, perhaps, half-hearted treatment of the mood disorder; failure to respond would then be blamed on the patient's "self-defeating character" or "resistance to getting well," thus exculpating the clinician.

Although more systematic research is needed on the complex interface of personality and mood disorders, clinically, they are often inseparable. As with alcohol and substance use disorders, it is generally preferable to diagnose mood disorders at the expense of personality disorders, which should not be difficult to justify in most cases that satisfy the validating strategies outlined previously. When features of personality and mood disorders coexist, it is good practice to defer Axis II diagnoses and to embark on competent treatment of the concurrent mood disorder. Although not all personality disturbances recede with the competent treatment of mood disorders, so many experienced clinicians have seen such disturbances melt away with the successful resolution of the mood disorder that erring in favor of mood disorders is justified.

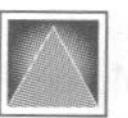

Table 13.6–39
Overlap of Borderline Personality Disorder and Mood Disorders

Familial
High rates of mood disorder
Phenomenology
Dysthymic disorder
Cyclothymic disorder
Bipolar II disorder
Mixed state
Pharmacological response
Worsening on tricyclic antidepressants
Stabilization on anticonvulsants
Prospective course
Major mood episodes
Suicide

Adapted from Akiskal H, Chen S, Davis G, et al.: Borderline: An adjective in search of a noun. *Clin Psychiatry.* 1985;46:41.

A 19-year-old single woman presented with the chief complaint that "all men are bastards." Since her early teens, with the onset of her menses, she had complained of extreme variability in her moods on a nearly daily basis; irritability with hostile outbursts was her main affect, although more protracted hypersomnic depressions with multiple overdoses and wrist slashings had led to at least three hospitalizations. She also had migrainous headaches that, according to the mother, had motivated at least one of those overdoses. Despite her tempestuous and suicidal moods that led to these hospitalizations, she complained of "inner emptiness and a bottomless void." She had used heroin, alcohol, and stimulants to overcome this troubling symptom. She also gave history of ice cream craving and frequent purging. She was talented in English and wrote much-acclaimed papers on the American confessional poet, Anne Sexton. She said that she was mentally disturbed because of a series of stepfathers who had all forced "oral rape" on her when she was between 11 and 15 years of age. She subsequently gave herself sexually to any man that she met in bars, no longer knowing whether she was a "prostitute" or a "nice little girl." On two occasions, she had inflicted cigarette burns inside her vagina "to feel something." She had also engaged in a "brief lesbian relationship" that ultimately left her "emptier" and guilt ridden; nonetheless, she now believed that she should burn in hell, because she could not get rid of "obsessing" about the excitement of mutual cunnilingus with her much older female partner. The patient's mother, who owned an art gallery, had been married five times and gave a history of unmistakable hypomanic episodes; a maternal uncle had died from alcohol-induced cirrhosis. The patient's father, a prominent lawyer known for his "temper and wit," had committed suicide. The patient was given phenelzine (Nardil), eventually raised to 75 mg per day, at which point the mother described her as "the sweet daughter she was before age 13." At her next premenstrual phase, the patient developed insomnia, ran away from home at night, started "dancing like a go-go girl, met an incredibly handsome man" of 45 years of age (actually, a pornography shop owner), and had a clandestine marriage to him. After many dosage adjustments, she is now maintained on a combination of lithium (900 mg per day) and divalproex (Depakote; 750 mg per day). The patient now attends college and has completed four semesters in art history. In addition to control of her irritable and suicidal moods, bulimic and migraine attacks have abated considerably. Her marriage has been annulled on the basis that she was not mentally competent at the time of the wedding. She is no longer promiscuous and now expresses fear of intimacy with men that she is attracted to. She is receiving individual psychotherapy for this problem.

This case illustrates the intimate relationship between atypical depression, borderline personality, and bipolar II disorder. These three conditions, listed as distinct nosological entities in the DSM-IV-TR, may nonetheless share an underlying psychobiological or genetic diathesis. The author often hears the complaint that, even when a mood disorder is diagnosed in a "borderline" patient, response to antidepressants is disappointing. The problem is that affective disorders in these patients usually conform to bipolar II disorder—often complicated by ultrarapid cycling—and many clinicians trained in an earlier era, including some with biological orientation, may lack sufficient experience in the art of pharmacologically managing patients who markedly deviate from classic bipolar I disorder. Recently, lamotrigine has shown promise for such patients.

Alcohol and Substance Use Disorders

The high comorbidity of alcohol and substance use disorders with mood disorders cannot be explained as merely the chance occurrence of two prevalent disorders. Self-medication for mood disorders is insufficiently appreciated by psychiatrists and other professionals who deal with addiction. Given the clinical dangers of missing an otherwise treatable disorder, mood disorder should be seriously considered as the primary diagnosis if marked affective manifestations persist or escalate after detoxification (e.g., 1 month). This consideration also pertains to cyclothymic disorder and dysthymic disorder, which appear particularly likely to invite self-medication. The clinical validating strategies listed perviously can further buttress a mood disorder diagnosis.

The DSM-IV-TR category of substance-induced mood disorder (Table 13.6–18) is difficult to validate clinically, because, in the absence of an affective diathesis, detoxification should, in principle, rapidly clear affective disturbances in persons whose primary problem is that of substance abuse. In the author's view, a dual diagnosis of a mood disorder and a substance use disorder is a more realistic clinical approach to this group of patients. Bipolarity, particularly bipolar II disorder, should be sought in the interface of mood and substance use disorders.

A 27-year-old married businessman employed in an international family venture owned by his father presented with a court-ordered request for psychiatric treatment. He had been found "bringing" cocaine across the U.S.–Mexican border and was briefly jailed. He had used stimulants since his late teens to enhance his already high level of energy. His family was rich, and he had no difficulty affording cocaine. During the previous year, he had needed more cocaine because of greater moodiness and fleeting suicidal ideation, which he linked to increasing tensions between him and his father: "My father was never satisfied with me and demanded greater and greater performance from me." His arrest by police was a major embarrassment for him and his family and motivated his compliance with psychiatric hospitalization to detoxify him. He had not had cocaine for 10 days, exhibited marked lability of mood, and gradually sank into a severe hypersomnic-retarded depression of stuporous proportions. He was treated in an inpatient unit with tranylcypromine (Parnate) 20 mg twice a day, and, within 10 days, he switched into hypomania, his mind "exploding with creativity and confidence," marked jocularity and witticisms that entertained other patients, and marked seductiveness toward the nurses. His wife recalled that the patient previously had several such periods naturally (i.e., "off cocaine"), which had strained their marriage due to "brief sexual liaisons." Reducing the tranylcypromine dosage by 50 percent did not eliminate the hypomanic behavior, and lithium, 900 mg a day, was added. He has since been maintained on a combination of tranylcypromine and lithium for 4 years; he has not relapsed into cocaine use, and, following few psychoeducational sessions involving father and spouse, relationships with family and spouse have been less tempestuous. (Since then, consultation was sought by the patient's 60-year-old mother, an attractive, sophisticated woman, who confessed that, for years, she had been engaged in "love relationships" with young artists, with, apparently, her husband's "tacit consent"; since at least her mid 20s, she, by history, would meet the criteria for bipolar II disorder, only treated "on the couch," and her sister and brother had received treatment for "alcohol excesses.") The patient states that pharmacotherapy, which did require adjustment now and then, has helped in balancing the "rough edges" of his "high-nervous temperament" and his "periodic lapse into paralyzing fatigue states that occurred at stressful times." If it had been assumed that these mood states were merely due to cocaine withdrawal, the patient's bipolar II disorder would never have been treated. DSM-IV-TR conventions in this regard unfortunately bias diagnosis in favor of substance use disorders and, more tragically, against the realistic chance of cure from substances.

There is emerging interest in treating dually diagnosed patients with anticonvulsant mood stabilizers and their judicious combination. Among the antidepressants, bupropion (Wellbutrin) is a suitable agent to "replace" stimulant craving; serotonin reuptake inhibitors can be useful for concurrent social phobia and anxious components. The intention is to attenuate any withdrawal phenomena from substances of abuse and to reduce craving, while treating any underlying or emerging bipolar diathesis.

Physical Disease

Somatic complaints are common in depressive disorders. Some, such as vegetative disturbances, represent the hypothalamic pathology that is believed to underlie a depressive disorder. Autonomic arousal, commonly associated with depression, could explain such symptoms as palpitations, sweating, and headache. In some instances, the physical symptoms might reflect delusional experiences. The clinician must be vigilant about the likelihood that somatic complaints in depression can also reflect an underlying physical illness. Table 13.6–40 lists the most common medical conditions that have been associated with depression. When depressive symptoms occur in the setting of physical illness, it is not always easy to determine whether they constitute a genuine depressive disorder. Before diagnosing depression, psychiatrists must ensure that they are not dealing with pseudodepression: (1) functional loss due to physical illness; (2) vegetative signs, such as anorexia and weight loss, as manifestations of such an illness; (3) stress and demoralization secondary to the hospitalization; (4) pain and discomfort associated with the physical illness; and (5) medication adverse effects. On the other hand, nonpsychiatric physicians who manage such patients must consider the diagnosis of depression in the presence of persistent anhe-

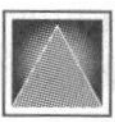

Table 13.6–40
Pharmacological Factors and Physical Diseases Associated with Onset of Depression

Pharmacological
- Steroidal contraceptives
- Reserpine (Serpalan), α-methyldopa
- Anticholinesterase insecticides
- Amphetamine or cocaine withdrawal
- Alcohol or sedative-hypnotic withdrawal
- Cimetidine (Tagamet), indomethacin (Indocin)
- Phenothiazine antipsychotic drugs
- Thallium, mercury
- Cycloserine (Seromycin)
- Vincristine, (Oncovin), vinblastine (Velban)
- Interferon

Endocrine-metabolic[a]
- Hypothyroidism and hyperthyroidism
- Hyperparathyroidism
- Hypopituitarism
- Addison's disease
- Cushing's syndrome
- Diabetes mellitus

Infectious
- General paresis (tertiary syphilis)
- Toxoplasmosis
- Influenza, viral pneumonia
- Viral hepatitis
- Infectious mononucleosis
- Acquired immune deficiency syndrome

Collagen
- Rheumatoid arthritis
- Lupus erythematosus

Nutritional
- Pellagra
- Pernicious anemia

Neurological
- Multiple sclerosis
- Parkinson's disease
- Head trauma
- Complex partial seizures
- Sleep apnea
- Cerebral tumors
- Cerebrovascular infarction (and disease)

Neoplastic
- Abdominal malignancies
- Disseminated carcinomatosis

[a]Cholesterol is not mentioned, because low levels as a factor in depression have been inconsistently reported.

donia; observed depressed mood with frequent crying; observed psychomotor retardation or agitation; indecisiveness; convictions of failure, worthlessness, or guilt; and suicidal ideation. The physician should also suspect clinical depression in all patients who refuse to participate in medical care.

Diagnosing depression in medically ill elderly patients can be particularly difficult. This task should be undertaken diligently, because it was recently reported that (especially in those with cardiovascular disease) mortality is accelerated by depression. Depressed elderly adults often deny being depressed but complain of anxiety, fatigue, and worsening memory. Hypochondriacal symptoms and pain are common. Patients may exhibit extreme negativism and querulousness when invited to participate in medical procedures; others develop poor fluid and food intake out of proportion to their physical conditions.

Another important diagnostic problem at the interface of mood disorder and physical disease is the rare development of malignancy in patients with an established mood disorder. Patients who had responded well to a given antidepressant during previous episodes now have an unsatisfactory response to the same medication. Even a small dose may cause such alarming symptoms as agitation, dizziness, depersonalization, and illusions, which might indicate an occult malignancy, perhaps in the abdomen or the brain. The psychiatrist should always be vigilant about the development of life-threatening physical diseases in patients with preestablished depressive disorder.

A 55-year-old woman had four previous episodes of severe depression that had responded to ECT, amitriptyline (Elavil), or a combination in her native city in the Middle East. She immigrated to the United States at 43 years of age and encountered several major stresses, including an unfamiliarity with English, her daughter dating a man of Chinese extraction, and a complicated series of operations for uterine prolapse. Then, her husband confessed that he had an affair with a much younger woman. For months, the patient had complained of intermittent fatigue and expressed hostility toward her husband. He had slapped her on her face on two occasions. Her ensuing fifth depressive episode (with pain localized to her face) appeared fully "understandable," but her physician's prescription of 25 mg of amitriptyline resulted in dizzy spells that culminated in syncope. Citalopram (Celexa), 10 mg, did not fare any better. An extensive medical workup revealed a retroperitoneal lymphoma. She died 6 months later.

Stupor Although less common today, stupor still raises a diagnostic problem in differentiating between a mood disorder and somatic disease, as well as other psychiatric disorders. Depressive stupor is relatively easy to distinguish from so-called hysterical mutism; in the latter, behavior is meaningfully directed to significant others in the patient's environment. The rubric of catatonic stupor is best reserved for a phase of schizophrenia; in such patients, the schizophrenic origin of the catatonia might be apparent from the patient's history. Otherwise, most acute-onset stupors are probably of affective origin. The main differential diagnosis here is from organic stupor (due to drugs or acute intracranial events); the physical and neurological examination is not always decisive in such cases, and diagnosis depends on a high index of suspicion of possible somatic factors.

Depressive Pseudodementia The geriatric equivalent of semistupor in younger persons with depressive disorder, depressive pseudodementia is distinguished from primary degenerative dementia by its acute onset without prior cognitive disturbance, a personal or family history of past affective episodes, marked psychomotor retardation with reduced social interaction, self-reproach, diurnal cognitive dysfunction (worse in the morning), subjective memory dysfunction in excess of objective findings, circumscribed memory deficits that can be reversed with proper coaching, and a tendency to improve with sleep deprivation.

Chronic Fatigue Syndrome Chronic fatigue syndrome is a complex differential diagnostic problem in view of the subtle immunological disturbances presumably associated with it. The following self-report by such a patient illustrates many of the uncertainties marking the present knowledge of the interface between the syndrome and mood disorders.

I am a 39-year-old, never-married woman, trained as a social worker but currently on disability. I have experienced extreme lethargy and fatigue for many years. I have always felt foggy headed and had trouble thinking and concentrating. My complaint is of fatigue not of depression. My body feels like lead and aches all over. My brain feels achy and sore. I feel much worse in the morning, and I can't get out of bed; I feel better at night. I feel bad every day. I ache all over, as though someone had beaten me up. Exercise has been prescribed to me, but it makes me worse. Also, I am very sensitive to hot and cold. My sexual drive is low. I have a general feeling of anhedonia. As far back as I remember—in junior high school—I was always exhausted. I always complained about fatigue, not depression, because that has been the overwhelming problem. I feel the depression is secondary to the fatigue. In high school, I was a compulsive overeater, and I was bulimic for a few years, but it was never severe, and I was only about 10 pounds overweight. In those days, I would sleep 10 or 12 hours a night on the weekend and still feel exhausted; I could not get up for school on Monday. As an adolescent, I felt inferior. I couldn't make decisions, I didn't want to go to camp or leave home for long periods of time—I felt so insecure. Recently, I had a sleep study done, which showed a short latency to stage REM sleep (49 minutes). I was diagnosed as having dysthymic disorder and began taking antidepressants. When I took tranylcypromine (Parnate), it was the first time in my life that I felt like a normal person. I could play sports, I had a sex drive, I had energy, and I was able to think clearly, but the benefits lasted for barely 2 months. My response was equally short-lived to phenelzine, imipramine (Tofranil), selegiline (Eldepryl), and bupropion. I have not responded to selective serotonin reuptake inhibitors (SSRIs) at all. I also wish to point out that I had never experienced high periods before I took antidepressants. My main problem has always been one of exhaustion. When I responded to medications, they worked very quickly (within a few days), and I felt great, but they all stopped working after a short time. The dose would be raised, and, again, I would feel better. Eventually, when I got to high doses, I either could not tolerate the high dose or the drug would no longer help. I have taken different combinations of drugs for 10 years, and I haven't been able to feel well for more than 6 weeks at a time. Recently, I went to an immunologist. He said I have an abnormality in regulating antibody production and recommended γ-globulin shots. They did not help, When I first started working, I always felt tired and foggy headed, so it was difficult to be sharp while at work. At times, I would close the door to my office and put my head down. Working has become increasingly difficult for me. I had two great jobs, which I blew. As of last year, I had to go on disability. I am desperate for relief, as my condition has drastically affected my life. Disability has been hard for me. I am single and have no other financial resources. I am very despondent, as I feel that my life is passing by without the hope of my ever really improving.

The foregoing clinical picture is compatible with a pseudo-unipolar or bipolar III disorder as described previously in this chapter. If so, mood stabilizer augmentation of the tranylcypromine would have been a therapeutic choice to pursue. Some biologists and immunologists, as well as some psychiatrists, believe that abnormal substances circulate in the bloodstream, supplying the brains of such patients. Industrial toxins have also been suggested. Although awaiting more definitive research on the etiology of chronic fatigue syndrome, the psychiatrist can cautiously consider certain patients for thymoleptic trials. That decision can be bolstered by the following considerations: The patient wakes up with fatigue and dread of facing the day; fatigue is part of a more generalized psychomotor inertia or lack of initiative; fatigue is associated with anhedonia, including sexual anhedonia; and fatigue coexists with anxious and pessimistic ruminations. Although none of the foregoing considerations alone is pathognomonic for depression, in aggregate, they point in that direction. The occurrence of hypomanic-like periods (as in the previous vignette) further supports the link between some cases of chronic fatigue and mood disorder. Several recent neuroendocrine challenge studies suggest that some chronic fatigue patients might have a strong anxiety substrate and could be managed accordingly. This is not to say that chronic fatigue is largely a matter of missed affective diagnoses with bipolar II and panic disorder features; yet, it would be a pity to miss potentially treatable diagnoses. A family or past personal history of classic affective illness or episodes should strongly weigh in this direction. Obviously definitive data are lacking on the essential nature of chronic fatigue, and practitioners should be guided by their own clinical experience with therapeutic trials of nonsedating thymoleptic agents, while awaiting new research developments.

Schizophrenia Despite some genetic overlap between schizophrenic and bipolar disorders, clinically, the two groups of disorders are in the main separate. Cross-sectionally, young patients with bipolar disorder might seem psychotic and disorganized and, thus, schizophrenic. Their thought processes are so rapid that they may seem loose, but, unlike those with schizophrenia, they display an expansive and elated affect, which is often contagious. By contrast, the severely retarded bipolar depressive person, whose affect may superficially seem flat, almost never exhibits major fragmentation of thought. The clinician, therefore, should place greater emphasis on the pattern of symptoms than on individual symptoms in the differential diagnosis of mood and schizophrenic psychoses. No pathognomonic differentiating signs and symptoms exist. Differential diagnosis should be based on the overall clinical picture, phenomenology, family history, course, and associated features. Because the two groups of disorders entail different combinations of pharmacological treatments on a long-term basis (mood stabilizers are usually needed as the mainstay in bipolar disorder), the differential diagnosis is of major clinical importance. Table 13.6–41 summarizes the author's clinical experience in the area and lists the most common pitfalls in diagnosis. In the past, many bipolar patients, especially those with prominent manic features at onset, were labeled as having *acute schizophrenia* or *schizoaffective schizophrenia.* In the past, such misdiagnoses (which typically led to long-term treatment with conventional neuroleptic agents) have been costly in terms of tardive dyskinesia, vocational and social decline, and even suicide. For instance, some patients with postpsychotic depressive disorder of schizophrenia in the DSM-IV-TR scheme (Table 13.6–25) have postmanic depressions that were treated with classic neuroleptic monotherapy without the benefit of more definitive thymoleptic agents.

Modern treatments—even with atypical antipsychotics—which tend to keep many persons with schizophrenia out of the hospital, do not always seem to prevent an overall downhill course in many cases. By contrast, the intermorbid periods in bipolar illness are relatively normal or even supernormal, yet, over time, some social impairment may result from the accumulation of divorces, financial catastrophes, and ruined careers. (Although rapid-cycling disorders, which have sharply risen during the past two decades, cause considerable social impairment, mood symptoms are so prominent that differentiation from schizophrenia is generally not difficult; also, such patients usually display more classic bipolar phases before the rapid cycling.)

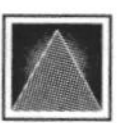

Table 13.6–41
Common Causes of Misdiagnosis of Mood Disorder as Schizophrenia

Reliance on cross-sectional rather than longitudinal picture
Incomplete interepisodic recovery equated with schizophrenic defect
Equation of bizarreness with schizophrenic thought disorder
Ascribing irritable and cantankerous mood to paranoid delusions
Mistaking depressive anhedonia and depersonalization for schizophrenic emotional blunting
Flight of ideas perceived as loose associations
Lack of familiarity with the phenomenological approach in assessing affective delusions and hallucinations
Heavy weight given to incidental schneiderian symptoms

Adapted from Akiskal HS, Puzantian VR: Psychotic forms of depression and mania. *Psychiatr Clin North Am.* 1979;2:419.

Postpsychotic depressions in persons with established schizophrenia are sometimes due to inadequate control of schizophrenic symptomology. In other patients, especially more intelligent young schizophrenic patients, they reflect the experience of losing one's ego and sanity. It would be more meaningful to give such patients a diagnosis of schizophrenia and a superimposed major depressive diagnosis and to treat the patient accordingly.

Schizoaffective Disorder As the previously mentioned considerations suggest, depression in the setting of a schizophrenic disorder does not necessarily constitute a distinct nosological entity. The concept of schizoaffective (or cycloid) psychosis should be restricted to recurrent psychoses, with full affective and schizophrenic symptoms occurring nearly simultaneously during each episode. This diagnosis should *not* be considered for a mood psychosis in which mood-incongruent psychotic features (e.g., schneiderian and bleulerian symptoms) can be explained on the basis of one of the following: (1) affective psychosis superimposed on mental retardation, giving rise to extremely hyperactive and bizarre manic behavior; (2) affective psychosis complicated by concurrent brain disease, substance abuse, or substance withdrawal, known to give rise to numerous schneiderian symptoms; or (3) mixed episodes of bipolar disorder (which are notorious for signs and symptoms of psychotic disorganization). Official diagnostic systems, such as DSM-IV-TR, use the category of schizoaffective disorder broadly. Thus, patients with clear-cut manic episodes receive a schizoaffective diagnosis if delusions or hallucinations occur in the interepisodic period in the absence of prominent affective symptoms. Many psychotic symptoms in mood disorders are often explanatory (albeit delusional), whereby the patient tries to make sense of the core experiences of the affective illness. In patients with recurrent episodes, delusional thinking can be carried over into the interepisodic period. Such patients are thus delusional in the absence of prominent mood symptoms and technically (i.e., by research diagnostic or DSM-IV-TR criteria) might be considered schizoaffective.

The author does not concur with that convention. Affective illness is typically a lifelong process, and limiting its features to discrete episodes is artificial. In the past, neuroleptic agents were prescribed on an as-needed basis to reduce the strong affective charge of those interepisodic delusions, but they did not effectively eliminate the affect-laden experiences. Atypical antipsychotic agents introduced during the 1990s are more likely to be beneficial in this regard. Augmenting with continued thymoleptic treatment (resorting to ECT, if necessary) and an empathic psychotherapeutic approach may prove more rewarding in the long run.

A 29-year-old female college graduate, mother of two children and wife of a bank president, had experienced several manic and retarded depressive episodes that had responded to lithium carbonate. She was referred to the author because she had developed the delusion that she had been involved in an international plot. Careful probing revealed that the delusion represented further elaboration, in a rather fantastic fashion, of a grandiose delusion that she had experienced during her last postpartum manic episode. She believed that she had played an important role in uncovering the plot, thereby becoming a national hero. Nobody knew about it, she contended, as the circumstances of the plot were top secret. She further believed that she had saved her country from the international scheme and suspected that she was singled out for persecution by the perpetrators of the plot. At one point, she had even entertained the idea that the plotters sent special radio communications to intercept and to interrupt her thoughts. As is typical in such cases, she was on a heavy dosage of a lithium-antipsychotic combination. The consultation was requested because the primary mood symptoms were under control, and, yet, she had not given up her grandiose delusion. She flippantly remarked that "I must be crazy to believe in my involvement in an international plot," but she could not help but believe in it. Over several months, seen typically in 60-minute sessions weekly, the patient had developed sufficient trust that the author could gently challenge her beliefs.

She was, in effect, told that her self-professed role in the international scheme was highly implausible and that someone with her superior education and high social standing could not entertain a belief, to use her own words, "as crazy as that." She eventually broke into tears, saying that everyone in her family was so accomplished and famous that to keep up with them she had to be involved in something grand; in effect, the international scheme, she said, was her only claim to fame: "Nobody ever gives me credit for raising two kids, and throwing parties for my husband's business colleagues: My mother is a dean, my older brother holds high political office; my sister is a medical researcher with five discoveries to her credit [all true] and who am I? Nothing. Now, do you understand why I need to be a national hero?" As she alternated, over subsequent months, between such momentary flashes of insight and delusional denial, antipsychotic medication was gradually discontinued. Maintained on lithium, she now only makes passing reference to the grand scheme. She was encouraged to pursue her career goal toward a master's degree in library science.

The vignette illustrates how phenomenological understanding, rational pharmacotherapy, and practical psychotherapeutic or vocational guidance can be fruitfully combined in the approach to patients with psychotic mood disorders. It also indicates that problems with insight are not necessarily state dependent in mood disorders. Cognitive disturbances have recently been described in all mood disorders, even when nonpsychotic. At a more fundamental level, the vignette suggests that clinical diagnoses cannot be based entirely on operational criteria; one's opinion of patients' illnesses is not infrequently changed by their response to treatment. In the author's view, DSM-IV-TR represents something good (operationalism of diagnostic criteria) carried to the extreme (arbitrary precision often divorced from clinical reality).

ICD-10

The ICD-10 criteria for mood disorders, which are used throughout the world, are listed in Table 13.6–42. Although the ICD-10 criteria

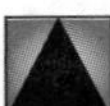

Table 13.6–42
ICD-10 Diagnostic Criteria for Mood (Affective) Disorders

Manic episode

Hypomania

A. The mood is elevated or irritable to a degree that is definitely abnormal for the individual concerned and sustained for at least 4 consecutive days.

B. At least three of the following signs must be present, leading to some interference with personal functioning in daily living:
  (1) Increased activity or physical restlessness
  (2) Increased talkativeness
  (3) Distractibility or difficulty in concentration
  (4) Decreased need for sleep
  (5) Increased sexual energy
  (6) Mild overspending, or other types of reckless or irresponsible behavior
  (7) Increased sociability or overfamiliarity

C. The episode does not meet the criteria for mania, bipolar affective disorder, depressive episode, cyclothymia, or anorexia nervosa.

D. *Most commonly used exclusion clause.* The episode is not attributable to psychoactive substance use or to any organic mental disorder.

Mania without psychotic symptoms

A. Mood must be predominantly elevated, expansive, or irritable, and definitely abnormal for the individual concerned. The mood change must be prominent and sustained for at least 1 week (unless it is severe enough to require hospital admission).

B. At least three of the following signs must be present (four, if the mood is merely irritable), leading to severe interference with personal functioning in daily living:
  (1) Increased activity or physical restlessness
  (2) Increased talkativeness (pressure of speech)
  (3) Flight of ideas or the subjective experience of thoughts racing
  (4) Loss of normal social inhibitions, resulting in behavior that is inappropriate to the circumstances
  (5) Decreased need for sleep
  (6) Inflated self-esteem or grandiosity
  (7) Distractibility or constant changes in activity or plans
  (8) Behavior that is foolhardy or reckless and that entails risks that the individual does not recognize, for example spending sprees, foolish enterprises, and reckless driving
  (9) Marked sexual energy or sexual indiscretions

C. There are no hallucinations or delusions, although perceptual disorders may occur (e.g., subjective hyperacusis and appreciation of colors as especially vivid).

D. *Most commonly used exclusion clause.* The episode is not attributable to psychoactive substance use or to any organic mental disorder.

Mania with psychotic symptoms

A. The episode meets the criteria for mania without psychotic symptoms with the exception of Criterion C.

B. The episode does not simultaneously meet the criteria for schizophrenia or schizoaffective disorder, manic type.

C. Delusions or hallucinations are present, other than those listed as typically schizophrenic in Criterion G1(1)b, c, and d for schizophrenia (i.e., delusions, other than those that are completely impossible or culturally inappropriate, and hallucinations that are not in the third person or giving a running commentary). The commonest examples are those with grandiose, self-referential, erotic, or persecutory content.

D. *Most commonly used exclusion clause.* The episode is not attributable to psychoactive substance use or to any organic mental disorder.

Specify whether the hallucinations or delusions are congruent or incongruent with the mood:

With mood-congruent psychotic symptoms (such as grandiose delusions or voices telling the individual that he or she has superhuman powers)

With mood-incongruent psychotic symptoms (such as voices speaking to the individual about affectively neutral topics or delusions of reference or persecution)

Other manic episodes

Manic episode, unspecified

Bipolar affective disorder

Note: Episodes are demarcated by a switch to an episode of opposite mixed polarity or by a remission.

Bipolar affective disorder, current episode hypomanic

A. The current episode meets the criteria for hypomania.

B. There has been at least one other affective episode in the past, meeting the criteria for hypomanic or manic episode, depressive episode, or mixed affective episode.

Bipolar affective disorder, current episode manic without psychotic symptoms

A. The current episode meets the criteria for mania without psychotic symptoms.

B. There has been at least one other affective episode in the past, meeting the criteria for hypomanic or manic episode, depressive episode, or mixed affective episode.

Bipolar affective disorder, current episode manic without psychotic symptoms

A. The current episode meets the criteria for mania without psychotic symptoms.

B. There has been at least one other affective episode in the past, meeting the criteria for hypomanic or manic episode, depressive episode, or mixed affective episode.

Specify whether the psychotic symptoms are congruent or incongruent with the mood:

With mood-congruent psychotic symptoms

With mood-incongruent psychotic symptoms

Bipolar affective disorder, current episode moderate or mild depression

A. The current episode meets the criteria for a depressive episode of mild or moderate severity.

B. There has been at least one other affective episode in the past, meeting the criteria for hypomanic or manic episode, depressive episode, or mixed affective episode.

Specify the presence of the *somatic syndrome* in the current episode of depression:

Without somatic syndrome

With somatic syndrome

Bipolar affective disorder, current episode severe depression without psychotic symptoms

A. The current episode meets the criteria for a severe depressive episode without psychotic symptoms.

B. There has been at least one well-authenticated hypomanic or manic episode or mixed affective episode in the past.

Bipolar affective disorder, current episode severe depression with psychotic symptoms

A. The current episode meets the criteria for a severe depressive episode without psychotic symptoms.

B. There has been at least one well-authenticated hypomanic or manic episode or mixed affective episode in the past.

Specify whether the psychotic symptoms are congruent or incongruent with the mood:

With mood-congruent psychotic symptoms

With mood-incongruent psychotic symptoms

(*continued*)

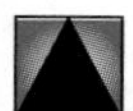

Table 13.6–42 (*continued*)

Bipolar affective disorder, current episode mixed

A. The current episode is characterized by a mixture or a rapid alternation (i.e., within a few hours) of hypomanic, manic, and depressive symptoms.

B. Both manic and depressive symptoms must be prominent most of the time during a period of at least 2 weeks.

C. There has been at least one well-authenticated hypomanic or manic episode, depressive episode, or mixed affective episode in the past.

Bipolar affective disorder, currently in remission

A. The current state does not meet the criteria for depressive or manic episode of any severity or for any other mood (affective) disorder (possibly because of treatment to reduce the risk of future episodes).

B. There has been at least one well-authenticated hypomanic or manic episode in the past and in addition at least one other affective episode (hypomanic or manic, depressive, or mixed).

Other bipolar affective disorders

Bipolar affective disorder, unspecified

Depressive episode

G1. The depressive episode should last for at least 2 weeks.

G2. There have been no hypomanic or manic symptoms sufficient to meet the criteria for hypomanic or manic episode at any time in the individual's life.

G3. *Most commonly used exclusion clause.* The episode is not attributable to psychoactive substance use or to any organic mental disorder.

Somatic syndrome

Some depressive symptoms are widely regarded as having special clinical significance and are here called *somatic.* (Terms such as *biological, vital, melancholic,* or *endogenomorphic,* are used for this syndrome in other classifications.)

A fifth character may be used to specify the presence or absence of the somatic syndrome. To qualify for the somatic syndrome, *four* of the following symptoms should be present:

(1) Marked loss of interest or pleasure in activities that are normally pleasurable
(2) Lack of emotional reactions to events or activities that normally produce an emotional response
(3) Waking in the morning 2 hours or more before the usual time
(4) Depression worse in the morning
(5) Objective evidence of marked psychomotor retardation or agitation (remarked on or reported by other people)
(6) Marked loss of appetite
(7) Weight loss (5 percent or more of body weight in the past month)
(8) Marked loss of libido

In *The ICD-10 Classification of Mental and Behavioral Disorders: Clinical Descriptions and Diagnostic Guidelines,* the presence or absence of the somatic syndrome is not specified for severe depressive episode, because it is presumed to be present in most cases. For research purposes, however, it may be advisable to allow for the coding of the absence of the somatic syndrome in severe depressive episode.

Mild depressive episode

A. The general criteria for depressive episode must be met.

B. At least two of the following three symptoms must be present:

(1) Depressed mood to a degree that is definitely abnormal for the individual, present for most of the day and almost every day, largely uninfluenced by circumstances, and sustained for at least 2 weeks
(2) Loss of interest or pleasure in activities that are normally pleasurable
(3) Decreased energy or increased fatigability

C. An additional symptom or symptoms from the following list should be present, to give a total of at least *four:*

(1) Loss of confidence or self-esteem
(2) Unreasonable feelings of self-reproach or excessive and inappropriate guilt
(3) Recurrent thoughts of death or suicide or any suicidal behavior
(4) Complaints or evidence of diminished ability to think or concentrate, such as indecisiveness or vacillation
(5) Change in psychomotor activity, with agitation or retardation (subjective or objective)
(6) Sleep disturbance of any type
(7) Change in appetite (decrease or increase) with corresponding weight change

A fifth character may be used to specify the presence or absence of the *somatic syndrome*:

Without somatic syndrome

With somatic syndrome

Moderate depressive episode

A. The general criteria for depressive episode must be met.

B. At least two of the three symptoms listed for the previously mentioned Criterion B must be present.

C. Additional symptoms from depressive episode, Criterion C, must be present, to give a total of at least *six.*

A fifth character may be used to specify the presence or absence of the *somatic syndrome*:

Without somatic syndrome

With somatic syndrome

Severe depressive episode without psychotic symptoms

Note: If important symptoms such as agitation or retardation are marked, the patient may be unwilling or unable to describe many symptoms in detail. An overall grading of severe episode may still be justified in such a case.

A. The general criteria for depressive episode must be met.

B. All three of the symptoms in Criterion B, depressive episode, must be present.

C. Additional symptoms from depressive episode, Criterion C, must be present, to give a total of at least *eight.*

D. There must be no hallucinations, delusions, or depressive stupor.

Severe depressive episode with psychotic symptoms

A. The general criteria for depressive episode must be met.

B. The criteria for severe depressive episode without psychotic symptoms must be met, with the exception of Criterion D.

C. The criteria for schizophrenia or schizoaffective disorder, depressive type, are not met.

D. Either of the following must be present:

(1) Delusions or hallucinations, other than those listed as typically schizophrenic in Criterion G1(1)b, c, and d for general criteria for paranoid, hebephrenic, catatonic, and undifferentiated schizophrenia (i.e., delusions other than those that are completely impossible or culturally inappropriate and hallucinations that are not in the third person or giving a running commentary); the commonest examples are those with depressive, guilty, hypochondriacal, nihilistic, self-referential, or persecutory content.
(2) Depressive stupor.

(*continued*)

Table 13.6–42 (*continued*)

A fifth character may be used to specify whether the psychotic symptoms are congruent or incongruent with mood:

With mood-congruent psychotic symptoms (i.e., delusions of guilt, worthlessness, bodily disease, or impending disaster, derisive or condemnatory auditory hallucinations)

With mood-incongruent psychotic symptoms (i.e., persecutory or self-referential delusions and hallucinations without an affective content)

Other depressive episodes

Episodes should be included here that do not fit the descriptions given for depressive episodes but for which the overall diagnostic impression indicates that they are depressive in nature. Examples include fluctuating mixtures of depressive symptoms (particularly those of the somatic syndrome) with nondiagnostic symptoms, such as tension, worry, and distress, and mixtures of somatic depressive symptoms with persistent pain or fatigue not due to organic causes (as sometimes seen in general hospital services).

Depressive episode, unspecified

Recurrent depressive disorder

G1. There has been at least one previous episode, mild, moderate, or severe, lasting a minimum of 2 weeks and separated from the current episode by at least 2 months that are free from any significant mood symptoms.

G2. At no time in the past has there been an episode meeting the criteria for hypomanic or manic episode.

G3. *Most commonly used exclusion clause.* The episode is not attributable to psychoactive substance use or to any organic mental disorder.

It is recommended that the predominant type of previous episodes is specified (mild, moderate, severe, or uncertain).

Recurrent depressive disorder, current episode mild

A. The general criteria for recurrent depressive disorder are met.

B. The current episode meets the criteria for mild depressive episode.

A fifth character may be used to specify the presence or absence of the *somatic syndrome* in the current episode:

Without somatic syndrome

With somatic syndrome

Recurrent depressive disorder, current episode moderate

A. The general criteria for recurrent depressive disorder are met.

B. The current episode meets the criteria for moderate depressive episode.

A fifth character may be used to specify the presence or absence of the *somatic syndrome* in the current episode:

Without somatic syndrome

With somatic syndrome

Recurrent depressive disorder, current episode without psychotic symptoms

A. The general criteria for recurrent depressive disorder are met.

B. The current episode meets the criteria for severe depressive episode without psychotic symptoms.

Recurrent depressive disorder, current episode severe with psychotic symptoms

A. The general criteria for recurrent depressive disorder are met.

B. The current episode meets the criteria for severe depressive episode with psychotic symptoms.

A fifth character may be used to specify whether the psychotic symptoms are congruent or incongruent with the mood:

With mood-congruent psychotic symptoms

With mood-incongruent psychotic symptoms

Recurrent depressive disorder, currently in remission

A. The general criteria for recurrent depressive disorder have been met in the past.

B. The current state does not meet the criteria for a depressive episode of any severity or for any disorder in mood (affective) disorders.

Comment

This category can still be used if the patient receives treatment to reduce the risk of further episodes.

Other recurrent depressive disorders

Recurrent depressive disorder, unspecified

Persistent mood [affective] disorders

Cyclothymia

A. There must have been a period of at least 2 years of instability of mood involving several periods of depression and hypomania, with or without intervening periods of normal mood.

B. None of the manifestations of depression or hypomania during such a 2-year period should be sufficiently severe or long-lasting to meet criteria for manic episode or depressive episode (moderate or severe); however, manic or depressive episodes may have occurred before or may develop after such a period of persistent mood instability.

C. During at least some of the periods of depression, at least three of the following should be present:

(1) Reduced energy or activity
(2) Insomnia
(3) Loss of self-confidence or feelings of inadequacy
(4) Difficulty in concentrating
(5) Social withdrawal
(6) Loss of interest in or enjoyment of sex and other pleasurable activities
(7) Reduced talkativeness
(8) Pessimism about the future or brooding over the past

D. During at least some of the periods of mood elevation at least three of the following should be present:

(1) Increased energy or activity
(2) Decreased need for sleep
(3) Inflated self-esteem
(4) Sharpened or unusually creative thinking
(5) Increased gregariousness
(6) Increased talkativeness or wittiness
(7) Increased interest and involvement in sexual and other pleasurable activities
(8) Overoptimism or exaggeration of past achievements

Note: If desired, time of onset may be specified as early (in late teens or the 20s) or late (usually between 30 and 50 years of age, after an affective episode).

Dysthymia

A. There must be a period of at least 2 years of constant or constantly recurring depressed mood. Intervening periods of normal mood rarely last for longer than a few weeks, and there are no episodes of hypomania.

B. None or few of the individual episodes of depression within such a 2-year period should be sufficiently severe or long-lasting to meet the criteria for recurrent mild depressive disorder.

C. During at least some of the periods of depression, at least three of the following should be present:

(1) Reduced energy or activity
(2) Insomnia
(3) Loss of self-confidence or feelings of inadequacy
(4) Difficulty in concentrating
(5) Frequent tearfulness
(6) Loss of interest in or enjoyment of sex and other pleasurable activities

(*continued*)

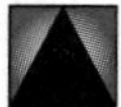

Table 13.6–42 (*continued*)

(7) Feeling of hopelessness or despair
(8) A perceived inability to cope with the routine responsibilities of everyday life
(9) Pessimism about the future or brooding over the past
(10) Social withdrawal
(11) Reduced talkativeness

Note: If desired, time of onset may be specified as early (in late teens or the 20s) or late (usually between 30 and 50 years of age, after an affective episode).

Other persistent mood (affective) disorders

This is a residual category for persistent affective disorders that are not sufficiently severe or long-lasting to fulfill the criteria for cyclothymia or dysthymia but that are nevertheless clinically significant. Some types of depression previously called *neurotic* are included here, provided that they do not meet the criteria for cyclothymia or dysthymia or for depressive episode of mild or moderate severity.

Persistent mood (affective) disorder, unspecified

Other mood (affective) disorders

There are so many possible disorders that could be listed that no attempt has been made to specify criteria, except for mixed affective episode and recurrent brief depressive disorder. Investigators requiring criteria more exact than those available in *Clinical Descriptions and Diagnostic Guidelines* should construct them according to the requirements of their studies.

Other single mood (affective) disorders

Mixed affective episode

A. The episode is characterized by a mixture or a rapid alternation (i.e., within a few hours) of hypomanic, manic, and depressive symptoms.
B. Manic and depressive symptoms must be prominent most of the time during a period of at least 2 weeks.
C. There is no history of previous hypomanic, depressive, or mixed episodes.

Other recurrent mood (affective) disorders

Recurrent brief depressive disorder

A. The disorder meets the symptomatic criteria for mild, moderate, or severe depressive episode.
B. The depressive episodes have occurred approximately once a month over the past year.
C. The individual episodes last less than 2 weeks (typically 2 to 3 days).
D. The episodes do not occur solely in relation to the menstrual cycle.

Other specified mood [affective] disorders

This is residual category for affective disorders that do not meet the criteria for any other categories mentioned previously.

From World Health Organization. *The ICD-10 Classification of Mental and Behavioural Disorders: Diagnostic Criteria for Research.* Geneva: World Health Organization; 1993, with permission.

in part derive from the DSM system of the American Psychiatric Association (APA), they are more flexible and clinician friendly: They do not pretend to impose arbitrary precision on the clinical universe of psychiatry. It is to be hoped that the current rapprochement of the APA and the World Psychiatric Association, as well as the WHO in the domain of classification, will serve as a ferment to come up with a classification system that combines the advantages of the DSM-IV-TR and ICD-10.

SUGGESTED CROSS-REFERENCES

Diagnosis and psychiatry are discussed in Chapter 7, the clinical manifestations of psychiatric disorders are covered in Chapter 8, and the classification of mental disorders is presented in Chapter 9. Schizophrenia is the subject of Chapter 12. The somatic treatment of mood disorders is discussed in Sections 13.7 and 13.8. Psychotherapy is covered in Section 13.9. Mood disorders and suicide in children are the topic of Chapter 45. Anxiety disorders are presented in Chapter 14, and mood disorders in geriatric psychiatry are discussed in Section 51.3d. Somatoform disorder, including neurasthenia and chronic fatigue syndrome, is further covered in Chapter 15.

REFERENCES

Akiskal HS: Toward a definition of generalized anxiety disorder as an anxious temperament type. *Acta Psychiatr Scand.* 1998;98[Suppl 393]:66–73.

Akiskal HS. Dysthymia, cyclothymia and related chronic subthreshold mood disorders. In: Gelder M, Lopez-Ibor J, Andreasen N, eds. *New Oxford Textbook of Psychiatry.* London: Oxford University Press; 2000:736–749.

Akiskal HS, Akiskal K: Re-assessing the prevalence of bipolar disorders: Clinical significance and artistic creativity. *Psychiatrie et Pyschobiologie.* 1998;3:29s–36s.

Akiskal HS, Azorin JF, Hantouche EG: A proposed multidimensional structure of mania: Beyond the euphoric-dysphoric dichotomy. *J Affect Disord.* 2003;73:7–18.

Akiskal HS, Benazzi F: Family history validation of the bipolar nature of depressive mixed states. *J Affect Disord.* 2003;73:113–122.

*Akiskal HS, Bourgeois ML, Angst J, Post R, Moller HJ, Hirschfeld RMA: Re-evaluating the prevalence of and diagnostic composition within the broad clinical spectrum of bipolar disorders. *J Affect Disord.* 2000;59[Suppl 1]:5S–30S.

Akiskal HS, Cassano GB, eds. *Dysthymia and the Spectrum of Chronic Depressions.* New York: Guilford Press; 1997.

Akiskal HS, Hantouche EG, Bourgeois ML, Azorin JM, Sechter D, Allilair JF, Chatenet-Duchene L, Lancrenon S: Toward a refined phenomenology of DSM-IV mania: Combining clinician-assessment and self-report in the French EPIMAN study. *J Affect Disord.* 2001;67:89–96.

Akiskal HS, Hantouche E, Bourgeois M, Azorin JM, Sechter D, Allilaire JF, Lancrenon S, Fraud JP, Chatenet-Duchene L: Gender, temperament and the clinical picture in dysphoric mixed mania: Findings from a French national study (EPIMAN). *J Affect Disord.* 1998;50:175–186.

Akiskal HS, Hantouche EG, Lancrenon S: Bipolar II with and without cyclothymic temperament: "Dark" and "sunny" expressions of soft bipolarity. *J Affect Disord.* 2003;73:49–57.

Akiskal HS, Mallya G: Criteria for the "soft" bipolar spectrum: Treatment implications. *Psychopharmacol Bull.* 1987;23:68–73.

Akiskal HS, Maser JD, Zeller P, Endicott J, Coryell W, Keller M, Warshaw M, Clayton P, Goodwin FK: Switching from "unipolar" to bipolar II: An 11-year prospective study of clinical and temperamental predictors in 559 patients. *Arch Gen Psychiatry.* 1995;52:114–123.

Akiskal HS, Pinto O: The evolving bipolar spectrum: Prototypes I, II, III, IV. *Psychiatr Clin North Am.* 1999;22:517–534.

Akiskal HS, Placidi GF, Signoretta S, Liguori A, Gervasi R, Maremmani I, Mallya G, Puzantian VR: TEMPS-I: Delineating the most discriminant traits of cyclothymic, depressive, irritable and hyperthymic temperaments in a nonpatient population. *J Affect Disord.* 1998;51:7–19.

Akiskal HS, Walker PW, Puzantian VR, King D, Rosenthal TL, Dranon M: Bipolar outcome in the course of depressive illness: Phenomenologic, familial, and pharmacologic predictors. *J Affect Disord.* 1983;5:115–128.

Angst J: The emerging epidemiology of hypomania and bipolar-II disorder: The Zurich study. *J Affect Disord.* 1998;50:143–151.

Armenian HK, Morikawa M, Melkonian AK, Hovanesian AP, Akiskal K, Akiskal HS. Risk factors for depression in the survivors of the 1988 earthquake in Armenia. *J Urban Health.* 2002;79:373–382.

Beard GM. *A Practical Treatise on Nervous Exhaustion (Neurasthenia): Its Nature, Sequences, and Treatment.* New York: Wood; 1881.

Beck AT, Steer RA, Beck JS, Newman CF: Hopelessness, depression, suicidal ideation, and clinical diagnosis of depression. *Suicide Life Threat Behav.* 1993;23: 139–145.

Benazzi F, Akiskal HS: Delineating bipolar II mixed states in the Ravenna–San Diego collaborative study: The relative prevalence and diagnostic significance of hypomanic features during major depressive episodes. *J Affect Disord.* 2001;67: 115–122.

Benazzi F, Akiskal HS: Refining the evaluation of bipolar II: Beyond the strict SCID-CV guidelines for hypomania. *J Affect Disord.* 2003;73:33–38.

Bottlender R, Sato T, Kleindienst N, Strauss A, Möller H-J: Mixed depressive features predict maniform switch during treatment of depression in bipolar I disorder. *J Affect Disord.* 2004;78:149–152.

Calabrese JR, Suppes T, Bowden CL, Sachs GS, Swann AC, McElroy SL, Kusumakar V, Ascher JA, Earl NL, Greene PL, Monaghan ET: A double-blind, placebo-controlled, prophylaxis study of lamotrigine in rapid-cycling bipolar disorder. Lamictal 614 Study Group. *J Clin Psychiatry.* 2000;61:841–850.

Clayton PJ: The sequelae and nonsequelae of conjugal bereavement. *Am J Psychiatry.* 1979;136:1530–1534.

Davidson JR, Miller RD, Turnbull CD, Sullivan JL: Atypical depression. *Arch Gen Psychiatry.* 1982;39:527–534.

Deisenhammer EA, Kramer-Reinstadler K, Liensberger D, Kemmler G, Hinterhuber H, Fleischhacker WW: No evidence for an association between serum cholesterol and the course of depression and suicidality. *Psychiatr Res.* 2004;121:253–261.

Dunner DL, Kai Tay L: Diagnostic reliability of the history of hypomania in bipolar II patients with major depression. *Compr Psychiatry.* 1993;34:303–307.

Ghaemi SN, Boiman EE, Goodwin FK: Diagnosing bipolar disorder and the effect of antidepressants: a naturalistic study. *J Clin Psychiatry.* 2000;61:804–808.

Hantouche EG, Angst J, Akiskal HS: Factor structure of hypomania: Interrelationships with cyclothymia and the soft bipolar spectrum. *J Affect Disord.* 2003;73:39–47.

James W. *The Varieties of Religious Experience.* New York: Random House; 1902.

*Judd LL, Akiskal HS, Maser JD, Zelle PJ, Endico HJ, Corey W, Parks MP, Kenovac JL, Leon AC, Mueller TJ, Rice JA, Keller MB: A prospective 12-year study of subsyndromal and syndromic depressive symptoms in unipolar major depressive disorders. *Arch Gen Psychiatry.* 1998;55:694–700.

Judd LL, Akiskal HS, Schettler PJ, Endicott J, Maser J, Solomon DA, Leon AC, Rice JA, Keller MB: The long-term natural history of the weekly symptomatic status of bipolar-I disorder. *Arch Gen Psychiatry.* 2002;59:530–537.

Karam EG: The nosological status of bereavement-related depressions. *Br J Psychiatry.* 1994;165:48–52.

Kendler KS, Karkowski LM, Corey LA, Neale MC: Longitudinal population-based twin study of retrospectively reported premenstrual symptoms and lifetime major depression. *Am J Psychiatry.* 1998;155:1234–1240.

Kendler KS, Neale MC, Kessler RC, Heath AC, Eaves LJ: Major depression and generalized anxiety disorder. Same genes, (partly) different environments? *Arch Gen Psychiatry.* 1992;49:716–722.

Klein DF: Endogenomorphic depression. A conceptual and terminological revision. *Arch Gen Psychiatry.* 1974;31:447–454.

*Koukopoulos A, Koukopoulos A: Agitated depression as a mixed state and the problem of melancholia. *Psychiatr Clin North Am.* 1999;22:547–564.

Koukopoulos A, Sani G, Koukopoulos AE, Minnai GP, Girardi P, Pani L, Albert MJ, Reginaldi D: Duration and stability of the rapid-cycling course: a long-term personal follow-up of 109 patients. *J Affect Disord.* 2003;73:75–85.

*Kraepelin E. In: Robertson GM ed. Barclay RM, transl. *Manic-Depressive Insanity and Paranoia.* Edinburgh, Scotland: Livingstone; 1921.

Licinio J, Bolis CL, Gold P. *Dysthymia: From Clinical Neuroscience to Treatment.* Geneva: World Health Organization; 1997.

Maj M, Pirozzi R, Magliano L, Bartoli L: Agitated depression in bipolar I disorder: Prevalence, phenomenology, and outcome. *Am J Psychiatry.* 2003;160:2134–2140.

Martinez-Arán A, Vieta E, Reinares M, Colom F, Torrent C, Sánchez-Moreno J, Benabarre A, Goikolea JM, Comes M, Salamero M: Cognitive function across manic or hypomanic, depressed, and euthymic states in bipolar disorder. *Am J Psychiatry.* 2004;161:262–270.

Mast BT, Neufeld S, MacNeill SE, Lichtenberg PA: Longitudinal support for the relationship between vascular risk factors and late-life depressive symptoms. *Am J Geriatr Psychiatry.* 2004;12:93–101.

McElroy SL, Pope HG Jr, Keck PE Jr, Hudson JI, Phillips KA, Strakowski SM: Are impulse-control disorders related to bipolar disorder? *Compr Psychiatry.* 1996;37:229–240.

Morley KI, Hall WD, Carter L: Genetic screening for susceptibility to depression: Can we and should we? *Aust N Z J Psychiatry.* 2004;38:73–80.

Pagani M, Lucini D: Chronic fatigue syndrome: A hypothesis focusing on the autonomic nervous syndrome. *Clin Sci.* 1999;96:117–125.

*Perugi G, Akiskal HS: The soft bipolar spectrum redefined: Focus on the anxious-sensitive, impulse-dyscontrol and binge-eating connection in bipolar II and related conditions. *Psychiatr Clin North Am.* 2002;25:713–737.

Perugi G, Akiskal HS, Lattanzi L, Cecconi D, Mastrocinque C, Patronelli A, Vignoli S: The high prevalence of soft bipolar (II) features in atypical depression. *Compr Psychiatry.* 1998;39:63–71.

Perugi G, Akiskal HS, Rossi L, Paiano A, Quilici C, Madaro D, Musetti L, Cassano GB: Chronic mania: Family history, prior course, clinical picture and social consequences. *Br J Psychiatry.* 1998;173:514–518.

Perugi G, Frare F, Madaro D, Maremmani I, Akiskal HS: Alcohol abuse in social phobic patients: Is there a bipolar connection? *J Affect Disord.* 2002;68:33–39.

Perugi G, Toni C, Travierso MC, Akiskal HS: The role of cyclothymia in atypical depression: Toward a data-based reconceptualization of the borderline–bipolar II connection. *J Affect Disord.* 2003;73:87–98.

Reynolds CF, Hoch CC, Kupfer DJ, Buysse DI, Hofick PR, Stack JA, Campbell DW: Bedside differentiation of depressive pseudodementia from dementia. *Am J Psychiatry.* 1988;145:1099–1103.

Rosenthal NE. *Winter Blues.* New York: Guilford Press; 1993.

Schatzberg AF, Rothschild AJ: Psychotic (delusional) major depression: Should it be included as a distinct syndrome in DSM-IV? *Am J Psychiatry.* 1992;149:733–745.

Tyrer P, Seivewright N, Ferguson B, Tyrer J. The general neurotic syndrome: A coaxial diagnosis of anxiety, depression and personality disorder. *Acta Psychiatr Scand.* 1992;85:201–206.

Widlocher DJ: Psychomotor retardation: Clinical, theoretical, and psychometric aspects. *Psychiatr Clin North Am.* 1983;6:27–40.

Winokur G, Turvey C, Akiskal HS, Coryell W, Solomon D, Leon A, Mueller T, Endicott J, Maser J, Keller M: Alcoholism and drug abuse in three groups—bipolar I, unipolars, and their acquaintances. *J Affect Disord.* 1998;50:81–89.

Zisook S, Shuchter SR, Pedrelli P, Sable J, Deaciuc SC. Bupropion sustained release for bereavement: Results of an open trial. *J Clin Psychiatry.* 2001;62:227–230.

▲ 13.7 Mood Disorders: Treatment of Depression

A. JOHN RUSH, M.D.

There are now many available options in the treatment of mood disorders. This section focuses on depressive disorders, which have enjoyed major therapeutic advances since the mid-1980s. The plethora of new treatment options presents clinicians with the issue of how to optimally organize these options for individual patients. Which types of treatment (i.e., strategies) should be selected, and in what order should they be implemented (strategic planning)? What delivery methods (tactics) (e.g., dose and duration) produce the best results for the greatest number of patients in the shortest period of time?

This chapter discusses the essential elements in treatment planning for managing major depressive and other forms of nonbipolar mood disorders, such as dysthymic disorder and double depression (i.e., coexisting major depressive and dysthymic disorder). Specification of the objectives to be met at each phase of treatment and careful, timely reappraisals of whether these treatment objectives are being met provide a clinically useful road map by which optimal outcomes for each patient may be obtained.

Each phase of treatment (i.e., acute, continuation, and maintenance) has specific objectives. These phases offer a strategic map for managing these patients. For depressive disorders, the initial treatment objectives are symptom remission (which may be accomplished in the acute phase) and restoration of psychosocial functioning (which may be accomplished in the acute or continuation phases). The prevention of a symptomatic relapse is also an objective of continuation phase treatment. Finally, prevention of new depressive episodes (i.e., recurrences) is the aim of maintenance phase treatment. Of course, only those patients with recurrent or chronic depressions are candidates for maintenance treatment.

STRATEGIES

When initiating acute phase treatment, practitioners select the setting in which the patient should be treated (e.g., outpatient, day hospital, or inpatient). The treatment setting is dictated by factors, such as (1) the imminent risk of suicide, (2) the capacity of the patient to recognize and to follow instructions or recommendations (adherence, psychosis), (3) the level of psychosocial resources, (4) the level of psychosocial stressors, and (5) the level of functional impairment.

Next, one chooses among the four common acute phase treatment groupings (medication, psychotherapy, the combination of medication and psychotherapy, or electroconvulsive therapy [ECT]). For some, light therapy alone or in combination with medications may also be an option.

In general, patients whose depressions respond to acute phase medication treatment (alone or combined with psychotherapy) are provided continuation phase medication at the same dose. Continuation phase ECT may also be indicated for acute phase ECT responders if continuation phase medication does not prevent relapse or if prior medications have been ineffective, although the efficacy of this approach rests only on open case series rather than on randomized controlled trials (RCTs) of continuation phase ECT.

A recent RCT of continuation phase cognitive therapy, as well as several open studies, suggests that patients who respond to acute phase psychotherapy alone may also further benefit from continuation phase psychotherapy at a less frequent interval for the subsequent 6- to 8-month period. Those most likely to benefit from continuation phase therapy appear to be those with earlier onset of the major depressive illness and those with residual symptoms at the end of acute phase treatment. The efficacy of the combination of medication and formal psychotherapy as continuation phase treatment has not been compared to continuation phase medication alone.

TACTICS

Tactics are selected to ensure an adequate treatment trial (e.g., adequate dose and duration of treatment). Only with adequate implementation can it be determined whether any strategic choice is correct. Adherence is the most important tactical issue. Low adherence may be due to side effects, the conscious or unconscious meaning of taking medication, or patients' desires to leave treatment once improved—perhaps owing to the shame and stigma that still surround psychiatric disorders.

A second key tactical issue is to adequately evaluate whether the objective (i.e., symptom remission) was met. Symptom severity may be gauged by careful interviewing or by the use of a rating scale. For mood disorders, a serious difficulty in acute phase treatment is the risk of accepting a response with residual symptoms or a partial response, rather than adjusting treatment tactics or even strategies to achieve complete symptom remission. A full symptomatic remission begets a better prognosis and is associated with better function than a response with residual symptoms.

In short, strategic issues involve what treatments to use, whereas tactical issues focus on how to optimally implement the treatments. The following sections address strategic (initial treatment selection, subsequent acute phase treatment revisions, and continuation and maintenance phase treatment planning) and tactical issues.

STRATEGIC CHOICES

Medication

The available antidepressants differ in their pharmacology, drug–drug interactions, short- and long-term side effects, likelihood of discontinuation symptoms, and ease of dose adjustment. They do not differ in overall efficacy, speed of response, or long-term effectiveness. There is substantial evidence that failure to tolerate or to respond to one medication does not imply that other medications will also fail. In fact, with a shift from one medication class to another, there is a 50-percent chance of response to the initial medication and to the next medication, should the first fail to provide a satisfactory response, although these estimates are largely based on open trial data.

A recent metaanalysis of studies comparing venlafaxine (Effexor) to selective serotonin reuptake inhibitors (SSRIs) suggested better efficacy for venlafaxine—especially in terms of achieving symptomatic remission. However, these trials were largely of 8-week durations or less, and subjects could have previously failed to achieve response with another SSRI, which limits the certainty of the findings. These findings have led some to assert that antidepressants that affect norepinephrine and serotonin may be more effective (or have more rapid onset of action) than more selective serotonin reuptake blocking agents. On the other hand, other studies comparing dual action agents (e.g., imipramine [Tofranil]) have not revealed greater efficacy than a comparator SSRI (e.g., sertraline [Zoloft]). Thus, the claim of differential efficacy of dual action agents needs further evaluation in longer term studies.

Clinical Management

General clinical management includes explanation of the diagnosis, treatment plan, treatment objectives, anticipated treatment period, counseling and management of adherence and side effects, and a regular assessment of whether the treatment objectives are being met. It may involve consulting the patient and significant others.

Psychotherapy

The objectives of formal psychotherapy, when used alone to treat mood disorders, are identical to those for medication: (1) symptom remission, (2) psychosocial restoration, and (3) prevention of relapse and recurrence. When used in combination with medication, psychotherapies can also achieve additional objectives, such as reducing the secondary psychosocial consequences of the disorder (e.g., marital discord and occupational difficulties) or increasing medication adherence. Formal psychotherapy to address the psychosocial consequences of the disorder may include individual, family, couples, or occupational approaches. These types of therapy, when used in combination with medication, result in improvement of the targeted difficulty (e.g., marital counseling improves marriages).

Although clinical management, in part, aims to increase adherence, formal psychotherapy can also be used to further enhance adherence. Individuals for whom more formal adherence counseling may be needed include those with significant prior or current adherence difficulties or those with relatively fixed negative attitudes toward a treatment that is clearly indicated.

Psychotherapy as the solo treatment for symptom remission has efficacy when contrasted to wait-list controls. These studies have generally included less severely or chronically ill, nonpsychotic, depressed outpatients. In addition, although some evidence suggests that psychotherapy alone as a maintenance treatment has some efficacy—by prolonging the well interval—in general, when maintenance treatment is anticipated, medications (alone or combined with psychotherapy) are preferred, given the larger number of randomized, controlled medication maintenance trials studies supporting efficacy.

Choosing Among the Psychotherapies

Three forms of time-limited therapy have demonstrated efficacy in reducing or eliminating depressive symptoms (interpersonal psychotherapy [IPT], cognitive therapy, and behavioral therapy). Recently, a new type of therapy (cognitive-behavioral analysis system of psychotherapy

[CBASP]) has been developed for the treatment of chronic depression, with efficacy demonstrated to be equivalent to the medication nefazodone (Serzone) in a controlled, 12-week acute phase trial. There are no established clinical predictors by which to select from the available psychotherapies. Cognitive therapy may be somewhat *less effective* (to a slight degree) in those with *more* dysfunctional attitudes, whereas IPT may be somewhat *less effective* in those with *more* interpersonal problems. However, these predictors lack the power needed for clinical usefulness. Time-limited therapies are usually preferred over time-unlimited therapies for depressive symptom reduction, because time-limited therapies have established efficacy in RCTs, whereas time-unlimited therapies do not, and because medication is an effective alternative if psychotherapy alone fails.

Some believe that reconstructive (time-unlimited) psychotherapies are more useful in the treatment of Axis II disorders, whereas reeducative therapies may be more useful with Axis I conditions. There is no evidence, however, that psychotherapy alone is preferred over medication when there is a concurrent Axis II disorder. On the other hand, different psychotherapeutic tactics may be called for in the medication management of depressed patients with Axis II conditions to ensure adherence. Logically, psychotherapy, if used alone, should be tried for a finite time period, and symptomatic outcomes should be evaluated, just as with any medication trial.

Declaration of psychotherapy failures is largely based on lack of efficacy, although a few patients discontinue treatment unilaterally. When to declare that psychotherapy is ineffective is a complex problem. Some patients respond early, whereas others may take 8 to 10 weeks. Thus, at least a 10-week trial of therapy seems warranted to determine if it is effective. Just as with medication, if a patient inappropriately discontinues treatment while symptomatic, it is advisable to actively attempt to reengage them, because the depression has not remitted, and, consequently, the prognosis is poor.

What treatment should follow if psychotherapy alone is ineffective? Medication, given its established efficacy, is the next best logical step. The psychotherapy may be continued or discontinued when medication is begun. Whether a different form of psychotherapy would be effective if the initial psychotherapeutic approach was not effective has not been evaluated.

Combined Treatment

Medication and formal psychotherapy are often combined in practice, although several randomized, controlled, acute phase trials in noncomplicated, nonchronic forms of depression failed to find that the combination predictably enhances the *symptom reducing effects* obtained with either treatment alone. On the other hand, the combination may have a broader spectrum (i.e., symptom reduction and psychosocial restoration), which provides an additional rationale for using the combined approach.

An important recent large multisite trial of chronically depressed outpatients revealed higher response and higher remission rates for the combination of nefazodone and therapy (CBASP) than with either treatment used alone. These findings support the use of combined treatment in chronic depression.

There are basically three paths to the development of a combined treatment: (1) the initiation of the combination as acute phase treatment; (2) the addition of formal psychotherapy to medication that has resulted in a partial response, particularly when there are residual cognitive, psychological, interpersonal symptoms or difficulties; or (3) the addition of medication when there is a partial response to psychotherapy alone.

The combination of medication and formal psychotherapy at the outset of acute phase treatment would be called for if (1) there is a chronic course to the depressive illness; (2) formal psychotherapy is used to increase adherence, while medications are used for symptom control; or (3) if the targets of each treatment were defined as somewhat distinct, and both were in need of early remediation (e.g., medication for depressive symptoms and psychotherapy for marital problems). In addition, clinical impression suggests that combination treatment may be preferable to treatment alone (1) when there is a coexisting Axis II disorder; (2) when the patient is discouraged and demoralized, as well as clinically depressed; or (3) when the depression is treatment resistant to medications alone based on prior history.

Because medication management itself requires time for patients and clinicians to collaborate to establish the optimal type and dose of medication, it is often simpler to initially begin with medication and clinical management or with psychotherapy alone, particularly for patients with minimal prior treatment without a chronic course. Then, depending on response to medication, formal psychotherapy may be added to achieve complete symptomatic remission or to address psychosocial problems unrelieved by medication, or, conversely, medication may be added to the therapy as the initial treatment to achieve complete symptom remission, if needed. For example, psychotherapy might be added when there is a partial medication response (e.g., persistence of cognitive and interpersonal difficulties).

Evidence suggests that psychosocial and occupational improvements occur during and for several weeks or longer after response to medication alone. Therefore, it may not be necessary to routinely use both treatments initially to achieve psychosocial restoration. Logically, the need for adjunctive psychotherapy to redress psychosocial difficulties becomes clearer the longer that symptom remission is present and the longer that the psychosocial problems persist with medication alone. A history of long-standing psychosocial difficulties, even during remission of chronic depression, may recommend beginning with combined treatment or adding psychotherapy shortly after symptom control has been achieved with medication.

When combined treatment does not produce a full response, a switch of medication classes or augmentation of the first medication with a second one (with continued psychotherapy) is a logical next step, given evidence that switching medication classes appears to be effective.

Electroconvulsive Therapy (ECT)

ECT is effective, even in patients who have not responded to one or several different medications or combined treatment. ECT is effective in psychotic and nonpsychotic forms of depression. Usually, eight to 12 treatments are needed to achieve symptomatic remission. Bilateral ECT is somewhat more effective than unilateral ECT, but it appears to have more cognitive side effects. Recent studies suggest that high-dose right unilateral (RUL) ECT achieves higher response rates than standard-dose RUL ECT.

Other Treatments

Light therapy has been most clearly evaluated in seasonal affective disorder, used alone or in combination with medication. Patients typically respond within 2 to 4 weeks.

STRATEGIC ISSUES

Role of Diagnosis in Treatment Selection

For dysthymic disorder, whether or not it is complicated by recurrent major depressive episodes, maintenance medication effectively prevents recurrences. Psychotic depressions usually require an antidepressant medication and a neuroleptic. Alternatively, ECT is useful in psychotic depression, as a first-line treatment or in those for whom medication has proven ineffective. For those with atypical symptom features, there is strong evidence that tricyclic agents are less effective than the monoamine oxidase inhibitors (MAOIs). There is some suggestive evidence for the efficacy of the SSRIs or bupropion (Wellbutrin) in atypical depression.

The concurrent presence of another disorder may also affect initial treatment selection. The presence of another nonmood Axis I disorder would suggest the recommendation of medications with demonstrated efficacy in the mood and nonmood disorders. For example, the treatment of obsessive-compulsive disorder (OCD) with or without depressive symptoms, if effective, usually results in remission of the depression. In this case, SSRIs would be preferred. Similarly, when panic disorder cooccurs with major depression, medications with demonstrated efficacy in both conditions are preferred (e.g., tricyclics and SSRIs). Thus, in general, the nonmood disorder dictates the choice of treatment.

Concurrent substance abuse raises the possibility of a substance-induced mood disorder, which must be evaluated by history or by requiring abstinence for several weeks, because abstinence results in remission of depressive symptoms in substance-induced mood disorders. For those with continuing significant depressive symptoms, even with abstinence, an independent mood disorder is diagnosed and treated.

Axis II disorders frequently accompany mood disorders, but the diagnosis of Axis II disorders remains tentative in the presence of a clinical depression. It is important not to mistake a chronic or recurrent major depressive disorder for an Axis II disorder, because treatment objectives and strategies are different in each case.

An Axis II disorder is not a contraindication to treating the mood disorder, but its presence may prolong the time to acute phase treatment response, may interfere with adherence, or may even preclude full symptomatic remission. In general, the presence of Axis II disorders suggests a less optimistic prognosis than their absence, because circumstantial evidence suggests that Axis II disorders are risk factors for subsequent relapse and recurrence.

Axis II disorders raise other tactical issues, such as adherence, the establishment of a therapeutic alliance, or the long-term management of these patients. In addition, the presence of an Axis II disorder appears to be associated with a slower or less complete response to medication or time-limited psychotherapy.

General medical conditions are established risk factors in the development of depression, and they are common accompaniments of mood disorders. Recent evidence indicates that the presence of a major depressive episode is associated with increased morbidity or mortality of many general medical conditions (e.g., cardiovascular disease, diabetes, cerebrovascular disease, and cancer).

Principles that apply to the treatment of depression without a general medical condition generally apply when these conditions are present. However, treatment strategies and tactics are more complex. The initial choice among the four main treatment options in the context of the general medical condition is influenced by prior response to antidepressant treatments, the relative medical safety of medications, and clinical judgment as to whether psychotherapeutic methods may be particularly beneficial for some of these patients. Selection among the available medications is affected by drug interactions, the pharmacological profile of the compound, the context of the general medical condition, and the drug dosing requirements.

Complex, ongoing significantly stressful life events or social contextual issues—often profoundly disturbing to patients—should not influence the decision as to whether medication is used. Often, patients in major depressive episodes who achieve symptom reduction with medication become less disabled from the mood disorder and are better able to manage these complex life circumstances. On the other hand, chronic, disturbing life circumstances (e.g., chronic marital discord and spousal abuse) logically argue for stronger consideration of combined treatment, initially or sequenced, to obtain symptom remission and psychosocial restoration. Table 13.7–1 summarizes the relationship between clinical diagnoses and treatment selection.

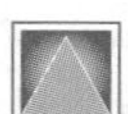

Table 13.7–1
Relationship of Diagnosis to Treatment Selection

Diagnosis	Treatment Recommendations
Major depressive disorder (mild to moderate severity)	Medication or time-limited, depression-targeted psychotherapies.[a]
Major depressive disorder (single episode)	No maintenance phase treatment.
Major depressive disorder, recurrent	Consider maintenance phase treatments.
Major depressive disorder with psychotic features	Antipsychotic plus antidepressant medication, ECT.
Major depressive disorder (severe or with melancholic features)	Medications are essential. Consider ECT.
Depression with atypical features	Nontricyclics are preferred. Monoamine oxidase inhibitors have established efficacy.
Depression with seasonal pattern	Light therapy or medications.
Dysthymic disorder	Medications or time-limited, depression-targeted psychotherapies, or a combination of the two. Consider maintenance phase therapy.
Complex or chronic depressions[b]	Medication plus psychotherapy.[c]

ECT, electroconvulsive therapy.
[a]Interpersonal psychotherapy, cognitive therapy, or behavior therapy.
[b]*Complex* refers to depression cooccurring with other Axis I or Axis II psychiatric conditions.
[c]Psychotherapy may aim at adherence enhancement, symptom reduction, relapse prevention, or psychosocial restoration.

Selecting Initial Treatment

In general, approximately 45 to 60 percent of all outpatients with uncomplicated (i.e., minimal psychiatric and general medical comorbidity), nonchronic, non–treatment-resistant, nonpsychotic major depressive disorder who begin treatment with medication or psychotherapy, or a combination of the two, respond (i.e., achieve at least a 50 percent reduction in baseline symptoms). Only 35 to 50 percent achieve remission (i.e., the virtual absence of depressive symptoms). Consequently, at least one-half of patients should anticipate a second treatment trial, should the initial treatment be poorly tolerated or ineffective.

Selection of the initial treatment depends on the chronicity of the condition, course of illness (a recurrent or chronic course is associated with increased likelihood of subsequent depressive symptoms without treatment), family history of illness and treatment response, symptom severity, concurrent general medical or other psychiatric conditions, prior treatment responses to other acute phase treatments, potential drug–drug interactions, and patient preference. In general, the less severe, less chronic, and less complex the depression (i.e., less current comorbidity), the greater the role for patient preference, because evidence to select between time-limited, depression-targeted psychotherapy and medication is lacking. Furthermore, it is believed that a combination of medication and formal psychotherapy is less likely to be needed in these milder, uncomplicated, nonchronic, non–treatment-resistant depressions.

For moderate to severe mood disorders with prominent chronicity or prior recurrences, the case for maintenance treatment is fairly clear. Because medications are the maintenance treatments with established efficacy, treatment with medication (alone or combined with psychotherapy) is recommended.

The evidence for the efficacy of medication alone in more severe depressions is clear, but psychotherapy alone is less well studied. For those with endogenous or melancholic symptom features, psychotherapy alone in outpatients may be less predictably effective than medication. Cognitive psychotherapy alone has recently been found to be as effective as MAOIs in outpatients with major depressions with atypical symptom features. Case series suggest that the SSRIs and bupropion may also be effective for this group.

Selecting Second Treatment Options

Should the first treatment fail, owing to intolerance or lack of efficacy, a strategic decision regarding the second treatment is called for, after the differential diagnosis (including occult general medical or substance abuse) has been reconsidered.

For those receiving medication initially, adjusting the dose, extending the period of the trial, switching to an alternative treatment (either medication or psychotherapy), or augmenting the current treatment with another are common options. Factors recommending dose escalations are (1) no side effects, (2) a prior history that is consistent with rapid drug metabolism, (3) low therapeutic blood levels, or (4) partial benefit at lower doses. However, blood levels do not relate to outcome for the newer generation medications, although they do relate to outcome for desipramine (Norpramin, Pertofrane), imipramine (Tofranil), and nortriptyline (Aventyl, Pamelor). Extending the initial trial further is indicated if (1) the initial trial is less than 6 weeks, (2) there is a partial response (≥25 percent reduction in pretreatment depressive symptom severity) by 6 weeks, or (3) prior medication trials have been unsuccessful and shorter than 6 weeks.

Similarly for psychotherapy, partial response by week 6 argues for further extending the trial period. Nonresponse by 8 to 10 weeks is typically indicative of an ultimately poor response. With regard to light therapy, extending a trial beyond 3 weeks in nonresponders has not been evaluated. Clinical experience and case series suggest that extending ECT beyond ten trials in the face of complete nonresponse is unlikely, in most cases, to yield a subsequent response.

The choice between switching from the initial single treatment to a new single treatment (as opposed to adding a second treatment to the first one) rests on the philosophy guiding the clinician, the patient's prior treatment history, the degree of benefit achieved with the initial treatment, other clinical issues, and patient preference. The best documented augmentation strategies involve inexpensive medicines (e.g., lithium [Eskalith] or thyroid hormone), and response, if it occurs, is often within 2 to 4 weeks. Conversely, a switching strategy, in some cases, involves a washout period (e.g., switching from fluoxetine [Prozac] to an MAOI) for safety reasons, as well as the need to wait longer than 2 weeks to attain a full effect. Alternatively, how long to continue augmentation is not clear, and lithium augmentation entails some expense and inconvenience (i.e., blood level monitoring).

If the initial trial is the patient's first treatment, and if other clinical or economic reasons favor a single treatment, switching rather than augmenting is preferred. On the other hand, augmentation strategies seem to be preferred with patients who have gained some benefit with the initial treatment but who have not achieved remission. Thus, switching might be preferable for those with only one or two prior treatment attempts or no meaningful benefit from the initial treatment, whereas augmentation may be preferable for those who have not benefited sufficiently from several single treatment trials. Recent reviews indicate that, if the initial medication is ineffective or cannot be tolerated, a reasonable step in primary care is to switch medication classes. In psychiatric settings, augmentation may be more likely to be called for, because more psychiatric patients have not benefited from several adequate prior single treatments.

The value of augmenting medication with psychotherapy has not been well evaluated. Many clinicians believe that, if the residual symptoms after a partial response to medication are largely cognitive or psychological in nature, augmenting with psychotherapy or prolonging the initial medication trial is preferred to switching medications or augmenting with another medication, based on the assumption that these symptoms represent residual psychosocial sequelae. On the other hand, if anhedonia persists after an initial medication trial, a strategic decision to switch or to augment with another medication rather than with psychotherapy is often seen as preferable, the assumption being that such symptoms suggest ongoing limbic and paralimbic system dysfunction. These suggestions, however, are largely based on clinical experience rather than on scientific evidence.

TACTICAL ISSUES

The strategic choices of treatment focus on selection of the initial therapy or, for those for whom the initial therapy has failed, the selection of a second or subsequent treatment options. Tactics focus on the optimal implementation of these strategies. Tactical issues include (1) careful attention to adherence, (2) careful evaluation of outcome, (3) proper dosing and duration of the trial, and (4) timely declaration of treatment failure.

Adherence

Treatment adherence is increased if patients are educated about anticipated treatment objectives and options. If fewer daily doses are required (e.g., once-a-day dosing versus three-times-a-day dosing), or if a personality disorder is not present, adherence is enhanced. Evidence also suggests that more frequent early visits (e.g., weekly versus monthly) improve adherence. Adherence is not related to gender, educational level, or socioeconomic status. The best predictor of future adherence is prior adherence. Whether other concurrent psychiatric conditions affect adherence is unclear.

Thus, general clinical management of medication treatment should include discussions with patients (and, potentially, significant others) of the nature and expected course of their depressive illness, objectives of treatment, treatment options, anticipated treatment period, adherence obstacles, and anticipated side effects. It is best to anticipate and to identify obstacles to adherence, even before prescribing medication or initiating psychotherapy, and to make adherence checks a routine part of each visit.

Initially, visit frequency should be often enough to ensure adherence and timely intervention, should untoward side effects occur. Several brief telephone contacts during the initial weeks of beginning a treatment help adherence by reassuring patients, ensuring that severe side effects are avoided, countering demoralization and pessimism that impair adherence, and providing information to overcome short-term concentration and recall problems that are part of depressive episodes.

Choosing Among Medications

If medication (alone or in combination with psychotherapy) is part of the first step, the practitioner must select among a variety of available compounds. Medications differ in their short- and long-term side effects, spectrum of action, drug–drug interactions, ease of dosing, and likelihood of symptoms on abrupt discontinuation but, in general, not in overall efficacy or speed of response. If maintenance medication is anticipated, long-term side effects play a greater role than short-term side effects in selecting the medication (e.g., tertiary tricyclics are associated with greater weight gain than SSRIs over the long run).

Table 13.7–2 lists and groups the antidepressant agents presently available in the United States. They are divided into groups based on their presumed mechanisms of action (e.g., presynaptic or postsynaptic activity, or both). However, as basic neuroscientific knowledge

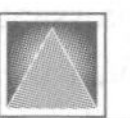

Table 13.7–2
Antidepressant Medications

Generic (Brand) Name	Usual Daily Dose (mg)	Common Side Effects	Clinical Caveats
NE reuptake inhibitors			
Desipramine (Norpramin, Pertofrane)	75–300	Drowsiness, insomnia, OSH, agitation, CA, weight ↑, anticholinergic[a]	Overdose may be fatal. Dose titration is needed.
Protriptyline (Vivactil)	20–60	Drowsiness, insomnia, OSH, agitation, CA, anticholinergic[a]	Overdose may be fatal. Dose titration is needed.
Nortriptyline (Aventyl, Pamelor)	40–200	Drowsiness, OSH, CA, weight ↑, anticholinergic[a]	Overdose may be fatal. Dose titration is needed.
Maprotiline (Ludiomil)	100–225	Drowsiness, CA, weight ↑, anticholinergic[a]	Overdose may be fatal. Dose titration is needed.
5-HT reuptake inhibitors			
Citalopram (Celexa)	20–60	All SSRIs may cause insomnia, agitation, sedation, GI distress, and sexual dysfunction	Many SSRIs inhibit various cytochrome P450 isoenzymes. They are better tolerated than tricyclics and have high safety in overdose. Shorter half-life SSRIs may be associated with discontinuation symptoms when abruptly stopped.
Escitalopram (Lexapro)	10–20		
Fluoxetine (Prozac)	10–40		
Fluvoxamine (Luvox)[b]	100–300		
Paroxetine (Paxil)	20–50		
Sertraline (Zoloft)	50–150		
NE and 5-HT reuptake inhibitors			
Amitriptyline (Elavil, Endep)	75–300	Drowsiness, OSH, CA, weight ↑, anticholinergic[a]	Overdose may be fatal. Dose titration is needed.
Doxepin (Triadapin, Sinequan)	75–300	Drowsiness, OSH, CA, weight ↑, anticholinergic[a]	Overdose may be fatal.
Imipramine (Tofranil)	75–300	Drowsiness, insomnia and agitation, OSH, CA, GI distress, weight ↑, anticholinergic[a]	Overdose may be fatal. Dose titration needed.
Trimipramine (Surmontil)	75–300	Drowsiness, OSH, CA, weight ↑, anticholinergic[a]	—
Venlafaxine (Effexor)	150–375	Sleep changes, GI distress	Higher doses may cause hypertension. Dose titration is needed. Abrupt discontinuation may result in discontinuation symptoms.
Pre- and post-synaptic active agents			
Nefazodone (Serzone)	300–600	Sedation	Dose titration is needed. No sexual dysfunction.
Mirtazapine (Remeron)	15–30	Sedation, weight ↑	No sexual dysfunction.
Dopamine reuptake inhibitor			
Bupropion (Wellbutrin)	200–400	Insomnia/agitation, GI distress	Twice-a-day dosing with sustained release. No sexual dysfunction or weight gain.
Mixed action agents			
Amoxapine (Asendin)	100–600	Drowsiness, insomnia/agitation, CA, weight ↑, OSH, anticholinergic[a]	Movement disorders may occur. Dose titration is needed.
Clomipramine (Anafranil)	75–300	Drowsiness, weight ↑	Dose titration is needed.
Trazodone (Desyrel)	150–600	Drowsiness, OSH, CA, GI distress, weight ↑	Priapism is possible.

Note: Dose ranges are for adults in good general medical health, taking no other medications, aged 18 to 60 years of age. Doses vary depending on the agent, concomitant medications, the presence of general medical or surgical conditions, age, genetic constitution, and other factors. Brand names are those used in the United States.
CA, cardiac arrhythmia; 5-HT, serotonin; GI, gastrointestinal; NE, norepinephrine; OSH, orthostatic hypotension; SSRI, selective serotonin reuptake inhibitor.
[a]Dry mouth, blurred vision, urinary hesitancy, and constipation.
[b]Not approved as an antidepressant in the United States by the U.S. Food and Drug Administration.

expands, actions now unknown about the currently marketed agents will likely be discovered. For example, the number of serotonin receptors has increased at a rate that has outstripped the ability to understand the physiological role played by many of them. A further caveat about dividing agents by mechanisms of action is that, for some (e.g., venlafaxine), the doses used (or levels attained in the central nervous system [CNS]) affect their pharmacological effects. Venlafaxine has a proportionally greater norepinephrine reuptake blockade than serotonin reuptake blockade at higher as opposed to lower doses.

Missing from Table 13.7–2 are commonly used drug combination treatments (e.g., lithium plus antidepressants, triiodothyronine [T_3] augmentation of tricyclics). A detailed discussion of these combinations is beyond the scope of this section. When, how, and whether to resort to combination treatment have recently been discussed.

Finally, Table 13.7–2 lists selected clinical caveats. This list is *not* exhaustive. A drug–drug interaction at the neuronal level (pharmacodynamics) or at the level of absorption, metabolism, and excretion (pharmacokinetics) is important information that affects selection of agents, their dosing, and, ultimately, the risk–benefit equation for individual patients.

Patients should be advised as to which side effects to anticipate and should be encouraged to report them as early as possible. Management of side effects may include lowering the dose, switching medications, or treating the side effects with an additional medication.

Among the tricyclic medications, the secondary amines (desipramine or nortriptyline) have fewer side effects but equivalent efficacy as the tertiary amines. Because nortriptyline has a well-established therapeutic window, it can be used with drug level monitoring to ensure that patients who need to have the *least* amount of medication exposure obtain a therapeutic level. Conversely, the upper limit of the nortriptyline window may be a disadvantage, because a blood level may be called in the face of nonresponse before switching or augmenting.

Choosing more sedating antidepressants (e.g., amitriptyline [Elavil, Endep]) for more anxious depressed patients or more activating agents (e.g., desipramine) for more psychomotor-retarded patients is not based on evidence of differential efficacy. However, some clinicians believe that such choices, based on side effect profile, increase adherence in the initial weeks of treatment. That is, patients with marked insomnia and anxiety feel some immediate relief from these associated symptoms before the full antidepressant effect of the drug appears, and they therefore are thought to be more likely to comply with acute phase treatment. These clinical observations are not supported by empirical data, however. In fact, attrition associated with paroxetine (Paxil) or fluoxetine (less sedating drugs) is lower in acute phase treatment than is attrition with imipramine or amitriptyline (more sedating drugs). In addition, the longer-term clinical impact of what may be a beneficial short-term side effect advantage must be considered. For example, initially sedating antidepressants often continue to be sedating in the longer run, which, in turn, may lead patients to prematurely discontinue continuation or maintenance phase treatment—thereby increasing the risk of relapse or recurrence.

Some practitioners use adjunctive medications (e.g., sleeping pills or anxiolytics) combined with antidepressants to provide more immediate symptom relief—routinely from the outset or when the need for such adjunctive medications is established in an individual patient. Adjunctive medications, if used briefly to provide quick symptomatic relief or to cover those side effects to which most patients ultimately adapt, can be useful. Conversely, discontinuing adjunctive medications can lead to some return of symptoms or side effects to which the patient has not adapted.

However, several disadvantages are associated with the *routine* use of adjunctive medications: (1) the potential risk, inconvenience, and expense of unnecessary medications (i.e., many patients may not require it), (2) difficulty identifying the cause of the medication intolerance or adverse side effects (e.g., an allergic rash) when the antidepressant and adjunctive medication(s) are begun at the same time, (3) and the masking of critical depressive symptoms by which to gauge the success of acute phase treatment, such that practitioners are unable to judge whether there is a full therapeutic response to the antidepressant medication alone, without discontinuing the adjunctive medication to see if the apparent response holds on the antidepressant alone. This effort may unnecessarily increase the number of visits or delay a timely revision in the treatment plan. (4) Finally, adjunctive medications may cover side effects, which, if observed, would lead to a dose reduction or to switching treatments. For example, a sedative hypnotic used in conjunction with an SSRI may inappropriately delay a strategic decision to decrease the dose or to switch to an alternative agent.

In addition to side effects, factors that affect medication choice include prior history of response, cross-sectional symptom features, patient preference, dosing convenience (which affects adherence), drug interactions (if patients are or will be taking other medications), presence of current general medical conditions (making one side effect profile preferred over another), and a family history of response.

A patient's prior treatment history is important, because prior response typically predicts current response. In addition, as noted previously, a documented failure on a properly conducted trial of a particular antidepressant class (e.g., SSRIs, tricyclics, or MAOIs) points in the direction, given the available data, of choosing an agent from an alternative class. Switching classes, for those who fail on one class, appears to be associated with roughly a 50 percent response rate with the second class of drugs, although open trial evidence also roughly suggests a 50 percent response rate when switching between different SSRIs.

The history of a first-degree relative responding to a tricyclics or an MAOI is associated with a better response to the same class of agents in the patient. Whether family history of response is an indicator among the newer antidepressant compounds is not known.

Dose and Duration Tactical issues surrounding medication use include dosing steps, drug metabolism, pharmacokinetics, drug interactions, and side effects. The tricyclics typically are started at lower doses and are elevated to find the maximally tolerated dose or, in the case of nortriptyline, until a therapeutic level is obtained. Gradual dose escalations are important to ensure adherence and to avoid severe initial side effects. Thus, the tricyclics are associated with a roughly once-a-week visit frequency for outpatients as doses are adjusted. With tricyclic blood level monitoring, dose adjustment time may be reduced. Dosing is less complicated for the SSRIs than for the tricyclics. Dose increments are fewer, and the proper dose is more easily attained earlier owing to better side effect profiles. For some newer agents (e.g., SSRIs and bupropion), fewer dose adjustments are needed, but, for others (e.g., venlafaxine and nefazodone), raising the dose increases the likelihood of response—so, several dose adjustments are often helpful.

Safety in overdose is an issue, especially early in treatment. Thus, a 1-week prescription is recommended (without refills) for medications with greater lethality in overdose (i.e., tricyclics and MAOIs), so patients return for frequent-enough medication visits at which time side effects and dose levels are managed. Tricyclics account for a greater percent of completed suicides than the newer agents, which are far safer in overdose.

Evaluation of Outcome The objective of acute phase treatment (with medication, psychotherapy, their combination, or ECT) is symptom remission, not just symptom reduction. Response with residual symptoms, as opposed to full remission, is associated with a more stormy prognosis and poorer daily function. Thus, careful interviewing for criterion depressive symptoms at each visit is essential. Self-reported or clinician-rated instruments can facilitate this assessment. In many cases, the patient is slower to recognize the early therapeutic effect of the treatment than is the clinician. Thus, a clinician-rated scale may be preferred over a self-reported instrument.

Timely Declaration of Treatment Failures Each treatment step should be applied in an optimal fashion (e.g., dosage and duration) to determine its effectiveness. There is a clinically important tension involved in the evaluation of the initial treatment—providing a sufficient amount of treatment for a long enough period of time to determine whether it is effective, while at the same time not unnecessarily prolonging exposure to a treatment that will ultimately be ineffective. Growing evidence indicates that acute phase medication trials should last 4 to 6 weeks to determine if meaningful symptom reduction will be attained. Most (but not all) patients who ultimately respond fully show at least a partial response (i.e., at least a 20 to 25 percent reduction in pretreatment depressive symptom severity) by week 4 if the dose is adequate during the initial weeks of treatment. Clinical impression and recent reports suggest that the lack of a partial response by 4 to 6 weeks (i.e., <20 percent reduction in symptoms) suggests that a treatment change is needed. That is, only approximately 20 percent of those without at least a modest signal of benefit by 6 weeks will respond over the next several weeks, assuming that an adequate dose was used in the initial 6 weeks. Longer time periods (e.g., 8 to 12 weeks or longer) are needed to define the ultimate full degree of symptom reduction achievable with a medication.

Medication dose obviously affects clinical outcome and side effect burden. Some patients may metabolize certain drugs more rapidly or more slowly than others. Slow metabolizers, especially for the more anticholinergic tricyclics, encounter side effects earlier in treatment or at lower doses. High blood levels of tricyclics may cause arrhythmias, seizures, or delirium. Fast metabolizers may be virtually absent of side effects and benefits, even with rather large doses. However, side effects, especially for desipramine and nortriptyline, are not good predictors of blood levels. Indeed, orthostatic hypotension can occur even with low blood levels. Such cases argue for the value of a therapeutic blood level to determine dosing strategies, especially when the tricyclics are used in the medically fragile.

Patients may not respond to a medication, because (1) they cannot tolerate the side effects, even in the face of a good clinical response; (2) an idiosyncratic adverse event may occur; or (3) the clinical response is not adequate. Idiosyncratic or serious adverse side effects (e.g. seizures and allergic reactions), although rare, are most likely encountered within the first several weeks of treatment and often occur with dose escalation or as medication levels rise to a steady state level. Some side effects are dose dependent (e.g., sedation) and can be reduced by decreasing the dose or slowing the rate of dose escalation. Moderate side effects, when encountered, argue for withholding further dose escalations and allowing time for physiological adaptation, which often results in lower side effects. Some side effects are less dose dependent (e.g., orthostatic hypotension), and tolerance to them is less likely. In these cases, gradual dose escalation is less useful, and a change in treatment is often indicated.

Lack of efficacy is the most common reason for medication failure, but this cannot be fully gauged until patients have had several weeks of treatment at adequate doses (4 to 6 weeks). Thus, careful evaluation of symptoms at visits during acute phase treatment, whether formally conducted with a rating scale or by clinical interview to assess each criterion symptom of the mood disorder, is essential to gauge the adequacy of medication response.

CONTINUATION TREATMENT

Continuation treatment typically lasts 4 to 9 months. In theory, the duration depends on an estimate of when the episode would have spontaneously remitted. Thus, patients with longer prior episodes (e.g., 9 to 15 months) who have had only 2 months of a current depression, for example, would be candidates for 5 to 11 months of continuation treatment, assuming that acute treatment lasted 2 months. For those with psychotic depressions, follow-up studies 1 year after acute phase treatment indicate a poorer prognosis than for nonpsychotic depression. Thus, continuation phase treatment for psychotic depressions should be longer.

When medication is used alone or combined with formal psychotherapy for acute phase treatment, continuation medication treatment is recommended, because early medication discontinuation is associated with higher relapse rates than later medication discontinuation. Continuation medication, whenever clinically feasible, should be at the same dose as that used during acute phase treatment. This recommendation is based on evidence from maintenance trials using lower dose tricyclics, suggesting a greater recurrence rate than that which occurs in those trials using full dose treatment.

Psychotherapy may be added to continuation phase medication if psychosocial residua do not remit with medication alone. Whether to continue psychotherapy after response to acute phase combined treatment is unclear and is left entirely up to clinical judgment at this time. Based on a recent randomized trial of continuation phase cognitive therapy, after response to acute phase cognitive therapy alone, continuation phase therapy is recommended for those who do not achieve remission with acute phase treatment and for those with longer-standing courses of illness (e.g., earlier age at onset of the first major depressive episode).

In a recent report of outcomes of continuation phase medication for chronic depressions, roughly 40 percent of those who attain a response, but with residual symptoms, at the end of 12 weeks of acute phase treatment achieve remission after 4 more months of medication alone. Conversely, a substantial number relapse during continuation phase medication. Thus, careful monitoring of symptom status during continuation phase treatment is recommended to facilitate early intervention, if needed.

Continuation phase medication treatment may end with a *gradual* taper of shorter half-life medications that block serotonin reuptake, discontinuation of other medications, and careful symptom assessment during and for several months after discontinuation, or entry into maintenance phase treatment.

MAINTENANCE TREATMENT

Strategic Issues

Maintenance treatment aims at preventing new episodes (recurrences). It is appropriate for recurrent or chronic depressions but not for single-episode major depressive disorder. Maintenance medication treatment has been documented to be effective in virtually all studies to date. There is strong evidence that those with three or more episodes should receive maintenance phase treatment, and, indeed, even at 5 years, maintenance medication has prophylactic efficacy.

Whether those with only two major depressive episodes should receive maintenance treatment is less clear. Information to inform this decision includes poor interepisode recovery between the two episodes, presence of two episodes within the last 3 years, or a positive family history for recurrent major depressive or bipolar disorder, any of which, when present, point toward a higher likelihood of an earlier new episode (recurrence) than for those without such histories. In any case, however, clinicians and patients need to decide collaboratively whether to initiate maintenance treatment or to provide more diligent monitoring with no treatment until the need is established by the development of a new episode. If a new episode develops when the patient is free of treatment, early intervention shortens the length of the new episode.

Tactical Issues

An important issue encountered in continuation and maintenance treatment is symptom breakthrough, which may be only modest and time limited, requiring minor shifts in the treatment plan (e.g., dose adjustment and reassurance). On the other hand, if symptom breakthrough is profound, prolonged, or unresponsive to dose adjustment and reassurance, it must be treated. Unfortunately, no RCTs addressing this issue are available. Perhaps the simplest approach is to augment the current medication with an additional one (e.g., lithium, thyroid hormone, or another antidepressant). Should this strategy prove effective, the augmenting medication may then be discontinued after a time (e.g., several months) to empirically evaluate whether it is necessary over the longer term. If the augmenting medication fails, then a switch in treatment to another medication may be needed.

If symptom breakthrough occurs, it could be remediated by psychotherapy, but this option has not been formally studied. Perhaps psychotherapy would be indicated if the symptoms were caused by disturbed interpersonal relationships or life events (e.g., divorce or unemployment).

Another tactical problem encountered in continuation and maintenance treatment is the management of the depression when pregnancy or intercurrent general medical illnesses requiring medication or surgery occur. For patients who need a window in time for surgery or pregnancy, medication discontinuation is preferred. Because pregnancy may last for a prolonged period of time, given the evidence for the efficacy of IPT alone as a maintenance treatment or cognitive therapy as continuation phase treatment, psychotherapy without medication may provide an extended drug-free period. The development of other general medical illnesses and the need for nonpsychotropic medications during continuation and maintenance treatment are common. These circumstances need to be managed, taking into account pharmacokinetics and drug–drug interactions between the psychotropic and nonpsychotropic agents.

When to discontinue maintenance medication treatment is unclear. As noted previously, RCT evidence indicates that those with highly recurrent depressions (e.g., more than three episodes) continue to be benefited by maintenance treatment for at least 5 years. Some patients may require prolonged periods (e.g., a decade) or even lifetime maintenance medication treatment. When discontinuation occurs, careful monitoring is needed, as the first 6 months after discontinuation appear to be a particular risk period for recurrences.

PATIENT PREFERENCE

It is important for patients to become informed about their depressive disorders and to collaborate in their treatment. Even so, some patients are adamantly opposed to medication, whereas others are equally opposed to psychotherapy. Patient preference can play a greater role when the evidence is not strong that the strategic choice between formal psychotherapy and medication is well-supported by data. Although patients may exercise their first preference initially, a contingency plan, should the first treatment be ineffective, is best developed early in the management of the patient, in case a second treatment trial is needed. Therefore, it may be wise, at the outset, to plan for at least two acute treatment trials, so that patients may avoid inappropriate discouragement and consequent premature attrition, should the initial treatment fail to provide full remission. Treatment tactics to obtain optimal outcome include attention to adherence, careful titration of medication to attain maximal benefit with minimal side effects, and careful symptom evaluation to ensure that remission, not just improvement, has occurred. Establishing explicit goals and following a step-wise plan to attain them can help practitioners and patients obtain the best outcomes.

TREATMENT GUIDELINES AND ALGORITHMS

Definition

In recent years, recommendations as to the appropriate treatment(s) for depression have been summarized in practice guidelines or specified in more detail in treatment algorithms. Guidelines review available treatment options, detail the nature and strength of the evidence available that supports each option, and make recommendations as to the type of patient best suited for each treatment option. Treatment algorithms (sometimes called *clinical pathways* or *disease management protocols*) offer more specific recommendations. They typically specify the treatments to be offered at the first, second, third, or subsequent treatment steps, and they provide tactical recommendations (e.g., what medication doses are to be used for what durations to determine if a meaningful clinical benefit will occur or to determine when the maximal therapeutic result has been achieved). Treatment algorithms often provide flow charts to specify the treatment steps to be implemented in sequence, depending on the patient's response to the treatment being tried. Algorithms rely on both scientific evidence and clinical consensus. Furthermore, the evidence on which to recommend specific treatment options available at the second, third, or subsequent treatment steps in these algorithms is, at best, modest. Several ongoing randomized, controlled trials will provide far greater documentation as to whether there are preferred "next-step" treatments in the context of previous, failed treatment trials. At the moment, such decisions still rest largely on clinician judgment.

As algorithms are more specific, they require clinicians to have a greater degree of sophistication and experience in their use (i.e., the users must decide when the specific recommendations must be ignored or modified to best suit the individual patient). For example, the algorithms may need to be modified to best serve older patients, those who are medically fragile, or those with specific difficulties in the use of previous treatments.

Development

A range of methods have been used to develop treatment guidelines and algorithms. Typically, they involve systematic reviews of published treatment trial reports, as well as a means by which to assess and synthesize clinical consensus when the published evidence is insufficient to make specific recommendations. The certainty of the evidence is typically rated (e.g., A, B, C) with the highest degree of certainty (A) resting on randomized, controlled trials.

The applicability of the evidence to the particular patient being treated must be judged by the clinician, because many randomized trials in depressed patients exclude those with substantial degrees of treatment resistance or comorbid Axis I or III conditions. Both guidelines and algorithms require regular updating as new evidence becomes available.

Implementation

The systematic implementation of guidelines or algorithms often requires changes in routine practice procedures. For example, the regular assessment of symptomatic outcomes (e.g., measurement of depressive symptom severity by self-report or clinician rating) that result from implementing each treatment option is recommended to gauge specifically whether a clinically significant benefit has been achieved, and, if so, whether symptom remission (the goal of treatment) has been reached. Often, the frequency of visits recommended may be greater than is typical in some practice settings. These guidelines and algorithms typically also call for systematic education of patient and families as part of a longer term chronic disease management program, especially for those with chronic or recurrent mood disorders. Practice procedure modifications may also entail reconfiguration of the organizational elements needed to deliver care—for example, the use of nonphysician staff to accomplish specific tasks, such as acquiring diagnostic information, assessing response, or providing education.

Effectiveness

Although a range of guidelines and algorithms have been developed, only recently have they been empirically evaluated. The evaluation of effectiveness to date has compared these approaches to treatment as usual. There are no direct, randomized comparisons of one algorithm (or guideline) versus another. For depressed patients, comparative evaluations have revealed better outcomes with algorithm- or guideline-based care than with treatment as usual in both primary and psychiatric practice settings. However, these improved outcomes (e.g., greater symptom resolution and improvements in daily function) have typically been associated with at least a modest increase in treatment costs (for the depression). Whether cost offsets are also achieved (e.g., less use of non–mental health services, greater work productivity) with these guidelines and algorithms is not yet clear. In addition, whether greater algorithm adherence by clinicians and patients further enhances clinical outcomes is not yet resolved.

SUGGESTED CROSS-REFERENCES

Classification of mental disorders is discussed in Section 9.1, treatment of mood disorders in Chapter 13, psychotherapies in Chapter 30, mood disorders in children and adolescents in Chapter 45, and diagnosis and treatment of psychiatric disorders in late life in Chapter 51.

REFERENCES

*American Psychiatric Association: Practice guidelines for major depressive disorder in adults. *Am J Psychiatry.* 1993;150[Suppl 4]:1.

*American Psychiatric Association Task Force: Tricyclic antidepressants—blood level measurements and clinical outcome. *Am J Psychiatry.* 1985;142:155.

American Psychiatric Association: Practice guidelines for the treatment of patients with major depressive disorder (revision). *Am J Psychiatry.* 2000;157[Suppl 4]:1.

Coryell W, Tsuang MT: Primary unipolar depression and the prognostic importance of delusions. *Arch Gen Psychiatry.* 1982;39:1181.

*Depression Guideline Panel. *Clinical Practice Guideline. Depression in Primary Care: Volume 2. Treatment of Major Depression.* Rockville, MD: U.S. Department of Health and Human Services, Public Health Service, Agency for Health Care Policy and Research; 1993; AHCPR Publication No. 93-0551.

Fava GA, Rafanelli C, Grandi S, Canastrari R, Morphy MA: Six-year outcome for cognitive behavioral treatment of residual symptoms in major depression. *Am J Psychiatry.* 1998;155:1443.

Fava GA, Rafanelli C, Grandi S, Conti S, Belluardo P: Prevention of recurrent depression with cognitive behavioral therapy: Preliminary findings. *Arch Gen Psychiatry.* 1998;55:816.

Fava M, Rush AJ, Trivedi MH, Nierenberg AA, Thase ME, Sackeim HA, Quitkin FM, Wisniewski S, Lavori PW, Rosenbaum JF, Kupfer DJ: Background and rationale for the Sequenced Treatment Alternatives to Relieve Depression (STAR*D) study. *Psychiatr Clin North Am.* 2003;26:457.

*Frank E, Kupfer DJ, Perel JM, Cornes C, Jarrett DB, Mallinger AG, Thase ME, McEachran AB, Grochocinski VJ: Three-year outcomes for maintenance therapies in recurrent depression. *Arch Gen Psychiatry.* 1990;47:1093.

Greden JF. Treatment of recurrent depression. In: Oldham JM, Riba MB, eds. *Review of Psychiatry Series.* Vol 20. Number 5. Washington, DC: American Psychiatric Publishing; 2001.

Hirschfeld RMA, Dunner DL, Keitner G, Klein DN, Koran LM, Kornstein SG, Markowitz JC, Miller I, Nemeroff CB, Ninan PT, Rush AJ, Schatzberg AF, Thase ME, Trivedi MH, Borian FE, Crits-Christoph P, Keller MB: Does psychosocial functioning improve independent of depressive symptoms? A comparison of nefazodone, psychotherapy, and their combination. *Biol Psychiatry.* 2002;51:123.

Jarrett RB, Kraft D, Doyle J, Foster BM, Eaves GG, Silver PC: Preventing recurrent depression using cognitive therapy with and without a continuation phase: A randomized controlled trial. *Arch Gen Psychiatry.* 2001;58:381.

Keller MB, McCullough JP, Klein DN, Arnow B, Dunner DL, Gelenberg AJ, Markowitz J, Nemeroff CB, Russell JM, Thase ME, Trivedi MH, Zajecka J, Blalock JA, Borian FE, DeBattista C, Fawcett J, Hirschfeld RMA, Jody DN, Keitner G, Kocsis JH, Koran LM, Kornstein SG, Manber R, Miller I, Ninan PT, Rothbaum B, Rush AJ, Schatzberg AF, Vivian D: A comparison of nefazodone, the cognitive behavioral-analysis system of psychotherapy, and their combination for the treatment of chronic depression. *N Engl J Med.* 2000;342:1462.

Kocsis JH, Schatzberg A, Rush AJ, Klein DN, Howland R, Gniwesch L, Davis SM, Harrison W: Psychosocial outcomes following long-term, double-blind treatment of chronic depression with sertraline vs. placebo. *Arch Gen Psychiatry.* 2002;59:723.

Koran LM, Gelenberg AJ, Kornstein SG, Howland RH, Friedman RA, DeBattista C, Klein D, Kocsis JH, Schaztberg AF, Thase ME, Rush AJ, Hirschfeld RMA, LaVange LM, Keller MB: Sertraline versus imipramine to prevent relapse in chronic depression. *J Affect Disord.* 2001;65:27.

*Kupfer DJ, Frank E, Perel JM, Cornes C, Mallinger AG, Thase ME, McEachran AB, Grochocinski VJ: Five-year outcome for maintenance therapies in recurrent depression. *Arch Gen Psychiatry.* 1992;49:769.

Miller IW, Keitner GI, Schatzerg AF, Klein DN, Thase ME, Rush AJ, Markowitz JC, Schlager DS, Kornstein SG, Davis SM, Harrison WM, Keller MB: The treatment of chronic depression, Part 3: Psychosocial functioning before and after treatment with sertraline or imipramine. *J Clin Psychiatry.* 1998;59:608.

Mintz J, Mintz LI, Arruda MJ, Hwang SS: Treatments of depression and the functional capacity to work. *Arch Gen Psychiatry.* 1992;49:761.

Nelson JC, Jatlow PI, Mazure C: Rapid desipramine dose adjustment using 24-hour levels. *J Clin Psychopharmacol.* 1987;7:72.

Nierenberg AA, DeCecco LM: Definitions of antidepressant treatment response, remission, nonresponse, partial response, and other relevant outcomes: A focus on treatment-resistant depression. *J Clin Psychiatry.* 2001;62[Suppl 16]:5.

Paykel ES, Scott J, Teasdale JD, Johnson AL Garland A, Moore R, Jenaway A, Cornwall PL, Hayhurst H, Abbott R, Pope M: Prevention of relapse in residual depression by cognitive therapy. A controlled trial. *Arch Gen Psychiatry.* 1999;56:829.

Reynolds CF III, Frank E, Perel JM, Imber SD, Cornes C, Miller MD, Mazumdar S, Houck PR, Dew MA, Stack JA, Pollock BG, Kupfer DJ: Nortriptyline and interpersonal psychotherapy as maintenance therapies of recurrent major depression: A randomized, controlled trial in patients older than 59. *JAMA.* 1999; 281:39.

Robinson DG, Spiker DG: Delusional depression: a one year follow-up. *J Affect Disord.* 1985;9:79.

Rosenbaum JF, Fava M, Nierenberg AA, Sachs G. Treatment-resistant mood disorders. In: Gabbard GO, ed. *Treatments of Psychiatric Disorders.* 3rd ed. Vol 2. Washington, DC: American Psychiatric Publishing; 2001.

Rush AJ. Pharmacotherapy and psychotherapy. In: Derogatis LR, ed. *Clinical Psychopharmacology.* Menlo Park, CA: Addison-Wesley Publishing Co; 1986.

Rush AJ. Guidelines for the treatment of major depression. In: Stein DI, Kupfer DJ, Schatzberg A, eds. *American Psychiatric Publishing Textbook of Mood Disorders.* Washington, DC: American Psychiatric Publishing; 2004 (*in press*).

Rush AJ, Crismon ML, Kashner TM, Toprac MG, Carmody TJ, Trivedi MH, Suppes T, Miller AL, Biggs MM, Shores-Wilson K, Witte BP, Shon SP, Rago WV, Altshuler KZ; TMAP Research Group: Texas Medication Algorithm Project, Phase 3 (TMAP-3): Rationale and study design. *J Clin Psychiatry.* 2003;64:357.

Rush AJ, Crismon ML, Toprac MG, Trivedi MH, Rago WV, Shon S, Altshuler KZ: Consensus guidelines in the treatment of major depressive disorder. *J Clin Psychiatry.* 1998;59[Suppl 20]:73.

Rush AJ, Kupfer DJ. Strategies and tactics in the treatment of depression. In: Gabbard GO, ed. *Treatments of Psychiatric Disorders.* 3rd ed. Vol 2. Washington, DC: American Psychiatric Press; 2001.

Rush AJ, Ryan ND. Current and emerging therapeutics for depression. In: Charney DS, Coyle JT, Davis KL, Nemeroff CB, eds. *Neuropsychopharmacology. The Fifth Generation of Progress.* Baltimore: Lippincott Williams & Wilkins; 2002.

Rush AJ, Thase ME. Psychotherapies for depressive disorders: A review. In: Maj M, Sartorius N, eds. *WPA Series. Evidence and Experience in Psychiatry.* Vol 1. *Depressive Disorders.* Chichester, UK: John Wiley and Sons; 1999.

Sackeim HA, Haskett RF, Mulsant BH, Thase, ME, Mann JJ, Pettinati HM, Greenberg RM, Crowe RR, Cooper TB, Prudic J: Continuation pharmacotherapy in the prevention of relapse following electroconvulsive therapy. A randomized controlled trial. *JAMA.* 2001;285:1299.

Schatzberg AF, Nemeroff CB: *American Psychiatric Press Textbook of Psychopharmacology.* 2nd ed. Washington, DC: American Psychiatric Press; 1998.

Segal Z, Vincent P, Levitt A: Efficacy of combined, sequential, and crossover psychotherapy and pharmacotherapy in improving outcomes in depression. *J Psychiatry Neurosci.* 2002;27:281.

Thase ME: When are psychotherapy and pharmacotherapy combinations the treatment of choice for major depressive disorder? *Psychiatr Q.* 1999;70:333.

Thase ME, Rush AJ. Treatment resistant depression. In: Bloom F, Kupfer DJ, eds. *Psychopharmacology: The Fourth Generation of Progress.* New York: Raven Press; 1995.

Thase ME, Rush AJ, Howland RH, Kornstein SG, Kocsis JH, Gelenberg AJ, Schatzberg AF, Koran LM, Keller MB, Russell JM, Hirschfeld RMA, LaVange LM, Klein DN, Fawcett J, Harrison W: Double-blind switch study of imipramine or sertraline treatment of antidepressant-resistant chronic depression. *Arch Gen Psychiatry.* 2002;59:233.

Trivedi MH, Rush AJ, Crismon ML, et al.: The Texas Medication Algorithm Project (TMAP): Clinical results for patients with major depressive disorder. *Arch Gen Psychiatry.* 2004 (*in press*).

Unützer J, Katon W, Callahan CM, Williams JW Jr, Hunkeler E, Harpole L, Hoffing M, Della Penna RD, Noel PH, Lin EH, Arean PA, Hegel MT, Tang L, Belin TR, Oishi S, Langston C; IMPACT Investigators: Improving Mood-Promoting Access to Collaborative Treatment: Collaborative care management of late-life depression in the primary care setting: A randomized controlled trial. *JAMA.* 2002;288:2836.

Wexler BE, Nelson JC: The treatment of major depressive disorders. *Int J Ment Health.* 1993;22:7.

▲ 13.8 Mood Disorders: Treatment of Bipolar Disorders

ROBERT M. POST, M.D., AND LORI L. ALTSHULER, M.D.

Bipolar I affective disorder occurs in approximately 1 percent of the population, which translates into 2.5 million people in the United States alone. Bipolar II disorder and bipolar disorder not otherwise specified (NOS) account for another 1 to 4 percent of the population. Twenty-five to 55 percent of patients with bipolar illness make a medically serious suicide attempt, and some 10 to 20 percent die of their illness by suicide. It is against this backdrop of a recurrent, potentially disabling medical illness that diagnosis and acute and long-term treatment approaches should be conceptualized.

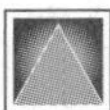

Table 13.8–1
Approach to the Treatment-Resistant Bipolar Patient

A. *Diagnostic clarification*
  1. Retrospective course (bipolar I disorder, bipolar II disorder, bipolar disorder not otherwise specified, recurrent brief mania, rapidity of cycling)
  2. Medication history (antidepressant-induced mania; tolerance or seasonal patterns)
  3. Family history of bipolar and other disorders and of medication response
  4. Comorbidities (alcohol and substance use, anxiety disorders)

B. *Maximize current treatment regimen*
  1. For acute manias: treatment first, blood levels and chemistries after
     For depression: start low and go slow
  2. Increase dose if side effects allow
  3. Change timing of dose (especially at night for increased sleep and compliance and decreased side effects)
  4. Address dose-limiting side effects:
     (a) Decrease dose to below side-effects threshold
     (b) Use another antimanic agent if possible (i.e., one with two-for-one return)
     (c) Treat side effect with another medication, i.e.:

Lithium	**Possible treatment**
Tremor	Propranolol (Inderal)
Polyuria	Amiloride (Midamor) and thiazide diuretics
Hypothyroidism	Thyroid replacement

     (d) Discontinuation (for severe or intolerable side effects)
  5. Address and treat comorbidities

C. *Augment:* especially with partial efficacy (i.e., do not discontinue ineffective but well-tolerated lithium without careful reconsideration of risk to benefit ratio, including its antisuicide and potential neurotrophic effects)
  1. As-needed high-potency benzodiazepine (clonazepam [Klonopin] or lorazepam [Ativan])
  2. Add second mood stabilizer (especially with acute efficacy)
  3. Use atypical antipsychotic or third mood stabilizer if needed
  4. Use atypical with best efficacy–to–side effect profile for target symptoms; consider clozapine (Clozaril) only for refractory mania and cycling
  5. Add drug with different mechanism of action, profile of efficacy, or side effects potential, for example:
     (a) Lamotrigine (Lamictal) (for recurrent depression)
     (b) Divalproex (Depakote, Depakene) (for migraine, panic disorder)
     (c) Carbamazepine (Tegretol) or oxcarbazepine (Trileptal) (for pain syndromes, alcohol comorbidity, bipolar II disorder, and mood-incongruent delusions)
     (d) Atypical antipsychotic (especially for psychosis and schizoaffective disorder)
     (e) Dihydropyridine calcium channel blocker (for ultradian cycling)

D. *Evaluate discontinuation of potential mania-inducing or cycle-inducing agents, such as:*
  1. Antidepressants and alprazolam (Xanax)
  2. Cocaine and related stimulants
  3. Steroids (if possible)

E. *Substitute* (if side effects are present, and the drug is ineffective)
  1. Consider drug with different side effect profile
  2. Consider drugs with different mechanisms of action

F. *Refocus on early warning system and prophylaxis*
  1. Mood chart, contract with patient for specific medication changes for mild symptoms and contact of physician for pronounced symptoms
  2. Provide education and address compliance
  3. Principle: maintain effective full prophylaxis in absence of side effects
     (a) Be conservative when good medication responses are achieved
     (b) Be more radical and make changes when adequate response is not achieved

The diagnosis and treatment of the mood disorders have reached a new level of sophistication based on a variety of advances. It is now widely recognized that bipolar illness is almost always recurrent and can be associated with severe morbidity and even mortality. Furthermore, there is recognition that bipolar affective disorders have a prominent genetic component interacting with environmental events. A host of neurobiological alterations have been documented biochemically and with functional brain imaging. Convergent with this growing knowledge about the classification, course, and mechanisms underlying acute episodes and their recurrences is an expanding array of effective psychotherapeutic and pharmacotherapeutic modalities. Accordingly, treatment approaches are beginning to be differentiated as a function of episode type, severity, and course and, like other chronic medical conditions, require careful longitudinal management and follow-up.

There is also an increasing consensus surrounding a series of new treatment principles. Early recognition and intervention in acute episodes and maintenance of effective long-term prophylaxis may not only save the patient months to years of pain and suffering, but also may be life saving. More careful assessment of a given agent in the individual patient within a short time frame and early revision of treatment if no improvement is shown are also new suggestions (Table 13.8–1). Consensus is growing that a patient with a first episode of bipolar illness, but in the context of a positive family history, is a candidate for continuation therapy and subsequent long-term prophylaxis after the resolution of that episode. However, education of patients and families about the need for long-term treatment even after several affective episodes is more easily said than done. It appears appropriate to reconceptualize the recurrent mood disorders not as a trivial illusory or mental phenomenon that can easily be modified by the patient's own will, but as serious and potentially life-threatening brain disorders that have clearly defined motor, mood, cognitive, somatic, neurophysiological, and neurochemical concomitants.

HISTORY

Over the course of the 20th century, a revolution has occurred in the treatment of bipolar illness. In the first half of the century, no adequate treatment was available; in the second half, lithium (Eskalith) emerged as a wonder drug for the acute and prophylactic management of the disorder. It is noteworthy, however, that oscillations in the assessment of lithium's safety, efficacy, and usefulness have persisted. The drug was initially abandoned as unsafe until adequate monitoring of blood levels was developed, virtually eliminating its most serious and potentially lethal cardiovascular and central nervous system (CNS) toxicities. However, concerns about long-term renal complications have not entirely dissipated, based largely on uncontrolled observations reported in the 1980s.

There is also greater recognition of lithium's efficacy limitations. As with penicillin, these limitations do not infer that lithium no longer works but only that a narrowing has occurred in the conceptualization of the incidence of complete therapeutic efficacy. It is now understood that more than 50 percent of patients in most academic centers do not show adequate, complete, or sustained response to lithium, even when adjunctive unimodal antidepressant and antimanic treatments are used.

Since the mid-1990s in the United States, new prescriptions for lithium have been superseded by those for valproic acid (Depakene) or divalproex (Depakote). Yet, lithium remains the only mood stabilizer with documented effectiveness in preventing suicide. It also normalizes the excess medical mortality that accompanies untreated recurrent affective illness.

Since the late 1990s, in vitro neurotrophic and in vivo neuroprotective effects of lithium have been documented. Not only does it keep cultured hippocampal, cerebellar, and cortical neurons alive, but it increases cell survival factors Bcl-2 and brain-derived neurotrophic growth factor (BDNF) and decreases levels of cell death factors, such as BAX and p53. In animal models of stroke and Huntington's chorea, pretreatment with lithium decreases lesion size and subsequent neurological deficit. These preclinical effects of lithium take place at clinically relevant concentrations, and preliminary evidence from patients also suggests that lithium treatment increases brain levels of *N*-acetylaspartate (NAA), a marker of neuronal integrity, and may also increase gray matter in a regionally selective fashion.

As decrements in CNS neural and glial cells are revealed in bipolar disorder, these neurotrophic mechanisms of action of lithium raise the possibility that they could be relevant to the delay or repair of such biochemical and structural alterations. Although this remains to be directly demonstrated, it would appear that one could make the case that lithium's pharmacological categorization should be transformed in physicians' and patients' conceptualizations from one that involves only neurotoxicities and thyroid and renal impairment to one that is potentially neurotrophic, neuroprotective, and medically life extending for those with bipolar illness.

In the middle of the last century, electroconvulsive therapy (ECT) emerged as the most effective approach to treat acute episodes. Antipsychotics (typical neuroleptics) rapidly became the mainstay of antimanic treatment, as well as for treatment of psychosis. In the 1960s, the first-generation nonselective monoamine oxidase inhibitors (MAOIs) and tricyclic antidepressants (TCAs) were introduced and widely used in conjunction with lithium. Now, selective serotonin reuptake inhibitors (SSRIs), bupropion (Wellbutrin), and venlafaxine (Effexor) have supplanted the TCAs because of their apparent equal efficacy and much greater safety in overdose. Mirtazapine (Remeron) and reversible inhibitors of monoamine oxidase type A (RIMAs) selective modalities are also available. Similarly, the typical antipsychotics of the phenothiazine, butyrophenone, and thiothixene classes have given way to the atypical antipsychotics (sequentially by chronological order of availability) clozapine (Clozaril), risperidone (Risperdal), olanzapine (Zyprexa), quetiapine (Seroquel), ziprasidone (Geodon), and aripiprazole (Abilify). These new major tranquilizers include drugs with novel structures and mechanisms of action and generally more benign CNS side effect profiles, although concerns about tardive dyskinesia with the original agents have been replaced by concerns about weight gain and its medical consequences with many of the atypicals. A new combination of olanzapine and fluoxetine (Symbyax) may also have a place in treatment of the illness.

As the limitations of lithium as a single mood stabilizer have been increasingly recognized, a variety of other mood stabilizers have become available, particularly the anticonvulsants carbamazepine (Tegretol), divalproex sodium (Depakote), and lamotrigine (Lamictal) and, perhaps, the dihydropyridine calcium channel blockers (CCBs). Other promising anticonvulsants are being explored as possible third-generation mood stabilizers, including oxcarbazepine (Trileptal). Mechanistically unique anticonvulsants levetiracetam (Keppra) and zonisamide (Zonegran) are just beginning to be studied. Vagus nerve stimulation (VNS), an approved treatment for refractory epilepsy, has shown promising preliminary results in bipolar as well as unipolar depressive illness, as have other physiological interventions, such as repeated transcranial magnetic stimulation (rTMS) of the brain.

This new range of available psychopharmacological agents raises a series of difficult issues for the clinician, particularly when these agents must be chosen on the basis of an inadequate literature on relative efficacy or clinical and biological markers of responsiveness (Table 13.8–2). Thus, the choice of agents is often based on their side effects profile and clinical lore regarding syndromic selectivity of response. There are imprecise guidelines for initially choosing among these agents, and guidelines are completely lacking for their use in dual or complex combination therapy, which is increasingly necessary to achieve remission and mood stability in bipolar illness. Moreover, in addition to unimodal antidepressants and antimanics and mood stabilizers, a whole host of adjunctive treatments have shown preliminary support for their usefulness in helping manage the illness. Precisely defining when and how and in what combination these treatments and adjuncts are used remains a considerable clinical challenge that is in need of systematic clinical study.

Thus, the clinician often has to resort to educated guesses and systematic and sequential clinical trials in individual patients to delineate optimal responsivity. Even with the availability of many new treatments, episodes of illness can often emerge through apparently successful pharmacoprophylaxis, necessitating further adjunctive measures (Fig. 13.8–1). The importance of complex combination therapies is well recognized in many other specialties and branches of medicine and is indispensable in the approach to tuberculosis, acquired immune deficiency syndrome (AIDS), congestive heart failure, or cancer chemotherapy. Systematic research of combination therapies has lagged markedly behind clinical practice and the clinician is often left to his or her own devices in finding the optimal algorithm for the large group of patients who are refractory to single standard treatment interventions.

This section therefore attempts not only to briefly summarize the knowledge base derived from systematic controlled clinical trials, but also to point beyond the current clinical consensus in new bipolar guidelines to possible novel treatment interventions that may be used when patients fail to respond to first-, second-, and third-line options. Although it is recognized that many of the recommendations contained in this chapter will be altered appropriately following the availability of more systematic research in the future, it is hoped that some of the principles elucidated will provide a more lasting series of guidelines to treating physicians that will assist in optimizing acute and long-term treatments for the bipolar patient.

INITIAL DIAGNOSTIC AND THERAPEUTIC APPROACHES

Impediments to Short- and Long-Term Treatment

Although bipolar mood disorders appear eminently treatable, a series of illness-related variables complicate diagnosis, access to treatment, and the ability of the patient to follow through with adequate long-term interventions. It is estimated that as many as 40 percent of bipolar I disorder patients in community surveys are not in treatment, and a disturbingly large number of those who are seeing physicians are receiving improper medicinal treatment. A series of recent studies suggests that 25 to 55 percent of patients with a unipolar major depressive diagnosis have a bipolar II disorder or bipolar disorder NOS illness. The Mood Disorder Questionnaire (MDQ) (Table 13.8–3) may be a useful screening device.

One-half of the persons with a diagnosis of bipolar illness have a depressive episode as their first sign of the illness, and time spent in depression over a lifetime with the disorder may exceed time spent in mania by a factor of three, even in intensively treated outpatients (Figs. 13.8–2 and 13.8–3). Many depressed individuals often do not recognize their symptoms as related to a constellation of a major depressive medical illness. Some of the symptoms themselves, such as motor retardation, loss of energy, a sense of inertia, and hopelessness, may also preclude the patient's seeking treatment. Thus, the patient's family, close friends, or general practitioner may have to play an active role in encouraging the patient into treatment.

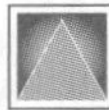

Table 13.8–2
Mechanistic Classes of Medications Used in Bipolar Illness: Preliminary Evidence of Spectrum of Efficacy in Mania or Depression

Class of Medication	Mania	Depression
Antimanics		
Typical antipsychotics block D_2 receptors		
Trifluoperazine (Stelazine)	+++	– –
Haloperidol (Haldol)	+++	– –
Molindone (Moban)	++	– –
High-potency benzodiazepines ↑ Cl^- influx, potentiate GABA		
Clonazepam (Klonopin)	++	±
Lorazepam (Ativan)	++	±
Atypical antipsychotics block mesolimbic D_1, D_2, and D_4 receptors and 5-HT type 2 receptors		
Clozapine (Clozaril)	+++	+
Risperidone (Risperdal)	+++	+
Olanzapine (Zyprexa)	+++	++
Quetiapine (Seroquel)	+++	+++
Ziprasidone (Geodon)	+++	+
Atypical antipsychotic partial agonist at D_1, D_2, D_3, 5-HT type 1A receptors		
Aripiprazole (Abilify)	+++	+
Possible mood stabilizers		
↓ Second messengers, G proteins, and inositol transport		
Lithium (Eskalith)	+++	++
Carbamazepine (Tegretol)	+++	++
Oxcarbazepine (Trileptal)	++	+
Valproate	+++	+
↑ Brain GABA		
Valproate	+++	+
Gabapentin (Neurontin)	0	±
Tiagabine (Gabitril)	0	±
Topiramate (Topamax)	0	+
↓ Glutamate release via (↓ Na_i^+)		
Carbamazepine	+++	++
Lamotrigine (Lamictal)	+	+++
Topiramate	0	+
Zonisamide (Zonegran)	++	+

Class of Medication	Mania	Depression
Possible mood stabilizers, continued		
Dihydropyridine ↓ L-type Ca^{2+}_i		
Nimodipine (Nimotop)	++	++
Isradipine (DynaCirc)	+	+
Amlodipine (Norvasc)	±	±
Phenylalkylamine ↓ L-type Ca^{2+}_i		
Verapamil (Calan)	++	0
Thyroid augmentation		
Triiodothyronine	±	++
High-dose thyroxine	+	+
Atypical antipsychotics (see above)		
Antidepressants		
Dopamine		
Bupropion (Wellbutrin)	0, –	++
Pramipexole (Mirapex)	0, –	++
5-HT selective serotonin reuptake inhibitors as a class	0, –	++
Fluoxetine (Prozac), Sertraline (Zoloft), Paroxetine (Paxil), Fluvoxamine (Luvox), Citalopram (Celexa)		
5-HT plus		
Nefazodone (Serzone)	0, –	++
Mirtazapine (Remeron)	0, –	++
NE		
Desipramine (Norpramin)	– –	++
Nortriptyline (Aventyl)	– –	++
Maprotiline (Ludiomil)	– –	++
Reboxetine (Edronax)	– –	0
Atomoxetine (Strattera)	– –	++
5-HT and NE		
Clomipramine (Anafranil)	– –	++
Venlafaxine (Effexor)	– –	++
Duloxetine (Cymbalta)	– –	++

– –, worsen; 0, –, ineffective, may worsen; 0, ineffective; ±, possibly effective; +, substantial open data; ++, much open and/or some controlled data; +++, good controlled data or wide use; D_1, dopamine type 1; D_2, dopamine type 2; D_3, dopamine type 3; GABA, γ-aminobutyric acid; 5-HT, serotonin; NE, norepinephrine.

The entire treatment context must be conducted against the backdrop of the patient's distorted depressive cognitions, hopelessness, and view of the untreatability of the illness. These need to be explained as symptoms of the illness that are not consistent with the physician's knowledge and optimism about treatment response based on the literature. Moreover, each phase of the treatment needs to be continually assessed in relation to the potential for suicide. The clinician's empirical basis for hope of recovery needs to be conveyed to the patient without the promise of immediate results, so that the expected lags in onset of treatment response are not further misinterpreted as a confirmation of the patient's worst fears of untreatability.

There are also major impediments to effective treatment of the manic phases of illness. In the early stages of hypomania, the sense of well-being, sociability, and increased energy and productivity may lead the patient to ignore more severe aspects of the illness, including irritability, argumentativeness, insomnia, poor judgment, and engagement in sexual and other high risk behaviors, without appropriate appreciation of the consequences. These deleterious activities may severely affect the patient's social structure, marriage, and employment. Recognition of these possibilities, as well as the denial of illness (agnosia) as the early components of bipolar illness itself, may be crucial to instituting appropriate treatment and preventing escalation to more destructive and full-blown manic episodes. Again, there is an important role for participation of the family in this treatment matrix, in the diagnostic evaluation and in the ongoing treatment of the patient. The family can assist in overcoming illness denial and thought disorder associated with hypomania and mania, which can be as problematic to receiving adequate treatment as the hopelessness and suicidal tendencies of depression.

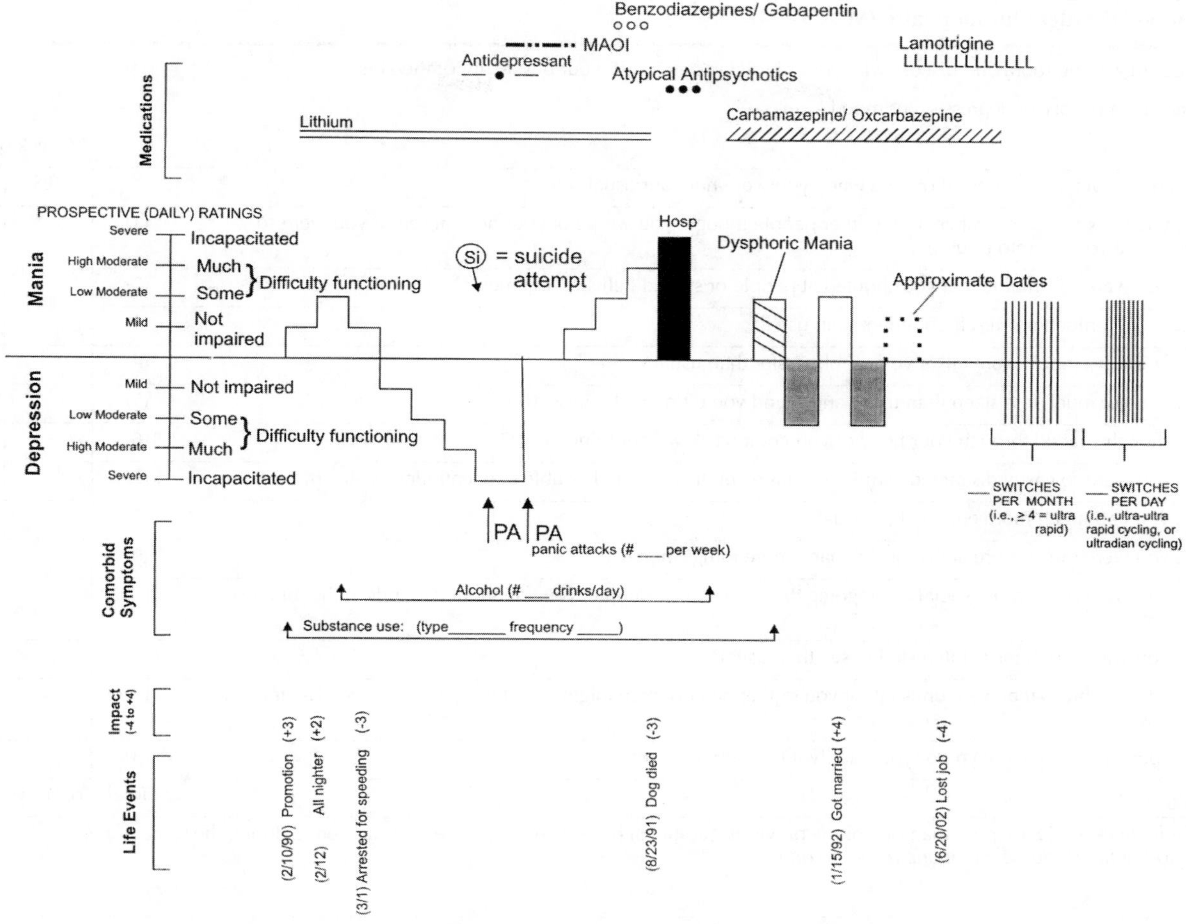

FIGURE 13.8–1 Schema for graphing the prospective course of mood disorders. MAOI, monoamine oxidase inhibitor; PA, panic attack; Si, suicide attempt. Hard copies of the National Institute of Mental Health Life Chart Method (NIMH-LCM) are available from http://www.bipolarnews.org.

Therefore, therapeutic activism, engagement of the family, and early and aggressive treatment of manic and depressive syndromes are of paramount importance. The individual patient and his or her family should receive important initial and ongoing informational support regarding the medical aspects of this illness, its potential course, and response to treatment, with the long-term goals of increasing compliance and medicalizing and destigmatizing the illness. Destigmatization may become a crucial issue later in therapy when one considers recommendations for long-term prophylaxis and when society's negative attitudes toward taking psychotropic maintenance medications (but not those for most other illnesses, such as digitalis, insulin, antihypertension, and viruses) may come forward. Conceptualizing the recurrent mood disorders as medical illnesses deserving the same attention, care, and long-term respect as disorders of other organ systems may be of considerable help to the patient and family in arriving at appropriate long-term treatment decisions.

During each successive phase of acute, continuation, and prophylactic treatment, the patient and his or her family should be assisted in their evaluation and reevaluation of the medical data and the potential impact of their actions on the illness course. It is important not to introduce all of these variables at once, but to approach them sequentially in each phase as is appropriate. For example, it may be more appropriate to emphasize the importance of long-term, if not lifelong, prophylaxis therapy once the patient has already begun to show an antimanic or antidepressant response, rather than to raise this issue with the acutely ill patient who may not be able to understand the rationales and data accurately.

Physician as Educator and Advocate Early education regarding the importance of long-term prophylaxis—with the appropriate graphic, statistical, and written, as well as verbal, presentation of the data to the patient and family—may be critical for ultimately achieving a positive outcome. It is worth noting that, even in an illness such as juvenile diabetes, in which the patient cannot survive without adequate insulin treatment, many adolescents nevertheless are still compelled to test directly or indirectly their need for insulin, the experience of hyperglycemic episodes, and, possibly, hospitalization. In a parallel fashion, it should be anticipated that patients with bipolar disorder are likely to be tempted to discontinue treatment, especially when the data regarding the morbid or lethal consequences are less well delineated. Nevertheless, the treating clinician has a critical educational role to play in providing patients and their families with the now overwhelming data of the high likelihood of a recurrence and of the ability of a variety of agents to prevent recurrences of manic and depressive episodes. These risks and benefits should be weighed against the likelihood of side effects, so that informed and data-based decision making can proceed.

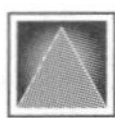

Table 13.8–3
Mood Disorder Questionnaire (MDQ)

Please fill out in waiting room and discuss with your physician's assistant, your physician, or therapist.

For patients with a history of depression or mood swings:

Check one box

			YES	NO
1.	Has there ever been a period of time when you were not your usual self and . . .		YES	NO
	. . . you felt so good or so hyper that other people thought you were not your normal self or you were so hyper that you got into trouble?	(1)		
	. . . you were so irritable that you shouted at people or started fights or arguments?	(2)		
	. . . you felt much more self-confident than usual?	(3)		
	. . . you were much more talkative or spoke faster than usual?	(4)		
	. . . you got much less sleep than usual and found you didn't really miss it?	(5)		
	. . . thoughts raced through your head or you couldn't slow your mind down?	(6)		
	. . . you were so easily distracted by things around you that you had trouble concentrating or staying on track?	(7)		
	. . . you had much more energy than usual?	(8)		
	. . . you were much more active or did many more things than usual?	(9)		
	. . . you were much more social or outgoing than usual, for example, you telephoned friends in the middle of the night?	(10)		
	. . . you were much more interested in sex than usual?	(11)		
	. . . you did things that were unusual for you or that other people might have thought were excessive, foolish, or risky?	(12)		
	. . . spending money got you or your family into trouble?	(13)		
		Total # of Yes ✔	_____	
2.	If you checked YES to more than one of the previous questions, have several of these ever happened during the same period of time? *Please circle one response only.* YES NO			
3.	How much of a problem did any of these cause you—having family, money, or legal troubles; getting into arguments or fights; or being unable to work? *Please circle one response only.* No problem Minor problem Moderate problem Severe problems			

If you scored yes on 7 or more of the 13 items in item No. 1 and checked yes on item No. 2, and these symptoms caused you moderate to serious problems in item No. 3, you should consult with your doctor about the possibility of a bipolar diagnosis.

From Hirschfeld RM, Williams JB, Spitzer RL, et al: Development and validation of a screening instrument for bipolar spectrum disorder: The Mood Disorder Questionnaire. *Am J Psychiatry.* 2000;157:1873–1875, with permission.

In bipolar illness, the high likelihood of relapse after discontinuation of effective lithium treatment (50 percent in the first 5 months and 80 to 90 percent within the first 1.5 years) is now well documented in metaanalyses and should be explained to the patient. Slower tapering of lithium reduces this risk only modestly. There is a sevenfold increased risk of suicide in those who discontinue lithium versus those who continue it, and this risk can be as much as 20 times higher in the first year of discontinuation. In addition, it has always been assumed that, if patients experience a relapse, they are as readily responsive as they were before, once their treatment has been reinstituted. Many investigators, but not all, have observed the phenomenon of lithium discontinuation–induced refractoriness in which a small percentage (10 to 15 percent) of patients who discontinue successful prophylactic lithium treatment and experience a relapse then fail to rerespond once the same treatment is reinstituted (Fig. 13.8–4). In other instances, patients may not respond as rapidly as they did initially, or they may require increased adjunctive antipsychotic medication.

With some prominent exceptions, a large number of studies report that lithium is less effective in patients who have had more than three or four (or, in one study, ten) prior episodes compared with those in whom prophylaxis is initiated earlier in the illness. Thus, the potential morbidity and mortality of an episode should be factored into the decision-making process for long-term prophylaxis, and the possibility that new episodes would not only convey their morbidity, but could also affect the subsequent course of the illness and its pharmacological responsivity. The physician should share this information with the patient when he or she is euthymic, so that the physician can be placed in the role of educator and advocate of the patient's long-term mental health.

PSYCHIATRIC HISTORY

A thorough medical history and examination are important, given the many syndromes that mimic manic and depressive syndromes. The older patient with late-onset illness, in particular, should be

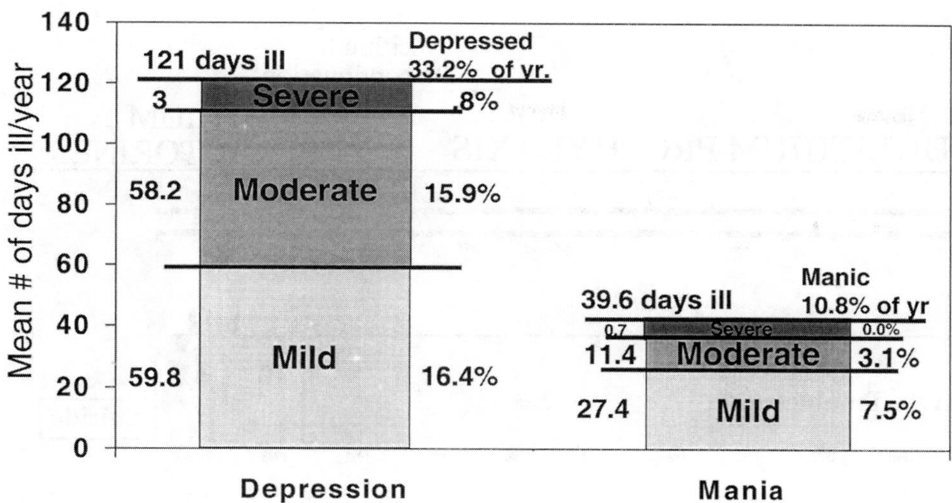

FIGURE 13.8–2 Greater amount of treatment-resistant depression (33.2 percent) than mania (10.8 percent) in 258 outpatients rated daily for 1 year in the former Stanley Foundation Bipolar Network. The depression-to-mania ratio is 2.9 in bipolar I and 3.6 in bipolar II patients.

approached with the possibility that an associated medical cause may exist. The physician should be alert to symptoms that are indicative of CNS neuropathology, underlying endocrinopathy, or other associated medical illness. Although these uncommon possibilities are to be ruled out, it may be helpful to emphasize that all of the observed physiological, endocrine, somatic, and vegetative symptoms are consistent with a typical primary affective illness.

The earliest parts of the history can be used for uncovering diagnostic clues and for the patient's initial education in the types of symptoms that are typical of the disorder, are associated with its natural course of spontaneous exacerbations and remission of episodes, and are likely to respond to somatic and pharmacological intervention. The medical history and examination should also be directed at uncovering evidence of comorbid cardiac, renal, or thyroid abnormalities that may help guide subsequent treatment choices. The physician should be aware that Axes I, II, and III comorbidities are common features of the illness as well.

The physician should uncover patients' own earliest signs and symptoms of an impending mood and depressive episode, thus providing target symptoms for future assessment of the efficacy of treatment interventions and monitoring of breakthrough symptoms. These symptoms are often highly characteristic for a given patient and can provide the basis for an early warning system (EWS) for illness detection and institution of additional treatment, as necessary.

A detailed family history of medical and psychiatric illness is also important in the initial diagnostic assessment of the patient. It is recommended that a formal family tree be graphically constructed and each first-degree relative be specifically inquired about, not only for their potential neuropsychiatric diagnosis, but also for their course of illness and response to therapy, because each of these may help guide the choice of therapies for the patient. A positive family history of bipolar illness may further support the recommendations for long-term prophylaxis with lithium, whereas a positive family history for one of the anxiety disorders may support a recommendation for lamotrigine or other anticonvulsants.

Childhood Onsets

A bipolar family history, especially if there is bilineal loading for affective disorder, should markedly raise suspicion of juvenile- or adolescent-onset bipolar illness in the offspring, even if its presentation is less than typical. The clinician should be aware of the problematic long lag, even in adult-onset bipolar illness, between affective symptom onset and first treatment. Moreover, in the prepubertal child, bipolar illness may present differently from the classic adult picture. Instead of showing discrete episodes that eas-

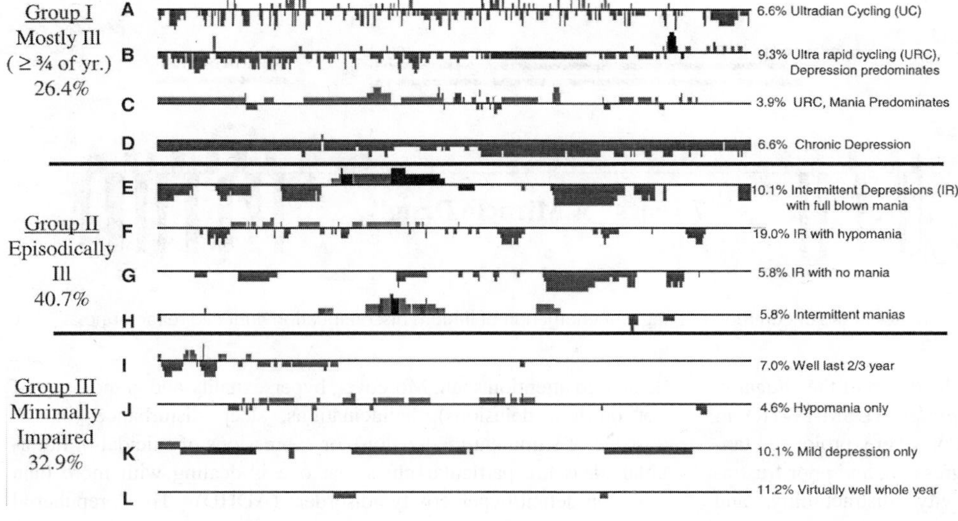

FIGURE 13.8–3 Life charts showing the varying patterns of illness among 258 outpatients treated and followed prospectively for 1 year. A through L are illness characteristics for that group. Individuals in group I were ill for at least three-fourths of the year. Those in group II were episodically ill, and patients in group III were only mildly ill.

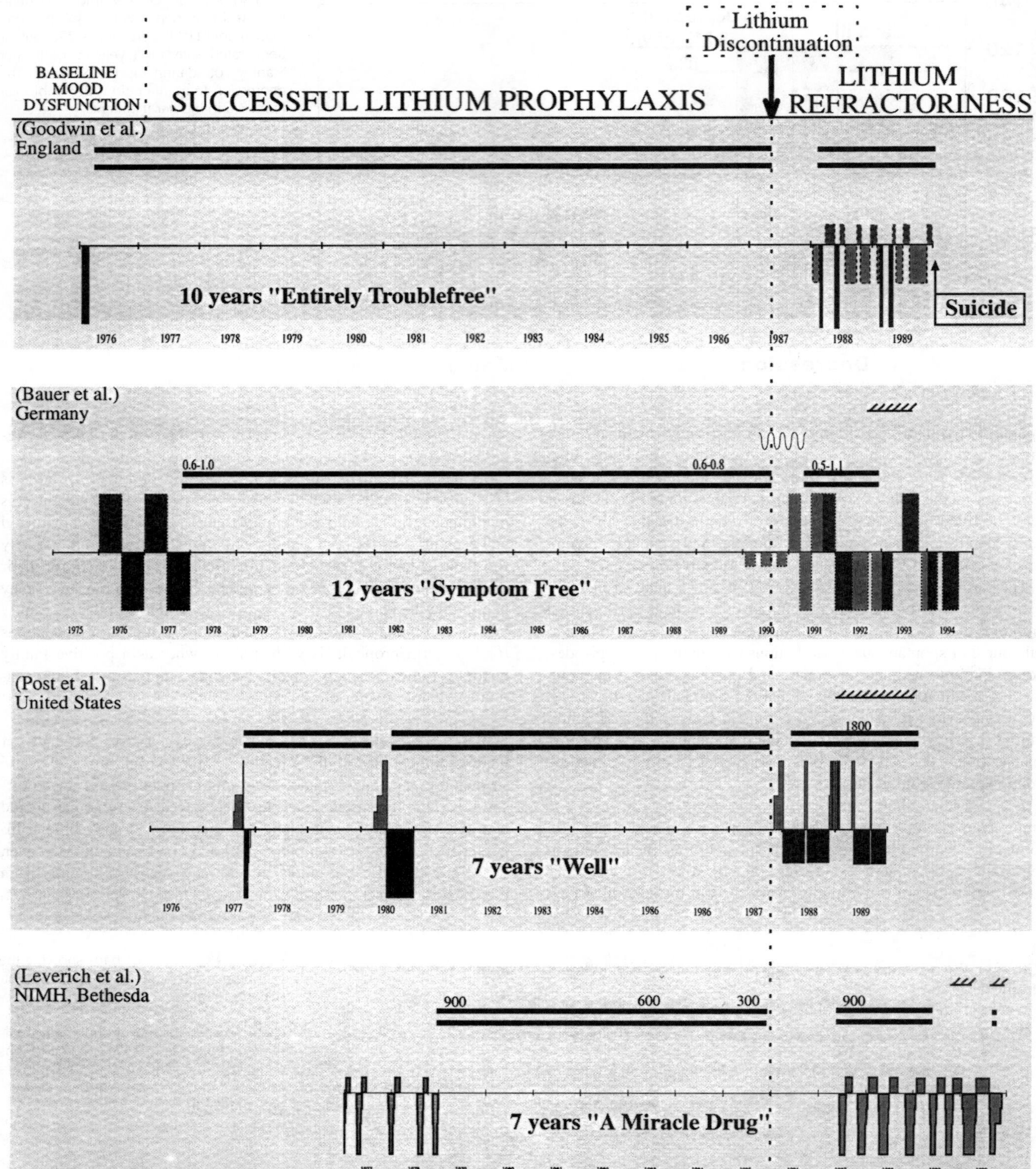

FIGURE 13.8–4 Life charts showing four examples of the uncommon but tragic phenomenon of lithium discontinuation–induced refractoriness.

ily meet duration criteria of the revised fourth edition of the *Diagnostic and Statistical Manual of Mental Disorders* (DSM-IV-TR) in prepubertal children, there may be a pattern of severe, prolonged tantrums, marked mood lability, irritability, aggression, and poor frustration tolerance, in addition to hyperactivity, distractibility, and decreased attention span. Moreover, hypersexuality and grandiosity (if not outright delusions), hallucinations, sleep disturbance (in the absence of stimulant medication), or expressions of suicidal or homicidal ideas are particular clues that one is dealing with more than attention-deficit/hyperactivity disorder (ADHD). The prepubertal

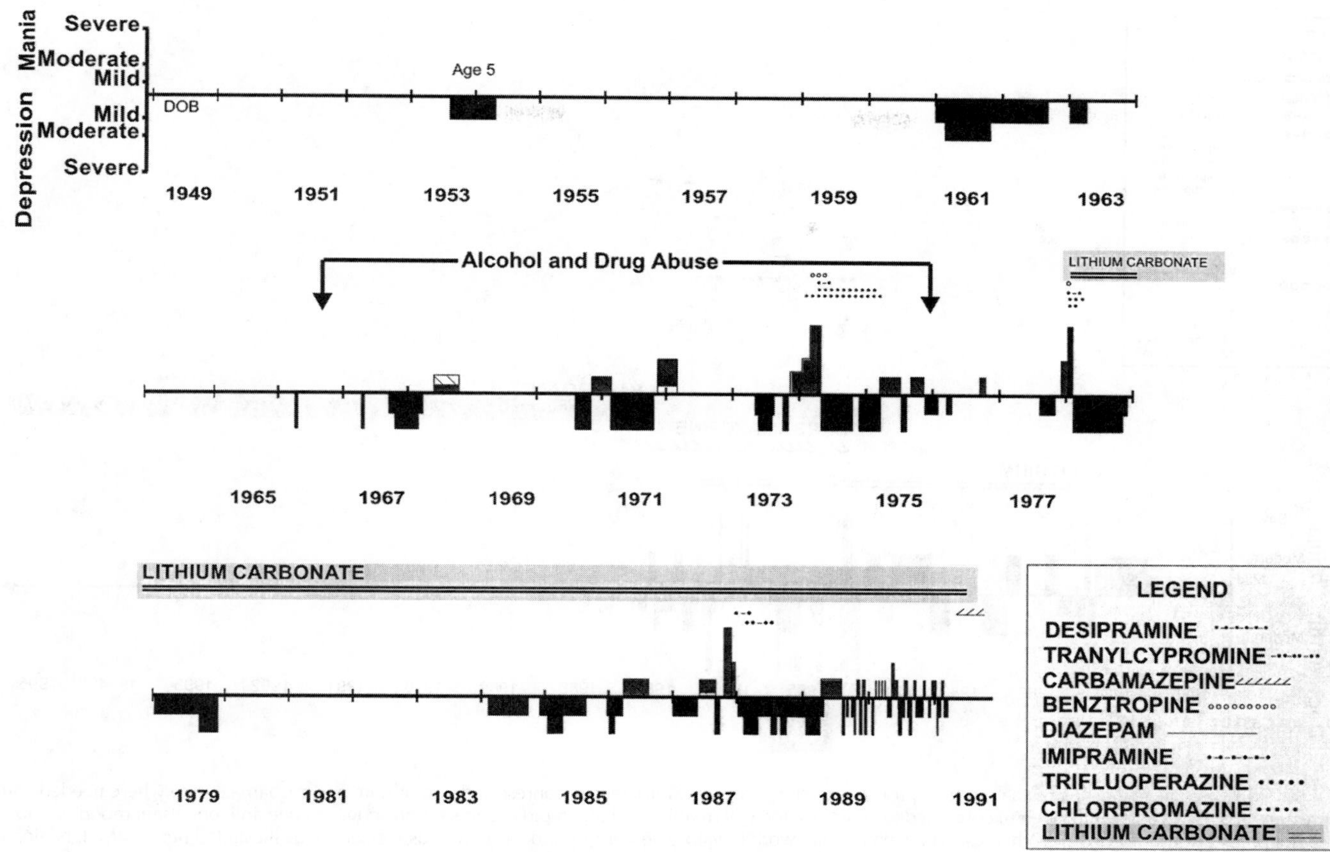

FIGURE 13.8–5 Life chart showing Kraepelinian illness progression (increasing severity and shorter well intervals), initial lithium response (1979 to 1984), and then the development of tolerance to the efficacy of lithium prophylaxis. This loss of responsiveness occurred despite adequate lithium intake and in the absence of renewed substance abuse. DOB, date of birth.

onset of a psychotic depression may herald the beginning of bipolar illness, because approximately 35 percent of such children switch into mania on treatment with antidepressants. Similarly, bipolar illness may present atypically in adolescence, with extremes of mood lability or with more psychotic and schizophreniform features. In prepubertal children and in adolescents with bipolar illness, stimulants and antidepressants may exacerbate the illness; instead, mood stabilizers, often given in combination, are required.

Graphing the Longitudinal Course

The authors suggest developing a graphic representation of the patient's prior (retrospective) course of illness (Figs. 13.8–4 and 13.8–5) and urging the patient to continue this on a daily prospective basis (Figs. 13.8–1 and 13.8–4). This graph forms a basis for evaluating the efficacy of previous treatments and the assessment of current and future prescription. Such a graph of the patient's longitudinal course of illness is useful for several reasons: (1) It provides a clear picture of the earlier illness course, which appears to be the best predictor of the future episode pattern; (2) it clarifies prior medication responsiveness, including loss of efficacy via tolerance; (3) it helps medicalize the patient's history and management process, as well as facilitate the recognition of low-level manic symptoms; and (4) it encourages the patient's collaboration and thus may enhance the doctor–patient relationship, bringing the patient into the process as an active partner rather than as a passive participant. Each of these factors may help compliance or treatment adherence.

The authors suggest that a rough graphic depiction of illness patterns be done as part of the initial intake session and be the primary mode of recording a patient's history, even preferable to an extensive written account. In this way, the patient and the physician are immediately and systematically focused on the longitudinal course of the illness and its variation over time, rather than being sidetracked by focus only on acute symptoms and their improvement. The graphic approach and its associated temporal landmarks can also facilitate recall of important events, dates, and even entire prior episodes that would otherwise be obscured or forgotten, as well as psychosocial precipitants. In this fashion, the mood chart may facilitate the formulation and institution of appropriate psychotherapeutic interventions as well.

Levels of Severity

Physicians can devise their own ways of plotting the course of illness or adopt the system of graphing three levels (mild, moderate, and severe) of episode severity based on the degree of manic or depressive symptom-driven functional incapacity (rated monthly) on the retrospective National Institute of Mental Health (NIMH) life chart method (NIMH-LCM) (Figs. 13.8–4 and 13.8–5).

In this system, mild severity level is one in which the patient or family member notes a distinct change in mood, but there is little or no impairment in social, educational, or employment roles. This state is readily recognized by depressed patients and may represent a low-level dysthymic baseline from which more severe episodes erupt (i.e., double depression). However, hypomanic patients resist categorization

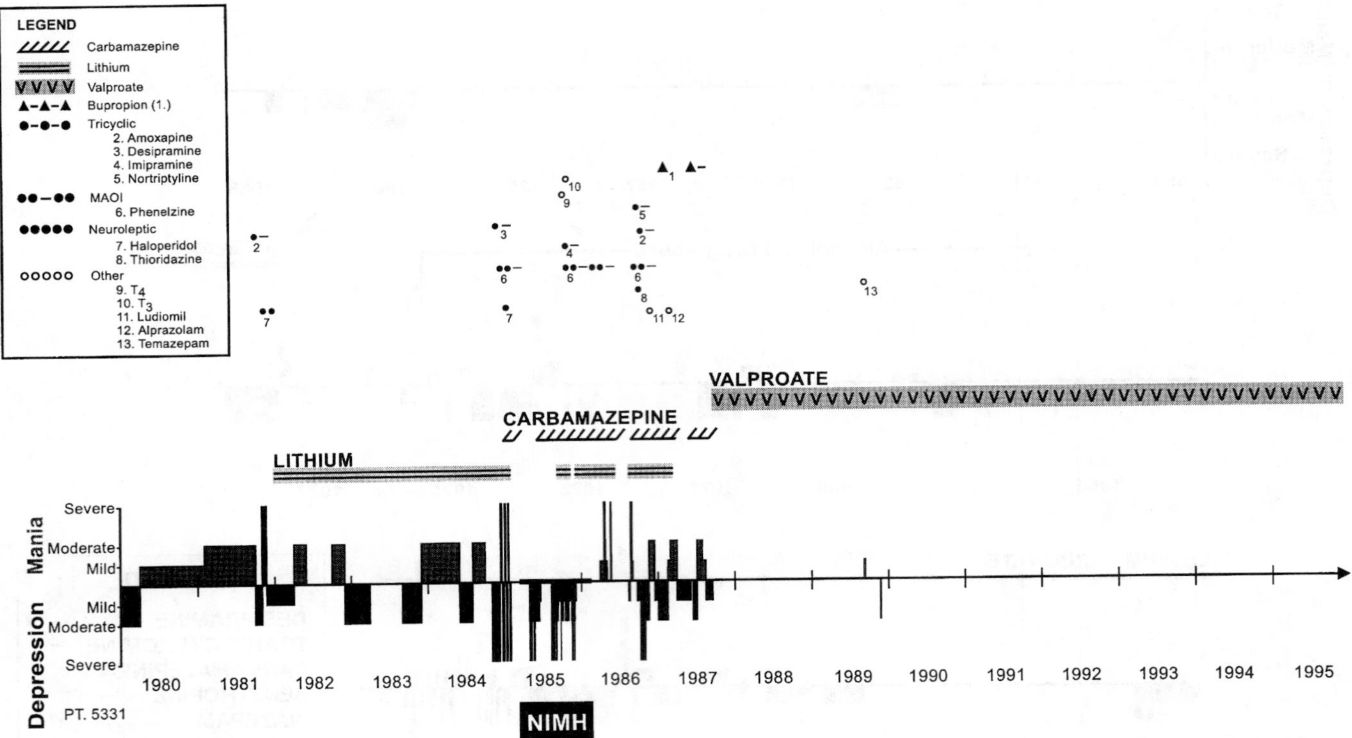

FIGURE 13.8–6 Life chart showing a complete prophylactic response to valproate in a nonresponder to lithium and carbamazepine where needed antidepressant treatments (Nos. 3 through 6) continued to be associated with manias and ultrarapid cycling. Nonresponse to one anticonvulsant mood stabilizer does not predict nonresponse to another. Carbamazepine may work in valproate nonresponders, as well as vice versa, as illustrated here. NIMH, National Institute of Mental Health; MAOI, monoamine oxidase inhibitor; T_3, triiodothyronine; T_4, thyroxine.

of their mood as abnormal, so that additional input from friends and family members is often important. This observation also reemphasizes the usefulness of a nonpsychoanalytical approach to the patient's diagnosis and treatment, including the participation and support of family members from the outset. This may be of value in gaining historical information and in managing potential suicidal tendency of depression and denial of the adverse consequences of hypomania. It may be helpful to explore for possible hypomania symptoms in a positive fashion with screening questions about previous periods of (1) increased energy and (2) decreased need for sleep. These periods, often associated with increased productivity and sociability, then become easier to explore as a positive part of the manic continuum.

Moderate levels of depression and mania represent phases associated with distinct functional impairment. Patients are able to continue their social or employment responsibilities, but only with obvious difficulties, such as not being able to perform some routine social, educational, or occupational tasks. In the prospective form of the NIMH-LCM using daily ratings, moderate mood-driven dysfunction has been divided into two separate categories of low-moderate and high-moderate severity representing *some* and *much* difficulty, respectively, in one's usual roles. For the manic patient, these levels of severity may be more easily revealed if one asks the patient whether coworkers, friends, or family members are commenting or complaining about the patient's behavior or directing them to seek help.

Severe impairment is when patients are essentially functionally incapacitated and unable to perform in their usual roles. Hospitalizations can be coded by shading in the severe manic or depressive episode on the graph. When the precise timing of an episode is unknown, it can be graphed with broken or dotted lines.

For prepubertal onsets, a kiddie-LCM is available that allows for the graphic depiction of symptom-driven dysfunction free from the diagnostic controversies of whether these often highly disturbed and dysfunctional young children meet the artificial duration criteria intended for classical adult presentations (see http://www.bipolarnews.org). Such documentation of what is now widely recognized as a more chronic continuous course of extreme mood lability of bipolar disorder NOS may be crucial to a child's receiving adequate pharmacological interventions. Professional and societal attitudes and stigma would also appear highly relevant here, as there is less concern about medications for children with epilepsy, rheumatoid arthritis, infections, malignancies, asthma, and many other medical illnesses with typical or atypical early onsets than for bipolar illness. Not only is childhood and adolescent onset bipolar illness prognostically more disabling than the adult variety in long-term outcome studies, but the illness also puts the child at increased risk for alcohol and other substance abuse and for other potentially deleterious high-risk behaviors. Moreover, adolescent suicide is one of the fastest growing categories of early mortality.

Graphing Psychopharmacological Interventions and Psychosocial Events Superimposed on this template of the severity of graphed mood fluctuations should be the history of prior psychopharmacological interventions plotted directly above the episodes, as illustrated in Figure 13.8–1 of the life chart schema and in the case example in Figures 13.8–5, 13.8–6, and 13.8–7. When graphed in this fashion, the partial efficacy of earlier treatments is often more precisely revealed. If it is found, one may want

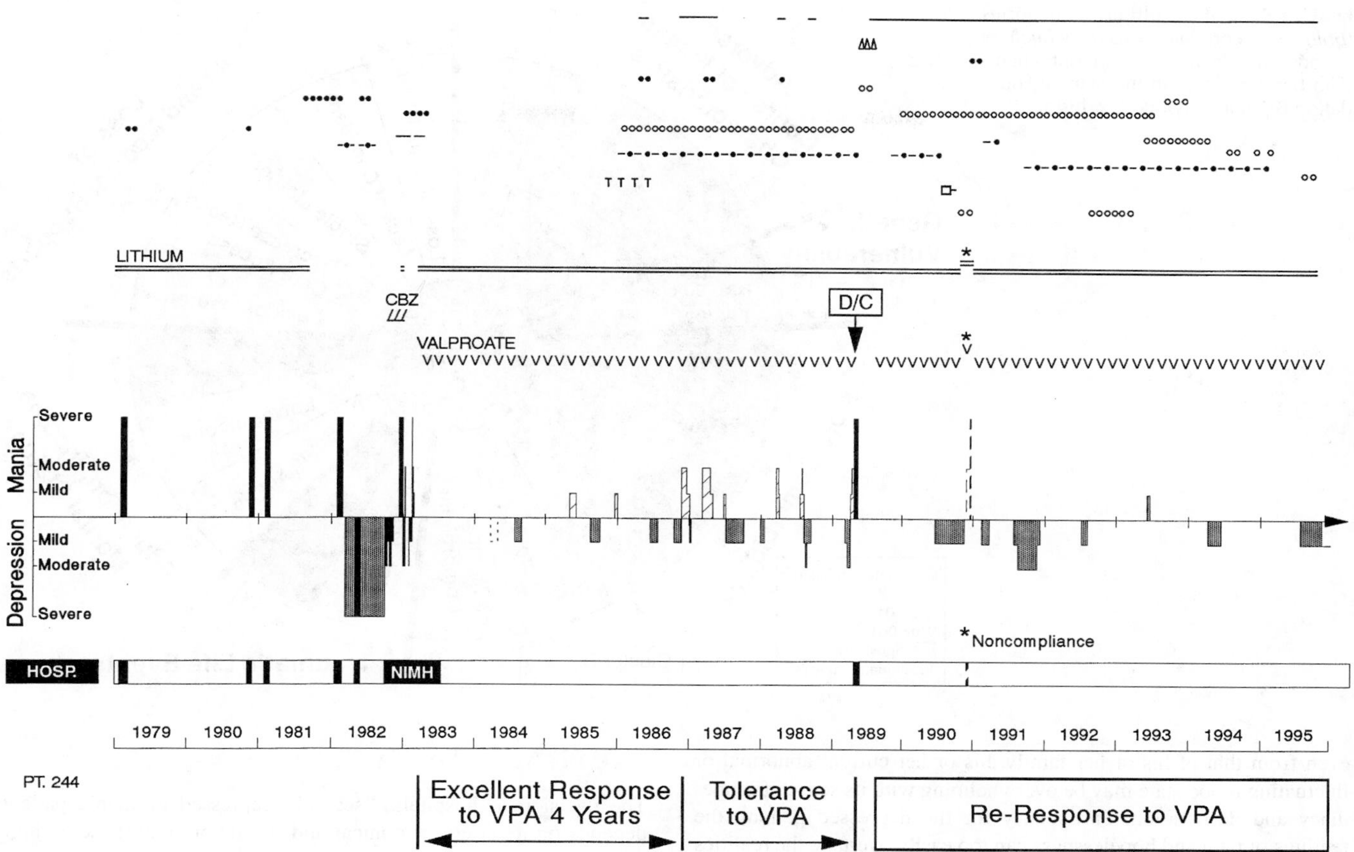

FIGURE 13.8–7 Apparent tolerance and reresponse to the prophylactic effects of valproate (VPA) combination treatment in a lithium monotherapy nonresponder (in 1979 to 1981 and in 1989 when VPA was discontinued). Note the increasing severity of both manic and depressive breakthrough episodes in 1984 to 1989 despite good lithium and VPA compliance and use of adjuncts (i.e., a pattern highly suggestive of loss of effectiveness via a process of pharmacodynamic tolerance). CBZ, carbamazepine; D/C, discontinuation; HOSP, hospitalizations (*shaded*); NIMH, National Institute of Mental Health.

to consider supplementing a partially effective and well-tolerated treatment rather than abandoning it altogether. Important psychosocial events (significant anniversaries, suicide attempts, etc.) and other notes about side effects (dosage, reasons for discontinuation of medications, etc.) can be noted below the mood graph.

Descriptive Symptoms The anamnestic account of specific symptoms and their associated degree of dysfunction in the initial consultation also provides the basis for following clinical improvement during an acute episode and during future possible episodes and provides the basis for an EWS. Should these or other residual symptoms break through during prophylaxis, they can be used as indicators of illness "roughening" and the need for more aggressive clinical management.

Clinicians should consider making a contract with their patients in advance about the appearance of specific symptoms or severities (for example, the number of hours of decreased sleep) that would trigger dosage changes or a call between visits.

Prospective Charting For the bipolar patient with several episodes or an unresolved or complicated course, the authors strongly suggest that this life chart process be continued by the patient prospectively on a daily basis. Mood, sleep, comorbid symptoms, and drug side effects can all be noted in a systematic manner that is unobtrusive and only takes seconds to complete. Pocket daily personal calendars for mood charting are also available from the Depression and Bipolar Support Alliance (DBSA). Mood rating, like self-assessment of urine glucose in the diabetic patient, may provide an important measure of how well the patient's illness is responding to a given treatment modality, and its dose, side effect, and efficacy ratios, and the need for drug titration. Ongoing prospective mood and medication charts may also help in future transfers of medical care, orientation of hospital staff, or consultation requests, should these be necessary.

TIME FRAME OF EDUCATION

Although a hopeful perspective about the treatability of a patient's episode should be maintained, a series of drugs or combinations may be needed before the best treatment regimen can be found. The evaluation of an acute antidepressant treatment response often requires 3 to 6 weeks, and a given agent's lack of efficacy should be treated as additional information about the patient's illness rather than as an indication that the illness is not responsive. Lack of some improvement in depression after 4 weeks or in mania after 1 week is a poor prognostic sign for eventual response, and augmentation approaches can be triggered at these early time frames.

Different time frame perspectives are available to the therapist and the patient. The physician is aware of the many treatment alternatives and the extended treatment course that often is required to achieve optimal efficacy. From the patient's perspective, and perhaps

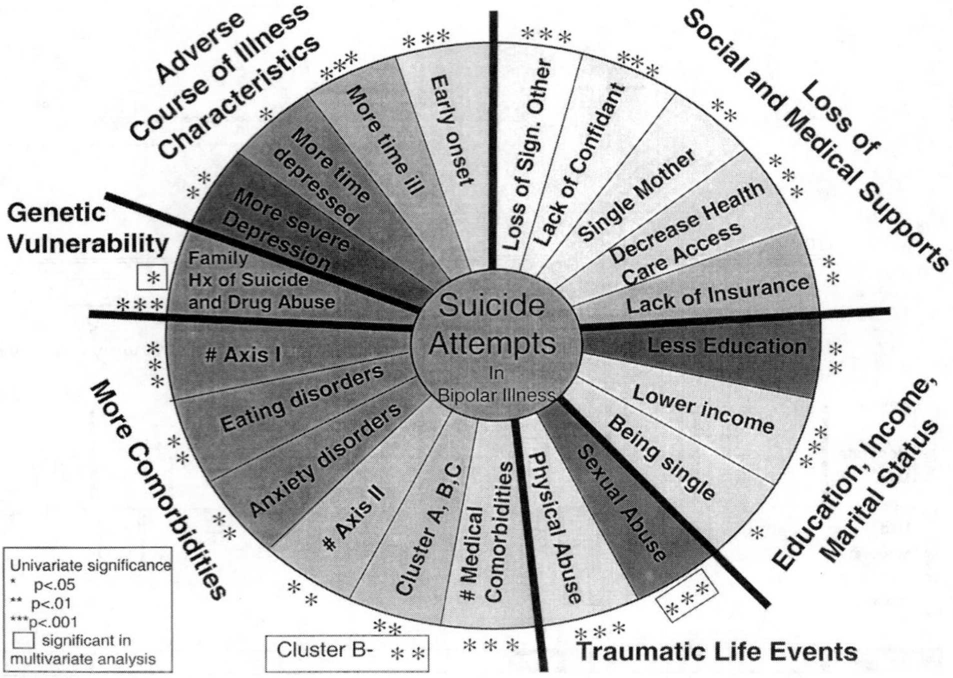

FIGURE 13.8–8 Multiple categories (*bold*) and correlates (*inside wheel*) of serious suicide attempts in outpatients with bipolar illness in the Stanley Foundation Bipolar Network. Hx, history.

even from that of his or her family, his or her current abnormal or fluctuating mood state may be overwhelming with its sense of immediacy and desperation. Particularly for the depressed patient, the feelings of pain and hopelessness can too easily overtake the realities of the situation and can increase the risk of suicide before a positive treatment outcome is achieved.

Reassurance without overpromising immediate therapeutic effect would thus appear to be an important part of the treatment process. A similar process may be required for the hypomanic patient, who also may see only the positive light of an acute response and not the longer-term perspective. The physician or therapist should encourage and help supply the ego for the longer-term view in both of these cases.

To this end, ongoing educational, supportive, interpersonal, and cognitive-behavioral approaches to the psychopharmacotherapy of bipolar disorder are essential. These adjunctive psychotherapeutic approaches have now been demonstrated as efficacious in multiple randomized, controlled trials and should be considered as a fundamental phase of treatment. Patients should also be counseled not to make crucial long-term decisions on the basis of a distorted view of themselves and their future during an acute depressive or manic episode.

Frequent visits with the patient may also help in assessing the progress of pharmacotherapy and the suicide risk (Fig. 13.8–8). In a depressed patient with severe pain and suffering, frequent meetings may facilitate the most rapid and maximal application of pharmacological leverage; regimens can be revised as appropriate at the shortest time frames (days to a week in mania, and several weeks in depression) if improvement is not forthcoming. Brief phone calls between face-to-face meetings at the initiation of a medical treatment to assess side effects, to provide continuity of support, to enhance compliance, and to decrease hopelessness in the patient are particularly helpful. Combined psychotherapeutic treatment may also be helpful in instances of partial response to pharmacotherapy, a protracted episode, poor interepisode recovery of function, an associated personality disorder, or the presence of past or acute psychosocial stressors.

HOSPITALIZATION

The decision to hospitalize severely depressed or manic patients depends on a variety of clinical and (disappointingly) increasingly economic issues. Hospitalization is often indicated for the acutely suicidal patient but may also be considered for the patient with associated medical problems or a complicated course requiring close monitoring or novel psychopharmacological regimens. For the knowledgeable patient and supportive family, one or more of a series of psychopharmacological approaches can often be accomplished on an outpatient basis, particularly if there is good coordination between the patient and physician regarding dosage, titration, side effects, and indicators of improvement. Despite many of the largely societal criticisms of the modern use of ECT, this modality should be considered for patients with extreme suicidal tendency, associated medical illnesses, or other medical emergency situations (such as malignant catatonia or hyperthermia) that demand the most rapid treatment response available.

For the recurrent manic patient who has or might be likely to refuse voluntary hospitalization at the height of an episode, obtaining an advance directive, that is, informed consent during a well interval for a future hospitalization and pharmacological treatment, may help avoid many of the cumbersome practical, medical, and legal difficulties surrounding involuntary hospitalization.

COMORBIDITY

Recent data from the former Stanley Foundation Bipolar Network (SFBN) have reaffirmed many other studies in the field indicating that outpatients with bipolar illness have a high incidence of comorbid psychiatric and medical problems. Forty percent of patients have an alcohol or substance abuse problem. There is a two- to threefold increased risk for alcohol abuse in men with bipolar illness compared with men in the general population, but, remarkably, a six- to eightfold increased risk in women with this disorder compared with women in the general population. The risk for women is associated with an

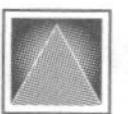

Table 13.8–4
Emerging Spectrum of Psychotropic Efficacy of Lithium and the Anticonvulsants

	AM		AD		
	Acute	Prophylaxis	Acute	Prophylaxis	Other Targets and Effects
AM > AD					
Lithium	+++	+++	++	++	Family history positive +++, suicidality +++
Divalproex (Depakote)	+++	(+++)	+	++	Migraine +++, panic disorder +
Carbamazepine (Tegretol)	+++	++	++	++	Paroxysmal pain syndromes +++, alcohol withdrawal ++, PTSD +
Oxcarbazepine (Trileptal)	++	±	±	±	Paroxysmal pain syndromes +++
Zonisamide (Zonegran)	+	±	±	±	Weight loss +++
AD > AM					
Lamotrigine (Lamictal)	±	++	+++	+++	Pain +, PTSD +
Not AM					
Topiramate (Topamax)	0	±	+	—	Weight loss +++, alcohol abstinence +++, pain +, migraine +, PTSD +
Gabapentin (Neurontin)	0, –	0, –	(+)	(+)	Pain +++, anxiety and social phobia +++, restless legs syndrome +, obsessive-compulsive disorder +, alcohol withdrawal +
Tiagabine (Gabitril)	0	0	±	±	Anxiety ±
Levetiracetam (Keppra)	±	±	±	±	—

0, none; –, none or worse; ±, equivocal; +, some uncontrolled evidence; ++, some controlled evidence; +++, clear evidence or wide use, acceptance; ( ), rating with qualifications or ambiguities; AD, antidepressant; AM, antimanic; PTSD, posttraumatic stress disorder.

increased number of prior depressive episodes, suggesting that some women attempt to self-medicate their affective disorder with alcohol.

Another 40 percent of subjects have had an anxiety disorder diagnosis; 42 percent of patients have had two or more lifetime comorbid medical conditions, and 24 percent have had three or more lifetime comorbid medical conditions. Recognition of these conditions and provision of treatments that simultaneously target the primary affective disorder and the comorbid symptoms, achieving a two-for-one beneficial effect with a given agent, should be sought (Table 13.8–4).

Another emerging comorbidity is overweight, obesity, and morbid obesity. One-half of the outpatient women in the SFBN and two-thirds of the men were overweight. Even so, more women than men were morbidly obese. The degree of overweight, as assessed by the body mass index (BMI), was associated with greater exposure to numbers of previous psychotropic medications associated with weight gain. Those who were obese were also more likely to have a variety of other medical comorbidities, including arthritis, hypertension, cardiovascular disease, and diabetes. Thus, awareness of the potential risks of psychotropic drug-induced or drug-facilitated weight gain (Table 13.8–5) is increasingly playing a role in the choice of pharmacotherapies of bipolar illness.

THEORETICAL RATIONALES AND ASSUMPTIONS: NEUROTRANSMITTER THEORIES

Because most of the effective treatments for mood disorders were discovered by serendipity, pharmacological agents have generally

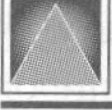

Table 13.8–5
Weight Gain Liability of Psychiatric Drugs Used in the Treatment of Bipolar Illness

Atypical Antipsychotics	Lithium and Anticonvulsants	Antidepressants
Clozapine (Clozaril) +++	Divalproex (Depakote) ++	Mirtazepine (Remeron) +++
Olanzapine (Zyprexa) +++	Lithium (Eskalith) ++	Tertiary amine TCAs
Risperidone (Risperdal) ++	Gabapentin (Neurontin) +	Amitriptyline (Elavil) ++
Quetiapine (Seroquel) + or ++	Carbamazepine (Tegretol) +	Imipramine ++
Ziprasidone (Geodon) 0	Oxcarbazepine (Trileptal) 0	Secondary amine TCAs
Aripiprazole (Abilify) 0	Lamotrigine (Lamictal) 0	Nortriptyline (Aventyl) +
	Levetiracetam (Keppra) 0	Desipramine (Norpramin) +
	Zonisamide (Zonegran) – –	Selective serotonin reuptake inhibitor 0 (acute treatment)→ +(chronic treatment)
	Topiramate (Topamax) – –	Venlafaxine (Effexor) 0 (acute treatment)→ +(chronic treatment)
		Bupropion (Wellbutrin) –

0, neutral; +, minor weight gain liability; ++, moderate weight gain liability; +++, high weight gain liability; –, minor weight loss; – –, moderate weight loss; TCA, tricyclic antidepressant.

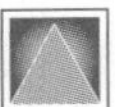

Table 13.8–6
Mechanisms of Action of Anticonvulsants

Anticonvulsant	GABA Levels	$GABA_A$ Receptor (Indirect)	↓ Na^+	↓ Ca^{2+} T	N	P	L	✓	*N*-methyl-D-aspartate Ca_1^{2+}	Other Mechanisms
Valproic acid (Depakene)	↑	—	+	T	—	—	—	✓	(↓)	↑ GABA synthesis and ↑ catabolism; ↑ K efflux; ↑ $GABA_B$ receptor, hippocampus; ↑ Bcl-2; ↑ histone deacetylase
Carbamazepine (Tegretol)	—	—	++	—	—	—	—	✓?	(↓)	↑ Arginine vasopressin effect; ↑ substance P; ↓ SRIF; ↓ dopamine turnover; ↓ α4 subunit muscarinic acetylcholine receptor; ↑ K efflux; ↑ $GABA_B$ receptor, hippocampus; ↓ adenosine A_1-receptor
Oxcarbazepine (Trileptal)	—	—	++	—	N	P	—	✓	—	↑ K efflux
Lamotrigine (Lamictal)	—	(↓)	++	—	N	P	—	✓	(↓)	—
Zonisamide (Zonegran)		↑	++	T	—	—	L	✓	—	↓↓CA; ↑, ↓ dopamine and serotonin, free radical scavenger
Phenytoin (Dilantin)	—	—	++	(T)	—	—	—	—	—	↓ SRIF
Topiramate (Topamax)	↑	↑	+	—	—	—	—	—	—	↓↓ CA; ↓ α-amino-3-hydroxy-5-methyl-4-isoxazolepropionic acid receptor
Gabapentin (Neurontin)[a]	↑	↑	—	—	—	—	L[a]	✓	—	↓ Strychnine insensitive glycine receptors, ↓ L-amino acid transporter
Tiagabine (Gabitril)	↑	—	—	—	—	—	—	—	—	GABA reuptake inhibitor
Levetiracetam (Keppra)	—	↑	—	—	N	—	—	✓	—	↓ Zn^{++} and beta carboline negative modulation of $GABA_A$ receptor; ↓ delayed K^+ rectifier, own central nervous system binding site

CA, carbonic anhydrase; GABA, γ-aminobutyric acid; $GABA_A$, γ-aminobutyric acid type A; $GABA_B$, γ-aminobutyric acid type B; L, N, and P, L-, N-, and P-type calcium channels; SRIF, somatotrophin release-inhibiting factor.
[a]Acts at α_2 δ subunit of L-type calcium channel.

propelled theoretical formulations, rather than vice versa. Neurotransmitter theories of the basis of depression have included serotonin (5-HT), norepinephrine (NE), acetylcholine (ACh), dopamine (DA), γ-aminobutyric acid (GABA), and, most recently, glutamate (Glu) theories, each based on presumed mechanisms of effective pharmacotherapeutic interventions. For example, the findings that drugs (which acutely potentiated catecholamines and indoleamines) were antidepressants and that reserpine (Serpalan) (which depleted these neurotransmitters) could exacerbate depression and treat mania led to the amine hypotheses of deficiencies in depression and excesses in mania.

Now that it appears that relatively selective manipulations of each of several different neurotransmitter systems (5-HT, NE, and DA) can be associated with antidepressant effects (Table 13.8–2), a critical psychopharmacological question is raised as to whether an individual may respond better to one type of treatment targeting a given neurotransmitter system but not to another. In the absence of definitive studies of this question, one is tempted to recommend the sequential use of drugs that act differently within the antidepressant class (e.g., changing from a 5-HT–selective to a 5-HT–NE reuptake blocker or to bupropion) or among classes (e.g., from reuptake blocker to an MAOI or to lithium, an anticonvulsant, or an atypical antipsychotic).

A similar strategy of using agents with different mechanisms of action sequentially or concurrently in mania may also be warranted (Tables 13.8–2 and 13.8–6). Although the precise mechanism of action resulting in decreased manic symptoms remains unknown, lithium, valproate, and carbamazepine each differentially alter dopaminergic, noradrenergic, and serotonergic function, commonly block inositol transport, and upregulate GABA type B receptors ($GABA_B$) in the hippocampus. They also target G protein systems, decrease protein kinase C (PKC) activity, and inhibit calcium influx through the Glu *N*-methyl-D-aspartate (NMDA) receptor. Lithium and valproate increase myristoylated alanine-rich C kinase substrate (MARCKS) and activator protein-1 (AP-1) binding, as well as messenger ribonucleic acid (mRNA) levels for Bcl-2 and BDNF, the latter two of which may be involved in the prevention of preprogrammed cell death (apoptosis).

A number of the new anticonvulsants increase brain GABA, including valproate, gabapentin (Neurontin), topiramate (Topamax), and tiagabine (Gabitril). However, because gabapentin, topiramate, and tiagabine do not have clear antimanic effects, one may surmise that the antimanic mechanisms of valproate lie elsewhere. Valproate, carbamazepine, lamotrigine, phenytoin (Dilantin), and topiramate decrease excitatory amino acid release as a consequence of their effects in blocking sodium channels. In addition, topiramate is a blocker of the Glu receptors of the α-amino-3-hydroxy-5-methyl-4-isoxazolepropionic acid (AMPA) kainate subtype, which are important for the maintenance of long-term potentiation, one of the best models for learning and memory. Interestingly, lithium, carbamazepine, valproate, and lamotrigine are all partial inhibitors of calcium influx through the NMDA receptor, raising this as a possible mechanism for their putative mood stabilizing effects.

TREATMENT OF ACUTE MANIA

Lithium Carbonate Lithium has been the paradigmatic treatment for acute mania and its prophylaxis. Because the onset of antimanic action with lithium can be slow, for the acutely deteriorating, aggressive, or psychotic manic patient, it usually is supplemented in the early phases of treatment. Until recently, this was accomplished with the typical antipsychotics, including the phenothiazines, thio-

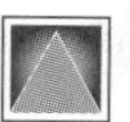

Table 13.8–7
Correlates of Relative Lithium Responsiveness

Factors	Good Response Rates (Approximately 60–80%)	Low Response Rates (Approximately 20–40%)	Strength of Evidence
Episode characteristics			
Rapid or faster cycling	No	Yes	+++ (12)
Episode contiguity	Intermittent, that is, with a well interval	Continuous, that is, no well interval	+
Sequence pattern	Mania→depression→well interval	Depression→mania→well interval	+++ (4)
Number of episodes before starting prophylaxis	Three or fewer	Four to ten or more	+++ (9)
Quality of mania	Euphoric	Dysphoric	+++ (4)
Comorbidities			
History of substance abuse	Negative	Positive	+
History of anxiety disorder	Negative	Positive	++
Genetic background			
Family history of anxiety disorder	Negative	Positive	++
Family history of bipolar illness and especially lithium (Eskalith) response	Positive	Negative	+++

+++, well-documented (number of supportive studies in literature); ++, reported in several studies; +, reported by several clinician observers.

thixenes, or butyrophenones such as haloperidol (Haldol). Because of the rapidly growing evidence for the parallel acute antimanic efficacy of all of the atypical antipsychotics, as well as the mood-stabilizing anticonvulsants carbamazepine and divalproex (Depakote), it is suggested that these alternative agents be the supplements along with high-potency benzodiazepines because of their better tolerability and lesser risk of tardive dyskinesia compared to the typical antipsychotics.

The typical clinical profile of the manic patient most responsive to lithium carbonate is one with a classic presentation of euphoric mania, rather than dysphoric mania; a pattern of mania (M) followed by a depression (D) and then a well interval (I) (M-D-I) rather than a D-M-I pattern or continuous cycling; a history of fewer prior episodes and a non–rapid-cycling course (i.e., fewer than four episodes a year); no comorbid anxiety or substance abuse disorder or schizoaffective illness; and a positive family history of primary affective illness in first-degree relatives, especially if there is a family history of a good response to lithium. These characteristics can make the difference between an approximately 70 percent response rate versus a 30 percent response rate (Table 13.8–7).

Lithium doses should be administered to achieve blood levels between 0.6 and 1.2 mEq/L. Although a high-dose strategy has been advocated by some investigators (levels to 1.5 mEq/L or greater), the authors have not seen many patients who, having failed to respond at more typical lithium blood levels, respond well when pushed to higher levels and greater toxicity. Dose-limiting side effects may include gastrointestinal (GI) disturbances and weight gain, as well as neuropsychiatric syndromes, including tremor, myoclonic twitches, and confusion (Table 13.8–8). Blood levels of lithium achieved at a given dose may also increase when the patient switches from mania to depression, leading to greater side effects. In those who tolerate lithium but are incompletely responsive to it, the authors generally recommend potentiation with other agents, rather than requiring a new agent to treat any additional symptoms related to lithium discontinuation. In this fashion, lithium's antisuicide and potential neurotropic and neuroprotective effects are also maintained.

The largest placebo-controlled study of lithium indicated that only 50 percent of patients achieved a 50 percent or greater degree of improvement by 3 weeks. However, even in the responsive group, many symptoms remained at the end of 3 weeks despite adequate and carefully monitored blood levels. Those with a prior anecdotal history of lithium nonresponse by self-report were particularly at risk for nonresponse in this controlled study. Thus, even without the increased pressures from managed care for rapid discharge from the hospital, most full-blown manic patients require adjunctive treatment to achieve a timely and more complete antimanic response. A broad range of such options is now available (Table 13.8–4).

Valproate (i.e., Valproic Acid [Depakene] or Divalproex Sodium [Depakote]) Typical dose levels of valproic acid are 750 to 2,500 mg per day, achieving blood levels between 50 and 120 μg per mL. Rapid oral loading with 15 to 20 mg/kg of divalproex sodium from day one of treatment has been well tolerated (Table 13.8–9) and associated with a rapid onset of response. Blood levels greater than 45 μg/mL have also been associated with earlier response. In several case series, patients with more typical manic syndromes and fewer schizoaffective symptoms appeared to show a high frequency of response. In contrast to lithium, those with a history of lithium nonresponse, dysphoric mania, or rapid cycling remain responsive to valproate (Table 13.8–7).

Carbamazepine (and Oxcarbazepine) Several preliminary studies have suggested that some of the variables associated with a poor response to or intolerance of lithium may be associated with a good, if not preferential, antimanic response to carbamazepine. Thus, the drug may be considered for lithium-nonresponsive manic patients. Individual patients may respond to carbamazepine and not valproate or vice versa.

Typical doses of carbamazepine to treat mania have ranged between 600 and 1,800 mg per day associated with blood levels of between 4 and 12 μg/mL. However, within this dose and blood-level range, there does not appear to be a clear relation to the degree of clinical response across patients. For an individual patient, however, clinical response and side effects are likely dose related. It is important to individualize doses of this anticonvulsant, as there is wide variability in the dose and blood level at which side effects occur. Furthermore, carbamazepine is metabolized by hepatic cytochrome P450 3A4 enzymes and induces its own metabolism within 2 to 3 weeks of treatment. Thus, doses may need to be increased to maintain initial treatment response. Increasing the dose to achieve a clinical effect and titrating the increases against the emergence of side

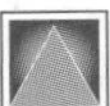

Table 13.8–8
Common Lithium Side Effects and Their Management

Side Effect	Possible Approaches (Most Not Based on Strong Evidence)
Tremor (C); usually worse under social scrutiny	Lower dose ++; use β-blocker, such as propanolol (Inderal) 10 mg four times daily ++
	Consider primidone (Mysoline) as alternative +
	Replace some of lithium (Eskalith) dose with dihydropyridine calcium channel blocker +
Gastrointestinal distress (O)	Lower dose +
	Switch lithium preparations ±
	Replace some of lithium dose with a calcium channel blocker ±
Weight gain (O)	Warn and treat in advance ±
	Avoid nondiet sodas +
	Consider weight loss adjuncts ++
Cognitive impairment (UC)	Treat residual depression +
	Check thyroid
	Even if euthyroid, consider treating with T_3 +++
Increased urination (C) (diabetes insipidus, i.e., blockage of vasopressin receptor response at level of decreased production of cyclic adenosine monophosphate)	If extreme or functionally impairing, treat with thiazide diuretics or amiloride (Midamor)
	Switch to other mood-stabilizing agents
	Carbamazepine (Tegretol) does not cause diabetes insipidus but does not correct lithium-related diabetes insipidus
Kidney function impairment (UC)	Reduce dose ±
	Monitor closely
	Discontinue drug if rise in creatinine is consistent ±
	Replace with other mood stabilizers +
Psoriasis (O, I)	Omega-3 fatty acid supplementation may help suppress lithium effect +
Acne (O)	Retinoic acid only for women not of childbearing age or men ++
	Tetracycline (Achromycin V), clindamycin (Cleocin) +
Hypothyroidism (O)	Replace with T_4 ++
	Use T_4 and T_3 combination if mood remains low +

+, likely works; ++, many case reports; +++, well-supported, controlled data; ±, questionable or hypothetical; C, common; I, idiosyncratic; O, occasional; T_3, triiodothyronine; T_4, thyroxine; UC, uncommon.

effects (Table 13.8–10) rather than frequent blood level monitoring are appropriate strategies for such wide individual variability in tolerability. Given carbamazepine's short half-life and requirement for twice-a-day to four-times-a-day dosing, and the availability of long-acting preparations, these latter are recommended and make single dosing at bedtime feasible and recommended. Two large, positive, placebo-controlled trials of Carbatrol in acute mania have resulted in the first U.S. Food and Drug Administration (FDA) approval for a carbamazepine preparation.

Carbamazepine and valproic acid have been used in combination to treat epilepsy, but only preliminary evidence for the efficacy of this combination in acute and prophylactic management of the refractory bipolar patient is available. When used in combination, valproate increases levels of carbamazepine and its active 10,11-epoxide metabolite, such that lower doses of carbamazepine are needed.

Although only preliminarily assessed in comparative studies, initial evidence suggests that the keto congener of carbamazepine, oxcarbazepine, may possess similar antimanic properties. Higher doses than those of carbamazepine are required, because 1,500 mg of oxcarbazepine approximates 1,000 mg of carbamazepine. In contrast to carbamazepine and its active 10,11-epoxide metabolite, neither oxcarbazepine nor its active monohydroxy metabolite is a potent inducer of hepatic enzymes, and it does not autoinduce. The only side effect that is more prominent with oxcarbazepine than carbamazepine is hyponatremia. Less frequent side effects are rash, white blood cell count suppression, and drug–drug interactions.

Clonazepam and Lorazepam

The high-potency benzodiazepine anticonvulsants studied in acute mania include clonazepam (Klonopin) and lorazepam (Ativan). Both may be effective and are widely used for adjunctive treatment of acute manic agitation, insomnia, aggression, and dysphoria, as well as panic. As noted previously, the safety and the benign side effect profile of these agents render them ideal adjuncts to lithium, carbamazepine, or valproate. The sedating side effects of clonazepam may be problematic in some outpatients, but this property can be used to advantage if given as a bedtime medication for insomniac manic and depressive patients.

Both of these two high-potency minor tranquilizers work rather selectively at the central-type benzodiazepine receptor; in contrast, carbamazepine is not active at this receptor and appears to act at the so-called peripheral-type (mitochondrial) benzodiazepine receptor. Classic central-type benzodiazepine receptors positively modulate GABA receptors that facilitate chloride influx and neuronal inhibition (Table 13.8–6). In contrast, the peripheral-type benzodiazepine receptor appears to be more closely associated with mitochondrial neurosteroid biosynthesis and calcium channels. These findings are noteworthy in regard to possible differential psychotropic responsiveness between these two classes of anticonvulsants.

Atypical and Typical Antipsychotics

Studies indicate that short-term use of typical antipsychotics in the treatment of mania results in the unintended and often unneeded persistence of neuroleptic use 6 months or more after the acute episode. Such intermittent to chronic maintenance treatment with traditional antipsychotics should be avoided, if possible, because bipolar patients are reported to be at high risk for extrapyramidal symptoms (EPSs) and tardive dyskinesia (20 to 40 percent of those exposed), that is, greater than that in patients with schizophrenia. The intermittency of antipsychotic use in bipolar illness, rather than being a protective factor, may be associated with an increased risk of tardive dyskinesia, according to clinical and preclinical studies.

The old strategy of rapid tranquilization with suprathreshold doses of antipsychotics also should be avoided. Many double-blind evaluations of this strategy in acute schizophrenia and one trial in manic patients have all shown the high-dosage strategy (40 to 60 mg per day of haloperidol) to be no more efficacious than traditional dosage regimens (10 mg per day) and only associated with greater side effects.

All of the atypical antipsychotics now have demonstrated antimanic efficacy in double-blind, placebo-controlled studies, although all are not yet FDA approved for this indication. However, no antipsychotic drug for schizophrenia has yet been found not to also possess antimanic efficacy.

The atypicals (Table 13.8–11) should be watched for their spectrum of efficacy in acute depression and prophylaxis to assess

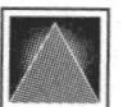

Table 13.8–9
Valproate Side Effects

Side Effect	Treatment	Comment
GI distress (O)	Switch to enteric coated preparation ++	—
	Add histamine 2 blocker +	—
	Give with meals or all at night +	—
Tremor (O)	↓ Dose +	—
	? Propanolol (Inderal) +	—
Weight gain (O)	Prophylactic diet and exercise instructions +	—
	Augment with topiramate (Topamax), sibutramine (Meridia) ++	—
Alopecia (UC)	Prophylaxis with zinc and selenium supplements ±	Straight hair may grow back curly
Polycystic ovary syndrome (UC)	Preventive treatment with oral contraceptives +	(May precede use of VPA)
	Switch to lamotrigine (Lamictal) ++	May be associated with ↑ testosterone
Hepatitic enzyme (O)	Monitor direction of change	Patient should advise physician if right upper-quadrant pain occurs or if fever, malaise fatigue, colored urine, or jaundice occurs
Elevation >3× normal	D/C VPA	
Hepatitis	D/C VPA	—
Pancreatitis (VR)	D/C VPA, monitor amylase	Patient should advise physician if severe GI pain, nausea, or vomiting occurs
Asymptomatic ↑ ammonia	↓ Dose, add l-carnitine ±	
Coarse, flapping tremor	↓ Dose, add l-carnitine ±	—
Encephalopathy	D/C VPA	—
Spina bifida 1–4% in in utero exposed fetus	Avoid pregnancy +	Avoid VPA and other anticonvulsants in combination (such as carbamazepine [Tegretol])
	Use birth control pill, other methods +	
	Use folate prophylactically in women of childbearing age +	

+, likely works; ++, many case reports; ±, questionable or hypothetical; D/C, discontinue; GI, gastrointestinal; O, occasional; UC, uncommon; VPA, valproate; VR, very rare.

whether they gain status as a new class of mood stabilizers. Their relatively positive side-effect profiles include less sedation (ziprasidone and aripiprazole), lack of prolactin increases (clozapine, quetiapine, ziprasidone, and aripiprazole), less anticholinergic side effects (quetiapine, ziprasidone, and aripiprazole), and less weight gain (risperidone and quetiapine) or no weight gain (ziprasidone and aripiprazole). Tables 13.8–11 and 13.8–12 summarize initial data on the atypical antipsychotics' mechanisms of action, side effects, and potential efficacy. These drugs are listed in order of the amount of data available in bipolar illness; the choice or sequencing remains an individual clinical decision.

Clozapine (Clozaril) Clozapine appears to have a particularly good spectrum of efficacy in refractory bipolar illness characterized by dysphoric mania or rapid cycling. Its efficacy in bipolar illness is equal to or greater than that in schizoaffective and schizophrenic illness as well. However, it has the considerable (several percent) liability of the risk of agranulocytosis, requiring weekly blood monitoring, with its associated inconvenience and cost. These liabilities and the increased risk for seizures at high doses, as well as a variety of other disconcerting side effects, such as drooling and weight gain, render it a second- or third-line atypical for refractory patients, even though its antimanic efficacy may be superior, and it has demonstrated antisuicide effects in schizophrenia.

Risperidone (Risperdal) Risperidone has been shown to be useful in acute mania, although, surprisingly, there are several case reports of depressed patients switching into mania when treated with higher doses. Low dosages are still associated with increases in prolactin and moderate weight gain, and higher dosages (≥8 mg per day) are associated with EPSs.

Olanzapine (Zyprexa) Olanzapine has a structure and biochemical profile that are most similar to clozapine, and preliminary evidence suggests that this newly approved agent will assume a similar role in the treatment of refractory bipolar patients. Trials of olanzapine in acute mania are positive, as are those, for the first time, in bipolar depression. In one randomized study, olanzapine was a more effective maintenance agent in preventing manic episodes than lithium. The drug appears generally well tolerated, except for the risk of considerable weight gain in some individuals and possible increased incidence of diabetes mellitus. Although the rate of weight gain slows after the initial months of treatment, it does not appear to plateau even after 6 months to 1 year of treatment.

Quetiapine (Seroquel) Quetiapine, a widely used atypical antipsychotic, has been demonstrated to be an effective monotherapy in acute mania and an adjunct to mood stabilizers compared to placebo in adult and adolescent patients with mania. Open studies suggested that it may have clinically relevant antidepressant effects, potentially of larger magnitude than those of risperidone or clozapine. Dramatic acute antidepressant effects in monotherapy have now been demonstrated in a randomized, controlled trial, making it the atypical with the best evidence of being a true bimodal agent.

Ziprasidone (Geodon) Ziprasidone is unique in relation to its lack of weight gain potential. It is also a blocker of NE and DA reuptake, raising hopes that it may be a particularly useful antidepressant, as well as antipsychotic. Not only is it not very sedating, but also some patients experience increased agitation with initial doses (20 to 40 mg) that, anecdotally, is reported not to occur at higher initial doses (80 to 160 mg). It also lengthens the QT interval, hypothetically making patients more vulnerable to serious arrhythmias, although this has not been reported to date.

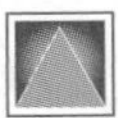

Table 13.8–10
Carbamazepine Side Effects and Their Management

Side Effect	Possible Approach	Comment
Dizziness, ataxia, diplopia (C,D)	Reduce peak dose effects by ↓ dose +++ or switching to sustained release +++ formation	Symptoms usually occur 2 hrs after dose.
Fatigue, sedation (C,I)	Switch more of dose to nighttime ++ ↓ Dose or wait for adaptation and autoinduction, or both ++	—
Benign rash (VC)	Discontinue drug +	Can restart slowly, under the cover of prednisone (Cordrol) +
Severe rash (VR) (S)	Discontinue drug +++	Obtain medical or dermatological consultation
Benign WBC suppression (VC) (D)	Lower dose +, add lithium (Eskalith) +++	Lithium increases CSF +++, whereas CBZ suppresses CSF; 3,000 WBC lower limit ±
Agranulocytosis (VR,I)	Discontinue drug +++	Medical support and consultation required
Aplastic amenia (VR,I)	Discontinue drug +++	—
Weight gain (O)	Switch to weight-neutral drug, such as lamotrigine (Lamictal) or oxcarbazepine (Trileptal) +	Consider topiramate (Topamax) augmentation +
Hyponatremia (O)	↓ Dose +++ Add lithium ++ Add demeclocycline (Demeclomycin) ++	Older women and use of higher doses are vulnerability factors
Thyroid hormone suppression (VC)	None needed, as ↓ thyroxine may correlate with better response	↓ Thyroxine and ↓ triiodothyronine may be additive with lithium
Hypothyroidism (VR)	Thyroid supplements rarely needed	No ↑ thyroid-stimulating hormone; no change in basal metabolic rate with CBZ
Tremor (VR)	↓ Dose +	Check ammonia levels when combined with valproic acid if tremor coarse and flappy
Teratogenic (O) Spina bifida 1–3% Cranial facial abnormality	Avoid use in pregnancy +++ ↑ Folate +	Avoid combination therapy if possible
Hepatitis (VR)	Discontinue if enzymes 3× normal, or if patient is symptomatic	—
Memory disturbance (O)	↓ Dose	Inherent potentiation of vasopressin receptors may help prevent ↓ memory

+, likely works; ++, many case reports; +++, well supported; controlled data; ±, questionable or hypothetical; C, common; CBZ, carbamazepine (Tegretol); CSF, colony-stimulating factor ; D, dose related; I, idiosyncratic; O, occasional; S, sensitivity may cross to other anticonvulsant; VC, very common; VR, very rare; WBC, white blood cell count.

Aripiprazole (Abilify) Aripiprazole is the most atypical of the atypical antipsychotic drugs. Whereas other classic and atypical antipsychotics block DA receptors, which is thought to account for their antipsychotic effects, aripiprazole is a partial agonist at DA type 1 (D_1), DA type 2 (D_2), DA type 3 (D_3), and 5-HT type 1A (5-HT_{1A}) receptors, as well as being a full 5-HT type 2A (5-HT_{2A}) receptor antagonist. The partial agonist activity at DA receptors provides for a relative balance mechanism wherein approximately 20 percent of the action of a full agonist is achieved by aripiprazole. At the same time, in the face of high levels of endogenous DA release, the drug acts as a relative antagonist because of its receptor occupancy. This lack of full DA receptor blockade (i.e., only 80-percent complete) accounts for the drug's good side effect profile and the lack of increases in serum prolactin, and prolactin levels actually decrease on the drug because of its weak agonist properties.

Accordingly, most side effects are not dose related, and a single dose of 15 to 20 mg per day appears sufficient for treatment of schizophrenic and manic psychoses. The drug causes few EPSs, even at high doses, and is weight neutral. However, bipolar patients may be particularly sensitive to akathisia on drug initiation, and lower starting doses are therefore recommended. Very young children should be started and treated at 2.5 to 5.0 mg per day. One trial in acute mania was positive, and, in another trial, it was better tolerated than haloperidol and more effective at week 12. It is hoped that the combination of weak DA agonist effects, the partial agonist effects at the 5-HT_{1A} receptor, and the antagonist effects on the 5-HT type 2 (5-HT_2) receptor will equate to a good antidepressant profile.

Overview The availability of a range of atypical antipsychotics with their equal efficacy but superior side effect profiles may change the algorithm for the treatment of acute mania (Table 13.8–13). The atypicals have a lesser liability for EPS and tardive dyskinesia; many do not increase prolactin. However, they have a wide range of substantial to no risk for weight gain (Table 13.8–5) with its associated problems of insulin resistance, diabetes, hyperlipidemia, hypercholesteremia, and cardiovascular impairment, which may influence the choice of drug for acute and long-term treatment.

L-Type Calcium Channel Blockers (CCBs) A series of preliminary reports and small controlled studies suggest that the phenyl alkylamine L-type calcium channel antagonist verapamil (Calan, Isoptin) has acute antimanic efficacy, although several recent studies suggest the superiority of lithium. One randomized study in acute depression

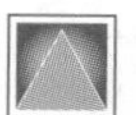

Table 13.8–11
Relative Strength of Receptor Activities Postulated Related to Positive and Negative Effects of Atypical Neuroleptics Relative to Haloperidol

	Receptor							
	D_1	D_2	5-HT Type 1A	5-HT Type 2B	α_1	α_2	Histamine 1	Muscarinergic 1–5
Negative side effects of receptor activity	↓ Motor activity, ↓ enabling effects on D_2 receptor activity	EPS (relative to 5-HT type 2 receptor); ↑ prolactin	—	Weight gain (5-HT type 2C receptor)	Reflex tachycardia, hypotension, dizziness	Block blood pressure effects of clonidine; panic attacks	Sedation, drowsiness, weight gain	↓ Memory (M_1), blurred vision, sinus tachycardia, dry mouth, constipation, glaucoma exacerbation
Positive effects of receptor activity	Block stress effects, ↑ signal to noise ratio	Antipsychotic	Antidepressant, anxiolytic	Antidepressant, ↓ EPS (5-HT type 2A receptor), ↑ slow wave sleep	—	Antipanic? Antidepressant?	—	↓ EPS; cognitive improvement (M_2)
Drug								
Haloperidol (Haldol) (butyrophenone)	+++	++++	0	+	+	NA	0	0
Clozapine (Clozaril) (dibenzodiazepine)	++	++	+	+++	+++	+++	+++	++++
Risperidone (Risperdal) (benzisoxazole)	++	++++	+	+++++	+++	+++	++	0
Olanzapine (Zyprexa) (thienobenzodiazepine)	++	+++	0	++++	+++	NA	+++	++++
Quetiapine (Seroquel) (dibenzothiazepine)	+	++	0	+	++++	+	+++	++
Ziprasidone (Geodon)	++	+++	+++	+++++	++	NA	+	0
Aripiprazole (Abilify)	↑, ↓, +	↑, ↓, ++++	↑, ↓	++++[a]	++	NA	++	0

0, none; +, weak; ++, mild; +++, moderate; ++++, strong; +++++, very strong; ↑, ↓, partial agonist; D_1, dopamine type 1; D_2, dopamine type 2; EPS, extrapyramidal side effects; 5-HT, serotonin; NA, not available.
[a]Full antagonist at 5-HT type 2A receptors.
Adapted from Pickar D: Prospects for pharmacotherapy of schizophrenia. *Lancet.* 1995;345:557–562.

indicated that verapamil was no more effective than placebo and less effective than routine antidepressant treatment. These data led to a search for a more effective CCB that might have a spectrum of antidepressant and prophylactic effects exceeding those of verapamil.

Several groups chose to study the dihydropyridine L-type CCB nimodipine (Nimotop) because of its (1) ability to penetrate the CNS, (2) relative lack of tolerance development in the treatment of migraine (in contrast to many other CCBs), (3) better profile in many types of animal models of seizures and depression compared to verapamil, and (4) its ability to block cocaine-induced hyperactivity and associated DA overflow.

One group reported in a double-blind study that ten of the first 30 treatment-refractory patients evaluated had a clinically relevant response to nimodipine, including patients with rapid- and ultradian-cycling frequencies. Responsivity was confirmed and reconfirmed in some of these patients in a double-blind, off-on-off-on design. This profile of efficacy may be shared by other dihydropyridines, such as isradipine or amlodipine, but this remains to be confirmed.

Lamotrigine (Lamictal)

The acute antimanic effects of lamotrigine have not been demonstrated in controlled studies, perhaps because lamotrigine should be initiated slowly with one 25-mg pill for the first 2 weeks and then 50 mg for 2 weeks, with slow increases thereafter to avoid a moderately high incidence of serious rash. The rate of increase should be cut in half if patients are on a regimen including valproate, which can markedly increase lamotrigine blood levels and the propensity for more serious dermatological complications. Conversely, carbamazepine decreases lamotrigine levels by approximately 50 percent, and one can start with approxi-

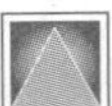

Table 13.8–12
Clinical Profiles of the Atypical Antipsychotics Relative to Haloperidol

Drug	Relative Potency, Chlorpromazine Equivalents	Weight Gain Liability	Sedation	Autonomic	Extrapyramidal Side Effects	Prolactin ↑	(Starting Dose)/Usual Clinical Range (mg/day)	Half-Life
Haloperidol (Haldol)	2	+	+	+	+++	+++	(1)/5–20	3 wks
Clozapine (Clozaril)	100	+++	+++	+++	±	0	(50)/100–600[c]	8 hrs
Risperidone (Risperdal)	1.5	++	++	++	++	++	(1)/4–12[c]	20 hrs
Olanzapine (Zyprexa)	4	+++	++	+	+	+	(2.5–5.0)/10–25	35 hrs
Quetiapine (Seroquel)	100	++	++	++	+	0	(25–100)/300–900 (limbic selective)	6.9 hrs (but single bedtime dose is feasible)
Ziprasidone (Geodon)	50	0	++[a]	++	++	+	(20)/80–200	5 hrs
Aripiprazole (Abilify)	15	0	+[b]	0	+	–	(5–15)/15–30	72 hrs

0, none; ±, equivocal; +, mild; ++, moderate; +++, severe; –, opposite.
[a]May cause activation; give in AM.
[b]Least sedating; can be given in AM.
[c]Modification from Richelson E: Preclinical pharmacology of neuroleptics: Focus on new generation compounds. *J Clin Psychiatry.* 1996;57[Suppl 11]:4–11.
Adapted from Gerlach J, Peacock L: New antipsychotics: The present status. *Int Clin Psychopharmacol.* 1995;10[Suppl 3]:39–48.

mately twice the usual doses of lamotrigine. Although lamotrigine is FDA approved only for the prevention of mood episodes, its slow initiation in the waning phases of mania may be appropriate.

The precise anticonvulsant or psychotropic mechanisms of action of lamotrigine remain to be delineated. However, it is of considerable interest that lamotrigine, like valproate, is a broad-spectrum anticonvulsant, effective not only in complex partial and generalized seizures, but also in absence and atonic seizures, in contrast to carbamazepine and phenytoin, which can exacerbate absence seizures. This is of considerable importance, as recent studies have suggested that carbamazepine and lamotrigine, as well as phenytoin, have highly similar properties in the blockade of type 2 sodium channels and consequent inhibition of release of excitatory amino acids, such as aspartate and Glu.

However, the differential clinical profile of these drugs in epilepsy and the preliminary data that lamotrigine may be effective in some patients who are inadequate responders to carbamazepine suggest that additional mechanisms not shared by carbamazepine will eventually be uncovered for lamotrigine, such as inhibition of N-type calcium channels. Although evidence suggests that lamotrigine blocks 5-HT reuptake and is active at 5-HT type 3 (5-HT_3) receptors, the high concentrations at which these effects are observed suggest that they are not clinically relevant. Preliminary data suggest that depressed patients with the classical topographical pattern of frontal hypoperfusion on positron emission tomography (PET) studies are likely responders to lamotrigine.

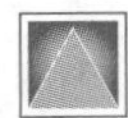

Table 13.8–13
Mania Algorithm

Hypomania	Acute Mania	Prophylaxis
MS, lithium (Eskalith), valproic acid (Depakene), carbamazepine (Tegretol), oxcarbazepine (Trileptal)	MS plus	MS
AA	AA plus	Second MS or AA
Bz	Bz	PM Bz
Insomnia	Combination MS	Alternative AA
Anxiety	Alternative MS	
Agitation		

AA, adjunctive antidepressant; Bz, benzodiazepine; MS, mood stabilizer.

Gabapentin and Tiagabine (Inefficacy in Acute Mania)

Gabapentin is an approved anticonvulsant for adjunctive therapy of partial epilepsies that may also have some usefulness in bipolar patients, according to open adjunctive studies. The drug appears to have positive effects on sleep and anxiety. However, a double-blind study in acute mania and another study of monotherapy in refractory affectively ill cyclic patients were not positive compared with placebo. The discrepancy between gabapentin's lack of efficacy in controlled trials and its positive effects when used adjunctively in open studies may be due to a requirement for combination with other mood stabilizers or its positive effects in many symptoms with which bipolar illness is comorbid. These include anxiety disorder, social phobia, obsessive-compulsive disorder (OCD), and pain and sleep syndromes. Whether gabapentin's prominent effects on the L-amino acid transport mechanism and resulting increases in brain GABA levels are related to its anticonvulsant, antinociceptive, or anxiolytic properties remains for further delineation.

Tiagabine is a potent and selective reuptake inhibitor for the major inhibitory neurotransmitter in the brain (GABA). As such, it potently increases the amount of GABA remaining in the synapse. This action is thought to account for its anticonvulsant effects, but, like gabapentin, which also increases brain GABA by a different mechanism, initial studies of tiagabine in bipolar illness are not promising.

Although there are a few positive case reports, Heinz Grunze and colleagues found none of eight manic patients responsive to tiagabine, and one patient without a history of previous seizures had a seizure while treated with the drug. Similarly, only partial degrees of improvement in three of 17 treatment-refractory patients were achieved when tiagabine was used adjunctively. Here, too, there were problems with tolerability; two patients had new-onset seizures, and a third patient required a visit to an emergency department.

The data with gabapentin and tiagabine suggest that merely increasing brain GABA levels is not sufficient to achieve antimanic or mood stabilizing effects. Although valproate increases brain GABA, many question whether this is relevant to its anticonvulsant actions; based on the inadequate efficacy of gabapentin and tiagabine in mania, GABAergic effects of valproate may not account for its antimanic actions either.

Topiramate (Inefficacy in Acute Mania) Topiramate, a recently approved add-on agent for treatment of refractory epilepsy, has been studied in an open add-on fashion in bipolar illness. Preliminary data from a range of uncontrolled studies had suggested that it may have antimanic or mood stabilizing properties in rapid cycling patients. However, four large, placebo-controlled monotherapy studies failed to find evidence of acute antimanic efficacy, whereas the active comparator lithium was effective.

A major potential asset of topiramate is its side effect of weight loss (Table 13.8–5), which contrasts with lithium, valproate, gabapentin, many antidepressants, and antipsychotics. It has also been reported highly effective versus placebo in primary alcoholism. As a carbonic acid inhibitor, it has a 1 percent risk of renal calculi (which respond well to emergency lithotripsy), and patients should be so informed. Cognitive slowing and difficulty with word finding may appear at even low doses and preclude the ability to dose escalate as needed for efficacy. Topiramate is a selective inhibitor of Glu AMPA receptors and also has indirect GABAergic actions and blocks Na^+ channels.

Other Anticonvulsants It is of considerable interest that two recent small studies suggest the potential acute antimanic and prophylactic efficacy of phenytoin. One study using phenytoin as an adjunct in a randomized, double-blind design compared to placebo suggested that phenytoin exerted antimanic effects. In a crossover study of 6 months of phenytoin versus 6 months of placebo, significantly better results were observed in the groups treated with phenytoin compared to placebo. These investigators postulated that sodium channel blockade, of which phenytoin is one of the most potent agents, could be a common mechanism of action of the effective antimanic drugs.

Acetazolamide (Diamox) has been reported to be effective in patients with atypical psychoses associated with dreamy, confusional states, as well as those occurring premenstrually or in the puerperium. Whether this profile will be shared by other carbonic acid-inhibitors, such as topiramate and zonisamide, remains to be assessed.

Zonisamide was reported to exert antimanic effects in one open study some years ago in Japan, but no controlled data are available. A recent study of open adjunctive zonisamide suggested useful, rapid onset; acute antimanic effects in 80 percent of patients; and a positive side effect of weight loss equal to that of topiramate. In addition to blocking sodium channels, zonisamide exerts dose-related biphasic effects on 5-HT and DA metabolism.

Levetiracetam has a unique mechanism of action, because it is not effective in classic epilepsy models of maximal electroshock seizures or pentylenetetrazole and does not act directly at any known neurotransmitter system. It does have its own binding site in the brain. Recent data suggest that it may enhance GABA inhibition by inhibiting negative modulation of benzodiazepine receptors by zinc and beta carbolines. Anecdotal data have not yet adequately elucidated its psychotropic profile.

Electroconvulsive Therapy Older clinical observations and controlled clinical trials have documented the efficacy of ECT in acute mania. Bilateral treatments appear required, as unilateral, nondominant treatments have been reported to be ineffective or to exacerbate manic symptoms in some studies. In light of the many effective pharmacological treatments noted previously and the usefulness of using the assessment of their acute antimanic efficacy as a surrogate marker for putative efficacy in long-term prophylaxis, ECT may be reserved for the rare refractory manic patient or for the patient with medical complications, as well as extreme exhaustion (lethal catatonia or malignant hyperthermia). One study has reported antimanic effects of a brief course of rTMS of the brain at 20 Hz versus 1 Hz over right frontal cortex; whether this well-tolerated nonconvulsive strategy will eventually have a role in clinical therapeutics remains for further examination.

Other Putative Antimanic Agents of Theoretical Interest

Antiadrenergic Drugs A series of other nonanticonvulsant compounds with some neurotransmitter selectivity have been reported efficacious in treating mania. Clonidine (Catapres), an α_2-adrenergic agonist, is used to treat hypertension. It acutely inhibits the firing of the noradrenergic locus ceruleus and has been reported to show acute antimanic efficacy in some, but not all, controlled trials. Response in the first few days of treatment may not be associated with an ultimate long-term response, however. Another agent that inhibits noradrenergic function is the β-adrenergic receptor antagonist propranolol (Inderal). Because high doses of this agent in the d- or l-isomer form have been effective, it is questionable whether the β-antagonist properties versus the membrane-stabilizing effects of this drug account for its acute antimanic efficacy. α-Methyl-p-tyrosine (AMPT), an inhibitor of DA and NE synthesis, also appears to have antimanic effects. Reserpine, which depletes these two catecholamines and also 5-HT, was one of the first used antimanics and antipsychotics.

Cholinomimetics High doses of choline (3 to 8 g per day) have been reported in one open study to possess antimanic and anticycling effects in refractory bipolar patients. Intravenous (IV) administration of the indirect cholinergic agonist physostigmine (Eserine Salicylate) has been demonstrated to have an almost immediate antimanic effect. Physostigmine inhibits ACh esterase function, making more ACh available at the synapse. Although this strategy can produce rapid decreases in manic symptomatology, it also has a rapid half-life and can be associated with rather marked increases in dysphoria and other side effects, such that its long-term usefulness is doubtful. The success of attempts to chronically increase cholinergic function through other methods, such as lecithin, deanol, or direct ACh agonists, has not been adequately delineated. Moreover, switches into mania have been observed in depressed patients when treated with the cholinesterase inhibitor donepezil (Aricept) for cognitive enhancement.

Neuropeptide and Other Mechanisms Alterations in endogenous neuropeptide function also have been postulated in mania. Although manipulations of opiates or cholecystokinin (CCK) have not revealed consistent results in psychotic schizophrenic patients, isolated reports that thyrotropin-releasing hormone (TRH) and calcitonin were successful in treating excited psychotic states, including mania, perhaps deserve replication.

A new approach examining common effects of chronic lithium and valproate has revealed inhibition of PKC as a putative target for antimanic effects. This idea has received preliminary support from the observations of rapid-onset acute antimanic effects in five of seven patients treated with the PKC inhibitor tamoxifen (Nolvadex). These findings raise the possibility that inhibition of other second messengers may prove a useful target for antimanic effects.

In this regard, new data indicate that lithium, carbamazepine, lamotrigine, and valproate all are partial inhibitors of Ca^{2+} influx through the Glu NMDA receptor, raising the theoretical rationale of using different mechanisms to block Ca^{2+} influx for more effective or complete effects in refractory patients. This is of particular interest, because multiple studies of blood cells (platelets and lymphocytes) show increased baseline or stimulant-induced increases in intracellular calcium.

As noted previously and in Tables 13.8–2 and 13.8–4, awareness of the multiple neurotransmitter approaches to the treatment of mania may be clinically useful in considerations of changing or combining treatments that target different systems in nonresponsive patients.

DRUG–DRUG INTERACTIONS OF ANTIMANIC AGENTS

As treatment of mania often involves use of drug combinations, some general principles derived from the information in Tables 13.8–6 and 13.8–14 are important. Carbamazepine and, to a lesser extent, topiramate are potent inducers of hepatic cytochrome P450 enzymes (especially CYP 3A4) and uridine diphosphate glucuronosyltransferases (UGTs). This induction results in approximate halving of the blood levels of lamotrigine and haloperidol and decreasing levels of the atypical antipsychotics clozapine, olanzapine, risperidone, quetiapine, and ziprasidone, as well as estrogen in oral contraceptives. These effects may translate into the need for higher doses of these compounds. Oxcarbazepine, in contrast to carbamazepine, has minimal effects on lamotrigine blood levels, so that one should not increase the rate of titration or the final dose of lamotrigine when combined with oxcarbazepine. (See a list of anticonvulsants that lower estrogen in Table 13.8–14.)

Conversely, valproate is a potent metabolic enzyme inhibitor (of CYP 2C9, GT, and epoxide hydroxylase), yielding an approximate doubling of lamotrigine and carbamazepine (via increases in the active 10,11-epoxide metabolite). Valproate can also increase antipsychotic levels and side effects, so antipsychotic doses may need to be titrated down when used in conjunction with valproate. The dose of lamotrigine initiation and maintenance should thus be halved, and the dose of carbamazepine should be decreased to avoid toxicity.

The CCBs verapamil and diltiazem (Cardizem) (but not nifedipine [Procardia] or nimodipine) also may double carbamazepine levels and induce toxicity. Many widely used nonantimanic compounds, including all of the macrolide antibiotics, isoniazid (Laniazid), propoxyphene (Darvon), fluoxetine (Prozac), and fluvoxamine (Luvox), may likewise increase carbamazepine levels. In these instances, patients should be advised to decrease their dose of carbamazepine to avoid toxicity.

ACUTE TREATMENT OF BIPOLAR DEPRESSION

The acute treatment of bipolar depression is more thoroughly addressed in the later section on depression breaking through prophylaxis, because the pharmacotherapy of bipolar depression almost always involves a mood stabilizer, with or without an adjunctive unimodal antidepressant. Some of the principles of treating unipolar depression are applicable to initiating treatment of acute bipolar depression but with four major caveats: (1) There is a critical role of concomitant treatment with mood stabilizers; (2) targeting the most characteristic components of bipolar depression—such as its atypicality or reverse vegetative symptoms of hypersomnia, increased appetite and weight, anergia and lethargy, and psychomotor retardation—also requires special attention; (3) the relative usefulness of unimodal antidepressants (Table 13.8–15) in bipolar illness, in general, and in rapid cycling and mixed states, in particular, remains controversial; and (4) the relative merits of using a mood stabilizer or an atypical antipsychotic rather than an antidepressant and a mood stabilizer are not well studied.

Acute Antidepressant Effects of Mood Stabilizers

Lithium's acute antimanic effects are better documented than its acute antidepressant properties. Nonetheless, a substantial series of controlled studies indicates that lithium in monotherapy is an effective acute antidepressant intervention for subjects with bipolar depression.

Lamotrigine's acute antidepressant efficacy in monotherapy has been demonstrated in one study (but not in others) with a dosage of 50 mg per day or 200 mg, significantly exceeding the efficacy of placebo. Similar results were observed in another study of refractory (primarily bipolar) patients wherein lamotrigine at dosages averaging approximately 200 mg per day was more effective in depression than gabapentin or placebo. An additional asset of lamotrigine is its otherwise favorable side effect profile for the reverse-vegetative presentation of bipolar depression. In contrast to many other putative mood stabilizers, it is mildly activating and usually not sedating. It is also weight neutral, and it does not cause the sexual dysfunction common with most SSRIs (Table 13.8–15). Its switch liability is low, comparable to placebo in controlled studies.

Carbamazepine's acute antidepressant effects have been less well delineated than its antimanic efficacy. A recent, double-blind, parallel-group, placebo-controlled trial indicated the efficacy of carbamazepine when used as the sole treatment in primary depression. These preliminary findings, taken with the more substantial emerging literature on the prophylactic efficacy of carbamazepine, raise the priority of using this agent as a supplement to lithium in depressive breakthroughs, particularly of the rapid-cycling variety.

Although only 17 of 54 acutely depressed, treatment-refractory patients responded in one study, the carbamazepine responders tended to be the patients with greater initial severity of depression and more clear prior histories of discrete episodes rather than chronic depression. Moreover, in a subgroup of ten of these initial good responders to carbamazepine, a second double-blind trial of the drug was instituted after a period of time off the drug associated with a recrudescence of depressive symptomatology. These ten patients then reresponded to reinstitution of carbamazepine on a double-blind basis with a time course and magnitude of response similar to that initially observed. Thus, these off-on-off-on data are highly supportive of the view that at least a subgroup of treatment-refractory mood disorder patients show an acute antidepressant response to carbamazepine monotherapy; this is confirmed by the relapse off the drug and the subsequent reresponse on the exposure to the blind medication.

When antidepressant response to carbamazepine was observed, it tended to occur with the typical lag observed with other antidepressant agents, so that only minor improvement was noted in the first and second weeks of treatment, but considerable improvement was observed after the third and fourth weeks. Surprisingly, the degree of antidepressant response was correlated with the degree of decrease

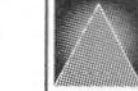

Table 13.8–14
Anticonvulsants: Doses, Levels, Kinetics, and Metabolism

Drug	Starting Dose	Usual Dose Range[a] (mg/day) (Typical)	Steady-State Blood Levels (μg/mL)	Nonlinear Kinetics	Percent Protein Bound	Enzyme	Metabolism	Half-Life (hrs) Acute (Chronic)	Half-Life (hrs) With Inducer[c]	↑ Metabolism and Clearance of Oral Contraceptives[b]
Valproic acid (Depakene)	250	500–2,500 (1,500)	50–120	d	90	Inhibitor	Liver, β oxidation[d]	6–16	2–12	—
Carbamazepine (Tegretol)	200	400–1,600 (600–1,200)	4–12	d	75	Inducer CYP 1A2, CYP 2C, CYP 3A4	Epoxide hydrolase CYP 3A4 metabolism	25–65 (12–17)	9–10	↑
Oxcarbazepine (Trileptal)	250	750–2,400	12–24	—	40	—	Glucuronidation of monohydroxy derivative	5–30	6–19	↑
Lamotrigine (Lamictal)	25	50–500 (200)	3–14	—	56	—	Glucuronide conjugation	50–70 (19–25)	9–12	—
Zonisamide (Zonegran)	25–100	100–600	15–40	e	60	—	CYP 3A4, glucuronidation, renal acetylation	57–68	27–37	—
Phenytoin (Dilantin)	100	300–600 (300)	10–20	d	90	Inducer CYP 1A2, CYP 2B, CYP 3A4	CYP 2C9 metabolism	7–42	7–42	↑
Topiramate (Topamax)	25	200–1,000 (100–200)	3–5?	—	15	Inducer CYP 3A4	Oxidation, renal excretion	19–25	9–12	↑
Gabapentin (Neurontin)	100	400–4,800 (1,200)	6–21	f	0	—	Renal excretion (no interactions)	5–9	?	—
Tiagabine (Gabitril)	1	4–32 (12)	—	—	98	—	CYP 3A4, oxidation, glucuronidation	4–13	2–5	—
Levetiracetam (Keppra)	250	500–3,000 (1,500–2,000)	~40?	—	0	—	Nonhepatic hydrolysis, renal excretion (no interactions)	6–8	?	—

[a]In epilepsy.
[b]Increases in metabolism and clearance of oral contraceptives should propel use of higher estrogen formulations or use of other types of contraception.
[c]Elimination of half-life when administered in conjunction with a liver cytochrome P450 enzyme inducer.
[d]Doubles carbamazepine epoxide → one-half dose of carbamazepine; doubles lamotrigine levels → one-half dose of lamotrigine.
[e]Due to saturation of metabolism.
[f]Due to saturation of gastrointestinal absorption.

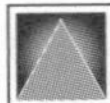

Table 13.8–15
Adverse Effects of Antidepressant Treatments Used in Bipolar Disorder Patients

Antidepressants (Dose in mg/day)	Manic Switch	Sedation	Hypo-tension	Anticho-linergic	NE/5-HT	Weight	Sexual Dysfunction	Lethality in Overdose	Other
Bupropion (Wellbutrin) (75–450)	+	±	0	+	+/0	0, ↓	±	Low	Seizures at high dosages; ↑ dopamine in caudate and nucleus accumbens
SSRIs	+	±	0	0	0/+++	↓, ↑	++	Low	Insomnia, headache
Olanzapine/fluoxetine (Symbyax) combination	0	+++	±	++	0/+++	↑↑	+++	Low?	—
Serotonin and noradrenaline reuptake inhibitor: Venlafaxine (Effexor) (37.5–250.0)	+++	+	—	±	+++/+++	↓, ↑	++	Low	↑ Blood pressure by several mm Hg
Trazodone (Desyrel) (50–600)	?	+++	+++	0	0/++	↑↑	++	Low	Priapism
Nefazodone (Serzone) (100–600)	?	++	0	0	0/+++	?	0	?	Increase in slow wave sleep; liver toxicity
Mirtazapine (Remeron) (15–45)	?	+++	—	—	++/+++	↑↑	0	?	α_2-Blocker; increases NE and 5-HT release
MAOIs	++?	+	+++	0	++/++	↑	++	High?	Off SSRIs by 1 mo, diet to avoid tyramine, avoid opiates
Reversible inhibitors of monoamine oxidase type A: Moclobemide (Manerix) (150–1,600)	+?	+	+	0	++/++	(↑)?	?	?	Not need diet? Less effective than MAOIs
Desipramine (Norpramin) (75–300)	+++	+	+++	+	+++/0	↓, 0	+	High	Switch rate higher than bupropion
Nortriptyline (Aventyl) (50–150)	++	++	++	++	+++/+	↑	+	High	Possible invert U-type blood concentration clinical response
Lithium (Eskalith) (600–1,500)	0	±	0	0	±	↑↑	0	Moderate	Especially for augmentation—may require thyroid supplementation
Lamotrigine (Lamictal)	±	0	0	0	?	0	0	Low	Rash
Electroconvulsive therapy (6–12 treatments)	+	+	—	++ (atropine)	++/++	0	0	Low N/A	Anesthesia; seizure, memory loss

0, none; ±, equivocal; +, minimal; ++, mild; +++, moderate; 5-HT, serotonin; MAOI, monoamine oxidase inhibitor; NE, norepinephrine; SSRI, selective serotonin reuptake inhibitor.

in thyroxine (T_4) and free T_4. Evidence of an abnormal electroencephalogram (EEG) or an increased number of psychosensory symptoms (possibly reflecting temporal lobe irritability) did not predict an acute response to carbamazepine's antidepressant or antimanic effects in a double-blind study but did in another open augmentation study. However, increased baseline metabolism in paralimbic areas, especially the insula, has been associated with a better antidepressant response to carbamazepine. Carbamazepine has been reported in one series to be effective in some patients who failed multiple traditional antidepressant trials, especially in those with a history of head trauma or EEG abnormalities. Patients with a history of alcohol abuse and problematic withdrawal episodes and those with comorbid paroxysmal pain syndromes may be particular candidates for carbamazepine prophylaxis.

One small placebo-controlled, randomized, parallel-group comparison of valproate to placebo suggested significantly greater reductions in depression rating scale scores during treatment with valproate compared to placebo, although the overall result was not significant on most measures.

Unimodal Antidepressants with a Mood Stabilizer Current consensus suggests that antidepressants augmented by a mood stabilizer or vice versa, a mood stabilizer augmented by an antidepressant, is the first-line treatment for a first or isolated episode of bipolar depression (Tables 13.8–15 and 13.8–16). If possible, one should start these two treatments nonsimultaneously to discriminate the one contributing to any emergent side effects. Use of an SSRI or

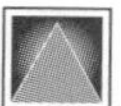

Table 13.8–16
Acute Depression Algorithm

	Depression Breaking through Ongoing MS Treatment	
Single Episode; No Medications	**Non–Rapid Cycling**	**Rapid Cycling to Ultrarapid Cycling**
1a. AD plus MS 1b. Versus LTG 1c. Start folate	1a. Add AD 1b. Add LTG 1c. ✓	1a. Add LTG or 1b. Li 1c. Folate
2. Li augmentation of AD if start 1a Add AD if start 1b	2. ✓	2. Add second MS (especially LTG) or Li
3. T_3 potentiation	3. ✓	3. T_3 3a. Add AA 3b. Add third MS 3c. Add AD
4. Add AA	4. ✓	4. Add one of two other 3a, 3b, or 3c options listed previously
5. Revise AD	5. ✓, consider serotonin and noradrenaline reuptake inhibitor	5. Revise AD, MS, AA
6. Revise MS	6. ✓	6. For ultraradian cycling, consider a dihydropyridine calcium channel blocker, such as amlodipine (Norvasc), isradipine (Dynacirc), or nimodipine (Nimotop)
7. High-potency benzodiazepine or gabapentin (Neurontin) augmentation for insomnia or anxiety	7a. Add serotonin and noradrenaline reuptake inhibitor plus bupropion (Wellbutrin) 7b. Add monoamine oxidase inhibitor after 4 wks off serotonin	7. High-dose T_4
8. Revise AD, MS, AA	8. Gabapentin for insomnia, anxiety, restless legs, and alcohol abuse	
9. Discontinue T_3 and add high-dose T_4	9. Carbamazepine for those with a history of alcohol abuse	
10. ECT or repetitive transcranial magnetic stimulation or VNS (if and when available)	10. ✓	

AA, atypical antipsychotic; AD, antidepressant; ECT, electroconvulsive therapy; Li, lithium (Eskalith); LTG, lamotrigine (Lamictal); MS, mood stabilizer; T_3, triiodothyronine; T_4, thyroxine; VNS, vagus nerve stimulation. Check mark indicates same as in Single Episode column.

bupropion appears high on the preference list, with venlafaxine just below. TCAs have been lowered to a second- or third-line status based on their (1) less than striking efficacy in bipolar depression; (2) less satisfactory side effect profile, including anticholinergic side effects and orthostatic hypotension; (3) likely higher liability for causing switches into mania; and (4) high lethality in overdose. Thus, the second-generation antidepressants—bupropion, SSRIs, or venlafaxine—appear to be the most highly recommended agents, although lamotrigine has been given equal status in the latest American Psychiatric Association (APA) treatment guidelines.

New data support the acute antidepressant effects of the atypical antipsychotics quetiapine and olanzapine and also the olanzapine-fluoxetine combination (Symbyax). Quetiapine compared with placebo had a rapid onset of action, improved sleep and anxiety, and a negligible switch rate. Thus, in instances in which concern about antidepressant-related switching is high, especially in rapid cyclers, one may prefer the use of atypical antipsychotics.

One randomized study suggested that the noradrenergic-active drug desipramine (DMI) (Norpramin) was equally acutely effective with the DA-active bupropion, but DMI showed a much higher incidence of manic switches during long-term continuation and prophylactic therapy. This raises the question of whether some inherent component of the TCAs or the noradrenergic selectivity of DMI accounts for the greater switch liability. Although many investigators have observed apparent switching and the induction of rapid cycling when cotreating with SSRIs, the data from controlled studies suggest that this is not a marked problem. One recent acute study found that treatment with paroxetine (Paxil) compared with placebo was no more likely to induce switches. At the same time, paroxetine only showed antidepressant efficacy in those with low baseline lithium levels. Two recent randomized studies have indicated a higher switch rate on venlafaxine compared with bupropion (or sertraline) or with paroxetine. These data suggest that it is the noradrenergic component of the dual actions of venlafaxine that account for the greater switch liability.

MAINTENANCE TREATMENT OF BIPOLAR ILLNESS

Lithium Prophylaxis Lithium carbonate originally appeared to be effective in some 70 to 80 percent of bipolar patients, but current estimates suggest that, even with adjunctive use of antidepressants and neuroleptics, a response rate of less than 50 percent in many lithium clinics is more accurate (Table 13.8–7).

Although the initial studies indicated the need for blood levels between 0.8 and 1.2 mEq/L, some case series have suggested that lower levels in the range of 0.5 to 0.8 mEq/L might also be effective in maintenance treatment. However, one controlled study has indicated that the lower levels of side effects are achieved at the cost of a three-times greater relapse rate when a low lithium-level range (0.4 to 0.6 mg/L) is used in comparison with higher levels (0.8 to 1.0 mg/L).

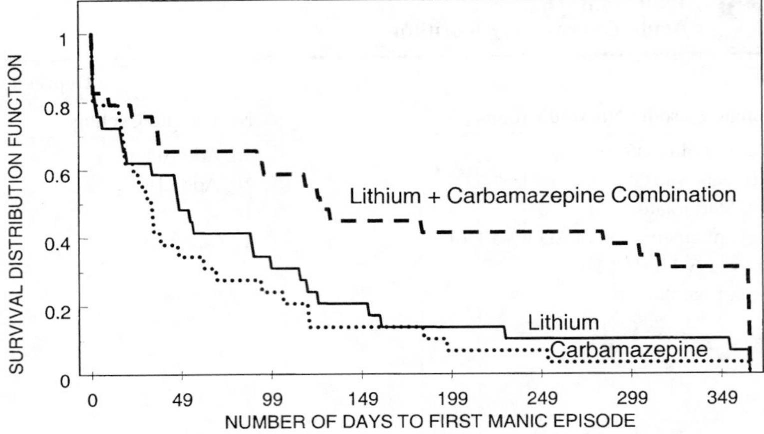

FIGURE 13.8–9 Mean survival time to first manic episode is longer on the combination of lithium and carbamazepine than with lithium or carbamazepine alone (N = 29).

Monitoring of trough levels (performed in the early morning with the AM dose withheld) at 1- to 2-month intervals or more frequently, if the patient's course is unstable, is recommended. One study reported that the greater the lithium-induced decreases in plasma free T_4 concentration (within the normal range), the greater the severity of depression and cycling during a 1-year controlled study. This study, and others indicating that thyroid augmentation (especially with T_3) may enhance cognitive function on lithium, suggest a possible role for more frequent thyroid hormone supplementation of lithium prophylaxis, but controlled studies are needed. Few controlled studies of T_3 augmentation in bipolar depression have been done.

Several studies with follow-up between 2 and 8 years have documented a protective effect of lithium against suicide attempts as well as completed suicide when used as a maintenance treatment for bipolar disorder.

Because of the substantial data on long-term efficacy and prevention of suicide with lithium treatment, it is important to consider preventive treatment after one manic episode, particularly if there is a positive family history of bipolar illness, and definitely after two episodes. The development of a life chart (outlined previously), so that the previous frequency, severity, and interval between episodes can be accurately assessed, may also assist in arriving at the decision for prophylaxis. If previous episodes were severe—socially incapacitating and requiring hospitalization—or associated with extremely adverse events for the patient and family, one would be more likely to consider prophylaxis earlier rather than later, despite the possibility of moderately long well intervals between initial episodes. These factors should be discussed with the patient during a euthymic interval, so that the appropriate risk to benefit ratios can be weighed carefully with adequate informed consent.

Data from nine different studies (but not a particular metaanalysis) indicate that greater numbers of prior episodes (more than three or four episodes in most studies and ten episodes in one study) are associated with a poor response to lithium prophylaxis, so that a delay in institution of prophylaxis may have consequences not only for morbidity during a recurrence, but also for ultimate treatment responsiveness. Whether greater numbers of prior episodes also predispose to the development of tolerance (Fig. 13.8–5) would be predicted on theoretical grounds but remains to be delineated directly.

Carbamazepine Whereas placebo controlled studies of carbamazepine prophylaxis are few and underpowered, a substantial number of randomized studies support the comparative efficacy of carbamazepine and lithium in the prophylaxis of bipolar episodes. Two studies reported fewer prophylactic antimanic effects of carbamazepine compared to lithium, however. Yet, one of these indicated a better response to carbamazepine in those with atypical presentations, that is, bipolar II rapid cycling, dysphoria, schizoaffective illness, and substance abuse comorbidity.

In a small series of patients who were inadequate responders to carbamazepine alone, one-half showed a rapid-onset antidepressant effect with lithium augmentation. Thus, the combination of carbamazepine and lithium appears to be helpful for a substantial subgroup of otherwise refractory patients. In one randomized study in bipolar outpatients with a high incidence of rapid cycling, response rates were less than 25 percent with lithium or carbamazepine monotherapy for 1 year, even when adjunctive antidepressants and antipsychotics were allowed, but greater than 50 percent with both drugs in combination (Fig. 13.8–9).

As noted previously, one alternative to traditional unimodal antidepressants for depressive breakthroughs is the addition of a first generation anticonvulsant mood stabilizer, such as carbamazepine, valproate, or the second-generation anticonvulsant lamotrigine.

Valproic Acid In many open series, valproic acid alone or in addition to lithium has been reported to be successful in the long-term treatment of a substantial subgroup of previously lithium- or carbamazepine-refractory patients, and high rates of response to valproate have been reported in a series of rapid-cycling patients studied by Joe Calabrese and colleagues (Figs. 13.8–6 and 13.8–7). One placebo-controlled study reported no advantage for valproate on the primary measure of prevention of manic episodes, but valproate was superior to placebo and lithium in lengthening the time to the first depressive episode. Because of the requirements for sustained remissions to enter this study and low relapse rates of the recruited population even on placebo, the mixed results of this controlled study should be viewed with some skepticism.

The acute antidepressant efficacy of valproic acid is much less well delineated than its antimanic efficacy, and the usefulness of this treatment for an acute depressive episode remains to be further elucidated. One small placebo-controlled, randomized, parallel-group comparison of valproate to placebo showed significantly greater reductions in depression rating scale scores during treatment with valproate compared to placebo, although the overall result was not significant on most measures. In another study, the addition of valproate to lithium appeared more effective than placebo.

The combination of lithium and valproate offers another option in the long-term management of bipolar patients who do not respond to lithium alone. Yet, in one controlled study of rapid-cycling patients responding to the combination of lithium and valproate (with the intent of later randomizing them to a comparative trial of each monotherapy), only 17 percent of the intent-to-treat cohort and 25 percent of the observed cases responded well enough to the combination to be included for randomization. This study indicates that, even with two of the best and most widely used prophylactic agents in combination, this subgroup of rapid-cycling patients is largely inadequately responsive. However, a similar combination study in childhood-onset mania showed much more positive results, with good mood stabilization in the majority of patients. When the adult responders were eventually randomized to monotherapy, 50 percent relapsed on either lithium or valproate before the end of the intended 1-year prophylactic study. The data in adults begin to suggest the potential usefulness of treating rapid cyclers with the combination of lithium and valproate or lithium and carbamazepine from the outset, rather than waiting for the expected high incidence of relapse on monotherapy in this poorly responsive subgroup.

A response to one anticonvulsant may not be predictive of a response to another, and positive long-term effects of valproic acid plus lithium have been noted in patients not responsive to lithium or carbamazepine prophylaxis (Fig. 13.8–6, Table 13.8–17).

Lamotrigine (Lamictal) A series of reports and four placebo-controlled trials suggest that lamotrigine has prophylactic antidepressant and, potentially, mood-stabilizing properties. In the largest open study, 67 patients were studied, usually with the drug as an add-on to other previously ineffective treatment regimens, and 27 out of 39 patients (69 percent) who presented in the depressed phase (as well as 19 out of 25 [76 percent] in the manic phase) showed moderate to marked acute improvement, which persisted on follow-up.

A randomized, double-blind study at the NIMH found good response in 15 of the first 31 patients (48 percent) randomized to blind lamotrigine monotherapy compared to gabapentin (29 percent) or placebo (20 percent). Several patients with refractory, unipolar depression were among those who showed a good response. However, patients with bipolar I disorder depression appeared to respond better than those with bipolar II disorder or unipolar depression. A multicenter study noted previously indicated that 50 mg per day and 200 mg per day of lamotrigine were superior to placebo in a 7-week trial in bipolar I disorder depressed patients, and, most importantly, the rate of switch into mania did not exceed that of placebo.

Two large, multicenter studies have now documented the prophylactic antidepressant effects of lamotrigine (200 mg per day) compared to placebo and, most surprisingly, lithium. One study started with those recently manic, and another started with those recently depressed. Lamotrigine was openly added, and other medications were tapered. This group of responsive patients was then randomized to placebo, lithium, or lamotrigine. Time to first intervention for depression was longer with lamotrigine than for lithium and placebo in each study (Fig. 13.8–10). When the two studies were combined, time to intervention for manic symptoms was longer for lamotrigine compared to placebo, but lithium's antimanic efficacy clearly surpassed that of lamotrigine.

Thus, lamotrigine is emerging as the first putative *mood stabilizer* (pending demonstration of its antimanic efficacy) that breaks the usual mode in which lithium, carbamazepine, and valproate are better antimanic agents than antidepressant agents. Lamotrigine, in contrast, appears to have superior acute and prophylactic antidepressant properties compared to antimanic properties. It is the first drug that the FDA approved for prophylaxis rather than for treatment of acute episodes.

This view of lamotrigine promises to change the usual treatment algorithm for bipolar illness in general and depression in particular. As in the new bipolar guidelines, lamotrigine is already considered a first-line option in addition to the traditional combination of a mood stabilizer and an antidepressant for bipolar depression. Given that breakthrough depressions are the most problematic phases of illness emergence during prophylaxis, lamotrigine's role is likely to expand substantially in this regard.

One can envision the combination of lithium and lamotrigine surpassing that of lithium and an antidepressant for usefulness in prophylaxis, particularly when more rapid-cycling patterns are evident at baseline. Dosing strategies of lamotrigine in prophylaxis have not yet been clearly delineated, and very slow titration increases to avoid a rash and to an efficacy end point would appear appropriate rather than targeting a specific dose. Two-hundred mg per day appears to be an average dose in many studies, but the dose-finding study of the large collaborative trial noted previously was underpowered for all groups other than 200 mg per day. Although higher doses of 400 to 500 mg per day are often used in the treatment of seizures, stopping at the lower dose when clinical response is achieved would appear prudent at the current time, allowing room for upward titration if breakthrough episodes occur.

Tolerance to the anticonvulsant effects of lamotrigine has been observed in animal models and only anecdotally reported for seizure and affective episode prophylaxis. Loss of efficacy via an apparent tolerance process has been observed in 20 to 40 percent of cohorts of previously treatment-refractory patients on most other pharmacological regimens (i.e., involving lithium, carbamazepine, and, to a lesser extent, valproate), and the extent to which this will emerge as a problem of clinical importance in routine clinical practice remains to be delineated.

These positive data on antidepressant effects of lamotrigine in two placebo-controlled studies, taken in conjunction with two long-term studies of prophylaxis, are indicative of the clinically useful antidepressant effects of lamotrigine. Although the drug has an acute rash rate of 3 to 8 percent, in most studies, this rate has not exceeded that of placebo in the controlled studies, and, with slow titration according to the *Physician's Desk Reference* (PDR) guidelines, the incidence of severe rash (i.e., Stevens-Johnson syndrome, a toxic epidermal necrolysis) is now thought to be approximately 2 in 10,000 adults and 4 in 10,000 children.

Atypical Antipsychotics Given their acute antimanic efficacy and their antipsychotic and therapeutic effects on the negative symptoms of schizophrenia in long-term studies, one would expect positive effects of the atypicals in the prevention of manic and psychotic episodes.

Initial studies support this view, with olanzapine having equal prophylactic antimanic effects to valproate in one study, and, in another, it had superior antimanic, but not antidepressant, effects compared to lithium. The more crucial unanswered question is whether this class of compounds will have prophylactic effects against depressive episodes, as data in acute depression might suggest (Fig. 13.8–11). One retrospective case series reported better antidepressant effects of open, add-on quetiapine than risperidone or clozapine on severe depression measured by the Inventory of Depressive Symptomatology (IDS) scale.

A recent, large, multicenter trial of quetiapine monotherapy versus placebo in acute depression found impressive rapid-onset effects ($P < .001$) for either the 300-mg or the 600-mg dose at week 1 and

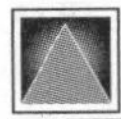

Table 13.8–17
Positive and Negative Selection Factors for Choice of Mood Stabilizer or Anticonvulsant

Mood Stabilizers: Better AM than AD

	Li	CBZ	VPA/DVPX
Target symptoms and auxiliary responsive syndromes	Euphoric ++++ Family history positive for Li response +++ Mania–depression–well interval pattern +++ Steroid induced ++ Suicidal risk +++ Intermittent episodes with well interval +	Euphoric mania +++ Dysphoric mania + Schizoaffective ++ Organic-affective +++ Aggressive +++ Alcohol abuse and withdrawal ++ Cocaine ± PTSD + Steroid induced ± Paroxysmal pain syndromes ++++ Hypermetabolism on positron emission tomography +	Dysphoric mania +++ Rapid cycling +++ Organic-affective ++ Panic + Migraine ++++ Alcohol + Cocaine ± PTSD +

	Choose Li	Avoid Li	Choose CBZ	Avoid CBZ	Choose VPA	Avoid VPA
Positive and negative side effect profiles	↑ White blood cell count (c) ↑ Ca^{++} (c) Renal excretion Nonsedating Bipolar I disorder mania prophylaxis	Weight gain (c) Tremor (c), DR Subjective (c), DR cognitive slowing ↓ Thyroid (c) ↓ Renal ↑ Diabetes insipidus (c) ↓ Glomerular filtration rate (r) Toxic in OD Cardiac (c) Cerebellar (r) Poor in multiple sclerosis and neurological illness Pregnancy? Ebstein's anomaly (vr)	Minimal cognitive changes Little weight gain Tolerated in OD	Many drug interactions! (c) ↓ Potency of birth control pills (c) Rash (10–15%) (c) Ataxia and sedation (c), DR Hyponatremia (r), DR Agranulocytosis (r), I Aplastic anemia (vr), I Allergy, I Pregnancy Spina bifida (1–3%) (r)	Few drug interactions Tolerated in OD Minimal cognitive changes	Weight gain (c) Gastrointestinal distress (c) Tremor (c), DR Alopecia (r), I Pancreatitis (vr), I Polycystic ovaries (?)↓ Platelets (c) ↑ Homocysteine Liver failure (vr) Child <2 yrs of age (vr) Pregnancy Spina bifida (2–6%) (r)

Anticonvulsants

	LTG: AD > AM	GPN: Not AM	TOP: Not AM
Target symptoms and auxiliary responsive syndromes	Rapid cycling ++ Continuous cycling + Treatment refractory ++ Pain syndromes + Anxiety disorder ++ Family history positive for anxiety disorder ++ Hypometabolism on positron emission tomography +	Insomnia ++ Social phobia +++ Anxiety +++, including obsessive-compulsive disorder + and PTSD + Pain syndromes +++ Alcohol withdrawal ++ Parkinsonian symptoms +	Bulimia +++ Alcohol craving +++ Overweight +++ PTSD ++

	Choose LTG	Avoid LTG	Choose GPN	Avoid GPN	Choose TOP	Avoid TOP
Positive and negative side effect profiles	Antidepressant Mood not set below baseline Nonsedating Weight neutral to weight loss	Rash (c): 5–10% Risk of severe rash (vr) 1 in 5,000 adults 1 in 2,500 children Slow titration required Avoid in children (if used, initiate at 12.5 mg every other day and exquisitely slow titration) ↑ Levels (× 2) with valproic acid and ↑ rash risk ↓ Levels (× 2) with carbamazepine (Tegretol) Weak antimanic effects	Renal excretion Few interactions Helps essential tremor, restless legs syndrome Wide dose range and safety Rapid titration possible Young age Shorter duration of illness	Not antimanic and may exacerbate mania Inhibits own uptake after a dose ≥1,200 mg, thus requires dosing 3 or 4 times a day High doses in older individuals	Sustained weight loss (c)	Not antimanic in monotherapy 1% incidence renal calculi (r) and paresthesias (o) Psychomotor slowing (r) Difficulty with word finding (o) Possible insomnia (o)

Note: Strength of evidence: ±, minimal, ambiguous, or inconsistent data; +, used, but no controlled data; ++, some controlled data; +++, positive and some controlled data; ++++, strong, widely used.

AD, antidepressant; AM, antimanic; (c), common; CBZ, carbamazepine (Tegretol); DR, dose related; DVPX, divalproex; GPN, gabapentin (Neurontin); I, idiosyncratic; Li, lithium (Eskalith); LTG, lamotrigine (Lamictal); (o), occasional; OD, overdose; PTSD, posttraumatic stress disorder; (r), rare; TOP, topiramate (Topamax); VPA, valproic acid; (vr), very rare.

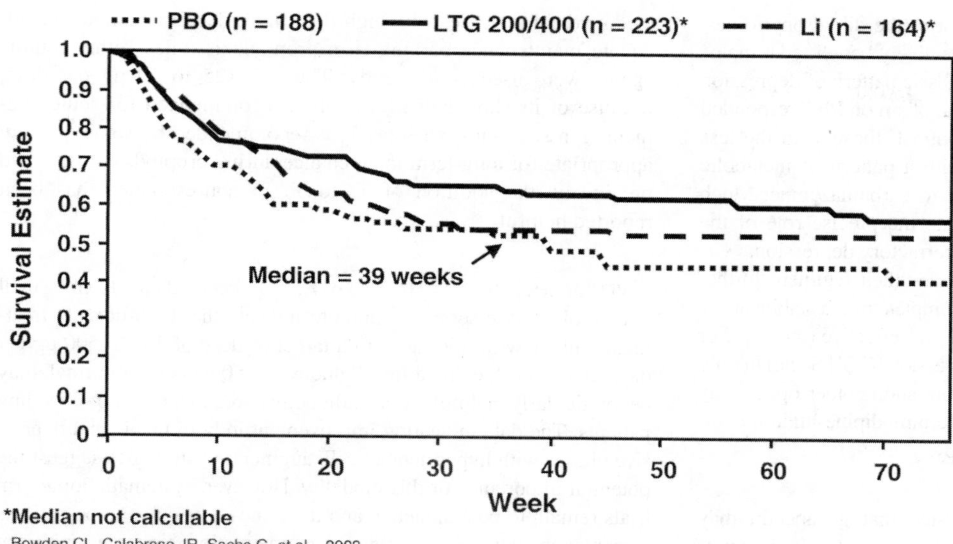

FIGURE 13.8–10 Time to intervention for depression in two combined double-blind, placebo (PBO)-controlled trials of lamotrigine (LTG) (N = 223), lithium (Li) (N = 164), or PBO (N = 188): lamotrigine was superior to lithium or placebo.

thereafter. Improvement in anxiety symptoms and self-rated sleep profile was also striking. Quetiapine monotherapy responses were of a similar magnitude to the olanzapine-fluoxetine combination group in Figure 13.8–11. The quetiapine depression data are the strongest to date, indicating that another atypical antipsychotic approved for acute mania will have true bimodal effects in both mood phases. The impact of using a mood stabilizer or an atypical instead of an antidepressant on the three-times-greater amount of depression, compared with mania, breaking through conventional treatment regimens deserves consideration and systematic evaluation.

Although efficacy differences among the atypical antipsychotics remain to be elucidated, one might consider tolerability as an important criterion in long-term prophylaxis. The relative proclivity of the atypical antipsychotics for weight gain and its associated liabilities of hypercholesterol, hyperlipidemia, insulin resistance, and perhaps diabetes are noted preliminarily in Tables 13.8–5 and 13.8–12.

Calcium Channel Blockers

As reviewed previously, the few uncontrolled studies of CCBs show promise as prophylactic treatments but may be less effective for depressive breakthroughs than for manias. Further controlled studies are sorely needed. Although data are limited to just one double-blind series at the NIMH, in several patients crossed over blindly from one L-type CCB to another, the dihydropyridine type may be preferred to phenyl alkylamine L-type CCBs because of their apparent better antidepressant and mood-stabilizing effects.

Of considerable interest were several patients in the blind study who were clear nimodipine responders to monotherapy or in combination with carbamazepine and transitioned from nimodipine on a double-blind basis to maximally tolerated doses of verapamil, without maintaining response. They later reresponded to nimodipine or to another dihydropyridine L-type CCB, such as isradipine (DynaCirc), not only further confirming the initial responsivity to this drug class, but also suggesting that responsivity might be better conferred by the dihydropyridine subtype of L-type CCBs (with its binding site deep inside the calcium channel) than by the phenyl alkylamine verapamil (which blocks at the outside of the channel).

Although there is some evidence that patients with extremely rapid-cycling fluctuations within a 24-hour period (ultra-ultra rapid

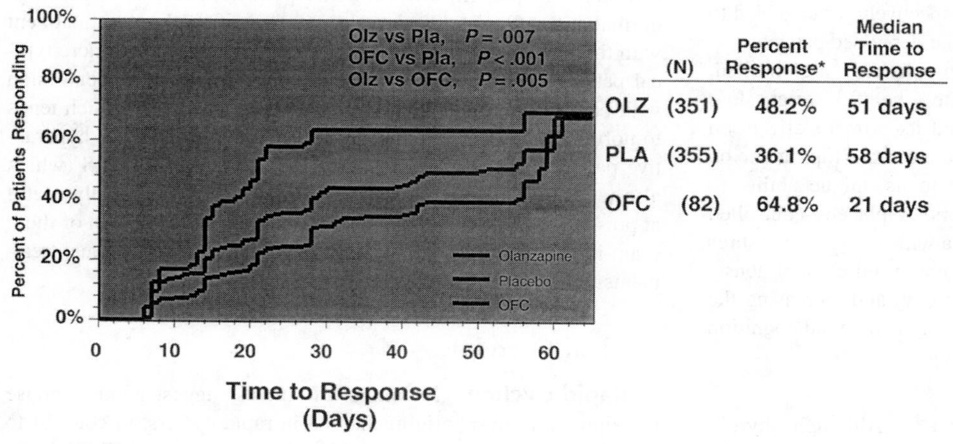

FIGURE 13.8–11 Antidepressant responses in bipolar depression to olanzapine (OLZ) and the olanzapine-fluoxetine combination (OFC). *50 percent improvement. PLA, placebo.

cycling) are among those who respond best to the dihydropyridines, the question of whether this subgroup is selectively benefitted remains to be further delineated. Patients with the classic pattern of depression associated with global and frontal hypometabolism on PET responded best to nimodipine (Table 13.8–17). In contrast, those with the less typical pattern of depression associated with a pattern of metabolic hyperactivity were more likely to respond to carbamazepine. Much work remains to be done to better delineate the precise role of the CCBs in the treatment sequence of bipolar refractory depression.

However, almost all of these patients needed their regimens further supplemented with another agent for more complete mood stabilization. Carbamazepine augmentation of nimodipine was effective (moderate or marked response on the Clinical Global Impression [CGI] Scale) in only 5 of 14 patients treated with the combination, and another open study suggested better prophylactic response to the nimodipine-lithium combination than with either drug in monotherapy.

Gabapentin Open trials have suggested that gabapentin may have positive effects on mood, anxiety, and sleep in 30 to 40 percent of bipolar patients with refractory depression, with higher rates when used in combination. In one double-blind study of treatment-refractory patients, gabapentin monotherapy was less effective than lamotrigine and equal to placebo for overall illness. Moreover, at higher doses of gabapentin, some patients showed exacerbations of the severity or frequency of manias, so its effectiveness as an acute antimanic agent or mood stabilizer has clearly not been demonstrated in controlled trials.

However, adjunctive gabapentin as a maintenance treatment with other anticonvulsants (carbamazepine, valproate, and lamotrigine) or mood stabilizers certainly deserves consideration for bipolar depressed patients with anxiety and social phobia or the profound sleep disturbance associated with a comorbid posttraumatic stress disorder (PTSD). If the patient has comorbid alcoholism, and benzodiazepines are to be avoided, gabapentin would appear to be a safe and easy-to-use alternative, especially because it is renally excreted and not metabolized in the liver.

Topiramate Topiramate, an anticonvulsant with unique mechanisms of action, although not effective in acute mania, has been reported to be a useful adjunct in a series of open, add-on studies in patients not adequately responsive to the more traditional regimens. Treatment initiated for mania or cycling appeared more effective than that for acute depression in one study. However, a recent randomized, single-blind study suggested an approximately 56 or 59 percent response rate to topiramate or bupropion, respectively, when added to a previous mood-stabilizer regimen for bipolar depressed patients.

Although more definitive studies in prophylaxis are awaited, many investigators believe that topiramate's helpful weight loss properties will be useful above and beyond its primary effects on mood. Open studies also suggest impressive effects of topiramate on PTSD symptoms, which could be related to its unique ability to block the AMPA subtype of Glu receptors. A placebo-controlled study documented very positive effects on a wide range of measures of topiramate's ability to treat those with comorbid alcohol abuse. Starting topiramate slowly (i.e., 25 mg per day) and increasing the drug slowly (i.e., 25 mg every 5 to 7 days) may help avoid cognition problems sometimes associated with the drug.

Adjunctive or Replacement Thyroid Although thyroid potentiation similar to that observed in unipolar depression can be attempted, treatment with greater than suppressive doses should be approached with caution. Several investigators have found associated medical toxicities with high-dose thyroid treatment and an inadequate maintenance of long-term prophylaxis unless other routine agents were used concurrently. Thus, T_3 (25 to 50 μg per day), because of its short half-life, is often recommended for acute augmentation strategies, whereas T_4 is recommended by some as more appropriate for long-term maintenance during prophylaxis. As noted previously, the addition of T_3 to T_4 in nonresponders has been reported helpful.

Hypermetabolic Doses of T_4 Recent data from small uncontrolled case series continue to indicate that high-dose T_4 treatment with slow titration toward a target of dose of 300 to 500 μg per day, aimed at achieving a free T_4 index of 150 percent of normal, may be particularly helpful as an adjunctive treatment in rapid-cycling patients. The data indicating improvement in both manic and depressive phases with hypermetabolic T_4 augmenting strategies suggest the potential importance of this modality. However, systematic long-term trials remain to be conducted, and the issue of whether some patients lose responsivity to such thyroid augmentation strategies with the development of tolerance also requires further exploration. Potential bone demineralization with this regimen has been feared but was not evident in one short-term follow-up study.

POTENTIAL CORRELATES OF RESPONSE TO THE MOOD STABILIZERS

Regional Brain Correlates of Clinical Response A question to be answered is whether the efficacy of carbamazepine, valproate, or the other putative mood-stabilizing anticonvulsants, such as lamotrigine, is related to their ability to stabilize neural excitability in temporal lobe and limbic structures (independent of whether a seizure disorder is found to underlie the mood disorder). Recent PET data suggest that patients with initial baseline hypermetabolism, particularly in the left insula, responded best to carbamazepine, whereas those with the more typical pattern of baseline hypometabolism responded best to nimodipine. During treatment, each drug tended to normalize the baseline alterations in the expected direction. Another initial study of valproate suggested that response was accompanied by normalization of baseline hyperactivity in medial basal frontal cortex.

However, patients with relative hypoperfusion at baseline tended to respond to lamotrigine or gabapentin and to show relative normalization of this pattern, whereas nonresponders tended to be closer to normal at baseline and then to decrease significantly with treatment with these agents. One preliminary study also linked this more typical pattern of baseline hypometabolism or perfusion in depression with better response to high-frequency (20 Hz) rTMS (which tends to normalize this pattern), whereas those with evidence of hyperactive patterns respond better to low-frequency (1 Hz) rTMS (which also tends to normalize this pattern). Although not clinically useful at present, one can only hope that replication and extension of these brain-imaging studies will assist in better matching individual treatments to individual patients.

Clinical Correlates

Rapid Cycling A number of studies suggest good response to valproate in dysphoric mania and in rapid cyclers, in contrast to the relatively poor response to lithium in these subtypes (Table 13.8–17). One small study in mania reported that responders to carbamazepine tended to be more dysphoric at baseline.

More than a dozen studies have reported a relatively poor response to lithium in rapid-cycling patients; only two studies have reported a good response, and five have reported no differential response in rapid-cycling patients versus non–rapid-cycling patients. When rapid-cycling patients were compared with non–rapid-cycling patients in two studies, both also found a higher prophylactic response rate to carbamazepine in non–rapid-cycling patients. Data from Japan are revealing: The 53 percent response rate to carbamazepine in those patients with a history of rapid cycling (compared to 76 percent in those without) was substantially higher than the 30 percent response rate observed for lithium in patients with a history of rapid cycling (compared to 64 percent in those without such a history).

Rapid cycling and prediction of response to valproate is less well studied, but open studies have reported a high incidence of excellent acute and prophylactic response with monotherapy or combination treatment. However, one study reported that a pattern of accelerating course of illness was a poor prognosis factor for predicting valproate response. In the group of rapid-cycling patients (discussed previously) who were treated with the combination of lithium and valproate to stabilize mood and, potentially, to enter these individuals into a double-blind randomization to monotherapy, it was observed that only one-fourth of the observed cases showed a good enough response to the combination to enter the clinical trial. These data further suggest that, even with the combination of lithium and valproate, rapid cycling is a relatively poor prognostic factor.

Rapid cycling appears to be a relatively poor prognostic indicator for monotherapy response to lithium, valproate, and carbamazepine. The data suggest the potential usefulness of starting rapid-cycling patients on the combination of lithium and carbamazepine from the outset (with its 53 percent response rate) in light of the poor response to monotherapy in rapid-cycling patients (28 percent response to lithium and 19 percent response to carbamazepine). A similar conclusion may be pertinent for the combination of lithium and valproate from the outset.

A small study suggested a number of discriminating features in patients responding to lithium compared to those who responded to lamotrigine. Response to lithium was less prominent in those with rapid-cycling patterns but was better in those using lamotrigine. Likewise, lamotrigine was more effective in those with anxiety symptoms. Interestingly, there was a higher incidence of positive family history of anxiety disorder and schizoaffective illness in family members of the lamotrigine-responsive probands compared to those who were lithium responsive. However, there was more unipolar depression in families of those who responded to lithium. Replication and confirmation of these data are eagerly awaited.

Family History A modicum of evidence suggests that a negative family history of affective illness may be associated with a good response to carbamazepine, whereas seven of eight studies reported that a positive family history of affective illness in first-degree relatives is associated with a positive response to lithium. These data, in conjunction with clinical case reports illustrating that patients with evidence of organic mental disorders show a relatively poor response to lithium, a high potential for toxicity, and a potentially good response to the anticonvulsants carbamazepine or valproate, suggest that the familial genetic subtype of affective illness may be more responsive to lithium than that subtype mediated through other nonhereditary pathophysiological mechanisms, which may be more responsive to the mood-stabilizing anticonvulsants. Possible pathophysiological mechanisms include neuronal and environmental insult related to birth trauma, infection, secondary affective illness, and substance abuse. Clearly, further study of this issue is required.

RELATIVE SIDE EFFECT PROFILES OF LITHIUM AND ANTICONVULSANTS: ROLE IN CHOICE OF PUTATIVE MOOD STABILIZER

Because only a modicum of data reviewed previously suggest currently available, potentially useful clinical or biological predictors of response to the mood stabilizers (Table 13.8–17), side effect profiles and tolerability in long-term prophylaxis (Tables 13.8–8 through 13.8–12) become important selection factors.

The general profile of lithium-induced side effects has proven to be relatively benign in the long-term maintenance treatment of bipolar patients. However, several of lithium's more prominent side effects deserve comment, as do the relative comparisons to and among the mood-stabilizing anticonvulsants.

Dose reduction may be a first maneuver in treating a variety of lithium-induced problems (tremor, weight gain, thirst, urinary frequency, diarrhea, or psychomotor slowing). If these lower doses are not adequate for prophylaxis, combination or alternative treatment, especially with carbamazepine (which has a different side effect profile), or other putative mood stabilizers may be indicated. It is noteworthy that the renal clearance of lithium appears to decrease with age, so that a lower dose may be adequate and necessary in the older patient on lithium maintenance.

Thyroid Function Lithium clearly can impair thyroid function by several different mechanisms; it has even been used to treat hyperthyroidism. Lithium uniformly lowers T_3 and T_4 levels circulating in the plasma, usually within the normal range. In some patients, lithium increases thyroid-stimulating hormone (TSH). TSH increases that are greater than normal can be taken to indicate that the hypothalamic-pituitary-adrenal (HPA) axis is working overtime to maintain normal levels of thyroid hormones. Lower levels of free T_4 (yet within the normal range) during lithium prophylaxis in one study were associated with increased severity of depression and more rapid mood fluctuation. Thus, one might consider thyroid replacement with T_4 when levels of TSH are elevated, even when thyroid hormone indices are still within their normal lower limits. Occasional checks of thyroid function at 6-month to 1-year intervals are wise in light of lithium's 4 percent rate of induction of hypothyroidism, as would be an earlier check if there was a breakthrough of depressive symptomatology during otherwise adequate lithium maintenance treatment. Treatment of underlying hypothyroidism can, in these instances, help alleviate a depression that is linked to this hormonal deficit. Whereas T_4 is generally used for suppression of TSH and replacement, anecdotal evidence suggests that the addition of T_3 to the T_4 replacement may help some patients with refractory depression or cycling.

Carbamazepine tends to decrease T_4, free T_4, and T_3 levels (as does lithium), and, in combination, the decreases are additive. During carbamazepine treatment, there is a negligible incidence of clinical hypothyroidism or greater than normal increases in TSH. Consequently, thyroid supplementation of carbamazepine is rarely needed. When the two drugs are used in combination, however, the lithium effect on TSH may override that of carbamazepine, and the patient may then require thyroid supplementation.

Renal and Electrolyte Function Current practice suggests that frequent monitoring of renal function during lithium treatment is not generally indicated, although periodic checks of serum creatinine levels at 6-month to once-yearly intervals are prudent. In patients with a history of or high risk for renal abnormalities, it would be useful to obtain baseline measures of renal function, including a creatinine clearance, before beginning lithium treatment. Patients should be cautioned to have adequate fluid intake to maintain appropriate fluid and electrolyte balance. Several cases have been reported in which high levels of lithium during intoxication have been associated with irreversible cerebellar toxicity. Thus, lithium levels or fluid and electrolyte status, or both, should be monitored closely during periods of febrile illness, decreased fluid intake, or greater than ordinary fluid loss, such as during extreme athletic stress or during GI illnesses with vomiting or diarrhea. The development of diabetes insipidus (DI) related to the inhibition of antidiuretic hormone (vasopressin) actions at the level of lithium's effects on adenylate cyclase is not uncommon and is virtually always reversible. It is unusual, however, for DI to reach the point of being clinically problematic rather than merely an inconvenience.

Amiloride (Midamor) (5 to 10 mg per day) has been useful in the treatment of lithium-induced polyuria or DI. If diuretics (furosemide [Lasix] or thiazides) or the nonsteroidal antiinflammatory agents (such as naproxen [Naprosyn]) are used, lower doses of lithium are indicated, because these agents increase lithium levels. Preliminary data suggest that less renal toxicity may occur in patients using single nighttime (HS) dosing (producing higher peaks, but lower nadirs) than that achieved with conventional dosing regimens. HS dosing may also reduce polyuria and facilitate compliance.

Because carbamazepine appears to act like a vasopressin agonist directly or by potentiating vasopressin effects at the receptor, it is not sufficient to reverse lithium-induced DI, which occurs by an action of lithium below the receptor level at the adenylate cyclase second-messenger system. The hyponatremic effects of the keto derivative oxcarbazepine (1 to 3 percent incidence) are more prominent than those of carbamazepine. Demeclocycline (Demeclomycin) and lithium counter the hyponatremic effects of carbamazepine, but their effects on oxcarbazepine have not been studied.

To the extent that some of the subjective sense of the minor cognitive impairments on lithium are related to its ability to impair vasopressin function in the brain, the inferences from the renal data would suggest that carbamazepine would be less likely to cause this impairment. In addition, during combination treatment, the side effects of lithium would override those of carbamazepine.

Carbamazepine tends to induce a benign hypocalcemia that is generally not associated with bone demineralization. In contrast, lithium often produces a transient increase in serum calcium and, with long-term use, has been rarely associated with hyperparathyroidism.

The biggest concern is lithium's long-term effects on renal function via glomerular toxicity, resulting in slowly progressing increases in serum creatinine and decreases in creatinine clearance. The incidence of this effect remains controversial, as do the appropriate clinical measures taken when initial creatinine increases are observed. Many would suggest a watchful course and increased frequency of monitoring, whereas others would try to find an alternative treatment. When lithium is discontinued, creatinine levels may stabilize (suggesting lithium involvement) or may continue to increase (suggesting other pathophysiological mechanisms were involved). Lithium should be tapered slowly to avoid the higher rates of relapse on rapid withdrawal and the subsequent confounding of the evaluation of the effectiveness of other treatments.

Tremor Tremor can be problematic for a small, but not insubstantial, percentage of patients treated with lithium. The tremor is frequently exacerbated by routine actions (e.g., bringing a cup to the mouth), social stress, or social scrutiny. When the tremor persists at doses near the lower end of the therapeutic range or at the minimum doses necessary for therapeutic efficacy, attempts can be made to treat it symptomatically. Some investigators find that a dose of 10 to 40 mg of the β-blocker propranolol in divided daily doses reduces lithium tremor. Relief may occur within 30 minutes and may last from 4 to 6 hours. More often, it is most practical to try to replace a portion of the lithium dose with another agent, such as a dihydropyridine CCB, which does not possess tremor inducing effects.

Valproate also has dose-related tremorogenic effects. Gabapentin, in contrast, has been used to treat essential tremor.

Gastrointestinal Effects GI side effects (diarrhea and indigestion) can also be problematic for many patients on lithium and valproate but may be attenuated by reducing the dose or giving it at meal times (for indigestion). Divalproex is less likely than valproate to cause gastrointestinal upset. Opiate-containing antidiarrheal agents should be restricted to acute treatment. Some CCBs may substitute for part or all of the dose of lithium for those who are intolerant of its side effects. Histamine 2 (H_2) blockers may help counter valproate's GI side effects.

Cognitive Effects Patients may express concern about the effects of lithium on their memory, spontaneity, or creativity. Although some impairment can be objectively delineated in some, but not all, types of detailed neuropsychological testing (specifically, tests of declarative memory and some tests of executive functioning), most patients do not experience this effect or do not find it unduly impairing. In fact, productivity and creativity may, overall, be enhanced during lithium treatment, because it prevents unproductive manic and depressive phases.

Although no adequate approach to the subjective cognitive effects of lithium has been demonstrated (other than reducing the dose), it is important to rule out associated causes for cognitive impairment, including possible subclinical hypothyroidism or an inadequately treated level of coexistent depression. T_3 augmentation has been reported to be a useful counter for this side effect, whether or not thyroid hormone levels are low initially. Donepezil has been reported to be helpful in isolated case reports, and this and other acetylcholinesterase inhibitors deserve further exploration and study.

Many so-called drug-related side effects are clearly evident during placebo treatment phases and thus appear more closely associated with illness-related variables rather than with a particular psychopharmacological treatment. This perspective on lithium maintenance treatment clearly needs to be explored with the patient to avoid premature discontinuation of treatment or noncompliance.

Carbamazepine and valproate are noted for their benign cognitive side effects in the epilepsies and may be better tolerated than lithium in some instances, although they too can be associated with word-finding difficulties. Valproate has been associated with a reversible organic brain syndrome with EEG slowing and a dementia-like presentation in isolated patients with epilepsy, but this has not been reported in psychiatric series. Lamotrigine does not appear to have these cognitive liabilities or problems with daytime sedation. On lamotrigine, some patients feel stabilized at a mood or energy level at or slightly over baseline (i.e., at or above 50 mm on the mood analog scale).

In contrast, topiramate is noted to clearly cause cognitive dysfunction and speech or word-finding difficulties in some patients. This can be avoided in patients with slow increases in the drug, but a small percentage is not able to tolerate even a single 25-mg dose.

Weight Gain Lithium-induced weight gain can be a vexing problem for a moderate percentage of patients and, in one study, was a correlate of better mood-stabilizing response to lithium. Thyroid indices should be rechecked, and the patient should be reminded not to use calorie-containing beverages when maintaining the necessary increased fluid intake associated with DI. Weight gain can also be problematic with valproate when used alone or, particularly, in combination with lithium. Topiramate has been used to help prevent or reverse weight gain induced with these agents. Its degree of weight loss parallels that of the FDA-approved drug sibutramine (Meridia).

Like most typical antipsychotics (with the exception of molindone [Moban]), the atypical antipsychotics can also be associated with moderate weight gain, and clozapine and olanzapine can be associated with substantial weight gain. However, ziprasidone and aripiprazole are weight neutral.

Topiramate has a strong tendency to help with weight loss, apparently by decreasing carbohydrate craving and possibly increasing metabolism as well. Another recently approved anticonvulsant, zonisamide, is also associated with weight loss. Oxcarbazepine, the L-type CCBs, and lamotrigine appear to be weight neutral (Table 13.8–5). In one 6-week study, patients lost approximately 2 lb on lamotrigine, showed no change on placebo, and gained approximately 2 lb on gabapentin.

Headache and Somatic Pain Many mood stabilizers, such as lithium, valproate, and the L-type CCBs, are reported to be effective in migraine prophylaxis. Carbamazepine increases substance P levels and sensitivity and may treat cluster headaches but can exacerbate migraine. Carbamazepine and oxcarbazepine are highly effective in a variety of paroxysmal pain syndromes, whereas gabapentin is widely used in neurology and internal medicine to adjunctively treat a variety of chronic pain syndromes. Lamotrigine may ameliorate or exacerbate headaches. Topiramate, lamotrigine, and levetiracetam may also be helpful in some pain syndromes.

Rash Lithium may precipitate or exacerbate psoriasis and acne. Isolated case reports suggest that the omega-3 fatty acid eicosapentaenoic acid (EPA) may ameliorate lithium-related psoriasis. Lamotrigine must be started extremely slowly to help avoid a serious rash; with rapid dose escalation, estimates suggest that one in 300 to 500 patients will progress to a severe, potentially lethal Stevens-Johnson syndrome or Lyell's syndrome. Using the now-conventional and mandated slow titration schedule, the risk for serious rash has decreased to 1 in 5,000 adults and 1 in 2,500 children. Risk factors, in addition to rate of titration and young age, include use with valproate (requiring a halving of the lamotrigine dose) and a history of severe rashes on other medications. If patients are off lamotrigine for more than 1 week, slow reinitiation and titration of the dose should again be used. Sudden large dose increases in the context of continuous ongoing treatment should also be avoided.

Carbamazepine may also produce a common pruritic rash (10 to 15 percent), but progression to a Stevens-Johnson syndrome may be less common than during lamotrigine treatment. Nonetheless, in most instances, carbamazepine should be discontinued with the onset of a rash. Sixty-five percent of those with a benign rash on carbamazepine do not rerash on oxcarbazepine. In cases that show evidence for the efficacy of carbamazepine, and if other effective treatments are not available, prednisone (Cordrol) has been reported to be effective in suppressing uncomplicated carbamazepine-induced rashes (i.e., those without evidence of systemic involvement with fever or lymphadenopathy) in a high percentage of patients. Whether a similar strategy would be effective for the benign lamotrigine rash remains unstudied.

Hepatitis and Pancreatitis Valproate has been associated with rare reports of severe hepatitis and pancreatitis in the neurological literature; most of the hepatic fatalities have been in children younger than 2 years of age, particularly those on polytherapy. Few serious hepatic side effects have been reported in adult psychiatric patients on valproic acid, but patients should be warned to report symptoms that might be referable to hepatitis, such as fever, right upper-quadrant pain, malaise, nausea, anorexia, Coca-Cola–colored urine, and jaundice. Symptoms of pancreatitis include severe abdominal pain and evidence of an acute abdomen, nausea, and anorexia, and an amylase level can be obtained to aid in the diagnosis. Benign elevation of liver function tests (LFTs) to two or three times normal is not uncommon on valproate, carbamazepine, and other anticonvulsants and can be followed without drug discontinuation. Zinc and selenium supplements are recommended with valproate, because they are suggested anecdotally to decrease the incidence of alopecia and, possibly, also hepatitis and pancreatitis. Rare cases of carbamazepine-induced hepatitis have also been reported, but routine monitoring for this side effect does not appear to be indicated. Because lithium and gabapentin are excreted by the kidney, they have no liability in those with evidence of liver pathology.

Hematological Effects The overall side effect profile of carbamazepine (Table 13.8–10) tends to be quite different from that of lithium or valproate (Tables 13.8–8 and 13.8–9). It is a useful rule of thumb that, whenever lithium and carbamazepine act on a common target system, the effects of lithium tend to override those of carbamazepine. In almost every instance, this is a clinical disadvantage, except in white-count suppression; in this case, the ability of lithium to increase the white count (via increases in colony-stimulating factor [CSF]) overrides the white-count–suppressing effects of carbamazepine (via decreasing CSF) and may be clinically useful in cases in which the absolute neutrophil count is below 1,500 cells.

However, lithium is effective in this regard only against carbamazepine's benign suppression of the white count, and its effects are doubtful if there is evidence of more problematic interference by carbamazepine in hematological function manifest in other cell lines, such as platelets or red cells, indicative of a possible pancytopenic or aplastic process. The risk of agranulocytosis and aplastic anemia on carbamazepine has been estimated to be from 1 in 10,000 to 1 in 100,000. Oxcarbazepine apparently does not possess these hematological liabilities. Valproate has been associated with thrombocytopenia; the potential impact of lithium on this syndrome has not been reported.

Teratogenicity The onset of bipolar illness often occurs during the childbearing years, and many women may already be on medication at the time of life when they want to conceive. Further, the postpartum period represents a time of high risk for relapse. The dilemma of taking medications must be considered in relation to the risks of being off medications. Cardiac anomalies (e.g., Ebstein's anomaly) have been reported to occur with a higher frequency than expected in patients treated with lithium during pregnancy compared to control populations, although recent studies suggest the risk may not be as great as originally reported. The best estimate of lithium-induced risk for Ebstein's anomaly is 10 to 20 times the baseline risk of 1 in 20,000 in the general population. This suggests that in utero exposure to lithium in the first trimester may result in a 1 in 1,000 chance of developing Ebstein's anomaly. This small risk must be weighed against the much higher risk of relapse of the mother if lithium is discontinued.

In some studies, risk of relapse has been estimated to be as high as 50 percent within the first 5 months after termination of lithium treatment. Thus, the previous recommendation against use of lithium during pregnancy is being reevaluated in the context of the risk of return of illness to a mother who discontinues her medication, especially if medications are stopped abruptly. In some instances in which the discontinuation of lithium would put the mother at high risk for a severe depression or mania, remaining on lithium may be appropriate, especially with increased ability for fetal monitoring. Neonate behavioral outcome from in utero lithium exposure suggests no long-term neurobehavioral sequelae in a few small studies.

An increased risk (2 to 5 percent) of spina bifida has been reported in relation to in utero exposure to valproate (which may be dose related), as well as a 1 to 3 percent risk for carbamazepine. Furthermore, minor congenital abnormalities (e.g., craniofacial anomalies) have been reported with both compounds. Folate supplements should be used to decrease this risk in instances in which the use of these agents cannot be avoided in pregnancy. These agents should be used only if other options are not possible. Even though folate has not been shown to reduce neural tube defects specifically in pregnant women on anticonvulsants, it has been shown to decrease risk for neural tube defects among the offspring of pregnant women in general. In light of folate's ability to potentiate the acute effects of antidepressants and the prophylactic effects of lithium, one would recommend folate supplementation (1 mg per day) in women of childbearing age and higher amounts during pregnancy. Vitamin K deficiencies have been reported with carbamazepine, and carbamazepine in utero could increase the risk of neonatal bleeding. It has been recommended by some to administer vitamin K 20 mg per day throughout pregnancy.

The North American Antiepileptic Drug Pregnancy Registry reports a rate of major malformations after first-trimester exposure to phenobarbital (12 percent) and valproate (8.6 percent). A retrospective registry of approximately 1,000 women reports a 1.8 percent rate on lamotrigine, which is similar to the 2 percent rate reported in the general population.

There are few data available for first trimester in utero exposure to gabapentin, but no specific teratogenic syndromes have been described. Topiramate causes some bone deformities in animals, but the risk for humans has not been described. ECT may have one of the lowest risks to the fetus among the somatic treatments and is sometimes recommended as an alternative intervention, if needed, in pregnancy, but the potential effects of maternal seizures on offspring have also not been systematically evaluated. The CCBs, such as verapamil and the dihydropyridines, have not shown fetal abnormalities, and these agents remain among the better candidates for continuation of a putative mood stabilizer during pregnancy.

Persisting biochemical alterations have been found in some animal studies of fetal exposure to typical antipsychotics, but their relevance to humans has not been systematically assessed. There is a slight but significantly increased risk for congenital abnormalities with first-trimester exposure to typical low-potency antipsychotic agents. Long-term neurobehavioral data, however, have not shown differences in behavior or intelligence quotient (IQ) in children exposed to antipsychotics in utero. Acute augmentation with atypical or higher-potency typical antipsychotics is often used, because no specific teratogenic effects of these agents have been reported. Studies of children with and without antipsychotic exposure show no differences in behavioral functioning or IQ when followed up to 5 years. The impact of benzodiazepine exposure in the first trimester as a risk for teratogenesis has been controversial but is probably associated with a small but significantly increased risk in congenital malformations.

Careful delineation of the known liabilities of carbamazepine and valproate for the major catastrophic congenital abnormality spina bifida and the much rarer incidence of lithium-related Ebstein's anomaly should be discussed with families in relation to close monitoring of the fetus along with an obstetrician, and these and other options should be considered when pregnancy is being sought.

Medication and Menstrual Irregularities

Lithium and carbamazepine do not appear to adversely affect the menstrual cycle. However, carbamazepine and other enzyme inducers may decrease levels of endogenous estrogens as well as the estrogens in oral contraceptives. Ongoing controversy surrounds the literature on the relationship of valproate to menstrual irregularities and polycystic ovary (PCO) syndrome. Several investigative groups have reported a higher incidence of the PCO syndrome (a constellation of endocrinological and clinical symptoms including overweight, menstrual irregularities, increased plasma testosterone, hirsutism, and PCOs) associated with long-term valproate use in women with epilepsy. Several investigators have studied whether the development of PCO syndrome occurs with long-term treatment with valproate in psychiatric patients. High rates of menstrual abnormalities in bipolar subjects using valproate have been reported. However, high rates of obesity and menstrual abnormalities have been found in general in subjects with bipolar disorder. To date, little direct evidence supports the idea that long-term valproate increases the risk for PCO syndrome in bipolar illness, but it may increase some of the elements of the syndrome, including increased levels of testosterone in one study but not in three others. Valproate increased levels of 17-hydroxyprogesterone and increased luteinizing hormone (LH)/follicle-stimulating hormone (FSH) ratios. The alterations and increases in prolactin associated with some antipsychotics could contribute to the increased rate of new-onset menstrual irregularities and anovulatory cycles on valproate.

Although it is still undetermined whether valproate use can cause PCO syndrome in women treated for bipolar disorder, if it were to occur, the syndrome appears reversible. When patients with epilepsy who developed PCO syndrome while taking valproate were switched to another anticonvulsant (lamotrigine), the syndrome reversed in a period of 6 months to 1 year after the switch. This indicates that the syndrome (as opposed to PCOs per se) can be reversed, even in those who have developed it on valproate. Furthermore, concomitant use of oral contraceptives has been reported to prevent the development of PCO syndrome in those taking valproate.

Although more definitive assessment of the role of valproate in the development of PCO syndrome symptoms in psychiatric patients is awaited, it would appear prudent to note the potential for these to occur in women of child-bearing age but not to preclude the use of this agent in women. If one does choose valproate as a therapeutic option, many psychotropics can cause weight gain, and the development of weight gain per se can result in the development of insulin resistance, high testosterone levels, and menstrual irregularities. One should also consider the concomitant use of birth control pills to help prevent or normalize the syndrome and encourage the development of regular menstrual cycles. Obtaining baseline weight and testosterone levels would further allow for observation of changes that might occur as a result of valproate treatment.

Osteoporosis

Women with affective illness appear to be at increased risk for osteoporosis in general. Reproductive-aged women with epilepsy taking carbamazepine, valproate, and phenytoin had decreased calcium levels compared with those taking lamotrigine, but only phenytoin was associated with increased bone turnover. Lithium increases calcium levels and may be associated with relative hyperparathyroidism.

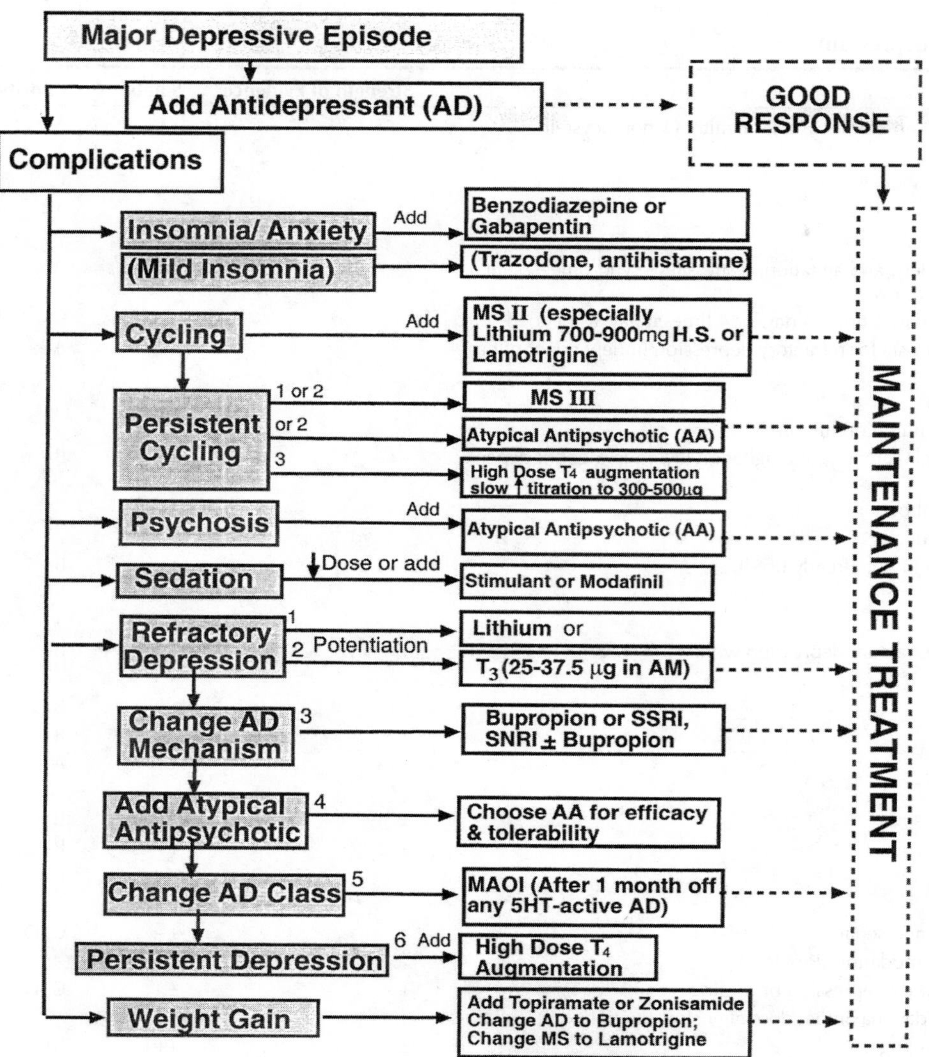

FIGURE 13.8–12 Options for treatment of bipolar depression emerging despite use of ongoing mood stabilizer (MS): possible treatment approaches to symptom targets. H.S., single nighttime; MAOI, monoamine oxidase inhibitor; SNRI, serotonin and noradrenaline reuptake inhibitor; SSRI, selective serotonin reuptake inhibitor; T_3, triiodothyronine; T_4, thyroxine.

Given the available data, women with bipolar illness should ingest adequate levels of calcium (1,200 mg per day) and vitamin D, engage in gravity-resisting exercise, and consider bone-density scans, repeated at 3- to 5-year intervals in premenopause, especially if they have been on long-term treatment with cabamazepine, valproate, or phenytoin.

TREATMENT OF BREAKTHROUGH DEPRESSIVE EPISODES DURING PROPHYLAXIS

Antidepressant Augmentation Although tricyclic and heterocyclic antidepressants, SSRIs, serotonin and noradrenaline reuptake inhibitors (SNRIs), and MAOIs are central treatments for the unipolar depressed patient, there is reason for caution in their use for the bipolar patient (Fig. 13.8–12, Tables 13.8–16 and 13.8–18). Some studies have reported an increased incidence of switches into hypomania or mania observed during TCA or MAOI therapy that is higher than expected for the patient's natural course of illness. Although there is still debate regarding whether this increased incidence of switching is sufficient to avoid the initial use of antidepressants in favor of mood stabilizers, there is evidence that these compounds can speed up the rate of cycling in rapid-cycling patients. Thus, a shorter depression may occur at the cost of the more rapid onset of the following manic episode, whereas withdrawal of TCAs and MAOIs has also been shown to slow this cycle acceleration in a small number of patients.

There are also uncontrolled observations that TCAs and related compounds may be implicated in the development of continuous-cycling phases (i.e., successive episodes without a well interval) (Fig. 13.8–12). This phase of the illness becomes difficult to treat and tends to be relatively lithium refractory. There is anecdotal evidence and one double-blind, randomized study indicating that bupropion may not be associated with the same tendency of switching as the TCA DMI. The role of the SSRIs in the switch phenomenon and in cycle induction may also be less than that of the tricyclics, but this too requires further investigation, because the use of SSRIs and the commencement of rapid or continuous cycling have been observed anecdotally.

As noted previously, a recent double-blind, randomized study revealed a lower switch rate for bupropion in comparison to venlafaxine, and an open, randomized study also found a higher switch rate for venlafaxine compared to paroxetine. The DMI and

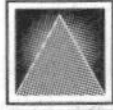

Table 13.8–18
Augmentation Strategies for Antidepressants

	Strength of Evidence[a]	Safety[b]	Priority[c]
1. *Folic acid* for antidepressant potentiation (and cardiovascular health) (↓ homocysteine)	+++	+++	A
800 μg–1 mg women			
1,600 μg–2 mg men			
2. *Ascorbate*	+	+++	A–
3,000 mg/day for depression and fatigue			
3. *Gabapentin* (Neurontin) for insomnia, anxiety, and agitation; restless legs syndrome; social phobia; pain syndromes; and alcohol withdrawal	++	+++	A–
100–400 mg at bedtime and then twice a day, 3 times a day, or 4 times a day, as needed			
4. T_3 (liothyronine [Cytomel]) 25.0–37.5 μg in AM for refractory depression (independent of baseline thyroid function)	++	++	A–
20–40% response in refractory depression			
May accelerate response and improve cognition on lithium			
5. High-potency *benzodiazepines* for insomnia, anxiety, and agitation (avoid in alcohol dependency)	+++	+++	B+
Clonazepam (Klonopin), 0.5–2.0 mg/day at bedtime			
Lorazepam (Ativan), 0.5–2.0 mg/day at bedtime			
6. *Lithium* (Eskalith) for refractory depression (if not already used)	+++	+	B+
600–900 mg/d at bedtime			
40–60% response in unipolar depression			
7. *Atypical antipsychotic* for psychosis and refractory depression with:	++	+ to +++	B+
Insomnia, anxiety, and anorexia			
Olanzapine (Zyprexa)	++	+	B
Risperidone (Risperdal)	±	++	B
Quetiapine (Seroquel)	+++	++	A–
Hypersomnia			
Ziprasidone (Geodon)	±	++	B+
Aripiprazole (Abilify)	±	+++	B+
8. *Inositol* for refractory depression	+	+++	B+
12–18 g			
9. *Stimulants* for AM retardation, immobility, and sedation	+	++	C, D
(Try bupropion [Wellbutrin] first; consider modafinil [Provigil])			
10. *Suprathreshold thyroid* hormone for refractory depression or cycling	++	±	C, D
T_4 (levothyroxine [Synthroid]) 300–500 μg/day maximum dose after slow titration			
11. *Omega-3 fatty acids* for depression and cycling	±	+++	B
1–2 g EPA (6 g not effective)			
6–9 g mixture of docosahexaenoic acid and EPA			
12. *Naltrexone* (ReVia) for alcohol craving (50 mg in AM)	+++	+++	B
Topiramate (Topamax) for alcohol craving	+++	++	B
13. *Naltrexone* for self-mutilation	+	+++	B
50 mg in AM			
14. *Acetylcholinesterase inhibitors* for cognitive dysfunction on antidepressants	+	±	C
5–10 mg donepezil (Aricept)			
15. *Memantine* (Namenda) for cognitive dysfunction or refractory depression	±	+++	B
30 mg/day, in divided doses			
16. *Glucocorticoid antagonists* for refractory (psychotic) depression	++	++	C, D
Ketoconazole (Nizoral), 400–800 mg/day			
Mifepristone (RU-486), 600 mg/day			

EPA, eicosapentaenoic acid.
[a]Strength: ±, equivocal; +, some open data; ++, much open data; +++, good controlled data or wide use.
[b]Safety: ±, Some serious reactions possible; +, relatively safe, some problematic side effects; ++, few problematic side effects; +++, essentially no side effects.
[c]Priority: A, no reason not to use; A–, promising approach; B+, use may be indicated; B, judicious use; C, careful assessment of risks; D, consider use late in algorithm because of possible difficulties relative to strength of efficacy data.

venlafaxine data implicate blockade of NE reuptake in the increased switch proclivity. Given the relative adverse side effect profile of the tertiary TCA compared with second- and third-generation antidepressants, these latter agents are recommended over the TCAs.

One study found that, once a switch has been observed on an MAOI, reexposure to even a different MAOI also led to a switch with an earlier onset than in the first instance, perhaps reflecting a sensitization phenomenon. Naturalistic data, however, raise questions about whether antidepressant-induced switches consistently occur on each exposure to these drugs. Moreover, it is unclear whether a drug-induced switch appears only in those predestined to have spontaneous switches or whether this occurrence actually predisposes the patient to develop further spontaneous manic episodes that do occur in a high percentage of patients. Patients with rapid-cycling presentations may be at higher risk for antidepressant-induced switching or cycle acceleration than those without.

However, it is acknowledged from the outset that a strong empirical database for recommendations on antidepressant use is lacking. Moreover, given the necessity for protracted clinical trials (of many weeks) to evaluate the clinical efficacy of each individual drug, it is recommended to attempt to potentiate a specific drug treatment once adequate doses or blood levels have been reached before switching treatment modalities (Table 13.8–18). Thus, thyroid or lithium potentiation deserves an earlier emphasis in the treatment sequence over multiple trials with single alternative agents. As noted previously, lamotrigine augmentation instead of a unimodal antidepressant has much to recommend it, especially if the patient is at high risk for antidepressant-induced mania, that is, with a history of rapid cycling or substance abuse, prior antidepressant-related switches, or a pattern of mania immediately preceding the depression being treated.

Rates of Switching into Hypomania or Mania in Acute Antidepressant Trials Switch rates into hypomania or mania in subjects acutely treated for bipolar depression have varied widely. Additional risk factors for switching include antidepressant type, absence of or subtherapeutic concomitant mood stabilizer dose or levels, bipolar I disorder, and treatment refractoriness. However, low switch rates in acute studies need to be distinguished from those occurring with longer-term observations during continuation treatment or prophylaxis.

Moreover, lower switch rates are consistently reported in studies that have excluded rapid-cycling patients. The natural switch rate into mania within 8 weeks after a depression, however, can be high and can lead to the incorrect conclusion that antidepressants precipitated the switch, when it was actually due to the illness itself. Data from one older study found a switch rate of 41 percent from depression to mania in bipolar inpatients taking no medications during hospitalization.

Four recent large, randomized, controlled treatment trials of non–rapid-cycling patients with bipolar I disorder depression have enhanced understanding of the natural versus drug-induced switch rate from bipolar depression into mania and the effect of different classes of antidepressants on the likelihood of switching. In a 7-week acute treatment trial of two doses of lamotrigine for the treatment of bipolar depression, clinical efficacy over placebo was found at both doses, with no greater acute switch rate on lamotrigine (5.4 percent) than on placebo (4.6 percent). The trial operationalized switching as an investigator-reported adverse event, in which the patient developed hypomania, mania, or a mixed state. In the other three randomized, controlled studies, there was no placebo group, but the acute switch rates on second-generation unimodal antidepressants were low (5 to 15 percent).

In relation to whether one group of antidepressants is more likely than another to induce an acute switch, six studies of non–rapid-cycling patients currently address the question. TCAs appear slightly more prone to cause switching than MAOIs, and, in one randomized study, the TCA DMI caused much higher switch rates than the second-generation antidepressant bupropion. In a recent 10-week acute treatment trial of 117 subjects with bipolar depression, 8 percent of patients receiving lithium plus TCA, 2 percent of patients receiving lithium plus placebo, and 0 percent of patients receiving lithium plus paroxetine switched into mania. Patients had a range of lithium levels, and it is not clear from the data presented if the patients who had switched into mania were those with lower levels of lithium.

A recent review of clinical trials also found a higher acute switch rate for TCAs (11.2 percent) compared to SSRIs (3.7 percent) or placebo (4.2 percent) (SSRI versus TCA, $P < .01$). If the 4.6 percent placebo switch rate from the lamotrigine study is used as a historical control of a natural switch rate in non–rapid-cycling patients, it appears that MAOIs may double the natural switch rate, and TCAs may triple the natural switch rate.

Switch rates were assessed in patients with bipolar depression entered into a trial of 10 weeks of double-blind treatment with the second-generation antidepressants sertraline (Zoloft), venlafaxine, or bupropion as adjunctive therapy to mood stabilizers. As a group, 9.1 percent of the trials of these medications were associated with an acute switch into hypomania, and another 9.1 percent of trials were associated with an acute switch into hypomania or mania (i.e., with some dysfunction). It is noteworthy that rapid cyclers were not excluded from this study, and that factor and the careful daily prospective rating might account for the higher acute switch rates in comparison with other studies of second-generation antidepressants noted above. The higher switch rate for venlafaxine than for bupropion (and intermediate for sertraline) has been noted previously.

Whether the concomitant use of mood stabilizers can block the induction of mania by heterocyclic antidepressants used acutely or chronically is a question that requires further study. Four prior studies suggest a lack of complete protection by a mood stabilizer against the mania-inducing properties of antidepressants, and four have suggested a protective effect.

Switch Rates during Longer Trials of Antidepressants In one review of 15 placebo-controlled long-term studies, data suggested a protective effect of a mood stabilizer against the proportion of switches that may be acutely antidepressant-induced. The incidence of hypomania and mania in the 158 patients specifically diagnosed as bipolar was 51 percent in the 49 patients treated with imipramine (Tofranil) alone, 21 percent in the 60 patients treated with lithium alone, 28 percent in the 36 treated with lithium and imipramine, and 23 percent in the 13 taking only placebo, suggesting that approximately one-half of the total switch rate for patients taking TCAs may be attributable to the TCAs and that lithium is able to attenuate this rate.

Optimal Duration of Antidepressant Treatment For bipolar subjects who have a successful antidepressant response when an antidepressant is added to an ongoing mood-stabilizer regimen for treatment of a depressive episode that did not respond to treatment with a mood stabilizer or that occurred despite ongoing mood-stabilizer treatment (e.g., a breakthrough depression), the risk of a depressive relapse may be increased by the common clinical practice of discontinuing the antidepressant soon after remission. Continuing antidepressants after remission of a depressive episode may protect against relapse into depression over the following year and does not appear, in one sample, to increase risk for manic relapse (Fig. 13.8–13). It should be noted that the majority of bipolar subjects given antidepressants do not respond or do not remain well. However, for the small subgroup that responds successfully to antidepressant augmentation and remains well or does not switch into mania within the first 2 months, continuation may reduce depressive relapses. Definitive results are awaited based on randomized prospective data, however.

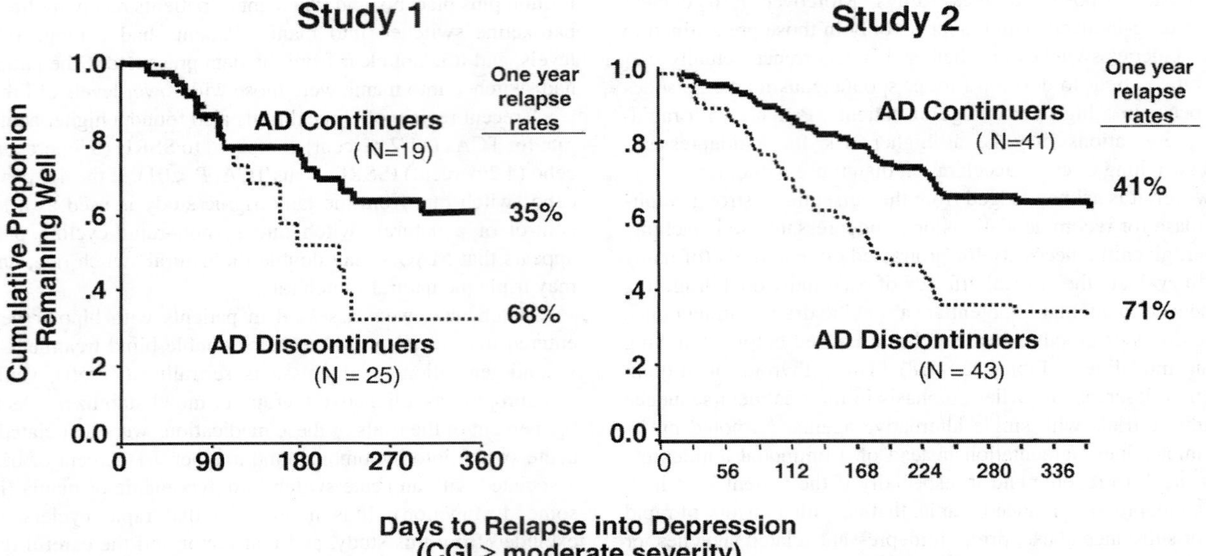

FIGURE 13.8–13 Increased rate of relapse into depression in bipolar patients who discontinued antidepressants (ADs) (with ADs as adjuncts to mood stabilizers). CGI, Clinical Global Impression. (From Altshuler L, Kiriakos L, Calcagno J, et al.: The impact of antidepressant discontinuation versus antidepressant continuation on 1-year risk for relapse of bipolar depression: A retrospective chart review. *J Clin Psychiatry.* 2001;62:612–616; and Altshuler L, Suppes T, Black D, et al.: Impact of antidepressant discontinuation after acute remission from bipolar depression on rates of depressive relapse at 1-year follow-up. *Am J Psychiatry.* 2003;160:1245–1250, with permission.)

If unimodal antidepressants are used for a bipolar depression, clinical lore had previously suggested that they should be tapered and discontinued as soon as possible to avoid the potential for drug-induced switches and cycle acceleration, because lithium and other mood stabilizers may not consistently be able to prevent switching. However, maintenance therapy with bupropion and lithium has been reported to be effective in rapid-cycling patients, and continuing to use the second-generation unimodal antidepressants in conjunction with the new putative mood stabilizers deserves consideration.

Potentiation of the Antidepressant

Antidepressant potentiation should be considered in the first or second antidepressant trial before switching antidepressants, even to a new category of agents. Thus, when a patient appears to be at maximally tolerated doses (or adequate blood levels of the drug) and has not responded adequately, one might consider the addition of thyroid hormones or lithium carbonate as potentiation strategies (Tables 13.8–16, 13.8–18, and 13.8–19). Alternatively, a second antidepressant with a different mechanism of action can be added to assess augmentation of the first.

Thyroid Hormone There is a sizable literature in unipolar depression regarding the efficacy of thyroid potentiation in converting (20 to 30 percent or higher) antidepressant nonresponders to responders. This effect appears to be independent of an initial clinical thyroid status or any evidence of hypothyroidism. A response to the addition of T_3 (25 to 37.5 μg per day in the AM) may occur within days, usually within the first week or two of treatment. Therefore, if there is no response in this time frame, the clinical trial of T_3 potentiation can be exchanged for other options, but, in practice, it is often continued for its potential usefulness on lithium-related cognitive side effects and prophylaxis of future episodes. T_3 can also be initiated at the onset of the antidepressant administration in hope of accelerating the rate of antidepressant responses, as reported in some series in unipolar depression. Side effects of T_3 are unusual but may include tachycardia, hypertension, anxiety, flushing, or sweating.

Lithium Augmentation A second option is potentiation of the antidepressant with lithium carbonate if lithium is not already part of the treatment regimen. An extensive literature, particularly in unipolar depression, documents that the addition of lithium carbon-

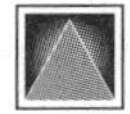

Table 13.8–19
Possible Augmentation Strategies for Circadian Dysregulation in Bipolar Depression

Circadian Dysregulation	Treatment	Strength of Evidence
Delayed to normal sleep onset—AM hypersomnia	Lamotrigine (Lamictal) in AM	++
	Bupropion (Wellbutrin) stimulants in AM	+
	High-intensity light in AM	++
	Sleep deprivation and phase advance	++
	Melatonin at bedtime	±
	Stimulant in AM	±
	AM atypical ziprasidone (Geodon)	+
Insomnia and early-morning awakening	PM high-potency benzodiazepine or gabapentin (Neurontin)	++
	PM valproic acid (Depakene), carbamazepine (Tegretol), and oxcarbazepine (Trileptal)	++
	PM atypical olanzapine (Zyprexa), risperidone (Risperdal), and quetiapine (Seroquel)	++
	Melatonin at bedtime	+
	Glucocorticoid antagonists	++
	High-intensity light in PM??	±

±, ambiguous data; +, some open data; ++, much open data.

ate to virtually any of the unimodal antidepressants is often (40 to 60 percent of the time) accompanied by clinical improvement. Response may begin within 24 to 48 hours but may be slower in onset and may stretch over 1 to 3 weeks. Doses of lithium that are slightly lower than those conventionally used for monotherapy are generally effective (i.e., 750 to 900 mg in a single HS dose may be sufficient to reach a target of 0.75 mEq/L, which is the level reported needed for potentiation in unipolar depression). When used in this fashion, the side effect profile of lithium appears to be quite benign. Lithium potentiation may be effective for all subtypes of depression.

Folate Augmentation One might consider folate augmentation (1 mg per day in women and 2 mg per day in men) for a variety of reasons. The U.S. diet is generally folate deficient, and one recent controlled study indicated folate (500 μg per day) was more effective than placebo in antidepressant augmentation. Folate at the higher doses mentioned are suggested by nutritional experts, and folate has other potential beneficial effects with no known liabilities. It may be useful in preventing myocardial infarction and perhaps in delaying onset of Alzheimer's dementia, based on its ability to decrease levels of homocysteine. Folate augmentation of valproate would appear to be indicated, as valproate increases levels of homocysteine.

Benzodiazepine Augmentation for Sleep and Anxiety Several case reports suggest that alprazolam (Xanax), like the TCAs, may also induce switches into hypomania and mania (even in unpredisposed patients), and this high-potency benzodiazepine should be avoided in favor of the long half-life compounds clonazepam and lorazepam, which do not appear to share the proclivity of the triazole benzodiazepine compounds for the induction of mania. These high-potency benzodiazepines may be useful adjuncts to the mood stabilizers; however, the rare patient may experience these classic benzodiazepines as mood destabilizing or even depressive. Gabapentin may also be a useful alternative to the benzodiazepines.

Shifting Antidepressant Classes: MAOIs One might consider shifting treatment from one type of antidepressant to another, should unacceptable side effects appear before adequate blood levels or a clinical response has been achieved. If adequate doses and blood levels have been achieved, but the response is inadequate, one may switch to a drug with a different biochemical profile within the same class or to a different class, such as an MAOI (Table 13.8–16). Problems with orthostatic hypotension may become more prominent in the second and third weeks of MAOI treatment. Salt loading, pressure stockings, and fludrocortisone (Florinef) may prove to be effective in the treatment of MAOI-induced hypotension. MAOIs can be given in single AM doses or in a divided dose. If marked insomnia occurs, nighttime doses of trazodone (Desyrel) have been recommended by some authorities, because it does not induce a 5-HT syndrome as will the SSRIs and related 5-HT–potent compounds. Irresistible daytime drowsiness and sedation may also become a problem. One might attempt to titrate the dose against side effects, as variations in dose or timing may be helpful on rare occasions.

The necessity of restricting substances that release tyramine or catecholamines and that can produce hypertensive crises during MAOI treatment should be emphasized to the patient. These crises may be clinically manifested as explosive headaches, flushing, palpitations, perspiration, and nausea. Some authorities suggest that patients carry a 10-mg nifedipine capsule with them that they could use sublingually or bite and swallow in the event of a hypertensive crisis while on the way to medical evaluation. Immediate treatment with a slow infusion of phentolamine (Regitine) (5 mg IV) in an emergency department has been a recommended treatment.

Some evidence suggests that the MAOIs, in general, may be less prone than the TCAs to induce switches. The MAOIs should be given relatively greater consideration, especially for the reversal of vegetative (anergic, hypersomnic, or hyperphagic) states in the bipolar patient. A substantially higher rate of antidepressant response has been reported in one controlled series for tranylcypromine (Parnate) (81 percent) compared with imipramine (48 percent) in bipolars. Clorgyline, a selective monoamine oxidase type A inhibitor that is not clinically available, has been reported to slow cycling frequency. The reversible inhibitor of monoamine oxidase type A (RIMA) moclobemide (Manerix) is widely available in Europe and Canada but not in the United States, and this drug is not believed to be as effective an antidepressant as the nonselective MAOIs tranylcypromine or phenelzine (Nardil). These MAOIs are unique in potentially all three amine systems (5-HT, NE, and DA). One could attempt such an equivalent effect by using venlafaxine (for its 5-HT and NE effects) in combination with bupropion (for its DA effects).

Adding a Second Mood Stabilizer or Atypical Antipsychotic The unimodal antidepressants should be used cautiously in conjunction with mood stabilizers for bipolar depressive episodes, particularly if there is a history of rapid- or ultrarapid-cycling and prior drug-induced switches. For the depressed bipolar patient, adding a second or even a third mood stabilizer (lithium, lamotrigine, carbamazepine, valproate, or an atypical antipsychotic) can be considered even before adding a standard unimodal antidepressant (Table 13.8–16). Which of the two approaches (adding two mood stabilizers versus adding an antidepressant to a mood stabilizer) is best for acute treatment and maintenance remains to be determined. One study by Trevor Young and colleagues found that the combination of lithium and valproate (two mood stabilizers) was equal in efficacy to a mood stabilizer–antidepressant combination, but patients on the former had more side effects. No other comparative efficacy study has been done to date. In the face of ultradian cycling, the dihydropyridine L-type CCBs may also be considered.

Dopamine Active Compounds and Other Treatments

Bupropion As noted previously, bupropion has shown promise in the acute and prophylactic management of bipolar patients, including rapid-cycling patients. Whereas it may be added to lithium or valproate prophylaxis without pharmacokinetic interactions, when used with carbamazepine, its blood levels are markedly decreased, and those of an active metabolite are increased.

Psychomotor Stimulants The role of psychomotor stimulants as an acute augmentation strategy has not been systematically explored, although it is apparently widely used by some experts in the field. However, Jan Fawcett has indicated that this is not a useful long-term strategy, because many patients appear to develop tolerance to this modality, and, therefore, this strategy should perhaps be reserved for temporary augmentation while awaiting more effective antidepressant response to other modalities (Table 13.8–19). The same investigator has also observed that tolerance does not appear to develop when the psychomotor stimulants are combined with MAOIs. This strategy should, perhaps, be reserved for the end of the treatment algorithm in only the most refractory patients, because the PDR lists an absolute contraindication to combining stimulants and MAOIs. Nonetheless, this appears to be a well-tolerated treatment in many small case series. In children with the bipolar disorder–ADHD comorbidity, stimulants in monotherapy can fuel an irritable dysphoric state, but small doses may be helpful for residual ADHD symptoms once mood has been stabilized with one or more mood stabilizers.

Dopamine Agonists Small clinical series have suggested some antidepressant efficacy of the direct DA agonist bromocriptine (Parlodel), which is used to treat parkinsonian patients. One double-blind study indicated that, compared to imipramine, it was equally effective. A related DA agonist, piribedil (Trivastal), has reportedly been effective for some refractory depressed patients. Pergolide (Permax) also has been reported as an effective augmenting agent in one series on refractory depression but not in another.

Pramipexole (Mirapex), a more potent D_3 than D_2 agonist recently approved for use in parkinsonism, is reported (at approximately 1 mg per day) to have antidepressant effects in unipolar depression equivalent to those of fluoxetine. A recent controlled study has now documented this in bipolar depressed individuals used at a mean dose of 1.7 mg per day. A second study has now confirmed these findings. The drug should be started at low doses and slowly titrated toward a target of 1 mg per day to avoid side effects such as nausea and orthostatic hypotension.

DA-active drugs had been reported to be more effective in those patients with low levels of the DA metabolite homovanillic acid (HVA) in their cerebrospinal fluid (CSF). A similar relation to low levels of the 5-HT metabolite 5-hydroxyindoleacetic acid (5-HIAA) and a better response to the 5-HT active compounds clomipramine (Anafranil) and sertraline have been reported. The results are inconclusive as to whether urinary levels of the NE metabolite 3-methoxy-4-hydroxyphenylglycol (MHPG) can predict the response to noradrenergically active antidepressants. Consistent biochemical markers of antidepressant response have not yet been identified.

Other Augmentation Strategies

Light in Morning and Melatonin at Night Systematic trials of augmentation with bright light (greater than 7,500 lux and the ideal of 10,000 lux) may also be worth considering in patients beyond those with seasonal affective disorder with marked disruption of circadian rhythmicity and the typical bipolar hypersomnia. In these instances, high-intensity light might be more useful in the AM, although this issue needs to be revisited with more systematic prospective randomized studies (Table 13.8–19).

An additional approach to altering sleep activity cycles (which are common in bipolar patients) might be to use melatonin adjunctively at night, although this too requires caution and prospective studies. In addition, there have been isolated reports of exacerbation of sleep or mood in some patients when using melatonin supplementation. Rather than the 1 to 5 mg often used, 40 μg may be sufficient.

Sleep Deprivation as an Acute-Acting Antidepressant Paradoxically, sleep deprivation may be an adjunctive procedure to hasten the onset of antidepressant response. An acute, but transient, antidepressant response to one night of sleep deprivation has been reported consistently in studies from many different laboratories. The response to sleep deprivation for bipolar subjects may be even greater (up to 80 percent) than that reported for unipolar subjects. Preliminary evidence suggests that deprivation of sleep in the last one-half of the night (from 3 to 7 AM) may be just as effective as total sleep deprivation and may thus be more convenient for clinical use and outpatient treatment.

Although many patients relapse after one night's recovery sleep, there is evidence that some modalities, especially lithium, may help sustain the sleep deprivation response. One recent report also indicates that progressive changes in the hours of sleep (from 5 PM to 2 AM on the sleep deprivation day, to 6 PM to 3 AM the next night, from 7 PM to 4 AM the next, etc. toward an 11 PM bedtime) also helps hold a sleep deprivation response.

The rapid onset of effects achieved in approximately one-half of severely depressed patients is different from the slower, but sustained, effects after selective deprivation of rapid eye movement (REM) sleep that is not amenable to easy clinical use. Response to sleep deprivation may be related to phase or duration of the depressive episode, with poor response occurring when sleep deprivation is attempted early in an episode and better response occurring when sleep deprivation is used toward the end of an episode. Several, but not all, studies indicate that the degree of antidepressant response to sleep deprivation is correlated with the degree of increase in AM plasma TSH, presumably driven by endogenous increases in TRH. In this regard, parenteral TRH administration (500 μg IV or subcutaneously) itself has also been reported to have rapid onset of antidepressant effects, and two case reports suggest more sustained effects when daily low doses (50 μg per day HS) are used.

Omega-3 Fatty Acids One randomized, double-blind study comparing the addition of omega-3 fatty acids (9 g per day) or an olive oil placebo in poorly controlled bipolar patients on inadequate mood stabilizers was terminated early at a planned interim analysis because of the marked superiority of the omega-3 fatty acid. Virtually all of the breakthrough depressive episodes occurred in the placebo control group, and almost none occurred in the active group. Several other studies in unipolar depression using 1 to 2 g per day of EPA have been positive. However, preliminary results from two large follow-up studies in bipolar depressed and cycling patients using 6 g of EPA versus placebo for 4 months were not positive. Explanations include use of too high an EPA dose, which paradoxically decreases arachidonic acid, or that only a subgroup of patients who have the expected increase in membrane docosahexaenoic acid (DHA) are responsive.

Inositol Inositol (12 to 16 g per day) has recently been reported to have antidepressant, antianxiety, and anti-OCD effects. Inositol is a membrane constituent that is generated in the phosphatidylinositol (PI) second messenger system used by many neurotransmitter receptor subtypes. The generation of inositol in the PI cycle is blocked by lithium. Therapeutic use of inositol remains to be more systematically explored in bipolar patients in light of one series reporting a 50 percent response rate (and no switches into mania) in patients who were concomitantly treated with lithium, carbamazepine, or valproate, and another study that found a much lower response rate. Theoretically, inositol should not only relieve some lithium-induced side effects, but could also potentially reverse its therapeutic efficacy to the extent that inositol depletion from reduced PI turnover is related to lithium's mechanism of action. *Myo*-inositol measured by magnetic resonance spectroscopy has been reported to be low in brains of bipolar patients (in proportion to the severity of their depression); lithium lowers it further. One would then predict that inositol augmentation might make carbamazepine even more effective, because carbamazepine has the opposite effects of lithium on the inositol 1-phosphatase enzyme. Lithium, carbamazepine, and valproate are all reported to inhibit the transporter for inositol that has recently been isolated and cloned.

Choline One open study, requiring replication, reported that potentiation with choline (3 to 8 g per day) may be helpful in stabilizing mood in those with refractory cycling.

Approaches to Suicidal Tendency Regular psychiatric visits during the prophylactic well phase are recommended on an interval ranging from weekly to biweekly in unstable patients to 1 to 4 months in better-stabilized patients, depending on a variety of ancillary circumstances, including completeness of response, lack of psychosocial crises, excellent history of compliance, lack of ambivalence about the process, absence of side effects, financial constraints, and the wishes of the patient. In addition to periodic assessment of all of these issues, regular treatment visits are recommended to assess the potential risks of suicide independently of the occurrence of discrete episodes. This is particularly important in instances in which there is a positive family history of suicide or other risk factors, including male gender, older age, early severe and concomitant psychosocial stressors, comorbid alcohol abuse, comorbid anxiety and eating disorders, prior suicide attempts, loss of social supports, and increased numbers of prior depressions (Fig. 13.8–8). Furthermore, in many bipolar subjects, there is a seasonal component to their affective episodes (commonly increased in fall and spring), and, in those subjects with predictable seasonal depressions or suicide attempts, close monitoring during these times may help prevent such episodes.

Suicidal impulses and acts may not always directly vary with severity of depression or reemergence of a full-blown episode requiring hospitalization and should be part of the careful ongoing clinical assessment of each patient throughout his or her treatment. Severe overwhelming psychic anxiety and agitation have been shown to be predictors of completed suicide, and, with the high comorbidity of panic disorder with either phase of bipolar illness, one should be particularly alert to this and other high risk factors (Fig. 13.8–8). Specific contracting (Table 13.8–20) for communication with the clinician on reemergence of suicidal thoughts should be considered in patients with some of the risk factors described previously.

ECT ECT may also be useful for bipolar depressed patients who do not respond to lithium or other mood stabilizers and their adjuncts, particularly in cases in which intense suicidal tendency presents as a medical emergency. Whether ECT would continue to help abbreviate recurrent depressive episodes in rapid-cycling patients or whether it would have sustained effects in long-term prophylaxis should be further investigated. The authors have observed several instances in which tolerance to the therapeutic effects of ECT develops, as well as rather profound degrees of sustained retrograde memory loss. The recent development of right unilateral high-dose ultrabrief pulse ECT parameters may help obviate this serious long-term side effect.

Anecdotal reports have indicated that the interval between ECT treatments can be gradually lengthened to find the longest intervals required to maintain response. One group reports success with the combination of clozapine and ECT for maintenance treatment in refractory bipolar patients, which would take advantage of clozapine's ability to lower seizure threshold (avoiding the need for caffeine pretreatment in those with elevated seizure thresholds) and ECT's ability to act as an anticonvulsant (putatively also for clozapine's proconvulsant effects).

COMPLEX COMBINATION THERAPY

As noted previously, the strategy supplementing the clinical effects of lithium or the mood-stabilizing anticonvulsants with the other modal-

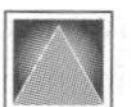

Table 13.8–20
Principles in the Treatment of Bipolar Disorders

Maintain dual treatment focus: (1) acute short term and (2) prophylaxis.
Chart illness retrospectively and prospectively.
Mania as medical emergency: Treat first, chemistries later.
Load valproate and lithium (Eskalith); titrate lamotrigine (Lamictal) slowly.
Careful combination treatment can decrease adverse effects.
Augment rather than substitute in treatment-resistant patient.
Retain lithium in regimen for its antisuicide and neuroprotective effects.
Taper lithium slowly, if at all.
Educate patient and family about illness and risk to benefit ratios of acute and prophylactic treatments.
Give statistics (i.e., 50 percent relapse in first 5 mos off lithium).
Assess compliance and suicidality regularly.
Develop an early warning system for identification and treatment of emergent symptoms.
Contract with patient as needed for suicide and substance use avoidance.
Use regular visits; monitor course and adverse effects.
Arrange for interval phone contact when needed.
Develop fire drill for mania reemergence.
Inquire about and address comorbid alcohol and substance abuse.
Targeted psychotherapy; use medicalization of illness.
Treat patient as a coinvestigator in the development of effective clinical approaches to the illness.
If treatment is successful, be conservative in making changes, maintain the course, and continue full-dose pharmacoprophylaxis in absence of side effects.
If treatment response is inadequate, be aggressive in searching for more effective alternatives.

ity is often more effective than using lithium or the anticonvulsant alone in rapid-cycling patients. By augmenting rather than substituting a mood stabilizer, withdrawal-induced exacerbations will not confound the evaluation of the next agent, and considerable time may be saved in the assessment of only one additional clinical trial of the combination rather than two sequential monotherapy trials (and then the combination). For patients who are unable to tolerate lithium carbonate, evidence does suggest that carbamazepine or valproate may be useful long-term maintenance treatments in preventing manic and depressive episodes. There is a rather substantial literature on open clinical trials with carbamazepine, and, now, multiple double-blind studies provide evidence of its prophylactic efficacy. Most of the prophylactic data on valproate are based on clinical case series, however. The choice of carbamazepine or valproate may depend on the development of clinical predictors or on the current assessment of their relative side effect profiles (Tables 13.8–9, 13.8–10, and 13.8–17). The data are even more preliminary for the L-type CCBs and the new putative mood-stabilizing agents, such as lamotrigine.

All of these agents have differential presumptive biochemical mechanisms of action. One can begin to use augmenting strategies, not only on the basis of empiricism, but also on the basis of combining agents with different actions (Tables 13.8–2 and 13.8–6), symptom targets (Table 13.8–4), side effect profiles (Tables 13.8–8 through 13.8–10), or benign pharmacokinetic and pharmacodynamic interactions (Table 13.8–14). It is unclear whether two drugs potentiating the action of the same neurotransmitter systems by two different molecular mechanisms will be less effective than simultaneously targeting two entirely different systems, such as simultaneously enhancing GABAergic inhibition and inhibiting glutamatergic excitation, but such a strategy is generally recommended.

Using several drugs in combination may actually help reduce the incidence of side effects by keeping each drug below its side effect threshold rather than pushing one drug to maximum doses for full therapeutic effect. It is also possible, based on preclinical evidence, that such a combination strategy will be less susceptible to the development of loss of effectiveness via tolerance. Optimally, one would like to use drugs with additive or synergistic therapeutic effects in the relative absence of side effects. As such, knowledge of pharmacokinetic as well as pharmacodynamic interactions is of considerable importance.

Data from a number of investigative groups indicate that increasing numbers of treatment-resistant patients require treatment with multimodal drug combinations. In one retrospective case series, patients in the years 1970 to 1974 required only monotherapy on discharge more than 75 percent of the time. This decreased to less than 25 percent of the time in the 1990s, and the average number of medications used at the time of discharge increased over the same time frame from one medication to more than three medications per patient. This increase was necessary to achieve the same high rate of improvement (75 to 80 percent) before discharge. Although these data, based on sequential augmentation strategies, did not involve a systematic randomized approach to therapeutics in this discharge phase of the hospitalization, they nonetheless reveal that many treatment-refractory patients can be managed with multiple mood stabilizers in combination, often with thyroid augmentation.

As in the late phases of other medical syndromes, complex combination treatment is often required for the treatment-refractory bipolar patient. Although, at first, it may seem inappropriate to consider a regimen with three, four, five, or more drugs for the treatment of refractory bipolar illness, this multidrug strategy is standard practice in many other areas of medicine, such as the treatment of malignancies, tuberculosis, AIDS, or congestive heart failure. In these instances, multiple therapeutic modalities with different mechanisms of action are often combined for optimal therapeutics. These types of approaches are driven by the clinical need to treat symptoms that are not responsive to more traditional evidence-based approaches and guidelines.

With the availability of a variety of agents for bipolar illness, it now befits the field to engage in a series of novel and systematic clinical trials to better delineate the optimal strategies for arriving at and comparing effective complex treatment algorithms, so that even the bipolar patients refractory to a host of more traditional approaches have an excellent chance at achieving and maintaining clinical remission. Whether one or more of the drugs used in these extreme regimens can be safely tapered and withdrawn without compromising the symptom remission is unknown, and whether this should be systematically attempted (in the absence of side effects) is also unclear.

Pharmacokinetic Interactions There do not appear to be major pharmacokinetic interactions among lithium and the other mood stabilizers. There have been occasional reports of neurotoxicity when lithium and carbamazepine are used together. Because both agents can cause these side effects at or below their own clinically accepted dose ranges or blood levels, neurotoxicity may occasionally occur from the combination treatment at these levels as well. In most studies, the combination appears to be well tolerated without more than additive side effects, that is, what would be expected when either agent is used alone. Many of the side effects reported in the literature appear to be caused by starting relatively large doses of carbamazepine (rather than slow increases) in combination with other agents and assuming that the attendant side effects are related to the combination treatment rather than to carbamazepine alone.

Carbamazepine enhances its own metabolism and other agents metabolized by the hepatic microsomal CYP 3A4 system, such as haloperidol or estrogen, and levels of these substances (as well as birth control pills) are markedly reduced by carbamazepine (Table 13.8–14). Despite a reduction in haloperidol blood levels, for example, most studies report improvement with carbamazepine supplementation, suggesting that carbamazepine might pharmacodynamically potentiate antipsychotic effects because of its action on systems other than DA receptor blockade. The only clinically relevant and pharmacokinetic effect of oxcarbazepine is to increase metabolism of estrogen in birth control pills, also necessitating the use of higher dosage forms. This is also required with the use of topiramate.

Agents commonly used in medical practice can markedly increase carbamazepine levels and can produce attendant toxicity. The most frequent dose-related toxic manifestations are dizziness, drowsiness, ataxia, diplopia, and confusion. These may occur in someone otherwise tolerating the drug well when other drugs are added. Erythromycin (E-Mycin), triacetyloleandomycin (Triocetin), isoniazid (but apparently not other MAOIs), fluoxetine and fluvoxamine, and the CCBs verapamil and diltiazem (but not nifedipine, nimodipine, amlodipine [Norvasc], or isradipine) increase carbamazepine levels. Less marked increases occur during cotreatment with propoxyphene and, transiently, with cimetidine (Tagamet). Carbamazepine lowers the blood levels of various agents (especially birth control pills) and interferes with some tests that are dependent on protein binding, including some pregnancy tests.

In contrast to the multiple pharmacokinetic interaction of carbamazepine with other drugs, based largely on its properties as an inducer of hepatic cytochrome P450 enzymes, valproate has fewer problematic effects, and they tend to be related to enzyme inhibition. If carbamazepine and valproate are used together, one should consider reducing the dose of carbamazepine (because valproate increases levels of the 10,11-epoxide metabolite) as well as increasing the free fraction of carbamazepine. Valproate increases lamotrigine levels by twofold or more and increases rash risk if not dealt with accordingly. Lithium and valproate are generally well tolerated in combination, but effects on tremor, weight gain, and GI distress may be additive.

Valproate approximately doubles blood levels of lamotrigine and thus increases the likelihood of a severe lamotrigine rash. If a rash does not occur, lamotrigine and valproate have excellent reported tolerability and efficacy in epilepsy (and perhaps in affective illness) when used in combination. In contrast, carbamazepine decreases lamotrigine levels by approximately one-half, and these two drugs may be less useful in combination because of their generally similar actions. When carbamazepine is discontinued, lamotrigine levels likely almost double over the next several weeks as hepatic enzymes are deinduced. Carbamazepine markedly reduces the level of bupropion but increases its active hydroxy metabolite. It can also decrease some antipsychotic agents (e.g., haloperidol), an action not shared by valproate.

Kinetic Interactions of the New Anticonvulsants

Fluoxetine and paroxetine are inhibitors of the isoform CYP 2D6, and levels of many agents, such as DMI and the secondary TCAs and phenothiazines, may be increased (Table 13.8–15). Fluvoxamine is a potent inhibitor of CYP 1A2 (potentially producing theophylline toxicity) and CYP 2C19 (increasing warfarin levels), as well as CYP 3A4. Nefazodone (Serzone) is also potent at CYP 3A4, producing cardiac arrhythmias with astemizole (Hismanal), cisapride (Propulsid), and terfenadine (Seldane).

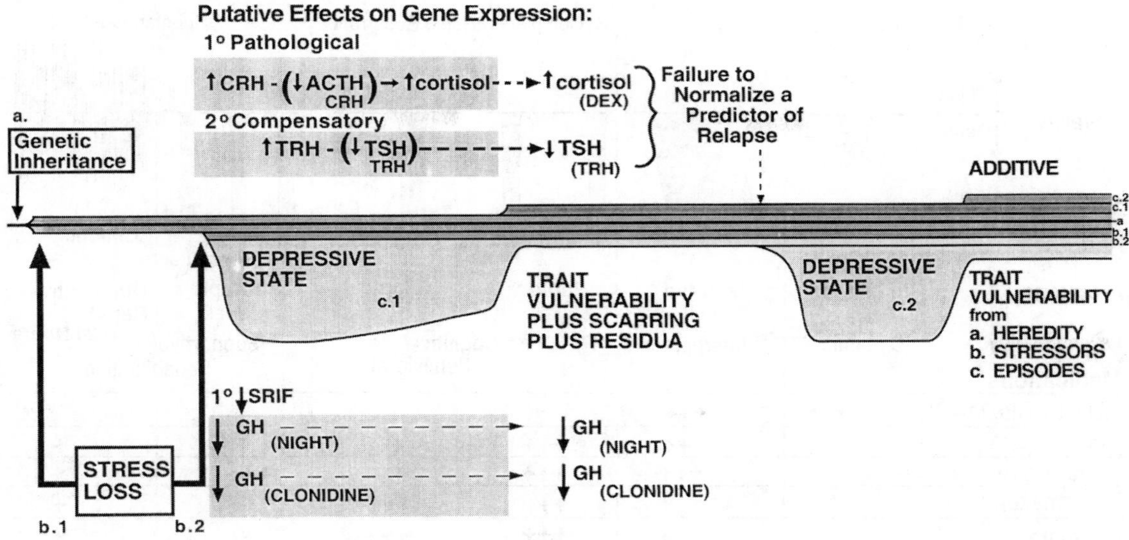

FIGURE 13.8–14 Accumulating experiential genetic vulnerability in recurrent affective illness. Schematic of how initial stressors (*b.1*) may leave behind trait vulnerabilities (at the level of alterations in gene expression). With appropriate reactivation by stress (*b.2*) of relevant neurobiological systems, the threshold for neuropeptide and hormonal changes associated with a depressive episode (*c.1*) may be exceeded. These episode-related alterations may be normalized with the termination of the episode but, in some instances, may persist and add further trait vulnerabilities toward recurrence (*c.2*) in addition to the genetic (*a*) and stressor (*b*) changes. ACTH, adrenocorticotropin-releasing hormone; CRH, corticotropin-releasing hormone; DEX, dexamethasone; GH, growth hormone; SRIF, somatotropin release-inhibiting factor; TRH, thyrotropin-releasing hormone; TSH, thyroid-stimulating hormone.

SENSITIZATION EFFECTS IN THE MOOD DISORDERS: IMPLICATIONS FOR PROPHYLAXIS

Early clinical observations and more recent systematic studies, with only a few exceptions, suggest that recurrent affective disorders can undergo a transition from initial episodes that are often precipitated by psychosocial stressors to later episodes that tend to occur more spontaneously. This transition occurs in the context of an overall pattern of cycle acceleration with a decreasing well interval between successive episodes that is most pronounced over the first several intervals (Figs. 13.8–14 and 13.8–15). Psychosocial stressors and recurrent affective episodes themselves are each probably associated with acute and longer-lasting biological perturbations based on alterations in gene expression that may convey increased vulnerability to relapse. Preliminary data from several groups suggest an association between early experiences of extreme stressors, such as physical or sexual abuse, and earlier onset and a more severe and comorbid course of bipolar disorders than in those without these early environmental adversities. The directional causality remains to be determined. However, sexual abuse appears to be associated with increased amounts of ultrarapid and ultradian cycling and suicide attempts (Fig. 13.8–8); physical abuse was associated with increased severity of mania.

Based on preclinical studies, the long-term effects of stressors are thought to result from a cascade of neurobiological effects. Acute neurotransmitter and second-messenger perturbations induce a variety of transcription factors, including the immediate early genes (IEGs) of a variety of classes, as well as a variety of neurotrophic factors. These transcription factors then influence the long-term regulation of transmitters, receptors, and neuropeptides—that is, late effector genes (LEGs). Adverse early life experiences have been associated with increases in corticotropin-releasing hormone (CRH) and hypercortisolemia and a variety of anxiety-related behaviors in adulthood, possibly modeling similar effects in humans related to depression vulnerability. Episodes themselves could similarly affect neurotransmitter function in a long-lasting fashion, also based on changes in gene expression.

If this conceptualization proves to be correct, it suggests the potential dual importance of preventing episodes of affective illness. Not only would episode-associated morbidity and potential mortality be prevented, but the longer-lasting neurobiological vulnerabilities associated with the experience of repeated affective episodes themselves (sensitization) might also be attenuated, possibly altering the course of illness in a more favorable direction. Although the mechanisms and causal relationships have not been clarified, greater numbers of prior affective episodes are associated with greater degrees of cognitive dysfunction and psychosocial impairment in euthymic bipolar outpatients, as well as greater treatment resistance to lithium, lamotrigine, and other approaches.

Thus, given the increasing evidence that greater numbers of affective episodes are a poor prognostic sign, the clinical and theoretical data speak to the importance of early institution and long-term maintenance of prophylaxis, particularly in patients already identified as being at high risk for recurrence (Figs. 13.8–1 and 13.8–8).

As in many other complex medical syndromes, the efficacy of treatment may vary as a function of the stage of illness evolution (Fig. 13.8–15). For example, pharmacotherapies such as lithium and unimodal antidepressants may be more effective in initial and middle phases of non–rapid-cycling bipolar illness, but, with the emergence of rapid and ultrarapid cycling, adjunctive treatments with the anticonvulsants, atypical antipsychotics, and other agents may be required. In the latest stages of illness evolution, complex combination pharmacotherapy may be required.

Similar transitions may take place in psychotherapeutic approaches in which insight-oriented and interpersonal psychotherapy may be effective in the earlier, stress-related episodes, but, with episode repetition, cognitive and behavioral techniques may play an increasingly important role in the later, more automatic shifts in mood. Regardless of the clinical and neurobiological constructs, numerous studies have now documented the efficacy of a variety of

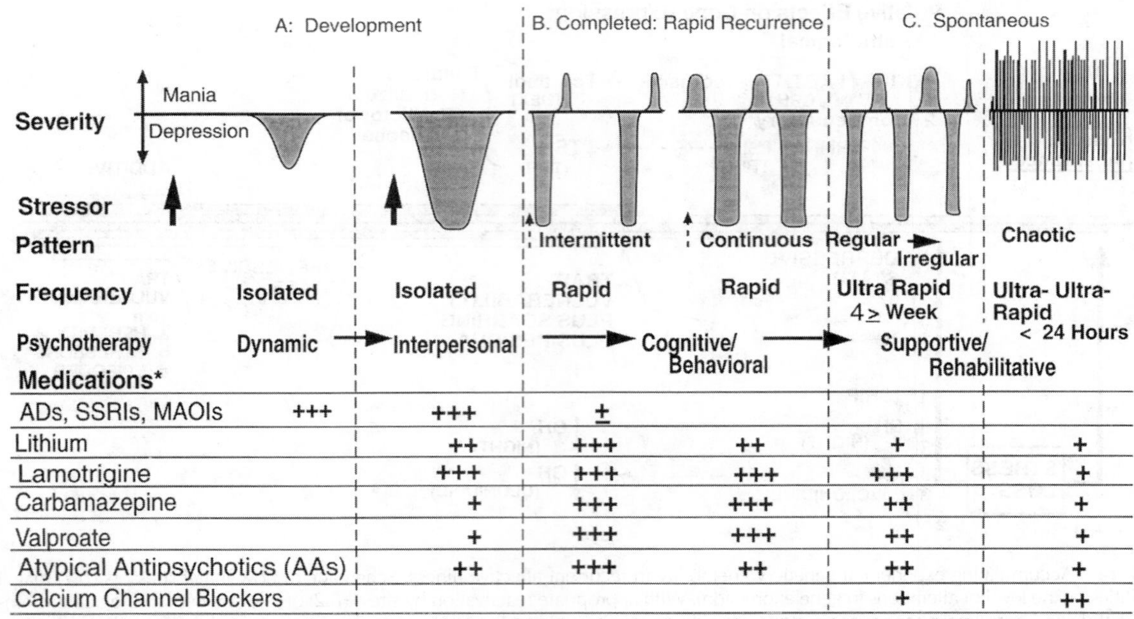

FIGURE 13.8–15 Hypothetical phases in evolution of mood cycling: potential relationship to treatment response. In an analogous fashion to kindling, episodes of affective illness may progress from triggered (*arrows*) to spontaneous and show different patterns and frequencies (*top*) as a function of stage of syndrome evolution. Just as different neural substrates are involved in different phases of kindling evolution, a similar principle is postulated in affective illness; these phases might also be responsive to different types of pharmacotherapies or psychotherapies. Although systematic and controlled studies have not examined the relationship of the illness phase to treatment response, anecdotal observations provide suggestive data that some treatments may be differentially highly effective (+++), moderately effective (++), possibly effective (+), or equivocally effective (±) as a function of course of illness. The principle of differential response as a function of stage may be useful and deserves to be specifically examined and tested. AD, antidepressant; MAOI, monoamine oxidase inhibitor; SSRI, selective serotonin reuptake inhibitor.

systematic psychotherapeutic and psychopharmacological educational approaches compared to treatment as usual. In addition, these therapeutic approaches also may help maintain a positive therapeutic alliance, enhance treatment compliance, and help prevent suicide.

The past several decades have demonstrated important advances in the understanding of the neurobiology of the unipolar and bipolar affective disorders. It is clear that these illnesses involve multiple pathways and areas of brain dysfunction and affect a variety of organ systems, involving alterations in not only mood, but also motor, cognitive, sleep, appetite, hedonic reward, and other somatic systems. Neurobiological alterations clearly occur at the level of endocrine dysfunction, as reflected in increases in glucocorticoid and neuropeptide dysregulation and in increased CRH and TRH and decreased somatotropin release-inhibiting factor (SRIF).

Some of these changes may involve episodic and cyclic alterations in gene transcription related to the primary pathology of the illness (such as increases in CRH), but others may be secondary and adaptive (such as increases in TRH) and may be endogenous attempts at antidepressant and mood-stabilizing effects. The authors have postulated that it is (at the level of changes in gene expression) the relative ratio of a host of pathological illness-related factors (such as increases in CRH and cortisol) to the endogenous adaptations (such as increases in TRH) that drive periods of illness versus well intervals. To the extent that exogenous medications can alter this ratio in a favorable direction by supplementing the endogenous adaptations or inhibiting pathological factors, short-term remissions would be achieved (Fig. 13.8–14). Sustained adequate treatment could also yield long-term prophylaxis, but marginal treatment may result in breakthrough episodes and a reinitiation of the pathological cascade. This conceptual model based on preclinical data also predicts that the development of tolerance would be delayed or prevented by (1) earlier, rather than later, treatment; (2) full sustained, rather than marginally effective, drug doses; (3) use of the most effective agents with a wide therapeutic margin; and (4) combinations of several agents with different mechanisms of action.

Structural and functional brain imaging studies have revealed differential patterns that may be linked to differences in clinical presentations and therapeutic outcome, as preliminarily suggested for differential response to carbamazepine versus nimodipine, which was noted previously. Ideally, in the future, these data can be used to aid in the differential diagnosis or treatment prognosis of patients to specific pharmacotherapies. Such studies are currently ongoing in many laboratories in the United States and elsewhere. The patient and the clinician should be reminded of this wealth of clinically relevant neurobiological evidence (Fig. 13.8–16) indicating that the mood disorders represent recurrent, potentially life-threatening, medical illnesses of the nervous system that are not different from those that afflict the other major organ systems of the body and, as such, should be treated with equal care and vigor.

FUTURE TRENDS

As the 21st century begins, one hopes for clearer definitions of the different pharmacotherapies and psychotherapies critical to successful therapeutic intervention in different individual patients with different severities, subtypes, patterns, and stages of illness. With magnetic resonance spectroscopy able to assess, in normal and ill individuals, regional brain levels of a variety of substances, including the major inhibitory transmitter GABA and the major excitatory neurotransmitter Glu, it is envisioned that one will be able to use these assessments to help choose and tailor individual drug treatment. The coming avail-

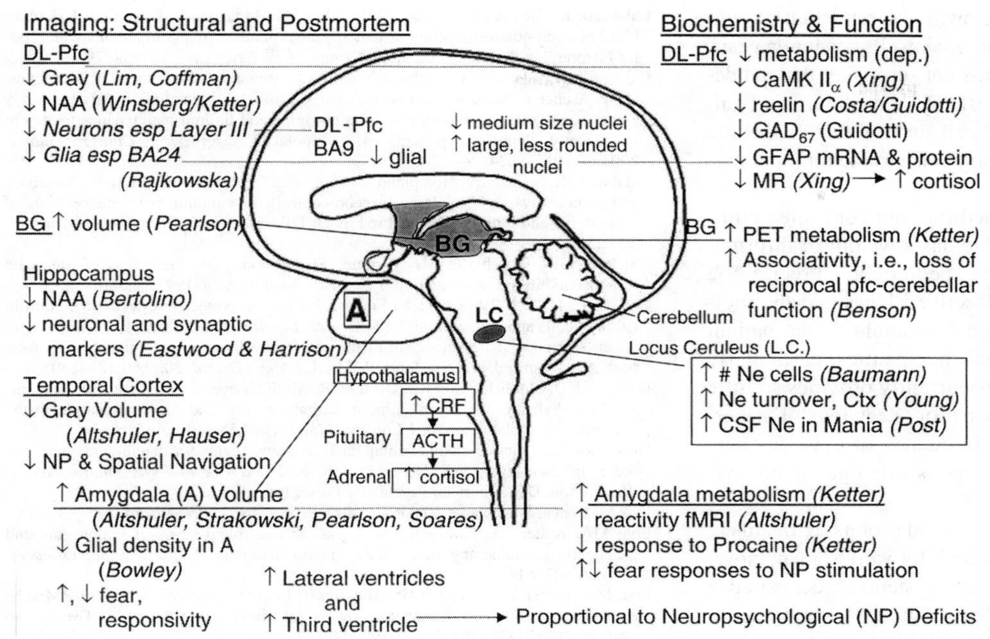

FIGURE 13.8–16 Convergence of structural (*left side*), biochemical, and functional (*right side*) abnormalities in bipolar illness. ACTH, adrenocorticotropin hormone; BA, Brodmann's area; BG, basal ganglia; CaMK-II, calcium calmodulin kinase II; CRF, corticotropin-releasing factor; CSF, cerebrospinal fluid; DL-Pfc, dorsolateral prefrontal cortex; fMRI, functional magnetic resonance imaging; GAD, glutamic acid decarboxylase; GFAP, glial fibrillary acidic protein; Gray, gray matter; mRNA, messenger ribonucleic acid; MR, mitochondrial receptors; NAA, *N*-acetylaspartate; Ne, norepinephrine; PET, positron emission tomography.

ability of assays of single nucleotide polymorphisms (SNPs) that are common gene variants (as opposed to rare mutations) should help supplement the precision of clinical and brain imaging predictors of individual responsiveness to a given treatment.

Since the last half of the 20th century, successive generations of pharmacotherapies have provided the critical neurobiological hypotheses for the mechanisms underlying the mood disorders, ranging from those sequentially involving aminergic neurotransmitters (1960s), endocrine alterations (1970s), receptor changes (1980s), second-messenger systems (1990s), and changes in gene transcription in the nucleus (2000). Such changes in which genes get turned on or off mediate some of the changes in brain biochemistry related not only to the illness (Fig. 13.8–16), but also to therapeutic interventions (Table 13.8–21). These changes in deoxyribonucleic

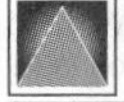

Table 13.8–21
Potential Neurotrophic and Neuroprotective Effects of Lithium and Antidepressants: Opposite Effects of Illness

	Stress	Glucocorticoids	Bipolar Illness	Lithium	Valproate	Antidepressants
Neurotrophic factors						
Brain-derived neurotrophic growth factor	↓	↓	↓ Neurons and glia, especially oligodendrocytes	↑		↑ (and block stress effects)
Bcl-2				↑	↑	
Cell death factors						
BAX, p53	↑	↑		↓		
Stroke model						
Severity	↑	↑	↑, ?	↓	↓	
Calcium signaling						
Ca_i (intracellular calcium)	↑		↑ Ca_i white blood cells	(↓)		
CaMK-II (calcium calmodulin kinase II)			↓ Prefrontal cortex CaMK-II			↑
Glucocorticoid receptors			↓ Glucocorticoid receptors			↑
Mineralocorticoid receptors			↓ Mineralocorticoid receptors			↑
New neurons and glia						
Neurogenesis	↓	↓	(↓ Neurons)	↑		↑
Gliogenesis			(↓ Glia)	↑		
Neuronal integrity						
N-acetylaspartate (prefrontal cortex > hippocampus)			↓ *N*-acetylaspartate	↑ Cortex		↑ Hippocampus
Gray matter on magnetic resonance imaging			↓ In prefrontal cortex, anterior cingulate	↑		
Clinical suicide	↑	(↑)	↑↑ Incidence	↓	?	↓?
Excess medical mortality if depressed		↑	↑ Incidence	↓	?	?

↑, increase; ↓, decrease; ?, unknown or not definite.

acid (DNA) expression also mediate growth and retraction of synapses necessary for learning and memory, as well as neurogenesis, cell survival, and cell death. It is perhaps not surprising that antidepressants increase gene expression of BDNF, and lithium and valproate increase Bcl-2 neurotrophic and cell survival factors that are critically involved in long-term memory, cell production, and survival (Table 13.8–21).

Not only is there much to be learned through controlled clinical trials research, but each patient also has a wealth of information to teach the practitioner and the theoretician. Precise life charting of the course of recurrent affective illness and the individual's response to treatment may be invaluable to the patient and the clinician in arriving at optimal therapeutics, particularly when evidence from controlled studies currently provides so little direction for the many crucial therapeutic decisions. Furthermore, patterns seen in the order and frequency of episodes may help predict the likelihood of the response to one or another mood stabilizer choice.

Although there are a host of well-tested and promising treatment alternatives now available, and one can look forward to many novel interventions in the future, a much wider systematic comparative clinical research base is urgently needed to guide the physician to the best therapeutic regimen for each individual bipolar patient. Such a research base needs to involve randomized comparisons of the efficacy and safety of different options, as well as the evaluation of the best algorithms for selecting treatment approaches for the nonresponders. It is hoped that some of the preliminary data and general guidelines and principles outlined in this chapter will assist in this process of helping patients achieve and sustain remission of this potentially disabling and lethal brain illness.

SUGGESTED CROSS-REFERENCES

Biological theories are discussed in Chapter 31. Section 13.7 provides a thorough discussion of the treatment of depressive (unipolar) disorders. OCD is covered in Chapter 14. The rest of Chapter 13 can be consulted for other aspects of mood disorders.

REFERENCES

Ahrens B, Muller-Oerlinghausen B, Schou M: Excess cardiovascular and suicide mortality of affective disorders may be reduced by lithium prophylaxis. *J Affect Disord.* 1995;33:6775.

*Altshuler L, Kiriakos L, Calcagno J, Goodman R, Gitlin M, Frye M, Mintz J: The impact of antidepressant discontinuation versus antidepressant continuation on 1-year risk for relapse of bipolar depression: A retrospective chart review. *J Clin Psychiatry.* 2001;62:612–616.

Altshuler L, Suppes T, Black D, Nolen WA, Keck PE Jr, Frye MA, McElroy S, Kupka R, Grunze H, Walden J, Leverich G, Denicoff K, Post R: Impact of antidepressant discontinuation after acute remission from bipolar depression on rates of depressive relapse at 1-year follow-up. *Am J Psychiatry.* 2003;160:1245–1250.

Baldessarini RJ, Tondo L, Hennen J: Effects of lithium treatment and its discontinuation on suicidal behavior in bipolar manic-depressive disorders. *J Clin Psychiatry.* 1999;60[Suppl 2]:77–84.

Basco MR, Rush AJ. *Cognitive-Behavioral Therapy for Bipolar Disorder.* New York: Guilford Press; 1996.

Benedetti F, Barbini B, Campori E, Fulgosi MC, Pontiggia A, Colombo C: Sleep phase advance and lithium to sustain the antidepressant effect of total sleep deprivation in bipolar depression: New findings supporting the internal coincidence model? *J Psychiatr Res.* 2001;35:323–329.

Bhagwagar Z, Goodwin GM: The role of lithium in the treatment of bipolar depression. *Clin Neurosci Responsivity.* 2002;2:222–227.

Bowden CL, Calabrese JR, Sachs GS, Yatham LN, Ashgar SA, Hompland M: A placebo controlled 18-month trial of lamotrigine and lithium maintenance treatment in recently manic or hypomanic patients with bipolar I disorder. *Arch Gen Psychiatry.* 2003;60:392–400.

Bowden CL, Calabrese JR, Sachs GS, Yatham LN, Ashgar SA, Hompland M, Montgomery P, Earl N, Smoot TM, DeVeaugh-Geiss J: A placebo-controlled 18-month trial of lamotrigine and lithium maintenance treatment in recently manic or hypomanic patients with bipolar I disorder. *Arch Gen Psychiatry.* 2003;60:392–400.

Calabrese JR, Bowden CL, Sachs GS, Ascher JA, Monaghan E, Rudd GD: A double-blind placebo-controlled study of lamotrigine monotherapy in outpatients with bipolar I depression. Lamictal 602 Study Group. *J Clin Psychiatry.* 1999;60:79.

Calabrese JR, Bowden CL, Sachs G, Yatham LN, Behnke K, Mehtonen OP, Montgomery P, Ascher J, Paska W, Earl N, DeVeaugh-Geiss J, Lamictal 605 Study Group: A placebo-controlled 18-month trial of lamotrigine and lithium maintenance treatment in recently depressed patients with bipolar I disorder. *J Clin Psychiatry.* 2003;64:1013–1024.

Calabrese JR, Soegaard J, Hompland M, Mehtonen OP, Ruetsch G, Paska W: Summary and meta-analysis of two large placebo-controlled 18-month maintenance trials of lamotrigine and lithium treatment in bipolar I disorder. *Int J Neuropsychopharmacol.* 2002;5:S58.

*Calabrese JR, Woyshville MJ, Kimmel SE, Rapport DJ: Predictors of valproate response in bipolar rapid cycling. *J Clin Psychopharmacol.* 1993;13:280.

Chuang DM, Chen RW, Chalecka-Franaszek E: Neuroprotective effects of lithium in cultured cells and animal models of diseases. *Bipolar Disord.* 2002;4:129–136.

Coppen A, Bailey J: Enhancement of the antidepressant action of fluoxetine by folic acid: A randomised, placebo controlled trial. *J Affect Disord.* 2000;60:121–130.

Denicoff KD, Smith-Jackson EE, Disney ER, Ali SO, Leverich GS, Post RM: Comparative prophylactic efficacy of lithium, carbamazepine, and the combination in the treatment of bipolar disorder. *J Clin Psychiatry.* 1997;58:470.

Dubovsky SL. Calcium channel antagonists as novel agents for manic-depressive disorder. In: Schatzberg AF, Nemeroff CB, eds. *Textbook of Psychopharmacology.* Washington, DC: American Psychiatric Press; 1995:377.

Fink M: Convulsive therapy: A review of the first 55 years. *J Affect Disord.* 2001;63:1–15.

Frye MA, Ketter TA, Kimbrell TA: A placebo-controlled study of lamotrigine and gabapentin monotherapy in refractory mood disorders. *J Clin Psychopharmacol.* 2000;20:607–614.

Frye MA, Ketter TA, Leverich GS, Huggins T, Lantz C, Denicoff KD, Post RM: The increasing use of polypharmacotherapy for refractory mood disorders: Twenty-two years of study. *J Clin Psychiatry.* 1999;60:152.

George MS, Nahas Z, Li X, Kozel FA, Anderson B, Yamanaka K: Potential new brain stimulation therapies in bipolar illness: Transcranial magnetic stimulation and vagus nerve stimulation. *Clin Neurosci Responsivity.* 2003;2:256–265.

Ghaemi SN, Rosenquist KJ, Ko JY, Baldassano CF, Kontos NJ, Baldessarini RJ: Antidepressant treatment in bipolar versus unipolar depression. *Am J Psychiatry.* 2004;161:163–165.

Goodwin FK, Fireman B, Simon GE, Hunkeler EM, Lee J, Revicki D: Suicide risk in bipolar disorder during treatment with lithium and divalproex. *JAMA.* 2003;290:1467–1473.

Goodwin FK, Jamison KR. *Manic-Depressive Illness.* New York: Oxford University Press; 1990.

Gould TD, Chen G, Manji HK: Mood stabilizer psychopharmacology. *Clin Neurosci Responsivity.* 2002;2:193–212.

Grunze H, Erfurth A, Marcuse A, Amann B, Normann C, Walden J: Tiagabine appears not to be efficacious in the treatment of acute mania. *J Clin Psychiatry.* 1999;60:759–762.

Gyulai L, Bowden CL, McElroy SL, Calabrese JR, Petty F, Swann AC, Chou JC, Wassef A, Risch CS, Hirschfeld RM, Nemeroff CB, Keck PE Jr., Evans DL, Wozniak PJ: Maintenance efficacy of divalproex in the prevention of bipolar depression. *Neuropsychopharmacol.* 2003;28:1374–1382.

Hirschfeld RM, Calabrese JR, Weissman MM, Reed M, Davies MA, Frye MA, Keck PE Jr, Lewis L, McElroy SL, McNulty JP, Wagner KD: Screening for bipolar disorder in the community. *J Clin Psychiatry.* 2003;64:53–59.

Judd LL, Akiskal HS, Schettler PJ, Endicott J, Maser J, Solomon DA, Leon AC, Rice JA, Keller MB: The long-term natural history of the weekly symptomatic status of bipolar I disorder. *Arch Gen Psychiatry.* 2002;59:530–537.

*Keck PE Jr, Buse JB, Dagogo-Jack S, D'Alessio DA, Daniels SR, McElroy SL, McIntyre RS, Sernyak MJ, Wirshing DA, Wirshing WC: Managing metabolic concerns in patients with severe mental illness. *Postgrad Med.* 2003;[Suppl 1]:1–89.

Kessing LV, Andersen PK, Mortensen PB, Bolwig TG: Recurrence in affective disorder. I. Case register study. *Br J Psychiatry.* 1998;172:23–28.

Ketter TA, Kimbrell TA, George MS: Baseline cerebral hypermetabolism associated with carbamazepine response, and hypometabolism with nimodipine response in mood disorders. *Biol Psychiatry.* 1999;46:1364–1374.

Ketter TA, Post RM. Clinical pharmacology and pharmacokinetics of carbamazepine. In: Joffe RT, Calabrese JR, eds. *Anticonvulsants in Mood Disorders.* New York: Marcel Dekker; 1994:147.

Koukopoulos A, Reginaldi D, Minnai G, Serra G, Pani L, Johnson FN: The long term prophylaxis of affective disorders. *Adv Biochem Psychopharmacol.* 1995;49:127.

Leverich GS, Perez S, Luckenbaugh DA, Post RM: Early psychosocial stressors: Relationship to suicidality and course of bipolar illness. *Clin Neurosci Responsivity.* 2002;2:161–170.

Leverich GS, Post RM: Life charting of affective disorders. *CNS Spectrums.* 1998;3:21–37.

McElroy SL, Altshuler LL, Suppes T: Axis I psychiatric comorbidity and its relationship to historical illness variables in 288 patients with bipolar disorder. *Am J Psychiatry.* 2001;158:420–426.

Morrell MJ: Reproductive and metabolic disorders in women with epilepsy. *Epilepsia.* 2003;44[Suppl 4]:11–20.

Muller-Oerlinghausen B, Ahrens B, Grof E: The effect of long-term lithium treatment on the mortality of patients with manic-depressive and schizoaffective illness. *Acta Psychiatr Scand.* 1992;86:218–222.

Obrocea GV, Dunn RM, Frye MA: Clinical predictors of response to lamotrigine and gabapentin monotherapy in refractory affective disorders. *Biol Psychiatry.* 2002;51:253–260.

Pande AC, Crockatt JG, Janney CA, Werth JL, Tsaroucha G: Gabapentin in bipolar disorder: A placebo-controlled trial of adjunctive therapy. Gabapentin Bipolar Disorder Study Group. *Bipolar Disord.* 2000;2:249–255.

Passmore MJ, Garnham J, Duffy A, MacDougall M, Munro A, Slaney C, Teehan A, Alda M: Phenotypic spectra of bipolar disorder in responders to lithium versus lamotrigine. *Bipolar Disord.* 2003;5:110–114.

Pazzaglia PJ, Post RM, Ketter TA, Callahan AM, Marangell LB, Frye MA, George MS, Kimbrell TA, Leverich GS, Cora-Locatelli G, Luckenbaugh D: Nimodipine monotherapy and carbamazepine augmentation in patients with refractory recurrent affective illness. *J Clin Psychopharmacol.* 1998;18:404–413.

*Post RM, Denicoff KD, Leverich GS, Altshuler LL, Frye MA, Suppes PM: Morbidity in 258 bipolar outpatients followed for 1 year with daily prospective ratings on the NIMH-LCM. *J Clin Psychiatry.* 2003;64:680–690.

Post RM, Leverich GS, Weiss SR, Zhang LX, Li H, Smith M. Psychosocial stressors as predisposing factors to affective illness and PTSD: Potential neurobiological mechanisms and theoretical implications. In: Cicchetti D, Walker E, eds. *Neurodevelopmental Mechanisms in Psychopathology.* New York: Cambridge University Press; 2001.

Post RM, Luckenbaugh DA: Unique design issues in clinical trials of patients with bipolar affective disorder. *J Psychiatr Res.* 2003;37:61–73.

Post RM, Speer AM, Obrocea GV, Leverich GS: Acute and prophylactic effects of anticonvulsants in bipolar depression. *Clin Neurosci Responsivity.* 2002;2:228–251.

Post RM, Weiss SRB: A speculative model of affective illness cyclicity based on patterns of drug tolerance observed in amygdala-kindled seizures. *Mol Neurobiol.* 1996;13:33.

Prudic J, Olfson M, Marcus SC, Fuller RB, Sackeim HA: Effectiveness of electroconvulsive therapy in community settings. *Biol Psychiatry.* 2004;55:301–312.

Ringel BL, Szuba MP: Potential mechanisms of the sleep therapies for depression. *Depress Anxiety.* 2001;14:29–36.

Rouillon F, Lejoyeux M, Filteau MJ: Unwanted effects of long-term treatment. In: Montgomery SA, Rouillon F, eds. *Long-Term Treatment of Depression.* Chichester: John Wiley & Sons, 1992:81–111.

Silverstone T: Moclobemide vs. imipramine in bipolar depression: A multicentre double-blind clinical trial. *Acta Psychiatr Scand.* 2001;104:104–109.

Stoll AL, Severus WE, Freeman MP: Omega 3 fatty acids in bipolar disorder: A preliminary double-blind, placebo-controlled trial. *Arch Gen Psychiatry.* 1999;56:407–412.

Szuba MP, Baxter LR Jr, Fairbanks LA, Guze BH, Schwartz JM: Effects of partial sleep deprivation on the diurnal variation of mood and motor activity in major depression. *Biol Psychiatry.* 1991;30:817–829.

Tennis P, Eldridge RR: Preliminary results on pregnancy outcomes in women using lamotrigine. *Epilepsia.* 2002;43:1161–1167.

*Thase ME, Sachs GS: The challenges of pharmacotherapy of bipolar depression. *Clin Neurosci Responsivity.* 2002;2:213–221.

Tohen M, Chengappa KN, Suppes T, Zarate CA Jr, Calabrese JR, Bowden CL, Sachs GS, Kupfer DJ, Baker RW, Risser RC, Keeter EL, Feldman PD, Tollefson GD, Breier A: Efficacy of olanzapine in combination with valproate or lithium in the treatment of mania in patients partially nonresponsive to valproate or lithium monotherapy. *Arch Gen Psychiatry.* 2002;59:62–69.

Tohen M, Vieta E, Calabrese J, Ketter TA, Sachs G, Bowden C, Mitchell PB, Centorrino F, Risser R, Baker RW, Evans AR, Beymer K, Dube S, Tollefson GD, Breier A: Efficacy of olanzapine and olanzapine-fluoxetine combination in the treatment of bipolar I depression. *Arch Gen Psychiatry.* 2003;60:1079–1088.

Zaretsky A: Targeted psychosocial interventions for bipolar disorder. *Bipolar Disord.* 2003;5[Suppl 2]:80–87.

▲ 13.9 Mood Disorders: Psychotherapy

JOHN R. MCQUAID, PH.D., AND STEPHEN R. SHUCHTER, M.D.

Knowledge regarding the treatment of mood disorders with psychotherapy varies greatly depending on the specific disorder. Although researchers have extensively studied the use of psychotherapy for treating major depression, research on the use of psychotherapy for treatment of bipolar disorders, manic symptoms, dysthymia, and other variations on mood disorders is much more limited. Several approaches to intervention, based on distinct models of the etiology and course of these disorders, have been efficacious in controlled trials. However, practicing clinicians frequently note that those trials are not sufficiently relevant to their needs. The current issues in psychotherapy for mood disorders involve applying the known technologies of treatment to the complex issues of patients, who often do not neatly fit into the categorical structure of the revised fourth edition of the *Diagnostic and Statistical Manual of Mental Disorders* (DSM-IV-TR). This section reviews the primary models of psychotherapy for mood disorders and the research literature regarding efficacy. The section then reviews in detail two treatment approaches. The first, cognitive-behavioral therapy (CBT), is the most extensively researched and used standardized treatment. The second, biologically informed psychotherapy for depression, provides an example of an integrative intervention that reflects the approach of many clinicians.

HISTORY OF PSYCHOTHERAPY FOR DEPRESSION

Psychotherapy for depression arose from psychoanalytical models. Early models conceptualized depression as internalized anger that arose from unconscious conflicts. Depression was conceptualized primarily as an intrapsychic phenomenon. Therefore, intervention was long-term, focused on developing awareness of these internal conflicts through identification and interpretation of historical experiences that reflected such conflicts. Intervention emphasized developing insight to these conflicts through the use of free association and the therapist's interpretations. This treatment also used the patient's projections onto the therapist (the transference neurosis) as a means of studying early object relationships and conflicts.

In contrast to psychodynamic approaches, behavioral therapy for depression emphasized training in specific skills to increase rewarding activities. Behavioral therapists developed interventions based on principles of operant and classical conditioning and applied scientific techniques to studying observable behaviors. Behaviorism, as elaborated by B. F. Skinner, rejected conscious thinking or unconscious drives as potential targets of intervention, because they could not be systematically observed and studied. Rather, behavioral therapists conceptualized depressive disorders as a consequence of decreased access to positive reinforcement, possibly due to loss of a relationship or rewarding activity. For example, Peter Lewinsohn developed a group intervention based on the conceptualization of depression arising from deficits in skills such as assertive communication and activity planning and scheduling. Intervention therefore involved skills training and increasing reinforcers in the patient's life.

Cognitive therapy (CT) models were primarily developed by clinicians attempting to develop an alternative to the limitations they perceived in psychoanalytic theory. The earliest cognitive model was that of Albert Ellis, the originator of rational-emotive therapy. Ellis attributed the development of depression and other mental disorders to the presence of absolute, rigid rules that are learned early in life. These rules, often described as *shoulds* or *musts*, lead individuals to believe that failure to act in a certain way (e.g., making everyone happy) leads to catastrophic outcomes (e.g., being worthless). Ellis argued that these rules often were unreasonable and unattainable, and, when people failed to live up to these expectations, they would become depressed. In developing treatment, Ellis looked to early Greek philosophers and the use of logical arguments to illuminate the flaws in the patient's beliefs. The core concept of rational-emotive therapy, that logic can be used to modify dysfunctional beliefs, is central to later cognitive models.

Aaron Beck used a somewhat similar approach in developing CT. He initially intended to test the assumptions of the psychoanalytic model of depression. In doing so, he started to develop a new model of cognitive structure. Beck proposed that depression is characterized by specific patterns of thinking. In response to a stimulus, depressed individuals tend to experience thoughts that were (as Ellis had noted) logically flawed. Beck labeled these cognitive responses to stimuli *automatic thoughts*. He proposed that the automatic thoughts in response to a situation (e.g., "I can't stand this" as a response to a relationship rejection) derive from assumptions that the patient holds about the self, the world, and the future. An individual who sees himself or herself as weak and dependent on others, the world as dangerous, and the future as uncertain would feel more threatened by the loss of a relationship than those who saw themselves as competent and the world as safe.

Beck proposed that depression also depended on the concept of a schema. A *schema* is an underlying cognitive structure that organizes information in memory and guides attention. It therefore determines which stimuli receive attention, are encoded in memory, and are remembered in specific situations. Beck proposed that some schemata could make a patient vulnerable to depression in response to specific situations. This stress-diathesis model of depression proposed that a depressogenic schema alone does not cause depression. However, when a matching stressful event occurs, the schema leads to an increase of depressive symptoms.

In CT, treatment emphasizes teaching the patient to test out the beliefs and assumptions that contribute to the depression. Techniques emphasize a collaborative approach between the therapist and the patient. The therapist provides the patient training in techniques for testing beliefs, and the patient practices these techniques. This approach, sometimes called *collaborative empiricism*, emphasizes using logical reasoning and hypothesis testing to question assumptions. As with the behavioral approaches, Beck emphasized the standardization of the treatment and the submission of the intervention to scientific evaluation. CT and variants are now the most researched form of psychotherapy in the world.

As emphasis on research-based treatments has increased, Gerald Klerman and colleagues developed interpersonal psychotherapy. They based their intervention on research in attachment theory and earlier interpersonal psychodynamic models of psychotherapy, such as those of Adolf Meyer and Harry Stack Sullivan. As the name implies, interpersonal psychotherapy differs from CBT and behavioral therapy because it focuses theoretically and practically on relationships. Interpersonal psychotherapy conceptualizes depression as arising from problematic patterns in relationships that stem from early development and establishment of attachment. The treatment therefore emphasizes patients learning to recognize their interpersonal patterns and to act more effectively in relationships. Interpersonal psychotherapy incorporates a variety of interventions in the service of understanding and modifying interpersonal behaviors and responses that contribute to depression. These interventions range from nondirective questioning and interpreting relationship patterns, in and out of therapy, to directive techniques, such as interpersonal skills training, psychoeducation, and role playing. Interventions are chosen to address one or more of four interpersonal domains (grief, interpersonal disputes, role transitions, and interpersonal deficits) that are relevant to the patient's current depressive episode.

Interpersonal psychotherapy shares many of the procedural aspects of cognitive and behavioral therapies. Intervention is focused and goal oriented. Sessions focus on experience in the present rather than exploration of the past. Therapy is time limited, because the goal is to reduce current symptoms rather than to modify personality dysfunction. As with CT, interpersonal psychotherapy emphasizes a research-based conceptualization of depression and the use of standardized assessment to evaluate outcome. Significantly, interpersonal psychotherapy is the first psychodynamic intervention to derive from research-based theory and to be submitted to rigorous scientific evaluation.

These different models have been greatly elaborated over time, in large part due to continuing integration among treatment interventions. *CT* is now often referred to as *CBT* (the term that is used for the rest of this section) in reflection of the integration of behavioral techniques. This is consistent with the extensive impact of social learning theory, which provided a unifying model that addressed behavioral and cognitive principles. CT also increasingly emphasizes interpersonal components, particularly in models addressing more complex cases.

There is also an increasing emphasis on incorporation of meditation techniques in psychotherapy. Mindfulness meditation, developed from Buddhist techniques, emphasizes two skills: observing one's perceived sensations and accepting and experiencing those sensations nonjudgmentally. In the application of this technique to depression, sensations include cognition and emotional states, as well as input through the five senses. Researchers such as Zindel Segal and John Teasdale propose that these techniques are relevant for three reasons. First, the training in observation facilitates gathering evidence, which is a central component in CBT. Second, learning to recognize thoughts as discrete, limited experiences that can be observed rather than imbuing them with special meaning can reduce the credence that patients give to dysfunctional thoughts. Third, the emphasis in meditation on nonjudgmental observing moves the treatment from being change focused to being acceptance focused. Several cognitive and behavioral clinicians argue that acceptance is a critical component of treatment, because the ability to accept and to tolerate distress is often one of the major difficulties experienced by patients with depression.

Another area of integration arises from the improved understanding of the biology of mood disorders. Ellen Frank and colleagues have incorporated the concept of social rhythms (i.e., the consistency of interpersonal activities) and the importance of such rhythms in a model of interpersonal psychotherapy for treating bipolar disorder. This model conceptualizes bipolar disorder as vulnerable to disruptions in circadian rhythms and identifies stable and consistent social rhythms as features that can protect against symptom exacerbation.

Stephen Shuchter and Sydney Zisook have developed biologically informed psychotherapy for depression, a psychotherapeutic approach to depression that has integrated a biological perspective with other psychotherapeutic models. Biologically informed psychotherapy for depression uses elements of education, coping skills training, and family involvement and includes the use of psychodynamic concepts, cognitive and behavioral techniques, and complementary psychopharmacological treatment. In contrast to other approaches that assume that psychological and cognitive etiologies of the affective disorders, biologically informed psychotherapy for depression assumes that depression develops out of a multifactorial matrix that leads to biological changes that operate autonomously. Although the etiology of depression remains unknown, numerous theories have been postulated, including genetic hypotheses, neurotransmitter hypotheses, neuroregulatory hypotheses, and others. Although biological changes are being treated psychopharmacologically, psychotherapeutic intervention in biologically informed psychotherapy for depression focuses on the influence of depression on the realms of personality functioning. The *language* of depression represents the translation of symptoms of depression to changes that occur in the depressed person's interpersonal functioning, productive capacities, and self-concept and identity. Biologically informed psychotherapy for depression conceptualizes these as state-dependent changes that are the consequence, rather than the course, of depression. The biologically informed psychotherapy for depression model is presented later in this section as a framework for treatment.

The next section briefly reviews the research literature on depression treatment. Two current models, CBT and biologically informed

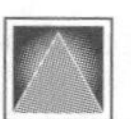

Table 13.9–1
Efficacious Treatments for Major Depression

Treatment	Conceptualization of Depression Etiology	Sample Interventions
Behavioral therapy	Deficit of reinforcers, including pleasant activities and positive interpersonal contacts	Increase activity level Structured goal setting Interpersonal skills training
Cognitive-behavioral therapy	Interaction of beliefs with matching stressor	Identify and challenge automatic thoughts Engage in activities that provide evidence disproving dysfunctional beliefs Modify core beliefs by reviewing evidence
Interpersonal psychotherapy	Interpersonal vulnerabilities arising from early attachment and learned relationship patterns	Develop awareness of patterns in primary relationships and the therapeutic relationship Interpersonal skills training Communication analysis
Behavioral marital therapy	Marital distress increases stress while impairing support resources	Assertive communication training Active listening exercises Problem-solving skills Increasing reinforcing behaviors toward spouse

psychotherapy for depression, are then described, and guidelines for clinicians are proposed based on the current state of knowledge.

REVIEW OF RESEARCH FINDINGS

Individual Psychotherapy

Arguably, the advancement in psychotherapy is as much one of evaluation as it is the development of novel interventions. Primary interventions in CT can be dated back to Socrates, and Sigmund Freud would recognize some interpersonal psychotherapy interventions (open-ended exploration and examination of the therapeutic relationship). The revolution in psychotherapy stems from the standardization of training (through manuals, as well as adherence and competency measures), the use of standard scientific methods for evaluating treatment, and the development of treatments using research-based conceptualizations of mood disorders. Because of these advances, there are now several interventions, shown in Table 13.9–1, known to be efficacious or probably efficacious for major depression. There are also promising treatments in chronic depression and bipolar disorders.

CBT has been evaluated in several randomized, controlled trials, and early studies of CT produced promising results. In several studies, CT provided outcomes as good or better than pharmacotherapy. Interpersonal psychotherapy also proved to be not significantly different from medications. However, several authors criticized these designs, pointing out, among other factors, the lack of an adequate placebo control to assure that medication was effectively administered. These concerns were addressed in the first large multisite study to compare CBT, interpersonal psychotherapy, medication (imipramine [Tofranil]), and a pill placebo: the National Institute of Mental Health (NIMH) Treatment of Depression Collaborative Research Program (TDCRP). The initial findings of the TDCRP suggested that interpersonal psychotherapy and imipramine were superior to placebo and were not significantly different from one another. CBT was not significantly different from interpersonal psychotherapy or imipramine but also was not significantly better than placebo. These findings have been extensively reviewed and discussed, with advocates for CBT arguing that the poor performance of CBT reflects problems in the study design (e.g., differences in CBT competence between study sites). Additional studies since that time that included control groups and medication have found CBT to be superior to placebo and equivalent to medication and other forms of psychotherapy.

In addition to initial treatment response, several investigators have examined whether psychotherapies may prevent recurrence of disorder. Although patients who respond to medication have high rates of relapse on discontinuation, patients who have responded to some forms of psychotherapy may have reduced risks of recurrence. These findings, although tentative, suggest that psychotherapy may be a more cost-effective intervention than some first-line medications, because the preventive effects do not require ongoing treatment.

Group and Couples Therapy

Other treatments that have been shown to be efficacious for depression include behavioral marital therapy (BMT) and Lewinsohn's coping with depression course, a group intervention. BMT for depression is administered to the couple and incorporates relationship skills training, including assertive communication, providing support, increasing rewarding interactions for each partner, and learning skills in acceptance of each partner's difference. Studies by Neil Jacobson and colleagues, as well as Steven Beach and colleagues, have demonstrated that, when individuals are depressed in the context of a distressed marriage, BMT is as effective as CBT in reducing depression. In addition, BMT leads to significantly greater improvement in marital functioning than CBT. In situations in which marital distress and depression are present, marital therapy is an important intervention to consider.

Several studies have found group therapy, particularly CBT and behavioral therapy, to be efficacious for major depression. Lewinsohn's course on coping with depression outperformed control groups, and a comparison between CBT and psychodynamic group therapies found that CBT was significantly more efficacious in reducing depression. In one small study group, CBT was significantly superior to group behavioral therapy, although both were superior to nondirective therapy and a control group. In addition, recent studies by Ricardo Muñoz and colleagues, as well as others, have suggested that group CBT may prevent the onset of a first episode of major depression, although these studies need replication. However, there are few studies comparing group to individual treatment or group treatment to pharmacotherapy, so the relative efficacy of group treatment relative to other validated treatments is not yet known.

Combined Psychotherapy and Pharmacotherapy

In addition to treatment response for psychotherapy alone, there have been a series of studies examining combined psychotherapy and medication for treating depression. In most studies, the effect size for combined treatment has not been significantly greater than that for separate treatments, calling into question the cost-effectiveness of combined treatment. However, a recent multisite study found that, for patients with chronic depression, a combination of nefazodone (Serzone) and cognitive behavioral analysis system of psychotherapy (a specific version of CBT for chronic depression) was significantly more effective than either treatment alone. The authors reported that 85 percent of the combined treatment sample achieved remission, in comparison to approximately 52 to 55 percent in either single treatment. This finding suggests that, for specific samples, combined treatments may be the intervention of choice.

APPLYING THE RESEARCH TO CLINICAL PRACTICE: WHAT TO MAKE OF THE DODO BIRD VERDICT

Several researchers have applied the Dodo Bird verdict from *Alice in Wonderland*, in which all participants were winners and deserving of prizes, to the results of psychotherapy outcome trials. At times, this seems to be the case with psychotherapies for major depression, with interpersonal psychotherapy and CBT appearing relatively efficacious, and with there being less evidence of superiority of one to the other. Because psychotherapy research is still quite early in development, many critical questions are largely unanswered, including which treatment is best for which patient, what are optimal doses (e.g., number and length of sessions), and whether continuation therapy is cost-effective. It is not clear how critical specific techniques associated with these interventions are for successful treatment of mood disorders. In particular, the few dismantling studies that have been completed have not demonstrated that particular techniques are necessary for change. A dismantling study of CBT that compared behavioral therapy, behavioral therapy plus thought challenging, and behavioral therapy plus thought challenging and schema change found no difference in outcomes between the three approaches. A study of the therapeutic process of interpersonal psychotherapy (i.e., the actual in-session behaviors of the therapist and patient) found that the process was more consistent with ideal CBT than ideal interpersonal psychotherapy. A metaanalysis examining comparisons between specific psychotherapies and placebo conditions found that the difference between treatments was related to the adequacy of the placebo design. Studies with placebo comparisons deemed adequate (e.g., using nonspecific therapy techniques for the placebo condition and matching for level of contact with therapists) showed smaller differences between active interventions and placebo than those studies with placebo conditions that were inadequate (e.g., less therapist contact, constraint of topics to issues not related to the patient's disorder). These findings suggest that differences between psychotherapy techniques may be less critical than some of the shared components (e.g., positive therapeutic relationship, shared goals, and facilitated behavior change). There are also no definitive answers regarding the underlying models of depression. Although behavior therapy, CT, and interpersonal psychotherapy are based on empirical models of psychopathology that all have supportive evidence, the development of these treatments and the conceptualization of depression are extrapolations beyond the available data.

Clinicians then are faced with how to use this knowledge in treating patients. Some researchers and clinicians argue for the exclusive use of empirically supported models. At the other end are those who argue for an integrative approach, drawing from what is known to be effective and applying those techniques based on clinical judgment and understanding of the research literature. The next section illustrates both approaches. CBT is described in detail and is illustrated with a case example, and then an integrative model (biologically informed psychotherapy for depression) is similarly described and illustrated.

COGNITIVE-BEHAVIORAL THERAPY

CBT is based on the assumption that dysfunctional beliefs, occurring in response to life experiences, lead to dysfunctional behavioral and emotional responses. Treatment therefore modifies these beliefs to reduce problematic responses and to increase functional responses. Patients learn to modify beliefs by first learning to observe their thinking, affect, and behavior and then evaluating how thoughts influence mood and actions. As the patient becomes aware of these processes, the therapist teaches skills in questioning and testing the validity of dysfunctional beliefs and developing alternative, more accurate, functional beliefs. The long-term goal of treatment is for patients to learn the skills to such an extent that they are able to be their own therapist.

Assessment and measurement, by the therapist and the patient, are central to effective CBT. The therapist teaches the patient to quantify the issues of concern. Patients learn to observe and to define their own assumptions that lead to depression and then to engage in a series of experiments to improve their mood. Patients learn to measure the effects of these experiments, so that they test the previous assumptions and can develop new, more constructive beliefs and actions that reduce depression and other problematic moods and behaviors.

A 23-year-old, unmarried, African American woman presented to a community mental health clinic. The patient was in the midst of her first semester at law school. Her primary physician had referred her to the clinic after the patient reported frequent crying and feeling hopeless. Symptoms included depressed mood nearly every day; crying spells "out of the blue"; anhedonia; early, middle, and late insomnia; decreased appetite; weight loss; difficulty concentrating; feeling worthless; thoughts of death; and suicidal ideation.

CBT, like most other psychotherapies, uses a case conceptualization approach to determining treatment for each patient. In CBT, the conceptualization is developed based on an understanding of how different aspects of cognition are related. Aaron Beck and, later, Judith Beck proposed that cognition could be divided into three levels: automatic thoughts, intermediate beliefs, and cognitive schemata. The most accessible, labeled, automatic thoughts represented the conscious response to stimuli. For example, the previously mentioned patient, when studying, often thought "I'll never understand this."

The second level, intermediate beliefs, is assumptions about the self, the world, and the future that led to the automatic thought occurring in response to a particular stimuli. Using the previous example, the patient believed that she was not competent and that she was not good enough; she perceived the world (in this case, professors and classmates) as attacking and critical. She anticipated that the future would be filled with failure. At times when things went well, she was not unduly distressed. However, in the face of failure or criticism, she quickly experienced self-critical thoughts that were consistent with these beliefs.

The content (e.g., the beliefs) and the organization of that content define the third level, cognitive schemata. An individual's schemata determine which stimuli are most likely noticed and encoded in memory, which stimuli are ignored or discounted, how encoded information is linked or associated in memory, and which memories are most easily recalled. For the previously mentioned patient, she may suffer from a schema that could be conceptualized as "I'm not good enough." She tends to notice information consistent with this belief and tends to ignore or to discount other information.

As the therapist completes an initial assessment and establishes a treatment plan, a central goal is to elaborate a case conceptualization that will facilitate treatment. By understanding the unique meaning of experiences to the patient, the therapist can be more effective in identifying interventions that truly test the beliefs and produce meaningful improvement.

Several authors have described models for developing case formulations in CBT, and they generally are based on gathering evidence to propose an underlying schema. Once the automatic thoughts, beliefs, and schemata are identified, interventions are chosen based on these hypothesized structures. The therapist continues to gather evidence throughout treatment, refining the formulation over time.

Initial Assessment Specificity and accurate data gathering are a key focus of CBT. In particular, assessment of diagnosis and symptoms is necessary. Primary assessment preferably includes standardized measures, including the Structured Clinical Interview for DSM-IV-TR (SCID), the Hamilton Rating Scale for Depression, and the Beck Depression Index (BDI). The assessment also needs to include the dimensions of functioning: interpersonal relationships, work and achievement, health, and recreation. As treatment progresses, a formulation is developed regarding the patient's case conceptualization, as well as particular cognitive and behavioral coping strategies that the patient uses.

The previously presented patient experienced impairments in several areas of functioning. The patient had not contacted family or friends for several weeks, which was unusual for her. She had no current close friends at her school and had not had a dating relationship for several years. She reported that she was skipping classes and that she believed she was failing her program. The patient made statements such as "I'm just a total loser" and "I don't belong." Despite excellent grades in college, she believed she was only accepted to law school due to her minority status. She primarily coped with stress by ruminating and had stopped many rewarding activities (e.g., exercise).

She had several relevant experiences from her early childhood. The patient had been adopted shortly after her birth by a white couple and was their only child. She grew up in an almost exclusively white neighborhood. She reported that, although she had some friends, she had no African American friends and that she often felt discriminated against by whites and the few African Americans with whom she had contact, who criticized her for "trying to be white." The patient described that, despite having devoted parents, she had a sense of not being good enough and being out of place since approximately 6 years of age, when she first started school.

Course of Therapy In the initial session, the therapist has several goals, including (1) orienting the patient to the treatment approach, (2) establishing rapport, (3) identifying problems and treatment targets, (4) assessing current symptom and problem severity, (5) providing some initial symptom relief, and (6) introducing an initial homework assignment. In reality, these components tend to overlap. For example, it is often helpful to illustrate the CBT model using a life experience of the patient and, in doing so, to provide a chance at some symptom relief. An example could be processing a situation such as being late to a first therapy appointment:

Therapist: You mentioned that you were upset because you were late. Can you tell me what you were thinking when you realized you were late?

Patient: I figured you'd be angry.

Therapist: Okay, and when you thought I'd be angry, how did you feel?

Patient: Pretty nervous.

Therapist: So that is what we will focus on in here, how your thinking in different situations influences how you feel. In this case, you were late, thought "he'll be angry," and felt nervous. Our goal is to test out the beliefs, like "he'll be angry," and change them when they aren't healthy or accurate. The great thing is, you sort of implicitly tested out the belief that I'll be angry by showing up. Was I angry?

Patient: You didn't seem angry.

Therapist: How anxious did you feel once we started talking?

Patient: Well, I'm feeling more comfortable.

Therapist: What thoughts do you have now about me being angry?

Patient: I don't think you're angry.

Therapist: So, this is an example of what we're going to be doing in therapy—I'll be helping you to identify thoughts that make you feel bad. We're then going to work together to come up with ways to check them out, and change them if they're not true or accurate. You checked out whether I was angry by observing me, and you changed your thought, and, now, I get the impression that you feel better.

In this example, the model of CBT is described for the patient and illustrated using her own thoughts, behaviors, and feelings. In particular, the effect of behavioral testing of beliefs (i.e., coming into session late and finding out if the therapist actually was angry) is pointed out. To increase her sense of efficacy, the therapist points out that her current actions can lead to mood change (feeling more relaxed after coming in late) and that she is already demonstrating some of the necessary skills to benefit from CBT.

To facilitate skills, an agenda is explicitly set forth and agreed on by the therapist and the patient every session. In the early sessions, the patient is oriented and trained in thought tracking and activity tracking. The decision of which thoughts or behaviors are targets for intervention is based on the specific needs of the patient, which the therapist assesses using the case formulation. In the case described, the patient reported feeling "miserable" when she arrived at class. The therapist used the situation to train the patient in using a thought record, as shown in Figure 13.9–1. The specific situation is identified, and the emotional response and the thought or thoughts are recorded, as well as the patient's belief in the thought.

Patients learn techniques for modifying unhelpful thinking, including identifying factual inaccuracies (e.g., "I don't understand anything" is all-or-nothing thinking) and biased information processing (ignoring evidence that she does know some things) and generating more accurate thoughts by the use of logic and testing beliefs.

Therapist: Okay, in this situation, you are feeling miserable at approximately 70 to 80. Now let's check this thought. What problems do you see with the thought "I don't understand anything"?

Patient: Well, it's pretty all or nothing, but it feels like it's true.

Therapist: Can you think of any times when you felt something was true and it wasn't?

Patient: Sure, I felt sure I wouldn't get into law school, or college for that matter.

Therapist: What does that tell you about this thought?

Patient: Well, it might not be true either.

Therapist: Okay, what would be other evidence that this thought isn't completely true?

Patient: Well, I do know some things.

Therapist: What is your evidence? Have you taken any tests or completed any assignments?

Patient: Yeah—and I got a B on the first test.

Therapist: So, what can we write in the rational responses column?

Patient: It isn't all or nothing; I do know some stuff.

Therapist: How miserable do you feel if you tell yourself that?

Patient: Well, a little less, maybe 50.

In this case, the patient experiences several types of distortion, including all-or-nothing thinking and emotional reasoning (i.e., "I feel it is true; therefore, it must be true"). The patient is asked to generate evidence that challenges the negative belief. The evidence reduces but does not eliminate the negative feeling. This is often the case, particularly when working with retrospective examples and patients experiencing significant depression. One approach to increase the efficacy of thought challenging and evidence gathering in CBT is by developing behavioral experiments to test the belief. In this case, the patient later conducted an experiment to test the "I don't know anything" belief. She wrote down her own answers to questions asked in the class, as well as the answers other students made. She found that her knowledge was on par with her classmates, and she was able to answer most of the questions. This experiment also addressed her "belonging," because she got evidence of her equivalence to her peers.

As treatment progresses, the therapist points out recurring themes and helps the patient to identify and to challenge core beliefs. In this example, the patient repeatedly experienced thoughts about not being good enough. She said that she felt this way all her life and attributed to her sense of being different from her parents and her European-American friends and her experience of several incidents of racism.

One approach to changing schemata is to generate alternative core beliefs and to help the patient identify behaviors and cognitions that are consistent with the new beliefs. In this case, a belief of "I belong just like everyone belongs; others may not believe it or act that way, but I do" was consistent with the patients' values and overriding experience. The therapist would therefore challenge thoughts by asking "is that the 'old self' or 'new self' talking?" This provided a shorthand for identifying dysfunctional thoughts and generating new ones consistent with the alternative schema.

Situation	Emotions (strength, 0-100)	Automatic Thoughts (strength of belief, 0-100)	Rational Responses	New Emotion (0-100)
ENTERING CLASS	MISERABLE (70-80)	I DON'T UNDERSTAND ANYTHING GOING ON IN THIS CLASS! (100)	THAT'S ALL-OR - NOTHING AND EMOTIONAL REASONING IN THE PAST, SOME THINGS I FELT WERE TRUE DIDN'T TURN OUT TO BE TRUE I DO KNOW SOMETHING, OR I WOULD NOT HAVE GOTTEN A B.	MISERABLE (50)

FIGURE 13.9–1 Thought record example.

In the final sessions, the tasks shift to reviewing progress, identifying potential future challenges, and the patient learning to administer interventions independently. Returning to the example, the patient showed significant improvement in her mood. Interventions that had been beneficial were attending the school gym on a regular schedule (activity scheduling), joining a study group (activity scheduling, assertiveness training, and social interaction), and gathering evidence regarding beliefs about being good enough and belonging (thought challenging and experiments). In addition, another student had invited the patient on several dates. At the end of therapy, the patient had a depression score on the BDI in the nondepressed range, her school attendance and grades had improved, and she had daily contact with friends and family.

In preparing for termination, it is important to identify the improvements that the patient has made, the skills that have been learned, and potential challenges that may arise in the future. This client identified her risk factors for increased depression as a rejection if she started dating or failure at school. She also noted that, although she now did not fear attending class, and she was doing well, she still was not talking in class unless she was called on.

Therapist: Is not answering questions in class a problem?

Patient: Yeah.

Therapist: Okay, you've been doing this a while, what do you think would be a good homework for you?

Patient: Well, I guess I could just plan to answer one or two questions in class, and see what happens.

Therapist: When you say "see what happens," what could you track?

Patient: Maybe how many I get right and my thoughts and feelings after each question.

Therapist: Sounds good. What are some things you can do to make that easy in the class setting?

Because CBT is a skills-based model, it is critical that the patient demonstrate an ability to use skills independently of the therapist. In this case, she is able to take on the role of therapist and to assign herself a task that can help her modify her beliefs and behavior.

BIOLOGICALLY INFORMED PSYCHOTHERAPY FOR DEPRESSION

Psychotherapy research has demonstrated the effectiveness of a number of approaches to treat depressive symptomatology and associated psychosocial morbidity. However, it is rare for such findings to be translated into clinical practice in its "whole cloth." Historically, the art of medicine has involved the incorporation and integration of general findings of scientific inquiry into practical applications: one patient at a time, use of the physician's best knowledge about a patient, the relevant factors to be addressed in that person's treatment, and the current available research literature.

Biologically informed psychotherapy for depression is an integrated approach that incorporates a number of psychological and behavioral technologies into a biological framework of affective illness. The integration of biological, psychological, and psychosocial treatments for depressive illnesses requires knowledge of the technologies to be applied and the individually determined areas of pathology (or problems in living) that require intervention. The authors have discussed the psychotherapeutic technologies that have been developed and studied. Specific biological treatments are not the focus of this section but are addressed at great length elsewhere in this text.

Biologically informed psychotherapy for depression is based on a number of research-derived assumptions:

- Mood disorders (major depressive disorders, dysthymic disorders, and bipolar spectrum disorders), are diatheses that, once initiated, have tendencies toward recurrence, chronicity, and, in general, autonomy (that is, a greater likelihood for recurrence without the same level of psychosocial stressors that precipitated episodes earlier in the course of illness). This implies the need for treatment strategies that have long-term application.
- Regardless of initial cause, there is a reciprocal relationship between depressive symptoms and impaired functioning: Each exacerbates the other.
- Efforts to prevent the onset of these illnesses, although promising, are only recently being developed and have uncertain efficacy. Therefore, treatment strategies must focus on alleviating pain and suffering that follow the onset of the disorder, limiting disruption of work and dysfunctional relatedness, and preventing suicide.
- Even when there has been relatively successful treatment defined by so-called remission, there is frequently some breakthrough of symptoms and some residue of illness to be treated.
- Most psychological and psychosocial interventions are likely to be done in periods of depression or euthymia, as individuals in states of mania are almost always inaccessible to such interventions, and even those in hypomanic states are compromised in their capacities to reflect and to use treatments.
- In the course of increasing understanding of the biology of mood disorders and the recognition that psychiatry remains largely ignorant of the ultimate *causes* of such disorders (albeit that they are multifactorial), the focus of treatment in psychiatry has shifted from trying to understand how someone got that way, in the hopes of reversing the process, to helping them understand what the impacts of such illnesses are on their lives and trying to minimize these effects.

Language of Depression

The language of depression represents the translation of its various symptoms into the problems of living encountered by people experiencing depressive phenomena, be they transitory mood changes associated with a life stressor or the serious ongoing sequelae of major psychiatric illness. The language of depression can be observed and assessed in each of the major arenas of functioning: (1) interpersonal relatedness, (2) productive capacities, and (3) identity and self-esteem. Because these arenas incorporate most of the problems of living with which patients struggle, they become a practical means of focusing on issues of assessment and treatment of depressive phenomenology.

Assessing State-Dependent versus Trait Phenomena

Of critical importance in assessing areas of dysfunction in the context of a mood disorder is the differentiation of qualities that are state dependent or state influenced from those qualities that are consistent traits and independent of mood state. There are important distinctions to make in helping clinicians and patients appreciate *who they are* as opposed to who they are when they are depressed. Here are examples that highlight such distinctions. A medical student with recurrent major depression describes, "I am not myself: I'm usually sure of myself, decisive, and gregarious," but, while depressed, she feels inadequate and socially avoidant. The regressed social behavior is understood as a manifestation of depression rather than the demonstration of permanent flaws that seem immutable. A contrasting example is a man in his 40s whose chronic depression has resulted in major impairments in his career and disruption of two marriages and whose views of himself and the world have been permanently altered by the impact of chronic illness. He may be unaware or unaccepting of what his strengths and capacities may be, having lived and deteriorated in the shadow of illness.

In the first of these two examples, reinstatement of euthymia (by time, medication, or psychotherapy) is likely to result in a full reversal of functioning and positive self-perceptions. In the second example, simply treating mood will not reverse the failures that have occurred or the perceptions that have accompanied them. A more schema-focused form of psychotherapy for this man would be useful.

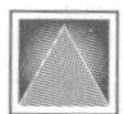

Table 13.9–2
Effects of Depression on Interpersonal Relationships

Social withdrawal and isolation
Irritability, bitterness, cynicism, and misanthropy
Lack of consideration and empathy
Infectiousness of mood
Resentment toward caregivers
Diminished resilience and flexibility, decreased coping
Emotional emptiness and unresponsiveness
Self-deprecation as a turnoff
Rejection sensitivity
Sensitivity to criticism
Distorted perspectives about significant others

Effects of Depression on Interpersonal Relationships

The impact of depression on interpersonal relationships can be profound and destructive. Table 13.9–2 includes a number of the changes that are seen in depressed patients. When they occur in marriages or other partnerships, with families, and with friends, these phenomena affect not only the person who is depressed, but also those around them. They are changes of substance and perspective and have a further impact of undermining the stability of and often threatening the existence of the relationship—from both sides.

To the extent that a patient is convinced of the reality of his or her experience, his or her misery allows or even encourages responding to significant others with anger, disappointment, criticism, or perceived rejection. Multiple offending issues interpreted through the distorting lens of depression may conspire to inform the individual that the relationship itself may be the source of his or her suffering and that reasonable adaptation would suggest limiting contact with others or even ending the relationship.

A common clinical example illustrates these issues.

> A middle-aged married man is experiencing a progressively worsening depression. He has been exquisitely sensitive to his wife's criticism (even in its absence). His anhedonia leaves him without feelings of affection or sexual interest. He believes his wife does not care for him, because he feels unlovable or because she is actually staying out of his way, because he is so irritable or inconsolable in his suffering. Through the prism of his negativity, he interprets her efforts at humor as sarcastic and mean spirited, her generosity as wastefulness, and her concern as intrusiveness. It is not a great leap for him to decide that his marriage is the source of his suffering and to feel quite justified in expressing his resentment for what his wife is doing to him. He does not possess the insight into his illness to appreciate depression's contribution to all of these factors that now provide him with ammunition to act out hostilely or to end the relationship.

Effects of Depression on Productive Capacities

The mechanisms by which depressive symptoms may undermine an individual's career, school, or other role functions are listed in Table 13.9–3. These include compromises in functioning based on impairments in energy, cognitive functioning, and altered motivational factors, as well as those already described interpersonal changes that enter into the workplace, school, or home and that may further undermine the individual's productive capacities. In this arena, impairments from each of these contributions are amplified and distorted by the tendency of depressed people to see themselves in their worst light. In a downward cyclical fashion, the depressed person is less able to function, is less likely to try, and, in an effort to escape from an increasingly overwhelming situation, often gives up and walks away from what may have been a promising career or school. Again, the person's justification may be reinforced by his or her depressively based experience, replete with distortions and unbalanced by perspective. Such disruptions are often commonplace in the experience of those with affective disorders and, after repeated failures or changes, make the possibilities for stability and continuity seem remote in their lives, leaving them with another level of reality-based demoralization.

A 45-year-old unmarried woman therapist with a history of recurrent major depression is treated with aggressive antidepressant therapy and psychotherapy but continues to manifest mild to moderate residual depression. Her mood is bearable, although unpleasant, and her depression is a daily struggle. She describes continuing difficulty in her work, as she has throughout her career when depressed. She often feels that she is just going through the motions and not experiencing much satisfaction from her work efforts. Her patients' problems seem overwhelming to her, and, when she starts to empathize with their suffering, her depression feels more intense. She finds herself creating more emotional distance than usual. She is more distracted and more preoccupied with her own problems. She is questioning the value of her work as a psychotherapist, denigrating herself as a "hired friend," and frequently feels like a fraud, despite fairly clear evidence of her continued effectiveness.

On a number of occasions in the past, she became convinced that she was simply "burned out" and that she should give up her career, believing that it was too stressful and that she was inadequate to the task. Acting on the distortions of her depression could have led to the loss of all of these positive elements in her life. Furthermore, she would still have had a major depressive disorder, and her life would likely have been much more miserable.

Such scenarios provide insight into the mechanisms of social and career deterioration that feed the morbidity of depression.

Effects of Depression on Identity and Self-Esteem

Identity and self-esteem represent those perceptions that individuals have of themselves: their place in the world, their capacities and personal qualities, and the sense of their own value. These views are complex, multifaceted, and fluid. These are perceptions that evolve with the development and maturation of the individual throughout life and its myriad experiences. Biologically informed psychotherapy for depression conceptualizes an individual's self-perceptions as contextual (i.e., feeling competent about one's work skills and inadequate about being a father). The impact of depression is invariably to create a regressive distortion of any of the depressed person's self-perceptions. This is true of almost any developmental issue, personal quality, or view of the world.

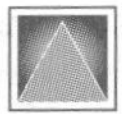

Table 13.9–3
Effects of Depression on Productive Capacities

Vegetative symptoms, especially insomnia and ↑ fatigue
↓ Physical and mental energy
Anhedonia leads to ↓ satisfaction
Pessimism leads to ↓ significance and value
Self-deprecation leads to ↓ confidence, ↓ decision making, and ↓ leadership
↓ Persistence and determination at tasks
Impaired formal cognitive processes: impaired concentration, distractibility, and disorganization
Interpersonal factors: irritability, withdrawal, impatience, and inflexibility

All mature adults have had the experiences of feeling inadequate, helpless, and fearful as normal elements of development. The most competent, self-assured, and fearless individual in the throes of depression usually regresses to earlier (developmentally) views of themselves. This reflects the negativity associated with degrees of anhedonia, as well as the reality-based observations of the various forms of impairment described previously.

A successful young attorney who experiences frequent alterations in mood has developed a different set of people with whom she communicates based on her mood state. When depressed, aware of her greater dependency and neediness, her self-deprecation, and her evolving pessimism about life, she calls her "loser" friends: women who are struggling with their lives, at times unsuccessfully, and who tolerate her self-pity and self-loathing and welcome an opportunity to give her support. They feel better helping her. In contrast, when her mood is euthymic or mildly elevated, her confidence, optimism, and expressiveness lead her to interact with a more competitive, self-assured group of people who are not at all receptive to her other self.

The biologically informed psychotherapy for depression model assumes all people experience similar kinds of regressive thinking in the context of the vicissitudes of living. These are associated with disappointments, rejections, losses, and unfavorable comparisons with others one has seen in the media. Under normal circumstances, and especially when *not* under the influence of a mood disorder, people quickly correct the distorted thinking that occurs. This is done in the interests of psychological homeostasis, and most people have some repertoire for dispelling cognitive dissonance. At times, this is through positive self-talk or reassurance from others, including a higher power, or even devaluation and deprecation of others for their own benefit. When people are depressed, these tools are not as available to them or it takes great effort to access them.

In extreme circumstances, the continuous onslaught of pain, self-deprecation, the pessimism about the future, and the sense of helplessness in the face of suffering leads the depressed to the logical (in their distorted perceptions) view that their suffering can only be relieved by their own death. They have no understanding of the extent that such views are driven by the depressed state, or (again influenced by depression) they have lost any hope that their depression can be relieved.

ELEMENTS OF BIOLOGICALLY INFORMED PSYCHOTHERAPY FOR DEPRESSION

Table 13.9–4 outlines the elements of integrated psychotherapy, which include education, psychodynamic understanding, coping

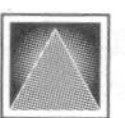

Table 13.9–4
Elements of Integrated Psychotherapy for Depression

Education about illness
Psychodynamic understanding
Coping skills, education, and training
Work with significant others
Development of therapeutic alliance

skills education and training, work with significant others, and development of a working therapeutic relationship.

Education Education about the illness is addressed at many different levels: Clinicians share their understanding of the nature of the illness. Physicians may include discussing a biological model using basic information about neurotransmitter functions. Depending on the patient's capacity, different kinds of literature may be provided. Because people often misattribute their mood symptoms, it is useful to examine their assumptions about why they are symptomatic and to correct common views identifying depression as a reflection of personal weaknesses, "badness," or even unresolved oedipal conflicts. Patients learn about the symptoms of depression and mania as a means of tracking their problems, seeking more help or support, or needing to change medication.

A critical element in patient education involves the identification, translation, and reinterpretation of the language of depression to prevent its misattribution and the potentially maladaptive consequences (i.e., helping the patient recognize how depression influences judgment). The following examples describe this principle in greater depth.

A depressed schoolteacher finds herself short-tempered and critical of her students, easily provoked, disorganized with her lesson plans, and greatly relieved when she gets home at night. Even at home, she avoids grading papers and preparing for her next class, choosing to watch television and to overeat, then berating herself. She decides that maybe she is not cut out for teaching, that students do not want to learn anyway and just need a baby-sitter (or jailer), and that she would not be as miserable as she feels if she just quit her job and found something less stressful. The therapist can help the patient by providing education about the state-dependent nature of emotions, cognitions, vulnerabilities, and behaviors as manifestations of depression. "It's the depression talking." This is the initial step in harm prevention.

When this same teacher arrives home and finds the dishes in the sink, her husband watching a ball game, and her teenage girls on the phone, she may feel inclined to yell at everyone for being inconsiderate or irresponsible, and, in her state of mind, she may have lost all sense of balance about others' motivations, interests, and inclinations and see them only in her highly personalized, critical, and irritable frame of mind. When she is in a euthymic state, however, she might respond constructively. "Captured" by depression, she likely feels justified in yelling at everyone (or perhaps she only feels out of control). Her therapist would like her to learn to recognize the impact of her depression on this situation, *if only* to undermine the moral authority of her acting out. This insight may not change her fundamental state, but it will help her avoid acting out in a way that may be destructive within her family and, in the long run, may worsen the depression. This may also save her from the embarrassment or humiliation that often follows such behavior. Over time, depressed patients are able to use such insight to protect their relationships or to persist with work in the face of otherwise debilitating symptoms.

One technique of education about depression involves the therapist helping reexamine the patient's life retrospectively through the prism of depression. For people who have had chronic forms of depression, reviewing the experiences with an understanding of the impact of depression on development may offer a kinder and gentler glimpse at life than patients usually have of themselves and their lives. An adult woman may have gone through adolescence depressed, yet thinking that she was lazy, unloving, and unlovable. Such review may help adult depressed patients who were highly critical of difficult parents develop an empathic appreciation for the same affective disorder in their parents that now afflicts them. A good deal of healing can occur when multiple family members examine their histories together from this perspective.

Psychodynamic Understanding and Learning History Historically, psychodynamic understanding was believed to be at the core of curing disorders whose etiology was viewed as conflict based. Although this view currently has limited value in biologically informed psychotherapy for depression, an examination of dynamic forces can help the patient with depression identify stressors in his or her life that may aggravate or complicate symptoms. There are universal and idiosyncratic dynamic responses to illness. These include struggles over loss of control and greater dependency, as well as other forces involved in the regression associated with depression. Psychodynamic issues are of central importance regarding acceptance of illness, compliance with medication, and the complications of the doctor–patient relationship.

A middle-aged man, who left home at an early age to escape his overly controlling and critical father, has dealt with his authority conflicts by becoming one (identification with the aggressor) and was the master of his universe in business and in his home life. Not surprisingly, he struggled with his teenage son's efforts at self-determination, but they both survived with few scars. The emergence of a major depressive episode after his wife's death was an anathema. He expected to suffer and was quite able to tolerate his grief in its most intense forms. What became unbearable and unacceptable was his cognitive dysfunction and the loss of control that this conferred on his daily life. Understanding the centrality of these dynamic issues allows the therapist to be more empathic and to intervene by helping this man appreciate the effects of depression and the time-limited nature of these overwhelming phenomena. Over time, cognitive approaches can also help this man examine the assumptions about the need to be in such control.

COPING SKILLS TRAINING

Even in cases in which mood symptoms are effectively treated with antidepressants and mood stabilizers, most patients with major depression, dysthymic disorders, or bipolar disorders experience breakthrough of symptoms as manifestations of an exacerbation, as transient depression, or as chronic residual depression. Developing the tools to deal with these states becomes a necessary component in treatment, and this is the arena in which the approaches of CBT, interpersonal psychotherapy, mindfulness, traditional meditation, guided imagery, and other therapeutic schools can be integrated. With the exception of mindfulness (whose goals are to recognize and to embrace all experiences whether positive or negative), the common thread of most such applications involves maneuvers to alter the pain and anguish of depression: to neutralize it, to deflect it, or to transform it into another state. First, simply by describing and discussing their experiences, patients are shifting from more affective to cognitive and intellectual processes. CBT methods include challenging underlying assumptions that shift cognitive processes that are negative and painful. Many therapeutic maneuvers try to capitalize on the reality that, with the exception of the most severely depressed (whose anhedonia is complete and whose hypothalamic mechanisms for experiencing pleasure are totally shut down), many depressed patients have some degree of hedonia or reactivity, and, placed in the right circumstances, they may feel better. Guided imagery, music, religious faith, cuddling with grandchildren, or other forms of socializing may help maximize positive experiences, even in cases in which motivational systems to achieve such goals may be compromised and require other forms of external motivation (e.g., a therapist's wishes, a commitment to participate in a treatment program, and the cajoling of loved ones). A corollary of this involves helping the affected person to persist with his or her work, school, social obligations, and other responsibilities wherever possible.

Distraction may neutralize depressive affects and may occur as a product of many kinds of mental and physical activity, jobs of all kinds, or even more passive distractions, such as television or radio. Sometimes, it may be therapeutic for patients to have permission to watch television if the only other option is to sit, to ruminate, and to suffer.

The tasks of the therapist include reviewing systematically the tools that patients have available, promoting the most adaptive tools (usually involving some focused activity or correcting distortions), suppressing the more maladaptive tools (eating, smoking, drinking alcohol, etc.), and developing new tools (guided imagery and assertiveness training), so that the periods in which depression does persist are less painful and more productive.

WORK WITH SIGNIFICANT OTHERS

Because of the enormous impact that mood disorders bring to the lives of those affected, bringing family members and other loved ones into treatment can have great practical benefit. Family involvement can include (1) assessment, (2) education, (3) support, (4) monitoring, and (5) treatment of relationship problems.

Assessment Assessment is often advanced through shared information by an outside observer: Depressed patients cannot always identify fully the impact of illness on themselves or others. In the throes of depression, individuals may be able to describe only their most distorted views of themselves, their lives, and their relationships. It may take a spouse to help a therapist appreciate how committed the patient has been to his or her work or how patient and understanding he or she is when not depressed.

Education Education about mood disorders can be as enlightening for families as it is for patients. The mysteries of changing moods, thought patterns, and behavior can be clarified, and order can be brought to the perception of chaos. Understanding that depression itself can cause sexual disinterest or a lack of emotional warmth or irritability can be reassuring to a loving family member who has taken such behavior personally or who feels helpless in the face of his or her best efforts to comfort the depressed. An awareness of the genetic vulnerability associated with the affective disorders may help explain the experience of other family members or sensitize parents to possible future illness in their children.

Support Support for the depressed individual often comes from family members. Incorporating significant others into a treatment plan to develop the healthiest means of coping with depression can make this process more efficient. In working with bipolar patients, in particular, this aspect of treatment can be crucial. Having family members involved in planning with the patient to develop contingencies in the event of a manic episode is sometimes the only form of control that can be exerted short of hospitalization (or jail) at the time of a full-blown manic episode. Prevention, or at least early intervention, in such circumstances almost always requires elaborate planning with family members.

Monitoring Monitoring the patient's mood states within families is a sometimes delicate, always conflictual, but occasionally necessary, function to allow for the wisest and safest interventions when a patient is at significant risk. This occurs most frequently around issues of suicide but also arises in evolving mania. Sessions with couples or families are best held early in treatment and, if possible, during periods of euthymia, during which the ground rules for communication between therapist and nonpatient family members can be discussed openly. The dilemmas for patient and therapist and family involve the undesirability of infantilizing the patient while maintaining safeguards for those periods when illness has compromised his or her rational capacities.

Treatment of Relationship Problems Treatment of relationship problems in the context of a depressive episode is complicated by the distorting effects of mood. Some conflicts hypertrophy, the means of solving them diminish, the motivations change, and the balance necessary for stability is absent. Although a therapist should always be prepared to listen to the complaints, it is often wisest to say: "Let's reexamine these issues between you once the depression has quieted down." During the acute phases of depression, it is more important for a couple to recognize the role depression is playing and to try to weather the storm. During euthymic states, marital therapy to resolve problems with money, sex, children, power, and others will likely proceed more efficiently. Occasionally, the issues that arise during depressed states dissolve once mood is normal.

PSYCHOTHERAPEUTIC RELATIONSHIP

The parallels between the affective disorders and many other chronic medical illnesses speak to the similar roles of the psychotherapist in relation to the chronically ill. Treatment requires an alliance between doctor and patient to fight the illness with whatever tools are available and to help the patient live most adaptively with whatever elements cannot be controlled. For the psychiatrist who provides an integrated treatment, this would include the use of psychopharmacology and psychotherapy to minimize symptoms, to prevent harm, to optimize function, and to cope adaptively with residual pain.

The demands of the psychiatrist and psychotherapist are numerous. He or she should have the capacity to establish a knowledgeable, empathically based alliance: Patients need to know that their therapist understands their experience and their disorder. The therapist should also be able to confront the distortions created by the illness. He or she must be active in teaching the patient about the impact of depression, and this alternation of empathy and confrontation is often a difficult orientation to develop.

Another essential psychotherapist function is to maintain the consistent vision by the therapist of the patient's healthy self undistorted by illness. This allows the therapist to maintain a conviction about the patient's identity even when the patient seems to have lost it. An extension of this role is that the therapist remain a bastion of hope regardless of the patient's state of mind.

The most difficult aspect of treating patients with affective disorders inevitably involves working with those whose illnesses have been relatively refractory to treatment. In such circumstances, powerful transference and countertransference issues arise: intensifying patient dependency, frustration, and desperation reflected by the therapists' sense of frustration, helplessness, anger, and blame. These are often situations in which a team approach may help spread out these difficult emotions and avoid demoralization or, occasionally, abandonment by the frustrated therapist. On the other hand, successful long-term work with such patients can be extraordinarily gratifying.

CONCLUSION

Some basic guidelines can be derived in treatment. In general, it is incumbent on the clinician to apply interventions for which there is empirical support. In the case of major depression, there are several psychotherapeutic options that have been reviewed, and there is an increase in options for other mood disorders (bipolar disorder and dysthymia). There are some patient characteristics that could recommend treatment, including the presence of significant marital distress, amenability to a particular validated treatment modality, and chronic depression.

The authors believe that an important component of good psychotherapy, regardless of model, is that the therapist has a treatment rationale that guides decisions regarding interventions. This is a shared theme of all the current validated treatments for mood disorders. However, such a model is not likely sufficient for effective treatment. Psychotherapies generally are built around mediational models of change, with modification of the target symptom (e.g., depressed mood) being achieved through intervention on a more accessible construct (e.g., an irrational belief, a rewarding activity, or a transference reaction in therapy). What distinguishes excellent clinicians, regardless of orientation, is their ability to hold a conceptual framework in mind and to apply that framework to the unique challenges of the patient.

SUGGESTED CROSS-REFERENCES

Information regarding related aspects of mood disorders is discussed further in the other sections of Chapter 13. Chapter 30 on psychotherapies also outlines behavioral and cognitive therapies and other psychosocial treatments. Psychiatric treatments of adolescents are reviewed in Chapter 48, and treatments in the elderly population are included in Section 51.4. Application of psychosocial treatment to schizophrenia may be found in Section 12.11.

References

Albon JS, Jones EE: Validity of controlled clinical trials of psychotherapy: Findings from the NIMH Treatment of Depression Collaborative Research Program. *Am J Psychiatry.* 2002;159:775–783.

Bandura A. *Principles of Behavior Modification.* London: Oxford Press; 1969.

Bandura A. *Social Learning Theory.* Englewood Cliffs, NJ: Prentice-Hall; 1977.

Baskin TW, Tierney SC, Minami T, Wampold BE: Establishing specificity in psychotherapy: A meta-analysis of structural equivalence of placebo controls. *J Consult Clin Psychol.* 2003;71:973–979.

Baucom DH, Shoham V, Mueser KT, Daiuto AD, Stickle TR: Empirically supported couple and family interventions for marital distress and adult mental health problems. *J Consult Clin Psychol.* 1998;66:53–88.

*Beck AT, Rush AJ, Shaw BF, Emery G. *Cognitive Therapy of Depression.* New York: Guilford Press; 1979.

Beck JS. *Cognitive Therapy: Basics and Beyond.* New York: Guilford Press; 1995.

*DeRubeis RJ, Crits-Cristoph P: Empirically supported individual and group psychological treatments for adult mental health problems. *J Consult Clin Psychol.* 1998;66:37–52.

DiMascio A, Weissman MM, Prusoff BA, Neu C, Zwilling M, Klerman GL: Differential symptom reduction by drugs and psychotherapy in acute depression. *Arch Gen Psychiatry.* 1979;36:1450–1456.

Elkin I, Shea MT, Watkins JT, Imber SD, Sotsky SM, Collins JF, Glass DR, Pilkonis PA, Leber WR, Doherty JP, Fiester SJ, Parloff MB: NIMH Treatment of Depression Collaborative Research Program: I. General effectiveness of treatments. *Arch Gen Psychiatry.* 1989;47:971–982.

Ellis A. *Reason and Emotion in Psychotherapy.* Oxford: Lyle Stuart; 1962.

Frank E, Swartz HA, Kupfer DJ: Interpersonal and social rhythm therapy: Managing the chaos of bipolar disorder. *Biol Psychiatry.* 2000;48:593–604.

Hollon SD, DeRubeis RJ, Evans MD, Wiemer MJ, Garvey MJ, Grove WM, Tuason VB: Cognitive therapy and pharmacotherapy for depression: Singly and in combination. *Arch Gen Psychiatry.* 1992;49:774–781.

Jacobson NS, Dobson KS, Truax PA, Addis ME, Koerner K, Gollan JK, Gortner E, Prince SE: A component analysis of cognitive-behavioral treatment for depression. *J Consult Clin Psychol.* 1996;64:295–304.

Jarrett RB, Schaffer M, McIntire D, Witt-Browder A, Kraft D, Risser RC: Treatment of atypical depression with cognitive therapy or phenelzine: A double-blind, placebo-controlled trial. *Arch Gen Psychiatry.* 1999;56:431–437.

Judd LL: The clinical course of unipolar major depressive disorders. *Arch Gen Psychiatry.* 1997;54:989–991.

Judd LL, Akiskal HS, Maser JD, Zeller PJ, Endicott J, Coryell W, Paulus MP, Kunovac JL, Leon AC, Mueller TI, Rice JA, Martin B: A prospective 12-year study of subsyndromal and syndromal depressive symptoms in unipolar major depressive disorders. *Arch Gen Psychiatry.* 1998;55:694–700.

Keller MB, McCullough JP, Klein DN, Arnow B, Dunner DL, Gelenberg AJ, Markowitz JC, Nemeroff CB, Russell JM, Thase ME, Trivedi MH, Zajecka J: A comparison of nefazodone, the cognitive behavioral-analysis system of psychotherapy, and their combination for the treatment of chronic depression. *N Engl J Med.* 2000;342:1462–1470.

*Klerman GL, Weissman MM, Rounsaville BJ, Chevron ES. *Interpersonal Psychotherapy of Depression.* New York: Basic Books; 1984.

Lewinsohn PM. A behavioral approach to depression. In: Friedman RJ, Katz MM, Martin M, eds. *The Psychology of Depression: Contemporary Theory and Research.* Oxford: John Wiley and Sons; 1974:318.

*Lewinsohn PM, Clarke GN: The coping with depression course. *Adv Behav Res Ther.* 1984;6:99–114.

Ma SH, Teasdale JD: Mindfulness-based cognitive therapy for depression: Replication and exploration of differential relapse prevention effects. *J Consult Clin Psychol.* 2004;72:31–40.

McCullough JP. *Treatment for Chronic Depression: Cognitive Behavioral Analysis System of Psychotherapy.* New York: Guilford Press; 2000.

Muñoz RF, Ying Y. *The Prevention of Depression.* Baltimore: The Johns Hopkins University Press; 1993.

Murphy GE, Simons AD, Wetzel RD, Lustman PJ: Cognitive therapy and pharmacotherapy. *Arch Gen Psychiatry.* 1984;41:33–41.

Persons JB. *Cognitive Therapy in Practice: A Case Formulation Approach.* New York: Norton; 1989.

Rush AJ, Beck AT, Kovacs M, Hollon S: Comparative efficacy of cognitive therapy and pharmacotherapy in the treatment of depressed patients. *Cogn Ther Res.* 1977;1:17–37.

Sanderson WC: Why empirically supported psychological treatments are important. *Behav Mod.* 2003;27:290–299.

Scott J, Palmer S, Paykel E, Teasdale J, Hayhurst H: Use of cognitive therapy for relapse prevention in chronic depression: Cost-effectiveness study. *Br J Psychiatry.* 2003;182:221–227.

Segal ZV, Williams JMG, Teasdale JD. *Mindfulness-Based Cognitive Therapy for Depression.* New York: Guilford Press; 2002.

*Shuchter SR, Downs N, Zisook S. *Biologically Informed Psychotherapy for Depression.* New York: Guilford Press; 1996.

Skinner BF. *Science and Human Behavior.* New York: Macmillan; 1953.

Swartz HA, Frank E: Psychotherapy for bipolar depression: A phase-specific treatment strategy? *Bipolar Disord.* 2001;3:11–22.

Watson JC, Gordon LB, Stermac L, Kalogerakos F, Steckley P: Comparing the effectiveness of process-experiential with cognitive-behavioral psychotherapy in the treatment of depression. *J Consult Clin Psychol.* 2003;71:773–781.

Zeiss AM, Lewinsohn PM, Munoz RF: Nonspecific improvement effects in depression using interpersonal skills training, pleasant activity schedules, or cognitive training. *J Consult Clin Psychol.* 1979;47:427–439.

14 Anxiety Disorders

▲ 14.1 Anxiety Disorders: Introduction and Overview

DENNIS S. CHARNEY, M.D.

Anxiety disorders are the most prevalent mental disorders in the general population. Approximately one in four adults in the U.S. population has an anxiety disorder at some point in his or her life. Similar to adults, anxiety disorders are the most common mental disorder in children and adolescents. However, the rates of specific childhood anxiety disorders suggest the importance of brain development in the phenotypic expression of anxiety proneness. This is reflected by the findings of prospective community-based investigations revealing differential peak periods of onset of specific anxiety disorders: separation anxiety disorder and specific phobias in middle childhood, overanxious disorder in late childhood, social anxiety disorder in middle adolescence, panic disorder in late adolescence, generalized anxiety disorder in young adulthood, and obsessive-compulsive disorder (OCD) in early adulthood. Gender differences in rates appear by 6 years of age when girls are significantly more likely to have an anxiety disorder than boys.

SELECTED PSYCHOLOGICAL CHARACTERISTICS RELATED TO THE RISK OF ANXIETY DISORDERS

Several psychological factors have been associated with increased risk for anxiety disorders. Among the most intensively researched has been the concept of anxiety sensitivity. *Anxiety sensitivity* has been defined as the individual response to physiological alterations associated with anxiety and fear. Patients with anxiety disorders have exaggerated psychological reactions that are reflective of misinterpretation of bodily cues, such that the patient misperceives these sensations inappropriately as being harmful and dangerous, leading in a circular fashion to increased anxiety and fear. Anxiety sensitivity is associated with a selective cognitive bias toward threat. Anxiety sensitivity predicts the frequency and intensity of panic attacks. There is evidence that parental concern about anxiety increases anxiety sensitivity in their children. Anxiety sensitivity appears to be a trait abnormality and increases the risk for anxiety disorders. Increased anxiety sensitivity can be reduced by cognitive-behavioral therapy (CBT).

Researchers have investigated whether specific temperamental factors affect the development of anxiety disorders in children and adolescents. It has become clear that some children have an inherited neurobiological predisposition to increased physiological reactivity and anxious symptoms in the context of unfamiliar environments and consequently are more vulnerable to one or more of the anxiety disorders. Jerome Kagan estimates that roughly 20 percent of healthy children are born with such a temperamental bias, which is termed *behavioral inhibition*. Environmental influences intersect with temperament, and, by adolescence, approximately one-third of behavioral inhibition children ultimately exhibit indications of serious social anxiety. In a recent study, behavioral inhibition was associated with social anxiety disorder in children whose parents had panic disorder. These data suggest that parental panic disorder and childhood behavioral inhibition could be used to identify children at high risk for social anxiety disorder.

Kagan has also suggested that behavioral inhibition children may be especially susceptible to anxiety or posttraumatic stress disorder (PTSD) after threatening events. Studies of children who developed anxiety after a traumatic event suggest that a prior avoidant personality was a major risk factor. However, it is noteworthy to point out that the majority of behavioral inhibition children do not develop anxiety disorders in later adult life, indicating the importance of other intervening biological and genetic factors.

The presence of behavioral inhibition and evidence of insecure attachment to caregivers are likely to contribute to the variance in the expression of anxious symptoms in preschoolers. This may be related to the findings that parental overprotection, excessive criticism, and lack of warmth are risk factors for the appearance of anxiety disorders in childhood. Environmental risk factors for the development of anxiety disorders (as well as depression) include poverty, exposure to violence, social isolation, and repeated losses of interpersonal significance.

The neurobiological phenotype and genotype associated with temperamental risk factors for anxiety disorders such as anxiety sensitivity and behavioral inhibition remain to be precisely defined. An example of the type of investigations needed is increases in amygdala responsiveness in adults categorized as behavioral inhibited as children.

GENETICS

The genetics of anxiety disorders is a relatively neglected area of research compared to other serious psychiatric disorders, such as schizophrenia and bipolar disorder. Despite increased age-adjusted morbidity in first-degree relatives of probands with most of the anxiety disorders, progress has been slow in defining specific regions of the human genome and, more importantly, specific genes associated with vulnerability to anxiety disorders. Thus far, endophenotypes for the anxiety disorders have not been reliably demonstrated with the possible exception of carbon dioxide–induced panic attacks in relatives of panic disorder patients.

In the future, it will be extremely important to relate the psychological and environmental risk factors for anxiety disorders to specific genotypes. The precise determination of gene–environment interactions relevant to anxiety disorders will greatly facilitate the discovery of novel preventative and therapeutic approaches.

CLINICAL AND NEUROBIOLOGICAL FEATURES

The overreliance on standardized diagnostic systems in genetic and neurobiological investigations of anxiety disorders has impeded progress. Daniel S. Pine and Erin B. McClure review the history and current classifications systems for anxiety disorders. They emphasize that the revised fourth edition of the *Diagnostic and Statistical Manual of Mental Disorders* (DSM-IV-TR) classification system for anxiety disorders is not based on etiology, pathophysiology, or treatment response. The tenth edition of the *International Statistical Classification of Diseases and Related Health Problems* (ICD-10) recognizes a broader category of *neurotic, stress-related and somatoform disorders* that includes each of the nine DSM-IV-TR anxiety disorders, as well as a number of disorders not considered anxiety disorders in DSM-IV-TR.

As currently described in DSM-IV-TR, the nine anxiety disorders described in this section represent a heterogeneous set of disorders. This probably accounts, in part, for the findings of neurotransmitter and neuropeptide studies implicating abnormalities in noradrenergic, benzodiazepine, corticotrophin-releasing hormone, and other neurotransmitter and neuropeptide systems across different diagnostic conditions, as reviewed by Alexander Neumeister, Omer Bonne, and Dennis S. Charney. Similarly, the neuroimaging studies of anxiety disorders have identified roles for a variety of brain structures, including the amygdala, hippocampus, cingulate, and medial and orbital prefrontal cortex, in the regulation of emotion and cognition relevant to anxiety disorders. However, neural circuits have not been identified that correspond specifically to standardized diagnostic criteria for anxiety disorders. A more fruitful approach may be to investigate the neural circuits and associated neurotransmitters and neuropeptides that mediate the neural mechanisms of fear conditioning, reward, and social interactions that are relevant to the symptoms that are relevant to all of the anxiety disorders. Furthermore, identification of the genes that contribute to the regulation of these circuits may lead to better diagnostic methods and novel targets for drug development.

TREATMENT OF ANXIETY DISORDERS

Given the high prevalence and morbidity of anxiety disorders in children, adolescents, and adults, more effective psychotherapeutic and psychopharmacological treatments are needed. Shawn P. Cahil and Edna B. Foa in their comprehensive review of CBT acknowledge that, although CBT is an effective treatment, there are many patients who respond incompletely or not at all. There is a need for new forms of psychotherapy that go beyond the tenets of CBT, particularly therapies that are sensitive to developmental considerations in children and adolescents with anxiety disorders. Murray B. Stein extensively reviews the current status of somatic treatments for anxiety disorders. The mainstay of drug treatments for anxiety disorders remains the monoamine reuptake inhibitors, monoamine oxidase inhibitors (MAOIs), and benzodiazepines. Psychiatrists eagerly await the results of ongoing or soon-to-be-commenced clinical trials with novel putative anxiolytic drugs, such as corticotrophin-releasing hormone antagonists, substance P antagonists, anxioselective benzodiazepines, glutamate release modulators, and vasopressin V1a receptor antagonists. Anxiety disorder research has not yet identified reliable descriptive, genetic, or neurobiological predictors of therapeutic response for any of the anxiety disorders. However, the tremendous advances in basic neuroscience relevant to the pathophysiology of anxiety disorders should facilitate substantial progress in these areas in the not-too-distant future. The emergence of a new neurobiology of anxiety disorders will redefine diagnostic classification, will more precisely delineate gene–environment interactions, will inform the choice of therapy, and will promote the discovery of more effective and selective classes of drugs for anxiety disorders.

SUGGESTED CROSS-REFERENCES

Neural sciences are covered in Chapter 1, and neuropsychiatry and behavioral neurology are covered in Chapter 2. The sections within Chapter 14 should serve as a guide to developments in research and treatment in the field of anxiety disorders: Epidemiology of anxiety disorders is discussed in Section 14.2; biochemical aspects of anxiety disorders in Sections 14.3, 14.4, and 14.5; genetics of anxiety disorders in Section 14.6; clinical features of anxiety disorders in Section 14.8; somatic treatment for anxiety disorders in Section 14.9; and psychological treatments for anxiety disorders in Section 14.10. Chapter 46 covers anxiety disorders in children, and Section 51.3c discusses anxiety disorders in the elderly.

REFERENCES

Doyle AC, Pollack MH: Establishment of remission criteria for anxiety disorders. *J Clin Psychiatry.* 2003;64[Suppl 15]:40–45.

Hariri AR, Mattay VS, Tessitore A, Kolachana B, Fera F, Goldman D, Egan MF, Weinberger DR: Serotonin transporter genetic variation and the response of the human amygdala. *Science.* 2002;297:400–403.

*Kagan J, Reznick JS, Snidman N: Biological bases of childhood shyness. *Science.* 1998;240:167–171.

Kagan J, Snidman N: Early childhood predictors of adult anxiety disorders. *Biol Psychiatry.* 1999;46:1536–1541.

Kagan J, Snidman N, Arcus D: Childhood derivatives of high and low reactivity in infancy. *Child Dev.* 1998;69:1483–1493.

Kagan J, Snidman N, Zentner M, Peterson E: Infant temperament and anxious symptoms in school age children. *Dev Psychopathol.* 1999;11:209–224.

*Keogh E, Dilon C, Georgiou G, Hunt C: Selective attentional biases for physical threat in physical anxiety sensitivity. *J Anxiety Disord.* 2001;15:299–315.

McNally RJ: Anxiety sensitivity and panic disorder. *Biol Psychiatry.* 2002;52:938–946.

Pigott TA: Anxiety disorders in women. *Psychiatr Clin North Am.* 2003;26:621–672.

Prior M, Smart D, Sanson A, Oberklaid F: Does shy-inhibited temperament in childhood lead to anxiety problems in adolescence? *J Am Acad Child Adolesc Psychiatry.* 2000;39:461–468.

*Pynoos RS, Frederick C, Neder K, Arroyo W, Steinberg A, Eth F: Life threat and posttraumatic stress disorder in school-age children. *Arch Gen Psychiatry.* 1987;44:1057–1063.

Rapee RM: The development and modification of temperamental risk for anxiety disorders: Prevention of a lifetime of anxiety? *Biol Psychiatry.* 2002;52:947–957.

*Schwartz CE, Snidman N, Kagan J: Adolescent social anxiety as an outcome of inhibited temperament in childhood. *J Am Acad Chld Adolesc Psychiatry.* 1999;38:1008–1015.

Schwartz CE, Wright CI, Shin LM, Kagan J, Rauch SL: Inhibited and uninhibited infants "grown up": Adult amygdala response to novelty. *Science.* 2003;300:1052–1053.

Stein MB: Attending to anxiety disorders in primary care. *J Clin Psychiatr.* 2003;64[Suppl 15]:35–39.

Vasey MW, Dadds MR. *The Developmental Psychopathology of Anxiety.* New York: Oxford University Press; 2001.

Velting ON, Setzer NJ, Albano AM: Update on and advances in assessment and cognitive-behavioral treatment of anxiety disorders in children and adolescents. *Professional Psychology—Research & Practice.* 2004;35:42–54.

Wittchen HU, Beesdo K, Bittner A, Goodwin RD: Depressive episodes: Evidence for a causal role of primary anxiety disorders? *Eur Psychiatry.* 2003;18:384–393.

▲ 14.2 Anxiety Disorders: Epidemiology

KATHLEEN RIES MERIKANGAS, PH.D.

Since the 1990s, there has been an increasing focus on the anxiety disorders that have emerged as the most prevalent mental disorders in the general population. According to the National Comorbidity Survey (NCS), a nationally representative sample of 8,098 adults in the United States, anxiety disorders affect nearly one in four adults in the U.S. population. In addition, international community surveys, such as the Zurich Cohort Study, the World Health Organization (WHO) World Mental Health 2000 Initiative (WMH 2000), and the Netherlands Mental Health Survey and Incidence Study (NEMESIS), have yielded comparable lifetime prevalence rates of anxiety disorders. The magnitude of anxiety disorders in youth is quite similar to that reported in adults, thereby indicating the importance of a life course approach to the study of anxiety.

Perhaps the most basic finding from these diverse investigations is the high prevalence of anxiety disorders in community residents. These investigations have added to psychiatry not only by portraying the natural history of these disorders in a descriptive sense, but also by raising important issues about the comparability of clinical and community samples concerning treatment use and the universal nature of psychiatric conditions.

Large-scale studies have also been launched that incorporate cross-national and cross-cultural samples, such as NEMESIS and the International Consortium in Psychiatric Epidemiology (ICPE), the latter of which was established to facilitate global research using the WHO Composite International Diagnostic Interview (CIDI). This effort has taken the critical step of moving psychiatric epidemiology beyond the United States and Europe to the global population and to minority populations within the United States. The work group is now coordinating the WMH 2000, which is collecting data on the prevalence, risk factors, correlates, and treatment patterns for mental disorders in more than 20 countries. These international and cross-cultural samples are essential for expanding understanding of the validity and correlates of psychiatric disorders.

ASSESSMENT AND DEFINITIONS OF ANXIETY DISORDER

This chapter considers *categorical anxiety disorders* as defined by the standardized diagnostic criteria of the American Psychiatric Association's *Diagnostic and Statistical Manual of Mental Disorders* (DSM) (i.e., the third edition of the DSM [DSM-III], the revised third edition of the DSM [DSM-III-R], and the text revision of the fourth edition of the DSM [DSM-IV-TR]). The subtypes of the anxiety states included are panic disorder, agoraphobia, specific phobia, social phobia, generalized anxiety or overanxious disorder, separation anxiety, obsessive-compulsive disorder (OCD), posttraumatic stress disorder (PTSD), and antisocial disorder. See Table 14.2–1 for a description of the key phenomenological features of the major anxiety disorders as defined by DSM-IV-TR.

Measures of anxiety assess symptoms on a continuum or disorders based on categorical classification of the presence of specified diagnostic criteria. The most commonly used symptom assessments include self-reported checklists of state and trait anxiety (e.g., Beck Anxiety Inventory and State Trait Anxiety Index), fears (e.g., Fear Survey Schedule, Revised, and Anxiety Sensitivity Index), phobias (e.g., Fear Questionnaire), and avoidance (e.g., Mobility Inventory), as well as clinician-administered symptom checklists (e.g., Hamilton Anxiety Rating Scale).

Despite the biological underpinnings of anxiety, there are no pathognomonic markers with which a presumptive diagnosis of an anxiety disorder may be made. Therefore, information for assessing the diagnostic criteria for anxiety disorders is strictly based on a direct clinical interview or observation of objective manifestations of anxiety. To identify the diagnostic criteria for specific anxiety disorders, several structured and semistructured diagnostic interviews have been developed. Community studies generally ascertain diagnostic criteria in tightly structured interviews (e.g., Diagnostic Interview Schedule [DIS]) administered by lay interviewers, whereas clinical studies use semistructured clinical interviews, such as the Structured Clinical Interview for the DSM-IV-TR (SCID), or the Schedule for Affective Disorders and Schizophrenia-Lifetime Anxiety (SADS-LA), administered by clinically experienced interviewers. Comparable interviews have also been developed to assess diagnostic criteria for anxiety disorders in youth. The Anxiety Disorders Interview Schedule, Revised (ADIS-R) is a semistructured interview designed to assess diagnostic criteria for childhood anxiety disorders, including separation anxiety, overanxious disorder, and phobic states. The more structured Diagnostic Interview Schedule for Children (DISC) can be administered by nonclinicians to ascertain diagnostic criteria for all of the major mental disorders experienced by children and adolescents. There are also several other structured diagnostic interviews that may be used to measure anxiety disorders in youth.

Several psychophysiological indicators of anxiety have also been used in adults and children. Experimental models that induce stress and measure autonomic output to test the human *fight-or-flight* response to threat have been used to study the range of triggers, correlates, and responses to fear-provoking situations. Behavioral tasks such as giving a speech or response to novelty have been used to experimentally induce anxiety states in control subjects, as well as in those with anxiety disorders. Measures of changes in pulse, galvanic skin response, heart rate, and temperature regulation, as well as self-reported, and observations of, facial expression, blushing, and other overt signs of anxiety are presumed to provide a more accurate depiction of the disorder than self-reports or interviews about typical response patterns to stress.

MAGNITUDE OF ANXIETY DISORDERS

Adults Table 14.2–2 presents methods from a variety of national and international community surveys of anxiety disorders in adults. Although the list is not exhaustive, these surveys provide a representative sample of the magnitude of anxiety disorders across cultures, age groups, and methods. The lifetime prevalence rates are presented whenever possible; however, data from studies that did not present lifetime prevalence were also included for completeness and are noted within the tables. When discussing panic, social phobia, and OCD, rates from several surveys were cited directly from the Cross-National Collaborative Study rather than from their individual sources to obtain data standardized for age and gender.

Panic Disorder Table 14.2–3 shows prevalence rates for panic disorder. Rates of panic disorder remained fairly consistent

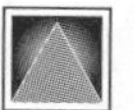

Table 14.2–1
Key Phenomenological Features of Major Anxiety Disorders As Defined by DSM-IV-TR

Panic disorder

- Recurrent unexpected panic attacks characterized by four or more of the following:
  - Palpitations
  - Sweating
  - Trembling or shaking
  - Shortness of breath
  - Feeling of choking (also known as *air hunger*)
  - Chest pain or discomfort
  - Nausea or abdominal distress
  - Feeling dizzy, lightheaded, or faint
  - Derealization or depersonalization
  - Fear of losing control or going crazy
  - Fear of dying
  - Numbness or tingling
  - Chills or hot flashes
- Persistent concern of future attacks
- Worry about the meaning of or consequences of the attacks (e.g., heart attack or stroke)
- Significant change in behavior related to the attacks (e.g., avoiding places at which panic attacks have occurred)
- ± Presence of agoraphobia

Agoraphobia

- Fear of being in places or situations from which escape might be difficult, embarrassing, or in which help may be unavailable in the event of having a panic attack
- Often results in avoidance of the feared places or situations, for example:
  - Crowds
  - Stores
  - Bridges
  - Tunnels
  - Traveling on a bus, train, or airplane
  - Theaters
  - Standing in a line
  - Small enclosed rooms

Social phobia

- Marked and persistent fear of one or more social or performance situations in which the person is concerned about negative evaluation or scrutiny by others, for example:
- Public speaking
- Writing, eating, or drinking in public
- Initiating or maintaining conversations
- Fears humiliation or embarrassment, perhaps by manifesting anxiety symptoms (e.g., blushing or sweating)
- Feared social or performance situations are avoided or endured with intense anxiety or distress

Specific phobia

- Marked and persistent fear that is excessive, unreasonable, cued by the presence or anticipation of a specific object or situation, for example:
  - Flying
  - Enclosed spaces
  - Heights
  - Storms
  - Animals (e.g., snakes or spiders)
  - Receiving an injection
  - Blood
- Provokes an immediate anxiety response
- Recognition that the fear is excessive or unreasonable
- Avoidance, anticipatory anxiety, or distress is significantly impairing

Obsessive-compulsive disorder

- Has obsessions or compulsions
  - *Obsessions* are defined as recurrent and persistent thoughts, impulses, or images that are experienced as intrusive and inappropriate, for example:
    - Contamination
    - Repeated doubts
    - Order
    - Impulses
    - Sexual images
  - *Compulsions* are defined as repetitive behaviors or mental acts whose goal is to prevent or to reduce anxiety or distress, for example:
    - Hand washing
    - Ordering
    - Checking
    - Praying
    - Counting
    - Repeating words
- Recognition that the fear is excessive or unreasonable
- Obsessions cause marked distress, are time consuming (more than 1 hour per day), or cause significant impairment in social, occupational or other daily functioning

Generalized anxiety disorder or overanxious disorder

- Excessive anxiety and worry about a number of events or activities (future oriented), occurring more days than not for at least 6 months
- Worry is difficult to control
- Worry is associated with at least three of the following symptoms:
  - Restlessness or feeling keyed up or on edge
  - Easily fatigued
  - Difficulty concentrating
  - Irritability
  - Muscle tension
  - Sleep disturbance
- Anxiety and worry cause significant distress and impairment in social, occupational, or other daily functioning

Separation anxiety disorder

- Developmentally inappropriate and excessive anxiety concerning separation from home or to an attachment figure. Characterized by three or more of the following:
  - Recurrent and excessive distress when separation from home or major attachment figure occurs or is anticipated
  - Persistent and excessive worry that major attachment figure will be lost or harmed
  - Persistent and excessive worry that an event will lead to separation from major attachment figure (e.g., getting kidnapped)
  - Persistent and recurring fear of being alone or without attachment figure at home
  - Reluctance or refusal to sleep away from home or without being near major attachment figure
  - Duration of at least 4 weeks
  - Age of onset before 18 years of age
  - Causes distress or impairment in functioning
  - Physical symptoms (e.g., headaches, stomachaches, nausea, and vomiting) when separation occurs or is anticipated

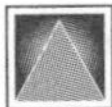

Table 14.2–2
Community Surveys of Anxiety Disorders in Adults

Study	Location	Age (Yrs)	N	Diagnostic Criteria	Diagnostic Interview	Period
United States						
National Comorbidity Survey	United States	15–54	8,098	DSM-III-R	CIDI	LT, 1 mo
Epidemiological Catchment Area Study	California, Connecticut, Maryland, Missouri, North Carolina	18+	20,861	DSM-III	DIS	LT, 12 mos
International						
Cross-National Collaborative Study		18+		DSM-III	DIS	LT, 12 mos
Edmonton Survey of Psychiatric Disorders	Edmonton, Canada		3,258			
Puerto Rico Study of Psychiatric Disorders	Puerto Rico		1,513			
French Study of Psychiatric Disorders	Savigny, France		1,746			
Munich, Germany Follow-up Study	West Germany		481			
Florence Community Survey of Anxiety Disorders	Florence, Italy		1,100			
Beirut War Events and Depression Study	Beirut, Lebanon		234			
Taiwan Psychiatric Epidemiology Project	Taiwan		11,004			
Korean Epidemiological Study of Mental Disorders	Korea		5,100			
Christchurch Psychiatric Epidemiological Study	New Zealand		1,498			
National Psychiatric Morbidity Survey	Great Britain	16–65	10,108	ICD-10	Clinical Interview Schedule-Revised	12 mos, 1 wk
Netherlands Mental Health Survey and Incidence Study	The Netherlands	18–64	7,076	DSM-III-R	CIDI	LT, 12 mos, 1 mo
World Health Organization Collaborative Study on Psychological Problems in General Health Care (all sites)	Brazil, Chile, China, England, France, Germany, Greece, India, Italy, Japan, the Netherlands, Nigeria, Turkey, United States	18–65	5,447	ICD-10	CIDI	Point, LT

CIDI, Composite International Diagnostic Interview; DIS, Diagnostic Interview Schedule; LT, lifetime.

across studies. The overall prevalence rates range from 0.4 percent (Taiwan) to 3.8 percent (Netherlands), with a median of 2.1 percent. In men, rates were low, with a range of 0.2 percent (Taiwan) to 2.0 percent (Zurich) and a median of approximately 1.3 percent. In women, the rates were higher, with a range of 0.6 percent (Taiwan) to 5.7 percent (Netherlands) and a median of 3.1 percent. As noted previously, rates from several of these studies came directly from the Cross-National Collaborative Study and have been standardized by age and gender.

Generalized Anxiety Disorder Rates of generalized anxiety disorder are shown in Table 14.2–4. The lifetime prevalence of generalized anxiety disorder is approximately 5 percent in both large-scale studies of the United States. However, there was a high degree of variability across the studies. Overall rates ranged from 2.3 percent (Netherlands) to 13.1 percent (Zurich), with a median of approximately 6.5 percent. The rates in men ranged from 1.6 percent (Netherlands) to 10.6 percent (Zurich). The rates of generalized anxiety disorder in women were slightly higher than those of men at all sites.

Agoraphobia Table 14.2–5 shows lifetime prevalence rates for agoraphobia in community samples. Rates varied slightly among the studies. Overall prevalence rates ranged from 1.3 percent in Italy to 6.9 percent in Puerto Rico, with a median of 4.2 percent. Rates in women were significantly higher than those in men, with a range from 3.3 percent in Korea to 9.0 percent in the NCS and a median of 7.8 percent. Conversely, the rates of agoraphobia in men ranged from 0.7 percent in Korea to 4.9 percent in Puerto Rico, with a median of 2.4 percent.

Social Phobia Table 14.2–6 shows the lifetime prevalence rates for social phobia from numerous international community studies using standardized diagnostic criteria. Rates from the Cross-National Collaborative Study reporting on DSM-III criteria from the United States (Epidemiological Catchment Area [ECA]), Canada, Puerto Rico, Korea, and Taiwan varied slightly, with the highest rates reported in the United States (2.6 percent) and the lowest appearing in the Asian countries (Korea, 0.5 percent; Taiwan, 0.6 percent). However, it cannot be distinguished if the differences in these rates are the result of methodological or translation inconsistencies rather than true cross-cultural differences. The NCS had the highest prevalence of social phobia, with a rate of 13.3 percent. The considerable difference in rates between this and other studies is likely linked to differences in the DSM-III-R and the inclusion of the fear of public speaking under social phobia in the NCS.

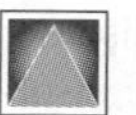

Table 14.2–3
Lifetime Prevalence of Panic Disorder in Community Surveys

Site	Men (%)	Women (%)	Total (%)
United States (National Comorbidity Survey)	1.9	5.1	3.5
United States (Epidemiological Catchment Area Study)	1.0	2.3	1.7
World Health Organization Collaborative Study (all sites)	—	—	1.1
Edmonton, Canada	0.9	1.9	1.4
Puerto Rico	1.4	1.8	1.7
Savigny, France	1.3	3.0	2.2
West Germany	1.4	3.8	2.6
Florence, Italy	1.2	3.9	2.9
Beirut, Lebanon	1.1	3.1	2.1
Taiwan	0.2	0.6	0.4
Korea	0.5	2.9	1.7
Christchurch, New Zealand	0.7	3.3	2.1
Great Britain	0.9	1.0	—
Zurich, Switzerland	2.0	4.7	3.4
The Netherlands	1.9	5.7	3.8

Specific Phobia The lifetime prevalence rates of specific phobias (Table 14.2–7) were quite consistent across sites, with approximately 10 percent of the samples reporting a specific fear associated with substantial distress or avoidance. The rates of specific phobias in women (13.6 to 16.1 percent) were double those of men (5.2 to 6.7 percent).

Obsessive-Compulsive Disorder The rates of OCD (Table 14.2–8) are fairly consistent across studies, with a range of lifetime rates from 0.7 percent (Taiwan) to 4.4 percent (Zurich). The median of 2.1 percent was representative of the majority of the rates across studies. There was no significant gender difference in the lifetime rates of OCD. In men, rates ranged from 0.5 percent (Taiwan) to 2.5 percent (Munich), with a median of 1.7 percent. The range of rates in women was 0.8 percent (Netherlands) to 6.5 percent (Zurich), with a median of 2.7 percent. Again, the rates cited were presented in the Cross-National Collaborative Study because of their standardization by gender and age.

Anxiety Disorders in Youth

Table 14.2–9 presents the methods of community studies of children and adolescents. There is an increasing number of studies during the past decade, although the methods across studies tend to be highly variable. Thus, it is difficult to draw conclusions across the aggregate data because of differences in diagnostic criteria and instruments, as well as variations in the source and age and gender composition of the sample.

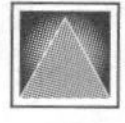

Table 14.2–4
Lifetime Prevalence of Generalized Anxiety Disorder in Community Surveys

Site	Men (%)	Women (%)	Total (%)
United States (National Comorbidity Survey)	3.6	6.6	5.1
United States (Epidemiological Catchment Area Study)[a]	1.9	3.4	2.7
World Health Organization (all sites)	—	—	7.9
Korea	2.4	4.3	3.6
Zurich, Switzerland	10.6	15.6	13.1
The Netherlands	1.6	2.9	2.3

[a]Only across three sites in the second wave.

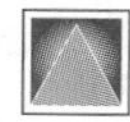

Table 14.2–5
Lifetime Prevalence of Agoraphobia in Community Surveys

Site	Men (%)	Women (%)	Total (%)
United States (National Comorbidity Survey)	4.1	9.0	6.7
United States (Epidemiological Catchment Area Study)	3.2	7.9	5.6
World Health Organization Collaborative Study (all sites)	—	—	1.5
Edmonton, Canada	1.5	4.3	2.9
West Germany	2.9	8.3	5.7
Puerto Rico	4.9	8.7	6.9
Korea	0.7	3.3	2.0
New Zealand	—	—	3.8
Florence, Italy	—	—	1.3
Zurich, Switzerland	1.8	6.6	4.2
The Netherlands	1.9	4.9	3.4

Similar to community studies of adults, anxiety disorders are the most common mental disorder in the general population of children and adolescents. However, there is a wide range in prevalence rates according to the specific anxiety subtypes, as well as according to the study methodology. In general, approximately 20 percent of youth experience one of the anxiety disorders, and one-half as many have impairment in functioning resulting from anxiety or phobias. The most common anxiety disorder is specific phobia, followed by social phobia, generalized anxiety disorder, and then all of the other anxiety disorder subtypes. Panic disorder has been shown to be extremely rare; most of the community studies identified no cases of panic disorder among youth (Table 14.2–10).

The rates of childhood anxiety disorders were lower than those of adulthood anxiety disorders. For example, rates of panic disorder ranged from 0.03 percent in the Great Smoky Mountain Study to 1.6 percent in the Early Developmental Stages of Psychopathology Study (EDSPS) in Munich, Germany, with a median (only three studies) of 0.8 percent (Oregon). The rates in boys (0.07 to 0.08 percent) were lower than those in girls (0 to 2.4 percent). Likewise,

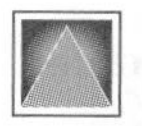

Table 14.2–6
Lifetime Prevalence of Social Phobia in Community Surveys

Site	Men (%)	Women (%)	Total (%)
United States (National Comorbidity Survey)	11.1	15.5	13.3
United States (Epidemiological Catchment Area Study)	2.1	3.1	2.6
Edmonton, Canada	1.3	2.1	1.7
Puerto Rico	0.8	1.1	1.0
Korea	0.1	1.0	0.5
Zurich, Switzerland	3.7	7.3	5.6
Taiwan	0.2	1.0	0.6
The Netherlands	5.9	9.7	7.8

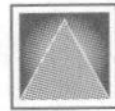

Table 14.2–7
Lifetime Prevalence of Specific Phobia in Community Surveys

Site	Men (%)	Women (%)	Total (%)
United States (National Comorbidity Survey)	6.7	15.7	11.3
United States (Epidemiological Catchment Area Study)	7.7	14.4	11.2
Puerto Rico	7.6	9.6	8.6
Edmonton, Canada	4.6	9.8	7.2
Korea	2.6	7.9	5.4
Zurich, Switzerland	5.2	16.1	10.7
The Netherlands	6.6	13.6	10.1

rates of generalized anxiety disorder in youth were quite low, affecting between 0.08 to 2.4 percent of the population. Overall, rates ranged from 0.8 percent (Munich) to 4.2 percent (Christchurch, New Zealand). The lifetime rates of overanxious disorder ranged from 1.3 percent (Oregon) to 2.9 percent (Dunedin, New Zealand), with a median of 1.7 percent. There were no consistent gender differences in this disorder. Finally, the most common disorders were overanxious disorder and separation anxiety disorder, which are specific anxiety disorders of childhood. There was a strong consistency of estimates of separation anxiety disorder, with a median of 3.5 percent. As described in the following discussion, rates of all of the anxiety disorders were more common in girls than among boys.

The rates of social phobia in children were fairly consistent across studies. Overall, rates ranged from 0.6 to 3.5 percent, with a median of approximately 1.3 percent. The lower rates of specific phobias than social phobias in youth were quite surprising. Overall, the rates ranged from 0.3 to 2.4 percent, with a median of 2.3 percent. Finally, lifetime rates of OCD in children were low, with overall rates ranging from 0.2 to 0.7 percent. In contrast to the other anxiety disorders, the gender ratio was nearly equal.

CLINICAL FEATURES

Age of Onset Retrospective reports of adults with anxiety disorders suggest that the onset generally occurs in childhood or adolescence. Although there is substantial variation across studies, the results of prospective community-based research reveal differential peak periods of onset of specific subtypes of anxiety: separation anxiety and specific phobias in middle childhood, overanxious disorder in late childhood, social phobia in middle adolescence, panic disorder in late adolescence, generalized anxiety disorder in young adulthood, and OCD in early adulthood.

Examining the age at which the gender difference in anxiety becomes apparent, as well as concomitant changes in the risk factors and correlates of anxiety across the period of risk for onset, may inform etiological pathways to anxiety disorders. Inspection of incidence curves reveals a sharp increase in girls beginning as early as 5 years of age, with a continuously increasing slope throughout adolescence. Although rates of anxiety among boys also increase throughout childhood and adolescence, the rise is far more gradual than that of girls, and rates begin to level in late adolescence. Thus, by 6 years of age, girls have significantly greater rates of anxiety than boys. Despite the far more rapid increase with age in girls than in boys, there is no gender difference in the mean age at onset of anxiety or in its duration.

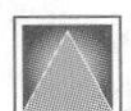

Table 14.2–8
Lifetime Prevalence of Obsessive-Compulsive Disorder in Community Surveys

Site	Men (%)	Women (%)	Total (%)
United States (Epidemiological Catchment Area Study)	1.7	2.8	2.3
Edmonton, Canada	2.0	2.7	2.3
Puerto Rico	2.3	2.7	2.5
Munich	2.5	1.9	2.1
Taiwan	0.5	0.9	0.7
Korea	1.7	2.0	1.9
New Zealand	0.9	3.4	2.2
Zurich, Switzerland	2.1	6.5	4.4
The Netherlands	0.9	0.8	0.9

Patterns of Comorbidity Comorbidity between anxiety disorders and other DSM-III-R or DSM-IV-TR disorders is even more common in adolescents than in adults. Anxiety disorders are associated with all of the other major classes of disorders, including other anxiety subtypes, depression, disruptive behaviors, eating disorders, and substance use. In older adolescents, anxiety disorders are more strongly associated with regular substance use, including cigarettes, alcohol, and illicit substances, in girls than in boys. A review of comorbid anxiety and depression suggests that these disorders may be part of the developmental sequence in which anxiety is expressed earlier in life than depression. Thus, although comorbidity between anxiety and depression and substance problems is quite common in children and adolescents, further research on the mechanisms for links between specific disorders is necessary.

Family and twin studies have been used to examine sources of overlap within the anxiety disorders and between the anxiety disorders and other syndromes, including depression, eating disorders, and substance abuse. Family studies have demonstrated the independence of familial aggregation of panic and phobias. With respect to comorbidity, whereas panic disorder, generalized anxiety, and depression have been shown to share common familial and genetic liability, there is substantial evidence for the independent etiology of anxiety disorders and substance use disorders. Similar results have emerged from studies of symptoms of anxiety and depression in youth in which anxiety and depression were found to result from a common genetic diathesis.

RISK FACTORS

The next section summarizes the evidence for broad domains of risk factors for the development of anxiety disorders, as shown in Table 14.2–11.

Gender Differences The results of community studies reveal that women have greater rates of almost all of the anxiety disorders. Despite differences in the magnitude of the rates of specific anxiety disorders across studies, the gender ratio is strikingly similar. Women have an approximately twofold elevation in lifetime rates of panic, generalized anxiety disorder, agoraphobia, and simple phobia compared to men in nearly all of the studies. The only exception is the nearly equal gender ratio in the rates of OCD and social phobia.

Studies of youth report similar differences in the magnitude of anxiety disorders among girls and boys. Similar to the gender ratio

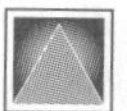

Table 14.2–9
Community Surveys of Anxiety Disorders in Children and Adolescents

Study	Location	Age (Yrs)	N	Diagnostic Criteria	Diagnostic Interview	Period
United States						
The Great Smoky Mountain Study of Youth	North Carolina	9, 11, 13	1,015	DSM-III-R	Child and Adolescent Psychiatric Assessment	3 mos
Oregon Adolescent Depression Project	Oregon	14–18	1,508	DSM-III-R	Schedule for Affective Disorders and Schizophrenia	PT, LT
Children in the Community Study	New York	9–18	776	DSM-III-R	DISC	PT, 12 mos
International						
Zurich Cohort Study	Switzerland	18–35	591	DSM-III, DSM-III-R, DSM-IV-TR	Structured Diagnostic Interview for Psychopathologic and Somatic Syndromes	12 mos, 20 yrs
Dunedin Multidisciplinary Health and Development Study	New Zealand	11	792	DSM-III	DISC (child version)	12 mos
Christchurch Health and Development Study	New Zealand	15	1,265	DSM-III-R	DISC	PT, 12 mos
Early Developmental Stages of Psychopathology	Munich, Germany	14–24	3,021	DSM-IV-TR	Composite International Diagnostic Interview	12 mos, LT

DISC, Diagnostic Interview Schedule for Children; LT, lifetime; PT, point.

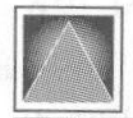

Table 14.2–10
Lifetime Rates of Anxiety Disorders in Community Samples of Children and Adolescents

		Anxiety (%)					Phobias (%)		
Study	Gender	Panic	Obsessive-Compulsive Disorder	Generalized Anxiety Disorder	Separation Anxiety Disorder	Overanxious Disorder	Agoraphobia	Social	Specific
United States									
Great Smoky Mountain Study[a]	Male	0.1	0.2	1.0	2.7	0.9	0.1	0.8	0.1
	Female	0	0.2	2.4	4.3	1.9	0	0.3	0.4
	Total	0.03	0.2	1.7	3.5	1.4	0.1	0.6	0.3
Oregon Adolescent Depression Project	Male	0.5	0.7	—	2.4	0.7	0.2	0.5	1.1
	Female	1.1	0.3	—	5.8	1.8	1.1	2.4	2.8
	Total	0.8	0.5	—	4.2	1.3	0.7	1.5	1.9
Children in the Community Study[b]	Male	—	—	—	7.7	3.6	—	6.7	7.7
	Female	—	—	—	9.5	18.0	—	10.1	17.8
International									
Dunedin Multidisciplinary Health and Development Study[c]	Male	—	—	—	2.1	3.6	—	0.2	1.7
	Female	—	—	—	5.0	2.1	—	1.6	3.2
	Total	—	—	—	3.5	2.9	—	0.9	2.4
Christchurch Health and Development Study[d]	Total	—	—	4.2	0.5	2.1	—	1.7	—
Munich Early Developmental Stages of Psychopathology Study[e]	Male	0.8	0.5	0.8	—	—	1.0	2.2	1.2
	Female	2.4	0.9	0.8	—	—	4.2	4.8	3.3
	Total	1.6	0.7	0.8	—	—	2.6	3.5	2.3

[a]Three-month prevalence rates.
[b]Rates taken from first episode.
[c]Twelve-month prevalence rates.
[d]Twelve-month prevalence rates; study uses child self-report.
[e]Rates for agoraphobia include only those without comorbid panic disorder.

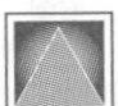

Table 14.2–11
Vulnerability Factors for Anxiety Disorders

Individual	Exogenous
Genetic factors	Exposure to stress or life events
Temperament	Drug use
Behavioral inhibition	Parenting
Anxiety sensitivity	Modeling
Preexisting psychiatric or medical disorder	Sensitization
Autonomic reactivity	
Respiratory sensitivity	
Neurobiological factors	
Neuroendocrine factors	

for adults, girls tend to have more of all subtypes of anxiety disorders, irrespective of the age composition of the sample. However, it has also been reported that, despite the greater rates of anxiety in girls across all ages, there is no significant difference between boys and girls in the average age at onset of anxiety.

Age-Specific Patterns of Expression

Anxiety disorders, particularly the phobias, tend to persist across the life course; however, there are major differences among the anxiety subtypes in terms of specificity and chronicity. Whereas the phobic states tend to be fairly stable and nonprogressive, generalized anxiety and panic tend to be less specific and less stable over time.

Several follow-up studies of children and adolescents have shown that anxiety symptoms and disorders in general tend to exhibit some stability but with substantial switching across categories of anxiety disorders over time. A recent 8-year follow-up study of a community sample of youth who were 9 to 18 years of age at study entry provides compelling evidence for the stability of the subtypes of anxiety disorders and yields some interesting gender differences in the stability of anxiety over time. The stability of social phobia and simple phobia was highly specific over time, whereas overanxious disorder was associated with major depression, social phobia, and generalized anxiety in early adulthood.

Epidemiological surveys of adults reveal that the female preponderance of anxiety disorders is present across all stages of life but is most pronounced throughout early and mid-adulthood. The rates of anxiety disorders in men are also rather constant throughout adult life, whereas the rates in women peak in the fourth and fifth decades of life and decrease thereafter. The increased rates in women are present across all ages and do not diminish as the rates of anxiety decrease in late life.

Social Class and Ethnicity

Community studies have consistently found that rates of anxiety disorders in general are greater among those at lower levels of socioeconomic status and education level. Anxiety disorders were negatively associated with income and education levels in the NCS. For example, there is almost a twofold difference between rates of anxiety disorders in individuals in the highest income bracket and those in the lowest and between those who completed more than 16 years of school and those who completed less than 11 years of school. In addition, certain anxiety disorders seem to be elevated in specific occupations. According to NEMESIS, anxiety disorders were higher in homemakers and those who were unemployed or had a disability. Similarly, the NCS found higher levels of generalized anxiety disorder and phobias in homemakers, students, and other unemployed persons. Several community studies have also yielded greater rates of anxiety disorders, particularly phobic disorders, among African Americans. The reasons for ethnic and social class differences have not yet been evaluated systematically; however, both methodological factors and differences in exposure to stressors have been advanced as possible explanations.

Familial and Genetic Factors

The familial aggregation of all of the major subtypes of anxiety disorders has been well established. The results of more than a dozen controlled family studies of probands with specific subtypes of anxiety disorders converge in demonstrating a three- to fivefold increased risk of anxiety disorders among first-degree relatives of affected probands compared to controls. The importance of the role of genetic factors in the familial clustering of anxiety has been demonstrated by numerous twin studies of anxiety symptoms and disorders. However, the relatively moderate magnitude of heritability also strongly implicates environmental etiological factors. Of the subtypes of anxiety, panic disorder is the anxiety syndrome that has been shown to have the strongest degree of familial aggregation, with an almost sevenfold elevation in risk. In addition, early-onset panic, panic associated with childhood separation anxiety, and panic associated with respiratory symptoms have each been shown to have a higher familial loading than other varieties of panic disorder. Likewise, twin studies also reveal that panic disorder has the highest heritability of all anxiety disorders.

Although there are far fewer controlled family and twin studies of the other anxiety subtypes, all of the phobic states (i.e., specific phobia and agoraphobia) have also been shown to be familial. The generalized type of social phobia appears to have the strongest magnitude of familial aggregation. Likewise, there are also few controlled family studies of OCD. The findings for familial clustering of OCD are less consistent; probands with an earlier age at onset and the presence of obsessions appear to have the strongest familial tendency.

Components of anxiety that may be inherited include somatic manifestations of anxiety, such as physiological responses, which include pulse, respiration rate, and galvanic skin response. Animal studies also reveal that anxiety or emotionality is under genetic control. Selective breeding experiments with mammals have demonstrated that emotional activity analogous to anxiety is controlled by multiple genes. These findings suggest that anxiety and fear states are highly heterogeneous and that future studies need to investigate the extent to which the components of anxiety result from common versus unique genetic factors and the role of environmental factors, biological or social, in potentiating or suppressing their expression.

Increased rates of anxiety symptoms and disorders have also been found among offspring of parents with anxiety disorders, which suggest that there may be underlying psychological or biological vulnerability factors for anxiety disorders in general that may already manifest in children before puberty. Previous research has shown that children at risk for anxiety disorders throughout life are characterized by behavioral inhibition, autonomic reactivity, somatic symptoms, social fears, enhanced startle reflex, and respiratory sensitivity.

Temperament and Personality

One of the earliest indicators of vulnerability to the development of anxiety is behavioral inhibition, characterized by increased physiological reactivity or behavioral withdrawal in the face of novel stimuli or challenging situations. Behavioral inhibition may be a manifestation of a biological predisposition characterized by overt behavioral and physiological measures.

Anxiety sensitivity is another potential sensitive and specific trait marker for the development of anxiety disorders. Anxiety sensitivity is characterized by beliefs that anxiety sensations are indicative of harmful physiological, psychological, or social consequences (e.g., fainting or an impending heart attack). Anxiety sensitivity has been shown to precede the development of anxiety symptoms and disorders and to have specificity in predicting the development of anxiety as opposed to depression.

Comorbid Disorders The magnitude of comorbidity in adults and adolescents with anxiety suggests that investigation of the role of other disorders in enhancing the risk for the initial development and persistence of anxiety disorders over time may be fruitful. The difficulty in dating the onset of specific disorders, particularly from retrospective data, diminishes the ability to determine temporal relations between disorders. Nevertheless, some prospective studies have examined the links between anxiety disorders and earlier expression of other forms of psychopathology.

Disorders that may enhance the risk for the development of anxiety disorders include eating disorders, depression, and substance use and abuse. In contrast, anxiety disorders have been shown to elevate the risk of subsequent substance use disorders and may comprise a mediator of the link between depression and the subsequent development of substance use disorders in a clinical sample. Conversely, some research suggests that substance use may trigger anxiety disorders in susceptible youth.

Medical Symptoms and Disorders Several studies have also suggested that there is an association between anxiety disorders and allergies, high fever, immunological diseases and infections, epilepsy, and connective tissue diseases. Likewise, prospective studies have revealed that the anxiety disorders may comprise risk factors for the development of some cardiovascular and neurological diseases, such as ischemic heart disease and migraine.

Life Events and Stressors The role of life experiences in the etiology of anxiety states, particularly phobias and panic disorder, has been widely studied. Life events have often been designated a causal role in the onset of phobias, which are linked inherently to particular events or objects. More broadly, life experiences that, to some extent, threaten one's notion of safety and security in the world are often perceived at least retrospectively to trigger or to precipitate the onset of anxiety disorders. In evaluating the evidence on the causal role of life experiences, it is critical to consider the subtypes of anxiety disorders separately. Although it is likely that life stress may exacerbate phobic and generalized anxiety states, phobic states resulting from exposure are far rarer than those that emerge with no apparent exposure. In contrast, PTSD is defined as a sequela of a catastrophic life event.

The major impediment to the evaluation of the causal role of life events in anxiety (or depression) is the retrospective nature of most research addressing this issue. Moreover, stressful life events may interact with other risk factors, such as a family history of depression, in precipitating episodes of panic. One of the few prospective studies did demonstrate a predictive relationship between life events during adolescence and depressive and generalized anxiety disorder symptoms. Interestingly, the association with anxiety was limited to women, consistent with differential vulnerability to stress across genders.

In terms of specific environmental risk factors, there has been abundant literature on the role of parenting in enhancing vulnerability to anxiety disorders. One widely held theory is that anxiety is a response to disruption in the mother–child relation; it has been postulated that maternal overprotection is related to anxiety, particularly separation anxiety. Another parental behavior that may enhance the risk of anxiety in offspring is parental sensitization of anxiety through enhancing cognitive awareness of the child to specific events and situations, such as bodily functions, social disapproval, the importance of routines, and the necessity for personal safety. In addition, another feature of the parental relationship that has received widespread attention in recent research has been the exposure to severe childhood trauma through separation or abuse. There is increasing animal research on the impact of early adverse experiences on brain systems and subsequent development.

FUTURE DIRECTIONS FOR RESEARCH ON ANXIETY

There are several directions that will be fruitful directions for future research. Better comprehension of the phenomenology of the specific anxiety disorders and their overlap should guide the development of the next phase of diagnostic categories of anxiety. In addition, as neuroscience and genetics inform knowledge regarding neural processes underlying anxiety disorders and the role of genetic and environmental factors in their evolution, studies of treatment and prevention strategies will assume increasing importance in reducing the magnitude and burden of this major source of mental disorders.

Some specific areas of future research should address the following issues:

- Establish more accurate and developmentally sensitive methods of assessment of anxiety with a focus on developing objective measures of the components of anxiety
- Apply within family design to minimize etiological heterogeneity and to refine diagnostic boundaries and thresholds
- Investigate specificity of putative markers with respect to other psychiatric disorders and the longitudinal stability of specific subtypes of anxiety disorders
- Examine the mechanisms for the onset of panic attacks associated with substance use
- Develop research on hormonally mediated neurobiological function to understand gender differences predisposing women to experience decreased resiliency to fear-provoking stimuli
- Investigate the mechanisms for comorbidity of specific medical disorders with anxiety symptoms and disorders

SUGGESTED CROSS-REFERENCES

Other relevant sections within the anxiety disorders chapter include genetics (Section 14.6), clinical features (Section 14.8), and treatments (Sections 14.9 and 14.10). Other related topics include epidemiology (Section 5.1), statistics and experimental design (Section 5.2), and classification of mental disorders (Section 9.1).

REFERENCES

Anderson JC, Williams S, McGee R, Silva PA: DSM-III disorders in preadolescent children: Prevalence in a large sample from the general population. *Arch Gen Psychiatry.* 1987;44:69.

Angst J: Comorbidity of anxiety, phobia, compulsion and depression. *Int Clin Psychopharmacol.* 1993;8[Suppl 1]:21.

Bijl RV, Ravelli A, van Zessen G: Prevalence of psychiatric disorder in the general population: Results of the Netherlands Mental Health Survey and Incidence Study (NEMESIS). *Soc Psychiatry Psychiatr Epidemiol.* 1998;33:587.

Bland RC, Orn H, Newman SC: Lifetime prevalence of psychiatric disorders in Edmonton. *Acta Psychiatr Scand.* 1988;77[Suppl 338]:24.

Brady E, Kendall P: Comorbidity of anxiety and depression in children and adolescents. *Psychol Bull.* 1992;111:244.

Canino GJ, Bird H, Shrout PE, Rubio-Stipec M, Bravo M, Martinez R, Sesman M, Guevara LM: The prevalence of specific psychiatric disorders in Puerto Rico. *Arch Gen Psychiatry.* 1987;44:727.

Canino G, Shrout PE, Rubio-Stipec M, Bird HR, Bravo M, Ramirez R, Chavez L, Alegria M, Bauermeister JJ, Hohmann A, Ribera J, Garcia P, Martinez-Taboas A: The DSM-IV rates of child and adolescent disorders in Puerto Rico: Prevalence, correlates, service use, and the effects of impairment. *Arch Gen Psychiatry.* 2004;61:85.

Cantwell D, Baker L: Stability and natural history of DSM-III childhood diagnoses. *J Am Acad Child Adolesc Psychol.* 1989;28:691.

Costello EJ, Angold A, Burns B, Stangl DK, Tweed DL, Erkanli A, Worthman CM: The Great Smoky Mountains Study of Youth: Goals, design, methods, and the prevalence of DSM-III-R disorders. *Arch Gen Psychiatry.* 1996;53:1129.

Fergusson DM, Horwood LJ, Lynskey MT: Prevalence and comorbidity of DSM-III-R diagnoses in a birth cohort of 15 year olds. *J Am Acad Child Adolesc Psychiatry.* 1993;32:1127.

Finn DA, Rutledge-Gorman MT, Crabbe JC: Genetic animal models of anxiety. *Neurogenetics.* 2003;4:109.

Fyer AJ, Mannuzza S, Chapman TF, Lipsitz J, Martin LY, Klien DF: Panic disorder and social phobia: Effects of comorbidity on familial transmission. *Anxiety.* 1996;2:173.

Groenink L, van Bogaert MJ, van der Gugten J, Oosting RS, Olivier B: 5-HT1A receptor and 5-HT1B receptor knockout mice in stress and anxiety paradigms. *Behav Pharmacol.* 2003;14:369.

Jenkins R, Lewis G, Bebbington P, Brugha T, Farrell M, Gill B, Meltzer H: The national psychiatric morbidity surveys of Great Britain—initial findings from the household survey. *Psychol Med.* 1997;27:775.

Kandel DB, Johnson JB, Bird HR, Canino G, Goodman SH, Lahey BB, Regier DA, Schwab-Stone M: Psychiatric disorders associated with substance abuse among children and adolescents: Findings from the Methods for the Epidemiology of Child and Adolescent Mental Disorders (MECA) study. *J Abnorm Child Psychol.* 1997;25:121.

Kessler RC, McGonagle KA, Zhao S, Nelson C, Hughes M, Eshleman S, Wittchen HU, Kendler K: Lifetime and 12-month prevalence of DSM-III-R psychiatric disorders in the United States. *Arch Gen Psychiatry.* 1994;51:8.

Lee CK, Kwak YS, Yamamoto J, Rhee H, Kim YS, Han JH, Choi JO, Lee YH: Psychiatric epidemiology in Korea: Part 1: Gender and age differences in Seoul. *J Nerv Ment Dis.* 1990;178:242.

*Lewinsohn PM, Hops H, Roberts R, Seeley JR, Andrews JA: Adolescents psychopathology: I. Prevalence and incidence of depression and other DSM-III-R disorders in high school students. *J Abnorm Psychol.* 1993;102:133.

Manfro GG, Otto MW, McArdle ET, Worthington JJ, Rosenbaum JF, Pollack MH: Relationship of antecedent stressful life events to childhood and family history of anxiety and the course of panic disorder. *J Affect Disord.* 1996;41:135.

Marks I: Genetics of fear and anxiety disorders. *Br J Psychiatry.* 1986;149:406.

*Merikangas KR, Avenevoli S. Epidemiology of mood and anxiety disorders in children and adolescents. In: Tsuang MT, Tohen M, eds. *Textbook in Psychiatric Epidemiology.* New York: Wiley-Liss; 2002.

Merikangas KR, Lieb R, Wittchen HU, Avenevoli S: Family and high-risk studies of social anxiety disorder. *Acta Psychiatr Scand (Suppl).* 2003;417:28.

Merikangas KR, Pollock RA. Anxiety disorders in women. In: Goldman MB, Hatch MC, eds. *Women and Health.* San Diego, CA: Academic Press; 2000.

Merikangas KR, Swendsen J: Genetic epidemiology of psychiatric disorders. *Epidemiol Rev.* 1997;19:1.

Merikangas KR, Zhang H, Avenevoli S, Acharyya S, Neuenschwander M, Angst J, Zurich Cohort Study: Longitudinal trajectories of depression and anxiety in a prospective community study: The Zurich Cohort Study. *Arch Gen Psychiatry.* 2003;60:993.

Murray C, Lopez A. *World Health Report 2002: Reducing Risks, Promoting Healthy Life.* Geneva: World Health Organization; 2002:192–197.

Ormel J, VonKorff M, Ustun TB, Pini S, Korten A, Oldehinkel T: Common mental disorders across cultures: Results from the WHO collaborative study on psychological problems in general health care. *JAMA.* 1994;272:1741.

Pine DS, Cohen E, Cohen P, Brook JS: Social phobia and the persistence of conduct problems. *J Child Psychol Psychiatry.* 2000;41:657.

Pine DS, Cohen P, Johnson JG, Brook JS: Adolescent life events as predictors of adult depression. *J Affect Disord.* 2002;68:49.

*Smoller J, Finn C, White C: The genetics of anxiety disorders: An overview. *Psychiatr Ann.* 2000;30:745.

Thaper A, McGuffin P: Anxiety and depressive symptoms in childhood: A genetic study of comorbidity. *J Child Psychol Psychiatry.* 1997;38:651.

*Weissman MM, Bland RC, Canino GJ, Faravelli C, Greenwald S, Hwu HG, Joyce PR, Karam EG, Lee CK, Lellouch J, Lepine JP, Newman SC, Oakley-Browne MA, Rubio-Stipec M, Wells JE, Wickramaratne PJ, Witthcen HU, Yeh EK: The cross-national epidemiology of panic disorder. *Arch Gen Psychiatry.* 1997;54:305.

Weissman MM, Bland RC, Canino GJ, Greenwald S, Hwu HG, Lee CK, Newman SC, Oakley-Browne MA, Rubio-Stipec M, Wickramaratne PJ, Wittchen HU, Yeh EK: The cross national epidemiology of obsessive compulsive disorder. *J Clin Psychiatry.* 1994;55[Suppl]:5.

*Weissman MM, Bland RC, Canino GJ, Greenwald S, Lee CK, Newman SC, Rubio-Stipec M, Wickramaratne PJ. The cross national epidemiology of social phobia: A preliminary report. *Int Clin Psychopharmacol.* 1996;11[Suppl]:9.

Wells EJ, Bushnell JA, Hornblow AR, Joyce PR, Oakley-Browne MA: Christchurch psychiatric epidemiology study, part 1: Methodology and lifetime prevalence for specific psychiatric disorders. *Aust N Z J Psychiatry.* 1989;23:315.

Wittchen H-U, Essau CA, von Zerssen D, Krieg JC, Zaudig M: Lifetime and six-month prevalence of mental disorders in the Munich follow-up study. *Eur Arch Psychiatry Clin Neurosci.* 1992;241:247.

Wittchen H-U, Nelson CB, Lachner G: Prevalence of mental disorders and psychosocial impairment in adolescents and young adults. *Psychol Med.* 1998;28:109.

▲ 14.3 Anxiety Disorders: Psychophysiological Aspects

CHRISTIAN GRILLON, PH.D.

Despite considerable research on the psychophysiology of anxiety and the abundance of physiological symptoms in anxiety disorders, psychophysiology remains essentially a research tool when it comes to psychopathology. Clinicians have not yet embraced psychophysiology as a useful adjunct to face-to-face interviews and to self-reports for diagnostic assessment. However, there is mounting evidence of the clinical usefulness of psychophysiology, at least for anxiety disorders with a strong physiological component.

Psychophysiology is a noninvasive tool used to quantify normal and abnormal physiological activity and reactivity. It is also a discipline that seeks to understand the biological basis of human behavior and mental processes. The psychophysiology of anxiety disorders is relevant on several accounts. First, physiological measures could help quantify and assess objectively anxiety symptoms. Second, psychophysiology could assist in identifying psychological and neurobiological dysfunctions. Finally, psychophysiology may help better characterize anxiety disorders, potentially leading to a redefinition of the different categories. This includes identifying endophenotypes that are not observable by diagnostic interviews. Markers of physiological vulnerability are crucial for identification of high-risk individuals in genetic linkage studies.

Historically, psychophysiology has relied on electrical signals generated from the body and recorded via electrodes placed on the skin (scalp, hands, and face). Examples of psychophysiological measures include palmar sweating (skin conductance), electromyographic and electrocortical activity, respiration, peripheral vasoconstriction, heart rate (HR), blood pressure, and reflexes. More recently, the field of psychophysiology incorporated neuroendocrine physiology and brain imaging (e.g., positron emission tomography [PET]). The present chapter focuses on measures of autonomic nervous system (ANS) and central nervous system (CNS) activity recorded via surface transducers.

The role of clinical psychophysiology as a diagnostic tool in psychiatry has been slow to evolve because of the claim that it has a limited capacity to discriminate clinical from nonclinical populations and to differentiate diagnostic categories. In addition, the low concordance between physiological measures and subjective reports of emotional experience and the low correlation among physiological measures of arousal have left the impression that physiological measures are unreliable. Paradoxically, physiological symptoms play a crucial role in the diagnostic profile of anxiety disorders, but symptom evaluation is based on verbal self-reports. It is well established that reports of physiological symptoms of fear and anxiety are frequently inaccurate and that they are influenced by misperception, erroneous interpretation, and catastrophically exaggerated state-

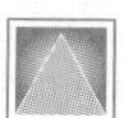

Table 14.3–1
Physiological Symptoms of Anxiety Disorders Explicitly Mentioned in DSM-IV-TR

Panic disorder
Palpitations, pounding heart, or accelerated heart rate
Sweating
Trembling or shaking
Sensation of shortness of breath or smothering
Feeling of choking
Chest pain or discomfort
Nausea or abdominal distress
Feeling dizzy, unsteady, lightheaded, or faint
Chills or hot flushes
Posttraumatic stress disorder
Physiological reactivity on exposure to trauma-related cues
Difficulties falling asleep or staying asleep
Exaggerated startle response
Generalized anxiety disorder
Muscle tension
Sleep disturbance
Acute stress disorder
Marked symptoms of arousal

ments. It is reasonable to assume that objective measures of physiological symptoms could contribute to the evaluation of patients and to the phenomenology of anxiety disorders. Table 14.3–1 lists physiological symptoms as explicitly stated in the revised fourth edition of the *Diagnostic and Statistical Manual of Mental Disorders* (DSM-IV-TR) for panic disorder, posttraumatic stress disorder (PTSD), generalized anxiety disorder, and acute stress disorder.

Most of these symptoms can be objectively evaluated via inexpensive and noninvasive psychophysiological techniques. Other physiological symptoms are not required by DSM-IV-TR to make a diagnosis (e.g., blushing in social phobia) but can be assessed with psychophysiological techniques. Finally, psychophysiology could help quantify psychological symptoms with a strong physiological component (e.g., of hyper- or hypoemotionality) and symptoms of abnormal attention (e.g., difficulty concentrating).

Neither the lack of concordance between self-report and physiological measures nor the low correlation among physiological measures of arousal is an impediment to the clinical use of psychophysiology for psychiatric assessments and investigations. Discordance between measures has been attributed to situational parameters and behavioral demands. Lack of concordance in physiological measures during anxiety may also be related to the intensity and to the imminence of threat. Low concordance and weak physiological arousal occur in response to weak and distal threat. Conversely, high levels of threat and imminent danger are characterized by parallel reports of fear and objective measure of physiological arousal. Discordance between self-report and physiological measures may reflect misperception of bodily symptoms rather than genuine autonomic disturbance. Hence, psychophysiology may provide information regarding the etiology of anxiety disorders. Objective monitoring of physiological activity can only contribute to the understanding of the nature of physiological complaints.

PSYCHOPHYSIOLOGY OF ANXIETY

Anxiety can be conceptualized as a normal and adaptive response to threat that prepares the organism for flight or fight. This preparation is accompanied by increased somatic and autonomic activity controlled by the interaction of the sympathetic and parasympathetic nervous systems. Anxiety becomes abnormal when it is excessive or its timing is inappropriate with regard to the threat. Pathological anxiety results in strong subjective feelings accompanied by similar physiological activation as normal anxiety, including muscle tension, shortness of breath, hyperventilation, heart palpitation or heart pounding, increased perspiration or cold sweat, and exaggerated startle. Some of these physiological changes, such as skin conductance (sweat), HR, muscle tension, and reflex potentiation, can be recorded easily and inexpensively. Other response systems, such as respiration volume and cardiac output, are more costly and cumbersome to record. An overview of the main physiological measures used in anxiety research is presented in the following sections. This is followed by a review of the main findings in clinical psychophysiology pertaining to the various anxiety disorders. Results in anxiety disorders with a strong physiological component (e.g., panic disorder and PTSD) are emphasized.

Electrodermal Activity

Unlike most autonomic functions, which are controlled by the interplay between sympathetic and parasympathetic activity, the electrodermal system is under control of the sympathetic branch of the ANS. Widespread focus on the role of sympathetic activity in response to threat has given center stage to electrodermal activity in anxiety research. Intense emotions, including fear and anxiety, are often accompanied by activation of sweat glands (e.g., moist hands). Recording devices can easily quantify this activation. Electrodermal activity is recorded as a change in electrical resistance after passage of an external small current across the skin. After activation of the eccrine glands, the previously dry skin becomes hydrated. Because electrical current is conducted better by wet skin than by dry skin, activation of the sweat ducts leads to a drop in skin resistance, which is recorded as a change in electrodermal activity. The recording of electrodermal activity is usually made from two electrodes placed on the inside of the hand or on the second phalanx of the second and third fingers of one hand.

The electrodermal activity can reflect tonic or phasic activity. *Tonic activity* is referred to as *skin conductance level.* Tonic activity has been linked to vigilance, sustained attention, anxiety, and arousal. Low skin conductance levels have been linked to depression. Phasic changes can be time locked to a specific stimulus and give rise to *skin conductance responses* (SCRs), or they can occur in the absence of a stimulus and are labeled *spontaneous fluctuations.* The SCR should be considered a measure of an attentional process (i.e., orienting response). In pavlovian aversive conditioning, several responses can be identified when the time interval between the conditioned stimulus and the unconditioned stimulus is long. The early, or first-interval, response (FIR) has been related to the orienting response. A second response, or second-interval response (SIR), is an emotional response linked to the emotional value of the unconditioned stimulus. A third-interval response (TIR) can be observed on test trial, when the unconditioned response is omitted. In general, the measure that is the most sensitive to conditioning is the FIR. The number of spontaneous fluctuations has been related to arousal and anxiety.

Cardiovascular Activity

Symptoms of cardiovascular abnormalities have been noted since initial studies of individuals with so-called irritable heart in the 1870s. Reports of prominent symptoms of tachycardia and heart palpitations accompanying anxiety and extreme fear have made cardiovascular activity an obvious focus of investigation. HR acceleration has been viewed as a sign of autonomic hyperreactivity or increased arousal, but this interpretation is too simplistic in light of the complex sympathetic and parasympathetic interactions that regulate cardiovascular activity. The heart receives innervations from the sympathetic and parasympathetic branches of the ANS. Parasympathetic fibers reach the heart via the vagus nerve. Their activation releases acetylcholine and leads to bradycardia (HR deceleration). Sympathetic fibers in the heart release norepinephrine, causing tachycardia (HR acceleration). Thus, tachycardia could be due to increased sympathetic activity or reduced parasympathetic activity, or both.

Heart Rate The HR is obtained by calculating the number of R waves of the QRS complex of the electrocardiogram (ECG). It is usually expressed in beats per minute. A convenient measure in the time domain is the interbeat interval, measured as the time between two consecutive R waves, expressed in milliseconds. HR and interbeat interval can be easily obtained using chest leads with one electrode on the sternum and the other on the left side of the heart. Various triggering devices (Schmitt device) now provide accurate detection of the R wave.

Heart Rate Variability The measure of heart rate variability (HRV) is becoming a prominent index of cardiovascular dysfunction in anxiety research. HRV is used to objectively assess cardiovascular dysfunction and to estimate sympathetic and parasympathetic influence on cardiovascular activity. The increasing amount of research on HRV is due to several factors. First, the use of HRV has helped reformulate biological theories of anxiety, shifting the focus of attention away from sympathetic nervous system disturbances in favor of a more balanced approach that considers the interaction between sympathetic activity and parasympathetic activity. Second, reduced HRV has been found in several anxiety disorders and in populations at high risk for anxiety disorders and may be associated with chronic worry. Third, prospective epidemiological studies have shown that a history of an anxiety disorder is associated with increased risk for coronary heart disease, including sudden cardiac death. Individuals with high levels of anxiety have a 4.5- to 6.0-fold increase in risk for sudden cardiac death, compared to individuals with no anxiety. This increased risk of sudden cardiac death has been linked to abnormal sympathovagal balance. Finally, there is emerging evidence that HRV may reflect attentional and affective regulation. A number of theories link deficits in attention (hypervigilance, scanning, and attentional bias for threat information) to deviant affective information processing. Flexibility in attention is necessary to shift from relevant to nonrelevant information in an ever-changing environment. The ineffective attentional processing of affective information leads to abnormal affective responses. HRV may index attentional flexibility and adaptability of the organism. In particular, low vagal tone is associated with impaired self-regulation and reduced attentional flexibility and with increased worry in healthy subjects and in patients with generalized anxiety disorder.

The influence of sympathetic and parasympathetic tone on cardiovascular activity can be assessed in the time domain and in the frequency domain via spectral analysis of HRV, the latter increasingly becoming the favored method of investigators. Fast Fourier transform of segment of ECG can be used to extract beat-to-beat variations in HR resulting in a high-frequency or respiratory sinus arrhythmia component (0.13 to 0.50 Hz, reflecting cardiac vagal tone) and a lower-frequency component (0.07 to 0.12 Hz) primarily due to baroreceptor-mediated regulation of blood pressure. High-frequency spectral power is often used to assess vagal tone. Low-frequency spectral power reflects sympathetic and parasympathetic influence but can be used as a marker of cardiac sympathetic activation under certain circumstances. Congestive heart failure and sudden death are marked by loss of high-frequency activity and increases in low-frequency activity, indicating a loss of cardiac vagal tone and a predominance of sympathetic control, respectively.

Respiration Respiratory psychophysiology may be one of the most underused variables in anxiety research. The identification of breathing problems in anxiety disorders has led to a renewed interest in respiratory psychophysiology, especially because hyperventilation can elicit panic attacks in susceptible individuals.

The principal function of the respiratory system is to supply oxygen to the organs of the body and to evacuate the body of carbon dioxide (CO_2). CO_2 is not only a waste product. It plays an important role in maintaining the acid–base balance within the internal milieu of the body. One common symptom associated with anxiety is hyperventilation, which lowers blood CO_2 (hypocapnia) and can result in dizziness, palpitations, and tingling in extremities.

Respiration rate can be measured with a strain gauge around the abdomen or the chest or with a thermistor, which is sensitive to differences in temperature between inhaled and exhaled air, taped to the nostril. Arterial partial pressure is difficult to measure. A good approximation is end-tidal partial pressure of CO_2 (PCO_2), which is the PCO_2 level reached at the end of a normal expiration.

Electrocortical Activity Measurement of the electrical activity of the brain has long been the only noninvasive measure of central activity available to clinicians. The electroencephalogram (EEG) and the event-related potentials (ERPs) have yielded important information about brain arousal and brain activity during cognitive and emotional tasks. Because anxiety has been considered a state of hyperarousal, the EEG has had a prominent place in anxiety studies. Although the electrophysiological recording of brain activity in psychiatry is being rapidly supplanted by functional imaging techniques, such as functional magnetic resonance imaging (fMRI) and PET, EEG and ERP are still highly useful. They are inexpensive and noninvasive functional tools with excellent temporal resolution that cannot be matched by any other techniques. The main disadvantage of EEG and ERP is poor spatial resolution.

Electroencephalography The EEG is a recording of brain wave electrical activity from the surface of the scalp. Not all structures contribute equally to the EEG. Deep structures, such as the amygdala or the hippocampus, do not contribute to the EEG as much as cortical structures. Power spectral analyses of EEG can be performed to provide an objective quantification of the EEG signal. After digitization, the raw signal is submitted to a fast Fourier transform that computes power for the traditional EEG frequency bands, delta (0.5 to 4.0 Hz), theta (4 to 7 Hz), alpha (8 to 12 Hz), and beta (13 to 30 Hz).

EEG is an excellent tool for the assessment of CNS arousal. The general observation is that greater cerebral and behavioral arousal is associated with reduced alpha activity and increased beta activity power in the EEG. This EEG pattern is reliably observed during fear and anxiety.

An important development in recent years is the assessment of asymmetrical patterns of EEG activity. Differential hemispherical activation is associated with basic dimensions of emotion. *Activation* commonly refers to a reduction in alpha power. It is calculated as the difference in alpha power over homologous sites of the two hemispheres.

Resting anterior functional brain asymmetry has been related to an approach and withdrawal dimension of behavior, with left and right frontal activation indexing approach- and withdrawal-related behaviors, respectively. Thus, anterior asymmetry is an index of responses to positive and negative emotions, including fear and anxiety. Because fear can lead to active withdrawal and behavioral inhibition, it is believed that right anterior activation is a marker of aversive states. Consistent with this view, chronically anxious and fearful monkeys show increased electrical activity in right frontal brain regions, as well as an increase in baseline cortisol levels. A potential pitfall of asymmetry studies is that alpha asymmetry is a relative measure. A given pattern of asymmetry can be attributed to increased alpha power in one hemisphere or reduced power in the other hemisphere, or a combination of the two.

Event-Related Potentials ERPs are time-locked electrical responses to specific events with excellent temporal resolution, making them a unique tool to investigate information processing. ERPs can be divided into sensory and cognitive components. The sensory components are sensitive to the physical characteristics (e.g., intensity) of the stimuli and arise in the first 100 milliseconds poststimulus. The cognitive components occur later and are sensitive to psychological processes such as attention and memory. They are labeled according to their polarity (negative or positive) and latency or order of appearance (e.g., *P300* is a positive waveform with a peak latency at approximately 300 milliseconds).

Because ERPs rely on averaging techniques, their usefulness is somewhat limited in studies that are interested in changes over time (e.g., orienting response, habituation, classical conditioning). ERPs have not been extensively used in anxiety disorders. This is surprising, given the relevance of attention processes (attentional bias for threat, hypervigilance, and distractibility) in various anxiety disorders. An emerging literature suggests that some characteristics of ERPs are sensitive to serotoninergic functions in humans.

Electromyogram

Skeletomotor System The electromyogram (EMG) could contribute substantially to the diagnosis in disorders that include somatic symptoms. The EMG is a recording of voltage changes resulting from multiple muscle action potentials traveling across many fibers when a muscle contracts. The EMG is best recorded with a bipolar electrode placement over the muscle of interest. The EMG signal consists of a series of discharges in the range from 20 to 1,000 Hz with an amplitude of approximately 100 to 1,000 μV. The frequency of interest is between 40 and 400 Hz. To facilitate analysis, a common technique of quantification is to rectify and to integrate the signal. To *rectify an electrical signal* means to align the positive and the negative spikes in a single direction. Integration provides a measure of total EMG output over a given period. The EMG of the forehead region is of interest for research on anxiety disorders, because anxious individuals report increased muscle tension in this area.

Startle or Eye-Blink Reflex In the last 10 years, the study of startle modification has had a profound impact on research on affective psychophysiology in general and, more particularly, on research on anxiety and anxiety disorders. The recent enthusiasm for the startle reflex methodology in anxiety research stems from the fact that (1) an exaggerated startle reflex is a symptom of PTSD, according to the DSM-IV-TR; (2) startle is sensitive to a number of psychological processes that have been implicated in anxiety disorders, such as habituation, sensitization, and fear potentiation; (3) startle is sensitive to anxiety and aversive states rather than a nonspecific index of arousal; and (4) the startle reflex is a cross-species response showing similar plasticity in humans and animals. Human research can benefit from neurobiological and psychopharmacological research on startle reactivity in animal models.

STARTLE REFLEX METHODOLOGY The startle reflex is a reflexive response to a sudden and intense stimulus, such as a loud sound (e.g., 100-dB, 40-millisecond duration white noise), an air puff to the face, or a flash of light. It consists of a forward thrusting of the head and a descending flexor wave reaction, extending through the trunk and the knees. The somatic startle reflex is typically measured by recording the eye-blink reflex, which is the most persistent component of the startle pattern. This can be accomplished by using miniature electrodes placed under one eye to record the EMG activity of the orbicularis oculi muscle, the muscle responsible for the closure of the eyelid. In addition to its somatic component, which occurs in the first 20 to 40 milliseconds, the startle reflex also elicits an intense ANS reaction consisting of a large SCR and a transient tachycardia that develops more slowly.

STARTLE REFLEX AND AVERSIVE STATES In humans and animals, similar methods designed to produce aversive states result in a facilitation of the amplitude of the startle reflex. There are three basic procedures relevant to anxiety disorders, namely, shock sensitization of startle, fear-potentiated startle, and the affective modulation of startle.

The *shock sensitization of startle* refers to the facilitation of the startle reflex after the administration of a shock. Michael Davis and his collaborators demonstrated that aversive foot shocks resulted in a transient facilitation starting 5 to 10 minutes after shock delivery and lasting as long as 1 hour. Although the duration of the shock sensitization of startle can be increased by increasing the intensity or number of shocks, the effect is never permanent. Startle can also be experimentally sensitized in humans after the administration of mildly unpleasant shocks. These observations suggest that startle could be a sensitive measure of sensitization processes after traumatic events, such as those that can lead to PTSD.

Fear-potentiated startle refers to the increased amplitude of the startle reflex by conditioned fear. Thus, startle is increased when it is elicited in the presence of a signal (e.g., a light) that has been previously paired with an aversive event (e.g., a shock). This effect, initially demonstrated in animals, has been replicated extensively in humans by using different techniques, ranging from cued fear conditioning to context conditioning to verbal threat.

One advantage of fear-potentiated startle, in addition to its value as an integrative research tool between psychological science and neuroscience, is that it nicely complements the traditional psychophysiological measure of conditioning, the SCR. Although the SCR measures cognitive or relational learning, fear-potentiated startle may be best described as an index of aversive learning.

The *affective modulation of startle* can be viewed as an extension of fear-potentiated startle. Startle can be facilitated not only by fear and anxiety, but also by more general negative affective moods. This effect can be obtained experimentally by having subjects view pictures depicting unpleasant scenes. The affective modulation of startle effect has been replicated in several laboratories by using different types of stimuli, such as movies, sounds, or odors, or by using affective imagery procedures.

PANIC DISORDER

Panic Attack: Ventilatory Abnormalities Panic attacks are the central feature of panic disorders. Panic attacks are accompanied by intense autonomic, especially cardiovascular and respi-

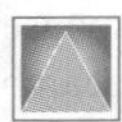

Table 14.3–2
Physiologic Measures: Mean (Standard Deviation) during 30 Minutes of Quiet Sitting

	Panic Disorder	Generalized Anxiety Disorder	Control Subjects	F	P	Post Hoc
Electrodermal and cardiovascular						
Skin conductance level (microsiemens)	7.80 (6.20)	7.14 (4.61)	4.50 (3.60)	2.14	—	—
Nonspecific skin conductance fluctuations (number per minute)	3.05 (2.63)	2.87 (2.64)	1.60 (1.64)	2.08	—	—
Heart rate (beats per minute)	70.1 (8.2)	76.8 (18.2)	69.0 (11.4)	0.88	—	—
Systolic blood pressure (mm Hg)	144.4 (31.5)	152.2 (33.1)	148.9 (23.1)	0.28	—	—
Diastolic blood pressure (mm Hg)	87.4 (25.1)	91.9 (18.7)	90.8 (16.8)	0.21	—	—
Stroke volume (mL)	61.5 (22.3)	64.4 (20.0)	60 (16.9)	0.21	—	—
Cardiac output (L per minute)	4.31 (1.40)	4.95 (1.20)	4.15 (1.42)	0.61	—	—
Systemic vascular resistance (dyne-second per cm^5)	1.32 (1.93)	1.24 (2.60)	1.37 (0.98)	0.26	—	—
Respiratory						
Respiratory rate (breaths per minute)	13.5 (2.5)	15.3 (3.1)	15.9 (2.5)	4.35	.02	P < C
Tidal volume (mL)	445 (123)	383 (63)	317 (70)	11.21	.0001	P > C
Tidal volume, sighs removed (mL)	369 (109)	343 (51)	291 (74)	4.77	.02	P > C
Duty cycle ratio	0.297 (0.037)	0.338 (0.062)	0.331(0.032)	4.39	.02	P < G = C
Inspiratory flow rate (mL per second)	301 (49)	279 (58)	241 (40)	8.50	.0007	P > C
End-tidal partial pressure of carbon dioxide (mm Hg)	33.8 (6.9)	38.2 (5.0)	39.5 (3.4)	5.22	.01	P < C
Sighs > 2 . normal (number per minute)	0.734 (0.384)	0.474 (0.31)	0.378(0.264)	5.25	.009	P > C
Apneas > 5 seconds (number per minute)	0.332 (0.443)	0.226 (0.291)	0.103(0.258)	1.98	—	—

Note: Physiological activity during 30 minutes of quiet sitting in patients with panic disorder or generalized anxiety disorder and in healthy controls. The electrodermal and cardiovascular measures did not differ among groups. Of the respiratory variables, end-tidal partial pressure of carbon dioxide, respiratory rate, and duty cycle were lower in the patients with panic disorder, compared to control subjects.
C, control patients; G, patients with generalized anxiety disorder; P, patients with panic disorder.
From Wilhelm FH, Traber W, Roth WT: Physiologic instability in panic disorder and generalized anxiety disorder. *Biol Psychiatry.* 2001;49:596, with permission.

ratory, reactions. These physiological measures have been used to inform on the nature of panic. Respiration has been an important topic of investigation in patients with panic disorder, not only because rapid breathing and dyspnea (shortness of breath) are prominent symptoms experienced during a panic attack, but also because of the *suffocation false alarm* theory proposed by Donald F. Klein. Unlike cardiovascular abnormalities, respiratory instability is specific to patients with panic disorder (Table 14.3–2). Respiratory instability includes hyperventilation syndrome and increased respiratory variability (Fig. 14.3–1). The close link between panic and respiratory manifestations raises questions about the significance of physiological changes in panic disorder. The presence of respiratory symptoms has led to the hypothesis that panic attacks represent a triggering of a false suffocation alarm. This view assumes that activation of suffocation mechanisms is etiological for panic disorder and that deviant respiration patterns represent compensatory responses.

An alternative is that there is nothing fundamentally abnormal in the basic brainstem respiratory control mechanisms of individuals with panic disorder. Rather, panic attacks are viewed as conditioned fear responses brought about by an oversensitive fear network (e.g., amygdala, prefrontal cortex, and hippocampus) that is responsible for the initial panic. In this conditioning model, individuals with panic disorder come to fear the panic attacks, which then play the role of unconditioned stimuli that have been associated with intense physiological responses. These physiological responses become the conditioned stimulus. According to this view, physiological changes are etiological to panic disorder, because they contribute to the perception of anxiety. This hypothesis can be traced back to the James-Lange theory that holds that emotional states are experienced because of physiological responses to provocative stimuli. Thus, panic patients become anxious not because of the identification of an objective danger, but because of the perception of bodily changes, especially respiratory instability.

An important problem with these models is that a significant proportion of panic patients experience panic attacks that are not accompanied by deviant physiological responses. Thus, large elevations in HR or respiratory instability may occur without the patient having a panic attack, and, conversely, naturally occurring panic attacks are not always accompanied by objective measures of hyperventilation or cardiovascular dysfunction.

One possibility to explain these discrepancies is that differences in cardiovascular and respiratory abnormalities reflect different subtypes of panic disorder. If so, then objective measures of cardiovascular and respiratory function may help distinguish between patients with specific types of panic and may improve diagnostic specificity and treatment efficiency.

Anticipatory Anxiety: Sustained Physiological Arousal Individuals with panic disorder exhibit enhanced *baseline* physiological arousal in laboratory settings (Fig. 14.3–2). A host of physiological measures distinguishes among patients and nonpatients. Patients with panic disorder exhibit abnormal respiratory measures, increased HR, heightened EMG activity, and enhanced levels of skin conductance together with a greater number of spontaneous skin conductance fluctuations.

At issue is whether heightened physiological activity is a persistent trait marker of chronic arousal or a transient change associated with threatening or new contexts. Ambulatory monitoring in real life situa-

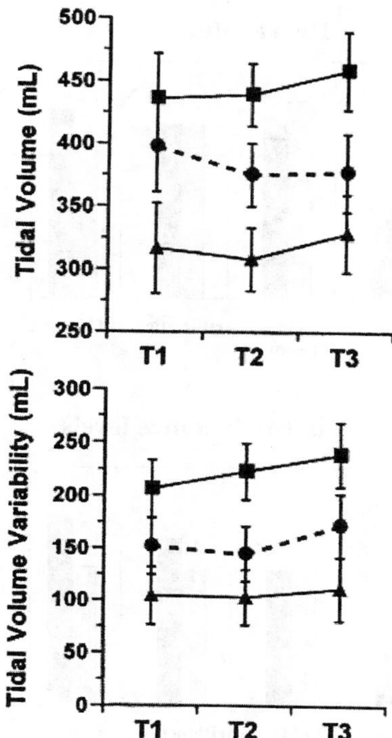

FIGURE 14.3–1 Means and standard errors of tidal volume **(top)** and tidal volume variability **(bottom)** for panic disorder patients (*black squares*), generalized anxiety disorder patients (*black circles*), and control subjects (*black triangles*) over three consecutive 10-minute epochs of the 30-minute quiet sitting period. (From Wilhelm FH, Traber W, Roth WT: Physiologic instability in panic disorder and generalized anxiety disorder. *Biol Psychiatry.* 2001;49:596, with permission.)

tions presents a promising methodological advance to address this issue. However, results are not as clear-cut as one would wish. Physiological measures of elevated arousal have been found in some studies but not in others (except for respiratory instability). One possibility is that chronic physiological arousal is present only in the more severely affected patients, especially those with intense or frequent unpredictable panic attack. In these individuals, physiological hyperactivity may represent high levels of chronic anxious apprehension caused by anticipatory anxiety about the recurrence of panic attacks.

Regardless of whether physiological arousal is or is not a chronic feature of panic disorder, there is substantial evidence indicating that panic patients are overly sensitive to challenging or stressful contexts. This is exemplified by the fact that their otherwise normal startle reflex is exaggerated in threatening contexts in which they anticipate future exposure to unpleasant shocks. Given that enhanced startle is rather specific to fear and anxiety, potentiated startle in this condition may reflect activation of a negative emotional state. This view is supported by measures of basic dimensions of emotion provided by EEG studies of anterior brain asymmetry. Patients with panic disorder exhibit EEG asymmetry with a pattern of right anterior activation (i.e., avoidance-withdrawal response). However, this laterality effect is present only during specific situations, before and during exposure to anxiety and panic-relevant situations, but not during exposure to emotionally challenging, but not panic-relevant, stimuli. A similar right anterior activation has been reported at rest in individuals with anxiety comorbid with depression, in internalizing preschoolers, in 8- to 11-year-old anxious children, and in behaviorally inhibited children.

Responses to Challenges: Autonomic Inflexibility

Despite prominent complaints of physiological symptoms and elevated baseline physiological activity in individuals with panic disorder, there is little evidence of heightened physiological arousal when confronted with nonspecific stressors such as mental arithmetic, threat of shock, cold pressor tests, postural challenges, and isometric exercise. There is growing consensus that, contrary to expectation, panic patients show autonomic inflexibility or autonomic rigidity. *Autonomic inflexibility* refers to the observation that panic patients show *less* physiological reactivity to nonspecific stressors, compared to normal control subjects.

The discovery of autonomic inflexibility in patients with anxiety disorders has sparked interest in the role of the parasympathetic nervous system in anxiety and has prompted a flurry of research on HRV as an index of sympathetic–parasympathetic balance. Most studies point to a reduction in the normal increase in HR during stressful challenges and lower HRV in panic disorder. Spectral analyses of HR have provided evidence of decreased high-frequency power and increased low-frequency power, suggesting that increased sympathetic activity is coupled with lower vagal or parasympathetic tone in these individuals. Reduced HRV has been reported during panic episodes and in their absence and in recent-onset panic disorder, as well as in panic patients with chronic conditions. Changes in cardiovascular measures that are suggestive of baroreflex modulation have also been associated with clinical recovery after psychopharmacological or cognitive therapy treatment.

Lower HRV in panic patients has meaningful implications for attention and emotion regulation and may explain the lack of ANS responsivity to external challenges and stimuli. Developmental studies point to the association between high HRV and adaptive responsivity to the environment. Low HRV is associated with impaired self-regulation, reduced attentional flexibility, and worry. Flexibility in attention is necessary to shift from relevant to nonrelevant information in an ever-changing environment. It is possible that the ineffective attentional processing of environmental cues indexed by low vagal tone contributes to abnormal physiological and affective responses in panic patients.

POSTTRAUMATIC STRESS DISORDER

PTSD may be the psychiatric condition that best illustrates the validity of psychophysiology for clinical assessment. Research has demonstrated a wide range of physiological alterations in PTSD. In particular, heightened physiological arousal has historically been an important symptom experienced by combat veterans with combat-related psychiatric sequelae. Early clinical observations of larger HR responses to stimuli reminiscent of the trauma in soldiers experiencing so-called irritable heart syndrome set the stage for current psychophysiological investigations.

Emotional Response to Trauma Reminders

PTSD patients show physiological arousal to cues that are reminders of the trauma (DSM-IV-TR symptoms, Criterion B.5). This symptom is typically assessed by using clinical interview, but there is no doubt that its quantification would greatly benefit from objective assessments. Research has consistently demonstrated increased physiological arousal after exposure to trauma reminders in individuals with PTSD (Fig. 14.3–3). Physiological arousal, which occurs across physiological systems, such as HR, skin conductance, blood pressure, and EMG activity, has been demonstrated for a variety of traumatic events (e.g., war, childhood sexual abuse,

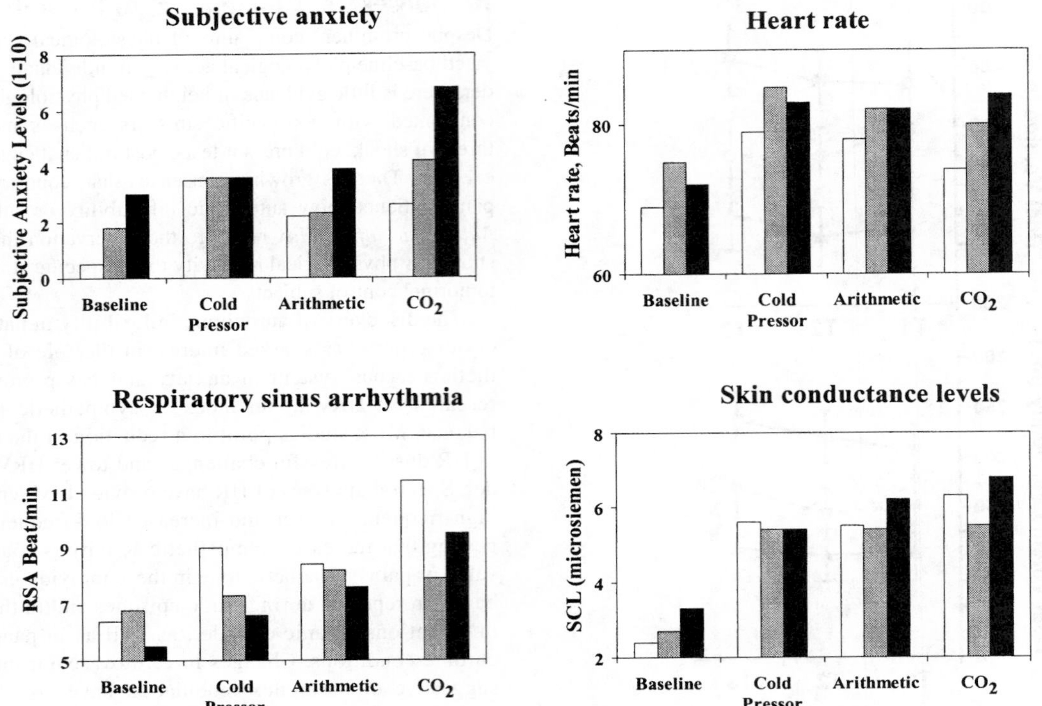

FIGURE 14.3–2 Mean subjective anxiety and physiological activity at rest and during three different stressors, including a panicogenic carbon dioxide (CO_2) stressor, in patients with panic disorders and in normal subjects (*white bars*). The patients are divided into individuals who experienced a panic attack (*black bars*) or did not experience a panic attack (*grey bars*) during the CO_2 stressor. Group differences in physiological activity and subjective anxiety were not restricted to the stress tests. They were already present at baseline. RSA, respiratory sinus arrhythmia; SCL, skin conductance level. (Adapted from Roth WT, Margraf J, Ehlers A, et al.: Stress test reactivity in panic disorder. *Arch Gen Psychiatry.* 1992;49:301.)

motor vehicle accident, and civilian events). Increased physiological reactivity in PTSD is specific to trauma-related cues, because nonspecific stressors elicit similar responses in PTSD and non-PTSD individuals.

The physiological responses to trauma reminders may be the area in which psychophysiological assessment is the most promising in terms of distinguishing PTSD individuals from non-PTSD individuals and in assessing treatment outcome. Findings from a collaborative study of more than 1,000 veterans at 15 different laboratories confirmed the heightened physiological reactivity to audiovisual cues of combat experiences, especially in veterans with the most severe symptomatology. Logistical regression of psychophysiological data correctly classified two-thirds of the participants as PTSD or non-PTSD veterans.

Baseline Physiological Activity According to current conceptualizations, PTSD should be associated with objective measures of *tonic* physiological arousal (DSM-IV-TR, symptom Criterion D). Some data support this concept. Elevated baseline HR, increased blood pressure, and excessive sweating have been reported in the context of trauma cue reactivity studies. Because these findings are based on recordings taken just before the presentation of

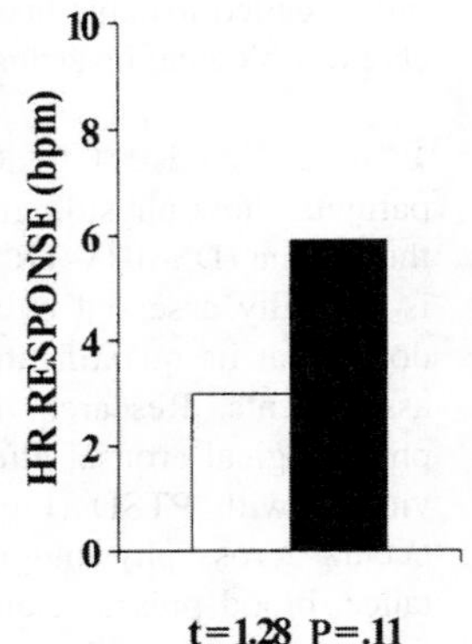

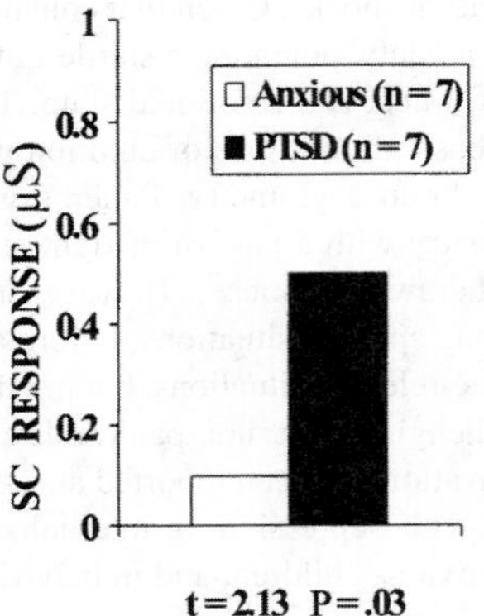

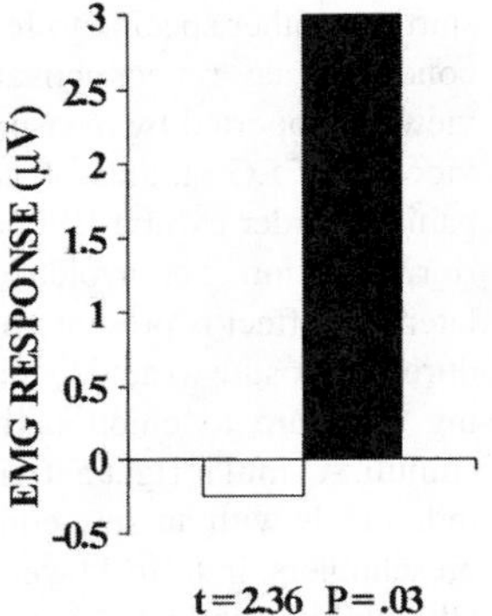

FIGURE 14.3–3 Mean heart rate (HR), skin conductance (SC), and electromyogram (EMG) response (changes scores) to individualized trauma script in Vietnam War veterans with current posttraumatic stress disorder (PTSD) or with current anxiety disorders but not current or past PTSD. The trauma script was based on the most stressful combat experience that the subject could recall. The control script was a neutral experience. bpm, beats per minute. (From Pitman RK, Orr SP, Forgue DF, et al.: Psychophysiologic assessment of posttraumatic stress disorder imagery in Vietnam combat veterans. *Arch Gen Psychiatry.* 1987;44:970, with permission.)

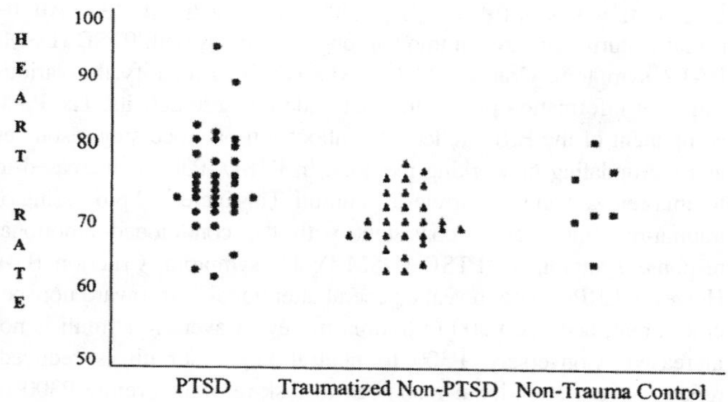

FIGURE 14.3–4 Metaanalysis of baseline heart rate in traumatized individuals with and without posttraumatic stress disorder (PTSD) and in nontraumatized controls. Each point represents individuals' study group mean value for heart rate as a function of diagnostic group. (From Buckley TC, Kaloupek DG: A meta-analytic examination of basal cardiovascular activity in posttraumatic stress disorder. *Psychosom Med.* 2001;63:585, with permission.)

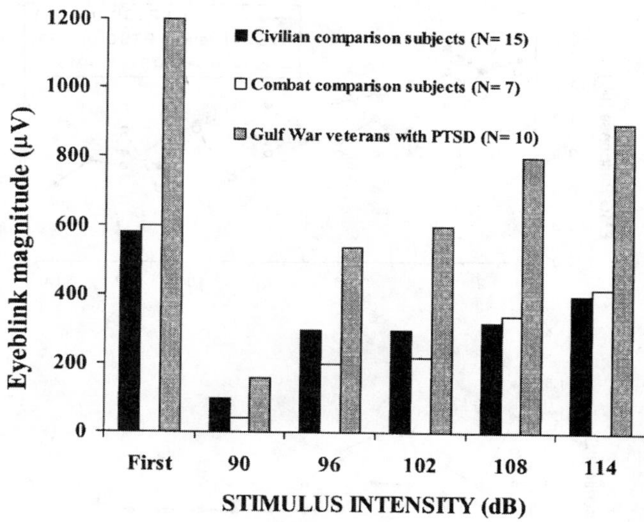

FIGURE 14.3–5 Magnitude of startle or eye-blink reflex to acoustic startle stimuli of different intensities in Gulf War veterans with and without posttraumatic stress disorder (PTSD). (From Morgan CA III, Grillon C, Southwick SM, et al.: Exaggerated acoustic startle reflex in Gulf war veterans with posttraumatic stress disorder. *Am J Psychiatry.* 1996;153:64, with permission.)

trauma reminders, it is possible that heightened physiological activity reflects only a phasic change due to anticipation of exposure to such stimuli. This hypothesis seems unlikely. Evidence from a metaanalysis study of 34 studies of baseline cardiovascular activity revealed a positive association between HR and PTSD (Fig. 14.3–4), which was not due to anticipatory anxiety. The chronicity of PTSD was a moderator of this association. The most chronic patients showed the largest HR elevation, suggesting that increased HR is a response to repeated stress. This finding has important clinical implications because of the risk of cardiovascular-related diseases associated with sustained elevation in HR.

The finding of elevated baseline HR activity is consistent with the hypothesis of tonic sympathetic nervous system arousal in PTSD. However, HRV studies have also reported reduced HRV and low vagal tone in PTSD. Thus, disturbance in ANS activity in PTSD is characterized by increased sympathetic and decreased parasympathetic tone. Preliminary evidence suggests that this autonomic imbalance can be normalized with selective serotonin reuptake inhibitor (SSRI) treatment.

CNS arousal can be assessed with EEG, but spectral analysis studies of EEG at tonic waking are scant and have not provided substantial evidence of abnormality in individuals with PTSD. Sleep disturbances are a hallmark of PTSD. Polysomnography, which is the standard EEG method to analyze sleep stages, has not revealed consistently different patterns of sleep EEG among PTSD and non-PTSD subjects.

Exaggerated Startle Exaggerated startle figures as an important symptom of hyperarousal in DSM-IV-TR (symptoms, Criterion D.5). Historically, the symptom of exaggerated startle was a prominent feature experienced by combat veterans with combat-related psychiatric disorder. So common was the symptom of exaggerated startle that it has long been considered a cardinal symptom of combat fatigue and traumatic neuroses. Although exaggerated startle is no longer viewed as a cardinal symptom of PTSD, it is still linked to trauma exposure and is reported in approximately 88 percent of PTSD sufferers. The presence of a physiological alteration accompanying a mental disorder provides the opportunity to obtain data that are more objective and more readily quantifiable than self-report data. In the case of the symptom of exaggerated startle, this alteration can also be linked to putative processes that have been implicated in the potentiation of startle in animal models.

Despite self-reports of exaggerated startle, there is no strong evidence indicating that the somatic (eye-blink) component of startle is increased in PTSD. Studies that have examined baseline levels have reported increased, reduced (in children), or normal startle or eyeblink response in PTSD groups compared to non-PTSD groups. Given that studies in animals have identified a number of processes by which the amplitude of startle can be increased, these discrepancies may reflect genuine differences in brain dysfunction among PTSD groups rather than methodological differences across laboratories. Exaggerated startle in PTSD may have multiple causes, reflecting innate vulnerability, evolution of the disease, or changes in symptoms over time, or a combination of these. Exaggerated startle in recent-onset PTSD may be due to a sensitization process (Fig. 14.3–5). In more chronic PTSD patients (e.g., in Vietnam veterans), exaggerated startle appears to reflect a transient aversive state elicited by anticipatory anxiety in threatening contexts. Because of the inconsistency in the results, and because the somatic startle reflex shows large variability across subjects, it is unlikely that startle can have widespread diagnostic usefulness. Nevertheless, the study of startle can be of considerable use and significance as a translational research tool across neuroscience, psychological science, and psychiatry.

Although the data on the somatic startle reflex are conflicting, studies that have assessed the autonomic component of startle have yielded more consistent evidence of elevated reactivity in PTSD. The findings of increased HR, larger SCRs, and slower skin conductance habituation to startling stimuli are well established (Fig. 14.3–6).

There are currently little data to address the specificity of these results to PTSD versus other anxiety disorders. However, there is preliminary evidence of heightened ANS reactivity to startling stimuli in patients with panic disorder. This hyperreactivity is consistent with findings of dysregulated autonomic function in anxiety disorders, especially when anxious patients are anticipating aversive stimuli.

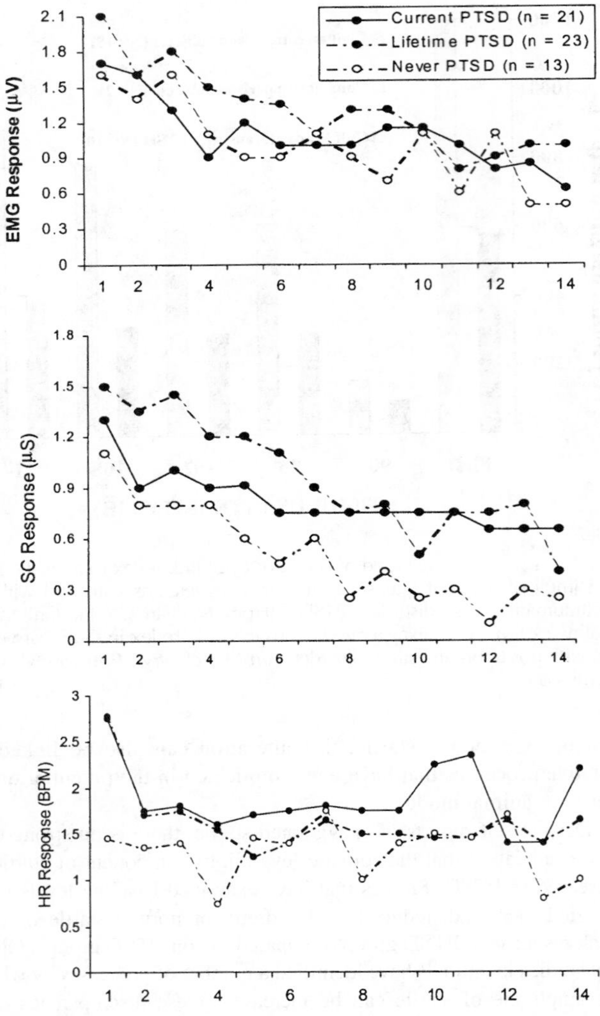

FIGURE 14.3–6 Group mean physiological responses to 15 acoustic startle stimuli (95-dB, 500-millisecond duration, 1,000-Hz pure tone) in women with current, lifetime, or no childhood sexual abuse–related posttraumatic stress disorder (PTSD). Electromyogram (EMG) data represent activity of the left orbicularis oculi. bpm, beats per minute; HR, heart rate; SC, skin conductance. (From Metzger LG, Orr SP, Berry NJ, et al.: Physiologic reactivity to startling tones in women with posttraumatic stress disorder. *J Abnorm Psychol.* 1999;108:347, with permission.)

Difficulty Concentrating and Hypervigilance Attentional disturbances are common among individuals with PTSD (DSM-IV-TR symptom, Criterion D.3). ERPs can help identify the various stages of information processing that underlie these deficits. The P300 component of the ERPs reflects the allocation of processing resources and the updating of working memory. In PTSD, P300 is increased to trauma-relevant and task-irrelevant stimuli. This increased processing of trauma-relevant cues is consistent with the conditioned emotional response symptom of PTSD (DSM-IV-TR symptom, Criterion B.4). However, ERPs do not reveal a general attentional bias toward nonspecific threat, because P300 to trauma-irrelevant aversive stimuli is not increased. Conversely, P300 to neutral target stimuli is reduced, reflecting less attentional resources to task-relevant events. P300 to trauma-relevant and trauma-irrelevant cues may have clinical application. In a recent study using visual trauma-reminder and target cues, P300 measures correctly classified 90 percent of the PTSD and 85 percent of the non-PTSD subjects.

Reduction in attentional resources could be caused by basic deficits in a preattentive sensory mechanism. This is suggested by the finding of reduced sensory gating of the P50 component and increased mismatch negativity (MMN) (Fig. 14.3–7). *Sensory gating of the P50 component* refers to the inhibition of P50 amplitude to the second of two stimuli delivered at close proximity. Lack of reduced sensory P50 gating is interpreted as a deficit in a hypothetical filtering mechanism that screens out sensory information. P50 sensory gating deficits have been reported in several psychiatric disorders, including obsessive-compulsive disorder (OCD), but more specifically in schizophrenia. Hence, sensory gating deficits are not specific to PTSD.

The MMN is an index of sensory echoic memory activated by stimulus deviation from a repetitive pattern. The MMN represents an unconscious process, but large MMN are followed by a P300 response, which reflects conscious processing of stimuli. Thus, it is conceivable that the process that promotes awareness of sensory stimuli is facilitated in PTSD. This could lead to stimulus flooding and increased distractibility because of the conscious perception of innocuous and irrelevant stimuli. The MMN is reduced in schizophrenia, but there are no available data of the specificity of increased MMN to PTSD versus other anxiety disorders.

Physiological Responses to Trauma An area that is receiving growing attention is that of the physiological responses to the trauma. Measures of physiological arousal shortly after the

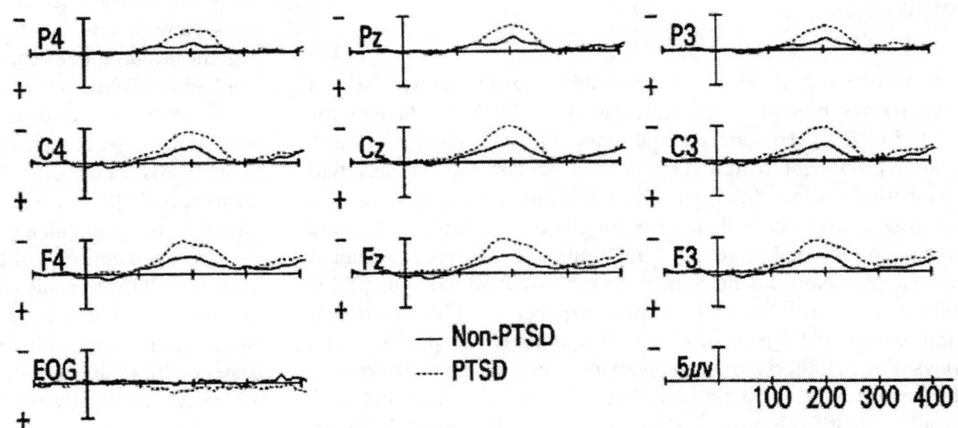

FIGURE 14.3–7 Mismatch negativity in women with sexual assault–related posttraumatic stress disorder (PTSD) and in control women. EOG, electrooculogram. (From Morgan CA III, Grillon C: Abnormal mismatch negativity in women with sexual assault-related posttraumatic stress disorder. *Biol Psychiatry.* 1999;45:827, with permission.)

trauma may provide an index of the intensity of the trauma and may become predictive of PTSD. Recent evidence indicates that elevation of HR in the emergency room or within a week after the trauma is associated with later development of PTSD. This psychophysiological assessment shortly after the trauma may help identify individuals at risk for developing PTSD.

SPECIFIC PHOBIAS

Individuals with specific phobias experience a marked, persistent, and unreasonable fear in the presence of or in anticipation of a clearly discernible object or situation. The somatic and ANS changes triggered by the phobic stimulus or situation play a significant role in the assessment of the disorder and in treatment outcome. Nevertheless, there is little research on the psychophysiology of phobias.

Emotional Response to Phobic Object Specific phobia is seen as an extreme fear response. As such, when confronted with their feared stimulus or situation, the phobic individual exhibits a surge of sympathetic activity, accompanied by the subjective experience of heightened arousal, reflecting a general mobilization for avoidance and escape behavior. Studies in animal phobics have examined psychophysiological responses to pictures or movies of the phobic object and have confirmed this physiological pattern of defense response. Spider phobics show increased HR and reduced HRV on exposure to a spider. The most intense physiological symptoms experienced by phobic individuals confronted with their specific stressor are tachycardia, tight muscles, hyperventilation, trembling, shortness of breath, cold hands, and a pounding sensation in the chest. Recent studies also indicate that the startle reflex is exaggerated on exposure to phobic objects.

In striking contrast to the tachycardia associated with animal phobic reactions, blood phobic reactions to blood, injuries, or wound situations are characterized by a biphasic cardiovascular pattern: sympathetic arousal followed quickly by parasympathetic hypotension and bradycardia that results in faintness and, ultimately, syncope. These data suggest that autonomic dysfunction in individuals with blood phobias is considerably different from that of other anxiety disorders, showing *more* vagal controls and *less* sympathetic modulation of the cardiac response.

Baseline Physiological Activity There is no evidence of chronic heightened physiological arousal in specific phobia. However, increased physiological arousal may occur during anticipation of exposure to phobic objects, in particular, when situational phobia can lead to panic attacks. There is also evidence of reduced HRV in nonclinical samples scoring high on phobic anxiety. Given that reduced HRV is a risk marker for sudden death, this result is consistent with the observation from epidemiological studies that phobic anxiety is associated with an increased risk of coronary artery disease.

Conditioning Processes Phobias, including social phobia, have been related to evolutionarily based unconscious conditioning processes. This hypothesis is based on results that fear conditioning, as indexed by the SCR, can be obtained with subliminal presentations of fear-relevant (e.g., spiders and faces), but not fear-irrelevant (e.g., flowers), stimuli. Accordingly, certain individuals may be predisposed to acquire unconscious conditioning to snakes or spiders, for example. In this conditioning model of phobia, ANS arousal plays a critical etiological role. Phobic stimuli would elicit physiological arousal before the stimulus comes into the focus of awareness. Perception of physiological arousal would trigger an uncontrollable anxiety response. Consistent with this hypothesis is the observation based on startle studies that initial physiological signs of fear during exposure to phobic stimuli appear faster in phobic individuals than in nonphobic individuals.

SOCIAL PHOBIAS

According to the DSM-IV-TR, social phobia, which is characterized by excessive and persistent fear of social or performance situations, is accompanied by substantial physiological symptoms of ANS dysfunction in the feared situation or even in anticipation of upcoming social situations. Although implicit in the description of social phobia, the presence of these physiological symptoms is not central to the diagnosis of this condition. Diagnosis of social phobia is largely based on history obtained from the patients. However, at examination, patients often exhibit physiological symptoms, including blushing and moist hands.

Emotional Response to Social Challenges There are contradictory reports as to whether social phobics exhibit exaggerated physiological responses during social challenges (e.g., social phobics asked to give a speech). Heightened ANS activity in anticipation of a social challenge has been documented in some, but not all, social phobics. Three types of social phobics have been identified. The two largest groups consist of individuals who show low or no physiological reactivity to phobic stressors but are characterized by high physiological perception or high cognitive reactivity. The third group is characterized by enhanced physiological reactivity with high physiological perception or high cognitive reactivity. Another distinction has been made between specific social phobics, whose fears are restricted to a single or a few specific situations (e.g., public speaking), and generalized social phobics, whose fears generalize to a broad range of social conditions. The specific social phobic demonstrates exaggerated increased physiological arousal to their phobic situations and may resemble patients with panic disorders. Like patients with panic disorder, they are caught in a vicious circle in which symptoms exacerbate through anticipatory anxiety. The generalized social phobics do not manifest substantial physiological arousal to their personally relevant feared situations. These results suggest that, for a majority of social phobics, the perception of physiological symptoms rather than the physiological symptoms themselves is crucial in eliciting anxiety. This is consistent with the view that social phobics focus more on internal sensations than do non–social phobic individuals. Alternatively, cognitive factors, such as attentional focus and dysfunctional appraisal of the self and social situations, may be more important than physiological symptoms in mediating social anxiety.

Blushing Blushing may be the most prominent and widespread symptom in social phobics, distinguishing individuals with this condition from individuals with other anxiety disorders. However, there is little evidence of an exaggerated propensity to blush in individuals who are high in fear of blushing. The coloration of the cheek can be reliably evaluated with a photoplethysmograph. Photoplethysmography studies have reported substantial increases in blushing in response to various social stressors. However, social phobics who are low and high in fear of blushing show equally intense blush responses. The factor that distinguishes the two groups is the perceived intensity of their blushing. Individuals who are high in fear of blushing report that they blush more than low-fear individuals, despite contrary evidence from photoplethysmography. This overestimation of blushing is consistent with cognitive theories that emphasize the role of attentional factors. According to these theories, interpersonal situations lead to increased self-focused attention, which intensifies the perception of physiological responses, and, in turn, further increases self-focused attention. However, the fact that social phobia can occur with and without complaints of blushing and with and without exaggerated physiological arousal suggests that there are several etiological mechanisms to this condition.

GENERALIZED ANXIETY DISORDER

The essential characteristics of generalized anxiety disorder are sustained and excessive anxiety and worry accompanied by a number of physiological symptoms. The psychophysiology of generalized anxiety disorder is poorly understood. There is no evidence of abnormal baseline physiological activity in individuals with generalized anxiety disorder. However, persons with generalized anxiety disorder show a restricted range of HR, SCR, and EMG reactivity to nonspecific stressors. This pattern of responses has been linked to worry. Indeed, worrisome thinking leads to a similar autonomic inflexibility, which has been attributed to low levels of vagal tone. However, this statement should be tempered by the fact that psychophysiological studies have focused mostly on ANS activity, whereas generalized anxiety disorder individuals complain essentially of symptoms of central origins (e.g., lack of concentration, insomnia, and restlessness), which may be best studied with measures of cortical activity.

OBSESSIVE-COMPULSIVE DISORDER

OCD is characterized by recurrent and disturbing thoughts or repetitive and stereotyped behaviors, or both, that the patient feels compelled to perform but recognizes as irrational. Although OCD is accompanied by physiological arousal, physiological symptoms do not play a prominent role in diagnostic assessment, and psychophysiological studies are relatively scant compared to studies in other anxiety disorders, such as panic disorder.

Emotional Response to Obsessive-Compulsive Stimuli OCD individuals are autonomically aroused when exposed to their obsessive-compulsive stimuli, but they are not abnormally overreactive to nonspecific stressors. Stimuli that evoke obsessive thoughts increase subjective anxiety in conjunction with an increase in ANS arousal. Conversely, OCD patients may be physiologically hyporeactive to nonspecific stressors. This reduced reactivity is not restricted to the ANS but also encompasses muscle activity.

Electrocortical Activity Because ANS dysfunction does not seem to be of key importance in OCD, psychophysiological research has focused on central dysfunction using EEG and ERP. There is no clear evidence regarding the nature of cognitive dysfunction in OCD, but neuropsychological and brain imaging studies have implicated frontal-striatal areas. Frontal structures have also been implicated by EEG studies. Research shows abnormalities in the lower-frequency EEG bands, especially excess theta power in frontal and frontotemporal regions. Deficits in OCD have been conceptualized in terms of reduced inhibitory or gating processes that are necessary to inhibit unwanted responses or for normal shifting ability. OCD patients demonstrate abnormalities in various ERP components associated with inhibitory processes attributed to frontal areas, such as the frontal P300 to no-go stimuli in a go–no-go task, and frontal negativity associated with the monitoring of action and the detection of error. However, these results should be interpreted with caution, given the poor spatial resolution of ERPs. Nevertheless, such evidence for inhibitory deficits is consistent with findings using prepulse inhibition (PPI) of the startle reflex as an index of gating mechanisms. The startle reflex is normally inhibited by weak sensory stimuli presented 30 to 500 milliseconds before the startle-eliciting stimulus. The gating startle circuitry includes corticostriatal substrates that have been implicated in OCD. The PPI effect is reduced in OCD, suggesting diminished gating processes. This finding is not specific to OCD. PPI deficits characterize patients who show disturbance in inhibitory function aimed at gating unwanted thoughts (e.g., schizophrenia) or movements (e.g., Huntington's disease and Tourette's syndrome).

FUTURE DIRECTIONS

The psychophysiology of anxiety disorders has been concerned with the examination of physiological activity in four main areas: (1) at rest, in innocuous environments; (2) at rest, before a stressful challenge; (3) during nonspecific stressors; and (4) during specific stressors, that is, during exposure to a stressor that is relevant to the disorder. Ambulatory monitoring studies suggest that anxious patients are not in a state of heightened arousal outside the laboratory. However, this conclusion should be taken with caution, because ambulatory monitoring provides only a limited range of physiological measures over limited periods of time. A consistent finding across anxiety disorders is the presence of enhanced physiological arousal in a laboratory setting before the confrontation with a specific or a nonspecific stressor. Baseline physiological activity before a stressor distinguishes patients with anxiety disorders from healthy controls. However, it lacks specificity with regard to the differentiation among disorders. An exception to this finding is the presence of respiratory abnormalities in patients with panic disorders. Symptoms of heightened ANS arousal in the laboratory are best understood in terms of anticipatory anxiety. A finding that also characterizes anxiety disorders in general is the relative lack of ANS reactivity to nonspecific stressors. This autonomic inflexibility may be due to low vagal tone or to preoccupation with personal stressors. An important question is whether autonomic inflexibility is due to comorbid conditions or to an underlying neurobiological dysfunction shared by all anxiety disorders. Autonomic inflexibility seems to be associated with the worry process. As such, it may represent a coping mechanism in response to chronic anxiety. However, the fact that it has also been reported in behaviorally inhibited children, who are at risk for anxiety disorders, may be indicative of a genetic predisposition. Finally, exposure to specific stressors leads to greater ANS differentiation between anxious patients and healthy controls, as well as among patients with various anxiety disorders.

There are limitations in using measures of ANS activity as an objective index of physiological symptoms. The lack of concordance between physiological measures and verbal complaint can be explained by the fact that the wrong physiological variable is assessed. For example, the symptom of heart pounding or racing is better reflected in stroke volume than in HR. In addition, no unique physiological measure can provide a direct index of ANS activity. Concurrent use of several measures may provide a better convergent index. Furthermore, technical advancement will soon permit recording of a multitude of physiological channels together with self-report items using unobtrusive monitoring devices. Ambulatory monitoring will help resolve the issue of the source of complaints about physiological symptoms. It will then be possible to relate physiological abnormalities to natural stressors.

Diagnosis and treatment outcome are areas of key interest in anxiety disorders. As psychophysiological techniques are refined, they should provide a fresh perspective into many aspects of anxiety disorders.

SUGGESTED CROSS-REFERENCES

The reader is encouraged to refer to the related anxiety disorders sections on clinical features (Section 14.8) and on applied electrophysiology (Section 1.14). Other related materials include the sections on stress and psychiatry (Section 24.9) and signs and symptoms in psychiatry (Section 7.4).

REFERENCES

American Psychiatric Association. *Diagnostic and Statistical Manual of Mental Disorders.* 4th ed. Washington, DC: American Psychiatric Association; 1994.

Attias J, Bleich A, Furman V, Zinger Y: Event-related potentials in post-traumatic stress disorder of combat origin. *Biol Psychiatry.* 1996;40:373.

Brown JS, Kalish HI, Farber IE: Conditioned fear as revealed by the magnitude of startle response to an auditory stimulus. *J Exp Psychol.* 1951;41:317.

Buckley TC, Kaloupek DG: A meta-analytic examination of basal cardiovascular activity in posttraumatic stress disorder. *Psychosom Med.* 2001;63:585.

Cuthbert BN, Lang JL, Strauss C, Drobes D, Patrick CJ, Bradley MB: The psychophysiology of anxiety disorders: Fear memory imagery. *Psychophysiology.* 2003;40:407.

*Davidson RJ: EEG measures of cerebral asymmetry: Conceptual and methodological issues. *Intern J Neurosci.* 1998;39:71.

Davis M: Sensitization of the acoustic startle reflex by foot shock. *Behav Neurosci.* 1989;103:495.

Davis M, Falls WA, Campeau S, Kim M: Fear-potentiated startle: A neural and pharmacological analysis. *Behav Brain Res.* 1993;58:175.

Grillon C: Startle reactivity and anxiety disorders: Aversive conditioning, context, and neurobiology. *Biol Psychiatry.* 2002;52:958.

Grillon C, Ameli R, Woods SW, Merikangas K, Davis M: Fear-potentiated startle in humans: Effects of anticipatory anxiety on the acoustic blink reflex. *Psychophysiol.* 1991;28:588.

Grillon C, Baas JM: A review of the modulation of startle by affective states and its application to psychiatry. *Clin Neurophysiol.* 2003;114:1557.

Hamm AO, Greenwald MK, Bradley MM, Lang PJ: Emotional learning, hedonic changes, and the startle probe. *J Abnorm Psychol.* 1993;102:453.

Hamm AO, Vaitl D: Affective learning: Awareness and aversion. *Psychophysiol.* 1996;33:698.

Hoehn-Saric R, McLeod DR: Anxiety and arousal: Physiological changes and their perception. *J Affect Disord.* 2000;61:217.

Hugdahl K. *Psychophysiology: The Mind-Body Perspective.* Cambridge, MA: Harvard University Press; 1995.

Kalin NH, Larson C, Shelton SE, Davidson RJ: Asymmetric frontal brain activity, cortisol, and behavior associated with fearful temperament in rhesus monkeys. *Behav Neurosci.* 1998;112:286.

Kardiner A. *War Stress and Neurotic Illness.* New York: Hoeber; 1947.

Kawachi I, Sparrow D, Vokonas PS, Weiss ST: Symptoms of anxiety and risk of coronary heart disease. The Normative Aging Study. *Circulation.* 1994;90:2225.

*Keane TM, Kaloupek DG, Blanchard EB, Hsieh FY, Kolb LC, Orr SP, Thomas RG, Lavori PW: Utility of psychophysiological measurement in the diagnosis of posttraumatic stress disorder: Results from a Department of Veterans Affairs cooperative study. *J Consult Clin Psychol.* 1998;66:914.

*Klein DF: False suffocation alarms, spontaneous panic, and related conditions: An integrative hypothesis. *Arch Gen Psychiatry.* 1993;50:306.

Lader MH: Palmar skin conductance measures in anxiety and phobic states. *J Psychosom Res.* 1967;11:271.

Lang PJ, Bradley MM, Cuthbert BN: Emotion, attention, and the startle reflex. *Psychol Rev.* 1990;97:1.

*Lang PJ, Davis M, Ohman A: Fear and anxiety: Animal models and human cognitive psychophysiology. *J Affect Disord.* 2000;61:137.

Mauss IB, Wilhelm FH, Gross JJ: Autonomic recovery and habituation in social anxiety. *Psychophysiology.* 2003;40:648.

Orr SP, Roth WT: Psychophysiological assessment: Clinical applications for PTSD. *J Affect Disord.* 2000;61:225.

Roth WT, Margraf J, Ehlers A, Taylor CB, Maddock RJ, Davies S, Agras WS: Stress test reactivity in panic disorder. *Arch Gen Psychiatry.* 1992;49:301.

Shalev AY, Sahar T, Freedman S, Peri T, Glick N, Brandes D, Orr SP, Pitman RK: A prospective study of heart rate response following trauma and the subsequent development of posttraumatic stress disorder. *Arch Gen Psychiatry.* 1998;55:553.

Thayer J, Friedman B, Borkovec T: Autonomic characteristics of generalized anxiety disorder and worry. *Biol Psychiatry.* 1996;39:255.

*Thayer JF, Lane RD: A model of neurovisceral integration in emotion regulation and dysregulation. *J Affect Disord.* 2000;61:201.

Wilhelm FH, Roth WT: The somatic symptom paradox in DSM-IV anxiety disorders: Suggestions for a clinical focus in psychophysiology. *Biol Psychol.* 2001;57:105.

▲ 14.4 Anxiety Disorders: Neurochemical Aspects

ALEXANDER NEUMEISTER, M.D., OMER BONNE, M.D., AND DENNIS S. CHARNEY, M.D.

The past decade has seen a rapid progression in knowledge of the neurobiological basis of fear and anxiety. Specific neurochemical and neuropeptide systems have been demonstrated to play important roles in the behaviors associated with fear and anxiety-producing stimuli. Long-term dysregulation of these systems appears to contribute to the development of anxiety disorders, including panic disorder, posttraumatic stress disorder (PTSD), and social anxiety disorder. These neurochemical and neuropeptide systems have been shown to have effects on distinct cortical and subcortical brain areas that are relevant to the mediation of the symptoms associated with anxiety disorders. Moreover, advances in molecular genetics portend the identification of the genes that underlie the neurobiological disturbances that increase the vulnerability to anxiety disorders. This chapter reviews clinical research pertinent to the neurobiological basis of anxiety disorders with particular emphasis on neurochemical aspects. The implications of this synthesis for the discovery of anxiety disorder vulnerability genes and novel psychopharmacological approaches are also discussed.

NEUROCHEMICAL BASIS OF FEAR AND ANXIETY

Specific neurotransmitters and neuropeptides act on brain areas that are believed to be involved in the mediation of fear and anxiety responses. These neurochemicals are released during stress, and chronic stress results in long-term alterations in function of these systems. Stress axis neurochemical systems prepare the organism for threat in multiple ways, through increased attention and vigilance, modulation of memory (to maximize the use of prior experience), planning, and preparation for action. In addition, these systems have peripheral effects, which include increased heart rate and blood pressure (catecholamines) and rapid modulation of the body's use of energy (cortisol). The neurobiological responses to threat and severe stress are clearly adaptive and have survival value, but they can also have maladaptive consequences when they become chronically activated. Examination of the preclinical data concerning neurochemical substrates of the stress response, the long-term impact of early life exposure to stress, and possible stress-induced neurotoxicity provides a context to consider clinical investigations of the pathophysiology of the anxiety disorders.

NORADRENERGIC SYSTEM

Stressful stimuli of many types produce marked increases in brain noradrenergic function (Table 14.4–1). Stress produces regional selective increases in norepinephrine (NE) turnover in the locus ceruleus (LC), the limbic regions (hypothalamus, hippocampus, and amygdala), and the cerebral cortex. These changes can be elicited with immobilization stress, foot-shock stress, tail-pinch stress, and conditioned fear. Exposure to stressors from which the animal cannot escape results in behavioral deficits termed *learned helplessness.* The learned helplessness state is associated with depletion of NE, probably reflecting the point at which synthesis cannot keep up with demand. These studies have been reviewed elsewhere in detail.

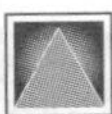

Table 14.4–1
Evidence for Altered Catecholaminergic Function in Anxiety Disorders

	Posttraumatic Stress Disorder	Panic Disorder
Increased resting heart rate and blood pressure	+/–	+/–
Increased heart rate and blood pressure response to traumatic reminders or panic attacks	+++	++
Increased resting urinary NE and epinephrine	+	+/–
Increased resting plasma NE or MHPG	–	–
Increased plasma NE with traumatic reminders or panic attacks	+	+/–
Increased orthostatic heart rate response to exercise	+	+
Decreased binding to platelet α_2 receptors	+	+/–
Decrease in basal and stimulated activity of cyclic adenosine monophosphate	+/–	+
Decrease in platelet monoamine oxidase activity	+	Not studied
Increased symptoms, heart rate and plasma MHPG with yohimbine (Actibine) noradrenergic challenge	++	+++
Differential brain metabolic response to yohimbine	+	+

–, One or more studies do not support this finding (with no positive studies) or the majority of studies do not support this finding; +/–, an equal number of studies support this finding and do not support this finding; +, at least one study supports this finding, and no studies do not support the finding, or the majority of studies support the finding; ++, two or more studies support this finding, and no studies do not support the finding; +++, three or more studies support this finding, and no studies do not support the finding; MHPG, 3-methoxy-4-hydroxyphenylglycol; NE, norepinephrine.

Neurons in the LC are activated in association with fear and anxiety states, and the limbic and cortical regions innervated by the LC are those thought to be involved in the elaboration of adaptive responses to stress. LC NE neurons in freely moving cats were activated twofold to threefold by confrontation with a dog or an aggressive cat, although exposure to other novel stimuli (such as a nonaggressive cat) did not increase the firing rate.

A series of investigations has shown that certain stressors elicit increased responsiveness of LC neurons to excitatory stimulation. Antagonism of α_2-adrenergic receptors with idazoxan or yohimbine (Actibine) increases the response of LC neurons to excitatory stimuli without altering their baseline firing rate. Acute cold restraint stress results in decreased density of α_2 receptors in the hippocampus and amygdala. Furthermore, in chronically cold-stressed rats, the release of NE produced by yohimbine or repeated stress in the hippocampus is enhanced. It has been hypothesized that a *functional blockade* of α_2 receptors is a consequence of NE depletion with inescapable stress, resulting in enhancement of LC neuron responsiveness to stimuli.

Chronic symptoms experienced by anxiety disorder patients, such as panic attacks, insomnia, startle, and autonomic hyperarousal, are characteristic of increased noradrenergic function. Potential drugs of abuse, such as alcohol, opiates, and benzodiazepines (but not cocaine), decrease firing of noradrenergic neurons. Increases in abuse of these substances parallel increases in anxiety symptoms, providing evidence for self-medication of these symptoms that is explainable based on animal studies of noradrenergic function. In addition, patients with anxiety disorders frequently report significant improvement of symptoms of hyperarousal and intrusive memories with alcohol, benzodiazepines, and opiates, which decrease LC firing, but worsening of these symptoms with cocaine, which increases LC firing.

There is strong evidence that function of the brain noradrenergic system is involved in mediation of fear conditioning. Neutral stimuli paired with shock (conditioned stimulus) produce increases in brain NE metabolism and behavioral deficits similar to those elicited by the shock alone, as well as increased firing rate of cells in the LC. An intact noradrenergic system appears to be necessary for the acquisition of fear-conditioned responses.

Many patients with anxiety disorders experience an increased susceptibility to psychosocial stress. Behavioral sensitization may account for these clinical phenomena. In the laboratory model of sensitization, single or repeated exposure to physical stimuli or pharmacological agents sensitizes an animal to subsequent stressors. For example, in animals with a history of prior stress, there is a potentiated release of NE in the hippocampus with subsequent exposure to stressors. Similar findings were observed in medial prefrontal cortex (mPFC). The hypothesis that sensitization is an underlying neural mechanism contributing to the course of anxiety disorders is supported by clinical studies demonstrating that repeated exposure to traumatic stress is an important risk factor for the development of anxiety disorders, particularly PTSD.

There is extensive clinical evidence that NE plays a role in human anxiety. Well-designed psychophysiological studies have been conducted that have documented heightened autonomic or sympathetic nervous system arousal in combat veterans with chronic PTSD. Because central noradrenergic and peripheral sympathetic systems function in concert, the data from these psychophysiology investigations are consistent with the hypothesis that noradrenergic hyperreactivity in patients with PTSD may be associated with the conditioned or sensitized responses to specific traumatic stimuli.

There is some evidence that baseline levels of NE are consistently altered in combat-related PTSD. Women with PTSD secondary to childhood sexual abuse had significantly elevated levels of catecholamines (NE, epinephrine [E], dopamine [DA]) and cortisol in 24-hour urine samples. Sexually abused girls excreted significantly greater amounts of catecholamine metabolites, metanephrine, vanilmandelic acid, and homovanillic acid (HVA) than nonsexually abused girls. Plasma levels of NE are elevated throughout a 24-hour collection period, as are cerebrospinal fluid (CSF) levels of NE in PTSD patients. Exposure to traumatic reminders in the form of combat films results in increased E and NE release.

Studies of peripheral NE receptor function have also shown alterations in α_2 receptor and cyclic adenosine monophosphate (cAMP) function in patients with PTSD. Decreases in platelet adrenergic α_2-receptor number, platelet basal adenosine, isoproterenol, forskolin-stimulated cAMP signal transduction, and basal platelet monoamine oxidase (MAO) activity have been found in PTSD. These findings may reflect chronic high levels of NE release that lead to compensatory receptor downregulation and decreased responsiveness.

Patients with combat-related PTSD had enhanced behavioral, biochemical, and cardiovascular responses to the α_2-antagonist yohimbine, which stimulates central NE release, compared to healthy controls. Moreover, a positron emission tomography (PET) study demonstrated that PTSD patients have a cerebral metabolic response to yohimbine that is consistent with increased NE release.

There is considerable evidence that abnormal regulation of brain noradrenergic systems is also involved in the pathophysiology of panic disorder. Panic disorder patients are sensitive to the anxiogenic effects of yohimbine in addition to having exaggerated plasma 3-methoxy-4-hydroxyphenylglycol (MHPG), cortisol, and cardiovascular responses. Children with a variety of anxiety disorders exhibit greater anxiogenic responses to yohimbine than normal comparison children. The responses to the α_2-adrenergic receptor agonist clonidine (Catapres) are also abnormal in panic disorder patients. Clonidine administration caused greater hypotension, greater decreases in plasma MHPG, and less sedation in panic patients than in controls.

Few studies have examined noradrenergic function in patients with phobic disorders. In patients with specific phobias, increases in subjective anxiety and increased heart rate, blood pressure, plasma NE, and E have been associated with exposure to the phobic stimulus. This finding may be of interest from the standpoint of the model of conditioned fear, reviewed previously, in which a potentiated release of NE occurs in response to a reexposure to the original stressful stimulus. Patients with social phobia have been found to have greater increases in plasma NE in comparison to healthy controls and patients with panic disorder. In contrast to panic disorder patients, the density of lymphocyte α-adrenergic receptors is normal in social phobic patients. The growth hormone response to intravenous (IV) clonidine (a marker of central α_2-receptor function) is blunted in social phobia patients.

HYPOTHALAMIC-PITUITARY-ADRENAL AXIS

There is consistent evidence that many forms of psychological stress increase the synthesis and release of cortisol. Cortisol serves to mobilize and to replenish energy stores and contributes to increased arousal, vigilance, focused attention, and memory formation; inhibition of the growth and reproductive system; and containment of the immune response. Cortisol has important regulatory effects on the hippocampus, amygdala, and prefrontal cortex. Glucocorticoids can enhance amygdala activity, can increase corticotropin-releasing hormone (CRH) messenger ribonucleic acid (mRNA) concentrations in the central nucleus of the amygdala (CEA), can increase the effects of CRH on conditioned fear, and can facilitate the encoding of emotion-related memory. Adrenal steroids, such as cortisol, have biphasic effects on hippocampal excitability and cognitive function and memory. These effects may contribute to adaptive alterations in behaviors induced by cortisol during the acute response to stress.

It is key, however, that the stress-induced increase in cortisol ultimately be constrained through an elaborate negative feedback system involving glucocorticoid receptors (GRs) and mineralocorticoid receptors (MRs). Excessive and sustained cortisol secretion can have serious adverse effects, including hypertension, osteoporosis, immunosuppression, insulin resistance, dyslipidemia, dyscoagulation, and, ultimately, atherosclerosis and cardiovascular disease.

Alterations in hypothalamic-pituitary-adrenal (HPA) axis function have been demonstrated in PTSD. Patients with chronic PTSD demonstrate increased suppression of cortisol with low-dose dexamethasone (DEX) (Decadron), the opposite pattern to that of depression. PTSD patients may also have an increased number of GRs on peripheral lymphocytes. It has been hypothesized that an increase in GR function in central brain structures such as the hypothalamus results in supersuppression to cortisol feedback and, therefore, decreased peripheral cortisol levels.

Male patients with combat-related PTSD were shown to have blunted adrenocorticotropic hormone (ACTH) response to corticotropin-releasing factor (CRF) in comparison to controls. However, a study of premenopausal women with PTSD revealed increased ACTH and cortisol response to CRH.

Twenty-four–hour measurements of urinary cortisol concentrations in PTSD patients have yielded mixed results. Two 24-hour studies measuring plasma cortisol levels revealed lower cortisol levels during the second half of the night.

In panic disorder patients, blunted ACTH responses to CRF have been reported in some studies and not in others. Normal and elevated rates of cortisol nonsuppression after DEX have been reported. The responsiveness of the HPA system to a combined DEX-CRF challenge test was found to be higher in panic disorder patients than in healthy controls but lower than in depressed patients. Urinary free cortisol results have been inconsistent. Elevated plasma cortisol levels were reported in one study but not in another. In a recent study of 24-hour secretion of ACTH and cortisol in panic disorder, only subtle abnormalities were seen. Patients had elevated overnight cortisol secretion and a greater amplitude of ultraradian secretory episodes. Patients with more severe panic disorder symptoms may be more likely to have elevated cortisol secretion.

CORTICOTROPIN-RELEASING HORMONE

CRH is one of the most important mediators of the stress response, coordinating the adaptive behavioral and physiological changes that occur during stress. Hypothalamic levels of CRH are increased by stress, resulting in activation of the HPA axis and increased release of cortisol and dehydroepiandrosterone (DHEA). Equally important are the extrahypothalamic effects of CRH. CRH-containing neurons are located throughout the brain, including the prefrontal and cingulate cortices, the CEA, the bed nucleus of the stria terminalis (BNST), the nucleus accumbens, the periaqueductal gray (PAG) matter, and the brainstem nuclei, such as the major NE-containing nucleus, the LC, and the serotonin (5-HT) nuclei in the dorsal and median raphe.

Increased activity of amygdala CRH neurons activates fear-related behaviors, whereas cortical CRH may reduce reward expectation. CRH also inhibits a variety of neurovegetative functions, such as food intake, sexual activity, and endocrine programs for growth and reproduction. It appears that early life stress can produce long-term elevation of brain CRH activity and that the individual response to heightened CRH function may depend on social environment, past trauma history, and behavioral dominance. Persistent elevation of hypothalamic and extrahypothalamic CRH contributes mightily to psychobiological allostatic load.

CRH-1 and CRH-2 receptors are found in the pituitary and throughout the neocortex (especially in prefrontal, cingulate, striate, and insular cortices), amygdala, and hippocampal formation in primate brain. The presence of CRH-1 (but not CRH-2) receptors within the LC, the nucleus of the solitary tract, the thalamus, and the striatum and of CRH-2 (but not CRH-1) receptors in the choroid plexus, certain hypothalamic nuclei, the nucleus prepositus, and the BNST suggests that each receptor subtype has distinct roles within the primate brain.

CRH-1–deficient mice display decreased anxiety-like behavior and an impaired stress response. In contrast, CRH-2–deficient mice display increased anxiety-like behavior and are hypersensitive to stress. Thus, evidence exists in favor of opposite functional roles for the two known CRH receptors; activation of CRH-1 receptors may be responsible for increased anxiety-like responses, and stimulation of CRH-2 may produce anxiolytic-like responses. Regulation of the relative contribution of the two CRH receptor subtypes to brain CRF pathways may be essential to coordinating psychological and physiological responses to stressors. Thus far, it has not been possible to evaluate CRH-1 and CRH-2 receptors in living human subjects, although efforts are ongoing to develop CRH receptor PET ligands. Increased cerebrospinal levels of CRH have been linked to PTSD.

J. Douglas Bremner and colleagues found increased levels of CRH in the CSF of patients with combat-related chronic PTSD based on a single lumbar puncture determination. Dewleen G. Baker and associates found elevations of CSF CRH throughout a 24-hour point. These findings are important to consider in the context of preclinical studies, which have demonstrated that basal CSF CRH is elevated in primates that have experienced early life stress, the effects of CRH on behavior occur in a context-dependent manner, and early life exposure of hippocampus to elevated levels of CRH is associated with hippocampal damage later in life. Intracerebroventricular injection of CRH produces an increase in hippocampal MR levels, suggesting that CRH is an important regulator of HPA axis regulation.

These findings implicate elevated CRH as related to the clinical observation that early life stress increases the risk for developing PTSD after traumatic stress exposure later in life. They also suggest that elevated CRH in the hippocampus may relate to the mechanism responsible for reduced hippocampal volume observed in PTSD. Finally, the ability of CRH to increase MR density may provide an explanation for the findings of elevated CSH and normal to low cortisol levels in some PTSD patients.

NEUROSTEROIDS

Steroids influence neuronal function through binding to intracellular receptors, which may act as transcription factors in the regulation of gene expression. Several neurosteroids, particularly 3α-reduced metabolites of progesterone and deoxycorticosterone, modulate ligand-gated channels via nongenomic mechanisms. They are positive modulators of γ-aminobutyric acid (GABA) type A ($GABA_A$) receptors. These neuroactive steroids have anxiolytic effects in animal models. They counteract the anxiogenic effects of CRH and reduce CRH gene expression. Studies in panic disorder patients indicate that 3α-reduced neurosteroids may serve as a counterregulatory mechanism against spontaneous panic attacks. Cholecystokinin (CCK)–4 and lactate-induced panic attacks are associated with a decrease in 3α,5α-tetrahydroprogesterone (THP) and 3α,5β-THP and on 3β,5α-THP (these changes may result in decreased GABA tone and do not occur in healthy subjects). The availability of synthetic analogs of 3α-reduced neuroactive steroids (ganaxolone) can test the concept that such compounds might have anxiolytic efficacy.

ARGININE VASOPRESSIN

CRH and arginine vasopressin (AVP) are the major secretagogs of the HPA-stress system. AVP, however, has been studied much less than CRH, and knowledge of the functional activity and pharmacology of AVP and its receptors in the regulation of HPA activity rests largely on studies conducted in rodents. AVP has ACTH-releasing properties when administered alone in humans, a response that may be dependent on the ambient endogenous CRH level. After the combination of AVP and CRH, a much greater ACTH response is seen, and both peptides are required for maximal pituitary-adrenal stimulation. The sensitivity of CRH and AVP transcription to glucocorticoid feedback apparently differs, and AVP-stimulated ACTH secretion may be refractory to glucocorticoid feedback. Vasopressinergic regulation of the HPA axis may therefore be critical for sustaining corticotroph responsiveness in the presence of high circulating glucocorticoid levels during chronic stress. Thus, in animals deficient for the CRH-1 receptor, a selective compensatory activation of the hypothalamic AVP system occurs that maintains basal ACTH secretion and HPA activity. Similar response patterns have been observed after chronic stress, leading to a hypothesis that CRH plays a predominantly permissive role in HPA regulation but that AVP represents the dynamic mediator of ACTH release.

AVP is produced by the parvocellular neurons of the paraventricular nucleus (PVN) and is secreted into the pituitary portal circulation from axon terminals projecting to the external zone of the median eminence. It is primarily released after a variety of stimuli, including increasing plasma osmolality, hypovolemia, hypotension, and hypoglycemia. Extrahypothalamic AVP-containing neurons have also been characterized in the rat, notably in the medial amygdala, and innervate limbic structures such as the lateral septum and the ventral hippocampus. In these latter structures, AVP was suggested to act as a neurotransmitter, exerting its action by binding to specific G-protein–coupled receptors, that is, vasopressin V1a and V1b receptors, which are widely distributed in the central nervous system (CNS), including the septum, cortex, and hippocampus. In addition to its role in fluid metabolism regulation, AVP has been implicated in learning and memory processes, pain sensitivity, synchronization of biological rhythms, and the timing and quality of rapid eye movement (REM) sleep. In recent years, AVP V1b antagonists have exhibited significant anxiolytic and antidepressant effect in various classic animal models.

In the only AVP-related study conducted in anxiety disorder patients, increased serum prolyl endopeptidase (an AVP-degrading enzyme) activity was found in PTSD, suggesting lower AVP concentration in PTSD, leading to decreased HPA axis activity in this disorder. This finding is of particular interest, given the discrepant findings of increased CSF-CRH levels and normal to low cortisol levels reported for PTSD. AVP may therefore play a pivotal role in PTSD. Additional studies of AVP function in other anxiety disorders are indicated.

NEUROPEPTIDE Y

Neuropeptide Y (NPY) is a highly conserved 36–amino acid peptide, which is among the most abundant peptides found in mammalian brain. There are four brain areas in which neurons containing NPY are densely concentrated: the LC and PVN of the hypothalamus, septohippocampal neurons, the nucleus of solitary tract, and the ventrolateral medulla. Moderate levels are found in the amygdala, the hippocampus, the cerebral cortex, the basal ganglia, and the thalamus.

Evidence suggesting the involvement of the amygdala in the anxiolytic effects of NPY is robust, and it probably occurs via the NPY-Y1 receptor. Microinjection of NPY into the CEA reduces anxious behaviors. The upregulation of amygdala NPY mRNA levels after chronic stress suggests that NPY may be involved in the adaptive responses to stress exposure. NPY may also be involved in the consolidation of fear memories; injection of NPY into the amygdala impairs memory retention in a foot-shock avoidance paradigm. The anxiolytic effects of NPY also involve the LC, possibly via the NPY-Y2 receptor. NPY reduces the firing of LC neurons. NPY also has behaviorally relevant effects on the hippocampus. Transgenic rats with hippocampal NPY overexpression have attenuated sensitivity to the behavioral consequences of stress and impaired spatial learning.

There are important functional interactions between NPY and CRH. NPY counteracts the anxiogenic effects of CRH, and a CRH antagonist blocks the anxiogenic effects of an NPY-Y1 antagonist. Thus, it has been suggested that the balance between NPY and CRH neurotransmission is important to the emotional responses to stress.

In general, brain regions that express CRH and CRH receptors also contain NPY and NPY receptors, and the functional effects are often opposite, especially at the level of the LC amygdala and the PAG.

These data suggest an important role for the NPY system in the psychobiology of resilience and vulnerability to stress. NPY has counterregulatory effects on CRH and LC-NE systems at brain sites that are important in the expression of anxiety, fear, and depression. Preliminary studies in special operations soldiers under extreme training stress indicate that high NPY levels are associated with better performance. Patients with PTSD have been shown to have reduced plasma NPY levels and a blunted yohimbine-induced NPY increase. Additionally, low levels of NPY have been found in depressed patients, and a variety of antidepressant drugs increase NPY levels.

GALANIN

Galanin is a peptide that, in humans, contains 30 amino acids. It has been demonstrated to be involved in a number of physiological and behavioral functions, including learning and memory, pain control, food intake, neuroendocrine control, cardiovascular regulation, and, most recently, anxiety.

Galanin is closely associated with ascending monoamine pathways. Approximately 80 percent of noradrenergic cells in the LC coexpress galanin. A dense galanin immunoreactive fiber system originating in the LC innervates forebrain and midbrain structures, including the hippocampus, hypothalamus, amygdala, and prefrontal cortex. Neurophysiological studies have shown that galanin reduces the firing rate of the LC, possibly by stimulating the galanin-1 receptor (Gal-R1), which acts as an autoreceptor.

Studies in rats have shown that galanin administered centrally modulates anxiety-related behaviors. Galanin-overexpressing transgenic mice do not exhibit an anxiety-like phenotype when tested under baseline (nonchallenged) conditions. However, these mice are unresponsive to the anxiogenic effects of the α_2-receptor antagonist, yohimbine. Consistent with this observation, galanin administered directly into the CEA blocked the anxiogenic effects of stress, which is associated with increased NE release in the CEA. Yohimbine increases galanin release in the CEA. Galanin administration and galanin overexpression in the hippocampus result in deficits in fear conditioning.

The mechanism by which galanin reduces NE release at LC projections to the amygdala, hypothalamus, and prefrontal cortex may be a direct action of galanin on these brain regions via galanin-synthesizing neurons or by stimulating galanin receptors in these regions. It is not known which galanin receptors are involved. Gal-R1 mRNA levels are high in the amygdala, hypothalamus, and BNST, and Gal-R1–deficient mice show increased anxiety-like behavior.

These results suggest that the noradrenergic response to stress can recruit the release of galanin in CEA and prefrontal cortex, which then buffers the anxiogenic effects of NE. Thus, the net behavioral response due to stress-induced noradrenergic hyperactivity may depend on the balance between NE and NPY and galanin neurotransmission. This hypothesis is consistent with evidence that release of neuropeptides preferentially occurs under conditions of high neurotransmitter activity. Galanin function has not been studied in anxiety disorder patients. Galanin and NPY receptor agonists may be novel targets for antianxiety drug development.

DOPAMINERGIC SYSTEM

Acute stress increases DA release and metabolism in a number of specific brain areas. However, the DA innervation of the mPFC appears to be particularly vulnerable to stress; low-intensity stress (such as that associated with conditioned fear) or brief exposure to stress increases DA release and metabolism in the prefrontal cortex in the absence of overt changes in other mesotelencephalic DA regions. Low-intensity electric foot shock increases in vivo tyrosine hydroxylase and DA turnover in the mPFC but not in the nucleus accumbens or striatum. Stress can enhance DA release and metabolism in other areas receiving DA innervation, provided that greater-intensity or longer-duration stress is used. Thus, the mPFC DA innervation is preferentially activated by stress compared to mesolimbic and nigrostriatal systems, and the mesolimbic DA innervation appears to be more sensitive to stress than the striatal DA innervation.

Uncontrollable stress activates mPFC DA release and inhibits nucleus accumbens DA release. Lesions of the amygdala pretraining and posttraining in a conditioned stress model block stress-induced mPFC DA metabolic activation, suggesting amygdala control of stress-induced DA activation and a role for integrating the behavioral and neuroendocrine components of the stress response. There is preclinical evidence that the susceptibility of the mesocortical DA system to stress activation may be, in part, genetically determined. It has been suggested that excessive mesocortical DA release by stressful events may represent a vulnerability to depression and may favor helpless reactions through an inhibition of subcortical DA transmission. These observations may be due to the effect of DA on reward mechanisms.

On the other hand, lesions of mPFC DA neurons delay extinction of the conditioned fear stress response (no effect on acquisition), indicating that prefrontal DA neurons are involved in facilitating extinction of the fear response. This suggests that reduced prefrontal cortical DA results in the preservation of fear produced by a conditioned stressor, a situation hypothesized to occur in PTSD. One way to reconcile these two sets of data is to suggest that there is an optimal range for stress-induced increases in mPFC cortical DA release to facilitate adaptive behavior responses. Too much mPFC cortical DA release produces cognitive impairment, and an inhibition in nucleus accumbens DA activity results in abnormalities in motivation and reward mechanisms. Insufficient prefrontal cortical DA release delays extinction of conditioned fear.

There has been little clinical research on DA function as it pertains to anxiety disorders. Several clinical investigations have reported increased urinary and plasma DA concentrations in PTSD. Roy Byrne and colleagues found a higher concentration of the DA metabolite HVA in plasma in panic disorder patients with high levels of anxiety and frequent panic attacks. Panic disorder patients were shown to have a greater growth hormone response to the DA agonist apomorphine (Zydis) than patients with depression. However, no alteration in CSF HVA levels in panic disorder patients and no correlations with anxiety severity or panic attacks have been found.

SEROTONIN

Different types of acute stress result in increased 5-HT turnover in the prefrontal cortex, nucleus accumbens, amygdala, and lateral hypothalamus. 5-HT release may have anxiogenic and anxiolytic effects, depending on the region of the forebrain involved and the receptor subtype activated. For example, anxiogenic effects are mediated via the 5-HT type 2A (5-HT_{2A}) receptor, whereas stimulation of 5-HT type 1A (5-HT_{1A}) receptors is anxiolytic and may even relate to adaptive responses to aversive events.

Understanding the function of the 5-HT_{1A} receptor is probably most pertinent to the current review. The 5-HT_{1A} receptors are found in the superficial cortical layers, hippocampus, amygdala, and raphe nucleus (primarily presynaptic). The behavioral phenotype of 5-HT_{1A} receptor knock-out mice includes increases in anxiety-like behaviors. These behaviors are mediated by postsynaptic 5-HT_{1A} receptors in the hippocampus, amygdala, and cortex. Of great interest is the recent finding that embryonic and early postnatal shutdown of 5-HT_{1A} receptor expression produces an anxiety phenotype that cannot be rescued with restoration of 5-HT_{1A} receptors. However, when 5-HT_{1A} receptor expression is reduced in adulthood and then reinstated, the anxiety phenotype is no longer present. These results suggest that altered function of 5-HT_{1A} receptors early in life can produce long-term abnormalities in the regulation of anxiety behaviors.

Postsynaptic 5-HT_{1A} receptor gene expression is under tonic inhibition by adrenal steroids, such as in the hippocampus, apparently mostly via activation of MR receptors. 5-HT_{1A} receptor density and mRNA levels decrease in response to stress, which is prevented by adrenalectomy.

Recent animal models have suggested a role of 5-HT_{1A} receptors in the development of chronic anxiety and have helped to generate animal models of anxiety-related disorders. However, it is not clear whether these models constitute relevant models for panic disorder in humans. The recent development of highly selective 5-HT_{1A} receptor radioligands such as [^{18}F]Trans-4-fluoro-N-2-[4-(2-methoxyphenyl)piperazin-1-yl]ethyl]-N-(2-pyridyl)cyclohexanecarboxamide (FCWAY) has now made it possible to assess central 5-HT_{1A} receptor binding in panic disorder, using PET. In the panic disorder patients, including those who also had depression, receptors were reduced by an average of nearly one-third in the anterior cingulate in the front middle part of the brain, the posterior cingulate, in the rear middle part of the brain, and in the raphe, also in the midbrain.

There may also be important functional interactions between the 5-HT_{1A} and benzodiazepine receptors. In one study of 5-HT_{1A} receptor knock-out mice, a downregulation of benzodiazepine GABA α1 and α2 receptor subunits, as well as benzodiazepine-resistant anxiety in the elevated plus maze, was reported. However, a subsequent study did not replicate these results when using mice with a different genetic background, raising the possibility that genetic background can affect functional interplay between 5-HT_{1A} and benzodiazepine systems.

These results suggest a scenario in which early life stress increases CRH and cortisol levels, which, in turn, downregulate 5-HT_{1A} receptors, resulting in a lower threshold for anxiogenic stressful life events. Alternatively, 5-HT_{1A} receptors may be decreased on a genetic basis. The density of 5-HT_{1A} receptors is reduced in depressed patients, when depressed and in remission. Examination of 5-HT_{1A} receptor density in patients with anxiety disorders is indicated.

Clinical studies of 5-HT function in anxiety disorders have had mixed results. Platelet imipramine (Tofranil) binding (a marker of the 5-HT reuptake site), which is generally reduced in depression, has been found to be normal in panic disorder, whereas platelet 5-HT uptake in panic disorder has been reported to be elevated, normal, or reduced. One study found that panic disorder patients had lower levels of circulating 5-HT in comparison to controls. Thus, no clear pattern of abnormality in 5-HT function in panic disorder has emerged from analysis of peripheral blood elements.

To date, pharmacological challenge studies of 5-HT in panic disorder have also been unable to establish a definite role for 5-HT in the pathophysiology of panic. Challenges with the 5-HT precursors L-tryptophan and 5-hydroxytryptophan (5-HTP) did not discriminate between panic disorder and controls on neuroendocrine measures. Conversely, tryptophan depletion was not anxiogenic in unmedicated panic disorder patients. However, challenge with the 5-HT–releasing agent fenfluramine has been reported to be anxiogenic and to produce greater increases in plasma prolactin and cortisol in panic disorder compared to controls. Studies with the 5-HT agonist meta-chlorophenylpiperazine (mCPP), a probe of postsynaptic 5-HT type 2 (5-HT_2) receptor function, have produced equivocal findings. Increases in anxiety and plasma cortisol in panic disorder patients, compared to controls, have been reported with oral but not IV administration of mCPP.

In a pharmacological challenge study, 5 out of 14 patients with PTSD had a panic attack, and four patients had a flashback after mCPP administration. In contrast, no patient had a panic attack, and one patient experienced a flashback after the infusion of placebo saline. Thus, a subgroup of patients with PTSD exhibited a marked behavioral sensitivity to serotoninergic provocation, raising the possibility of pathophysiological subtypes among traumatized combat veterans.

BENZODIAZEPINE SYSTEM

Benzodiazepine receptors are present throughout the brain, with the highest concentration in cortical gray matter. Benzodiazepines potentiate and prolong the synaptic actions of the inhibitory neurotransmitter GABA. Central benzodiazepine receptors and $GABA_A$ receptors are part of the same macromolecular complex. These receptors have distinct binding sites, although they are functionally coupled and regulate each other in an allosteric manner. The hypothesis that alterations in benzodiazepine receptor function play a role in the pathophysiology of the anxiety disorders is supported by several lines of preclinical evidence, such as studies using uncontrollable acute and chronic stress or studies using genetically altered animals.

Despite the preclinical support for the involvement of benzodiazepine systems in stress, clinical investigations of the function of this system in patients with anxiety disorders have been limited. Pharmacological challenge studies support a role for benzodiazepine function in anxiety in normal human subjects. The benzodiazepine receptor inverse agonist FG 7142 induces severe anxiety resembling panic attacks and biological characteristics of anxiety in healthy subjects. Administration of the benzodiazepine receptor antagonist flumazenil (Romazicon) to patients with panic disorder results in an increase in panic attacks and subjective anxiety in comparison to controls. Oral and IV flumazenil has been shown to produce panic in a subgroup of panic disorder patients but not in healthy subjects. Benzodiazepine-induced changes in sedation and cortisol levels, as well as saccadic eye movement velocity, have been suggested to be indicative of benzodiazepine receptor-mediated actions. Panic disorder patients were found to be less sensitive than controls to diazepam (Valium), using saccadic eye movement velocity as a dependent measure, suggesting a functional subsensitivity of the GABA–benzodiazepine supramolecular complex in brainstem regions controlling saccadic eye movements.

Neuroimaging studies reveal reduced cortical and subcortical benzodiazepine receptor binding in patients with PTSD and panic disorder and reduced cortical GABA levels in panic disorder. The relevant question of whether the downregulation of benzodiazepine receptor binding is a consequence of exposure to stress or whether a preexisting low level of benzodiazepine receptor density may be a genetic risk factor for the development of stress-related anxiety disorders remains to be elucidated.

CHOLECYSTOKININ

CCK is an anxiogenic neuropeptide present in the gastrointestinal (GI) tract, as well as the brain, that has recently been suggested as a neural substrate for human anxiety. Neurons containing CCK-containing neurons are found with high density in the cerebral cortex, the amygdala, and the hippocampus. They are also found in the midbrain, including the PAG, substantia nigra, and raphe nuclei. Iontophoretic administration of CCK has depolarizing effects on pyramidal neurons, suggesting that it may serve as an excitatory neurotransmitter. CCK-4 through CCK-8 have stimulatory effects on action potentials in the dentate gyrus of the hippocampus. Activation of hippocampal neurons is suppressed by low-dose benzodiazepines. CCK agonists are anxiogenic in a variety of animal models of anxiety, whereas CCK antagonists have anxiolytic effects in these tests. Panic disorder patients were found to be more sensitive to the anxiogenic effects of CCK-4 and a closely related peptide, pentagastrin, and these effects were blocked by CCK antagonists. In a small sample of PTSD patients, CCK-4 had enhanced anxiogenic effects compared to responses in healthy subjects. Imipramine also antagonizes the panicogenic effects of CCK-4 in panic disorder patients. The mechanism is unclear but may relate to the ability of imipramine to downregulate β-adrenergic receptors, because propranolol antagonizes the anxiogenic actions of CCK-4. Levels of CCK in the CSF are lower in panic disorder patients than normal subjects, raising the possibility of enhanced function of CCK receptors. The mechanism responsible for the enhanced sensitivity to CCK-4 has not been elucidated. Patients may have an elevated production or turnover of CCK or increased sensitivity of CCK receptors. Because CCK has important functional interactions with other systems implicated in anxiety and fear (noradrenergic, dopaminergic, and benzodiazepine), these interactions should be evaluated in panic disorder patients. CCK-β receptor antagonists have potential as antipanic drugs.

OPIOID PEPTIDES

One of the primary behavioral effects of uncontrollable stress is analgesia, which results from the release of endogenous opiates. Significant analgesia is observed after uncontrollable, but not controllable, stress and also is seen after presentation of neutral stimuli previously paired with aversive stimuli. There is also evidence that sensitization occurs because reexposure to less intense shock in rats previously exposed to uncontrollable shock also results in analgesia. These effects are likely to be mediated, in part, by a stress-induced release of endogenous opiates in the brainstem. Moreover, opiate peptides are elevated after acute uncontrollable shock, and uncontrollable, but not controllable, shock decreases the density of μ-opiate receptors. Given these facts, it is reasonable to study opiate systems in the anxiety disorders.

Only a few studies have looked at opiate function in PTSD. L. Hoffman and colleagues reported significantly lower AM and PM plasma beta-endorphin levels in 21 PTSD patients compared to 20 controls. The results were viewed as support for Bessel A. van der Kolk's hypothesis that patients with PTSD have a chronic depletion of endogenous opiates, which causes them to seek out recurrent stressors to increase opiate release. Another study found no differences in plasma levels of methionine-enkephalin between PTSD patients and controls, although degradation half-life was significantly higher in the PTSD group. In a pharmacological challenge of the opiate system, PTSD patients showed reduced pain sensitivity, compared to veterans without PTSD, after exposure to a combat film. This was reversible by the opiate antagonist naloxone (Narcan). These findings could be explained by increased release of endogenous opiates with stress in PTSD. This is supported by a recent report of elevated levels of CSF beta-endorphin in PTSD.

Whether alterations in endogenous opiates contribute to the core symptoms seen in PTSD is not clear. It has been hypothesized that symptoms of avoidance and numbing are related to a dysregulation of opioid systems in PTSD. Furthermore, it has been suggested that the use of opiates in chronic PTSD may represent a form of self-medication. Consistent with this hypothesis, in structured interviews, Bremner and colleagues found that a significant number of patients with combat-related PTSD reported that opiates made their symptoms of hyperarousal better. Animal studies have shown that opiates are powerful suppressants of central and peripheral noradrenergic activity. If, as suggested previously in this section, some PTSD symptomatology is mediated by noradrenergic hyperactivity, then opiates may serve to treat or to dampen that hypersensitivity and accompanying symptoms. On the other hand, during opiate withdrawal, when opiates are decreased, and noradrenergic activity is increased, PTSD symptoms may become acutely exacerbated. In fact, many symptoms of PTSD are similar to those seen during opiate withdrawal. Additional studies of opiate receptor function and its functional interaction with monoamine systems in anxiety disorders are indicated.

FUTURE DIRECTIONS

There is emerging evidence that indicates the role of genetic factors in the vulnerability to stress-related psychopathology, such as PTSD. An investigation of twin pairs from the Vietnam Twin Registry reported that inherited factors accounted for as much as 32 percent of the variance of PTSD symptoms, above and beyond the contribution of trauma severity. The molecular neurobiological abnormalities that underlie these findings have not been elucidated. Two relatively small association studies which evaluated DA type 2 (D_2) receptor polymorphisms in PTSD yielded contradictory results. A preliminary study found an association between the dopamine transporter (DAT) polymorphism and PTSD. Volumetric magnetic resonance imaging (MRI) investigations demonstrated a smaller hippocampal volume in PTSD patients. A study of monozygotic twins discordant for trauma exposure found evidence that smaller hippocampal volume may constitute a risk factor for the development of stress-related psychopathology. The recent identification of functional polymorphisms for GR, the α_{2C}-adrenergic receptor subtype, and NPY synthesis provides opportunities to investigate the genetic basis of the neurochemical response patterns to stress.

Work is commencing to examine the genetic basis of the neural mechanisms of fear conditioning. There have been several recent advances in understanding the genetic contribution and molecular machinery related to amygdala-dependent learned fear. A gene encoding gastrin-releasing peptide (GRP) has been identified in the lateral amygdala. The GRP receptor (GRPR) is expressed in GABAergic interneurons and mediates their inhibition of principal neurons. In GRPR knock-out mice, this inhibition is reduced and long-term potentiation (LTP) enhanced. These mice have enhanced and prolonged fear memory for auditory and contextual cues, indicating that the GRP signaling pathway may serve as an inhibitory feedback constraint on learned fear. The work further supports the role of GABA in fear and anxiety states and suggests that the genetic basis of vulnerability to anxiety may relate to GRP, GRPR, and GABA. Other preclinical studies indicate that there may be a genetically determined mesocortical and mesoaccumbens DA response to stress that relates to learned helplessness. Recently, it was demonstrated that healthy subjects with the 5-HT transporter polymorphism, which has been associated with reduced 5-HT expression and function and increased fear and anxiety behaviors, exhibit increased amygdala neuronal activity in response to fear-inducing stimuli. The preclinical and clinical data (Table 14.4–2) suggest that multidisciplinary studies that use neurochemical, neuroimaging, and genetic approaches have the potential to clarify the

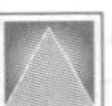

Table 14.4–2
Neural Mechanisms Related to Pathophysiology and Treatment of Anxiety Disorders

Mechanism	Neurochemical Systems	Brain Regions	Pathophysiology	Treatment Development
Pavlovian (cue specific) fear conditioning	Glutamate, NMDA receptors, VGCCs	Medial prefrontal cortex, sensory cortex, anterior cingulate, dorsal thalamus, lateral amygdala, and central nucleus of amygdala	May account for common clinical observation in panic disorder and posttraumatic stress disorder that sensory and cognitive stimuli associated with or resembling the frightening experience elicit panic attacks, flashbacks, and autonomic symptoms.	Treatment with NMDA receptor antagonist and VGCC antagonist may attenuate acquisition of fear.
Inhibitory avoidance (contextual fear)	NE, β-adrenergic receptor, cortisol, glucocorticoid receptor, CRH, GABA, opioids, acetylcholine	Medial prefrontal cortex, basolateral amygdala, hippocampus, bed nucleus of the stria terminalis, entorhinal cortex	Excessive stress-mediated release of CRH, cortisol, and NE facilitates development of indelible fear memories. Chronic anxiety and phobic symptoms may result from excessive contextual fear conditioning.	CRH antagonists and β-adrenergic receptor agonists may have preventative effects.
Reconsolidation	Glutamate, NMDA receptors, NE, β-adrenergic receptors, cyclic adenosine monophosphate response element binding protein	Amygdala, hippocampus	Repeated reactivation and reconsolidation may further strengthen the memory trace and may lead to persistence of trauma- and phobia-related symptoms.	Treatment with NMDA receptor and β-adrenergic receptor antagonists after memory reactivation may reduce the strength of the original anxiety-provoking memory.
Extinction	Glutamate, NMDA receptors, VGCCs, NE, dopamine, GABA	Medial prefrontal cortex, sensory cortex, amygdala	Failure in neural mechanisms of extinction may relate to persistent traumatic memories, reexperiencing of symptoms, autonomic hyperarousal, and phobic behaviors.	Psychotherapies need to be developed that facilitate extinction through the use of conditioned inhibitors and the learning of new memories. The combination of extinction-based psychotherapy and D-cycloserine may be a particularly effective treatment.
Sensitization	Dopaminergic, noradrenergic NMDA receptors	Nucleus accumbens, amygdala, striatum, hypothalamus	May explain the adverse effects of early life trauma on subsequent responses to similarly stressful events. May play a role in the chronic course of many anxiety disorders and, in some cases, the worsening of the illness over time.	Suggests the efficacy of treatment may vary according to the state of evolution of the disease process. Emphasizes the importance of early treatment intervention.

CRH, corticotrophin-releasing hormone; GABA, γ-aminobutyric acid; NE, norepinephrine; NMDA, *N*-methyl-D-aspartate; VGCC, voltage-gated calcium channels.

complex relationships among genotype, phenotype, and psychobiological responses to stress.

SUGGESTED CROSS-REFERENCES

Monoamine neurotransmitters are discussed in Section 1.4, and neuropeptide neurotransmitters are discussed in Section 1.6. Genome, transcriptome, and proteome are covered in Section 1.10, population genetic methods are covered in Section 1.17, and genetic linkage analysis of psychiatric disorders is discussed in Section 1.18.

REFERENCES

Allen YS, Adrian TE, Allen JM, Tatemoto K, Crow TJ, Bloom SR, Polak JM: Neuropeptide Y distribution in the rat brain. *Science.* 1983;221:877–879.

Aston-Jones G, Shipley MT, Chouvet G, Ennis M, VanBockstaele EJ, Pieribone V, Shiekhattar R: Afferent regulation of locus coeruleus neurons: Anatomy, physiology and pharmacology. *Prog Brain Res.* 1991;88:47–75.

Baker DG, West SA, Orth DN, Hill KK, Nicholson WE, Ekhator NN. Bruce AB, Wortman MD, Keck PE, Geracioti JD: Cerebrospinal fluid and plasma beta endorphin in combat veterans with post traumatic stress disorder. *Psychoneuroendocrinology.* 1997;22:517–529.

Bale TL, Contarino A, Smith GW, Chan R, Gold LH, Sawchenko PE, Koob GF, Vale WW, Lee KF: Mice deficient for corticotrophin-releasing hormone receptor-2 display anxiety-like behavior and are hypersensitive to stress. *Nat Genet.* 2000;24;410–414.

*Bale TL, Picetti R, Contarino A, Koob GF, Vale WW, Kuo-Fen L: Mice deficient for both corticotrophin-releasing factor receptor 1 (CRFR1) and CRFR2 have an impaired stress response and display sexually dichotomous anxiety-like behavior. *J Neurosci.* 2002;22:193–199.

Blanchard EB, Kolb LC, Prins A, Gates S, McCoy GC: Changes in plasma norepinephrine to combat-related stimuli among Vietnam veterans with post traumatic stress disorder. *J Nerv Ment Dis.* 1991;179:371–373.

Bradwejn J, Koszycki D: Imipramine antagonism of the panicogenic effects of CCK-4 in panic disorder patients. *Am J Psychiatry.* 1994;151:261–263.

Bradwejn J, Koszycki D, Couetoux du Tetre A, van Megen H, den boer J, Westenberg H, Annable L: The panicogenic effects of CCK-4 are antagonized by L-365-260, a CCK receptor antagonist, in patients with panic disorder. *Arch Gen Psychiatry.* 1994;51:486–493.

Bremner JD, Innis RB, Ng CK, Staib L, Duncan J, Bronen R, Zubal G, Rich D, Krystal JH, Dey H, Soufer R, Charney DS: PET measurement of central metabolic correlates of yohimbine administration in posttraumatic stress disorder. *Arch Gen Psychiatry.* 1997;54:246–256.

Bremner JD, Innis RB, White T, Fujita M, Silbersweig D, Goddard AW, Staib L, Stern E, Cappiello A, Woods S, Baldwin R, Charney DS: SPECT [I-123] iomazenil measurement of the benzodiazepine receptor in panic disorder. *Biol Psychiatry.* 2000;47:96–106.

Bremner JD, Licinio J, Darnell A, Krystal JH, Owens M, Southwick SM, Nemeroff CB, Charney DS: Elevated CSF corticotropin-releasing factor concentrations in posttraumatic stress disorder. *Am J Psychiatry.* 1997;154:624–629.

*Britton KT, Akwa Y, Spina MG, Koob GF: Neuropeptide Y blocks anxiogenic-like behavioral action of corticotrophin-releasing factor in an operant conflict test and elevated plus maze. *Peptides.* 2000;21:37–44.

Brunson KL, Eghbal-Ahmadi M, Bender R, Chen Y, Baram TZ: Long-term, progressive hippocampal cell loss and dysfunction induced by early-life administration of corticotrophin-releasing hormone reproduce the effects of early-life stress. *Proc Natl Acad Sci U S A.* 2001;98:8856–8861.

Cassens G, Kuruc A, Roffman M, Orsulak P, Schildkraut JJ: Alterations in brain norepinephrine metabolism and behavior induced by environmental stimuli previously paired with inescapable shock. *Behav Brain Res.* 1981;2:387–407.

Charney DS, Deutch A: A functional neuroanatomy of anxiety and fear: Implications for the pathophysiology and treatment of anxiety disorders. *Crit Rev Neurobiol.* 1996;10:419–446.

Charney DS, Drevets WD. Neurobiological basis of anxiety disorders. In: Davis KL, Charney D, Coyle JT, Nemeroff C, eds. *Neuropsychopharmacology: The Fifth Generation of Progress.* Baltimore: Lippincott Williams & Wilkins; 2002.

Charney DS, Heninger GR, Breier A: Noradrenergic function in panic anxiety: Effects of yohimbine in healthy subjects and patients with agoraphobia and panic disorder. *Arch Gen Psychiatry.* 1984;41:751–763.

Charney DS, Woods SW, Goodman WK, Heninger GR: Serotonin function in anxiety. II. Effects of the serotonin agonist MCPP in panic disorder patients and healthy subjects. *Psychopharmacology.* 1987;92:14–24.

Consolo S, Baldi G, Russi G, Civenni G, Bartfai T, Vezzani A: Impulse flow dependency of galanin release in vivo in the rat ventral hippocampus. *Proc Natl Acad Sci U S A.* 1994;91:8047–8051.

Coplan JD, Andrews MW, Rosenblum LA, Owens MJ, Friedman S, Gorman JM, Nemeroff CB: Persistent elevations of cerebrospinal fluid concentrations of corticotropin-releasing factor in adult nonhuman primates exposed to early-life stressors: Implications for the pathophysiology of mood and anxiety disorders. *Proc Natl Acad Sci U S A.* 1996;20:1619–1623.

Coplan JD, Papp LA, Martinez MA, Pine P, Rosenblum LA, Cooper T, Liebowitz MR, Gorman JM: Persistence of blunted human growth hormone response to clonidine in fluoxetine-treated patients with panic disorder. *Am J Psychiatry.* 1995;152:619–622.

Coplan JD, Pine D, Papp L, Martinez J, Cooper T, Rosenblum LA, Gorman JM: Uncoupling of the noradrenergic-hypothalamic-pituitary adrenal axis in panic disorder patients. *Neuropsychopharmacology* 1995;13:65–73.

Coste SC, Kesterson RA, Heldwein KA, Stevens SL, Heard AD, Hollis JH, Murray SE, Hill JK, Pantely GA, Hohimer AR, Hatton DC, Phillips TJ, Finn DA, Low MJ, Rittenberg MB, Stenzel P, Stenzel-Poore MP: Abnormal adaptations to stress and impaired cardiovascular function in mice lacking corticotrophin-releasing hormone receptor-2. *Nat Genet.* 2000;24;403–409.

DeRijk RH, Schaaf M, de Kloet ER: Glucocorticoid receptor variants: Clinical implications. *J Steroid Biochem Mol Biol.* 2002;81:103–122.

Dorow R, Horowski R, Paschelke G, Amin M, Braestrup C: Severe anxiety induced by FG7142, a beta-carboline ligand for benzodiazepine receptors. *Lancet.* 1983;2:98–99.

Drevets WC, Frank JC, Kupfer DJ, Holt D, Greer PJ, Huang Y, Gautier C, Mathis C: PET imaging of serotonin 1A receptor binding in depression. *Biol Psychiatry.* 1999;46:1375–1387.

Drugan RC, Morrow AL, Weizman R, Weizman A, Deutsch SI, Crawley JN, Paul SM: Stress-induced behavioral depression in the rat is associated with a decrease in GABA receptor-mediated chloride ion flux and brain benzodiazepine receptor occupancy. *Brain Res.* 1989;487:45–51.

Garpenstrand H, Annas P, Ekblom J, Oreland L, Fredrikson M: Human fear conditioning is related to dopaminergic and serotonergic biological markers. *Behav Neurosci.* 2001;115:358–364.

Gentleman SM, Falkai P, Bogerts B, Herrero MT, Polak JM, Roberts GW: Distribution of galanin-like immunoreactivity in the human brain. *Brain Res.* 1989;505:311–315.

Gilbertson MW, Shenton ME, Ciszewski A, Kasai K, Lasko NB, Orr SP, Pitman RK: Smaller hippocampal volume predicts pathologic vulnerability to psychological trauma. *Nat Neurosci.* 2002;5:1242–1247.

Goddard AW, Mason GF, Almai A, Rothman DL, Behar KL, Petroff OA, Charney DS, Krystal JH: Reductions in occipital cortex GABA levels in panic disorder detected with 1h-magnetic resonance spectroscopy. *Arch Gen Psychiatry.* 2001;58:556–561.

Goddard AW, Sholomskas DE, Augeri FM, Walton KE, Charney DS, Heninger GR, Goodman WK, Price LH: Effects of tryptophan depletion in panic disorders. *Biol Psychiatry.* 1994;36:775–777.

*Grammatopoulos DK, Chrousos GP: Functional characteristics of CRH receptors and potential clinical applications of CRH-receptor antagonists. *Trends Endocrinol Metab.* 2002;13:436–444.

Griebel G, Simiand J, Serradeil-Le Gal LC, Wagnon J, Pascal M, Scatton B, Maffrand JP, Soubrie P: Anxiolytic-and antidepressant-like effects of the non-peptide vasopressin V1b receptor antagonist, SSR149415, suggest an innovative approach for the treatment of stress-related disorders. *Proc Natl Acad Sci U S A.* 2002;99:6370–6375.

Gross C, Zhuang X, Stark K, Ramboz S, Oosting R, Kirby L: Serotonin 1A receptor acts during development to establish normal anxiety-like behavior in the adult. *Nature.* 2002;416:396–400.

Gurvits TV: Magnetic resonance imaging study of hippocampal volume in chronic, combat-related posttraumatic stress disorder. *Biol Psychiatry.* 1996;40:1091–1099.

Gustafson EL, Smith KE, Durkin MM, Gerald C, Branchek TA: Distribution of a rat galanin receptor mRNA in rat brain. *Neuroreport.* 1996;7:953–957.

Hamon M, Gozlan H, El Mestikawy S, Emerit M, Bolanos F, Schechter L: The central 5-HT1a receptors; Pharmacological biochemical, functional, and regulatory properties. *Ann N Y Acad Sci.* 1990;600:114–129.

Hariri AR, Mattay VS, Tessitore A, Kolachana B, Fera F, Goldman D, Egan MF, Weinberger DR: Serotonin transporter genetic variation and the response of the human amygdala. *Science.* 2002;297:400–403.

Heilig M: Antisense inhibition of neuropeptide Y (NPY)-Y1 receptor expression blocks the anxiolytic-like action of NPY in amygdala and paradoxically increases feeding. *Regul Pept.* 1995;59:201–205.

Heisler L, Chu H-M, Brennan T, Danao J, Bajwa P, Parsons L: Elevated anxiety and antidepressant-like responses in serotonin 5-HT1A receptor mutant mice. *Proc Natl Acad Sci U S A.* 1998;95:15049–15054.

Holmes A, Kinney JW, Wrenn CC, Li Q, Yang RJ, Vishwanath J, Saavedra M, Innerfield CE, Jacoby AS, Shine J, Lismaa TP, Crawley JN: Galanin GAL-R receptor null mutant mice display increased anxiety-like behavior specific to the elevated plus-maze. *Neuropsychopharmacology.* 2003;28:1031–1044.

Holmes A, Yang RJ, Crawley JN: Evaluation of an anxiety-related phenotype in galanin overexpressing transgenic mice. *J Mol Neurosci.* 2002;18:151–165.

Holmes PV, Crawley JN. Coexisting neurotransmitters in central noradrenergic neurons. In: Bloom FE, Kupfer DJ, eds. *Psychopharmacology: The Fourth Generation of Progress.* New York: Raven Press; 1995:347–353.

Holsboer F, vonBardeleben U, Buller R, Heuser I, Steiger A: Stimulation response to corticotropin-releasing hormone (CRH) in patients with depression, alcoholism and panic disorder. *Horm Metab Res.* 1987;16[Suppl]:80–88.

Illes P, Finta EP, Nieber K: Neuropeptide Y potentiates via Y2-receptors the inhibitory effect of noradrenaline in rat locus coeruleus neurons. *Nauyn Schmiedebergs Arch Pharmacol.* 1993;348:546-548.

Ishikawa-Brush Y, Powell JF, Bolton P, Miller AP, Francis F, Willard HF, Lehrach H, Monaco AP: Autism and multiple exostoses associated with an X-8 translocation occurring within the GRPR gene and 3' to the SDC2 gene. *Hum Mol Genet.* 1997;6:1241–1250.

Kallio J, Personen U, Kaipio K, Karvonen MK, Heinonen OJ, Uusitupa MI, Koulu M: Altered intracellular processing and release of neuropeptide Y due to leucine 7 to proline 7 polymorphism in the signal peptide of preproneuropeptide Y in man. *FASEB J.* 2001;15:1242–1244.

Karlamangla AS, Singer BH, McEwen BS, Rowe JW, Seeman TE: Allostatic load as a predictor of functional decline: Mac Arthur studies of successful aging. *J Clin Epidemiol.* 2002;55:696–710.

Kask A, Harro J, von Horsten S, Redrobe JP, Dumont Y, Quiron R: The neurocircuitry and receptor subtypes mediating anxiolytic-like effects of neuropeptide Y. *Neurosci Behav Rev.* 2002;26:259–283.

Kellner M, Wiedemann K, Yassouridis A, Levengood R, Guo LS, Holsboer F, Yehuda R: Behavioral and endocrine response to cholecystokinin tetrapeptide in patients with posttraumatic stress disorder. *Biol Psychiatry.* 2000;47:107–111.

Kent JM, Mathew SJ, Gorman JM: Molecular targets in the treatment of anxiety. *Biol Psychiatry.* 2002;52:1008–1030.

Khoshbouei H, Cecchi M, Dove S, Javors M, Morilak DA: Behavioral reactivity to stress: Amplification of stress-induced noradrenergic activation elicits a galanin-mediated anxiolytic effect in central amygdala. *Pharmacol Biochem Behav.* 2002;71:407–417.

Kinney JW, Starosta G, Holmes A, Wrenn CC, Yang RJ, Harris AP, Long KC, Crawley JN: Deficits in trace cued fear conditioning in galanin-treated rats and galanin-overexpressing transgenic mice. *Learn Mem.* 2002;9:178–190.

Lopez JF, Chalmers DT, Little KY, Watson SJ: A.E. Bennett Research Award. Regulation of serotonin1A, glucocorticoid, and mineralocorticoid receptor in rat and human hippocampus: Implications for the neurobiology of depression. *Biol Psychiatry.* 1998;43:547–573.

Lydiard RB, Ballenger JC, Laraia MT, Fossey MD, Beinfeld MC: CSF cholecystokinin concentrations in patients with panic disorder and normal comparison subjects. *Am J Psychiatry.* 1992;149:691–693.

Maes M, Lin AH, Delmeire L, Van Gastael A, Kenis G, De Jongh R, Bosmans E: Elevated serum interleukin-6 (IL-6) and IL-6 receptor concentrations in posttraumatic stress disorder following accidental man-made traumatic events. *Biol Psychiatry.* 1999;45:833–839.

Makino S, Baker RA, Smith MA, Gold PW: Differential regulation of neuropeptide Y mRNA expression in the accurate nucleus and locus coeruleus by stress and antidepressants. *J Neuroendocrinol.* 2000;12:387–395.

Malizia AL, Cunningham VJ, Bell CJ, Liddle PF, Jones T, Nutt DJ: Decreased brain GABA(A)-benzodiazepine receptor binding in panic disorder: Preliminary results from a quantitative PET study. *Arch Gen Psychiatry.* 1998;55:715–720.

Martins AP, Maras RA, Guimaraes FS: Anxiolytic effect of a CRH receptor antagonist in the dorsal periaqueductal gray. *Depress Anxiety.* 2001;12:99–101.

Mathe HH: Early life stress changes concentrations of neuropeptide Y and corticotrophin-releasing hormone in adult rat brain. Lithium treatment modifies these changes. *Neuropsychopharmacology.* 2002;27:756–764.

Moller C, Sommer W, Thorsell A, Heilig M: Anxiogenic-like action of galanin after intra-amygdala administration in the rat. *Neuropsychopharmacology.* 1999;21:507–512.

Morgan CA, Wang S Mason J, Southwick SM, Fox P, Hazlett G, Charney DS, Greenfield G: Hormone profiles in humans experiencing military survival training. *Biol Psychiatry.* 2000;47:891–901.

Morrow BA, Elsworth JD, Rasmusson AM, Roth RH: The role of mesoprefrontal dopamine neurons in the acquisition and expression of conditioned fear in the rat. *Neuroscience.* 1999;92:553–564.

Nesse RM, Curtis GC, Thyer BA, McCann DS, Huber-Smith MJ, Knopf RF: Endocrine and cardiovascular responses during phobic anxiety. *Psychosom Med.* 1985;47:320.

*Neumeister A, Bain E, Nugent AC, Carson R, Bonne O, Luckenbaugh DA, Eckelman W, Herscovitch P, Charney DS, Drevets WC: Reduced serotonin type 1A receptor binding in panic disorder. *J Neurosci.* 2004 (*in press*).

Nisenbaum LK, Abercrombie ED: Presynaptic alterations associated with enhancement of evoked release and synthesis of NE in hippocampus of chemically cold stressed rats. *Brain Res.* 1993;608:280–287.

Nutt DJ, Glue P, Lawson C, Wilson S: Flumazenil provocation of panic attacks: Evidence for altered benzodiazepine receptor sensitivity in panic disorder. *Arch Gen Psychiatry.* 1990;47:917–925.

Overstreet DH, Commissaris RC, De La Garza R 2nd, File SE, Knapp DJ, Seiden LS: Involvement of 5-HT_{1A} receptors in animal tests of anxiety and depression: Evidence from genetic models. *Stress.* 2003;6:101–110.

Parks C, Robinson P, Sibille E, Shenk T, Toth M: Increased anxiety of mice lacking the serotonin 1A receptor. *Proc Natl Acad Sci U S A.* 1998;95:10734–10739.

Pattij T, Groenink L, Oosting RS, van der Gugten J, Maes RAA, Olivier B: $GABA_A$-benzodiazepine receptor complex sensitivity in 5-HT1A receptor knockout mice on a 129/Sv background. *Eur J Pharmacol.* 2002;447:67–74.

Pazos A, Probst A, Palacios J: Serotonin receptors in the human brain III. Autoradiographic mapping of serotonin-1 receptors. *Neuroscience.* 1987;21:97–122.

Perez SE, Wynic D, Steiner RA, Mufson EJ: Distribution of galaninergic immunoreactivity in the brain of the mouse. *J Comp Neurol.* 2001;434:158–185.

Perry BD, Giller EL, Southwick SM: Altered platelet $alpha_2$ adrenergic binding sites in posttraumatic stress disorder. *Am J Psychiatry.* 1987;144:1511–1512.

Pichot W, Annsseau M, Moreno AG, Hansenne M, Von Frenckell R: Dopaminergic function in panic disorder: Comparison with major and minor depression. *Biol Psychiatry.* 1992;32:1004–1011.

Pieribone VA, Brodin L, Friberg K, Dahlstrand J, Soderberg C, Larhammar D, Hokfelt T: Differential expression of mRNAs for neuropeptide Y-related peptides in rat nervous tissues: Possible evolutionary conservation. *J Neurosci.* 1992;12:3361–3371.

Pitman RK, van der Kolk BA, Orr SP, Greenberg MS: Naloxone reversible analgesic response to combat-related stimuli in posttraumatic stress disorder. *Arch Gen Psychiatry.* 1990;47:541–544.

Rasmusson AM, Hauger RI, Morgan CA, Bremner JD, Charney DS, Southwick SM: Low baseline and yohimbine-stimulated plasma neuropeptide Y (NPY) levels in combat-related PTSD. *Biol Psychiatry.* 2000;47:526–539.

Risold PY, Swanson LW: Chemoarchitecture of the rat lateral septal nucleus. *Brain Res Rev.* 1997;24:91–113.

Roozendaal B: Glucocorticoids and the regulation of memory consolidation. *Psychoneuroendocrinology.* 2000;25:213–238.

Roy-Byrne PP, Wingerson DK, Radant A, Greenblatt DJ, Cowley DS: Reduced benzodiazepine sensitivity in patients with panic disorder: Comparison with patients with obsessive compulsive disorder and normal subjects. *Am J Psychol.* 1996;153:1444–1449.

Rupprecht R: Neuroactive steroids: Mechanism of action and neuropharmacological properties. *Psychoneuroendocrinology.* 2003;28:139–168.

Sajdyk TJ, Vandergriff MG, Gehlert DR: Amygdala neuropeptide Y Y1 receptors mediate the anxiolytic-like actions of neuropeptide Y in the social interaction test. *Eur J Pharmacol.* 1999;368:143–147.

Sallee FR, Sethuraman G, Sine L, Liu H: Yohimbine challenge in children with anxiety disorders. *Am J Psychiatry.* 2000;157:1236–1242.

Sanchez MM, Young LJ, Plotsky PM, Insel TR: Autoradiographic and in situ hybridization localization of corticotrophin-releasing factor 1 and 2 receptors in nonhuman primate brain. *J Comp Neurol.* 1999;408:365–377.

Schruers K, vanDiest R, Nicolson N, Griez E: L-5-Hydroxytryptophan induced increase in salivary cortisol in panic disorder patients and healthy volunteers. *Psychopharmacology.* 2002;161:365–369.

Shepard JD, Barron KW, Myers DA: Corticosterone delivery to the amygdala increases corticotrophin-releasing factor mRNA in the central amygdaloid nucleus and anxiety-like behavior. *Brain Res.* 2000;861:288–295.

Sheriff S, Dautzenberg FM, Mulchahey JJ, Pisarska M, Hauger RL, Chance WT, Balasubramaniam A, Kasckow JW: Interaction of neuropeptide Y and corticotrophin-releasing factor signaling pathways in AR-5 amygdala cells. *Peptides.* 2001;22:2083–2089.

Sibille E, Pavlides C, Benke D, Toth M: Genetic inactivation of the serotonin1A receptor in mice results in downregulation of major $GABA_A$ receptor α subunits, reduction of $GABA_A$ receptor binding, and benzodiazepine-resistant anxiety. *J Neurosci.* 2000;20:2758–2765.

Smagin GN, Harris RB, Ryan DH: Corticotropin-releasing factor receptor antagonist infused into the locus coeruleus attenuates immobilization stress-induced defensive withdrawal in rats. *Neurosci Lett.* 1996;220:167–170.

Small KM, Wagoner LE, Levin AM, Kardia SLR, Liggett ST: Synergistic polymorphisms of β_1 and α_{2C} adrenergic receptors and the risk of congestive heart failure. *N Engl J Med.* 2002;347:1135–1142.

*Southwick SM, Krystal JH, Bremner JD, Morgan CA, Nicolaou A, Nagy LM, Johnson DR, Heninger GR, Charney DS: Noradrenergic and serotonergic function in posttraumatic stress disorder. *Arch Gen Psychiatry.* 1997;54:749–758.

Stein MB, Tancer ME, Uhde TW: Heart rate and plasma norepinephrine responsivity to orthostatic challenge in anxiety disorders. Comparison of patients with panic disorder and social phobia and normal control subjects. *Arch Gen Psychiatry.* 1992;49:311–317.

Strohle A, Romeo E, DiMichele F, Pasini A, Herman B, Gajewsky G, Holsboer F, Rupprecht R: Induced panic attacks shift γ-aminobutyric acid type A receptor modulatory neuroactive steroid composition in patients with panic disorder. *Arch Gen Psychiatry.* 2003;60:161–168.

Strome EM, Trevor GHW, Higley JD, Liriaux DL, Suomi SJ, Doudet DJ: Intracerebroventricular corticotrophin-releasing factor increased limbic glucose metabolism and has social context dependent behavioral effects in nonhuman primates. *Proc Natl Acad Sci U S A.* 2002;99:15749–15754.

Stuckey J, Marra S, Minor T, Insel TR: Changes in μ opiate receptors following inescapable shock. *Brain Res.* 1989;476:167–169.

Thorsell A, Carlsson K, Ekman R, Heilig M: Behavioral and endocrine adaptation, and up-regulation of NPY expression in rat amygdala following repeated restraint stress. *Neuroreport.* 1999;10:3003–3007.

Thorsell A, Michalkiewicz M, Dumont Y, Quirion R, Caberlotto L, Rimondini R, Mathe AA, Helig M: Behavioral insensitivity to restraint stress, absent fear suppression of behavior and impaired spatial learning in transgenic rats with hippocampal neuropeptide Y overexpression. *Proc Natl Acad Sci U S A.* 2000;97:12852–12857.

True WR, Rice J, Eisen SA, Heath AC, Goldberg J, Lyons MJ, Nowak J: A twin study of genetic and environmental contributions to liability for posttraumatic stress symptoms. *Arch Gen Psychiatry.* 1993;50:257–264.

Ventura R, Cabib S, Puglisi-Allegra S: Genetic susceptibility of mesocortical dopamine to stress determines liability to inhibition of mesoaccumbens dopamine and to behavioral despair in a mouse model of depression. *Neuroscience.* 2002;115:999–1007.

Walker DL, Davis M: Involvement of NMDA receptors within the amygdala in short-versus long-term memory for fear conditioning as assessed with fear-potentiated startle. *Behav Neurosci.* 2000;114:1019–1033.

Weizman A, Weizman R, Kook KA, Vocci F, Deutsch SI, Paul SM: Adrenalectomy prevents the stress-induced decrease in in vivo [^{3}H]Ro 15-1788 binding to GABAA benzodiazepine receptors in the mouse. *Brain Res.* 1990;519:347–350.

Xu ZQ, Tong YG, Hokfelt T: Galanin enhances noradrenaline-induced outward current on locus coeruleus noradrenergic neurons. *Neuroreport.* 2001;12:1179–1182.

Yehuda R: Posttraumatic stress disorder. *N Engl J Med.* 2002;346:108–114.

Yehuda R, Boisoneau D, Lowy MT, Giller EL Jr: Dose response changes in plasma cortisol and lymphocyte glucocorticoid receptors following dexamethasone administration in combat veterans with and without posttraumatic stress disorder. *Arch Gen Psychiatry.* 1995;52:583–593.

Yehuda R, Levengood RA, Schneidler J, Wilson S, Guo LS, Gerber D: Increased activation following metyrapone administration in post-traumatic stress disorder. *Psychoneuroendocrinology.* 1996;21:1–16.

Yeragani VK, Berger R, Pohl R, Srinivasan K, Balon R, Ramesh C, Weinberg P, Berchou R: Effects of yohimbine on heart rate variability in panic disorder patients and normal controls. *J Cardiovasc Pharmacol.* 1992;20:609–618.

Zubieta JK, Heitzeg MM, Smith YR, Bueller JA, Xu K, Xu Y, Koeppe RA, Stohler CS, Goldamn D: COMT *val*^{158}*met* genotype affects μ-opioid neurotransmitter response to a pain stressor. *Science.* 2003;299:1240–1243.

▲ 14.5 Anxiety Disorders: Neuroimaging

WAYNE C. DREVETS, M.D., AND DENNIS S. CHARNEY, M.D.

The 1990s have witnessed tremendous progress in the acquisition of knowledge about the neuroanatomical, cellular, and molecular correlates of fear and anxiety. Advances in neuropharmacology, molecular biology, and genetic engineering have enabled elucidation of neurotransmitter systems that play roles in fear and anxiety behavior. The anatomical circuits in which these transmitters participate in mediating and modulating fear and anxiety are also being illuminated through convergent information from lesion analysis and neurophysiological mapping techniques, each of which has become more informative through advances in brain imaging technology. The findings from investigations applying these techniques are beginning to elucidate how dysfunction within these neurochemical and anatomical systems may result in pathological anxiety syndromes, such as panic disorder, posttraumatic stress disorder (PTSD), and phobic disorder.

This chapter reviews the neuroimaging data pertaining to the neural substrates and the receptor pharmacology underlying healthy and pathological anxiety states. Interpretation of the neurophysiological and structural imaging findings in anxiety disorders is facilitated by understanding the literature derived from basic science studies of fear, anxiety, and stress in experimental animals, so these data are also reviewed here. The parallel literature regarding the neurochemical basis of anxiety disorders, which is additionally germane to interpretation of the receptor imaging data in anxiety disorders that are presented herein, is, in contrast, reviewed elsewhere in other chapters of this volume.

ANATOMICAL CORRELATES OF FEAR AND ANXIETY

Fear and anxiety normally constitute adaptive responses to threat or stress. These emotional and behavioral sets arise in response to exteroceptive sensory stimuli and to interoceptive visceral and autonomic input. Anxiety may also be produced by cognitive processes mediating the anticipation, interpretation, or recollection of perceived stressors and threats.

Emotional processing in general can be divided into evaluative, expressive, and experiential components. Evaluation of the emotional salience of a stimulus involves appraisal of its valence (e.g., appetitive versus aversive) and its relationship to previous conditioning and behavioral reinforcement experiences and to the environmental context in which the stimulus arises. *Emotional expression* conveys the range of behavioral, endocrine, and autonomic manifestations of the emotional response, whereas *emotional experience* describes the subjective feeling accompanying the response. To optimize their capacity for guiding behavior, each of these aspects of emotional processing is modulated by complex neurobiological systems that prevent fear or anxiety responses from becoming persistent, excessive, or inappropriate to reinforcement contingencies.

Anatomical Correlates of Fear Processing: Preclinical Studies in Experimental Animals The design and interpretation of functional imaging studies of human anxiety have relied heavily on information about the neural circuits supporting fear and anxiety behavior from studies of experimental animals. Most of these preclinical studies investigated the anatomical correlates of emotional processing within the context of pavlovian fear conditioning, fear-potentiated startle (FPS), and other putative anxiety-related paradigms in rodents. The former two types of *fear learning* constitute experience-dependent forms of neural plasticity in an extended anatomical network centering on the critical involvement of the amygdala. Structures that function in concert with the amygdala during fear learning include other mesotemporal cortical structures, the sensory thalamus and cortex, the orbital and medial prefrontal cortex (mPFC), the anterior insula, the hypothalamus, and multiple brainstem nuclei. This network participates in the general processes of learning that a sensory stimulus (referred to as a *conditioned stimulus* [CS]) or operant behavior temporally predicts the occurrence of an emotionally salient stimulus (the *unconditioned stimulus* [UCS]), recognizing the CS when it recurs, organizing the behavioral and visceral response to the CS, and modulating these responses as reinforcement contingencies change.

Role of the Amygdala in Fear Learning and Expression The anatomical systems supporting fear learning are organized to permit rapid responses to simple perceptual elements of potentially threatening stimuli and longer-latency responses to more highly processed information about complex sensory stimuli and environmental contexts. The former processes depend on monosynaptic projections from the sensory thalamus to the amygdala, whereas the latter involve projections from sensory association cortices and anatomically related mesotemporal cortical structures to the amygdala. These networks also respond to visceral input received directly through the nucleus paragigantocellularis and the nucleus tractus solitarius of the vagus nerve and indirectly through the locus ceruleus (LC), the anterior insula, and the infralimbic and prelimbic cortices. Finally, neural activity within the amygdala is modulated by cortisol, norepinephrine (NE), acetylcholine, and other neurotransmitters and by mnemonic input related to previous conditioning and reinforcement experiences conveyed via projections from mesotemporal and prefrontal cortical structures.

The lateral nucleus of the amygdala (LA) serves as the primary sensory interface of the amygdala, receiving sensory information from the sensory thalamus and cortices. Single neurons within the LA respond to auditory, visual, and somatic stimuli, and information within these domains about the CS and the UCS converges in the LA. In contrast, olfactory input enters the periamygdaloid cortex via direct projections from the olfactory bulb through the olfactory tract. Although the periamygdaloid cortex neurons project to deeper amygdaloid nuclei, the specific pathways conveying olfactory information through the amygdala have not been delineated. The olfactory tract also carries projections to the pyriform cortex and entorhinal cortex, areas that share reciprocal anatomical connections with the amygdala.

In addition to its role in conditioning to explicit sensory stimuli, the amygdala is involved in the development of emotional responses to environmental context. Projections from the hippocampal formation to the amygdala via the fornix have been specifically implicated in spatial contextual conditioning. For example, lesioning these projections specifically prevents fear conditioning to the chamber or the position within a maze in which aversive stimulation previously occurred. Other structures that participate in the modulation of contextual fear include the rostral perirhinal cortex, the ventrolateral prefrontal cortex (VLPFC), and the anterior insula. Lesions of the latter two regions reduce fear reactivity to contextual stimuli but do not affect CS acquisition or response extinction. In contrast, lesions placed in the rostral perirhinal cortex after fear conditioning interfere with the expression of conditioned fear responses elicited by visual and auditory stimuli when these stimuli are presented in contexts that differ from the initial conditioning context.

The projections from sensory thalamus to the LA are thought to support rapid conditioning to simple auditory or visual stimuli (i.e., bypassing cortical processing), enabling fear responses below the level of conscious awareness. Thus, lesioning the auditory cortex before conditioning does not prevent conditioning to single auditory tones. In contrast, projections to LA from the primary sensory and sensory association cortices appear essential for some aspects of conditioned responding to more complex sensory stimuli. These relationships are modality specific, such that disruption of the projections from the auditory thalamus and the auditory cortex to the LA specifically prevents acquisition of fear conditioning to auditory stimuli and fear-conditioned responses to previously conditioned auditory stimuli.

After sensory input enters the LA, the neural representation of the stimulus is distributed in parallel to various amygdaloid nuclei, where it is modulated by diverse functional systems, such as those conveying mnemonic information about past experiences or interoceptive input related to ongoing homeostatic states. The most extensive amygdala projections of the LA consist of reciprocal projections to the basal and accessory basal nuclei and the central nucleus of the amygdala (CEA). Lesions of the LA or CEA—but not of other amygdala nuclei—disrupt fear conditioning to a tone CS, suggesting that the direct projection from the LA to the CEA is sufficient to mediate conditioning to simple sensory stimuli.

The projections from LA to the basal amygdaloid nuclei also participate in forming long-lasting memory traces for fear conditioning. Functional inactivation of the lateral and basal amygdaloid nuclei before pavlovian fear conditioning interferes with acquisition of learning, whereas inactivation immediately after conditioning has no effect on memory consolidation. The basal nuclei have widespread intranuclear connections and also project to other amygdala nuclei, including the CEA and LA. The basal nuclei also share extensive, reciprocal projections with the orbital prefrontal cortex (PfC) and mPFC, through which they appear to modulate neuronal responses of the PfC and the LA and the CEA.

The plasticity within the amygdala that constitutes memory for conditioning experiences involves long-term potentiation-like associative processes. Plasticity related to fear learning also occurs in cortical areas, presumably making possible the establishment of explicit or declarative memories about the fear-related event through interactions with the medial temporal lobe memory system. The influence of the amygdala on cortically based memories has been most clearly characterized with respect to late plastic components of the auditory cortex neuronal responses to a CS. Single-unit recordings during fear conditioning indicate that some auditory cortex neurons, which, before conditioning, did not respond to the CS tone, develop late-conditioned responses (i.e., 500 to 1,500 milliseconds after CS onset) that anticipate the UCS and show extinction-resistant memory storage. These late-conditioned auditory cortical neuronal responses take more trials to learn and respond more slowly than LA neurons within trials, and their late development is prevented by amygdala lesions. Thus, although rapid conditioning of fear responses to potentially dangerous stimuli depends on plasticity in the amygdala, learning involving higher cognitive (i.e., mnemonic and attentional) processing of fear experiences may depend on plasticity involving cortical neurons that is influenced by neural transmission from the amygdala.

Other auditory cortex neurons show an early (<50 milliseconds after stimulus onset) plastic component during fear conditioning, in which the preexisting electrophysiological responses of auditory cortex neurons to the CS become enhanced by conditioning. This short-latency plasticity within the auditory cortex appears to depend on input from the auditory thalamus and is unaffected by amygdala lesions. Nevertheless, such short-latency responses extinguish more quickly (i.e., during repeated exposure to the CS alone) in animals with amygdala lesions, implying that the amygdala is involved in preventing extinction of these responses.

Activation of the amygdala during other types of emotional events enhances the strength of long-term memory for emotional stimuli represented in other cortical memory circuits as well. These circuits presumably involve the medial temporal lobe memory system, which has extensive anatomical connections with the amygdala, through which interactions between storage and explicit recall of affectively salient memories are supported. For at least some types of emotional learning, memory consolidation is critically dependent on noradrenergic stimulation of β- and α_1-adrenergic receptors in the basolateral nucleus of the amygdala. Acquisition of fear-conditioned responses thus requires an intact central noradrenergic system. The activation of NE release during emotional learning is facilitated by glucocorticoid effects on noradrenergic neurons.

Role of the Amygdala in Organizing Emotional Expression The amygdaloid output nuclei, especially the CEA, receive convergent information from multiple amygdala regions and organize behavioral responses that are thought to reflect the sum of neuronal activity produced by different amygdaloid nuclei. The CEA comprises the interface between the amygdala and the motor, autonomic, and neuroendocrine systems involved in expressing fear behavior. The CEA projects to nuclei in the hypothalamus, midbrain, and medulla that mediate the neuroendocrine, autonomic, and behavioral responses associated with fear and anxiety. For example, the amygdala facilitates stress-related corticotropin-releasing hormone (CRH) release via intrinsic CRH-containing neurons and bisynaptic (double γ-aminobutyric acid [GABA]ergic) anatomical projections to the paraventricular nucleus (PVN) of the hypothalamus. Electrical stimulation of the CEA produces responses similar to those elicited by fear-conditioned stimuli, and lesions of the CEA prevent the expression of fear responses of various types. In contrast, lesioning of specific structures efferent to the CEA, such as the lateral hypothalamus or the periaqueductal gray (PAG) matter, produces selective deficits in cardiovascular or somatomotor behavioral fear responses, respectively.

The amygdala also sends projections to the thalamus, the nucleus accumbens, the ventromedial caudate, and parts of the ventral putamen, which participate in organizing motor responses to threatening stimuli. For example, activation of the amygdala projections to the ventral striatum arrests goal-directed behavior in experimental animals, suggesting a possible neural mechanism for the cessation of motivated or reward-directed behavior during anxiety and panic. The amygdala may also influence motor behavior via projections through the hypothalamus and the PAG. For example, in experimental animals, stimulation of the lateral PAG produces defensive behaviors, sympathetic autonomic arousal, and hypoalgesia, whereas stimulation of the ventrolateral PAG produces social withdrawal and behavioral quiescence (as in response to deep injury or visceral pain).

Role of the Amygdala in Innate Fear and Evaluation of Emotional Salience of Social Behavior The amygdala also appears to play important roles in mediating innate fear and processing affective elements of social interactions. Amygdala lesions cause rats to lose their fear of cats and monkeys to lose their fear of snakes. In monkeys, amygdala lesions reduce aggression, as well as fear, and cause animals to become more submissive to dominant animals. Nevertheless, amygdala-lesioned monkeys appear oblivious to socially significant signals conveyed by the behavior or facial expressions of other monkeys (e.g., attempting to engage in sexual behavior with nonreceptive animals or without regard to dominance hierarchy) and, presumably as a consequence, are killed relatively rapidly by other monkeys in wild (i.e., natural setting) primate colonies.

Correspondence to Neuroimaging, Neurophysiological, and Lesion Analysis Data in Humans Consistent with evidence from electrophysiological and lesion analysis studies of experimental animals, functional imaging studies of humans demonstrate that hemodynamic activity increases in the amygdala during exposures to fear-conditioned stimuli and other types of emotionally aversive or arousing sensory stimuli, although the spatial resolution of imaging technologies applied to date has not permitted delineation of specific amygdaloid nuclei. Moreover, during repeated, unreinforced exposures to the same CS, single-trial functional magnetic resonance imaging (fMRI) studies show that the initial elevation of hemodynamic activity attenuates and subsequently decreases below baseline. This biphasic pattern resembles that seen in electrophysiological studies of neuronal habituation during extinction learning.

The relationship between amygdala activation during an emotional event and the enhancement of long-term memory for that event has also been studied using neuroimaging. As healthy humans read stories of differing emotional valence, the magnitude of physiological activation in the amygdala correlates with the negative emotional intensity and the subsequent recall performance of the story's content. Physiological activity in the amygdala and the hippocampus measured during memory encoding reportedly correlates with enhanced episodic memory for pleasant, as well as aversive, visual stimuli, and the amygdala's role in modulating emotional memory may depend more generally on the degree of arousal or the behavioral salience associated with target information.

Human neuroimaging, electrophysiological, and lesion analysis studies have also demonstrated that the amygdala is involved in the recall of emotional or arousing memories. In humans, bursts of electroencephalogram (EEG) activity have been recorded in the amygdala during recollection of specific emotional events. Moreover, electrical stimulation of the amygdala in humans can evoke the experience of fear or anxiety and the recollection of emotionally charged life events from remote memory.

Finally, the involvement of the amygdala in evaluating social behavior with respect to the emotional information conveyed by human facial expression or voice intonation has been demonstrated in humans. Humans with amygdala lesions are impaired in their ability to recognize fear or sadness in facial expression and fear and anger expressed in spoken language. In positron emission tomography (PET) and fMRI studies, hemodynamic activity increases in the amygdala as humans view faces expressing fear or sadness. The automatic nature of this response is evident by its occurrence even when the fearful face is shown so briefly (e.g., for 30 milliseconds using backward masking techniques) that subjects are unaware of having seen the fearful face.

Other Temporal Cortical Structures The hippocampus and perirhinal cortex interact with the amygdala in the development of emotional responses to environmental context. Projections from the hippocampal formation to the amygdala via the fornix have been specifically implicated in spatial contextual conditioning. For example, lesioning these projections specifically prevents fear conditioning to the chamber or the position within a maze in which aversive stimulation previously occurred. Other structures that participate in the modulation of contextual fear include the anterior perirhinal cortex, the ventrolateral PfC (VLPFC), and the anterior insula. Lesions of the latter two regions reduce fear reactivity to contextual stimuli but do not affect CS acquisition or response extinction. In contrast, lesions placed in the anterior perirhinal cortex after fear conditioning interfere with the expression of conditioned fear responses elicited by visual and auditory stimuli when these stimuli are presented in contexts that differ from the initial conditioning context.

The perirhinal cortex shares reciprocal anatomical connections with the amygdala and is thought to play a role in conveying information about complex visual stimuli to the amygdala during presentation of fear-conditioned visual stimuli. Lesions of the anterior perirhinal cortex, the basolateral nucleus of the amygdala, or the CEA can each completely eliminate FPS during exposure to some conditioned visual stimuli. In contrast, complete removal of the entire visual cortex, insular cortex, mPFC, and posterior perirhinal cortex produces no significant effect on the magnitude of FPS, and lesions of the frontal cortex only partly attenuate FPS. The perirhinal cortex receives input regarding conditioned visual stimuli from the lateral geniculate nucleus, and lesions of this structure can also block FPS. Finally, the anterior perirhinal cortex receives afferent projections from the visual cortices, as well as from the anterior cingulate cortex (ACC), the infralimbic cortex, and the parietal cortex, structures implicated in modulating behavioral responses to fear-conditioned stimuli.

The temporopolar cortex has been implicated in modulating autonomic aspects of emotional responses and in processing emotionally provocative visual stimuli. Electrical stimulation of various sites within the temporopolar cortex can alter a variety of autonomic nervous system functions. In humans with simple phobias or PTSD, physiological activity increases in the anterior temporopolar cortex during experimentally induced exacerbations of anxiety involving visual exposure to phobic stimuli or word scripts describing traumatic events, respectively. Blood flow also increases in the anterior temporopolar cortex of healthy humans during exposure to emotionally provocative visual stimuli, whether the stimuli convey sad, disgusting, or happy content, relative to conditions involving exposure to emotionally neutral visual stimuli and to conditions in which corresponding emotional states are elicited via recall of autobiographical information. Portions of the temporopolar cortex may thus function as sensory association areas that participate in evaluating the emotional salience of actual or anticipated stimuli and in modulating autonomic responses to such stimuli.

Bed Nucleus of the Stria Terminalis: Hypothesized Role in Anxiety The hypothalamic and brainstem structures that mediate the expression of emotional behavior can be activated directly via the CEA or the bed nucleus of the stria terminalis (BNST). Anxiety-like responses elicited by exposure to a threatening environment for several minutes or by intraventricular administration of CRH appear to be specifically mediated via the BNST, rather than the CEA. This system is thus hypothesized to play a role in mediating anxiety during exposure to less explicit or less well-defined sensory cues or to contexts that occur over a longer duration, or both.

Anatomical Structures Mediating Neuroendocrine and Autonomic Responses of Fear or Stress The peripheral hormonal and autonomic responses to threat mediated by the hypothalamic-pituitary-adrenal (HPA) axis and the sympathetic and parasympathetic autonomic nervous systems facilitate the generation of adaptive responses to threat or stress. Stimulation of the lateral nucleus of the hypothalamus by afferent projections from the CEA, the BNST, or the ventral striatum activates the sympathetic system, producing increases in blood pressure and heart rate, sweating, piloerection, and pupillary dilation. Stress stimulates release of CRH from the PVN of the hypothalamus and amygdala. The CRH secretion from the PVN in turn increases peripheral adrenocorticotropic hormone (ACTH) levels, which stimulate the adrenal glands to secrete cortisol. The ACC, anterior insula, and posterior orbital cortex send anatomical projections to the hypothalamus that participate in modulating or inhibiting cardiovascular and endocrine responses to threat and stress.

Regional differences in the regulation of CRH function by glucocorticoid receptor stimulation and stress appear to play major roles in the mediation of fear and anxiety. Feedback inhibition of CRH release by glucocorticoid receptor stimulation (i.e., to suppress HPA axis activity) occurs at the level of the PVN of the hypothalamus, at which systemically administered glucocorticoids reduce CRH expression, and the anterior pituitary, at which glucocorticoids decrease CRH receptor expression. In contrast, neither glucocorticoid administration nor restraint stress alters the CRH receptor expression or CRH release in the CEA of the amygdala or the BNST. The positive feedback of glucocorticoids on extrahypothalamic CRH function in the amygdala or the BNST may thus contribute to the production of anxiety symptoms.

The vagus and splanchnic nerves constitute the major efferent projections of the parasympathetic nervous system to the viscera. The vagal nuclei receive afferent projections from the lateral hypothalamus, the PVN, the LC, the amygdala, the infralimbic cortex, and the prelimbic portion of the ACC. The splanchnic nerves receive afferent connections from the LC. The innervation of the parasympathetic nervous system from these limbic structures is thought to mediate visceral symptoms associated with anxiety, such as gastrointestinal (GI) and genitourinary disturbances.

Functional Interactions Involving Noradrenergic, HPA, and CRH Systems Coordinated functional interactions between the HPA axis and the noradrenergic systems play major roles and are critical to the production of adaptive responses to some types of stress, anxiety, or fear. The secretion of CRH increases LC neuronal firing activity, resulting in enhanced NE release in a variety of cortical and subcortical regions. Conversely, NE release stimulates CRH secretion in the PVN (the nucleus containing the majority of CRH-synthesizing neurons in the hypothalamus). During chronic stress, in particular, the LC is the brainstem noradrenergic nucleus that appears to preferentially mediate NE release in the PVN. Conversely, as CRH release in the PVN stimulates ACTH secretion from the pituitary and thereby increases cortisol secretion from the adrenal glands, the rise in plasma cortisol concentrations acts through a negative feedback pathway to decrease CRH and NE synthesis at the level of the PVN. Glucocorticoid-mediated inhibition of NE-induced CRH stimulation may be evident primarily during stress, rather than under resting conditions, as an adaptive response that restrains stress-induced neuroendocrine and cardiovascular effects mediated by the PVN. NE, cortisol, and CRH are thus tightly linked as a functional system that offers a homeostatic mechanism for responding to stress.

In experimental animals, alterations of brain catecholamine and glucocorticoid levels affect the consolidation and retrieval of emotional memories. Glucocorticoids influence memory storage via activation of glucocorticoid receptors in the hippocampus, whereas NE effects are mediated in part through β-adrenoreceptor stimulation in the amygdala. In humans, adrenocortical suppression blocks the memory-enhancing effects of amphetamine and epinephrine, and propranolol (Inderal) impairs memory for an emotionally provocative story but not for an emotionally neutral story. The acute release of glucocorticoids and NE in response to trauma would thus modulate the encoding of traumatic memories.

Prefrontal Cortical Structures in Modulating Fear and Anxiety Behavior

Multiple areas of the mPFC and orbital PfC participate in modulating anxiety and other emotional behaviors. These structures are putatively involved in interpreting the higher-order significance of experiential stimuli, modifying behavioral responses based on competing reward-versus-punishment contingencies, and predicting social outcomes of behavioral responses to emotional events. These areas share extensive, reciprocal projections with the amygdala, through which the amygdala modulates PfC neuronal activity, and the PfC can modulate amygdala-mediated responses to emotionally salient stimuli.

Areas within the orbital PfC and mPFC and the anterior insula also participate in modulating peripheral responses to stress, including heart rate, blood pressure, and glucocorticoid secretion. The neuronal activity within these PfC areas is, in turn, modulated by a variety of neurotransmitter systems that are activated in response to stressors and threats. For example, the noradrenergic, dopaminergic, and serotoninergic systems play roles in enhancing vigilance, modulating goal-directed behavior, and facilitating decision making about probabilities of punishment versus reward by modulating neuronal activity in the PfC.

Medial Prefrontal Cortex (mPFC) The mPFC areas implicated in anxiety- and fear-related behavior in humans and experimental animals include the infralimbic cortex, the ACC, and a more anterior mPFC region extending from the rostral ACC (Brodmann's areas [BAs] 24 and 32) toward the frontal pole. The reciprocal projections between the amygdala and the mPFC are hypothesized to play critical roles in attenuating fear responses and extinguishing behavioral responses to fear-conditioned stimuli that are no longer reinforced. Lesions of the ACC in rats enhance freezing to a fear-conditioned tone, suggesting that this mPFC region is involved in fear reduction. In addition, neurons in the rat prelimbic cortex (thought to be homologous to the ACC located ventral to the genu of the corpus callosum or subgenual in humans) reduce their spontaneous firing activity in the presence of a conditioned, aversive tone to an extent that is inversely proportional to the magnitude of fear. This suppression of prelimbic cortex neuronal firing activity is inversely correlated with increases in amygdala neuronal activity. Finally, lesions of the infralimbic cortex specifically interfere with the recall of extinction processes after long delays between the acquisition of extinction learning and reexposure to the initial CS. Extinction does not appear to occur by erasing memory traces of the CS–UCS association but rather by new learning through which the behavioral response to the CS is actively inhibited.

In humans, the pregenual ACC (i.e., anterior to the genu of the corpus callosum) shows areas of elevated hemodynamic activity during a variety of anxiety states elicited in healthy or anxiety disordered subjects. Electrical stimulation of this region elicits fear, panic, or a sense of foreboding in humans and vocalization in experimental animals. Nevertheless, physiological activity also increases in the ACC during the generation of positive emotions in healthy humans and during depressive episodes in major depressive disorder.

The subgenual ACC has been implicated in healthy sadness, major depression, mania, and PTSD. In familial unipolar and bipolar depressives, reductions in cerebral blood flow (CBF) and metabolism were associated with left-lateralized reductions in the volume of the corresponding cortex. The subgenual ACC activity shows a mood state dependency in which the metabolism is higher in the depressed phase than the remitted phase of major depressive disorder, which is consistent with the findings that blood flow increases in this region in healthy, nondepressed humans during experimentally induced sadness and in PTSD subjects during internally generated imagery of past trauma.

The subgenual and pregenual ACCs share reciprocal anatomical connections with areas implicated in emotional behavior, such as the posterior orbital cortex, amygdala, hypothalamus, nucleus accumbens, PAG, VTA, raphe, LC, and nucleus tractus solitarius. Humans with mPFC lesions that include the pregenual and subgenual ACCs show abnormal autonomic responses to emotionally provocative stimuli, inability to experience emotion related to concepts, and inability to use information regarding the probability of aversive social consequences versus reward in guiding social behavior. In rats, bilateral or right-lateralized lesions of the ventral mPFC comprised of infralimbic, prelimbic, and ACC cortices attenuate corticosterone secretion, sympathetic autonomic responses, and gastric stress pathology during restraint stress or exposure to fear-conditioned stimuli. In contrast, left-sided lesions of this cortical strip increase sympathetic arousal and corticosterone responses to restraint stress. Finally, the ventral ACC contains glucocorticoid receptors that, when stimulated, inhibit stress-induced corticosterone release in rats.

Physiological activity also increases in more anterior mPFC areas in healthy humans as they perform tasks that elicit emotional responses or that require emotional evaluations. During anxious anticipation of an electrical shock, CBF increases in the rostral mPFC (vicinity of anterior BA24, BA32, and rostral BA9), and the magnitude of the change in CBF correlates inversely with changes in anxiety ratings and heart rate. In rats, lesions of the rostral mPFC result in exaggerated heart rate responses to fear-conditioned stimuli, and stimulation of these sites attenuates defensive behavior and cardiovascular responses evoked by amygdala stimulation. In primates, whereas BA24 and BA32 have extensive reciprocal connections with the amygdala through which they may modulate emotional expression, the BA9 cortex has only sparse projections to the amygdala. Nevertheless, all three areas send extensive efferent projections to the PAG and the hypothalamus, through which cardiovascular responses associated with emotional behavior may be modulated.

In the depressed phase of major depressive disorder and bipolar disorder, metabolic activity is abnormal in the dorsomedial and dorsal anterolateral PfC (in the vicinity of rostral BA9). Postmortem studies of these regions have shown abnormal reductions in the size of glia and neurons in major depressive disorder. Given the preclinical and neuroimaging evidence presented previously indicating that this area may modulate anxiety, it is conceivable that dysfunction of this mPFC area contributes to the development of anxiety symptoms in mood disorders.

Orbital and Anterior Insular Cortices Other areas of the PfC that are implicated in studies of fear or anxiety in human and nonhuman primates are the posterior and lateral orbital cortex, the anterior insula, and the VLPFC. Physiological activity increases in these areas during experimentally induced anxiety states in healthy subjects and in subjects with obsessive-compulsive disorder (OCD), simple phobia, and panic disorder. The baseline metabolic activity is also abnormally elevated in these regions in unmedicated subjects with primary major depressive disorder and OCD who were scanned while resting with eyes closed. The elevated activity in these areas in major depressive disorder and OCD appears state dependent, and effective antidepressant or antiobsessional treatment results in decreases in CBF and metabolism in the medicated-improved relative to the unmedicated-symptomatic phase.

A complex relationship exists between physiological activity and anxiety or depressive symptoms in the orbital cortex and the VLPFC. In major depressive disorder, although CBF and metabolism increase in these areas in the depressed relative to the remitted phase, the magnitude of these measures correlates inversely with ratings of depressive ideation and severity. Similarly, posterior orbital cortex flow increases in OCD and animal phobic subjects during exposure to phobic stimuli and in healthy subjects during induced sadness, but this change in CBF correlates inversely with changes in obsessive thinking, anxiety, and sadness, respectively.

These data appear consistent with electrophysiological and lesion analysis data showing that the orbital cortex participates in modulating behavioral and visceral responses associated with fearful, defensive, and reward-directed behavior as reinforcement contingencies change. Nearly one-half of the orbital cortex pyramidal neurons alter their firing rates during the delay period between stimulus and response, and this firing activity relates to the presence or absence of reinforcement. These cells are thought to play roles in extinguishing unreinforced responses to aversive or appetitive stimuli. The posterior and lateral orbital cortex and the amygdala send projections to each other and to overlapping portions of the striatum, hypothalamus, and PAG, through which these structures modulate each other's neural transmission. For example, the defensive behaviors and cardiovascular responses evoked by electrical stimulation of the amygdala are attenuated or ablated by concomitant stimulation of orbital sites, which, when stimulated alone, exert no autonomic effects.

Humans with orbital cortex lesions show impaired performance on tasks requiring application of information related to punishment or reward, perseverate in behavioral strategies that are unreinforced, and exhibit difficulty shifting intellectual strategies in response to changing task demands. Likewise, monkeys with surgical lesions of the lateral orbital cortex and VLPFC demonstrate *perseverative interference*, which is characterized by difficulty in learning to withhold prepotent responses to nonreinforced stimuli as reinforcement contingencies change. Activation of the orbital cortex during anxiety or obsessional states may thus reflect endogenous attempts to attenuate emotional expression or to interrupt unreinforced aversive thought and emotion. Conversely, dysfunction of the orbital cortex may contribute to pathological anxiety and obsessional states by impairing the ability to inhibit nonreinforced or maladaptive emotional, cognitive, and behavioral responses to social interactions and sensory or visceral stimuli.

Posterior Cingulate Cortex Many functional imaging studies report that exposure to aversive stimuli of various types increases physiological activity in the retrosplenial cortex and other portions of the posterior cingulate gyrus. Posterior cingulate cortical flow and metabolism have also been found abnormally elevated in some studies of depressed subjects with major depressive disorder. The posterior cingulate cortex appears to serve as a sensory association cortex and may participate in processing the affective salience of sensory stimuli. The posterior cingulate cortex sends a major anatomical projection to the ACC, through which it may relay such information into the limbic circuitry.

Other Regions Changes in regional CBF associated with anxiety in other structures have been less consistently replicated. Several studies have reported anxiety-associated, hemodynamic changes in the lateral temporal and inferior parietal cortical areas or in the striatum. Some of these cortical areas appear to reflect sensory association cortices, and physiological activity in these regions during anxiety may reflect sensory processing of the anxiety-provoking stimuli or feedback to these regions by the amygdala or other subcortical regions.

Medial cerebellar CBF consistently increases during experimentally induced anxiety or sadness in healthy or anxiety disordered subjects. One metaanalysis of PET studies investigating the anatomical correlates of multiple types of anxiety found two regions in which CBF increased across all normal and pathological anxiety states studied, namely, the medial cerebellum and the midbrain (in the vicinity of the PAG). The medial cerebellum contains a set of nuclei that serve as functional complements to the hypothalamus in the modulation of autonomic responses. In addition, most or all areas of the cerebral cortex form closed, multisynaptic circuits through the cerebellum, although the functional significance of these anatomical loops remains unclear.

ANATOMICAL CORRELATES OF ANXIETY DISORDERS

Neuroimaging studies have assessed neurophysiological abnormalities in anxiety-disordered samples in the baseline, resting condition and during symptom provocation. These data converge with those obtained from studies of healthy subjects and of experimental animals to implicate the limbic, paralimbic, and sensory association areas reviewed previously in the functional anatomy of anxiety and fear. Nevertheless, the results of most of the imaging studies reviewed herein await replication, and the data they provide do not clearly establish whether the differences observed between anxiety-disordered and control subjects reflect physiological correlates of anxiety symptoms or instead constitute trait-like biological abnormalities underlying the vulnerability to anxiety syndromes.

Panic Disorder The baseline state in panic disorder is characterized by mild to moderate levels of chronic anxiety (termed *anticipatory anxiety*). In this state, abnormalities of CBF and metabolism have been reported in the vicinity of the hippocampus and the parahippocampal gyrus. Abnormal resting asymmetries (left less than right) of blood flow and metabolism have been reported in the vicinity of the hippocampus and the parahippocampal gyrus. Resting flow is also elevated in the midbrain in the vicinity of the PAG, which has been implicated in lactate-induced panic, other acute anxiety states, and animal models of panic attacks.

Subjects with panic disorder have also been imaged during panic elicited by using a variety of chemical challenges. Panic attacks induced in panic disorder subjects by intravenous (IV) sodium lactate infusion were associated with regional CBF increases in the anterior insula, the anteromedial cerebellum, and the midbrain. Blood flow also increased in these regions in animal phobic subjects during exposure to phobic stimuli and in healthy subjects during the threat of a painful electrical shock, suggesting that these CBF changes reflect the neurophysiological correlates of fear processing in general. Consistent with this hypothesis, anxiety attacks induced in healthy humans using cholecystokinin-4 (CCK-4) were also associated with CBF increases in the insular-amygdala region and the anteromedial cerebellum.

Preliminary evidence suggests that the neurophysiological responses in the PFC during challenge with panic-inducing chemical agents may differ between panic disorder subjects and healthy controls in the ACC. The ACC blood flow increased in healthy subjects but not in panic disorder subjects during fenfluramine challenge in a study in which fenfluramine induced panic attacks in 56 percent of panic disorder subjects but only 11 percent of controls. Compatible with these data, panic attacks induced by CCK-4 administration were associated with CBF increases in the ACC in healthy humans, but flow did not significantly change in the ACC in panic disorder subjects during lactate-induced panic.

Structural magnetic resonance imaging (MRI) studies have not established the existence of morphometric or morphological abnormalities in panic disorder. One study reported qualitative abnormalities of temporal lobe structure in panic disorder, but these findings have not been replicated. Another reported a reduction of the entire temporal lobe volume in panic disorder, but this finding was difficult to interpret, because, when normalized to whole brain volume, the mean temporal lobe measure in the panic disorder sample was essentially the same as that of the control sample.

Phobias In simple animal phobias, phobic anxiety has been imaged by acquiring blood flow scans during exposures to the feared animal. During the initial fearful scans, flow increases bilaterally in the lateral orbital and anterior insular cortex, the pregenual ACC, and the anteromedial cerebellum, areas in which CBF also increases in other anxiety states. During the development of habituation to phobic stimuli, the magnitude of the hemodynamic responses to the phobic stimulus diminished in the anterior insula and the medial cerebellum but increased in the infralimbic cortex and left posterior orbital cortex in an area in which flow had not changed during exposures that preceded habituation. The magnitude of the CBF increase in this latter region was inversely correlated with the corresponding changes in heart rate and anxiety ratings. As discussed previously, the infralimbic cortex has been implicated in extinction learning in experimental animals, and the posterior orbital cortex was a site at which CBF increased in OCD subjects during exposure to phobic stimuli, with the increase in flow being inversely correlated with ratings of obsessive and anxious ideation.

In social anxiety disorder, an aversive conditioning paradigm (in which the UCS was an aversive odor, and the CS was a picture of a human face) showed that hemodynamic activity decreased in the amygdala and hippocampus during repeated CS presentations in healthy controls but increased in social phobic subjects. Interpretation of these data was confounded by the problem that human faces and aversively conditioned stimuli normally activate the amygdala, so it remained unclear which of the stimuli produced abnormal responses in social phobia. Nevertheless, these data appear conceptually intriguing, given the role of hippocampal-amygdala projections in mediating contextual fear and the possibility that deficits in the transmission of information regarding context may be involved in the pathogenesis of phobias.

Posttraumatic Stress Disorder (PTSD) PTSD is hypothesized to involve the emotional-learning circuitry associated with the amygdala, because the traumatic event constitutes a fear-conditioning experience, and subsequent exposure to sensory, contextual, or mnemonic stimuli that recall aspects of the event elicits psychological distress and sympathetic arousal. Potentially consistent with this expectation, some studies demonstrated activation of the amygdala as PTSD subjects listened to auditory scripts describing the traumatic event or to combat sounds (in combat-related PTSD) or generated mental imagery related to the traumatic event in the absence of sensory cues. However, other PET studies found no significant changes in amygdala CBF as PTSD subjects listened to scripts describing the traumatic event or viewed trauma-related pictures, and studies comparing CBF responses to trauma-related stimuli have not shown significant differences between PTSD subjects and trauma-matched, non-PTSD controls in the amygdala. The extent to which these negative findings reflect limitations in PET's spatial or temporal resolution awaits investigation in provocation studies involving larger subject samples that use fMRI (which can more accurately assess amygdala responses to the task stimuli before the development of habituation). In this regard, it is noteworthy that a preliminary fMRI study found exaggerated hemodynamic changes in the amygdala in PTSD subjects relative to trauma-matched, non-PTSD controls during exposure to pictures of fearful faces presented preconsciously by using a backward masking technique. If replicated, this observation suggests that the emotional dysregulation associated with PTSD may involve elevated amygdala responses to emotional stimuli of various types.

Other limbic and paralimbic cortical structures have also been implicated in provocation studies of PTSD. In PTSD subjects and trauma-matched, non-PTSD controls, CBF increases in the posterior orbital cortex, anterior insula, and temporopolar cortex during exposure to trauma-related stimuli, but these changes have generally not differentiated between PTSD and control samples. In contrast, the pattern of CBF changes elicited in the mPFC by traumatic stimuli may differ between PTSD and control subjects. During exposure to trauma-related sensory stimuli, flow decreased in the left pregenual ACC but increased in the right pregenual ACC in PTSD, potentially consistent with the evidence from experimental animals that the role of the mPFC in emotional behavior is lateralized. In the right pregenual ACC, however, CBF increased significantly more in non-PTSD, trauma-matched controls than in PTSD subjects. Moreover, in the infralimbic cortex, CBF decreased in combat-related PTSD subjects but increased in combat-matched, non-PTSD controls during exposure to combat-related visual and auditory stimuli.

Given evidence that the ACC and the infralimbic cortex play roles in extinguishing fear-conditioned responses, the observation that PTSD subjects fail to activate these structures to a similar extent as traumatized, non-PTSD controls during exposure to traumatic cues suggests that neural processes mediating extinction to trauma-related stimuli are impaired in PTSD. Compatible with this hypothesis, PTSD samples have been shown to acquire de novo conditioned responses more readily and to extinguish them more slowly than control samples. Such impairment could conceivably be related to the vulnerability of developing PTSD, because PTSD occurs in only 5 to 20 percent of individuals exposed to similar traumatic events.

Structural MRI studies of PTSD have identified subtle reductions in the volume of the hippocampus in PTSD samples relative to healthy or traumatized, non-PTSD control samples. Although limitations existed in these studies in the matching of alcohol use and abuse between PTSD and control samples, the reductions in hippocampal volume did not correlate with the extent of alcohol exposure in the PTSD samples, and no volumetric differences were found between PTSD and control samples in the amygdala, the entire temporal lobe, the caudate, the whole brain, or the lateral ventricles.

Although the magnitude of the reduction in hippocampal volume only ranged from 5 to 12 percent in the PTSD samples relative to trauma-matched controls, these abnormalities were associated with short-term memory deficits in some studies.

It remains unclear whether the difference in hippocampal volume reflects a result of the chronic stress associated with PTSD or a biological antecedent that may confer risk for developing PTSD. In support of the latter hypothesis, a study of monozygotic twins who were discordant for trauma exposure showed that, of twin pairs in which one twin developed severe PTSD, the trauma-exposed twin and the trauma-unexposed co-twin had smaller hippocampal volumes than control twin pairs in whom trauma exposure had not resulted in PTSD. Furthermore, illness severity in the PTSD subjects exposed to trauma was negatively correlated with the hippocampal volume of the PTSD subjects and their trauma-unexposed co-twins.

Obsessive-Compulsive Disorder The anatomical circuits involved in the production of obsessions and compulsions have been elucidated by converging evidence from functional neuroimaging studies of OCD, analysis of lesions resulting in obsessive-compulsive symptoms, and observations regarding the neurosurgical interventions that ameliorate OCD. PET studies of OCD show that resting CBF and glucose metabolism are abnormally increased in the orbital cortex and the caudate nucleus bilaterally in primary OCD. With symptom provocation via exposure to relevant phobic stimuli (e.g., skin contact with contaminated objects for OCD subjects with germ phobias), flow increased further in the orbital cortex, the ACC caudate, the putamen, and the thalamus. During effective pharmacotherapy, orbital metabolism decreased toward normal, and drug treatment and behavioral therapy were associated with a reduction of caudate metabolism. The areas of baseline hypermetabolism in the orbital cortex and caudate may thus reflect physiological concomitants of obsessive thoughts or chronic anxiety, or both, and, conversely, the reduction in caudate metabolism associated with effective (but not ineffective) treatment may reflect a physiological correlate of symptom resolution rather than a primary mechanism of treatment.

Based on the evidence reviewed previously from electrophysiological and lesion analysis studies indicating that the orbital cortex participates in the correction of behavioral responses that become inappropriate as reinforcement contingencies change, posterior orbital areas may specifically activate as an endogenous attempt to interrupt patterns of nonreinforced thought and behavior in OCD. Compatible with this hypothesis, the posterior orbital cortex CBF increases during symptom provocation in OCD, but the magnitude of this increase correlates inversely with the corresponding rise in obsession ratings. In contrast, flow also increased in an area of the right anterior orbital cortex implicated in a variety of types of mnemonic processing, and the change in CBF in this region correlated positively with changes in obsession ratings.

The neurological conditions associated with the development of secondary obsessions and compulsions also provide evidence that dysfunction within circuits formed by the basal ganglia and the PfC may be related to the pathogenesis of OCD. Such conditions involve lesions of the globus pallidus and the adjacent putamen, Sydenham's chorea (a poststreptococcal autoimmune disorder associated with neuronal atrophy in the caudate and putamen), Tourette's syndrome (an idiopathic syndrome characterized by motoric and phonic tics that may have a genetic relationship with OCD), chronic motor tic disorder, and lesions of the ventromedial PfC. Several of these conditions are associated with complex motor tics (repetitive, coordinated, involuntary movements occurring in patterned sequences in a spontaneous and transient manner). It is conceivable that complex tics and obsessive thoughts may reflect homologous, aberrant neural processes manifested within the motor and cognitive-behavioral domains, respectively, because of their origination in distinct portions of the cortical-striatal-pallidal-thalamic circuitry.

In contrast to the regional metabolic abnormalities observed in primary OCD, imaging studies of obsessive-compulsive syndromes arising in association with Tourette's syndrome or secondary to basal ganglia lesions have not found elevated blood flow and metabolism in the caudate and, in some cases, have found reduced metabolism in the orbital cortex in such subjects relative to controls. The differences in the functional anatomical correlates of primary versus secondary OCD are consistent with a neural model in which dysfunction arising at various points within the ventral prefrontal cortical-striatal-pallidal-thalamic circuitry can produce pathological obsessions and compulsions. This circuitry has been generally implicated in switching of response strategies, habit formation, stereotypic behavior, and organizing internally guided behavior toward a reward.

These circuits have also been implicated in the pathophysiology of major depressive disorder, another illness in which intrusive, distressing thoughts recur to an extent that the ability to switch to goal-oriented, rewarding, cognitive-behavioral sets is impaired. Although major depressive disorder and OCD appear distinct in their course, prognosis, genetics, and neurochemical concomitants, substantial comorbidity exists across these syndromes. Major depressive episodes occur in approximately one-half of patients with OCD, pathological obsessions commonly arise in primary major depressive disorder, and the pharmacological interventions that ameliorate OCD also effectively treat major depressive disorder. Moreover, the neurosurgical procedures that can reduce obsessive-compulsive and depressive symptoms in intractable cases of OCD and major depressive disorder interrupt white matter tracts carrying neural projections between the frontal lobe, basal ganglia, and thalamus. The clinical comorbidity across these two disorders may thus reflect involvement of an overlapping neural circuitry by otherwise distinct pathophysiological processes.

NEURORECEPTOR IMAGING IN ANXIETY DISORDERS

The anatomical circuits supporting fear and anxiety processing are modulated by a variety of chemical neurotransmitter systems. These systems involve the peptidergic neurotransmitters, such as CRH, neuropeptide Y, substance P and a variety of opioids, the monoaminergic transmitters, NE, serotonin (5-HT) and dopamine (DA), the amino acid transmitters, GABA and glutamate, and adrenal steroids such as cortisol. These neurochemical systems subserve important adaptive functions in preparing the organism for responding to threat or stress by increasing vigilance, modulating memory, mobilizing energy stores, and elevating cardiovascular function but can become maladaptive if chronically or inappropriately activated.

The neuroimaging literature regarding these neurochemical concomitants of stress and fear and their potential relevance to the pathophysiology of anxiety disorders are reviewed in the following discussion. This literature is limited by the paucity of PET radioligands available for in vivo investigation of neurochemical systems in anxiety-disordered humans. For example, among the neurotransmitter systems that have been best studied in experimental animals in association with responses to stress or threat are the central noradrenergic system and the HPA axis. However, PET radioligands for noradrenergic, glucocorticoid, or CRF receptors are thus far unavailable for human imaging, so limited information exists on these receptor systems in human anxiety disorders.

Central Benzodiazepine–γ-Aminobutyric Acid (GABA) Receptor System Several lines of preclinical and clinical evidence have established that benzodiazepine (BZD) receptor agonists exert anxiolytic effects and suggest that BZD receptor function is altered in anxiety disorders. Central BZD receptors are expressed throughout the brain but are most densely concentrated in the cerebral cortex. The BZD and GABA type A ($GABA_A$) receptors form parts of the same macromolecular complex, and, although they constitute distinct binding sites, they are functionally coupled and regulate each other in an allosteric manner. Central BZD receptor agonists potentiate and prolong the synaptic actions of the inhibitory neurotransmitter, GABA, by increasing the frequency of GABA-mediated chloride channel openings. Microinjection of BZD receptor agonists in limbic and brainstem regions such as the amygdala and the PAG exerts antianxiety effects in animal models of anxiety and fear. Conversely, administration of BZD receptor inverse agonists produces behaviors and increases in heart rate, blood pressure, plasma cortisol, and catecholamines that are similar to those seen in anxiety and stress, and these effects are blocked by administration of BZD receptor agonists.

Receptor imaging studies using PET and single photon emission computed tomography (SPECT) have assessed central BZD receptor binding in panic disorder and PTSD. In panic disorder, multiple SPECT studies reported reduced uptake of the selective BZD receptor radioligand, [^{123}I]iomazenil, in the frontal cortex, left hippocampus, lateral temporal cortex, and occipital cortex in panic disorder relative to control samples. One SPECT-iomazenil study additionally reported that the BZD receptor binding in the frontal cortex was inversely correlated with panic anxiety ratings in unmedicated panic disorder subjects. The central BZD receptor binding has also been assessed in panic disorder by using PET imaging and [^{11}C]flumazenil. One study reported a global reduction in BZD receptor binding in panic disorder subjects relative to healthy controls, with the most prominent decreases evident in the right orbitofrontal cortex and insula, but the other found no differences in the receptor density, dissociation constant (K_d), or bound and free values for [^{11}C]flumazenil in any brain region in unmedicated panic disorder subjects relative to healthy controls. In PTSD, the BZD receptor binding was reported to be decreased in the rostral mPFC in the vicinity of BA9 and BA10 in PTSD subjects relative to healthy controls in a SPECT-[^{123}I]iomazenil study and a PET-[^{11}C]flumazenil study.

The imaging data showing differences in central BZD binding in panic disorder are noteworthy in light of evidence that the behavioral sensitivity to pharmacological challenges involving this system is altered in panic disorder. Oral or IV administration of the BZD receptor antagonist, flumazenil (Romazicon), produces panic attacks and increases anticipatory anxiety in a large proportion of subjects with panic disorder but not in healthy controls. In addition, the effects of diazepam (Valium) on saccadic eye-movement velocity are abnormally reduced in panic disorder, implying that the functional sensitivity of the $GABA_A$-BZD supramolecular complex is diminished in brainstem regions controlling saccadic eye movements. Similarly, panic disorder subjects also show abnormally reduced sensitivity to the suppressant effects of diazepam on plasma NE, epinephrine, and heart rate.

The neuroimaging findings of reduced BZD receptor binding in the PfC in panic disorder and PTSD also appear consistent with evidence that stress downregulates BZD receptor binding in the frontal cortex and the hippocampus of experimental animals. In rats exposed to inescapable stress in the form of cold swim or foot shock, the BZD receptor binding decreases in the frontal cortex, shows less consistent reductions in the hippocampus and hypothalamus, and does not change in the occipital cortex, striatum, midbrain, thalamus, or cerebellum. When such stressors are administered repeatedly or chronically, BZD receptor binding additionally decreases in the hippocampus (i.e., in addition to frontal cortex) and may also decrease in the cerebellum, midbrain, and striatum but remains unaltered in the occipital cortex.

Serotoninergic System Acute exposure to a variety of severe stressors, including restraint stress, tail shock, tail pinch, and high level foot shock, results in increased 5-HT turnover in the mPFC, nucleus accumbens, amygdala, and lateral hypothalamus in experimental animals. During exposure to fear-conditioned stimuli, the 5-HT turnover in the mPFC appears particularly sensitive to the severity of stress, increasing as the aversiveness of the UCS and the magnitude of the conditioned fear behavioral response increase. In contrast, repeated exposure to electric shocks sufficient to produce learned helplessness is associated with reduced in vivo release of 5-HT in the frontal cortex. Preadministration of BZD receptor agonists or tricyclic antidepressant drugs prevents this stress-induced reduction in 5-HT release and interferes with the acquisition of learned helplessness, whereas infusion of 5-HT into the frontal cortex after stress exposure reverses learned helplessness behavior. The effect of stress in activating 5-HT turnover may stimulate anxiogenic and anxiolytic pathways within the forebrain, depending on the region that is involved and the 5-HT receptor subtype that is predominantly stimulated. For example, microinjection of 5-HT into the amygdala enhances conditioned fear, whereas 5-HT injection into the PAG inhibits unconditioned fear.

In panic disorder, the results of pharmacological challenge studies suggest that alterations in some individual 5-HT receptors may play a role in the pathophysiology of panic disorder, although abnormalities of serotoninergic function in general may not exist in panic disorder. For example, neuroendocrine responses to challenge with the 5-HT precursors, L-tryptophan and 5-hydroxytryptophan (5-HTP), did not differentiate panic disorder subjects from healthy controls, and tryptophan depletion did not prove anxiogenic in unmedicated panic disorder subjects. Nevertheless, challenge with the 5-HT–releasing agent, fenfluramine, produced greater increases in anxiety, plasma prolactin, and cortisol in panic disorder compared to control subjects. In a PET-[O-15]water study, fenfluramine challenge resulted in reduced CBF in the left posterior parietal-superior temporal cortex in panic disorder subjects relative to healthy controls, although it was unclear whether this abnormality reflected dysfunction of the serotonergic system or a physiological correlate of fenfluramine-induced anxiety, because more panic disorder subjects (56 percent) developed panic attacks than control subjects (11 percent).

Studies of the sensitivity of specific 5-HT receptor subtypes implicated 5-HT type 1A ($5\text{-}HT_{1A}$) receptor function in the pathophysiology of panic disorder. The elevation of plasma corticotrophin (ACTH) and cortisol and the hypothermic responses to the $5\text{-}HT_{1A}$ receptor partial agonist, ipsapirone, were blunted in panic disorder relative to healthy control samples. Consistent with this blunted sensitivity to $5\text{-}HT_{1A}$ receptor agonist challenge, a PET study using a selective, $5\text{-}HT_{1A}$ receptor radioligand reported that the $5\text{-}HT_{1A}$ receptor binding potential (proportional to density × affinity) is decreased in the hippocampus and raphe nucleus of panic disorder subjects relative to healthy controls. Similar abnormalities have also been demonstrated in major depressive disorder and bipolar disorder. Notably, $5\text{-}HT_{1A}$ receptor knockout mice show a marked elevation of anxiety and fear behaviors, as well as behavioral despair responses, which can all be reversed if rescued by administration of $5\text{-}HT_{1A}$ receptor agonists, as long as these agents are administered before a critical developmental period.

These findings regarding the $5\text{-}HT_{1A}$ receptor system may conceivably reflect effects of repeated or chronic stress on the genetic expression of $5\text{-}HT_{1A}$ receptors. Postsynaptic $5\text{-}HT_{1A}$ receptor gene expression is under tonic inhibition by adrenal steroids in the hippocampus and other regions in which mineralocorticoid receptors are expressed. Thus, $5\text{-}HT_{1A}$ receptor density and messenger ribonucleic acid (mRNA) levels decrease in response to chronic stress or cortisol administration and increase after adrenalectomy. The stress-induced downregulation of $5\text{-}HT_{1A}$ receptor expression is prevented by adrenalectomy, showing the importance of circulating adrenal steroids in mediating this effect. Conversely, 5-HT type 2A (5-HT_{2A}) receptor expression is upregulated during chronic stress and cortisol administration and downregulated in response to adrenalectomy. In view of evidence that chronic administration of $5HT_{1A}$ receptor partial agonists and 5-HT_{2A} receptor antagonists each exert anxiolytic effects in a variety of chronic anxiety states, it is conceivable that these stress- and corticosteroid-mediated effects on 5-HT_{1A} and 5-HT_{2A} receptor expression are relevant to the pathophysiology of anxiety.

Dopaminergic System Acute stress increases DA release and turnover in multiple brain areas. The dopaminergic projections to the mPFC appear particularly sensitive to stress, as brief or low-intensity stressors (e.g., exposure to fear conditioned stimuli) increase DA release and turnover in the mPFC in the absence of corresponding changes in other mesotelencephalic dopaminergic projections. For example, in rats, low-intensity electric foot shock increases tyrosine hydroxylase activity and DA turnover in the mPFC but not in the nucleus accumbens or caudate-putamen. In contrast, stress of greater intensity or longer duration additionally enhances DA release and metabolism in other areas as well. The regional sensitivity to stress thus appears to follow a pattern in which dopaminergic projections to the mPFC are more sensitive to stress than the mesoaccumbens and nigrostriatal projections, and the mesoaccumbens dopaminergic projections are more sensitive to stress than the nigrostriatal projections.

PET-[^{11}C]raclopride imaging studies of dynamic DA release during administration of dopaminergic drugs have permitted correlation between the amount of DA released in the striatum and associated changes in anxiety and euphoria ratings in humans. In healthy humans, the amount of DA released during dextroamphetamine administration correlates negatively with anxiety and positively with euphoria in the ventral striatum but not in the dorsal striatum. Consistent with this observation, DA depletion induced by α-methyl-para-tyrosine administration results in increased anxiety responses to moderately severe stressors in healthy humans.

Although there is little evidence that dopaminergic dysfunction plays a primary role in the pathophysiology of human anxiety disorders, two preliminary SPECT studies involving small subject samples reported abnormal reductions in DA binding sites in social phobia. One of these found a significant reduction in methyl 3β-(4-iodo-phenyl)tropane-2β-carboxylate (β-CIT) binding in the striatum in social phobics relative to healthy control samples, presumably reflecting a reduction in DA transporter binding. The other reported reduced uptake of the DA type 2 and 3 receptor radioligand, [^{123}I] iodobenzamide (IBZM), in social phobics relative to healthy control subjects. Both findings await replication.

Imaging and the Central Noradrenergic System in Fear and Anxiety Exposure to stressful stimuli of various types increases central noradrenergic function. For example, exposure to fear-conditioned stimuli, immobilization stress, foot shock, or tail pinch increases NE turnover in the LC, hypothalamus, hippocampus, amygdala, and cerebral cortex. The firing activity of LC neurons also increases during exposure to fear-conditioned stimuli and other stressors or threats. Repeated exposure to severe stressors from which the animal cannot escape, in contrast, results in a reduction of NE release that is associated with the behavioral pattern termed *learned helplessness*.

The responsiveness of LC neurons to future novel stressors can be enhanced by chronic exposure to some stressful experiences. In rats, the amount of NE synthesized and released in the hippocampus and the mPFC in response to a novel stressor or to local depolarization is exaggerated after repeated exposure to chronic cold stress. This effect of chronic stress on noradrenergic responses to subsequent, novel stressors may constitute a form of *behavioral sensitization*, in which single or repeated exposures to aversive stimuli or pharmacological agents can increase the behavioral sensitivity to subsequent stressors.

Subjects with PTSD and panic disorder show evidence of heightened peripheral sympathetic nervous system arousal, which, because of the correlation between peripheral sympathetic activity and central noradrenergic function, is compatible with the hypothesis of increased central NE activity in these disorders. Panic disorder has been specifically associated with elevations of α_2-adrenoreceptor sensitivity and nocturnal urinary NE excretion, although β-adrenoreceptor function, baseline heart rate and blood pressure, and other measures reflecting central NE secretion are not consistently altered in panic disorder. In addition, administration of the α_2-adrenoreceptor antagonist, yohimbine (Actibine) (which stimulates NE release by antagonizing presynaptic α_2-adrenoreceptors), produces exaggerated anxiogenic and cardiovascular responses and enhanced plasma 3-methoxy-4-hydroxyphenylglycol (MHPG) and cortisol increases in panic disorder relative to control subjects. One SPECT [^{99m}Tc]-hexamethyl propyleneamine oxime imaging study reported that yohimbine administration resulted in reduced relative frontal cortex perfusion in panic disorder subjects but not in controls. It remains unclear, however, whether this difference reflected a differential physiological sensitivity to yohimbine or an effect of greater anxiety in the panic disorder subjects, as all of the panic disorder subjects, but only one control subject, developed increased anxiety in response to yohimbine.

The sensitivity of α_2-adrenoreceptors also appears to be increased in PTSD. Subjects with combat-related PTSD show increased behavioral, chemical, and cardiovascular responses to yohimbine, relative to healthy controls. Potentially compatible with these observations, a PET-fluorodeoxyglucose study of glucose metabolic responses to yohimbine administration found differences in glucose metabolism activity in the orbital, temporal, parietal, and prefrontal cortices in PTSD subjects relative to healthy controls.

Opioid Peptides Acute, uncontrollable shock increases secretion of opiate peptides and decreases μ-opiate receptor density in rodents. The elevation of opioid peptide secretion may contribute to the analgesia observed after uncontrollable stress and exposure to fear-conditioned stimuli. This analgesic effect shows evidence of sensitization, as subsequent exposure to less intense shock in rats previously exposed to uncontrollable shock also results in analgesia.

Potentially consistent with these data, PTSD subjects show reduced pain sensitivity compared to veterans without PTSD after exposure to a combat film, an effect that is reversed by the opiate antagonist naloxone (Narcan) (suggesting mediation by endogenous opiate release during symptom provocation). In the baseline state, the cerebrospinal fluid (CSF) beta-endorphin levels were abnormally elevated in PTSD relative to control samples. In addition, a preliminary study of μ-opioid receptor binding in PTSD observed that [^{11}C]carfentanil binding was increased in the amygdala, ACC, and anterior insula of PTSD subjects relative to healthy controls and that the magnitude of the μ-opioid receptor binding potential in the amygdala correlated inversely with ratings of PTSD and anxiety severity.

FUTURE DIRECTIONS

The application of neuroimaging technology to investigation of the neurobiological basis of anxiety disorders is yielding seminal information about the functional anatomical and neurochemical correlates of normal and pathological anxiety and fear states. In some cases, the inconsistency in the results of neuroimaging studies of anxiety disorders highlights the importance of addressing the neurobiological heterogeneity inherent within criteria-based, psychiatric diagnoses. Elucidating this heterogeneity will be facilitated by the application of newer neuroimaging technologies and radioligands and the integration of neuroimaging data with information obtained from genetic and neurochemical approaches to refine anxiety disorder phenotypes and to elucidate the genotypes associated with these phenotypes. Pursuit of these experimental approaches will also facilitate research aimed at elucidating the mechanisms of antianxiety therapies.

SUGGESTED CROSS-REFERENCES

The basic principles of nuclear magnetic resonance imaging (nMRI) are discussed in Section 1.15, and the basic principles of radiotracer imaging are discussed in Section 1.16.

References

Adolphs R, Tranel D, Damascio H, Damascio AR: Fear and the human amygdala. *J Neurosci.* 1995;15:5879–5891.

Bandler R, Shipley MT: Columnar organization in the midbrain periaqueductal grey: Modules for emotional expression? *Trends Neurosci.* 1994;17:379–389.

Bremner JD, Innis RB, Southwick SM, Staib LH, Zoghbi S, Charney DS: Decreased benzodiazepine receptor binding in prefrontal cortex in combat-related posttraumatic stress disorder. *Am J Psychiatry.* 2000;157:1120–1126.

Bremner JD, Narayan M, Staib LH, Southwick SM, McGlashan T, Charney DS: Neural correlates of memories of childhood sexual abuse in women with and without posttraumatic stress disorder. *Am J Psychiatry.* 1999;156:1787–1795.

Bremner JD, Staib LH, Kaloupek D, Southwick SM, Soufer R, Charney DS: Neural correlates of exposure to traumatic pictures and sounds in Vietnam combat veterans with and without posttraumatic stress disorder: A positron emission tomography study. *Biol Psychiatry.* 1999;45:806–816.

Charney DS, Drevets WC. The neurobiological basis of anxiety disorders. In: Davis K, Charney DS, Coyle J, Nemeroff CB, eds. *Psychopharmacology: The Fifth Generation of Progress.* New York: Lippincott Williams & Wilkins; 2002:901–930.

Damasio AR, Tranel D, Damasio H: Individuals with sociopathic behavior caused by frontal damage fail to respond autonomically to social stimuli. *Behav Brain Res.* 1990;41:81–94.

Davis M: Are different parts of the extended amygdala involved in fear versus anxiety? *Biol Psychiatry.* 1998;44:1239–1247.

Dioro D, Viau V, Meaney MJ: The role of the medial prefrontal cortex (cingulate gyrus) in the regulation of hypothalamic-pituitary-adrenal responses to stress. *J Neurosci.* 1993;3:3839–3847.

Drevets WC, Raichle ME: Reciprocal suppression of regional cerebral blood flow during emotional versus higher cognitive processes: Implications for interactions between emotion and cognition. *Cogn Emotion.* 1998;12:353–385.

Drevets WC, Simpson JR, Raichle ME: Regional blood flow changes in response to phobic anxiety and habituation. *J Cereb Blood Flow Metab.* 1995;15:S856.

Ferry B, Roozendaal B, McGaugh JL: Role of norepinephrine in mediating stress hormone regulation of long-term memory storage: A critical involvement of the amygdala. *Biol Psychiatry.* 1999;46:1140–1152.

Frysztak RJ, Neafsey EJ: The effect of medial frontal cortex lesions on cardiovascular conditioned emotional responses in the rat. *Brain Res.* 1994;643:181–193.

*Garcia R, Vouimba R-M, Baudry M, Thompson RF: The amygdala modulates prefrontal cortex activity relative to conditioned fear. *Nature.* 1999;402:294–296.

*Gilbertson MW, Shenton ME, Ciszewski A, Kasai K, Lasko NB, Orr SP, Pitman RK: Smaller hippocampal volume predicts pathologic vulnerability to psychological trauma. *Nat Neurosci.* 2002;5:1242–1247.

Gloor P, Olivier A, Quesney LF, Andermann F, Horowitz S: The role of the limbic system in experiential phenomena of temporal lobe epilepsy. *Ann Neurol.* 1982;12:129–144.

LaBar KS, Gatenby JC, Gore JC, LeDoux JE, Phelps EA: Human amygdala activation during conditioned fear acquisition and extinction: A mixed trial fMRI study. *Neuron.* 1998;20:937–945.

LaPlane D: Obsessive-compulsive and other behavioural changes with bilateral basal ganglia lesions. *Brain.* 1989;112:699–725.

LeDoux J: Fear and the brain: Where have we been, and where are we going? *Biol Psychiatry.* 1998;44:1229–1238.

Lesch KP, Wiesmann M, Hoh A: 5-HT1A receptor-effector system responsivity in panic disorder. *Psychopharmacology.* 1992;106:111–117.

Liberzon I, Taylor SF, Amdur R, Jung TD, Chamberlain KR, Minoshima S, Koeppe RA, Fig LM: Brain activation in PTSD in response to trauma-related stimuli. *Biol Psychiatry.* 1999;45:817–826.

López JF, Chalmers DT, Little KY, Watson SJ: Regulation of serotonin$_{1A}$, glucocorticoid, and mineralocorticoid receptor in rat and human hippocampus: Implications for the neurobiology of depression. *Biol Psychiatry.* 1998;43:547–573.

Maddock RJ: The retrosplenial cortex and emotion: New insights from functional neuroimaging of the human brain. *Trends Neurosci.* 1999;22:310–316.

Makino S, Gold PW, Schulkin J: Effects of corticosterone on CRH mRNA and content in the bed nucleus of the stria terminalis; comparison with the effects in the central nucleus of the amygdala and the paraventricular nucleus of the hypothalamus. *Brain Res.* 1994;657:141–149.

Malizia AL, Cunningham VJ, Bell CJ, Liddle PF, Jones T, Nutt DJ: Decreased brain GABA$_{A-}$benzodiazepine receptor binding in panic disorder: Preliminary results from a quantitative PET study. *Arch Gen Psychiatry.* 1998;55:715–720.

McEwen BS: Stress and hippocampal plasticity. *Ann Rev Neurosci.* 1999;22:105–122.

Milad MR, Quirk GJ: Neurons in medial prefrontal cortex signal memory for fear extinction. *Nature.* 2002;420:70–74.

Morgan MA, LeDoux JE: Contribution of ventrolateral prefrontal cortex to the acquisition and extinction of conditioned fear in rats. *Neurobiol Learn Mem.* 1999;72: 244–251.

Neumeister A, Bain E, Nugent A, Carson RE, Bonne O, Luckenbaugh D, Eckelman W, Herscovitch P, Charney DS, Drevets WC: Reduced serotonin type 1A receptor binding in panic disorder. *J Neurosci.* 2004;24:589–591.

Nutt DJ, Glue P, Lawson C, Wilson S: Flumazenil provocation of panic attacks: Evidence for altered benzodiazepine receptor sensitivity in panic disorder. *Arch Gen Psychiatry.* 1990;47:917–925.

Phillips ML, Drevets WC, Rauch SL, Lane RD: The neurobiology of emotion perception I: Towards an understanding of the neural basis of normal emotion perception. *Biol Psychiatry.* 2003;54:504–514.

Phillips ML, Drevets WC, Rauch SL, Lane RD: The neurobiology of emotion perception II: Implications for understanding the neural basis of emotion perceptual abnormalities in schizophrenia and affective disorders. *Biol Psychiatry.* 2003;54: 515–528.

Pitman RK, van der Kolk BA, Orr SP, Greenberg MS: Naloxone-reversible analgesic response to combat-related stimuli in posttraumatic stress disorder. Arch Gen Psychiatry. 1990;47:541–544.

*Quirk GJ, Russo GK, Barron JL, Lebron K: The role of the ventromedial prefrontal cortex in the recovery of extinguished fear. *J Neurosci.* 2000;20:16.

*Ramboz S, Oosting R, Amara DA, Kung HF, Blier P, Mendelsohn M, Mann JJ, Brunner D, Hen R: Serotonin receptor 1A knockout: An animal model of anxiety-related disorder. *Proc Natl Acad Sci U S A.* 1998;95:14476–14481.

Rauch SL, Savage CR, Alpert NM, Fischman AJ, Jenike MA: The functional neuroanatomy of anxiety: A study of three disorders using positron emission tomography and symptom provocation. *Biol Psychiatry.* 1997;42:446–452.

Rauch SL, Whalen PJ, Shin LM, McInerney, Macklin ML, Lasko NB, Orr SP, Pitman RK: Exaggerated amygdala response to masked facial stimuli in posttraumatic stress disorder: A functional MRI study. *Biol Psychiatry.* 2000;47:769–776.

Reiman EM, Raichle ME, Robins E, Mintun MA, Fusselman MJ, Fox PT, Price JL, Hackman K: Neuroanatomical correlates of a lactate-induced anxiety attack. *Arch Gen Psychiatry.* 1989;46:493–500.

Roozendaal B: Glucocorticoids and the regulation of memory consolidation. *Psychoneuroendocrinology.* 2000;25:213–238.

Schneider F, Weiss U, Kessler C, Muller-Gartner HW, Posse S, Salloum JB, Grodd W, Himmelmann F, Gaebel W, Birbaumer N: Subcortical correlates of differential classical conditioning of aversive emotional reactions in social phobia. *Biol Psychiatry.* 1999;45:863–871.

Schneier FR, Liebowitz MR, Abi-Dargham A, Zea-Ponce Y, Lin SH, Laruelle M: Low dopamine D(2) receptor binding potential in social phobia. *Am J Psychiatry.* 2000;157:457–459.

*Shin LM, McNally RJ, Kosslyn SM, Thompson WL, Rauch SL, Alpert NM, Metzger LJ, Lasko NB, Orr SP, Pitman RK: Regional cerebral blood flow during script-driven imagery in childhood sexual abuse-related PTSD: A PET investigation. *Am J Psychiatry.* 1999;156:575–584.

Sullivan RM, Gratton A: Lateralized effects of medial prefrontal cortex lesions on neuroendocrine and autonomic stress responses in rats. *J Neurosci.* 1999;19:2834–2840.

Vythilingam M, Heim C, Newport J, Miller AH, Anderson E, Bronen R, Brummer M, Staib L, Vermetten E, Charney DS, Nemeroff CB, Bremner JD: Childhood trauma associated with smaller hippocampal volume in women with major depression. *Am J Psychiatry.* 2002;159:2072–2080.

Weizman A, Weisman R, Kook KA, Vocci F, Deutsch SI, Paul SM: Adrenalectomy prevents the stress-induced decrease in in vivo [^{3}H]Ro 15-1788 binding to GABA$_A$ benzodiazepine receptors in the mouse. *Brain Res.* 1990;519:347–350.

Woods SW, Charney DS, Silver JM, Krystal JH, Heninger GR: Behavioral, biochemical, and cardiovascular responses to the benzodiazepine receptor antagonist flumazenil in panic disorder. *Psychiatry Res.* 1988;36:115–124.

▲ 14.6 Anxiety Disorders: Genetics

FRANCIS J. MCMAHON, M.D., AND LAYLA KASSEM, PSY.D.

Anxiety is a mood state characterized by a markedly negative affect and somatic symptoms of tension in which people apprehensively anticipate future danger. The study of anxiety disorders poses a challenge because anxiety can be manifested through a variety of phenomena: a subjective sense of unease; a set of behaviors, such as avoidance and restlessness; or a physiological response originating in the nervous system, such as increased heart rate, perspiration, and muscle tension. These phenomena are not in themselves abnormal, but are considered "disorders" when they lead to marked distress or impairment in function. Even within the realm of anxiety disorders, the subjective experience of anxiety differs markedly. In panic disorder and generalized anxiety disorder, the anxiety is unfocused; phobias and posttraumatic stress disorder (PTSD) involve a fear aroused by specific, identifiable objects or situations; and in obsessive-compulsive disorder (OCD), anxiety occurs when the patient *resists* a thought or behavior. Furthermore, anxiety disorders often cooccur with a variety of other psychiatric illnesses, especially mood disorders.

This multiplicity in both the phenomena and experience of anxiety complicates research aimed at uncovering the genetic basis of anxiety disorders. Heredity has been recognized as a predisposing factor in the development of anxiety disorders since at least the late 19th century. Despite this early insight, psychodynamic and learning theories dominated etiological research in anxiety disorders up until the 1980s. Although psychodynamic and learning theories remain significant, recent decades have been marked by a growing interest in and focus on genetic contributions to the etiology of anxiety disorders, particularly panic disorder. What is currently known about the role of genetics in the etiology of the anxiety disorders is based on data gathered from family, twin, and adoption studies, as well as more recent genetic linkage and association studies. Studies of model organisms have provided some promising leads, but much remains to be learned.

In the 1970s, three anxiety disorders were recognized, and all were considered to be under the rubric of "neurosis": phobia, obsessional neurosis, and anxiety neurosis, which included panic attacks. The revised fourth edition of the *Diagnostic and Statistical Manual of Mental Disorders* (DSM-IV-TR) divides anxiety disorders into six groups: panic disorder with or without agoraphobia, generalized anxiety disorder, specific phobia, social phobia, OCD, and PTSD. Of these, panic disorder has been the subject of the most genetic studies. Evidence of a genetic contribution to the other anxiety disorders can certainly be found in the literature, but it is weaker and less extensive than that which is available for panic disorder.

METHODS AND TERMINOLOGY

Genetics is still a rather specialized science, so a brief review of genetic methods and terminology is provided. The focus of human genetics research ranges widely, from populations (population genetics and genetic epidemiology) to molecules (cellular and molecular genetics), unified by a common focus on biological variation in traits, such as susceptibility to disease (Table 14.6–1). *Complex genetics* refers to the study of diseases that do not display simple, Mendelian patterns of inheritance. Non-Mendelian inheritance is seen when there is no direct, one-to-one relationship between gene and disease, usually due to the influence of other genes and of nongenetic (environmental) factors. Most common diseases with a genetic basis—including most anxiety disorders—display non-Mendelian patterns of inheritance.

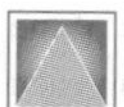

Table 14.6–1
Methods of Study in Human Genetics

Method	Key Variable
Family study	Familiality
Twin study	Heritability
Adoption study	Genetic transmission
Cytogenetics	Chromosomal abnormalities
Genetic linkage	Cosegregation of marker and disease
Genetic association	Allele frequencies
Gene expression	Relative abundance of transcript

Genetic epidemiological investigations take the form of family, twin, and adoption studies, which establish the importance of genetics in the etiology of a disease. Although the methods of genetic epidemiology help parse the genetic and nongenetic contributions to disease, genetic epidemiology is an observational, rather than experimental, science, thus limiting the conclusions that can be drawn from genetic epidemiological data.

In *twin studies*, the relative genetic contribution to an illness (*heritability*) can be estimated by comparing identical (monozygotic) twins with fraternal (dizygotic) twins. Because monozygotic twins share all genes while dizygotic twins share, on average, only half, monozygotic twins should be more alike, or concordant, for a trait with a substantial genetic contribution. Although twin studies cannot definitively establish a genetic etiology for a disease, they are a fundamental starting point.

Family studies reveal the familial nature of a disease: its mode of inheritance, the range of clinical or phenotypic expression within the family, and the intergenerational differences resulting from dynamic genes and environments. The classic family study design requires the collection of a large sample of unrelated cases, or probands, followed by the systematic evaluation of relatives. A properly collected family sample is valuable for many kinds of studies. Segregation analysis attempts to model the mode of inheritance. Studies of the rates of illness among relatives can help define traits that belong to the range of clinical expression for that illness, or its phenotypic spectrum.

Because familial traits are not necessarily genetic, the genetic basis of a familial trait is best demonstrated by *adoption studies*. In the simplest adoption study design, the rates of a disease are compared in the biological and the adoptive parents of adoptees who are affected by that disease. Diseases due more to genetic influences will tend to occur in biological parents of the adoptees, whereas diseases due more to environmental influences will tend to occur in the adoptive parents. Adoption study designs are the best way to control for environmental influences in human genetics.

Twin, family, and adoption studies form a kind of three-part account of the genetic basis of disease that is often viewed as a prerequisite for molecular genetic studies, although this may change as molecular methods become ever more powerful. Unlike bipolar disorder and schizophrenia, remarkably few anxiety disorders have so far been subjected to all three kinds of genetic epidemiological investigations.

Molecular genetic studies can be conveniently grouped into studies of linkage, association, and gene expression. In *linkage studies*, genetic markers whose locations on each chromosome are known with some precision are used to track the transmission of disease within a family. Diseases that are consistently transmitted together with a particular genetic marker are likely to be caused by a gene residing near that same marker. A linkage study can identify the general location of a gene, not the gene itself. The final localization of the gene depends on a potentially laborious process of elimination, studying each gene in the linked segment for evidence of changes associated with disease.

It is at the stage of pinpointing a particular disease gene that association studies come into play. *Association studies* look for the cooccurrence of marker and disease in populations. Association studies can be used to evaluate the potential role of a particular known gene in a disease, as in candidate gene studies. Association studies are also useful for the fine mapping of disease genes because association signals extend a short distance across a chromosome in most populations. Association studies are often performed in a sample of cases and controls. Such a design can be powerful, but it is subject to spurious findings due to genetic differences between cases and controls unrelated to the disease of interest. For this reason, family-based designs that determine the proportion of marker alleles transmitted by heterozygous parents to affected offspring are often preferred.

Direct studies of gene expression and function are usually necessary to definitively establish the role of particular gene or set of genes in disease. *Gene expression studies* have benefited enormously in recent years from the introduction of micro-array technology. This technology is now beginning to be applied in the field of anxiety disorders. A set of expressed genes (complementary deoxyribonucleic acid [cDNA]) is placed onto a solid chip, then exposed to messenger ribonucleic acid (mRNA) from a region of the brain. Highly sensitive tags allow for a precise determination of the relative degree of hybridization between the test mRNA molecules and each cDNA molecule. In this way, the full range of genes represented on the chip can be tested for increased or decreased expression in brain. Comparisons between cases and controls may reveal differences, but it is important to consider drug exposures and other confounding variables in interpreting the changes seen.

PANIC DISORDER

Worldwide, the lifetime prevalence of panic disorder ranges between 1 and 3 percent. Women are affected approximately twice as often as men. Panic disorder is most common in young adulthood. Studies have focused on the possible role of environmental as well as genetic factors, and some have attempted to elucidate the interaction between developmental, environmental, and genetic influences. The many different studies conducted on panic disorder suggest that familial contributions appear strong; however, the exact genetic mechanisms involved remain elusive. The four main methods used to study the influence of heredity on panic disorder have been family, twin, linkage, and association studies.

Family Studies

Panic disorder has been the subject of several family studies, all of which have revealed increased rates of panic disorder among the first-degree relatives of probands compared with relatives of subjects with no mental illness. The age-adjusted morbidity risk to first-degree relatives of probands with panic disorder ranges from 7 to 20 percent, approximately two to four times higher than the risk to relatives of unaffected control probands (Table 14.6–2). The risk for other disorders is also increased among the relatives of probands with panic disorder, including phobias, alcoholism, and possibly major depression. Panic disorder may also be increased among the relatives of probands with comorbid panic and mood disorder.

Some family studies have focused on age at onset. As with other complex genetic disorders, probands with an earlier onset of panic disorder tend to have higher rates of panic disorder among their relatives. Conversely, probands from families with at least one additional case of panic disorder among close relatives tend to have an earlier age at onset than probands who have no affected relatives. This suggests a greater burden of familial risk factors in early-onset panic disorder, some of which are probably genetic.

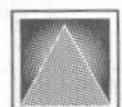

Table 14.6–2
Familial Relative Risks in Selected Anxiety Disorders

Disorder	Population Prevalence (%)	Familial Relative Risk[a]
Panic disorder	1–3	2–20
Generalized anxiety disorder	3–5	6
Obsessive-compulsive disorder	1–3	3–5

[a]Ratio of risk to relatives of cases versus risk to relatives of controls.

Segregation analyses have failed to reveal a consistent mode of inheritance for panic disorder. Some studies seem to support single locus models, but the majority of studies are most consistent with multifactorial or polygenic transmission of panic disorder in families. Several studies suggest that relatives of probands with panic disorder display increased sensitivity to inhaled carbon dioxide or to lactate (a metabolic product of carbon dioxide) infused intravenously (IV). This increased sensitivity manifests as anxiety or panic attacks, even among relatives who deny ever having had panic attacks before. This suggests that carbon dioxide or lactate sensitivity may be an alternative manifestation of panic disorder in susceptible individuals, a familial marker of an inherited susceptibility to panic disorder. Indeed, one segregation analysis that utilized the sensitivity phenotype found that the familial transmission pattern was compatible with a Mendelian model with incomplete penetrance—that is, a single gene that failed to manifest clinically in some relatives. Additionally, data from the same analysis suggested that families of probands with panic disorder and carbon dioxide sensitivity differed from other families. Additional research is needed to further elucidate these findings.

Twin Studies

There is a large twin literature in panic disorder. The results of several twin studies conducted over the years indicate that monozygotic twins are at least two to three times more likely to be concordant for panic disorder than dizygotic twins. The Virginia Twin Registry studies found that 24 percent of monozygotic twins were concordant for narrow definitions of panic disorder, compared to 11 percent of dizygotic twins. The best-fitting model suggested that genes jointly influence the risk of phobia, bulimia nervosa, and panic disorder, with the expression of a particular disease in a particular person largely determined by individual environmental factors. Similar concordance rates were observed in the Norwegian Twin Registry studies and in several smaller studies, all of which differ in phenotype definition, ascertainment methods, and sample sizes.

Linkage and Association Studies

Linkage and association studies of panic disorder have only commenced in the 1990s and are still in the early phases. The three genome-wide genetic linkage studies of panic disorder published so far were all inconclusive, but several genetic linkage studies of panic disorder are under way.

Association studies have focused on genes whose function can be plausibly related to panic attacks, including genes that encode neurotransmitter receptors, transporters, and related genes. Some studies implicate genes encoding the serotonin transporter, monoamine oxidase A, or catechol methyltransferase (COMT), but definitive findings have not yet emerged.

Other Studies

Chromosomal (cytogenetic) abnormalities have been reported in a few individuals and some families with panic disorder and related phenotypes. Further molecular work is needed to clarify whether these cytogenetic abnormalities play a causative role in these cases, and, if they do, which genes are involved.

GENERALIZED ANXIETY DISORDER

Generalized anxiety disorder is marked by the presence of diffuse, chronic, and continuous fear or apprehension, with feelings of tension and restlessness. Generalized anxiety disorder is differentiated from panic disorder (with which it often cooccurs) by the absence of spontaneous panic attacks. Genetic investigation of generalized anxiety disorder has been ongoing for less than a decade, but a few family and twin studies have been published. Those studies indicate possible genetic contributions to generalized anxiety disorder, but the results remain inconclusive, and further genetic epidemiologic investigations are needed. There are no published genetic linkage or association studies in people with generalized anxiety disorder.

Family Studies Several family studies have found an increased rate of generalized anxiety disorder among the relatives of probands with generalized anxiety disorder. A metaanalysis of selected family studies concluded that the familiality of generalized anxiety disorder was statistically significant, with an overall odds ratio of approximately 6 (Table 14.6–2).

Twin Studies The large twin studies present a mixed picture for generalized anxiety disorder. Whereas some studies suggest at least moderate heritability, others do not. Heritability seems to depend strongly on how cases are ascertained and defined in a particular study. In contrast, relatively high heritability estimates have come from twin studies that measure so-called trait anxiety, usually operationalized as high scores on standardized personality tests for anxiety-related personality traits or neuroticism.

Other Studies Several molecular genetic studies have focused on serotonin-related genes, in particular, the serotonin transporter, which contains a genetic polymorphism that reduces expression of the transporter protein in cells. Taken together, these studies suggest that the low-expression allele of the serotonin transporter accounts for at least a small portion of individual variation in trait anxiety. This same polymorphism may also modulate individual responses of the amygdala to fearful stimuli. It is likely that many genes, each of small effect, contribute to individual variation in anxiety, but that this correlates only loosely with the current definitions of anxiety disorder.

OBSESSIVE-COMPULSIVE DISORDER

Long considered a learned behavior, OCD is now recognized as having an important genetic basis. However, the variability of the clinical phenotype and lack of understanding of the molecular mechanism have complicated attempts to define specific genetic contributions to this common disorder. Several family studies have been conducted, showing clear familiality of OCD and indicating that several clinically similar conditions might be alternative expressions of the disorder. Twin studies show that most of the familiality of OCD has a genetic basis. Intriguing genetic linkage and association findings are beginning to appear in the literature but await confirmation by replication in other samples.

Family Studies Relatives of probands with OCD consistently have a three- to fivefold higher probability of having OCD or obsessive-compulsive features than families of control probands (Table 14.6–2). Some studies suggest that certain clinical features of OCD, such as hoarding behavior, are more familial than others, and that early age at onset predicts higher rates of illness among relatives. Some studies also demonstrate increased rates of a variety of conditions among relatives of OCD probands, including generalized anxiety disorder, tic disorders, body dysmorphic disorder, hypochondriasis, eating disorders, and habits such as nail-biting. These findings suggest that these conditions share familial, perhaps genetic, determinants in common with OCD.

Segregation analyses have proven more fruitful in OCD than in other anxiety disorders. Single locus and major gene effects have been suggested by more than one study, especially when OCD is broken down into its component clinical features and late-onset cases are excluded.

Twin Studies Data from twin studies of OCD suggest that OCD is heritable, with higher concordance rates for monozygotic twins than for dizygotic twins. However, all twin studies published to date suffer from significant methodological limitations.

Linkage and Association Studies One genome-wide genetic linkage study has been performed in families of probands with OCD. So far, no conclusive evidence of linkage has been found, but sample sizes have been too small to detect genes of small effect. Candidate gene association studies of OCD have so far failed to produce strong and widely replicated findings, but intriguing results with several functional candidates have appeared in the literature.

PHOBIAS

Phobias have been less studied genetically than the other anxiety disorders. Some family studies have been published that suggest that phobias are familial and predict higher rates of a variety of anxiety disorders in relatives. Twin studies indicate that at least some of the familiality of phobias is due to genetic factors, but some kinds of phobias (e.g., social phobia) appear to be more heritable than others. No genome-wide genetic linkage studies of phobias have been published. A few candidate gene linkage and association studies have appeared but did not have conclusive results.

POSTTRAUMATIC STRESS DISORDER

PTSD is a condition marked by the development of symptoms after exposure to traumatic life events. It was first introduced as a psychiatric diagnosis in the late 1980s but has probably existed as long as there have been wars and other severe traumatic experiences. The lifetime incidence of PTSD is estimated to be 9 to 15 percent. In spite of the moderately high incidence of this disorder, there is a paucity of data regarding its etiology. PTSD develops only after exposure to events that are fortunately rather unusual, which complicates genetic studies that rely on the availability of multiple cases per family or on large sample sizes.

Family and Twin Studies Family studies have shown that relatives of World Wars I and II veterans had a higher incidence of psychiatric disorders than families of controls. Another study concluded that paternal PTSD was associated with an increased risk for PTSD in offspring. Higher rates of PTSD are also found in families that show a predisposition toward depression and anxiety disorders. Although these results are consistent with the well-known association between PTSD and some other psychiatric disorders, they do not present a strong argument in support of a genetic basis for PTSD.

The first and largest study attempting to determine the genetic contribution to PTSD came out of the Vietnam Veterans Twin Registry. Two other twin studies have been published, both with small sample sizes. Taken together, these studies indicate that the heritability of PTSD ranges between 0.21 and 0.37.

Genetic Linkage and Association Studies There have been no genetic linkage studies conducted on people with PTSD. Only a few candidate gene association studies have been published, with no established findings to date. A number of interesting traits have been associated with PTSD in case control studies, including abnormalities of the pituitary-adrenal axis and of the startle response. These traits might be excellent endophenotypes for future genetic linkage and association studies of PTSD.

SUGGESTED CROSS-REFERENCES

The reader is encouraged to refer to the related sections on genetics (Sections 1.17 and 1.18), anxiety disorder epidemiology (Section 14.2), and anxiety disorder clinical features (Section 14.8).

REFERENCES

Breslau N, Davis GC, Andreski P, Peterson E: Traumatic events and posttraumatic stress disorder in an urban population of young adults. *Arch Gen Psychiatry*. 1991;48:216–222.

Bromet E, Sonnega A, Kessler RC: Risk factors for DSM-III-R posttraumatic stress disorder: Findings from the National Comorbidity Survey. *Am J Epidemiol*. 1998;147:353–361.

Chantarujikapong SI, Scherrer JF, Xian H, Eisen SA, Lyons MJ, Goldberg J, Tsuang M, True WR: A twin study of generalized anxiety disorder symptoms, panic disorder symptoms and post-traumatic stress disorder in men. *Psychiatry Res*. 2001;103:133–145.

Connor KM, Davidson JR: Familial risk factors in posttraumatic stress disorder. *Ann N Y Acad Sci*. 1997;821:35–51.

Crowe RR, Goedken R, Samuelson S, Wilson R, Nelson J, Noyes R Jr: Genomewide survey of panic disorder. *Am J Med Genet*. 2001;105:105–109.

Finn CT, Smoller JW. The genetics of panic disorder. *Curr Psychiatry Rep*. 2001;3:131–137.

Gelernter J, Bonvicini K, Page G, Woods SW, Goddard AW, Kruger S, Pauls DL, Goodson S: Linkage genome scan for loci predisposing to panic disorder or agoraphobia. *Am J Med Genet*. 2001;105:548–557.

Hamilton SP, Fyer AJ, Durner M, Heiman GA, Baisre de Leon A, Hodge SE, Knowles JA, Weissman MM: Further genetic evidence for a panic disorder syndrome mapping to chromosome 13q. *Proc Natl Acad Sci U S A*. 2003;100:2550–2555.

Hariri AR, Mattay VS, Tessitore A, Kolachana B, Fera F, Goldman D, Egan MF, Weinberger DR: Serotonin transporter genetic variation and the response of the human amygdala. Science 2002;297:400–403.

Hettema JM, Annas P, Neale MC, Kendler KS, Fredrikson M: A twin study of the genetics of fear conditioning. *Arch Gen Psychiatry*. 2003;60:702–708.

Hettema JM, Neale MC, Kendler KS: A review and meta-analysis of the genetic epidemiology of anxiety disorders. *Am J Psychiatry*. 2001;158:1568–1578.

Hopper JL, Judd FK, Derrick PL, Burrows GD: A family study of panic disorder. *Genet Epidemiology*. 1987;4:33–41.

Kaufman J, Charney D: Comorbidity of mood and anxiety disorders. *Depress Anxiety*. 2000;12(Suppl 1):69–76.

Kendler KS, Neale MC, Kessler RC, Heath AC, Eaves LJ: A population-based twin study of major depression in women: The impact of varying definitions of illness. *Arch Gen Psychiatry*. 1992;49:257–266.

*Kendler KS, Neale MC, Kessler RC, Heath AC, Eaves LJ: Panic disorder in women—a population-based twin study. *Psychol Med*. 1993;23:397–406.

Kendler KS, Walters EE, Truett KR, Heath AC, Neale MC, Martin NG, Eaves LJ: A twin-family study of self-report symptoms of panic-phobia and somatization. *Behav Genet*. 1995;25:499–515.

Knowles JA, Fyer AJ, Vieland VJ, Weissman MM, Hodge SE, Heiman GA, Haghighi F, De Jesus GM, Rassnick H, Preudhome-Rivelli X, Austin T, Cinjak J, Mick S, Fine JD, Woodley KA, Das K, Maier W, Adams PB, Freimer NB, Klein DF, Gilliam TC: Results of a genome-wide genetic screen for panic disorder. *Am J Med Genet*. 1998;81:139.

Koenen KC, Lyons MJ, Goldberg J, Simpson J, Williams WM, Toomey R, Eisen SA, True WR, Cloitre M, Wolfe J, Tsuang MT: A high-risk twin study of combat-related PTSD comorbidity. *Twin Res*. 2003;6:218–226.

Lesch KP, Bengel D, Heils A, Sabol S, Greenberg B, Petri S, Benjamin J, Muller C, Hamer D, Murphy D: Association of anxiety-related traits with a polymorphism in the serotonin transporter gene regulatory region. *Science*. 1996;274:1527–1531.

*Mazzanti CM, Lappalainen J, Long JC, Bengel D, Naukkarinen H, Eggert M, Virkkunen M, Linnoila M, Goldman D: Role of the serotonin transporter promoter polymorphism in anxiety-related traits *Arch Gen Psychiatry*. 1998;55:936–940.

*Pauls DL, Bucher KD, Crowe RR, Noyes R: A genetic study of panic disorder pedigrees. *Am J Hum Genet*. 1980;32:639–644.

*Risch N: Linkage strategies for genetically complex traits. *Am J Hum Genet*. 1996;46:229–241.

Sack WH, Clarke GN, Seeley J: Posttraumatic stress disorder across two generations of Cambodian refugees. *J Am Acad Child Adolesc Psychiatry*. 1995;34:1160–1166.

*Skre I, Onstad S, Torgersen S, Lygren S, Kringlen E: A twin study of DSM-III-R anxiety disorders. *Acta Psychiatrica Scand*. 1993;88:85–92.

Skre I, Onstad S, Torgersen S, Philos DR, Lygren S, Kringlen E: The heritability of common phobic fear: A twin study of a clinical sample. *J Anxiety Disord*. 2000;14:549–562.

Smoller JW, Tsuang MT: Panic and phobic anxiety: Defining phenotypes for genetic studies. Am *J Psychiatry*. 1998;155(9):1152–1162.

Spielman RS, McGinnis RE, Ewens WJ: Transmission test for linkage disequilibrium: The insulin gene region and insulin-dependent diabetes mellitus (IDDM). *Am J Hum Genet*. 1996;52:506–516.

Stein MB, Chartier MJ, Lizak MV, Jang KL: Familial aggregation of anxiety-related quantitative traits in generalized social phobia: Clues to understanding "disorder" heritability? *Am J Med Genet*. 2001;105:79–83.

Stein MB, Jang KL, Livesley WJ: Heritability of anxiety sensitivity: A twin study. *Am J Psychiatry*. 1999;156:246–251.

Teng J, Risch N: The relative power of family-based and case-control designs for linkage disequilibrium studies of complex human diseases. II. Individual genotyping. *Genome Res*. 1999;9:234–241.

van den Heuvel OA, van de Wetering BJ, Veltman DJ, Pauls DL: Genetic studies of panic disorder: A review. *J Clin Psychiatry*. 2000;61:756–766.

▲ 14.7 Anxiety Disorders: Psychodynamic Aspects

JOHN CASE NEMIAH, M.D.

HISTORICAL PRELUDE

During the second week of August, 1889, the newly organized International Congress of Experimental Psychology held its first meeting in Paris. The congress's president, Jean-Martin Charcot, was "prevented from being present by indisposition," but the proceedings were ably convened by the organization's other officers, among them the vice president, Théodule Ribot, a distinguished psychologist and an editor of the *Revue Philsophique*. Some 100 individuals attended the congress, having traveled from North and South America as well as from all of Europe, including among them many distinguished scholars and clinical investigators such as William James, Hippolyte Bernheim, and Pierre Janet.

In his report of the congress's proceedings, written for the members of the British Society for Psychical Research, A. T. Myers paints a vivid picture of a lively series of debates on hypnosis dominated, if not overwhelmed, by Bernheim. If Myers' reporting is accurate, Janet's active participation was minimal. He is mentioned only once as having commented that hypnotizability was "a sign of mental and moral weakness."

DEVELOPMENT OF A THEORY

Pierre Janet Although Janet's comment earned him several sharp rejoinders, it reflected a basic concept of the human psyche that he had presented in detail in his first major work, *l'Automatisme Psychologique,* which had been published shortly before the Paris congress. Every human being, Janet postulated, is genetically endowed with a given quantity of psychological energy, the function of which is to bind together in an integrated whole the entire spectrum of mental functions—sensorimotor, cognitive, emotional, and volitional. In the normal human being, there are no unconscious mental processes. However, in those individuals who are endowed with an insufficiency of mental energy or in those whose quantum of such energy is reduced below a critical level as a result of emotionally traumatic stress, specific mental functions escape the control of the ego and, thus "dissociated," operate independently as ego-alien psychiatric symptoms.

Janet's initial formulation of a deficiency of psychic energy and a degeneration of psychological functioning was based on the study of a relatively small number of individuals with major hysterical disorders. In the decade that followed that formulation, Janet turned to a far more extensive and ambitious analysis of the symptoms of the whole spectrum of neurotic disorders. In particular, he focused his attention on a large number of individuals with anxiety disorders whose symptoms, he postulated, were the result of a loss of emotional control by an ego weakened by psychological trauma. Janet's investigations involved the study of many scores of patients whose clinical histories, published in several massive volumes, were often wonderfully vivid. Indeed, Janet may with justice be considered the master portrait painter of the neuroses. Consider for example, B. U., a man of 52 years, who was, as Janet writes, in *Les Obsessions et la Psychasthénie*:

> about 25 when what he himself calls the business of spaces first started. He was going across the place de la Concorde, alone it should be noted, when he suddenly experienced a strange feeling of dread. His breathing became rapid, he felt as if he were suffocating, his heart beat violently, and his legs went limp as if half-paralyzed. He could move neither forward nor backward, and it took a tremendous effort for him, bathed in sweat, to reach the other side of the square. Since that first incident he has taken a great dislike to the place de la Concorde and has decided not to risk going there alone again. However, some time later the same feeling of anxiety returned on the Invalides bridge, and then again on a street that, although narrow, was long and seemed to be rather too steep.
>
> It was at that point that the patient consulted Legrand du Saulle, who considered him to be a typical case of agoraphobia and treated him with douches and a daily dose of four to five grams of bromide. . . . After leaving the hospital the patient remained better for a decade.
>
> The illness, however, was not cured and continued to develop slowly. The anxiety that he experienced when he had to venture forth on a square of any width was such that he could not master it, and he could no longer succeed in getting across the square. It was about ten years ago that he had been charged with escorting a young woman to her home. As long as she was with him, all went well, but once she had left him, he did not know how to get home. At the end of five hours, noticing that it was getting late, that it was raining, and that he had not yet come home, his wife became worried and went out to hunt for him. She found him, pale as a ghost and trembling with cold on the edge of the place de la Concorde, which he had been unable to cross.
>
> After that dreadful experience, they no longer allowed him to go out alone. That was exactly what he wanted and thus his crises continued. Whenever he approached a square, he would begin to shake and breathe heavily; he would develop tics, and would repeat the following absurd phrase: 'Maman, ratan, bibi, btaque, I am going to die!' His wife would then have to grab him firmly by his arm and he would cross the square without too much difficulty. It is now necessary that she accompany him everywhere, even when he goes to the toilet. When she succeeds in encouraging him, and particularly when she gets him to do a little work, he feels better. The poor woman has discovered that she herself is the best therapy. (author's translation)

With the exception, perhaps, of the elegance of his Parisian surroundings, B. U. presents the classic picture of agoraphobia with panic attacks, and, at the same time, he strikingly demonstrates the loss of control of its functions by a pathologically weakened ego that was for Janet the central factor in the pathogenesis of neurotic disorders. Janet's formulation, however, overlooks a remarkable fact: When B. U.'s wife is with him, he suddenly regains the functions he had lost when he was alone. His phobic deficits are not permanently fixed by internal structural changes but vary in severity with the nature of his external circumstances and relationships. Clearly, a more complex theoretical model than that offered by Janet was needed to do justice to all the facts, and it was not long in coming from yet another participant in that memorable congress: Sigmund Freud.

Sigmund Freud Freud was, at the time of the congress, undergoing a change in his clinical interests and activities. In his earlier years, he had been deeply involved in neuropathological studies and research, but during a period of study with Charcot, he had been introduced to the concepts and clinical manifestations of traumatic hysteria, an experience that led him eventually to the use of hypnosis in his clinical practice and to an intensive study of Bernheim's theories and therapeutic applications of hypnotic suggestion. At that point, Freud embarked on a collaborative study with Josef Breuer of a small number of patients with hysteria, reported in his first psychoanalytic publication, "On the Psychical Mechanism of Hysterical Phenomena: Preliminary Communication." The publication was written jointly with Breuer, and it was in this context that Freud first observed the relation of hysterical symptoms to unconscious traumatic memories. In a close partnership such as that between Breuer and Freud, it is, of course, difficult to assign credit for the creative ideas that emerged from their collaboration. It appears certain, however, that Freud was responsible for introducing the concepts of "defence" (*abwehr*) and repression, as well as for the concepts of psychic structure, psychological conflict, and the various forms of psychological defenses that underlie the clinical manifestations of the neuroses.

Freud's conception of psychological functioning and symptom formation differs markedly from that held by Janet. Both men, it is true, ascribed neurotic symptoms to environmental stress, but they differed radically in their conceptions of the nature of the individual's psychological response to that stress. In Janet's view, traumatic stress so seriously lowers the ego's quantum of psychological energy that it loses its capacity to activate and coordinate its functions and lapses into a state of passive helplessness. In Freud's theoretical conception, on the other hand, the ego is viewed as having sufficient strength and resiliency to defend itself against the damaging effects of the trauma by repressing both the memory and the associated painful affect of the traumatic episode and by transforming them by a number of psychodynamic defensive maneuvers into psychoneurotic symptoms.

Not surprisingly, these differences in Freud's and Janet's formulation of the pathogenesis of psychoneurotic symptoms led to differences in the therapeutic measures that they used in the early phases of their clinical studies. Janet relied heavily on combatting symptoms directly by therapeutic suggestion, hypnotic and otherwise, whereas Freud, in what he called "cathartic treatment," emphasized the importance of raising unconscious traumatic memories into consciousness, along with a full and vigorous conscious discharge of the pathogenic emotions associated with them.

The two men differed as well in their classification of neurotic disorders. Janet divided neurotic illness into two major categories: hysteria, which he had delineated in detail in *l'Automatisme Psychologique*, and paraphrenia, a diagnostic category to which he assigned patients who manifested a variety of individual disabling symptoms such as phobias, obsession, and compulsions. If Janet was a "lumper," Freud was a "splitter" when it came to delineating diagnostic categories. In a series of publications during the 1890s, including the *Studies on Hysteria* written jointly with Josef Breuer, Freud delineated the "psychoneuroses of defence," whose clinical characteristics and nomenclature were determined by the psychodynamic process underlying them.

In the light of these innovative and creative psychological investigations and theories, it is surprising that, when Freud turned his attention to a study of clinical anxiety, he concluded that it was a purely physiological phenomenon. Observing that anxiety was common in individuals who practiced coitus interruptus, he concluded that anxiety was the result of a physiological transformation of blocked, undischarged libido. To emphasize its purely physiological character, Freud designated pathological anxiety as an "actual" neurosis and referred to its clinical manifestations as "anxiety neurosis" rather than "psychoneurosis," the categorical term he had applied to the other emotional disorders in his purview. Throughout the subsequent development of Freud's discoveries and theoretical formulations, anxiety remained outside the pale of psychodynamic theory. It was not until 30 years later, with the publication of "Inhibitions, Symptoms, and Anxiety," that anxiety finally achieved psychological status as "signal anxiety."

In this new formulation, anxiety is seen as playing an important role in the production of psychoneurotic disorders. It is now conceived of as an "ego affect," constituting the ego's response to sexual and aggressive drives that run counter to the moral and ethical standards of the superego. A consideration of the case histories that follow will perhaps help to bring life and meaning to that starkly cognitive formulation.

CLINICAL OBSERVATIONS

Generalized Anxiety

D. B., a 26-year-old married woman, was admitted to the hospital for the evaluation of persistent anxiety that had begun 8 months earlier and was becoming increasingly disabling. Especially disturbing to the patient was the spontaneous intrusion of intermittent images in her mind's eye of her father and herself locked in a naked sexual embrace. The images were not only frightening, but they puzzled her greatly, for she had always disliked her father intensely. Not only was he "poison" to her, but she tried to avoid any contact with him and found it difficult to talk to him if she was forced to be in his company.

As the patient described the difficulty of her relationship with her father, she suddenly recalled the fact that her anxiety had begun at a time when her father was seemingly being more intrusive than ever as he tried to help her and her husband over a period of financial difficulty.

As the patient continued to revile her father, she suddenly commented that her mother had told her that her father "had been good to me when I was little and he used to sing songs to me and take me on his lap, but I don't remember. I only remember when he was mean to me. I just am glad when he keeps on talking mean to me the way he always has. I just wouldn't know what to do if he was nice to me." When asked by the interviewer if there might have been a time when she *had* wanted him to be nice to her, the patient replied, "When I was little, I just wanted to know that he did love me a little. I guess I always wanted him to be nice to me. But when I stop to think about it, I guess I didn't want him to be nice to me." The doctor then commented, "It sounds as if a part of you wants to be close to your father." In response, the patient burst into agitated sobs and blurted out, "I don't know how to be close to my father! I am too old to care about my father now!"

When the patient regained her composure, she recalled the memory of an event she had not thought of since it had occurred 15 years earlier. When she was 11, she reported, while in the living room with her father, she had suddenly had the mental image of being in a sexual embrace with him. Terrified, she had run into the kitchen to find her mother. There had been no recurrence of that image until the onset of the current illness, and the incident had remained forgotten until its recall during the interview. Its emergence into consciousness amplified the history of the patient's illness and disclosed an earlier transient outbreak of the same symptoms she had experienced as an adult. After the patient had recovered her composure, she recalled further hitherto forgotten memories. She had slept in her parents' bedroom until she was 6, during which period her father, on one occasion, had taken her into bed and told her stories and, on another, had yelled at her very angrily as she lay in her crib.

During a clinical interview the next day, the patient revealed a fact that she had forgotten in her earlier account of her illness: At the end of the period during which her father had been making the friendly overtures that had so deeply troubled her, and the night before the sudden onset of her symptoms, she had had a nightmare. She was, she dreamed, at a zoo. It was night, and she heard strange noises in the darkness. She asked an attendant standing next to her what the noises were. "Oh," the attendant replied casually, "that's only the animals mating." She then noticed a large, gray elephant lying on its right side in the grass in front of her. As she watched, she noticed the creature moving its left hind leg up and down as if it were trying to get to its feet. At that point she awoke from the dream with a feeling of terror and, afterward, during the morning, experienced the first episode of the frightening imagery of sexual activity with her father.

In direct association to the dream, the patient recalled a long-forgotten childhood memory of an incident that had occurred during her fourth or fifth year. She had awoken one night while in her crib in her parents' bedroom to observe her parents having sexual intercourse. They suddenly became aware of her watching them and sprang apart. The patient remembered seeing her mother hastily pulling up the bedclothes around her to cover her nakedness. Her father, meanwhile, rolled over half on his back, half on his left side. The patient noticed his erection and then saw him lift up his left leg as he sat up and yelled at her angrily to go to sleep.

It was not easy for the patient to communicate these memories. She spoke haltingly, in a low voice and was visibly ashamed and anxious throughout the whole recital of the dream and its associations. She discharged a great quantity of affect, but after doing so appeared considerably relaxed, relieved, and composed. On her return to the psychiatric ward, she was observed to be cheerful and outgoing with the ward personnel and other patients. Of particular note was the fact that she no longer experienced any anxiety and had no recurrence of the sexual images involving her father that had previously been so deeply distressing. The patient was discharged a short while later after a further series of psychotherapeutic interviews, and when seen for a follow-up visit 2 months later, she reported continued emotional calm and comfort, without recurrence of psychiatric symptoms.

By the end of this patient's treatment, it was evident that her generalized anxiety disorder was the surface manifestation of an unconscious psychological conflict associated with her relationship with her father. It was also apparent that her adult illness was the final act in a series of anxiety-provoking memories and images going back in time to her pathogenic childhood experience in her parents' bedroom. Finally, it is notable that, in the course of psychotherapy, the patient was able to recall the repressed traumatic memories and to discharge the associated painful affects with a resolution of her clinical symptoms.

Anxiety Verging on Panic

J. P. was a married man in his early 30s who had been admitted to a psychiatric unit for the evaluation of a puzzling ataxia that kept him confined to a wheelchair. Because his home was a considerable distance from the hospital, he had remained there over Christmas day. The following afternoon, he came to his doctor's office for an interview. His appearance was arresting. He was trembling, sweating, and breathing heavily and deeply. In a voice that was distressed and distressing, he blurted out, "Boy! This is the roughest day yet!" Then he proceeded to describe in detail how anxious he felt—worse than anything he had ever experienced in his life. As he talked, he gradually became calmer and quieter and began describing his Christmas day on the psychiatric ward. The place was like a tomb; he had missed being at home with his wife and children for the holiday and had gone to bed lonely and crying. When he awoke that morning, he felt tense and nervous, a feeling that had intensified during the day. Suddenly, in the midst of his repetitions and expressions of anxiety, he exclaimed, "I think if I could throw something, I would feel better." From that point on, he alternated expressions of anxious distress with descriptions of strange impulses that had suddenly seized him during the day. At lunch, for example, he suddenly had the urge to pick up a water pitcher and heave it at the person across the table from him. "No one in his right mind would do something like that. I don't know what the hell it is," he continued, "but I think if I went back to the ward now, I would enjoy having a fight with someone or banging things or tearing my bed all to pieces. It's a terrible feeling to have, and I don't know what would happen if I should give ground to these feelings. If I got hold of someone, would I be satisfied to smack him in the face or really do a job on him—go berserk! It's a horrible feeling! I'm scared of what I'll do!"

The sequence of the patient's associations is interesting and instructive. He begins with the vigorous complaint about his extreme and painful anxiety, and then, as noted, suddenly interjects into this litany of *feelings* a fantasy of an *action*—"throwing something." As the interview progresses, he describes more and more fantasies of action that become more vigorous, more violent, and more destructive as he progresses.

A comparison of the clinical features of D. B. and J. P. reveals a major similarity and a significant difference. On examination, both manifest anxiety that is deeply distressing and disrupting, but the similarity ends there. D. B.'s anxiety is a response to libidinal feelings and imagery, whereas aggressive fantasies and impulses are immediately associated with J. P.'s almost overwhelming anxious despair. Furthermore, examination readily reveals the source of D. B.'s anxiety in her sexual fantasies about her father. In the case of J. P., however, the origin of his aggression is a mystery that is perhaps partially solved by further psychological exploration.

As the interview progressed, J. P. began to feel calmer and more comfortable and shifted the focus of his communications to an account of his previous day on the ward. It being Christmas, there were only four patients there. J. P. was very lonely and thinking of home and had the faintest thought that his wife might call. She had not said that she would call, but J. P thought she might. He had told the nurse he "didn't expect a call from his wife, but if she did, could the call be put through to the ward?" and then he forgot about the whole thing. It wasn't that J. P.'s wife and children had forgotten about him—there were many people at the house for Christmas dinner and they were busy—but it would have been nice if they had called. He said he never thought "Why the hell didn't you call—you had all day to do it!" And so the day passed slowly, and J. P. began to realize that, since his injury and disability, his wife and children had become the most important thing in the world to him, and he went to bed feeling lonely and bawled himself to sleep.

One wonders why the patient spends so much time talking about a phone call he did not expect and his wife had not planned to make. Under those circumstances, why did he go out of his way to make excuses for his wife's not calling? Why does he deny having thought "Why the hell didn't you call—you had all day to do it!" when no one suggested he had had such a thought? Perhaps he "doth protest too much." Perhaps the angry feelings and fantasies that had so frightened him earlier that day were a displacement of the rage against his wife that he could not yet allow himself to feel. Therein lay a hint for the focus of exploration in later therapeutic sessions.

Phobia

C. E. was a married woman of 28 years suffering from a severe and highly incapacitating phobia of boats. The mere sight of a boat would throw her into a state of utter terror, accompanied by feelings of suffocation, a pounding heart, sweating, and trembling. The patient could not remember the time or circumstances of the onset of these symptoms, but it was only recently that their severity had increased enough to motivate her to seek professional help. The patient could not remember the date of onset of her phobia or recall the circumstances in which it first occurred but reported that it had become more frequent and more disabling in recent months, during which time her husband had been pressuring her, against her strongest opposition, to become pregnant.

During the first phase of treatment, the patient focused on her great fear and dislike of sexuality and her predominant perception of men as being sexually demanding and dangerously and destructively sadistic in their sexual behavior. In this context, she suddenly recalled a memory of an event that had occurred when she was 17 that had been forgotten for many years. She had become attached in a friendly way to a young man of her age, Jim, who owned a sailboat on which they spent many companionable hours. One day, however, on Jim's initiative, they indulged in minor but clearly arousing sexual play. At this point in her recital of the episode, the patient was overcome with sudden panic and could not proceed with her account for several minutes. When she was able to talk, she blurted out, "The terrible thing was that I liked it!" She then revealed that, after that incident, she had developed a profound fear that she would become pregnant and that her mother would discover what had occurred and be furious. Overwhelmed by this anxiety, the patient had broken off her relationship with Jim and never saw him again.

The retrieval of this long-buried memory ushered in a new and final phase of the patient's psychotherapy. The focus of her attention and associations was on her neurotic ambivalence toward her mother. The result was a deeper, more satisfying, and more supportive relationship for them both. At the same time, the patient came emotionally closer to her husband, began to share his wish for a family, and became pregnant. When the therapy ended shortly before the patient's delivery of a baby boy, she was asymptomatic and remained so through the delivery of her baby and beyond. She had, she wrote, "never been happier," and a follow-up 2 years after the conclusion of therapy indicated that she was continuing to do well.

A comparison of symptom formation in D. B. and C. E. reveals similarities and differences. In both individuals, libido is a source of painful anxiety, and, in both, it is accordingly defensively repressed from conscious awareness and expression. At that point, however, D. B. and C. E. differ in the further defensive mechanisms they use. D. B. avoids all contact with her father, whose mere presence arouses considerable anxiety despite her defensive repression. C. E., on the other hand, travels a different route. The entire set of memories of her relationship with Jim is completely repressed, and, at the same time, the powerful emotional charge and forbidden drives are displaced to a cognitive fragment of the entire structure of memories—the image of boats, which became the phobic symbol of the entire structure of the neurotic conflict.

A Phobia That Grew

Nearly a century ago, a woman of 40 years consulted a noted Boston neuropsychiatrist, Morton Prince, because of an intense and irrational fear of towers and church steeples and, as it turned out, of the ringing of church bells in particular. No amount of exploration during clinical interviews gave the slightest clue as to the origin or meaning of this incapacitating phobia, and Prince at length induced automatic writing, a remarkable dissociative hypnotic phenomenon in which the subject's hand, without any conscious volition on the part of the writer, automatically writes sentences whose subject matter is unknown to the writer until they are read. In this manner, Prince's patient wrote: "G.M. church. . . and they cut my mother. I cried and prayed all the time that she would live and the church bells were always ringing and I hated them." Although quite unaware of what she was writing, the patient was visibly very anxious and fearful but had no idea as to why she was so distressed.

On being wakened from hypnosis, the patient rapidly regained her composure. On reading what she had written automatically, she immediately recalled the events to which the writing referred. Indeed, she had never forgotten the events during that period of her life, but it had never occurred to her to report them during her clinical interviews with Dr. Prince. She now, however, proceeded to recount the events surrounding her mother's death, which occurred during her adolescence when she and her parents were visiting England. Her mother had suddenly been taken ill and had died after surgery in a provincial town. During the first days of this ordeal, the patient had spent many hours in her hotel room tearfully praying for her mother's recovery against the backdrop of the bells in the neighboring church, which rang every quarter of an hour.

Of particular interest in the patient's account of her distress was the emergence of the fact that, not only had she been desperately grief-stricken, but also that she felt a haunting sense of guilty responsibility for her mother's death. She had, on one occasion, omitted praying for her mother and was convinced that her mother's death had resulted from that delinquency. More than that, the patient confessed, she had a deeper sense of guilty responsibility for her mother's death. Many months before, while the family was still at home, she had left the house one day in defiance of her mother's orders to stay home. She then caught a cold and developed a chronic cough, as the result of which, on doctor's orders, her parents took her to Europe. Had she been obedient, the patient was convinced, her mother would still be alive. Moreover, the patient revealed, behind the specific instances of self-accusation and guilt was a deep, pervasive sense of guilty responsibility for anything and everything that went wrong around her, and whenever she was away from home for even a short time she would be plagued with a haunting fear that something bad was going to happen that she would have been able to prevent had she stayed at home.

A comparison of this patient with C. E. reveals similarities and differences. Both present themselves clinically with the same kind of leading complaint—a striking and classic phobia. Whereas the libidinal drive is the primary source of C. E.'s anxiety, in Prince's patient, it is her aggressive drive that is the central focus of conflicts and anxiety. Furthermore, whereas C. E.'s basic psychopathological mechanisms are those of displacement and phobic avoidance, in Prince's patient, guilty, self-accusatory obsessions and compulsive acts of prevention and undoing predominate.

Obsessive-Compulsive Disorder

P. S. was a single man of 27 years who was obsessed with the fear that he had accidentally bumped others as he passed, causing them to fall and hurt themselves. Walking down the street, he frequently would have to stop, turn around, and look to see if anyone was lying injured on the sidewalk. The obsession was particularly vivid and terrifying when he was in a subway station. As he put it, "I have this terrible fear that I have bumped somebody and they have fallen into the pit and been run over by a train. Not on purpose—no! Just that accidentally I bumped someone and they lost their balance and fell off the platform. It's a terrible feeling to have!" At times, indeed, he would be so distraught that he would call the local transit authority to inquire whether any such incident had been reported. At this point in the interview, the patient, who had been growing increasingly agitated, paused and looked anxiously at the interviewer (who had been smoking a pipe) and then suddenly blurted out, "You didn't drop a spark on your pants, did you, doctor?" After being reassured that all was well, the patient continued. "That's another worry I have, doctor. I'm terribly worried about fires. Maybe it's because of my father." His father, he continued, had been a fireman and, when the patient was a little boy, had had a terrible fall while on duty and had died shortly thereafter from his injuries. As the patient recalled these memories, he burst into deep sobs of grief. When he was able to speak again, he expressed surprise at his feelings, which he did not remember ever having experienced before. The feelings were, however, an important clinical finding. They indicated the presence of a lively and active affect behind the patient's rigid obsessional defenses. Furthermore, the circumstances of the father's death suggested a connection between that event and the patient's obsession with fire and with lethal falls—a constellation of factors strongly warranting further psychological investigation and psychotherapeutic intervention.

Angoisse Diffuse

C. S. was a woman of 38 years who, as Janet writes in *Les Obsessions et la Psychasthénie*, "was a remarkable example of anxiety neurosis in the diffuse form of the disorder. . . . During her youth, she already gave evidence of being easily excitable, and her emotions often got in the way of her carrying out simple actions. She was, for example, very timid. When she attempted to do things in public (which, as we know, are the most difficult of all), she would experience a sensation of suffocation, her heart would pound, and she could neither say nor do what she wanted to. These disturbances were not, however, considered to be particularly serious, and she remained simply an impressionable person until she was 30. At the age of 31, she had her third child. She was recovering from a difficult delivery, which had occurred two days before, when the attendant made an unlikely and stupid blunder. As she stood looking at the patient's baby, she suddenly began to scream and cried out, 'Madame! He doesn't seem to be breathing! Is he dead?' Needless to say, the baby was merely sleeping quietly and began to howl when his mother grabbed him up violently. She herself was thrown into complete confusion and felt an alteration in her entire being that she could not describe. . . .

For several months the patient remained in a dreadful state; she was ceaselessly anxious, sighing and incapable of applying herself to anything. She gradually improved, however, especially when she recovered her physical health several months after the delivery. A year later she consulted her doctor for some pains she was experiencing. He quite innocently requested a urine sample for analysis. 'Why?' she asked, already frightened. 'I want to know whether there is albumin present,' the doctor replied. This word, which vaguely recalled to her the illness of a neighbor, had the same baneful effect as the phrase uttered previously by the attendant: headaches, generalized uneasiness, attacks of anxiety. She could scarcely get back home, and from that point her illness recurred in full force.

Let us examine the state in which she now finds herself. The illness appears to progress in small stages. The symptoms are not continuously present. The patient is often calm enough, sleeps reasonably well during the night, although she claims the contrary; she eats adequately, and though she has neurasthenic digestive complaints, she digests her food tolerably well. From time to time you will find her playing checkers or dominos with her attendant in the most innocent manner in the world. But at intervals the scene changes: a dozen times a day. . . . you will observe the patient to be extremely agitated. She cannot stay put in one place; she gesticulates and pounds on the furniture. Simultaneously, her face is flushed, she appears to breathe with difficulty, is short of breath, and her heart beats violently. But above all, internal sufferings are added to these physical symptoms. She constantly complains, 'Oh! I've got such a headache in the back of my head and my temples! I have such a pain in my neck, my throat, my stomach, my heart, my belly! I'm lost, I shall never get well, I'm going to die! Help me!' and so on. Nothing whatsoever can quiet these jeremiads and these cries. They are shrill enough to upset a whole household, and they last two or three hours at a stretch. Then the patient gradually calms down and is unconcerned about what has happened or the exhaustion of the attendants. She then remains reasonably quiet, though she remembers everything, and then in a half-hour she begins all over again. This is the kind of life the patient has led and has inflicted on her relatives over the course of many years." (author's translation)

C. S.'s clinical biography graphically delineates the characteristics of generalized anxiety disorder and reveals the chronic, debilitating course that patients with anxiety disorders are often fated to follow.

CONCLUDING CLINICAL AND THEORETICAL REFLECTIONS

A review of the clinical histories recorded above reveals an interesting and significant difference between those written by Janet and those reported a generation later by a psychodynamically oriented American psychiatrist. In his case reports, Janet shows himself to be a dispassionate observer. He watches and records his patients' observable patterns of behavior and relationships, and the external manifestations of their emotions. The psychodynamically oriented psychiatrist, on the other hand, focuses his attention on his patients' inner life—their thoughts, their feelings, their fantasies, their perceptions, their memories and lapses thereof. In essence, he attempts to empathize with his patients, to share their inner experiences, at the same time, however, maintaining a thoughtful and reflective distance on all that they are experiencing. The psychodynamic psychiatrist views anxiety as a marker of underlying psychological conflicts to be explored and resolved, whereas, for the phenomenologically minded Janet, anxiety is a psychiatric symptom that defines the diagnostic class of anxiety disorders.

Finally, it should be noted that the same differences between Janet and the psychodynamic clinician are observable in the distinctly different character of their clinical evaluations. Janet restricts himself to the conventional medical history of the onset, course, and characteristics of the patient's symptoms, with the aim of arriving at an accurate diagnostic classification, whereas the psychodynamic clinician goes beyond a structured clinical interview to use techniques designed to explore the nature of the patient's psychological conflicts and their potential for resolution by psychodynamic psychotherapy. Both of those methods of eliciting information are essential components of the clinical evaluation of patients with anxiety disorders.

SUGGESTED CROSS-REFERENCES

Section 6.1 on psychoanalysis provides a discussion of psychoanalytic theory in general that puts the psychodynamic view of anxiety in perspective. Section 14.8 on the clinical features of anxiety disorders describes the clinical and diagnostic aspects of the individual anxiety disorders as defined in the revised fourth edition of the *Diagnostic and Statistical Manual of Mental Disorders* (DSM-IV-TR). Section 30.1 on psychoanalysis and psychoanalytic psychotherapy gives a general view of analytically oriented psychotherapy that serves as a background for its specific application to the individual anxiety disorders.

REFERENCES

*Breuer J, Freud S. On the psychical mechanism of hysterical phenomena: Preliminary communication. *Standard Edition of the Complete Psychological Works of Sigmund Freud.* Vol. 2. London: Hogarth Press; 1953–1964:3.

Ellenberger H. *The Discovery of the Unconscious.* New York: Basic Books; 1970.

*Freud S. On the grounds for detaching a particular syndrome from neurasthenia under the description "Anxiety Neurosis." *Standard Edition of the Complete Psychological Works of Sigmund Freud.* Vol 3. London: Hogarth Press; 1953–1964:90.

*Freud S. Inhibitions, symptoms and anxiety. *Standard Edition of the Complete Psychological Works of Sigmund Freud.* Vol 20. London: Hogarth Press; 1953–1964:87.

Janet P. *Les Obsessions et la Psychasthénie.* 2nd ed. Paris: Félix Alcan; 1908.

Janet P. *l'Automatisme Psychologique* (1889). Noveau Edition. Paris: la Sociétá Pierre Janet; 1989.

Myers A: International Congress of Experimental Psychology. *Proc Soc Psychical Res.* 1889–1890;6:71.

*Nemiah J. *Foundations of Psychopathology.* New York: Oxford Press; 1961.

Prince M. *The Unconscious.* 2nd ed. New York: Macmillan; 1925.

*Sifneos P. *Short-Term Dynamic Psychotherapy.* 2nd ed. New York: Plenum; 1987.

▲ 14.8 Anxiety Disorders: Clinical Features

DANIEL S. PINE, M.D., AND ERIN B. MCCLURE, PH.D.

Since the 1970s, clinical research on a group of mental conditions labeled *anxiety disorders* in the revised fourth edition of the *Diagnostic and Statistical Manual of Mental Disorders* (DSM-IV-TR) has increased dramatically. Although the term *anxiety* has been applied to diverse phenomena in the psychoanalytical, learning-based, and neurobiological literature, in the clinical psychopathological literature, it is used to refer to the presence of fear or apprehension that is out of proportion to the context of the life situation. Hence, extreme fear or apprehension can be considered *clinical anxiety* if it is developmentally inappropriate (i.e., fear of separation in a 12-year-old child) or inappropriate to an individual's life circumstances (i.e., a successful banker worrying about supporting his or her family). Since the 1970s, clinical research has led to a progressive refinement of the nosology for clinical anxiety disorders. Although these disorders were broadly conceptualized in the early 20th century, narrower definitions have arisen, partially stimulated by Donald Klein's observations on pharmacological distinctions between *panic* and *nonpanic* anxiety.

Consensus has emerged on the view of anxiety disorders as a family of related but distinct mental disorders. This consensus is reflected in the relatively minor changes to the broad categorization of anxiety disorders since the 1980s, encompassed in the third edition of the DSM (DSM-III) and DSM-IV-TR. It is also of note that both DSM-IV-TR and the tenth edition of the *International Statistical Classification of Diseases and Related Health Problems* (ICD-10) recognize similar groups of syndromes as discrete diagnostic entities. There is some disagreement, however, on whether all of these syndromes are most properly considered anxiety disorders. Although DSM-IV-TR considers a group of nine disorders to be the primary "anxiety disorders," ICD-10 adopts a broader category of neurotic, stress-related, and somatoform disorders that includes each of the conditions in DSM-IV-TR, as well as a number of disorders not considered anxiety disorders in DSM-IV-TR. DSM-III brought a relatively major revision to the nosology of mental disorders in the United States. Before it, anxiety disorders were classified in a group of conditions that included many of the disorders currently listed in DSM-IV-TR, in addition to a set of disorders that have been reclassified. Such reclassified disorders included affective disorders, formerly classified as *depressive neurosis*; somatoform and dissociative disorders, formerly classified as *hysterical neurosis*; and neurasthenia, a disorder that was eliminated from DSM-III.

DSM-III placed a strong emphasis on empiricism and the validity of nosological categories. This led to the reclassification of anxiety disorders into categories that were quite similar to the disorders included in the current anxiety section of DSM-IV-TR, which include panic disorder with and without agoraphobia, agoraphobia with and without panic disorder, specific phobia, social phobia, obsessive-compulsive disorder (OCD), posttraumatic stress disorder (PTSD), acute stress disorder, and generalized anxiety disorder. This section reviews the clinical features of these nine conditions, as conceptualized in DSM-IV-TR. This includes the primary symptomatology, history, epidemiology, differential diagnosis, and course of each disorder, in addition to a clinical vignette designed to capture the essential features of each disorder as it typically presents in the clinic. Because this section is primarily devoted to a discussion of clinical features, other aspects of these disorders, such as theories on etiology, family and genetics, and treatment are discussed elsewhere. Similarly, DSM-IV-TR recognizes substance-induced anxiety disorder and anxiety disorder due to a general medical condition as distinct anxiety disorders. These conditions are discussed in the respective chapters on substance use disorders and on the psychiatric complications of medical conditions. Finally, DSM-IV-TR includes a residual category for conditions with prominent anxiety that do not conform to the criteria for any of the above disorders. Given the focus on clinical anxiety disorders commonly treated by the mental health professional, these conditions will not be discussed in this chapter.

PANIC DISORDER AND AGORAPHOBIA

Symptomatology Recurrent panic attacks represent the hallmark feature of panic disorder. The *panic attack* is defined as an episode of abrupt intense fear accompanied by at least four autonomic or cognitive symptoms listed in Table 14.8–1. Such episodes of abrupt fear occur in many situations. For example, a healthy person might experience a panic attack when confronted with sudden extreme danger, and an individual with a phobia of spiders might experience a panic attack when seeing such an insect during a walk through the woods.

DSM-IV-TR recognizes three types of panic attacks: *spontaneous*, *situationally bound*, and *situationally predisposed.* Whereas unexpected or spontaneous panic attacks occur without cue or warning, situationally bound and situationally predisposed panic attacks occur upon exposure to or in anticipation of exposure to a feared stimulus. If a patient almost inevitably experiences panic attacks in the presence of a situational trigger, such as a spider, then his or her attacks are situationally bound. Patients for whom an environmental cue increases the likelihood of an attack but does not inevitably precipitate one experience situationally predisposed attacks. In panic disorder, panic attacks occur spontaneously, arising without any trigger or environmental cue. This does not imply that all such attacks

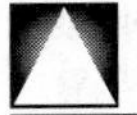

Table 14.8–1
DSM-IV-TR Criteria for Panic Attack

Note: Panic attack is not a codable disorder. Code the specific diagnosis in which the panic attack occurs.

Panic attack is a discrete period of intense fear or discomfort in which four (or more) of the following symptoms develop abruptly and reach a peak within 10 minutes:

1. Palpitations, pounding heart, or accelerated heart rate
2. Sweating
3. Trembling or shaking
4. Sensations of shortness of breath or smothering
5. Feeling of choking
6. Chest pain or discomfort
7. Nausea or abdominal distress
8. Feeling dizzy, unsteady, lightheaded, or faint
9. Derealization (feelings of unreality) or depersonalization (being detached from oneself)
10. Fear of losing control or going crazy
11. Fear of dying
12. Paresthesias
13. Chills or hot flashes

From American Psychiatric Association. *Diagnostic and Statistical Manual of Mental Disorders.* 4th ed. Text rev. Washington, DC: American Psychiatric Association; 2000, with permission.

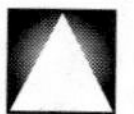

Table 14.8–2
DSM-IV-TR Criteria for Agoraphobia

Note: Agoraphobia is not a codable disorder. Code the specific disorder in which the agoraphobia occurs.

A. Anxiety about being in places or situations from which escape might be difficult (or embarrassing) or in which help may not be available in the event of having an unexpected or situationally predisposed panic attack or panic-like symptoms. Agoraphobic fears typically involve characteristic clusters of situations that include being outside the home alone; being in a crowd or standing in a line; being on a bridge; and traveling in a bus, train, or automobile.

Note: Consider the diagnosis of specific phobia if the avoidance is limited to one or only a few specific situations, or social phobia if the avoidance is limited to social situations.

B. The situations are avoided (e.g., travel is restricted), are endured with marked distress or anxiety about having a panic attack or panic-like symptoms, or require the presence of a companion.

C. The anxiety or phobic avoidance is not better accounted for by another mental disorder, such as social phobia (e.g., avoidance limited to social situations because of fear of embarrassment), specific phobia (e.g., avoidance limited to a single situation, such as elevators), obsessive-compulsive disorder (e.g., avoidance of dirt in someone with an obsession about contamination), posttraumatic stress disorder (e.g., avoidance of stimuli associated with a severe stressor), or separation anxiety disorder (e.g., avoidance of leaving home or relatives).

From American Psychiatric Association. *Diagnostic and Statistical Manual of Mental Disorders.* 4th ed. Text rev. Washington, DC: American Psychiatric Association; 2000, with permission.

occur spontaneously but that such attacks have occurred at some point in the development of the disorder. As shown in Table 14.8–2, panic disorder requires the presence of at least two spontaneous panic attacks, at least one of which is associated with concern about additional attacks, worry about attacks, or changes in behavior.

Patients with panic disorder present with a number of comorbid conditions, but there has been particular interest in the relationship between panic disorder and agoraphobia, which refers to fear of or anxiety regarding places from which escape might be difficult (Tables 14.8–2, 14.8–3, and 14.8–4). There has, in fact, been some debate as to whether agoraphobia is best conceptualized as a complication of panic disorder or as a separate condition. This controversy centers on the frequency with which patients develop agoraphobia in the absence of panic disorder or panic attacks. DSM-IV-TR suggests that such patients do exist, noting the existence of both panic disorder with and without agoraphobia (Table 14.8–3). However, even in "agoraphobia without history of panic disorder," agoraphobia is thought to relate to the fear of developing "panic-like" symptoms.

Like most anxiety disorders, panic disorder often cooccurs with a number of mental conditions besides agoraphobia, particularly anxiety and depressive disorders. These include specific and social phobia, generalized anxiety disorder, and major depressive disorder. Some data also suggest associations with substance use disorders, bipolar disorder, and suicidal behavior. The high degree of comorbidity seen in the clinic at least partially reflects referral bias. Nevertheless, considerable comorbidity with these anxiety and depressive disorders is also found in epidemiological studies. This suggests that panic disorder, as it occurs in the community, is frequently compounded by comorbid mental conditions.

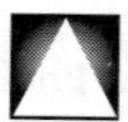

Table 14.8–3
DSM-IV-TR Criteria for Panic Disorder with and without Agoraphobia and Agoraphobia without History of Panic Disorder

Criteria for panic disorder without agoraphobia (300.01)

A. Both (1) and (2)
  1. Recurrent unexpected panic attacks
  2. At least one of the attacks has been followed by 1 month (or more) of one (or more) of the following:
    a. Persistent concern about having additional attacks
    b. Worry about the implications of the attack or its consequences (e.g., losing control, having a heart attack, "going crazy")
    c. A significant change in behavior related to the attacks

B. Absence of agoraphobia.

C. The panic attacks are not due to the direct physiological effects of a substance (drug of abuse, a medication) or a general medical condition (e.g., hyperthyroidism).

D. The panic attacks are not better accounted for by another mental disorder, such as social phobia (e.g., occurring on exposure to feared social situations), specific phobia (e.g., occurring on exposure to a specific phobic situation), obsessive-compulsive disorder (e.g., occurring on exposure to dirt in someone with an obsession about contamination), posttraumatic stress disorder (e.g., occurring on exposure to stimuli associated with a severe stressor), or separation anxiety disorder (e.g., occurring on response to being away from home or close relatives).

Criteria for panic disorder with agoraphobia (300.21)

A. Both (1) and (2)
  1. Recurrent unexpected panic attacks
  2. At least one of the attacks has been followed by 1 month (or more) of one (or more) of the following:
    a. Persistent concern about having additional attacks
    b. Worry about the implications of the attack or its consequences (e.g., losing control, having a heart attack, "going crazy")
    c. A significant change in behavior related to the attacks

B. Presence of agoraphobia.

C. The panic attacks are not due to the direct physiological effects of a substance (drug of abuse, a medication) or a general medical condition (e.g., hyperthyroidism).

D. The panic attacks are not better accounted for by another mental disorder, such as social phobia (e.g., occurring on exposure to feared social situations), specific phobia (e.g., occurring on exposure to a specific phobic situation), obsessive-compulsive disorder (e.g., occurring on exposure to dirt in someone with an obsession about contamination), posttraumatic stress disorder (e.g., occurring on exposure to stimuli associated with a severe stressor), or separation anxiety disorder (e.g., occurring on response to being away from home or close relatives).

Criteria for agoraphobia without history of panic disorder (300.22)

A. The presence of agoraphobia related to fear of developing panic-like symptoms (e.g., dizziness or diarrhea).

B. Criteria have never been met for panic disorder.

C. The disturbance is not due to the direct physiological effect of a substance (e.g., a drug of abuse, a medication) or a general medical condition.

D. If an associated general medical condition is present, the fear described in Criterion A is clearly in excess of that usually associated with the condition.

From American Psychiatric Association. *Diagnostic and Statistical Manual of Mental Disorders.* 4th ed. Text rev. Washington, DC: American Psychiatric Association; 2000, with permission.

History and Comparative Nosology

Although the term *panic disorder* was first coined in DSM-III, a syndrome characterized by recurrent episodes of spontaneous fear has been recognized for more than 100 years. This syndrome has been given various labels throughout history, including *DaCosta's syndrome* in the late 19th century and *effort syndrome*, or *neurocirculatory asthenia*, in the earlier part of the 20th century. Even Freud's descriptions of "anxiety neurosis" invoked many of the key features of panic disorder.

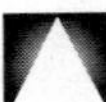

Table 14.8–4
DSM-IV-TR Criteria for Specific Phobia and Social Phobia

Criteria for specific phobia (300.29)

A. Marked and persistent fear that is excessive or unreasonable cued by the presence or anticipation of a specific object or situation (e.g., flying, heights, animals, receiving an injection, seeing blood).

B. Exposure to the phobic stimulus almost invariably provokes an immediate anxiety response, which may take the form of a situationally bound or situationally predisposed panic attack. **Note:** In children, the anxiety may be expressed by crying, tantrums, freezing, or clinging.

C. The person recognizes that the fear is excessive or unreasonable. **Note:** In children, this feature may be absent.

D. The phobic situation(s) is avoided or is endured with intense anxiety or distress.

E. The avoidance, anxious anticipation, or distress in the feared situation(s) interferes significantly with the person's normal routine, occupational (or academic) functioning, or social activities or relationships, or there is marked distress about having the phobia.

F. In individuals under the age of 18 years, the duration is at least 6 months.

G. The anxiety, panic attacks, or phobic avoidance associated with the specific object or situation are not better accounted for by another mental disorder, such as obsessive-compulsive disorder (e.g., fear of dirt in someone with an obsession about contamination), posttraumatic stress disorder (e.g., avoidance of stimuli associated with a severe stressor), separation anxiety disorder (e.g., avoidance of school), social phobia (e.g., avoidance of social situations because of fear of embarrassment), panic disorder with agoraphobia, or agoraphobia without history of panic disorder.

Specify type:

Animal type

Natural environment type (e.g. heights, storms, water)

Blood–injury type

Situational type (e.g., airplanes, elevators, enclosed places)

Other type (e.g., phobic avoidance of situations that may lead to choking, vomiting. or contracting an illness; in children, avoidance of loud sounds or costumed characters)

Criteria for social phobia (300.23)

A. A marked or persistent fear of one or more social or performance situations in which the person is exposed to unfamiliar people or to possible scrutiny by others. The individual fears that he or she will act in a way (or show anxiety symptoms) that will be humiliating or embarrassing. **Note:** In children, there must be evidence of the capacity for age-appropriate social relationships with familiar people, and the anxiety must occur in peer settings, not just in interactions with adults.

B. Exposure to the feared social situation almost invariably provokes anxiety, which may take the form of a situationally bound or situationally predisposed panic attack. **Note:** In children, the anxiety may be expressed by crying, tantrums, freezing, or shrinking from social situations with unfamiliar people.

C. The person recognizes that the fear is excessive or unreasonable. **Note:** In children, this feature may be absent.

D. The feared social or performance situations are avoided or are endured with intense anxiety or duress.

E. The avoidance, anxious anticipation, or distress in the feared social or performance situation(s) interferes significantly with the person's normal routine, occupational (academic) functioning, or social activities or relationships, or there is marked distress about having the phobia.

F. In individuals under age 18 years, the duration is at least 6 months.

G. The fear or avoidance is not due to the direct physiological effects of a substance (e.g., a drug of abuse, a mediation) or a general medical condition and is not better accounted for by another mental disorder (e.g., panic disorder with or without agoraphobia, separation anxiety disorder, body dysmorphic disorder, a pervasive developmental disorder, or schizoid personality disorder).

H. If a general medical condition or another mental disorder is present, the fear in Criterion A is unrelated to it (e.g., the fear is not of stuttering, trembling in Parkinson's disease, or exhibiting abnormal eating behavior in anorexia nervosa or bulimia nervosa).

Specify if:

Generalized: if the fears include most social situations (also consider the additional diagnosis of avoidant personality disorder).

From American Psychiatric Association. *Diagnostic and Statistical Manual of Mental Disorders.* 4th ed. Text rev. Washington, DC: American Psychiatric Association; 2000, with permission.

A major change to the DSM conceptualization of anxiety occurred in 1980, when DSM-III first recognized panic disorder as a distinct entity. Between 1980 and 1994, one significant change to the conceptualization of the disorder involved a refining of the view of panic disorder and agoraphobia as tightly linked constructs. As conceptualized in DSM-IV-TR, agoraphobia invariably involves at least some form of spontaneous crescendo anxiety, even if such episodes do not meet formal criteria for panic attacks (Table 14.8–3). In the earlier versions of the DSM and ICD-10, agoraphobia is considered less closely linked to panic disorder. Indeed, ICD-10 classifies agoraphobia as one of many phobic disorders and does not emphasize the relationship with panic disorder to the same degree as DSM-IV-TR does.

Differential Diagnosis Panic disorder with or without agoraphobia must be differentiated from a number of medical conditions that produce similar symptomatology. Panic attacks are associated with a variety of endocrinological disorders, including both hypo- and hyperthyroid states, hyperparathyroidism, and pheochromocytomas. Episodic hypoglycemia associated with insulinomas can also produce panic-like states, as can primary neuropathological processes. These include seizure disorders, vestibular dysfunction, neoplasms, or the effects of both prescribed and illicit substances on the central nervous system (CNS). Finally, disorders of the cardiac and pulmonary systems, including arrhythmias, chronic obstructive pulmonary disease, and asthma, can produce autonomic symptoms and accompanying crescendo anxiety that can be difficult to distinguish from panic disorder. Clues of an underlying medical etiology to panic-like symptoms include the presence of atypical features during panic attacks, such as ataxia, alterations in consciousness, or bladder dyscontrol; onset of panic disorder relatively late in life; and physical signs or symptoms indicative of a medical disorder.

Panic disorder also must be differentiated from a number of psychiatric disorders, particularly other anxiety disorders. Panic attacks occur in many anxiety disorders, including social and specific phobia, PTSD, and even OCD. The key to correctly diagnosing panic disorder and differentiating the condition from other anxiety disorders involves the documentation of recurrent spontaneous panic attacks at some point in the illness. Differentiation from generalized anxiety disorder can also be difficult. Classically, panic attacks are characterized by their rapid onset (within minutes) and short duration (usually less than 10 to 15 minutes), in contrast to the anxiety associated with generalized anxiety disorder, which emerges and dissipates more slowly. This distinction can be difficult, however, as the anxiety surrounding panic attacks can be more diffuse and slower to dissipate than is typical. Because anxiety is a frequent concomitant of many other psychiatric disorders, including the psychoses and affective disorders, discrimination between panic disorder and a multitude of disorders can also be difficult.

Epidemiology The best data on the prevalence and incidence of all anxiety disorders, including panic disorder with and without agoraphobia, are derived from a series of epidemiological studies completed since the early 1980s. In the United States, these include the Epidemiological Catchment Area (ECA) and National Comorbidity studies. Both are large-scale, community-based studies that relied on standardized interviews and sophisticated sampling designs that provide the most valid, generalizable data on the prevalence of and risk factors for psychopathology.

The lifetime prevalence of panic disorder is in the 1 to 4 percent range, with 6-month prevalence approximately 0.5 to 1.0 percent. Epidemiological studies also suggest continuity between panic disorder and more common but less severe conditions, such as syndromes of isolated panic attacks or even "subclinical" panic attacks. These conditions are at least twice as common as "full-blown" panic disorder in the community and have been shown in the ECA to predict the development of panic disorder over time.

Estimates of agoraphobia prevalence are somewhat more controversial, varying between 2 to 6 percent across studies. This relates to disagreement about the conceptualization of agoraphobia's relationship to panic disorder. For example, at least half of all cases of agoraphobia in epidemiological settings occur in the absence of panic disorder, a finding that is inconsistent with the DSM-IV-TR's view of a tight relationship between agoraphobia and panic disorder. This finding might relate to the misdiagnosis of specific or social phobias as agoraphobia in epidemiological settings.

Course Panic disorder typically has its onset in late adolescence or early adulthood, although cases of childhood-onset and late adulthood–onset disorder have been described. There are only tentative data on the natural course of panic disorder. The best evidence on the course of any disorder, including panic disorder, is derived from prospective epidemiological research, as both retrospective and clinically based studies are vulnerable to biases that preclude firm conclusions on course. Unfortunately, few such studies exist. Research from retrospective or clinical studies suggest that panic disorder tends to exhibit a fluctuating course, with varying levels of persistence over the life span. Approximately one-third to one-half of patients appear psychiatrically healthy at follow-up, with the majority of these patients living relatively normal lives, despite either fluctuating or recurrent symptoms. Typically, patients with chronic disorders exhibit a pattern of exacerbation and remissions rather than chronic disability.

Ms. S. was a 25-year-old student who was referred for a psychiatric evaluation from the medical emergency department at a large university-based medical center. Ms. S. had been evaluated in this emergency department three times over the preceding 3 weeks. Her first visit was prompted by a paroxysm of extreme dyspnea and terror that occurred while she was trying out for the volleyball team. The dyspnea was accompanied by palpitations, choking sensations, sweating, shakiness, and a strong urge to flee. Ms. S. thought that she was having a heart attack, and she immediately went to the emergency room. She received a full medical evaluation, including an electrocardiogram (ECG) and routine blood work, which revealed no sign of cardiovascular, pulmonary, or other illness. Ms. S. was given the number of a local psychiatrist, but she did not make a follow-up appointment, because she did not think that her episode would recur. She developed two other episodes of a similar nature—one while she was on her way to visit a friend and a second that woke her up from sleep. She immediately went to the emergency department after experiencing each paroxysm and received full medical work-ups that showed no sign of illness.

PHOBIAS

Symptomatology The term *phobia* refers to an excessive fear of a specific object, circumstance, or situation. Phobias are classified based on the nature of the feared object or situation, and DSM-IV-TR recognizes three distinct classes of phobia: agoraphobia (which is discussed above as it is considered to relate closely to panic disorder), specific phobia, and social phobia. Criteria for specific and social phobia are shown in Table 14.8–4. Both specific and social phobias require the development of intense anxiety to the point of even situationally bound panic when exposed to the feared object or situation. Both conditions also require the fear to either interfere with an individual's functioning or cause marked distress. Finally, both conditions require that an individual recognize the fear as excessive or irrational and that the feared object or situation be either avoided or endured with great difficulty.

Specific Phobia Specific phobia is divided into four subtypes (animal type, natural environment type, blood–injury type, and situational type) in addition to a residual category for phobias that do not clearly fall into any of these four categories. The key feature in each type of phobia is that the fear is circumscribed to a specific object, both temporally and with respect to other objects. Hence, an individual with specific phobia becomes immediately frightened when presented with a feared object. This fear may relate to concern about harm from a feared object, concern about embarrassment, or fear of consequences of exposure to the feared object. For example, individuals with blood–injury phobia may be afraid of fainting when exposed to blood, and individuals with fear of heights may be afraid of becoming dizzy at high elevations.

Specific phobia often involves fears of more than one object, particularly within a specific subcategory of phobia. For example, it is common for an individual with a phobia of thunderstorms to also have a phobia of water—both phobias are classified as natural environment type phobias. Further, in the clinical setting, specific phobia often occurs with other anxiety or mood disorders. Because it is rare for patients to seek treatment for an isolated phobia, some of the comorbidity seen in the clinic reflects referral bias. Community-based studies also suggest that specific phobia is associated with other anxiety disorders, although at lower rates than seen in the clinic. It is sometimes difficult to quantify the degree of impairment associated with a specific phobia, as the comorbid disorders typically tend to cause more impairment than specific phobia does and individuals with isolated specific phobia are rarely seen in the clinic. Impairment associated with specific phobia typically takes the form of restricting the social or professional activities of the individual.

Social Phobia As indicated in the DSM-IV-TR criteria in Table 14.8–4, social phobia, or social anxiety disorder, involves fear of social situations, including situations that involve scrutiny or contact with strangers. Individuals with social phobia typically fear embarrassing themselves in social situations, such as at social gatherings, during oral presentations, or when meeting new people. They may have specific fears about performing certain activities, such as writing, eating, or speaking in front of others, or they may experience a vague nonspecific fear of embarrassing themselves. DSM-IV-TR provides a specifier for the diagnosis of social phobia. Individuals with social phobia who fear most social situations are considered to have generalized social phobia. Such individuals are fearful of initiating conversations in many settings, dating or participating in most group activities or social gatherings, and speaking with authority figures.

The clinician should recognize that many patients exhibit at least some degree of social anxiety or self-consciousness. In fact, community studies suggest that approximately one-third of all people consider themselves to be far more anxious than other people in social situations. Moreover, such concerns may appear particularly heightened during particular developmental stages, such as adolescence, or after lifestyle changes, such as marriage or a change of occupation, which bring new demands for increasing social interaction. Such anxiety only becomes social phobia when the anxiety either prevents an individual from participating in desired activities or causes marked distress in such activities. Individuals with the more specific form of social phobia fear specific, circumscribed social situations. For example, extreme anxiety about public speaking that interferes with an individual's ability to perform his or her job is a common type of specific social phobia. Such a phobia would not be considered generalized social phobia unless it was associated with fears related to many other social situations in addition to public speaking.

Like many anxiety disorders, social phobia frequently cooccurs with other mood and anxiety disorders. The association of social phobia with both panic disorder and major depression has received considerable attention in recent literature. Major questions remain concerning the degree to which childhood or adolescent social phobia represents a risk factor for later adult-onset major depression. Associations with substance use disorders and childhood conduct problems have also been documented.

History and Comparative Nosology

Phobias have been recognized as incapacitating mental disorders for more than 100 years. The prominent place of phobia in the history of modern mental health science is indicated by the central role that case histories of phobic patients played in the development of both psychoanalytical and cognitive therapies. The category *phobia* has undergone progressive refinement since the 1980s, as research has focused on each of the specific classes of phobia described above. Much of this refinement crystallized in DSM-III, which was based on emerging evidence that phobias represented a group of related but distinct conditions rather than one heterogeneous disorder. Such evidence included Isaac Mark's work on differentiating social and specific phobias. The fine-tuning in DSM-III produced the categorization of agoraphobia as a condition closely related to panic disorder and the distinct categorization of social and simple phobia, which was relabeled specific phobia in DSM-IV-TR.

There have been some changes to the view of phobias since the DSM-III was published. Although discussion of agoraphobia has emphasized the role of panic since DSM-III, DSM-IV-TR also contains descriptions of "panic-like" phenomena in both the specific and social phobia sections, as well as in the discussion of agoraphobia. Beyond this change, the most significant other change for specific phobia between DSM-III and DSM-IV-TR involved the inclusion of the four subcategories of phobia described above based on research noting distinct physiology and demographics of each subtype. For social phobia, the most significant other change occurred with DSM-III-R, which distinguished between generalized and more specific forms of social phobia. This change was based on descriptive phenomenology, epidemiology, and pharmacology studies that validated the two variants of the condition. Growing evidence also suggests that social phobia represents a condition distinct from specific phobia. This view is partially reflected in DSM-IV-TR, in which the label *social anxiety disorder* accompanies the label *social phobia*.

The approach to categorization of phobias in the ICD system is similar to the approach in DSM-IV-TR. ICD-10 recognizes specific phobia as a distinct category and includes the subtypes from DSM-IV-TR. Social phobia is also classified in ICD-10, although without the qualifier in DSM-IV-TR. As discussed above, perhaps the primary difference between DSM-IV-TR and ICD-10 in the consideration of phobia relates to agoraphobia. Whereas DSM-IV-TR emphasizes a close relationship between panic disorder and agoraphobia, ICD-10 restricts the term *panic disorder* to cases without phobia and applies the term *agoraphobia* to all cases that meet the criteria, regardless of the presence or absence of panic attacks.

Differential Diagnosis

Specific phobia is usually easily distinguished from anxiety stemming from primary medical problems by the focused nature of the anxiety, as such specificity is not typical of anxiety disorders related to medical problems. The most difficult diagnostic issues related to specific phobia involve differentiating the condition from other anxiety disorders. As DSM-IV-TR emphasizes the presence of panic-like symptoms (including situationally bound panic attacks) with specific phobia, specific phobia must be differentiated from panic disorder, in which panic attacks occur without a cue. Specific phobia can occasionally be confused with PTSD, because both conditions can involve focused fears of specific objects or situations. The two disorders are most easily differentiated based on the other features of PTSD, such as the reexperiencing of the trauma, avoidance, and enhanced startle, that are markedly absent in specific phobia. Similarly, specific phobia can be confused with generalized anxiety disorder, as both conditions may involve worry about exposure to specific situations. The two disorders are differentiated based on the focused nature of the fear, both over time and with respect to objects, in specific phobia.

Like specific phobia, *social phobia* is rarely confused with anxiety that stems primarily from medical disorders. However, as a number of psychiatric disorders are associated with social withdrawal, it can be difficult to correctly diagnose social phobia. Perhaps the most difficult distinction involves the differentiation of social phobia and agoraphobia, as both conditions involve fear of situations in which people typically gather. The key distinction between the disorders centers on the nature of the feared object. Patients with social phobia are specifically afraid of encountering people. In contrast, individuals with agoraphobia do not specifically fear people; rather, they are afraid of situations from which escape would be difficult. Hence, whereas an individual with agoraphobia might find the presence of other people reassuring, provided the physical properties of the location are suitable, an individual with social phobia flees other people. The clinician might also encounter difficulty in distinguishing social phobia from the social isolation that accompanies a number of psychiatric disorders, including major depression and the early stages of psychosis. Two factors are essential in making this distinction. First, the individual with social phobia must experience anxiety or fear in social situations, whereas individuals who are isolated due to depression or indolent psychosis often isolate themselves for other reasons. Second, in social phobia, symptomatology is restricted to fears of social situations, whereas, in other disorders, social isolation is accompanied by a broad array of symptoms not found in social phobia.

Epidemiology Circumscribed fears of specific objects are exceedingly common, such that a large minority of individuals possess at least one such fear. The key factor in labeling such a circumscribed fear as a specific phobia is the degree of impairment associated with the fear. A circumscribed fear is only considered a phobia when it interferes with activities or causes marked distress. Approximately 10 percent of individuals in the United States meet criteria for specific phobia, but there has been some variation in prevalence estimates, based on differences across studies in the impairment threshold criteria. The condition is more commonly diagnosed in women than in men, and onset is typically in childhood or adolescence, with animal phobias particularly prominent in children.

Social phobia is also an exceedingly common mental disorder. As with specific phobias, a large minority of individuals possesses at least some fear of social situations. Only some of these individuals, however, meet the impairment threshold for a diagnosis of social phobia. Because different studies have used different impairment thresholds, prevalence estimates of social phobia vary widely, from 2 to approximately 15 percent. Like specific phobia, social phobia exhibits a female preponderance, although the gender ratio in the clinic may be more equal, and the disorder frequently has its onset in childhood or adolescence.

Course Specific phobia exhibits a bimodal age of onset, with a childhood peak for animal phobia, natural environment phobia, and blood–injury phobia, and an early-adulthood peak for other phobias, such as situational phobia. There are limited prospective epidemiological data on the natural course of specific phobia. Because patients with isolated specific phobias rarely present for treatment, there is also little research on the course of the disorder in the clinic. The limited information that is available suggests that the majority of specific phobias that begin in childhood and persist into adulthood will continue to persist for many years. The severity of the condition is thought to remain relatively constant, which contrasts with the waxing and waning course seen in other anxiety disorders.

Mr. A. was a successful businessman who presented for treatment after a change in his business schedule. Although he had formerly worked largely from an office near his home, a promotion led to a schedule of frequent out-of-town meetings requiring weekly flights. Mr. A. reported being "deathly afraid" of flying. Even the thought of getting on an airplane led to thoughts of impending doom in which he envisioned his airplane crashing to the ground. These thoughts were associated with intense fear, palpitations, sweating, clamminess, and stomach upset. Although the thought of flying was terrifying enough, Mr. A. became nearly incapacitated when he went to the airport. Immediately before boarding, Mr. A. would often have to turn back from the plane, running to the bathroom to vomit.

Social phobia tends to have its onset in late childhood or early adolescence. Social phobia tends to be a chronic disorder, although there are limited prospective epidemiological data to support this observation. Both retrospective epidemiological and prospective clinical studies suggest that the disorder can profoundly disrupt an individual's life over many years. This can include disruption of school or academic achievement, interference with job performance, and impedance of social development.

Ms. S. was a successful secretary working in a law firm. Although she reported a long history of feeling uncomfortable in social situations, Ms. S. only came for treatment when she began to feel that her uneasiness was interfering with her social life and job performance. Ms. S. reported that she noticed herself feeling increasingly nervous whenever she met a new person. For example, upon meeting a new member of the law firm, she described feeling suddenly tense and sweaty and noticing that her heart was beating very fast. She had the sudden thought that she would say something very foolish in these situations or commit a terrible social gaffe that would cause people to laugh at her. At social gatherings, she described similar feelings that led her to either leave the gathering very early or even decline invitations to attend.

OBSESSIVE-COMPULSIVE DISORDER

Symptomatology Obsessions and compulsions are the essential features of OCD. As shown in Table 14.8–5, an individual must exhibit either obsessions or compulsions to meet DSM-IV-TR criteria. DSM-IV-TR recognizes obsessions as "persistent ideas, thoughts, impulses, or images that are experienced as intrusive and inappropriate," causing distress. Obsessions provoke anxiety, which accounts for the categorization of OCD as an anxiety disorder. However, they must be differentiated from excessive worries about real-life problems and associated with efforts to either ignore or suppress the obsessions. Typical obsessions associated with OCD include thoughts about contamination ("my hands are dirty") or doubts ("I forgot to turn off the stove").

Compulsions are defined as repetitive acts, behaviors, or thoughts that are designed to counteract the anxiety associated with an obsession. The key characteristic of a compulsion is that it reduces the anxiety associated with the obsession. Although many compulsions are acts associated with specific obsessions, such as hand washing or checking, compulsions can also manifest as thoughts. For example, a patient with the obsession that he or she has committed a sin might relieve the anxiety from this obsession by repetitively saying a silent prayer to him or herself.

Obsessions and compulsions must cause an individual marked distress, consume at least 1 hour per day, or interfere with functioning to be considered above the diagnostic threshold. During at least some point in the illness, adult patients must recognize symptoms of OCD as unreasonable, although there is great variability in the degree to which this is true, both across individuals and in a given individual over time. For example, early in the course of the disorder, patients may recognize their hand washing as excessive or irrational, but, over a number of years, this recognition may no longer exist. DSM-IV-TR recognizes a "poor insight" subtype of OCD when an individual fails to recognize the irrational or unreasonable nature of the obsessions. This subtype of OCD has been labeled the "psychotic subtype" in some of the clinical literature, prompting trials of neuroleptic therapy. The criterion related to insight does not apply to children, who

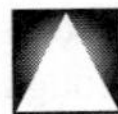

Table 14.8–5
DSM-IV-TR Criteria for Obsessive-Compulsive Disorder (OCD)

A. Either obsessions or compulsions:
Obsessions are defined by (1), (2), (3), and (4):
1. Recurrent and persistent thoughts, impulses, or images that are experienced at some time during the disturbance as intrusive and inappropriate and that cause marked anxiety or distress
2. The thoughts, impulses, or images are not simply excessive worries about real-life problems
3. The person attempts to ignore or suppress such thoughts, impulses, or images, or to neutralize them with some other thought or action
4. The person recognizes that the obsessional thoughts, impulses, or images are a product of his or her own mind (not imposed from without as in thought insertion)

Compulsions are defined by (1) and (2)
1. Repetitive behaviors (e.g., hand washing, ordering, checking) or mental acts (e.g., praying, counting, repeating words silently) that the person feels driven to perform in response to an obsession, or according to rules that must be applied rigidly
2. The behaviors or mental acts are aimed at preventing or reducing distress or preventing some dreaded event or situation; however, these behaviors or mental acts either are not connected in a realistic way with what they are designed to neutralize or prevent or are clearly excessive

B. At some point during the course of the disorder, the person has recognized that the obsessions or compulsions are excessive or unreasonable. **Note:** This does not apply to children.

C. The obsessions or compulsions cause marked distress, are time consuming (take more than 1 hour a day), or significantly interfere with the person's normal routine, occupational (or academic) functioning, or usual social activities or relationships.

D. If another Axis I disorder is present, the content of the obsessions or compulsions is not restricted to it (e.g., preoccupation with food in the presence of an eating disorder, hair pulling in the presence of trichotillomania, concern with appearance in the presence of body dysmorphic disorder, preoccupation with drugs in the presence of a substance use disorder, preoccupation with having a serious illness in the presence of hypochondriasis, preoccupation with sexual urges or fantasies in the presence of a paraphilia, or guilty ruminations in the presence of major depressive disorder).

E. The disturbance is not due to the direct physiological effects of a substance (e.g., a drug of abuse, a medication) or a general medical condition.

Specify if:

With poor insight: if, for most of the time during the current episode, the person does not recognize that the obsessions and compulsions are excessive or unreasonable.

From American Psychiatric Association. *Diagnostic and Statistical Manual of Mental Disorders.* 4th ed. Text rev. Washington, DC: American Psychiatric Association; 2000, with permission.

either may lack adequate insight to recognize the unreasonableness of their condition or may be too embarrassed to discuss the condition as unreasonable.

OCD frequently cooccurs with other disorders. The association with major depression is particularly prominent, although comorbidity with panic disorder, phobias, and eating disorders is also not uncommon. Finally, OCD exhibits a particularly interesting association with Tourette's syndrome. Approximately half of all patients with Tourette's syndrome meet criteria for OCD, although less than 10 percent of patients with OCD meet criteria for Tourette's syndrome. There is also evidence of cotransmission of Tourette's syndrome, OCD, and chronic motor tics within families.

History and Comparative Nosology Patients with a syndrome of recurrent obsessions and compulsions were described in the 19th century, when these conditions were viewed as a form of depressive state. Descriptions of OCD also played a prominent role in Sigmund Freud's writings, as evidenced in the case history of the Rat Man and in early learning-based theories that attempted to apply treatments developed for patients with phobias to patients with OCD. A major change in research on OCD emerged with the ECA Study in the early 1980s. Before this study, OCD was recognized as a discrete but rare entity and stimulated only a modest degree of research. The ECA Study noted OCD to have a prevalence in excess of 1 percent in the population and to be associated with marked impairment. This observation led to extensive research on all aspects of OCD, including its phenomenology.

The main change in OCD from DSM-III to DSM-IV-TR involved the conceptualization of compulsions. Whereas DSM-III-R viewed compulsions exclusively as behaviors, DSM-IV-TR recognizes compulsions as either behaviors or mental acts designed to reduce the anxiety-provoking nature of an obsession. The conceptualization of OCD in the ICD and DSM systems is generally similar, with a few exceptions in the emphasis on specific features of the condition. For example, ICD-10 emphasizes that a compulsive act must not be pleasurable. ICD-10 also stipulates that obsessions or compulsions must be present most days for 2 weeks, a requirement not included in DSM-IV-TR, and ICD-10 does not quantify the amount of time a patient must spend on compulsions. Perhaps the primary difference between the DSM-IV-TR and ICD-10 views of the disorder involves categorization with respect to other anxiety disorders. DSM-IV-TR recognizes OCD as one of the nine anxiety disorders discussed in this section. There has been some debate, both in the United States and in Europe, as to whether OCD is more properly classified in a distinct category. ICD-10 has adopted such a scheme, using the term *OCD* as a label for a group of syndromes considered distinct from anxiety disorders.

Differential Diagnosis A number of primary medical disorders can produce syndromes bearing a striking resemblance to OCD. In fact, the current conceptualization of OCD as a disorder of the basal ganglia derives from the phenomenological similarity between idiopathic OCD and OCD-like disorders that are associated with basal ganglia diseases, such as Sydenham's chorea and Huntington's disease. Hence, neurological signs of such basal ganglia pathology must be assessed when considering the diagnosis of OCD in a patient presenting for psychiatric treatment. It should also be noted that OCD frequently develops before age 30 years, and new-onset OCD in an older individual should raise questions about potential neurological contributions to the disorder. Finally, among children, there is some evidence of an association between an immune reaction to streptococcal infections and either initial manifestations or dramatic exacerbation of OCD. This syndrome appears to emerge relatively acutely, in contrast to a more insidious onset in other cases of childhood OCD. Hence, in children with acute presentations, the role of such an infectious process should be considered.

Obsessive-compulsive behavior is also found in a host of other psychiatric disorders, and the clinician must also rule out these conditions when diagnosing OCD. OCD exhibits a superficial resemblance to obsessive-compulsive personality disorder, which is associated with an obsessive concern for details, perfectionism, and other similar personality traits. The conditions are easily distinguished by the fact that only OCD is associated with a true syndrome of obsessions and compulsions, as described above.

Psychotic symptoms often lead to obsessive thoughts and compulsive behaviors that can be difficult to distinguish from OCD with poor insight, in which obsessions border on psychosis. The keys to distinguishing OCD from psychosis are (1) patients with OCD can almost always acknowledge the unreasonable nature of their symptoms, and (2) psychotic illnesses are typically associated with a host of other features that are not characteristic of OCD. Similarly, OCD can be difficult to differentiate from depression, as the two disorders often occur comorbidly, and major depression is often associated with obsessive thoughts that, at times, border on true obsessions like those that characterize OCD. The two conditions are best distinguished by their courses. Obsessive symptoms associated with depression are only found in the presence of a depressive episode, whereas true OCD persists despite remission of depression.

Finally, as noted above, OCD is closely related to Tourette's syndrome, as the two conditions frequently cooccur, both in individuals over time and within families. In its classic form, Tourette's syndrome is associated with a pattern of recurrent vocal and motor tics that bears only a slight resemblance to OCD. However, the premonitory urges that precede tics often strikingly resemble obsessions, and many of the more complicated motor tics are very similar to compulsions.

Epidemiology As noted above, although OCD was once considered relatively rare, recent epidemiological studies place the prevalence in the range of 2 to 3 percent. The prevalence of the disorder is approximately equal in men and women, although men tend to have an earlier onset than women do.

Course OCD typically begins in late adolescence, although onset in childhood is not uncommon. The disorder tends to exhibit a waxing and waning course over the life span, with periods of relatively good functioning and limited symptoms punctuated by periods of symptomatic exacerbation. Small minorities of patients exhibit either complete remission of their disorder or a progressive, deteriorating course.

Ms. B. presented for psychiatric admission after being transferred from a medical floor where she had been treated for malnutrition. Ms. B. had been found unconscious in her apartment by a neighbor. When brought to the emergency department by an ambulance, she was found to be hypotensive and hypokalemic. At psychiatric admission, Ms. B. described a long history of recurrent obsessions about cleanliness, particularly related to food items. She reported that because she often had the thought that a food item was dirty, it was difficult for her to eat any food unless she had washed it three or four times. She reported that washing her food decreased the anxiety she felt about its dirtiness. Although Ms. B. reported that she had occasionally tried to eat food that she had not washed (e.g., in a restaurant), she found that she became so worried about becoming ill from eating such food that she could no longer dine in restaurants. Ms. B. reported that her obsessions about the cleanliness of food had become so extreme over the past 3 months that she could eat very few foods, even if she washed them excessively. She recognized the irrational nature of these obsessive concerns, but either could not bring herself to eat or became extremely nervous and nauseated after eating.

POSTTRAUMATIC STRESS AND ACUTE STRESS DISORDERS

Symptomatology Both PTSD and acute stress disorder are characterized by the onset of psychiatric symptoms immediately after exposure to a traumatic event. As noted in Table 14.8–6, DSM-IV-TR explicitly notes that such a traumatic event involves either witnessing or experiencing threatened death or injury or witnessing or experiencing threat to physical integrity. Further, the response to the traumatic event must involve intense fear or horror. Such traumatic experiences might include being involved in or witnessing a violent accident or crime, military combat, assault, being kidnapped, being involved in natural disasters, being diagnosed with a life-threatening illness, or experiencing systematic physical or sexual abuse. Both PTSD and acute stress disorder also require characteristic symptoms after such trauma. There is evidence of a dose–response relationship between the degree of trauma and the likelihood of symptoms. The greater the proximity and intensity of the trauma, the greater the probability of developing symptomatology.

In PTSD, the individual develops symptoms in three domains: reexperiencing the trauma, avoiding stimuli associated with the trauma, and experiencing symptoms of increased autonomic arousal, such as an enhanced startle. Flashbacks, in which the individual may act and feel as if the trauma were recurring, represent the classic form of reexperiencing. Other forms of reexperiencing include distressing recollections or dreams and either physiological or psychological stress reactions when exposed to stimuli that are linked to the trauma. An individual must exhibit at least one reexperiencing symptom to meet criteria for PTSD. Symptoms of avoidance associated with PTSD include efforts to avoid thoughts or activities related to the trauma, anhedonia, reduced capacity to remember events related to the trauma, blunted affect, feelings of detachment or derealization, and a sense of a foreshortened future. An individual must exhibit at least three such symptoms. Symptoms of increased arousal include insomnia, irritability, hypervigilance, and exaggerated startle. An individual must exhibit at least two such symptoms. Finally, the diagnosis of PTSD is only made when symptoms persist for at least 1 month; the diagnosis of acute stress disorder is made in the interim. DSM-IV-TR acknowledges three subtypes of PTSD, differentiating among syndromes with varying time courses. *Acute PTSD* refers to an episode that lasts less than 3 months, whereas *chronic PTSD* refers to an episode lasting 3 months or longer. *PTSD with delayed onset* refers to an episode that develops 6 months or more after exposure to the traumatic event.

The diagnosis of acute stress disorder is applied to syndromes that resemble PTSD but last less than 1 month after a trauma. Acute stress disorder is characterized by reexperiencing, avoidance, and increased arousal, much like PTSD. Acute stress disorder is also associated with at least three of the dissociative symptoms listed in Table 14.8–6.

Because individuals often exhibit complex biological and behavioral responses to extreme trauma, the clinician must identify other medical and psychiatric conditions in the traumatized patient. The clinician must always evaluate whether neurological etiologies underlie trauma-related symptoms, particularly after traumatic events that involve physical injury. Traumatized patients also can develop mood disorders, including dysthymia and major depression, as well as other anxiety disorders, such as generalized anxiety disorder or panic disorder, and substance use disorders. Finally, recent research suggests that some psychiatric features of posttraumatic syndromes can relate to a patient's state before the trauma. For example, patients with premorbid anxiety or affective syndromes may be more likely to develop posttraumatic symptoms than individuals who are free of mental illness before the trauma. As a result, the clinician should consider the premorbid mental state of the trauma-

Table 14.8–6
DSM-IV-TR Criteria for Posttraumatic Stress Disorder and Acute Stress Disorder

Criteria for posttraumatic stress disorder (PTSD)

A. The person has been exposed to a traumatic event in which both of the following were present:
   1. The person experienced, witnessed, or was confronted with an event that involved actual or threatened death or serious injury, or a threat to the physical integrity of self or others.
   2. The person's response involved intense fear, helplessness, or horror. **Note:** In children this may be expressed, instead, by disorganized or agitated behavior.

B. The traumatic event is persistently reexperienced in one (or more) of the following ways:
   1. Recurrent and intrusive distressing recollections of the event, including images, thoughts, or perceptions. **Note:** In young children, repetitive play may occur in which themes or aspects of the trauma are expressed.
   2. Recurrent distressing dreams of the event. **Note:** In children, there may be frightening dreams without recognizable content.
   3. Acting or feeling as if the traumatic event were recurring (includes a sense of reliving the experience, illusions, hallucinations, and dissociative flashback episodes, including those that occur on awakening or when intoxicated). **Note:** In young children, trauma-specific reenactment may occur.
   4. Intense psychological distress at exposure to internal or external cues that symbolize or resemble an aspect of the traumatic event.
   5. Physiological reactivity on exposure to internal or external cues that symbolize or resemble an aspect of the traumatic event.

C. Persistent avoidance of stimuli associated with the trauma and numbing of general responsiveness (not present before the trauma), as indicated by three (or more) of the following:
   1. Efforts to avoid thoughts, feelings, or conversations associated with the trauma
   2. Efforts to avoid activities, places, or people that arouse recollections of the trauma
   3. Inability to recall an important aspect of the trauma
   4. Markedly diminished interest or participation in significant activities
   5. Feeling of detachment or estrangement from others
   6. Restricted range of affect (e.g., unable to have loving feelings)
   7. Sense of a foreshortened future (e.g., does not expect to have a career, marriage, children, or a normal life span)

D. Persistent symptoms of increased arousal (not present before the trauma), as indicated by two (or more) of the following:
   1. Difficulty falling or staying asleep
   2. Irritability or outbursts of anger
   3. Difficulty concentrating
   4. Hypervigilance
   5. Exaggerated startle response

E. Duration of the disturbance (symptoms in Criteria B, C, and D) is more than 1 month.

F. The disturbance causes clinically significant distress or impairment in social, occupational, or other important areas of functioning.

Specify if:
   Acute: if duration of symptoms is less than 3 months
   Chronic: if duration of symptoms is 3 months or more
   With delayed onset: if onset of symptoms is at least 6 months after the stressor

Criteria for acute stress disorder

A. The person has been exposed to a traumatic event in which both of the following were present:
   1. The person experienced, witnessed, or was confronted with an event that involved actual or threatened death or serious injury, or a threat to the physical integrity of self or others.
   2. The person's response involved intense fear, helplessness, or horror.

B. Either while experiencing or after experiencing the distressing event, the individual has three (or more) of the following dissociative symptoms:
   1. A subjective sense of numbing, detachment, or absence of emotional responsiveness
   2. A reduction in awareness of his or her surroundings (e.g., "being in a daze")
   3. Derealization
   4. Depersonalization
   5. Dissociative amnesia (i.e., inability to recall an important aspect of the trauma)

C. The traumatic event is persistently reexperienced in at least one of the following ways: recurrent images, thoughts, dreams, illusions, flashback episodes, or a sense of reliving the experience, or distress on exposure to reminders of the traumatic event.

D. Marked avoidance of stimuli that arouse recollections of the trauma (e.g., thoughts, feelings, conversations, activities, places, people).

E. Marked symptoms of anxiety or increased arousal (e.g., difficulty sleeping, irritability, poor concentration, hypervigilance, exaggerated startle response, motor restlessness).

F. The disturbance causes clinically significant distress or impairment to social, occupational, or other important areas of functioning or impairs the individual's ability to pursue some necessary task, such as obtaining necessary assistance or mobilizing personal resources by telling family members about the traumatic experience.

G. The disturbance lasts for a minimum of 2 days and a maximum of 4 weeks and occurs within 4 weeks of the traumatic event.

H. The disturbance is not due to the direct physiological effects of a substance (e.g., a drug of abuse, a medication) or a general medical condition, is not better accounted for by brief psychotic disorder, and is not merely an exacerbation of a preexisting Axis I or Axis II disorder.

From American Psychiatric Association. *Diagnostic and Statistical Manual of Mental Disorders.* 4th ed. Text rev. Washington, DC: American Psychiatric Association; 2000, with permission.

tized patient to enhance understanding of symptoms that develop after a traumatic event.

History and Comparative Nosology Astute clinicians have recognized the juxtaposition of acute mental syndromes and traumatic events for more than 200 years. Observations of trauma-related syndromes were documented after the Civil War and early psychoanalytical writers, including Freud, noted the relationship between neurosis and trauma. Considerable interest in posttraumatic mental disorders was stimulated by observations of battle fatigue, shell shock, and soldier's heart in both World War I and World War II. Moreover, increasing documentation of mental reactions to the Holocaust, to a series of natural disasters, and to assault contributed to the growing recognition of a close relationship between trauma and psychopathology.

The syndrome of PTSD was first recognized in the DSM nosology with DSM-III in 1980, whereas acute stress disorder was first identified in DSM-IV-TR in 1994. The recognition of acute stress disorder came after observations suggesting that many individuals exhibit mental syndromes immediately after trauma and that such individuals might face an elevated risk for PTSD. The original DSM-III definition of PTSD required only one symptom of reexperiencing, two symptoms of "psychic numbing," and one symptom from a list of miscellaneous items, with no duration criteria. DSM-III-R added a number of symptoms to the DSM-III definition and removed the DSM-III symptom of guilt. DSM-III-R also adopted the symptom groupings that are found in DSM-IV-TR, in which symptoms are classified as manifestations of either reexperiencing, avoidance, or hyperarousal. The major change to the definition in DSM-IV-TR involved the definition of trauma. Whereas DSM-III-R emphasized trauma as an event that was "outside of normal experience," a number of field studies suggested that the typical traumatic precipitants of PTSD were relatively common events. As a result, DSM-IV-TR emphasizes the threat and fear-provoking nature of a trauma, without reference to "normal experience."

There are some differences between the DSM-IV-TR and ICD-10 definitions of PTSD and acute stress disorder. Whereas ICD-10 acknowledges the same core group of symptoms for PTSD than DSM-IV-TR does, including exposure to a trauma, reexperiencing, avoidance, and increased arousal, ICD-10 provides considerably less detail for each of the criteria than DSM-IV-TR does. For example, unlike DSM-IV-TR, ICD-10 provides only brief examples of reexperiencing or avoidance symptoms. The broader views of PTSD and acute stress disorder also differ between the DSM and ICD systems. As it does with OCD, ICD-10 groups PTSD and acute stress reaction in a distinct category, *stress-related disorders*, rather than grouping them with other anxiety disorders.

Differential Diagnosis Because patients often exhibit complex reactions to trauma, the clinician must be careful to exclude other syndromes as well when evaluating patients presenting in the wake of trauma. It is particularly important to recognize potentially treatable medical contributors to posttraumatic symptomatology. For example, neurological injury after head trauma can contribute to the clinical picture, as can psychoactive substance use disorders or withdrawal syndromes, either in the period immediately surrounding the trauma or many weeks after the trauma. Medical contributors can usually be detected through a careful history and physical examination, as long as the clinician remembers to consider such factors.

Symptoms of PTSD can be difficult to distinguish from both panic disorder and generalized anxiety disorder, as all three syndromes are associated with prominent anxiety and autonomic arousal. Keys to correctly diagnosing PTSD involve a careful review of the time course relating the symptoms to a traumatic event. Further, PTSD is associated with reexperiencing and avoidance of a trauma, features typically not present in panic or generalized anxiety disorder. Major depression is also a frequent concomitant of PTSD. Although the two syndromes are not usually difficult to distinguish phenomenologically, it is important to note the presence of comorbid depression, as this may influence treatment of PTSD. Finally, PTSD must be differentiated from a series of related disorders that can exhibit phenomenological similarities, including borderline personality disorder, dissociative disorders, and factitious disorders.

Epidemiology As acute stress disorder represents a new disorder in DSM-IV-TR, there has been minimal research on its prevalence. Research on the psychological response to trauma, however, shows that psychological reactions that resemble acute stress disorder are very common with exposure to extreme trauma at close proximity. Estimates of PTSD prevalence depend on the population studied, as exposure to trauma varies widely across communities. Recent studies generally estimate the prevalence in the community to be between 2 and 15 percent.

Course Much of the recent research on the course of psychological reactions to trauma has focused on the time course of symptoms immediately after a trauma. The likelihood of developing symptoms, the severity of such symptoms, and the duration of the symptoms are each proportional to the proximity, duration, and intensity of the trauma. Many individuals develop acute stress reactions when faced with close, persistent, and intense trauma. Moreover, many individuals who develop PTSD exhibit features of the acute stress syndrome before developing PTSD, although many individuals with acute stress syndromes do not develop PTSD. Finally, the full syndrome of PTSD also exhibits a variable course, with some evidence that this also relates to the nature of the trauma. A large minority of patients develop complete remissions, whereas another large group exhibits only mild symptoms. PTSD is persistent or chronic in approximately 10 percent of patients with the disorder.

> Mr. F. sought treatment for symptoms that he developed in the wake of an automobile accident that had occurred approximately 6 weeks before his psychiatric evaluation. While driving to work on a mid-January morning, Mr. F. lost control of his car on an icy road. His car swerved out of control into oncoming traffic, collided with another car, and then hit a nearby pedestrian. Mr. F. was trapped in his car for 3 hours while rescue workers cut through the car door. After referral, Mr. F. reported frequent intrusive thoughts about the accident, including nightmares of the event and recurrent intrusive visions of his car slamming into the pedestrian. He reported that he had altered his driving route to work to avoid the scene of the accident and that he found himself switching the TV channel whenever a commercial for snow tires appeared. Mr. F. described frequent difficulty falling asleep, poor concentration, and an increased focus on his environment, particularly when he was driving.

GENERALIZED ANXIETY DISORDER

Symptomatology Generalized anxiety disorder is characterized by a pattern of frequent, persistent worry and anxiety that is out of proportion to the impact of the event or circumstance that is the focus of the worry, as shown in Table 14.8–7. For example, although college students often worry about examinations, a student who persistently worries about failure despite consistently getting outstanding grades shows a pattern of worry that is typical of generalized anxiety disorder. Patients with generalized anxiety disorder may not acknowledge the excessive nature of their worries, but they must be bothered by their degree of worry. This pattern must occur more days than not for at least 6 months. Patients must find it difficult to control this worry and must report at least three of six somatic or cognitive symptoms. Such symptoms include feelings of restlessness, fatigue, muscle tension, and insomnia. Finally, worry is a ubiquitous feature of many anxiety disorders, as patients with panic disorder often worry about panic attacks, patients with social phobia worry about social encounters, and patients with OCD worry about their obsessions. The worries in generalized anxiety disorder must exceed in breadth or scope the worries that characterize these other anxiety disorders. Children with marked and persistent worry can also be diagnosed with generalized anxiety disorder, but, unlike

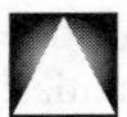

Table 14.8–7
DSM-IV-TR Criteria for Generalized Anxiety Disorder

A. Excessive anxiety and worry (apprehensive expectation) about a number of events or activities (such as work or school performance) occurring more days than not for at least 6 months.

B. The person finds it difficult to control the worry.

C. The anxiety and worry are associated with three (or more) of the following six symptoms (with at least some symptoms present for more days than not for the past 6 months). **Note:** Only one item is required in children.
   1. Restlessness or feeling keyed up or on edge
   2. Being easily fatigued
   3. Difficulty concentrating
   4. Irritability
   5. Muscle tension
   6. Sleep disturbance (difficulty falling or staying asleep, or restless unsatisfying sleep)

D. The focus of the anxiety and worry is not confined to features of an Axis I disorder—e.g., the anxiety or worry is not about having a panic attack (as in panic disorder), being embarrassed in public (as in social phobia), being contaminated (as in obsessive-compulsive disorder), being away from home (as in separation anxiety disorder), gaining weight (as in anorexia nervosa), having multiple physical complaints (as in somatization disorder), or having a serious illness (as in hypochondriasis), and the anxiety or worry does not occur exclusively during posttraumatic stress disorder.

E. The anxiety, worry, or physical symptoms cause clinically significant distress or impairment in social, occupational, or other important areas of functioning.

F. The disturbance is not due to the direct physiological effects of a substance (e.g., a drug of abuse, a medication) or a general medical condition (e.g., hypothyroidism) and does not occur exclusively during a mood disorder, a psychotic disorder, or a pervasive developmental disorder.

From American Psychiatric Association. *Diagnostic and Statistical Manual of Mental Disorders.* 4th ed. Text rev. Washington, DC: American Psychiatric Association; 2000, with permission.

adults, they must only meet one of the six somatic or cognitive symptom criteria.

History and Comparative Nosology

Clinicians have documented symptoms of generalized anxiety disorder for more than 100 years. Many of the syndromes that are considered related to panic disorder, such as DaCosta's syndrome or neurocirculatory asthenia, also bear a close resemblance to generalized anxiety disorder. In fact, before DSM-III, panic disorder and generalized anxiety disorder were both subsumed under the broader category of anxiety neurosis.

The conceptualization of generalized anxiety disorder has changed gradually from DSM-III to DSM-IV-TR. The disorder was originally conceived as a residual category in DSM-III for anxiety disorders that did not fulfill criteria for another disorder. DSM-III only required a 1-month duration of symptoms, and concerns arose about the low reliability of the diagnosis. DSM-III-R increased the duration criterion to 6 months, placed more emphasis on the symptom of worry, and added a list of 18 symptoms, out of which patients had to exhibit at least 6. DSM-III-R also removed some of the hierarchical rules in DSM-III that had limited the diagnosis to individuals who were free of other specific disorders. Finally, DSM-IV-TR brought further revisions to the diagnosis. The list of associated symptoms was narrowed from 18 to 6, of which adult patients had to exhibit at least three. More emphasis was also placed on the pervasiveness of the patient's worry. DSM-IV-TR attempted to expand this emphasis on worry across development. Whereas DSM-III-R included the diagnosis of overanxious disorder for use among children, DSM-IV-TR integrated this DSM-III-R diagnosis with generalized anxiety disorder, with the caveat that minor threshold differences apply when making the diagnosis in children rather than in adults.

ICD-10 includes the diagnosis of generalized anxiety disorder and emphasizes the distinction between generalized anxiety and panic disorders. Although ICD-10 places a similar emphasis on worry to that in DSM-IV-TR, it approaches the other symptoms of generalized anxiety disorder in a way that more closely resembles DSM-III-R than DSM-IV-TR. For example, in ICD-10, the diagnosis requires four associated symptoms from a list of 22 symptoms.

Differential Diagnosis

Like other anxiety disorders, particularly panic disorder, generalized anxiety disorder must be differentiated from both medical and psychiatric disorders. Neurological, endocrinological, metabolic, and medication-related disorders similar to those considered in the differential diagnosis of panic disorder must be considered in the differential diagnosis of generalized anxiety disorder. Common cooccurring anxiety disorders also must be considered. These include panic disorder, phobias, OCD, and PTSD. To meet criteria for generalized anxiety disorder, patients must not only exhibit the full syndrome, but their symptoms also cannot be explained by the presence of a comorbid anxiety disorder. To diagnose generalized anxiety disorder in the context of other anxiety disorders, it is most important to document anxiety or worry related to circumstances or topics that are either unrelated or only minimally related to other disorders. Hence, proper diagnosis involves both definitively establishing the presence of generalized anxiety disorder and properly diagnosing other anxiety disorders. Patients with generalized anxiety disorder frequently develop major depressive disorder. As a result, this condition must also be recognized and distinguished. Again, the key to making a correct diagnosis is documenting anxiety or worry that is unrelated to the depressive disorder.

Epidemiology

It is difficult to provide a definitive estimate of the prevalence of generalized anxiety disorder, given the changes to the diagnostic criteria since the 1990s. In general, most community-based studies place the prevalence in the range of 2 to 5 percent, with the ECA suggesting a lifetime prevalence as high as 8 percent. The disorder tends to be more common in women and usually has its onset in late adolescence or early adulthood. However, cases are commonly seen in older adults. There is also some evidence suggesting that the prevalence of generalized anxiety disorder is particularly high in primary care settings.

Course

The lack of prospective epidemiological studies precludes firm conclusions about the course of generalized anxiety disorder. Moreover, there is also insufficient prospective research even among clinical samples. The most complete data on the course of the disorder are derived from retrospective epidemiologically based studies. These studies suggest that generalized anxiety disorder is chronic, as most patients report symptoms for many years before assessment. Given the possible biases in such studies, no definitive statement on the course of the disorder can be made.

Ms. X. was a successful, married, 30-year-old attorney who presented for a psychiatric evaluation to treat mounting symptoms of worry and anxiety. For the preceding 8 months, Ms. X. noted that she had become increasingly worried about her job performance. For example, although she had always been a superb litigator, she found herself worrying more and more about her ability to win cases. Similarly, although she had always been in outstanding physical condition, she increasingly worried that her health had begun to deteriorate. Ms. X. noted frequent somatic symptoms that accompanied her worries. For example, she often felt restless while she worked and while she commuted to her office, at which time she tended to think about the upcoming challenges of the day. She reported feeling increasingly fatigued, irritable, and tense. She noted that she had increasing difficulty falling asleep at night as she worried about her job performance and impending trials.

Three other anxiety disorders will be discussed in less detail. Anxiety disorder not otherwise specified will only be discussed briefly due to the limited research on this condition. Substance-induced anxiety and anxiety disorder due to a general medical condition are only discussed briefly, as these topics are considered in more detail in other chapters.

ANXIETY DISORDER NOT OTHERWISE SPECIFIED

Anxiety represents one of the most common psychiatric symptoms encountered in various settings, including primary care settings, and it is relatively common to encounter patients who exhibit impairment from anxiety but do not meet criteria for one of the disorders discussed in the preceding sections. These patients are appropriately classified as having *anxiety disorder not otherwise specified.*

Two clinical features of this disorder must be recognized to properly identify the condition. First, the anxiety described by the patients must be distressing, interfering with some aspect of functioning. Second, the anxiety must not be attributable to another psychiatric condition. For example, patients with generalized anxiety disorder may not initially report sufficient associated symptoms to meet criteria for this condition. However, on further probing, such symptoms may be identified. It is important to establish that another anxiety disorder does not account for the complaints, particularly in patients with long-standing anxiety. Perhaps the most consistent research on this condition examines patients with *mixed anxiety-depressive disorder*, a condition described in the Appendix of DSM-IV-TR.

Patients with mixed anxiety-depressive disorder exhibit symptoms of both depression and anxiety that do not meet criteria for another mood or anxiety disorder. Such patients must show signs of consistent low mood for at least 1 month, accompanied by additional symptoms that include prominent worries. Longitudinal studies find a relatively high risk for later mood or anxiety disorders with this condition, particularly major depression. Due to the paucity of data on treatment for the condition, clinicians often use approaches that are effective in other mood or anxiety disorders. Anxiety concerning an embarrassing medical problem or scenario is another frequently encountered form of anxiety disorder not otherwise specified. For example, patients who exhibit excessive concern regarding a dermatological condition might exhibit symptoms of this syndrome.

SUBSTANCE-INDUCED ANXIETY AND ANXIETY DUE TO A GENERAL MEDICAL CONDITION

Each of these conditions is characterized by prominent anxiety that arises as the direct result of some underlying physiological perturbation. Hence, for patients with substance-induced anxiety, clinically significant symptoms of panic, worry, phobia, or obsessions emerge in the context of substance use—this can refer to either prescribed or illicit substances. For example, both prescribed and illicit sympathomimetic substances can often produce relatively marked degrees of anxiety. Similarly, for anxiety due to a general medical condition, symptoms develop in the context of an identifiable medical syndrome. For example, panic attacks have been tied to various medical conditions, including endocrinological, cardiac, and respiratory illnesses.

The first step in identifying an anxiety disorder due to either a medical condition or substance is to confirm the presence of one or the other complicating factor. Clearly, practitioners should routinely document the medical and substance use status of all patients. However, the clinician should be particularly wary when encountering a patient with an unusual symptomatic presentation. For example, changes in consciousness or neurological function almost never occur in acute anxiety states unless there is also an underlying medical component to the syndrome. In cases in which there is a suspicion of such complicating factors, the presence of substance use or medical problems first must be definitively confirmed by obtaining the necessary medical history or evaluative procedures. Next, the clinician must determine that this underlying problem is the cause of the ongoing anxiety symptoms. Although there is no definitive test to establish such a causal relationship, at least three factors can be helpful—the timing of the symptoms, the existing literature pertaining to the strength of the association between anxiety and the potential complicating factor, and signs or symptoms (e.g., changes in consciousness) that are atypical for an anxiety disorder. Finally, even more suggestive evidence can be provided if alleviation of the complicating medical factor produces an amelioration of the anxiety symptoms.

SUGGESTED CROSS-REFERENCES

Other aspects of these disorders are discussed elsewhere within this chapter, such as theories on etiology (Sections 14.3, 14.4, 14.5, 14.6, and 14.7) and treatment (Sections 14.9 and 14.10). Similarly, substance-induced anxiety disorder and anxiety disorder due to a general medical condition as distinct anxiety disorders are also discussed in Chapter 11, on substance use disorders, and Chapter 10, on the psychiatric complications of medical conditions.

REFERENCES

Angst J, Vollrath M: The natural history of anxiety disorders. *Acta Psychiatr Scand.* 1991;84:446.

Ballenger JC, Fyer AJ: DSM-IV in progress: Examining criteria for panic disorder. *Hosp Community Psychiatry.* 1993;44:226.

*Barlow DH. *Anxiety and Its Disorders: The Nature and Treatment of Anxiety and Panic.* New York: Guilford; 1988.

*Breslau N, Davis GC, Andreski P, Peterson E: Traumatic events and posttraumatic stress disorder in an urban population of young adults. *Arch Gen Psychiatry.* 1991;48:216.

Carden E, Speigel D: Dissociative reaction to the San Francisco Bay Area earthquake of 1989. *Am J Psychiatry.* 1993;150:474.

Davidson JRT, Foa EB: Diagnostic issues in posttraumatic stress disorder: Considerations for the DSM-IV. *J Abnorm Psychol.* 1991;100:346.

Davidson JRT, Hughes DL, George LK, Blazer DG: The epidemiology of social phobia. Findings from the Epidemiologic Catchment Area Study. *Psychol Med.* 1993;23:709.

Freud S. Inhibitions, symptoms and anxiety. In: *Standard Edition of the Complete Psychological Works of Sigmund Freud.* Vol 20. London: Hogarth Press; 1966:77.

Freud S. Obsessions and phobias. In: *Standard Edition of the Complete Psychological Works of Sigmund Freud.* Vol 3. London: Hogarth Press; 1966:71.

Fyer AJ, Mannuzza S, Chapman T, Liebowitz MR, Klein DF: A direct interview family study of social phobia. *Arch Gen Psychiatry*. 1994;50:286.
Gorman JM, Papp LA: Chronic anxiety: Deciding the length of treatment. *J Clin Psychiatry*. 1990;51(Suppl):11.
Gorman JM, Papp LA, eds. Anxiety disorders. In: Tasman, ed. *Annual Review of Psychiatry*. Vol 11A. Washington, DC: American Psychiatric Association Press; 1992.
Horwath E, Wolk SI, Goldstein RB, Wickramaratne P, Sobin C, Adams P, Lish JD, Weissman MM: Is the comorbidity between social phobia and panic disorder due to familial cotransmission or other factors? *Arch Gen Psychiatry*. 1995;52:574.
Jarrell MP, Ballenger JC: Psychiatric comorbidity in patients with generalized anxiety disorder. *Am J Psychiatry* 1993;150:1216.
Jenike MA, Baer L, Minichiello WE. *Obsessive-Compulsive Disorders: Theory and Management*. 2nd ed. Chicago: Yearbook Publishing; 1990.
Keller MB: The lifelong course of social anxiety disorder: A clinical perspective. *Acta Psychiatr Scand Suppl*. 2003;417:85–94.
Kessler RC, Sonnega A, Bromet E, Hughes M, Nelson CB: Posttraumatic stress disorder in the national comorbidity survey. *Arch Gen Psychiatry*. 1995;52:1048.
Klein DF: Delineation of two drug-responsive anxiety syndromes. *Psychopharmacology*. 1964;5:397.
Klein DF: False suffocation alarms, spontaneous panics, and related conditions: An integrative hypothesis. *Arch Gen Psychiatry*. 1993;50:306.
Klein DF, Rabkin JG, eds. *Anxiety: New Research and Changing Concepts*. New York: Raven Press; 1981.
Klerman GL, Weissman MM, Ouellette R, Johnson J, Greenwald S: Panic attacks in the community: Social morbidity and health care utilization. *JAMA*. 1991;265:742.
*Liebowitz MR, Gorman JM, Fyer AF, Klein DF: Social phobia: Review of a neglected anxiety disorder. *Arch Gen Psychiatry*. 1985;42:729.
*Magee WJ, Eaton WW, Wittchen HU, McGonagle KA, Kessler RC: Agoraphobia, simple phobia, and social phobia in the National Comorbidity Survey. *Arch Gen Psychiatry*. 1996;53:159.
*Marks IM. *Fears, Phobias, and Rituals: Panic, Anxiety, and Their Disorders*. New York: Oxford University Press; 1988.
McFarlane AC. The phenomenology of post-traumatic stress disorders following a natural disaster. *J Nerv Ment Dis*. 1988;176:22.
Merikangas KR, Zhang H, Avenevoli S, Acharyya S, Neuenschwander M, Angst J: Longitudinal trajectories of depression and anxiety in a prospective community study: The Zurich Cohort Study. *Arch Gen Psychiatry*. 2003;60:993–1000.
Pigott TA: Anxiety disorders in women. *Psychiatr Clin North Am*. 2003;26:621–672.
Rapee RM, Barlow DH, eds. *Chronic Anxiety*. New York: Guilford; 1991.
Rapoport JL: *The Boy Who Couldn't Stop Washing*. New York: Dutton; 1989.
Stein MB, Walker JR, Forde DR: Public-speaking fears in a community sample: Prevalence, impact on functioning, and diagnostic classification. *Arch Gen Psychiatry*. 1995;53:169.
Weissman MM: Panic and generalized anxiety: Are they separate disorders? *J Psychiatr Res*. 1990;24(2 Suppl):157.

▲ 14.9 Anxiety Disorders: Somatic Treatment

MURRAY B. STEIN, M.D.

Anxiety disorders are among the most common psychiatric syndromes, affecting approximately 25 percent of persons in the general population during their lifetimes. The psychosocial and economic impact of anxiety disorders is substantial, with an estimated $40 billion per year spent primarily on medical services. The toll on individuals, in terms of suffering and functional disability, is enormous. Moreover, it is being increasingly recognized that anxiety disorders often start early in life and provide a template on which other forms of comorbidity (e.g., major depression, substance abuse) and adverse health outcomes (e.g., suicidal ideation) are layered. For all these reasons, anxiety disorders are finally being recognized as serious public health problems.

HISTORY

Treatment of anxiety disorders has markedly evolved since the 1950s. Until the middle of the 20th century, anxiety disorders were treated with psychoanalysis or barbiturates. Psychoanalysis, while offering the promise of a deep understanding of the roots of anxiety, has yet to be empirically demonstrated to be efficacious for anxiety disorders. Barbiturates, although powerful in their antianxiety and sedating effects, were no doubt misused and overused, resulting in physical dependence and substantial risk of overdose for some. Benzodiazepines, partial agonists of the γ-aminobutyric acid type A ($GABA_A$) receptors, were discovered in the 1960s and achieved prominence in the pharmacological treatment of anxiety. These agents continue to be widely used because of their high degree of therapeutic efficacy and good safety profile.

Another milestone in the pharmacological treatment of anxiety disorders came in the early 1960s when Donald Klein and colleagues determined that a tricyclic antidepressant, imipramine (Tofranil), reduced the frequency of spontaneous panic attacks in anxious-depressed patients. This observation sparked interest in the pharmacological dissection of anxiety, which was a key factor in the development of a nosology of anxiety disorders that featured discrete "anxiety disorders" as opposed to anxiety and phobic "neuroses." Although some investigators might argue that this separation was premature, it had the monumental impact of stirring interest in the treatment of anxiety with compounds other than barbiturates, benzodiazepines, or neuroleptics (e.g., thioridazine [Mellaril]). Although tricky to use because of anxious patients' sensitivity to their side effects, tricyclic and heterocyclic antidepressants assumed a prominent role in the treatment of panic disorder and related syndromes. In the mid-1980s, the arrival of the selective serotonin reuptake inhibitor (SSRI) fluoxetine (Prozac) heralded a next stage in the treatment of anxiety disorders with antidepressants. Although sometimes associated with initial worsening of anxiety, the use of SSRIs, beginning with low doses and gradually working upward, rapidly became a mainstay of the pharmacotherapy of anxiety disorders whose influence has not yet ebbed.

In the past two decades, hundreds of large-scale clinical trials have been conducted to test the efficacy of new therapeutic agents for anxiety disorders. These studies have led to the development of a burgeoning evidence base for the pharmacotherapy of anxiety disorders. In parallel, cognitive-behavioral therapists have developed and empirically verified the utility of a cadre of potent psychological therapies for anxiety disorders. For the most part, the best pharmacological therapies rival the best psychological (i.e., cognitive-behavioral) therapies in terms of overall efficacy, although the latter seem to confer more long-lasting therapeutic benefits. Current knowledge of what medications work has so far outstripped knowledge of how they work in the treatment of anxiety disorders. It is presumed that the mechanism of action of antidepressants in treating anxiety is similar (perhaps identical) to their mechanism of action in treating depression; this is thought to involve alterations in neuronal serotonin metabolism with accompanying changes in receptor sensitivity. Actions on other neurotransmitter systems in specific neuronal circuits (e.g., involving the amygdala) or on neurotrophic factors in specific brain regions (e.g., hippocampus) are also possibilities that are currently the subject of much research. The good news for consumers is that, even though researchers' understanding of mechanisms of action lag behind the awareness of what works, they now have at their disposal a sizable menu of empirically proven treatments from which to choose.

APPROACH TO TREATMENT

Medical Evaluation Before initiating any treatment, appropriate diagnosis is mandatory. Physicians must recognize that physiological causes for anxiety are legion, and that it is their job to rule out other medically treatable conditions before resorting to symptomatic treatment of an anxiety disorder.

Ms. A. C., a 43-year-old married mother of two, had seen her family doctor approximately 2 years before her death with the complaints of anxiety and insomnia. Her family doctor queried her about her psychosocial circumstances and learned that she had been experiencing substantial marital distress as a result of her husband's numerous extramarital affairs. He prescribed alprazolam (Xanax)—which the patient did not take because she did not like the idea of taking medication for "psychological troubles"—and referred her to a counselor.

Ms. A. C. saw the counselor intermittently over the ensuing 2 years and saw her family doctor several times for mostly unrelated complaints. At several visits, the physician's case notes revealed that she was continuing to experience "anxiety and stress" and that additional counseling was recommended. No laboratory tests or additional investigations were ordered at any visit.

Ms. A. C. was found dead on the couch by her husband upon his return from work. Autopsy determined that the cause of death was thyrotoxicosis ("thyroid storm") from Graves' disease.

The list of medical conditions that may present with or feature anxiety includes thyroid disease, hypoglycemia, pheochromocytoma (a tumor of the adrenal medulla), hypoparathyroidism, seizure disorders, arrhythmias and other cardiac conditions, asthma, and chronic obstructive pulmonary disease. Most of these conditions can be ruled out by history and physical examination, with the exception of thyroid disease, which can be occult and yet is easily detected with an ultrasensitive thyroid-stimulating hormone (TSH) blood test. When treatment does not proceed as expected, or if there is a change in the character or intensity of established anxiety symptoms, then reconsideration of the diagnosis, along with further examinations (as appropriate) should be undertaken.

Substance use may also contribute to anxiety symptoms.

Mr. J. T., a 28-year-old business executive, reported to his physician that he had been experiencing anxiety attacks for the previous 3 months. These occurred "out of the blue" and were associated with tachycardia and shortness of breath. The most recent attack occurred while he was driving to work and necessitated that he pull his car over to the side of the freeway and call 911 for assistance.

In the history, Mr. J. T. revealed to his physician that he had increased his coffee intake during a period of increased pressure at work. He reported that he began the morning with two cups of cappuccino brewed on his home espresso maker, followed by a "cup" (which, on further questioning, was revealed to be a 36-oz travel mug) of coffee in the car on the way to work. He drank coffee from the office coffee machine all morning long, had one or two 16-oz caffeinated beverages with lunch, and typically had a double espresso in the late afternoon "to restore my energy late in the day." He refilled his travel mug for the trek back home on the freeway after work, and then had one or two cups of cappuccino with his dessert after dinner.

Using the approximate rule of thumb of 100 mg of caffeine per cup (8 oz) of coffee, Mr. J. T.'s physician estimated that he was consuming, on average, 2,000 mg of caffeine per day. He recommended to Mr. J. T. that he cut down by one cup of coffee per day until he was consuming no more than four cups of coffee per day. He recommended that he drink half-decaffeinated and half-caffeinated cups to make the transition easier. Mr. J. T. returned to see his physician 4 weeks later and reported that his anxiety attacks had ceased (and that he was sleeping better and feeling less "stressed" overall).

Taking a caffeine history should become a routine part of the evaluation of anxious patients. Indeed, patients with panic disorder may be exquisitely sensitive to caffeine and other stimulants, such that doses that might not bother the average individual can exacerbate panic attacks. Persons with panic disorder (or a family history thereof) should be cautioned to limit their daily caffeine intake to 200 mg (i.e., no more than two or three 8-oz cups) per day. Other stimulants (e.g., ephedrine, contained in many over-the-counter cold remedies), including illicit drugs such as cocaine or methamphetamine, can result in pathological anxiety symptoms, as can alcohol abuse (particularly during withdrawal). Careful history taking, supplemented if appropriate with drug testing, can sort out this differential diagnosis in most cases. Once a nonpsychiatric medical etiology has been ruled out, the clinician can then proceed with treatment based on the primary considerations of diagnosis and patient preference.

Choosing a Treatment Modality

For most patients, pharmacotherapy, empirically proven psychotherapy (e.g., cognitive-behavioral therapy [CBT]), or some combination thereof are appropriate initial treatment options. Which of these, then, should be instituted for a given patient? This becomes an issue of individual choice, negotiated between the physician and the patient, but there are some considerations that may help guide this process. If a patient is seriously depressed in addition to experiencing pathological anxiety, then some experts would argue that pharmacotherapy with an antidepressant should be instituted (either alone or with CBT). If a patient has a prior history of good response to pharmacotherapy (or a family history thereof), then serious consideration should be given to restarting that particular medication, with the expectation that a similarly good outcome will be obtained. (Costs and formulary restrictions may also, by necessity, influence the selection of treatment modality. Here, it should be remembered that CBT, although more expensive in the short term, might be very cost-effective in the long run.) Beyond that, patient preference and physician experience should together form the basis for an informed decision about which route (i.e., pharmacotherapy or empirically proven psychotherapy) to take. Some patients are of the opinion that taking a medication for emotional problems should be avoided, and although education by the physician can help change these beliefs, it is usually an uphill battle. For such patients, many of whom are much more comfortable with the idea of actively participating in a course of learning tools and techniques for coping with anxiety, CBT may be a much better choice. On the other hand, some patients will espouse a strong belief that their anxiety is biological and that a medication designed to correct their "chemical imbalance" is just the ticket. For such patients, beginning with pharmacotherapy is eminently reasonable. Either way, patients (and physicians) should keep in mind the fact that they are not wed to a particular treatment. If the initially chosen treatment modality, after a reasonable course of treatment (usually several months in the case of either CBT or most forms of pharmacotherapy for anxiety disorders), is not yielding the expected symptom resolution and improvement in functioning, then a switch to another treatment modality (or an alternate form of the same modality, e.g., switch to a different class of anxiolytic medication) should be made.

PHARMACOTHERAPY

Once a decision is made to proceed with pharmacotherapy (either alone or in conjunction with CBT or some other form of psychotherapy), numerous choices of medication class and type are available. Ideally, decisions about which medication to use will be based on a good understanding of the patient's personal and family history of response to psychopharmacologic agents, in conjunction with a strong awareness of the evidence base for use of particular medications for particular anxiety disorders. To the extent that randomized controlled trials are available for these indications, the following information emphasizes information garnered from such studies. This information will be supplemented with the author's clinical experience over the past 20 years in treating patients with anxiety disorders. Readers are also encouraged to read some of the treatment guidelines and algorithms (e.g., for panic disorder, published by the American Psychiatric Association [APA]) that have become available in recent years and to stay attuned to anticipated updates to these guidelines as the evidence base changes over time to reflect newly accrued data.

Medications for Anxiety in Predictable Situations

There are basically two different ways to use medications for anxiety. One is to use them on an as-needed (or prn) basis. Only certain medications can be used this way, however, and only for certain indications, and the medication can only be used when the situation is predictable and arises only occasionally.

Mr. A. Z. is a 49-year-old salesman with a major hirsutism relief organization, Werewolves Anonymous. He presents to his family doctor asking for something to help him with his fear of flying. He admits that he has coped with his fear in the past by imbibing copious quantities of alcohol before and during flights, but that he is traveling with his boss and does not want to come across "like a lush." The flight is tomorrow.

After cautioning him against combining anxiolytic medication with alcohol, the physician provides Mr. A. Z. with a prescription for a benzodiazepine (lorazepam [Ativan], 0.5 mg) to be taken 1 hour before the flight and, if necessary, once during the flight. She also provides Mr. A. Z. with a referral to a therapist with a good reputation for helping people overcome their fear of flying using a combination of behavioral techniques and exposure supplemented with virtual reality therapy. She encourages Mr. A. Z. to contact the therapist upon his return to work to overcome his fear in anticipation of future flights.

Specific phobias are often treated with as-needed benzodiazepines, but exposure therapy is recommended if the goal is to eventually overcome the phobia. Another example where as-needed medication may be used is for social phobia (also known as *social anxiety disorder*), in those instances in which the individual's symptoms are limited to anxiety only in performance situations, such as speaking in front of large crowds. (Many patients with social phobia have the generalized type of the disorder and fear and avoid many situations in addition to public speaking. For those individuals, as-needed medication is usually insufficient.) A reasonable approach would be to recommend that the individual participate in a local Toastmasters group or similar self-help organization. If this has already been tried (or will be tried in the future, but something more immediate is required because of an impending speaking engagement), then the use of as-needed benzodiazepines or β-adrenergic antagonists may be recommended.

β-Adrenergic Receptor Antagonists β-Blockers can be useful on an as-needed basis for performance anxiety. β-Blockers that are sometimes used for this purpose include propranolol (Inderal) and atenolol (Tenormin). Some clinicians recommend titrating the dose to yield an approximate 10-beats-per-minute reduction in heart rate compared to pretreatment, whereas others simply try one or two fixed doses (typical starting doses are 20 to 40 mg per dose for propranolol and 25 to 50 mg per dose for atenolol). β-Adrenergic antagonists are believed to work for performance anxiety by reducing tachycardia (racing heart) and tremor (shaking). Some people with performance anxiety have a heightened awareness of their heart racing or their hands shaking, which makes them even more nervous. By reducing some of these symptoms of social anxiety, the β-blockers can help some individuals focus less on their bodily symptoms and more on the task at hand—for example, speaking in public. β-Blockers are sometimes used by people in oral test-taking situations (e.g., medical students before their practical examinations) or by professional musicians (e.g., concert violinists). β-Blockers are typically taken 30 to 60 minutes before the performance situation. Although the published literature suggests that β-blockers have a high success rate for public speaking anxiety, the author's experience is that they are helpful in fewer than 50 percent of cases. When they do not work, prn short-acting benzodiazepines (e.g., lorazepam, 0.5 to 1.0 mg) may provide a reasonable alternative for most patients.

β-Blockers used on an as-needed basis are generally well tolerated with few side effects. Occasionally, however, they can result in feelings of dizziness, lightheadedness, or fatigue. It is important to ask patients to try the medication on one or two occasions before the real performance situation to determine how it affects them and to find the right dose. β-Blockers should not be prescribed to patients with bradycardia or heart block, asthma or chronic obstructive pulmonary disease, angle-closure glaucoma, or diabetes.

Benzodiazepines Another option to help with performance anxiety is a relatively short- or intermediate-acting benzodiazepine, such as lorazepam or alprazolam. Like β-blockers, benzodiazepines can be used on an as-needed basis to treat performance anxiety and are typically taken 30 to 60 minutes before the performance situation. The potential for abuse and misuse has led to this class of medication becoming notoriously disliked in the medical community. In fact, when used to treat anxiety under appropriate medical supervision, benzodiazepines are often an excellent choice given their high safety margin (e.g., in overdose) and their overall excellent efficacy and rapid onset of action. If an individual has a history of alcohol or other substance abuse, however, then benzodiazepines (with some exceptions, e.g., if other classes of medications have been tried first and not worked) should not be prescribed. Adverse effects of the benzodiazepines are generally few and mild. The main side effects are sedation and dizziness, which usually go away with time or with dosage adjustment. Caution must be exercised when using heavy or dangerous machinery or when driving, especially when first starting the medication or when the dosage is changed. Benzodiazepines should not be used in combination with alcohol, as they can intensify its effects.

Medications for Chronic Recurrent or Unpredictable Anxiety

Most anxiety disorders are characterized by chronic recurrent anxiety (e.g., generalized anxiety disorder, posttraumatic stress disorder [PTSD], generalized social anxiety disorder, or obsessive-compulsive disorder [OCD]) or unpredictable

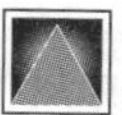

Table 14.9–1
Commonly Used Medications for Treating Chronic or Unpredictable Anxiety Syndromes

Medication	Brand Name	Daily Dosage[a]
Antidepressants[b]		
Fluoxetine	Prozac	20–80 mg/day
Fluvoxamine	Luvox	100–300 mg/day
Paroxetine	Paxil	20–50 mg/day
	Paxil CR	25–75 mg/day
Sertraline	Zoloft	50–200 mg/day
Citalopram	Celexa	20–60 mg/day
Escitalopram	Lexapro	10–30 mg/day
Venlafaxine	Effexor XR	75–225 mg/day
Phenelzine	Nardil	45–90 mg/day
Benzodiazepines[c]		
Alprazolam	Xanax	2–6 mg/day[e]
Clonazepam	Klonopin	1–4 mg/day
Lorazepam	Ativan	1–3 mg/day[e]
Azapirone[d]		
Buspirone	BuSpar	30–60 mg/day

[a]Some individuals will require higher or lower dosages than those listed here.
[b]Useful as a primary treatment for panic disorder (where lower starting doses are usually used) with or without agoraphobia, generalized anxiety disorder, generalized social anxiety disorder, and posttraumatic stress disorder. All except phenelzine are useful as a primary treatment for obsessive-compulsive disorder.
[c]Useful as a primary treatment for panic disorder with or without agoraphobia, generalized anxiety disorder, and generalized social anxiety disorder. May be a useful adjunct to antidepressants in the treatment of posttraumatic stress disorder or obsessive-compulsive disorder.
[d]Useful as a primary treatment for generalized anxiety disorder.
[e]Total daily dosage that is divided across 3–4 doses/day.

attacks of anxiety (e.g., panic disorder with or without agoraphobia). Given the nature of these illnesses, the use of as-needed medication is almost always insufficient, and the regular use of medication to control or prevent the occurrence of symptoms is strongly preferred. The aforementioned anxiety disorders—as well as major depression and dysthymia, with which they are frequently comorbid—share responsiveness to medications that have presynaptic serotonin reuptake blockade as one of their properties. This grouping includes all of the SSRIs, the serotonin–norepinephrine reuptake inhibitors (SNRIs) (also known as *dual reuptake inhibitors*), and several cyclic antidepressants (e.g., clomipramine [Anafranil]). The evidence base is stronger for particular compounds used for particular disorders, but this is almost certainly a reflection of how decisions were made to test and market particular compounds, rather than real differences in utility. Rather than repeat nearly identical prescribing information on a disorder-by-disorder basis, the next section of this chapter describes the use of these compounds to treat the aforementioned set of disorders as a group. Where applicable, differences among disorders are described.

Table 14.9–1 lists some of the commonly used medications for treating chronic or unpredictable anxiety syndromes.

Antidepressants for Anxiety Disorders Antidepressants are among the most effective antianxiety agents available. Many nonpsychiatrist physicians have experience using these medications with their depressed patients, so they are familiar with them and comfortable prescribing them. Although nonpsychiatrist physicians may be relatively unfamiliar with some of the anxiety disorders, they can readily translate their knowledge of how to treat depression with medications to the treatment of most of the anxiety disorders. Increasingly, the treatment of the most common anxiety disorders (i.e., panic disorder, social anxiety disorder, generalized anxiety disorder, and, to a lesser extent, PTSD) is falling into the hands of primary care practitioners. The role of the psychiatrist is to support the appropriate use of these medications (along with adequate counseling and education) by their primary care physician colleagues, to make recommendations in difficult-to-treat cases, and, in some cases, to assume direct care of patients who require more specialized psychotherapeutic or pharmacotherapeutic management.

SELECTIVE SEROTONIN REUPTAKE INHIBITORS (SSRIS) The SSRIs are a class of antidepressant medication that came to the market in the United States and Canada in the mid-1980s. The first medication of this class to be marketed in the United States was fluoxetine, soon to be followed by sertraline (Zoloft), paroxetine (Paxil), fluvoxamine (Luvox), citalopram (Celexa), and the S-enantiomer of citalopram, escitalopram (Lexapro). These medications, as a group, have been shown to help reduce or prevent various forms of anxiety, including panic anxiety, obsessive-compulsive symptoms, generalized anxiety, posttraumatic stress symptoms, and social anxiety. Most treatment algorithms begin treatment of each of these disorders with an SSRI. Effective dosages are essentially the same as for the treatment of depression, although it is customary to start with lower initial doses than in depression (to minimize an initial anxiolytic effect, which is almost always short-lived) and to titrate upward somewhat more slowly toward a therapeutic dosage. Typical duration of a therapeutic trial (i.e., before the decision is made to switch to another medication due to lack of efficacy) is 8 to 12 weeks, and perhaps even longer for OCD, in which it is believed that the time course of response is somewhat slower than for the other disorders. Although this practice is not strongly supported by randomized, controlled trials, it is the author's experience that patients will very often do better at higher doses, and that medication dose should generally be titrated upward to achieve an optimal balance between efficacy and adverse effects. A common error on the part of practitioners is to settle for partial response, which can often be easily achieved at a starting dose of an SSRI, rather than to aim for a more complete response. Patients who are only partially treated are at greater risk for recurrence of symptoms and for persistent psychosocial dysfunction. It is therefore incumbent on treating physicians to aim for as complete a response (i.e., remission) as possible.

Although certain of these medications have been tested more extensively for one indication or another within this spectrum of anxiety problems, and some have indications for the treatment of certain disorders with the U.S. Food and Drug Administration (FDA), they are all more or less effective for each condition. If the first SSRI tried is ineffective or results in intolerable adverse effects, it is possible to switch to a different SSRI and have a reasonable expectation of a better outcome. Although this strategy of switching between SSRIs (or, alternatively, from an SSRI to an antidepressant in another class) is better substantiated in the case of major depression, clinical experience supports this strategy for the anxiety disorders as well.

The SSRIs are generally very well tolerated. Although there are some differences between the SSRIs in their adverse event profiles, in general they can cause sleep problems, drowsiness, lightheadedness, nausea, diarrhea, and sexual dysfunction. Many of these adverse effects improve with continued use, but sexual dysfunction, consisting mainly of delayed ejaculation for men and difficulty in reaching orgasm for women (although diminished sexual desire and erectile problems are also seen) often do not diminish with time and are among the most common causes for noncompliance or medication discontinuation. If an individual is having problems with side effects from a particular SSRI, very often it is possible to switch to another SSRI and achieve a better balance between side effects and efficacy. Once again, though, sexual side effects often do not conform to this pattern and persist despite a switch between SSRIs (or from an SSRI to an SNRI). Many strategies have been proposed to deal with sexual dysfunction in patients taking SSRIs. These include the adjunctive use of yohimbine, bupropion (Wellbutrin), nefazodone (Serzone), mirtazapine (Remeron), and a host of other agents. These tend to be useful in only a minority of patients. There is stronger evidence to suggest that SSRI dosage reduction or the adjunctive use of sildenafil (Viagra) can be helpful.

Use of SSRIs to Treat Anxiety Disorders in Children Several randomized, controlled trials now provide conclusive evidence that SSRIs are useful in the treatment of certain anxiety disorders in children and adolescents. At present, the evidence base is strongest for the treatment of OCD, generalized social anxiety disorder, separation anxiety disorder, and panic disorder in youth. These treatments are generally reserved for children who do not respond to psychosocial interventions. Given the serious functional morbidity associated with chronic anxiety and avoidance in children and adolescents, the use of pharmacotherapy should not be unduly withheld in these situations.

DUAL (SEROTONIN–NOREPINEPHRINE) REUPTAKE INHIBITORS At the time of this writing, the only dual reuptake inhibitor on the U.S. market is venlafaxine extended-release (Effexor XR), although others are expected to become available in the near future. Venlafaxine extended-release has been shown in randomized, controlled trials to be as effective as SSRIs in the treatment of generalized anxiety disorder and generalized social anxiety disorder, and data for panic disorder and PTSD are expected to be forthcoming. Venlafaxine extended-release has a similar side-effect profile to the SSRIs. At the upper end of the therapeutic range (e.g., 225 mg per day or higher), routine blood pressure monitoring is warranted, as some patients (probably <5 percent) experience dose-related hypertension. In the treatment of depression, there is currently controversy over whether dual reuptake inhibitors are slightly superior to SSRIs in terms of overall efficacy. For the anxiety disorders, no such controversy exists: the extant data show them to be comparable. Dual reuptake inhibitors can be used as initial treatment for these disorders, or they can be used as a class to switch to in the case of SSRI failures.

TRICYCLIC AND HETEROCYCLIC ANTIDEPRESSANTS The discovery in the 1960s that imipramine would prevent panic attacks marked a major breakthrough in the treatment (and classification) of anxiety disorders. Until the advent of the SSRIs in the mid-1980s, imipramine, desipramine (e.g., Norpramin), and other tricyclic and heterocyclic compounds (e.g., doxepin [Sinequan]) were widely used for treating panic disorder with or without agoraphobia and, to a lesser extent, generalized anxiety disorder. Although effective for these conditions (and probably ineffective for social anxiety disorder, although this is not entirely clear), some anxious patients (especially those with panic disorder) experience an initial "jitteriness" syndrome when treatment is initiated. This adverse effect can often be minimized by beginning with very low doses (e.g., 5 mg of imipramine) and then titrating upward very slowly (e.g., by 5 or 10 mg every 3 to 4 days) until therapeutic doses are reached. But, for the same reasons (i.e., mainly anticholinergic and adverse cardiac effects) that these types of antidepressants are infrequently used in the treatment of major depression, they have fallen out of favor for the treatment of anxiety disorders since the arrival of the SSRIs. An exception is OCD, for which clomipramine is still widely used as a monotherapy or as an adjunct to SSRIs.

MONOAMINE OXIDASE INHIBITORS The monoamine oxidase inhibitors (MAOIs) have been known for more than two decades to be effective in treating the phobic neuroses, which, using revised fourth edition of the *Diagnostic and Statistical Manual of Mental Disorders* (DSM-IV-TR) terminology, would include panic disorder with or without agoraphobia and the generalized type of social anxiety disorder. Their utility in the treatment of other anxiety disorders is less clear. Some experts believe that MAOIs are qualitatively superior to any other antidepressant class for treating panic disorder or social anxiety disorder, but because of their side effect profile (which features postural hypotension, insomnia, and weight gain) and the need for a special (very low tyramine) diet to reduce the risk of a hypertensive crisis, they are usually reserved for nonresponders to other treatments.

The two most commonly used MAOIs in the United States and Canada are phenelzine (Nardil) and tranylcypromine (Parnate). Phenelzine has been more extensively studied for treating anxiety disorders (especially generalized social phobia), although the author's clinical experience is that tranylcypromine can also be effective, sometimes even when phenelzine has failed. Most authorities recommend a minimum 2-week washout period when switching to an MAOI from a tricyclic antidepressant, an SSRI (6 weeks for fluoxetine), or another MAOI.

Mr. S. R. is a 43-year-old teacher's aide with a lifelong history of social anxiety and avoidance. He reports being extremely shy in grade school and high school and would frequently cut classes when oral presentations were scheduled. In his early 20s, he found that "a drink or two" before social occasions helped reduce his anxiety, and he soon developed severe alcoholism, resulting in the loss of several jobs and a driving-under-the-influence conviction. He had been treated by psychiatrists for depression over the years and recalled experiencing relief in his social anxiety when he was taking fluoxetine several years previously, but this was stopped after 6 months when his depression remitted, resulting in the recurrence of his social anxiety and avoidance. At present, he works part-time as a teacher's aide in a local high school, hoping to eventually get a teaching degree. Although comfortable in the classroom, he was terrified of interacting with the other teachers and aides and reported that they viewed him to be a snob because of his reluctance to join them for conversations or after-work social outings.

Mr. S. R. tried several SSRIs under the care of his new psychiatrist but experienced intolerable adverse effects (including diarrhea and severe nausea) that could not be managed with dosage reduction or other methods. A dual reuptake inhibitor at full therapeutic dosage for 12 weeks improved his social avoidance considerably, but he still experienced residual fears that interfered significantly with his functioning. His psychiatrist was reluctant to prescribe a benzodiazepine because of his history of substance abuse. She recommended a therapeutic trial of an MAOI, carefully explaining to Mr. S. R. the pros and cons, including the need for careful dietary monitoring to reduce the risk of a hypertensive crisis.

He was started on phenelzine, 15 mg each morning, and after 1 week his dosage was increased to 30 mg per day. He was held at this dosage for 3 weeks, during which time he reported some reduction in his level of self-consciousness when in the company of peers. His dosage was increased to 45 mg per day, after which he experienced some mild postural hypotension that was managed conservatively by exercising caution, arising slowly from a lying or seated position, and maintaining good hydration. After an additional 2 weeks, Mr. S. R. reported to his psychiatrist that he had felt comfortable enough at work that he had joined in several conversations with staff in the school lunchroom and was planning to attend a weekend party with a few colleagues. His psychiatrist advised him to remain on this dose of phenelzine and encouraged him to increase his number of social outings and to push himself to engage in conversations with parents of his students. After 3 more months, Mr. S. R. was doing sufficiently well that he completed an application for teacher's college for the following September.

REVERSIBLE INHIBITORS OF MONOAMINE OXIDASE TYPE A Reversible inhibitors of monoamine oxidase type A (RIMAs) are unavailable in the United States, although one (moclobemide [Manerix in Canada]) is available in Canada and Mexico and a number of countries outside North America. Moclobemide has been shown to be effective for social anxiety disorder in some studies, and ineffective in others. Overall, it does not seem to be as effective as irreversible MAOIs (e.g., phenelzine or tranylcypromine) but, in the author's experience, it has been helpful for some patients. Its advantage over irreversible MAOIs is that no special diet is required. It also tends to have a very different side effect profile than SSRIs or dual reuptake inhibitors. When side effects do occur, they consist mainly of sleep problems, dizziness, and nervousness; most are transient and go away with time. In countries where they are available, RIMAs such as moclobemide are probably a reasonable alternative to SSRIs or dual reuptake inhibitors for the treatment of generalized social anxiety disorder, particularly in patients who have tried one or more of these agents and experienced problematic side effects.

OTHER ANTIDEPRESSANTS Nefazodone (Serzone), mirtazapine (Remeron), and bupropion (usually prescribed in sustained-release form as Wellbutrin SR) are other newer antidepressants on the market. Their efficacy for any of the anxiety disorders is not supported by large, randomized, controlled trials, although they may be somewhat useful for depression with comorbid anxious symptoms. Mirtazapine has achieved some clinical notoriety for use in the anxious elderly, although the published literature is largely restricted to treatment of major depression, rather than to any of the anxiety disorders. Use of any of these agents for treating DSM-IV-TR anxiety disorders should be considered on a case-by-case basis, probably after better-substantiated treatments have been tried and failed. The author's experience is that nefazodone or mirtazapine may also be useful in low doses as adjuncts to SSRIs or dual reuptake inhibitors, with the main target of reducing insomnia that may be associated with either of those treatments.

Benzodiazepines The benzodiazepines, taken on an as-needed basis, were discussed earlier in the context of performance anxiety. This class of medications also can be used on a regular (rather than an as-needed) basis to treat generalized anxiety disorder, panic disorder with or without agoraphobia, and generalized social anxiety disorder. They are not indicated as a primary treatment for OCD or PTSD. The benzodiazepines are also very frequently used as an adjunct to an antidepressant, either to improve the therapeutic effect or to help relieve side effects from the antidepressant (e.g., insomnia).

It is not entirely clear whether all of the benzodiazepines are similarly effective for these conditions. In the case of panic disorder (with or without agoraphobia) or social phobia, the most extensively studied are alprazolam and clonazepam (Klonopin). For treatment of chronic or unpredictable anxiety syndromes, alprazolam is usually taken 3 to 4 times daily, whereas clonazepam, with its longer half-life, is usually taken 1 to 2 times daily. Although some authorities believe that benzodiazepines can be used as initial treatments for these anxiety disorders, it is the author's preference to reserve the use of benzodiazepines for patients who have less-than-optimal responses to antidepressants. In those cases, a benzodiazepine may be added to an antidepressant to achieve a better overall effect with the combination. At other times, use of a benzodiazepine alone can be justified when other treatments have failed or cannot be tolerated. Patients who have been on benzodiazepines for many years and continue to have good therapeutic responses to chronic benzodiazepine use, with no evidence of misuse or abuse, should generally be permitted to stay on the benzodiazepine if that is their preference. Switching stable patients merely for the sake of "getting them off a benzodiazepine" generally does not make good clinical sense. Another well-supported indication for benzodiazepines is in the initial treatment of panic disorder.

H. T. is a 21-year-old college student who presents to the Student Health Clinic for help with anxiety. She reports the recent onset of unpredictable attacks of anxiety characterized by shortness of breath, tachycardia, sweating, and the fear that she was going crazy. She experienced five or six such attacks in the past week, once while in the classroom and subsequently before leaving her dormitory room to attend class. She also experienced several attacks that had woken her from sleep, usually in the early part of the night. As a result of these symptoms, she had begun missing classes and was having a friend bring her notes and assignments to the room. She worried that if this pattern persisted, she would miss so much class that she would have to drop her classes for the semester and lose her scholarship in the process.

After a careful history (including caffeine and drug use habits) and medical evaluation, which revealed no other explanation for her anxiety attacks, the physician at the student health clinic made a tentative diagnosis of panic disorder. He explained to H. T. that panic disorder was quite common in her age group and that it often comes on during periods of stress. He reassured her that this was a treatable condition, and he provided her with the address for a Web site so she could learn more about the disorder. He also started H. T. on 0.5 mg of lorazepam, to be taken three times daily on a regular basis (i.e., not just when she felt anxious), and arranged to see her 1 week later.

At that time, H. T. reported that she was sleeping better and that she had experienced only two less severe panic attacks since the last visit. She had not missed any classes. The physician explained that he wanted to keep her on the lorazepam, if possible, for only a relatively short period, and that he would be starting treatment with an SSRI, a class of medications known to be useful in preventing anxiety attacks. He started her on 10 mg of paroxetine at bedtime and continued the lorazepam at the same dose for another week. At that time, he increased the dosage of paroxetine to 20 mg at bedtime and tapered the dosage of lorazepam by reducing it to 0.25 mg three times daily for 4 days, then stopping it. After a total of 4 weeks, H. T. was taking paroxetine monotherapy at 20 mg per day and was free of panic attacks and phobic avoidance. The physician recommended that H. T. continue taking the medication at this dose for the remainder of the school year (another 7 months), and that she work with a psychiatrist in her home town during the summer to consider if and when to discontinue the medicine and to discuss the possibility of CBT.

Other Antianxiety Medications Buspirone (BuSpar) is effective in the treatment of chronic anxiety states, but its usefulness for this group of disorders is probably limited to the treatment of generalized anxiety disorder. There are published placebo-controlled trials showing that buspirone was not effective in treating social anxiety disorder or panic disorder. Buspirone, an azapirone, is effective in dosages ranging from 30 to 60 mg per day, usually given in three divided doses. The time course of response to buspirone is similar to that of antidepressants, usually taking at least several weeks, and sometimes several months, to reach full therapeutic efficacy. There is some evidence, most of it anecdotal, to suggest that buspirone may be useful as an adjunct to antidepressants in the treatment of anxiety disorders other than generalized anxiety disorder.

Hydroxyzine (Atarax) is an antihistamine that is efficacious in the treatment of generalized anxiety disorder. In one randomized, controlled trial at a fixed dose of 50 mg per day, it was superior to placebo and equally efficacious as a benzodiazepine (bromazepam, 6 mg per day). It may be a good alternative to benzodiazepines for some patients.

An anticonvulsant, gabapentin (Neurontin), has shown some promise as a treatment for social anxiety disorder. It may turn out to be a popular form of treatment for this and other anxiety disorders, because it has very few drug–drug interactions, and because it may have less potential for abuse than benzodiazepines. The author's experience is that gabapentin may be most useful as an adjunct to other antianxiety medications. Another anticonvulsant, divalproex (Depakote) may be useful for treating some forms of resistant panic disorder. Other anticonvulsants, including topiramate (Topamax), lamotrigine (Lamictal), and levetiracetam (Keppra), have shown some preliminary promise in the treatment of PTSD.

The practice of adding low-dose antipsychotics (e.g., pimozide [Orap] or haloperidol [Haldol]) to SSRIs or clomipramine for patients with OCD who have psychotic symptoms (or chronic tics) is well established. Several atypical antipsychotic medications, such as olanzapine (Zyprexa), risperidone (Risperdal), quetiapine (Seroquel), and aripiprazole (Abilify) are showing some very early potential as adjunctive therapies for patients whose anxiety disorders (e.g., PTSD) are refractory to other forms of treatment. Although randomized, controlled trial data are quite limited, the practice of adding an atypical neuroleptic in low dose to enhance SSRI response has already achieved fairly widespread clinical notoriety. It is hoped that the evidence base will accrue to support this practice. In this regard, although it is believed that the risk of tardive dyskinesia with these compounds is very low, this should be demonstrated specifically in patients with anxiety disorders.

Prazosin (Minipress), an α_1-adrenergic antagonist, has shown some promise in the treatment of PTSD. It may be especially useful for the treatment of sleep-related problems, including nightmares, which are so common in PTSD and yet are often resistant to established therapies such as SSRIs.

EXPECTED OUTCOMES WITH PHARMACOTHERAPY

Response rates to pharmacotherapy differ somewhat among the anxiety disorders. The absolute rates depend in large part on the definition of response used in a given study. The goal of treatment in panic disorder is to have the patient free of panic attacks; additional foci of treatment should be anticipatory anxiety and phobic avoidance, reducing these to levels where their impact on functioning is minimal. Panic disorder is among the most treatment-responsive anxiety disorder, with response rates of 60 to 70 percent not uncommon for most effective treatments. Patients with comorbid agoraphobia may be somewhat more difficult to treat, in some cases requiring higher doses of medication or, more often, benefiting from concomitant CBT. OCD is generally regarded as the least treatment responsive of the anxiety disorders. Indeed, most randomized, controlled trials define "response" in OCD as a 30 percent or greater reduction in obsessive-compulsive symptom scores, and only 30 to 40 percent of patients might achieve this response. This may appear to be trifling, but even a 10 to 20 percent reduction in obsessions and compulsions can make a dramatic difference in a patient's life. Still, this observation points to the need to develop better treatments for OCD. Response rates to effective somatic therapies in generalized anxiety disorder, generalized social anxiety disorder, and PTSD are intermediate between those for panic disorder and OCD, with 50 to 60 percent of patients having a good clinical outcome.

Duration of Pharmacotherapy

Empirical data on the optimal duration of pharmacotherapy are lacking for most of the anxiety disorders. A number of controlled studies do show, however, that between 20 and 50 percent of patients with chronic anxiety disorders experience a recurrence of clinically significant symptoms within several months of discontinuing SSRI pharmacotherapy. This has led to the development of guidelines for most chronic anxiety disorders specifying that patients be treated for at least a year before consideration is given to dosage reduction or discontinuation.

Combining Pharmacotherapy and Psychotherapy

Combinations of pharmacotherapy and psychotherapies (such as CBT) have been little studied in randomized, controlled trials. For the most part, studies have not shown consistent benefits of routinely combining pharmacotherapy and CBT; this may be because either treatment modality alone is sufficiently good so that showing an additive (or better) effect is difficult without enormous sample sizes. It is the author's experience, however, that some patients receiving pharmacotherapy make substantially larger gains when they participate in CBT. This seems to be particularly true for patients with OCD and PTSD, for whom pharmacotherapy very often seems to provide sizable, but incomplete, resolution of compulsive and avoidant behaviors, respectively. Some authorities recommend that pharmacotherapy and CBT be started simultaneously. It is the author's experience, however, that the routine provision of formal CBT is unnecessary for many patients, particularly if the treating physician is adept at making recommendations for in vivo exposure and the patient is motivated to use self-help tools (e.g., books and online information). For those patients who begin with pharmacotherapy and fail to achieve remission, *sequential* provision of CBT is the authors' preferred modus operandi.

Ms. C. L., a 52-year-old self-employed, married woman, was referred by her family doctor for treatment of recurrent obsessions and compulsions. History confirmed that she had been plagued by these symptoms for several decades—she had seen a psychiatrist in the past but did not follow up on his recommendations for therapy—but she had been able to keep them "in check" by keeping very busy with her work and family life. Quite recently, apparently precipitated by her youngest child leaving for college, she found that her obsessions about germs and her compulsion to wash had begun to consume more and more of her energy and time. At the time of referral, she was spending approximately 3 hours per day showering and washing and countless other hours worrying about and engineering ways to avoid contamination. She admitted that "nearly every waking moment" was occupied by worrying about whether she would become ill if she were to touch, eat, or drink contaminated substances.

After discussing treatment alternatives, Ms. C. L. and her psychiatrist opted to begin treatment with an SSRI, fluoxetine, at 20 mg each morning. The psychiatrist also suggested that Ms. C. L. and her husband read a self-help book on OCD, for which the psychiatrist provided several of his favorite titles. The phone number and Web address of a local anxiety support group were also provided. Her dosage of fluoxetine was increased to 30 mg each morning 1 month later, at which time a definite reduction was noted in the frequency of obsessive thoughts and in the urgency to perform compulsions. The dose was increased to 40 mg each morning, at which point Ms. C. L. began to complain of insomnia and anorgasmia. She agreed to continue taking the medication but at the lower dose of 30 mg per day. At this point, her psychiatrist pointed out that, although she was doing much better, she still had considerable residual symptoms—mainly compulsive rituals and avoidance behaviors—that would be excellent targets for CBT.

Not having a lot of experience himself in the provision of CBT for OCD, the psychiatrist referred Ms. C. L. to a psychologist in the community who had a good reputation in treating OCD with CBT. He continued to manage her medication and spoke with the psychologist at intervals to receive an update on Ms. C. L.'s progress. After 15 weekly sessions of CBT (which were provided in a combination of group and individual sessions), Ms. C. L. reported the near cessation of obsessive thoughts and compulsive behaviors and overall minimal interference with her day-to-day functioning.

For any patient with an anxiety disorder (indeed, with *any* mental disorder), pharmacotherapy should not be provided in a vacuum. Education about the illness (which can be effectively provided by referring the patient to high-quality sources of information, such as Web sites sponsored by federal or state governments, or reputable self-help organizations), recommendations for combating problem behaviors (such as phobic avoidance or compulsions), and advice about how to maximize the response to medication (e.g., "Once you are feeling less anxious, you should push your limits and improve your confidence by starting to do things you have not been able to do in a long time) are all mandatory components of providing pharmacotherapy for patients with anxiety disorders.

HERBAL AND OTHER "NATURAL" REMEDIES

Many consumers have used herbal or other "natural" remedies to help reduce their anxiety. A recent study in Canada showed that more than 50 percent of people with social anxiety had tried one or more of these alternative therapies. Included among the plethora of "natural" substances with purported antianxiety properties are kava kava, valerian root, Gotu Kola (*Centella asiatica*), and St. John's wort. The available scientific evidence that any of these are effective for treating anxiety disorders is sparse, but well-controlled randomized, controlled trials are currently under way that should help clarify their role in this regard. Physicians should query their patients about their use of herbals to reduce the risk of untoward interactions with other medications that they may be taking.

PSYCHOSURGICAL TECHNIQUES

Patients with severe OCD whose symptoms are refractory to extensive pharmacological and behavioral management may be considered for psychosurgery. Recent studies suggest that approximately one-third of patients with previously intractable OCD have meaningful improvement (although rarely complete remission of symptoms) after cingulotomy. Other surgical procedures (e.g., subcaudate tractotomy, also known as *capsulotomy*) have also been used for this purpose, and these are all increasingly being performed using magnetic resonance imaging (MRI)-guided stereotactic techniques. When psychosurgery is being contemplated for OCD, referral to one of the handful of centers with extensive experience in this area should be strongly considered. Psychosurgery for anxiety indications other than OCD has not been systematically studied.

NOVEL THERAPEUTICS FOR ANXIETY

The neuroscience of anxiety is advancing in leaps and bounds. Currently in development and testing are new compounds for treating anxiety that have novel mechanisms of action. These include corticotrophin-releasing factor antagonists, neurokinin-1 antagonists, and metabotropic glutamate receptor agonists. Medications that target various serotonin receptor subtypes, some of which have been specifically implicated in the etiology of anxiety-related behaviors, are also in development, as are a number of compounds originally developed as anticonvulsants (e.g., levetiracetam [Keppra] and pregabalin). Time will tell whether these new medications will prove to be safe, well tolerated, and, of course, efficacious for the treatment of anxiety disorders.

Several specific anxiety disorders have new treatments in development that deserve mention. Some children with OCD-like symptoms are thought to have acquired their illness through an immune-mediated pathway activated by infection with streptococcus type A. Plasma exchange is being studied as a treatment for this illness, which is sometimes referred to as *PANDAS* (*p*ediatric *a*utoimmune *n*europsychiatric *d*isorders *a*ssociated with *s*treptococcal infections). Preventive treatments for PTSD are also in development. There is very preliminary evidence to suggest that β-blockers (e.g., propranolol) administered in close temporal proximity to acute psychological trauma may reduce eventual rates of PTSD development. These treatment strategies are still in the experimental stages and should not be attempted until results of the clinical trials become available.

SUGGESTED CROSS-REFERENCES

More detailed discussion of medications used in anxiety disorders can be found in Chapter 31. Side effects, interactions, pharmacokinetics and pharmacodynamics are described in Section 31.1. The neurobiology of anxiety disorders and the hypothesized basis of the efficacy of antianxiety medications is given in Section 14.3. Detailed diagnostic description of various anxiety disorders is given in Section 14.8. The epidemiology of anxiety disorders is discussed in Section 14.2. More detailed discussion of psychosurgery for mental disorders is discussed in Section 31.31. Additional discussion of pharmacotherapy for children and adolescents with anxiety disorders is discussed in Chapter 46.

REFERENCES

*Barlow DH, Gorman JM, Shear MK, Woods SW: Cognitive-behavioral therapy, imipramine, or their combination for panic disorder: A randomized controlled trial. *JAMA*. 2000;283:2529–2536.

Birmaher B, Axelson DA, Monk K, Kalas C, Clark DB, Ehmann M, Bridge J, Heo J, Brent DA: Fluoxetine for the treatment of childhood anxiety disorders. *J Am Acad Child Adolesc Psych*. 2003;42:415–423.

*Brady KT, Pearlstein T, Asnis GM, Baker DG, Rothbaum BO, Sikes CR, Farfel GM: Efficacy and safety of sertraline treatment of posttraumatic stress disorder: A randomized controlled trial. *JAMA*. 2000;283:1837–1844.

Bruce SE, Vasile RG, Goisman RM, Salzman C, Spencer M, Machan JT, Keller MB: Are benzodiazepines still the medication of choice for patients with panic disorder with or without agoraphobia? *Am J Psychiatry*. 2003;160:1432–1438.

Davidson JRT, Connor KM. *Herbs for the Mind*. New York: Guilford Press; 2000.

Davidson JRT, Potts NL, Richichi E, Krishnan KR: Treatment of social phobia with clonazepam and placebo. *J Clin Psychopharmacol.* 1993;13:423–428.

Davidson JRT, Rothbaum BO, van der Kolk BA, Sikes CR, Farfel GM: Multicenter, double-blind comparison of sertraline and placebo in the treatment of posttraumatic stress disorder. *Arch Gen Psychiatry.* 2001;58:485–492.

Dougherty DD, Baer L, Cosgrove GR, Cassem EH, Price BH, Nierenberg AA, Jenike MA, Rauch SL: Prospective long-term follow-up of 44 patients who received cingulotomy for treatment-refractory obsessive-compulsive disorder. *Am J Psychiatry.* 2002;159:269–275.

Gelenberg AJ, Lydiard RB, Rudolph RL, Aguiar L, Haskins JT, Salinas E: Efficacy of venlafaxine extended-release capsules in nondepressed outpatients with generalized anxiety disorder: A 6-month randomized controlled trial. *JAMA.* 2000;283:3082–3088.

Goddard AW, Brouette T, Almai A, Jetty P, Woods SW, Charney DS: Early co-administration of clonazepam with sertraline for panic disorder. *Arch Gen Psychiatry.* 2001;58:681–686.

Greenberg PE, Sisitsky T, Kessler RC, Finkelstein SN, Berndt ER, Davidson JRT, Ballenger JC, Fyer AJ: The economic burden of anxiety disorders in the 1990s. *J Clin Psychiatry.* 1999;60:427–435.

Heimberg RG, Liebowitz MR, Hope DA, Schneier FR, Holt CS, Welkowitz LA, Juster HR, Campeas R, Bruch MA, Cloitre M, Fallon B, Klein DF: Cognitive behavioral group therapy vs phenelzine therapy for social phobia. *Arch Gen Psychiatry.* 1998;55:1133–1141.

Kessler RC, McGonagle KA, Zhao S, Nelson CB, Hughes M, Eshleman S, Wittchen H-U, Kendler KS: Lifetime and 12-month prevalence of psychiatric disorders in the United States: Results from the National Comorbidity Survey. *Arch Gen Psychiatry.* 1994;51:8–19.

*Klein DF: Delineation of two drug-responsive anxiety syndromes. *Psychopharmacology.* 1964;5:397–408.

Leinonen E, Lepola U, Koponen H, Turtonen J, Wade A, Lehto H: Citalopram controls phobic symptoms in patients with panic disorder: Randomized controlled trial. *J Psychiatry Neurosci.* 2000;25:24–32.

Llorca PM, Spadone C, Sol O, Danniau A, Bougerol T, Corruble E, Faruch M, Macher JP, Sermet E, Servant D: Efficacy and safety of hydroxyzine in the treatment of generalized anxiety disorder: A 3-month double-blind study. *J Clin Psychiatry.* 2002;63:1020–1027.

March JS, Biederman J, Wolkow R, Safferman A, Mardekian J, Cook EH, Cutler NR, Dominguez R, Ferguson J, Muller B, Riesenberg R, Rosenthal M, Sallee FR, Wagner KD: Sertraline in children and adolescents with obsessive-compulsive disorder: A multicenter randomized controlled trial. *JAMA.* 1998;280:1752–1756.

Mendlowicz MV, Stein MB: Quality of life in individuals with anxiety disorders. *Am J Psychiatry.* 2000;157:669–682.

Nurnberg HG, Hensley PL, Gelenberg AJ, Fava M, Lauriello J, Paine S: Treatment of antidepressant-associated sexual dysfunction with sildenafil: A randomized controlled trial. *JAMA.* 2003;289:56–64.

Otto MW, Pollack MH, Maki KM: Empirically supported treatments for panic disorder: Costs, benefits, and stepped care. *J Consult Clin Psychol.* 2000;68:556–563.

Pande AC, Crockatt JG, Feltner DE, Janney CA, Smith WT, Weisler R, Londborg PD, Bielski RJ, Zimbroff DL, Davidson JR, Liu-Dumaw M: Pregabalin in generalized anxiety disorder: A placebo-controlled trial. *Am J Psychiatry.* 2003;160:533–540.

Perlmutter SJ, Leitman SF, Garvey MA, Hamburger S, Feldman E, Leonard HL, Swedo SE: Therapeutic plasma exchange and intravenous immunoglobulin for obsessive-compulsive disorder and tic disorders in childhood. *Lancet.* 1999;354:1153–1158.

Pollack MH, Zaninelli R, Goddard A, McCafferty JP, Bellew KM, Burnham DB, Iyengar MK: Paroxetine in the treatment of generalized anxiety disorder: Results of a placebo-controlled, flexible-dosage trial. *J Clin Psychiatry.* 2001;62:350–357.

Raskind MA, Peskind ER, Kanter ED, Petrie EC, Radant A, Thompson CE, Dobie DJ, Hoff D, Rein RJ, Straits-Troster K, Thomas RG, McFall MM: Reduction of nightmares and other PTSD symptoms in combat veterans by prazosin: A placebo-controlled study. *Am J Psychiatry.* 2003;160(2):371–373.

Roy-Byrne PP, Katon W, Cowley DS, Russo J: A randomized effectiveness trial of collaborative care for patients with panic disorder in primary care. *Arch Gen Psychiatry.* 2001;58:869–876.

Sareen J, Stein MB: Pharmacotherapy for anxiety disorders in the new millennium. *Psychiatr Clin North Am.* 2000;7:173–186.

Stahl SM, Gergel I, Li D: Escitalopram in the treatment of panic disorder: A randomized, double-blind, placebo-controlled trial. *J Clin Psychiatry.* 2003;64:1322–1327.

Stein DJ: Obsessive-compulsive disorder. *Lancet.* 2002;360:397–405.

*Stein MB: A 46-year-old man with anxiety and nightmares after a motor vehicle collision. *JAMA.* 2002;288:1513–1522.

Stein MB: Attending to anxiety disorders in primary care. *J Clin Psychiatry.* 2003;64[Suppl 15]:35–39.

Stein MB, Fuetsch M, Muller N, Höfler M, Lieb R, Wittchen H-U: Social anxiety disorder and the risk of depression: A prospective community study of adolescents and young adults. *Arch Gen Psychiatry.* 2001;58:251–256.

Stein MB, Kline NA, Matloff JL: Adjunctive olanzapine for SSRI-resistant combat-related posttraumatic stress disorder: A double-blind, placebo-controlled study. *Am J Psychiatry.* 2002;159:1777–1779.

Stein MB, Liebowitz MR, Lydiard RB, Bushnell W, Gergel IP: Paroxetine treatment of generalized social anxiety disorder (social phobia): A randomized controlled trial. *JAMA.* 1998;280:708–713.

*The Research Unit on Pediatric Psychopharmacology Anxiety Study Group: Fluvoxamine for the treatment of anxiety disorders in children and adolescents. *N Engl J Med.* 2001;344:1279–1285.

Walker JR, Van Ameringen MA, Swinson R, Bowen RC, Chokka PR, Goldner E, Johnston DC, Lavallie YJ, Nandy S, Pecknold JC, Hadrava V, Lane RM: Prevention of relapse in generalized social phobia: Results of a 24-week study in responders to 20 weeks of sertraline treatment. *J Clin Psychopharmacol.* 2000;20:636–644.

▲ 14.10 Anxiety Disorders: Cognitive-Behavioral Therapy

SHAWN P. CAHILL, PH.D., AND EDNA B. FOA, PH.D.

The term *anxiety* can have several different meanings. At the broadest level, anxiety refers to a normal emotion that most people experience at different times in their lives. At a somewhat more restricted level, anxiety may refer to a sign or symptom of some underlying medical or psychological condition or a substance-induced state, such as when someone ingests too much caffeine. The interest of the present section, however, rests at the level of anxiety as a psychiatric disorder and its treatment through cognitive-behavioral therapy (CBT). The fourth revised edition of the *Diagnostic and Statistical Manual of Mental Disorders* (DSM-IV-TR) specifies eight primary anxiety disorders: phobias, panic disorder (with and without agoraphobia), agoraphobia without panic disorder, obsessive-compulsive disorder (OCD), social anxiety disorder, posttraumatic stress disorder (PTSD), acute stress disorder, and generalized anxiety disorder. Common to the anxiety disorders is the emotion of anxiety and associated cognitions related to present and future threat of harm, physiological arousal when confronted with anxiety-relevant stimuli, and behavioral tendencies to escape from or avoid anxiety triggers and to prevent anticipated harm. Pathological anxiety is distinguished from normal anxiety in that the anxiety and avoidance must cause significant impairment in normal functioning or cause the individual substantial distress about having the various symptoms.

Each of the various anxiety disorders are distinguished from one another by the focus of the anxiety and specific symptom clusters. Panic attacks, for example, are discrete episodes of intense anxiety associated with several physiological (e.g., rapid heart rate, chest pain, cold chills, or hot flashes) and cognitive (e.g., thoughts that one is going to die, go crazy, or lose control) symptoms that may occur in up to 30 percent of the general population in a given year, yet only 2.3 percent of the population has a diagnosable panic disorder over the same period. The diagnosis of panic disorder requires, in addition to recurrent unexpected panic attacks, the development of an enduring anxiety about the occurrence of the next panic attack or concerns about the implications of such attacks for one's well-being. The central feature of panic disorder, therefore, is the fear of one's own fight-or-flight reaction, or the "fear of fear." Further, agoraphobic avoidance may develop to prevent the individual from experiencing the next panic attack.

By contrast, the focus of concern for individuals with PTSD is the anxiety caused by recollections and reminders of a previously experienced life-threatening event, such as physical or sexual assault, a severe accident, or combat. Although individuals with PTSD may experience panic attacks and often develop extensive behavioral avoidance, the panic tends to be cued by memories and reminders of the trauma, and the behavioral avoidance is designed to prevent activation of the trauma memory and prevent the occurrence of additional traumatic events.

Taken as a group, the anxiety disorders are among the most prevalent mental disorders, with an incidence rate (past 12 months) of 17 percent, compared to 11 percent for substance use disorders and affective disorders. The lifetime incidence of the anxiety disorders and substance use disorders are each approximately 25 percent and

20 percent for affective disorders. Anxiety disorders are frequently comorbid with one another and with mood and substance abuse disorders. Moreover, the onset of one of the anxiety disorders frequently precedes the onset of mood and substance abuse disorders and may thus play a role in their etiology. Thus, anxiety disorders are a significant mental health problem. Fortunately, effective pharmacological and psychological treatments have been developed for all of the primary anxiety disorders. This section describes the theory and practice of CBT for anxiety disorders and reviews evidence of its efficacy.

EMOTIONAL PROCESSING THEORY: A PSYCHOLOGICAL MODEL OF ANXIETY DISORDERS AND THEIR TREATMENT

Before describing the components of CBT and its efficacy in the treatment of the various anxiety disorders, a general psychological model of anxiety disorders and the conditions necessary for successful treatment are presented. In his influential model of information processing in fear-related imagery, Peter Lang proposed that the phenomenological, physiological, and behavioral components of anxiety reflect the activation of an underlying cognitive structure, called a *fear structure*, that contains stimulus, response, and meaning information that serves as a blueprint to avoid or escape from danger. Activation of the fear structure happens when environmental input matches some of the information stored in the structure. The environmental stimuli activate the matching information in the fear structure, and then the activation spreads throughout the rest of the structure via associative connections, thereby recruiting prior memories of the feared stimulus and the physiological and behavioral responses associated with the fight-or-flight reaction. Lang suggested, but with little elaboration, that activation of a fear structure is a necessary condition for altering it.

Building on Lang's work, Edna Foa and Michael Kozak's theory of emotional processing distinguished between normal and pathological fear structures, further specified the necessary conditions for the therapeutic modification of pathological fear structures, and specified indicators of emotional processing.

Pathological Fear Structures A fear structure is adaptive if the stimuli represented in it are objectively harmful and the responses represented in it lead to effectively avoiding, escaping, or coping with the threat. A fear structure is pathological when the associations among stimulus, response, and meaning representations do not accurately reflect reality, such that harmless stimuli or responses are erroneously interpreted as being dangerous. The characteristic features of each anxiety disorder, which differentiate them from one another, are thought to reflect the operation of specific pathological fear structures. For example, the fear structure for a specific small animal phobia would include associations among representations of the feared animal; meaning representations of the animal as being dangerous and uncontrollable; and responses such as physiological arousal and various defensive behaviors (e.g., calling for help, running away).

In contrast, the fear structure in panic disorder is characterized by fear of physical sensations associated with panic symptoms (e.g., rapid breathing, heart palpitations) and interpretation of these sensations as a heart attack or as signs of going crazy. As a result of the erroneous meaning associated with these sensations, people with panic disorder avoid situations that will give rise to panic or cause similar sensations, such as intense physical activity. In PTSD, the fear structure involves associations among trauma-related harmful stimuli and similar but nonharmful stimuli, inaccurate interpretations of safe stimuli as dangerous (e.g., all men are rapists), and unhelpful interpretations of one's reactions as indicators of being incompetent (e.g., "My symptoms mean I can't cope with this").

Emotional Processing We use the term *emotional processing* to refer to changes in a pathological fear structure that result in long-term fear reduction and resolution of the anxiety disorder. Foa and Kozak proposed that two conditions are necessary for emotional processing to take place. First, the fear structure must be activated either through a direct match with stimuli in the environment (e.g., confronting the feared stimulus) or through symbolic means (e.g., imagining or thinking about the feared stimuli). Second, new information that is *incompatible* with the pathological aspects of the fear structure must be available and incorporated into the structure, thereby altering the structure and creating a more realistic, or "nonfear" structure.

Emotional processing theory was explicitly designed to explain the efficacy of exposure therapy in the treatment of anxiety. Although Foa and Kozak advanced the hypothesis that any psychological treatment that was effective in the treatment of anxiety achieved its results through the same mechanisms, research investigating predictions derived from emotional processing theory has predominately focused on exposure therapy. Thus, it will be easier to initially describe emotional processing theory in terms of exposure therapy. Accordingly, exposure therapy involves helping patients to systematically confront feared but otherwise safe stimuli in a manner that promotes eventual fear reduction. The efficacy of exposure therapy in reducing anxiety has been widely demonstrated, and exposure procedures are a basic component of nearly every CBT program that has been shown to be effective in the treatment of the various anxiety disorders. The relevance of emotional processing theory to other treatments for anxiety, specifically anxiety management training and cognitive therapy, is addressed later in the chapter.

Emotional processing theory is offered as an explanation for fear reduction; therefore, it is important to distinguish observations that serve as indicators of emotional processing from treatment outcome to avoid circular reasoning. To avoid this problem, Foa and Kozak specify three indicators of emotional processing that can be measured separately from treatment outcome. Following from the proposal that activation of the fear structure is necessary for change in the structure to occur, one indicator of emotional processing is emotional engagement, as reflected in facial reactions, self-reports of fear and anxiety, or physiological reactions such as increased skin conductance or heart rate when the person confronts or thinks about the feared stimulus.

A second indicator of emotional processing is a gradual reduction in these indexes of emotional engagement over the course of a therapy session. In the context of exposure therapy, this is called *within-session habituation*. However, acute fear reduction can occur for reasons other than habituation, such as distraction, engaging in compulsions, or other safety behaviors. Although such methods of fear reduction may be partially effective when used to cope with exposure to feared stimuli, they can interfere with long-term fear reduction. Theoretically, such measures limit emotional engagement and prevent exposure to disconfirming information, thereby preventing therapeutic changes from taking place in the fear structure. For example, if a person with OCD who fears contamination touches a public toilet, thus activating the fear structure, but then immediately washes to prevent contracting an illness, he or she will not have the opportunity to learn that simply touching a toilet seat will not lead to a fatal disease.

The third indicator of emotional processing is reduction in the levels of fear experienced across repeated sessions, or *between-session habituation*. Fear reduction obtained in one session that does not at least partially transfer to a subsequent session (i.e., the lack of between-session habituation) indicates that the fear structure was not altered and suggests that any previously observed fear reduction may have been brought about by some kind of compulsion, safety behavior, or other form of defensive maneuver. By contrast, fear reduction that does transfer across sessions strongly suggests that the previous experiences have led to some enduring change in the fear structure.

These indicators of emotional processing are distinguishable from treatment outcome, which is a broader construct that encompasses variables not specifically targeted in treatment. For example, PTSD is defined by the presence of symptoms from each of three symptom clusters: reexperiencing the trauma, avoidance or numbing, and hyperarousal. Although emotional engagement would overlap with increased distress and physiological arousal in response to trauma memories and reminders (two of the reexperiencing symptoms), the other symptoms of PTSD are separate from the indicators of emotional processing. Moreover, a full assessment of treatment outcome would include aspects of the person's functioning, such as the quality of job performance, personal relationships, and degree of life satisfaction.

Several studies conducted across a range of disorders, including specific phobias, OCD, and PTSD, have investigated the relationship between indicators of emotional processing and treatment outcome of exposure therapy. For example, in a study of systematic desensitization for simple phobias, Lang and colleagues found three variables that predicted successful treatment: greater initial heart rate reactivity during fear-relevant imagery, greater concordance between self-reported distress and heart rate elevation during fear-relevant imagery, and systematic decline in heart rate reactivity with repetition of the imagery.

Studying exposure therapy for OCD, Foa and colleagues found that within-session habituation predicted between-session habituation. They also found that the effect of within-session habituation on outcome was mediated through the relationship between within- and between-session habituation: Individuals who displayed the best outcome were those who obtained a pattern of both within- and between-session habituation. Emotional engagement in this study, however, was negatively correlated with within-session habituation and treatment outcome. In a second study of OCD, Kozak and colleagues found that emotional engagement and between-session habituation were both positively correlated with treatment outcome, although there was no relationship of within-session fear reduction to treatment outcome.

In a study of students with a fear of public speaking, Ellen Chaplin and Bruce Levine provided participants with two 25-minute exposure exercises per session for four sessions. One group of participants received the exposures one immediately after the other (massed trials condition), whereas the other group had a 10-minute interval between the two exposures (spaced trials condition). Participants in both groups showed successive reductions in fear across sessions. However, only participants in the massed trials condition showed within-session habituation. On a measure of treatment outcome, participants in the massed trials reported greater improvement than those in the spaced trials condition.

Foa and colleagues investigated whether emotional engagement, as measured by facial reactions of fear during an early imaginal exposure session, would predict subsequent treatment outcome of PTSD in female assault victims. In addition, based on earlier evidence that anger in the acute aftermath of an assault is associated with less natural recovery, Foa and colleagues hypothesized that anger would inhibit emotional engagement with fear and thereby reduce treatment efficacy. The results revealed that high levels of PTSD at pretreatment were predictive of greater self-reported distress and greater facial fear reactions during exposure therapy, which in turn was predictive of greater improvement. However, levels of pretreatment anger were negatively correlated with facial fear reactions during imaginal exposure. Thus, anger appears to dampen fear reactivity during imaginal exposure, thereby reducing the effectiveness of the treatment.

In another study of exposure therapy for female assault victims with PTSD, Lisa Jaycox et al. submitted self-reports of anxiety and distress obtained during each of six imaginal exposure therapy sessions to a cluster analysis. This procedure yielded three distinct patterns that were differentially associated with treatment outcome. One group, termed *high engagers/habituators*, displayed a pattern of high distress during the first session, followed by a systematic decline over the subsequent sessions. A second group, termed *high engagers/nonhabituators*, showed similar levels of distress during the first session, but little decline across sessions. The third group, termed *low engagers/nonhabituators*, displayed a pattern of significantly lower levels of distress during the first session than either of the high-engager groups and little distress across the subsequent sessions. At the final exposure session, distress levels for the high engagers/nonhabituators were significantly greater than for the low engagers/nonhabituators, which in turn were significantly greater than levels for the high engagers/habituators. On outcome assessment of PTSD symptoms, high engagers/habituators reported significantly lower levels of reexperiencing symptoms than high engagers/nonhabituators and significantly lower arousal symptoms than group low engagers/nonhabituators.

Roger Pitman et al. investigated the three indicators of emotional processing in veterans undergoing exposure therapy. Self-report measures of emotional processing in this study assessed fear, sadness, arousal, guilt, and anger. Psychophysiological measures of emotional processing were heart rate, skin conductance, and facial electromyography (EMG). Emotional engagement and within-session habituation were observed for all, and between-session habituation was observed for heart rate and self-reported arousal, sadness, anger, and fear. The magnitude of heart rate activation was positively correlated with reduced self-monitored intrusions after treatment. Within- and between-session habituation of heart rate reactivity was correlated with reductions in the frequency of posttreatment reexperiencing of symptoms.

Sources of Corrective Information and Conditions That Interfere with Emotional Processing It is relatively easy to see how exposure therapy promotes emotional engagement, as patients are helped to think and talk about feared thoughts, images, and memories; to confront feared things and situations; and to engage in feared activities. It may not be as easy to see what sources of corrective or fear-disconfirming information is contained in an exposure exercise.

One important source of corrective information is within-session habituation, which provides new response information about the *absence* of physiological responding in the presence of feared stimuli that is incompatible with prior response information. Physiological habituation can also provide corrective information to modify erroneous associations between physiological responses and certain meaning representations or interpretations. For example, the experience of habituation disconfirms the common belief that anxiety will persist unless the person escapes the situation and corrects misperceptions that physiological responses associated with the fight-or-flight system are evidence of a heart attack or of going crazy.

Repeated and prolonged exposure may also provide corrective information as to the realistic likelihood or significance of feared consequences. Anxious people frequently overestimate the probability of feared events and the significance of those consequences, should they happen. For example, a person with OCD with obsessional fears related to illness may make an unrealistically high estimate of the probability of nausea, diarrhea, and vomiting as a result of eating certain foods (e.g., spicy foods, food prepared at a "greasy diner"). Repeated exposure allows the person to test whether the feared consequence happens. Moreover, even if it does happen—for example, the person feels nauseous or develops a case of diarrhea—the person has the opportunity to learn that these consequences, although unpleasant, are not catastrophic.

Exposure to intrusive and unwanted thoughts can help a person to distinguish between unpleasant thoughts that occur in his or her mind and reality or to separate thoughts from overt actions. For example, some individuals with OCD experience intrusive images of inflicting harm on people around them and are afraid they will act on these images by attacking someone. Exposure therapy allows these individuals to learn that they can think these upsetting thoughts without acting on them. In cases of PTSD, individuals may experience the memory of the trauma as if it were the same as actually reexperiencing the trauma. However, no matter how severe the trauma was or how distressing the memory may be, it is not physically harmful. Exposure to the trauma memory can help the person to differentiate between a past event that was objectively threatening or harmful in some way and the current safe experience of remembering the trauma.

Failures of Emotional Processing If repeated exposure to feared stimuli contains corrective or fear-disconfirming information, then why do most anxiety disorders have a chronic course? An important feature of all anxiety disorders, in addition to the experience of intense distress on exposure to feared stimuli, is a strong tendency to escape from feared situations or avoid them altogether. To the extent that such escape and avoidance strategies are effective, they are strengthened through the principle of negative reinforcement, making it even more likely the person will engage in escape or avoidance in the future. At the same, successful escape or avoidance limits the person's exposure to fear-disconfirming information. For example, a person who is afraid of and successfully avoids dogs, even friendly dogs, will not have the opportunity to learn that dogs can not only be safe but also fun to play with.

Two procedures studied in the context of exposure therapy that have been found to promote acute reductions in distress while in the presence of feared stimuli but that interfere with between-session habituation are distraction and the use of benzodiazepine medications. Several studies have investigated the effects of distraction on exposure. These studies have differed substantially in how distraction was manipulated, the population that was studied, and the duration of the exposure sessions, which may account for some of the variability in results across studies. Moreover, the pattern of results emerging from these studies strongly indicates that the acute effects of manipulations designed to focus attention toward or away from feared stimuli must be distinguished from their long-term effects. For example, Michelle Craske et al. tested snake- and spider-phobic individuals under three conditions. All participants first underwent a brief natural exposure test in which no specific instructions were provided. Participants then underwent brief exposure tests under focused and distracting conditions, in counter-balanced order. In the focused condition, participants listened to an audiotape that contained prompts to attend to the characteristics of the snake or spider and their own bodily reactions. In the distracted condition, participants listened to irrelevant tape-recorded passages that were followed by multiple-choice questions on their content. Compared to baseline, self-reported anxiety increased during each of the three test conditions. However, anxiety was greater in the focused-attention condition than in either the neutral or distracted conditions, which were not different from one another.

F. Dudley McGlynn, Michael Rose, and colleagues conducted a series of studies comparing brief stimulus-focused trials, in which participants were instructed to attend to the feared animal (snakes and various insects), with response-focused trials, in which participants were instructed to attend to their own bodily reactions. Results of these studies yielded a consistent pattern of greater anxiety under the stimulus-focused instructions compared to response-focused instructions. These studies illustrate that focusing on the feared object has the acute effect of increasing anxiety, whereas turning attention away from the feared object may have the acute effect of reducing anxiety. However, studies reviewed previously suggest that exposure therapy is most effective when people are emotionally engaged with the feared object. This would suggest that distraction procedures should reduce between-session habituation.

In a recent study, Kyla Penfold and Andrew Page used a between-group design to study distraction among mildly blood- and injury-phobic individuals. In the first phase of the study, participants completed a relevant behavioral approach test. In phase two, participants were randomly assigned to a 10-minute exposure test under one of three conditions: exposure plus focusing (discussion about the features of exposure stimulus), exposure plus distraction (discussion about irrelevant topics), or exposure alone (no discussion). Individuals in the distracted exposure condition reported significantly less anxiety during and immediately after exposure than the other two groups. However, there were no differences among groups in a subsequent behavioral approach test. Indeed, anxiety during the test was numerically highest in the condition that previously underwent distracted exposure, although the differences were not statistically significant.

Jonathan Grayson et al. tested the effects of distraction on both within- and between-session habituation in the treatment of OCD. These authors used a crossover design to compare distraction and attention-focusing conditions on fear reduction during 90-minute in vivo sessions. In the distraction condition, participants each held a "contaminated" object in one hand while playing a video game with their therapist with their other hand. In the attention-focusing condition, the participants held the contaminated object but engaged in a conversation with their therapist about the object and their reactions to it. Within-session fear reduction occurred under both distracting and attention-focusing conditions; however, between-session fear reduction was observed on the second day only for those participants who received focused exposure on the first day.

These studies show that, under some circumstances, distraction can produce acute reductions in anxiety, although it may not always be successful. Moreover, fear reduction obtained through distraction does not transfer to subsequent tests in the absence of the distraction strategy. Not only does fear reduction via distraction appear to not promote between-session fear reduction, Grayson et al. demonstrated that distraction techniques can interfere with between-session habituation.

When taken shortly before exposure to a feared stimulus, benzodiazepines can significantly reduce anxiety. As with distraction, however, the fear reduction that occurs with the medication does not transfer to subsequent tests in a nonmedicated condition and, indeed, appears to interfere with the normal process of between-session habituation. Frank Wilhelm and Walton Troth demonstrated this among a group of patients undergoing treatment for the fear of flying that involved taking two flights scheduled 1 week apart. Ninety minutes before taking the first flight, half of the patients took the high-potency benzodiazepine alprazolam (Xanax), and the remaining patients took a placebo. Patients taking the active medication reported significantly less anxiety during the first trip than patients who took the placebo. Before the second trip, all patients were given a placebo pill. Patients who had taken the placebo before the first flight showed a reduction in their anxiety on the second flight, whereas those who had taken the active medication showed an increase in anxiety on the second flight.

COGNITIVE-BEHAVIORAL THERAPY PROCEDURES FOR ANXIETY DISORDERS

Most CBT programs for anxiety disorders begin with an assessment, patient education, and specific treatment planning. The actual treatment procedures involve at least one of four components: (1) exposure to thoughts, objects, situations, and physiological sensations that are not dangerous but are nonetheless feared, avoided, or endured with great distress; (2) training in general anxiety or stress management techniques; (3) use of cognitive therapy techniques; and (4) training in specific skills, such as heterosocial dating skills, assertiveness, and so forth.

Assessment, Psychoeducation, and Treatment Planning CBT begins with a thorough assessment of the patient's presenting complaints using empirically validated assessment procedures. Self-report and interviewer rating measures have been developed for the diagnosis and assessment of severity for each anxiety disorder. The assessment may also include measures of related psychopathology, such as depression and general anxiety, and specific theoretically relevant variables associated with the disorder of interest, such as trauma-related cognitions in PTSD and anxiety sensitivity in panic disorder. Typically, assessments are repeated over the course and at the end of treatment for the purpose of establishing a diagnosis, selecting treatment procedures, monitoring the process of treatment, and evaluating treatment outcome.

The next step of CBT is psychoeducation. Patients are typically provided with information about their specific diagnoses, a description of treatment options, and specific treatment recommendations. If the patient decides to continue in therapy, the therapist usually provides greater details about the specific procedures being recommended along with an appropriate theoretical rationale or treatment model. The treatment model helps the patient to understand the important factors associated with the development and maintenance of their symptoms and how the treatment procedures are thought to alleviate their symptoms.

As part of the initial assessment and patient education, the therapist and patient work together to identify specific targets for treatment and to work out the details of the treatment plan. An example of this is the development of a hierarchy for conducting in vivo exposure exercises. In addition, expectations are set that the patient will engage in homework between sessions to increase mastery of the therapy skills and self-monitoring procedures for symptoms.

Exposure Therapy Exposure therapy involves intentionally confronting feared, but otherwise not dangerous, objects, situations, thoughts, memories, and physical sensations for the purpose of reducing fear reactions associated with the same or similar stimuli. Systematic desensitization was the first exposure therapy technique to undergo scientific investigation. Although an effective treatment for some anxiety disorders, it has generally fallen out of use among researchers and cognitive-behavioral therapists. The contemporary use of exposure therapy may be usefully divided into three classes of procedures: in vivo exposure, imaginal exposure, and interoceptive exposure.

Systematic Desensitization Systematic desensitization requires initial training in progressive muscle relaxation and the development of one or more carefully constructed hierarchies of feared stimuli. Treatment then involves the pairing of mental images of the lowest items on the hierarchy with relaxation until the image can be held in mind without it producing significant distress. This process is then repeated with each item on the hierarchy. Although systematic desensitization has been found to be effective in the treatment of specific phobias and social anxiety, it is generally no longer used among contemporary cognitive-behavioral therapists and researchers. This is due to the convergence of two lines of research. First, studies of the systematic desensitization procedures failed to produce convincing evidence that the unique features of this procedure, related to Joseph Wolpe's theory of reciprocal inhibition, are necessary for good outcome. For example, treatment need not begin at the bottom of the hierarchy, and it is not necessary to pair the fear-relevant images with relaxation for fear reduction to occur. Indeed, rather than reducing anxiety, the primary role of relaxation procedures in the effects of systematic desensitization appears to be the enhancement of image vividness, thereby increasing physiological reactivity to the image. These results are contrary to hypothesis that the efficacy of systematic desensitization is brought about by relaxation inhibiting anxiety but are consistent with the tenets of emotional processing theory.

Second, alternative procedures entailing repeated, prolonged exposure to stimuli of moderately high levels of anxiety, particularly in vivo, until the anxiety decreases without the use of any specific anxiety management techniques were being developed. In particular, the prolonged exposure approach was found to have beneficial effects in the treatment of OCD and agoraphobia, two conditions that were minimally responsive to systematic desensitization. Subsequently, direct comparisons also found these more intense forms of exposure therapy to be as effective as or more effective than systematic desensitization in the treatment of simple phobias.

In Vivo Exposure In vivo exposure involves helping patients to directly confront feared objects, activities, and situations. It is usually conducted in a graduated fashion according to a mutually agreed-on (between patient and therapist) hierarchy. For example, a hierarchy for a specific animal phobia, such as a snake or spiders, may begin with looking at pictures and other representations of the feared animal, followed by looking at the actual animal kept in a cage, first at a distance and then gradually moving closer. Depending on the animal, subsequent steps may involve touching and handling the animal, perhaps first while wearing a glove and then without the glove. These steps may be repeated across several different examples of the animal, differing in such dimensions as size and activity level.

In the case of OCD, in vivo exposure is explicitly combined with response prevention, in which the patient agrees to not engage in compulsions or rituals designed to reduce anxiety when exposed to an object that elicits obsessional fears or designed to control feared harmful consequences. For example, a person with fears of contamination may be asked to touch and use a variety of common objects such as door knobs, public phones, and public restrooms while intentionally refraining from washing or taking specific measures to limit the spread of contamination (e.g., using a tissue as a barrier between the skin and the contaminated object). In the case of PTSD, patients are asked to confront reminders of the traumatic event. However, because this disorder is the result of actually experiencing a traumatic event, the therapist needs to use good judgment in assessing whether trauma reminders are objectively safe. For example, victims of interpersonal crime (e.g., rape, physical assault) may have experienced their trauma in a relatively dangerous setting, such as an abandoned building late at night. Such realistically high-risk situations would not be a part of their treatment—rather, the goal would be to identify situations and activities that are objectively low risk but are nonetheless avoided or only tolerated with great distress.

Imaginal Exposure Imaginal exposure typically involves having the patient close his or her eyes and imagine feared stimuli as vividly as possible. Imaginal exposure has two general uses. The primary use is to help patients confront feared thoughts, images, and memories. For example, individuals with OCD may experience obsessional thoughts and images about causing harm to people they love. In addition, they may have fearful thoughts about long-term consequences of their current actions, such as contracting human immunodeficiency virus (HIV) from a public toilet seat. For these conditions, imaginal exposure to these feared thoughts and consequences is used to promote habituation of emotional reactivity to the image and to help the patient distinguish between thoughts of committing harm or contracting a serious illness and reality, in which they do not act on those thoughts or do not actually have the illness. In the case of PTSD, imaginal exposure is used to help the patient confront his or her memory of the traumatic event. Here again, the procedure promotes habituation to the memory and helps the patient to distinguish between the actual traumatic event, which was dangerous, and the current memory of the event, which, although distressing, is not harmful.

A second use of imaginal exposure is in lieu of in vivo exposure when arranging direct contact with the feared situation is not safe or feasible or as a preparatory exercise to facilitate subsequent in vivo exposures. In these cases, the patient imagines confronting the feared object or engaging in the feared task. When the patient's level of anticipatory anxiety is reduced, in vivo exposure may be conducted with the actual feared object or task, assuming it is both safe and available.

Interoceptive Exposure Interoceptive exposure is the most recent form of exposure therapy to be introduced. This procedure is designed to induce feared physiological sensations under controlled circumstances. Interoceptive exposure exercises are most commonly used in the treatment of panic disorder and certain specific phobias, for example, the fear of vomiting, in which internal cues such as those associated with physiological arousal (e.g., rapid heart rate, dizziness, tingling in the finger tips) or gastric upset (e.g., after eating a spicy meal) elicit fear, anxiety, and further arousal.

A number of specific exercises have been developed to induce specific panic-like sensations. For example, the step-up exercise, in which the patient repeatedly steps up and down on a single step as rapidly as possible, produces rapid heart rate and shortness of breath. Spinning in a chair or spinning in place produces dizziness and, in some people, mild nausea. Hyperventilating produces shortness of breath, dizziness, and tingling in the fingers and around the mouth and can produce a sense of unreality. Breathing through a thin straw produces the sensation of not getting enough air. Other possible activities include consuming mild stimulants (e.g., eating chocolate-covered espresso beans), engaging in various forms of vigorous activity, going on amusement park rides (e.g., the roller coaster), and eating spicy foods. The goal is to find an activity that produces similar sensations to the ones that patients find unduly distressing and attempt to avoid. As with other forms of exposure, the purposes for inducing these sensations are to promote habituation of fear in response to them (i.e., the fear of fear or anxiety sensitivity) and to distinguish these sensations, which are normal responses to the various exercises, from physiological sensations that may actually signal a significant health problem.

Anxiety Management and Stress Inoculation Training

Anxiety management training is a general approach to treating anxiety, of which Meichenbaum's stress inoculation training is one specific example. Emotions in general, and stress and anxiety in particular, reflect the activity of three loosely coupled and interacting "channels," or modes, of responding: cognitive–phenomenological, physiological, and behavioral. Stress inoculation training involves training patients in the application of specific skills and techniques designed to address each of these response modes in a flexible manner that is tailored to the individual's needs. For example, spiraling negative cognitions that often occur during times of stress may be interrupted by the use of thought stopping, in which the patient thinks the word "stop" in their mind while vividly imagining the word stop and then replaces it with positive or coping self-statements. The physiological manifestations of anxiety and stress (e.g., hyperventilation and its consequences, muscle tension, and gastric symptoms) may be addressed through training in diaphragmatic breathing and progressive muscle relaxation (e.g., Jacobson's "tense and relax") method). Changes in overt behavior are promoted through the use of role playing and covert rehearsal, in which patients practice new behaviors while executing other coping skills either with another person or in their mind. Exposure to feared situations either in vivo or in the imagination is frequently a part of stress inoculation training, but is usually for the purpose of practicing new skills and is accompanied by the use of other coping skills.

From the perspective of emotional processing theory, stress inoculation training involves altering response information in the fear structure. These new responses are typically first learned in the relative safety of the therapist's office but are then applied in stressful or anxiety-producing situations. Thus, this new response information has the opportunity to be incorporated and thereby alter the fear structure. In addition, successful coping with fear and anxiety provides new meaning information related to personal competence that counters typical fear-related beliefs related to self-incompetence.

Cognitive Therapy

The basic assumption of cognitive therapy is that people's beliefs and appraisals of events and situations are at least as important in determining their emotional reactions as the actual events and situations. Problematic emotions such as anxiety are frequently the result of unrealistic and unhelpful beliefs about the world, the self, and others. The goal of cognitive therapy is to help patients to identify unhelpful cognitions and cognitive errors (e.g., all-or-nothing thinking, overgeneralization, only considering evidence that is consistent with existing beliefs) and to modify them. Three of the most common traditional cognitive therapy procedures are (1) the use of Socratic dialogue, in which the therapist uses a series of questions to help the patient identify and challenge unhelpful beliefs or to uncover evidence disconfirming fear-related beliefs; (2) the downward arrow technique, in which the therapist helps to uncover deeper beliefs and meanings by repeatedly asking for greater clarification; and (3) the use of thought records, in which patients record automatic beliefs, list evidence for and against those beliefs, review potential cognitive errors that may be reflected in those beliefs, and then generate more realistic and helpful beliefs.

A fourth technique that is frequently used in the treatment of anxiety disorders is the behavioral experiment, which has features overlapping with in vivo exposure. The goal of a behavioral experiment is to test beliefs about the nature and probability of feared consequences under conditions that will optimize exposure to and the encoding of disconfirming information. For example, before conducting a behavioral experiment, the patient makes detailed predictions about what he or she believes will happen under a particular set of circumstances and then conducts the relevant experiment to see what happens. For example, a person with OCD who fears accidentally causing harm to others may be afraid that normal use of a razor has a high probability of causing the blade to fall out and that the lost blade will go unnoticed until an unsuspecting child finds it and gets injured. A behavioral experiment to test predictions about the likelihood of the razor blade falling out might involve throwing the razor blade a number of times and then checking to see if the blade is still present. Each time the razor is tossed without the blade falling out, the patient is confronted with evidence that disconfirms his or her beliefs about the probability that it will fall out. The conceptual emphasis in cognitive therapy on changing beliefs through exposure to disconfirming evidence is consistent with the tenets of emotional processing theory. The practical and empirical issues involve determining the best ways to accomplish this goal.

Social Skills Training

According to the social skills deficit model, people with social anxiety lack important skills to interact effectively with others. Consequently, they experience fewer interpersonal rewards and more punishments, leading them to avoid social interactions when possible, thereby further limiting their ability to acquire effective social skills. Accordingly, comprehensive treatment for social anxiety would provide explicit training to help patients acquire and use appropriate social skills and thereby reverse the negative cycle. In the absence of appropriate social skills, the punitive interactions with others only serve to strengthen the fear structure.

EFFICACY OF COGNITIVE-BEHAVIORAL THERAPY

Phobias and Agoraphobia

The key features of phobias are the presence of persistent and intense fear and avoidance of specific objects or situations that the individual recognizes as being excessive or unreasonable. If avoidance is not possible, the feared stimulus is endured with great distress. To qualify as a phobia, the fear and avoidance must significantly interfere with the person's social or occupational functioning or the person must experience marked distress about the fears. Although the range of phobic situations is potentially quite broad, the most common are animal phobias (e.g., dogs, insects), natural environment phobias (e.g., heights, storms, water), blood or injury phobias (including receiving or viewing injections), and situational phobias (e.g., bridges, flying, enclosed spaces). *Agoraphobia* is a pattern of pervasive avoidance of places and situations. If such places and situations cannot be avoided, then they are endured with great distress— the person with agoraphobia is afraid that he or she may experience a full-blown or symptom-limited panic attack and perceives that help is unavailable. Common agoraphobic situations include various crowded public places (e.g., malls, restaurants, and theaters) and enclosed spaces (e.g., closets, elevators, and cars).

A large body of research beginning in the mid-1960s has clearly demonstrated the efficacy of several exposure therapy protocols in the treatment of simple phobias and fear of public speaking. This research establishes exposure therapy as the treatment of choice for these conditions. The earliest studies focused on systematic desensitization. In the first controlled study, Lang and David Lazovik compared systematic desensitization with a waitlist control condition in the treatment of students with a fear of snakes. In the first phase of the study, participants in the desensitization group separately practiced relaxation and created a hierarchy. In the second phase, participants in the desensitization group paired the feared images from the hierarchy with relaxation. Neither group showed any changes during the first phase, but the desensitization group showed significant improvement across the second phase, whereas the control group showed no change.

In a follow-up study, desensitization was found to be superior to a pseudotherapy that, like desensitization, included training in relaxation and hierarchy construction. After the initial preparation, participants in the desensitization group paired the feared images with relaxation, whereas the pseudotherapy group engaged in positive imagery during relaxation. Gordon Paul compared the efficacy of five sessions of systematic desensitization for the public speaking fears and other forms of social anxiety with waitlist and two alternative treatment conditions (insight-oriented psychotherapy and an attention-placebo condition in which subjects were given a placebo pill but told it was a drug that reduced anxiety in stressful situations and then conducted a task that was said to be stressful but actually induced drowsiness). Results revealed that all three treatments were superior to waitlist and that systematic desensitization was superior to the alternative treatments, which did not differ from one another. This pattern of outcome was maintained up to 2 years after the completion of treatment.

Research beginning in the 1970s began to investigate the "flooding" approach to imaginal and in vivo approaches, which involved repeated and prolonged exposure to fear cues of high intensity without including relaxation. Results from the earliest of these studies provided evidence for efficacy of all three approaches (systematic desensitization, imaginal exposure, and in vivo exposure) but provided mixed results regarding the relative efficacy among the treatments. For example, a crossover study comparing desensitization and imaginal exposure found that the two treatments were equally effective in the treatment of specific phobias, but imaginal exposure was more effective in the treatment of agoraphobia. Michael Gelder et al. found that both systematic desensitization and imaginal exposure were more effective than a nonspecific treatment control condition among a mixed sample of patients with specific phobias and patients with agoraphobia. However, they did not replicate the finding of superiority of imaginal exposure over desensitization for agoraphobia.

Similarly conflicting results were reported for early studies comparing the efficacy of imaginal and in vivo exposure in the treatment of agoraphobia. The research group at Oxford University compared 16 weekly sessions of in vivo exposure alone with eight weekly sessions of imaginal exposure followed by eight weekly sessions of in vivo exposure and 16 weekly sessions that included both imaginal and in vivo exposure. All three treatments produced comparable improvements. By contrast, Paul Emmelkamp and Hemmy Wessels, working in the Netherlands, found that four sessions of in vivo exposure with or without additional imaginal exposure were superior to four sessions of imaginal exposure alone.

A more consistent pattern of outcome in favor of a particular form of in vivo exposure, called *participant modeling* or *guided mastery*, over other forms of exposure therapy in the treatment of phobias and agoraphobia has been reported in series of studies by Albert Bandura and colleagues. In participant modeling, the therapist actively models handling the feared object for the patient and may make use of various "response induction aids" to help the patient successfully handle the feared object. For example, in treating a patient with a spider phobia, the therapist may first demonstrate how to touch, handle, and control a tarantula. The therapist then coaches the patient in performing the same behaviors, first while wearing protective gloves and then without gloves. This active approach to in vivo exposure may be contrasted with more passive approaches in which the patient may be instructed to sit and observe a snake in a cage and attempt contact with the object when their fear at the earlier step has decreased.

Bandura et al. compared systematic desensitization with participant modeling and a variation called *symbolic modeling* in the treatment of individuals with a fear of snakes. Symbolic modeling consisted of watching a movie of several different models interacting with snakes, but participants in this group did not receive any in vivo exposure. All three treatments were superior to a waitlist condition. Among the active treatments, however, both forms of modeling were superior to desensitization and participant modeling was superior to symbolic modeling.

In a series of three similarly designed studies, S. Lloyd Williams and colleagues compared participant modeling with passive in vivo exposure in which the therapist did not model successful performance or actively assist subjects in completing the therapeutic activities. The therapist's primary role was to monitor and record the patients' performance and their self-reported levels of distress during the task. One study included a mixed group of driving phobics and acrophobics, another studied acrophobics only, and another studied agoraphobics. In all three studies, the active treatments were found to be superior to waitlist, and participant modeling was found to be superior to passive exposure. Extending this work to group treatment, Lars Ost et al. found that group participant modeling was superior to other forms of group exposure therapy in the treatment of spider phobia.

Systematic desensitization, prolonged imaginal exposure, and prolonged in vivo exposure have all been found to be effective in the treatment of phobias. In addition, systematic desensitization and imaginal exposure may be of some limited effectiveness in treating agoraphobia. Prolonged in vivo exposure is at least as effective as, and often more effective than, desensitization and prolonged imaginal exposure. The participant modeling variation of in vivo exposure has been found to be particularly effective in treating a range of phobias, including small animal phobias, acrophobia, and agoraphobia.

Obsessive-Compulsive Disorder

People with OCD have one or more obsessions or compulsions or both. *Obsessions* are recurrent thoughts, images, or impulses that are experienced as intrusive and unwanted and cause extreme distress. *Compulsions* are thoughts or behaviors that are usually carried out in response to an obsession or according to rigid rules, with the goal of reducing distress associated with an obsession or to prevent some feared consequence.

Exposure and Response Prevention

Although OCD was previously thought to be particularly resistant to treatment, one study reported successful outcome in two cases of OCD with a combination of prolonged exposure to obsession-related cues combined with the prevention of compulsive rituals. Further success was reported in a series of 10 out of 15 cases similarly treated, with only two cases of relapse over the course of a 5-year follow-up period. In 1996, Foa and Kozak summarized 13 studies that reported short-term outcome and 16 studies that reported long-term outcome for the use of exposure and response prevention in the treatment of OCD. Overall, 83 percent of subjects (N = 330) were classified as responders after 10 to 25 sessions (N = 15). After an average follow-up interval of 29 months, 76 percent of 376 subjects were classified as responders.

The efficacy and specificity of exposure and response prevention has been tested in a number of studies and found to be superior to placebo medication, relaxation, and anxiety management training. One study used a crossover design to investigate whether the separate components of exposure and response prevention have differential effects on obsessions and compulsions. Half of the participants received 2 weeks of treatment with exposure but no response prevention, followed by an additional 2 weeks of treatment with response prevention but no formal exposure. The remaining patients received the same treatments in reverse order. Results indicated that exposure produced greater reductions in fear during an in vivo test, whereas response prevention produced a greater reduction in the time spent engaged in compulsions. This finding was replicated in a study with a between-group design that found that the combination was superior to either component alone.

Andrew Rabavilas et al. compared imaginal with in vivo exposure and found, contrary to studies of phobias and agoraphobia, that these two modalities produced comparable outcome. Foa and colleagues obtained a similar result. They compared the combination of imaginal and in vivo exposure plus response prevention with in vivo exposure plus response prevention. Treatments produced comparable outcome immediately after treatment; however, there was a tendency towards greater relapse for the group that did not include imaginal exposure. A more recent study failed to replicate this finding.

Cognitive Therapy

Researchers have also investigated the efficacy of variations of cognitive therapy for the treatment of OCD and compared them with exposure and response prevention. One study compared the efficacy of exposure and response prevention with rational-emotive therapy. Both treatments resulted in significant improvement, with no statistically significant differences between them. Another study compared more traditional Beck-style cognitive therapy that incorporated behavioral experiments with exposure and response prevention. Both treatments resulted in improvement. At the end of treatment, 50 percent of patients receiving cognitive therapy were judged to be recovered, compared to 28 percent in the exposure condition. However, the effect of exposure therapy in this study was smaller than reported in other studies. A 2001 study also compared cognitive therapy with group exposure and response prevention. Both treatments were superior to waitlist. Exposure therapy was numerically superior to cognitive therapy, but the differences were not statistically significant.

Exposure and response prevention is the best-established psychological treatment for OCD. Imaginal exposure is used to help patients confront obsessional thoughts and feared consequences, whereas in vivo exposure is used to help patients confront feared objects, situations, and activities. Response prevention is used to decrease the frequency of compulsions and interrupt the cycle of negative reinforcement that serves to maintain the OCD. Optimal treatment includes both exposure and response prevention. More recently, cognitive therapy has also been found to be effective in the treatment of OCD. In general, direct comparisons have found few differences between the efficacy of these two treatment strategies. However, the inclusion of behavioral experiments in cognitive therapy reduces somewhat the distinctiveness of the two therapies, thereby complicating their direct comparison.

Posttraumatic Stress Disorder and Acute Stress Disorder

Acute stress disorder and PTSD are reactions that may develop after exposure to an event involving physical harm or threat to life in which the person's response involved intense terror, horror, or helplessness. Both disorders are characterized by symptoms of reexperiencing the trauma (e.g., intrusive thoughts, nightmares), avoidance of trauma reminders and related thoughts and feelings, and hyperarousal (e.g., difficulties sleeping and concentrating, exaggerated startle). In addition, the diagnosis of acute stress disorder requires the presence of dissociative symptoms (e.g., flashbacks). Acute stress disorder is diagnosable only within the first month after the trauma. For the diagnosis of PTSD, the symptoms must be present for at least 1 month. When the symptoms persist for 3 months or longer, it is designated as *chronic PTSD*.

Prospective longitudinal studies of a variety of traumatized populations indicate that high levels of PTSD symptoms along with general anxiety, depression, and disruption in social adjustment are common immediately after the traumatic event. Over the subsequent weeks and months, however, the majority of individuals experience a pattern of natural recovery in which their symptom levels decline faster during the period immediately after the assault and more slowly thereafter. This pattern of natural recovery has been observed for female rape victims, male and female victims of nonsexual assault, and victims of motor vehicle accidents. These same studies, however, also show that a significant minority of trauma victims do not display this pattern of natural recovery. Meeting criteria for acute stress disorder in the month after the trauma is a risk factor for chronic PTSD. In one prospective longitudinal study of motor vehicle accident survivors, 78 percent of people diagnosed with acute stress disorder in the month after the accident met full criteria for PTSD 6 months after the accident.

Prevention of PTSD and Treatment of Acute Stress Disorder In a 1995 study, recent rape victims meeting symptom criteria for PTSD were provided with four 90- to 120-minute sessions of brief CBT. The treatment included education about trauma reactions, breathing and relaxation training, imaginal exposure to the trauma memory and in vivo exposure to trauma reminders, thought stopping, and cognitive restructuring of trauma-related cognitions. Treatment was started 2 to 4 weeks after the assault and accelerated patients' recovery. Fewer women in the treatment condition (10 percent) met criteria for PTSD after the intervention than in a matched assessment-only control group (70 percent). However, there were no group differences at the follow-up assessment 5.5 months after the assault (11 percent and 22 percent for treatment and control groups, respectively).

In another study, five sessions of the same treatment package were provided to male and female survivors of motor vehicle and industrial accidents who met criteria for acute stress disorder. Significantly fewer patients who received the CBT met criteria for PTSD immediately after treatment (8 percent) and at 6-month follow-up (17 percent) than patients who received supportive counseling (83 percent and 67 percent at posttreatment and follow-up, respectively). The superiority of the CBT program over supportive counseling was again found in another study that further compared the full treatment program with a treatment program in which the stress management and cognitive restructuring components were removed. There were no differences in effectiveness between the full package and the package that focused primarily on the exposure components. A 2003 study replicated the efficacy of the full treatment package among individuals with mild brain injury and acute stress disorder.

Treatment of Chronic PTSD Several cognitive-behavioral approaches have demonstrated efficacy in the treatment of PTSD, including exposure therapy, stress inoculation training (a form of anxiety management training), cognitive therapy, and a more recently developed treatment called *eye movement desensitization and reprocessing*. In summary, studies have demonstrated the efficacy of all four of these treatments across a range of different trauma populations. However, exposure therapy has received the most systematic investigation and is the only treatment that has been compared with all of the other treatment options. Therefore, exposure therapy is the best standard for comparison.

Exposure therapy for chronic PTSD typically combines imaginal exposure to the memory of the trauma with in vivo exposure to safe, but otherwise avoided, people, places, things, and activities that remind the survivor of the trauma and trigger intense negative emotional reactions. However, some researchers have used exposure interventions limited to imaginal exposure. In addition, some programs have focused on exposure as the primary treatment component, and others have combined exposure with significant elements of anxiety management training, cognitive therapy, or both. The superiority of variations of exposure therapy over several control conditions has been demonstrated for waitlist, supportive counseling, and relaxation. Moreover, the efficacy of variations of exposure therapy has been demonstrated in a range of populations, including male Vietnam-era combat veterans, female victims of sexual and nonsexual assault, female survivors of abuse in childhood, female victims of domestic violence, male and female refugees, male and female survivors of motor vehicle accidents, and mixed-gender samples of a variety of traumatic events.

Two studies have compared exposure therapy with stress inoculation training and waitlist. Both treatments in both studies were superior to waitlist, but neither treatment was significantly better than the other. Two studies compared exposure therapy with cognitive therapy and either waitlist or relaxation control groups. In both studies, active treatments were superior to control conditions, but neither treatment was superior to the other on measures of PTSD severity. A third study used an assessment-only run-in phase before randomly assigning patients to either imaginal exposure or cognitive therapy. Both treatments were associated with significant improvement, but there were no differences between groups. Three studies have compared exposure therapy with eye movement desensitization and reprocessing and either waitlist or relaxation control groups. Two studies found both treatments were superior to waitlist, with no significant differences between groups. In a 2003 study, exposure therapy, but not eye movement desensitization and reprocessing, was found to be superior to relaxation. Two additional studies compared exposure therapy with eye movement desensitization and reprocessing but did not include an additional control group. One used a run-in phase before randomly assigning patients to exposure plus stress inoculation training or eye movement desensitization and reprocessing. Both treatments were associated with significant improvement. The only posttreatment difference between treatments was that eye movement desensitization and reprocessing produced greater improvement on reexperiencing symptoms. In a second study, patients were randomly assigned to either exposure therapy or eye movement desensitization and reprocessing. Both treatments were associated with improvement, but there were no differences between the treatments.

Three studies have compared exposure therapy (imaginal plus in vivo) alone with exposure therapy combined with either stress inoculation training or cognitive therapy and either waitlist or relaxation control groups. In all three studies, both active treatments were superior to controls, but there were no significant differences between treatments. In a fourth study, patients were randomly assigned to either exposure therapy alone or exposure therapy plus cognitive therapy. Both treatments were associated with improvement, but there were no differences between groups. The only study to find an effect of augmenting exposure therapy with additional interventions found that adding cognitive therapy to imaginal exposure was superior to imaginal exposure alone. The elimination of in vivo exposure from the protocols is important to note because there is independent evidence that in vivo exposure adds to treatment outcome over imaginal exposure alone.

Several CBTs have been evaluated for the treatment of PTSD, including exposure therapy, anxiety management training, cognitive therapy, combinations of the preceding components, and eye movement desensitization and reprocessing. All treatments have been found to be more effective than waitlist or some kind of minimal treatment control condition such as relaxation or supportive counseling. Direct comparisons between active treatments have generally found comparable results for the different interventions, and studies evaluating the effects of combining treatments have not found evidence for superiority of combined treatments over the individual components. One exception to this generalization is that imaginal exposure plus in vivo exposure or imaginal exposure plus cognitive restructuring appear to be more effective than imaginal exposure alone. Studies of treatment for acute traumatic stress reactions and the prevention of chronic PTSD have yielded a similar pattern of results. Specifically, exposure therapy, with and without training in anxiety management techniques, is superior to waitlist. However, combined treatment is not superior to exposure therapy alone.

Panic Disorder A panic attack is a sudden, intense rush of fear, anxiety, or impending doom that reaches a peak very quickly and is associated with at least 4 of 13 physical and cognitive symptoms (e.g., shortness of breath, dizziness, heart palpitations, fear of dying, fear of going crazy or losing control). Panic attacks may be cued by a specific situation, as when someone who is afraid of snakes encounters one, or they may be unexpected and perceived by the individual as coming out of the blue. For the diagnosis of panic disorder, a person must experience repeated unexpected panic attacks that result in persisting (at least 1 month) concerns about having additional attacks or worries about the physical or psychological consequences of the attack (e.g., having a heart attack, going crazy).

According to the cognitive-behavioral model of panic disorder, a consequence of experiencing unexpected panic attacks for some individuals is the development of a vicious cycle. The cycle begins with hypervigilance for somatic cues indicative of a panic attack which, if detected, are interpreted negatively (e.g., as an indicator of having a heart attack or going crazy). The negative interpretation of somatic sensations results in increased anxiety and arousal, spiraling into a panic attack. Agoraphobic avoidance may also develop as an attempt to avoid experiencing panic attacks in situations in which help may not be available. Cognitive-behavioral treatments based on this model contain several components: (1) psychoeducation regarding the cognitive-behavioral model of panic disorder, (2) training in techniques to reduce anxiety such as diaphragmatic breathing and progressive muscle relaxation, (3) cognitive restructuring to challenge catastrophic cognitions about the likelihood and significant of panic attacks, (4) interoceptive exposure to feared somatic sensations to reduce the "fear of fear," and (5) in vivo exposure to avoided cues, particularly in cases in which agoraphobic avoidance has developed.

The efficacy of CBT programs based on this model has been demonstrated in a series of four well-controlled studies. Between 41 and 87 percent of patients receiving CBT were panic free after treatment compared to 36 percent receiving relaxation only, 50 percent receiving alprazolam, 20 percent receiving imipramine (Tofranil), 13 to 36 percent receiving placebo, and 30 to 33 percent for waitlist. In the one study that combined imipramine with CBT, the combination treatment was found to be no more effective than CBT alone or combined with placebo. Several other research groups have investigated variations of CBT with similar results, replicating the superiority of CBT over relaxation, imipramine, supportive counseling, and waitlist.

Several studies have attempted to identify which components add to treatment outcome. Two studies found that adding cognitive restructuring to in vivo exposure substantially improved outcome, although other researchers have not been able to replicate this. Another study compared CBT consisting of education, cognitive restructuring, and interoceptive exposure with the same program plus relaxation and found that adding relaxation did not improve outcome. A 1997 study compared two treatments that incorporated cognitive restructuring and in vivo exposure. In addition, one included interoceptive exposure, and the other group substituted breathing retraining. Both treatments were associated with improvement, but the group receiving interoceptive exposure had superior outcome on panic frequency at posttreatment and follow-up assessments. In a study using a crossover design, patients were assigned to receive four sessions of cognitive therapy followed by four sessions of interoceptive exposure or the reverse. Both treatments were associated with improvement, and more improvement was observed for the first intervention administered, but there was no difference in the efficacy of the two components. Another study compared education, cognitive restructuring, and in vivo exposure with or without the inclusion of breathing retraining and found no reduction in treatment efficacy. Three variations of self-conducted exposure therapy—in vivo exposure, interoceptive exposure, and the combination of in vivo plus interoceptive exposure—were compared with a waitlist control in another study. All three treatments were superior to the waitlist condition, but there were no significant differences among treatment conditions.

Treatment for panic disorder has largely consisted of multicomponent packages consisting of education about the cognitive-behavioral model of panic along with one or more of the following: diaphragmatic breathing, relaxation, cognitive therapy, in vivo exposure, and interoceptive exposure. Dismantling studies have been partially successful in identifying the active ingredients, which seem to be cognitive restructuring combined with in vivo or interoceptive exposure. Indeed, the addition of interoceptive exposure may be particularly helpful. In a metaanalysis of 43 controlled studies of treatment for panic disorder, the largest mean effect size was obtained for the combination of cognitive therapy plus interoceptive exposure (.88), followed by CBT without interoceptive exposure (.68), CBT plus medication (.56), and medication alone (.47). Moreover, dropout rates from CBT were lower than dropout rates from medication conditions (alone or in combination with therapy), and a more recent trial suggested greater resistance to relapse for CBT in comparison to medication.

Social Anxiety Disorder Individuals with social anxiety disorder experience marked and persistent fear and avoidance of one or more social or performance situations. The person may fear doing or saying something embarrassing or fear manifesting the signs of anxiety (e.g., blushing, sweating, trembling) in such situations. Most individuals with social anxiety disorders fear and avoid multiple situations, falling within the generalized subtype of social anxiety disorder.

Treatments for social phobia have generally consisted of exposure therapy, cognitive therapy, the combination of exposure plus cognitive therapy, and social skills training. A metaanalysis summarized the outcome of 25 studies of treatments for social phobia, yielding 42 within-group effect sizes across four active treatments (exposure, cognitive therapy, exposure plus cognitive therapy, and social skills training) and two control conditions (waitlist and pill placebo). All active treatments were superior to waitlist, and there were no significant differences among active treatments. However, exposure plus cognitive therapy was the only condition found to be superior to placebo. The results of individual dismantling studies yield a similarly ambiguous picture. In the first such study, exposure alone was compared with exposure plus cognitive therapy. Although both groups improved, outcome was somewhat better for the combined treatment, particularly at the 3-month follow-up assessment. In a second study by the same group, the efficacy of each component alone, as well as the combination of the two, was compared with a waitlist control group. Compared to the waitlist control group, all three treatments were found to be effective in reducing social anxiety. Again, however, outcome was best among subjects who received the combined treatment. By contrast, another study did not find evidence for superiority of combined treatment over exposure alone. On some measures, patients who received exposure only had numerically better outcome than those who received the combined program.

One particular treatment program that has received considerable research attention is Richard Heimberg's cognitive-behavioral group therapy (CBGT), consisting of in-session exposure to feared social situations and cognitive restructuring and corresponding homework.

The group format not only serves to make treatment more affordable, it is believed that group treatment provides a great resource for conducting exposures, obtaining feedback, and learning vicariously. One study found CBGT to be superior to waitlist, and three studies have found CBGT to be superior to a group attention control condition, in which patients received education about social anxiety and nondirective group therapy. Heimberg and colleagues also compared CBGT with phenelzine (Nardil) and placebo. Although there were no differences between CBGT and phenelzine immediately after treatment, there were more instances of relapse for patients receiving phenelzine during the 6-month follow-up. Another study also compared CBGT with the same treatment components administered individually and found the two methods to be comparable. However, using a somewhat different CBT program with a strong emphasis on eliminating safety behaviors and shifting attention outward from the self, one study found individually administered treatment to be superior to group treatment.

Generalized Anxiety Disorder The key feature of generalized anxiety disorder is the presence of excessive worry accompanied by anxiety and symptoms of physiological arousal. The content of the worry must encompass a range of domains (e.g., school or work performance, personal finances) and not be limited to features of another specific disorder, such as worrying about having a panic attack (as in panic disorder). The worry, anxiety, and arousal symptoms must be present more days than not over a minimum period of 6 months. Pathological worry, as occurs in generalized anxiety disorder, is distinguished from normal worry in that the frequency, intensity, and duration of the worry in addition to the attendant anxiety and arousal greatly exceed the actual probability or impact of the feared event and that the worry is experienced as difficult to control.

CBT packages for generalized anxiety disorder have typically included training in relaxation and cognitive therapy. In addition, some packages have included some form of exposure therapy to the worry content. Relaxation alone, cognitive therapy alone, and their combination (with and without the further addition of exposure) have all been found to be effective in reducing worry and anxiety compared to waitlist. Four studies have made a direct comparison between cognitive therapy and relaxation, with no differences between groups immediately after treatment; however, one study found cognitive therapy to be superior to relaxation at follow-up. In a recent study, cognitive therapy alone was compared to relaxation plus self-control desensitization—a form of exposure in which the patient imagines coping with the feared situation while simultaneously applying coping strategies such as relaxation—and their combination. All three treatments were associated with significant improvement, but there were no differences among treatments.

FUTURE DIRECTIONS

The above literature review demonstrates the efficacy of CBT programs in the treatment of anxiety across the full range of anxiety disorders. Exposure in vivo to feared but otherwise safe stimuli and imaginal exposure to unwanted and upsetting thoughts are essential components to most CBT programs for anxiety. The addition of explicit response prevention is necessary for optimal outcome in the treatment of OCD, and the addition of interoceptive exposure appears to make a significant contribution to the treatment of panic disorder. Exposure alone or exposure with response prevention has been shown to be helpful as a stand-alone treatment for all of the anxiety disorders, except perhaps for generalized anxiety disorder, for which relaxation training may be the primary component. Anxiety management training and cognitive therapy have also been shown to be effective in the treatment of PTSD. Cognitive therapy that includes behavioral experiments, which inherently involves at least limited in vivo exposure, may also be an effective treatment for OCD.

Several researchers have demonstrated the efficacy of multicomponent CBT packages that include components of anxiety management, cognitive therapy, and exposure. To date, however, few of the relevant dismantling studies have shown significantly improved outcome for these combined treatments as compared to the individual components. This may, to some extent, reflect low statistical power to detect the additive effects of treatments that individually are effective. Consistent with this hypothesis, metaanalyses have sometimes detected evidence for the superiority of combined treatments that were not as evident in individual studies.

Despite the success of CBT in the treatment of anxiety disorders, it is important to acknowledge two limitations. First, not everyone is responsive to treatment, and many people judged to have responded to treatment continue to experience significant residual symptoms. Thus, one avenue for future research is to identify ways to enhance existing treatments or to develop new treatments that are more effective. As noted above, however, attempts thus far to augment one psychological component with another treatment have not generally been very successful at significantly enhancing treatment outcome.

Another approach to potentially improving outcome is to combine psychotherapy with pharmacotherapy. This section did not provide coverage of the many studies that have investigated the efficacy of combining medication and CBT. Foa and colleagues reviewed all of the studies that met basic methodological standards (e.g., clearly established diagnosis, reliable and valid assessment measures, randomization) and provided an unambiguous test of the hypothesis that combined treatment would be superior monotherapy. They concluded that, at present, there is no clear evidence that adding medication to CBT improves treatment outcome for OCD, social anxiety disorder, or generalized anxiety disorder. Although combined treatment appeared to have slightly better immediate outcome for panic disorder, it was associated with greater relapse on discontinuation of treatment. There are no published studies on the effect of adding medication to CBT in the treatment of acute stress disorder or PTSD. Most studies of combined treatments, whether combining two forms of CBT or combining CBT with medication, have implemented both treatments simultaneously. This strategy may actually serve to minimize the ability to detect the effects of combined treatments when the individual treatments are generally effective. An alternative strategy would be to use an augmentation strategy, in which partial responders to one active treatment are then randomized to continue with the original treatment alone or to add a second treatment.

The second limitation of CBT is its relative inaccessibility to people who do not live in large cities or near a university-based medical school or graduate program in clinical psychology. Greater research is needed to determine the factors that limit the use of CBT among community-based clinicians and the development of models for the dissemination of these treatments to make them more widely available.

SUGGESTED CROSS-REFERENCES

Other psychotherapies are of use in dealing with anxiety disorders. The reader is referred to Section 30.4 on group psychotherapy and combined individual and group therapy; Section 30.7 on interpersonal therapy; Section 30.1 on psychoanalysis and psychoanalytic psychotherapy; Section 30.9 on intensive short-term psychotherapy; and Section 30.12 on combined psychotherapy and psychopharmacology.

References

Abramowitz JS, Foa EB, Franklin ME: Exposure and ritual prevention for obsessive-compulsive disorder: Effects of intensive versus twice-weekly sessions. *J Consult Clin Psychol.* 2003;72:394–398.

Abramowitz JS, Franklin ME, Schwartz SA, Furr JM: Symptom presentation and outcome of cognitive-behavioral therapy for obsessive-compulsive disorder. *J Consult Clin Psychol.* 2003;72:1049–1057.

Angst J, Vollrath M, Merikangas KR, Ernst C. Comorbidity of anxiety and depression in the Zurich Cohort Study of Young Adults. In: Maser JD, Clonginger RC, eds. *Comorbidity of Mood and Anxiety Disorders.* Washington, DC: American Psychiatric Press; 1990:123–137.

*Bandura A. *Principles of Behavior Modification.* New York: Holt, Rinehart & Winston; 1969.

Barlow DH. *Anxiety and Its Disorders: The Nature and Treatment of Anxiety and Panic.* 2nd ed. New York: Guilford; 2002.

*Beck AT. *Cognitive Therapy and the Emotional Disorders.* New York: International University Press; 1976.

Chambless DL, Baker MJ, Baucom DH, Beutler LE, Calhoun KS, Crits-Christoph P, Daiuto A, DeRubeis R, Deweiler J, Haaga DF, Johnson SB, McCurry S, Mueser KT, Pope KS, Sanderson WC, Shoham V, Stickle T, Williams DA, Woody SR: Update on empirically validated therapies II. *Clin Psychol.* 1998;51:3–16.

Chaplin EW, Levine BA: The effects of total exposure duration and interrupted versus continuous exposure in flooding therapy. *Behav Ther.* 1981;12:360–368.

Clark DM, Ehlers A, McManus F, Hackmann A, Fennell M, Campbell H, Flower T, Davenport C, Louis B: Cognitive therapy versus fluoxetine in generalized social phobia: A randomized placebo-controlled trial. *J Consult Clin Psychol.* 2003;72:1058–1067.

Craske MG, DeCola JP, Sachs AD, Pontillo DC: Panic control treatment for agoraphobia. *J Anxiety Disord.* 2003;17:321–333.

Craske MG, Street LL, Jayaraman J, Barlow DH: Attention versus distraction during in vivo exposure: Snake and spider phobias. *J Anxiety Disord.* 1991;5:199–211.

Dugas MJ, Ladouceur R, Leger E, Freeston MH, Langolis F, Provencher MD, Boisvert J: Group cognitive-behavioral therapy for generalized anxiety disorder: Treatment outcome and long-term follow-up. *J Consult Clin Psychol.* 2003;72:821–825.

Emmelkamp PMG, Wessels H: Flooding in imagination vs. flooding in vivo: A comparison with agoraphobics. *Behav Res Ther.* 1975;13:7–15.

Foa EB, Franklin ME, Moser J: Context in clinic: How well do cognitive-behavioral therapies and medication work in combination? *Biol Psychiatry.* 2002;52:987–997.

*Foa EB, Kozak MJ: Emotional processing of fear: Exposure to corrective information. *Psychol Bull.* 1986;99:20–35.

Foa EB, Kozak MJ. Psychological treatment for obsessive compulsive disorder. In: Mavissakalian MR, Prien RP, eds. *Long-Term Treatments of Anxiety Disorders.* Washington, DC: American Psychiatric Press; 1996:285–309.

Foa EB, Riggs DS, Massie ED, Yarczower M: The impact of fear activation and anger on the efficacy of exposure treatment for posttraumatic stress disorder. *Behav Ther.* 1995;26:487–499.

Gelder MG, Banchcroft JHJ, Gath DH, Johnston DW, Matthews AM, Shaw PM: Specific and nonspecific factors in behavior therapy. *Br J Psychiatry.* 1973;123:309–319.

Grayson JB, Foa EB, Steketee G: Habituation during exposure treatment: Distraction versus attention focusing. *Behav Res Ther.* 1982;20:323–328.

Harvey AG, Bryant RA, Tarrier N: Cognitive-behavior therapy for posttraumatic stress disorder. *Clin Psychiatr Rev.* 2003;23:501–522.

Heimberg RG, Becker RE. *Cognitive-Behavioral Group Therapy for Social Phobia: Basic Mechanisms and Clinical Strategies.* New York: Guilford Press; 2002.

Heimberg RG, Turk CL, Mennin DS. *Generalized Anxiety Disorder: Advances in Research and Practice.* New York: Guilford; 2004.

Jaycox LH, Foa EB, Morral AR: Influence of emotional engagement and habituation on exposure therapy for PTSD. *J Consult Clin Psychol.* 1998;66:185–192.

Kenardy JA, Dow MGT, Johnston DW, Newman MG, Thomson A, Taylor CB: A comparison of delivery methods of cognitive-behavioral therapy for panic disorder: An international multicenter trial. *J Consult Clin Psychol.* 2003;71:1068–1075.

Lang PJ: A bio-informational theory of emotional imagery. *Psychophysiology.* 1979;16:495–512.

Lang PJ, Lazovik AD: Experimental desensitization of a phobia. *J Abnorm Soc Psychol.* 1963;66:519–525.

McGlynn FD, Mealiea WL, Landau DL: The current status of systematic desensitization. *Clin Psychol Rev.* 1981;1:149–179.

McGlynn FD, Rose MP, Jacobson N: Effects of control and of attentional instructions on arousal and fear during exposure to phobia-cue stimuli. *J Anxiety Disord.* 1995;9:451–461.

Meichenbaum D. *Cognitive Behavior Modification.* Morristown, NJ: General Learning Press; 1974.

Ost LG, Ferebee I, Furmark T: One-session group therapy of spider phobia: Direct versus indirect treatments. *Behav Res Ther.* 1997;8:721–732.

Paul GL. Outcome of systematic desensitization II: Controlled investigations of individual treatment, technique variations, and current status. In Franks CM, ed. *Behavior Therapy: Appraisal and Status.* New York: McGraw-Hill; 1969:105–159.

Penfold K, Page AC: The effect of distraction on within-session anxiety reduction during brief in vivo exposure for mild blood-injection fears. *Behav Ther.* 1999;30:607–621.

Pitman RK, Orr SP, Altman B, Longpre RE, Poire RE, Macklin ML, Michaels MJ, Steketee GS: Emotional processing and outcome of imaginal flooding therapy in Vietnam veterans with chronic posttraumatic stress disorder. *Compr Psychiatry.* 1996;37:409–418.

Rabavilas AD, Boulougouris JC, Stefanis C: Duration of flooding sessions in the treatment of obsessive-compulsive patients. *Behav Res Ther.* 1976;14:349–355.

Shapiro F. *Eye Movement Desensitization and Reprocessing: Basic Principles, Protocols, and Procedures.* 2nd ed. New York: Guilford; 2001.

*Stangier U, Heidenreich T, Peitz M, Lauterbach W, Clark DM: Cognitive therapy for social phobia: Individual versus group treatment. *Behav Res Ther.* 2003;41:991–1007.

Wilhelm FH, Troth WT: Acute and delayed effects of alprazolam on flight phobics during exposure. *Behav Res Ther.* 1997;35:831–841.

Williams SL. Therapeutic changes in phobic behavior are mediated by changes in perceived self-efficacy. In: Rapee RM, ed. *Current Controversies in the Anxiety Disorders.* New York: Guilford; 1996:344–368.

*Wolpe J. *Psychotherapy by Reciprocal Inhibition.* Stanford, CA: Stanford University Press; 1958.

15

Somatoform Disorders

MICHAEL A. HOLLIFIELD, M.D.

There are seven somatoform disorders in the revised fourth edition of the *Diagnostic and Statistical Manual of Mental Disorders* (DSM-IV-TR), two of which are subsyndromal or nonspecific disorders (Table 15–1). This nosology overlaps with the tenth edition of the *International Statistical Classification of Diseases and Related Health Problems* (ICD-10) classification (Table 15–2), yet there are important differences that are apparent from the criteria. The DSM-IV-TR has conversion disorder and body dysmorphic disorder in its classification, whereas the ICD-10 does not, but instead specifies somatoform autonomic dysfunction and other somatoform disorders. In the ICD-10, conversion is classified as a dissociative disorder, and somatoform autonomic dysfunction is similar to the symptoms associated with anxiety and depressive disorders in the DSM-IV-TR. In the ICD-10, body dysmorphic disorder is subsumed under hypochondriacal disorder. Nonetheless, the two classification systems are more similar than different in how they represent the core phenomenology and the history that links the somatoform disorders together. Somatization disorder is the prototype and has the best evidence for being a discrete, impairing, and stable illness over time. The other somatoform disorders are linked together by certain core features, yet also have features that call into question their fit in this category of illness. For example, there is support for classifying conversion disorder as a dissociative disorder and subsets of hypochondriacs and body dysmorphics as monosymptomatic delusional disorders or anxiety disorders. The history and phenomenology of the specific somatoform disorders have much in common.

BRIEF HISTORY

Somatoform means taking the form of (or in) soma, which implies that these illnesses are nonsomatic. *Somatoform* is thus a misnomer and reflects the historical and current lack of knowledge about the physiology of these disorders. With respect to the epistemological problems of mind–body dualism, the general category of somatoform disorders is better thought of as *unexplained symptoms*, a class of illnesses that have changed in their presumed etiology over time. The earliest notions about unexplained symptoms were focused on disturbances of organs and body systems. Hippocrates and the Greeks believed that abdominal organs were the source of emotional disorders. The word *hypochondrium*, being the part of the body just caudal to the rib cage, arose from this era. This body area was to be distinguished from the *praecordia*, which was the chest over the heart. The Greek view, prominent well into the second millennium, held that the hypochondrium pertained to digestive symptoms and emotional disturbances and that the praecordia was the seat of melancholia, which had little connection to depressive illness as it is now known. Before the Renaissance, *hysteria* was a disorder of the uterus, which could wander through the body and even cause suffocation by pressing on the organs of respiration. Treatment included physical manipulation of the uterus and applications of ointments to vulvar tissues.

The 1600s brought increased understanding of the central nervous system (CNS) and ideas that unexplained symptoms were a product of the brain. The father of neurology, Thomas Willis (1621 to 1675), regarded hysteria in women and hypochondriasis in men as nervous disorders of the brain and advocated hitting affected patients with a stick to the head as one treatment. Thomas Sydenham (1624 to 1689) may have had the most impact on the shift to consider hysteria and hypochondriasis as psychological diseases of the mind and not the body. However, he did recommend treatments integrating physical and psychological modalities, consisting of regular exercise, psychological strengthening, and purification of the blood, as well as tending to the overall welfare of the patient. The 1700s saw continued sophistication of terms to describe unexplained symptoms as nervous disorders. George Cheyne (1671 to 1743) coined the term *English malady*, and many great writings about this disorder were produced. Debate raged about the mechanism of hypochondriasis in men and hysteria in women, which continued to be considered nervous disorders of the brain or mind, or both.

William Cullen (1712 to 1790) is widely quoted as having coined the term *neurosis*, and he wrote that all disorders considered to be related to hypochondriasis and hysteria were of just one primary, idiopathic species, namely *hypochondriasis melancholia*. Hysteria, he held, was a separate disorder that had been confused with hypochondriasis. Later, in the 1800s, hypochondriasis was considered to be a form of insanity, which could begin in the abdominal organs but would progress to cause a general inflammation of all organs, including the brain. Postmortem cases suggested that hypochondriasis might be associated with cortical plaques and softening of the brain. However, when pathological studies in the 19th century failed to demonstrate anatomical abnormalities of the body or brain, hypochondriasis and hysteria began to be considered subtle or *functional*. Jean-Martin Charcot and his pupils were certain that hysteria in women and hypochondriasis in men were disorders of the nervous system and it centers throughout the body, but they were not sure of its nature or location. Physical therapies, such as manipulation of the hypochondrium or pressure on the ovaries, paralleled this line of thinking. Other writers began to consider this set of disorders as problems of sensation, in which the combined mind and body had some function in overfeeling or oversensing.

The early 20th century brought about a paradoxical shift in which unexplained physical symptoms were thought of as primarily psychological. It was paradoxical because it was the students of Charcot, including Sigmund Freud, who were the impetus for this shift. They were certain that these were disorders of the CNS and were

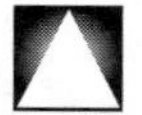

Table 15–1
DSM-IV-TR Somatoform Disorders Diagnostic Criteria

300.81 Somatization disorder

A. A history of many physical complaints beginning before 30 years of age that occur over a period of several years and result in treatment being sought or significant impairment in social, occupational, or other important areas of functioning.

B. Each of the following criteria must have been met, with individual symptoms occurring at any time during the course of the disturbance:

(1) *Four pain symptoms.* A history of pain related to at least four different sites or functions (e.g., head, abdomen, back, joints, extremities, chest, rectum, during menstruation, during sexual intercourse, or during urination).

(2) *Two gastrointestinal symptoms.* A history of at least two gastrointestinal symptoms other than pain (e.g., nausea, bloating, vomiting other than during pregnancy, diarrhea, or intolerance of several different foods).

(3) *One sexual symptom.* A history of at least one sexual or reproductive symptom other than pain (e.g., sexual indifference, erectile or ejaculatory dysfunction, irregular menses, excessive menstrual bleeding, or vomiting throughout pregnancy).

(4) *One pseudoneurological symptom.* A history of at least one symptom or deficit suggesting a neurological condition not limited to pain (conversion symptoms, such as impaired coordination or balance, paralysis or localized weakness, difficulty swallowing or lump in throat, aphonia, urinary retention, hallucinations, loss of touch or pain sensation, double vision, blindness, deafness, and seizures; dissociative symptoms, such as amnesia; or loss of consciousness other than fainting).

C. Either (1) or (2):

(1) After appropriate investigation, each of the symptoms in Criterion B cannot be fully explained by a known general medical condition or the direct effects of a substance (e.g., a drug of abuse, a medication).

(2) When there is a related general medical condition, the physical complaints or resulting social or occupational impairment are in excess of what would be expected from the history, physical examination, or laboratory findings.

D. The symptoms are not intentionally produced or feigned (as in factitious disorder or malingering).

300.81 Undifferentiated somatoform disorder

A. One or more physical complaints (e.g., fatigue, loss of appetite, or gastrointestinal or urinary complaints).

B. Either (1) or (2):

(1) After appropriate investigation, the symptoms cannot be fully explained by a known general medical condition or the direct effects of a substance (e.g., a drug of abuse or a medication).

(2) When there is a related general medical condition, the physical complaints or resulting social or occupational impairment is in excess of what would be expected from the history, physical examination, or laboratory findings.

C. The symptoms cause clinically significant distress or impairment in social, occupational, or other important areas of functioning.

D. The duration of the disturbance is at least 6 months.

E. The disturbance is not better accounted for by another mental disorder (e.g., another somatoform disorder, sexual dysfunction, mood disorder, anxiety disorder, sleep disorder, or psychotic disorder).

F. The symptom is not intentionally produced or feigned (as in factitious disorder or malingering).

300.11 Conversion disorder

A. One or more symptoms or deficits affecting voluntary motor or sensory function that suggest a neurological or other general medical condition.

B. Psychological factors are judged to be associated with the symptom or deficit, because the initiation or exacerbation of the symptom or deficit is preceded by conflicts or other stressors.

C. The symptom or deficit is not intentionally produced or feigned (as in factitious disorder or malingering).

D. The symptom or deficit cannot, after appropriate investigation, be fully explained by a general medical condition or by the direct effects of a substance, or as a culturally sanctioned behavior or experience.

E. The symptom or deficit causes clinically significant distress or impairment in social, occupational, or other important areas of functioning or warrants medical evaluation.

F. The symptom or deficit is not limited to pain or sexual dysfunction, does not occur exclusively during the course of somatization disorder, and is not better accounted for by another mental disorder.

Specify the type of symptom or deficit:

With motor symptom or deficit

With sensory symptom or deficit

With seizures or convulsions

With mixed presentation

Pain disorder

A. Pain in one or more anatomical sites is the predominant focus of the clinical presentation and is of sufficient severity to warrant clinical attention.

B. The pain causes clinically significant distress or impairment in social, occupational, or other important areas of functioning.

C. Psychological factors are judged to have an important role in the onset, severity, exacerbation, or maintenance of the pain.

D. The symptom or deficit is not intentionally produced or feigned (as in factitious disorder or malingering).

E. The pain is not better accounted for by a mood, anxiety, or psychotic disorder and does not meet criteria for dyspareunia.

Code as follows:

307.80 Pain disorder associated with psychological factors: Psychological factors are judged to have the major role in the onset, severity, exacerbation, or maintenance of the pain. (If a general medical condition is present, it does not have a major role in the onset, severity, exacerbation, or maintenance of the pain.) This type of pain disorder is not diagnosed if criteria are also met for somatization disorder.

Specify if:

Acute: duration of less than 6 months

Chronic: duration of 6 months or longer

307.89 Pain disorder associated with both psychological factors and a general medical condition: Both psychological factors and a general medical condition are judged to have important roles in the onset, severity, exacerbation, or maintenance of the pain. The associated general medical condition or anatomical site of the pain (see the following discussion) is coded on Axis III.

Specify if:

Acute: duration of less than 6 months

Chronic: duration of 6 months or longer

Note: The following is not considered to be a mental disorder and is included here to facilitate differential diagnosis.

Pain disorder associated with a general medical condition: A general medical condition has a major role in the onset, severity, exacerbation, or maintenance of the pain. (If psychological factors are present, they are not judged to have a major role in the onset, severity, exacerbation, or maintenance of the pain.) The diagnostic code for the pain is selected based on the associated general medical condition if one has been established or on the anatomical location of the pain if the underlying general medical condition is not yet clearly established—for example, low back (724.2), sciatic (724.3), pelvic (625.9), headache (784.0), facial (784.0), chest (786.50), joint (719.4), bone (733.90), abdominal (789.0), breast (611.71), renal (788.0), ear (388.70), eye (379.91), throat (784.1), tooth (525.9), and urinary (788.0).

(*continued*)

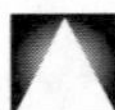

Table 15–1 *(continued)*

300.7 Hypochondriasis

A. Preoccupation with fears of having, or the idea that one has, a serious disease based on the person's misinterpretation of bodily symptoms.

B. The preoccupation persists despite appropriate medical evaluation and reassurance.

C. The belief in Criterion A is not of delusional intensity (as in delusional disorder, somatic type) and is not restricted to a circumscribed concern about appearance (as in body dysmorphic disorder).

D. The preoccupation causes clinically significant distress or impairment in social, occupational, or other important areas of functioning.

E. The duration of the disturbance is at least 6 months.

F. The preoccupation is not better accounted for by generalized anxiety disorder, obsessive-compulsive disorder, panic disorder, a major depressive episode, separation anxiety, or another somatoform disorder.

Specify if:

With poor insight: if, for most of the time during the current episode, the person does not recognize that the concern about having a serious illness is excessive or unreasonable

300.7 Body dysmorphic disorder

A. Preoccupation with an imagined defect in appearance. If a slight physical anomaly is present, the person's concern is markedly excessive.

B. The preoccupation causes clinically significant distress or impairment in social, occupational, or other important areas of functioning.

C. The preoccupation is not better accounted for by another mental disorder (e.g., dissatisfaction with body shape and size in anorexia nervosa).

300.81 Somatoform disorder, not otherwise specified

This category includes disorders with somatoform symptoms that do not meet the criteria for any specific somatoform disorder. Examples include

1. Pseudocyesis: a false belief of being pregnant that is associated with objective signs of pregnancy, which may include abdominal enlargement (although the umbilicus does not become everted), reduced menstrual flow, amenorrhea, subjective sensation of fetal movement, nausea, breast engorgement and secretions, and labor pains at the expected date of delivery. Endocrine changes may be present, but the syndrome cannot be explained by a general medical condition that causes endocrine changes (e.g., a hormone-secreting tumor).
2. A disorder involving nonpsychotic hypochondriacal symptoms of less than 6 months' duration.
3. A disorder involving unexplained physical complaints (e.g., fatigue or body weakness) of less than 6 months' duration that are not due to another mental disorder.

Adapted from American Psychiatric Association. *Diagnostic and Statistical Manual of Mental Disorders.* 4th ed. Text rev. Washington, DC: American Psychiatric Publishing; 2000.

due to repressed physical energy caused by psychological conflict. The paradoxical shift occurred because of the lack of good physical treatments and the development of psychological treatments, including psychoanalysis, which demonstrated treatment success. Once the province of general medicine and neurology, unexplained medical symptoms now became entrenched in the burgeoning field of psychiatry. With psychiatry's movement away from the rest of somatic medicine in the early 20th century, so too moved the disorders of unexplained symptoms.

Formal psychiatric classification divided unexplained physical symptoms in the second edition of the DSM (DSM-II) (1968) into the categories *neuroses*, *psychophysiologic disorders* (ten types), and *special symptoms*. Neuroses were further divided into *hysterical neuroses* (divided into conversion and dissociative types), *neurasthenia*, *depersonalization*, *hypochondriasis*, and *other neuroses*. There was also a *hysterical personality disorder*. The third edition of the DSM (DSM-III) (1980) made the shift to separating the *disorders with physical symptoms* (subtyped *organic mental disorders* and *somatoform disorders*) from the *dissociative disorders*, a new category. Hysterical personality disorder was replaced with *histrionic personality disorder*. Conversion disorder was classified with somatization, psychogenic pain, and hypochondriasis under somatoform disorders.

There remains a fair debate about the relevance of the category of somatoform disorders, the way in which diagnoses are constructed, and the usefulness of specific diagnostic entities. Somatoform disorders overlap with anxiety, affective, dissociative, and personality disorders. Somatic symptoms are more common manifestations of anxiety, depression, and trauma syndromes throughout the world than are psychological symptoms. Inclusion of a broader range of international and cultural conceptualization is needed. However, there is not much debate about the importance of this set of disorders to psychiatry and the rest of medicine. Unexplained physical symptoms associated with high distress and high health care use are a common problem for clinical medicine. More than one-half of the most common symptoms in primary care are not adequately explained by a current biomedical paradigm.

GENERAL PHENOMENOLOGY

Embodiment Expressing general distress bodily is common worldwide. Psychologizing of general distress seems to be a variant born of Western intellectual commitments to mind–body dualism. Many body systems are used to determine the source of distress and the requisite action to counter it. Sensory and motor systems are activated during threat, appraisal, and resolution of threat. During normal conditions, a person accurately appraises the source of threat and the behavior needed to counter it, and successful resolution quiets systems back to normal. Thus, although sensory systems are always active, they are not consciously felt if there is an appraisal of no threat.

Various elements of human psychobiology create conditions in which a person perceives ongoing threats that are felt in the body. Temperament may influence the degree to which a child is focused on sensory systems as a cue for danger. For example, young children of parents with panic disorder are more likely than children of parents without panic disorder to inhibit their exploring behavior in novel situations. Second, there is strong evidence that young children learn how to express their distress. Many investigators describe case reports and case studies in which a child comes to medical care talking about pain in one or another body system that is similar to how a parent expresses his or her distress. Third, psychiatric disorders are associated with an increase in bodily sensation, and successful treatment of the disorder, such as an anxiety or affective illness, can markedly reduce the somatic preoccupation and distress. Fourth, ongoing life stressors coupled with poor coping skills lead to gener-

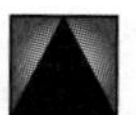

Table 15–2
ICD-10 Somatoform Disorders Diagnostic Criteria

F45.0 Somatization disorder

A. There must be a history of at least 2 years' complaints of multiple and variable physical symptoms that cannot be explained by any detectable physical disorders. (Any physical disorders that are known to be present do not explain the severity, extent, variety, and persistence of the physical complaints, or the associated social disability.) If some symptoms clearly due to autonomic arousal are present, they are not a major feature of the disorder in that they are not particularly persistent or distressing.

B. Preoccupation with the symptoms causes persistent distress and leads the patient to seek repeated (three or more) consultations or sets of investigations with primary care or specialist doctors. In the absence of medical services within the financial or physical reach of the patient, there must be persistent self-medication or multiple consultations with local healers.

C. There is persistent refusal to accept medical reassurance that there is no adequate physical cause for the physical symptoms. (Short-term acceptance of such reassurance, i.e., for a few weeks during or immediately after investigations, does not exclude this diagnosis.)

D. There must be a total of six or more symptoms from the following list, with symptoms occurring in at least two separate groups:

Gastrointestinal symptoms

(1) Abdominal pain
(2) Nausea
(3) Feeling bloated or full of gas
(4) Bad taste in mouth or excessively coated tongue
(5) Complaints of vomiting or regurgitation of food
(6) Complaints of frequent and loose bowel motions or discharge of fluids from anus

Cardiovascular symptoms

(7) Breathlessness without exertion
(8) Chest pains

Genitourinary symptoms

(9) Dysuria or complaints of frequency of micturition
(10) Unpleasant sensations in or around the genitals
(11) Complaints of unusual or copious vaginal discharge

Skin and pain symptoms

(12) Blotchiness or discoloration of the skin
(13) Pain in the limbs, extremities, or joints
(14) Unpleasant numbness or tingling sensations

E. *Most commonly used exclusion clause.* Symptoms do not occur only during any of the schizophrenic or related disorders (F20 through F29), any of the mood (affective) disorders (F30 through F39), or panic disorder (F41.0).

F45.1 Undifferentiated somatoform disorder

A. Criteria A, C, and E for somatization disorder (F45.0) are met, except that the duration of the disorder is at least 6 months.

B. One or both of Criteria B and D for somatization disorder (F45.0) are incompletely fulfilled.

F45.2 Hypochondriacal disorder

A. Either of the following must be present:

(1) A persistent belief, of at least 6 months' duration, of the presence of a maximum of two serious physical diseases (of which at least one must be specifically named by the patient).
(2) A persistent preoccupation with a presumed deformity or disfigurement (body dysmorphic disorder).

B. Preoccupation with the belief and the symptoms causes persistent distress or interference with personal functioning in daily living and leads the patient to seek medical treatment or investigations (or equivalent help from local healers).

C. There is persistent refusal to accept medical reassurance that there is no physical cause for the symptoms or physical abnormality. (Short-term acceptance of such reassurance, i.e., for a few weeks during or immediately after investigations does not exclude this diagnosis.)

D. *Most commonly used exclusion clause.* The symptoms do not occur only during any of the schizophrenic and related disorders (F20 through F29, particularly F22) or any of the mood (affective) disorders (F30 through F39).

F45.3 Somatoform autonomic dysfunction

A. There must be symptoms of autonomic arousal that are attributed by the patient to a physical disorder of one or more of the following systems or organs:

(1) Heart and cardiovascular system
(2) Upper gastrointestinal tract (esophagus and stomach)
(3) Lower gastrointestinal tract
(4) Respiratory system
(5) Genitourinary system

B. Two or more of the following autonomic symptoms must be present:

(1) Palpitations
(2) Sweating (hot or cold)
(3) Dry mouth
(4) Flushing or blushing
(5) Epigastric discomfort, "butterflies," or churning in the stomach

C. One or more of the following symptoms must be present:

(1) Chest pains or discomfort in and around the precordium
(2) Dyspnea or hyperventilation
(3) Excessive tiredness on mild exertion
(4) Aerophagy, hiccough, or burning sensations in chest or epigastrium
(5) Reported frequent bowel movements
(6) Increased frequency of micturition or dysuria
(7) Feeling of being bloated, distended, or heavy

D. There is no evidence of a disturbance of structure or function in the organs or systems about which the patient is concerned.

E. *Most commonly used exclusion clause.* These symptoms do not occur only in the presence of phobic disorders (F40.0 through F40.3) or panic disorder (F41.0).

A fifth character is to be used to classify the individual disorders in this group, indicating the organ or system regarded by the patient as the origin of the symptoms:

F45.30 Heart and cardiovascular system
Includes: cardiac neurosis, neurocirculatory asthenia, and Da Costa's syndrome.

F45.31 Upper gastrointestinal tract
Includes: psychogenic aerophagy, hiccough, and gastric neurosis.

F45.32 Lower gastrointestinal tract
Includes: psychogenic irritable bowel syndrome, psychogenic diarrhea, and gas syndrome.

F45.33 Respiratory system
Includes: hyperventilation.

F45.34 Genitourinary system
Includes: psychogenic increase of frequency of micturition and dysuria.

F45.38 Other organ or system

F45.4 Persistent somatoform pain disorder

A. There is persistent severe and distressing pain (for at least 6 months, and continuously on most days), in any part of the body that cannot be explained adequately by evidence of a physiological process or a physical disorder and that is consistently the main focus of the patient's attention.

(*continued*)

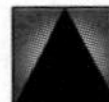

Table 15–2 *(continued)*

B. *Most commonly used exclusion clause.* This disorder does not occur in the presence of schizophrenia or related disorders (F20 through F29), or only during any of the mood (affective) disorders (F30 through F39), somatization disorder (F45.0), undifferentiated somatoform disorder (F45.1), or hypochondriacal disorder (F45.2).

F45.8 Other somatoform disorders

In these disorders, the presenting complaints are not mediated through the autonomic nervous system and are limited to specific systems or parts of the body, such as the skin. This is in contrast to the multiple and often changing complaints of the origin of symptoms and distress found in somatization disorder (F45.0) and undifferentiated somatoform disorder (F45.1). Tissue damage is not involved.

Any other disorders of sensation not due to physical disorders, which are closely associated in time with stressful events or problems or which result in significantly increased attention for the patient, personal or medical, should also be classified here.

F45.9 Somatoform disorder, unspecified

Adapted from *ICD-10 Classification of Mental and Behavioural Disorders.* Geneva: World Health Organization; 1993:105–109.

alization across multiple situations of the general stress response and the flight, fight, or freeze response. This generalizing phenomenon is strongly conditioned by the intermittent and random nature of the life stressors and is mitigated by resolution of the fear response by adequate coping. Fifth, early-life adverse experiences may cause changes in psychobiology, such as persistent hyperadrenalism and hyper- or hypocortisolism, which have an impact on sensory perception and reflex behavior. There is good evidence in animal and human research indicating that adverse experiences, such as maternal separation, isolation, and deprivation, and overt forms of trauma influence the development and functioning of central and peripheral nervous system components and the immune system and are associated with worse health perception and worse health by objective measures. The phenomenon of reexperiencing in posttraumatic stress disorder (PTSD) is perhaps the best example of how trauma becomes embodied. It has been known since the late 1980s that there is a heightened autonomic response to general threat cues in people with PTSD and that this response is incrementally larger to greater specificity of trauma cue. Recently, investigators have determined that the sensory cortex associated with specific body areas is stimulated as seen on positron emission tomography (PET) in response to a cue of a past trauma to that body area. The integration of memory of past events with perception of current events occurs in sensory pathways just as it does in cognitive pathways. These memories are designed to be protective but, as in all organic systems, can become pathological and maladaptive. In any case, as past events are learned and stored in brain, they are also learned and stored in those sensory circuits that extend from brain that are called *body*.

Perception and Cognition Many studies have demonstrated that certain perceptual and cognitive styles are associated with somatoform disorders. People with somatization and hypochondriasis have a lower threshold for perceiving certain physiological processes and think that minor physical complaints may be catastrophic physical events. They often have high negative self-appraisal and self-concepts of being weak and unable to tolerate stress. People with somatoform disorders generally are more accurate in distinguishing between smaller increments of sensory stimuli than people without these disorders, although there are a few mitigating studies about this. People with these disorders tend to overreport symptoms during minor illnesses and during medical tests, such as pulmonary function tests, and notice symptoms more often when they read about them. People with hypochondriasis differ from normal subjects and anxiety patients in their perception and their misinterpretation of normal bodily sensations, and this may be due to fluctuations in emotion.

Amplification Bodily sensations are felt, thought about, appraised for meaning, and acted on. Many investigators have noted the interactive relationship and mutual reinforcement between sensation, cognitive appraisal, and behavior in people with somatoform disorders. These reinforcing interactions have been termed *somatosensory amplification*, a process in which a person learns to feel body sensations more acutely, sometimes more accurately, and may catastrophically distort the meaning of those sensations by equating them with illness. This phenomenon is likely part of a cognitive style of abnormal self-observation coupled with selective perception and amplification of physical sensations, which lead to excessive perception of body vulnerability and overestimation of the likelihood of being ill.

Interaction with Anxiety and Depression Unexplained somatic symptoms are highly prevalent in anxiety and affective disorders and diminish significantly with adequate treatment of the anxiety or depressive disorder. There are numerous hypotheses about how this occurs, including selective perception, amplification, and increased autonomic nervous system activity. Eighty-eight to 95 percent of people who come to primary care settings around the world and who are subsequently diagnosed with an anxiety or depressive disorder present with only somatic symptoms as their chief complaint. This may be because somatic symptoms are actually prominent in these disorders because of their psychobiology or because people use somatic symptoms as the most acceptable currency to obtain care, or both.

Primary and Secondary Disorders It is thought that C. F. Michea (1815 to 1882) was the first to postulate an idiopathic (primary or true) form and a secondary form of hypochondriasis, which he called *manie triste* (sad monomania). These forms are important conceptually for purposes of classification and for determining treatment and predicting outcomes. Primary forms are when the somatoform disorder is the only condition of concern or, when there is comorbidity, the somatoform disorder precedes the other disorder and is responsible for the unexplained physical symptoms. The secondary form occurs when another disorder precedes the onset of the somatoform disorder, and the unexplained physical symptoms are thought to be due to, or secondary to, the other illness. Somatoform disorders may be secondary to other psychiatric or other medical illness. There is empirical support for the importance of both forms.

Relationship to Factitious and Malingering Disorders There is often confusion about the relationship between somatoform disorders and factitious and malingering disorders. This is partly because they are all viewed as the faking of symptoms in common medical parlance. However, they are different processes, with overlap between them, with features that are critical for the general psychiatrist to be familiar with.

A concept that helps distinguish between them is how a symptom is produced and whether it is really being felt and not faked. It is not a critical feature of these disorders that the physician believe in the authenticity of the symptoms, as this is not a reliable feature for diagnosis. Physicians often only consider symptoms *authentic* if they can be measured in the context of the biomedical culture. In fact, the realness of a given symptom has to do with whether it is produced consciously or unconsciously by the patient. In somatoform disorders, symptoms are produced unconsciously and are thus as authentic as a symptom of diabetes mellitus. The somatoform-disordered patient is not making the symptom up for any reason for which he or she is aware, and he or she is rightfully offended when it is suggested that the symptom is being faked. In factitious disorders, the patient has some awareness that he or she intentionally produces the symptom, although this awareness is usually less than complete. In malingering disorders, the person is clearly and consciously fabricating the symptom to obtain external incentives.

The other concept that helps distinguish these conditions is the reason for, or the gain produced by, the symptom, regardless of the nature of symptom production. In somatoform disorders, the patient has no awareness of why this symptom has been produced, even if psychological factors are responsible for its production. In this regard, the reason for the symptom is said to be for primary gain. This implies that the patient has no external incentives for the symptoms, which may be due to psychophysiological variables that are out of the awareness of the patient. The gain in somatoform disorders is generally primitive—the patient who has the symptoms simply hopes that there is someone who can help him or her feel better. However, because the somatoform patient feels sick, he or she often requests the physical or social benefits of illness, such as time off from duties or disability benefits. In factitious disorders, the reason for the symptoms is also generally unconscious and is thought to be due to the need to assume the sick role and to obtain the benefits that go along with being ill. These benefits are usually primary, or about the internal self, but these needs and benefits may also extend to the physical or social world of the patient. As long as this gain remains partially or fully unconscious to the patient, a factitious, not a malingering, disorder is present. In malingering, the person is fully aware of why he or she is producing the illness, and the gain is said to be secondary, or external, to the self. The malingering person is conscious of using symptoms to obtain money or medications or to avoid duties. One problem for the clinician is that all three conditions can result in the person asking for assistance with things external to the self, and, thus, all three often get equated with being faked for external gain. The difference is that the somatoform and factitious patient thinks they deserve what they are requesting to gain based on an illness, whereas the malingerer has no illusions that symptoms are the reason for the attempted gain.

Figure 15–1 demonstrates the relationship of symptom production and gain between these three disorders. Clinically, there is a spectrum between these disorders of how symptoms are produced and for what gain, and it is the expertise of the clinician that allows him or her to best classify a person who has symptoms that are not explained by known biomedical cause. Somatoform and factitious disorders imply the presence of psychopathology or illness, whereas malingering implies the absence of psychopathology and the presence of sociopathy.

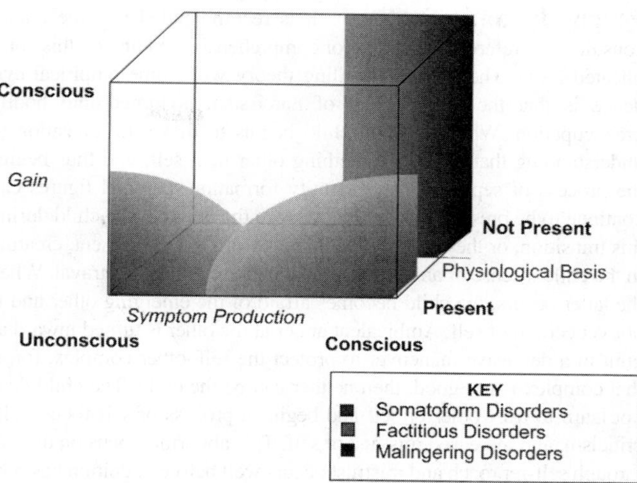

FIGURE 15–1 Somatoform, factitious, and malingering disorders: a comparison of symptom production, gain, and physiological basis.

GENERAL ETIOLOGIES

The etiologies of all somatoform disorders are unknown. There are theories and some physiological data to support some of these theories.

Genetic There is no direct evidence of a genetic etiology for any of the somatoform disorders. The few family and twin studies that have been conducted support a familial etiology for somatization disorder but not for hypochondriasis. There is support for a familial component for somatic anxiety from a general population twin study. Adoption studies demonstrate a weak, but present, familial relationship for the somatization phenomenon. Taken as a whole, it appears that a small amount of the variance for developing a preoccupation with body sensation or a propensity to amplify bodily sensations is genetically determined.

Learning and Sociocultural A large body of research supports the idea that early experiences and learning are the primary etiological factors of somatic sensitivity and bodily preoccupation. Children's symptoms are often a copy of other family members' symptoms. Adult somatoform symptoms are similar to those symptoms that were given attention by parents in childhood. Habitual attention to a given body part improves the ability of a person to detect sensations in that body part. Research has demonstrated that people can be trained to improve perception of bodily sensation.

Sociocultural construction of body and mind has an impact on how people feel emotion and how it manifests. There is evidence for differential conditioning of physiological arousal across different cultural groups. Culture also teaches people what is acceptable to express and what is not, and this influences the manifestation of emotion and body sensation. Socioeconomic class, education level, and subculture influence the rates of expressing emotional distress as somatic complaint.

Psychodynamic Factors It is recommended that the reader consult cross-reference material for comprehensive reading on this complicated issue. The most compelling theory with some empirical evidence is that the development of narcissism is turned into bodily preoccupation. When a young child begins to make the transition to understanding that there is something other than self, and thus begins the process of separation and identity formation, parental figures can continue to be present and to acknowledge the needs of the child during this transition, or they can be intermittently present and absent, creating in the child a sense of anxiety, fear of abandonment, and betrayal. When the latter occurs, the child becomes afraid of the emerging other and is not yet certain of self. Ambivalent anger at the other is turned inward as guilt in a defensive maneuver to protect the self–other complex, for, if that complex is not good, then neither can be the child. The child does not learn to trust other or self and begins a process of self-focus, self-criticism, and increased mistrust of self. This abnormal focus on the self through self-reproach and mistrust occurs well before cognition has substantially developed and thus becomes associated with body sensations and perception, as well as with affect. The self–other complex has betrayed the child, and there remains a fear throughout life that the body as self may abandon and betray the individual at any time. The individual, who has learned how to focus on the body self, begins to do so more often as a defense against a catastrophe of body betrayal.

Stressors and Coping The late 20th century brought improved understanding of the relationship between life events, trauma, and subsequent somatic symptoms and physical health. Adverse life events provide multiple stimuli to which a person responds, and that response, often somatic due to autonomic nervous system and endocrine activation, can become conditioned as memory. This memory is intended to serve the person to remember the event and to learn to avoid other such events. However, in pathological trauma syndromes in which memory systems are altered, body memory may be reexperienced in response to stimuli that are reminders of earlier stressors and trauma. This phenomenon is considered more fully later in the chapter.

Day-to-day stressors also create somatic experiences that may be learned by continued selective perception to the sensation. Coping style then predicts individual response to stressors. If stressors are many, persistent, or of high-impact quality, somatic responses occur and may be learned. If one's coping style is inadequate to resolve the physiological consequences of the stressors, then persistent somatic responses may be learned. Individuals who are burdened with an unusually high number of persistent and high-impact stressors and poor coping mechanisms are at the highest risk of somatoform disorders, as well as some other psychiatric disorders. Anger, impulsivity, hostility, isolation, and lack of confiding in others are some coping styles that have been associated with an increased risk for somatic symptoms and somatoform disorders. There are many empirical reports that link anger and hostility to somatization. Hostility, in particular, is associated with cardiovascular reactivity and a greater increase in blood pressure in response to stress compared to nonhostile subjects and, along with cynicism, is the component of the type A personality that is predictive of developing cardiovascular disease. This provides indirect evidence that this coping style is linked to physiological reactivity, which is associated with somatic sensation and amplification.

TREATMENT PRINCIPLES

Patient–Physician Relationship and Structure of Treatment Perhaps there is no set of disorders that better highlights the importance of the therapeutic relationship between doctor and patient and of treatment structure than the somatoform disorders. The doctor–patient relationship is the primary element of diligent and committed doctoring and is the foundation of all medical practice. It partly imbues the physician with power to hurt or to heal, dependent on how the relationship unfolds. Particularly with the somatoform-disordered patient, there are three elements of this relationship that make or break other specific treatment effects.

The first of these elements is attention. It has been written that one difference between doctors of today and of the past is that, with the advent of and reliance on technology, physicians today have forgotten how to attend to and to *see* the patient. It is not the disease, but the man or the woman, who needs to be seen and treated. Attending primarily to laboratory values or to the abdomen or the heart only leads to worsening of the patient with a somatoform disorder and failure on the part of the physician. Attention—that simple yet hard-to-conduct behavior of looking, watching, and listening—if present, allows doctor and patient to move toward care and treatment and, if absent, promotes dislike and anger between doctor and patient and disallows any effective care.

The second important element is unconditional care. It is the role of the physician to understand the illness and the patient who has the illness and to provide care. It is not the job of the patient to understand and to care for the doctor. In a patient with a somatoform disorder, the astute physician understands that he or she must know the patient to provide unconditional care, which is characterized by

- Acceptance and respect for the person, his or her symptoms, and how the symptoms are adversely affecting the person, which is why he or she comes to the doctor as a patient.
- Hearing what is being said by listening to words, skillfully eliciting words that are not said, and intentional watching of body posture, movement, and affect.
- Reflecting back to the patient what has been said via all forms of communication and letting him or her know that he or she is attended to.
- Not expecting or needing appreciation, as many patients with somatoform disorders assumed a parental role early in life for parent or other authority figure. Requiring this of a somatoform patient may make his or her symptoms worse.

The third element is skillful treatment. Specific treatments are considered later in this chapter in each section. General treatment elements in all somatoform disorders are essential to encourage the patient to engage in specific treatments. Some of these elements are referred to as *nonspecific* variables of treatment. However, some are general modalities that are more specific to somatoform disorders than to other psychiatric illness.

- Attend to transference and countertransference. The former allows treatment to occur, and the latter can destroy treatment. Patients with somatoform disorders generally do not appreciate their providers, are unsatisfied with care, are not loyal patients, and are attached to their symptoms and not to their doctor and his or her caring. Effective treatment begins by the doctor managing his or her countertransference, which, if not done effectively, may result in the physician avoiding or firing the patient or rescuing him.
- Formulate without labels when the diagnosis is uncertain. The somatoform patient is standing ready to hear the doctor tell him or her that "it is all in your head." Unfortunately, the somatoform patient is easily able to interpret that this is being said, regardless of physician behavior. This cue likely acts as the stimulus that recreates scenes in which the patient was not seen, not heard, not respected, and not cared for.

- Evaluate appropriately with standard and limited workup. Take the history. Conduct an examination. Order tests that one might order for any patient with the signs and symptoms of the patient being treated. Consider not ordering a test that is requested by a patient, but order it if one would otherwise. Do not pursue the vanishing symptom. Do not order repeat tests before they are reasonably due.
- Frame and make boundaries. Once diagnosed, it is in the best interest of the patient to know his or her diagnosis and the treatment plan of the physician. It is important to conduct the psychosocial history and to discuss its relevance to the disorder in a slow, deliberate, and rational way. This helps the physician to restrain the impulse to rapidly translate the physical into the psychological and gradually allows the patient to understand and to integrate information about the role of psychosocial factors in his or her disorder.
- Connect for the patient the languages of psyche and soma. This is perhaps the single most important general skill that allows the therapeutic relationship to move on to specific treatment. Most people do not have a problem with the idea that the mind and body are connected, and, in fact, patients generally wish that doctors would think this way more often. However, most people also have a hard time understanding how the mind and body are connected and how symptoms are created. Draw pictures of brain centers and how they are connected to and influence peripheral organ functioning. Give patients homework, consistent with their educational level, to better understand these relationships and to teach the doctor about them. Ask the patient to keep diaries and logs about the relationship of body symptoms to external events. Give them scientific information about psychophysiology and somatic symptom production. Also, do not be afraid to discuss what is not known about his or her disorder; just do so in a competent and confident way.
- Reassure appropriately and sparingly. This topic is discussed more in this chapter's section on hypochondriasis. Reassured too much, the somatoform-disordered patient is certain that the physician is not attending to the so-called real illness, and, if reassured too little, the patient is convinced that the doctor is hiding information about the ominous medical disorder that is lurking.
- Communicate clearly. Volumes have been written on this subject. Suffice it to say that the physician needs to be clear with the somatoform patient on what is said and what is being heard without being pedantic or demeaning. Take time to hear from the patient what issues were discussed during each session, and reframe this information for the patient if it is incorrect.

Finally, the structure of treatment is an essential part of treatment of the somatoform patient. Follow-up appointments should be time contingent, not symptom contingent. Discussing the follow-up schedule, its intervals, and its changes is necessary. Each appointment might best begin by discussing gains in functioning or changes in emotion or life events. Time should be set aside to attend to symptoms with history or physical examination, or both. Each appointment should end by verifying the next scheduled appointment and how to use urgent care systems. Once diagnosed properly, referral to other specialists should be prudently restrained. There is always an urge to refer, and this urge should always be viewed in relation to the countertransference. Thus, the best thing that the doctor can do for the somatoform patient is to commit to the therapeutic relationship rather than to zealous workup or treatment of individual symptoms.

Reassurance Reassurance is discussed in this chapter's section on hypochondriasis, and the reader is also referred to the reference section. Reassurance is a general technique for all of medicine and is also a specific technique to be used skillfully with the somatoform-disordered patient.

Cognitive-Behavioral and Other Psychotherapies

The value of the psychotherapies for somatoform disorders are just beginning to be understood. The reader should be aware that the rubric *cognitive-behavioral therapy* (CBT) represents many modalities that are usually delivered over a relatively brief period of time, such as 8 to 20 sessions. Psychoanalysis was, as discussed in the history, partly responsible for the categorization of the hysterias because of its success in the hands of some.

There have been more than 30 controlled trials to date designed to evaluate the efficacy of CBT in patients with somatization or symptom syndromes. Most of these studies targeted a specific syndrome, such as chronic fatigue or irritable bowel disorder, although eight focused on more general somatization or hypochondriasis. The most common outcomes measured were physical symptoms, psychological distress, and functional status. Physical symptoms appeared to be the most responsive to treatment, as the CBT-treated patients had greater improvement than control subjects in more than two-thirds of the studies, and there were trends toward improvement in approximately 10 percent of the studies. Psychological distress was definitely improved by CBT compared to control subjects in approximately 40 percent of the studies, with trends toward improvement in approximately 10 percent of the studies. Functional status was definitely helped by CBT in approximately 50 percent of the studies, and trends toward improvement were shown in approximately 25 percent of the studies. Health care use seems to be decreased by approximately 25 percent in two studies. In studies that followed up participants, gains were generally maintained at 12 to 18 months after treatment completion.

Randomized, controlled studies to date also support the efficacy of individual CBT for the treatment of hypochondriasis, body dysmorphic disorder, and undifferentiated somatoform disorders, which include medically unexplained symptoms, chronic fatigue syndrome, and noncardiac chest pain. Group CBT has been shown effective for the treatment of body dysmorphic disorder and somatization disorder.

Long-term and dynamic therapies were the first treatments available for disorders of unexplained symptoms in the late 19th century and early 20th century. There is some modern empirical evidence that supports their use in somatoform disorders, and some suggest that dynamic therapy is a contraindication (i.e., in conversion disorder) until more basic psychosocial issues have been addressed. One problem with assessing outcomes of this group of therapies is that there is a range of modalities labeled as *dynamic*, and these therapies also variably overlap with modalities called *CBT*. Methods sections in some studies of somatoform disorders often do not describe the kind of therapy conducted or, better, what was actually done and for how long. It will be critical in the coming decade to identify the specific and nonspecific ingredients of therapies that are useful for somatoform disorders.

Pharmacotherapy There is mounting evidence for the usefulness of antidepressant medications in somatoform disorders. Conversely, it has been argued that, in these studies, the somatoform symptoms are often secondary to mood or anxiety disorders, and these comorbid disorders are being effectively treated, decreasing the somatoform symptoms. One critical diagnostic feature to determine the choice of pharmacotherapy is whether the somatoform disorder is primary or secondary and, if primary, whether there is a comorbid psychiatric condition present. Information is presented in individual disorder sections of this chapter on current pharmacological approaches, which should be interpreted in light of the problems with classification and diagnosis.

Combination Therapies

As in all of medicine, a prudent clinical approach that first does no harm is always warranted. Somatoform disorders are distressing, impairing, and costly but are usually not emergencies. This gives the clinician time to diagnose, to formulate, and to plan treatment. In most cases, given the epidemiology, comorbidity, and current treatment knowledge, combination therapies of modalities discussed previously are used. Furthermore, there are emerging data that combination therapies are likely to be the most efficacious for the treatment of somatoform disorders.

SOMATIZATION DISORDER

Definition

Somatization disorder is an illness of multiple somatic complaints in multiple organ systems that occurs over a period of several years and results in significant impairment or treatment seeking, or both. Somatization disorder is the prototypic somatoform disorder and has the best evidence of any of the somatoform disorders for being a stable and reliably measured entity over many years in individuals with the disorder.

History

The term *somatization* was first used by Wilhelm Stekel in 1943. Briquet's syndrome was the DSM-III predecessor to current somatization disorder, which was named in the revised third edition of the DSM (DSM-III-R).

Comparative Nosology

In the ICD-10, somatization syndromes of the DSM-IV-TR are distributed among the somatoform disorders (F45), the dissociative disorders (F44), and neurasthenia (F48).

Epidemiology

Studies report widely variable lifetime prevalence rates of somatization disorder, ranging from 0.2 to 2.0 percent among women and less than 0.2 percent in men. However, there is evidence that less restrictive diagnostic criteria than the current DSM-IV-TR criteria carry prevalence rates of as great as 5 percent with similar levels of impairment in this population. Approximately 5 percent of primary care patients meet diagnostic criteria for the disorder, but many more somatize psychosocial distress. Recent work demonstrated that 9 percent of hospitalized general medical patients had somatization disorder, and 12 percent of chronic pain patients and 17 percent of outpatients with irritable bowel syndrome met the diagnostic criteria. Differences in prevalence rates depend on whether the interviewer is a physician, on the method of assessment, and on the demographic variables in the samples studied. In epidemiological studies, nonphysician interviewers diagnose somatization disorder more frequently than physicians. The onset is before 25 years of age in 90 percent of people with the disorder, but initial symptoms generally develop during adolescence. Risk factors for children to develop somatization disorder are living with a family member who has the disorder and parental substance abuse and antisocial symptoms. The female to male ratio ranges from 5 to 1 to 20 to 1.

Somatization disorder is relatively more common in rural areas and in people who are nonwhite and unmarried and who have less education. The type and frequency of somatic symptoms in somatization disorder, as in mood and anxiety disorders, may differ across cultures. For example, burning hands and feet or nondelusional symptoms of insects crawling under the skin are symptoms that may be more common in Africa and South Asia than in North America. Accordingly, diagnosis must take into account cultural norms. The DSM-IV-TR lists symptoms in order of frequency as found in research within the United States. Cultural factors may also influence the gender ratio, as there is a higher reported frequency in Greek and Puerto Rican men than in North American men.

Somatization disorder is observed in 10 to 20 percent of female first-degree biological relatives of women who have the disorder. The male relatives of women with somatization disorder show an increased risk of antisocial personality disorder and substance-related disorders. Having a biological or adoptive parent with any of these three disorders increases the risk of developing antisocial personality disorder, a substance-related disorder, or somatization disorder.

Somatization disorder is not highly prevalent but is proportionally costly. These patients seek care approximately three times more often than the U.S. norm, and they incur between 6 and 14 times the national average for health care expenditures for physician and hospital services.

Etiology

The etiology for somatization disorder is considered in the section General Etiologies.

A 34-year-old female temporary clerk presented with chronic and intermittent dizziness, paresthesias, pain in multiple areas of her body, and intermittent nausea and diarrhea. On further history, the patient said that the symptoms had been present most of the time, although they had been undulating since she was approximately 24 years of age. In addition to the symptoms previously mentioned, she had mild depression, was disinterested in many things in life, including sexual activity, and had been to many doctors to try to find out what was wrong with her. Even though she had seen many doctors and had many tests, she stated that "no one can find out what's wrong" with her. She wanted another opinion. She commented that she had been "sick a lot" since childhood and had been on various medications on and off. Physical examination revealed a normotensive, slightly overweight female in no acute distress. She had diffuse and mild abdominal tenderness, without true guarding or rebound tenderness. Her neurological examination was normal. She winced when physical examination was conducted on various parts of her body, although this wincing went away when the physician was speaking with her while conducting the examination.

Diagnosis and Clinical Features

The essential feature of somatization disorder is persistent or recurring somatic complaints in multiple organ systems that cause medical treatment or significant impairment in social, occupational, or other important areas of functioning. Physician-rated legitimacy of the symptoms is not an essential criterion of the disorder. The symptoms begin before 30 years of age and occur over several years (Criterion A), although the type and severity of symptoms may change over time. The multiple symptoms are not fully explained by another medical condition or by a substance, or, if they do occur as part of another medical condition, the physical complaints or resulting impairment is in excess of what would be expected from the history, physical examination, or laboratory tests (Criterion C). Further diagnostic criteria include pain in at least four different anatomical sites, at least two gastrointestinal (GI) symptoms other than pain, at least one sexual or reproductive symptom other than pain, and at least one symptom, other than pain, that suggests a neurological condition (Criterion B). The most common pain symptoms in U.S. populations are located in the head, the back, the abdomen, the joints or extremities, the chest, and the rectum, and pain is often present during menstruation and with intercourse. The most common GI symptoms are nausea and abdominal bloating, but vomiting, diarrhea, and food intolerance are less common. Sexual and reproductive symptoms may consist of irregular menses, menorrhagia, or vomiting throughout pregnancy in women. Men are most likely to have erectile or ejaculatory dysfunction. Women and men may have sexual indifference. The pseudoneurological symptoms commonly include impaired coordination or balance described by the patient as dizziness, paralysis, paresthesias or localized weakness, difficulty swallowing, aphonia, urinary hesitancy or retention, hallucinations, diminished or loss of touch or pain sensation, double vision, diminished hearing, amnesia, or loss of consciousness other than fainting.

As mentioned previously, a less restrictive form of somatization that requires fewer symptoms for diagnosis is more prevalent than DSM-IV-TR somatization disorder. This abridged form has moderate to strong empirical support for being a sound diagnosis by demonstrating similar levels of impairment and health care use as the full DSM-IV-TR disorder. This also highlights the spectral nature of somatization and the resultant diagnostic difficulties.

People with somatization disorder consider themselves to be ill and are usually reluctant to entertain the idea that the cause of their symptoms arises from psychological or social distress. Partly because of the undulating nature of the disorder, people with somatization are usually poor historians, and they seem to exaggerate various symptoms each at different times. They often defy good medical care by attending various clinics and by getting multiple opinions from different doctors. Furthermore, people with this disorder often do not report overall improvement, even when specific symptoms have been addressed by a physician and have improved. In fact, the improved symptom seems to be forgotten, and the patient moves to being bothered by another symptom. This has led to the idea that symptom substitution occurs in these patients, in which one symptom develops in place of another that has improved. These clinical features of the patient do not engender the affection of physicians. In fact, one study indicated that patients who somatize are among the four illness types who are the least liked by doctors, the others being people with substance abuse, with neurological deficits, and with personality disorders. One common feature of these four disorders is that they are not as well understood and treated by Western medicine as are many other disorders. The somatizing patient often frustrates physicians, as if the patient is challenging the education and good skill of the doctor.

This frustration alludes to a weakness in the scientific and clinical medical education of U.S.-trained physicians, which is the lack of education about how mind and body are integrated in their function. As discussed previously, general distress can be embodied as somatic complaint, which is more common around the world than is psychological distress. The embodiment of distress is at cultural odds with much of Western medical care, which views bodily symptoms as evidence that there should be an identifiable illness in peripheral organs. When the search for this proposed illness ends without explanation, the symptoms and the patient are logically deemed to be inauthentic. This clinical feature, which becomes part of the countertransference of physician to patient, can cause an adversarial relationship between doctor and patient.

Psychiatric comorbidity is high in somatization disorder. Prominent anxiety and mood symptoms are common and are usually the reasons for being seen in mental health settings. Major depressive disorder, panic disorder, and substance-related disorders are commonly associated Axis I disorders, and histrionic, borderline, and antisocial personality disorders are the most commonly associated Axis II disorders. There may be impulsive behavior, suicide threats and attempts, and marital discord. The lives of these individuals are often as chaotic and complicated as their symptoms. Frequent and intermittent use of medications may lead to side effects and substance-abuse disorders. People with somatization disorder are at relatively high risk of iatrogenic harm owing to their increased health care use, numerous medical examinations, diagnostic procedures, surgeries, and hospitalizations.

Pathology There is no known tissue pathology in somatization disorder. Experimental studies demonstrate that somatizing patients are more somatically sensitive and often are more accurate in distinguishing between small differences in stimuli compared to normal control subjects. For example, somatizing subjects are more likely to feel pain at lesser amounts of barium in the colon and can detect smaller volumes of inflation of a balloon at the end of an esophageal endoscope than normal control subjects. Somatic amplification is thus the primary pathological finding in this disorder, but these phenomena are not easily used in clinical medicine for diagnosis. Physical examination elicits different signs on different examinations and is remarkable for the absence of objective findings to fully explain the degree of the subjective complaints of patients with this disorder. Laboratory test results are remarkable for the absence of findings to support the subjective complaints.

Differential Diagnosis Table 15–3 shows the vast differential diagnosis for somatization phenomena. There are three features that most suggest a diagnosis of somatization disorder instead of *another medical disorder*, and those are the involvement of multiple organ systems, early onset and chronic course without development of physical signs or structural abnormalities, and absence of laboratory abnormalities that are characteristic of the suggested medical condition. In the process of diagnosis, the astute clinician considers other medical disorders that are characterized by vague, multiple, and confusing somatic symptoms, such as *thyroid disease*, *hyperparathyroidism*, *intermittent porphyria*, *multiple sclerosis* (MS), and *systemic lupus erythematosus.* Of course, other medical disorders may be comorbid with somatization disorder and, in fact, are risk factors for developing somatization. The onset of multiple physical symptoms late in life must be considered to be another medical condition until proven otherwise.

Given the nature of the multiple somatic complaints in somatization disorder, there are many other possible somatoform and psychiatric disorders in the differential diagnosis. When full criteria are not met, *undifferentiated somatoform disorder* is diagnosed if the duration of the syndrome is 6 months or longer, and *somatoform disorder not otherwise specified* (NOS) is diagnosed for presentations of shorter duration. As noted in the previous discussion on the core phenomenology of somatoform disorders, there is overlap between these disorders and *factitious* and *malingering* disorders, dependent on whether the symptom production is volitional and on the nature of the gain. When these elements are mixed, somatization disorder and a factitious disorder or malingering can be diagnosed. *Mood* and *anxiety disorders* often, but not always, have prominent somatic symptoms, which do not exist separately from the mood or anxiety disorder. However, somatization disorder may be diagnosed as a comorbid condition with mood and anxiety disorders. *Schizophrenia* and other *psychotic disorders* with multiple somatic delusions need to be differentiated from the nondelusional somatic complaints of individuals with somatization disorder. Hallucinations can occur as pseudoneurological symptoms and must be distinguished from the typical hallucinations seen in

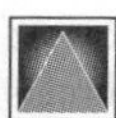

Table 15–3
Differential Diagnosis of the Somatizing Patient

Psychophysiological symptoms
- Psychological factors affecting physical illness
- Nonpathological, transient psychogenic somatic symptoms (all are acute but may become chronic)
  - Grief and bereavement, with physical symptoms
  - Fear, with physical symptoms
  - Exaggeration or elaboration of physical symptoms (e.g., postaccident, when litigation or compensation is involved)
  - Sleep deprivation, with physical symptoms
  - Sensory overload or deprivation, with physical symptoms

Psychiatric syndromes (other than somatoform disorders)
- Mood disorders (e.g., major depression and dysthymia)
- Anxiety disorders (e.g., panic disorders)
- Substance use, abuse, and withdrawal
- Psychotic disorders (e.g., schizophrenia, psychotic depression, and monosymptomatic hypochondriasis)
- Adjustment disorders with anxiety or depression, or both
- Personality disorders
- Dementias

Somatoform disorders
- Somatization disorder
- Hypochondriasis
- Body dysmorphic disorder
- Somatoform pain disorder
- Conversion disorder
- Somatoform disorder, not otherwise specified

Voluntary psychogenic symptoms or syndromes
- Factitious, with physical symptoms (e.g., Munchausen syndrome)
- Malingering, with physical symptoms

Adapted from Rubin RH, Voss C, Derksen DJ, et al., eds. *Medicine: A Primary Care Approach.* Philadelphia: WB Saunders; 1996:390.

schizophrenia. Somatization disorder symptoms are usually easier to distinguish from psychotic disorders than is the case for *hypochondriasis*, the disease fears of which can reach delusional quality.

Course and Prognosis Somatization disorder is a chronic, undulating, and relapsing disorder that rarely remits completely. It is unusual for the individual with somatization disorder to be free of symptoms or help seeking for greater than 1 year. Research has indicated that a person diagnosed with somatization disorder has approximately an 80 percent chance of being diagnosed with this disorder 5 years later. Although patients with this disorder consider themselves to be medically ill, there is good evidence that they are no more likely to develop another medical illness in the next 20 years than people without somatization disorder.

Treatment The primary mainstay of treatment is managing symptoms and helping the patient understand that symptom does not equal disease. Promoting function is a key component of education and treatment. An early study demonstrated that sending a consultation letter to primary care physicians suggesting how to treat identified patients with somatization disorder resulted in increased physical functioning and decreased health care costs for those patients. Recent work shows promise for cognitive and behavioral therapies. One uncontrolled study using group CBT that focused on patient education and stress reduction demonstrated moderate but significant improvement of physical symptoms, somatic preoccupation, hypochondriasis, and health care use compared to a control group of untreated patients. Another uncontrolled trial of ten sessions of individual CBT demonstrated patient-reported significant improvement in symptomatology and physical functioning between baseline and posttreatment, as well as between baseline and follow-up 8 months later. One randomized controlled clinical trial of group therapy with 70 patients demonstrated significantly better patient-reported physical and mental health in a 1-year period during and after therapy. The more group sessions attended, the greater the improvement in general and mental health. There was also a 52 percent net savings in health care charges in the year after treatment compared to the year before.

Pharmacological treatment for somatization disorder is not well understood. In one prospective, 8-week, open-label study, 15 patients diagnosed with full or abridged somatization disorder were treated with nefazodone (Serzone). Fourteen of the 15 patients achieved the target dosage of 300 mg per day and completed the trial, and 73 percent of the patients were rated as globally improved and significantly improved on functional abilities as measured by the Medical Outcomes Study Short Form-36 (SF-36).

HYPOCHONDRIASIS

Definition *Hypochondriasis* is characterized by 6 months or more of a general and nondelusional preoccupation with fears of having, or the idea that one has, a serious disease based on the person's misinterpretation of bodily symptoms. This preoccupation causes significant distress and impairment in one's life, it is not accounted for by another psychiatric or medical disorder, and a subset of individuals with hypochondriasis has poor insight about the presence of this disorder.

History Confusion and conceptual change epitomize the history of hypochondriasis. Issy Pilowsky was the first modern investigator to identify the three dimensions of bodily preoccupation, disease phobia, and disease conviction with a failure to respond to medical evaluation and reassurance that now comprise hypochondriasis. Multiple investigators have replicated the validity of these dimensions.

Comparative Nosology ICD-10 *hypochondriacal disorder* is similar to DSM-IV-TR hypochondriasis, but also includes body dysmorphophobia as one potential "A" criterion, which is not possible by DSM-IV-TR criteria. DSM-IV-TR hypochondriasis highlights the element of misinterpretation of body symptoms.

Epidemiology There are no good community epidemiological data about hypochondriasis. The Epidemiological Catchment Area Study and the National Comorbidity Survey failed to include hypochondriasis. This reinforces the notion that hypochondriasis is considered less important than other psychiatric disorders or that it is considered diagnostically invalid or unreliable, or that both are true. For whatever reason, this has rendered knowledge of the epidemiology of this disorder deficient. Early researchers suggested community prevalence rates between 4 and 25 percent. Robert Kellner pioneered the Illness Attitudes Scales and determined a 2 to 13 percent prevalence of disease phobia in many nonclinical settings, including employee panels, community samples, and medical and law students. Best current estimates are that there is a 1.1 to 4.5 percent prevalence of hypochondriasis in the community and an additional 10 percent of people who have hypochondriacal fears and beliefs.

Data from nonpsychiatric medical settings have relied primarily on screening instruments for prevalence studies and have used both dimensional and categorical scoring to determine rates. Hypochondriasis is probably more common in these settings with a prevalence between 0.8 and 10.3 percent. Medical specialty clinics, such as gastroenterology, otolaryngology, neurology, and endocrinology, have a higher rate of hypochondriacs. The prevalence is approximately 12 to 22 percent in psychiatric outpatients and 30 to 45 percent in psychiatric inpatients, although people with other psychiatric disorders are uncommonly diagnosed with hypochondriasis.

The onset of the disorder is most commonly in the third or fourth decade of life, and the symptoms at different ages do not differ significantly, except for a higher prevalence of depression in the elderly. Hypochondriasis is equally common in men and women. Studies suggest a slightly higher prevalence in people with lower education and income levels and in African Americans after controlling for socioeconomic status. Physical disease does not appear to be associated with hypochondriasis. Disease does not predict the onset nor do people with hypochondriasis develop more physical disease over many years after diagnosis. Little is known about other factors predisposing people to hypochondriasis, although there is a suggestion that certain personality features and adverse life events may contribute to the genesis of this disorder.

Etiology The etiology of hypochondriasis is considered in the section General Etiologies.

Diagnosis and Clinical Features The critical diagnostic feature of hypochondriasis is at least 6 months of impairment caused by preoccupation with fears of having, or the idea that one has, a serious disease based on a misinterpretation of one or more bodily signs or symptoms (Criteria A, D, and E), and the preoccupation persists despite medical reassurance (Criterion B). For hypochondriasis to be diagnosed when another medical condition is present, the physical signs or symptoms cannot fully account for the person's preoccupation with disease. The disease phobia present in hypochondriasis is not of delusional intensity and is not restricted to a circumscribed concern about appearance, as seen in *body dysmorphic disorder* (Criterion C). The preoccupation is not better accounted for by other psychiatric disorders considered in the following discussion of differential diagnosis (Criterion F). The Whiteley Index and the Illness Attitude Scales have demonstrated sensitivity/specificity of 71/80 percent and 72/79 percent, respectively, to clinical diagnosis.

There are rational doubts about hypochondriasis as a distinct entity. Investigators have established internal validity based on DSM criteria and external and concurrent validity to measures of fear, anxiety, depression, vulnerability to illness, somatic amplification, and health care service use. Three studies have demonstrated predictive validity, demonstrating that 50 to 70 percent of hypochondriacs continue to have the diagnosis after 1 to 5 years and that those who no longer meet diagnostic criteria still have more bodily preoccupation than control subjects. However, family and twin studies have failed to demonstrate a genetic basis for hypochondriasis. Rather, hypochondriacal probands have a stronger family association to *somatization disorder*. Discriminant validity for hypochondriasis is less sound than internal and concurrent validity.

The preoccupation in hypochondriasis may be with bodily functions, minor physical abnormalities, or ambiguous physical sensations. The person attributes these symptoms or signs to a suspected disease and is concerned with their meaning and cause. The concerns may involve several body systems or may be about a specific organ or a single disease. Examinations, diagnostic tests, and reassurance from the physician do not generally reassure the hypochondriac, especially in chronic conditions and when these examinations and tests are conducted in a manner perceived as flippant by the patient. For example, an individual preoccupied with having MS may not be reassured by the repeated lack of findings on physical examination or neuroimaging studies. In fact, showing radiological pictures to a hypochondriacal patient may elicit heightened distress when the patient sees a normal structure and firmly interprets it as being abnormal. The actual preoccupation with disease may be so prominent that specific symptoms are not the central concern or are absent. However, hypochondriacal patients do report more symptoms than healthy control subjects. People with hypochondriasis are also highly thanatophobic, and this degree of death fear is greater than in people with *somatization disorder*.

Thanatophobia is a central clinical feature of hypochondriasis and highlights the relationship to and embodiment of personality features. Hypochondriacs focus so much on their own body that there is a marked decrease of interest in other people or other matters outside of their body. They obsessionally focus on thoughts about having a disease, first this one and then maybe that one to the exclusion of, or marked reduction in, thoughts about anything other than self. Investigators have noted this conflictual relationship of the hypochondriac to his or her body, having severe fears of somatic uncertainty coupled with rigid certainty about the state of his or her health. This manifests in inappropriate help seeking and attention to details of symptoms that are irrelevant to their overall health coupled with rejecting help for real health problems and inattention to adaptive health behaviors. For example, a hypochondriac may be certain that he or she has heart disease, even when a reasonable evaluation is negative, yet he or she may ignore suggestions to prevent possible heart disease through exercise, a low-fat diet, and cholesterol-lowering medications. They are persistent seekers of explanations rather than of treatment, are largely unsatisfied with their medical care, and often feel that physicians have not recognized their needs. In this way, hypochondriasis is the embodiment of neurotic, obsessional, and narcissistic personality features, which are the personality traits with the most empirical support in their relationship to hypochondriasis. Classical and contemporary authors have emphasized how hypochondriasis develops from, or is part of, a defective ego structure, possibly as a result of poor object relations and insecure attachments during development, and how narcissistic injury results in a defensive focus on the body self. This defensive concern with perfect health results in amplified and selective somatic perception, cognitive distortions about the meaning of symptoms, and fear of illness and death because of the belief that inner badness may cause the body to suddenly and perhaps fatally betray the individual at any time.

Pathology There is no known somatic pathology specific to hypochondriasis. Nineteenth-century investigators who conducted postmortem examinations on hypochondriacs debated whether there was inflammation and congestion in the upper GI tract. This was refuted.

Differential Diagnosis The most common condition in the differential diagnosis of hypochondriasis is *transient preoccupation with the fear of having a disease*. This is a commonly discussed phenomenon that may occur during the course of medical training, known as *the medical student syndrome*. This syndrome has been reported in two studies to occur with a 70 to 79 percent prevalence in medical students. However, another study compared medical students with law students, who had the same level of hypochondriacal fears and beliefs and took only slightly less precautions about their

FIGURE 15–2 Somatization and hypochondriasis. (Data from Hollifield M, Tuttle L, Paine S, Kellner R: Hypochondriasis and somatization related to personality and attitudes toward self. *Psychosomatics.* 1999;40:387.)

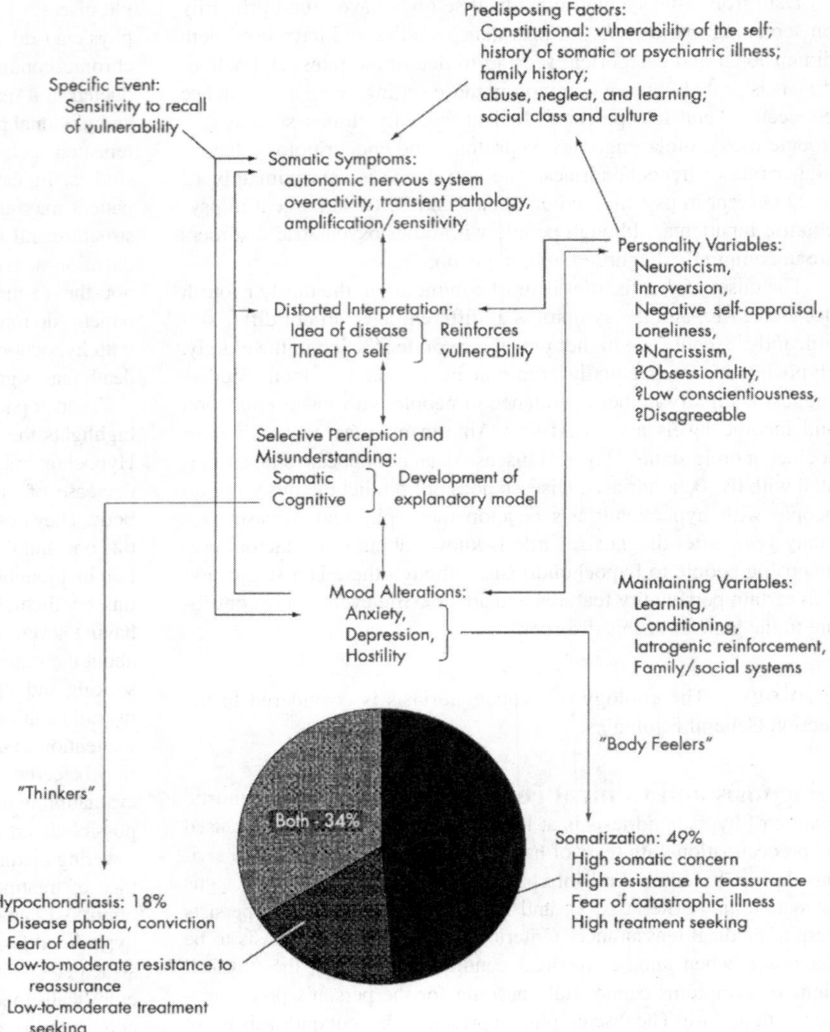

health and paid only slightly less attention to somatic symptoms. Thus, *transient fears of having a disease* are not limited to medical students but are most likely to occur when a person has some experience with major transition, disease, or death, such as when one's family member dies or when one's friend contracts a serious illness.

The most important set of conditions to consider in the differential diagnosis of hypochondriasis is another *medical condition.* Before the use of improved diagnostic techniques and instruments, it may have been common for early, undetected medical disorders to be thought to be a form of hypochondriasis, perhaps in as many as 30 percent of people diagnosed as hypochondriacal. Today, approximately 2 to 5 percent of people diagnosed with hypochondriasis are symptomatic of another medical disorder that is subsequently diagnosed. However, there are no good prospective studies on this issue, and the purported hypochondriacal symptoms could be symptoms of many subsequent medical conditions, at least one of which everyone, at some time, acquires. There are no typical diseases that should be considered in the differential diagnosis. The physician is implored to think clearly about other insidious diseases that could be the cause of the patients' symptoms, such as those in the endocrine, neurological, autoimmune, and malignant categories. However, a physician should also not promote iatrogenic harm by conducting tests without good rationale. The presence of another medical condition does not rule out coexisting hypochondriasis. In fact, people with chronic medical illness are more likely than those without chronic illness to have a comorbid somatoform disorder, usually hypochondriasis or somatization disorder. Even if the patient has a known medical illness, the diagnosis of hypochondriasis can be made if it can be definitively established that the symptoms and preoccupation with the fear of having disease are out of proportion to the seriousness of the organic pathology. However, given the variability in normal response to illness and disease, the diagnosis of hypochondriasis in the context of other known medical pathology should be reserved for individuals who are able to benefit from the diagnosis by having an explanation for the degree of their suffering and by being able to benefit from treatment for hypochondriasis.

Other somatoform disorders are in the differential diagnosis. *Somatization disorder* occurs in 7 to 40 percent of individuals diagnosed with hypochondriasis. Much of the descriptive literature to date considers somatization disorder and hypochondriasis together in their genesis and phenomenology. A few recent studies conclude that they are separate entities and that people with somatization disorder are more concerned with actual symptoms, have more abnormal personality characteristics and more depression and anxiety, and are more likely to seek treatment, whereas people with hypochondriasis are more afraid of death. Figure 15–2 depicts a model of hypochondriasis and somatization that helps identify shared and different characteristics, as well as places to intervene with treatment. People with *body dysmorphic disorder* and hypochondriasis share elements of obsessive preoccupation with their body associated with specific overvalued ideas. However, the difference is that people with body dysmorphic disorder focus on specific, presumed defects, are not as fearful of having a disease or of death, and are more likely to seek specific medical care, such as cosmetic surgery or dermatological advice.

Other psychiatric disorders are also in the differential diagnosis of hypochondriasis. A *psychotic disorder*, such as a *delusional disorder*, a *major affective disorder with psychotic features*, and *schizophrenia*, must be ruled out before establishing the diagnosis of hypochondriasis. It may be difficult to distinguish between disease phobia, disease conviction, and a psychotic process. Many people with hypochondriasis have a firm conviction that they have a disease, and there is a fair debate about whether delusional thoughts are part of hypochondriasis. However, an individual with hypochondriacal delusions has a fixed, unfounded belief that a disease is present. Furthermore, those with hypochondriacal delusions often have bizarre explanations for their belief or gross impairment of reality, or both, such as being convinced they have been poisoned, that their organs have somehow moved, or that someone or something outside of self has agency over their organs and health. Hypochondriacal beliefs accompany *depression* in at least a great minority of people with significant depressive symptoms. There are no good studies that determine whether hypochondriacal beliefs are more common in major depression than in dysthymia or depression in the context of bipolar affective disorder. A diagnosis of a major affective disorder is more likely if the hypochondriacal preoccupations begin in later life. Treatment of depression is likely to diminish or to ablate hypochondriacal fears that are secondary to the depression, whereas comorbid primary hypochondriasis is much less likely to abate with successful treatment of comorbid depression. *Anxiety disorders* are highly comorbid with hypochondriasis. Individuals with hypochondriasis have intrusive thoughts about the fear of having a disease and also may have associated compulsive behaviors (e.g., checking their blood pressure). The relationship between hypochondriasis and obsessional personality is well known. However, although this bodily preoccupation in hypochondriasis is distressing, the patient believes that he or she has a disease, and, in that sense, the disease conviction is not ego-dystonic. Thus, a separate diagnosis of *obsessive-compulsive disorder* (OCD) is warranted only when the obsessions or compulsions are not restricted to concerns about illness and meet other criteria for the disorder, including that the symptoms are ego-dystonic. *Specific phobias* are generally not limited to the body but should be considered in the person with hypochondriasis. *Panic disorder* and *generalized anxiety disorder* are highly comorbid with hypochondriasis. Approximately 50 percent of patients diagnosed with *panic disorder* have significant hypochondriacal preoccupations. Conversely, one study demonstrated that more than 50 percent of patients with hypochondriasis had panic disorder. *Generalized anxiety disorder* is probably less common in hypochondriasis than in panic disorder, but studies about this comorbidity are scarce. These two anxiety disorders share common features with hypochondriasis, such as pathological fear and worry and behaviors designed to diminish anxiety. However, in people with hypochondriasis, the fear and worry are limited to the idea of disease, and they do not necessarily have the autonomic symptoms associated with panic or generalized anxiety disorder.

Malingering and *personality disorders* are in the differential diagnosis of hypochondriasis and are considered more fully in other parts of this chapter.

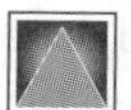

Table 15–4
Elements of Effective Reassurance in Hypochondriasis

Thorough examination of medical records and history
Acceptance of the patient, his or her complaints, and their legitimacy
Scheduling regular visits with a clear goal
Using clear and simple language with unambiguous terms
Providing relevant information and explanations
Fostering the patient's responsibility for his or her treatment
Shifting attention from physical symptoms to underlying psychological and social problems and focusing on patient assets
Adjusting a reassuring style in a way that is effective for a given patient
Providing repeated reassurance
Performing appropriate examinations and tests with adequate explanation

Adapted from Starcevic V. Reassurance in the treatment of hypochondriasis. In: Lipsitt D, Starcevic V, eds. *Hypochondriasis: Modern Perspectives on an Ancient Malady.* Oxford, UK: Oxford University Press; 2001:299–308.

Course and Prognosis The course of hypochondriasis is usually intermittent and chronic. Approximately two-thirds of people diagnosed with hypochondriasis continue to have the disorder 1 year later, and those who are not diagnosable have persistent hypochondriacal symptoms. Poor prognostic factors include severity and duration of symptoms, comorbid psychiatric disorders, and neuroticism, including affective instability and interpersonal vulnerability. Acute onset, medical comorbidity, the absence of a current or past Axis I or II psychiatric disorder, and the absence of secondary gain are favorable prognostic indicators. Risk factors for developing transient hypochondriasis are a past psychiatric history, personality pathology, and an underlying sensitivity to somatic sensations.

Well-devised reassurance, consisting of the development of a shared explanatory model between doctor and patient, education, and the rational use of examination and laboratory testing can improve the prognosis in more than one-half of people with hypochondriasis, particularly those with transient or short duration of symptoms and with other positive prognostic factors.

Treatment

Reassurance A thorough description of the definition and use of reassurance in hypochondriasis has recently been well discussed. Discussion with the hypochondriacal patient about the false nature of his or her illness is not successful. However, reassurance that is delivered confidently by a competent doctor using multiple modalities, including skillful examination, effective communication, and helpful education, is the cornerstone of treatment of the hypochondriacal patient. Without successful reassurance, more specific treatments are not likely to be accepted or adhered to by the patient. Important elements of effective reassurance are shown in Table 15–4.

It is important that all therapies work to diminish the preoccupation with the fear of having a disease. Thus, reassurance is effective when preoccupation decreases and is harmful when it gets worse. This can happen, for example, when examinations and tests iatrogenically reinforce the notion that a disease is present. Another example is when the patient believes that a doctor is not competent to find the disease that is believed to be present or that the doctor is dismissing the patient's concerns by shifting attention to emotional or social issues. However, when there is a therapeutic relationship that is trusting due to the competence and skill of the physician, then examinations, tests, and shifting attention to important psychosocial issues in the patient's life may encourage the patient to focus on relevant features of the illness and not on the disease phobia.

Cognitive-Behavioral Therapy (CBT) Uncontrolled case series have demonstrated promising results of CBT in hypochondriasis. Two controlled studies are also supportive for CBT being effective in hypochondriasis. Psychoeducation and cognitive therapy aimed at changing the thoughts that there is a disease present have been the standard of treatment for many years. Poor prognostic factors for successful CBT include worse hypochondriasis, more somatic symptoms, psychiatric comorbidity, more dysfunctional thoughts about body functions, and higher levels of health care use and social impairment.

Pharmacological Selective serotonin reuptake inhibitors (SSRIs) and serotonin norepinephrine reuptake inhibitors (SNRIs) have been shown to be useful for hypochondriasis in a few small, open-label studies. Larger clinical trials were under way at this writing.

CONVERSION DISORDER

Definition

Conversion disorder is an illness of symptoms or deficits that affect voluntary motor or sensory functions, which suggest another medical condition, but that is judged to be due to psychological factors because the illness is preceded by conflicts or other stressors. The symptoms or deficits of conversion disorder are not intentionally produced, are not due to substances, are not limited to pain or sexual symptoms, and the gain is primarily psychological and not social, monetary, or legal.

History

Conversion disorder is one of many disorders that stem from early concepts of hysteria, which was considered previously in this chapter.

Comparative Nosology

DSM-IV-TR conversion disorder is considered a dissociative disorder in ICD-10. Approximately 30 percent of inpatients diagnosed with DSM-IV-TR conversion disorder have a comorbid dissociative disorder, all of whom report a history of childhood neglect and sexual abuse.

Epidemiology

Reported rates of conversion disorder vary from 11 out of 100,000 to 300 out of 100,000 in general population samples. Five to 16 percent of all psychiatry consultation patients in a general hospital setting have symptoms that are consistent with conversion disorder. Conversion disorder is the focus of treatment in 1 to 3 percent of outpatient referrals to mental health clinics. Some studies suggest a lifetime risk of approximately 33 percent for transient or longer-term conversion symptoms. By contrast, conversion disorder represents less than 1 percent of all admissions to psychiatric hospitals and is infrequently diagnosed in emergency departments. Conversion disorder appears to be more frequent in women than in men, with reported ratios varying from 2 to 1 to 10 to 1. Symptoms are more common on the left than on the right side of the body in women. Women who present with conversion symptoms are more likely to subsequently develop somatization disorder than women who have not had conversion symptoms. There is an association between conversion disorder and antisocial personality disorder in men. The onset of conversion disorder is generally from late childhood to early adulthood and is rare before 10 years of age or after 35 years of age, but onset as late as the ninth decade of life has been reported. When symptoms suggest a conversion disorder onset in middle or old age, the probability of an occult neurological or other medical condition is high. Conversion symptoms in children younger than 10 years of age are usually limited to gait problems or seizures.

Conversion disorder seems to be more common in rural populations, developing nations and regions, people in lower socioeconomic class, and people with less general education and medical knowledge. The form of conversion symptoms may reflect cultural ideas about acceptable ways to express distress. Falling or an alteration of consciousness is a feature of some culture-specific syndromes. On the other hand, behaviors resembling conversion or dissociative symptoms are aspects of certain culturally sanctioned religious and healing ceremonies. Thus, cultural norms are important to consider in making the diagnosis.

Limited data suggest that conversion symptoms are more frequent in relatives of people with conversion disorder. An increased risk of conversion disorder in monozygotic, but not dizygotic, twin pairs has been reported.

Etiology

The term *conversion* arose from the hypothesis that a symptom or deficit represents a symbolic playing out of an unconscious psychological conflict aimed at reducing anxiety about the conflict and serving to keep the conflict out of awareness (primary gain). The individual may also derive secondary gain from the conversion symptom, but these external benefits are generally not the aim of the conversion symptom or deficit. This hypothesis has support from studies that demonstrate that psychotherapy aimed at helping the patient gain insight about the conflict can make the physical conversion worse, and treatment aimed at rehabilitation, allowing the patient to further avoid the conflict, helps resolve the symptoms.

Mr. J. is a 28-year-old single man who is employed in a factory. He was brought to an emergency department by his father, complaining that he had lost his vision while sitting in the back seat on the way home from a family gathering. He had been playing volleyball at the gathering but had sustained no significant injury except for the volleyball hitting him in the head a few times. As was usual for this man, he had been reluctant to play volleyball because of the lack of his athletic skills, and was placed on a team at the last moment. He recalls having some problems with seeing during the game, but his vision did not become ablated until he was in the car on the way home. By the time he got to the emergency department, his vision was improving, although he still complained of blurriness and mild diplopia. The double vision could be attenuated by having him focus on items at different distances.

On examination, Mr. J. was fully cooperative, somewhat uncertain about why this would have occurred, and rather nonchalant. Pupillary, oculomotor, and general sensorimotor examinations were normal. After being cleared medically, the patient was sent to a mental health center for further evaluation.

At the mental health center, the patient recounts the same story as he did in the emergency department, and he was still accompanied by his father. He began to recount how his vision started to return to normal when his father pulled over on the side of the road and began to talk to him about the events of the day. He spoke with his father about how he had felt embarrassed and somewhat conflicted about playing volleyball and how he had felt that he really should play because of external pressures. Further history from the patient and his father revealed that this young man had been shy as an adolescent, particularly around athletic participation. He had never had another episode of visual loss. He did recount feeling anxious and sometimes not feeling well in his body during athletic activities.

Discussion with the patient at the mental health center focused on the potential role of psychological and social factors in acute vision loss. The patient was somewhat perplexed by this but was also amenable to discussion. He stated that he clearly recognized that he began seeing and feeling better when his father pulled off to the side of the road and discussed things with him. Doctors admitted that they did not know the cause of the vision loss and that it would likely not return. The patient and his father were satisfied with the medical and psychiatric evaluation and agreed to return for care if there were any further symptoms. The patient was appointed a follow-up time at the outpatient psychiatric clinic.

Diagnosis and Clinical Features

The essential feature of conversion disorder is that psychological factors are judged to be proximal to and responsible for the presence of symptoms or deficits affecting voluntary motor or sensory function that suggest a neurological or other general medical condition, because the initiation or exacerbation of the symptom or deficit is preceded by conflicts or other stressors (Criteria A and B). The symptoms are not intentionally produced or feigned (Criterion C), and the disorder is not diagnosed if the symptoms or deficits are fully explained by a neurological or other medical condition, by the direct effects of a substance, or as a culturally sanctioned behavior or experience (Criterion D). It is not diagnosed if symptoms are limited to pain or sexual dysfunction, occur only during the course of somatization disorder, or are better accounted for by another mental disorder (Criterion F). The symptoms or deficits cause marked distress, impairment, or the seeking of medical care (Criterion E).

Motor symptoms or deficits include impaired coordination or balance, paralysis or localized weakness, tremor or flaccidity, difficulty swallowing or a sensation of a lump in the throat, aphonia, and urinary retention. Sensory symptoms or deficits include loss of touch or pain sensation, hyperesthesia and paresthesia, double vision, blindness, deafness, and hallucinations. Thus, the clinician can specify two types of conversion disorder: (1) with motor symptom or deficit and (2) with sensory symptom or deficit. Movements that mimic a form of seizures may also occur, but there is a rich academic debate about whether these symptoms are best classified as conversion or as dissociative, and this debate is highlighted by conversion proponents adding a third type: (3) with seizures or convulsions. The clinician can also specify a fourth type: (4) with mixed presentation.

It is perhaps obvious that a diagnosis of conversion disorder should be made only after a thorough medical investigation has been performed to rule out another medical condition as etiological for symptoms or deficits. However, it is only recently that research has demonstrated that misdiagnosis is uncommon, perhaps reflecting increased awareness of the disorder, as well as improved knowledge and diagnostic techniques. Early studies found other medical etiologies to be responsible for the purported illness in approximately one-fourth to one-half of persons initially diagnosed with conversion symptoms. These studies were beset by different methodologies and the problem of attributing causality. Nonetheless, there has been concern among physicians for years that attributing symptoms or deficits to the diagnosis of conversion disorder is deprecatory and medically risky for the patient and lessens the stature of the physician owing to his or her inability to find something real. This attitude can be helpful to a patient because of the insistence to find organic pathology where it is eventually found but, at other times, can relegate a patient to becoming a subject of the obsessive and insecure physician's search for the Holy Grail. The diagnosis of conversion disorder is not just one of exclusion and should be made firmly and tentatively at the same time, with an ever-present eye to the overall biopsychosocial context of patient and symptoms. When the diagnosis is made with too much certainty, other medical illness is missed. When too tentative, multiple and irrational medical evaluations are conducted, and iatrogenic reinforcement and harm are produced.

History and physical examination must be used together to diagnose conversion disorder. As this disorder is not a diagnosis of exclusion, there must be positive data on history and examination that the symptoms or deficits, or both, are functional and possibly transient and not from a stable organic lesion or illness. Taking care to understand history in the context of a thorough examination and vice versa is critical to make or to exclude the diagnosis of conversion disorder. There are no *sine qua non* historical events to make the diagnosis, and there are usually conflicting signs on examination. Table 15–5 demonstrates that historical data generally thought to be helpful for diagnosis have not actually been found to be specific markers. Thus, as a working differential diagnosis is being developed, each diagnosis is proposed and worked through sequentially with history and examination, sometimes in an iterative fashion. Determining that a symptom or deficit is being experienced in the absence of findings consistent with other organic disease and is not being intentionally produced can be difficult. It must be inferred from a careful evaluation of the symptom contextualized by its development, its potential external rewards, or the assumption of the sick role. A history of other unexplained somatic or dissociative symptoms increases the likelihood that the symptoms or deficits are due to conversion disorder, especially if criteria for somatization disorder have been met in the past. A positive history for other medical disorders does not lessen the risk for a conversion disorder unless the current symptoms are clearly of that medical disorder. In fact, a medical illness is a risk factor for conversion disorder, as it is for other somatoform disorders.

A phenomenological problem with conversion disorder is that, although the diagnosis requires that psychological factors be judged proximal to and responsible for the symptoms or deficits, there are no good data that recent psychosocial stressors are sensitive or specific predictors of a conversion reaction. It may be that there are stressors that are associated with conversion disorder, but empirical data about this are lacking. The alternative is that there is no natural

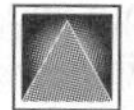

Table 15–5
Relative Diagnostic Validity of Criteria for Conversion Symptoms

Diagnostic Criterion	Validation[a]	Reference(s)[b]
Somatization disorder	3+	7, 8
Associated psychopathology	3+	9
Model for the symptom	2+	8,10
Emotional stress before the onset of symptoms	1+	—
Disturbed sexuality	0–1+	11
Sibling position	0–1+	12, 13
Symptom as symbolism (primary gain)	0	14
Secondary gain	0	8
Hysterical personality	0	—
La belle indifférence	0	8, 15

[a]Expressed on a scale of 0 to 3+, according to established validity.
[b]Reference number in original article.
Adapted from Lazare A: Current concepts in psychiatry. Conversion symptoms. *N Engl J Med.* 1981;305:745.

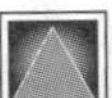

Table 15–6
Distinctive Physical Examination Findings in Conversion Disorder

Condition	Test	Conversion Findings
Anesthesia	Map dermatomes.	Sensory loss does not conform to recognized pattern of distribution.
Hemianesthesia	Check midline.	Strict half-body split.
Astasia-abasia	Walking, dancing.	With suggestion, those who cannot walk may still be able to dance; alteration of sensory and motor findings with suggestion.
Paralysis, paresis	Drop paralyzed hand onto face.	Hand falls next to face, not on it.
	Hoover test.	Pressure noted in examiner's hand under paralyzed leg when attempting straight leg raising.
	Check motor strength.	Give-away weakness.
Coma	Examiner attempts to open eyes.	Resists opening; gaze preference is away from doctor.
	Ocular cephalic maneuver.	Eyes stare straight ahead and do not move from side to side.
Aphonia	Request a cough.	Essentially, normal coughing sound indicates that cords are closing.
Intractable sneezing	Observe.	Short nasal grunts with little or no sneezing on inspiratory phase; little or no aerosolization of secretions; minimal facial expression; eyes open; stops when asleep; abates when alone.
Syncope	Head-up tilt test.	Magnitude of changes in vital signs and venous pooling does not explain continuing symptoms.
Tunnel vision	Visual fields.	Changing pattern on multiple examinations.
Profound monocular blindness	Swinging flash light sign (Marcus Gunn).	Absence of relative afferent papillary defect.
	Binocular visual fields.	Sufficient vision in "bad eye" precludes plotting normal physiological blind spot in good eye.
Severe bilateral blindness	"Wiggle your fingers, I'm just testing coordination."	Patient may begin to mimic new movements before realizing the slip.
	Sudden flash of bright light.	Patient flinches.
	"Look at your hand."	Patient does not look there.
	"Touch your index fingers."	Even blind patients can do this by proprioception.

Adapted from Sadock BJ, Sadock VA. *Kaplan and Sadock's Comprehensive Textbook of Psychiatry.* 7th ed. Philadelphia: Lippincott Williams & Wilkins; 2000:1512.

relationship between stressors and conversion reactions. An epistemological problem surrounds the concept of *psychosocial stress.* Although this concept has been much discussed through medical history and across disease states, measuring it outside of experimental conditions remains as crude as it is difficult. Thus, in spite of the lack of experimental evidence, the notion that recent stressors are causal to conversion is a long-standing intellectual commitment for psychiatry, one that has been developed over centuries from a plethora of theoretical writings from forceful thinkers, and one that is thus difficult to abandon. DSM-IV-TR sits firmly on this fragile fence by not using the words "cause" or "responsible for" in Criterion B. Rather, the phrase "psychological factors are judged to be associated with the symptom or deficit" supports history and science by indicating that there is believed to be a relationship between stressors and conversion reactions, even though science has not yet proven it.

This paradox is also present with the concept of *la belle indifférence*, which, since the time of Pierre Janet, has been used to characterize the lack of concern about profound symptoms or deficits seen in these patients. This is a striking phenomenon to observe and goes by the synonym *denial* in the patient with myocardial infarction and *neglect* in the neurologically impaired patient. Although *la belle indifférence* is also hard to measure, there is no good evidence that it is more common in conversion disorder than in other medical disorders.

Pathology The lack of tissue pathology and symptoms and signs that do not correlate well is the pathology seen in conversion disorder. Conversion symptoms typically do not conform to known anatomical pathways and physiological mechanisms but instead follow the individual's conceptualization of his or her illness. Table 15–6 shows examples of various conversion symptoms and their physical examination findings that demonstrate that conversion patterns do not conform to anatomically known patterns and may change on multiple examinations and with suggestion. Expert skill with examination procedures is indispensable for the proper diagnosis of conversion disorder, and there are multiple text chapters on how to conduct such examinations. However, knowledge of anatomical and physiological mechanisms is incomplete, and available methods of objective assessment have limitations. This is highlighted in a study of patients with psychogenic nonepileptic seizures (PNESs), comparing them to subjects with other somatoform disorders and healthy controls. The subjects with PNESs reported more minor head injuries in the past than did the two comparison groups, and the PNES group had more nonspecific electroencephalogram (EEG) dysrhythmias on EEG. The mean number of comorbid psychiatric diagnoses was higher in the PNES group (1.9 ± 0.3 compared to 1.5 ± 0.5 in the somatoform group). Ten of 23 PNES patients also had a somatoform pain disorder, and seven had an undifferentiated somatoform disorder.

No specific laboratory abnormalities are associated with conversion disorder. In fact, the absence of findings supports the diagnosis of conversion disorder. However, laboratory findings consistent with another medical condition do not exclude the diagnosis of conversion disorder, because the diagnosis requires that the symptoms or deficits not be fully explained by the other medical condition.

Experimental psychophysiology has suggested two abnormalities in conversion disorder. First, when given increasingly higher anxiogenic stimuli, conversion subjects have increasing levels of sympathetic nervous system (SNS) discharge, as measured by skin conductance, up to a moderately high level, and then SNS discharge levels off. In contrast, anxiety disorder subjects continue to have higher SNS discharge to higher levels of anxiogenic stimuli. Second, conversion subjects may have more rapid cortical evoked potential spikes in contralateral sensory cortex than in ipsilateral cortex to

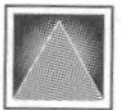

Table 15–7
Medical Disorders in the Differential Diagnosis of Conversion Disorder

Myasthenia gravis
Systemic lupus erythematosus
Periodic paralysis
Brain tumor
Multiple sclerosis
Optic neuritis
Partial vocal cord paralysis
Guillain-Barré syndrome
On-off syndrome of Parkinson's disease
Degenerative neurological diseases
Acquired myopathies
Idiopathic and sarcoma-induced osteomalacia
Subdural hematoma
Acquired, hereditary, and drug-induced dystonias
Creutzfeldt-Jakob (prion) disease
Early manifestations of acquired immune deficiency syndrome

physical stimuli, suggesting that the affected paralytic limb is actually more sensitized to stimuli, even though the subject states that he or she has no sensation.

Other psychopathology that is commonly comorbid with conversion disorder includes mood and anxiety disorders on Axis I in approximately 25 to 50 percent of patients and Cluster B personality disorders on Axis II in approximately 10 to 40 percent of patients.

Differential Diagnosis

The most important conditions in the differential diagnosis are *neurological* or other *medical disorders* and *substance-induced disorders*. Appropriate evaluation for these conditions includes a careful history of the current symptoms and context, a thorough medical history, complete neurological and general physical examinations that focus on detection of signs to include or to exclude medical illness, and appropriate laboratory studies, which may include urine or serum toxicology. Thorough documentation of the history, examination, context, laboratory tests, and clinician impression of the factors ruling in or out various medical conditions is important to alleviate further unnecessary medical evaluations. Table 15–7 lists some of the more frequent neurological, other medical, and substance conditions that need to be considered in the differential diagnosis. *Partial complex seizure disorders* and *autoimmune disorders* may be misdiagnosed for years, given the variability in symptomatology and the undulating nature of the illnesses. Approximately 30 percent of systemic lupus erythematosus cases present with predominantly neuropsychiatric symptoms or deficits, or both, usually mania or psychosis.

Other somatoform and psychiatric disorders are prominent in the differential diagnosis of conversion. If the symptoms or deficits are limited to pain or sexual function, then a *pain disorder* or a *sexual disorder* is diagnosed instead of conversion disorder. An additional diagnosis of conversion disorder is not made if the symptoms or deficits occur only during the course of *somatization disorder.* The differential must include *body dysmorphic disorder*, for which the emphasis is on a preoccupation with an imagined or slight defect in appearance, rather than a change in voluntary motor or sensory function. *Hypochondriasis* must be considered in the differential, although it distinguishes itself from conversion by disease phobia, not necessarily symptoms or loss of function. *Factitious* and *malingering disorders* need to be considered. Both of these disorders share the feature of intentionally produced symptoms, which distinguish them from conversion disorder. However, determining whether symptoms are volitional is usually not an easy task. The presence of catatonia or somatic delusions must bring to consideration *schizophrenia* or other *psychotic disorders*, including a *mood disorder with psychotic features*. It is controversial whether hallucinations should be considered as the presenting symptom of conversion disorder. When they do occur in conversion disorder, they generally present without other psychotic symptoms, often involve more than one sensory modality, and often have a vague or fantastic content. High anxiety states are associated with multiple somatic symptoms or deficits that are sometimes sudden in onset. For example, difficulty swallowing may be associated with a panic attack in the course of *panic disorder* or a *phobic disorder*. It is becoming increasingly understood that early adverse life experiences can lead to a chronic and undulating course of *PTSD*, which may be associated with symptoms or loss of function in body areas that were involved in the traumatic experience. Thus, a careful history of trauma type and residual posttrauma symptoms is essential when thinking about the differential diagnosis of conversion disorder.

Conversion disorder shares features with *dissociative disorders*. Both involve symptoms that suggest neurological involvement, they may have antecedent stressors, and the history may be difficult to obtain, partly because of the nature of the symptoms. At present, if a patient meets criteria for conversion and dissociative symptoms, both diagnoses can be made.

Course and Prognosis

The onset of conversion disorder is usually acute, but a crescendo of symptomatology may also occur. Symptoms or deficits are usually of short duration, and approximately 95 percent of acute cases remit spontaneously, usually within 2 weeks in hospitalized patients. If symptoms have been present for 6 months or greater, the prognosis for symptom resolution is less than 50 percent and diminishes further the longer that conversion is present. Recurrence occurs in one-fifth to one-fourth of people within 1 year of the first episode. Thus, one episode is a predictor for future episodes. A good prognosis is heralded by acute onset, presence of clearly identifiable stressors at the time of onset, a short interval between onset and the institution of treatment, and above average intelligence. Paralysis, aphonia, and blindness are associated with a good prognosis, whereas tremor and seizures are poor prognostic factors.

Treatment

In acute cases without a previous history of conversion, accurate reassurance coupled with reasonable rehabilitation to fit the symptoms is warranted. The longer the symptoms remain, the more aggressive the rehabilitation should be. Confrontation of the patient about the so-called false nature of the symptoms is contraindicated. Psychotherapy is a relative contraindication, but attention to the patient's psychosocial needs is likely to be a valuable contribution to symptom resolution. In acute cases with a history of conversion, reassurance and suggestion of recovery coupled with early rehabilitation are the treatments of choice. If symptoms continue, more aggressive rehabilitation is indicated.

Chronic cases are more difficult to treat. As with acute cases, comorbid psychiatric illnesses need to be treated aggressively. Treatment then needs to begin with another thorough and rational evaluation, open explanation to the patient about the findings, and education aimed at helping the patient understand that, although the symptoms are real and are causing impairment, there is hope for a full recovery. This education focuses on the real, although not well-understood, psychophysiological mechanisms that are likely contributing to the illness and how rehabilitation can change these mechanisms back to normal, because the physiological pathways in question are likely intact. Three specific treatments must then be considered.

First, psychomotor and sensory rehabilitation is useful when aggressively pursued by an experienced multidisciplinary team consisting of physiatrists, psychiatrists, and physical and occupational therapists. Early rehabilitation aimed at the dysfunction coupled with motivational interviewing, reassurance, and suggestion may be followed by the ethical use of placing the patient in a *double-bind* if the initial treatment is not successful. The double-bind works on the principle that the patient's symptoms or deficits are being maintained to avoid psychological or social conflict, or both, and that the unconscious will do anything, even get better, to avoid discussing the conflict. Thus, lack of progress is interpreted to the patient as being due to one of three possible reasons: (1) The patient is not trying to get better, which constitutes a reason to end treatment; (2) the symptoms are caused by excessive overstimulation and fatigue, which would necessitate periods of deep rest without stimulation of any kind; or (3) the continued symptoms are due to deep-seated psychological conflicts, which would necessitate long-term psychotherapy and discussion of these conflicts. The patient agrees that the second choice is the most likely cause, because he or she neither wants to lose the therapeutic relationship nor wants to engage in interpersonal therapy. Treatment proceeds to have the patient work hard with intermittent periods of deep rest, which means no reading, no television watching, and no social contact. This encourages the patient to engage in treatment sessions to avoid deep rest periods and to gain rightful discharge. If the patient likes the deep rest periods, then the alternative explanations for failure to improve need to be discussed again. This technique has proven useful to refractory cases when conducted on an inpatient rehabilitation unit.

Second, pharmacotherapy may be useful. Anxiolytic and antidepressant medications may decrease some of the symptoms to allow the patient to engage in physical rehabilitation or psychotherapy. Medication-induced sedation therapy, such as an amobarbital (Amytal) interview, may be useful to gain information about early or hidden conflicts and may facilitate integration of this information by the patient under skilled therapeutic supervision. Infusion of 50-mg doses of amobarbital is administered in a dextrose 5 percent in water (D5W) solution over 5 minutes every 30 to 40 minutes, until the patient is sleepy, usually requiring between 100 and 700 mg per interview. Standard practice is that another person in addition to the therapist is present and that a crash cart is available for use by a capable clinician in the event of severe respiratory depression. The interview is meant to relate symptoms to events, proximal or remote, and to elicit from the patient ways to ameliorate the symptoms or conflicts. Videotaping may be useful as feedback to the patient, when appropriate, to augment therapist interpretation.

Finally, psychotherapy may be useful but also may be contraindicated in a patient who remains highly resistant to it or who gets worse when it is initiated. Therapy is directed at increasing function and having the patient demonstrate to himself or herself that the symptom or deficit is alterable and that it is also related to psychological or social phenomena, or both. There is no strong support for any given type of psychotherapy, and further empirical work is needed to improve knowledge about how and when to apply psychological therapies.

BODY DYSMORPHIC DISORDER

Definition *Body dysmorphic disorder* is characterized by a preoccupation with an imagined defect in appearance that causes clinically significant distress or impairment in important areas of functioning. If a slight physical anomaly is actually present, the person's concern with the anomaly is excessive and bothersome.

History Body dysmorphic disorder was initially classified in the United States as the atypical somatoform disorder *dysmorphophobia* in DSM-III in 1980. It has been described in many parts of the world with various names over the past 150 years. Over this history, body dysmorphic disorder has often been described as a disorder with obsessive and neurotic features about one's body coupled with intense shame and self-loathing.

Comparative Nosology Body dysmorphic disorder is included in the ICD-10 diagnosis of *hypochondriacal disorder*.

Epidemiology The epidemiology of body dysmorphic disorder is not well understood. In a cross-sectional sample of 318 depressed and 658 nondepressed women between 36 and 44 years of age who were selected from seven Boston metropolitan area communities, the overall point prevalence was 0.7 percent and was significantly associated with the presence of major depression and anxiety disorders. Other studies estimate community prevalence between 1.0 and 2.2 percent and prevalence in dermatology and cosmetic surgery clinics between 6 and 15 percent.

Etiology The neurobiology of body dysmorphic disorder is not known. Given the high comorbidity of depression and obsessive features and the reputed benefits of SSRI medication in body dysmorphic disorder, it is assumed that frontal, serotonin pathways are involved in body dysmorphic disorder. Sociocultural bases for body dysmorphic disorder are more clear. The epidemiology varies between geographical region and gender, as do concepts of body normality, perhaps making body dysmorphic disorder the somatoform disorder with the strongest sociocultural basis. There is an extensive literature describing how culture influences individual experience of psychopathology, and the clinical manifestations, course, diagnosis, treatment, and treatment outcomes of psychiatric illness. Predominant social contexts become internalized as psychobiology, and pathogenesis is influenced by an ongoing sociocultural fabric and a biogenetic substrate. This is why excessive bodily preoccupation varies in type, clinical manifestation, and consequent behavior across the world.

Ms. J., a 30-year-old single unemployed woman, presents to a psychiatrist with this chief complaint: "My biggest wish is to be invisible so that no one can see how ugly I am. My biggest fear is that people are laughing at me thinking I'm ugly." In reality, Ms. J. is an attractive woman who has been preoccupied with her supposed ugliness since 12 years of age. At that time, she became "obsessed" with her nose, which she thought was too "big and shiny." Before the onset of this concern, Ms. J. had been confident, a good student, and socially active. However, as a result of her fixation on her nose, she became socially withdrawn and was unable to concentrate in school; her grades plummeted from As to Ds and Fs.

At age 18 years, Ms. J. dropped out of school because of her concern about her nose. Shortly after this, she took a job she disliked and, at that time, also became excessively focused on her minimal acne. She frequently picked at her few "blemishes"—sometimes all night long—with tweezers and needles, a behavior she found difficult to resist. Over the following years, Ms. J. developed additional excessive preoccupations with the appearance of her hair, which "wasn't smooth and neat enough"; her breasts, which she thought were too small; her supposedly thin lips; and her supposedly large buttocks. Ms. J. thinks about her "defects" nearly all day long and states that "I always have two tapes playing—one saying not to worry and the other saying I'm ugly."

Ms. J. frequently checks her supposed defects in mirrors and other reflecting surfaces, such as windows, car bumpers, and spoons. Before she can leave her house, she asks her family members "at least 30 times" whether she looks OK, but she cannot be reassured by their responses. She also combs her hair excessively and attempts to camouflage her supposed defects with clothing, posture, and elaborate makeup that takes several hours a day to apply. Despite her efforts to hide her "ugliness," Ms. J. thinks that others are probably taking special notice of her, staring at her or laughing at her behind her back. She sometimes drives through red lights, because she is "unable to tolerate people looking at me." On one occasion, when she was stuck in a traffic jam, Ms. J. became so anxious over her belief that other drivers were staring at her nose, skin, and hair that she fled her car and left it in the middle of the highway.

Ms. J. thinks that her view of her appearance and her belief that others are ridiculing her are probably accurate. However, she is able to acknowledge that she has "a small amount of doubt" about her beliefs, noting that it is possible—although unlikely—that she has a distorted view of her defects. Nonetheless, Ms. J. occasionally briefly feels "100 percent" convinced that she is hideously ugly and is "completely certain" that others are taking special notice of her, as happened when she abandoned her car. At these times, she firmly believes that the neighbors are staring at her through binoculars, and she hides where she thinks they cannot see her.

As a result of her preoccupation with her appearance, Ms. J. has been able to work only briefly and intermittently. She became increasingly socially isolated and avoided dating and other social interactions. As her concern intensified, Ms. J. began to go out only at night when she could not be seen. Finally, after more than a decade of symptoms, Ms. J. stopped working altogether and went on disability. She also became completely housebound, even hiding when relatives came to visit. As she explains, "I didn't leave my house because I didn't want people to see how ugly I was." Although Ms. J. relies on her family members to buy her clothes, food, and other necessities, she is unable to tell them about her concerns about her appearance, because she is too embarrassed. She has become increasingly depressed, with poor sleep, appetite, and energy, and has suicidal ideation. As a result of her social isolation and her feelings of hopelessness about her appearance, Ms. J. has made two suicide attempts and has been hospitalized on several occasions.

Before she became housebound, Ms. J. received antibiotics from several dermatologists, but this did not alleviate her concerns about her appearance. She was refused a rhinoplasty by a plastic surgeon she consulted. Ms. J. also sought outpatient psychiatric treatment but was never able to discuss her preoccupations with her therapist, because she was too embarrassed to do so.

Diagnosis and Clinical Features The critical feature to make the diagnosis of body dysmorphic disorder is preoccupation with an imagined defect in one's body or any of its parts or markedly excessive concern about a slight physical defect (Criterion A). To meet diagnostic criteria, as in other disorders, this critical feature (dysmorphophobia) must cause significant distress or impairment in social, occupational, or other important areas of functioning (Criterion B) and must not be better accounted for by another mental disorder (Criterion C). Assessment instruments with acceptable psychometric properties have been developed to specifically assess body dysmorphic disorder (e.g., the Body Dysmorphic Disorder Examination and the Yale-Brown Obsessive-Compulsive Scale modified for Body Dysmorphic Disorder).

Determining Criterion C, that dysmorphophobia is not due to another mental disorder, can be challenging. People with *anorexia nervosa* have the perception that they are obese when they are not. It is common for people with *schizophrenia* to think that a part or parts of their body are distorted or defective when there is no objective evidence of a defect. Highly anxious and depressed people or those with *PTSD* believe that something is wrong with their body, and this may take the form of dysmorphophobia. Effective treatment of these other disorders does not always make the concern with body abate. Finally, body dysmorphic disorder is highly comorbid with anxiety, affective, and eating disorders, although this epidemiology is not well known.

Imagined or exaggerated flaws of the face and head are the most common symptoms in body dysmorphic disorder, such as wrinkles and scars, vascular markings, paleness or redness of the complexion, swelling, acne and other lesions, facial asymmetry or disproportion, hair thinning, or excessive facial hair. Other imagined or exaggerated defects include the size or shape of the nose, eyes or their components, ears, mouth, lips, teeth, jaw, chin, cheeks, or head. Other body parts may be the dysmorphobic focus as well, and this may include highly specific parts, such as the shape of a finger; larger body areas, such as the shape of the hips; or even the size or shape of the whole body. Pathological preoccupation may focus on several body parts simultaneously. Getting an accurate history may be challenging owing to the high level of embarrassment that some people have about their imagined defects, the person's perception and description of the defects, and the fear by the person that physicians will not take them seriously. Thus, they avoid describing their imagined or real, slight defects in detail and may instead refer only to the general shame or ugliness of their body.

The most common personality features associated with body dysmorphic disorder include obsessional and avoidant traits, although any cluster of traits may be present, and no single personality trait or disorder dominates as comorbid with body dysmorphic disorder. These patients are shy, have a history of being highly sensitive to remarks about their body, and can often remember a single event in which negative comments about their body were associated with the onset of bothersome preoccupation with body image. If the disorder begins in early adolescence, it is likely followed by a history of having fewer friends than others, dating less than others, and being more isolated than their peers.

Many individuals with this disorder describe their preoccupations as being intensely painful. Ideas of reference related to the imagined defect are also common, in which people with this disorder think that others are taking special notice of their reported flaw. Some individuals are preoccupied with thoughts that their flawed body part will fail them. Thus, the preoccupations are bothersome and not desired, but the belief about the presence of the imagined defect is ego-syntonic. In fact, body dysmorphic disorder patients have difficulty controlling their bodily preoccupations, and they usually make little or no attempt to resist them because they believe that they have the imagined defect. As with hypochondriasis, a subset of people with body dysmorphic disorder cannot easily be convinced or reassured that the imagined defect is not present. Thus, there is a debate about whether there is a subset of body dysmorphic disorder patients that should more accurately be diagnosed with a *delusional disorder*.

As a result of this conflictual relationship between the dislike of the preoccupation and the belief that they are defective, people with body dysmorphic disorder often spend hours a day thinking about their defect, and these thoughts and subsequent behaviors may dominate their lives. Checking the defect in any available reflecting surface may consume many hours of their day. Some individuals use magnifying glasses to scrutinize their defect and conduct excessive grooming behavior. These mental and physical behaviors are intended to diminish anxiety about the defect, but, as in all pathological anxiety states, the behaviors actually reinforce and intensify not only the anxiety, distress, and isolation, but also the frequency and strength of the behaviors. Consequently, this disorder becomes so distressing that some people with body dysmorphic disorder then spend a lot of time and energy avoiding mirrors and other checking accoutrements and further isolate to prevent anxiety. They may instead try to camouflage the defect by using excessive makeup or padded clothing. In severe cases, individuals may leave their homes only at night so that they cannot be seen, or may become housebound. They may quit their jobs, drop out of school, or work below their capacity in an attempt to hide. Further maladaptive behaviors ensue. The distress and dysfunction associated with body dysmorphic disorder, although variable, can lead to repeated hospitalization, suicide attempts, and completed suicide.

Some people with body dysmorphic disorder try to solve the conflict and distress by getting help in medical, not psychiatric, settings. They may first go for frequent requests for diagnosis of or reassurance about the defect, but such reassurance leads to only temporary, if any, relief. After engaging in a pattern of comparing their body to those of others by observing others in the natural environment or in magazines or on television, they often decide to obtain medical or surgical care, or both. In cases in which self-evaluation has been highly distorted, and the expectations for medical or surgical care are inappropriately high, such treatment may cause the disorder to worsen, leading to intensified or new preoccupations. This may lead to further unsuccessful procedures, so that these individuals eventually have a synthetic-looking body part. As with all psychopathology, the very elements of the disorder that are intended to be used as a helpful defense become maladaptive, and, in the case of body dysmorphic disorder, the psychopathology is literally worn on the patient's sleeve, or on the nose, face, or breasts, as it were. It is one of the disorders in psychiatry in which the maladaptive psychological defense may become visible.

Body dysmorphic disorder is highly comorbid with affective, anxiety, substance use, and eating disorders. Studies about the epidemiological and pathogenesis of these disorders are lacking. There is some evidence that high anxiety states more commonly predate body dysmorphic disorder, whereas depression and substance use disorders are more a result of chronic body dysmorphic disorder, but more investigation of these relationships is needed.

Pathology There is no known neurobiological pathology in body dysmorphic disorder. One preliminary study showed caudate asymmetry similar to that seen in OCD. The psychopathology was described previously and also demonstrates a strong relationship to anxiety disorders.

Differential Diagnosis The primary condition in the differential diagnosis is somewhat excessive, but nonpathological, concerns with body features and appearance. Unlike *normal concerns about appearance*, the preoccupation with appearance and specific imagined defects in body dysmorphic disorder and the changed behavior because of the preoccupation are excessively time consuming and are associated with significant distress or impairment. There is a significant lay and academic literature about the quest for certain body types and body features in modern U.S. culture. There is also evidence that, for some individuals, exercise, body shaping, and cosmetic surgery designed to change body appearance can be helpful psychologically. Conversely, there is also evidence that these behaviors can be maladaptive and harmful to an individual's psychological and social development.

The diagnosis of body dysmorphic disorder should not be made if the excessive bodily preoccupation is better accounted for by another psychiatric disorder. Excessive bodily preoccupation is generally restricted to concerns about being fat in *anorexia nervosa*, to discomfort with or a sense of wrongness about his or her primary and secondary sex characteristics occurring in *gender identity disorder*, and to mood-congruent cognitions involving appearance that occur exclusively during a *major depressive episode*. Individuals with *avoidant personality disorder* or *social phobia* may worry about being embarrassed by imagined or real defects in appearance, but this concern is usually not prominent, persistent, distressing, or impairing. *Taijin kyofu-sho*, a diagnosis in Japan, is similar to *social phobia* but has some features that are more consistent with body dysmorphic disorder, such as the belief that the person has an offensive odor or body parts that are offensive to others. Although individuals with body dysmorphic disorder have obsessional preoccupations about their appearance and may have associated compulsive behaviors (e.g., mirror checking), a separate or additional diagnosis of *OCD* is made only when the obsessions or compulsions are not restricted to concerns about appearance and are ego-dystonic. An additional diagnosis of *delusional disorder, somatic type* can be made in people with body dysmorphic disorder only if their preoccupation with the imagined defect in appearance is held with a delusional intensity.

Course and Prognosis Body dysmorphic disorder usually begins during adolescence, although it may begin later after a protracted dissatisfaction with body. Age of onset is not well understood because there is variably long delay between symptom onset and treatment seeking. The onset may be gradual or abrupt. The disorder usually has a long and undulating course with few symptom-free intervals. The part of the body on which concern is focused may remain the same or may change over time.

The prognosis with and without treatment is not well understood. Reassurance is not thought to be effective, but it may be that adolescents with a gradual onset are reassured in their home or social context quite often and never are detected by the medical profession. It is also not clear whether an abrupt or gradual onset of the disorder is a higher risk for symptom continuation.

Treatment It appears that many individuals with body dysmorphic disorder receive nonpsychiatric medical treatment and surgery. One study that assessed this issue in 289 individuals (250 adults and 39 children and adolescents) with DSM-IV-TR body dysmorphic disorder found that 66 percent of adults received nonpsychiatric treatment. Dermatological treatment was most often received (45 percent), followed by surgery (23 percent). These treatments rarely improved body dysmorphic disorder symptoms. Results were similar in children and adolescents. These findings suggest that a majority of patients with body dysmorphic disorder receive nonpsychiatric treatment and tend to have a poor outcome.

Randomized, controlled studies support the efficacy of individual and group CBT for the treatment of body dysmorphic disorder. Research on the pharmacotherapy of body dysmorphic disorder is limited. There is evidence from one open-label study and one placebo-controlled study that SSRIs may be effective for body dysmorphic disorder. In a published chart-review study of 90 patients with DSM-IV-TR body dysmorphic disorder treated for as long as 8 years by the authors in their clinical practice, 87 subjects received an adequate dose of an SSRI, and 63 percent had improvement in body dysmorphic disorder symptoms. Similar response rates were obtained for each type of SSRI. Discontinuation of an effective SSRI resulted in relapse in 84 percent of cases. Augmentation of the SSRI with clomipramine (Anafranil), buspirone (BuSpar), lithium (Eskalith), methylphenidate (Ritalin), or antipsychotics improved the response rate between 15 and 44 percent.

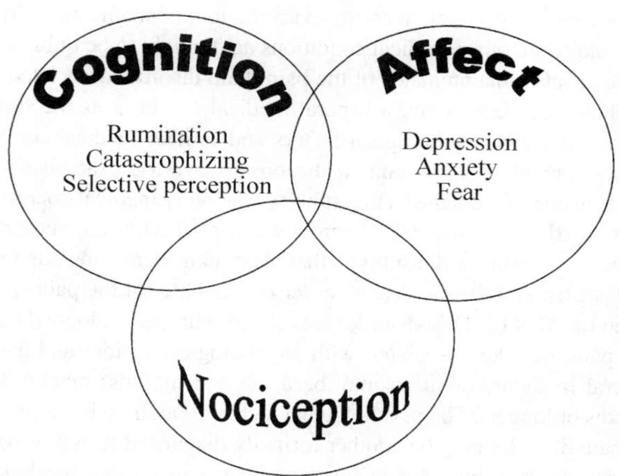

FIGURE 15–3 Elements of pain perception.

PAIN DISORDER

Definition

A *pain disorder* is characterized by the presence of and focus on pain in one or more body sites and is severe enough to come to clinical attention. Psychological factors are necessary in the genesis, severity, or maintenance of the pain, which causes significant distress or impairment, or both. The physician does not have to judge the pain to be "inappropriate" or "in excess of what would be expected," as these DSM-III criteria are not reliably applied. Rather, the phenomenological and diagnostic focus is on the importance of psychological factors and the degree of impairment caused by the pain.

Comparative Nosology

The ICD-10 has a similar category called *persistent somatoform pain disorder*, which is not divided into subtypes by the presumed role of psychological factors as in the DSM-IV-TR. The ICD-10 excludes back pain, tension and migraine headache, and general muscle tension from the diagnosis. The ICD-10 retains an approach similar to the DSM-III-R in which psychological factors are judged to be the primary cause of the pain, whereas the DSM-IV-TR now specifies genesis, severity, or maintenance of pain, or a combination of these, as different elements of the pain disorder on which the important psychological factors may act.

The Subcommittee on Taxonomy of the International Association for the Study of Pain proposed a five-axis system for categorizing chronic pain according to (1) anatomical region, (2) organ system, (3) temporal characteristics of pain and pattern of occurrence, (4) the patient's statement of intensity and time since the onset of pain, and (5) etiology. This five-axis system focuses primarily on the physical manifestations of pain. It provides for psychological factors on the second axis, where a mental disorder can be coded, and on the fifth axis, where possible etiologies include *psychophysiological* and *psychological*.

Epidemiology

The prevalence of pain disorder appears to be common. Recent work indicates that the 6-month and lifetime prevalence is approximately 5 percent and 12 percent, respectively. It has been estimated that 10 to 15 percent of adults in the United States have some form of work disability due to back pain alone in any year. Approximately 3 percent of people in a general practice have persistent pain with at least one day per month of activity restriction due to the pain.

Pain disorder may begin at any age. The gender ratio is unknown. Pain disorder is associated with other psychiatric disorders, especially affective and anxiety disorders. Chronic pain appears to be most frequently associated with depressive disorders, and acute pain appears to be more commonly associated with anxiety disorders. The associated psychiatric disorders may precede the pain disorder, may cooccur with it, or may result from it. Depressive disorders, alcohol dependence, and chronic pain may be more common in relatives of individuals with chronic pain disorder. Individuals whose pain is associated with severe depression and those whose pain is related to a terminal illness, such as cancer, are at increased risk for suicide. There may be differences in how various ethnic and cultural groups respond to pain, but the usefulness of cultural factors for the clinician remains obscure to the treatment of individuals with pain disorder because of a lack of good data and because of high individual variability.

Etiology

The cause of pain in general is complicated and is not pertinent to this chapter. What is important are the mechanisms thought to underlie how pain is physiologically and perceptually enhanced by psychological factors, such as emotion and cognition. Figure 15–3 demonstrates a relationship between nociception, cognition, and affect, in which all three interact to either enhance or diminish pain perception. There is physiological evidence to support the interaction between these three elements in the gating and learning theories of pain perception. Furthermore, treatment such as mindfulness meditation and pain medication has been shown to change these relationships, as if the three circles are being pulled apart from each other, diminishing the interaction that enhances pain perception.

Diagnosis and Clinical Features

The critical diagnostic feature of pain disorder is that pain is the predominant focus of the clinical presentation and is of sufficient severity to warrant clinical attention (Criterion A) and that psychological factors are considered significant in the onset, severity, exacerbation, or maintenance of the pain (Criterion C). As in all psychiatric disorders, the pain causes significant distress or impairment in important areas of functioning (Criterion B) and is not due to other disorders considered in the discussion of differential diagnosis (Criteria D and E).

The diagnosis of pain disorder is divided into subtypes that best characterize the factors involved in the etiology and maintenance of the pain. Pain disorder associated with psychological factors is the subtype diagnosed when psychological factors are judged to have the major role in the onset, severity, exacerbation, or maintenance of the pain and when other medical conditions are thought to be unimportant to the onset or maintenance of the pain. Pain disorder associated with psychological factors and a general medical condition is the subtype diagnosed when psychological factors and another medical condition are thought to be important to the onset, severity, exacerbation, or maintenance of the pain. In this subtype, the other medical condition is an Axis III diagnosis. Pain disorder associated with another general medical condition is the subtype that is not considered an Axis I mental disorder, and the medical disorder responsible for the pain is diagnosed on Axis III. Pain disorder associated with psychological factors and pain disorder associated with psychological factors and another general medical condition may be acute (<6 months) or chronic (6 months or longer). The psychological factors thought to be responsible for pain disorder may be another formally diagnosed Axis I or Axis II disorder or may be other factors that do not reach the threshold for another diagnosis (e.g., personality traits or reactions to social stressors). Examples of diagnostic levels of impairment resulting from the pain include diminished capacity or attendance at school or work, high or expensive use of health care, and interpersonal and social problems, such as marital disruption or discord in the social environment due to pain behavior.

Illness behavior is the observed manifestation of pain disorder, because pain is a reported subjective phenomenon. Clinicians may use any of various pain scales available to help determine the severity, place, and quality of pain. These scales may also help the clinician determine if there is a reliably reported pattern of pain, and, in this way, scales may help with the differential diagnosis. However, the interpersonal and social nature of the disability is the most reliably measured aspect of pain disorder, and treatment is best aimed at improving function and not necessarily ablating pain. Observing the quality and quantity of the many severe disruptions in various aspects of daily life—such as unemployment, family problems, and dependence and addiction on medications and other substances—and their association to various psychological gains and losses is an important measure in the development of a therapeutic plan.

It is important to commence treatment aimed at decreasing inactivity and social isolation as aggressively and as soon as possible to diminish the risk of further psychological and social problems.

Pathology In pain disorder associated with psychological factors and another general medical condition, testing may reveal pathology that is associated with the medical condition that is partly responsible for the pain (e.g., finding of a herniated lumbar disc on a magnetic resonance imaging [MRI] scan in an individual with low-back pain). There is no known histopathology for pain disorder associated with psychological factors.

Differential Diagnosis The most important conditions in the differential diagnosis are *other medical disorders* causing pain that have been overlooked. It is well established that the ability to measure pain from the variety of sources and mechanisms is not adequate. It is not uncommon for pain to be present because of a disorder that cannot be well detected or due to a mechanism for which enough is not yet known. This is reflected in the fact that *dyspareunia*, for example, is excluded from the diagnosis of pain disorder. There is evidence that people may develop pain in early stages of illnesses such as rheumatoid arthritis or malignancies that are clinically below detection methods. *Myofascial pain* syndromes are common, are often overlooked in general medical practice, and are evaluated by a skilled musculoskeletal examination. Thus, in the early stages of the diagnostic process for pain disorder, the clinician is well advised to carefully revisit the possibility of other medical disorders while not iatrogenically reinforcing the pain disorder and misperceptions of its cause by the patient.

Other somatoform disorders are to be considered in the differential diagnosis of pain disorder. Pain symptoms may be part of the symptomatology in *somatization disorder.* However, if the pain occurs exclusively during the course of *somatization disorder*, an additional diagnosis of pain disorder associated with psychological factors is not made. Pain complaints may also be prominent in individuals with *conversion disorder*, but, by definition, conversion disorder is not limited to pain symptoms. Pain symptoms may be intentionally produced or feigned in *factitious disorder* or *malingering*.

Pain symptoms are commonly associated with other psychiatric disorders, such as *major depression*, *anxiety disorders*, and *psychotic disorders*, in which pain may be partly due to nociceptive phenomena or may be delusional. An additional diagnosis of pain disorder should be considered only if the pain is an independent focus of clinical attention and meets other diagnostic criteria for pain disorder. The relationship between other psychiatric disorders and pain has received much theoretical and empirical attention. Pain disorder is not a somatic analog of depression, but depression interacts with pain disorder to worsen the course and prognosis. Anxiety is not thought to cause pain but can increase catecholamines and corticotropin-releasing factor, both of which are associated with enhanced pain perception. Because of the common comorbidity and the relationship between some of the mechanisms of pain disorder and other psychiatric disorders, empirical treatment of the diagnosed psychiatric disorder is important to diminish pain and to determine which disorder is primary.

Course and Prognosis Acute pain disorders have a more favorable prognosis than chronic pain disorders. There is a wide range of variability in the onset and course of chronic pain disorder. In many cases, the pain has been present for many years by the time the individual comes to psychiatric care, owing to the reluctance of patient and physician to see pain as a psychiatric disorder. People with pain disorder who resume participation in regularly scheduled activities despite the pain have a more favorable prognosis than people who allow the pain to become the determining factor in their lifestyle.

Treatment A metaanalysis of 11 studies showed that antidepressants decreased pain intensity significantly more than placebo in patients with psychogenic pain or somatoform pain disorder. The overall effect sizes were moderate (mean Cohen's d, 0.48; range, 0 to 0.91). Positive effects of autogenic relaxation training in at least three studies were found for somatoform pain disorder, unspecified type, and tension headache and migraine, as well as for mild to moderate essential hypertension, coronary heart disease, asthma, Raynaud's disease, anxiety disorders, mild to moderate depression and dysthymia, and functional sleep disorders.

There are single or uncontrolled studies that indicate possible benefit for other treatments. In one, fluvoxamine (Luvox) was significantly more likely than placebo to reduce pain intensity and to normalize urinary flow rates in men with prostatodynia. This therapeutic effect could not be attributed to change in mood, as the two groups did not differ with respect to affective ratings at the end of the study. The fluvoxamine-treated group also had significantly lower final scores on the General Health Questionnaire, indicating an overall benefit from pain relief. In two other studies, inpatient rehabilitation aimed at improving functioning was shown to decrease pain, to increase functioning, and to decrease short-term health care use. Another feature of one of these studies of 200 people with chronic back pain was the high rate of comorbid psychiatric illnesses and their temporal relationship to back pain. The results indicated that certain psychiatric syndromes appear to precede chronic low-back pain (substance abuse and anxiety disorders), whereas others (specifically, major depression) develop before or after the onset of chronic low-back pain. One literature review concluded that exercise may reduce pain, but further studies are needed to examine this relationship. One study did not support the clinical practice of adding low-dose neuroleptics to low-dose antidepressants in the treatment of somatoform pain disorder. Mindfulness meditation has been shown to reduce pain significantly and to increase functioning in approximately 70 percent of people with chronic pain that has been refractory to prior treatment.

UNDIFFERENTIATED SOMATOFORM DISORDER

Definition *Undifferentiated somatoform disorder* is characterized by one or more unexplained physical symptoms of at least 6 months' duration, which are below the threshold for a diagnosis of somatization disorder. These symptoms are not due to or fully explained by another medical, psychiatric, or substance abuse disorder, and they cause clinically significant distress or impairment.

Comparative Nosology The category of undifferentiated somatoform disorder is also in the ICD-10, and it is virtually identical to the DSM-IV-TR category. Neurasthenia (Table 15–8) is an ICD-10 diagnostic syndrome characterized by at least 3 months of exhaustion, fatigue and weakness, and an inability to recover from the fatigue with rest and is classified in the DSM-IV-TR as an undifferentiated somatoform disorder if symptoms have persisted for longer than 6 months. However, neurasthenia is of disorder status in many other parts of the world, and there are empirical data that support the validity of the construct.

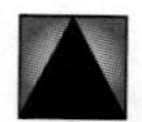

Table 15–8
ICD-10 Diagnostic Criteria for Neurasthenia

F48.0 Neurasthenia

A. Either of the following must be present:
  (1) Persistent and distressing complaints of feelings of exhaustion after minor mental effort (such as performing or attempting to perform everyday tasks that do not require unusual mental effort).
  (2) Persistent and distressing complaints of feelings of fatigue and bodily weakness after minor physical effort.

B. At least one of the following symptoms must be present:
  (1) Feelings of muscular aches and pains
  (2) Dizziness
  (3) Tension headaches
  (4) Sleep disturbance
  (5) Inability to relax
  (6) Irritability

C. The patient is unable to recover from the symptoms in Criterion A (1) or (2) by means of rest, relaxation, or entertainment.

D. The duration of the disorder is at least 3 months.

E. *Most commonly used exclusion clause*. The disorder does not occur in the presence of organic emotionally labile disorder (F06.6), postencephalitic syndrome (F07.1), postconcussional syndrome (F07.2), mood (affective) disorders (F30 through F39), panic disorder (F41.0), or generalized anxiety disorder (F41.1).

Adapted from *ICD-10 Classification of Mental and Behavioural Disorders*. Geneva: World Health Organization; 1993:109–110.

Epidemiology As undifferentiated somatoform disorder is considered a category that is residual to somatization disorder, there is little epidemiology about its prevalence. One study of a representative community sample in Germany found a 19.7 percent prevalence using a German version of the DSM-IV–adapted Composite International Diagnostic Interview. Javier Escobar and his colleagues have demonstrated that somatization disorder may be described as a spectrum on a somatic symptom index, and that four symptoms in men and six symptoms in women predict similar levels of impairment and help seeking as a 13-item index or as full somatization disorder. The prevalence of this subsyndromal disorder is as much as 100 times higher than that for somatization disorder. Many other investigators have argued for less restrictive criteria for somatization disorder, which is why the DSM-IV-TR is less restrictive than the DSM-III-R. Further work on the most parsimonious classification of somatization is required and is being considered by many investigators.

Etiology No specific etiology for undifferentiated somatoform disorder is known.

Diagnosis and Clinical Features The critical feature of undifferentiated somatoform disorder is the presence of one or more unexplained physical symptoms (Criterion A) that persist for 6 months or longer (Criterion D) but do not meet full diagnostic criteria for somatization disorder and are not due to another defined illness (Criteria B and E). This is a residual category for persistent symptoms that do not meet the full criteria for somatization or another somatoform disorder. However, that does not imply a less severe illness. As in all psychiatric disorders, symptoms must cause clinically significant distress or impairment in social, occupational, or other important areas of functioning (Criterion C). Furthermore, as in other somatoform disorders, symptoms are not intentionally produced or feigned (as in factitious disorder or malingering) (Criterion F). Common complaints are chronic fatigue, loss of appetite, and GI or genitourinary symptoms, but an array of other symptoms may also occur. One diagnostic challenge is to distinguish between normal symptomatic distress and a somatoform process. It is normal for people to experience some bodily distress even while in good health, and somatic symptoms are more common than psychological symptoms in random community samples. Approximately 80 percent of healthy individuals experience somatic symptoms in any given week. However, only a fraction of these go on to have persistent symptoms that are distressing and unexplained. It has been estimated that more than 4 percent of people in U.S. communities have chronic somatic complaints.

A second diagnostic challenge is in distinguishing between an unexplained symptom and a symptom that may be due to another medical or psychiatric disorder. Symptoms comprising an undifferentiated disorder are not directly due to or cannot be fully explained by any known general medical or psychiatric condition or the direct effects of a substance. Thus, if the symptoms are related to another disorder, but the physical complaints or resultant impairment is grossly in excess of what would be expected from the history, physical examination, or laboratory findings, an undifferentiated somatoform disorder may exist. This highlights the fact that somatoform disorders are not diagnoses of exclusion nor are they mutually exclusive of other medical illnesses. In fact, medical and psychiatric illnesses are risk factors for also having unexplained distressing somatic symptoms. The challenge lies in proving that there is no significant underlying medical disorder that is causing the symptoms without reinforcing the idea of illness to a patient by conducting multiple diagnostic evaluation tests. Excluding significant medical illness does not mean that there is no physical cause for the symptoms. The literature is replete with descriptions of altered *heightened* physiological responses in people with somatoform disorders. Trying to verbally convince a patient—just like trying to convince him or her with medical technology—that there is nothing wrong with him or her may make the somatoform disorder worse. Both kinds of attempted reassurance may cause iatrogenic reinforcement of the illness because there is no explanation for the felt symptoms.

A third diagnostic challenge is that unexplained physical symptoms and worry about illness may constitute culturally shaped *idioms of distress* that are used to express concerns about a broad range of personal and social problems, without necessarily indicating psychopathology. Unexplained physical complaints occur with high frequency in young women of low socioeconomic status, although these symptoms are not limited to any age, gender, or sociocultural group.

Pathology There is no specific histopathology for undifferentiated somatoform disorder.

Differential Diagnosis Because physical complaints are so common in everyday life, the differential diagnosis for undifferentiated somatoform disorder is large and broad. Other psychiatric disorders are in the differential diagnosis. *Somatization disorder* requires more symptoms of several years' duration and an onset before 30 years of age. *Somatoform disorder NOS* is diagnosed when the physical complaints have persisted for less than 6 months but are not due to another medical, psychiatric, or substance use disorder. *Hypochondriasis* is often expressed with somatic complaints, but preoccupation with the fear of having a disease or the belief that one has a disease coupled with resistance to reassurance is more prominent in hypochondriasis than in undifferentiated somatoform disorder. *Chronic pain* and *somatoform pain disorders* are diagnosed when the unexplained somatic symptoms are exclusively pain related. However, pain may be part of an undifferentiated somatoform disorder. The medical literature has multiple accounts and studies of increased unexplained somatic symptoms in *affective disorders*, *anxiety disorders*, some *psychotic disorders*, *substance use disorders*, *adjustment disorders*, and *personality disorders*.

Chronic medical illnesses make it more likely that a person will develop a comorbid somatoform disorder. Chronic illness is reasonably perceived as a threat, which in turn causes heightened vigilance and scanning of bodily functions, leading to amplification of somatic sensation and perception. Diagnosing a somatoform disorder in the context of chronic medical illness should be a prudent and thorough process, balancing the need to obtain objective data with the need to do no harm to the patient.

Transient unexplained somatic symptoms are normal. Amplification of somatic sensations may occur in times of personal stress or loss or even with positive events that cause a person to become more aware of bodily sensations, such as in the "medical student syndrome." The common theme of the personal context in each case is the perception of some threat, resulting in a hypervigilant survey of bodily systems.

Course and Prognosis The course of unexplained physical symptoms is unpredictable. Given the time criteria for undifferentiated somatoform disorder, there is resolution or the eventual diagnosis of another medical or psychiatric disorder.

Treatment There is no specific treatment for undifferentiated somatoform disorder. Reassurance by interpreting the threat and the physiology of heightened arousal and perception is the treatment of choice in these cases and is successful in more than 95 percent of the cases.

SOMATOFORM DISORDER NOT OTHERWISE SPECIFIED

Definition *Somatoform disorder NOS* is diagnosed in people with somatoform symptoms that do not meet the criteria for any of the specific somatoform disorders and that are not due to another psychiatric, medical, or substance use disorder. The epidemiology and etiology of this category are not studied.

Comparative Nosology The ICD-10 has a similar residual category called *other somatoform disorders*, but it specifies that the symptoms are not mediated through the autonomic nervous system and are not persistent as they are in somatization disorder.

Diagnosis and Clinical Features This diagnostic category includes somatoform symptoms that do not meet the criteria for any specific somatoform disorder. Examples provided in the DSM-IV-TR include

1. Pseudocyesis: a false belief of being pregnant that is associated with objective signs of pregnancy, such as abdominal enlargement without umbilical eversion, reduced menstrual flow or amenorrhea, nausea, breast engorgement and secretions, subjective sensation of fetal movement, and labor pains at the expected date of delivery. Pseudocyesis may be associated with endocrine changes that cannot be explained by another medical condition.
2. Nonpsychotic hypochondriacal symptoms of less than 6 months' duration. Hypochondriacal symptoms may occur separate from other disorders and also occur in people with high somatic sensitivity and with other specific psychiatric disorders. Although these hypochondriacal symptoms may be transient, even if they are severe, they may progress to a primary or secondary form of hypochondriasis or may remit with reassurance or treatment of comorbid conditions.
3. Unexplained physical symptoms of less than 6 months' duration that are not due to another illness or substance use disorder.

Pathology There are no known cellular or histopathological pathology features of unexplained physical symptoms. There is ample evidence for physiological activity that is accentuated by stress and emotions, which may cause unexplained symptoms.

Smooth and Striated Muscle Contraction Abnormalities of smooth muscle contraction, such as abnormal motility of the esophagus and intestinal tract, may cause symptoms in the chest and the right upper quadrant and middle or lower quadrants of the abdomen. Striated muscle contracts and also returns to baseline more slowly during various emotional states. Different emotional states affect various muscle groups differently. Anxiety and depression are associated with higher electromyographic (EMG) activity in some muscle groups. Clinical research has demonstrated a relationship between specific types of pain, such as headache and low-back pain, increased aversive emotional states, and increased EMG activity.

Blood Flow and Endocrine Physiology Psychophysiology research has demonstrated significant adrenergic and corticosteroid changes associated with various emotional states, particularly fear and anger. Increased sympathetic adrenergic tone in response to fear and anger may cause heightened blood pressure, an increase in heart rate and stroke volume, increased respiration, and redistribution of blood flow away from visceral organs and toward striated muscle. Furthermore, this increased tone in response to fear and anger may be responsible for vascular spasm, transient ischemic attacks, and instability of blood flow regulation in some people. The cardiologist Bernard Lown demonstrated changes in vascular tone, blood flow, and even atherogenesis and sudden death in response to severe emotional distress. Although death is not to be equated with unexplained physical symptoms, the point is that these physiological changes in response to emotional distress are spectral, and some people have symptoms due to these changes that are not necessarily measurable in the routine clinical setting. Other symptoms and signs caused by stress and emotional mechanisms include cold sensitivity of the Raynaud's type, acrocyanosis and erythromelalgia, and, perhaps, nutcracker esophagus.

Physiological Arousal and Symptoms There is a demonstrated association between arousal, the perception of this arousal, and experiencing this arousal in various somatic areas. Individuals have an idiosyncratic and recurrent pattern of physiological response to stress, which may explain the recurring unexplained somatic symptoms in individuals during different stress episodes. However, healthy subjects and anxious subjects with predominantly psychological symptoms may have somatic sensations that correlate poorly with physiological arousal. On the other hand, anxious patients with predominantly somatic symptoms have physiological arousal that correlates with their physical sensations.

Differential Diagnosis As with *undifferentiated somatoform disorder*, the differential diagnosis for somatoform disorder NOS primarily includes other *somatoform*, *affective*, and *anxiety disorders*, *undiagnosed medical illness*, and *transient* and *normal somatic symptoms*.

When other psychiatric, medical and substance use disorders are excluded, the primary diagnoses to be considered are *undifferentiated somatoform disorder* and *transient amplification of normal symptoms*. There are no empirical data about how to best distinguish between these three categories. It is likely that there is a continuum between transient amplification, the NOS category, the undifferentiated category, and full-blown somatoform disorders in terms of symptom number, severity, and associated distress. The NOS category is the only somatoform disorder that does not have explicit language in the DSM-IV-TR diagnostic criteria about causing significant clinical distress. This does imply that the NOS category is most like transient distressing somatic symptoms. Thus, this diagnosis can be made when the patient has one or more distressing somatic symptoms and when the clinician is not certain if this is transient or if the symptoms are beginning to form part of a somatoform disorder. If the symptoms persist for longer than 6 months and are not due to another medical disorder, the diagnosis of undifferentiated somatoform disorder becomes appropriate.

Course, Prognosis, and Treatment Approximately 95 percent of new-onset distressing symptoms remit with competent reassurance. Once symptoms become chronic, the diagnosis should be changed to one of the more specific somatoform disorders.

The most appropriate first-line treatment is reassurance. If the presenting somatoform symptoms become distressing, then two treatments are indicated. First, cognitive and behavioral therapies can be used to help the patient maintain functioning and not equate symptoms with being an illness or disease. Education about the nature of symptom amplification and its physiological basis is important, so that the patient does not think that the physician is lying or not competent. Familiarizing the patient with the concept of cognitive distortions is crucial for the patient to learn that symptoms do not mean that there is an illness or disease present and that symptoms can create catastrophizing cognitions that are inaccurate. Prudent examination and testing procedures should be used only when the physician truly believes that further clinical investigation is warranted. If the patient demands laboratory or radiological examinations that are unwarranted, the physician must review the symptoms, their meaning, and the need for testing rather than just send the patient for testing out of frustration. The latter maneuver reinforces the patient's belief that his or her body may fail at any time and that the doctor is not competent. The patient can be instructed to keep a behavioral log to enhance learning about how certain activities change symptoms. Exercise is also a reasonable behavioral approach. Stretching and strengthening specific muscle groups is the treatment of choice for myofascial pain syndromes, which are a common problem in people with somatoform symptoms. This may be prescribed through physical therapy programs or through yoga or meditation classes, or both. Furthermore, aerobic exercise has demonstrated efficacy for depression and some anxiety disorders, which are highly comorbid with somatoform symptoms.

The second treatment is the prudent use of medications combined with patient education. Anxiolytics, antidepressants, muscle relaxants, and hypnotics may be warranted to assist with symptom relief if the patient understands the meaning and value of this treatment and if there are no contraindications to their use.

SPECIAL CONSIDERATIONS

Presentations in Different Settings

The paradox that unexplained somatic symptoms became considered psychological and entrenched in psychiatry has one remaining paradoxical twist. The patients did not know about this nor have they accepted it. They primarily present to nonpsychiatric settings.

Primary Care Somatoform disorders in primary care are common, ranging from 0.8 to 14.0 percent of all visits. These patients have abnormal body sensations and authentically come for help to understand and to manage them. They also have characteristics that are different from nonsomatoform patients. For example, hypochondriacal patients in primary care present with more pain and higher levels of psychological distress, have less consistent health maintenance, and more often present owing to anxiety or fear than nonhypochondriacal patients. They worry about their health and their emotional state, but they usually only share the somatic complaints with their doctor. This is often assumed by doctors to be because of the patient's somatization and lack of psychological mindedness, yet a high number of patients report that they wish that their doctor would talk with them about emotional and spiritual issues.

Other Tertiary Settings Somatoform disorders have a prevalence of 5 to 40 percent in some subspecialty clinics, such as gastroenterology, neurology, cardiology, and endocrinology. Unexplained physical symptoms not meeting diagnostic criteria are even more common in these settings. Patients with somatoform disorders who are not satisfied with their primary care often seek an explanation from a specialist physician. These patients are often disappointed that the specialist finds nothing wrong with them.

Inpatient Consultation-Liaison Psychiatry Reports about the prevalence of somatoform disorders in patients referred to consultation psychiatry services vary widely. The two largest studies found that 16 and 55 percent of all referred patients have a somatoform disorder, respectively. These patients tend to be older and have more active medical problems than patients in primary care with somatoform disorders. This highlights the particular challenge in the consultation-liaison setting of making the diagnosis of a somatoform disorder in older and more medically ill patients.

Psychiatry Other psychiatric illnesses are highly comorbid with somatoform disorders, which are rarely the focus of clinical attention. Rather, unexplained physical symptoms are subsumed under diagnoses of major depression, panic disorder, schizophrenia, and other illnesses. Although there is little doubt that other psychiatric disorders have a risk of increased somatic complaints, somatoform disorders themselves are considered less often than other disorders, and patients are often encouraged to see their primary care doctor for complaints about their stomach, head, heart, or back. Psychiatrists see their limits in the practice of general medicine, yet the primary care physician has referred the patient because of the concern of a somatoform process, and the psychiatrist's approach places the patient firmly between doctors and systems. Thus, somatoform patients are at high risk of being lost to care, which may reinforce narcissistic and obsessional traits that are so common in these patients.

Cross-Cultural Disorders

This chapter is not about the authenticity of culture-bound disorders or the range of cultural effects on the process of somatization. Rather, this section is here to stress the importance of cultural variables to body sensation and expression. A few examples are given that highlight how symptoms may occur and what the impetus for the symptoms might be.

***Pibloqtoq* (and Other Arctic Hysterias)** This disorder, one of the *arctic hysterias* (others include *amos, akek, kajat, matamuk, kalagik, sanraq, montak, sautak, tesogat,* and *nirik*), originated from observations made during a series of expeditions by Robert Peary and expedition doctors to Ellesmere Island and northwestern Greenland between 1891 and 1909. The historian Lyle Dick noted that this syndrome was described in 40 of 150 polar Eskimo tribe members by expedition members. The only commonality between the numerous professional investigators who have since described this syndrome is that none of them has witnessed an episode of this intermittent disorder. *Pibloqtoq* has been described as intermittent episodes of withdrawal, followed by singing or screaming; rolling on the ground; making noises like the birds, dogs, or seals, with subsequent clonic movements; and carpopedal spasms while "walking on the sky," followed by up to an hour of trembling with resultant weakness and dazedness. The native treatment approach for an episode is generally for men not to intervene, unless the episode occurs in a wife, and for women to soothe another woman who has an attack. Expedition members and doctors took a more interventional and authoritative approach, including prescriptions for sleep, brandy and whiskey ingestion, emetics, and injections of mustard water. More recent workers believe that this phenomenon is multifactorial and not necessarily culture bound, with possible etiologies including partial complex seizures, vitamin A excess, infections, somatoform phenomena, and a social protest resulting from power differences in the contact between native and expedition people.

Koro *Koro*, a so-called culture-bound syndrome, occurs primarily in Southeast Asia and may be related to body dysmorphic disorder and hypochondriasis. However, *koro* has been diagnosed and successfully treated with SSRIs in the United States. It occurs primarily in men and is characterized by a belief that the penis or testicles will shrink and disappear into the abdomen, resulting in death. When *koro* occurs in women, the belief is usually that the labia or nipples will involute and result in death. *Koro* differs from body dysmorphic disorder by its usually brief duration, different associated features (primarily acute anxiety and fear of death), more of a positive response to reassurance, and occasional occurrence as an epidemic.

Other Medical Disorders Likely to Masquerade as a Somatoform Disorder

Any medical disorder that presents with vague or nonclassic symptoms may be taken to be a somatoform disorder. One problem is that most medical illness presents nonclassically a large minority of the time. When debating whether symptoms are due to another medical illness or a somatoform disorder, the clinician should consider the diagnoses of thyroid diseases; parathyroid disease; uncommon infections, such as syphilis; other infections, such as human immunodeficiency virus (HIV) and disseminated gonococcus; nervous system disorders, such as MS or tumor; and autoimmune disorders, such as lupus erythematosus or myasthenia gravis.

Children and Adolescents

During childhood, people learn to integrate affect and body sensation with cognition to express themselves. During infancy, body sensation is the primary feeling used to learn about the self in relation to other things. Early childhood continues by pairing precognitive affect with somatic sensations. Late childhood brings thought and cognition to the person in his or her expression about the self and its relation to the outside world. Somatic complaint or pleasure is thus the first, primary modality of expressing displeasure or joy about the self and its relation to the world. Affect and then cognition are later, secondary modalities that are learned parallel to somatic sensation. Early concepts of self and its relation to others are thus all wrapped up in body-feeling, and the expression of somatic complaint in children is the expression of displeasure with the self or one's relationship to other people or other things. That displeasure may be due to any number of noxious agents, including virus, physical injury, tumor, or learned general sensation that all is not right with the self in its world. It is the task of the physician to determine the source of displeasure.

Somatic symptoms in children are common, although the prevalence in the community, schools, or primary care is not known. School is a common place for expression of somatic distress, which can influence the child's attendance and grades. There may be gender differences in childhood somatization, with some evidence that girls have a higher prevalence of abdominal pain and that boys a higher prevalence of chest and back pain. Because somatic symptoms are common in children, the clinician should be more concerned with the social and psychological context that may be responsible for the symptoms than with diagnosis. Somatization disorder or hypochondriasis diagnoses should be held in reserve, unless the child has a prolonged course of unexplained symptoms in multiple body systems or preoccupation with having a serious illness.

Body dysmorphic disorder is an underrecognized and underdiagnosed problem that is relatively common among adolescents and may be becoming more common with the increase in media depicting unattainable ideals of beauty and perfection. Body dysmorphic disorder has a high rate of comorbidity with depression and suicide, which argues for prompt diagnosis and treatment in adolescents. Effective treatment options include CBT and pharmacotherapy with SSRIs.

Geriatric Populations Research about somatoform disorders in the elderly is limited. The late onset of a somatoform disorder should be considered another medical disorder until clearly proven otherwise. However, the astute clinician realizes that somatoform disorders may be comorbid with other medical disorders and that bodily preoccupations and fears of debility may be frequent in elderly persons. The multiple losses that occur with aging may cause heightened distress, which may interact with the pains of chronic illness. The onset of preoccupation with health concerns in old age is more likely to be realistic or to be associated with an affective disorder or poor social support, or both, than to be a specific somatoform disorder.

Relationship of Personality to Somatoform Disorders There are some data, given throughout this chapter, about the relationship of somatoform disorders to specific personality traits and disorders. There are also attitudes and traits, such as defense and resolution of conflict, communication style, hostility and anger, and certain cognitive styles, that have been studied and written about in their relationship to somatoform disorders. As is evident from the history of somatoform disorders, the relationship between somatoform disorders as personality constructs—stable characteristics of the person—and as disorders that develop later in life is a lively academic debate. The primary problem with this debate is the inability to distinguish between inherent traits of the person (i.e., temperament) and traits that develop into disorders. For psychiatry, separating Axis I from Axis II disorders is problematic. They are both characterized by symptoms and enduring patterns of internal experience and behavior that develop over time, becoming chronic and pervasive parts of the individual. The trend of transforming chronic Axis I disorders into personality disorders because of their duration is already evident with other disorders, such that social phobia is thought of as avoidant personality disorder, and dysthymia is considered a depressive personality disorder. This is in light of the fact that personality disorders have little empirical support as discrete entities.

The state–trait problem is no more evident than in hypochondriasis. There is support for considering this disorder a personality disorder. However, the state personality construct and the trait disorder are more alike than different. They are both defined by rigid preoccupation with amplified bodily symptoms, the belief that these symptoms equal illness, and behaviors designed to refute these frightening beliefs but that reinforce them because of the rigidity of the conviction. Furthermore, both constructs can be viewed as the result of abnormal cognitive processing that includes amplification and misinterpretation of bodily symptoms and the behavioral outcomes of help seeking coupled with resistance to reassurance. However, a view that is alternative to the state–trait dichotomy exists. This view uses a developmental and life span approach to demonstrate that somatoform disorders develop in the context of developmental tasks. Early childhood experiences interact with temperament and culture to come together in adulthood as somatization—a process in which bodily distress is one way in which a person can express that something is not right with one's relationship to self or to things outside of the self. This developmental view more accurately describes how somatoform disorders occur without forcing distinctions that have little or no empirical support.

Relationship of Trauma to Somatoform Disorders

There is evidence that chronic stress and trauma are associated with increased physical symptoms. The majority of the studies that examine this relationship have been conducted in veterans of war. The presence of unexplained physical symptoms is associated with acute psychological distress at the time of trauma; ongoing psychopathology; alcohol, tobacco, and medication use; and symptoms of PTSD. Combat veterans with PTSD have higher rates of cardiovascular, neurological, GI, audiological, and pain symptoms compared to combat veterans without PTSD. There is mounting evidence that physical symptoms are a part of PTSD and also may be a nonspecific response to trauma that is independent of PTSD. It has been documented that pain symptoms are often localized to the site of previous trauma in people with PTSD.

Somatization and hypochondriasis are associated with the presence of self-reported traumatic experiences. There are numerous reports about the increased history of trauma in people with somatization disorder. There are two studies about this relationship in hypochondriasis. In one study, there was a three- to fourfold higher risk for having experienced traumatic sexual contact, physical violence, or major parental upheaval before 17 years of age in hypochondriacal people compared to normal control subjects. The other study validated an interpersonal model of hypochondriasis, which posits that early adverse experiences lead to insecure and fearful attachment styles, high levels of physical symptoms and illness phobia, and interpersonal problems in daily life and in medical care. There is also mounting evidence that people with body dysmorphic disorder, dissociative conversion reactions, and pain disorders experience a higher number of early adverse experiences than normal control subjects.

The mechanisms for unexplained physical symptoms in people who have experienced trauma are unclear. Neuroimaging studies in trauma survivors with PTSD demonstrate dysfunction of the anterior cingulate with a failure to inhibit amygdala activation or an intrinsically lower threshold of amygdala response to fearful stimuli, or both. There is also some evidence that somatosensory cortex and Brodmann's areas 1 through 4 and 6 have increased regional blood flow during traumatic recall and that this activation is associated with self-reports of physical sensations. Some investigators are proposing that subcortical memory systems help determine this neurobiological response to trauma recall. It is well established that memory function is changed in PTSD and that cognitive and somatosensory processing is abnormal. Multiple physiological systems are activated or inhibited with stress, and chronic stress can produce lasting changes in autonomic nervous, immune, and hypothalamic-pituitary-adrenal (HPA) axis systems. Furthermore, trauma produces increases of cortisol and epinephrine levels, both of which have adverse effects on brain and body when unchecked.

Perhaps the most parsimonious theory is that of Hans Selye who observed in medical school that there was a nonspecific "syndrome of just being sick" that was similar across various medical illnesses. Selye went on to conduct elegant laboratory work with animals to define the *general adaptation syndrome* (GAS), which occurs with multiple stressors, such as behavioral stress, heat, cold, infection, trauma, hemorrhage, and other stimuli. The GAS has three stages: (1) the alarm reaction, (2) resistance and defense, and (3) exhaustion. If the stress is not resolved, then chronic changes begin to occur after days and weeks, including fatigue, sleep disorders, symptoms of depression and anxiety, and an increased risk for infection and respiratory and cardiovascular compromise. The involvement of central memory and somatosensory processing, the HPA axis involving cortisol and epinephrine, and diminished immunity results in physiological changes in nearly every body system. Thus, physical sensations are more prominent in those exposed to stressors that activate the GAS. Without rapid resolution of the stress response, physiology can become so profoundly altered that it would be surprising if an individual did not experience ongoing physical sensations.

FUTURE DIRECTIONS

Psychiatrists need improved training about recognition and treatment of individual somatoform disorders, as well as somatoform disorders that are comorbid with other psychiatric and medical illnesses. Particularly when a patient is referred to psychiatry for care, it is best for the psychiatrist to conduct relevant examinations and laboratory studies and to obtain the relevant history to make or to exclude a somatoform disorder. This may include knowledge and skill of a focused, thorough neurological examination to determine if conversion disorder is present or if there is pathology to support another medical disorder in the differential diagnosis. This is where psychiatry can be at its best and where psychiatrists best maintain their identities as doctors capable of diagnosing and treating the whole person. If this training is not improved, then patients with somatoform disorders will continue to receive suboptimal care and to be dismissed as "crocks."

Primary care physicians require further education about the known physiology of somatoform disorders; the distinction between somatoform, factitious, and malingering disorders; and pharmacological and psychotherapeutic treatment principles and modalities. Excluding other medical disorders is only one-half of the equation in the care of the somatoform-disordered patient. The other half is to make a positive diagnosis and to use standard, helpful, nonspecific and specific treatment modalities that have been shown effective for this group of disorders.

Psychiatrists and primary care physicians need to forge further multidisciplinary relationships and care models appropriate for the care of the somatoform-disordered patient. These patients need a place to be seen and to be taken seriously rather than being shunted back and forth between clinics. Psychosomatic and medical-psychiatric paradigms need to be introduced further into curricula and systems of care, so that the patient's illness is not being perpetuated by first being viewed through a biomedical paradigm and then a psychological one, mimicking the mind–body split in Western culture that is so elemental to their disorder.

The public will benefit from education about the high prevalence of unexplained physical symptoms and the fact that, although these are not necessarily life threatening, they can be disabling. The public should also know that there are treatments available for these disorders.

Finally, research about somatoform disorders should not be neglected. These disorders are impairing to patients and costly to society, and medicine needs to better understand the pathogenesis, phenomenology, and treatment options for somatoform disorders.

SUGGESTED CROSS-REFERENCES

Related disorders are discussed in Chapter 16 on factitious disorders and Chapter 17 on dissociative disorders. Section 24.11 on consultation-liaison psychiatry, Section 30.12 on noncompliance with treatment, and Section 26.1 on malingering also have information relevant to somatoform disorders.

REFERENCES

*Barsky AJ: Patients who amplify bodily symptoms. *Ann Intern Med.* 1979;91:63.

Barsky AJ, Wool C, Barnett MC, Cleary PD: Histories of childhood trauma in adult hypochondriacal patients. *Am J Psychiatry.* 1994;151:397.

Bass C, ed. *Somatization: Physical Symptoms & Psychological Illness.* Oxford, UK: Blackwell Science; 1990.

Bass C, Murphy M: Somatoform and personality disorders: Syndromal comorbidity and overlapping developmental pathways. *J Psychosom Res.* 1995;39:403.

Burton R: *The Anatomy of Melancholy.* London: Oxford University Press; 1883.

*Escobar J, Canino G: Unexplained physical complaints: Psychopathology and epidemiological correlates. *Br J Psychiatry.* 1989;154[Suppl 4]:24.

Fabrega H. Cultural and historical foundations of psychiatric diagnosis. In: Mezzich JE, Kleinman A, Fabrega H, Parron DL, eds. *Culture and Psychiatric Diagnosis: A DSM-IV Perspective.* Washington, DC: American Psychiatric Press; 1996.

*Ford CV. *The Somatizing Disorders: Illness as a Way of Life.* New York: Elsevier Science; 1983.

Ford CV: The somatizing disorders. *Psychosomatics.* 1986;27:327.

Foulks E. In: Maybury-Lewis D, ed. *The Arctic Hysterias of the North Alaskan Eskimo. Anthropological Studies, No. 10.* Washington, DC: The American Anthropological Association; 1972.

Frances A, Ross R. *DSM-IV Case Studies: A Clinical Guide to Differential Diagnosis.* Washington, DC: American Psychiatric Press; 1996:208.

Freud S. On narcissism: An introduction. In: *Standard Edition of the Complete Psychological Works of Sigmund Freud.* London: Hogarth Press; 1955.

Grabe HJ, Meyer C, Hapke U, Rumpf HJ, Freyberger HJ, Dilling H, John U: Specific somatoform disorder in the general population. *Psychosomatics.* 2003;44:304.

Hiller W, Rief W, Fichter MM: Dimensional and categorical approaches to hypochondriasis. *Psychol Med.* 2002;3:707.

Hollifield M. Hypochondriasis and personality disturbance. In: Starcevic V, Lipsitt DR, eds. *Hypochondriasis: Modern Perspectives on an Ancient Malady.* Oxford, UK: Oxford University Press; 2001.

Hollifield M, Tuttle L, Paine S, Kellner R: Hypochondriasis and somatization related to personality and attitudes toward self. *Psychosomatics.* 1999;40:387.

Katon W, Kleinman A, Rosen G: Depression and somatization: A review. Part I. *Am J Med.* 1982;77:101.

*Kellner R. *Somatization and Hypochondriasis.* New York: Praeger; 1986.

Kellner R. *Abridged Manual of the Illness Attitude Scales.* Albuquerque, NM: Department of Psychiatry, University of New Mexico School of Medicine; 1987.

Kellner R. *Psychosomatic Syndromes and Somatic Symptoms.* Washington, DC: American Psychiatric Press; 1991.

Kirmayer LJ, Robbins JM: Three forms of somatization in primary care: Prevalence, co-occurrence and sociodemographic characteristics. *J Nerv Ment Dis.* 1991;179:647.

Kraus R. *Pibloqtoq Revisited.* Paper presented at: The annual meeting of The Society for the Study of Psychiatry and Culture; October 19, 2002; Charlottesville, VA.

Ladee GA. *Hypochondriacal Syndromes.* Amsterdam: North-Holland Publishing; 1966.

Lipowski ZJ: Somatization: The concept and its clinical application. *Am J Psychiatry.* 1988;145:1358.

Lipsitt DR. The patient-physician relationship in the treatment of hypochondriasis. In: Starcevic V, Lipsitt DR, eds. *Hypochondriasis: Modern Perspectives on an Ancient Malady.* Oxford, UK: Oxford University Press; 2001.

Looper KJ, Kirmayer LJ: Behavioral medicine approaches to somatoform disorders. *J Consult Clin Psychol.* 2002;70:810.

Morrison J: Childhood sexual histories of women with somatization disorder. *Am J Psychiatry.* 1989;146:239.

Noyes R Jr, Holt CS, Happel RL, Kathol RG, Yagla SJ: A family study of hypochondriasis. *J Nerv Ment Dis.* 1997;185:223.

Noyes R Jr, Kathol RG, Fisher MM, Phillips BM, Suelzer MT, Holt CS: The validity of DSM-III-R hypochondriasis. *Arch Gen Psychiatry.* 1993;51:961.

Noyes R Jr, Stuart SP, Langbehn DR, Happel RL, Longley SL, Muller BA, Yagla SJ: Test of an interpersonal model of hypochondriasis. *Psychosom Med.* 2003;65:292.

Phillips KA. *Somatoform and Factitious Disorders.* Washington, DC: American Psychiatric Publishing, Inc.; 2001.

Phillips KA, Albertini RS, Rasmussen SA: A randomized placebo-controlled trial of fluoxetine in body dysmorphic disorder. *Arch Gen Psychiatry.* 2002;59:381.

*Pilowsky I: Dimensions of hypochondriasis. *Br J Psychiatry.* 1967;113:89.

Pilowsky I: Primary and secondary hypochondriasis. *Acta Psychiatr Scand.* 1970;46:273.

Selye H. *The Stress of Life.* New York: McGraw-Hill; 1978.

Smith GR. *Somatization Disorder in the Medical Setting.* Washington, DC: American Psychiatric Press; 1991.

Smith GR, Rost K, Kashner M: A trial of the effect of standardized psychiatric consultation on health outcomes and costs in somatizing patients. *Arch Gen Psychiatry.* 1995;52:238.

Starcevic V. Reassurance in the treatment of hypochondriasis. In: Starcevic V, Lipsitt DR, eds. *Hypochondriasis: Modern Perspectives on an Ancient Malady.* Oxford, UK: Oxford University Press; 2001.

Stekel W. *The Interpretations of Dreams: New Developments and Technique.* New York: Liveright; 1943.

Stolorow RD: Defensive and arrested developmental aspects of death anxiety, hypochondriasis and depersonalization. *Int J Psychoanal.* 1979;60:201.

Tezcan E, Atmaca M, Kuloglu M, Gecici O, Buyukbayram A, Tutkun H: Dissociative disorders in Turkish inpatients with conversion disorder. *Comp Psychiatry.* 2003;44:324.

Torgersen S: Genetics of somatoform disorders. *Arch Gen Psychiatry.* 1986;43:502.

Tyrer P. *The Role of Bodily Feelings in Anxiety.* London: Oxford University Press; 1976.

Tyrer P: Somatoform and personality disorders: personality and the soma. *J Psychosom Res.* 1995;39:395.

Weintraub MI. *Hysterical Conversion Reactions: A Clinical Guide to Diagnosis and Treatment.* New York: SP Medical and Scientific Books; 1983.

16 Factitious Disorders

DORA WANG, M.D., DEEPA N. NADIGA, M.D., AND JAMES J. JENSON, M.D.

According to the American Heritage Dictionary, the word *factitious* means "artificial; false," derived from the Latin *facticius,* which means "made by art." Those with factitious disorder simulate, induce, or aggravate illness, often inflicting painful, deforming, or even life-threatening injury on themselves or those under their care. Unlike malingerers who have material goals, such as monetary gain or avoidance of duties, factitious disorder patients undertake these tribulations primarily to gain the emotional care and attention that comes with playing the role of the patient. In doing so, they practice artifice and art, creating hospital drama that often causes frustration and dismay. Clinicians may exclaim, "He's not really sick! He's doing it to himself!" and thus dismiss, avoid, or refuse to treat factitious disorder patients. Strong countertransference of clinicians can be major obstacles toward the proper care of these patients who arguably are among the most psychiatrically disturbed.

Significant morbidity or even mortality often occurs. Therefore, even though presenting complaints are falsified, the medical and psychiatric needs of these patients must be taken seriously. Factitiously produced wounds can result in infection and osteomyelitis and can even necessitate amputation. One woman factitiously complained of an extensive family history of breast cancer, incurring a medically unnecessary bilateral mastectomy. Cases resulting in death are not uncommon. A 21-year-old operating room technician, the daughter of a physician, repetitively injected herself with pseudomonas, causing multiple bouts of sepsis and bilateral renal failure before her death.

For patients with factitious disorder, unmet emotional needs are so great that even imperilment of life or limb can be merited. Factitious illness behavior often represents a severe underlying psychiatric disturbance, such as a personality disorder. Ironically, even those presenting with factitious psychological complaints, such as bereavement or psychosis, usually have another psychiatric disturbance for which they are not seeking help.

Treatment involves harm reduction and efforts to steer patients toward the psychiatric care that they need, in face-saving, nonthreatening ways.

Despite potentially high stakes, relatively little empirical knowledge is available about the etiology, epidemiology, course and prognosis, and effective treatment of factitious disorders. Most knowledge comes from case reports, information that is frequently suspect, given the false, unreliable nature of the information these patients give. Methodological problems are inherent in the study of these deceptive patients, as they are difficult to identify, and, when found out, they often flee to avoid charges of fraud from the hospital and insurance companies. Systematic studies of factitious disorder are few, and federally funded investigation is nonexistent, despite the substantial human and financial cost imposed by the disorder.

However, the situation is not as grim as previously assumed. Munchausen syndrome, the prototypical factitious disorder and the first to engender wide medical interest, is now known to be a chronic, severe variant, comprising only a small portion of all factitious disorders. Factitious illness behavior represents a wide spectrum and, at one end, represents normal behavior, such as when children exaggerate distress from scrapes and bruises to gain parental attention. It is important to remember that not all factitious illness behavior is as refractory or as chronic as that demonstrated by Munchausen syndrome patients.

DEFINITION

The main clinical feature is the intentional production or feigning of physical or psychological signs or symptoms with the motivation of assuming the sick role. The definition of *factitious disorder*, according to the revised fourth edition of the *Diagnostic and Statistical Manual of Mental Disorders* (DSM-IV-TR), is given in Table 16–1.

Munchausen syndrome, a colorful name coined by Richard Asher in his landmark 1951 publication, is also known as *chronic factitious disorder with predominantly physical signs and symptoms*. The two terms are used interchangeably. These cases are a small subset of the most severe cases of factitious disorder in which factitious illness behavior becomes a lifestyle, usually precluding stable relationships or employment. Constantly seeking medical care and hospitalization, these patients often assume grandiose, false identities, sometimes claiming to be royalty, relatives of celebrities, or figures in important historical events. They travel from hospital to hospital seeking medical care, and, when they become well-known in town, take their act on the road to another locale, where they begin the behavior anew. The nicknames *hospital hoboes*, *hospital addicts*, and *professional patients* have been applied to them. Two distinguishing features of Munchausen syndrome are *pseudologica fantastica*, the telling of tall lies and fascinating but untrue tales, and *peregrination*, as these patients tend to be well traveled.

Munchausen syndrome comprises only approximately 10 percent of all cases of factitious disorder, and the two should be distinguished. Not all those with factitious disorder have the same poor prognosis as the small minority of Munchausen syndrome patients.

In factitious disorder by proxy, a person intentionally simulates illness in another person who is under that individual's care. Most commonly, the perpetrator is a mother causing illness in her own child so that that she gains the emotional gratification of the sick role vicariously. In other cases, factitious disorder by proxy may be committed by one adult against another adult, such as an elder or spouse. Medical personnel have committed factitious disorder by proxy on patients, causing epidemics of hospital deaths. Perpetrators usually gain the admiration of others, appearing like self-sacrificing ideal caretakers. Because factitious disorder by proxy almost always constitutes child abuse or a criminal act, the forensic terms *perpetrator*

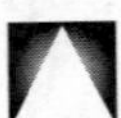

Table 16–1
DSM-IV-TR Diagnostic Criteria for Factitious Disorder

A. Intentional production or feigning of physical or psychological signs or symptoms.
B. The motivation for the behavior is to assume the sick role.
C. External incentives for the behavior (such as economic gain, avoiding legal responsibility, or improving physical well-being, as in malingering) are absent.

Code based on type:

300.16 With predominantly psychological signs and symptoms: if psychological signs and symptoms predominate in the clinical presentation.

300.19 With predominantly physical signs and symptoms: if physical signs and symptoms predominate the clinical presentation.

300.19 With combined psychological and physical signs and symptoms: if psychological and physical signs and symptoms are present, but neither predominates the clinical presentation.

From American Psychiatric Association. *Diagnostic and Statistical Manual of Mental Disorders.* 4th ed. Text rev. Washington, DC: American Psychiatric Association; 2000, with permission.

and *victim* are used even in the medical literature. Factitious disorder by proxy currently falls under the category of factitious disorder not otherwise specified (NOS), according to DSM-IV-TR. It is listed as a criteria set deserving of further study, and its research criteria are listed in Table 16–2. The terms *factitious disorder by proxy* and *Munchausen syndrome by proxy* are used interchangeably, and, at the current time, there is no clear distinction between the terms. Although, by DSM-IV-TR criteria, the term *factitious disorder by proxy* refers to the perpetrator, not the victim, there is some variance of this in the literature.

HISTORY

Self-inflicted illness occurs throughout historical literature. In the second century AD, the Greek-born physician Galen wrote of patients inducing or simulating symptoms such as vomiting or rectal bleeding. The Bible relates accounts of people self-inflicting injury. In the European middle ages, *hysterics* reportedly put leeches in their mouths to simulate hemoptysis and abraded their skin to reproduce skin conditions. However, judging historical accounts through contemporary mindsets is often problematical, and it is difficult to say if these accounts actually represent factitious disorder.

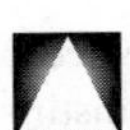

Table 16–2
DSM-IV-TR Research Criteria for Factitious Disorder by Proxy

A. Intentional production or feigning of physical or psychological signs or symptoms in another person who is under the individual's care.
B. The motivation for the perpetrator's behavior is to assume the sick role by proxy.
C. External incentives for the behavior (such as economic gain) are absent.
D. The behavior is not better accounted for by another mental disorder.

From American Psychiatric Association. *Diagnostic and Statistical Manual of Mental Disorders.* 4th ed. Text rev. Washington, DC: American Psychiatric Association; 2000, with permission.

In 1838, the Scottish military physician Hector Gavin published his essay, "On the Feigned and Factitious Diseases of Soldiers and Seamen, on the Means Used to Simulate or Produce Them, and on the Best Modes of Discovering Impostors." Although most of Gavin's subjects were malingering, aiming to escape duty in the high casualty Napoleonic Wars, Gavin also noted that the motive of some was simply "to excite compassion or interest" and that "some soldiers, indeed, without any ulterior object, seem to experience an unaccountable gratification in deceiving their officers, comrades, and surgeon."

Jean-Martin Charcot, in approximately 1890, used the term *mania operativa activa* to describe a young girl who continually sought surgery for pain in a knee joint, until she found a surgeon who amputated the leg. Subsequently, no pathology was found in the leg. In 1901, the Swiss physician Henri F. Secretan described a peculiar syndrome, to which he lent his name, of nonhealing traumatically induced edema of the dorsum of the hand. George Reading, in 1980, confirmed that Secretan's syndrome is factitiously produced. In 1934, Karl Menninger described *polysurgical addiction.*

Interest in factitious disorder increased markedly when the term *Munchausen syndrome* was coined in a 1951 publication by British physician Richard Asher. Asher wrote

> Here is described a common syndrome which most doctors have seen, but about which little has been written. Like the famous Baron von Munchausen, the persons affected have always traveled widely; and their stories, like those attributed to him, are both dramatic and untruthful. Accordingly, the syndrome is respectfully dedicated to the baron, and named after him.

Asher's provocative paper described three patients with false abdominal complaints, all of whom used multiple identities and sought care at a number of hospitals. The paper inspired much correspondence and subsequent reports.

The Baron Karl Friedrich Hieronymus von Munchhausen (1720 to 1797) was an honorable nobleman who served the Russian army in war against the Turks (Fig. 16–1). After retirement, he entertained friends with embellished stories of his war adventures. The peregrinating, pseudological figure was in fact the Baron's friend, Rudolph Eric Raspe, who was forced to flee Germany for England after he was caught embezzling from a museum. Seeking to pay off debts, Raspe published an account of the baron's tales in 1785.

In 1968, Herzl R. Spiro noted that, of the 38 cases of Munchausen syndrome then published, none involved a detailed psychiatric workup and less than one-half were evaluated by a psychiatrist. He advocated greater understanding of these patients and presented the first detailed psychiatric case study, confirming information with collateral sources. He called the Munchausen syndrome label "facetious" and recommended the less pejorative term *chronic factitious symptomatology*.

Factitious disorder with psychological symptoms was first described by Alan J. Gelenberg in 1977, who mused that, although other factitious disorder patients avoided psychiatrists, his patient, a war veteran, gained admission to more than 30 psychiatric hospitals within a few years, usually feigning depression and suicidal tendency under various pseudonyms.

The term *Munchausen syndrome by proxy* was first used in 1976 by John Money and June Werlwas, who reported two cases of child abuse and deprivation that resulted in psychosocial dwarfism. The motive of assuming the sick role was not a feature of these cases. The term *Munchausen syndrome by proxy* as it is used today was first applied in 1977 by British pediatrician Roy Meadow who published the widely read article, "Munchausen's by Proxy; The Hinterland of Child Abuse," which detailed the accounts of a mother

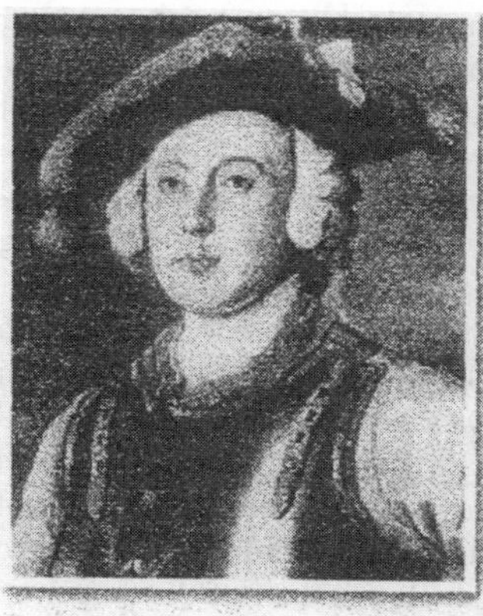
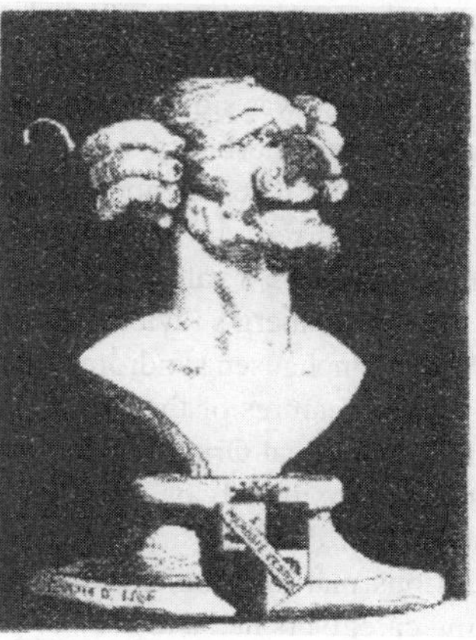

FIGURE 16–1 The Baron Karl Friedrich Hieronymus von Munchhausen (1720 to 1797). **Left:** The Baron wears military armor in this 1750 portrait by G. Bruckner. An honorable nobleman who served in the Russian army in war against the Turks, the Baron entertained friends in his retirement with embellished stories of his war adventures. His tales gained fame when published by Rudolph E. Raspe. **Right:** The Baron appears as a caricature in this drawing by 19th-century artist Gustave Dore. Like the Baron, patients with factitious disorders are persons deserving of respect, even though they often present themselves as caricatures. (Portrait courtesy of Bernhard Wiebel, http://www.muenchhausen.ch. The actual portrait was lost in World War II. Caricature from *The Adventures of Baron Munchausen: One Hundred and Sixty Illustrations by Gustave Dore*. New York: Pantheon Books, Inc.; 1944, with permission.)

who caused salt poisoning in her child and another who fabricated urinary tract infections in her daughter. The latter case was of a 6-year-old girl who had undergone 12 hospitalizations, more than 150 urine cultures, six examinations under anesthesia, five cystoscopies, and seven major X-ray procedures. When the girl was admitted for observation, the diagnosis of Munchausen syndrome by proxy was made based on urine samples that were bloody when they were collected by the mother but normal when they were collected by the nurse. Of note, the mother had also sought medical treatment for factitiously induced urinary tract infections in herself.

COMPARATIVE NOSOLOGY

The third edition of the *Diagnostic and Statistical Manual of Mental Disorders* (DSM-III) in 1980 was the first edition of the DSM to recognize factitious disorder. Munchausen syndrome was called the *prototype* of all factitious disorders, and, accordingly, emphasis was placed on chronic factitious disorder with physical symptoms. Factitious disorder with psychological symptoms was recognized, as was atypical factitious disorder, which included disorders that would now fall into the DSM-IV-TR category of factitious disorder with predominantly physical signs and symptoms.

Subsequent editions of the DSM increasingly recognized the rarity of Munchausen syndrome and accordingly placed more emphasis on a greater spectrum of factitious disorders. The revised third edition of the DSM (DSM-III-R) recognized factitious disorder with physical symptoms and factitious disorder with psychological symptoms. The emphasis on Munchausen syndrome was lessened. Factitious disorder with combined physical and psychological symptoms made its appearance under the category of factitious disorder NOS.

In contrast, the fourth edition of the DSM (DSM-IV) chose to espouse a single category, factitious disorder, with three types: (1) with predominantly psychological signs and symptoms, (2) with predominantly physical signs and symptoms, and (3) with combined psychological and physical signs and symptoms. Factitious disorder NOS was exemplified by factitious disorder by proxy, a disorder named as a category deserving of more research, with research criteria listed. The DSM-IV-TR criteria for factitious disorders are unchanged in comparison with DSM-IV criteria.

When the diagnosis of factitious disorder by proxy is made, it should be coded as factitious disorder NOS. The diagnosis applies to the perpetrator, not the victim. Physical abuse of child for the caregiver and physical abuse of child for the child should also be coded.

Emphasizing the personality disorder aspect of factitious disorders, the tenth revision of the *International Statistical Classification of Diseases and Related Health Problems* (ICD-10) lists factitious disorder under the category *other disorders of adult personality and behavior*. Two subsets corresponding with common notions of factitious disorder are identified: (1) elaboration of physical symptoms for psychological reasons and (2) intentional production or feigning of symptoms or disabilities, physical or psychological (factitious disorder). Under the second subtype, hospital hopper syndrome, Munchausen syndrome, and peregrinating patient are listed. The ICD-10 excludes "person feigning illness (with obvious motivation)," just as DSM-IV-TR excludes malingering. The ICD-10 makes no mention of factitious disorder by proxy.

Limitations exist in the DSM-IV-TR and ICD-10 nosologies. Both classification systems specify that symptoms of factitious disorder are intentionally or consciously produced. However, in reality, intent can be difficult to discern, and consciousness may represent a spectrum of awareness. Likewise, the DSM-IV-TR and the ICD-10 exclude cases in which there are obvious or external motivations. Motive, however, can also be difficult to determine. Criteria of intent and motivation are completely subject to the clinician's opinion. Even though the DSM-IV-TR and the ICD-10 exclude malingering, the reality is that factitious disorder and malingering can coexist, as when patients who habitually gratify themselves in the sick role discover that they can also receive disability payments or pleasurable pain medications at the same time.

Neither the current DSM-IV-TR nor the ICD-10 accommodates the growing literature about perifactitious disorder by proxy diagnoses in which parents impose their psychiatric disorders or emotional needs on their children. For example, *hypochondriasis by proxy* can result in repetitive pediatric visits and unnecessary tests and procedures for a child, but without fabrication of induction of illness. *Anorexia nervosa by proxy* and *malingering by proxy* are other examples.

Interestingly, although the psychiatric nosology remains equivocal about the existence of factitious disorder by proxy as a disease entity, the legal system has decided. All 50 states require reporting of Munchausen syndrome by proxy to child protective services as a form of child abuse. Munchausen syndrome by proxy is well established in the legal literature, with an abundance of representation in case law.

EPIDEMIOLOGY

No comprehensive epidemiological data on factitious disorder exist, as traditional epidemiological methods would be problematical with this deceptive population. Because factitious disorder may be difficult to detect, its prevalence may be underestimated. On the other hand, prevalence might be overestimated, as many of these patients seek care at multiple venues. Furthermore, those with factitious disorders may not present to a health care setting but may play the sick role with family, friends, or coworkers. For example, a fan of the Broadway musical *Rent* feigned terminal illness and suicidal tendency, rallying the sympathies of fellow fans and even the cast, who dedicated songs to her during performances. Internet bulletin boards and chat groups provide new opportunities to fabricate illness and to play the sick role in cyberspace.

Limited studies indicate that factitious disorder patients may comprise approximately 0.8 to 1.0 percent of psychiatry consultation patients. Of 1,288 medical inpatients referred for psychiatric consultation at a large Toronto teaching hospital, 0.8 percent were diagnosed with factitious disorder. At a New York City hospital, 1 percent of psychiatry consultation patients were diagnosed with factitious disorders.

Fever is one of the most commonly detected factitious symptoms, and studies indicate that 2.2 to 9.3 percent of fevers of unknown origins may be factitious. A Stanford University study showed that, of 506 cases, 2.2 percent were factitious. On the other hand, more than four times that percentage, a remarkable 9.3 percent of 343 cases at the National Institute for Allergy and Infectious Disease, were found factitious. Other estimates include 3.5 percent in a study of 199 cases in the 1980s and 6.5 percent of 200 cases at the National Institutes of Health. In a study of urinary calculi, 3.5 percent of stones brought in by patients were factitious, consisting of materials such as quartz and feldspar. Factitious disorders may play a larger role than expected in health care use and may be an underrecognized confounding factor in medical research.

Various authors agree that approximately two-thirds of patients with Munchausen syndrome are male. They tend to be middle-aged, unemployed, unmarried, and without significant social or family attachments. For those with non–Munchausen syndrome factitious disorders with predominantly physical signs and symptoms, women outnumber men, with a ratio of 3 to 1. They are usually 20 to 40 years of age with a history of employment or education in nursing or a health care occupation. In a 10-year retrospective study, 28 of 41, or 68 percent, of hospitalized patients with factitious disorders had worked in medically related fields, 15 as nurses. Factitious physical disorders usually begin for patients in their 20s or 30s, although the literature contains cases ranging from 4 to 79 years of age. Reported cases are almost exclusively about whites, although two African-American men with Munchausen syndrome have been reported. International reports have come from Europe and Africa.

Far less information is available about the epidemiology of factitious disorders with predominantly psychological signs and symptoms. Dinesh Bhugra estimated psychiatric Munchausen syndrome at 0.5 percent of adult psychiatric admissions who were younger than 65 years of age, based on four diagnoses of Munchausen syndrome out of 775 admissions. In a study of 4,500 visits to a psychiatric emergency room (ER), seven visits, or 0.15 percent, represented factitious disorder. Similarly, a 1994 study estimated the prevalence at 0.14 percent in a community sample.

Factitious disorder by proxy is most commonly perpetrated by mothers against infants or young children. Rare or underrecognized, it accounts for less than 0.04 percent, or 1,000 of three million cases of child abuse reported in the United States each year. Good epidemiological data are lacking. Of infants brought to an Australian clinic for apparently life-threatening episodes, an estimated 1.5 percent represented factitious disorder by proxy. A clinical practice at Great Ormond Street in England reported that, in 20 years, 43 children from 37 families were diagnosed as having induced illnesses.

Donna A. Rosenberg's review of 117 cases revealed valuable information. Male and female children were equally victimized. The mean age of a child at diagnosis was 3.3 years of age, with the onset of symptoms being a mean of 1.24 years earlier. All perpetrators were mothers, with 98 percent being biological mothers and 2 percent being adoptive mothers. Paternal collusion was suspected in only 1.5 percent of the cases. In one-half of the cases, illness was actively produced and inflicted on the child, whereas, in 25 percent, illness was simulated without direct infliction on the child. In 25 percent, illness was simulated and produced. Interestingly, in 25 percent of the cases, morbidity on the child was iatrogenic only, through procedures and investigations. Surprisingly, 70 percent of produced illness occurred in the hospital, making investigation during hospitalization a valuable diagnostic option.

In Rosenberg's review, 10 percent of perpetrators were thought to have Munchausen syndrome themselves, whereas another 14 percent showed features of the syndrome. On the other hand, data collected from the Great Ormond Street clinic over a 20-year period indicated that approximately one-third of perpetrating mothers had a history of factitious disorder themselves. Nearly one-half of them described serious marital problems. Approximately one-half of the perpetrating caregivers had a history of psychiatric symptoms; approximately one-third gave histories of emotional neglect or physical abuse. Fathers were generally absent or peripheral.

ETIOLOGY

The etiology of factitious disorder is not known, and a variety of causes likely explain the wide spectrum of factitious illness behavior. Although factitious illness behavior is, by definition, consciously produced, the underlying motivations for the behaviors are largely considered to be unconscious. Two factors underlie most cases of factitious disorder: (1) an affinity to the medical system and (2) poor, maladaptive coping skills.

A majority of factitious disorder patients have training in medicine, and many work as nurses. In a review of six case series comprising a total of 165 patients, Peter Reich and Lili A. Gottfried found that 60 percent worked in the medical profession. Motives behind medical career choices appeared to be lifelong preoccupations with health rather than access to information to deceive. Indeed, many with factitious disorder see health care providers as allies, not adversaries. In this case series, many patients had personal ties with their physicians, having worked in their offices or having baby-sat for them.

Coping deficits are widely noted. Patients often have immature coping skills, not falling into any current category of personality disorder. This is consistent with observations that many factitious disorder patients come from large families or have been neglected as children, therefore lacking the nurturing conducive to the development of mature coping. This is also consistent with the fact that children often demonstrate factitious illness behavior that is not considered pathological, for example, feigning a stomachache to gain parental attention. On the other end of the spectrum, poor coping may be part of a personality disorder, such as borderline personality or antisocial personality disorder. Dependent and narcissistic personality traits may also be evident.

An underlying psychiatric diagnosis may predispose to factitious illness behavior. Many case reports indicate lessening or alleviation of factitious illness behavior when major depression is treated. Other case reports point to hypochondriasis as an underlying factor. For example, a 27-year-old physician simulated insulinoma by insulin injections. When insulin and a syringe were found in the toilet tank, he confessed a preoccupation that he had pancreatic cancer and that he was trying to provoke further investigation. A 15-year-old boy, convinced that he had a lesion in his urogenital system, simulated hematuria to encourage investigation. Substance abuse, psychotic disorders, and mental retardation have also been implicated.

No genetic or familial inheritance pattern has been shown. No substantial evidence of a biological etiology has been found, despite scattered reports of abnormal brain scans and deficits in neuropsychological testing in a few patients. Indeed, a great percentage of factitious disorder patients achieve advanced degrees, maintain high-functioning jobs as medical professionals, and demonstrate great cognitive astuteness in their manipulations of medical signs and symptoms.

Psychodynamic theories have focused on the concepts of mastery, masochism, and mothering. Achieving mastery may be especially true for factitious disorder patients with predominantly psychological signs and symptoms. For example, as those who present with factitious psychosis often progress to develop a genuine psychotic disorder, the feigning of psychosis may actually be a way of feeling in control of initial psychotic symptoms. As for physical factitious disorder, many of these patients experienced traumatic illnesses as children, and their adult factitious illness behavior may allow them to master situations and to feel control that they never did as children. They demand or refuse procedures and leave the hospital against medical advice when they feel that they are losing control. Masochism may be involved when patients repetitively endure painful or deforming surgeries and procedures, such as amputations of limbs and fingers, or exploratory abdominal surgeries that result in scars and even the gridiron stomach that Asher described as a classic symptom of Munchausen syndrome. The theory here is that the patient relives childhood physical or emotional abuse in a repetition compulsion. The physician and the medical system at large become symbolic parents against whom the patient reenacts dependency, idealization, and anger. The system responds with caring but also with physical and emotional abuse and, too often, ultimately with derision and abandonment. Indeed, for those with chronic factitious disorder, the medical system becomes the main object relation in the patient's life, a substitute mother. The medical system may be a place to experience caring, while avoiding emotional intimacy.

Factitious illness behavior often occurs in the setting of a loss, such as the death of a relative or an occupational loss. Securing the attention of medical clinicians, family, and friends may be a way of obtaining emotional solace without directly confronting the loss. Dependency and narcissistic needs are fulfilled.

Factitious illness behavior may organize some patients, giving them a role and identity. They acquire the role of patient and masterful orchestrator of medical drama. Through pseudologica fantastica, they might even construct desirable and interesting identities.

Behavioral theories postulate that, early in life, these patients received positive reinforcement while in the sick role. Many experienced childhood illnesses and gained nurturing from the medical community that they did not receive at home. Perhaps, they learned to see the medical system as a source of caring and emotional support. Alternatively, many of these patients came from neglectful, large families and became the center of focus when they were ill.

In factitious disorder by proxy, psychodynamic explanations predominate. A common view is that caretakers often have a profound sense of loss, sometimes a history of early abandonment particularly by the father, or loss of contact with another child. Controversy exists regarding the likelihood of a history of abuse for the mothers, as many have reported histories of abuse that were later disqualified by collateral sources. The objectification of the child to serve the parent's psychological needs characterizes all variations of the disorder. A *disorder of empathy* among perpetrating mothers was recognized by Rosenberg, along with pervasive themes of loneliness and isolation, often under circumstances of uninvolved or absent husbands. Through the ill child, the mother seeks a relationship with the physician, the idealized parent, who substitutes for the uninvolved husband. The relationship with the physician is a highly ambivalent one in which the caregiver seeks closeness, although often belittling the physician in some contexts. The more severe the child's illness, the more the mother is needed, and the more she fulfills her own need for caretaking, vicariously through the child and more directly in her relationship with the physician. Fathers tend to be uninvolved or distant. D. Mary Eminson and Robert J. Postlethwaite argue that two axes play a role in factitious disorder by proxy: the desire to consult and the inability of the parent to distinguish parental needs from the child's needs. Herbert A. Schreier and Judith A. Libow call Munchausen syndrome by proxy a *perversion of mothering* in which the child is dehumanized and instead is seen by the mother as a fetishistic object through which her own dependency needs are met.

DIAGNOSIS AND CLINICAL FEATURES

Factitious Disorder with Predominantly Physical Signs and Symptoms Early diagnosis and intervention can minimize physical harm to the patient and iatrogenic complications. Therefore, the diagnosis of factitious disorder should be actively pursued.

Diseases of every organ system have been simulated, including rare illnesses, such as Goodpasture's syndrome and panhypopituitarism. Disease simulation is limited only by the patient's creativity and knowledge and the technological means available. As they tend to have medical training, the factitious patient's knowledge of the disease may exceed that of his or her physicians. This is especially true, as they often present to hospital ERs or clinics during evenings or weekends when less experienced staff or resident physicians are on duty.

Factitious symptoms can be (1) *fabricated*, for example, by giving a false history of cancer, acquired immune deficiency syndrome (AIDS), or another illness; (2) *feigned*, for example, by faking symptoms such as pain or seizures; (3) *induced*, by actively producing symptoms through self-infliction of injury or through injection or ingestion; or (4) *aggravated*, such as manipulating a wound so that it will not heal.

Table 16–3 lists various reported presentations of factitious disorders along with the means used to produce the symptoms and possible means of detection. Viewing the list, one can appreciate the creativity and resourcefulness of these patients, as well as their willingness to undergo pain, injury, and inconvenience for the sake of satisfying emotional needs.

Table 16–4 lists clues that should trigger suspicion of factitious disorder. Factitious disorder should be suspected whenever medical signs or symptoms defy conventional medical understanding or when they do not respond to usual medical treatment, for example, when a wound refuses to heal or when test results show a pattern that is inconsistent with usual disease presentation. Factitious disorder patients may also demonstrate an exceptional eagerness to undergo invasive or extensive testing. They may deny access to collateral sources of information, refusing to sign releases of information and refusing to give contact information for family or friends. An extensive medical history, evidence of multiple surgeries, and reports of multiple drug allergies may also provide clues for the astute clinician. These patients often have jobs in a medical profession, have few visitors, and often have been known to forecast the progression of their symptoms.

Simply raising the suspicion of factitious disorder is the first important step toward diagnosis. After this, information supporting the diagnosis should be collected. A review of past medical records may reveal inconsistencies. Gathering collateral information from family, friends, or other health care providers may likewise show inconsistencies. Ward clerks may be the first to notice waxing and waning levels of distress, depending on when the patient thinks cli-

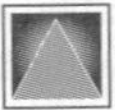

Table 16–3
Presentations of Factitious Disorder with Predominantly Physical Signs and Symptoms with Means of Simulation and Possible Methods of Detection

Symptom	Means of Simulation That Have Been Reported	Possible Methods of Detection
Autoimmune		
Goodpasture's syndrome	False history, adding blood to urine	Bronchoalveolar lavage negative for hemosiderin-laden cells
Systemic lupus erythematosus	Malar rash simulated through cosmetics, feigning joint pain	Negative antinuclear antibody test, removability of rash
Dermatological		
Burns	Chemical agents, such as oven cleaner	Unnatural shape of lesions, streaks left by chemicals, minor injury to fingers
Excoriations	Self-infliction	Found on accessible parts of the body or, for example, a preponderance of left-sided lesions in a right-handed person
Lesions	Injection of exogenous material, such as talc, milk, or gasoline	Puncture marks left by needles, discovery of syringes
Endocrine		
Cushing's syndrome	Steroid ingestion	Evidence of exogenous steroid use
Hyperthyroidism	Thyroxine or L-iodothyronine ingestion	24-hr iodine-131 uptake is suppressed in factitious disease and increased in Graves' disease
Hypoglycemia or insulinoma	Insulin injection	Insulin to C-peptide ratio is greater than one, detection of serum insulin antibodies
	Ingestion of oral hypoglycemics	Serum levels of hypoglycemic medication
Pheochromocytoma	Epinephrine or metaraminol injection	Analysis of urinary catecholamines may reveal epinephrine only or other suspicious findings
Gastrointestinal		
Diarrhea	Phenolphthalein or castor oil ingestion	Testing of stool for laxatives, increased stool weight
Hemoptysis	Contamination of sputum sample, self-induced trauma, such as cuts to tongue	Collect specimen under observation, examine mouth
Ulcerative colitis	Laceration of colon with knitting needle	—
Hematological		
Aplastic anemia	Self-administration of chemotherapeutic agents to suppress bone marrow	Hematology-oncology consultation
Anemia	Self-induced phlebotomy	Blood studies
Coagulopathy	Ingestion of warfarin or other anticoagulants	—
Infectious disease		
Abdominal abscess	Injection of feces into abdominal wall	Unusual pathogens in microbiology tests
Acquired immune deficiency syndrome	False history	Collateral information
Neoplastic		
Cancer	False medical and family history, shaving head to simulate chemotherapy	Collateral information, examination
Neurological		
Paraplegia or quadriplegia	Feigning, fictitious history	Imaging studies, electromyograms
Seizures	Feigning, fictitious history	Video electroencephalogram
Obstetric and gynecological		
Antepartum hemorrhage	Vaginal puncture wounds, use of fake blood	Examination, test blood
Ectopic pregnancy	Feigning abdominal pain while self-injecting hCG	Ultrasound
Menorrhagia	Using stolen blood	Type blood
Placenta previa	Intravaginal use of hat pin	Examination
Premature labor	Feigned uterine contractions, manipulation of tocodynamometer	Examination
Premature rupture of membranes	Voiding urine into vagina	Examine fluid
Trophoblastic disease	Addition of hCG to urine	—
Vaginal bleeding	Self-mutilation with fingernails, nail files, bleach, knives, tweezers, nut picks, glass, and pencils	Examination
Vaginal discharge	Applying cigarette ash to underwear	Examination

(continued)

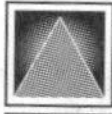

Table 16–3 (*continued*)

Symptom	Means of Simulation That Have Been Reported	Possible Methods of Detection
Systemic		
Fever	Warming thermometer against a light bulb or other heat source, drinking hot fluids, friction from mouth or anal sphincter, false recordings, injection of pyrogens such as feces, vaccines, thyroid hormone, or tetanus toxoid	Simultaneous taking of temperature from two different locations (orally and rectally), recording temperature of freshly voided urine, cool skin despite high thermometer readings, normal white blood cell count, unusually high or inconsistent temperatures
Urinary		
Bacteriuria	Contamination of urethra or specimen	Unusual pathogen
Hematuria	Contamination of specimen with blood or meat, warfarin ingestion, foreign bodies in bladder (pins)	Collect specimen under observation
Proteinuria	Inserting egg protein into urethra	—
Stones	Feigning of renal colic pain, bringing in stones made of exogenous materials or inserting them into urethra	Pathology report

hCG, human chorionic gonadotropin.

nicians are observing. Collection of laboratory specimens under close observation can minimize contamination or manipulation of samples. Sometimes, laboratory values can provide important diagnostic clues, such as in the case of high insulin and low C-peptide levels in patients simulating insulinoma through self-administration of insulin or when microbiology reports reveal unusual pathogens.

Conclusive confirmation of factitious disorder can be difficult. Surveillance techniques, such as covert observation, covert video, or searching the patient's belongings for syringes or illness-inducing substances, have been used. When these techniques are considered, it is essential to involve legal counsel as the patient's right to privacy, as well as constitutional protections against searches and seizures, is at stake. In some cases, court orders should be obtained. Consultation from a bioethics team can help weigh the benefits and risks of these violations of privacy versus morbidity from factitious disorder. This phase of acquiring information to confirm a diagnosis is often a time of conflict for staff who may have split opinions about the patient and about the means being used to confirm diagnosis. Regular interdisciplinary meetings are helpful.

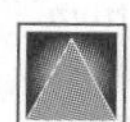

Table 16–4
Clues That Should Trigger Suspicion of Factitious Disorder

- Unusual, dramatic presentation of symptoms that defy conventional medical or psychiatric understanding
- Symptoms do not respond appropriately to usual treatment or medications
- Emergence of new, unusual symptoms when other symptoms resolve
- Eagerness to undergo procedures or testing or to recount symptoms
- Reluctance to give access to collateral sources of information, that is, refusing to sign releases of information or to give contact information for family and friends
- Extensive medical history or evidence of multiple surgeries
- Multiple drug allergies
- Medical profession
- Few visitors
- Ability to forecast unusual progression of symptoms or unusual response to treatment

Chronic Factitious Disorder with Predominantly Physical Signs and Symptoms (Munchausen Syndrome) Because of more dramatic, exaggerated presentations, chronic factitious disorders with predominantly physical signs and symptoms are often more easily diagnosed than those with less chronic factitious disorder, even if treatment and management can be far more challenging. As these patients are prone to peregrination, they often arrive new in town. They demonstrate pseudologia fantastica, with grandiose and far-fetched tales. They often appear eerily comfortable in hospital settings, immediately talking to nurses, physicians, and medical staff as peers. Many show up for hospital admission wearing surgical scrubs. One patient, who claims to be the son of a famous golfer, arrives at the University of New Mexico Hospital each spring seeking medical or psychiatric admission, having made his rounds at other hospitals across several states, using various pseudonyms. The cost of this disorder can be tremendous, as illustrated by the British report of a "million-dollar man" who, over a 13-year period, spent 1,300 days in psychiatric units, 556 days in prison, and 354 days in medical care for 261 hospital admissions.

All diagnostic considerations that apply to factitious disorder also apply here. As the risk of morbidity and mortality may be higher in these patients, it may be prudent to involve bioethics consultations and hospital legal counsel early.

Mr. S. was a 25-year-old, right-handed, married white man who was admitted for square-shaped burns on his left forearm. Because of the odd shape of the burns, factitious disorder was suspected, and psychiatry consultation was promptly obtained. Two weeks earlier, the patient was admitted for necrotizing fasciitis of the left forearm. During that hospitalization, his wife gave birth to an infant son. Factitious disorder was not suspected at that time. Mr. S. reported a past medical history of juvenile-onset diabetes from 1 year of age, asthma, and accidental hot water burns to his left forearm and left lateral thigh at 10 years of age. He reported allergies to 13 medications.

Mr. S. presented in a dramatic manner to the psychiatry consultants saying, "I'm safe nowhere! They happen even while I'm here in the hospital!" He pulled open his hospital gown to reveal a square-shaped burn on his upper back. He reported being the 15th of 16 children born to a Mormon family. He described his childhood as "good," and he denied a history of physical or sexual abuse. He said that his father died of a fall when he was 10 years of age. Mr. S. proudly stated that, even though he was diabetic, he was admitted to the Air Force at 16 years of age in which he worked as a mechanic and an emergency medical technician. Subsequently, he worked at commercial airlines, which took him to live in four different states over 4 years. He stated that his current marriage was his second and that he had lost a son, a daughter, and his first wife all on the same day. As his 4-year-old daughter was dying in the hospital of a brain tumor, his 7-year-old son was killed in a motor vehicle accident while crossing the street to visit her. Under the stress of losing both children, his wife left him that same day. His second wife had schizoaffective disorder and heroin dependence in remission. She was known to the psychiatry consult team who evaluated her after the birth of her son.

The diagnosis of factitious disorder was made, and the patient was informed in a nonconfrontational manner that emphasized that he must have been under great emotional distress to have inflicted such physical pain on himself. The birth of his son, childhood neglect, and traumatic experiences that he may not have disclosed were cited as possible sources of stress. He was referred to psychiatric services.

The week after discharge, the patient returned to seek out the consulting psychiatrist who had confronted him. He voiced concern that his wife was having auditory hallucinations telling her that she was the next bride of Christ. His eagerness to seek treatment for his wife was noted in the context of his reports of the deaths of his first two children. The vague possibility of Munchausen syndrome by proxy was first entertained at this time.

Mr. S. sought psychiatric services, as directed by the psychiatry consultation team. At the psychiatric clinic, he was prescribed nefazodone (Serzone) and later was switched to sertraline (Zoloft) to target depressive disorder NOS, with the primary symptom being irritability toward his wife, with occasional urges to strike her. Periodically, he presented to the psychiatric emergency services complaining of urges to be violent with his wife.

He spent most of the next 4 months admitted to various hospitals in town. Of note, the records of one of the hospitals stated that Mr. S. told them that he had been an F-15 fighter pilot. Two days after discharge from that hospital, he was readmitted to the university hospital for necrosis of a skin graft that he had received. The burn surgery team initially refused to treat him, stating that he was doing it to himself and that they suspected that he was seeking narcotics. They agreed to accept care only after conversation with the psychiatry consultation team. During this admission, his arm was placed in a cast, and it began to heal.

The next month, he was readmitted with worsening of the necrotizing fasciitis with possible osteomyelitis. He asked for amputation of the arm, citing his long treatment course and stating that he wanted to be rid of the pain. Physical therapists noted that his arm healed whenever placed in a cast that precluded tampering of the wounds but that it worsened when placed in looser casts that allowed access to the wounds. At this time, because of the endangerment of losing his arm, he was admitted to the psychiatric hospital involuntarily for close observation. He was informed of a new treatment plan that, whenever he was admitted for a factitious illness, involuntary admission to the psychiatric hospital would follow. On the psychiatric ward, the patient accepted psychotherapy and continued with sertraline. He continued to deny that his wounds were self-inflicted but inquired about treatment for Munchausen syndrome. At one point, when the inpatient psychiatrist asked him, "Why do you do this?" he replied, "I don't know why I do it either." Of note, during the psychiatric hospitalizations, he required no sliding-scale insulin, and he rarely required it while in the medical hospital.

One other admission to the university hospital occurred for worsening of his wounds. He was transferred to the psychiatric hospital according to plan. After this, he ceased seeking admission to the university hospital. Within 1 month, outpatient physical therapy notes indicated that the wound was 90-percent healed, and, within another month, it was near closure.

Approximately 6 months later, he presented to the psychiatric emergency services complaining of difficulty containing his anger toward his wife. Shortly after that, his wife relapsed on heroin and left Mr. S. alone to care for their 1-year-old son. Since his birth, pediatricians had recognized the precarious situation of this child and had been seeing him for scheduled biweekly visits. Child Protective Services were already involved. During a visit with family in another state, the patient brought his son to an ER seeking admission. His son was not admitted and died the next day. Munchausen syndrome by proxy was suspected. An autopsy was performed, but no charges were ever filed against the patient.

One year later, near the anniversary of the son's death, Mr. S.'s then ex-wife presented to the psychiatric emergency services for relapse on heroin and worsening auditory hallucinations telling her that she would be the next bride of Christ. She stated that she too found it suspicious that three of Mr. S.'s children had died. She had recently seen him at a bus stop. His arm was healed, and he appeared healthy. He insisted to her that the university physicians had confirmed that his wounds had indeed been caused by spider bites.

DISCUSSION

Mr. S. showed the classic features of Munchausen syndrome: peregrination, pseudologica fantastica, and the presentation of unusual symptoms that were self-inflicted. His case also illustrates the overlap of different types of factitious disorder, as he sought psychological treatment and demonstrated activity consistent with factitious disorder by proxy. Lastly, his case demonstrates that even Munchausen syndrome, which generally has a grim prognosis, is not completely refractory to intervention.

Self-infliction was suspected, because the square-shaped burns defied usual medical understanding, and because they did not heal with usual treatment. That the nonhealing wounds healed when in a cast and inaccessible was virtually diagnostic of self-infliction. Mr. S. sought care from various hospitals locally, demonstrating peregrination. He had also recently lived in several other states in which he may have sought medical care. Notably, he sought hospitalization in the same month that he moved to town. Pseudologica fantastica was demonstrated in his bragging about admission to the Air Force, even though he was diabetic (the Air Force does not accept diabetics). His tale of losing two children and his first wife on the same day seemed exaggerated and also had the hint of pseudologica fantastica. Although the patient sought narcotic pain medication, he had access to narcotics without needing to endanger his arm or to incur pain, as his wife was a heroin user. His primary motive appeared to be to gain care and attention by assuming the patient role.

Like many others with factitious disorder, Mr. S. reported being from a large family in which he was possibly neglected. Other characteristics present that are common in factitious disorder patients included an affinity to a medical profession (he claimed he was an emergency medical technician), a history of childhood illness (burns at 10 years of age that injured his left arm), and multiple medication allergies. Like others with factitious disorder, he sought medical care at a time of interpersonal loss. With the birth of his son, he faced loss of his wife's attention, in addition to facing other stresses of fatherhood.

Comorbidity with other psychiatric disorders is more the rule than the exception. Mr. S. was treated for depressive disorder NOS. Opiate abuse was also diagnosed. Malingering for opiates may also have been part of his motivation.

His eagerness to procure psychiatric treatment for his wife may have demonstrated genuine concern, but, in the context of the death of his son and the possible deaths of two other children, it is quite likely that Mr. S. also had factitious disorder by proxy. The comorbidity of factitious disorder and factitious disorder by proxy is estimated to be from 10 to 30 percent, and there is an extremely high likelihood of siblings being victimized, usually serially.

Mr. S. sought psychiatric treatment after referral from the psychiatry consultation team. Often, he went to the psychiatric emergency services complaining of anger and potential violence toward his wife. Although there is no clear evidence that he feigned or fabricated psychiatric symptoms, he clearly enjoyed the attention of receiving psychiatry services.

Intervention from the psychiatry consultation team consisted of gentle, nonaccusatory confrontation and psychiatric referral, which the patient accepted. Later, when he was in danger of losing his arm, the behavioral intervention of involuntary psychiatric hospitalization deterred the course of self-injury, and the wounds began to heal consistently. Although morbid consequences ensued with the death of the patient's son, at least intervention was able to prevent amputation of his arm.

Factitious Disorder with Predominantly Psychological Signs and Symptoms Factitious psychological symptoms are more challenging to diagnose because of the lack of clear objective markers for psychiatric disorders. Methods of confirmation applicable with factitious physical disorders, such as contradictory laboratory tests or findings on room searches, do not apply here. Nevertheless, certain features of the patient's presentation can alert the psychiatrist that the patient may be simulating illness. As with physical factitious disorders, the patient may present with unusual symptoms that fail to correspond to any recognizable diagnosis. For example, one patient reported no other psychotic symptoms except seeing the entire cast of a television show emerge from her closet. Other features include worsening of symptoms when the patient is aware of being observed, inconsistencies in the patient's story over time, and the patient's over-eagerness to recount symptoms of the illness. The patient is often suggestible and readily admits to additional symptoms on questioning. The patient may refuse to cooperate with obtaining collateral information, and untraceable prior health care providers are not unusual. On admission to the ward, patients may reveal familiarity with hospital routine, although denying previous hospitalizations. They may exhibit dramatic and unusual reactions to medications. They may demonstrate attention-getting tactics by breaking ward rules. Visitors are usually few or absent.

In contrast to patients with physical factitious disorders who tend to avoid psychiatric care, these patients actively seek contact with the psychiatric system and readily acknowledge the presence of a psychiatric disorder, even if it may not be the one that the patient actually has. Feigned bereavement and then psychosis appear to be the most common presenting symptoms. Ironically, one patient sought psychiatric admission for his Munchausen syndrome, claiming that he feigned physical illness when, in fact, there was no evidence of this.

In a series of 20 patients who presented with factitious bereavement, 15 also exhibited a history of factitious physical symptoms. A majority of them met criteria for other psychiatric disorders. They typically reported recent, dramatic, violent, and, often, multiple deaths of loved ones, whereas collateral information showed that, in fact, no deaths had occurred. Another series of 12 cases of factitious bereavement yielded similar findings of complaints of violent, dramatic deaths and referral from medical wards for supposed physical illness. Although the complaints of bereavement were factitious, these patients exhibited prominent symptoms of depression. A theory about factitious bereavement is that patients are expressing the underlying truth of their emotional state, if not the factual truth. In contrast to the stigma associated with psychiatric illness, sympathy and care are usually offered to those in mourning. This may be why factitious bereavement is the most commonly seen factitious psychological disorder. One patient stated that she had fabricated the complaint of bereavement to rationalize her depression.

In a series of 219 consecutive cases of psychosis, nine (0.04 percent) met criteria for factitious disorder. All nine patients demonstrated severe personality disorder. These patients were doing poorly when followed up 4 to 7 years later, with multiple hospitalizations and poor quality of life. Their outcome was no better than for schizophrenics that were concurrently followed. In another study of six patients who presented with feigned psychosis to the University Hospital of South Manchester, five of the six had developed schizophrenia when followed up 3 months to 10 years later. Consistent with psychodynamic theories about factitious disorders being an attempt to feel mastery, feigning psychosis may have been a way for these patients to feel in control over early psychotic symptoms. These studies show that factitious psychosis may bode as poor a prognosis as genuine psychosis.

Posttraumatic stress disorder (PTSD) can be fabricated through the reporting of subjective symptoms, without requiring the patient to feign or to act. Factitious PTSD can be elucidated through collateral sources of information about alleged trauma, for example, by checking military records for actual tours of duty.

Ms. M. A. was 24 years of age when she first presented in 1973 after an overdose. She gave a history of recurrent overdoses and wrist-slashing attempts since 1969, and, on admission, she stated that she was controlled by her dead sister who kept telling her to take her own life. Her family history was negative.

She was found to be carrying a list of schneiderian first-rank symptoms in her handbag; she behaved bizarrely, picking imaginary objects out of the wastepaper basket and opening imaginary doors in the waiting room. She admitted to visual hallucinations and offered four of the first-rank symptoms on her list, but her mental state reverted to normal after 2 days. When she was presented at a case conference, the consensus view was that she had been simulating schizophrenia but had a gross personality disorder; however, the consultant in charge dissented from that general view, feeling that she was genuinely psychotic.

On follow-up, this turned out to be the case. She was readmitted in 1975 and was mute, catatonic, grossly thought disordered, and the diagnosis was changed to that of a schizophrenic illness. She has been followed up regularly since and now presents the picture of a mild schizophrenic defect state; she takes regular depot medication but still complains of auditory hallucinations, hearing her dead sister's voice. She is a day patient.

DISCUSSION

Ms. M. A.'s diagnosis was factitious disorder with predominantly psychological signs and symptoms, along with a personality disorder. Although her initial psychotic symptoms were elaborate and feigned, 2 years after her initial presentation, she developed psychotic symptoms believed to be genuine by clinicians, even after continued observation as a day patient.

This case illustrates that, even if psychotic symptoms are factitious, they are often a sign of serious psychopathology, such as a severe personality disorder, or a prodrome to a genuine psychotic disorder.

Factitious Disorder with Combined Psychological and Physical Symptoms Factitious disorder with combined psychological and physical symptoms is the appropriate diagnosis for patients who present with psychological and physical signs and symptoms of factitious disorder, with neither dominating the clinical picture.

Mr. M. T. was a man who appeared to be middle-aged but who arrived at a children's psychiatric hospital claiming to be 17 years of age and suicidal. As he held a gun to his head, staff called security officers who promptly recognized him as the Munchausen syndrome patient who arrived in early May each year. He was denied admission.

Late that evening, he presented to the ER of the main hospital claiming that he was diabetic, dizzy, and weak. Intern physicians found his blood glucose to be low and immediately admitted him. Hospital staff on the wards recognized him as "that Munchausen syndrome patient," and a psychiatric consultation was requested. The patient continued to insist that he was 17 years of age and that he was the son of famous golfer Lee Trevino. Hospital legal counsel revealed that he used at least two other pseudonyms and social security numbers and was wanted for health insurance fraud in at least two other states.

When the psychiatry consultants greeted him with familiarity, the patient immediately claimed suicidal tendency, but, when denied psychiatric admission, he left the hospital against medical advice. An inquisitive medical student called local pharmacies, which informed him that, if a customer claimed to be diabetic, traveling, and without insulin, they would give the customer insulin even without a prescription to avoid liability. In this manner, Mr. M. T. could have procured insulin to induce hypoglycemia.

At a care conference, a psychiatry consultant expressed that, in the past, common practice was to call ERs in town to alert them to Munchausen syndrome patients, giving all possibly helpful descriptions and information. However, because of heightened attention to confidentiality rights, she now instead advocated calling ERs and simply warning them about the possible appearance of a patient with factitious hypoglycemia. An ER physician, however, stated that he would go ahead and give a detailed description of the patient to friends in each ER in town. The May of the following year, the patient failed to appear for the first time in several years.

DISCUSSION

This case demonstrates an almost exaggerated example of peregrination and pseudological fantastica, typical among Munchausen syndrome patients. The debilitating consequences of the disorder are also demonstrated, with his life, by all indications, consisting of short hospital stays across many states, precluding stable relationships or employment. The case also illustrates the complexity of legal and ethical issues involved in the management of factitious disorder in regard to privacy.

As he sought hospitalization for psychological and physical disorders equally in this instance, Mr. M. T.'s diagnosis was factitious disorder with combined psychological and physical signs and symptoms.

Factitious Disorder by Proxy Also called *Munchausen syndrome by proxy*, the essential feature of factitious disorder by proxy is the intentional feigning or production of physical or psychological symptoms in another person who is under an individual's care. The perpetrator's motive is to assume the sick role by proxy. Mothers of young, preverbal children are the most common perpetrators, however, fathers, grandmothers, foster mothers, stepmothers, and even baby-sitters have also been implicated. Victims can also be spouses, elderly parents, or anyone under the care of the perpetrator. In an unusual case of adult factitious disorder by proxy, a 34-year-old man drugged his wife with sleeping pills in her coffee, then injected gasoline into her skin to cause lesions from which she eventually died. Subsequently, he repeated his actions with a female baby-sitter whom he hired to care for his children. In each case, he assumed the role of the concerned caretaker in the center of hospital drama. Factitious disorder by proxy has also been cited as the etiology for death epidemics at hospitals and nursing homes. Perpetrators have largely been nurses and nurses' aides who produced illness through various means, such as injection of insulin, lidocaine, digoxin, or other substances.

By and large, however, reported cases have involved mothers and their children. Difficulties in recognizing deception and diagnosing this condition are illustrated by two unfortunate examples. First Lady Nancy Reagan presented an award to an apparently valorous foster mother of extremely ill children. The woman was later suspected of having killed her children through factitious disorder by proxy. Sudden infant death syndrome (SIDS) was initially thought to have a strong genetic component, as it often occurred in siblings. Today, when siblings die of SIDS, infanticide is suspected. A study of 81 children who died at the hands of parents but who were initially thought to have died of SIDS or natural causes showed that one-half of the perpetrating parents had factitious disorder or another somatizing disorder. In both of these examples, as in other cases, perpetrators were initially regarded with sympathy and respect.

The variety of medical presentations of factitious disorder by proxy is impressive. In the first comprehensive review of the disorder published in 1987, Rosenberg described 68 different induced or fabricated signs or symptoms. The most common presentations were bleeding (44 percent), seizures (42 percent), central nervous system (CNS) depression (19 percent), apnea (15 percent), diarrhea (11 percent), vomiting (10 percent), fever (10 percent), and rash (9 percent). Many children had more than one presentation. Twenty-five percent of cases involved simulation of illness, 50 percent involved illness production, and, in the remaining 25 percent, simulation and production of illness were concurrent.

Perpetrating caregivers usually appear concerned and interested in every aspect of their children's care. They are exemplary in their interactions with medical staff, enlisting support and sympathies, often crossing professional boundaries by helping nurses with duties or eating meals with staff. They may demonstrate unusual willingness or even excitement at the prospect of invasive procedures for their children.

Factitious disorder by proxy should not be considered a diagnosis of exclusion. Confirmatory evidence should be actively pursued, so as to lessen risk to the child. Safety of the child should be ensured at the same time. The gold standard for confirming factitious disorder by proxy is covert video surveillance that may record evidence of a parent causing harm to a child. Covert video has also shown cases in which mothers, who appear concerned in the presence of staff, behave indifferently toward their children when they are not aware of being watched. Covert video should only be undertaken after consultation with legal counsel. A court order may need to be obtained, and a bioethics consultation may be helpful to weigh the potential benefits to the child versus compromises of privacy for the parent.

Other means of confirming factitious disorder by proxy include searching the mother's belongings for illness-inducing agents, reviewing collateral information and past medical records for inconsistencies, gathering information on siblings, recording temporal associations between parental visits and the child's signs and symptoms, observing the child's well-being when removed from the parent's care for extended periods, and analyzing specimens taken in the presence of the parent compared to those taken in the parent's absence.

The international literature on Munchausen syndrome by proxy indicates that the signs and symptoms appear consistent across the world. Perpetrators are usually mothers, and serial abuse of children is common. This does not appear to be a phenomenon that is exclusive to medicalized societies.

B. C. was a 1-month-old girl admitted for evaluation of temperature elevation. Psychiatric consultation was requested owing to inconsistencies in the mother's reporting of medical information, despite her initial presentation as a knowledgeable and caring mother who worked as an emergency medical technician. B. C.'s mother said that she was diagnosed with ovarian cancer at 3 months' gestation with B. C., that she had had a hysterectomy during the cesarean section, and that she had been getting radiation therapy at a local hospital since B. C.'s birth. The pediatrician called the local hospital with the mother's permission and found that she had a corpus luteum cyst removed at 3 months' gestation and mild hydronephrosis, but no cancer and no hysterectomy. B. C.'s mother, when confronted with this, stated only that she might need a kidney transplant for the hydronephrosis.

On further exploration, it was discovered that the mother had pursued care for her children in multiple ERs and had reported inaccurate histories that resulted in excessive testing. For example, she told clinicians that her 2-year-old son had lupus and hypergammaglobulinemia and, at another time, that he had asthma and seizures. She also pursued a minor cosmetic surgical procedure for her son against the recommendation of his pediatrician. No clinicians suspected that B. C.'s mother had produced symptoms in any of her children, but rather that she had intentionally fabricated symptoms by raising the temperature on B. C.'s thermometer. She had been faithful in keeping medical appointments. Her children appeared healthy and well cared for, despite her descriptions of illness. The mother denied a psychiatric history but gave permission for clinicians to call the local psychiatric hospital to inquire. Her record there showed a history of depression, anorexia, and panic disorder and included a psychiatric hospitalization after a suicide attempt. Subsequently, she received psychotherapy and psychopharmacotherapy, which she stopped a few months before this presentation. During B. C.'s admission for temperature elevation, her mother agreed to resume treatment with her previous psychiatric clinicians. A social services referral was also made, and the children's pediatrician agreed to coordinate regularly scheduled follow-up visits and monitoring of the children.

DISCUSSION

B. C.'s case illustrates several common features of factitious disorder by proxy. This mother, who had medical training, simulated fever in her child in the hospital as a means of maintaining contact with the hospital system and obtaining the sympathy of clinicians. She had a psychiatric history that, in this case, included depression, anorexia, and panic disorder. Shortly before this presentation, she had lost the support of her psychiatric clinicians, which may have exacerbated her need for contact with the medical system. Several of her children had been the victims of her simulations of illness, as is common in factitious disorder by proxy.

A less common aspect of this case was the mother's easy willingness to engage in treatment. The medical team's supportive, nonaccusatory approach most likely helped enable her to cooperate as much as she did. Ambivalence toward clinicians, including overt praise and cooperation alternating with covert rage and belittling, is more common. Acceptance of psychiatric treatment recommendations is not often so smooth.

PATHOLOGY AND LABORATORY REPORTS

No laboratory or pathology tests are diagnostic of factitious disorders, although they may be useful in demonstrating deception and helping to confirm diagnosis.

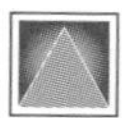

Table 16–5
Urine Samples Confirming Munchausen Syndrome by Proxy from a 6-Year-Old Girl with Unexplained Hematuria

Time	Appearance	Collection
5:00 PM	Normal	By nurse
6:45 PM	Bloody	By mother
7:15 PM	Normal	By nurse
8:15 PM	Bloody	By mother
8:30 PM	Normal	By nurse

Adapted from Meadow R: Munchausen syndrome by proxy: The hinterland of child abuse. *Lancet.* 1977;2:343.

In the first Munchausen syndrome by proxy article published in 1977, Meadow reported the case of a 6-year-old girl with unexplained hematuria. Table 16–5 displays urine samples collected during one evening that helped establish the diagnosis.

DIFFERENTIAL DIAGNOSIS

A true physical or psychiatric disorder is the main consideration in the differential diagnosis of a suspected factitious disorder. This is particularly true of psychological factitious disorders, as they are most often a manifestation of, or a prodrome to, an actual psychiatric illness.

Comorbid physical or psychiatric disorders are more the rule than the exception in factitious disorder. For example, most patients who feign pseudoseizures have true underlying seizure disorders. Those who manipulate blood sugars to produce symptoms are usually diabetics. Munchausen syndrome patients who compulsively seek the sick role for emotional reasons may also become addicted to narcotics or learn to seek disability payments, thereby also demonstrating substance abuse and malingering. A woman who consciously produced cellulitis by smearing feces on a leg wound was sometimes also seen in a dissociative state, unconsciously picking at wounds. Often, factitious disorder patients aggravate an actual physical illness. Furthermore, even factitiously produced physical symptoms, such as infections or poisonings, must be treated seriously, as, once the symptoms are induced, they are all too real. In all cases of factitious disorder, underlying psychopathology should be suspected.

Other special considerations in the differential diagnosis are detailed in the following sections.

Factitious Disorder with Predominantly Physical Signs and Symptoms Figure 16–2 provides an algorithm for the differential between factitious disorder, malingering, and somatoform disorders.

If the primary goal is not to play the patient role but is material, such as procuring disability payments, narcotics, or an excuse from work, the diagnosis is malingering. If the symptoms are manifest unconsciously, then the following somatoform disorders should be considered. In *conversion disorder*, neurological symptoms, such as paralysis or pseudoseizures, are unconsciously manifested, usually in response to stresses. In *somatization disorder*, the patient has a pattern of multiple unexplained medical complaints in four categories: at least four pain symptoms, four gastrointestinal (GI) symptoms, one sexual symptom, and one neurological symptom. For those with unexplained physical complaints that last 6 months or longer but who do not meet the threshold for the diagnosis of somatization disorder, *undifferentiated somatoform disorder* should be

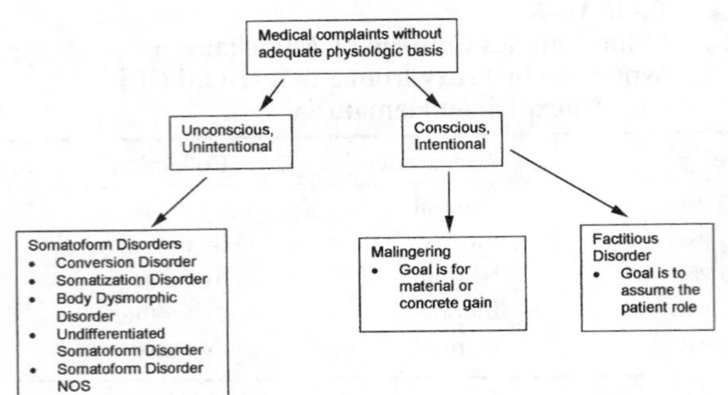

FIGURE 16–2 Differential diagnosis of factitious disorder with predominantly physical signs and symptoms. NOS, not otherwise specified.

diagnosed. In *pain disorder*, psychological factors contribute to the exacerbation or onset of pain. Those with *hypochondriasis* are preoccupied with the fear of illness and are vigilant about bodily symptoms, falsely believing that they are ill. Those with *body dysmorphic disorder* are preoccupied with an imagined or exaggerated defect in bodily appearance. *Somatoform disorder NOS* should be diagnosed for patients who unconsciously manifest physical symptoms but who do not meet criteria for the previously mentioned disorders.

In actuality, whether a symptom has conscious or unconscious origins can be difficult to discern. Furthermore, whether the patient's primary motive is to assume the sick role or to avoid a court date of which the clinician is unaware can also be difficult to discern. These judgments are completely dependent on the subjective opinion of the clinician. For these reasons, Marc D. Feldman, James C. Hamilton, and Holly N. Deemer argue that these disorders fall along a continuum: "There is little to be gained, and much to be lost, by the use of the current practice of viewing the somatoform disorders, factitious disorder, and malingering as discreet and distinct clinical entities."

Factitious Disorder with Predominantly Psychological Signs and Symptoms

With psychological factitious symptoms, it can be especially difficult to separate conscious from unconscious production of symptoms. For this reason, Richard Rogers questions the legitimacy of this diagnostic category. Furthermore, many authors propose that consciousness and unconsciousness constitute a continuum and are not distinct entities.

Ganser syndrome, first described in 1897, consists of twilight states, memory disturbances, and *vorbeireden*, a German term loosely translated as "talking at cross purposes." An example would be answering "65" to the question of "How much is eight times eight?" Ganser syndrome is thought to be dissociative in nature or due to organic causes.

Again, comorbidity should be strongly considered, as these patients often have coexisting personality disorders. Factitious psychological symptoms can often be a prodrome to true psychiatric illness, as in the case studies of factitious psychosis evolving into schizophrenia.

Factitious Disorder by Proxy

Factitious disorder and malingering at the initiation of the child should also be considered, especially in older children and teenagers. Other *by-proxy* disorders should be considered. Children can be made to manifest the psychopathologies of their parents. For example, in hypochondriasis by proxy, a hypochondriac mother is preoccupied with the health of her child and repetitively seeks pediatric care, putting her child at risk for unnecessary procedures and iatrogenic illness. In anorexia nervosa by proxy, an anorexic mother restricts her child's food owing to unfounded fears of excessive weight in her child. One mother with malingering by proxy put her child through multiple evaluations to maintain disability payments. A paranoid father with a history of psychosis feared that his son was being poisoned by breast milk and insisted that the ER check his son's hair for mercury. Other by-proxy syndromes described in the literature include *masquerade syndrome* (in which illness fabrication results in the child's increasing dependency on the mother), *mothering to death* (confining a child to a sick role as if the child were ill, while avoiding physicians and agencies), *extreme illness exaggeration* (when a parent exaggerates the child's symptoms in an effort to increase a pediatrician's attention to the child), and *achievement by proxy* (as in youth sports).

Clinicians should also keep in mind the wide range of normal behavior in parents who seek medical care for their children. According to Meadow, "exaggeration and mild deception are part of everyday behavior."

To aid in differential diagnosis, it is helpful to keep in mind that, in factitious disorder by proxy, illnesses tend to have exotic, dramatic presentations, and parents often exhibit a remarkable lack of relief as the child's condition improves.

COURSE AND PROGNOSIS

Factitious Disorder with Predominantly Physical Signs and Symptoms

The wide spectrum of factitious disorder with predominantly physical signs and symptoms should be remembered when considering course and prognosis. At the more benign end of the spectrum, factitious illness behavior can be considered normal, as when a child exaggerates distress from a knee scrape to gain attention or when a mother magnifies her child's symptoms to seek reassurance. Further along the spectrum, factitious illness behavior can be a maladaptive way of coping with stress and does not necessarily imply an ongoing factitious disorder.

An underlying mood, anxiety, or substance abuse disorder that is treatable bodes for a better prognosis, whereas an underlying personality disorder, especially antisocial personality disorder, bodes for a poorer prognosis. Most patients with factitious disorder experience remission at approximately 40 years of age, corresponding to the age of remission for many with borderline personality disorder.

Munchausen syndrome or chronic factitious disorder with predominantly physical signs and symptoms, on the other hand, has an unremitting, refractory course. Management and treatment are directed toward harm reduction, rather than remission or cure.

Factitious Disorder with Predominantly Psychological Signs and Symptoms

Psychological factitious disorder is also thought to forebode a poor prognosis. A 1982 study of patients with factitious psychosis showed that at follow-up 4 to 7 years later, the functioning of these patients was comparable to the functioning of schizophrenic patients in the same study. Other studies found that feigned psychosis is commonly a precursor to actual psychosis, leading one investigator, Hays, to comment: "Acting crazy may bode more ill than being crazy." In general, factitious disorder with predominantly psychological signs and symptoms is thought to have a poor prognosis comparable to that of Munchausen syndrome.

Factitious Disorder by Proxy

For victims of factitious disorder by proxy, the estimated mortality rate is from 6 to 22 percent, usually through suffocation or poisoning. In Rosenberg's 1987 review, 10 of the 117 children in the review died, a mortality rate of 9 percent, and the youngest were the most vulnerable to death. A sobering statistic is that, in 20 percent of the deaths, caretakers were confronted with the diagnosis of Munchausen syndrome by proxy, but the children were sent back to them, subsequently to die. Of the survivors, 8 percent had long-term morbidity, including impairment of GI functioning, destructive joint changes, limp, cerebral palsy, cortical blindness, and serious psychiatric problems. In 75 percent of the cases, morbidity was caused by the medical staff and the perpetrator. In 25 percent of the cases, however, morbidity was solely iatrogenic, caused by procedures and investigations.

Siblings of victims of factitious disorder by proxy are at great risk. Studies indicate that 9 to 29 percent of siblings die, underscoring the vital importance of investigating the siblings of suspected factitious disorder by proxy patients. The involvement of different children tends to occur serially rather than simultaneously, so one must always be on the alert for additional victims. In 1990, Meadow studied 27 young children suffocated by their mothers. Over 13 years, nine died, and one had severe brain damage. These 27 children had 18 siblings who had died "suddenly and unexpectedly in early life." In another study of 32 children presenting with factitious epilepsy, 21 percent of siblings (7 of 33) had died of SIDS. Similarly, in a separate study of suffocation cases, 21 percent of siblings (3 of 14) had died unexpectedly. In another study of 56 victims of Munchausen syndrome by proxy, 39 percent of siblings were subjected to illness fabrication. Among Rosenberg's review of 117 cases, ten siblings had died under "unusual circumstances."

TREATMENT AND MANAGEMENT

Guidelines for the treatment and management of factitious disorder are given in Table 16–6. There are three major goals in the treatment and management of factitious disorders: (1) to reduce the risk of morbidity and mortality, (2) to address the underlying emotional needs or psychiatric diagnosis underlying factitious illness behavior, and (3) to be mindful of legal and ethical issues.

Management of countertransference is also a major issue, as strong negative feelings on the part of clinicians can interfere with appropriate patient care. Allowing the patient to save face is essential to establishing a therapeutic alliance and preventing the patient from simply taking the factitious illness behavior elsewhere. This is especially true, as factitious disorder patients usually have immature personalities or personality disorders that make them especially sensitive to narcissistic injury. Legal disincentives might be pursued. In Arizona, a woman with factitious disorder was prosecuted for fraudulent procurement of medical, psychiatric, and dental services, and she pled guilty.

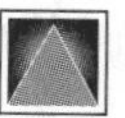

Table 16–6
Guidelines for Management and Treatment of Factitious Disorder

Active pursuit of a prompt diagnosis can minimize the risk of morbidity and mortality.
Minimize harm. Avoid unnecessary tests and procedures, especially if invasive. Treat according to clinical judgment, keeping in mind that subjective complaints may be deceptive.
Regular interdisciplinary meetings to reduce conflict and splitting among staff. Manage staff countertransference.
Consider facilitating healing by using the double-bind technique or face-saving behavioral strategies, such as self-hypnosis or biofeedback.
Steer the patient toward psychiatric treatment in an empathic, nonconfrontational, face-saving manner. Avoid aggressive direct confrontation.
Treat underlying psychiatric disturbances, such as Axis I disorders and Axis II disorders. In psychotherapy, address coping strategies and emotional conflicts.
Appoint a primary care provider as a gatekeeper for all medical and psychiatric treatment.
Consider involving risk management professionals and bioethicists from an early point.
Consider appointing a guardian for medical and psychiatric decisions.
Consider prosecution for fraud, as a behavioral disincentive.

Factitious Disorder with Predominantly Physical Signs and Symptoms

The hippocratic doctrine of "first do no harm" should be kept firmly in mind. Prompt recognition of factitious disorder can reduce the risk of morbidity or mortality. Therefore, active pursuit of the diagnosis and timely management are essential. For example, in the case of the woman who sought prophylactic mastectomy for an extensive family history of breast cancer, early recognition of the factitious disorder may have prevented the bilateral mastectomies that were performed. Recognition of factitious asthma or arthritis prevents the prescribing of potentially harmful steroid medications. Likewise, invasive and potentially harmful tests, procedures, and treatments can be minimized. Once symptoms are confirmed or agreed on as factitious, clinicians should administer medical treatment according to their own clinical judgment, weighing objective evidence and keeping in mind that subjective complaints and requests from the patient can be deceptive. Of course, in many instances, the patient has induced illness, so that invasive treatments must be administered.

In a medical setting, psychiatric consultation should be promptly obtained. Involvement of risk management and bioethicists is usually prudent. As these patients are prone to cause confusion and splitting of caretakers, good communication between all involved is essential. Regular interdisciplinary meetings are helpful.

Several strategies have been successfully used to facilitate the healing of factitiously produced symptoms in face-saving ways. Stuart J. Eisendrath has advocated a *double-bind* technique, whereby patients are told that, if the physical or psychological symptoms are genuine, then they should improve with the treatment being administered. If the symptoms do not improve, then they are factitious. This technique can be used with nonhealing wounds, factitious paralysis, or psychological factitious symptoms that should improve with medications. For example, factitious patients who chronically induce or worsen wounds can be informed, "this treatment should heal your wound. If it doesn't, we have no choice but to conclude that this is due to a factitious disorder."

Self-hypnosis and biofeedback can also allow the patient to relinquish factitious behavior while saving face. For example, a patient can be told that, under self-hypnosis, blood flow to a wound can be increased and therefore promote healing. In this manner, the patient can take control of healing the wound, rather than seek control by worsening symptoms. Positive feedback should be given to patients when their efforts result in healing. Biofeedback can be used in a similar way.

On an outpatient basis, all medical care should be directed through a single primary care physician through whom all care is coordinated. This can minimize unnecessary repetition of tests and treatments. However, it should be remembered that the patient may seek care from clinicians in another system, in another city, or even in another state or country. Appointments with the gatekeeping primary care physician should be regular and frequent and not dependent on medical crises.

This fosters object constancy while minimizing the patient's need to induce illness to seek medical attention.

Once the factitious disorder is confirmed, or suspicions are deemed sufficient, the patient should be gently and artfully steered toward ongoing psychiatric treatment in a face-saving, sympathetic manner that the patient can accept. The patient can be told that the factitious illness behavior is an expression of great emotional need or distress. The clinician can make empathic statements about the neglect, abuse, or trauma that the patient has undergone. This allows the patient to save face, while promoting insight about probable origins of the patient's factitious behavior. The patient should then be steered toward seeking care in a psychiatric setting in which underlying psychiatric issues can be addressed and in which the risk of morbidity and mortality is substantially less. Personality-disordered patients usually crave to be understood and to have their emotional needs recognized. This type of understanding confrontation that focuses on the patient's genuine, rather than factitious, needs can be well accepted by patients.

Direct or aggressive confrontation is generally not effective. The patient usually responds with anger and denial and may leave against medical advice only to perpetuate the factitious illness behavior elsewhere, the need for mastery through deception now amplified. Clinicians should remember that confession is not a necessary aspect of management or treatment.

Psychiatric treatment should first focus on the treatment of underlying Axis I disorders. Although rare, the presence of a comorbid Axis I disorder, such as a mood disorder, an anxiety disorder, or substance abuse disorder, bodes a better prognosis. Pharmacological and psychotherapeutic treatments should be used according to the diagnosis. Other than targeting comorbid psychiatric disorders, there is no standard pharmacological treatment for factitious disorder. Comorbid Axis II disorders are more common than Axis I disorders. Borderline personality disorder is the most common comorbid diagnosis. Antisocial personality traits are also common, especially in those exhibiting pseudologica fantastica and Munchausen syndrome. Psychiatric treatment should be directed at these underlying disorders.

Psychiatrists should be aware of their own countertransference and then should help medical clinicians cope with their countertransference, so that they do not let negative feelings interfere with treating these patients who may falsify symptoms but who also have genuine needs. Negative countertransference can lead to therapeutic nihilism, nonemergent breaches of confidentiality, or denial of care. Countertransference feelings of frustration and anger should be used constructively, as a way of understanding the patient's long-standing feelings.

Once in psychiatric treatment, relapses should be expected in a similar manner as for substance abusers. Clinicians should not be disappointed at relapses but should see them as opportunities for further understanding about the patient. For example, if a patient has a pattern of relapsing under conditions of new romantic involvements or arguments with authority figures, then this provides valuable insight into the patient's vulnerabilities, and these issues can be addressed in psychotherapy.

Legal and ethical issues play prominently in the management of factitious disorder patients, and, for this reason, risk management professionals and bioethicists should be involved from an early point. Confidentiality, the right to privacy, and the constitutional protection against unwarranted searches and seizures are major issues. The once-common practice of alerting all ERs about factitious disorder patients is now not routinely practiced because of heightened sensitivity about confidentiality rights. Nevertheless, this kind of widespread alerting can be done with the consent of the patient. For example, once a patient acknowledges having factitious disorder, the patient can be asked, "I'd like to minimize harm to you. Can I have your permission to alert ERs and some doctors in the community?" Likewise, the patient's right to confidentiality should be respected when gathering collateral information in nonemergent situations. Verbal permission or, preferably, signed releases of information should be obtained before contacting collateral sources, except in emergency situations. Clinicians should be careful about revealing information to the patient's employers, friends, or family. The diagnosis of factitious disorder must never be revealed, even to spouses or significant others, without the explicit permission of the patient. Searching a patient's hospital room or personal belongings for illness-inducing means may facilitate the diagnosis of factitious disorder and may lessen morbidity, but this should only be done after consulting with risk management or other legal counsel, as it may violate a patient's constitutional protections. Likewise, covert surveillance, such as covert video, should only be undertaken after careful legal consultation. It should also be remembered that, simply because an action is legal, it is not necessarily ethical. Therefore, the involvement of bioethicists can be helpful.

Factitious Disorder with Predominantly Psychological Signs and Symptoms The most widely used strategy is empathic communication that the feigned illness represents intrapsychic distress that can be alleviated through proper psychiatric treatment. Brief but regular contacts on a time-contingent, rather than a distress-contingent, basis are the mainstay of therapy. Consistent long-term psychotherapy is aimed at enabling patients to express their feelings, to gain insight and coping skills, and to provide a reliable and supportive outlet for communication.

The double-bind approach can be applied. Patients are told that their conditions should improve with certain medications and psychotherapy and that, if they do not improve, factitious disorder will be suspected.

A critical aspect of treatment in an inpatient setting is the management of staff reaction, which can include hostile and negative countertransference. It is essential to preserve good staff communication and to formulate a clear management plan involving the whole team, to minimize splitting. The psychiatrist or psychotherapist may also be prone to negative countertransference, arising from feelings of being duped or manipulated. The clinician must take care to manage possible feelings of therapeutic nihilism and other feelings that may interfere with the ability to form a therapeutic alliance.

Comorbid mental illnesses must be recognized and treated appropriately. For example, most cases of feigned bereavement are comorbid with major depression. One patient claimed to have feigned bereavement to justify depression. Another claimed to have recently been raped and sought help for PTSD. Although she was not recently raped, she had experienced long-standing childhood sexual abuse. Feigned mental illnesses may express an emotional truth for the patient, if not a factual truth.

Factitious Disorder by Proxy Protection of the child is the first priority in factitious disorder by proxy. Active pursuit of the diagnosis and then prompt intervention are essential toward minimizing the risk of morbidity and mortality to the vulnerable child. In the process of gathering clinical information and evidence, clinicians should keep in mind that, if the mother feels that suspicions are raised or that she is losing control of the situation, she is likely to take the child out of the medical setting and to seek care elsewhere. When the diagnosis of factitious disorder by proxy is confirmed, or as evidence is sufficient so that clinicians are convinced, parents should be confronted together. In this way, the father's involvement in the perpetration, as well as his possible role as an ally, can be assessed. In advance of confrontation, Child Protective Services should be involved, and a legal hold should be instituted to prevent parents from fleeing with the child. In all 50 states, reporting of factitious disorder by proxy to child abuse protection authorities is mandatory.

In Rosenberg's review of cases, 20 percent of children who died of factitious disorder by proxy were sent home with their parents, after parents were confronted with the diagnosis. Given the high rate of mortality and morbidity in these cases, the child should be removed from the parents until treatment and further assessment indicate that it is safe for the family to be reunited. Child Protective Services usually take responsibility for this action. When this is done, there is a high likelihood that the mother will need intervention for suicidal ideation. Investigation into possible abuse of siblings should also be initiated.

After separation, the child must be treated for ongoing medical problems, as well as for psychological problems. For many children, long-standing refractory medical illnesses resolve, once they are separated from perpetrators. Psychologically, many children experience PTSD and should be treated. As is typical of those with PTSD, many victims avoid medical care as adults. On the other hand, others develop factitious disorder themselves. By adolescence, many victims of factitious disorder by proxy collude with parents in perpetrating deception.

The perpetrator, usually the mother, should also undergo treatment. Underlying psychiatric disorders should be addressed. The mother should be evaluated to determine whether it is likely that she will ever achieve good enough parental status and whether reunification with the child is a realistic goal. Those who actively induce illness in their children are less likely to ever be adequate parents. If reunification is unrealistic, then psychotherapy should focus on the mother's underlying psychopathology, as well as her loss of the child. If reunification is the goal, then treatment should address emotional maturation of the mother, the ability to put the child's needs before her own, relinquishing the defense of denial, and learning to seek help and to express herself in appropriate ways. The mother should also work on boundary issues and should learn to distinguish her own needs from the needs of the child.

If reunification occurs, careful monitoring should follow. Child Protective Services should be involved. A primary pediatrician should act as a gatekeeper who monitors and approves all medical care.

Although the literature on factitious disorder by proxy is cast in the shadow of the most severe cases, mild cases do occur. Meadow advocates that, in these mild cases, mothers should be supported and prevented from putting their children through needless investigations and treatments. Psychotherapy should be undertaken. The prognosis in these cases may not be so grim.

There is little literature on the treatment of factitious disorder by proxy between adults. In these cases, removal of the victim through legal means is usually not an option, as the victim is an adult. The victim must usually be responsible for initiating separation. In cases in which health care providers are suspected of perpetrating illness among their patients, removal of the health care provider is essential, and legal prosecution should be considered.

FUTURE DIRECTIONS

Clearly, the entire area of factitious disorder would benefit from more research, as little empirical evidence is available, and virtually no controlled studies have been done. The deceptive nature of the illness makes systematic study difficult.

At the current time, factitious disorder by proxy is not an official DSM diagnosis but is considered a diagnosis deserving of further study. Acceptance as an official DSM and ICD-10 diagnosis should increase its recognition in the clinical setting and should lead to decreased morbidity and mortality. Within the realm of factitious disorder by proxy, perifactitious disorders, such as hypochondriasis by proxy and other by-proxy disorders that result in excessive medical care for children, should also be further considered.

SUGGESTED CROSS-REFERENCES

Somatoform disorders are discussed in Chapter 15. Malingering is the subject of Section 26.1. Personality disorders are addressed in Chapter 23. Psychotherapy is discussed in Chapter 30.

References

Adshead G, Brooke B, eds. *Munchausen's Syndrome by Proxy: Current Issues in Assessment, Treatment and Research.* London: Imperial College Press; 2001.

Aduan RP, Fauci AS, Dale DD: Factitious fever and self-induced infection: A report of 32 cases and review of the literature. *Ann Intern Med.* 1979;90:230.

Allison DB, Roberts MS. *Disorder Mother of Disordered Diagnosis? Munchausen by Proxy Syndrome.* Hillsdale, NJ: The Analytic Press; 1998.

*Asher R: Munchausen's syndrome. *Lancet.* 1951;1:339.

Ayoub CC, Alexander R: Definitional issues in Munchausen by proxy. *APSAC Advisor.* 1998;11:7.

Bhugra D: Psychiatric Munchausen's syndrome: Literature review with case reports. *Acta Psychiatr Scand.* 1988;77:497.

Edi-Osagie EC, Hopkins RE, Edi-Osagie NE: Munchausen's syndrome in obstetrics and gynecology: A review. *Obstet Gynecol Surv.* 1998;53:45.

Eisendrath SJ: Factitious physical disorders: Treatment without confrontation. *Psychosomatics.* 1989;30:383.

Eisendrath SJ, McNeil DE: Factitious disorders in civil litigation: Twenty cases illustrating the spectrum of abnormal illness-affirming behavior. *J Am Acad Psychiatry Law.* 2002;30:391.

Eminson DM, Postlethwaite RJ: Factitious illness: Recognition and management. *Arch Dis Child.* 1992;67:1510.

Feldman MD, Eisendrath SJ, eds. *The Spectrum of Factitious Disorders.* Washington, DC: American Psychiatric Press; 1997.

*Feldman MD, Hamilton JC, Deemer HN. Factitious disorder. In: Phillips KA, ed. *Somatoform and Factitious Disorders.* Washington, DC: American Psychiatric Publishing; 2001.

Folks DG: Munchausen's syndrome and other factitious disorders. *Neurol Clin.* 1995;13:2.

Ford CF. *The Somatizing Disorders: Illness as a Way of Life.* New York: Elsevier Science; 1983.

Gavin H. *On the Feigned and Factitious Diseases of Soldiers and Seamen, on the Means Used to Simulate or Produce Them, and on the Best Modes of Discovering Impostors.* Edinburgh: University Press; 1838.

Gelenberg AJ: Munchausen's syndrome with a psychiatric presentation. *Dis Nerv Syst.* 1977;38:378.

Hay GG: Feigned psychosis: A review of the simulation of mental illness. *Br J Psychiatry.* 1983;143:8.

Krahn LE, Li H, O'Connor MK: Patients who strive to be ill: Factitious disorder with physical symptoms. *Am J Psychiatry.* 2003;160:1163.

*Meadow R: Munchausen syndrome by proxy: The hinterland of child abuse. *Lancet.* 1977;2:343.

Meadow R: Management of Munchausen syndrome by proxy. *Arch Dis Child.* 1985;60:385.

Meadow R: Unnatural sudden infant death syndrome. *Arch Dis Child.* 1999;80:7.

Phillips MR, Ward NG, Ries RK: Factitious mourning: Painless patienthood. *Am J Psychiatry.* 1983;147:1057.

Pope HG, Jonas JM, Jones B: Factitious psychosis: Phenomenology, family history, and long-term outcome of nine patients. *Am J Psychiatry.* 1982;139:1480.

*Reich P, Gottfried LA: Factitious disorders in a teaching hospital. *Ann Intern Med.* 1983;99:240.

Rogers R, Bagby RM, Rector N: Diagnostic legitimacy of factitious disorder with psychological symptoms. *Am J Psychiatry.* 1989;146:1312.

*Rosenberg DA: Web of deceit: A literature review of Munchausen syndrome by proxy. *Child Abuse Neglect.* 1987;11:547.

Schrier H: Munchausen by proxy defined. *Pediatrics.* 2003;110:958.

Schreier HA, Libow JA. *Hurting for Love: Munchausen by Proxy Syndrome.* New York: Guilford Press; 1993.

Snowdon J, Solomons R, Druce H: Feigned bereavement: Twelve cases. *Br J Psychiatry.* 1978;133:15.

Spiro HR: Chronic factitious illness: Munchausen's syndrome. *Arch Gen Psychiatry.* 1968;18:569.

Sutherland AJ, Rodin GM: Factitious disorders in a general hospital setting: Clinical features and a review of the literature. *Psychosomatics.* 1990;31:392.

Wallach J: Laboratory diagnosis of factitious disorders. *Arch Intern Med.* 1994;154:1690.

Wise MG, Ford CV: Factitious disorders. *Primary Care.* 1999;26:2.

17 Dissociative Disorders

RICHARD J. LOEWENSTEIN, M.D., AND
FRANK W. PUTNAM, M.D.

DISSOCIATION AND DISSOCIATIVE PHENOMENA

Introduction According to the text revision of the fourth edition of the *Diagnostic and Statistical Manual of Mental Disorders* (DSM-IV-TR), "the essential feature of the dissociative disorders is a disruption in the usually integrated functions of consciousness, memory, identity, or perception of the environment. The disturbance may be sudden or gradual, transient or chronic." The DSM-IV dissociative disorders are dissociative identity disorder, depersonalization disorder, dissociative amnesia, dissociative fugue, and dissociative disorder not otherwise specified (NOS). In the following section, many issues that are common to all the dissociative disorders are discussed together, with separate sections on the different disorders to follow.

Diagnostic Criteria: DSM and ICD The study of the dissociative disorders began at the end of the 18th century. However, the modern notion that these conditions are a distinct group of disorders, with systematic research about them, did not really begin until the advent of the third edition of the DSM (DSM-III) in 1980. Although the first edition of the DSM (DSM-I) distinguished *dissociative reactions* from other *reactions*, the second edition of the DSM (DSM-II) subsumed dissociative conditions under the superordinate category of hysterical neurosis. The latter was conceptualized as a conversion or dissociative subtype.

In DSM-III, conditions that developed from the 19th century construct of *hysteria* were distributed among different diagnostic categories: dissociative disorders, somatoform disorders (especially conversion disorder and somatization disorder), posttraumatic stress disorder (PTSD) (in the anxiety disorder section), and histrionic and borderline personality disorders. The DSM-III took the stance that the label *hysteria* had become so imprecise and variously defined that it had become meaningless. The DSM-III took the approach that these conditions would be defined and organized separately, so that systematic, empirical research could better clarify their reliability and validity.

The tenth edition of the *International Statistical Classification of Diseases and Related Health Problems* (ICD-10) classifies the dissociative disorders among the *neurotic*, *stress-related*, and *somatoform disorders*. The ICD-10 explicitly states that the term *hysteria* should be avoided because of its lack of precision. The ICD-10 dissociative [conversion] disorders include dissociative amnesia, dissociative fugue, dissociative stupor, trance and possession disorder, and dissociative disorders of movement and sensation (roughly equivalent to the DSM-IV-TR conversion disorder diagnosis). The latter includes dissociative motor disorders, dissociative convulsions, and dissociative anesthesia and sensory loss. Ganser syndrome and multiple personality disorder are classified under *other* dissociative disorders. Depersonalization disorder is classified separately. The ICD-10 diagnostic criteria for these disorders are found in Table 17–1.

Controversies about Dissociative Disorders The DSM-IV-TR and the ICD-10 take divergent approaches to the relationship of conversion disorders to dissociative disorders. The former treats them as separate conditions, and the latter treats them as conditions with similar underlying mechanisms. This difference symbolizes only one of the many passionate disagreements that surround the disorders that have evolved from classic hysteria. Indeed, it is unlikely that any other group of disorders in psychiatry can evoke so much heated controversy, conflict, and fervent debate than the conditions derived from the hysteria concept, particularly the dissociative disorders. This is especially ironic, because, since the 1980s, there is finally an increasingly rigorous body of research data on many of the DSM-IV-TR dissociative disorders, as well as the phenomenon of dissociation, itself.

Why should there be such a passionate debate? Why should appeals to the results of scientific research not resolve it? More so than other psychiatric conditions, these disorders touch on many complex and contentious aspects of personal, political, philosophical, and even religious beliefs. These include the nature of memory, volition, and consciousness and the responsibility of individuals for their own behavior. Indeed, the debate touches on fundamental questions about the nature of the mind, the self, and the most intimate human behaviors.

When viewed within a larger sociopolitical perspective, dissociation theory intersects with many of the most controversial social issues of modern times. Recent systematic research consistently has found a robust relationship between dissociation and traumatic experiences. The role of trauma in Western culture, particularly intergenerational violence and sexual abuse, crosses into historically taboo subjects, such as rape, incest, child abuse, and domestic violence, and their actual prevalence in Western society. In addition, the study of trauma leads into larger legal, social, and cultural questions related to peace and war, the meaning of violence in Western society, and even varying religious views about the relationship between men, women, and children and the nature of the family.

In psychiatry and psychology, these disorders are the focus of controversies that include the long-standing debates between mentalists and behaviorists, between *psychodynamically oriented* and *biologically oriented* clinicians, between various researchers in cognitive psychology, between cognitive researchers and clinical researchers and practitioners, and between different theoretical schools at odds over the nature of hypnosis. Some fundamentalist Christian clinicians even have viewed demonic possession as part of the differential diagnosis of dissociative disorders.

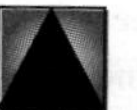

Table 17–1
ICD-10 Diagnostic Criteria for Dissociative (Conversion) Disorders

G1. There must be no evidence of a physical disorder that can explain the characteristic symptoms of this disorder (although physical disorders may be present that give rise to other symptoms).

G2. There are convincing associations in time between the onset of symptoms of the disorder and stressful events, problems, or needs.

Dissociative amnesia

A. The general criteria for dissociative disorder must be met.

B. There must be amnesia, partial or complete, for recent events or problems that were or still are traumatic or stressful.

C. The amnesia is too extensive and persistent to be explained by ordinary forgetfulness (although its depth and extent may vary from one assessment to the next) or by intentional simulation.

Dissociative fugue

A. The general criteria for dissociative disorder must be met.

B. The individual undertakes an unexpected yet organized journey away from home or from the ordinary places of work and social activities, during which self-care is largely maintained.

C. There is amnesia, partial or complete, for the journey, which also meets Criterion C for dissociative amnesia.

Dissociative stupor

A. The general criteria for dissociative disorder must be met.

B. There is profound diminution or absence of voluntary movements and speech and of normal responsiveness to light, noise, and touch.

C. Normal muscle tone, static posture, and breathing (and often limited coordinated eye movements) are maintained.

Trance and possession disorders

A. The general criteria for dissociative disorder must be met.

B. Either of the following must be present:

(1) *Trance.* There is temporary alteration of the state of consciousness, shown by any two of the following:

(a) Loss of the usual sense of personal identity

(b) Narrowing of awareness of immediate surroundings or unusually narrow and selective focusing on environmental stimuli

(c) Limitation of movements, postures, and speech to repetition of a small repertoire

(2) *Possession disorder.* The individual is convinced that he or she has been taken over by a spirit, power, deity, or other person.

C. (1) and (2) of Criterion B must be unwanted and troublesome, occurring outside, or being a prolongation of, similar states in religious or other culturally accepted situations.

D. *Most commonly used exclusion clause.* The disorder does not occur at the same time as schizophrenia or related disorders, or mood (affective) disorders with hallucinations or delusions.

Dissociative motor disorders

A. The general criteria for dissociative disorder must be met.

B. Either of the following must be present:

(1) Complete or partial loss of the ability to perform movements that are normally under voluntary control (including speech)

(2) Various or variable degrees of incoordination or ataxia, or inability to stand unaided

Dissociative convulsions

A. The general criteria for dissociative disorder must be met.

B. The individual exhibits sudden and unexpected spasmodic movements, closely resembling any of the varieties of epileptic seizure but not followed by loss of consciousness.

C. The symptoms in Criterion B are not accompanied by tongue biting, serious bruising or laceration due to falling, or urinary incontinence.

Dissociative anesthesia and sensory loss

A. The general criteria for dissociative disorder must be met.

B. Either of the following must be present:

(1) Partial or complete loss of any or all of the normal cutaneous sensations over part or all of the body (specify: touch, pin prick, vibration, heat, cold)

(2) Partial or complete loss of vision, hearing, or smell (specify)

Mixed dissociative (conversion) disorders

Other dissociative (conversion) disorders

This residual code may be used to indicate other dissociative and conversion states that meet Criteria G1 and G2 for dissociative (conversion) disorders but do not meet the criteria for the dissociative disorders listed previously.

Ganser syndrome (approximate answers)

Multiple personality disorder

A. Two or more distinct personalities exist within the individual, only one being evident at a time.

B. Each personality has its own memories, preferences, and behavior patterns and, at some time (and recurrently), takes full control of the individual's behavior.

C. There is inability to recall important personal information, which is too extensive to be explained by ordinary forgetfulness.

D. The symptoms are not due to organic mental disorders (e.g., in epileptic disorders) or psychoactive substance-related disorders (e.g., intoxication or withdrawal).

Transient dissociative (conversion) disorders occurring in childhood and adolescence

Other specified dissociative (conversion) disorders

Specific research criteria are not given for all disorders mentioned previously, because these other dissociative states are rare and not well described. Research workers studying these conditions in detail should specify their own criteria according to the purpose of their studies.

Dissociative (conversion) disorder, unspecified

From World Health Organization. *The ICD-10 Classification of Mental and Behavioural Disorders: Diagnostic Criteria for Research.* Geneva: World Health Organization; 1993, with permission.

Issues here include the significance of early trauma for human psychopathology; the existence of *unconscious* mental life and *intrapsychic defenses*, such as *repression*; the nature of memory; and the nature of hypnosis and whether it involves altered states of consciousness. Furthermore, the existence of dissociative amnesias and delayed recall of traumatic events raise difficult-to-answer questions about the reliability of traumatic memory. The latter issue has been a significant controversy in the psychiatric community that has spilled over into the courts and the popular media, arenas in which dispassionate scientific inquiry is unlikely to be the central concern of the participants.

A particularly contentious debate has evolved over the relationship of dissociative disorders to psychological trauma. This idea has been the subject of systematic research, generally showing a repeated, robust relationship between trauma and dissociative phenomena and disorders. In fact, this research led the American Psychiatric Association (APA) DSM-IV Advisory Committee on PTSD to include dissociative amnesia, dissociative fugue, and dissociative identity disorder/multiple personality disorder among the disorders most strongly related to an antecedent history of traumatic or stressful experiences, or both.

Alternatively, another group of psychiatric clinicians and researchers has decried the emphasis on trauma in the conceptualization of dissociative disorders. These authors doubt the relationship between traumatic circumstances and the development of dissociative disorders, particularly in regard to dissociative amnesia and dissociative identity disorder. They dispute the notion that there is a strong association between the development of dissociative identity disorder and early childhood maltreatment. Similarly, they insist that amnesia for trauma does not occur, particularly for childhood sexual abuse.

Some of these critics have argued that dissociative identity disorder and dissociative amnesia are not valid disorders at all and should be dropped from the DSM-IV-TR. Others have proposed a resurrection of the term *hysteria* to account for these conditions. Others have conceptualized them as factitious conditions, related to patient suggestibility and clinician naïveté. Some relate the development of these disorders to underlying personality disorders, particularly borderline personality disorder. In this view, the personality disorder is seen as the primary disorder, with the dissociative disorder developing secondary to *sociocognitive* factors.

The clash of views about these issues has been particularly notable in the debate over *repressed* or *recovered* memory that has divided the mental health community since the 1990s. High-profile legal cases have been the center of this debate. In one incarnation, so-called victims alleging delayed recall for childhood maltreatment have been given standing to sue or to bring criminal actions based on the *delayed discovery* rule, overcoming the statute of limitations.

In the alternative form, accused parents or recanting former victims, or both, have sued mental health providers alleging malpractice or alienation of affections, or both, based on the notion that there is no such thing as dissociation, amnesia, repression of memory, and dissociative disorders. These cases have been the subject of considerable media attention.

Dissociation and the Media From the middle of the 19th century to the present, the popular media has nurtured public fascination with various forms of dissociation, especially multiple personality. Accounts of 19th century cases were carried in popular magazines such as *Harpers*, and famous cases, such as Morton Prince's Miss Beauchamps (1905), became the subjects of books and plays. Robert Lewis Stevenson's *The Strange Case of Dr. Jekyll and Mr. Hyde* (1886) is the most well-known of these works. Other popular 19th century novels and plays focused on fugue, amnesia, and crimes committed under the influence of hypnosis or in somnambulistic states. From at least the 1930s onward, sensational reports of patients with generalized dissociative amnesia or fugue, or both, were featured in the daily newspapers. Similar cases are still periodically featured in the news when amnestic patients are found who cannot be identified.

In the late 20th century, popular accounts of multiple personality, such as *The Three Faces of Eve*, *Sybil*, and a recent spate of similar first-person accounts, continued in this vein. The widespread use of multiple personality as a fictional plot device—generally to give a bizarre twist to the story—has contributed to the public and professional confusion that surrounds this disorder. Similarly, amnesia for life circumstances and for trauma is also a recurrent story mechanism in contemporary novels, films, and television—almost never portrayed accurately. Media stereotyping occurs for many forms of mental illness, but the distortions typical in most fictional depictions of dissociative disorders are particularly misleading.

Highly publicized criminal and civil cases, such as the Hillside Strangler, the Franklin murder case, the Ramona case, and many others, have brought additional media attention to claims of multiple personality, amnesia, and recovered memory. These contentious cases, with their warring academic experts and sensationalized media depictions, have also fueled popular stereotyping of dissociative disorders. Media spin about these cases has often been inaccurate and misleading.

Because of all this, one commentator ruefully observed that most clinicians get the bulk of their training about dissociation and dissociative disorders from television. For the foreseeable future, because of the complexity of the social, cultural, philosophical, and political issues that these conditions evoke, it is unlikely that debates about them will remain purely in the academic arena.

History The study of hysteria and dissociation begins at the end of the 18th century with shift of interest in these phenomena from the religious to the medical realm. Paracelsus, writing in 1646, is credited with the first medical report of an individual with alternating selves. In 1791, Eberhardt Gmelin described a German woman who alternately exchanged her peasant personality for that of an aristocratic French lady, each amnesic for the other's existence.

By the early 19th century, such cases, with diagnoses of dual, double, or duplex consciousness, were being regularly reported on both sides of the Atlantic. In 1811, Benjamin Rush, considered the father of American psychiatry, included a classic example in his medical school lectures. Rush proposed that dual personality reflected a functional disconnection between the two cerebral hemispheres. In the same year, the case of Mary Reynolds, who became the American archetype of dissociative identity disorder for the remainder of the century, was first published.

In Europe, disciples of Franz Anton Mesmer developed the first systematic descriptions of what is now called *hypnosis*. These thinkers developed an interest in *magnetic diseases* (from Mesmer's theories of animal magnetism): amnesia, fugue, somnambulistic states, and alternating or multiple personality that could be treated with *artificial somnambulism*, that is, hypnosis. These *magnetizers* were mostly outside the mainstream of European academic medicine, and their works are not widely known. Among them, Antoine Despine, a French family doctor, wrote systematic case studies and reports about several series of multiple personality patients, including child and adolescent cases. Most of these 19th century patients also had extensive conversion and somatoform symptoms as part of the clinical presentation.

Psychiatric historians have charted the shift in interest from somnambulism to multiple personality to hysteria and back over the course of the 19th century, with hysteria finally seen as a unifying concept for all these conditions. Many contemporary debates about dissociation were prefigured by those in the 19th century. For example, Paul Briquet, who wrote a famous study of hysteria in the mid-19th century, disputed the prevailing notion that the disorder was caused by sexual frustration. He believed that traumatic, overwhelming, and grief-engendering experiences led to the development of hysteria.

The famous 19th century French psychiatrist, Jean-Martin Charcot, synthesized the teachings of the magnetizers with those of the more accepted medical and psychiatric establishment, including Briquet's etiological theories. Charcot influenced major figures in psychiatry and neurology, such as Sigmund Freud, Pierre Janet, Georges Gilles de la Tourette, and Joseph Babinski. As is well known, he gave public demonstrations of hysterical patients and hypnosis at his hospital, La Salpetriere. Unknown to the careless Charcot, however, many patients were readily prompted in various ways to perform spectacularly for him. Some were magnetized (i.e., hypnotized) on the wards or encouraged by sycophantic followers of Charcot to act as dramatically as possible for the great man. In addition, Charcot's methods of demonstrating his patients abundantly cued them to the expected responses.

After his death, two of Charcot's most important successors, Babinski and Janet, took divergent views of hysteria. Babinski took the radically nihilistic view that all hysteria was caused by *suggestion* and could be removed by persuasion or countersuggestion. He coined the term *pithiatism* as a substitute for hysteria. In addition, the Nancy school of hypnosis, led by Hippolyte Bernheim, believed that hypnosis was not necessarily a sign of pathology, as Charcot believed, but an effect of suggestion. Babinski and Bernheim believed that the symptoms of Charcot's patients were artifacts of suggestion and contagion, not of bone fide disorders. This view continues today, most prominently in the thinking of Paul McHugh, a vehement critic of the current trauma-based theories of dissociation.

At the end of the 19th century, Pierre Janet in France, Prince and William James in the United States, and others across Europe were engaged in a lively transatlantic discussion about possible psychological and neurological mechanisms underlying cases of multiple personality, amnesia, and fugue. Medical models of the time invoked phenomena such as sleep and dreams, hypnosis and somnambulism, epilepsy, and disconnections between the cerebral hemispheres to explain multiplicity. Pierre Janet's research and clinical theory, in particular, his emphasis on the role of traumatic antecedents of dissociation, are widely regarded as the foundation for modern views of dissociation.

As the 20th century began, however, interest in dissociation waned, and alternative theories, like psychoanalysis, began their ascendance. However, clinical interest in dissociative phenomena has reoccurred in every war since the turn of the century with the observation of amnesia, fugues, and conversion symptoms in traumatized soldiers. Subsequently, these observations tended to be forgotten by the psychiatric community, as the wars themselves fade from memory.

For example, Babinksi's ideas had considerable influence on European psychiatrists until the onset of World War I. At that time, with the development of the concept of *shell shock*, psychiatrists systematically reported that virtually all of the symptoms of dissociation, amnesia, automatism, and hysteria could be found among battle traumatized soldiers, plainly contradicting Babinski's ideas and supporting those of Janet.

Janet and Freud Janet is generally regarded as the founder of modern approaches to dissociation and dissociative disorders. He was also the first psychiatrist to provide systematic, modern descriptions of obsessive-compulsive disorder (OCD), phobias, and anorexia nervosa. He was deeply knowledgeable of the works of the magnetizers and their early papers on dissociation, hysteria, and multiple personality. He developed theories of hysteria and dissociation, suggesting that many cases of hysteria are based on covert, dissociated aspects of the personality that were engendered by traumatic experiences in susceptible individuals. He believed that the fundamental lesion in hysteria was the *narrowing of consciousness* in which the hysterical person is unable to perceive aspects of subjective or objective phenomena. These then become dissociated, independent-agent aspects of the mind. Janet also posited a kind of *stress-diathesis* model in which constitutional and environmental factors coincided to produce the psychopathological dissociative outcome.

Janet developed a sort of cognitive behavioral psychotherapy for his patients, involving hypnosis and a search for a hierarchy of hidden traumatic memories and related *fixed ideas* going back in the patient's history. Janet also used hypnotic suggestion, imagery, and creative engagement with his patients to modify their bizarre hallucinations, disturbed perceptions, and hysterical alterations of consciousness. Janet worked intensely with the hysterical crises of the patients and, despite intense symptomatic storms and suicidal crises, found that the patients improved after this work. In addition, intellectual tasks and work were prescribed for the patient. Janet also described many issues in the process of therapy that have been rediscovered by contemporary students of the dissociative disorders. These include a kind of addiction to altered states of consciousness and intense involvement with the therapist, leading to therapeutic stalemate.

Janet was attacked by followers of Babinksi and Berheim as a credulous disciple of the discredited ideas of Charcot. His critics notwithstanding, Janet himself was distressed by the contamination of patients under Charcot's hospital administration; Charcot's failure to fully understand the work of prior scholars, such as the magnetizers; and the factitious nature of many of the patients' symptoms. For the most part, he refused to work with former patients of Charcot and took careful histories of patients' prior treatments to uncover potential therapeutic shaping of symptoms.

Freud and Joseph Breuer's revered *Studies in Hysteria* (1893) referenced Janet's work, and used similar notions of fixed ideas and traumatic etiology, and introduced the cathartic method of cure for hysteria. Anna O., the archetypal Freudian hysteric, is clearly described as having a dual personality and a plethora of dissociative symptoms, such as complex amnesias for current and historical experience; spontaneous age regressions and trances; depersonalization; fluctuations in handwriting, handedness, and language; and alternating states of consciousness.

However, as time went on, many psychoanalysts excoriated Janet, asserting that he dishonestly claimed priority for these ideas related to hysteria, even though Janet's work clearly antedated Freud's. Janet, for his part, was uncharacteristically publicly angry at this failure to acknowledge his work. Throughout his career, he remained critical of Freud and psychoanalytic ideas.

Despite the janetian ideas found in early freudian works on hysteria, freudian theories of hysterical and dissociative phenomena differ in important ways from those of Janet. Freud posited the ideas of the dynamic unconscious, intrapsychic conflict, and intrapsychic defense related to unacceptable thoughts, wishes, ideas, and memories. Later, he developed theories of transference and countertransference. After Freud repudiated the seduction theory and developed a new and different theory of mental life, he and his followers increasingly focused on the somatoform aspects of hysterical phenomena, to the neglect of the dissociative ones. David Rappaport, Merton Gill, Margaret Brenman, Charles Fischer, and Elisabeth Geleerd, among others, wrote important psychoanalytic papers on fugue, amnesia, and dissociation in the 1940s and 1950s. However, psychoanalytic thinkers have largely ignored this work.

It is unfortunate that disputes over primacy of ideas led to a schism between Janet and the freudians. Modern conceptualization of dissociative disorders often involves a synthesis of janetian ideas and freudian ones. For example, current theories of treatment include the janetian notions of systematic work with traumatic memories using adjunctive hypnotic and imagery techniques, work with posttraumatic cognitive distortions, using cognitive and behavioral psychotherapy, psychoeducation, and building of life skills. The psychoanalytic concepts of transference, countertransference, object relations, intrapsychic defense, and conflict, among others, are also essential to understanding modern therapy of dissociative patients.

Janet continued to be active in psychology and psychiatry until his death in 1947, writing on many different clinical, theoretical, and philosophical subjects. Janet never developed a formal school of psychology nor a group of disciples committed to his theories. He was deeply concerned with the protection of patient confidentiality, perhaps in part as a reaction to the excesses of the Charcot era. Accordingly, he had his library of detailed case histories, including those of the most famous classic hysterics, destroyed at his death. Because of this, and because of the primacy of the psychoanalytic theories in the latter part of the 20th century, his work was largely neglected until the recent resurgence of interest in dissociation.

Janet's contributions to modern dissociation theory include (1) recognition of the causal role of trauma in dissociation in a stress-diathesis model; (2) the taxonometric approach—Janet believed that dissociation was not on a continuum from normal psychological experience; (3) recognition that the underlying mental mechanisms of somatoform and dissociative disorders were similar; (4) the role of *fixed ideas* in dissociative disorders and attempts to find the most fundamental ideas that influence the patient's behavior; (5) treatment using a multimodal approach with hypnotic and trauma-focused methods combined with cognitive therapy, behavioral therapy, and life-skills building.

World Wars I and II and after Clinicians treating battlefield casualties in World Wars I and II readily noted dissociative symptoms, such as amnesia, fugue, automatisms, and somatoform symptoms, in traumatized soldiers as part of *traumatic war neurosis*, as it came to be known in World War II. The extent of amnesia described in psychiatric battlefield casualties in World War II ranged from relatively brief periods of time to complete amnesia for life history (generalized amnesia), as well as fugue episodes.

Treatment of these World War II amnesia cases included hypnosis, narcosynthesis with sodium amobarbital (Amytal), or individual and group psychotherapy, or a combination of these. Attempts were made to treat these soldiers on the front lines and to return them rapidly to combat. Detailed case descriptions of dissociative amnesia and fugue can be found in clinical studies from that time. Soldiers from the Korean conflict also were noted to have amnesia as part of the posttraumatic syndromes related to combat experiences and were treated with similar modalities.

The observations of these military psychiatrists were mostly lost until the resurgence of interest in trauma and dissociation in the 1970s and 1980s. Authorities cite several social and cultural factors leading to this revival. These include the return of the Vietnam veterans and the systematic academic study of their psychiatric problems; the recognition of the prevalence of childhood physical and sexual abuse with its associated mandated reporting; development of clinical attention to, mandated reporting of, and research on child abuse and family violence; the rise of feminism with its critique of psychological theories that ascribed sexual abuse reports to fantasy; increased academic rigor in theories about hypnosis, such as Earnest Hilgard's *neodissociation* theory, and greater acceptance of academic hypnosis research; popular interest in multiple personality owing to works, such as *Sybil*; and the DSM-III, with its promulgation of diagnostic criteria for the dissociative disorders and PTSD.

Later History Since the publication of the DSM-III in 1980, a large body of systematic research has developed about dissociative disorders, particularly dissociative identity disorder, dissociative amnesia, and depersonalization disorder. Many academic studies have also investigated dissociation as a quantifiable trait in clinical and nonclinical samples. Studies have also looked at the prevalence and phenomenology of amnesia, particularly as it relates to the question of delayed recall for traumatic experiences.

As noted previously, the study of the dissociative disorders appears to be inseparable from the social and cultural ambiance in which it occurs. Academic interest in trauma and its clinical outcomes has been paralleled by social and religious movements focusing on self-identification as a victim of childhood abuse, and the seeking of recovery through a variety of therapeutic and self-help modalities. Furthermore, some feminist theorists opined that healing from childhood sexual abuse mandated confrontation with alleged perpetrators in personal meetings or in the courts, or both.

Legal theorists, concerned that victims of childhood maltreatment did not have standing to sue for damages or to bring criminal actions under usual statutes of limitations, lobbied state legislatures to expand the length of time that victims could seek legal redress. This was based on the idea that many survivors had amnesia for abuse or did not recognize the harm that had been done to them until many years after the abuse had occurred, or both.

Many states did alter the statute of limitations for childhood sexual abuse, allowing the statute to begin to toll after the person recovered memory of the abuse or, alternatively, after recognizing the harm that had been done whether amnesia was present or not. A number of successful legal actions were brought under these theories, with courts accepting expert testimony concerning the validity of "repressed memory" for childhood maltreatment.

In the 1980s, clinicians working with dissociative disorders began to report patient accounts of multiperpetrator, multivictim abuse in the context of supposed underground cult groups. These frightening and chilling accounts were amplified by highly publicized day care abuse cases that alleged multiple perpetrators, in some cases with elements of occultism and ritualized abuse. Several state governments developed commissions to investigate allegations of ritual abuse and claimed to have found evidence of these activities. Needless to say, the media also developed an intense interest in these reports, with publication of popular autobiographical accounts of patients with reported histories of "ritual abuse," as well as frequent news stories and television specials on this and related topics.

Unfortunately, some clinicians working with these dissociative patients chose to respond to their patients' reports in a highly publicized and sensationalized manner, rather than subjecting them to dispassionate and rigorous scrutiny. Some of these clinicians painted themselves as crusaders against a vast criminal conspiracy that threatened the nation, presenting themselves and their patients on television and in the newspapers. Patients on some specialized dissociative disorders units shared detailed recollections of trauma in group therapy and in the hospital milieu, with relatively little concern for possible cross-contamination or confusion about the origin of accounts of trauma. Cautionary or critical voices among dissociative disorders researchers and clinicians were ignored or rebuked. Forensic and clinical research was disregarded that cast doubts on the veracity of these patients' accounts and suggested alternative mechanisms for many of these ritual abuse narratives.

Ultimately, an extensive backlash occurred that focused broadly on a large number of claims related to childhood maltreatment. This included a wholesale debunking of the day care criminal cases, even those that had resulted in convictions and for which there was solid proof. There was increased skepticism about the reliability of children's reports of childhood maltreatment, particularly for childhood sexual abuse. Popular works that encouraged readers to work on recovery from abuse were castigated as suggesting abuse to millions when none had occurred. Allegations of delayed recall for childhood trauma in clinical and forensic cases were disparaged as based on erroneous views of human memory and cognition. The dissociative disorders construct was dismissed completely as engendered by suggestion and sociocognitive factors. Therapy based on working with traumatic memories was discounted as risky. The reports of an extensive prevalence of childhood abuse in the general population and its actual impact on psychopathology were questioned. Some critics raised doubts about the validity of the diagnostic construct of PTSD.

As always, the print and television media, looking for a new angle on an old story with which to increase revenue or viewer and reader interest, devoted extensive space to these critiques. Where they once had devoted hours to crying child abuse victims, they now showed hours of crying wrongfully accused parents, day care providers, and recanting former victims.

A significant impact on this debate was produced by the False Memory Syndrome Foundation, founded in 1992 by parents whose psychologist daughter had privately accused her father of sexual abuse, reportedly recalled only in adulthood. These parents sought out other families with similar histories, some of whom had had successful criminal or civil judgments brought against them because of their children's allegations of abuse. The organization sought to publicize the claims of its founders and members that their adult children's accounts of trauma were confabulations caused by psychotherapy. This organization, accompanied by several attorneys, developed a legal theory that was a direct counterpoint to that developed by the feminist clinicians and attorneys who had sought legal confrontation with alleged abusers.

In this theory, there was no such thing as delayed recall for trauma. Instead, clinicians who were ignorant of the complexities of human memory engaged in risky clinical strategies, such as hypnosis or *guided imagery*. They convinced credulous patients that their difficulties were all based on a history of repressed childhood abuse and engaged in therapeutic techniques that led patients to believe that these confabulations were accurate. The patients then made these abuse accounts the explanatory center of their lives, ascribing all problems to their alleged early maltreatment. The patients were urged to confront or to stop all contact with family members accused of sexual abuse, ritual abuse, and other forms of maltreatment.

A group of attorneys and a coterie of academic expert witnesses sought out patients and ex-patients to bring civil cases throughout the country in which therapists were sued for malpractice or were subject to licensing board complaints, or both, based on diagnoses of dissociative identity disorder and dissociative amnesia and engagement in therapy involving work with apparent traumatic memories. Many of these cases were settled without ever ending up in court. Several resulted in jury findings for the plaintiffs with significant damage awards. Others concluded with juries finding for the defendant doctors. A federal mail fraud case against several clinicians ended in a mistrial before the prosecution's case had concluded, with the prosecution declining to retry the case.

Only one published study has looked systematically at retractors of abuse allegations, amnesia, and dissociative identity disorder. It found that virtually all of these individuals had long psychiatric histories, with PTSD and dissociative symptoms predating contact with defendant clinicians. Virtually all of these patient-plaintiffs had significant personality disorders in which they readily took the victim role and looked to forces outside themselves for explanation of their problems. Factitious elements were prominent in many patients' presentations. With treatment, most had actually *improved* with respect to their dissociative psychopathology, but the other Axis I and Axis II difficulties remained substantial. Later, usually after termination of treatment by their clinicians, the patients shifted their perception of victimization from their parents to their prior therapists, now putting their attorneys in the role of rescuer, usually with the promise of large sums of money if they prevailed in their lawsuits.

Despite its popularity in the media, *false memory syndrome* as a clinical construct has never been operationalized or studied using methods to validate it as a construct. Virtually no research has been done on this entity as a clinical disorder. However, a number of experiments on memory have been performed by cognitive psychology researchers, subsequent to the naming of the false memory syndrome, that support or cast doubts on whether memory is permanently altered by various forms of misinformation and suggestion. Studies are discrepant regarding whether memory is easy to modify for a variety of types of experiences. Studies vary with the population studied, the type of information (or misinformation) provided, and the research paradigm to test memory fallibility. Often presented as a simple problem in research that has been definitively solved, the opposite is more accurate: This is a complex area of research on a set of highly complex phenomena in which a number of competing paradigms exist.

Nonetheless, the experience of many experts suggests, however, that some therapies that resulted in false memory lawsuits could have been subject to malpractice litigation without this factor. Although many such treatments were exemplary, others resulted in a positive outcome, despite clinicians' difficulties in managing transference and countertransference, therapeutic limits and boundaries, and overinvolvement with the patient. A case example suggests the complexity of many of these cases.

Ms. C., a single woman in her mid-20s, brought a malpractice suit against her former primary therapist, several clinicians who had seen her as a hospital patient, and a hospital system that has a specialty trauma disorders and women's program. Ms. C.'s psychiatric history began in adolescence. She ran away from home repeatedly, resulting in a social service investigation. She was removed from her parental home based on her reports of physical, sexual, and emotional abuse primarily perpetrated by her father. She subsequently recanted these accusations, and her father was not prosecuted. Attempts to return her home were unsuccessful, however, and she lived in a succession of foster placements. Sporadic contact with her family continued, usually associated with clinical deterioration. She was treated with multiple trials of outpatient, inpatient, and day hospital care throughout her adolescence and early adulthood. She received many different diagnoses and was treated unsuccessfully with several different psychopharmacological regimens. She reported amnesia, fugue, automatic writing, and a sense of shifting internal states to several treating clinicians who documented a dissociative disorder diagnosis in the chart. The patient was terrified of this diagnosis and was reluctant to cooperate with assessing it.

Eventually, she was hospitalized in the women's trauma unit and became the patient of Dr. Z., a clinical psychologist. Ms. C. developed an intense therapeutic relationship with Dr. Z., who made the diagnosis of dissociative identity disorder based on switching to defined alter identities and the presence of dissociative amnesia. Dr. Z. rapidly became overinvolved with Ms. C., telling her that she loved her and considered her to be like one of her daughters. In addition to treatment sessions, for which Ms. C. was not billed for insurance copayments, Dr. Z. saw Ms. C. outside of sessions in several social venues. They also engaged in a voluminous e-mail correspondence on a daily basis. Ms. C. began to report a bizarre history of multiperpetrator occultist abuse, based in her family and rural hometown. Some of these accounts appeared to be fanciful and unlikely to be possible in physical reality. Despite this, Dr. Z. repeatedly reassured Ms. C. that she believed her accounts. Dr. Z. would screen Ms. C.'s voice mail messages, lest evil "cult programming" calls reached her. Dr. Z. also helped Ms. C. financially.

The treatment lasted several years. Despite the boundary problems, Dr. Z. insisted that the patient work on maintaining herself free from self-harm and out of the hospital. Ms. C. was gradually more able to do this. Her social function improved, with a more consistent performance at school and work. She did require periodic hospitalization, but these became less frequent. Her alter identities worked on becoming less separate and many of them fused, with decreased dissociative symptoms and better functioning. As the therapy wore on, however, Dr. Z. found herself increasingly enervated by the extensive demands that Ms. C. continued to place on her for out-of-session contacts, e-mail, crisis management, and personal support. Dr. Z. consulted with more senior clinicians who suggested more rigorous boundaries and attention to transference and countertransference issues. When Dr. Z. attempted to change the therapy framework according to these suggestions, Ms. C. reacted catastrophically to this as a profound rejection. Finally, Ms. C. physically attacked Dr. Z. in her office, resulting in summary termination of the therapy.

Ms. C. eventually began treatment with a clinician who debunked the dissociative identity disorder and recovered memory ideas and encouraged Ms. C. to sue Dr. Z. and other clinicians to right the so-called wrongs that had been done to her. Eventually, the case was settled out of court for a relatively small sum from Dr. Z.

As the previous discussion indicates, these academic and social debates of the *memory wars* parallel many of those that polarized the field in the days of Babinski and Janet. Like Janet, modern authorities on the dissociative disorders generally accept the trauma-based etiology of dissociative conditions and the validity of the trauma-dissociation construct. This model most completely and rigorously accounts for the current data about these patients. Like Janet, sophisticated modern students of the dissociative disorders have a healthy respect for the kinds of phenomenological and psychotherapeutic complexity that many dissociative patients embody and the multilayering of pathologies that may appear in their treatment.

For example, there is a broad spectrum of dissociative individuals. At one extreme are high-functioning patients with significant adaptive resources and relatively circumscribed and treatment-responsive personality disorder symptoms. At the other extreme are patients with major multiaxial difficulties, factitious and antisocial clinical features, significant substance abuse, enmeshment in criminal subgroups, and major life problems in most spheres of function. The current polarization of the psychiatric community about dissociative disorders makes it more difficult to develop research that dispassionately evaluates these subgroups. A comprehensive model for evaluating this complexity could include genetic factors of relative vulnerability or resilience, or both, psychobiological developmental factors, the differential effects of trauma and neglect, restitutive environmental factors, and the impact of differing forms of family chaos and dysfunction on the individual.

Scientific Investigation of Dissociation

The scientific investigation of dissociation dates to the experiments of Prince in 1908 using a crude polygraph to measure galvanic skin resistance (GSR) across the alter personality states of a dissociative identity disorder patient—a physiological measure that remains of interest today. Prince reported seeing differential GSR reactivity to words that were emotionally laden for one alter personality state but not for another. Over the next century, several dozen psychophysiological and cognitive performance studies were added to the literature. Many of these reported findings suggesting differential responses across dissociative identity disorder alter personality states. The small sample sizes—often only a single case—and the frequent lack of controls limit their credibility, however. The few studies with larger samples and better controls generally support the earlier findings of differences across alter personality states. The scattering of experimental methodologies and the often idiosyncratic differential responses elicited in dissociative identity disorder subjects have limited opportunities for replication. Nonetheless, investigation of differential psychophysiological responses and cognitive performance across alter personality states of dissociative identity disorder patients continues to be an important source of information about the nature of dissociation.

The advent of reliable and valid measures of dissociation opened up a new avenue of experimental investigation. The correlation of scale scores with a variety of physiological, neuroendocrine, cognitive, and brain imaging data facilitates examination of the biological underpinnings of dissociation and the impact of dissociation on physical and mental functioning. By dividing subjects into high and low dissociative subgroups, investigators have identified significant differences in the way in which highly dissociative individuals perform on physiological and cognitive measures. Measures such as the Clinician-Administered Dissociative States Scale (CADSS) document pharmacologically induced dissociative-like experiences in normal controls and in clinical populations, such as PTSD patients. These studies primarily focus on traumatized individuals, most of whom do not have a diagnosable dissociative disorder but often have PTSD or trauma-associated psychopathology. Much of what has been learned since the 1990s is a result of the large numbers of studies including measures of dissociation in their assessment.

Dissociation Scales and Diagnostic Interviews

Following the example set by affective and anxiety disorder researchers, dissociation screening measures and DSM-based structured diagnostic interviews were developed in parallel. After approximately a decade of clinical and research application, the best of these instruments equal the levels of reliability and validity established for measures of depression, anxiety, and PTSD. Reliable and valid measurement of dissociation has proven particularly important in neurobiological studies, as well as for understanding the clinical contribution of dissociation to trauma-associated disorders. Many of these instruments are now available on the Internet or are reproduced in articles and books. A number have been modified by others and then circulated under names similar to the original, so provenance should be established to ensure that a properly validated version is being used.

SYMPTOM SCREENING MEASURES

Several general dissociation screening scales exist. The best known of these is the Dissociative Experiences Scale (DES), developed by Eve Bernstein Carlson and Frank Putnam in the mid-1980s and now included in hundreds of studies. There are 28 items, which primarily tap amnesias, identity alteration, depersonalization, derealization, and absorption. The overall DES score can range from 0 to 100. Several studies using receiver operating characteristic (ROC) methodology converge on DES scores of 30 or greater as the cut-point for identifying pathological levels of dissociation. Studies comparing high- and low-scoring subjects typically use an overall DES score of 30 or a score of 30 on the eight-item, DES taxon (DES-T) subscale as the dividing line. The DES has high coefficients of internal and test-retest reliability across multiple studies, and DES scores are highly correlated with other dissociation measures and dissociative disorder structured interview scores. Factor analyses with clinical samples generally produce trifactorial solutions with subscales for amnesia, depersonalization, and absorption. Gender, socioeconomic status, and, within reason, intelligence quotient (IQ), do not appear to have significant confounding effects on DES scores. The DES has been translated into more than 40 languages, and studies across cultures reveal strong similarities for Western and non-Western samples, attesting to the universality of the dissociation.

The Peritraumatic Dissociative Experiences Questionnaire (PDEQ) developed by Charles R. Marmar and colleagues assesses dissociative experiences at the time of the traumatic event. Several versions exist, with the PDEQ ten-item self-report version (PDEQ-10-SRV) now widely used for research and clinical screening. A metaanalytical study established that peritraumatic dissociation is the single best predictive factor for the subsequent development of PTSD. The 20-item Somatoform Dissociation Questionnaire (SDQ-20) developed by Ellert R. S. Nijenhuis taps many of the somatosensory and conversion symptoms common in dissociative patients. These include motor inhibitions, loss of function, anesthesias and analgesias, pain, and problems with vision, hearing, and smell. The SDQ-20 has good reliability and validity for discriminating dissociative disorder patients. The five-item SDQ (SDQ-5) provides a quick screening measure. The CADSS by J. Douglas Bremner is administered by a clinician, usually in the context of an experimental study, to assess symptoms of amnesia, depersonalization, and derealization. The CADSS has proven particularly useful in pharmacological studies and in military stress studies. It has good convergent validity with other measures of dissociation and high interrater and test-retest reliability.

Two other self-report inventories, the Multiscale Dissociation Inventory (MDI) and the Multiaxial Inventory of Dissociation (MID), have been developed to assess pathological dissociative symptoms and to assist in differential diagnosis of dissociative disorders.

Three primary dissociation measures exist for children and adolescents. The Child Dissociative Checklist (CDC) is a parent-caretaker-teacher 20-item report measure that uses a three-point scale. The CDC is a reliable and valid screen for dissociation in children who are 5 to 12 years of age. Scores can range from 0 to 40, with scores of 12 or greater indicative of pathological levels of dissociation. A dissociative subscale has also been extracted by several investigators from the popular Child Behavior Checklist (CBCL) and has proven useful in research studies, although its clinical usefulness has not, as yet, been tested with dissociative patients. The Adolescent Dissociative Experiences Scale (A-DES) is an adolescent-oriented version of the DES with differences in item content but similar constructs of amnesia, identity alteration, depersonalization, and derealization. This 30-item instrument uses a 0-to-10 answer format and has good reliability and validity as a research tool and a clinical screening instrument.

DIAGNOSTIC INTERVIEWS Two DSM-based structured interviews have been developed for the formal diagnosis of dissociative disorders, the Structured Clinical Interview for DSM-IV-TR Dissociative Disorders, Revised (SCID-D-R) and the Dissociative Disorders Interview Schedule (DDIS). The SCID-D-R by Marlene Steinberg is widely regarded as the gold standard for research studies requiring a diagnosis. It is a semi-structured clinician-administered interview that assesses the presence and severity of amnesias, identity confusion and alteration, depersonalization, and derealization and renders a DSM-IV diagnosis for all five dissociative disorders and for acute stress disorder. It includes 276 questions and rates the severity of each symptom on a four-point scale. For dissociative disorder patients, administration time typically ranges from 1 to 2 hours but is much briefer for nondissociative psychiatric patients. The SCID-D-R has good to excellent interrater and test-retest reliability and well-established validity in numerous studies. It has been translated into at least a dozen languages with similar results in different cultures.

The DDIS by Colin Ross is primarily a clinical diagnostic instrument and is sometimes used as a screen for pathological dissociation. It inquires about a wide range of phenomena in addition to dissociative symptoms, including child abuse history, major depression, somatic complaints, substance abuse, and paranormal experiences. It requires approximately 30 to 60 minutes to administer to dissociative identity disorder patients. Except for depersonalization disorder, interrater reliability is acceptable, and convergent validity includes strong correlations with the DES and clinical diagnoses of dissociative disorders.

Memory and Cognitive Dysfunctions Dysfunctions of memory are a central feature of the dissociative disorders. Dissociative identity disorder, with its apparent web of directional amnesias among alter personality states, was the focus of early attempts at experimental investigation. Many of the case studies that followed also sought to document these amnesias. A 1985 National Institute of Mental Health (NIMH) study used nine dissociative identity disorder patients and ten matched controls, who were tested as themselves and in a simulated alter personality state. They tested the separateness of memory between pairs of reportedly mutually amnesic alter personality states by measuring intrusions from categorically similar word lists learned by the other alter personality states. The dissociative identity disorder patients were more likely to compartmentalize the stimuli learned, whereas those mimicking dissociation showed far less evidence of information partitioning. Subsequent studies suggested that dissociation had differential impacts on the domains of implicit and explicit memory.

Conversely, in some recent studies of memory and amnesia in dissociative identity disorder, cognitive researchers have not been able to document claimed amnesia between subjectively mutually amnestic alters using a variety of implicit and explicit memory paradigms. In one study, feigning control subjects familiar with dissociative identity disorder showed lack of priming in an implicit memory task because they "knew" they were supposed to be amnestic, although actual dissociative identity disorder subjects *did* show normal priming. On the other hand, in another study, researchers could not document supposed transfer of information between alters claiming to be "co-conscious" using implicit and explicit memory tasks.

Accordingly, some researchers have questioned the actuality of dissociative identity disorder amnesias. However, the failure of transfer of information in supposedly co-conscious alters suggests other possible implications of these studies. These include that dissociative identity disorder patients may not always be reliable reporters of either amnesia or coawareness between alter self-states. For example, in a single case study, a dissociative identity disorder subject was randomly signaled by a beeper and filled out mood and activity rating scales, as well as information pertaining to the personality state who was "out." Rating scales filled out in real time were discrepant with the alters' self-professed mood and activity reports during clinical interviews.

Finally, it may be more useful to devise studies using autobiographical memory paradigms and to more globally and naturalistically study dissociative identity disorder patients' memory problems and switching behaviors without necessarily devoting specific attention to which alter does or does not have recall at a given time.

However, the existence of differential and directional amnesias across dissociative identity disorder alter personality states has been found in most studies to date. The more rigorous studies, however, also document considerable leakage or transfer of information across alter personality states, which report being completely amnesic for one another. The most parsimonious neuropsychological explanation put forward, that these amnesias are examples of state-dependent learning and retrieval, was first articulated by Theodule Ribot at the end of the 19th century. The degree of amnesia demonstrated in dissociative identity disorder patients, however, exceeds that typically seen in experimental studies of state dependent memory.

Studies show that memory tasks can be constructed such that highly dissociative individuals perform better or worse than control subjects. Memory tasks that involve division of attention or compartmentalization of highly similar information seem to favor highly dissociative individuals. Memory tasks that demand focused attention place them at a significant disadvantage. These attentional and memory differences, perhaps together with other yet-unrecognized cognitive differences, operating during critical periods of development and over the life span of the individual, could lead to considerable deviation from normal developmental trajectories, as described in the section on the developmental model.

Psychophysiology of Dissociation Clinical observations of differences in handedness; visual acuity; sensitivity to various visual, tactile, olfactory, and auditory stimuli; and energy level date to some of the earliest case descriptions and became a staple of 19th century case reports. In a study measuring a battery of autonomic nervous system indices, including GSR, eight of nine dissociative identity disorder patients consistently manifested physiologically distinct personality states over a several week period. Three of the five simulating controls could, by using hypnosis or deep relaxation, also manifest distinct *personality states*, although these differed physiologically from those produced by the patients.

Case reports continue to report electroencephalogram (EEG) differences across dissociative identity disorder alter personality states, but, increasingly, investigators are turning to the newer brain imaging technologies in their efforts to document these. A functional magnetic resonance imaging (fMRI) study of 12 switches among three alter personality states found changes in brain activity bilaterally in the hippocampus and in the right parahippocampal and medial temporal regions. In a study comparing 15 dissociative identity disorder patients to eight controls, the patients showed significant hypoactivity bilaterally in the orbitofrontal region and increased left lateral temporal activity. No differences were found between alter personality states, however. An EEG study of alpha wave coherence using five simulator controls and five dissociative identity disorder subjects found significant differences between personality states for alpha wave coherence in six brain regions, whereas there were no differences for the controls. Another study compared event-related potentials elicited by words learned in the same or a different alter personality state for four dissociative identity disorder patients. Here, little support was found for the existence of amnesia between personality states, when compared to controls from another study who had deliberately concealed knowledge of previously learned words.

Using script-driven traumatic imagery to evoke dissociative states in PTSD patients, one fMRI study found significantly increased activation in the superior and middle temporal gyri (Brodmann's area [BA] 38), the inferior frontal gyrus (BA47), the occipital lobe (BA19), the parietal lobe (BA7), medial frontal gyrus (BA10), the medial cortex (BA9), and the anterior cingulate (BA24 and BA32).

A recent study used positron emission tomography (PET) to investigate the functional anatomical representation of autobiographical self-awareness in 11 dissociative identity disorder patients. Subjects were tested with personally relevant script-driven imagery of traumatic versus neutral narratives. Dissociative identity disorder subjects were tested in self-states that reported subjective ownership of a traumatic event with accompanying emotional reactivity (Traumatic Personality State [TPS]) and, in alternation, in self-states that denied emotional reactivity to the event and denied that the event had happened to them (Neutral Personality State [NPS]).

Comparison of subjects in various conditions, such as TPS-neutral script, NPS-neutral script, TPS-traumatic script, and NPS-traumatic script, in various trials showed that TPS subjects responded to trauma scripts with changes in perfusion of right hemisphere frontal, visual association, and parietal integration areas similar to those of normal subjects responding to autobiographical episodic memory retrieval. TPS subjects showed activation of areas related to regulation of emotion and pain. NPS subjects did not show changes in perfusion between neutral and traumatic scripts, consistent with their failure to recognize the trauma scripts as autobiographical. The authors conclude that the results are consistent with a single human brain/mind generating at least two distinct states of self-awareness with differing access to autobiographical memory primarily related to differential activation of medial prefrontal cortex (MPFC) areas and posterior association areas.

Similarly, another group used fMRI to study script-driven imagery in traumatized subjects with and without PTSD. Functional connectivity analysis showed significantly different patterns of activation between the PTSD and non-PTSD groups with script-driven imagery. PTSD subjects experienced the trauma scripts as producing flashbacks with strong emotional, somatic, and sensory responses. Non-PTSD subjects experienced recall as personal narratives without intense emotion. Non-PTSD subjects showed a more left-hemisphere activation pattern including verbal association areas. PTSD subjects showed a right-hemisphere dominance pattern with increased blood flow to right brain frontal, posterior association, subcortical, and paralimbic areas similar to the findings in the PET study of dissociative identity disorder subjects and prior PET and fMRI studies of PTSD subjects.

fMRI has also recently been used to study a laboratory paradigm of memory suppression/repression using subjects instructed to either think or not think of the second member of a pair of words previously seen. Subsequent cued recall of suppression items was inferior to recall of baseline items and actually generalized to novel test cues. Neural networks implicated in this suppression response involved bilateral prefrontal cortex, paralimbic, subcortical, and parietal integration areas. In addition, suppression reduced activation bilaterally in hippocampal areas. Hippocampal activation patterns differed from trials involving ordinary forgetting compared with those involving suppression-induced forgetting. Hippocampal activation was increased in suppression-induced forgetting compared to that found in suppression items that were recalled. The authors concluded that activation of a broad neural network was involved in memory suppression, including interrelation of the dorsolateral prefrontal cortex, hippocampus, anterior cingulate cortex, medial-temporal lobe, dorsal premotor cortex, presupplementary motor area, and intraparietal areas. In addition, the authors stated that these findings strongly suggest a neurobiological model for memory control in response to trauma, including the possibility that these networks are involved in producing lasting amnesia in response to traumatic events.

A few individual case studies of patients with global dissociative amnesia and with dissociative fugue with loss of personal identity have shown unusual metabolic and activation patterns using PET scanning and single photon emission computed tomography (SPECT). These included reversal of the usual patterns of right and left hemisphere activation during autobiographical and semantic recall, respectively, with similarities to some individuals with traumatic brain damage and related memory deficits. A recent review of these studies suggested that disruptions or functional disconnections between major neural networks may be etiological in dissociative amnesia syndromes.

The strategy of dividing traumatized subjects into high and low dissociative subgroups has also yielded interesting results for psychophysiological measures. Several studies of rape victims, subjects with PTSD using script driven imagery, and sexually abused girls compared to controls on a measure of *most traumatic life experience* have found a unique pattern of psychophysiological responding in high dissociatives. Using indicators of subjective distress, heart rate, and GSR, high dissociatives showed *decreased* heart rate and GSR with highest reported subjective distress. This combination of increased distress and decreased heart rate predicted more PTSD symptoms, blunted emotion, and poorer outcome.

Two studies have found an inverse relationship between dissociation scores and urinary catecholamines. Douglas Delahanty and colleagues collected 15-hour urine from 59 motor vehicle accident victims on hospital admission. In men, peritraumatic dissociation was correlated with epinephrine but not norepinephrine, whereas women showed a reversed pattern of significance. Using DSM-IV depersonalization disorder subjects, Daphne Simeon and colleagues found strong negative correlations between urinary norepinephrine and depersonalization scores. These results are congruent with the physiological data, suggesting that high levels of dissociation act to suppress arousal in the face of stressors but do little or nothing to dampen subjective distress.

Neurobiology of Dissociation Understanding of the neurobiology of dissociation is based on two primary sources of information. The first is a body of case reports describing dissociative reactions in the context of illicit drug use or as a side effect of medications. Drugs that can precipitate dissociative-like reactions include alcohol, barbiturates and related hypnotics, benzodiazepines, scopolamine (Transderm-Scop), β-adrenergic blockers, marijuana, other psychedelics, and anesthetics, such as ketamine (Ketalar) and its relatives. The array of implicated drugs and their range of activities would suggest that many neurotransmitter systems might be involved in producing dissociative reactions.

The second source is data from placebo-controlled, drug challenge studies using a range of dissociative drugs. Challenge studies that have elicited depersonalization or other dissociative phenomena include marijuana, infusions of lactate, yohimbine (Actibine), metachlorophenylpiperazine (mCPP), and ketamine. These studies appear to narrow down the number of neurotransmitter systems that are likely to make significant contributions to dissociative states. Increasing evidence suggests that the *N*-methyl-D-aspartate (NMDA) glutamate receptor plays a central role in dissociative symptoms.

A series of studies, using ketamine, an NMDA antagonist that increases glutamate release, found that the drug produced dose-dependent increases in dissociation scores. High doses of ketamine produced slowed perception of time, tunnel vision, derealization, and depersonalization, similar to that described by trauma victims. Pretreatment with a benzodiazepine or lamotrigine (Lamictal), an anticonvulsant that decreases glutamate release, reduced but did not entirely eliminate the dissociative effects of ketamine. These studies suggest that dissociation, heretofore widely regarded as virtually impervious to medication, may be responsive to certain classes of drugs.

Neurobiological theories of dissociation draw on preclinical data indicating that stress increases the release of glutamate and the similarity of the hyperglutamatergic effects of NMDA antagonists with stress- and trauma-induced dissociative symptoms. In summary, it postulates that NMDA blockade decreases inhibitory tone, leading to increased glutamate release and subsequent dissociative symptoms. This theory also accounts for the structural brain changes in the hippocampus found in magnetic resonance imaging (MRI) studies of PTSD subjects and controls. In two studies, dissociation measures strongly correlated with volume loss in key brain regions implicated in PTSD.

Glutamate has a well-documented role in neuroplasticity, and increased glutamate release can lead to neurotoxic cellular events. It should be noted, however, that challenge studies with marijuana and mCPP implicate serotonin, and studies with yohimbine suggest that noradrenergic systems may play roles in dissociation and PTSD symptoms. Also, in two studies of military subjects undergoing high stress training, a strong negative relationship was found between neuropeptide Y (NPY) levels and dissociative symptoms.

Comparative Nosology This section discusses nosological issues for all of the dissociative disorders, although issues related to the specific disorders are described briefly in the individual sections. The disorders are discussed together, because most of the major nosological issues bear on the group of disorders and their relationship to other DSM-IV-TR disorders. The early DSM definitions and ICD-10 criteria have been reviewed in the introduction. Scales and measures for the assessment of dissociation and dissociative disorders are also discussed.

History The DSM-III criteria for dissociative disorders were established by expert consensus. By the time the DSM-III-R was published, there was a body of systematic research on the dissociative disorders. Little changed in the diagnostic criteria for depersonalization disorder, psychogenic amnesia, and psychogenic fugue. However, the criteria for multiple personality disorder changed considerably to make them more flexible, less reified, and more compatible with research findings about the phenomenology of alter identities.

In the DSM-IV revision, the names of most of the disorders were changed; for example, *psychogenic amnesia* and *psychogenic fugue* became, respectively, *dissociative amnesia* and *dissociative fugue*, and *multiple personality disorder* became *dissociative identity disorder*. The criteria for dissociative amnesia now specified that the amnesia usually occurred for traumatic or stressful circumstances. Dissociative fugue now could be diagnosed even if there were no assumption of another identity. Amnesia was added back as a criterion symptom for dissociative identity disorder. The disorders were structured to reflect pathologies of memory, identity, and perception, respectively.

Dissociation and Trauma The current diagnostic categories for dissociative disorders developed from nosological systems based on the hysteria concept, not on modern research showing a robust relationship between dissociation and trauma. Furthermore, the complexity and overlapping nature of the phenomenology of dissociative amnesia, dissociative fugue, and dissociative identity disorder were not appreciated. In particular, the complexity of the phenomenology of dissociative identity disorder was not understood with its multifaceted amnesias, fugues, and depersonalization and derealization symptoms.

In addition, the DSM-IV work group for PTSD unsuccessfully proposed adding to DSM-IV the diagnosis of disorders of extreme stress NOS. This construct was developed to describe a group of multiply traumatized individuals with problems of affect regulation, dissociation, somatization, and relationship, identity, and safety problems. Despite its lack of inclusion in the DSM-IV, PTSD researchers have begun to systematically study this complex form of PTSD to help differentiate patients with single acute traumas from those with multiple types of trauma and life adversity. For example, recent studies have shown that the complex PTSD paradigm more rigorously conceptualizes traumatized borderline patients than the borderline personality disorder construct. Most patients with dissociative identity disorder, dissociative disorder NOS, and dissociative amnesia fit readily into the disorders of extreme stress NOS or complex PTSD paradigms, or both. Many trauma researchers consider these constructs to be slightly dissimilar ways of conceptualizing the same spectrum of patients. Recent neurobiological studies of dissociative identity disorder patients show similarities on neurobiological variables to PTSD patients without severe dissociation.

Accordingly, some members of the DSM-IV work groups for PTSD and the dissociative disorders proposed that the DSM-IV create a section of posttraumatic or stress-related disorders (trauma spectrum disorders) that would include PTSD, acute stress disorder, the dissociative disorders, and, possibly, other disorders, such as conversion disorder, somatization disorder, and borderline personality disorder.

A trauma spectrum disorders category would help more logically integrate multiple lines of research showing different psychopathological outcomes to trauma and would help better organize future research efforts. Furthermore, such a category would help with conceptual confusion; for example, amnesia is a criterion symptom for the avoidance cluster of DSM-IV PTSD and for somatization disorder, not just for dissociative amnesia and dissociative identity disorder. Finally, such a classification would be more helpful for the clinician confronted with typical patients with mixtures of posttraumatic, dissociative, and somatoform symptoms who now frequently wind up in NOS categories.

It would be more logical to combine the DSM-IV-TR dissociative disorders and PTSD work groups as subgroups of a single trauma and stress disorders work group for the fifth edition of the DSM (DSM-V). This group could devise nosological categories that better define the broad spectrum of posttraumatic conditions, from acute to chronic, from simple to complex, and from those with marked dissociation to those with minimal dissociation.

Many of these suggested changes would involve radical restructuring of several DSM diagnostic categories. This might involve negotiations among several different groups of clinicians and researchers who otherwise work relatively separately from one another. However, the data strongly suggest that, at the least, a unifying trauma spectrum disorders section, including PTSD and the dissociative disorders, would be the most logical classification of apparently disparate disorders related to trauma.

Revisions to Dissociative Disorder Categories Even if this radical perspective is not adopted, major critiques have been launched at the current dissociative disorders classification. In general, these involve the relatively greater complexity and pleomorphism of dissociative, PTSD, and somatoform symptoms in dissociative patients. For example, patients with dissociative amnesia, dissociative fugue, and dissociative identity disorder may exhibit or describe a number of significant symptoms that are not included in the current diagnostic criteria.

Dissociative identity disorder patients commonly complain of spontaneous autohypnotic phenomena, depersonalization, derealization, PTSD symptoms, somatoform symptoms, and pseudopsychotic symptoms, in addition to complex amnesias and switching to alter self-states. In clinical evaluation of dissociative identity disorder, these associated symptoms are frequently essential in arriving at a correct diagnosis.

Many patients with dissociative amnesia or dissociative fugue describe depersonalization, derealization, alterations of consciousness, somatoform and conversion symptoms, and autohypnotic symptoms along with the DSM-IV-TR criterion symptoms. Accordingly, many of these patients may be placed in the dissociative disorder NOS category, because they have a number of dissociative symptoms that go beyond the current diagnostic criteria for dissociative amnesia and dissociative fugue, although some of these are described in the text as associated features. This creates the awkward situation in which the clinician must wrestle with the problem that a large number of typical patients potentially will be classified as NOS.

Many patients with acute dissociative amnesia and dissociative fugue may actually be in an episode of dissociative identity disorder amnesia. Modern clinical assessment of such patients frequently finds a much more chronic history of multiple types of dissociative symptoms, including partial or full alter identities or personality states.

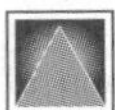

Table 17–2
Prevalence of Dissociative Disorders in the General Population of Winnipeg, Canada (N = 502)

Diagnosis	Subjects (%)
Dissociative amnesia	6.0
Dissociative fugue	0
Dissociative identity disorder	1.3
Depersonalization disorder	2.8
Dissociative disorder not otherwise specified	0.2
All dissociative disorders	12.2

From Ross CA. *Dissociative Identity Disorder: Diagnosis, Clinical Features, and Treatment of Multiple Personality.* New York: John Wiley & Sons; 1997:109, with permission.

Accordingly, several critics have suggested developing new diagnostic criteria based on the data sets already acquired using the SCID-D-R, the DDIS, the MID, the DES, and similar instruments, along with data sets from clinical case series. Some have proposed radical restructuring of the dissociative disorders category to reflect the phenomenological data. Others have proposed more a conservative position maintaining the current diagnostic structure but moving to a polythetic classification system with additional symptom categories as part of the diagnostic criteria for most disorders.

Epidemiology

There is only one systematic general population study of the prevalence of dissociative disorders. Ross and colleagues studied a random sample of 1,055 adults in Winnipeg, Canada. They were given the DES, and a representative subsample of 502 respondents was subsequently reevaluated with the DDIS. Table 17–2 gives the findings for the various dissociative disorders.

This study has significant limitations and needs to be replicated. These include the lack of validating clinical interviews, the unknown validity of the DDIS in nonclinical samples, the relatively small sample size from only one city, and the lack of other diagnostic instruments given to the participants.

The DES findings, however, have been replicated in other studies. These include the finding that dissociation is found in a left-skewed distribution, indicating that most individuals in the general population experience few dissociative symptoms. A small subset of the population, 3 to 5 percent, endorses many forms of pathological dissociative experience. A taxonometric reanalysis of the data of Ross and colleagues found that 3.3 percent of the population showed *pathological dissociation* and could be completely discriminated from nondissociative psychiatric controls and normal subjects.

Etiological Theories

This section discusses etiological theories about dissociation and dissociative disorders. A comprehensive etiological model involves integration of data from several of these models and theories.

Taxon Model of Pathological Dissociation Recent interest in the *taxon model* resurrects a century-old debate about whether dissociation occurs along a continuum proceeding from normal to pathological or whether pathological dissociation, such as dissociative identity disorder, represents a different type (a taxon) of psychological organization. Janet favored the latter, believing that constitutional factors, suggestibility, and powerful emotional events contributed to creation of a group of individuals who were fundamentally different from normal individuals. James and Prince argued for a continuum model, ranging from so-called normal dissociative

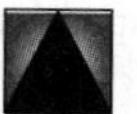

Table 17–3
Dissociative Experiences Scale Items That Make Up the Dissociative Experiences Scale Taxon Score

Subjects are asked to rate the percentage of time, from 0 to 100 percent, that they have the experience.

3. Some people have the experience of finding themselves in a place and having no idea how they got there.
5. Some people have the experience of finding new things among their belongings that they do not remember buying.
7. Some people sometimes have the experience of feeling as though they are standing next to themselves or watching themselves do something, and they actually see themselves as if they were looking at another person.
8. Some people are told that they sometimes do not recognize friends or family members.
12. Some people have the experience of feeling that other people, objects, and the world around them are not real.
13. Some people have the experience of feeling that their body does not seem to belong to them.
22. Some people sometimes find that, in one situation, they may act so differently compared to another situation that they feel almost as if they were two different people.
27. Some people sometimes find that they hear voices inside their head that tell them to do things or comment on things that they are doing.

From Waller NG, Putnam FW, Carlson EB: Types of dissociation and dissociative types: A taxonometric analysis of dissociative experiences. *Psychol Methods.* 1996;1:300–321, with permission.

phenomena, such as absorption, to pathology, such as amnesias, fugues, and multiple personalities. The continuum theory carried the day, although some hypnosis researchers continued to caution about possible discontinuities between normal consciousness and some deep trance phenomena.

As data with dissociation measures accrued across clinical and normal populations, it became apparent that there existed a distinct group of high-scoring individuals. Different diagnostic groups contained different percentages of these high scorers, yielding different diagnostic group mean scores. The greater the percentage of high scorers, the greater the elevation of the group's mean score relative to the group's modal score. On the DES, for example, high scorers cluster around a mean score of 45, with the rest of the sample clustering around 8.

These observations led to a statistical study directly investigating the possibility that there exists a dissociative type of individual who differs significantly on dissociation measures from other individuals, irrespective of their psychiatric status. Using newly developed taxonometric approaches, researchers examined item-response data for manifestations of a latent class variable. They identified eight DES items, composing the DES-T subscale, that could robustly differentiate dissociative disorder patients from other psychiatric patients and normal controls, who almost never endorsed these items. These items are listed in Table 17–3.

Studies have subsequently affirmed that a taxonic approach is a clinically useful way to cull out a distinct subgroup of dissociative patients within any given diagnosis who differ on symptoms and features from the rest of the group. In psychophysiological investigations of dissociation, simply dividing samples into high and low scorers has proven fruitful in identifying distinctly different physiological and cognitive responses to stimuli that serve as traumatic reminders.

The taxon model implies a significantly different developmental scenario than the continuum model, as well as a different approach to treatment. The typological differences between high dissociators and virtually everyone else would have to lie in a strong genetic predisposition or a fundamentally different early developmental trajectory, or both, that essentially wires their brains differently. A convincing genetic difference remains to be demonstrated, but research linking dissociation with type D attachment disturbances offers a potential mechanism for the latter.

In a continuum model of dissociation, a positive treatment response would be conceptualized as moving a dissociative individual more toward the normal dissociation segment of the continuum. By contrast, a positive treatment outcome in a taxon model implies changing an individual's type from the dissociative to the nondissociative category. The clinical lore on fusion or integration of dissociative identity disorder alter personalities into a unified personality hints at this possibility. However, beyond these clinical accounts, no empirical data exist to confirm that integration produces a taxonic clinical change. The few studies of dissociative identity disorder that include pretreatment and posttreatment dissociation measures show moderate (but significant) decreases in scale scores rather than a significant taxonic shift from the dissociative to nondissociative categories. The taxonic model has proven valuable in spurring researchers to compare high and low dissociators on a variety of measures, but its clinical usefulness as a index of treatment success remains to be demonstrated.

Dissociation As a Response to Trauma Since the 1980s, research has elucidated multiple lines of evidence linking dissociative disorders with antecedent trauma. In aggregate, these separate lines of evidence constitute a strong case for significant trauma as a necessary antecedent to the development of pathological dissociation.

The most basic set of these lines of evidence involves quantification of Janet's early clinical observations. For each of the DSM-IV-TR dissociative disorders, there now exist multiple independent case series, including non-Western samples, documenting unusually high rates of trauma in dissociative disorder patients (although this linkage is notably weaker for depersonalization disorder). Although critics often point out that these studies are retrospective, and, thus, the accuracy of the reports of trauma cannot be established, several case series exist in which the majority of subjects had one or more traumas verified.

Several hundred peer-reviewed studies have found significantly higher levels of dissociation, as measured by well-validated instruments, such as the DES, in traumatized groups compared to nontraumatized clinical and general population samples. The frequency of this finding for many different forms of traumatic experience (e.g., combat, rape, natural disasters, child abuse, and Cambodian holocaust, among others) and across many cultures indicates the universality of the association between trauma and dissociation. Measures of trauma severity, for example, combat intensity or rape severity scales, are approximately equally correlated with PTSD and dissociation measures ($r \sim .025$ to .40), indicating a weak to moderate dose effect–like relationship. The lack of a stronger correlational relationship between trauma and PTSD and dissociation may reflect the difficulties in quantifying the subjective elements of traumatic experience. Although these findings significantly link dissociation with antecedent trauma, they are not sufficient to demonstrate that the trauma actually causes the dissociation.

More sophisticated statistical approaches are uncovering new lines of evidence indicating that increased dissociation is instrumental in shaping outcomes related to traumatic experience and psychophysiological responses to future stress and trauma. Peritraumatic dissociation, measured proximal to the trauma in some studies and retrospectively in others, has been found to predict the subsequent development of PTSD. This predictive power is important for identifying individuals at risk for developing PTSD after an acute trauma. A smaller number of studies has demonstrated that dissociation qualifies as a mediator of the relationship between antecedent trauma and subsequent psychopathology, including PTSD. This means that, if the level of dissociation is statistically controlled, the strength of the relationship between trauma and psychopathology is significantly decreased or disappears. High levels of dissociation also alter the psychophysiological responses of traumatized individuals to traumatic reminders.

Not every study measuring peritraumatic dissociation finds that it predicts subsequent PTSD, nor have there, as yet, been a sufficient number of replications for the physiological and statistical mediation studies to be unquestionably accepted. These findings do suggest, however, that trauma-associated dissociation may serve as an important mechanism mediating the transformation of traumatic experiences into subsequent psychopathology.

The remarkable studies of Charles A. Morgan and colleagues conducted on military special operations units under extremely stressful conditions are as close as one can ethically come to an experimental model of trauma-induced dissociation. Working with units undergoing forms of simulated combat, such as survival school, Morgan examined the neurobiological and psychological effects of intense stress uniformly applied to drug-free, healthy, nonclinical subjects. Stressors included semi-starvation, exhaustion, sleep deprivation, lack of control over hygiene and bodily functions, and control over movement, social contact, and communication. The neuroendocrine stress effects measured in these soldiers was equal to or exceeded those reported for individuals subjected to life-threatening experiences. There were significant differences between pretest and posttest scores on the CADSS overall and for virtually all scale items, with the greatest effects for depersonalization items, such as looking at the world through a fog, feeling time slow down, and spacing out. Life threat from a prior trauma was significantly correlated with prestress and poststress dissociative symptoms. Dissociation scores also accounted for 41 percent of the variance in health complaints after the stress experience.

Morgan's systematic studies are congruent with observational reports of the high frequency of dissociation, especially depersonalization symptoms, in normal individuals exposed to life-threatening stress. The ubiquity of increased acute levels of dissociation during extreme stress indicates that other factors, perhaps the experience of prior life-threatening trauma, are operative in the peritraumatic dissociation–PTSD linkage discussed previously. The highest dissociation scores were associated with intense subjective appraisal of life threat from past trauma. One highly traumatized subgroup, Special Forces soldiers, had low life-threat appraisals of their past trauma and, consequently, the lowest prestress and poststress change in dissociation scores. This stress-hardy group underscores the importance of psychological adaptation to prior trauma on responses to current stressors. The significant relationship ($r = .67$) between the prestress-poststress change in dissociation score and somatic symptoms is congruent with many clinical studies reporting linkages between somatization and dissociation.

In summary, a number of independent lines of evidence point to a causal relationship between trauma and dissociation. This relationship is apparent for many forms of trauma and has been found across all cultures in which it has been investigated. Significant levels of dissociation in the immediate aftermath of a trauma appear to predispose an individual to developing PTSD and related psychopathology, although additional factors related to psychological appraisal of prior trauma also appear to be involved. Dissociation appears to serve as a major mediating process between traumatic experiences and subsequent psychopathology and thus is an important target for prevention and early intervention efforts. Stress-resistant individuals can be characterized, in part, by their lack of dissociative responses to significant stressors.

Discrete Behavioral States Model The discrete behavioral states (DBS) model postulates that dissociative disorders belong to a group of psychiatric conditions characterized by rapid—often environmentally triggered—discrete shifts in state of consciousness. Examples include rapid-cycling bipolar disorder, panic disorder, periodic catatonia, and PTSD. Although these disorders differ in many respects, a central feature of their pathology is abrupt switches between two or more distinct states of consciousness, at least one of which is pathological in some fashion. Panic attacks and the abreactions and flashbacks of PTSD are examples of dysfunctional behavioral states, often triggered by specific stimuli or interactions, that rapidly reorganize an individual's emotions, thinking, and behavior. Bipolar patients often cycle through a spectrum of distinct affective states extending from deep depression to psychotic mania.

The concept of a state of consciousness—as a distinct unit of behavioral organization—has been part of the psychological vocabulary for several centuries. Ribot's speculations that state-dependent learning and memory explained the phenomena seen in dissociative identity disorder arose in the context of widespread interest and clinical experimentation with hypnosis, somnambulism, and trance-like states. In his 1896 Lowel lectures on exceptional mental states, James often referred to altered states of consciousness as underlying multiple personality, fugues, conversion symptoms, and other hysterical symptoms. Modern state theory owes much to psychologist Charles Tart, who advocated for a science of discrete states of consciousness. Hilgard's neodissociation theory, which he traces in part to Janet, conceptualizes hypnosis as a set of altered states of consciousness characterized by increased suggestibility, enhanced imagery, decreased planning capacity, and a reduction in reality testing. Research with drug-induced altered states and meditation has also contributed to current theory and understanding.

It remained, however, for a group of child psychologists and psychiatrists to formally operationalize the study of DBS of consciousness. Heinz Prechtl, Robert Emde, Robert Harmon, and Peter Wolff empirically validated a multidimensional classification system used in the study of normal infants. By using as few as four or five independent variables, such as heart rate, respiratory rate, extremity muscle tone, skin perfusion, vocalization, or facial expression, researchers were able to delineate a basic set of DBS shared by most full-term, newborn infants. As the child matures, additional behavioral states are added, and the pathways of connections among the distinct states grow more complex—corresponding to an increased behavioral repertoire on the part of the child. The ability to self-modulate the expression of these DBS and to integrate the many additional states created with growth and development is regarded as fundamental to establishing healthy emotional regulation.

The DBS model conceptualizes dissociative phenomena as the manifestations of alternations among distinct states of consciousness that differ in terms of the individual's sense of identity, access to explicit, implicit, and autobiographical memory, and psychophysiological reactivity. Identity disturbances are the nucleus around which other features of the dissociative state organize in much the same fashion as distinct affects serve to organize the DBS of a bipolar patient. Dissociative disturbances of memory are viewed as extreme examples of state-dependent learning, storage, and retrieval. Alterations in psychophysiological sensitivity in dissociative disorders reflect state-dependent changes in autonomic nervous system and neuroendocrine function. Changes of equal magnitude have been measured in laboratory studies of panic attacks and PTSD flashbacks.

The DBS model of dissociation postulates that early childhood trauma or disturbances in attachment, or both, disrupt the processes essential to self-modulation and the developmental integration of new behavioral states. The DBS model postulates three levels of psychopathology inherent in such *state* disorders. The first is intrinsic to the nature of the pathological states per se, for example, anxiety, depression, mania, catatonia, or depersonalization. The second level results from the individual's inability to self-modulate the expression of these dysfunctional states or to better integrate them into their lives. The third level results from the consequences of maladaptive attempts to block the often painful experiences of these pathological states, for example, attempts to self-medicate depression or social withdrawal to avoid triggering flashbacks. The increased psychiatric comorbidity commonly noted in these patients is a consequence of the second and third levels of psychopathology. The DBS model predicts that effective treatment should facilitate better self-modulation of intense or dysphoric states and should address the state dependency of dysfunctional perceptions, cognitions, and assumptions.

Developmental Model of Dissociation Modern interest in a developmental model of dissociative disorders, especially dissociative identity disorder, can be traced to pioneers with child cases, such as Cornelia Wilbur and Richard Kluft. Subsequently, long-forgotten case reports were discovered in which 19th century clinicians used Latin phrases to hint at incest and unspeakable familial trauma. Small case series and reviews of childhood dissociative disorders appeared in the mid- to late 1980s, with more systematic studies coming in the last decade. As with the adult case series, histories of severe trauma were commonly noted.

The core phenomenology of child cases is, for the most part, similar to adult cases with the corresponding dissociative disorder diagnosis. As is the case for most childhood manifestations of lifelong psychiatric disorders, the day-to-day manifestation of core symptoms varies with the child's age. In general, older children and adolescents are more overtly symptomatic than younger children. In part, this may reflect the ability of older children to better report subjective distress, as well as their greater opportunity to manifest psychopathology in a variety of settings.

In a pooled sample of 177 child and adolescent dissociative disorder cases, amnesias, identity disturbances, and auditory hallucinations increased with age, whereas trance-like and spacey behavior was ubiquitous across all age groups. Related psychopathology, such as suicidal ideation, self-mutilation, and somatization, increased with age in parallel with dissociative symptoms. Boys and girls did not differ on dissociative symptoms, but girls were significantly more symptomatic for anxiety and phobic symptoms, PTSD, sleep disturbances, sexual acting out, and somatization. These findings closely parallel the gender differences in adult clinical profiles. Children and adolescents diagnosed with dissociative identity disorder were the most symptomatic across all age groups, which is consonant with the clinical belief that dissociative identity disorder is the most severe of the dissociative disorders.

Validated child and adolescent dissociation measures have been administered to a variety of clinical and nonclinical samples. Scores were significantly higher for traumatized (typically child abuse) versus nontraumatized subjects across all age groups. Higher levels of dissociation were also significantly associated with more general psychopathology. Among maltreated preschoolers, there were robust correlations with externalizing and internalizing behavior problems for boys and girls. A comparison of these maltreated preschoolers with demographically and family constellation-matched, nontraumatized preschoolers found that the maltreatment group had significantly increased levels of dissociation a year later, with the physically abused children accounting for the greatest increase in scores. The controls showed substantial decreases in their dissociation scores over the same period, in line with the often reported decrease in dissociation scores with age in normal children.

Studies have explored the possible mediating role of dissociation in the development of psychopathology in sexually abused children and adolescents. Measuring psychopathology with a variety of standard measures, the main effect of sexual abuse on behavioral problems disappeared when levels of dissociation were controlled for, as measured by a self-report measure (A-DES) or by observer report (CDC). The possibility that dissociation is a critical mediating variable for subsequent psychopathology has significant implications for early intervention with maltreated and traumatized children. Assessment of dissociation should be a standard part of the evaluation of traumatized children and adolescents, and significant elevations should be addressed as part of the treatment plan.

SEARCH FOR DEVELOPMENTAL PRECURSORS AND SUBSTRATES OF DISSOCIATION

Imaginary Companionship The focus on child dissociative identity disorder led clinical investigators to initially focus on childhood fantasy phenomena, such as imaginary companionship, as possible developmental precursors for dissociative disorders. Imaginary companions are reported in 20 to 60 percent of normal children, depending on the age of the child and the definition used. Normal imaginary companionship is widely regarded as benign and is commonly considered to be a sign of creativity in young children, but it becomes increasingly suspect in older children and adolescents and is thought to be always pathological in adults. In dissociative children, the rates of imaginary companionship range from 42 to 84 percent, with the highest rates reported for children diagnosed with dissociative identity disorder.

Studies comparing normal children's imaginary companions with those of maltreated boys show striking differences. The maltreated boys averaged 6.4 entities compared to 2.5 entities for the normal boys. The latter first appeared between 2 and 4 years of age and had all disappeared by 8 years of age. The imaginary companions reported by the boys in residential treatment, however, served other functions, including (1) helpers and comforters, (2) powerful protectors, and (3) family members. In some cases, the boys reported feeling as if they had lost control, and their imaginary companions took over their behavior. The maltreated boys reported that their imaginary companions were still present at a mean age of 10.6 years, well after they had disappeared in the normal boys. The imaginary companions of the maltreated boys often had names such as *God*, *the devil*, and *guardian angel*. A number of authorities theorize that some of the imaginary companions found in maltreated children eventually evolve into the alter personality states that personify dissociative identity disorder. As yet, no one has documented this transformation, but dissociative identity disorder patients sometimes report that this happened with them.

Type D Attachment Type D attachment is characterized by the child exhibiting disorganized and conflicting movement patterns when the primary caregiver returns to the room after a period of enforced separation during the *strange situation*, a standardized procedure for assessing attachment in preverbal children. The child may exhibit contradictions in intention, lack of orientation to the environment, and sudden immobility associated with a dazed expression or a trance-like state, termed *stilling* in the attachment literature. Type D attachment disturbances are common in maltreated infants and toddlers and are thought to result when the child periodically experiences the primary caretaker as frightening. Studies show that the best predictor of type D attachment is a high DES score in the mother. It is hypothesized that an infant with multiple incompatible models of self and other resulting from intermittent frightening experiences with the caretaker would rapidly switch back and forth between attachment models when confronted with a stressful interaction involving the primary caretaker, such as the strange situation.

In a prospective longitudinal study, 168 high-risk children were followed over a 19-year period, examining whether trauma, sense of self, quality of early mother–child relationship, temperament, intelligence, and dissociation measured at four time points were related to subsequent dissociative symptomatology with a clinical measure (CDC). Age of onset, chronicity, and severity of trauma were highly correlated and were predictive of dissociation. Two forms of attachment disorders, avoidant and type D attachment, were strong predictors of subsequent dissociation. A subsequent structural equation model analysis found that type D attachment acted as a mediating variable, accounting for 15 percent of the variance in dissociation scores (DES) at 19 years of age.

Developmental Mediation of Psychopathology by Dissociation The negative effects of high levels of dissociation on child development are postulated to operate through impacts on the development of sense of self, emotional regulation, impulse control, and impairments in information processing and coping with stressors. Children assemble and seek to integrate a complex, multidimensional sense of self over the course of development. Dissociative components, such as autobiographical amnesias, depersonalization, and passive influence experiences, interfere with the integration of self and the development of a unified sense of self-agency.

Dissociative amnesias also disrupt the child's understanding of cause-and-effect sequences, so that negative or risky behaviors may not appear to be connected to their subsequent consequences, which may be experienced as coming from out of the blue. Conversely, consequences may not be well related to the behaviors that caused them, so that dissociative children have a great deal of difficulty learning from experience. The impact of dissociation on the metacognitive function of self-monitoring one's behavior is thought to disrupt the integration of experience across contexts, further complicating the child's ability to learn and to practice self-control, particularly in the context of stressors. Increased dissociation is well correlated with increased aggression, impulsivity, and poorer social skills in a number of child and adolescent studies.

Prospectively comparing sexually abused girls with carefully matched controls, studies have found that dissociation is negatively associated with competent learning and overall classroom performance and is strongly predictive of school avoidance. The combination of cognitive dysfunctions and negative school trajectories puts the dissociative child at an academic disadvantage, which has profound implications for adult attainment.

Chronic depersonalization, closely associated with emotional numbing in PTSD patients, is thought to promote a sense of detachment from self that fosters risky and self-destructive behavior, such as self-mutilation. Self-mutilation has been strongly associated with increased dissociation in numerous studies. Dissociative patients often describe self-inflicting pain in attempts to break through profound states of depersonalization. At other times, they report feeling nothing as they cut or burn themselves. Alienation from self is also thought to play a role in the high rate of suicide attempts in dissociative patients. In addition, dissociation has been implicated in predisposing an individual to revictimization. In aggregate, these experiences expose dissociative individuals to further traumatization, which takes a cumulative toll over the individual's life.

Identification of environmental protective factors may help stimulate intervention models that prevent the development of significant dissociation in acutely traumatized children.

Hypnotic Model In its basic form, the hypnotic model hypotheses that a traumatized individual uses his or her innate hypnotic capacity to induce autohypnosis as a defense against overwhelming or repetitive traumatic experiences. With continued use, the autohypnotic state is transformed into an independent alter personality state. Several lines of evidence are said to support the autohypnotic hypothesis. The first is that dissociative, especially dissociative identity disorder, patients are highly hypnotizable. Second, many of the clinical phenomena associated with pathological dissociation, such as trance states, age regression, auditory hallucinations, and amnesias, can be produced in normal individuals using hypnosis. Finally, a pair of studies suggested that childhood trauma might increase hypnotizability.

More systematic research has dispelled the notion that childhood trauma generally increases hypnotizability. At least six studies found no differences between traumatized and nontraumatized adult or child samples, nor are there discernible dose effects between measures of trauma severity and hypnotizability in clinical and general population samples. However, a small group of individuals, termed *double dissociators*, score high on measures of dissociation and hypnotizability. These individuals generally have histories of earlier and more severe trauma. This observation is most compatible with the taxonic model of pathological dissociation and may explain the greater hypnotizability of dissociative identity disorder patients. Hypnotizability studies have shown that there may be different types of hypnotizability, with high dissociators making up a distinct type. They are in contrast to other subgroups of highly hypnotizable people, like the *fantasy-prone personality*, a specific construct in normal people elucidated in hypnotizability research studies.

Autohypnosis is not the only pathway to dissociative symptoms, but it remains a possible contributing mechanism in some individuals.

Neurological Models Two basic neurological explanations of dissociation have been repeatedly proposed over the last century and a half: the epileptic model and the hemispheric laterality model. Variants of these two models continue to be offered as explanations for dissociation, although recent empirical tests have not provided substantial support for either.

The epileptic model originates from the clinical observation that dissociative symptoms such as depersonalization; amnesias for complex behavior, such as fugue episodes; and phenomena such as autoscopy are sometimes associated with ictal and preictal states in seizure patients. Several cases series of seizure patients with dissociative identity disorder–like or dissociative disorder NOS–like clinical profiles have been published, and abnormal EEGs, particularly temporal slow waves, may be more common in dissociative disorder patients than in psychiatric patients in general. Yet, the vast majority of seizure patients score in the normal range on dissociation scales.

The strongest finding to emerge from these investigations thus far is that high levels of child abuse and dissociation, as measured by high DES scores, are common in patients diagnosed with pseudoseizures. More than 12 studies have documented this relationship in well-diagnosed patient samples in which genuine seizure patients had low DES scores and low clinical levels of dissociative symptoms. However, recent studies have identified abnormal EEG activity, particularly left-hemisphere slowing, as significantly more common in abused children than in nonabused psychiatric inpatients or normal controls. Thus, there may be an effect of child abuse on the developing brain that accounts for the high rates of EEG abnormalities seen in dissociative identity disorder patients.

The hemispheric laterality model was stimulated by early clinical observations of differences in the dominant handedness of alter personality states. Such handedness changes are still frequently reported today. Several modern single-case studies document apparent shifts in laterality using indirect measures, such as the GSR. One study of two dissociative identity disorder patients with seizures involved anesthetizing each cerebral hemisphere individually with an intracarotid injection of amobarbital (the Wada test). They reported emergence of different alter personality states seemingly related to inactivation of one or the other cerebral hemispheres. EEG monitoring during these procedures revealed no epileptiform activity associated with the alter personality states. The largest sample and only controlled study to examine the laterality hypothesis, however, did not find evidence of shifts in laterality across alter personality. Studies of split-brain patients who had commissurotomies for intractable epilepsy do not find evidence of alter personality–like phenomena. In short, intriguing as the shifts in dominant handedness are, shifts in laterality or differences in hemispheric laterality do not readily account for many of the clinical features of dissociative identity disorder patients.

Iatrogenic and Sociocognitive Models of Dissociative Disorders Some authorities believe that dissociative identity disorder and dissociative amnesia are not authentic psychiatric disorders but rather the product of suggestion on susceptible individuals that leads them to believe that they have a dissociative disorder and to enact the role of a person with multiple selves or amnesia for childhood maltreatment. This has been called the *iatrogenic* or *sociocognitive model* (SCM). Caution should be used concerning the term *iatrogenic*, however. This term is rarely defined rigorously and frequently is used pejoratively. The term is almost never operationalized, and its boundaries are unclear with respect to other untoward aspects of clinical encounters, such as side effects, complications, misdiagnosis, or acceptance by clinicians of factitious or malingered presentations, or a combination of these.

The SCM posits several interrelated factors that account for the phenomenon. The first, a susceptible patient, is commonly described as being highly suggestible, highly hypnotizable, or having a fantasy-prone personality, or a combination of these. In the clinical literature, these patients usually are described as having personality disorders characterized by dependent, borderline, or histrionic traits, or a combination of these, and who are conceptualized as desperate to find acceptance or a sense of identity, or both.

The second factor is a therapist who unwittingly, or through an ideological belief in the existence of dissociative identity disorder or amnesia for traumatic experiences, engages in a therapy that implicitly or explicitly encourages the patient to undertake the role of the dissociative identity disorder patient or the patient with so-called recovered memories for abuse. Accordingly, the condition is worsened by paying attention to the apparent dissociative disorder and engaging therapeutically with the alter identities. The patient develops a real, albeit iatrogenic disorder, now truly believing in the roles that he or she enacts.

A third factor has to do with broader cultural and social influence, often promulgated by the mass media, self-help books, or victim support groups in which people, primarily in North America, come to accept the possibility of multiple identity enactments or a history of forgotten childhood victimization, or both, as part of an established social role. In this view, therapy may not be a necessary factor in the development of a dissociative disorder; a susceptible person could do so simply through social influence.

Recent comprehensive reviews of the SCM for dissociative disorders have made several points. Virtually no empirical, scientific studies have been performed in clinical populations to attempt to examine the SCM or related ideas. The original database supporting this construct comes from a small, heterogeneous group of studies done in the 1940s and 1950s, mostly uncontrolled, quasi-experimental, anecdotal case reports. These demonstrated that some degree of role enactment of an alternative identity occurred with hypnosis, automatic writing, and strong repeated suggestions. Some of the subjects were the students of the researchers and were knowledgeable of the goals of the studies. The role enactments were limited to the experimental situation. In fact, one of the researchers, studying a traumatized soldier, concluded that hypnosis allowed access to authentic, previously dissociated self-aspects, not to artifacts of the procedure.

Studies of thousands of subjects undergoing hypnosis research over several decades have shown that a subgroup of highly hypnotizable individuals can exhibit limited, temporary alter self-states with hypnotic suggestions. These were dissimilar phenomenologically to clinical cases of dissociative identity disorder and were limited to the experimental situation. The researchers noted that they could not determine whether these procedures uncovered previously existing dissociated aspects of the mind or created them de novo.

A small series of studies on college student volunteers in a variety of hypnotized and nonhypnotized conditions found that highly hypnotizable, fantasy-prone students would enact the role of a dissociative identity disorder murderer with amnesia when given a series of robustly explicit suggestions to do so. Hypnosis was not a necessary or sufficient condition for this finding. These latter studies have been critiqued on a variety of grounds, including the lack of controls (e.g., enacting another psychiatric disorder, such as a murderer with schizophrenia); lack of equivalence of the research design with the clinical situation; conflation of dissociative identity disorder with role enactments, rather than the complex polysymptomatic picture described in the clinical and research literature; failure to produce alter behavior and reactivity typical of dissociative identity disorder; lack of control for strong expectancies and demand characteristics of the research design; role enactments limited to the experimental situation; and failure to control for preexisting dissociated self-states and traumatic experiences.

Finally, it is generally agreed among dissociative disorders authorities, beginning with Janet, that the shaping of bona fide dissociative identity disorder usually does occur in the clinical situation, although this phenomenon itself has never been subject to systematic research. In this model, the core symptoms of dissociative identity disorder are not created in the therapeutic encounter. A variety of developmental, social, cultural, intrapsychic, interpersonal, and cognitive factors, which can include psychotherapy, are hypothesized to account for the secondary structuralization of the dissociative process into the individualized dissociative identity disorder alter identities characteristic of a given person.

Little research has been conducted on clinical dissociative disorders patients to assess factors such as fantasy-prone personality and other forms of suggestibility. A recent report studied 17 dissociative identity disorder patients with the Gudjonsson Suggestibility Scale (GSS), an inventory developed to assess susceptibility to making false confessions to crimes. It tests memory for an event and liability to interpersonal pressure to change one's story about the event. In this study, dissociative identity disorder patients scored *lower* in overall suggestibility than control groups with PTSD, borderline personality disorder, and trauma victims without PTSD. Dissociative identity disorder subjects were *more* resistant than the other clinical groups to interpersonal persuasion. In another study of patients with so-called recovered memories of childhood sexual abuse, these patients also had lower GSS scores when compared to nonabused control psychiatric patients.

Furthermore, psychological assessment of large numbers of dissociative identity disorder patients using the Rorschach test and other assessment instruments did not show a personality profile typical of borderline or histrionic personality types. Rather, dissociative identity disorder individuals show a unique personality structure characterized by obsessional features, traumatic reactivity, complexity of response, introversion, unusual thinking at times, and insightfulness.

It remains a researchable question whether fully autonomous clinical dissociative identity disorder can be produced in susceptible individuals by sociocognitive factors alone. These studies would be difficult to design from an ethical standpoint. However, to be definitive, they would have to rigorously demonstrate a lack of preexisting dissociative psychopathology or history of trauma, or both; similarity of the experimental to the clinical situation with respect to the interactions of researchers and subjects; production of the extensive clinical phenomenology of dissociative identity disorder reported in the literature, not just role enactments; automatization of the symptoms outside the experimental situation; use of control populations enacting other psychiatric disorders; control for researcher bias; and extensive longitudinal follow-up.

DISSOCIATIVE AMNESIA

According to DSM-IV-TR (Table 17–4), the essential feature of dissociative amnesia is an inability to recall important personal information, usually of a traumatic or stressful nature, that is too extensive to be explained by normal forgetfulness.

The disturbance does not occur exclusively during the course of dissociative identity disorder, dissociative fugue, PTSD, acute stress disorder, or somatization disorder and is not due to the direct physiological effects of a substance or a neurological or other general medical condition. *Dissociative amnesia* can be more broadly defined as a reversible memory impairment in which groups of memories for personal experience that would ordinarily be available for recall to the conscious mind cannot be retrieved or retained in a verbal form (or, if temporarily retrieved, cannot be wholly retained in consciousness). This disturbance may be based on neurobiological changes in the brain caused by traumatic stress. However, the disorder manifests itself as a potentially reversible form of psychological inhibition.

The diagnosis of dissociative amnesia generally connotes four factors. First, relatively large groups of memories and associated affects have become unavailable, not just single memories, feelings, or thoughts. Second, the unavailable memories usually relate to day-to-day information that would ordinarily be a more or less routine part of conscious awareness: who a person is, what he or she did, where he or she went, what happened, with whom he or she spoke, what was said, what he or she thought and felt at the time, and so forth. Third, the ability to remember new factual information, general cognitive functioning, and language capacity are usually intact, although, in extreme cases, the dissociative process can interfere with retrieval of procedural memory information and registration of new memories. Finally, the dissociated memories often indirectly reveal their presence in more or less disguised form, such as intrusive visual images, flashbacks, somatoform symptoms, nightmares, conversion symptoms, and behavioral reenactments. That is, in most cases, dissociative amnesia must be understood as a part of the spectrum of memory dysfunction related to traumatic stress, often alternating with forms of hyperamnesia or a derealized awareness in which the person experiences detachment or estrangement from elements of autobiographical memory, or both.

There are two basic presentations of dissociative amnesia. The first is a dramatic, sudden disturbance in which extensive aspects of memory for personal information are not available to conscious verbal recall. These patients are often seen in emergency departments or general medical or neurological services, because the sudden development of memory loss requires medical assessment. In addition, during an acute amnestic episode, some of these individuals may demonstrate disorientation, perplexity, alterations in consciousness, somatoform symptoms, or purposeless wandering, or a combination of these.

Table 17–4
DSM-IV-TR Diagnostic Criteria for Dissociative Amnesia

A. The predominant disturbance is one or more episodes of inability to recall important personal information, usually of a traumatic or stressful nature, that is too extensive to be explained by ordinary forgetfulness.

B. The disturbance does not occur exclusively during the course of dissociative identity disorder, dissociative fugue, posttraumatic stress disorder, acute stress disorder, or somatization disorder and is not due to the direct physiological effects of a substance (e.g., a drug of abuse, a medication) or a neurological or other general medical condition (e.g., amnestic disorder due to head trauma).

C. The symptoms cause clinically significant distress or impairment in social, occupational, or other important areas of functioning.

From American Psychiatric Association. *Diagnostic and Statistical Manual of Mental Disorders.* 4th ed. Text rev. Washington, DC: American Psychiatric Association; 2000, with permission.

A 45-year-old, divorced, left-handed, male bus dispatcher was seen in psychiatric consultation on a medical unit. He had been admitted with an episode of chest discomfort, light headedness, and left-arm weakness. He had a history of hypertension and had a medical admission in the past year for ischemic chest pain, although he had not suffered a myocardial infarction. Psychiatric consultation was called, as the patient complained of memory loss for the previous 12 years, behaving and responding to the environment as if it were 12 years previously (e.g., he didn't recognize his 8-year-old son, insisted that he was unmarried, and denied recollection of current events, such as the current president). Physical and laboratory findings were unchanged from the patient's usual baseline. Brain computed tomography (CT) scan was normal.

On mental status examination, the patient displayed intact intellectual function but insisted that the date was 12 years earlier, denying recall of his entire subsequent personal history and of current events for the last 12 years. He denied awareness of his current address, life circumstances, job, recent political events, and so forth. He was perplexed by the contradiction between his memory and current circumstances. The patient described a family history of brutal beatings and physical discipline. He was a decorated combat veteran, although he described amnestic episodes for some of his combat experiences. In the military, he had been a champion golden glove boxer noted for his powerful left hand.

He was educated about his disorder and given the suggestion that his memory could return as he could tolerate it, perhaps overnight during sleep or perhaps over a longer time. If this strategy was unsuccessful, hypnosis or an amobarbital interview was proposed.

On the subsequent examination, the patient reported that his memory had returned. Before the amnestic episode, he described an escalating series of conflicts at work, in his marriage, and with his son. His wife was discussing a separation and had asked him to discuss this with his son. He felt completely responsible for his coworkers and for the care of his relatives. He had felt panicked, overwhelmed, and enraged. He had felt violently angry at his wife but had vowed in the past that he would "beat to death anybody who tried to hurt her." He stated that he would have attempted suicide, but he "couldn't," because he had too many people relying on him. The amnesia developed after he felt a kind of "paralysis" in his left arm. His wife had rushed him to the hospital and had been extremely concerned about his well-being.

He was aware that none of these problems existed 12 years before and that he had unconsciously returned to a less stressful time by losing his memory. The patient was treated with supportive psychotherapy in the hospital, and coordination of care was arranged with his cardiologist. The patient was referred for marital and individual psychotherapy and for psychopharmacological intervention.

Despite its relative rarity, this type of dissociative amnesia is featured in the media and in most textbooks as representative of the condition. However, a far more prevalent form of dissociative amnesia is a deletion from conscious memory of significant aspects of the personal history. Ordinarily, patients do not complain of this, and it is usually only discovered in taking a careful life history. Dissociative amnesia typically has a clear-cut onset and offset, so that the person is subjectively aware of a gap in continuous memory. For example, a patient may report that she does not remember being in third grade, although having clear memory for other school years. Usually such symptoms are associated with traumatic circumstances, for example, the patient reports that she has been told that, during third grade, she was kidnapped by her estranged father in a custody dispute, held by him for a number of months, and was sexually abused by him during that time. In extreme cases, the patient may deny recall for his or her entire childhood or other major life epochs.

Dr. G. is a 33-year-old clinical psychologist who was admitted to the hospital because of repeated acts of severe self-mutilation. She reported chronic depressed mood, anxiety, and interpersonal problems with inability to form intimate relations. She had periods of bulimia and anorexia requiring hospital treatment during her early 20s and ongoing struggles with eating. She described a variety of OCD symptoms, including recurrent checking "to make sure" that the doors were locked to her home, arranging things to "prevent harm from befalling me," and repeated rituals of counting and singing in her mind. Medications and intensive outpatient psychotherapy had helped moderate some of her symptoms, but she had become increasingly demoralized by her overall failure to improve in treatment. Mental status revealed an oddly cheerful, cerebral woman who could not explain the profound impulses that she felt to harm herself or to commit suicide. She was articulate and spoke in intellectualized psychodynamic formulations.

When asked about her childhood history, she described virtually no recall for her life between 5 and approximately 13 years of age. Her siblings would joke with her about her inability to recall family holidays, school events, and vacation trips. She described her relationship with her family as "great," reporting a warm, supportive relationship with her parents. On further questioning, however, she revealed that her father had been an alcoholic throughout her childhood, only achieving sobriety in her early adolescence. She had reported several episodes of "weird sexual" touching by him to her seventh grade teacher, resulting in a social service investigation. Her father had acknowledged these episodes at the time and received treatment for alcoholism and "sex addiction." He denied any other episodes of sexual abuse toward his children. The children were not removed from the home. Dr. G. denied any feelings about these episodes, stating that "he took care of the problem. Now, he's a great support. I have no reason to be mad at him." She explained her amnesia by saying that "maybe nothing important happened and that's why I don't remember."

Treatment focused on establishing safety from self-injury. Cognitive therapy focused on the patient's self-blame, lack of affect, minimization of self-harm, and a profoundly negative view of herself. The patient was provided with education about her disorders and was taught symptom management skills. The patient increasingly became aware of affects of shame, anger, hurt, and betrayal related to having been abused. These seemed to precede episodes of self-harm. The latter also occurred after phone conversations with her parents. As therapy progressed, the patient began to spontaneously remember other episodes of abuse that her father had not acknowledged, such as episodes of oral and vaginal sex. As this occurred, she had more intrusive PTSD symptoms, including nightmares, flashbacks, and intrusive images and bodily sensations. She remembered that, as a child, she would arrange things obsessively in the belief that, by doing so, she could prevent her father's nocturnal visits. During the abuse, she recalled that she sang and counted in her head to distance herself from the experience. She also began to recall much more serious conflict and chaos in the family related to her father's alcoholism during the years for which she had been amnestic. Dr. G. reported intense distress at the conflict between the attachment to her parents and family and the implications of these emerging memories. She became increasingly aware of the extent to which she avoided thinking about the abuse, her response to it, and its impact on her life.

Following Janet, several different patterns of dissociative amnesia have been identified. These are listed in Table 17–5.

Epidemiology As noted in the overview, *dissociative amnesia*, as defined by DSM-IV-TR, has been reported in approximately 6 percent of a general population sample in Winnipeg Canada, studied with the DES and the DDIS. There is no known difference in incidence between men and women. Cases generally begin to be reported in late adolescence and adulthood. Dissociative amnesia may be especially difficult to assess in preadolescent children because of their more limited ability to describe subjective experience. It may be confused with daydreaming, inattention, anxiety, oppositional behavior, learning disorders, and psychotic disturbances. Adolescents are better able to verbalize the experience of amnesia. For example, one teenager said, "I skip time" to describe the amnesia experience. Patients may describe more than one amnesia episode.

A variety of studies have looked at the prevalence of amnesia for specific types of traumatic experiences: combat, sexual abuse, physical abuse, and emotional abuse. Other studies have reported amnesia along with other symptoms of PTSD in various traumatized groups.

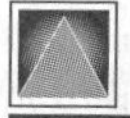

Table 17–5
Types of Dissociative Amnesia

Localized amnesia
Inability to recall events related to a circumscribed period of time
Selective amnesia
Ability to remember some, but not all, of the events occurring during a circumscribed period of time
Generalized amnesia
Failure to recall one's entire life
Continuous amnesia
Failure to recall successive events as they occur
Systematized amnesia
Amnesia for certain categories of memory, such as all memories relating to one's family or to a particular person

Across several studies, the prevalence of amnesia during combat reported among several thousand active duty soldiers in World War II ranged from 5 to 14.4 percent. Only a small percentage of these soldiers were reported to have suffered significant head injuries. In one study of 1,000 soldiers, 35 percent of the group exposed to the most intense combat had amnesia. Past or family history of dissociation or hysterical symptoms was associated with amnesia in soldiers with minimal battlefield exposure.

Structured interview data using the SCID-D-R have shown significantly higher amnesia scores in Vietnam era veterans with PTSD compared to combat veteran controls without PTSD. Studies of Nazi Holocaust survivors, Korean War veterans, and Vietnam era combat veterans with PTSD and adult survivors of childhood sexual abuse have repeatedly documented deficits in explicit memory on standardized memory tests as compared to matched controls.

Forty percent of a sample of 50 randomly selected survivors of the Cambodian Holocaust endorsed amnesia on PTSD diagnostic inventories. The average DES score in this group of severely traumatized individuals was 37.1. Amnesia was reported in 3 to 10 percent of Holocaust survivors assessed with a PTSD inventory. The highest prevalence was found in tattooed survivors of Auschwitz. Studies of natural disasters, such as the San Francisco earthquake in 1989, have found that 3 to 5 percent of survivors report amnesia for at least some aspects of these events.

With respect to delayed recall of sexual or physical abuse, or both, more than 70 studies have confirmed this finding in clinical, community, and forensic populations, including retrospective, prospective, and longitudinal study designs. In various studies of clinical populations and individuals who identified themselves as survivors of abuse, 16 to almost 100 percent reported amnesia for the abuse at some time in their lives, averaging approximately 30 percent across studies. Lower prevalence was found in outpatients. In studies of college undergraduates and women in the community, prevalence of amnesia for abuse ranged from 13 to more than 50 percent.

A random sample of 505 men and women in the general population found that approximately 21 percent reported a history of childhood sexual abuse. Of these, 20 percent described full amnesia, and 22 percent reported partial amnesia for the abuse at some time in their lives.

Somewhat lower rates of amnesia for physical and emotional abuse have been reported in clinical and nonclinical samples: Approximately 20 percent of subjects endorse this finding across studies.

Longitudinal and prospective studies, primarily following up large samples of individuals with documented prior childhood sexual trauma from court or medical reports, have found that almost 40 percent of respondents failed to recall a forensically or medically documented episode of childhood sexual abuse when interviewed 20 years or more later, even though, in some cases, other episodes of trauma or maltreatment were recalled. Some respondents denied any history of maltreatment at all.

In a recent 10-year follow-up study of children of various ages involved in criminal prosecution against their sexual abuse perpetrators, 19 percent of this highly selected sample appeared unable or unwilling to describe the abuse at a later time. Factors thought to predispose to amnesia for trauma are listed in Table 17–6. However, none of these factors has been shown to exclusively distinguish those with amnesia for trauma from those without amnesia.

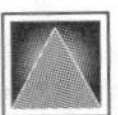

Table 17–6
Factors Leading to Dissociative Amnesia after Traumatic Experiences

Trauma caused by human assault rather than natural disaster
Repeated traumatization as opposed to single traumatic events
Longer duration of trauma
Fear of death or significant harm during trauma
Trauma caused by multiple perpetrators
Close relationship between perpetrator and victim
Betrayal by a caretaker as part of abuse
Threats of death or significant harm by perpetrator if the victim discloses his or her identity or information regarding the traumatic experience
Violence of trauma (i.e., physical injury caused by the trauma)
Earlier age at onset of trauma

Note: No factor has exclusively been associated with dissociative amnesia.
Adapted from Loewenstein RJ. Dissociative amnesia and dissociative fugue. In: Gabbard GO, ed. *Treatment of Psychiatric Disorders,* 3rd ed. Vol 2. Washington, DC: American Psychiatric Press; 2001:1625.

Etiology

Several different theories have been developed to explain dissociative amnesia. A unified theory combines several of these.

Behavioral State and Information Processing Model

In the behavioral state and information processing model, dissociation is conceptualized as a basic part of the psychobiology of the human response to life-threatening danger: a protective activation of altered states of consciousness that change perception, pain sensation, time sense, and sense of self. Memories and affects relating to the trauma are encoded during these altered states. When the person returns to the baseline state, there is relatively less access to the dissociated information, leading, in many cases, to dissociative amnesia for at least some part of the traumatic events. However, the dissociated memories and affects can manifest themselves in nonverbal forms: posttraumatic nightmares, reenactments, intrusive imagery, and somatoform symptoms. Not only is there amnesia for the trauma, but the person also frequently has dissociated that certain basic assumptions about the self, relationships, other people, and the nature of the world have been altered by the trauma.

This model does not posit that trauma is forgotten. Furthermore, the model does not necessitate that psychic pain is the controlling variable in the onset of amnesia, although the latter may be a factor in inhibiting retrieval of dissociated information. Rather, it suggests that trauma is encoded and remembered but remains relatively verbally inaccessible owing to difficulty in retrieving information across different DBS. Some authorities have made the analogy between posttraumatic dissociative amnesia and experimentally produced hypnotic amnesia. In both cases, implicit memory for the material can usually be demonstrated. Following Janet, some have hypothesized that amnesia occurs when there is a relative decrease in executive control or synthesis among groups of psychic or memory elements and the inhibition of control elements that can give access to information that is stored in memory.

The results of recent neuroimaging studies of small groups of trauma survivors support this model by indicating possible neurobiological substrates of dissociative amnesia. For example, PET and fMRI studies of PTSD subjects have shown that stimulation of trauma recall by script driven imagery is associated with activation of nondominant hemisphere areas, limbic areas, and the occipital lobe with relative suppression of left-brain language areas, such as Broca's area, and inhibition of the prefrontal cortex.

Some researchers have focused on the finding of significant reduction of hippocampal volume in various traumatized populations as a marker for pathological processes involving memory in posttraumatic disorders. Also, studies using ketamine, a noncompetitive antagonist of the NMDA receptor, result in increases in dissociative symptoms as measured by the CADSS, including amnesia.

Amnesia and Extreme Intrapsychic Conflict

Acute, florid amnestic episodes and the chronic covert amnesias generally occur after severe, overwhelming, life-threatening traumas, such as combat, childhood sexual assault, adult rape, threats of death or physical violence, and other similarly overwhelming events. However, in many cases of acute dissociative amnesia, the psychosocial environment out of which the amnesia develops is not traumatic per se, but, rather, massively conflictual, with the patient experiencing intolerable emotions of shame, guilt, despair, rage, and desperation. These are usually reported to result from conflicts over unacceptable urges or impulses, such as intense sexual, suicidal, or violent compulsions. Thus, these patients are conceptualized as experiencing massive psychological conflict from which fight or flight seems impossible or psychologically unacceptable. However, most of the latter cases have prior histories of severe trauma predating the episode of amnesia. The loss of memory in some of these individuals has been conceptualized as an alternative to suicide. Indeed, premature therapeutic efforts to overcome amnesia have been reported to result in successful suicide in some cases.

Betrayal Trauma A related explanatory model is derived from social psychological principles and from developmental attachment theory. *Betrayal trauma* attempts to explain amnesia by the intensity of trauma and by the extent that a negative event represents a betrayal by a trusted, needed other. This betrayal is thought to influence the way in which the event is processed and remembered. For example, in this model, a child is more likely to develop amnesia when subjected to abuse by a family member or another person whom the child trusts or on whom the child is dependent. The amnesia is protective of the child's developmentally mediated need for attachment, allowing for preservation of overall emotional and cognitive growth, despite the abuse. In this model, information about the abuse is not linked to mental mechanisms that control attachment and attachment behavior.

Lack of shareability of trauma experiences is also thought to contribute to amnesia for trauma. That is, in addition to the neurobiological factors that inhibit verbal access to such events, they are less likely to be shared with others because of threats, shame, lack of developmental ability to have words for the experience, and intense confusion and emotional arousal engendered by the abuse. Thus, it is theorized that traumas involving betrayal are processed differently cognitively from other autobiographical experiences, leading to subjective memory deficits. Betrayal trauma theory also helps to explain the lower prevalence of amnesia for wartime trauma, natural disasters, and the Nazi Holocaust, among others, as compared to that for childhood sexual or physical abuse.

Various studies have supported the betrayal trauma model. In one study of college undergraduates, abuse by a caretaker was a better predictor of memory impairment related to the abuse than age at the time of the abuse or duration of the abuse. Stroop test data have also shown that high DES subjects who report more trauma and more betrayal trauma, compared to low DES subjects, may actively inhibit threatening information, but not neutral information, from being accessed consciously.

A unified information processing and betrayal model predicts the relative likelihood of amnesia under varying circumstances, such as high threat and low betrayal, high threat and high betrayal, and so forth.

Validity of Dissociative Amnesia Studies that address the validity of dissociative amnesia have primarily centered on the existence of the phenomenon, not on the study of the clinical disorder. As noted previously, all of the studies that have attempted to investigate the presence of amnesia for trauma have reported that it occurs.

Alternative hypotheses about trauma and memory claim that trauma virtually always causes an indelible inscribing of memory in the brain and that dissociative amnesia is a myth. The debate about the existence of dissociative amnesia has also focused in part on hypothesized psychological mechanisms for the reported amnesia, such as repression or dissociation. Critics have suggested that more mundane processes, such as failure to report, cognitive avoidance, or ordinary forgetting, might account for the apparent delayed recall, although it is difficult to understand how these alternative mechanisms could account for the findings of amnesia during acute trauma, such as combat.

Data from a variety of research studies show that individuals who report problems with recall of trauma may describe several subjective processes. Some experience inability to recall some or all of traumatic life events or life epochs in which the trauma occurred. Others report deliberate attempts to avoid thinking about the traumas because of the subjective distress or shame that they experience when they try to do so. Another group describes lack of ability to appreciate the abusive nature of trauma until they were older or more emancipated from abusive social milieus, or both. In clinical practice, all of these mechanisms may help account for aspects or apparent dissociative amnesia in an individual patient.

Many studies have found corroboration for the abuse and trauma recalled by individuals with dissociative amnesia. Types of corroboration have included medical records, social service records, church diocesan records, verbal or written admission by perpetrators, criminal convictions or civil judgments against perpetrators, reports of family members, and information from witnesses or other victims of the same perpetrator. Also, studies have shown no significant differences in the accuracy of delayed recall of trauma compared to accounts of individuals who report continuous memory for trauma.

Like continuous memories, delayed memories may be shown by corroboration to be generally accurate, partially accurate, or completely confabulated. Reliable corroboration, which may be very difficult to obtain, particularly in cases of reported childhood maltreatment or intimate-partner violence, is the only way to resolve the extent to which a memory is generally accurate.

Diagnosis and Clinical Features As described in prior sections, there are two major clinical presentations of dissociative amnesia.

Classic Presentation Classically presenting patients are the textbook cases that form the image of dissociative disorders for most mental health professionals. The classic disorder is an overt, florid, dramatic clinical disturbance that frequently results in the patient being brought quickly to medical attention specifically for symptoms related to the dissociative disorder. The paradigmatic case is that of the individual who is found without memory for identity or life history, sometimes leading to media reporting of the case. Less extreme forms of amnesia, such as acute amnesia for recent traumatic circumstances, such as combat or rape, also fall into this category.

This presentation of amnesia is frequently found in those who have experienced extreme acute trauma. However, it also commonly develops in the context of profound intrapsychic conflict or emotional stress. For example, a terrified soldier in combat experiences excruciating conflict over his or her urge to flee and his or her belief that "all cowards should be shot."

There are little systematic modern data about patients with this form of dissociative amnesia. Patients may present with intercurrent somatoform or conversion symptoms, or both, alterations in consciousness, depersonalization, derealization, trance states, spontaneous age regression, and even ongoing anterograde dissociative amnesia. Depression and suicidal ideation are reported in many, but not all, cases. No single personality profile or antecedent history is consistently reported in these patients, although a prior personal or family history of somatoform or dissociative symptoms has been shown to predispose individuals to develop acute amnesia during traumatic circumstances. Case reports suggest that many of these patients have histories of prior adult or childhood abuse or trauma. However, in the wartime cases, as in other forms of combat-related posttraumatic disorders, the most important variable in the development of dissociative symptoms appears to be the intensity of combat.

Factors relating to avoidance of responsibility may be prominent in some of these cases, with sexual indiscretions, legal difficulties, financial problems, or fear of anticipated combat being part of the clinical matrix that surrounds the amnesia. There is a possible association in some cases with an antecedent history of head trauma with or without loss of consciousness, although this finding has never been studied rigorously using adequate controls. There are no data on the prevalence of PTSD symptoms in these patients.

If carefully questioned, some of these patients give a history of recurrent episodes of amnesia or fugue. Some actually meet criteria for dissociative identity disorder or dissociative disorder NOS. In the dissociative identity disorder cases, the amnesia occurs when the person creates a new alter self state that experiences itself as unaware of some or all of the past history of the person to cope with overwhelming or traumatic circumstances.

In most of the acute dissociative amnesia cases, the amnesia resolves within hours to months, spontaneously or through psychotherapy, hypnotherapy, pharmacologically facilitated interviews, or combinations of these modalities. However, in rare cases, a chronic course develops, with the patient seemingly unable to tolerate recall of the events that surrounded the onset of the amnesia.

Ms. M. is a 55-year-old woman who was seen in psychiatric consultation because of the sudden, complete loss of memory for her entire life history. For the several years preceding this event, the patient had been seeking "meaning" in her life subsequent to the last of her children leaving home. She had been involved in a number of community activities in her home city but began to seek inner understanding through psychotherapy. She explored a reported history of neglect, emotional abuse, and physical abuse in her family of origin and a history of childhood sexual abuse involving several women outside her family. She became friends with a female psychotherapist who encouraged the patient to seek training as a counselor, herself. The friend declared a sexual attraction to the patient, although the patient apparently did not reciprocate this attraction.

The two became involved in therapy training and similar activities, culminating in their attendance at a new age–oriented therapy workshop in a distant city. They shared a room, and the friend began to pressure the patient sexually. The patient remains uncertain whether she rebuffed these advances. On one hand, she was terrified that her friend would be "mad" about her refusal. On the other hand, she was panicked lest her family find out about the sexual pressures from her friend. The workshop consisted of a number of group sessions involving movement, imagery, "inner child work," artwork, and similar experiences. During an intense session involving picturing oneself going back in time and being reborn, the patient appeared to enter a deep trance state. At the conclusion of the session, she remained in a fetal position. When questioned, she could not identify who she was, where she was, or anything else about herself or her situation.

Instead of seeking psychiatric help, the workshop organizers took the patient back to her hotel room, lit candles, and provided aromatherapy. At the end of several days, there was no change in the patient's condition, and the members of the workshop and the patient's companion left. The patient's family found her in a dazed, confused, and disoriented state, unable to recognize them or to provide any history of recent events. She had difficulty learning new information, seemingly forgetting it as it was provided. She was panicked and complained of not "feeling in my body." In addition to loss of autobiographical memory, she appeared to have difficulty dressing herself until shown how, did not know how to put in her contact lenses, and was confused about a number of activities of daily living.

Brought to neuropsychiatric attention, the patient was given an extensive neurological and neuropsychological workup, all of which showed that the cognitive deficits were consistent with a psychologically based amnesia, not a neurological process. On mental status examination, the patient presented as a scared, confused, neatly dressed woman who frequently entered trance states, staring off and losing track of the conversation. She had relearned a variety of information, including the identities of her children and spouse but had no sense that she had known any of this before being recently taught it. She "knew" about a variety of family events but had no sense of first-hand memory for them. She complained of ongoing amnesia, spontaneous trances, and periods of intense depersonalization and derealization. She was unable to perform daily functions, such as driving and cooking, having no recall of these skills. Mood was depressed, with periods of intense suicidal preoccupation. In reviewing the history with family members, the patient's former psychotherapists, and the patient herself, significant marital conflicts and family conflicts between the patient, her siblings, and her elderly mother were described.

As treatment progressed, the patient began to describe the subjective experience of different self-states, although it was quite difficult to determine if they met DSM-IV-TR criteria for a dissociative identity disorder alter identity. She described the belief that "the old M." had been unable to cope with the family, marital, and personal conflicts preceding the amnesia "and just crumbled into pieces." The workshop exercises that preceded the memory loss uncannily recreated features of some of the patient's reported childhood trauma, about which she had written extensively before the onset of the amnesia. At times, she experienced herself as "the little girl" who recalled horrifying episodes of sadistic childhood maltreatment and was terrified lest they recur. At other times, she experienced herself as the "new M." who had to relearn her entire life history. She was rediagnosed as dissociative disorder NOS.

After several years, despite individual psychotherapy using supportive, psychodynamic and cognitive-behavioral modalities, hypnotherapy, couples therapy, family therapy, and antidepressant medication, the patient continues to experience amnesia, although she has "relearned" enough to manage her day-to-day life. Mood has improved, and the patient has made some adjustment to her difficult family situation. Settlement of a lawsuit against the workshop organizers did not result in any clinical change. She has repeatedly refused an amobarbital interview.

Nonclassic Presentation The nonclassic dissociative amnesia patients can be said to have a *covert* dissociative syndrome, because their primary complaints infrequently relate directly to amnesia. Chronic, recurrent, or persistent dissociative amnesia, or a combination of these, is the most common symptom in these cases, although some may also describe a history of fugue-like states. Commonly, patients with the nonclassic presentations of amnesia do not reveal the presence of dissociative symptoms unless directly asked about them. These patients are often uncomfortable when amnesia is inquired about and may minimize the presence or rationalize the importance of the symptom.

In these patients, the amnesia manifests itself as a circumscribed memory gap or series of memory gaps for the life history, primarily for times when traumatic events occurred, such as childhood or wartime.

These patients frequently come to treatment for a variety of symptoms, such as depression or mood swings, substance abuse, sleep disturbances, somatoform symptoms, anxiety and panic, suicidal or self-mutilating impulses and acts, violent outbursts, eating problems, and interpersonal problems. Self-mutilation and violent behavior in these patients may also be accompanied by amnesia. Amnesia may also occur for flashbacks or behavioral reexperiencing episodes related to trauma.

Only one systematic study exists that has examined the characteristics of these patients. In a small, highly selected sample referred for consultation at a specialty clinic for dissociative disorders, most dissociative amnesia patients were women. Almost all had a prior history of childhood or adult physical, sexual, or emotional abuse and neglect, or a combination of these. The trauma history was less severe than has been reported in patients with dissociative identity disorder. Duration of reported amnesia ranged from minutes to years. Slightly less than one-half of the sample had recurrent episodes. Traumatic precipitants of the amnesia were most common, although, in 30 percent of cases, amnesia was present for problematic behaviors, such as sexual indiscretions and self-mutilation. The most common comorbid conditions were mood disorders, PTSD, and a mixed personality disorder. Patients differed from dissociative identity disorder patients in that they had lower rates of substance abuse, self-mutilation, hallucinations, fugues, sexual dysfunction, and somatoform symptoms. DES scores averaged lower than those of dissociative identity disorder patients. Family history was characterized by alcoholism and mood disorders.

Pathology and Laboratory Examination Dissociative amnesia can be diagnosed with the DDIS or the SCID-D-R, or both. Dissociative amnesia patients have been reported to have high hypnotizability, as measured with standardized hypnosis scales.

Differential Diagnosis

Ordinary Forgetfulness and Nonpathological Amnesia The DSM-IV-TR diagnostic criteria for dissociative amnesia specify that the disturbance must be "too extensive to be explained by normal forgetfulness." Furthermore, nonpathological forms of amnesia have been described, such as infantile and childhood amnesia, amnesia for sleep and dreaming, and hypnotic amnesia.

Most forms of dissociative amnesia are thought to primarily involve difficulties with episodic and autobiographical memory, not implicit or semantic memory. Several studies have confirmed the clinical observation that subjects with pathological dissociative amnesia for their life history can demonstrate implicit autobiographical memory while amnesic. When asked to free associate, to imagine, or to make up a story or when exposed to projective tests, patients with dissociative amnesia include in their productions elements that contain autobiographical information without necessarily being consciously aware of this.

Amnesic patients may also have intense reactions to stimuli that are emotionally significant, without knowing consciously the reason for the reaction or the significance of the stimulus, such as when a patient with PTSD has a flashback without consciously knowing what triggered it and often without clear recall later of the memory being evoked.

Studies of autobiographical memory in several populations support the notion that infantile and childhood amnesia can be experimentally documented. However, there is now a substantial body of data being accumulated on preverbal learning and memory in young children. Amnesia may result in later years owing to the difficulty in translating this preverbal memory into verbal form. However, experiments designed to overcome this factor in young children have shown that children can later report preverbal memories accurately in verbal form under suitable experimental conditions.

Studies demonstrate that normal adult autobiographical memory has a retention gradient for memory for the most recent 20 to 30 years of the subject's life, often with a subjective sense of wearing away of memories for the past, in contrast to the subjective gaps in memory typical of dissociative amnesia. Elderly patients in autobiographical memory studies have been shown to have a relative decrease in recent autobiographical memories and a *reminiscence component* for the subject's youth. Subtle cumulative memory difficulties may be a feature of normal aging, often with decreased ability to retain new information, increased time to recall already learned information, or both, resulting in *age-related cognitive decline*, also known as *benign forgetfulness of the elderly*.

Memories for repeated routine events, such as going to work or school every day, may not be encoded as discrete memories for each day, but rather as broad memory categories for the events that repeatedly reoccur. This is also thought to occur with some traumatic experiences, such as repeated episodes of childhood sexual abuse that happen recurrently over many years.

Clinically, patients with dissociative amnesia may describe exaggerated or extended forms of childhood amnesia. This finding has been documented in an experimental study of a cognitively normal dissociative identity disorder patient who, unlike normal controls, showed a virtual absence of memories for the first 10 years of her life. In another study, a patient with a global dissociative amnesia after a rape was evaluated with cognitive testing while amnesic and after memory recovery. As compared to an organically impaired control, the dissociative amnesia patient was able to recall memories from various parts of the life history without the temporal gradient that characterized the retrograde amnesia of the organic patient. Recall of autobiographical information during dissociative amnesia seemed related to life events with positive affects that were unconnected with the traumatic events precipitating the amnesia. Implicit autobiographical memory phenomena were documented as well in this patient. Similar phenomena have been described in posthypnotic amnesia, with implicit demonstration that the memories for which amnesia has been suggested have been encoded and stored, but without their being accessible directly for retrieval.

Dementia, Delirium, and Organic Amnestic Disorders There is no single test or examination that can establish absolutely whether a memory disorder is dissociative, organic, malingered, or of mixed etiology. The clinician evaluating the amnesic patient must have a reasonable index of suspicion about any of these. In ambiguous cases, there should be careful reassessment of the clinical situation on an ongoing basis. However, most cases of dissociative amnesia present differently from other disorders with memory impairment (Table 17–7).

The evaluation of acute dissociative amnesias is described in Table 17–8.

In patients with dementia, organic amnestic disorders, and delirium, the memory loss for personal information is embedded in a far more extensive set of cognitive, language, attentional, behavioral, and memory problems. Loss of memory for personal identity is usually not found without evidence of a marked disturbance in many domains of cognitive function. Confabulation may be present to various degrees and is usually implausible or bizarre. Causes of organic amnestic disorders include Korsakoff's psychosis, cerebral vascular accident (CVA), postoperative amnesia, postinfectious amnesia, anoxic amnesia, and transient global amnesia. Electroconvulsive therapy (ECT) may also cause a marked temporary amnesia, as well as persistent memory problems in some cases. Here, however, memory loss for autobiographical experience is unrelated to traumatic or overwhelming experiences and seems to involve many different types of personal experience, most commonly that occurring just before or during the ECT treatments.

Posttraumatic Amnesia In posttraumatic amnesia due to brain injury, there is usually a history of a clear-cut physical trauma, a period of unconsciousness or amnesia, or both, and

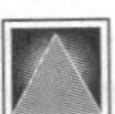

Table 17–7
Differential Diagnosis of Dissociative Amnesia

Ordinary forgetfulness
- Age-related cognitive decline

Nonpathological forms of amnesia
- Infantile and childhood amnesia
- Amnesia for sleep and dreaming
- Hypnotic amnesia

Dementia

Delirium

Amnestic disorders

Neurological disorders with discrete memory loss episodes
- Posttraumatic amnesia
- Transient global amnesia
- Amnesia related to seizure disorders

Substance-related amnesia
- Alcohol
- Sedative-hypnotics
- Anticholinergic agents
- Steroids
- Marijuana
- Narcotic analgesics
- Psychedelics
- Phencyclidine
- Methyldopa (Aldomet)
- Pentazocine (Talwin)
- Hypoglycemic agents
- β-Blockers
- Lithium carbonate
- Many others

Other dissociative disorders
- Dissociative fugue
- Dissociative identity disorder
- Dissociative disorder not otherwise specified

Acute stress disorder

Posttraumatic stress disorder

Somatization disorder

Psychotic episode
- Lack of memory for psychotic episode when returns to nonpsychotic state

Mood disorder episode
- Lack of memory for aspects of episode of mania when depressed and vice versa or when euthymic

Factitious disorder

Malingering

objective clinical evidence of brain injury. In general, the length of the posttraumatic amnesia is a reasonable predictor of cognitive outcome. Retrograde amnesia may also occur. An extensive retrograde amnesia out of proportion to the extent of the head injury suggests that an investigation for dissociative factors may be warranted.

Seizure Disorders In most seizure cases, the clinical presentation is quite different from that of dissociative amnesia, with clear-cut ictal events and sequelae. Patients with pseudoepileptic seizures may also have dissociative symptoms, such as amnesia and an antecedent history of psychological trauma. Rarely, patients with recurrent complex partial seizures may present with ongoing bizarre behavior, memory problems, irritability, or violence, leading to a differential diagnostic puzzle. In some of these cases, the diagnosis can only be clarified by telemetry or ambulatory EEG monitoring.

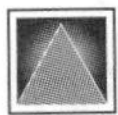

Table 17–8
Evaluation of Acute Amnesia

Complete history (to the extent that this can be gathered)
- Medical history
- Psychiatric history
- Trauma history (combat, violence, childhood maltreatment, etc.)
- Developmental history
- Collateral informants (if available)
  - Family and concerned others
  - Medical, military, police, and social service records
- Sequential clinical observation

Physical and neurological examination
- Baseline physical and laboratory examination
- Full mental status examination
- Mini-Mental State Examination
- Dementia workup
- Electrocardiogram
- Electroencephalogram
  - Telemetry in unusual cases
- Brain imaging
- Neuropsychological assessment

Substance-Related Amnesia A variety of substances and intoxicants have been implicated in the production of amnesia. Common offending agents are listed in Table 17–7.

In most cases, a careful history from the patient and ancillary sources, sequential clinical observation, and objective testing clarify the substance-related nature of the amnesia. In some instances of pathological intoxication, in which a small amount of alcohol or similar substance produces a major behavioral disinhibition, the alcohol may be producing its effect by facilitating the onset of a dissociative episode in a susceptible individual. This may be analogous to the disinhibition that occurs in a clinical amobarbital interview. Subjects may report amnesia for violent or other out-of-character behavior during such an episode.

The most difficult differential diagnostic problem usually involves patients with a history of substance-induced and dissociative memory problems. Some of these patients may minimize dissociative amnesia and vice versa. Clinically, the relative contribution of the substance abuse and the dissociation may only be fully clarified by sequential clinical observation once the patient has achieved sobriety.

Transient Global Amnesia Transient global amnesia may be mistaken for a dissociative amnesia, especially because stressful life events may precede either disorder. However, in transient global amnesia, there is the sudden onset of complete anterograde amnesia and learning abilities; pronounced retrograde amnesia; preservation of memory for personal identity; anxious awareness of memory loss with repeated, often perseverative, questioning; overall normal behavior; lack of gross neurological abnormalities in most cases; and rapid return of baseline cognitive function, with a persistent short retrograde amnesia. The patient usually is older than 50 years of age and shows risk factors for cerebrovascular disease, although epilepsy and migraine have been etiologically implicated in some cases.

Dissociative Disorders As noted previously, dissociative identity disorder patients can present with acute forms of amnesia and fugue episodes. However, dissociative identity disorder patients are characterized by a plethora of symptoms, only some of which are usually found in patients with dissociative amnesia. With respect to amnesia, most dissociative identity disorder patients and patients with dissociative disorder NOS with dissociative identity disorder features report multiple forms of complex amnesia, including recurrent blackouts, fugues, unexplained possessions, and fluctuations in skills, habits, and knowledge.

Acute Stress Disorder, Posttraumatic Stress Disorder, and Somatoform Disorders As discussed in the introductory nosology section, most forms of dissociative amnesia are best conceptualized as part of a group of trauma spectrum disorders that includes acute stress disorder, PTSD, and somatization disorder. Many dissociative amnesia patients meet full or partial diagnostic criteria for acute stress disorder, PTSD, or somatization disorder, or a combination of these. Amnesia is a criterion symptom of each of the latter disorders. DSM-IV-TR stipulates that, to be diagnosed, the dissociative amnesia must be distinct from the course of acute stress disorder, PTSD, or somatization disorder. In practice, clinical judgment usually determines whether the extent of the amnesia warrants a separate dissociative diagnosis.

Malingering and Factitious Amnesia Feigned amnesia is more common in patients presenting with the acute, classic forms of dissociative amnesia. However, in one recent forensic case, an adult individual attempting to sue an admitted abuser using the delayed discovery rule was shown to have falsified delayed recall for trauma in an attempt to overcome the statute of limitations. Investigations showed that the patient had discussed the abuse with others on many occasions before the purported delayed recall. On the other hand, some patients may have secondary amnesia for having remembered and discussed traumatic experiences in the past.

There is no absolute way to differentiate dissociative amnesia from factitious or malingered amnesia. Malingerers have been noted to continue their deception even during hypnotically or barbiturate-facilitated interviews. As noted previously, many of the classical cases were described as occurring in a clinical context of financial, sexual, and legal problems or in soldiers who wished to escape from combat.

On the other hand, in the clinical case reports, many malingerers quickly confessed their deceptions spontaneously or when confronted by the examiner. In these nonforensic reports, the malingered amnesiacs were frequently pathetic individuals whose deception was transparent. It was often unclear where the conscious deception began and the unconscious defenses ended.

In the current clinical environment, a patient who presents to psychiatric attention asking to recover repressed memories as a chief complaint is most likely to have a factitious disorder or to have been subject to suggestive influences. Most of these individuals actually do not describe bona fide amnesia when carefully questioned but are often insistent that they must have been abused in childhood to explain their unhappiness or life dysfunction.

Clinical Course and Prognosis

Little is known about the clinical course of dissociative amnesia. Acute dissociative amnesia frequently spontaneously resolves once the person is removed to safety from traumatic or overwhelming circumstances. At the other extreme, there are patients who develop chronic forms of generalized, continuous, or severe localized amnesia who are profoundly disabled and require high levels of social support, such as nursing home placement or intensive family caretaking.

Those with nonclassic dissociative amnesia may have a persistent form of the disorder that does not cause them overt distress, and, thus, they do not seek clinical attention. Some of these individuals may be understood as being in an episode of PTSD characterized primarily by avoidant symptoms. In some cases, a later traumatic event or stress, even a relatively minor one, precipitates a florid episode of PTSD with alternations of reexperiencing and avoidant or amnesia symptoms.

Studies have shown that recall of previously dissociated memory frequently occurs outside of therapeutic settings, triggered by a variety of stimuli, including one's own children reaching an age at which one was abused, one's child being abused, media accounts of trauma or abuse, death of an abusive parent, a variety of sensory cues, and feeling safe in one's life situation, among others.

Treatment

The treatment of dissociative amnesia became controversial in the 1990s. Controversy exists not only for the existence of dissociative amnesia, but also for how to treat it. Critics of the dissociative amnesia construct have invented the term *recovered memory therapy* (RMT) to characterize treatment in which clinicians are thought to make aggressive efforts to have patients recall so-called forgotten traumas as the central focus of treatment. RMT does not represent a known school of therapy or of scholarly research. It may more accurately describe individual fringe practitioners or media or layperson views of trauma treatment. In fact, reviews of the literature on trauma treatment report that the predominant model for work on traumatic memories involves a focus on integration of posttraumatic memories, beliefs, cognitions, affects, somatic representations, and object relations, not on memory recall per se.

Phase-Oriented Treatment Phase-oriented treatment is the current standard of care for the treatment of trauma disorders, including dissociative amnesia. Treatment of the acute classical dissociative amnesia patient follows a similar phasic model. However, here, memory recall is a central issue, because loss of memory for personal identity and large gaps in current autobiographical memory are acutely disabling symptoms that require relatively rapid intervention.

In general, three basic phases are recognized. This structure is heuristic to some extent, because aspects of each phase may be worked on during another. First, there is a stabilization phase, with a focus on safety, symptom control, containment of affects and impulses, and education about trauma treatment. Once adequate personal safety and clinical stability are established, if indicated, the individual may engage in a second phase, the focus of which is the integration of traumatic material in greater depth. This processing may involve attempts to overcome persistent amnesia symptoms and to resolve material that is not dissociated or less completely dissociated. Finally, there is a third phase of *resolution* or *reintegration*, in which the traumatized person is reconnected to ordinary life. In this phase, the focus is less on the trauma per se and more on the development of a renewed, reinvigorated life apart from the lack of freedom imposed by symptoms of the trauma disorder and the domination of the person's psychology by issues related to traumatization.

Safety in Acute Dissociative Amnesia In the case of the patient with an acute stress disorder primarily characterized or accompanied by dissociative amnesia, the establishment of the person's physical safety is the first concern. This involves removing the individual from the traumatizing environment (e.g., acute combat), evaluating and treating medical problems, and providing shelter, food, and sleep. Sedative medications, such as the benzodiazepines, may be indicated to assist the patient with sleep. Patients with acute amnesia for personal identity or life circumstances, or both, frequently have a relatively rapid spontaneous remission of symptoms once brought to the safety of the hospital or other protected environment.

If immediate spontaneous remission does not occur in patients with acute amnesia after removal from traumatic environments, symptoms may abate later simply in the course of the clinician's taking a psychiatric history or merely with suggestions and reassurance.

Safety in Nonclassic Dissociative Amnesia Patients with nonclassic, covert amnesia presentations generally should be managed within the framework of a longer-term psychotherapy directed at resolution of the complex psychological sequelae of the events producing the amnesia, usually severe traumatization due to childhood abuse, combat, rape, domestic violence, or other forms of adult victimization, or a combination of these.

Here, too, the first tasks of treatment are restoration of the patient's physical well-being and safety and establishment of a working alliance. The clinician must be prepared to intervene actively if the patient is acutely dangerous to self or others or is abusing substances in an uncontrollable way, or both. Typically, these patients' difficulties involve suicide attempts, self-mutilation, eating disorders, alcohol or substance abuse, involvement in abusive or destructive relationships, episodes of rage or violence, abuse of the individual's own children or family members, and lack of adequate food, clothing, or shelter. Hospitalization may be necessary to stabilize such patients, as may referral to specialty resources, such as treatment for substance abuse or eating disorders.

In individuals with severe intrusive PTSD symptoms alternating with amnesia, containment and management of intrusive recollections rather than detailed processing of the traumatic material are usually the goal in the stabilization phase of treatment. This may be accomplished with supportive psychotherapy, pharmacotherapy, imagery or hypnotic techniques for containment and symptom control, or cognitive therapy techniques, or a combination of these. There is no pharmacological agent that specifically targets dissociative amnesia. However, specific psychopharmacological treatment of the patient's PTSD, affective, dyscontrol, psychotic, obsessive-compulsive, or anxiety symptoms with medications may help stabilize severe symptoms that prevent the patient's meaningful participation in psychotherapy.

Long-term treatment for these patients is focused on the manifold dimensions of dysfunction that chronic trauma engenders. These include problems with mood, anxiety, and impulse regulation, disordered attachment schemas engendering troubled relationships and problems with interpersonal boundaries, spontaneous altered states and dissociation, memory problems, cognitive distortions and disordered meaning systems, perceptual abnormalities, problems with the sense of self and body image, somatoform symptoms, and self-destructiveness.

Treatment of Amnesia Treatment of patients with nonclassic forms of dissociative amnesia necessitates that the clinician familiarize himself or herself with the current controversies about trauma and memory to provide adequate informed consent to the patient.

In general, studies of treatment outcome in survivors of rape and childhood sexual abuse have shown better outcome when patients directly discuss trauma material in the context of a carefully designed, phasically structured individual or group psychotherapy. Nonetheless, it is a matter of clinical judgment and the patient's individual decision whether the patient has achieved sufficient stability and has sufficient ego strength to move from the stabilization phase of treatment to the phase of memory integration. Factors that usually contraindicate intensive memory integration work are listed in Table 17–9.

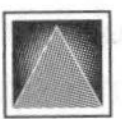

Table 17–9
Contraindications to the Integration Phase of Amnesia Treatment

Has not achieved safety from high-risk behaviors
Current substance abuse or dependence
Has not achieved symptom stabilization
Severe, uncontrolled, intrusive posttraumatic stress disorder symptoms
Severe, uncontrolled dissociative episodes
Dysregulated mood symptoms
Dysregulated anxiety symptoms
Inadequate therapeutic alliance
Current or ongoing abusive relationship
Acute life crisis or times of life transition (divorce, job change, etc.)
Severe physical illness or infirmity
Severe personality disorder symptoms, regression, psychosis
Current involvement in litigation
Impending absence of therapist

Adapted from Loewenstein RJ. Dissociative amnesia and dissociative fugue. In: Gabbard GO, ed. *Treatment of Psychiatric Disorders,* 3rd ed. Vol 2. Washington, DC: American Psychiatric Press; 2001:1633.

Free Recall Patients with the acute and chronic forms of dissociative amnesia may respond well to free recall strategies in which they allow memory material to enter into consciousness. The clinician is supportive and nondirective but focuses on reluctance or resistance to allowing free recall to take place. Classic free-association suggestions are often the most helpful in understanding factors that interfere with recall and for allowing recall to occur at a pace that the patient can tolerate. In general, it is believed that memory accuracy is improved if the clinician asks nonleading questions of the patient, whether in a free-recall situation or with methods that facilitate memory recall.

Transference Interpretations Studies of transference in patients with combat-related PTSD and severe dissociative disorders indicate that a traumatic transference is usually the predominant initial transference theme in these individuals. This is a set of unconscious perceptions of the clinician, based on relationships formed in traumatic circumstances: The therapist becomes the buddy who was killed next to the patient in battle, the persecutory abusive parent, the incompetent officer who sent the patient into battlefield disaster, the neglectful relative unconcerned about the patient's abuse, or the patient himself or herself who is subject to the sadistic, abusive behaviors of an implacable other. Identification of the overt patterns of traumatic transference observed by the therapist may be another route to undoing amnesia. A recent study of corroborated trauma memory found that transference-based recall was more accurate than other forms of facilitated recall.

Cognitive Therapy Cognitive therapy may have specific benefits for individuals with trauma disorders. Identifying the specific cognitive distortions that are based in the trauma may also provide an entrée into autobiographical memory for which the patient experiences amnesia. As the patient is more able to correct cognitive distortions, particularly about the meaning of prior trauma, more detailed recall of traumatic events may occur.

Facilitated Recall of Trauma Material A hierarchy of techniques for facilitation of recall has been described for dissociative amnesia. Research suggests that each of these may successively introduce the potential for greater error rates for what is recalled. These include (1) context-reinstatement, that is, attempts to focus the patient on time periods for which there is amnesia; (2) state-dependent recall, that is, intensification and focus on affects or somatic sensations that appear to be related to trauma, such as terror, horror, confusion, rage, or feeling suddenly nauseated or dizzy; and (3) specialized adjunctive techniques, such as hypnosis, relaxation, imagery, or pharmacologically assisted interviews. Each of these may facilitate recall of dissociated memory information in classic and nonclassic forms of dissociative amnesia. In each of these, the clinician should use nonleading, nonsuggestive questions to minimize concern about inaccurate or confabulated recall.

Hypnosis for Amnesia Hypnosis has frequently played an important adjunctive role in the treatment of individuals with dissociative amnesia and dissociative fugue. Hypnosis is not a treatment in itself; rather, it is a set of adjunctive techniques that facilitate certain psychotherapeutic goals. The construct of hypnosis encompasses a wide and complex domain of phenomena and responses that have been applied to a diverse array of therapies offered to a variety of individuals. Concern about inaccuracies in hypnotically facilitated recall cite research studies of memory for nontraumatic information recalled with hypnosis that have shown that hypnosis increases the subject's confidence in what is recalled, even if it is erroneous. However, critical reviews have noted the complexity of this research problem, the inconsistency in findings among studies, and the many variables related to hypnosis and nonhypnotic factors that appear to influence this and related phenomena. The critical reviews have emphasized that memory confabulation is related to techniques of social influence on suggestible subjects, not to hypnosis per se.

The use of hypnosis for memory recall in no way ensures the veracity, or lack of veracity, of the information produced. The clinician should be well aware of the reconstructive nature of memory and should avoid suggestions to the contrary. Thus, in addition to obtaining the patient's informed consent for the use of hypnosis, it is currently considered prudent to also obtain informed consent concerning the reliability or possible lack thereof for autobiographical information revealed during hypnosis. Studies also suggest that educating patients about the controversies regarding hypnosis and memory and informing them of the need to critically evaluate any memory material that they recall during hypnosis or at any other time in treatment reduce the likelihood of credulous acceptance of potentially inaccurate information.

Also, clinicians should be aware that, in some states, individuals who have been exposed to therapeutic hypnosis may be enjoined from giving testimony as a witness in court. This may be so even if the hypnosis had little relationship to the events at legal issue. The clinician should attempt to discuss fully these issues with the patient and his or her legal counsel.

Finally, the use of hypnosis as part of a *forensic* examination should proceed only after obtaining consent from the patient after he or she has consulted with relevant legal authorities and attorneys involved in criminal or civil litigation. Training in forensic hypnosis is mandatory in this context. Should hypnosis be used in this way, electronic recording of all hypnosis sessions, preferably on videotape, should be used.

Hypnosis can be used in a number of different ways in the treatment of dissociative amnesia. In particular, hypnotic interventions can be used to contain, modulate, and titrate the intensity of symptoms; to facilitate controlled recall of dissociated memories; to provide support and ego strengthening for the patient; and, finally, to promote working through and integration of dissociated material.

In addition, the patient can be taught self-hypnosis to apply containment and calming techniques in his or her everyday life. Successful use of containment techniques, whether hypnotically facilitated or not, also increases the patient's sense that he or she can more effectively be in control of alternations between intrusive symptoms and amnesia.

In the acutely amnestic patient, a few sessions to help the patient experience trance successfully and to explore containment and distancing techniques may be sufficient to allow focused hypnotic work on the material for which the patient is amnestic. However, in nonclassic cases of severe, long-standing, posttraumatic disorders, the amnesia itself should be addressed only gradually, in the context of a longer-term psychotherapy in which life stability and function are the basic foci.

Clinicians since World War I have recognized the importance of the patient's repeatedly processing dissociated material in a number of different sessions, often at different levels of affective intensity, to complete the process of integrating the material.

In cases of acute amnesia, the first session for memory processing may necessarily be explorative. Here, again, the initial goal is to gain an overview of the information for which the patient is amnestic. As in cases of chronic amnesia, subsequent sessions then focus on reworking the material in greater detail.

It is useful to try to account systematically for different dimensions of the traumatic experience: sensory, affective, cognitive, and behavioral, so as to ensure that all key components have been identified and reconstructed. It is likewise useful to attempt to account systematically for a variety of dysphoric affects that are commonly experienced during traumatic experiences: despair, sorrow, grief, horror, shame, helplessness, rage, guilt, confusion, anguish, and the like. Not all of these may be present in a given patient; however, it is useful for the clinician to keep track of which affects seem most readily described by the patient and which seem less available. Inquiry about these other affects may be quite helpful in resolving the amnesia. In particular, shame, horror, helplessness, and overwhelming confusion are emotions that patients may have the most trouble identifying without assistance from the therapist.

The treatment process is similar when the acute amnesia results not from traumatic experiences, but rather from aspects of their current behavior that are in conflict with deeply held moral values or behavioral standards. Treatment in such instances seeks to help the patient tolerate these affects and conflicts without resorting to dissociative defenses. Frequently, these patients describe a developmental history characterized by a rigid family moral code enforced with harsh physical discipline. These experiences often appear to be the traumatic underpinning of the dissociative diathesis. Psychotherapy and hypnotherapy in these patients are directed in part at reducing the patient's brutally unreasonable, and often conflicting, expectations of himself or herself and the guilt and shame that so often accompany acute dissociation. Furthermore, these patients may have tremendous difficulty tolerating anger or violent impulses, because such affects tend to trigger recall of earlier experiences with physical abuse or similar traumas, often as a flashback experience. Thus, psychotherapy may serve not only to focus on the conflicts that led to the acute amnesia, but also to explicate and to work through the patient's thoughts, feelings, and self-perceptions related to the antecedent traumatic events.

Somatic Therapies There is no known pharmacotherapy for dissociative amnesia other than pharmacologically facilitated interviews. A variety of agents have been used for this purpose, including sodium amobarbital, thiopental (Pentothal), oral benzodiazepines, and amphetamines. At present, no adequately controlled studies have been conducted that assess the efficacy of any of these agents in comparison with one another or with other treatment methods. A single placebo-controlled study of the barbiturate-facilitated interview did not find superiority of sodium amobarbital over placebo in producing more clinically useful information. In more systematic World War II studies of barbiturate-facilitated interviews for amnesia and conversion reactions, this treatment was described as leading to more rapid recovery, especially for amnesia, although little overall difference was found in recovery in comparison to subjects treated with psychotherapy alone or with hypnotherapy.

Amobarbital narcosynthesis is a term devised to underscore the need for material uncovered in a pharmacologically facilitated interview to be processed by the patient in his or her usual conscious state. Pharmacologically facilitated interviews are used primarily in working with acute amnesias and conversion reactions, among other indications, in general hospital medical and psychiatric services. This procedure is also occasionally useful in refractory cases of chronic dissociative amnesia when patients are unresponsive to other interventions.

The current standard of care is that this procedure must be performed in settings in which resuscitation equipment is available in case of respiratory arrest, a possible, albeit rare, complication. The interview usually is audiotaped or videotaped to replay for the patient, because amnesia generally is present for material produced. Although in some cases repeated procedures may be helpful, in other cases, repeated procedures may lead to the patient's developing a dependence on pharmacologically facilitated interviews.

The current controversies over delayed recall for traumatic experiences have also focused on the use of pharmacologically facilitated interviews for patients with reported amnesia for childhood maltreatment. No modern systematic data exist on memory fallibility or accuracy in those undergoing pharmacologically facilitated interviews. As discussed previously, pharmacologically facilitated interviews were used extensively in World War II for the treatment of combat-related dissociation. Although wartime memories recovered with pharmacologically facilitated interviews were generally considered to be accurate, some subjects were reported to dissemble completely or withhold crucial information, or both, despite barbiturate treatment.

Given the current controversies, the clinician should give a similar informed consent regarding the nature of memory to the patient contemplating a pharmacologically facilitated interview for amnesia symptoms as that given to the patient considering hypnosis. The clinician should emphasize that these drugs are not a truth serum; whatever apparently new information emerges under the drug condition should be regarded no differently with respect to accuracy than any other material that emerges in the course of treatment.

Group Psychotherapy for Amnesia During World War II, group psychotherapy and group hypnotherapy were among the treatments given to promote recovery in traumatic war-related amnesia. Highly supportive, structured, reassuring, and reeducative approaches were often used by therapists in such cases in an attempt to accomplish return of the patient to functional status and to prevent chronic disability.

Time-limited and longer-term group psychotherapies have been reported to be helpful for combat veterans with PTSD and for survivors of childhood abuse. During group sessions, some authors report that patients may recover memories for which they have had amnesia. Supportive interventions by the group members or the group therapist, or both, may facilitate integration and mastery of the dissociated material.

On the other hand, concern has been raised about memory contamination in such group therapy settings, as it has for patients' involvement in 12-step or self-help groups for trauma survivors.

EMDR Eye movement desensitization and reprocessing (EMDR) is a set of structured procedures for working on specific traumatic memories in PTSD. Originally, therapist-facilitated eye movements were thought to be an essential part of the technique for EMDR. However, subsequent research has shown this to be a nonspecific factor compared to the structured approach for work on specific reported traumas. Studies have shown greater immediate efficacy of EMDR compared to waiting list and other similar control conditions, especially for individuals reporting single traumas. However, comparison of EMDR to other forms of structured, multistaged trauma treatment has not been performed, especially for individuals with multiple traumas and complex comorbidities. Longitudinal studies of such cases have not shown a persistent improvement with EMDR.

Because *EMDR* is defined as a procedure for helping with resolution of consciously recalled traumatic memories, no data have been presented on its efficacy for reducing dissociative amnesia.

DEPERSONALIZATION DISORDER

For many years, the ubiquity of depersonalization as a psychiatric symptom obscured its broader recognition as a disorder. Recent research has identified clinical features, course and prognosis, and neurobiological correlates that distinguish it from other psychiatric disorders with symptoms of depersonalization. Valid and reliable instruments exist for screening and diagnosis. Research with these measures is advancing understanding of this often unrecognized condition.

Definition The DSM-IV-TR identifies the essential feature of depersonalization as the persistent or recurrent feeling of detachment or estrangement from one's self. The individual may report feeling like an automaton or as if in a dream or watching himself or herself in a movie. According to DSM-IV-TR, "there may be a sensation of being an outside observer of one's mental processes, one's body, or parts of one's body." There is often a sense of an absence of control over one's actions.

History First described by Maurice Krishnaber in 1872, depersonalization was formally named in 1898 by Ludovic Dugas, who sought to convey "the feeling of loss of ego." Freud, Janet, Eugen Bleuler, and other 19th century authorities reported patients with symptoms of depersonalization and derealization. A monograph by Paul Schilder in 1914 is regarded as a turning point in psychiatric interest. Classic studies followed by Wilhelm Mayer-Gross in 1939, Harold Shorvonn in 1946, and Jerome Saperstein in 1949 furthered the delineation of a syndrome of chronic depersonalization. Brian Ackner enumerated the essential features of current diagnostic definitions in 1954. These include "(1) the feeling of unreality or strangeness apropos the self; (2) the retention of insight and lack of delusional elaboration; (3) the lack of affective response ('numbness') except for the discomfort regarding depersonalization; and (4) the unpleasant property that may vary in intensity inversely with the subject's familiarity with the phenomenon." In the last decade, research by Eric Hollander, Simeon, and colleagues has significantly

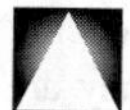

Table 17–10
DSM-IV-TR Diagnostic Criteria for Depersonalization Disorder

A. Persistent or recurrent experiences of feeling detached from, and as if one is an outside observer of, one's mental processes or body (e.g., feeling like one is in a dream).

B. During the depersonalization experience, reality testing remains intact.

C. The depersonalization causes clinically significant distress or impairment in social, occupational, or other important areas of functioning.

D. The depersonalization experience does not occur exclusively during the course of another mental disorder, such as schizophrenia, panic disorder, acute stress disorder, or another dissociative disorder, and is not due to the direct physiological effects of a substance (e.g., a drug of abuse, a medication) or a general medical condition (e.g., temporal lobe epilepsy).

From American Psychiatric Association. *Diagnostic and Statistical Manual of Mental Disorders*. 4th ed. Text rev. Washington, DC: American Psychiatric Association; 2000, with permission.

increased understanding of depersonalization disorder with systematic case series, medication trials, brain imaging, and improved measurement.

Comparative Nosology

The DSM has classified depersonalization as a separate dissociative disorder since its first inclusion in 1980. The current DSM-IV-TR definition of depersonalization disorder is found in Table 17–10.

The ICD-10 (Table 17–11), however, lists depersonalization-derealization syndrome under other neurotic disorders. The ICD-10 requires concurrent experiences of derealization in addition to symptoms of depersonalization. The ICD-10 and the DSM require that the affected individual must have intact reality testing and must retain good insight into the psychological nature of his or her symptoms.

Some authorities disagree with the classification of depersonalization as a dissociative disorder. They argue that the absence of amnesia and its occurrence across so many different psychiatric and organic conditions make it likely that depersonalization is a final common pathway process rather than a specific disorder. The DSM criteria focus instead on the dissociative alteration in sense of self that is inherent in the persistent or recurrent experiences of feeling detached from one's own body or mind. It is this profound, but not psychotic, division in sense of self that qualifies it as a dissociative disorder. Depersonalization disorder does differ in some important ways from the other dissociative disorders, but it may prove an informative exception. Its ubiquity as a symptom and the ability to experimentally induce it in laboratory settings provide unique opportunities for research that may shed light on dissociation in general.

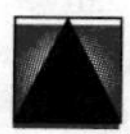

Table 17–11
ICD-10 Diagnostic Criteria for Depersonalization-Derealization Syndrome

For a definite diagnosis, there must be either or both (a) and (b), plus (c) and (d):

(a) Depersonalization symptoms, that is, the individual feels that his or her own feelings or experiences, or both, are detached, distant, not his or her own, or lost

(b) Derealization symptoms, that is, objects, people, or surroundings, or a combination of these, seem unreal, distant, artificial, colorless, or lifeless

(c) An acceptance that this is a subjective and spontaneous change, not imposed by outside forces or other people (i.e., insight)

(d) A clear sensorium and absence of toxic confusional state or epilepsy

From World Health Organization. *The ICD-10 Classification of Mental and Behavioural Disorders. Clinical Descriptions and Diagnostic Guidelines.* Geneva: World Health Organization; 1992:172, with permission.

Epidemiology

Transient experiences of depersonalization and derealization are extremely common in normal and clinical populations. They are the third most commonly reported psychiatric symptoms, after depression and anxiety. A survey of a random sample of 1,000 adults in the rural South found a 1-year prevalence of 19 percent for depersonalization and 14 percent for derealization. Not uncommon in seizure patients and migraine sufferers, they can also occur with use of psychedelic drugs, especially marijuana, lysergic acid diethylamide (LSD), and mescaline, and less frequently as a side effect of some medications, such as anticholinergic agents. They have been described after certain types of meditation, deep hypnosis, extended mirror or crystal gazing, and sensory deprivation experiences. They are common after mild to moderate head injury, where there is little or no loss of consciousness, but are significantly less likely if unconsciousness lasts for more than 30 minutes. One study estimated that at least 20 percent of minor head injury patients experience significant depersonalization and derealization. They are also common after life-threatening experiences, with or without serious bodily injury.

Psychiatric case series typically have two to four times more women than men. However, a recent, rigorously diagnosed series of 117 patients showed a 1 to 1 gender ratio. Head injury and seizure disorder samples are generally equally divided. Several studies have identified age as a significant factor for transient experiences of depersonalization and derealization, with adolescents and young adults reporting the highest rates in normal population samples. Approximately one-half of college students (46 percent) in one study reported at least one significant episode of depersonalization within the prior year.

Etiology

Psychodynamic

Traditional psychodynamic formulations have emphasized the disintegration of the ego or have viewed depersonalization as an affective response in defense of the ego. These explanations stress the role of overwhelming painful experiences or conflictual impulses as triggering events. The high rates in normal adolescents and in patients conceptualized as having borderline or narcissistic personality organizations are cited as evidence that ego immaturity or ego deficits are predisposing factors. More recently, attention has been drawn to the similarities between depersonalization and obsessive-compulsive symptoms. Depersonalization disorder patients often display obsessive-like behaviors with respect to their symptoms. The split between an observing and a participating self is likened to the division of intellect and emotional experience in obsessive patients. Both groups respond to serotonin reuptake inhibitors, although the therapeutic response for depersonalization disorder patients is usually less robust.

Traumatic Stress

A substantial proportion, typically one-third to one-half, of patients in clinical depersonalization case series report histories of significant trauma. Several studies of accident victims find as much as 60 percent of those with a life-threatening experience report at least transient depersonalization during the event or immediately thereafter. Military training studies find that symptoms of depersonalization and derealization are commonly evoked by stress and fatigue and are inversely related to performance. One of the few controlled, clinical studies found significantly more childhood trauma, especially emotional abuse, in well-diagnosed depersonalization disorder patients compared with normal subjects.

In approximately 20 percent of a sample of chronic depersonalization patients, there was a first-degree relative with a severe psychotic illness, either schizophrenia or bipolar disorder. It was hypothesized that the chronic fear engendered by the psychotic relative was etiological in the subsequent development of the depersonalization disorder. For example, one patient reported that, throughout her childhood, she was left alone by her father and older brother to handle her violent, schizophrenic mother whenever the mother had psychotic episodes. The patient recalled waiting in a state of terror and dread until the emergency workers came and hospitalized her mother.

In general, the trauma reported by the depersonalization patients was less severe than that typically reported by other dissociative disorder patients. A large general population study found that individuals with chronic pain were three times more likely to have episodes of depersonalization, but there was only a weakly significant association with dangerous or upsetting experiences. A substantial number of individuals with depersonalization disorder do not identify a traumatic antecedent and report that the onset of their disorder occurred without a clear precipitant. On the other hand, nontraumatic stressors, such as interpersonal, financial, or occupational losses, have been associated with the onset or exacerbation of depersonalization disorder. In addition, chemical stressors, such as marijuana, hallucinogens, and stimulants, have been known to precipitate chronic depersonalization in some people. These individuals can be conceptualized as having a neurobiological or genetic vulnerability to chronic depersonalization after drug use.

Temporal Lobe and Limbic Theories

In the epilepsy literature, there is a long-standing clinical association between symptoms of depersonalization and derealization and temporal lobe and limbic system dysfunction. Wilder Penfield reported depersonalization symptoms elicited during neurosurgery by stimulation of the superior and middle temporal gyri. Brain imaging studies have likewise found differential activation of these areas. The only study to date restricted to depersonalization patients found decreased activity in the right superior and middle temporal gyri and increased brain glucose metabolism bilaterally in the parietal BA7B. Dissociation and depersonalization scale scores were strongly correlated with increased parietal metabolic activity. Imaging studies of dissociative states in PTSD patients find activation in all of these areas, as well as the medial frontal gyrus and anterior cingulate gyrus. Mauricio Sierra and German Berrios propose that depersonalization involves a corticolimbic disconnection, such that left medial prefrontal activation reciprocally inhibits the left amygdala, producing detachment and decreased arousal, whereas right dorsolateral prefrontal activation with concomitant right amygdala inhibition leads to attentional problems and feelings of emptiness.

Neurobiological Theories

The association of depersonalization with migraines and marijuana, its generally favorable response to selective serotonin reuptake inhibitor (SSRI) drugs, and the increase in depersonalization symptoms seen with the depletion of L-tryptophan, a serotonin precursor, point to serotoninergic involvement. Depersonalization is the primary dissociative symptom elicited by the drug-challenge studies described in the section on neurobiological theories of dissociation. These studies strongly implicate the NMDA subtype of the glutamate receptor as central to the genesis depersonalization symptoms. It seems likely that serotoninergic and glutamate systems are involved in clinical depersonalization. Two recent twin studies are discordant for a genetic contribution to the development of depersonalization disorder.

Diagnosis and Clinical Features

Patients experiencing depersonalization often have great difficulty expressing what they are feeling. Trying to express their subjective suffering with banal phrases, such as "I feel dead," "nothing seems real," or "I'm standing outside of myself," depersonalized patients may not adequately convey to the examiner the distress they experience. While complaining bitterly about how this is ruining their life, they may nonetheless appear remarkably undistressed. Accordingly, clinicians may not take the severity of this disorder as seriously as they should. Despite this outward appearance of lack of distress, depersonalization disorder patients are enduring an intensely unpleasant, and often disabling, subjective experience. Many say that they would gladly exchange the depersonalization for physical pain, which would at least reconnect them with their body.

There are a number of distinct components to the experience of depersonalization. These include a sense of bodily changes, a sense of duality of self as observer and actor, a sense of being cut off from others, and a sense of being cut off from one's own emotions. On the other hand, *derealization*, coined by William Mapother, is the sense that the world appears strange, foreign, or dream-like. It is conceptualized as a dissociative alteration in the perception of the environment. Objects may appear as if viewed from a great distance and as if they are two dimensional, without depth or substance. Sounds come from a distance, muffled and distorted. Objects feel strange to the touch. Colors dim and lose their vitality. The faces of others change, becoming unfamiliar and frightening. The world and all action and behavior lose meaning and purpose.

Ms. R. was a 27-year-old, unmarried, graduate student with a Masters in Biology. She complained about intermittent episodes of "standing back," usually associated with anxiety-provoking social situations. When asked about a recent episode, she described presenting in a seminar course. "All of a sudden, I was talking, but it didn't feel like it was me talking. It was very disconcerting. I had this feeling, 'who's doing the talking?' I felt like I was just watching. Watching someone else talk. Listening to words come out of my mouth, but I wasn't saying them. It wasn't me. It went on for a while. I was calm, even sort of peaceful. It was as if I was very far away. In the back of the room somewhere—just watching myself. But the person talking didn't even seem like me really. It was like I was watching someone else." The feeling lasted the rest of that day and persisted into the next, during which time it gradually dissipated. She thought that she remembered having similar experiences during high school but was certain that they occurred at least once a year during college and graduate school. Although she said that she usually felt detached and sometimes peaceful during the experience, she was upset at the thought that she would likely have more episodes. She complained that the sudden onset, the eeriness of seemingly watching an almost unrecognizable version of herself from a distance, and the sense of not "being in the world" were almost unbearable in retrospect.

As a child, Ms. R. reported frequent intense anxiety due to overhearing or witnessing the frequent violent arguments and periodic physical fights between her parents. She remembered lying awake in bed, listening to her parents, imagining the terrible things that were occurring, or about to occur, between them. In addition, the family was subject to many unpredictable dislocations and moves owing to the patient's father's intermittent difficulties with finances and employment. The patient's anxieties did not abate when the parents divorced when she was a late adolescent. Her father moved away and had little further contact with her. Her relationship with her mother became increasingly angry, critical, and contentious. She was unsure if she experienced depersonalization during childhood while listening to her parents' fights.

Differential Diagnosis The variety of conditions associated with depersonalization complicate the differential diagnosis of depersonalization disorder. Depersonalization may result from a medical condition or neurological condition, intoxication or withdrawal from illicit drugs, or as a side effect of medications or may be associated with panic attacks, phobias, PTSD, or acute stress disorder, schizophrenia, or another dissociative disorder. A thorough medical and neurological evaluation is essential, including standard laboratory studies, an EEG, and any indicated drug screens. Drug-related depersonalization is typically transient, but persistent depersonalization may follow an episode of intoxication with a variety of substances, including marijuana, cocaine, and other psychostimulants. A range of neurological conditions, including seizure disorders, brain tumors, postconcussive syndrome, metabolic abnormalities, migraine, vertigo, and Ménière's disease, have been reported as causes. Depersonalization caused by organic conditions tends to be primarily sensory without the elaborated descriptions and personalized meanings common to psychiatric etiologies.

Course and Prognosis Depersonalization after traumatic experiences or intoxications commonly remits spontaneously after removal from the traumatic circumstances or ending of the episode of intoxication. Depersonalization accompanying mood, psychotic, or other anxiety disorders commonly remits with definitive treatment of these conditions.

Depersonalization disorder itself may have an episodic, relapsing and remitting, or chronic course. The latter is most common. Many patients with chronic depersonalization may have a course characterized by severe impairment in occupational, social, and personal functioning. Mean age of onset is thought to be in late adolescence or early adulthood in most cases. Most depersonalization disorder patients are initially treated for secondary anxiety and mood disorder symptoms. The primary nature of the depersonalization disorder is usually only recognized later on. Traumatic or stressful events may exacerbate depersonalization disorder symptoms. Symptom exacerbations are commonly related to negative affects; high levels of sensory input; and threatening, stressful, or unfamiliar situations.

Treatment Clinicians working with depersonalization patients often find them to be a singularly clinically refractory group. There is some systematic evidence that SSRI antidepressants, such as fluoxetine (Prozac), may be helpful to depersonalization patients. However, two recent, double-blind, placebo-controlled studies found no efficacy for fluvoxetine (Luvox) and lamotrigine, respectively, for depersonalization disorder. Clinical experience suggests that many depersonalization patients respond at best sporadically and partially to the usual groups of psychiatric medications, singly or in combination: antidepressants, mood stabilizers, typical and atypical neuroleptics, anticonvulsants, and so forth.

Many different types of psychotherapy have been used with depersonalization patients: psychodynamic, cognitive, cognitive-behavioral, hypnotherapeutic, and supportive. No systematic data exist that compare these modalities. Clinical experience suggests that many depersonalization patients do not have a robust response to these specific types of standard psychotherapy. A recent large case series of severely ill depersonalization patients found that stress management strategies, distraction techniques, reduction of sensory stimulation, relaxation training, and physical exercise may be somewhat helpful in some patients.

Nonetheless, many severely impaired depersonalization patients may require long-term supportive treatment, with the clinician being acutely aware of the depersonalization patient's interpersonal sensitivity, distress, and sense of hopelessness about the condition.

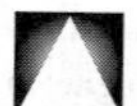

Table 17–12
DSM-IV-TR Diagnostic Criteria for Dissociative Fugue

A. The predominant disturbance is sudden, unexpected travel away from home or one's customary place of work, with inability to recall one's past.
B. Confusion about personal identity or assumption of a new identity (partial or complete).
C. The disturbance does not occur exclusively during the course of dissociative identity disorder and is not due to the direct physiological effects of a substance (e.g., a drug of abuse, a medication) or a general medical condition (e.g., temporal lobe epilepsy).
D. The symptoms cause clinically significant distress or impairment in social, occupational, or other important areas of functioning.

From American Psychiatric Association. *Diagnostic and Statistical Manual of Mental Disorders*. 4th ed. Text rev. Washington, DC: American Psychiatric Association; 2000, with permission.

DISSOCIATIVE FUGUE

Dissociative fugue is the least studied and most poorly understood of the dissociative disorders. The symptoms of the disorder are similar to those of dissociative amnesia and dissociative identity disorder.

Definition The essential feature of dissociative fugue (Table 17–12) is described as sudden, unexpected, travel away from home or one's customary place of daily activities, with inability to recall some or all of one's past (Criterion A). This is accompanied by confusion about personal identity or even the assumption of a new identity (Criterion B). The disturbance does not occur exclusively during the course of dissociative identity disorder and is not due to the direct physiological effects of a substance or a general medical condition (Criterion C). The symptoms must cause clinically significant distress or impairment in social, occupational, or other important areas of functioning (Criterion D).

History In the 19th century, the magnetic disorders included nocturnal somnambulism and its waking counterpart, the ambulatory automatism or fugue. In these conditions, the person performed activities that were complex and coordinated but apparently "cut off from the continuity of consciousness" with resultant amnesia. Charcot and his contemporaries reported a number of these cases and studied them intensively. Charcot divided the cases into those with epileptic, traumatic, or hysterical etiology, although a modern reading of the cases suggests that some of those diagnosed with epileptic or traumatic fugues would be more readily classified as having a dissociative disorder today.

Outside Europe, during this time, there was interest in similar phenomena as well. In the United States, James described one of the paradigmatic cases of fugue with change of personal identity, that of Ansel Bourne. Bourne, an itinerant preacher, disappeared from his home in Providence, Rhode Island, in January 1887, after withdrawing $500 from his bank account to pay some bills. Two months later, he "awoke," finding himself in Norristown, Pennsylvania, where had been living quietly under the name of A. J. Brown and working as a shopkeeper. Subsequently, he had no memory for the time between his disappearance and his return to the Bourne identity. Under hypnosis, he could communicate as Brown and described his activities during the fugue but could not unify his memory with that of Bourne. During the fugue, Bourne apparently behaved normally and did not attract unusual attention.

Janet also studied fugue states in his classic studies of dissociation and hysteria. Janet hypothesized that fugue was based on dissociation of more complex groups of mental functions than occurred in amnesia and was usually organized around a powerful emotion or feeling state that linked many trains of associations accompanied by a wish to run away.

Dissociative fugue was also described by World Wars I and II military psychiatrists. Important papers describing case studies of dissociative fugue in civilian and military populations were written in the 1940s by the psychoanalytic authors David Rappaport, Charles Fischer, Elisabeth Geleerd, Merton Gill, and Margaret Brenman, among others. However, many of these cases would be classified as dissociative amnesia, dissociative disorder NOS, or, possibly, dissociative identity disorder by contemporary diagnostic criteria.

Nosology There are insufficient data to validate dissociative fugue as a disorder distinct from dissociative amnesia, dissociative identity disorder, or other trauma spectrum conditions. Further research is needed to clarify whether dissociative fugue should be considered a separate disorder rather than a symptom of other disorders.

Individuals with various culturally defined *running* syndromes may have symptoms that meet diagnostic criteria for dissociative fugue. These conditions are characterized by a sudden onset of a high level of activity, trance-like states, potentially dangerous behavior in the form of running or fleeing, and ensuing exhaustion, sleep, and amnesia for the episode. They include *pibloktoq* among native peoples of the Arctic, *grisi siknis* among the Miskito of Honduras and Nicaragua, *latah* and *amok* in Western Pacific cultures, and Navajo frenzy witchcraft.

Etiology Traumatic circumstances, leading to an altered state of consciousness dominated by a wish to flee, are thought to be the underlying cause of most fugue episodes. These have included combat, rape, recurrent childhood sexual abuse, massive social dislocations, and natural disasters. In most other cases, there has been a similar antecedent history, although a psychological trauma was not present at the onset of the fugue episode. In these cases, instead of, or in addition to, external dangers or traumas, the patients were usually struggling with extreme emotions or impulses, such as overwhelming fear, guilt, shame, or intense incestuous, sexual, suicidal, or violent urges, or a combination of these, that were in conflict with the patient's conscience or ego ideals. Thus, the patients were also described as experiencing massive psychological conflict from which fight or flight was experienced as impossible or psychologically unacceptable, resulting in dissociation in which the patient could flee without consciously acknowledging doing so.

Shortly after the end of the Gulf War, a soldier was brought to a military psychiatric facility after emerging from a movie in a disoriented and disorganized state. Eventually, the police were called and determined that he had no apparent awareness of his identity or life history and that he was disoriented to current circumstances.

At the hospital, a complete medical, toxicological, and neurological workup was within normal limits, and a psychiatric consultation was requested. The patient presented as a perplexed, disoriented, healthy young man who described complete amnesia for personal identity and life history, depersonalization, derealization, confusion, and anxiety and fear at his predicament. Military records were located that showed the patient to have been in combat in the Gulf War. He had been subject to a friendly fire incident in which several of his buddies were killed and he himself barely escaped severe injury or death. He was treated at a military hospital and was airlifted back to the United States, where he was treated at another military facility, was adjudged healthy, and, at his request, was discharged back to active duty.

He was noted to have gone absent without leave (AWOL) at this point and only resurfaced in the movie theater, 3 months later, 2,000 miles from where he was supposed to have reported back for duty. When family and friends visited, he experienced them as "familiar" but did not recall who they were.

The patient's father was a decorated veteran of World War II who had physical disabilities and PTSD subsequent to his service. He enforced brutal physical discipline on his children but was a charismatic, complex man otherwise, deeply loved by his children, who protected and defended him. He had died suddenly, shortly before the patient entered military service. The son had vowed to follow in his father's footsteps.

The patient did not respond to attempts to help him regain his memory by free recall strategies, and a course of hypnosis was begun. Over a series of hypnosis sessions, the patient was given age-regression suggestions, taking him back to the beginning of the fugue, the time during the fugue, the point of loss of awareness of personal identity, and the events during the war.

The events were reconstructed as follows: The patient had not shown it at the time but had been profoundly traumatized by the friendly fire incident. He felt guilt at surviving his friends, horror at the carnage that had taken place around him, terrified at what had happened, and furious at his own military and government for its failures in the occurrence of the friendly fire event. He was enraged at his superiors, his branch of service, and his country, all of whom he felt had failed him and his friends by needlessly attacking them. At the same time, he was deeply patriotic, loved his country, and identified with his father's wish for him to be a "good soldier."

After discharge from the state-side hospital, he believed that he needed to get back to his unit and put the past behind him. Unconsciously, however, he felt vengeful toward the military and had violent fantasies of retaliation against his superiors. During his travels across the country, he had the overriding conviction that he had to get back to join his unit, although traveling thousands of miles in the opposite direction. He assumed another name and apparently attracted no attention during his wanderings. In the city in which he was found, he met several people who suggested that he attend a movie with them. The movie plot centered around a friendly fire episode during the Vietnam War. The patient became emotionally overwhelmed, entered an altered state, and eventually was brought to clinical attention.

Over the course of several months of hypnotherapy and psychotherapy, the patient was able to regain his memory and to better integrate his response to the wartime traumas and began to work out and tolerate his mixed feelings about his father. At times, recall of the wartime and childhood traumas was associated with intense affects of sadness, anger, horror, and confusion. He responded well to addition of an SSRI antidepressant to help modulate symptoms of PTSD, dysphoria, depression, and anxiety. As therapy progressed, the patient was more able to tolerate these emotions and was less overwhelmed by them.

He also began to report a much more chronic history of dissociative symptoms, with persistent imaginary companions until late adolescence, fugue and amnesia episodes in childhood and adolescence, and a subjective sense of inner division into multiple self-states. He received a medical discharge from the military with diagnoses of PTSD, dissociative disorder NOS, and mood disorder NOS.

Epidemiology As noted previously, no case of dissociative fugue was diagnosed in a random general population sample in Winnipeg, Canada. The disorder is thought to be more common during natural disasters, wartime, or times of major social dislocation and violence, although no systematic data exist on this point. Most of the pre–DSM-III cases are difficult to assess, because the diagnostic conventions are so different. Most cases in the literature describe men with dissociative fugue, primarily in military samples. However, no adequate data exist to demonstrate a gender bias to this disorder. Dissociative fugue is usually described in adults.

Diagnosis and Clinical Features Dissociative fugues have been described to last from minutes to months. Some patients report multiple fugues. However, in most cases in which this was described, a more chronic dissociative disorder, such as dissociative identity disorder, was not ruled out.

In some extremely severe cases of PTSD, nightmares may be terminated by a waking fugue in which the patient runs to another part of the house or runs outside, for example. Children or adolescents may be more limited than adults in their ability to travel. Thus, fugues in this population may be brief and involve only short distances. Some cases of children or adolescents who precipitously run away actually may be cases of dissociative fugue, with the child escaping from an abusive or violent home situation. No systematic research exists on this point.

A teenage girl was continually sexually abused by her alcoholic father and another family friend. She was threatened with perpetration of sexual abuse on her younger siblings if she told anyone about the abuse. The girl became suicidal but felt that she had to stay alive to protect her siblings. She precipitously ran away from home after being raped by her father and several of his friends as a "birthday present" for one of them. She traveled to a part of the city where she had lived previously with the idea that she would find her grandmother with whom she had lived before the abuse began. She traveled by public transportation and walked the streets, apparently without attracting attention. After approximately 8 hours, she was stopped by the police in a curfew check. When questioned, she could not recall recent events or give her current address, insisting that she lived with her grandmother. On initial psychiatric examination, she was aware of her identity, but she believed that it was 2 years earlier, giving her age as 2 years younger and insisting that none of the events of recent years had occurred.

Classically, three types of fugue have been described: (1) fugue with awareness of loss of personal identity; (2) fugue with change of personal identity; and (3) fugue with retrograde amnesia. In stage I, there is thought to be generation of an altered state of consciousness during which complex activities may be engaged in, sometimes over long periods of time. A single idea that symbolizes or condenses, or both, a number of important ideas and emotions frequently dominates the patient's thinking in this stage. In stage II, the patient becomes aware of the amnesia or loss of personal identity, at which point he or she frequently is brought for treatment. In this stage, amnesia is usually present for the first stage. In stage III, the patient returns to his or her baseline state, usually with amnesia for the first stage and sometimes for the second as well. An alternative view describes stage II as a return to the baseline state with amnesia for stage one or to a state in which there is (1) awareness of loss of personal identity, (2) change in personal identity, or (3) return to a chronologically earlier period of life, similar to a spontaneous hypnotic age regression.

During a fugue, patients often appear without psychopathology and do not attract attention. On the other hand, some individuals may display overtly bizarre, disorganized, or dangerous behavior, such as a soldier in the midst of battle who began a fugue episode by standing up and walking away from the front lines, exposing himself to intense enemy fire.

After the termination of a fugue, the patient may experience perplexity, confusion, trance-like behaviors, depersonalization, derealization, and conversion symptoms, in addition to amnesia. Some patients may terminate a fugue with an episode of generalized dissociative amnesia. They may be brought to media attention in an attempt to discover who they are and from where they have come.

As the dissociative fugue patient begins to become less dissociated, he or she may display mood disorder symptoms, intense suicidal ideation, and PTSD or other anxiety disorder symptoms. In the classic cases, an alter identity is created under whose auspices the patient lives for a period of time. Many of these latter cases are better classified as dissociative identity disorder or dissociative disorder NOS with features of dissociative identity disorder.

Pathology and Laboratory Examination Patients with dissociative fugue tend to have high scores on standardized measures of hypnotizability and dissociation. Dissociative fugue can be diagnosed with the DDIS or the SCID-D-R. Because dissociative fugue may be a response to sexual trauma, clinicians should have an index of suspicion for sexually transmitted diseases and genital or rectal trauma. Physical and laboratory examinations should be directed at ruling out medical causes of dissociative fugue.

Differential Diagnosis Individuals with dissociative amnesia may engage in confused wandering during an amnesia episode. However, in dissociative fugue, there is *purposeful* travel away from the individual's home or customary place of daily activities, usually with the individual preoccupied by a single idea that is accompanied by a wish to run away.

Patients with dissociative identity disorder may have symptoms of dissociative fugue, usually recurrently throughout their lives. Dissociative identity disorder patients have multiple forms of complex amnesias and, usually, multiple alter identities that develop starting in childhood.

In complex partial seizures, patients have been noted to exhibit wandering or semi-purposeful behavior, or both, during seizures or in postictal states, for which there is subsequent amnesia. However, seizure patients in an epileptic fugue often exhibit abnormal behavior, including confusion, perseveration, and abnormal or repetitive movements. Other features of seizures are typically reported in the clinical history, such as an aura, motor abnormalities, stereotyped behavior, perceptual alterations, incontinence, and a postictal state. Stressful life events may be associated with an increase in seizure frequency in some susceptible patients. Thus, this factor alone is not sufficient as a differential diagnostic indicator. Serial or telemetric EEGs, or both, usually show abnormalities associated with behavioral pathology.

Wandering behavior during a variety of general medical conditions, toxic and substance-related disorders, delirium, dementia, and organic amnestic syndromes could theoretically be confused with dissociative fugue. However, in most cases, the somatic, toxic, neurological, or substance-related disorder can be ruled in by the history, physical examination, laboratory tests, or toxicological and drug screening. Use of alcohol or substances may be involved in precipitating an episode of dissociative fugue.

Wandering and purposeful travel may occur during the manic phase of bipolar disorder or schizoaffective disorder. Manic patients may not recall behavior that occurred in the euthymic or depressed state and vice versa. In purposeful travel due to mania, however, the patient is usually preoccupied with grandiose ideas and often calls attention to himself or herself owing to inappropriate behavior. Assumption of an alternate identity does not occur.

Similarly, peripatetic behavior may occur in some patients with schizophrenia. Memory for events during wandering episodes in such patients may be difficult to ascertain owing to the patient's thought disorder. However, dissociative fugue patients do not demonstrate a psychotic thought disorder or other symptoms of psychosis.

Malingering of dissociative fugue may occur in individuals who are attempting to flee a situation involving legal, financial, or personal difficulties, as well as in soldiers who are attempting to avoid combat or unpleasant military duties. These precipitating factors may be present as well in bona fide dissociative fugue, however. There is no test, battery of tests, or set of procedures that invariably distinguish true dissociative symptoms from those that are malingered. Malingering of dissociative symptoms, such as reports of amnesia for purposeful travel during an episode of antisocial behavior, can be maintained even during hypnotic or pharmacologically facilitated interviews. Many malingerers confess spontaneously or when confronted. In the forensic context, the examiner should always give careful consideration to the diagnosis of malingering when fugue is claimed.

Course and Prognosis Most fugues are relatively brief, lasting from hours to days. Most individuals appear to recover, although refractory dissociative amnesia may persist in rare cases. Some studies have described recurrent fugues in the majority of individuals presenting with an episode of dissociative fugue. However, no systematic modern data exist that attempt to differentiate dissociative fugue from dissociative identity disorder with recurrent fugues.

Treatment Dissociative fugue is usually treated with an eclectic, psychodynamically informed psychotherapy that focuses on helping the patient recover memory for identity and recent experience. Hypnotherapy and pharmacologically facilitated interviews are frequently necessary adjunctive techniques to assist with memory recovery. Therapy should be carefully paced, following the phasic approach discussed in prior sections. The initial phase is centered on establishing clinical stabilization, safety, and a therapeutic alliance using supportive and educative interventions. Patients may need medical treatment for injuries sustained during the fugue, food, and sleep.

Once stabilization is achieved, subsequent therapy is focused on helping the patient regain memory for identity, life circumstances, and personal history. During this process, extreme emotions related to trauma or severe psychological conflict, or both, may emerge that require working through. In general, the therapist should maintain a supportive and nonjudgmental stance, especially if the fugue has been precipitated by intense guilt or shame over an indiscretion. At the same time, it is important for the therapist to balance this with being a spokesperson for the patient, taking realistic responsibility for misbehavior.

Clinicians should be prepared for the emergence of suicidal ideation or self-destructive ideas and impulses as the traumatic or stressful prefugue circumstances are revealed. Psychiatric hospitalization may be indicated if the patient is an outpatient.

In this phase of treatment, hypnotherapy may be helpful in containing intense affects and impulses, titrating the pace of returning memory, and processing and integrating the memory material. Patients may need specific psychopharmacological interventions for mood, anxiety, and dyscontrol symptoms as the acute dissociative symptoms are reduced and the patient becomes consciously aware of his or her actual life situation.

Some dissociative fugue patients may resist uncovering their actual identity even with hypnosis or pharmacologically assisted interviews. Appeals through the local (or even regional) media may not alert the patient's concerned others if the patient has wandered a substantial distance from home. In one case, the patient was asked to randomly select numbers on a phone key pad. This resulted in the patient's tapping out a phone number—apparently outside of conscious awareness—that allowed the treating clinician to find the patient's family hundreds of miles away.

Family, sexual, occupational, or legal problems, or a combination of these, that were part of the original matrix that generated the fugue episode may be substantially exacerbated by the time the patient's original identity and life situation are detected. Thus, family treatment and social service interventions may be necessary to help resolve such complex difficulties.

Rarely, in the most extreme cases, the fugue patient has established a new identity, occupation, and social relationships in a different location. When the original identity is discovered, often by accident, a variety of predicaments may ensue regarding the real-world complications of the situation. In response to these, the patient may become acutely suicidal, overwhelmed, or confused, or a combination of these. Also, the patient may display other extreme or bizarre dissociative symptoms, such as the Ganser symptom of approximate answers (e.g., the question "What color is snow?" is answered with "green") or attempt to engage in another fugue to escape the situation.

When dissociative fugue involves assumption of a new identity, it is useful to conceptualize this entity as psychologically vital to protecting the person. Traumatic experiences, memories, cognitions, identifications, emotions, strivings, or self-perceptions, or a combination of these, have become so conflicting and, yet, so peremptory that the person can resolve them only by embodying them in an alter identity. The therapeutic goal in such cases is neither suppression of the new identity nor fascinated explication of all its attributes. As in dissociative identity disorder, the clinician should appreciate the importance of the psychodynamic information contained within the alter personality state and the intensity of the psychological forces that necessitated its creation. In these cases, the most desirable therapeutic outcome is fusion of the identities, with the person working through and integrating the memories of the experiences that precipitated the fugue.

Once the fugue had resolved, the problem of responsibility for illegal acts may become an issue (e.g., having married without divorcing a prior spouse, financial indiscretions). The treating psychiatrist may become involved with police and legal agencies, military authorities, and others who may be brought into these complex cases.

It is prudent for the treating clinician to try to balance in a commonsense way the patient's real responsibility for his or her behavior, as well as the psychopathological issues that may be mitigating factors. Attempts to find a mediated agreement among the contending parties rather than punishment alone may be best in situations in which sexual, marital, or financial misdeeds, or a combination of these, complicate the clinical situation. However, it is important that, whatever resolution is found, it should focus on real responsibility for misconduct being accepted by the patient.

DISSOCIATIVE IDENTITY DISORDER

Dissociative identity disorder, previously called *multiple personality disorder*, has been researched most extensively of all the dissociative disorders. It is the paradigmatic dissociative psychopathology in that the symptoms of all the other dissociative disorders are commonly found in patients with dissociative identity disorder: amnesias, fugues, depersonalization, derealization, and similar symptoms.

According to DSM-IV-TR, dissociative identity disorder "is characterized by the presence of two or more distinct identities or

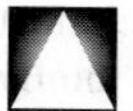

Table 17–13
DSM-IV-TR Diagnostic Criteria for Dissociative Identity Disorder

A. The presence of two or more distinct identities or personality states (each with its own relatively enduring pattern of perceiving, relating to, and thinking about the environment and self).
B. At least two of these identities or personality states recurrently take control of the person's behavior.
C. Inability to recall important personal information that is too extensive to be explained by ordinary forgetfulness.
D. The disturbance is not due to the direct physiological effects of a substance (e.g., blackouts or chaotic behavior during alcohol intoxication) or a general medical condition (e.g., complex partial seizures). **Note:** In children, the symptoms are not attributable to imaginary playmates or other fantasy play.

From American Psychiatric Association. *Diagnostic and Statistical Manual of Mental Disorders*. 4th ed. Text rev. Washington, DC: American Psychiatric Association; 2000, with permission.

personality states that recurrently take control of the individual's behavior accompanied by an inability to recall important personal information that is too extensive to be explained by ordinary forgetfulness." The identities or personality states, sometimes called *alters*, *self-states*, *alter identities*, or *parts*, among other terms, differ from one another in that each presents as having "its own relatively enduring pattern of perceiving, relating to, and thinking about the environment and self" (Table 17–13).

History After the extraordinary interest in multiple personality throughout the 19th century, the study of dissociative identity disorder mostly waned after the beginning of the 20th century. Authorities suggest that this was related to a variety of factors, including the rising dominance of freudian paradigms of hysteria; the disrepute into which hypnosis fell at this time; the rise of the bleulerian construct of schizophrenia, which may have subsumed dissociative patients; and the loss of interest in the works of Janet, Prince, and others who had been so crucial in the development of models of dissociation. A number of case studies, such as the famous *Three Faces of Eve*, continued to be published in the professional and popular literature. In addition, periodic systematic reviews of the literature continued to support the validity of the diagnostic construct.

The modern era in the study of multiple personality disorder began with the work of Arnold Ludwig and colleagues at the University of Kentucky during the 1970s. This included their extensive work on the psychobiology of single cases of dissociative identity disorder and multiple personality disorder, studying the differential findings among the alter identities. Cornelia Wilbur, widely identified with the case of *Sybil*, was influential in describing the clinical features of the modern construct of dissociative identity disorder and identifying the role of childhood trauma as a major factor in the etiology of the disorder. Wilbur, Richard Kluft, and others began the articulation of a systematic modern treatment approach.

Beginning in the 1980s, Putnam, Eve Carlson, Judith Armstrong, Ross, Phillip Coons, Steinberg, Onno van der Hart, Suzette Boon, Nel Draijer, Vedet Sar, and other researchers in the United States, Canada, Europe, Latin America, Turkey, and Japan began systematic research studies on the phenomenology, epidemiology, psychobiology, and treatment of dissociative identity disorder in children, adolescents, and adults. Despite this, controversy continues over the validity of the disorder, with a vocal minority of clinicians subscribing to the SCM of dissociative identity disorder.

Validity of the Dissociative Identity Disorder Construct Debate about the existence of dissociative identity disorder has waxed and waned for more than a century. However, sufficient data on pathological dissociation, in general, and on dissociative identity disorder, in particular, have accrued to judge this condition by the same standards that are applied to the validity of other psychiatric diagnoses.

The most widely accepted standards are based on a set of criteria first articulated by Eli Robins and Samuel Guze and subsequently refined by others. In essence, a psychiatric diagnosis is considered valid if it satisfies three basic requirements: content validity, criterion-related validity, and construct validity. Content validity requires a detailed clinical description of the disorder that is repeatedly independently replicated. More than a dozen clinical phenomenological studies of dissociative identity disorder, including those from North America, South America, Europe, Turkey, and Asia, document the presence of a core dissociative psychopathology in dissociative identity disorder patients that fulfills this requirement. Criterion-related validity requires that laboratory tests or reliable psychological tests are consistent with the defined clinical picture. This stipulation is met by the reliable and valid diagnostic interviews and scales that have increasingly been used in dissociation research, as well as psychological testing protocols that discriminate dissociative identity disorder patients from normals, schizophrenics, and depressed patients, among others.

Construct or discriminant validity requires that the disorder be differentiable from other disorders. This has been empirically demonstrated for dissociative identity disorder with respect to disorders such as schizophrenia, borderline and other personality disorders, and affective disorders. Also, dissociative identity disorder patients can be discriminated from normal individuals and other psychiatric patient groups, including those with personality disorders, PTSD, and dissociative disorder NOS, by structured interviews such as the SCID-D-R. Psychological test batteries and experimental cognitive and psychophysiological studies have discriminated dissociative identity disorder patients from other subjects including simulators. In addition, recent reviews of the dissociative identity disorder construct, using a number of different psychiatric validity paradigms, found that dissociative identity disorder met all current criteria for a valid diagnosis in psychiatry.

Recent psychobiological studies have shown that a variety of variables, such as salivary cortisol, urinary catecholamines, low-dose dexamethasone-suppression test (DST), and MRI measurements of hippocampal and amygdala volume, discriminate dissociative identity disorder from patients with borderline personality disorder and trauma controls (TCs). However, there were only subtle biological differences between dissociative identity disorder and PTSD subjects, although the two groups differed significantly in several measures of dissociation, such as the CADSS and the DES. On the GSS, a robust measure of susceptibility to external pressure to produce confabulated narrative accounts, the dissociative identity disorder subjects scored as *less* suggestible than patients with PTSD, borderline personality disorder, and traumatized controls. These findings support the notion that dissociative identity disorder is best conceptualized as a posttraumatic psychopathology, not an iatrogenic condition or an epiphenomenon of borderline personality disorder or other disorders.

Accordingly, dissociative identity disorder satisfies widely accepted standards for psychiatric validity and should be regarded as a legitimate disorder requiring an informed diagnostic and treatment approach.

Epidemiology Few systematic epidemiological data exist for dissociative identity disorder. One study yielded a prevalence rate of 3.1 percent for a stratified sample (N = 1,055) of the general population of Winnipeg, Canada, although a more conservative analysis of these data suggests a prevalence of approximately 1.3 percent for dissociative identity disorder. Independent analysis of the DES data collected on the same sample found a prevalence rate of 3.3 percent for *pathological dissociation*, a construct including DES items for amnesia, depersonalization, derealization, identity confusion and alteration, and inner voices (pseudohallucinations), a symptom profile typical of clinical dissociative identity disorder patients. Several studies have examined the prevalence rate of dissociative identity disorder in general psychiatric patient samples. Results from the United States, Canada, Turkey, and several Western European countries using structured interview data suggest that between 1 and 20 percent of adolescent and adult psychiatric inpatients meet diagnostic criteria for dissociative identity disorder, with an average estimate of 3 to 5 percent across studies. Higher rates were found in substance abuse treatment populations and inpatient adolescents. Available epidemiological data are insufficient, and a large-scale, population-based study is necessary to resolve controversies about the prevalence of dissociative identity disorder.

Clinicians have long noted gender differences in the frequency of dissociative identity disorder. Clinical studies report female to male ratios between 5 to 1 and 9 to 1 for diagnosed cases. Research with measures such as the DES, however, finds no evidence of gender differences in the propensity or capacity to dissociate. Developmental studies indicate that the ratio of female to male dissociative identity disorder cases steadily increases from 1 to 1 in early childhood to approximately 8 to 1 by late adolescence. Reasons proposed for the increased numbers of female dissociative identity disorder patients relative to male patients include gender-related differences in the types, age of onset, and duration of maltreatment experienced by men and women; differences in clinical presentations, such that male cases are more likely to be missed; and the possibility that more male dissociative identity disorder cases end up in the criminal justice or alcohol and drug treatment systems, or both, rather than the mental health system.

Etiology Theories of the etiology of dissociative disorders have been extensively discussed in the introductory section on dissociative phenomena. This section briefly summarizes the theories that are most relevant to dissociative identity disorder and that are best supported by empirical data.

Dissociative identity disorder is strongly linked to severe experiences of early childhood trauma, usually maltreatment, in all studies—in Western and non-Western cultures—that have systematically examined this question. The rates of reported severe childhood trauma for child and adult dissociative identity disorder patients range from 85 to 97 percent of cases across a wide variety of studies. Physical and sexual abuse, usually in combination, are the most frequently reported sources of childhood trauma in clinical research studies, although other kinds of trauma have been reported, such as multiple painful medical and surgical procedures during childhood and wartime trauma. Critics have raised questions about the validity of dissociative identity disorder patients' self-reports of childhood trauma. Recent studies, including large samples of maltreated children with dissociative disorders and intensively validated case studies, have provided rigorous independent corroboration of the patients' reports of maltreatment. These studies continue to strongly support a developmental linkage between childhood trauma and dissociative identity disorder.

Early life experiences resulting in disturbances in attachment relationship with the primary caregiver and other abnormal family processes have been implicated in the genesis of pathological levels of dissociation and the development of dissociative identity disorder. Recent research indicates that a high level of dissociation in mothers is associated with disturbed, often dissociative-like, attachment behavior in their children. In another study, early presence of these attachment disturbances prospectively predicted higher levels of dissociation in late adolescence. The contribution of genetic factors is only now being systematically assessed, but preliminary studies have not found evidence of a significant genetic contribution. One small study did find an elevated prevalence of dissociative identity disorder and other dissociative disorders in the first-degree relatives of dissociative identity disorder patients.

Autohypnotic Model The autohypnotic model is widely subscribed to by clinicians working with dissociative identity disorder patients. It postulates that pathological dissociation is an extreme form of self-hypnosis or autohypnosis. Autohypnosis is postulated to be adaptive in the immediate context of trauma or abuse but subsequently becomes maladaptively elaborated into dissociative alter personality states. Proponents point to similarities between the phenomenology of deep trance states and some of the clinical phenomenology seen in dissociative identity disorder. Also, adjunctive hypnotherapeutic interventions can be quite helpful in the treatment of many dissociative identity disorder patients. In addition, studies of hypnotizability using standardized scales have shown that dissociative identity disorder patients have the highest hypnotizability compared to patients with other diagnoses, such as affective disorders, panic disorder, personality disorders, and schizophrenia, among others, as well as normal controls.

On the other hand, more than a dozen studies find only low correlations between measures of hypnotizability and dissociation in clinical and nonclinical subjects. A history of trauma is not *necessarily* associated with increased hypnotizability, although a subgroup of traumatized individuals shows high levels of hypnotizability clinically and on standardized measures. These findings indicate that hypnotizability and clinical dissociation, as defined by standard measures, are different processes. Although high hypnotizability may be a correlate of traumatization in some patients, the autohypnotic model of the etiology of dissociative identity disorder does not by itself appear to account for the disorder. However, autohypnotic abilities and phenomena may be involved in shaping the clinical presentation of dissociative identity disorder.

Discrete Behavioral State Model The DBS model conceptualizes dissociative identity disorder as a developmental failure by a traumatized child to consolidate a core sense of identity. Drawing on research demonstrating the key role of DBS in the patterning and organization of normal early childhood behavior and affect regulation, the behavioral state model postulates that trauma disrupts unification of identity in a least two key ways. The first is through the creation of DBS associated with the mitigation of and restitution from repetitive traumatic experiences, such as incest. These dissociative behavioral states psychologically encapsulate intolerable memories and affects through cognitive mechanisms, such as state-dependent learning and memory retrieval, described previously. Second, repetitive traumatic experiences, together with disturbed caretaker–child attachment and parenting, disrupt the development of normal metacognitive processes involved in the elaboration and consolidation of a unified sense of self. These metacognitive processes, which flower between 1 to 6 years of age, enable the child to integrate the different experiences of self that normally occur across different contexts, for example, with parents, peers, and others. A corollary of this notion is the idea that the failure of integration of self may preserve aspects of parent–child attachment necessary for development, because the child may continue to perceive the caretaker as good, despite mistreatment or neglect (as in betrayal trauma therapy). Encapsulation of traumatic experiences may also permit more normal maturation in other developmental dimensions, such as educational and intellectual tasks, interpersonal relations, and artistic endeavors.

Overall, however, the long-term outcome of these developmental deficits and deformations operating over childhood and adolescence is an individual with multiple, relatively concretized, quasi-independent senses of self, which are often in psychological conflict with each other. The secondary structuring of these self-states, due to a variety of developmental pressures and intrapsychic needs, results in the concrete elaboration of the alter identities with names, personal descriptors, and variable ways of presenting themselves to others. These secondary elaborations are *not* the core aspect of the disorder. However, they may be highly invested in by some dissociative identity disorder individuals and thus may be quite resistant to change. At the other extreme, some dissociative identity disorder patients may show significant liability to influence and suggestion in outward presentational features of the alters.

Virtually no empirical data in any clinical or research population exist to support the sociocognitive or iatrogenesis theory of the etiology of dissociative identity disorder.

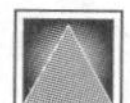

Table 17–14
Amnesia and Memory Symptoms

Blackouts or time loss
Disremembered behavior
Fugues
Unexplained possessions
Inexplicable changes in relationships
Fluctuations in skills, habits, and knowledge
Fragmentary recall of entire life history
Chronic mistaken identity experiences
Microdissociations

Mental status examination questions for dissociative amnesia

If answers are positive, ask the patient to describe the event.

Make sure to specify that the symptom does not occur during an episode of intoxication.

(1) Do you ever have blackouts? Blank spells? Memory lapses?
(2) Do you lose time? Have gaps in your experience of time?
(3) Have you ever traveled a considerable distance without recollection of how you did this or where you went exactly?
(4) Do people tell you of things you have said and done that you do not recall?
(5) Do you find objects in your possession (such as clothes, personal items, groceries in your grocery cart, books, tools, equipment, jewelry, vehicles, weapons, etc.) that you do not remember acquiring? Out-of-character items? Items that a child might have? Toys? Stuffed animals?
(6) Have you ever been told or found evidence that you have talents and abilities that you did not know that you had? For example, musical, artistic, mechanical, literary, athletic, or other talents? Do your tastes seem to fluctuate a lot? For example, food preference, personal habits, taste in music or clothes, etc.
(7) Do you have gaps in your memory of your life? Are you missing parts of your memory for your life history? Are you missing memories of some important events in your life? For example, weddings, birthdays, graduations, pregnancies, birth of children, etc.?
(8) Do you lose track of or tune out conversations or therapy sessions as they are occurring? Do you find that, while you are listening to someone talk, you did not hear all or part of what was just said?
(9) What is the longest period of time that you have lost? Minutes? Hours? Days? Weeks? Months? Years? Describe.

Adapted from Loewenstein RJ: An office mental status examination for chronic complex dissociative symptoms and multiple personality disorder. *Psychiatr Clin North Am.* 1991;14:567–604.

Diagnosis and Clinical Features

Table 17–13 lists the DSM-IV-TR criteria for dissociative identity disorder. The comparable ICD-10 disorder, multiple personality disorder, falls under the other dissociative (conversion) disorder category. The DSM-IV-TR and ICD-10 criteria are virtually identical. Both require that organic disorders (e.g., general medical conditions, substance abuse) be ruled out. DSM-IV-TR adds that, in children, the symptoms cannot be attributable to imaginary playmates or other fantasy play.

Dimensions of Trauma

Traditional characterizations of dissociative symptoms largely derive from 19th century formulations and do not incorporate recent understanding of the psychiatric effects of trauma. Comparative study of psychiatric symptoms associated with different types of trauma suggests that a number of common dimensions underlie traumatic sequelae. Affect modulation is frequently disturbed, giving rise to mood swings, depression, suicidal tendency, and generalized irritability. Impulse control is often impaired, leading to risk taking, substance abuse, and inappropriate or self-destructive behaviors. High levels of anxiety and panic are common. A variety of disturbances in sense of self, from the identity diffusion seen in borderline patients to the alter identities of dissociative identity disorder, reflects disruptions in the psychological integration of traumatic and nontraumatic aspects of self. Eating disorders are common in a subgroup of trauma patients and may also relate to disorders of body image and identity. Frequent somatization, conversion, and psychophysiological disorders may represent disruptions in the integration of psychic and somatic representations of overwhelming recollections, intolerable affects, posttraumatic cognitive schema, and intrapsychic conflicts. In addition, studies suggest that childhood sexual abuse survivors with psychophysiological disorders, when compared to controls, are more likely to have a lower threshold for experiencing physiological phenomena as noxious or painful.

Consequently, initial clinical presentations in trauma victims of all kinds may encompass or mimic a variety of psychiatric conditions, including affective and anxiety disorders, somatoform disorders, personality disorders, and psychosis. Some of these disorders may also be comorbidly associated with dissociative identity disorder, especially PTSD, affective disorders, somatoform disorders, substance use disorders, and a mixed personality disorder, most commonly with some combination of avoidant, obsessive-compulsive, dependent, and borderline traits. All systematic studies of the clinical phenomenology of dissociative identity disorder emphasize the polysymptomatic presentations of these patients. Therefore, the detection and diagnosis of dissociative identity disorder involve looking behind a confusing plethora of symptoms for core dissociative symptoms of functional amnesias, depersonalization and derealization, passive influence experiences, and identity alterations. Tables 17–14, 17–15, and 17–16 describe the symptom clusters that are most commonly found in dissociative identity disorder patients and some of the mental status questions that may elicit these symptoms in suspected dissociative identity disorder patients.

Memory and Amnesia Symptoms

Dissociative disturbances of memory are manifest in several basic ways and are frequently observable in clinical settings (Table 17–14). As part of the general mental status examination, clinicians should routinely inquire about experiences of losing time, black-out spells, and major gaps in the continuity of recall for personal information. Patients rarely spontaneously report these experiences and require active

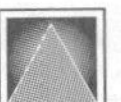

Table 17–15
Dissociative Identity Disorder Process Symptoms

	Mental status examination questions for dissociative identity disorder process symptoms

Presence of dissociative identity disorder alter identities
Switching behaviors (identity alteration)
Identity confusion
Passive influence symptoms/interference phenomena between alters
  Made feelings from alter identity
  Made impulses from alter identity
  Made actions by alter identity
  Thought insertion from alter identity
  Thought withdrawal by alter identity
  Alters' voices commenting on behavior
  Alters' voices arguing
Multimodal hallucinations or pseudohallucinations (may occur in a flashback)
  Visual
  Auditory
  Tactile
  Olfactory
  Gustatory
  Somatoform
Dissociative or posttraumatic thought disorder
Posttraumatic stress disorder–based cognitive distortions
Trance logic
Other thought process abnormalities
  Disorganization due to switching, passive influence
  Posttraumatic suspiciousness
  Literal and concrete alternating with abstract
Linguistic usage: refers to self as we, they, us, him, her, etc.
Depersonalization and derealization symptoms
  Depersonalization
  Out-of-body experiences
  Derealization
  Déjà vu
  Jamais vu
  Déjà vécu
  Dream-like states
	If answers are positive, ask the patient to describe the event.
	Make sure to specify that the symptom does not occur during an episode of intoxication.
	(1) Do you act so differently in one situation compared to another situation that you feel almost like you were two different people?
	(2) Do you ever feel that there is more than one of you? More than one part of you? Side of you? Do they seem to be in conflict or in a struggle?
	(3) Does that part (those parts) of you have its (their) own independent way(s) of thinking, perceiving, and relating to the world and the self? Have its (their) own memories, thoughts, and feelings?
	(4) Does more than one of these entities take control of your behavior?
	(5) Do you ever have thoughts or feelings, or both, that come from inside you (outside you) that you cannot explain? That do not feel like thoughts or feelings that you would have? That seem like thoughts or feelings that are not under your control (passive influence)?
	(6) Have you ever felt that your body was engaged in behavior that did not seem to be under your control? For example, saying things, going places, buying things, writing things, drawing or creating things, hurting yourself or others, etc.? That your body does not seem to belong to you?
	(7) Do you ever feel you have to struggle against another part of you that seems to want to do or to say something that you do not wish to do or to say?
	(8) Do you ever feel that there is a force (pressure, part) inside you that tries to stop you from doing or saying something?
	(9) Do you ever hear voices, sounds, or conversations in your mind? That seem to be discussing you? Commenting on what you do? Telling you to do or not do certain things? To hurt yourself or others? That seem to be warning you or trying to protect you? That try to comfort, support, or soothe you? That provide important information about things to you? That argue or say things that have nothing to do with you? That have names? Men? Women? Children?
	(10) I would like to talk with that part (side, aspect, facet) of you (of the mind) that is called the "angry one" (the Little Girl, Janie, that went to Atlantic City last weekend and spent lots of money, etc.). Can that part come forward now, please?
	(11) Do you frequently have the experience of feeling like you are outside yourself, inside yourself? Beside yourself, watching yourself as if you were another person?
	(12) Do you ever feel disconnected from yourself or your body as if you (your body) were not real?
	(13) Do you frequently experience the world around you as unreal? As if you are in a fog or a daze? As if it were painted? Two-dimensional?
	(14) Do you ever look in the mirror and not recognize yourself? See someone else there?

Adapted from Loewenstein RJ: An office mental status examination for chronic complex dissociative symptoms and multiple personality disorder. *Psychiatr Clin North Am.* 1991;14:567–604.

inquiry by the interviewer to uncover amnesia. Positive responses should be documented with specific examples provided by the patient. In some instances, patients report coming to or waking up in the midst of some activity with little or no recall of how they came to be involved in that activity. In other instances, patients find evidence of having done or acquired things for which they have no recall. Friends and family members may tell them about significant things that they have said or done that they cannot remember. Patients may find that they have unknowingly traveled some distance (a fugue episode) or that days or even weeks have passed for which the patients cannot account. Dissociative time loss experiences are too extensive to be explained by normal forgetting and typically have sharply demarcated onsets and offsets. It is important to establish that such time loss experiences occur in the absence of intoxication or substance abuse, although high rates of drug and alcohol abuse in dissociative patients may complicate this determination.

Patients with severe dissociative memory disturbances also report perplexing fluctuations in skills, habits, or well-learned abilities, such as fluency in a foreign language or athletic abilities. Patients report drawing a complete blank for skills or knowledge at times, whereas, at other times, they easily and reliably access the information in question. This perplexing forgetfulness is believed to be related to the dissociative state-dependent disturbances of implicit memory functions that have been documented in laboratory settings.

Dissociative patients often report significant gaps in autobiographical memory, especially for childhood events. Dissociative gaps in autobiographical recall are usually sharply demarcated and do not fit the normal decline in autobiographical recall for younger ages. For example, a patient may complain that he or she cannot recall anything between 8 and 12 years of age, while reporting readily available memories before and afterward. Another patient may report having no memories available for the first 10 years of

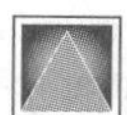

Table 17–16
Autohypnotic Symptoms

Spontaneous trance
Deep enthrallment
Spontaneous age regression
Negative hallucinations
Hidden observer phenomenon
Trance logic (tolerance of logical inconsistency during a trance state)
Voluntary analgesia/anesthesia
Eye roll, eye blinking, etc., with switching

Mental status examination questions for spontaneous autohypnotic symptoms

(1) Do you frequently space out, trance out, block out, withdraw from the world around you? Perhaps by putting yourself in a pleasant scene or place in your mind? By focusing your attention on something inside or outside of you? (spontaneous trance)

(2) Do you get so wrapped up in a book or a movie that you can completely block out everything else around you? As if the world could end, and you would still be completely engrossed in that activity? (enthrallment)

(3) Do you feel that you are different ages at different times? Do you ever feel like you get little? Like you become a child or an adolescent again? When this happens, does it feel like your body changes in size? Do you experience it in your mind only, or does your whole perception of yourself and the world change also? (spontaneous age regression)

(4) Do you ever *not* see or hear what is going on around you? Do you or can you block out people and things altogether? (negative hallucinations)

(5) Are you able to block out (ignore) physical pain if you want to? Wholly? Partly? Always? Sometimes? (voluntary analgesia)

Adapted from Loewenstein RJ: An office mental status examination for chronic complex dissociative symptoms and multiple personality disorder. *Psychiatr Clin North Am.* 1991;14:567–604.

life. Available autobiographical memories may have a depersonalized quality, such that recalled events seem to be memories of a dream or as if the patient had seen them happen to someone else.

Ms. A. is a 33-year-old married woman, employed as a librarian in a school for disturbed children. She presented to psychiatric attention after discovering her 5-year-old daughter "playing doctor" with several neighborhood children. Although this event was of little consequence, the patient began to become fearful that her daughter would be molested. Ms. A. became panicked and increasingly obsessed with this idea, much to the bafflement of her husband. The patient was seen by her internist and was treated with antianxiety agents and antidepressants, but with little improvement. Ms. A. became increasingly anxious, phobic, depressed, and preoccupied. She sought psychiatric consultation from several clinicians, but repeated, good trials of antidepressants, antianxiety agents, and supportive psychotherapy resulted in limited improvement. After the death of her father from complications of alcoholism, the patient became more symptomatic. He had been estranged from the family since the patient was approximately 12 years of age, owing to his drinking and associated antisocial behavior.

Ms. A. developed a variety of somatic complaints, including headaches, abdominal pain, menstrual and gastrointestinal (GI) problems, back pain, and sleep difficulties. Repeated medical workup was unrevealing, leading to diagnoses such as fibromyalgia, irritable bowel syndrome, and premenstrual tension. Family and marital difficulties increased as the patient withdrew from her husband and was increasingly dysfunctional in taking care of her children. Work function also deteriorated. Psychiatric hospitalization was precipitated by the patient's arrest for disorderly conduct in a nearby city. She was found in a hotel, in revealing clothing, engaged in an altercation with a man. She denied knowledge of how she had come to the hotel, although the man insisted that she had come there under a different name for a voluntary sexual encounter.

On psychiatric examination, the patient described dense amnesia for the first 12 years of her life, with the feeling that her "life started at 12 years old." She reported that, for as long as she could remember, she had an imaginary companion, an elderly black woman, who advised her and kept her company. She reported hearing other voices in her head: several women and children, as well as her father's voice repeatedly speaking to her in a derogatory way. She reported that much of her life since 12 years of age was also punctuated by episodes of amnesia: for work, for her marriage, for the birth of her children, and for her sex life with her husband. She reported perplexing changes in skills; for example, she was often told that she played the piano well but had no conscious awareness that she could do so. Her husband reported that she had always been "forgetful" of conversations and family activities. He also noted that, at times, she would speak like a child; at times, she would adopt a southern accent; and, at other times, she would be angry and provocative. She frequently had little recall of these episodes.

Questioned more closely about her early life, the patient appeared to enter a trance and stated, "I just don't want to be locked in the closet" in a child-like voice. Inquiry about this produced rapid shifts in state between alter identities who differed in manifested age, facial expression, voice tone, and knowledge of the patient's history. One identified itself by a diminutive of the patient's name and appeared child-like. Another spoke in an angry, expletive-filled manner and appeared irritable and preoccupied with sexuality. She discussed the episode with the man in the hotel and stated that it was she who had arranged it. A third alter identified itself as a protective entity, experiencing itself as an elderly African-American woman who commented sadly and philosophically about "this whole situation." Gradually, the alters described a history of family chaos, brutality, and neglect during the first 12 years of the patient's life, until her mother, also alcoholic, achieved sobriety and fled her husband, taking her children with her. The patient, in the alter identities, described episodes of physical abuse, sexual abuse, and emotional torment by the father, her siblings, and her mother.

Family sessions with the mother and siblings confirmed many of these reports, with the family recalling episodes of maltreatment that the patient did not recollect. The patient's mother had bid the family never to speak of the earlier difficulties, hoping that everyone would "just forget the whole thing." After additional assessment of family members, the patient's mother also met diagnostic criteria for dissociative identity disorder, as did her older sister, who also had been molested. A brother met diagnostic criteria for PTSD, major depression, and alcohol dependence.

The patient improved significantly with psychotherapy directed at stabilization of her dissociative identity disorder and PTSD. She responded well to clomipramine (Anafranil) with a marked reduction in obsessive-compulsive and depressive symptoms. Family therapy was helpful in stabilizing the patient's marriage and helping her husband with the aftermath of the hospitalization and its precipitants. The husband also reported a family history of abuse, although primarily directed at his mother and siblings. He had always seen himself as the family protector. The patient's mother and siblings were already in treatment but were helped by the opening up of the family history and clarification of their diagnoses. At 3-year follow-up, the patient reported fusion of most alters and marked diminution in dissociative, somatoform, and PTSD symptoms, although she still required clomipramine for stabilization of mood and OCD symptoms.

Process Symptoms Dissociative process symptoms include depersonalization and derealization, dissociative hallucinations, passive influence and interference experiences, and dissociative cognition (Table 17–15). Some authorities include dissociative alterations in identity under this category. Symptoms of depersonalization and derealization are commonly reported by dissociative identity disorder patients and may include profound out-of-body experiences. Patients frequently report feeling spaced out or disconnected from themselves and others. The world is perceived as distant or unreal, with a hazy or foggy quality. Patients may report feeling, at times, as if they exist in a waking dream state. Out-of-body experiences commonly take the form of watching oneself from a distance (inner, as well as outer), as if observing another person, with little or no ability to affect their actions.

Dissociative auditory hallucinations commonly take the form of voices heard as originating from within the person (pseudohallucinations), as opposed to coming from outside. Individual hallucinated voices typically have distinctive age and gender attributes. They may comment negatively about the patient, argue with each other, command the patient to perform certain acts, discuss neutral topics, or sometimes provide useful information or comfort, or a combination of these. Patients generally recognize that the voices are hallucinations and may be reluctant to reveal their existence for fear of being considered psychotic. Many patients report some ability to ignore or disregard hallucinations, unless they are stressed. Hallucinated voices often come to be identified with specific alter personality states. Visual hallucinations typically take the form of detailed images with traumatic or frightening content. Other visual hallucinations may be understood as depicting the alter identities or may even have a complex artistic quality. Tactile, gustatory, and olfactory hallucinations may also occur, leading to misdiagnoses of seizure disorder or other organic mental disorders. Intrusive posttraumatic flashbacks and images may also be experienced as complex multimodal hallucinations.

Negative hallucinations, in which external percepts and stimuli are not consciously registered, are not uncommon. Patients also report the volitional ability to block out various perceptions or sensations, including pain. Most hallucinations, pseudohallucinations, and negative hallucinations in dissociative identity disorder patients are likely homologous to phenomena that can be experienced in deep trance states among highly hypnotizable individuals and are not a manifestation of a process psychosis.

Passive influence and interference symptoms include many first-rank schneiderian symptoms, such as audible thoughts, voices arguing with each other, influences playing on the body, thought withdrawal and insertion, and made feelings, impulses, and actions. These symptoms were once considered to be pathognomonic of schizophrenia, but they can also be found in patients with affective, organic, and dissociative disorders. Passive influence symptoms now have been demonstrated to be more common in dissociative identity disorder patients than in psychotic mental disorders. However, in dissociative identity disorder, the agents of the passive influence symptoms are usually experienced as internal, not external, as in psychotic disorders. In addition, patients may report strong affects or impulses that they experience without a sense of personal ownership, but with a peremptory sense of intrusion and control. Dissociative identity disorder patients generally do not have delusional explanations for these experiences. They may feel confused, puzzled, or ashamed of them. Personification is commonly part of the explanation, such as "I feel like someone else wants to cry with my eyes."

The recognition that dissociative patients frequently manifest subtle, but often clinically significant, cognitive impairments emerges from clinical research with psychological and cognitive test batteries. Research using projective testing finds distinctive cognitive process markers, including evidence of confusing and contradictory responses to the same stimulus. Distinctive responses to standardized projective testing can often be helpful in distinguishing dissociative patients from other diagnostic groups, such as patients with affective disorders, nondissociative forms of PTSD, personality disorders, psychotic disorders, and factitious disorders.

Dissociative Alterations in Identity Clinically, dissociative alterations in identity may first be manifested by odd first-person plural or third-person singular or plural self-references. In addition, patients may refer to themselves using their own first names or make depersonalized self-references, such as "the body," when describing themselves and others; for example, "The father hurt the body so she was upset. We tried to protect her, but it didn't work." Patients often describe a profound sense of concretized internal division or personified internal conflicts between parts of themselves. In some instances, these parts may have proper names or may be designated by their predominate affect or function, for example, "the angry one" or "the wife." Patients may suddenly change the way in which they refer to others, for example, "the son" instead of "my son."

A set of behaviors, collectively referred to as *switching behaviors*, may be manifest during evaluation or therapy sessions. Switching behaviors include intrainterview amnesias, in which the patient does not seem to recall or is confused about the process and content of that session. These microdissociative episodes may be manifested by abrupt shifts in train of thought or sudden inexplicable changes in affect or in rapport. A variety of physical signs, including pronounced upward eye rolls or bursts of rapid blinking and eyelid fluttering, may occur in conjunction with microdissociative episodes. The patient's tone of voice and manner of speaking, posture, and demeanor may show marked alteration. When clinicians encounter evidence of possible microdissociative episodes, they should seek to clarify what the patient is experiencing and can recall with nondirective, open-ended questions

These cognitive, behavioral, and physical shifts are manifestations of alter personality switching or overlap and interference between alter states, or both. The alter personalities of dissociative identity disorder patients are best conceptualized as DBS, each organized around a prevailing affect, sense of self (often including a distinct body image), a set of state-dependent autobiographical memories, and a limited behavioral repertoire. Authorities have long cautioned that alter personalities should not be regarded as separate people. Rather, the alter personalities are conceptualized as relatively stable and enduring patterns of behavior that are largely unintegrated with each other and are often in direct conflict.

The set of alter personality states, usually referred to as the *personality system*, constitutes the personality of the individual. Most psychotherapeutic work is directed toward this larger personality system and thus toward the individual as a whole. Much has been made of the psychological and physiological differences among the alter personality states of individuals with dissociative identity disorder, and popular accounts emphasize the presentational differences among alters. Laboratory studies support clinical accounts of significant differences; however, much general information and many functions and abilities are shared in common across alter personality states and indicate the fundamental unity of the mental processes of the dissociative individual. This provides the foundation for therapeutic efforts directed at the development of a more consciously integrated sense of self in the dissociative identity disorder patient.

Apparent differences in the organization and dynamics of alter personality systems have been used to classify dissociative identity disorder patients into various categories for more than a century. The validity of these classifications remains to be proven, but, as a group, dissociative identity disorder patients show considerable variability in the complexity and therapeutic tractability of their alter personality systems. Several alter personality types are commonly reported, including child alter personalities; internalized persecutory alters, who inflict pain and may attempt to kill the individual; and depleted and depressed host personality states, who function as the primary identity with respect to the world at large. Alter personality states often reflect painful psychological issues for the individual and frequently take the form of polarized pairs representing antithetical positions, although alters representing more neutral and conflict-free processes also commonly occur. In some dissociative identity disorder individuals, virtually every aspect of mental life is structuralized and personified in this form.

Symptoms Related to Spontaneous Autohypnotic Phenomena Dissociative identity disorder patients commonly exhibit or describe symptoms of involuntary autohypnotic phenomena, consistent with their high scores on standardized hypnotizability scales (Table 17–16). These include spontaneous trance states that can be clinically disabling, spontaneous or voluntary anesthesia and analgesia, negative hallucinations, spontaneous age regressions, and the *trance logic* or literal-mindedness of the hypnotized subject. Other similar symptoms overlap with dissociative process symptoms (hallucinations, thought disorder, child alter identities) and PTSD symptoms (behavioral reexperiencing episodes with multimodal hallucinations and age regression to the time of the trauma).

Other Associated Symptoms Because dissociative identity disorder is conceptualized as a trauma spectrum disorder, it is not surprising that the majority of these patients also meet diagnostic criteria for PTSD by clinical criteria or by using standardized measures and diagnostic inventories (Table 17–17). Depending on the study, 70 to 100 percent of dissociative identity disorder patients have been shown to meet diagnostic criteria for PTSD by DSM-III-R, DSM-IV, and DSM-IV-TR criteria.

Dissociative identity disorder patients commonly exhibit multiple types of psychophysiological, somatoform, and conversion symptoms. For example, across studies, 40 to 60 percent of dissociative identity disorder patients also meet diagnostic criteria for somatization disorder, and many others meet diagnostic criteria for undifferentiated somatoform disorder, somatoform pain disorder, or conversion disorder, or a combination of these.

Finally, numerous recent studies have shown a robust relationship between certain forms of affective disorders and an antecedent history of trauma, particularly childhood sexual abuse. Depression is increasingly understood as one of the outcomes following traumatic experiences. Accordingly, most dissociative identity disorder patients meet criteria for a mood disorder, usually one of the depression spectrum disorders. Frequent, rapid mood swings are common, but these are usually due to posttraumatic and dissociative phenomena, not a true cyclic mood disorder. There may be considerable overlap between PTSD symptoms of anxiety, disturbed sleep, and dysphoria and mood disorder symptoms.

Obsessive-compulsive symptoms are also commonly found in individuals with PTSD. Obsessive-compulsive personality traits are common in dissociative identity disorder, and intercurrent OCD symptoms are regularly found in dissociative identity disorder patients, with a subgroup manifesting severe OCD symptoms. OCD symptoms commonly have a posttraumatic quality: checking repeatedly to be sure that no one can enter the house or the bedroom, compulsive washing to relieve a feeling of being dirty because of abuse, and repetitive counting or singing in the mind to distract from anxiety over being abused, for example.

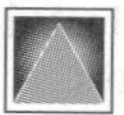

Table 17–17
Dissociative Identity Disorder-Associated Symptoms Commonly Found in Dissociative Identity Disorder

Posttraumatic stress disorder symptoms
- Intrusive symptoms
- Hyperarousal
- Avoidance and numbing symptoms

Somatoform symptoms
- Conversion and pseudoneurological symptoms
- Seizure-like episodes
- Somatization disorder or Briquet's syndrome
- Somatoform pain symptoms
- Headache, abdominal, musculoskeletal, pelvic pain
- Undifferentiated somatoform disorder
- Psychophysiological symptoms or disorders
- Asthma and breathing problems
- Perimenstrual disorders
- Irritable bowel syndrome
- Gastroesophageal reflux disease
- Somatic memory

Affective symptoms
- Depressed mood, dysphoria, or anhedonia
- Brief mood swings or mood lability
- Suicidal thoughts and attempts or self-mutilation
- Guilt and survivor guilt
- Helpless and hopeless feelings

Obsessive-compulsive symptoms
- Ruminations about trauma
- Obsessive counting, singing
- Arranging
- Washing
- Checking

Child and Adolescent Presentations A growing clinical research literature documents the diagnosis and treatment of child and adolescent dissociative disorders, including dissociative identity disorder. In many respects, children and adolescents manifest the same core dissociative symptoms and secondary clinical phenomena as adults. Age-related differences in autonomy and lifestyle, however, may significantly influence the clinical expression of dissociative symptoms in youth. For example, dissociative amnesias and perplexing forgetfulness are more apparent in school situations rather than work or family life. Younger children, in particular, have a less linear and less continuous sense of time and are often not able to self-identify dissociative discontinuities in their behavior. Fortunately, there are often additional informants, such as teachers and relatives, available to help document dissociative behaviors.

A number of normal childhood phenomena, such as imaginary companionship and elaborated daydreams, must be carefully differentiated from pathological dissociation in younger children. For example, preadolescent children with dissociative identity disorder may manifest less in the way of gross switching behaviors than adolescents or adults. The clinical presentation may be that of an elaborated or autonomous imaginary companionship, with the imaginary companions taking control of the child's behavior, often experienced through passive influence experiences or auditory pseudohallucinations, or both, that command the child to behave in certain ways.

Pathology and Laboratory Examination A clinical mental status examination based on the various symptom clusters described in Tables 17–14 through 17–17 can be helpful in the diagnosis of dissociative identity disorder. Questioning about amnesic, autohypnotic, PTSD, affective, and somatoform symptoms usually precedes detailed inquiry about more overt symptoms related to the alter identities. Careful in-depth questioning about these phenomena may readily bring forth information about dissociative identity disorder process symptoms. For example, discussion of complex amnesia experiences may readily lead to questions about how purposive behaviors can occur without apparent memory. Discussion of PTSD symptoms may lead to manifestations of alter identities related to traumatic experiences.

The development and increasing use of screening instruments and standardized diagnostic interviews have contributed to the increase in numbers of identified dissociative identity disorder cases seen over the last decade. Dissociative identity disorder patients commonly score over 30 on the DES and the DES-T. However, this is a screening instrument and cannot be used to make a clinical diagnosis. The SCID-D-R is currently considered the gold standard for diagnosis of dissociative disorders. The major drawback of the SCID-D-R is that it can take several hours to administer, especially if the patient has many positive responses. Accordingly, some clinicians rely on the shorter DDIS for its ease and speed of administration. The MID is a self-report inventory that may assist in diagnosis of dissociative identity disorder and other dissociative disorders.

The CDC and A-DES are two commonly used screening measures for assessment of dissociation in children and adolescents, respectively. They are reliable and valid measures in clinical and research populations.

Before the development of these clinical and psychometric assessment tools, hypnotic or amobarbital interviews were often used to attempt diagnosis of dissociative identity disorder. Due to the current academic and forensic controversies surrounding dissociative disorders and trauma memory, it is prudent to reserve these interventions for emergency situations when other methods of assessment have failed, for example, in a female patient who is emergently hospitalized after engaging in repeated, dangerous nocturnal fugues and who cannot account for these behaviors, despite intensive interviewing. These interventions should optimally be conducted by a clinician experienced in their use and in the differential diagnosis of dissociative disorders. Clear, informed consent should be obtained for use of these interventions for diagnosis of dissociative identity disorder and recall of traumatic experiences.

Differential Diagnosis On average, more than 6 years pass between first psychiatric contact and the diagnosis of dissociative identity disorder. Although often portrayed as flamboyant hysterics, only a small minority of dissociative identity disorder patients present in this way. Dissociative identity disorder patients are typically reticent about revealing their dissociative symptoms, especially hallucinations, amnesia, and identity divisions. They most commonly present as relatively inhibited and obsessional, with affective and somatic complaints, and typically acquire three or more psychiatric diagnoses before their dissociative identity disorder is recognized. A subgroup of dissociative identity disorder patients show interpersonal dynamics that are reminiscent of borderline personality disorder, for which some dissociative identity disorder patients qualify as a secondary diagnosis once PTSD and dissociative symptoms are stabilized. The presence of auditory hallucinations, disturbed thinking and behavior, confusion due to amnesic gaps, and schneiderian first-rank symptoms contributes to the misdiagnosis of schizophrenia in approximately one-half of dissociative identity disorder patients at some point in their psychiatric histories. Rapid changes in affect associated with alter personality switching may suggest a rapid-cycling affective disorder or schizoaffective disorder. Table 17–18 lists the most common disorders that must be differentiated from dissociative identity disorder. However, because many of these disorders may coexist with dissociative identity disorder, as well as being mimicked by dissociative identity disorder, differential diagnosis may be a complex process.

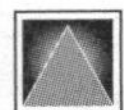

Table 17–18
Differential Diagnosis of Dissociative Identity Disorder

Comorbidity versus differential diagnosis
Affective disorders
Psychotic disorders
Anxiety disorders
Posttraumatic stress disorder
Personality disorders
Cognitive disorders
Neurological and seizure disorders
Somatoform disorders
Factitious disorders
Malingering
Other dissociative disorders
Deep-trance phenomena, such as the hidden observer or ego states

Factitious, Imitative, and Malingered Dissociative Identity Disorder Concerns about factitious and malingered dissociative identity disorder are common. Recently, there are increasing reports of individuals claiming to have dissociative identity disorder who do not meet diagnostic criteria for dissociative identity disorder when carefully assessed clinically or with structured interviews, such as the SCID-D-R. There may be a mixture of factors leading to this presentation, including misdiagnosis, factitiousness, and assumption of a social role of an abuse victim or a dissociative identity disorder patient. Dutch researchers have named this *imitative dissociative identity disorder* when there does not appear to be conscious simulation. Patients may build their lives around their diagnosis and are commonly supported by concerned others and by their therapists in so doing.

Indicators of falsified or imitative dissociative identity disorder are reported to include those typical of other factitious or malingering presentations. These include symptom exaggeration, lies, use of symptoms to excuse antisocial behavior (e.g., amnesia only for bad behavior), amplification of symptoms when under observation, refusal to allow collateral contacts, legal problems, and pseudologia fantastica. Genuine dissociative identity disorder patients are usually confused, conflicted, ashamed, and distressed by their symptoms and trauma history. The nongenuine patients frequently show little dysphoria about their disorder.

These imitative and factitious patients actually fit the SCM of dissociative identity disorder, with one exception: Rigorous diagnostic efforts show that they do not meet actual diagnostic criteria for dissociative identity disorder.

The SCID-D-R has been used to help distinguish genuine from bogus dissociative identity disorder in clinical and forensic contexts. In addition, psychological assessment by a psychologist experienced in evaluation of trauma, PTSD, and dissociation may also be quite helpful in differential diagnosis. On the SCID-D-R, fabricated dissociative identity disorder patients tend not to describe the typical comorbid conditions and symptoms associated with dissociative identity disorder, such as amnesia, identity confusion, and identity alteration, although they may report high levels of depersonalization and derealization. They often describe symptoms in a jargon filled way ("I'm dissociating" or "I'm switching") and cannot readily explain their subjective experience on follow-up questions on the SCID-D-R or in clinical interviews.

There are no absolute clinical indicators to differentiate imitative, factitious, or malingered dissociative identity disorder from the actual disorder. Some bona fide dissociative identity disorder patients become invested in a dissociative identity disorder identity or that of being a trauma survivor as their main social role. There is a subgroup of dissociative identity disorder patients who present in a dramatic, histrionic fashion, unlike the majority of dissociative identity disorder patients who are reticent and secretive about their illness. There are also genuine dissociative identity disorder patients who report factitious histories, produce factitious crises, and create factitious alter identities. Some dissociative identity disorder patients report that their only happy childhood experiences were while medically hospitalized. Like more typical factitious disorder patients, they seek out and try to maintain themselves as hospital patients in psychiatric and medical settings. Munchausen syndrome and Munchausen syndrome by proxy also have been reported in dissociative identity disorder patients and in their first-degree relatives.

Ms. F., a 48-year-old divorced mother of three, was referred to a trauma disorder inpatient unit by her managed care company for a consultation about diagnosis and treatment. Ms. F. had been diagnosed with dissociative identity disorder after doing "inner child work" with her outpatient therapist, Dr. Q., to whom Ms. F. reported an extensive history of childhood neglect, as well as physical and sexual abuse. Ms. F. had numerous hospitalizations for suicidal ideation, as well as for episodes of superficial self-mutilation. Ms. F. was on disability. She did not care for her children adequately and had been investigated several times by her state division of child welfare, who had recently placed her children in foster care.

On arrival in the trauma unit, Ms. F. proclaimed to patients and staff that, "I have dissociative identity disorder. I was sexually abused." She did not seem distressed by either of these ideas. She repeatedly stated, "I'm switching, I'm switching," although staff members, experienced with dissociative identity disorder patients, did not observe any of the typical signs of dissociative identity disorder switches. Staff noted that they had never observed a dissociative identity disorder patient announce switches in this way. Ms. F. became irritable when staff attempted to dissuade her from speaking in such a dramatic and graphic way in the milieu.

Ms. F. was evaluated clinically, observed by nursing staff in the ward milieu, and given a battery of psychological tests, including the DES, the SCID-D, assessments of PTSD, and personality assessments. On the clinical evaluation, Ms. F. did not endorse complex chronic amnesia symptoms, amnesia for her life history, spontaneous self-hypnosis, passive influence symptoms, or inner voices. She endorsed episodes of depersonalization and derealization. She reported only "child and baby alters" but could describe little about them when questioned. She would say things like, "See, now I'm like a child. Can't you tell? That's one of my littles." She did not endorse any sense of fear, shame, conflict, or inner struggle around switching nor were any of the typical phenomena of switching noted at these times (e.g., eye roll; eye blinking; subtle shifts in voice, posture, and facial expression; momentary confusion; intrainterview amnesia, and so forth). Supposed alter identities did not seem to have relatively independent ways of thinking, relating, perceiving, or remembering.

Ms. F. described a history of childhood chaos and neglect in detail but became more stereotypically, perseveratively vague when discussing other types of childhood adversity: "The man hurt me. I'm here to recover from it. It's just like what happened to K. (a friend of the patient's from the incest survivors' group). Dr. Q. says I have a long way to go in my healing. That's all. Isn't that enough?" She did not seem distressed, hesitant, or ashamed when discussing the alleged history of childhood sexual abuse. She became angry when confronted with contradictions in her accounts, the dramatic nature of her presentation, and discrepancies between her history and her emotional reactions.

Ms. F. appeared uninterested in individual or group psychotherapy that sought to teach her more effective ways to manage symptoms and to increase effective coping. She was angry when nursing staff attempted to get her to take responsibility for managing her symptoms of anxiety and regression in a more proactive and adult fashion. She was infuriated when the unit social worker did not see her role as attempting to find Ms. F. alternative housing or intervening with the state child welfare system on her behalf.

Staff contacted Dr. Q., who became angry and affronted when questions were raised about the patient's clinical presentation and authenticity of her sexual abuse history.

On psychological and diagnostic testing, Ms. F. did not endorse most items consistent with clinical dissociation, other than depersonalization and derealization. She did not display typical PTSD or dissociative reactivity to inquiries about the abuse history, nor did she meet diagnostic criteria for PTSD. She did not show behaviors typical of dissociative identity disorder patients on stressful test batteries or during a serendipitous event while being tested, when another patient suddenly required aggression management on the ward near the testing room. Other patients reacted with PTSD and dissociative symptoms: panic, marked startle, spontaneous trance, hiding, loss of reality orientation, assumption of a fetal position, rocking with hands over the face, entrance into flashback, and so forth. Ms. F. blithely continued her testing with minimal reaction.

At the conclusion of the assessment, Ms. F. was diagnosed with factitious disorder with psychological symptoms, mood disorder NOS, and personality disorder NOS with histrionic, borderline, and dependent features. The staff struggled with the factitious diagnosis, because Ms. F. did not appear to be consciously feigning dissociative identity disorder in the strict sense and actually seemed to believe in her self-reports of switching and alter identities. Ms. F. and Dr. Q. were both resistant to the new diagnostic formulation. Dr. Q. stated that she would insist that the managed care company seek another expert opinion to correctly diagnose her patient.

Course and Prognosis Little is known about the natural history of untreated dissociative identity disorder. A few case studies of partially treated patients followed up many years later suggest that the disorder becomes less overt over time, with a decrease in florid dissociative symptoms and less intrapsychic conflict among the alter personality states. These cases, however, are too few and too selected to generalize. Small studies of dissociative identity disorder patients diagnosed in middle age and in geriatric populations have shown that severe dissociative identity disorder symptoms can persist or can appear in older-age patients. A relapsing and remitting course is common. Also, patients can more or less successfully mask or suppress symptoms for periods of time. Both of these latter phenomena may be mistaken for complete spontaneous remission of the disorder.

Some untreated dissociative identity disorder individuals are thought to continue involvement in abusive relationships or violent subcultures, or both, that may result in the traumatization of their children, with the potential for additional family transmission of the disorder. Many authorities believe that some percentage of undiagnosed or untreated dissociative identity disorder patients die by suicide or as a result of their risk-taking behaviors. Experience with a large number of dissociative identity disorder cases suggests that there are several subgroups of dissociative identity disorder individuals. These range from those who function at quite high levels for long periods of time to others who have severely impaired and dysfunctional life trajectories often beginning early in development.

Patient presentations and prognosis vary somewhat across the life span. Children with dissociative identity disorder show many dissociative symptoms and behaviors but typically have fewer and less crystallized alter personality states that are less invested in their individuality. If diagnosed early, children often have an excellent prognosis, and many seem to have relatively spontaneous resolutions when removed from abusive and neglectful environments. In adolescence, alter personality states become more distinct and more invested in their autonomy. Additional alter personalities associated with life stresses, such as academic, athletic, social, or sexual challenges, may appear, and the personality system dynamics become more complicated and polarized. In general, adolescents have a poorer prognosis than children or adults, in part because they are often not invested in their treatment. Better outcome with dissociative identity disorder adolescents has been reported when the patients' families were successfully engaged in treatment. Young adults typically present in crisis and have a layering of affective, somatic, posttraumatic, and personality disorder symptoms in addition to their core dissociative pathology.

First dissociative identity disorder presentations in older dissociative identity disorder patients frequently involve a life event, such as the loss of a job, death of a parent, or a revictimization, such as a rape, that reactivates earlier conflicts and destabilizes the alter personality system. Achieving sobriety in a substance-abusing dissociative identity disorder patient may precipitate overt dissociative identity disorder and PTSD presentations. In adult patients, there appear to be treatment-responsive and treatment-refractory subgroups of dissociative identity disorder patients. Time course of improvement also may vary, with some patients improving relatively quickly and others requiring intensive treatment efforts over long periods of time.

Prognosis is poorer in patients with comorbid organic mental disorders, psychotic disorders (*not* dissociative identity disorder pseudopsychosis), and severe medical illnesses. Refractory substance abuse and eating disorders also suggest a poorer prognosis. Other factors that usually indicate a poorer outcome include significant antisocial personality features, current criminal activity, ongoing perpetration of abuse, and current victimization, with refusal to leave abusive relationships. Repeated adult traumas with recurrent episodes of acute stress disorder may severely complicate clinical course. Boundary violations and abuse by a therapist or psychiatrist may severely prolong the treatment course, because the setting of treatment now feels unsafe and precipitates intense posttraumatic reactivity. Severe personality disorders with overinvestment in multiplicity as a way of life, engagement in psychotherapy primarily to seek gratification, and a refusal to take responsibility for behavior change and symptom management are also generally associated with a poorer prognosis. Number of alter personality states, however, has only a moderate effect on treatment course.

Treatment

Stages and Goals Current treatment approaches to dissociative identity disorder have evolved considerably with the conceptualization of dissociative identity disorder as a complex developmental trauma disorder and as the spectrum of dissociative identity disorder patients has been better appreciated. Appropriate treatment of the dissociative identity disorder patient follows a phasic model that is the current standard of care for posttraumatic disorders. The phases include (1) a phase of symptom stabilization, (2) an optional phase of focused, in-depth attention to traumatic material, and (3) a phase of integration or reintegration in which the dissociative identity disorder patient moves more completely away from a life adaptation based on chronic traumatization and victimization. Obviously, these phases are relatively heuristic, and aspects of each may be part of the others.

Stabilization of the dissociative identity disorder patient is vital to permit more successful negotiation of all aspects of treatment. Stabilization focuses on safety, stability, and management of core dissociative identity disorder and comorbid symptoms. The vast majority of dissociative identity disorder patients engage in some form of self-destructive behavior, including suicide attempts, self-mutilation, eating disorders, substance abuse, promiscuity, risk-taking activities, and involvement in abusive, violence-based relationships. Many male, and some female, dissociative identity disorder patients have difficulty with aggression, violence, and homicidal tendency, including perpetration of child abuse. It is incumbent on the clinician to make these issues the basic focus of treatment. In general, cognitive and behavioral approaches are used, framing these behaviors as part of a set of quasi-addictive, trauma-related, homeostatic mechanisms. Experienced clinicians find that many dissociative identity disorder patients can bring self-destructive and high-risk behaviors under control. Cognitive and behavioral methods are used to develop therapeutic agreements (also called *safety contracts*), so that patients have a repertoire of techniques to manage their difficulties instead of by self-destruction. Eating disorders, severe substance abuse, enmeshment in abusive relationships, and perpetration of violence may be more refractory to these methods and may require concurrent specialty treatment interventions and involvement of police, social service, and community agencies.

Stabilization of severe symptoms generally involves work with posttraumatic stress and dissociative symptoms. Dissociative identity disorder patients frequently present with highly disturbing PTSD symptoms, such as intrusive thoughts, imagery, somatic sensations, hyperarousal, and flashbacks. The latter may present as acute behavioral reexperiencing episodes with loss of reality orientation or more subtle and pervasive reliving experiences, or both. Patients may be overwhelmed by dissociative hallucinations, amnesia and fugue episodes, passive influence experiences, or profound identity confusion and disorganization. Sorting out genuinely comorbid disorders from the plethora of posttraumatic, anxiety, affective, and somatic symptoms commonly manifested by dissociative patients in crisis is important, as some disorders, for example, affective disorders, require additional treatment interventions. Assessment of available family and community supports is also important.

Psychotherapy A survey of more than 300 clinicians treating dissociative identity disorder patients found that the vast majority considered psychotherapy to be their primary and most efficacious treatment modality. Successful psychotherapy for the dissociative identity disorder patient requires the clinician to be comfortable with a range of psychotherapeutic interventions and a willingness to actively work to structure the treatment. These modalities include psychoanalytic psychotherapy, cognitive therapy, behavioral therapy, hypnotherapy, and a familiarity with the psychotherapy and psychopharmacological management of the traumatized patient. Comfort with family treatment and systems theory is helpful in working with a patient who subjectively experiences himself or herself as a complex system of selves with alliances, family-like relationships, and intragroup conflict. A grounding in work with patients with somatoform disorders may also be helpful in sorting through the plethora of somatic symptoms with which these patients commonly present.

Therapeutic Engagement with Alter Identities Effective stabilization in most dissociative identity disorder patients requires psychotherapeutic work with individual alter personality states. Many dissociative identity disorder patients are not able to stabilize symptoms in the long term if the alter identities who control these symptoms are not therapeutically engaged. Clinicians new to dissociative identity disorder are frequently uncomfortable or perplexed by the need to work with individual alters and how to do this without producing a chaotic regression. Certain basic principles are important to understand. No alter is any more or less real than any other alter or more good or bad than another. All are aspects of a single human being and have adaptive, psychological importance that needs to be heard and respected. All alters are held accountable and responsible for the behavior of any part, even if experienced with amnesia or lack of subjective ownership. In the context of psychotherapy, alters can be understood as developmentally concretized, trauma-based metaphors or forms of organizing and mobilizing mental contents. These unusual metaphors have many problematic cognitions and affects, as well as adaptive attributes, such as the alter personality state-dependent memory data described previously. As such, the fullest participation of all mental symbols and sources of knowledge, skills, and adaptations is likely to produce the best outcome in psychotherapy.

Concerns about iatrogenesis are often raised in this context. Understanding the alters as forms of intrapsychic symbolization reduces this concern to a more routine psychotherapeutic task of understanding the meaning of mental contents, rather than a suppression of some mental states as less authentic than others. At the same time, the clinician must also be able to appreciate the patient's subjective reality in which the alter self-states are experienced as distinct selves or even as separate persons. The therapist must be able to tolerate engaging with the alters *as if* they are separated entities, while simultaneously maintaining the understanding that the alters represent the structuring of psychological processes in personified form within a single human mind.

The continuity, stability, and respectful impartiality of the therapist toward the different alter personalities provide an important therapeutic experience that helps the patient experience, examine, and integrate these dissociated aspects of self. The processing of negative life events, often from the multiple perspectives of different alter personality states, is an important part of the narrative reorganization of the patient's fragmented identity into a more coherent whole. The therapist usually is actively involved in negotiating between and among the various alter identities to achieve therapeutic goals. These can include negotiation of agreements to stop self-destructive behaviors, to allow more adaptive interidentity function and communication, and to permit certain alters to participate more fully in therapy.

Initial Phase of Dissociative Identity Disorder Treatment The initial phase of treatment of the dissociative identity disorder patient involves a number of simultaneous and sequential tasks.

EDUCATION AND INFORMED CONSENT It is important to educate the dissociative identity disorder patient about the disorder, its comorbidities, and the course of treatment. Educative interventions help decrease anxiety about symptoms that are often frightening and overwhelming, build a therapeutic alliance, and provide information that is the basis for a meaningful consent for treatment. Furthermore, it is necessary to educate the patient about the contentious and divisive debates that surround the diagnosis and treatment of dissociative identity disorder in contemporary psychiatry and psychology.

Other major issues in informed consent include advising the patient of potential risks and benefits of the treatment, alternative approaches, and their potential risks and benefits. The patient should also be informed about the current controversies about traumatic memory and its retrieval and explication in therapy. Additional informed consent should be obtained if formal hypnosis is used and for administration of medications. The patient should be counseled that symptomatic worsening may occur during treatment, particularly during phases in which memory material is worked with in depth (second phase of treatment). Simultaneously, however, subjective amelioration of other symptoms may occur, with the patient achieving a better sense of control, mastery, and self-coherence as the patient successfully works through painful material.

This sort of dialectical process is common in dissociative identity disorder treatment. It is often helpful to point this out as part of the informed consent process. For example, at times, the patient may feel a sense of subjective unity, and the idea of having dissociative identity disorder seems unreal and impossible. At other times, the patient's sense of himself or herself as divided and enacting alter identity roles seems so compelling and overwhelming that no other diagnosis seems possible.

Similarly, like many obsessional individuals, dissociative identity disorder patients often respond positively to learning that the dissociative and PTSD symptoms that they experience have a name and an organizing framework for diagnosis and treatment. There is often relief at a diagnosis that fits the patient's subjective and life experience, especially if there has been a long prior history of unsuccessful psychiatric treatment for other disorders. At the same time, patients may respond with distress at the dissociative identity disorder diagnosis, partly because of media and popular stereotypes, partly because it brings into sharper relief the meaning of painful symptoms, and partly because it brings more focus to the distressing history of early trauma and problematic relationships with family members.

Dissociative identity disorder patients may need to be informed that treatment does not attempt to suppress or to destroy alter identities, but rather to allow therapeutic engagement with them as vital aspects of the mind. Patients usually want to get rid of alter identities and are also terrified that the therapist will attempt to do so. Most experienced clinicians educate patients that treatment is geared toward optimal function and adaptation and that there are usually too many variables at the beginning of treatment to predict whether it will necessarily ultimately result in unification of all self-divisions. At the same time, most experienced clinicians see unification of all alter self-states as usually providing the best long-term outcome in dissociative identity disorder.

The education and informed consent process is an ongoing one throughout treatment. Many of these issues need to be revisited as treatment proceeds and as the patient changes over treatment time.

Boundaries and Treatment Frame Most dissociative identity disorder patients report that their traumatic life experiences usually occur over long periods of time in the context of close personal relationships with those who have hurt them. Furthermore, dissociative identity disorder patients often report many boundary violations in subsequent relationships with teachers, therapists, medical professionals, and social service workers, among others. For these patients, the role description of significant others does not necessarily predict their behavior, and relationships are often seen as up for grabs. The patient expects and fears that the clinician will violate boundaries. There may be a subtle (or not so subtle) pull in the transference for the therapist to change the frame of treatment. Patients may experience this as trying to make the inevitable happen, so that they do not have to endure the agony of waiting for things to go wrong. Accordingly, clinicians working with these patients must pay careful attention to issues of the treatment frame and appropriate and consistent boundaries. These include firm limits on the length of therapy sessions, acceptable behavior during sessions, the extent of extra session contacts, and payment of fees, among many others. Interpretation of the patient's fears over the perceived inevitability of boundary violations is preferable to enacting them. Clinicians working with dissociative identity disorder patients should avoid boundary changes that make the patient "special," even if the patient insists that only these interventions will help. These include holding or hugging the patient, holding the patient's hand, accepting more than a token gift such as a card or a small piece of artwork, giving the patient gifts, phoning the patient while on vacation, and going for walks or other out-of-office contacts with the patient, among many others. The dissociative identity disorder patient may implore the therapist to make these sorts of interventions. Clinicians who feel overwhelmed by the treatment of these patients are more likely to accede to these importunings. It is important to recognize that the patient's reported history of abuse often involved being special to the abuser in some way. Thus, these boundary transgressions recreate this double-edged situation for the patient. Once again, education of the patient about appropriate boundaries is the most helpful clinical strategy.

Many of the clinical and conceptual issues that help make treatment workable with these patients are not taught in standard training programs for mental health professionals. Consultation should be considered by clinicians who are new to working with this patient population, or if stalemates or unsolvable predicaments develop in treatment.

Development of Skills to Manage Symptoms Experienced therapists commonly rapidly introduce a variety of symptom management strategies into the treatment. This necessitates active structuring of sessions to work on containment of severe symptoms and skill building This may involve imagery techniques to attenuate the intensity of PTSD, somatoform, and dissociative symptoms, successful stabilization of alter identities who embody or are experienced as creating symptoms, and encouragement of collaboration, communication, and empathy among alter identities. In particular, experienced clinicians work to attenuate the impact of PTSD intrusions, rather than opening up this material prematurely.

The clinician should be clear that the ultimate responsibility for symptom and behavioral management outside of sessions lies with the patient, who is viewed as an active partner in the treatment. In this regard, dissociative identity disorder patients often respond well to therapeutic contracting, taking more active responsibility for safety or behavioral control between sessions. The therapist may prescribe homework for the patient to work on symptom management and internal communication between sessions. These strategies are often essential in countering the patient's tendency toward regression and demoralization. Patients often use journal writing as a helpful adjunctive treatment strategy that allows more controlled expression and communication among alter identities, fulfillment of homework assignments, and a more attenuated and distanced way of handling overwhelming subjective experiences.

Cognitive Therapy Dissociative identity disorder patients may experience a multitude of cognitive errors and distortions based on traumatic life experiences and the ability of dissociation to interfere with reality testing. Typical cognitive distortions include (but are hardly limited to) the insistence that alters inhabit separate bodies and are unaffected by the actions of one another (delusional separateness), that the patient is helpless to control himself or herself and requires the clinician to manage all difficulties, that the clinician is completely untrustworthy and must be not be allowed any access to the patient's mind, that the patient is bad and deserved or caused childhood sexual abuse to occur, that anger and violence are the same, that love and sex are the same, that self-injury is safety, and that, because trauma and abuse are inevitable, it is best to invite them or enact them oneself, so that at least their timing and intensity can be better controlled.

Behind these cognitive distortions frequently lie exceptionally painful realizations and recollections. For example, if the patient gives up the idea of blameworthiness for childhood incestuous experiences, the reality must be faced that a beloved relative has done the patient grievous harm and has treated the patient as an object, not a person. Accordingly, many cognitive distortions are only slowly responsive to cognitive therapy techniques, and successful cognitive interventions may lead to additional dysphoria.

A subgroup of dissociative identity disorder patients does not progress beyond a long-term supportive treatment entirely directed toward stabilization of their multiple multiaxial difficulties. To the extent that they can be engaged in treatment at all, these patients require a long-term treatment focus on symptom containment and management of their overall life dysfunction, as would be the case with any other severely and persistently ill psychiatric patient population.

Transference and Countertransference Dissociative identity disorder patients often manifest a complex multilayered transference as a whole, as a system of personality states, and as individual alter personality states. Commonly, transference is dominated by themes of trauma and abuse, with the therapist most commonly experienced as potentially exploitative and abusive or uninvolved or uncaring about the patient's difficulties or as a helpless victim, like the patient faced with an implacable other. Dissociative identity disorder alters may literally envision the clinician as the embodiment of an abusive figure from the past, requiring active interventions to help the patient separate the past from the present.

Countertransference responses may vary as well, with overinvolvement, detached hostile skepticism, or a sense of being exasperated, overwhelmed, and deskilled being quite common. Clinicians may experience countertransferential autohypnotic and dissociative phenomena during dissociative identity disorder treatment that need to be recognized and managed. Burnout and secondary PTSD have been reported for therapists and treatment teams working with dissociative identity disorder patients, unless adequate attention is paid to limit setting, boundaries, and assistance to clinicians adversely experiencing reports of extreme abusive trauma or overwhelmed by work with dissociative identity disorder patients.

Second Phase: Work on Traumatic Memories For patients who can stabilize and form a reasonable working alliance in treatment, longer-term treatment goals involve the detailed, affectively intense, psychotherapeutic processing of life experiences, especially traumatic experiences, and the transformation of the meaning of these experiences for the individual. Authorities emphasize that, in most cases, intensive, detailed psychotherapeutic work

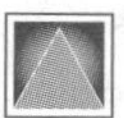

Table 17–19
Medications for Associated Symptoms in Dissociative Identity Disorder

- Medications and somatic treatments for PTSD, affective disorders, anxiety disorders, and OCD
  - Selective serotonin reuptake inhibitors (no preferred agent, except for OCD symptoms)
  - Fluvoxamine (Luvox) (for OCD presentations)
  - Clomipramine (Anafranil) (for OCD presentations)
  - Tricyclic antidepressants
  - Monoamine oxidase inhibitors (if patient can reliably maintain diet safely)
  - Electroconvulsive therapy (for refractory depression with persistent melancholic features across all dissociative identity disorder alters)
  - Mood stabilizers (more useful for PTSD and anxiety than mood swings)
  - Divalproex (Depakote)
  - Lamotrigine (Lamictal)
  - Gabapentin (Neurontin)
  - Topiramate (Topamax)
  - Carbamazepine (Tegretol)
  - Benzodiazepines
  - Clonazepam (Klonopin) and lorazepam (Ativan) have best track records
  - Atypical neuroleptics
  - Typical neuroleptics (if patient fails trials of atypicals)
  - β-Blockers (for PTSD hyperarousal symptoms)
  - Clonidine (Catapres) (for PTSD hyperarousal symptoms)
  - Prazosin (Minipress) (for PTSD nightmares)
- Medications for thought disorder
  - Atypical neuroleptics preferred
- Medications for acute dyscontrol
  - Oral or intramuscular neuroleptics
  - Oral or intramuscular benzodiazepines
- Medications for sleep problems
  - Low-dose trazodone (Desyrel)
  - Low-dose mirtazapine (Remeron)
  - Low-dose tricyclic antidepressants
  - Low-dose neuroleptics
  - Benzodiazepines (often less helpful for sleep problems in this population)
  - Zolpidem (Ambien)
  - Anticholinergic agents (diphenhydramine [Benadryl], hydroxyzine [Vistaril])
  - Chloral hydrate (Aquachloral Supprettes) (primarily for inpatient use)
- Medications for self-injury, addictions
  - Naltrexone (ReVia)

OCD, obsessive-compulsive disorder; PTSD, posttraumatic stress disorder.

with traumatic memories should only be initiated after the patient has demonstrated the ability to use symptom management skills independently, after the alter identity system can work together in a reasonably cooperative way, and after a solid therapeutic relationship has been established. The patient should be able to give informed consent and should have a realistic understanding of the potential risks and benefits of intensive focus on traumatic material. Potential risks may include acute worsening of PTSD, affective, somatoform, and self-destructive symptoms and short-term interference with daily activities. Long-term benefits may include significant amelioration of dissociative and PTSD symptoms, decreases in subjective self-division, fusion of alter identities, and freeing of psychological energy for daily life. The patient must be able to understand that the goal is integration of dissociated thoughts, feelings, recollections, and perceptions, not the exhumation of memories per se.

Furthermore, the patient should not be in the midst of an acute life crisis or major life change, comorbid medical and psychiatric disorders should be stabilized, the patient must have the ego strength and psychosocial resources to withstand the rigors of the process, and there must be adequate resources, such as support by significant others, to support the patient for additional sessions (Table 17–9).

Experienced clinicians attempt to structure carefully affectively intense sessions focused on traumatic material, with attention being given to affect modulation, restabilization of the patient before concluding the session, and reasonable availability to assist the patient supportively between sessions. In addition, many sessions may be needed to explicate fully the cognitive and emotional meaning of traumatic events, so that they may become part of the patient's repertoire of nondissociated, ordinary memories for life experience.

Traumatic Memories Media attention and legal cases have led to concerns over the authenticity of traumatic recollections of dissociative identity disorder patients. Recent rigorous case series have supported the experience of clinicians, who have found corollary information to corroborate recollections of dissociative identity disorder patients or who have even unearthed data about traumas that the patient does not recall. Based on corollary information, however, some dissociative identity disorder patients can be shown to misinterpret and misrepresent contemporary information or confabulate aspects of their past history. In addition, dissociative patients are hardly immune to ordinary human emotions, such as greed, envy, wishes for revenge, wishes to evade consequences for misbehavior, and desires to placate significant others. All of these may complicate the patient's veracity, especially in situations of potential financial gain, media attention, evasion of legal consequences, and possible loss of family contacts, among others. Conversely, collateral informants, such as family members, may be subject to the same sources of unreliability as the index patient, and their input should be weighed accordingly.

Dissociative identity disorder patients typically oscillate from regarding their recollections as all true to all false. Specific alter identities may take opposing positions. The clinician is best served by maintaining a stance of neutrality toward the patient's recollections of his or her life. In this regard, it is generally most helpful for the clinician to identify for the dissociative identity disorder patient his or her internal conflicts over the veracity of recollections and to invite an open airing of all points of view. Repeated discussion of the complex factors that may impact autobiographical recall may need to be part of an ongoing informed consent process as treatment progresses.

The therapist should respond respectfully and thoughtfully to all clinical material brought by the dissociative identity disorder patient. Patients can be helped not to come to premature closure about their views of events. Some dissociative identity disorder patients come to understand life events quite differently as they become less dissociative over the course of treatment. Consequently, clinicians must avoid validating memories for the patient or dismissing them out of hand, in the absence of reliable collateral information. Therapy is most successful for the dissociative identity disorder patient if the clinician maintains the role of therapist, not personal advocate, detective, or derisive skeptic.

Third Phase: Fusion, Integration, Resolution, and Recovery Over the course of treatment, significant unification of dissociated mental processes may be observed. Alters lose distinctness and decrease compartmentalization of thoughts, memories, and affects. The patient develops a more unified sense of self. Transference is modified consistent with these changes. Amnesia and switching become less apparent. Fusion of alters results in psychological merging of two or more entities at a point in time, with a subjective experience of loss of all separateness. The term *integration* is sometimes used synonymously with *fusion* but is more generally defined as the process of undoing all forms of dissociative division during treatment. Some patients proceed to what appears to be a complete fusion of all alters, with a shift in self-representation from that of a dissociative identity disorder individual to one with a consistent and continuous sense of self across all behavioral states. Many patients never attain a complete fusion of their alter personalities but leave treatment when they have achieved a therapeutic *resolution*: relative stability, adequate function, and some measure of internal harmony among self-states.

As this integrative process occurs, PTSD symptoms usually improve significantly. Patients often experience a freeing of energy toward everyday life and away from trauma-focused ways of living. Cognitive distortions frequently substantially subside. At the same time, nondissociative and integrative coping strategies must be identified and substituted for dissociative responses to life stressors. Losses must be mourned, and the patient must be helped to connect and cope with the larger world in a more functional manner.

Hypnosis Despite the controversy about its use, hypnosis was endorsed by approximately two-thirds of respondents as a psychotherapeutic adjunct in dissociative identity disorder treatment. Hypnotherapeutic interventions can often alleviate self-destructive impulses or reduce symptoms, such as flashbacks, dissociative hallucinations, and passive-influence experiences. Teaching the patient self-hypnosis may help with crises outside of sessions. Hypnosis may be useful for accessing specific alter personality states and their sequestered affects and memories. Hypnosis is also used to create relaxed mental states in which negative life events can be examined without overwhelming anxiety. Clinicians using hypnosis should be trained in its use in general and in trauma populations. Clinicians should be aware of current controversies over the impact of hypnosis on accurate reporting of recollections and should use appropriate informed consent for its use.

Psychopharmacological Interventions Pharmacotherapy was the third most commonly endorsed treatment modality. Although double-blind, controlled clinical trials have not been conducted, a variety of medications are considered clinically effective with many dissociative identity disorder patients. Guidelines for the use of medications with dissociative patients emphasize the need to identify specific treatment-responsive symptoms rather than attempting to treat the dissociation per se. Medications may be helpful in attenuating symptoms to assist the patient in stabilizing during treatment. Patients should be advised that medication response is likely to be partial, devising the best shock absorber system for the patient at a given time. In general, success is more likely if medication target symptoms are present across a range of alter personality states rather than confined to one or a few personality states.

Among the target symptoms considered most responsive to medication are affective symptoms. In many instances, these are secondary symptoms and show a more heterogeneous and less robust response than primary affective disorders. Nonetheless, antidepressant medications are often important in the reduction of depression and stabilization of mood. A variety of PTSD symptoms, especially intrusive and hyperarousal symptoms, are partially medication responsive. Guided by clinical experience and research with PTSD patients, clinicians report some success with SSRI, tricyclic, and monamine oxidase (MAO) antidepressants, β-blockers, clonidine (Catapres), anticonvulsants, and benzodiazepines in reducing intrusive symptoms, hyperarousal, and anxiety in dissociative identity disorder patients. Sleep disturbances and traumatic nightmares may also be improved by medications, although patients should be cautioned that dissociative identity disorder and PTSD sleep disturbances may be particularly refractory to medications and respond best to cognitive and behavioral interventions directed at patients' severe PTSD reactivity to nighttime or even to sleeping. Recent research suggests that the α_1-adrenergic antagonist, prazosin (Minipress), may be helpful for PTSD nightmares. Case reports suggest that aggression may respond to carbamazepine in some individuals if EEG abnormalities are present. Many dissociative identity disorder patients show significant obsessive-compulsive symptoms. These patients may preferentially respond to antidepressants with antiobsessive efficacy. Open-label studies suggest that naltrexone (ReVia) may be helpful for amelioration of recurrent self-injurious behaviors in a subset of traumatized patients.

Questions are often raised about the efficacy of neuroleptic medications, particularly for symptoms such as hallucinations. Although neuroleptics are only minimally effective for quasi-psychotic symptoms, such as hallucinations, in many dissociative identity disorder patients, low doses may be useful in some cases for severe anxiety and for the subtle cognitive slippage found in some dissociative identity disorder patients. The newer atypical neuroleptics, such as risperidone (Risperdal), quetiapine (Seroquel), ziprasidone (Geodon), and olanzapine (Zyprexa), may be more effective and better tolerated than typical neuroleptics for overwhelming anxiety and intrusive PTSD symptoms in dissociative identity disorder patients. Occasionally, an extremely disorganized, overwhelmed, chronically ill dissociative identity disorder patient, who has not responded to trials of other neuroleptics, responds favorably to a trial of clozapine (Clozaril).

In general, to date, dissociative memory and process symptoms, as psychopharmacological targets in and of themselves, have proven refractory to medications. Dissociative-like symptoms and behaviors, however, can be induced in some PTSD patients and normal individuals with drugs (e.g., phencyclidine [PCP], cannabinoids), suggesting the presence of pharmacologically sensitive neurobiological mechanisms that may lead to future medications that may target dissociative symptoms per se.

Electroconvulsive Therapy During their long psychiatric careers of misdiagnosis and treatment failure, many dissociative identity disorder patients receive unsuccessful trials of ECT. This led to the view that ECT was not an effective treatment in the patient population. One small clinical study of severely depressed dissociative disorder patients, primarily with dissociative disorder NOS, suggested that, for some patients, ECT was helpful in ameliorating refractory mood disorders and did not worsen dissociative memory problems as measured by the DES. Clinical experience in tertiary care settings for severely ill dissociative identity disorder patients suggests that a clinical picture of major depression with persistent, refractory melancholic features across all alter states may predict a positive response to ECT. However, this response is usually only partial, as is typical for most successful somatic treatments in the dissociative identity disorder population.

Target symptoms and somatic treatments for dissociative identity disorder are listed in Table 17–19.

Inpatient Treatment As with patients with other psychiatric diagnoses, inpatient hospitalization is most commonly used for treatment of dissociative identity disorder patients who are acutely unsafe or completely destabilized, or both. Less commonly, in the age of managed care, hospitalization can be used to provide a safe environment in which to do intensive work with painful affects and memories. For a number of reasons, overt dissociative identity disorder patients can have disruptive effects on the milieu of general psychiatric units and often stimulate division and conflict among staff about the best way in which to relate to the patient and the alter personalities. Typically, the split is between the believers and the skeptics, often paralleling the larger societal debates as well as the subjective conflict within the patient about belief in the dissociative identity disorder diagnosis and the authenticity of traumatic memories. Inpatient programs specializing in the treatment of dissociative and PTSD patients may be more successful, because they provide a unified treatment approach in which rigorous boundaries and firm limit setting are combined with specific supportive treatment interventions to assist with dissociative and PTSD symptoms. Inpatient treatment on general hospital units is most successful if there is an attempt to bridge different opinions about dissociative identity disorder to focus on a unified approach for ameliorating specific target symptoms to allow the patient to resume outpatient treatment in safety.

In specialty and general hospital units, the patient should be expected to respond to his or her legal name, or at least one specific name, in the hospital milieu and in all therapeutic interactions, except individual psychotherapy or individual interactions with designated hospital staff. The patient should be expected to be able to present in a reasonably functional adult mode in the hospital, with regressed, dysfunctional, or child alters restricted to designated one-on-one encounters or private time in the patient's room or quiet room. The patient's activities in the hospital (e.g., group therapy) should be limited to those in which the patient can participate while following these guidelines. Some dissociative identity disorder patients may be so overwhelmed or overstimulated in the hospital that they need time in the quiet room. However, this can become a permanent berth for the patient, who may need to be weaned back into more routine hospital activities to prevent a major regression.

Dissociative identity disorder patients may experience hospital crisis management strategies, such as quiet room, all-staff call, or restraints, as abusive. Because of this, the patient should be urged to work proactively with staff to find reasonable clinical alternatives to help with possible dyscontrol. However, hospital staff may need to use restraints or similar measures if the dissociative identity disorder patient is acutely dangerous to self or others and if less restrictive alternatives have failed to deescalate the situation. In specialty units, restraints are often used less frequently with these patients than on general hospital units. Specialty unit staff are usually trained in helping dissociative identity disorder patients use symptom management and containment strategies to handle potential crises to minimize use of physical interventions to control behavior. Single doses of intramuscular (IM) neuroleptics, such as 2 to 5 mg of haloperidol (Haldol) or fluphenazine (Prolixin), with or without 1 to 2 mg of IM lorazepam (Ativan), may be helpful for management of acute dyscontrol in dissociative identity disorder patients by inducing sleep to allow a change in state once the patient reawakens. Sublingual olanzapine or intramuscular ziprasidone is a more costly alternative for this indication, assuming monitoring for cardiac side effects of ziprasidone. Anecdotal clinical reports suggest that the latter drugs have lower rates of oversedation and extrapyramidal (EPS) symptoms compared with older typical neuroleptics when used in this way.

As with other types of patients, discharge from hospital usually occurs when the acute crisis has been negotiated, the patient has made adequate gains in symptom management skills and internal communication to handle problems more adaptively, medications have been adjusted to provide better treatment of comorbid disorders, the outpatient psychosocial environment has restabilized sufficiently, or a treatment agreement for outpatient safety has been reached that is consistent with discharge to the next level of care, or a combination of these. To some extent, tertiary care specialty trauma disorders programs may be given more leeway by third-party providers to help patients develop a broader array of symptom management skills and to have time to work more intensively to stabilize symptomatic alter identities. Patients referred to these centers have commonly failed to improve, despite multiple previous general hospital stays. Because of this, third-party payers may be slightly more open to a longer specialty inpatient stay to reduce the potential for additional hospitalization.

Partial Hospitalization Partial hospital treatment can be an effective modality for the dissociative patient if clinical interventions target trauma-based issues and adaptations. Specialized trauma partial hospital programs with groups emphasizing symptom containment, cognitive and behavioral interventions, development of life skills, and psychoeducation can be effective in helping stabilize the more severely and persistently ill dissociative patients, as well as providing an intensive stabilization experience for higher-functioning dissociative identity disorder patients.

Adjunctive Treatments

GROUP THERAPY Authorities agree that, in therapy groups including general psychiatric patients, the emergence of alter personalities can be disruptive to the group process by eliciting excess fascination or by frightening other patients. Therapy groups composed only of dissociative identity disorder patients are reported to be more successful, although the groups must be carefully structured, must provide firm limits, and should generally focus only on here-and-now issues of coping and adaptation.

FAMILY THERAPY Family or couples therapy is often important for long-term stabilization and to address pathological family and marital processes that are common in dissociative identity disorder patients and their family members. Education of family and concerned others about dissociative identity disorder and dissociative identity disorder treatment may help family members cope more effectively with dissociative identity disorder and PTSD symptoms in their loved ones. Group interventions for education and support of family members have also been found helpful. In particular, family members should be discouraged from interacting with individual alters, calling them out, and relating to them as separate individuals. Family members should be helped to support the goal of the dissociative identity disorder patient becoming a functional adult in adult relationships and a functional parent to children. Sex therapy may be an important part of couple's treatment, as the dissociative identity disorder patient may become intensely phobic of intimate contact for periods of time, and spouses may have little idea how to deal with this in a helpful way.

Family therapy with the family of origin of the dissociative identity disorder patient is often extremely distressing to the dissociative identity disorder patient. Care must be exercised in setting up such meetings, because some interactions with family members may lead to an acute decompensation in the dissociative identity disorder patient. Accordingly, such contacts should be carefully structured for defined therapeutic purposes, and the patient should be well prepared for potential adverse reactions. However, such meetings may be helpful in clarifying or resolving the conflictual emotions that dissociative identity disorder patients frequently experience toward family members. Confrontation of family members about past traumas in an accusatory manner almost invariably has a disastrous outcome for the dissociative identity disorder patient and family members. Accordingly, there is usually little place for such interventions in dissociative identity disorder treatment.

EYE MOVEMENT DESENSITIZATION AND REPROCESSING (EMDR) EMDR is a treatment that has recently been advocated for adjunctive treatment of PTSD. There are disagreements in the literature about the usefulness and efficacy of this modality of treatment, and published efficacy studies are discrepant. No systematic studies have been done in dissociative identity disorder patients using EMDR. Case reports suggest that some dissociative identity disorder patients may be destabilized by EMDR procedures, with acutely increased PTSD and dissociative symptoms. Some authorities believe that EMDR can be used as an helpful adjunct for later phases of treatment in well-stabilized dissociative identity disorder outpatients.

SELF-HELP GROUPS Dissociative identity disorder patients usually have a negative outcome to self-help groups or 12-step groups for incest survivors. Accordingly, most experienced clinicians strongly discourage dissociative identity disorder patients' participation in these modalities. A variety of problematic issues occur in these settings, including intensification of PTSD symptoms due to discussion of trauma material without clinical safeguards, exploitation of the dissociative identity disorder patient by predatory group members, contamination of the dissociative identity disorder patient's recall by group discussions of trauma, and a feeling of alienation even from these other reputed sufferers of trauma and dissociation.

EXPRESSIVE AND OCCUPATIONAL THERAPIES Expressive and occupational therapies, such as art and movement therapy, have proven particularly helpful in treatment of dissociative identity disorder patients. Art therapy may be used for help with containment and structuring of severe dissociative identity disorder and PTSD symptoms, as well as to permit dissociative identity disorder patients safer expression of thoughts, feelings, mental images, and conflicts that they have difficulty verbalizing. Movement therapy may facilitate normalization of body sense and body image for these severely traumatized patients. Occupational therapy may help the patient with focused, structured activities that can be completed successfully and may help with grounding and symptom management.

Outcome Studies Single-case descriptions of successful treatments for dissociative identity disorder date back more than a century. Systematic outcome studies, however, have only appeared within the past few years. The first such study followed up 20 dissociative identity disorder patients at an average of 3 years after intake. The majority were in treatment with therapists who were unfamiliar with dissociative identity disorder. Nonetheless, two-thirds of the clinicians reported moderate to great improvement in their patients. A history of severe retraumatization during the course of treatment was associated with poorer outcomes. In the Netherlands, a chart review study of 101 dissociative disorder patients in outpatient treatment for an average of 6 years found that clinical improvement was related to the intensity of the treatment, with more comprehensive therapies having better outcomes. A study using the DES to track treatment progress of 21 dissociative identity disorder inpatients found a significant drop in overall scores over a 4-week hospitalization.

The largest and most systematic treatment outcome study reevaluated 54 dissociative identity disorder inpatients 2 years after discharge to outpatient treatment. As a group, there were significant overall decreases in psychopathology, including number of Axis I and Axis II disorders, decreased DES scores, decreased depression on the Beck Depression Index and the Hamilton Depression Scale, and decreased dissociative symptoms on all of the DDIS subscales. Patients who were reported integrated according to rigorous criteria were the most improved. Two studies investigating cost efficacy of dissociative identity disorder treatment have concordant findings suggesting that outcome depends on clinical subgroup. The more treatment-responsive group of dissociative identity disorder patients showed significant remission of symptoms within 3 to 5 years of beginning appropriate treatment. A second group with more alters and more personality disorder features showed good outcome but required hospitalizations in addition to outpatient treatment. A third group, characterized by the longest period of treatment before dissociative identity disorder diagnosis, largest number of alters, and most personality disorder problems, had a much longer, more costly, and more difficult course. Overall, however, treatment approaches specifically targeting dissociative identity disorder showed reductions in overall psychiatric treatment cost after the first year, compared to prior treatment for these patients. Some health maintenance organization (HMO) groups report that more intensive treatment benefits for dissociative identity disorder patients have not only reduced overall psychiatric costs, but also reduced costs for medical use for somatoform symptoms.

These preliminary studies have notable limitations, including the diverse and nonstandardized nature of the therapy and lack of comparison groups. Nonetheless, in aggregate, they indicate that many dissociative identity disorder patients improve with treatments focused on their dissociative symptoms and that overall treatment costs may be saved in the long term by using the phasic trauma treatment model for these patients.

DISSOCIATIVE DISORDER NOT OTHERWISE SPECIFIED

The category of dissociative disorder NOS covers all of the conditions characterized by a primary dissociative response that do not meet diagnostic criteria for one of the other DSM-IV-TR dissociative disorders. Dissociative disorder NOS cases must also fail to exclusively meet diagnostic criteria for acute stress disorder, PTSD, or somatization disorder, which all include dissociative symptoms among their criteria. Thus, dissociative disorder NOS is regarded clinically as a heterogeneous collection of dissociative reactions, some of which are common expressions of distress in other cultures but are relatively rare in Western societies.

There are few systematic studies of dissociative disorder NOS patients. Most authorities believe that there are two major dissociative disorder NOS subgroups. First is a group of patients similar in clinical presentation, life history, clinical course, and treatment response to those with dissociative identity disorder but whose sense of subjective self-division does not meet the first DSM-IV-TR criterion for a dissociative identity disorder alter identity or personality state. Rarely, a patient may present with the first two DSM-IV-TR criteria for dissociative identity disorder, but without apparent amnesia. Most of these dissociative identity disorder–like patients ultimately meet full criteria for dissociative identity disorder, but some never exhibit clear alter identities or demonstrate dissociative amnesia and continue to be diagnosed with dissociative disorder NOS.

The other dissociative disorder NOS subgroup is a heterogeneous collection of patients with a variety of dissociative symptoms and multiple comorbidities, usually accompanied by a past history of severe trauma at some time in life. One study found that the dissociative disorder NOS patients had DES scores that were intermediate between those of patients with dissociative amnesia and those diagnosed with dissociative identity disorder.

Mr. P. is a 22-year-old unmarried man admitted to a psychiatric hospital for assessment and treatment after a serious suicide attempt following an altercation with his girlfriend.

On admission history and mental status examination, Mr. P. reported extensive involvement in an inner fantasy world to which he retreated when life became overwhelming. He had done poorly in school, despite his documented high intelligence, because of "spacing out," losing track of class work owing to intense daydreaming. Sometimes, his inner world was filled with frightening and confusing images, but, mostly, it was a place of retreat. He reported rapid changes in his sense of age, acting child-like, adolescent, and adult in alternation. He reported amnesia for many years of his childhood, although he could recall some of it. He described ongoing amnesia experiences with disremembered behavior, inexplicable changes in abilities, repeatedly spacing out while driving, and loss of time. He denied the existence of fully developed alter identities but felt subdivided into "colors" that represented different emotions and age states. He did not experience loss of sense of self across these state changes but experienced himself and was observed to behave differently when he reported changes in these states. He reported chronic dysphoric mood, anxiety, fear of falling asleep, nightmares, and panic when physically touched in certain ways, although he could not explain why this was. He had significant OCD symptoms, compulsively arranging things in particular ways and panicking if they were changed.

He grew up in a family of "workaholic alcoholics." All adult members of his own and extended family drank heavily, although Mr. P. experienced them as "more pleasant" when drinking than when preoccupied with work. Family members frequently teased him brutally because of his emotional sensitivity and anxiety. He denied intrafamilial sexual abuse or frequent physical discipline, although he reported occasionally being beaten or struck by his parents. For the most part, he was left to himself. From 4 years of age to approximately 12 years of age, he was sent to religious schools, day care, and camps. He reported inexplicable obsessive preoccupations with those experiences, although he could not recall much about them, including whether anything distressing, overwhelming, or traumatic had occurred in these settings. During the years in which he attended these schools and camps, he developed repeated unexplained rectal bleeding from anal fissures and hepatitis B. No medical explanation was reportedly found for these illnesses.

An intensive psychological assessment battery, including the Minnesota Multiphasic Personality Inventory (MMPI), personality inventories, projective tests, intelligence tests, and the SCID-D-R, supported a diagnosis of dissociative disorder NOS, intense preoccupation with traumatic imagery similar to PTSD patients, but without a clear history of trauma, and a subtle atypical thought disorder. Hypnotizability testing showed that Mr. P. scored high on standardized hypnosis scaling.

Treatment included a variety of cognitive behavioral strategies to provide alternatives to fantasy withdrawal when experiencing dysphoria or strong affects. He was taught self-hypnosis to increase control over spontaneously occurring hypnotic experiences. He responded well to trials of 150 mg of fluvoxamine daily and 20 mg of ziprasidone twice a day for mood, anxiety, OCD, and thought confusion symptoms. He began to have more recall of aspects of his early life for which he had been amnestic, including frightening images with sexual content related to the religious school. Family meetings were held with his parents to review the developmental history, for Mr. P. to address his concerns about his treatment during childhood, and to help improve his relationship with his parents. He was discharged with diagnoses of dissociative disorder NOS, anxiety disorder NOS, and mood disorder NOS. Personality configuration was thought to include avoidant, dependent, and schizotypal features.

A Japanese study of 19 dissociative patients, compared to normal and psychiatric controls, diagnosed with Japanese versions of the DES and SCID-D-R, found a similar pattern of DES scores as in non-Japanese samples. However, more dissociative disorder NOS subjects and fewer dissociative identity disorder subjects than expected were diagnosed on the SCID-D-R, although the highest DES scores were found in the dissociative disorder NOS patients. The authors speculated that different cultural attributions and meanings of the subjective self and normal Japanese encouragement of highly developed social and private selves might account for more dissociative disorders NOS being diagnosed on the SCID-D-R in Japanese subjects.

Cultural Variants of Dissociative Disorders

Included within dissociative disorder NOS are the many cultural variants of dissociative trance. Anthropologists have identified forms of dissociation within every culture that they have examined. In some instances, this takes the form of specific trance state disorders; in others, it is manifest in religious rites and rituals; and, in still others, it is manifest in the form of traditional healing practices. All of these forms of dissociation are common in many non-Western societies. Increasingly, measures such as the DES and SCID-D-R are being adapted for these cultures and used to investigate these conditions.

The DSM-IV-TR also includes under dissociative disorder NOS (Table 17–20) those dissociative reactions elicited by coercive persuasive practices, such as torture, brainwashing, thought reform, mind control, and indoctrination intended to induce an individual to relinquish basic political, social, or religious beliefs in exchange for antithetical ideas and beliefs. Finally, Ganser syndrome, a rare and poorly understood condition, characterized by the giving of approximate answers, is also included in this category.

The ICD-10 (Table 17–1) classifies all dissociative (conversion) disorders in one section, which includes the conditions (trance and possession disorders, dissociative convulsions, and Ganser syndrome) that are carried under dissociative disorder NOS in the DSM-IV-TR.

Dissociative Trance Disorder

Definition

Dissociative trance disorder is manifest by a temporary, marked alteration in the state of consciousness or by loss of the customary sense of personal identity without the replacement by an alternate sense of identity (Table 17–21). There is often a narrowing of awareness of the immediate surroundings or a selective focus on stimuli within the environment and the manifestation of stereotypical behaviors or movements that the individual experiences as beyond his or her control. A variant of this, possession trance, involves single or episodic alternations in the state of consciousness, characterized by the exchange of the person's customary identity by a new identity usually attributed to a spirit, divine power, deity, or another person. In this possessed state, the individual exhibits stereotypical and culturally determined behaviors or experiences being controlled by the possessing entity. There must be partial or full amnesia for the event. The trance or possession state must not be a normally accepted part of a cultural or religious practice and must cause significant distress or functional impairment in one or more of the usual domains. Finally, the dissociative trance state must not occur exclusively during the course of a psychotic disorder and is not the result of any substance or general medical condition.

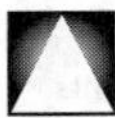

Table 17–20
DSM-IV-TR Diagnostic Criteria for Dissociative Disorder Not Otherwise Specified

This category is included for disorders in which the predominant feature is a dissociative symptom (i.e., a disruption in the usually integrated functions of consciousness, memory, identity, or perception of the environment) that does not meet the criteria for any specific dissociative disorder. Examples include the following:

(1) Clinical presentations similar to dissociative identity disorder that fail to meet full criteria for this disorder. Examples include presentations in which (a) there are not two or more distinct personality states or (b) amnesia for important personal information does not occur.

(2) Derealization unaccompanied by depersonalization in adults.

(3) States of dissociation that occur in individuals who have been subjected to periods of prolonged and intense coercive persuasion (e.g., brainwashing, thought reform, or indoctrination while captive).

(4) Dissociative trance disorder: single or episodic disturbances in the state of consciousness, identity, or memory that are indigenous to particular locations and cultures. Dissociative trance involves narrowing of awareness of immediate surroundings or stereotyped behaviors or movements that are experienced as being beyond one's control. Possession trance involves replacement of the customary sense of personal identity by a new identity, attributed to the influence of a spirit, power, deity, or other person and associated with stereotyped involuntary movements or amnesia, and is perhaps the most common dissociative disorder in Asia. Examples include *amok* (Indonesia), *bebainan* (Indonesia), *latah* (Malaysia), *pibloktoq* (Arctic), *ataque de nervios* (Latin America), and possession (India). The dissociative or trance disorder is not a normal part of a broadly accepted collective cultural or religious practice.

(5) Loss of consciousness, stupor, or coma not attributable to a general medical condition.

(6) Ganser syndrome: the giving of approximate answers to questions (e.g., 2 + 2 = 5) when not associated with dissociative amnesia or dissociative fugue.

From American Psychiatric Association. *Diagnostic and Statistical Manual of Mental Disorders.* 4th ed. Text rev. Washington, DC: American Psychiatric Association; 2000, with permission.

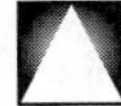

Table 17–21
DSM-IV-TR Research Criteria for Dissociative Trance Disorder

A. Either (1) or (2):

(1) Trance, that is, temporary marked alteration in the state of consciousness or loss of customary sense of personal identity without replacement by an alternate identity, associated with at least one of the following:

(a) Narrowing of awareness of immediate surroundings or unusually narrow and selective focusing on environmental stimuli

(b) Stereotyped behaviors or movements that are experienced as being beyond one's control

(2) Possession trance, a single or episodic alteration in the state of consciousness characterized by the replacement of customary sense of personal identity by a new identity. This is attributed to the influence of a spirit, power, deity, or other person, as evidenced by one or more of the following:

(a) Stereotyped and culturally determined behaviors or movements that are experienced as being controlled by the possessing agent

(b) Full or partial amnesia for the event

B. The trance or possession trance state is not accepted as a normal part of a collective cultural or religious practice.

C. The trance or possession trance state causes clinically significant distress or impairment in social, occupational, or other important areas of functioning.

D. The trance or possession trance state does not occur exclusively during the course of a psychotic disorder (including mood disorder with psychotic features and brief psychotic disorder) or dissociative identity disorder and is not due to the direct physiological effects of a substance or a general medical condition.

From American Psychiatric Association. *Diagnostic and Statistical Manual of Mental Disorders.* 4th ed. Text rev. Washington, DC: American Psychiatric Association; 2000, with permission.

Ataque de Nervios

Diagnosis and Clinical Features *Ataque de nervios* is the best studied example of the dissociative trance state disorder form of dissociative disorder NOS. It is characterized by somatic symptoms, such as fainting, numbness and tingling, fading of vision, seizure-like convulsive movements, palpitations, and sensations of heat rising through the body. Individuals may moan, cry out, curse uncontrollably, attempt to harm themselves or others, or fall down and lie with death-like stillness. During the episode, there is a narrowing of consciousness and a lack of awareness of the larger environment. After the episode, the individual usually reports partial or full amnesia for the events and their actions. Attacks may occur only once, may be episodic, or occasionally may become chronically recurring with significant functional impairment. Frequency of *ataques* was correlated with DES scores in one study.

Etiology Triggers seem most often to involve family, marital, or other interpersonal conflicts or losses. Alcohol, physical or sexual violence, financial loss, or stress and fear may also precipitate an attack. Histories of physical and sexual abuse are common but are not well correlated with frequency or severity of episodes. The triggering event may initially evoke a sense of being overwhelmed, hopeless, and helpless. This is followed by an abrupt shift in state of consciousness, with a narrowing of consciousness and the development of more florid symptoms. Attacks can last from minutes to days but are usually a few hours in duration.

Epidemiology Contributing demographic factors include being female; being 45 years of age or older; being divorced, separated, or widowed; having less than a high school education; and living in poverty. In Puerto Rico, there is an estimated lifetime prevalence rate of approximately 14 percent for *ataque de nervios*.

Differential Diagnosis There is often significant comorbidity with depression, anxiety disorders, agoraphobia, and PTSD. *Ataque de nervios* is differentiated from these disorders by its dissociative alterations in consciousness and somatosensory motor disturbances. This condition may be a manifestation of dissociative identity disorder.

Treatment Episodes usually end with the intervention of others, who may restrain the victim if he or she is in danger or assaultive or may otherwise calm him or her. Praying, rituals, use of herb or alcohol rubs, or other folk medicine interventions are common. In addition, the individual's distress and symptoms usually elicit increased social support or prompt interventions to reduce the stressors that precipitated the attack. In most instances, professional help is not sought. In cases in which the triggering stressors are deemed minor by the victim's significant others or there are concerns about chronicity, the patient may be brought for psychiatric treatment. No clinical trials have been conducted as yet, but some success is reported with antidepressant and antianxiety medications.

Possession Trance

Diagnosis and Clinical Features Although the Greeks believed in divine possession, it was not part of their explanation for mental illness, which was largely subsumed under the label of melancholia, thought to be a disorder of the black bile. Demonic possession, as an explanation for psychological distress and mental illness, appears to date to the first century AD in Palestine and was common in New Testament writings. During the Middle Ages, demonic possession was widely regarded as the cause of lunacy and epilepsy. Canon law forbade the ordination of any individual who had been publicly possessed for this reason. Even as the medical nature of mental illness and epilepsy became increasingly documented, rejection of the diabolical notion of possession proceeded surprisingly slowly and unevenly. Today, there are numerous religious subcultures within the United States that believe in possession, demonic and divine, and practice exorcism or spirit possession rituals. Possession trance is common in many third-world cultures. Anthropological studies suggest that possession and exorcism occur most commonly in oppressive societies in which there is alienation from the establishment, and protest or direct action is dangerous or unacceptable.

The initial onset of possession trance is often similar to that of dissociative trance state, with an acute triggering stressor followed shortly thereafter by convulsive or uncontrolled movements, trembling, flailing, or fainting. Then, the individual may lapse into a stupor or may appear to be struggling in the grip of an unseen force, when, suddenly, a distinctly different personality emerges. A dramatic physical and psychological transformation may occur in the individual's face, voice, demeanor, and behavior.

The personality may identify itself as external to and distinct from the personality of the possessed individual. Sometimes, it has to be tricked or coaxed into revealing itself. It may claim to be a deity, demon, spirit, ghost, deceased relative, or historic individual. This personality, imbued with these attributes, now focuses attention on the conflicts or stressors that triggered the possession. It may make demands or may suggest structural realignment within the social group to ease the precipitating conditions. If these demands are met, then the possession entity agrees to relinquish control of the victim. During the period of possession, the individual may exhibit unusual strength, agility, or other abilities or may behave in a dangerous or threatening fashion. Possession episodes usually last hours to days. In some instances, it can become chronically disabling.

Spirit possession, although not a disorder where it is religiously sanctioned, shares many similarities with possession trance. Known to occur in many regions of the world, especially western Africa, the Caribbean, and South America, spirit possession is usually induced through rituals characterized by rapid, loud drumming, feverish dancing, and, sometimes, native intoxicants. As the spirit begins to catch, there is often a dramatic transformation. The individual may stagger, sway, or fall into the arms of bystanders. The body may tremble or convulse. The face may change, the voice may deepen, and another personality becomes apparent. Bystanders may further the transformation by dressing the individual in clothing appropriate for the identified spirit or otherwise addressing it in a worthy fashion. While possessed, the individual may dance with even greater agitation and force or may circulate among the crowd, addressing people, questioning their health, or making pointed suggestions. Sometimes, the individual becomes childish, may stutter or speak with a lisp, may soil him- or herself, or may use vulgar language.

Ceremonially induced spirit possession typically lasts minutes to hours, with an average duration of approximately 1 hour in one review. As with dissociative trance state disorder, the individual is largely amnesic for his or her behavior and the events of the possession episode. In some instances, the individual acts as a messenger of the powers. With one foot in the world of the deities and the other among men and women, the messenger exists in a halfway state between full possession and normal behavior and usually retains memory for the events of the possession.

Etiology

Anthropological studies strongly implicate personal crisis as a common precipitant. In such cases, special attention is paid to the messages and advice given by the power as reported and interpreted by the audience. Dreams or visions may also precipitate possession, although these are generally more fleeting events. Spiritual leaders may seek spirit possession as a source of guidance for their communities or to locate lost individuals or sacred objects. Sometimes, spirit possession is experienced as a punishment for profaning a sacred site or angering a deity. In most instances, possession trance appears to be in the service of reducing overwhelming stressors or resolving an acute crisis in the individual's life. It also provides an opportunity to express forbidden impulses, to behave in socially unacceptable ways, to assume cross-gender roles, and to influence people important to the possessed.

Epidemiology

Possession trance disorders have been described in many third-world countries. The Indian psychiatric literature contains the most systematic descriptions and largest number of cases. In India, possession syndrome or hysterical possession is the most common form of dissociative disorder, whereas dissociative identity disorder is thought to be exceedingly rare. Prevalence of possession trance in India has been estimated to range from 1 to 4 percent of the general population, but the data on which this estimate is based may not truly be representative. Epidemics of possession syndrome have been reported in the context of larger social crises.

Differential Diagnosis

Possession trance differs from dissociative identity disorder in that (1) it is generally a sharply time-limited condition (usually hours), (2) it is usually related to immediate stressors, (3) the possessing personality seeks to differentiate itself as external to the victim, and (4) the possessing personality is usually recognizable to its audience by its stereotypical speech and behavior. Possession trance may be mistaken for a psychotic state when clinicians are not familiar with the cultural traditions of an individual's ethnic group.

In the United States, some religious groups view the alter identities in dissociative identity disorder as manifestations of demonic possession. Dissociative identity disorder patients from these subcultures may feel torn between the religious pressure from their family and friends and the views of their treating clinicians. Commonly, these dissociative identity disorder individuals have alter identities who subscribe to the religious view of their social group and other alters who do not. An additional complexity is that dissociative identity disorder patients from these sociocultural milieus, and from other backgrounds as well, not uncommonly have self-states that identify themselves as demonic, angelic, or of other spiritual types. In one study of dissociative identity disorder patients who had been subjected to exorcism, the outcome was uniformly negative, with marked clinical worsening, increased mistrust of religious and clinical caregivers, and a more difficult overall treatment course.

Treatment

Individuals with possession trance or spirit possession seldom seek treatment outside of the individual's family or ethnic group. Intervention is most likely to come from family or traditional healers, who may perform an exorcism if the individual appears to be in great distress or spiritual danger. When psychiatric help is sought, the presence of dissociative identity disorder, a psychotic disorder, PTSD, or an affective disorder should be assessed.

Brainwashing

Definition

The concept of *brainwashing* or *thought reform* emerged from Western reactions to the Soviet Communist show trials of the late 1940s and alarm over Communist Chinese methods of coercive political reeducation that were central to the ideology of Mao Tse-Tung. These fears intensified during the Korean conflict after many American prisoners of war made anti-American statements. In 1950, a journalist, Edward Hunter (later identified as a Central Intelligence Agency [CIA] agent) proposed that the Chinese Communists had discovered techniques to modify mental attitudes and beliefs, a process that he called *brainwashing*.

After the Armistice, a team of psychiatrists and psychologists, including Robert J. Lifton and Edgar Schein, interviewed the returning prisoners. Similar studies done for the CIA also obtained information from Communist interrogators and former Soviet and Chinese prisoners. These studies concluded that the apparent brainwashing of these prisoners, as well as of the victims of the Russian show trials, was the result of extreme police interrogation techniques involving severe physical and psychological deprivation, followed by rewarding the severely deprived prisoners with the possibility of the end of their ordeal, as well as food and warm clothing. The reports concluded that the basic attitudes of the American prisoners in Korea had not, in fact, been altered.

However, the subsequent release of another group of prisoners (missionaries, businessmen, doctors, and students) caught in China at the beginning of the war did seem to suggest that some form of thought reform had occurred with these individuals, several of whom continued to falsely insist that they were spies. In a second round of studies, Lifton, Schein, and others concluded that changes in an individual's basic beliefs could occur in the context of extreme physical, psychological, and social coercion. The use of extreme group persuasion methods by the Chinese Communists on political prisoners may have been influential in this outcome. Clinical presentations of individuals subjected to extreme forms of coercive persuasion may resemble those of survivors of other sorts of torture.

One legacy of the fear of Communist brainwashing was the unfortunate misuse of psychiatry and psychology by the CIA and other U.S. government agencies from the late 1940s and onward to develop methods of behavioral control, which was revealed in release of government documents and Congressional hearings in the 1970s. In an effort to combat or to preempt potential Communist use of mind control, the CIA studied or supported studies of psychedelic drugs and other toxins and intoxicants, radiation, hypnosis, sensory deprivation, repeated ECT treatments, and bizarre conditioning experiments, among others, often on unwitting civilian or military subjects. At least one subject killed himself during an LSD experiment, and other psychiatric casualties have brought suits against the U.S. and Canadian governments because of damage caused them during CIA-funded experiments.

According to reviews of CIA documents, some CIA officials apparently believed in the possibility of using hypnosis to create assassins or spies with hypnotically induced alter identities or amnesia, or both, who could thus resist interrogation and torture. However, it has been reported that other CIA officials in charge of mind control experiments doubted that this could be done successfully. Because CIA officials destroyed many documents relating to these activities, it is not known to what extent these experiments were ever attempted. Popularized accounts continue to suggest that the U.S. government attempted to create multiple-personality spies. However, a careful reading of cases purported to demonstrate this show that, based on available information, most bear little similarity to clinical dissociative identity disorder.

Allegations of brainwashing or mind control resurfaced in the late 1960s and 1970s in the context of counterculture religious movements. This theory was also advanced by a group of defense psychiatric experts that included Louis J. West, Lifton, Martin Orne, and Margaret T. Singer in the famous case of Patty Hearst, the heiress who was kidnapped, tortured, sexually abused, and held in prolonged solitary confinement by a radical cult-like group. After many months of this treatment, Hearst was said to have transformed her identity into that of the revolutionary Tania, who aided her captors in criminal acts, including bank robbery and murder. The Patty Hearst jury was not convinced, however, and convicted Hearst despite the arguments of the defense psychiatric experts.

Singer subsequently widely publicized her ideas about conditioning techniques that she believed were used by religious cults to render their members incapable of complex rational thought and unable to make decisions. In a series of lawsuits by ex-members against various religious cults, she testified that these techniques were capable of overpowering a person's free will and that the group's control over a member could be total. These often sensational trials instilled in the public the notion of brainwashing as a common practice in religious cults.

In response, a group of academics, primarily psychologists and sociologists, challenged Singer, pointing out that members often came from dysfunctional families and joined cults to avoid the anxieties and responsibilities of independence. Psychiatrist Marc Galanter reframed the religious cult mind-control debate by advocating the more neutral term *charismatic religious sects* and pointing out that an individual's behavior within such a social group may reflect psychological adaptation rather than psychopathology. Surveys and studies of ex-cult members indicated that the manner of leaving the group, voluntarily or by being involuntarily deprogrammed, was a significant determinant of their subsequent assessment of whether they had been brainwashed, with the latter the most likely to express this belief.

In the context of a particularly sensational case, the American Psychological Association and American Sociological Association submitted *amicus* briefs refuting the concept of brainwashing as lacking scientific validity, which has had the larger effect of essentially nullifying its legal status. Although the academic community has largely avoided the topic in the last decade, the notion of brainwashing, in which individuals are rendered hypersuggestible through hypnosis, drugs, or physical stressors, and their belief systems are transformed by special conditioning techniques, continues to fascinate the public and to be invoked by a few psychotherapists and others as evidence of occult or government conspiracies.

At the same time, some researchers on destructive cults have continued to suggest that cult membership produces an ego state or dissociated self-aspect that allows the person to function ego-syntonically within the cult milieu. This entity is not conceptualized as meeting diagnostic criteria for a dissociative identity disorder alter identity but suggests a diagnosis of dissociative disorder NOS. Research studies to attempt to fully explicate such issues are likely to be exceptionally difficult to perform.

The military stress studies of Morgan and colleagues prove, however, that combinations of pain, hunger, cold, fatigue, fear, sensory deprivation, and control over bodily functions and social communication can profoundly alter an individual's state of consciousness, producing prominent dissociative symptoms. The accompanying degree of identity alteration induced by such techniques remains to be empirically established, but it seems possible that dissociative reactions could account for many of the psychological changes reported in captive individuals subjected to coercive interrogation and persuasion.

Diagnosis and Clinical Features Individuals who have been subjected to extreme coercive techniques are at risk for persistent depersonalization and, possibly, other dissociative symptoms, including amnesias, trance-like behaviors, and emotional numbing. They may exhibit reduced cognitive flexibility, behavioral regression, and profound changes in values, attitudes, beliefs, and sense of self. In some instances, an alter self state may emerge that identifies with former tormentors and behaves in a fashion contrary to the individual's prior behavior. This alter self usually disappears or weakens significantly when the individual is returned to safety and security but may be transiently reactivated by circumstances reminiscent of the traumatic events.

Treatment There are no empirical studies of the treatment of individuals subjected to extreme coercion applied in the service of indoctrination of a belief system or an attempt at identity alteration. The basic principles of phased trauma treatment would seem to provide an organizing framework for treatment of these individuals, as it has for victims of other forms of torture. This begins with the creation of safety and symptom stabilization, along with educational information to help normalize the individuals' response. This is followed, when and if appropriate, by a supportive but nonsuggestive exploration of the events and experiences to desensitize their memory and to integrate them better into the individuals' transformed sense of self. Any preexisting psychopathology likely is exacerbated by such experiences and should be addressed as the dissociative symptoms abate. Family interventions may be necessary as a result of the duress and disruption accompanying the precipitating events and the social effects of the profound changes in the individuals' attitudes, behaviors, and beliefs.

Ganser Syndrome

Definition Ganser syndrome is a poorly understood condition, reclassified from a factitious disorder to a dissociative disorder in the DSM-III, characterized by the giving of approximate answers (paralogia) together with a clouding of consciousness, and frequently accompanied by hallucinosis and other dissociative, somatoform, or conversion symptoms. First described by Dr. S. J. M. Ganser in an 1897 lecture entitled "A Peculiar Hysterical State," who observed that the "most obvious sign consists of their inability to answer correctly the simplest questions which are asked to them even though by many of their answers, they indicate that they have grasped a large part of the sense of the question." Ganser offered the example of a patient who, when asked how many noses he had, replied "I don't know if I have a nose."

Diagnosis and Clinical Features The symptom of *passing over* (*vorbeigehen*) the correct answer for a related, but incorrect one, is the hallmark of Ganser syndrome. The approximate answers often just miss the mark but bear an obvious relation to the question, indicating that it has been understood. When asked how old she was, a 25-year-old woman answered, "I'm not five." Another patient, when asked how many legs a horse had, replied "three." If asked to do simple calculations (e.g., $2 \times 2 = 5$), for general information (the capital of the United States is New York), to identify simple objects (a pencil is a key), or to name colors (green is grey), the Ganser patient gives erroneous but comprehensible answers.

There is also a clouding of consciousness, usually manifest by disorientation, amnesias, loss of personal information, and some impairment of reality testing. Visual and auditory hallucinations occur in roughly one-half of the cases. Many of the case reports include histories of head injuries, dementia, or organic brain insults. Neurological examination may reveal what Ganser called *hysterical stigmata*, for example, a nonneurological analgesia or shifting hyperalgesia. Many authorities make a distinction between Ganser symptoms of approximate answers, which may occur in a number of psychiatric and neurological conditions, and Ganser syndrome, which must be accompanied by other dissociative symptoms, such as amnesias, conversion symptoms, or trance-like behaviors.

Epidemiology Cases have been reported in a variety of cultures, but the overall frequency of such reports has declined with time. This may reflect trends in diagnosis, case reporting, or a genuine decline in cases. In the clinical literature, men outnumber women by approximately 2 to 1. Three of Ganser's first four cases were convicts, leading some authors to consider it to be a disorder of penal populations and, thus, an indicator of potential malingering. Ganser believed that he had adequately ruled out this possibility, and most authorities are convinced that these patients have a genuine disorder. Subsequent case series indicate that it occurs in other settings and is not unique to prisoners.

Etiology Some case reports identify precipitating stressors, such as personal conflicts and financial reverses, whereas others note organic brain syndromes, head injuries, seizures, and medical or psychiatric illness. Psychodynamic explanations are common in the older literature, but organic etiologies are stressed in more recent case studies. It is speculated that the organic insults may act as acute stressors, precipitating the syndrome in vulnerable individuals. Some patients have reported significant histories of childhood maltreatment and adversity.

Differential Diagnosis Given the reported frequent history of organic brain syndromes, seizures, head trauma, and psychosis in Ganser syndrome, a thorough neurological and medical evaluation is warranted. Differential diagnoses include organic dementia, depressive pseudodementia, the confabulation of Korsakoff's syndrome, organic dysphasias, and reactive psychoses. Dissociative identity disorder patients occasionally may also exhibit Ganser-like symptoms.

Treatment There have been no systematic treatment studies, given the rarity of this condition. In most case reports, the patient has been hospitalized and has been provided with a protective and supportive environment. In some instances, low doses of antipsychotic medications have been reported to be beneficial. Confrontation or interpretations of the patient's approximate answers are not productive, but exploration of possible stressors may be helpful. Hypnosis and amobarbital narcosynthesis have also been used successfully to help patients reveal the underlying stressors that preceded the development of the syndrome, with concomitant cessation of the Ganser symptoms. Usually, there is a relatively rapid return to normal function within days, although some cases may take a month or more to resolve. The individual is typically amnesic for the period of the syndrome.

FORENSIC ISSUES AND DISSOCIATIVE DISORDERS

Individuals with dissociative disorders present a variety of problems in criminal and civil law. In criminal law, defendants claiming to have dissociative identity disorder have been associated with highly publicized cases, primarily seeking exculpation through the insanity defense. However, dissociative identity disorder individuals have also appeared as alleged victims or witnesses in criminal actions. Many of these cases have been subject to intense media coverage. Malingered dissociative identity disorder and amnesia are major concerns when claims of not guilty by reason of insanity (NGRI) or diminished capacity for criminal acts are broached. However, less publicized dissociative identity disorder defendants have been accused of driving while intoxicated (DWI), shoplifting, theft, check kiting, embezzlement, credit card fraud, child abuse and neglect, stalking, and many other crimes. They also may be plaintiffs, particularly in cases involving interpersonal aggression: domestic violence, stalking, and rape.

Dissociative individuals also commonly appear in civil law cases. They may be plaintiffs in a variety of tort suits, commonly malpractice litigation, sexual harassment, and therapist misconduct complaints. They also may appear in workers' compensation matters, disability litigation, and family law related to divorce and child custody evaluations, among many others. Some dissociative disorder patients have sued alleged abusers, usually parents, claiming damages for previously forgotten childhood abuse using the delayed discovery rule. Conversely, individuals diagnosed with dissociative disorders—usually dissociative identity disorder—have sued for malpractice, alleging that the diagnosis was erroneous or iatrogenically created and that the plaintiff was harmed by therapy focused on therapeutically induced false memories of childhood maltreatment based on a belief in repressed memory. Some of the latter plaintiffs had previously sued or prosecuted their parents for abuse before recanting and suing their therapists!

State jurisdictions may differ among themselves and with the federal courts on a variety of legal issues, such as NGRI, diminished capacity, criminal intent, competence, statutes of limitations, capacity to give testimony, and allowance of testimony about amnesia for trauma. Different jurisdictions have been divergent in their approach to dissociative individuals as well. At least one district court rejected dissociative identity disorder as a valid diagnosis to be considered for an insanity defense plea, but this ruling was reversed on appeal. Other courts have diverged in findings of criminal responsibility for dissociative identity disorder individuals, based on differing ways of viewing which alter was responsible for the criminal acts.

In the criminal arena, *mens rea*, the state of mind indicating culpability for criminal acts, may seem hard to determine in an individual who claims dense amnesia for crimes or who experiences himself or herself as self-states that variously profess or deny responsibility for criminal behavior. Some legal scholars have suggested that dissociative disorders in the criminal courts raise issues related to an *actus reus* defense, based on the inability to control involuntary actions, as in crimes committed in epileptic or somnambulistic states. In this regard, in one recent high-profile criminal case, depersonalization was used successfully as a basis for a finding of lack of criminal responsibility due to involuntary action, claimed by a defendant who shot and wounded an alleged past abuser.

Dissociative Identity Disorder and the Law The intersection between the diagnosis of dissociative identity disorder and the legal system has proven to be exceedingly controversial. The contentious dispute over its existence, the often sensationalized media attention, and the need to rule out simulation or malingering have made the forensic evaluation of dissociative identity disorder difficult to perform and to defend. In criminal matters, the most common claims are that (1) dissociative identity disorder defendants do not have control over or are not conscious of their alter personalities and therefore cannot be held responsible for their actions; (2) dissociative identity disorder defendants are not competent, because they cannot recall the actions of their alter self-states and therefore cannot participate in their own defense; and (3) a diagnosis of dissociative identity disorder makes it impossible for a defendant to conform to the law or to know right from wrong. Evidentiary questions, including the admissibility of material gathered with hypnotic or amobarbital interviews and the reliability or relative independence of testimony by different alter identities, have raised difficult legal questions.

In general, trial and appeals courts in state and federal jurisdictions have ruled that dissociative identity disorder meets Frye or Daubert criteria, or both, so that it may be used legitimately as a criminal defense, and so that dissociative identity disorder individuals can testify in court in alter identities and in dissociative states.

In many cases, courts have struggled with the reification of the alter identities, confusing their cognitions and behaviors with those of separate persons and failing to view the alters as *mental constructs* with relatively independent cognitions, affects, and memory systems with a capacity for behavioral and role enactment.

In fact, one extreme legal theory has posited that dissociative identity disorder self-states *should* be treated like separate individuals, so that those uninvolved in criminal behavior would, by definition, be absolved of responsibility, and a finding of not guilty by reason of insanity would be mandated. Conversely, clinicians experienced in the treatment of dissociative identity disorder have found that holding the whole human being responsible for the behavior of any part is far more likely to lead to clinical progress and increased function. An attempt to absolve or to excuse the patient of responsibility for maladaptive or antisocial behaviors is apt to lead to spiraling regression and escalating dysfunction.

Accordingly, these authorities have recommended that the *clinical standard* of holding the whole human being responsible for the behavior of any part be the foundation for any legal consideration of diminished responsibility for criminal conduct in the dissociative identity disorder individual. An *affirmative* case should be made that the dissociative identity disorder defendant meets the standard for legal insanity or diminished capacity, just as would be the case for any psychiatric defense.

Similarly, forensic commentators have argued that it is vital not to confuse the behavior of an individual experiencing himself or herself as an alter identity with the mental states and behaviors of separate persons. These authorities suggest careful attention to avoid reification of the dissociative identity disorder alters and a focus on the symptoms and mental state of the whole individual at the time of the criminal act.

There is no pathognomonic presentation of dissociative identity disorder in the criminal setting. However, authorities suggest that genuine dissociative identity disorder defendants are more likely to show a complex alter system, not just a good–bad alter dichotomy. Bona fide dissociative identity disorder individuals may have bizarre explanations for why and how they (in alter identities) committed crimes, not just "the bad one did it." Authorities also describe a number of dissociative identity disorder defendants as *minimizing* their psychiatric symptoms and attempting to *avoid* being labeled psychiatrically ill, although a few exaggerate bona fide dissociative identity disorder symptoms. Genuine dissociative identity disorder defendants may behave in self-defeating and problematic ways that may undermine the success of their defenses.

Mr. A. was arrested and charged with the murder of his long-time gay lover. The circumstances of the case were complex and bizarre. Mr. A. called the police on the night of the murder claiming that his lover was holding him hostage and was going to kill him. He stated that his lover was heavily armed and was prepared to kill police officers if they stormed the house. A Special Weapons and Tactics (SWAT) team was dispatched, contacted Mr. A. by phone, and spent the next several hours attempting to talk him out of the house. He spoke with them in a child-like voice, identified himself by a diminutive of his actual name, and described hiding in a closet with his pet. He appeared completely terrified, repeatedly stating that he was going to be killed, that "the man" was dangerous and armed, and that he would be shot if he attempted to flee. Eventually, the police stormed the house, located Mr. A. hiding behind a couch, and found his lover in the bedroom, dead of multiple gunshot wounds. Ballistics tests and other forensic evidence indicated that Mr. A. had shot his lover, who had been killed before the phone call to the police was initiated. At the time of his arrest, Mr. A. claimed no memory of the shooting, although he did describe a frightening altercation earlier in the evening in which he stated that his lover had threatened to kill him for an alleged infidelity (which Mr. A. denied).

Mr. A.'s attorney sought a finding of incompetence, because Mr. A. could not assist in his defense owing to lack of recall of the shooting. A court-appointed forensics team had Mr. A. transferred to a state forensics facility for assessment. There, Mr. A. engaged in a variety of bizarre, confusing, and self-defeating behaviors. He was alternately overly compliant, defiant and oppositional, child-like and confused, and provocative and angry. On occasion, he identified himself by different names. Diagnosed with a personality disorder and PTSD related to the shooting, he was declared competent, even though he continued to claim amnesia for the crime. The defense attempted to portray the shooting as self-defense but could offer no direct information about it because of the reported amnesia. The court limited psychiatric testimony concerning Mr. A.'s amnesia.

Mr. A. was convicted of murder, although, as the trial progressed, his behavior became increasingly bizarre in the courtroom. He threw water at the district attorney, stood up and shouted at the judge, and became combative with the court guards, resulting in additional charges of assault. In the course of the sentencing proceeding, he became even more confused, child-like, and inappropriate. During a jailhouse conference with his attorney, Mr. A. apparently began to switch states, identified himself by different names, and referred to himself in the third person singular and the first person plural. He began to recount a bizarre history of the shooting in which several alter identities claimed responsibility for "protecting the little guy" (an alleged child alter) from the murderous assault of the dead lover. Mr. A. recounted a long history of infidelity and physical, sexual, and emotional torment by the lover. He hinted at a history of childhood maltreatment by his father.

The alters switched rapidly back and forth, with the "host," Mr. A., apparently unable to recall what was said by the other alters. He appeared terrified, insisting that this was not happening to him and demanding that his attorney not bring this material into court. Mr. A. began to claim that his attorney was untrustworthy and not helping him adequately in his legal defense. When in the alter states, Mr. A. described fears of other prisoners in the jail. He elaborated a variety of paranoid ideas about plots against him and vowed to defend himself against the other prisoners.

Defense investigators found only limited evidence supporting the claims of maltreatment or infidelity by the murdered lover. The defendant's family side-stepped questions about childhood abuse, although they confirmed that the father was a violent, rageful, alcoholic who experienced war-related PTSD and had been arrested several times for violent behavior.

Additional defense forensic assessment, including extensive psychiatric evaluation, psychological diagnostic assessment, and formal assessment of malingering, resulted in an opinion supporting a diagnosis of dissociative identity disorder. The alter identities were particularly bizarre and paranoid in their thinking. Based on all the evidence, it was unclear if the lover was shot owing to Mr. A.'s paranoia or under conditions of actual threat, or both. Under state law, the defense forensic evaluation supported a finding of incompetence owing to Mr. A.'s inability to control dysfunctional switching, and paranoia, leading to inability to assist his attorney in the sentencing procedure. The court rejected the claim of incompetence. Mr. A. was sentenced to 50 years in prison. Appeals are proceeding claiming that, under state law, an insanity defense should have been allowed at trial.

Mr. B. was arrested and charged with rape and attempted murder approximately 48 hours after he released his victim to her home. He had kidnapped the victim after knocking her unconscious and driving her to his house. There, he tortured her bizarrely over 10 hours, culminating in a series of sexual acts, the last of which was a vaginal rape. After this, his mood seemed to change, and the victim found him less malevolent than he had been. Up until then, she had been certain that she would be killed. She somehow persuaded him to release her with a promise that she would not call the police. She did not keep this promise, and Mr. B. was quickly found and arrested.

All police contacts during the arrest and initial interrogation were audiotaped or videotaped. Mr. B. admitted the assault to the police and become increasingly despondent and distressed. Eventually, he was transferred to a state hospital forensics unit because of fear that he would commit suicide. Subsequently, Mr. B. was implicated in two other attempted rapes in the previous year, which he also admitted. In the course of assessment by state and defense psychiatrists and psychologists, Mr. B. began to describe a "bad person" who lived inside him and who had "taken over" and "made him" commit the crimes of which he was accused. He described a complex series of hallucinations, preoccupation with rape fantasies done by the "bad person," and loss of interest in life over the year preceding the rape. He claimed that he was so preoccupied by these fantasies that he ignored many basic aspects of daily life. Defense mental health experts made a diagnosis of dissociative identity disorder, sexual sadism, and major depression. They opined that the defendant was not guilty by reason of insanity, based on the "bad person" doing the crimes and the defendant's loss of contact with reality in the year before arrest.

Review of Mr. B.'s past revealed a documented history of severe physical abuse, emotional abuse, and neglect perpetrated by his mentally ill mother and alcoholic father. Mr. B.'s history was noteworthy for a virtually lifelong psychiatric disturbance characterized by a preoccupation with rape, sexual sadism, and murder. He hinted that he might have attempted rapes at other times in his life.

Additional experts hired by the state evaluated Mr. B. over several days. They performed the SCID-D-R and other psychometric diagnostic assessments. In neither the clinical nor the psychometric assessment did Mr. B. describe typical dissociative identity disorder phenomena, such as amnesia, depersonalization, spontaneous autohypnotic phenomena, switching, internal voices, internal passive influence, or somatization nor did he report PTSD symptoms. The personified entities in his mind did not have relatively independent ways of thinking, behaving, or remembering nor did they clearly take control of Mr. B.'s behavior. They were more like fantasy characters, rather than alter self-states. Mr. B. described ideas of influence and reference at times emanating from others in his environment, periodic paranoid thinking, and social isolation. Unusual and idiosyncratic thinking was observed at times during the interviews. He proclaimed remorse for his crimes but, on closer questioning, actually seemed rather pleased with himself for completing the rape. The history of recent, extreme social withdrawal was belied by the defendant's acknowledgment that he had traveled out of state, dated several women, and actually prepared his house for sale in the year preceding his arrest. He acknowledged knowing the difference between right and wrong and taking evasive actions to avoid arrest, in all alleged states of mind. Prosecution experts made DSM-IV Axis I diagnoses of schizotypal personality disorder with antisocial personality traits; dissociative disorder NOS, due to the bizarre fantasy preoccupations; sexual sadism; and major depressive disorder, in partial remission. They concluded that Mr. B. did not meet criteria for a diagnosis of dissociative identity disorder nor did he meet state criteria for NGRI. Mr. B. pled guilty and is now serving 25 to 50 years in state prison.

Therapists may find themselves treating dissociative identity disorder patients who face criminal charges for minor crimes, such as shoplifting, check forgery, credit card fraud, and DWI. It may be impossible for the patient to hire an independent forensic expert. In these cases, the clinician may be unable to avoid providing a written report or appearing in court to testify at the request of the patient or the patient's attorney. The clinician should educate himself or herself about the role of the treating professional testifying on behalf of a patient. The clinician should be clear with the attorney and the patient on the differing roles of the forensic expert and the treating clinician and the potential risks that may ensue if the primary therapist is made to testify. It may be difficult for the therapist to separate the roles of the advocate for a disturbed patient from that of a forensic examiner. However, the clinician should take seriously the importance of protecting the public from the patient. Clinically, the forensic situation may be useful to underscore for the patient the responsibility of the whole person for behavior committed in dissociated states of consciousness and to gain better adherence to responsible behavior from antisocial alter identities.

Amnesia for Criminal Behavior From a legal standpoint, amnesia alone is generally not considered a sufficient factor to generate a finding of incompetence to stand trial or a verdict of not guilty by reason of insanity. Accordingly, it is disadvantageous for a malingerer to make amnesia claims in the hopes of achieving a successful psychiatric defense. Case series have found that perpetrators claimed dissociative amnesia in 30 to 40 percent of homicide cases and in a lesser percentage of other violent crimes. Although malingering is often suspected in such cases, many of these individuals did little to avoid being charged with a crime, and some even called the authorities themselves. In general, the cases with apparent true dissociative amnesia were characterized by an unpremeditated assault in a state of high emotional arousal on a victim closely related to the perpetrator.

There is no absolute way to differentiate true dissociative amnesia from malingering. Malingerers have been noted to continue their deception even during hypnotically or barbiturate-facilitated interviews. Malingered amnesia is more common in individuals presenting with dramatic forms of generalized or circumscribed dissociative amnesia or fugue, or both. Many of the amnesia cases in the classical literature were described as occurring in a clinical context of financial, sexual, and legal problems or in soldiers who wished to escape from combat. On the other hand, in the clinical case reports, many malingerers quickly confessed their deceptions spontaneously or when confronted by the examiner.

A variety of procedures have been suggested to differentiate objectively between actual and malingered amnesia. At this point, none has achieved a definitive status in differentiating among these conditions. The forensic approach outlined in the following discussion should be used to assess individuals claiming dissociative amnesia in the criminal court context, buttressed, when indicated, by specific diagnostic assessment measures, including psychometric scales to detect malingering.

Individuals with dissociative fugue may also be involved in legal issues. The fugue may occur in the context of severe psychosocial stressors, such as combat, financial or marital indiscretions, fears of violent behavior toward others, and so on. When the individual is discovered, he or she may face a variety of legal problems on return home.

Forensic Assessment of Dissociative Disorders

In the assessment of possible dissociative disorder in criminal defendants, as well as plaintiffs or defendants in the civil arena, a number of guidelines may be helpful: (1) Follow basic principles of rigorous independent forensic assessment. (2) Undertake a comprehensive assessment of all available documentary materials concerning the defendant and the case. (3) Review all available past psychiatric, social service, and related materials. (4) It is often best to perform a standard diagnostic assessment on the defendant before introducing specialized testing. In some cases, it may be desirable to videotape or audiotape the interview following forensic guidelines; the latter may be mandatory in some states if hypnosis is involved in the assessment. (5) Avoid suggestive or leading questions during forensic assessment of possible dissociative disorders. (6) A longitudinal life-history interview may be useful in cases in which malingered amnesia or dissociative identity disorder is suspected: Ask the defendant to relate his or her entire life history, beginning with the first memory and proceeding forward up to the present time, following up information as necessary in a neutral manner. (7) After completion of the basic clinical assessment, formal psychological testing, including interviews assessing malingering, specialized dissociative disorders interviews (e.g., the SCID-D-R), or neuropsychiatric testing, or a combination of these, may be done. (8) Interviews with corollary sources (e.g., friends, family) may be necessary to corroborate the history in addition to written records. (9) Use forensic guidelines for hypnotically facilitated or drug-facilitated interviews. Guidelines for hypnotically facilitated forensic interviews have been published by the American Society for Clinical Hypnosis. These should only be performed by forensic examiners trained in their use.

Dissociative-Disordered Plaintiff

In the few cases in which the issue has been litigated, several state trial and appeals courts have allowed testimony of dissociative identity disorder plaintiffs, despite their testifying in dissociative or self-hypnotic states. Nonetheless, involvement of adult dissociative patients as plaintiffs in legal cases frequently results in an adverse impact on the patient's clinical course. This may be due to the negative effect of the adversarial system on the patient, who may have a highly idealized view of what will occur; an increased sense of loss of control due to the continual delays inherent in the legal process; the opening up of the patient's psychiatric history and clinical status in the courts; and, sometimes, the inherent difficulties in proving allegations of crimes or civil wrongs with a severely psychiatrically ill, periodically amnestic, complaining witness who may become overwhelmed, confused, or unconvincing during deposition or in court. Highly symptomatic patients in the stabilization phase of therapy may have a particularly difficult time in the legal system.

Clinicians should carefully review with the patient the potential clinical risks and benefits of proceeding with legal cases. In addition to the concerns enumerated previously, therapy for the issues that brought the patient to treatment mostly gets put on hold, except insofar as it illuminates the patient's struggles in the legal system. The primary focus becomes a supportive treatment based on helping the patient maintain relative stability during the case. The patient may need ongoing education about the nature of the adversarial process, the purpose of specific legal procedures, such as depositions, and the role of various participants. The clinician may also need to act as an intermediary with attorneys and the police, to help them understand the patient's psychopathology and relative strengths and liabilities during various parts of the proceedings. It is inadvisable for the clinician to act as an expert witness in such a context, although the clinician may be examined as a fact witness.

Some patients elect not to go forward with criminal or civil proceedings, such as prosecuting a rape, because of their realistic dread of the difficulty that they will face in court. Some prosecutors and police also shy away from going forward in such matters because of the inherent difficulties in these cases, even without a dissociative plaintiff. They drop charges, or, when possible, seek a plea bargain to avoid a court proceeding.

In the civil arena, dissociative patients have brought a variety of tort actions, most commonly malpractice claims against prior psychiatric and medical treaters. Some patients have reluctantly decided not to go forward because of the previously mentioned issues. When the statute of limitations permits, some patients have postponed litigation until they were clinically better stabilized.

In the current legal climate, tort suits against family members for abuse, based on delayed recall, are likely to be bitterly contested, even when there is independent, reliable confirmatory evidence of the abuse. From a clinical perspective, there is no requirement that adults who recall childhood abuse confront their alleged abusers or prosecute them to heal. Unless carefully thought out clinically, these sorts of confrontations often result in a poor outcome for accusers and accused. The long-term clinical focus is usually more appropriately placed on the patient's resolving his or her conflicted, ambivalent attachment to the accused abusive relative. When this is better resolved, the pressure for confrontation frequently diminishes substantially, or, if disclosure to family members occurs, it is handled in a way that is more likely to lead to resolution, not exacerbation of difficulties.

False Memory Litigation

The premises of false memory litigation are severalfold: (1) It is always below the standard of care to diagnose and to treat dissociative identity disorder or dissociative amnesia, or both, because these disorders do not exist, and (2) clinicians should have known this and should have informed patients of this before undertaking their treatment. (3) The underlying premise of treatment of dissociation and amnesia is to recover memories of abuse by whatever means necessary. (4) Adjunctive therapeutic techniques, such as imagery, hypnosis, journaling, and amobarbital interviews, are inherently high-risk procedures that are liable to contaminate the memories of patients and to produce iatrogenically dissociative identity disorder or dissociative amnesia, or both. (5) Inpatient specialty treatment for these disorders leads to contamination of patient autobiographical accounts and a contagion of iatrogenically created dissociative identity disorder.

To be sure, some treatments of apparent dissociative disorders, both inpatient and outpatient, have been characterized by misdiagnosis; failure of informed consent; focus on recall of trauma memories to the exclusion of symptom stabilization and proper treatment staging; misuse of hypnosis, medications, imagery, or pharmacologically facilitated interviews; failure to appreciate the complexities of human memory; continual infliction of the therapist's ideology on the patient (e.g., fundamentalist Christianity, belief in certain conspiracy theories); failure to manage inpatient milieus to minimize intensive discussion of trauma material among patients; and lack of appropriate therapeutic boundaries.

Nonetheless, the extreme false-memory hypotheses ignore the abundant recent research on dissociation and trauma and disregard the complexity of the issues related to trauma, memory, and dissociation reviewed in prior sections.

Most of these cases are handled by a small group of attorneys and plaintiffs' experts who join with local counsel to develop the case. It is important to alert defense attorneys and insurance companies that these are not regular malpractice cases, but a specialized type of litigation that usually requires a specialized defense, using experts familiar with these cases. Many attorneys and insurance companies are unaware of the forensic track record of the attorneys and experts that typically are involved in these cases. On the other hand, insurance companies often choose to settle these cases, even if there is a reasonable defense, rather than risk the uncertain financial exposure of litigation. Unfortunately, this tactic may actually encourage similar suits, because plaintiffs' attorneys often prefer the certainty of settlement to the vagaries of trial.

SUGGESTED CROSS-REFERENCES

Alcohol-related disorders are described in Section 11.2. Amnestic disorders, other cognitive disorders, and mental disorders due to a general medical condition are discussed in Chapter 10. Neuropsychiatric aspects of head trauma are presented in Section 2.5. Dissociative mechanisms are also discussed in Chapter 6 on psychoanalytic theory. Dissociative disorders in children and adolescents are discussed in Section 49.7. The diagnostic distinction between dissociative disorders and other mental disorders is clarified in Chapter 12 on schizophrenia and in Chapter 14 on anxiety disorders. Chapter 15 on the somatoform disorders provides a detailed description of the somatic symptoms that, in this chapter, are viewed as manifestations of dissociation. Expanded descriptions of the various psychotherapeutic approaches appear in Chapter 30, and biological therapies are described in Chapter 31. Culture-bound syndromes are discussed in Chapter 27.

REFERENCES

*Anderson MC, Ochsner KN, Kuhl B, Cooper J, Robertson E, Gabrieli SW, Glover GH, Gabrieli JDE: Neural systems underlying the suppression of unwanted memories. *Science.* 2004;303:232–235.

Behnke SH: Confusion in the courtroom: How judges have assessed the criminal responsibility of individuals with multiple personality disorder. *Int J Law Psychiatry.* 1997;20:293–310.

Bremner JD, Marmar CR. *Trauma, Memory, and Dissociation.* Vol 54. Washington, DC: American Psychiatric Press; 1998.

Brown D, Scheflin AW, Hammond DC. *Memory, Trauma, Treatment, and the Law.* New York: Norton; 1998.

Brown DW, Frischholz EJ, Scheflin AW: Iatrogenic dissociative identity disorder: An evaluation of the scientific evidence. *J Psychiatry Law.* 1999;27:549–638.

Brown DW, Scheflin AW, Whitfield CL: Recovered memories: The current weight of the evidence in science and in the courts. *J Psychiatry Law.* 1999;27:5–156.

Chambers RA, Bremner JD, Moghaddam B, Southwick SM, Charney DS, Krystal JH: Glutamate and post-traumatic stress disorder: Toward a psychobiology of dissociation. *Semin Clin Neuropsychiatry.* 1999;4:274–281.

Coons PM: Dissociative disorders not otherwise specified: A clinical investigation of 50 cases with suggestions for typology and treatment. *Dissociation.* 1992;5:187–195.

Dorahy M: Dissociative identity disorder and memory dysfunction: The current state of experimental research and its future directions. *Clin Psychol Rev.* 2001;5:771–795.

Ellenberger HF. *The Discovery of the Unconscious.* New York: Basic Books; 1970.

Fisher C: Amnesic states in war neurosis: The psychogenesis of fugue. *Psychoanal Q.* 1945;14:437–468.

Freyd JJ. *Betrayal Trauma: The Logic of Forgetting Childhood Abuse.* Cambridge, MA: Harvard University Press; 1996.

Gleaves DH, May MC, Cardena E: An examination of the diagnostic validity of dissociative identity disorder. *Clin Psychol Rev.* 2001;21:577–608.

Kisiel C, Lyons J: Dissociation as a mediator of psychopathology among sexually abused children and adolescents. *Am J Psychiatry.* 2001;158:1034–1039.

Kluft RP. Dissociative identity disorder. In: Gabbard GO, ed. *Treatment of Psychiatric Disorders.* 3rd ed. Vol 2. Washington, DC: American Psychiatric Press; 2001:1653–1693.

*Lanius RA, Williamson PC, Boksman K, Densmore M, Gupta M, Neufeld RWJ: Brain activation during script-driven imagery induced dissociative responses in PTSD: A functional magnetic resonance imaging investigation. *Biol Psychiatry.* 2002;52:305–311.

Lanius RA, Williamson PC, Densmore M, Boksman K, Neufeld RWJ, Gati JS, Menon R: The nature of traumatic memories: A 4-T fMRI functional connectivity analysis. *Am J Psychiatry.* 2004;161:36–44.

Lewis DO, Yaeger CA, Swica Y, Pincus JH, Lewis M: Objective documentation of child abuse and dissociation in 12 murderers with dissociative identity disorder. *Am J Psychiatry.* 1997;154:1703–1710.

Markowitsch HJ: Psychogenic amnesia. *Neuroimage.* 2003;20:S132–S138.

*Morgan CA, Hazlett G, Wang S, Richardson EG, Schnurr PP, Southwick SS: Symptoms of dissociation in humans experiencing acute, uncontrollable stress: A prospective investigation. *Am J Psychiatry.* 2001;158:1239–1247.

Nijenhuis ERS. *Somatoform Dissociation: Phenomena, Measurement, and Theoretical Issues.* Assen, Netherlands: van Gorcum; 1999.

Putnam FW. *Diagnosis and Treatment of Multiple Personality Disorder.* New York: Guilford; 1989.

Putnam FW. *Dissociation in Children and Adolescents: A Developmental Perspective.* New York: Guilford; 1998.

Reinders AA, Nijenhuis ERS, Paans AMJ, Korf J, Willemsen ATM, den Boer JA: One brain, two selves. *Neuroimage.* 2003;20:2119–2125.

Silberg JL: Fifteen years of dissociation in maltreated children: Where do we go from here? *Child Maltreat.* 2000;5:119–136.

*Simeon D, Knutelska M, Nelson D, Guralnik O: Feeling unreal: A depersonalization disorder update of 117 cases. *J Clin Psychiatry.* 2003;64:990–997.

Spiegel DE. The dissociative disorders. In: Tasman A, Goldfinger S, eds. *American Psychiatric Press Annual Review of Psychiatry.* Vol 10. Washington, DC: American Psychiatric Press; 1991.

Steinberg M. *Handbook for the Assessment of Dissociation: A Clinical Guide.* Washington, DC: American Psychiatric Press; 1995.

van Ijzendoorn MH, Schuengel C: The measurement of dissociation in normal and clinical populations: Meta-analytic validation of the Dissociative Experiences Scale (DES). *Clin Psychol Rev.* 1996;16:365–382.

*Vermetten E, Loewenstein RJ, Zdunek C, Wilson K, Bremner JD: Cortisol, memory and the hippocampus in PTSD and DID. *Biol Psychiatry.* 2002;51(Suppl):114S–145S.

18 Normal Human Sexuality and Sexual and Gender Identity Disorders

18.1a Normal Human Sexuality and Sexual Dysfunctions

VIRGINIA A. SADOCK, M.D.

Sexual behavior is diverse and determined by a complex interaction of factors. It is affected by one's relationship with others, by life circumstances, and by the culture in which one lives. An individual's sexuality is enmeshed with other personality traits, with his or her biological makeup, and with a general sense of self. It includes the perception of being a man or a woman and reflects developmental experiences with sex throughout the life cycle. Sexuality encompasses all those thoughts, feelings, and behaviors connected with sexual gratification and reproduction, including the attraction of one person to another.

A rigid definition of normal sexuality is difficult to draw and is clinically impractical. It is easier to define *abnormal sexuality*—sexual behavior that is destructive to oneself or others, that is markedly constricted, that cannot be directed toward a partner, that excludes stimulation of the primary sex organs, and that is inappropriately associated with guilt or anxiety.

There have been myriad advances in the field of sexuality in the areas of pharmacology and psychology and in the study of the interaction of sex and the social milieu. Significant new developments are the availability of medications that enable men to gain and maintain erections later in their lives and hormonal therapies that allow women to have pleasurable coitus postmenopausally. These medications have helped breach the taboo against sex in elderly adults. Theories on the psychology of sex have examined compulsive sexual behavior—not an official diagnosis in the revised fourth edition of the *Diagnostic and Statistical Manual of Mental Disorders* (DSM-IV-TR). The last major study of sex in the United States was conducted in 1994, consisting of a survey of sexual practices that placed the sexual behavior of Americans in a social context.

HISTORY

Cultural mores regarding sexual behavior have varied throughout the history of Western civilization. Attitudes have oscillated between the liberal and the puritanical, between the acceptance and the repression of human sexuality. Since the 1960s, the prevalent attitudes toward sex in the United States have been markedly liberal. However, recent studies indicate a trend toward accepting more conservative values. That shift is attributed largely to the fear of acquired immune deficiency syndrome (AIDS). One poll reported that 40 percent of Americans are concerned about contracting AIDS and are altering their sexual behavior because of that fear. The greatest concern was expressed by young adults, who are now more likely to use condoms as a precaution and to choose their sexual partners with greater care. In 1997, the rate of teenage pregnancy declined for the first time in 40 years, and, in 1998, the number of teenagers who had sexual intercourse fell below 50 percent for the first time in a decade. Nonetheless, currently, one in five teenagers has sex before the age of 15 years. Conservative segments of society emphasize abstinence before marriage as the answer to the fear of AIDS. The recurrence of conservative attitudes in response to the threat of illness has parallels in history. The sexual liberality of the Renaissance ended when syphilis swept the European continent and became a major argument for chastity among proponents of the Reformation. Other factors that predispose to more restrictive mores are periods of economic recession that tend to bring people to more puritanical positions. Few of these issues have been resolved definitively in the form of new social mores, however, and the permissive legacies of the sexual revolution of the 1960s and 1970s exert a strong effect on current sexual behavior.

The advent of effective birth control methods and legalized abortion clearly differentiated the pleasure of sexual activity from its procreative function. The feminist movement attacked the double standard for acceptable sexual behavior for men and women, encouraged women to accept sexual responsibility for the gratification of their needs, and challenged society to reevaluate stereotyped male and female roles. The women's movement also focused attention on rape and incest. Gerontologists and elderly people alike have drawn attention to the sexual needs of the aged. Middle-class adolescents became sexually active, and gay rights groups urged acceptance of their sexual orientation and succeeded in 1980 when homosexuality was dropped as a diagnostic category in the third edition of the DSM (DSM-III).

Concurrent with the cultural changes of the sexual revolution was the growth in scientific research into sexual physiology and sexual dysfunctions. William Masters and Virginia Johnson published their pioneering work on the physiology of sexual response in 1966 and reported on their program for treating sexual complaints in 1970. Most medical centers now have programs specifically geared to the treatment of sexual dysfunctions.

Historically, problems of sexual conflict and sexual dysfunction have been the province of psychiatry. Such pioneers as Havelock Ellis (Fig. 18.1a–1), Richard Krafft-Ebing (Fig. 18.1a–2), and Sigmund Freud focused broadly on human sexuality. Later, others focused more intensively on sexual physiology and dysfunctions. The work of Alfred Charles Kinsey (Fig. 18.1a–3), who published *Sexual Behavior in the Human Male* in 1948 and its companion volume, *Sexual Behavior in the*

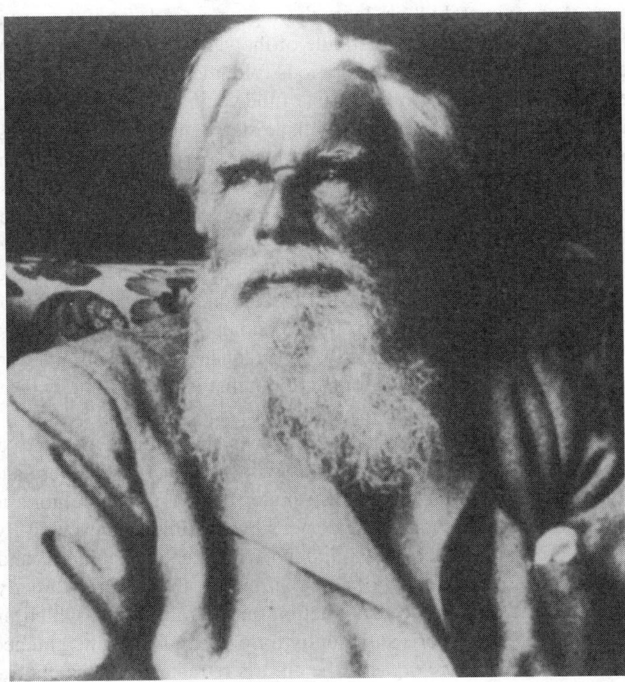

FIGURE 18.1a–1 Havelock Ellis, 1859–1939. In his book, *Studies in the Psychology of Sex* (1896), Ellis recorded examples of normal and abnormal sexuality. It remains a classic in the field of sexology. (Courtesy of New York Academy of Medicine.)

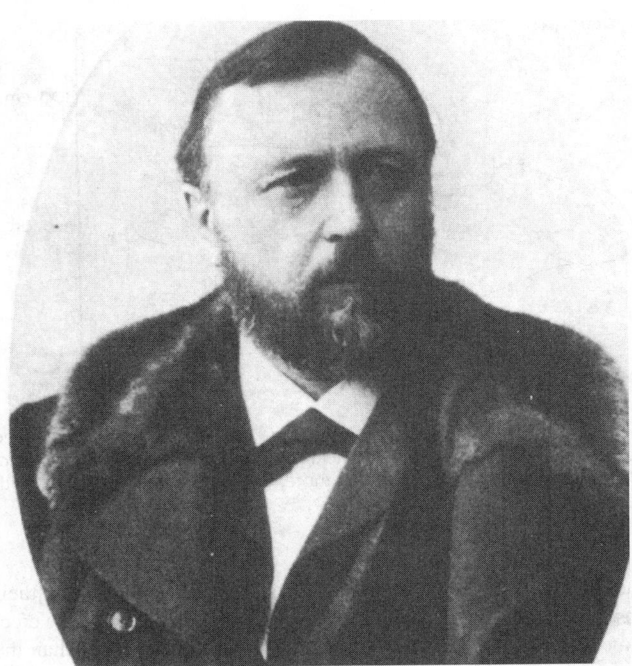

FIGURE 18.1a–2 Richard von Krafft-Ebing (1840–1903), a psychiatrist who published a classic text, *Psychopathia Sexualis* (1898), in which he documented every variation in sexuality, including zoophilia, necrophilia, urolagnia, and lust murder, among others. Case reports were so lurid and detailed that early editions were published in Latin. (Courtesy of New York Academy of Medicine.)

Human Female, 5 years later, was the most extensive study performed in human sexuality in America up to that time. The current approach to sexual dysfunctions reflects the cultural and scientific developments of recent years, the development of specific techniques for the treatment of these problems, the historical interest of psychiatry in this area, and the recognition of its importance in psychiatric practice.

NORMAL SEXUALITY

Anatomical and Physiological Bases

Knowledge about the organs of sexuality and the normal physiological sequence of male and female response is necessary for an informed understanding of the sexual dysfunctions. In fact, since the 1990s, greater emphasis has been placed on the genetic, neuroanatomical, and neurochemical model of human sexuality than on psychological and social factors. Research in sexual differentiation, including the genetics of gonadal development and hormonal influences on sexuality is of great interest, and new findings in these areas of sexual development are occurring rapidly.

Male Anatomy

The external genitalia of the normal adult man include the penis, scrotum, testes, epididymis, and parts of the vas deferens. Internal components include the vas deferens, ejaculatory ducts, and prostate gland.

Freud referred to the penis as the executive organ of sexuality. Since antiquity, culture has represented the penis in a variety of art forms. In ancient Greece, the cults of Dionysus, Priapus, and the satyrs used the phallus as a recurrent symbol of fertility and rejuvenation. The word *penis* has been traced from the Latin, meaning variously "tail" or "to hang" and refers to the pendant position of the organ in its resting or flaccid state. The size of the penis varies within a fairly constant range, but sex researchers over the years have disagreed on the dimensions of the range. All agree, however, that concern over the size of the penis is practically universal among men. Masters and Johnson report a range of 7 to 11 cm in the flaccid state

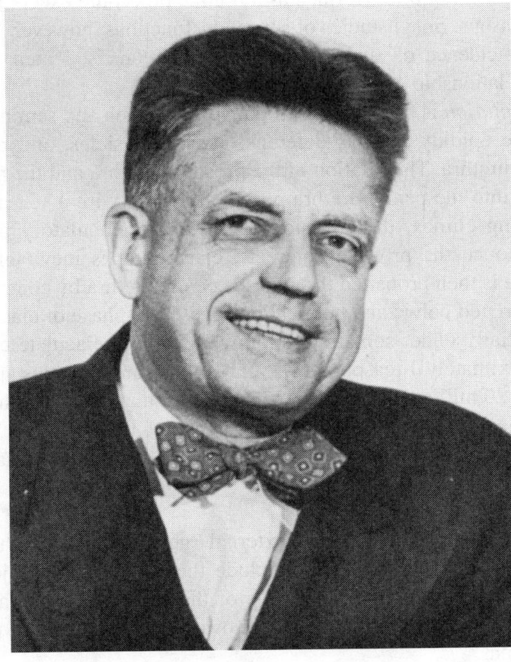

FIGURE 18.1a–3 Alfred Kinsey. (Courtesy of Institute for Sex Research, Bloomington, IN.)

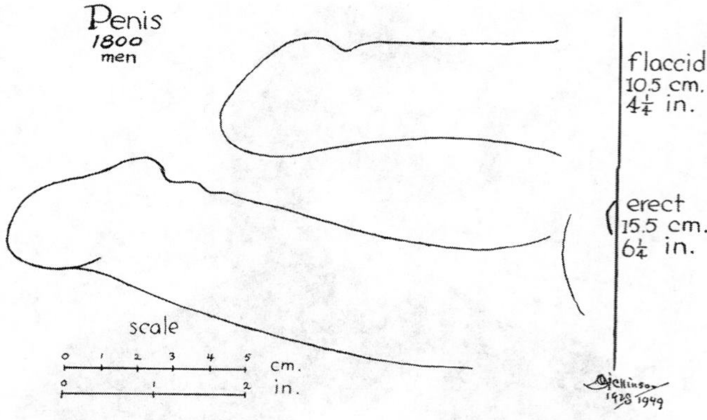

FIGURE 18.1a–4 The penis in the flaccid and erect state, with average size as surveyed and drawn by Dickinson. (From Dickinson RL. *Atlas of Human Sex Anatomy*. 2nd ed. Baltimore: Williams & Wilkins; 1949, with permission.)

and 14 to 18 cm in the erect state. Of particular interest was their observation that the flaccid dimension bears little relation to the erect dimension, as the smaller penis erects proportionally more than the larger one (Fig. 18.1a–4).

Circumcision, a procedure in which the prepuce is surgically removed, has been practiced for centuries as a religious rite by Jews and Moslems and is a common medical procedure in the United States today. The circumcised penis, with its exposed glans, was once believed to be less sensitive because of cornification of the epithelium. In laboratory studies, however, researchers have found no difference in tactile threshold between the circumcised penis and the uncircumcised penis. Intravaginally, the prepuce of the uncircumcised penis remains retracted behind the glans during penile thrusting, dispelling the myth that premature ejaculation may be more common in uncircumcised men because of increased stimulation caused by preputial movements. In 1999, the American Academy of Pediatrics recommended that male circumcision not be performed as a routine procedure except for religious reasons. Some studies of sexual dysfunctions, however, found a higher incidence of such problems in uncircumcised men, but no causal relationship was determined.

Ejaculation is the forceful propulsion of semen and seminal fluid from the epididymis, vas deferens, seminal vesicles, and prostate into the urethra. The dilation of the prostatic urethra and the passage of fluid into the penile urethra provide the man with a sensation of impending climax, the emission phase of the ejaculatory process. Indeed, once the prostate contracts, ejaculation is inevitable. The ejaculate is then propelled through the penile urethra by contractions of the striated pelvic and perineal muscles. This phase of ejaculation is essentially under somatic efferent control. The ejaculate consists of approximately 1 teaspoon (2.5 mL) of fluid and contains approximately 120 million sperm cells. It is believed that the larger the ejaculate, the more pleasurable the orgasm, but this belief is highly subjective. The sense of pleasure that accompanies orgasm is thought to be a cortical experience.

Female Anatomy The external genitalia of the normal woman, also called the *vulva,* include the mons pubis, major and minor lips, clitoris, glans, vestibule of the vagina, and vaginal orifice. The internal system includes the ovaries, fallopian tubes, uterus, and vagina.

The word *vagina* comes from the Latin word meaning "sheath." The vagina is usually collapsed, a potential rather than an actual space. Approximately 8 cm long, the vagina extends from the cervix of the uterus above to the vestibule of the vagina or vaginal opening below. In most virgins, a membranous fold, the hymen, separates the vestibule and opening from the rest of the vaginal canal. The mucous membrane lining the vaginal walls rests in numerous transverse folds. To accommodate the penis during sexual intercourse, the vagina expands in both length and width. After menopause, because circulating estrogen concentrations decrease, the vagina loses much of its elasticity.

Hippocrates first described the clitoris in the medical literature, referring to it as the site of sexual excitation. Masters and Johnson described the clitoris as the primary female sexual organ, because orgasm depends physiologically on adequate clitoral stimulation. Anatomically, the clitoris has a nerve net that is proportionally three times as large as that of the penis.

Alfred Kinsey found that when women masturbate, most prefer clitoral stimulation. That finding was refined further by Masters and Johnson, who reported that women prefer the shaft of the clitoris to the glans, because the glans is hypersensitive if stimulated excessively.

The clitoral prepuce is contiguous with the labia minora, and, during coitus, the penis does not stimulate the clitoris directly. Rather, penile thrusting exerts traction on the minor lips, which, in turn, stimulate the clitoris sufficiently for orgasm. During heightened excitement, just before orgasm, the clitoris retracts under the clitoral hood because of contraction of the ischiocavernosus muscles. Retracting, the clitoris moves away from the vaginal barrel, which makes clitoral–penile contact impossible. The size of the clitoris varies considerably and is unrelated to the sexual responsiveness of a particular woman.

In 1950, Ernst Graefenberg described an area surrounding the female urethra in the anterior wall of the vagina that has come to be called the *G spot*. Approximately 0.5 to 1.0 cm in size, it becomes engorged during sexual stimulation. Many women report that stimulation of the area is highly pleasurable and, in some, can induce orgasm. Graefenberg believed that the tissue here was analogous to the prostate and might account for the spurt of fluid during orgasm reported by some women, similar to male ejaculation.

Innervation of Sex Organs Innervation of the sexual organs is mediated primarily through the autonomic nervous system (ANS). Penile tumescence occurs through the synergistic activity of two neurophysiological pathways. A parasympathetic (cholinergic) component mediates reflexogenic erections via impulses that pass through the pelvic splanchnic nerves (S2, S3, and S4). A thoracolumbar, mainly sympathetic pathway transmits psychologically induced impulses. Both parasympathetic and sympathetic mechanisms are thought to play a part in relaxing the smooth muscles of the penile corpora cavernosa, which allows the penile arteries to dilate and causes the inflow of blood that results in penile erection. Relaxation of cavernosal smooth muscles is aided by the release of nitric oxide, an endothelium-derived relaxing factor. Clitoral engorgement and vaginal lubrication also result from parasympathetic stimulation that increases blood flow to genital tissue.

Evidence indicates that the sympathetic (adrenergic) system is responsible for ejaculation. Through the hypogastric plexus, adrenergic impulses innervate the urethral crest, the muscles of the epididymis, and the muscles of the vas deferens, seminal vesicles, and prostate. Stimulation of the plexus causes emission. In women, the sympathetic system facilitates the smooth muscle contraction of the vagina, urethra, and uterus that occurs during orgasm.

The ANS functions outside of voluntary control and is influenced by external events (e.g., stress, drugs) and internal events (hypotha-

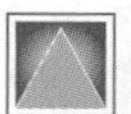

Table 18.1a–1
Responses of Sex Organs to Autonomic Nerve Impulses

	Adrenergic Impulses		Cholinergic Impulses
Effector Organs	**Receptor Type**	**Responses**	**Responses**
Urinary bladder			
Detrusor	β_2	Relaxation (usually)	Contraction
Trigone and sphincter	α_1	Contraction	Relaxation
Ureter			
Motility and tone	α_1	Increase	Increase (?)
Uterus	α_1, β_2	Pregnant: contraction (α_1), relaxation (β_2); nonpregnant: relaxation (β_2)	Variable
Sex organs, male	α_1	Ejaculation	Erection
Skin			
Pilomotor muscles	α_1	Contraction	
Sweat glands	α_1	Localized secretion	Generalized secretion

Adapted from Goodman Gilman A, Rall TW, Nies AS, Taylor P, eds. *Goodman and Gilman's The Pharmacological Basis of Therapeutics.* 8th ed. New York: Pergamon; 1990.

lamic, limbic, and cortical stimuli). Considering these influences, it is not surprising that erection and orgasm are so vulnerable to dysfunction (Table 18.1a–1).

Endocrinology From the time of conception, hormones play a major role in human sexual development. Unlike the fetal gonads, which are under chromosomal influence, the fetal external genitalia are very susceptible to hormones. Testosterone mediates the development of the undifferentiated mesodermal wolffian ducts into the male vas deferens, epididymis, and seminal vesicles. Dihydrotestosterone, produced from testosterone, induces the penis and scrotum. The raphe in men corresponds to the anatomical location of the vaginal orifice in women (Fig. 18.1a–5).

Exogenous hormonal administration can cause external genital development inconsistent with the fetal sex gland development. For instance, if the pregnant mother receives sufficient exogenous androgen, a female fetus possessing an ovary can develop external genitalia resembling those of a male fetus. Fetal, maternal, or exogenous hormones administered to a pregnant woman may all affect development of the external genitalia of the fetus. Deprived of male and female gonads and the respective hormones, testosterone and estrogen, the human adult does not develop normal secondary sexual characteristics, is incapable of reproduction, and, in the case of the woman, does not develop a menstrual cycle.

Testosterone is the hormone believed to be connected with libido in both men and women. In men, stress is inversely correlated with testosterone blood concentration. Other factors, such as sleep, mood, and lifestyle, influence circulating levels of the hormone. The release of testosterone in men is under the control of the hypothalamic-gonadal-pituitary axis. The hormone is secreted in a pulsatile manner and in a diurnal rhythm, with the highest levels occurring in the morning and the lowest levels in the evening. Normal concentrations range from 270 to 1,100 ng/dL. Decreased testosterone concentrations are apparent by age 50 years and decrease at the rate of approximately 100 ng/dL per decade. However, many healthy, aging men never become hypogonadal. It has also been suggested that the sensitivity of androgen receptor sites decreases in aging men.

Androgen administered to men complaining of loss of potency and loss of libido is usually unsuccessful unless testosterone concentrations are below normal, and administration to women may precipitate disturbing virilization. Many clinicians correct the hormone deficiency of the postmenopausal period with estrogen replacement therapy. Testosterone has been used in combination with estrogen in women who do not respond to estrogen alone. The combination is especially useful in treating headache, depression, and reduced libido. Oxytocin, secreted by the hypothalamus, stimulates lactation and uterine contractions and may enhance sexual activity. Plasma oxytocin concentrations increase in men and women during orgasm. Diethylstilbestrol (DES), an androgenic steroid, was prescribed in the 1950s and 1960s for pregnant women with threatened abortion. However, the drug had untoward effects on the children (especially female children) born to these mothers. Reports of cervical and uterine abnormalities were reported in women and reproductive tract abnormalities were reported in men. The children (called *DES*

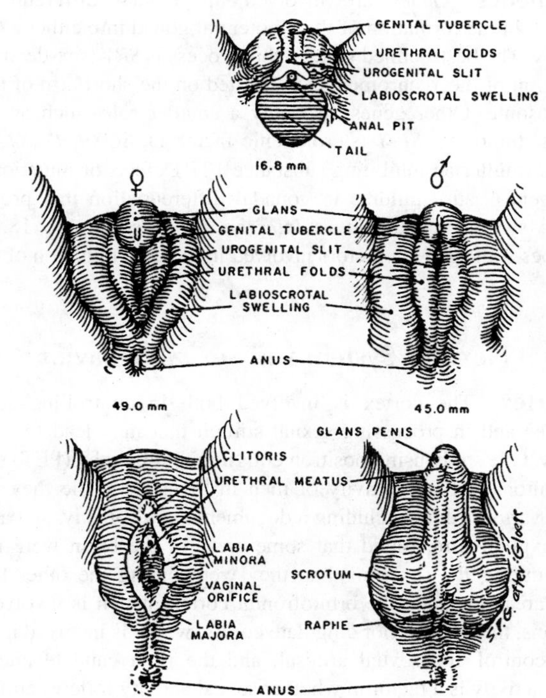

FIGURE 18.1a–5 Differentiation of male and female external genitalia from indifferent primordia. Male differentiation occurs only in the presence of androgenic stimulation during the first 12 weeks of fetal life. (From Van Wyk and Grumbach, 1968. Reprinted from Brobeck JR, ed: *Best and Taylor's Physiological Basis of Medical Practice.* 9th ed. Williams & Wilkins, Baltimore; 1973, with permission.)

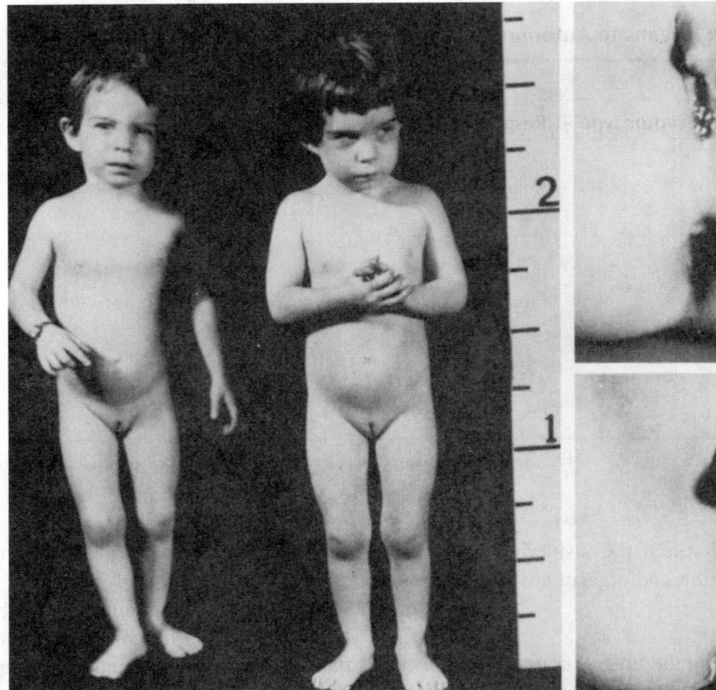

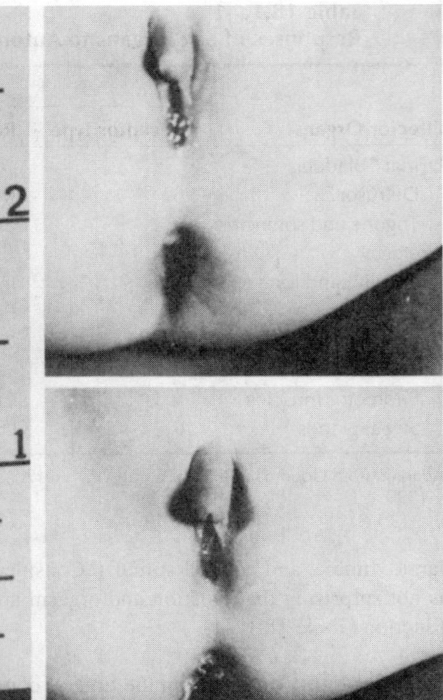

FIGURE 18.1a–6 Twins born to a mother who received ethisterone during pregnancy. Note the enlarged clitoris in each child. (Courtesy of Robert B. Greenblatt, M.D., and Virginia McNamarra, M.D.)

daughters and sons) organized a National DES Education Program sponsored by the National Cancer Institute to provide information on the potential medical problems confronting those born to DES mothers (Fig. 18.1a–6).

Genetics Genes are involved in gonadal differentiation, resulting in the formation of the bipotential gonad into either a testis or ovary. The best-defined gene in this process is *SRY* (sex-determining region of the Y chromosome), located on the short arm of the Y chromosome. Other genes also play a smaller role, such as *WT1* (Wilms' tumor 1), *SF-1* (steroidgenic factor 1), *SOX9*, *DAX1*, and *MIS-12* (müllerian inhibiting substance 12). Defects or mutations in these genes cause failures in gonadal differentiation that produce clinical syndromes known as *intersex disorders*. Figure 18.1a–7 describes some genetic factors involved in the determination of male sex.

Central Nervous System and Sexual Behavior

Cortex The cortex is involved both in controlling sexual impulses and in processing sexual stimuli that may lead to sexual activity. One study using positron emission tomography (PET) scans to monitor the brain activity of men in their 20s while they were shown various films, including a documentary, a comedy, and a sexually explicit film, found that some areas of the brain were more active during the sex film than they were during the other films. These areas included the orbitofrontal cortex, which is involved in emotions, the left anterior cingulate cortex, which is involved in hormone control and sexual arousal, and the right caudate nucleus, whose activity is a factor in whether sexual activity follows arousal.

Limbic System Experimentation with animals has demonstrated that the limbic system is directly involved with elements of sexual functioning. In all mammals, the limbic system is involved in behavior required for self-preservation and the preservation of the species.

Chemical or electrical stimulation of various sites of the limbic system, the lower part of the septum and the contiguous medial preoptic area, the fimbria of the hippocampus, the mammillary bodies, and the anterior thalamic nuclei have all elicited penile erection.

The hippocampus is believed to influence genital tumescence and affect the regulation of the release of gonadotropins. Stimulation of the amygdala in primates initiates oral (chewing, lip smacking) and then genital (penile erection) behavior. Researchers have stated that the closeness of these functions may derive from the evolutionary fact that the olfactory sense was strongly involved in both feeding and mating. They speculate that the evolution of the third subdivision of the limbic system may reflect a shift in importance from olfactory contact to visual communication in sociosexual behavior.

Brainstem Brainstem sites exert inhibitory and excitatory control over spinal sexual reflexes. One site, the nucleus paragigantocellularis, has been identified as important in inhibitory control of climax-like responses in men and is suspected to be involved in female physiology as well. This nucleus projects directly to pelvic efferent neurons in the lumbosacral spinal cord, apparently causing them to secrete serotonin, which is known to inhibit orgasms. The lumbosacral cord also receives strong projections from other serotonergic nuclei in the brainstem, the raphe nuclei, pallidus, magnus, and parapyramidal region.

Brain Neurotransmitters A vast array of neurotransmitters is produced by the brain, including dopamine, epinephrine, norepinephrine, and serotonin, among others. All affect sexual function. For example, an increase in dopamine is presumed to increase libido. Serotonin produced in the upper pons and midbrain is presumed to have an inhibitory effect on sexual function. Oxytocin, the neurohormone involved in the milk ejection reflex, is also released with orgasm and is believed to reinforce pleasurable activities. Basic science and clinical research on brain neurotransmitters and their effects on behavior (including sex) are rapidly expanding fields.

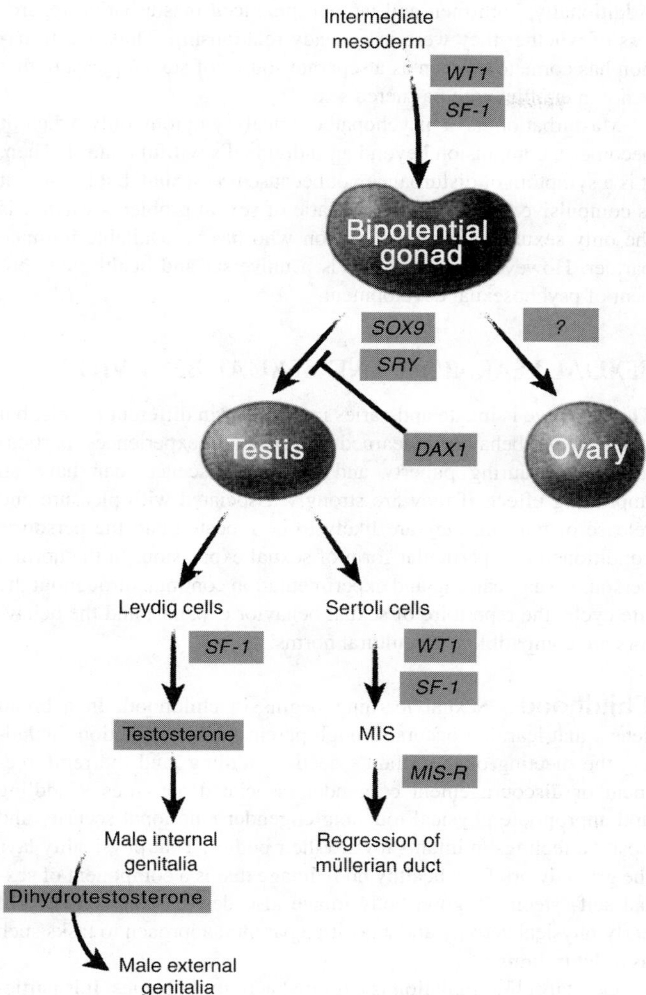

FIGURE 18.1a–7 A complex series of steps must occur in gonadal differentiation. A number of genes are critical to appropriate male genital development. *SRY* (sex-determining region of the Y chromosome), a gene on the short arm of the Y chromosome, is a testis-determining factor. The *SOX9* gene is also important in male sexual differentiation. *DAX1*, an orphan member of a nuclear hormone receptor family located on the X chromosome, interacts with steroidogenic factor 1 (*SF-1*). Other genes involved in male gonadal differentiation include the tumor-suppressor gene *WT1* (Wilms' tumor 1), and the müllerian inhibiting substance gene (*MIS*) and its receptor, MIS-R. (From Federman DD: Perspective: Three facets of sexual differentiation. *N Engl J Med.* 2004;350:323–324, with permission.)

Spinal Cord As described in the innervation of sex organs, sexual arousal and climax are ultimately organized at the spinal level. Sensory stimuli related to sexual function are conveyed via afferents from the pudendal, pelvic, and hypogastric nerves. These afferents terminate in the medial portions of the dorsal horn and in the medial central gray matter of the spinal cord. Several separate experiments suggest that sexual reflexes are mediated by spinal neurons in the central gray region of the lumbosacral segments.

PSYCHOSEXUALITY

Sexuality and total personality are so entwined that it is virtually impossible to speak of sexuality as a separate entity. The term *psychosexual* is therefore used to describe personality development and functioning, as these are affected by sexuality. *Psychosexual* applies to more than sexual feelings and behavior, and it is not synonymous with libido in the broad Freudian sense.

Freud's generalization that all pleasurable impulses and activities are originally sexual has given lay people a somewhat distorted view of sexual concepts and has given psychiatrists a confused picture of motivation. For example, some oral activities are directed toward obtaining food, and others are directed toward achieving sexual gratification. Both activities are pleasure-seeking and use the same organs, but they are not, as Freud contended, both necessarily sexual. Labeling all pleasure-seeking behaviors *sexual* obviates specifying precise motivation. People may also use sexual activities to gratify nonsexual needs, such as dependency, aggression, power, and status. Although sexual and nonsexual impulses may jointly motivate behavior, the analysis of behavior depends on understanding the underlying individual motivation and their interactions. Sexuality is something more than physical sex, coital or noncoital, and something less than all behaviors directed toward gaining pleasure.

Psychosexual Factors Sexuality depends on four interrelated psychosexual factors: sexual identity, gender identity, sexual orientation, and sexual behavior. These factors affect personality, development, and functioning.

Sexual identity is the pattern of a person's biological sexual characteristics: chromosomes, external and internal genitalia, hormonal composition, gonads, and secondary sex characteristics. In normal development, these characteristics form a cohesive pattern that leaves individuals in no doubt about their sex.

Gender identity is an individual's sense of maleness or femaleness. By the age of 2 or 3 years, almost everyone has a firm conviction that "I am a boy" or "I am a girl." Gender identity results from an almost infinite series of clues derived from experiences with family members, peers, and teachers, and from cultural phenomena. For instance, male infants tend to be handled more vigorously and female infants tend to be cuddled more. Fathers spend more time with their infant sons than with their daughters, and they also tend to be more aware of their sons' adolescent concerns than of their daughters' anxieties. Boys are more likely to be physically disciplined than girls are. A child's sex affects parental tolerance for aggression and reinforcement or extinction of activity and of intellectual, aesthetic, and athletic interests. Physical characteristics derived from a person's biological sex (e.g., physique, body shape, and physical dimensions) interrelate with an intricate system of stimuli, including rewards, punishment, and parental gender labels, to establish gender goals. Recent studies of children with intersex conditions have drawn attention to a physiological basis for gender identity. In particular, they have focused on the masculinization or feminization of the fetal brain.

Sexual orientation describes the object of a person's sexual impulses: heterosexual (opposite sex), homosexual (same sex), or bisexual (both sexes). The overwhelming majority of people have a heterosexual orientation. In the United States, 2.8 percent of men and 1.4 percent of women identify themselves as homosexual. These numbers are compatible with figures from Western European countries as well. However, a higher percentage of persons have had at least one same-sex experience in their lives. Additionally, homosexuals congregate in urban areas, so the incidence of homosexuality in some large cities is as high as 8 or 9 percent.

Sexual behavior includes desire, fantasies, pursuit of partners, autoeroticism, and all the activities engaged in to express and gratify sexual needs. It is an amalgam of psychological and physiological responses to internal and external stimuli.

Masturbation Masturbation usually is a normal precursor of object-related sexual behavior and a form of sexual pleasure that generally lasts throughout a person's lifetime. No other form of sexual activity has been as universally practiced in spite of being severely condemned by many cultures for long periods of time.

In the classical period, Greco-Roman writers and medical authorities, such as Galen, recommended masturbation as a healthful practice for both men and women. The categorization of masturbation as sinful in Western culture derives from Judeo-Christian attitudes. Masturbation is sometimes called *onanism* after Onan in the Old Testament, who was slain for spilling his seed upon the ground. Many biblical scholars today posit that this punishment was not a result of his masturbation, but because he did not obey Jehovah's commandment to take his brother's wife as his own. The prohibition against masturbation was reinforced by Christian Church fathers, particularly by St. Augustine, who preached celibacy and held that sex was appropriate only for purposes of procreation. Ambivalence about masturbation also existed in Eastern cultures. Some Hindus and the ancient Chinese believed that loss of semen resulted in reduction of a vital male essence. However, the prohibitive emphasis was on ejaculation and not on manipulation of the genitalia. Female masturbation was better tolerated or ignored.

For many years, science held attitudes toward masturbation that were as negative as many religious views. What had been viewed as sinful came to be seen as pathological (Fig. 18.1a–8). For example, in the 1800s, Krafft-Ebing believed that masturbation could lead to insanity. Currently, and in the second half of the 20th century, a liberal attitude toward sexual behavior, including masturbation, has prevailed. Research by Kinsey in the 1940s into the prevalence of masturbation indicated that nearly all men and three-fourths of all women masturbate sometime during their lives. Masters and Johnson discussed techniques of masturbation in the 1960s and identified the shaft of the clitoris as the preferred site of masturbation for women. In the 1990s, a study of sexual practices in America found that masturbation was the first postpubertal sexual practice of most men and of approximately 50 percent of women. Studies in Europe noted an increased incidence in masturbatory activity in both young men and women in the 1980s and, especially, in the 1990s, as compared to the 1960s. In these studies, most of the women had experienced masturbation before their first coital experience, following a pattern of sexual development that has long been typical for men.

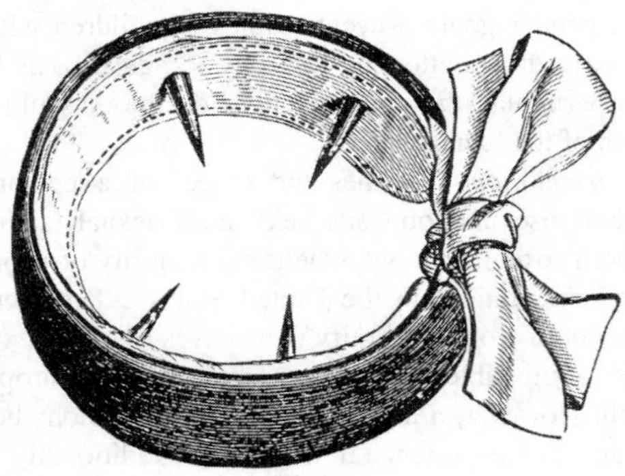

FIGURE 18.1a–8 A four-pointed urethral ring, which was used to prevent masturbation during the 19th century. This engraving shows how the ring was tied to the penis. (From Sadock BJ, Kaplan HI, Freedman AM. *The Sexual Experience*. Baltimore: Williams & Wilkins; 1976, with permission.)

Additionally, both men and women practiced masturbation regardless of whether they were in a steady relationship. Thus, masturbation has come to be seen as a separate source of sexual pleasure that is not in conflict with partnered sex.

Masturbation is a psychopathological symptom only when it becomes a compulsion beyond an individual's willful control. Then, it is a symptom of disturbance not because it is sexual, but because it is compulsive. It is also symptomatic of sexual problems when it is the only sexual activity of a person who has an available intimate partner. However, masturbation is a universal and healthy component of psychosexual development.

SEXUAL LEARNING AND SEXUAL BEHAVIOR

The sex drive is innate and varies in intensity in different people, but much sexual behavior is learned. Early sexual experiences, particularly those during puberty and early adolescence, can have an imprinting effect. If they are strongly associated with pleasure and release of tension, they are likely to be repeated and the person is conditioned to a particular form of sexual expression. In the normal person, sexual learning and experimentation continue throughout the life cycle, the repertoire of sexual behavior expands, and the behaviors are compatible with cultural norms.

Childhood Sexual learning begins in childhood. In a broad sense, that learning occurs through parent–child interaction, including the meeting of the infant's needs, cuddling, and the reinforcement or discouragement of gender-associated activities. Cuddling and appropriate physical touching engender emotional security and positive feelings in infants toward their bodies. That physicality lays the groundwork for a healthy body image that is a component of sexual self-esteem. A good body image also derives from mastery of early physical activity and a positive parental approach to tasks such as toilet training.

Genital self-stimulation is a normal activity of babies. It is particularly pronounced between the ages of 15 and 19 months, and it is part of the general interest of children in their bodies. The activity is reinforced by the pleasurable sensations it produces. As youngsters acquire playmates, curiosity about their own and others' genitalia motivates episodes of exhibitionism or genital exploration. Unless the child is unduly shamed, such experiences contribute to continued pleasure from sexual stimulation.

Children also learn by watching the interaction of their parents. They observe demonstrations of physical affection (although usually not the sex act itself), and they are sensitive to the sexual undertone of flirtation, bantering, or seductive interchange.

Sexual learning in childhood is adversely affected by exploitative, abusive adults. Incestuous activity, with or without penetration, or sexual abuse by other adults (babysitter, other older relatives, teachers, coaches, etc.) is damaging to the child. It may precipitate sexual dysfunction in adult life, as well as promiscuity and problems with intimacy. It may produce delinquent activities and behavioral problems in adolescence, as well as learning problems in school.

Some children are inappropriately stimulated short of outright incest or genital fondling. They are the objects of extremely seductive parents. Termed *eroticized children*, they frequently become sexually precocious.

Children who view the *primal scene*—the term Freud used to describe a child seeing sex between their parents—may be traumatized. This is particularly the case if they interpret coital sounds and movements as a physical aggression between the parents.

Adolescence With the approach of puberty, the upsurge of sex hormones, and the development of secondary sex characteristics, sexual curiosity is intensified. Adolescents are physically capable of coitus and orgasm but are usually inhibited by social restraints. The dual, often conflicting pressures of establishing their sexual identities and controlling their sexual impulses produce a strong physiological sexual tension in teenagers that demands release, and masturbation is a normal way to reduce this tension. In general, boys learn to masturbate to orgasm earlier than girls and masturbate more frequently. Consequently, many boys integrate their sexuality as an autonomous characteristic earlier than some girls. An important emotional difference between the adolescent and the younger child is the presence of coital fantasies during masturbation in the adolescent. These fantasies are an important adjunct to the development of sexual identity; in the comparative safety of the imagination, the adolescent learns to perform the adult sex role. Fantasies that accompany masturbation vary and reflect individual psychodynamics; however, in general, fantasies differ for the sexes. Boys respond to visual stimuli of nude or barely dressed women and images of explicit physical acts. Girls report responding to romantic stories in which a man demonstrates intense passion for and commitment to a woman. Their fantasies focus more on touching, emotions, and the partner's response than on visualizing an explicit sexual act.

In addition to masturbation, adolescents learn sexually through caressing and kissing with partners. In early adolescence, sex play may involve a partner of the same sex for a short period of time for heterosexuals and for homosexuals. Adolescence is also when one's body image becomes more definitive and a sense of sexual adequacy and sexual desirability begins to develop. Peer acceptance by the same sex and by the opposite sex is of paramount importance. Engaging in sexual talk and jokes, kissing, touching genitalia, experimenting with degrees of nudity, and experimenting with different partners or with one partner are part of the process of learning about sexuality. These experiences reinforce the adolescent's sense of being a sexual boy or girl.

First Coitus The first coitus is a rite of passage for both sexes. The modal age for first coitus in the United States is 16 years for boys and 17 years for girls. Currently, both considerable peer pressure and individual sex drive impel adolescents or young adults to participate in their first coital experience. In the past, virginity conferred status on the young person. Today, many young people feel embarrassed or inadequate if they are virgins. A small backlash is present in some groups in which adolescents sign premarital chastity pledges in a public forum. Also, a survey by the Centers for Disease Control reported that 49 percent of male teenagers had intercourse in 1998, down from 57 percent in 1991. The corresponding number for girls was 48 percent, down from 51 percent. Many adolescents are choosing to have oral sex instead of coitus in their intimate relations.

For boys, anxiety about first coitus relates to performance. Will he be able to get an erection, to penetrate the vagina, to last for some period of time before he ejaculates? He is vulnerable in his masculine pride and may fear being judged inadequate by his female partner and his male peers.

First coitus for a girl has been surrounded by cultural ambivalence and concern about the meaning of her loss of virginity and her assumption of the risk of pregnancy and responsibility for the next generation. That risk has been eased by the availability of contraceptive methods. Development of the birth control pill in the 1960s changed societal attitudes about premarital sex for women and created a more permissive climate. The cohort of women who came of age sexually after the late 1960s report a much higher frequency of premarital intercourse than women before that time. However, only 30 percent of young women use contraception with their first sexual mate and many use it inconsistently. In effect, many young women deny that they are planning to have sex by not being prepared in terms of contraception, reflecting cultural ambivalence about their sexual activity.

Studies have shown that first coitus is most likely to be a positive experience for girls with strong feelings for their partners. In general, women report a greater need to experience sex in the context of an affectionate relationship than do boys.

Adulthood By their late 20s, 70 percent of men and 85 percent of women have formed a union, either exclusive cohabitation or marriage. The sexual impulse is catalytic in forming and maintaining adult love relationships. Ideally, a mature sexual relationship encompasses the capacity for intimacy and love for one's partner.

As sexual access ceases to be problematic, more attention is focused on the activity itself. Interference with sexual activity arises from the time and energy required for the pursuit of careers, child rearing, and other family and community obligations. Nonetheless, studies reveal a much higher frequency of sexual interaction among married persons than among single persons. The modal frequency for married persons is three times a month, with many couples relating sexually twice a week. The highest frequency of sexual interaction, four or more times a week, exists among cohabiting couples.

Kissing, intercourse, and masturbation are frequent sexual activities. Even after a permanent sexual relationship has been established, masturbation remains a healthy practice during the illness or absence of a partner or when intercourse is unsatisfactory. Masturbation should only be considered maladaptive when it is a compulsive activity or when it is preferred to partner interaction. Many adults have some experience with oral sex. Studies show that, although it is not a regular activity for most couples, many people are likely to engage in it occasionally throughout their lifetimes. The incidence of the practice of cunnilingus and fellatio are the same; the lifetime prevalence is 75 percent of sexually active people. Anal sex is not part of the repertoire of regular sexual activities for most men and women in the United States. Although a sizable minority (25 percent of men and 20 percent of women) report one experience of anal sex, very few repeat the practice. In general, a graph of sexual practices does not form a bell curve. Most curves of sexual behavior are strongly skewed, with many persons indulging in a particular behavior or, conversely, very few people doing so.

Middle Age During middle age, the frequency of marital intercourse may decline. The rates of interaction depend more on male interest, and the middle-aged man may devote much of his energy to his career at this point. The decline in sexual interaction often reflects deeroticization of the woman because of her wife–mother role. Familiarity also contributes to a decreased passion, and some men have difficulty connecting marital sexual activity with the erotic scripts they elaborated during their adolescence. Conversely, a couple's experience of each other makes them comfortable and augments their skill at mutual arousal. For women, interest in sexual competence typically increases at this time. A woman's erotic pleasure and sexual commitment are strongly connected to feelings of attachment toward her partner and the security of being in a loving relationship.

With late middle age, the biological drive decreases in intensity. It takes the man longer to reach orgasm, he has a longer refractory period, and he requires more stimulation to achieve an erection. The woman must adjust to the hormonal fluctuations of her perimenopausal years, and she, too, requires more stimulation to become aroused. Although medications are available to address these specific physiological changes, they do not eliminate all need to adjust to the aging process. In terms of family dynamics, children often leave the house for work or further education at this time. This fact plus freedom from concern regarding unwanted pregnancy may enhance sexual activity for persons who have more time to direct attention toward each other and renew their life as a couple.

However, middle age is the period of rising extramarital activity, although the frequencies of such occurrences are low—75 percent of men and 85 percent of women remain faithful throughout the lifetime of their marriages. Daniel Offer has explained that the patterning of extramarital sexual activity for both sexes continues to express earlier patterns of psychosexual development:

> For men, it predominantly has the capacity for detachment that in adolescence was directly related to the pursuit of sexual fantasies and the homosocial validation of masculinity. For women, on the other hand, it resembles a quest for circumstances that justify and confirm a romantic self-image rather than a quest for orgasms.

In the context of a loving, communicative, and committed relationship, a decreased frequency of sexual interaction does not herald the onset of extramarital affairs or threaten the stability of the marriage.

Old Age An estimated 70 percent of men and 20 percent of women over age 60 years are sexually active; sexual activity is usually limited by the absence of an available partner. Longitudinal studies have found that the sex drive does not decrease as men and women age; in fact, some report an increased sex drive. Masters and Johnson reported sexual functioning among those in their 80s. Expected physiological changes in men include a longer time for erection to occur, decreased penile turgidity, and ejaculatory seepage; in women, decreased vaginal lubrication and vaginal atrophy are associated with lower estrogen levels. Medications can also adversely affect sexual behavior. A significant finding was that the more active a person's sex life was in early adulthood, the more likely it is to be active in old age.

CURRENT TRENDS

A study conducted by the University of Chicago in 1994, The National Health and Social Life Survey, was the latest and the most authoritative sex survey. Based on a representative U.S. population between the ages of 18 and 59 years, it found the following:

1. Eighty-five percent of married women and 75 percent of married men are faithful to their spouses.
2. Forty-one percent of married couples have sex twice a week or more, compared with 23 percent of single persons.
3. Cohabiting single persons have the most sex of all, twice a week or more.
4. The median number of sexual partners over a lifetime for men is six; for women, two.
5. A homosexual orientation was reported by 2.8 percent of men and 1.4 percent of women, with 9 percent of men and 5 percent of women reporting that they had at least one homosexual experience after puberty.
6. Vaginal intercourse was considered the most appealing type of sexual experience by 83 percent of men and 78 percent of women.
7. Among married partners, 93 percent are of the same race, 82 percent are of similar educational level, 78 percent are within 5 years of each other's age, and 72 percent are of the same religion.
8. Both men and women who, as children, had been sexually abused by an adult were more likely, as adults, to have had more than 10 sex partners, to engage in group sex, to report a homosexual or bisexual identification, and to be unhappy.
9. Less than 8 percent of the participants reported having sex more than four times a week, approximately two-thirds said they had sex a few times a month or less, and approximately three in ten have sex a few times a year or less.
10. Approximately one in four men and one in ten women masturbate at least once a week, and masturbation is less common among those 18 to 24 years of age than among those 24 to 34 years of age.
11. Three-quarters of the married women said they usually or always had an orgasm during sexual intercourse, compared with 62 percent of the single women. Among men, married or single, 95 percent said they usually or always had an orgasm.
12. More than half of the men said that they thought about sex every day or several times a day, compared with only 19 percent of the women.
13. More than four in five Americans had only one sexual partner or no partner in the past year. Generally, African Americans reported the most sexual partners and Asian Americans the fewest.

Another report, based on the same data and published in 2001 discussed sexual dysfunction and sexual behavior and public health policies. Findings include the following:

1. Thirty-nine percent of men and 41 percent of women have a sexual dysfunction and have experienced decreased well-being and quality of life as a result.
2. Fifteen percent of male respondents, single before marriage or after a divorce, who experimented widely sexually, had multiple partners, and sought multiple areas of stimulation (e.g., erotic videos, nude beaches, paid sex) composed the core group implicated in the maintenance of sexually transmitted disease in the population at large.
3. The likelihood of a pregnant girl younger than 18 years of age opting to have an abortion increased dramatically with the educational level of her parents.

PHYSIOLOGICAL RESPONSES

Normal men and women experience a sequence of physiological responses to sexual stimulation. In the first detailed description of these responses, Masters and Johnson observed that the physiological process involves increasing vasocongestion and myotonia tumescence and subsequent release of the vascular activity and muscle tone as a result of orgasm detumescence. Tables 18.1a–2 and 18.1a–3 describe the female and male sexual response cycles, respectively. DSM-IV-TR defines a four-phase response cycle: phase I, desire; phase II, excitement; phase III, orgasm; phase IV, resolution.

Phase I: Desire Phase I is a psychological phase distinct from any identified solely through physiology and reflects the psychiatrist's fundamental concern with motivations, drives, and personality. It is characterized by sexual fantasies and the conscious desire to have sexual activity.

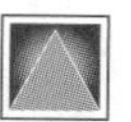

Table 18.1a–2
Female Sexual Response Cycle[a]

Organ	Excitement Phase	Orgasmic Phase	Resolution Phase
Mental	Lasts several minutes to several hours; heightened excitement before orgasm, 30 secs to 3 mins	3–15 secs	10 –15 mins; if no orgasm, 0.5 to 1 day
Skin	Just before orgasm: sexual flush inconsistently appears; maculopapular rash originates on abdomen and spreads to anterior chest wall, face, and neck; can include shoulders and forearms	Well-developed flush	Flush disappears in reverse order of appearance; inconsistently appearing film of perspiration on soles of feet and palms of hands
Breasts	Nipple erection in two-thirds of women, venous congestion and areolar enlargement; size increases to one-fourth more than normal	Breasts may become tremulous	Return to normal in approximately 0.5 hour
Clitoris	Enlargement in diameter of glans and shaft; just before orgasm, shaft retracts into prepuce	No change	Shaft returns to normal position in 5–10 secs; detumescence in 5–30 mins; if no orgasm, detumescence takes several hours
Labia majora	Nullipara: elevate and flatten against perineum Multipara: congestion and edema	No change	Nullipara: increase to normal size in 1–2 mins Multipara: decrease to normal size in 10–15 mins
Labia minora	Size increase two to three times more than normal; change to pink, red, deep red before orgasm	Contractions of proximal labia minora	Return to normal within 5 mins
Vagina	Color change to dark purple; transudate appears 10–30 secs after arousal; elongation and ballooning; lower third constricts before orgasm	3–15 Contractions of lower third at intervals of 0.8 sec	Ejaculate forms seminal pool in upper two thirds; congestion disappears in seconds or, if no orgasm, in 20–30 mins
Uterus	Ascends into false pelvis; labor-like contractions begin in heightened excitement just before orgasm	Contractions throughout orgasm	Contractions cease, and uterus descends to normal position
Other	Myotonia A few drops of mucoid secretion from Bartholin's glands during heightened excitement Cervix swells slightly and is passively elevated with uterus	Loss of voluntary muscular control Rectum: rhythmic contractions of sphincter Hyperventilation and tachycardia	Return to baseline status in seconds to minutes Cervix color and size return to normal, and cervix descends into seminal pool

[a]A desire phase consisting of sex fantasies and desire to have sex precedes the excitement phase.

Phase II: Excitement Phase II is brought on by psychological stimulation (fantasy or the presence of a love object), physiological stimulation (stroking or kissing), or a combination of the two. It consists of a subjective sense of pleasure and objective signs of sexual excitement. The excitement phase is characterized by penile tumescence leading to erection in men and vaginal lubrication in women. The nipples of both sexes become erect, although nipple erection is more common in women than in men. The woman's clitoris becomes hard and turgid, and her labia minora become thicker as a result of venous engorgement. Initial excitement may last several minutes to several hours. With continued stimulation, the man's testes increase in size 50 percent and elevate. The woman's vaginal barrel shows a characteristic constriction along the outer third, known as the *orgasmic platform.* The clitoris elevates and retracts behind the symphysis pubis; hence, it is not easily accessible. However, stimulation of the area causes traction on the labia minora and the prepuce, and there is intrapreputial movement of the clitoral shaft. Breast size in the woman increases 25 percent. Continued engorgement of the penis and vagina produces specific color changes, particularly in the labia minora, which become bright or deep red. Voluntary contractions of large muscle groups occur, rate of heartbeat and respiration increases, and blood pressure rises. Heightened excitement lasts 30 seconds to several minutes.

Phase III: Orgasm Phase III consists of peaking sexual pleasure, with release of sexual tension and rhythmic contraction of the perineal muscles and pelvic reproductive organs. A subjective sense of ejaculatory inevitability triggers the man's orgasm, and forceful emission of semen follows. The male orgasm is also associated with four to five rhythmic spasms of the prostate, seminal vesicles, vas, and urethra. In women, orgasm is characterized by 3 to 15 involuntary contractions of the lower third of the vagina and by strong, sustained contractions of the uterus, flowing from the fundus downward to the cervix. Both men and women have involuntary contractions of the internal and external anal sphincter. These and the other contractions during orgasm occur at 0.8-second intervals. Other manifestations include voluntary and involuntary movements of the large muscle groups, including facial grimacing and carpopedal spasm. Blood pressure rises 20 to 40 mm (both systolic and diastolic), and the heart rate increases up to 160 beats per minute. Orgasm lasts from 3 to 25 seconds and is associated with a slight clouding of consciousness.

Phase IV: Resolution Resolution consists of the disgorgement of blood from the genitalia (detumescence), which brings the body back to its resting state. If orgasm occurs, resolution is rapid; if it does not occur, resolution may take 2 to 6 hours and be associated with irritability and discomfort. Resolution through orgasm is characterized by a subjective sense of well-being, general relaxation, and muscular relaxation. After orgasm, men have a refractory period that may last from several minutes to many hours; in this period, they cannot be stimulated to further orgasm. The refractory period does not exist in women, who are capable of multiple and successive orgasms.

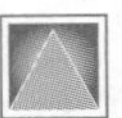

Table 18.1a–3
Male Sexual Response Cycle[a]

Organ	Excitement Phase	Orgasmic Phase	Resolution Phase
Mental	Lasts several minutes to several hours; heightened excitement before orgasm, 30 secs to 3 mins	3–15 secs	10–15 mins; if no orgasm, 0.5 to 1 day
Skin	Just before orgasm: sexual flush inconsistently appears; maculopapular rash originates on abdomen and spreads to anterior chest wall, face, and neck, and can include shoulders and forearms	Well-developed flush	Flush disappears in reverse order of appearance; inconsistently appearing film of perspiration on soles of feet and palms of hands
Penis	Erection in 10–30 secs caused by vasocongestion of erectile bodies of corpus cavernosa of shaft; loss of erection may occur with introduction of asexual stimulus—e.g., loud noise; with heightened excitement, size of glans and diameter of penile shaft increase further	Ejaculation: emission phase marked by three to four contractions of 0.8 sec of vas, seminal vesicles, prostate; ejaculation proper marked by contractions of 0.8 sec of urethra and ejaculatory spurt of 12–20 in. at age 18, decreasing with age to seepage at 70	Erection: partial involution in 5–10 secs with variable refractory period; full detumescence in 5–30 mins
Scrotum and testes	Tightening and lifting of scrotal sac and elevation of testes; with heightened excitement, 50% increase in size of testes over unstimulated state and flattening against perineum, signaling impending ejaculation	No change	Decrease to baseline size because of loss of vasocongestion; testicular and scrotal descent within 5–30 mins after orgasm; involution may take several hours if no orgasmic release takes place
Cowper's glands	2–3 Drops of mucoid fluid that contain viable sperm are secreted during heightened excitement	No change	No change
Other	Breasts: inconsistent nipple erection with heightened excitement before orgasm Myotonia: semispastic contractions of facial, abdominal, and intercostal muscles Tachycardia: up to 175 beats/min Blood pressure: rises to 20–80 mm systolic; 10–40 mm diastolic Respiration: increased	Loss of voluntary muscular control Rectum: rhythmic contractions of sphincter Heart rate: up to 180 beats/min Blood pressure: up to 40–100 mm systolic; 20–50 mm diastolic Respiration: up to 40 respirations/min	Return to baseline state in 5–10 mins

[a]A desire phase consisting of sex fantasies and desire to have sex precedes the excitement phase.

Sexual response is a true psychophysiological experience. Arousal is triggered by both psychological and physical stimuli, levels of tension are experienced both physiologically and emotionally, and, with orgasm, there is normally a subjective perception of a peak of physical reaction and release. Psychosexual development, psychological attitude toward sexuality, and attitudes toward one's sexual partner are directly involved with and affect the physiology of human sexual response.

ABNORMAL SEXUALITY AND SEXUAL DYSFUNCTIONS

Seven major categories of sexual dysfunction are listed in DSM-IV-TR: (1) sexual desire disorders, (2) sexual arousal disorders, (3) orgasm disorders, (4) sexual pain disorders, (5) sexual dysfunction due to a general medical condition, (6) substance-induced sexual dysfunction, and (7) sexual dysfunction not otherwise specified.

Definition In DSM-IV-TR, sexual dysfunctions are categorized as Axis I disorders. The syndromes listed are correlated with the sexual physiological response, which is divided into the four phases discussed above. The essential feature of the sexual dysfunctions is inhibited in one or more of the phases, including disturbance in the subjective sense of pleasure or desire or disturbance in objective performance or experience (Tables 18.1a–4 and 18.1a–5). Either type of disturbance can occur alone or in combination. Sexual dysfunctions are diagnosed only when they are the major part of the clinical picture. They can be lifelong or acquired, generalized or situational, and due to psychological factors, physiological factors, or combined factors. If they are attributable entirely to a general medical condition, substance use, or adverse effects of medication, then sexual dysfunction due to a general medical condition or substance-induced sexual dysfunction is diagnosed.

According to the tenth revision of *International Statistical Classification of Diseases and Related Health Problems* (ICD-10), *sexual dysfunction* refers to a person's inability to "participate in a sexual relationship as he or she would wish." The dysfunction is expressed as a lack of desire or of pleasure or as a physiological inability to begin, maintain, or complete sexual interaction. Because sexual response is psychosomatic, it may be difficult to determine "the relative importance of psychological and/or organic factors."

Sexual dysfunction such as lack of desire can occur in both men and women, but women more often complain of the "subjective quality" of the experience than of the "failure of a specific response." ICD-10 advises looking "beyond the presenting complaint to find the most appropriate diagnostic category." Table 18.1a–6 presents the ICD-10 diagnostic criteria.

With the possible exception of premature ejaculation, sexual dysfunctions are rarely found separate from other psychiatric syndromes. Sexual disorders may lead to or result from relational problems, and patients invariably develop an increasing fear of fail-

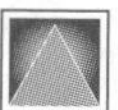

Table 18.1a–4
DSM-IV-TR Phases of the Sexual Response Cycle and Associated Sexual Dysfunctions[a]

Phases	Characteristics	Dysfunction
1. Desire	Distinct from any identified solely through physiology and reflects the patient's motivations, drives, and personality; characterized by sexual fantasies and the desire to have sex.	Hypoactive sexual desire disorder; sexual aversion disorder; hypoactive sexual desire disorder due to a general medical condition (man or woman); substance-induced sexual dysfunction with impaired desire
2. Excitement	Subjective sense of sexual pleasure and accompanying physiological changes; all physiological responses noted in Masters and Johnson's excitement and plateau phases are combined in this phase.	Female sexual arousal disorder; male erectile disorder (may also occur in stages 3 and 4); male erectile disorder due to a general medical condition; dyspareunia due to a general medical condition (man or woman); substance-induced sexual dysfunction with impaired arousal
3. Orgasm	Peaking of sexual pleasure, with release of sexual tension and rhythmic contraction of the perineal muscles and pelvic reproductive organs.	Female orgasmic disorder; male orgasmic disorder; premature ejaculation; other sexual dysfunction due to a general medical condition (man or woman); substance-induced sexual dysfunction with impaired orgasm
4. Resolution	A sense of general relaxation, well-being, and muscle relaxation; men are refractory to orgasm for a period of time that increases with age, whereas women can have multiple orgasms without a refractory period.	Postcoital dysphoria; postcoital headache

[a]DSM-IV-TR consolidates the Masters and Johnson excitement and plateau phases into a single excitement phase, which is preceded by the desire (appetitive) phase. The orgasm and resolution phases remain the same as originally described by Masters and Johnson.

ure and self-consciousness about their sexual performance. Sexual dysfunctions are frequently associated with other mental disorders, such as depressive disorders, anxiety disorders, personality disorders, and schizophrenia. In many instances, a sexual dysfunction may be diagnosed in conjunction with another psychiatric disorder; in other cases, however, it is only one of many signs or symptoms of the psychiatric disorder.

A sexual disorder can be symptomatic of biological problems, intrapsychic conflicts, interpersonal difficulties, or a combination of these factors. Sexual function can be affected by stress of any kind, by emotional disorders, and by a lack of sexual knowledge.

Taking a Sexual History

As with all psychiatric interviews, taking a sexual history not only is a time to gather information, but it also permits the development of a positive doctor–patient relationship. The development of rapport requires an accepting atmosphere and a nonjudgmental attitude on the part of the therapist toward the patients' sexual values, ideas, and practices.

The sexual history is more structured than the rest of the psychiatric interview, although patients are encouraged to take their own lead in areas of great personal significance. In general, the therapist structures the interview so that both recent and early sexual histories are covered. The therapist must ascertain the specific current sexual complaint, the patient's sexual practices and pattern of interaction with partners, the patient's sexual goal and fantasies, the patient's masturbatory history, the presence or extent of extramarital relationships, and the degree of commitment to the marriage or the partner. Patients describe their view of the problem and when it began. If married, the courtship, honeymoon, and reproductive history are examined in detail. Premarital expectations, mutual physical attraction, periods of separation, the type of contraception used, and the effect of children on the couple's sexual life are covered. The satisfying aspects of the marriage must also be discussed. The patient is particularly asked to evaluate the partner's contribution to the present distress.

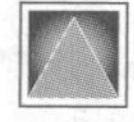

Table 18.1a–5
Sexual Dysfunction Not Correlated with Phases of the Sexual Response Cycle

Category	Dysfunctions
Sexual pain disorders	Vaginismus (woman) Dyspareunia (woman and man)
Other	Sexual dysfunctions not otherwise specified. Examples: 1. No erotic sensation despite normal physiological response to sexual stimulation (e.g., orgasmic anhedonia) 2. Female analog of premature ejaculation 3. Genital pain occurring during masturbation

Early sexual development and education are also thoroughly discussed. The interviewer asks for the patient's view of the parents' marriage as seen in retrospect and as perceived in childhood. Relationships to peers, siblings, and important familial figures other than parents are also explored. Particular attention is paid to ways in which affection was expressed in the family and the degree of physical contact between family members. The sexual climate in which the patient grew up is seen through reported parental attitudes, memories of sexual games played as a child, the way in which the patient learned sexual facts, the specifics of religious training, reactions to masturbation and nocturnal emissions or the menarche, dating patterns, an adolescent rebellious phase, and any significant premarital involvements. Ethnic background and the socioeconomic level of the patient's primary family are also taken into account. As the interview progresses, the patient's self-image emerges. The interviewer must be sensitive to any event that was exceptional in the patient's sexual life in either a destructive or a highly pleasant manner and should take particular note of the people who contributed to the patient's sexual education, identity, and mores.

The interviewer must also ask specific questions to elicit information that may be outside the patient's view of the socially acceptable, such as premarital and extramarital affairs, group sex, homosexual involvements, and abortions. The sexual orientation of the person being interviewed should be ascertained, and questions related to same-sex interactions explored. All interviews should review high-risk sexual behavior regardless of sexual orientation, as transmission of the human immunodeficiency virus (HIV) occurs in all groups. Additionally, the issue of sexual abuse must be explored, particularly because a history of abuse predisposes to the development of sexual dysfunction.

Similar disorders exist among both homosexual and heterosexual partners, with variations imposed by anatomical differences. For example,

Table 18.1a–6
ICD-10 Diagnostic Criteria for Sexual Dysfunction, Not Caused by Organic Disorder or Disease

G1. The subject is unable to participate in a sexual relationship as he or she would wish.

G2. The dysfunction occurs frequently, but may be absent on some occasions.

G3. The dysfunction has been present for at least 6 months.

G4. The dysfunction is not entirely attributable to any of the other mental and behavioral disorders in ICD-10, physical disorders (such as endocrine disorder), or drug treatment.

Comments

Measurement of each form of dysfunction can be based on rating scales that assess severity as well as frequency of the problem. More than one type of dysfunction can coexist.

Lack or loss of sexual desire

A. The general criteria for sexual dysfunction must be met.

B. There is a lack or loss of sexual desire, manifest by diminution of seeking out sexual cues, of thinking about sex with associated feelings of desire or appetite, or of sexual fantasies.

C. There is a lack of interest in initiating sexual activity either with a partner or as solitary masturbation, resulting in a frequency of activity clearly lower than expected, taking into account age and context, or in a frequency very clearly reduced from previous much higher levels.

Sexual aversion and lack of sexual enjoyment

Sexual aversion

A. The general criteria for sexual dysfunction must be met.

B. The prospect of sexual interaction with a partner produces sufficient aversion, fear, or anxiety that sexual activity is avoided, or, if it occurs, is associated with strong negative feelings and an inability to experience any pleasure.

C. The aversion is not the result of performance anxiety (reaction to previous failure of sexual response).

Lack of sexual enjoyment

A. The general criteria for sexual dysfunction must be met.

B. Genital response (orgasm and/or ejaculation) occurs during sexual stimulation but is not accompanied by pleasurable sensations or feelings of pleasant excitement.

C. There is no manifest and persistent fear or anxiety during sexual activity (see sexual aversion).

Failure of genital response

A. The general criteria for sexual dysfunction must be met.

In addition, for men:

B. Erection sufficient for intercourse fails to occur when intercourse is attempted. The dysfunction takes one of the following forms:

(1) full erection occurs during the early stages of lovemaking but disappears or declines when intercourse is attempted (before ejaculation if it occurs);

(2) erection does occur, but only at times when intercourse is not being considered;

(3) partial erection, insufficient for intercourse, occurs, but not full erection;

(4) no penile tumescence occurs at all.

In addition, for women:

B. There is failure of genital response, experienced as failure of vaginal lubrication, together with inadequate tumescence of the labia. The dysfunction takes one of the following forms:

(1) general: lubrication fails in all relevant circumstances;

(2) lubrication may occur initially but fails to persist for long enough to allow comfortable penile entry;

(3) situational: lubrication occurs only in some situations (e.g., with one partner but not another, or during masturbation, or when vaginal intercourse is not being contemplated).

Orgasmic dysfunction

A. The general criteria for sexual dysfunction must be met.

B. There is orgasmic dysfunction (either absence or marked delay of orgasm), which takes one of the following forms:

(1) orgasm has never been experienced in any situation;

(2) orgasmic dysfunction has developed after a period of relatively normal response:

(a) general: orgasmic dysfunction occurs in all situations and with any partner;

(b) situational:

for *women:* orgasm does occur in certain situations (e.g., when masturbating or with certain partners); for *men,* one of the following can be applied:

i) orgasm occurs only during sleep, never during the waking state;

ii) orgasm never occurs in the presence of the partner;

iii) orgasm occurs in the presence of the partner but not during intercourse.

Premature ejaculation

A. The general criteria for sexual dysfunction must be met.

B. There is an inability to delay ejaculation sufficiently to enjoy lovemaking, manifest as either of the following:

(1) occurrence of ejaculation before or very soon after the beginning of intercourse (if a time limit is required: before or within 15 seconds of the beginning of intercourse);

(2) ejaculation occurs in the absence of sufficient erection to make intercourse possible.

C. The problem is not the result of prolonged abstinence from sexual activity.

Nonorganic vaginismus

A. The general criteria for sexual dysfunction must be met.

B. There is spasm of the perivaginal muscles, sufficient to prevent penile entry or make it uncomfortable. The dysfunction takes one of the following forms:

(1) normal response has never been experienced;

(2) vaginismus has developed after a period of relatively normal response:

(a) when vaginal entry is not attempted, a normal sexual response may occur;

(b) any attempt at sexual contact leads to generalized fear and efforts to avoid vaginal entry (e.g., spasm of the adductor muscles of the thighs).

Nonorganic dyspareunia

A. The general criteria for sexual dysfunction must be met.

In addition, for women:

B. Pain is experienced at the entry of the vagina, either throughout sexual intercourse or only when deep thrusting of the penis occurs.

C. The disorder is not attributable to vaginismus or failure of lubrication; dyspareunia of organic origin should be classified according to the underlying disorder.

In addition for men:

B. Pain or discomfort is experienced during sexual response. (The timing of the pain and the exact localization should be carefully recorded.)

C. The discomfort is not the result of local physical factors. If physical factors are found, the dysfunction should be classified elsewhere.

Excessive sexual drive

No research criteria are attempted for this category. Researchers studying this category are recommended to design their own criteria.

Other sexual dysfunction, not caused by organic disorder or disease

Unspecified sexual dysfunction, not caused by organic disorder or disease

From World Health Organization. *The ICD-10 Classification of Mental and Behavioural Disorders: Diagnostic Criteria for Research.* Geneva: World Health Organization; 1993, with permission.

although penile–vaginal dysfunction cannot be described among homosexuals, penile–anal dysfunction may occur. Regardless of sexual orientation, each phase of the sex cycle applies equally to same-sex and heterosexual partners, and the methods and principles for treatment are essentially similar. Taking a sex history is summarized in Table 18.1a–7.

Rating Scales

In addition to the interview, several questionnaires are available to assess sexual function. They were developed primarily to evaluate illness or medication-related effects on sexual functioning. The most commonly used scales are the Arizona Sexual Experience Scale, the Brief Sexual Function Questionnaire, the Changes in Sexual Functioning Questionnaire, the Derogatis Sexual Function Inventory, and the Rush Sexual Inventory. The scales vary in length, reliability, validity, and method of administration. Some are rated by the patients themselves, others by the therapist. The formats include structured and semistructured approaches. The scales differ in number of symptoms assessed, the dysfunctions they target, and the time frame they cover.

Sexual Desire Disorders

DSM-IV-TR divides sexual desire disorders into two classes: hypoactive sexual desire disorder, characterized by a deficiency or lack of sexual fantasies and desire for sexual activity, and sexual aversion disorder, characterized by an aversion to and avoidance of genital contact with a sexual partner. The former condition is more common than the latter.

Hypoactive Sexual Desire Disorder

Hypoactive sexual desire disorder (Table 18.1a–8) is experienced by both men and women; however, they may not be hampered by any dysfunction once they are involved in the sex act. Conversely, hypoactive desire may be used to mask another sexual dysfunction. Lack of desire may be expressed by decreased frequency of coitus, perception of the partner as unattractive, or overt complaints of lack of desire. Upon questioning, the patient is found to have few or no sexual thoughts or fantasies, a lack of awareness of sexual cues, and little interest in initiating sexual experiences.

Sometimes, biochemical correlates are associated with hypoactive desire. A recent study found markedly low serum testosterone concentrations in men complaining of this dysfunction when they were compared with normal controls in a sleep laboratory situation. Also, a central dopamine blockage is known to decrease desire. The need for sexual contact and satisfaction varies among different persons, as well as in the same person over time. In a group of 100 couples with stable marriages, 8 percent reported having intercourse less than once a month. In another group of couples, one-third reported lack of sexual relations for periods averaging 8 weeks. In a survey of a general medical practice in England, 25 percent of that sample reported no sexual activity most of the time. It has been estimated that 20 percent of the total population have hypoactive sexual desire disorder. The complaint is more common among women.

Patients with desire problems often have good ego strengths and use inhibition of desire defensively to protect against unconscious fears about sex. Lack of desire can also result from chronic stress, anxiety, or depression. Abstinence from sex for a prolonged period sometimes suppresses the sexual impulse. Desire problems may also be an expression of hostility toward the partner or signal a deteriorating relationship.

The presence of desire depends on several factors: biological drive, adequate self-esteem, previous good experiences with sex, the availability of an appropriate partner, and a good relationship in nonsexual areas with one's partner. Damage to any of those factors may result in diminished desire.

Hypoactive sexual desire disorders often become manifest during puberty and may remain a lifelong condition. A general medical workup should be conducted to rule out a medical cause, which, if present, would be, according to DSM-IV-TR, diagnosed as male or female sexual desire disorder due to a general medical condition.

Mr. and Mrs. K. presented for therapy because of the wife's complaints regarding lack of sexuality in their marriage. Mr. K. stated that he rarely felt sexual desire at all and that this problem was not restricted to the marriage or lack of desire for his wife. In the course of the workup, the couple proved to have multiple sexual dysfunctions, including dyspareunia on the part of the wife and erectile disorder on the part of the husband, as well as lack of desire. Mr. and Mrs. K. were in their early 50s, had been married for 18 years, and had no children. Mrs. K. had had some psychotherapy and was currently on medication for recurrent depression. The couple had similar backgrounds—both were immigrants from an Eastern European country. Husband and wife had both attained Ph.D.s, valued education highly, and were successful in their respective fields.

Mrs. K. had emigrated with her family. She was the oldest of five children and had been responsible for taking care of her younger siblings. She received little nurturing herself and had been the recipient of considerable emotional abuse from her mother. Of particular importance, she had been sexually abused by an elderly neighbor. She discussed this in therapy for the first time since the incident occurred. Mr. K. had come to the United States alone in his late adolescence. He had been separated from his parents in early childhood and was raised by distant relatives. In spite of their lack of intimacy, the couple had a strong sense of loyalty to each other and shared a similar culture and values.

They practiced the behavioral exercises as directed, and Mrs. K. was very pleased by the touching and attention she received. She practiced using size-graduated dilators for her dyspareunia and eventually allowed digital penetration of her vagina by her husband. Mr. K. became freer in his discussions of sex, including voicing his feeling that it was dirty. He used 50 mg of sildenafil (Viagra) to facilitate his erections and felt much better about himself when he was able to maintain them. The couple approached therapy as they had approached school, diligently and conscientiously. Although their sexual interaction remained rather rigid—planned for the same time each week—they were pleased with their progress individually and as a couple. They were able to experience sexual pleasure manually and have had some episodes of intercourse.

Sexual Aversion Disorder

Sexual aversion disorder (Table 18.1a–9) is defined in DSM-IV-TR as a "persistent or recurrent and extreme aversion to, and avoidance of, all or almost all, genital sexual contact with a sexual partner." Some researchers consider the line between hypoactive desire disorder and sexual aversion disorder blurred, and, in some cases, both diagnoses are appropriate. Low frequency of sexual interaction is a symptom common to both disorders. The clinician should think of the words "repugnance" and "phobia" in relation to the patient with sexual aversion disorder. Freud conceptualized sexual aversion as the result of inhibition during the phallic psychosexual phase and unresolved oedipal conflicts. Some men, fixated at the phallic stage of development, fear the vagina and believe that they will be castrated if they approach it (a concept Freud called *vagina dentata*), because they believe unconsciously that the vagina has teeth. Hence, they avoid contact with the female genitalia entirely.

The disorder may result from a traumatic sexual assault, such as rape or childhood abuse, from repeated painful experiences with coi-

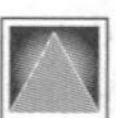

Table 18.1a–7
Taking a Sex History

- I. Identifying data
  - A. Age
  - B. Sex
  - C. Occupation
  - D. Relationship status—single, married, number of times previously married, separated, divorced, cohabiting, serious involvement, casual dating (difficulty forming or keeping relationships should be assessed throughout the interview)
  - E. Sexual orientation—heterosexual, homosexual, or bisexual (this may also be ascertained later in the interview)
- II. Current functioning
  - A. Unsatisfactory to highly satisfactory
  - B. If unsatisfactory, why?
  - C. Feelings about partner satisfaction
  - D. Dysfunctions?—e.g., lack of desire, erectile disorder, inhibited female arousal, anorgasmia, premature ejaculation, retarded ejaculation, pain associated with intercourse (dysfunction discussed below)
    1. Onset—lifelong or acquired
       - a. If acquired, when?
       - b. Did onset coincide with drug use (medications or illegal recreational drugs), life stresses (e.g., loss of job, birth of child), interpersonal difficulties?
    2. Generalized—occurs in most situations or with most partners
    3. Situational
       - a. Only with current partner
       - b. In any committed relationship
       - c. Only with masturbation
       - d. In socially proscribed circumstance (e.g., affair)
       - e. In definable circumstance (e.g., very late at night, in parental home, when partner initiated sex play)
  - E. Frequency—partnered sex (coital and noncoital sex play)
  - F. Desire/libido—how often are sexual feelings, thoughts, fantasies, dreams, experienced (per day, week, etc.)?
  - G. Description of typical sexual interaction
    1. Manner of initiation or invitation (e.g., Verbal or physical? Does same person always initiate?)
    2. Presence, type, and extent of foreplay (e.g., kissing, caressing, manual or oral genital stimulation)
    3. Coitus? Positions used?
    4. Verbalization during sex? If so, what kind?
    5. Afterplay? (whether sex act is completed or disrupted by dysfunction); typical activities (e.g., holding, talking, return to daily activities, sleeping)
    6. Feeling after sex: relaxed, tense, angry, loving
  - H. Sexual compulsivity? (intrusion of sexual thoughts or participation in sexual activities to a degree that interferes with relationships or work, requires deception, and may endanger the patient)
- III. Past sexual history
  - A. Childhood sexuality
    1. Parental attitudes about sex—degree of openness or reserve (assess unusual prudery or seductiveness)
    2. Parents' attitudes about nudity and modesty
    3. Learning about sex
       - a. From parents (Initiated by child's questions or parent volunteering information? Which parent? What was child's age?)? Subjects covered (e.g., pregnancy, birth, intercourse, menstruation, nocturnal emission, masturbation)?
       - b. From books, magazines, or friends at school or through religious group?
       - c. Significant misinformation
       - d. Feeling about information
    4. Viewing or hearing primal scene—Reaction?
    5. Viewing sex play or intercourse of person other than parent
    6. Viewing sex between pets or other animals
  - B. Childhood sex activities
    1. Genital self-stimulation before adolescence—Age? Reaction if apprehended?
    2. Awareness of self as boy or girl—Bathroom sensual activities (regarding urine, feces, odor, enemas)?
    3. Sexual play or exploration with another child (playing doctor)—Type of activity (e.g., looking, manual touching, genital touching)? Reactions or consequences if apprehended (by whom?)?
- IV. Adolescence
  - A. Age of onset of puberty—development of secondary sex characteristics, age of menarche for girl, wet dreams or first ejaculation for boy (preparation for and reaction to)
  - B. Sense of self as feminine or masculine—body image, acceptance by peers (opposite sex and same sex), sense of sexual desirability, onset of coital fantasies
  - C. Sex activities
    1. Masturbation—Age begun? Ever punished or prohibited? Method used, accompanying fantasies, frequency (questions about masturbation and fantasies are among the most sensitive for patients to answer)?
    2. Homosexual activities—Ongoing or rare and experimental episodes? Approached by others? If homosexual, has there been any heterosexual experimentation?
    3. Dating—casual or steady; description of first crush, infatuation, or first love
    4. Experiences of kissing, necking, petting ("making out" or "fooling around"), age begun, frequency, number of partners, circumstances, type(s) of activity
    5. Orgasm—When first experienced (may not be experienced during adolescence)? With masturbation, during sleep, or with partner? With intercourse or other sex play? Frequency?
    6. First coitus—age, circumstances, partner, reactions (may not be experienced during adolescence), contraception and/or safe sex precautions used
- V. Adult sexual activities (may be experienced by some adolescents)
  - A. Premarital sex
    1. Types of sex play experiences—frequency of sexual interactions, types and number of partners
    2. Contraception and/or safe sex precautions used
    3. First coitus (if not experienced in adolescence)—age, circumstances, partner
    4. Cohabitation—age begun, duration, description of partner, sexual fidelity, types of sexual activity, frequency, satisfaction, number of cohabiting relationships, reasons for breakup(s)
    5. Engagement—age; activity during engagement period with fiancé(e), with others; length of engagement
  - B. Marriage (if multiple marriages have occurred, explore sexual activity, reasons for marriage, and reasons for divorce in each marriage)
    1. Types and frequency of sexual interaction—describe typical sexual interaction (see above). Satisfaction with sex life? View of partner's feeling
    2. First sexual experience with spouse—When? What were the circumstances? Was it satisfying? Disappointing?
    3. Honeymoon—Setting, duration, pleasant or unpleasant, sexually active? Frequency? Problems? Compatibility?
    4. Effect of pregnancies and children on marital sex
    5. Extramarital sex—Number of incidents, partner, emotional attachment to extramarital partners? Feelings about extramarital sex
    6. Postmarital masturbation—Frequency? Effect on marital sex?
    7. Extramarital sex by partner—effect on interviewee
    8. Ménage à trois or multiple sex (swinging)
    9. Areas of conflict in marriage (e.g., parenting, finances, division of responsibilities, priorities)

(*continued*)

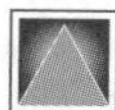

Table 18.1a–7 (*continued*)

VI. Sex after widowhood, separation, divorce—celibacy, orgasms in sleep, masturbation, noncoital sex play, intercourse (number of and relationship to partners), other

VII. Special issues
- A. History of rape, incest, sexual or physical abuse
- B. Spousal abuse (current)
- C. Chronic illness (physical or psychiatric)
- D. History or presence of sexually transmitted diseases
- E. Fertility problems
- F. Abortions, miscarriages, or unwanted or illegitimate pregnancies
- G. Gender identity conflict—(e.g., transsexualism, wearing clothes of opposite sex)
- H. Paraphilias—(e.g., fetishes, voyeurism, sadomasochism)

tus, or from early developmental conflicts that have left the patient with unconscious connections between the sexual impulse and overwhelming feelings of shame and guilt. The disorder may also be a reaction to a perceived psychological assault by the partner and to relationship difficulties.

Mr. and Mrs. J. were 38 and 36 years old, respectively, when they presented for treatment, stating they had not had coitus for 3 years. Three years previously, Mrs. J. revealed that she had been having an extramarital affair for 2 months, which she then ended. At that time, she told her husband that she had been unhappy with their lovemaking.

Upon hearing of her affair, the husband was angry and refused to approach his wife sexually. When he finally did so, she would allow caressing of her body but not her genitalia, although she was willing to stimulate him sexually. At this point, the husband also had an affair, but stopped when he realized it would not solve his problems with his wife, and she then agreed to enter sex therapy. When they presented for sex therapy, their sexual interaction consisted of mutual kissing and her manual stimulation of his penis until he reached orgasm.

In the individual interviews that were part of the evaluation of the case, Mrs. J. reiterated that she found her husband's lovemaking unsatisfactory but did not have a problem allowing other men to caress her genitalia and could have coitus with other men. Mr. J. had been traumatized by his wife's rejection and sexual betrayal, and he, in turn, was averse to touching her genitalia or attempting intromission.

This was a case in which both partners suffered from sexual aversion disorder. The husband feared touching his wife in an explicitly sexual way, the wife was averse to his touching her genitalia, and both spouses avoided coitus. For both partners, the dysfunction was acquired and situational.

Sexual Arousal Disorders

DSM-IV-TR divides the sexual arousal disorders into (1) female sexual arousal disorder, characterized by the persistent or recurrent partial or complete failure to attain or maintain the lubrication–swelling response of sexual excitement until the completion of the sexual act, and (2) male erectile disorder, characterized by the recurrent and persistent partial or complete failure to attain or maintain an erection until the completion of the sex act. The diagnosis takes into account the focus, the intensity, and the duration of the sexual activity in which the patient engages. If sexual stimulation is inadequate in focus, intensity, or duration, the diagnosis should not be made.

Female Sexual Arousal Disorder

Women who have excitement phase dysfunction often have orgasmic problems as well. In one series of relatively happily married couples, 33 percent of the women described difficulty in maintaining sexual excitement. Other data indicate that 14 to 19 percent of women have chronic lubrication difficulties, whereas 23 percent have intermittent problems with lubrication. In studies of postmenopausal women, complaints of persistent or intermittent lubrication difficulties increase to 44 percent. Numerous psychological factors are associated with female sexual inhibition. These conflicts may be expressed through inhibition of excitement or orgasm and are discussed under orgasmic phase dysfunctions. In some women, arousal disorders are associated with dyspareunia or lack of desire.

Less research has been done on physiological components of dysfunction in women than of dysfunction in men, and there have been conflicting results. Masters and Johnson found normally responsive women to desire sex premenstrually. Dysfunctional women, however, tended to be more responsive immediately after their periods. Another group of dysfunctional women felt the greatest sexual excitement at the time of ovulation. Some evidence indicates that dysfunctional women are less aware of physiological responses in their bodies, such as vasocongestion, during arousal.

There are some medical causes for female sexual arousal disorder. Alterations in testosterone, estrogen, prolactin, and thyroxine concentrations have been implicated. Medications with antihistaminic or anticholinergic properties lessen vaginal lubrication and interfere with arousal. Also, postmenopausal women require longer

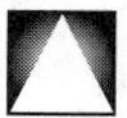

Table 18.1a–8
DSM-IV-TR Diagnostic Criteria for Hypoactive Sexual Desire Disorder

A. Persistently or recurrently deficient (or absent) sexual fantasies and desire for sexual activity. The judgment of deficiency or absence is made by the clinician, taking into account factors that affect sexual functioning, such as age and the context of the person's life.

B. The disturbance causes marked distress or interpersonal difficulty.

C. The sexual dysfunction is not better accounted for by another Axis I disorder (except another sexual dysfunction) and is not due exclusively to the direct physiological effects of a substance (e.g., a drug of abuse, a medication) or a general medical condition.

Specify type:
- **Lifelong type**
- **Acquired type**

Specify type:
- **Generalized type**
- **Situational type**

Specify:
- **Due to psychological factors**
- **Due to combined factors**

From American Psychiatric Association. *Diagnostic and Statistical Manual of Mental Disorders.* 4th ed. Text rev. Washington, DC: American Psychiatric Association; 2000, with permission.

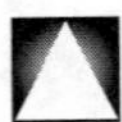

Table 18.1a–9
DSM-IV-TR Diagnostic Criteria for Sexual Aversion Disorder

A. Persistent or recurrent extreme aversion to and avoidance of all (or almost all) genital sexual contact with a sexual partner.
B. The disturbance causes marked distress or interpersonal difficulty.
C. The sexual dysfunction is not better accounted for by another Axis I disorder (except another sexual dysfunction).

Specify type:
Lifelong type
Acquired type

Specify type:
Situational type
Generalized type

Specify:
Due to psychological factors
Due to combined factors

From American Psychiatric Association. *Diagnostic and Statistical Manual of Mental Disorders*. 4th ed. Text rev. Washington, DC: American Psychiatric Association; 2000, with permission.

stimulation for lubrication to occur, and there is generally less vaginal transudate after menopause. An artificial lubricant is frequently useful in this situation.

Table 18.1a–10 presents the diagnostic criteria for female sexual arousal disorder.

Male Erectile Disorder Male erectile disorder (Table 18.1a–11) is also called *erectile dysfunction* and *impotence*. A man with lifelong male erectile disorder has never obtained an erection sufficient for vaginal insertion. In acquired male erectile disorder, however, the man successfully achieved vaginal penetration at some time in his sexual life but, later, cannot do so. In situational male erectile disorder, the man can have coitus in certain circumstances but not in others—for example, a man may function effectively with a prostitute but not with his wife. Kinsey estimated that a few men (2 to 4 percent)

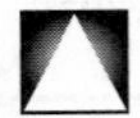

Table 18.1a–10
DSM-IV-TR Diagnostic Criteria for Female Sexual Arousal Disorder

A. Persistent or recurrent inability to attain, or to maintain until completion of the sexual activity, an adequate lubrication–swelling response of sexual excitement.
B. The disturbance causes marked distress or interpersonal difficulty.
C. The sexual dysfunction is not better accounted for by another Axis I disorder (except another sexual dysfunction) and is not due exclusively to the direct physiological effects of a substance (e.g., a drug of abuse, a medication) or a general medical condition.

Specify type:
Lifelong type
Acquired type

Specify type:
Generalized type
Situational type

Specify:
Due to psychological factors
Due to combined factors

From American Psychiatric Association. *Diagnostic and Statistical Manual of Mental Disorders*. 4th ed. Text rev. Washington, DC: American Psychiatric Association; 2000, with permission.

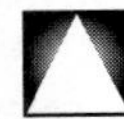

Table 18.1a–11
DSM-IV-TR Diagnostic Criteria for Male Erectile Disorder

A. Persistent or recurrent inability to attain, or to maintain until completion of the sexual activity, an adequate erection.
B. The disturbance causes marked distress or interpersonal difficulty.
C. The erectile dysfunction is not better accounted for by another Axis I disorder (other than a sexual dysfunction) and is not due exclusively to the direct physiological effects of a substance (e.g., a drug of abuse, a medication) or a general medical condition.

Specify type:
Lifelong type
Acquired type

Specify type:
Generalized type
Situational type

Specify:
Due to psychological factors
Due to combined factors

From American Psychiatric Association. *Diagnostic and Statistical Manual of Mental Disorders*. 4th ed. Text rev. Washington, DC: American Psychiatric Association; 2000, with permission.

are dysfunctional at age 35 years but 77 percent are dysfunctional at age 80 years. Ten percent of the men in the University of Chicago study reported an experience with erectile dysfunction in the past year, and between 15 and 20 percent experienced anxiety about performing. More recently, it was estimated that the incidence of erectile dysfunction in young men is approximately 8 percent. However, this sexual dysfunction may first appear later in life. Masters and Johnson reported a fear of impotence in all men over 40 years of age, which the researchers believed reflects the masculine fear of loss of virility with advancing age. (As it happens, however, erectile dysfunction is not a regularly occurring phenomenon in aged men; good health and an available sexual partner are more closely related to continuing potency than is age per se.) The chief complaint of between 35 and 50 percent of all men treated for sexual disorders is erectile dysfunction.

In general, the psychological conflicts that cause erectile dysfunction are related to an inability to express the sexual impulse because of fear, anxiety, anger, or moral prohibition. Lifelong dysfunction is a more serious but less common condition than acquired erectile disorder and is less amenable to treatment.

Many developmental factors have been cited as contributing to erectile disorder. Any experience that hinders the ability to be intimate, that leads to a feeling of inadequacy or distrust, or that develops a sense of being unloving or unlovable may result in this problem. Erectile dysfunction in an ongoing relationship may reflect difficulties between the partners, particularly if one person cannot communicate his or her needs or angry feelings in a direct and constructive manner. Successive episodes of impotence are reinforcing, with the man becoming increasingly anxious about his next sexual encounter. Regardless of the original cause of the dysfunction, his anticipatory anxiety about achieving and maintaining an erection interferes with his pleasure in sexual contact and his ability to respond to stimulation, thus perpetuating the problem.

Mr. Y. came for therapy after his wife complained about their lack of sexual interaction. The patient avoided sex because of his frequent erectile dysfunction and painful feelings of inadequacy he suffered after his "failures." He presented as an articulate, gentle, and self-blaming man.

He was faithful to his wife but masturbated frequently. His fantasies involved explicit sadistic components, including hanging and biting women. The contrast between his angry, aggressive fantasies and his loving, considerate behavior toward his wife symbolized his conflicts about his sexuality, his masculinity, and his mixed feelings about women. He was diagnosed with erectile dysfunction, situational type.

Orgasmic Disorders *Female orgasmic disorder* (also known as *inhibited female orgasm*, or *anorgasmia*) is defined as the recurrent and persistent inhibition of the female orgasm, manifested by the absence or delay of orgasm after a normal sexual excitement phase that the clinician judges to be adequate in focus, intensity, and duration. Women who can achieve orgasm with noncoital clitoral stimulation but cannot experience it during coitus in the absence of manual clitoral stimulation are not necessarily categorized as anorgasmic.

Physiological research on the female sexual response has demonstrated that orgasms caused by clitoral stimulation are physiologically identical to those caused by vaginal stimulation. Freud's theory that women must give up clitoral sensitivity for vaginal sensitivity to achieve sexual maturity is now considered misleading, although some women say that they gain a special sense of satisfaction from an orgasm precipitated by coitus. Some attribute that to the psychological feeling of closeness engendered by the act of coitus, but others maintain that the coital orgasm is a physiologically different experience. Many women achieve orgasm during coitus by a combination of manual clitoral stimulation and penile vaginal stimulation.

Lifelong female orgasmic disorder exists when a woman has never experienced orgasm by any kind of stimulation. Acquired orgasmic dysfunction exists if a woman has previously experienced at least one orgasm regardless of the circumstances or means of stimulation, whether by masturbation or during sleep while dreaming. Kinsey found that the proportion of married women over 35 years of age who had never achieved orgasm by any means was only 5 percent. The incidence of orgasm increases with age. According to Kinsey, the first orgasm occurs in late adolescence in approximately 50 percent of women. The rest usually experience orgasm by some means as they get older. Lifelong female orgasmic disorder is more common among unmarried women than among married women; 39 percent of the unmarried women over age 35 years in Kinsey's study had never experienced orgasm. Increased orgasmic potential in women older than 35 has been explained on the basis of less psychological inhibition, greater sexual experience, or both. Also, orgasmic consistency has been correlated with marital happiness, although cause and effect have not been determined. In the University of Chicago study, three-fourths of the married female respondents usually or always experienced orgasm during sex, compared with two-thirds of the single women. One woman in ten complained of difficulty in achieving orgasm.

Mr. and Mrs. Z. were a childless couple, both in their late 20s. She was a college instructor, and he was a freelance writer. The couple had been married for 4 years and came to therapy with a mutual complaint of steadily lessening sexual frequency.

During the year before they were seen, they had had intercourse six times. In the initial interview, Mrs. Z. stated that she had never been able to have an orgasm with her husband and had never experienced an orgasm during intercourse. Her frustration made her increasingly reluctant to have coitus and caused her to reject her husband sexually. Mrs. Z. could masturbate to orgasm while indulging in masochistic fantasies, but she did so very infrequently.

She was the oldest of four children, raised by rigid, intellectual, and undemonstrative parents. She stated that she had been a very docile child and adolescent but openly rebelled in marrying her husband. Her parents disapproved of him because he came from a different religious background. Mrs. Z.'s father particularly objected, and relations between Mr. Z. and his father-in-law were strained. Mrs. Z. stated that she often felt caught between them.

Mr. Z. was the middle child and the only boy in a family of three siblings. There was a 20-year age difference between his parents, and the father was not actively involved with the children. He felt that he had always been his mother's favorite.

Mr. and Mrs. Z. met in college, and, although neither was sexually experienced, they were strongly attracted to one another and indulged in enjoyable sexual play short of intercourse. Mrs. Z. perceived her husband as a very assertive man and was impressed by the way he stood up to her family. When he completed school a year ahead of Mrs. Z., he broke off the relationship with her. During that year, Mrs. Z. became involved with another man and enjoyed sexual play with him. She did not have intercourse with him but sometimes came to orgasm through manual manipulation. At the time of her graduation, she ended this relationship and managed to regain Mr. Z.'s attention. The couple married 6 months after her graduation. Intercourse was a disappointment to Mrs. Z. from the beginning. She felt unfulfilled, and her husband felt rejected and inadequate.

In therapy, the couple's premarital expectations were discussed. In effect, each had expected more assertiveness from the other, and, in reality, each had some problem with passivity. Several sessions were also spent dealing with relations with the in-laws. Mrs. Z. was encouraged to give priority to her relationship with her husband, and Mr. Z. was encouraged to face and restrain his competitiveness with her father. They responded to the behavioral exercises that were prescribed. At the time of their discharge from therapy, the couple was having intercourse one to two times a week. Mrs. Z. could not reach orgasm during intercourse but could frequently achieve climax after coitus through manual stimulation.

Acquired female orgasmic disorder is a common complaint in the clinical population. One clinical treatment facility described nonorgasmic women as approximately four times more common in its practice than patients with all other sexual disorders. In another study, 46 percent of the women complained of difficulty in reaching orgasm, and 15 percent described an inability to have orgasm. The overall prevalence of inhibited orgasm in women is estimated to be 30 percent.

Numerous psychological factors are associated with female sexual inhibition—fears of impregnation, rejection by the sexual partner, or damage to the vagina; hostility toward men; and feelings of guilt regarding sexual impulses. Some women equate orgasm with loss of control or with aggressive, destructive, or violent behavior. Fear of those impulses may be expressed through inhibition of excitement or orgasm. The expression of orgasmic inhibition varies. Some women feel unentitled to gratify themselves and cannot masturbate to climax. Others enjoy self-stimulation but cannot reach orgasm with a partner present. Cultural expectations and societal restrictions on women are also relevant. Nonorgasmic women may be otherwise symptom-free or may experience frustration in a variety of ways, including such pelvic complaints as lower abdominal pain, itching, and vaginal discharge, as well as increased tension, irritability, and fatigue. The diagnostic criteria for female orgasmic disorder are presented in Table 18.1a–12.

Table 18.1a–12
DSM-IV-TR Diagnostic Criteria for Female Orgasmic Disorder

A. Persistent or recurrent delay in, or absence of, orgasm after a normal sexual excitement phase. Women exhibit wide variability in the type or intensity of stimulation that triggers orgasm. The diagnosis of female orgasmic disorder should be based on the clinician's judgment that the woman's orgasmic capacity is less than would be reasonable for her age, sexual experience, and the adequacy of sexual stimulation she receives.
B. The disturbance causes marked distress or interpersonal difficulty.
C. The orgasmic dysfunction is not better accounted for by another Axis I disorder (except another sexual dysfunction) and is not due exclusively to the direct physiological effects of a substance (e.g., a drug of abuse, a medication) or a general medical condition.

Specify type:
 Lifelong type
 Acquired type
Specify type:
 Generalized type
 Situational type
Specify:
 Due to psychological factors
 Due to combined factors

From American Psychiatric Association. *Diagnostic and Statistical Manual of Mental Disorders*. 4th ed. Text rev. Washington, DC: American Psychiatric Association; 2000, with permission.

Male Orgasmic Disorder In male orgasmic disorder (previously called *inhibited male orgasm*; also called *retarded ejaculation*), a man achieves climax during coitus with great difficulty, if at all. A man is considered to have lifelong orgasmic disorder if he has never ejaculated during coitus. The disorder is diagnosed as acquired if it develops after previous normal functioning (Table 18.1a–13).

Some suggest that orgasm and ejaculation should be differentiated. Certainly, inhibited orgasm must be differentiated from retrograde ejaculation, in which ejaculation occurs but the seminal fluid passes backward into the bladder. This condition always has an organic cause. Retrograde ejaculation can develop after genitourinary surgery and is also associated with medications that have anticholinergic adverse effects, such as the phenothiazines, particularly thioridazine (Mellaril).

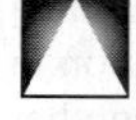

Table 18.1a–13
DSM-IV-TR Diagnostic Criteria for Male Orgasmic Disorder

A. Persistent or recurrent delay in, or absence of, orgasm after a normal sexual excitement phase during sexual activity that the clinician, taking into account the person's age, judges to be adequate in focus, intensity, and duration.
B. The disturbance causes marked distress or interpersonal difficulty.
C. The orgasmic dysfunction is not better accounted for by another Axis I disorder (except another sexual dysfunction) and is not due exclusively to the direct physiological effects of a substance (e.g., a drug of abuse, a medication) or a general medical condition.

Specify type:
 Lifelong type
 Acquired type
Specify type:
 Generalized type
 Situational type
Specify:
 Due to psychological factors
 Due to combined factors

From American Psychiatric Association. *Diagnostic and Statistical Manual of Mental Disorders*. 4th ed. Text rev. Washington, DC: American Psychiatric Association; 2000, with permission.

The incidence of male orgasmic disorder is much lower than the incidences of premature ejaculation and erectile dysfunction. Masters and Johnson reported only 3.8 percent in one group of 447 sexual dysfunction cases. This problem is more common among men with obsessive-compulsive disorders (OCDs) than among others. Male orgasmic disorder may have physiological causes and can occur after surgery of the genitourinary tract, such as prostatectomy. Male orgasmic dysfunction may also be associated with Parkinson's disease and other neurological disorders involving the lumbar or sacral sections of the spinal cord. The antihypertensive drugs guanethidine monosulfate (Ismelin) and methyldopa (Aldomet) have been implicated in retarded ejaculation. Phenothiazines have also been associated with the disorder, as have almost all the antidepressants. Transient retarded ejaculation may occur with excessive alcohol intake or with hyperglycemia. Strictly organic cases and problems that are symptomatic of other Axis I psychiatric syndromes are not to be included in the diagnosis.

Primary male orgasmic disorder indicates a more severe psychopathology. The man often comes from a rigid, puritanical background; he perceives sex as sinful and the genitals as dirty and may have conscious or unconscious incest wishes and guilt. Usually, difficulties with closeness exist that extend beyond the area of sexual relations.

Some cases involve men with adult attention-deficit disorder. It is as though these men are so easily distracted that they cannot focus on the pleasurable sensations of arousal consistently enough to attain a degree of excitement necessary for orgasm. Another theory holds that men with retarded ejaculation are preoccupied with sex, unusually voyeuristic, and easily aroused. However their elaborate fantasies of exceptionally beautiful or lust-driven women and atypical sexual activities require them to work unusually hard to achieve orgasm in more routine sexual encounters.

In an ongoing relationship, secondary ejaculatory inhibition frequently reflects interpersonal difficulties. The disorder may be the man's way of coping with real or fantasized changes in the relationship. Those changes may include plans for a pregnancy about which the man is ambivalent, the loss of sexual attraction to the partner, or demands by the partner for greater commitment as expressed by sexual performance. In some men, the inability to ejaculate reflects unexpressed hostility toward women.

In a version of the dysfunction, some men experience partial inhibition of ejaculation. These men experience a slow dribbling of ejaculation (not related to age) rather than an ejaculatory spurt. They usually do not experience the pleasurable sensations of orgasm.

A couple presented with the man as the identified patient suffering from an inability to ejaculate with intercourse. The problem was of recent onset and had started shortly after the couple decided to have a baby. The man was 43 years of age and the woman was 39 years of age. Although they had been married for 2 years and had agreed to have children when they married, the husband had put off trying to have a child. He had started a new business at the time the couple married and felt a great deal of financial pressure. The wife had been sympathetic to his anxieties, but, as her 40th birthday loomed, she insisted that they try to conceive. The husband expressed his understanding and agreed but promptly developed the symptoms of retarded ejaculation. He was diagnosed with male orgasmic disorder, acquired type.

Premature Ejaculation In *premature ejaculation*, the man recurrently achieves orgasm and ejaculates before he wishes to do so. There is no definite time frame within which to define the dysfunction. The diagnosis is made when the man regularly ejaculates before or immediately after entering the vagina or after minimal sexual stimulation. The clinician should consider factors that affect duration of the excitement phase, such as age, novelty of the sexual partner, and the frequency and duration of coitus. Masters and Johnson conceptualized the disorder in terms of the couple and considered a man a premature ejaculator if he could not control ejaculation long enough during intravaginal containment to satisfy his partner in at least half of their episodes of coitus. This definition assumes that the female partner is capable of an orgasmic response. As with other dysfunctions, the disturbance is diagnosed only if it is not caused exclusively by medical factors or is not symptomatic of any other Axis I syndrome.

Premature ejaculation is more common today among college-educated men than among men with less education and is thought to be related to their concern for partner satisfaction. It is estimated that 30 percent of the male population have the dysfunction, and approximately 40 percent of men treated for sexual disorders have premature ejaculation as the chief complaint.

Difficulty in ejaculatory control may be associated with anxiety regarding the sex act. Both anxiety and ejaculation are mediated by the sympathetic nervous system. Other psychological factors that have been noted include sexual guilt, a history of parent–child conflict, interpersonal hypersensitivity, and perfectionism or unrealistic expectations about sexual performance.

Current research also suggests that a subgroup of premature ejaculators (particularly those with a lifelong history of premature ejaculation) may be biologically predisposed to this dysfunction. Some researchers believe that certain men are constitutionally more vulnerable to sympathetic stimulation, hence, they ejaculate rapidly. Others have found a shorter bulbocavernosus reflex nerve latency time in men with lifelong premature ejaculation than in men who had acquired the dysfunction.

Premature ejaculation also may result from negative cultural conditioning. The man who has most of his early sexual contacts with prostitutes, who demand that the sex act proceed quickly, or in situations in which discovery would be embarrassing, such as in an apartment shared with roommates or in the parental home, may become conditioned to achieving orgasm rapidly. In ongoing relationships, the partner has some influence on the premature ejaculator. A stressful marriage exacerbates the disorder. Table 18.1a–14 gives the diagnostic criteria for premature ejaculation.

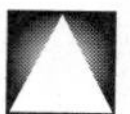

Table 18.1a–14
DSM-IV-TR Diagnostic Criteria for Premature Ejaculation

A. Persistent or recurrent ejaculation with minimal sexual stimulation before, on, or shortly after penetration and before the person wishes it. The clinician must take into account factors that affect duration of the excitement phase, such as age, novelty of the sexual partner or situation, and recent frequency of sexual activity.
B. The disturbance causes marked distress or interpersonal difficulty.
C. The premature ejaculation is not due exclusively to the direct effects of a substance (e.g., withdrawal from opioids).

Specify type:
Lifelong type
Acquired type

Specify type:
Generalized type
Situational type

Specify:
Due to psychological factors
Due to combined factors

From American Psychiatric Association. *Diagnostic and Statistical Manual of Mental Disorders*. 4th ed. Text rev. Washington, DC: American Psychiatric Association; 2000, with permission.

Sexual Pain Disorders

Dyspareunia *Dyspareunia* refers to recurrent and persistent pain during intercourse in either a man or a woman. In women, the dysfunction is related to and often coincides with vaginismus. Repeated episodes of vaginismus may lead to dyspareunia and vice versa, but, in either case, somatic causes must be ruled out. Dyspareunia should not be diagnosed as such when a medical basis for the pain is found or when (in a woman) it is associated with vaginismus or with lack of lubrication.

The true incidence of dyspareunia is unknown, but it has been estimated that 30 percent of surgical procedures on the female genital area result in temporary dyspareunia. Additionally, among women seen in sex therapy clinics, the complaint is more common in women with a history of rape or childhood sexual abuse.

Dynamic factors are usually considered causative, although situational factors probably account for more secondary dysfunction. Painful coitus may result from tense vaginal muscles. The pain is real and makes intercourse unbearable or unpleasant. Anticipation of further pain may cause the woman to avoid coitus altogether. If the partner proceeds with intercourse regardless of the woman's state of readiness, the condition is aggravated.

Dyspareunia can also occur in men, but it is uncommon and usually associated with a medical condition such as Peyronie's disease, prostatitis, or gonorrheal or herpetic infections. Vasocongestion during sexual activity without orgasmic release also may lead to discomfort. Rarely, some men experience pain on ejaculation (postejaculatory pain disorder). This pain is caused by an involuntary spasm of the perineal muscles that may be due to psychological conflicts about the sex act or may be an adverse effect of some antidepressant medications. Table 18.1a–15 lists the diagnostic criteria for dyspareunia. In DSM-IV-TR, *dyspareunia due to a general medical condition* is used when the medical condition is the sole or major causal factor.

Vaginismus *Vaginismus* is an involuntary and persistent constriction of the outer one-third of the vagina that prevents penile insertion and intercourse. The response may be demonstrated during a gynecological examination when involuntary vaginal constriction prevents introduction of the speculum into the vagina, although some women only have vaginismus during coitus. The diagnosis is not made if the dysfunction is caused exclusively by medical or surgical factors or if it is symptomatic of another Axis I psychiatric syndrome (Table 18.1a–16). Vaginismus is less prevalent than anorgasmia. It most often afflicts highly educated women and those in the higher socioeconomic groups. A milder form of the dysfunction, in which some vaginal tightness makes penile entry difficult, is experienced by more women on an intermittent or chronic basis.

A woman suffering from vaginismus may consciously wish to have coitus but unconsciously prevents penile entrance into her body. A sexual trauma, such as rape, may result in vaginismus. Women who have experienced pain with nonsexual bodily traumas, through accidents or because of illness or surgery, may become sensitized to the idea of penetration. Women with psychosexual con-

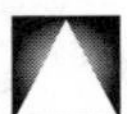

Table 18.1a–15
DSM-IV-TR Diagnostic Criteria for Dyspareunia

A. Recurrent or persistent genital pain associated with sexual intercourse in either a man or a woman.
B. The disturbance causes marked distress or interpersonal difficulty.
C. The disturbance is not caused exclusively by vaginismus or lack of lubrication, is not better accounted for by another Axis I disorder (except another sexual dysfunction), and is not due exclusively to the direct physiological effects of a substance (e.g., a drug of abuse, a medication) or a general medical condition.

Specify type:
Lifelong type
Acquired type

Specify type:
Generalized type
Situational type

Specify:
Due to psychological factors
Due to combined factors

From American Psychiatric Association. *Diagnostic and Statistical Manual of Mental Disorders.* 4th ed. Text rev. Washington, DC: American Psychiatric Association; 2000, with permission.

flicts may perceive the penis as a dangerous weapon. Pain or the anticipation of pain at the first coital experience causes vaginismus in some women. A strict religious upbringing that associates sex with sin is frequently noted in such cases. Others have problems in the dyadic relationship; a woman who feels emotionally abused by her partner may protest in this nonverbal fashion.

Miss B. was a 27-year-old, single woman who presented for therapy because of an inability to have intercourse. She described episodes with a recent boyfriend in which he had tried vaginal penetration but had been unable to enter. The boyfriend did not have erectile dysfunction. Miss B. experienced desire and was able to achieve orgasm through manual or oral stimulation. For almost a year, she and her boyfriend had sex play without intercourse. However, he complained increasingly about his frustration at the lack of coitus, which he had enjoyed in previous relationships. Miss B. had a conscious fear of penetration and dreaded going to the gynecologist, although she was able to use tampons when she menstruated. She was diagnosed with vaginismus, lifelong type.

Sexual Dysfunction Due to a General Medical Condition

The category sexual dysfunction due to a general medical condition covers sexual dysfunction that results in marked distress and interpersonal difficulty when there is evidence from the history, physical examination, or laboratory findings of a general medical condition judged to be causally related to the sexual dysfunction (Table 18.1a–17).

Male Erectile Disorder Due to a General Medical Condition

Many studies have focused on the relative incidences of psychological and organic male erectile disorder. Statistics indicate that 50 to 80 percent of men with erectile disorder have an organic basis for the disorder. Physiologically, erectile dysfunction may be due to a variety of medical causes (Table 18.1a–18). In the United States, it is estimated that two million men cannot gain erections because they suffer from diabetes mellitus; an additional 300,000 are dysfunctional because of other endocrine diseases; 1.5 million are dysfunctional as a result of vascular disease; 180,000 because of multiple sclerosis; 400,000 because of traumas and fractures leading to pelvic fractures or spinal cord injuries; and another 650,000 as a result of radical surgery, including prostatectomies,

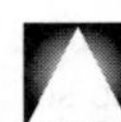

Table 18.1a–16
DSM-IV-TR Diagnostic Criteria for Vaginismus

A. Recurrent or persistent involuntary spasm of the musculature of the outer third of the vagina that interferes with sexual intercourse.
B. The disturbance causes marked distress or interpersonal difficulty.
C. The disturbance is not better accounted for by another Axis I disorder (e.g., somatization disorder) and is not due exclusively to the direct physiological effects of a general medical condition.

Specify type:
Lifelong type
Acquired type

Specify type:
Generalized type
Situational type

Specify:
Due to psychological factors
Due to combined factors

From American Psychiatric Association. *Diagnostic and Statistical Manual of Mental Disorders.* 4th ed. Text rev. Washington, DC: American Psychiatric Association; 2000, with permission.

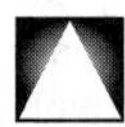

Table 18.1a–17
DSM-IV-TR Diagnostic Criteria for Sexual Dysfunction Due to a General Medical Condition

A. Clinically significant sexual dysfunction that results in marked distress or interpersonal difficulty predominates in the clinical picture.
B. There is evidence from the history, physical examination, or laboratory findings that the sexual dysfunction is fully explained by the direct physiological effects of a general medical condition.
C. The disturbance is not better accounted for by another mental disorder (e.g., major depressive disorder).

Select code and term based on the predominant sexual dysfunction:

Female hypoactive sexual desire disorder due to . . . [indicate the general medical condition]: if deficient or absent sexual desire is the predominant feature

Male hypoactive sexual desire disorder due to . . . [indicate the general medical condition]: if deficient or absent sexual desire is the predominant feature

Male erectile disorder due to . . . [indicate the general medical condition]: if male erectile dysfunction is the predominant feature

Female dyspareunia due to . . . [indicate the general medical condition]: if pain associated with intercourse is the predominant feature

Male dyspareunia due to . . . [indicate the general medical condition]: if pain associated with intercourse is the predominant feature

Other female sexual dysfunction due to . . . [indicate the general medical condition]: if some other feature is predominant (e.g., orgasmic disorder) or no feature predominates

Other male sexual dysfunction due to . . . [indicate the general medical condition]: if some other feature is predominant (e.g., orgasmic disorder) or no feature predominates

Coding note: Include the name of the general medical condition on Axis I (e.g., male erectile disorder due to diabetes mellitus); also code the general medical condition on Axis III.

From American Psychiatric Association. *Diagnostic and Statistical Manual of Mental Disorders.* 4th ed. Text rev. Washington, DC: American Psychiatric Association; 2000, with permission.

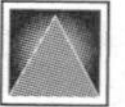

Table 18.1a–18
Diseases and Other Medical Conditions Implicated in Erectile Dysfunction

Infectious and parasitic diseases	Neurological disorders
Elephantiasis	Multiple sclerosis
Mumps	Transverse myelitis
Cardiovascular disease	Parkinson's disease
Atherosclerotic disease	Temporal lobe epilepsy
Aortic aneurysm	Traumatic and neoplastic spinal cord diseases
Leriche's syndrome	Central nervous system tumor
Cardiac failure	Amyotrophic lateral sclerosis
Renal and urological disorders	Peripheral neuropathy
Peyronie's disease	General paresis
Chronic renal failure	Tabes dorsalis
Hydrocele and varicocele	Pharmacological contributants
Hepatic disorders	Alcohol and other dependence-inducing substances (heroin, methadone, morphine, cocaine, amphetamines, and barbiturates)
Cirrhosis (usually associated with alcohol dependence)	Prescribed drugs (psychotropic drugs, antihypertensive drugs, estrogens, and antiandrogens)
Pulmonary disorders	Poisoning
Respiratory failure	Lead (plumbism)
Genetic disorders	Herbicides
Klinefelter's syndrome	Surgical procedures
Congenital penile vascular and structural abnormalities	Perineal prostatectomy
Nutritional disorders	Abdominal–perineal colon resection
Malnutrition	Sympathectomy (frequently interferes with ejaculation)
Vitamin deficiencies	Aortoiliac surgery
Endocrine disorders	Radical cystectomy
Diabetes mellitus	Retroperitoneal lymphadenectomy
Dysfunction of the pituitary-adrenal-testis axis	Miscellaneous
Acromegaly	Radiation therapy
Addison's disease	Pelvic fracture
Chromophobe adenoma	Any severe systemic disease or debilitating condition
Adrenal neoplasia	
Myxedema	
Hyperthyroidism	

colostomies, and cystectomies. In addition, the clinician should be aware of the possible pharmacological effects of medication on sexual functioning. The increased incidence of organic causes for erectile dysfunction in the past 15 years may partly reflect the increased use of psychotropic and antihypertensive medications. Adverse effects of medication may impair male sexual functioning in a variety of ways. Castration (removal of the testes) does not always lead to sexual dysfunction, depending on the person. Erection may still occur after castration via a reflex arc that passes through the sacral cord erectile center. It is triggered when the inner thigh is stimulated.

PHYSIOLOGICAL TESTS A number of procedures, benign and invasive, are used to help differentiate psychogenic erectile dysfunction. The procedures include monitoring nocturnal penile tumescence (erection that occurs during sleep) normally associated with rapid eye movement; monitoring tumescence with a strain gauge; measuring blood pressure in the penis with a penile plethysmograph or an ultrasound (Doppler) flow meter, both of which assess blood flow in the internal pudendal artery; and measuring pudendal nerve latency time. Neurological impairment of penile function may be indicated by decreased vibratory perception in the penis. Other diagnostic tests that delineate organic bases for erectile disorder include glucose tolerance test, plasma hormone assays, liver and thyroid function tests, prolactin and follicle-stimulating hormone (FSH) determinations, and cystometric examinations. Invasive diagnostic studies include penile arteriography, infusion cavernosonography, and radioactive xenon penography. Invasive procedures require expert interpretation and are used only for patients who are candidates for vascular reconstructive procedures.

MEDICAL VERSUS PSYCHOGENIC CAUSES A good history is crucial to determining the cause of the male erectile disorder. If a man reports having spontaneous erections at times when he does not plan to have intercourse, having morning erections or only sporadic erectile dysfunction, or having good erections with masturbation or with partners other than his usual one, then organic causes for his disorder can be considered negligible, and costly diagnostic procedures can be avoided. When a medical basis for erectile dysfunction is found, psychological factors often contribute to the dysfunction, and psychiatric treatment may be helpful. Some diabetics, for instance, may experience psychogenic erectile dysfunction.

Dyspareunia Due to a General Medical Condition

An estimated 30 percent of all surgical procedures on the female genital area result in temporary dyspareunia. In addition, 30 to 40 percent of women with the complaint who are seen in sex therapy clinics have pelvic pathology. Organic abnormalities leading to dyspareunia and vaginismus include infected hymenal remnants or congenitally imperforate or unusually thick hymens; episiotomy scars; Bartholin's glands infections; various forms of vaginitis and cervicitis; testosterone deficiency; vulvodynia; vaginal treatment, such as radiation or surgery that has caused scarring; dermatological disorder, such as lichens sclerosis or lichens planus; and endometriosis. Postcoital pain reported by women with myomata and endometriosis

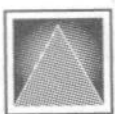

Table 18.1a–19
Neurotransmitter Effects on Sex Function

	Dopamine	Serotonin	Adrenergic	Cholinergic	Clinical Correlation
Erection	+ +	+/–	α, β – +	+/–	Antipsychotics (dopamine receptor antagonists) may lead to erectile dysfunction; dopaminergic drug agonists may lead to enhanced erection and libido; priapism with trazodone (α_1 block); β-adrenergic receptor antagonists may lead to impotence.
Ejaculation and orgasm	+/–	+	+ α_1	+/–	α_1-Adrenergic receptor antagonists, tricyclic drugs, MAOIs, thioridazine may lead to impaired ejaculation; serotonergic agents may inhibit orgasm.

+/– minimal or no effect; + facilitates effect; – inhibiting effect; MAOI, monoamine oxidase inhibitor.

is attributed to the uterine contractions during orgasm. Postmenopausal women may have dyspareunia because of thinning of the vaginal mucosa and reduced lubrication.

Dyspareunia can also occur in men, but it is uncommon and is usually associated with an organic condition such as Peyronie's disease, which consists of sclerotic plaques on the penis that cause penile curvature.

Hypoactive Sexual Desire Disorder Due to a General Medical Condition Desire commonly decreases after major illness or surgery, particularly when body image is affected after such procedures as mastectomy, ileostomy, hysterectomy, and prostatectomy. Illnesses that deplete a person's energy, chronic conditions that require physical and psychological adaptation, and serious illnesses that may cause the person to become depressed can all result in a marked lessening of sexual desire in both men and women. In some cases, biochemical correlates are associated with hypoactive sexual desire disorder (Table 18.1a–19). A recent study found markedly lower serum testosterone concentrations in men complaining of low desire than in normal controls in a sleep laboratory situation. Drugs that depress the central nervous system (CNS) or decrease testosterone production can decrease desire.

Other Male Sexual Dysfunction Due to a General Medical Condition The category *other male sexual dysfunction due to a general medical condition* is used when some dysfunctional feature other than those discussed above predominates (e.g., orgasmic disorder) or no feature predominates. Male orgasmic dysfunction may have physiological causes and can occur after surgery on the genitourinary tract, such as prostatectomy. It may also be associated with Parkinson's disease and other neurological disorders involving the lumbar or sacral sections of the spinal cord. The antihypertensive drug guanethidine monosulfate, methyldopa, the phenothiazines, the tricyclic drugs, and serotonin reuptake inhibitors, among others, have been implicated in retarded ejaculation. Male orgasmic disorder must also be differentiated from retrograde ejaculation, in which ejaculation occurs but the seminal fluid passes backward into the bladder. Retrograde ejaculation always has an organic cause. As mentioned above, it can develop after genitourinary surgery and is also associated with medications with anticholinergic adverse effects, such as the phenothiazines.

Other Female Sexual Dysfunction Due to a General Medical Condition The category *other female sexual dysfunction due to a general medical disorder* is used when some feature other than those discussed above (e.g., orgasmic disorder) predominates or no feature predominates. Some medical conditions—specifically, such endocrine diseases as hypothyroidism, diabetes mellitus, and primary hyperprolactinemia—can affect a woman's ability to have orgasms.

Substance-Induced Sexual Dysfunction The diagnosis *substance-induced sexual dysfunction* is used when evidence from the history, physical examination, or laboratory findings indicates substance intoxication or withdrawal when dysfunction follows the use of prescribed medication. Distressing sexual dysfunction occurs within a month of significant substance intoxication or withdrawal (Table 18.1a–20). Specified substances include alcohol; amphetamines or related substances; cocaine; opioids; sedatives, hypnotics, or anxiolytics; and other or unknown substances.

Abused recreational substances affect sexual function in various ways. In small doses, many substances enhance sexual performance by decreasing inhibition or anxiety or by temporarily elevating mood. However, continuous use impairs erectile, orgasmic, and ejaculatory capacities. The abuse of sedatives, anxiolytics, and, particularly, opioids nearly always depresses desire. Alcohol may foster the initiation of sexual activity by removing inhibitions, but it impairs performance. Cocaine and amphetamines produce similar effects. Although no direct evidence indicates that sexual drive is enhanced by stimulants, the user initially has a feeling of increased energy and may become sexually active. Ultimately, dysfunction occurs. Men usually go through two stages: prolonged erection without ejaculation and then a gradual loss of erectile capacity.

Recovering substance-dependent patients may need therapy to regain sexual function. In part, this is one piece of psychological readjustment to a nondependent state. Many substance abusers have always had difficulty with intimate interactions. Others have missed the experience that would have enabled them to learn social and sexual skills because they spent their crucial developmental years under the influence of some substance.

Pharmacological Agents Implicated in Sex Dysfunction

Many pharmacological agents, particularly those used in psychiatry, have been associated with an effect on sexuality. In men, these effects include decreased sex drive, erectile failure (impotence), decreased volume of ejaculate, and delayed or retrograde ejaculation. In women, decreased sex drive, decreased vaginal lubrication, inhibited or delayed orgasm, and decreased or absent vaginal contractions may occur. Drugs may also enhance the sexual response and increase the sex drive, but this effect is less common than are inhibiting effects.

Antipsychotic Drugs Antipsychotic drugs that block adrenergic and cholinergic receptors are accompanied by adverse sex effects. Chlorpromazine (Thorazine), thioridazine, trifluoperazine (Stelazine), and haloperidol (Haldol) are potent anticholinergic agents that impair erection and ejaculation in men and inhibit vaginal lubrication and orgasm in women. Chlorpromazine and thioridazine also block adrenergic receptors. Thioridazine has a particular adverse

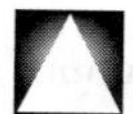

Table 18.1a–20
DSM-IV-TR Diagnostic Criteria for Substance-Induced Sexual Dysfunction

A. Clinically significant sexual dysfunction that results in marked distress or interpersonal difficulty predominates in the clinical picture.
B. There is evidence from the history, physical examination, or laboratory findings that the sexual dysfunction is fully explained by substance use as manifested by either (1) or (2):
 (1) the symptoms in Criterion A developed during, or within a month of, substance intoxication
 (2) medication use is etiologically related to the disturbance
C. The disturbance is not better accounted for by a sexual dysfunction that is not substance-induced. Evidence that the symptoms are better accounted for by a sexual dysfunction that is not substance-induced might include the following: the symptoms precede the onset of the substance use or dependence (or medication use); the symptoms persist for a substantial period of time (e.g., approximately a month) after the cessation of intoxication, or are substantially in excess of what would be expected given the type or amount of the substance used or the duration of use; or there is other evidence that suggests the existence of an independent non–substance-induced sexual dysfunction (e.g., history of recurrent non–substance-related episodes).

Note: This diagnosis should be made instead of a diagnosis of substance intoxication only when the sexual dysfunction is in excess of that usually associated with the intoxication syndrome and when the dysfunction is sufficiently severe to warrant independent clinical attention.

Code [Specific substance]-induced sexual dysfunction:
 Alcohol; amphetamine [or amphetamine-like substance]; cocaine; opioid; sedative, hypnotic, or anxiolytic; other [or unknown] substance

Specify if:
 With impaired desire
 With impaired arousal
 With impaired orgasm
 With sexual pain

Specify if:
 With onset during intoxication: if the criteria are met for intoxication with the substance and the symptoms develop during the intoxication syndrome

From American Psychiatric Association. *Diagnostic and Statistical Manual of Mental Disorders*. 4th ed. Text rev. Washington, DC: American Psychiatric Association; 2000, with permission.

effect of causing retrograde ejaculation, in which the seminal fluid backs up into the bladder rather than being propelled through the penile urethra. Patients still have a pleasurable sensation of orgasm, but it is dry. When urinating after orgasm, the urine may be milky white because it contains the ejaculate. The condition is startling but harmless and may occur in up to 50 percent of patients taking the drug. Paradoxically, rare cases of priapism have been reported with antipsychotics. Second-generation antipsychotic drugs, such as quetiapine (Seroquel), have a lower incidence of sexual side effects.

Selective Serotonin Reuptake Inhibitors The most commonly prescribed group of antidepressants are the selective serotonin reuptake inhibitors (SSRIs). Adverse sexual effects may occur with this group of drugs because of increased serotonin concentration. A lowering of the sex drive and difficulty reaching orgasm occur in both sexes. Of the SSRIs, the most frequent sexual adverse effects are seen with paroxetine (Paxil), next with fluoxetine (Prozac), and the least with sertraline (Zoloft). Similar symptoms have been associated with fluvoxamine (Luvox), citalopram (Celexa), and escitalopram (Lexapro). Reversal of negative sexual side effects has been achieved with cyproheptadine (Periactin), an antihistamine with antiserotonergic effects; amantadine (Symmetrel), a dopamine agonist; yohimbine (Yocon), a central α_2-adrenergic receptor antagonist used in treating male erectile disorder; and methylphenidate (Ritalin) and dextroamphetamine (Dexedrine), which are dopaminergic and have adrenergic effects. There are reports of sildenafil (Viagra), a nitric oxide enhancer used to treat erectile dysfunction, overcoming orgasmic problems associated with the SSRIs. Buspirone (BuSpar) helps some patients overcome adverse sexual effects of SSRIs, possibly because it is 5-hydroxytryptamine type A (5-HT_A) agonist or because it suppresses SSRI-induced elevation of prolactin.

Heterocyclic Antidepressants The tricyclic and tetracyclic antidepressants have anticholinergic effects that interfere with erection and delay ejaculation. Because the anticholinergic effects vary among the cyclic antidepressants, those with the fewest side effects (e.g., desipramine [Norpramin]) produce the fewest sexual side effects. The effects of the heterocyclic drugs in women have not been studied sufficiently; however, few women seem to complain of any effects. Selegiline (Eldepryl) is a selective monoamine oxidase type B (MAO_B) inhibitor reported to increase sex drive, possibly by dopaminergic activity and increased production of norepinephrine.

Some men report a pleasurable increased sensitivity of the glans with this class of drugs that does not interfere with erection, although it delays ejaculation. In some cases, however, the tricyclic drug causes a painful ejaculation, perhaps as the result of interference with seminal propulsion caused by interference with urethral, prostatic, vas, and epididymal smooth muscle contractions. Clomipramine (Anafranil) has been reported to increase sex drive in some individuals.

Monoamine Oxidase Inhibitors (MAOIs) The MAOIs affect biogenic amines broadly. Accordingly, they produce impaired erection, delayed or retrograde ejaculation, vaginal dryness, and inhibited orgasm. Tranylcypromine (Parnate) has a paradoxical sexually stimulating effect in some individuals, possibly as a result of its amphetamine-like properties.

General Effects of Antidepressants Because depression is associated with a decreased libido, varying levels of sexual dysfunction and anhedonia are part of the disease process. This phenomenon makes assessment of dysfunction as a result of sexual side effects difficult in patients taking the drugs. Some patients report improved sexual function as their depression improves with antidepressant medication. Sometimes, sexual side effects disappear with time, perhaps because a biogenic amine homeostatic mechanism comes into play. In many cases, antidepressants without associated side effects of sexual dysfunction are substituted, such as bupropion (Wellbutrin), nefazodone (Serzone), or mirtazapine (Remeron). There have been rare, individual reports of orgasmic dysfunction with the latter two drugs.

Mrs. J. presented with the complaint of inability to achieve orgasm. Her problem dated from the time, 18 months previously, when she had been placed on fluoxetine. Before that time, she had been able to achieve orgasm through masturbation and in the majority of her sexual interactions with her husband.

Mrs. J. tried several other SSRIs, as well as venlafaxine (Effexor), but the side effect of anorgasmia persisted. Unfortunately, none of the usual antidotes to SSRI-induced anorgasmia proved effective, and the patient did not respond well to antidepressants of other categories. Mrs. J. was able to achieve orgasm with the aid of a vibrator, even while she was on an SSRI. Sex therapy, in this case, required encouraging her husband to accept inclusion of the vibrator in their sex play and reassuring him that its use was not a reflection of his lovemaking skills. Mrs. J. was diagnosed as having substance-induced sexual dysfunction.

Lithium Lithium regulates mood and, in the manic state, may reduce hypersexuality, possibly via dopamine antagonism. Some patients have reported impaired erection.

Psychostimulants Psychostimulants are sometimes used in the treatment of depression and include such drugs as amphetamine and methylphenidate, which raise plasma concentrations of norepinephrine and dopamine. Libido is increased; however, with prolonged use, men may experience a loss of desire and erections. One study found that ephedrine sulfate facilitated arousal in functional women.

α-Adrenergic and β-Adrenergic Receptor Antagonists Adrenergic receptor antagonists are used to treat hypertension, angina, and certain cardiac arrhythmias. They diminish tonic sympathetic nerve outflow from vasomotor centers in the brain. As a result, they can cause impotence, decrease the volume of ejaculate, and produce retrograde ejaculation. Changes in libido have been reported in both sexes. Suggestions have been made to use the side effects of drugs therapeutically. Thus, a drug that delays or interferes with ejaculation (such as fluoxetine) might be used to treat premature ejaculation.

Anticholinergics The anticholinergics block cholinergic receptors and include such drugs as amantadine and benztropine (Cogentin). They can produce dryness of the mucous membranes (including those of the vagina) and erectile dysfunction.

Antihistamines Drugs such as diphenhydramine (Benadryl) have anticholinergic activity and are mildly hypnotic. As a result, they may inhibit sexual function. Cyproheptadine, although an antihistamine, also has potent activity as a serotonin antagonist. It is used to block the serotonergic adverse sexual effects produced by SSRIs, such as delayed orgasm and erectile dysfunction.

Antianxiety Agents The major class of antianxiety drugs is the benzodiazepines (e.g., diazepam [Valium]). They act on the γ-aminobutyric (GABA) receptors, which are believed to be involved in cognition, memory, and motor control. Because they decrease plasma epinephrine concentration, they diminish anxiety, thus improving sexual function in individuals inhibited by anxiety.

Alcohol Alcohol suppresses CNS activity generally and, hence, can produce erectile disorders in men. Alcohol has a direct gonadal effect that decreases testosterone concentrations in men; paradoxically, it can produce a slight increase in testosterone concentrations in women. This may account for increased libido in women after drinking small amounts of alcohol. Long-term use of alcohol reduces the ability of the liver to metabolize estrogenic compounds; in men, this produces signs of feminization (e.g., gynecomastia as a result of testicular atrophy).

Opioids Opioids such as heroin have such adverse sexual effects as erectile failure and decreased libido. Altered consciousness may enhance the sexual experience in occasional users.

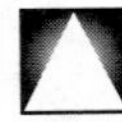

Table 18.1a–21
DSM-IV-TR Diagnostic Criteria for Sexual Dysfunction Not Otherwise Specified

This category includes sexual dysfunctions that do not meet criteria for any specific sexual dysfunction. Examples include

1. No (or substantially diminished) subjective erotic feelings despite otherwise normal arousal and orgasm
2. Situations in which the clinician has concluded that a sexual dysfunction is present but is unable to determine whether it is primary, due to a general medical condition, or substance induced

From American Psychiatric Association. *Diagnostic and Statistical Manual of Mental Disorders.* 4th ed. Text rev. Washington, DC: American Psychiatric Association; 2000, with permission.

Hallucinogens The hallucinogens include lysergic acid diethylamide (LSD), phencyclidine (PCP), psilocybin (from some mushrooms), and mescaline (from peyote cactus). In addition to inducing hallucinations, these drugs cause loss of contact with reality and an expanding and heightening of consciousness. Some users report that the sexual experience is similarly enhanced; others experience anxiety, delirium, or psychosis, which clearly interferes with sex function.

Cannabis The altered state of consciousness produced by cannabis may enhance sexual pleasure for some individuals. Its prolonged use depresses testosterone concentrations.

Barbiturates and Similarly Acting Drugs Barbiturates are sedative-hypnotics that may enhance sexual responsiveness in persons who are sexually unresponsive because of anxiety. They have no direct effect on the sex organs, but they do alter consciousness, which some individuals find pleasurable. They are subject to abuse and may be fatal when combined with alcohol or other CNS depressants. Methaqualone (Quaalude) acquired a reputation as a sexual enhancer that had no biological basis in fact. It is no longer marketed in the United States.

Sexual Dysfunction and Sexual Disorder Not Otherwise Specified

DSM-IV-TR uses two categories—sexual dysfunction not otherwise specified and sexual disorder not otherwise specified. The diagnostic criteria are listed in Tables 18.1a–21 and 18.1a–22, respectively. The distinction between the two categories is unclear, however, and there is overlap between them. Many sexual disorders are not classifiable as sexual dysfunctions or as paraphilias. These unclassified disorders are rare, poorly documented, not easily classified, or not specifically described in DSM-IV-TR. ICD-10 has a similar residual category for problems related to sexual development or preference (Table 18.1a–23).

Examples of such unclassified disorders include individuals who experience the physiological components of sexual excitement and orgasm but report no erotic sensation or even anesthesia and the male experience of orgasm with a flaccid penis. The orgasmic woman who desires but has not experienced multiple orgasms can be classified under this heading as well. Also, disorders of excessive rather than inhibited function, such as compulsive masturbation, might be diagnosed under atypical dysfunction. Other sexual practices exist that are not listed in DSM-IV-TR—for example, behaviors that attempt to enhance sexual arousal by oxygen deprivation (hypoxyphilia) or other deviant methods. Atypical dysfunction also might be used to cover complaints engendered by couple, rather than

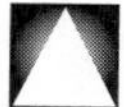

Table 18.1a–22
DSM-IV-TR Diagnostic Criteria for Sexual Disorder Not Otherwise Specified

This category is included for coding a sexual disturbance that does not meet the criteria for any specific sexual disorder and is neither a sexual dysfunction nor a paraphilia. Examples include

1. Marked feelings of inadequacy concerning sexual performance or other traits related to self-imposed standards of masculinity or femininity
2. Distress about a pattern of repeated sexual relationships involving a succession of lovers who are experienced by the individual only as things to be used
3. Persistent and marked distress about sexual orientation

From American Psychiatric Association. *Diagnostic and Statistical Manual of Mental Disorders*. 4th ed. Text rev. Washington, DC: American Psychiatric Association; 2000, with permission.

individual, dysfunction—for example, a couple in which one partner prefers morning sex and the other functions more readily at night or a couple with unequal frequencies of desire.

Compulsive Sexual Behavior The concept of compulsive sexual behavior (Table 18.1a–24), or sex addiction, was developed in the 1980s to describe persons who compulsively seek out sexual experiences and whose behavior becomes impaired if they cannot gratify their sexual impulses. The concept of sex addiction is derived from the model of addiction to drugs such as heroin or addiction to behavioral patterns such as gambling. Addiction implies psychological dependence, physical dependence, and a withdrawal symptom if the substance (e.g., the drug) is unavailable or the behavior (e.g., gambling) is frustrated.

DSM-IV-TR does not use the terms *sex addiction* or *compulsive sexual behavior,* nor is this disorder universally recognized or accepted. Nevertheless, the person whose entire life revolves around sex-seeking behavior and activities, who spends an excessive amount of time in such behavior, and who often tries to stop such behavior but cannot do so is well known to clinicians. Such persons show repeated and increasingly frequent attempts to have a sexual experience, and deprivation evokes symptoms of distress. In the author's view, sex addiction is a useful concept heuristically because it can alert the clinician to seek an underlying cause for the manifest behavior.

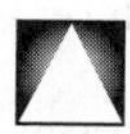

Table 18.1a–23
DSM-IV-TR Diagnostic Criteria for Psychological and Behavioral Disorders Associated with Sexual Development and Orientation

This section is intended to cover those types of problems that derive from variations of sexual development or orientation, when the sexual preference per se is not necessarily problematic or abnormal.

Sexual maturation disorder

The patient suffers from uncertainty about his or her gender identity or sexual orientation, which causes anxiety or depression.

Ego-dystonic sexual orientation

The gender identity or sexual preference is not in doubt, but the individual wishes it were different.

Sexual relationship disorder

The abnormality of gender identity or sexual preference is responsible for difficulties in forming or maintaining a relationship with a sexual partner.

Other psychosexual development disorders

Psychosexual development disorder, unspecified

From American Psychiatric Association. *Diagnostic and Statistical Manual of Mental Disorders*. 4th ed. Text rev. Washington, DC: American Psychiatric Association; 2000, with permission.

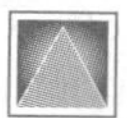

Table 18.1a–24
Signs of Sexual Addiction or Compulsive Sexual Behavior

1. Out-of-control behavior
2. Severe adverse consequences (medical, legal, interpersonal) due to sexual behavior
3. Persistent pursuit of self-destructive or high-risk sexual behavior
4. Repeated attempts to limit or stop sexual behavior
5. Sexual obsession and fantasy as a primary coping mechanism
6. Need for increasing amounts of sexual activity
7. Severe mood changes related to sexual activity (e.g., depression, euphoria)
8. Inordinate amount of time spent in obtaining sex, being sexual, or recovering from sexual experience
9. Interference of sexual behavior in social, occupational, or recreational activities

Data from Carnes P. *Don't Call It Love*. New York: Bantam Books, 1991.

Postcoital Dysphoria Postcoital dysphoria is not listed in DSM-IV-TR. It occurs during the resolution phase of sexual activity, when individuals normally experience a sense of general well-being and muscular and psychological relaxation. Some individuals, however, experience postcoital dysphoria—after an otherwise satisfactory sexual experience, they become depressed, tense, anxious, and irritable and show psychomotor agitation. They often want to get away from the partner and may become verbally or even physically abusive. The incidence of the disorder is unknown, but it is more common in men than in women. Its several causes relate to the person's attitude toward sex in general and the partner in particular. It may occur in adulterous sex and with prostitutes, when there is a profound fear of intimacy, or when individuals cannot experience sex without consequent strong feelings of guilt. The fear of sexually transmitted disease causes some persons to experience postcoital dysphoria. Treatment requires insight-oriented psychotherapy to help patients understand the unconscious antecedents to their behavior and attitudes.

Unconsummated Marriage A couple involved in an unconsummated marriage have never had coitus and are typically uninformed and inhibited about sexuality. Their feelings of guilt, shame, or inadequacy are increased by their problems, and they experience conflict between their need to seek help and their need to conceal their difficulty. Couples present with the problem after having been married several months or several years. Masters and Johnson reported an unconsummated marriage of 17 years' duration.

Frequently, the couple does not seek help directly, but the woman may reveal the problem to her gynecologist on a visit ostensibly concerned with vague vaginal or other somatic complaints. On examining her, the gynecologist may find an intact hymen. In some cases, however, the wife may have undergone a hymenectomy to resolve the problem. Inquiry by a physician who is comfortable in dealing with sexual problems may be the first opening to a frank discussion of the couple's distress. Often, the pretext of the medical visit is a discussion of contraceptive methods or even a request for an infertility workup. Once presented, the complaint often can be successfully treated. The duration of the problem does not significantly affect the prognosis or the outcome of the case.

The causes of unconsummated marriage are varied: lack of sex education, sexual prohibitions overly stressed by parents or society, problems of an oedipal nature, immaturity in both partners, overdependence on primary families, and problems in sexual identification. Religious orthodoxy, with severe control of sexual and social development or the equation of sexuality with sin or uncleanliness, has also been cited as a dominant cause. Many women involved in an unconsummated marriage have distorted concepts about their vaginas. They may fear that the vagina is too small or too soft, or they may confuse the vagina with the rectum, leading to feelings of being unclean. The man may share in those distortions about the vagina and, in addition, perceive it as dangerous to himself. Similarly, both partners may have distortions about the man's penis, perceiving it as a weapon, as too large, or as too small. Many patients can be helped by simple education about genital anatomy and physiology, by suggestions for self-exploration, and by correct information from a physician. The problem of the unconsummated marriage is best treated by seeing both members of the couple. Dual-sex therapy has been markedly effective. However, other forms of conjoint therapy, marital counseling, traditional psychotherapy on a one-to-one basis, and counseling from a sensitive family physician, gynecologist, or urologist are all helpful.

Body Image Problems Some individuals are ashamed of their bodies and experience feelings of inadequacy related to self-imposed standards of masculinity or femininity. They may insist on sex only during total darkness, not allow certain body parts to be seen or touched, or seek unnecessary operative procedures to deal with their imagined inadequacies. Body dysmorphic disorder should be ruled out.

Don Juanism Some men who appear to be hypersexual, as shown by their need to have many sexual encounters or conquests, use their sexual activities to mask deep feelings of inferiority. Some have unconscious homosexual impulses, which they deny by compulsive sexual contacts with women. After having sex, most Don Juans are no longer interested in the woman. The condition is also referred to as *satyriasis* or as a form of sex addiction.

Nymphomania Nymphomania signifies excessive or pathological desire for coitus in a woman. There have been few scientific studies of the condition. Those patients who have been studied usually have had one or more sexual disorders, usually including female orgasmic disorder. The woman often has an intense fear of loss of love. She attempts to satisfy her dependency needs rather than to gratify her sexual impulses through her actions. It is sometimes classified as a form of sex addiction.

Fantasies Other atypical disorders are found in individuals who have one or more sexual fantasies about which they obsess, feel guilty, or are otherwise dysphoric. As indicated in Table 18.1a–25, however, the range of common sexual fantasies is broad.

Persistent and Marked Distress about Sexual Orientation Distress about sexual orientation is usually characterized by dissatisfaction with homosexual arousal patterns, a desire to increase heterosexual arousal, and strong negative feelings about being homosexual. Occasional statements to the effect that life would be easier if the person were not homosexual do not constitute persistent and marked distress about sexual orientation.

Treatment of sexual orientation distress is controversial. One study reported that with a minimum of 350 hours of psychoanalytic therapy, approximately one-third of approximately 100 bisexual and homosexual men achieved a heterosexual reorientation at 5-year follow-up, but that study was challenged and never replicated. Behavior therapy and avoidance conditioning techniques have also been used, but a basic problem with behavioral technique is that the behavior may be changed in the laboratory setting but not outside the laboratory. Prognostic factors weighing in favor of heterosexual reorientation for men include being younger than 35 years, having some experience of heterosexual arousal, and having a high motivation for reorientation.

Another style of intervention is directed at enabling the person with persistent and marked distress about sexual orientation to live comfortably as a homosexual without shame, guilt, anxiety, or depression. Gay counseling centers are engaged with patients in such treatment programs. At present, outcome studies of such centers have not been reported in detail.

Few data are available about the treatment of women with persistent and marked distress about sexual orientation, and those are primarily single-case studies with variable outcomes.

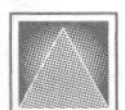

Table 18.1a–25
Common Sexual Fantasies[a]

Men	Women
Heterosexual	
Replacement of established partner	Replacement of established partner
Forced sexual encounters with women	Forced sexual encounters with men
Observing sexual activity	Observing sexual activity
Sexual encounters with men	Idyllic encounters with unknown men
Group sex	Sexual encounters with women
Homosexual	
Images of male anatomy	Forced sexual encounters with women
Forced sexual encounters with men	Idyllic encounters with established partner
Sexual encounters with women	Sexual encounters with men
Idyllic encounters with unknown men	Memories of past sexual experiences
Group sex	Sadistic imagery

[a]Listed in order of occurrence. A 1994 study found that one in five persons experienced a same-sex sexual fantasy at some time in their lives.
Adapted from Masters W, Schwartz M: The Masters and Johnson treatment program for dissatisfied homosexual men. *Am J Psychiatry*. 1984;141:173.

Postcoital Headache Postcoital headache is a headache immediately after coitus and may last for several hours. It is usually described as throbbing and is localized in the occipital or frontal area. The cause is unknown but may be vascular, due to muscle contraction (tension), or psychogenic. Coitus may precipitate migraine or cluster headaches in predisposed persons.

Orgasmic Anhedonia Orgasmic anhedonia is a condition in which the person had no physical sensation of orgasm, even though the physiological component (e.g., ejaculation) remains intact. Medical causes, such as sacral and cephalic lesions that interfere with afferent pathways from the genitalia to the cortex, must be ruled out. Psychic causes usually relate to extreme guilt about experiencing sexual pleasure—these feelings produce a type of dissociative response that isolates the affective component of the orgasmic experience from consciousness.

Female Premature Orgasm Data on female premature orgasm are lacking; no separate category for premature orgasm in women is included in DSM-IV-TR. However, in the University of Chicago study, 10 percent of women felt they reached orgasm too quickly.

Masturbatory Pain Some individuals may experience pain during masturbation. Organic causes should always be ruled out. A small vaginal tear or early Peyronie's disease may produce a painful sensation. The condition should be differentiated from compulsive masturbation. People may masturbate to the extent that they do physical damage to their genitals and eventually experience pain during subsequent masturbatory acts.

Certain masturbatory practices have resulted in what has been called *autoerotic asphyxiation*, which is usually classified as a paraphilia (hypoxyphilia). The practices may involve masturbating while hanging by the neck to heighten erotic sensations and the intensity of the orgasm through the mechanism of mild hypoxia. Although they intend to release themselves from the noose after orgasm, an estimated 500 to 1,000 persons a year accidentally kill themselves by hanging. Most who indulge in the practice are men; transvestism is often associated with the habit, and most deaths occur among adolescents. Such masochistic practices are usually associated with severe mental disorders, such as schizophrenia and major mood disorders.

TREATMENT

The treatment of sexual disorders has evolved significantly since the 1970s, when Masters and Johnson focused the attention of the psychiatric community on sexual disorders. Innovations in treatment reflect the results of research and changes in the patient population. For example, in the late 1960s, most cases of erectile dysfunction were considered psychological in origin, with approximately 20 percent of erectile problems having an organic cause. Currently, the numbers are reversed, with the majority of cases considered to result from a physiological problem. Actually, many cases are of mixed origin. Similarly, early patients in sex therapy were assumed to suffer, in part, from lack of sexual information and culturally reinforced negative attitudes toward sex. Since the 1970s, the public has received a great deal of accurate information about sex through the media, and cultural attitudes regarding sexual behavior have become markedly more liberal. Patients now have more knowledge and greater sexual sophistication. Their dysfunctions have a complex etiology frequently involving psychodynamic and relational issues. Problems of desire are seen with increasing frequency and are among the most challenging cases for therapists. Couple issues involve problems of trust, intimacy, lack of sexual attraction, and struggles for dominance. Finally, along with the rest of psychiatry, sex therapy has experienced medicalization. Biological treatment approaches have developed rapidly. An eclectic approach that allows the use of several techniques sequentially or in combination may be necessary.

Before entering therapy, the patient should have a thorough medical evaluation, including a medical history, physical examination, and appropriate laboratory studies when necessary. If a medical cause for the disorder is found, treatment should be directed toward ameliorating that cause.

Before 1970, the most common treatment of sexual dysfunction was individual psychotherapy. Classic psychodynamic theory considers sexual inadequacy to have its roots in early developmental conflicts, and the sexual disorder is treated as part of a more pervasive emotional disturbance. Treatment focuses on the exploration of unconscious conflicts, motivation, fantasy, and various interpersonal difficulties. Therapy assumes that removal of the conflicts will allow the sexual impulse to become structurally acceptable to the patient's ego and thereby find appropriate means of satisfaction in the environment. Unfortunately, the symptom of sexual dysfunction frequently becomes secondarily autonomous and persists after resolution of the other problems evolving from the patient's pathology. The addition of behavioral techniques is often necessary to cure the sexual problem.

Dual-Sex Therapy

The theoretical basis of the dual-sex therapy approach is the concept of the marital unit or dyad as the object of therapy. The method of dual-sex therapy was originated and developed by Masters and Johnson. Dual-sex therapy does not accept the idea of a sick half of a patient couple. Both individuals are involved in a relationship in which there is sexual distress, and, thus, both must participate in the therapy program.

The sexual problem often reflects other areas of disharmony or misunderstanding in the marriage. The marital relationship as a whole is treated, with emphasis on sexual functioning as a part of that relationship. Improved communication in sexual and nonsexual areas is a specific goal of treatment. Psychological and physiological aspects of sexual functioning are discussed with an educational attitude. Suggestions are followed in the privacy of the couple's home.

Initial histories are taken to determine suitability for this type of treatment. Evidence of major underlying psychopathology suggests further psychiatric evaluation, and participation in the program may be deferred until the patient seems better able to benefit from it. Concurrent psychotherapy with a psychiatrist while participating in dual-sex therapy is sometimes recommended.

Each patient is interviewed individually early in the course of treatment. A complete sexual history is obtained, which is later reflected back to the couple to help them understand their present problem. The individual sessions also help the therapist understand the patients' lifestyle and allow for suggestions that fit into that lifestyle.

Behavioral Exercises Treatment is short term and behaviorally oriented. Specific exercises are prescribed to help the couple with their particular problem. Sexual dysfunction often involves a fear of inadequate performance; thus, couples are specifically prohibited from any sexual play other than that prescribed by the therapist. Initially, intercourse is interdicted, and couples learn to give and receive bodily pleasure without the pressure of performance. Beginning exercises usually focus on heightening sensory awareness to touch, sight, sound, and smell.

During these exercises, called *sensate focus exercises,* the couple is given much reinforcement to lessen anxiety. They are urged to use fantasies to distract them from obsessive concerns about performance, which is termed *spectatoring.* The needs of both the dysfunctional partner and the nondysfunctional partner are considered. If either partner becomes sexually excited by the exercises, the other is encouraged to bring him or her to orgasm by manual or oral means. This procedure is important to keep the nondysfunctional partner from sabotaging the treatment. Open communication between the partners is urged, and the expression of mutual needs is encouraged. Resistances, such as claims of fatigue or not enough time to complete the exercises, are common and must be dealt with by the therapist. Genital stimulation is eventually added to general body stimulation. The couple is sequentially taught to try various positions for intercourse without necessarily completing the act and to use varieties of stimulating techniques before they are permitted to proceed with intercourse.

The specific exercises vary with differing presenting complaints, and special techniques are used to treat the various dysfunctions. In cases of vaginismus, for instance, the woman is advised to dilate her vaginal opening with her fingers or with size-graduated vaginal dilators as part of the therapy. In cases of premature ejaculation, an exercise known as the *squeeze technique* is used to raise the threshold of penile excitability. In this exercise, the man or the woman stimulates the erect penis until the earliest sensations of impending orgasm and ejaculation are felt. Penile stimulation is then stopped abruptly, and the coronal ridge of the penis is forcibly squeezed for several seconds. The technique is repeated several times. A variation is the *stop–start technique*, in which stimulation is interrupted for several seconds but no squeeze is applied. Masturbation to the point of imminent orgasm raises the threshold of excitability to a more tolerant stimulation level. The man is encouraged to focus on sensations of excitement rather than distract himself from them. This makes him more familiar with his excitement pattern and lets him feel in control rather than overwhelmed by sensations of arousal. Communication between the partners is improved because the man must let his partner know his level of sexual excitement so that she can squeeze the penis before the ejaculatory process has started. Sex therapy has been successful with some premature ejaculators; however, a subgroup of dysfunctional men may need pharmacotherapy as well.

A man with sexual desire disorder or erectile disorder is sometimes told to masturbate to demonstrate that full erection and ejaculation are possible. A woman with lifelong female orgasmic disorder is directed to masturbate, sometimes using a vibrator. Kegel's exercises may be introduced to strengthen the pubococcygeal muscles—that is, the woman is encouraged to contract her abdominal and perineal muscles during masturbation and coitus. When a man has erectile disorder, the woman may be instructed to stimulate or tease his penis. The same technique is used with men who suffer from retarded ejaculation, with stimulation sometimes involving a vibrator. Retarded ejaculation is managed by extravaginal ejaculation initially and gradual vaginal entry after stimulation to the point of near ejaculation.

Treatment Goals The overall goal of treatment is to initiate an educational process, to diminish the fears of performance felt by both sexes, and to facilitate communication in sexual and nonsexual areas. Therapy sessions follow each new exercise period, and problems and satisfactions (both sexual and nonsexual) are discussed. Specific instructions and new exercises geared to the individual couple's progress are reviewed in each session. Gradually, the couple gains confidence and learns (or relearns) to communicate verbally and sexually. Dual-sex therapy is most effective when the sexual dysfunction exists apart from other psychopathology.

Hypnotherapy Hypnotherapists focus specifically on the anxiety-producing symptom—that is, the particular sexual dysfunction. Successful use of hypnosis helps the patient gain control over the symptom that has been lowering self-esteem and disrupting psychological homeostasis. Patient cooperation is first obtained and encouraged during a series of nonhypnotic sessions with the therapist, designed to develop a secure doctor–patient relationship and a sense of physical and psychological comfort on the part of the patient and to establish mutually desired treatment goals. During that time, the therapist assesses the patient's capacity for the trance experience. The nonhypnotic sessions also permit the clinician to take a careful psychiatric history and do a mental status examination before beginning hypnotherapy. Treatment focuses on symptom removal and attitude alteration. In a trance state, patients can entertain ideas incongruent with their usual (nonhypnotized) perceptions of reality. Patients are instructed in developing alternative means of dealing with the anxiety-provoking situation (i.e., the sexual encounter).

For example, a woman with vaginismus is given the posthypnotic suggestion that she will feel no pain during intercourse and will be able to relax the muscles surrounding her vagina. If compliance with the suggestion is successful, she can deal with the anxiety produced by the sex act. She is also taught new attitudes, such as being entitled to sexual pleasure. Under hypnosis, her fear or anger at sexual contact can be examined, and she learns how her emotions are expressed by involuntary vaginal spasms.

Some patients respond particularly well to the use of self-hypnosis and indirect suggestion. These techniques allow them to retain a greater sense of control over their situation. Typically, patients are instructed to conjure up images and develop ideas antithetical to their dysfunctional responses. For example, a woman with an arousal disorder may first agree to concentrate on imagery that causes her to salivate. She is then told that, just as she has made her mouth water by focusing on stimulating images, she can effect the lubricating response of her vagina by focusing on images she finds erotic or romantic. At the same time, the therapist helps her deal with her anxieties about a positive sexual response. Patients are also taught relaxing techniques to use before sexual relations. With these methods to alleviate anxiety, the physiological responses to sexual stimulation can more readily result in pleasurable excitation and discharge. Hypnosis may be added to a basic individual psychotherapy program to accelerate the impact of psychotherapeutic intervention.

Behavior Therapy Behavior therapists assume that sexual dysfunction is learned, maladaptive behavior. Behavioral approaches were initially designed to treat phobias. In cases of sexual dysfunction, the therapist sees the patient as phobic of sexual interaction. Using traditional techniques, the therapist sets up a hierarchy of anxiety-provoking situations for the patient, ranging from the least threatening to the most threatening. Mild anxiety may be experienced at the thought of kissing, and massive anxiety may be felt when imagining penile penetration. The behavior therapist helps the patient master the anxiety through a standard program of systematic desensitization. The program is designed to inhibit the learned anxious response by encouraging behaviors antithetical to anxiety. The patient first deals with the least anxiety-producing situation in fantasy and progresses by steps to the most anxiety-producing situation. Medication, hypnosis, or special training in deep muscle relaxation is sometimes used to help with the initial mastery of anxiety.

Assertiveness training helps teach patients to express their sexual needs openly and without fear. Exercises in assertiveness are given in conjunction with sex therapy, and patients are encouraged both to make sexual requests and to refuse to comply with requests perceived as unreasonable. Sexual exercises may be prescribed for patients to perform at home, and a hierarchy may be established, starting with activities that proved most pleasurable and successful in the past.

One treatment variation involves the participation of the patient's sexual partner in the desensitization program. The partner, rather than the therapist, presents the hierarchical items to the patient. In such situations, a cooperative partner is necessary to help the patient carry gains made during treatment sessions to sexual activity at home.

Behavior therapy techniques have been particularly effective in treating women with severe inhibition of excitement and orgasm when such feelings were accompanied by strong feelings of anxiety, anger, or disgust.

Group Therapy Methods of group therapy have been used to examine both intrapsychic and interpersonal problems in patients with sexual disorders. The therapy group provides a strong support system for patients who feel ashamed, anxious, or guilty about a particular sexual problem. It is a useful forum in which to counteract sexual myths, correct misconceptions, and provide accurate information regarding sexual anatomy, physiology, and varieties of behavior.

Groups for the treatment of sexual disorders can be organized in several ways. Members may all share the same problem, such as premature ejaculation; members may all be of the same sex and have different sexual problems; or groups may be composed of both men and women who are experiencing different sexual problems. Group therapy may be an adjunct to other forms of therapy or the prime mode of treatment. Groups organized to cure a particular dysfunction usually have a behavioral approach. For example, patients with anorgasmia may participate with others who have the same problem in a short-term, intensive group experience. Sexual histories, feelings of inadequacy, and concerns about body image are shared. Specific physiological information, sometimes with the aid of audiovisual materials, is presented to the group members. Members are given homework assignments (e.g., they may be instructed to masturbate). A combination of group support and group pressure helps some of the participants complete assignments they might otherwise avoid. As the short-term group process nears termination, members are encouraged to talk about their experiences with their partners.

Groups have also been effective when composed of sexually dysfunctional married couples. The group provides an opportunity to gather accurate information, provides consensual validation of individual preferences, and enhances self-esteem and self-acceptance. Such techniques as role-playing and psychodrama may be used in treatment. These groups are not indicated for couples in which one partner is uncooperative, has severe depression or psychosis, or has a strong repugnance for explicit sexual audiovisual materials or a strong fear of groups.

Integrated Sex Therapy One of the most effective treatment modalities is the use of sex therapy integrated with supportive, psychodynamic, or insight-orientated psychotherapy. Adding psychodynamic conceptualizations to the behavioral techniques used to treat sexual dysfunctions allows treatment of patients with sex disorders associated with other psychopathology. Also, this type of therapy is appropriate for patients with hypoactive desire disorders. Insight-oriented therapy helps them deal with problems in their interpersonal relationships or intrapsychic conflicts that frequently are at the root of the problem. The themes and dynamics that emerge in patients in analytically oriented sex therapy are the same as those that emerge in psychoanalytic therapy—relevant dreams, fear of punishment, aggressive feelings, difficulty with trusting the partner, fear of intimacy, oedipal feelings, and fear of genital mutilation. Two cases follow that demonstrate some of these dynamics.

A 34-year-old widow presented for therapy with a chief complaint of vaginismus. Her marriage of 3 years, which had been unconsummated, ended when her husband was killed in a car accident. Approximately 1 year after she lost her husband, the patient became involved with a married man. She was very attracted to him and became highly aroused during their sexual encounters. Although she could reach orgasm through manual or oral stimulation, she could not tolerate penetration. Although she never considered therapy when she was married, in spite of her husband's requests to do so, she was motivated to seek help for her problem, because she felt sure her lover would leave his wife for her if they could share a more complete sexual experience.

The patient's vaginismus resulted partly from unresolved developmental conflicts. Her parents had been loving but constricted people who came from different socioeconomic backgrounds. Their values often conflicted, and they frequently fought over their daughter as she entered adolescence. The mother insisted that she take an academic course in high school to prepare for college, whereas the father pushed a "more practical" business program. The patient sided with her mother and felt that her father, whom she had always perceived as cold, became more distant than before.

Some of her difficulties were due to unresolved oedipal problems; both her husband and her lover were more than 20 years older than she was, and her lover (reflecting her parental situation) was married to a woman who was more successful than he was. In addition, she had identified with some of her mother's negative feelings about men. The mother had once told the patient she hoped that she would be spared marriage. Vaginismus protected the patient from the closeness with men that she consciously wanted but unconsciously perceived as hurtful and dangerous.

A 56-year-old man came for treatment because of an erectile disorder. In general, he functioned better in extramarital affairs than in his marriage. Although he loved his wife and considered her an attractive woman, he believed that she was not interested in sex. He could rarely achieve an erection with her, and he gradually stopped approaching her sexually. His wife felt deprived by their lack of sexual relations and frequently masturbated.

The patient had been a sickly child, with a mother he described as devoted but smothering. He remembered her cuddling him in bed until he was 8 years old, and he felt that she was inappropriately affectionate in general ("she embarrassed me"). At the same time, he remembered his father as an earthy man and had a childhood recollection of hearing his mother ask his father, "How could you, how could you?" The patient believed it had been his mother's response to a sexual overture or act. In part, his disorder derived from his unconscious oedipal associations to his wife, which made her taboo for him as a sex partner. The women to whom he responded had to be blatantly sexual and signal their acceptance of him before he would risk an advance. Therapy involved both individual sessions with the patient and joint sessions with him and his wife. Communication, which had been strained partly because of the sexual distance between them, was encouraged, and a behavioral approach was used to reestablish some physical interaction. Individual work focused on his deeper psychological problems.

The dynamics and the emotional difficulties evident in these vignettes are seen every day by psychiatrists. Psychiatrists can readily absorb the techniques of sex therapy into their treatment armamentarium, just as they have modified and absorbed any number of specialized techniques, from classic analytical dynamic formulations to the use of pharmacotherapy, group therapy techniques, and behavioral and other directive modalities. The combined approach of individual and sex therapy is used by the general psychiatrist, who carefully judges the optimal timing of sex therapy and the ability of patients to tolerate the directive approach that focuses on their sexual difficulties.

Biological Treatment Methods Biological treatments, including pharmacotherapy and surgery, have applications in specific cases of sexual disorder. Advances in biological treatment methods, particularly pharmacological methods of treating sexual dysfunction have significantly augmented the therapist's catalogue of therapeutic approaches. Most of the recent advances involve male sexual dysfunctions. Current studies are under way to test pharmacological treatment of sexual dysfunctions in women.

Pharmacotherapy A variety of drugs have been explored in the treatment of sexual dysfunction. The major new medications are nitric oxide enhancers such as sildenafil (Viagra); oral prostaglandin (Vasomax); alprostadil (Caverject), an injectable phentolamine; and a transurethral alprostadil (MUSE), all used in the treatment of erectile disorder.

Nitric Oxide Enhancers Nitric oxide enhancers facilitate the inflow of blood to the penis necessary for an erection. The physiological mechanism of penile erection involves release of nitric oxide in the corpus cavernosum during sexual stimulation. Nitric oxide activates the enzyme guanylate cyclase, which increases cyclic guanosine monophosphate concentration and produces smooth muscle relaxation in the corpus cavernosum that allows the penile vessels to dilate and admit blood. The first drug developed, sildenafil, enhances the effect of nitric oxide by inhibiting the enzyme that degrades cyclic guanosine monophosphate. Thus, sildenafil augments the natural process involved in gaining and maintaining an erection during sexual stimulation. The drug takes effect approximately 1 hour after ingestion, and its effect can last up to 4 hours. Sildenafil has no effect in the absence of sexual stimulation.

The most common adverse events associated with sildenafil are headaches, flushing, and dyspepsia. Some sildenafil users see things in a blue tint for several hours after taking the medication; because of this, airline pilots have been prohibited from taking the drug so that this visual artifact does not interfere with safe landings. The use of sildenafil is contraindicated for people taking organic nitrates. The concomitant action of the two drugs can result in large, sudden, and sometimes fatal drops in systemic blood pressure. The U.S. Food and Drug Administration (FDA) has posted 130 deaths in which sildenafil was listed as an associated medication and advises caution in prescribing sildenafil to men with a recent (6-month) history of myocardial infarction, stroke, life-threatening arrhythmia, significant hypotension or hypertension, cardiac failure, angina, or retinitis pigmentosa. However, the FDA has reiterated that it is a safe drug. Sildenafil is not effective in all cases of erectile dysfunction. It fails to produce an erection rigid enough for penetration in approximately 50 percent of men who have had radical prostate surgery or in those with long-standing, insulin-dependent diabetes. It is also ineffective in certain cases of nerve damage.

Two new nitric oxide enhancers similar to sildenafil—vardenafil (Levitra) and tadalafil (Cialis)—have been developed. Tadalafil has an effective therapeutic window of 36 hours compared to sildenafil and vardenafil, which are effective for approximately 4 hours.

Oral phentolamine has proved effective as a potency enhancer in men with minimal erectile dysfunction. It may prove useful for men with cardiac problems, as sildenafil is contraindicated for men using organic nitrates, but it is not currently approved by the FDA. Apomorphine is also being tested as an oral remedy for erectile dysfunction.

Alprostadil In contrast to the oral medications, injectable and transurethral alprostadil act locally on the penis and can produce erections in the absence of sexual stimulation. Alprostadil contains a naturally occurring form of prostaglandin E. Prostaglandins are composed of complex hydroxy fatty acids, and they have wide biological influences. Although some prostaglandins are vasoconstrictive, prostaglandin E_1, found in alprostadil, is a powerful vasodilating agent, especially in local vascular areas, such as the corpus cavernosum of the penis. The drug causes direct smooth muscle relaxation of penile vessels and erectile tissue; this reaction lowers the vascular resistance of the corpus and significantly increases blood flow to the penis. The firm erection produced within 2 to 3 minutes by increased blood flow may last as long as 1 hour. Treatment consists of the patient's self-injection of alprostadil into the corpus before coitus. This technique is easily taught and relatively painless. Infrequent adverse effects include penile bruising and changes in liver function test results, which are readily reversible when a man stops the injections. However, possible hazardous sequelae exist, including priapism and sclerosis of the small veins of the penis. Another substance being tried is vasoactive intestinal polypeptide (VIP). Intracavernous injection of VIP causes erection and has a parasympathomimetic effect. Some researchers speculate that this substance, which has been found in the hypothalamus and the female genital organs, is the essential factor in male and female arousal. In Europe, phenoxybenzamine (Dibenzyline) is used to produce erections by injection into the penis. Serious adverse effects include priapism and pain accompanying the injection, and the drug is not allowed as a therapy in the United States.

Alprostadil can also be delivered via the urethra, eliminating the need for self-injection. Some men prefer the local, nonsystemic effects of alprostadil to oral sildenafil; others prefer sildenafil because it seems more like a nonpharmacologically aided response to them and their partners. A small trial found a topical cream effective in alleviating erectile dysfunction. The cream consists of three vasoactive substances that are a mixture of ergot alkaloids. Alprostadil is a useful treatment for patients in whom nitric oxide enhancers are contraindicated (e.g., patients who are taking nitrate-containing medication). It is also of use in patients who do not tolerate the side effects of other drugs.

The pharmacological treatments described above are useful in treatment of erectile dysfunction of various causes: psychogenic, neurogenic, arterial insufficiency, venous leakage, and mixed. The following case demonstrates the use of pharmacotherapy to treat erectile dysfunction of psychogenic origin.

Mr. B. and Ms. C. (his fiancée) presented for sex therapy, with Mr. B. having experienced erectile dysfunction for 7 months, as well as a lifelong history of premature ejaculation. Mr. B. was a 42-year-old professional, and Ms. C. was a 38-year-old corporate executive. She had never been married; it was to be his second marriage.

Mr. B.'s sexual history was remarkable for a late first coitus (age 25) and a general sexual insecurity that contrasted with his professional confidence and social poise. Ms. C. was sexually responsive, in spite of a history of anxiety attacks for which she had been treated in the past. Their early sexual activity together had been frequent and satisfying to both, in spite of his prematurity. After a few months, however, she began to complain about both the premature ejaculation and the secrecy of their relationship. Although Mr. B. was legally separated when they became involved, he was worried about divorce negotiations if his spouse learned about his new relationship. Treatment revealed that he found the secrecy in their relationship exciting.

The two were treated with integrated sex therapy, a combination of behavioral and insight-oriented techniques, and made substantial progress. They successfully controlled the premature ejaculation by practicing the squeeze technique (i.e., forcibly squeezing the coronal ridge of the penis before ejaculation to increase the threshold of penile sensitivity). In genital-caressing sessions. Mr. B.'s erections returned, and he could maintain a good erection to climax, with manual and oral stimulation. However, he continued to lose his erection when he attempted vaginal penetration. It was decided to supplement psychotherapy with intracavernosal injections of alprostadil (sildenafil was not yet available). Ms. C. was present when he was instructed in the injection technique and supported the process. Mr. B. was delighted with the results, and, after 1 month of pharmacologically assisted coitus, he successfully achieved penetration without assistance. Currently, he has coitus once a week, with occasional use of sildenafil rather than intracavernosal injection when he is feeling stressed. The availability of a medication to treat his erectile problem significantly relieves his performance anxiety.

Erectile dysfunction of psychological or mixed origin should not be treated by medication alone, even though the dysfunction can be corrected pharmacologically. The drugs should be used in conjunction with, not as a replacement for, sex therapy. In some cases, erectile dysfunction serves as a defense against unconscious conflicts that must be faced when the sexual symptom is removed as result of medication. In some cases, the patient deals with his conflicts by simply not using the medications prescribed for his erectile problem. Also, patients in long-standing or marital relationships require the cooperation of their partners for this treatment to be effective. Although most women are very accommodating to their partner's desire for treatment, several concerns occur with some frequency: the element of romance is an important part of sexual interaction for many women, and pharmacological assistance of erections may eliminate that sense of romance; the woman, or the couple, may bemoan the lack of spontaneity when pharmacotherapy is part of the sex act; and some women feel deprived of feedback about their desirability. Joint sessions help the couple cope with these issues.

Sildenafil Use in Women The physical sign of sexual excitement in women is vaginal lubrication. That lubrication is a transudate believed to result from increased vasocongestion of the extensive capillary net in the vaginal walls. The same physiological mechanism—vasocongestion—results in erection in the man. Researchers believe that sildenafil may facilitate blood flow in women just as it does in men and, thus, give women with inhibited excitement of psychological or physiological origin a pharmacological remedy for their dysfunction. Some reports suggest that women find it preferable to apply sildenafil in a cream base to the clitoris, labia, and vagina. However, as in men, pharmacological treatment may need to be combined with psychological modalities to be effective.

Recognition of sexual excitement may be more complex for women than it is for men. For example, in studies of response to pornography, men and women underwent physiological measurements of excitement after visual stimuli. In these studies, men were more accurate in correlating their subjective sense of arousal (i.e., erection) than were women (i.e., lubrication).

Other Pharmacological Agents

Numerous other pharmacological agents have been used to cure the various sexual disorders. Intravenous methohexital sodium (Brevital) has been used in desensitization therapy. Antianxiety agents may have some application in tense patients, although these drugs can also interfere with the sexual response. The side effects of antidepressants, particularly the SSRIs and tricyclic drugs, which include delayed orgasm, have been used to prolong the sexual response in patients with premature ejaculation. This approach is particularly useful in patients refractory to behavioral techniques or who may have physiologically determined premature ejaculation. The use of antidepressants has been advocated in the treatment of patients who are phobic of sex and in those with a posttraumatic stress disorder (PTSD) after rape. The risks of taking such medications must be carefully weighed against their possible benefits. Bromocriptine (Parlodel) is used in the treatment of hyperprolactinemia, which is frequently associated with hypogonadism. Such cases are first worked up to rule out pituitary tumors. Bromocriptine, a dopamine agonist, may improve sexual function impaired by hyperprolactinemia.

Yohimbine is an α-adrenergic receptor antagonist that may cause dilation of the penile artery and improve erections. Recreational drugs, including cocaine, amphetamines, alcohol, and cannabis, are considered enhancers of sexual performance. Although they may provide the user with an initial benefit because of their tranquilizing, disinhibiting, or mood-elevating effects, consistent or prolonged use of any of these substances impairs sexual functioning.

Ginseng has been reported to have androgenic effects. One report described the case of a mother who ingested large amounts of ginseng during her pregnancy, resulting in androgenization of the neonate, who was born with pubic hair and enlarged testes.

Other drugs that have been used by women to alleviate arousal dysfunction include oral phentolamine, topical prostaglandin E, oral oxytocin, ginkgo biloba, and various psychostimulants, including caffeine. Many of these drugs have not been approved for treatment of female sexual dysfunction and must be prescribed with caution.

Dopaminergic agents have been reported to increase libido and improve sex function. Those drugs include L-dopa, a dopamine precursor, and bromocriptine, a dopamine agonist. The antidepressant bupropion has dopaminergic effects and has increased sex drive in some patients. Selegiline, an MAOI, is selective for MAO_B and is dopaminergic. It improves sexual functioning in older persons.

Hormone Therapy Androgens increase the sex drive in women and in men with low testosterone concentrations. Women may experience virilizing effects, some of which are irreversible (e.g., deepening of the voice). In men, prolonged use of androgens may produce hypertension and prostatic enlargement. Testosterone is most effective when given parenterally; however, effective transdermal preparations are available. Oral preparations are associated with increased risk of hepatotoxicity.

Gonadotrophin-releasing hormone (GnRH), also known as *luteinizing hormone-releasing hormone* (LHRH), stimulates the release of luteinizing hormone, which increases testosterone secretion in both sexes. GnRH is used as an inhalant in Europe. It stimulates desire and increases potency. Because GnRH is released normally in a pulsatile fashion, portable infusion pumps have been developed that simulate pulsatile delivery. An excess of GnRH suppresses estrogen and testosterone; thus, the therapeutic use of GnRH is limited by a narrow therapeutic window.

Women who use estrogens for replacement therapy or for contraception may report decreased libido; in such cases, a combined preparation of estrogen and testosterone has been used effectively. Estrogen itself prevents thinning of the vaginal mucous membrane and facilitates lubrication.

Testosterone is given to women around the world in the form of tablets, implants, patches, and creams. In the United States, methyltestosterone pills and compounded creams are the primary methods of administration. Testosterone is primarily administered to postmenopausal (occurring surgically or naturally) women, but testosterone deficiency also exists in premenopausal women.

Mrs. M. presented for therapy alone with a chief complaint of pain on intercourse dating from the onset of menopause 14 months before coming for treatment. Her husband knew of her visit but did not accompany her, as he was away on one of many routine and frequent business trips.

Sexual intercourse was infrequent because of his heavy travel schedule, but their sex play was varied and, before menopause, Mrs. M. had enjoyed sex. Mrs. M. found her sexual interactions with her husband gratifying. She had a strong libido and would masturbate when Mr. M. was away.

Mrs. M. was on oral hormone replacement therapy, which had helped but had not eliminated the pain she had with intercourse. In consultation with her gynecologist, the occasional use of hormone cream was added to her treatment regimen. Additionally, she was instructed to use vaginal dilators routinely when Mr. M. was away. This was not for purposes of masturbation, which for her involved clitoral stimulation, but for routine stretching of the vagina. Nonhormonal vaginal cream was prescribed for the couple to use with intercourse. The combination of oral hormone replacement therapy, vaginal creams, and the routine use of vaginal dilators served to eliminate Mrs. M.'s pain. She was diagnosed with dyspareunia, acquired type.

Pheromones are sexual scents that are found in animals and may be present in humans. They produce dramatic sex-seeking behavioral patterns in animals (e.g., male deer following female deer in estrus, mounting behavior in primates). Human pheromones are believed to be short-acting fatty acids present in vaginal secretions and male sweat. In one study, women were consistently more attracted to items impregnated with a chemical derived from male sweat (α-androstenol) than to control items. In another study, the sweat of women was preserved in underarm pads they changed daily, and the date each pad was worn was correlated with the women's menstrual cycle. A second group of women was asked to smell these pads as they were rubbed above their upper lips, without knowing what they were and recognizing no scent but the alcohol preservative used on the pads. Depending on whether they were exposed to pads from the early or late part of the first group's (the wearers) menstrual cycle, the second group (the sniffers) saw their own menstrual cycles shortened or lengthened. This area is still being researched.

Antiandrogens and Antiestrogens Estrogen and progesterone are antiandrogens that have been used to treat compulsive sexual behavior in men, usually in sex offenders.

Medroxyprogesterone acetate (Depo-Provera), used primarily as a contraceptive in women, inhibits the secretion of gonadotrophins. It is used in men with compulsive sexual behavior to reduce libido by lowering testosterone levels. Cyproterone acetate is a strong antiandrogen used in Europe to treat sex offenders. At dosages of 100 to 200 mg a day, the sex drive disappears within 2 weeks.

Tamoxifen (Nolvadex) is used to treat breast cancer and has antiestrogenic properties. In some women, increased libido may result from the unopposed testosterone levels. Clomiphene (Clomid) is an ovulatory stimulant used in women with ovulatory menstrual cycles desiring pregnancy. Clomiphene increases release of pituitary gonadotrophins, and some women may report increased libido. Neither of these drugs, however, is used as a treatment for decreased libido in women.

Mechanical Treatment Approaches

Steal Syndrome In male patients with arteriosclerosis (especially of the distal aorta, known as *Leriche's syndrome*), the erection may be lost during active pelvic thrusting. The need for increased blood in the gluteal muscles and others served by the ilial or hypogastric arteries takes blood away (steals) from the pudendal artery and, thus, interferes with penile blood flow. Relief may be obtained by decreasing pelvic thrusting, which is also aided by the woman-superior coital position.

Vacuum Pump Vacuum pumps are mechanical devices that patients without vascular disease can use to obtain erections. The blood drawn into the penis after the creation of the vacuum is kept there by a ring placed around the base of the penis. This device has no adverse effects, but it is cumbersome, and partners must be willing to accept its use. Some women complain that the penis is redder and cooler than when erection is produced by natural circumstances, and they find the process and the result objectionable.

A vacuum pump with the marketing name *Eros* was devised for women to precipitate a clitoral erection. It works similarly to the vacuum pump used to create penile erections in men, although no band is placed around the clitoris once erection is obtained. The pump is not necessary for intercourse to occur; it was devised to enhance female excitement, but its effectiveness has not been studied rigorously.

Surgical Treatment

Male Prostheses Surgical treatment is infrequently advocated, but improved penile prosthetic devices are available for men with inadequate erectile response who are resistant to other treatment methods or who have medically caused deficiencies. There are two main types of prosthesis: a semirigid rod prosthesis that produces a permanent erection that can be positioned close to the body for concealment and an inflatable type that is implanted with its own reservoir and pump for inflation and deflation. The latter type is designed to mimic normal physiological functioning. Placing a penile prosthesis in a man who has lost the ability to ejaculate or to have an orgasm as a result of medical causes will not restore those functions. Men with prosthetic devices have generally reported satisfaction with their subsequent sexual functioning, but their wives report much less satisfaction. Presurgical counseling is strongly recommended so that the couple has a realistic expectation of what the prosthesis can do for their sex lives. Postsurgical counseling may also be necessary to help the couple adapt to their rediscovered ability to have intercourse. They may experience a high level of anxiety if their sex life had been inactive for a prolonged period before surgery. Prosthetic devices have been associated with severe adverse effects, including perforation, infection, urinary retention, and persistent pain.

Some surgeons are attempting revascularization of the penis as a direct approach to treating erectile dysfunction resulting from vascular disorders. Such surgical procedures are indicated in patients with corporal shunts that allow normally entrapped blood to leak from the corporal spaces, leading to inadequate erections (steal syndrome). Limited reports exist of prolonged success with the technique. Endarterectomy can be of benefit if aortoiliac occlusive disease is responsible for the erectile dysfunction.

Another medical treatment being studied for erectile disorders is electrostimulation at the base of the penis. Initial reports indicate minimal physical discomfort in patients receiving this therapy. However, response to treatment is inconsistent, and a problem exists in terms of maintaining erections. At the present time, the treatment seems to have no benefits.

Female Procedures Surgical approaches to female dysfunctions include hymenectomy in the case of dyspareunia in an unconsummated marriage, vaginoplasty in multiparous women complaining of lessened vaginal sensations, or freeing clitoral adhesions in women with inhibited excitement. Such surgical treatments have not been carefully studied and should be considered cautiously.

Outcome Demonstrating the effectiveness of the varieties of sex therapy is just as difficult as assessing the effectiveness of outpatient psychotherapy in treating other psychological problems. As with other disorders, the more severe the psychopathology associated with a problem of long duration, the more adverse the outcome is likely to be.

Masters and Johnson first reported positive results for their behavioral treatment approach in 1970. They studied the failure rates of their patients (defined as failure to initiate reversal of the basic symptom of the presenting dysfunction). They compared initial failure rates with 5-year follow-up findings for the same couples. Although some have criticized their definition of the percentage of presumed successes, other studies have confirmed the effectiveness of their approach.

The most difficult treatment cases involve couples with severe marital discord. Cases involving problems of fear of intimacy, excessive dependency, or excessive hostility are also complex. Other challenges are posed by patients with impulse disorders, unresolved homosexual conflicts, or fetishistic defenses. Patients phobic of sex also present treatment difficulties, as do patients diagnosed with lifelong dysfunctions. Desire disorders are particularly difficult to treat. They require longer, more intensive therapy than some other disorders, and their outcomes are very variable.

When behavioral approaches are used, empirical criteria that are supposed to predict outcome are more easily isolated. Using these criteria, for instance, couples who regularly practice assigned exercises appear to have a much greater likelihood of successful outcome than do more resistant couples or those whose interaction involves sadomasochistic or depressive features or mechanisms of blame and projection. Flexibility of attitude is also a positive prognostic factor. Overall, younger couples tend to complete sex therapy more often than older couples. Couples whose interactional difficulties center on their sex problems, such as inhibition, frustration, or fear of performance failure, are also likely to respond well to therapy.

In general, methods that have proved effective singly or in combination include training in behavioral sexual skills, systematic desensitization, directive marital counseling, traditional psychodynamic approaches, group therapy, and pharmacotherapy. Although most prefer to treat a couple for sexual dysfunctions, treatment of individual persons has also been successful. The frequency of sessions is not a significant factor in treatment success. Thus, whether patients have intensive daily therapy over a period of 2 weeks, weekly therapy, or biweekly therapy appears to have little effect on the outcome of treatment. Also, the use of one therapist to treat a couple instead of a dual-sex cotherapy team is nearly as effective and certainly more practical.

Patients seen today are frequently older when they present for therapy, more informed about sex, and more likely to have disorders of mixed etiology than were those seen in the mid-1970s. Moreover, numerous new biological treatments are now available for incorporation into sex therapy treatment programs. Today, a multimodal treatment regimen and an eclectic approach to sexual disorders will result in a favorable outcome in the great majority of cases.

SUGGESTED CROSS-REFERENCES

Homosexuality is discussed in Section 18.1b, paraphilias are discussed in Section 18.2, and gender identity disorders are discussed in Section 18.3. Sexual addiction is covered in Section 18.4. The neuropsychological and neuropsychiatric aspects of HIV infection are covered in Section 2.8. Couples therapy is discussed in Section 30.5, and biological and other pharmacological therapies are discussed in Chapter 31. The physical and sexual abuse of children, including incest, is covered in Section 49.3.

REFERENCES

Araoz DL: Uses of hypnosis in the treatment of psychogenic sexual dysfunctions. *Psychiatr Ann.* 1986;16:102.

Assalian P, Margolese H: Treatment of antidepressant induced side effects. *J Sex Marital Ther.* 1996;22:3.

Brady JP: Behavior therapy and sex therapy. *Am J Psychiatry.* 1976;133:896.

Chessick RD: Thirty unresolved psychodynamic questions pertaining to feminine psychology. *Am J Psychother.* 1988;42:86.

*Delgardo PL, McGauey CA, Moreno FA, Laukes C, Gelenberg AJ: Treatment strategies for depression and sexual dysfunction. *J Clin Psychiatry.* 1999;17:22.

Ellis A. *Studies in the Psychology of Sex.* New York: Preston House; 1936.

Federman DD: Perspective: Three facets of sexual differentiation. *N Engl J Med.* 2004;350:323–324.

Goldstein I, Lue T, Padma-Nathatan H, Rosen R, Steers WD, Wicker PA: The sildenafil study group, oral sildenafil in the treatment of erectile dysfunction. *N Engl J Med.* 1996;338:1397.

Herman J, LoPiccolo J: Clinical outcome of sex therapy. *Arch Gen Psychiatry.* 1983;40:443.

Kegeles SM, Adler NE, Irwin CE: Sexually active adolescents and condoms: Changes over one year in knowledge, attitudes and use. *Am J Public Health.* 1988;78:460.

Koppelman M, Parry BL, Hamilton JA, Alogna SW, Loreaux PL: Effect of bromocriptine on affect and libido in hyperprolactinemia. *Am J Psychiatry.* 1987;144:1037.

Koren G: Maternal ginseng use associated with neonatal androgenization. *JAMA.* 1990;264:2866.

Krafft-Ebing R. *Psychopathia Sexual.* Munich: Matthes & Seitz; 1984.

*Laughman E, Gagnon J, Michael R, Michaels S. *Sex in America.* Chicago: University of Chicago Press; 1994.

Leitenberg H, Detzer M, Srebnik D: Gender differences in masturbation and the relation of masturbation experience in preadolescence and/or early adolescence to sexual behavior and sexual adjustment in young adulthood. *Arch Sex Behav.* 1993;22:87.

Linet OI, Ogrinc FG (for the Alprostadil Study Group): Efficacy and safety of intracavernosal alprostadil in men with erectile dysfunction. *N Engl J Med.* 1996;334:875.

Loosen PT, Purdon SE, Pavlou SN: Effects on behavior of modulation of gonadal function in men with gonadotropin-releasing hormone antagonists. *Am J Psychiatry.* 1994;151:271.

MacLaughlin DT, Donahoe PK: Mechanisms of disease: Sex determination and differentiation. *N Engl J Med.* 2004;350:369.

*Masters WH, Johnson VE. *Human Sexual Inadequacy.* Boston: Little, Brown; 1970.

*Masters WH, Johnson VE. *Human Sexual Response.* Boston: Little, Brown; 1970.

Padma-Nathan H, Hellstrom WJG, Kaiser FE, Labasky RF, Lue TF, Nolten WE, Norwood PC, Peterson CA, Shabsigh R, Tam PY, Place VA, Gesundheit N (for the Medicated Urethral System for Erection [MUSE] Study Group): Treatment of men with erectile dysfunction with transurethral alprostadil. *N Engl J Med.* 1997;336:1.

*Purnine DM, Carey MP, Jorgensen RS: Gender differences regarding preferences for specific heterosexual practices. *J Sex Marital Ther.* 1994;20:271.

Rhoden EL, Morgentaler A: Risks of testosterone-replacement therapy and recommendations for monitoring. *N Engl J Med.* 2004;350:482.

*Riley AJ: Life-long absence of sexual drive in a woman associated with 5-dihydrotestosterone deficiency. *J Sex Marital Ther.* 1999;25:13.

*Rosen RC, Lane RM, Menza M: Effects of SSRIs on sexual function: A critical review. *J Clin Psychopharmacol.* 1999;19:67.

*Sadock VA. The treatment of psychosexual dysfunctions: An overview. In: Grinspoon L, ed. *Psychiatry 1982. The American Psychiatric Association Annual Review.* Washington, DC: American Psychiatric Press; 1982.

Sadock VA. Group psychotherapy of psychosexual dysfunctions. In: Kaplan HI, Sadock BJ, eds. *Comprehensive Group Psychotherapy.* Baltimore: Williams & Wilkins; 1983:286.

Seagraves RT, Seagraves KB: Human sexuality and aging. *J Sex Educ Ther.* 1995;21:88.

Semans JH: Premature ejaculation: A new approach. *South Med J.* 1956;49:353.

Shrainer-Engel P, Schiavi R: Lifetime psychopathology in individuals with low sexual desire. *J Nerv Ment Dis.* 1986;174:646.

Stein DJ, Hollander E, Anthony DT, Schneier FR: Serotonergic medications for sexual addictions, and paraphilias. *J Clin Psychiatry.* 1992;53:267.

Sternbach H: Age associated testosterone decline in men: Clinical issues for psychiatry. *Am J Psychiatry.* 1998;155:10.

Thase M, Reynolds C, Glanz L, Jennings JR, Sweitz DE, Kupper DJ, Frank E: Nocturnal penile tumescence in depressed men. *Am J Psychiatry.* 1987;144:89.

Waldinger MD, Hengeveld WH, Zwinderman A, Olivier B: Effect of SSRI antidepressants on ejaculation: A double-blind, randomized, placebo-controlled study with fluoxetine, fluvoxamine, paroxetine and sertraline. *J Clin Psychopharmacol.* 1998;189:274.

Wiley D, Borts WM: Sexuality and aging—usual and successful. *J Gerontol.* 1996;51:22.

▲ 18.1b Homosexuality, Gay and Lesbian Identities, and Homosexual Behavior

JACK DRESCHER, M.D., TERRY S. STEIN, M.D., AND WILLIAM M. BYNE, M.D., PH.D.

There have been many psychiatric theories about homosexuality's origins, its social and personal meanings, its diagnostic implications, and what constitutes correct clinical approaches toward it. In 1973, the American Psychiatric Association (APA) officially accepted a normal variant model and removed homosexuality per se from its *Diagnostic and Statistical Manual of Mental Disorders* (DSM). In 1992, the World Health Organization (WHO) followed the American example and made a similar change in the *International Classification of Diseases* (ICD).

Psychiatry and medicine's nosological changes reflect a dramatically increased social acceptance of openly gay, lesbian, and bisexual individuals in Western societies. This acceptance is a rapidly evolving social phenomenon. In 2003, the U.S. Supreme Court ruled that state sodomy laws, which criminalized homosexual behavior, were discriminatory and unconstitutional. At the time of this chapter's writing, same-sex marriage is legal in Belgium and the Netherlands. Some other form of recognized civil union has become a viable option in several Western European countries (Croatia, Denmark, Finland, France, Germany, Hungary, Iceland, Norway, Portugal, Sweden, and Switzerland), in the U.S. state of Vermont, and in the Canadian provinces of British Columbia, Ontario, and Quebec. Civil unions are expected to become the law in all of Canada. Countries that extend some benefits to same-sex partners, or contain jurisdictions that do so, include Argentina, Australia, Brazil, Canada, Colombia, Costa Rica, Israel, Italy, New Zealand, South Africa, and Spain. In addition, numerous corporations throughout the United States, Europe, and Canada offer some form of domestic partnership rights for same-sex couples. In 2003, the most populous state in the United States, California, passed a domestic partnership law almost as broad in scope as Vermont's civil unions. Also, in 2003, the Supreme Judicial Court of Massachusetts ruled that the state was required to grant same-sex couples the right to marry. National and state governments are increasingly addressing the rights of same-sex couples to adopt and to act as foster parents to children. This section offers a historical view of the evolution of psychiatry's conceptualizations of homosexuality, as well as contemporary perspectives on the mental health issues related to gay, lesbian, and bisexual populations.

DEFINITIONS

Sexual orientation refers to a person's erotic response tendency or sexual attractions, be they *homosexual, bisexual, or heterosexual.* Sexual orientation can be assessed through such parameters as the proportion of dreams and fantasies directed to one or the other sex, the sex of one's sexual partners, and the extent of physiological response to erotic stimuli associated with one or both sexes. *Sexual orientation* and *sexual preference* are sometimes used interchangeably; however, the former term has a wider currency in contemporary professional and popular usage. Sexual orientation is generally used by experts to refer more narrowly to a person's involuntary, erotic response tendency, whereas sexual preference sometimes implies a volitional component. In this chapter, *sexual orientation* is used to refer to erotic response tendency as it is more commonly used in the psychiatric, scientific, and social science literature. Sexual orientation consists of three components—desire, behavior, and identity—that may be congruent in an individual. The Kinsey heterosexual-homosexual scale—a 7-point continuous scale, with 0 representing exclusive heterosexuality, 6 representing exclusive homosexuality, and 3 representing equal amounts of both—is the most widely used instrument for describing sexual orientation. The Kinsey scale has been criticized for its unidimensional and bipolar conceptualization of sexual orientation, suggesting a diminished attraction toward one sex may be proportional to an increased attraction to the other sex.

Homosexuality was first introduced as a medical term in the second half of the 19th century to describe erotic desire for persons of the same sex. *Heterosexuality*, previously thought of as just normal, was later coined as a scientific term to describe erotic desire for persons of the other sex. A third category of sexual orientation, *bisexuality*, was used to describe an attraction to members of both sexes. The terms *homosexuality, heterosexuality*, and *bisexuality* are not applied consistently in theoretical, research, or popular discourse; depending on the context, these terms have been used to refer to a wide range of differing constructs. These include the categories of sexual desire, gender role attributes, forms of sexual behavior, personal and social identities, types of personalities and persons, degrees of normality and abnormality, and the presence or absence of mental illness. For example, in the 19th century, *bisexuality* referred to the hypothetical ability of an organism to physiologically develop as a male or female of its species. Scientists had observed the capacity in some species to reproduce as a male or female. When it was discovered that the external genitalia of human embryos did not differentiate as male or female until the 12th week of gestation, it was believed that human beings carried a bisexual potential in them as well. In that era, scientists still believed that ontogeny, the development of an individual in utero, reproduced phylogeny, the evolution of that individual's species. Sigmund Freud, among others, took this paradigm one step further and hypothesized that human beings are psychologically bisexual. Such conceptual shifts in which old words take on new meanings are not uncommon in the medical and scientific literature. Many theorists work from an underlying assumption that the concept of sexual orientation refers to some unitary quality within different individuals. This assumption, among others, has complicated efforts to understand the complex personal and social meanings of sexual desire and relationships.

In this chapter, *homosexuality* refers to an erotic desire for someone of the same biological sex; its presence in an individual does not necessarily imply or dictate the concurrent existence of any other characteristics. When used as an adjective, *homosexual* is intended to refer to sexual ideation or activity involving members of the same sex. Thus, for example, a woman may engage in homosexual behavior, may demonstrate typical feminine gender role characteristics, may be married to a man, and may experience a heterosexual identity; a man may have homosexual desire and fantasies, may have sex only with women, and may show gender role nonconformity. These different characteristics have distinct developmental and expressive pathways in each individual. However, as the result of socialization and because of possible predisposing biological factors, their development is interactive and reinforcing in some individuals.

Bisexuality can also refer to an erotic propensity, an individual identity, or a pattern of sexual behaviors. It may occur sequentially (expressed as an attraction to or relationship with both sexes, albeit at different times in one's life) or simultaneously (attraction or relationships to both sexes at the same time). Some believe bisexuality to be a transitional state toward the development of a more stable heterosexual, gay, or lesbian identity. However, there are a large number of men and women who, at some point in their lives, maintain a stable and persistent bisexual identity. In this chapter, references to bisexuality and bisexual persons are often, although not always, included, because there are frequent parallels in the experiences of gay men, lesbian women, and bisexual men and women. However, a full discussion of the topic of bisexuality is beyond the scope of this section.

In the latter part of the 20th century, the terms *gay*, *gay man*, *lesbian*, and *bisexual* began to be used to refer to men and women whose sexual identity, to some degree, openly recognized their homosexual or bisexual attractions. Although *gay* is sometimes used as a politically inclusive term for men and women, there are significant differences between these groups in their development and experiences. Being gay or lesbian is not the same thing as being a *homosexual*. The latter is a medical term—often with pejorative connotations—that takes one aspect of a person's identity, his or her sexual attractions, and treats it as if it were the sum of the person's entire identity. In much of the early psychological and psychoanalytic literature, *homosexual* was used as a noun to designate a person with same-sex desire or behavior; however, the noun is used increasingly less often in the scientific and popular literature. For example, recognizing the wide range of sexual identities in those populations at risk, much of the recent literature on human immunodeficiency virus (HIV) and acquired immune deficiency syndrome (AIDS) refers to *men who have sex with men* (MSM). MSM do not necessarily think of themselves as gay, or even as homosexual for that matter. In some cultures, only a receptive sexual partner is considered gay or homosexual, whereas an insertive man who also has sex with women is not culturally defined as homosexual. Thus, scientific categories to classify behaviors often come into conflict with cultural and subjective experiences of the meaning of homosexuality.

Homosexual, or lesbian and gay, and bisexual *identities* are constituted by the subjective experiences of having significant or exclusive homosexual or bisexual desires or attractions. These identities also involve some measure of self-acceptance of one's homosexual or bisexual feelings. The acquisition of lesbian, gay, and bisexual identities is often conceptualized as a developmental process that occurs over time. Models of lesbian, gay, and bisexual identity development usually portray a series of linear progressive stages involving tasks such as *coming out* (the process of recognizing one's homosexual or bisexual attraction and acknowledging it to oneself and to others); involvement in lesbian, gay, and bisexual communities; establishing same-sex relationships; and integrating one's sexual identity into other aspects of the self.

However, it is important to note that not all persons who experience homoerotic desire or who participate in homosexual behavior follow such a linear path or develop a stable lesbian, gay, or bisexual identity. In other words, a *sexual identity* is not always equivalent to a *sexual orientation*. For example, an individual with a homosexual orientation may not accept having same-sex feelings. Such an individual might reject a gay identity, choosing instead to marry a member of the other sex and to maintain an ostensibly heterosexual identity. Such persons may never lose their homosexual desires but might nevertheless still think of themselves as heterosexual. The subjectivity of such a *non–gay-identified* individual does not have a common cultural definition as yet. Such persons may be aware of their same-sex feelings and may have even acted on them, but they cannot or will not accept any meanings that might naturalize them. Such a person may have even experimented with the possibility of being gay but has no wish to come out any further. Such an individual may seek religious or professional help to change his or her sexual orientation. In recent years, some of these individuals have come refer to themselves as *ex-homosexual* or *ex-gay*. Whether they have actually changed their sexual orientation is not well studied; they have, however, changed their public identities.

These differing attitudes toward one's own homosexuality should not be thought of as existing on a developmental continuum or as being associated with more or less psychopathology. Thus, the clinician must be careful, when assessing a patient's sexuality, to inquire about all of the components of sexual orientation: desire, behavior, and identity. One cannot assume congruence between all three of these components based solely on information regarding one or two of them. To repeat, the presence of homosexual desires in an individual does not mean that the person has a gay or lesbian identity. It should further be emphasized that sexual identities are neither diagnostic nor immutable. Although a sexual orientation may be difficult, if not impossible, to change, sexual identities may be more flexible, because they are shaped by individual and cultural factors. There is a wide range of psychosocially constructed attitudes and responses that individuals may develop toward their own homosexuality. A woman with homosexual feelings may come out and may identify herself as lesbian but then may regret that decision and return to her earlier practices of hiding her feelings. Another may choose a nongay identity and may seek to change her homosexuality but then later may accept her homosexual feelings and come out. A self-identified heterosexual man might sexually perform insertively with other men while in prison, but this would not necessarily mean that he thinks of himself as gay or bisexual nor would he necessarily accept the assignment of such an identity from others.

A *heterosexual identity* refers, in theory, to the subjective experience of those men and women who primarily are aware of attraction to persons of the other sex. However, as a social construct, this identity is not as well developed as lesbian, gay, and bisexual identities. In Western society, unless one has ongoing contact with nonheterosexual identities, a heterosexual identity is not consciously experienced as anything other than what is expected. Where a heterosexual developmental outcome is assumed to be the norm, it is assumed that most people have a heterosexual identity unless they disavow it or proclaim an alternative identity. Consequently, there is no parallel in the development of a heterosexual identity to the experience of coming out as gay, lesbian, or bisexual.

The following terms do not directly pertain to contemporary theories of homosexuality. However, they are presented here for two reasons. The first is historic; some of these terms were not yet coined in early scientific reports and were therefore conflated with homosexuality. Second, some of these concepts are often blurred in the popular imagination with homosexuality.

Although *sex* refers to the biological attributes of being male or female, *gender identity* refers to a persistent sense of oneself as being male or female. Many historical discussions of homosexuality erroneously linked a homosexual orientation with an abnormal gender identity. These theories presumed the cause of homosexuality to be a confusion about one's own gender identity, which was then thought to subsequently cause confusion about the gender to which one was attracted. *Gender role* refers to overtly displayed gender-associated social behavior that establishes one's position—for oneself and for others—as a member of one gender or the other. It represents the perception of an individual's ability to act as a man or a woman should conventionally behave in public. Although *gender identity* describes an inner, subjective experience of being male or female, *gender role* and *social sex role* are the external markers of masculinity, femininity, or androgyny. Most people, regardless of their sexual orientation, have a gender identity and gender role that is consistent with their biological sex, although social attitudes in some gay and lesbian communities often do permit a greater degree of gender role flexibility.

Gender stability, a term from the child developmental literature, refers to a child's understanding that one's gender at birth remains the same throughout life, that is, an understanding that girls are born as girls and grow up to be women and that boys grow up to be men. *Gender constancy* refers to a child's understanding that external changes in appearance or activity do not change one's gender. For example, a boy learns that, even if he changes his physical appearance by putting on a dress or growing long hair, he remains a boy.

The presence of cross-gender characteristics in a person is one of the most salient criteria of the revised fourth edition of the DSM (DSM-IV-TR) diagnosis of *gender identity disorder.* There is also a DSM-IV-TR diagnosis of *gender identity disorder of childhood. Transsexualism* consists of a strong and persistent cross-gender identification, discomfort with one's biological sex, and a wish to acquire the characteristics of the other sex, eventually leading to *sex-reassignment surgery.* An individual born a man who *transitions* to being a woman is called a *male to female* (MTF) *transsexual.* This is a much more common phenomenon than a woman being surgically reassigned as a man, or a *female to male* (FTM) *transsexual.* There is a great deal of popular confusion between transsexualism and homosexuality. However, it is extremely rare for those who stably identify as gay, lesbian, or bisexual to have the intense cross-gender identifications associated with transsexualism or to seek sex-reassignment surgery. Complicating matters further, cross-gender identifications give little indication of a transsexual person's eventual sexual orientation. For example, depending on the individual, a fully transitioned, postoperative MTF transsexual may have sexual feelings for a man (heterosexual MTF) or a woman (homosexual MTF).

Paralleling the homosexual protests of the mid-20th century, there is now an increasing number of cross-gender identified individuals who challenge the characterization of their feelings as symptoms of a mental disorder. Furthermore, not all individuals with cross-gendered identifications desire, seek, or obtain transsexual surgery. Some may undergo a *partial transition,* by wearing the clothing or accessories of the *nonnatal gender* or by taking hormone supplements to acquire secondary sexual characteristics of the other gender. *Transgendered* has become an umbrella term used to describe any individual who identifies with and adopts the gender role of a member of the other biological sex. The term, as currently used, includes transsexuals and individuals with gender discordant feelings who do not fully transition. Again, depending on the individual, a partially transitioned MTF may identify as homosexual, heterosexual, or bisexual.

Transvestitism consists of sexual urges and fantasies involving cross-dressing. When the behavior is distressing to a patient or brought to the attention of a psychiatrist, it may be diagnosed as *transvestic fetishism,* which the DSM-IV-TR classifies as a *paraphilia.* Cross-dressing is strongly linked in the popular imagination with homosexuality, although most fetishistic cross-dressers are heterosexual men who do so in private. These men are often married to women who may not know about their cross-dressing interests. Most gay men and women do not cross-dress. However, there are social venues within gay and lesbian communities that allow for public cross-dressing. These may include socially performative events (gay pride, Halloween, or Mardi Gras parades) or cross-dressing as a form of paid entertainment (drag shows).

THEORIES

The meanings of homosexual behavior appear to vary according to time, place, and culture. Homosexual practices played an important role for men in ancient Greece and other cultures, whereas homosexual acts have been ritualized and prohibited in various societies. Plato's *Symposium* told a creation myth with three original sexes—man, woman, and *androgyne*—each a symmetrical being split in two for defying the gods. The split-off aspects all look for their other halves. Men who were originally from the androgyne seek women and vice versa. Women who seek women and men who seek men were instead part of the original male and female beings. In the Judeo-Christian tradition, biblical prohibitions against homosexuality can be found in Genesis 19, Leviticus 18:7, 18:22, and 20:13, Judges 19, I Kings 22:46, II Kings 23:7, Romans 1:27, I Corinthians 6:9, and I Timothy 1:9. The historian John Boswell has convincingly argued that contemporary intolerance of homosexuality was not an essential factor of Christianity itself but only became a prevailing church attitude in the second millennium AD. Postmodern historians in the tradition of Michel Foucault argue that the idea of identifying *a type* or *a category of person* based on homosexual behavior or identity is a relatively new cultural phenomenon that coincides with the medicalization of homosexuality during the 19th century. Historians like Boswell, on the other hand, believe that a category of homosexually identified person, although not entirely equivalent to a modern gay identity, has always existed across time and cultures. Regardless of how one interprets the historical data, the study of the forms and meanings of homosexual behavior in different cultures and historical periods is a vastly rich and growing field. This literature has expanded knowledge about the transcultural and transhistoric range of sexual practices and types of gender-based relationships. Nevertheless, the forms of socialization and identity development associated with homosexuality in contemporary society are generally considered to be unique. The history of the development of present forms of homosexual identity is the focus of the following review of theoretical perspectives about homosexuality.

History The origin of the modern view of homosexuality can be traced to the second half of the 19th century when European sexologists, including several prominent psychiatrists, began the study of homosexuality from a scientific and medical perspective. Through much of the 20th century, this intellectual enterprise was dominated by a predominance of biological and psychological, particularly psychoanalytic, theories. Most theories of the first half of the 20th century, with a few exceptions, regarded homosexuality as a form of psychopathology or as a developmental arrest. In the latter half of the 20th century, however, theories that characterized homosexuality as a normal variant of human sexuality began to predominate. This view emerged from a wide range of social and scientific perspectives outside medicine and psychiatry and eventually supplanted earlier theories of homosexual pathology and immaturity. This modern *normal variant* view began gaining influence around the time of the publication of the two Alfred Kinsey volumes on male and female sexuality—in 1948 and 1953, respectively—and culminated in the APA's removal of homosexuality from its list of mental disorders, the DSM, in 1973. The ascendancy of the normal variant model presaged the postmodern academic interest in homosexuality that emerged in the last part of the 20th century and that continues today.

Medicalization of Homosexuality: From Morality to Pathology

LATE 19TH AND EARLY 20TH CENTURY BIOLOGICAL VIEWS During the second half of the 19th century, researchers in Europe began to scientifically study homosexuality. This was part of a wider shift away from earlier religious and moral views that held that homosexual acts and other forms of socially stigmatized behaviors were an expression of sin. The term *homosexual* was first coined by the Hungarian physician Károli Mária Kertbeny in 1869 and was later adopted by the influential German psychiatrist Richard von Krafft-Ebing in his classic *Psychopathia Sexualis.* The conceptual basis for homosexuality arose from the early scientific belief that the two sexes, male and female, had dichotomous characteristics and that each was mutually exclusive of the other. Thus, most modern attempts to make sense of homosexuality primarily derived from attempts to use the categories of male and female as explanatory devices. This led to an early conceptualization of the homosexual as a person of one biological sex characterized by the sexual longing of the other sex. A famous early advocate of this position was the German jurist and homosexual rights' advocate Karl Heinrich Ulrichs. In the 1860s, he described a male homosexual as a female soul trapped in a male body. However, Ulrichs believed that, for some people, this was a natural state of affairs, or what today might be referred to as *biologically determined homosexuality*. He hypothesized the existence of separate male and female "love drives" in the brain—which develop in *Urninge* (male homosexuals) and *Urninden* (female homosexuals) in opposite directions to their genital sex.

The psychiatrists Carl Westphal and Krafft-Ebing adopted many of Ulrichs' ideas; however, they deemed unnatural the traits the latter described as normal. Magnus Hirschfeld, a German physician and sexual emancipator, was an openly homosexual psychiatrist who also believed that there was a genetic basis for homosexuality. Although he considered homosexuality to be a malformation in development, presumed to have a number of different biological etiologies, he nevertheless asserted that the condition was natural. Similarly, the English sex reformer Havelock Ellis thought of homosexuality as a biological variation. Although he attributed it to "imperfect sexual differentiation," he nevertheless considered homosexuality to be nonpathological, because it did not cause any illness in the individual himself. Other biological bases for homosexuality began to be examined during this period. These included studies of anatomical structures in the brains and the nerve structures in the rectums of homosexual men. Endocrinological hypotheses led to experiments in which the supposedly atrophied or abnormal testicles of homosexual men were removed and replaced with what were believed to be the normal testicles of heterosexual men. However, this experiment did not make the homosexual men heterosexual.

Early biological theories, with their emphasis on heredity, endocrinological influences, and anatomical or structural differences between homosexual and heterosexual persons, heralded many of the current efforts to find a biological basis for homosexuality. Biological theories, however, also provided a rationalization for subsequent eugenic efforts in Nazi Germany to eradicate homosexual persons. In the 1970s, East German surgeons unsuccessfully tried to eliminate homosexuality in men by operating on the hypothalamus, where the cause of homosexuality was presumed to lie. It should be noted that an almost exclusive emphasis on the study of homosexuality in men parallels later 20th century biological research that mostly ignores homosexuality in women. Biological arguments, in addition, contributed to creating the notion of a homosexual person in hypothesizing fundamental constitutional differences between those attracted to persons of the same sex and those attracted to persons of the other sex. The conflation of behavior with personhood is a conceptual precursor to the later development of modern gay and lesbian identities.

PSYCHOANALYTICAL APPROACHES Like some biological theorists of his time, Freud believed that homosexuality could be the natural outcome of normal development in some people. However, he did not view homosexuality, or *inversion*, as he called it, as a sign of illness, by which he meant a symptom arising from psychic conflict. Instead, he saw homosexuality as the unconflicted expression of an innate instinct. He noted that homosexuality could occur in individuals who had no other signs of deviation and no impairment in their functioning. Freud believed in *constitutional bisexuality*, that, in every individual, there was a certain component of *masculine* (active) as well as *feminine* (passive) *tendencies*. A homosexual tendency did not necessary imply a homosexual behavior. Although bisexual tendencies were universal, Freud believed some people were constitutionally endowed with more of one tendency than the other. He believed that life experiences, particularly traumatic ones (environmental factors), could have an impact on the development and expression of one's innate instincts (biological factors). Under normal and nontraumatic circumstances, the component instincts that determine the sex of one's final object choice should be consistent with one's anatomical sex. That is to say that an anatomic man should ideally express the masculine component instinct and should obtain sexual satisfaction from women. However, Freud also believed that even adult heterosexuals retain the homosexual component, albeit in sublimated form. For Freud, adult homosexuality represented an arrest in development on the road from the instinctual bisexuality of childhood to mature heterosexuality. His *theory of immaturity* comprised an alternative category that was neither religion's sin nor medicine's disease. By maintaining that homosexuality could be a normal part of everyone's heterosexual experience, his was a more inclusive paradigm. Freud did not endorse so-called third-sex theories. His theory allowed for the possibility that the adult homosexual person might sufficiently mature and, if sufficiently motivated, become heterosexual. However, late in his life, Freud was pessimistic about the possibility of changing adult homosexuality to heterosexuality in most people.

After Freud's death, however, Sandor Rado's theories eventually held greater sway on psychoanalytical theorizing about homosexuality than those of Freud himself. In the 1940s, Rado argued that the theory of bisexuality was based on a faulty analogy with anatomical bisexuality. That is, underlying Freud's theory was a 19th century belief in embryonic hermaphroditism, the hypothesis that the potential to become an anatomical man or a woman was present in every embryo. Rado claimed that this theory had been disproved, which led to his claim that heterosexuality is the only nonpathological outcome of human sexual development. He viewed homosexuality as an illness, specifically, a phobic avoidance of the other sex caused by parental prohibitions against childhood sexuality. Almost all of the mid-20th century psychoanalytic theorists who pathologized homosexuality followed Rado's theory in one form or another. The psychoanalytic community's shift from Freud's model of immaturity (homosexuality as a normal developmental step toward adult heterosexuality) to Rado's model of pathology (homosexuality as a sign of development gone awry) led some analysts to optimistically claim that they could cure homosexuality.

The work of the psychoanalyst Irving Bieber and his associates was particularly influential in its portrayal of a pathogenic family type—a detached and rejecting father and a close-binding and domineering mother—that presumably led to homosexuality in the 106 adult homosexual men that they studied. This theory of familial etiology, however, is not supported by research of larger, nonpatient gay male populations. Bieber and his colleagues claimed a 27 percent cure rate of the patients in their study. The Bieber study was criticized for its methodology and for the fact that the authors were unable to provide any long-term follow-up on their subjects or to produce any patients to support their claims of change. Finally, although some discussion of the etiology of female homosexuality existed in the early psychoanalytic literature, the primary emphasis in psychoanalysis, as in the biological sciences, was on male homosexuality; often, the causes and types of homosexuality in women were simply treated as mirror images of those for male homosexuality.

EARLY THEORETICAL ASSUMPTIONS Late 19th and early 20th century theories of homosexuality, whether biological, medical, or psychoanalytic, largely relied on a dichotomous model of human nature that used categories of male or female, masculine or feminine, and heterosexual or homosexual. Whatever the etiological theories of homosexuality hypothesized, all were based on similar assumptions about gender, sexuality, and sexual orientation polarities that shaped research in the biological sciences during that period. Whether the theorist held homosexuality to be a normal variant, a form of pathology, or a form of immaturity, the theory usually relied on the assumption that some intrinsic quality of one gender had made its way into a person of another gender. Even psychoanalysis, with its emphasis on combined intrapsychic and interpersonal development, made basic assumptions about homosexuality that were derived from the same materialistic beliefs on which the biological theories rested: that the wide range of human sexuality could be understood when reduced to the two component parts of male and female. Thus, the studies of homosexuality within the medical and the psychoanalytic fields during this period led to similar outcomes: removing responsibility for defining homosexuality from the realms of morality and religion and securing it within science and medicine; creating a category of person, the homosexual, in contrast to the moral or religious belief that homosexuality was a behavior rather than a source of identity; and perpetuating the social stigma of homosexuality by taking it out of the realm of sin and immorality and placing it within the realm of pathology and immaturity. Ironically, these developments would also eventually set the stage for the transition toward normalizing homosexuality that began to take shape in the middle of the 20th century.

Normalization of Homosexuality: From Diagnosis to Normality

INFLUENCE OF RESEARCH FINDINGS FROM SEXOLOGY, CROSS-CULTURAL, ANIMAL, AND PSYCHOLOGICAL STUDIES The publication of two volumes on male and female sexuality by Alfred Kinsey and his colleagues in 1948 and 1953, respectively, was a scientific and cultural watershed. Their appearance marked the beginning of a cultural shift away from the view of homosexuality as pathology and toward viewing it as a normal variant of sexual desire and behavior. Despite his studies' own methodological flaws, Kinsey's finding of a widespread presence of same-sex feelings and behaviors among his samples of several thousand American men and women changed the general impression that homosexuality was an isolated and aberrant phenomenon. His homosexuality-heterosexuality scale, which conceptualized sexual orientation on a continuum, expanded on the binary model used by earlier theorists. In his nominalist world view, "the world is not to be divided into sheep and goats. Not all things are black nor all things white. It is a fundamental of taxonomy that nature rarely deals with discrete categories. Only the human mind invents categories and tries to force facts into separated pigeon-holes."

Cleland Ford and Frank Beach's work, published in 1951, between the two Kinsey studies, found homosexuality to be common across cultures and documented its existence in almost all nonhuman primate species. The interpretation of these findings supported the notion that homosexuality was natural (as opposed to being caused by civilized decadence) and widespread. In 1957, psychologist Evelyn Hooker published a groundbreaking study that compared projective test results from 30 nonpatient homosexual men to those of 30 nonpatient heterosexual men. Her study found that experienced judges, unaware of whose test results they were interpreting, could not distinguish between the two groups. Most of the medical and psychiatric literature of that time that regarded homosexuality as pathological was based on evaluations of individuals in treatment who were troubled about their sexuality. Hooker's study of *nonpatient subjects* was a serious challenge to the then-prevailing psychoanalytic theory that held that homosexuality was always associated with mental illness or serious psychopathology. The impact of this significant finding was to draw attention to the a priori assumption of many clinical papers that homosexuality was itself pathological. In the 1960s, psychiatrists including Judd Marmor—a psychoanalyst and future president of the APA and the American Academy of Psychoanalysis—gave serious consideration to the nonpsychiatric perspectives offered in these newer research findings. They began publishing books and articles that helped to move the psychiatric profession away from the perspective of homosexuality as a form of mental disorder. The perspectives offered in this newer research, particularly as articulated by spokespersons for an increasingly vocal gay rights' movement, eventually led to the next phase of development in theorizing about and attitudes toward homosexuality.

DECLASSIFICATION BY THE AMERICAN PSYCHIATRIC ASSOCIATION Homosexuality had been officially classified as a mental disorder with the publication of the APA's first edition of the DSM (DSM-I) in 1952. There it was designated as a "sociopathic personality disturbance." Unlike the contemporary DSM, that diagnostic label was based on the presence of certain behaviors rather than on subjective distress or objective dysfunction. Classifying homosexuality as a mental illness was not controversial at the time of the DSM-I's publication; societal attitudes of that time coincided with prevailing medical views that homosexuality was an aberration. In 1968, the second edition of the DSM (DSM-II) still listed homosexuality as a sexual deviation, but sexual deviations were no longer categorized as a sociopathic personality disturbance.

This revision coincided with a time of great social ferment by gay rights' activists. These activists found their most powerful symbol in the 1969 Stonewall riots in New York City. Having successfully fought off police and government attempts to shut down the public places where gay people congregated, the gay rights movement was prepared to challenge psychiatric authority as well. This inevitably led to an increasingly vocal opposition to modern psychiatry's classification of homosexuality as a mental disorder. Before that time, many homophile organizations, in the United States and abroad, had accepted the medical view of homosexuality as a mental disorder. Accepting the view of homosexuality as disease meant treating it as a disability, a category intended to replace moral and religious judgments with scientific, objective, and humane attitudes. However, in most instances, medical and psychiatric portrayals of homosexuality were as problematic as the religious views that they supplanted. For example, a homosexual individual could be denied the right to immigrate to the United States on the grounds that the person had a mental disorder. Gay men and lesbians were discharged from the military as medically unfit. To gay activists of that period, the psychiatric designation of homosexuality as a mental disorder had exacerbated antihomosexual societal prejudices rather than ameliorated them, as originally intended. These activists found a receptive audience among an increasing numbers of psychiatrists who were familiar with research findings showing that homosexuality occurred in large numbers of people, in persons who demonstrated normal psychological adjustment, and across a wide range of cultures.

Gay activists began to confront the APA about its position on homosexuality. After a series of dramatic encounters between gay rights' advocates and psychiatrists at annual meetings of the APA between 1970 and 1972, the APA officially began to reevaluate the status of homosexuality as a mental disorder. After considerable political activity and significant scientific study of the issue, the Nomenclature Committee of the APA proposed that homosexuality be eliminated from the DSM. The proposal was approved by the APA's Council on Research and Development, its Reference Committee, and by the Assembly of District Branches before being accepted by the APA's Board of Trustees in December 1973. This marked the end of the classification of homosexuality per se as an illness. Other major mental health professional organizations, including the American Psychological Association and the National Association of Social Workers, soon endorsed the APA action. The decision to declassify homosexuality was accompanied by passage of a position statement by the APA that supported the protection of the civil rights of homosexual persons:

> Whereas homosexuality in and of itself implies no impairment in judgment, stability, reliability, or vocational capabilities, therefore, be it resolved that the American Psychiatric Association deplores all public and private discrimination against homosexuals in such areas as employment, housing, public accommodations, and licensing, and declares that no burden of proof of such judgment, capacity, or reliability shall be placed on homosexuals greater than that imposed on any other persons. Further, the APA supports and urges the enactment of civil rights legislation at local, state, and federal levels that would insure homosexual citizens the same protections now guaranteed to others. Further, the APA supports and urges the repeal of all legislation making criminal offenses of sexual acts performed by consenting adults in private.

Some psychiatrists, primarily psychoanalysts who continued to adhere to pathologizing views of homosexuality, criticized the Board of Trustees and challenged their action by calling for a referendum of the entire APA membership. The decision to remove homosexuality was upheld by a 58 percent majority of voting APA members.

The original scientific and clinical rationale for removing homosexuality from the DSM was based, in part, on a new formulation of the definition of a mental disorder by the Nomenclature Committee's Chair, Robert Spitzer, M.D. To be classified as a disorder, a condition had to meet the criteria of an experience of subjective distress or of a generalized, objective impairment in social effectiveness or functioning resulting from the condition itself. Neither of these criteria applied to homosexual persons who were satisfied with their sexual orientation and who did not demonstrate impaired functioning. In recognition of the opposition to the diagnostic change, however, the APA did not fully embrace a normal variant model of homosexuality; instead, it made a compromise. The DSM-II diagnosis of *sexual orientation disturbance* replaced *homosexuality*. As a result, individuals who were comfortable with their homosexuality were no longer considered mentally ill. According to sexual orientation disturbance criteria, only those who were "bothered by" or "in conflict with" or who "wished to change" their homosexuality had a mental disorder. Sexual orientation disturbance, however, had two significant conceptual problems. First, the diagnosis could also apply to heterosexuals, a solution to APA's internal debate that did not concur with clinical reality. There were no reported cases of unhappy heterosexual individuals seeking psychiatric treatment to become homosexual. This problem of diagnostic overinclusiveness was resolved in the 1980 the third edition of the DSM (DSM-III), in which sexual orientation disturbance was replaced by *ego-dystonic homosexuality*. The name change, however, did not resolve a thornier conceptual issue, which was that of making patients' subjective experiences of their own homosexuality the *determining factor* of their illness. To rely on patient subjectivity alone was now incongruous with the new evidence-based approach that psychiatry had embraced. This ultimately led, in 1987, to ego-dystonic homosexuality being removed from the revised edition of DSM-III (DSM-III-R). Then, in 1992, the WHO followed suit and also removed homosexuality from the ICD.

For two decades after the 1973 APA decision, the meetings and publications of the American Psychoanalytic Association were among the few American forums in which pathological views of homosexuality continued to be expressed. Eventually, however, normal variant views of homosexuality prevailed in the APsaA as well. In 1991, the organization issued a nondiscrimination statement to allow training of gay and lesbian psychoanalytic candidates and the promotion of qualified gay and lesbian individuals to the position of training and supervising analyst. In 1997, the APsaA became the first mental health organization to support the right to same-sex marriage. Psychoanalytic views that pathologized homosexuality nevertheless could still be found in the international psychoanalytic community. However, in 2002, the APsaA's influence in the International Psychoanalytical Association (IPA) led the latter to issue a statement prohibiting discrimination in the selection of openly gay and lesbian candidates or in the promotion of gay and lesbian faculty.

All of these actions represented the definitive acknowledgment by the psychiatric, psychoanalytic, medical, and mental health professions that homosexuality, in itself, was not a mental disorder. Not only did this change in the mental health professions' view of homosexuality represent wider acceptance of a newer scientific view of homosexuality, it also symbolized a dramatic conceptual shift in the cultural meaning and significance of homosexual behavior within Western society. This shift set the stage for an outpouring of publications and a profusion of new theory and research findings about homosexuality and gay men and lesbians.

Postmodern Theories: Essentialist and Constructivist Arguments The 1973 declassification of homosexuality per se from its list of mental illnesses and the elimination of ego-dystonic homosexuality from the DSM in 1987 coincided with a significant cultural shift in approaches to epistemology and knowledge. The late 20th century saw the emergence of *postmodernism*, an intellectual movement characterized by a challenging attitude toward fixed beliefs and received categories of knowledge. Postmodern academics use constructivist methods to unravel and to elucidate the particular historical and social influences that influence language and understanding. Postmodernists often seek to identify the origins of knowledge from social and political influences.

The biomedical field—focused on biology, the physical sciences, and the body—continues to rely on more traditional materialist approaches to studying and viewing the world. Postmodernism, on the other hand, has had its strongest influence within the humanities and the social sciences. During the latter part of the 20th century, traditional and postmodern methods for the study of homosexuality were bridged in debates between *essentialist* and *constructivist* (also known as *social constructionist*) theorists. These debates originated within the fields of philosophy, feminism, and identity politics and built on the critiques of sex, gender, and racial categories developed by feminist and civil rights' thinkers. Led in the 1970s by the work of French historian and philosopher Michel Foucault and others, constructivists criticized classical theories of sexuality that posit inherent and immutable qualities associated with sex, gender, and sexual orientation. They, instead, maintain that there is no inner sexual drive, arguing that the human potential for thinking and acting is shaped by social forces of regulation and categorization into various types of sexual desire at different times in history and in different societies. From this perspective, a homosexual (or gay or lesbian or bisexual) identity is constructed from available cultural meanings of sexuality, rather than being a reflection of an innate (homo- or bi-) sexual orientation. Constructivist approaches in the humanities, particularly as they question and examine contemporary notions of gender and sexuality, including homosexuality, are sometimes referred to as *queer theory*.

Essentialism, on the other hand, refers to the view that sexual desires and identities are fixed, personal characteristics. Essentialists, for example, believe that a sexual orientation is inherent, objective, transcultural, and transhistorical. The American gay man of today, from this perspective, would have homosexual counterparts in other cultures and time periods, albeit different cultures and times might not permit an identical expression of those innate qualities. Essentialism treats masculinity and femininity as a biological bedrock that is capable of explaining sexual differences; masculinity and femininity, in turn, serve as the basis for understanding all sexual categories and identities. In regard to sexual orientation, essentialist theorists hold that fundamental differences in sexual desire are the basis for creating three major categories of persons: the homosexual, the heterosexual, and the bisexual.

To a certain extent, the debate between essentialists and constructivists parallels earlier debates within psychiatry regarding the relative influences of nature and nurture in causing mental illness or in determining the etiology of homosexuality. However, the scope of the postmodern debate encompasses more than questions of origins or etiology alone. It offers challenges to many of the ways in which one makes sense of sexuality, in general, and of homosexuality, in particular. Although essentialist and constructivist arguments are often framed in terms of their oppositional positions, thoughtful adherents of both perspectives usually subscribe to a continuum of contributions from biological and environmental factors. In addition, criticisms of both views are useful in understanding the limitations of each model.

Homosexuality: Innate versus Constructed An example of the polarized debate is the belief that homosexuality is innate (an expression of biological factors) versus the belief that homosexuality is constructed (an expression of cultural or other external influences). These two positions represent a fundamental distinction between, respectively, essentialist and constructivist views. An essentialist assumption is the notion that homosexual persons exist and that they can be defined by their homoerotic desire alone. Another corollary belief is that these homosexual persons have shared fundamental characteristics throughout history and in different cultures. The essentialist belief that homosexuality is innate is represented most dramatically in scientific attempts to find a biological basis for homosexuality and that some quality of one gender has found its way into a person of the other gender. For example, one study done in the 1990s claimed to have found a genetic marker of homosexuality on the Xq28 region of the X, or female, chromosome. To date, these findings have not been replicated. Nevertheless, a key concept in this hypothesis is the *mistaken crossover* of some deoxyribonucleic acid (DNA) from a Y chromosome to a daughter or from an X chromosome to a son. The study's authors believe this suggests a *genetic crossover* between the male and female sex chromosomes that is related to the *behavioral crossover* between heterosexuality and homosexuality.

This essentialist theory draws on several unproven assumptions about homosexuality. First, the *behavioral crossover* to which the authors allude assumes that an attraction to women is a male trait and that an attraction to men is a female trait, a variation of the cultural belief that a homosexual man crosses a gender boundary by acting like a girl. It is also consistent with the essentialist assumption that there are only two biological genders, male and female. According to this theory, the physiological antecedents of sexual attractions are encoded in the so-called sex chromosomes. The argument rests on the semantic equation of two expressions of sexual attraction, one to men and the other to women, with two kinds of sex chromosomes, one male (Y) and the other female (X). The theory is also based on the everyday belief that a gay man has feminine qualities. In fact, although the technology of the research has greatly advanced, many modern efforts to find the biological origins of homosexuality are based on gender concepts that are identical to those first proposed in the19th century: For example, Ulrichs believed that a male homosexual had a female spirit trapped in a man's body. Scientific researchers of his time sought to identify a source for male homosexuality in a so-called feminized brain or other parts of the body. During the early part of the 20th century, endocrinologists searched for possible hormonal causes of homosexuality—female hormones in male bodies and vice versa. To date, no evidence of any anatomical, physiological, or hormonal gender crossing has been found to explain homosexuality.

In contrast, constructivist theorists following Foucault argue that different forms of sexual desire and expression arise as the result of social forces that vary across time and cultures. Thus, although the individual may experience same-sex desire and even some sense of being lesbian or gay, these experiences are viewed as the product of larger social forces—such as the market place, urbanization, and government regulation—that influence sexual desire and behavior. The implications of this belief include the idea that homosexual desire and gay and lesbian identity are variable and fluid in their origins and expression. This position would argue that there is no biological basis for homosexuality, because the category of homosexuality is entirely a social construction. However, other historians, particularly those working in the tradition of Boswell, argue that a homosexual category, although not specifically labeled as such, has existed across time and cultures. Boswell has convincingly argued, for example, that homosexual individuals in pre-Renaissance Europe had official church recognition of their same-sex relationships. This interpretation of the historical data is at odds with the postmodern belief that an identity based on same-sex attractions is only a modern phenomenon.

Homosexuality: Fixed versus Mutable Another dimension of the debate between essentialist and constructivist positions involves beliefs about the extent to which homosexuality is fixed or mutable. There is considerable variability in the positions represented by essentialists and constructivists on this matter, and any distinction between the two schools of thought cannot be collapsed into disagreement about the possibility of changing sexual orientation. For example, persons believing that homosexuality should be changed through psychotherapy or other means hold an essentialist view that heterosexuality is the normal, default setting of human sexuality. At the same time, they see the causes of homosexuality as environmental—normally considered to be a constructivist view. Many who endorse a postmodern constructivist conceptualization of sexuality may nevertheless recognize that most individuals are unable to alter their adult sexual attractions.

Scientific debates on this matter are further complicated by a political debate—colloquially known as the *culture wars*—that surrounds the issue of homosexuality's immutability. Opposing sides argue from the belief that (1) homosexuality is normal and acceptable or that (2) homosexuality is neither normal nor acceptable. The contradictory values and beliefs separating these two sides stand in sharp relief. The first position argues from a *normal-identity model,* which regards homosexuality as a normal variation of human expression, analogous with left-handedness. Adherents of the normal-identity model believe that homosexuality is biologically based and therefore fixed and immutable. It views the acceptance of an essential homosexual orientation as a distinguishing feature of a gay or lesbian identity. It further defines individuals with a gay or lesbian identity as members of a sexual minority. As minority group members, this position holds, gay men and lesbians need protection from the discriminatory practices and beliefs of the heterosexual majority. Among those protections are changing laws based on characterizations of homosexuality as an illness or an immoral choice.

The opposing position in this debate argues from an *illness-behavior model.* One of its central tenets is to challenge the essentialist rationale that often underlies belief in the normal-identity model. Adherents of the illness-behavior model regard any open expressions of homosexuality as (1) behavioral symptoms that are pathognomonic of psychiatric illness, (2) a moral failing, or (3) some combination of both. This position maintains that illness or immorality cannot provide a foundation for creating a normal identity, let alone serve as a basis for defining a sexual minority. Thus, according to this view, those who engage in homosexual behavior do not merit the kinds of modern legal protections afforded to racial, ethnic, or religious minorities. One corollary of this position is a belief that homosexual feelings and behaviors are not innate but are learned behaviors that can be reversed, through some kind of psychotherapy or through faith healing.

Both sides in the culture wars intermingle scientific theories in the political debates about what constitutes a natural category of human experience. Thus, it is entirely possible to believe that sexual orientation is innate without believing that this is pertinent to granting gay and lesbian civil rights, such as same-sex marriage. It is also possible to believe that, even if homosexuality is socially constructed, gay people are nevertheless in need of civil protections. In cultural debates that appropriate the language of science, the fixed-mutable dimension of sexual orientation is often conflated with other clinical issues: These include concerns about attempts to coercively change a homosexual or bisexual orientation to a heterosexual orientation, the question of the degree of individual freedom in relation to choosing a particular sexual orientation, and the ethics of clinicians who provide services not endorsed by the mental health mainstream, to name a few. Thus, it is difficult to disentangle any scientific discussion of the degree to which a sexual orientation is fixed or mutable from the moral questions of how change can or should be accomplished and to what extent individuals choose their sexual desire, behavior, and identity.

The belief that homosexuality is a stable phenomenon, relatively resistant to change, derives from several sources. These include the experiences of many people who are lesbian, gay, and bisexual and who have consistent same-sex attractions, some of whom have tried and failed to change their sexual attractions; the empirical finding that homosexuality rarely changes as the result of psychotherapy or other external attempts to alter it; the subjective experience of many gay men and women that their sexual orientation is the outer representation of some constitutionally determined inner characteristic; the political stance that external agents should not attempt to alter sexual orientation; and a deterministic assumption that individuals have no choice regarding the ultimate direction of their adult sexual desire.

In contrast, the idea that sexual orientation can change for some persons derives from a different set of observations about sexual orientation. These include the experiences of some people who report fluctuations in their sexual attractions over the course of their lives, a belief that heterosexuality is the natural, biological expression of sexuality throughout history and in different cultures, and an unwillingness to accept homosexuality as part of a normal identity.

Toward an Interactionist Model An important distinction between essentialist and constructivist approaches to homosexuality is the manner in which they conceptually organize the phenomena they address. Strict essentialists often assume that homosexuality is a unitary phenomenon comprised of similar experiences and behaviors that fundamentally represent the same characteristic. As a result, observations that are at variance with a unitary notion of homosexuality may not be viewed by strict essentialists as part of the subject under study. For example, people who experience fluctuations in their sexual desire for one or the other sex may be considered to be bisexual, and only persons who go through certain developmental stages or who demonstrate certain biological markers may be described as *true homosexuals*. As a result of demarcating this conceptual boundary, other essentialist assumptions that homosexuality is innate, fixed, and uniform are reinforced. By excluding variations and focusing on means, a more discrete descriptive category can be created.

In contrast, constructivists tend to focus on variability and to see multiple phenomena within the construct of homosexuality. The constructivist methods of analyzing and deconstructing fixed categories and ideas result in the recognition of multiple layers and types of experiences that are associated with same sex desire, behavior, and identity in different cultures and periods and that vary for some individuals across the life span. The result of this perspective may be that the constructivist draws attention to the dehumanizing effects of narrow categorization and labeling but may also be speaking about something that is different from what the essentialist is addressing. Essentialists, for example, often try to create general categories that are capable of being scientifically studied. Constructivists, instead, try to draw attention to the exception that disproves the essentialist rule.

The apparent contradictions that are represented between the essentialist and constructivist positions, like those in earlier arguments about nature and nurture, may reflect complementary aspects of the complex phenomena that are associated with sexual orientation and sexual identity. When differences between the two theoretical stances are highlighted, the focusing lens of the essentialist and the dispersing crystal of the constructivist can be used to help view different aspects of what contemporary society calls *homosexuality*. Like the blind men describing an elephant, however, each one may be looking at only part of the whole picture. When taken together, these different vantage points may foster new thinking and research in understanding human sexuality in general and homosexuality in particular.

FREQUENCY

Studies that purport to demonstrate the extent of homosexuality in a population have generally failed to distinguish between the various components of sexual orientation: desire, behavior, and identity. One methodological difficulty is that an interview or survey question may simply ask if a person is gay or lesbian or homosexual. Respondents who only have sexual relations with other persons of the same sex but do not identify themselves as gay or lesbian may deny that they are gay or lesbian. In some cases, the stigma associated with homosexuality may interfere with full disclosure. Similarly, persons who are not open about their sexual orientation may also fail to respond fully or accurately to questions about their sexual behavior or identity. Even when questions about sexual orientation are constructed in a manner that takes into account such problems of definition and disclosure, it may be difficult to obtain a representative sampling of individuals with different sexual orientations. Studies have shown that self-reports of sexual orientation vary significantly across age groups, for example, from early to late teenage years, and in different geographical locations. These variations are compounded when frequency rates are compared cross-culturally because of the variable meanings of sexual behaviors and practices in different cultures.

Given these limitations in the existing studies of the frequency of homosexuality, it is impossible to determine definitively the number of persons who have same-sex desire, behavior, or identity in the United States today. The 1948 Kinsey study of male sexuality, based on a sample of men between 16 and 55 years of age, found that 4 percent of the men were exclusively homosexual, 50 percent were exclusively heterosexual, and 46 percent were somewhere in between. The Kinsey study has subsequently been criticized for its sampling errors, which are believed to have led to inflated estimates of the extent of homosexual and bisexual behavior. Later studies of the frequency of same-sex sexual contacts between men, using results from national surveys conducted in 1970 and 1988, determined that 20 percent of men had sexual contact to orgasm with another man at some time in their lives. It was also found that 5 to 7 percent of men had such behavior in adulthood but that only one-fourth to one-half of these men also reported having such contact in the preceding 12 months. Because of problems in reporting and with missing data, these figures were considered to be the lower bounds of actual frequency of same-sex behavior among men. Although reports about the frequency of homosexuality among women in the United States have been almost absent since the publication of Kinsey's 1953 volume on sexuality in women, the number of women reporting same-sex sexual contact or identifying themselves as lesbian is generally considered to be considerably lower than for men, often one-half of, or less, the number of men.

A large-scale study of sexuality in the United States published in 1994 by Edward Laumann and his colleagues provides the most reliable current estimates of the prevalence of homosexuality in the United States. This study used more precise definitions of homosexuality and heterosexuality, inquiring about individual desire, behavior, and identity, and obtained a carefully stratified representative sampling of the general population. The total number of persons reporting at least one of the components of homosexuality was only 293 in a total sample of 3,159—150 of 1,749 women and 143 of 1,410 men. Consequently, the number of persons reporting same-sex desire, behavior, and identity in specific age groups, in different geographical locations, and in other demographic categories was rather small. This study showed that, of the total sample, 1.3 percent of the women and 2.7 percent of the men participated in same-sex sexual behavior during the preceding year, and 4.1 percent of women and 4.9 percent of men had done so since 18 years of age; 7.5 percent of women and 7.7 percent of men reported the presence of sexual desire for someone of the same sex, and 1.4 percent of the women and 2.8 percent of the men reported a homosexual or bisexual identity. These figures varied considerably across groups based on age, marital status, education, religion, race, and place of residence.

These later studies demonstrate that the figure of one in ten, or 10 percent, often used to describe the number of persons who are gay and lesbian, was an overestimate of the actual number of persons who report same-sex desire or behavior or who acknowledge a gay or lesbian identity. Historically, there has been a political dimension to the issue of how prevalent homosexuality is in the population. Proponents and opponents of gay rights have attempted to respectively exaggerate or diminish the importance of the gay and lesbian presence in the population at large. However, it is nevertheless clear from the results of these studies that a larger number of persons report the existence of same-sex desire without associated behavior or identity and that, in certain population groups—for example, individuals living in the 12 largest U.S. cities—the number of gay and lesbian persons does approach the 10 percent figure. For the clinician, it is important to understand the variable prevalence dependent on which component of homosexuality and which social or demographic groups are being considered. Studies of prevalence of homosexuality in other Western countries show similar trends, but estimates of the extent of homosexuality in a given country must take into consideration factors such as the degree of social repression of homosexuality and the cultural meaning of same-sex desire, behavior, and identity.

ORIGINS OF HOMOSEXUALITY

Four areas in which research on the origins of homosexuality have been focused are biology, cross-cultural studies, psychological development, and the acquisition of gay and lesbian identities.

Biological Studies

Since the emergence of the concept of sexual orientation within Western medical discourse, there has been a debate as to whether it is primarily determined by biological or psychosocial factors. As it is currently unknown which contribution is more important, this section suggests some alternative pathways through which biological and experiential factors might interact. Before reviewing the biological research into sexual orientation, this section begins by describing three basic models for conceptualizing the possible contributions of biological factors, as well as the ways in which these factors may influence and interact with psychological and social factors.

Biological Models to Explain Homosexuality

The *model of direct biological effects*, on which most biological research regarding sexual orientation has been premised, is called *direct* because the arrow of causation goes directly from biological factors to sexual orientation. That is, the actions of biological factors, such as genes or hormones, would directly influence the organization or activity of brain circuits that mediate sexual orientation. According to this model, the brain would have an intrinsic (i.e., constitutional) sexual orientation or predisposition, the expression of which could nonetheless be subsequently modified by experience.

In a *model of permissive biological effects*, biology primarily plays a permissive role by providing the neural machinery through which sexual orientation is inscribed by formative experience. In addition, biological factors could also delimit the developmental stage during which the relevant formative experience must occur. For example, many songbirds must learn their species' song by hearing it during a restricted period of early development. Although the song is clearly acquired through experience, biology determines the critical period during which that experience must occur. Once a particular song has been acquired, that is the bird's song for life; it will not be able to unlearn that song or to acquire another. This is not to imply that sexual orientation might be acquired by simple mimicry. Instead, it suggests that a particular experience or set of experiences might have a greater or lesser impact on sexual orientation, depending on the developmental period during which it occurs. This example also shows that phenomena acquired through experience may nonetheless be immutable and therefore militates against the widespread notion that sexual orientation must be innate if it is impervious to change.

The *model of indirect biological effects* addresses the contribution of individual differences, some of which may be constitutionally influenced. In this model, biological factors influence sexual orientation only indirectly. Rather than acting directly on sexual orientation itself, the more direct or immediate action of biological factors would be on temperament or other personality traits. From birth, these personality or temperamental traits would then influence how an individual subsequently experiences, interacts with, and modifies the environment. This would include how the individual shapes the relationships and experiences thought to influence the development of a sexual orientation. Although similar to the model of permissive biological effects, the model of indirect biological effects goes farther and suggests that the relevant formative experiences may, themselves, be strongly affected by biologically influenced personality variables.

The existing biological data relevant to causation of sexual orientation are equally compatible with the direct and indirect models. The distinction between these models can be appreciated in their differing interpretations of three of the more robust findings in the sexual orientation literature. The first of these findings is that the propensity to engage in *rough-and-tumble play* appears to be influenced by prenatal exposure to male hormones. Second, compared to heterosexual men, more, but not all, homosexual men recall a childhood aversion to competitive rough-and-tumble play. Third, compared to heterosexual men, more, but not all, homosexual men recall their fathers as having been distant or rejecting.

In the direct model interpretation, the aversion to rough-and-tumble play represents the childhood expression of a brain that has been prewired for homosexuality. This is the position of Richard Isay, a psychoanalyst who suggests that biological factors wire the brain for sexual orientation and consequently reverse the polarity of the oedipal complex. According to this model, in addition to shunning rough-and-tumble play, prehomosexual boys are erotically interested in their fathers during the oedipal period. Fathers might recoil from their prehomosexual sons' gender nonconformity or sexual inclinations. Even if the father did not recoil, Isay speculates that, in adulthood, gay men might nevertheless recall their fathers as having been cold or distant to avoid conscious awareness of their earlier sexual attractions to them.

Alternatively, an indirect model interpretation postulates that a biologically influenced aversion to rough-and-tumble play does not necessarily imply prewiring for homosexuality. Instead, such an aversion becomes a potent factor predisposing to homosexual development in particular environments—perhaps where this behavior is stigmatized as sissy behavior and therefore causes the boy to see himself as different from his father and male peers. In this scenario, the father's withdrawal from his son would contribute to, rather than result from, his homosexuality. Significantly, an aversion to rough-and-tumble play would arguably have different consequences in environments in which this is acceptable, perhaps making no contribution to sexual orientation at all. This example does not suggest that a distant or rejecting father (whether real or projected) is a feature of all or even the majority of pathways to male homosexuality. Based on the indirect model, one might conjecture how any number of biologically influenced personality variants could influence sexual orientation. A given variant might predispose to homosexuality in one environment and to heterosexuality in another, while making no contribution to sexual orientation in others.

Neuroendocrine Research Historically, much biological research begins with the premise that the constitution of gay men and lesbians is somehow intermediate between that of their male and female heterosexual counterparts. This assumption led to investigations of various attributes for evidence of sexual atypicality in gays and lesbians, including chromosomes, genitalia, skeletal proportions, and facial hair. No features distinguishing gays and lesbians from heterosexual individuals emerged from those studies. From the 1950s into the 1970s, considerable research examined the endocrine system for atypical levels of the so-called sex hormones in gays and lesbians. An overwhelming majority of such studies failed to demonstrate any correlation between sexual orientation and adult hormone levels. In fact, androgens, frequently referred to as *male hormones*, although they are present in both sexes, have been found to increase sexual desire in men and women with no effect on sexual orientation. Moreover, sexual orientation does not change in adults when hormone levels are altered by gonadal malignancies, trauma, or surgical removal.

PRENATAL HORMONAL HYPOTHESIS The *prenatal hormonal hypothesis* is currently a major focus of sexual orientation research. It posits that (1) the brains of heterosexual men and women differ from each other structurally and functionally and that (2) those differences result from early hormonal influences on the developing fetus. This perspective also views sexual orientation as derivative of a hormonally mediated developmental process leading to sexual differentiation of the brain. Consequently, the brains of homosexual individuals are expected to exhibit characteristics that would be considered more typical of the other sex. This is sometimes referred to as the *intersex hypothesis* of homosexuality.

The prenatal hormonal hypothesis draws on observations of rodents in which the balance between male and female patterns of mating behaviors is strongly influenced by the amount and timing of early androgen exposure. The period of maximal sensitivity to these organizing effects of androgen varies from one species to the next. The rat has been used extensively in such research, because the period of brain sexual differentiation extends into the early postnatal period (which corresponds to the mid-trimester of human gestation). Thus, the hormonal exposure of the rat's brain can be experimentally manipulated by perinatal gonadectomies and injections of various hormones. Such research has revealed that many effects of androgens are mediated by conversion to estrogens by aromatase enzymes within the brain. Subsequently, these brain-derived estrogens interact with estrogen receptors within the brain. Various hypotheses have been advanced to explain why the brains of female fetuses are not masculinized by estrogens of maternal origin or those that originate from their own ovaries. One hypothesis is that peripheral estrogens are bound by proteins and are prevented from crossing the blood–brain barrier.

It is problematic to make assumptions about human sexual psychology based on extrapolations from rodent behaviors caused by experimental, perinatal endocrine manipulation. For example, a neonatally castrated male rat that shows *lordosis*—presenting with an arched back to permit mounting—when mounted by another male rat is sometimes considered to be homosexual, as is the perinatally androgenized female rat that mounts others. The male rat that mounts another male rat is sometimes considered to be heterosexual, as is the female rat that displays lordosis when mounted by another female rat. Thus, in this particular laboratory paradigm, sexual orientation is defined in terms of specific behaviors and postures. In contrast, human sexual orientation is defined not by the motor patterns of copulation but by one's pattern of erotic responsiveness and the gender of one's preferred sex partner.

Because of the problems in equating rodent behavior with human sexual orientation, researchers have begun to use a variety of strategies to assess partner preference in animals. This is sometimes done by seeing whether a test animal chooses to approach a male or a female stimulus animal placed in opposite arms of a T-maze. Although some unaltered laboratory animals spontaneously direct most of their sexual behaviors toward their own sex, animal studies of sexual orientation are usually carried out on animals that have been experimentally manipulated. For example, a genetically male rodent may be castrated as a neonate, depriving his developing brain of androgens, or particular androgen-responsive regions of his brain may be destroyed. However, to activate the display of female-typical behaviors and preferences in such male animals, estrogen injections are also required in adulthood. Because adult homosexual men and women have hormonal profiles that are indistinguishable from those of their heterosexual counterparts, it remains unclear how findings based on such hormonally abnormal animals reveal anything about human sexual orientation.

Ethical constraints make it impossible to test the prenatal hormonal hypothesis in humans; one cannot experimentally manipulate the prenatal hormonal exposure of human fetuses to study their effects on subsequent sexual orientation. However, there are alternative strategies. These include assessing sexual orientation in individuals with known or suspected prenatal hormonal abnormalities and assessing presumed correlates of prenatal hormonal exposure in known homosexual and heterosexual individuals. These strategies are discussed in turn.

ORIENTATION AFTER DOCUMENTED PRENATAL HORMONAL ABNORMALITIES: HUMAN INTERSEXES The prenatal hormonal hypothesis would predict that a large proportion of men with medical conditions known to involve prenatal androgen deficiency or insensitivity would be homosexual or transsexual. The same is true of a large proportion of women exposed prenatally to excess androgens. Because androgens are required for the development of the external male genitalia, such individuals may be born with genitals that are intermediate in morphology between those of normal males and females. Such individuals, historically referred to as *hermaphrodites*, are now referred to as *intersexes*, because their sexual differentiation is, in some respects, intermediate between male and female.

Regardless of their genetic sex or the nature of their prenatal hormonal exposure, the current published consensus is that intersexes usually become heterosexual in accordance with the gender that they are assigned—provided that gender assignment is made early and that rearing is unambiguous with respect to that assignment. However, several studies suggest that the incidence of homosexuality (relative to the assigned gender) may be increased among intersex individuals. Interpretation of these results, however, is complicated by many complex variables. For example, in many cases, the rearing of individuals born with genital ambiguity may not be unambiguous with regard to the assigned gender, despite the intentions of physicians and parental figures. This may occur when the affected individual has had multiple surgeries in an attempt to construct more normal-appearing genitalia. Even surgeries performed so early that the individual has no memory of them may leave physical scars or other anomalies that give rise to concerns about gender. Moreover, parents may remain ambivalent about the gender of the child and may communicate this unwittingly and nonverbally to the child. Thus, studies that detect an increased incidence of homosexual identity, behavior, or fantasy in intersex individuals do not provide unequivocal support for direct-model hormonal effects on sexual orientation. Adequate long-term follow-up studies of sexual orientation in intersex individuals are lacking and, in many cases, may not be feasible. Many of these individuals are not aware of their intersex status, because their family and physicians have withheld that knowledge as detrimental to normal psychosexual development. Such individuals have therefore been lost to follow-up studies of adult sexual orientation. The gender assignment and other aspects of the medical management of intersex individuals pose many ethical dilemmas (e.g., the withholding of medical information and informed consent for surgical gender reassignment) that have only recently begun to receive careful scrutiny.

PRESUMED CORRELATES OF PRENATAL HORMONAL EXPOSURE IN HOMOSEXUAL INDIVIDUALS Another strategy in attempting to establish a link between prenatal hormonal exposure and sexual orientation has been to examine presumed correlates of such exposure in known homosexual and heterosexual individuals. The most obvious correlates would be abnormalities of testicular or ovarian function and abnormalities in the differentiation of the external genitalia. Such variations are rare in homosexual individuals and lend no support to the prenatal hormonal hypothesis; however, the androgens could influence the differentiation of the external genitalia and the brain during different periods of development. Animal research suggests two additional correlates of early androgen exposure that have been explored in humans as possible correlates of sexual orientation: the pattern of luteinizing hormone secretion elicited by estrogen and neuroanatomical sexual dimorphisms.

In rats, exposure of the developing hypothalamus to aromatized androgens determines the signal that the adult's brain relays to the pituitary gland in response to high levels of estrogen in the bloodstream. If rats do not experience high levels of aromatized androgens at a certain early phase of development (as in normal females), the adult brain responds to estrogen by directing the pituitary to increase its secretion of luteinizing hormone, a phenomenon referred to as *positive feedback*. However, if the developing rat brain is exposed to high androgen levels (as in normal males), it is not able to support this positive feedback response. Thus, in rats, the presence or absence of this positive feedback response can be used to infer the pattern of the brain's early androgen exposure. Specifically, the positive feedback response can be elicited in adulthood from normal females and from males that were castrated during the critical period of sexual differentiation of the brain but not from normal males or from females that were experimentally exposed to high androgen levels in early development.

These observations generated speculation that, in humans, the luteinizing hormone response to an injection of estrogen would also indicate the sexually differentiated state of the brain and would correlate with sexual orientation. Empirical research in this area has produced conflicting results; however, the current consensus opinion is that the feedback response in humans does not correlate with sexual orientation. Moreover, in humans and other primates, convincing research suggests that the brain mechanism regulating luteinizing hormone is the same in both sexes, rather than taking two sexually distinct forms as it does in rodents. If there is no sex difference in the feedback mechanism, it cannot be argued logically that the mechanism should exhibit atypical sexual differentiation in gays and lesbians. Because the positive feedback response is required for cyclical ovarian function and fertility in women, the growing number of lesbian mothers also supports this interpretation.

Several anthropometric characteristics have been explored in relation to sexual orientation. Most of these studies have been executed with the expectation that homosexual individuals would exhibit characteristics intermediate between those of heterosexual men and women, or that are more typical of heterosexuals of the other sex. Such measures have included not only height and weight, but also the amount and distribution of facial hair, the ratio of shoulder width to hip width, the size of the genitalia, and, more recently, dematoglyphic (fingerprint) characteristics and finger length ratios (ratio of length of index to ring finger). Most of these studies have been flawed in one or more ways that make their findings difficult to interpret. Some of these flaws include reliance on small self-selected samples, relying on self-reports of subjects rather than on objective measures, or on measures obtained by raters who were not blind to the sexual orientation status of the subjects. The finger length ratio appears to be a sexually dimorphic phenomenon, but whether it truly varies with sexual orientation remains to be established by further investigation. Moreover, it remains to be demonstrated that the sex difference in finger length ratio is a function of early androgen exposure. Recent research suggests that cell-autonomous mechanisms (e.g., sex differences in gene dosing due to incomplete inactivation of one X chromosome in female cells) contribute more to the establishment of sexual dimorphism than previously appreciated. Finally, one laboratory has reported that lesbian women exhibit masculinized otoacoustic emissions (an echo-like waveform emitted by the inner ear in response to brief sounds). Replication by independent laboratories is required to substantiate these results.

Neuroanatomical Sexual Dimorphism Since the early 1980s, sex differences have been confirmed in the size of several brain structures in a variety of laboratory animals. These findings have generated speculation concerning the existence of parallel differences in the human brain associated not only with sex, but also with sexual orientation.

Most of the structural sex differences identified involve specific cell groups within a broad region of the rodent hypothalamus that participates in regulating a variety of functions, including sexually dimorphic copulatory behaviors. Like the sex differences in copulatory behaviors, several structural sex differences in the rodent brain have been demonstrated to develop in response to sex differences in early androgen exposure: High androgen levels at the appropriate time lead to male-typical anatomy, whereas low levels lead to female-typical anatomy. Consequently, behavioral sex differences are thought to be mediated, at least in part, by structural differences.

The best-studied anatomical sex difference in the rodent brain involves a cell group straddling the medial preoptic and anterior regions of the hypothalamus—the sexually dimorphic nucleus of the preoptic area (SDN-POA). In the rat, in which it was initially described, this structure is five to eight times larger in male rats than in female rats. Damage to the preoptic region has been demonstrated to decrease mounting behavior in laboratory animals, whereas electrical stimulation of the region elicits mounting behavior. These observations, as well as the finding that the size of the SDN-POA correlates positively with the frequency of mounting behavior displayed by male rats, have established the belief that the SDN-POA participates in regulating male sex behavior.

The belief that the SDN-POA participates in regulating male sex behavior in rats has led the search for a comparable nucleus in humans. The human third interstitial nucleus of the anterior hypothalamus (INAH3) has been identified as the most promising candidate. This nucleus is much larger and contains substantially more neurons in presumed heterosexual men than in women, and, by extrapolation from animal work, this sex difference is widely believed to reflect sex differences in early hormone exposure. The AIDS epidemic has made it possible to study this nucleus in individuals whose medical records indicated homosexual behavior as the HIV risk factor. (Unless someone dies from complications of AIDS, there is usually no documentation of sexual orientation in the medical records available for autopsy studies.) These studies suggest that the volume of INAH3 may be smaller in homosexual men than in heterosexual men but that the number of neurons within the nucleus does not vary with sexual orientation. The suggestion of volume reduction must be viewed skeptically for a variety of technical reasons, including the confounding of sexual orientation and AIDS (i.e., all of the brains of gay men were from AIDS victims). In addition, tissue shrinks in the process of fixation for histological analysis. This shrinkage influences measures of size but not measures of cell number. Thus, the finding of equal numbers of neurons in homosexual and heterosexual men may be a more reliable finding than the suggestion of a difference in the volume of the nucleus. Additional studies are needed to clarify these issues. It is, therefore, premature to accept the finding of decreased volume of INAH3 in homosexual men or the hypothesis that such volume reduction reflects decreased early androgen exposure.

In addition, speculation regarding the function of INAH3 has been based on the assumption that it is the homolog of the rat's SDN-POA. However, the function of the rat's nucleus has eluded researchers. The rat's nucleus can be destroyed by electrolytic lesions without any discernible effect on mounting behavior. After larger lesions that included the region surrounding the SDN-POA, however, male rats could be induced to display a female copulatory response if they were also injected with estrogen and progesterone. This observation suggests that the SDN-POA may act to inhibit the display of particular female-typical copulatory behaviors. This further illustrates the previously mentioned problems of extrapolating from animal behaviors to sexual orientation in humans.

In addition to the hypothalamus, researchers have sought to identify variation with sex and sexual orientation in the brain commissures, the fiber bundles that connect the left and right hemispheres of the brain. The rationale underlying these studies was drawn from speculation regarding the neuroanatomical basis for observed statistical sex differences in the lateralization of particular cognitive functions within the brain. Briefly, several lines of investigation suggest that women are more likely to exhibit bilaterally symmetrical hemispheric activation in the performance of particular cognitive tasks, whereas men are more likely to exhibit asymmetrical activation. A popular hypothesis holds that this sex difference in brain activity reflects increased interhemispherical communication in women compared to men and that this is due to more interhemispherical fibers and, therefore, larger interhemispherical commissures in women. Of approximately 50 studies examining the corpus callosum, the largest of the brain's commissures, the vast majority has not confirmed sexual dimorphism. No study has described morphometric variation in the corpus callosum as a function of sexual orientation. A few studies have examined the anterior commissure, a small bundle of fibers connecting portions of the left and right temporal lobes. These studies have produced conflicting results regarding variation with sex and sexual orientation. To date, there is no compelling evidence of sexual atypicality in the cerebral commissures of homosexuals.

Genetic Research As in the neuroendocrinological research, some genetic studies have also been premised on the intersex hypothesis. Some of these studies attempt to show that gays and lesbians have chromosomal material that is typical of the other sex in their cells. Other studies seek to link homosexuality with genetically controlled aberrations in the process of sexual differentiation. No such genetic links have been demonstrated. More recent studies examine the heritability of sexual orientation. Although several studies have suggested that homosexuality runs in families, such studies are not helpful in distinguishing between genetic and environmental influences, because most related individuals share environmental influences, as well as genes.

FAMILY STUDIES A first step toward disentangling genetic and environmental influences can be made by studying sexual orientation in identical and fraternal twins. One such study assessed sexual orientation not only in the identical and fraternal twins, but also in the nontwin biological brothers and the unrelated adopted brothers of homosexual men. The concordance rate for identical twins (52 percent) in that study was much higher than the rate for the fraternal twins (22 percent). Assuming that environmental influences would be the same for all brothers reared together, the higher concordance rate in the identical twins is consistent with a genetic effect, as identical twins share all of their genes, whereas fraternal twins, on average, share only one-half of their genes.

It would be a mistake, however, to attribute the increased concordance rate in identical twins to increased gene sharing alone. If there were no environmental effect on sexual orientation, then the rate of homosexuality among the adopted brothers should have equaled the rate of homosexuality in the general population. Recent studies place the rate of homosexuality in men between 2 and 5 percent. That the concordance rate in adopted brothers was 11 percent (two to five times higher than in the general population) suggests a major environmental contribution. The rate for homosexuality among nontwin biological brothers was only 9 percent, a figure that is statistically indistinguishable from the 11 percent recorded for adopted brothers. If the concordance rate for homosexuality among nontwin brothers is the same regardless of whether the brothers are genetically related, then the concordance rate cannot be explained exclusively by genetics.

When considered together, the data from the studies of twins and adopted brothers suggest that the increased concordance in the identical twins may be due to a combination of genetic and environmental influences. From another perspective, perhaps the most interesting finding to emerge from twin studies is that approximately 50 percent of identical twins are discordant for sexual orientation, even when they are reared together. The discordance for sexual orientation among genetically identical individuals reared in identical environments has been consistent across studies and underscores just how little is actually known about the origins of sexual orientation.

LINKAGE STUDIES The notion of a *gay gene* has captured the popular imagination. It is worth underscoring, however, that gay genes are not required for homosexuality to run in families or for researchers to determine that homosexuality is heritable. *Heritability* has a precise technical meaning and is defined as the ratio between genotypic variation (genetic variation) and phenotypic variation (observable expressed variation in a trait). Thus, heritability reflects only the *degree* to which a given trait is *associated* with genetic factors. It says nothing about the specific genetic factors involved or about the mechanisms through which they exert their influence. Furthermore, the concept of heritability provides no information about how a particular trait might change under different environmental conditions. Thus, homosexuality could be highly heritable, even if genes influenced sexual orientation entirely through indirect pathways.

However, genes alone cannot directly determine any behavior or psychological phenomenon. Instead, genes direct a particular pattern of ribonucleic acid (RNA) synthesis that, in turn, specifies the production of a particular protein that then may influence behavior. There are necessarily many intervening pathways between a gene and a specific behavior and even more intervening variables between a gene and a pattern that involves thinking and behaving. The term *homosexual gene* is therefore without meaning, unless one proposes that a particular gene, perhaps through a hormonal mechanism, directs the brain to develop in such a way that an individual can only be erotically attracted to others of the same gender. Evidence in support of such a simple and direct link between genes and sexual orientation is lacking.

As previously mentioned, a highly publicized study presented statistical evidence that genes influencing sexual orientation reside on a portion of the X chromosome known as the *q28 region*. However, the statistical significance of that study rests on the assumption that the rate of male homosexuality in the population at large is 2 percent. If the base rate is actually 4 percent or higher, the linkage described in that study is not statistically significant. It can be argued that the data gathered in that study itself support the 4 percent estimate, rendering the linkage nonsignificant. An independent research team has been unable to duplicate the Xq28 finding in men by using a comparable experimental design, and no group has found evidence that Xq28 is linked to sexual orientation in women.

Cross-Cultural Studies

Anthropological studies of human sexuality have demonstrated an enormous variation in gender and sexual organization and behavior in different cultures. These studies provide evidence for the fluidity and complexity of sexual behavior and experience at individual and social levels. The findings from ethnographic studies of gender and sexuality among different cultural groups have drawn attention to a cultural bias inherent in many developmental theories of homosexuality. Building on the work of Margaret Mead, Ruth Benedict, and other anthropologists, researchers have been able to classify structural types of sexual development and forms of homosexual organization in different cultures. Gilbert Herdt, in particular, has explicated cross-cultural models based on his study of ritualized homosexuality among the Sambia tribe of Papua New Guinea and on his review of findings from other anthropological studies of sexual practices. Traditional developmental theory posits a presumed continuity in sexual development across the life span. Herdt suggests instead the idea of *discontinuity* in sexual development to explain variation in the psychological experience and symbolic meaning of sexuality. He also explores the cultural aspects of fluidity in experience and expression of sexual orientation that have defined much of the theoretical discourse on bisexuality.

Herdt has theorized three types of sexual development that occur cross-culturally—linear, sequential, and emergent—which explain variations in patterns of sexual orientation. *Linear development* refers to sexual behavior that occurs without significant change in behavior or orientation across a lifetime. *Sequential development* describes a developmental pattern that incorporates important change at different life stages. One example of sequential development could be found in Victorian England—and perhaps to some extent modern America—in which children were assumed to be sexually naïve, but adults were expected to have a fully developed range of sexual practices. Another example are the Sambia of Papua New Guinea, in which men practice ritualized homosexual behavior during childhood and yet only function heterosexuality as adults. *Emergent development* occurs in societies that allow some degree of ambiguity and uncertainty in adult sexual outcomes based on childhood socialization. Emergent development can be identified in societies that have undergone massive social change leading to changes in traditional sexual norms and values and in segments of modern American society that allow a range of adult sexual options. Each of these patterns of sexual development can be shown to significantly influence the forms and expression of sexual orientation that exist in different cultures.

Herdt also describes a typology of homosexuality based on a cross-cultural organization of same-sex behavior. The first type is *age-structured homosexuality*, usually involving older and younger men and generally including a sequential pattern of childhood same-sex practices that yield to primarily heterosexual behaviors in adults. An example would be the male homosexual practices of classical Greece. Another form of homosexuality is *gender-reversed homosexuality*, which refers to a reversal in the normative sex-role dress and behavior. An example of such gender-reversed homosexuality is the Native-American *berdache*, a man who is permitted to assume the gender role of a woman. The third type identified by Herdt is *role-specialized homosexuality*, in which same-sex sexual activity is restricted to certain social roles and positions. This type occurs among the shamans of some Native-American tribes who—in following dreams or visions revealing their special status—cross-dress and engage in homosexual behavior. Role-specialized homosexuality was also found among certain working-class women in 19th century China. Finally, Herdt describes the *modern gay movement*, consisting of egalitarian same-sex practices, as a fourth type of homosexual organization. Although acknowledging that hierarchical relationships still exist in parallel with traditional forms of heterosexual relationships, he states that homosexuality in contemporary America has arisen as a new form of homosexual practice that comprises a sexual orientation, a social identity, and a political movement.

Cross-cultural studies of sexuality and homosexuality highlight the limits of any single explanation for the development and experience of homosexuality in a particular society. There are enormous variations in the organization and meaning of same-sex practices across cultures, and changes within a given society over time have been amply demonstrated. The universality of same-sex sexual expression has been matched by the constancy of change and variation in its organization and meaning. Future cross-cultural studies can further explicate the social factors, such as industrialization, urbanization, religion, and class stratification, that influence the structural forms into which individual sexual desire and behavior are shaped within cultures.

Psychosocial Studies of Development

Classical theories of psychological development posit the origins of adult personality and identity in childhood experience. These theories often assume linear pathways of development that progress sequentially from childhood to adulthood. In the latter part of the 20th century, however, greater attention was paid to the distinct processes of development during adulthood itself. The result has been a refutation of the view that homosexuality can be explained as due to circumstances occurring in the first 3 years of life. Instead, the development of a sexual orientation can be better understood on examination of psychological and interpersonal events throughout the life cycle, and such understanding must incorporate assumptions of continuous and discontinuous patterns of development. Consequently, when applied to sexuality, in general, and to sexual orientation, in particular, any model of development must be sensitive to the physical, cognitive, and emotional maturation that occurs across the life span without making the a priori assumption that early childhood behaviors, awareness, and feelings are the definitive precursors of adult behaviors, awareness, and feelings. It should be further noted that early psychological studies of homosexuality were often based on unrepresentative populations, such as psychiatric patients, prison populations, and military personnel. Most psychosocial studies continue to be plagued by problems of sampling. Although they may no longer be limited to these special populations, studies have tended to focus on white, urban, openly identified, and community-affiliated gay men and lesbians. It is not known whether one can generalize the development and experience of the latter group to the experience of individuals coming from other ethnic, racial, or culturally diverse groups.

Findings from psychosocial studies may also vary depending on the research methodology followed. For example, in early retrospective studies of adult homosexual patients in psychoanalysis, the stories these individuals told of their upbringing were often consistent with cultural notions of homosexuality. In other words, how these individuals viewed their early childhood may have resulted from social learning of popular theories of homosexuality, before or during their psychoanalytic treatment, with subsequent internalization of the theory as part of their life scripts. In addition, many studies of purported childhood precursors of adult homosexuality often focus too narrowly on selected characteristics, such as effeminacy in boys, that are associated with stereotyped notions of adult homosexuality. Consequently, such studies tend to ignore the enormous individual variability in patterns of development toward and characteristics associated with adult sexual identity.

The prospective examination of potential childhood and adolescent antecedents of adult homosexuality is a relatively recent endeavor. However, empirical studies of homoeroticism in American society before puberty are nonexistent, and only a few studies of same-sex desire during adolescence have been published. Currently, disapproving social attitudes toward acknowledging sexual attractions and behaviors, particularly same-sex desire and behavior, during childhood have made scientific inquiry into this area difficult, if not impossible. Consequently, one finds instead a profusion of models of development that are derived from a retrospective reconstruction of childhood experiences. The only perspective that has been readily available to examine the psychosocial origins of homosexuality in American society is that of the clinician. However, using that approach to understand normal development is often compromised by the tendency to focus on dysfunction, pathology, and abnormality in the clinical setting. As a result, until recently, children with severely atypical gender behavior (gender identity disorder of childhood) and disturbed homosexual adults have often continued to serve as the primary source of statistics about and models for the psychological development of homosexuality. The potential psychosocial understanding that might derive from ethnographic and other social science approaches to studying sexuality in children has been applied only in other cultures and has thus not been used as a tool for the study of the development of sexual orientation in American society.

Current knowledge about the psychosocial contributions to homosexuality has thus largely been acquired through studies of children who demonstrate early gender-role nonconformity, reconstruction within psychotherapy of childhood histories, and a small number of empirical reports about sexuality and homosexuality in adolescence. The origins of adult gay, lesbian, and bisexual identities in Western society have been described in theoretical models of identity acquisition and in the findings from a limited number of empirical studies of the specific behaviors and events associated with establishing these identities.

Origins of Homosexuality in Childhood and Adolescence Early attempts to describe childhood psychosocial antecedents of adult homosexuality consisted primarily of psychoanalytic formulations derived from the histories of psychiatric patients. These usually depicted trauma, loss, and disturbed family relationships in childhood as causal mechanisms. In psychoanalysis, this was true not only for homosexuality, but also for all conditions under analytical scrutiny. However, the analytical model does not adequately explain the multiple forms of same-sex desire and behavior in psychologically healthy and disturbed individuals. Modern sexologists in the tradition of Kinsey have sought alternative explanations for the development of a variety of forms of normal sexual expression and identity. Current explorations into homosexuality in childhood are often guided by essentialist views of sexual orientation that assume that a particular personality characteristic or specific behavior is a reliable predictor of adult sexual orientation. It remains to be seen, however, whether a single set of characteristics or some unitary pathway leading to adult homosexuality will be identified.

The most robust finding in studies of childhood factors associated with adult homosexuality is early gender nonconformity *and* the recollection of an awareness of being different. The appearance of early gender nonconformity, femininity in boys and masculinity in girls, appears to be correlated with the development of homosexuality in adulthood for some individuals. Similarly, many adult gay men and lesbians report a recollection of an awareness of feeling different from others during childhood. These characteristics seem to be more common among children who will become homosexual than in those who will become heterosexual.

Findings from large-scale surveys of sexual attraction during adolescence show that younger adolescents tend to be less aware of same-sex feelings and to identify themselves less often as lesbian, gay, or bisexual than older adolescents. Reports of same-sex attraction range from 7.5 to 18.0 percent in teenage girls and from 7.7 to 21.0 percent in boys, with an estimate of approximately 15 percent of youth overall experiencing some same-sex attraction. Fewer youth report same-sex sexual activity, and even fewer identify themselves as gay, lesbian, or bisexual, although this latter figure increases with age. Although exact figures are unavailable for comparison, a larger number of youth currently identify themselves as bisexual or uncertain about their sexual orientation than previous generations. This is likely a reflection of the greater awareness of flexibility in sexual expression and of the diminishing social stigma associated with a bisexual identity when compared to lesbian and gay identities.

The study of homoeroticism and of the development of homosexual or bisexual identities in adolescence continues to be difficult because of strong peer pressures to conform to heterosexual norms, ongoing and significant societal stigmatization of same-sex desire and behavior, and institutional and familial repression and denial of the existence of same-sex sexual feelings and behaviors in youth. Recent studies have focused on the adjustment, health, and mental health issues present for young people who self-identify as gay, lesbian, or bisexual and who present to community centers providing services for these individuals. As a result of increased access and attention paid to this segment of the youth population, more is being learned about the problems experienced by youth with an emerging or solidified gay, lesbian, or bisexual identity than is known about the normative events associated with such a developmental pathway.

Acquisition of Gay and Lesbian Identities Much of the contemporary discussion about the psychosocial development of homosexuality has taken place within the field of identity development. There, it has flourished as a primary theme in the broader discourse of social constructionism and its analysis of the political and social meaning of identities in late 20th-century postindustrial Western society. Thus, it is useful not only to understand the theoretical description of gay, lesbian, and bisexual identity development in an individual, but also to appreciate the meaning of personal identities at a cultural level. From this perspective, the appearance of lesbian, gay, and bisexual identities—and the detailed description of their emergence and multifaceted expression within society and the individual—can be seen as an outcome of personal growth and development for the individual and of the cultural evolution of the concept of the *homosexual person.* It could be reasonably argued that the self-acceptance of fully developed gay, lesbian, and bisexual identities in individual men and women is an outgrowth of the creation and social acceptance of the 19th-century biomedical belief that sexual desire and behavior are core characteristics defining selfhood.

The view of gay, lesbian, and bisexual identities as personal narratives and cultural constructions does not detract from the recognition of their centrality in organizing the subjective experiences of individual women and men. However, there is always a possibility that the clinician's own adherence to theoretical models of development and categories of understanding sexual orientation may objectify or simplify the enormous range of individual experiences associated with sexuality. It is more helpful if the clinician, in working with persons who talk about their experiences of becoming gay or lesbian, understands these personal stories as framed within a contemporary language intended to make meaning of their experience. Understanding and acceptance of the language used to encapsulate these subjective experiences can be helpful in the clinical setting.

Many theoretical descriptions of lesbian, gay, and bisexual identity acquisition are inconsistent, as they sometimes fail to distinguish between the concepts of identity, self, and self-concept. However, the experience of these identities by lesbians, gay men, and bisexuals is widespread and subjectively meaningful. For this reason, it is important for the psychiatrist to be familiar with the narratives of identity development that are relevant for these men and women. Models of lesbian, gay, and bisexual identity acquisition describe an intrapsychic and interpersonal process whereby a subjective experience of oneself as lesbian, gay, or bisexual becomes increasingly congruent with other people's perception of that identity. This process is generally conceived of as occurring over time, in sequential stages, and in a manner that leads to an increasing integration of one's experience of being lesbian, gay, or bisexual into other aspects of one's sense of self. Gay, lesbian, and bisexual identity development has generally been conceived of as consisting of a series of stages. The first is a period of homosexual self-awareness, a growing awareness and possible confusion about the presence and meaning of same-sex erotic attractions. In people who become gay, lesbian, or bisexual, the period of homosexual self-awareness is followed by a time during which the individual considers accepting these feelings and begins to incorporate them into experiences. In many cases, this phase is followed by an extended phase of growing acceptance of and perhaps even pride in the new identity.

The process of identity development leads to different outcomes for different individuals; it is influenced by interpersonal effects and consequences and feedback from others and may be interrupted or terminated at any point. Most models of gay, lesbian, and bisexual identity development incorporate the completion of several events or tasks: coming out, or becoming aware of same-sex attraction and disclosing it, at some point, to others; forming relationships with other gay and lesbian persons; engaging in same-sex sexual behaviors; becoming involved in gay and lesbian activities and communities; establishing primary relationships with persons of the same sex; and learning how to integrate one's sexual orientation identity into other aspects of the self.

Models of gay and lesbian identity acquisition sometimes present an image of progressive elaboration and synthesis of homosexual orientation with other aspects of the self. However, individuals vary considerably in the degree to which they follow such models. In some persons, the development of a gay, lesbian, or bisexual identity may be inhibited in response to a number of factors. These include a punitive or harsh internal or environmental response to openly expressing aspects of such an identity or a redirection of one's focus on other developmental tasks, such as schooling or career development. Because of what may be a greater potential fluidity in their sexual orientation, women may be less likely than men to adhere to some ideal of identity development; instead, they may focus on an existing relationship, regardless of the sex of their partner. Similarly, because models of gay, lesbian, or bisexual identities have been developed based on experiences of urban white persons, individuals who live in situations that do not provide reinforcement for adopting these identities (for example, rural areas and some communities of color) may participate in same-sex sexual activities without ever acquiring an identity associated with these behaviors.

Individual variations in the extent of development of gay, lesbian, and bisexual identities may result from prohibitive factors, internal or external, that interfere with optimal personal growth and from normative psychosocial influences reflecting diverse individual experiences and different adaptational needs. The tasks for any clinician working with these individuals are to appreciate the individuality of identity development in each patient, to understand their particular psychological and social resources and needs in this area, and to appreciate the risks and benefits in differing pathways of development. Ultimately, each individual develops her or his own identity; the clinician can only help optimize the understanding of the meaning of various options and establish opportunities for maximizing freedom in making choices about often conflicting outcomes.

Homosexuality and Nongay Identities The complexities involved in establishing a gay, lesbian, or bisexual identity require a psychiatrist to be tolerant, respectful, and sophisticated regarding sexual matters. The different kinds of subjectivities that one may encounter in working with gay and lesbian patients can be understood and appreciated within such concepts as hiding and revealing, awareness and unawareness, and self-acceptance and self-nonacceptance. Patients with same-sex feelings can be helped to understand that their own sexuality is, in part, shaped by the meanings attributed to homosexuality by a predominantly heterosexual world. The subjectivity of a sexual identity is shaped by culture and language, often with little or no regard to prevailing scientific categories of sexuality. Some broad subjectivities are identified to provide clinicians with a way to understand the range of ways in which patients may manage their same-sex feelings.

Closeted individuals are unable to acknowledge to themselves or to others that they have homoerotic feelings and fantasies. From a behavior perspective, the popular terms *closeted* or *in the closet* may refer to a person who is actively engaging in homosexual acts but is concealing them. However, from the retrospective accounts of many gay men and lesbians, the experience of being in the closet is often more psychologically complex. The feeling of same-sex attraction is often unacceptable and, as a result, is unavailable to conscious awareness or integration into the individual's public persona. It may therefore be hidden from the self, as well as from others. A closeted individual may not act on the feeling at all or may do so only in a dissociated state. These feelings are not unconscious, as in the classical concept of latent homosexuality, but they are out of awareness and only sometimes accessible to consciousness at certain times or in certain situations. Subjectively, a closeted man may tell himself that he really does not have same-sex feelings, or, if he is aware of the feelings, he hopes that they have some other meaning besides homosexuality.

Homosexually self-aware individuals acknowledge to themselves the existence of their homoerotic feelings and attractions. Subjectivities and behaviors may vary from individual to individual. A person may choose not to act on the feelings or may act on them in a secretive way. Some behaviorally closeted individuals are homosexually self-aware and some are not. Some homosexually self-aware individuals consider the possibility of accepting and integrating these feelings into their public persona. For many individuals, this subjectivity may be a normative phase in eventually coming out and affirmatively accepting a gay or lesbian identity. Others may not accept these feelings, as in the example of a homosexually self-aware individual seeking a celibate lifestyle as a way of binding and avoiding a problematic gay or lesbian identity. For a clinician to assume that a patient is gay but does not know it is an external judgment that offers little insight into an individual's subjective experience. Such a phrase could describe a closeted woman or man who is truly unaware of her homoerotic feelings; it could just as well describe a homosexually self-aware woman or man who knows that she or he has these feelings but is trying to prevent others from knowing that she or he has them; finally, it could describe a lesbian or gay man who is out to a limited circle of individuals and recognizes her or his own sexual feelings but is selective about revealing them.

A new subjectivity, one that does not yet have a common cultural definition is that of *non–gay-identified individuals.* These individuals struggle against accepting any meanings that might naturalize their homosexual feelings. Because almost all gay men and lesbians who come out go through a phase of rejecting their own homosexual feelings before accepting their own gay or lesbian identity, it is sometimes assumed that all individuals overcome this period of rejection. However, this is not always the case, and some individuals may never accept their homosexual feelings or a gay or lesbian identity. In an effort to disidentify with homoerotic feelings and activities, such individuals may refer to themselves as *ex-homosexual* or *ex-gay* and may seek out ways to change their sexual orientation. In many ways, this is a new cultural subjectivity that grows out of response to the growing presence of openly gay, lesbian, and bisexual identities.

These different subjectivities should not be thought of as existing on a developmental continuum or as being associated with more or less psychopathology. It should also be emphasized that this approach does not view sexual identities as offering any diagnostic information about an individual. In addition, these subjectivities are not mutually exclusive—there is overlap between them and differing motivations within them—nor are these sexual subjectivities immutable. Although it may be difficult, if not impossible, to change one's sexual orientation, it is entirely possible to change attitudes about one's sexuality. As the subjectivities outlined previously are shaped by individual and cultural factors, there may be a wide range of psychosocially constructed attitudes and responses that individuals may develop toward their own homosexuality. Furthermore, the homosexual subjectivities outlined previously have no exact heterosexual equivalents, as having to hide one's interest in the other sex is usually not intrinsic to forming a heterosexual identity.

LIFE CYCLE AND DEVELOPMENTAL ISSUES

All men and women are faced, at different ages, with important developmental tasks. These include establishing a sense of trust in themselves and others, respecting their own identities, creating and maintaining intimate relationships, learning how to lead productive lives and to have fun, and sustaining a sense of generativity and personal integrity in old age. Success in completing such tasks is dependent on many factors, including biological and environmental resources, the impact of larger social and historical events, personal opportunities and traumas, and individual personality characteristics. Each of these factors interacts at different developmental stages to shape a unique life for each person. Whereas the day-to-day lives of lesbians and gay men may often be similar to those of heterosexual cohorts, the former also face unique developmental tasks throughout the life cycle. For example, during childhood and adolescence, young people who become aware of significant attractions to someone of the same sex need to understand what makes them different from the majority of people around them. Some choose to disclose their homosexuality to others through the process of coming out. Some wait until they are older to do so, and some never come out. During adulthood, these men and women confront unique challenges as they try to establish close relationships and to create families. They may do so even without traditional, formal rituals that celebrate their relationships or laws to protect their families. However they navigate the life cycle, gay men and lesbians and bisexual men and women need to contend with the adversity of having a stigmatized sexual identity, as well as the potentially life-affirming factors associated with finding one's true self, finding one's true partner, and being part of a community in which one can be oneself.

Antihomosexual Attitudes

Antihomosexual attitudes were once considered normative in most social and institutional settings, including schools, police departments, the military, and religious organizations. However, as the cultural foundations of antihomosexual attitudes have shifted, many traditionally antihomosexual groups and organizations have changed their positions. As a consequence of increasing cultural debates about homosexuality, many high schools and universities now offer clubs—gay-straight alliances—for students of all sexual identities to socialize. Many Western countries now allow openly gay and lesbian personnel to serve in their armed forces and police departments. Some religious denominations now appoint openly gay and lesbian priests, ministers, and rabbis to serve their congregations. Despite these changes, antihomosexual attitudes are still widespread, and it is helpful to identify their potential impact on gay, lesbian, and bisexual patients.

The terms *antihomosexual attitudes* or *antigay and antilesbian attitudes* are used here to refer to a wide range of critical and disapproving beliefs and feelings about homosexuality, gay men, and lesbians. The term *homophobia* was coined by George Weinberg in 1972. This refers to the fear or hatred of homosexuality and of gay and lesbian persons (*external homophobia*) or the self-hatred that gay people feel for themselves (*internal homophobia*). All lesbian, gay, and bisexual persons, to some extent, contend with *internalized homophobia.* A developing gay or lesbian person psychologically incorporates disapproving societal views of homosexuality and then experiences these feelings and beliefs in the form of a critical self-evaluation.

Mr. A. was a middle-aged gay man who had recently ended a 10-year relationship and was dating other men. He had identified himself as a gay man for years and appeared comfortable with his homosexuality. He was anxious about a weekend home that he had jointly purchased with his former partner before their relationship had ended. Mr. A. had received the property in the separation agreement but had come up against some legal complications in his efforts to sell it. Although he was usually a focused person who finished most of the tasks that he took on, Mr. A. was having difficulty taking care of this project. He was reluctant to speak with his lawyer or to address the issue at all, even though he felt that holding onto the house kept him from getting on with his life. His stated reason for entering treatment was to try to overcome what he felt was an unwelcome inhibition.

After some exploration of this issue, Mr. A.'s therapist remarked that the feelings evoked in Mr. A. when he thought about selling the property seemed difficult to tolerate. The therapist helped Mr. A. identify those feelings as a mixture of anger, despair, and anxiety. Mr. A. feared that he was going "crazy. I'm crazy. I think I was psychotic when we bought that property." The therapist asked for clarification. Mr. A. and his ex-partner were already having difficulties in their relationship when they acquired the house. It was Mr. A.'s idea to buy it, because he thought that having a weekend place in the country might reduce the tensions between them. "It was crazy, psychotic." The therapist suggested that it was possible that Mr. A. had not considered all of the implications in making the purchase, but why was that psychotic? Nevertheless, Mr. A. persisted in his strong belief that he was "crazy."

The therapist asked Mr. A. how buying a weekend house to save a relationship was any different from a couple trying to save their marriage by having a baby. Although trying to have a baby to save a marriage might be ill advised, it was hardly psychotic. Mr. A.'s anxiety suddenly diminished as he became silent and said, "I never thought of that." As the therapist helped Mr. A. contextualize his behavior within a normal frame of reference, Mr. A. recalled that, when his relationship had ended, he had felt it was because "gay relationships cannot last." The therapist thought it was a terrible burden for Mr. A. to bear if he believed that the end of his relationship also represented an indictment of his sexuality. The therapist, who was gay himself, then wondered aloud if heterosexuals, when they divorce, felt that the dissolution of their marriages meant that heterosexual relationships do not work. He went on to suggest that, given a 50 percent divorce rate in the United States, such beliefs could mean the end of sex as we know it. This comment made Mr. A. laugh, and he told the therapist that he found the ironic perspective useful.

This therapeutic intervention revealed how Mr. A. had dissociated from his own internalized homophobia, embodied in his belief that "gay relationships cannot last." After several more sessions in which he explored this belief, Mr. A. moved vigorously to resolve his legal difficulties. He sold the house and became more involved with a new boyfriend. Three years later, Mr. A. and his new partner moved into a house that they bought together.

The effects of internalized homophobia on the development of one's sexual orientation differ widely at an individual level. Among other things, however, these feelings can lead to the suppression or closeting of awareness of one's own same-sex attraction, can impair the acceptance of one's homosexuality, and can interfere with the integration of one's homosexual orientation into other aspects of identity. For many gay men and lesbians, internalized homophobia is experienced as a feeling of devaluation and limitation in relation to their homosexuality; for some, it may produce a variety of psychiatric and behavioral symptoms, including depression, anxiety, denial, and, sometimes, even suicide. Internalized homophobia may produce a unique interaction in each gay and lesbian person, but its common roots lie in anxieties about being criticized and shamed.

The term *homophobia* has gained widespread popular currency and has been generally, if inexactly, applied to a range of antihomosexual attitudes. The term has been criticized for suggesting that the existence of antihomosexual attitudes in an individual indicates the presence of a phobia or a formal psychiatric diagnosis. However, cultural attitudes in general fall outside the purview of psychiatric classification. Thus, the occurrence of antihomosexual attitudes does not necessarily represent the existence of a mental illness, distressing as they may be to individuals who hold them or those around them. Early research on homophobic attitudes demonstrated that they are correlated with certain demographic and personality characteristics, including sex, geographical location, religious beliefs, and degree of authoritarianism. Studies have also shown that some individuals with antihomosexual attitudes may regard same-sex behaviors as a threat to their cherished personal values.

Heterosexism has been defined as an ideological system that denies, denigrates, and stigmatizes any nonheterosexual form of behavior, identity, relationship, or community. This system regards heterosexuality as *normal* and *natural* and treats gay and lesbian people as outsiders who are neither. Heterosexism organizes experience from a point of view that naturalizes and idealizes heterosexuality and dismisses or ignores a gay subjectivity. Heterosexist beliefs can serve to enforce the maintenance of *compulsory heterosexuality* in society. Some common expressions of heterosexism include valuing heterosexual relationships over homosexual ones, an intensely felt opposition to gay and lesbian parenting—regardless of individuals' actual parenting qualities—and the belief that lesbians and gay men are unsuited for certain professions. Heterosexist attitudes are pervasive in Western cultures in which most books, plays, movies, and print and television ads contain naturalized depictions of heterosexuality. Heterosexism is not necessarily motivated by fear or hatred; in many ways, it is primarily self-referential. However, in the experience of many gay people, heterosexism is frequently experienced as antihomosexual, which is why it is sometimes confused with homophobia.

Heterosexism does not necessarily imply malice or ill will toward lesbians and gay men. Nevertheless, in extremis, it may equate the nonheterosexual with the immoral and unnatural and can rationalize the condemnation of same-sex feelings and behaviors. *Moral condemnations of homosexuality* treat homosexual acts as intrinsically harmful to the individual, to the individual's spirit, and to the social fabric. Those who condemn same-sex activities believe that heterosexist traditions of philosophical, legal, and religious opposition to homosexuality are, in and of themselves, sufficient reason to forbid its open expression in the modern world. This reasoning led a U.S. Supreme Court majority to uphold the state of Georgia's right to ban same-sex acts in the 1986 case of *Bowers versus Hardwick.* The justices stated that their decision did "not require a judgment on whether laws against sodomy are wise or desirable" but was based on the "ancient roots" of proscriptions against consensual homosexual activity and a long-standing condemnation of those practices in "Judeo-Christian" moral and ethical standards. This decision justified the censure of homosexuality in the present, because it has been censured in the past, and argued that antihomosexual laws are permissible, because they have always existed. Ironically, more than a decade later, that same statute was overturned by the Georgia Supreme Court in the case of a heterosexual, male defendant accused of engaging in so-called unnatural sexual practices with a woman. However, in 2003, the U.S. Supreme Court reversed its own 1986 ruling in the case of *Lawrence and Garner versus Texas*, declaring that state sodomy laws were unconstitutional.

Many contemporary, antihomosexual religious authorities speak of embracing the homosexual person but not the person's homosexuality. This antihomosexual attitude is sometimes referred to as *loving the sinner and hating the sin.* It derives from a cultural belief that one *chooses* to be *a homosexual* despite social and biblical prohibitions. Antihomosexual religious authorities believe that sinners can be saved and that there is a duty to care about those who make immoral choices. It should be underscored that *choice* has become a charged word in the moral debates surrounding homosexuality. For example, at the other end of this cultural debate, gay people believe that they *choose* to act on their homoerotic feelings to avoid the choice of suffering in the closet.

Antihomosexual attitudes—in the form of homophobia, heterosexism, and moral condemnations of homosexuality—serve to shape important aspects of development and day-to-day experience in the lives of lesbians and gay men. Antihomosexual attitudes can ultimately lead to *antigay* or *antilesbian violence*. Even in the absence of overt violence, however, antihomosexual attitudes impinge on the completion of normative developmental tasks in some gay men and lesbians and may delay or prevent successful adaptation and achievement of an integrated sense of self. The psychiatrist can be helpful by recognizing the influence of these factors on the personalities and experiences of gay, lesbian, and bisexual persons and by carefully identifying their intrapsychic and interpersonal impact. It is also reasonable for psychiatrists and other clinicians to acknowledge the everyday dangers that gay men and lesbians face or may have faced. If a gay person has been assaulted, that experience is internalized, and working through that trauma is inevitably part of any therapy that might be undertaken. Even if they have not been physically assaulted themselves, gay men and lesbians are sensitized to the ways in which members of the dominant culture, in positions of authority or on its margins, feel that they can make threats and do as they please. In addition, many individuals have had verbal assaults directed against them for being gay or lesbian. For some, experiences of verbal abuse can have traumatic consequences as well. A psychiatrist can be most helpful by being sensitive to patient anxieties regarding antihomosexual attitudes, as gay patients can be retraumatized when clinicians deny or minimize the extent to which the phenomenon colors their lives and affects their self-esteem. Finally, in this culture, antihomosexual attitudes are ubiquitous, and no one is free of them, not even psychiatrists. This obliges clinicians to understand and to be aware of the ways in which these attitudes may have affected the development of their own identities and belief systems. Such awareness can help psychiatrists come to a greater empathic appreciation of the impact of antihomosexual attitudes on the gay, lesbian, or bisexual patient whom they are treating.

Coming Out and Meaning of Disclosure

Coming out, previously defined as the process of recognizing one's homosexuality and disclosing it to oneself and to others, is an essential concept in understanding the lives of lesbians, gay men, and bisexual persons. Coming out, however, is not synonymous with identity development. One way of understanding the difference between these two concepts is to view coming out as one part of a process whose outcome may lead to forming a lesbian or gay identity. Behaviors associated with coming out reflect underlying cognitive and affective transformations that occur as part of identity development. Thus, coming out to oneself—a subjective experience of inner recognition that previously unacceptable feelings or desires are part of one's self—may facilitate disclosure of these feelings to others in the hope of finding social reinforcement and support. Some gay men and lesbians may only come out in certain spheres of their lives, for example, within friendship groups, but remain closeted in other areas, such as in the work setting or within families.

An extensive literature on coming out views the process as the most basic and clear expression of being openly gay or lesbian. Coming out is usually contrasted with remaining in the closet or hiding one's homosexuality from oneself or from others. Historically, early gay liberation publications portrayed the distinction between coming out and being closeted as a political struggle between liberation and oppression. In the social science literature, *coming out* has been defined as a psychological and social process that can help the gay person to overcome self-hatred and other adverse effects of internalized homophobia.

Coming out is an ongoing process, because gay and lesbian persons must repeatedly choose whether to inform others of their identity. People are generally assumed to be heterosexual, unless they declare themselves to be otherwise. Usually, disclosure of one's homosexuality involves *telling* someone else that one is gay or lesbian or *displaying* some commonly accepted signal of a homosexual identity. Adoption of certain styles of dress or behavior, residence in neighborhoods in which other gay men and lesbians live, entrance into gay and lesbian communities, and involvement in relationships with persons of the same sex may serve to confirm the identity of a gay or lesbian person. For some, these activities are signifiers of coming out, performed to show others that one is gay or lesbian. However, it should also be noted that many young people with stable, heterosexual identities often play with gender ambiguity. Nontraditional gender performances are not necessarily a sign of homosexuality, and interpreting them superficially may lead to confusion about or an inaccurate assessment of a person's actual sexual orientation.

Most empirical studies of coming out describe the ages at which gay men have reported events associated with coming out; fewer studies report on the process for lesbians. However, those studies show, in general, that women, when compared to men, tend to have first sexual experiences and to come out later. Younger lesbians may experience stronger prohibitions against coming out because of intense expectations of heterosexual dating for women. More recent studies have also suggested that coming out, much like the age of the first sexual experience, is occurring at progressively earlier ages among adolescents and that there is significant variation in the process based on a variety of factors in addition to sex, such as socioeconomic status, education, and ethnicity. The study of various cultures also demonstrates variation in the coming out process based on the degree of sexual restrictiveness of a society.

Coming out is a complicated process that involves internal and external dimensions, occurs across a lifetime, and may vary in different domains of a person's life. Coming out can mean increased comfort with one's own feelings, and this is integral to social and psychological development. Greater ease in expressing one's feelings, to oneself and to others, can lead to enrichment of work and relationships. The clinician should also be aware that even persons who appear to be gay or lesbian may have never verbally disclosed their sexual orientation and that others who provide no stereotypical indications of being gay or lesbian may have disclosed their identity to most of their family, friends, and coworkers. Some persons who are fully aware of their homosexuality may never disclose this fact to others. Furthermore, the time frame between awareness of same-sex attraction and self-labeling as gay or lesbian may range from less than 1 year to decades. Psychiatrists should understand that each individual's coming out process is unique and multidimensional.

Impact of Diversity

Homosexuality and its various forms of expression develop in relation to other aspects of the self, which are influenced by a variety of individual and group characteristics. Commensurate with their presence in the general population, lesbians and gay men can be found in those groups defined by race, religion, ethnicity, age, and class. Their experiences as gay men and lesbians, however, may be significantly shaped by membership in these other groups. For example, being an older woman of color in a long-term relationship with another woman generally leads to a completely different identity construction than that of a young, Latino gay man. Thus, understanding the development and experiences of lesbians, gay men, and bisexuals often requires appreciation of their multiple affiliations and identifications, including, but not limited to, their sexual orientation. Membership in these other groups may involve additional experiences of discrimination, not only from members of the racial, ethnic, or religious majority, but also from heterosexual members of one's own minority group. For some lesbians and gay men, identification with another group may be a more important determinant of their identity than their sexual orientation. It is helpful for the psychiatrist to understand the diverse meanings of sexual orientation within these groups.

Sex and Gender

Kinsey remarked that "although there can be no objection to designating relations between females by a special term [lesbian], it should be recognized that such activities are quite the equivalent of sexual relations between males." Yet, the most important group characteristic affecting different expressions of sexual orientation is biological sex. Men and women have different experiences of being homosexual, because sex and gender are profound determinants of identity. In some cases, sexism, or prejudice against women, can have as much or more of an impact on a lesbian's development as antihomosexual attitudes. Consider, as well, that the existing body of research and theory about homosexuality focuses largely on homosexuality in men and may have much less relevance for lesbians. Therefore, although lesbians and gay men may share common psychological qualities and interests, this assumption must be tempered with the recognition that lesbian psychology and development may relate as much to female development as it does to the psychology of gay men.

Growing up as a boy or girl in Western society influences the experience of sexuality and sexual orientation in two general ways. The first is through the development of different gender characteristics associated with men and women. The second is through differing expectations for men and women, expectations that may limit women's choices or may lead to sex discrimination. Gender socialization of boys and girls profoundly influences the quality of their social interactions, and, as a result, men and women generally behave in different ways. Consequently, a variety of features of same-sex relationships are influenced by the gender characteristics of the partners. When compared to heterosexuals, however, gay men and lesbians may conform less to traditional gender stereotypes and may express more variability in their manifestations of gender-related characteristics.

As previously stated, gay men and lesbians have been historically portrayed as persons with the gender characteristics of the other biological sex. Another disproved historical assumption is that same-sex couples divide up the stereotypical roles of heterosexual couples, with one partner playing the role of the man and the other the role of the woman. In fact, there is a wide range of gender attributes in gay men and lesbians, and gay relationships are as varied as those of heterosexuals. The psychiatrist working with gay men, lesbians, and bisexuals should appreciate the significant role of gender socialization in shaping the personalities of all men and women. It is important to consider the effect of this socialization on gay men and lesbians and on the dynamics of their relationships. It is also helpful to assess the specific gender-related issues that might be present for a particular individual or couple. It is also generally helpful to set aside preconceived notions of any patient's gender role characteristics, regardless of their sexual identity.

Age and Generation

The age at which an individual came out, the era during which he or she grew up, and the length of time since he or she came out significantly affect his or her experiences of being gay, lesbian, or bisexual. Comparisons between a 50-year-old man or woman who came out at 20 years of age, a 50-year-old person who came out at 45 years of age, and a young person coming out today are inevitably different and reveal vastly different external reactions to their homosexuality. Generally, older lesbians and gay men were confronted with much more social disapproval of their homosexuality than are young people today. Those who remain closeted during their adolescence and much of their adulthood generally feel a greater sense of loss in relation to their homosexuality than those who come out and establish a gay or lesbian identity at an earlier age.

A person's age does not necessarily tell much about his or her gay or lesbian identity. There are disparities between people of similar ages who came out relatively earlier and later. These disparities reflect not only changes in social responses to homosexuality during different historical periods, but also the interaction between an individual's developmental maturation and the acquirement of a gay or lesbian identity. For example, the impact of coming out is different for the individual who establishes an openly gay or lesbian identity before involvement in an intimate, primary same-sex relationship than it is for someone who comes out after being involved with another person in a heterosexual relationship; the impact of coming out is altogether different for someone who has avoided any expression of same-sex intimacy out of fear of being identified as gay or lesbian. In addition to diverse developmental factors, in American society, differing historical periods have been characterized by different kinds of responses to homosexuality. The shift in the last 30 years has been from the invisibility of gay people to the creation of increasing numbers of social structures and organizations available to them. Access to these structures and organizations varies considerably as a function not only of the historical period, but also of the chronological age and geographical location of the individual. In addition, many settings and groups within the gay and lesbian community are age specific and may not be welcoming to persons who are older or struggling with their sexual identity.

The psychiatrist should carefully evaluate the influences of age and generation on the individual gay man, lesbian, or bisexual. Most young people growing up gay or lesbian today are exposed to a vastly different set of social depictions of homosexuality than people who came of age decades ago. Today's portrayals of homosexuality are not always affirmative and may, in fact, arise from sources that are disapproving of gay and lesbian people. Nevertheless, where once silence and invisibility prevailed, there is now a much greater public discussion of homosexuality and a greater visibility of possible role models for young people. In addition, many high schools and universities provide space for clubs, gay or gay-straight alliances, as supervised settings for young people. In contrast, an older person who struggles with coming out today often has more deeply ingrained internalized homophobia with which to contend. Paradoxically, for some older people, increased gay and lesbian visibility and social supports can lead to increased frustration and lowered self-esteem; their internalized inhibitions not only interfere with their ability to access potential supports but also lead to self-recrimination about their social isolation and inadequacy. Such variable responses must be carefully assessed in doing clinical work with lesbians and gay men of differing ages and of differing developmental pathways.

Race and Ethnicity

When considering a particular race or ethnic background of a gay, lesbian, or bisexual individual, consideration must be given to two additional issues: attitudes within that particular racial or ethnic group toward sexuality and homosexuality and the types of prejudice directed toward that racial or ethnic group by the larger society. These two factors may compound the experiences of stigma and discrimination of gay and lesbian racial and ethnic minority members. For example, a combination of racism in the gay community and homophobia within the African American community may lead to inadequate coping techniques and poor self-concepts among some African American gay men. Finding support within the African American or gay and lesbian communities may be difficult, and integration of potentially conflictual identities based on race and sexual orientation may be an important need for persons from these groups. Similar issues may arise for persons from other racial and ethnic groups. Latino men and Latina women are often influenced by antihomosexual religious attitudes, as well as by traditional, heterosexist gender role and family expectations. Native peoples' concepts of gender, sexuality, and sexual orientation often diverge considerably from European notions of these constructs and may incorporate beliefs about spirituality as well. Because Asian American gay men and lesbians come from many differing cultural groups with diverse attitudes toward homosexuality and gay, lesbian, and bisexual persons, it is impossible to generalize about their experiences. Thus, although membership in a particular group may assist in predicting family, religious, and social reactions to homosexuality, the diversity of backgrounds within many legally designated minority groups requires careful assessment of each individual's experience, degree of cultural identity, and level of acculturation.

The expression of sexual attraction and identity may be strongly influenced by racial and ethnic identity. When these identities are experienced as conflictual, an individual may maintain complete secrecy about homoerotic feelings; may adopt a bisexual, rather than a gay or lesbian, identity; or may feel it necessary to choose between cultural and sexual orientation identities. For some persons, the conflict between identities may lead to profound confusion and alienation from both groups. The integration of potentially oppositional identities may be extremely difficult to achieve, and the difficulty of this struggle must be appreciated and understood by psychiatrists who work among multicultural gay and lesbian populations.

Religion The impact of religion on the lives of gay men and lesbians reflects its importance in an individual's history and in society at large. Individuals from different religious backgrounds may have had exposure to a wide range of attitudes toward homosexuality, and they may maintain ties to the religions of their families of origin. At a social level, religion influences gay men and lesbians who belong to religious groups that present supportive, tolerant, or disapproving views of homosexuality. Religion also has an impact on all gay and lesbian persons, because it contributes to shaping cultural and political attitudes toward homosexuality. Many gay men and lesbians attempt to avoid disapproving or condemnatory religious teachings about homosexuality by eschewing any contact with organized religion; others work within their religious groups to try to change traditional, unaccepting attitudes about homosexuality; still others stay attached to, while perhaps feeling powerless to change, religions that reinforce their own antihomosexual attitudes. Many gay men and lesbians have actively sought a reconciliation between their sexual identity and their spirituality within traditional religious groups; some have been successful in doing so. Others have moved to create new churches and spiritual settings that affirm their sexual identities and their relationships.

Increasingly, religious institutions within American society have been forced to deal with the meanings of homosexuality, as a personal issue for their members and as an issue of ongoing theological contention. A growing number of religious groups have moved toward positions that tolerate or actively embrace gay men and lesbians; some are ordaining priests, ministers, and rabbis. Other, socially conservative, religious organizations have loudly reaffirmed their traditional opposition to open expressions of homosexuality. They criticize the morality not only of individuals who adopt gay, lesbian, and bisexual identities, but also of the heterosexual individuals who accept those identities as well. Regardless of one's personal relationship to religion or one's involvement with a specific religious group, all gay men and lesbians are profoundly affected by religious teachings and beliefs about homosexuality.

Disapproving religious views of homosexuality often become internalized in lesbians and gay men and may have an effect on their psychosexual development, particularly inhibiting sexual expression and the development of relationships. Religious beliefs that disapprove of homosexuality constitute substantive, ongoing themes in psychotherapy with some gay and lesbian patients. Many of these themes are intertwined with issues regarding family relationships, particularly in gay men and lesbians who have had strict, fundamentalist, or orthodox religious upbringings. Gay men and lesbians who grow up in communities in which social and religious activities are deeply intertwined may stop participating in religious activities and may become estranged from their families. They may be deeply concerned about the moral implications of being gay or lesbian and about their alienation from their co-religionists. Spiritual development itself may be affected by an inability to reconcile the conflicting internal and external messages concerning the erotic and spiritual aspects of the self. Gay men and women who are able to overcome disapproving, religiously based self-evaluations may nevertheless find it difficult to be comfortable with their sexual identity. Even when faced with denigrating judgments of their homosexuality, some individuals may not be able to disengage, nor do they wish to disengage, from their religions. Many others struggle to establish a connection to a different, more affirming spiritual community. The psychiatrist working with gay men and lesbians must understand the important need felt by some gay and lesbian persons to resolve these dilemmas without totally cutting themselves off from their religious groups or families. As the desire to retain connections to such groups can be strong, it is essential to provide ongoing support for those individuals who are unable to extricate themselves from this situation. Even when a separation occurs, psychological sequelae may interfere with the integration of spirituality and sexuality. As a consequence, conflicts between religion and sexuality are usually an important focus in clinical work with religious lesbians and gay men.

Interaction of Sexual Orientation with Stage of Development

Having a homosexual orientation leads to a variety of tasks, challenges, and opportunities for gay men and lesbians at different points in their lives. The factors involved include an individual's level of biological and psychosocial maturation, as well as where the individual is in the process of coming out and of acquiring a gay or lesbian identity. In general, many of the psychosocial and physical issues confronting gay men and lesbians during different developmental stages are the same as those for heterosexual persons. However, there are issues specific to being gay or lesbian that occur during childhood, adolescence, young adulthood, mid-life, and old age. Developmental tasks across the life cycle do not take place at the same age for all persons. Nevertheless, most gay men and lesbians have to confront certain tasks during each stage of development.

Childhood Based on retrospective accounts from adults, children who grow up to be gay or lesbian often struggle with feelings of being different; for some of these children, there is an additional and perhaps related issue of atypical gender role behavior. Feeling different can lead to a sense of alienation that may result in social isolation. Boys who are not stereotypically masculine may be shunned, humiliated, and derided by their peers in school and other social settings, leading to future difficulties with self-esteem. Girls are less subject to this process, as tomboy behaviors in girls are usually better tolerated than so-called effeminacy in boys. Nevertheless, children with gender-atypical behavior are often criticized or otherwise devalued within their own families and, sometimes, even by mental health professionals. Some parents may forcefully try to shape developmental outcomes toward more typical gender role behaviors in their children. Others may ignore or distance themselves from children who fail to conform to parental expectations of conventional, heterosexual development. These experiences can lead children who grow up to be gay to internalize the rejecting reactions of others as they come to devalue aspects of their selves that they associate with atypical sexuality and gender. In cases in which this process is accompanied by incidents of overt discrimination or violence, the child may experience adult impairment in the capacity for psychological, social, and work adaptation.

Adolescence Adolescence is a particularly vulnerable time for most young people. It is during this period that they must establish a coherent identity, separate from their families of origin, and practice patterns of relating and working that are further developed in early adulthood. Many gay and lesbian youth first become aware of their same-sex attraction during puberty, when they begin to mature physically. Again, from retrospective accounts, gay and lesbian adults often recall a budding cognitive awareness of their same-sex attractions during adolescence. Most gay and lesbian youth are involved in heterosexual relationships during this time. However, some of them may enter the early stages of establishing a gay or lesbian identity, as they begin to have affectionate and physical relationships with persons of the same sex. Some adolescents may go on to develop connections with community structures, such as gay-straight alliances, gay and lesbian youth groups, and adult gay and lesbian community centers. These activities can be inhibited or facilitated by the reactions of families, relatives, teachers, religious leaders, and peers.

Most gay and lesbian adolescents, consciously or unconsciously, delay some aspect of the development of their sexual identity until they are older. Often, they obtain a greater degree of safety and support by going away to school, by moving to an urban environment that allows more anonymity and acceptance, or by creating a hometown network of friends who are accepting of a gay or lesbian identity. Some adolescents may suppress any awareness of their same-sex attractions, others may defensively attempt to establish a heterosexual identity and relationships, and still others may consciously avoid any outward display of a gay or lesbian identity. Less often, but with increased frequency in urban settings, gay and lesbian youth may openly identify their sexual orientation at an early age, may disclose their feelings to others, and may complete significant aspects of gay and lesbian identity formation during adolescence. Even outside of urban settings, this process has also been greatly facilitated by access to the Internet, where gay and lesbian youth can more easily find each other. It remains to be seen whether future generations of gay and lesbian youth will follow in the footsteps of an older generation whose members often entered into unsatisfactory heterosexual relationships and eschewed intimate relationships with persons of the same sex out of fear of disclosure of being gay or lesbian.

Despite the rapid social changes taking place, there is still ongoing stigma associated with being gay or lesbian. When there are few adult role models and inadequate resources for support, discrimination and violence are often directed against visible gay and lesbian youth in schools. In the absence of recognition and affirmation from parents and other adult figures in their lives, most pregay and prelesbian adolescents undoubtedly continue to experience significant difficulty in developing a stable gay or lesbian identity. Whatever the setting, the psychiatrist should be aware of these adverse influences for gay and lesbian youth and should be sensitive to the potential effects of these factors on their mental health.

Young Adulthood The period of transition from adolescence to adulthood is a time when many lesbians and gay men have their first opportunity to come out and to establish gay and lesbian identities independent of their families of origin. Gay men and lesbians in their 20s and 30s confront the same developmental tasks as heterosexual peers. These include developing a career, establishing a social identity, developing intimate relationships, and, increasingly for some, raising children. However, for gay men and lesbians, when compared to heterosexual cohorts, these tasks may be accomplished in different ways and at different times than for their heterosexual cohorts. Although heterosexual men and women may be seriously dating, getting engaged, and getting married, closeted gay men and lesbians may be pretending to be heterosexuals as they date members of the other sex. Such hiding activities may cause a delay in the consolidation of an integrated sexual identity. Others may sublimate their sexual energies entirely and may invest greater efforts in careers. The delays and omissions that follow the secrecy surrounding gay adolescence can have developmental consequences. For example, many young gay men and lesbians in their 20s and 30s may appear to behave, from a developmental perspective, more like adolescents. In some urban settings, such individuals form cliques, in groups, and out groups with a strong emphasis on style, conformity to standards of dress, and a hierarchy of popularity based on looks, athleticism, and affability, as well as opportunities for experimentation with sex and drugs. For some individuals, this *delayed gay adolescence* provides opportunities missed when they actually were adolescents: to learn same-sex peer and social skills and to experiment in public enactments of their sexual identities. The psychiatrist should understand that these relational patterns are understandable for those who, in adolescence, had to hide their sexual identities and behaviors.

During early adulthood, many heterosexual persons marry and have children. Gay men and lesbians may also form long-term relationships at this age. Many of them do, in fact, enter into primary relationships at some point. In previous generations, a significant proportion of young adult men and women with same-sex attractions adopted a heterosexual identity and entered into conventional marriages; many of these individuals also had children and raised families. However, more relational options are currently available to gay and lesbian people. These include living in gay communities with supportive friendship networks, forming primary same-sex relationships, and choosing to conceive or to adopt children. Many young gay and lesbian adults experience limitations in their choices as a result of discrimination and the effects of internalized homophobia. Among sexually active gay men, the threat of HIV infection and AIDS has created new barriers to establishing a sense of well-being and to forming intimate relationships.

In the areas of creativity and work, gay men and lesbians may, in some instances, choose careers during early adulthood that tend to assure greater acceptance of their sexual identity. Although gay men and lesbians are employed, whether openly or in secret, in every type of profession, often, they may feel more comfortable working in fields in which they can be visible. Nonetheless, discrimination in hiring and promotion may be a problem for gay men and lesbians, and a lack of legal protection creates considerable work-related stress for many of them.

Middle Life For gay men and lesbians, the mid-life decades of the 40s and 50s are characterized, as they are for heterosexual men and women, by consolidation of career identity, concerns about generativity, emerging problems with one's own health and aging, and care for aging and dying parents. Gay and lesbians baby boomers who are currently in middle age represent the first generation to have openly come out in significant numbers. As a result, new scripts for a modern gay mid-life are still being written.

Mid-life lesbians are considerably more likely to be employed in professional or technical and managerial positions when compared to other women, although their incomes are not always commensurate with their level of experience. Lesbians and gay men may have to struggle with integration of their identities into the workplace, and many are confronted with limitations on their advancement at work because of antihomosexual discrimination.

Many lesbians and gay men have begun raising children in mid-life. These children may come from a previous heterosexual marriage, or they may be adopted or conceived by a single gay parent or two people in a committed same-sex relationship. As many of these parents may not receive the same support from their extended families as their heterosexual cohorts, they may often rely much more heavily on friendship networks and paid child care.

Gay men and lesbians share the same mid-life health concerns as their heterosexual cohorts. Some, however, may receive suboptimal health care, because they fear disclosing their sexual orientation to health care providers. As a result of high rates of HIV infection, a large number of gay men are confronted during mid-life with issues of death and dying. Increasingly, as HIV treatments become more effective, many gay men find themselves living with a chronic illness that creates its own ongoing uncertainties about one's health status.

Old Age Individuals who are 60 years of age or older have a wide range of experiences in relation to aging; some develop serious illnesses and become incapacitated, whereas others live healthy lives for several more decades. In addition, the commercial worship of youth often tends to stigmatize all elderly people. All older persons need to deal with the approach of death. Yet, older gay men and lesbians face additional concerns. For example, they must confront a widespread stereotype that older gay people are always lonely and unhappy. Studies, however, have shown older gay men and lesbians to be as well adjusted as their heterosexual counterparts. In addition, they may sometimes be better able than younger gay people to contend with the critical reactions to their sexual identities, as they may no longer be concerned about disclosure at work, or they may have come to accept their sexuality.

The best predictors of psychological adjustment in older gay men appear to be a stable sexual identity and integration into a gay community. Older gay men generally prefer to associate with their age peers, and many of them report being in relationships. A large majority of older gay men and lesbians report being happy, deny significant concerns about loneliness or fear of death, and describe good integration into social networks.

Specific problems for older gay men and lesbians include a lack of adequate resources, a widespread reluctance to disclose one's homosexual orientation to health care and other providers, and an almost total invisibility regarding the needs of older gay and lesbian persons, whether single or in relationships, within institutions and agencies that provide care for the aged. Failing to recognize older gay men and lesbians is a function of the denial of sexuality in older people in general and an unwillingness to recognize relationships that are not legally sanctioned. Same-sex partners and gay and lesbian friends may often be excluded from health care settings, which may significantly compromise the quality of life and the care received by the older gay or lesbian patient. In some cases, this may reawaken old psychological wounds. It is always helpful for the psychiatrist working with older gay and lesbian patients to acknowledge and to affirm their sexual identities, as well as their partnerships and friendships.

Families and Relationships

Gay, lesbian, and bisexual persons usually grow up in families that do not acknowledge or affirm their children's emerging homosexual attractions or provide them with positive, adult gay and lesbian role models. Those who come out as adults often do not find acceptance from their families of origin. In some cases, they do not come out to their families at all. Consequently, many single gay men and lesbians often create what have been called *families of choice* or friendship networks. These provide interpersonal bonds, acceptance, adult friendships, and resources unobtainable from their families of origin. Many gay men and lesbians go on to form new family structures in their ongoing, romantic same-sex relationships, long-term cohabiting relationships, and single or coparent households with children. The findings from a growing body of research have begun to describe these couples and families.

Families of Choice

Many gay men and lesbians grow up in families that ignore, disapprove, or openly denigrate their homosexual feelings and emerging identities; some report significant physical and emotional harm in families who condemn their homosexual orientation. The reactions of parents and other family members to a young person coming out, whether deliberately or inadvertently, can significantly influence the self-esteem and self-acceptance of gay and lesbian youth. It may irreparably shape the young person's expectations of acceptance or rejection by others outside the family. In the past, gay and lesbian youth could expect no more than tolerance within their families; few would receive active acceptance or empathic support for the experiences and concerns that occur in relation to their emerging sexualities. Greater social acceptance of homosexuality appears to be changing some parents' attitudes toward an increasing acceptance of their gay and lesbian children, but this is still a distinctly minority position.

Consequently, once most gay and lesbian young people achieve sufficient separation from their families of origin, they often create networks of friends and acquaintances who provide them with the support and respect they lacked or were denied within their families. For a single gay or lesbian person, families of choice are extremely important; they serve the functions of an extended family. They may help a person pass through developmental crises, are present at celebrations and rituals, and provide a source of comfort and intimacy. In a community that, until recently, has had little recognition of their primary affectionate relationships, these friendships may even be more enduring than romantic relationships, and some even take on greater day-to-day importance than a lover or partner in the life of a particular gay man or lesbian. Understanding and accepting the importance of these friendship networks are essential for the clinician working with gay and lesbian individuals.

Couples

In 2003, the Supreme Judicial Court of Massachusetts ruled that the state had no legal basis for denying marriage rights to same-sex couples. Consequently, at the time of this writing, same-sex marriage has become a contentious social and legal issue in the United States. Although the 1996 Federal Defense of Marriage Act (DOMA) already defines marriage as a union only between people of different sexes, the issue of adopting a constitutional amendment to ban same-sex marriage is being debated intensively in all public and legal forums. Only one state—Vermont—recognizes same-sex civil unions, although California passed a broad domestic partnership law in 2003. According to Human Rights Watch, same-sex marriage is now legal in several Canadian provinces, Belgium, and the Netherlands; several Western European countries (Croatia, Denmark, Finland, France, Germany, Hungary, Iceland, Norway, Portugal, Sweden, and Switzerland) offer some form of same-sex civil union. Despite these severe legal restrictions, many gay men and women nevertheless choose to live in enduring relationships. A majority report being in a committed romantic relationship, with surveys indicating that 45 to 80 percent of lesbians and 40 to 60 percent of gay men are in such relationships. From 8 to 14 percent of lesbian couples and from 18 to 25 percent of gay male couples report that they have lived together for more than 10 years. The growing research on gay and lesbian couples reveals several findings. First, lesbian couples tend to be more sexually exclusive than male couples. When compared with heterosexual couples, gay male couples and, even more so, lesbian couples have more equality in their relationships and do not divide household duties based on gender stereotypes. Gay men and lesbians report the same degree of global satisfaction in their relationships as heterosexual men and women.

Gay and Lesbian Parents and Their Children

Many lesbians and gay men have had children. In the past, this usually took place within a heterosexual marriage that ended when a closeted gay or lesbian partner came out. However, the 1990s saw the start of a gay baby boom in which single or coupled gay men and lesbians began raising children they adopted or conceived through alternative insemination (using known or unknown donors) or surrogacy. Consequently, in recent years, there has been a greater visibility of families with gay and lesbian parents, and many younger gay men and lesbians today seriously consider the option of having children.

There are numerous studies that describe the characteristics of gay and lesbian families and the impact of having a gay or lesbian parent on children. This research was initially undertaken in the late 1970s to evaluate antihomosexual psychological and judicial beliefs about the presumed harm done to children raised by gay and lesbian parents. For example, it was not uncommon—and, in some states, it is still common—to award custody of children to a nongay parent in a divorce if the other parent comes out as gay or lesbian. These custody decisions were not based on results of empirical studies but on the belief that gay parents were, by nature, unfit or would influence the eventual sexual identity of their own children. However, an overwhelming body of research findings shows that having a lesbian or gay parent has no adverse psychological consequences for children, nor does having a gay or lesbian parent influence the eventual gender identity, gender role, or sexual orientation of children when compared to the children of heterosexual parents. In addition, studies show that children with two parents do better than children with one parent, regardless of the sexual orientation of the parent.

These early studies did reveal some differences. The children of divorced lesbian mothers had much more contact with their fathers and a great deal more contact with men than the children of divorced, heterosexual mothers. The lesbian mothers made greater efforts to be sure that their children had male companionship, because they did not intend to remarry, as did the heterosexual mothers. Gay and lesbian parents and their children also have to confront the fact of being different from heterosexual families and may experience stigma or antihomosexual bias as a result. In addition, the ability of both same-sex parents to be legally recognized as parents is prohibited in most states. Consequently, the children in families with same-sex parents are often denied parental benefits from one of the partners, including clear inheritance rights, death benefits, or the right to be covered by a nonbiological parent's health insurance. In response to the needs of these children, in 2001, the American Academy of Pediatrics issued a position statement in support of legal adoption by a second same-sex parent. The psychiatrist treating the children or parents in gay-parented families should be aware of the complex social barriers that they often face.

CLINICAL APPROACHES

In most circumstances, the psychiatric issues of lesbians, gay men, and bisexuals resemble those of the general population, and the clinical work, including assessment and treatment, is like that done with other patients. In addition, the psychiatrist should also be aware of unique aspects of the clinical work with this patient population.

General Considerations

Some mental health professionals, including psychiatrists, continue to believe that homosexuality is associated with mental illness and dysfunction, report feelings of discomfort with gay and lesbian individuals, and admit to varying degrees of bias toward these men and women. Some even engage in attempts to change a person's homosexual orientation. Because they have encountered disapproval, discrimination, insensitivity to their concerns, or even abusive treatment within clinical settings, many gay, lesbian, and bisexual patients are reluctant to disclose their sexual orientation or even to enter treatment without some clear demonstration by the clinician of a nonjudgmental and accepting attitude. Because medical doctors have been strongly identified with heterosexual authority, psychiatrists—in comparison to psychologists and social workers—were often perceived as the mental health professionals least likely to accept a gay man or lesbian's sexual identity. This perception appears to be changing, particularly with the increased visibility of openly gay and lesbian psychiatrists. Regardless of the psychiatrist's own sexual identity, optimal evaluation and treatment require a respectful and thorough assessment of all aspects of sexual orientation, a potentially volatile and painful topic.

Inclusive and Special Clinical Settings

Gay men and lesbians are usually treated in the same inpatient, outpatient, and residential clinical settings as other patients. In recent years, a small number of specialized units have been developed for working with gay, lesbian, and bisexual persons—community health centers intended to serve the needs of the local lesbian and gay communities or units geared toward particular problems, such as HIV infection or substance abuse. Whether services are provided in general or specialized settings, staff should be trained in the delivery of sensitive and unbiased care to gay men and lesbians. Such training should include knowledge about the special concerns of this population.

The clinical setting and staff with whom the patient comes into contact are important determinants in creating a climate of inclusiveness for gay, lesbian, and bisexual patients. Explicit and implicit communications of acceptance in these settings can ensure successful psychiatric treatment. For example, the language and behavior of psychiatrists and other staff should convey that they do not presume that all individuals and families are heterosexual. Questions about relationships should be open ended and nonjudgmental when inquiring about the sex of a patient's partner. One should not assume that all married persons are heterosexual or sexually exclusive with their spouses. Questions regarding sexuality should distinguish between desire, behavior, and identity. The presence of gay-friendly publications in the waiting area and self-reporting forms for patients that neutrally inquire about diverse sexual orientations and family arrangements can help reassure a gay, lesbian, or bisexual person—as well as those uncertain about their sexual orientation—of acceptance in this clinical setting and that they can talk openly about their concerns.

Another important strategy in clinical work with gay and lesbian patients is to routinely include, when appropriate, references to significant friends and members of nontraditional families during evaluation and treatment. When necessary, same-sex partners and children in these families should be involved in the care of gay and lesbian patients. For example, it may be important to obtain corroborative information from partners, to identify potential sources of a patient's problems within the context of the couple or family, or to include a partner in maintaining compliance. In addition, issues of confidentiality and decision making in working with heterosexual families should also apply to working with gay and lesbian families.

Sexual Orientation of the Psychiatrist

The impact of the psychiatrist's sexual orientation and the impact of disclosing this orientation to the patient are complex. The heterosexist assumption that everyone is heterosexual usually means that a psychiatrist's sexual orientation does not come up in treating most patients. However, this assumption does not hold when treating a gay, lesbian, or bisexual patient. A heterosexual psychiatrist trained to be nondisclosing may refuse to answer questions about his or her sexual orientation and may turn the question back on the patient. In general, this would be a technical error with many gay, lesbian, and bisexual patients, as it would generally be taken to mean that the psychiatrist is not entirely comfortable speaking about sexual identities.

When the lesbian or gay patient works with a psychiatrist who is openly gay or lesbian, there are several possible benefits and risks to self-disclosure. The benefits of working with a psychiatrist of the same sexual orientation may include an easier rapport, greater efficiency resulting from shared knowledge about experiences associated with being lesbian or gay, and affirmative role modeling when a therapist has established a secure gay or lesbian identity. Possible risks for such therapeutic dyads include unwarranted assumptions about shared experiences or personal characteristics based on sexual orientation alone, transferential or countertransferential overidentification of the therapist or patient with each other, and a shared, unconscious collusion to avoid discussing painful events or affects associated with gay or lesbian development.

How a gay or lesbian psychiatrist's sexual orientation is disclosed to a patient may vary. Sometimes the patient has requested to work with an openly gay or lesbian therapist and has this knowledge before beginning treatment. In other cases, this information becomes known after treatment has begun, as the result of self-disclosure by the psychiatrist or through some outside source. When self-disclosure is involved, the timing of the disclosure may have a significant impact on facilitating or inhibiting the work in therapy. In some cases, it may have no effect at all. It is useful for the gay or lesbian psychiatrist to be able to identify those individuals and the clinical situations in which working with an openly gay or lesbian therapist might be most helpful.

In general, the psychiatrist's sexual orientation should not be the most significant factor in determining clinical outcomes. Any therapist working with gay men and lesbians needs to maintain conscious awareness of his or her own antihomosexual attitudes and heterosexist assumptions; to possess a reasonable knowledge base about lesbian, gay, and bisexual issues; to apply gay-sensitive and gay-affirmative approaches to psychotherapy; and to obtain adequate supervision, peer supervision, or outside consultation when necessary.

Sexual orientation may be far less significant than other personal characteristics in determining the effectiveness of a psychiatrist in working with gay, lesbian, and bisexual patients. A gay or lesbian therapist who has not fully come out or established a comfortable identity may have trouble working with patients struggling with similar concerns. A therapist of any sexual orientation who is uncomfortable talking about sexual problems has more trouble being helpful to gay and lesbian patients with a sexual concern. Ultimately, the degree of empathy experienced and expressed by the therapist for the patient is, in most cases, an important factor in determining the effectiveness of treatment.

Assessment of Sexual Orientation

Sexual orientation is multifaceted, and there are a variety of scales that can be useful in its assessment. However, when undertaken at all, an assessment often does not go beyond designating a person as *homosexual*, *bisexual*, or, less commonly, *heterosexual*, which is usually assumed unless otherwise stated. Existing assessment scales look at different components of sexual orientation, including desire, behavior, and identity, and evaluate the relative degree of each component. Additional variables may include changes over time in an individual's sexual orientation, social and emotional preference for one gender or the other, lifestyle choices, and gender role identity. Sexological research regarding sexual orientation may involve psychophysiological quantification of sexual attraction through techniques such as penile and vaginal plethysmography.

The usefulness to the individual psychiatrist of these assessments depends on the extent to which information about a patient's sexual orientation may be relevant to the ongoing treatment. In any event, an assessment of sexual orientation along several dimensions can help in better understanding the meaning and purpose of sexuality in an individual's life. In making these assessments, it is important for the psychiatrist to individualize his or her approach to patients. Among other things, this means avoiding superficial responses to patients who come in anxiously questioning whether they are gay, straight, or bisexual. For example, although some questioning patients may be confused about their sexual identities, they can readily describe their sexual behaviors and fantasies. Such incongruities between a patient's desire, behavior, and identity are not uncommon, nor are they necessarily psychopathological. Instead, they usually reflect the complex processes involved in integrating a gay identity within a cultural milieu that disapproves of homosexuality.

In evaluating sexual orientation, the psychiatrist must balance the need to obtain relevant information with sensitivity and tact about inquiring into an area in which a patient may feel vulnerable or defensive. It is helpful to approach a patient's sexual orientation not solely as a sexual matter, but as a factor that involves relational patterns, family structures, friendship and support networks, and community and cultural activities in which he or she is participating. The consideration of each of these psychosocial dimensions can facilitate therapeutic rapport.

Special Concerns

There are certain concerns that are unique to lesbians, gay men, and bisexuals. The presentation of other concerns that do not directly relate to sexual orientation may also be shaped by the fact that a person is gay, lesbian, or bisexual, and, for some persons, being a member of a sexual minority group may interfere with, and even prevent, interactions with the health care system.

Societal and Domestic Violence

The problem of *antigay* or *antilesbian violence* is widespread. In 1990, the federal government passed a law ordering a study of hate crimes, including attacks on gay men and women, the first time a federal, U.S. civil rights' law covered sexual orientation. Gay bashing is a common form of violence in which gangs of young men descend on neighborhoods in which gay people meet. Armed with bats, clubs, or other weapons, they attack anyone they believe to be gay. The most sensational case of antigay violence in the United States was the death of Matthew Shepard, a young man from Wyoming, who was killed because he was gay by two other young men in 1998. The trial of his killers, as well as increasing publicity surrounding gay-bashing incidents in general, has provoked the open articulation of previously unspoken cultural beliefs. One of these is the belief that violence is an excusable response to an unwanted sexual advance from a gay man. Another is that gay people are responsible for provoking any violence that occurs as a response to coming out. Gay men and lesbians who have been the objects of violence or sexual or domestic abuse may have difficulties in reporting their experiences and seeking help; they often fear disclosing their sexual identities or receiving judgmental responses—even harassment—from police or social service workers.

Antigay violence appears to be an underreported phenomenon, because its victims are often reluctant to come forward and to face reprisals from the authorities to whom such incidents are reported. It has also been argued that antigay violence is the inevitable outgrowth of the unexamined beliefs associated with homophobia, heterosexism, and moral condemnations of homosexuality. Thus, those who marginalize homosexuality may be directly or indirectly responsible for the brutality aimed at gay men and lesbians. Inevitably, gay men and lesbians may have legitimate concerns about potential physical attacks. The problem of violence directed against lesbians and gay men is widespread and well documented and ranges from verbal abuse to homicide. Violence against gay people may be committed by strangers, family members, gangs, fellows soldiers within the military, and, sometimes, authority figures, such as the police.

Although some therapists believe that childhood sexual abuse causes homosexuality, studies show no causal connection between the phenomenon and the adult development of a gay, lesbian, or bisexual identity. Studies show that sexual abuse of gay men and lesbians during childhood appears to occur at approximately the same rate as in the general population. Studies of domestic violence and abuse in lesbian and gay male relationships demonstrate that physical abuse occurs at approximately the same rate as in heterosexual relationships.

The impact of violence on gay men and lesbians, as on other victims of violence, includes posttraumatic stress disorder (PTSD), depression, and a range of other psychological and emotional problems. These include feelings of inadequacy, embarrassment, or shame. In addition, there may be specific symptoms associated with being part of a stigmatized minority group. For example, the victims of antigay or antilesbian violence may hold themselves responsible and may believe that their homosexuality caused the assault. The experience of violence can lead an individual to deny a gay or lesbian identity and to avoid other gay and lesbian individuals. The psychiatrist should be prepared to respond to the immediate crisis after an incident of abuse or violence, the potential long-term effects of these events on the individual, and the ongoing concerns of all gay men and lesbians about potential violence being directed against them.

Suicide Determining the rate of suicide attempts and completed suicide among lesbian, gay, and bisexual persons is difficult. Factors complicating this research include the absence of information identifying sexual orientation on death certificates, the reluctance of many individuals distressed about their same-sex feelings to discuss them with mental health professionals, an inadequate assessment of sexual orientation in most health care settings, and the inability to obtain representative samples. In spite of methodological difficulties, results from recent studies suggest that gay, lesbian, or bisexual youth have an increased risk for attempted suicide. Among all youth, regardless of sexual orientation, young women are more at risk for attempting suicide, and young men are at greater risk for completing suicide. Suicide rates among gay, lesbian, and bisexual youth may also vary on the basis of other risk factors, such as mental illness, substance abuse, rejection by family, and, perhaps, degree of gender role nonconformity. It has also been suggested that, for all age groups, an increased risk of suicide may accompany struggles with internalized homophobia, problems with coming out, and difficulty in establishing a firm gay, lesbian, or bisexual identity.

Determination of the exact numbers of gay, lesbian, bisexual, or uncertain people who attempt or complete suicide may be less important than understanding the characteristics that contribute to a risk for suicide. For gay youth, enforced invisibility and a lack of adequate resources to address their physical and mental health needs can prevent adequate assessment of their concerns or can interfere with developing specialized programs for prevention and treatment. In the United States, this problem is exacerbated by the fact that, in a socially conservative political climate, efforts to identify the mental health needs of gay, lesbian, and bisexual individuals are sometimes labeled as an endorsement of homosexuality. This has hindered public funding and research efforts to study suicide among gay, lesbian, and bisexual young people.

Any young person in distress should be carefully evaluated for concerns about sexuality and sexual identity. The psychiatrist should ensure that assessment and treatment do not place young people at further risk of suicide when they disclose their sexual orientation. For example, premature coming out, sometimes precipitated by a conversation with a mental health professional, can increase the possibility of rejection by peers and family. The potential risk of suicide for persons of any age who are struggling with coming out and establishing a gay, lesbian, or bisexual identity should be recognized. Clinical services appropriate for managing suicidal feelings and behaviors and for providing support to suicidal persons should be available as needed.

Alcohol and Substance Abuse Research findings about alcohol and substance abuse in the gay and lesbian community vary considerably. Controlled studies comparing groups of heterosexuals with lesbians and gay men are absent. Nevertheless, alcohol and other substance use and abuse appear to be greater among some segments of the gay and lesbian communities, with an estimated incidence that is perhaps as much as two to three times higher than that of the general population. Some attribute this increased usage to the psychosocial stressors associated with being lesbian, gay, and bisexual. In many cities, bars and clubs in which one can enter freely and anonymously are often the first and only point of entry for some individuals into the wider gay and lesbian community. Although lesbians and gay men are more likely to use or abuse substances at different points in their lives than the general population, they do not appear to have greater rates of drug or alcohol dependency. In general, rates of substance abuse appear to be equally high among lesbians as compared to gay men.

In recent years, recreational or club drugs have become increasingly popular among some segments of the gay and lesbian community. Among these are 3,4-methylenedioxymethamphetamine (MDMA), also known as *Ecstasy*, which can induce depression and panic attacks in those who use it. Ketamine, or *Special K*, is a disassociative anesthetic that induces feelings of unreality and may cause catatonia. γ-Hydroxybutyrate (GHB) is a naturally occurring biological substance whose effects mimic alcohol. In modest doses, it can cause sleep and coma, and, in overdose, some cases have been fatal. The psychiatrist working with gay men and lesbians who are involved in the club scene or circuit parties should be aware of these particular substances and their dangers.

Mood-altering substances are often used to disinhibit prohibitions on sexual expression, and, as a result, many lesbians and gay men begin coming out by using drugs or alcohol. For some people, their gay or lesbian identities are strongly associated with alcohol or substance abuse. Awareness of this linkage is useful in planning adequate approaches when treating substance abuse among gay men, lesbians, and bisexuals. There are numerous specialized programs, inpatient and outpatient, that simultaneously address substance use problems while respecting the sexual identities of gay, lesbian, and bisexual persons. There are also 12-step and other self-help programs that provide special groups for gay men and lesbians that allow for a more comfortable and open discussion of sexual identity and substance use issues.

The psychiatrist should be prepared to identify a potential overlap between problems with acceptance of one's sexual orientation and substance abuse. Gay, lesbian, and bisexual patients with addiction problems often show signs of a poorly integrated or a self-loathing identity. Like addicts in general, such persons may exhibit denial, fear, anger, guilt, helplessness, hopelessness, dishonesty, low self-esteem, self-hatred, and social isolation and alienation. Assessment of these traits and an awareness of how addiction and internalized homophobia may reinforce each other are helpful in providing adequate treatment. Furthermore, it is difficult to treat substance abuse problems in this population without addressing concomitant sexual identity problems. As a result, substance abuse programs that are gay sensitive and gay affirming work best for treating substance abuse disorders among gay men and lesbians. Prevention or reduction of substance abuse among this population must include the development of settings for socializing without alcohol or drugs.

Sexual Problems and Sexual Dysfunction Most problems of gay men and lesbians' sexual functioning are similar to those for the heterosexual population. However, as psychiatrists and other health professionals are often uncomfortable talking about sexuality in general, dealing with the specific sexual behaviors and concerns of gay men and lesbians may be particularly difficult. Problems may result from unfamiliarity with and disapproval of same-sex behaviors. The psychiatrist should be able to discuss the sexual concerns of gay and lesbian patients in an objective and comprehensive manner and should be aware of special diagnostic issues and approaches to sex therapy with these men and women. Descriptions of existing diagnostic categories for sexual dysfunction and disorders have a heterosexist bias, often leading to an avoidance or omission of same-sex couples' concerns. These include problems with anal intercourse and concerns about HIV infection among gay men and affectionate and orgasmic difficulties among lesbians. Some gay men with HIV have low serum testosterone and may seek treatment because of a loss of sexual drive. Some gay men may struggle with issues of sexual compulsivity, and bisexual men and women may have difficulty mastering safer sex practices.

Patterns of same-sex sexuality have been shown to be different from those in heterosexual couples, with female couples having decreased sexual interaction and male couples initially having increased amounts of sexual interaction in comparison to heterosexual couples. Typologies of male couples have sometimes described them in terms of their degree of sexual exclusivity and openness, and some male couples present with problems related to sexual exclusivity. In contrast, female couples present more often with problems related to decreased sexual desire.

The psychiatrist working with the sexual problems of gay and lesbian individuals and couples should consider organic, developmental, interpersonal, and social etiologies. Assessment and treatment can adapt traditional, heterosexually oriented paradigms of sexuality to include consideration of issues related to gay and lesbian development and the dynamics of same-sex relationships. Special attention should be given to cultural factors that may contribute to sexual problems among gay men and lesbians. These include a lack of readily available and accurate information about same-sex practices, as well as the inevitable internalization of judgmental societal attitudes about homosexuality.

Physical Problems Although often presenting with the same medical problems as the general population, lesbians and gay men have unique problems as well. One is psychosocial: Gay men and lesbians often have to deal with judgmental attitudes from health care personnel. This may not be as great a problem in some urban settings with large gay and lesbian communities in which clinicians, in private practice or public settings, have experience in caring for lesbian and gay patients. However, even in large urban settings, not all gay and lesbian patients have access to health care personnel who are sensitive and knowledgeable about their concerns or their increased risk for some diseases. Finally, knowledge of patients' current gay or lesbian sexual orientation and behaviors should not exclude a careful clinical inquiry about their current or past heterosexual relationships and experiences that could also put them at risk for certain diseases.

There are no gynecological problems that are unique or occur more frequently among lesbians than among heterosexual women. Lesbians, however, may be at greater risk for undetected disease, as studies show that they often undergo fewer pelvic exams and Pap smears. Sexually transmitted diseases are rare among women who are sexually active only with other women, and there are few cases of HIV infection in these women. The risk for some types of cancer in women may be affected by factors such as history of sexual intercourse with men, number of pregnancies, and breast-feeding. Historically, lesbians have had a lower number of pregnancies than heterosexual women. However, an increasing number of lesbians are choosing to have children through alternative insemination (from anonymous or known donors). It is important to consider the special needs of these women, a higher proportion of whom may seek care from nonmedical providers, such as midwives.

In general, when compared to heterosexual men, gay men have increased rates of sexually transmitted diseases, HIV infection, and use of certain substances, such as inhaled nitrites (poppers). Since the 1980s, the influence of HIV infection and AIDS on individual lives and the communities of gay men has been enormous and has affected almost every aspect of the personal and public experience of being gay. Public health campaigns to reduce infection among gay male populations do appear to work for some time in reducing the rate of infection. However, as younger gay men enter the community, educational strategies tailored to older men do not reach the new arrivals, and public health responses to their needs have not always been effective. For example, some young gay men believe that only older gay men are infected with HIV and that they are safe from HIV infection if they only have sex with men their own age. In fact, HIV infection—being infected or knowing someone with the virus—is a potential problem in the life of any gay man who enters the health care system. Health issues related to HIV include testing for infection; ensuring early treatment intervention in infected individuals; preventing further HIV infection; responding to reasonable and irrational fears about contracting the disease; dealing with the chronic stress resulting from illness, multiple losses, or both; and having to take care of someone else who is infected. For many gay men, associating HIV infection with their sexual identity exacerbates their own internalized homophobia.

Although recent advances in treating HIV infection have changed its course from an almost universally fatal diagnosis to a chronic medical condition for many of those infected, almost all gay men are profoundly affected by the epidemic. Among other things, the psychiatrist can play an important role in differentiating functional and organic symptoms that occur in HIV-infected patients, for example, diagnosing the clinical depression that may occur as a result of low testosterone levels. Psychiatrists can also treat the psychiatric sequelae of the disease, including depression, bipolar disorder, anxiety disorders, psychosis, and dementia.

Physical illness in gay men and lesbians may interact with experiences associated with their sexual identity. Lifestyle factors, family structures, and social networks can determine the extent and type of support available. The stress of being ill may evoke psychological reactions that affect the capacities for intimacy, affection, and sexuality. The psychiatrist should be sensitive to the unique issues that may arise for the gay man or lesbian when confronted with physical problems.

Psychotherapy The topic of psychotherapy with gay men and lesbians has been explored in a large number of publications that identify the special problems of these men and women and describe effective approaches to treatment. Treatment modalities include individual, couples, family, and group therapies. Since the 1970s, much of the literature has been written from the perspective of *gay and lesbian affirmative psychotherapy*, described by Alan Malyon as a "theoretical disposition (that) regards homosexuality as a non-pathological human potential." Gay and lesbian affirmative psychotherapy recognizes the centrality of sexual attraction, behaviors, and identity in a person's life but also appreciates that sexual orientation is only one aspect of personality and, depending on the patient's needs and goals, may not be a central focus of therapeutic work.

Historically, psychoanalytic approaches to psychotherapy with gay men and lesbians in the mid-20th century focused on homosexuality as a developmental arrest or a neurotic symptom. Since the 1990s, however, newer psychoanalytic approaches emerged. These see the therapist as an agent of the gay patient, rather than a representative of the patient's heterosexual social milieu. In addition, psychoanalytic psychotherapy with gay and lesbian patients has touched on many contentious issues in the modern psychoanalytic world. These include, but are not limited to, psychoanalytic epistemology, one-person versus two-person psychologies, the developmental influences of nature and nurture, the role of analytic neutrality, the existence of neutrality, the role of subjectivity, the discovery of meaning versus the creation of meaning, the influence of the therapist's beliefs on the conduct and outcome of a psychotherapy or analysis, the primacy of the Oedipus complex, the meaning of a developmental line, the nature of the unconscious, the uses of countertransference, therapist self-revelation, the psychoanalytic understanding of affects, and psychoanalytic pluralism.

Gay and Lesbian Affirmative Psychotherapy Acceptance, acknowledgment, and affirmation of gay, lesbian, and bisexual persons are essential elements in psychotherapeutic work with these men and women. These therapeutic stances reflect the therapist's regard and empathy for patients' sexual feelings and for their same-sex relationships. The therapist's attitudes represent a contrast to the social denial and derogation with which these aspects of the patient have previously been met. Ultimately, as with any patient, the psychiatrist working with gay and lesbian patients should maintain a position of neutrality that helps contain the struggles of the patient and, at the same time, serves to convey a recognition of the ongoing adverse impact of social prejudice against gay and lesbian persons. Lack of awareness about and failure to explicitly acknowledge the effects of the antihomosexual interpersonal and social forces working against the expression of same-sex desire may suggest to the patient an agreement on the part of the psychiatrist with these attitudes.

Being lesbian, gay, or bisexual represents a fundamental experience of feeling different and frequently alienated from mainstream culture. Often the sexual, romantic, and affectionate expressions of gay and lesbian patients have been ridiculed and rejected. For many gay men and lesbians, speaking with a therapist may represent the first chance that they have had to discuss their stigmatized sexuality with another person. The fundamental importance in therapy of having these feelings listened to without judgment, having them acknowledged as real by a person in authority, and having them affirmed as commonly felt and normal cannot be emphasized enough. The tolerance and validation of such feelings by the therapist allow the patient to express his or her own antihomosexual feelings as well, such as a fear of the reactions of others, disapproving feelings about being gay or lesbian, and regret of losses associated with being gay or lesbian. At these times, the therapist should not reassure patients prematurely, but, rather, should allow them to express and to come to terms with these experiences—which are often manifestations of internalized homophobia—at their own pace.

Contemporary Psychoanalytic Approaches to Gay and Lesbian Patients Psychotherapeutic work with gay and lesbian patients draws attention to aspects of the therapy process that are sometimes overlooked in psychotherapy with nongay patients. This work offers insights into some general principles of psychoanalysis, as well as basic psychoanalytic beliefs and practices, including the nature of the psychotherapeutic frame, the values and risks of therapist self-disclosure, the limitations of psychoanalytic data to support theories of etiology, how adherence to theoretical preconceptions restricts or inhibits a therapist's clinical listening, experience-near versus experience-distant responsiveness from the therapist, the therapist's entrenchment in cultural preconceptions and how they have an impact on treatment, the role of the patient's and the therapist's subcultural identities and how they coconstruct narratives in treatment, and the meanings and therapeutic uses of countertransference. Developing one's own therapeutic stance in treating gay and lesbian patients depends on specialized training in psychotherapy, continuing education, the therapist's own personal analysis, and ongoing self-analysis. Furthermore, the therapist's stance does not just entail what one knows, it also includes what the therapist does not know and requires an ability to allow a dynamic interplay of knowing and not knowing in the patient, the therapist, and the transitional space between them.

A therapist should create a therapeutic holding environment, a space in which all of a patient's feelings and ideas are allowed to emerge. As in gay and lesbian affirmative psychotherapy, the analyst's job is to remain open to hearing the patient's complaints, sexual or otherwise. In the atmosphere of the holding environment, meanings are discovered, created, and deciphered. All patients, not just gay ones, can benefit from a therapeutic holding environment based on respectful principles. Respect for the patient is essential. By itself, however, it is not enough. The subject of homosexuality often evokes uncomfortable feelings and denigrated meanings. When these emerge in treatment, they certainly need to be tolerated and respected by the therapist. In addition, a prerequisite for psychotherapy with gay men and lesbians is for therapists themselves to be able to accept their patients' homosexuality as a normal variation of human sexuality and to value and respect same-sex feelings and behaviors as well. It should again be noted that, for some gay men and lesbians, being treated with such respect by a therapist is a novel experience.

In addition to respect, this newer psychoanalytic stance focuses on the meanings, rather than the origins, of human sexuality. The therapist who searches for the causes of homosexuality ultimately mistakes its meanings to the patient for something else. Alternatively, this contemporary therapeutic stance instead shifts its focus to the affective meanings of the language of the patient, as well as those of the therapist, and to their transferential and countertransferential implications. From this perspective, it is important to understand that there are consequences to a therapist's taking sides in a gay or lesbian patient's interpersonal struggles with family and friends. Ideally, everyone whom a patient discusses should be treated respectfully, including those for whom the patient expresses disapproval. This therapeutic stance allows for a wider exploration of a patient's conflictual feelings and identifications with those who accept the patient's sexual identity and those who do not. Patients may try to resolve inner conflicts about being gay or lesbian by selectively inattending to their own antihomosexual identifications. This is sometimes seen in gay men and lesbians who preach rigid doctrine to themselves to affirm their homosexuality. Unable to tolerate conflictual feelings about homosexuality, these individuals sound as if they are trying to convince themselves that "it is OK to be gay." However, this strategy only reverses the feelings and identifications of a former state of mind. In the subjectivity of a closeted identity, heterosexuality is idealized, and homosexuality is dissociated. After coming out, being gay can become idealized, whereas disapproving feelings are denied. For example, a patient's internalized religious beliefs may not be limited to condemnations of homosexuality. They also include moral and ethical beliefs that are integral to the adult self. Patients cannot simply rid themselves of self-condemnatory attitudes without severing their attachments to other important identifications. The psychotherapeutic challenge is to integrate patients' adult feelings and understanding of sexuality, ethics, and morality with their internalized childhood beliefs. Therapeutic holding entails being able to contain all of those aspects of the patient, so that greater integration of all the patient's feelings can take place.

Sexual Conversion Therapies Some individuals with same-sex feelings may believe that a heterosexual social identity will expand their freedom of movement. Usually for religious reasons, although not always, these individuals are unable or unwilling to accept their homoerotic feelings as normal, natural, or moral. Toward that end, they may seek support from family members and friends, coreligionists, and professional colleagues who also disapprove of homosexuality. Such individuals may seek clinicians who practice *sexual conversion* (so-called reparative) *therapy* or religiously based ex-gay groups out of a legitimate wish to live as a heterosexual in a heterosexual world. Nonetheless, according to a 2000 position taken by the APA's Commission on Psychotherapy by Psychiatrists:

> To date, there are no scientifically rigorous outcome studies to determine either the actual efficacy or harm of reparative treatments. There is sparse scientific data about selection criteria, risks versus benefits of the treatment, and long-term outcomes of reparative therapies. The literature consists of anecdotal reports of individuals who have claimed to change, people who claim that attempts to change were harmful to them, and others who claimed to have changed and then later recanted those claims.
>
> With little data about patients, it is [still] possible to evaluate the theories which rationalize the conduct of "reparative" or [sexual] conversion therapies. . . . [These theories] are at odds with the scientific position of the American Psychiatric Association which has maintained, since 1973, that homosexuality per se, is not a mental disorder.
>
> . . . Until there is such research available . . . ethical practitioners refrain from attempts to change individuals' sexual orientation, keeping in mind the medical dictum to, first, do no harm.

In 2003, in response to the APA position statement, Robert L. Spitzer published his study of 200 individuals (143 men and 57 women) who reported once having had a predominantly homosexual orientation—about which they felt conflicted—and who claimed, due to some kind of "therapy," to have sustained some change to a heterosexual orientation for at least 5 years. Therapy was defined in this study as seeing a mental health professional, attending an ex-gay or other religious support group, reading the Bible, repeated meetings with a heterosexual role model, or "changing one's relationship with God."

The study's subjects, primarily recruited from religious, ex-gay organizations or referred by clinicians who regard homosexuality as an illness, were asked 114 questions about their sexual function in a 45-minute telephone interview. The author claimed that 65 percent of the males and 44 percent of the females reported a heterosexual reorientation. However, methodological criticisms of the study included its reliance on self-report, the biased selection of the sample, the study's retrospective design, and the use of a telephone interview as the only data collection method. There were no follow-up interviews of the study's subjects. Physiological indicators of change, such as penile or vaginal photoplethysmography, were not performed, according to the author, due to inadequate funding. Finally, the study's author, commenting on the difficulty he had in finding his 200 subjects, concluded that changing one's sexual orientation is a "rare or uncommon outcome of reparative therapy."

The study made no effort to assess the issue of harm raised by the APA position statement. In fact, the study's subject recruitment process made it unlikely that individuals who had been harmed by these treatments would be solicited. However, in calling for a moratorium on sexual conversion treatment, it was organized psychiatry's intent to protect patients who may be harmed by those procedures. This is because other recent studies indicate that unsuccessful conversion therapies may cause depression, intimacy avoidance, and sexual dysfunction. Furthermore, in calling for a moratorium on sexual conversion treatment, organized psychiatry has acted to protect patients who may be harmed by those procedures. Recent studies indicate that unsuccessful conversion therapies may cause depression, intimacy avoidance, and sexual dysfunction. Furthermore, in calling for further research on the risks versus benefits of such treatments, the APA recognizes that some individuals may still wish to change their sexual orientation for religious or other reasons. Clinical exploration of the irrational aspects of patients' internalized antihomosexual attitudes does not always lead to acceptance of their homosexuality. Thus, even if homosexuality per se is not a mental disorder, psychiatry and other mental health professions may wish to find a way to help individuals who wish to rid themselves of same-sex feelings. However, this cannot be done by simply redefining homosexuality as an illness. If psychiatry is to play a role in assisting such patients, perhaps the field of plastic surgery might serve as a model: Plastic surgeons devote much time, energy, and resources to treating nonpathological, but socially stigmatized, physical conditions.

Plastic surgeons, however, use standards of care that are not matched by those of sexual conversion therapists, who have not developed scientifically and clinically sound selection criteria for patients. It also is not certain that more exacting standards of care can be developed by today's sexual conversion therapists. After the mental health mainstream endorsed a normal variant model for homosexuality and its social acceptance increased, the professional training, credentials, and standing of sexual conversion therapists diminished. For example, a recent study showed that conversion therapists regularly violated professional codes of conduct regarding informed consent, confidentiality, pretermination counseling, and provision of referrals after treatment failure. A field once dominated by medically trained practitioners is now primarily the province of less rigorously trained clinicians, pastoral counselors, and self-help groups. Many reparative therapists work primarily within a faith-healing model. Therefore, it remains to be seen whether they can successfully develop scientific and clinical selection criteria to distinguish individuals who have a reasonable prospect of changing their sexual orientation from those who may be harmed by sexual conversion treatments. Until reparative therapists are able to generate more rigorous selection standards, the dictum to "first do no harm" should be kept in mind for those concerned about the well-being and the quality of care for all patients, regardless of their eventual sexual orientation.

Special Issues Gay men and lesbians present in psychotherapy with the same concerns as other patients, seeking help with a wide range of mental disorders and adjustment to interpersonal, work, and social situations. In many cases, the sexual feelings, behaviors, or identity of the individual may be incidental to treatment; in other cases, these issues may be central to the treatment. For example, some gay and lesbian patients, who may have no problems with their sexual feelings or identity, present with symptoms of sexual dysfunction, whereas others seek help directly because of confusion about their attraction to someone of the same sex or because of struggles with coming out or identity formation. It is helpful for the psychiatrist to be aware of several special treatment issues relevant to psychotherapy with lesbians and gay men. These issues can be clustered into general topics that have been discussed in other sections of this chapter: developmental experiences, including problems of youth, coming out, and acquiring a gay or lesbian identity; effects of heterosexism and antihomosexual attitudes, including violence and internalized homophobia; families and relationships, including families of origin and families of choice, same-sex relationships, and having children; and physical and mental problems, such as alcohol and substance abuse, sexual dysfunction, and HIV infection.

ETHICAL AND LEGAL ISSUES

Principle I of *The Principles of Medical Ethics: With Annotations Especially Applicable to Psychiatry* states that "a physician shall be dedicated to providing competent medical service with compassion and respect for human dignity," and the annotation goes on to say that "a psychiatrist should not be a party to any type of policy that excludes, segregates, or demeans the dignity of any patient because of ethnic origin, race, sex, creed, age, socioeconomic status, or sexual orientation." There are several ethical and legal issues that may come up in doing psychiatric work with lesbians, gay men, and bisexuals. These include confidentiality of medical records; a potential for abuse in military and other settings that discriminate against gay, lesbian, and bisexual patients; and maintenance of standards of care. Information about sexual feelings, behaviors, identity, and relationships should only be entered into the medical record when it is relevant to the evaluation and treatment of the patient and must always be treated in a confidential manner. Recent court decisions have upheld confidentiality between a therapist and a patient to be as important as lawyer–client privilege. Nevertheless, confidentiality regarding an individual's sexual orientation is an ongoing concern because of the risk of discrimination that lesbians, gay men, and bisexuals may face when their sexual identity is known within the health care setting or by health insurers. In addition, as same-sex relations remain illegal in some states with antisodomy laws, a medical record that finds its way into court could lead to criminal charges against a gay man or lesbian. Similarly, a medical record that indicates that a parent is gay or lesbian could be used by a court to deny that parent custody privileges. Although a clinician's knowledge of a patient's sexual identity is essential to quality care, it is problematic to record this information in an unprotected medical record (as in a public clinic or managed care setting) without informing the patient that this is being done. Nonclinical communications to others (a clinic's clerical staff, managed-care case managers, school officials, etc.) about a patient's sexual identity or sexual behavior without the informed consent of the patient are always unethical. When treating patients in settings in which total confidentiality cannot be assured, it is usually best if the psychiatrist discusses with the patient what can and cannot be kept confidential before personal data are entered into the chart. When the patient does not wish this information to be recorded, and the psychiatrist does not believe that this information should be withheld, a referral to another clinician or clinical setting is highly recommended.

There are institutional settings, such as the armed forces, prisons, or antihomosexual religious universities, where public knowledge of a person's sexual orientation could have adverse consequences for a patient. As in the public sector, the psychiatrist in these settings is employed by an institution and not directly by the patient. Nevertheless, at least in nonmilitary settings, the ethical constraints on the psychiatrist are similar to those in the public mental health sector: The confidentiality of the patient, with the exception of potential harm to self or others, always takes precedence over any other institutional needs. Psychiatrists in the military, however, are faced with a difficult ethical dilemma. Under the current "don't ask, don't tell" policy, a gay or lesbian patient who reveals his or her sexual identity to a military psychiatrist faces possible discharge. The APA currently has no official position on what response it would take toward a psychiatrist who violates confidentiality and reports a gay or lesbian patient's statements regarding his or her sexual orientation. Informed consent may provide a partial solution for military psychiatrists who find themselves in a bind between their ethical responsibilities as psychiatrists to maintain patient confidentiality and their official responsibilities to uphold the rules of the military. All patients in the military should be informed when they enter treatment that the psychiatrist is bound by other obligations that take precedence over patient confidentiality. Obviously, withholding information about one's sexuality is less than optimal in meeting the mental health needs of gay, lesbian, and bisexual military personnel. However, such an informed consent approach by psychiatrists prevents military personnel from inadvertently revealing information to a psychiatrist that may lead to their discharge.

Appropriate standards of care in treating gay, lesbian, and bisexual patients require that psychiatrists monitor their own antihomosexual bias when providing assessment and treatment. In this culture, antihomosexual attitudes are ubiquitous, and, consequently, no one is free of them, not even gay and lesbian psychiatrists. This obliges the psychiatrist to understand and to be aware of the ways in which these attitudes have had an impact on the development of their own identities. This can help a psychiatrist come to a greater empathic appreciation of the impact of such attitudes on a gay, lesbian, or bisexual patient. Psychiatrists and other practitioners who continue to treat homosexuality as a form of mental illness do so outside of the mental health mainstream and risk ethical sanctions, particularly if they violate professional codes of conduct regarding informed consent, confidentiality, pretermination counseling, and provision of referrals after treatment failure. Closeted gay and lesbian psychiatrists struggling with their own identity issues may need to refrain for a period of time from working with patients who have similar problems. All psychiatrists, regardless of their own sexual identity, should undertake training to keep them informed about the concerns of gay, lesbian, and bisexual patients and the ethical issues that may arise when caring for them.

TRAINING AND RESEARCH NEEDS

As previously mentioned, traditional concepts of sexuality, sexual identity, and sexual orientation have shifted significantly in the second half of the 20th century. Training medical students and psychiatric residents about contemporary theories of sexuality helps them develop skills that allow them to interact sensitively and competently with persons of all sexual orientations. Instruction about the lives and mental health needs of gay men, lesbians, and bisexual persons should not be restricted to classes on human sexuality but should be integrated into the cross-cultural curriculum. In addition, lesbian, gay, and bisexual residents benefit from support during their training, whereas all residents benefit from contact with respected psychiatrist role models who are openly gay, lesbian, and bisexual. Medical schools and professional organizations should increase the opportunities available for training about the clinical concerns of sexual minorities and should encourage gay and lesbian faculty and other leaders to be visible and active in a wide range of professional activities.

There is still much to be understood about sexual orientation and its development. Although accepting attitudes toward gay, lesbian, and bisexual individuals are increasing, antihomosexual bias is widespread. There is further need of psychosocial research to understand the impact that these attitudes have, not only on the development of gay and lesbian identities, but also on society as a whole.

Preliminary research has been undertaken to describe variations in sexual desire, behavior, and identity associated with a range of demographic and personal characteristics, such as biological sex, age, race, class, geographical location, and religion. Many studies continue to focus on white, urban, middle-class men, and there is a need to study sexual diversity in other groups as well. There is also a need for ongoing longitudinal studies about the development and experience of sexual orientation and sexual identity over time and across the life span. Longitudinal studies can also expand understanding about those childhood characteristics that contribute to the development of an adult sexual orientation, as well as those factors that shape individual expression of desire and behavior. Future research will inevitably expand beyond traditional biological and psychosocial approaches and will use constructivist methodologies to account for the role of fluctuating cultural and other historical forces in shaping individual lives and experience.

SUGGESTED CROSS-REFERENCES

Normal child development is discussed in Section 32.2, and normal adolescent development is discussed in Section 32.3. Normal human sexuality, other than homosexuality and homosexual behavior, and sexual dysfunctions are discussed in Section 18.1a. Gender identity disorders are discussed in Section 18.3. The psychotherapies are discussed in Chapter 30. Neuropsychiatric aspects of HIV infection and AIDS are discussed in Section 2.8. Contributions of the sociocultural sciences are discussed in Chapter 4. The psychiatric interview is discussed in Section 7.1. Substance-related disorders are discussed in Chapter 11. Ethics in psychiatry are discussed in Section 54.2.

References

American Psychiatric Association: Commission on Psychotherapy by Psychiatrists (COPP): Position statement on therapies focused on attempts to change sexual orientation (Reparative or conversion therapies). *Am J Psychiatry.* 2000;157:1719.

Arnold P, Agate RJ, Carruth LL: Hormonal and nonhormonal mechanisms of sexual differentiation of the brain. In: Legato M, ed. *Principles of Gender Specific Medicine.* San Diego: Elsevier Science, 2004:84.

*Bayer R. *Homosexuality and American Psychiatry: The Politics of Diagnosis.* Princeton, NJ: Princeton University Press; 1987.

Bell AP, Weinberg MS, Hammersmith FK: *Sexual Preference: Its Development in Men and Women.* Bloomington, IN: Indiana University Press; 1981.

Boswell J. *Same-Sex Unions in Premodern Europe.* New York: Villard Books; 1994.

*Byne W: The biological evidence challenged. *Sci Am.* 1994;270:50–55.

Byne W, Parsons B: Human sexual orientation: The biologic theories reappraised. *Arch Gen Psychiatry.* 1993;50:228.

Byne W, Sekaer C: The question of psychosexual neutrality at birth. In: Legato M, ed. *Principles of Gender Specific Medicine.* San Diego: Elsevier Science, 2004:155.

*Cabaj RP, Stein TS. *Textbook of Homosexuality and Mental Health.* Washington, DC: American Psychiatric Press; 1996.

D'Augelli AR, Patterson CJ. *Lesbian, Gay, and Bisexual Identities Over the Lifespan: Psychological Perspectives.* New York: Oxford University Press; 1995.

DeCecco JP, Parker DA, eds. *Sex, Cells, and Same-Sex Desire: The Biology of Sexual Preference.* New York: Haworth Press; 1995.

*Drescher J. *Psychoanalytic Therapy and the Gay Man.* Hillsdale, NJ: The Analytic Press; 1998.

Ford CS, Beach FA. *Patterns of Sexual Behavior.* New York: Harper & Row; 1951.

Foucault M. *The History of Sexuality, Volume 1: An Introduction.* Hurley R, trans. New York: Pantheon; 1978.

Freud S. Three essays on the theory of sexuality. In: *Standard Edition of the Complete Psychological Works of Sigmund Freud.* Vol 7. London: Hogarth Press; 1996.

Greenberg DF. *The Construction of Homosexuality.* Chicago: University of Chicago Press; 1988.

Guss JF, Drescher J, eds. *Addictions in the Gay and Lesbian Community.* New York: Haworth Press; 2000.

Herdt G. *Guardians of the Flutes: Idioms of Masculinity.* Chicago: University of Chicago Press; 1994.

Herek GM, Berrill KT, eds. *Hate Crimes.* Newbury Park, CA: Sage Publications; 1992.

Hooker EA: The adjustment of the male overt homosexual. *J Projective Techniques.* 1957;21:17.

Isay R. *Being Homosexual: Gay Men and Their Development.* New York: Farrar, Straus and Giroux; 1989.

Kernberg OF: Unresolved issues in the psychoanalytic theory of homosexuality and bisexuality. *J Gay Lesb Psychother.* 2002;6:9.

Kinsey AC, Pomeroy WB, Martin CE. *Sexual Behavior in the Human Male.* Philadelphia: WB Saunders; 1948.

Kinsey AC, Pomeroy WB, Martin CE, Gebhard P. *Sexual Behavior in the Human Female.* Philadelphia: WB Saunders; 1953.

Lasco M, Jordan T, Edgar M, Petito C, Byne W: A lack of dimorphism of sex or sexual orientation in the human anterior commissure. *Brain Res.* 2002;936:95.

Laumann EO, Gagnon JH, Michael RT, Michaels S. *The Social Organization of Sexuality: Sexual Practices in the United States.* Chicago: University of Chicago Press; 1994.

LeVay S, Hamer DH: Evidence for a biological influence in male homosexuality. *Sci Am.* 1994;270:44–49.

Lingiardi V, Drescher J, eds. *The Mental Health Professions and Homosexuality: International Perspectives.* New York: Haworth Press; 2003.

Magee M, Miller D. *Lesbian Lives: Psychoanalytic Narratives Old and New.* Hillsdale, NJ: The Analytic Press; 1997.

Malyon A: Psychotherapeutic implications of internalized homophobia in gay men. *J Homosex.* 1982;1:59.

McWhirter DP, Sanders SA, Reinisch, eds. *Homosexuality/Heterosexuality: Concepts of Sexual Orientation.* New York: Oxford University Press; 1990.

Mustanski BS, Chivers ML, Bailey JM: A critical review of recent biological research on human sexual orientation. *Annu Rev Sex Res.* 2002:89.

Sandfort TGM: Studying sexual orientation change: A methodological review of the Spitzer study, "Can some gay men and lesbians change their sexual orientation? *J Gay Lesbian Psychother.* 2003;7:15.

*Shidlo A, Schroeder M, Drescher J, eds. *Sexual Conversion Therapy: Ethical, Clinical and Research Perspectives.* New York: Haworth Press; 2001.

Spitzer RL: Can some gay men and lesbians change their sexual orientation? 200 subjects reporting a change from homosexual to heterosexual orientation. *Arch Sex Behav.* 2003;32:403.

Stein TS, Cohen CJ, eds. *Contemporary Perspectives on Psychotherapy with Lesbians and Gay Men.* New York: Plenum Publishing; 1986.

Weinberg MS, Williams CJ, Pryor DW. *Dual Attraction: Understanding Bisexuality.* New York: Oxford University Press; 1994.

▲ 18.2 Paraphilias

Ethel Spector Person, M.D.

Sexual symptoms fall readily into two groups; they are pleasure inhibitors or pleasure facilitators, and the sexual disorders can be classified accordingly. In the first group, referred to as *sexual dysfunctions*, the patient experiences an impairment, most often an inhibition, in the initiation of the sexual cycle, in sexual arousal, or in the ability to achieve orgasm. In other words, there is impairment of desire, sexual arousal, or orgasm. In the second group, the *paraphilias* (previously labeled as *perversions* or *deviations*), the sexual response is preserved, but the symptom, a significant deviation in the erotic stimulus or in the activity itself, is the precondition for sexual excitement and orgasm.

In the paraphiliac, sexual excitement is contingent on the invocation or enactment, or both, of a specific fantasy that is unusual or sometimes even bizarre. Conversely, sexual excitement and arousal do not occur or are diminished if, for whatever reason, the accompanying paraphiliac fantasies are suppressed. This is at the heart of the difficulty in curing or controlling paraphilias; it is hard for people to give up sexual pleasure with no assurance that new routes to sexual gratification will be secured. Moreover, the paraphiliac sexual scripts often serve other vital psychic functions. They may assuage anxiety, bind aggression, or stabilize identity.

Sigmund Freud originally described *perversion* (paraphilia) as comprising a distortion in sexual aim, that is, in the nature of the activity, for example, urolagnia, urinating on the object as a prerequisite to arousal. He broadened the definition to include distortions in the choice of the sexual object. Distortions in the aim or the object constitute a paraphilia only when they are prerequisite to the sexual act, that is when they are obligatory rather than elective. For example, if a man achieves sexual excitement only in response to a sheep as an object (in fantasy or actuality), his sexuality would be considered perverse. In contrast, the sexual behavior of a herdsman who resorts to intercourse with a sheep in the absence of an appropriate object might be considered to be engaged in a sexual variation rather than in acting out a paraphiliac desire. Even so, because masturbation (with its attendant fantasy) always exists as a sexual outlet, the choice of an animal object might suggest that the herdsman had some minor perverse strain. It may be of some interest that *The Goat*, Edward Albee's play, which depicts the unraveling of a marriage when the husband falls in love with a goat, won the 2002 Tony Award for the best dramatic play. Albee expressed his pleasure that a love story should have taken first prize.

With the possible exception of sadism and masochism, the paraphilias are relatively rare compared to sexual dysfunctions. Yet, paraphilias have claimed just as much attention as the sexual dysfunctions. In part, this may be because so many people have strands of perverse interest woven into their sexual makeup that fly just under the radar of consciousness but that express themselves in self-evident interest in films and books that feature one or another paraphilia. This interest can be inferred from a quick look at the bestseller lists, which often feature books depicting masochistic surrender or serial sexual murders. Moreover, newspapers, magazines, and television play to this interest with stories of sex crimes, some of which, like pedophilia, are paraphilias.

To fully understand the clinical presentation of the paraphilias, the fundamental definitions and conceptualizations of sex and sexuality and their interrelationship should be considered. *Sex* refers to biological sexuality and is defined by six component parts: chromosomes, gonads, internal genitalia, external genitalia, sex hormones, and secondary sexual characteristics. *Sexuality,* in contrast to biological sex, refers to erotic excitement, genital arousal, and orgasm. It is expressed in fantasy and behavior, object choice, subjective desire, arousal, preferred activities, and orgasmic discharge.

Each individual, whether paraphiliac or not, develops a characteristic pattern of sexual expression—sometimes called a *sex print* or *love map*. This pattern constitutes an erotic signature, signifying that the individual's sexual potential has been progressively narrowed between infancy and adulthood. It conveys more than just a preference for a particular sexual object and activity; it also indicates that an individualized script, that is, a specific fantasy or group of fantasies is the most reliable and, sometimes, the necessary prerequisite to elicit erotic desire. From the subjective point of view, such preferences are almost always thought of as deep rooted and stemming from a person's nature rather than as conditioned by experience. Consequently, the sex print or love map often forms part of a person's conscious identity or sense of self and, as such, may be regarded as sexual identity. Although the *sex print* or *love map* refers to sexual fantasies and observable sexual practices and preferences, *sexual identity* refers to the internal experience of sexual arousal patterns and self-labeling.

For most heterosexuals and homosexuals, male or female, the sex print encompasses an evolving series of several different fantasies. In contrast, in paraphiliacs, the sex print is much narrower. Similarly, although most heterosexuals and homosexuals can achieve sexual arousal under a fairly wide set of circumstances, in a full-blown paraphilia, a stereotypical paraphiliac fantasy, its depiction in pornography, or its enactment is almost always prerequisite to arousal. Although most paraphiliacs favor one fantasy, some rotate interest among several different paraphiliac fantasies.

The study of paraphilias stands on its own, but it has also proved relevant to theories of sexual development. The study of the perversions (paraphilias) was decisive in Freud's formulations of normal psychosexual development and culminated in his publication of *Three Essays on the Theory of Sexuality*. Analogously, the study of the gender identity disorders, particularly transsexualism, later played a pivotal role in contemporary reconceptualizations of gender. These are both examples of how the study of a phenomenon that, at first, appears to be marginal sometimes opens up new vistas of knowledge.

DEFINITION

In the classical case of paraphilia, paraphiliac fantasies or stimuli are obligatory to erotic arousal. However, a paraphiliac preference may occur episodically, especially during stress, whereas, at other times, the same individual may be able to function sexually without the benefits of paraphiliac fantasies or stimuli. According to the revised fourth edition of the *Diagnostic and Statistical Manual of Mental Disorders* (DSM-IV-TR), to diagnose a paraphilia, the patient must have recurring, intensely arousing fantasies, sexual urges or behaviors that involve nonhuman objects; that involve the suffering or humiliation of oneself, one's partner, children, or nonconsenting others; and that occur over a period of at least 6 months (Criterion A). In addition, the behavior, sexual urges, and fantasies must cause clinically significant distress or impairment in social, occupational, or other important areas of functioning (Criterion B). What this definition fails to do is delineate the difference between paraphilias that are harmful to others and that may even be criminal, including pedophilia, exhibitionism, voyeurism, frotteurism, and those that are not necessarily physically or psychologically harmful to others. This is an important distinction for practical, as well as theoretical, reasons. The two groups generally receive different therapeutic interventions, and the genesis of their disorders is understood somewhat differently. It is the group of paraphilias that causes harm that stigmatizes the whole group and leads one to think of paraphilias as invariably pernicious. In fact, some well-known and productive individuals have had perversions, including the sexologist Havelock Ellis, who wrote in his autobiography of his urolagnia.

The paraphilias include *exhibitionism* (exposure of one's genitals), *fetishism* (use of nonliving objects), *frotteurism* (rubbing against or touching a nonconsenting person), *pedophilia* (sexual fantasy preoccupation or sexual activity with prepubescents), *sexual masochism* (seeking humiliation or suffering), *sexual sadism* (inflicting humiliation or suffering), *transvestic fetishism* (the obligatory use of clothing of the opposite sex to achieve arousal), and *voyeurism* (arousal through viewing another person's undressing, toileting, or sexual activity). There is a residual category, *paraphilia not otherwise specified*, that includes less frequently encountered paraphilias. It includes such behaviors as *infantilism* (dressing in diapers or requiring a partner who does so) or the requirement that a sexual partner has an amputated limb. In fact, more than 40 conditions qualify as paraphilias.

Some paraphiliacs eschew intercourse in favor of masturbation; for example, voyeurs and exhibitionists may favor masturbation accompanying the pornographic act to any sexual congress, heterosexual or homosexual. Transvestic fetishists, too, show a diminished, although not absent, interest in sexual intercourse. Some individuals are polymorphous perverse and use a number of different paraphiliac fantasies that coexist, whereas others may have paraphiliac preferences that migrate from one paraphilia to another over the course of time. If an individual's preferences meet the criteria for more than one paraphilia, all must be diagnosed.

Associated Features and Disorders

Although paraphilias are predominantly disorders of sexuality, they are sometimes associated with some deviation in gender role identity. Paraphilias and gender identity disorders sometimes exist on a continuum. For example, a transvestic fetishist may use cross-dressing primarily fetishistically—that is, to achieve sexual arousal—in which case, his disturbance would be diagnosed as a paraphilia, whereas, to the degree that a transvestic fetishist progresses to complete cross-dressing to relieve his anxiety and to stabilize his identity, his disturbance would be more likely to be diagnosed as a cross-gender disorder.

HISTORY

Sex has always been regarded as a force that must be reckoned with. Before the subject of sex was medicalized and became the object of study of sexologists and psychiatrists, it was regulated by religious precepts. Under religious auspices, deviation from the norm was regarded as sinful or criminal rather than pathological. In today's world, the precepts of various religions continue to determine what is thought of as acceptable, although, to some degree, the authority of religion has been eroded by the findings in the burgeoning field of sex research.

The scientific study of sex began in the late 19th century. Although various paraphilias have existed as long as recorded history, they enter into the scientific dialogue courtesy of the psychiatrist Richard von Krafft-Ebing (1840 to 1902), who labeled *sadistic* behavior as such, deriving the term from the writings of the Marquis de Sade, an 18th-century French nobleman. Leopold von Sacher-Masoch, an Austrian born in the 19th century, wrote novels that dealt with masochistic themes, and it is from his name that the term *masochism* is derived. It is through Krafft-Ebing's detailed clinical descriptions of a range of sexual disorders that the scientific study of sex was born. In 1895, the psychologist Albert von Schrenk-Notzing linked sadism and masochism together into the term *algolagnia*, emphasizing the connection between sexual excitement and pain. In 1938, Freud affirmed this association through his invocation of the term *sadomasochism*. In 1966, John Money created a research program for the psychohormonal treatment of *perversions* (paraphilias) and sex-offender syndromes. This was the same year that William Masters and Virginia Johnson published their landmark book on normal human sexuality.

Paraphilias, or *sexual deviations*, as they are frequently called, imply a deviation from normative patterns. However, there is a fundamental problem in delineating the paraphilias in this way: No definitive description of what entails normal can be established, because definitions of normality change over time. One of the most striking examples is the psychiatric profession's reversal of its views on homosexuality in the late 1960s. Although homosexuality was long considered an aberration, it was first labeled as a paraphilia in 1968 in the second edition of the DSM (DSM-II). However, psychiatrists shortly reversed themselves on grounds that there was no evidence that homosexuality was anything more than a sexual variation, that is, that it was not invariably associated with any discernible disabilities different from those of heterosexuals. This turnaround in the United States occurred in the context of the gay liberation movement of the 1960s. Only in 1978 did the sexologists Alan P. Bell and Martin S. Weinberg confirm through a large-scale study of homosexuals that there were no significant differences in the psychological disabilities attached to homosexuals and heterosexuals. However, not all psychiatrists and psychoanalysts worldwide have accepted this change in thinking. For example, a large number, and perhaps the majority, of psychoanalysts in Latin America still consider homosexuality to be perverse.

Freud had come close to the North American position a half century earlier. He asserted the normality of homosexuals, declaring that inverts were a group of individuals who might be quite sound in all other respects. (Note, however, the implication that homosexuals were not sound in one respect.) Although the psychiatric profession's turnaround (before Bell and Weinberg's study) has been widely applauded, and rightly so, it nonetheless suggests that the psychiatric profession's criteria for classification of the paraphilias are not altogether based on scientific criteria. In essence, the exemption of homosexuality as a paraphilia raises questions about the methodology by which what constitutes a perversion is judged.

Paraphilias, unlike neurotic symptoms, provide pleasure of the highest order and may sometimes be ego-syntonic. The question necessarily arises as to why some sexual fantasies and behaviors are considered pathological rather than merely different. Some liberation groups, such as sadomasochism liberation (based on the model of gay liberation), question whether the psychiatric profession is labeling some sexual behaviors perverse or deviant on moral grounds in the guise of medical ones. A number of sexologists have pointed out that there is a major difference in paraphilias that are limited to an eccentric expression of sexuality (for example, fetishism) and those that may be harmful to others (for example, pedophilia).

Despite the medical, psychiatric, and legal interest in paraphilia, its scientific study is limited by access to subjects. Most ideas on paraphilias are based on information gathered from patients whose paraphilia troubles them or from paraphiliacs who have run afoul of the law. It is not reliably known what percentage of the population might be diagnosed as paraphiliacs.

The major limitation to any absolute claim of abnormality in paraphiliacs is the failure of psychiatrists to study large groups of nonpatient paraphiliacs. To scientifically conclude the degree to which a particular paraphilia is connected to psychological disabilities would depend on large-scale studies of nonpatient populations. These results would then need to be compared to psychological disabilities in a nonparaphiliac sample. This research could only be done through field work in which investigators identified a large sample of nonpatient paraphiliacs. Some such studies have been conducted with transvestites—now called *transvestic fetishists*. The existence of a transvestic subculture made access to research subjects relatively easy. Several studies of nonpatient transvestites support the contention that the full-blown transvestic syndrome is associated with disabilities and impairment that warrant the designation of disorder, for example, the hyposexuality that so often accompanies it and the high incidence of depression often linked to it. However, comparable studies have not yet been systemically carried out with respect to most of the other sexual deviations. Alfred Kinsey's sexual surveys were so important precisely because he studied sexuality in a nonpatient population. This methodology, of course, was what made Bell and Weinberg's study on homosexuality so compelling. There are suggestions that so-called perverse interests may be more extensive than may be thought. One hint of this comes from the Internet, which has generated any number of sexual sites devoted to a variety of sexual deviations.

COMPARATIVE NOSOLOGY

The criteria for diagnosing paraphilias have been revised time and again over the past 50 years. In the first edition of the DSM (DSM-I) (1952), sexual deviations were grouped with psychopathic personality disturbances. Such a classification reflected the fact that the enactments of certain paraphilias are legal offenses (e.g., pedophilia and exhibitionism), but the classification also suggests the possibility that the society held pejorative attitudes toward all deviations. At that time, homosexuality was included among the sexual deviations. In DSM-II (1968), sexual deviations were classified with the personality disorders. By 1980, with the publication of the third edition of the DSM (DSM-III), the term *paraphilia* was substituted for the term *perversion*. In part, the name change was made because the term *paraphilia* is descriptive. As noted in DSM-III, "The deviation (para) is in that to which the individual is attracted (philia)." But the name change was also meant to be nonjudgmental, because it was felt that the term *perversion* carried a negative connotation. The whole group of paraphilias was reclassified under the category of psychosexual disorders, which also included gender identity disorders, psychosexual dysfunctions, and ego-dystonic homosexuality. These changes reflect a shift in attitude among psychiatrists and the general public as well—the unwillingness to stigmatize a patient for symptoms beyond his or her control, particularly because not all of the paraphilias come within the purview of current law.

A major change in the revised edition of the DSM-III (DSM-III-R) was to retract the idea that, to make the diagnosis of paraphilia, the paraphiliac acts had to be the preferred or exclusive means of achieving sexual pleasure. The diagnosis was extended to those who might prefer heterosexual intercourse but who had entertained significant paraphiliac fantasies over the past 6 months.

DSM-IV-TR diagnoses paraphilias on the basis that they may entail interference with "the capacity for reciprocal, affectionate sexual activity." To make the diagnosis, the individual must have acted out his or her paraphiliac fantasy or must be distressed by the fantasy for at least 6 months.

To qualify as a DSM-IV-TR diagnosis, the sexual patterns must have persisted for a period of at least 6 months (Criterion A) and must have caused clinically significant distress or impairment in social, occupational, or other important areas of function (Criterion B). DSM-IV-TR emphasizes that, although, for some individuals, the paraphiliac fantasies are merely stimulating, for others, they are obligatory to arousal and are always included in sexual activity. In some other cases, these preferences occur only episodically, particularly during periods of stress; that is, there are times when the individual can function sexually without such fantasies or stimuli. The changes made in DSM-IV-TR go a long way toward addressing the critique that labeling one or another sexual preference as a paraphilia is arbitrary. They argue that the diagnosis of paraphilia must rest on the existence of some disability or impairment that attaches to the sexual act so designated. The downside here is that the paraphilias may fail to be seen as a spectrum in which harmless perversions are incorporated into productive lives. Havelock Ellis might serve as an example here.

DSM-IV-TR draws special attention to the paraphiliac fantasies and imagery that are acted out with a nonconsenting partner. Sexual sadism and pedophilia are generally thought to be injurious to the partner. (It should be noted, however, that sexual sadism is often enacted with a consenting partner, whose sexual pleasure is dependent on masochistic gratification.) The paraphiliac enactment can lead to arrests and imprisonment. Sexual offenses against children account for a large proportion of all reported criminal sex acts. Exhibitionists and voyeurs, along with pedophiles, make up most of those sex offenders who are arrested. Although not creating as much devastation in their victims as do pedophiles, exhibitionists, voyeurs, and frotteurists often frighten their victims.

No classification is without its contradictions. Several experts have observed that paraphiliacs who are sexual offenders are more stressed by the discovery of their crimes than by guilt over the harm that they inflict. This is unlike that group of paraphiliacs who seek therapy because of psychic pain or stress within the family. This bifurcation suggests that the paraphilias may encompass at least two different groups of disorders. The classification of paraphiliacs might be improved by distinguishing between those who pose a threat to others and those who do not.

DSM-IV-TR may also go awry in relabeling transvestism as *transvestic fetishism* and in subsuming it entirely within the paraphilias as distinct from the disorders of gender identity. A significant number of transvestic fetishists evolve into transsexuals, and, in most transvestic fetishists, there is a component of cross-gender identification. It is clear, for example, that three different categories of patients may evolve into transsexuals: transvestites, extreme cross-dressing homosexuals, and a category that is generally referred to as *primary transsexuals*.

Rationale for the Classification

An evolutionary value system is no longer held in which sexuality must be tied to reproduction to be considered normal and in which all other sexuality is considered suspect. However, there are grounds for preserving the concept and classification of paraphilias without invoking an evolutionary imperative. Two lines of argument have been invoked to demonstrate the legitimacy of this classification, one philosophic, the other psychiatric.

Philosophers have observed that the fact that humans even possess a concept of sexual perversion tells something about sex. Social disapproval is insufficient to label something as perverse. Thus, although adultery may be viewed as a moral outrage, it has not been labeled as perverse. Although some religions believe that masturbation is a sin, no one claims it is perverse. This suggests that paraphilias convey something unnatural rather than immoral. How to distinguish what is natural from what is unnatural is at the heart of the problem. Some sexual activities, such as heterosexual intercourse, are clearly normal, whereas such sexual acts as shoe fetishism are clearly paraphilias. Still other sexual behaviors may fall somewhere in between.

The argument in DSM-IV-TR, similar to the philosophical perspective, is that people with paraphilias have some impairment in their capacity for reciprocal affectionate sexual activity. This argument, however, is permeated with value biases, evident in the fact that it is not universally applied. Compulsive promiscuity is not listed among the paraphilias, and neither is lovelessness in couples. The boundary between perverse and normal sexuality is not always clear cut.

The validity of the classification of paraphilias must rest on specific criteria. To make the diagnosis of perversion, there must be evidence that the perverse fantasy or activity permeates mental life to an unusual degree, that its suppression yields high-level anxiety or dysphoric affect, or that it is connected with some other personality dysfunction. In the more overt cases, those usually seen in clinical practice, these claims appear to be adequately demonstrated. However, there are many instances in which perverse elements are subsumed into sexuality in such a minor key that the diagnosis of perversion is not warranted.

EPIDEMIOLOGY

Gender Ratio

One characteristic feature of the distribution of the paraphilias is remarkable: the enormous predominance of paraphilias in men. Except for sadism and masochism, almost all of the reported cases are in men. This preponderance in men is characteristic not just of the paraphilias, but also, to a much lesser degree, of the gender disorders. Any attempt to explain this discrepancy must be related to understanding of the etiology of the paraphilias. Insofar as etiology has not been conclusively demonstrated, explanations can only be tentative.

Prevalence

Insofar as a paraphilia yields pleasure, many individuals so affected do not seek psychiatric intervention. Even those who feel anguished may avoid confiding in a doctor or psychiatrist out of profound shame. Restricted to studying a psychotherapy patient population or a population convicted of sexual crimes, relatively little is known about the incidence and distribution of the paraphilias or about the natural history of the course of any given paraphilia over time.

Some paraphilias appear to be more common than others. In an individual psychiatric practice, masochism, sadism, and fetishism appear to be the most commonly encountered paraphilias, whereas the excretory perversions are rarely seen. In contrast, in clinics that specialize in the treatment of sex offenders against whom criminal charges have been raised, the most commonly encountered paraphilias are pedophilia, voyeurism, and exhibitionism.

It has long been thought that, because some paraphilias depend on the participation of nonconsenting individuals and come to the attention of the courts (e.g., pedophilia and exhibitionism), they might be overrepresented in attempts to determine relative frequencies. Yet, as it turns out, many pedophiles have been sheltered from the law. Pedophilia has recently exploded onto the world stage by virtue of the crisis within the Catholic Church; the Church is being criticized for its reluctance to acknowledge the sexual abuse perpetrated by priests, the most egregious of these abuses being pedophilia. Given that the actual incidence of paraphilias involving nonconsenting individuals or the number of paraphiliacs who fail to seek psychiatric help is not known, the incidence of any one of the paraphilias is clearly underreported.

Something is known about the range of sexual behaviors, the variety of sexual fantasies, and the high incidence of sadomasochistic fantasies in a nonpatient population. For example, one study elicited the male and female responses of 193 university students to questions about sexual experience and sexual fantasies. The study differentiated recent and cumulative behaviors and recent sexual fantasies and cumulative sexual fantasies.

Sexual behavior showed only a modest degree of gender influence. Because the population was predominantly heterosexual, it was no surprise that there was a close correlation between male and female behaviors. Most behavioral items referred to interpersonal consensual activity. Those behaviors most frequently enacted were romantic, traditional, nongenital sexual encounters, closely followed by sexual intercourse and its variations.

In their report of recent sexual experiences, 1 percent of the women and 1 percent of the men reported being tortured, 1 percent of women and 1 percent of men reported being whipped or beaten by a partner, 1 percent of women and 1 percent men reported degrading a sexual partner, 1 percent of women and 3 percent of men reported forcing a partner to submit, 0 percent of women and 4 percent of men reported exhibiting their body in public, and 0 percent of women and 2 percent of men reported whipping or beating a partner. A few cumulative sexual experiences were statistically significant for gender differences: Thirteen percent of women and 4 percent of men reported being forced to submit, and 8 percent of women and 21 percent of men reported exhibiting their body in public.

Greater differences between men and women emerged in their self-reports of fantasies, which was not an unanticipated finding, because fantasies, by virtue of being independent, are more likely to reveal individual desires.

Twenty percent of women in the study reported recent sexual fantasies of being forced to submit, 20 percent reported being tied or bound during sexual activity, 12 percent reported being sexually degraded, 10 percent reported being prostituted, 9 percent reported being tortured by a sexual partner, 8 percent reported being whipped or beaten by a partner, 5 percent reported forcing a partner to submit, 1 percent reported whipping or beating a partner, and 1 percent reported degrading a sex partner. Comparable percentages in men were 15 percent reporting being forced to submit, 15 percent reporting being tied or bound, 5 percent reporting being degraded, 5 percent reporting being prostituted, 5 percent reporting being tortured, 5 percent reporting being whipped or beaten, 31 percent reporting forcing to submit, 7 percent reporting whipping or beating, and 7 percent reporting degrading. Six percent of men also reported fantasies of torturing a sex partner.

In the cumulative sexual fantasies, both genders reported the same level of ongoing masochistic fantasies: being tortured by a sex partner (10 percent of women, 11 percent of men), being whipped (15 percent of women, 14 percent of men), being brought into a room against one's will (20 percent of women, 15 percent of men), being tied or bound during sex activities (30 percent of women, 31 percent of men), and being forced to submit (31 percent of women, 27 percent of men). The one item that may suggest a female tendency to passivity or masochism is the fantasy of being rescued from danger by one who will become a lover. However, the fantasy preoccupation with domination showed significant gender differences. Forty-four percent of the men reported the fantasy of forcing a sexual partner to submit. A smaller number reported other sadistic fantasies: whipping, 20 percent; degrading, 15 percent; and torturing, 12 percent.

Of the significant minority of subjects who had sadomasochistic fantasies, more men reported sadistic content, whereas both genders reported similar levels of masochistic content. However, the study was not designed so as to estimate how many of the subjects might be classified as paraphiliacs. What is certain is that, although both genders have a significant fantasy preoccupation with sadism and masochism, enactments are infrequent. Nonetheless, the relatively high incidence of sadomasochistic fantasies compared to other kinky fantasies suggests that power issues in growing up lend themselves to widespread incorporation of sadomasochistic concerns into fantasy life.

ETIOLOGY

The etiology of the paraphilias is not definitively known. Brain abnormalities or biological predispositions, identification with parents who have paraphilias, developmental adversity of a greater or lesser degree, and psychological conflict have all been proposed as potential etiologies for paraphilias, whether singly or in concert.

The inability to explain etiology in paraphilias is not so odd when it is considered that the etiology of heterosexuality or homosexuality is not fully understood. The argument for an exclusive biological causality is difficult to support. Kinsey and colleagues pointed out that the argument that homosexuality was biological could not account for the fact that there were no replicable distinguishing data (such as hormone assays) and, moreover, that homosexuality and heterosexuality were not mutually exclusive but could coexist in all combinations. Similarly, when the etiology of preferential heterosexual choice is considered, the best data suggest that it may be the result of postnatal experience. This having been said, it should be reiterated that the etiology of heterosexuality and homosexuality, like that of the paraphilias, remains unknown.

Brain Abnormalities or Biological Predispositions

Some studies indicate that, among sex offenders seeking treatment, those with congenital or acquired brain damage are overrepresented. Similarly, clinicians have observed that, after brain damage, whether the result of accidents, surgery, epilepsy, or toxic substances, anomalous sexual behaviors, including paraphilias, may emerge. Investigators have observed a link between sexually anomalous behavior and temporal lobe impairment or temporal lobe epilepsy. Different theories have been proposed to explain what the connection might be between brain abnormalities and paraphilias. They include the idea that a brain abnormality diminishes the individual's control over preexisting paraphiliac impulses, that it releases impulses otherwise repressed, that it disadvantages the individual thus afflicted, that it leads to paraphiliac substitutions, or that it may be a direct result of damage to cerebral wiring. It certainly may be that some biological vulnerability or predisposition facilitates a pattern of variant psychosexual development. Even if some biological predisposition is ultimately implicated, its influence would be mediated in interaction with cognitive, affective, and experiential development.

Identification with Parents There is some evidence that there may be an inclination to paraphilia or atypical gender identity in the offspring of a paraphiliac parent. In one study of boys displaying femininity (considered at risk for atypical gender development, including transvestism), of a sample of 20, two fathers were transvestites, and two mothers were lesbians. However, it might also be argued on the basis of the same data that some hereditary factor might be at play. Psychoanalysts and psychotherapists have observed that sadistic patients often report that their parents were brutal or sadistic, whereas masochistic patients may report that their parents were sadistic or masochistic. The child may identify with a sadistic or masochistic parent or may eroticize being abused.

Developmental Adversity and the Offender as Victim Some psychoanalysts and psychotherapists have suggested that a spectrum of early experiences is common in the histories of patients with particular paraphilias and that they appear to be symbolically or actually reenacted in the perverse fantasy. For example, the transvestic fetishist sometimes gives a history in which his mother dressed him in girls' clothes when he was a child, and the sadist gives a history that he was beaten. However, the question has not been settled as to whether such histories reflect real events, retrospective and unconscious falsification, or childhood misperception.

It has been observed that, among those paraphilias that constitute sexual abuse, as much as 30 percent of the paraphiliacs may themselves have been victims of sexual abuse before they were 18 years of age. The mechanism by which a victim becomes an abuser is understood as identification with the aggressor, that is, reliving a trauma but placing oneself in the power position.

Psychogenic Origin It is possible to reconstruct the psychodynamics in some paraphiliac patients and to assess the role of early childhood experiences in the construction of the perverse fantasy. Although psychodynamic formulations are crucial to understanding the structure and meaning of the perverse fantasy, they do not, in and of themselves, establish etiology.

Freud originally postulated that neuroses and perversions were inversely related, with neuroses representing symbolic displacement from perverse fixations, whereas perversions were direct expressions of preoedipal psychosexual fixations. Most psychoanalysts have revised this early formulation and now regard perversion, too, as a defensive compromise.

Psychoanalysts also believed that perversion in the man primarily served as a defense against castration anxiety by symbolizing an illusory female phallus. The fetish was viewed as the prototypical perversion and was literally equated with the illusory female phallus. It was thought to deny the sexual distinction and, thereby, the fear of castration anxiety. Freud made no effort to explain why castration anxiety sometimes led to perversion and, at other times, to homosexuality but most commonly was resolved with no untoward influence.

By and large, the hypothesis that the fetish is an illusory female phallus has become much less influential. More recent formulations have addressed the sources of any disposition to intensified castration anxiety, and, consequently, they have focused on factors occurring early in development. Problems in the separation-individuation phase seem to form the matrix within which perverse formation becomes more likely. Such problems include the development of a poorly defined and unstable body image and the twin fears of engulfment and abandonment by the mother, usually with some oscillation between them. As a defensive maneuver against separation anxiety, it is theorized that the boy invokes a compensatory identification with his mother. The sight of the maternal genital then becomes frightening, because it serves to emphasize the difference between the boy and his mother. At the same time, the feminine identification leaves him vulnerable to an exaggerated threat of castration anxiety in the oedipal period, because he already doubts his masculinity. In this formulation, the fetish is sometimes viewed as a bridge to the mother (a symbolic representation of her) that allays separation anxiety, rather than as a representation of the female phallus.

In addition to anxiety and preoedipal conflicts with the mother as codeterminants of perversion, analysts have emphasized the central role of aggression in erotic excitement. Some analysts have remarked on the transformation of dependent relationships into aggressively destructive ones. Undoubtedly, the dispositions of aggression and power in early developmental life enter into the genesis of paraphilias. This is explicit in sadomasochism. Interviews with sadomasochists show how much they focus on assuming control or giving it away. Paradoxically, masochists may find a feeling of control in submission, something generally acknowledged in the sadomasochistic community in which it is the convention that bottom rules. Others describe masochism as freedom from the demands of the ego. Power is clearly an issue in dominance, which is manifest by the impulse to exert complete control over another's reality. Paradoxically, then, both the masochist and the sadist can achieve a sense of power in the sadomasochistic encounter. These power issues are the residue of conflicts encountered between parent and child, as the child attempts to achieve a sense of agency and independence that mandates the overthrow of parental authority.

To date, no psychodynamic formulation fully addresses the question of why one particular perverse fantasy is selected. The perverse fantasy or act is frequently described as a scenario in which the perverse script symbolizes the sexualization of and triumph over a real or imagined trauma of childhood. Thus, the perversion is believed to undo an actual trauma from an early childhood period, often using real life occurrences as its narrative structure. Sometimes it appears to be an identification or counteridentification with a parent.

There is general agreement among psychoanalysts that the function of the paraphilia often goes beyond the facilitation of sexual potency. It may stabilize personality, in helping to patch over flaws in reality testing or in warding off psychoses. Aggressive wishes, deriving from the traumatic experiences of the preoedipal period, are bound and controlled in the perverse structure. Some authors may go too far in emphasizing how playful, imaginative, and creative the perverse solution is. They ignore the fact that the various perversions are not original creations but are stereotypical and constricting solutions to intrapsychic problems that frequently limit ego development.

DIAGNOSIS AND CLINICAL FEATURES

The term *paraphilia* denotes the presence of an obligatory behavior or fantasy that is deviant in respect to the *object* of the sexual instinct or its *aim*. DSM-IV-TR emphasizes that the use of perverse sexual imagery and acts must be unusual or bizarre:

> The essential features of a Paraphilia are recurrent, intense sexually arousing fantasies, sexual urges, or behaviors generally involving (1) nonhuman objects, (2) the suffering or humiliation of oneself or one's partner, or (3) children or other nonconsenting persons, that occur over a period of at least 6 months (Criterion A). For some individuals, paraphiliac fantasies or stimuli are obligatory for erotic

arousal and are always included in sexual activity. In other cases, the paraphiliac preferences occur only episodically (e.g., perhaps during periods of stress), whereas at other times, the person is able to function sexually without paraphiliac fantasies or stimuli. The behavior, sexual urges, or fantasies cause clinically significiant distress or impairment in social, occupational, or other important areas of functioning (Criterion B).

Accurate diagnosis depends on eliciting the paraphiliac fantasy and ritualized behavior. To make the diagnosis, the achievement of sexual excitement must be dependent on the mental elaboration or behavioral enactment of the deviant fantasy.

The diagnosis of the specific paraphilia depends on the nature of the deviant fantasy, imagery, and behavior. The overt clinical syndrome most often begins shortly after puberty and follows a chronic course. In the paraphilias, by definition, the deviant fantasy and behavior must be the precondition for orgasmic discharge. Therefore, it is obvious that the diagnosis can only be made in adolescence or later. Even though there is evidence for antecedent psychological maladjustments or affective discomfort during childhood, these are not specific to or pathognomonic for the paraphilia and are therefore not predictive. For example, although most transvestites engaged in cross-dressing in childhood, not all cross-dressing boys grow up to be transvestites.

Each of the subclassifications of paraphilias or any specific paraphilia is distinguished by its central imagery and fantasy. Although many individuals who have paraphilias favor one single paraphilia, many are *polymorphous perverse*, that is, they engage in more than one paraphilia.

Although there are many theories that attempt to explain the meaning of each perversion, the following sections are limited to an exposition of the clinical features that are descriptive of each. Their symbolic meanings were alluded to in the section on etiology.

Exhibitionism Table 18.2–1 lists the DSM-IV-TR diagnostic criteria for exhibitionism. In men, sexual arousal is produced by exposure of the genitals to an unknown woman or girl, usually in a public place. It is the experience of the exhibitionistic urge as an irresistible impulse that defines it as pathological. The exhibitionist often, but not always, masturbates as part of his exposure. Exhibitionism, identified in the law as *indecent exposure*, counts for approximately one-third of the sexual offenses in the English-speaking world. As much as 30 or 40 percent of women may have been exposed to exhibitionism. Sexologists sometimes refer to these women as *victims*.

Exhibitionism is primarily reported in men, some of whom may be married and have regular sexual contact with their wives. Obscene phone calls accompanied by masturbation, as a sexual outlet, constitute a related perversion. In fact, exhibitionism, voyeurism, and telephone scatologia are frequently combined.

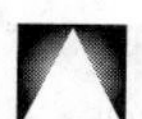

Table 18.2–1
DSM-IV-TR Diagnostic Criteria for Exhibitionism

A. Over a period of at least 6 months, recurrent, intense, sexually arousing fantasies, sexual urges, or behaviors involving the exposure of one's genitals to an unsuspecting stranger.
B. The person has acted on these sexual urges, or the sexual urges or fantasies cause marked distress or interpersonal difficulty.

From American Psychiatric Association. *Diagnostic and Statistical Manual of Mental Disorders*. 4th ed. Text rev. Washington, DC: American Psychiatric Association; 2000, with permission.

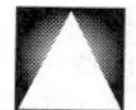

Table 18.2–2
DSM-IV-TR Diagnostic Criteria for Fetishism

A. Over a period of at least 6 months, recurrent, intense, sexually arousing fantasies, sexual urges, or behaviors involving the use of nonliving objects (e.g., female undergarments).
B. The fantasies, sexual urges, or behaviors cause clinically significant distress or impairment in social, occupational, or other important areas of functioning.
C. The fetish objects are not limited to articles of female clothing used in cross-dressing (as in transvestic fetishism) or devices designed for the purpose of tactile genital stimulation (e.g., a vibrator).

From American Psychiatric Association. *Diagnostic and Statistical Manual of Mental Disorders*. 4th ed. Text rev. Washington, DC: American Psychiatric Association; 2000, with permission.

Occasionally, women are flashers. For example, a woman may go out wearing only a raincoat and open it to expose herself. Here, however, the thrill is often reported as a sense of exposure accompanied by humiliation and is not invariably accompanied by sexual arousal.

Fetishism In the case of fetishism, an inanimate object (e.g., a shoe or a handkerchief) or a part-object (e.g., a foot or a partner wearing high-heeled shoes) is required for sexual arousal (Table 18.2–2). The fetish may itself be the only object of sexual interest, in which case, genital discharge is achieved through masturbation, or, alternatively, the fetish may be incorporated into sexual activity with a partner who embodies or wears the fetish. Fetishes often have particular textural characteristics, for example, rubber, leather, and velvet are favored fetishistic materials. The fetish is most commonly associated in some way with humans or their bodily adornments, not something so far removed as furnishings or impersonal belongings. Although some fetishists favor a single fetish, others favor a small variety of objects. A particular fetish or group of fetishes is generally favored for long periods of time. One hospitalized patient favored urinals as his fetishistic object, but he was clearly in the psychotic range, and his perversion, as such, merged with the excretory perversions.

Fetishism has been reported only in men, homosexual and heterosexual, and often exists in combination with other perversions. For example, some transvestites are easily aroused by wearing tightly bound rubber underpants or prefer leather clothing.

Occasionally, women report being a victim of a fetishistic impulse. One woman vividly remembers riding in the subway, sitting next to a man who reached over and took the fabric of her skirt between his two fingers, raised it off her knee, and lowered it without ever making contact with her actual flesh. She said nothing, and he soon got off the train. (His behavior might also be considered kin to frotteurism.)

Frotteurism *Frotteurism* is defined by fantasies and impulses to touch or to rub against an unconsenting female (Table 18.2–3). The full-blown perversion involves a man positioning himself next to a woman in a crowded situation (for example, the subway or bus) to take advantage of the crowding and the movement to rub his genitals against her crotch, thighs, buttocks, or some other body part. Some frotteurists may fantasize that this constitutes a consenting sexual encounter. One sexologist proposed the term *toucherism* to refer to a man's touching a woman on her breasts or buttocks. In a clinical practice, one hears about as much about frotteurism from the female object as from the perpetrator. A woman may be stunned when a strange man passes her on the street, reaches out, touches her

Table 18.2–3
DSM-IV-TR Diagnostic Criteria for Frotteurism

A. Over a period of at least 6 months, recurrent, intense, sexually arousing fantasies, sexual urges, or behaviors involving touching and rubbing against a nonconsenting person.
B. The person has acted on these sexual urges, or the sexual urges or fantasies cause marked distress or interpersonal difficulty.

From American Psychiatric Association. *Diagnostic and Statistical Manual of Mental Disorders.* 4th ed. Text rev. Washington, DC: American Psychiatric Association; 2000, with permission.

breast, and keeps on moving. She may find this sufficiently disturbing that it triggers an anxiety reaction.

Pedophilia To make the diagnosis of pedophilia, the patient's preferred route to sexual excitement must be fantasied or enacted sex with prepubescent children. There must be an age differential of at least 5 years between the perpetrator and the victim (Table 18.2–4). The activity includes exposure of genitals, masturbation with or without the child's awareness or participation, manual manipulation of the child, oral or anal contact, or penetration. The pedophile may seduce, bribe, or coerce the child into masturbating or otherwise pleasuring him. The enactment may take place with an unknown child but may also occur within the home. Pedophilia is differentiated through specifying which gender the perpetrator prefers (male or female, or both), his relationship to the victim (incestuous or nonincestuous), and whether the sexual pattern is obligatory, that is, whether the pedophile is attracted exclusively to children or may be able to have other sexual contacts as well. In one study, heterosexual molesters (nonincestuous) reported an average of 20 victims, whereas homosexual child molesters (nonincestuous) had an average of 150 offenses. Pedophilia has been reported in heterosexual and homosexual men, more frequently among heterosexuals. However, it is not clear whether this is simply because there are more heterosexual males. Occasionally, a woman is a pedophile. Psychotic distortions of the pedophiliac urge may be enacted: One father maneuvered his infant daughter to nurse on his penis; a woman became excited by biting her daughter's vagina. Although this woman was disturbed by her behavior, she experienced it as a compulsion that she was unable to control.

A distinction needs to be made between the pedophile, on the one hand, and the child molester, on the other hand. Pedophiles prefer children as their sexual partners. Child molesters are motivated not by preference but by the unavailability of another adult or by the use of some substance that disinhibits control. For the child molester, his sexual preference is not sex with children, and he targets children simply because of convenience. Some studies show that more than one-half of child molesters were themselves victims of sexual abuse during their childhoods. Some rationalize their behavior by a belief that it may be good for the child, that the child enjoys it, or, at the very least, that the child is not troubled by it. Frequently overlooked is hebephilia, which targets young adolescents rather than children.

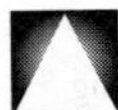

Table 18.2–4
DSM-IV-TR Diagnostic Criteria for Pedophilia

A. Over a period of at least 6 months, recurrent, intense, sexually arousing fantasies, sexual urges, or behaviors involving sexual activity with a prepubescent child or children (generally 13 years of age or younger).
B. The person has acted on these sexual urges, or the sexual urges or fantasies cause marked distress or interpersonal difficulty.
C. The person is at least 16 years of age and at least 5 years older than the child or children in Criterion A.
Note: Do not include an individual in late adolescence involved in an ongoing sexual relationship with a 12- or 13-year-old.

Specify if:
Sexually attracted to males
Sexually attracted to females
Sexually attracted to both

Specify if:
Limited to incest

Specify type:
Exclusive type (attracted only to children)
Nonexclusive type

From American Psychiatric Association. *Diagnostic and Statistical Manual of Mental Disorders.* 4th ed. Text rev. Washington, DC: American Psychiatric Association; 2000, with permission.

Sexual Masochism Table 18.2–5 presents the diagnostic criteria for sexual masochism. The masochist fantasizes being humiliated, beaten, bound, or made to suffer and has impulses to enact these fantasies. Some women like to fantasize about being hookers and being paid to do whatever humiliating behavior is required. Although some masochists may fantasize about being tortured, only a few fantasize about being mutilated or killed. Masochistic elaborations of other paraphilias are common; for example, the erotic preference for being straddled and urinated on combines an excretory and masochistic perversion.

Sexual Sadism Sexual sadism is in some ways a mirror image of sexual masochism. It consists of sexual fantasies and urges that involve the infliction of psychological or physical suffering, or both, on a partner (Table 18.2–6). Fantasies and enactments include verbal and physical humiliation, bondage, forceful restraint, and spanking and, at the extreme, may include torture, mutilation, and killing. The partner's involvement may be fully consenting (as is the case in ongoing sadomasochistic relationships), or the partner may exhibit a complete lack of consent (as sometimes can occur in violent initial sexual encounters).

Masochism and sadism are distinguished from the other paraphilias in two ways and are therefore of special interest. First, although, like the other paraphilias, they occur among heterosexuals and homosexuals, they are the only paraphilias that occur in large numbers in both genders. Second, they merge more perceptibly into aspects of normal sexuality. Indeed, in DSM-III, it was suggested that "the diagnosis of sexual masochism is made only if the individual engages in masochistic sexual acts, not merely fantasies." This

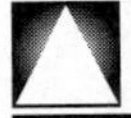

Table 18.2–5
DSM-IV-TR Diagnostic Criteria for Sexual Masochism

A. Over a period of at least 6 months, recurrent, intense, sexually arousing fantasies, sexual urges, or behaviors involving the act (real, not simulated) of being humiliated, beaten, bound, or otherwise made to suffer.
B. The fantasies, sexual urges, or behaviors cause clinically significant distress or impairment in social, occupational, or other important areas of functioning.

From American Psychiatric Association. *Diagnostic and Statistical Manual of Mental Disorders.* 4th ed. Text rev. Washington, DC: American Psychiatric Association; 2000, with permission.

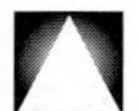

Table 18.2–6
DSM-IV-TR Diagnostic Criteria for Sexual Sadism

A. Over a period of at least 6 months, recurrent, intense, sexually arousing fantasies, sexual urges, or behaviors involving acts (real, not simulated) in which the psychological or physical suffering (including humiliation) of the victim is sexually exciting to the person.

B. The person has acted on these sexual urges with a nonconsenting person, or the sexual urges or fantasies cause marked distress or interpersonal difficulty.

From American Psychiatric Association. *Diagnostic and Statistical Manual of Mental Disorders*. 4th ed. Text rev. Washington, DC: American Psychiatric Association; 2000, with permission.

exemption is not applied to the other paraphilias, including sadism. This may be indicative of how widespread masochistic fantasies are and certainly suggests that the border between normal and deviant may be porous.

Beginning with Freud, it has been recognized that masochism and sadism are often linked, that is, that although an individual is usually preferentially a sexual masochist or sadist, he or she can occasionally enact the other role. These observations suggest that the masochist and sadist often identify with the sadomasochism transaction, not exclusively with one role. Some psychiatrists prefer the term *sadomasochism*, rather than *sadism* and *masochism* separately, to make the point that pure sadism is generally laced with masochism, and pure masochism is laced with sadism.

It is unusual to see any patient whose sexual life is predominantly sadistic or masochistic who does not enact some form of sadomasochism in the nonsexual arena. Sadomasochism is particularly complicated, because it can be embedded in the overlapping spheres of the sexual and the relational. In the sexual situation, aggression in the form of controlled sadism or masochism can be experienced as pleasurable, but this is far less true in the case of relational sadomasochism, particularly for battered wives.

In some individuals, the need for sadistic behavior escalates and may result in sadistic rape, lust murder, or serial murders. Far more common, however, is the clinical finding that sadistic men may inhibit themselves sexually, because they are reluctant to engage in those enactments that are requisite to arousal, particularly with their wives. These individuals give up sexuality rather than run the risk of indulging the fantasy or the behavior or seek out prostitutes. It might be argued that those who do not engage in any sadistic behavior and who suppress the fantasy, when possible, are not perverse. However, in terms of personality organization and preoccupation, they are close psychological kin to sadists who exhibit the overt syndrome.

Although it is commonly believed that masochism predominates among women, the reports of gender ratios vary considerably. For example, almost all of Krafft-Ebing's reported cases were in men. Curiously enough, Freud derived the concept of feminine masochism from analyzing the masochistic perversion in men. The enacted fantasy may well be more common in men, although it is still an open question as to whether obligatory masochistic fantasies predominate in one gender or the other.

Common is the sexual sadomasochist who is sadistic in one relationship and masochistic in another (or dismissive in one, yearning in the other), reprising Arthur Schnitzler's famous play, *La Ronde*. Mr. B., a successful 45-year-old businessman, splits his emotional life between a wife whom he oppresses and his assistant, Ms. J., with whom he is enthralled and whom he placates moment to moment. When Ms. J. tells him she is involved with a younger man, one who works in a position subservient to her, Mr. B. suffers, but his sexual desire for her explodes. The minute that she is out of his sight, he begins to obsess in a kind of masochistic perseveration about whether she is at that moment sleeping with the other man. Mr. B. holds a dominant position in the business world, but, in his psychic world, he is under the spell of Ms. J. In his sexual life, he will do whatever is demanded of him, including limiting his own preferences, to please her. He allows himself to experience orgasm only with her consent. In contrast, he dominates and humiliates his wife. His cruelty towards her is expressed in his reluctance to sleep with her, in his emotional coldness toward her, and in sadism on the rare occasions when he sleeps with her out of sexual need or out of anger that Ms. J. is with another man. Then he slaps her around. Even when he is not sexually abusive, he verbally expresses contempt for her body and her erotic skills. The more he feels humiliated by Ms. J., the more he humiliates his wife. This kind of split appears to be an enactment of a split relationship with one or another parent. Mr. B.'s angry dominating stance toward his wife appears to be a derivative of the rage he felt toward his neglectful mother; he now wishes to dominate and to humiliate his wife, just as he felt his mother had done to him. In parallel, his subordination to Ms. J. appears to echo the intermittent but abject longing for his mother's love, which he experienced in childhood, but which was forthcoming only in brief moments.

Transvestic Fetishism

Transvestic fetishism literally means cross-dressing. In psychiatry, however, the term was used not only phenomenologically, but also diagnostically. It was defined as heterosexual cross-dressing in which pieces of clothing were used fetishistically for sexual arousal. Because of the fetishistic component, the term *transvestic fetishism* has come to be substituted for the term *transvestite*. The cross-dressing may be used to promote sexual excitement that can lead to masturbation or heterosexual intercourse. Although the cross-dressing may begin in childhood, it usually becomes sexualized only in adolescence. In the predominant pattern, the child spontaneously cross-dresses, using the garments of his mother or sister, and the activity most often remains surreptitious. In some instances, it is reported to have been initiated by the mother or mother surrogate. Cross-dressing can start with a desire to promote a sense of self-soothing and well-being and then becomes sexualized, or it can be erotic from the outset. It is sporadic at first and, in most transvestic fetishists, remains so. In some, however, it becomes a daily occurrence. Table 18.2–7 lists the DSM-IV-TR diagnostic criteria for transvestic fetishism.

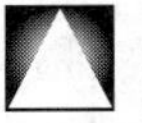

Table 18.2–7
DSM-IV-TR Diagnostic Criteria for Transvestic Fetishism

A. Over a period of at least 6 months, in a heterosexual man, recurrent, intense, sexually arousing fantasies, sexual urges, or behaviors involving cross-dressing.

B. The fantasies, sexual urges, or behaviors cause clinically significant distress or impairment in social, occupational, or other important areas of functioning.

Specify if:

With gender dysphoria: if the person has persistent discomfort with gender role or identity.

From American Psychiatric Association. *Diagnostic and Statistical Manual of Mental Disorders*. 4th ed. Text rev. Washington, DC: American Psychiatric Association; 2000, with permission.

Transvestic fetishists are, by definition, preferential heterosexuals. Fetishistic arousal can be intense, but interpersonal sexuality is almost always attenuated. It is typical for a transvestic fetishist to report his entire sexual experience as limited to one or two partners. In adulthood, his behavior may be masculine in male clothes, effeminate in female clothes. Many are employed in hypermasculine professions (e.g., race care driving, munitions experts). Some transvestic fetishists carry photographs of themselves dressed as women; others habitually wear hidden female undergarments. These are mini symbols of cross-dressing and enhance the illusion of being a woman even while dressed as a man.

In the pornography favored by transvestic fetishists, the initiation into cross-dressing is usually forced on the novice by a dominant, big-breasted, corseted, booted, phallic woman who enslaves him or by a kindly protective woman who does so to save his life. Such initiation fantasies permeate the collective fantasy life of transvestic fetishists.

Some transvestic fetishists fall in love with transsexuals and, as a consequence, give up cross-dressing altogether. This relationship appears to be based on projective identification; that is, the transvestic fetishist projects his fantasy of being female onto the transsexual and then reincorporates it by identifying with "her."

Mr. H. is 46-year-old married transvestic fetishist, a successful lawyer who loves his work. He and his wife have two grown children, who no longer live at home. Ambitious and competitive, he masks his aggression behind a gentle facade. He views himself as helpful to other people and is proud of his ability to assert himself when necessary.

Mr. H. was the youngest of two siblings with a sister who was 3 years older. His parents had a tempestuous marriage and, after multiple separations, ultimately divorced when Mr. H. was 7 years of age. During the separations, and after the divorce, he and his sister stayed with their maternal grandparents. Mr. H. was living with them on a consistent basis even before his parents finally divorced. He saw his mother only irregularly. He has obliterated all memory of his father. His mother was outgoing and loving to Mr. H. when she saw him, but, with each separation, he feared he might never see her again and was overwhelmed with sadness. As he grew older, his grandparents left him on his own. He would disappear and stay with friends for several days, and no one questioned why. Although he sometimes recounts this as a positive experience, the fact is that he felt abandoned throughout childhood, commenting that he largely raised himself. He was never effeminate, and he never played with girls. He was a good student, and, after college, he went to law school.

His aunt's ministrations were tender and, at times, seductive. She fondled him, combed his hair, and rubbed him down with oil. He remembers an early attachment to her mohair blankets but denies that she ever cross-dressed him. He began to cross-dress in his aunt's clothes at 8 years of age. It was always in secret, and he was never discovered. Cross-dressing was initially nonerotic and produced a safe form of relaxation—like alcohol. Only in adolescence did he begin to eroticize female clothing and to have spontaneous ejaculations while cross-dressed. In his late teens, he had sexual intercourse for the first time with an older female neighbor whom he married while he was still in his early 20s.

His cross-dressing escalated after the birth of his first child. At the same time, his sexual drive toward his wife began to diminish. He continues to have an increasing urge to cross-dress under stress. He entered treatment, because the cross-dressing preoccupied him more and more, and his wife was threatening divorce in response to his loss of sexual interest in her. Like many other transvestic fetishists, he continues to have a pronounced interest in masculine activities.

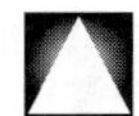

Table 18.2–8
DSM-IV-TR Diagnostic Criteria for Voyeurism

A. Over a period of at least 6 months, recurrent, intense, sexually arousing fantasies, sexual urges, or behaviors involving the act of observing an unsuspecting person who is naked, who is in the process of disrobing, or who is engaging in sexual activity.
B. The person has acted on these sexual urges, or the sexual urges or fantasies cause marked distress or interpersonal difficulty.

From American Psychiatric Association. *Diagnostic and Statistical Manual of Mental Disorders*. 4th ed. Text rev. Washington, DC: American Psychiatric Association; 2000, with permission.

Voyeurism *Voyeurism* is defined as a preference for masturbating while observing nude women who are unaware of being seen (Table 18.2–8). Men may achieve sexual arousal by looking at strange women in situations that they construe as sexual (e.g., spying on a woman who is undressing—the proverbial Peeping Tom). Voyeurs do not otherwise accost the women observed. Excitement may sometimes be purely psychic. Voyeurism has been reported only in men, and it often takes priority over any wish for sexual intercourse.

Voyeurism may be one of the least researched forms of paraphilia. It has been reported that the voyeur seeks no sexual contact with the victim, yet, in one study, one-third of the subjects had committed rape. A number of voyeurs are married but nonetheless have fears of approaching women sexually.

One man, best described as polymorphous perverse, spent the early years of his marriage avoiding sex with his wife while sneaking glances of a woman across the courtyard dressing and undressing. This man, like many other voyeurs, had a number of coexisting paraphilias; he preferred watching his spouse insert the tube of an enema bag into her vagina, so as to masturbate rather than having intercourse with her. He associated this preference to having once seen his mother naked in her bathroom, holding a douche bag or an enema bag. In his therapy sessions, he frequently closed his eyes. He eventually disclosed that, during such moments, he had flash fantasies in which he visualized women in a number of erotic poses.

Paraphilias Not Otherwise Specified Paraphilias not otherwise specified include telephone scatologia (obscene phone calls), necrophilia (corpses), partialism (exclusive focus on part of the body), coprophilia (feces), klismaphilia (enemas), and urophilia (urine). Although sporadic sexual relationships with animals can be elicited by history, it is rare that this is the preferential route of sexual discharge. Some authors distinguish zoophilia (sexual excitement experienced with stroking or fondling animals) from bestiality (a sex act between an individual and an animal).

LABORATORY EXAMINATION

The penile plethysmograph is used as a diagnostic parameter, and it may also be used in some desensitization therapies. Its therapeutic use is discussed in the section on therapy. As a diagnostic tool, it helps delineate paraphiliac response by measuring penile volume assessment or penile circumference (the newer measure) in response to suggestive films of sexual scenes. Originally used to identify compulsive homosexuality, it was later applied to paraphiliacs. Although it was initially thought that penile circumference assessments would have results comparable to those of penile volume assessment, this may not be the case.

The difference in the two procedures is in the length of the subjects' exposure to sexual films. With the earlier technology, exposure was for the duration of only 10 to 13 seconds. The newer technology uses 2-minute video clips. The issue is whether with the newer technology—penile circumference—the test result can be faked or is resistant to faking. Penile circumference assessment inevitably requires longer exposure to erotic stimuli, because the blood flow that accompanies penile tumescence cannot maintain penile circumference while maintaining the rapid increase in penile length. The longer time needed to assess circumference may allow the subject to suppress his response to the erotic material being shown; that is, he can fool the researcher. The questions raised about the validity of this test have importance insofar as it is used in outcome studies to measure change after therapy with sex offenders, including, for example, pedophiles.

DIFFERENTIAL DIAGNOSIS

Differential diagnosis is usually relatively easy. Occasionally, there is some confusion between paraphilias and the gender identity disorders or psychoses.

Characteristics Essential to the Diagnosis of Paraphilia The following features are essential to the diagnosis of the paraphilias and are common to them all.

- The deviation appears fixed. Unusual fantasies or behaviors are persistent and repetitive and permeate mental life. They are ritualized and stereotypical.
- The deviant fantasy must have been pervasive for the preceding 6 months, or the impulse must be imperative and insistent.
- Perverse behavior generally occurs in two distinct phases. The perverse activity is usually followed by a heterosexual or homosexual encounter or by masturbation. Sexual excitement and potency appear to be facilitated by the preceding perverse behavior. Therefore, most perverse behavior terminates with genital orgasm. It must be emphasized that neither the perverse behavior nor the sexual act necessarily requires another person. For example, transvestism and fetishism are considered perversions, even when the deviant activity is solitary, and the genital activity is masturbation.
- The deviation may be ego-syntonic or ego-dystonic. When the individual is under the pressure of seeking orgasmic release, it is most often experienced as ego-syntonic. However, there may be a marked ego-dystonic reaction after the enactment of the perverse activity. There may also be long periods in which the individual makes the attempt to disavow the perverse fantasy and enactment.
- Suppression of the perverse fantasy becomes difficult, if not impossible. Enactment is often triggered by anxiety or some other dysphoric emotion. After the fantasy is enacted, it sometimes results in depression, the feeling of profound emptiness, or the reemergence of anxiety.

The question arises as to whether the presence of pervasive perverse fantasies that are not enacted is adequate for the diagnosis of paraphilias. DSM-IV-TR suggests that it is. Thus, although the behavioral manifestations of sexuality may appear normal, the patients are aware of, if not alarmed by, the obligatory and sometimes obsessive nature of their fantasy lives. However, if the perverse fantasies are incidental or occasional, they can be understood as part of normal sexuality and not of decisive psychological significance.

Features Commonly Associated with the Paraphilias Although some characteristics are common to all the paraphilias, individual cases vary in terms of personality integration, associated pathology, and overall adaptation.

- Some married individuals enact the paraphilia only outside of the marital sexual situation, although the perverse fantasy may fuel the marital sexual encounter. Excitement is invariably greater with the deviant enactment.
- In some instances, the perverse activity tends to escalate over time. This seems particularly true of transvestic fetishism and, perhaps, sadomasochism.
- Aside from the paraphiliac fantasy, which is obsessional and intrusive in nature, there is a diminution in other kinds of sexual fantasies and in nonsexual fantasies. Dreaming is sometimes scant.
- Patients may regard their behavior as essentially normal, although they know that their preferences are unusual. Despite their claims of normality, they often feel humiliation, guilt, shame, and fear of legal entanglement. Insofar as they wish to suppress their perverse behaviors, they experience dysphoric affects, if they are successful, and a feeling of lack of control, if they are not.
- Paraphilias are not invariably mutually exclusive. For example, one may see combinations of transvestism and sexual masochism. The paraphilias frequently coexist with sexual dysfunctions.
- Although perversion may be associated with a borderline personality organization, most contemporary therapists and sexologists observe that paraphilias may have higher or lower levels of personality integration. In the higher levels of integration, the perversion serves primarily to facilitate sexual functioning. It is among these individuals that perverse fantasies, rather than enactments, may suffice to facilitate potency. In the lower ranges of integration, the paraphilia is not only used to promote pleasurable sexual function, but also to maintain ego boundaries and the sense of self and to bind aggression.
- The nature of the paraphilia is not indicative of the level of personality integration. Sometimes, it has been assumed that certain paraphilias must be associated intrinsically with greater ego disturbance than others; for example, some observers have suggested that, to the extent that the object is a part-object or denigrated, the overall personality is more primitive. Yet, this is not necessarily so. Each syndrome comprises individuals exhibiting a wide diversity of personality integrations.
- Although the DSM-IV-TR calls attention to the fact that there is often impairment in the capacity for reciprocal affectionate sexual activity, this is variable. Within the higher levels of personality organization, the individual is more often able to achieve reciprocal affectionate sexual relationships, sometimes of a dependent nature, and to maintain meaningful nonsexual relations.
- Paraphiliacs are depression prone: The depression often takes the form of an ongoing empty depression. Alcoholism or drug addiction is widely observed and may represent a maladaptive attempt at self-medication of the depression.
- Perverse behavior often entails interpersonal complications that themselves become the source of depression and anxiety; for example, it may be the source of discord in a marriage and may lead the paraphiliac to enter into other relationships, with a more tolerant girlfriend or with a prostitute. Perverse behaviors with nonconsenting individuals may lead to legal entanglements.

Disorders That Are Sometimes Confused with the Paraphilias Although some transvestic fetishists use cross-dressing almost exclusively to achieve sexual excitement, nevertheless, there are also a significant number of transvestic fetishists for whom the purpose of cross-dressing evolves or changes over time. In this latter group, the cross-dressing becomes the purpose in and of itself, to assuage anxiety and to assert a partial female gender identity; its importance as a prerequisite to sexual arousal takes second place to the increasing urgency to self-identify as a woman. DSM-

IV-TR takes no account of the frequent evolution of transvestic fetishists into transsexuals. In fact, transvestic fetishists are one of three diagnostic entities that feed into the transsexual diagnosis. (The other two consist of cross-dressing homosexuals and primary transsexuals.) Although DSM-IV-TR attempts to address differences in transvestic fetishists by suggesting that the diagnosis specify if the transvestic fetishism is accompanied by gender dysphoria, it is important to emphasize that, in many cases, there is a metamorphosis, such that the primary emphasis becomes sex change rather than the facilitation of a sex act.

The gender identity disorders are distinguished by an impairment of core gender. It is not altogether clear why transsexualism and cross-gender identifications in children are classified as identity disorders, whereas transvestic fetishism is grouped with the paraphilias.

In some patients, an obsessive sexual fantasy in an otherwise neurotic patient may mimic a paraphilia. Although perverse fantasies may surface in the course of an in-depth psychotherapy, they do not invade conscious life to the same degree as in the paraphilias nor are such obsessive fantasies necessarily associated with any preemptive urge to enact the fantasy.

Certain behaviors are classified as paraphilias by some experts but not by others. The most confusing category may involve sexual acts that infringe on the welfare of others. For example, sexual assault, which, along with child molestation, may commonly result in imprisonment, is not classified as paraphilia. Although some clinicians consider rape to be paraphilia, most do not. For most rapists, rape is neither the preferred sexual activity nor a consistent fantasy preoccupation, and these remain the hallmarks requisite to the diagnosis of a paraphilia. It is true that rape perpetrated against enemy women in war time or in gang rapes is far different from the psychologically driven sexual enactments classified as paraphilias. In contrast, serial rapists are often acting out some powerful impulse or fantasy. Part of the problem in labeling compulsive rapists as paraphiliacs may be a legal one; that is, if something is diagnosed as a paraphilia, such a psychological or medical diagnosis might protect the perpetrator against criminal action. However, this is not the case with pedophilia. As previously noted, a related problem is the question of whether a distinction should be made between paraphilias that inflict harm and those that do not.

Homosexuality was declassified as a paraphilia in the context of gay liberation. The declassification was warranted because of the following compelling reasons. First, the central imagery of homosexuals is not generally bizarre. Second, the homosexual impulse, like the heterosexual one (but unlike the deviant one), may not be driven. Third, homosexual behavior need not be ritualized or stereotypical in the way that the paraphilias invariably are. Fourth, fantasy life is not impoverished. Fifth, and most importantly, it has not been demonstrated that homosexual ideation invariably permeates mental life to an excessive degree, that the suppression of any one homosexual act yields high-level anxiety or dysphoric affect, or that homosexuality is connected to personality dysfunction any more than heterosexuality is. However, homosexuals are no more immune from paraphilias than are heterosexuals. Homosexuality and paraphilias may coexist just as heterosexuality and paraphilia coexist.

COURSE AND PROGNOSIS

The sexual fantasies that are at the core of the paraphilias generally begin to take shape in childhood but are elaborated and become more precise throughout adolescence and early adulthood. Although many paraphiliacs revise and edit their fantasies throughout their lifetimes, some rotate between a few favorite paraphiliac fantasies. The pressure to enactment varies over time, usually increasing at times of external stress. To the degree that opportunities to enact the paraphilia present themselves, interest in it may grow. For some people, the paraphilias decline with age and a decreased interest in sexuality.

The frequency and intensity of paraphiliac fantasies and enactments increase in proportion to involvement in networks of people similarly inclined. For example, in transvestic fetishism, the man uses a piece of female clothing or dresses in female clothes to facilitate sexual arousal and masturbation. Immersion in a transvestic subculture, an activity first facilitated through magazines such as *Transvestia,* generally promotes an evolution in intensity. Insofar as a transvestic fetishist is involved in a subculture, his cross-dressing tends to escalate. Immersion in such a subculture normalizes the behavior and appears to reduce some of the internal resistance to compulsive dressing.

Whenever there is communication among people who share the same paraphilia, the usual outcome is to normalize the paraphilia and thereby to increase the individual's likelihood of enacting it. The Internet provides virtual groups that have the same effect.

Because the preconditions for the paraphilia—whether they are biological or psychological—are laid down so early in the paraphiliac's life, they become part of his or her identity and the source of sexual pleasure. Paraphilias, like all behaviors that yield pleasure, are difficult to relinquish. This is more so for the paraphilias than for, say, smoking or drinking, because the paraphiliac fantasy is so closely woven into the paraphiliac's identity and sense of self. At the same time, paraphiliacs often feel shame or are disturbed by the compulsive nature of their sexuality and may make the attempt to give up the paraphiliac behavior. This is generally successful for only a short period of time, so that psychiatrists who follow their patients for a number of years observe cycles of activity and inactivity—of pleasure in the paraphilia and revulsion toward it. During one of the cycles of inactivity, the paraphiliac patient may feel that he or she has conquered the problem but nonetheless remains susceptible to its reoccurrence, particularly during times of stress. Clinicians, too, may be prematurely seduced into believing that they have secured a cure. Some researchers may display the same naïveté, confusing cycles of renunciation with permanent cure.

TREATMENT

Treatment is extremely difficult, because the symptom yields pleasure and, as a consequence, is hard to relinquish. Renunciation may be even more difficult when the paraphilias are associated with a borderline personality. Patients with paraphilias are subject to many kinds of secondary crises, including depressions. Although the treatment of paraphilia itself is invariably difficult, the secondary crises can be successfully treated by a variety of means.

At least three different kinds of psychiatric modalities are used to assist the paraphilia patient in establishing internal control over the enactment of a paraphiliac fantasy. These include cognitive-behavioral therapy and group therapy, often coupled with relapse prevention, medication to reduce sexual drive, and dynamic psychotherapy or psychoanalytic psychotherapy. Although there have been attempts to empirically evaluate the first two modes of therapy, outcome studies on patients treated by psychotherapists and psychoanalysts depend on the individual case reports of the therapist. However, there should be a disclaimer for the validity of follow-up studies, no matter what the mode of therapy. Relapse often occurs after the evaluations have been completed, particularly if evaluations are done within a short time after the treatment.

In those instances in which sexual victimization is part of the paraphiliac fantasy, the urgent need is not for any of the three treatment modalities, but for the establishment of external controls to prevent the victimization of others.

Finally, therapists need to treat comorbid conditions that affect the urgency of the paraphiliac fantasy and enactment.

The choice of treatment depends, in part, on the presumed etiology and on the urgency of controlling the enactment of potentially dangerous paraphilias. In reality, most paraphiliac enactments that entail a victim are designated as sex offenses, and the perpetrators receive cognitive-behavioral therapy or psychopharmacological treatment. Those who are self-referred and who seek individual treatment are more likely to receive dynamic psychotherapy and, sometimes, cognitive-behavioral therapy.

Cognitive-Behavioral Therapy Cognitive-behavioral therapy consists of direct, behavioral interventions rather than an exploration of the possible early developmental factors and interpersonal conflicts that may be part of the etiology. The behavior therapies aim to teach patients techniques that they can use to decrease deviant sexual urges and to maintain control of their behaviors. These include olfactory aversion, covert sensitization, various masturbatory reconditioning techniques, modified aversive behavioral rehearsal, and imaginal desensitization training. In covert sensitization, the patient is trained in relaxation. Once he is relaxed, he is asked to visualize his deviant behavior and then to introduce a negative event. For example, one expert suggested the following sequence: An exhibitionist is asked to picture himself in a car, exposing himself to school girls. As part of the story, he is asked to imagine calling the girls over to his car while he masturbates. It is then suggested to him that, as the girls are staring at him, he experiences a pain, the result of his penis getting stuck in his pants zipper. He is unable to yank it free, only hurting himself more. His penis starts to bleed, and he loses his erection. The girls are laughing, and a policeman is coming over. The resolution is that he is finally able to zip up his pants and drive off, whereon he begins to relax and to breathe more easily. The directed fantasy is structured in such a way that it starts with the build-up of deviant sexual arousal, which is interrupted by a negative consequence. The patient is able to escape only by renouncing his deviant stimulus. By introducing an adverse event into an established sexual scenario, it is hoped that deconditioning takes place. This and similar techniques may be carried out between therapist and patient in one-on-one therapy, or they may be implemented within a group format.

It has been suggested that different kinds of cognitive-behavioral treatments are more effective with different subgroups; for example, those that focus on relational problems may work relatively well with exhibitionists. However, even in treatments with the best outcomes, patients are vulnerable to relapse. Some patients may become lax out of wishful thinking that their cure is permanent. Therefore, part of the treatment should be concerned with relapse rehearsal.

Relapse therapy is a program designed to help the paraphiliac or offender become aware of danger signs and cope with them. Warning signals include the reappearance of the paraphiliac fantasies or decisions that may place him in a high-risk situation. Relapse rehearsal is exactly what the name suggests; the paraphiliac is asked to fantasize a relapse, to conjure up the negative feelings sometimes associated with it, including guilt, shame, and self-blame. He is encouraged to use those coping strategies and self-controls that he has already mastered, to visualize himself controlling the situation, rather than succumbing to it. The positive feelings that he conjures up in response to his successful handling of the situation reinforces his feeling of self-control. Without such an intervention, recidivism rates may reach 55 percent. (Some observers would consider the recidivism rate to be much higher.) Outcome is sometimes assessed by means of a penile plethysmograph, in which a posttherapy patient is exposed to erotic stimuli known to have previously aroused him.

Psychopharmacological Treatment to Reduce the Sexual Drives Aversion therapy and treatment with antiandrogenic medication have been attempted with sex offenders and with paraphiliac patients. Sometimes called *chemical castration*, this misnomer may give the impression that treatment is definitive. Quite the contrary. Short-term control is easier to obtain than fundamental long-term change. Among the main antiandrogens used is cyproterone acetate (CPA), which acts on the androgen receptors to block intracellular testosterone intake and intracellular metabolism of androgen. Erections, ejaculates, and spermatogenesis are all decreased and, interestingly, so are sexual fantasies. Medroxyprogesterone acetate (MPA) has long been the leading drug studied in treating sexual offenders in North America. The principal action is through its stimulus to testosterone-A-reductase in the liver, which enhances the metabolic clearance of testosterone, thus reducing its plasma level. Its side effects include weight gain, decreased sperm production, and some gastrointestinal (GI) symptoms. Relapse generally follows the cessation of the medicine.

It is still debated whether paraphiliac behavior can be understood as part of the obsessive-compulsive spectrum of disorders. In this framework, the paraphiliac fantasies are considered to be to obsessions what paraphiliac enactments are to compulsions. In other words, the paraphilia is enacted when internal resistance is overwhelmed by the compulsion. It has been demonstrated that the same drugs that are effective in the treatment of some impulse control disorders, such as kleptomania, may have some effect in the paraphilias. These are drugs that are selective serotonin reuptake inhibitors (SSRIs). One advantage of this group of drugs is that they can be safely given to adolescents. None of the psychopharmacological treatments, however, constitutes a cure.

Dynamic Psychotherapy Although there are individual case reports of good results, there are no long-term follow-up studies and few large-scale studies. Not many psychotherapists would claim a high percentage of cure in patients with full-blown perverse syndromes. The patient's overall adaptation may well improve, but permanent change in the perverse structure is more problematical. The patient may learn how to identify situations that lead to increased anxiety or depression and to the escalation of paraphiliac fantasy and enactment, and he may learn how to avoid them. Outcome depends on the underlying personality organization. Insofar as the major function of the perversion is to facilitate sexual excitement more than to preserve the integrity of the ego, there is a greater opportunity for a successful treatment intervention. To the degree that borderline features are more prominent, the outcome is generally less favorable.

Some patients learn how to manage their lives so that perverse enactments are kept out of their intimate relationships. They may act out their perverse impulses with call girls or with willing extramarital partners. This, of course, only works with paraphilias that are nonthreatening to the welfare of their sexual partners.

External Controls External controls are indicated when paraphiliac behavior threatens sexual victimization of others. In the case of abuse within the family, adults other than the abuser and children must be protected by being instructed as to the danger. To the degree that these constraints are ineffective, the offender must be removed from the home.

Treatment of Comorbid Conditions Various comorbid conditions may tilt a paraphilia toward escalating enactments. Chief among these are depressive reactions, loss of key relationships through divorce or death, loss of jobs or positions within the community, and self-medication with alcohol or recreational drugs. In addition, the paraphilias may be complicated by their coexistence with other psychological disorders: major depressive disorders, psychoses, or psychotic decompensation. When present, treatment for these conditions or counseling must become part of the treatment plan.

Treatment Results It is difficult to compare outcome results between the treatment of sex offenders (often including groups other than paraphiliacs) and the treatment of paraphiliacs seen in private practice. The two venues not only use different treatment modalities, but also deal with different patients.

The complaint against psychodynamically oriented clinicians is largely that there are few, if any, follow-up studies, and this is a valid criticism. In fact, as the following case demonstrates, analysts may believe that a patient is cured and may publish a case report to that effect, only to witness an exacerbation that goes far beyond the original problem.

A patient diagnosed as a transvestite (the terminology then used to describe what is now called a *transvestic fetishist*) engaged in a long psychoanalysis with a distinguished psychoanalyst, one of whose subspecialties was the paraphilias. The analyst well understood the patient's dynamics and worked through them with the patient. The patient married and had a child. At a certain point, the analyst came to believe that the patient's problems were resolved. This, of course, turned out to be a rather naïve assumption. In fact, several years later, the patient underwent a sex reassignment surgery and now lives full time as a woman. Such cases are cautionary tales. They show that the internal struggle between yielding to a paraphilia and resisting it can sometimes mislead psychotherapists and sexologists, who may mistake a pendulum swing to renunciation for a genuine resolution.

Nonetheless, psychodynamic treatment does provide considerable support to many paraphiliacs, particularly those who are not sex offenders. Therapists can intervene by addressing issues of stress and relational problems that may reduce anxiety within the home and by identifying those stresses that inevitably lead to an escalation of the paraphiliac impulse.

Unlike psychotherapy, which is conducted by therapists who generally see relatively few full-blown paraphiliac cases, cognitive-behavioral therapy, followed by relapse rehearsal and psychopharmacological treatment, has the advantage that some of its practitioners are immersed in the treatment of paraphiliacs under the auspices of programs to treat sex offenders.

The limitation to the treatment with antiandrogenic medications is the patient's noncompliance in continuing to take the medication. This limitation is a direct product of its mode of operation: It acts by reducing sexual desire and erections, not by selectively inhibiting deviant impulses. Over the course of months or years, patients may be unwilling to give up sexual pleasure. (An analogous problem is seen in some manic-depressives who stop taking their medication, because they are unwilling to forego manic bursts of energy.) Other reasons for noncompliance include side effects, such as weight gain, testicular atrophy, and hypertension.

Most of the investigators and therapists working with paraphiliac patients use some combination of cognitive-behavioral therapy along with relapse prevention programs. It is believed that this is the most viable combination of treatment for paraphiliacs who have committed sex offenses. Many of these therapists formalize follow-up studies. Most of the follow-up studies show continuing improvement in the majority of treated patients for several years. Ultimately, the measure of success or failure is linked to rates of recidivism. The limitation to these follow-up studies is their duration; most of them do not follow the patients for a sufficiently long period of time, sometimes for just a few years. Given the nature of paraphilias, follow-up studies of only several years' duration are not good indicators of ultimate treatment outcomes. Because recidivism rates increase over time, long-term outcome studies are essential. Relapse rehearsal can be viewed as a mode of self-control. However, as several investigators have pointed out, this model does not focus on cure, but rather focuses on a prevention model of change.

Paraphilia needs to be viewed as a chronic condition that can be controlled rather than eradicated. In this context, stress management becomes an important component of any treatment plan. One can maintain some optimism, as long as the goal is control rather than cure, with the realization that results are much better if no sex offense is implicated, if there is a single paraphilia, if there is a stable home environment, and if the therapeutic relationship can be carried out consistently with the same person no matter what the modality of treatment. (Most reports stress that individual, rather than group, therapy is most beneficial.) That there seldom appears to be a cure should not discourage those in the field from seeking partial therapeutic success.

There are a good number of paraphiliac patients who have minor perversions and who live extremely productive lives. These are the paraphiliacs who seldom come to attention and whose paraphilias are contained within the boundaries of a relationship.

One often reads in the literature accounts of a successful and devoted pairing between individuals with complementary perversions. Therefore, there appear to be a number of self-described ongoing, gratifying relationships between sexual sadists and sexual masochists, some of whom extend sadomasochistic interactions to behaviors outside the sexual realm and who are known as *relational sadomasochists*. It is difficult to evaluate these claims, because these are the people who do not seek therapy. It does seem possible that sometimes consensual sadomasochistic relationships serve the needs of both people. Furthermore, minor perversions can be embraced within the context of an ongoing committed relationship.

SUGGESTED CROSS-REFERENCES

Gender identity disorder is discussed in Section 18.3, personality disorders are discussed in Chapter 23, and sexual dysfunctions are discussed in Section 18.1a. The discussions of pervasive developmental disorders in Chapter 38 and separation anxiety disorders in children in Section 46.3 are also relevant. Child abuse is covered in Section 49.3.

REFERENCES

Abel GG, Hoffman J, Warberg B, Holland CL: Visual reaction time and plethysmography as measures of sexual interest in child molesters. *Sex Abuse J Res Treat.* 1998;10:81–95.

Abel GG, Rouleau JL. The nature and extent of sexual assault. In: Marshall WL, Laws DL, Barbaree HA, eds. *Handbook of Sexual Assault: Issues, Theories, and Treatments of the Offender.* New York: Plenum Publishing; 1990.

Bak R: Fetishism. *J Am Psychoanal Assoc.* 1953;1:285–298.

Baker SW. Biological influences on human sex and gender. In: Stimpson CR, Person ES, eds. *Women: Sex and Sexuality.* Chicago: University of Chicago Press; 1980.

Barbaree HE: Evaluating treatment efficacy with sexual offenders: The insensitivity of recidivism studies to treatment effects. *Sex Abuse J Res Treat.* 1997;9:111–128.

Barbaree HE, Seto MC. Pedophilia assessment and treatment. In: Laws DR, Donohue WO, eds. *Sexual Deviance: Theory, Assessment and Treatment.* New York: Guilford Press; 1997.

Bell AP, Weinberg MS. *Homosexuality: A Study of Diversity Among Men and Women.* New York: Simon and Schuster; 1978.
Berlin FS, Abel GG, Levis, DJ, Clancy, J: Aversion therapy applied to taped sequence of deviant behavior in exhibitionism and other sexual deviations: A preliminary report. *J Behav Ther Exp Psychiatry.* 1970;1:59–66.
Berlin FS, Meinecke CF: Treatment of sex offenders with antiandrogenic medication: Conceptualization, review of treatment modalities, and preliminary findings. *Am J Psychiatry.* 1981;138:601–607.
*Bradford JMW. Pharmacological treatment of the paraphilias. In: Oldham JM, Riba MB, eds. *Review of Psychiatry.* Vol 14. Washington, DC: American Psychiatric Press; 1995.
Brame D, Jacobs J. *Different Loving: The World of Sexual Domination and Submission.* New York: Villard; 1996.
*Chasseguet-Smirgel J. *Creativity and Perversion.* New York: Norton; 1984.
Dimen M. Perversion is us? Eight notes. In: *Sexuality, Intimacy, Power.* Hillsdale, NJ: The Analytic Press; 2003:257–291.
Freud S. Three essays on the theory of sexuality. In: Strachey J, ed. *The Standard Edition of the Complete Works of Sigmund Freud.* Vol 7. London: Hogarth Press; 1905.
Freud S. The economic problem of masochism. In: Strachey J, ed. *The Standard Edition of the Complete Works of Sigmund Freud.* Vol 19. London: Hogarth Press; 1961.
Glover E: The relation of perversion formation to the development of reality sense. *Int J Psychoanal.* 1953;14:486–504.
Hirigoyen MF. *Stalking the Soul: Emotional Abuse and the Erosion of Identity.* New York: Helen Marx Books 2000; 1998.
Jacobson L: On the use of "sexual addiction": The case for "perversion." *Contemp Psychoanal.* 2003;39:107–113.
*Kernberg O. A theoretical frame for the study of sexual perversions. In: *Aggressive Personality Disorders and Perversions.* New Haven: Yale University Press; 1992.
Kinsey A, Pomeroy W, Martin CE. *Sexual Behavior in the Human Male.* Philadelphia: WB Saunders; 1948.
Krafft-Ebing R. *Psychopathia Sexualis.* Klaff SS, trans. New York: Stein and Day; 1965.
*Maletzky BM. The paraphilias: Research and treatment. In: Nathan PE, ed. *A Guide to Treatments that Work.* New York: Oxford University Press; 1998.
McConaghy N: Methodological issues concerning evaluation of treatment for sexual offenders: Randomization, treatment dropouts, untreated controls, and within-treatment studies. *Sex Abuse J Res Treat.* 1998;11:183–193.
*McConaghy N: Unresolved issues in scientific sexology. *Arch Sex Behav.* 1999;28:285–318.
McDougall J: Identifications, neoneeds, and neosexualities. *Int J Psychoanal.* 1986;67:19–31.
McNulty RD, Adams HE, Dillon J. Sexual deviation: Paraphilias. In: Sutker PB, Adams HE, eds. *Comprehensive Handbook of Psychopathology.* New York: Kluwer Academic Publishers; 2001.
Meltzer D. *Sexual States of Mind.* Perthshire, Scotland: Clunie Press; 1973.
Nagel T: Sexual perversion. *J Philosophy.* 1969;66:5–17.
Ostow M, Greenacre P: Perversions: General considerations concerning their genetic and dynamic background. In: *Emotional Background.* Vol 1. New York: International Universities Press; 1968.
Ovesey L, Person ES: Transvestism: A disorder of the sense of self. *Int J Psychoanal Psychother.* 1976;5:219–236.
Paul GCN: Sexual offender recidivism revisited: A meta-analysis of recent treatment studies. *J Consult Clin Psychol.* 1995;63:802–809.
Person ES. *The Sexual Century.* New Haven: Yale University Press, 1999.
Person ES, Terestman N, Myers WA, Goldberg EL, Salvadori C: Gender differences in sexual behaviors and fantasies in a college population. *J Sex Marital Ther.* 1989;15:187–198.
Person ES. Sadomasochism: Interpersonal power corrupted by aggression. In: *Feeling Strong: The Achievement of Authentic Power.* New York: William Morrow; 2002:155–179.
Richards AK: A fresh look at perversion. *JAPA.* 2003;51:1199–1218.
Stoller RJ. *Perversion: The Erotic Form of Hatred.* New York: Pantheon Books; 1975.

▲ 18.3 Gender Identity Disorders

RICHARD GREEN, M.D., J.D.

DEFINITIONS

The fourth edition of the *Diagnostic and Statistical Manual of Mental Disorders* (DSM-IV) and the revised fourth edition of the DSM (DSM-IV-TR) define *gender identity disorders* as a group whose common feature is a strong, persistent preference for living as a person of the other sex. The affective component of gender identity disorders is gender dysphoria, discontent with one's designated birth sex and a desire to have the body of the other sex, and to be regarded socially as a person of the other sex. *Gender identity disorder in adults* was referred to in early versions of the DSM as *transsexualism*.

In the current DSM-IV-TR, no distinction is made for the overriding diagnostic term *gender identity disorder* as a function of age. In children, it may be manifested as statements of wanting to be the other sex and as a broad range of sex-typed behaviors conventionally shown by children of the other sex.

In 1960, the author cowrote a paper describing behaviors in children that were consistent with the later described gender identity disorder of childhood. In 1974, the author published a text describing a few dozen boys with sexual identity conflict. Drawing on this clinical experience, the psychosexual disorders advisory committee of the DSM that was to become the third edition (DSM-III), on which the author served, introduced the diagnostic entity *gender identity disorder of childhood* in 1980.

Interest in gender identity disorders grew from several sources. Behaviors distinguished between male and female children are a focus of developmental psychologists studying conventional patterns of psychosexual differentiation. Work with sexually atypical adults, including transsexuals and homosexuals who recalled extensive cross-gender behavior in childhood, brought clinical interest to this area. Transsexuals became popularly known with the sex change of George Jorgensen into Christine Jorgensen in 1952. The 1966 book by Harry Benjamin, the pioneer who evaluated or treated many hundreds of patients, and the introduction of sex reassignment surgery at The Johns Hopkins Hospital in that same year were great strides in transsexualism's medical recognition and treatment.

COMPARATIVE NOSOLOGY

Gender identity disorders first entered the American Psychiatric Association's nomenclature in DSM-III. They were included in the category of psychosexual disorders along with paraphilias and sexual dysfunctions. In the revised third edition of the DSM (DSM-III-R), gender identity disorders were placed in the section on disorders usually first evident in infancy, childhood, or adolescence. In DSM-IV, gender identity disorders were placed in a separate section called *sexual and gender identity disorders*.

Number of Major Categories

In DSM-III, two specific categories of gender identity disorder were coded, each with its diagnostic criteria, that is *transsexualism* and *gender identity disorder of childhood*. The DSM-III-R had a third category, *gender identity disorder of adolescence or adulthood, nontranssexual type* to apply to persons with mild or fluctuating gender dysphoria.

DSM-IV reversed the trend to greater differentiation by reducing the number of major diagnostic categories to one, *gender identity disorders*. The objective of the change was to unify the diagnostic criteria for children, adolescents, and adults. However, the DSM-IV diagnostic criteria for nonadults did not fully parallel those for adults.

Subtypes

DSM-III and DSM-III-R classified patients additionally by their sexual orientation. The heterosexual subtype of gender identity–disordered person was attracted to a person of the other genetic sex, the homosexual subtype was attracted to a person of the same genetic sex, and the asexual subtype was attracted to neither. DSM-IV continued the subtype classifications and added bisexuality but coded the individuals as sexually attracted to males, females, both, or neither, without calling the attraction homosexual or heterosexual.

DSM-IV-TR Diagnostic Criteria

Current diagnostic criteria for children and adults are organized under two main groupings: *cross-gender identification* and *discomfort with assigned gender role*. The arrangement promotes a questionable distinction between the two categories. Criterion A for children includes the intense desire to participate in the games and pastimes of the other sex, whereas Criterion B includes rejection of gender-conventional toys and games.

For all ages, the presence of an intersexed state precludes the diagnosis. Exclusion of a physical intersex condition assumes, not always correctly, that when the symptoms of gender identity disorder are manifested by a child with some form of intersex, the behaviors are due to the intersex. It also assumes that children without obvious intersex have no physiological basis for their disorder, which may ultimately be proven false.

ICD Classification Schemes

In the ninth revision of the *International Classification of Diseases* (ICD-9), *gender identity disorders*, without diagnostic criteria, were placed in the section on sexual deviations and disorders. The tenth edition of the ICD (ICD-10) includes, under the category gender identity disorders, *transsexualism, dual role transvestism,* and *gender identity disorder of childhood. Gender identity disorders* are placed in the section on disorders of adult personality and behavior, although including gender identity disorder of childhood.

EPIDEMIOLOGY

Prevalence in Children

The prevalence of gender identity disorder of childhood can only be estimated, because no epidemiological studies have been published. A rough estimate can be obtained from two items on Thomas Achenbach's Child Behavior Checklist (CBCL) that are consistent with components of the diagnosis, that is "behaves like opposite sex" and "wishes to be child of opposite sex."

Among a sample of 4- to 5-year-old boys referred for a range of clinical problems, the reported desire to be the opposite sex was 15 percent. Among 4- to 5-year-old boys not referred for behavioral problems, it was only 1 percent. For boys 6 to 7 years of age, the rates were 2.7 and 0 percent; for boys 8 to 9 years of age, the rates were 5.1 and 0 percent; and for 10 to 11 years of age, the rates were 1.1 and 2.3 percent. For clinically referred girls, there was more uniformity across age, with the highest rate, 8 percent, at 9 years of age and the lowest rate, 4 percent. For clinically nonreferred girls, the highest rate was 5 percent at 4 to 5 years of age and then less than 3 percent for other ages.

Parents reported cross-gender behavior for 16 percent of clinically referred boys at 4 to 5 years of age and for approximately 10 percent in other age groups. Among nonreferred boys, rates were approximately 5 percent. With clinically referred girls, nearly 19 percent of parents reported that their daughters showed cross-gender behaviors at 4 to 5 years of age, and between 9 and 14 percent reported these behaviors in the other age groups. With nonreferred girls, the rate was approximately 11 percent for all ages.

It is problematic to extrapolate from these data to prevalence of gender identity disorder in children, because these items do not assess the longitudinal persistence of the reported behavior and do not elucidate what constitutes "behaves like opposite sex."

Another way to estimate grossly the prevalence of gender identity disorder in children is the percentage of adults with predominant or exclusive homosexual orientation. Adult rates can then be compared to the percentage of homosexual men and women who report childhood cross-gender behavior. Predominant or exclusive homosexuality is estimated at approximately 2 percent in men and 1.0 to1.5 percent in women. Estimates for homosexual men recalling childhood cross-gender behavior are between 50 and 65 percent, and estimates for homosexual women are approximately 50 percent. However, methodological problems here are the validity of retrospective reports contaminated by time and the differing criteria from study to study. Furthermore, retrospective reports rarely address the key item of wanting to be the other sex as a young child. Notwithstanding, based on imprecise assumptions, an estimate is reached of approximately 1.0 percent of boys and 0.5 percent of girls.

Sex Ratio in Children

In most clinical programs, the sex ratio of referred children is four to five boys for each girl. Several explanations are offered. First, there is greater parental concern with cross-gender behavior in boys, called *sissiness*, than there is with cross-gender behavior in girls, called *tomboyism*. Greater peer group stigma attaches to substantial cross-gender behavior in boys. Thus, there may be an equal prevalence of gender identity disorder in the two sexes but a differential referral rate. Another possibility is that a genuine disparity results from men's more perilous developmental course. The fundamental mammalian state is female. No sex hormones are required for prenatal female anatomical development, whereas adequate sex hormone levels are required at critical developmental times for male anatomical differentiation. If mechanisms of behavioral development track anatomical development, then the masculine behavioral system also requires adequate levels of sex hormone at appropriate times for normative expression.

Elements of diagnosis of gender identity disorder should distinguish between gender atypical children without, what would be termed in adults, *gender dysphoria*. Thus, non–rough-and-tumble, sensitive boys and athletic girls preferring utilitarian clothing rather than traditionally feminine clothes would not be diagnosed with gender identity disorder.

Age of Onset in Children

Most children with gender identity disorder are referred for clinical evaluation in early grade school years. However, parents typically report that the cross-gender behaviors were apparent before 3 years of age.

Controversy over Gender Identity Disorder Diagnosis in Children

In November 1996, the San Francisco Board of Supervisors passed a resolution calling on the American Psychiatric Association to abolish the diagnosis of gender identity disorder for children and adolescents. Arguments included statements that researchers had "created the pre-adult gender identity disorder diagnosis with motivations including the preservation of ongoing government funding, career enhancing studies and treatment of those who in reality were simply 'gender non-conforming' children and adolescents." In reply, a child psychiatrist transgendered male, describing himself as a person struggling with gender dysphoria since 4 years of age, wrote

> With allies like the supervisors and the gender identity disorder abolitionists, trans-gendered children would be even less well served by mental health clinicians than they are now. I know from my own experience as a gender identity disorder child, gender identity disorder adolescent and gender identity disorder adult that gender dysphoria hurts real bad and it is not adequately described as simple effeminacy in a boy or masculinity in a girl nor is it non-conformity in the gender-independent youth who is exercising free choice in selecting from a varied menu of alternative roles. I truly envy the gen-

der non-conformist because they don't have gender identity disorder. A deficient damaged and/or anatomically incongruent gender identity cannot make its vital contribution during childhood to the development and maintenance of a cohesive, integrated sense of self. . . . "Sissy boys" and "tomboys" in the large majority of gender variant children are not DSM-IV kids.

Gender identity conflict issues may be found more commonly among some intersex conditions, such as congenital adrenal hyperplasia in women and partial androgen insensitivity in men who are reared as girls. Therefore, the history taken should include questions addressed to physical signs of intersex or endocrine status.

Prevalence in Adults The best estimate of gender identity disorder or transsexualism in adults emanates from the Netherlands and appears to represent national population data. There, the prevalence appears to be 1 in 11,000 men and 1 in 30,000 women.

Sex Ratio in Adults Most clinical centers report a sex ratio of three to five male patients for each female patient. Exceptions have been reported from some Eastern European centers at which the sex ratio is one of parity or even sex-reversed. Reasons for a greater number of male patients can be, as suggested previously, the more perilous route of male psychosexual differentiation, and the greater cosmetic and functional success of surgical intervention for male-to-female transsexuals. Vaginoplasty has been far more effective than phalloplasty. However, in recent years, significant advances have been made in the creation of a cosmetically satisfactory and, to some extent, functional neophallus, and this may influence the number of female-to-male transsexuals coming for treatment. Also, historically, there has been more publicity given to male-to-female transsexuals. However, in recent years, female-to-male transsexual community support groups have been organized, so more patients may be expected to request treatment.

Age of Onset in Adults At clinical interview, most adults with gender identity disorder report having felt different from other children of their same sex, although, in retrospect, many could not identify the source of that difference. Many report feeling extensively cross-gender identified from the earliest years, with the cross-gender identification becoming more profound in adolescence and young adulthood. Some cynicism meets these lifelong histories of gender dysphoria in that patients may be educated to know that they should be presenting such a history to be taken seriously with respect to treatment geared to changing their sex. However, it is hard to understand how a profound cross-gender identification would commence in adulthood without some substantial prodromata in earlier years.

Many adults with gender identity disorder may well have qualified for gender identity disorder in childhood. However, the author's longitudinal study of several dozen boys with gender identity disorder found some three-fourths to emerge as homosexual or bisexual young men and only one-fourth to emerge as probably transsexual. Gender dysphoric adult men who are sexually attracted primarily to women, and who perhaps evolve through a period of fetishistic cross-dressing, typically present at clinics to change sex a decade or more later than patients who have been sexually attracted to persons of their same anatomical sex and who have not evolved through fetishistic transvestism.

Age of onset and age of presentation at a clinical center can be quite disparate from patient to patient. Many persons attempt to suppress gender dysphoria through a range of devices, including marriage and children. Only after all attempts at suppression fail do they present clinically asking for treatment to change their sex.

ETIOLOGY

The development of atypical sexuality, homosexuality, or gender identity disorders has taken on an increasingly biological basis in research.

Genetic Influence Unlike studies of homosexuality in which there have been large samples of monozygotic and dizygotic twin pairs, male and female, studied for concordance rates, the relative rarity of transsexualism makes such study unlikely. However, the author identified ten pairs of patients, closely related, in which there is concordance for gender identity disorder or gender dysphoria from a pool of some 1,500 patients at a gender identity clinic. For concordant gender identity disorder, there are one set of male monozygotic twins, three sets of nontwin brothers, one brother and sister pair, one set of sisters, and one father and son. For gender identity disorder and transvestism, there are one transsexual father with a gender dysphoric transvestite son, one transvestite father with a gender dysphoric transvestite son, and one transvestite father with a transsexual daughter. Father and child coexisting gender identity disorder or gender identity disorder and transvestism could not be explained simply by evoking role modeling. This is because the children did not know of the father's atypical gender behavior before they themselves manifested atypical gender behavior.

Hormonal Influence Evidence for hormonal influence in gender identity disorder derives from several sources. Substantial data show the effect on early childhood sex-typed play behaviors of prenatal androgen in the girl. Girls with congenital virilizing adrenal hyperplasia overproduce adrenal androgen in utero, and, as girls, they are more rough and tumble in play, less interested in dolls, and more likely to be considered tomboys than girls who do not have the disorder. Conversely, there is limited evidence that prenatal exposure of boys to estrogenic or progestational agents may reduce the expression of conventional boy-type behaviors.

Atypical levels of sex hormones before birth and the attendant effects on specific sex-typed behaviors may modify the child's early social experiences. Boys disinclined to rough-and-tumble play or who play with dolls have different father–son and mother–son relationships and a different peer group experience than more conventionally masculine boys. Similarly, girls who prefer rough-and-tumble activity and sports to doll play have a different early socialization experience with parents and peers than girls who are conventionally feminine. These experiences may influence gender identity and may manifest subsequently as gender dysphoria during later years.

Rodent studies have shown that prenatal exposure to the anticonvulsants phenobarbital (Barbita) and phenytoin (Dilantin) alters sex-steroid hormone levels, resulting in unmasculinized sexual differentiation. In a few human case studies, an increased number of genital malformations was reported in male infants prenatally exposed to phenobarbital and phenytoin. Therefore, humans exposed prenatally via their mothers to these anticonvulsants were studied for gender development and sexual orientation. There was a trend for more prenatally anticonvulsant-exposed subjects to report current or past cross-gender behavior, gender dysphoria, or both. Extraordinarily, three out of 243 prenatally exposed anticonvulsant subjects were transsexuals and had undergone sex-reassignment surgery. Contrary to expectation, one was a male-to-female transsexual, and two were female-to-male transsexuals.

Additionally, two exposed men had exclusively homosexual experiences compared to none in the control group. The male-to-female transsexual had been born with bilateral undescended testes. One woman who reported gender dysphoria had a transverse vaginal septum. She had been a tomboy with gender dysphoria in childhood before the anomaly was recognized.

Reports describe polycystic ovaries as more common in female-to-male transsexuals than in the typical female population. In one series, 25 percent were found to have polycystic ovary syndrome. In another series, one-half had symptoms of polycystic ovary syndrome, and most had a pelvic ultrasound diagnosis of polycystic ovaries. However, the endocrine profiles of the patients were not markedly abnormal, although, in another series, there was a significant elevation in plasma testosterone.

Findings of polycystic ovaries on ultrasound may be found in 20 percent of the normal population. Furthermore, the precise cause of polycystic ovary syndrome is unknown. Additionally, gender dysphoria reported by female-to-male transsexuals usually becomes evident before puberty, long before the consequences of polycystic ovaries are likely to be expressed. It may be that a basic underlying common denominator for both conditions operates in fetal or early extrauterine life.

Brain and Central Nervous System (CNS) Involvement One brain area that shows a sex difference has been found to differ in a sample of six male-to-female transsexuals compared to male nontranssexuals. The size of a small area of the bed nucleus of the stria terminalis (BNST) was the same in male-to-female transsexuals as in nontranssexual females. Whether the male transsexuals were sexually attracted to male or female partners was not relevant to the size. Evidence against the size difference being a result of long-term estrogen treatment was that men with prostate cancer treated with estrogens had a normal male subdivision size. Additionally, there was one female-to-male transsexual in whom the size of the subdivision was typical of men.

A follow-up study on the BNST in the same subjects discerned whether the first reported difference was based on a neuronal count difference or was a reflection of a difference in vasoactive intestinal polypeptide (VIP) innovation from the amygdala, which was used as a marker. The number of somatostatin-expressing neurons of male-to-female transsexuals was similar to that of women. For a female-to-male transsexual, the number was in the typical male range. These are postmortem studies and are necessarily limited in number. Confirmation and extension await technological advancement, perhaps with functional magnetic resonance images (MRIs) to identify these subnuclei in a living subject.

Because of the difficulties with direct observation and assessment of brain areas that might show a sex difference and that could reflect prenatal sex steroid organization, the author's research has looked at indirect markers of prenatal sex steroids and other biologically related phenomena.

Fingerprint Asymmetry The different number of fingerprint ridges on the left hand compared to the right hand originates in the first trimester of pregnancy. It may be sex-steroid influenced. Leftward asymmetry, that is, more ridges on the left, is more common in women. Men have a higher total ridge count for both hands. Two-hundred and seventy male-to-female transsexuals and 54 female-to-male transsexuals were compared along with 220 male and female controls. Male controls had a higher ridge count than female controls. Male and female controls did not differ on directional asymmetry. However, on directional asymmetry, male transsexuals sexually attracted to male partners differed from male controls. Male transsexuals sexually attracted to male partners and female transsexuals attracted to female partners, combined, differed from male and female heterosexual controls, combined. Heterosexual male and female transsexuals attracted to persons of the opposite birth sex, combined, did not differ from heterosexual controls. Thus, an association was found between dermatoglyphics and sexual orientation but not with transsexualism per se.

However, another study of dermatoglyphic characteristics of transsexuals looking at total ridge count and fingerprint asymmetry in 184 male-to-female transsexuals and 110 female-to-male transsexuals found different results. There was a trend for a sex difference in total ridge count between male and female controls, and no difference was found in directional asymmetry. The total ridge count and finger ridge asymmetry of transsexuals were similar to their genetic sex controls. Directional asymmetry was not related to sexual orientation.

Hand Use Preference An indicator of cerebral lateralization, hand use preference, has been assessed in patients with gender identity disorder. Handedness is manifest during the first trimester of pregnancy, and there is evidence that it is related to prenatal sex steroid levels.

In earlier series of small samples of male and female transsexuals compared to controls, transsexuals of both birth sexes were found to be less exclusively right handed. The author studied 443 male-to-female transsexuals and 93 female-to-male transsexuals for the use of the right or left hand in six common, one-handed tasks. Male and female transsexuals were more often non–right handed than male and female controls.

With 205 boys with gender identity disorder and 205 patient control boys referred for other psychiatric reasons, boys with gender identity disorder were significantly more likely to be non–right handed than control boys, 19.5 versus 8.3 percent.

Sibling Sex Order Substantial research by Ray Blanchard has found homosexual males to be later in the birth order, with more older brothers but not with more older sisters. The author studied a sample of 442 male-to-female transsexuals subdivided by sexual partner preference plus 100 female-to-male transsexuals. Male-to-female transsexuals sexually attracted to male partners had a later than expected birth order and more older brothers than other subgroups of male-to-female transsexuals. Each older brother increased the odds that a male transsexual was sexually attracted to male partners by 40 percent. The hypotheses explaining these findings include a progressive maternal immunization to the male fetus through the H-Y antigen or protein-bound testosterone or alterations in fetal androgen levels in successive pregnancies, all modifying the later-born male's psychosexual development.

The sibling sex ratio of boys with gender identity disorder from a multicenter study was calculated for 444 boys. They had a significant excess of brothers to sisters, 131 to 100. This replicated a previous study in which the sibling sex ratio was 140 to 100.

Birth weight of gender identity disorder boys was compared to control boys because of a previous finding that homosexual men with older brothers weighed less at birth than heterosexual men with older brothers. Feminine boys with two or more older brothers weighed 385 g less at birth than control boys with two or more older brothers. However, feminine and control boys with fewer than two older brothers did not differ in birth weight.

Birth order in girls with gender identity disorder has also been studied in a smaller sample. Here, probands were significantly more likely to be early born than non–gender identity disorder controls and were born early compared to sisters but not to brothers. Thus, these findings are the inverse of the studies of boys.

Maternal Aunt to Uncle Ratio Earlier research showed a significant skewing in the sex ratio in favor of women for families of homosexual men, such that there were fewer maternal uncles than aunts. The author extended this study to a large series of transsexual families. Four hundred seventeen male-to-female transsexuals and 96 female-to-male transsexuals were assessed. Male-to-female transsexuals had a significant excess of maternal aunts to uncles. No differences from expected parity were found for female-to-male transsexuals or on any paternal side. A putative explanation for these findings by Barry Keverne invokes genomic imprinting. Here, there is a grand parental retention on the epigenotype on the X chromosome. The first generation is characterized by a failure to erase paternal imprints on the paternal X chromosome. Daughters of the second generation produce sons with an X chromosome from the father and the mother. Those from the father result in one-half of the sons being lost in early pregnancy, whereas daughters survive by virtue of inheriting two X chromosomes. In the third generation, sons inheriting the paternal X factor at the second passage through the female germ line survive, but one-half inherit the feminizing X from the paternal line–imprinted genes. This results in atypical male psychosexual differentiation. This is a theoretical explanation that is compatible with the findings.

Psychoanalytic Theories

Few direct psychoanalytic observations of children developing gender identity disorder and of interactions with parents are available for practical reasons. A small retrospective series described excessive mother–son symbiosis in the early years, replete with extensive mother–son skin-to-skin contact, appearing in conjunction with later significant feminine behavior. That was attributed to the inability of the son to differentiate psychologically from the mother. In small samples, again primarily retrospective, male-identified women have been reported to have mothers who are removed in affect from their children, frequently by depression, and fathers who do not support their daughter's femininity. In some cases, the girl was seen as being a substitute husband to treat the mother.

Additional psychodynamic models propose factors that increase the child's insecurity or anxiety about the self. These include a constitutional reactivity to stress, early attachment difficulties, and familial or situational factors that increase the child's anxiety. Factors that make a child likely to develop gender identity disorder may reside in dynamic factors within the parents that permit them to tolerate the child's cross-gender behavior and, perhaps, within the child, for example, activity levels and sensitivity, which make cross-gender activities more salient.

Transsexualism can be seen in men as originating from unresolved separation anxiety during the separation-individuation phase of infantile development. To cope with this anxiety, the child resorts to a reparative fantasy of psychological fusion with mother. Adult transsexualism may be understood in that theory as an attempt to master that anxiety through sex reassignment surgery for which the transsexual acts out this unconscious fantasy and symbolically becomes mother.

Another theory would explain the etiology of transsexualism in men who are sexually attracted to men. It begins with the grandmother of the future transsexual, who treats her daughter coldly and neither encourages nor models femininity for her. The grandfather has a closer relationship with the daughter, but he encourages masculinity in her. As a consequence, the mother of the future transsexual develops a mild gender identity disorder of her own. In adolescence, she abandons her conscious transsexual wishes of someday being a man but, at the unconscious level, retains strong penis envy. The transsexual's mother eventually enters an empty marriage, and the final path of the atypical gender process becomes operative when the mother gives birth to an infant son whom she perceives as particularly beautiful and graceful. The boy represents her feminized phallus and fulfills her lifelong wish for a penis. Mother–son interaction includes excessively close and prolonged body contact. The transsexual boy's early experiences produce an overidentification with mother and eventually a feminine gender identity.

Social Learning Theories

Social learning theories focus on differential reinforcement of sex-typed behavior by parents, starting shortly after birth. That reinforcement shapes conduct into conventional masculinity and femininity. However, cause and effect are hard to distinguish. On the one hand, sex differences are reported early in life, probably before any major differential impact of parental reinforcement. On the other hand, mothers and fathers may treat male and female newborns differently.

In *Baby X* experiments, adults are told, sometimes incorrectly, the sex of a clothed child and asked to describe its attributes. The infants are then provided with toys. Perceived boys are encouraged more to physical action and are given more whole body stimulation than perceived girls. Perceived girls are initially offered a doll; perceived boys are offered a hammer.

Fathers are equally likely to give a 1-year-old daughter a truck as a doll but are more likely to give their son a truck than a doll. However, when children are given dolls, boys play with them less than girls do. Fathers, more than mothers, give negative responses to boys playing with dolls. Boys receive more positive responses for playing with blocks, and girls receive more positive responses for playing with dolls.

At 1 year of age, boys may be more exploratory and active, and toy preferences may differ. Girls were found to prefer soft toys and dolls, whereas boys preferred transportation toys and robots. A preference for same-sex playmates emerges early. When children 3.5 to 4.5 years of age were shown photographs of boys and girls and asked to select those with whom they would like to play, boys preferred boys, and girls preferred girls. By 2 to 3 years of age, boys appeared to be more aggressive toward peers and to show more rough-and-tumble play.

In a sample of 66 boys with gender identity disorder, the author found a positive correlation between the extent to which parents supported the early cross-gender behaviors in their sons and the extent of that cross-gender behavior. In most of the families, at least initially, there was no discouragement of cross-gender behaviors.

Across ten samples of boys with gender identity disorder, the rate of father absence, owing to separation or divorce, was 34 percent. The author's study found that fraternal separation occurred earlier in families with gender identity disorder boys than in families with control boys. Additionally, fathers of gender identity boys, in father-present and father-separated families, recalled spending less time with their sons than did fathers of control boys. This was found at 2 years of age, 3 to 5 years of age, combined, and at time of assessment.

Earlier research by the author showed that boys with gender identity disorder were perceived by their parents as having been "beautiful" during infancy, as judged by masked raters reading interview transcripts of parents of boys with gender identity disorder and control boys. This may influence parent–child interactions.

More recently, facial photographs of boys with gender identity disorder were judged by adults to be more stereotypically feminine and less stereotypically masculine than male controls. Pictures of boys taken from the chest up were rated on the traits attractive, beautiful, cute, handsome, and pretty. With the exception of handsome, the traits were intentionally selected with a somewhat stereotypically feminine connotation. Attractive, beautiful, handsome, and pretty were judged to be significantly more characteristic of boys with gender identity disorder compared to same-sex controls.

With girls, ratings were also made for five traits: attractive, beautiful, cute, pretty, and ugly. Attractive, beautiful, cute, and pretty were judged to be less characteristic of the girls with gender identity disorder compared to same-sex controls.

Relative to same-sex controls, the physical appearance of boys with gender identity disorder is associated with lower trait ratings of adjectives with stereotypically masculine connotations, whereas the physical appearance of girls with gender identity disorder, relative to same-sex controls, is associated with higher masculine trait ratings.

Explanations for these findings are not clear. There may be a contribution from the manner in which the children present themselves, for example with hair length and clothing style or color.

Parents of gender identity disorder boys may manifest more psychopathology than parents of boys without gender identity disorder. More than one-half of mothers had two or more psychiatric disorders on the Diagnostic Interview Schedule, with depressive episodes and recurrent major depression being most common. Among fathers, depression and alcohol abuse have been reported as common.

Nature versus Nurture Research on intersexed children points to the early-life emergence of gender identity as being influenced largely by environment. In the seminal studies of John Money, Joan Hamson, and John Hamson, the range of anatomical features discordant with the gender of rearing was reported to be less relevant to the adoption of a male or female identity than the gender of rearing.

Studies of matched pairs of intersex children demonstrate that, with females with congenital adrenal hyperplasia, a newborn girl who is considered to be male in consequence of prenatal virilization of the genitalia and who is designated male matures with a male identity, although having the female XX chromosomal pattern, ovaries, and a uterus. However, questions have been raised about the ability to generalize to nonintersex children because of the atypical prenatal endocrine environment and other atypical genetic influences.

Studies of children born with normal sex characteristics who undergo gender reassignment early in life may be a more relevant test of nature versus nurture. In two cases, penile amputation through negligent circumcision resulted in boys, presumably with normal prenatal androgen levels, being sex reassigned early in life as girls. In one celebrated case of a twin pair, earlier reports indicated that the sex-reassigned twin living as a girl had developed a feminine identity. However, subsequent reports revealed that, by mid-adolescence, this individual was clearly male identified and soon reverted to living as a male. The reassigned twin married a woman. The other man studied, who was not a twin and who was raised as a girl, has retained a female identity and is bisexual in orientation. An effort to reconcile these two reports looks to the age at which sex reassignment was instituted. In the twin case, it was not until late in the second year, whereas, in the singleton case, it was late in the first year. A critical period may be operant with respect to gender identity.

More recent interest has focused on children born with cloacal exstrophy. The genital birth defect for males is so considerable that many are reassigned to female status at birth and raised as girls. A recent report of 14 such children found that 10 have now requested to live as males. However, a yet-unpublished series from another medical center reports that most such sex-reassigned children are accepting their female status.

DIAGNOSIS AND CLINICAL FEATURES

Children The author's longitudinal study of 66 boys provides a picture of gender identity disorder in children. The age range at initial evaluation was 4 to 12 years. One-third of the boys frequently stated that they wished to be girls. Three quarters cross-dressed frequently. The age of onset of cross-dressing was before the fifth birthday. A female-typed doll, such as Barbie, was the favorite toy for one-fifth of the boys, and was a frequently played-with toy for another two-fifths. Three-fifths of the boys regularly took a female role in playing house. More than four-fifths had a primarily female peer group.

The full prepubertal age range for evaluating gender identity disorders in children yields a variety of presenting behaviors. Younger children, 3 to 5 years of age, may believe that they are of the other sex or that they can easily become the other sex. At older ages, 6 to 9 years of age, children's gestures and mannerisms may be cross-sex stereotypes. Older children have often been subjected to peer teasing and so may have gone underground with cross-gender behaviors, particularly cross-dressing.

Gender identity disorder diagnosis has been subjected to factor analysis with respect to the statement of wishing to be the opposite sex and whether this should be a separate criterion in the diagnosis or clustered with other behaviors. One database was the author's study of 66 feminine boys. Analysis assessed whether the stated wish to be of the opposite sex loaded on the same factor as other traits or was part of a separate factor. Within the feminine boy group, the database was also divided as a function of whether the boys stated the wish to be a girl. Approximately 15 percent of that sample did not. One strong factor accounting for 51 percent of the variance was found, and the wish to be the opposite sex was one of several behavioral variables that loaded on this factor. Thus, there was support for the argument against separating identity statements from other behavioral variables of cross-gender identification. The stated wish to be of the opposite sex was more prevalent in the younger age group, that is, boys who were 3 to 9 years of age as opposed to those who were 9 to 12 years of age.

Case Histories of Children

The parents of a 7-year-old boy came for consultation, because the boy had told his parents on several occasions that he would like to be a girl. From 2 to 3 years of age, he showed interest in dressing in his older sister's clothing. Initially, both parents thought that their son's interest in his sister's and, occasionally, his mother's clothes was cute. They made no effort at discouraging it, considering it to be a passing phase. They were reassured of its transient nature by their family doctor. Preschool teachers told them that many boys dress up and that it was normal. When his parents kept the clothes from him, he would improvise with a towel for long hair and a large t-shirt for a dress. When playing mother-father games, he would be mother, and he imitated female characters from children's stories. Pictures drawn included only women. Most playmates were girls. He played often with his sister's discarded dolls and did not like sports. At school, he was teased by age-mates, notably boys, for cross-gender activities. Mother more than father was concerned with his cross-gender behavior. Father's long work hours precluded much time available for his son except on weekends, and then the boy's disinterest in sports resulted in their not sharing in many activities. At consultation, father was concerned that his son would grow up to be gay. Mother was less concerned with this potential but was more worried that he was becoming a loner and unhappy at school in consequence of peer stigma.

The parents of an 11-year-old girl came for consultation, because the girl had told her parents that she was unhappy being a girl. For years, she had refused to wear a skirt or dress. Her playmates were all boys. She had never played with dolls but preferred conventionally boy-type toys. She imitated men from the media. She was moderately accepted by male age-mates but not by female age-mates. The parents, during earlier years, considered her to be a typical tomboy. However, her continued insistence on boy-type activities and clothing and her saying that she wanted to be a boy and to become a man caused concern. She did not want to develop breasts or to menstruate. The parents were a bit worried about transsexualism in their daughter's future but were more concerned that she would be lesbian.

Associated Features Boys with gender identity disorder in some reports manifest greater general psychopathology than nonclinical control boys. With the CBCL, boys with gender identity disorder had levels of psychopathology similar to a clinic-referred group used in the instrument standardization. However, another report did not find more behavioral problems than among concurrently assessed demographically comparable clinical controls.

Child and adolescent patients with gender identity disorder were compared on the CBCL and a measure of peer relations. Adolescent samples showed significantly more general behavioral disturbance than the child sample, although both groups had scores that fell within the clinical range. The adolescent sample had significantly poorer peer relations.

The author's clinical experience argues that many of the behavioral problems seen in gender atypical boys are secondary to discomfort over gender and the consequent peer ostracism and teasing. That ostracism is the basis of psychopathology in cross-gendered boys is supported by a finding that CBCL symptoms increase with the age of the child, when stigma increases. Girls with gender identity disorder also experience some peer-group teasing.

Some clinicians have found separation anxiety disorder in boys with gender identity disorder. The claim is that separation anxiety disorder precedes feminine behavior, with cross-gender behavior emerging to restore the emotional tie with a mother perceived as unavailable. A study using liberal criteria for diagnosing separation anxiety disorder found a correlation between the two disorders. However, owing to the absence of convincing data demonstrating that separation anxiety disorder precedes gender identity disorder, and because most children with separation anxiety disorder do not have a gender identity problem, the connection remains tenuous.

Psychological Tests No psychological test is diagnostic of gender identity disorder in children. However, the author has demonstrated that two tests, the It-Scale for Children and the Draw-A-Person test, discriminate boys with gender identity disorder from gender typical boys.

The It-Scale presents a child with a neuter stick figure (It). The child then has It select from a series of cards depicting gender-typed accessories and activities. Cross-gendered boys more often select feminine or girl-typed cards. The Draw-A-Person test, in its basic format, requires a child to draw a person. Most gender-typical children draw a person of their sex. By contrast, the majority of cross-gendered boys draw a girl first. Conversely, with a sample of nonclinical tomboys, the majority drew a boy first in contrast to a matched sample of nontomboys.

Gender constancy is the piagetian construct of the constancy of gender and its possibility to change by altering superficial characteristics. There is an age-related stage-like sequence in gender constancy development, with children first self-categorizing the gender of self and others—gender identity—then appreciating its invariance over time—gender stability—and finally understanding that invariance in the face of superficial transformations of gender, such as changing sex-typed clothing or hair length. Children with gender identity disorder performed more poorly than controls at the three stage levels. Children who failed the gender identity or gender stability stages were more likely to draw an opposite-sex person first on the Draw-A-Person test.

Differential Diagnosis of Children Children with a gender identity disorder must be distinguished from other gender-atypical children. For girls, tomboys without gender identity disorder prefer functional and gender-neutral clothing. By contrast, gender identity–disordered girls adamantly refuse to wear girls clothes and reject gender-neutral clothes. Many girls may prefer shirts and pants to dresses, may enjoy rough-and-tumble play or sports, and may show little interest in doll play. They may say that it is better to be a boy because of perceived social advantages. Those girls do not necessarily have a gender identity disorder. What distinguishes girls who do is their repeated statements of being or wanting to be a boy and wanting to grow up to be a man, along with repeated cross-sex fantasy play, so that, in mother-father games or other games imitating characters from mass media, they are male. This accompanies a marked aversion to traditionally feminine activities.

For boys, the differential diagnosis must distinguish those who do not conform to traditional masculine sex-typed expectations but do not show extensive cross-gender identification and are not discontent with being male. It is not uncommon for boys to reject rough-and-tumble play or sports and to prefer nonathletic activities or occasionally to role play as a girl, to play with a doll, or to dress up in girl's or women's costumes. Such boys do not necessarily have a gender identity disorder. This must be stressed to parents, especially to fathers, who may have vigorous athletic expectations for their sons. What distinguishes boys who do have a gender identity disorder is stating a preference for being a girl and for growing up to become a woman, along with repeated cross-sex fantasy play, as in mother-father games, a strong preference for traditionally female-typed activities, cross-dressing, and a female peer group.

Because the diagnosis of gender identity disorder excludes children with anatomical intersex, a medical history needs to be taken with the focus on any suggestion of hermaphrodism in the child. When there is doubt, referral to a pediatric endocrinologist is indicated.

Adults

Clinical Presentation Nearly all adult patients presenting to a clinician make their self-diagnosis of being transsexual and prescribe their own treatment, cross-sex hormones, and sex reassignment surgery. Insistence by the patient of a self-proclaimed diagnosis and treatment regimen presents management issues for the clinician, who may be seen as an unnecessary obstacle in the patient's path to a better life.

Psychotic persons, typically experiencing schizophrenia, may develop the delusion that they are changing sex. This is accompanied by delusions of body changes or the conviction of having hidden internal organs of the other sex. Such beliefs are not expressed by patients with only gender identity disorder. At times, however, patients present with diagnoses of schizophrenia and gender identity disorder. When this occurs, and it becomes clear that the extent of gender identity disorder does not wax and wane in synchrony with the psychosis, then they are distinct clinical phenomena and should be treated distinctly.

Case Histories of Adult Transsexuals

A 27-year-old anatomical woman referred to a gender identity clinic reported having felt different as a child from other girls, although unable then to identify its source. As a young girl, she enjoyed playing sports with girls and boys but generally preferred the companionship of boys. She preferred wearing unisex or boyish clothes and resisted wearing a skirt or dress. Everyone referred to her as a tomboy. Pubertal changes were unwelcome. She tried to hide her breast development by wearing loose fitting tops and stooping forward. Menses were embarrassing and poignantly reminded her of her femaleness, which was becoming increasingly alienating. As sexual attractions evolved, they were exclusively directed to female partners. In her late teens, she had one sexual experience with a man, and it was aversive. She began socializing in lesbian circles but did not feel comfortable there and did not consider herself lesbian but more a man. For sexual partners, she wanted heterosexual women and wanted to be considered by the partner as a man. As gender dysphoric feelings became increasingly pronounced, she consulted transsexual sites on the Internet and contacted a female-to-male transsexual community support group. She then set into motion the process of clinical referral. She transitioned to living as a man, had a name change, and was administered androgen injections. Voice deepened, facial and body hair grew, menses stopped, and sex drive increased, along with clitoral hypertrophy. After 2 years, the patient underwent bilateral mastectomy and is on the wait list for phalloplasty and hysterectomy-ovariectomy. Employment as a man continues, as does a 3-year relationship with a female partner. The partner has a child from a previous marriage.

A 37-year-old anatomical man referred to a gender identity clinic was currently married and the father of two children. He reported always having been aware of wanting to be female but keeping it secret as a child. When he had the opportunity, he would dress in his mother's or sister's clothes but was never found out. Boys and girls were his playmates. He did not enjoy sports, except swimming. Cross-dressing became more frequent in early teens and was accompanied by sexual arousal. Sexual relations were satisfactory with a woman, although sex drive was low. To enhance sexual arousal with a partner, he would frequently imagine himself to also be female. He found men only minimally sexually attractive. He married at 24 years of age and did not tell his wife of his cross-dressing. In the first year or so of marriage, he did not experience any great drive to continue cross-dressing, but it gradually returned over the next few years as sexual contact with his wife waned. He would cross-dress secretly when the opportunity arose. Eventually, his wife discovered his cross-dressing and was angered. He attempted to involve her in the cross-dressing, but she refused and was worried that their children would find out. By now, the cross-dressing was no longer sexually arousing, and the desire to live full-time as a woman was increasing. The couple separated, the children remaining with their mother. He began living as a woman on weekends, although continuing to work as a man. He then presented requesting female hormone treatment with the goal of sex-reassignment surgery. The transition process was slow. There were problems regarding his career in effecting a full-time gender transition. After another year, he left his place of employment and sought different work. He began facial hair removal. After a name change and full-time living socially as a woman, he was administered estrogens. Vocal retraining was undertaken to enhance social passing as a woman. The children were introduced to their father's new role and were moderately accepting. The patient secured work in the voluntary sector as a woman and reported being happier than at any time previously. Sexual interest diminished with hormone treatment, and the patient reported finding men somewhat sexually attractive. Breast development was moderate and pleased the patient. After 2 years of successfully living as a woman, referral was made for genital sex-reassignment surgery. The patient was not in a sexual relationship but hoped that a partner would be found, preferably a man.

Associated Features Gender identity disorders may be associated with other diagnoses. Although some gender identity–disordered patients have a history of major psychosis, including schizophrenia or major affective disorder, most do not. When a diagnosis of gender identity disorder is made, as well as another DSM Axis I diagnosis, it is clinically considered whether the diagnoses are distinct. A variety of Axis II personality disorders may be found in patients with gender identity disorder, particularly borderline personality, but none is specific. A proportion of nonhomosexual, gender identity–disordered men report a past history of erotic arousal in association with cross-dressing, and some would still qualify for a concurrent diagnosis of fetishistic transvestism. Some are more sexually aroused by imagining themselves with a female body or by seeing themselves cross-dressed in a mirror (autogynephilia) than by items of women's clothing per se.

Course in Adulthood Adult, male, gender dysphoric patients sexually attracted to male partners may have a continuous development of gender dysphoria from childhood. However, some manifestations of their gender dysphoria may be driven underground in an effort, during their teens and, perhaps, early 20s, to merge with the larger community. They may also hope or think that their gender dysphoria will disappear. Sexual interest in male partners begins in early puberty, and some may consider themselves to be homosexual. However, they find that they do not integrate effectively into the gay community. In their sexual relationships, they may see their interaction as heterosexual, because they see themselves as women and typically report that their partners see them as women. Approximately two-thirds of adult men with gender identity disorder are sexually attracted to men only.

Gender identity disorders in men sexually attracted to females partners may be characterized as more progressive disorders with insidious onset. The course is fairly continuous in some cases; in others, the intensity of symptoms fluctuates. Some experience a lifelong struggle with feminine identification that changes in intensity from time to time and may temporarily recede in the face of conflicting desires, such as marriage and family. In most cases, the first outward manifestation is cross-dressing in childhood, dressing in mother's or sister's clothing, and many patients report that they first began wishing to be female during that period. However, the extent of their cross-gender behavior in childhood does not usually warrant diagnosis of gender identity disorder. At puberty, cross-dressing is typically sexually arousing, and, for the next few years or even decades, the individual may qualify for a diagnosis of fetishistic transvestism. However, over time, usually in the 20s or 30s, penile responsivity to cross-dressing wanes, and the desire to have a woman's body becomes stronger. Most men with gender identity disorder who are sexually attracted to women or who are sexually attracted to men and women marry and father children. Those who fall in love with women often report that, during the early phases of the romance, they lose interest in cross-dressing or in becoming women. However, over time, the desire to cross-dress or to live as women reemerges.

Female patients may experience adolescence in which they initially consider themselves lesbian because of sexual attraction to female partners. However, they come to define themselves as distinct from lesbians, as they consider themselves to be men in their relationships with women. They insist that their partners treat them as men and that the partners are heterosexual women. Female patients are often, more often than male patients, in a romantic or sexual relationship at the time of initial clinical assessment.

In earlier clinical experience, it was the rare female-to-male transsexual who reported sexual attractions to male partners. This has changed. In the author's gender identity clinic, approximately one-tenth of patients born female report a sexual partner orientation to men and consider themselves to be gay men.

IMPAIRMENT AND COMPLICATIONS

Children Peer ostracism can make school attendance difficult, particularly for boys with gender identity disorder. They may drop out without qualifications or adequate training. Lack of education and job skills contributes to chronic underemployment. Social rejection, anxiety, or guilt over their gender identity disorder may lead to alcohol or other drug abuse.

Adults Intercourse with a female partner may require the gender identity–disordered man to fantasize that he is the woman and the partner is a man or that they are both women. The clinical picture commonly results in marital breakdown, because the husband wishes to be free to pursue sex reassignment, or because the marital partner can no longer tolerate the husband's cross-dressing. These men often experience considerable guilt about the effects of the behavior on their children and anxiety regarding continued access to them. There can be a legally contested issue of child contact with the gender-transitioning parent.

Children of Transsexual Parents An early report by the author described seven children raised by male-to-female transsexuals and nine children raised by female-to-male transsexuals. These children were typical on childhood gender behavior, and those old enough to report sexual orientation were heterosexual. Since that time, a larger series of some 20 children of patients transitioning in gender or who have transitioned in gender has been assessed. None shows gender identity disorder. They are still too young to assess sexual orientation.

TREATMENT

Children In the author's prospective study, a subsample of boys with gender identity disorder was treated by a variety of approaches from several therapists, including psychoanalysis, family therapy, individual psychotherapy, and behavior modification. With each intervention, or without, most boys showed lessening of cross-gender behaviors. At follow-up, none of the treated boys expressed a desire to be female. Only one nontreated boy expressed such an interest. However, the rates of homosexual or bisexual orientation in these treated boys did not differ from those who had no formal treatment.

The treatment strategy was eclectic. The child's interaction with each parent and the child's social environment at home were addressed. The child's perception of sex roles and relations to peers was also addressed. Typically, for a period of 1 year or more, parents observed behaviors in their child that constituted gender identity disorder. During that time, one parent may have taken a firmer stand on some behaviors, but, for the most part, the children were not interrupted in these activities. Parents were typically uncertain or ambivalent about their meaning, and, until recently, if at all, the child was not aware that the parents objected to the atypical behaviors. A child may interpret a parent's neutral stance to atypical behaviors as positive. Some parents may begin to be concerned, but they have been advised by preschool teachers or friends or relatives that the behaviors are normal and should not be discouraged. A parent who is concerned about the excessive nature of the child's cross-gender behaviors may have difficulty convincing other adults of the child's special needs, notwithstanding any ideal of androgyny. Initial limit setting by the parents usually meets with considerable resistance and testing by the child. It may result in the behaviors continuing in secret.

One strategy of therapy looks at the child's level of cognitive development. Young children paint the world in black and white. In the area of gender, there are no grays. A child who does not like the activities usually associated exclusively with his or her sex concludes that being the other sex is the only solution. A girl will say that only boys play sports, or a boy will say that boys play too rough. Grays should be introduced. Boys need to know that they can participate in sedentary play with other children, boys and girls. Girls need to know that girls can play sports and can be as good as or better than many boys. Parents should find children who demonstrate these behaviors to play with their child.

Many parents are motivated to the initial clinical evaluation by fears that their children will become transsexual or homosexual. Parents should be redirected from the hypothetical concerns of decades ahead to the immediacy of the child's life. At present, the child is unhappy being a boy or a girl. The focus should be on helping the child be more content with who he or she is. In the immediate term, the child is experiencing social stigma. The child should be integrated more effectively into the peer group.

A boy with a gender identity disorder typically has a strained relationship with his father. The author's study of cross-gendered boys found the extent of father–son involvement in the early years to be related to later sexual orientation. The association emerged not only between the two groups of boys studied (gender identity disorder and control), but also within the subgroup of boys with gender identity disorder. Thus, for the clinic-referred boys, the less time the father and son shared in preschool years, the higher the later Kinsey score for homosexuality.

Identifying cause and effect in the distant father–son relationship is difficult. Some fathers are not available to their sons in the early years, and the boy gravitates toward his mother's activities. Then, the father finds that the boy does not respond to his belated attempts to engage him in sports or other activities. Alternatively, a father may be available from the outset, but the child is temperamentally attuned to his mother's activities. The father becomes discouraged, and the attention is focused elsewhere, perhaps to another sibling with whom he shares interests.

The need for a positive father–son experience must be emphasized to fathers. Nonathletic activities can be mutually enjoyable. Taking the son to work from time to time provides a better image of who father is. Board games, video games, and computer games can be helpful. Father's busy work schedule must be compromised, lest the best years of their relationship be sacrificed, irrespective of any influence on later sexual orientation.

The child may believe that the parents wanted a child of the other sex. Sometimes, the parents did and conveyed the wish to a child. Parents and therapists should convey the message to the child that this is not so (if it ever was) and that they are happy having a child of that sex.

Children should know that sex is irreversible. Not yet having achieved gender constancy at 4 to 6 years of age, younger children may think that cross-dressing or changing hair length will change their sex. They should know the anatomical differences between the sexes and that superficial change will not achieve their goal. Older children who are aware of genital differences and who are cognitively more advanced may also be sophisticated about sex-change surgery. They may have seen transsexuals on television. Thus, the clinician's statement of irreversibility of sex can be challenged by the child.

The same treatment strategies used for boys with gender identity disorder are applicable to girls. Parental responses that have been supportive of behaviors causing the girl to be stigmatized should be interrupted. Same-sex peer-group experiences are to be encouraged.

At present, there is no convincing evidence that psychiatric or psychological intervention for children with gender identity disorder affects the direction of subsequent sexual orientation. Transsexualism, however, may be affected. Transsexuals or adults with gender identity disorder are unable to cope socially as persons of their anatomical birth sex. The treatment of gender identity disorder in children is directed largely at developing social skills and comfort in the sex role expected by birth anatomy. To the extent that treatment is successful, transsexual development may be interrupted. The low prevalence of transsexualism in the general population, however, even in the special population of cross-gender children, thwarts the testing of this assumption.

No hormonal or psychopharmacological treatments for gender identity disorder in childhood have been identified.

Adolescents Adolescents whose gender identity disorder has persisted beyond puberty present unique treatment problems. One is how to manage the rapid emergence of unwanted secondary sex characteristics. Thus, a new area of treatment management has evolved with respect to slowing down or stopping pubertal changes expected by anatomical birth sex and then implementing cross-sex body changes with cross-sex hormones.

Young persons whose previous gender identity disorder has remitted may experience new conflicts should homosexual feelings emerge. This may be a source of anxiety in the adolescent and may cause conflict within the family. Teenagers should be reassured about the prevalence and nonpathological aspects of a same-sex partner preference. Parents must also be informed of the nonpathological nature of same-sex orientation. The goal of family intervention is to keep the family stable and to provide a supportive environment for the teenager.

Adults Adult patients coming to a gender identity clinic usually present with straightforward requests for hormonal and surgical sex reassignment. No drug treatment has been shown to be effective in reducing cross-gender desires per se. When patient gender dysphoria is severe and intractable, sex reassignment may be the best solution.

Attitudes toward sex change have changed. As opposed to an earlier U.S. study in the 1960s by the author, in which the majority of physicians would allow a patient to commit suicide rather than be granted sex-reassignment surgery, a recent study of attitudes shows a marked liberalization. The majority of Swedish respondents supported the possibility for transsexuals undergoing sex reassignment. However, two-thirds thought that the individual should bear the expense. A majority support transsexuals' right to marry in their new sex. The right to adopt and to raise children was supported by 43 percent, whereas 41 percent opposed this right. Respondents who believe that transsexualism is caused by biological factors hold a less restrictive view.

There is controversy regarding inclusion of gender identity disorder in adults in the DSM. The International Conference of Transgender Law and Employment Policy and the National Center for Lesbian Rights issued a statement on gender identity disorder and the transgender movement. With respect to adults, they acknowledged that self-identified transsexuals must receive the diagnosis to get hormone treatment and surgeries and, in some cases, reimbursement for transition-related care. Furthermore, gender identity disorder has also been used to gain legal protection for transgendered people, sometimes under laws prohibiting discrimination against people with psychiatric disabilities. Therefore, their statement did not advocate an immediate blanket elimination of gender identity disorder in a vacuum, without an alternative means of ensuring continued access to and reimbursement for medical treatment. They believed that the best long-term solution was to eliminate gender identity disorder as a psychiatric disorder and to redefine transsexualism as a medical condition.

An extensive set of clinical management guidelines for treatment of adults with gender identity disorder is published by the Harry Benjamin International Gender Dysphoria Association. It has gone through several revisions since 1979, with the current, sixth revision, completed in 2001.

There is controversy with respect to the timing of introducing endocrine treatment of transsexuals. Many clinics require that the patient begin the *Real Life Test* or *Real Life Experience* before endocrine treatment. This is a full-time social transition to living in the desired gender, which may include name change and change of work status. The treatment philosophy is to proceed with reversible procedures before those that are irreversible. Once the social transition has been effected, hormone treatment can be introduced. For the psychiatric clinician not experienced in this regard, this intervention should be supervised by an endocrinologist.

The Real Life Test is typically 1 to 2 years of full-time cross-gender living, including at least 1 year of employment in the desired gender role and 1 year on high doses of cross-sex hormones. The work requirement, which can also be that of a full-time student, is intended to demonstrate that the patient is capable of interacting successfully with members of the general public in the new gender role.

Persons born male are typically treated with daily doses of oral estrogen. This may be conjugated equine estrogens or ethinylestradiol or estrogen patches. These hormones produce breast enlargement, the amount being largely determined by genetic predisposition, which continues for approximately 2 years. Other major effects of estrogen treatment are testicular atrophy, decreased libido, and diminished erectile capacity. There also may be a decrease in the density of body hair and, perhaps, an arrest of male pattern baldness. Side effects of endocrine treatment can be elevated levels of prolactin, blood lipids, fasting blood sugar, and hepatic enzymes. Patients should be monitored with appropriate blood tests. Smoking is a contraindication of endocrine treatment, as it increases the risk of deep vein thrombosis and pulmonary embolism. There is no effect on voice. Facial hair removal is required by laser treatment or electrolysis.

Histological change in the mammary glands of male-to-female transsexuals induced by chemical and surgical castration and estrogen therapy has been examined. Combined progestatonal or antiandrogens and estrogens are helpful for genetically male breast tissue to mimic the histology of the female breast but may not affect the size of the breasts. Apocrine metaplasia may occur in breasts of male-to-female transsexuals, but only four cases of breast cancer have been documented.

Biological women are treated with monthly or three weekly injections of testosterone. Because the effects of exogenous testosterone are more profound than those of estrogen, clinicians should be more cautious about commencing female patients on hormone treatment. The pitch of the voice drops permanently into the male range as the vocal cords thicken. The clitoris enlarges to two or three times its pretreatment length and is often accompanied by increased libido. Hair growth changes to the male pattern, and a full complement of facial hair may grow. Menses cease. Male pattern baldness may develop, and acne may be a complication.

Ethinylestradiol in male-to-female transsexuals increases regional fat depots and thigh muscle mass. Conversely, female-to-male transsexuals receiving testosterone may have increased thigh muscle and reduced subcutaneous fat deposition. Thus, cross-sex steroid hormones affect general body fat and muscle distribution, as well as promoting breast development in patients born male.

Sex reassignment surgery for a person born anatomically male consists principally of removal of the penis, scrotum, and testes, construction of labia, and vaginoplasty. Operative techniques vary mainly in the method of obtaining material to line the neovagina. Standard methods involve lining with penile skin flaps, scrotal skin flaps, and free grafting from the thigh and various combinations. One technique uses a section of the intestine. Some clinicians attempt to construct a neoclitoris from the former frenulum of the penis. The neoclitoris may have erotic sensation. Postoperative complications include urethral strictures, rectovaginal fistulas, vaginal stenosis, and inadequate width or depth.

There is uncertainty and controversy with respect to the capacity for sexual arousal by the patient postsurgery. Some patients maintain that they are orgasmic. They describe the sensation of orgasm as more gradual and attenuated than their orgasms preoperatively. On the other hand, some patients report little sexual responsivity postsurgery. To date, there are no adequate assessments of the physiological functioning of postoperative male-to-female transsexuals with respect to the human sexual response cycle. However, many patients report satisfaction with being able to have vaginal intercourse with a male partner.

Some male patients who do not have adequate breast development from years of hormone treatment may elect augmentation mammaplasty. Some also have thyroid cartilage shaved to reduce the male-appearing thyroid cartilage. Patients need to undergo vocal retraining, and those who do not have a fully effective response may undergo a cricothyroid approximation procedure, which can raise vocal pitch. The results of these operations are variable.

Female-to-male patients typically first undergo bilateral mastectomy. Until the last few years, the construction of a neophallus has been quite unsatisfactory with respect to its appearance, as well as its function sexually, and for urination. However, technology has improved substantially. There are several approaches. One is metoidioplasty, which is essentially freeing up the enlarged clitoris, which creates a micropenis, and suture of the labia, with insertion of prosthetic testes. This may allow the patient to stand to urinate. However, the phallic appearance is not deemed satisfactory for most patients. Another approach is an abdominal flap with construction of a neophallus. This can be adapted for creation of a urethra within the neophallus, so that the patient can stand to urinate, and, additionally, it is possible to implant a hydraulic pump or semirigid rods to allow penile vaginal intercourse. The problem here is the extent to which there is sensation in the neophallus, with some risk of perforation from the implant if sensation is not adequate. The most elaborate technique involves removal of nerve and substantial tissue from the forearm. These are free radial forearm osteocutaneous flaps. This results in the most cosmetically effective neophallus, perhaps with adequate erotic sensation as well, when the arm nerve is grafted to the nerve in the inguinal area. Concurrently with the phalloplasty, patients may undergo hysterectomy and ovariectomy. Because of increased technical skills in phalloplasty, more female-to-male patients are now electing these procedures.

Consideration is being given to storing spermatozoa for male-to-female transsexuals before they start female hormonal therapy and oocysts or ovarian tissue, possibly obtained at the time of oophorectomy, from female-to-male transsexuals. Thus, they could biologically parent children.

Treatment Outcome: Adults Numerous studies have investigated the postoperative adjustments of sex-reassigned transsexuals. Most of these patients have been assessed and approved for surgery by established gender identity clinics. Therefore, the findings are generalized only to properly screened patients. In a study cowritten by the author of a 10-year search of English language medical literature, based on a gross category of whether the reassignment was considered satisfactory by the patient and without regret, some 87 percent of male-to-female patients and 97 percent of female-to-male patients met that criterion of success. Notwithstanding the gross classification utilized, the extent is not known to which these patients represent a random sample of the sex-reassigned population. Clinicians are less likely to report poor outcomes in their patients, thus shifting the reporting bias to positive results. Additionally, some successful patients who wish to blend into the community as men or women do not make themselves available for follow-up. Also, some patients who are not happy with their reassignment may be more known to clinicians as they continue clinical contact.

For male-to-female transsexuals, the cosmetic and functional adequacy of surgical interventions affects self-image. Generally, the better the surgical result, other things being equal, the better the postoperative psychological adjustment.

There has been, however, only one outcome study that included a random assignment as surgically treated and a waiting-list control group. The finding supports postoperative improvement in social integration, sexual adjustment, and psychological symptomatology with surgical intervention.

Regrets after sex-reassignment surgery are reported. Nine male-to-female transsexuals and one female-to-male transsexual are described. They had applied for sex reassignment surgery at average of 35 years of age and had undergone a Real Life Test of more than 2 years. The first significant signs of disturbed reassignment became clear approximately 1.5 years after operation. Six male-to-female transsexuals and one female-to-male transsexual reported to have, at some point, changed their gender identity toward their former birth status. Seven, including the female-to-male transsexual, decided to live permanently in their former gender role. Seven reported having doubts before or during the sex reassignment procedures, but only five expressed them preoperatively, because they were afraid that, if they shared them with their clinicians, they would have put their sex reassignment surgery at risk. With the exception of one male-to-female and one female-to-male transsexual, none had shown distinct atypical gender role behavior during childhood. Postoperative analysis led to the conclusion that eight had not experienced extreme gender dysphoria related to a genuine, irreversible cross-gender identity before surgery. Risk factors appear to be a history of fetishistic cross-dressing, psychological instability, or social isolation.

Treatment Outcome: Adolescents A retrospective study on postoperative functioning of 22 adolescent transsexuals who had undergone sex-reassignment surgery 2.5 years earlier concluded that starting sex-reassignment procedures before adulthood resulted in positive postoperative functioning, provided that there were careful diagnosis and strict criteria for initiating the procedures. Twelve began hormone treatment between 16 and 18 years of age. There were 15 female-to-male transsexuals and seven male-to-female transsexuals. Ages, on average, were 17.5 years of age at pretest and 22 years of age at follow-up. Nine started the Real Life Test supported by hormone treatment before 18 years of age. Early antiandrogen treatment blocked facial hair growth and kept voice from deepening, which enabled postoperative male-to-female transsexuals to pass more effectively as women.

A prospective follow-up study of 20 adolescents with gender identity disorder used hormone therapy between 16 and 18 years of age in two phases. First, hormones with reversible effects, that is, antiandrogens for male-to-female transsexuals and progestins for female-to-male transsexuals, were administered, and, second, estrogens to feminize the male-to-female transsexual and androgens to masculinize the female-to-male transsexual were administered. There were 13 female-to-male transsexuals and seven male-to-female transsexuals, and they were assessed 1 year after surgical treatment. They reported less gender dysphoria in follow-up. No person expressed regret about sex reassignment. Postoperatively, they functioned socially and psychologically well and scored in the normal range. Patients selected were the most psychologically stable and had a supportive family background.

Follow-Up and Outcome: Children In the author's 15-year prospective study, 44 of 66 cross-gendered boys, most of whom would be diagnosed today with gender identity disorder, were followed to late adolescence or young adulthood. Sexual orientation was determined by interviews addressing erotic fantasies and erotic behaviors. Fantasies were determined from questioning about masturbation content, erotic nocturnal dreams, and experiences of arousal when seeing pornography or sexually attractive persons. Behaviors were assessed by reports of interpersonal genital sexuality.

On the dimension of erotic fantasy, 33 of 44 previously gender-atypical boys were bisexual to homosexual (rated 2 to 6 on the Kinsey 7-point scale of sexual orientation, where 0 is exclusive heterosexuality, and 6 is exclusive homosexuality). Regarding behavior, 24 of 30 were bisexual to homosexual. One boy at 18 years of age was gender dysphoric and probably diagnosable as transsexual. Another boy reported sexual arousal to cross-dressing. Since that study, two additional previously cross-gendered boys have come to the author's attention. Both are homosexual.

Although only one of the author's gender identity disorder boys later expressed gender dysphoria, in a follow-up in adolescence by Kenneth Zucker, of 45 children initially assessed for gender identity disorder, 20 percent continued to exhibit gender dysphoria, six of whom were requesting sex reassignment.

Several possible reasons exist for the considerable behavioral change from the time of initial evaluation to adolescence in these boys with or without formal treatment. When deciding to seek professional counsel, parents have usually concluded or may conclude after consultation that their child's extensive cross-gender behaviors should be limited or eliminated. Also, the child is receiving negative reaction from age-mates for cross-gendered activities. This may result in greater gender conformity. The developmental course of sex-typed activity preferences in conventional children also dictates change. Because even typical girls play less with dress-up dolls as they get older, cross-gendered boys can also be expected to show lessened interest.

No large studies of gender atypical females evolving into adolescence or young adulthood have been conducted. A nonclinical sample of 50 tomboys was generated in collaboration with others in which the girls shared some, but not all, features with girls with gender identity disorder. However, federal research funding was not forthcoming, so no systematic follow-up data are available. However, the author has become aware of two of these girls, now young women, who are female-to-male transsexuals.

INTERSEX

According to DSM-IV-TR, intersex conditions are diagnosed, when gender dysphoria is present, as *gender identity disorder not otherwise specified*.

CONGENITAL VIRILIZING ADRENAL HYPERPLASIA

Congenital virilizing adrenal hyperplasia was formerly called the *adrenogenital syndrome*. An enzymatic defect in the production of adrenal cortisol, beginning prenatally, leads to overproduction of adrenal androgens and virilization of the female fetus. Postnatally, excessive adrenal androgen can be controlled by steroid administration.

With early diagnosis, children develop a gender identity that is consistent with chromosomal and gonadal sex. However, girls show more tomboyish behavior than controls, including unaffected relatives. Higher rates of bisexual or homosexual behavior in adulthood have been reported.

Four patients with congenital adrenal hyperplasia were recently described who changed gender from female to male in a gradual process extending into adulthood. Medical histories included delay beyond infancy or lack of surgical feminization of genitalia and progressive virilization with inconsistent or absent hormonal replacement therapy. All were sexually attracted to women only.

ANDROGEN INSENSITIVITY SYNDROME

Androgen insensitivity syndrome was formerly called *testicular feminization*. In these persons with the XY karyotype, tissue cells are unable to use testosterone or other androgens. Therefore, the person appears to be a normal female at birth and is raised as a girl. Breasts develop as female owing to conversion of testosterone to estradiol.

Fourteen women with complete androgen insensitivity syndrome have been recently assessed at a mean of 45 years of age, all of whom were raised as female. They reported a high degree of femininity, along with a low degree of masculinity, throughout psychosexual development. They all reported satisfaction being women. Ninety-three percent were heterosexual. However, partial androgen insensitivity syndrome has been associated with gender change from female to male during adulthood.

TURNER'S SYNDROME

In Turner's syndrome, one sex chromosome is missing, such that the sex karyotype is simply X. Children have female genitalia and, possibly, anomalies such as a shield-shaped chest and a webbed neck. They are short. As a consequence of dysfunctional ovaries, they require exogenous estrogen to develop female secondary sex characteristics. Gender identity is female.

KLINEFELTER'S SYNDROME

An extra X chromosome is present in Klinefelter's syndrome, such that the karyotype is XXY. At birth, patients appear to be normal males. There may be excessive gynecomastia in adolescence. Testes are small, usually without sperm production. They are tall, and body habitus is eunuchoid. Reports suggest a higher rate of gender identity disorder.

5-α-REDUCTASE DEFICIENCY

In 5-α-reductase deficiency, an enzymatic defect prevents the conversion of testosterone to dihydrotestosterone, which is required for prenatal virilization of the genitalia. At birth, the affected person appears to be female, although there is some visible anomaly. In earlier generations, before childhood identification of the disorder was common, these persons, raised as girls, virilized at puberty and changed their gender identity to male. Later generations were expected to virilize and thus may have been raised with ambiguous gender. Recently, there are reports of a small number of patients for whom early removal of the testes and socialization as girls have resulted in a female gender identity.

EARLY LIFE SURGERY FOR INTERSEX CHILDREN

Controversy has developed over surgery of the genitalia for anatomically intersexed children. For decades, it was considered appropriate to modify the genitalia early to conform with the sex of rearing. This is because a professional consensus was that socialization as a boy or girl would prevail over other variables of sex, such as chromosome configuration as XX or XY. Also, it would prevent peer group stigmatization in consequence of the atypical genitalia. More recently, some intersex persons, now adults, argue that their surgery was mutilating and limited full erotic arousal. Others report that surgery was in accord with the wrong early decision for sex of rearing. Currently, there is some professional movement toward delay in implementing surgery, if at all, until the child involved can contribute to the decision.

SUGGESTED CROSS-REFERENCES

Related discussions include Section 18.1a on normal human sexuality and sexual dysfunctions, Section 18.1b on homosexuality, Section 32.2 on normal child development, and Section 32.3 on normal adolescent development. Transvestic fetishism is discussed in Section 18.2 on paraphilias, and intersex disorders are discussed in Section 24.6 on endocrine and metabolic disorders.

REFERENCES

Bailey J. *The Man Who Would Be Queen: The Science of Gender Bending and Transsexualism.* Washington, DC: John Henry Press; 2003.

Benjamin H. *The Transsexual Phenomenon.* New York: Julian Press; 1966.

*Blanchard R, Steiner B, eds. *Clinical Management of Gender Identity Disorders in Children and Adults.* Washington, DC: American Psychiatric Press; 1990.

Blanchard R, Zucker K, Bradley S, Hume C: Birth order and sibling sex ratio in homosexual male adolescents and probably pre-homosexual feminine boys. *Develop Psychol.* 1995;31:22.

Bradley S, Oliver G, Chernick A, Zucker K: Experiment of nurture: Ablatio penis at 2 months, sex reassignment at 7 months, and a psychosexual follow-up in young adulthood. *Pediatrics.* 1998;102:e9.

Coates S, Person E: Extreme boyhood femininity: Isolated behavior or pervasive disorder. *J Am Acad Child Psychiatry.* 1985;24:702.

Cohen-Kettenis P, Van Goozen S: Sex reassignment of adolescent transsexuals: A follow-up study. *J Am Acad Child Adolesc Psychiatry.* 1997;36:263.

Dessens A, Cohen-Kettenis P, Mellenbergn G, Poll N, Koppe J, Boer K: Prenatal exposure to anticonvulsants and psychosexual development. *Arch Sex Behav.* 1999;28:31.

*Diamond M, Sigmundson H: Sex reassignment at birth: Long-term review and clinical implications. *Arch Pediatr Adolesc Med.* 1997;151:298.

Futterweit W, Weiss R, Fagerstrom R: Endocrine evaluation of forty female-to-male transsexuals. Increased frequency of polycystic ovarian disease in female transsexualism. *Arch Sex Behav.* 1986;15:69.

*Green R. *Sexual Identity Conflict in Children and Adults.* New York: Basic Books; 1974.

Green R. *The "Sissy Boy Syndrome" and the Development of Homosexuality.* New Haven, CT: Yale University Press; 1987.

Green R: Birth order and ratio of brothers to sisters in transsexuals. *Psychol Med.* 2000;30:789.

Green R, Fleming D: Transsexual surgery follow-up: Status in the 1990's. *Ann Rev Sex Res.* 1990;1:63.

Green R, Keverne B: The disparate maternal aunt-uncle ratio in male transsexuals. An explanation invoking genomic imprinting. *J Theor Biol.* 2000;202:55.

*Green R, Money J, eds. *Transsexualism and Sex Reassignment.* Baltimore: Johns Hopkins Press; 1969.

Green R, Young R: Fingerprint asymmetry in male and female transsexuals. *Person Ind Diff.* 2000;29:933.

Green R, Young R: Hand preference, sexual preference and transsexualism. *Arch Sex Behav.* 2001;30:567.

Harry Benjamin International Gender Dysphoria Association. *Standards of Care.* 6th version. Minneapolis, MN: Harry Benjamin International Gender Dysphoria Association; 2001.

Intersex Society of North America: http://www.isna.org.

Kruijver F, Zhou J-N, Pool C, Hofman M, Gooren L, Swaab D: Male-to-female transsexuals have female neuron numbers in limbic nucleus. *J Clin Endocrinol Metab.* 2000;85:2034.

*Mate-Kole C, Freschi M, Robin A: A controlled study of psychological and social change after surgical gender reassignment in selected male transsexuals. *Br J Psychiatry.* 1990;157:261.

Money J, Hampson J, Hampson J: An examination of some basic sexual concepts. *Bull John Hopkins Hosp.* 1955;97:301.

Person E, Ovesey L: The transsexual syndrome in males. I. Primary transsexualism. II. Secondary transsexualism. *Am J Psychother.* 1974;28:4.

Reiner W, Gearhart J: Discordant sexual identity in some genetic males with cloacal exstrophy assigned to female sex at birth. *N Engl J Med.* 2004;350:333.

Sidocowic L, Lunney G: Baby X revisited. *Sex Roles.* 1980;6:67.

Smith Y, Van Goozen S, Cohen-Kettenis P: Adolescents with gender identity disorder who were accepted or rejected for sex reassignment surgery: A prospective follow-up study. *J Am Acad Child Adolesc Psychiatry.* 2001;40:472.

Stoller R. *Sex and Gender.* New York: Science House; 1968.

Zucker K, Beaulieu N, Bradley S, Grimshaw G, Wilcox A: Handedness in boys with gender identity disorder. *J Clin Psychol Psychiatry.* 2001;42:767.

Zucker K, Green R, Coates S, Zuger B, Cohen-Kettenis P, Zecca G, Letora V, Money J, Hahn-Burke S, Bradley S, Blanchard R: Sibling sex ratio of boys with gender identity disorder. *J Child Psychol Psychiatry.* 1997;38:543.

Zucker K, Wild J, Bradley S, Lowry C: Physical attractiveness of boys with gender identity disorder. *Arch Sex Behav.* 1993;22:23.

▲ 18.4 Sexual Addiction

PATRICK J. CARNES, PH.D.

Since James Orford's classic article on sexual dependency appeared in the *British Journal of Addictions* in the late 1970s, there has been a growing awareness among medical professionals of sexual behavior that was problematic yet did not fit traditional categories, such as the paraphilias. In these cases, sexual behavior had similar patterns to substance abuse, pathological gambling, and compulsive eating and frequently cooccurred with these problems. Loss of control, significant adverse consequences, and continuation despite consequences emerged as beginning criteria for patient identification. Compulsive sexual patterns, coupled with extreme preoccupation, characterized these patients who often incorporated diverse normal and abnormal behavior. Cultural changes worked to reveal and to accentuate the problem. Public awareness and accountability connected to sexual exploitation and harassment in religious, political, military, and business contexts generated more patients seeking help. Furthermore, the acquired immune deficiency syndrome (AIDS) epidemic brought more patients who were behaving in self-destructive ways counter to their own wishes. Finally, Internet sex dramatically escalated the frequency of patients seeking help from clinicians. Al Cooper's landmark studies reveal that 6 percent of Internet users manifest problematic online behavior. Many of those in trouble with cybersex probably would not have had a problem without the Internet. Parallel to sexual awareness, 12-step groups, such as Sex Addicts Anonymous (SAA), have grown dramatically as an adjunct to therapy.

With growing recognition of the problem, clinicians have used varying terminology depending on their professional orientation. *Hypersexuality*, *sexual compulsivity*, *sexual impulsivity*, *sexual addiction*, and *nonparaphilic sex addiction* have been the most commonly used terms. In the addiction field, one of the key signs of addiction is compulsive use. One of the recent formulations of that position is Alan Leshner's description of addiction as a *hijacked brain*. He explains addiction as a brain disease that manifests as compulsive behavior. In practice, some professionals may make distinctions between *addiction* and *compulsion*, others may use the terms interchangeably.

The term *sex addiction* has several advantages conceptually and practically. First, it discerns the difference between compulsively accessing the pleasure centers of the brain and nonpleasure behavior that is more typical of obsessive-compulsive behavior. Second, the frequency, similarity, and interaction with other comorbid addictive behaviors argue strongly for common etiology. Finally, the addiction model leads to clear-cut, successful intervention strategies, including nationwide networks of self-help support groups. Currently, an inclusive national effort is under way to develop comprehensive diagnostic criteria that are being tested on large samples for prevalence data. Researchers gathering statistical evidence by using advanced neuroimaging technology may add clarifying data about the biology of the condition, which, in turn, may redefine terminology.

PROBLEM RECOGNITION

The nature of sexually compulsive behavior interferes with problem recognition. Patients are not candid about their behavior nor are they likely to reveal that specific behaviors are actually part of a consistent, self-destructive pattern. Patients frequently hide the severity of the problem from others, delude themselves about their ability to control their behavior, and minimize the impact on others. Their shame extends to being deceptive with their physician. Sometimes, their role as leaders in church, business, community, or political settings compounds the problem, because they are expected to exhibit behavior that is beyond reproach. Usually, some event precipitates a visit to the physician. The incident is presented as a one-time event, as a moral lapse, or as an event precipitated by marital problems. Careful assessment and data assembling may reveal a much deeper pattern that requires specific therapy for sexual compulsion. These deeper patterns may emerge in diversified forms, including compulsive masturbation, compulsive prostitution, cybersex, and affairs. They may extend to include exhibitionism, voyeurism, and criminal sexual misconduct. Seldom is there just one pattern, but rather there is a collage of patterns affected by hierarchies of preference, situation, combination, and opportunity. For example, pornography on the Internet may serve as a portal to other addictive sexual behaviors, including prostitution and affairs, or it may be a gateway to solicitation and stalking of underaged girls. The following scenarios would prompt the clinician to assess the patient for the presence of sex addiction:

- *The patient volunteers a long-term pattern of problematic sexual behavior.* Usually, this occurs because the patient has hit a level of despair or is suicidal. He or she knows that he or she simply cannot continue living this way.
- *The clinician has evidence of a long-term problem.* If the patient history shows frequent consequences due to sexual acting out, a pattern may emerge. If the clinician learns of chronic affairs, and the spouse discovers evidence of pervasive prostitution use, such compulsive behavior may signal an addictive pattern.
- *Some sexual event occurs, and the clinician has evidence of other compulsive or addictive behaviors.* Patient issues with drug use, gambling, and food point to the larger problem of a loss of control. Many times these issues cooccur and amplify each other.
- *The patient's behavior involving abuse of power should prompt a thorough evaluation.* Sex with children, congregants, employees, patients, or other persons under the authority of the patient usually involve at least a temporary removal of the person from his or her position and may require reporting in some jurisdictions.
- *Unexplained problems accompanying compulsive sexual behavior necessitate delving deeper.* Unexplained absences, failure to perform expected tasks, and the disappearance of large sums of money could result.

An inappropriate sexual incident does not always mean the presence of addictive illness. A long-term, extramarital affair, for example, may be a problem for a spouse but does not represent a compulsive pattern. Likewise, exploitive or even violent behavior does not indicate a sexually addictive illness. In a recent study of sex offenders, only 72 percent of pedophiles and 38 percent of rapists fit the criteria for sexual addiction. The following cases illustrate the diversity and complexity of sexually addictive behavior:

A 48-year-old woman comes to treatment for alcoholism and heard a lecture on sexual addiction. She reveals to her counselor that she has been married four times, and, each time, the marriage has ended because of her infidelity. In each marriage, she was always involved in at least one affair and, at times, several affairs. At the time of one of her weddings, she was having an affair with a member of the wedding party. She still does not know who fathered one of her children. She informs her counselor that she can no longer deny the truth about herself. She decided that romance is preferable to alcohol. Her story to her counselor revealed that she would have periods of abstinence from alcohol in which her sexual behavior would escalate. She would relapse with alcohol, because her sexual behavior was creating such chaos in her life. During treatment, she identified her father's sexually abusive behavior toward her as part of the genesis of her inability to establish boundaries with men. She was referred to an extended care facility with a special track for sex addicts who had experienced significant trauma.

A 35-year-old police officer is placed on leave, pending an investigation of accusations that he demanded sex in return for not giving speeding tickets. He reveals to his psychiatrist that he also has a compulsive prostitution habit that costs approximately 1,500 dollars per week. He has been accepting bribes to support his habit. He has had several affairs over which his wife had left him 1 year earlier. His physician referred him to an inpatient facility specializing in sexual compulsion.

An anesthesiologist is suspended for viewing Internet pornography on the hospital computer system: pictures of adolescent girls. Being quite gifted technologically, he reveals in therapy that he is the Webmaster of a site that hosts pornography involving older and young women. He had been molested by a neighbor woman and had had a pornography problem from the age of approximately 9 years of age. He would find his father's pornography, and then he would be severely beaten for having it. He found escorts on the Internet with whom he had sex and from whom he purchased amphetamines.

A businessman in his late 30s was having sex with street prostitutes and had three arrests. He told his therapist that, out of the previous 365 days, he had been with a prostitute for 357 of those days. Many days, it was two times a day and, on occasion, three times a day. The idea of being with a woman he knew and cared for was beyond his imagination. Sex with someone he knew would be unbearable. In therapy, he reported significant physical and sexual abuse.

A 71-year-old chief executive officer of a successful office products manufacturing company received two sexual harassment complaints in a matter of a few weeks. The company hired an outside investigator to do a company-wide sexual harassment audit. More than 70 women (past and current employees) came forward with stories of constant propositions, fondling, and affairs. The investigation further uncovered similar stories among vendors, trade people, family friends, and an unfortunate incident with his daughter-in-law.

By the time he was 18 years of age, a patient had been viewing Internet pornography for 10 years. He was caught viewing underage pictures by a computer repairman and was reported when he was in the eighth grade. His parents made efforts to police his Internet behavior, but he was more savvy than they were and could hide his tracks. He flunked out of his first year of college, because he was spending an average of 40 hours per week masturbating while online. His parents' first warning came when his second-semester tuition had gone unpaid. Their son had expended in strip bars all of the tuition money he had been given.

Clinicians notice that sexual compulsion surfaces in many guises. Common to them all is that patients report a loss of control and life consequences. Age or sex excludes no one. The ratio of men to women is 3 to 1, which parallels alcoholism and problem gambling. The notable exception is problematic online sexual behavior, for which 40 percent of patients are women. The Internet has also pushed boundaries: Younger and elderly people are becoming involved in compulsive cybersex. Some additional factors complete a profile that might signal a need for clinical intervention. In a large survey (N = 953), patients in recovery reported the following: Seventeen percent had attempted suicide, and 72 percent obsessed about it because of their sexual behavior. (More than 50 percent of hospital admissions with a diagnosis of sex addiction also had significant depression.)

The majority of sex addicts (65 percent) routinely ran the risk of sexually transmitted diseases (STDs). Thirty-eight percent of the men and 45 percent of the women contracted STDs as a result of their addictive behavior.

Sex addicts recognized AIDS as the most lethal complication of their illness. (Yet, a recent University of Georgia study revealed that, although 87 percent of health practitioners were aware of sexually compulsive behavior, only 13 percent screened for human immunodeficiency virus [HIV].) Many sex addicts have lost a partner or spouse (40 percent) and most have experienced severe marital or relationship problems (70 percent) because of their behavior.

Female sex addicts report deep grief over abortions (36 percent) and unwanted pregnancies (42 percent). More than 58 percent reported severe financial consequences. Some reported losing the opportunity to work in the career of their choice (27 percent). Most sex addicts (79 percent) talk of serious losses in job productivity; 11 percent were demoted. Thirty-eight percent experienced some physical injury as part of sexual acting out. Nineteen percent of the men and 21 percent of the women were involved in automobile accidents as part of acting-out behavior. Sixty percent of the women were physically abused during sex; 50 percent were raped. Men also reported physical battering (16 percent) and dangerous situations (44 percent). Sixty-five percent reported sleep disorders related to shame, fear, and despair over their behavior.

Mary L. Gannon and other specialists have made the case that, each year, urologists, surgeons, gynecologists, and emergency room physicians examine patients who have self-inflicted genital trauma or who have inserted objects into their urethras, bladders, rectums, and external genitalia. These patients have experienced serious injury due to unusual or risky sexual practices. Sex addiction specialists routinely do grand rounds for these specialties, because they quickly become primary referents.

ETIOLOGY

Addiction is a complex biosocial illness. More than 87 percent of sex addicts also report having other addictions, which add to the complexity. Searching for the biological precursors has been a touchstone of addiction medicine research. Many hypotheses are being explored to explain susceptibility to multiple avenues of addiction and compulsion. For example, addiction researchers have noted that the Taq 1A1 allele of D2 receptor gene is associated with increased risk of alcoholism, drug abuse, smoking, obesity, compulsive behaviors, and Tourette's syndrome. Although sex addiction is relatively new in attracting researchers' interest at this level, it has been clearly shown that sex addicts come from families with multiple addictions. For example, 22 percent of mothers, 40 percent of fathers, and 56 percent of siblings are known to have more than one addiction.

A clear picture has emerged in families of sex addicts in addition to the presence of addictive pathology. Using assessments based on the circumplex model of family systems, most addicts come from families that are rigid (77 percent). These families are characterized by extreme efforts to control and minimal negotiation. Offspring from this family type often have difficulty with accountability and authority. They are also prone to secret lives out of the purview of the family. This *double-life* phenomenon is especially strong when adolescents discover that parents do not live up to their proclaimed values. If parents proclaim sexual fidelity, for example, and that turns out to be untrue, it deepens defiance and secrecy. These families also tend to have negative attitudes toward sexuality in general, which tend to increase shame and obsession.

Sex addicts also tend to originate in *disengaged* families (87 percent). This family type makes a great effort to look good for appearances but has little intimacy. Family members are "ships passing in the night." Some have argued that addiction is a result of a failure to adequately bond. Mark F. Schwartz and colleagues, using an attachment perspective, propose that sex addiction is, in fact, an intimacy disorder. The net effect is that these patients do not trust relationships. More than two-thirds of these patients come from families that are rigid and disengaged. The challenge in treatment is that they distrust authority and accountability, and they have little confidence in relationships or intimacy. The difficulties that propel them into addiction become the factors that make them difficult to engage in therapy.

Trauma also appears to contribute to sex addiction. Eighty-one percent report a history of sexual abuse, 72 percent report a history of physical abuse, and 97 percent identify various forms of emotional abuse. One study by Patrick J. Carnes and David Delmonico shows that the amount of physical and sexual abuse is a substantive factor in the number of addictions as an adult. Addiction becomes a solution for the distress of the reactivity that typifies posttraumatic stress disorder (PTSD). Bessel van der Kolk and others point to the neurochemical shifts that occur in which trauma victims actually repeat their trauma compulsively. Clinicians note that sex addicts incorporate significant scenarios and even actual behaviors from their abuse experiences into their acting-out cycles. Ken Adams and others point to enmeshment with specific parents (surrogate spouse) and covert eroticization as common phenomena in sex addiction.

Another common pattern is high-risk behaviors that result in severe consequences, such as loss of career or arrest. Children who were sexually abused often integrate fear into their arousal patterns. For sex to work for these adults, it has to have a fear component, which results in risk-seeking sex. One of the most common stories that clinicians hear are sex addicts who knew that their behavior would be disastrous but did it anyway. An example is an addict who strongly believes that the street prostitute is a police decoy and notices a squad car down the street but proceeds to solicit sex anyway.

Onset of sex addiction also appears to be triggered by stressful events. Addicts report this stress in terms of specific events (deaths, accidents, severe losses, and trauma) or catalytic or specific demanding environments (medical school, seminary, and developmental business). Catalytic events and environments activate trauma memories and compulsive behavior. Addiction also appears to be a repressive mechanism, because, when behaviors stop, memories of abuse begin to return. Most clinicians also notice an extreme ability to compartmentalize and to dissociate from reality, which becomes incorporated into addictive behavior as part of escapism. Family systems and rules that result in secrecy combined with trauma survivors' capacity to compartmentalize are the building blocks of the addict's secret life.

The result is an implicit dishonesty and failure to live up to values, which creates a chronic sense of shame. Almost all addicts admit to strong feelings of guilt and shame (96 percent), strong feelings of isolation and loneliness (94 percent), feelings of hopelessness and despair (91 percent), and acting against personal values and beliefs (90 percent). Merl A. Fossom and Marilyn Mason created a conceptual framework to explain the role of shame in binge-and-purge behavior across all addictions. The inability to meet personal standards leads to an *acting-in* mode that calls for extreme abstinence. Because of these excessively high standards, there is progressive *acting out*. A good example is clergymen who preach against promiscuity or some sexual behavior only to be discovered engaging in that behavior or being arrested for it. Investigation reveals a chronic pattern of that behavior. In public pronouncements, they are purging, and, in private behavior, they are bingeing. This dichotomy underlies the roles of shame and compartmentalization. A hospital-based survey of sexual disorders revealed that 72 percent of sex addicts identified with a binge-and-purge pattern.

Comorbidity Few of these patients have only a sexual problem. For example, 41 percent have problems with drugs or alcohol, and 38 percent have an eating disorder. Other problems include pathological gambling, nicotine abuse, and compulsive working. In addiction medicine, the term *addiction interaction* is used to describe how addictions more than coexist but actually reinforce or amplify one another. Frequently, the term *fusing* is used when two addictions are almost always used at the same time. An example would be cocaine and sex addiction. Arnold Washton and others have documented that 50 to 70 percent of cocaine addicts also exhibit sexually compulsive behavior. Most acquisition of cocaine is connected to some form of sexual behavior. One frequent subset is an addict combining cocaine and extended masturbation, which lasts as long as 15 to 20 hours. Patients report that the goal is not to ejaculate, because that brings a severe migraine-like headache. Rather, the goal is to preserve this feeling. These patients *fuse* their behavior. They never masturbate without cocaine; they never use cocaine without masturbation.

Other examples of interaction would include

- Using alcohol to disinhibit for specific high-risk sex
- Combining the hyperventilation of tobacco smoke and compulsive masturbation
- Arousal activities, such as risky sex and amphetamines or crystal meth followed by numbing activities, such as overeating, alcohol, and masturbation (a common scenario of PTSD victims)
- Merging of cruising rituals to pick up partners and drinking (bars) or drug using (raves and dances)
- Going to a topless casino to drink, to gamble, and to be sexual

Compulsive spending and debts (sometimes part of a cluster of behaviors called the *financial disorders*) are frequently noted (27 percent). Although many have experienced great financial losses as part of their sex addiction, some actually eroticize money. For example, it is estimated that 1.6 million men use prostitutes compulsively. Of men seeking treatment, two-thirds report significant financial problems related to prostitution. Patients are able to tell the clinician the dollar amount of cash or credit that precipitates acting out. The financial issues in many cases extend beyond their sexual behaviors. They frequently spend more than they can afford or earn and amass significant debt as a result. These patients need help beyond treatment for their sexual disorder.

Sexual aversion (International Classification of Diseases diagnosis number 302.79) also is a common problem that may seem ironic, given the amount of sexual experience that these patients have. Usually, it is trauma and family related. One pattern is long periods of bingeing followed by long periods of sexual abstinence. Another common issue is bingeing outside of a primary relationship (usually with high-risk or unknown people) but being compulsively nonsexual within the relationship. Sexual avoidance also appears in spouses of sex addicts, providing the addict with an excuse for outside activities. Sexual aversion and addiction parallel the eating disorders in that the extremes and bingeing and purging are a family of issues with common etiology. Similarly, in the case of food disorders, one does not give up food but learns how to eat differently. The clinical risk of undiagnosed aversion is that patients slip into sexual avoidance, as opposed to focusing on sexual health for themselves. Usually, compulsive sexual behavior is part of an intricate weave of addictive and avoidant behaviors to manage internal distress.

Sexual Behavior Patterns In 1985, an extended survey of more than 170 behaviors revealed that sex addicts tended to cluster into ten distinct types of behavior. These typologies have a specific erotic focus that seems to correlate with distinct phases of courtship that have become distorted through the addicts' development.

Table 18.4–1 summarizes these ten *archetypes*. They are useful to the clinician, because the behavioral clusters help reveal the addict's arousal patterns. For example, intrusive sex includes patients who compulsively use frotteurism and toucherism. The goal of those behaviors is to touch people sexually without them being aware of the behavior or without being caught. If they exhibit those behaviors, they are also likely to make obscene phone calls. If they make obscene calls, they also are likely to insert inappropriate sexual humor into conversations. If they are professionals, such as physicians, dentists, clergy, or therapists, they touch patients inappropriately under the guise of their professional tasks.

The clinician looks for the *erotic moment*. In intrusive sex, the erotic moment is to invade the space of others in ways that make it difficult for

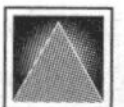

Table 18.4–1
Sexual Behavior Patterns

Fantasy sex: sexually charged fantasies, relationships, and situations
Arousal depends on sexual possibility. Neglecting responsibilities to engage in fantasy or to prepare for the next sexual episode, or both, is common among fantasy sex addicts.

Seductive role sex: seduction of partners
Arousal is based on conquest and diminishes rapidly after initial contact. Arousal can be heightened by increasing risk or the number of partners, or both.

Voyeuristic sex: visual arousal
The use of visual stimulation to escape into an obsessive trance. Arousal may be heightened by masturbation, risk (e.g., peeping), or violation of boundaries (e.g., voyeuristic rape), but, for arousal to be maintained, it must be illicit somehow and must be visual.

Exhibitionistic sex: attracting attention to the body or sexual parts of the body
Sexual arousal stems from reaction to viewer shock or interest.

Paying for sex: purchase of sexual services
Arousal is connected to payment for sex, and, with time, the arousal actually becomes connected to money itself. Payment creates an entitlement and a sense of power over meeting needs, but the arousal starts with having money and the search for someone in the business.

Trading sex: selling or bartering sex for power
Arousal is based on gaining control of others by using sex as leverage.

Intrusive sex: boundary violation without discovery
Sexual arousal occurs by violating boundaries with no repercussions.

Anonymous sex: high-risk sex with unknown persons
Arousal involves no seduction or cost and is immediate. The arousal has no entanglements or obligations associated with it and often is accelerated by unsafe or high-risk environments, such as bars, beaches, parks, and restrooms.

Pain exchange sex: being humiliated or hurt as part of sexual arousal or sadistic hurting or degrading another sexually, or both
Arousal is built around specific scenarios or narratives of humiliation and shame.

Exploitive sex: exploitation of the vulnerable
Arousal patterns are based on target types of vulnerability. Certain types of vulnerable persons (e.g., clients or patients of professionals, children or adolescents, or distressed persons) become the focus of arousal.

people to react or to hold the addict accountable. Empirical evidence shows that the behaviors are related. For the clinician, it becomes a guide to the internal world of the addict. In intrusive sex, the courtship distortion has to do with fear of rejection and having somehow to steal sex, even in fleeting ways. It also reveals *eroticized anger*, common in sex addiction, wherein the patient notices the sex but not the anger.

Sex addicts are often active in more than one cluster of behaviors. They may, in fact, shift focus. An exhibitionist who wishes to avoid arrest may go to a massage parlor, because it is a safer place to be seen. Compulsive affairs may replace prostitution. Most often, there is a variety of ways to act out, including paraphilic and offending behaviors. One of the distinct advantages of the addiction paradigm is that it allows clinicians to see that not only do currents of compulsive behavior transcend specific categories, but they also have the same common self-destructive results and obsessional purposes. The key for clinicians is to understand the escalation factor. Addicts act out using more of the behaviors, add risk and danger, or seek new behaviors, often with great risk and danger. Escalation is tempered with plateaus, efforts to reduce risk, and sexually aversive periods. Most addicts are able to pinpoint moments of escalation and resulting consequences.

Core to the treatment process is identification of the arousal template. In 1985, John Money used the term *love map* to describe the internal guide as to what was erotic. This arousal template is more dynamic than a map, for it usually contains a scenario based on an abuse experience, a fantasy, or something historical. Clinicians approach this issue by having the patient identify the *ideal fantasy*—if acting out were perfect, what would it look like? Therapy is about tracing back the origins of the arousal, understanding its functional and dysfunctional parts, and reimaging healthy sexual practice. In this way, the *organizing principles* of the compulsion are exposed and, with psychological distance, can lose their power.

Cybersex: Crack Cocaine of Sex Addiction One of the greatest escalators of sexual addiction is the Internet. Cybersex has been termed the *crack cocaine of sex addiction*. In 2002, sex-related sites became the number one economic sector of the Internet, recording sales that exceeded that of software and computers. Pornography alone has become a problem in the workplace. Seventy percent of Internet pornography traffic occurs between 9 AM and 5 PM. Seventy-two percent of companies that have faced Internet misuse reported that 69 percent of those cases were related simply to pornography. Leading software publishers estimate as much as 83 billion dollars per year in lost productivity for American companies. Serious researchers showed in large samples that one in six employees was now having trouble with sexual behavior online.

Researchers have noted problems with compulsive and addictive behavior online, especially in the areas of gambling and sexuality. Others have noted behaviors such as online trading, gaming, and compulsive computer use. In addition to Cooper's original articles, others who work with compulsive sexual behavior patients documented problematic online sexual behavior in which people's daily ability to function was being affected by their cybersex activities. Specific patterns of arousal emerged in these online compulsive scenarios. Among them were

Rapid escalation of amount and variety. Patients report consistently that they experienced a rapid increase in the amount of the behavior and the diversity of sexual behavior. People who have significant problems often find that the problems start almost immediately. Consider the clergyman who started viewing pornography on July 4th. By the time that he was discovered only 5 weeks later, he had already embezzled 8,000 dollars from the church to pay for his online activities. That pattern, although not true of all cases, is common enough to be noticed by clinicians. Factors that contribute to escalation include the appearance of anonymity and ease of access. Also, a pattern of denial quickly emerges in which the behavior is seen as having no consequences, even though clear consequences are inevitable (such as discovery of embezzled funds).

Escalation becomes obsessional, with new, specific behaviors becoming quickly fixated. Patients report that they become obsessed with specific behaviors that they had never experienced or even knew of before their Internet experiences. This pattern is intriguing, given that sexual science has long taken the position that the arousal template or *love map* is established early. John Money suggests that arousal patterns are firmly established between 5 and 11 years of age. Patients, however, report being unable to stop thinking about behaviors that they did not know existed until they were in their 60s and on the computer. Thus, under the influence of the computer, users are experiencing high degrees of arousal of which they have no history and that are difficult to stop. This finding also counters much of the traditional addiction and compulsion literature that traces obsessive behavior in adults to experiences of childhood or adolescent sexual abuse.

Relational regression occurs, in which absorption in Internet sexual activities results in serious withdrawal from sexual contact with partners and withdrawal from overall intimacy. Patients report that sex with spouses or partners declines in frequency and appeal. Furthermore, they note a withdrawal from social contact with family, friends, and colleagues. In part, that is a result from many hours spent on the computer and the emotional depletion that accompanies Internet bingeing. There also appears to be a shame component that leads to isolation and despair. Although some have reported that pornography in general leads to a decline in intimate sexual interaction, the intimacy avoidance with cybersex appears to be quite profound and needs to be studied systematically.

Internet sexual behavior can accelerate existing addictive and compulsive behavior and can precipitate new compulsive off-line behavior. A common finding is that patients who are already having trouble with compulsive sexuality found the Internet to be a significant behavior intensification catalyst. The Internet not only intensifies the problematic eroticization but also adds new resources. If compulsive prostitution was a problem, it became even more so as a result of Internet activity. Some patients report having had no history of compulsive sexual behavior until they discovered the Internet. When their sexual behavior escalated online, they started behaviors off-line that became compulsive as well.

One theory of explanation for escalation, intensity of arousal, and compulsive behavior is that, through the Internet, patients *access the unresolved*. All people have sexual experiences that leave them unfinished. Sexual play as a child, for example, may leave a person with unfinished experiences. As a person matures, he or she realizes that he or she no longer has an interest in that behavior or that those experiences are no longer appropriate for adults. Yet, a person might experience the right image or story that is an absolute overlay of something unfinished from childhood or adolescence. The nature of marketing for pornography sites is to bombard potential clients with a variety of images to stimulate the purchase of memberships. When that which is unfinished is accessed, the individual begins to search for more of the same genre. The marketing loops of sex sites are literally labyrinthine; each choice may bring a person closer to the types of images that most closely fit that unresolved, unfinished aspect of the sexual self. Patients often report the phenomenon of a *burned-in image*—a specific scene out of their Internet experience about which they cannot stop thinking. This phenomenon is similar to the intrusive images that PTSD patients describe. Patients report that preoccupation with a specific image became so troublesome that they would delete it from their files only to go back to the original source and retrieve it. This happens over and over again.

DIFFERENTIAL DIAGNOSIS

Summarizing the previously stated material, sex addiction patients are characterized by being in some type of sexual crisis. They are typically distrustful of authority, have significant intimacy deficits, and have a history of some type of trauma. Their behavior patterns are hidden and varied but are extensive. Their sexual behavior is clouded by other cooccurring addictions and compulsions. There is a history of crises and consequences around the patient's sexual behavior. Many times, the therapist literally has to be like a detective piecing together the story, because it comes in classic dribs and drabs.

Two principles are extremely important at this stage. First, if there is any written complaint (lawsuit, arrest record, or company harassment complaint), it is critical to review these documents with the patient. This saves time and discovery effort. Second, if there are family members involved, they often have a wealth of data, which add to the picture. Interviewing family members independently may reveal significant gaps and inconsistencies in the patient's story, adding depth and insight to the impact of the patient's behavior.

Currently, there is a large-scale effort to validate diagnostic criteria and to collect prevalence data. Sponsored by the Compass Point Addiction Foundation, this project was initiated in 2001 and is scheduled to be completed in 2005. Strong position statements were made for different conceptualizations of this disorder, including statements by Aviel Goodman who termed it *addiction*, Mart Kafka who used the term *nonparaphilic hypersexuality*, Reid Finlayson who called it *problematic hypersexuality*, Eli Coleman who argued for *compulsive sexual behavior*, and William Marshall and William Marshall who used the term *excessive sexual desire disorder*. Terminology aside, remarkable agreement exists on the basic elements of loss of control, continuation despite consequences, and obsession.

The term *sex addiction* does not appear in the revised fourth edition of the *Diagnostic and Statistical Manual of Mental Disorders* (DSM-IV-TR). However, the criteria listed for various addictive disorders, such as substance dependence and pathological gambling, can be condensed into the same three key elements: (1) *loss of control (compulsivity)*: "There is a persistent desire or unsuccessful efforts to cut down or control substance use"; the patient "has persistent unsuccessful efforts to control, cut back, or stop gambling." (2) *Continuation despite adverse consequences*: "The substance use is continued despite knowledge of having a persistent or recurrent physical or psychological problem that is likely to have been caused or exacerbated by the substance use"; the patient "has committed illegal acts such as forgery, fraud, theft, or embezzlement to finance gambling." (3) *Obsession or preoccupation*: "A great deal of time is spent in activities necessary to obtain the substance, use the substance, or recover from its effects"; the patient "is preoccupied with gambling." When a set of sexual behaviors fulfill the same three criteria, the person can be considered to have a sexual addiction. Note that tolerance and withdrawal are not mentioned in this discussion: Many drugs of abuse are not associated with tolerance and do not have specific withdrawal symptoms, so these features are not essential for the diagnosis of addiction.

However, many clinicians have noted withdrawal symptoms parallel to those experienced by cocaine addicts in withdrawal, including extreme irritability, sleeplessness, and anxiety. Usually, these patterns intensify and then wane over a 3-week period.

The value of the addiction model is that it leads to a specific treatment approach, which is described in the following discussion. For many affected patients, the more traditional treatments, such as psychoanalysis, insight-oriented therapy (in the belief that once the behavior is understood, it stops), or even punishment (such as incarceration), have failed. It is well accepted that psychotherapy for alcohol dependence is likely to fail until the drinking problem has been directly addressed and stopped. The addiction model posits that the same is true for many persons whose sexual behavior is compulsive.

Any sexual activity can be compulsive, including those considered normal and healthy, such as masturbation and consensual sexual intercourse. However, some sexual behaviors are considered abnormal. These are listed in the DSM-IV-TR under the heading of paraphilia. The chief feature of a paraphilia is that which is desired sexually is objectified: What matters is the particular body part (e.g., a foot), item of clothing (e.g., an undergarment), or age (e.g., a child), or a sequence of activities. These behaviors may be episodic, situational, or compulsive. They also may reflect culture, disordered courtship patterns, and perversity (arousal dependent on rule breaking). Thus, sex addiction might include paraphilia. Because someone has an unusual preference does not mean that an addictive or compulsive behavior is present.

Another major advantage of the addiction approach is that such patients tend toward many types of sexual activities, normal and abnormal. They engage in several behaviors simultaneously or in a specific hierarchy of preference. Clinical diagnoses based on specific behaviors such as the paraphilias miss the dynamic and interactive quality of patient behavior patterns. Nor do the paraphilias account for normal behaviors that have become excessive, self-destructive, or dysfunctional. Addiction manifested in compulsive behavior extends through paraphilic and nonparaphilic, abnormal and normal, perverse and diverse.

John Sealey, Kafka, and others have observed the importance of pharmacological interventions, which have helped reduce patient symptoms. Monoamine neurotransmitters such as serotonin, norepinephrine, and dopamine serve a modulatory role in human and mammalian sexual motivation, appetitive, and consummatory behaviors. Pharmacological agents that enhance serotonergic and dopaminergic function have been shown to be helpful to patients in reducing obsession, modifying behavior, and utilizing therapy. Monoamine neurotransmitters have long been associated with other compulsive behaviors, including compulsive drug use, gambling, and eating. The addiction model has long defined addiction as present when there is compulsive behavior. Carnes has also made the case that not only does sex addiction involve multiple sexual behaviors, but it is highly interactive with other comorbid disorders that have common underpinnings.

Historically, clinicians have used criteria similar to those used for substance abuse and pathological gambling. These criteria are based on the three standard principles of evaluation of addictive disorders as listed previously. Ten elaborated criteria are used. Table 18.4–2 summarizes those criteria. Two data sets are supplied: (1) patients who identified with the specified criteria on admission to an inpatient sex addiction program and (2) patients who had been in recovery for a substantial amount of time. The patients who had been in recovery over time reported higher concurrence with the criteria.

Other diagnoses must be considered in the differential diagnosis of excessive sexual activity, including the following:

- Impulse control disorders
- Bipolar affective disorder
- PTSD
- Adjustment disorder (a temporary change of behavior)
- Substance-induced disorders
- Dissociative disorders
- Delusional disorders (erotomania)
- Obsessive-compulsive disorder (OCD)
- Gender identity disorder
- Delirium, dementia, or other cognitive disorder
- Personality disorders

A number of authors (Jennifer P. Schneider, Richard R. Irons, John Sealey, and Nancy Raymond) have described how these disorders can be expressed as excessive sexual behavior. For example, a hypersexual patient who is in the manic phase of bipolar illness usually demonstrates other features of the disorder, such as grandiose thinking, rapid speech, excessive activity, and short attention span. A person whose sexual behavior has been disinhibited by a high concentration of alcohol in the brain is likely to exhibit other signs of intoxication. A patient whose sexual behavior has been disinhibited by Alzheimer's disease shows other cognitive deficits. As for adjustment disorder, this is a temporary situation related to current stresses or events in a person's life. For example, a person who is in the midst of a divorce may demonstrate significant, but temporary, behavior changes. In contrast, an addiction is a pervasive pattern of behavior that is present for months and years.

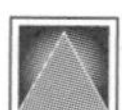

Table 18.4–2
Diagnostic Criteria and Patients in Initial and Long-Term Treatment Who Fit These Criteria

Criteria	Initial Treatment (%)	Long-Term Duration (%)
Recurrent failure (pattern) to resist sexual impulses to engage in specific sexual behavior	73	94
Frequent engaging in those behaviors to a greater extent or over a longer period of time than intended	66	93
Persistent desire or unsuccessful efforts to stop, to reduce, or to control behaviors	67	88
Inordinate amount of time spent in obtaining sex, being sexual, or recovering from sexual experiences	58	94
Preoccupation with the behavior or preparatory activities	37	77
Frequent engaging in the behavior when expected to fulfill occupational, academic, domestic, or social obligations	52	87
Continuation of the behavior despite knowledge of having a persistent or recurrent social, financial, psychological, or physical problem that is caused or exacerbated by the behavior	63	85
Need to increase the intensity, frequency, number, or risk of behaviors to achieve the desired effect or diminished effect with continued behaviors at the same level of intensity, frequency, number, or risk	36	74
Giving up or limiting social, occupational, or recreational activities because of the behavior	51	87
Distress, anxiety, restlessness, or irritability if unable to engage in the behavior	55	98

Courtesy of P. J. Carnes, Ph.D.

Finally, characterological disorders can be the primary cause of excessive sexual behaviors. For example, persons with antisocial or narcissistic personality disorder may have sexual contact with multiple partners, but the reason is that the other person is viewed simply as an object to be used for one's own sexual pleasure, not because there is loss of control.

TREATMENT PROCESS

Carnes headed a research team and initiated a study in the mid-1980s in an effort to understand recovery from sexual compulsion. For the study, recovering sex addicts and their partners were asked to complete a number of instruments, including an extensive life status inventory and a month-by-month history of their recovery. The team also interviewed people with extended recovery in a stage-by-stage fashion and analyzed their responses. The following overview of a 5-year recovery process is based on changes in quality-of-life variables. (See Table 18.4–3 for a summary of findings.)

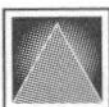

Table 18.4–3
Categories of Recovery over Time

Worse		Better
Second 6 Mos	**Yrs 2 and 3**	**Yr 3 Plus**
Relapse	Financial situations[a]	Healthy sexuality
Health status	Coping with stress[a]	Primary relationships
	Spirituality	Life satisfaction
	Self-image	Relationship with family of origin
	Career status[a]	
	Friendships[a]	

[a]Continued to improve after 3 years or more.
Courtesy of P. J. Carnes, Ph.D.

First 5 Years of Recovery

First Year In the first year, there was no measurable improvement, and, yet, most sexual addicts reported that life was "definitely better." The apparent contradiction might be explained by one respondent's comment: "When you are hitting your head against the wall, even stopping the hitting helps." According to the research team's assessments, some aspects of functioning actually became worse. Most slips tended to occur in the second 6-month period of recovery. Furthermore, all health indicators—accidents, sickness, and visits to physicians—showed the second 6 months to be the worst over the 5 years. The first year appeared to be characterized by turmoil, which tests the person's resolve to change. Some of the consequences of sexual addiction continued, and the change itself was difficult.

Second and Third Years Once the addicts were through the first year, significant rebuilding began. There was measurable improvement occurring in many areas, including finances, ability to cope with stress, spirituality, self-image, career status, and friendships. These indicators reflected a period of intense personal work, which resulted in more productivity, stability, and a greater sense of well-being.

Beyond Year Three Once the personal base of recovery was established, healing occurred in the sexual addicts' relationships. Often, dramatic improvement occurred in their relationships with children, parents, siblings, and partners, with some exceptions. Approximately 13 percent found that unresolved issues with their family of origin could not be healed, because the family was abusive or was threatening to recovery. Also, some marriages were casualties of the recovery process. Most importantly, sex addicts reported shifts toward more healthy and satisfying sexual expression. With improved relationships, overall life satisfaction improved dramatically.

Six Stages of Recovery A series of content analyses were also conducted in the study, which enabled the discernment of six stages in which these quality-of-life changes occur. The stages are summarized as follows.

Developing Stage (Lasts up to 2 Years) The sexual addict's problems mount and create an awareness that something needs to be done. The person may seek therapy or may attend a 12-step group and then drop out. It was also noted that many therapists failed to see the problem of sexual acting out or, if they did see it, failed to follow through on it. Even knowledgeable therapists felt shame at this stage because the patient dropped out of therapy. They would tell themselves that, if they had been better therapists, the patient might have persisted.

Research showed that, no matter what therapists try at this stage, patients still might not be ready. Persons with compulsive sexual behavior have a growing appreciation of the reality of the problem but tend to minimize the problem or to believe they can handle it themselves. Some persons temporarily curtail their behaviors or substitute other behaviors (e.g., switching from exhibitionism to use of prostitutes).

Crisis and Decision Stage (1 Day to 3 Months) At some point, the addict crosses a line at which there is a fundamental commitment to change. This is often precipitated by a personal crisis. This crisis may include all kinds of events, such as arrests, diagnosis of an STD, a spouse (or partner) leaving, a positive human immunodeficiency virus test, a sexual harassment lawsuit, loss of a professional license, a car accident involving death or injury, or a suicide attempt. For example, sometimes a crisis is precipitated by a therapist or employer who refuses to continue enabling destructive behaviors (e.g., an employer who will no longer run the risk of sexual harassment suits or pay for cybersex on a company computer). For some respondents, the commitment to change was not about crisis, but rather about choice. They simply were no longer willing to exist in the old way. They reflected the old aphorism from Alcoholics Anonymous (AA) of "being sick and tired of being sick and tired" and became willing to go to any lengths to get better.

Shock Stage (First 6 to 8 Months) Once they admit the problem, addicts enter a stage that parallels what happens to anyone who has experienced deep loss and change. Disbelief and numbness alternate with anger and feelings of separation. Addicts describe physical symptoms of withdrawal that are, at times, agonizing. They also report disorientation, confusion, numbness, and inability to focus or to concentrate. Feelings of hopelessness and despair become more intense as their sense of reality grows. Sexual addicts become reactive to limits set by therapists, sponsors, or family members. When they join a recovery group, they experience a sense of belonging and a realization that recovery was the right decision for them. The time-honored 12-step wisdom, distilled in slogans such as "keep it simple" and "one day at a time," appears to be appropriate at this point. They report feelings of relief and acceptance once the double life is over.

Grief Stage (Second 6 Months of First Year) As they emerge further from their shock, patients become aware of emotional pain. Their suffering has several components. First, there is awareness of all the losses caused by their sexual addiction, including jobs, relationships, children, time, money, and physical well-being. Second, there is a sense of loss as the sexual addiction ceases to serve as friend, comforter, and emotional high. Third, the sexual addiction has masked deeper hurts, usually stemming from early childhood abuse or neglect. Without the cover of the addictive process, memories return, and clarity about those early wounds emerges. Understanding the level of suffering at this point helps explain why the relapse rate was so high during this time period in this study.

Repair Stage (18 to 36 Months) Sexual addicts who successfully negotiated the rigors of the previous stage move from pain into a deep, internal restructuring. Belief systems about self, sex, family, and values are overhauled. New patterns of behavior develop. Systems theory would describe this stage as a *paradigm shift*. It is a second-order change in which the programming or internal rules are different, whereas first-order change is characterized by using old solutions with greater energy (trying harder). However, when the paradigm changed, improvements were dramatic. It was noted that sexual addicts took responsibility for themselves in all areas of life, including career, finances, and health. They reported a new ability to express their needs

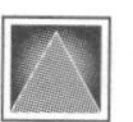

Table 18.4–4
Treatment Choices of 190 Persons Asked to Note the Helpfulness of Various Treatment Options

Type of Treatment	Helpful (%)	Not Helpful (%)
Inpatient	35	2
Outpatient group	27	7
After care (hospital)	9	5
Individual therapy	65	12
Family therapy	11	3
Couples therapy	21	11
Twelve-step group (for sexual addiction)	85	4
Twelve-step group (other)	55	8
Sponsor	61	6
Partner support	36	6
Higher power	87	3
Friends' support	69	4
Celibacy period	64	10
Exercise and nutrition	58	4

Courtesy of P. J. Carnes, Ph.D.

and to work to meet them. A common thread in this study was the deepening of new bonds with others. Sexual addicts also reported efforts to complete projects (e.g., degrees, projects, and work) and to be dependable (e.g., being on time, following through, and responding to requests).

Growth Stage (2 Years Plus) As sexually compulsive persons achieve more balance in their lives and develop a greater sense of themselves, they become more available to others. Relationships with partners, friends, children, and family go through a period of renewal. Here, too, is where life-satisfaction measures showed improvement in the study. Sexual addicts reported expressing more compassion for themselves and others. They developed a new trust for their own boundaries and integrity in relationships.

Treatment and Support Options

Participants in the study who had achieved a significant amount of time in recovery (N = 190) were presented with a list of treatment and support resources and asked to indicate whether they had used them and if they were helpful. The participants were also asked to indicate anything else that they had tried and whether that, too, was useful. Table 18.4–4 summarizes the results of this portion of the survey. A number of factors stood out as being helpful in recovery, including the following:

- Inpatient treatment
- Group treatment
- Long-term individual therapy
- Participation in 12-step programs
- An active and knowledgeable sponsor
- An ongoing spiritual life
- The support of friends
- A period of celibacy
- Regular exercise and balanced nutrition

The results indicate that recovery is a long-term process. Brief interventions, including therapy, medication, or limited hospital stays, did not produce the desired results. Because compulsive sexual behavior often results from a combination of powerful family forces, neurochemical interactions, and early childhood trauma, there is no quick fix. In addition, it became clear that success was dependent on patient follow-through. If the patient did not follow the treatment plan, success was marginal. This changes perceptions about measuring outcomes. For example, completing steps 1 through 3 of a 12-step program at an inpatient facility but never actively completing further steps or attending further therapy lessens the chance of success, no matter how effective the program. Similarly, individual therapy without the support of the patient's partner or a 12-step fellowship significantly reduces desired outcomes.

Diagnosis and Treatment Path

Figure 18.4–1 provides a schematic overview of the diagnosis and treatment path involved in therapy with the sexually compulsive or addictive patient. When the patient presents sexual issues involving a loss of impulse control, the physician conducts an in-depth sexual history. If the situation has escalated to the point at which the family, the employer, or the legal system is involved, all the data should be gathered. To rely on the patient alone with respect to these sensitive issues does not help because of characteristic denial. Interviewing family members or obtaining copies of lawsuits, legal charges, or company complaints is vital. Comparing what the clinician learns with the patient's version is often the beginning of therapy. The physician needs to confront the patient about discrepancies, so that a clear picture emerges.

The physician then must decide whether the sexually excessive behavior is situational or part of a pattern. If situational, then the focus is on the patient's response to the situation. If it is a pattern, there is a repetitive set of recursive sexual events in which there is significant loss of control. This pattern may be punctuated with periods of sexual aversion followed by bingeing. The physician then must make the decision that the behavior is about compulsivity and not other mental health issues. Sexual impulsivity may be found with bipolar or borderline conditions, as well as with alcohol and drug abuse. Therefore, it is important to rule out other mental disorders that would explain the behavior. If the behavior fits the criteria for sexual addiction and compulsion, including the essential elements of repetition and the inability to control one's behavior despite causing significant life problems, a compulsive pattern exists.

The next decision is the level of intervention. Some patients are appropriate for inpatient settings, particularly if they are suicidal or are at significant risk to themselves or others. Failure at an outpatient level may also indicate the need for hospitalization. A patient who continues high-risk, life-threatening sexual practices despite all outpatient efforts is a candidate for inpatient treatment. Signs of a good prognosis on an outpatient basis are a significant commitment to therapy; an involved, intact, supportive family; and significant periods of time in which the patient is able to abstain from self-destructive behavior.

Three Phases of Treatment

Treatment can be divided into three phases, whether it is outpatient or inpatient (Table 18.4–5). The first phase is about intervening in the cyclical compulsive process. The physician must extend the patient's sexual history to include all aspects of the problematic behavior. This survey is important, because it gives the patient and the physician an awareness of the extent of the problem. The physician's inquiry helps the patient understand the severity of the problem, and the physician most likely may be less surprised by unpleasant disclosure that occurs later in therapy; however, sometimes surprises happen regardless of what preventative measures are taken.

During the initial phase of treatment, therapy focuses on teaching the patient about the illness. In addition to coaching from the therapist, the patient must read and learn about the problem. The next section provides a list of resources from which patients can obtain such infor-

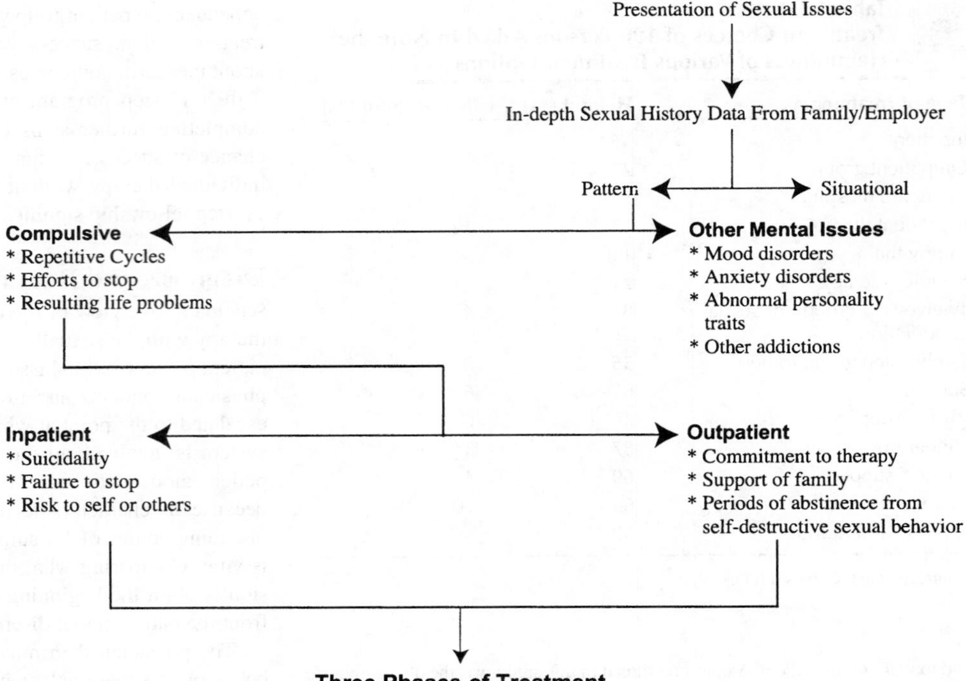

FIGURE 18.4–1 Diagnosis and treatment pattern for compulsive sexual behavior.

mation. The initial phase of treatment is also the time to refer the patient to a local 12-step group for sex addiction or sexual compulsion. As the patient starts to trust the therapist and becomes more familiar with the disorder, it is time to start confronting areas of significant denial in the patient. The best place to start is with the most obvious and the most dangerous areas. Clearly self-destructive behaviors, such as exhibitionism in a shopping mall, unprotected sex with prostitutes, or sex with dangerous persons, have to stop. At this point, the therapist develops a behavioral contract with the patient about behaviors from which the patient will abstain while in therapy. For example, if exhibitionism in a shopping center is a problem, or if compulsive use of prostitutes occurs in a certain area of town, the patient agrees not only to refrain from these behaviors, but also to avoid going to these areas alone. The patient also agrees to report any problems.

Once this foundation is in place, the second phase of treatment can begin. The following strategies are typically used at this time (during the first 4 to 8 weeks of treatment) for inpatient or outpatient treatment:

- *Completion of the first step.* The 12-step program starts with a first step in which patients acknowledge problems that, on their own, they have been unable to stop. Inventories of efforts to stop and consequences of sexual behavior are used to break through denial. This step is presented in the support group and in therapy.
- *Written abstinence statement.* This is a carefully scrutinized list with three parts: (1) the destructive behaviors from which the patient agrees to abstain, (2) the boundaries needed to avoid those behaviors, and (3) a full statement of the positive sexual behaviors that the patient wishes to cultivate. All of these are carefully reviewed in therapy and in the support groups.
- *Relapse prevention plan.* With the therapist's help, the patient prepares a comprehensive plan to prevent relapse, including understanding triggers (specific items or events that activate patient's rituals and addiction obsession) and precipitating situations (e.g., extreme stress or a fight with spouse) that are not directly related to sex, as well as performing addiction fire drills (i.e., automatic responses to prevent relapse).
- *Celibacy period.* The patient is asked to make a commitment to celibacy, which includes masturbation, for 8 to 12 weeks. If the person is part of a couple, his or her partner must also commit to this process. This period is designed to reduce sexual chaos and to teach how sex has been used as a

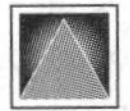

Table 18.4–5
Three Phases of Treatment

Phase I: Intervention
Survey extent of problematic behavior
Teach about illness
Referral to 12-step program
Confront denial
Agree on behavior contract
Phase II: Initial treatment
Twelve-step program attendance
Complete first step of 12-step process
Agree on writing an abstinence definition
Written relapse prevention plan
Complete a period of celibacy
Develop a sex plan
Partner and family involvement
Multiple addiction assessment
Trauma assessment
Group therapy
Shame reduction
Phase III: Extended therapy
Complete steps 2–4 of 12-step process
Developmental issues
Family-of-origin issues
Grief resolution
Marital and family therapy
Career issues
Trauma therapy

coping mechanism. It also creates a window in which patient and partner can explore conceptually what constitutes sexual health. Often, during this period, the patient experiences memories of early childhood sexual and physical abuse.

- *Sex plan*. At the conclusion of the celibacy period, the therapist and patient create a sex plan, which further articulates the difference between destructive and healthy sexuality.
- *Partner and family involvement*. Partners and family members go through therapy about the impact of the behavior. This is to further confront denial, but also to help those close to the patient engage in therapy for themselves.
- *Multiple addiction assessment*. Addictions and compulsions work together in various ways. The therapist helps the patient see that addictions, compulsions, and deprivations are all part of the repetitive pattern. The relapse prevention plan and sex plan are adjusted accordingly.
- *Trauma assessment*. A complete assessment of abuse and assault is done by the physician. This assessment helps clarify the goals of long-term therapy. For many patients whose behavior stems from early abuse, this becomes the key to understanding their behavior as the acting out of a scenario and provides important psychological distance from the addictive pattern.
- *Group therapy*. Patients participate in an ongoing group. Optimally, this would be a group whose members share the same issues, but follow-up studies have indicated that any ongoing group makes a substantial difference.
- *Shame reduction*. The therapist works with the patient in using various strategies to reduce sexual shame and shame about past behavior.

Once a period of relapse-free behavior has taken place, the third phase of treatment may begin. This phase focuses on underlying developmental issues and family-of-origin issues (as they are reflected in the patient's sexual acting out). If substantial abuse is part of the picture, therapy to deescalate reactivity and to defuse sexual triggers to inappropriate behavior is required. Furthermore, physicians find substantial amounts of unresolved grief, which requires attention. As noted previously, sometimes grief leads to slips into old behavior patterns. Unattended grief can precipitate total relapse. During this period, the patient must continue working the steps of the 12-step program. In an unpublished outcome study, Carnes and colleagues found that only 23 percent of patients actually completed steps 1 through 9 of the 12 steps in 18 months. Among these patients, relapse was rare.

Many patients' careers have been adversely affected by their behavior. As previously noted, some may never return to the career for which they were trained. This becomes an issue that must also be dealt with therapeutically. Similarly, marriage partners and family members require extended therapy to overcome feelings of betrayal and loss, as well as to understand the role of family dysfunction in the compulsive cycles. Helping professions, including physicians and clergy, also require special intervention and monitoring.

Finally, if the behavior involved criminal sexual misconduct and was part of a compulsive pattern, treatment time is usually extended dramatically. In part, this is usually a developmental issue requiring other therapeutic components, which promote victim empathy and accountability.

SUGGESTED CROSS-REFERENCES

Normal human sexuality and sexual dysfunctions are discussed in Sections 18.1a and 18.2. Substance-related disorders are discussed in Chapter 11, and mood disorders are discussed in Chapter 13.

REFERENCES

Black DW, Kehrberg L, Flumerfelt D, Schlosser S: Characteristics of 36 subjects reporting compulsive sexual behavior. *Am J Psychiatry.* 1997;154:243.

Blanchard G: Differential diagnosis of sex offenders: Distinguishing characteristics of the sex addict. *Am J Prevent Psychol Neurol.* 1991;2:45.

*Carnes PJ. *Contrary To Love: Helping the Sexual Addict.* Center City, MN: Hazelden Educational Materials; 1989.

*Carnes PJ. *Don't Call It Love.* New York: Bantam Books; 1991.

Carnes PJ: Addiction or compulsion: politics or illness? *Sex Addict Compuls J Treat Prevent.* 1996;3:127.

Carnes PJ: Sexual addiction and compulsion: Treatment and recovery. *CNS Spectrums.* 2000;5:53.

*Carnes PJ, Adams K. *Clinical Management of Sex Addiction.* New York: Brunner-Rutledge; 2002.

Carnes PJ, Murray R, Charpantier L. Addiction interaction disorder. In: Combs RH, ed. *Handbook of Addictive Disorders: A Practical Guide to Diagnosis and Treatment.* Hoboken, NJ: John Wiley & Sons, Inc.; 2004:31.

Carnes PJ, Nonemaker D, Skilling N: Gender difference in normal and sexually addicted populations. *Am J Prevent Psychiatry Neurol.* 1991;3:16.

Coleman E, Raymond N, McBean A: Assessment and treatment of compulsive sexual behavior. *Minn Med.* 2003;86:42.

Comings DE, Blum K: Reward deficiency syndrome: Genetic aspects of behavioral disorders. *Prog Brain Res.* 2000;126:325.

Cooper AL, Putnam D, Planchon LA, Boies SC: Online sexual compulsivity: Getting tangled in the net. *Sex Addict Compuls J Treat Prevent.* 1999;6:79.

*Earle MR, Earle RH, Osborn K. *Sex Addiction: Case Studies and Management.* New York: Brunner/Mazel Publishers; 1995.

Evans K, Sullivan J. *Treating Addicted Survivors of Trauma.* New York: Gilford Press; 1995.

Fossom MA, Mason M. *Facing Shame: Families in Recovery.* New York: Norton; 1986.

Gannon ML: Physical complications of sexual addiction. *Am J Prevent Psychiatry Neurol.* 1990;2:19.

*Goodman A. *Sexual Addiction: An Integrated Approach.* Madison, CT: International Universities Press; 1998.

Gordon LJ, Fargason P, Kramer J: Sexual behaviors of patients in a residential chemical dependency program: Comparison of sexually compulsive physicians and nonphysicians. *Sex Addict Compuls J Treat Prevent.* 1995;2:233.

Griffin-Shelly E, Benjamin L, Benjamin R: Sex addiction and dissociation. *Sex Addict Compuls J Treat Prevent.* 1995;2:295.

Hollander E, Wong C: Body dysmorphic disorder, pathological gambling, and sexual compulsion. *J Clin Psychiatry.* 1995;6:10.

Kafka MP: The monoamine hypothesis for the pathophysiology of paraphilic disorders: An update. *Ann N Y Acad Sci.* 2003;989:86.

Kafka MP: Sex offending and sexual appetite: The clinical and theoretical relevance of hypersexual desire. *Int J Offender Ther Comp Criminol.* 2003;47:439.

Kafka MP, Hennen J: Hypersexual desire in males: Are males with paraphilias different from males with paraphilia-related disorders? *Sex Abuse.* 2003;15:307.

Leshner A: Science-based views of drug addiction and its treatment. *JAMA.* 1999;282:1314.

Money J. *Lovemaps.* New York: Irvington; 1985.

Nestler EJ: Psychogenomics: Opportunities for understanding addiction. *J Neurosci.* 2001;21:8324.

Nestler EJ, Malenka RC: The addicted brain. *Sci Am.* 2004;290:78.

Raymond NC, Coleman E, Miner MH: Psychiatric comorbidity and compulsive/impulsive traits in compulsive sexual behavior. *Compr Psychiatry.* 2003;44:370.

Schneider JP, Irons RR: Differential diagnosis of addictive sexual disorders using the DSM-IV. *Sex Addict Compuls J Treat Prevent.* 1996;3:7.

Schwartz MF: Reenactments related to bonding and hypersexuality. *Sex Addict Compuls J Treat Prevent.* 1996;3:195.

Schwartz MF: Reenactments, trauma, and compulsive behavior. *Sex Addict Compuls J Treat Prevent.* 1996;3:195.

Sealy J: Psychopharmacologic intervention in addictive sexual behavior. *Sex Addict Compuls J Treat Prevent.* 1995;2:257.

van der Kolk B: The trauma spectrum: The interaction of biological and social events in the genesis of the trauma response. *J Trauma Stress.* 1988;1:273–290.

Wang GJ, Volkow ND: Brain dopamine and obesity. *Lancet.* 2001;357:354.

Washton A: Cocaine may trigger sexual compulsivity. *U S J Drug Alcohol Depend.* 1989;13:8.

Washton A: Cruising and using: Compulsive sex and substance abuse. *Professional Counselor.* 1998;13:6.

Wines D: Exploring the applicability of criteria for substance dependence to sexual addiction. *Sex Addict Compuls J Treat Prevent.* 1997;4:195.

Yehuda R, ed. *Treating Trauma Survivors with PTSD.* Washington, DC: American Psychiatric Publications; 2002.

19 Eating Disorders

Arnold E. Andersen, M.D, and Joel Yager, M.D.

Eating disorders are disorders of eating behavior deriving primarily from an overvaluation of the desirability of weight loss that result in functional medical, psychological, and social impairment. These disorders represent dysfunctional, emotional, cognitive, and behavioral strategies for coping with issues in development, mood disturbances, interpersonal relationships, and intrapsychic conflicts, becoming self-sustaining illnesses, usually in the context of overvalued beliefs internalized from sociocultural norms promoting the benefits of thinness or shape change. Despite their often innocuous, culturally syntonic origins, eating disorders have undoubtedly been present in various forms for thousands of years, but their prevalence has increased substantially since the 1950s. They now present as common serious clinical syndromes. Eating disorders have some of the highest rates of premature mortality in psychiatry—up to 19 percent within 20 years of onset among those initially requiring hospitalization. The syndrome bulimia nervosa was first described as part of the eating disorders spectrum only in 1979, but hindsight suggests it has been present as long as anorexia nervosa, often occurring below the level of common recognition because of the lack of visible starvation. The official recognition of binge-eating disorder is even more recent, although forms of compulsive overeating have been recognized throughout history.

A few principles concerning eating disorders will guide the discussion. First, eating disorders are syndromes, clusters of symptoms that have a fairly predictable course and sometimes well-established treatments, but they are not understood at the fundamental level of a specific proven etiology. Second, as with some other psychiatric disorders, diagnosing eating disorders involves imposing categorical limits on what are dimensional features, such as degrees of weight loss and attitudes toward weight and shape. Although eating disorders as formally defined by the revised fourth edition of the *Diagnostic and Statistical Manual of Mental Disorders* (DSM-IV-TR) afflict approximately 3 to 5 percent of the female population and approximately one-third as many men, subsyndromal forms of eating disorders are widely present and cause great distress, especially in the quality of life of adolescents who struggle to achieve the widespread overvalued norm for thinness in women and lean muscularity in men. Furthermore, eating disorders are culture-bound disorders with varying prevalence according to social norms in different cultures and countries—a vastly different situation from schizophrenia or manic-depressive illness, whose rates of prevalence are essentially uniform around the world. Third, eating disorders rarely present as sole diagnostic entities; they are almost always accompanied by significant comorbid disorders on Axis I and Axis II.

Clinicians have made rapid progress in earlier recognition of eating disorders, and several evidence-based treatments have been validated. Families, teachers, athletic and dance coaches, and clinicians are all more aware of these disorders than they were before the early 1980s when anorexia nervosa first became a media topic, and the syndrome of bulimia nervosa was just becoming widely publicized. Before this time, anorexia nervosa, especially, was considered a rare and obscure disorder, at times dismissed as a willful and voluntary fad, afflicting upper-class white girls. Anorexia nervosa before 1980 was only slowly recognized, if at all, usually after extensive "rule-out" medical investigations. The death of the singer Karen Carpenter in 1983 represents a watershed in public awareness, as her death from anorexia nervosa engraved on public consciousness the presence and seriousness of the disorder.

DEFINITIONS

The two major categories of eating disorders are anorexia nervosa and bulimia nervosa, but partial and subclinical syndromes abound, and transitions from one to another form of these disorders—for example, from anorexia nervosa to bulimia nervosa, or full syndromes to subclinical syndromes—is common.

The term *anorexia nervosa* is derived from the Greek term for "loss of appetite" and a Latin word implying nervous origin. The words used to label anorexia nervosa, and eating disorders in general, vary greatly from language to language, with rich implications. The German term for anorexia nervosa, *pubertetsmaigresucht* (thinness seeking of adolescents), captures only a portion of the disorder but, in some ways, is a clearer term linguistically than anorexia nervosa, the term now embedded in the English language. The French have called anorexia nervosa *anorexie mentale* (mental anorexia) and *anorexie hysterique* (hysterical anorexia) and define eating disorders as "disorders of alimentation."

Anorexia nervosa is a syndrome characterized by three essential criteria. The first is a self-induced starvation to a significant degree—a *behavior*. The second is a relentless drive for thinness and/or a morbid fear of fatness—a *psychopathology*. (The essential psychopathology seems tightly linked to overvalued beliefs, primarily the overvaluation of thinness. The drive for thinness psychopathological motif has been emphasized more by Americans, beginning with Hilde Bruch, whereas the morbid fear of fatness, the phobic avoidance of normal weight, has been emphasized more by the British.) The third criterion is the presence of medical signs and symptoms resulting from starvation—a *physiological symptomatology*. (In the past, amenorrhea for three or more months consecutively was specifically required. A sounder approach is to document significant general medical symptomatology secondary to starvation rather than only reproductive hormone abnormality). Anorexia nervosa is often, but not always, associated with disturbances of body image, the perception that one is distressingly large despite obvious medical starvation. The distortion of body image is disturbing when present, but not pathognomic, invariable, or required for diagnosis. A more summary integrative transdiagnostic theme in all anorexia nervosa subtypes and subsyndromal variants is the highly disproportionate emphasis placed on thinness as a vital source, sometimes the only source, of self-esteem, with weight, and to a lesser degree, shape, becoming the overriding and consuming day-long preoccupation of thoughts, mood, and behaviors.

Two subtypes of anorexia nervosa exist with much overlap and frequent transitions between them, especially from the restricting subtype to the binge and/or purge subtype. In the classic historical form of anorexia nervosa, present in approximately 50 percent of cases, food intake is highly restricted (usually with attempts to consume fewer than 300 to 500 calories per day and no fat grams), and the patient may be relentlessly and compulsively overactive, with overuse athletic injuries. In the second subtype, binge and/or purge, patients alternate attempts at rigorous dieting with intermittent binge or purge episodes, with the binges, if present, being either subjective (more than the patient intended, or due to social pressure, but not enormous) or objective. Purging represents a secondary compensation for the unwanted calories, most often accomplished by self-induced vomiting, frequently by laxative abuse, less frequently by diuretics, and occasionally with emetics. Sometimes repetitive purging occurs without prior binge eating, after ingesting only relatively few calories.

The term *bulimia nervosa* derives from the terms for "ox-hunger" in Greek and "nervous involvement" in Latin. Bulimia nervosa represents in many ways a failed attempt at anorexia nervosa, sharing the goal of becoming very thin, but occurring in an individual less able to sustain prolonged semi-starvation or severe hunger as consistently as classic restricting anorexia nervosa patients. These eating binges provoke panic as individuals feel that their eating has been out of control. They experience significant panic-laden conflict between their physiologically driven eating behavior from hunger, on the one hand, and the deep-seated desire to be thin on the other hand, with the anxiety heightened by the pervasive morbid fear of fatness. The unwanted binges, creating psychological and physical distress, in turn lead to secondary attempts to avoid the feared weight gain by a variety of compensatory behaviors, such as purging or excessive exercise. Later, the binges tend to be more typically initiated by dysphoria and often become intractable at that point. Occasionally, a bulimia nervosa patient begins directly by purging, often after media information describes purging in detail, sometimes after inappropriate teaching efforts focusing on symptoms, or after receiving a "tip" from a friend suggesting that purging is a quick way to lose weight.

Binge episodes (defined as repeated episodes of overeating large quantities of food that is generally of dense caloric content rapidly and usually privately, leading to guilt, anxiety about becoming fat, low self-esteem, and frequently gastric distress) are behaviors shared among several eating disorder subtypes. Regular binge and/or purge episodes may occur with low body weight (in which case it is classified as a subtype of anorexia nervosa), in normal weight individuals (most typically bulimia nervosa), or in overweight persons as manifestations of binge-eating disorder (without any compensation). In bulimia nervosa, compensation for binge episodes is carried out most commonly by purging through self-induced vomiting or laxative abuse (approximately 80 percent of cases), but, in a second subtype of bulimia nervosa (20 percent), it is carried out by "other compensation"—usually intensified, even stricter dieting or heroic exercise or both.

Patients who binge eat but do not compensate in any way after binge eating are often medically overweight or obese, generally somewhat older (30s to 50s), and are as likely to be male as female. These patients meet criteria for binge-eating disorder, an eating disorder subtype currently considered a research diagnosis within "atypical" eating disorders not otherwise specified, a category more logically constituting a third subtype of bulimia nervosa, not a residual or "atypical" category. In general, patients presenting with bulimia nervosa for specialized treatment differ from those untreated in the community, where rates of nonpurging syndromes equal those of the purging forms.

The term *binge*, essential for the diagnosis of binge-eating syndromes, presents challenges in definition, although these may be more pertinent for research purposes than for actual clinical practice. The exact distinction between a *subjective binge* (eating more than one ostensibly desires or physiologically requires, even if a small amount) and an *objective binge* (eating what anyone would consider to be abnormally large amounts [often 2,000 to 5,000 calories] of food that is usually sweet and high in fat; food is eaten quickly to the point of medical and/or psychological distress, often in private, and is most times associated with secrecy or shame) is undecided, as they blend into each other.

Subsyndromal eating disorders and variants that lack some required diagnostic feature of the current criteria are considered to belong to the category of *eating disorder not otherwise specified.* This category is overly large, often representing 30 to 50 percent of admissions to experienced eating disorder programs. Patients with eating disorder not otherwise specified are no less ill and no less responsive to treatment than those with anorexia or bulimia nervosa, but the category is confusing in its terminology and implication. Currently, approximately 80 percent of patients with eating disorder not otherwise specified would fit into a slightly revised, more evidence-based scientific approach to diagnosis of anorexia nervosa, primarily, and bulimia nervosa to a lesser extent.

Understanding definitions of eating disorders requires appreciating the concept of overvalued beliefs. Although many clinicians alternately view the psychopathology underlying the abnormal eating of eating-disordered patients as being either obsessive-compulsive in nature or deriving from delusional beliefs, neither concept adequately captures or represents the characteristic and essential psychopathology seen most commonly in eating disorders. Overvalued beliefs, which are behind most acts of world terrorism, are also the driving force behind most eating disorders. *Overvalued beliefs* are defined as culturally normative beliefs that have been assigned disproportionate and ruling passion in an individual's life and come to dominate that individual's thinking, emotions, and behaviors. The behaviors resulting from these overvalued beliefs are, at their extremes, risky and life threatening, whether the behaviors are dangerous to the individual (anorexia nervosa) or to others (terrorism). These beliefs are not fixed and false, as are beliefs found in delusions, nor are they ego-dystonic thoughts or behaviors as required for a diagnosis of obsessive-compulsive disorder (OCD). Thinking about losing weight is culturally normative in American society. However, regulating one's every waking moment and mood around the overriding importance of slimness and how to achieve it represents a psychopathological category best described as an overvalued belief. Understanding the nature and definition of overvalued beliefs seems essential for treating eating disorders in a comprehensive and enduring manner.

Using this functional definition of eating disorders—abnormalities of eating behavior driven by overvalued beliefs that lead to medical, social, and psychological consequences—eating disorders have a long history. The Roman practice of gorging and vomiting in "purgatoriums" at fancy dinners was not an eating disorder, but simply culturally condoned gluttony. Closer to real eating disorders were the fasting practices of the Gnostic sect of Christian men in the fourth century who self-starved because of the belief that material objects, including food, were evil. In the practice of their asceticism, they spent years on top of pillars in the desert consuming very little food, to the point of severe self-starvation. During the Middle Ages, women were generally treated as second-class citizens, with the exception of those demonstrating exceptional holiness. Female holiness in that era was most commonly manifest by denial of the body through chastity, self-denial, and, especially, fasting to the point of emaciation. In these instances, the patterns of restrictive eating became self-sustaining and ego-syntonic, immune to pleas or threats to change from those around, forming the core of lifelong identities, even if life was shortened by these acts.

Reasonable attempts to assign eating disorder diagnoses through biographical analysis to historical figures such as Lord Byron are interesting exercises, but these diagnoses are distinctly less secure than those based on early medical reports of specific cases. Richard Morton, physician to the court of England, described two cases in 1689—a boy and a girl—that conformed reasonably well to current diagnostic criteria for anorexia nervosa. These two patients were young people with "cares of the mind" who took to fasting and were noted to suffer emaciation without medical causation.

Although more contemporary medical identification of anorexia nervosa was hinted at in several reports from physicians in the early 1800s, it was most clearly described, almost at the same time, by Sir William Gull in London and Dr. Charles Lasègue in France in the 1860s and 1870s. Both physicians described cases of self-starvation, primarily in upper-class young girls, but "occasionally seen . . . in males at the same age," "distinguishing them clearly from cases with medical causation." Sir William described anorexia nervosa with the clarity possible only in an era in which treatments were less available and time for clinical observation was greater. In his words, "The want of appetite is, I believe, due to a morbid mental state." He prescribed "food. . . administered at intervals varying inversely with the exhaustion and emaciation. The inclination of the patient must be in no way consulted. The patient should be fed at regular intervals and surrounded by persons who would have moral [i.e. psychological] control over them, relations and friends being generally the worst attendants." The keen observation may still be applicable in certain instances.

Lasègue captured the dilemma of a family of anorexics, noting that the patient was not responsive to either "entreaties or menaces," sound counsel to contemporary families and physicians. The social isolation of these patients was captured as well: "the circle within which revolved the ideas and sentiments of the patient become more narrowed . . . what dominates in the mental condition is . . . almost a condition of contentment truly pathological . . . she is not ill-pleased with her condition." He anticipated the future warning of Hilde Bruch to avoid letting patients quickly "eat their way out of hospital" by cautioning that "as a general rule we must look forward to a change for the better only taking place slowly."

In the late 1800s, anorexia nervosa was temporarily confused with postpartum pituitary necrosis, leaving a lasting, even if disproved, assumption that some primary abnormality of endocrine function was implicated in the origin of anorexia nervosa.

Early in the 20th century, the pendulum of etiological assumptions swung toward early, primitive psychoanalytic hypotheses, leading to searches for psychoanalytic themes, such as "fear of oral impregnation," and then to attempts to work through these sexual conflicts with psychoanalytic methods. A much more contemporary, psychodynamically oriented approach was initially formulated by Hilde Bruch in the 1950s. In the 1960s, the modem era of phenomenological description and pragmatic treatment of anorexia nervosa relatively free of theoretical bias was initiated in England by Gerald Russell, Arthur Crisp, Pierre Beumont, and others.

Russell described bulimia nervosa in 1979, using the term *nervosa* to unite the two forms of the eating disorders spectrum—the self-starving syndrome of anorexia nervosa and the newly recognized binge–purge disorder—psychopathologically. Bulimia nervosa was initially described as "an ominous variant of anorexia nervosa," but later descriptions incorporated the syndrome of bulimia nervosa at normal weight.

The recognition of bulimia nervosa was hidden for a number of reasons, including the shame and secrecy of sufferers, who were reluctant to reveal these symptoms even while being treated for other related comorbid disorders, such as depression; the seemingly normal weight of most bulimic patients; and the lack of requests for help. The "night-eating binge syndrome," characterized by often unremembered binge eating while still in some stage of sleep, is even more difficult to diagnose, but increasingly is recognized as a true variant. Despite the relatively recent formal description of bulimia nervosa, evidence-based treatment strategies have emerged quickly and have proven more effective than those for anorexia nervosa.

The recent history of eating disorders has focused on several areas, including (1) better delineation of the noncompensating binge-eating disorder, (2) clearer descriptions of the prevalence and syndrome characteristics of eating disorders in men, and (3) studies recognizing the contributions of genetic and other predisposing neurobiological factors interacting with sociocultural norms. Only recently has there been recognition that the overvalued beliefs driving men with eating disorders may vary considerably from those driving women. It is almost entirely in men that a still-evolving diagnostic subtype—a mirror image of anorexia nervosa called *reverse anorexia nervosa*—is found, characterized by the distorted perception that one is too thin, too small, and not muscular enough despite even heroic and outwardly successful efforts at muscular development.

Historical trends in food availability have shifted significantly. In the 18th and 19th centuries, food was readily available only to the prosperous. In general, there was less social pressure for extreme thinness, except in upper-class families in which women corseted themselves mercilessly to achieve impossibly thin waists. By the late 20th century, fatty, palatable foods were available to most populations in Western countries, and, paradoxically, high-fat foods became particularly cheap and available for many low-income populations. Obesity has become much more prominent among all social classes, particularly poorer populations. Concurrently, pressures to be thin, weight control efforts, and eating disorders as clinical problems have become increasingly associated with affluent societies. It has been hypothesized that there has always been a small number of cases of anorexia nervosa that are primarily genetic in origin, and this core group has been augmented substantially by the influence of sociocultural norms that mandate thinness, resulting in the current prevalence of anorexia nervosa, which represents a blend of genetic and sociocultural factors.

NOSOLOGY

Nosology, the art and science of classification, remains challenging in eating disorders for several reasons. Eating disorders are, first of all, culture-bound disorders occurring primarily within cultures that promote specific norms for body weight and shape. Their core features are somewhat uniform across cultures, but, unlike schizophrenia, their prevalence varies widely across cultures. Second, eating disorders are best described as syndromes, not as more fundamentally understood diseases with proven etiologies and mechanisms. Questions regarding the etiology and pathophysiological mechanisms of eating disorders are still hotly debated without clear agreement as to the relative contributions of psychosocial and biomedical factors. In general, a multifactorial causation is accepted.

Complexities in classification of eating disorders can be appreciated by recognizing the different names used for anorexia nervosa in different languages and over time. Although the term *anorexia nervosa* derives from Sir William Gull's presentation to the clinical society of London in 1873, this appellation represents only one attempt at capturing the nature of the disorder by a name suggesting an etiology. Many countries now use the term *anorexia nervosa* but, for the essential meaning of the disorder, they rely on the prevailing criteria listed in either DSM-IV-TR or the tenth revision of the *International Statistical Classification of Diseases and Related Health Problems* (ICD-10).

Although labeling the self-starving form as anorexia nervosa is, for now, a *fait accompli*, the propriety of this term is in question, as the disorder does not result from true "anorexia," or loss of appetite, especially at the onset, in contrast to the anorexia of cancer or acquired immune deficiency syndrome (AIDS). No abnormality of brain mechanism mediates any initial loss of appetite, starting the process leading to the full syndrome of anorexia nervosa; appetite loss occurs only in the severe state of emaciation, sustained perhaps by ketosis, but the degree of medical anorexia is quite variable. The term *anorexia nervosa* is embedded in the English language, however, until there is consensus for a more useful descriptive English phrase. The term *bulimia nervosa* better captures the core behavioral feature of that syndrome. Even the location of eating disorders in the DSM-IV-TR has reflected changing views on classification. In third edition of the DSM (DSM-III) and the revised third edition of the DSM (DSM-III-R), eating disorders were classified under disorders of childhood or adolescence, perhaps, in part, contributing to previous underdiagnosis of later-onset cases. It was only in DSM-IV-TR that eating disorders were moved to a separate and independent section.

The case could be made that all subtypes of eating disorders could be most usefully regarded as part of an overarching unitary syndrome—simply, eating disorders—in view of the common natural history of transitions from one subtype of eating disorder to another. A transdiagnostic approach appreciates the shared underlying features of all eating disorders—an overvaluation of thinness or shape change, sustained abnormal eating behavior, and functional impairment medically, socially, and psychologically. A transdiagnostic approach also can shape an integrative treatment approach to all eating disorders, with layered additional specifics for each subtype. There is also merit, however, in retaining some identity among the several eating disorder variants based on differences in predisposition and clinical course. The "lumping" versus "splitting" approaches to the classification of eating disorders both have merits and drawbacks. Ultimately, a more scientific approach to classification must await more fundamental understanding of etiology and mechanism.

Previous efforts to classify eating disorders as subtypes of mood disorders have been found wanting because eating disorders "breed true," without evolving into mood disorders or other disorders. Attempts to understand eating disorders as primary forms of OCD have also faltered. They have resisted classification as psychotic disorders, despite hints at this etiology in earlier writings before more rigorous modern definitions of schizophrenia, such as the U.S.–U.K. study of schizophrenia. Although incompletely understood, eating disorders, as a unitary group or as separate subtypes, are clearly distinct psychiatric disorders not subsumed into any other psychiatric disorder.

EPIDEMIOLOGY

Epidemiology concerns the prevalence and incidence of a disorder, as well as the sum of factors associated with the onset and course of that disorder. The thorniest issues related to accurate epidemiology of eating disorders have been threefold: (1) the changing definition of what constitutes an eating disorder, (2) the previous presentation of eating disorders by their physical consequences in *forme frustes* as medical disorders, and (3) the lack of recognition by health professionals until fairly recently of even clear cases of eating disorders because of widespread lack of clear diagnostic criteria and reliable assessment methods, especially for the nonstereotypical cases in males, minorities, and matrons. The underlying issue for determining the epidemiology of eating disorders, as with a number of other disorders, is deciding where to draw the line separating the large majority of women and men who are merely dissatisfied with their weight and shape from those who have the full syndromes. Seventy percent of young women, by high-school age, not only desire thinness, but also practice dieting behavior. With young men, equal dissatisfaction with body size and shape reigns, but the desire to increase weight in the form of lean muscle mass matches the desire to lose weight. It is simply normative for most women, and increasingly for men, to at least give lip service to the need to lose weight.

Defining eating disorders epidemiologically involves problems similar to those that occur when defining hypertension, another disorder that involves using somewhat arbitrarily imposed categories—presumably built on statistical probabilities of current and future impairment and risk—to separate clinically significant cases from others. A helpful trend in general medicine has been to move from hypertensive versus not hypertensive or diabetic versus not diabetic cases to the spectrum of normal to prehypertensive to clear clinical hypertension. With these caveats and examples in mind, there is general consensus that approximately 1 percent of young women have classic anorexia nervosa and that 2 to 4 percent of young women meet criteria for bulimia nervosa as defined in DSM-IV-TR. The healthiest end of the spectrum is composed of individuals with normal eating and no preoccupation with weight or shape (approximately 15 percent; "normal controls" are difficult to find for research on eating behavior), and then there are those who are simply preoccupied with weight and body image (70 percent of the general population), and finally there are distinctly disordered individuals with partial or full eating disorders interfering with normal development or daily life. Approximately 20 percent of college women experience transient bulimic symptoms at some point during their college years, and approximately 5 percent have mild forms of anorexia nervosa. Likewise, approximately 17 percent of high school boy wrestlers meet short-term criteria for an eating disorder during their active sports season. Although the number of college students with eating disorders remains relatively constant, the specific individuals who have an eating disorder on admission to college are not always the individuals who have features of an eating disorder on graduation. Transient eating disorder symptoms are common.

The lifetime prevalence of individuals with an eating disorder is approximately three times that of current point prevalence. Much argument has taken place about whether eating disorders are increasing in incidence. The bulk of studies suggest a true increase in new cases, especially of bulimia nervosa, recognizing that the higher current prevalence rates probably represent a combination of actual new cases and better recognition of previously undiagnosed cases.

The largest background epidemiological factor predisposing to eating disorders is a culture that values slimness and, in the case of men, lean muscularity. This preoccupation can only take place in large numbers in a population when there is sufficient food to make obesity possible, and, concomitantly, when social norms stigmatize overweight individuals. There is little psychological purchase to be gained from self-starvation in a poor, developing country in which starvation is common. As a society becomes more prosperous, with increased availability of densely caloric foods (fats and sugar), and increasingly values slimness and lean muscularity, eating disorders increase in prevalence, starting with a few individuals who are perhaps genetically predisposed, such as appears to be the case in medieval days, and progressing to a much larger contemporary ill population who come to see dieting as a seemingly obligatory rite of passage to a state of thinness perceived to be mandatory for success or happiness.

Obesity is much more common in lower- than upper-socioeconomic classes in American society, and stigmatization of obesity is common, suggesting that, although anorexia nervosa is becoming more widely distributed among cultures and social classes, some women still see anorexia nervosa as a badge of upper-class status. However, this thesis does not hold for bulimia nervosa. Recent studies suggest that bulimic symptomatology is equally present in all socioeconomic classes.

Eating disorders are among the most gender-divergent disorders in psychiatry, but the divergence is substantially narrower than previously believed. Previous estimates of the ratio of men to women for eating disorders were typically 1 in 20 to 1 in 10. Excellent recent community-based epidemiological studies, however, found a ratio of two women to one man for the combination of full- and partial-syndrome anorexia nervosa, and a ratio of three to one for bulimia nervosa.

This study suggests that a large unidentified population of men with eating disorders exists in American society and that the gender ratios present in clinical settings do not reflect actual community prevalence. The trend for men during the 1970s to follow women in increasingly valuing slimness appears to have been reversed in the 1980s, perhaps because of the increasingly common media pictures of emaciated gay males with AIDS that began appearing in the media at that time. Since then, in both the gay and heterosexual male communities, there has been an increasing value placed on lean muscularity rather than on thinness alone, with the ideal in the gay community being more lean muscularity rather than the caricature of huge muscular development. Being a gay man is a documented risk factor for developing an eating disorder, but the mediating variable relates to the ideal body image of virtually impossible physical perfection, not the sexual orientation or behavior of the man. Recently, clinicians have come to recognize a still incompletely defined but clinically significant disorder, occurring primarily in men, that is in many ways the mirror image of typical anorexia nervosa, called *reverse anorexia*, *bigarexia* (linguistically ugly, albeit descriptive), *body dysmorphic disorder* (most common), or, most sensationally, *the Adonis complex*. In these disorders, which are often accompanied by steroid abuse, men perceive that they are still too small in size or too thin, despite huge objective muscle development. This variant of life-dominating body dysmorphic disorder is characterized by a desire for impossibly low body fat along with huge, clearly defined muscle mass.

Binge-eating disorder appears in approximately 25 percent of patients who seek medical care for obesity and in 50 to 75 percent of those with stage III obesity. It is in some ways the most subtle eating disorder and the latest to be described because of patients' lack of dramatic thinness or purging behavior, seemingly blending in with obesity that is erroneously, but commonly, attributed to lack of will. Although eating disorders have been described in patients ranging from prepubertal ages to those in the ninth decade of life, peak onsets most commonly occur in the early and late teens. Extremely early cases—in those younger than 5 to 7 years—almost certainly represent patterns of abnormal eating behaviors that differ from true anorexia nervosa and bulimia nervosa and are due to other causes, such as medical or neurological conditions. They may also represent childhood behavioral expressions of anger, defiance, and fear or may represent attempts to control family dynamics, such as occurs with breath holding. Sadly, some emaciated young children without obvious medical illness may suffer from parental deprivation of food (Munchausen syndrome by proxy). Lastly, finicky appetites can be taken too seriously by worried parents. Although worries about weight and shape, with resulting dieting behaviors, are being seen at earlier ages, true anorexia nervosa and, less commonly, bulimia nervosa, as defined here, do not occur below the age at which children can internalize fat phobias or overvalue social norms of slimness. A type of imitative eating disorder occurs in young children who behaviorally mirror abnormal eating behaviors seen in parents, such as stepping on a scale frequently or trying to induce vomiting after a meal.

A final epidemiological theme is that eating disorders are rarely seen as solitary psychiatric disorders. They are almost invariably associated with two to four additional comorbid diagnoses on Axis I and Axis II of DSM-IV-TR, especially mood, anxiety, obsessive-compulsive, body dysmorphic, and substance abuse disorders on Axis I and personality vulnerabilities and disorders on Axis II. Anorexia nervosa, restricting subtype, is usually associated with Cluster C personality disorder, whereas bulimia nervosa is more likely to occur with Cluster B traits or disorders. The probability of having some diagnosable personality disorder is significantly greater in individuals with eating disorders than it is in the general population. The course and prognosis of any given case is strongly influenced by these comorbid conditions, particularly the nature and intensity of any personality disorders or preexisting mood disorders, anxiety disorders, or OCDs.

Mood disorders are especially common in bulimia nervosa, with estimates of 50 to 70 percent comorbidity being typical. Causal relationships and interactions, including the possibility of some shared vulnerabilities between mood disorders and eating disorders, are complex and controversial. In approximately equal numbers does depression precede bulimia nervosa, bulimia nervosa precede depression, and the two conditions appear concomitantly. Classic studies have documented that emotional blunting, social isolation, and frank depression may result from severe weight loss alone. Table 19–1 summarizes some of the epidemiological factors related to eating disorders.

ETIOLOGY

Current etiological thinking about eating disorders involves several principles and an integrating paradigm. First, eating disorders are disorders of eating behavior. All other factors may be present (overvaluation of thinness, body image distortion), but, without abnormal eating, there is no diagnosable disorder. Eating disorders represent in some ways a "highjacking" of normal neurobiologically regulated eating behaviors, which become distorted and overridden until the abnormal eating pattern becomes autonomous, responding to the continued drive for thinness and the neurobiological fear conditioning about normal weight. Second, although the analogy may easily

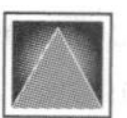

Table 19–1
Epidemiological Risk Factors Related to Eating Disorders

Cultural: Societal endorsement of weight loss and dieting

Gender: Women > men (2:1 to 3:1 in community; 10:1 to 20:1 in clinical series)

Age: Peaks occur at early and late teen years, but onset can be prepubertal through 8th decade.

Prevalence: Anorexia nervosa, approximately 1% of young women; bulimia nervosa, 2–4% of young women (full syndromes, DSM-IV-TR/ICD-10)

Family disorders: Eating disorders, affective disorders, obesity

Family patterns: Enmeshed or disengaged

Socioeconomic class: Anorexia, possibly ↑ with social class; bulimia, independent of social class

Personality role: ↑ probability of a personality disorder; anorexia, ↑ with Cluster C; bulimia, ↑ with Cluster B

Prior psychiatric disturbance: Childhood and early-adolescent anxiety, mood, and obsessive-compulsive disorders

Pubertal age: ↑ with early puberty, especially pubertal obesity, for girls

Monozygotic to dizygotic ratio: 3:1

Monozygotic twin concordance: ≥50%

Rural vs. urban: ↑ with move from rural to urban setting

Sexual orientation: ↑ with gay orientation; possibly ↓ with lesbian orientation

Medical comorbidity: Possible ↑ with type I diabetes mellitus (controversial)

Prior physical, emotional, or sexual abuse: Nonspecific ↑ in all psychiatric disorders, not specifically eating disorders

Premature mortality: 0–19% on 10- to 20-yr follow-up after hospitalization (medical causes, closely followed by suicide); anorexia nervosa plus insulin-dependent diabetes mellitus ↑ mortality 10 times either anorexia or diabetes alone

Vocational, avocational risks: Ballet, modeling, amateur wrestling, visual media roles, appearance sports (female gymnastics, figure skating), thinness sports (jockey, cross-country running, lightweight crew)

be overdone, similarities exist between eating disorders and drug abuse in that abnormal eating, whether self-starvation or binge–purge behaviors, produce significant immediate emotional changes that include initial relief of dysphoria and production of excitement but subsequently result in more dysphoria, a vicious circle. Third, although biological theories are popular and are being actively researched, no convincing evidence yet exists that eating disorders derive primarily from preillness structural or functional abnormalities of the brain; eating disorders, however, do result in profound consequences to the brain, not necessarily all fully reversible. The search for brain abnormalities as the cause of eating disorders is understandable but may prove too simplistic. A more complex, multifactorial etiological approach may better account for current data. Genetic contributions are certainly involved, estimated from 40 to 60 percent, but less so in a deterministic manner, as with Huntington's chorea or even bipolar disorder, and more likely in a contributory manner, by increasing the presence and strength of risk factors, such as persevering, sensitive, fearful, or impulsive personality traits, or through more easily disrupted regulation of serotoninergic mechanisms when dieting occurs.

Thus, eating disorders may presently be best conceptualized as probabilistic, as overdetermined disorders with multiple contributing causes, none of which—besides dieting behavior—is now known to be absolutely essential. The most compelling perspective is a recognition that eating disorders probably derive from a cluster of predisposing vulnerability factors (imagine kindling wood) reacting to precipitating events, especially those occurring during vulnerable "windows" in development (the match for the fire to start), and are maintained by sustaining social, psychological, and biomedical reinforcements (the wind, oxygen, and lack of rain that keep the fire burning).

VULNERABILITY: PREDISPOSING FACTORS

It is doubtful that individuals who are not predisposed with typical known risk factors can develop true sustained eating disorders, even with dieting behavior. For example, an extroverted young woman with an internal rather than external locus of control who grew up in a balanced, supportive family, who possesses high assertiveness, has a self-accepting body image, is average in weight, and has no family history of affective disorder or obesity is a doubtful candidate for an eating disorder, even if she practices brief dieting to meet job (e.g., modeling) or avocational (e.g., ballet) requirements.

Biological Vulnerability Biological theories of the etiology of eating disorders began hundreds of years ago and culminated in the late 1800s with the pronouncement that anorexia nervosa was caused by postpartum pituitary necrosis. Although this theory was soon disproved, a variety of subsequent theories have been advanced focusing on putative biological underpinnings—for example, the hypothesis that some predisposing hypothalamic abnormality exists, evidenced by amenorrhea. However, convincing studies have demonstrated in volunteers willing to starve themselves to 15 percent or more below their normal weights that virtually all the endocrine abnormalities characteristic of anorexia nervosa are absent before self-starvation, only appear as weight declines, and return to normal when weight is restored.

Several lines of evidence suggest genetic vulnerability, including high rates of familial transmission. Twin studies demonstrate a high concordance in monozygotic twins, approximately three times higher than in dizygotic twins, suggesting that both genetic and psychosocial contributions are operative. Monozygotic twins are documented to have a 50 to 80 percent concordance rate for eating disorders. Exactly what is being inherited remains controversial. Genetic factors definitely contribute, probably through multiple effects on temperament, cognitive style, personality, mood-regulating tendencies, set points for weight, and predispositions toward physical activity. Restricting-type anorexia nervosa, in contrast to bulimia nervosa, may require a specific genetic endowment of perseverance, sensitivity, perfectionism, and low impulsivity to allow development of sustained food restriction and maintenance of a severely starved state, impossible for most people who are offered options to eat. Impulsive and extroverted personality styles increase the probability of binge eating–purging dieting cycles. Personality, a highly heritable variable, plays a major role in the probability of developing any eating disorder and its specific subtype.

The identification of genetically derived animal models of anorexia nervosa is also intriguing. Take, for example, "thin sow" disease. During breeding experiments, hyperactive sows that starved themselves produced thinner overactive hogs. Active searches are under way to identify specific genes that may contribute to the development of animal models, including research on knock-out gene models, increasing or decreasing genes related to fear and avoidance. The complexity of the task of identifying specific genetic contributions to eating disorders is enormous. To date, more than 200 genes have been identified that contribute to eating, activity, and weight regulation alone in simple species, with new regulatory genes or gene interactions such as daf-2 constantly being described.

Contemporary theories have pointed to putative serotonin mechanisms, largely based on observations that individuals with anorexia nervosa have abnormal cerebrospinal fluid (CSF) serotonin levels when ill, levels that may not completely reverse on partial weight gain. To date, no firm data are available showing that serotonin abnormalities exist in vulnerable populations before the onset of an eating disorder. However, these hints have stimulated studies into the possibility that variations in genetically mediated serotonin regulation may be important predisposing factors, perhaps increasing vulnerability to stressful situations, a more indirect and interactive mechanism of diathesis interacting with events during vulnerable periods.

Although molecular genetic research of these disorders is in its infancy, promising areas for investigation have already pointed to the potential importance of serotonin mechanisms, among others. Genetically interesting loci and polymorphisms have been associated with genes for the 5-hydroxytryptamine type 1B (5-HT_{1B}), type 2A (5-HT_{2A}), and type 2C (5-HT_{2C}) receptors, uncoupling proteins 2 (UCP2) and 3 (UCP3), beta-type estrogen receptor, hSKCa3 potassium channel, and human agouti protein. To illustrate, a polymorphism in the coding region of the gene for the 5-HT_{2C} receptor subtype resulting in a cysteine to serine substitution has been reported in 23.7 percent of adolescent girls reporting weight loss compared to 7.7 percent of normal-weight girls. In studies of the human agouti-related protein gene (related to an orexigenic neuropeptide), two alleles have been found to be in complete linkage disequilibrium and are significantly enriched in anorectic patients (11 percent; $P = .015$) compared to controls (4.5 percent). Several large-scale linkage and association studies are under way. To date, areas of particular interest have been identified on at least chromosomes 1, 2, and 13. But, on the whole, the percentage of occurrence explained by these specific genetic associations is still quite small. Population studies suggest that genetic factors may, overall, contribute approximately 50 percent or more to the appearance of anorexia nervosa and bulimia nervosa.

Theories regarding potentially preexisting functional or structural brain dysfunctions have been proposed, but, as yet, no convincing preexisting abnormalities have been revealed or replicated. More research in this area can be expected with the availability of sophisticated imaging technology, with the goal of eventual prospective studies of the brain imaging and neurobiological functioning of individuals who later develop eating disorders.

The most notable biological vulnerability factors are those related to dieting and its attendant undernutrition. Dieting itself is a major stressor to the nervous system, one for which the typical individual is evolutionarily prepared with multiple mechanisms to defend life in the setting of famine, but it is nonetheless stressful in that it involves rearranging virtually every aspect of cognition and metabolism.

Temperament, Psychological, and Social Vulnerability Family transmission represents a major vulnerability factor for eating disorders, with a family history of eating disorders, affective spectrum disorders, anxiety disorders, OCDs, and obesity contributing approximately equally. Mood disorders are approximately four times more common in families of eating-disordered individuals than in the community at large. The exact mechanism by which this family history predisposes to eating disorders is unknown.

Mood and anxiety disorders and OCDs in childhood and the early appearance of perfectionistic personality traits appear to be major vulnerability factors for the development of eating disorders, especially anorexia nervosa. In young girls with shaky self-esteem, teasing by family or friends, or comments and directives from authority figures (doctors, nurses, teachers, coaches) regarding need to change weight and shape contribute to vulnerability. Not uncommonly, children are weighed in class or by a school nurse for no credible reason, with frequent long-term distress resulting. Overall, twin studies suggest that approximately 17 to 46 percent of the variance in both anorexia nervosa and bulimia nervosa can be accounted for by nonshared environmental factors.

Vocational and avocational interests interact with other vulnerability factors to increase the probability of developing eating disorders. In young women, participation in strict ballet schools increases the probability of developing anorexia nervosa at least sevenfold. In high school boys, wrestling is associated with a prevalence of full or partial eating-disordered syndromes during wrestling season of approximately 17 percent, with a minority developing an eating disorder and not improving spontaneously at the end of training. Although these athletic activities probably select for perfectionistic and persevering youth in the first place, pressures regarding weight and shape generated in these social milieus reinforce the likelihood that these predisposing factors will be channeled toward eating disorders.

The influence of family functioning style as a potential predisposing factor remains controversial. No single, specific family functioning style appears to be either a necessary or sufficient requirement for developing an eating disorder. As in most psychiatric disorders, various family dysfunctional styles appear to act as nonspecific vulnerability factors and also hamper recovery. Thankfully, routine blaming of families or the assumption that they are causative factors for an eating disorder in a child has receded along with the invidious concept of the "schizophrenogenic" mother or the autism-promoting parents. Given the presence of other vulnerability factors, enmeshed families that provide youth little room to individuate may be more likely to foster the emergence of adolescents with anorexia nervosa. So-called negative expressed emotion in families, in which blame and criticism are heaped on the patient by other family members, may add considerable nonspecific stresses to other vulnerabilities.

Trauma arising from childhood or adolescent physical, emotional, or sexual abuse clearly contributes to the likelihood that these abused individuals will later develop some psychiatric disorder, but not specifically an eating disorder. There is no evidence that sexual abuse alone is a major cause of bulimia nervosa. The unscientific practices of assuming that sexual abuse underlies bulimia nervosa and using "recovered memories" to support this theory have produced much suffering and malpractice. Of course, when present, a sexual abuse history requires thorough and sympathetic attention and decisions about "uncovering" versus "working through" techniques, often with expert guidance.

The extent to which media simply mirror society or play active roles in contributing to societal overvaluation of thinness and dieting and the increased prevalence of eating disorders remains controversial. Recent studies from Fiji suggest that the introduction of popular television programs highlighting slimness and stigmatizing obesity launched widespread dieting behavior and new eating-disordered cases in populations that were previously unconcerned with these issues.

Racial and ethnic factors per se offer no protection or predisposition to eating disorders. The only vulnerability conferred by specific racial or ethnic groups is related to the degree to which those groups promote weight loss or shape change. A gay orientation in men is a proven predisposing factor, not because of sexual orientation or sexual behavior per se, but because norms for slimness, albeit muscular slimness, are very strong in the gay community, only slightly lower than for heterosexual women. In contrast, a lesbian orientation may be slightly protective, as lesbian communities may be more tolerant of higher weights and a more normative natural distribution of body shapes than their heterosexual female counterparts.

The potential contribution of insulin-dependent diabetes as a predisposing factor to eating disorders remains uncertain. The largest studies suggest no actual increase in eating disorders in young individuals with type I diabetes, but data are controversial, and the presence of insulin-dependent diabetes mellitus in a patient with anorexia nervosa may disguise the eating disorder, and it certainly complexifies treatment.

PRECIPITATING FACTORS

Although no single predisposing factor is necessary or sufficient by itself to lead to an eating disorder, the likelihood that an eating disorder will occur seems to be related to the number and severity of predisposing risk factors. In almost all patients, a sympathetic and trained history will reveal one or a small number of precipitating events (often engraved indelibly in the patient's memory) that interacted with these predisposing factors to launch the illness when the patient reacted to the event(s) with dieting behavior—usually with food restriction, often with exercise in addition, and rarely with initial purging only. In approximately 95 percent of cases, the eating disorder is precipitated by dieting. In approximately 5 percent of cases, initial weight loss may be inadvertent (automobile accident requiring jaw wiring, flu, ulcer, etc.), but after some weight loss occurs for medical reasons, social praise or self-observation with a scale or mirror soon reinforces the desirability of the weight loss, and the patient now actively directs further weight loss by voluntary dieting. Even less common is an iatrogenic onset, but this seldom happens in teenagers. Once eating disorder patients have firmly internalized a morbid fear of fatness based on the overvalued belief in the necessity for slimness, the disorder is locked in until it becomes, in practice, autonomous and self-perpetuating. Furthermore, blending excessive exercise with dieting behavior appears to create a particularly risky combination. In another animal model of activity anorexia, rats that are simultaneously food restricted and given unrestricted access to an exercise wheel often run themselves to death rather than eat.

Numerous events have been identified as frequent precipitating factors for eating disorders. The most common include events around puberty, especially if puberty is early and accompanied by higher-than-average body weight and the individual is sensitive to criticism. Repugnance toward menses and sexuality in general is historically recognized to predispose to anorexia nervosa. Many patients can identify the specific place, time, and content of the teasing, criticism, or even well-intentioned remarks about weight that launched the eating disorder. These defining moments remain clearly etched in the individual's mind, usually accompanied by feelings of shame or humiliation and followed by determination to reduce body weight. After much contemplation of the hurtful remarks or comparison with others who are thinner, the future eating-disordered patient experiences growing dissatisfaction with body image, and dieting with or without intense physical activity begins in earnest. Depending on the temperament, persevering traits, and impulsivity of the individual, the subtype of the eating disorder is generally predictable.

A move to a new location, changes in schools, social or academic competition with peers, romantic disappointments, family illness or death, and the urging of coaches, teachers, or physicians to lose weight are all common precipitating factors. Sexual abuse may be a precipitating event for a number of psychiatric disorders, including eating disorders. Family discord, the onset of a mood disorder leading to a self-critical and worsened body image, or spurts of weight gain from any source may stimulate dieting behavior as a means of increasing one's sense of personal control, sustaining factors for continued weight loss attempts.

SUSTAINING FACTORS

Most individuals who initiate severe dieting and experience various degrees of subclinical eating disorder symptoms do not go on to develop full-blown, sustained eating disorders meeting full diagnostic criteria. Many serious dieters experience early, transient eating disorder symptoms and either retreat to intermittent or subsyndromal symptoms or stop the abnormal eating behaviors completely as a learning experience. The major sustainers of sustained eating disorders involve a combination of external social reinforcements and internal, psychological, or physiological reinforcers.

Social praise commonly provides external reinforcement for further weight loss in self-critical, self-doubting, perfectionistic, persevering individuals who have lost some weight through dieting or exercise or both. Successful weight loss may offer the first sense of internally effective self-control when the process of puberty is overwhelming, when childhood is mourned, when adulthood appears unattractive and fearful, and when perfectionistic tendencies prove inadequate for the challenges of adolescence. Anorexia nervosa is an implicitly sanctioned pseudosolution to the existential challenges of adolescence. With rigid control of weight, the process seems to be more controllable. After significant weight has been lost through dieting or purging, attempts at healthy eating may, in fact, engender uncomfortable medical symptoms in the short run, such as gastric bloating or fluid retention, that, in turn, lead to renewed dieting based on the experience that normal eating is painful and impossible. The exact mechanisms by which altered physiological processes sustain eating disorders are only speculative. They putatively involve changes in opioids, neuropeptides, serotonin, leptin, ghrelin, cholecystokinin, neuropeptide Y, and other neurobiological molecules involved in the regulation of eating, hunger, satiety, and body weight.

Negative expressed emotion in families may contribute to poor prognosis by offering anorexia nervosa as a moderator of disturbing family emotions and functioning; anorexia can act as a regulator of family dynamics, unconsciously reinforcing its role as a necessity for survival in certain families. Factors that sustain anorexia nervosa and bulimia nervosa differ to some extent. In some instances, bulimia nervosa appears to represent failed attempts at restricting anorexia nervosa in individuals who have less perseverance and less perfectionism than those who purely restrict. In response to severe hunger, binge eating is naturally compensatory, and it is more likely to occur when dietary discipline is not sustainable, particularly in individuals with impulsive traits. In other instances, binge eating initially occurs in response to frustration and dysphoric moods in attempts to quell or soothe these distressing emotional states. Purging episodes, similarly, may offer brief periods of dissociative-like states that temporarily remove the individual from other plaguing negative thoughts and moods. What appears to sustain bulimia nervosa is that binges and purges become elaborated into all-purpose mechanisms for dealing with dysphoric states of any kind. After being used repeatedly to deal with hunger and dysphoric states, bingeing and purging behaviors simply become ingrained habits.

Biochemically, animal studies suggest that intermittent, excessive sugar intake may induce mechanisms causing endogenous changes in opioid regulation, and these processes may also contribute to sustaining binge-eating behavior.

INITIATING AND SUSTAINING PSYCHOPATHOLOGY

Anorexia nervosa often appears to serve as a long-term strategy for coping maladaptively with maturational fears, including pressures to develop a personal identity, and with difficult situations in family and social functioning. Eating disorders of adolescent onset are most commonly pseudosolutions to core challenges of adolescence as delineated by Erik Erikson—in other words, the challenge of developing a coherent personal identity rather than experiencing role diffusion. Some early adolescents are rudely surprised when coping mechanisms they had previously been using to successfully contend with preadolescent issues of work and task completion no longer adequately manage adolescent challenges and chaos. In response, some of the more sensitive, perfectionistic, and compulsive adolescents may develop identities oriented around having anorexia nervosa. They succumb to one type of "quick fix" for developing an adolescent identity, devoting themselves to becoming thin or, in the case of boys, lean and muscular. The motivations behind eating disorders are always "normal," in that they involve attempts to deal with the process of development, emotions, family dynamics, social relationships, and internal self-regulation.

Although early psychoanalytic theories regarding fear of oral impregnation and other historically fanciful formulations appear irrelevant, if not quaint, more recent psychodynamic theories seem more applicable to eating disorders, especially those based on object relations and self-psychology. However, they still remain more difficult to systematically operationalize and have not yet been adequately validated. Therapies based on these formulations have been proposed and may have promise, but, at least in research circles, they have not yet achieved the wider support accorded to cognitive-behavioral therapies or interpersonal therapy.

Psychodynamic conflicts almost certainly contribute to eating disorders as predisposing and sustaining factors, but adequately elucidating these phenomena has remained methodologically hard to pin down. Key psychodynamic components vary from patient to patient, family to family, and between genders. A relatively appealing, although not firmly proven, hypothesis is that a cluster of psychodynamic themes is causally connected to the majority of eating disorders. For example, maturational and existential fears are very commonly involved with eating disorders, and restricting-type anorexia nervosa seemingly provides escape from onrushing negative visions of the emerging sexuality and other biological and social challenges of adolescence.

Concurrently, other psychodynamic themes concern how sensitive personalities deal with childhood narcissistic injuries, seeking safety and avoiding injury from repeated physical, emotional, and sexual abuse through self-starvation and disappearing into "nothingness," detaching from the material world. Gender-associated psychodynamics reveal that boys not only fear the existential anguishes of adolescents, but also fear mortality far beyond medical reality, perhaps more than girls do.

Both bingeing and purging offer short-term solutions and problem solving (or problem avoidance) before they insidiously turn into long-term sources of medical and psychological distress. Despite being ego-dystonic in most individuals, bulimic symptoms have to be understood as coping mechanisms, albeit ineffective ones, for dealing with real issues in mood regulation, such as anxiety, depression, anger, boredom, loneliness, and ennui; interpersonal relations; self-protection; family functioning; and continued worries over body weight.

Later-onset disorders differ thematically from those with earlier onsets. For example, older adult men may initially slim to increase their sexual desirability to extramarital partners, enhance their upward mobility at work, or improve their image in visual media. Some men slim to become more acceptable to gay partners. Later onset in women may represent attempts at emotional self-regulation when previously unresolved issues present themselves, such as fractured relationships, perceived loss of attractiveness, or feelings of ineffectiveness or lack of control.

Although much disagreement pervades psychodynamic understanding of eating disorders, the phenomenology of eating disorders, especially the core psychopathology involving overvalued beliefs in the desirability of weight loss for some reason, has not changed since its first description. The psychopathology of eating disorders involves overvalued beliefs, but the content of these overvalued beliefs may differ in different cultures. A chronic and sustained eating disorder is as much a "friend" as an "enemy." Eating disorders may satisfy fundamental human needs, albeit in a manner that ultimately fails, and simultaneously provides a "profession," an identity, and an organizing principle for daily life. Basically, overvalued beliefs reflect the psychology of the fundamentalist zealot—in the case of eating-disordered patients, these beliefs are centered around shape, weight, and fear of fat in society. They may take on religious tones in some individuals that hearken back to earlier eras when asceticism was praised.

Generally, the overvalued ideas are not entirely impervious to challenge with evidence-based psychological methods and do not generally attain the level of incorrigible, unfalsifiable truth of fixed delusions. Rather, they are more fluid with time. Depending on the patient's level of insight and motivation to change, the ability to objectively reflect on these overvalued ideas shifts. Ultimately, recovery requires the capacity to sense these ideas as intrusive and unwanted, as pseudosolutions rather than failures. The core abnormal beliefs of eating disorders have the potential for being challenged and discarded in favor of adaptive coping skills and healthy methods of internal self-regulation.

DIAGNOSIS AND CLINICAL FEATURES

The diagnosis of an eating disorder is straightforward and can be confidently accomplished with moderate knowledge and experience by directly identifying the eating disorder through the psychiatric history and mental status examination, without extensive medical evaluation. Anorexia nervosa is present when (1) an individual voluntarily reduces and maintains an unhealthy degree of weight loss or fails to gain weight proportional to growth; (2) an individual experiences an intense fear of becoming fat and/or a relentless drive for thinness despite obvious medical starvation; (3) an individual experiences significant starvation-related medical symptomatology, often, but not exclusively, abnormal reproductive hormone functioning, but also hypothermia, bradycardia, orthostasis, and severely reduced body fat stores; and (4) the behaviors and psychopathology are present for at least 3 months.

A distorted body image is common but not essential or invariable in eating disorders. When patients are asked how other people see them, they almost always acknowledge that they are objectively too thin to others but insist that they perceive themselves as fat. Especially as the initial illness wears on, more insightful patients often recognize their thinness but persist in remaining phobically avoidant of healthy weight. The term *atypical anorexia nervosa* has been applied to patients who recognize their thinness, in contrast to those with typical anorexia nervosa, who insist that their body image distortions represent objective fact. These are not truly atypical cases, only more insightful individuals. Prognostically, those with recognition of their extreme thinness have better responses to treatment and more favorable outcomes because they are not constantly fighting an inaccurate view of themselves as heavy. In most patients, body weight is tightly tied to self-esteem. Even when patients intellectually appreciate that their weight is within the normal range, the conviction that they weigh more than they desire leads to plummeting self-esteem and fears of even thin-normal weights as being too fat.

Where self-induced starvation and the core drive for thinness or fear of fatness exist, a diagnosis of anorexia nervosa can be confidently made. Medical disorders may be present as consequences of starvation by food restriction and other methods of weight loss (especially purging) or may be incidental or preexisting findings, but they are never primary causes when the core psychopathology is present and dieting was self-initiated. In these cases, delaying the diagnosis of eating disorders while waiting for extensive work-ups to rule out a primary gastrointestinal, neurological, endocrine, or other suspected underlying medical disorder to account for the weight loss or purging behavior is contraindicated. Such testing delays treatment and harms patients.

Although the contemporary DSM and ICD approaches to psychiatric diagnosis, in all of their serial iterations, represent vast improvements over previous vague and impressionistic approaches to diagnosis, they are both works in progress, with the criteria for various disorders varying from mostly scientific in origin to substantially based on minority opinions. Over the years, new studies and changing opinions have produced different criteria regarding how much weight loss, for example, is required for anorexia nervosa to be diagnosed. The third edition of the DSM (DSM-III) required a weight of less than 75 percent of "normal." In contrast, DSM-IV-TR requires less than 85 percent of a healthy weight, achieved either by weight loss or failure to increase weight along with normal growth. The DSM-IV-TR requires amenorrhea, thereby technically excluding men, and ignores studies disproving the need or value of amenorrhea. The specific weight-loss requirement of less than 85 percent of a healthy weight is also problematic at best and unscientific at worst. The decrement from a prior, usually normal, weight to an unhealthy, significantly lower weight by dieting, exercise, and/or purging is the key concept, not the attainment of a specific percentage of some population average. Because weight, like height, is bell shaped in its natural distribution, a self-induced loss from 120 percent of a population weight, or an "ideal" weight, to 90 percent of that norm can be as indicative of anorexia nervosa as a reduction from a normal 90 percent of ideal weight to 84 percent of that ideal. Psychobiologically, anorexia nervosa is present whenever a decrement from a self-sustaining "set point" to a substantially lower weight causes starvation-related medical symptomatology. Relegating cases in which the final weight is not less than 85 percent of "expected" weight to the category of eating disorders not otherwise specified is scientifically disproved and a source of the overly large and unnecessary number of eating disorders not otherwise specified diagnoses, which are confusing clinically because of the implied "atypicality," and often refused reimbursement because of the assumption that they are not as serious. The diagnostic Criterion A for anorexia nervosa in DSM-IV-TR for amount of weight loss for a diagnosis of anorexia nervosa gives 85 percent of expected weight as an *exemplia gratia*, but the number is taken as an absolute requirement, not simply an example.

A young woman who weighed 20 percent above the average weight but was otherwise healthy, functioning well, and working hard on a rural farm, left home and entered university. She joined a sorority, started to perceive herself as fat compared to her sorority sisters, started to diet, and reduced weight to 90 percent of the "ideal weight" for her age and gender. At her point of maximum weight loss, she felt cold, dizzy, apathetic, and morbidly afraid of becoming fat. She started to restrict her food choices even more, exercised compulsively, and saw herself as still in need of further weight loss. Her menstrual periods became lighter and briefer but did not cease. She was not taking oral contraceptives.

Although, using strict DSM-IV-TR criteria, she would be diagnosed as having an eating disorder not otherwise specified because she did not reach less than 85 percent of "expected weight" and had some menstrual functioning, clinical experts would diagnose her with incontestable anorexia nervosa. She meets all of the core clinical psychopathological and behavioral criteria for anorexia nervosa. She responded to standard treatment for anorexia nervosa.

Anorexia nervosa has been divided into two subtypes—the food-restricting category and the binge-eating or purging category. In the binge-eating or purging subtype, little objective binge eating may actually occur. Some patients purge after only eating small amounts of food. Overexercising and perfectionistic traits are common in both types. Table 19–2 lists current diagnostic criteria for anorexia nervosa according to DSM-IV-TR. Table 19–3 shows the slightly different, but substantially similar, criteria of ICD-10.

Bulimia nervosa is present when (1) episodes of binge eating occur relatively frequently (twice a week or more) for at least 3 months; (2) compensatory behaviors are practiced after binge eating to prevent weight gain, primarily self-induced vomiting, laxative abuse, diuretics, or abuse of emetics (80 percent of cases), and, less commonly, severe

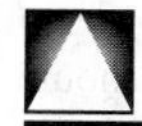

Table 19–2
DSM-IV-TR Diagnostic Criteria for Anorexia Nervosa

A. Refusal to maintain body weight at or above a minimally normal weight for age and height (e.g., weight loss leading to maintenance of body weight less than 85% of that expected, or failure to make expected weight gain during period of growth, leading to body weight less than 85% of that expected).

B. Intense fear of gaining weight or becoming fat, even though underweight.

C. Disturbance in the way in which one's body weight or shape is experienced, undue influence of body weight or shape on self-evaluation, or denial of the seriousness of the current low body weight.

D. In postmenarcheal women, amenorrhea, i.e., the absence of at least three consecutive menstrual cycles. (A woman is considered to have amenorrhea if her periods occur only following hormone, e.g., estrogen, administration.)

Specify type:

Restricting type: during the current episode of anorexia nervosa, the person has not regularly engaged in binge-eating or purging behavior (i.e., self-induced vomiting or the misuse of laxatives, diuretics, or enemas)

Binge-eating or purging type: during the current episode of anorexia nervosa, the person has regularly engaged in binge-eating or purging behavior (i.e., self-induced vomiting or the misuse of laxatives, diuretics, or enemas)

From American Psychiatric Association. *Diagnostic and Statistical Manual of Mental Disorders.* 4th ed. Text rev. Washington, DC: American Psychiatric Association; 2000, with permission.

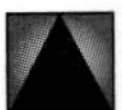

Table 19–3
ICD-10 Diagnostic Criteria for Anorexia Nervosa

Anorexia nervosa

A. There is weight loss or, in children, a lack of weight gain, leading to a body weight at least 15% below the normal or expected weight for age and height.

B. The weight loss is self-induced by avoidance of "fattening foods."

C. There is self-perception of being too fat, with an intrusive dread of fatness, which leads to a self-imposed low weight threshold.

D. A widespread endocrine disorder involving the hypothalamic-pituitary-gonadal axis is manifest in women as amenorrhea and in men as a loss of sexual interest and potency. (An apparent exception is the persistence of vaginal bleeds in anorexic women who are on replacement hormonal therapy, most commonly taken as a contraceptive pill.)

E. The disorder does not meet Criteria A and B for bulimia nervosa.

Comments

The following features support the diagnosis but are not essential elements: self-induced vomiting, self-induced purging, excessive exercise, and use of appetite suppressants or diuretics.

If onset is prepubertal, the sequence of pubertal events is delayed or even arrested (growth ceases—in girls, the breasts do not develop and there is a primary amenorrhea; in boys, the genitals remain juvenile). With recovery, puberty is often completed normally, but the menarche is late.

Atypical anorexia nervosa

Researchers studying atypical forms of anorexia nervosa are recommended to make their own decisions about the number and type of criteria to be fulfilled.

From World Health Organization. *The ICD-10 Classification of Mental and Behavioural Disorders: Diagnostic Criteria for Research.* Geneva: World Health Organization; 1993, with permission.

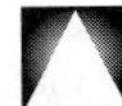

Table 19–4
DSM-IV-TR Diagnostic Criteria for Bulimia Nervosa

A. Recurrent episodes of binge eating. An episode of binge eating is characterized by both of the following:

(1) eating, in a discrete period of time (e.g., within any 2-hour period), an amount of food that is definitely larger than most people would eat during a similar period of time and under similar circumstances

(2) a sense of lack of control over eating during the episode (e.g., a feeling that one cannot stop eating or control what or how much one is eating)

B. Recurrent inappropriate compensatory behavior in order to prevent weight gain, such as self-induced vomiting; misuse of laxatives, diuretics, enemas, or other medications; fasting; or excessive exercise.

C. The binge eating and inappropriate compensatory behaviors both occur, on average, at least twice a week for 3 months.

D. Self-evaluation is unduly influenced by body shape and weight.

E. The disturbance does not occur exclusively during episodes of anorexia nervosa.

Specify type:

Purging type: during the current episode of bulimia nervosa, the person has regularly engaged in self-induced vomiting or the misuse of laxatives, diuretics, or enemas

Nonpurging type: during the current episode of bulimia nervosa, the person has used other inappropriate compensatory behaviors, such as fasting or excessive exercise, but has not regularly engaged in self-induced vomiting or the misuse of laxatives, diuretics, or enemas

From American Psychiatric Association. *Diagnostic and Statistical Manual of Mental Disorders.* 4th ed. Text rev. Washington, DC: American Psychiatric Association; 2000, with permission.

dieting and strenuous exercise (20 percent of cases); (3) weight is not severely lowered as in anorexia nervosa; and (4) the patient has a morbid fear of fatness and/or a relentless drive for thinness and/or a disproportionate amount of self-evaluation depends on body weight and shape. When making a diagnosis of bulimia nervosa, clinicians should explore the possibility that the patient has experienced a brief or prolonged prior bout of anorexia nervosa, present in approximately half of bulimia nervosa patients. Tables 19–4 and 19–5 list the DSM-IV-TR and ICD-10 criteria for bulimia nervosa.

The eating disorders not otherwise specified category is broad and best used where identification of the core psychopathology is lacking or where behaviors differ substantially from requirements for anorexia nervosa or bulimia nervosa (Table 19–6). For example, eating disorders not otherwise specified may properly describe patients who show only occasional binges or purges, repeated short episodes of severe dieting, chewing and spitting out food as the predominant form of disordered eating, or binge eating in a semi- or unaware state during sleepwalking episodes.

Experts are currently working on suggested modifications for the current criteria for future editions of the DSM and ICD to better account for current knowledge about such issues as variability of impairment associated with varying degrees of weight loss, variability of menstrual function, male physiology, binge-eating disorder, and night-eating syndromes, among others.

Because shame is prominent in eating-disordered patients, symptoms are often concealed, and some diagnostic detective work may be needed to elicit the diagnosis. Although the biggest reason for failing to diagnose an eating disorder is the failure to ask pertinent questions, patients sometimes deny eating disorders, especially bulimia nervosa at normal weight, even when clinicians inquire directly about them. Concealed bulimia nervosa may be suspected in the presence of loss of dental enamel, gastroesophageal reflux disease in a young person, abrasions on the knuckles (from self-induced vomiting), and puffy cheeks or upper-neck soft tissue in otherwise thin or normal-weight individuals (resulting from parotid and salivary gland hypertrophy). Others may report the presence of vomitus in the home in the absence of gastroenteritis or food poisoning, finding unexpected laxatives or diuretics, or habitual departure to the bathroom immediately after meals. Unexpected laboratory tests that raise suspicion include unexplained low serum potassium and, occasionally, bizarre findings, such as a toothbrush in the stomach on X-ray.

Many young individuals with eating disorders are resistant to or ambivalent about presenting themselves for diagnostic assessment, fearing that they will be forced to gain weight against their will or that they will be additionally shamed and scorned. Collateral information from parents or other close persons is extremely valuable and should be sought when an eating disorder is suspected.

The most commonly overlooked categories of patients with eating disorders are men, matrons, and minorities, largely because clinicians rarely think of eating disorder diagnoses when assessing these populations. Men should be asked about desire for muscularity, fear of being too small, concern with body image from the waist up (in contrast to women, who are primarily concerned with waist down), and use of steroids to enhance weight gain and desired shape.

Among older patients, especially those with onset in their 40s and 50s, mixtures of true eating disorder symptoms may coexist with separate medical or psychiatric disorders. The core diagnostic features confirm or reject the diagnosis of an eating disorder. Similarly, eating disorders should not be excluded from consideration in indi-

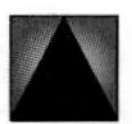

Table 19–5
ICD-10 Diagnostic Criteria for Bulimia Nervosa

A. There are recurrent episodes of overeating (at least twice a week over a period of 3 months) in which large amounts of food are consumed in short periods.
B. There is persistent preoccupation with eating and a strong desire or a sense of compulsion to eat (craving).
C. The patient attempts to counteract the "fattening" effects of food by one or more of the following:
(1) self-induced vomiting
(2) self-induced purging
(3) alternating periods of starvation
(4) use of drugs such as appetite suppressants, thyroid preparations, or diuretics; when bulimia occurs in diabetic patients, they may choose to neglect their insulin treatment
D. There is self-perception of being too fat, with an intrusive dread of fatness (usually leading to underweight).

Atypical bulimia nervosa

Researchers studying atypical forms of bulimia nervosa, such as those involving normal or excessive body weight, are recommended to make their own decisions about the number and type of criteria to be fulfilled.

From World Health Organization. *The ICD-10 Classification of Mental and Behavioural Disorders: Diagnostic Criteria for Research.* Geneva: World Health Organization; 1993, with permission.

viduals with borderline low or mild mental retardation or in the developmentally impaired.

DIAGNOSTIC COMORBIDITIES

The diagnostic challenges of eating disorders are only partly addressed when a specific eating disorder is identified, because, in the large majority of cases, comorbid psychiatric disorders accompany the eating disorder, with two to four separate additional diagnoses on Axis I or II of DSM-IV-TR commonly seen. In addition to identifying Axis I mood, anxiety, obsessive-compulsive, and substance abuse disorders and Axis II personality vulnerabilities and disorders, the temporal relationship of these disorders to the eating disorder should be noted. Mood disorders that precede eating disorders differ significantly from those that first occur after the eating disorder is initiated. Mood disorders starting before eating disorders usually require separate and specific treatment, whereas those starting in the wake of an eating disorder often improve on their own during recovery from the eating disorder. In the setting of an eating disorder, vulnerable personality traits may be amplified into what appear to be primary personality disorders but are actually secondary personality disturbances. As with Axis I disorders, how personality traits vary in relation to the onset of the eating disorder influences the prognosis of the Axis II component. Premorbid obsessional traits, for example, may appear to be full-blown obsessive-compulsive states when an individual is malnourished but may improve with weight restoration—this differs from conditions in which frank obsessional symptoms were present in childhood before the eating disorder.

Table 19–7 shows data from one of several studies that have documented the high comorbidity of Axis I diagnosis in one study of hospitalized eating-disordered patients. Although the specific percentages vary with populations studied, the high comorbidity is common.

Well-diagnosed schizophrenia is rarely seen together with a typical eating disorder, although, in rare cases, it may cooccur as a statistical coincidence. The phrase "perceptual distortion of delusional proportion," used in older literature to describe body image distortions in some eating-disordered patients, is a reminder that borders between delusional perceptions and strongly held body image distor-

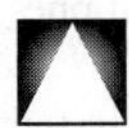

Table 19–6
DSM-IV-TR Diagnostic Criteria for Eating Disorder Not Otherwise Specified

The eating disorder not otherwise specified category is for disorders of eating that do not meet the criteria for any specific eating disorder. Examples include

1. For females, all of the criteria for anorexia nervosa are met except that the individual has regular menses.
2. All of the criteria for anorexia are met except that, despite significant weight loss, the individual's current weight is in the normal range.
3. All of the criteria for bulimia nervosa are met except that the binge eating and inappropriate compensatory mechanisms occur at a frequency of less than twice a week or for a duration of less than 3 months.
4. The regular use of inappropriate compensatory behavior by an individual of normal body weight after eating small amounts of food (e.g., self-induced vomiting after the consumption of two cookies).
5. Repeatedly chewing and spitting out, but not swallowing, large amounts of food.
6. Binge-eating disorder: recurrent episodes of binge eating in the absence of the regular use of inappropriate compensatory behaviors characteristic of bulimia nervosa.

From American Psychiatric Association. *Diagnostic and Statistical Manual of Mental Disorders.* 4th ed. Text rev. Washington, DC: American Psychiatric Association; 2000, with permission.

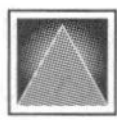

Table 19–7
Frequency of Comorbid Axis I Diagnoses in Eating Disorder Subgroups

Diagnosis	Restricting-Type Anorexia Nervosa	Binge-Eating and Purging Type Anorexia Nervosa	Bulimia Nervosa
Any affective disorder	57%	100%	100%
Intermittent depressive disorder	29%	44%	25%
Major depression	57%	66%	100%
Minor depression	0	11%	0
Mania/hypomania	0	33%	25%
Any anxiety disorder	57%	67%	50%
Phobic disorder	43%	11%	0
Panic disorder	29%	22%	0
Generalized anxiety disorder	14%	11%	50%
Obsessive-compulsive disorder	14%	56%	50%
Any substance abuse/ dependence	14%	33%	50%
Drug	14%	22%	0
Alcohol	0	33%	50%
Schizophrenia	0	0	0
Any codiagnoses	71%	100%	100%
3 or more codiagnoses	71%	100%	100%
No. of codiagnoses ($x \pm$ SD)	2.3 ± 2.5	3.8 ± 1.4	3.2 ± 1.5
Female	100%	89%	100%
Single	71%	89%	100%
Age ($x \pm$ SD)	23.6 ± 10.8	25.0 ± 6.4	19.8 ± 5.6

SD, standard deviation.

tions, obsessional beliefs, and unshakable overvalued ideas have not been definitively clarified and that additional research is necessary to further illuminate these distinctions. For example, there is a high comorbidity of anorexia nervosa with body dysmorphic disorder—estimated at 20 percent—in which patients additionally have obsessional preoccupations regarding specific body parts not related to weight or shape in particular. Body dysmorphic disorder occurs in delusional and nondelusional forms, depending on the extent to which the obsessions are ego-alien and recognized as unrealistic or the extent to which the individual firmly believes that the obsessional concerns are realistically justified.

LABORATORY EXAMINATION AND CLINICAL PATHOLOGY

Pathophysiology in eating disorders results from (1) the amount and rate of starvation, (2) the means used to produce weight loss (dieting alone, with or without over exercising, self-induced vomiting, laxatives, diet pills, diuretics), and (3) binge eating. Eating disorder patients die from either the medical consequences of starvation (cardiac muscle loss and arrhythmia, sometimes related to hypokalemia) or suicide. The physical examination should include height; postvoiding weight in a simple hospital gown observed for hidden weights; vital signs, with particular attention to pulse rate and orthostatic blood pressure changes; a complete examination of skin, muscle, and subcutaneous fat (noting the degree of starvation); a neurological examination (which is, in general, completely normal); and a photograph of the patient if notably thin.

Laboratory tests are helpful for assessing the severity of eating disorders and their medical consequences, but not for chasing after obscure nonpsychiatric etiologies. It should be remembered that anorexia nervosa patients may die with completely normal laboratory test results. Abnormal laboratory findings document the presence of pathophysiological processes and may also be helpful in enhancing motivation. Physiological measures can largely be divided into those that reflect nonspecific consequences of starvation and that are generally self-ameliorating, such as mild bradycardia, and those that require urgent medical intervention, such as a prolonged QT interval on electrocardiogram (EGG) or marked hypokalemia. Medical specialist consultation should be regularly used in the comanagement of these patients. Table 19–8 lists suggested laboratory tests for patients with anorexia nervosa or bulimia nervosa, with judgment regarding the full extent of workup for individual patients based on weight loss, severity of illness, subtype, and comorbidity. For example, laboratory studies in anorexia nervosa binge-eating and purging type and bulimia nervosa often include determination of electrolytes and serum amylase, which are more likely to be abnormal in these disorders than in the restricting type of anorexia nervosa. The elevated levels of amylase derive from salivary gland rather than pancreatic sources, unless alcoholism is comorbidly present. Where abnormal serum amylase is found, fractionation can identify the origin as salivary, although this is usually unnecessary in clinical practice.

Patients who have been abusing diuretics require renal function tests. Many malnourished patients with anorexia nervosa develop a euthyroid sick syndrome, in which decreased levels of thyroid-stimulating hormone (TSH), total thyroxine (T_4), and total triiodothyronine (T_3) may be seen, free T_4 and free T_3 are usually unchanged, and reverse T_3 (rT_3) is elevated. Generally, these endocrine abnormalities represent energy-conserving consequences of starvation that improve spontaneously with refeeding. They do not require immediate treatment but are to be followed with a repeat determination in approximately 3 weeks to determine if improvement occurs with refeeding.

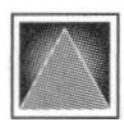

Table 19–8
Suggested Laboratory Studies for Patients with Eating Disorders

All
Complete blood count (anemia is frequent)
Electrolytes
Blood urea nitrogen, creatinine
Thyroid-stimulating hormone, free thyroxine
Electrocardiogram
Total protein and prealbumin
Fasting glucose
Amylase if purging occurs
Serum phosphate
Bulimic syndromes
In addition to above, amylase (fractionated if abnormal to determine parotid/salivary gland origin vs. pancreatic origin)
If amenorrhea >3 mos
Bone mineral density (dual energy X-ray absorptiometry)
In men with weight loss
Testosterone

Low estrogen and progesterone levels in anorexia nervosa are associated with the energy-conserving role of central hypothalamic hypogonadism; low levels of luteinizing hormone and follicle-stimulating hormone are also seen, in contrast to elevated luteinizing hormone and follicle-stimulating levels resulting from failing ovaries, as in postmenopausal patients.

In men, testosterone levels decrease in proportion to weight loss. A man with anorexia nervosa is not fully restored to a normal weight until testosterone is in the normal range, provided no other causes, such as congenital testicular insufficiency, exist. The restoration of normal testosterone is a necessary but not sufficient criterion to assess adequate weight improvement in men.

When drug abuse is suspected, urine and blood screens are indicated. A fair number of teenage girls using stimulant drugs, such as methamphetamine, do so to control appetite and promote weight loss in addition to seeking excitement. Stool tests for the presence of phenolphthalein may reveal occult, nondisclosed laxative abuse.

Bone mineral density should be regularly assessed in the initial workup of patients with anorexia nervosa or bulimia nervosa with a history of amenorrhea in women or weight loss with low testosterone in men. Because amenorrhea has been associated with negative calcium balance, with loss of skeletal calcium in the range of 4 percent per year, many eating disorder patients have significant bone mineral deficiency—usually osteopenia but occasionally as severe as osteoporosis—by their late teens and early twenties, with bones similar to those of elderly women. Osteopenia occurs when bone density is one standard deviation below mean age-adjusted scores; osteoporosis occurs when bone density is at least two and a half standard deviations below these scores. These deficiencies cannot be assessed by physical examination. Dual-energy X-ray absorptiometry (DEXA) scans entail very low levels of radiation, are relatively inexpensive, and are helpful in alerting patients to the realistic medical consequences of their disorders and in guiding clinicians' recommendations concerning nutrition and participation in high-impact activities. The mechanisms of osteopenia/osteoporosis in anorexia nervosa are more complex than in postmenopausal osteoporosis, and treatments useful in postmenopausal women do not necessarily help in anorexia nervosa. Estrogen supplementation in anorexia nervosa has been shown to offer no benefit in bone mineral density while the patient is still low in weight.

Ovarian sonograms, preferably transvaginal, can be particularly useful in assessing individuals who have been adopted (and for whom early growth charts are unavailable) or have grown substantially and when a healthy target weight is uncertain. Ovarian changes occur in a dose–response relationship to the degree of starvation. Multiple small follicles are present when an individual is extremely starved; several small cysts (normal polycystic, not abnormal polycystic) are seen with partial weight restoration. When a woman is close to normal menstruation, a single dominant cyst is present. Thus, the status of the ovarian follicles may be a useful guide to the amount of weight restoration indicated. *Healthy target weight*, defined as the weight at which ovulation can spontaneously occur, is achieved when weight is approximately 5 lb greater than the weight at which a single dominant cyst can be present. On the average, the weight at which menses reoccur is approximately 92 percent of healthy weight for an individual woman.

The structural and functional neuropathology of anorexia nervosa is increasingly well documented by magnetic resonance imaging (MRI), computed tomography (CT), functional MRI (fMRI), positron emission tomography (PET), and single photon emission CT (SPECT) scans. Decreases in total brain volume and sulcal complexity and increases in brain ventricular size are usually seen, but normal brain structural studies may also be seen in some very malnourished patients. The neuropathology of anorexia nervosa reverses substantially with refeeding and weight gain. However, although white matter deficits recover, gray matter changes resulting from starvation may not completely return to normal, even many months after weight restoration. These abnormalities are often reflected in corresponding deficits seen in neuropsychological testing. Approximately 40 percent of typical anorexia nervosa patients score in an abnormal range on two or more neuropsychological tests in standard batteries, suggesting that these patients may have difficulties using cognitive-behavioral therapies and other psychotherapies in these states. The extent to which long-term improvement in neuropsychological abnormalities may occur in proportion to weight restoration and cessation of binge–purge activity over a prolonged period of stability is not yet clear. Functional imaging studies have suggested unusual degrees of temporal lobe vascular flow asymmetry in adolescent anorexia nervosa patients, with persistent abnormalities after weight restoration in some patients, but these studies await extension, replication, and confirmation. In usual clinical practice, neuroimaging is not necessary, but, in patients with atypical features, especially if other findings suggest that a brain lesion may be present, imaging studies may be of value.

Laboratory tests should not be used to frighten patients. However, many individuals with anorexia nervosa, especially those who minimize or deny its seriousness, benefit from frank discussions of laboratory abnormalities. Sympathetically shared results from bone mineral density and other laboratory examinations may help patients reassess and take their disorders more seriously.

DIFFERENTIAL DIAGNOSIS

Differential diagnosis per se is not generally difficult when a full history and mental state examination indicate typical findings of an eating disorder and the core psychopathology is present. It has been suggested that eating disorders primarily represent indirect manifestations of mood disorders, but this hypothesis has been robustly rejected by several sources of evidence, including family studies. On their own, mood disorders lack a drive for thinness and a morbid fear of fat, but severe depression may produce significant weight loss, lack of appetite, and many of the nonspecific symptoms of weight loss, such as irritability, apathy, and fatigue. Because mood disorders commonly cooccur within eating disorders, starting either before, coincident with, or after their onset, their presence needs to be carefully delineated, and the time course and temporal sequence relating these disorders must be noted. Most commonly, depressive symptoms emerge gradually after the eating disorder has started and almost never have melancholic or psychotic features.

Some studies suggest a higher-than-expected concurrence of type II bipolar illness in both anorexia nervosa in and bulimia nervosa. Patients with bulimia nervosa who have concurrent seasonal affective disorder and patterns of atypical depression (with overeating and oversleeping in low-light months) may manifest seasonal worsening of both bulimia nervosa and depressive features. In these cases, binges are typically much more severe during winter months. Bright light therapy (10,000 lux for 30 minutes, in early AM, at 18 to 22 inches from the eyes) may be a useful component of comprehensive treatment of an eating disorder with seasonal affective disorder.

Similarly, anxiety disorders may be present before or accentuated during the emergence of eating disorders. Eating disorders themselves do not conform either to generalized anxiety or to panic disorder diagnostic criteria, although these are frequent comorbid syndromes. In some instances, a case might be made that anorexia nervosa substantially results from a phobic anxiety disorder (with fear of fatness as the core of the psychopathology). Some confusion may occur in which previously unrecognized choking episodes and food avoidance result in substantial weight loss due to fear of recurrent choking, a form of specific phobia. Careful histories may elicit previous episodes of choking on food, often in childhood, that are not previously recalled and may be confirmed by a parent. A small number of patients, usually socially phobic, sensitive personalities, fear vomiting in public, sometimes based on previous experiences. Such fear of losing control in public may lead to substantial food inhibition, but these individuals manifest the core psychopathology of anxiously anticipating uncontrolled vomiting rather than primarily desiring thinness or fearing fatness. Additionally, actual vomiting episodes, in the form of psychophysiological reactions, often do occur in the context of specific types of social phobias, such as stage fright and performance anxieties.

Eating disorders have been identified primarily as OCDs. Although OCD as an Axis I comorbidity may occur in 15 to 25 percent of patients with anorexia nervosa, eating disorders are separate disorders. By definition, OCDs involve ego-alien thoughts or behavioral urges that are resisted, but the process of resisting generates anxiety. Self-starvation in anorexia nervosa is usually, at least initially, ego-syntonic and based on overvalued beliefs of the benefits of weight loss rather than on ego-alien thoughts and behaviors, such as excessive hand-washing or checking behaviors. More likely to be present in anorexia nervosa than Axis I OCD as a state are obsessive-compulsive traits and obsessive-compulsive personality disorder, marked by perseverance, perfectionism, inflexibility, and emotional hypersensitivity in the face of failure or disappointment with performance. In body dysmorphic disorder, obsessions focus on specific body parts, not on the body as a whole or on weight or shape.

Substance abuse, especially of stimulants, can produce substantial weight loss. The use of stimulants by eating disorder patients may be usefully divided into cases in which the stimulants are used primarily to promote weight loss and those in which substances are used for hedonic experiences or mood improvement. Alcohol abuse is much more common in bulimia nervosa than in restricting-type anorexia nervosa. When present, it may disinhibit restraint and allow the individual to eat some otherwise impermissible calories or release underlying hunger and dysphoria, resulting in binge behavior followed by purging.

Among bulimia nervosa patients, a substantial minority—perhaps 15 percent—have multiple comorbid impulsive behaviors, including substance abuse, and lack of ability to control themselves in such diverse areas as money management (resulting in impulse buying and compulsive shopping) and sexual relationships (often resulting in brief, passionate attachments and promiscuity). They exhibit self-mutilation, chaotic emotions, and chaotic sleeping patterns. They often meet criteria for borderline personality disorder and other mixed personality disorders and, not infrequently, bipolar II disorder.

Occasionally, delusional disorders or other psychotic conditions associated with fear that food is being poisoned may result in food avoidance, but the differential diagnosis is usually not difficult.

Although clinicians who are not familiar with eating disorders often confuse eating disorders with primary gastrointestinal or endocrine medical diagnoses, such confusion almost always disappears when core psychopathology is assessed. In more than 60 cases at the National Institutes of Health, where extensive medical and laboratory examinations were made, not a single individual was later found to have a primary medical cause for his or her weight loss when core eating disorder psychopathology was present. This principle has been confirmed in several thousand additional cases. Occasional coincidental medical disorders may be present—for example, a higher-than-expected incidence of irritable bowel syndrome occurs in patients with anorexia nervosa. Furthermore, eating disorders may certainly produce profound medical consequences in many cases, such as compression of the superior mesenteric arteries in emaciated patients resulting in significant intermittent abdominal pain and symptoms of small-bowel obstruction (Wilkie's syndrome) or the superior mesenteric artery syndrome (Table 19–9). However, the medical symptomatology is never the cause of the eating disorder. In occasional case reports about brain tumors misdiagnosed as anorexia nervosa, the nonspecific weight loss, amenorrhea, and apathy seen in such cases are never accompanied by self-induced starvation or a morbid fear of fatness.

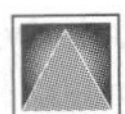

Table 19–9
Potential Medical Consequences of Eating Disorders

Disorder and System Affected	Consequence
Anorexia nervosa	
Vital signs	Bradycardia, hypotension with marked orthostatic changes, hypothermia, poikilothermia
General	Muscle atrophy, loss of body fat
Central nervous system	Generalized brain atrophy with enlarged ventricles, decreased cortical mass, seizures, abnormal electroencephalogram
Cardiovascular	Peripheral (starvation) edema, decreased cardiac diameter, narrowed left ventricular wall, decreased response to exercise demand, superior mesenteric artery syndrome
Renal	Prerenal azotemia
Hematologic	Anemia of starvation, leukopenia, hypocellular bone marrow
Gastrointestinal	Delayed gastric emptying, gastric dilatation, decreased intestinal lipase and lactase
Metabolic	Hypercholesterolemia, nonsymptomatic hypoglycemia, elevated liver enzymes, decreased bone mineral density
Endocrine	Low luteinizing hormone, low follicle-stimulating hormone, low estrogen or testosterone, low/normal thyroxine, low triiodothyronine, increased reverse triiodothyronine, elevated cortisol, elevated growth hormone, partial diabetes insipidus, increased prolactin
Bulimia nervosa and binge-eating and purging type anorexia nervosa	
Metabolic	Hypokalemic alkalosis or acidosis, hypochloremia, dehydration
Renal	Prerenal azotemia, acute and chronic renal failure
Cardiovascular	Arrhythmias, myocardial toxicity from emetine (ipecac)
Dental	Lingual surface enamel loss, multiple caries
Gastrointestinal	Swollen parotid glands, elevated serum amylase levels, gastric distention, irritable bowel syndrome, melanosis coli from laxative abuse
Musculoskeletal	Cramps, tetany

COURSE AND PROGNOSIS

The course of eating disorders is extremely varied in duration and severity. They are truly spectrum disorders, especially bulimia nervosa. Some broad perspectives concerning the natural history of the eating disorders are as follows. Outcome reports describing the natural history of eating disorders depend greatly on how the disorders are defined. Using a fairly rigorous definition of anorexia nervosa that includes a history of hospital care, high mortality rates have been reported, with studies reporting up to 19 percent death rates in patients who received relatively little posthospital care on 20-year follow-up. Other studies, from centers using very structured inpatient treatment programs to full weight restoration and with intensive group and family psychotherapy, document no premature deaths on 10- to 15-year follow-up. Although this study excluded dropouts from treatment completion, it represents the best results published in patients younger than 18 years. Some studies suggest that death rates among young women with anorexia nervosa may be as much as 12 times higher than age-matched community comparison groups and up to twice as high as other female psychiatric populations. Death in chronically ill or relapsed patients occurs in a steady progression, in proportion to the number of years out of hospital.

Most recent outcome studies involve follow-up after some form of treatment. No data currently exist on which treatment methods result in the lowest morbidity and highest rates of global improvement. The best outcomes, consisting of no deaths and complete absence of eating disorder symptoms in 70 percent of patients on follow-up, were found in adolescents initially treated with intensive inpatient acute treatment in a multidisciplinary program followed by 4 years of intensive relapse prevention emphasizing carefully conducted, evidence-based, informed psychotherapy. Follow-up studies of anorexia nervosa patients that encompass a broad range of ages, initial severity, and subsequent chronicity reveal that, overall, approximately 30 percent are well, 30 percent are partially improved, 30 percent are chronically ill, and 10 percent have died. Many continue to have chronic mood, anxiety, and personality disorders.

Long-term studies show higher-than-expected subsequent rates of an assortment of medical conditions among those with adolescent eating disorders. Of increasing concern and only recently documented is the fact that long-term osteopenia and osteoporosis are commonly found even in young anorectic patients. The sobering implication is that these female patients will enter the postmenopausal phase, even if they return to normal gonadal function, with amounts in the "bone bank" insufficient for the inevitable additional decline after menstrual function ceases. Of more concern is the demonstration that estrogen is ineffective in restoring bone density in starved patients. The worst outcome of any eating disorder involves a combination of anorexia nervosa and type I diabetes mellitus, with this group accounting for a disproportionately high number of deaths on follow-up. Mortality for patients with comorbid type I diabetes and anorexia nervosa is 34.8 percent compared to 6.5 percent for type I diabetes alone and 2.5 percent for anorexia nervosa alone.

A common finding on follow-up is the transition from anorexia nervosa to bulimia nervosa—seen in 50 percent of bulimia nervosa cases—but the opposite transition may occur, and many patients move in and out of complete or partial syndromes of these disorders. An encouraging finding suggests that, on long-term follow-up, it is completely possible for many intensively treated adolescents to show complete cure with the absence of any diagnosable eating disorder on follow-up years later. These findings are consistent with other studies, suggesting that, in general, young age of onset and earlier treatment intervention to attain and maintain full weight restoration are associated with better prognosis.

The best prognostic signs in anorexia nervosa for excellence in outcome are completely normal weight at discharge from acute treatment, intensive follow-up by experienced teams, less rather than more psychiatric comorbidity, less severe decrease in weight at admission, shorter duration of illness, and average age of onset in early to mid-teens rather than very young age or onset later than 25 years. Maleness by itself confers no greater risk for poor outcome. Men with some degree of sexual fantasy or activity before anorexia nervosa have a better outcome.

Bulimia nervosa is a more variable disorder than anorexia nervosa in its severity, comorbidity, and treatment outcome. Although much more recently described than anorexia nervosa, it has been better studied because of its higher prevalence, its lack of severe weight loss requiring hospitalization, and the relative ease of completing outpatient treatment studies comparing and contrasting psychotherapeutic and pharmacological interventions. In general, bulimia nervosa is characterized by higher rates of partial and full recovery compared to anorexia nervosa. As noted in the treatment section, treated cases fare much better than untreated cases. Untreated cases tend to remain chronic or may show small but generally unimpressive degrees of improvement with time. In a 10-year follow-up study of patients who had previously participated in treatment programs, the number of women who continued to meet full criteria for bulimia nervosa declined as the duration of follow-up increased. Approximately 30 percent continued to engage in recurrent binge-eating or purging behaviors. A history of substance use problems and a longer duration of the disorder at presentation predicted worse outcome. Depending on definitions, 38 to 47 percent of women were fully recovered at follow-up.

Often, the type of psychiatric comorbidity defines the outcome of treatment more than the illness itself. Recent cluster analysis studies have suggested three coherent prototypes based on eating disorder symptoms and personality profiles: a high-functioning or perfectionistic group with reasonably good prognosis, a constricted or overcontrolled group for which the condition is usually chronic, and an emotionally dysregulated or undercontrolled group least likely to recover. For example, among patients with bulimia nervosa, those with multiple impulsive behaviors and borderline personality disorders have much less likelihood of sticking with treatment and of recovering than those with no significant comorbidity or only mild depressive symptoms.

Maleness has not proved to be a predictor of adverse outcome in either anorexia nervosa or bulimia nervosa. Among men, as in women, the best outcomes occur in adolescents with good sexual adjustment for their age before the onset of illness, with supportive families, who have had less initial weight loss and less psychiatric comorbidity.

Binge-eating disorder, still in a process of definition, appears to have less mortality on follow-up than anorexia nervosa. Long-term outcome studies related to specific methods of treatment are lacking, but early studies are encouraging. Severe obesity augurs worse health outcomes, especially class II obesity (body mass index >35) and class III obesity (body mass index of more than 40). Even less well-defined in outcome is reverse anorexia, which overlaps with the newly defined spectrum of body dysmorphic disorders in men.

The outcome of psychiatric comorbidity in eating disorders is variable. The responsiveness or refractoriness of comorbid Axis I mood and anxiety disorders and OCDs depends largely on whether these syndromes preceded the onset of eating disorders or occurred in their wake. Severe mood and anxiety disorders and OCDs existing before the eating disorders generally remain long-term problems requiring specific additional treatment, but, even without specific treatments for them, obsessive and depressive symptoms often improve substantially when weight is restored to normal in anorexia nervosa patients and when bulimia nervosa abates. The most common outcome after weight recovery and behavioral improvement for vulnerable personality traits worsened by starvation, such as perfectionism, perseverance, and avoidance, is the return to preillness levels. For all eating disorders, the greatest risk of relapse occurs in the first 12 months after successful treatment.

TREATMENT OF EATING DISORDERS

The four essential components of treatment are sound principles, evidence-based practices (to the extent that studies have been published), a spectrum of care appropriate to the intensity of illness, and a skilled multidisciplinary team for serious cases. The core treatment goals for all eating disorders are straightforward and transdiagnostic: (1) attaining and maintaining a normal, healthy, individualized, stable body weight; (2) stopping all abnormal eating behaviors, such as food restricting, binge eating, or purging, and associated abnormal behaviors, especially compulsive exercise; (3) dismantling the core overvalued beliefs and unhealthy cognitive "schemas" of automatic cognitive distortions, replacing them with healthy, balanced views of self (not primarily dependent on body weight or shape) and the capacity for emotional and behavioral self-regulation; (4) treating the comorbid conditions, psychiatric and medical; and (5) planning for ongoing relapse prevention for approximately 5 years after acute improvement. The methods of treatment include medical, nutritional, psychotherapeutic, behavioral, and pharmacological components. Treatment planning requires matching the intensity of treatment to the severity of illness. After initial outpatient comprehensive assessment, patients will be referred to appropriate levels of intensity of care, ranging from medical/pediatric intensive care units for the medically unstable; specialty eating disorder inpatient units for the majority of serious cases of eating disorders; step-down or step-up to partial hospital (full-day) programs—to long-term residential community programs where needed or to outpatient treatment for less severe cases; or relapse prevention. Treatment of severe eating disorders usually requires transitions between several steps in the spectrum, with steps up and steps down according to response to the initial location of treatment. Outreach and prevention programs in school and community settings round out resources.

Studies show that outcomes are generally better for patients treated in specialty eating disorder units than in general psychiatry units that lack specialty programs and are considerably better for anorexia nervosa cases restored to full normal weight.

Treatment of Anorexia Nervosa

Inpatient care is indicated not only for physiological abnormalities, but also to provide 24-hour treatment, management, and containment for the intensively ingrained behavioral abnormalities, such as starving, compulsive exercising, and purging, which often have failed to respond to even full-day programs. At weights below 20 percent less than healthy, except under unusual circumstances, most patients require inpatient care; especially if the eating disorder is recurrent or associated with significant psychological or medical comorbidity. Even full day or partial hospital programs may not provide adequate containment to produce recovery but are increasingly used in the spectrum of care.

Controversy exists concerning the propriety and use of treating treatment-reluctant patients on an involuntary basis through legal commitment. Approximately 10 to 15 percent of cases in large treatment programs require involuntary treatment. In life-threatening cases, involuntary treatment is appropriate when persuasion alone fails to get the patient to agree to accept treatment. Studies show that involuntarily committed patients have approximately the same outcomes as voluntarily committed patients during acute hospitalization, almost always subsequently appreciate the intervention, and rarely persist in feeling angry or litigious.

Reluctance of some third-party payers to authorize ongoing care for severely ill anorexia nervosa patients presents a formidable challenge to patients, families, and clinicians. As lengths of stay have decreased for anorexia nervosa due to insurance restrictions, relapse rates have increased. Effective state and federal parity laws, as well as judicial decisions, may help. A federal district court–level decision ruling that medical benefits should be made available to patients with anorexia nervosa until they reach 85 percent of healthy weight has been underutilized as a precedent for accessing medical benefits for the starvation associated with anorexia nervosa. The judge reasoned that malnutrition is a medical diagnosis and that medical benefits, regardless of the cause of a medical disorder, are legally mandated.

Typical anorexia nervosa patients can transition to partial hospital from inpatient care at 85 percent of healthy weight, but exceptions occur. Those with chronic and repeated bouts of illness, comorbid diabetes, or severe comorbidities on Axis I and Axis II may require higher weights and more prolonged inpatient stays. The essential difference between partial hospital and inpatient care is the length of treatment during the 24-hour day, not the intensity of treatment or the adequacy of a multidisciplinary staff. Short-term successful treatment appears directly related to the number of hours per day and number of days per week of containment and treatment. Going from 5 to 4 days per week in day programs has resulted in approximately 25 percent less effectiveness.

Regarding exceptions to hospital care, research is currently under way to examine the effectiveness of supervised family-based outpatient treatment, in which highly motivated, involved, carefully instructed, and closely supervised parents may supervise the refeeding of young adolescent patients—the so-called Maudsley model, now protocolized and often successful. Data from these studies may influence treatment practices in the future.

Weight Restoration

The initial short-term goal is to restore patients fully, safely, and promptly to the ideal healthy range as specified in population weights for age, height, and gender or the weight at which there is a 50 percent chance of return of menses for adolescent girls. The ultimate goal, not always achieved during initial inpatient or partial hospital treatment, is to restore each person to biological health—for women, the weights at which they will menstruate and ovulate without artificial inducements and, for men, the weights at which normal sexual physiology and function returns. Accordingly, some patients will not achieve normal biological function until they reach higher weights than they desire. The concept of a bell-shaped distribution of heights is widely accepted, but similar acceptance is lacking by many clinicians and most eating-disordered patients for body weights.

Methods of achieving weight restoration vary, but available evidence suggests that nursing-supervised refeeding of normal food in appropriate amounts and composition as directed by a dietitian promptly and safely restores weight. For women receiving inpatient care, approximately 3 lb per week are restored and, for men, up to 4 lb per week; up to 2 lb per week are restored in partial hospital programs. In outpatient treatment, a minimum weight restoration of 1 lb per week is readily achievable with motivated patients. Although nasogastric feedings are not ordinarily recommended or endorsed, some adolescent medicine and pediatric programs use voluntary overnight gastric gavage to supplement, but not replace, oral feedings in an effort to achieve desired weights more efficiently. Hyperalimentation by central venous lines is usually contraindicated and often fraught with severe medical complications.

Failure to fully restore weight adversely affects future outcome. Hunger, even in mildly underweight patients, often serves to trigger binge-eating episodes. In general, patients above 70 percent of healthy weight can start at 1,500 calories per day, which can be increased 500 calories per day every 4 days during inpatient or partial hospital treatment or each week in outpatient care. Typically, women require a maximum of 3,500 calories per day, while men may need 4,000 calories or more. These levels of energy intake are varied according to individual response and medical complications, the most common of which are refeeding edema, gastric bloating, and, invariably, constipation. Any goal of less-than-fully-normal weight is substandard. Refeeding hypophosphatemia is an occasional finding even in purely food-restricting anorexia nervosa patients during treatment and requires correction.

Other Treatment Goals and Strategies

The treatment challenge of eating disorders is enabling patients to start eating normally and stop compulsive exercise, binge eating, purging, and other compensatory behaviors. Evidence suggests that the most effective way to change abnormal behaviors, whenever possible, is to completely interrupt them from the beginning of treatment and replace them with healthy alternatives.

Medication

When experienced eating disorder inpatient units provide comprehensive care for anorexia nervosa, adding psychotropic medications—specifically, selective serotonin reuptake inhibitors (SSRIs) or atypical antipsychotics—appears to offer no added advantage in typical cases. Furthermore, low-weight patients are more likely to experience medication side effects, particularly from tricyclic antidepressants (TCAs). Several mechanisms contribute to the sensitivity of malnourished patients to medications—for example, depletion of body protein, particularly albumin, can increase the percentage of unbound or free drug in blood, and depletion of body fat can decrease the volume distribution of fat-soluble medications, leading to increases in steady-state plasma levels. The use of these medications in other settings or for more treatment-resistant cases has not been fully explored. When severe major depression, anxiety disorders, or OCD precede the onset of anorexia nervosa, concurrent pharmacological treatment of those conditions may be helpful. On occasion, antianxiety medications may enable patients to deal with the anticipatory anxiety of confronting meals. Two studies have demonstrated that SSRIs are not more effective than placebo in decreasing depressive symptomatology or improving weight restoration in starved anorexia nervosa patients during nutritional rehabilitation. It is not clear yet whether the atypical neuroleptics play any role in treatment of eating disorders, or whether they provoke ego-dystonic appetite and the metabolic syndrome. Zinc (50 to 100 mg elemental zinc) has been shown to more rapidly improve weight restoration in anorexia nervosa.

Once weight has been restored, fluoxetine (Prozac) has been shown to reduce relapse in anorexia nervosa, compared to placebo, all other factors being equal. Of caution, one outpatient study found that adolescents with anorexia nervosa lost weight on citalopram (Celexa) plus psychotherapy versus psychotherapy alone.

Psychotherapies In addition to restoring weight and interrupting abnormal eating and exercise behaviors, treatment requires addressing the core psychopathology of the eating disorders. Psychotherapies aimed at modifying and altering core pathological beliefs and other contributing psychopathological issues are key elements of treatment. Available evidence strongly favors treatments based on cognitive-behavioral therapies, similar to those robustly demonstrated to be effective in bulimia nervosa, but less well proven in anorexia nervosa because of the medical status of starved patients and the ethical unacceptability of random assignment to no psychological treatment. Additional alternative psychotherapeutic interventions based on interpersonal therapies, family therapies, or psychodynamically informed psychotherapies—particularly those using self-psychology and "focal analytical" approaches—may also be beneficial. Simply changing the abnormal behaviors through behavioral contingencies of reward and punishment has been disproved as being effective for more than the short term, as it essentially lets patients "eat their way out of hospital," without change in the overvalued beliefs and distorted cognitions. The core of psychotherapeutic treatment is successfully engaging and relating to patients, increasing their own self-awareness and motivation for change and persuading and helping them to recognize, challenge, and replace their overvalued beliefs regarding the desirability of weight loss and their phobic fear of fatness with acceptance of healthy, normal, individualized body weights and the skills for self-regulation. For adolescent patients with anorexia nervosa, studies show that family involvement is essential for good outcomes, with various elements of family education, counseling, instruction, and therapy incorporated into treatment. Individual, group, and family contexts for psychotherapy are all effective, and the blend of these contexts is decided on a programmatic or age-appropriate basis.

Treatment of Bulimia Nervosa

Psychiatric hospitalization is only occasionally indicated for the treatment of normal-weight patients with bulimia nervosa. Exceptions are the presence of intractable symptoms producing significant physiological impairment, repeated failure to respond to competent outpatient treatment, suicidality, and the presence of complicating comorbidities, especially borderline personality disorder, substance abuse, and mood disorders. Fifteen percent of recent and less severe cases of bulimia nervosa have responded to four sessions of psychoeducation emphasizing healthy nutrition with relief of bulimic symptoms and behaviors. Up to 20 percent respond to guided self-help programs using professionally prepared manuals, psychoeducation, and cognitive-behavioral principles. For the average, moderately severe case of bulimia nervosa, cognitive-behavioral therapy has been clearly documented as an effective treatment that is superior to other forms of psychotherapy or psychopharmacology alone. Of concern is the fact that relatively few clinicians have currently received adequate training in cognitive-behavioral psychotherapy skills. Cognitive-behavioral therapy has been effective in both individual and group formats, with short-term abstinence reported by 40 to 50 percent of cases treated with cognitive-behavioral therapy and symptom reduction to a lesser degree reported in higher percentages. If patients show little response to cognitive-behavioral therapy after approximately eight sessions, studies suggest that adding an SSRI will improve outcome. At times, other psychotherapies, especially interpersonal psychotherapy, may be most useful. Psychodynamically informed psychotherapies have not yet been well studied for bulimia nervosa, but experienced clinicians value psychotherapeutic tactics derived from psychodynamic perspectives, particularly relational therapies, self-psychology, and focal analytic therapies. Enhancing motivation is a key early treatment element.

Antidepressants have been shown to be effective for symptom reduction in bulimia nervosa, with approximately 60 percent experiencing some symptom reduction. However, their use as a sole therapy is not adequate to effectively treat most patients, as relatively few patients become abstinent of binge eating and purging on medication alone, and most relapse if the medication is discontinued. Fluoxetine has been the most extensively studied, and higher doses—60 to 80 mg per day—appear to be more effective than the 20- to 40-mg-per-day traditional antidepressant dose if there are OCD components. In addition, TCAs and monoamine oxidase inhibitors (MAOIs) have been effective, although generally more problematic due to side effects and potential for suicide by overdose. Surprisingly, results using fluvoxamine (Luvox) have not been better than placebo. Bupropion (Wellbutrin) is relatively contraindicated due to an increased risk for seizures in patients with bulimia nervosa. In practice, if results from the initial medication trials are inadequate, clinicians have found that empirically trying several medications in sequence yields better results. If results are beneficial, a minimum of 6 months to a year on medication is suggested, preferably in conjunction with CBT.

Studies in which bulimic patients have been treated with both evidence-based psychotherapy and conjoint psychopharmacology show small but important benefits over cognitive-behavioral therapy alone and, especially, over pharmacology alone.

Cognitive-Behavioral Therapy Cognitive-behavioral therapy for bulimia nervosa consists of several phases. The first focuses on educating patients about bulimia nervosa, helping them to increase the regularity of eating and resist urges to binge or purge, in part, through careful self-monitoring and recording. The second phase uses various structured procedures and homework assignments to help patients broaden their food choices and identify and correct dysfunctional attitudes, beliefs, and avoidance behaviors. Next, patients are taught to identify interpersonal stressors and deal more effectively with them by employing more adaptive coping styles. Finally, after symptoms have abated, relapse prevention strategies are used to reduce the likelihood of relapses by anticipating and preparing for stressful situations and setbacks likely to be encountered in the future. A list of guided self-help cognitive-behavioral therapy–oriented workbooks for patients and clinicians appears in the reference list.

Patients with difficult-to-manage multiimpulsive bulimia nervosa are currently being treated with combinations of dialectical behavioral therapy, intensive psychotherapies, and medications. Controlled studies are under way to examine the effectiveness of such treatment approaches for these patients.

Treatment of Binge-Eating Disorder Because binge-eating disorder and nonpurging bulimia nervosa clearly overlap, systematic research on binge-eating disorder has been designed based on observations of bulimia nervosa and non–binge-eating forms of obesity, and current treatment recommendations derive from information from all of these fields. General treatment principles suggest that binge-eating behavior should be addressed before weight reduction for obesity is attempted. Treatment of the binge-eating behaviors is usually best accomplished via treatment with cognitive-behavioral therapy, and some studies show that, for the control of binge-eating behaviors, medications add little to well-conducted cognitive-behavioral therapy. However, because only approximately 50 percent of patients stop binge eating after cognitive-behavioral therapy and because the addition of antidepressants has been shown to increase weight loss and sometimes increase abstinence rates when added to cognitive-behavioral therapy, the addition of antidepressant medication is often useful. In addition to cognitive-behavioral therapy, interpersonal therapy has also shown effectiveness for binge-eating disorder. A randomized clinical trial showed that both therapies administered in group settings were similarly effective in achieving binge-eating recovery (73 to 79 percent posttreatment and 62 to 59 percent at 1 year).

Symptoms of binge eating per se appear to benefit from medication treatment with several different SSRIs, desipramine (Norpramin), imipramine (Tofranil), and, most recently, topiramate (Topamax). Open studies suggest that inositol and sibutramine (Meridia) may be useful. Most, but not all, studies show that medication added to cognitive-behavioral therapy is much more effective than medication alone. Older studies showed that high-dose SSRI treatment (e.g., fluoxetine at 60 to 100 mg) often initially resulted in weight loss. However, the weight loss was ordinarily short lived, even when medication was continued, and weight always returned when medication was stopped.

Treatment of the obesity associated with binge-eating disorder requires both nutritional modification with calorie reduction and an increase in aerobic exercise. For severe obesity, especially class III, medical supervision and, on occasion, gastric surgery are required.

Self-Help Groups Evidence indicates that self-help groups—often lay-led—can be beneficial for those who have a variety of medical and psychiatric disorders. Some reports suggest that malnourished anorexia nervosa patients may have difficulty participating in groups and that adverse consequences of group participation may include competition for being the thinnest patient and learning new maladaptive, "pro-anorexia" techniques. There is general agreement that groups can be helpful for bulimia nervosa. A spectrum of professionally mediated to entirely lay-led groups exists. Although data are sparse, some reports indicate that a subpopulation of patients with bulimia nervosa and binge-eating disorder find organizations such as Overeaters Anonymous (OA) to be helpful (with experience varying from group to group and individual to individual). For the treatment of moderate obesity, organizations such as Weight Watchers can be extremely helpful and are free of common fads or "quick-fixes."

Relapse Prevention Risk of relapse is most common the first several years of recovery. Ongoing treatment requires attention both to preventing relapse and to enhancing the biopsychosocial development and adaptability of recovering patients. In addition to monitoring for signs of symptom return, clinicians attempt to guide patients to work toward developing age-appropriate behaviors and mature coping skills; satisfying involvement in school, work, and social relationships; and an identity based on healthy core factors rather than on an eating disorder. Major challenges face individuals whose identities have centered around their eating disorders and who cannot imagine life without anorexia nervosa or bulimia nervosa. In relapse prevention work, common crises can be anticipated, such as the return to school, family, holidays involving food, special occasions, complexities in relationships, moves, and unexpected disappointments. Prevention requires building alternative coping skills and methods of stress reduction so that stressors do not automatically trigger regression to maladaptive, ineffective eating disorder–related modes of reaction. Methods include ongoing psychotherapy incorporating basic elements of cognitive-behavioral therapy, as well as interpersonal and other psychotherapies. The focus remains on continuing normal weight and eating behaviors and moderate exercise. For weight-restored anorexia nervosa patients in posthospital follow-up, patients receiving fluoxetine—averaging 40 mg per day—experienced less weight loss and fewer episodes of depression and rehospitalization in the subsequent year than those not receiving medication.

The clinicians who are most effective with eating-disordered patients combine nonpossessive warmth; freedom from controlling or hierarchical relationships based on power; a sound knowledge of technical psychotherapeutic skills, normal human development, family dynamics, and sociocultural influences; an understanding of the neurobiology of food and weight regulation and the medical symptomatology of eating behaviors; and the capacity to work as a team member and leader. Although objectively not important, the gender of the therapist may be subjectively very important to individual patients. Specific training in eating disorders confers clinical advantages. Generally well-trained clinicians who lack specific training with eating-disordered patients do not necessarily do well with these patients.

SUGGESTED CROSS-REFERENCES

Some of the specific syndromes that can be associated with eating disorders are found in Chapter 13 on mood disorders, in Chapter 14 on anxiety disorders, in Chapter 15 on somatoform disorders, in Chapter 11 on substance-related disorders, in Chapter 21 on impulse-control disorders not elsewhere classified, in Section 24.6 on endocrine and metabolic disorders, and in Section 7.4 on typical signs and symptoms of psychiatric illness. Personality disorders are discussed in Chapter 23, and the relationship between eating disorders and feeding in childhood, rumination, and pica are discussed in Chapter 41. Other areas that relate to this chapter include consultation-liaison psychiatry (Section 24.11), relational problems (Chapter 25), psychodynamic therapy (Section 30.1), and psychiatric treatment of infants, children, and adolescents (Chapter 48). Sections on genetics and psychiatry (Section 1.18), psychopharmacology (Chapter 31), and family therapy (Section 30.5) provide more detailed background to understanding eating disorders.

REFERENCES

Agras WS, Apple RF. *Overcoming Eating Disorders Client Workbook: A Cognitive-Behavioral Treatment for Bulimia Nervosa.* New York: Academic Press; 1999.

Agras WS, Walsh BT, Fairburn CG, Wilson GT, Kraemer HC: A multicenter comparison of cognitive-behavioral therapy and interpersonal psychotherapy. *Arch Gen Psychiatry.* 2000;54:459–465.

*American Psychiatric Association Work Group on Eating Disorders: Practice guideline for the treatment of patients with eating disorders (revision). *Am J Psychiatry.* 2000;157(1 Suppl):1–39.

Andersen AE, ed.: Eating disorders. *Psychiatr Clin North Am.* 2001;24(2).

Attia E, Haiman C, Walsh BT, Flater SR: Does fluoxetine augment the inpatient treatment of anorexia nervosa? *Am J Psychiatry.* 1998;155:548–551.

Bachar E, Latzer Y, Kreitler S, Berry EM: Empirical comparison of two psychological therapies. Self psychology and cognitive orientation in the treatment of anorexia and bulimia. *J Psychother Pract Res.* 1999;8:115–128.

Baran SA, Weltzin TE, Kaye WH: Low discharge weight and outcome in anorexia nervosa. *Am J Psychiatry.* 1995;152(7):1070–1072.

Bergh C, Eriksson M, Lindberg G, Sodersten P: Selective serotonin reuptake inhibitors in anorexia nervosa. *Lancet.* 1997;348(9023):339–340.

Birmingham CL, Goldner EM, Bakan R: Controlled trial of zinc supplementation in anorexia nervosa. *Int J Eat Disord.* 1994;15:251–255.

Colantuoni C, Rada P, McCarthy J, Patten C, Avena NM, Chadeayne A, Hoebel BG: Evidence that intermittent, excessive sugar intake causes endogenous opioid dependence. *Obes Res.* 2002;10(6):478–488.

Dare C, Eisler I, Russell G, Treasure J, Dodge L: Psychological therapies for adult patients with anorexia nervosa: a randomised controlled trial of outpatient treatments. *Br J Psychiatry.* 2001;178:216–221.

Devlin B, Bacanu SA, Klump KL, Bulik CM, Fichter MM, Halmi KA, Kaplan AS, Strober M, Treasure J, Woodside DB, Berrettini WH, Kaye WH: Linkage analysis of anorexia nervosa incorporating behavioral covariates. *Hum Mol Genet.* 2002;11(6): 689–696.

de Zwaan M, Roerig J. Pharmacological treatment, in evidence and experience in psychiatry. In: Halmi KA, Maj M, eds. *Eating Disorders.* Vol 6. World Psychiatric Association, John Wiley (*in press*).

Eastwood H, Brown KM, Markovic D, Pieri LF: Variation in the ESR1 and ESR2 genes and genetic susceptibility to anorexia nervosa. *Mol Psychiatry.* 2002;7(1): 86–89.

*Eisler I, Dare C, Russell GFM, Szmukler GI, le Grange D, Dodge E: Family and individual therapy in anorexia nervosa. A 5-year follow-up. *Arch Gen Psychiatry.* 1997; 54:1025–1030.

Fairburn C. *Overcoming Binge Eating.* New York: Guilford; 1995.

Fairburn CG, Cooper Z, Doll HA, Welch SL: Risk factors for anorexia nervosa: three integrated case-control comparisons. *Arch Gen Psychiatry.* 1999;56:468–476.

Fairburn CG, Norman PA, Welch SL, O'Connor ME, Doll HA, Peveler RC: A prospective study of outcome in bulimia nervosa and the long-term effects of three psychological treatments. *Arch Gen Psychiatry.* 1995;52:304–312.

Fairburn CG, Welch SL, Doll HA, Davies BA, O'Connor ME: Risk factors for bulimia nervosa: a community-based case-control study. *Arch Gen Psychiatry.* 1997;54:509–517.

Garfinkel PE, Lin E, Goering P, Spegg C, Goldbloom D, Kennedy S, Kaplan AS, Woodside DB: Should amenorrhoea be necessary for the diagnosis of anorexia nervosa? Evidence from a Canadian community sample. *Br J Psychiatry.* 1996;168(4):500–506.

Garner DM, Garfinkle PE, eds. *Handbook of Treatment for Eating Disorders.* 2nd ed. New York: Guilford; 1977.

Gordon I, Lask B, Bryant-Waugh R, Christie D, Timimi S: Childhood-onset anorexia nervosa: towards identifying a biological substrate. *Int J Eat Disord.* 1997;22(2):159–165.

*Grice DE, Halmi KA, Fichter MM, Strober M, Woodside DB, Treasure JT, Kaplan AS, Magistretti PJ, Goldman D, Bulik CM, Kaye WH, Berrettini WH: Evidence for a susceptibility gene for anorexia nervosa on chromosome 1. *Am J Hum Genet.* 2002; 70(3):787–792.

Howard WT, Evans KK, Quintero-Howard CV, Bowers WA, Andersen AE: Predictors of success or failure of transition to day hospital treatment for inpatients with anorexia nervosa. *Am J Psychiatry.* 1999;156(11):1697–1702.

Hu X, Murphy F, Karwautz A, Li T, Freeman B, Franklin D, Giotakis O, Treasure J, Collier DA: Analysis of microsatellite markers at the UCP2/UCP3 locus on chromosome 11q13 in anorexia nervosa. *Mol Psychiatry.* 2002;7(3):276–277.

Johnson JG, Cohen P, Kasen S, Brook JS: Eating disorders during adolescence and the risk for physical and mental disorders during early adulthood. *Arch Gen Psychiatry.* 2002;59(6):545–552.

Keel PK, Mitchell JE, Miller KB, Davis TL, Crow SJ: Long-term outcome of bulimia nervosa. *Arch Gen Psychiatry.* 1999;56:63–69.

Kendler KS, Maclean C, Neale M, Kessler R, Heath A, Eave L: The genetic epidemiology of bulimia nervosa. *Am J Psychiatry.* 1991;148:1627–1637.

Lambe EK, Katzman DK, Mikulis DJ, Kennedy SH, Zipursky RB: Cerebral gray matter volume deficits after weight recovery from anorexia nervosa. *Arch Gen Psychiatry.* 1997;54(6):537–542.

Levitan RD, Kaplan AS, Masellis M, Basile VS, Walker ML, Lipson N, Siegel GI, Woodside DB, Macciardi FM, Kennedy SH, Kennedy JL: Polymorphism of the serotonin 5-HT1B receptor gene (HTR1B) associated with minimum lifetime body mass index in women with bulimia nervosa. *Biol Psychiatry.* 2001;50(8):640–643.

Lock J, le Grange D, Agras WS, Dare C. *Treatment Manual for Anorexia Nervosa.* New York: Guilford Press; 2002.

Mitchell JE, Fletcher L, Hanson K, Mussell MP, Seim H, Crosby R, Al-Banna M: The relative efficacy of fluoxetine and manual-based self-help in the treatment of outpatients with bulimia nervosa. *J Clin Psychopharmacol.* 2001;21:298–304.

*Palmer RL, Birchall H, McGrain L, Sullivan V: Self-help for bulimic disorders: a randomised controlled trial comparing minimal guidance with face-to-face or telephone guidance. *Br J Psychiatry.* 2002;181:230–235.

Pierce DW, Epling FW: Activity-based anorexia: a biobehavioral perspective. *Int J Eat Disord.* 1988;7:475–485.

Piran N, Kaplan AS, ed. *A Day Hospital Group Treatment Program for Anorexia Nervosa and Bulimia Nervosa.* New York: Brunner/Mazel; 1990.

Ratnasuriya RH, Eisler I, Szmukler GI, Russell GF: Anorexia nervosa: outcome and prognostic factors after 20 years. *Br J Psychiatry.* 1991;158:495–502.

Robb AS, Silber TJ, Orrell-Valente JK, Valadez-Meltzer A, Ellis N, Dadson MJ, Chatoor I: Supplemental nocturnal nasogastric refeeding for better short-term outcome in hospitalized adolescent girls with anorexia nervosa. *Am J Psychiatry.* 2002;159(8):1347–1353.

Safer DL, Telch CF, Agras WS: Dialectical behavior therapy for bulimia nervosa. *Am J Psychiatry.* 2001;158:632–634.

Schmidt U, Treasure J. *Getting Better BitE by BitE: A Survival Kit for Sufferers of Bulimia Nervosa and Binge Eating Disorders.* London: Psychology Press; 1993.

Strober M, Freeman R, Lampert C, Diamond J, Kay W: Controlled family study of anorexia nervosa and bulimia nervosa: evidence of shared liability and transmission of partial syndromes. *Am J Psychiatry.* 2000;157:393–401.

Strober M, Freeman R, Morrell W: Atypical anorexia nervosa: separation from typical cases in course and outcome in a long-term prospective study. *Int J Eat Disord.* 1999;25(2):135–142.

Sullivan PF: Mortality in anorexia nervosa. *Am J Psychiatry.* 1995;152(7):1073–1074.

Treasure JL, Owen JB: Intriguing links between animal behavior and anorexia nervosa. *Int J Eat Disord.* 1997;21(4):307–311.

Treasure J, Schmidt U. *Anorexia Nervosa. Clinical Evidence 7.* London: BMJ Publishing Group; 2002:161–162.

Vannatta JB, Cagas CR, Cramer RI: Superior mesenteric artery (Wilkie's) syndrome: report of three cases and review of the literature. *South Med J.* 1976;69(11):1461–1465.

Villapiano M, Goodman LJ. *Eating Disorders: A Time For Change: Plans, Strategies, and Worksheets.* New York: Brunner-Routledge; 2001.

Vink T, Hinney A, van Elburg AA, van Goozen SH, Sandkuijl LA, Sinke RJ, Herpertz-Dahlmann BM, Hebebrand J, Remschmidt H, van Engeland H, Adan RA: Association between an agouti-related protein gene polymorphism and anorexia nervosa. *Mol Psychiatry.* 2001;6(3):325–328.

Walsh BT, Agras WS, Devlin MJ, Fairburn CG, Wilson GT, Kahn C, Chally MK: Fluoxetine for bulimia nervosa following poor response to psychotherapy. *Am J Psychiatry.* 2000;157:1332–1334.

Watson TL, Bowers WA, Andersen AE: Involuntary treatment of eating disorders. *Am J Psychiatry.* 2000;157(11):1806–1810.

Westberg L, Bah J, Rastam M, Gillberg C, Wentz E, Melke J, Hellstrand M, Eriksson E: Association between a polymorphism of the 5-HT2C receptor and weight loss in teenage girls. *Neuropsychopharmacology.* 2002;26(6):789–793.

Westen D, Harnden-Fischer J: Personality profiles in eating disorders: rethinking the distinction between axis I and axis II. *Am J Psychiatry.* 2001;158(4):547–562.

Wilfley DE, Welch RR, Stein RI, Spurrell EB, Cohen LR, Saelens BE, Dounchis JZ, Frank MA, Wiseman CV, Matt GE: A randomized comparison of group cognitive-behavioral therapy and group interpersonal psychotherapy for the treatment of overweight individuals with binge-eating disorder. *Arch Gen Psychiatry.* 2002;59(8):713–721.

*Wolk SL, Devlin MJ. Stage of change as a predictor of response to psychotherapy for bulimia nervosa. *Int J Eat Disord.* 2001;30:96–100.

20 Sleep Disorders

WALLACE MENDELSON, M.D.

In traditional psychiatric practice, a complaint about the consequences of the illness often leads to discovery of the underlying disorder. Thus, a patient who comes in to the office because of difficulties at the job, or with his or her spouse, may be found to have a previously unrecognized depression. In a similar manner, the search for underlying sleep disorders usually begins with a complaint about consequences, usually insomnia or daytime sleepiness. Just as an important aspect of helping the patient whose problem at first appeared to be job-related is to give a specific treatment for an underlying condition, so, in treating sleep complaints, one must first recognize and give specific remedies for underlying processes. This chapter reviews the pathophysiologies of sleep, emphasizing those likely to be seen in psychiatric practice.

Before beginning, it should be mentioned that, of course, there are many other fascinating aspects of sleep that have only passing relevance to the clinical sleep disorders presented here and, hence, are not covered in detail. Among these is the continuing mystery of the ultimate functions of sleep. Like most drive behaviors, sleep probably has multiple functions, just as breathing, for instance, facilitates gas exchange but, in addition, provides a mechanism for speech and more complex behaviors, such as playing a musical instrument. So, too, sleep may have originated to serve some basic need, superimposed on which are additional functions. From an evolutionary point of view, the observation that it involves a controlled loss of consciousness, which, at face value, makes an organism vulnerable to the dangers of the environment, suggests that its beneficial functions are important indeed. Among those that have been proposed are energy conservation, restoration of cellular energy stores, emotional regulation, consolidation of memory, and preservation of context in which to organize memory of new stimuli.

As with the enigma of the functions of sleep, the nature of dreaming is beyond the current scope of this chapter. In summary, interest in sleep and dreaming as aspects of health goes back to the earliest times. The Egyptian Imhotep, who may be the earliest recorded physician in history and who was later worshipped as a god himself, incorporated *temple sleep* in his treatment regimen in the third millennium BC. By Ptolemaic times, many Egyptian temples had sanatoria in which patients slept; it was believed that, while they dreamed, they were approached and healed by the resident deity. In ancient Greece, Asclepius asked his patients to sleep on the floor in his temple (although one wonders how comfortable this might be, given the proximity of the native snake population from which his symbol, and, ultimately, the badge of the medical profession, was derived). In both cases, patients were encouraged to talk about their dreams, which were likely influenced by the atmosphere of the temple setting and the religious beliefs of patient and priest.

Theories of functions of dreams in modern times are many, ranging from views that they represent manifestations of unconscious conflicts or mechanisms for assimilating stressful events or that they represent a delirium-like state. Positron emission tomography (PET) studies of rapid eye movement (REM) sleep suggest that there is activation of the pontine brainstem, as well as limbic and paralimbic cortical structures mediating emotional responses, accompanied by a reduction in activity of dorsolateral prefrontal cortical structures regulating executive and mnemonic cognitive processes. Two clinical sleep disorders associated with dreaming, nightmares and night terrors, are discussed later in this chapter.

PRIMARY AND SECONDARY SLEEP DISORDERS

Sleep may, of course, be disturbed as a consequence of some other disorder. In the example used previously, a patient reported insomnia as a result of depression. Similarly, sleep may be disturbed owing to pain or discomfort from a medical illness. In terms of the revised fourth edition of the *Diagnostic and Statistical Manual of Mental Disorders* (DSM-IV-TR), such cases are considered to be *secondary sleep disorders*. In contrast, *primary sleep disorders* result from conditions inherent to the mechanisms by which sleep is regulated. Although this is a useful clinical distinction in organizing one's thoughts about a specific patient, ultimately, these two categories are less clear. In the case of sleep disturbance due to depression, for instance, it is possible that fundamental alterations in biogenic amine metabolism that alter mood states may also lead to sleep disturbance. The manifestation of primary sleep disorders may also be strongly influenced by nonsleep conditions. Sleepwalking in children, for instance, often comes out during periods of stress or family disturbance. Although secondary sleep disturbances are not the focus here, sleep in affective disorders is discussed for the reasons given previously, and the increased rate of insomnia during periods of societal stress is mentioned in passing. Indeed, severe trauma, such as that faced by those who survived the Holocaust, may be associated with reports of altered sleep and dreaming for decades. External stimuli can, of course, also disturb sleep, as is reflected by the observation that the rate of issuing prescriptions for sleeping pills (hypnotics) rises in areas surrounding major airports. On the other hand, the overall frequency of reported insomnia is approximately the same in urban and rural areas, reflecting the universality of disturbance in basic sleep mechanisms and, incidentally, perhaps dispelling the fantasy held by city dwellers of the blissful country life.

The DSM-IV-TR divides primary sleep disorders into *dyssomnias* and *parasomnias*. The dyssomnias, disorders of quantity or timing of sleep, are, in turn, divided into *insomnia* and *hypersomnia.* Insomnia is a perceived disturbance in the quantity or quality of sleep, which, depending on the specific condition, may be associated with disturbances in objectively measured sleep. Forms of insomnia include the primary insomnias and circadian rhythm sleep disturbances. Hypersomnias represent conditions that are clinically expressed as excessive sleepiness. Again, this distinction is not as sharp in practice as this classification suggests. Some circadian sleep disorders, such as delayed sleep-phase syndrome, for instance, may present as a complaint of insomnia at night, as well as morning sleepiness. Similarly, periodic leg movement disorder may present as a complaint of insomnia or hypersomnia. Parasomnias are abnormal behaviors during sleep or the transition between sleep and wakefulness. Often, they reflect the appearance of normal sleep processes at inappropriate times. In a sense, they are analogous to sexual parapraxias, in which a fundamentally normal, but often minor, activity in the context of overall sexual behavior comes to dominate and to disturb other aspects of sex.

PRIMARY INSOMNIA

Inadequate Sleep Hygiene A common finding is that a patient's lifestyle leads to sleep disturbance. This is usually phrased as *inadequate sleep hygiene*, referring to a problem in following generally accepted practices to aid sleep. These include, for instance, keeping regular hours of bedtime and arousal, avoiding excessive caffeine, not eating heavy meals before bedtime, and getting adequate exercise. For example, a patient might come to clinic complaining of difficulty getting off to sleep. A closer examination of his history revealed that he got home from his commute at 7:00 PM, ate a hasty dinner, kissed the kids goodnight, did some work for a few hours, and then was surprised to find that he could not sleep. In this case, the problem (or one of them) was that his life no longer contained an evening in which to relax and to prepare for sleep. Alternatively, a school teacher might spend the evening grading papers and then find himself or herself wide awake at bedtime. In this case, the intervention might be to teach him or her better time-management skills to use during the daytime, so that his or her evening will be free for relaxation. A patient who complains of awakening after only a few hours might turn out to be a disco aficionado, whose extremely irregular bedtimes have disrupted the rhythm of sleep and waking. In this case, guidance in keeping more regular hours may be important. A variation on this problem is the patient whose work and social activities lead him or her to become progressively more sleep deprived as the week progresses; he or she then crashes and sleeps in on the weekends. Again, education about the importance of keeping relatively regular hours would likely be useful.

Two caveats are in order when helping to educate a patient about sleep hygiene. The first is that these are general principles and are not applicable to all patients. In general, for instance, napping is discouraged, except in elderly and debilitated patients, but a small group of insomniacs may actually sleep better at night when they take brief daytime naps. The second is that when trying to modify a patient's behavior, it is usually better to focus on one or two changes at a time, rather than assaulting him or her with a panoply of desired changes, which can come across as overwhelming. In a way, this is a specific case of a general principle: When a task seems so large as to be daunting, it can help to break it down into individual doable pieces.

Psychophysiological Insomnia Psychophysiological insomnia typically presents as a primary complaint of difficulty in going to sleep. A patient may describe this as having gone on for years and usually denies that it is associated with stressful periods in his or her life. A typical comment is "I don't understand it; things are actually going pretty well for me right now. If I could just get over this problem in going to sleep." Often, the patient seems to be focused on the sleep disturbance and how it is affecting his or her life. While lying in bed before sleep, the patient typically ruminates about issues on his or her mind, often thinking through the battles of the preceding day or planning strategies for problems to be faced tomorrow. He or she typically says that he or she works at going to sleep and feels frustrated that his or her efforts are not rewarded. Characteristically, the patient describes sleeping better when away from home. When asked, the patient reports that he or she can fall asleep when not trying to, for instance, when watching television. A typical story is that the patient is dozing in the living room in front of the television; the spouse then comes in and wakes him or her up, saying that it is time to go to bed. Then, when the patient gets into pajamas and climbs into bed, he or she feels wide awake and unable to sleep.

It is thought that patients with psychophysiological insomnia have developed a conditioned state of heightened arousal that has become associated with the act of going to bed or the environment in which sleep typically occurs—the bedroom. The genesis of this conditioned response is not always certain, but, often, after getting to know the patient, one discovers that the sleep disturbance began after some emotionally traumatic event, which the patient has long since forgotten or which he or she no longer associates with the sleep difficulty. A typical history would be that, some years before, the patient had an upsetting breakup with a girlfriend or boyfriend. In the short term, of course, he or she experienced sleep difficulty as part of a grief or separation reaction. In many individuals, the emotional upset gradually works its way through in the next few weeks, and, as things settle down, sleep returns to normal. In these individuals, however, the emotional upset resolves, but the sleep problem persists and seems to take on a life of its own. The patient becomes worried about the poor sleep and works hard to overcome it. Over time, the original association with the traumatic event is forgotten.

One model of psychophysiological insomnia suggests that it can be considered to have three components—a predisposition, a precipitating cause, and factors that maintain the sleep disturbance. Little is known about why these patients may be more vulnerable to sleep disturbance. The maintaining factors, however, appear to include the excessive worry about poor sleep. It is a little bit like Franklin Roosevelt's remark that "the only thing we have to fear is fear itself." In this case, the worry about not sleeping becomes one of the causes of poor sleep. In effect, the patient associates the act of entering the bedroom or going to bed with an uncomfortable condition generating anxiety and heightened arousal, which are incompatible with sleep. (Because of the arousal response on entering the bedroom, the patient sometimes reports that he or she sleeps better when in a strange environment—such as a hotel room—than when at home.) Often, he has found that, in most areas of life, working harder leads to rewards, so he tries even harder to sleep; sadly, this is one of the few areas in which trying hard does not work and may, indeed, complicate the problem.

When a patient with psychophysiological insomnia has a sleep study, the polysomnogram (PSG) usually indicates objectively disturbed sleep with a relatively long sleep latency (the time from when the lights are turned out until sleep onset), shortened total sleep time, or frequent awakenings during the night. When asked in the morning to estimate how long it took him or her to fall asleep and how long he or she slept, the patient is usually fairly accurate. This finding of good concordance between objective and subjective measures of sleep is crucial to the distinction between psychophysiological insomnia and sleep state misperception. Treatment of psychophysiological insomnia is usually oriented to decathecting the powerful emotional focus that the patient has placed on his sleep problem, reducing the tendency to work hard at going to sleep, and removing the conditioned response of anxiety and heightened arousal that has become associated with the act of trying to go to sleep.

It should be noted that the kind of conditioned response seen in these patients is a special case of a phenomenon seen in many different areas of medicine. One example is the cancer patient who becomes nauseous while driving to the chemotherapy clinic. Finally, it should be remembered that, although psychophysiological insomnia may be a disorder in its own right, many patients develop a conditioned arousal and anxiety response as a complicating factor on top of insomnia owing to some other reason. A patient whose sleep is disturbed due to pain or who has the sleep difficulty associated with depression, for instance, may begin to worry excessively about his or her sleep and may develop an arousal response when entering the bedroom. This illustrates a broader problem, which is that, in evaluating patients with chronic insomnia, one often discovers multiple causes, each of which needs to be treated.

Sleep State Misperception Recognition of sleep state misperception (also known as *subjective insomnia*) arose in response to a common—and often frustrating—clinical phenomenon. A patient would present at the sleep center describing sleeping only for 1 or 2 hours each night and, in colorful terms, would describe the agony of lying in bed awake for endless hours. Shortly after the lights are turned out in the laboratory, the patient closes his or her eyes and lies still with the quiet, regular respirations of sleep. The electroencephalogram (EEG) appears that of a normal sleeper. In the morning, when the doctor enters the bedroom, the patient opens his or her eyes and, with bewildering sincerity, says "See doctor, I told you I wouldn't sleep a wink." Later, when the PSG is completely analyzed, the study indicates a relatively normal night's sleep. In contrast, the patient's morning estimate of the previous sleep describes a poor night, which contrasts sharply with these polygraphic results. This is different from the morning report of a patient with conditioned insomnia, a report which shows good concordance with the sleep recording.

Subjective insomnia, then, is characterized by a dissociation between the patient's experience of sleeping and the objective polygraphic measures of sleep. The ultimate cause of this dissociation is not yet understood, although it appears to be a specific case of a general phenomenon seen in many areas of medicine. One example is the sensation of dyspnea. On the one hand, one can see patients with severe chronic obstructive pulmonary disease (COPD) and markedly poor blood gases who report no trouble breathing; in contrast, an apparently healthy young man with normal pulmonary function tests can come in reporting a sensation of not being able to get enough air. Similarly, in the gastrointestinal (GI) literature, there are reports of a wide variation in the subjective recognition of a sensation of satiety when the stomach is distended, and it is thought that at least one aspect of the complex phenomena that led to obesity is that some obese patients have decreased recognition of this sensation of satiety.

One hint at the genesis of subjective insomnia comes from a landmark study by L. J. Monroe, who reported that, when poor sleepers were awakened in early stage II sleep, they said that they felt that they had previously been awake, in contrast to good sleepers, who believed that they had been asleep. This seemed to suggest that some insomniacs may have a different subjective experience of sleep and wakefulness than good sleepers. This disturbance does not appear to be due to being light sleepers, as insomniacs, as a group, are no more easily aroused by an auditory stimulus than good sleepers. This phenomenon has also been explored in terms of the way that hypnotic medication may act to improve sleep. The author and colleagues found that, after receiving a placebo, subjective insomniacs tend to report that they had been awake, when asked after being awakened from nonrapid eye movement (NREM) sleep by an auditory tone. After receiving a hypnotic, such as zolpidem (Ambien) or flurazepam (Dalmane), however, the same patients respond like good sleepers, saying that they believed that they had been asleep. This suggests that one aspect of the mechanism by which hypnotics act may be that they have a cognitive effect; that is, they change a patient's perception of whether he or she is awake or asleep. Such a cognitive action may help explain why, clinically, many hypnotics seem to offer a great deal of relief to insomniacs (at least acutely), whereas drug-induced increases in EEG measures, such as total sleep time, are often relatively modest (in one review, the mean increase in total sleep induced by a variety of hypnotics was approximately 30 minutes). The underlying physiological basis for this disorder remains unclear. One promising hypothesis is that at least some insomniacs are in a state of hyperarousal, which is supported by data indicating that they may have increased metabolic rate.

One common mistake in dealing with patients with subjective insomnia is to tell them that (based on the polygraphic data) there is nothing wrong with their sleep. There is always a temptation to do this, with the hope that the patient will be relieved to hear this good news. In practice, telling the patient that he or she is sleeping normally flies in the face of his or her experience, and most likely leads to alienating him and losing his cooperation. It is better—although harder—to respect the patient's symptom, explaining that there is a disparity between what he or she is experiencing and what the polygraph seems to be showing.

Idiopathic Insomnia Among primary insomnia patients, there remains a group that appears to have neither a conditioned sleep disturbance nor a dissociation between subjective experience and polygraphic data. They are classified as having idiopathic insomnia. Typically, a history of trouble going to sleep or of awakening during the night goes back to childhood or even infancy, and the patient's complaint is confirmed by the sleep study, which may show an increased sleep latency, decreased total sleep, or increased arousals. There have been many hypotheses to explain the genesis of this disturbance, including the possibility that there may be a dysregulation of biogenic amine metabolism, alterations in basal forebrain function, an altered response to γ-aminobutyric acid type A ($GABA_A$)–benzodiazepine receptor activity, or reduced levels of endogenous sleep-promoting substances. Psychodynamic theories have suggested that these patients failed to have a normal erotization of sleep as infants or that they received conflicting messages from their mothers as to the safety of sleeping alone.

Finally, before examining issues of therapy, it should be mentioned that primary insomnia is probably not the same as light sleep or sleep deprivation. As mentioned previously, there is significant evidence that insomniacs, as a group, do not awaken in response to an auditory tone more easily than good sleepers. Moreover, they are not excessively sleepy during the daytime, at least as assessed by the Multiple Sleep Latency Test (MSLT); indeed, if anything, they may be hyperaroused. Neuropsychological testing studies suggest that their pattern of deficits is different from that typically seen in sleep deprivation. Insomniacs do not seem to estimate time differently from good sleepers. Thus, it appears that the problem of insomnia is more complex than first meets the eye, and the solutions for it are probably different from merely increasing the number of minutes of EEG-measured sleep.

Treatment Treatments for insomnia include nonpharmacological and pharmacological approaches.

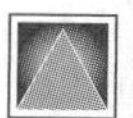

Table 20–1
Sleep Hygiene

Maintain regular hours of bedtime and arising. Try to avoid a lifestyle of progressive sleep deprivation during the week and then crashing on the weekends.

Do not eat heavy meals near bedtime. A light snack, in contrast, may be helpful.

In general, it is best to avoid napping during the daytime. (Exceptions are made for the elderly or debilitated.)

Exercise daily. This is best in the late afternoon or early evening. Exercise later in the evening may disturb sleep.

Minimize caffeine intake and cigarette smoking within 8 hrs of bedtime.

Do not look at the clock during the night. If an alarm clock is needed, put it in a drawer by the bed, so that it can be heard but not seen.

If there is something that is worrisome while lying in bed, write it down on a piece of paper and promise to look at the paper in the morning. Let it go until then.

Make the bedroom comfortable. In general, it is better to be slightly cool than to be too warm.

Do not use alcohol to help in going to sleep.

Nonpharmacological Treatments Nonpharmacological treatments include some general recommendations for all patients and more specific behavioral and cognitive approaches.

General *sleep hygiene* principles are summarized in Table 20–1. As mentioned previously, it is important to remember that these are general guidelines, and they may not fit all patients. When presenting these to a patient, it is usually better to help him or her focus on only one or two of these principles at a time and to work slowly through the entire list, rather than making global recommendations that may feel overwhelming. It should also be noted that, although it has long since become part of the accepted tradition in lectures on sleep disorders to begin with sleep hygiene, there are minimal long-term outcome data to support its use.

Among specific behaviorally oriented therapies is *stimulus control*, developed by Richard Bootzin. It suggests that an important cause of sleep disturbance is that the patient has come to associate behaviors that are incompatible with sleep with the act of trying to go to sleep and the setting in which sleep is to take place. The goal, then, is to remove all behaviors from the bedroom, except sleep and loving. Thus, the patient is instructed to conduct all other activities in another room. For example, it would not be appropriate to have a small desk at which one pays household bills in the bedroom. Some couples with children retreat to the bedroom as one of the few places that they can have a fight behind closed doors. Obviously, if a patient comes to associate the bedroom with the act of having frank discussions with the spouse, this does not aid sleep. Finally, it is important that the patient not come to think of the bedroom as a place of discomfort. For this reason, he or she is told that whenever he or she finds himself lying in bed unable to sleep, he or she should get up, go in another room, and not to return to bed until he or she feels ready to sleep.

Sleep restriction therapy, developed by Arthur Spielman, addresses the concern that one of the factors that maintains a sleep disturbance is the relatively inefficient sleep resulting from the patient staying in bed for unnecessarily long periods. In practice, the patient is asked to keep a sleep diary for, perhaps, 2 weeks and to bring it to the office. There, the patient and therapist summarize the average time that the patient is in bed each night and the average amount that he or she estimates is spent asleep. If, for instance, the patient estimates that he or she is in bed 9 hours nightly but sleeps only 5 hours, he is instructed to stay in bed only 5 hours and to continue to keep the sleep diary. When his subsequent estimates of sleep time indicate that he has been asleep 85 percent of the 5 hours, the duration in bed is increased to 5.5 hours; again, this is increased in 0.5-hour intervals each time the estimated sleep rises to 85 percent of the time in bed. Eventually, the patient's time in bed approaches more conventional amounts, while sleep efficiency is improved.

Although stimulus control and sleep restriction address different aspects of the factors that maintain poor sleep, it should be noted that, like most behaviorally oriented therapies, they share many qualities. Typically, they are performed with what Peter Hauri and others refer to as the *co-scientist model*. This approach avoids the situation in which the therapist is an authority figure who dispenses knowledge or instructions to a patient who is a passive recipient. Rather, the therapist says, in effect, "We are each experts in certain parts of the common problem that we have before us. I am an expert in the principles of sleep regulation but know less about you. You, on the other hand, are the person most knowledgeable about your own behavior and habits. Let's work together, then, and each bring our own expertise to this problem that we face together." The therapist encourages the patient to take an active role in the process, rather than passively receiving guidance. In part, this is in response to the observation that insomniacs often have a passive view of their affliction. From the patient's perspective, it can sound as if the heavens had inexplicably opened up and struck him or her down with this affliction, which, from his or her perspective, has no relationship to events in his or her present or past life. One goal of these therapies is to encourage the patient to take a much more active stance and to be actively engaged in the resolution. This includes giving well-earned credit to the patient when there is improvement.

Another method of encouraging active involvement in the previously mentioned therapies is to negotiate with the patient what an acceptable outcome would be. Before beginning treatment, the therapist considers possible outcomes. He might ask the patient what he or she hopes to gain from therapy. If the patient gives an unrealistically high expectation, the therapist might say something like this: "It sounds like the best thing that could happen here would be that you would come here for two or three visits, and, from then, on you would sleep perfectly for the rest of your life. I wish this would happen, but it doesn't seem likely to me that such a miraculous cure will take place. On the other extreme, probably, the worst thing that might happen would be that you would come weekly for a year, and improve only, let's say, by 5 percent. We need to find a balance, somewhere in the middle, that each of us will agree is likely and that would be acceptable." By negotiating such an outcome, the therapist helps dispel unrealistic expectations and helps the patient take a more active role in the process.

Cognitive-behavioral therapy (CBT) emphasizes the role of dysfunctional thoughts in the maintenance of primary insomnia. It suggests, for instance, that incorrect beliefs (e.g., that there is nothing one can do about poor sleep or that one night of poor sleep has disastrous consequences) may lead to anxiety that perpetuates the disorder and that insomniacs tend to have more emotion-oriented coping strategies to stressors. It has been reported that as few as six weekly sessions can modify a patient's beliefs and that this change correlates significantly with PSG measures of reduced wakefulness and improved sleep efficiency at 6-month follow-up. It has also been demonstrated to aid in discontinuation of benzodiazepines in older insomniacs, with benefits evident for up to 1 year.

Other behaviorally oriented therapies have been adapted for dealing with insomnia, although, unlike the former, they lack long-term efficacy studies. In *systematic desensitization by reciprocal inhibition*, the patient is asked to construct a hierarchy of situations that, in his or her experience, are associated with poor sleep. This preliminary part of the treatment often seems useful in itself, as the insomniac patient's tendency is often to state that the sleep disturbance is not associated in any way with events in his or her life. In the meantime, the patient is taught a basic relaxation technique, such as Jacobsonian muscle relaxation. After the hierarchy is constructed, the patient is asked to visualize the lowest ranking situation associated with poor sleep (e.g., going to bed the night before a trip) and then to pair this visualization with the relaxation response. When this is successful, he or she moves up the ladder to the second least stressful situation, and so on. The goal is to desensitize the patient to these experiences, so that, when they occur, they carry less anxiety.

In passing, it should be mentioned that, when working with the patient to construct the hierarchy and dealing with his or her statement that events in his or her life do not seem associated with poor sleep, a technique sometimes used in the psychotherapy of pain patients can be useful. In the case of pain management, a cancer patient, for instance, says, in effect, "My pain comes from cancer; what can you, as a psychiatrist, do about something like that?" The therapist's response can be to ask the patient whether his or her pain is exactly the same every day or whether it is worse some days, and it is better some days. Typically, a patient agrees that the severity may vary on different days. Then the therapist suggests that "our job, then, is to see what is different about the good days and the bad days." An analogous process can be used when dealing with sleep disturbance.

In *paradoxical intention*, the patient is asked to try not to sleep. As he or she finds out how difficult it is to stay awake intentionally, he or she comes to recognize the potency of homeostatic sleep regulation. The therapist can then suggest to the patient that his or her body will not allow him or her to miss too much sleep. Other techniques focus on breaking up the ruminative thought processes that typically occur while an insomniac lies awake in bed. This is presumably the mechanism by which the old folk remedy of counting sheep may have some benefit. A more formal way of achieving this end is used in *cognitive focusing*, in which the patient prepares in advance a series of reassuring thoughts and images on which he or she is asked to concentrate, should he or she wake up during the night. Other techniques emphasize somatic relaxation, including muscle relaxation procedures, and electromyographic (EMG) biofeedback. In general, their efficacy has been minimal.

RELATIONSHIP BETWEEN DIFFERENT THERAPIES The relation of nonpharmacological and pharmacological approaches for chronic insomnia also needs to be considered. The limited number of studies comparing the two have been inconsistent. Those in favor of nonpharmacological therapy report improvement in 70 to 80 percent of patients and suggest that it takes longer to show benefit initially but that the effects are more durable. Those in favor of medication point to the generally lower cost and also emphasize that, in the major studies of nonpharmacological therapy, only a small number of potential patients screened for the projects agreed to participate in the fairly rigorous programs and that many patients drop out. Indeed, some of the studies showing long-term efficacy of nonpharmacological approaches present data only for those who completed the trial and appeared for follow-up.

Similarly, studies examining the efficacy of combining pharmacological and nonpharmacological treatments have been inconsistent, ranging from those showing potentiation to at least one suggesting that the use of medication may inhibit the effectiveness of behavioral therapies. In the absence of conclusive data, the clinical impression is that the two are not mutually inconsistent and, indeed, may aid each other. For example, if a patient is given a supply of medicine sufficient for use two or three times a week, the therapist may inquire on which nights the patient took the medicine and may try to determine what was different about these days that led the patient to be concerned that he or she might not sleep at night. Similarly, when assessing how deeply a patient slept while using a behavioral technique, the therapist may use the medicine as a kind of benchmark, asking how the night felt in comparison to the medication night. A more conclusive answer as to whether combined therapy is more efficacious than either approach alone awaits the performance of appropriate outcome studies.

Pharmacological Treatments Pharmacological agents for primary insomnia are considered elsewhere in this volume and hence are not discussed in detail here. Some broad comments about their use are in order, however.

USE IN ACUTE VERSUS CHRONIC INSOMNIA Virtually all prescription hypnotics are efficacious for acute insomnias due to upsetting events or change in environment (e.g., a night in the hospital or on a trip). In general, short-acting agents may be more desirable, because they improve sleep on the first night, whereas long-acting agents, such as flurazepam, may not show clear benefit until the second or third night of administration. Hence, most therapeutic issues are with the management of chronic primary insomnia, which is the focus here. In passing, some therapists believe that the use of sedatives or hypnotics after upsetting experiences may not be desirable, because they might prevent the patient from processing the recent events and working through the problems facing him or her. The counterargument has been that, if a patient gets a good night's sleep, he or she may be more alert and effective in dealing with difficulties the next day.

LONG-ACTING VERSUS SHORT-ACTING HYPNOTICS The original benzodiazepine sedative-hypnotics, such as flurazepam, chlordiazepoxide (Librium), and diazepam (Valium), were relatively long-acting agents, with active metabolites showing half-lives of 50 to 100 hours or more. Flurazepam, the first benzodiazepine specifically approved for sleep, rapidly replaced the older barbiturates in the 1970s and is representative of the most widely used agents for the following decade. It came to be recognized, however, that flurazepam and related compounds had several significant limitations, specifically, that they did not reach full potency until the second or third night and that, because of their long half-lives, they also caused daytime sedation. The later introduction of the short-acting triazolam (Halcion) (half-life of 2 to 5 hours) seemed to correct both of these problems, but concerns arose that, along with these benefits, it might have introduced a new difficulty, namely, increased memory disturbance. In addition, it was thought by some to lead to more discontinuation sleep disturbance than the longer-acting agents, which were, in effect, self-tapering. Newer nonbenzodiazepine hypnotics, including zolpidem (half-life of 2.6 hours) and, later, zaleplon (Sonata) (half-life of 1 hour), appear to be relatively free of daytime sedation, act on the first night, and have less significant memory effects. At the time of this writing, the short-acting zolpidem is by far the most widely prescribed prescription hypnotic in the United States. Overall trends for drugs given with the intention of improving sleep, however, show a 10-year decline in prescription hypnotics and an increase in the use of sedating antidepressants.

Unless daytime sedation is specifically desired (as it may be in some cases of insomnia secondary to anxiety), shorter-acting agents are probably the treatments of choice. Their most significant limitation is the transient appearance of discontinuation sleep disturbance with the short-acting benzodiazepines, and even this is ameliorated by giving a half dose for two or three nights before stopping the medication. Another issue that arises is whether the short half-life of zaleplon may make it more desirable, specifically for those cases of insomnia in which the difficulty is primarily in going to sleep, as it has minimal effects on total sleep time. This short duration of action may also lead to new methods of administration, however; it may be useful to give it during the middle of the night when the patient awakens.

LONG-TERM ADMINISTRATION Although chronic insomniacs experience sleep disturbance for months (by definition) and, often, for years, prescription hypnotics are officially recommended for brief periods of time, generally 7 to 10 days. The main concern about long-term use has been that tolerance might develop, a view founded in studies of long-acting benzodiazepines in the 1970s. More recently, a growing body of studies that examine the nonbenzodiazepine zolpidem in nightly use for 6 months has shown no evidence of tolerance, as have open-label studies of zaleplon for as long as 1 year. Eszopiclone, which is under review for approval for clinical use at the time of this writing, has been reported to maintain efficacy for 6 months. If these studies continue to be borne out, it seems likely that the widespread view that hypnotics are effective only in the short term will need to be reconsidered.

ALTERNATIVE ADMINISTRATION STRATEGIES Traditionally, most studies of hypnotics have been based on nightly administration of medicine, although, in practice, many patients take these compounds irregularly. The minimal data that are available, which include use of quazepam (Doral) and triazolam every other night or zolpidem in nonnightly use for 8 weeks, have suggested that these may be viable alternative strategies. The short half-life of zaleplon (1 hour) has led to a new approach in administration as well—the notion that the patient can take the medication when he or she awakens during the night, rather than the traditional approach of taking before bedtime in anticipation of later sleep difficulty. The only caveat to this practice is that, even with the short half-life, it is recommended that the patient take zaleplon only if he or she plans to remain in bed for an additional 4 hours.

ALTERNATIVES TO PRESCRIPTION HYPNOTICS A number of studies have indicated that, although insomniacs infrequently go to their doctors for help, they are a treatment-seeking group. Indeed, as many as 40 percent consume alcohol, over-the-counter (OTC) hypnotics, or both to aid their sleep. The former is undesirable, because it exposes them to the risk of alcohol abuse, and it is relatively ineffective as an oral hypnotic owing to disturbed sleep toward the next morning. The latter, usually *antihistamines*, such as diphenhydramine (Benadryl), have significant daytime sedative properties, may impair daytime functioning, and are relatively ineffective as nighttime hypnotics. In addition to laboratory studies, which are minimal and conflicting, a survey of persons in the community by the Consumer's Union indicated that many fewer considered them "very helpful" compared to those who took prescription hypnotics.

Many insomniacs take *melatonin* and herbal remedies for sleep. Although melatonin has clock-resetting properties that may make it helpful in treating sleep disturbance due to jet lag or irregular sleep cycle disturbances in the blind, its usefulness in primary insomnia is a matter of controversy. Among the few well-controlled laboratory-based studies is one indicating that 1 and 5 mg of melatonin given at 11:30 PM to healthy volunteers had no significant effects, whereas dosing at 6:30 PM, before endogenous secretion occurs, did alter sleep. Higher doses (5 mg) may even disturb sleep and, when given in the daytime, may impair performance on such measures as tracking and reaction time. Its safety also is an issue, particularly its actions at melatonin receptors in the vasculature of the coronary and cerebral arteries. In rats, melatonin has been reported to cause vasoconstriction in the middle cerebral artery and reduced cerebral blood flow. The Consumer's Union study mentioned previously found that persons taking melatonin ranked it "very helpful" much less frequently than prescription hypnotics and gave it the rating "not at all helpful" more frequently than any other treatment.

Valerian derivatives, taken from the root stock of *Valeriana officinalis*, are representative of herbal preparations for sleep. It is listed in pharmacopoeias in some European countries, although, in practice, it is used primarily in folk medicine. There is some rationale for its use, as one of its components, the lignan hydroxypinoresinol, interacts with the benzodiazepine receptor.

Although its use as a sedative goes back to ancient times, actual studies evaluating its benefits are limited and have mixed results. Studies in elderly poor sleepers and psychophysiological insomniacs showed no effects on sleep latency or wake time, although slow wave sleep was increased. A single study of a mixture of valerian extract and hops given to PSG-screened insomniacs showed an improvement in sleep latency, wake time, and sleep efficiency, as well as improved subjective reports, after 2 weeks. On the positive side, there appears to be minimal or no daytime residual effects on several neuropsychological tests. In the last 2 years, a combination of valerian and hops has entered the U.S. marketplace as an OTC sleep agent manufactured by a major pharmaceutical house, and how it will be received remains to be seen.

Antidepressants are often used to aid sleep; the one that is by far the most widely prescribed for this purpose is *trazodone* (Desyrel), the number of prescriptions for which are approximately the same as those for the leading prescription hypnotic, zolpidem. Despite this remarkably widespread use, there are few studies evaluating its possible benefits. A multicenter study found that patients reported that it had some benefits for sleep, although less than those of zolpidem. Two recent sleep laboratory studies found that 100 mg given for one night had no benefits in dysthymic patients complaining of sleep disturbance, although it improved sleep in patients with major depression. Its usefulness may be limited by its side effects, which include aggravation of ventricular arrhythmias, QT interval prolongation, and priapism. Given the limited data about its effectiveness, the reasons behind its widespread use are not entirely clear, although, certainly, ease of prescribing (unlike prescription hypnotics, it is not a class IV restricted agent) may be one factor. *Mirtazapine* (Remeron) is sometimes prescribed for sleep, although its benefits are often offset by daytime sedation. Blood dyscrasias appearing in roughly one in 1,000 patients should also be considered in weighing the risk to benefit ratio of its use in nondepressed patients.

NEW HYPNOTIC COMPOUNDS The last few years have seen the development of various hypnotic compounds that are neither benzodiazepines nor nonbenzodiazepines acting at the $GABA_A$-benzodiazepine receptor. Although none is approved for commercial use at the time of this writing, it seems likely that some will appear in the next few years. Among these compounds are melatonin receptor agonists (the goal of which is to achieve the possibly sedative effects of melatonin with a more desirable side effect profile), neurosteroids, antagonists to serotonin receptor subtypes, and substance P antagonists. New methods of administration, including an intranasal spray of antihistamines, are being considered.

CIRCADIAN RHYTHM SLEEP DISTURBANCES

The presence and consistency of the circadian pacemaker throughout evolution indicate its vital biological functions. In mammals, many tissues have the capability of rhythmic behavior, but the fundamental pacemaker is located in the suprachiasmatic nuclei (SCNs) in the anterior hypothalamus. As described by Charles Czeisler and others, the SCN pacemaker can be considered to have four fundamental characteristics: phase, amplitude, period, and resetting capacity. The latter, in which the inherent rhythmicity of SCN cells is coordinated with external time cues indicating whether it is day or night, is made possible by input from a subset of retinal ganglion cells that use the neuromodulator melanopsin. The output ultimately reaches the pineal gland, where it influences the release of melatonin. The SCN, in turn, is sensitive to melatonin, which decreases its waking signal. Melatonin, discussed previously as a possible sedative-hypnotic, has been hypothesized to have two main functions: resetting the SCN pacemaker with information about daylight and promoting processes associated with sleep. Various aspects of these circadian processes can go awry, resulting in several clinical states that can be manifested as insomnia or hypersomnia.

Delayed Sleep-Phase Syndrome

In delayed sleep-phase syndrome, the circadian system is operating in a delayed, but stable, relationship to the day-night cues of the external world. Hence, a patient complains of being unable to fall asleep until perhaps 2:00 to 3:00 AM, as it is only then that his circadian system is at a point reached by the general population at 11:00 PM to midnight. In the morning, the patient has a difficult time getting up until late morning or complains of hypersomnia in the morning, because it is only then that the circadian system reaches a state that is expressed in most individuals at 8:00 or 9:00 AM. A sleep study begun before midnight shows a long sleep latency (often as long as 2 to 3 hours) but then a relatively normal sleep pattern and total sleep time. The patient often senses that his or her sleep is relatively normal, although altered in timing. Thus, when taking a history, one can say "I know, of course, that you have many constraints on when you can sleep and get up—your job or schoolwork, for instance. But if you could live a life in which you go to bed as late as you like, and get up when you feel ready, do you think your sleep would be okay?" The patient usually says that he or she would do just fine under those circumstances. Similarly, one can ask if there was ever a time in his or her life in which he or she could choose his or her hours of sleep, and, if so, how did he or she do? Often, he or she says, yes, when he or she was in college, he or she would stay up late and sleep late into the morning and felt well and energetic during that period. Many of these patients are drawn to jobs in which they can choose their own hours of sleep and waking, for instance, working from home as freelance computer programmers. For most, however, the constraints of the working world lead to distress.

Originally, delayed sleep-phase syndrome was hypothesized to arise from a decreased ability of the resetting capacity of the pacemaker, such that information from the retina was only partially successful in coordinating the daylight–night signal from the external world with the inherent rhythmicity of the SCN. More recently, the possibility that these are patients with unusually long cycle periods has been suggested. Others focus on the role of the patient's behavior in the genesis of this syndrome.

The first major therapy for delayed sleep-phase syndrome was chronotherapy, in which the patient is instructed to shift his or her hours of sleep and waking progressively later each night, until he or she has moved around the clock to a point at which he or she has a more traditional bedtime. (It may seem paradoxical to ask him or her to use a progressive delay in his or her sleep to adjust to the new earlier bedtime; this is done because it takes advantage of the inherent period of the pacemaker, which is slightly longer than 24 hours.) Once the patient has achieved his or her new earlier bedtime, one has to emphasize the importance of faithfully keeping these new hours; only a few nights of going to bed later can disrupt the newly established pattern. In practice, it is difficult to keep the patient doing this. Many a therapist has heard the patient come in with poor sleep again, giving elaborate explanations as to why he or she had had to stay up late the last several nights (e.g., "my friend in California just got divorced, and she keeps calling me to talk, at all hours"). Indeed, one could speculate that the many reasons patients give for shifting back to a much later bedtime represent logical rationales for obeying a biological impulse. In any event, the difficulty in having a patient move his or her sleep time around the clock and the difficulty in maintaining the new hours led to the quest for new approaches.

An alternative approach for managing delayed sleep-phase syndrome is bright-light therapy. In this case, the patient is exposed to bright artificial light in the early morning. Various commercial fluorescent lights can be used for this purpose, and typical treatments might be 30 minutes or more at 3,000 to 10,000 lux. This results in a phase advance of the pacemaker, such that the sleep–waking signal is reset to more traditional hours. This is a generally benign and effective therapy, although one should be aware of the rare possibility of phototoxicity to retinal receptors, particularly in the macula, or of solar retinopathy.

Advanced Sleep-Phase Syndrome Advanced sleep-phase syndrome is similar in principle to delayed sleep-phase syndrome, except that, in this case, the rhythm of sleep and waking is advanced relative to traditional hours of bedtime and arising. Thus, it is manifest as sleepiness early in the evening and then awakening in the early morning hours with an inability to go back to sleep. It is particularly common in the elderly, who have a phase advance of approximately 1 hour in terms of their temperature and melatonin rhythms. This condition can be treated by administering bright light in the early evening, resulting in a phase delay of the pacemaker, such that the sleep–wake signal is in closer concert with traditional hours for bedtime and arising.

Non–24-Hour Sleep–Wake Cycle In a non–24-hour sleep–wake cycle, a patient may report intermittent insomnia that periodically recurs. It is usually found in blind individuals and results from a complete failure of the resetting mechanism of the pacemaker. The patient then begins to live with a propensity to have a sleep–wake rhythm with the inherent and uncorrected period of the internal pacemaker, approximately 24.15 hours. In a world in which day and night follow a 24.0-hour cycle, this means that the patient's propensity for sleep is constantly shifting forward relative to what would be appropriate to his or her surroundings. The result is that he or she experiences insomnia, which is periodically exacerbated when his or her internal rhythm is most out of phase with the environment and which improves as he or she moves more in phase with his surroundings. Melatonin administration has been demonstrated to be useful in regulating sleep in these individuals.

Shift Work Shift work can induce sleep disturbances, as well as other difficulties, including accidents due to sleepiness during nighttime working hours and, in more extreme cases, a *shift-work syndrome* characterized by GI and cardiovascular disorders. A common experience among night shift workers is to come home in the early morning, to go to bed feeling exhausted, to sleep only 2 to 3 hours, and to awaken feeling unrefreshed but unable to continue sleeping. The treatments for shift work are complex and vary with the type of work schedule (*shift work* is, of course, a general term that can include a wide variety of schedules: fixed work on an evening shift, progressively cycling shifts from day to evening to night shifts, and so on). Various strategies, including napping before going into work in the evening or taking a scheduled nap during nighttime work hours, may be helpful. Using bright light at night and avoiding light during the day have been proposed. It may be helpful, for instance, for a night-shift worker driving home in the morning to wear sunglasses, so as not to get a large light exposure immediately before going to bed. It has been demonstrated that using circadian principles to design industrial work schedules can reduce absenteeism and medical difficulties. Treatment with melatonin has been found to be less successful than timed bright light exposure in aiding adjustment to shift work.

Jet Lag Jet lag sleep disorder is similar to that of shift work in that it represents a dyssynchrony between one's internal sleep–wake rhythm and that of the external world; in this case, however, the dyssynchrony results from rapidly changing one's location to a new environment. After westward travel, one is phase advanced relative to the environment; that is, one wants to go to bed earlier and to get up earlier than what is appropriate for the new location. Eastward travel results in being phase delayed relative to one's surroundings—

the tendency is to stay up later and to get up later than what is needed. A number of strategies have been proposed for dealing with jet lag. One can, for instance, slowly adjust to the new hours before leaving on the trip. Before traveling westward, for instance, one can progressively go to bed later and get up later while still at home. Special diets have been proposed, but their effects seem relatively modest. Maximizing light exposure during the new daytime and minimizing light during the new nighttime are helpful, and there is evidence that timed melatonin administration may aid adjustment. In jet lag and shift work, the use of short-acting hypnotics can aid sleep at the new bedtime, but there is no evidence that this leads to more rapid adjustment to the new time schedule. A number of investigators and pharmaceutical houses are trying to develop chronobiotics, medications that help reset the pacemaker, although none has yet reached the prescription drug market with this indication.

Irregular Sleep–Wake Rhythm Irregular sleep–wake rhythm is characterized by constantly shifting hours of sleepiness and wakefulness. It is generally an affliction of disco aficionados and others who maintain a highly irregular schedule, although it is sometimes seen in persons who have had tumors or other pathology of the hypothalamus. Treatment is organized around altering behavior, encouraging the patient to keep regular hours of bedtime and arising and to avoid napping.

PERIODIC LIMB MOVEMENT SYNDROME

Periodic limb movement syndrome (PLMS) (also known as *nocturnal myoclonus*), along with restless legs syndrome, would be considered to be in the *dyssomnia not otherwise specified* category in terms of the DSM-IV-TR. A patient with PLMS is neurologically normal while awake but, during sleep, manifests periodic stereotyped movements of the limbs (usually the legs). These movements include extension of the toes, as well as flexion of the ankle and knee. The patient is usually unaware that these movements occur, although the bed partner may be only too aware. The result of these events is usually insomnia, although hypersomnia may also appear.

PLMS is associated with renal disease, as well as iron and vitamin B_{12} anemia; some investigators believe that it is exacerbated by tricyclic antidepressants, although there are differing views on this issue. The disorder tends to be a problem of middle age in both sexes, with increasing frequency with advancing age. Childhood cases have been reported, and there is some evidence that it is associated with attention-deficit/hyperactivity disorder (ADHD). It is not clear whether the sleep disruption associated with the movements leads to sleepiness, manifested in children as hyperactivity, or whether both result from a common underlying etiology. Periodic limb movements (PLMs) are commonly seen in sleep studies of narcoleptics. One study found a PLM index of greater than five in 61 percent of obstructive sleep apnea (OSA) patients; the PLMs and the disordered breathing events had different periodicities, however, suggesting that they have different pacemakers. The ultimate etiology is uncertain, although it has been hypothesized that it results from hyperactivity in some areas of the spinal column, particularly in the lumbosacral and cervical segments, triggered by a poorly understood supraspinal sleep-related mechanism. Although most authors emphasize the role of the PLMs in disrupting sleep, others speculate that they are, in fact, responses to sleep that is disturbed for some other reason. This latter view would explain the high frequency of PLMs in narcolepsy, which is characterized by multiple awakenings in nocturnal sleep, and in sleep apnea, in which sleep is disturbed by arousals resulting from disordered breathing events. Others have questioned whether the frequent appearance of PLMs in end-stage renal disease is associated with the sense of disturbed sleep in these patients.

On the PSG, PLMs are 0.5 to 5.0 seconds in duration and occur every 20 to 40 seconds (Fig. 20–1) during periods of NREM sleep. Often, they are accompanied by a K complex or brief arousal signal in the EEG channels of a PSG. Clinicians differ as to whether to count only those that are accompanied by EEG evidence of arousal or to count all PLMs regardless of EEG consequences. A diagnosis of PLMS requires a PLM index of at least five per hour.

The traditional treatment for PLMS has been clonazepam (Klonopin) in doses of 0.5 to 2.0 mg per day. Interestingly, this often brings a subjective sense of improved sleep to the patient but is usu-

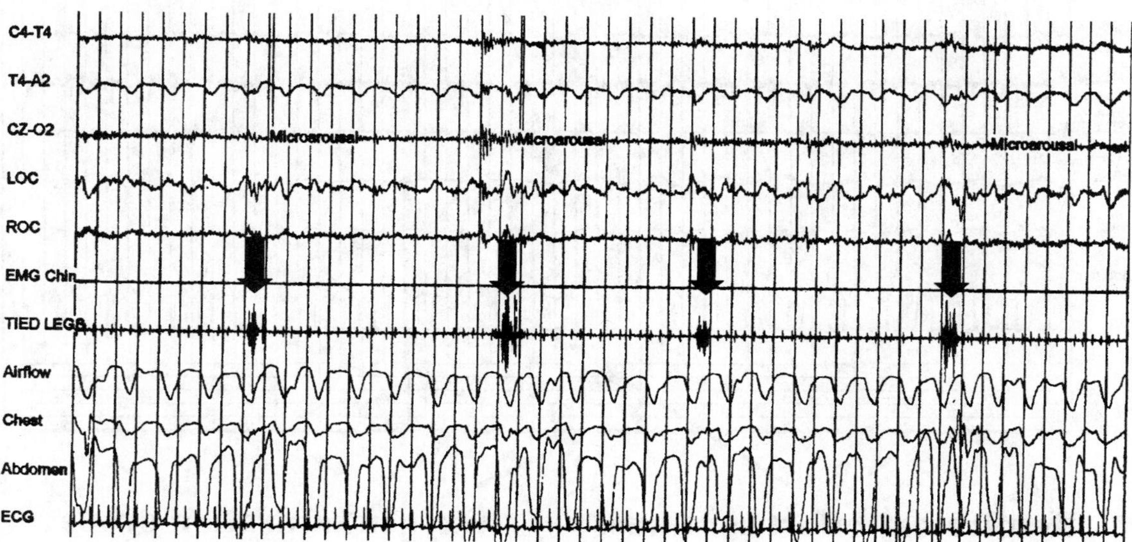

FIGURE 20–1 Example of periodic leg movements (*arrows*) as seen on the polysomnogram. CZ-02, electroencephalogram channel; ECG, electrocardiogram; EMG, electromyogram; LOC, left electrooculogram; ROC, right electrooculogram.

ally not associated with decreased numbers of PLMs on the PSG. This has suggested to some investigators that the mechanism of action of clonazepam may be to decrease the arousal response to the movement. Effectiveness is often limited by the complaint of daytime sedation, which has led many clinicians to administer shorter-acting benzodiazepines. Another approach is to administer low doses of L-dopa (Larodopa), although others are hesitant to do this because of the possibility of bringing out movement disorders or dopaminergic psychosis. Although no specific evidence is known, some clinicians believe that the need for medications is reduced over time if patients enter stress-management programs or similar anxiety-relieving programs.

RESTLESS LIMBS SYNDROME

Restless limbs syndrome (RLS) (also known as *Ekbom syndrome*) is an uncomfortable subjective sensation of the limbs, usually the legs, sometimes described as a "creepy crawly" feeling or as the sensation of ants walking on the skin. It tends to be worse at night, and (in contrast to claudications) is relieved by walking or moving about. It appears as a cause of sleep initiation insomnia, as the patient may find it difficult to lie still in bed, needing to get up to relieve the discomfort. The ultimate cause is unknown, but it appears often in pregnancy, iron or vitamin B_{12} deficiency anemia, and renal disease.

There are no specific findings on the PSG, although one often sees increased movement artifact on the EMG channel before sleep onset. Most patients with RLS also have PLMS, although most patients with PLMS do not have RLS.

The first step in treatment is looking for anemia and treating it, if found. Benzodiazepines are relatively ineffective. The off-label use of L-dopa and carbidopa (Sinemet), bromocriptine (Parlodel), and pergolide (Permax) is often helpful. In rare patients who are severely affected, the off-label use of narcotic analgesics can help when other treatments have been tried and have failed.

SLEEP-DISORDERED BREATHING

Sleep-disordered breathing may present as hypersomnia or insomnia. OSA, the most common and relevant disorder for this chapter, is characterized by periods of functional obstruction of the upper airway during sleep, resulting in decreases in arterial oxygen saturation and a transient arousal, after which respiration (at least briefly) resumes normally. It tends to occur in patients who snore (although the majority of snorers do not have sleep apnea) and results in a sensation that sleep has not been refreshing. Many, although by far not all, patients are overweight, and it appears more frequently in patients with smaller jaws or true micrognathia, acromegaly, and hypothyroidism. Studies of the upper airway suggest that, as a group, these patients have smaller airways than normal sleepers, but there is a great deal of overlap. Medical consequences include cardiac arrhythmias, systemic and pulmonary hypertension, and decreased sexual drive or function. The exact relationship of obesity, OSA, and hypertension is a matter under investigation, some arguing that hypertension is a consequence of OSA, whereas others believe that OSA and hypertension can best be viewed as difficulties arising from a common etiology, including obesity. It tends to be an illness of middle age, primarily in men, but can occur at any age, including children.

On the PSG, episodes of OSA in adults are characterized by multiple periods of at least 10 seconds in duration in which nasal and oral airflow ceases completely (an apnea) or partially (a hypopnea), while the abdominal and chest expansion leads indicate continuing efforts of the diaphragm and accessory muscles of respiration to move air through the obstruction (Fig. 20–2). The arterial oxygen

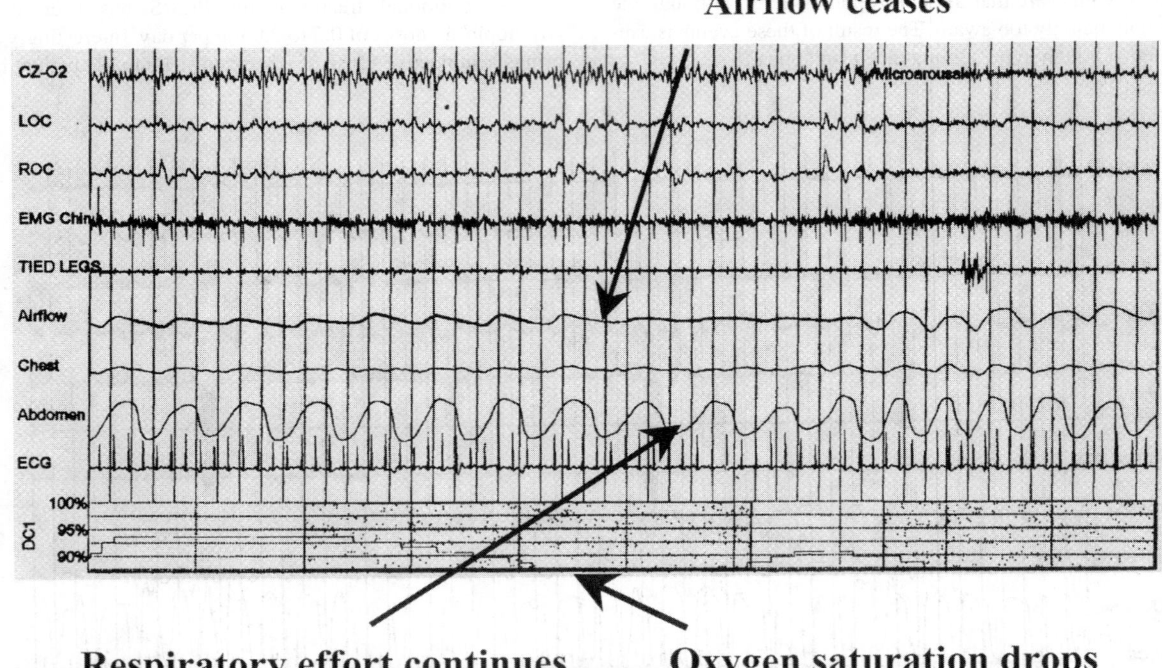

FIGURE 20–2 Example of an obstructive sleep apnea event on the polysomnogram. CZ-O2, electroencephalogram channel; ECG, electrocardiogram; EMG, electromyogram; LOC, left electrooculogram; ROC, right electrooculogram.

saturation drops, and, often, there is a bradycardia that may be accompanied by other arrhythmias, such as premature ventricular contractions. At the end, an arousal reflex takes place, seen as a waking signal and possibly as a motor artifact on the EEG channels. At this moment, sometimes called the *breakthrough*, the patient can be observed making brief restless movements in bed. The patient then returns to sleep, with normal respirations. These events can occur in NREM or REM sleep, the former usually more frequent, the latter usually more severe. Different laboratories require different numbers of events to make a diagnosis, usually five or ten disordered breathing events per hour of sleep. Many laboratories use a scale of the number of disordered breathing events per hour to classify OSA as mild, moderate, or severe. Such a classification based solely on the frequency of events may be less helpful than first supposed, as the true severity should include consideration of the degree of arterial oxygen saturation, the presence or absence of cardiac arrhythmias, and other factors.

Central sleep apnea (CSA), which tends to occur in the elderly, results from periodic failure of central nervous system (CNS) mechanisms that stimulate breathing. The original teaching was that OSA results in a complaint of excessive sleepiness, whereas CSA is manifest as insomnia, but later case series have emphasized that either symptom may appear in either disorder. The PSG features of CSA are similar to those of OSA, except that, during the periods of apnea, a cessation of respiratory effort is seen in the abdominal and chest expansion leads.

Several features of OSA and CSA are significant in psychiatric practice. These include decreased ability to concentrate, decreased libido, memory complaints, and deficits in neuropsychological testing. Many or even most patients have dysthymic features, and, although many patients manifest OSA and major depression, it is not certain that this occurs more often than would be seen by chance. One study has indicated that, among OSA patients, those with a history of treatment for affective disorder show greater decrements in ventilatory measurements. Although systematic data are minimal, many clinicians have the impression that, in cases of refractory depression, if OSA is found and treated, the depressive symptoms may improve. Neuropsychological testing indicates that most, but not all, deficits can be relieved by treatment.

Patients sometimes awaken from apneas with a sensation of being unable to breathe, and these episodes need to be distinguished from nocturnal panic attacks. In taking a history, it should be noted that perhaps one-third of patients with daytime panic attacks also have these episodes during sleep, but it is rare to have panic attacks purely at night. Similar awakenings can occur in cases of paradoxical vocal cord movement, but, in this situation, there is usually a history of trauma or surgery of the neck. Sleep apnea episodes also need to be distinguished from nocturnal laryngospasm, in which patients report that they are unable to speak or can only whisper for a few minutes after awakening.

Another reason for awareness of sleep-disordered breathing in psychiatric practice is that patients who complain of insomnia and who have unrecognized OSA may develop respiratory depression if given most traditional hypnotics. The benzodiazepines have such mild respiratory depressant qualities that their effects are clinically insignificant in persons with normal ventilation; on the other hand, they can significantly exacerbate OSA and other ventilatory disorders. This appears to be particularly true of the longer-acting agents. Studies of short-acting agents have been mixed, and one study even suggested slight improvement in CSA. The newer nonbenzodiazepines appear to share these respiratory depressant qualities, although in milder form. The important thought to keep in mind is that, if a patient with sleep disturbance appears oversedated in the daytime after being given a hypnotic, there should be at least two considerations: (1) that this represents daytime residual sedation as a direct effect of the drug or (2) that the drug has exacerbated previously unrecognized sleep apnea. When a sedative is needed for patients with sleep apnea, one can give low doses of sedating tricyclic antidepressants (an off-label use), as they do not suppress respiration and may have mild stimulatory effects. When a daytime anxiolytic is desired, it should be noted that buspirone (BuSpar) does not appear to adversely affect respiration.

In addition to OSA and CSA, some patients are found to have mixed-type apneas, in which the early part of the disordered breathing event appears central in nature (i.e., there is an absence of respiratory effort), whereas the latter part of the event appears obstructive. Clinically, there is little or no difference between what is seen in this form and what is seen in OSA. Upper airway resistance syndrome (UARS) is an interesting condition in which the patient manifests the sleepiness, fatigue, and other features of OSA, but the PSG fails to reveal specific apneic events. More elaborate testing with measures of intraesophageal pressure (a surrogate for intrapleural pressure) reveals that, owing to increased upper airway resistance, the patient must generate much greater negative pressures to produce airflow. Treatment with continuous positive airway pressure (CPAP) has been shown to improve daytime alertness and other symptoms.

The major treatments for OSA are CPAP and surgical approaches. CPAP is performed by administering room air at low pressures (usually less than 15 cm of water pressure) through a nasal mask or small cushioned nasal cannulae during sleep. It is remarkably effective acutely and has the advantage of sparing the patient from a surgical procedure, although it carries the disadvantage that it must be used for long periods of time, or even the lifetime of the patient. A Belgian study has indicated that 70 to 80 percent of patients who try CPAP accept it, and 90 percent of them (usually those who derive subjective benefit initially) continue to use it in the long term. Devices that automatically titrate and deliver the correct pressure have been developed; initial data indicate that they may be better tolerated, although the degree of improvement in daytime sleepiness is approximately the same as for conventional CPAP. Minor complications of CPAP include irritation of the eyes from air leaks around the mask and nasal dryness or congestion. In rare cases, pneumomediastinum or pneumocephalus can occur. Alternative devices for treating OSA include tongue-retaining devices or systems for advancing the mandible. Their effectiveness remains under investigation.

The original surgical treatment for OSA was chronic tracheotomy, which is extremely effective (and may be the gold standard of effectiveness). The concerns, of course, are that it is, in some senses, a disfiguring procedure, that it requires maintenance, and that it can have complications, such as infection. Later, a modified procedure, the uvulopalatopharyngoplasty (UPPP) was developed, in which portions of the uvula and soft palate are removed and the upper airway is widened. Its advantage is that (if successful) it is a one-time procedure (in contrast to the continuing need to use CPAP), but its disadvantage is that it is a major surgical procedure requiring hospitalization and a certain amount of initial discomfort. More importantly, even in the best of surgical hands, the success rate, in the range of 60 to 70 percent, is much lower than that of CPAP. Rare complications can include changes in the voice and nasal regurgitation of liquids when swallowing. A number of more sophisticated surgical approaches, including mandibular advancement or selective widening of specific portions of the airway, are performed as well, although selection procedures to determine which patient is likely to benefit from which procedure are still under investigation. For patients with snoring without sleep apnea, an outpatient laser-based technique (laser-assisted uvuloplasty [LAUP]) is available.

Medical remedies for sleep apnea are of limited benefit and probably should be considered treatments of second choice. Perhaps the best studied is off-label use of protriptyline (Vivactil), 5 to 20 mg, which decreases REM sleep (which is usually associated with the more severe apneas) and increases genioglossus muscle tone. Its benefits are often limited by its anticholinergic side effects. Low doses of medroxyprogesterone acetate (Provera) (again, an off-label use) may have beneficial effects, although, in rare cases, apneas may be exacerbated owing to uneven stimulation of the diaphragm and accessory muscles of respiration. Other compounds that have been tried experimentally but are less widely used are the off-label use of fluoxetine (Prozac) and buspirone. Low-flow nasal oxygen has had mixed results; it is generally of little benefit in uncomplicated sleep apnea, although it is indicated in cases of apnea complicating other respiratory conditions.

In addition to these specific procedures, a number of general precautions and behavioral interventions should be used in all patients. Certainly, weight loss should be encouraged in all obese patients, and, in extreme cases, gastric surgical procedures can be considered. Significant weight loss can widen the upper airway and can lead to proportionate reduction in required CPAP pressure. The patient should be encouraged to learn not to sleep on his or her back and to avoid alcohol and drugs that are respiratory depressants. He or she should be cautioned about driving, as OSA patients have been found to have a higher rate of automobile accidents.

NARCOLEPSY

Narcolepsy is a condition characterized by excessive sleepiness, as well as auxiliary symptoms that represent the intrusion of aspects of REM sleep into the waking state. It typically begins in the teens or 20s but can occur earlier or later. Once it appears, it is a lifelong condition. The sleep attacks of narcolepsy represent episodes of irresistible sleepiness, leading to perhaps 10 to 20 minutes of sleep, after which the patient feels refreshed, at least briefly. In helping separate sleep attacks from daytime sleepiness of other causes, it is helpful to ask about episodes of sleep that have appeared at unusual or inappropriate times, for instance, during intense conversations or sex. In addition to sleep attacks, patients develop one or more additional symptoms, usually over the course of the next few years after the appearance of the sleepiness. The most common of these is *cataplexy*, the sudden onset of weakness of the weight-bearing muscles, lasting for a minute or less and occurring in association with the expression of emotion, such as anger or laughter. (Cataplexy should be distinguished from catalepsy, the waxy flexibility of the limbs in catatonic schizophrenia.) Cataplectic episodes may be as mild as a sudden sensation of needing to sit down or may be so severe that the patient collapses helplessly to the ground. Often, the patient remains awake during the episode, although visual hallucinations may appear in longer ones lasting more than 1 minute. Other symptoms include sleep paralysis or hypnagogic hallucinations. The former is characterized by a brief period of paralysis that occurs as the patient is drifting off to sleep or awakening in the morning. Hypnagogic hallucinations are vivid dream-like experiences that occur when the patient is drifting off to sleep or is in the process of awakening in the morning (hypnopompic hallucinations). Sleep paralysis and hypnagogic hallucinations can be accompanied by a sensation of a weight on the chest and anxiety. Their appearance in narcolepsy, in combination with sleep attacks and cataplexy, should be distinguished from occasional episodes in the absence of daytime sleepiness, which can occur as isolated events in persons without narcolepsy. Some patients describe episodes that are suggestive of automatic behavior, in which they have done inexplicable things, such as putting dishes in the clothes washer, for which they have no memory. These probably represent actions taken during a period of sleepiness, which are not later recalled. Finally, and somewhat paradoxically, these sleepy individuals typically complain of difficulty with nighttime sleep, which is characterized by frequent awakenings.

On the PSG, sleep is indeed disturbed, with frequent arousals, and, often, there are significant numbers of periodic leg movements. The diagnosis is made from a specialized daytime sleep recording, the MSLT, in which a patient is given four or five opportunities to sleep for as long as 20 minutes, at 2-hour intervals across the day. The mean time to fall asleep is calculated, and it is determined whether the patient has marked sleepiness (usually defined as a mean sleep latency of less than 5 minutes). In addition to sleepiness, however, during these naps, the narcoleptic patient typically shows two or more episodes of REM sleep, a phenomenon that is unlikely in other conditions of excessive sleepiness. This observation of *REM onset sleep* is diagnostic, as well as suggestive, of the pathophysiology of narcolepsy, which appears to involve the intrusion of aspects of REM sleep (muscle atonia and dreams) into wakefulness. Hence, cataplexy and sleep paralysis can be seen as representing the atonia that occurs in REM, whereas hypnagogic hallucinations may be an expression of the dreaming that is characteristic of REM.

Although there is some understanding of this dysregulation of REM sleep in narcolepsy, the underlying pathophysiology is still being investigated. An association with certain genetic human leukocyte antigen (HLA) markers has been found, but these can also occur in asymptomatic individuals. The child of a narcoleptic is approximately 20 times more likely to have narcolepsy than the general population, but there is no simple Mendelian mode of transmission. Recent work suggests that the sleepiness of narcolepsy may result from abnormalities in the function of the neuromodulator orexin/hypocretin in the hypothalamus. Occasional cases of a narcolepsy-like condition (secondary narcolepsy) have been reported in patients with various CNS pathologies, including children with suprasellar tumors and hypothalamic obesity.

The medical treatment of narcolepsy is oriented to the target symptoms. For the sleepiness, the traditional treatment has been the use of stimulants, such as amphetamines. Tolerance may appear, and some clinicians believe that the use of weekly drug holidays decreases its likelihood. More recently, modafinil (Provigil) has been found to increase wakefulness, while demonstrating a more benign side effect profile than the traditional analeptics. Cataplexy is usually responsive to the tricyclic antidepressants. In this off-label use, compounds such as imipramine are given in much lower doses than are used for depression, for example, 50 mg, and the patient often shows improvement within one or two nights. Other tricyclics, such as protriptyline, and selective serotonin reuptake inhibitors (SSRIs), such as fluoxetine, may benefit cataplexy in this off-label use.

In addition to medical treatments, a number of behavioral and educational interventions are important in managing narcolepsy. Because patients often awaken refreshed from brief naps, it is helpful to work with the patient, employer, or both to arrange for periods of scheduled sleep during the day. Symptoms are usually exacerbated during sleep deprivation, which should be avoided. The consequences of narcolepsy are such that patients have often not achieved as much in life as their intelligence and drive might otherwise have produced; often, they have been told by teachers and employers that they are lazy, when, in fact, they are pathologically sleepy. Not surprisingly, these experiences can lead to poor self-esteem, which can further inhibit the patient's ability to achieve. Hence, education about the disorder and reassurance, for the patient and family, can be important.

Many patients with narcolepsy are dysthymic. In contrast, a number of clinicians comment on the simultaneous occurrence of major depression and narcolepsy, but population studies indicate that these are common illnesses, and their coexistence appears no more often than would be expected by chance. In psychiatric practice, it is also important to distinguish between hypnagogic hallucinations and visual hallucinations from other causes and to consider narcolepsy in the differential diagnosis when hearing about a patient who exhibits episodes that are suggestive of automatic behavior.

IDIOPATHIC HYPERSOMNIA

Idiopathic hypersomnia is a condition characterized by excessive sleepiness and naps from which the patient does not awaken refreshed. The MSLT confirms significant sleepiness, without evidence of REM onset sleep episodes. Nocturnal sleep studies show no characteristic pattern, although slow wave sleep may sometimes be elevated. It usually begins in young adulthood and becomes a chronic condition lasting a lifetime. Some cases appear to be familial and are associated with specific HLA antigens, whereas others begin after viral infections, and a residual group develops these symptoms but has neither family history nor postviral status. Treatment is empirical, usually involving use of amphetamines or other psychostimulants. There are also *recurrent hypersomnias* that appear in distinct episodes weeks apart. An example of these is Kleine-Levin syndrome, usually found in male adolescents and characterized by periods of sleepiness and excessive eating.

PARASOMNIAS

Parasomnias, abnormal behaviors during sleep, are often divided into forms associated with slow wave sleep or REM sleep. The former includes sleep terror and sleepwalking disorder, whereas the latter includes nightmare disorder and REM behavior disorder.

Sleep Terrors

Sleep terrors are episodes in which a child awakens confused and upset, with marked autonomic stimulation seen clinically as rapid pulse and diaphoresis. There is no report of dreaming, and, eventually, the seemingly inconsolable child returns to sleep, with no memory of the event in the morning. The PSG shows that these episodes appear out of slow wave sleep, and the overall night may have hypersynchronous delta activity. Sleep terrors can occur in as much as 3 percent of children and tend to go away in adolescence.

Sleepwalking Disorder

Sleepwalking disorder tends to occur between 4 to 8 years of age and, like night terrors, tends to dissipate in adolescence. Episodes occur out of slow wave sleep; during them, patients appear confused and disoriented. In rare cases, they may become violent if aroused, but, usually, they can be guided back to bed. This benign condition needs to be distinguished from the rarer, but more clinically significant, problem of nocturnal seizures. Although a clinical EEG is the ultimate way of distinguishing these two disorders, some features of the history are of help: (1) Patients with sleepwalking usually return to bed, whereas those with seizure disorder may awaken in the morning in another room. (2) Although it is good practice to help protect sleepwalkers from accidental harm, they rarely injure themselves; in contrast, the patient with seizure disorder may have a history of falling down the stairs or walking into a window. (3) The sleepwalker can usually be guided back to bed, whereas the seizure patient is not responsive to guidance during the episode.

If an episode is captured on the polygraph, it is seen as an awakening and motor artifact appearing during slow wave sleep. If a patient with night terrors or sleepwalking does not have an episode during a particular sleep recording, one suggestive piece of evidence is the presence of arousals out of slow wave sleep, which are fairly uncommon in the absence of a parasomnia.

Night terrors and sleepwalking are benign conditions, and treatment consists primarily of educating and reassuring the parents. Although both can be exacerbated by periods of stress or sleep deprivation, in childhood, neither is associated with psychiatric illness. Some cases of sleepwalking may be induced by medication. Medical intervention is rarely needed for typical night terrors or sleepwalking. In difficult cases, some clinicians try the off-label use of benzodiazepine sedatives, which decrease slow wave sleep.

Nightmares

Nightmares are vivid dreams that become progressively more anxiety producing, ultimately resulting in an awakening. They can occur occasionally in as much as one-half of children in the range of 3 to 6 years of age. In contrast to night terrors, the child is not confused, does not exhibit the massive autonomic signs, and describes having had a scary dream. Nightmares in children are not associated with psychiatric illness; in contrast, approximately one-half of the roughly 1 percent of adults who experience frequent nightmares are found to have disorders, including borderline personality and schizophrenia. Nightmares are sometimes brought out by REM-suppressing drugs, in which case, the treatment is to gradually discontinue the medication, if possible. Some authors suggest that nightmares occur more frequently in persons with certain personality traits, including those with thin boundaries and more creative individuals. There is no widely accepted medical intervention.

REM Behavior Disorder

REM behavior disorder is characterized by episodes of complex, often violent, behavior and is thought to represent a patient acting out his or her dreams. It is more common in older men, and there is often a history of a small stroke or other CNS insult in the last months or year. It may also appear as an early event in the evolution of Parkinson's disease. If an episode is captured on the polygraph, it shows motor artifact appearing out of REM sleep. If a patient with REM behavior disorder does not have an episode while in the laboratory, the sleep study may show a failure of the normal hypotonia of the weight-bearing muscles during REM sleep. In cats, a syndrome that is suggestive of REM behavior disorder can be induced by lesions of the areas surrounding the locus ceruleus, a brainstem noradrenergic center. The initial view was that the clinical disorder represents a malfunction of the descending pathway to the spinal cord, which produces atonia during REM; its prevalence in the elderly and in parkinsonian patients has suggested that there may be a more complex etiology involving alteration of function in pontine areas, including the nucleus pedunculopontine, where integration of sleep–wake regulation with locomotor systems takes place. The most widely used treatment for REM behavior disorder is the off-label administration of clonazepam.

Sleep Disturbances in Psychiatric Disorders

Sleep disturbances in psychiatric disorders are described in the chapters of this volume devoted to the specific disorders. Several epidemiological studies have pointed to the association of insomnia and psychiatric disorder; indeed, one suggests that if a person with no known illness complains of insomnia at initial interview and does so again at 1-year follow-up, he or she is almost 40 times as likely as the general population to have a diagnosable psychiatric disorder. In the sleep center setting, approximately one-third of persons coming in complaining of insomnia are found to have a psychiatric disorder, which is major depression in approximately one-half the cases. There are also several studies indicating that affectively normal insomniacs have a much higher rate of subsequently developing major depression in the next several years. It is not yet known whether therapeutic interventions for the insomnia will reduce this increased risk.

Perhaps 80 percent of patients with major depression complain of insomnia. Roughly 10 percent of depressed patients describe hypersomnia, and this usually represents those with atypical or bipolar depression. Sleep studies in major depression reveal some combination of prolonged sleep latency, shortened total sleep, and increased arousals during the night. Slow wave sleep is usually reduced. In addition, a number of features of REM sleep are characteristic: (1) The first REM episode often occurs 60 minutes or less after sleep onset (a *short REM latency*), substantially earlier than the roughly 90- to 110-minute REM latency seen in asymptomatic normal young adults; (2) instead of the normal progression in duration of REM episodes across the night, they are all of roughly equal length; and (3) the first REM episode may have a particularly high number of eye movements. The short REM latency has been interpreted by some to be a biological marker of depression. The underlying pathophysiology behind the short REM latency is not clear. Possible interpretations are that it is a consequence of heightened sensitivity of muscarinic cholinergic receptors, that it represents an altered ratio of cholinergic activity to adrenergic activity in the brainstem, or that it is a consequence of a possibly phase-advanced oscillator in the circadian regulatory system.

A number of investigators have suggested that sleep disturbance is more than an epiphenomenon resulting from depression and may instead be involved in its genesis. Support for this notion comes from the observation that several manipulations of sleep (total or partial sleep deprivation or REM sleep deprivation) represent potent (although time consuming and not always practical) treatments for depression. In treating the sleep disturbance in depressed patients, several therapeutic options are available. One approach is to change to a more sedating antidepressant, for instance, from imipramine (Tofranil) to amitriptyline (Elavil). Among the SSRIs and newer mixed-action agents, this could be done by changing, for instance, from fluoxetine or paroxetine (Paxil) to the sedating mirtazapine. (In using the latter, however, one should be aware of the rare, but potentially serious, blood dyscrasias that can appear.) If an antidepressant is of clinical benefit but disturbs sleep, as can happen with fluoxetine, some clinicians add low doses of trazodone, although, in rare cases, confusional states can result. There are some data to suggest that initially adding the newer nonbenzodiazepine hypnotics to the antidepressant regimen can give symptomatic relief for the depressed patient's poor sleep, although this issue is still under investigation.

Posttraumatic Stress Disorder Posttraumatic stress disorder (PTSD) patients typically describe poor sleep, and, indeed, the DSM-IV-TR incorporates two aspects (nightmares and a hyperarousal state manifested as insomnia) in the diagnostic criteria. A study of car accident victims suggests that those who have persistent insomnia and daytime sleepiness for months after the trauma are more likely to later develop PTSD. Many patients complain of difficulty initiating and maintaining sleep, and some have anxiety dreams. Increased REM density and elevated arousal thresholds from REM have been reported. In general, however, laboratory findings have been inconsistent, and interpretation is complicated by not fully considering comorbid psychiatric conditions. Clinically, many of these patients also have major depression and are receiving various antidepressants. There are some data to suggest that the off-label use of the anticonvulsant gabapentin (Neurontin) or the α_1-adrenergic antagonist prazosin (Minipress) may improve their sleep.

SUGGESTED CROSS-REFERENCES

The basic science of sleep is discussed in Section 1.20. Mood disorders are covered in Chapter 13, and anxiety disorders are discussed in Chapter 14. Light therapy, sleep deprivation, and sleep delay are discussed in Section 31.32, and sleep disorders among the elderly are discussed in Section 51.3b.

REFERENCES

Antrobus J. Theories of dreaming. In: Kryger MH, Roth T, Dement WC, eds. *Principles and Practice of Sleep Medicine.* Philadelphia: WB Saunders; 2000:472–481.

Baillargeon L, Landreville P, Verreault R, Beauchemin JP, Gregoire JP, Morin CM: Discontinuation of benzodiazepines among older insomniac adults treated with cognitive-behavioural therapy combined with gradual tapering: A randomized trial. *CMAJ.* 2003;169:1015–1020.

Bassiri AG, Guilleminault C. Clinical features and evaluation of obstructive sleep apnea-hypopnea syndrome. In: Kryger MH, Roth T, Dement WC, eds. *Principles and Practice of Sleep Medicine.* Philadelphia: WB Saunders; 2000:869–878.

Bootzin RR: Stimulus control treatment for insomnia. *Proceedings of the 80th Annual Convention of the American Psychological Association.* 1972;7:395–396.

Capsoni S, Stankov BM, Fraschini F: Reduction of regional cerebral blood flow by melatonin in young rats. *Neuroreport.* 1995;6:1346–1348.

Consumers Union: Overcoming insomnia. *Consumer Report.* 1997;62:10–13.

Czeisler CA, Duffy JF, Shanahan TL, Brown EN, Mitchell JF, Rimmer DW, Ronda JM, Silva EJ, Allan JS, Emens JS, Dijk D-J, Kronauer RE: Stability, precision, and near-24-hour period of the human circadian pacemaker. *Science.* 1999;284:2177–2181.

Dawson D, Van Den Heuvel CJ: Integrating the actions of melatonin on human physiology. *Ann Med.* 1998;30:95–102.

Gillin JC, Dow BM, Thompson P, Parry B, Tandon R, Benca R: Sleep in depression and other psychiatric disorders. *Clin Neurosci.* 1993;1:90–96.

Hobson JA, Stickgold R, Pace-Schott EF: The neuropsychology of REM sleep dreaming. *Neuroreport.* 1998;9:R1–R14.

*James SP, Mendelson WB: Herbal preparations for sleep. *Sleep Hypnosis.* (*in press*).

James SP, Mendelson WB: The use of trazodone as a clinical hypnotic: A critical review. *J Clin Psychiatry.* (*in press*).

Krystal A, Walsh J, Roth T, Amato DA: The sustained efficacy and safety of eszopiclone over six months of nightly treatment: A placebo-controlled study in patients with chronic insomnia. *Sleep.* 2003;26[Suppl]:A310.

Mendelson WB. *Human Sleep: Research and Clinical Care.* New York: Plenum Press; 1987:1–436.

*Mendelson WB. Do studies of sedative/hypnotics suggest the nature of chronic insomnia? In: Montplaisir J, Godbout R, eds. *Sleep and Biological Rhythms: Basic Mechanisms and Applications to Psychiatry.* New York: Oxford University Press; 1990: 209–218.

Mendelson WB. Drugs which alter sleep and sleep-related respiration. In: Kuna ST, ed. *Sleep and Respiration in Aging Adults.* New York: Elsevier Science; 1991:49–54.

*Mendelson WB: Effects of flurazepam and zolpidem on the perception of sleep in insomniacs. *Sleep.* 1995;18:92–96.

Mendelson WB: The relationship of sleepiness and blood pressure to respiratory variables in obstructive sleep apnea. *Chest.* 1995;108:966–972.

Mendelson WB: Are periodic leg movements associated with clinical sleep disturbance? *Sleep.* 1996;19:219–223.

Mendelson WB. Hypnotics: Basic mechanisms and pharmacology. In: Kryger MH, Roth T, Dement WC, eds. *Principles and Practice of Sleep Medicine.* Philadelphia: WB Saunders; 2000:407–413.

Mendelson WB. Insomnia. In: *Conn's Current Therapy.* Philadelphia: WB Saunders; 2001:31–34.

Mendelson WB, Caruso C. Pharmacology in sleep medicine. In: Poceta JS, Mitler MM, eds. *Sleep Disorders: Diagnosis and Treatment.* Totowa, NJ: Humana Press; 1998:137–160.

Mendelson WB, Garnett D, Gillin JC, Weingartner H: The experience of insomnia and daytime and nighttime functioning. *Psychiatr Res.* 1984;12:235–250.

*Mendelson WB, James SP, Garnett D, Sack D, Rosenthal NE: A psychophysiological study of insomnia. *Psychiatr Res.* 1986;19:267–284.

Monroe LJ: Psychological and physiological differences between good and poor sleepers. *J Abnorm Psychol.* 1967;72:255–264.

*Morin CM, Culbert JP, Schwartz SM: Nonpharmacological interventions for insomnia: A meta-analysis of treatment efficacy. *Am J Psychiatry.* 1994;151:1172–1180.

Morin CM, Rodrigue S, Ivers H: Role of stress, arousal, and coping skills in primary insomnia. *Psychosom Med.* 2003;65:259–267.

Pelayo R, Guilleminault C. Narcolepsy and excessive daytime sleepiness. In: Poceta JS, Mitler MM, eds. *Sleep Disorders: Diagnosis and Treatment.* Totowa, NJ: Humana Press; 1998:95–116.

Provini F, Vetrugno R, Meletti S, Plazzi G, Solieri L, Lugaresi E, Coccagna G: Motor pattern of periodic limb movements during sleep. *Neurology.* 2001;57:300–304.

Ray JD. Cults. In: Redford DB, ed. *The Ancient Gods Speak.* Oxford, UK: Oxford University Press; 2002:61–91.

Schweitzer PK, Walsh JK: Ten-year trends in the pharmacologic treatment of insomnia. *Sleep.* 1998;21:247(abst).

Spielman AJ, Saskin P, Thorpy MJ: Treatment of chronic insomnia by restriction of time in bed. *Sleep.* 1987;10:45–56.

Stone BM, Turner C, Mills SL, Nicholson AN: Hypnotic activity of melatonin. *Sleep.* 2000;23:663–669.

Turek FW, Dugovic C, Zee PC: Current understanding of the circadian clock and the clinical implications for neurological disorders. *Arch Neurol.* 2001;58:1781–1787.

21 Impulse-Control Disorders Not Elsewhere Classified

HARVEY ROY GREENBERG, M.D.

The category of *impulse-control disorders, not elsewhere specified,* includes impulse-related conditions that are not subsumed under other diagnostic categories in the revised fourth edition of the *Diagnostic and Statistical Manual of Mental Disorders* (DSM-IV-TR). The expansion of this chapter over earlier discussions in *Kaplan and Sadock's Comprehensive Textbook of Psychiatry* reflects an increasing awareness that these disorders, taken together, account for a substantial proportion of psychiatric illnesses.

The feature common to this group is the repeated inability to resist an intense impulse, drive, or temptation to perform a particular act that is obviously harmful to self or others, or both. Before the event, the individual usually experiences mounting tension and arousal, sometimes—but not consistently—mingled with conscious anticipatory pleasure.

Completing the action brings immediate gratification and relief. Within a variable time afterward, the individual experiences a conflation of remorse, guilt, self-reproach, and dread. These feelings may stem from obscure unconscious conflicts or awareness of the deed's impact on others (including the possibility of serious legal consequences in syndromes such as kleptomania). Shameful secretiveness about the repeated impulsive activity frequently expands to pervade the individual's entire life, often significantly delaying treatment.

Sigmund Freud declared that artists discovered the Oedipus complex long before psychoanalysis. Analogously, powerful portraits of impulse-ridden personalities were drawn by Sophocles and William Shakespeare, long before 19th century French psychiatrist Jean-Etienne Esquirol described patients whose irresistible impulsiveness demonstrated "all the features of passion, elevated to the point of delirium." Since Esquirol, maladies of impulse control have eluded definitive classification—let alone effective means of treatment.

In contemporary nosology, the category of *impulse-control disorders not elsewhere classified* entered the third edition of the DSM (DSM-III) in 1980. By DSM-IV-TR, this basket of syndromes has been expanded to encompass pathological gambling, trichotillomania, kleptomania, intermittent explosive disorder, pyromania, and impulse-control disorders not otherwise specified. The latter addresses syndromes waiting in the wings for definitive inclusion or exclusion.

The category of *habit and impulse disorder* in the 1992 tenth edition of the *International Statistical Classification of Diseases and Related Health Problems* (ICD-10) (Table 21–1) is analogous to the DSM-IV-TR's *impulse-control disorders, not elsewhere specified.* Intermittent explosive disorder is not mentioned per se in the ICD-10 schema. Habitual use of alcohol or drugs, as well as addictive or otherwise pathological sexual and eating disorders, is specifically excluded.

The ICD-10's habit and impulse disorders are characterized by repeated acts with no clear rational motive that cannot be controlled by the patient and are usually harmful to the interests of self and others. ICD-10 states the causes of these conditions are unknown, further asserting that they are only grouped together because of broad descriptive similarities, "not because they are known to share any other important features."

Over the past several decades, numerous studies have probed the complex phenomenology and etiology of the impulse-control disorders. Considerable progress has been made in conceptualization and treatment. Diverse, apparently disparate, conditions are now widely believed to have common epidemiological, genetic, psychological, neurobiological, and therapeutic features. These are shared not only within the group, but often with other serious psychiatric illnesses (notably depressive and addictive disease) as well. Interconnections are complex and vary enormously from one impulse-ridden patient to another.

The blurring of diagnostic boundaries between impulse-control disorders and other Axis I and Axis II conditions is often cited in the literature and regularly challenges the clinician. Studies suggest that a significantly high comorbidity exists between the impulse-control disorders, substance abuse disorders, affective disorders, obsessive-compulsive disorder (OCD), and obsessive-compulsive personality disorder. Other important comorbid conditions include borderline personality, antisocial personality, and narcissistic personality disorders; one or another type of pathological aggression; attention-deficit disorder; eating disorders; and paraphilias.

From a genetic perspective, family histories of individuals with impulse-control problems are replete with depression, bipolarity, substance abuse, and personality disorders. *Mutatis mutandis*, the family trees of patients with the latter problems often reveal a statistically meaningful presence of one or another impulse-control disorders.

Neurobiological research suggests that compromised frontal lobe function may contribute to the disinhibition of some impulse-disordered patients. Similarities in serotoninergic and other neurotransmitter dysregulation have also been discovered across the entire spectrum of impulse disorders. Improvement with selective serotonin reuptake inhibitors (SSRIs), mood regulators, and opioid antagonists points to common neurobiological attributes between the impulse-control syndromes, which are variably displayed in their comorbid illnesses.

From a behavioral and cognitive viewpoint, whatever the other origins of impulse-control disorders may be, the frequent repetition of impulsive behavior *sui generis* is regarded as a major cause of its installation within the psyche. Behavioral strategies useful in treating substance abuse disorders and obsessional states have been applied to a gamut of impulsive behaviors with reasonable success.

Given this intricate web of intersections in etiology and treatment, researchers have attempted to ascertain some "figure in the

Table 21–1
ICD-10 Diagnostic Criteria for Habit and Impulse Disorders

Pathological gambling

A. Two or more episodes of gambling occur over a period of at least 1 year.

B. These episodes do not have a profitable outcome for the individual but are continued despite personal distress and interference with personal functioning in daily living.

C. The individual describes an intense urge to gamble which is difficult to control and reports that he or she is unable to stop gambling by an effort of will.

D. The individual is preoccupied with thoughts or mental images of the act of gambling or the circumstances surrounding the act.

Pathological fire setting (pyromania)

A. There are two or more acts of fire setting without apparent motive.

B. The individual describes an intense urge to set fire to objects, with a feeling of tension before the act and a feeling of relief afterward.

C. The individual is preoccupied with thoughts or mental images of fire setting or of the circumstances surrounding the act (e.g., abnormal interest in fire engines or in calling out the fire service).

Pathological stealing (kleptomania)

A. There are two or more thefts in which the individual steals without any apparent motive of personal gain or gain for another person.

B. The individual describes an intense urge to steal, with a feeling of tension before the act and a feeling of relief afterward.

Trichotillomania

A. Noticeable hair loss is caused by the individual's persistent and recurrent failure to resist impulses to pull out hairs.

B. The individual describes an intense urge to pull out hairs, with mounting tension before the act and a sense of relief afterward.

C. There is no preexisting inflammation of the skin, and the hair pulling is not in response to a delusion or hallucination.

Other habit and impulse disorders

This category should be used for other kinds of persistently repeated maladaptive behaviors that are not secondary to a recognized psychiatric syndrome and for which it appears that there is repeated failure to resist impulses to carry out the behavior. There is a prodromal period of tension with a feeling of release at the time of the act.

Habit and impulse disorder, unspecified

From World Health Organization. *The ICD-10 Classification of Mental and Behavioural Disorders: Diagnostic Criteria for Research.* Geneva: World Health Organization; 1993, with permission.

carpet," a central organizing schema for the impulse disorders that may also explain the link between them and their comorbid conditions. One theory postulates a constellation of *obsessive-compulsive spectrum disorders*, with varying degrees of overlapping features in each case between three subgroups: (1) impulse-control disorders, (2) disorders of physical appearance and sensation (e.g., body dysmorphic disorder and hypochondriasis), and (3) neurological disorders hallmarked by repetitive bursts of tics, spasms, or other pathological movements (e.g., Tourette's syndrome and Sydenham's chorea) (Fig. 21–1).

It has been further suggested that the syndromes within the obsessive-compulsive spectrum could notionally be located along an axis according to the approximate degree that each disorder is driven by risk aversiveness on the one hand (compulsive syndromes), or

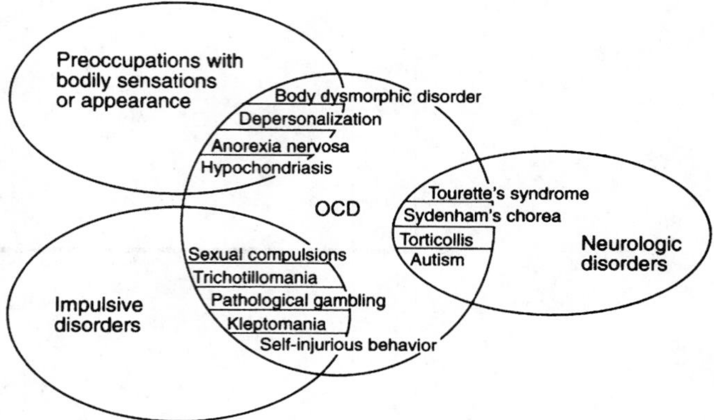

FIGURE 21–1 Obsessive-compulsive–related disorders. (From Hollander E, Kwon JH, Stein DJ, et al.: Obsessive-compulsive and spectrum disorders: Overview and quality of life issues. *J Clin Psychiatry.* 1996;57[Suppl]:3, with permission.)

risk seeking (impulsive syndromes) on the other (Fig. 21–2). Psychological contributing factors aside, the amplitude of risk seeking or risk avoidance may be mediated by serotonin, with other neurotransmitters playing a lesser part.

Another important line of inquiry stems from the conspicuous comorbidity of impulse-control disorders with unipolar and—most notably—with bipolar illness (common features of bipolarity and impulse-control difficulties include pleasurable and dangerous behaviors, onset in adolescence or early adulthood, episodic versus chronic course, similar abnormalities in neurotransmission, and improvement with mood stabilizers and SSRIs) (Fig. 21–3).

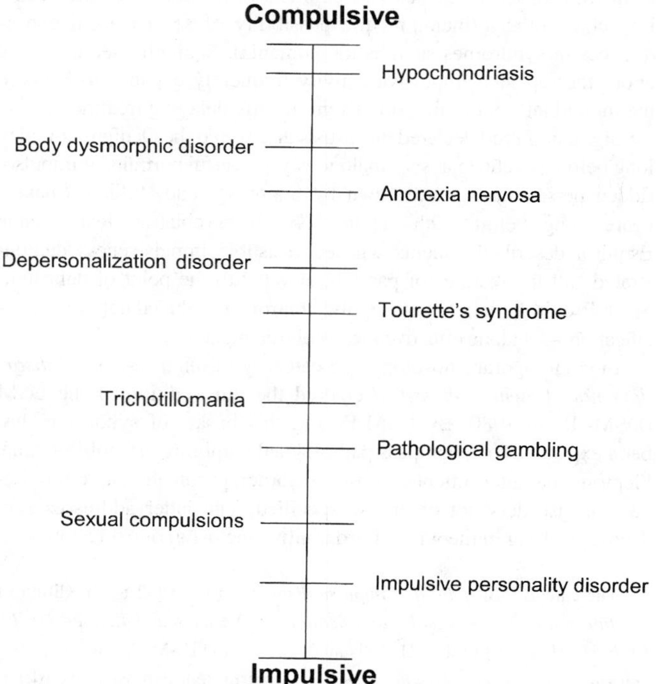

FIGURE 21–2 Compulsivity–impulsivity dimension. (From Hollander E: Treatment of obsessive-compulsive disorders with SSRIs. *Br J Psychiatry.* 1998;25[Suppl]:7, with permission.)

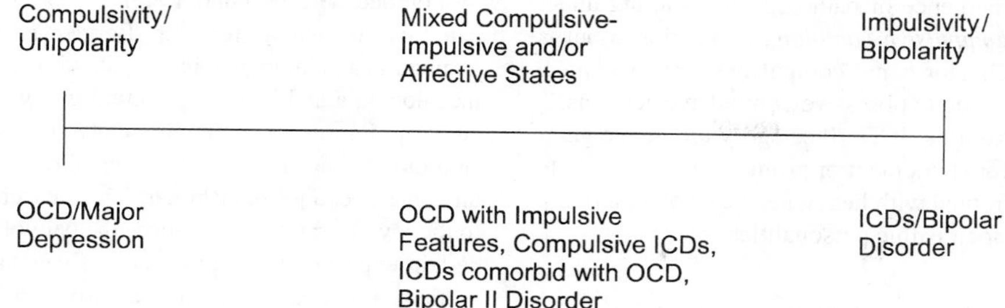

FIGURE 21–3 Hypothesized relationship between compulsivity, impulsivity, unipolarity, and bipolarity along a single dimension. The compulsivity-unipolarity end of the spectrum is characterized by harm-avoidant behaviors, inhibited thinking and behavior, insight into senselessness of symptoms, resistance to impulses and behaviors, and absence of pleasure. The impulsivity-bipolarity end of the spectrum is characterized by harmful behaviors, disinhibited or spontaneous thinking and behavior, little insight into dangerousness of symptoms, little resistance to impulses and behaviors, and pleasurable feelings. ICD, impulse-control disorder; OCD, obsessive-compulsive disorder. (From McElroy S, et al. Are impulse control disorders related to bipolar disorder? *Compr Psychol.* 1996;37:229, with permission.)

On this basis, a class of *affective spectrum disorders* has been hypothesized that embraces affective, obsessive, and impulsive disorders. These conditions are notionally located on an inferred axis according to their different degrees or combinations of compulsivity and unipolarity or impulsivity and bipolarity. The schema elegantly accounts for patients presenting a perplexing mixture of impulsivity and obsession (these *liminal* cases presumably would be situated at the midpoint of the axis).

Such formulations are neither definitive nor mutually exclusive. They are best contemplated as touchstones, signifying that the truth about the deep structures of the impulse-control disorders is finally being glimpsed, as through a glass darkly. The increasing volume and sophistication of research will surely shed more light on these intriguing maladies.

Freud famously predicted that psychiatry's future would manifest a swing of the pendulum between psychodynamically and somatically oriented theories about mental illness. Current research into impulse-control disorders overwhelmingly explores their materiality—neurobiology, heredity, and psychopharmacology. In the context of this latest oscillation, the astute clinician will not neglect psyche for soma. One's attentiveness to genetic loading and serotonin fluctuations should not preclude receptiveness to the impulsive patient's inner world, to past trauma, and to dysfunctional family and social circumstances. There is, after all, a search for authenticity and meaning embedded within the molecules of human beings.

PATHOLOGICAL GAMBLING

Pathological gambling is the most common impulse disorder in this category. It afflicts several million Americans, constituting a major, increasing public health problem; hence, significant space is devoted to it here.

History

Archeological and anthropological research bear eloquent testimony to the ubiquity of gambling, normative and pathological, in every time and place.

Gambling may well have had religious origin: Perhaps attempts to divine the will of the Gods or Fates eventually gave way to betting on more tangible outcomes. Wagering on the speed and strength of man or beast arguably dates back to human prehistory. Dice have been found in the tombs of Egypt. Encamped soldiers of yore upended chariots and bet on the turn of their wheels. The ancient Chinese are said to have staked digits or limbs on games of chance, the American Mojave Indians risked their wives, and the Germanic barbarians of Julius Caesar's day wagered life or freedom. Predecessors of modern card games, craps, and gaming machines go back several hundred years to several thousand years. Every manner of gambling was wildly popular in Renaissance and Enlightenment Europe. Despite the Puritan ethic, the gamut of European gambling quickly found favor amongst the first American colonists, especially horse racing.

As the American frontier expanded, gamblers followed the farmer, the rancher, and the entrepreneur. Gambling flourished in the marginal milieus of cattle towns and mining camps, on Mississippi riverboats, and in the slums and salons of major cities. By the mid-19th century, gambling had established an increasingly ominous association with criminal elements in western towns and eastern cities. Corruption of law enforcement officials and politicians inevitably accompanied the consolidation of gambling interests. A powerful gangster and gambler coalition was forged by the 1930s and 1950s, with gangland muscle and cash backing illegal gambling and legitimate businesses behind the scenes.

In the last two decades, major entertainment corporations in Las Vegas, Atlantic City, and Native American casinos have reaped vaster profit from legitimate gaming than from their mob antecedents. Corporate strategies are increasingly—and successfully—aimed at low-stake, family gambling. The new wave of gaming is further fueled by states and churches with straitened budgets. Internet gambling Web sites are plentiful: This global casino may well prove to be the greatest source of gaming revenue in history. The current total take of legal and illegal gaming is estimated to be at least 0.5 trillion dollars yearly.

The chaotic life and times of the pathological gambler have proven perennially fertile ground for artists. One of the most powerful and clinically accurate depictions of the disorder is found in Fyodor Dostoevsky's novella, *The Gambler*, based on the author's own descent into gaming hell.

Nosology

Pathological gambling was first designated as a separate diagnostic entity in DSM-III. Parameters were revised in the revised DSM-III (DSM-III-R), redefined yet again for DSM-IV, and essentially retained in DSM-IV-TR. The current definition emphasizes the afflicted individual's overwhelming preoccupation and obsession with gambling, tolerance and withdrawal in the progress of the condition, difficulty in controlling gambling activity and chasing behavior, the use of gambling to alleviate dysphoric emotional states, and the devastating impact of gambling on vocation, social, and family life.

ICD-10 delineates *pathological gambling* as a "disorder of frequent, repeated episodes of gambling that dominate the patient's life, to the detriment of social, occupational, material, and family values and commitments." Like DSM-IV-TR, ICD-10 notes the patient's obsessive preoccupation with and inability to control gambling behavior, as well as the emergence of pathological gambling under stress. An alternate term, *compulsive gambling*, is mentioned but is dismissed, "because the behavior is not compulsive in the technical sense, nor is the disorder related to obsessive-compulsive neurosis."

Specifically excluded from the ICD-10 category are manic gambling episodes; gambling for excitement or profit by those "likely to curb their habit when confronted with heavy losses, or other adverse effects"; and gambling by sociopathic personalities.

Epidemiology Although comprehensive worldwide statistics have yet to be compiled, excellent local studies all point to a 3 to 5 percent rate of problem gamblers in the general population and an approximate 1 percent rate of individuals meeting the requirements for pathological gambling.

In the United States, the combined population of problem and pathological gamblers is estimated at 5 million. Their combined losses run into the billions, with an average individual indebtedness of $30,000. Wealthy pathological gamblers with the means to sustain a huge habit may owe hundreds of thousands or even millions of dollars. Collateral losses due to time away from work, total unemployability, and erosion of savings as a result of gambling are staggering.

The typical patient in treatment studies is a white man from a comfortable economic background, 35 to 50 years of age. However, surveys of more extensive nontreatment populations indicate that pathological gambling cuts across every ethnic, class, age, and occupational divide (according to anonymous casino personnel, physicians are amongst their most consistent heavy players and losers).

As every type of gambling has become increasingly accessible over the past few decades, the rate of normal and pathological gambling has risen spectacularly, especially in locales with legalized gaming. Escalation has been noted in the poor, notably poor minorities; adolescents; elderly retirees; and women. One out of three pathological gamblers is now female: It has been suggested that women are gambling more because an increased presence in the workplace gives them more cash. These groups are all still greatly underserved with regard to research and treatment.

Family histories of pathological gamblers show an increased rate of substance abuse (particularly alcoholism) and depressive disorders. A parent or influential relative of the patient often has been a problem or pathological gambler. The family circle is likely to be competitively and materialistically oriented, evincing intense admiration for money and associated symbols of success. In this respect, compulsive gambling has been called the dark side of the American dream.

Comorbidity Significant comorbidity occurs between pathological gambling and mood disorders (especially major depression and bipolarity) and substance abuse disorders (notably alcohol and cocaine abuse and caffeine and nicotine dependence). Comorbidity also exists with attention-deficit/hyperactivity disorder (ADHD) (particularly in childhood), various personality disorders (notably narcissistic, antisocial, and borderline personality disorders), and other impulse-control disorders. Although many pathological gamblers have obsessive personality traits, full-blown obsessive-compulsive disorder is uncommon.

Etiology Considerable differences in precipitating factors are discovered from one patient to another and within the pathological gambler's lifetime as well. The disorder—like others in its class—is best conceptualized not as a monolithic entity, but as a condition encompassing subsets of dysfunctional behavior with diverse articulation of diverse etiologies.

For decades, Edmund Bergler's *compulsive loser* theory dominated psychoanalytic research. Bergler asserted that the pathological gambler is a pathological narcissist, who resents the loss of childhood megalomania and bears a profound grudge against parents and other authority figures for reining in inflated infantile omnipotence. Aggression directed against sundry agents of deprivation occasions guilt and an intense need for punishment. The pleasures of gambling are related to the joy of grandiose rebellion; the pain of gambling is related to the certain expectation of punishment. Eventually, the anguish of loss is eroticized and elaborated into a chronic masochistic stance, wherein the patient savors victimhood, relishes injustice collecting, and revels in self-pity and spurious righteous indignation.

Bergler's views have largely been superseded by more nuanced formulations, notably by Ralph Greenson and successors. Greenson believed that pathological gambling gratified multiple pregenital and genital conflicts, rooted in oral-receptive, anal-sadistic, and, especially, oedipal strivings. Greenson was one of the first clinicians to speculate that gambling might defend against depressive affect.

Hearkening back to the possible theological origins of gambling, the pathological gamblers' relentless devotion to play comprises a kind of spilt religion, betokened by a host of superstitions and rituals pitched at beating the odds. Analytical therapy often reveals a covert, devastating fear of death, suggesting that these patients may be courting the erratic favors of Lady Luck in aid of the ultimate score—winning over mortality itself.

Many studies indicate that the makeup of most pathological gamblers does not conform to tidy psychoanalytic paradigms. Research efforts have been directed at elucidating other causes—none of which necessarily negates the importance of psychological factors.

The family history of problem gambling in pathological gamblers has already been mentioned. Twin studies further suggest that the dysfunctional gambler, besides identifying with a gambling relative, may have inherited a genetic potential for the illness.

Behavioral-cognitive studies conceptualize pathological gambling as a learned, disastrous habit.

Many pathological gamblers exhibit exquisite sensitivity to a gamut of reinforcers directly or indirectly related to wagering. An example of direct or *primary* reinforcement is the slot-machine jackpot's lure of high magnitude of return for a *low-response*, supposedly small, investment (ignoring cumulative loss). An example of indirect or secondary reinforcement would be the "comps" offered by casinos, such as special room rates and free drinks. Overall, casino design and management suggest an elegantly sinister deployment of virtually every behavioral stimulus to encourage betting over one's head.

Cognitive studies indicate that many pathological gamblers are prone to characteristic cognitive biases and distortions. These include discounting the sum of many small bets made at great cost toward achieving a big score, such as a jackpot; magnifying one's own skills while minimizing the talents of others; losing sight of the amount of gambling time necessary to make up losses; selectively privileging memories of wins over losses; and the absolute conviction that a chain of losses heralds an impending win (the so-called *gambler's fallacy*).

Promising recent research has probed the neurobiology of the pathological gambler, although more questions have been raised than answered. Patients with lesions in a neural system whose pathways involve the ventromedial (VM) prefrontal cortex, amygdala, and other structures show denial or unawareness of various problems calling for common-sense judgments. This type of injury also seems to predispose patients to pursue actions with short-term rewards but long-term negative consequences.

The VM regulatory system is believed to activate various somatic markers, which then provide covert or overt signals heralding the need for appropriate decision making. Investigators speculate that substance abusers and, possibly, pathological gamblers, who have analogous problems in seeking short-term gratification over long-term pain, may have a lack of warning makers due to dysfunction of the VM regulating apparatus.

Various studies suggest that complex, articulating neurotransmitter dysregulation may exist in pathological gamblers, similar to abnormalities in substance abusers and patients with other behavioral and impulsive problems. Imbalances in serotoninergic, noradrenergic, and dopaminergic mediation have all been postulated to subvert the mechanisms underpinning appropriate behavioral arousal, initiation, disinhibition, and reward and reinforcement.

In normal subjects exposed to high-risk and low-risk gambling experiments, individuals who preferred stimulus-rich environments consistently sought *long shots*, wagering more to win more. One conjectures that—given the presence of other predisposing factors—such people might easily be attracted to social and even problematic gambling.

Much has been written about one or another culture's supposed gambling predilections—the English, for blood sports; Texans, for high-stakes poker. These notions are largely anecdotal and, often, frankly prejudicial. As noted, the entire United States is experiencing an unparalleled explosion of legal and illegal gambling, regardless of the bettor's race, creed, or national origin.

A connection has definitely been established between the arrival of a casino and the rise of pathological gambling in the surrounding area, with a lag of approximately 3 to 5 years before the increase occurs. At least most casinos are situated some distance away from most American towns or cities. Sadly, the greater accessibility of other betting opportunities, such as bingo games, lotteries, and off-track parlors where none existed before, may well activate a vast legion of problem gamblers who never knew they had a problem. The destructive potential of ever more available Internet gambling looms especially ominous.

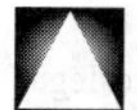

Table 21–2
DSM-IV-TR Diagnostic Criteria for Pathological Gambling

A. Persistent and recurrent maladaptive gambling behavior as indicated by five (or more) of the following:
   (1) The patient is preoccupied with gambling (e.g., preoccupied with reliving past gambling experiences, handicapping or planning the next venture, or thinking of ways to get money with which to gamble).
   (2) The patient needs to gamble with increasing amounts of money to achieve the desired excitement.
   (3) The patient has had repeated unsuccessful efforts to control, to cut back, or to stop gambling.
   (4) The patient is restless or irritable when attempting to cut down or to stop gambling.
   (5) The patient gambles as a way of escaping from problems or of relieving a dysphoric mood (e.g., feelings of helplessness, guilt, anxiety, and depression).
   (6) After losing money gambling, the patient often returns another day to get even ("chasing" one's losses).
   (7) The patient lies to family members, therapist, or others to conceal extent of involvement with gambling.
   (8) The patient has committed illegal acts, such as forgery, fraud, theft, or embezzlement, to finance gambling.
   (9) The patient has jeopardized or lost a significant relationship, job, or educational or career opportunity because of gambling.
   (10) The patient relies on others to provide money to relieve a desperate financial situation caused by gambling.

B. The gambling behavior is not better accounted for by a manic episode.

From American Psychiatric Association. *Diagnostic and Statistical Manual of Mental Disorders.* 4th ed. Text rev. Washington, DC: American Psychiatric Association; 2000, with permission.

Diagnosis, Course, and Prognosis

The typical individual meeting the DSM-IV-TR criteria for pathological gambling (Table 21–2) is in his or her mid-30s to 40s, married or divorced, and vocationally successful. A strong gambling interest has frequently paralleled his or her ordinary life since adolescence or young adulthood. Contrary to Bergler's theories, the potential sufferer usually has excellent gaming knowledge and skills and may be a reasonably consistent winner.

In the setting of life stress or a big win or without obvious cause, the previously successful gambler begins to fall behind. Instead of stopping and cutting losses, he or she begins to *chase*—spending ever more time and money, expanding his or her wagering repertoire to include multiple gaming opportunities. Over several months to years of chasing losses, he or she becomes embroiled in an escalating, tightening, and frightening spiral of options, which inevitably extend outside gambling itself. Business and family resources are raided, loan sharks are used, and criminal enterprises are undertaken, although usually as a last recourse. Male gamblers commonly turn to embezzlement, scams, and credit card fraud; women may be drawn into prostitution.

When every option is exhausted, the pathological gambler is exposed, often to the horrified surprise of significant others. The experience is devastating: Bankruptcy, divorce, imprisonment, and even suicide may follow. However, exposure can have a positive outcome through the *bail-out*, such as a rescue by family or friends paying off debts or remission of indebtedness by bank, bookmaker, or loan shark.

Once exposed, some pathological gamblers get help and quit betting. Unfortunately, the patient more often grows bored and restless, begins associating with other gamblers, commences wagering, and soon is engaged in chasing anew. Many pathological gamblers undergo repeated episodes of spiraling, exposure, bail-out, and relapse, with gradual deterioration of personal relationships and career until, at the end stages of the illness, their lives lie in utter ruin.

Morris Chafetz's classification of *reactive* and *addictive* alcoholism usefully applies to many pathological gamblers. The *reactive* gambling type has a stable, productive social and vocational life. His or her normal gambling behavior typically involves one or two wagering modalities but periodically shades over into binges of compulsive play, often precipitated by obvious external stressors. The patient keeps recovering his or her stride, usually without treatment, until he or she loses control definitively.

The *addicted* pathological gambler, on the other hand, is intensely involved with every aspect of gambling and goes out of control much earlier. By his or her 20s, gambling pervades every aspect of an idiosyncratic, marginal lifestyle, hallmarked by chronic instability in work and social relationships. One emphasizes that prolonged spirals of pathological gambling by a healthier reactive type eventually produce a deteriorated end-stage clinical picture that is indistinguishable from that of the addicted type.

Regardless of typology, a craving for action is central to the behavior of most pathological gamblers. Although they may ascribe their driven modus vivendi to an obvious need for cash, the arousal afforded by action itself draws them ever deeper into the gaming vortex, or, once caught up, action sustains them as an independent attraction.

Action may spin out of a gaming situation's peculiar ambiance—for example, the steamy milieu of the race track, polluted by rumor and false report, or the eternal glittering daylight of the casino with the seductive click of a roulette wheel and the jingle of slot machines. The *action high* can be found far from ordinary gambling locales, in bowling alleys, bars, and legal and illegal betting parlors in which any form of play can be instantly arranged. In time, the harried search for ever more elusive sources of financing itself becomes part of the action.

Regardless of social background, ethnicity, or comorbidity, many pathological gamblers exhibit strikingly similar personality traits. They tend to be intelligent (although not deeply intellectual) and overconfident to the point of abrasiveness. They are perennial optimists, deniers, and rationalizers. By turns, they are touchingly loyal or horridly insensitive—notably when chasing. They possess an ironic gallows wit and appear superficially quite gregarious but are often inwardly beset by profound feelings of loneliness. They do not easily express their feelings; indeed, they may be so unable to get in touch with an inner life as to be considered alexithymic (a feature of patients with other impulse-control disorders).

Both pathological and successful professional gamblers typically evince a curious grandiose elitism. They are absolutely certain that they "know the score" about gambling, as well as life in the wider world—for which gambling is held as a dog-eat-dog metaphor. The pride of pathological gamblers in their idiosyncratic vocation, even at its disastrous end stage, is especially poignant, defying the enormous suffering entailed.

The course of the pathological gambler is often influenced for the worse by comorbid conditions, notably substance abuse and affective illness. The easy accessibility of drugs and alcohol in gambling environments often disinhibits the pathological gambler, resulting in wilder play, or the heavy burden of indebtedness precipitates depression, which, in turn, triggers off more gambling binges.

Many pathological gamblers are paradoxically hypochondriacal and dreadfully neglectful of their physical well-being. They eat poorly and often excessively, are sleep deprived and underexercised, and are excessive consumers of caffeine and nicotine. Hard statistics are lacking, but anecdotal evidence suggests that they may be more vulnerable than general populations to hypercholesterolemia, cardiopulmonary disease, and peptic ulcer.

Differential Diagnosis

Pathological gambling should be distinguished from the social gambling practiced in one form or another by a majority of the population (estimated at approximately 85 percent). Normative gambling is based on the desire for relaxation and profit, the inherent pleasure in exercising a variety of ego functions, risk taking in a controlled setting, and the satisfaction of other obscure, possibly conflict-related, drives. Unpathological gamblers usually play on designated occasions, with a notion of predetermined acceptable losses. Their pleasure is highly predicated on the companionable social milieu that gambling frequently offers.

For professional gamblers, play is business—often one of many businesses. Contrary to the conception of the glamorous high roller, professionals usually avoid the limelight to avoid taxes. They know specific games thoroughly, are prepared to take requisite risks, coolly acknowledge the losing streaks that come with the territory, and are prepared to weather them without losing control. However, reactive professional gamblers—and, to a lesser extent, social gamblers—may slip into pathological gambling, often in the context of some environmental stressor.

Acute substance abuse, notably acute alcoholism, may precipitate a gambling bout in an individual without other signatures of pathological gambling.

Gambling binges are occasionally seen in the context of a schizophrenic's delusional system (e.g., being convinced that God has told one to wager one's life's savings in aid of saving mankind). Excessive wagering may occur during the manic phase of bipolarity, in patients not otherwise inclined to gamble.

The relationship between bouts of gambling and vicissitudes of mood is more problematic in pathological gamblers with comorbid affective illness—especially hypomania and mania. The latter often seem wired to the universe, like the manic, and fairly crackle with tension as they pursue their dizzy dance over the abyss. Yet, they return quickly to a more temperate state of mood once play has ceased, may be reactively elated after a win, or appropriately depressed after a loss. In any case, most pathological gamblers wager chronically whether high, low, or relatively euthymic, with or without obvious precipitating cause. It is moot whether mood swings precipitated by biological dysfunction per se can escalate gambling.

The antisocial personality frequently presents with collateral gambling behavior that reflects the individual's inherent criminality and lack of empathy. He (or, less often, she) does anything possible to win and is often a chronic cheater. Loss stimulates blame rather than remorse and may precipitate violent retaliation. Unlike antisocial gamblers, the majority of pathological gamblers have a better work record, a more stable family life, and a higher moral set before the disruptions caused by chronic chasing begin. When they commit crimes or scams, it is out of desperation, with a humiliating loss of pride, in a last-ditch effort to get money to cover losses or to keep on gambling. Unlike the morbid ego-alien preoccupations of the obsessive-compulsive patient, the pathological gambler's overweening preoccupation with play is, in most cases, completely ego-syntonic.

Treatment

Virtually every mental health modality has been directed at the pathological gambler. For decades, the results were ungratifying, and relapse rates were high. Better understanding of the patient's psychology and neurobiology now contributes to improved outcomes. Chances for success hinge on careful individualizing of treatment for each case. Combined approaches are often useful. Most pathological gamblers make difficult patients, regardless of the type of therapy. Like adolescents—whom they much resemble—they rarely seek help on their own and, indeed, may bitterly oppose treatment. They are usually forced into consultation after many years of gambling, after exposure precipitates an ultimatum that the gambler gets help or suffers divorce or prosecution, for example.

The pathological gambler's enormous pride, formidable denial, lack of introspection, impatience, and incurable optimism all militate against the formation of a working alliance in psychoanalytically oriented therapy (as well as other therapies). Besides their gambling, patients often present a host of serious problems and symptoms—depersonalization, hypochondriasis, obesity, panic attacks, and profound depression—that do not yield readily to talking therapies.

Pathological gamblers expect magical interventions and are likely to leave when miracles are not forthcoming. They may go through the motions of patienthood and yet remain inwardly convinced that a turn in luck and adequate funding will provide the solution to their problems. They are notably contemptuous about gambling inexpertise. The therapist who is a gambling tyro can occasionally use ignorance to good advantage by having the client teach him or her the ropes.

Psychotherapy with a pathological gambler is likely to be stormy—marked by missed sessions, relapses, and financial crises leading to disruption or cessation of treatment. These patients especially require a tolerant, noncritical attitude. With their testy pride and razor-keen intuition of rejection, they do not remain long in an atmosphere with the smallest tincture of moralizing or contempt. Firm but kind limit setting, which may include payment at each session, is often necessary. Greater responsibility in handling fees can be an important signal of improvement.

The attractiveness of group techniques for pathological gamblers is not surprising, given their extraversion. Group, family, and couples therapy have all been helpful. The distressing impact of gambling on significant others often becomes clearer and registers more potently on the patient in family sessions than in individual therapy alone.

Gamblers Anonymous (GA) is an international self-help organization administered by abstinent pathological gamblers, with branches in nearly every large city and many small towns across the world. GA is run along 12-step lines analogous to Alcoholics Anonymous (AA), with similar collateral groups for relatives, which are especially worthwhile when a pathological gambler refuses help. Clients are encouraged to confront their problems in the company of others thoroughly acquainted with every turn and twist of chasing. Sponsors can be provided; organizing financial restitution is a crucial aspect of treatment. Unfortunately, the GA drop-out rate is high, especially for first-time clients and when GA (or individual therapy, for that matter) is the sole source of help.

Once deemed ineffective, medication now figures regularly in the treatment of many pathological gamblers. Studies indicate stabilization of affect and modification of aberrant gambling behavior with mood stabilizers (notably lithium [Eskalith]) and antidepressants (notably SSRIs and clomipramine [Anafranil]). Improvement is most likely in dual diagnosis patients with significant comorbid affective illness. The close relationship of pathological gambling to drug and alcohol addiction has led to treatment trials with the opioid antagonist naltrexone (ReVia) to specifically block gambling urges, with a measure of success.

Educational, behavioral, and cognitive strategies appeal to the pathological gambler's inherent pragmatism—particularly in patients who are highly resistive to analytically oriented treatment. Simple instruction about their condition by an instruction manual and class work has enabled many patients to stop or to reduce excessive gambling. More intricate cognitive-behavioral approaches aim at undoing the habituating impact of specific gambling milieus and decreasing or redirecting the need for action. Patients are instructed in relaxation exercises to decrease tension, to identify specific gambling triggers, and to substitute gambling with competing rewards, for example.

Gambling programs are especially useful in assaying and coordinating multiple modalities; these are steadily increasing across the United States. Treatment of the pathological gambler usually takes place in an outpatient setting. However, it may be necessary to break a debilitating gambling cycle by hospitalization, using a stay of several days to weeks to organize an effective outpatient treatment plan. Intriguingly, hospitalized pathological gamblers may show signs of physiological, as well as emotional, distress analogous to hospitalized drug addicts undergoing detoxification. Given the pathological gambler's chronically poor health habits, many patients need a complete physical examination, appropriate laboratory studies, and thorough evaluation of nutritional and exercise status.

Gambling and the Law

State and federal legal systems are still primarily concerned with the punishment of pathological gamblers, rather than their rehabilitation. Some 60 percent of pathological gamblers commit illegal acts over their careers. These crimes are overwhelmingly nonviolent—bouncing checks, financial scams, and prostitution. It is not generally appreciated that incarceration can paradoxically become a disguised bail-out, forestalling or eliminating requirements for restitution. Prison life itself is often ridden with gambling, for cigarettes, drugs, and other items and services.

Experts believe that rather than jailing most pathological gamblers outright—particularly the majority without antisocial pathology—the offender should be offered the option to discontinue gambling, to make restitution, and to undergo some form of treatment as a condition of probation.

To date, a few states have actually set up agencies and programs to deal with pathological gambling—even as most states have been quick to allow lotteries, race tracks, and casinos to replenish their coffers. It is the height of hypocrisy for powerful gaming interests, backed by the powers that be, to tell the pathological gambler to "bet with your head, not over it," while failing to redress the psychological disasters that they are facilitating.

Frank was a 32-year-old businessman whose uncle was a compulsive horse player. His maternal grandmother committed suicide with sleeping pills. He was an avid card player and sports bettor since his early teens, taking pride in being a small but steady winner. Frank found formal education boring and dropped out of college in his freshman year to take over his father's appliance store. He expanded the business to a chain of electronic equipment outlets. Over the next decade, he prospered, married happily, had three children, and lived in substantial luxury.

During the same time, Frank's inveterate gambling slowly increased. Besides his weekly poker game and weekend sports betting, he enjoyed occasional Saturday outings with his poker buddies to a casino that had opened at a nearby Indian reservation. He mostly broke even or sustained small losses, but he was immensely exhilarated by several big scores at blackjack and craps, games that he had not played much before.

After his father's sudden death from a stroke, Frank began traveling more often to the casino and started playing at higher stakes. Soon, he found himself betting hundreds, then thousands, of dollars on the turn of a card or the throw of the dice. The size of sports betting similarly increased. He visited the casino most weekends and many weekday nights, lying about his whereabouts to colleagues and family.

Within 2 years, Frank accumulated several million dollars in gambling debts. Now, he gambled not to win but to catch up—still fervently believing that "one streak would put me straight." He invaded business and personal finances, juggled accounts, charged his credit cards beyond the maximum limit, and borrowed money from loan sharks at exorbitant rates. He had always shielded his wife and family from his problem. Profoundly depressed, he considered killing himself in a car accident, so that "everyone would be taken care of." He used cocaine to alleviate his despair.

The grim reality of Frank's indebtedness and its cause was unmasked when his wife discovered that he had plundered the children's college funds to pay off a loan shark who had threatened to have his family killed. At first, she wanted to divorce him, but then her wealthy father intervened and bailed Frank out. He swore that he would never gamble again, entered GA, and, within a few months, was back at the casino.

Several more episodes of recovery and relapse did lead to divorce and left Frank penniless. He finally entered a pilot program for pathological gamblers, where he was diagnosed as also having atypical bipolar disorder. Treatment has included individual and group counseling, medication with an antidepressant and mood regulator, family therapy (his wife is now willing to see him, but not to live with him), and a program of restitution. He works as a delicatessen clerk, has been abstinent for 6 months, and says that "not a day goes by that I don't miss the action."

TRICHOTILLOMANIA

History and Description

Trichotillomania is a chronic disorder characterized by repetitive hair pulling, driven by escalating tension and causing variable hair loss that is usually—but not always—visible to others. The disorder was known at least as far back as the 12th century. Formation of *trichobezoars*—hairballs accumulating in the alimentary tract from hair pulling and swallowing—was described in the late 18th century. The term *trichotillomania* was coined by a French dermatologist, Francois Hallopeau, in 1889.

Trichotillomania was once deemed rare, and little about it was described beyond phenomenology. The condition is now regarded as more common. With a substantial increase in research, treatment has greatly improved since the 1980s.

Nosology

Trichotillomania was first recognized in the DSM-III-R. DSM-III-R classified trichotillomania as an impulse-control disorder, chiefly because of the typical cycle of mounting tension, the inability to resist the urge to pull hair, and the release and gratification afterwards. DSM-IV then specifically excluded hair pulling secondary to medical conditions or other psychiatric disorders from the diagnosis. The criterion of significant distress or impairment *in social, occupational, or other important areas of functioning* was added and was subsequently maintained in DSM-IV-TR.

ICD-10 classifies trichotillomania under *habit and impulse disorders*, as a condition "characterized by noticeable hair loss due to a recurrent failure to resist impulses to pull out hairs, preceded by mounting tension and . . . followed by a sense of relief or gratification." The diagnosis should not be made if "pre-existing inflammation of the skin" exists or if hair pulling occurs "in response to a delusion or hallucination." "Stereotyped movement disorder with hair-plucking (F98.4)" is also specifically excluded.

Epidemiology

The prevalence of trichotillomania may be underestimated because of accompanying shame and secretiveness. The diagnosis encompasses at least two categories of hair pullers differing in incidence, severity, age of presentation, and gender ratio. Other subsets may exist.

The potentially most serious, chronic form of the disorder usually begins in early to mid-adolescence, with a lifetime prevalence ranging from 0.6 percent to as high as 3.4 percent in general populations and with a female to male ratio as high as 9 to 1. The number of men may actually be higher, because men are even more likely than women to conceal hair pulling. A chronic trichotillomania patient is likely to be the only or oldest child in the family.

A childhood type of trichotillomania occurs approximately equally in girls and boys. It is said to be more common than the adolescent or young adult syndrome and is generally far less serious dermatologically and psychologically.

The family history of trichotillomania patients is weighted toward OCD and obsessive-compulsive personality disorder, anxiety and affective disorders (notably depressive), and tics. Although a strong history of trichotillomania has not been discovered in family members, one study demonstrated a 25 percent rate of unspecified alopecia in relatives of childhood hair pullers.

An estimated 33 to 40 percent of trichotillomania patients chew or swallow the hair that they pull out at one time or another. Of this group, approximately 37.5 percent develop potentially hazardous bezoars.

Comorbidity

Significant comorbidity is found between trichotillomania and OCD (as well as other anxiety disorders); Tourette's syndrome; affective illness, especially depressive conditions; eating disorders; and various personality disorders—particularly obsessive-compulsive, borderline, and narcissistic personality disorders. Comorbid substance abuse disorder is not encountered as frequently as it is in pathological gambling, kleptomania, and other disorders.

Etiology

The precise causes of trichotillomania are still unknown. Psychoanalytically oriented theories cite childhood loss or separation as precipitants. The child-like appearance of some adolescent patients resulting from hair pulling supposedly betokens the wish to regress to an infantile state and to avoid the burgeoning pressure of adolescent sexuality. Erotic, sadomasochistic, and symbolic masturbatory aspects of hair pulling have been discussed in the analytical literature.

The frequent hair twisting and hair patting of infants and young children (often combined with thumb sucking) are said to represent attempts to recuperate the absent mother's presence via the child's own body. Intriguing analogies may be drawn between human hair manipulation and various animal and avian grooming behaviors that appear to facilitate homeostasis, when alone, and social bonding via mutual grooming. Under this rubric, trichotillomania has a distinctively tactile, self-soothing quality for many patients.

A specific family constellation has been described in a predominantly female cohort of adolescent and young adult patients with chronic trichotillomania. Although found in other psychiatric disorders, these family dynamics are peculiarly inflected by the role played by early experiences centered around hair and, later, by hair pulling itself.

One parent, usually the mother, is dominating and intrusive. Her aggressive facade conceals considerable fear and neediness. Often, her child has shown anxious clinging since infancy, possibly on a constitutional basis. Mother and child become increasingly embroiled in an intense, hostile-dependent relationship that interferes with the child's healthy separation. An uncanny mutual preoccupation with the beauty of the daughter's hair—its styling and grooming—develops early on and may involve other family members.

With the onset of trichotillomania during puberty, the mother's attempts to make her daughter stop pulling her hair are countered by the youngster's stubborn resistance. This tangled partnership has been deemed a *hair-pulling symbiosis*: The symptom becomes a battleground for acting out conflicts over individuation. On tactful probing, adult patients may reveal an earlier hair-pulling symbiosis. One emphasizes that the constellation is not encountered in every case—or may exist in a more benign version. Chronic trichotillomania may share biological features, as well as comorbidity with obsessional and affective illness. Trichotillomania and obsessive-affective illness respond to serotoninergic drugs. Because many chronic hair pullers do not respond as robustly or at all to serotoninergic agents, other neurobiological dysregulation could be implicated.

From a cognitive-behavioral perspective, chronic hair pulling is an intensely self-reinforcing activity, eventually acquiring an intense, habitual life of its own.

Diagnosis, Clinical Features, and Course

Chronic trichotillomania is hallmarked by complex behaviors before, during, and after epilation (Table 21–3). The urge to pull customarily develops during solitary activity—relaxing, reading, and watching television, for example. Alternately, it arises in the context of anxiety or frustration related to external stress. Some patients state that antecedent tingling or burning sensations in the scalp compel them to seek relief by pulling.

A favorite private location is often used for hair pulling, especially the patient's bedroom or bathroom (the masturbatory connotation of these locales is obvious). The prodromal period may last for a few moments, but, more commonly, tension builds over a longer time, until it consumes the patient's thoughts, and epilation begins. Tension may be experienced as pleasurable or painful, or a meld of both. The hair-pulling episode lasts minutes to several hours.

Most patients pluck at a particular site—typically the crown or side of the scalp, with variable spread into adjacent areas in time (Fig. 21–4). Besides—or instead of—the scalp, hair may be pulled from the eyebrows, armpits, and pubic region (denuding the latter is a notable cause of embarrassment) (Fig. 21–5). Men pull hair from beards and moustaches or from arm and leg hair growth.

The hair root is a favored target of hair-pulling. Patients describe an idiosyncratic pleasure in getting the root, particularly in stripping

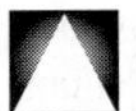

Table 21–3
DSM-IV-TR Diagnostic Criteria for Trichotillomania

A. Recurrent pulling out of one's hair resulting in noticeable hair loss.
B. An increasing sense of tension immediately before pulling out the hair or when attempting to resist the behavior.
C. Pleasure, gratification, or relief when pulling out the hair.
D. The disturbance is not better accounted for by another mental disorder and is not due to a general medical condition (e.g., a dermatological condition).
E. The disturbance causes clinically significant distress or impairment in social, occupational, or other important areas of functioning.

From American Psychiatric Association. *Diagnostic and Statistical Manual of Mental Disorders.* 4th ed. Text rev. Washington, DC: American Psychiatric Association; 2000, with permission.

it away from a plucked hair. Some state that they hear a special popping sound or otherwise know that the root has been extracted. The hair is often nibbled and swallowed while pulling or after a sufficient quantity of hair has been collated. The root may be conspicuously savored.

When the bout ends, pleasure is succeeded by shame, remorse, and disgust—particularly over hair swallowing. Shame and frustration are especially intense when an area is denuded that had been left alone for awhile, so that new growth could take place.

Hair loss from trichotillomania can be concealed from family and friends for a considerable time, as long as epilation is confined to a small area. Concealment is maintained by careful combing, use of hair extensions, or wearing hats or kerchiefs on one pretext or another. Inevitably, loss becomes obvious to others, although the patient does not easily admit its cause at home or in a doctor's office. Treatment for other alopecias is typically undertaken with a profusion of remedies and healers, until a firm diagnosis is finally made—usually by a knowledgeable dermatologist.

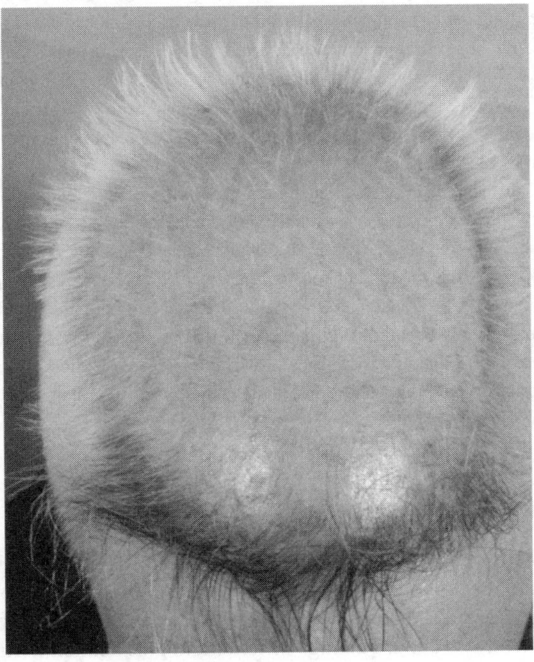

FIGURE 21–4 Example of plucking of the hair of the scalp due to trichotillomania. (See Color Plate.)

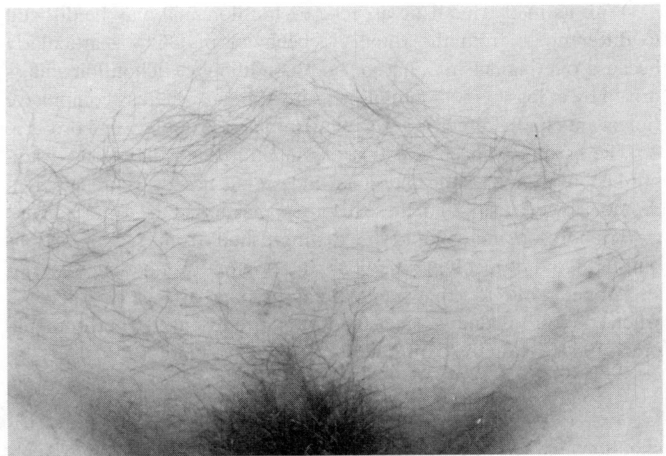

FIGURE 21–5 Example of plucking of the pubic hair due to trichotillomania.

Permanent cessation of severe trichotillomania after exposure is the exception rather than the rule. The course is sometimes marked by little change in hair loss or even gradual improvement, but, more often, frequent remissions and serious exacerbations occur over many years. Using a wig is common; occasionally, hair is plucked from it, too. Chronic trichotillomania can be associated with permanent follicular damage and baldness.

The long-term psychological outcome of trichotillomania does not simply hinge on the seriousness of hair loss per se. The prognosis often depends on the extent to which hair pulling is conflated with comorbid psychopathology. On its own, trichotillomania spins off abundant despair and diminished self-esteem. These problems can articulate with major depression, borderline or narcissistic personality problems, or eating disorders to create a malignant feedback loop, with substantial deterioration in quality of life.

The progression of childhood trichotillomania is usually benign compared to the adolescent and young adult variety. A hair-pulling symbiosis is notably lacking in most cases. Epilation is more akin to a transient habit, analogous in duration and limited impact to the brief episodes of phobic or compulsive symptoms common in childhood.

The formation of a trichobezoar is always a potential complication in trichotillomania. Impacted hair can cause anemia due to nutritional deficiencies, intestinal obstruction, pancreatitis, peritonitis, small or large bowel perforation, and, rarely, acute appendicitis. Symptoms appear insidiously or acutely, depending on the location and extent of the trichobezoar. Presenting problems include epigastric discomfort associated with meals, altered bowel habits, weakness, weight loss, anorexia, nausea, and vomiting, with or without hematemesis.

Weight preoccupation without a full-fledged eating disorder is commonly associated with trichotillomania, particularly during adolescence.

Differential Diagnosis

True trichotillomania should be distinguished from childhood or adolescent hair twirling and twisting without actual hair plucking, which is found more frequently in girls than boys.

Hair pulling can develop ex nihilo during an acute psychotic illness—schizophrenic or affective—as a response to command hallucinations or a specific delusional system or as a tangible expression of the hyperbolic despair and self-loathing of psychotic depression. Epilation usually ceases with remission of the acute psychosis, although it may occasionally be noted in chronic psychosis.

With its many ritualistic aspects, trichotillomania may be difficult to differentiate from the ritualistic behavior of OCD—particularly because one patient may harbor both conditions. Trichotillomania is driven by at least a modicum of pleasure seeking, whereas compulsive rituals are chiefly directed at relieving intolerable anxiety and dread.

The usually planned epilation of trichotillomania should be distinguished from spasmodic muscular and verbal tics of Tourette's syndrome. However, as noted, these disorders may afflict the same patient.

Trichotillomania should be distinguished from factitious hair pulling in aid of receiving medical attention and sympathy.

Alopecia due to other medical causes must always be ruled out when trichotillomania is suspected. It is rare to find trichotillomania precipitated by or coexisting with organic alopecia.

Laboratory Studies If necessary, the clinical diagnosis of trichotillomania can be confirmed by punch biopsy of the scalp. In patients with a trichobezoar, blood count may reveal a mild leukocytosis and hypochromic anemia due to blood loss. Appropriate chemistries and radiological studies should also be performed, depending on the bezoar's suspected location and impact on the gastrointestinal (GI) tract.

Treatment Most cases of childhood trichotillomania respond well to brief therapy, using support, simple behavioral strategies, and issue-focused stress management for family and patient, when necessary.

By contrast, the treatment of severe adolescent or adult trichotillomania is likely to be prolonged and arduous and requires a combination of modalities. Clinicians should be aware that patients are deeply ashamed of their hair pulling, easily frightened, and intensely denial prone. Many have avoided help for years. In teenagers with trichotillomania, resistances are compounded by puberty's native opposition to adult intervention. An unpressured, unintrusive stance is especially helpful during the initial workup. Much comfort derives from simple education, from discovering that hair pulling does not automatically make one weird or crazy and that others share the problem and successfully deal with it.

Psychoanalytically oriented psychotherapy yields mixed results. Improved understanding and esteem may lead to improved relationships and educational and vocational success, although hair pulling itself persists stubbornly. Individual therapy is especially problematic with teenagers embroiled in the tangled web of a hair-pulling symbiosis. Effective work cannot proceed in the office when a patient is constantly being cajoled, bribed, or criticized vis à vis hair pulling at home.

The predictable repercussion of parental persuasion, however well intended, is what one youngster called "screw-you" hair pulling, further hair loss and reinforcement of a negative self-image. Some sort of family intervention is needed in this setting by the primary therapist or a collateral therapist, if forging an effective working alliance with the patient precludes intensive contact with family members. Healthier families may require counseling and support to weather the stress imposed by a youngster's trichotillomania per se.

Virtually every class of psychotropic medication has been directed at chronic hair pulling. Serotoninergic agents, particularly SSRIs and clomipramine, have figured prominently in recent years, reflecting investigation of the relationship between trichotillomania and OCD or affective disorder. Case studies and anecdotal reports predominate over controlled large-scale outcome studies. Some patients do well and consistently maintain improvement. Others do not respond at all, or an early robust response fades over time.

Tricyclics, lithium, and buspirone (BuSpar) have been used along with or for augmentation of SSRIs. Improvement has been occasionally reported with clonazepam (Klonopin) and monoamine oxidase inhibitors (MAOI). Preliminary work indicates that the opioid antagonist naltrexone may be helpful in disrupting the rush that is experienced in hair-pulling attacks.

Cognitive-behavioral therapy has shown increasing promise. For instance, in habit reversal training (HRT), the therapist assembles a package of individualized strategies to address hair pulling, such as fostering awareness of specific affective and situational triggers, instruction in relaxation and stopping techniques, development of competing responses, and the use of journals to document progress. Individual HRT is combined with HRT group meetings for teaching, as well as social support. As with other modalities, relapse after initial success is common, so patients should be counseled to see past a temporary defeat.

Anecdotal reports indicate some effectiveness of hypnosis on a short-term basis.

Ignorance and shame about trichotillomania continue to prevent patients from getting help. Awareness of the problem has been enhanced by local and national support groups.

Kathy was a 24-year-old editor who had suffered from trichotillomania since 17 years of age. Typical hair-pulling behavior began during junior year at a highly competitive private high school in the setting of increasing torment by ruminations about not getting into the "right" college. She plucked, chewed, and swallowed hair from the top and sides of her scalp, as well as her eyebrows. She concealed hair pulling from her family and friends, because she thought "I was going nuts." She finally blurted out her symptoms to a trusted pediatrician during a routine office visit.

Kathy's parents were professionals who made intense academic demands on all of their children; family life was otherwise not notably problematic. As a child, she was extremely critical of herself and afraid of failure. Her father experienced mild periodic depression since college. One brother developed obsessions and compulsions during his late teens. Both responded well to fluoxetine (Prozac).

Kathy had received analytic psychotherapy, behavioral therapy, and medication (recently fluoxetine and clomipramine) elsewhere. Although she made reasonably good progress psychologically, she was never able to stop pulling her hair long enough for it to grow back. She had a wide circle of friends but still kept romance at arm's length, fearing that a potential lover would be frightened off if he found out her "secret." She could not bring herself to replace the "ratty" wig that she had been wearing since her late teens. "It makes me look dowdy," she said, "but buying a new one would be like telling myself I'll never get better."

Kathy sought treatment chiefly for regulation of her medication but quickly proved amenable to weekly psychotherapy sessions. Her clomipramine was increased, while she explored the sense of damage and "freakiness" that made her fend off men who liked her. She was much helped by weekly meetings at a trichotillomania support group. After 6 months, her self-esteem had improved, she had fewer bouts of hair pulling and had begun dating hesitantly. She arrived at her last session displaying an attractive new wig, stating ironically: "It isn't my real hair yet, but at least it's better than my old rug."

KLEPTOMANIA

Definition and History The defining behavior of kleptomania is the repetitive theft of items that are usually of little monetary value and are not realistically needed. Increasing tension is experienced before stealing. Feelings of relief and gratification during and after the act eventually give way to guilt, remorse, and self-loathing, compounded by the fear of arrest. Kleptomania is profoundly repug-

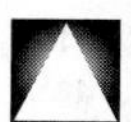

Table 21–4
DSM-IV-TR Diagnostic Criteria for Kleptomania

A. Recurrent failure to resist impulses to steal objects that are not needed for personal use or for their monetary value.
B. Increasing sense of tension immediately before committing the theft.
C. Pleasure, gratification, or relief at the time of committing the theft.
D. The stealing is not committed to express anger or vengeance and is not in response to a delusion or a hallucination.
E. The stealing is not better accounted for by conduct disorder, a manic episode, or antisocial personality disorder.

From American Psychiatric Association. *Diagnostic and Statistical Manual of Mental Disorders.* 4th ed. Text rev. Washington, DC: American Psychiatric Association; 2000, with permission.

nant to many sufferers, inconsistent with their otherwise ethical behavior and beliefs (Table 21–4).

The diagnosis of kleptomania was first coined in 1838 by Esquirol and Charles-Chretien-Henri Marc and was grounded on Phillipe Pinel's earlier concept of a *manie sans delire*—insanity without delusion or clouding of consciousness. Esquirol subsumed kleptomania under the *instinctive monomanias*—conditions in which a single, *irresistible* impulse was acted out.

Subsequent investigation during the 19th century was largely descriptive. Psychoanalytic exploration of single or few cases of kleptomania throughout the 20th century yielded valuable insights and some headway in treatment. Since the 1980s, interest in kleptomania has increased, paralleling research into the psychobiology of other impulse-control disorders, as well as affective and obsessive illness. Nevertheless, no large cohort of kleptomania patients has been studied to date.

Nosology

Kleptomania was mentioned *passim* in the first edition of the DSM (DSM-I). It was omitted from the second edition of the DSM (DSM-II), arguably because it was viewed as a constituent symptom of other conditions, rather than a separate disorder. It was listed as a viable diagnosis in DSM-III and, subsequently, in DSM-III-R, DSM-IV, and DSM-IV-TR, with several changes along the way.

DSM-III-R emphasizes that the stolen object is not needed for personal use. Associated tension specifically occurs "immediately before committing the theft." Criterion D of DSM-III-R newly stipulates that stealing "is not committed to express anger or vengeance" and is not a response "to a delusion or hallucination." The absence of planning and collaboration in connection with theft as a qualifier is dropped in DSM-III-R. Criterion D—"the stealing is not due to conduct disorder or anti-social personality disorder"—is thus reframed in DSM-IV: "The stealing is not better accounted for by Conduct disorders, a Manic episode, or Antisocial Personality Disorder." DSM-IV-TR continues these exclusions.

ICD-10 designates kleptomania as "pathological stealing" hallmarked by "repeated failure to resist impulses to steal objects that are not acquired for personal use or monetary gain. The objects may be discarded, given away, or hoarded." The typical cycle of tension before stealing, "a sense of gratification during and immediately after, the act," and the solitary nature of thefts are noted. "Anxiety, despondency, and guilt" between episodes of stealing do "not prevent repetition." Excluded from the diagnosis are recurrent acts of carefully planned shoplifting for personal gain; organic mental disorder, in which payment for goods is overlooked "as a consequence of poor memory and other kinds of intellectual deterioration"; and "depressive disorder with stealing."

Epidemiology

Kleptomania was once thought to be extremely rare: For instance, in a 1947 study of arrested shoplifters, less than 4 percent showed evidence of the disorder. Many experts in the field now believe that kleptomania is substantially underreported owing to the reluctance of ashamed patients to seek help, as well as their not-unwarranted fear of prosecution.

Failure to document kleptomania may also stem from lack of education or prejudice about the condition by law enforcement officials and health professionals. When kleptomania is seen as a criminal, rather than a medical, issue, many patients are sure to be misdiagnosed—and written off—as antisocial personalities, to be accordingly sanctioned.

Although it is widely held that kleptomania is predominantly a disorder of women, the high female to male ratio (approximately 3 to 1) may reflect the fact that more women seek or are compelled to use psychiatric services than men. For instance, once under court supervision, a female shoplifter is likely to be sent for a psychiatric evaluation, whereas a male offender is dispatched to jail.

Several of the kleptomaniacs described by Marc and Esquirol were royals, such as King Victor of Sardinia and King Henry IV of France. A lion's share of interest in the disorder is commanded by patients from favored backgrounds because of the discrepancy, absurd or poignant, between their wealth and power and the mean objects that they filch. Nevertheless, there is no evidence that kleptomania is a special affliction of the rich.

Limited data suggest that higher rates of affective illness and obsessive-compulsive traits occur in first-degree relatives of kleptomania patients. Families also may be pervaded by the same preoccupation with financial success and material acquisition encountered in the relatives of pathological gamblers.

Comorbidity

Patients with kleptomania are said to have a high lifetime comorbidity of major affective illness (usually, but not exclusively, depressive) and various anxiety disorders. Associated conditions also include other impulse-control disorders (notably pathological gambling and compulsive shopping), eating disorders, and substance abuse disorders, alcoholism in particular.

Etiology

Psychoanalytic speculation about kleptomania has been abundant relative to the small number of patients treated. Analysts conceptualize compulsive stealing as a highly overdetermined act, exquisitely balanced between gratification and punishment. Stealing is intended to restore intrapsychic equilibrium and to redress sundry childhood traumata, intrapsychic distortions, or both. The syndrome has been interpreted as an attempt to rectify actual or perceived neglect and narcissistic injuries of childhood via vengeful attack, to stave off formidable feelings of low self-esteem through aggressive acquisition, and to gratify forbidden infantile sexual wishes and masturbatory fantasies. With the omnipresent threat of retaliation, stealing often comes to possess a peculiar masochistic sizzle.

The stolen object has been construed as a talisman of recuperated loss across the stages of child development—oral, anal, and genital. According to the developmental level of the patient's fixation, it may symbolize milk, feces, breast, penis, or child.

In some patients, compulsive stealing is strongly inflected by the familial superego lacunae described in childhood and adolescent conduct disturbances by Adelaide Johnson and Samuel Szurek: An apparently upright, ethical parent projects unconscious delinquent wishes on the child, who proceeds to act out the disavowed parental behavior.

Since the 1980s, analytical theories have been superseded by speculation on the neurobiology of kleptomania. The significant comorbidity of the condition with affective disorders and obsessive-compulsive pathology has been emphasized, as well as the meaningful occurrence of affective disorder and OCD in close relatives. Although substantive confirmation is yet to come, kleptomania has been theorized as an obsessive-compulsive spectrum disturbance and affective spectrum disturbance.

From a behavioral and cognitive perspective, compulsive stealing—like other impulse-control disorders—is powerfully self-reinforcing by virtue of its repetitive and highly ritualistic aspects.

Clinical Features and Course

Most episodes of kleptomania seem to occur spontaneously and suddenly, with little, if any, premeditation. However, deeper probing often reveals that theft ensued in the setting of a recent stress—an argument with a business colleague or a lover's quarrel—accompanied by frustration, anger, and an ambiguous sense of neediness.

Patients report a mixture of dread and pleasure before stealing. Some feel agonizingly caught between the urge to relieve intolerable tension versus moral scruples and fear of capture. Others plunge directly into action without a moment's hesitation, especially when a well-defined pattern of stealing has developed over repeated episodes.

Most bouts of kleptomania take place in public, at stores, supermarkets, and malls, for example. Stealing at private parties or social events is less common. Stolen objects usually have negligible value; in any case, they are not needed or could be easily afforded. The items vary, or the same object is stolen each time (especially undergarments). Some patients hoard and examine pilfered goods: Their kleptomania possesses a distinctly fetishistic aspect. More frequently, stolen material is hidden without subsequent attention; given away, thrown out, or donated to charity by way of restitution; surreptitiously replaced at the point of origin; or returned with a jury-rigged explanation or with an admission of guilt and a plea for forgiveness.

Patients are intensely ashamed of stealing and strive mightily to keep it secret and under control. They avoid stores pilfered in the past; they even warn stores in advance or cease shopping altogether. Patients feel good psychologically and morally when they are able to free themselves of stealing for a while; they feel devastated and despairing when they backslide.

Kleptomania classically begins in late adolescence to the mid-20s, often emerges in the context of compulsive shopping, and can remain undetected for years (in one study, first involvement with the legal system occurred at 35 years of age for women and at 50 years of age for men). Stealing bouts may occur sporadically, with quiescent periods, or may relentlessly escalate until the patient's inevitable arrest and prosecution.

Exposure precipitates crushing humiliation, akin to the trauma experienced by pathological gamblers when their losses are revealed. Although exposure usually compels the individual to seek help, it may also—as in the course of gamblers—provide an unhelpful bail-out, through deals struck with compassionate store owners, restitution by the patient or relatives, or adjudication for lesser offenses on condition of treatment, and so forth.

Kleptomania is likely to be a chronic illness, hallmarked by repeated relapses over decades. Statistics on outcome are lacking. By anecdotal report, some patients find relief through therapeutic or spiritual intervention, or both; others simply burn out or continue stealing indefinitely. Imprisonment and suicide to avoid incarceration are meaningful possibilities.

The course of kleptomania is decisively influenced by serious comorbid conditions. Individuals with compulsive shopping disorder often begin compulsive stealing earlier, the former condition easily shading over into the latter. Episodes of kleptomania are also precipitated by the disinhibiting influence of substance abuse.

Although there is no consistent kleptomania personality type, many patients manifest obsessive-compulsive and narcissistic tendencies. Lacunae in judgment about stealing may extend into other life areas. Patients experience genuine contrition and deeply fear arrest; yet, they can also appear strangely incapable of grasping the actual legal consequences of their actions and feel obscurely unempathic, wronged, and entitled vis à vis their victims' injured feelings:

> A woman pilfered her best friend's favorite paperweight during a party and then returned it the next day and revealed her kleptomania. She was offended and angry because her friend did not immediately express what she considered to be the proper degree of sympathy and forgiveness about her problem.

Differential Diagnosis

Episodes of theft occasionally occur during psychotic illness, for example, acute mania, major depression with psychotic features, or schizophrenia. Psychotic stealing is obviously a product of pathological elevation or depression of mood or command hallucinations or delusions.

Theft in individuals with antisocial personality disorder is deliberately undertaken for personal gain, with some degree of premeditation and planning, often executed with others. Antisocial stealing regularly involves the threat of harm or actual violence, particularly to elude capture. Guilt and remorse are distinctively lacking, or patients are patently insincere. In contrast, kleptomania is a solitary activity, directed at property rather than person, and stealing occasions shows of genuine remorse after the event.

Shoplifting has become a national epidemic. Few shoplifters have true kleptomania; the majority are teenagers and young adults who "boost" in pairs or small groups for "kicks," as well as goods, and do not have a major psychiatric disorder.

Acute intoxication with drugs or alcohol may precipitate theft in an individual with another psychiatric disorder or without significant psychopathology.

Patients with Alzheimer's disease or other dementing organic illness may leave a store without paying owing to forgetfulness, rather than larcenous intent.

Malingering kleptomania is common in apprehended antisocial types, as well as nonantisocial youthful shoplifters. Given a sufficiently intelligent perpetrator, the fictive version can be quite difficult to distinguish from the genuine disorder.

Episodes of stealing are commonplace in childhood, for example, taking change from a parent's purse or pockets. The overwhelming majority of these are transient and reflect no serious psychological disturbance.

Treatment

The majority of patients avoid help until they become involved with the law, and some form of psychological assistance is made a condition of remaining free. By that time, the disorder is likely to be entrenched, and therapy is correspondingly difficult. Complex therapeutic issues are often raised by the implied threat of prosecution if treatment is not sought or maintained.

No controlled treatment studies of kleptomania have been undertaken. Multiple modalities are common. Success has been reported on an anecdotal basis with various outpatient talking approaches, including psychoanalysis, group, and family work. Individual psychotherapy alone is often insufficient to control acting out. Indeed, stealing may actually be precipitated by the transferential vicissitudes of insight-oriented treatment.

A panoply of behavioral and cognitive strategies and medications have addressed kleptomania, with the usual anecdotal reports of success. Antidepressants and mood stabilizers may be particularly helpful in cases in which kleptomania clearly occurs against a background of serious affective illness. Naltrexone has shown some promise in specifically blocking the impulse to steal.

Very few 12-step programs exist for kleptomania per se, arguably owing to tremendous shame combined with unwillingness to go public, because of fear of legal consequences. Individuals with comorbid substance abuse or gambling difficulties indicate that stealing is often remediated by AA and GA participation, even when they choose not to reveal their thieving. Some nonabusing kleptomania patients claim that they have obtained relief simply by attending 12-step meetings without direct participation or self-revelation.

Uncontrollable kleptomania can occasionally be broken by brief hospitalization, although securing insurance coverage presents a formidable problem. Hospitalization in a dual-diagnosis program that accepts patients with kleptomania is particularly helpful, if one can be found.

An unwary therapist can easily become overinvolved in the patient's attempts to avoid legal action. One does well to remember that relapses are common and must be dealt with realistically, while making authorities duly aware of the pathological nature of the problem. The process of adjudication that is so desperately feared by patients may occasionally turn out to be an unexpected adjuvant to treatment. Regular check-ins with a competent, compassionate probation officer can help strengthen the patient's impaired superego function.

Jane was a 42-year-old, highly successful, single executive from a wealthy background. She called herself a "shop-'til-you-drop type" and had always been able to afford the expensive designer clothing that she loved. Since college, her "legit" shopping had been paralleled by "boosting" cheap panties and brassieres from discount stores. She did not wear the stolen items; indeed, she considered them "sleazy." She could never bring herself to get rid of them either and kept boxes filled with pilfered lingerie in a storage facility.

Jane talked or bought her way out of trouble until her 30s, when she was arrested while stealing pantyhose from the same K-Mart for the third time in as many months. As a condition of probation, she was ordered to see a psychiatrist. Her attendance was sporadic, and several more thefts occurred over the next 2 years. She also experienced substantial depression, which she tried to alleviate by heavy drinking.

Jane finally began taking her problem seriously after yet another arrest precipitated a suicidal gesture. She began keeping appointments regularly and consented to taking citalopram (Celexa) and naltrexone. She believes that her participation in an AA group for high-pressured executives has been at least as effective—if not more so—in controlling her stealing.

PYROMANIA

Definition and History

Pyromania is defined as recurrent, deliberate fire setting (Table 21–5). Controversy continues over whether the condition should be classified under the impulse-control disorders or, indeed, whether it comprises a separate entity at all.

Like kleptomania, pyromania evolved out of Pinel's concept of *la manie sans delire*—madness without delusion or clouding of the sensorium, with substantive preservation of reasoning power. Early 18th century French psychiatrists Marc and Esquirol categorized pyromania as a *monomanie incendiare*—another of the *instinctive monomanias* in which a patient acts out one irresistible impulse.

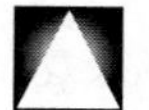

Table 21–5
DSM-IV-TR Diagnostic Criteria for Pyromania

A. Deliberate and purposeful fire setting on more than one occasion.
B. Tension or affective arousal before the act.
C. Fascination with, interest in, curiosity about, or attraction to fire and its situational contexts (e.g., paraphernalia, uses, and consequences).
D. Pleasure, gratification, or relief when setting fires or when witnessing or participating in their aftermath.
E. The fire setting is not done for monetary gain, as an expression of sociopolitical ideology, to conceal criminal activity, to express anger or vengeance, to improve one's living circumstances, in response to a delusion or hallucination, or as a result of impaired judgment (e.g., in dementia, mental retardation, or substance intoxication).
F. The fire setting is not better accounted for by conduct disorder, a manic episode, or antisocial personality disorder.

From American Psychiatric Association. *Diagnostic and Statistical Manual of Mental Disorders.* 4th ed. Text rev. Washington, DC: American Psychiatric Association; 2000, with permission.

Nosology

Pyromania was mentioned *passim* in DSM-I and was omitted altogether in DSM-II, under the tacit assumption that it did not merit consideration as a new diagnosis. It was so acknowledged for the first time in DSM-III; was categorized under impulse-control disorders, not elsewhere specified; and was described as a

> recurrent failure to resist impulses to set fires, intense fascination with the setting of fires, and seeing fires burn. Prior to setting the fire, there is a build-up of tension. Once the fire is under way, the individual experiences intense pleasure or release. Although the fire-setting results from a failure to resist an impulse, there may be considerable advance preparation.

DSM-III-R redefined and otherwise modified several of the DSM-III parameters. The phrase "recurrent failures to resist impulses to set fires" was eliminated and was replaced by "deliberate and purposeful fire setting on more than one occasion." Criterion C ("fascination with") elaborates further on psychological preoccupations related to fire setting. The exclusions of DSM-III's Criterion E were augmented to indicate that pyromania cannot be diagnosed if fire setting is clearly a response to psychotic delusions or hallucinations. The revised Criterion F further states that the diagnosis cannot be made when fire setting occurs in the setting of a manic episode, conduct disorder, or antisocial personality disorder. All DSM-III-R criteria for pyromania are maintained in DSM-IV and DSM-IV-TR.

The ICD-10 characterizes pyromania as "multiple acts of, or attempts at setting fire to property or other objects, without apparent motive." Incendiary activity is said to be accompanied by tension and excitement over its course. Also noted are persistent preoccupations with fire-related subjects, fire-fighting equipment, and calling out the fire service. Excluded from the diagnosis are fire setting for obvious reasons and fire setting by "a young person with conduct disorder," by "an adult with 'sociopathic personality disorder,'" and by individuals with schizophrenia or organic psychiatric disorders.

Epidemiology

No major study of pyromania has been conducted since Nolan D. Lewis and Helen Yarnell's 1951 examination of nonprofit incendiary cases from the files of the National Board of Fire Underwriters and since J. L. Geller's 1992 overview of adult pathological fire setting. Only 3 to 4 percent—some 50 of the 1,594 fire setters—of the Lewis and Yarnell population fit DSM-IV-TR criteria for pyromania. Given the persistent paucity of literature, assertions about epidemiology and, indeed, any other aspects of pyromania are tentative.

The condition is supposedly rare. Most patients are male, with a male to female ratio of approximately 8 to 1.

Fire setting by children and adolescents continues to pose enormous problems, resulting in substantial damage to property and danger to life. More than 40 percent of arrested arsonists are younger than 18 years of age. One stresses that few meet formal criteria for pyromania, although differential diagnosis is often difficult.

By anecdotal report, the families of pyromania patients show increased psychiatric problems, similar to the family derangements of other impulse-control disordered patients, such as affective illnesses; substance abuse, particularly alcoholism; and various personality disorders.

Comorbidity Pyromania is significantly associated with substance abuse disorder (especially alcoholism); affective disorders, depressive or bipolar; other impulse control disorders, such as kleptomania in female fire setters; and various personality disturbances, such as inadequate and borderline personality disorders. Attention-deficit disorder and learning disabilities may be conspicuously associated with childhood pyromania; this constellation frequently persists into adulthood.

Etiology The few in-depth explorations of pyromania have been conducted by psychoanalysts. Freud famously inferred an articulation between fire, ambition, and *urethral eroticism*; he also theorized that pyromania represented a masturbatory equivalent. Subsequent investigators describe fire setting and its related preoccupations as highly overdetermined activities expressing repressed childhood sexual or aggressive drives, or both, aimed at redressing a panoply of real or perceived early traumata, in the context of a dysfunctional, chaotic early family life.

Pyromania has been variously interpreted as a striving to exact revenge against rejecting, abusive parents or other adult figures, to acquire power in the context of chronic feelings of helplessness and inadequacy, or to master traumatic memories of the primal scene. Some young pyromania patients are said to act out projected, disavowed incendiary impulses of a parent or other family member with superego lacunae.

There has been little research on the biological and cognitive-behavioral features of pyromania. The lack reflects not only the disorder's inherent rareness, but also an unwillingness to be identified that is even more formidable than the resistance of trichotillomania and kleptomania patients. Preliminary studies hint at serotoninergic and other neurotransmitter dysfunction, as well as disordered glucose regulation with the possibility of a hypoglycemic trigger.

Abundant clinical and phenomenological similarities between pyromania and other impulse-control *disorders of desire* warrant the consideration of pathological fire setting as an affective spectrum disturbance or an obsessive-compulsive spectrum disturbance.

Clinical Features and Course A typical episode of pyromania begins with rising tension linked to thoughts of fire setting. Tension often possesses a distinctly erotic quality and may be accompanied by restlessness, headaches, palpitations, and tinnitus. Dissociated feelings and alcohol intoxication before fire setting have been reported. In some cases, preparation for setting a fire is painstaking; in others, it is perfunctory. The incendiary's pleasure over the conflagration derives from several sources: watching the flames themselves, which may engender sexual arousal that is so intense (pyrolagnia) as to lead to masturbation, and watching activities connected with the fire, including the conflagration's escalating material devastation, its impact on others, and, especially, the firemen's activities as they go about extinguishing the blaze.

Pyromania patients often strongly identify with the firefighter's strength and competence. In addition to lighting fires, they may undertake volunteer duties at firehouses or may become volunteer firefighters themselves, then taking delight in putting out the blazes that they have lit. Women are less likely to become involved with the firefighting community.

Many patients prolong their idiosyncratic enjoyment by lingering in the vicinity of a fire that they have set. It is in the context of a perennial return to the scene or inability to leave it that they are frequently apprehended by vigilant police or arson squad detectives. They then regularly display striking denial, even after being presented with the most damning evidence (unlike individuals with kleptomania, who readily confess when caught).

Tension drops after a fire-setting episode, and the patient may fall into a deep, relaxed sleep. The overwhelming guilt and remorse of individuals with kleptomania or trichotillomania do not seem to plague pyromania patients as consistently. Some even seem eerily indifferent toward the destruction that they have wrought.

Episodes of pyromania may occur sporadically, with prolonged impulse-free intervals. Other patients are afflicted by daily urges to set fire over many years. One's clinical impression is that a majority of fire-setting episodes occur at night—a time that offers greater possibilities for concealment and that may also possess potent sexual and aggressive associations.

> A 28-year-old fire setter said that he was tremendously aroused by the sight of flames against the background of a black night sky. He remembered being awakened at 6 years of age by ominous noises coming from his teenage sister's bedroom. He peeked through her open door and was profoundly shocked—and aroused—by the stark vision of her and a boyfriend, lit by a pool of bright lamplight, having passionate sex.

Pyromania usually begins in mid- to late adolescence, but earlier onset is not unusual. The typical patient is said to be intellectually limited; comes from an underprivileged social background and a dysfunctional, violence-prone family; and often has significant learning and socialization handicaps in childhood. Child or adolescent fire setting and preoccupations with fire may be unaccompanied by other symptoms. Pyromaniac behavior is more likely to be part of a cluster of petty delinquent behaviors that includes running away, truancy, and thieving, making the primary diagnosis uncertain (vide infra). Fire setting at home frequently occurs in the youngster's room or the parental bedroom. If behavioral problems are serious enough to require institutionalization, incendiary behavior is likely to carry over to residential treatment centers, training schools, and other inpatient settings, causing enormous problems.

The typical adult patient with pyromania supposedly is a vocational underachiever, has difficulty in sustaining relationships, and may lead a marginal existence. However, this notionally average patient may comprise only one subtype, if the most common, of the condition. Other patients come from more stable families and exhibit better achievement levels vocationally and socially. Their parallel life of fire setting remains a shameful secret.

No definitive data about the course of pyromania exist. On anecdotal evidence, some patients continually set fires throughout their lives, despite repeated incarcerations, or end up permanently imprisoned. Others persist in their fire setting indefinitely, keeping it surreptitious and limited enough to avoid arrest. For still others, a gradual burnout of the disorder takes place in later decades. One surmises that the progression of pyromania is considerably inflected by comorbid conditions, especially substance abuse disorders and affective illness.

Most self-immolations are obviously a function of psychosis or nonpsychotic social protest. However, it seems reasonable to assume that some pyromaniacs terminate their lives by setting fire to themselves, accidentally (particularly when intoxicated) or deliberately, in the context of profound depression.

Differential Diagnosis

Despite the DSM-IV-TR's exclusionary criteria, it is often extremely difficult to differentiate true pyromania from the fire setting of other syndromes, especially adolescent conduct disturbances.

Fire setting in schizophrenia or manic-depressive disorder is clearly a function of flagrant thought disturbance, precipitated by command hallucinations or delusions.

Pyromania should not be diagnosed if fire setting is caused by acute intoxication with alcohol or other substances, lacking other parameters of the disorder.

Fire setting in severe mental retardation or organic dementia clearly stems from impaired judgment based on cerebral deficit:

An 80-year-old man with Alzheimer's disease forgot that he had left a cigarette burning on the edge of a night table while looking for an ashtray. The cigarette fell into a wastebasket filled with combustible material, causing a major conflagration.

Fire setting by individuals with antisocial disorder reflects their criminal, unempathic, and remorseless natures. Incendiary acts are clearly aimed at revenge, profit, or concealing a crime. The triad of violence to animals, fire setting, and bedwetting in childhood is widely held to be a marker for particularly violent antisocial behavior in adolescence and adulthood.

Pyromania should be distinguished from setting fires as a means of political protest or sabotage, of bringing attention to some personal wish or need, or of gaining some other recognition in a nonpsychotic context.

Children with no psychiatric disturbance may set fires inadvertently as a function of ordinary experimentation. Playing with matches or lighters in this context is occasionally catastrophic but nevertheless does not warrant a diagnosis of pyromania or other psychiatric disorder.

Little is known about the professional arsonist or *torch*. Law enforcement sources suggest that career arsonists are overwhelmingly male, pride themselves on their highly specialized expertise, and—if only to avoid more punitive prosecution—go to great lengths to ensure that their work does not cause physical harm.

The torch's criminality is usually confined to fire setting, and he or she may not always fit the tidy paradigms of the antisocial personality disorder. One speculates that some torches embody yet another subset of pyromania, in which pathological incendiary impulses are rationalized and acted out under the aegis of doing a job for hire.

Treatment

Treatment of pyromania continues to be problematic owing to a lack of a willing clientele, even when fire setters are incarcerated. Despite anecdotal reports of success with psychoanalytic methods, most pyromania patients are hardly apt candidates for insight-oriented therapy owing to their profound denial, heavy drinking, and an alexithymic inability to identify and to work through feelings.

With so little data available on any sort of therapy, and no definitive cure in sight, one can only advocate the multimodal approach that is characteristic of treatment for other impulse-control disorders: flexible deployment of various psychotherapies, cognitive and behavioral work, and drug intervention according to the unique presentation of each patient.

Childhood fire setting must always be taken seriously, especially when episodes are repeated, damage is substantial, the family structure notably is dysfunctional, and the patient is substantially inarticulate. Under these circumstances, family therapy combined with individual treatment may be particularly helpful.

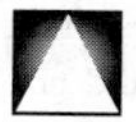

Table 21–6
DSM-IV-TR Diagnostic Criteria for Intermittent Explosive Disorder

A. Several discrete episodes of failure to resist aggressive impulses that result in serious assaultive acts or destruction of property.
B. The degree of aggressiveness expressed during the episodes is grossly out of proportion to any precipitating psychosocial stressors.
C. The aggressive episodes are not better accounted for by another mental disorder (e.g., antisocial personality disorder, borderline personality disorder, a psychotic disorder, a manic episode, conduct disorder, or attention-deficit/hyperactivity disorder) and are not due to the direct physiological effects of a substance (e.g., a drug of abuse or a medication) or a general medical condition (e.g., head trauma or Alzheimer's disease).

From American Psychiatric Association. *Diagnostic and Statistical Manual of Mental Disorders.* 4th ed. Text rev. Washington, DC: American Psychiatric Association; 2000, with permission.

INTERMITTENT EXPLOSIVE DISORDER

Definition

Intermittent explosive disorder is characterized by repeated failure to resist aggressive impulses, resulting in punctate explosions of aggression that cause serious physical harm or damage, or both, to property. The eruption of violence is typically far out of proportion to the precipitating stress (Table 21–6).

Comparative Nosology

Intermittent explosive disorder arguably is the most controversial entity of this group. The diagnosis emerged out of several decades of debate about whether a syndrome consisting of repeated explosive episodes should be classified as a psychiatric illness in the first place and, assuming this syndrome exists, about where to place it nosologically. Investigators have particularly disagreed over whether a disorder such as this could be indicative of some kind of neurophysiological dysfunction, although still being separated diagnostically from other syndromes with obvious organically induced aggression.

A patient meeting current DSM-IV-TR criteria for intermittent explosive disorder would have been diagnosed in DSM-I as a *passive-aggressive personality, aggressive type*. DSM-II replaced the latter with *explosive personality*, which, in turn, was eliminated by DSM-III in favor of *intermittent explosive disorder.*

The new diagnosis was advanced to account for patients with so-called episodic dyscontrol syndrome, in which sudden episodes of violent behavior erupted without notable intervening psychopathology. A diagnosis of *isolated explosive disorder* was also added to the group: Its salient feature was a single episode of violent behavior with catastrophic consequences. The DSM-III version of intermittent explosive disorder allowed for but did not require an organic etiology to support the diagnosis. It was noted that, in some cases, "features suggesting an organic disturbance may be present such as nonspecific EEG [electroencephalogram] abnormalities or minor neurological signs and symptoms thought to reflect subcortical or limbic system dysfunction." The assumption was implicit, however, that psychosocial factors alone could cause the disorder.

During the fashioning of DSM-III-R, intermittent explosive disorder was, at first, deleted and then restored. Those favoring elimination believed that repetitive violent outbursts should not be subsumed within a discrete psychiatric entity or thought that, when a substantive neurophysiological etiology could be proven, explosive episodes would be best classified under the rubric of an organic mental disorder. Concern was voiced at that time—and still exists today—about standardizing a nonorganic psychiatric diagnosis that could then be used as a legal defense in cases of violent crime.

The restored DSM-III-R diagnosis reflected the final conclusion of evaluators that psychosocial and environmental factors played a conclusive role in some cases of intermittent violent behavior. However, another exclusionary category was created—organic personality syndrome, explosive type—to account for intermittent explosive cases with a definitive history of central nervous system (CNS) dysfunction.

DSM-IV and DSM-IV-TR retain the DSM-III-R's *intermittent explosive disorder*; eliminate *organic personality syndrome, explosive type*; and redefine the exclusionary criteria: The diagnosis now should not be made in the presence of manic episode, ADHD, and any "general medical condition (e.g. head trauma, Alzheimer's disease)."

Intermittent explosive disorder is not recognized as a distinct diagnosis in ICD-10. It is mentioned under *other habit and impulse disorders* (F63.8), without spelling out specific parameters.

Epidemiology

Intermittent explosive disorder is believed to be relatively rare, although the condition may be underreported. The few studies available indicate a male preponderance as high as 80 percent. Family histories, particularly in first-degree relatives, show a high rate of one or more comorbid mood disorders, anxiety disorders, substance abuse disorders, and impulse-control disorders—including intermittent explosive disorder itself.

Comorbidity

A major association has been noted between intermittent explosive disorder and mood disturbances—particularly bipolar disorder (more than 50 percent in one study). Meaningful comorbidity is also described with anxiety disorders, substance abuse disorders, eating disorders, personality disorders, attention-deficit disorder, and other impulse-control disorders.

Etiology

Although research has been limited, it is generally assumed that intermittent explosive disorder—like other impulse-control disturbances—is caused by a varying confluence of psychosocial and neurobiological factors.

Patients regularly describe chaotic family backgrounds, rife with explosive behavior and verbal and physical abuse, often in the context of acute alcohol intoxication. *Identification with the aggressor* is a common defense mechanism, in which the explosive violence of a parent or close relative is internalized. This sinister coping strategy replicates the acts of stormy violence to which patients have been exposed during their formative years.

Situations that realistically or symbolically evoke memories of early oppression and trauma may spark explosive episodes. Typically, an acute sense of narcissistic injury, a lowered self-esteem, and profound feelings of shame and humiliation are evoked:

> A 28-year-old man had been repeatedly brutalized by his alcoholic mother throughout childhood and early adolescence. He felt particularly humiliated when she would slap his face during frequent bouts of uncontrollable anger. One evening, while they were drinking at a local tavern, a friend playfully slapped his cheek. The patient suddenly "saw red," broke a beer bottle over the man's head, and then mauled him severely.

Modest neurobiological studies point to possible deranged serotonin neurotransmission in patients identified with intermittent explosive disorder; low cerebrospinal fluid (CSF) levels of 5-hydroxyindoleacetic acid (5-HIAA) in some impulsive, temper-prone individuals; and lowered levels of platelet serotonin reuptake in patients with episodic rage. A connection has also been inferred between elevated CSF testosterone levels and aggressive or openly violent behavior.

Patients may show *soft* neurological signs (e.g., asymmetry of reflexes) and nonspecific EEG findings (e.g., diffuse slow activity). An element of genetic loading is suggested by the fact that blood relatives are more likely to have characteristic outbursts of explosive behavior compared to adoptive relatives.

In an overview of 27 cases, Susan L. McElroy and colleagues concluded that intermittent explosive disorder could be classified as an affective spectrum disturbance based on the strong comorbidity of bipolar disorder, a high familial rate of mood disturbances, disturbed circadian rhythms, and responsiveness to thymoleptics.

Clinical Features, Diagnostic Considerations, and Course

An explosive episode may be preceded by a period of escalating tension and aggressive feelings or may ignite in a flash with little or no inciting cause. The attack itself is often accompanied by irritability, rage, mood elevation, increased energy, and racing thoughts. Feelings of mild dissociation and depersonalization, without later amnesia for the event, are described. Physical symptoms may antedate or may occur during the outburst—for example, tingling, tremor, palpitations, chest tightness, tinnitus, and head pressure or headaches. After the episode, relief is quickly followed by remorse, fatigue, and depression. A migraine-type headache may be carried over from the attack or may develop de novo. Explosive eruptions usually last approximately 10 to 20 minutes; they may occur frequently, in clusters; or weeks to months may intervene before another episode. Some patients exhibit no aggressive tendencies between outbursts, but the majority exhibit some type of chronic impulsive or aggressive behavior. Patients are often perceived by others—and view themselves—as perennially angry. Many experience *subthreshold* states, in which serious aggression is headed off by exercising shaky control or by engaging in less dangerous behavior—screaming, pounding a table, or punching a wall. Against the background of severe family dysfunction, the childhood of individuals with intermittent explosive disorder is hallmarked by temper tantrums and sundry behavioral difficulties—stealing or fire setting. The youngster's problems are often compounded by defective attention, concentration, and hyperactivity.

Intermittent explosive disorder characteristically begins during late childhood to the early 20s, with a mean age of onset of 18.3 years of age. Course is dependent on the frequency and severity of explosive episodes. Severe cases show poor school performance, employment problems, and stormy interpersonal relationships. Divorce, injury to self or others from fights and accidents (e.g., during attacks of road rage), and sundry financial and legal problems (including incarceration) are common. Narcissistic, obsessive, paranoid, or schizoid personality traits may especially predispose patients to aggressive outbursts.

Although there is no extensive study of outcome, the long-term history of the disorder may be episodic or chronic. A prolonged course with markedly deteriorated quality of life is likely when explosive behavior occurs regularly, with serious consequences, in the presence of severe comorbid conditions—especially substance abuse disorders, mood disorders, and substantive character pathology.

When intermittent explosive disorder is suspected, the patient must be painstakingly evaluated to rule out one of the many medical or neurological conditions that can cause aggressive episodes. A basic workup includes thorough neurological examination; blood chemistries to assay the possibility of diabetes, liver disease, kidney disease, thyroid disease, syphilis, alcohol, and lead or other poisoning; urinalysis with toxicology screen; and skull X-rays. Further study may use EEG, magnetic resonance imaging (MRI), computed tomography (CT), and positron emission tomography (PET) scanning.

Differential Diagnosis DSM-IV-TR stresses that intermittent explosive disorder can only be diagnosed after *all* other medical and psychiatric causes of intemperate aggression are absolutely ruled out. When it can be proven definitively that the aggressive behavior is directly caused by a medical or organic condition (e.g., postconcussion syndrome), a diagnosis of *personality change due to a general medical condition, aggressive type*, is made, rather than *intermittent explosive disorder*.

Aggressive outbursts are common in delirium and cease when the underlying cause has been resolved. Aggressive explosions are rarely seen in epilepsy, notably in frontal and temporal lobe seizures.

Aggression due to substance intoxication or withdrawal is diagnosed by a history of abuse (not always easy to obtain), as well as by appropriate blood and urine studies. Alcohol remains the most common cause of intoxicated aggressive behavior. Amongst street drugs, phencyclidine (PCP) is especially known to precipitate extreme, violent behavior. Intermittent explosive disorder can only be diagnosed in a violence-prone substance abuser if other criteria of the former disorder are completely met.

Aggressive outbursts associated with various personality disorders usually have a more planned, premeditated quality. However, antisocial personality disorder and borderline personality disorder occasionally present with serious, deliberate aggressive acts, as well as outbursts of unpremeditated violence. Given the fulfillment of other criteria, intermittent explosive disorder can then be diagnosed together with the requisite personality disorder. Attacks of anger associated with autonomic arousal (e.g., tachycardia and flushing), related to terrifying feelings of being out of control, can occur in major depressive disorder and panic disorder. DSM-IV-TR allows the additional diagnosis of intermittent explosive disorder when aggressive and destructive outbursts clearly do not take place during periods of depression or a panic attack, and other criteria are satisfied.

Aggressive outbursts associated with schizophrenic illness or a manic psychotic state are obviously related to other psychotic phenomena, such as command hallucinations or delusions of persecution.

Individuals with violent antisocial tendencies may malinger symptoms of intermittent explosive disorder to escape punishment.

Intentional violent behavior without any mental disorder is distinguished by obvious motivation and hope for gain through aggressive action.

Display of anger in the context of frustrating life events, standard environmental pressures, or posttraumatic stress disorder (PTSD), precipitated by extraordinary stress, shows a response appropriate to the cause of distress—unlike the rage on little provocation that is characteristic of intermittent explosive disorder.

Amok is a culturally inflected eruption of exhibitionistic violence. The perpetrator, typically a man with no previous pattern of violence, slashes or shoots at random victims, often in a crowded public place, until he is subdued or killed. He appears to be in a dissociated state; if he survives, he is amnesic for the episode. The practice of *running amok* is traditionally attributed to various southeast Asian countries but has been reported elsewhere.

Treatment Most individuals with intermittent explosive disorder do not seek treatment. Instead, they are compelled to get help by family pressure or legal circumstances. Psychoanalytic psychotherapy is not likely to be undertaken and is problematic because of the average patient's limited capacity for insight, brittleness of defenses, and alexithymia. A long-term supportive relationship combined with other modalities is generally more helpful. Simply knowing that one can call a concerned therapist when destructive impulses threaten can greatly help a patient exert successful control. Group *rage management* sessions specifically directed at impulse control are also useful.

The psychopharmacological treatment of intemperate aggression is still in its infancy, and is largely predicated on single or small case studies. Improvement has been reported with diverse medications; using drugs from more than one class has become increasingly common. These include anticonvulsants (e.g., carbamazepine [Tegretol], phenytoin [Dilantin], gabapentin [Neurontin], lamotrigine [Lamictal]); antianxiety agents (e.g., benzodiazepines); mood regulators (e.g., lithium); β-adrenergic receptor antagonists (e.g., propranolol [Inderal]); and antidepressants. Several studies indicate that SSRIs can reduce anger and irritability, with improvement rates as high as 60 percent. Solid research is clearly needed in this area.

When prescribing drugs of the benzodiazepine family to buffer anxiety related to explosive behavior, the clinician should be aware of their potential for causing disinhibition and consequent escalation of aggression in some patients (notably with clonazepam at higher doses).

Various cognitive-behavioral strategies can help patients bring aggressive impulses under control. For instance, deep relaxation is used in systematic flooding of imagined explosive situations to decrease angry responses. After mastery of imaginal flooding, the patient uses relaxation to neutralize anger in carefully graded real-life circumstances.

IMPULSE-CONTROL DISORDERS NOT OTHERWISE SPECIFIED

The conditions within the category of *impulse-control disorders not otherwise specified* do not satisfy the criteria for any of the previously mentioned impulse-control disorders or do not fit the paradigm of any other psychiatric disorder involving impulse-control problems described in the DSM-IV-TR (e.g., paraphilias and substance abuse disorders) (Table 21–7).

This heterogenous group includes compulsive sexual behavior that is unclassifiable elsewhere, compulsive nail and cuticle biting (onychotillomania), face picking, delicate self-cutting and other

Table 21–7
DSM-IV-TR Diagnostic Criteria for Impulse-Control Disorder Not Otherwise Specified

This category is for disorders of impulse control (e.g., skin picking) that do not meet the criteria for any specific impulse-control disorder or for another mental disorder having features involving impulse control described elsewhere in the manual (e.g., substance dependence or a paraphilia).

From American Psychiatric Association. *Diagnostic and Statistical Manual of Mental Disorders.* 4th ed. Text rev. Washington, DC: American Psychiatric Association; 2000, with permission.

forms of self-mutilation, and compulsive buying. The last two syndromes warrant further discussion, because compulsive shopping is now considered to be a major mental health problem, and delicate self-cutting appears to be on the rise. A future DSM will possibly recognize one or both as viable diagnostic entities to be listed with *impulse control disorders not elsewhere specified.*

ICD-10 contains two categories analogous to the DSM-IV-TR's *impulse control disorders not otherwise specified*. The first—*other habit and impulse disorders*—accommodates disorders of "persistently maladaptive behavior" that are clearly not associated with "a recognized psychiatric syndrome," characterized by "repeated failure to resist impulses to carry out the behavior," prodromal tension, and "a feeling of release at the time of the act." Intermittent explosive (behavior) disorder is the only entity listed in this group without comment. No criteria are listed, and no examples are given for the second category—*habit and impulse disorders, unspecified*.

Compulsive Buying The irresistible compulsion to buy was well known to the ancients. Petronius' *Satyricon* ironically delineates the insensate greed for acquisition that gripped wealthy Romans. Nineteenth century nosology termed the condition *oniomania*; it was also classified as one of the *impulsive insanities*. The inordinate buying habits of wealthy addicts—like wealthy kleptomaniacs—has always commanded public attention. However, like pathological gambling, compulsive buying cuts across the entire social spectrum and is ominously on the rise. Estimates of prevalence range from 1 percent to as high as 5 percent of the general population. Most patients—80 to 90 percent—are female.

Compulsive buyers feel rising tension and excitement during a variable prodromal period and experience release and satisfaction during a shopping binge, followed by depressive deflation. Guilty despair may seem obviously related to ruinous overspending. Yet, many well-to-do excessive buyers still report agonizing postshopping remorse, self-loathing, and a terrible sense of emptiness.

Most patients shop alone, for themselves. Buying impulses vary in frequency, length, and duration. A typical bout lasts several hours; however, some patients describe sprees that consume a day or several days. During intervening periods, thinking is often invaded by fantasies about shopping, as patients wrestle frantically for control. They may deliberately confine themselves outside to store-free areas or may stay at home to quell their buying—where they are tempted by catalogues and television shopping networks.

Items purchased are often related to personal adornment: clothes, perfume, makeup, and shoes. Clothing may be worn a few times or never at all and is hoarded. Male patients favor electronic and automobile equipment, hardware, or tools. However, essentially any object for sale may be sought obsessively. Impulse purchasing is common.

Compulsive buying gradually consumes ever more of the individual's time and money, with calamitous impact on vocational performance and social life:

After several years of increasing shopping binges, Janet, a 35-year-old attorney, began attending weekend auctions. At first, she only bid on jewelry but soon became so caught up in the action that she found herself impulsively placing bids on objects that she neither needed nor wanted. She ran up more than $200,000 of debt and invaded business resources. Her marriage and friendships deteriorated. She was hounded by loan sharks and considered killing herself, yet still kept attending auctions until she was barred for failure to make good on her purchases. She sought help only when threatened with bankruptcy, and her husband said that he wanted a divorce.

The similarity of compulsive buying to the driven behavior of pathological gambling and kleptomania is obvious. Comorbidity for kleptomania is especially high—frequently, but not exclusively, related to financial difficulties. Other significant comorbid conditions include mood disorders, substance abuse disorder, eating disorder (bulimia in particular), OCD, attention-deficit disorder, and various personality disturbances. Family histories are positive for mood, substance abuse, and impulse-control disorders.

Compulsive buying usually begins in late adolescence and develops insidiously, until it is unmasked in the late 20s to early 30s. The course thereafter is episodic and more favorable or chronic and severe, with attendant job loss, bankruptcy, family dysfunction, divorce, and even suicide or imprisonment. Serious comorbid pathology—especially related to bulimia, mood disorder, and drug abuse—militates for a poorer prognosis.

The etiology of the condition is multifaceted. Psychoanalysts speculate that compulsive buying represents a complex symbolic restitution, variously redressing low self-esteem, female castration anxiety (purchase equals penis), fear of death, and depressive emptiness, for example. Behaviorist theory underscores similarities between compulsive buying and other addictions regarding the intense reinforcement of repeated shopping binges and the development of tolerance with the need for more purchases to obtain relief, to name a few.

Neurobiologists conjecture that compulsive buying may be yet another affective spectrum disorder or obsessive spectrum disorder by virtue of its phenomenology, its familiar comorbidity pattern, and its family history. Analogous dysregulation within the serotoninergic and other neurotransmitter systems has been postulated but not yet proven.

It is commonplace that Western society is intensely consumerist. Enormous advances in the technology of consumption, ever more sophisticated advertising, and the ubiquity of Internet marketplaces all combine to escalate compulsive buying in the afflicted and even, perhaps, to create a legion of new shopping addicts in those predisposed by chemistry, conflict, and character.

With regard to differential diagnosis, compulsive and noncompulsive shoppers feel energized and happy while buying. This transitory well-being should not be confused with the prolonged elation propelling the febrile purchasing of bipolarity, accompanied by other manic stigmata. Devotees of unpathological so-called shop-'til-you-drop sprees occasionally overspend but do not shop as frequently and are not obsessed with shopping, nor does purchasing have the pervasive destructive impact characteristic of the compulsive buyer. However, quotidian shopping may insidiously escalate into compulsive buying. Suspicions on this score warrant the clinician's deeper exploration of shopping behavior and shopping-related preoccupations.

There have been no large-scale treatment studies of compulsive buying. Case reports suggest that a combination of therapies is favored and more effective than a single modality. Success has been achieved with psychoanalytically oriented and supportive therapy, as well as cognitive techniques, for example relaxation and imaginal work. The results of pharmacotherapy are ambiguous; variable improvement has been reported with antidepressants, mood stabilizers, anxiolytics, and antipsychotics, and combinations thereof. Debtors Anonymous (DA) meetings or other self-help groups have proven effective in controlling buying impulses, alone or combined with other therapies.

Delicate Self-Cutting The term *delicate self-cutting* was coined by Paul Pao in 1969 to delineate a syndrome of precise self-mutilation, predominantly afflicting adolescent and young adult women, which exhibits the hallmarks of other impulse-control disorders. Its prevalence has not been established, but many clinicians believe that the syndrome is not rare and has been increasing significantly.

The condition is characterized by shallow, meticulous cutting into the skin, using a razor blade or sharp knife, often in a series of slices. The most favored locations are the wrist and lower arms. Cutting elsewhere, such as the breasts, abdomen, pubic area, is said to be associated with even more serious psychopathology. Cutting is *not* a suicidal act but is connected with the release of tension and anger, with or without the attempt to stabilize frightening feelings, such as fragmentation.

Borderline personality disorder is arguably associated more consistently with delicate self-cutting than is the case with any other impulse-control disorders. Additional significant comorbid conditions include OCD, affective disorder, dissociative or depersonalization disorder, body dysmorphic disorder, and eating disorders. Families are extraordinarily dysfunctional, with high rates of affective and anxiety disorders.

Most theories about etiology derive from psychoanalytic work. A substantial number of patients have experienced illness, injury, or abuse by family members in childhood. Analytical investigators describe difficulties in affective regulation, with early failure to internalize appropriate self-soothing mechanisms; chronic anxiety about ego disintegration, loss of control, and maintaining ego boundaries; disturbances in body image; and intense fear of sexual arousal and vaginal sensations. Bizarre and frightening as self-cutting appears, to the patients themselves, it is a profoundly reparative means for restoring psychic equilibrium. Little is written about the neurobiological and behavioral features of delicate self-cutting. The condition may qualify as an obsessive spectrum disorder or affective spectrum disorder (especially the former), with possible dysregulation of several neurotransmitter systems. Behaviorists stress the formidable reinforcing potential of the symptom, based on the immense relief it provides.

Delicate self-cutting typically begins in early adolescence, around menarche. Patients may hide the disorder for years, adroitly concealing their wounds with long-sleeved clothing. The condition is episodic in some patients, fading away with time. The outcome is far more problematic once behavior is firmly entrenched as a coping strategy, particularly when delicate self-cutting is associated with severe borderline personality disorder and mood disorders. In chronic cases, dysfunction and marginalization of life is extensive, with multiple hospitalizations and suicidal tendency.

Regarding differential diagnosis, single or multiple suicide attempts in major depressive disorder may be confused with delicate self-cutting; the former diagnosis is made on the basis of the obvious guilt-ridden intention to kill or, at least, to injure oneself, as well as obviously depressed mood and vegetative symptoms. Self-mutilation in schizophrenia is often bizarre (e.g., castration and ocular enucleation) and is responsive to command hallucinations or delusions.

Malingered cutting, notably encountered in incarcerated prisoners or psychiatric inpatients with no previous history (especially adolescents), has an obvious, manipulative purpose or can occur during an epidemic of copy-cat acting out. The wrist cutting and other self-mutilations of mentally retarded or autistic institutionalized patients lack the complex intrapsychic symbolic meanings of delicate self-cutting.

Lesch-Nyhan syndrome is a rare X-linked recessive genetic disorder that usually presents with the hallmark symptoms of severe, involuntary self-mutilation, occasionally including self-cutting. Associated with the disease are cognitive impairment, choreoathetosis, and hyperuricemia. Most patients are male.

Success has been reported in treating delicate self-cutting with psychoanalysis. Insight-oriented therapy is not to be undertaken lightly with these patients and is often prolonged and stormy, with a substantial risk of dangerous transferential distortions. Anecdotal reports note improvement with SSRIs, mood regulators, and various cognitive-behavioral techniques.

Whatever treatments are used, delicate self-cutters often make enormous emotional demands on the therapist because of their unshakable need for attention, even as they push help away. Too much involvement may be perceived as a frightening intrusion by a patient whose sensibility is also finely tuned to the least hint of rejection and who is prone to act out in either case. Balanced compassion is requisite.

SUGGESTED CROSS-REFERENCES

As abundantly described, many other disorders are comorbid with the impulse-control disorders, may present with impulsive features, and may be contemplated as alternatives during differential diagnosis. The reader is therefore directed to discussions of OCD (Chapter 14); mood disorders, notably bipolar disorder (Chapter 13); anxiety disorders (Chapter 14); and substance abuse and dependency disorders (Chapter 11; also, see Section 11.2 for a discussion of conditions associated with alcoholism); eating disorders, notably bulimia (Chapter 19); dissociative disorders, notably fugue states (Chapter 17); personality disorders, notably antisocial and borderline personality disorders (Chapter 23); paraphilias, compulsive sexual behavior, and sexual addiction (Chapter 18); and various neurological and medical conditions associated with impulsivity (dementias, Section 10.3).

References

Baudamant M: Description de deux masses de cheveux trouvee dans l'estomac et les intestines d'un jeune garcon age de 16 ans. *Hist Soc Roy Med.* 1779;2:262.

Black DW: Compulsive buying: a review. *J Clin Psychiatry.* 1996;57[Suppl]:50.

Blaszczynski A. *Overcoming Compulsive Gambling: A Self-Help Guide Using Cognitive-Behavioral Techniques.* London: Robinson; 1998.

Brady KT, Myrick H, McElroy S: The relationship between substance use disorders, impulse control disorders, and pathological aggression. *Am J Addict.* 1998;7:221.

Brower C, Stein DJ: Trichobezoars in trichotillomania: case report and literature overview. *Psychosom Med.* 1998;60:658.

Chambers RO, Potenza MN: Neurodevelopment, impulsivity, and adolescent gambling. *J Gambl Stud.* 2003;19:53.

*Christenson GA, Crow SJ: The characterization and treatment of trichotillomania. *J Clin Psychiatry.* 1996;57[Suppl]:42.

Christenson GA, Faber RJ, de Zwaan M, Raymond NC, Specker SM, Ekern MD, Mackenzie TB, Crosby RD, Crow SJ, Eckert ED, Mussel MP, Mitchell JF: Compulsive buying: descriptive characteristics and psychiatric comorbidity. *J Clin Psychiatry.* 1994;55:5.

Cohen IJ, Stein DJ, Simeon D, Spadaccini E, Rosen J, Aronowitz B, Hollander E: Clinical profile, comorbidity, and treatment history in 123 hairpullers: a survey study. *J Clin Psychiatry.* 1995;56:319.

*Crockford DN, el-Guebaly N: Pathological gambling: a critical review. *Can J Psychiatry.* 1998;43:43.

Cunningham-Williams RM, Cottler LB: The epidemiology of pathological gambling. *Semin Clin Neuropsychiatry.* 2001;6:155.

Dannon PN: Topirmate for the treatment of kleptomania: a case series and review of the literature. *Clin Neuropharmacol.* 2003;26:1.

Dickerson MG, Hinchy J, England S: Minimal treatments and problem gamblers: a preliminary investigation. *J Gambling Studies.* 1990;6:87.

Doctors S. The symptom of delicate self-cutting in adolescent females: a developmental view. In: Feinstein SC, Looney JG, Schwartzberg AZ, Sorosky AD, eds. *Adolescent Psychiatry: Developmental and Clinical Studies.* Vol 9. Chicago: University of Chicago Press; 1981:443.

*Durst R, Katz G, Teitelbaum A, Zislin J, Dannon PN: Kleptomania: Diagnosis and treatment options. *CNS Drugs.* 2001;15:185.

Esquirol E. *Mental Maladies: A Treatise on Insanity.* Philadelphia: Lea and Blanchard; 1845.

Felthous AR, Bryant SG, Wingerter CB: The diagnosis of intermittent explosive disorder in violent men. *Bull Am Acad Psychiatry Law.* 1991;19:71.

*Geller JL: Pathological firesetting in adults. *Intl J Law Psychol.* 1992;15:283.

Geller JL, Bertsch G: Fire-setting behavior in the histories of a state hospital population. *Am J Psychiatry.* 1985;142:465.

Grant JE, Kim SW, Potenza MN: Advances in the pharmacological treatment of pathological gambling. *J Gambl Stud.* 2003;19:85.

*Greenberg HR, Sarner CA: Trichotillomania: symptom and syndrome. *Arch Gen Psychiatry.* 1985;12:482.

Hollander E, Begaz T, DeCaria C: Pharmacologic approaches in the treatment of pathological gambling. *CNS Spectrums.* 1998;3:72.

Hollander E, Kwon JH, Stein DJ, Broatch J, Rowland CT, Himelein CA: Obsessive-compulsive and spectrum disorders: overview and quality of life issues. *J Clin Psychiatry.* 1996;57[Suppl]:3.

Kammerer T, Singer L, Michel D: The incendiaries: criminological, clinical and psychological study of 72 cases. *Ann Med Psychol.* 1967;1:687.

Keuthen NJ, O'Sullivan RL, Sprich-Buckminster S: Trichotillomania: current issues in conceptualization and treatment. *Psychother Psychosom.* 1998;67:202.

Kim SW, Grant JE: The psychopharmacology of pathological gambling. *Semin Clin Neuropsychiatry.* 2001;3:184.

Lejoyeux MJ, Ades J, Tassain V, Solomon J: Phenomenology and psychopathology of uncontrolled buying. *Am J Psychiatry.* 1996;153:1524.

Leong GB: A psychiatric study of persons charged with arson. *J Forensic Sci.* 1995;37:1319.

Lesieur HR, Rosenthal RJ: Pathological gambling: a review of the literature. *J Gambling Studies.* 1991;7:5.

Lewis ND, Yarnell H: Pathological firesetting (pyromania). *Nerv Ment Dis Mon.* 1951;82:8.

Lion JR: The intermittent explosive disorder. *Psychiatr Ann.* 1992;22:64.

Mansueto CA, Townsley-Sternberger RM, McCombs-Thomas A, Goldfinger-Golomb R: Trichotillomania: a comprehensive behavioral model. *Clin Psychol Rev.* 1997;17:567.

Marc H: Considerations medico-legales sur la monomanie et particularement incendiare. *Ann Hyg Publ Med Leg.* 1833;10:367.

McElroy SL, Hudson JI, Pope HL Jr, Keck PE Jr, Aizley HG: The DSM-III-R impulse control disorders not elsewhere classified: clinical characteristics and relations to other psychiatric disorders. *Am J Psychiatry.* 1992;149:318.

McElroy SL, Keck PE Jr, Phillips KA: Kleptomania, compulsive buying, and binge-eating disorder. *J Clin Psychiatry.* 1995;56:14.

McElroy SL, Pope HG Jr, Keck PE Jr: Are impulse control disorders related to bipolar disorder? *Compr Psychiatry.* 1996;37:229.

McElroy SL, Soutullo CA, DeAnna BA, Taylor P Jr, Keck PE: DSM-IV intermittent explosive disorder: a report of 27 cases. *J Clin Psychiatry.* 1998;59:203.

Pao P: The syndrome of delicate self-cutting. *Br J Med Psychol.* 1969;42:195.

Petry NM, Armentano C: Prevalence, assessment, and treatment of pathological gambling: a review. *Psychiatr Serv.* 1999;50:1021.

Petry NM, Roll JM: A behavioral approach to understanding and treating pathological gambling. *Semin Clin Neuropsychiatry.* 2001;6:177.

Potenza MN: The neurobiology of pathological gambling. *Semin Clin Neuropsychiatry.* 2001;3:217.

Reist C, Nakamura K, Sagart E, Sokolski KN, Fujimoto KA: Impulsive aggressive behavior: open-label treatment with citalopram. *J Clin Psychiatry.* 2003;64:81.

Spunt B, DuPont I, Lesieur H, Liberty HJ, Hunt D: Pathological gambling and substance misuse: a review of the literature. *Subst Use Misuse.* 1998;33:2535.

Stein DJ, Hollander E, Liebowitz MR: Neurobiology of impulsive behavior and the impulse control disorders. *J Neuropsychiatry Clin Neurosci.* 1993;5:9.

Stein DJ, Simeon D, Cohen LJ, Hollander E: Trichotillomania and obsessive-compulsive disorder. *J Clin Psychiatry.* 1995;56[Suppl]:28.

Sylvan C, Ladouceur R, Boisvert JM: Cognitive and behavioral treatment of pathological gambling: A controlled study. *J Consult Clin Psychol.* 1997;65:727.

Tavares H, Zilberman ML, el-Guebaly N: Are there cognitive and behavioural approaches specific to the treatment of pathological gambling? *Can J Psychiatry.* 2003; 48:22.

Toneatto T: Cognitive pathology of problem gambling. *Subst Use Misuse.* 1999;34: 1593.

Winchell RM: Trichotillomania: presentation and treatment. *Psychiatr Ann.* 1992; 22:84.

Index

Page numbers followed by *t* and *f* indicate tables and figures, respectively. Page numbers in boldface indicate major discussions.

B

C

D

H

J

K

N

O

V